KU-632-184

TIETZ *Textbook of* Clinical Chemistry AND Molecular Diagnostics

CARL A. BURTIS, Ph.D.
Senior Technical Specialist
Health Services Division
Oak Ridge National Laboratory
Oak Ridge, Tennessee;
Clinical Professor of Pathology
University of Utah School of Medicine
Salt Lake City, Utah

EDWARD R. ASHWOOD, M.D.
Professor of Pathology
University of Utah School of Medicine,
Chief Medical Officer/Laboratory Director
ARUP Laboratories
Salt Lake City, Utah

DAVID E. BRUNS, M.D.
Professor of Pathology
University of Virginia Medical School,
Director of Clinical Chemistry and Associate Director of Molecular Diagnostics
University of Virginia Health System
Charlottesville, Virginia;
Editor, *Clinical Chemistry*
Washington, D.C.

FOURTH EDITION

with **944** *illustrations and* **12** *color plates*

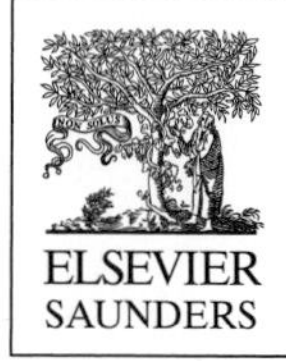

ELSEVIER
SAUNDERS

11830 Westline Industrial Drive
St. Louis, Missouri 63146

TIETZ TEXTBOOK OF CLINICAL CHEMISTRY AND MOLECULAR DIAGNOSTICS

ISBN-13: 978-0-7216-0189-2
ISBN-10: 0-7216-0189-8

Publishing Director: Andrew Allen
Managing Editor: Mindy Hutchinson
Developmental Editor: Ellen Wurm
Publishing Services Manager: Pat Joiner
Senior Project Manager: Rachel E. Dowell
Senior Designer: Teresa McBryan

Printed in the United States of America

Last digit is the print number: 9 8 7 6 5 4 3 2

To

Marvel, Candice, and **Liz,**

our friends and companions in life,

for their understanding, encouragement, and patience,

especially during our many absences—the mental as well as the physical.

And to the memory of **David J. Newman,**

a good friend and valued colleague.

Contributors

CONSTANTIN ALIFERIS, M.D., Ph.D.
Assistant Professor of Biomedical Informatics,
Director, Discovery Systems Laboratory
Department of Biomedical Informatics
Vanderbilt University School of Medicine
Nashville, Tennessee
Clinical Evaluation of Methods

THOMAS ANNESLEY, Ph.D.
Professor of Clinical Chemistry
University of Michigan Medical School
Ann Arbor, Michigan
Mass Spectrometry

FRED S. APPLE, Ph.D.
Medical Director, Clinical Laboratories
Hennepin County Medical Center,
Professor of Laboratory Medicine & Pathology
University of Minnesota School of Medicine
Minneapolis, Minnesota
Cardiac Function

DOMINIK ARONSKY, M.D., Ph.D.
Department of Biomedical Informatics
Vanderbilt University Medical Center
Assistant Professor of Biomedical Informatics & Emergency Medicine
Vanderbilt University
Nashville, Tennessee
Clinical Evaluation of Methods

EDWARD R. ASHWOOD, M.D.
Professor of Pathology
University of Utah School of Medicine,
Chief Medical Officer/Laboratory Director
ARUP Laboratories
Salt Lake City, Utah
Clinical Chemistry of Pregnancy; Clinical Chemistry of Pregnancy Appendix

MALCOLM BAINES, F.R.S.C., F.R.C.Path.
Principal Clinical Scientist
Royal Liverpool University Hospital
Liverpool, United Kingdom
Vitamins and Trace Elements; Vitamins and Trace Elements Appendix

RENZE BAIS, Ph.D.
Principal Hospital Scientist
Department of Clinical Biochemistry
Pacific Laboratory Medicine Services
Royal North Shore Hospital
Senior Clinical Associate
Department of Medicine
University of Sydney
Sydney, NSW, Australia
Principles of Clinical Enzymology; Enzymes; Enzymes Appendix

EDWARD W. BERMES, Jr., Ph.D.
Professor Emeritus, Department of Pathology
Loyola University Medical Center
Maywood, Illinois
Introduction to Principles of Laboratory Analyses and Safety; Introduction to Principles of Laboratory Analyses and Safety Appendix; Specimen Collection and Processing; Preanalytical Variables and Biological Variation

ERNEST BEUTLER, M.D.
Chairman, Department of Molecular and Experimental Medicine
The Scripps Research Institute
La Jolla, California
Hemoglobin, Iron, and Bilirubin; Hemoglobin, Iron, and Bilirubin Appendix

RONALD A. BOOTH, Ph.D.
Assistant Professor, University of Ottawa,
Clinical Biochemist, The Ottawa Hospital
Ottawa, Ontario, Canada
Tumor Markers

PATRICK M.M. BOSSUYT, Ph.D.
Head, Department Clinical Epidemiology and Biostatistics,
Professor of Clinical Epidemiology
Academic Medical Center
University of Amsterdam
Amsterdam, The Netherlands
Introduction to Laboratory Medicine and Evidence-Based Laboratory Medicine; Introduction to Laboratory Medicine and Evidence-Based Laboratory Medicine Appendix

JAMES C. BOYD, M.D.
Department of Pathology
University of Virginia Medical Center
Charlottesville, Virginia
Automation in the Clinical Laboratory; Automation in the Clinical Laboratory Appendix; Selection and Analytical Evaluation of Methods—With Statistical Techniques; Selection and Analytical Evaluation of Methods—With Statistical Techniques Appendix

DAVID E. BRUNS, M.D.
Professor of Pathology
University of Virginia Medical School,
Director of Clinical Chemistry and Associate Director of Molecular Diagnostics
University of Virginia Health System
Charlottesville, Virginia;
Editor, *Clinical Chemistry*
Washington, D.C.
Introduction to Laboratory Medicine and Evidence-Based Laboratory Medicine; Introduction to Laboratory Medicine and Evidence-Based Laboratory Medicine Appendix; Reference Information for the Clinical Laboratory

BONNY LEWIS BUKAVECKAS, Ph.D.
Assistant Professor, Department of Pharmacy
Virginia Commonwealth University
Richmond, Virginia
Pharmacogenetics

MARY F. BURRITT, Ph.D.
Director, Metals Laboratory
Medical Co-Director, Central Clinical Laboratory
Mayo Clinic,
Professor of Laboratory Medicine
Associate Dean, Mayo School of Health Sciences
Mayo Clinic College of Medicine
Rochester, Minnesota
Toxic Metals; Toxic Metals Appendix

CARL A. BURTIS, Ph.D.
Senior Technical Specialist
Health Services Division
Oak Ridge National Laboratory
Oak Ridge, Tennessee;
Clinical Professor of Pathology
University of Utah School of Medicine
Salt Lake City, Utah
Chromatography; Reference Information for the Clinical Laboratory

JOHN BUTZ, B.A.
Supervisor, Metals Laboratory
Department of Laboratory Medicine and Pathology
Mayo Clinic
Rochester, Minnesota
Toxic Metals; Toxic Metals Appendix

ANGELA M. CALIENDO, M.D., Ph.D.
Associate Professor of Pathology and Laboratory Medicine
Emory University School of Medicine,
Vice Chair, Clinical Pathology
Emory University Hospital
Atlanta, Georgia
Molecular Methods in Diagnosis and Monitoring of Infectious Diseases

DANIEL W. CHAN, Ph.D., D.A.B.C.C., F.A.C.B.
Professor of Pathology, Oncology, Radiology, and Urology
Johns Hopkins University School of Medicine,
Director, Clinical Chemistry Division
Johns Hopkins Hospital
Baltimore, Maryland
Tumor Markers

ROSSA W.K. CHIU, M.B.B.S., Ph.D., F.R.C.P.A.
Associate Professor
Department of Chemical Pathology
The Chinese University of Hong Kong
Hong Kong SAR
Principles of Molecular Biology and Approaches to Nucleic Acid Isolation

ALLAN C. DEACON, B.Sc., Ph.D., Dip.C.B., F.R.C.Path.
Consultant Clinical Scientist
King's College Hospital
Denmant Hill, London, England
Porphyrins and Disorders of Porphyrin Metabolism; Porphyrins and Disorders of Porphyrin Metabolism Appendix

MICHAEL P. DELANEY, B.Sc., M.D., M.R.C.P.
Consultant Nephrologist
Renal Unit, Kent & Canterbury Hospital
East Kent Hospitals NHS Trust
Canterbury, Kent, United Kingdom
Kidney Disease

LAURENCE M. DEMERS, Ph.D., F.A.C.B., D.A.B.C.C.
Director, Clinical Chemistry, Core Endocrine Laboratory, GCRC Core Laboratory
M.S. Hershey Medical Center
Distinguished Professor of Pathology and Medicine
Penn State University College of Medicine
Hershey, Pennsylvania
Pituitary Function; The Adrenal Cortex; The Thyroid: Pathophysiology and Thyroid Function Testing

ELEFTHERIOS P. DIAMANDIS, M.D., Ph.D.
Professor and Head, Division of Clinical Biochemistry
University of Toronto,
Section Head of Clinical Biochemistry
Mount Sinai Hospital
Toronto, Ontario, Canada
Tumor Markers

PAUL D'ORAZIO, Ph.D.
Director, Sensor Development
Instrumentation Laboratory
Lexington, Massachusetts
Electrochemistry and Chemical Sensors

BASIL T. DOUMAS, Ph.D.
Professor Emeritus
Department of Pathology
Medical College of Wisconsin
Milwaukee, Wisconsin
Hemoglobin, Iron, and Bilirubin; Hemoglobin, Iron, and Bilirubin Appendix

D. ROBERT DUFOUR, M.D.
Chief, Pathology and Laboratory Medicine Service (retired)
Veterans Affairs Medical Center, Washington DC,
Professor of Pathology
George Washington University Medical Center
Washington DC;
Adjunct Professor of Pathology
Uniformed Services University of the Health Sciences
Bethesda, Maryland
Liver Disease

GRAEME EISENHOFER, Ph.D.
Staff Scientist, Clinical Neurocardiology Section
National Institute of Neurological Disorders and Stroke
National Institutes of Health
Bethesda, Maryland
Catecholamines and Serotonin; Catecholamines and Serotonin Appendix

GEORGE H. ELDER, M.D.
Emeritus Professor
Department of Medical Biochemistry and Immunology
Unversity of Wales College of Medicine
Cardiff, United Kingdom
Porphyrins and Disorders of Porphyrin Metabolism; Porphyrins and Disorders of Porphyrin Metabolism Appendix

KOJO S.J. ELENITOBA-JOHNSON, M.D.
Associate Professor of Pathology
University of Utah School of Medicine,
Director, Molecular Pathology Fellowship Training Program
Director, Molecular Hematopathology and Proteomics
ARUP Laboratories
Salt Lake City, Utah
Molecular Genetics and Diagnosis of Hematopoietic Neoplasms

DAVID B. ENDRES, Ph.D.
Professor of Clinical Pathology
Keck School of Medicine
University of Southern California,
Consultant, Chemistry
Los Angeles County University of Southern California Medical Center
Los Angeles, California
Mineral and Bone Metabolism

GORDON S. FELL, Ph.D., F.R.C.Path.
Emeritus Professor of Pathological Biochemistry
University of Glasgow
Glasgow, Scotland
Vitamins and Trace Elements; Vitamins and Trace Elements Appendix

ANDREA FERREIRA-GONZALEZ, Ph.D.
Associate Professor of Pathology
Virginia Commonwealth University,
Director, Molecular Diagnostics Laboratory
Medical College of Virginia Hospitals
Richmond, Virginia
Molecular Methods in Diagnosis and Monitoring of Infectious Diseases

ELIZABETH L. FRANK, Ph.D., D.A.B.C.C., F.A.C.B.
Assistant Professor (Clinical)
Department of Pathology
University of Utah Health Sciences Center,
Medical Director, Analytic Biochemistry
ARUP Laboratories
Salt Lake City, Utah
Catecholamines and Serotonin Appendix

ANN M. GRONOWSKI, Ph.D.
Assistant Professor
Washington University School of Medicine,
Assistant Medical Director, Chemistry
Barnes-Jewish Hospital
St. Louis, Missouri
Reproductive Related Disorders

SIHOUN HAHN, M.D., Ph.D.
Co-director, Biochemical Genetics Laboratory,
Associate Professor of Laboratory Medicine and Pathology
Mayo Clinic College of Medicine
Rochester, Minnesota
Inborn Errors of Amino Acid, Organic Acid, and Fatty Acid Metabolism; Inborn Errors of Amino Acid, Organic Acid, and Fatty Acid Metabolism Appendix

DORIS M. HAVERSTICK, Ph.D.
Associate Professor
University of Virginia, Department of Pathology
Charlottesville, Virginia
Specimen Collection and Processing

CHARLES D. HAWKER, Ph.D., M.B.A., F.A.C.B.
Associate Professor of Pathology (Adjunct)
University of Utah School of Medicine,
Scientific Director, Automation and Special Projects
ARUP Laboratories
Salt Lake City, Utah
Automation in the Clinical Laboratory; Automation in the Clinical Laboratory Appendix

SHANNON HAYMOND, Ph.D.
Department of Pathology
Washington University School of Medicine
St. Louis, Missouri
Reproductive Related Disorders

TREFOR HIGGINS, M.Sc.
Associate Clinical Professor
University of Alberta,
Co-Director of Clinical Chemistry
Dynacare Kasper Medical Laboratory
Edmonton, Alberta, Canada
Hemoglobin, Iron, and Bilirubin; Hemoglobin, Iron, and Bilirubin Appendix

PETER G. HILL, Ph.D., C. Chem., F.R.S.C., F.R.C.Path.
Consultant Clinical Scientist
Department of Clinical Pathology
Derby Hospitals NHS Foundation Trust
Derby, United Kingdom
Gastric, Pancreatic, and Intestinal Function

ALLAN S. JAFFE, M.D.
Consultant in Cardiology/Internal Medicine and Laboratory Medicine and Pathology
Professor of Medicine
Mayo Clinic and Mayo Medical School
Rochester, Minnesota
Cardiac Function

A. MYRON JOHNSON, M.D.
Clinical Professor of Obstetrics and Gynecology
University of North Carolina
Chapel Hill, North Carolina
Amino Acids, Peptides, and Proteins

STEPHEN E. KAHN, Ph.D.
Professor
Pathology, Cell Biology, Neurobiology and Anatomy
Vice Chair
Laboratory Medicine Director
Core Laboratory Operations Section Chief and Director
Clinical Chemistry, Toxicology and Near Patient Testing
Loyola University Medical Center
Maywood, Illinois
Introduction to Principles of Laboratory Analyses and Safety; Introduction to Principles of Laboratory Analyses and Safety Appendix

MALEK KAMOUN, M.D., Ph.D.
Professor of Pathology and Laboratory Medicine
University of Pennsylvania School of Medicine,
Director, Clinical Immunology Lab
Hospital of the University of Pennsylvania
Philadelphia, Pennsylvania
Identity Assessment

RAYMOND KARCHER, Ph.D.
Clinical Chemist, William Beaumont Hospital
Royal Oak, Michigan,
Adjunct Associate Professor
Oakland University
Rochester, Michigan
Electrophoresis

ANTHONY A. KILLEEN, M.D., Ph.D.
Director of Clinical Laboratories
Fairview-University Medical Center,
Associate Professor
Department of Laboratory Medicine and Pathology
University of Minnesota
Minneapolis, Minnesota
Design and Operation of the Molecular Diagnostics Laboratory

GEORGE G. KLEE, M.D., Ph.D.
Chair, Division of Experimental Pathology
Department of Laboratory Medicine and Pathology,
Professor of Laboratory Medicine
Mayo Clinic College of Medicine
Rochester, Minnesota
Quality Management

MICHAEL KLEEREKOPER, M.D., F.A.C.E., F.A.C.B.
Professor of Medicine and Pathology
Wayne State University School of Medicine
Endocrine Division
Detroit, Michigan
Hormones

JAMES STACEY KLUTTS, M.D., Ph.D.
Department of Pathology and Immunology
Washington University School of Medicine
St. Louis, Missouri
Electrolytes and Blood Gases; Electrolytes and Blood Gases Appendix; Physiology and Disorders of Water, Electrolyte, and Acid-Base Metabolism

GEORGE J. KNIGHT, Ph.D.
Director, Prenatal Screening Laboratory
Director, Medical Genetics Laboratory
Foundation for Blood Research
Scarborough, Maine
Clinical Chemistry of Pregnancy; Clinical Chemistry of Pregnancy Appendix

L.J. KRICKA, D.Phil., F.A.C.B., C. Chem., F.R.S.C., F.R.C.Path.
Professor of Pathology and Laboratory Medicine
Director, General Chemistry Department of Pathology and Laboratory Medicine
University of Pennsylvania Medical Center
Philadelphia, Pennsylvania
Optical Techniques; Principles of Immunochemical Techniques

MARK M. KUSHNIR, M.S.
Senior Scientist
ARUP Institute for Clinical & Experimental Pathology
ARUP Laboratories
Salt Lake City, Utah
Catecholamines and Serotonin Appendix

NORIKO KUSUKAWA, Ph.D.
Adjunct Associate Professor of Pathology
University of Utah School of Medicine
Assistant Vice President
ARUP Laboratories,
Salt Lake City, Utah
Nucleic Acid Techniques

EDMUND LAMB, Ph.D.
Consultant Clinical Scientist
Department of Clinical Biochemistry
East Kent Hospitals NHS Trust
Kent and Canterbury Hospital
Canterbury, Kent, United Kingdom
Kidney Function Tests; Kidney Disease

JAMES P. LANDERS, Ph.D.
Professor of Chemistry
University of Virginia,
Associate Professor of Pathology
University of Virginia Health System
Charlottesville, Virginia
Electrophoresis

VICKY A. LeGRYS, D.A., M.T.(A.S.C.P.), C.L.S.(N.C.A.)
Professor
Division of Clinical Laboratory Science
University of North Carolina at Chapel Hill
Chapel Hill, North Carolina
Electrolytes and Blood Gases; Electrolytes and Blood Gases Appendix

MARK W. LINDER, Ph.D.
Associate Professor of Pathology and Laboratory Medicine,
Associate Director
Pharmacogenetics Diagnostic Laboratory
University of Louisville School of Medicine
Louisville, Kentucky
Pharmacogenetics

KRISTIAN LINNET, M.D.
Professor
The Department of Forensic Chemistry
Institute of Forensic Medicine
University of Copenhagen
Copenhagen, Denmark
Selection and Analytical Evaluation of Methods—With Statistical Techniques; Selection and Analytical Evaluation of Methods—With Statistical Techniques Appendix

Y.M. DENNIS LO, M.A., D.M., D.Phil., F.R.C.P., F.R.C.Path.
Professor of Chemical Pathology
The Chinese University of Hong Kong
Department of Chemical Pathology
Prince of Wales Hospital
Shatin, New Territories
Hong Kong SAR
Principles of Molecular Biology and Approaches to Nucleic Acid Isolation

T.D.G. LYON, B.Sc, Ph.D.
Principal Scientist
Department of Clinical Biochemistry
Glasgow Royal Infirmary
Glasgow, Scotland
Vitamins and Trace Elements; Vitamins and Trace Elements Appendix

MARK J. MAGERA, B.S., M.A.
Development Coordinator, Biochemical Genetics Laboratory
Department of Laboratory Medicine and Pathology
Mayo Clinic College of Medicine
Rochester, Minnesota
Catecholamines and Serotonin Appendix

DIETRICH MATERN, M.D.
Assistant Professor of Laboratory Medicine
Mayo Clinic College of Medicine
Rochester, Minnesota
Catecholamines and Serotonin Appendix; Inborn Errors of Amino Acid, Organic Acid, and Fatty Acid Metabolism; Inborn Errors of Amino Acid, Organic Acid, and Fatty Acid Metabolism Appendix

GWENDOLYN A. McMILLIN, Ph.D., D.A.B.C.C.
Assistant Professor (Clinical) of Pathology
University of Utah School of Medicine,
Medical Director, Toxicology, Trace Elements, Pharmacogenomics
ARUP Laboratories
Salt Lake City, Utah
Pharmacogenetics; Reference Information for the Clinical Laboratory

MARK E. MEYERHOFF, Ph.D.
Philip J. Elving Professor of Chemistry
Department of Chemistry
The University of Michigan
Ann Arbor, Michigan
Electrochemistry and Chemical Sensors

ANABELA MOTA PINTO, Ph.D.
Director of General Pathology Institute
Faculty of Medicine,
Professor of Pathophysiology
University of Coimbra
Coimbra, Portugal
Cytokines

THOMAS P. MOYER, Ph.D.
Chair, Division of Clinical Biochemistry and Immunology
Department of Laboratory Medicine and Pathology
Mayo Clinic,
Professor of Laboratory Medicine
Mayo College of Medicine
Rochester, Minnesota
Therapeutic Drugs and Their Management; Therapeutic Drugs and Their Management Appendix; Toxic Metals; Toxic Metals Appendix

DAVID J. NEWMAN, Ph.D.
Consultant Clinical Scientist and Scientific Director
South West Thames Institute for Renal Research
St Helier Hospital
Carshalton, Surrey, United Kingdom
Kidney Function Tests; Kidney Disease

MAURO PANTEGHINI, M.D.
Chair of Clinical Biochemistry and Clinical Molecular Biology
Department of Clinical Sciences "Luigi Sacco"
University of Milan Medical School
Milan, Italy
Principles of Clinical Enzymology; Enzymes; Enzymes Appendix

WILLIAM H. PORTER, Ph.D.
Professor
Pathology and Laboratory Medicine
University of Kentucky Medical Center,
Director of Clinical Chemistry, Toxicology, and Core Laboratories
University of Kentucky
Lexington, Kentucky
Clinical Toxicology; Clinical Toxicology Appendix

CHRISTOPHER P. PRICE, Ph.D.
Vice President, Outcomes Research
Diagnostics Division, Bayer HealthCare
Strawberry Hill
Newbury, Berkshire,
United Kingdom
Point-of-Care Testing; Introduction to Laboratory Medicine and Evidence-Based Laboratory Medicine; Introduction to Laboratory Medicine and Evidence-Based Laboratory Medicine Appendix; Kidney Function Tests; Kidney Disease

NADER RIFAI, Ph.D.
Director, Clinical Chemistry
Department of Laboratory Medicine
Children's Hospital Boston,
Associate Professor
Harvard Medical School
Boston, Massachusetts
Lipids, Lipoproteins, Apolipoproteins, and Other Cardiovascular Risk Factors; Lipids, Lipoproteins, Apolipoproteins, and Other Cardiovascular Risk Factors Appendix

PIERO RINALDO, M.D., Ph.D.
Professor of Laboratory Medicine
Mayo Clinic College of Medicine
Rochester, Minnesota
Catecholamines and Serotonin Appendix; Inborn Errors of Amino Acid, Organic Acid, and Fatty Acid Metabolism; Inborn Errors of Amino Acid, Organic Acid, and Fatty Acid Metabolism Appendix

WILLIAM L. ROBERTS, M.D., Ph.D.
Associate Professor of Pathology
University of Utah School of Medicine,
Medical Director, Automated Core Laboratory
ARUP Laboratories
Salt Lake City, Utah
Reference Information for the Clinical Laboratory

ALAN L. ROCKWOOD, Ph.D.
Scientific Director for Mass Spectrometry,
Adjunct Associate Professor of Pathology
University of Utah School of Medicine
Salt Lake City, Utah
Mass Spectrometry

THOMAS G. ROSANO, Ph.D.
Professor of Pathology and Laboratory Medicine
Albany Medical College,
Director of Clinical Laboratory Services
Albany Medical Center Hospital
Albany, New York
Catecholamines and Serotonin; Catecholamines and Serotonin Appendix

ROBERT K. RUDE, M.D.
Professor of Medicine
Director, Clinical Pathology Training Program
University of Southern California
Los Angeles, California
Mineral and Bone Metabolism

DAVID B. SACKS, M.B., Ch.B., F.R.C.Path.
Associate Professor of Pathology Harvard Medical School
Medical Director of Clinical Chemistry
Director, Clinical Pathology Training Program
Brigham and Women's Hospital
Boston, Massachusetts
Carbohydrates; Carbohydrates Appendix

MANUEL SANTOS ROSA, Ph.D.
Director of Immunology Institute
Faculty of Medicine,
Professor of Immunology
University of Coimbra
Coimbra, Portugal
Cytokines

MITCHELL G. SCOTT, Ph.D.
Professor of Pathology and Immunology
Department of Pathology and Immunology
Washington University School of Medicine
St. Louis, Missouri
Electrolytes and Blood Gases; Electrolytes and Blood Gases Appendix; Physiology and Disorders of Water, Electrolyte, and Acid-Base Metabolism

LESLIE M. SHAW, Ph.D.
Professor,
Director, Toxicology Laboratory and Xenobiotic Toxicokinetics Research Laboratory
Department of Pathology and Laboratory Medicine
University of Pennsylvania Medical Center
Philadelphia, Pennsylvania
Therapeutic Drugs and Their Management; Therapeutic Drugs and Their Management Appendix

ALAN SHENKIN, Ph.D.
Professor
Department of Clinical Chemistry
University of Liverpool,
Consultant Chemical Pathologist
Department of Clinical Biochemistry and Metabolic Medicine
Royal Liverpool University Hospital
Liverpool, England
Vitamins and Trace Elements; Vitamins and Trace Elements Appendix

NICHOLAS E. SHERMAN, Ph.D.
Assistant Professor for Research
University of Virginia
Department of Microbiology
Charlottesville, Virginia
Mass Spectrometry

EDWARD K. SHULTZ, M.D., M.S.
Associate Professor, Biomedical Informatics
Vanderbilt University,
Director, Information Technology Integration
Vanderbilt University Medical Center
Nashville, Tennessee
Clinical Evaluation of Methods

RAVINDER JIT SINGH, Ph.D.
Assistant Professor of Pathology
Division of Clinical Biochemistry and Immunology
Department of Laboratory Medicine and Pathology
Mayo Clinic
Rochester, Minnesota
Catecholamines and Serotonin Appendix

HELGE ERIK SOLBERG, M.D., Ph.D.
Quality and IT Manager, Retired
Department of Clinical Chemistry
Rikshospitalet
Oslo, Norway
Establishment and Use of Reference Values

KENT A. SPACKMAN, M.D., Ph.D.
Professor of Pathology and Medical Informatics
Oregon Health and Science University
Portland, Oregon
Clinical Laboratory Informatics

CAROLE SPENCER, Ph.D.
Professor of Medicine
Department of Medicine
University of Southern California
Los Angeles, California
The Thyroid: Pathophysiology and Thyroid Function Testing

ANDREW ST. JOHN, Ph.D., M.A.A.C.B.
Consultant
ARC Consulting
Mt Lawley 6050
Perth
W Australia
Point-of-Care Testing

M. DAVID ULLMAN, Ph.D.
Research Biochemist
VA Hospital
Bedford, Massachusetts;
Research Associate Professor
University of Massachusetts Medical School
Worcester, Massachusetts
Chromatography

MARY LEE VANCE, M.D.
Professor of Internal Medicine and Neurosurgery
Division of Endocrinology and Metabolism
School of Medicine
University of Virginia
Charlottesville, Virginia
Pituitary Function

WOUTER W. VAN SOLINGE, Ph.D.
Director
Department of Laboratory Medicine
University Medical Center Utrecht
Utrecht, The Netherlands
Enzymes; Enzymes Appendix

CINDY L. VNENCAK-JONES, Ph.D.
Associate Professor of Pathology and Pediatrics,
Director, Molecular Genetics Laboratory
Vanderbilt University Medical Center
Nashville, Tennessee
Inherited Diseases

G. RUSSELL WARNICK, M.S., M.B.A.
President
Pacific Biometrics Research Foundation
Seattle, Washington
Lipids, Lipoproteins, Apolipoproteins, and Other Cardiovascular Risk Factors; Lipids, Lipoproteins, Apolipoproteins, and Other Cardiovascular Risk Factors Appendix

VICTOR W. WEEDN, M.D., J.D.
Principal Research Scientist,
Director of Biotechnology and Health Initiatives
Carnegie Mellon University
Pittsburgh, Pennsylvania
Identity Assessment

JAMES O. WESTGARD, Ph.D.
Professor
Department of Pathology and Laboratory Medicine
University of Wisconsin Medical School
Madison, Wisconsin
Quality Management

SHARON D. WHATLEY, Ph.D.
Principal Biochemist
University Hospital of Wales
Cardiff, United Kingdom
Porphyrins and Disorders of Porphyrin Metabolism; Porphyrins and Disorders of Porphyrin Metabolism Appendix

RONALD J. WHITLEY, Ph.D.
Professor
Department of Pathology and Laboratory Medicine
University of Kentucky
Associate Director of Clinical Chemistry
University of Kentucky Medical Center College of Medicine
Lexington, Kentucky
Catecholamines and Serotonin; Catecholamines and Serotonin Appendix

PETER WILDING, Ph.D., F.R.C.Path., F.R.S.C., H.C.L.D.(A.B.B.)
Professor Emeritus
Department of Pathology and Laboratory Medicine
University of Pennsylvania Medical Center
Philadelphia, Pennsylvania
Nanotechnology and Microfabrication

THOMAS M. WILLIAMS, M.D.
Professor of Pathology
University of New Mexico, Department of Pathology,
Director, Genetics and Cytometry Division
TriCore Reference Laboratories
Albuquerque, New Mexico
Identity Assessment

CARL T. WITTWER, M.D., Ph.D.
Professor of Pathology
University of Utah School of Medicine,
Medical Director of the Advanced Technology Group
ARUP Laboratories
Salt Lake City, Utah
Nucleic Acid Techniques

DONALD S. YOUNG, M.B., Ph.D.
Pathology and Laboratory Medicine
University of Pennsylvania School of Medicine
Philadelphia, Pennsylvania
Introduction to Principles of Laboratory Analyses and Safety; Introduction to Principles of Laboratory Analyses and Safety Appendix; Specimen Collection and Processing; Preanalytical Variables and Biological Variation

Reviewers

GRANT C. BULLOCK, M.D., Ph.D.
Department of Pathology
University of Virginia
Charlottesville, Virginia

GORDON H. GUYATT, M.D.
Clinical Epidemiology and Biostatistics and Medicine
McMaster University
Hamilton, Ontario, Canada

DORIS M. HAVERSTICK, Ph.D.
Department of Pathology
University of Virginia
Charlottesville, Virginia

MANI S. MAHADEVAN, M.D.
Department of Pathology
University of Virginia
Charlottesville, Virginia

MELINDA D. POULTER, Ph.D.
Department of Pathology
University of Virginia
Charlottesville, Virginia

ALISON PRESLEY, M.D.
Department of Pathology
University of Virginia
Charlottesville, Virginia

JOHN SAVORY, Ph.D.
Department of Pathology
University of Virginia
Charlottesville, Virginia

LAWRENCE M. SILVERMAN, Ph.D.
Department of Pathology
University of Virginia
Charlottesville, Virginia

KARL V. VOELKERDING, M.D.
Medical Director, Molecular Development Group
ARUP Laboratories
University of Utah
Salt Lake City, Utah

Foreword

During the last 10 years, new results of biomedical research and new developments in biotechnology entered the medical sciences and changed traditional orientations. The identification of human genes and the cellular functions of gene products resulted in new concepts in the explanation of several diseases, especially in malignant transformation and cancer. Developments in communication technology with fast information exchange between researchers and clinicians globally led to fundamental changes in several medical disciplines and integration of new knowledge into the practice of medicine. The surgeon using endoscopic procedures, the radiologist employing magnetic resonance in metabolism investigations, and the anatomic pathologist applying molecular biology and immunohistochemistry staining in diagnostics are a few examples of these rapid changes. This is also true for clinical chemistry and laboratory medicine, whose objectives now extend beyond diagnosis and monitoring to include risk assessment and prevention. For clinicians and laboratorians, it is pertinent in a time of "managed patient care" to decide as a team on the most efficient diagnostic strategy for a patient that combines clinical information with laboratory results.

The fourth edition of the famous *Tietz Textbook* recognizes new areas requiring greater recognition and understanding from clinical chemists as they strive to be laboratory medicine consultants, linking science and medicine for the benefit of patients and the health of the community. The most immediate change is in the name, which has been enlarged to the *Tietz Textbook of Clinical Chemistry and Molecular Diagnostics*. The importance of this change is highlighted by the introduction of a section dedicated to molecular diagnostics and genetics. Understanding the principles of molecular biology in hematology, infectious disease, and genetics, together with the rapidly expanding area of pharmacogenetics, clearly emphasizes how the clinical laboratory must link technology and clinical understanding and then translate the results of such investigations into terms understandable by clinicians and patients.

It is a notable achievement for any book to become an internationally recognized reference work that successfully appeals to professionals from different medical disciplines and cultures while still managing to overcome the barriers that are raised by language differences. All over the world the *Tietz Textbook of Clinical Chemistry* has been acknowledged as an outstanding, broadly based source of knowledge and information for our profession. It provides guidance for the youngest to the oldest, whether neophyte or laboratory-tested veteran, thus bridging generation gaps. It is a tool not only for the education of those training to be clinical laboratory professionals but for the continuing education of those who may have acquired specific expertise and recognition, yet who need to keep current with an extensive understanding of our present and future scientific, technological, and organizational development.

Such recognition for a reference book is not easily attained or maintained and requires considerable talent and effort to have its reputation enhanced. This fourth edition once again faces up to the challenge of freshness and relevance in what to introduce and what to leave out. The judicious selection of subjects and authors, together with their integration into an up-to-date, coherent, and balanced text, is the responsibility of the editors. Following the excellent first edition, which reflected the science and personality of Dr. Norbert Tietz, the second and third editions were edited by Dr. Carl A. Burtis and Dr. Edward R. Ashwood. The fourth edition benefits once again from their experience, complementary skills, and knowledge of science and technology as applied to clinical chemistry and laboratory medicine. Dr. David E.

Bruns, widely known and respected as the Editor of *Clinical Chemistry,* is the new addition to the editorial group. Making a strong editorial team even stronger is a far-sighted move that inspires confidence.

This edition is notable also for the large number of new authors and the challenge given to them to respond to significant regroupings of chapters and subjects, thus introducing room for new information and discussion of new topics. The principles of evidence-based laboratory medicine are addressed. The basic science, its application and management in the clinical laboratory, allied with the interpretation and use of the information produced, are all components of the evidence base. This new edition reflects the continuing maturity of an excellent textbook that will be an extremely useful aid for clinicians and laboratory professionals in their daily work.

Professor Matthew McQueen
Department of Pathology and Molecular Medicine
McMaster University,
Director, Hamilton Regional Laboratory Medicine Program
Hamilton, Ontario, Canada

Professor Mathias Müller
Institute of Laboratory Diagnostics
Kaiser Franz Josef Hospital
Vienna, Austria

Preface

The goal of the editors of the prior three editions of the *Tietz Textbook of Clinical Chemistry* (1986, 1994, 1999) was to produce an authoritative textbook that provided a current and comprehensive overview of the discipline of clinical chemistry. We have set the same goal for this fourth edition. Meeting this goal has become a greater challenge with each edition as technical and medical advances expand the discipline in both depth and breadth and blur the traditional boundaries between clinical chemistry and other disciplines of laboratory medicine.

To meet this challenge and yet keep the book manageable and in one volume has necessitated extensive revision of the format of the fourth edition and additions to its content. The first major change was to add eight new chapters on molecular diagnostics, a change reflected in amending the title of the fourth edition to the *Tietz Textbook of Clinical Chemistry and Molecular Diagnostics.* A second major change was the addition of Professor David E. Bruns as a co-editor to our editorial team. The two editors of the previous edition found that his wealth of knowledge and experience and his superb editing skills were invaluable in producing this new edition.

As a result of adding new chapters and the retirement of several authors who had participated in earlier editions, many new authors have joined our team of core veterans from previous editions. In fact, 66 of the 97 authors represented in the fourth edition are new to the effort. These knowledgeable and enthusiastic new authors coupled with core veterans have produced chapters that are timely and reflect the state-of-the-art in their respective fields. The international flavor of the book and the international nature of the field are more evident than ever before in the list of countries represented by this outstanding group of colleagues.

In addition to the eight new chapters on molecular diagnostics (Chapters 36-43), other new chapters include those on Nanotechnology and Microfabrication (Chapter 10), Point-of-Care Testing (Chapter 12), Introduction to Laboratory Medicine and Evidence-Based Laboratory Medicine (Chapter 13), and Inborn Errors of Amino Acid, Organic Acid, and Fatty Acid Metabolism (Chapter 55). We have also removed a few chapters and combined elements from them into new chapters including Selection and Analytical Evaluation of Methods—With Statistical Techniques (Chapter 14), Vitamins and Trace Elements (Chapter 30), and Hemoglobin, Iron, and Bilirubin (Chapter 31). The fourth edition now contains 56 chapters, a large increase when compared with the 20 chapters of the first edition. These 56 chapters include over 10,000 references, 900 figures, and 500 tables and boxes. We have grouped these chapters into seven sections entitled Laboratory Principles, Analytical Techniques and Instrumentation, Principles of Laboratory Medicine, Analytes, Molecular Diagnostics and Genetics, Pathophysiology, and Reference Information. As in previous editions, the reader will find that the distinction between "Analytes" and "Pathophysiology" is indistinct as several analytes are discussed in the chapters included in the Pathophysiology section and the pathophysiologies of several disorders are discussed in chapters placed in the Analytes section.

A major addition to the fourth edition is a companion website (http://evolve.elsevier.com/Tietz/textbook/), which contains analytical methods, case studies, and supplementary information. We plan to periodically include updated and new information on this website, including corrections when errors are found in the textbook. We invite readers to call such errors to our attention so that corrections can be made and subsequent printings of the textbook will reflect the process of continuous improvement for which we strive. All of the reference citations in the book are also listed in the Evolve website where they are linked electronically to the PubMed database of articles and abstracts. Because PubMed has links to on-line journals, readers can access the full texts of many cited articles with two clicks of a mouse.

Information technology played a much-increased role in the preparation and production of the fourth edition. Each chapter was submitted, edited, and typeset electronically. As with the third edition of the *Textbook,* many of the figures, especially those that included chemical structure were drawn or revised by one of us (EA) using ChemWindows software (http://www.softshell.com). This resulted in a uniform representation of chemical structures and facilitated the integration of figures with the text while reducing errors. The Internet also helped authors and editors to find the latest information and sources of products. Readers will note that references to web-based sources of information are found throughout the text.

We greatly appreciate the opportunity provided to us by Elsevier to participate in the preparation of the fourth edition of this textbook. It has been an exciting, challenging, and educational experience. We have endeavored to ensure that this edition will live up to the reputation and success of its distinguished predecessors. We have enjoyed working with the team of dedicated authors who have spent countless hours preparing comprehensive chapters that are authoritative and timely. We believe that they have produced a textbook that is reflective of the diverse, technical, and practical nature of the current practice of clinical laboratory science and medicine.

We have also benefited from and enjoyed working with the Elsevier staff, especially Managing Editor, Mindy Hutchinson; Developmental Editor, Ellen Wurm; and Senior Project Manager, Rachel Dowell. Their patience, warm cooperation, sound advice, and professional dedication are gratefully acknowledged.

Carl A. Burtis
Edward R. Ashwood
David E. Bruns

Contents

Color insert follows page 1468.

SECTION III
PRINCIPLES OF LABORATORY MEDICINE

SECTION I

Laboratory Principles

CHAPTER 1

Introduction to Principles of Laboratory Analyses and Safety*

Edward W. Bermes, Jr., Ph.D., Stephen E. Kahn, Ph.D., and Donald S. Young, M.B., Ph.D.

To reliably perform qualitative and quantitative analyses on body fluids and tissue, the clinical laboratorian must understand the basic *principles and procedures* that affect the analytical process and operation of the clinical laboratory. These include the knowledge of: (1) the concept of solute and solvent, (2) units of measurement, (3) chemicals and reference materials, (4) basic techniques, such as volumetric sampling and dispensing, centrifugation, measurement of radioactivity, gravimetry, thermometry, buffer solution, and processing of solutions, and (5) safety.[†]

CONCEPT OF SOLUTE AND SOLVENT

Many analyses in the clinical laboratory are concerned with the determination of the presence of or measurement of the concentration of substances in solutions, the solutions most often being blood, serum, urine, spinal fluid, or other body fluids (see Chapter 2).

DEFINITIONS

A *solution* is a homogeneous mixture of one or more *solutes* dispersed molecularly in a sufficient quantity of a dissolving *solvent.* In laboratory practice, solutes are typically measured and are frequently referred to as *analytes.* A solution may be gaseous, liquid, or solid. A clinical laboratorian is concerned primarily with the measurement of gases or solids in liquids, where there is always a relatively large amount of solvent in comparison with the amount of solute.

EXPRESSING CONCENTRATIONS OF SOLUTIONS

The concentration of a solute in a solution may be expressed in different ways (Table 1-1). In the United States, laboratory data typically are reported in terms of mass of solute per unit volume of solution, usually the deciliter. However, the Système International d'Unités (SI) recommends the use of moles of solute per volume of solution for analyte concentrations (substance concentrations), whenever possible, and the use of liter as the reference volume. Although considered incorrect and inappropriate by metrologists, mass concentration also is reported in terms of grams percent or percent. This is typically how concentrations of ethanol in blood are expressed. This terminology indicates an amount of solute per mass of solution (e.g., grams per 100 g) and would be appropriate only if reference materials against which the unknowns were compared were also measured in the same terms. An exception to the general expression of analyte con-

*The authors gratefully acknowledge the original contributions of Drs. Edward R. Powsner and John C. Widman on which the Measurement of Radioactivity portion of this chapter is based.

[†]Note: Additional discussions on the topics of (1) Chemicals, Reference Materials, and Related Substances, (2) General Laboratory Supplies, (3) Calibration of Volumetric Pipettes, (4) Centrifugation, (5) Procedures for Concentrating Solutions, (6) Separatory Funnels and Extraction Procedures, (7) Laboratory Mixers and Homogenizers, and (8) Filtration are found in the Appendix of this chapter located in the Evolve site that accompanies this book at http://evolve.elsevier.com/Tietz/textbook and in the previous edition of this textbook (Bermes EW, Young DS. In: Burtis CA, Ashwood ER, eds. Tietz textbook of clinical chemistry, 3rd ed. Philadelphia: W.B. Saunders, 1999:3-41.)

TABLE 1-1 Concentration Quantities and Units

Name and Quantity	Definition	Unit
Substance concentration (of a given solute component)	Amount of substance of a solute divided by volume of solution	mol/m^3; mol/L
Molality (of a given solute component)	Amount of substance of a solute divided by mass of solvent	mol/kg
Mole fraction (or substance fraction) [of a given component]	Amount of substance of a component divided by amount of substance of mixture (i.e., all components of the system)	mol/mol
Mole ratio (or substance ratio) [of a given solute component]	Amount of substance of a solute divided by amount of substance of the solvent	mol/mol
Mass concentration (of a given component)	Mass of a component (e.g., solute) divided by volume of system (e.g., solution)	kg/m^3; kg/L
Mass fraction (of a given component)	Mass of a component divided by mass of system (mixture)	kg/kg
Volume fraction (of a given component)	Volume of a component divided by volume of system (mixture)	m^3/m^3; L/L
Number concentration	Number of specified particles or elementary entities divided by volume of system (mixture)	m^{-3}; L^{-1}
Number fraction	Number of specified particles or elementary entities divided by total number of particles or entities in the system (mixture)	1 (a ratio)
Substance content (of a given component)	Amount of substance of a component divided by mass of system (mixture)	mol/kg

From The SI for the Health Professions, World Health Organization, 1977.

centrations in terms of volume of solution is the measurement of osmolality, in which concentrations are expressed in terms of mass of solvent (mOsmol/kg or mmol/kg).

When the solution and solvent are both liquids, as in alcohol solutions, the concentration of such a solution is frequently expressed in terms of volume per volume (vol/vol).[33] By adding 70 mL of alcohol to a flask and mixing it to 100 mL with water, a solution whose concentration is 700 mL/L would be achieved. The expression "700 mL/L" is preferred to the alternatives of 70 volumes percent or 70% (vol/vol).

The following equations define the expressions of concentrations:

$$\text{Mole} = \frac{\text{mass (g)}}{\text{gram molecular weight (g)}}$$

$$\text{Molarity of a solution} = \frac{\text{number of moles of solute}}{\text{number of liters of solution}}$$

$$\text{Molality of a solution} = \frac{\text{number of moles of solute}}{\text{number of kilograms of solvent}}$$

$$\text{Normality of a solution} = \frac{\text{number of gram equivalents of solute}}{\text{number of liters of solution}}$$

$$\text{Normality (in oxidation–reduction reaction)} = \text{molarity} \times \text{difference in oxidation state}$$

$$\text{Gram equivalent weight (as oxidatant or reductant)} = \frac{\text{formula weight (g)}}{\text{difference in oxidation state}}$$

For example, using these equations, a 1 *molar* solution of H_2SO_4 contains 98.08 g H_2SO_4 per liter of solution. (Note: The symbol M, to denote molarity, is no longer acceptable and has been replaced by mol/L.) A *molal* solution contains 1 mol of solute in 1 kg of solvent. Molality is properly expressed as mol/kg.

Likewise, a one *normal* solution contains 1 g equivalent weight of solute in 1 L of solution; for example, 1 mol HCl, 0.5 mol H_2SO_4, and 0.33 mol H_3PO_4, each in 1 L of solution, are one normal solutions. The use of normality is limited in that a given solution may have more than one normality, depending on the type of reaction for which the solution is used. The molarity of a solution, however, is a fixed number because there is only one molecular mass for any substance. Normality is no longer recommended to express concentrations. Nevertheless, the term is included here because it remains in common usage and is related to the equivalent concept sometimes favored for serum electrolyte concentrations in the United States and some other countries.

A milligram equivalent of a substance is its equivalent weight expressed in milligrams. The equivalent mass of H_2SO_4 is 49.04 g; therefore 1 mg equivalent of H_2SO_4 =

49.04 mg H_2SO_4. Because substances may react on the basis of their valence, 1 mol calcium (atomic weight = 40), which is bivalent, has twice the combining power of 1 mol sodium (atomic weight = 23). Forty mg calcium is therefore equivalent to 46 mg sodium.

An older unit of measurement used to express the concentration of electrolytes in plasma is the milliequivalent (mEq), which is one thousandth of an equivalent.

$$\text{Milliequivalents (mEq)} = \frac{\text{weight (g)}}{\text{milliequivalent mass (g)}}$$

Milligrams per 100 mL (deciliter) can be converted to mEq per liter using the following formula:

$$\text{mEq/L} = \frac{\text{mg/dL} \times 10 \times \text{valence}}{\text{mg atomic mass}}$$

Example: If the serum sodium concentration is 322 mg/dL, then the serum contains 3220 mg/L. The equivalent mass of sodium is 23, and the valence is 1; therefore:

$$\text{mEq/L} = \frac{322 \times 10 \times 1}{23} = 140$$

The *recommended* units for sodium concentration in plasma are millimoles per liter (mmol/L). In the previous example, the concentration of sodium is:

$$\text{mmol/L} = \frac{\text{mg/L}}{\text{mg molecular mass}} = \frac{322 \times 10 \times 1}{23} = 140$$

In chemical terms, the *titer* of a solution is the mass of a substance equivalent to a unit volume of the solution.

$$\text{Titer} = \frac{\text{grams of substance}}{\text{liters of solution}} = \frac{\text{mg substance}}{\text{mL solution}}$$

However, in clinical laboratory practice, a titer is more commonly thought of as the lowest dilution at which a particular reaction takes place. Titer is customarily expressed as a ratio, for example, 1:10 or 1 to 10.

Regarding gases in solution, Henry's law states that the solubility of a gas in a liquid is directly proportional to the pressure of the gas above the liquid at equilibrium. Thus as the pressure of a gas is doubled, its solubility is also doubled. The relationship between pressure and solubility varies with the nature of the gas. When several gases are dissolved at the same time in a single solvent, the solubility of each gas is proportional to its partial pressure in the mixture. The solubility of most gases in liquids decreases with an increase in temperature and indeed boiling a liquid frequently drives out all dissolved gases. Traditionally the unit used to describe the concentration of gases in liquids has been percent by volume (vol/vol). Using the SI, gas concentrations are expressed in moles per cubic meter (mol/m^3).

UNITS OF MEASUREMENT

A meaningful measurement is expressed with both a number and a unit. The unit identifies the dimension—mass, volume, or concentration—of a measured property. The number indicates how many units are contained in the property.

Traditionally, measurements in the clinical laboratory have been made in metric units. In the early development of the metric system, units were referenced to length, mass, and time. The first absolute systems were based on the centimeter, gram, and second (CGS) and then the meter, kilogram, and second (MKS). The SI is a different system that was accepted internationally in 1960. The *units of the system* are called SI units.

The SI takes its origin from the Conférence Générales des Poids et Mesures (CGPM), which since 1889 has functioned as the international authority for measurement. Operating under CGPM is the Comité International des Poids et Mesures (CIPM), whose prime responsibilities are to define units and to direct the Bureau International des Poids et Mesures (BIPM). The BIPM, established in 1875, serves as the international reference laboratory and has the responsibility for ensuring uniformity of physical measurements.

TABLE 1-2 SI Base Units

Quantity	Name	Symbol
Length	meter	m
Mass	kilogram	kg
Time	second	s
Electric current	ampere	A
Thermodynamic temperature	kelvin	K
Amount of substance	mole	mol
Luminous intensity	candela	cd
Catalytic amount	katal	kat

INTERNATIONAL SYSTEM OF UNITS[38]

There are three classes of SI units: base, derived, and supplemental units. A *base unit* was decreed by the CGPM for each of eight fundamental but dimensionally independent physical quantities. These units are listed in Table 1-2. A *derived unit* is derived mathematically from two or more base units (Table 1-3). A *supplemental unit* is a unit that conforms to the SI but that has not been classified as either base or derived. At present only the radian (for plane angles) and the steradian (for solid angles) are classified this way.

The CGPM recognizes that some units outside the SI continue to be important and useful in particular applications. An example is the liter as the reference volume in clinical analyses. Liter is the name of the submultiple (cubic decimeter) of the SI unit of volume, the cubic meter. Considering that 1 cubic meter represents some 200 times the blood volume of an adult human, the SI unit of volume is neither a convenient nor a reasonable reference volume in a clinical context. Nevertheless, the CGPM recommends that such exceptional units as the liter should not be combined with SI units and preferably should be replaced with SI units whenever possible.

TABLE 1-3 Examples of SI-Derived Units Important in Clinical Medicine, Expressed in Terms of Base Units

Quantity	Name	SI Symbol	Expression in Terms of Other SI Units	Expression in Terms of SI Base Units
Volume	cubic meter	m^3		m^3
Mass density	kilogram per cubic meter	kg/m^3		kg/m^3
Concentration of amount of substance	mole per cubic meter	mol/m^3		mol/m^3
Frequency	hertz	Hz		s^{-1}
Force	newton	N		$m{\cdot}kg{\cdot}s^{-2}$
Pressure	pascal	Pa	N/m^2	$m^{-1}{\cdot}kg{\cdot}s^{-2}$
Energy, work, quantity of heat	joule	J	N•m	$m^2{\cdot}kg{\cdot}s^{-2}$
Power	watt	W	J/sec	$m^2{\cdot}kg{\cdot}s^{-3}$
Electric potential, potential difference, electromotive force	volt	V	$W{\cdot}A^{-1}$	$m^2{\cdot}kg{\cdot}s^{-3}{\cdot}A^{-1}$

TABLE 1-4 Non-SI Units Retained for Use with the SI

Quantity	Unit	Symbol	Value in SI Units
Time	minute	min	1 min = 60 s
	hour	h	1 h = 3600 s
	day	d	1 d = 86,400 s
Plane angle	degree	°	1° = π/180 rad
	minute	′	1′ = π/10,800 rad
	second	″	1″ = π/648,000 rad
Volume	liter	L	1 L = 1 dm^3 or 10^{-3} m^3
Mass	tonne	t	1 t = 1000 kg

The minute, hour, and day have had such long-standing use in everyday life that it is unlikely that new SI units derived from the second could supplant them. Some other non-SI units are still accepted, although they are rarely used by most individuals in their daily lives but have been very important in some specialized fields. Examples of such units are the nautical mile, knot, and hectare. Examples of non-SI units retained for use with the SI are illustrated in Table 1-4.

Decimal Multiples and Submultiples of SI Units

In practical application of SI units, certain values are too large or too small to be expressed conveniently in the base or derived units. Numerical values can be brought to convenient size when the unit is appropriately modified by official SI prefixes. In general the prefixes are such that the value of the unit changes 1000-fold. However, certain common previously accepted multiples or submultiples, such as deci- and hecto-, are still accepted in the SI framework. The SI prefixes are listed in Table 1-5 together with their symbols.

The International Organization for Standards (ISO) recommends that prefix symbols be printed in Roman (upright) type without spacing between the prefix symbol and the unit symbol, thus mL rather than m L. Furthermore, an exponent attached to a symbol containing a prefix indicates that the multiple or submultiple of the unit is raised to the power expressed by the exponent (e.g., cm^3 is $10^{-6}\,m^3$). Compound prefixes formed by the juxtaposition of two or more SI prefixes are not to be used. Thus 1 nm is appropriate, whereas 1 mμm is not. Likewise, the appropriate unit of mass is the megagram (Mg) rather than the kilokilogram (kkg).

Applications of SI in Laboratory Medicine

Many international clinical laboratory organizations and national professional societies have accepted the SI units in its broad application. The World Health Organization has also recommended its adoption. These organizations have accepted the liter as the preferred unit of volume. For multiples and submultiples of units, including derived units, only one prefix should be used. The prefix should preferably be confined to the numerator, except in the case of the kilogram. Units of concentration should use the liter as denominator. Use of the milli-, micro-, or femtoliter for reporting of test values requires little alteration in thinking when liter is used for reporting mass concentrations, provided that the numerator unit is changed by a similar factor. The numerator unit is usually adjusted so that clinically probable values are less than 1000. When liter is used instead of deciliter for reporting of results, their numerical value is increased by a factor of 10. Such values, when considered in conjunction with the patient's clinical status, should be understandable.

Use of the liter as reference volume causes little confusion in interpretation of test results. However, introduction of the concept of amount of substance expressed as mole (mol) and

TABLE 1-5 Metric Prefixes of SI Units*

Factor	Prefix	Symbol	Factor	Prefix	Symbol
10^{24}	yotta	Y	10^{-1}	deci	d
10^{21}	zetta	Z	10^{-2}	centi	c
10^{18}	exa	E	10^{-3}	milli	m
10^{15}	peta	P	10^{-6}	micro	μ
10^{12}	tera	T	10^{-9}	nano	n
10^{9}	giga	G	10^{-12}	pico	p
10^{6}	mega	M	10^{-15}	femto	f
10^{3}	kilo	k	10^{-18}	atto	a
10^{2}	hecto	h	10^{-21}	zepto	z
10^{1}	deka†	da	10^{-24}	yocto	y

From The International System of Units [SI]. Washington, DC, National Institute of Standards and Technology, 1991.

*The Eleventh Conférence Générale des Poids et Mésures (CGPM) (1960, Resolution 12) adopted a first series of prefixes and symbols of prefixes to form the names and symbols of the decimal multiples and submultiples of SI units. Prefixes for 10^{-15} and 10^{-18} were added by the twelfth CGPM (1964, Resolution 8), those for 10^{15} and 10^{18} by the fifteenth CGPM (1975, Resolution 10), and those for 10^{21}, 10^{24}, and 10^{-24} were proposed by the CIPM (1990) for approval by the nineteenth CGPM (1991).

†Outside the United States, the spelling "deca" is used extensively.

TABLE 1-6 Typical Values for Analytes and Reporting Increments

	Conventional Units	Recommended Units	Rounded Recommended Units	Smallest Recommended Reporting Increment
Albumin	3.8 g/dL	550.6 μmol/L	550.0 μmol/L	10.0 μmol/L
Bilirubin	0.2 mg/dL	3.42 μmol/L	3 μmol/L	2 μmol/L
Calcium	9.8 mg/dL	2.45 mmol/L	2.45 mmol/L	0.02 mmol/L
Cholesterol	200 mg/dL	5.17 mmol/L	5.2 mmol/L	0.05 mmol/L
Creatinine	0.8 mg/dL	90.48 μmol/L	90 mmol/L	10 μmol/L
Glucose	90 mg/dL	5.00 mmol/L	5.0 mmol/L	0.1 mmol/L
Phosphorus	3.0 mg/dL	0.97 mmol/L	1.0 mmol/L	0.05 mmol/L
Thyroxine	7.0 μg/dL	90.09 nmol/L	90 nmol/L	10 nmol/L
Triglycerides	100 mg/dL	1.14 mmol/L	1.15 mmol/L	0.05 mmol/L
Urea nitrogen*	10 mg/dL	3.57 mmol/L	3.5 mmol/L	0.05 mmol/L
Uric acid	5.0 mg/dL	297 μmol/L	300 μmol/L	10 μmol/L

*Urea nitrogen is reported as urea (mmol/L) when SI units are used.

its decimal fractions of mmol, μmol, nmol, and so on, could lead to confusion because of general lack of familiarity with these units in comparison with more traditional units. The SI does not mandate the use of amount of substance (moles) or substance concentration (moles per liter) instead of mass of substance (kilograms) or mass concentration (kilograms per liter). However, in those countries in which the SI has been introduced into medical practice, amounts of constituents of body fluids are usually reported as substance concentrations rather than mass concentrations, for example, 2.5 mmol/L instead of 10 mg/dL for calcium and 3.9 mmol/L instead of 70 mg/dL for glucose. The rationale for this change is that compounds react on a molar basis, and expression of amounts of substances in such terms allows a better understanding of the relative proportion of compounds. Even though physicians initially have little comprehension of the meaning of results when expressed in units of substance concentration, experience in other countries has shown that they soon adjust to the previously unfamiliar units. Nevertheless, during and after the transition from one set of units to another, it is essential that numbers be unequivocally associated with units. There is therefore no cause for misinterpretation. A comparison of results of some of the commonly measured serum constituents, at a concentration found in healthy individuals, is shown in Table 1-6.

Problem Areas in the Use of SI Units

Problems in the implementation of SI units in the clinical laboratory have been encountered in the following areas.

Expressing Acidity

Some individuals have advocated reporting of *acidity* of body fluids in terms of hydrogen ion concentration instead of pH. Their rationale is that pH is a measure of the chemical potential of hydrogen ions rather than a measure of the concentration of the ions. Because chemical potential is a function of the activity coefficient, which is not known with certainty, the antilog of pH cannot be assumed to equal the hydrogen ion concentration. pH values should be treated as primary variables and reported as measured.

Expressing Enzyme Units

The base unit katal (symbol kat), mol/sec, is the *catalytic amount* of any catalyst, including enzymes, that catalyzes a reaction rate of 1 mol per second in an assay system.* The kind of quantity measured is identified as catalytic amount. There is a constant relationship between the international unit (1 μmol/min) and the katal (1 mol/sec); to convert a value in international units to nmol/sec, the value is multiplied by 16.67. Note, however, that dependence on reaction conditions applies to SI units in the same way as to international units; therefore data reported in the same units but obtained under different conditions may not be comparable. Replacement of the international unit for reporting enzyme activity is likely to be slow; even units that antedated the international unit are sometimes used in clinical laboratory practice. (See Chapters 8 and 21 for further details on the expression of enzyme activity.)

Expressing Protein Concentration

For some *proteins* whose molecular weight is uncertain, debate continues as to the appropriate unit for reporting test results. Nevertheless, because substance concentration gives a better indication of the relative amount of a protein, substance concentration units are still preferred, even if the molecular weight of the protein is not exactly known. The molecular weight actually used for the substance concentration should be included as part of the test description. The concentration of *hormones* should also be reported as substance concentration. Units of activity, such as international units related to a consensus standard, should be avoided. Again, where uncertainty in the correct molecular weight of the hormone exists, an approximate value may be used without introducing a major error in the reported results. Even though the molecular weight of hemoglobin is known, there is no agreement as to whether the monomer Hb(Fe), or the tetramer $Hb_4(Fe_4)$, should be used to report values as substance concentration. Until agreement is reached, the International Committee for Standardization in Hematology (ICSH) recommends that hemoglobin results be reported in terms of mass concentration, i.e., grams per liter (g/L).

Expressing Drug Concentration

Although it is probable that *drugs* will be prescribed and administered in mass units for the immediate future, it is still desirable that the concentration of a drug in a body fluid be expressed in terms of substance concentration rather than mass concentration. Substance concentration allows the concentration of a drug to be understood in comparison with the concentrations of proteins, to which drugs are largely bound, and of other compounds with which drugs compete for protein-binding sites. For drugs it is essential that units be clearly stated to prevent dangerous misinterpretations of test values, which might occur when drugs are administered and measured in body fluids in different units.

Expressing Osmolality

The osmole is not an SI unit and therefore theoretically is not suitable for reporting results of measurements of the concentration of osmotically active particles. The appropriate alternatives would be to record the depression of freezing point, whose unit is kelvin or degree Celsius, or the change in vapor pressure in pascals. But because the units would be method dependent, some of the benefits of using the osmole would be lost. The current recommendation is to report osmolality in moles per kilogram (mol/kg). If osmolarity is reported, the preferred unit remains moles per liter (mol/L).

Expressing Units of Energy

Implementation of the SI requires the use of the joule (J) to replace the calorie as the unit of *energy.* The calorie, as now used, is an ill-defined unit. The terms "calorie" and "Calorie," widely used in nutrition practice, actually relate to the thermochemical kilocalorie. Thus replacement of calorie by joule would prevent confusion and introduce a uniform practice. Resistance to conversion from calories to joules is based on the same arguments that have been used against the change from other traditional units to SI units. The arguments, in the case of energy units, also cite the lack of published tables of nutrition information in SI units. It is recommended that dietary allowances be presented in megajoules rather than kilojoules, because the smaller number probably has some psychological benefit to the dieter. A 2000-kilocalorie diet seems more acceptable when expressed as 8.37 MJ than as 8370 kJ.

Expressing Units of Pressure

The correct unit for reporting *pressure,* whether it is the partial pressure of blood gases or blood pressure, is the pascal. Because the numerical values expressed in pascals are too small to be used for most clinically important pressure

*In 1999, with passage of Resolution 12 of the 21st CGPM, the katal became an official international unit. With its formal adoption, metrologists expect that the katal will eventually replace the non-SI "unit." However, currently, "units" are more commonly used than the katal.

measurements, the kilopascal is a more convenient unit. Thus kilopascal replaces mm Hg or torr. The present common units for gas concentrations in blood are volume percent (vol%) or mmol/L. The carbon dioxide content of blood is expressed in mmol/L. If all the carbon dioxide in the blood were in the form of bicarbonate, mEq/L of bicarbonate and mmol/L of carbon dioxide would be identical. Because carbon dioxide exists in the blood as a mixture of free CO_2, HCO_3^-, and H_2CO_3, concentrations of carbon dioxide are best reported in mmol/L.

Conversion Rules

To convert from conventional units to SI units, the following scheme may be used:

1. Mass concentration (mass units/dL) to mass concentration (mass units/L):

$$\text{Numerical value in mass units/dL} \times 10 = \text{mass units/L}$$

$$\text{e.g., Serum albumin, } 4.0\,\text{g/dL} \times 10 = 40\,\text{g/L}$$

2. Mass concentration to substance concentration:

$$\frac{\text{Numerical value in mass concentration/dL}}{\text{molecular mass}} \times 10 = \text{substance units/L}$$

$$\text{e.g., Serum albumin, } 4.0\,\text{g/dL} = \frac{4.0 \times 10}{69{,}000\,\text{mol/L}} = 580\,\mu\text{mol/L}$$

3. Mass amount to amount of substance:

$$\frac{\text{Numerical value in mass units}}{\text{molecular mass}} = \text{amount of substance}$$

$$\text{e.g., Urine albumin, } 150\,\text{mg/d} = (150/69{,}000)\,\text{mmol/d} = 2.2\,\mu\text{mol/d}$$

$$\text{Urine urate, } 600\,\text{mg/d} = 600/168 = 3.6\,\text{mmol/d}$$

In some cases, a factor of 1000 may be required so that values in SI units generally fall between 1 and 1000. To convert from SI to conventional units the reverse process of that shown previously is used.

The factors for converting from traditional to SI units for many of the constituents of body fluids commonly measured in the clinical laboratory are listed in the table of reference intervals in Chapter 56.

Standardized Reporting of Test Results

To describe test results properly, it is important that all necessary information be included in the test description. Systems developed for expressing the results produced by the clinical laboratory include the Logical Observation Identifier Names and Codes (LOINC) system and the International Federation of Clinical Chemistry/International Union of Pure and Applied Chemistry (IFCC)/IUPAC system.

LOINC System

The LOINC system is a universal coding system for reporting laboratory and other clinical observations to facilitate electronic transmission of laboratory data within and between institutions (http://www.loinc.org).[13,23] This set of codes was developed by an ad hoc group of clinical chemists, clinical pathologists, and representatives from the diagnostic industry. It was supported in part by grants and contracts from the John A. Hartford Foundation of New York, the U.S. National Library of Medicine, the Agency for Health Care Policy and Research, and the Regenstrief Institute for Healthcare. These codes are intended to be used in context with existing standards, such as ASTM E1238 (American Society for Testing and Materials),[2] HLV Version 2.2. (Health Level Seven),[19] and the Systematized Nomenclature of Medicine, Reference Technology (SNOMED-RT).[52] A similar standard, known as CEN ENV 1613, is being developed by the European Committee for Standardization of the Comité Européen de Normalisation (CEN) Technical Committee 251[10] (http://www.cenorm.be).

The LOINC data base currently carries records for greater than 30,000 observations.[23] For each observation, there is a code, a long formal name, a short 30-character name, and synonyms. A mapping program termed "Regenstrief LOINC mapping assistant" (RELMA) is available to map local test codes to LOINC codes and to facilitate searching of the LOINC data base. Both LOINC and RELAM are available at no cost from http://www.regenstrief.org/loinc/.

IFCC/IUPAC System[50]

The IFCC/IUPAC system recommends that the following items be included with each test result:

1. The name of the system or its abbreviation
2. A dash (two hyphens)
3. The name of the analyte (never abbreviated) with an initial capital letter
4. A comma
5. The quantity name or its abbreviation
6. An equal sign
7. The numerical value and the unit or its abbreviation

The following example illustrates a correct description of a test result in complete and abbreviated forms for the IFCC/IUPAC system:

Plasma from fasting patient – glucose, substance concentration = 5.5 millimoles per liter.

Fasting patient(fPt) P-Glucose, substance concentration (substc) = 5.5 mmol/L.

This is not the type of abbreviated information that would appear on a report. This would be:

FPt P-Glucose (substc) = 5.5 mmol/L

The *system* represents the material that is examined. It should be described to the greatest extent necessary to make interpretation of results unambiguous. The system may be the patient, a body fluid, or a component of a body fluid. Although spelling out the system is preferable, certain abbreviations have been recommended by IFCC and IUPAC. The abbreviations may be combined to build up a complete description (e.g., fPt and aB for fasting patient or arterial blood, respectively). The abbreviations recommended by the

TABLE 1-7 Recommended Abbreviations for Systems and Prefixes

a	arterial
Amf	amniotic fluid
B	blood
c	capillary
d	24 hours (diem)
Df	duodenal fluid
Erc	erythrocyte
Ercs	erythrocytes
f	fasting
F	feces
Gf	gastric fluid
Lkc	leukocyte
Lkcs	leukocytes
P	plasma
Peritf	peritoneal fluid
Plf	pleural fluid
Pt	patient
S	serum
Semf	seminal fluid
Sf	spinal fluid
Synf	synovial fluid
T	tissue
U	urine
v	venous

IFCC, IUPAC, and other organizations are listed in Table 1-7. The different kinds of quantities used and their accepted abbreviations are listed in Table 1-8.

CHEMICALS AND REFERENCE MATERIALS

The quality of the analytical results produced by the laboratory is a direct indication of (1) the purity of the chemicals used as analytical reagents and (2) the availability and quality of the reference materials used to calibrate assays and to monitor their analytical performance. Laboratory chemicals are available in a variety of grades. The solutes and solvents used in analytical work are *reagent grade chemicals,* among which water is a solvent of primary importance. IUPAC has established criteria for "primary standards." The National Institute of Standards and Technology (NIST; http://ts.nist.gov/ts/htdocs/230/232/232.htm) has a number of Standard Reference Materials (SRMs) available for the clinical chemistry laboratory. The National Committee for Clinical Laboratory Standards (NCCLS; http://www.ncccls.org) has established a standard for reagent grade water[34] and has published several documents that describe and discuss the use of reference materials in clinical laboratory medicine and their role in the National Reference System for the Clinical Laboratory.[29-31] Certified reference materials of clinical relevance are also available from the Institute for Reference Materials and Measurements (IRMM) in Geel, Belgium (http://www.irmm.jrc.be/)[49] and the World Health Organization (WHO; http://www.who.int/biologicals/IBRP/Catalogue.htm).

TABLE 1-8 Abbreviations for Names of Quantities

ams.	amount of substance
diff.	difference
equil.	equilibration
massc.*	mass concentration
massfr.†	mass fraction
molal.	molality
numc.	number concentration
numfr.	number fraction
rel.	relative
substc.	substance concentration
substfr.	substance fraction
vol.	volume
volfr.	volume fraction

*Previously masc.
†Previously masfr.

Reagent Grade Water

The preparation of most reagents and solutions used in the clinical laboratory requires "pure" water. In the distant past, the term "distilled" has been used to mean "pure," because distillation was the principal procedure used to remove the impurities that water contains in its natural state. Now there are alternative, cost effective, methods to produce "pure" water. In fact single-distilled water fails to meet the specifications for Type I Clinical Laboratory Reagent Water put forward by the NCCLS.[34]

Since the term "deionized water" and the term "distilled water" describe preparation techniques, they should be replaced by *reagent grade water,* followed by designation of the Type (I through III), which better defines the specifications of the water and is independent of the method of preparation (Table 1-9).

In general no single process of purification produces water that meets the rigid specifications for reagent grade water type I set forth by the NCCLS. The following processes or any combination of these may be used in the preparation of reagent grade water as long as the final product meets the specifications. The combination selected is usually dictated in part by the quality of the source water and in part by the intended use of the water. In reality most clinical laboratories use reagent water that exceeds the NCCLS specifications.

Preparation of Reagent Grade Water

Distillation, ion exchange, reverse osmosis, and ultraviolet oxidation are processes used to prepare reagent grade water. In practice, water is often filtered before any of these processes are used.

TABLE 1-9 NCCLS Specifications for Reagent Grade Water

	Type I	Type II	Type III
*Microbiological content,** colony forming units per mL, cfu/mL (maximum)	10	10^3	N.A.
pH	N.A.	N.A.	5.0-8.0
Resistivity,† MΩ per centimeter (MΩ-cm), 25 °C	10 (in line)	2.0	0.1
Silicate, mg SiO_2/L (maximum)	0.05	0.1	1.0
Particulate matter‡	Water passed through 0.2-μm filter	N.A.	N.A.
Organics	Water passed through activated carbon	N.A.	N.A.

From National Committee for Clinical Laboratory Standards: Preparation and Testing of Reagent Water in the Clinical Laboratory. 3rd ed. Approved Standard. NCCLS Document C03-A3. Wayne, PA, National Committee for Clinical Laboratory Standards, 1997.

**Microbiological content.* The microbiological content of viable organisms, as determined by total colony count after incubation at 36 ± 1 °C for 14 hr, followed by 48 hr at 25 ± 1 °C, and reported as colony forming units per mL (cfu/mL).

†*Specific resistance or resistivity.* The electrical resistance in ohms measured between opposite faces of a 1-cm cube of an aqueous solution at a specified temperature. For these specifications, the resistivity will be corrected for 25 °C and reported in MΩ/cm. The higher the amount of ionizable materials, the lower the resistivity and the higher the conductivity.

‡*Particulate matter.* When water is passed through a membrane filter with a mean pore size of 0.2 μm, it is considered to be free of particulate matter.
Organic material. When water is passed through a bed of activated carbon, it is considered to contain minimum organic material.

Distillation

Distillation is the process of vaporizing and condensing a liquid to purify or concentrate a substance or to separate a volatile substance from less volatile substances. It is the oldest method of water purification. Problems with distillation for preparing reagent water include the carryover of volatile impurities and entrapped water droplets that may contain impurities into the purified water. This will result in contamination of the distillate with volatiles, sodium, potassium, manganese, carbonates, and sulfates. As a result, water treated by distillation alone does not meet the specific conductivity requirement of type I water.

Ion Exchange

Ion exchange is a process that removes ions to produce mineral-free *deionized water.* Such water is most conveniently prepared using commercial equipment, which ranges in size from small, disposable cartridges to large, resin-containing tanks. Deionization is accomplished by passing feed water through columns containing insoluble resin polymers that exchange H^+ and OH^- ions for the impurities present in ionized form in the water. The columns may contain cation exchangers, anion exchangers, or a "mixed-bed resin exchanger," which is a mixture of cation- and anion-exchange resins in the same container.

A single-bed deionizer generally is capable of producing water that has a specific resistance in excess of 1 MΩ/cm. When connected in series, mixed-bed deionizers usually produce water with a specific resistance that exceeds 10 MΩ/cm.

Reverse Osmosis

Reverse osmosis is a process by which water is forced through a semipermeable membrane that acts as a molecular filter. The membrane removes 95% to 99% of organic compounds, bacteria, and other particulate matter and 90% to 97% of all ionized and dissolved minerals but fewer of the gaseous impurities. Although the process is inadequate for producing reagent grade water for the laboratory, it may be used as a preliminary purification method.

Ultraviolet Oxidation

Ultraviolet oxidation is another method that works well as part of a total system. The use of ultraviolet radiation at the biocidal wavelength of 254 nanometers eliminates many bacteria and cleaves many ionizing organics so they can be removed by deionization.

Quality, Use, and Storage of Reagent Grade Water

Type III water may be used for glassware washing. (Final rinsing, however, should be done with the water grade suitable for the intended glassware use). It may also be used for certain qualitative procedures, such as those used in general urinalysis.

Type II water is used for general laboratory testing not requiring type I water. Storage should be kept to a minimum; storage and delivery systems should be constructed to ensure a minimum of chemical or bacterial contamination.

Type I water should be used in test methods requiring minimal interference and maximal precision and accuracy. Such procedures include trace metal, enzyme, and electrolyte measurements, and preparation of all calibrators and solutions of reference materials. This water should be used immediately after production. No specifications for storage systems for type I water are given because it is not possible to maintain the high resistivity while drawing off water and storing it.

Testing for Water Purity

At a minimum, water should be tested for microbiological content, pH, resistivity, and soluble silica,[1,7,34] and the maximum interval in the testing cycle for purity of reagent water should be 1 week. It should be noted that measurements taken at the time of production may differ from those at the time and place of use. For example, if the water is piped a long distance, consideration must be given to deterioration en route to the site of use. To meet the specifications for high-performance liquid chromatography (HPLC), in some instances it may be necessary to add a final 0.1-µm membrane filter. The water can be tested by HPLC using a gradient program and monitoring with an ultraviolet (UV) detector. No peaks exceeding the analytical noise of the system should be found.

Reagent Grade or Analytical Reagent Grade (AR) Chemicals

Chemicals that meet specifications of the American Chemical Society (ACS) are described as reagent or analytical reagent grade. Currently, ACS is the only organization in the world that sets requirements and develops validated methods for determining the purity of reagent chemicals. These specifications have also become the de facto standards for chemicals used in many high-purity applications. These are available in two forms: (1) lot-analyzed reagents, in which each individual lot is analyzed and the actual amount of impurity reported and (2) maximum impurities reagents, for which maximum impurities are listed. The Committee on Analytical Reagents of the ACS periodically publishes "Reagent Chemicals" listing specifications.[48] Manufacturers of ACS chemicals check each lot in a control laboratory and place "ACS" on the labels only of those lot chemicals that meet the society's published specifications. These reagent grade chemicals are of very high purity and are recommended for quantitative or qualitative analyses.

Ultrapure Reagents

Gas and high-performance liquid chromatographic, fluorometric, electrophoretic, trace metal, and molecular diagnostic analyses frequently call for reagents whose purity exceeds the specifications of those described previously. Manufacturers offer selected chemicals that have been especially purified to meet specific requirements. There is no uniform designation for these chemicals and organic solvents. Terms such as "spectrograde," "nanograde," and "HPLC pure" have been used. Data of interest to the user (e.g., absorbance at a specific UV wavelength) are supplied with the reagent.

Other designations of chemical purity include Chemically Pure *(CP)*; USP and NF Grade (chemicals produced to meet specifications set down in the United State Pharmacopeia [USP] or the National Formulary [NF]). Chemicals labeled purified, practical, technical, or commercial grade should not be used in clinical chemical analysis without prior purification.

Reference Materials

Primary reference materials[29] are highly purified chemicals that are directly weighed or measured to produce a solution whose concentration is exactly known. The IUPAC has proposed a degree of 99.98% purity for primary reference materials.

These highly purified chemicals may be weighed out directly for the preparation of solutions of selected concentration or for the calibration of solutions of unknown strength. They are supplied with a certificate of analysis for each lot. These chemicals must be stable substances of definite composition that can be dried, preferably at 104 ° to 110 °C, without a change in composition. They must not be hygroscopic, so that water is not absorbed during weighing.

Secondary reference materials are solutions whose concentrations cannot be prepared by weighing the solute and dissolving a known amount into a volume of solution. The concentration of secondary reference materials is usually determined by analysis of an aliquot of the solution by an acceptable reference method, using a primary reference material to calibrate the method.

Certified Reference Standards (Standard Reference Materials, SRMs) for clinical laboratories are available from the NIST[39] and the IRMM.[49] Cholesterol, the first SRM developed by the NIST, was issued in 1967. Today, the lists from the NIST and IRMM are extensive (Table 1-10 and Table 1-11, respectively). Not all standard reference materials have the properties and the degree of purity specified for a primary standard, but each has been well characterized for certain chemical or physical properties and is issued with a certificate that gives the results of the characterization.[29-31] These may then be used to characterize other materials.

BASIC TECHNIQUES AND PROCEDURES

Basic practices used in the clinical and molecular diagnostic laboratories include optical, chromatographic, electrochemical, electrophoretic, mass spectrometric, enzymatic, and immunoassay techniques. These techniques are discussed in detail in Chapters 3-9. The specialized techniques used in molecular diagnostic laboratories are discussed in Chapters 36, 37, and 41. Here we discuss the basic techniques of volumetric sampling and dispensing, centrifugation, measurement of radioactivity, gravimetry, thermometry, buffer solutions, and processing solutions.

Volumetric Sampling and Dispensing

Clinical chemistry procedures require accurate volumetric measurements to ensure accurate results. For accurate work, only Class A glassware should be used. Class A glassware is certified to conform to the specifications outlined in NIST circular C-602.[40]

Pipettes

Pipettes are used for the transfer of a known volume of liquid from one container to another. They are designed

TABLE 1-10 Standard Reference Materials (SRMs) Available from the National Institute of Standards and Technology (www.nist.gov).

Analyte	SRM Number
Antiepilepsy drug level assay (phenytoin, ethosuximide, phenobarbital, and primidone)	900
Human serum	909b
Sodium pyruvate	910
Cholesterol	911b
Urea	912a
Uric acid	913a
Creatinine	914a
Calcium carbonate	915a
Bilirubin	916a
D-Glucose (dextrose)	917b
Potassium chloride	918a
Sodium chloride	919a
D-Mannitol	920
Cortisol (hydrocortisone)	921
Lithium carbonate	924a
VMA (4-hydroxy-3-methoxymandelic acid)	925
Bovine serum albumin	927c
Lead nitrate	928
Magnesium gluconate (clinical)	929
Iron metal (clinical)	937
4-Nitrophenol	938
Lead in blood	955b
Electrolytes in frozen human serum	956a
Glucose in frozen human serum	965
Toxic elements in blood	966
Fat-soluble vitamins, carotenoids, and cholesterol in human serum	968c
Ascorbic acid in frozen human serum	970
Angiotensin 1 (human)	998
Bone ash	1400
Bone meal	1486
Marijuana metabolite in urine	1507b
Benzoylecgonine (cocaine metabolite) in urine	1508b
Palmitin	1595
PCBs, pesticides, and dioxin/furans in human serum	1589c
Inorganic constituents in bovine serum	1598
Anticonvulsant drug level assay (valproic acid and carbamazepine)	1599
Ethanol-water solution	1828
Lipids in frozen human serum (freeze dried)	1951a
Cholesterol in human serum (freeze dried)	1952a
Gallium melting point	1968
Drugs of abuse in human hair I	2379
Drugs of abuse in human hair Ii	2380
Morphine glucuronide	2382
Amino acids/hydrochloric acid	2389
Toxic metals	2670
Urine fluoride (freeze dried)	2671a
Urine mercury (freeze dried)	2672a
Cotinine in human urine (freeze dried)	8444

TABLE 1-11 Reference Materials (RMs) Available from the Institute for Reference Materials and Measurements (www.irmm.jrc.be)

Analyte	RM Number
Lyophilized human serum	BCR-304
Creatinine in human serum	BCR-573, 574, & 575
Latex spheres of certified size (blood cell size)	BCR-165; 166; & 167
Cortisol reference panel	IRMM/IFCC-451
Progesterone in human serum	BCR-347
Estradiol in human serum	BCR-576; 577; 578
Lead and cadmium in blood	BCR-194; 195; 196
Creatine kinase (human placenta)	BCR-299
Gamma-glutamyltransferase (pig kidney)	BCR-319; IRMM/IFCC-452
Alkaline phosphatase (pig kidney)	BCR-371
Lactate dehydrogenase (human isoenzyme)	BCR-404; IRMM/IFCC-453
Prostatic acid phosphatase (human prostate)	BCR-410
Alanine aminotransferase (pig heart)	BCR-426; IRMM/IFCC-454
α-Amylase (human pancreas)	BCR-476; IRMM/IFCC-456
Creatine kinase (human heart)	BCR-608; IRMM/IFCC-455
Adenosine deaminase (human erythrocytes)	BCR-647
Cortisol in human serum	BCR-192; 193
Serum proteins	BCR-470
Glycated hemoglobin	BCR-405
Hemiglobincyanide	BCR-522
Prostate specific antigen	BCR-613
Thromboplastins	BCR-148; 149S
Apolipoproteins	BCR-393; 394
Alpha fetoprotein	BCR-486
Thyroglobulin	BCR-457

BCR, Bureau Communautaire de Reference (Community Bureau of Reference); *IRMM*, Institute for Reference Materials and Measurements; *IFCC*, International Federation of Clinical Chemistry.

either to contain (TC) a specific volume of liquid or to deliver (TD) a specified volume. Pipettes used in clinical, molecular diagnostic, and analytical laboratories include manual transfer and measuring pipettes, micropipettes, and electronic and mechanical pipetting devices. Developments in improved design of pipetting systems include robotic automation, the capability to provide electronic and personal computer (PC) control of pipetting devices, and careful attention to advanced ergonomic design features. There are also automatic photometric pipette calibration systems available[24] that can reduce the time to periodically check pipettes and potentially provide more efficient use of personnel.

Transfer and Measuring Pipettes

A transfer pipette is designed to transfer a known volume of liquid. Measuring and serological pipettes are scored in units such that any volume up to a maximum capacity is delivered. Table 1-12 shows examples of tolerances of various types of these pipettes.

Transfer Pipettes. *Transfer pipettes* include both volumetric and Ostwald-Folin pipettes. They consist of a cylindrical bulb joined at both ends to narrower glass tubing. A calibration mark is etched around the upper suction tube, and the lower delivery tube is drawn out to a gradual taper. The bore of the delivery orifice should be sufficiently narrow so that rapid outflow of liquid and incomplete drainage cannot cause measurement errors beyond tolerances specified.

A volumetric transfer pipette (Figure 1-1, *A*) is calibrated to deliver accurately a fixed volume of a dilute aqueous solution. The reliability of the calibration of the volumetric pipette decreases with a decrease in size, and therefore special micropipettes have been developed.

Ostwald-Folin pipettes (Figure 1-1, *B*) are similar to volumetric pipettes but have their bulb closer to the delivery tip and are used for the accurate measurement of viscous fluids, such as blood or serum. In contrast to a volumetric pipette, an Ostwald-Folin pipette has an etched ring near the mouthpiece, indicating that it is a blow-out pipette. With the use of a pipetting bulb, the liquid is blown out of the pipette only after the blood or serum has drained to the last drop in the delivery tip. When filled with opaque fluids, such as blood, the top of the meniscus must be read. Controlled slow

TABLE 1-12 Accuracy Tolerances of Various Types of Pipettes

	Volumetric Transfer Pipettes		Measuring & Serological Pipettes	
	Tolerances, ± mL*			
Capacity, mL	Class A‡	Class B‡	Capacity, mL	Tolerances, ± mL† Class B‡
0.5	0.006	0.012	0.1	0.005
1.0	0.006	0.012	0.2	0.008
2.0	0.006	0.012	0.25	0.008
3.0	0.01	0.02	0.5	0.01
4.0	0.01	0.02	0.6	0.01
5.0	0.01	0.02	1.0	0.02
10.0	0.02	0.04	2.0	0.02
15.0	0.03	0.06	5.0	0.04
20.0	0.03	0.06	10.0	0.06
25.0	0.03	0.06	25.0	0.10
50.0	0.05	0.10		
100.0	0.08	0.16		

Modified from Dean JA. Analytical chemistry handbook. New York: McGraw-Hill. 1995: 1.56.
*Accuracy tolerances for volumetric transfer pipettes are given by ASTM Standard E969.02 "Standard Specification for Glass Volumetric (Transfer) Pipets," West Conshohocken, PA: American Society for Testing of Material, 2003 and Federal Specification NNN-P-395.
†Accuracy tolerances for measuring pipettes are given by Federal Specification NNN-P-350 and for serological pipettes by Federal Specification NNN-P-375.
‡Class A pipettes are manufactured to the highest tolerances. Class B pipettes have tolerances approximately twice that of Class A pipettes.

drainage is required with all viscous solutions so that no residual film is left on the walls of the pipette.

Measuring Pipettes. The second principal type of pipette is the *graduated* or *measuring pipette* (Figure 1-1, *C*). This is a piece of glass tubing that is drawn out to a tip and graduated uniformly along its length. Two kinds are available; the Mohr pipette is calibrated between two marks on the stem, whereas the serological pipette has graduated marks down to the tip. The serological pipette (Figure 1-1, *D*) must be blown out to deliver the entire volume of the pipette and has an etched ring (or pair of rings) near the bulb end of the pipette signifying that it is a blow-out pipette. Mohr pipettes require a controlled delivery of the solution between the calibration marks. Serological pipettes have a larger orifice than do the Mohr pipettes and thus drain faster. In practice, measuring pipettes are principally used for the measurement of reagents and are not generally considered sufficiently accurate for measuring samples and calibrators.

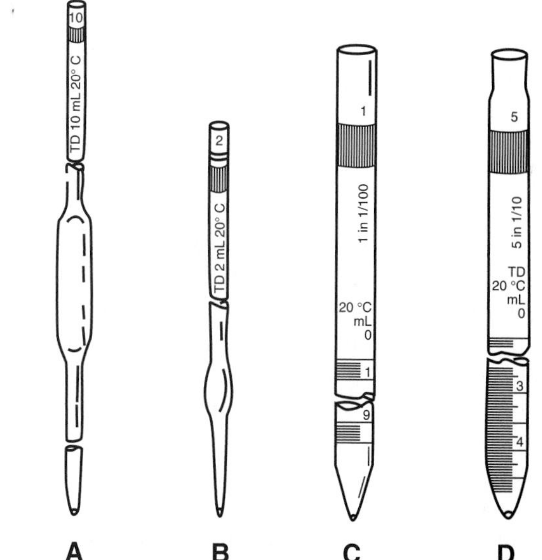

Figure 1-1 Pipettes. **A,** Volumetric (transfer). **B,** Ostwald-Folin (transfer). **C,** Mohr (measuring). **D,** Serological (graduated to the tip).

Pipetting Technique

There are general pipetting techniques that apply to the pipettes described above. For example, pipetting bulbs should always be used, and pipettes must be held in a vertical position when adjusting the liquid level to the calibration line and during delivery. The lowest part of the meniscus, when it is sighted at eye level, should be level with the calibration line on the pipette. The flow of the liquid should be unrestricted when using volumetric pipettes, and the tips should be touched to the inclined surface of the receiving container for 2 seconds after the liquid has ceased to flow.

With graduated pipettes, the flow of liquid may have to be slowed during delivery. Serological pipettes are calibrated to the tip, and the etched glass ring on top of the pipette signifies that it is to be blown out. The pipette is first allowed to drain, and then the remaining liquid is blown out.

TABLE 1-13 Tolerances for Micropipettes

Capacity μL	Accuracy* %	Precision* %	Capacity μL	Accuracy* %	Precision* %
10	1.2	0.4	100	0.5	0.2
40	0.6	0.2	250	0.5	0.15
50	0.5	0.2	500	0.5	0.15
60	0.5	0.2	600	0.5	0.15
70	0.5	0.2	900	0.5	0.15
80	0.5	0.2	1000	0.5	0.15

Modified from Dean JA. Analytical chemistry handbook. New York: McGraw-Hill. 1995: 1.56.
*Tolerances given by ASTM Standard E193-94(1999) "Standard Specification for Laboratory Glass Micropipets." West Conshohocken, PA: American Society for Testing of Material, 1999.

Micropipettes

Micropipettes are pipettes used for the measurement of microliter volumes. In such devices, the remaining volume that coats the inner wall of a pipette can cause notable error. For this reason, most micropipettes are calibrated to contain (TC) the stated volume rather than to deliver it. Proper use requires rinsing the pipette with the final solution after delivering the contents into the diluent. Volumes are expressed in microliters (μL); the older term *lambda* is no longer recommended. (One lambda [λ] = 1 μL = 0.001 mL.) Micropipettes are generally available in small sizes, ranging from 1 to 500 μL but can be obtained for volumes as low as 0.2 μL. Tolerances for several Eppendorf micropipettes are listed in Table 1-13.

Semiautomatic and Automatic Pipettes and Dispensers

Figures 1-2, *A* and *B* illustrate two types of adjustable micropipetting devices that also demonstrate unique ergonomic design features. These devices are programmable and can be used for dispensing aliquots of liquid into multiple wells at the same time. In practice, using disposable plastic tips, they allow simultaneous aspiration and delivery of solutions to multiple sample micro wells. Each channel is piston driven to allow the user to pipette with as few or as many tips as necessary. Aliquots of liquid as small as 0.2 μL can be dispensed at three different aspiration or dispense rates.

Semiautomatic manual and electronic versions of pipettes and dispensers are available in sizes from 0.5 μL to 10 mL. Figure 1-2, *C* illustrates an electronically operated, positive-displacement multi-channel pipettor. This device draws up and dispenses its predefined volumes (from 0.5 to 200 μL) when its plunger is moved through a complete cycle. Its disposable, fluid containment tips are made of a plastic material that tends to retain less inner surface film than does glass. Such pipettes avoid the risk of cross contamination among samples, eliminate the necessity for washing between samples, and improve the precision of measurements. Models that allow for digital adjustment of the volume aspirated and dispensed are available.

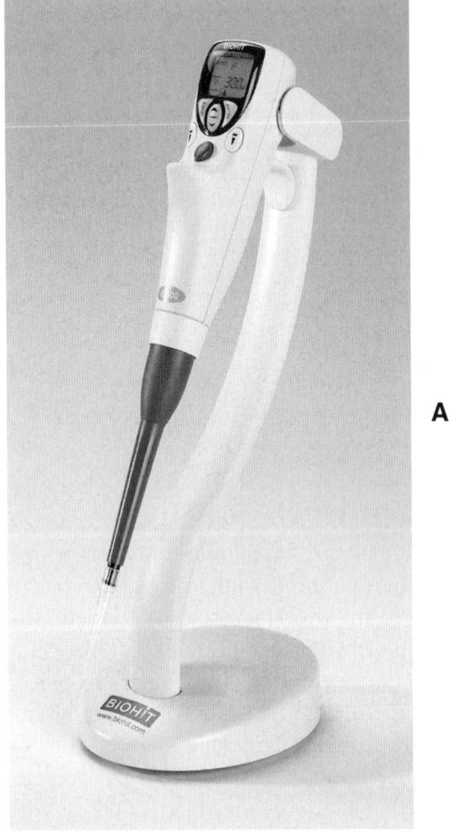

Figure 1-2 A, Adjustable volume micropipetting device with ergonomic design.

Figure 1-3, *A* shows an automatic dispensing apparatus that aspirates and dispenses preset volumes of two different liquids by means of two motor-driven syringes, one for metering a volume of the sample and one for metering a volume of the diluent. This device can be adjusted to aspirate as little as 1 μL of one liquid and to deliver it with as much as 999 μL of the other. This type of device, available as a dilutor or dispenser, can be obtained as a manual, electronic, and computer-controlled device. The device is microprocessor controlled and is easily programmed.

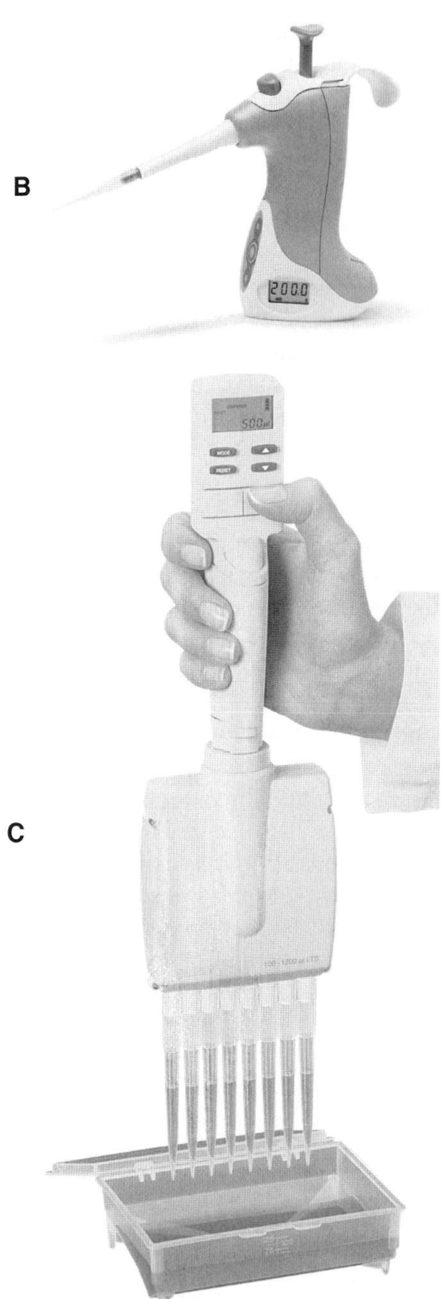

Figure 1-2, Cont'd B, Adjustable volume electronic micropipetting device with ergonomic design. **C,** Electronic programmable multi-channel pipette. *(**A** Courtesy Biohit Plc. **B** Courtesy VistaLab Technologies, Inc.* **C** *Courtesy Rainin Instrument Co.)*

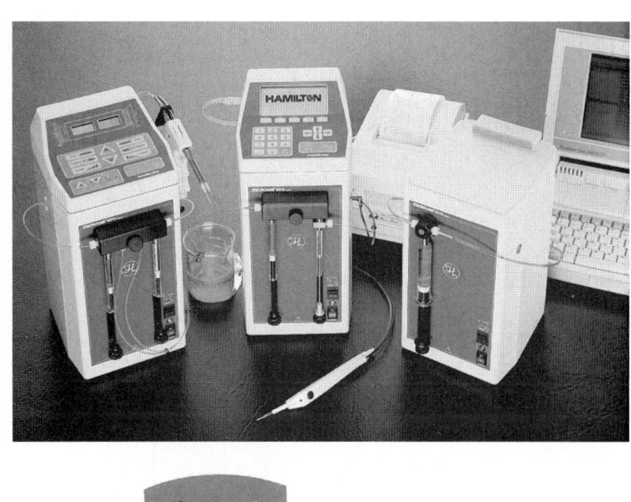

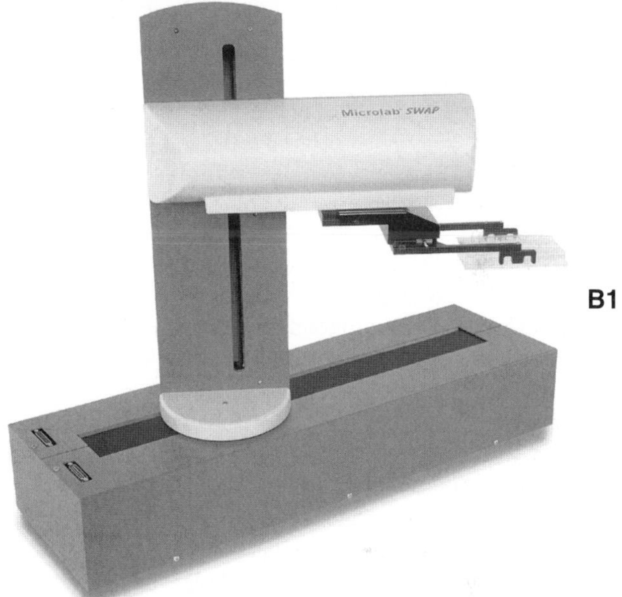

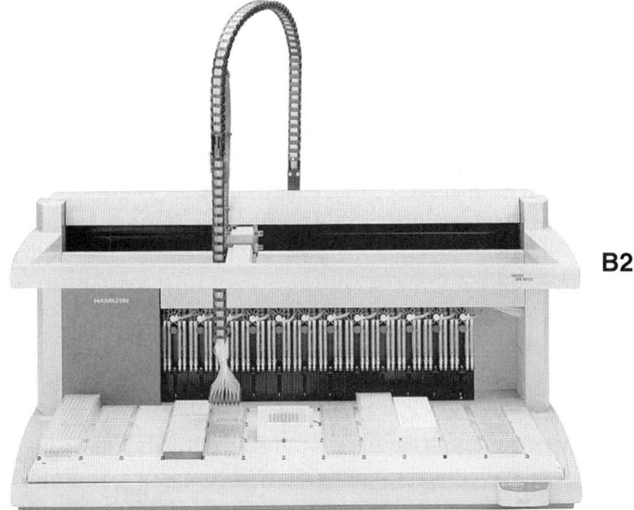

Figure 1-3 A, PC-controlled diluting and/or dispensing apparatus that aspirates and dispenses preset volumes of either one or two different liquids, such as a diluent and sample by means of motor-driven syringes. *(Courtesy Hamilton Co.)* **B,** Robotic liquid handling workstations. *(Courtesy Hamilton Co.)*

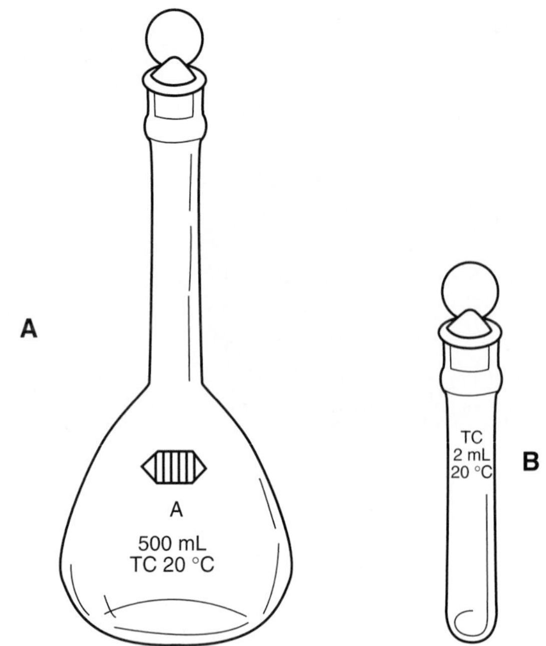

Figure 1-4 Volumetric flasks. **A,** Macro. **B,** Micro.

Twenty-one dispensing programs can be stored in memory and retrieved. This type of liquid dispensing device can also be obtained as a computer-controlled system.

A more versatile piece of equipment is the robotic liquid handling workstation shown in Figure 1-3, *B*, which can be used for clinical chemistry, genomic, proteomic, and other applications. This automated pipetting station can be used with individual reaction tubes and 96- and 384-well microtiter plates. Depending on the design of the system, either a single probe or multiple probes are used rapidly to transfer programmed volumes of solution from one container to microtiter plates (e.g., so that the transfer to all 96 wells can be completed in 1 minute). In some systems, liquid sensing is incorporated into the sample probes to minimize contact with sample and reagents even though automatic washing of the probes is performed between specimens. Two-dimensional (X-Y) movement of probes and tubes or microtiter plates is built into the pipetting stations to minimize the necessity for operator intervention. This device dispenses programmed volumes from 0.5 μL to 1000 μL in serial dilutions from 4 to 16 channels employing an autoloaded system with barcodes for positive identification.

Volumetric Flasks

Volumetric flasks (Figure 1-4) are used to measure exact volumes; they are commonly found in sizes varying from 1 to 4000 mL. In practice, they are primarily used in preparing solutions of known concentration, and they are available in various grades. The most accurate are certified to meet standards set forth by the NIST.

An important factor in the use of volumetric apparatus is the requirement for an accurate adjustment of the meniscus. A small piece of card that is half black and half white is most useful. The card is placed 1 cm behind the apparatus with the white half uppermost and the top of the black area about 1 mm below the meniscus. The meniscus then appears as a clearly defined, thin black line. This device is also useful in reading the meniscus of a burette.

Volumetric equipment should be used with solutions equilibrated to room temperature. Solutions diluted in volumetric flasks should be repeatedly mixed during dilution so that the contents are homogeneous before the solution is made up to final volume. Errors caused by expansion or contraction of liquids on mixing are thereby minimized.

Volumetric flasks should be thoroughly cleaned and dried before calibration. The flask is then weighed and filled with carbon dioxide–free deionized water until just above the graduation mark. The neck of the flask just above the water level should be kept free of water. The meniscus mark is set at the graduation line by removing excess water, and the flask is reweighed. The final weight is corrected for the equilibrated water and air temperature to obtain the volume of the flask. Flasks may also be calibrated by the spectrophotometric technique described below.

Maintenance and Care of Volumetric Glassware

Volumetric glassware and glass apparatus must be absolutely clean to ensure that the volumes measured are accurate, and that the subsequent chemical reactions are not adversely affected. One method that may be used to test for cleanliness is to fill the vessel with distilled water and then empty it and examine the walls to see whether they are covered by a continuous, thin film of water. Imperfect wetting or the presence of discrete droplets of water indicates that the vessel is not sufficiently clean. Obviously, this criterion cannot be used for nonwettable plastics. A test for residual acid or alkaline detergents is the measurement of the pH of water added to the glassware. A dilute solution of an acid-base indicator applied to the surface is another method to check for residual alkaline detergents. The number of pieces of glassware checked depends on the workload and number of pieces cleaned, but at least one piece of randomly selected glassware should be checked each day.

Calibration of Volumetric Pipettes

Accurate calibration and verification of calibration of pipettes, dispensers, and dilutors are important components of a clinical laboratory's quality assurance program. In the past, the gravimetric measurement of the volume of mercury dispensed was the classic procedure used to calibrate such devices. However, owing to the environmental and safety hazards involved with the handling of mercury, this procedure is no longer recommended for use in routine clinical laboratories and has been replaced with gravimetric and spectrophotometric procedures that use aqueous solutions. With the gravimetric procedure, dispensed aliquots of water are weighed with density correction.[18] As an alternative to gravimetric calibration, a spectrophotometric procedure can be used in which aliquots of a compound that absorbs light are pipetted into known volumes of diluent and the absorbance of the diluted liquid measured (e.g., p-nitrophenol at 401 nm). The volumes of the dispensed aliquots are then computed to verify the calibration of the pipette. In addition, calibration services can be purchased from vendors who advertise their services on the Internet. Examples of gravimetric and spectrophotometric procedures can be found in an earlier edition of this chapter[4] or on the Evolve site that accompanies this book.

CENTRIFUGATION

Centrifugation is the process of using centrifugal force to separate the lighter portions of a solution, mixture, or suspension from the heavier portions. A *centrifuge* is a device by which centrifugation is effected.

In the clinical laboratory, centrifugation is used to:

1. Remove cellular elements from blood to provide cell-free plasma or serum for analysis (see Chapter 2).
2. Concentrate cellular elements and other components of biological fluids for microscopic examination or chemical analysis.
3. Remove chemically precipitated protein from an analytical specimen.
4. Separate protein-bound or antibody-bound ligand from free ligand in immunochemical and other assays (see Chapter 9).
5. Extract solutes in biological fluids from aqueous to organic solvents.
6. Separate lipid components such as chylomicrons from other components of plasma or serum, and lipoproteins from one another (see Chapter 26).

Types of Centrifuges

Horizontal-head or swinging-bucket, fixed-angle or angle-head, ultracentrifuge, and axial are the four types of centrifuges used in the clinical laboratory. In addition, the development of automatic balancing centrifuges, which use hydraulic principles based on Archimedes' and Pascal's laws, has enabled centrifugation to be incorporated as an integral step in the total automation of laboratory testing.[9] As discussed in Chapter 11, such centrifuges are incorporated in various robotized analytical systems that are commercially available.

Horizontal-Head or Swinging-Bucket Centrifuges

This type of centrifuge allows the tubes placed in the cups of the rotor to assume a horizontal plane when the rotor is in motion and a vertical position when it is at rest. During centrifugation, particles travel in a constant manner along the tube while the tube is at right angles to the shaft of the centrifuge; thus the sediment is distributed uniformly against the bottom of the tube. The surface of the sediment is flat (parallel to the shaft of the centrifuge) and remains so, with a column of liquid on top of it when the rotor stops, and the tube assumes a vertical position. Supernatant liquid is removed by a pipette with negligible disturbance of the packed sediment. If the sediment is well packed, the supernatant is decanted.

The spinning rotor of a horizontal-head centrifuge offers considerable resistance to rotation and generates heat as a result of air friction. This resistance is lessened if the swinging buckets are enclosed in a windshield.

Fixed-Angle or Angle-Head Centrifuge

In the rotor of an angle-head centrifuge, tubes are held in a fixed position at angles from 25° to 40° to the vertical axis of rotation. Upon centrifugation, particles are driven outward horizontally but strike the side of the tube so that the sediment packs against the side and bottom of the tube with the surface of the sediment parallel to the shaft of the centrifuge. As the rotor slows down and then stops, gravity causes the sediment to slide down the tube; usually a poorly packed pellet is formed.

Ultracentrifuge

An ultracentrifuge is a very high-speed centrifuge that usually uses fixed-head rotors. The most common application of an ultracentrifuge in the clinical laboratory is the separation of lipoproteins (see Chapter 26). Because the separation may require hours or days and may generate considerable heat as a result of friction at high speeds, ultracentrifugation requires a refrigerated chamber. Ultracentrifuges are available in both analytical and preparative models. A tabletop model is available that is a miniature air turbine with a small rotor capable of achieving a centrifugal force of 165,000 times gravity ($\times\ g$). It is used in the clinical laboratory to clear serum of chylomicrons so that accurate analyses may be performed on the infranatant.

Axial Centrifuge

An *axial centrifuge* is based on a centrifugal concept that allows tubes of blood to be spun in a vertical orientation as opposed to the horizontal orientation used in traditional centrifuges.[6,12,15,16,45]

Principles of Centrifugation

The correct term to describe the force required to separate two phases in a centrifuge is *relative centrifugal force* (RCF), also called *relative centrifugal field.* Units are expressed as number of times greater than gravity (e.g., $500 \times g$).

RCF is calculated as follows:

$$\text{RCF} = 1.118 \times 10^{-5} \times r \times rpm$$

where

1.118×10^{-5} = an empirical factor

r = radius in centimeters from the center of rotation to the bottom of the tube in the rotor cavity or bucket during centrifugation

rpm = the speed of rotation of the rotor in revolutions per minute

The RCF of a centrifuge may also be determined from a nomogram distributed by manufacturers of centrifuges. RCF is derived from the distance from the rotor center to the bottom of the tube, whether the tube is horizontal to, or at an angle to, the rotor center. The RCF as calculated above is the maximum RCF. However, not all of the contents of a tube are subjected to the maximum RCF. The minimum RCF, calculated in the same way but from the center of rotation to the surface of the liquid, may be several hundred g less than the maximum value. Note also that RCF applied to a tube in a fixed-angle head is much less than that applied to the same tube in a horizontal-head rotor, because the tube in a fixed-angle head is unable to swing outward.

The time required to sediment particles depends on the rotor speed, the radius of the rotor, and the effective path length traveled by the sedimented particles, that is, the depth of the liquid in the tube. Duplication of conditions of centrifugation is often desirable. The following is a useful formula for calculating speed required of a rotor whose radius differs from the radius with which a prescribed RCF was originally defined:

$$\text{rpm (alternate rotor)} = 1000 \times \sqrt{\frac{\text{RCF, original rotor}}{11.18 \times r\,(\text{cm}),\ \text{alternate rotor}}}$$

The length of time for centrifugation can also be calculated so that running with an alternate rotor of a different size is equivalent to running with the original rotor:

$$\text{time (alternate rotor)} = \frac{\text{time} \times \text{RCF (original rotor)}}{\text{RCF (alternate rotor)}}$$

Note, however, that it may not be possible to reproduce conditions exactly when a different centrifuge is used. Descriptions of times of centrifugation include the time for the rotor to reach operating speed (which may vary from instrument to instrument) and do not include deceleration time, during which sedimentation is still occurring but less efficiently. Even with maximal braking, deceleration may take as long as 3 minutes in some centrifuges.

Operation of the Centrifuge

For proper operation of a centrifuge, only those tubes recommended by their manufacturer should be used. The material used for the tube must withstand the RCF to which the tube is likely to be subjected. Polypropylene tubes are generally capable of withstanding RCFs of up to 5000 ×g. The tubes should have a tapered bottom, particularly if a supernatant is to be removed, and should be of a size to fit securely into the rack to be centrifuged. The top of the tube should not protrude so far above the bucket that the swing into a horizontal position is impeded by the rotor.

For smooth operation of the centrifuge, the rotor must be properly balanced. The weight of racks, tubes, and their contents on opposite sides of a rotor should not differ by more than 1% or by an acceptable limit established by the manufacturer. The smaller the difference in weight is, the smoother the centrifugation. Before centrifuging any laboratory specimens, pairs of adapters and specimen tubes should be placed on opposite pans of a balance, and the tubes rearranged so that the weights are equal and the placement of tubes is symmetrical. Tubes filled with water may also be used to equalize the weights. The total weight of each rack should not exceed the limits stated by the centrifuge manufacturer at a rated speed. As discussed earlier, centrifuges that automatically balance their rotors are now available.[9]

Tubes of collected blood should be centrifuged before being unstoppered to reduce the probability of an aerosol being produced when the tube is opened. The practice of using a wooden applicator to release a clot stuck to the top of the tube or to its stopper should be avoided; it is a potential cause of hemolysis. Centrifugation at an appropriate RCF usually ensures that the clot is released from the tube wall and drawn to the bottom of the tube.

Despite years of experience with centrifuges, there are just a few specific recommendations for RCF or time for centrifugation of blood specimens. For example, NCCLS standard H18-A[25] proposes an RCF of 1000 to 1200 × *g* for 10 ± 5 minutes. Standards have not been established for centrifugation of other specimens, such as serum to which a protein precipitant has been added.

Operating Practice[54]

Cleanliness of a centrifuge is important in minimizing the possible spread of infectious agents, such as hepatitis viruses. With proper operation of a centrifuge, few tubes break. In case of breakage, the racks and chamber of the centrifuge must be carefully cleaned. Any spillage should be considered a possible blood-borne pathogen hazard. Gray dust arising from the sandblasting of the chamber by fragments of glass indicates tube breakage and possible contamination, necessitating cleaning of the chamber. Broken glass embedded in cushions of tube holders may be a continuing cause of breakage if cushions are not inspected and replaced in the cleanup procedure.

The speed of a centrifuge should be checked at least once every 3 months. The procedure should use a stroboscopic light or a vibrating-reed external tachometer of known accuracy. The measured speed should not differ by more than 5% from the rated speed under specified conditions. All the speeds at which the centrifuge is commonly operated should be checked. The centrifuge timer should be checked weekly against a reference timer (such as a stopwatch) and should not be more than 10% in error. Commutators and brushes should be checked at least every 3 months. Brushes (where used) should be replaced when they show considerable wear. However, in many modern induction-drive motors, brushes have been eliminated thus removing a source of dust that can cause motor failure.

Because centrifuges generate heat, the temperature in the chamber in many centrifuge models may increase by as much as 5 °C after a single run. The change in temperature depends on the initial ambient temperature in the centrifuge chamber, rotor speed, duration of centrifugation, and rotor design. These factors affect the concentration of analytes in a specimen because of loss of water caused by evaporation. A large chamber around the rotor dissipates heat. When the material to be centrifuged has a labile temperature, a refrigerated centrifuge should be used. In the simplest form, a refrigerator unit is mounted beside the centrifuge, and cold air is blown into the rotor chamber. This approach is usually inadequate to stabilize the low temperature. In more sophisticated centrifuges, refrigeration coils around the chamber make it possible to maintain a preset temperature within ±1 °C. The temperature of a refrigerated centrifuge should be measured monthly under reproducible conditions and should be within 2 °C of the expected temperature.

MEASUREMENT OF RADIOACTIVITY

With the development of radioimmunoassays (RIAs) in the 1960s that used radioactive isotopes as labels (see Chapter 9), the measurement of radioactivity became a common and important practice in clinical laboratories. However, concerns about, and problems with, the safe handling and disposal of radioactive reagents and waste have led to the development of immunoassays that use nonisotopic labels (see Chapter 9). The rapid acceptance and extensive use of nonisotopic immunoassays by the clinical laboratory have resulted in a decreased use of RIA and ultimately a decreased requirement for them to measure radioactivity. Because of this deemphasis on the necessity to measure radioactivity, only a brief discussion of the topic is presented here. Readers requiring more detail on this topic are referred to the chapter entitled "Basic Principles of Radioactivity and Its Measurement" that is included in a prior edition of this textbook.[46]

Basic Concepts

An *atom* is the smallest unit of an element having the properties of that element. An individual atom consists of a positively charged nucleus around which revolve negatively charged electrons. The *nucleus* is composed of positively charged protons and neutral neutrons. The *atomic number* (Z) of an element is the number of protons in its nucleus; the total number of nucleons, protons plus neutrons, is its *mass number* (A). A *nuclide* is an atomic species with a given atomic number and a given mass number. *Isotopes* are nuclides with the same atomic number but different mass numbers. These represent various nuclear species of the same element. Radionuclides used in the clinical laboratory are listed in Table 1-14.

Radioactive Decay

Isotopes of a given element have nuclei with the same number of protons but different numbers of neutrons. Some isotopes are stable; however radioisotopes are unstable, disintegrate, and decay by alpha or beta decay, electron capture, or gamma emission and internal conversion.

Radioactive decay is a property of the atomic nucleus and is evidence of nuclear instability. The rate of decay is unaffected by temperature, pressure, concentration, or any other chemical or physical condition but is characteristic of each individual radionuclide.

Alpha Decay. To achieve stable configurations, heavy elements, particularly those with atomic numbers above 70, may shed some of their nuclear mass by emitting a two-proton, two-neutron fragment identifiable after emission as a helium nucleus. Because nuclear radiations were observed before their identity was known, this fragment was called an *alpha* (α-) *particle,* and its emission is termed α-decay. Alpha particles are relatively large in mass, interact strongly with matter, but are absorbed by as little as a sheet of paper. However, because they are so heavy, even with low velocity,

TABLE 1-14 Radiation Properties of Some Radionuclides Used in the Clinical Laboratory

Nuclides	Half-life	Decay Type	MAXIMUM ENERGY OF RADIATION (MeV)†	
			Beta	Gamma
^{3}H	12.3 y	β^-	0.186	None
^{14}C	5730 y	β^-	0.155	None
^{32}P	14.3 d	β^-	1.71	None
^{35}S	87 d	β^-	0.167	None
^{51}Cr	27.7 d	EC	None	0.320
^{57}Co	272 d	EC	None	0.122, 0.136, 0.014
^{58}Co	71 d	EC, β^+	0.474	0.811, annihilation photons only
^{59}Fe	45 d	β^-	0.475, 0.273	1.10, 1.29
^{99}Mo	66 h	β^-	1.21, 0.450	0.740, 0.181, 0.778
^{99m}Tc	6.0 h	IT	None	0.141
^{125}I	60 d	EC	None	0.035
^{131}I	8.04 d	β^-	0.607, 0.336	0.364, 0.637, 0.284

*β^-, β^+, EC, and IT refer to β-decay, positron decay, electron capture, and isomeric transition, respectively. Where a nuclide is known to have more than one mode of decay, they are listed in the order of their prevalence.

†Energies are given only for the more prevalent β- and γ-radiations and are in approximate order of prevalence. Electron capture (EC) decay also yields the characteristic x-rays of the daughter; the energies of the x-rays are not included in this listing. As noted in the gamma column, positron decay (β^+) is accompanied by annihilation radiation, which consists principally of a pair of 0.511 MeV photons.

their momentum is high. Consequently, they do not travel far, but when they collide with other molecules they do a lot of damage; therefore α-emitters are considered to be quite hazardous.

Beta Decay. For some heavy nuclides and for almost all those with atomic numbers below 60, stability is achieved by a rearrangement of the nucleus in which the total number of nucleons is unchanged. In terms of the neutron-proton model of the nucleus, this rearrangement is the conversion of a neutron to a proton or vice versa. During such conversions, the nucleus emits either a negative electron or its positive equivalent, a *positron.* The emission of the negative electron, named the *beta* (β-) *particle,* is what is usually meant by the term *β-decay.*

The emission of a negative β-particle leaves the nucleus with one additional positive charge, a neutron is converted to a proton, and the nucleus assumes the next higher atomic number. Negative β-emission is characteristic of a nucleus that has more neutrons than required by its protons for stability. For example, tritium is an unstable isotope of hydrogen (^3H), consisting of a proton, an electron, and two neutrons. When an atom of tritium decays, one of the neutrons is converted to a proton, one β-particle and one neutrino are released, and a helium isotope (^3He) remains. Tritium is called a "soft" β-emitter, because its β-particles have relatively low velocities. A hard β-emitter, such as *phosphorus* 32 (^{32}P) is more hazardous because its β-particles carry more kinetic energy; however, it is easier to detect.

Other examples of nuclides that decay by negative β-emission are carbon-14(^{14}C), iron-59 (^{59}Fe), and iodine-131 (^{131}I). Negatively charged β-particles are smaller in mass and interact less with matter than β-particles, easily penetrate paper and cardboard, but are absorbed by metal sheets.

Electron Capture. An alternative decay process to the emission of positive β-particles is the capture of an electron. In this process, an orbital electron is "absorbed" by the nucleus. The end effect on nuclear structure is the same; a proton appears to have changed into a neutron, the atomic number decreases by one, and the atomic mass remains the same. For example, ^{125}I decays exclusively by electron capture to tellurium-125 ($^{125}_{53}I \rightarrow {}^{125}_{52}Te$).

Gamma Radiation and Internal Conversion. The original observations of naturally occurring radioactive nuclides disclosed a third radiation, the *gamma* (γ-) *ray.* Its ability to penetrate materials that blocked γ- and β-radiation distinguished this radiation. Gamma radiation is high-energy electromagnetic radiation that resemble x-rays. An example of a γ-emitter is ^{131}I. Gamma radiation may accompany either α- or β-particle emission. After either α- or β-decay or after electron capture, the nucleus may be left in an excited state from which it goes to the ground state by shedding the excess energy either through the emission of a γ-photon or through the ejection of an orbital electron *(conversion electron).* In either case the energy emitted equals the energy released in deexcitation. Deexcitation may occur in one or in multiple steps. Each step produces a photon of corresponding energy. For every radionuclide, the deexcitation steps and the corresponding γ-ray energies provide a unique *γ-ray spectrum,* which can be used to identify unknown nuclides. Because γ-rays are high-energy photons, they interact with matter much less strongly than do α- and β-particles and consequently their penetrating power is very high and more difficult to shield.

Activity and Half-life

The rate of decay of a radioactive source is called its *activity* and is simply the rate at which radioactive parent atoms decay to more stable daughter atoms. The relationship between the initial activity (A_0) at time zero and the activity (A) after an elapsed time *t*, is given by:

$$A = -\frac{dN}{dt} = A_0 e^{-\lambda t}$$

where N is the number of atoms present at time t and λ is the decay constant characteristic of a given nuclide.

In practice, it is often convenient to describe the rate of decay in terms of *half-life* ($t_{1/2}$), the time required for a nuclide's e activity to decrease to half its initial value:

$$t_{1/2} = \frac{\ln 2}{\lambda} = \frac{0.693}{\lambda}$$

This equation is useful in planning experiments and in the disposal of radioactive waste. For disposal, a rule of thumb is that a decay time of seven half-lives reduces the activity to less than 1% of its original value ($2^{-7} = 1/128 =$ 0.78%), and that after 10 half-lives, to less than 0.1%.

Units of Radioactivity

The *becquerel* (Bq) is the SI unit of radioactivity and is defined as one decay per second (dps). Because 1 Bq is a very small amount of activity, the activity of typical chemistry samples is often expressed in kilobecquerels (kBq). The *curie* (Ci) is the older, *conventional unit;* it is defined as 3.7×10^{10} dps. One curie equals 37 gigabecquerels (GBq). Because the becquerel is inconveniently small and the curie very large, they are typically used as their multiples or submultiples, for example, megabecquerels (MBq) and millicuries (mCi). One mCi equals 37 MBq.

Specific Activity

The term "specific activity" has several meanings. It may refer to any one of the following: radioactivity per unit mass of an element, radioactivity per mass of labeled compound, or radioactivity per unit volume of a solution. The denominator of reference must be specified. In terms of radioactivity per unit mass, the maximum specific activity attainable for each radionuclide is that for the pure radionuclide. For example, pure ^{14}C has a specific activity of 62 Ci/mol or 4400 Ci/kg. As usually available, ^{14}C is a tracer for compounds in which it represents only a small fraction of the total carbon, most of which is the naturally occurring mixture of stable ^{12}C and stable ^{13}C. If there is no stable element present, the radionuclide is said to be *carrier free.*

Detection and Measurement of Radioactivity

Autoradiography, gas ionization detectors, and fluorescent scintillation are the basis for techniques used to detect and measure radioactivity in the clinical laboratory.

Autoradiography

In autoradiography a photographic emulsion is used to visualize molecules labeled with a radioactive element. For example, this technique is used to visualize nucleic acids and fragments that have been hybridized with nucleic acid probes labeled with ^{32}P (see Chapter 37). With such techniques, nucleic acid probes labeled with radioactive ^{32}P are incubated with target nucleic acid. After hybridization, hydrolysis, and separation of fragments by gel electrophoresis, a photographic film is applied to the covered gel and allowed to incubate. Alternatively the nucleic acid fragments are transferred to a nylon membrane and the photographic film applied to the membrane (see Chapter 5). With either, the film is developed with the resulting image reflecting the radioactivity of the target nucleic acid fragments.

Gas-Filled Detectors

Detectors filled with certain gases or gas mixtures are designed to capture and measure the ions produced by radiation within the detector. Gas-filled detectors used to measure radioactivity include the: (1) *ionization chamber*, (2) *proportional counter*, and (3) *Geiger counter*. Of the three, the Geiger counter is used in the clinical chemistry laboratory as a portable radiation monitor.

Scintillation Counting

In both scintillator and gas detectors, the absorption of radiation causes excitation and ionization; however with the scintillation process, the absorbed energy produces a flash of light, rather than a pulse of current. The principal types of scintillation detectors found in the clinical chemistry laboratory are the sodium iodide *crystal scintillation detector* and the *organic liquid scintillation detector*. Because of the crystal detector's relative ease of operation and economy of sample preparation, most clinical laboratory procedures have been developed to measure nuclides, such as ^{125}I, which can be counted efficiently in a crystal detector. A liquid scintillation detector is used to measure pure β-emitters, such as tritium or ^{14}C.

Crystal Scintillation Detector. The *well detector* is a common type of a crystal scintillation detector and has a hole drilled in the end or side of the cylindrical crystal to accept a test tube. Because it is hygroscopic, the crystal is hermetically sealed in an aluminum can with a transparent quartz window at one end through which the blue-violet (420 nm) scintillations are detected. The photons of gamma emitters, such as ^{51}Cr, ^{57}Co, ^{59}Fe, ^{125}I, and ^{131}I (Table 1-14) in the sample easily penetrate the specimen tube and the thin, low-density can and enter the crystal where they are likely to be absorbed in the thick, high-density sodium iodide. A well counter is not suitable for measuring β-radiation, because it cannot penetrate the sample container and aluminum lining of the wall.

The crystal itself is usually a circular cylinder machined from a single crystal of sodium iodide that was carefully grown to ensure optical clarity for efficient light collection. A small amount of thallium is added to the mother liquor to improve performance. The high atomic number of iodine and the density of sodium iodide (3.7 g/cm^3) favor the absorption of γ-radiation. For this reason, a well counter is often referred to as a γ-counter. For a typical well detector, the counting efficiency for ^{125}I, expressed as the percentage of decays that produces counts, approximates 70%.

Liquid Scintillation Detector. This detector measures radioactivity by recording scintillations occurring within a transparent vial that contains the unknown sample and liquid scintillator. Because the radionuclide is intimately mixed with, or actually dissolved in, the liquid scintillator, the technique is ideal for the pure β-emitters, such as ^3H, ^{14}C, and ^{32}P. Typical efficiencies for liquid scintillation counting in the absence of significant quenching are 60% for tritium and 90% for ^{14}C.

The liquid scintillator is known as the *scintillation cocktail* and contains at least two components (the primary solvent and the primary scintillator). The *primary solvent* is usually inexpensive and chosen for its efficiency in absorbing and transferring radiation energy. It is usually one of the aromatic hydrocarbons: toluene, xylene, or pseudocumene (1,2,4-trimethyl benzene). The *primary scintillator* absorbs energy from the primary solvent and converts it into light. The usual material is PPO (2,5-diphenyl oxazole) used in a concentration of 3 to 6 g/L. PPO emits ultraviolet light of 380 nm. In addition, other components added to the liquid scintillator include: (1) a *secondary solvent* to improve the solubility of aqueous samples, (2) a surfactant to stabilize or emulsify the sample, (3) a *secondary scintillator*, sometimes referred to as a wavelength shifter, to absorb the ultraviolet photons of the primary scintillator and reemit the energy at a longer wavelength, which facilitates the response of some photomultiplier tubes, and (4) one or more *adjuvants*, such as suspension agents, solubilizers for biological tissue, and antifreezes, to prevent freezing and separation of water at low temperatures.

Other Components and Techniques. Other components of a liquid scintillator detector include: (1) electronics, (2) a photomultiplier tube, (3) a preamplifier, and (4) a pulse-height analyzer. Description of these components and discussion of relevant topics such as (1) efficiency of scintillation counting, (2) quenching, (3) counting statistics, (4) assay optimization, and (5) radiation safety can be found in an earlier edition of this textbook.[46]

GRAVIMETRY

Mass is an invariant property of matter. Gravimetry is the process used to measure the mass of a substance. Weight is a function of mass under the influence of gravity, a relationship expressed by the equation:

$$\text{Weight} = \text{mass} \times \text{gravity}$$

Two substances of equal weight and subject to the same gravitational force have equal masses. The determination of mass is made using a balance to compare the mass of an unknown with that of a known mass. This comparison is called *weighing*, and the absolute standards with which masses are compared are called *weights*. In practice, the terms *mass* and *weight* are used synonymously.

The classic form of a balance is a beam poised on an agate knife-edge fulcrum, with a pan hanging from each end of the beam and a rigid pointer hanging from the beam at the poise point. With the object to be weighed on one pan and weights of equal mass on the other pan, the pointer comes to rest at an equilibrium or balance point between the extremes of the path of excursion. The weight required to achieve the equilibrium is therefore equal to the weight of the substance being weighed.

Although the classic form of the balance is of great antiquity, modern balances—both mechanical and electronic—continue to apply the principle of equilibrium in a variety of ingenious ways. More than one type of balance is required for a clinical laboratory because there is a necessity to weigh, for example, 3 kg of timed urine output and microgram amounts of drug for a reference solution. Coarse balances of large capacity (up to 5 kg) have a detection limit of 0.1 g. The typical analytical balance has a capacity of 200 g and a detection limit of about 10 µg. Microbalances may have a maximum capacity of as little as 5 g and detection limit of 0.1 µg.

All balances require a vibration-free location. The more sensitive a balance, the more protection it requires, not only from vibration but also from air currents that can disturb the equilibrium between the weighed object and weights. The zero or null point of the balance (the rest point in the absence of either weights or an object to be weighed) must be known or kept adjusted. Scrupulous attention to cleanliness is essential. Chemical substances being weighed should never be placed in direct contact with the pans. Disposable plastic weighing boats come in various sizes and are convenient for weighing most chemicals. They have largely replaced weighing bottles and weighing paper for most uses. Loose crystals of chemicals or liquids with corrosive vapors should not be permitted to remain on or around the immediate area of the pans. Good weighing technique for samples weighing less than 1 g calls for handling weights with forceps and weighed objects with suitable utensils to prevent deposition of moisture, oils, or salts from an analyst's skin.

Principles of Weighing

Direct comparison and substitution are the two operations used in weighing. In weighing by *direct comparison*, weights are added to one side of the beam to counterbalance the weight of the object on the other side. This approach is more common. In weighing by *substitution*, weights are removed from the side of a balance to which the object to be weighed has been added to restore equilibrium.

In practice, two modes of weighing are used: (1) analytical weights are added to equal the weight of the object being weighed or (2) the material to be weighed is added to a balance pan to achieve equilibrium with a preset weight. This second mode is used more commonly in clinical laboratories, where the major necessity is to weigh a fixed quantity of chemical so that a calibrator or reagent solution of known concentration may be prepared. Before weighing a sample of the chemical, the weight of the container must be determined to subsequently allow for deducting the weight of the container from the gross weight of the container plus sample to obtain the net weight of the sample: a process called "taring." When taring is impractical, the weight of the empty container must be subtracted from the combined weight of the container and the material to obtain the weight of the material alone.

Types of Balances

Double- and single-pan and electronic balances are frequently used in the clinical laboratory.

Double-Pan Balance

A double-pan balance conforms to the classic design, consisting of a single beam with arms of equal length. Standard weights are usually added by hand to the right-side pan to counterbalance the weight of the object on the other, but in some models, a dial or vernier with chain is used to make fine adjustments to the mass associated with the right-side pan. In *single-pan* balances, the arms are of unequal length. The object to be weighed is placed on the pan attached to the shorter arm. A restoring force is applied mechanically or electronically to the other arm to return the beam to its null position. Double- and triple-beam balances are forms of the unequal-arm balance. A single pan on a short arm is balanced about a fulcrum by a larger arm consisting of two or three parallel beams to which weights or poises of different weights are attached. In general these balances are designed to weigh bulk reagents and have relatively low accuracy.

Single-Pan Balance

The single-pan balance is a commonly used balance in the clinical laboratory. It is most often electronically operated and self-balancing. Such a balance may be coupled directly to a computer or recording device. In the electronic single-pan balance, a load on the pan causes the beam to tilt downward. A null detector senses the position of the beam and indicates when the beam has deviated from the equilibrium point.

Electronic Balance

In an electronic balance, an electromagnetic force is applied to return the balance beam to its null position. The electromagnetic force takes the place of weights in a two-pan balance. The restoring force is proportional to the weight on the pan and is applied through a solenoid or torque motor. The current required to produce the force is displayed digitally by liquid crystals or light-emitting diodes in a form equivalent to the mass on the balance pan. The accuracy of an electronic balance depends on the linearity of both the digital voltmeter and the torque motor. Almost all electronic balances have a built-in provision for taring so that the mass of the container is subtracted easily from the total mass measured. Thus operation of an electronic balance is very simple. It entails switching on the balance, placing a container to hold the material to be weighed on the balance pan, taring off the weight of the container, transferring the material to be weighed to the container, and recording the mass of the material as shown on the digital display. In many modern balances, a built-in microprocessor compensates for changes in temperature and provides both automatic zero tracking and calibration.

Analytical Weights

Analytical weights are used to counterbalance the weight of objects weighed on two-pan balances and to verify the performance of both single- and two-pan balances. The NIST recognizes the following five classes of analytical weights:

1. Class M weights are of primary standard quality and are used only to calibrate other weights.
2. Class S weights are used for calibrating balances. In the clinical laboratory, balances should be calibrated at least monthly and before conducting very accurate analytical work.
3. Class S-1 weights have greater tolerance than class S weights and are used for routine analytical work.
4. Class P weights have even tighter tolerances.
5. Class J weights are intended for microanalytical work and range from 0.05 to 50 mg, in contrast to the range of 1 mg to 100 g of the other classes.

Class S weights are typically made from brass or stainless steel and are lacquered or plated for protection. The fractional weights of a set of class S standards are usually made of platinum or aluminum. Tolerances of the different weights have been defined by the NIST. For class S weights from 1 to 5 g, the tolerance is ± 0.054 mg, from 500 to 100 mg it is ± 0.025 mg, and from 1 to 50 mg it is ± 0.014 mg.

THERMOMETRY

In the clinical chemistry laboratory, measurements of temperature are made primarily to verify that devices measure within the prescribed temperature limits. Water baths or heated cells where reactions take place are examples of such devices, as are refrigerators, whose temperatures must be measured and recorded daily to meet laboratory regulatory requirements.

The two most popular types of thermometers in the chemistry laboratory are liquid-in-glass thermometers and thermistor probes. A thermistor made of a transition metal oxide whose resistance changes with temperature is the most common of the latter type.

All thermometers must be verified against a certified thermometer before being placed into use. For example, the NIST SRM 934 is a mercury-in-glass thermometer with calibration points at 0 °C, 25 °C, 30 °C, and 37 °C. Some manufacturers supply liquid-in-glass thermometers that have ranges greater than the SRM thermometer and are verified to have been calibrated against the NIST thermometers. Details of the verification of the calibration of a thermometer have been described in a NCCLS standard.[26]

The NIST also supplies several materials that melt at a known temperature. For example, gallium (SRM 1968) and rubidium (SRM 1969), which melt at 29.7723 °C and 39.3 °C, respectively, are particularly useful in the clinical laboratory (see Table 1-10).

BUFFER SOLUTIONS

Buffers are defined as substances that resist changes in the pH of a system. All weak acids or bases, in the presence of their salts, form buffer systems. The action of buffers and their role in maintaining the pH of a solution can best be explained with the aid of the Henderson-Hasselbalch equation, which may be derived as follows.

The ionization of a weak acid, HA, and of a salt of that acid, BA, can be represented as:

$$\mathrm{HA} \leftrightarrows \mathrm{H^+ + A^-}$$

$$\mathrm{BA} \longrightarrow \mathrm{B^+ + A^-}$$

The dissociation constant for a weak acid (K_a) may be calculated from the following equation:

$$K_a = \frac{[\mathrm{H^+}][\mathrm{A^-}]}{[\mathrm{HA}]}$$

Thus

$$[\mathrm{H^+}] = K_a \times \frac{[\mathrm{HA}]}{[\mathrm{A^-}]}$$

or

$$\log[\mathrm{H^+}] = \log K_a + \log\frac{[\mathrm{HA}]}{[\mathrm{A^-}]}$$

where brackets indicate the concentration of the compound contained within. Now multiplying throughout by −1:

$$-\log[\mathrm{H^+}] = -\log K_a - \log\frac{[\mathrm{HA}]}{[\mathrm{A^-}]}$$

By definition, pH = −log [H^+], and pK_a = −log K_a, therefore

$$\mathrm{pH} = \mathrm{p}K_a + \log\frac{[\mathrm{A^-}]}{[\mathrm{HA}]}$$

Because A^- is derived principally from the salt, the equation may, for practical purposes, be written:

$$\mathrm{pH} = \mathrm{p}K_a + \log\frac{[\text{salt}]}{[\text{undissociated acid}]}$$

or simply:

$$pH = pK_a + \log\frac{[salt]}{[acid]}$$

where [salt] = $[A^-]$ = concentration of dissociated salt and [acid] = [HA] = concentration of undissociated acid.

Consequently, the pH of the system is determined by the pK_a of the acid and the ratio of $[A^-]$ to [HA]. The buffer has its greatest buffer capacity at its pK_a, that is, that pH at which the $[A^-]$ = [HA]. This entered into the preceding equation gives:

$$pH = pK_a + \log 1$$

$$pH = pK_a + 0$$

The capacity of the buffer decreases as the ratio deviates from 1. In general buffers should not be used at a pH greater than 1 unit from their pK_a. If the ratio is beyond 50/1 or 1/50, the system is considered to have lost its buffering capacity. This point is approximately 1.7 pH units to either side of the pK_a of the acid, because

$$pH = pK_a + \log\frac{50}{1} + \log\frac{1}{50}$$

or

$$pH = pK_a \pm 1.7$$

Buffers commonly used in clinical and molecular diagnostic laboratories include acetate, boric acid–borate, carbonate-bicarbonate, citrate diethanolamine, glycine-glycinate, phosphate, phthalate, tris(hydroxymethyl) aminomethane, and veronal–sodium veronal, and the so-called "Good" buffers (Table 1-15).

Procedures for Processing Solutions

Several procedures are routinely used to process solutions in the clinical laboratory, including those for diluting, concentrating, and filtering solutions.

TABLE 1-15 Biological Buffers Commonly Used in the Laboratory*

Trivial Name	Chemical Name	pK_a†	Useful pH Range
ACES	N-(2-Acetamido)-2-aminoethane-sulfonic acid	6.8	6.1-7.5
ADA	N-(2-Acetamido)iminodiacetic acid	6.6	6.0-7.2
AMP	2-Amino-2-methyl-propanol	9.7	9.0-10.5
AMPSO	3-([1,1-Dimethyl-2-hydroxyethyl]amino)-2-hydroxypropanesulfonic acid	9.0	8.3-9.7
BES	N,N-Bis(2-hydroxyethyl)-2-aminoethane sulfonic acid	7.1	6.4-7.8
BICINE	N,N′-Bis(2-hydroxyethyl)glycine	8.3	7.6-9.0
BIS-TRIS	2-(Bis[2-hydroxyethyl]amino)-2-(hydroxymethyl)-1,3-propanediol	6.5	5.8-7.2
BIS-TRIS PROPANE	1,3-Bis(tris[hydroxymethyl]methylamino)propane	6.8 & 9.0	6.3-9.0
CAPS	3-(Cyclohexylamino)propane sulfonic acid	10.4	9.7-11.1
CAPSO	3-(Cyclohexylamino)-2-hydroxy-1-propanesulfonic acid	9.6	8.9-10.3
CHES	2-(Cyclohexylamino)ethane-2-sulfonic acid	9.3	8.6-10.0
DIPSO	N,N-Bis(2-hydroxyethyl)-3-amino-2-hydroxypropanesulfonic acid	7.6	7.0-8.2
EPPS/HEPPS	N-(2-Hydroxyethyl)piperazine-N′-(3-propanesulfonic acid)	8.0	7.3-8.7
HEPBS	N-(2-Hydroxyethyl)piperazine-N′-(4-butanesulfonic acid)	8.3	7.6-9.0
HEPES	N-(2-Hydroxyethyl)piperazine-N′-2-ethanesulfonic acid	7.5	6.8-8.2
HEPPSO	N-(2-Hydroxyethyl)piperazine-N′-3-propanesulfonic acid	7.8	7.1-8.5
MES	Morpholinoethane sulfonic acid	6.1	5.5-6.7
MOBS	4-(N-Morpholino)butane sulfonic acid	7.6	6.9-8.3
MOPS	Morpholinopropane sulfonic acid	7.2	6.5-7.9
PIPES	Piperazine-N,N′-bis(2-ethane sulfonic acid)	6.8	6.1-7.5
POPSO	Piperazine-N,N′-bis(2-hydroxypropanesulfonic acid)	7.8	7.2-8.5
TABS	N-tris(Hydroxymethyl)methyl-4-aminobutanesulfonic acid	8.9	8.2-9.6
TAPS	N-Tris(hydroxymethyl)methyl-3-aminopropane sulfonic acid	8.4	7.7-9.1
TES	N-Tris(hydroxymethyl)methyl-2-aminoethane sulfonic acid	7.5	6.8-8.2
TRICINE	N-Tris(hydroxymethyl)methylglycine	8.1	7.4-8.8
TRIS	2-Amino-2-(hydroxymethyl)-1,3-propane	8.1	7-9

*These buffers are known collectively as "Good" buffers. (Good NE, Winget GD, Winter W, et al, Hydrogen ions buffers for biological research. Biochemistry 1966; 5:467-77.)

†Data obtained at 25 °C.

Dilution

Dilution is the process whereby the concentration or activity of a given solution is decreased by the addition of solvent. In laboratory practice, most dilutions are made by transferring an exact volume of a concentrated solution into an appropriate flask and then adding water or other diluent to the required volume, with appropriate mixing to ensure homogeneity. A serial dilution is a sequential set of dilutions in mathematical sequence. A given dilution is expressed as the amount, either volume or weight, of a solute (analyte) in a specified volume. For example, a 1:5 volume to volume (vol/vol) dilution contains one volume in a total of five volumes (one volume plus four volumes).

To prevent errors that arise when two liquids of very different composition are mixed, the technique of diluting to volume is used. Instead of adding 90 mL water to 10 mL concentrated solution, the 10-mL concentrated solution should be pipetted into a 100-mL volumetric flask, and water is added to bring the volume to the 100-mL mark on the neck of the flask.

When performing a dilution, the following equation is used to determine the volume (V_2) necessary to dilute a given volume (V_1) of solution of a known concentration (C_1) to the desired lesser concentration (C_2):

$$C_1 \times V_1 = C_2 \times V_2$$

or

$$V_2 = \frac{C_1 \times V_1}{C_2}$$

Likewise, the equation is also used to calculate the concentration of the diluted solution when a given volume is added to the starting solution.

Evaporation

Evaporation is a process used to convert a liquid or a volatile solid into vapor. It is used in the clinical laboratory to remove liquid from a sample thereby increasing the concentrations of analyte(s) left behind.

Lyophilization

Lyophilization (freeze drying) is used in laboratory medicine for the preparation of calibrators, control materials, reagents, and to a lesser extent individual specimens for analysis. Lyophilization first entails freezing a material at −40 °C or less and then subjecting it to a high vacuum. Very low temperatures cause the ice to sublime; solid nonsublimable material, initially locked in an ice matrix, remains behind in a dried state.

Filtration

Filtration is defined as the passage of a liquid through a filter and is accomplished by gravity, pressure, or vacuum. *Filtrate* is the liquid that has passed through the filter. The purpose of filtration is to remove particulate matter from the liquid. Many filtrations in the clinical laboratory are carried out with *filter paper* and with plastic *membranes* of controlled pore size.

Membrane filters are used under vacuum, with positive pressure, or with gravity. Filters have been incorporated into certain disposable tips for use with semiautomatic pipettes. These filters minimize the exchange of aerosol droplets between the tips and the pipette. This is of particular importance for DNA amplification and microbiological procedures. Other membrane filters are designed for ultrafiltration and are available with a variety of pore sizes for selective filtration. *Ultrafiltration* is a technique for removing dissolved particles using an extremely fine filter. It is used to concentrate macromolecules, such as proteins, because smaller dissolved molecules pass through the filter.

SAFETY

In the United States, the Federal Occupational Safety and Health Act of 1970 was the beginning of the formal regulatory oversight of employee safety. Since 1970 the Occupational Safety and Health Administration (OSHA) and the Centers for Disease Control and Prevention (CDC) have published numerous safety standards that apply to clinical laboratories. Each year as the Joint Commission on Accreditation of Healthcare Organizations (JCAHO) and the College of American Pathologists (CAP) revise their guidelines, more attention is devoted to safety. Consideration for the health and responsibility for the safety of employees are now accepted as obligations of all employers and laboratory directors. In May of 1988, OSHA expanded the Hazard Communication Standard to apply to hospital workers. Part of this standard is frequently referred to as the "Lab Right to Know Standard."

There are many aspects to the safe operation of a clinical laboratory. Key elements for safety in the clinical laboratory include:

1. A formal safety program
2. Documented policies and effective use of mandated plans and/or programs in the areas of chemical hygiene, control of exposure to blood-borne pathogens, tuberculosis control, and ergonomics
3. Identification of significant occupational hazards, such as biological, chemical, fire, and electrical hazards and clearly identifying and documenting policies for employees to deal with each type of hazard (e.g., packaging and shipping of diagnostic specimens and infectious substances)
4. Recognition that in the twenty-first century clinical laboratory, there are additional important and relevant safety areas of concern. These areas include effective waste management policies for the identification and disposal of regulated and nonregulated waste streams with the intent of ensuring compliance with all federal and state agency mandates, and bioterrorism and chemical terrorism response plans in the event of potential threats or casualties involving these types of agents.

Safety Program

Every clinical laboratory must have a comprehensive and effective formal safety program. Regardless of the size of the clinical laboratory, it is an accepted and strongly recommended practice to assign a specific individual the title of "Safety Officer" or "Chair of the Safety Committee." Safety is each employee's responsibility, but responsibility for the entire program begins with the laboratory leadership (directors, administrative directors, supervisors, managers, etc.) and is delegated through the leadership to the safety officer or safety committee. This individual or committee then has the duties of providing guidance to laboratory leadership on matters relating to the provision of a safe workplace for all employees. The duties and responsibilities of the safety officer and/or safety committee are important. Although a small institution may have one individual who deals with all safety-related matters for all departments including the laboratory, OSHA[41] mandates that the laboratory specifically have a chemical hygiene officer who is designated based on training or experience to provide technical guidance in the development of the chemical hygiene plan (CHP) discussed later.

An integral part of the laboratory safety program is the education and motivation of all laboratory employees in all matters relating to safety. Each new employee should be given a copy of the general laboratory safety manual as part of his or her orientation. Each employee should know the location of available fire-fighting equipment and how to use it and where the evacuation routes are. The continuing education program of the laboratory should include periodic talks on safety. Several audiovisual resources are available from a variety of sources to support the continuing educational part of the safety program. These include videotapes adapted from selected NCCLS documents relating to laboratory safety.[27,32]

Another important part of the laboratory safety program relates to ensuring that the laboratory environment meets accepted safety standards. This effort would include, but not be limited to, attention to such items as proper labeling of chemicals, types and location of fire extinguishers, hoods that are in good working order, proper grounding of electrical equipment, ergonomic issues (which include equipment, such as pipetting devices, laboratory furniture, and prevention of musculoskeletal disorders) and providing means for the proper handling and disposal of biohazardous materials, including all patient specimens. As noted previously, effective waste management is a key aspect of laboratory safety. NCCLS has an approved guideline that deals in detail with management of clinical laboratory waste.[28]

Provision of all required safety equipment, regularly scheduled employee training sessions (including relevant documentation and certification, if necessary, such as with the federally mandated packaging and shipping regulations for infectious specimens), and scheduling of periodic inspections are all necessary activities to ensure that the laboratory staff is complying with the various mandates of the safety program.

Safety Equipment

A large and growing number of safety items are available for employees of the laboratory. OSHA requires that institutions provide employees with all necessary personal protective equipment (PPE). Many safety items are shown and described in a Safety Products Reference Manual.[51] Key important safety items are clothing (such as laboratory coats, gowns, and/or scrubs), gloves, and eye protection. These safety items should be used in areas where they are appropriate. Eye washers or face washers should be available in every chemistry laboratory. Many types are available, and some simply connect to existing plumbing. A hand-held eye and/or face safety spray is a requisite safety device and can be consistently placed in a position next to each sink while using only a few inches of space. Safety showers, strategically located in the laboratory, must be available and should be tested on a regular schedule.

Heat-resistant (nonasbestos) gloves should be available for handling hot glassware and dry ice. Safety goggles, glasses, and visors, including some that will fit conveniently over regular eyeglasses, are available in many sizes and shapes. Personnel wearing contact lenses should be aware of the danger of irritants getting under a lens; wearing such lenses can make it difficult to irrigate the eye properly. Shatterproof safety shields should be used in front of systems posing a potential danger because of implosion (vacuum collapse) or pressure explosions. Desiccator guards should be used with vacuum desiccators. Hot beakers should be handled with tongs. Inexpensive polyethylene pumps are available to pump acids from large bottles. Spill kits for acids, caustic materials, or flammable solvents come in various sizes. Such kits and the other appropriate safety materials should be located in convenient and appropriate sites in the laboratory.

A chemical fume hood is a necessity for every clinical chemistry laboratory. The fume hood is the only safe place to open any container of a material that gives off harmful vapors, to prepare reagents that produce fumes, and to heat flammable solvents. In the event of an explosion or fire in the hood, closing its window contains the fire.

Safety Inspections

It is good laboratory practice to organize a safety inspection team from the laboratory staff. This team is then responsible for conducting periodic and scheduled safety inspections of the laboratory.[32]

In the United States there are several regulatory, private accreditation, state, and federal organizations that may conduct a safety inspection of the laboratory. Some of these safety inspections may occur unannounced. From an external perspective, OSHA inspectors have the authority to enter a clinical laboratory unannounced and, on presentation of credentials, inspect it. The inspection may be regular or as a result of a complaint. In addition, the Commission on Inspection and Accreditation of the CAP inspects clinical laboratories and uses various safety checklists (available to the laboratory before inspection) when evaluating a laboratory for accreditation. These inspections are carried out on a regular basis. Although the JCAHO will accept CAP accreditation of a laboratory, it may still conduct a safety inspection of the laboratory when it inspects the hospital. The JCAHO is also planning to conduct their accreditation inspections, which may include a full laboratory or laboratory safety component, unannounced.

Depending on the group designated responsible for accrediting a particular laboratory, selected laboratories may be subject to inspections for the purposes of accreditation and/or safety only by state agencies or local Center for Medicare and Medicaid Services (CMS) groups. Inspections may also be made on a regular basis by state or local health departments or by local fire departments to determine conformance to their particular safety requirements. Currently a laboratory that meets federal or state OSHA requirements is likely to satisfy the standards of any other inspecting agency.

Mandated Plans

In 1991 OSHA mandated that all clinical laboratories in the United States must have a chemical hygiene plan (CHP)[41] and an exposure control plan.[42] OSHA has since updated their requirements for the exposure control plan to provide new examples of engineering controls and to place significantly greater responsibilities on employers to minimize and manage employee occupational exposure to blood-borne pathogens.[43] The CAP and other groups require that an accredited laboratory must have a documented tuberculosis exposure control plan conforming with biosafety guidelines published by the CDC.[5,17] There has been a resurgent recognition that the workplace setting of a clinical laboratory does expose employees to the occupational risk of having various musculoskeletal disorders. As a result, the focus of OSHA on laboratories having an effective ergonomics program has led to federal, state, and private accreditation groups addressing this area of occupational safety. Unfortunately, there has been considerable controversy in implementing a final ergonomics rule as one was published in 2001 and then withdrawn.[11,44]

Chemical Hygiene Plan

Major elements of a CHP plan include listing of responsibilities for employers, employees, and a chemical hygiene officer. Also among the items that have to be covered in the plan is the stipulation that every laboratory must have a complete chemical inventory that is updated annually. A copy of the Material Safety Data Sheet (MSDS), which defines each chemical as toxic, carcinogenic, or dangerous, must be on file and readily accessible and available to all employees 24 hours a day, 7 days a week. The MSDS contains important information for the benefit of laboratory employees. The chemical manufacturer's information as supplied on the MSDS is used to ascertain whether a certain chemical is hazardous. Each MSDS must give the product's identity as it appears on the container label and the chemical and common names of its hazardous components. The MSDS also provides physical data on the product, such as boiling point, vapor pressure, and specific gravity. Easily recognized characteristics of the chemical are also listed on the line for "appearance and odor." Information about hazardous properties is given in detail on the MSDS; this includes fire and explosion hazard data and health-related data, including the threshold limit value (TLV), exposure limits, and toxicity values. The TLV is the exposure allowable for an employee during one 8-hour day. It also notes effects of overexposure and provides first-aid procedures. Each MSDS also provides information on spill and disposal procedures and protective personal gear and equipment requirements. Originally there was no standard format for MSDSs, which made information hard to find. In June 1993 the American Standards Institute (ANSI) approved a new standard that specified a standard format for MSDSs.[53]

Exposure Control Plan

OSHA regulations[42,43] require that each laboratory develop, implement, and adhere to a plan that ensures the protection of laboratory workers against potential exposure to blood-borne pathogens[27,32,42] and to ensure that the medical wastes produced by the laboratory are managed and handled in a safe and effective manner.[28,32] OSHA regulations also place responsibility on employers for implementing new developments in exposure control technology; to solicit the input of employees directly involved in patient care in the identification, evaluation, and selection of these work practice controls; and in certain instances to maintain a log for employee percutaneous injuries from sharp devices, such as syringe needles.[43] Organizationally the plan should include sections on (1) purpose, (2) scope, (3) applicable references, (4) applicable definitions, (5) definition of responsibilities, and (6) detailed procedural steps.

When implementing the plan, each laboratory employee must be placed into one of three groups. The three classifications are as follows:

Group I: A job classification in which **ALL** employees have occupational exposure to blood or other potentially infectious materials.

Group II: A job classification in which **SOME** employees have occupational exposure to blood or other potentially infectious materials. Employees in this group would be those whose performance of their duties as defined by their job classification, or whose special assigned tasks, put them at risk for *possible* exposure to human blood or other potentially infectious materials. An example of an employee who would fit into this classification would be an instrument technician whose duties require routine maintenance or repair of an instrument in which blood or other potentially infectious materials might be encountered. These individuals must receive the same training and orientation as employees in Group I.

Group III: A job classification in which employees do **NOT** have **ANY** occupational exposure to blood or other potentially infectious materials. It is not mandatory that employees who qualify in this group receive training on the OSHA Bloodborne Standard. It is imperative, however, that these employees are never asked to perform any procedure that would subject them to occupational exposure. If at any future date an employee in this group has any additional duties added to his or her job that would include any exposure-prone tasks, then this employee needs to be added to the Group II list. Training of this employee in all aspects of the OSHA Bloodborne Standard **MUST** be completed before his or her actual performance of these new duties. In addition, this employee must be offered vaccination for hepatitis B within 10 working days of initial assignment to a position involving exposure.

Tuberculosis Control Plan[17]

The purpose of the tuberculosis control plan is to prevent the transmission of tuberculosis (TB), which occurs when an individual inhales a droplet that contains *Mycobacterium tuberculosis. M. tuberculosis* is aerosolized when an infected individual sneezes, speaks, or coughs. Transmission of TB and exposure to TB can be greatly diminished with early identification and isolation of patients at risk, environmental controls, appropriate use of respiratory protection equipment, education of laboratory employees, and when necessary early initiation of therapy.

An effective tuberculosis control plan will include determination of exposure at regular intervals for all employees who are at occupational risk. Engineering and work practice controls are particularly important in laboratory areas, such as surgical pathology and microbiology. But there is clearly a risk of exposure from specimens of patients with suspected or confirmed tuberculosis in every section of the laboratory, including chemistry.

Ergonomics Program

More than one third of occupational related injuries or illnesses reported by employees to the U.S. Bureau of Labor Statistics are estimated to be caused by musculoskeletal disorders. In 2003 federal regulations based on occupational management guidelines that are 15 years old are still not finalized as a result of OSHA continuing to work with Congress and small business advocacy groups to complete a rule that is deemed fair to both employees and employers.[11,37,44]

There are several areas of occupational risk for development of musculoskeletal disorders in the clinical laboratory.[36] These include routine laboratory activity, functionality of the workspace (including laboratory floor matting, bright lighting, and noise generation), and equipment design (computer keyboards and displays, workstations, and chairs). One particular laboratory function, pipetting and related pipette design, has received considerable attention. As depicted in Figure 1-2, pipettes are being designed with a goal of reducing an employee's risk of having cumulative stress disorders caused by awkward posture, repetitive motion, and the repeated use of force. An example of an ergonomically engineered laboratory work chair is shown in Figure 1-5.

The CAP requires accredited laboratories to have a comprehensive and defined ergonomics program that is designed to prevent work-related musculoskeletal disorders through prevention and engineering controls. The documented ergonomics plan should include elements of employee training regarding the areas of risk, engineering controls to minimize or eliminate risks, and an assessment process to identify problematic issues for documentation and remediation.[14]

Hazards in the Laboratory

Various types of hazards are encountered in the operation of a clinical laboratory. These hazards must be identified and labeled, and work practices developed for dealing with them. The major categories of hazards encountered include biological, chemical, electrical, and fire hazards.

Identification of Hazards

Clinical laboratories deal with each of the nine classes of hazardous materials. These are classified by the United Nations (UN) as (1) explosives, (2) compressed gases,[8] (3) flammable liquids, (4) flammable solids, (5) oxidizer materials, (6) toxic materials, (7) radioactive materials, (8) corrosive materials, and (9) miscellaneous materials not elsewhere classified. Shipping and handling of Class (6) toxic materials,

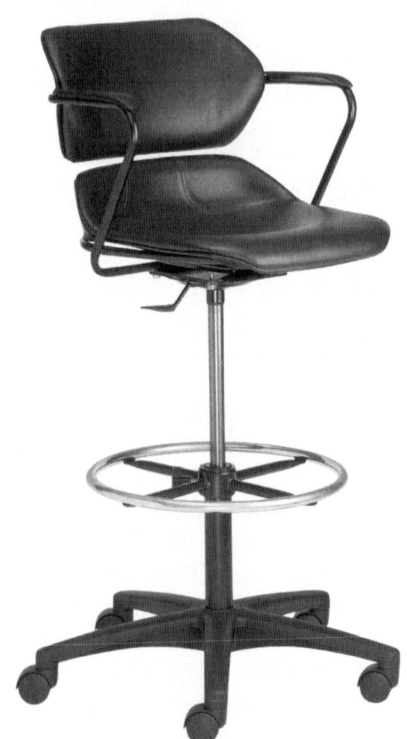

Figure 1-5 A example of an ergonomically designed laboratory chair. *(Courtesy MarketLab Inc.)*

specifically biological and potentially infectious materials, has received considerable attention. In 2002 the U.S. Department of Transportation (DOT) released a revised rule with standards for infectious substance hazardous material handling.[3,20] The impact and requirements of these regulations are described in the section on biological hazards.

Warning labels aid in the identification of chemical hazards during shipment. Under regulations of the DOT, chemicals that are transported in the United States must carry labels based on the UN classification. DOT placards or labels are diamond shaped with a digit imprinted on the bottom corner that identifies the UN hazard class (1 to 9). The hazard is identified more specifically in printed words placed along the horizontal axis of the diamond. Color coding and a pictorial art description of the hazard supplement the identification of hazardous material on the label; the artwork appears in the top corner of the diamond (Figure 1-6, *A*).

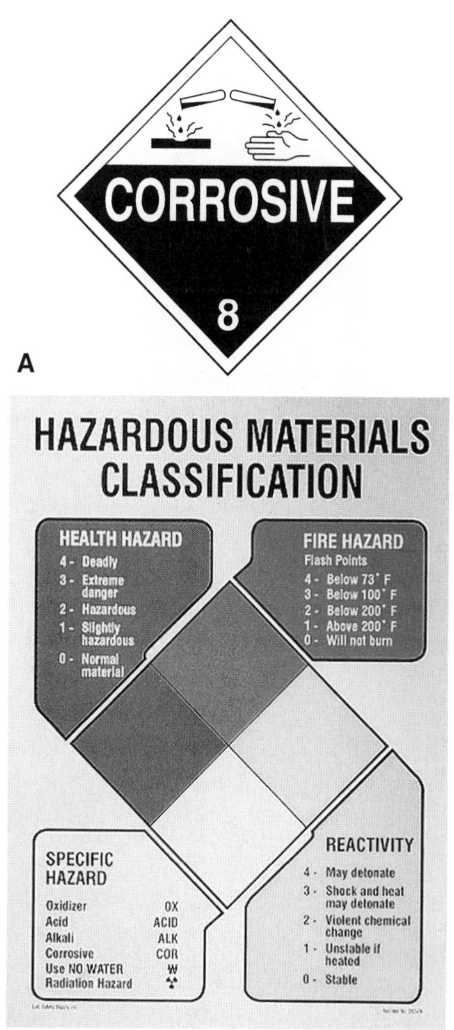

Figure 1-6 A, Department of Transportation label for corrosives. **B,** Labeling identification system of the National Fire Protection Association. *(Courtesy Lab Safety Supply Inc., Janesville, Wis.)*

The upper half of the label for corrosive materials shows a metallic bar and a hand, both of which are being eaten away by drops of fluid; the black bottom half of the label is lettered "corrosive" in white. The bottom corner shows the digit "8."

The system is used by the DOT for shipping hazardous materials; however, when the hazardous material reaches its destination and is removed from the shipping container, this identification is lost. The laboratory must then label each individual container. Usually the information necessary to classify the contents of the container appropriately is contained on the shipping label and should be noted. Important first-aid information is also usually provided on this label.

Even though OSHA prescribes the use of labels or other appropriate warnings at present, no single uniform labeling system for hazardous chemicals exists for clinical laboratories. Appropriate hazard warnings include any words, pictures, symbols, or combinations that convey the health or physical hazards of the container's contents and must be specific as to the effect of the chemical and the specific target organs involved.[21] The National Fire Protection Association (NFPA) has developed the 704-M Identification System, which classifies hazardous material from 0 to 4 (most hazardous) according to flammability and reactivity (instability). This system uses diamond-shaped labels, which are available from most companies that sell laboratory safety equipment. The labels are color coded and are divided into quadrants. Three of the quadrants have a characteristic color and represent a type of hazard. A number in the quadrant indicates the degree of the hazard. The fourth (lower) quadrant contains information of special interest to firemen; for example, "W" indicates a water-ignitable material (Figure 1-6, *B*). Some chemicals require labels using two or three of the quadrants to convey the necessary information.

Descriptive labels, such as "corrosive," "flammable," "poison," and "explosives" may also be used. Obviously, some containers may require two or three labels because several types of hazard are involved.

Kits of assorted safety signs are available from most laboratory supply dealers. These contain most general labels necessary in a clinical laboratory. Some examples of the contents of one kit are "eye wash," "use in hood," "safety shower," "empty cylinder," and "wear eye protection in this area."

Biological Hazards

To operate a clinical laboratory safely, it is essential to minimize the exposure of laboratory workers to infectious agents, such as the hepatitis viruses and the human immunodeficiency virus (HIV). Exposure to infectious agents results from (1) accidental puncture with needles, (2) spraying of infectious materials by a syringe or spilling and splattering of these materials on bench tops or floors, (3) centrifuge accidents, and (4) cuts or scratches from contaminated vessels. Any unfixed tissue, including blood slides, must also be treated as potentially infectious material.

As discussed earlier in this section, OSHA has mandated that all U.S. laboratories have an exposure control plan.[42] In addition, the National Institute for Occupational Safety and Health (NIOSH), a functional unit of the CDC, has prepared and widely distributed a document entitled Universal Precautions that specifies how U.S. clinical laboratories handle infectious agents.[35] In general it mandates that clinical laboratories treat all human blood and other potentially infectious materials as if they were known to contain infectious agents, such as HBV, HIV, and other blood-borne pathogens. These requirements apply to all specimens of blood, serum, plasma, blood products, vaginal secretions, semen, cerebrospinal fluid, synovial fluid, and concentrated HBV or HIV viruses. In addition, any specimen of any type that contains visible traces of blood should be handled using these Universal Precautions.

Universal Precautions also specify that barrier protection must be used by laboratory workers to prevent skin and mucous membrane contamination from specimens. These barriers, also known as PPE, include gloves, gowns, laboratory coats, face shields or mask and eye protection, mouth pieces, resuscitation bags, pocket masks, or other ventilator devices. Soon it was noted that latex allergy can be a problem when using latex gloves for barrier protection. By September 1992, 1100 reactions and 15 fatalities related to latex allergy had been reported to the Food and Drug Administration (FDA).[22] If latex gloves are to be used, they should be powder-free, low-allergen latex. A variety of medical grade nonlatex gloves made of materials such as vinyl, nitrile, neoprene or thermoplastic elastomer is available. The cost varies considerably.

New products for increasing employee protection against needle sticks include an array of novel sharps containers and biological safety disposal bags and needle sheaths that may be closed following venipuncture without physically touching the needle or the sheath. Although additional studies are required on their efficacy and effects on laboratory test results, microlaser devices are now available for piercing a patient's skin to collect a capillary blood specimen.

The NCCLS has also published a similar set of recommendations,[27,32] several of which are specified as requirements in the OSHA exposure control plan. They include:

1. Never perform mouth pipetting and never blow out pipettes that contain potentially infectious material.
2. Do not mix potentially infectious material by bubbling air through the liquid.
3. Barrier protection, such as gloves, masks, and protective eye wear and gowns, must be available and used when drawing blood from a patient and when handling all patient specimens. This includes the removal of stoppers from tubes. Gloves must be disposable, nonsterile latex, or of other material to provide adequate barrier protection. Phlebotomists must change gloves and adequately dispose of them between drawing blood from different patients.
4. Wash hands whenever gloves are changed.
5. Facial barrier protection should be used if there is a significant potential for the spattering of blood or body fluids.
6. Avoid using syringes whenever possible and dispose of needles in rigid containers (Figure 1-7, *A*) without handling them (Figure 1-7, *B*).
7. Dispose of all sharps appropriately.
8. Wear protective clothing, which serves as an effective barrier against potentially infective materials. When leaving the laboratory, the protective clothing should be removed.
9. Strive to prevent accidental injuries.

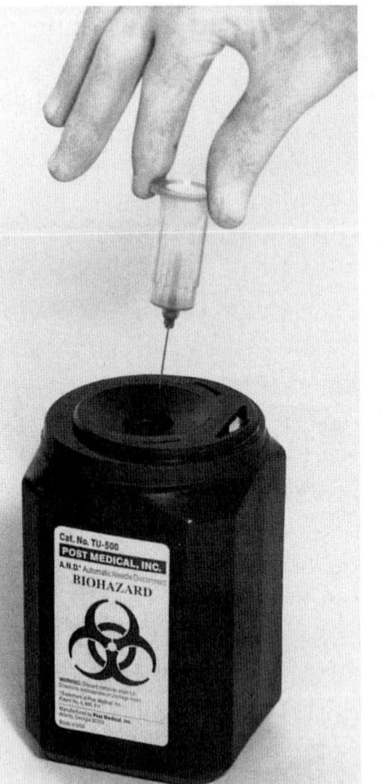

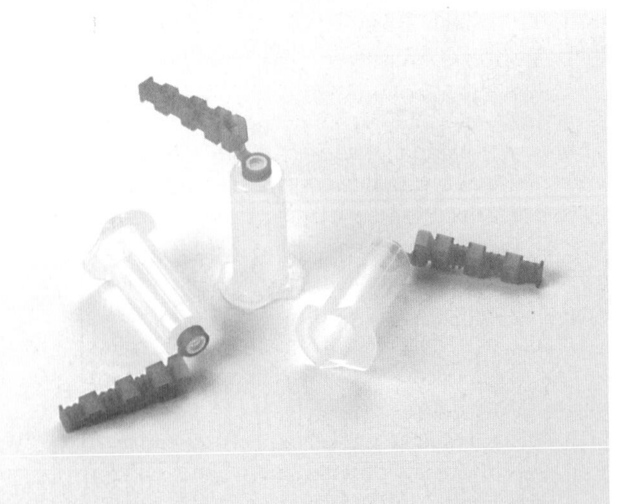

Figure 1-7 A, Convenient needle disposal system for sharps. **B,** Needle sheathing devices for prevention of body contact with needle. *(**B** Courtesy MarketLab Inc.)*

10. Encourage frequent hand washing in the laboratory; employees must wash their hands whenever they leave the laboratory.
11. Make a habit of keeping your hands away from your mouth, nose, eyes, and any other mucous membranes. This reduces the possibility of self-inoculation.
12. Minimize spills and spatters.
13. Decontaminate all surfaces and reusable devices after use with appropriate U.S. Environmental Protection Agency (EPA)–registered hospital disinfectants. Sterilization, disinfection, and decontamination are discussed in detail in NCCLS publication M29-T2.[27]
14. No warning labels are to be used on patient specimens since all should be treated as potentially hazardous.
15. Biosafety level 2 procedures should be used whenever appropriate.
16. Before centrifuging tubes, inspect them for cracks. Inspect the inside of the trunnion cup for signs of erosion or adhering matter. Be sure that rubber cushions are free from all bits of glass.
17. Use biohazard disposal techniques (e.g., "Red Bag").
18. Never leave a discarded tube or infected material unattended or unlabeled.
19. Periodically, clean out freezer and dry-ice chests to remove broken ampoules and tubes of biological specimens. Use rubber gloves and respiratory protection during this cleaning.
20. OSHA requires that hepatitis B vaccine be offered to all employees at risk of potential exposure as a regular or occasional part of their duties. CDC's Advisory Committee on Immunization Practices (ACIP) recommends that medical technologists, phlebotomists, and pathologists be vaccinated with hepatitis B vaccine. It is a regulatory mandate that all of the above laboratory employees at a minimum at least be given the option to freely receive the hepatitis B vaccine.

Investigation of tragic air accidents in the late 1990s by the U.S. National Transportation Safety Board (NTSB) led to the DOT, in cooperation with the International Air Transport Association (IATA) and the International Civil Aviation Organization (ICAO), developing revised and strict requirements for the shipping and handling of hazardous materials.[3,20] With the continued awareness of the necessity for Universal Precautions, the risk of blood-borne pathogens and the potentially adverse consequences of serious infection, the shipping and handling of Class 6 toxic materials—biological materials—is a critical safety issue.

The federal shipping and packaging guidelines[51] divide potentially infectious specimens or substances into the following risk groups:

1. A microorganism unlikely to cause human or animal disease. Materials containing only such microorganisms are not subject to the requirements of these regulations. The risk to individuals and the community is very low.
2. A pathogen that can cause human or animal disease, but is unlikely to be a serious hazard and, although capable of causing serious infection on exposure, for which there are effective treatments and preventive measure available and the risk of spread of infection is limited. Risk to individuals is moderate, but the risk to the community is low.
3. A pathogen that usually causes serious human or animal disease but does not ordinarily spread from one infected individual to another, and for which effective treatments and preventive measures are available. Risk to individuals is high, but risk to the community is low.
4. A pathogen that usually causes serious human or animal disease and that can be readily transmitted from one individual to another, directly or indirectly, and for which effective treatments and preventive measures are not usually available. Risk to the individual and the community is high.

These regulations place particular emphasis on the Hazardous Material (HAZMAT) training that must be given to laboratory employees when shipping and handling infectious substances. Elements include general awareness and familiarization, function-specific, and safety training. Proper training, particularly in the areas of package labeling and documentation (including a shipper's declaration of contents for dangerous goods), is mandatory with documented certification required from employers that the relevant employees have appropriate training programs. Although the adverse impact of improper training can be reflected most by potential human morbidity and mortality, identified violations of these regulations also carry large financial fines and penalties for both the infringing individual and the employer or institution.

Chemical Hazards

The proper storage and use of chemicals is necessary to prevent dangers, such as burns, explosions, fires, and toxic fumes. Thus knowledge of the properties of the chemicals in use and of proper handling procedures greatly reduces dangerous situations. Bottles of chemicals and solutions should also be handled carefully, and a cart should be used to transport a heavy or a multiple number of containers from one area to another. Glass containers with chemicals should be transported in rubber or plastic containers that protect them from breakage and, in the event of breakage, contain the spill. Appropriate spill kits should be available in strategic locations. A general spill kit, such as the Sasco Solidifier Spill Response Kit, should contain specific materials to be used with spills of acid or of caustic or organic materials. Directions for use of these materials are contained in the kit.

Spattering from acids, caustic materials, and strong oxidizing agents probably represents the greatest hazard to clothing and eyes and is a potential source of chemical burns. A bottle should never be held by its neck but instead firmly around its body with one or both hands, depending on the size of the bottle. Acids must be diluted by slowly adding them to water while mixing; water should never be added to concentrated acid. When working with acid or alkali solutions, safety glasses should be worn. Acids, caustic materials, and strong oxidizing agents should be mixed in the sink. This provides water for cooling and for confinement of the reagent in the event the flask or bottle breaks.

All bottles containing reagents must be properly labeled. It is good practice to label the container before adding the reagent, thus preventing the possibility of having an unlabeled reagent. The label should bear the name and concentration of the reagent, the initials of the person who made up the reagent, and the date on which the reagent was prepared. When appropriate, the expiration date should also be included. The labels should be color coded or an additional label added to designate specific storage instructions, such as the requirement for refrigeration or special storage related to a potential hazard. All reagents found in unlabeled bottles should be disposed of using the appropriate procedures and precautions.

Strong acids, caustic materials, and strong oxidizing agents should be dispensed by a commercially available automatic dispensing device. Under no circumstances is mouth pipetting permitted.

In some instances, all waste materials are not collected in the same container. With certain pieces of equipment, strong acids or other hazardous materials are pumped directly into the drain. This should always be accompanied by a steady flow of water from the faucet. Safety glasses should be used by instrument operators when acids are pumped under pressure.

Perchloric acid, because it is potentially explosive in contact with organic materials, requires careful handling. Perchloric acid should not be used on wooden bench tops, and bottles of this acid should be stored on a glass tray. Disposal may be accomplished by adding the acid dropwise (using a splatter shield) to at least 100 volumes of cold water and pouring the diluted acid down the drain with large amounts of additional cold water. Special perchloric acid hoods, with special wash-down facilities, should be installed if large amounts of this acid are used.

Special care is necessary when dealing with mercury. Even small drops of mercury on bench tops and floors may poison the atmosphere in a poorly ventilated room. The element's ability to amalgamate with a number of metals is well known. After an accidental spillage of mercury, the spill area should be cleaned carefully until there are no droplets remaining. All containers of mercury should be kept well stoppered.

The EPA controls the disposal of nonradioactive hazardous wastes.[47] The Resource Conservation and Recovery Act of 1976 (RCRA) states that disposal of materials classifiable within any of the nine UN hazardous materials classes is enforced in such a way that health and safety professionals involved in the disposal of such materials are personally liable for each individual violation.

A NCCLS publication[28] covers hazardous waste disposal; however, many municipalities and states have their own regulations. The agencies should be contacted by the laboratory for specifics.

Volatile chemicals and compressed gases pose specific hazards.

Hazards from Volatiles

The use of organic solvents in a clinical laboratory represents a potential fire hazard and hazards to health from inhalation of toxic vapors or skin contact. These solvents should be used in a fume hood. Storage of organic solvents is regulated by rules set down by OSHA (Table 1-16). However, some local fire department rules are more stringent. Solvents should be stored in an OSHA-approved metal storage cabinet that is properly vented. The maximum working volume of flam-

TABLE 1-16 Maximum Allowable Size of Containers for Storage of Solvents Inside Buildings (OSHA)

	Maximum Allowable Size of Containers			
Container Type	**Class IA**	**Class IB**	**Class IC**	**Classes II and III**
Glass or approved plastic	1 pt	1 qt	1 gal	1 gal
Safety cans*	1 gal	2 gal	5 gal	5 gal
Metal drums (DOT)	60 gal	60 gal	60 gal	60 gal

Definitions of Classes	
IA	Flash point below 22.8 °C and boiling point below 37.8 °C
IB	Flash point below 22.8 °C and boiling point above 37.8 °C
IC	Flash point between 22.8 °C and 37.8 °C
II	Flash point between 37.8 °C and 60 °C
III	Flash point above 60 °C

OSHA, Occupational Safety and Health Administration; *DOT*, Department of Transportation.

*Safety cans are metal or plastic containers having a spring-closing spout cover designed to relieve internal pressure when subjected to the heat of fire and prevent leakage if tipped over. They are also equipped with a flame-arrester screen. Portable safety cans range in size from 1 pint to 5 gallons and are made in numerous styles with faucets, pouring spouts, or dispensing hoses. Only FM (Factory Mutual Engineering Corporation of the Factory Mutual System) or UL (Underwriters Laboratories, Inc.) recognized safety cans should be used, because these cans have been tested and approved by these agencies.

mable solvents allowed outside storage cabinets is 5 gallons per room. No more than 60 gallons of type I and II solvents may be stored in a single cabinet. No more than three cabinets may be located in each 5000 sq ft of laboratory space. Larger amounts than shown in Table 1-16 must be stored in special refrigerated storage rooms or in outside storage buildings.

Vaporization is the major problem in the ignition and spread of fires. Vapors from flammable and combustible liquids and solids form a flammable mixture with air. They are characterized by their flash point, where the flash point is defined as the lowest temperature at which a solvent gives off flammable vapors in the close vicinity of its surface. The mixture at its flash point ignites when exposed to a source of ignition. At temperatures below the flash point, the vapor given off is considered too lean for ignition.

Disposal of flammable solvents in storm sewers or sanitary sewers is, in general, not allowed. Exceptions are small amounts of those materials that are miscible with water, but even disposal of these should be followed by large amounts of cold water. Other solvents should be collected in safety cans. Separate cans should be used for ether and for chlorinated solvents; all other solvents may be combined in a third can. The cans should be stored, in keeping with storage quantity rules, in a safety cabinet until pickup by a waste-disposal firm. A more economical approach is to transfer the solvents to larger cans or drums in an outside storage facility so that pickup could be less frequent. Some large institutions have their own in-house disposal facilities.

Hazards from Compressed Gases

The DOT regulations cover the labeling of cylinders of compressed gases that are transported by interstate carriers. The diamond-shaped labels described previously are used on all large cylinders and on any boxes containing small cylinders. Some general rules for handling large cylinders of compressed gas are:

1. Always transport cylinders using a hand truck to which the cylinder is secured.
2. Leave the valve cap on a cylinder until the cylinder is ready for use, at which time the cylinder should have been secured by a support around the upper one third of its body. Disconnect the hose or regulator, shut off the valve, and replace the cap before the cylinder is completely empty to prevent the possibility of the development of a negative pressure. Place an "empty" sign or label on the cylinder.
3. Chain or secure cylinders at all times even when empty.
4. Always check cylinders for the composition of their contents before connection.
5. Never force threads; if a regulator does not thread readily, something is wrong.

The precautions cited for large refillable gas cylinders also apply to small cylinders that are not refillable. Propane cylinders of the type frequently secured to a flame photometer and cylinders of calibrating gases for blood gas equipment are examples of disposable cylinders. Cylinders in floor-standing base supports require the additional security of a chain or strap attached to a wall or fixed piece of furniture. Local fire department regulations (which vary considerably from place to place) govern the disposal of exhausted cylinders.

Electrical Hazards

Wherever there are electrical wires or connections, there is a potential for shock or fire hazard. Worn wires on all electrical equipment should be replaced immediately; all equipment should be grounded using three-prong plugs. OSHA regulations stipulate that the requirements for grounding of electrical equipment of the National Electrical Code (published by NFPA) be met. If grounded receptacles are not available, a licensed electrician should be consulted for proper alternative grounding techniques. Some local codes are more stringent than OSHA requirements and do not allow for two-pole mating receptacles with adapters for a three-pole plug.

Use of extension cords is prohibited. This standard is more stringent than any other existing regulation. In some instances, an extension cord may have to be used temporarily. In such cases, the cord should be less than 12 feet in length, have at least 16 American Wire Gauge (AWG) wire, be approved by the Underwriters Laboratory (UL), and have only one outlet at the end. If several outlets are necessary in an area, a power strip with its own fuse or circuit breaker may be installed at least 3 inches above bench top level. Several manufacturers now sell devices to check for high resistance in neutral or ground wiring or excess voltage in the neutral wiring.

Electrical equipment and connections should not be handled with wet hands, nor should electrical equipment be used after liquid has been spilled on it. The equipment must be turned off immediately and dried thoroughly; a fan or hair dryer will speed up the drying process. In case of a wet or malfunctioning electrical instrument that is used by several people, the plug should be pulled and a note cautioning co-workers against use should be left on the instrument.

Fire Hazards

The ideal solution to the problem of fires and indeed to all laboratory accidents is prevention. However, all fires cannot be prevented, so provisions must be made for those that do occur. NFPA and OSHA publish standards covering subjects from emergency exits (including means of egress) to safety and firefighting equipment. NFPA also publishes the National Fire Codes. Many state and local agencies have adopted these codes (some of which are more stringent than OSHA requirements) and thus make them legally enforceable.

Every laboratory should have the necessary equipment to put out or to confine a fire in the laboratory and to put out a fire on the clothing of an individual. Easy access to safety showers is essential. A safety shower should have a pull chain

TABLE 1-17 Classification of Fires and Fire Extinguisher Requirements

Type of Hazard	Class of Fire	Recommended Extinguisher Agents
Ordinary combustibles: Wood, cloth, paper	A	Water, dry chemical foam, loaded steam
Flammable liquids and gases: Solvents and greases Natural or manufactured gases	B	Dry chemical, carbon dioxide, loaded steam, Halon 1211 or 1301 foam
Electrical equipment: Any energized electrical equipment. If electricity is turned off at source, this reverts to a Class A or B	C	Dry chemical, carbon dioxide, Halon 1211 or 1301
Combinations of: Ordinary combustibles and flammable liquids and gases	A & B	Dry chemical, loaded steam, foam
Combinations of: Ordinary combustibles and electrical equipment	A & C	Dry chemical
Combinations of: Flammable liquids and gases and electrical equipment	B & C	Dry chemical, carbon dioxide, Halon 1211 or 1301
Combinations of: Ordinary combustibles, flammable liquids and gases, and electrical equipment	A, B, & C	Triplex dry chemical

either attached to the wall at a convenient height or hanging down from the shower head; the chain should have a large ring attached so that the shower may be easily activated, even with eyes closed. Fire blankets for smothering fire on clothing should be available in an easily accessible wall-mounted case. The blanket is unrolled from the case and rolled around the body by taking hold of the rope that is attached to the blanket and turning the body around. The location of this equipment and the locations of fire alarms and maps of evacuation routes are dictated by the local fire marshal.

Various types of fire extinguishers are available. The type to use depends on the type of fire. Because it is impractical to have several types of fire extinguishers present in every area, dry chemical fire extinguishers are among the best all-purpose extinguishers for laboratory areas. An extinguisher should be provided near every laboratory door and, in a large laboratory, at the end of the room opposite to the door. Everyone in the laboratory should be instructed in the use of these extinguishers and any other firefighting equipment. All fire extinguishers should be tested by qualified personnel at intervals specified by the manufacturer. The three classes of fires and the type of fire extinguisher to be used for each are listed in Table 1-17. Every fire extinguisher is labeled as to the type of fire it should be used to extinguish.

Two additional types of fires, designated "D" and "E," should be handled only by trained personnel. Type "D" fires include those involving powdered metal materials (e.g., magnesium). A special powder is used to fight this hazard. A type "E" fire is one that cannot be put out or is liable to result in a detonation (such as an arsenal fire). A type "E" fire is usually allowed to burn out while nearby materials are being appropriately protected.

Many clinical laboratories now have a computer that is housed in a temperature- and humidity-controlled room. The most popular automatic fire control system used for these rooms is Halon 1301 (bromotrifluoromethane). Although this is the least toxic of the halons, NFPA regulations require a warning sign at the entrance to the room and availability of self-contained breathing equipment.

REFERENCES

1. American Society for Testing and Materials. ASTM Standards 11.01-Water and 11.02-Water 2. Philadelphia: American Society for Testing and Materials, 1991.
2. American Society for Testing and Materials. ASTM Standard E1238-94. Standard specification for transferring clinical observations between independent computer systems. Philadelphia: American Society for Testing and Materials, 1994.
3. Bennett C. HAZMAT Training 101. Adv Admin Lab 2003;12:42-5.
4. Bermes EW Jr, Young DS. General laboratory techniques and procedures. In Burtis CA, Ashwood ER eds, Tietz textbook of clinical chemistry 3rd ed. Philadelphia: W B Saunders, 1999:3-41.
5. Biosafety in microbiological and biomedical laboratories 4th Ed. Washington, DC: Department of Health and Human Services, Centers for Disease Control and Prevention and the National Institutes of Health. US Government Printing Office, May, 1999.
6. Columbus RL, Palmer HJ. The integrated blood-collection system as a vehicle into complete clinical laboratory automation. Clin Chem 1991;37:1548-58.
7. Commission on Laboratory Inspection and Accreditation. Reagent water: Specifications. Skokie, IL: College of American Pathologists, 1985.
8. Compressed Gas Association, Inc: Handbook of compressed gases 2nd ed. New York: Reinhold Publishing Corporation, 1981.

9. Dudley AW, Lin,JJ, Leu NC. Automatic balancing centrifuge (ABC). Am J Clin Pathol 1994;101:399.
10. ENV 1613. Messages for Exchange of Clinical Laboratory Information. Brussels: Comite Europeen de Normalization, 1994.
11. Ergonomics program. Final rule; removal. Occupational Safety and Health Administration (OSHA). Fed Reg 2001; 666:20403.
12. Estey CA, Felder RA: Clinical trials of a novel centrifugation method: Axial separation. Clin Chem 1996; 42:402-9.
13. Forrey AW, McDonald CJ, DeMoor G, et al. Logical observation identifier names and codes (LOINC) database: A public use set of codes and names for electronic reporting of clinical laboratory test results. Clin Chem 1996; 42:81-90.
14. Gile TJ: Ergonomics in the laboratory. Lab Med 2001; 32: 263-7.
15. Goldophin W, Bodtker K, Uyeno D, Goh LO: Automated blood- sample handling in the clinical laboratory. Clin Chem 1990; 36:1551-5.
16. Godolphin W, Bodker K.: Automation and simulation of central processing in clinical laboratories: Chemometrics and intelligent laboratory systems. Laboratory Information Management 1993; 21:181-8.
17. Guidelines for preventing the transmission of tuberculosis in health care facilities. Centers for Disease Control and Prevention. Fed Reg 1993; 58: 52810-54.
18. Handbook of chemistry and physics. 78th ed. Linde DR ed. Boca Raton, FL: The Chemical Rubber Co, 2003-2004: D-141.
19. Health Level Seven. An Application Protocol for Electronic Data Exchange in Healthcare Environments. Version 2.2, Ann Arbor, MI, Health Level Seven, 1994.
20. Hazardous materials: Revision to standards for infectious substances. Final Rule. Department of Transportation. Fed Reg 2002; 67 (157): 53118-44.
21. Inspection Procedures for the Hazard Communication Standard (29 Code of Federal Regulations 1910.1200). United States Department of Labor, Office of Health Compliance Assistance, OSHA Instruction CPL 2-2.38C, October 22, 1990.
22. Landwehr L, Boguniewicz M. Current perspectives on latex allergy. Pediatrics 1996; 128:305-12.
23. McDonald CJ, Huff SM, Suico JG, Hill G, Leavelle D, et al. LOINC, a Universal Standard for Identifying Laboratory Observations: A 5-Year Update. Clin Chem 2003; 49:624-33.
24. Mowery C: Calibration system reduces pipette checking time. Clin Lab Prod 2000; 29, May.
25. National Committee for Clinical Laboratory Standards. Procedures for the Handling and Processing of Blood Specimens: Approved Guideline. 2nd ed. NCCLS Document H18-A2. Wayne, PA: National Committee for Clinical Laboratory Standards, 1999.
26. National Committee for Clinical Laboratory Standards. Temperature Calibration of Water Baths, Instruments, and Temperature Sensors: Approved Standard. 2nd ed. NCCLS Document 12-A2. Wayne, PA: National Committee for Clinical Laboratory Standards, 1990.
27. National Committee for Clinical Laboratory Standards. Protection of Laboratory Workers from Occupationally Acquired Infections: Approved Guideline. 2nd ed. NCCLS Document M29-A2. Wayne, PA: National Committee for Clinical Laboratory Standards, 2001.
28. National Committee for Clinical Laboratory Standards. Clinical Laboratory Waste management: Approved Guideline. 2nd ed. NCCLS Document GP5-A2. Wayne, PA: National Committee for Clinical Laboratory Standards, 2002.
29. National Committee for Clinical Laboratory Standards. Terminology and Definitions for Use in NCCLS Documents: Approved Standard. NCCLS Document NRSCL08-A. Wayne, PA: National Committee for Clinical Laboratory Standards, 1998.
30. National Committee for Clinical Laboratory Standards. Source Book of Reference Methods, Materials, and Related Information for the Clinical Laboratory: Proposed Guideline. NCCLS Document NRSCL12-P. Wayne, PA: National Committee for Clinical Laboratory Standards, 1994.
31. National Committee for Clinical Laboratory Standards. The Reference System for the Clinical Laboratory: Criteria for Development and Credentialing of Methods and Materials for Harmonization of Results: Approved Guideline. NCCLS Document NRSCL13-A. Wayne, PA: National Committee for Clinical Laboratory Standards, 2000.
32. National Committee for Clinical Laboratory Standards. Clinical Laboratory Safety: Approved Guideline. NCCLS Document GP17-A. Wayne, PA: National Committee for Clinical Laboratory Standards, 1996.
33. National Committee for Clinical Laboratory Standards. Blood Alcohol Testing in the Clinical Laboratory: Approved Guideline. NCCLS Document T/DM6-A. Wayne, PA: National Committee for Clinical Laboratory Standards, 1997.
34. National Committee for Clinical Laboratory Standards. Preparation and Testing of Reagent Water in the Clinical Laboratory. Approved Guideline. 3rd ed. NCCLS Document C03-A3. Wayne, PA: National Committee for Clinical Laboratory Standards, 1997.
35. National Institute for Occupational Safety and Health. Guidelines for Prevention of Transmission of Human Immunodeficiency Virus and Hepatitis B Virus of Health-Care and Public Safety Workers. DHSS (NIOSH) Publication No. 89-107. Washington DC:

Department of Health and Social Services, February, 1989.

36. National Institute for Occupational Safety and Health (NIOSH): Elements of ergonomics programs. A primer based on workplace evaluations of musculoskeletal disorders. Centers for Disease Control (NIOSH) Publication No. 97-117. Atlanta, GA: Centers for Disease Control, March, 1997.
37. National Institute for Occupational Safety and Health (NIOSH). Musculoskeletal disorders and workplace factors: A critical review of epidemiologic evidence for work-related musculoskeletal disorders of the neck, upper extremities, and low back. Centers for Disease Control (NIOSH) Publication No. 97-141. Atlanta, GA: Centers for Disease Control, July, 1997.
38. National Institute of Standards and Technology. The International System of Units (SI). NIST Special Publication 811. Gaithersburg, MD: National Institute of Standards and Technology (http://www.nist.gov), 1994.
39. National Institute of Standards and Technology. Standard Reference Materials. Publication No. 260. Washington DC: U.S. Department of Commerce, 1996.
40. National Institute of Standards and Technology. Testing of Glass Volumetric Apparatus, NBS C-602. Washington, DC, US Department of Commerce, 1959.
41. Occupational Exposure to Hazardous Chemicals in the Laboratory. Occupational Safety and Health Administration (OSHA). Document 29 CFR, Part 1910. Fed Reg 1991; 55:3300-35.
42. Occupational Exposure to Bloodborne Pathogens. Occupational Safety and Health Administration (OSHA) Final Rule. Fed Reg 1991; 56:64004-182.
43. Occupational exposure to bloodborne pathogens; needle sticks and other sharps injuries; Final Rule. Occupational Safety and Health Administration (OSHA). Fed Reg 2001; 66:5318-25.
44. Occupational injury and illness recording and reporting requirements. Final Rule. Occupational Safety and Health Administration (OSHA). Fed Reg 2001; 66: 5916-6135.
45. Perkins SL, Adams GA. Evaluation of the DuPont axial separation system. Clin Chem 1996; 42:1467-73.
46. Powsner ER, Widman JC. Basic Principles of Radioactivity and Its Measurement. In: Burtis CA, Ashwood ER, eds. Tietz textbook of clinical chemistry, 3rd ed. Philadelphia: W B Saunders, 1999:113-132.
47. Protection of Environment, Code of Federal Regulations, Environmental Protection Agency, *40:* Parts 260-299. Rockville MD: Government Institutes Inc 1990.
48. Reagent Chemicals, 10th Edition, Washington DC: American Chemical Society, 2005. (*http://pubs.acs.org/reagents/*)
49. Reference Samples/Reference Materials. Geel, Belgium: Institute for Reference Materials and Measurements, European Commission, Joint Research Center, 1996. (*http://www.irmm.jrc.be/*)
50. Rigg JC, Brown SS, Dybkaer R, Olesen H eds. The Silver Book: *Compendium of terminology and nomenclature of properties in clinical laboratory sciences* (recommendations 1995). London: Blackwell Science, 1995.
51. Safety Products Reference Manual. Pittsburgh, Fisher Scientific Co, 1992.
52. Spackman KA. Integrating sources for a clinical reference terminology: experience linking SNOMED to LOINC and drug vocabularies. Medinfo 1998; 9 Pt 1:600-3.
53. Turk AR. New MSDS could make safety data easier to understand Material Management in Health Care 1993; 2:14-15.
54. Uldall A, Damgaard PT, Magnussen E, et al. Guidelines for the use of centrifuges. J Anal Chem 1989; 11:28-31.

ADDITIONAL READING

General

Dean JA. Analytical chemistry handbook. New York: McGraw-Hill, 1995.

Calibration and Standardization

American Society for Testing and Materials. ASTM Standard E542-94 Calibration of Laboratory Volumetric Apparatus. Philadelphia: American Society for Testing and Materials, 1996.

Curtis RH. Performance verification of manual action pipettes. Part I. Am Clin Lab 1994; 12:8-9.

Curtis RH. Performance verification of manual action pipettes. Part II. Am Clin Lab 1994; 12:16-17.

Skeen GA, Ashwood ER. Using spectrophotometry to evaluate volumetric devices. Lab Med 2000; 31:478-9.

Laboratory Safety

Beckala HR.: Regulations for packaging and shipping laboratory specimens. Lab Med 1999; 30(10): 663-7.

Bendixen H, Manning F, Sparacino L. Blood and blood products: Safety and Risk. Washington DC: National Academy Press, 1996.

Committee on Hazardous Substances in the Laboratory. Prudent practices for handling hazardous chemicals in laboratories: National Research Council. Washington DC: National Academy Press, 1985.

Fleming DO, Richardson JH, Tulis JJ, Velsey D. Laboratory safety 2nd ed. Washington DC:ASM Press, 1995.

Laboratory safety: Principles and practices. Washington DC: American Society for Microbiology, 1994.

Montgomery L. Health and safety guidelines for the laboratory, Chicago: ASCP Press, 1995.

National Committee for Clinical Laboratory Standards. Clinical Laboratory Safety: Approved Guideline. NCCLS

Document GP17-A. Wayne, PA: National Committee for Clinical Laboratory Standards, 1996.

National Committee for Clinical Laboratory Standards. Implementing a needle stick and sharps injury prevention program in the clinical laboratory; A report. NCCLS Document X3-R. Wayne, PA: National Committee for Clinical Laboratory Standards, 2003.

Stricoff RS, Walters DB. Handbook of laboratory health and safety. New York: John Wiley & Sons, 1995.

Radioactivity

Gilmore G, Hemingway JD. Practical gamma-ray spectrometry. New York, John Wiley & Sons, 1st ed. 1995: 322 pp.

Knoll GF. Radiation detection and measurement. New York, John Wiley & Sons; 3rd ed. 1999: 802 pp.

L'Annunziata MF, Kessler MJ eds. Handbook of radioactivity analysis. San Diego: Academic Press; 1st ed. 1998: 771 pp.

Powsner RA, Powsner ER.: Essentials of nuclear medicine physics. Malden, MA: Blackwell Science Inc, 1998: 199 pp.

Ross H, Noakes JE, Spaulding JD. Liquid scintillation counting and organic scintillators. New York: Lewis Publishers, Inc., 1991: 752 pp.

Shackett, P, Shackett P. Nuclear medicine technology: Procedures and quick reference. Philadelphia: Lippincott Williams & Wilkins, 2000: 473 pp.

Units and Terminology

Burtis CA, Geary TD. Glossary of bioanalytical nomenclature. Pure Appl Chem 1994; 66:2587-2604.

Inczedy J, Lengyel T, Ure AM: The Orange book: Compendium of analytical nomenclature, 3rd ed. London: http://www.iupac.org/publications/books/order.htmlBlackwell Science, 1998.

McNaught AD, Wilkinson A. The Gold book: Compendium of chemical terminology, 2nd ed. London: http://www.iupac.org/publications/books/order.htmlBlackwell Science, 1997.

Rigg JC, Brown SS, Dybkaer R, Olesen H eds. The Silver Book: Compendium of terminology and nomenclature of properties in clinical laboratory sciences (recommendations 1995). London: Blackwell Science, 1995.

Young DS, Huth EJ. SI units for clinical measurements. Philadelphia: American College of Physicians, 1997.

CHAPTER 2

Specimen Collection and Processing

Donald S. Young, M.B., Ph.D.,
Edward W. Bermes, Jr., Ph.D.,
and Doris M. Haverstick, Ph.D.

In this chapter, we discuss proper specimen collection techniques, processing, and storage of common sample types and the aspects of these activities that affect test values and their interpretation.

SPECIMEN COLLECTION

Many errors can occur during the collection, processing, and transport of biological specimens. Minimizing these errors will result in more reliable information for use by healthcare professionals. Examples of biological specimens that are analyzed in clinical laboratories include whole blood; serum; plasma; urine; feces; saliva; spinal, synovial, amniotic, pleural, pericardial, and ascitic fluids; and various types of solid tissue. The National Committee for Clinical Laboratory Standards (NCCLS) has published several procedures for collecting many of these specimens under standardized conditions.[9-12,14] In addition, the NCCLS has published documents related to sample collection and analysis for specialized tests, such as sweat chloride (see also Chapter 27).

BLOOD

Blood for analysis may be obtained from veins, arteries, or capillaries. Venous blood is usually the specimen of choice, and *venipuncture* is the method for obtaining this specimen.[12] In young children and for many point-of-care tests, *skin puncture* is frequently used to obtain what is mostly capillary blood; *arterial puncture* is used mainly for blood gas analyses.

Venipuncture

In the clinical laboratory, venipuncture is defined as all of the steps involved in obtaining an appropriate identified blood specimen from a patient's vein.[12]

Preliminary Steps

Before any specimen is collected, the phlebotomist must confirm the identity of the patient. (See Chapter 11 for discussion of techniques used for identification.) This entails the patient stating his or her name and the phlebotomist verifying information on the patient's wrist band, if the patient is hospitalized. If the patient is an outpatient, the phlebotomist must ask the patient to state his or her name and confirming information on the test requisition form with identifying information provided by the patient. At least three items of identification should be used (e.g., name, medical record number, date of birth, room location if the patient is hospitalized or address if the patient is an outpatient). In specialized situations, such as tests for alcohol or other tests of medicolegal importance, establishment of a chain of custody for the specimen may require additional patient identification, such as a photo. Before collection of a specimen, a phlebotomist should be properly dressed in personal protective equipment, such as an impervious gown and gloves. If the phlebotomist is to collect a specimen from a patient in isolation in a hospital, the phlebotomist should notify one of the patient's nurses that he or she is about to collect a blood specimen and must put on a clean gown and gloves and a face mask and goggles before entering the patient's room. The face mask limits the spread of potentially infectious droplets, and the goggles limit the possible entry of infectious material into the eye. The extent of the precautions required will vary with the nature of a patient's illness and the institution's policies and bloodborne pathogen plan (see Chapter 1), to which a phlebotomist must adhere. If airborne precautions are indicated, the phlebotomist must wear a N95 TB respirator.

If appropriate the phlebotomist should verify that the patient is fasting. The patient should be comfortably seated or supine, if sitting is not feasible, and should have been in this position for 20 minutes before the specimen is drawn. This standardization minimizes differences in concentrations of blood constituents caused by variations in blood volume (hemoconcentration or hemodilution). Either of the patient's arms should be extended in a straight line from the shoulder to the wrist. An arm with an inserted intravenous line should be avoided, as should an arm with extensive scarring or a hematoma at the intended collection site. If a woman has had a mastectomy, arm veins on that side of the body should not be used because the surgery may have caused lymphostasis, affecting the blood composition. If a woman has had double mastectomies, blood should be drawn from the arm of the side on which the first procedure was done. If the surgery was done within 6 months on both sides, a vein on the back of the hand or at the ankle should be used.

Before performing a venipuncture, the phlebotomist should estimate the volume of blood to be drawn and select the appropriate number and types of tubes for the blood, plasma, or serum tests requested. An appropriate needle must also be selected. The most commonly used sizes are gauges 19 to 22. The larger the gauge size is, the smaller the bore. The usual choice for an adult with normal veins is gauge 20; if veins tend to collapse easily, a size 21 is preferred. For volumes of blood from 30 to 50 mL, an 18-gauge needle may be required to ensure adequate blood flow. A needle is typically 1.5 inches (3.7 cm) long, but 1-inch (2.5-cm) needles are also used. All needles must be sterile, sharp, and without barbs. If blood is drawn for trace element measurements, the needle should be stainless steel and known to be free from contamination. For trace element determinations, all apparatus coming in contact with the specimen should be acid washed or known to be free of trace metal contamination (see Chapter 30).

Location

The median cubital vein in the antecubital fossa, or crook of the elbow, is the preferred site for collecting venous blood in adults because the vein is both large and close to the surface of the skin. Veins on the back of the hand or at the ankle may be used, although these are less desirable and should be avoided in diabetics and other individuals with poor circulation. It is appropriate to collect blood through a cannula that is being inserted for long-term fluid infusions at the time of first insertion to avoid a second stick. In severely ill individuals or those requiring many intravenous injections, an alternative blood-drawing site should be chosen. Selection of a vein for puncture is facilitated by palpation. An arm containing a cannula or arteriovenous fistula should not be used without consent of the patient's physician. If fluid is being infused intravenously into a limb, the fluid should be shut off for 3 minutes before a specimen is obtained and a suitable note made in the patient's chart and on the result report form. Specimens obtained from the opposite arm or below the infusion site in the same arm may be satisfactory for most tests except for those analytes that are contained in the infused solutions (e.g., glucose or electrolytes).[16]

Preparation of Site

The area around the intended puncture site should be cleaned with a prepackaged alcohol swab or with a gauze pad saturated with 70% isopropanol. Cleaning of the puncture site should be done with a circular motion and from the site outward. The skin should be allowed to dry in the air. No alcohol should remain on the skin, because traces may cause hemolysis and invalidate test results. When specimens are to be collected for ethanol determinations, the skin should be cleaned with a benzalkonium chloride solution (Zephiran Chloride solution, 1:750) that is free of alcohol. Povidone-iodine should be avoided as a cleaning agent because it may interfere with several chemistry procedures. Once the skin has been cleaned, it should not be touched until after the venipuncture has been completed.

Timing

The time at which a specimen is obtained is important for those blood constituents that undergo marked diurnal variation (e.g., corticosteroids and iron) and for those used to monitor drug therapy (see Chapter 33). Furthermore, timing is important in relation to specimens for alcohol or drug measurements in association with medicolegal considerations.

Venous Occlusion

After the skin is cleaned, either a blood pressure cuff or a tourniquet is applied 4 to 6 inches (10 to 15 cm) above the intended puncture site. This obstructs the return of venous blood to the heart and distends the veins. When a blood pressure cuff is used as a tourniquet, it is usually inflated to approximately 60 mm Hg (8.0 kPa). Tourniquets are typically made from precut soft rubber strips or from Velcro type of bands. It is rarely necessary to leave a tourniquet in place for longer than 1 minute, but even within this short time the composition of blood changes. Although the changes that occur in 1 minute are slight, marked changes have been observed after 3 minutes (Table 2-1).

The composition of blood drawn first—that is, the blood closest to the tourniquet—is most representative of the composition of circulating blood. The first-drawn specimen should therefore be used for those analytes such as calcium that are pertinent to critical medical decisions. Blood drawn later shows a greater effect from venous stasis. Thus the first tube may show a 5% increase of protein, whereas the third

TABLE 2-1 Changes in Composition of Serum When Venous Occlusion Is Prolonged from 1 Minute to 3 Minutes*

Increase	%	Decrease	%
Total protein	4.9	Potassium	6.2
Iron	6.7		
Total lipids	4.7		
Cholesterol	5.1		
Aspartate aminotransferase	9.3		
Bilirubin	8.4		

From Statland BE, Bokelund H, Winkel P: Factors contributing to intraindividual variation of serum constituents: 4. Effects of posture and tourniquet application on variation of serum constituents in healthy subjects. Clin Chem. 1974;20:1513-19.
Mean values obtained from 11 healthy individuals
*To estimate the probable effect of a factor on results, relate percent increase or decrease shown (or intimated) in table to analytical variation (± % CV) routinely found for analytes.

tube may show a 10% change.[8] The concentration of protein-bound constituents is also influenced by stasis. Prolonged stasis may increase the concentration of protein or protein-bound constituents by as much as 15%. A uniform procedure for order of draw for tests should therefore be established (see below). If it is possible to collect only a small volume of blood, the priority of which tests to perform should be established.

The increase in activity of creatine kinase and aspartate aminotransferase in serum seen after venipuncture may be caused by hemoconcentration, by the slight trauma to tissue as the needle pierces the skin, and by stasis of blood in the tissue.

Pumping of the fist before venipuncture should be avoided because it causes an increase in the plasma potassium, phosphate, and lactate concentrations. The lowering of the blood pH by accumulation of lactate causes the plasma ionized calcium concentration to increase. The ionized calcium concentration reverts to normal 10 minutes after the tourniquet is released.

Stress associated with blood collection can have effects in patients at any age. As a consequence, plasma concentrations of cortisol and growth hormone may increase. Stress occurs particularly in young children who are frightened, struggling, and held in physical restraint. Collection under these conditions may cause adrenal stimulation leading to an increased plasma glucose concentration or create increases in the serum activities of enzymes that originate in skeletal muscle.

Collection with Evacuated Blood Tube

Evacuated blood tubes are usually considered to be less expensive and more convenient and easier to use than syringes. There are several types of evacuated tubes used for venipuncture collection. They vary by the type of additive added and volume of the tube. The different types are identified by the color of the stopper used (Table 2-2). Some glass tubes are siliconized to reduce adhesion of clots to walls or stoppers and to decrease risk of hemolysis. Blood collected into a tube containing one additive should never be transferred into other tubes, because the first additive may interfere with tests for which a different additive is specified. Thrombin is added to some tubes to accelerate clotting. However, the silicone-coated wall may also activate and accelerate the clotting mechanism.

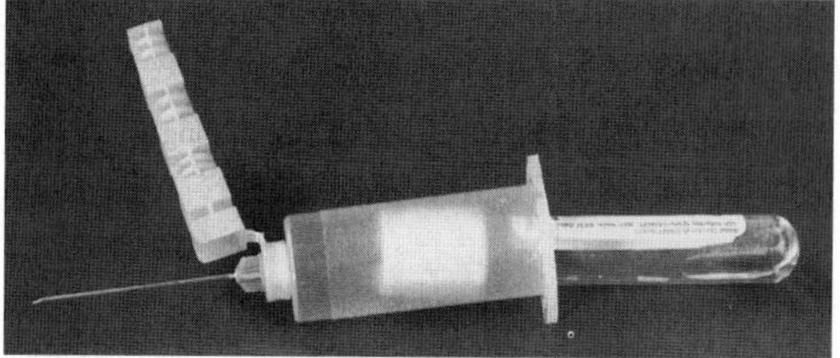

Figure 2-1 Assembled venipuncture set. *(From Flynn, JC: Procedures in Phlebotomy. 3rd ed. Saunders, St Louis, 2005, p 84.)*

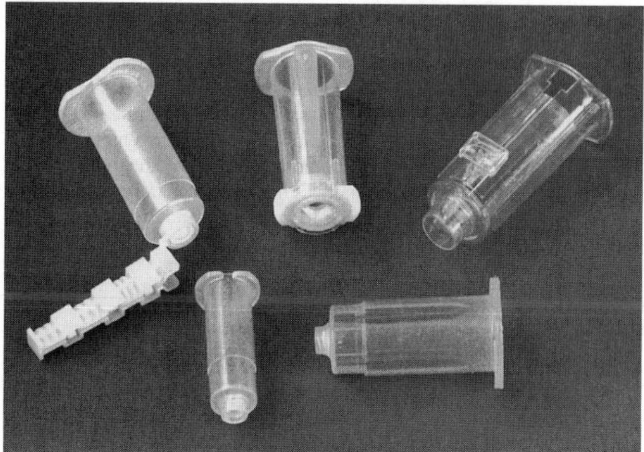

Figure 2-2 Various tube holders used in venipuncture. *(From Flynn, JC: Procedures in Phlebotomy. 2nd ed. W. B. Saunders, Philadelphia, 1999, p79.)*

A typical system for collecting blood in evacuated tubes is shown in Figure 2-1. This is an example of a recently introduced single-use device that incorporates a cover that can be safely placed over the needle when sample collection is complete. A needle is screwed into the collection tube holder (Figure 2-2), and the tube is then gently inserted into this holder. Before use, the tube should be gently tapped to dislodge any additive from the stopper before the needle is inserted into a vein; this prevents aspiration of the additive into the patient's vein. Both single-draw and multidraw needles are available.

After the skin is cleaned, the needle should be guided gently into the patient's vein (Figure 2-3); once the needle is in place, the tube should be pressed forward into the holder

TABLE 2-2 Coding of Stopper Color to Indicate Additive in Evacuated Blood Tube

Tube Type	Additive	Stopper Color	Alternative
Gel separation tubes	Polymer gel/silica activator	Red/black	Gold
	Polymer gel/silica activator/lithium heparin	Green/gray	Light gray
Serum tubes (nonadditive)	Silicone-coated interior	Red	Red
	Uncoated interior	Red	Pink
Serum tubes (with additives)	Thrombin (dry additive)	Gray/yellow	Orange
	Particulate clot activator	Yellow/red	Red
	Thrombin (dry additive)	Light blue	Light blue
Whole blood/plasma tubes	K_2EDTA (dry additive)	Lavender	Lavender
	K_3EDTA (liquid additive)		
	Na_2EDTA (dry additive)		
	Citrate, trisodium (coagulation)	Light blue	Light blue
	Citrate, trisodium (erythrocyte sedimentation rate)	Black	Black
	Sodium fluoride (antiglycolic agent)	Gray	Light (lt) gray
	Heparin, lithium (dry or liquid additive)	Green	Green
	Potassium oxalate	Light gray	Light gray
	Lithium iodoacetate	Light gray	Light gray
Special chemistry tubes			
Lead	Heparin, sodium (liquid additive)	Brown	Brown
	Heparin, sodium (dry additive)	Royal blue	Royal blue
Trace elements	Silicone-coated interior (serum tube)	Royal blue	Royal blue
Stat chemistry	Thrombin	Gray/yellow	Orange
Plasma preparation tube*	K_2EDTA (dry additive)/polymer gel/silica activator	Opalescent white	Opalescent white

Modified from the National Committee for Clinical Laboratory Standards: Evacuated Tubes and Additives for Blood Specimen Collection: Approved Standard H1-A4. 4th ed. Wayne PA:National Committee for Clinical Laboratory Standards, 1996 and information listed in the Becton Dickinson Web page (http://www.bd.com/).

*The Plasma Preparation Tube™ (Becton Dickinson, Franklin Lakes, New Jersey) is a plastic evacuated tube used for the collection of venous blood that upon centrifugation separates undiluted plasma for use in molecular diagnostic test methods.

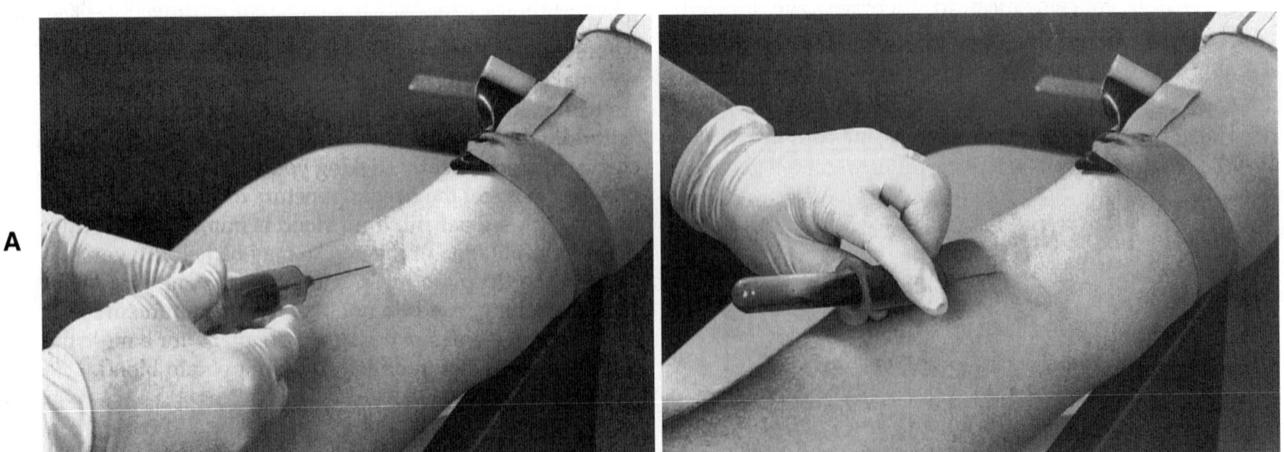

Figure 2-3 Venipuncture. *(From Flynn, JC: Procedures in Phlebotomy. 2nd ed. W. B. Saunders, Philadelphia, 1999, p94.)*

to puncture the stopper and release the vacuum. When blood begins to flow into the tube, the tourniquet should be released without moving the needle. The tube is filled until the vacuum is exhausted, and the tube can then be withdrawn from the holder and replaced by another tube, if this is necessary. Other tubes may be filled if required using the same technique with the holder in place. When several tubes are required from a single blood collection, a shut-off valve—consisting of rubber tubing that slides over the needle opening inside the tube—is used to prevent spillage of blood during exchange of tubes.

Serum separator tubes are available (Table 2-2) that contain an inert, thixotropic, polymer gel material with a specific gravity of approximately 1.04.[5] Aspiration of blood into the tube and subsequent centrifugation displace the gel, which settles like a disk between cells and supernatant when the tube is centrifuged. Relative centrifugal force (RCF) must be at least 1100 ×g for gel release and barrier formation. Release of intracellular components into the supernatant is prevented by the barrier for several hours or, in some cases, for a few days. These separator tubes may be used as primary containers from which serum can be directly aspirated by a number of analytical instruments.

Evacuated blood tubes may be made of soda-lime or borosilicate glass or plastic (polyethylene terephthalate). Because of the decreased likelihood of breakage and hence exposure to infectious materials, many laboratories have converted from glass tubes to plastic tubes. Tubes made from the soda-lime glass may release trace elements, particularly calcium and magnesium, into solutions. Special tubes are available for trace element determination (Table 2-2).

Stoppers may contain zinc, invalidating the use of evacuated blood tubes for zinc measurement, and TBEP (tris[2-butoxyethyl] phosphate), a constituent of rubber, which may interfere with the measurement of certain drugs. With time, the vacuum in evacuated tubes is lost and their effective draw diminishes. The silicone coating also decays with age. Therefore the stock of these tubes should be rotated and careful attention paid to the expiration date. Problems with evacuated blood tubes also arise when too little blood is collected into the tubes (short draw). Although an incorrect draw is of little consequence when clotted blood is required, a disproportionate ratio of blood to anticoagulant may affect some hematology and other special tests. Therefore some tubes from each batch should be checked for volume of draw before the lot is put in use.

In a few patients, backflow from blood tubes into veins occurs owing to a decrease in venous pressure. The dangerous consequences of this occurrence may be prevented if only sterile tubes are used for collection of blood. Backflow is minimized if the arm is held downward and blood is kept from contact with the stopper during the collection procedure. To minimize problems if backflow should occur and to optimize the quality of specimens—especially to prevent cross contamination with anticoagulants—blood should be collected into tubes in the following order: (1) blood cultures, (2) nonadditive tubes (red stopper), (3) coagulation- or citrate-containing tube (blue stopper), (4) serum separator tube containing gel (red stopper with black flecks), (5) heparin-containing tube (green stopper), (6) EDTA-containing tube (lavender stopper) and oxalate-fluoride–containing tube (gray stopper).

Blood Collection with Syringe

Syringes are customarily used for patients with difficult veins. If a syringe is used, the needle is placed firmly over the nozzle of the syringe and the cover of the needle is removed. If the syringe has an eccentric nozzle, the needle should be arranged with the nozzle downward but the bevel of the needle upward. The syringe and needle should be aligned with the vein to be entered and the needle pushed into the vein at an angle to the skin of approximately 15° (Figure 2-3). When the initial resistance of the vein wall is overcome as it is pierced, forward pressure on the syringe is eased, and the blood is withdrawn by gently pulling back the plunger of the syringe. Should a second syringe be necessary, a gauze pad may be placed under the hub of the needle to absorb the spill; the first syringe is then quickly disconnected and the second put in place to continue the draw. After removal of the needle from the syringe, drawn blood should be quickly transferred by gentle ejection into tubes prepared for its receipt. The tubes should then be capped if they contain an additive or anticoagulant, and then gently mixed (5 to 10 inversions).

Vigorous suction on a syringe during collection or forceful transfer from the syringe to the receiving vessel may cause hemolysis of blood. Hemolysis is usually less when blood is drawn through a small-bore needle because turbulence of the blood is less than when a larger-bore needle is used.

Completion of Collection

When blood collection is complete and the needle withdrawn, the patient is instructed to hold a dry gauze pad over the puncture site, with the arm raised to lessen the likelihood of leakage of blood. The pad can subsequently be held in place by a bandage, which can be removed after 15 minutes. The phlebotomist must separate the needle from the syringe or collection tube and discard it into a sharps container. On completion of the collection, the phlebotomist must dispose of his or her gloves in a hazardous waste receptacle before proceeding to the next patient.

Venipuncture in Children

The techniques for venipuncture in children and adults are similar. However, children are likely to make unexpected movements, and assistance in holding them still is often desirable. Either a syringe or evacuated blood tube system may be used to collect specimens. A syringe should be either the tuberculin type or a 3-mL-capacity syringe, except when a large volume of blood is required for analysis. A 21- to 23-gauge needle or 20- to 23-gauge butterfly needle with attached tubing is appropriate to collect specimens.

Skin Puncture

Skin puncture is an open collection technique in which the skin is punctured by a lancet[10] and a small volume of blood collected into a microdevice, such as a capillary tube. In practice it is used in situations where (1) sample volume is limited (e.g., pediatric applications), (2) repeated venipunctures have resulted in severe vein damage, or (3) patients may have been burned or bandaged and veins are therefore unavailable for venipuncture. This technique is also commonly used when the sample is to be applied directly to a testing device in a point-of-care testing situation, such as whole blood glucose or hemoglobin testing. It is most often performed on the tip of a finger, on an earlobe, and on the heel or big toe of infants. For example, in an infant younger than 1 year of age, the lateral or medial plantar surface of the foot should be used for skin puncture; suitable areas are illustrated in Figure 2-4. In older children, the plantar surface of the big toe may also be used, although blood collection should be avoided on ambulatory patients from anywhere on the foot. The proper procedure for collecting blood from infants is described in the NCCLS standard H4-A4.[10]

To collect a blood specimen by a skin puncture, the phlebotomist first thoroughly cleans the skin with a gauze pad saturated with 70% isopropanol. All alcohol must be allowed to evaporate from the skin so that hemolysis does not occur. When the skin is dry, it is quickly punctured by a sharp stab with a lancet. The depth of the incision should be less than 2.5 mm to avoid contact with bone.[1] To minimize the possibility of infection, a different site should be selected for each finger puncture. The finger should be held in such a way that gravity assists the collection of blood on the finger tip. Massage of the finger to stimulate blood flow should be avoided, because it causes the outflow of debris and of tissue fluid, which does not have the same composition as plasma. To improve circulation of the blood, the finger may be warmed by application of a warm, wet washcloth for 3 minutes before pricking. The first drop of blood is wiped off, and subsequent drops are transferred to the appropriate collection tube by gentle contact. Filling should be done rapidly to prevent clotting, and introduction of air bubbles should be avoided.

Blood may be collected into capillary blood tubes by capillary action. A variety of collection tubes is commercially available (Figure 2-5). Such containers can be purchased with different anticoagulants, such as sodium and ammonium heparin, and some can be obtained in brown glass for collection of light-sensitive analytes, such as bilirubin. There are also many small plastic or glass tubes that can be used to collect blood. A disadvantage of some of the collection devices shown in Figure 2-5 is that blood tends to pool in the mouth of the tube and must be flicked down the tube with a risk of hemolysis. Drop-by-drop collection should be avoided because it increases hemolysis.

For the collection of blood specimens on filter paper for neonatal screening and, increasingly, molecular genetics testing, the skin is cleaned and punctured as described previously. Then the filter paper is gently touched against a large drop of blood, which is allowed to soak into the paper to fill the marked circle. Only a single application per circle should be made. The paper is examined to verify that there has been complete penetration of the paper. The procedure is repeated to fill all the circles. Avoid milking or squeezing of the foot, because this procedure contributes tissue fluids. The filter papers should be air dried. Blood should not be transferred onto filter paper after it has been collected in capillary tubes because partial clotting may have occurred.

Arterial Puncture

Arterial puncture requires considerable skill and is usually performed only by physicians or specially trained technicians or nurses. The preferred sites of arterial puncture are, in order, the (1) radial artery at the wrist, (2) brachial artery in the elbow, and (3) femoral artery in the groin. Because leakage of blood from the femoral artery tends to be greater, especially in the elderly, sites in the arm are most often used. The proper technique for arterial puncture is described in NCCLS Standard H11-A3.[11]

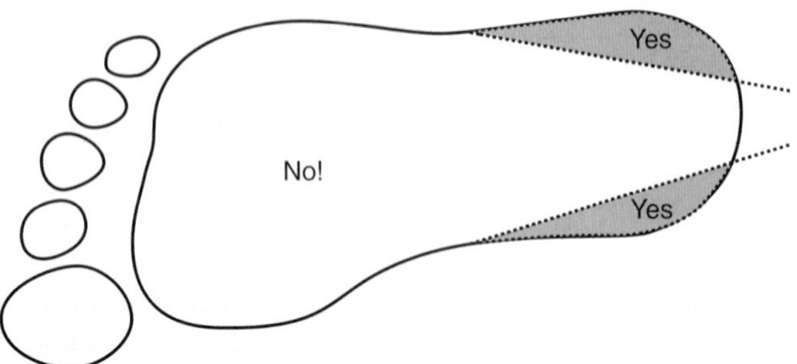

Figure 2-4 Acceptable sites for skin puncture to collect blood from an infant's foot. *(Modified from Blumenfeld TA, Turi GK, Blanc WA. Recommended site and depth of newborn heel punctures based on anatomical measurements and histopathology. Reprinted with permission from Elsevier [The Lancet 1979, 1, 230-233].)*

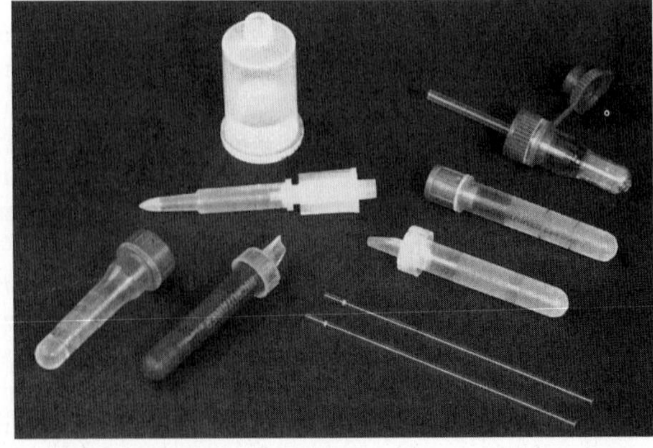

Figure 2-5 Microcollection tubes. *(From Flynn, JC: Procedures in Phlebotomy. 3rd ed. Saunders, St Louis, 2005, p 78.)*

In the neonate, an indwelling catheter in the umbilical artery is best to obtain specimens for blood gas analysis. In the older child or adult in whom it is impossible to perform an arterial puncture, a capillary puncture may be performed to obtain *arterialized capillary blood.* Such a specimen yields acceptable values for pH and PCO_2, but not always for PO_2. In the older child or adult, the preferred puncture site is the earlobe; in the young child or infant, it is the heel. Capillary blood specimens are particularly inappropriate when the blood circulation is poor and thus should be avoided when a patient has reduced cardiac output, hypotension, or vasoconstriction. For each capillary puncture, the skin should first be warmed with a hot, moist towel to improve the circulation. The puncture itself should be performed as described previously; a free flow of blood is essential. Heparinized capillary tubes containing a small metal bar are used to collect the blood. Tubes should be sealed quickly and the contents mixed well by using a magnet to move the metal bar up and down in the tube so that a uniform specimen is available for analysis.

Anticoagulants and Preservatives for Blood

Serum is the specimen of choice for many assay systems. Sometimes considerable differences may be observed between the concentrations of analytes in serum and plasma as shown in Table 2-3.[4] However, some assay systems require a whole blood or plasma specimen. If so an anticoagulant must be added to the specimen during the collection procedure. A number of anticoagulants are used including heparin, EDTA, sodium fluoride, citrate, oxalate, and iodoacetate.

Heparin

Heparin is the most widely used anticoagulant and causes the least interference with tests,[7] except for tests performed using polymerase chain reaction (PCR). It is a mucoitin polysulfuric acid and is available as sodium, potassium, lithium, and ammonium salts. This anticoagulant accelerates the action of antithrombin III, which neutralizes thrombin and thus prevents the formation of fibrin from fibrinogen. Most blood tubes are prepared with approximately 0.2 mg heparin for each milliliter of blood (1000 units/mL) to be collected. The heparin is usually present as a dry powder that is hygroscopic and dissolves rapidly.

Heparin has the disadvantage of high cost and temporary action, and it produces a blue background in blood smears that are stained with Wright's stain. In addition, heparin is said to inhibit acid phosphatase activity and to interfere with the binding of calcium to EDTA in analytical methods for calcium involving complexing with EDTA. It has also been reported to affect the binding of triiodothyronine and thyroxine to their carrier proteins, thus producing higher free concentrations of these hormones.

EDTA

EDTA is a chelating agent that is particularly useful for hematological examinations because it preserves the cellular components of blood. It is used as the disodium, dipotassium, or tripotassium salt, the last two being more soluble. It is effective at a final concentration of 1 to 2 g/L of blood. Higher concentrations hypertonically shrink the red cells. EDTA prevents coagulation by binding calcium, which is essential for the clotting mechanism. Blood collection tubes are prepared by adding a 0.1% solution of an EDTA salt followed by evaporation of water at room temperature.

EDTA, probably by chelation of metallic cofactors, inhibits alkaline phosphatase, creatine kinase, and leucine aminopeptidase activities. Because it chelates calcium and iron, EDTA is unsuitable for specimens for calcium and iron analyses using photometric or titrimetric techniques. As an

TABLE 2-3 Differences in Composition Between Plasma and Serum*

Plasma Value Greater Than Serum Value (%)		No Difference Between Serum and Plasma Values	Plasma Value Less Than Serum Value (%)	
Calcium	0.9	Bilirubin	Albumin	1.3
Chloride	0.2	Cholesterol	Alkaline phosphatase	1.6
Lactate dehydrogenase	2.7	Creatinine	Aspartate aminotransferase	0.9
Total protein	4.0		Bicarbonate	1.8
			Creatine kinase	2.1
			Glucose	5.1
			Phosphorus	7.0
			Potassium	8.4
			Sodium	0.1
			Urea	0.6
			Uric acid	0.2

From Ladenson JH, Tsai L-MB, Michael JM, et al: Serum versus heparinized plasma for eighteen common chemistry tests. Am J Clin Pathol 1974;62:545-52. Copyright 1974 by the American Society of Clinical Pathologists. Reprinted with permission.

*To estimate the probable effect of a factor on results, relate percent increase or decrease shown (or intimated) in table to analytical variation (±% CV) routinely found for analytes.

TABLE 2-4 Difference in Composition of Capillary and Venous Serum*

Capillary Value Greater Than Venous Value (%)	No Difference Between Capillary and Venous Values	Capillary Value Less Than Venous Value (%)
Glucose 1.4	Phosphate	Bilirubin 5.0
Potassium 0.9	Urea	Calcium 4.6
		Chloride 1.8
		Sodium 2.3
		Total protein 3.3

From Kupke IR, Kather B, Zeugner S: On the composition of capillary and venous blood serum. Clin Chim Acta 1981;112:177-85.
*To estimate the probable effect of a factor on results, relate percent increase or decrease shown (or intimated) in table to analytical variation (±% CV) routinely found for analytes.

anticoagulant, it has little effect on other clinical tests although the concentration of cholesterol has been reported to be decreased by 3% to 5%.

Sodium Fluoride

Sodium fluoride is a weak anticoagulant but is often added as a preservative for blood glucose. As a preservative, together with another anticoagulant such as potassium oxalate, it is effective at a concentration of approximately 2 g/L blood. It exerts its preservative action by inhibiting the enzyme systems involved in glycolysis. Most specimens are preserved at 25 °C for 24 hours or at 4 °C for 48 hours. Without an antiglycolytic agent, the blood glucose concentration decreases approximately 100 mg/L (0.56 mmol/L) per hour at 25 °C. The rate of decrease is faster in newborns because of the increased metabolic activity of their erythrocytes and in leukemic patients because of the high metabolic activity of the white cells. Sodium fluoride is poorly soluble, and blood must be well mixed before effective antiglycolysis occurs.

When sodium fluoride is used alone for anticoagulation, three to five times greater concentrations than the usual 2 g/L are required. This high concentration and the inhibition of the glycolytic cycle are likely to cause fluid shifts and a change in the concentration of some analytes. Fluoride is also a potent inhibitor of many serum enzymes and in high concentrations also affects urease, used to measure urea nitrogen in many analytical systems.

Citrate

Sodium citrate solution, at a concentration of 34 to 38 g/L in a ratio of 1 part to 9 parts of blood, is widely used for coagulation studies because the effect is easily reversible by addition of Ca^{2+}. Because citrate chelates calcium, it is unsuitable as an anticoagulant for specimens for measurement of this element. It also inhibits aminotransferases and alkaline phosphatase but stimulates acid phosphatase when phenylphosphate is used as a substrate. Because citrate complexes molybdate, it decreases the color yield in phosphate measurements that involve molybdate ions and produces low results.

Oxalates

Sodium, potassium, ammonium, and lithium oxalates inhibit blood coagulation by forming rather insoluble complexes with calcium ions. Potassium oxalate ($K_2C_2O_4 \cdot H_2O$), at a concentration of approximately 1 to 2 g/L of blood, is the most widely used oxalate. At concentrations of greater than 3 g oxalate per liter hemolysis is likely to occur.

Combined ammonium and/or potassium oxalate does not cause shrinkage of erythrocytes. However, other oxalates can cause shrinkage by drawing water into the plasma. Reduction in hematocrit may be as much as 10%, causing a reduction in the concentration of plasma constituents of 5%. As fluid is lost from the cells, an exchange of electrolytes and other constituents across the cell membrane occurs. Oxalate inhibits several enzymes, including acid and alkaline phosphatases, amylase, and lactate dehydrogenase, and may cause precipitation of calcium as the oxalate salt.

Iodoacetate

Sodium iodoacetate at a concentration of 2 g/L is an effective antiglycolytic agent and a substitute for sodium fluoride. Because it has no effect on urease, it can be used when glucose and urea tests are performed on a single specimen. It inhibits creatine kinase but appears to have no notable effects on other clinical tests.

Influence of Site of Collection on Blood Composition

Blood obtained from different sites differs in composition. Skin puncture blood is more like arterial blood than venous blood. Thus there are no clinically significant differences between freely flowing capillary blood and arterial blood in pH, PCO_2, PO_2, and oxygen saturation. The PCO_2 of venous blood is up to 6 to 7 mm Hg (0.8-0.9 kPa) higher. Venous blood glucose is as much as 70 mg/L (0.39 mmol/L) less than the capillary blood glucose.

Blood obtained by skin puncture is contaminated to some extent with interstitial and intracellular fluids. The major differences between venous serum and capillary serum are illustrated in Table 2-4.

TABLE 2-5 Influence of Collection Site on Composition of Plasma*

	Arterial	Central Venous	Peripheral Venous
Alanine aminotransferase (U/L)	62	61	81
Albumin (g/L)	36	37	39
Alkaline phosphatase (U/L)	114	113	107
Amylase (U/L)	149	148	177
Aspartate aminotransferase (U/L)	20	20	21
Calcium (mg/L)	81	82	83
Chloride (mmol/L)	99	97	101
Creatine kinase (U/L)	82	73	91
Creatinine (mg/L)	14	13	12
γ-Glutamyltransferase (U/L)	13	14	14
Potassium (mmol/L)	4.0	3.9	3.8
Sodium (mmol/L)	144	145	144
Total protein (g/L)	66	68	77
Urea nitrogen (mg/L)	320	310	250
Uric acid (mg/L)	81	81	79

From Rommel, K., Koch, C-D., Spilker, D.: Einfluss der Materialgewinnung auf klinisch-chemische Parameter in Blut, Plasma und Serum bei Patienten mit stabilem und zentralisiertem Kreislauf. J. Clin. Chem. Clin. Biochem., *16*:373-80, 1978.

*To estimate the probable effect of a factor on results, relate percent increase or decrease shown (or intimated) in table to analytical variation (±% CV) routinely found for analytes.

Collection of Blood from Intravenous or Arterial Lines

When blood is collected from a central venous catheter or arterial line, it is necessary to ensure that the composition of the specimen is not affected by the fluid that is infused into the patient. The fluid is shut off using the stopcock on the catheter, and 10 mL of blood is aspirated through the stopcock and discarded before the specimen for analysis is withdrawn. Blood properly collected from a central venous catheter and compared with blood drawn from a peripheral vein at the same time shows notable differences in composition. A comparison of arterial blood with central and peripheral venous blood is illustrated in Table 2-5.

Blood may be collected from the veins of an arm below an intravenous line without interference from the fluid being infused, because retrograde blood flow does not occur in the veins, and the fluid that is infused must first circulate through the heart and return to the tissue before it reaches the sampling site.

Hemolysis

Hemolysis is defined as the disruption of the red cell membrane and results in the release of hemoglobin. Serum shows visual evidence of hemolysis when the hemoglobin concentration exceeds 200 mg/L. Slight hemolysis has little effect on most test values. Severe hemolysis causes a slight dilutional effect on those constituents present at a lower concentration in the erythrocytes than in plasma. However, a notable effect may be observed on those constituents that are present at a higher concentration in erythrocytes other than in plasma. Thus plasma activities or concentrations of aldolase, total acid phosphatase, lactate dehydrogenase, isocitrate dehydrogenase, potassium, magnesium, and phosphate are particularly increased by hemolysis. The inorganic phosphate in serum increases rapidly as the organic esters in the cells are hydrolyzed. Aspartate aminotransferase activity is increased by 2% for each 100 mg of hemoglobin per liter. One hundred milligrams hemoglobin per liter increases serum lactate dehydrogenase activity by 10% and serum potassium concentration by 0.6%. An additional band caused by hemoglobin may be observed on serum protein electrophoresis.

Although the amount of free hemoglobin could be measured and a calculation made to correct test values affected by hemoglobin,[2] this practice is undesirable because factors other than hemoglobin could contribute to the altered test values, and it would be impossible to assess their impact. Hemolysis may affect many unblanked or inadequately blanked analytical methods.[19]

URINE

The type of urine specimen to be collected is dictated by the tests to be performed. Untimed or random specimens are suitable for only a few chemical tests; usually, urine specimens must be collected over a predetermined interval of time, such as 1, 4, or 24 hours. A *clean, early morning, fasting specimen* is usually the most concentrated specimen and thus is preferred for microscopic examinations and for the detection of abnormal amounts of constituents, such as proteins, or of unusual compounds, such as chorionic gonadotropin. The *clean timed specimen* is one obtained at specific times of the day or during certain phases of the act of micturition. Bacterial examination of the first 10 mL of urine voided is most appropriate to detect urethritis, whereas the midstream specimen is best for investigating bladder disorders. The *double-voided specimen* is the urine excreted during a timed period after a complete emptying of the bladder; it is used, for example, to assess glucose excretion during a glucose tolerance test. Its collection must be timed in relation to the ingestion of glucose. Similarly, in some metabolic disorders, urine must be collected during or immediately after symptoms of the disease appear (see Chapter 32 on porphyrins).

When they are to be tested for their alcohol and drugs of abuse content, urine specimens are collected under rigorous conditions requiring chain of custody documentation. (See Chapter 34 for details of such a collection.)

Catheter specimens are used for microbiological examination in critically ill patients or in those with urinary tract obstruction but should not normally be obtained just for examination of chemical constituents. The *suprapubic tap specimen* is a useful alternative, because the tap is unlikely to cause infection. After appropriate cleaning of the skin over the full bladder, a 22-gauge spinal needle is passed through a small wheal made by a local anesthetic. The bladder is penetrated and the urine withdrawn into the syringe.

Even though tests in the clinical laboratory are not usually affected by lack of sterile collection procedures, the patient's genitalia should be cleaned before each voiding to minimize the transfer of surface bacteria to the urine. Cleansing is essential if the true concentration of white cells is to be obtained. Details of collection of urine specimens are contained in an NCCLS guideline.[14]

Timed Urine Specimens

The collection period for timed specimens should be long enough to minimize the influence of short-term biological variations. When specimens are to be collected over a specified period of time, the patient's close adherence to instructions is important. The bladder must be emptied at the time the collection is to begin, and this urine is discarded. Thereafter all urine must be collected until the end of the scheduled time. If a patient has a bowel movement during the collection period, precautions should be taken to prevent fecal contamination. If a collection has to be made over several hours, urine should be passed into a separate container at each voiding and then emptied into a larger container for the complete specimen. This two-step procedure prevents the danger of a patient's splashing himself or herself with a preservative, such as acid. The large container should be stored at 4 °C in a refrigerator during the entire collection period.

Before beginning a timed collection, a patient should be given written instructions with regard to diet or drug ingestion if appropriate to avoid interference of ingested compounds with analytical procedures. Thus instructions for collection of specimens for 5-hydroxyindoleacetic acid measurements should specify avoidance of avocados, bananas, plums, walnuts, pineapples, eggplant, acetaminophen, and cough syrups containing glyceryl guaiacolate (guaifenesin). The dietary components are sources of 5-hydroxytryptamine and should be avoided for this reason; the other compounds interfere with certain analytical procedures but may not interfere with highly specific analytical methods. The staff of each laboratory should determine its own requirements. See also specimen information for specific analytes in the respective chapters.

For 2-hour specimens, a prelabeled 1-L bottle is generally adequate. For a 12-hour collection, a 2-L bottle usually suffices; for a 24-hour collection, a 3- or 4-L bottle is appropriate for most patients. A single bottle allows adequate mixing of the specimen and prevents possible loss of some of the specimen if a second container does not reach the laboratory. Urine should not be collected at the same time for two or more tests requiring different preservatives. Aliquots for an analysis such as a microscopic examination should not be removed while a 24-hour collection is in process. Removal of aliquots is not permissible even when the volume removed is measured and corrected because the excretion of most compounds varies throughout the day, and test results will be affected. Appropriate information regarding the collection, including warnings with respect to handling of the specimen, should appear on the bottle label.

Collection of Urine from Children

Collection of a timed specimen from an infant is difficult, but fortunately such specimens are rarely required. The scrotal or perineal area is first cleaned and dried, and any natural or applied skin oils are removed. For an untimed specimen, a plastic bag (U-bag, Hollister Inc, Chicago IL; or Tink-Col, C.R. Bard, Inc, Murray Hill, NJ) is placed around the infant's genitalia and left in place until urine has been voided.

A metabolic bed is used to collect timed specimens from infants. The infant lies on a fine screen above a funnel-shaped base containing a drain under which a container is placed to receive urine. The fine screen retains fecal material. Nevertheless, the urine is likely to be contaminated, to some extent, by such material.

To obtain a sterile urine specimen for culture from an infant, a suprapubic tap is performed. The collection of specimens from older children is done as in adults, using assistance from a parent when this is necessary.

Urine Preservatives

The most common preservatives and the tests for which the preservatives are required are listed in Table 2-6. Preservatives have different roles but are usually added to reduce bacterial action or chemical decomposition or to solubilize constituents that might otherwise precipitate out of solution. Another application is to decrease atmospheric oxidation of unstable compounds. Some specimens should not have *any* preservatives added because of the possibility of interference with analytical methods.

One of the most acceptable forms of preservation of urine specimens is *refrigeration* immediately after collection; it is even more successful when combined with chemical preservation. Urinary preservative tablets that contain a mixture of

TABLE 2-6 Commonly Used Urine Preservatives

Analyte	None	Freeze	Glacial Acetic Acid	Boric Acid	Concentrated Hydrochloric Acid	Mild Base (pH 8-9)	Petroleum Ether	Nitric Acid
Aldosterone			X	X				
Amino acids					X			
5-Aminolevulinic acid			X			X		
Calcium					X			
Catecholamines			X		X			
Citrate				X				
Copper	X				X			
Cortisol (free)	X		X	X				
Cystine		X		X				
Estrogens			X	X				
hCG	X			X				
Homogentisic acid	X							
Homovanillic acid			X	X	X			
5-Hydroxyindoleacetic acid				X	X			
Hydroxyproline					X			
17-Ketosteroids			X	X				
Magnesium	X				X			
Mercury	X				X			X
Metanephrines			X		X			
Nitrogen	X				X			
Osmolality	X	X						
Oxalate	X				X			
Porphyrins						X		
Pregnanetriol			X	X				
Uric acid						X		
Urobilinogen	X	X					X	
Vanillylmandelic acid				X	X			
Zinc	X				X			

hCG, Human chorionic gonadotropin.

chemicals, such as potassium acid phosphate, sodium benzoate, benzoic acid, hexamethylene tetramine, sodium bicarbonate, and mercuric oxide (Starplex Scientific, Inc, www.starplexscientific.com), have been used for chemical and microscopic examination. Because these tablets contain sodium and potassium salts among others, they should not be used for analysis of these analytes. The preservative tablets act mainly by lowering the pH of the urine and by releasing formaldehyde. *Formalin* has also been used for preserving specimens, but in large amounts it precipitates urea and inhibits certain reactions (e.g., the dipstick esterase test for leukocytes). Acidification to below pH 3 is widely used to preserve 24-hour specimens and is particularly useful for specimens for calcium, steroids, and vanillylmandelic acid (VMA) determinations (10 mL HCl, 6 mol/L, per 24-hour excretion). However, precipitation of urates will occur, thereby rendering a specimen unsuitable for measurement of uric acid.

Sulfamic acid (10 g/L urine) has also been used to reduce pH. *Boric acid* (5 mg/30 mL) has been used, but it too causes precipitation of urates. Although *thymol* and *chloroform* were widely used in the past to preserve specimens for chemical and microscopic urinalysis, it is now recognized that specimens for these tests should be analyzed immediately, and that the addition of preservatives is both largely ineffective and a source of interference with several analytical methods. *Toluene* is the only organic solvent that is still used as a preservative. When present in a large enough amount, it acts as a barrier between the air and the surface of the specimen. Toluene, however, does not prevent the growth of anaerobic microorganisms and, because of its flammable nature, is a safety hazard. A mild base, such as *sodium bicarbonate* or a small amount of sodium hydroxide (NaOH), is used to preserve porphyrins, urobilinogen, and uric acid. A sufficient quantity should be added to adjust the pH to between 8 and 9.

When a timed collection is complete, the specimen should be delivered without delay to the clinical laboratory, where the volume should be measured. This may be done by using graduated cylinders or by weighing the container and urine when preweighed or uniform containers are used. The mass in grams may be reported as if it were the volume in milliliters. There is rarely a need to measure the specific gravity of a weighed specimen because errors in analysis usually exceed the error arising from failure to correct the volume of urine for its mass. Nevertheless, it is relatively easy to apply a simple mathematical correction based on an average specific gravity or to measure the specific gravity and to derive a correct volume for each specimen.

Before a specimen is transferred into small containers for each of the ordered tests, it must be thoroughly mixed to ensure homogeneity because the specific gravity, volume, and composition of the urine may all vary throughout the collection period. The small container into which an aliquot is transferred should not be a plastic bottle if toluene or another organic compound has been used as a preservative; metal-free containers must be used for trace metal analyses.

Feces

Small aliquots of feces are frequently analyzed to detect the presence of "hidden" blood, so-called *occult blood,* which is recognized as one of the most effective clues to the presence of a bleeding ulcer or malignant disease in the gastrointestinal tract. The utility of screening for occult blood is that it is included as part of many periodic health examinations. Tests for occult blood should be done on aliquots of excreted stools rather than on material obtained on the glove of a physician doing a rectal examination, because this procedure may cause enough bleeding to produce a positive result. In other instances, the small amount of stool present on the glove may not be representative of the whole, so that bleeding may not be recognized. Patients have even been encouraged to recover, by means of a spatula, small parts of feces that have been excreted into a toilet bowl and apply them directly to the reagent-impregnated slides used for the detection of blood. These specimens are then mailed or delivered to a laboratory for analysis (see also Chapter 48).

Feces from children may be screened for tryptic activity to detect cystic fibrosis. In the infant, fecal material for these tests is usually recovered from the child's diaper. See Chapter 21 for a discussion of the measurement of trypsin in feces.

In adults, measurement of fecal nitrogen and fat in 72-hour specimens is used to assess the severity of malabsorption; measurement of fecal porphyrins is occasionally required to characterize the type of porphyria (see Chapter 32).Usually, no preservative is added to the feces, but the container should be kept refrigerated throughout the collection period and care should be taken to prevent contamination from urine. When the collection is complete, the container and feces are weighed, and the mass of excreted feces is calculated. The specimen is homogenized and aliquotted so that the amount of fat or nitrogen excreted per day and the proportion of dietary intake excreted can be calculated.

For metabolic balance studies, collections of stool are usually made over a 72-hour period. Many balance studies are carried out in conjunction with research on the metabolism of such elements as calcium. It is important for such studies that a patient be on a controlled diet for a sufficiently long time before the commencement of the study, so that a steady state has been attained.

Spinal Fluid

Spinal fluid is normally obtained from the lumbar region, although a physician may occasionally request analysis of fluid obtained during surgery from the cervical region or from a cistern or ventricle of the brain. Spinal fluid is examined when there is a question as to the presence of a cerebrovascular accident, meningitis, demyelinating disease, or meningeal involvement in malignant disease. Lumbar punctures should always be performed by a physician. The physician thoroughly cleans the skin of the lumbar region below the termination of the spinal cord where the cauda equina goes through the spinal canal. He or she makes a small bleb in the skin over the space between the third and fourth or fourth and fifth lumbar vertebrae with 2% procaine and then introduces a spinal needle (22-gauge, 3.5 inches [9 cm] long) through the bleb into the spinal canal. He or she measures the pressure with a manometer and then allows 3 to 4 mL of fluid to drip into plain tubes. The tubes should be sterile, especially if microbiological tests are required. Because the initial specimen may be contaminated by tissue debris or skin bacteria, the first tube should be used for chemical or serological tests, the second for microbiological tests, and the third for microscopic and cytological examination. The same procedure is used for infants and children, but the volume of fluid withdrawn should be the minimum for the requested tests.

Up to 20 mL of spinal fluid can be safely removed from an adult, although this amount is not usually required. Antiglycolytic agents usually are not added to the tube for glucose measurement; rapid processing of specimens, a clinical requirement for tests on spinal fluid, ensures that little metabolism of glucose occurs even in the presence of many bacteria. To allow proper interpretation of spinal fluid glucose values, a simultaneous blood specimen should be obtained.

Synovial Fluid

The technique of obtaining synovial fluid for examination is called *arthrocentesis.* Synovial fluid is withdrawn from joints to aid characterization of the type of arthritis and to differentiate noninflammatory effusions from inflammatory fluids. Normally, only a very small amount of fluid is present in any joint, but this volume is usually very much increased in the presence of inflammatory conditions. Arthrocentesis should be performed by a physician using sterile procedures, and the technique must be modified from joint to joint depending on the anatomical location and size of the joint. The skin over the joint is cleaned with an antiseptic, such as iodine, and then anesthetized with an agent like ethyl chloride. A needle of appropriate size is introduced into the joint and the required amount of fluid aspirated into the syringe. The physician should establish priorities for the tests to be performed in case the available volume is insufficient for all tests. Sterile plain tubes should be used for culture and for glucose and protein measurements; an EDTA tube is necessary for a total leukocyte, differential, and erythrocyte count. Microscopic slides are prepared for staining with Gram's or other stains indicated and for visual inspection.

Amniotic Fluid (Amniocentesis)

Amniocentesis is performed by a physician for prenatal diagnosis of congenital disorders, to assess fetal maturity, or to look for Rh isoimmunization or intrauterine infection. Although ultrasound is not essential, amniocentesis is best performed with its assistance to aid localization of the placenta and to determine the presentation of the fetus. The best sites for obtaining amniotic fluid are behind the neck of the fetus, below its head, or from other unoccupied areas of the amniotic cavity.

The skin is cleaned and anesthetized as for other similar procedures, and 10 mL of fluid is aspirated into a syringe connected to the spinal needle that is typically used. Sterile containers such as polypropylene test tubes or urine cups are used to transport the fluid to the laboratory. If a specimen is for the determination of the lecithin-sphingomyelin (L/S) ratio, the container is immediately placed in ice; if it is for spectrophotometric analysis, the specimen should be transferred to a brown tube or bottle to prevent photodegradation of bilirubin. Alternatively the specimen container may be wrapped in aluminum foil.

There are few complications from amniocentesis. Occasionally a bloody tap is made. The blood may come from the uterine wall, the placenta, or even the fetus. Determination of fetal hemoglobin can be used to help ascertain the source if it is important to do so.

Pleural, Pericardial, and Ascitic Fluids

The pleural, pericardial, and peritoneal cavities normally contain a small amount of serous fluid that lubricates the opposing parietal and visceral membrane surfaces. Inflammation or infections affecting the cavities cause fluid to accumulate. The fluid may be removed to determine if it is an effusion or an exudate, a distinction made possible by protein or enzyme analysis. The collection procedure is called *paracentesis.* When specifically applied to the pleural cavity, the procedure is a *thoracentesis;* if applied to the pericardial cavity, a *pericardiocentesis.* Paracenteses should be performed only by skilled and experienced physicians. Pericardiocentesis has now been largely supplanted by echocardiography.

The skin over the intended puncture site should be cleaned with 70% isopropanol and then allowed to dry in the air. A spinal needle is then inserted into the body cavity through a small bleb in the skin raised by injection of a local anesthetic. Fluid is then withdrawn by a syringe and transferred to appropriate tubes for analysis. Paracentesis is rarely associated with complications. Occasionally, blood-stained fluid is obtained because of puncture of a small blood vessel. If adhesions are present between the intestine and abdominal wall, a part of the intestine could be perforated by a peritoneal tap. With a thoracentesis, pneumothorax and bronchopleural fistulas are potential complications.

Saliva

Although measurements of concentrations of certain analytes in saliva have been advocated, the clinical application of methods using saliva has been limited. Exceptions are the measurement of blood group substances to determine secretor status and the genotype. Measurement of a drug in saliva (see Chapter 34) has been suggested to estimate the free, pharmacologically active concentration of the drug in serum. There is, however, a considerable difference in pH between saliva and serum, and ratios of bound-free drug would not be the same. Fortunately, ultrafiltration techniques are now available that facilitate the processing of serum for free drug analysis.

Several slightly different techniques have been devised for the collection of saliva. Usually an individual is asked to rinse out his or her mouth with water and then chew an inert material, such as a piece of rubber or paraffin wax, from 30 seconds to several minutes. The first mouthful of saliva is discarded; thereafter the saliva is collected into a small glass bottle.

Swabs

Although most commonly used for collection of specimens for microbiological testing, swabs are sometimes used to collect epithelial cells of the cheek for molecular genetics testing. A sterile Dacron or rayon swab with a plastic shaft is preferred because calcium alginate swabs or swabs with wooden sticks may contain substances that inhibit PCR-based testing. After collection, the swab may be stored in an air-tight plastic container or immersed in liquid, such as phosphate-buffered saline (PBS) or viral transport medium.

Solid Tissue

The solid tissue most often analyzed in the clinical laboratory is malignant tissue from the breast for estrogen and progesterone receptors. During surgery, at least 0.5 to 1 g tissue should be removed and trimmed of fat and nontumor material. The tissue should be quickly frozen, preferably in liquid nitrogen or in a mixture of dry ice and alcohol. The time between collection and freezing should be less than 20 minutes. A histological section should always be examined at the time of analysis of the specimen to confirm that the specimen is indeed malignant tissue. The same procedure may be used to obtain and prepare solid tissue for toxicological analysis; however, when trace element determinations are to be made, all materials used in the collection or handling of the tissue should be made of plastic or materials known to be free of contaminating trace elements (see also Chapter 30).

Hair and Finger Nails

Hair and finger or toe nails have been used for trace metal analyses. However, collection procedures have been poorly standardized, and quantitative measurements are better obtained on blood or urine. Hair specimens have also been analyzed for their drug content (see Chapter 34).

HANDLING OF SPECIMENS FOR TESTING

Maintenance of Specimen Identification

Valid test results require a representative, properly collected, and properly preserved specimen. Proper identification of the specimen must be maintained (see Chapter 11 for discussion on the use of bar codes to identify specimens). Every specimen container must be adequately labeled even if the specimen must be placed in ice or if the container is so small that a label cannot be placed along the tube, as might happen with a capillary blood tube. Direct labeling of a capillary blood tube by folding the label like a flag around the tube is preferred; a less satisfactory alternative is to label a larger container into which the capillary tube can be placed. For small volumes of urine submitted in a screw-cap urine cup and any specimen submitted in a screw-cap test tube or cup, the label should be placed on the cup or tube directly, not to the cap. The minimum information on a label should include a patient's name, location, identifying number, and the date and time of collection. All labels should conform to the laboratory's stated requirements to facilitate proper processing of specimens. No specific labeling should be attached on specimens from patients with infectious diseases to suggest that these specimens should be handled with special care. All specimens should be treated as if they are potentially infectious. However, labels suggesting special handling for other purposes are sometimes indicated.

Preservation of Specimens in Transit

Although delays of a specimen in transit from a patient in a hospital to the laboratory are usually short, the time elapsing from the separation of serum and cells until analysis may be considerable. The specimen must be properly treated both during its transport to the laboratory and from the time the serum has been separated until it is analyzed. For some tests, specimens must be kept at 4 °C from the time the blood is drawn until the specimens are analyzed, or until the serum or plasma is separated from the cells. Examples are specimens for ammonia and blood gas determinations, such as PCO_2, PO_2, and blood pH (see Chapter 27). Transfer of these specimens to the laboratory must be done by placing the specimen container in ice water. Specimens for acid phosphatase, lactate and pyruvate, and certain hormone tests (e.g., gastrin and renin activity) should be treated the same way. A notable decrease in pyruvate and increase in lactate concentration occurs within a few minutes at ambient temperature (see Chapter 25).

For all test constituents that are thermally labile, serum and plasma should be separated from cells in a refrigerated centrifuge. Specimens for bilirubin or carotene and some drugs, such as methotrexate, must be protected from both daylight and fluorescent light to prevent photodegradation. Some special handling requirements are listed in Table 2-7.

Although transport of specimens from the patient to the clinical laboratory is often done by messenger, pneumatic tube systems have been used to move the specimens more rapidly over long distances within the hospital. Hemolysis may occur in these systems unless the tubes are completely filled and movement of the blood tubes inside the specimen carrier is prevented.[17] The pneumatic tube system should be designed to eliminate sharp curves and sudden stops of the specimen carriers, because these factors are responsible for much of the hemolysis that may occur. With many systems, however, the plasma hemoglobin concentration may be increased, and the serum activity of red cell enzymes, such as lactate dehydrogenase, may also be increased. Nonethe-

TABLE 2-7 Selected Blood Constituents Requiring Special Collection and Storage Conditions*†

Constituent	Anticoagulant	Handling Requirements
S-Acetone, acetoacetate†‡		Freeze; stopper
S-Acid phosphatase		Add citrate (10 g/L); freeze
P-ACTH (corticotropin)	Heparin, 0.2 g/L	Freeze within 15 min of collection
S-Alcohol		Add NaF (10 g/L) to serum
S-Aldolase		Freeze
P,S-Aldosterone		Add boric acid (25 g/L) or freeze
P-Amino acids	Heparin, 0.2 g/L	Freeze
S-Androstenedione		Draw sample in AM (0000-1200 hr)
S-Ascorbic acid		Freeze
S-Barbiturates		Do not use heparin
S-Bile acids		Freeze

TABLE 2-7 *Continued*

Constituent	Anticoagulant	Handling Requirements
S-C-peptide		Draw from fasting patient, freeze
S-Calcitonin		Freeze
P-Carcinoembryonic antigen (CEA)	EDTA, 2 g/L	
B-Cholinesterase	Heparin, 0.2 g/L	
S-Citric acid		Freeze
S-Complement		Freeze
P-Cortisol	Heparin, 0.2 g/L	Separate immediately
S-Creatine		Freeze
S-Creatine kinase isoenzymes		Freeze
S-Creatinine		Freeze
S-Cryoglobulins		Keep above 20 °C
P-11-Deoxycortisol	Heparin, 0.2 g/L	Separate immediately
P,S-Digitoxin		Draw 6-12 hr postadministration
S-Digoxin		Draw 8 hr postadministration
P-Estradiol	Heparin, 0.2 g/L	Freeze
P-Fatty acids (free and esterified)	Heparin, 0.2 g/L	Freeze
P-Fibrinogen	Citrate, ~4 g/L	Do not use heparin
S,B-Fluoride		Do not collect in glass container
P-Folate (tetrahydrofolate)		Freeze
B-Galactose	Heparin, 0.2 g/L	NaF (10 g/L) added with heparin
S-Gastrin		Collect from fasting patient; freeze
B-Glucose-6-phosphate dehydrogenase[†]	EDTA, 2 g/L	
P-HDL-cholesterol	EDTA, 2 g/L	Collected after 12-14 hr fast, freeze
B-Hemoglobins (for quantitation and electrophoresis)	EDTA, 2 g/L	
S-Histidine		Freeze
S-17-Hydroxyprogesterone		Draw between 0900 and 1100 hr
S-Insulin		Collect from fasting patient, freeze
S-Isocitrate dehydrogenase		Freeze
B-Lactate		Immediately dilute with an equal volume of 5% (50 g/L) perchloric acid, shake and mix
B-Lead	Heparin, 0.2 g/L	Collect in lead-free tube containing heparin
S-Lipoprotein phenotyping		Freeze
S-Lysozyme		Freeze
S-Magnesium		Separate immediately
S-Parathyroid hormone (PTH)		Freeze
S-Pepsinogen		Freeze
S-Placental lactogen		Freeze
S-Prolactin		Freeze
S-Prostaglandin $F_{2\alpha}$		Freeze
P-Pyridoxal phosphate (vitamin B_6)	EDTA, 2 g/L	Protect from light
B-Pyruvate		Immediately dilute with an equal volume of 5% (50 g/L) perchloric acid, shake and mix
P-Renin	EDTA, 2 g/L	Chill during collection, centrifugation
S-Vitamin A		Protect from light
S-Zinc		Use only acid-washed glass, prevent hemolysis

From Winsten S, Gordesky SE: Transportation of specimens. *In:* Selected methods of clinical chemistry. Vol. 9. Faulkner WR, Ed. Washington, DC, AACC Press, 1982:11-15.

P, Plasma; *S,* serum; *B,* whole blood; *EDTA,* ethylenediaminetetraacetate.

*All specimens listed, except those to be assayed for cryoglobulins, should be transported at temperatures below 15 °C, except as noted.

†A sealable styrofoam container with "freezer packs" is usually sufficient to keep specimen frozen for 12 hr. Solid CO_2 is necessary for longer periods.

‡There is some question as to whether this constituent remains stable even with this procedure.

less, the amount of hemolysis is usually so small that it can be ignored. In special cases, such as in a patient undergoing chemotherapy whose cells are fragile, samples should be centrifuged before being placed in the pneumatic tube system or identified as "messenger delivery only."

For specimens that are collected in a remote facility with infrequent transportation by courier to a central laboratory, proper specimen processing must be done in the remote facility so that appropriately separated and preserved plasma or serum is delivered to the laboratory. This necessitates that the remote facility has ready access to all commonly used preservatives and wet ice.

Separation and Storage of Specimens

Plasma or serum should be separated from cells as soon as possible and certainly within 2 hours.[6] Premature separation of serum, however, may permit continued formation of fibrin and lead to obstruction of sample probes in testing equipment. Coagulation in plain or silicone-coated glass tubes is usually complete in 20 to 30 minutes but is prolonged in plastic containers. If it is impossible to centrifuge a blood specimen within 2 hours, the specimen should be held at room temperature rather than at 4 °C to decrease hemolysis. If the specimens cannot be analyzed at once, the separated serum should usually be stored in capped tubes at 4 °C until analysis, both to maintain stability of the specimen and to reduce evaporation. If a specimen for a particular test is sufficiently unstable at 4 °C, the serum specimen should be held at −20 °C in a freezer capable of maintaining this temperature. Frost-free freezers should be avoided because they have a wide temperature swing during the freeze-thaw cycle. Note, however, that 4 °C or −20 °C is not the optimum storage temperature for all tests; some lactate dehydrogenase isoenzymes, for instance, are more stable at room temperature than at 4 °C. Although changes in concentration of test constituents have been observed when serum is stored in a serum separator tube in a refrigerator for 24 hours, the changes do not appear to be large enough to be of clinical significance.

Specimen tubes should be centrifuged with stoppers in place. Closure reduces evaporation, which occurs rapidly in a warm centrifuge with the air currents set up by centrifugation. Stoppers also prevent aerosolization of infectious particles. Specimen tubes containing volatiles, such as ethanol, *must* be stoppered while they are spun. Centrifuging specimens with the stopper in place maintains anaerobic conditions, which are important in the measurement of carbon dioxide and ionized calcium. Removal of the stopper before centrifugation allows loss of carbon dioxide and an increase in blood pH. Control of pH is especially important for the enzymatic measurement of acid phosphatase, which is labile under alkaline conditions engendered by CO_2 loss. Indeed, once the serum is separated for acid phosphatase tests, a tablet of disodium citrate should be added to stabilize the pH at about 6.2.

Transport of Specimens

Before a referral laboratory is used for any tests, the quality of its work should be verified by the referring laboratory. Guidelines for selection and evaluation of a referral laboratory have been published.[15] The specimen handling requirements of the referral laboratory must be observed, and test results reported by a referral laboratory must be identified as such when they are filed in a patient's chart.

It should be assumed that transport from a referring laboratory to a referral laboratory may take as long as 72 hours. Under optimal conditions, a referring laboratory should retain enough specimen for retesting should an unanticipated problem arise during shipment. The tube used for holding a specimen *(primary container)* should be so constructed that the contents do not escape if the container is exposed to extremes of heat, cold, or sunlight.[18] Reduced pressure of 0.50 atmosphere (50 kPa) may be encountered during air transportation, together with vibration, and specimens should be protected by a suitable container from these adverse conditions. Variability of temperature is a significant factor in causing instability of test constituents.[3]

Polypropylene and polyethylene containers are usually suitable for specimen transport. Glass should be avoided because of its tendency to break. Polystyrene is also unsuitable because it may crack when frozen. The containers must be leak proof and should have a Teflon-lined screw cap that does not loosen under the variety of temperatures to which the container may be exposed. The materials of both stopper and container must be inert and must not have any effect on the concentration of the analyte.

The shipping or *secondary container* used to hold one or more specimen tubes or bottles must be constructed to prevent the tubes from knocking against each other. Corrugated, fiberboard, or styrofoam boxes designed to fit around a single specimen tube may be used. A padded shipping envelope provides adequate protection for shipping single specimens. When specimens are shipped as drops of blood on filter paper (e.g., for neonatal screening), the paper should be enclosed in a plastic bag that then can be mailed in a regular envelope.

For transportation of *frozen* or *refrigerated* specimens, a styrofoam container should be used. The container walls should be 1 inch (2.5 cm) thick to provide effective insulation. The container should be vented to prevent buildup of carbon dioxide under pressure and a possible explosion. Solid carbon dioxide (dry ice) is the most convenient refrigerant material for keeping specimens frozen, and temperatures as low as −70 °C can be achieved. The amount of dry ice required in a container depends on the size of the container and the efficiency of its insulation and the time for which the specimens must be kept frozen. One piece of solid dry ice (about 3 inches × 4 inches × 1 inch) in a container with 1-inch styrofoam walls and a volume of 125 cubic inches (2000 cm^3) will maintain a single specimen frozen for 48 hours.

Various laws and regulations apply to the shipment of biological specimens. Although they theoretically apply only to etiological agents (known infectious agents), all specimens should be transported as if the same regulations applied.[13] Airlines have rigid regulations covering the transport of specimens. The airlines deem dry ice a hazardous material; therefore the transport of most clinical laboratory specimens is affected by the regulations.

The various modes of transport of specimens influence the shipping time and cost. Priority mail service is usually adequate within the United States if a delay of up to 3 days is acceptable. Express mail service ensures delivery within 24 hours, but it is available only between certain cities. Small-package service is available from many airlines, as is service by bus lines and train.

The cost of specimen transport is often included in the fee of a referral laboratory for each test. Many referral laboratories either provide their own courier service or contract with large national companies to provide such services.

The director of a referring laboratory has the responsibility to ensure that specimens will be adequately transported to the referral laboratory. He or she should determine the benefits of different services and should keep in mind that the fastest service is usually the most expensive. He or she should also know that specimens should not be sent to a referral laboratory at the end of the week, because more delays in transit occur during weekends than during the working week and deterioration of specimens is more likely.

REFERENCES

1. Blumenfeld TA, Turi GK, Blanc WA. Recommended site and depth of newborn heel skin punctures based on anatomic measurements and histopathology. Lancet, 1979;1:230-33.
2. Caraway WT. Chemical and diagnostic specificity of laboratory tests. Am J Clin Pathol 1962;37:445-64.
3. Felding P, Hyltoft Petersen P, Horder M. The stability of plasma and serum constituents during simulated transport. Scand J Clin Lab Invest 1981;41:35-40.
4. Ladenson JH. Nonanalytical sources of variation in clinical chemistry results. *In:* Gradwohl's Clinical Laboratory Methods and Diagnosis. 8th ed. AC Sonnenwirth and L Jarett, Eds. St. Louis:CV Mosby Co, 1980:149-92.
5. Laessig RH, Hassemer DJ, Westgard JO, et al. Assessment of the serum separator tube as an intermediate storage device within the laboratory. Am J Clin Pathol 1976;66:653-7.
6. Laessig RH, Indriksons AA, Hassemer DJ, et al. Changes in serum chemical values as a result of prolonged contact with the clot. Am J Clin Pathol, 1976;66:598-604.
7. Lum G, Gambino SR. A comparison of serum versus heparinized plasma for routine chemistry tests. Am J Clin Pathol 1974;61:108-13.
8. McNair P, Nielsen SL, Christiansen C, et al. Gross errors made by routine blood sampling from two sites using a tourniquet applied at different positions. Clin Chim Acta 1979;98:113-8.
9. National Committee for Clinical Laboratory Standards. Evacuated Tubes and Additives for Blood Specimen Collection: Approved Standard H1-A4. 4th ed. Wayne, PA, National Committee for Clinical Laboratory Standards, 1996.
10. National Committee for Clinical Laboratory Standards. Procedures and Devices for the Collection of Diagnostic Blood Specimens by Skin Puncture: Approved Standard H4-A4. 3rd ed. Wayne, PA, National Committee for Clinical Laboratory Standards, 1999.
11. National Committee for Clinical Laboratory Standards. Procedures for the Collection of Arterial Specimen: Approved Standard H11-A3. 3rd ed. Wayne, PA, National Committee for Clinical Laboratory Standards, 1999.
12. National Committee for Clinical Laboratory Standards. Procedures for the Collection of Diagnostic Blood Specimens by Venipuncture: Approved Standard H3-A4. 4th ed. Wayne PA:National Committee for Clinical Laboratory Standards, 1998.
13. National Committee for Clinical Laboratory Standards. Procedures for the Handling and Transport of Domestic Diagnostic Specimens and Etiologic Agents: Approved Standard H5-A3. 3rd ed. Wayne, PA, National Committee for Clinical Laboratory Standards, 1994.
14. National Committee for Clinical Laboratory Standards. Routine Urinalysis and Collection, Transportation, and Preservation of Urine Specimens: Approved Guideline GP16-A2. 2nd ed. Wayne, PA, National Committee for Clinical Laboratory Standards, 2001.
15. National Committee for Clinical Laboratory Standards. Selecting and Evaluating a Referral Laboratory: Approved Guideline GP9-A. Wayne PA:National Committee for Clinical Laboratory Standards, 1998.
16. Ong YY, Boykin SF, Barnett RN. You can draw blood from the "IV arm" below the intravenous needle if you put a tourniquet in between. Am J Clin Pathol 1979;72:101-2.
17. Steige H, Jones JD. Evaluation of pneumatic tube system for delivery of blood specimens. Clin Chem 1971;17:1160-4.
18. Wollner GC. Handling, storing and transporting diagnostic specimens. Lab Med 1980;11:87-91.
19. Young DS. Effects of preanalytical variables on clinical laboratory tests. 2nd edition. Washington DC:AACC Press, 1997.

ADDITIONAL READING

Banfi G, Bauer K, Brand W, Buchberger M, Deom A, Ehret W, Enger WD, da Fonesca-Wollheim F et al. Use of anticoagulants in diagnostic laboratory investigations and stability of blood, plasma and serum samples. Geneva, Switzerland, World Health Organization, 2002.

Calam RR. Reviewing the importance of specimen collection. J. Am Med Technol 1997;39:297-302.

Flynn JC. Procedures in Phlebotomy, 3rd ed. St Louis: Saunders, 2005.

Guder WG, Narayanan S, Wisser H, Zawta B. Samples from the patient to the laboratory. 3rd ed. Weinheim, Germany:Wiley-VCH Verlag, 2003.

Slockbower JM, Blumenfeld TA, Eds. Collection and Handling of Laboratory Specimens. Philadelphia:JB Lippincott Co, 1983.

Wilding P, Zilva JF, Wilde C. Transport of specimens for clinical chemistry analysis. Ann Clin Biochem, 1977;14:301-6.

SECTION II

Analytical Techniques and Instrumentation

CHAPTER 3

Optical Techniques*

L.J. Kricka, D.Phil., F.A.C.B., C.Chem., F.R.S.C., F.R.C.Path.

Many determinations made in the clinical laboratory are based on measurements of radiant energy emitted, transmitted, absorbed, scattered, or reflected under controlled conditions. The principles involved in such measurements are considered in this chapter.

NATURE OF LIGHT

Electromagnetic radiation includes radiant energy that extends from cosmic rays with wavelengths as short as 10^{-9} nm up to radio waves longer than 1000 km. However, in this chapter the term *light* is used to describe radiant energy from the visible and ultraviolet portions of the spectrum (180 to 800 nm).

The wavelength of light, the distance between two peaks as the light travels in a wavelike manner, is expressed in nanometers (nm) for wavelengths commonly used in photometry. Other units include:

$$1\,\text{nm} = 1\,\text{millimicrons}\,(\text{m}\mu) = 10\,\text{Angstroms}\,(\text{Å}) = 10^{-9}\,\text{m}$$

In addition to possessing wavelength characteristics, light also has properties that indicate it is composed of discrete energy packets called *photons*. The relationship between the energy of photons and their frequency is given by the equation:

$$E = h\nu \qquad (1)$$

where E = energy in ergs, ν = frequency of light in cycles per second, and h = Planck's constant (6.62×10^{27} erg seconds). The frequency of light (ν) is related to the wavelength by an equation:

$$\nu = \frac{c}{\lambda} \qquad (2)$$

where c = speed of light in a vacuum (3×10^{10} cm/s), and λ = wavelength in centimeters. Combining equations (1) and (2) results in:

$$E = \frac{hc}{\lambda} \qquad (3)$$

This equation shows that the energy of light is inversely proportional to the wavelength. For example, ultraviolet (UV) radiation at 200 nm possesses greater energy than infrared (IR) radiation at 750 nm.

The human eye responds to radiant energy with wavelengths between about 380 and 750 nm, but modern instrumentation permits measurements at both shorter wavelength (UV) and longer wavelength (IR) portions of the spectrum. Sunlight, or light emitted from a tungsten filament, is a mixture or spectrum of radiant energy of different wavelengths that the eye recognizes as "white." Table 3-1 shows approximate relationships between wavelengths and color characteristics for the UV, visible, and short IR portions of the spectrum. Thus a solution will appear green when viewed against white light if it transmits light maximally between 500 and 580 nm but absorbs light at other wavelengths. Similarly a solid object appears green if it reflects light in this region (500 to 580 nm) but absorbs light at other portions of the spectrum. In general, if we compare the intensity of light transmitted by a colored solution to that of a blank or reference solution over the entire spectrum, we obtain a typical spectral transmittance curve characteristic for that spectrum. Such curves are shown in Figure 3-1 for solutions of nickel sulfate *(a)* and potassium permanganate *(b)*. Inspection of the curves should lead us to predict that the color of solution *A* is green because light is transmitted maximally near the green portion of the spectrum. Curve *B*, on the other hand, illustrates the spectrum of a solution that transmits light maximally in the blue, violet, and red portions of the spectrum. The eye recognizes this mixture of colors as purple.

*The author gratefully acknowledges the original contributions by Dr. Merle A. Evenson and Dr. Thomas O. Tiffany, upon which portions of this chapter are based.

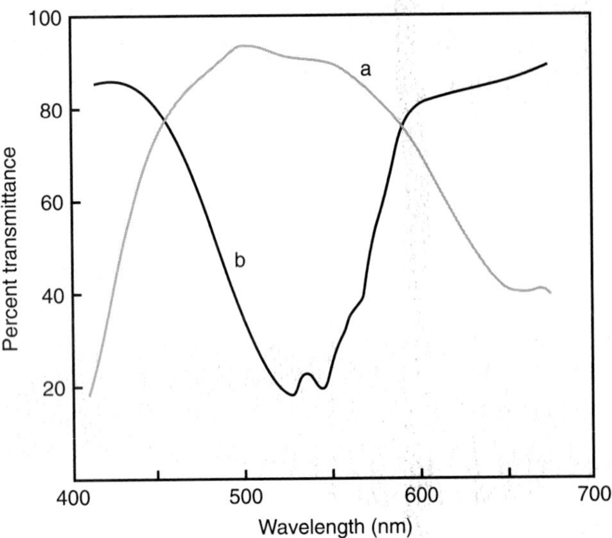

Figure 3-1 Spectral transmittance curves of nickel sulfate *(a)* and potassium permanganate *(b)*. Arbitrary concentrations, read versus water as a blank. *(Beckman DB-G spectrophotometer.)*

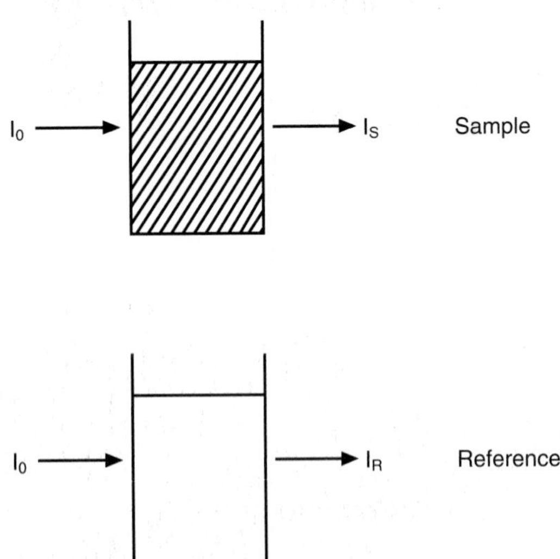

Figure 3-2 Transmittance of light through sample and reference cells. Transmittance of sample versus reference = $\frac{I_S}{I_R}$. I_0 = intensity of incident light; I_S = intensity of transmitted light for compound in solution; I_R = intensity of transmitted light through reference cell.

TABLE 3-1 Ultraviolet, Visible, and Short Infrared Spectrum Characteristics

Wavelength (nm)	Region Name	Color Observed*
<380	Ultraviolet†	Invisible
380-440	Visible	Violet
440-500	Visible	Blue
500-580	Visible	Green
580-600	Visible	Yellow
600-620	Visible	Orange
620-750	Visible	Red
800-2500	Near-infrared	Not visible
2500-15,000	Mid-infrared	Not visible
15,000-1,000,000	Far-infrared	Not visible

*Owing to the subjective nature of color, the wavelength intervals shown are only approximations.

†The ultraviolet (UV) portion of the spectrum is sometimes further divided into "near" UV (200-380 nm) and "far" UV (<220 nm). This arbitrary distinction has a practical basis, because silica used to make cuvets transmits light effectively at wavelengths ≥220 nm.

SPECTROPHOTOMETRY

Photometry is defined as the measurement of light; *spectrophotometry* is defined as the measurement of the intensity of light at selected wavelengths. Spectrophotometric analysis is a widely used method of quantitative and qualitative analysis in the chemical and biological sciences; it is accurate and sensitive. The method depends on the light absorbing properties of either the substance or a derivative of the substance being analyzed. The intensity of transmitted light passing through a solution containing an absorbing substance (chromogen) is decreased by the absorbed fraction. This fraction is then detected, measured, and used to relate the light transmitted or absorbed to concentration of the analyte in question.

Basic Concepts

Consider an incident light beam with intensity I_0 passing through a square cell containing a solution of a compound that absorbs light of a certain wavelength, λ (Figure 3-2). Given that the intensity of the transmitted light beam I_S is less than I_0, the transmittance (T) of light is defined as:

$$T = \frac{I_S}{I_0} \quad (4)$$

A portion of the incident light, however, may be reflected by the surface of the cell or absorbed by the cell wall or solvent. To focus attention on the compound of interest, elimination of these factors is necessary. This is achieved using a reference cell identical to the sample cell, except that the compound of interest is omitted from the solvent in the reference cell. The transmittance (T) through this reference cell is I_R divided by I_0; the transmittance for the compound in solution then is defined as I_S divided by I_R. In practice the reference cell is inserted and the instrument adjusted to an arbitrary scale reading of 100 (corresponding to 100% transmittance), after which the percent transmittance reading is made on the sample. As we increase the concentration of the compound in solution, we find that transmittance varies inversely and logarithmically with concentration. Consequently, it is more convenient to define a new term, absorbance (A), that will be directly proportional to con-

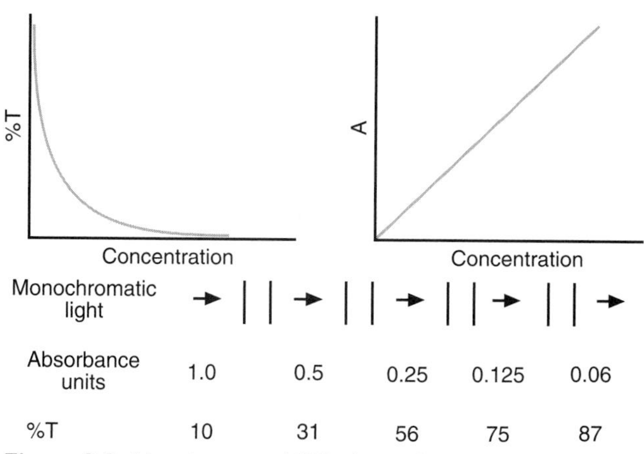

Figure 3-3 Absorbance and %*T* relationship.

TABLE 3-2 Spectrophotometry Nomenclature

Name	Symbol	Definition
Absorbance	A	$\log T$ or $\log I_0/I$
Absorptivity	a	A/bc (c in g/L)
Molar absorptivity	ε	A/bc (c in mol/L)
Path length	b	Internal cell or sample length, in cm
Transmittance	T	I/I_0*
Wavelength unit	nm	10^{-9} m
Absorption maximum	λmax	Wavelength at which a maximum absorption occurs

*I/I_0 is the ratio of the intensity of transmitted light to incident light.

centration. Thus the amount of light absorbed (A) as the incident light passes through the sample is equivalent to

$$A = -\log\frac{I_S}{I_R} = -\log T \quad (5)$$

Analytically, the amount of light absorbed or transmitted is related mathematically to the concentration of the analyte in question by Beer's law.

Beer's Law—Relationship between Transmittance, Absorbance, and Concentration

Beer's law (also known as the Beer-Lambert law) states that the concentration of a substance is directly proportional to the amount of light absorbed or inversely proportional to the logarithm of the transmitted light (Figure 3-3). Mathematically, Beer's law is expressed as

$$A = abc \quad (6)$$

where

A = Absorbance
a = Proportionality constant defined as absorptivity
b = Light path in centimeters
c = Concentration of the absorbing compound, usually expressed in grams per liter

This equation forms the basis of quantitative analysis by absorption photometry. When b is 1 cm and c is expressed in moles per liter, the symbol ε is substituted for the constant a. The value for ε is a constant for a given compound at a given wavelength under prescribed conditions of solvent, temperature, pH, etc., and is called the molar absorptivity. The nomenclature of spectrophotometry is summarized in Table 3-2. Values for ε are useful to characterize compounds, establish their purity, and compare sensitivities of measurements obtained on derivatives. Pure bilirubin, for example, when dissolved in chloroform at 25 °C, has a molar absorptivity of 60,700 ± 1600 at 453 nm. The molecular weight of bilirubin is 584. Hence a solution containing 5 mg/L (0.005 g/L) should have an absorbance of

$$A = (60{,}700) \times (1) \times (0.005/584) = 0.520$$

The molar absorptivity of the complex between ferrous iron and *s*-tripyridyltriazine is 22 600, whereas that with 1,10-phenanthroline is 11 000. Thus for a given concentration of iron, *s*-tripyridyltriazine produces a complex with an absorbance about twice that of the complex with 1,10-phenanthroline. Consequently, *s*-tripyridyltriazine is a more sensitive reagent to use in the measurement of iron.

Application of Beer's Law

In practice, the direct proportionality between absorbance and concentration must be established experimentally for a given instrument under specified conditions. Frequently a linear relationship exists up to a certain concentration or absorbance. When this relationship occurs, the solution is said to obey Beer's law up to this point. Within this limitation, a calibration constant (K) may be derived and used to calculate the concentration of an unknown solution by comparison with a calibrating solution. Rearranging equation (6) gives:

$$a = \frac{A}{bc} \quad (7)$$

Therefore

$$\frac{A_1}{b_1 c_1} = \frac{A_2}{b_2 c_2} \quad (8)$$

Because the light path (b) remains constant in a given method of analysis with a fixed cuvet size ($b_1 = b_2$), Equation (8) then becomes

$$\frac{A_1}{c_1} = \frac{A_2}{c_2} \quad \text{or} \quad \frac{A_c}{c_c} = \frac{A_u}{c_u} \quad (9)$$

where subscripts c and u indicate the absorbance (A) and concentration (c) of calibrating and unknown solutions, respectively.

Solving for the concentration of unknown

$$c_u = \frac{A_u}{A_c} \times c_c \quad (10)$$

or the equivalent expression

$$c_u = A_u \times \frac{c_c}{A_c} = A_u K \qquad (11)$$

where $K = \frac{c_c}{A_c}$. The value of the constant K is obtained through measurement of the absorbance (A_c) of a calibrator of known concentration (c_c).

Certain precautions must be observed with the use of such calibration constants. Under no circumstances should the constant be used when either the calibrator or unknown readings exceed the linear portion of the calibration curve, a condition when the curve no longer obeys Beer's law. At least two and preferably more calibrators should be included in each series of determinations to permit direct comparison of unknown with calibrator or to calculate the calibration constant because variations in reagents, working conditions, cell diameters, and deterioration or changes in instruments may result in day-to-day changes of the absorbance value for the calibrator. A nonlinear calibration curve may be used if a sufficient number of calibrators of varying concentrations is included to cover the entire range encountered for readings on unknowns.

In some cases a pure reference material may not be readily available, and constants may be provided that were obtained on pure materials and reported in the literature. In general, published constants should be used only if the method is followed in detail and readings are made on a spectrophotometer capable of providing light of high spectral purity at a verified wavelength. Use of broader-band light sources usually leads to some decrease in absorbance. The absorbance of NADH at 340 nm, for example, frequently is used as a reference for the determination of enzyme activity, based on a molar absorptivity of 6.22×10^3 (see Chapter 8). This value is acceptable only under the carefully controlled conditions previously described and should not be used unless these conditions are met. Published values for molar absorptivities and absorption coefficients should be used only as guidelines until they are verified by readings on pure reference materials for a given instrument. In addition, Beer's law is followed only if the following conditions are met:

- Incident radiation on the substance of interest is monochromatic.
- The solvent absorption is insignificant compared with the solute absorbance.
- The solute concentration is within given limits.
- An optical interferant is not present.
- A chemical reaction does not occur between the molecule of interest and another solute or solvent molecule.

INSTRUMENTATION

Modern instruments isolate a narrow wavelength range of the spectrum for measurements. Those that use filters for this purpose are referred to as *filter photometers;* those that use prisms or gratings are called *spectrophotometers.* Spectrophotometers are classified as being either single or double-beam.

The major components of a *single-beam spectrophotometer* are shown schematically in Figure 3-4. In such an instrument, a beam of light is passed through a monochromator that isolates the desired region of the spectrum to be used for measurements. Slits are used to isolate a narrow beam of the light and improve its chromatic purity. The light next passes through an absorption cell (cuvet), where a portion of the radiant energy is absorbed, depending on the nature and concentration of the substance in the solution. Any light not absorbed is transmitted to a detector (photocell or phototube), which converts light energy to electrical energy that can be registered on a meter or recorder or digitally displayed.

In operation, an opaque block is substituted for the cuvet, so that no light reaches the photocell, and the meter is adjusted to read 0% *T.* Next a cuvet containing a reagent blank is inserted and the meter is adjusted to read 100% *T* (zero absorbance). The composition of the reagent blank should be identical to that of calibrating or unknown solutions except for the substance to be measured. Calibrating solutions containing various known concentrations of the substance are inserted, and readings are recorded. Finally, a reading is made of the unknown solution, and its concentration is determined by comparison with the readings obtained on the calibrators. In most spectrophotometers, digital hardware and software are integral components and perform these functions automatically.

Figure 3-5 illustrates schematically a typical double-beam-in-space system in which all components are duplicated except the light source. Another approach is a double-beam-in-time instrument that uses a light-beam chopper (a rotating wheel with alternate silvered sections and cutout sections) inserted after the exit slit (Figure 3-6). A system of mirrors passes the portions of the light reflected

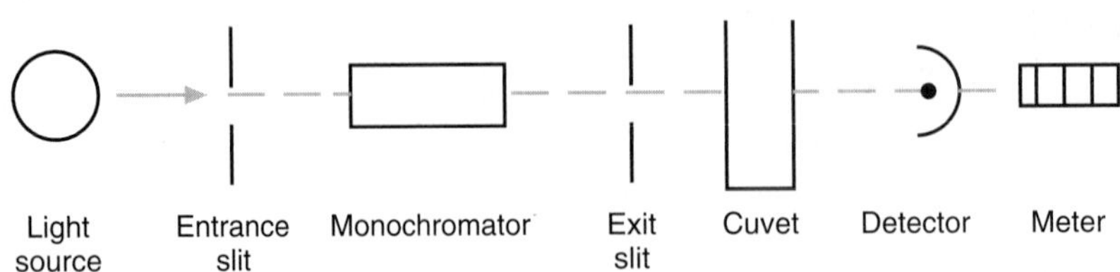

Figure 3-4 Major components of a single-beam spectrophotometer.

off the chopper alternately through the sample and a reference cuvet onto a common detector. The chopped-beam approach, using one detector, compensates for light source variation and for sensitivity changes of the detector.

Components

The basic components of a spectrophotometer include (1) a light source; (2) a means to isolate light of a desired wavelength; (3) fiber optics; (4) cuvets; (5) a photodetector; (6) a readout device; (7) a recorder; and (8) a microprocessor.

Light Sources

Types of light sources used in spectrophotometers include incandescent lamps and lasers.

Incandescent Lamps. The light source for measurements in the visible portion of the spectrum is usually a tungsten light bulb. The lifetime of a tungsten filament is greatly increased by the presence of a low pressure of iodine or bromine vapor within the lamp. An example is the *quartz-halogen* lamp, which has a fused-silica envelope and which provides high-intensity light over a wide spectrum and for extended operating periods (2000 to 5000 hours before replacement is necessary). The tungsten lamp is acceptable for making measurements of moderately dilute solutions in which the change in absorbance varies significantly with small changes in concentration.

A tungsten light source does not supply sufficient radiant energy for measurements below 320 nm. In the UV region of the spectrum, a low-pressure mercury-vapor lamp that emits a discontinuous or line spectrum is useful for calibration purposes but is not very practical for absorbance measurements, because it can be used only at certain wavelengths. Hydrogen and deuterium lamps provide sources of continuous spectra in the UV region with some sharp emission

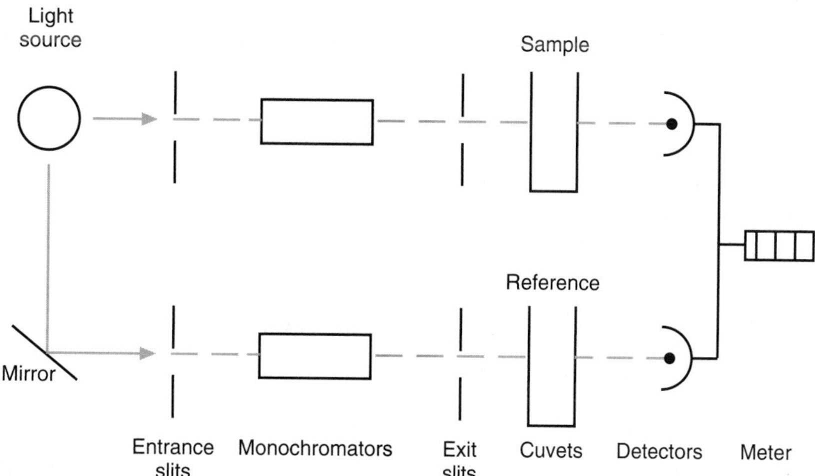

Figure 3-5 Double-beam-in-space spectrophotometer.

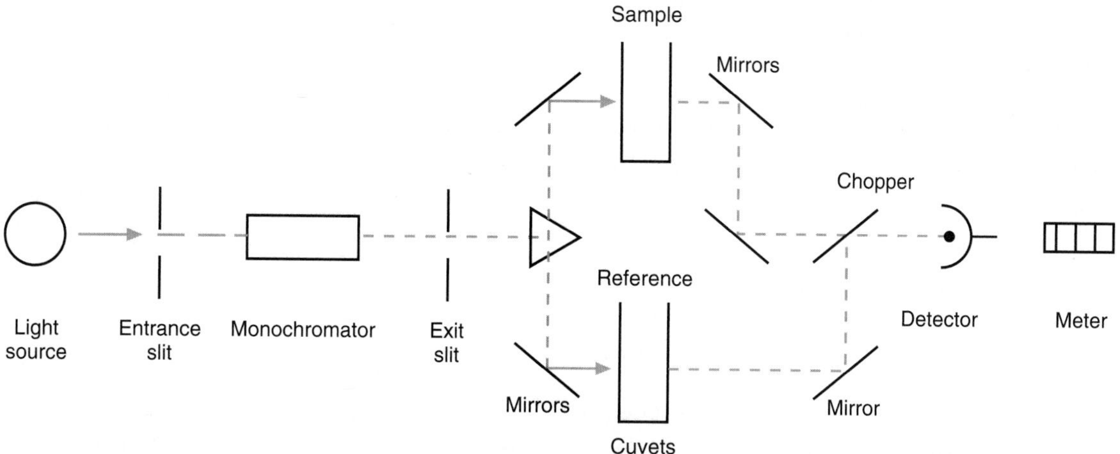

Figure 3-6 Double-beam-in-time spectrophotometer.

lines, as do high-pressure mercury and xenon arc lamps. These sources are more commonly used in UV absorption measurements. A deuterium lamp is more stable and has a longer life than a hydrogen lamp.

A widely used photometer used as a high-pressure liquid chromatographic (HPLC) detector uses the intense 254-nm resonance line produced by a mercury arc lamp (see Chapter 6). Others employ a miniature hollow cathode lamp as a very-narrow-wavelength intense source. For example, a zinc hollow cathode lamp gives a line at 214 nm that is adequately close to the maximum wavelength of peptide bond absorption (206 nm) so that it can be used to measure peptides and proteins. Details on the hollow cathode lamp are found in the section on Atomic Absorption Spectrophotometry. The hollow cathode lamp also has a long, useful lifetime if a lower-current, nonpulsed power supply is used.

Laser Sources. A laser (light amplification by stimulated emission of radiation) is a device that controls the way that energized atoms release photons; they are used as light sources in spectrophotometers as they provide intense light of a narrow wavelength. These devices are based on certain materials having the capability of absorbing energy and storing all or part of it. If the loss of absorbed energy is forbidden by quantum mechanical rules, the material will remain in an excited state. The delayed and slow release of energy from such materials in some cases may be called phosphorescence. If this excited material has more energy pumped into it, either at the phosphorescence wavelength or by electrical energy pumping, then there may be a rapid decay to lower energy with the emission of highly quantified light. Because of kinetic mechanisms of decay to lower energy, a highly coherent beam of light that has minimum scatter and is nearly monochromatic is produced. By selection of different materials, different wavelength(s) of light are emitted by different types of lasers (Table 3-3).

Three properties of laser sources distinguish them from "conventional" sources: (1) spatial coherence is a property of lasers that allows beam diameters in the range of several microns; (2) lasers produce monochromatic light; and (3) lasers have pulse widths that vary from microseconds (flash lamp-pulsed lasers) to nanoseconds (nitrogen lasers) to picoseconds or less (mode-locked lasers) in duration. Air-cooled argon ion lasers produce about 25 mW of energy output at 488 nm and have plasma tube lifetimes of 6000 hours or more. Continuous-wave dye lasers typically use an argon ion laser with an output of 1 W or less as an energy pump and use different fluorescent dyes to achieve excitation wavelength ranges of 400 to 800 nm. Helium-neon and helium-cadmium lasers are useful because of their low cost and ease of operation and because they emit a number of excitation wavelengths, but for helium-neon lasers power output has been limited to about 2 mW at 594 nm.

Infrared diode lasers are used in compact disc players and laser printers, and in bar code readers (see Chapter 11). They are solid-state devices, typically constructed of gallium arsenide, and energy is pumped into them at a low potential of ~1.5 V. Depending on its construction, the wavelength output of the laser ranges from 550 to 1810 nm. The development of inexpensive near-IR lasers has led to interest in using reflective techniques in the near-IR region of the spectrum (0.8 to 2.5 μm wavelength) for noninvasive monitoring of glucose. With this technique, a near-IR light source is focused on the skin of a patient. By measuring the relative absorbance differences at several lines of the near-IR spectrum—by computer subtraction of blank signals and by computer-mathematical enhancement of the signal-to-noise ratios (Fourier transform)—it is possible to measure the glucose concentration of the patient.[22]

TABLE 3-3 Various Types of Lasers and the Wavelengths at which They Operate

Laser	Wavelength(s) (nm)
Argon fluoride	193
Argon fluoride	248
Helium-cadmium	325 or 442
Nitrogen	337
Argon (blue)	488
Argon (green)	514
Helium-neon (green)	543
Light emitting diode—GaP	550 or 700
Rhodamine 6G dye (tunable)	570-650
Laser diode (AlGaInP, GaAlAs)	633-1,660
Helium-neon (red)	633
Ruby ($CrAlO_3$) (red)	694
Light emitting diode—GaAs	880
Light emitting diode—Si	1100
Neodymium-YAG (yttrium aluminum garnet)	1064
Carbon dioxide	9300, 9600, 10,300, or 10,600

Spectral Isolation

A system for isolating radiant energy of a desired wavelength and excluding that of other wavelengths is called a *monochromator.* There are various ways of accomplishing this, including the use of filters, prisms, and diffraction gratings. Combinations of lenses and slits may be inserted before or after the monochromatic device to render light rays parallel or to isolate narrow portions of the light beam. Variable slits may be used to permit adjustments in total radiant energy reaching the photocell.

Filters. The simplest type of filter is a thin layer of colored glass. Certain metal complexes or salts, dissolved or suspended in glass, produce colors corresponding to the predominant wavelengths transmitted. Strictly speaking, a glass filter is not a true monochromator because it transmits light over a relatively wide range of wavelengths. The spectral

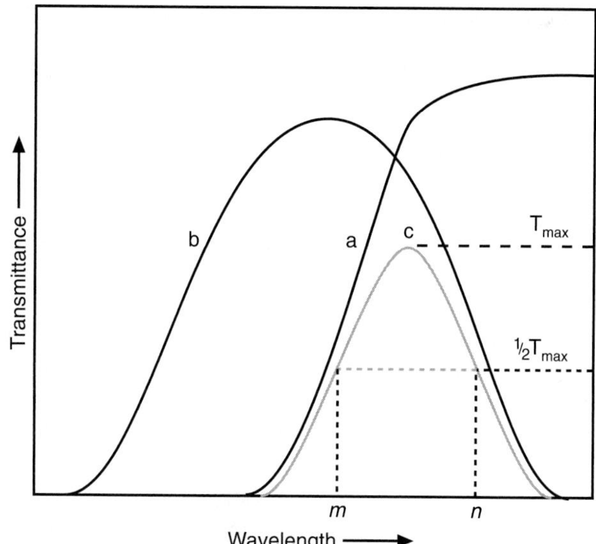

Figure 3-7 Spectral characteristics of a sharp-cutoff filter *(a)* and a wide-bandpass filter *(b)*. The narrow-bandpass filter *(c)* is obtained by combining filters *a* and *b*. The spectral bandwidth of filter c (distance *n-m*) is defined as the width in nanometers of the spectral transmittance curve at a point equal to one half of maximum transmittance.

purity of a filter or other monochromator is usually described in terms of its *spectral bandwidth*. This is defined as the width, in nanometers, of the spectral transmittance curve at a point equal to one half the peak transmittance (Figure 3-7). Commonly used glass filters have spectral bandwidths of approximately 50 nm and are referred to as *wide-bandpass filters*.

Other glass filters include the narrow-bandpass and sharp-cutoff types (see Figure 3-7). As shown, a cutoff filter typically shows a sharp rise in transmittance over a narrow portion of the spectrum and is used to eliminate light below a given wavelength. Narrow-bandpass filters may be constructed by combining two or more sharp-cutoff filters or regular filters; however, the availability of high-intensity light sources now favors the use of narrow-bandpass interference filters.

Another approach for construction of narrow-bandpass filters is to use a dielectric material of controlled thickness sandwiched between two thinly silvered pieces of glass. The thickness of the layer determines the wavelength of energy transmitted. These filters have narrow spectral bandwidths, usually from 5 to 15 nm, and are referred to as *interference filters*. Because they also transmit harmonics, or multiples, of the desired wavelength, accessory glass filters are required to eliminate these undesired wavelengths. Thus an interference filter designed for 620 nm will also transmit some radiation at 310 and 1240 nm unless accessory cutoff filters are provided to absorb this undesired stray light.

Prisms and Gratings. Prisms and diffraction gratings are also widely used as monochromators. A *prism* separates white light into a continuous spectrum by refraction with shorter wavelengths being bent, or refracted, more than longer wavelengths as they pass through the prism. A *diffraction grating* is prepared by depositing a thin layer of aluminum-copper alloy on the surface of a flat glass plate, then ruling many small parallel grooves into the metal coating. Better gratings contain 1000 to 2000 lines/mm and must be made with great care. These are then used as molds to prepare less expensive replicas for general use in instruments.

Modern holographic gratings are made using a laser in a "high-precision machining" mode. The focused beam of the laser is accurately scanned over a photosensitive material termed a "photoresist." After multiple lines have been scribed on the photoresist, chemicals are used to dissolve and elute the exposed photoresist to create the channels that become the lines of the grating. A layer of a highly reflective material is then sputtered onto the surface of the laser-etched channels, and the grating is ready for use. Either a flat photoresistive surface or a concave surface can be used to make this type of grating. These types of gratings are extremely accurate, have low light scatter, and are widely used in the spectrophotometers used in clinical chemistry instruments. For example, most UV-visible spectrophotometers and virtually all IR spectrophotometers use reflective gratings. In addition, HPLC detectors frequently use a concave holographic reflective grating in their optical system.

Each line ruled on the grating, when illuminated, gives rise to a tiny spectrum. Wave fronts are formed that reinforce those wavelengths in phase and cancel those not in phase. The net result is a uniform linear spectrum. Some instruments contain diffraction gratings that produce spectral bandwidths of 20 nm or more; higher-priced instruments may have a resolution of 0.5 nm or less.

The flat surface grating discussed above is called a plane *transmission grating*. Lines are engraved on the surface of a mirror, which may be either a polished metal slab or a glass plate on which a thin, metallic film has been deposited. A grating may also be ruled at a specified angle, so that a maximum fraction of the radiant energy is directed into wavelengths diffracted at a selected angle. This type of grating is called an *echelette* and is said to have been given a *blaze* at a particular angle or to have been blazed at a certain wavelength (e.g., 250 nm).

Selection of a Monochromator. The type of monochromator chosen depends on the analytical purpose for which it is to be used. For example, narrow-bandpass filters are typically used in flame photometry to isolate emission energy at a given wavelength. Alternately, narrow spectral bandwidths are required in spectrophotometers for resolving and identifying sharp absorption peaks that are closely adjacent. Lack of agreement with Beer's law will occur when a part of the spectral energy transmitted by the monochromator is not absorbed by the substance being measured. This is more commonly observed with wide-bandpass instruments.

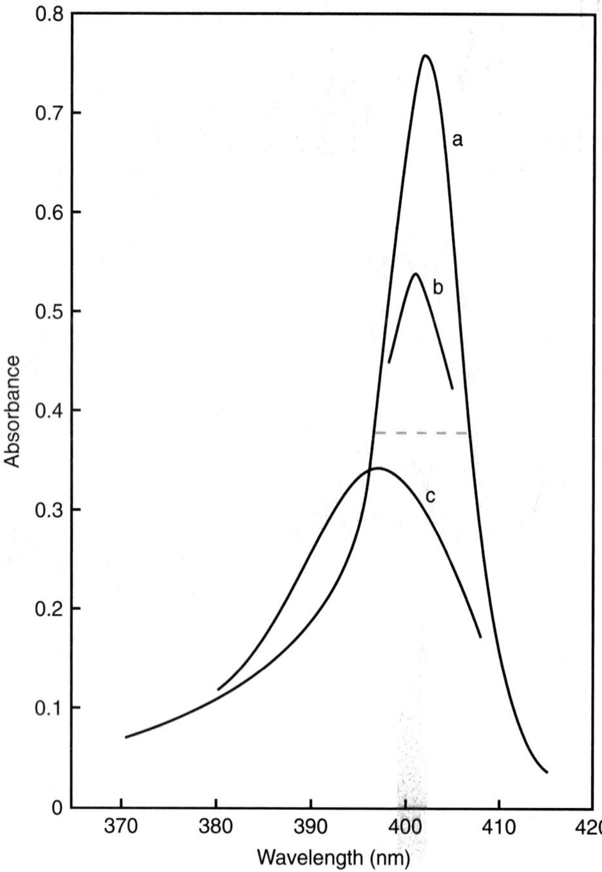

Figure 3-8 Effect of spectral bandwidth (SBW) on the absorption spectrum of coproporphyrin I. Nominal concentration, 1 µg/mL in HCl, 0.1 mol/L. SBW: *curve a,* 1 nm, Beckman DB-G spectrophotometer; *curve b,* 10 nm; and *curve c,* 20 nm, Beckman DB spectrophotometer. The *dotted horizontal line* shows a natural bandwidth of 10 nm for coproporphyrin I when scanned at a spectral bandwidth of 1 nm. The shift of A_{max} to lower wavelengths as SBW is increased is related to skewness of the absorption spectrum to the left.

Some increase in absorbance and improved linearity with concentration is usually observed with instruments that operate at narrower bandwidths of light. This is especially true for substances that exhibit a sharp peak of absorption. Spectral absorbance curves for a solution of coproporphyrin I (Figure 3-8) demonstrate the marked decrease in maximum absorbance as the spectral bandwidth is increased from 1 to 20 nm. The *natural bandwidth* of an absorbing substance is defined as "the bandwidth of the spectral absorbance curve at a point equal to one half of the maximum absorbance." Curve A in Figure 3-8, scanned at a *spectral* bandwidth of 1 nm, shows a *natural* bandwidth of approximately 10 nm. As a general rule, for peak absorbance readings to be within 99.5% of true values, the spectral bandwidth should not exceed 10% of the natural bandwidth. For example, many chemistry procedures used in the clinical laboratory produce an absorbing species for which the natural bandwidth ranges from 40 to over 200 nm. The natural bandwidth of NADH is 58 nm ($\lambda max = 339$ nm). Therefore, for accurate measurements of this compound, we should use a spectral bandwidth of 6 nm or less. Actual studies have shown that use of a 10-nm spectral bandwidth at 340 nm produces absorbance values approximately 98% of those obtained with a 1-nm spectral bandwidth.

In practice, the wavelength selected is usually at the peak of maximum absorbance to achieve maximum sensitivity; however, it may be desirable to choose another wavelength to minimize interfering substances. For example, turbidity readings on a spectrophotometer are greater in the blue region than in the red region of the spectrum, but the latter region is chosen for turbidity measurements to avoid absorption of light by bilirubin (460 nm) or hemoglobin (417 and 575 nm). The absorbing species developed in the alkaline picrate procedure for creatinine produces a relatively flat peak in the visible region of the spectrum at approximately 480 nm, but the reagent blank itself absorbs light strongly below 500 nm. A compromise is made by selecting a wavelength at 520 nm to minimize the contribution of the blank. Blank readings should, of course, be kept to a minimum. A small difference between two large numbers is subject to greater uncertainty; hence minimizing absorbance of the blank improves precision and accuracy. The linear working range of a method can be expanded also by not measuring at the peak absorbance. However, measurements should not be taken on the steep slope of an absorption curve, because a slight error in wavelength adjustment would introduce a significant error in absorbance readings.

Fiber Optics

In the single- and double-beam spectrophotometers shown diagrammatically in Figures 3-4 through 3-6, the positioning of the individual components dictates the path that the light beam must follow as it travels from the source to the detector. This approach places certain restrictions on the design, size, and cost of such instruments. To overcome these restrictions, fiber optics are now integrated into the optical design of spectrophotometers.[15] Fiber optics, also known as *light pipes,* are bundles of thin, transparent fibers of glass, quartz, or plastic that are enclosed in material of a lower index of refraction and that transmit light throughout their lengths by internal reflections. The use of fiber optics in spectrophotometers offers the advantage of better directional control of the beam of light within the geometrical confines of an instrument; this allows for the design and manufacture of miniature and inexpensive optical subsystems for use in automated instruments. For example, a single light source can be multiplexed with multiple detectors by fiber optics for optimal positioning of the source and detectors in an automated system (see Chapter 11). Disadvantages of fiber optics include greater amounts of stray light; refractive index changes in the glass, quartz, or plastic rods; and the loss of transmitted energy after continued use in the UV region of the spectrum. This loss of energy is known as solarization and results in a decrease in the optical sensitivity of an instrument.

Cuvets

A cuvet (also often termed a cuvette) is a small vessel used to hold a liquid sample to be analyzed in the light path of a spectrometer. Cuvets may be round, square, or rectangular and are constructed from glass, silica (quartz), or plastic. Square or rectangular cuvets have plane-parallel optical surfaces and a constant light path. The most popular have a 1.0-cm light path, held to close tolerances. Ordinary borosilicate glass cuvets are suitable for measurements in the visible portion of the spectrum. For readings below 340 nm, however, quartz cells are usually required. Some plastic cells have good clarity in both the visible and UV range but can present problems relating to tolerances, cleaning, etching by solvents, and temperature deformations. Many of the plastic cuvets are designed for disposable, single-use applications.

Cuvets must be clean and optically clear, as etching or deposits on the surface affect absorbance values. Cuvets used in the visible range are cleaned by copious rinsing with tap water and distilled water. Alkaline solutions should not be left standing in cuvets for prolonged periods, because alkali slowly dissolves glass and produces etching. Cuvets may be cleaned in mild detergent or soaked in a mixture of concentrated HCl : water : ethanol (1:3:4). Cuvets should never be soaked in dichromate cleaning solution, because the solution is hazardous and tends to adsorb onto and discolor the glass.

Cuvets used for measurements in the UV region should be handled with special care. Invisible scratches, fingerprints, or residual traces of previously measured substances may be present and absorb significantly. A good practice is to fill all such cuvets with distilled water and measure the absorbance for each against a reference blank over the wavelengths to be used. This value should be essentially zero.

Photodetectors

Photodetectors are devices that convert light into an electric signal that is proportional to the number of photons striking its photosensitive surface. The photomultiplier tube is a commonly used photodetector for measuring light intensity in the UV and visible regions of the spectrum. Photodiodes are solid-state devices that are also used in modern instruments. In older instruments, barrier layer cells (also known as photovoltaic cells) were used as photodetectors, because they were rugged and less expensive.[5]

Photomultiplier Tubes. A photomultiplier tube (PMT) contains a cathode, a light-sensitive metal, and a series of dynodes all of which are enclosed in an evacuated glass enclosure. As many as 10 to 15 stages or dynodes are present in common photomultipliers. Photons that strike the photoemissive cathode emit electrons that are accelerated toward the dynodes. Additional electrons are generated at each dynode. This cascading effect creates 10^5 to 10^7 electrons for each photon hitting the first cathode depending on the number of dynodes and the accelerating voltage. This amplified signal is finally collected at the anode where it can be measured.

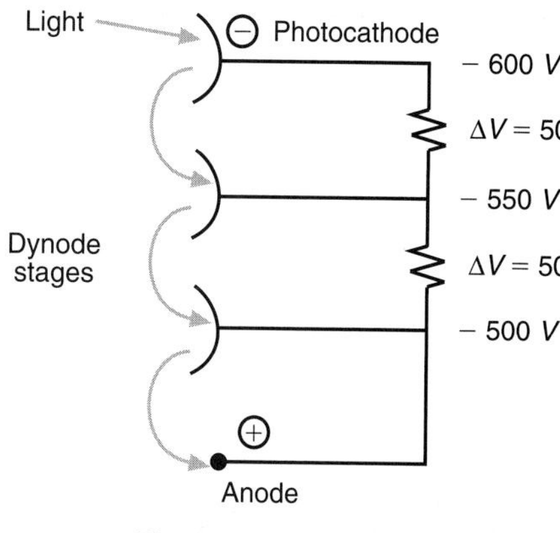

Figure 3-9 Schematic diagrams of a glass photomultiplier tube.

When operating such a tube, voltage is applied between the photocathode and each successive stage. The normal increment of voltage increase of each photomultiplier stage is from 50 to 100 V larger than that of the previous stage (Figure 3-9). Typically, a conventional PMT tube has approximately 1500 V applied to it.

PMTs have extremely rapid response times, are very sensitive, and are slow to fatigue. Because these tubes have excellent sensitivity and rapid response, they must be carefully shielded from all stray light and daylight. A PMT with the voltage applied should never be exposed to room light because it will burn out. Because of the fast response time of the PMT, this detector is readily used with interrupted light beams such as those produced by choppers, and it therefore has significant advantages when used as a UV-visible detector in spectrophotometers. The rapid response times are needed when a spectrophotometer is being used to determine an absorption spectrum of a compound. PMTs also have adequate sensitivity over a wide range of wavelengths.

When voltage is applied to a PMT in the absence of any incident light, some current is usually produced. This current is called *dark current.* It is desirable to have the dark current of a PMT at its lowest level because this current is also amplified and appears as background noise.

Photodiodes. Photodiodes are solid-state photodetectors that are fabricated from photosensitive semiconductor materials such as silicon, gallium arsenide, indium antimonide, indium arsenide, lead selenide, and lead sulfide. These materials absorb light over a characteristic wavelength range (e.g., 250 nm to 1100 nm for silicon). Their development and use as detectors in spectrophotometers have resulted in instruments capable of measuring light at a multitude of wavelengths. When a photodetector consists of two-dimensional arrays of diodes, each of which responds to a specific wavelength, it is known as photodiode array. For example, photodiode arrays have been designed to have a 2-nm resolution per diode from 200 to 340 nm, and a 1-nm resolution per diode from 340 to 800 nm.

In practice, all diodes are initially charged to 5 V, and they discharge when they are struck by light. Each diode is then sequentially scanned and recharged to 5 V. The amount of energy required for recharging is proportional to the quantity of light striking that diode. Because scan time for all diodes is in the millisecond range, many scans can be taken. The resultant data can be processed using a variety of algorithms, including signal averaging, background subtraction, and correction for scattered light. Consequently, an optical spectrum of an ongoing chemical reaction can be monitored as a function of time with a high degree of resolution and accuracy.

Readout Devices

Electrical energy from a detector is displayed on some type of meter or readout system. In the past analog devices were widely used as readout devices in spectrophotometers. However, they have been replaced by digital readout devices that provide a visual numerical display of absorbance or converted values of concentrations. These operate on the principle of selective illumination of portions of a bank of light-emitting diodes (LEDs), controlled by the voltage signal generated. Visible LEDs incorporate gallium as the major component, and at present, $GaAs_xP_x$ diodes that emit red light are most widely used. Compared with meters, the digital readout devices have faster response and are easier to read.

Microprocessors

Microprocessors are incorporated into both photometers and spectrophotometers. With a resident microprocessor and software, output from a calibrator is digitally stored, digital signals from blanks are subtracted from calibrators and unknowns, and the concentration of unknowns automatically calculated. Data from multiple calibrators may be used to store a complete calibration curve, display or print out the curve for visible inspection, and calculate results of unknowns based on the curve or some mathematical transformation of the data. A microprocessor and its resident software are also used to convert kinetic data into concentration or enzyme activity.

Recorders

Spectrophotometers may be equipped with recorders in addition to or instead of a digital display. These are synchronized to provide line traces of transmittance or absorbance as a function of either time or wavelength. When a continuous tracing of absorbance versus wavelength is recorded, the resultant figure is called an *absorption spectrum*. If a substance absorbs light, distinct peaks of absorbance will be observed (see Figure 3-1). Measuring the absorption spectra of an unknown sample and comparing them with spectra from known compounds is very useful for qualitative purposes. For example, this type of procedure is especially useful for identification of drugs that absorb in the UV region. Several criteria are used, including determination of those wavelengths showing maximum and minimum absorbance in both dilute acid and alkaline solutions; absorptivity at the wavelength of maximum absorbance; and ratios of absorbance at two wavelengths. Finally, the entire spectrum is compared with that of a known sample of the suspected drug.

Performance Parameters

In most spectrophotometric analytical procedures, the absorbance of an unknown is compared directly with that of a calibrator or series of calibrators. Under these circumstances, minor errors in wavelength calibration, variation in spectral bandwidths, or presence of stray light are compensated for and do not usually contribute serious errors. Use of a series of calibrators covering a wide range of concentrations also provides a measure of linearity (i.e., agreement with Beer's law for a given procedure and instrument). When calculations are based on published or previously determined values for molar absorptivities or absorption coefficients, however, the spectrophotometer must be checked more rigorously. Performance verification of spectrophotometers on a periodic basis also improves reliability of routine comparative analyses.

To verify that a spectrophotometer is performing satisfactorily, the device must be shown to be able to operate within the specifications provided for it. Parameters to be tested include (1) wavelength accuracy, (2) spectral bandwidth, (3) stray light, (4) linearity, and (5) photometric accuracy.

The National Institute of Standards and Technology (NIST), formerly the National Bureau of Standards (NBS), provides several standard reference materials (SRMs) for spectrophotometry that are useful in the calibration or verification of the performance of photometers or spectrophotometers (e.g., SRM 930e is for the verification and calibration of the transmittance and absorbance scales of visible absorption spectrometers) (see http://www.nist.gov).

The Institute for Reference Materials and Measurements (IRMM), a metrology institute that belongs to the European Commission, also provides reference materials for verification of the performance of photometers or spectrophotometers. These materials are listed in the IRMM BCR Reference Materials Catalogue (http://www.irmm.jrc.be/).

Wavelength Calibration

For many analytical purposes, the calibration wavelength chosen may be satisfactory if it is close to the λ_{max} of the chromogen being measured and the wavelength is reproducible. Most filters fall into this category and are quite satisfactory because unknowns are compared with calibrators at a fixed wavelength and spectral bandwidth. With prisms

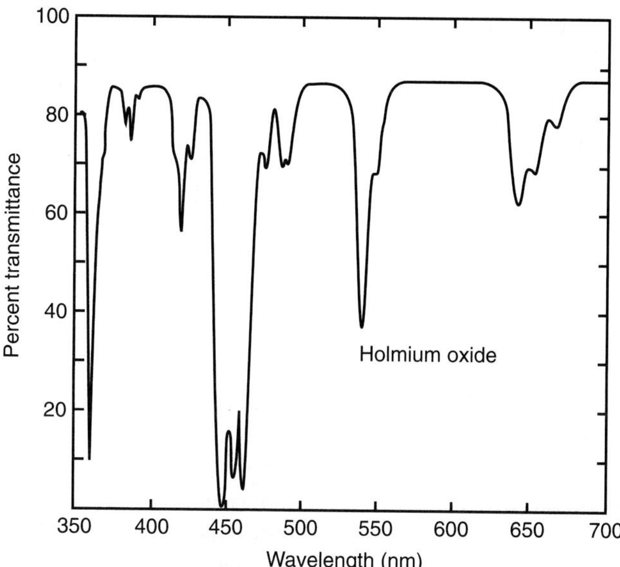

Figure 3-10 Spectral transmittance curve of holmium oxide filter.

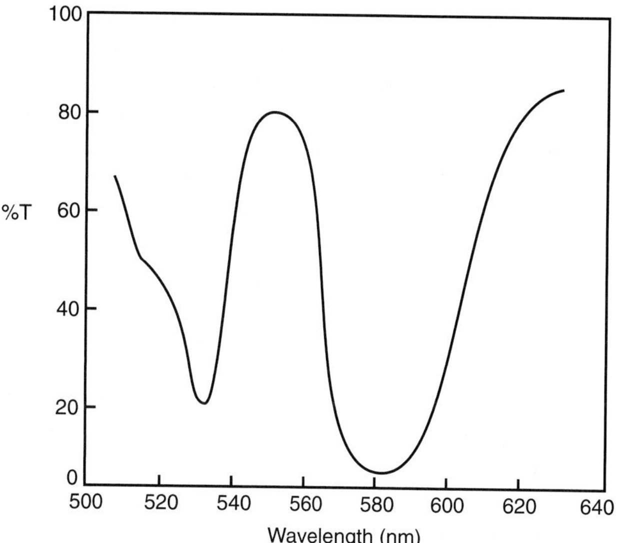

Figure 3-11 Spectral transmittance curve of a didymium filter. *(Perkin-Elmer Model 35 spectrophotometer, 8-nm nominal spectral bandwidth.)*

and diffraction gratings, however, a continuous choice of wavelengths is available, and it becomes necessary to verify their accuracy and reproducibility. Knowledge of exact wavelength becomes critical when using published molar absorptivities for identification of substances in toxicological studies and in the use of differential absorption techniques. Enzyme assays using the NAD-NADH reaction, for example, are based on a molar absorptivity constant for NADH of 6.22 $\times 10^3$ at 339 nm (340 nm). The wavelength settings therefore must be accurate and reproducible, and the instrument must show spectrophotometric accuracy if the constant is to be used in results calculation.

For the narrow-spectral-bandwidth instruments, a *holmium oxide glass* may be scanned over the range of 280 to 650 nm. This material shows very sharp absorbance peaks at defined wavelengths, and the operator may compare the wavelength scale readings that produce maximum absorbance with established values. Should these not coincide, a calibration curve can be constructed to relate scale readings to true wavelengths. A typical spectral transmittance curve for holmium oxide glass is shown in Figure 3-10. Selected absorption peaks for this filter, which are suitable for calibration purposes, occur at the following wavelengths: 279.3, 418.5, 287.6, 536.4, 333.8, 637.5, and 360.8 nm. Solutions of holmium oxide in dilute perchloric acid have also been recommended and may be used with any spectrophotometer.

With broader-bandpass instruments, a didymium filter may be used to verify wavelength settings. This filter should show a minimum percent transmittance at 530 nm against an air blank (Figure 3-11). Because didymium has several absorption peaks, the setting should be verified grossly by visual examination of transmitted light. This light should appear green at 530 nm.

Spectral Bandwidth

The spectral bandwidth of a spectrophotometer is measured by use of a mercury-vapor lamp, which shows a number of sharp, well-defined emission lines between 250 and 580 nm. The apparent width of an emission band at half-peak height is taken to be the spectral bandwidth of the instrument (see Figure 3-7). The spectral bandwidth may also be calculated from the manufacturer's specifications. Interference filters with spectral bandwidths of 1 to 2 nm are available and may be used to check those instruments with a nominal spectral bandwidth of 8 nm or more.

Stray Light

Stray light, in general terms, is radiation of wavelengths outside the narrow band nominally transmitted by the monochromator. A perfect monochromator would transmit light only within its passband. In practice, scattering and diffraction inside the monochromator introduce light of other wavelengths into the exit beam. This light is further modified by other components of the spectrophotometer and by the sample itself. Stray light is usually defined as a ratio or percent of the stray light to the total detected light.

Other sources of unwanted light include light leaks and fluorescence of the sample. Light leaks should be excluded by covering the cell compartments. Light arising from fluorescence can increase the signal to the detector and cause an apparent decrease in absorbance. These sources of light are not included in the usual definition of stray light.

The major effect of stray light on the performance of a spectrophotometer is an absorbance error, especially in the upper end of the absorbance range of the instrument. Most spectrophotometers are equipped with one or more stray-light filters. Thus a blue filter is used with a tungsten lamp for wavelength settings below about 400 nm. When the spectrophotometer is set to 350 nm, for example, most of the stray light is of wavelengths in the visible range. The blue filter absorbs most of the visible light but transmits well in this UV portion of the spectrum. By analogy, a red filter is used for wavelengths in the range of 650 to 800 nm.

A cutoff filter is satisfactory for the detection of stray light. These may be of glass, similar to the stray-light filters discussed previously, and produce a sharp cut in the spectrum with almost complete absorption on one side and high transmittance on the other. Liquid cutoff filters are satisfactory and convenient in the UV range where stray light is usually more of a problem. A 50 g/L aqueous solution of sodium nitrite should show essentially 0% T when read against water over the range of 300 to 385 nm. Acetone, read against water, should show 0% T over the range of 250 to 320 nm.

Linearity

For a spectrophotometer to give accurate absorbance measurements throughout its absorbance range, a linear relationship should exist between the light absorbed and the instrument readout. Various liquid solutions have been used to check instrument linearity. Several sources of error may be encountered in this type of reference material, such as dilution errors and errors from lack of stability, shifts in pH, and temperature effects. An alternative procedure is to use a solid glass filter that, at a given wavelength, has an absorbance that is a small fraction of the total linear range of the instrument. The didymium filter in Figure 3-11 has an absorbance of approximately 0.09 at 550 nm and is satisfactory for establishing linearity. Linearity is satisfactory as long as the ΔA increments remain constant. The same general procedure may be used with a suitable filter on those spectrophotometers in which the blank reference settings can be adjusted in steps up to approximately 1 unit of absorbance.

Photometric Accuracy

Solutions of potassium dichromate ($K_2Cr_2O_7$) are also used for overall checks on photometric accuracy. These also provide an indication of wavelength calibration, linearity, cuvet light path, and freedom from stray light in the UV region.

In practice, analytical reagent grade $K_2Cr_2O_7$ is dried at 110 °C for 1 hour. The following solutions in 0.005 mol/L sulfuric acid are prepared:

Solution A: 0.0500 g/L for the absorbance range from 0.2 to 0.7

Solution B: 0.1000 g/L for the absorbance range from 0.4 to 1.4

Measurements should be made in 10-mm cells with the temperature controlled in the range of 15 to 25 °C, using 0.005 mol/L sulfuric acid as the reference. Table 3-4 gives the expected values for the two absorbance maxima and minima of the solutions based on literature values. Because the natural bandwidth of solution A at 350 nm is approximately 63 nm, the values shown apply strictly to spectrophotometers with a spectral bandwidth of 6 nm or less.

Multiple-Wavelength Readings

Background interference can often be eliminated or minimized either by inclusion of blanks or by reading absorbance at two or three wavelengths. In one approach, termed "bichromatic," absorbance is measured at two wavelengths, one corresponding to peak absorbance and another at a point near the base of the peak to serve as a baseline. The difference in absorbance at the two wavelengths is related to concentration. In effect, this provides a blank reference point for each individual sample. Another method to correct for background interference is to measure absorbance at the peak wavelength and at two other wavelengths equidistant from the peak. Values for the latter are averaged to obtain a baseline under the peak, which is then subtracted from the peak reading. The value thus obtained is known as a "corrected" absorbance and can be related to the concentration, provided that the background absorbance is linear with wavelength over the region in which readings are made. This correction also must be applied to absorbances obtained from calibrators.

Before the correction is used, knowledge of the shape of the absorption curve for the substance of interest and of the interference is required. The linearity of the baseline shift should be verified by measuring the absorption spectrum of commonly encountered interferences. Care should be exercised in the use of the correction because if it is not properly used, it may introduce larger errors than would be observed without correction. For example, such a situation may occur if the background reading is not linear over the region measured.

REFLECTANCE PHOTOMETRY

In *reflectance photometry,* diffuse reflected light is measured.[5] The reflected light results from illumination, with diffused light, of a reaction mixture in a carrier or from the diffusion

TABLE 3-4 Recommended Absorbance Values for Acidic Potassium Dichromate Solutions

Wavelength (nm)	Absorbance	
	Solution A	Solution B
235 (min)	0.626 ± 0.009	1.251 ± 0.019
257 (max)	0.727 ± 0.007	1.454 ± 0.015
313 (min)	0.244 ± 0.004	0.488 ± 0.007
350 (max)	0.536 ± 0.005	1.071 ± 0.011

of light by a reaction mixture in an illuminated carrier. The intensity of the reflected light from the reagent carrier is compared with the intensity of light reflected from a reference surface. Because the intensity of reflected light is nonlinear in relation to the concentration of the analyte, either the Kubelka-Munk equation or the Clapper-Williams transformation is commonly used to convert the data into a linear format (see Chapter 11). The electro-optical components used in reflectance photometry are essentially the same as those required for absorbance photometry. Reflectance photometry is used as the measurement method with dry-film chemistry systems (see Chapter 11).

FLAME EMISSION SPECTROPHOTOMETRY

Flame emission spectrophotometry is based on the characteristic emission of light by atoms of many metallic elements when given sufficient energy, such as that supplied by a hot flame. The wavelength to be used for the measurement of an element depends on the selection of a line of sufficient intensity to provide adequate sensitivity and freedom from other interfering lines at or near the selected wavelength. For example, lithium produces a red, sodium a yellow, potassium a violet, rubidium a red, and magnesium a blue color in a flame. These colors are characteristic of the metal atoms that are present as cations in solution. Under constant and controlled conditions, the light intensity of the characteristic wavelength produced by each of the atoms is directly proportional to the number of atoms that are emitting energy, which in turn is directly proportional to the concentration of the substance of interest in the sample. Although this technique once was widely used for the analysis of sodium, potassium, and lithium in body fluids, it now has been replaced largely by electrochemical techniques.

For additional information on this technique, the reader is referred to an earlier version of this chapter.[5]

ATOMIC ABSORPTION SPECTROPHOTOMETRY

Atomic absorption (AA) spectrophotometry is used widely in clinical laboratories to measure elements such as aluminum, calcium, copper, lead, lithium, magnesium, zinc, and other metals.

BASIC CONCEPTS

Atomic absorption is an emission technique in which an element in the sample is excited and the radiant energy given off measured as the element returns to its lower energy level. However, the element is not appreciably excited in the flame, but is merely dissociated from its chemical bonds (atomized) and placed in an unexcited or ground state (neutral atom). Thus, the atom is at a low energy level in which it is capable of absorbing radiation at a very narrow bandwidth corresponding to its own line spectrum. A hollow cathode lamp with the cathode made of the material to be analyzed is used to produce a wavelength of light specific for the material. Thus, if the cathode were made of sodium, sodium light at predominantly 589 nm would be emitted by the lamp. When the light from the hollow-cathode lamp enters the flame, some of it is absorbed by the ground-state atoms in the flame, resulting in a net decrease in the intensity of the beam from the lamp. This process is referred to as *atomic absorption*.

The process is analogous to absorption spectrophotometry. For example, a specific hollow-cathode lamp serves as the light source, and the sample heated in the flame replaces the sample in the cuvet. The pathlength of the flame is analogous to the light path through the cuvet. As noted previously, only a small fraction of the sample in the flame contributes emission energy, and only a fraction of this is transmitted to the detector. Hence, most of the atoms are in the ground state and are able to absorb light emitted by the cathode lamp. In general, AA methods are approximately 100 times more sensitive than flame emission methods. In addition, owing to the unique specificity of the wavelength from the hollow-cathode lamp, these methods are highly specific for the element being measured.

INSTRUMENTATION

Figure 3-12 shows the basic components of an AA spectrophotometer. The basic component of such an instrument is the hollow-cathode lamp made of the metal of the substance to be analyzed and is different for each metal analysis. In some cases, an alloy is used to make the cathode, resulting in a multielement lamp.

The hollow-cathode lamp usually contains argon or neon gas at a pressure of a few millimeters of mercury. An argon-filled lamp produces a blue-to-purple glow during operation, and the neon produces a reddish-orange glow inside the hollow-cathode lamp. Quartz, or special glass that allows transmission of the proper wavelength, is used as a window. A current is applied between the two electrodes inside the hollow-cathode lamp, and metal is sputtered from the cathode into the gases inside the glass envelope. When

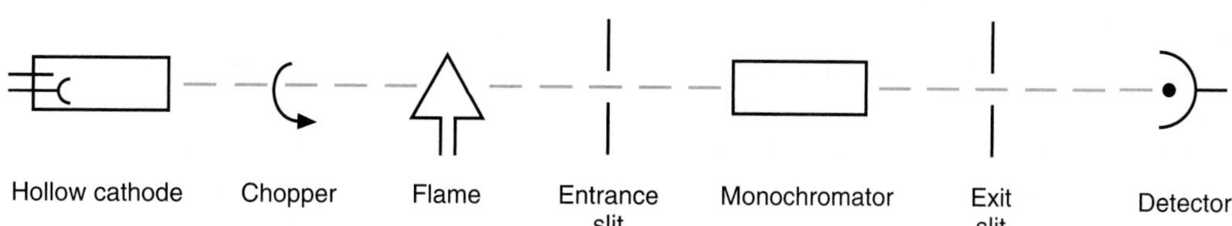

Figure 3-12 Basic components of an atomic absorption spectrophotometer.

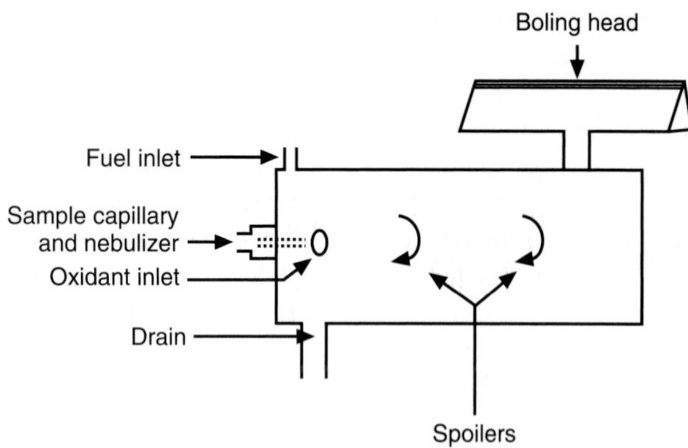

Figure 3-13 Laminar flow burner.

the metal atoms collide with the neon or argon gases, they lose energy and emit their characteristic radiation. Calcium has a sharp, intense, analytical emission line at 422.7 nm, which is most frequently used for calcium analysis. In an interference-free system, only calcium atoms absorb the calcium light from the hollow cathode as it passes through the flame.

An electric beam chopper and a tuned amplifier are incorporated into most AA instruments. Operationally, the power to the hollow-cathode lamp is pulsed so that the light is emitted by the lamp at a certain number of pulses per second. On the other hand, all of the light coming from the flame is continuous. When light leaves the flame, it is composed of pulsed, unabsorbed light from the lamp and a small amount of unpulsed flame spectrum and sample emission. The detector senses all light, but the amplifier is electrically tuned to accept only pulsed signals. In this way, the electronics in conjunction with the monochromator discriminate between the flame spectrum and sample emission.

Figure 3-13 shows a laminar flow premix burner and illustrates how the sample is aspirated, volatilized, and burned. Note that the gases are mixed and the sample is atomized before being burned. An advantage of this system is that the larger droplets go to waste while the fine mist enters the flame, thus producing a less noisy signal. In addition, the path length through the flame of the burner is longer than that of the total consumption burner. This produces a greater absorption and increases the sensitivity of the measurement. A disadvantage of the premix burner is that the flame usually is not as hot as that of the total consumption burner, and thus it cannot sufficiently dissociate certain metal complexes in the flame (e.g., calcium-phosphate complexes).

In *flameless AA* techniques (carbon rod or "graphite furnace"), the sample is placed in a depression on a carbon rod in an enclosed chamber. Strips of tantalum or platinum metal may also be used as sample cups. In successive steps, the temperature of the rod is raised to dry, char, and finally atomize the sample into the chamber. The atomized element then absorbs energy from the corresponding hollow-cathode lamp. This approach is more sensitive than the conventional flame methods and permits determination of trace metals in small samples of blood or tissue.

With flameless AA, a novel approach has been used to correct for background absorption called the Zeeman correction.[17] In Zeeman background correction, either the light source or the atomizer is placed in a strong magnetic field. In practice, because Zeeman correction requires special lamps, the analyte is placed in the magnetic field. The intense magnetic field splits the degenerate (i.e., of equal energy) atomic energy levels into two components that are polarized parallel and perpendicular to the magnetic field, respectively. The parallel component is at the resonance line of the source, whereas the two perpendicular components are shifted to different wavelengths. The two components interact differently with polarized light. A polarizer is placed between the source and the atomizer, and two absorption measurements are taken at different polarizer settings. One measures both analyte and background absorptions, A_t, the other only the background absorption, A_{bc}. The difference between the two absorption readings is the corrected absorbance.

The major advantage of the Zeeman correction method is that the same light source at the same wavelength is used to measure the total and the background absorption. The implementation is complex and expensive, and the strength of the magnetic field needs to be optimized for every element, but the method gives more accurate results at higher background levels than the other correction techniques.

Interferences in Atomic Absorption Spectrophotometry

Interferences in AA spectroscopy are divided into spectral and nonspectral interferences.

Spectral Interferences

Spectral interferences include absorption by other closely absorbing atomic species, absorption by molecular species, scattering by nonvolatile salt particles or oxides, and background emission (which can be electronically filtered). Absorption by other atomic species usually is not a problem because of the extremely narrow bandwidth (0.01 nm) used in the absorption measurements. Absorption and scattering by molecular species are particularly problematic at lower atomizing temperatures.

Nonspectral Interferences

Nonspectral interferences are either nonspecific or specific. *Nonspecific interferences* affect the nebulization by altering the viscosity, surface tension, or density of the analyte solution, and consequently the sample flow rate. Certain contaminants also decrease the desolvation and atomization efficiency by lowering the atomizer temperature. *Specific interferences* are also called chemical interferences because they are more analyte dependent. *Solute volatilization inter-*

ference refers to the situation when the contaminant forms nonvolatile species with the analyte. An example is the phosphate interference in the determination of calcium that is caused by the formation of calcium-phosphate complexes. The phosphate interference is overcome by adding a cation, usually lanthanum or strontium, that competes with calcium for the phosphate. Enhancement effects are also observed in which the addition of contaminants increases the volatilization efficiency. Such is the case with aluminum, which normally forms nonvolatile oxides but in the presence of hydrofluoric acid forms more volatile aluminum fluoride. *Dissociation interferences* affect the degree of dissociation of the analyte. Analytes that form oxides or hydroxides are especially susceptible to dissociation interferences. *Ionization interference* occurs when the presence of an easily ionized element, such as K, affects the degree of ionization of the analyte, which leads to changes in the analyte signal. In case of *excitation interference*, the analyte atoms are excited in the atomizer, with a subsequent emission at the absorption wavelength. This type of interference is more pronounced at higher temperatures.

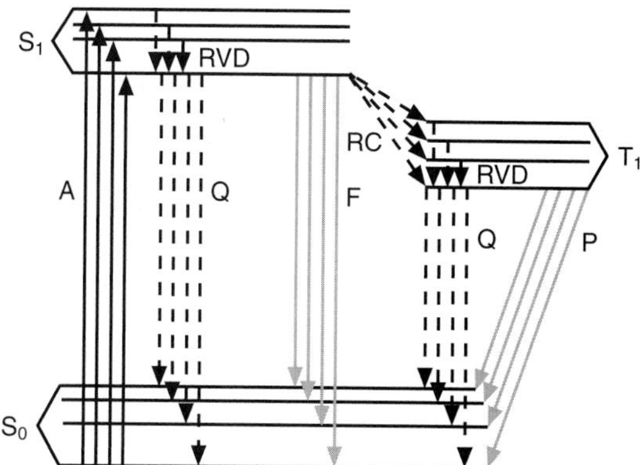

Figure 3-14 Luminescence energy-level diagram of typical organic molecule. S_0 is the ground level singlet state; S_1 is the first excited singlet state; A is the absorption process; T_1 is the first excited triplet state; and RVD is the radiationless vibrational deactivation. Q is quenching of the excited singlet or triplet state. F is the fluorescence process from the first excited singlet state. P is the phosphorescence process from the first excited triplet state. RC is the radiationless crossover from the first excited singlet state to the first excited triplet state.

FLUOROMETRY

Fluorescence occurs when a molecule absorbs light at one wavelength and reemits light at a longer wavelength. An atom or molecule that fluoresces is termed a fluorophore. *Fluorometry* is defined as the measurement of the emitted fluorescence light. Fluorometric analysis is a widely used method of quantitative analysis in the chemical and biological sciences; it is accurate and very sensitive.

BASIC CONCEPTS

Figure 3-14 diagrammatically illustrates the relationship between absorption, fluorescence, and phosphorescence. As indicated, each molecule contains a series of closely spaced energy levels. Absorption of a quantum of light energy by a molecule causes the transition of an electron from the singlet ground state to one of a number of possible vibrational levels of its first singlet state. The actual number of molecules in the excited state under typical reaction conditions and excited with a typical 150-W light source is very small and is estimated to be about 10^{-13} mole per mole of fluorophore. Once the molecule is in an excited state, there are several ways it can return to its original energy state. These include radiationless vibrational equilibration, the fluorescence process, quenching of the excited singlet state, radiationless crossover to a triplet state, quenching of the first triplet state, and the phosphorescence process.

As shown in Figure 3-14, vibrational equilibration before fluorescence results in some loss of the excitation energy. The emitted fluorescence light is therefore of less energy or has a longer wavelength than the excitation light. The difference between the maximum wavelength of the excitation light and the maximum wavelength of the emitted fluorescence light is a constant referred to as the "Stokes shift." This constant is a measure of the energy lost during the lifetime of the excited state (radiationless vibrational deactivation) before return to the ground singlet level (fluorescence emission).

Time Relationships of Fluorescence Emission

The time required for a molecule to absorb radiant energy and to be promoted to an excited state is approximately 10^{-15} s. The length of time for vibrational equilibration to occur to the lowest excited state is of the order of 10^{-14} to 10^{-12} s. The length of time required for fluorescence emission to occur is of the order of 10^{-8} to 10^{-7} s. Relatively speaking, there is a considerable time delay between the absorption of light energy, the return to the lowest excited state, and the emission of fluorescence light. This time relationship is shown in Figure 3-15. Phase I in Figure 3-15 represents the time period between absorbance of light energy and radiationless loss of energy during vibrational rearrangement to the lowest excited energy state. This time period is represented by the up and down arrows in the diagram. Phase II shows the emission and decay of a short-lived (b) and a longer-lived (a) fluorophore. If the fluorescence emission is measured over time following a pulse of light from an excitation source, such as a xenon lamp or laser, the intensity of the emitted light decays as a first-order process similar to radioactive decay (i.e., phase II of Figure 3-15). The time required for the emitted light to reach 1/e of its initial intensity, where e is the Naperian base 2.718, is called the average lifetime of the excited state of the molecule, or the fluorescence decay time.

The time delay between absorption of quanta of energy and fluorescence is used in fluorescence instrumentation called time-resolved fluorometers.[9] The advantage of a time-resolved fluorometer is the elimination of background light

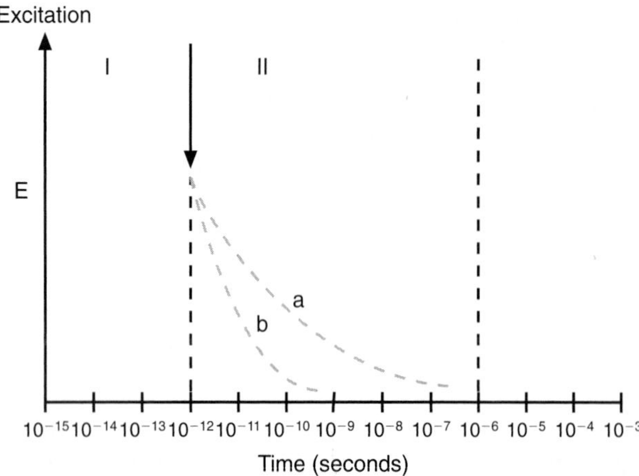

Figure 3-15 Fluorescence decay process: E is the absorption of energy; I is the vibrational deactivation time phase; II is the fluorescence emission time phase; a is long fluorescence decay time; and b is short fluorescence decay time.

scattering due to Rayleigh and Raman signals and short-lived fluorescence background with consequent dramatic increase in signal-to-noise and detection sensitivity.

Time-resolved fluorometry[3] falls into one of two categories, depending on how the fluorescence emission response is measured: (1) pulse fluorometry, in which the sample is illuminated with an intense brief pulse of light and the intensity of the resulting fluorescence emission is measured as a function of time with a fast detector system, or (2) phase fluorometry, in which a continuous-wave laser illuminates the sample, and the fluorescence emission response is monitored for impulse and frequency response.[9]

Relationship of Concentration and Fluorescence Intensity

The relationship of concentration to intensity of fluorescence emission is derived from the Beer-Lambert law. By expansion through a Taylor series, rearrangement, logarithm base conversion, and basic assumptions about dilute solutions, the following equation is obtained:

$$F = \phi I_0 abc \tag{12}$$

where

F = relative intensity

ϕ = fluorescence efficiency (i.e., the ratio between quanta of light emitted and quanta of light absorbed)

I_0 = initial excitation intensity

a = molar absorptivity

b = volume element defined by geometry of the excitation and emission slits

c = the concentration in mol/L

Equation (12) indicates that fluorescence intensity is directly proportional to the concentration of the fluorophore and the excitation intensity. This relationship holds only for dilute solutions, where absorbance is less than 2% of the exciting radiation; the fluorescence intensity becomes nonlinear as the absorbance of the solution increases above 2% of the exciting radiation. This phenomenon is called the *inner filter effect*, and it is discussed in more detail in a later section. Other factors influencing the measurement of fluorescence intensity are the sensitivity of the detector and the degree of background light scatter seen by the detector.

Fluorescence intensity measurements are more sensitive than absorbance measurements. The magnitude of absorbance of a chromophore in solution is determined by its concentration and the path length of the cuvet. The magnitude of fluorescence intensity of a fluorophore is determined by its concentration, the path length, and the intensity of the light source. The sensitivity of fluorescence measurements can be 100 to 1000 times greater than the sensitivity of absorbance measurements through the use of more intense light sources, digital signal filtering techniques, and sensitive emission photometers. All of these are incorporated in conventional spectrofluorometric instrumentation, described later in this chapter.

Frequently, fluorescence measurements are expressed in relative intensity units. The word relative is used because the intensity measured is not an absolute quantity. It is a small part of the total fluorescence emission, and its magnitude is defined by the instrument slit width, detector sensitivity, monochromator efficiency, and excitation intensity. Because these are instrument-related variables, establishing an absolute intensity unit for a given concentration of a fluorophore that is valid from instrument to instrument is difficult, if not impossible.

Fluorescence Polarization

Light is composed of electrical and magnetic waves at right angles to each other. Light waves produced by standard excitation sources have their electrical vectors oriented randomly. Light waves, passed through certain crystalline materials (polarizers), have their electrical vectors oriented in a single plane and are said to be plane-polarized. Fluorophores absorb light most efficiently in the plane of their electronic energy levels. If their rotational relaxation (Brownian movement) is slower than their fluorescence decay time, as is the case for large fluorescent-labeled molecules, the emitted fluorescence light will be polarized. Because small molecules have rotational relaxation times that are much shorter than their fluorescence decay time, their emitted fluorescence light is depolarized. However, if the small fluorescent molecule is attached to a macromolecule or if it is placed in a viscous solution, the small molecule will emit polarized light. Fluorescence polarization, P, is defined by the following equation:

$$P = \frac{(I_v - I_h)}{(I_v + I_h)} \tag{13}$$

where

I_v = intensity of the emitted fluorescence light in the vertical plane

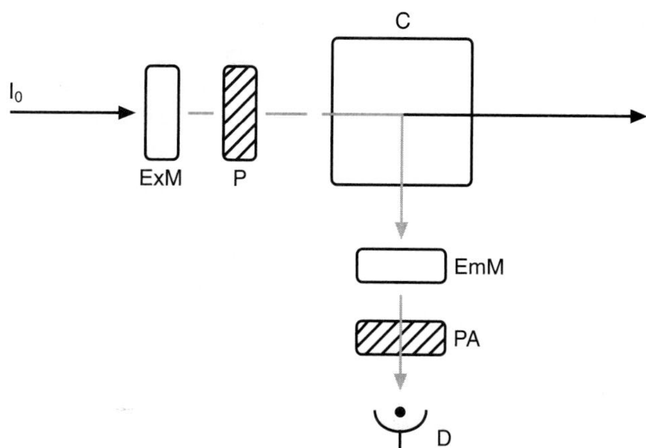

Figure 3-16 Schematic diagram of a fluorescence polarization analyzer. P is the polarizer to provide polarized excitation light. PA is the polarizer analyzer, which is rotated to provide the measurement of parallel and perpendicular polarized fluorescence-emission intensity. ExM is the excitation monochromator, EmM is the emission monochromator, D is the detector, and C is the reaction cell or cuvet.

I_h = intensity of the emitted fluorescence light in the horizontal plane

As indicated, P is the difference between the two observed intensities divided by their sum. Fluorescence polarization is measured by placing a mechanically or electrically driven polarizer between the sample cuvet and the detector. A diagram of a fluorescence polarization measurement system is shown in Figure 3-16. In the normal instrumentation mode, the sample is excited with polarized light to obtain maximum sensitivity. The polarization analyzer is positioned first to measure the intensity of the emitted fluorescence light in the vertical plane (I_v), and then the polarization analyzer is rotated 90° to measure the emitted fluorescence light intensity in the horizontal plane (I_h). P is then calculated manually or automatically by use of equation (13).

Fluorescence polarization is used to quantitate analytes by use of the change in fluorescence depolarization following immunological reactions (see Chapter 9). Quantitation is accomplished by adding a known quantity of fluorescent-labeled analyte molecules to a reaction solution containing an antibody specific to the analyte. The labeled analyte binds to the antibody and causes a change in its rotational relaxation time, resulting in fluorescence polarization. The addition of a nonlabeled analyte, such as an unknown quantity of a therapeutic drug in a serum specimen, will result in a competition for binding to the antibody with the fluorescent-labeled analyte. This change in binding of the fluorophore-labeled analyte causes a change in fluorescence polarization that is inversely proportional to the amount of analyte contained in a given sample. Because the change in fluorescence polarization is a direct response to the reaction mixture, the bound fluorophore need not be separated from free fluorophore. Thus fluorescence polarization is applicable to homogeneous assays of low-molecular-weight analytes, such as therapeutic drugs.[11]

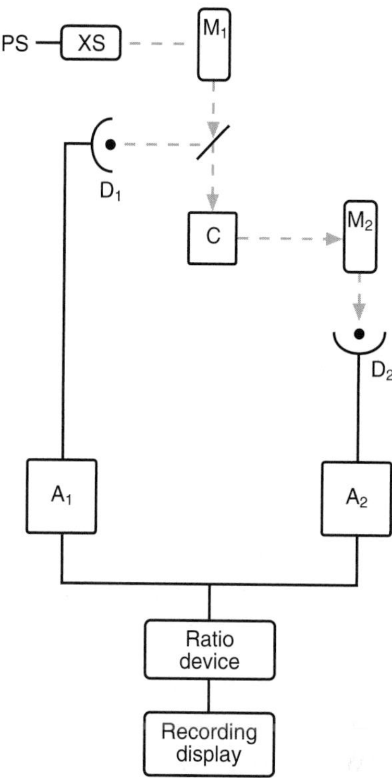

Figure 3-17 Block diagram of a typical spectrofluorometer: XS is the xenon source; PS is the power supply; M_1 is the excitation monochromator; C is the sample cell; M_2 is the emission monochromator. D_1 and D_2 are detectors; D_1 monitors the variation in excitation intensity and D_2 measures fluorescence emission intensity. A_1 and A_2 are excitation signal and emission signal amplifiers, respectively.

INSTRUMENTATION

Fluorometers and spectrofluorometers are used to measure fluorescence. Operationally, a fluorometer uses interference filters or glass filters to produce monochromatic light for sample excitation and for isolation of fluorescence emission, whereas a spectrofluorometer uses a grating or prism monochromator.

Components

Basic components of fluorometers and spectrofluorometers include (1) an excitation source, (2) an excitation monochromator, (3) a cuvet, (4) an emission monochromator, and (5) a detector. In Figure 3-17, these components are shown as they would be configured in a 90° optical system.

Excitation Source

The absorption spectra of most fluorescent compounds of interest are in the spectral region of 300 to 700 nm. The fluorescence emission intensity is proportional to the initial excitation intensity and to concentration and size of the volume element being measured in the sample cell. Therefore, an intense lamp capable of emitting radiant energy over a large spectral region is desirable. Excitation sources used in fluorometers and spectrophotometers include xenon, quartz halogen, and mercury arc lamps and lasers. Some provide high-intensity spectra at one or more wavelengths, while others provide a continuum over the spectral range of interest.

Xenon Lamp. The xenon lamp is a popular excitation source as it provides a continuum of relatively high-intensity radiant energy over the spectral region of 250 to 800 nm. It is widely used for certain fluorescence applications because of its high energy output, stability of lamp flashes, and higher ultraviolet and visible spectral output. These flash lamps can be pulsed at rates up to 2500 pulses per second. Light output is typically in the 0.01- to 0.1-J interval, with a spectral distribution ranging from 250 to 800 nm. The life of flash lamps varies from 10^6 to 10^9 flashes, with the spectral stability being maintained throughout the life of the flash lamp. A limitation of xenon lamps for analytical use is arc wandering or flicker. However, the use of current-stabilized power supplies has minimized this problem and improved the performance of fluorescence instrumentation using xenon lamps.

Lasers. Laser sources (discussed earlier in the Spectrophotometry section) are widely used in fluorescence applications in which highly intense, well-focused, and essentially monochromatic light is required. Examples of these applications include time-resolved fluorometry, flow cytometry, pulsed laser confocal microscopy, laser-induced fluorometry, and light-scattering measurements for particle size and shape. Several different types of lasers are available as an excitation source for fluorescence measurements (see Table 3-3).

Excitation and Emission Monochromator

Monochromators used in fluorescence instrumentation include interference filters, colored glass filters, gratings, and prisms. Most modern analytical instruments using interference filters use the all-dielectric multicavity filter or a hybrid Fabry-Perot coupled-dielectric-layer filter (a filter with metal reflective layers). Either type of filter is combined with appropriate sharp cutoff glass filters to form a single filter package, which removes undesired transmission of higher orders and provides narrow bandwidth, higher peak wavelength transmission, and increased band slope. The increased slope of the spectral band makes the transition from peak transmission to nontransmission more abrupt, which is very important for the spectral separation of excitation and emission bands with a small Stokes shift.

Colored glass filters selectively absorb certain wavelengths of light. These filters have been used for both excitation and emission wavelength selection, but they are more susceptible to transmitting stray light and unwanted fluorescence.

Grating monochromators are devices that isolate regions of the spectrum. The spectral resolution of the light at the slit is a function of the slit width and the resolution of the grating. Spectrofluorometers generally use larger slit widths than absorbance spectrophotometers to obtain higher excitation intensities. An advantage of the grating monochromator is that it provides a selectivity of the excitation and emission wavelengths required when working with new fluorophores with absorbance and emission maxima for which specially fabricated interference filters may not exist. The rotation of the grating is digitally controlled when spectral scans of fluorescence excitation and emission are automated. In the conventional operation of a spectrofluorometer, either the excitation wavelength or the emission wavelength is held constant, and the other is scanned. With more automated instrumentation, both the excitation and emission monochromators are synchronized and scanned together at programmed rates. This provides a change in emission intensity as a function of change in excitation and emission wavelength and gives an additional dimension of specificity to fluorescence measurements. Due to their high degree of monochromaticity, lasers are being used as both the excitation light source and monochromator. When a laser is used as a combination excitation source and monochromator, a narrow-band interference filter is usually placed before the detector to eliminate additional orders of emission.

Cuvet

As with spectrophotometers, cuvets are used in fluorometers and spectrofluorometers to hold the liquid sample to be analyzed. However, with fluorescence instruments, the cuvets used are typically square or rectangular and are constructed from a material that allows the excitation and emitting light to pass (glass or plastic for visible light; quartz for ultraviolet light). However, some plastic cuvets contain ultraviolet absorbers that fluoresce, causing unwanted background signal and loss of sensitivity.

With fluorometers and spectrofluorometers, the placement of the cuvet and excitation beam relative to the photodetector is critical in establishing the optical geometry for fluorescence measurements. As fluorescence light is emitted in all directions from a molecule, several excitation/emission geometries are used to measure fluorescence (Figure 3-18). Most commercial spectrofluorometers and fluorometers use the right angle–detector approach, because it minimizes the background signal that limits analytical sensitivity. The end-on approach allows the adaptation of a fluorescence detector to existing 180° absorption instruments. Its sensitivity is limited by the quality of the excitation and/or emission interference filter pair, the excitation and/or emission spectral band overlap, and the inner filter effect. The front surface approach provides the greatest linearity over a broad range of concentration because it minimizes the inner filter effect.

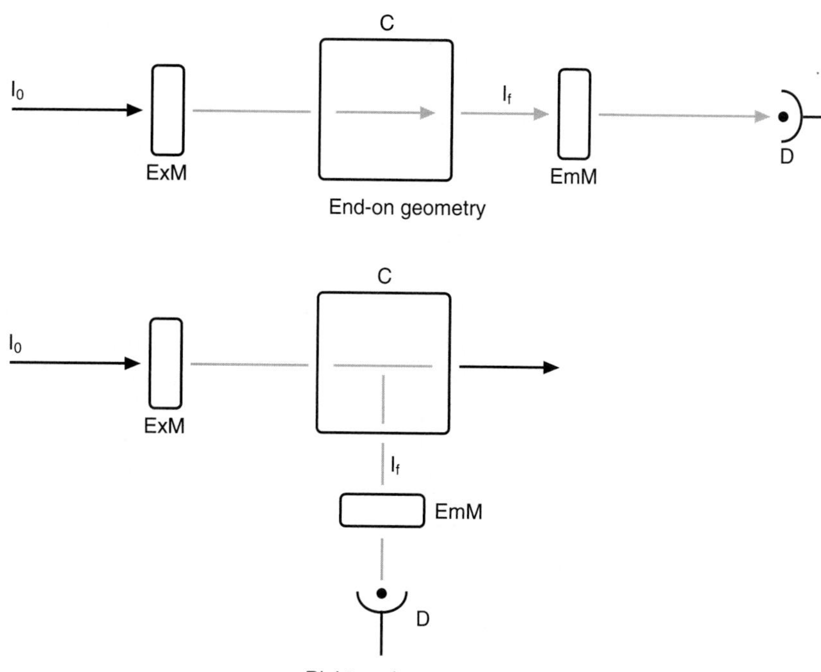

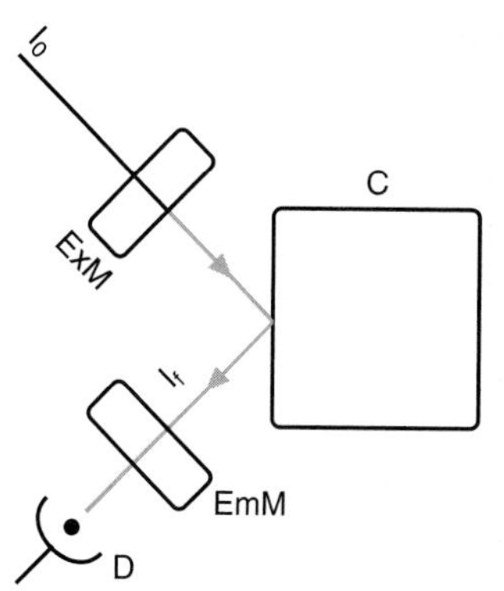

Figure 3-18 Fluorescence excitation/emission geometries: I_0 is the initial excitation energy; ExM is the excitation monochromator; C is the sample cuvet; I_f is the fluorescence intensity; EmM is the emission monochromator; and D is the detector.

The front surface approach shows similar sensitivity to the right angle detectors but is more susceptible to background light scatter. Front surface fluorometry has been widely applied to heterogeneous solid-phase fluorescence immunoassay systems.

To accommodate these different geometries, the sample cell is oriented at different angles in relation to the excitation source and the detector. The major concerns related to the geometry of the sample cell are light scattering, the inner filter effect, and the sample volume element seen by the detector. Figure 3-19 shows the sample cell and slit arrangement for a conventional fluorescence spectrophotometer with the excitation and emission slits oriented at a right angle. S_1 and S_2 designate the excitation and emission slits, respectively. The position of the emission slit and the width of the slit are important. If the emission slit is located near the front edge of the sample cell, as shown in Figure 3-19, *B*, the inner filter effect is minimized. If the emission slit width is increased, sensitivity will increase, but specificity may decrease.

Photodetectors

As with spectrophotometric instruments, a number of devices are used as photodetectors in fluorometric instruments, including the photomultiplier tube (PMT) and charged-coupled detector (CCD). In addition, visual observation is used for some applications.

Visual Observation. Because the human eye is a very sensitive detector with a wide range of spectral recognition, qualitative fluorescent thin-layer methods in the clinical laboratory use short- and long-wavelength ultraviolet lamp source coupled with visual observation.

Photomultiplier Tube. For quantitative assays, the most commonly used detector in fluorometers and spectrofluo-

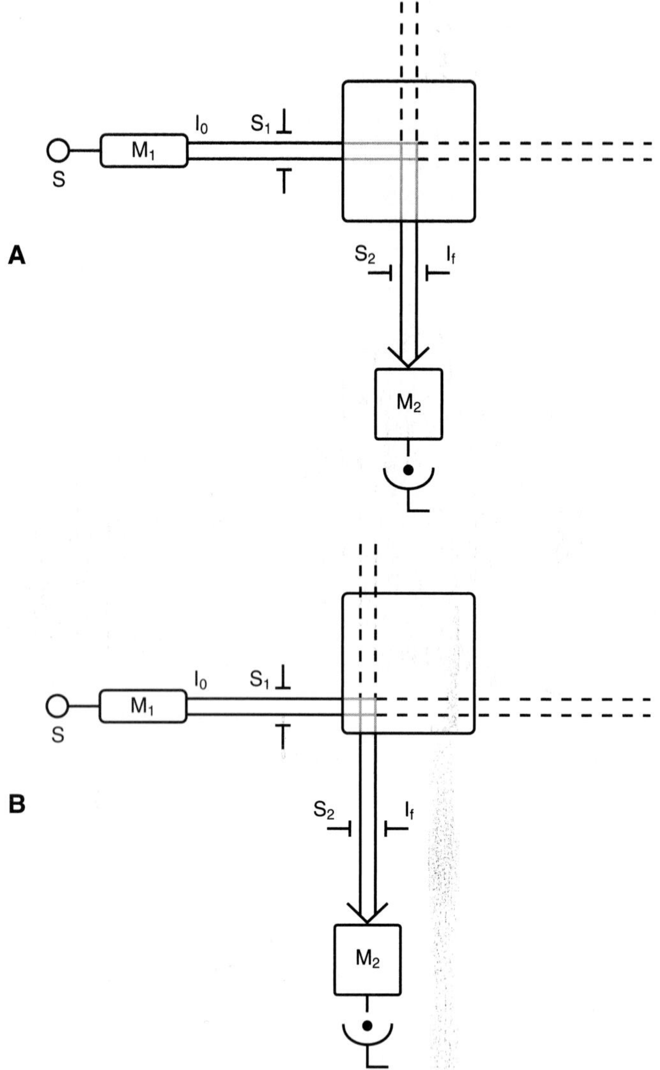

Figure 3-19 Two right angle fluorescence sample cuvet positions. **A** is the standard 90° configuration. **B** is the offset positioning of the cuvet to minimize the inner filter effect.

rometers is the PMT. The important features of the PMT for fluorescence measurements are a wide choice of spectral responses, rapid photon response time (i.e., nanosecond response time), and sensitivity. Sensitivity is due to the possible gain of 10^6 electrons at the anode of the photomultiplier tube for each incident photon hitting the photo cathode.

Depending on the light level (photon flux) striking the PMT cathode and the desired sensitivity, the measurement of electron flow at the PM tube anode is accomplished in different ways. At high light intensities, analog techniques for measurement of PMT current are used. The analog signal is then converted to a digital signal for computer use or for panel digital display. At low light levels, spikes or pulses generated at the cathode of the PMT are counted. The number of pulses that occur per unit of time is directly proportional to the intensity of emitted fluorescence light striking the PMT. This method is called *photon counting.* The use of photon counting increases the signal-to-noise ratio and the sensitivity of the measurement of fluorophores at very low concentrations.

Charge-Coupled Detector. CCDs are multichannel devices having dynamic range and a signal-to-noise ratio that are superior to those of photomultiplier tubes.[4,23] These solid-state devices are composed of a large number of photodetecting shift registers that are read horizontally and vertically. CCD were first used for astronomy applications and in ground-based optical telescopes in which sensitive low-light measurements are required. Because of their ability to detect very low levels of light, they have been used for molecular fluorescence measurement of very low concentrations of fluorescent molecules[23] and as a quantitative electronic imager for quantitative confocal microscopy.[12] A data-reading technique called binning has been developed that allows multielement devices to have functional elements linked together much like rectangular slit widths. A fluorometer has been built using a CCD and a 30-W mercury pen lamp as its light source. With this instrument, detection limits have been decreased by one order of magnitude.

Performance Verification

As with spectrophotometers, NIST provides a number of SRMs for use in the calibration or verification of the performance of fluorometers or fluorospectrophotometers. These include SRM 936a (quinine sulfate dihydrate) for calibrating such instruments and SRM 1932 (fluorescein) for establishing a reference scale for fluorescence measurements (see http://www.nist.gov).

Types of Fluorometers and Spectrofluorometers

Fluorometers and fluorescence spectrophotometers are available that offer a variety of features. These features include ratio referencing, microprocessor-controlled excitation and emission monochromators, pulsed xenon light sources, photon counting, rhodamine cell for corrected spectra, polarizers, flow cells, front-surface viewing adapters, multiple cell holders, and microprocessor-based data reduction systems.

In addition, to the basic spectrofluorometer discussed earlier (see Figure 3-17), other types of fluorometric instruments include a ratio-referencing spectrofluorometer, time-resolved fluorometer, flow cytometer, and hematofluorometer.

Ratio-Referencing Spectrofluorometer

A typical ratio-referencing spectrofluorometer is illustrated in Figure 3-20. Basically, this is a simple right angle instrument that uses two monochromators (M1 and M2), two photomultiplier tube detectors (D1 and D2, the reference and sample PMTs), and a xenon lamp source. The light from the exciter monochromator (M1) is split, and a small portion (10%) is directed to the reference PMT (D1) for ratio refer-

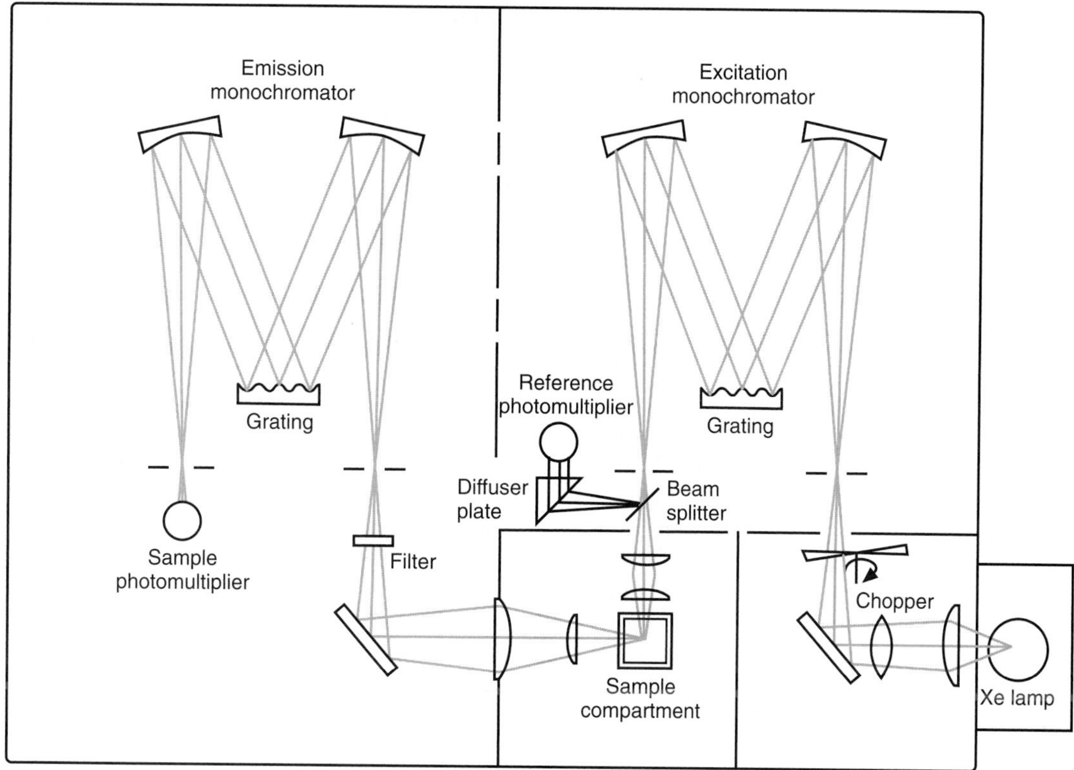

Figure 3-20 Diagram of a typical ratio-referencing spectrofluorometer.

encing purposes. The remaining excitation light is focused into the sample cuvet (C). Emission optics are positioned at a right angle to the excitation optics. An emission monochromator (M2) is used to select or scan the desired portion of the emission spectra, which is directed to the sample PMT (D2) for measurement of the emission intensity. The output signals from the reference and the sample PMTs are amplified (A1 and A2), and a ratio of the sample to the reference signal is provided by a digital display or a chart recorder. The operational mode of a ratio fluorometer is similar to that of the spectrofluorometer; however, only discrete excitation and emission wavelengths are available, and the use of this type of instrument is precluded from scanning fluorophores to obtain emission and excitation spectra. The ratio filter fluorometer is most useful for obtaining concentration measurements at defined excitation and emission wavelengths.

The ratio-referencing spectrofluorometer is operated at either fixed excitation and emission wavelength settings for concentration measurements or used to measure the excitation or emission spectrum of a given compound. The measurement of concentration of unknowns is accomplished in a similar manner as with a single-beam fluorometer. A blank and a calibrating solution are first measured, and then the unknown samples are measured. The ratio-referencing spectrofluorometer in Figure 3-20 provides two advantages over single-beam spectrofluorometers. First, it eliminates short- and long-term xenon lamp energy fluctuations (i.e., arc flicker and lamp decay) and thus minimizes the need for frequent calibration of the instrument during analysis. Second, it provides "essentially" corrected excitation spectra by compensating for wavelength-dependent energy fluctuations.

Time-Resolved Fluorometers

The time-resolved fluorometer was introduced in the mid-1970s when Weider developed a pulsed nitrogen laser fluorometer in conjunction with a lanthanide-based immunoassay system to measure the fluorescence decay of lanthanide chelates as a means of eliminating background interferences from light scatter and short decay time fluorescence compounds.[26] The time-resolved fluorometer[3,18] is similar to the ratio-referencing fluorometer with the exception that the light source is pulsed and that the detector monitors, in a fast photon-counting mode, the exponential decay of the fluorescence signal after the excitation. Time-resolved fluorometry requires the use of long-lived fluorophores, such as the lanthanide (rare earth) metal ions europium (Eu^{3+}) and samarium (Sm^{3+}). Whereas most fluorescence compounds have decay times of 5 to 100 ns, europium chelates decay in 0.6 to 100 s. Thus time-resolved fluorescence assays take advantage of the difference in the lifetimes of fluorophore and the background fluorescence by measuring the decaying fluorescence signal. This eliminates background interferences and at the same time averages the signal to improve the precision of measurement. Detection limits of approximately 10^{-13} mol/L can be achieved with time-resolved fluorometry; this is an improvement of about four orders of magnitude compared with conventional fluorometric measurements. For example, Eu^{3+}-labeled nanoparticles in combination with time-resolved fluorometry have been used to develop a highly sensitive immunoassay for free and total prostate specific antigen having a functional sensitivity of 0.5 ng/L.[8,19,20]

Flow Cytometer

Cytometry refers to the measurement of physical and/or chemical characteristics of cells, or, by extension, of other biological particles. Flow cytometry is a process in which such measurements are made while the cells or particles pass, preferably in single file, through the measuring apparatus in a fluid stream. Flow sorting extends flow cytometry by using electrical or mechanical means to divert and collect cells with one or more measured characteristics falling within a range or ranges of values set by the user.[14,16]

Operationally, flow cytometry combines laser-induced fluorometry and particle light scattering analysis that allows different populations of molecules, cells, or particles to be differentiated by size and shape using low-light and right angle light scattering. The use of a laser is ideally suited for low-angle light scattering. These cells, molecules, or particles are labeled with different specific fluorescent labels, such as β-phycoerythrin, fluorescein isothiocyanate, rhodamine-6G, and dye-labeled antibodies. As they flow through the flow cell, simultaneous fluorescence and light scattering measurements are automatically performed by the flow cytometer. Most flow cytometers incorporate two or more fluorescence emission detection systems so that multiple fluorescent labels can be used. In this manner, molecules, cells, or particles can be classified by size, shape, and type according to their light-scattering and fluorescent properties. A schematic diagram of a flow cytometer is shown in Figure 3-21. An optical stop is placed in the 180° beam after the flow capillary to block the main laser beam and permit low-angle forward light scattering measurements. The 90° emission signal is split and directed to two PMTs to determine right angle light scattering and detect at least two separate fluorescence emission signals. Two narrow-bandpass interference filters (530 nm and 596 nm) are placed in front of the two 90° fluorescence emission PMTs. A computer with substantial resident software is employed to reduce the acquired data to appropriate histograms for final result reporting. Cell-sorting electrodes are shown in the schematic drawing. Most commercial flow cytometers use a single argon ion laser (488 nm), which excites fluorescein isothiocyanate and phycoerythrin. When excited, fluorescein isothiocyanate–labeled cells emit green light (E_{max} = 530 nm), and phycoerythrin-labeled cells emit orange light (E_{max} = 596 nm).

Flow cytometers are able to measure multiple parameters, including cell size (forward scatter), granularity (90° scatter), DNA content, RNA content, DNA (A + T)/(G + C) nucleotide ratios, chromatin structure, antigens, total protein content, cell receptors, membrane potential, and calcium ion concentration as a function of pH. These parameters are used in hematology, immunology (e.g., in T-cell subsets, tissue typing, lymphocyte stimulation, and antigen-antibody reactions), oncology (e.g., in diagnosis, prognosis, and treatment monitoring), microbiology (e.g., in bacterial identification and antibiotic sensitivity), virology, genetics

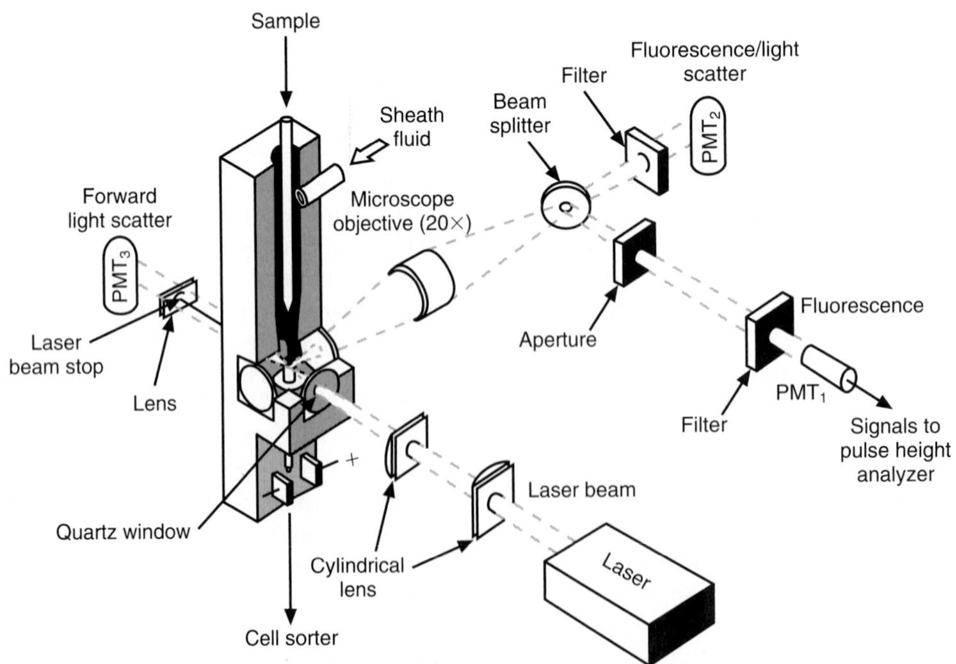

Figure 3-21 Schematic diagram of a flow cytometer.

(e.g., in karyotyping and carrier state detection), parasitology, reproduction and fertility studies, and possibly may have application in cervical cytology. Flow cytometry also has potential applications for the development of sensitive laser-induced fluoroimmunoassays. Phycoerythrin is a large phycobiliprotein molecule (MW = 250,000) with the fluorescence emission equivalent of 25 rhodamine-6G molecules, a quantum yield of 0.98, a broad emission spectrum of 530 to 630 nm, and low photodecomposition. It is an excellent label for cells and possibly for use in new fluoroimmunoassays.

Of particular note has been the development and use of particle-based flow cytometric assays. With this technology, a flow cytometer is combined with microspheres that are used as the solid support for conventional immunoassay, affinity assay, or DNA hybridization assay.[25] The resultant system is very flexible and has led to the development of multiplexed assays that simultaneously measure many different analytes in a small sample volume.

Hematofluorometer

The *hematofluorometer* is a single-channel front surface photofluorometer dedicated to the analysis of zinc protoporphyrin in whole blood (see Chapter 32). A typical hematofluorometer uses a quartz tungsten lamp, a narrow bandpass excitation filter (420 nm), front surface optics, a narrow bandpass filter (594 nm), and a PM tube. A drop of whole blood is placed on a small rectangular glass slide that serves as a cuvet.

Limitations of Fluorescence Measurements

Factors that influence fluorescence measurements include concentration effects (e.g., inner filter effect and concentration quenching), background effects (due to Rayleigh and Raman scattering), solvent effects (e.g., interfering nonspecific fluorescence and quenching from the solvent), sample effects (e.g., light scattering, interfering fluorescence, and sample adsorption), temperature effects, and photodecomposition (bleaching) of the sample.

Inner Filter Effect

The linear relationship between concentration and fluorescence emission (equation [12]) is valid when solutions are used that absorb less than 2% of the exciting light. As the absorbance of the solution increases above this amount, the relationship becomes nonlinear, a phenomenon known as the "inner filter effect." It is caused by a loss of excitation intensity across the cuvet path length as the excitation light is absorbed by the fluorophore. Thus as the fluorophore becomes more concentrated, the absorbance of the excitation intensity increases, and the loss of the excitation light as it travels through the cuvet increases. This effect is most often encountered with a right angle fluorescence instrument, in which the emission slits are set to monitor the center of the sample cell where the absorbance of excitation light is greater than at the front surface of the cuvet. Therefore it is less problematical if a front surface fluorescence instrument is used. However, most fluorescence measurements are made on very dilute solutions and the inner filter effect is therefore not a problem.

Concentration Quenching

Another related phenomenon that results in a lower quantum yield than expected is called *concentration quenching.* This can occur when a macromolecule, such as an antibody, is heavily labeled with a fluorophore, such as fluorescein isothiocyanate. When this compound is excited, the fluorescence labels are in such close proximity that radiationless energy transfer occurs. Thus, the resulting fluorescence is much lower than expected for the concentration of the label. This is a common problem in flow cytometry and laser-induced fluorescence when attempting to enhance detection sensitivity by increasing the density of the fluorescing label.

Light Scattering

Light scattering, both Rayleigh and Raman, limit the use of fluorescence measurements. Rayleigh scattering occurs with no change in wavelength. For fluorophores with small Stokes shifts, the excitation and emission spectra overlap and are particularly susceptible to loss of sensitivity because of background light scatter. Rayleigh-type light scatter is controlled by the use of well-defined emission and excitation interference filters or by appropriate monochromator settings and by the use of polarizers.

Raman scattering occurs with a lengthening of wavelength. This type of light scattering is independent of excitation wavelength and is a property of the solvent. Because Raman light scattering appears at longer wavelengths than the exciting radiation, it is a difficult interference to eliminate when working at very low fluorophore concentrations. As an example, the wavelength shift in water is ~50 nm at an excitation wavelength of 365 nm and ~75 nm at an excitation wavelength of 436 nm. The shift would represent a problem if the excitation maximum of a fluorophore was 365 nm and the emission maximum was 415 nm. Raman light scattering is controlled by setting the excitation and emission wavelengths far enough apart to prevent the Raman scatter. Also, it is controlled by narrowing the slit width on the excitation monochromator. However, both options tend to decrease sensitivity.

Cuvet Material and Solvent Effects

Certain quartz glass and plastic materials that contain ultraviolet absorbers will fluoresce. Some solvents, such as ethanol, are also known to cause appreciable fluorescence. It is therefore important when developing a fluorescence assay to assess the background fluorescence of all components of the reaction mixture. Fluorescence grade solvents and cuvets with minimum fluorescence emission, which minimize these types of fluorescence background problems, are commercially available.

Quenching by the solvent can be a problem and should be investigated when setting up a new fluorometric method. Quenching is related to the interaction of the fluorophore with the solvent or with a solute dissolved in the solvent. Such interaction results in a loss of fluorescence owing to energy transfer or other mechanisms, but there is no effect on the absorbance spectrum of the fluorophore. An example of quenching is the loss of fluorescence when halides are added to quinine in dilute sulfuric acid. Quenching can be a useful tool for studying molecular structure, because fluorescence emission is sensitive to and specific for changes in atomic and molecular structure.

Sample Matrix Effects

A serum or urine sample contains many compounds that fluoresce. Thus the sample matrix is a potential source of unwanted background fluorescence and must be examined when new methods are developed. The most serious contributors to unwanted fluorescence are proteins and bilirubin. However, because protein excitation maxima are in the spectral region of 260 to 290 nm, their contribution to overall background fluorescence is minor when excitation occurs above 300 nm.

The light scattering of proteins and other macromolecules in the sample matrix has been known to cause unwanted background fluorescence. Lipemic samples, for example, are noted for their intense light scattering, and the relative contribution of lipids to the background signal of a fluorescence measurement should be investigated when setting up a new method.

In addition to background interferences, dilute solutions of some fluorophores in the concentration range of 10^{-9} mol/L and below will absorb to the walls of glass cuvets and other reaction vessels. Also, dilute solutions of fluorophores, when excited over long periods of time, are susceptible to photodecomposition by intense excitation light. Operationally, these problems are avoided by selecting proper reaction vessels, adding wetting agents, and minimizing the length of time a sample is exposed to the excitation light.

Temperature Effects

The fluorescence quantum efficiency of many compounds is sensitive to temperature fluctuations. Therefore, the temperature of the reaction must be regulated to within ±0.1°C. In general, fluorescence intensity decreases with increasing temperature by approximately 1% to 5% per degree Celsius. Furthermore, collisional quenching decreases with increasing viscosity, thus reducing quenching of fluorescence. Operationally, fluorescence intensity is therefore enhanced by either increasing reaction viscosity or lowering solvent temperature. Temperature effects are minimized by controlling reaction temperature and warming samples or reagents, or both, if they have been refrigerated.

Photodecomposition

In conventional fluorometry, excitation of weakly fluorescing or dilute solutions with intense light sources will cause photochemical decomposition of the analyte (photobleaching).

The following steps help to minimize photodecomposition effects:

1. Always use the longest feasible wavelength for excitation that does not introduce light-scattering effects.
2. Decrease the duration of excitation of the sample by measuring the fluorescence intensity immediately after excitation.
3. Protect unstable solutions from ambient light by storing them in dark bottles.
4. Remove dissolved oxygen from the solution.

In addition, highly intense laser light sources with an energy output greater than 5 to 10 mW that are used for flow cytometry, fluorescence microscopy, and laser-induced fluorescence measurements will rapidly photodecompose some fluorescence analytes. This decomposition introduces nonlinear response curves and loss of the majority of the sample fluorescence. Fluorescence-based assays for analytes at ultralow concentrations require optimization of laser intensity and the use of a sensitive detector.

PHOSPHORESCENCE

Phosphorescence is the luminescence produced by certain substances after absorbing radiant energy or other types of energy.[24] Phosphorescence is distinguished from fluorescence in that it continues even after the radiation causing it has ceased. The decay time of emission of phosphorescence light is longer (10^{-4} – 10^{2} s) than the decay time of fluorescence emission. Decay times are expressed in a time range of several orders of magnitude and vary with the molecule and its solution environment. Phosphorescence shows a larger shift in emitted light wavelength than does fluorescence.

CHEMILUMINESCENCE, BIOLUMINESCENCE, AND ELECTROCHEMILUMINESCENCE

Chemiluminescence, bioluminescence, and *electrochemiluminescence* are types of luminescence in which the excitation event is caused by a chemical, biochemical, or electrochemical reaction and not by photoillumination.

Basic Concepts

The physical event of the light emission in chemiluminescence, bioluminescence, and electrochemiluminescence is similar to fluorescence in that it occurs from an excited singlet state, and the light is emitted when the electron returns to the ground state.

Chemiluminescence and Bioluminescence

Chemiluminescence is the emission of light when an electron returns from an excited or higher energy level to a lower energy level. The excitation event is caused by a chemical reaction and involves the oxidation of an organic compound, such as luminol, isoluminol, acridinium esters, or luciferin, by an oxidant (e.g., hydrogen peroxide, hypochlorite, or oxygen); light is emitted from the excited product formed in the oxidation reaction. These reactions occur in the presence of catalysts, such as enzymes (e.g., alkaline phosphatase, horseradish peroxidase, and microperoxidase), metal ions or metal complexes (e.g., Cu^{2+} and Fe^{3+} phthalocyanine complex), and hemin.[2,6,7,13,27]

Bioluminescence is a special form of chemiluminescence found in biological systems. In bioluminescence, an enzyme or a photoprotein increases the efficiency of the luminescence reaction. Luciferase and aequorin are two examples of these biological catalysts. The quantum yield (e.g., total photons emitted per total molecules reacting) is approximately 0.1% to 10% for chemiluminescence and 10% to 30% for bioluminescence.

Chemiluminescence assays are ultrasensitive (attomole to zeptomole detection limits) and have wide dynamic ranges. They are now widely used in automated immunoassay and DNA probe assay systems, (e.g., acridinium ester and acridinium sulfonamide labels and 1,2-dioxetane substrates for alkaline phosphatase labels and the enhanced-luminol reaction for horseradish peroxidase labels [see Chapter 9]).

Electrochemiluminescence

Electrochemiluminescence differs from chemiluminescence in that the reactive species that produce the chemiluminescent reaction are electrochemically generated from stable precursors at the surface of an electrode.[1] A ruthenium (Ru^{2+}), tris(bipyridyl) chelate is the most commonly used electrochemiluminescence label and electrochemiluminescence is generated at an electrode via an oxidation-reduction–type reaction with tripropylamine. This chelate is very stable and relatively small and can be used to label haptens or large molecules (e.g., proteins or oligonucleotides). The electrochemiluminescence process has been used in both immunoassays and nucleic acid assays. The advantages of this process are improved reagent stability, simple reagent preparation, and enhanced sensitivity. With its use, detection limits of 200 fmol/L and a dynamic range extending over six orders of magnitude can be obtained.

Instrumentation

Luminometers are instruments used to measure chemiluminescence and electrochemiluminescence.[2,27] The basic components are (1) the sample cell housed in a light-tight chamber, (2) the injection system to add reagents to the sample cell, and (3) the detector. The detector is usually a photomultiplier tube. However, a CCD, x-ray film, or photographic film has been used to image chemiluminescence reactions on a membrane or in the wells of a microplate. For electrochemiluminescence, the reaction vessel incorporates an electrode at which the electrochemiluminescence is generated.

Limitations of Chemiluminescence and Electrochemiluminescence Measurements

Light leaks, light piping, and high background luminescence from assay reagents and reaction vessels (e.g., plastic tubes exposed to light) are common factors that degrade analytical performance. The extreme sensitivity of chemiluminescence assays requires stringent controls on the purity of reagents and the solvents (e.g., water) used to prepare reagent solutions. Efficient capture of the light emission from reactions that produce a flash of light requires an efficient injector that provides adequate mixing when the triggering reagent is added to the reaction vessel. Chemiluminescent and electrochemiluminescent assays have a wide linear range, usually several orders of magnitude, but very high intensity light emission can lead to pulse pile-up in photomultiplier tubes and this leads to a serious underestimate of the true light emission intensity.

NEPHELOMETRY AND TURBIDIMETRY

Light scattering is a physical phenomenon resulting from the interaction of light with particles in solution. Nephelometry and turbidimetry are analytical techniques used to measure scattered light. Light-scattering measurements have been applied to immunoassays of specific proteins and haptens. Specific applications are described in Chapters 9, 20, and 26.

Basic Concepts

Light scattering occurs when radiant energy passing through a solution encounters a molecule in an elastic collision, which results in the light being scattered in all directions. Unlike fluorescence emission, the scattered light is of the same frequency as the incident light.

Factors that influence light scattering include the effect of particle size, wavelength dependence, distance of observation, effect of polarization of incident light, the concentration of the particles, and the molecular weight of the particles.

Particle Size

The Rayleigh scattering equation (see next section) applies to the scattering of light from small particles with much smaller dimensions than the wavelength of incident light (e.g., particle size $<\lambda/10$). When the dimensions of the particles are much smaller than the wavelength of the incident light, each particle is subjected to the same electric field strength at the same time. The reradiated or scattered light waves from the small particle are in phase and reinforce each other. As the particles become larger than the incident light wave, the radiated light waves are no longer all in phase.

Reinforcement of radiation occurs in some directions, and destructive interference occurs in others. The scattering patterns from these large particles are characteristic of the size and shape of the particle.

Wavelength Dependence of Light Scattering

In 1871 Lord Rayleigh derived the following equation that demonstrates the relationship of the intensity (I_s) of scattered light to the intensity (I_0) of the incident light:

$$\frac{I_s}{I_0} = \frac{16\pi^2\, a \sin^2\theta}{\lambda^4 r^2} \tag{14}$$

where

I_s = intensity of scattered light
I_0 = intensity of the excitation light
a = polarizability of the small particle
θ = angle of observation
λ = wavelength of the incident light
r = distance from light scattering to the detector

As indicated, the intensity of light scattering increases by the fourth power of the wavelength as the wavelength of the incident light is decreased. Another useful observation from equation (14) is the fact that the light intensity decreases by the square of the distance r from the light-scattering particles to the detector. Thus, the detector should be located close to the analytical cell either by the juxtaposition of the cell to the detector or by the use of good collection optics.

Concentration and Molecular Weight Factors in Light Scattering

The direct relationship of light scattering to the concentration of the particles and to the molecular weight of the particles is derived from equation (14) showing that:

$$\frac{I_S}{I_0} = \frac{4\pi^2\,(dn/dc)^2\, Mc \sin^2\theta}{N_a \lambda^4 r^2} \tag{15}$$

where

I_S = intensity of scattered light from small particles excited by polarized light
I_0 = incident intensity
dn/dc = change in refractive index of the solvent with respect to change in solute concentration
M = molecular weight (g/mol)
c = concentration (g/mL) of the particles
θ = angle of observation
N_a = Avogadro's number
λ = wavelength of the incident light
r = distance from light scattering to the detector

The important observation to be made from equation (15) is the direct relationship of light scattering to the concentration of the particles and to the molecular weight of the particles.[24]

The Effect of Polarized Light on Light Scattering

Equations (14) and (15) are different forms of the Rayleigh expression for light scattering from small particles if excited by polarized light. Figure 3-22, *A* shows the effect of polarized and nonpolarized light on light-scattering intensity from small particles as a function of scattering angle. Curve 2 shows a spherically symmetrical intensity diagram as predicted by equation (14). Curve 3 is the resultant intensity diagram when curves 1 and 2 are summed and is the scattering angular intensity diagram obtained when light scatters from small particles excited with nonpolarized light. Curves 1 and 2 represent intensity diagrams from vertically and horizontally polarized light components that are considered to be comprising nonpolarized light. The Rayleigh light-scattering expression for small particles excited by nonpolarized light is given by equation (16):

$$\frac{I_S}{I_0} = \frac{2\pi^2\,(dn/dc)^2\, Mc(1+\cos\theta)}{N_a \lambda^4 r^2} \tag{16}$$

There are two important observations to be made from equation (16) and Figure 3-22, *A*. First, the total light scattered by small particles is less when excited by polarized light than by nonpolarized light, and a reduction of background signal from light scattering in fluorescence measurements is achieved if an appropriately oriented polarizer is used in front of the emission detector. Second, the light-scattering

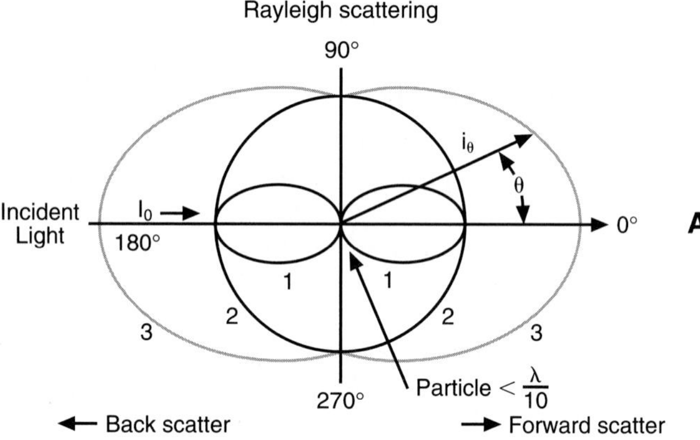

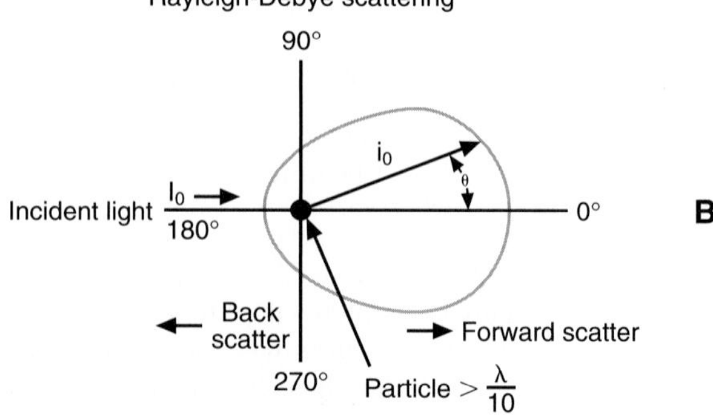

Figure 3-22 The angular dependence of light-scattering intensity with nonpolarized and polarized incident light for small particles **(A)** and the angular dependence of light scattering with nonpolarized light for larger particles **(B).**

intensity from small particles excited by nonpolarized light shows a symmetrical angular dependence of light scattering about the 90° axis (refer to Figure 3-22, *A*, curve 3).

The Angular Dependence of Light Scattering

The angular dependence of light scattering from small particles (i.e., less than $\lambda/10$), as indicated in the previous section, is represented by Figure 3-22, *A*. Examination of Figure 3-22, *A* (curve 3) shows that the light scatter intensity for forward scatter and back scatter (I_0 at 0° and 180°) from small particles excited by nonpolarized light is equal. However, light scatter intensity at 90° is much less. As the size of particles becomes larger (e.g., $>\lambda/10$), the angular dependence of light scatter takes on the dissymmetrical relationship shown in Figure 3-22, *B*. In this situation, the light-scattering intensities at forward and back angles are not equal; the forward scatter intensity is much larger. Also, the light-scattering intensity at 90° is much less than the intensity at the forward (0°) angle. As particles become even larger, this dissymmetry increases even further. This dissymmetry and the change of angular dependence of light scattering with change in the size of particles is very useful for characterization and differentiation of various classes of macromolecules and cells. As was previously mentioned, this property of light scattering is being used in the design of flow cytometers. These instruments measure near forward light scattering and right angle light scattering from cellular particles flowing through an optical cell and excited by a high-intensity laser. The ratio of the near forward light scattering intensity to the right angle light intensity is used in these instruments to distinguish different cell sizes.

Light Scattering and Plasma Proteins

The expression for light scattering given in equation (14) holds true in dilute solution for small particles if the largest dimension is less than one tenth of the wavelength of the incident light. Thus the upper limit on size of particles exhibiting Rayleigh scattering is about 40 nm when using visible light at 400 nm. Many of the plasma proteins—such as immunoglobulins, β-lipoproteins, and albumin—are below this limit. For larger particles (~40 to 400 nm), the angular dependence of the scattered light loses the symmetry around the 90° axis as seen in Figure 3-22, *A* and *B* and shows an increase in forward scattering. Some plasma proteins of the immunoglobulin M class, chylomicrons, and aggregating immunoglobulin/antigen complexes fall into this size category. The scattering from particles in this size range is known as Rayleigh-Debye scattering, and the equation for this type of scattering becomes more complex. Particles, such as red blood cells and bacteria, are larger yet (i.e., 7000 to 40,000 nm). These particles show a complex angular dependence of light scattering, and this type of scattering from very large particles is called Mie scattering. These large particles produce a predominance of scattered light in a narrow angular region in the forward direction.

Measurement of Scattered Light

Turbidimetry and nephelometry are methods used to measure scattered light. Their measurement has proven useful for the quantitation of serum proteins (see Chapters 9 and 20).

Turbidimetry

Turbidity decreases the intensity of the incident beam of light as it passes through a solution of particles. The measurement of this decrease in intensity is called turbidimetry. Analogous to absorption spectroscopy, the turbidity is defined as:

$$I = I_0 e^{-bt} \qquad (17)$$

or

$$t = \frac{1}{b}\ln\frac{I_0}{I} \qquad (18)$$

where

t = turbidity
b = path length of the incident light through the solution of light-scattering particles
I = intensity of transmitted light
I_0 = intensity of incident light

Turbidity is measured at 180° from the incident beam, or more simply, in the same manner as absorbance measurements are made in a spectrophotometer. Turbidity can be measured on most spectrophotometers and automated clinical chemistry analyzers. The stability and resolution of modern microprocessor-driven spectrophotometers and photometers have greatly improved the ability to measure turbidity with accuracy and precision.

Nephelometry

Nephelometry is defined as the detection of light energy scattered or reflected toward a detector that is not in the direct path of the transmitted light.[10] Common nephelometers measure scattered light at right angles to the incident light. The ideal nephelometric instrument would be free of stray light and neither light scatter nor any other signal would be seen by the detector when the solution in front of the detector is free from particles. However, because of stray light-generating components in the optical system and in the sample cuvet or sample itself, a truly dark field situation is difficult to obtain when making nephelometric measurements. Some nephelometers are designed to measure scattered light at an angle other than 90° to take advantage of the increased forward-scatter intensity caused by light scattering from larger particles (e.g., immune complexes).

Selection of Method

The choice between turbidimetry and nephelometry depends on the application and the available instrumentation. Nephelometry, however, still offers some advantage in sensitivity when measuring low-level antigen-antibody reactions.[10]

INSTRUMENTATION

Turbidimeters and nephelometers are used to measure the intensity of light scattering.

Turbidimeter

Turbidimetric measurements are easily performed on photometers or spectrophotometers and require little optimization. The principal concern of turbidimetric measurements is signal-to-noise ratio. Photometric systems with electro-optical noise in the range of ±0.0002 absorbance unit or less are useful for turbidity measurements.

Nephelometer

Although light scattering can be measured with standard analytical fluorometers or photometers, the angular dependence of light-scattering intensity has resulted in the design of special nephelometers. These devices place the PMT detector at appropriate angles to the excitation light beam. The design principle of a nephelometer is similar to the design principle applied in fluorescence measurements. The major operational difference between the fluorometer and the nephelometer is that the excitation and detection wavelengths will be set to the same value. The principal concerns of light scatter instrumentation are excitation intensity, wavelength, distance of the detector from the sample cuvet, and minimization of external stray light. As shown in Figure 3-23, the basic components of a nephelometer include (1) a light source, (2) collimating optics, (3) a sample cell, and (4) collection optics, which include light-scattering optics, detector optical filter, and a detector. The schematic diagram also shows the different angles from the incident light beam where the detector, filter, and optics are placed to measure light scattering. Figure 3-23, *A* is the straight-through arrangement for turbidimetry, whereas Figure 3-23, *B* and *C* are arrangements frequently found in nephelometers. The detector arrangement shown in Figure 3-23, *B* is for measurement of forward scatter at 30°, the optical arrangement used in some commercial nephelometers.

Operationally, the optical components used in turbidimeters and nephelometers are similar to those used in fluorometers or photometers. For example, the light sources commonly used are quartz halogen lamps, xenon lamps, and lasers. He-Ne lasers, which operate at 633 nm, have typically been used for light-scattering applications, such as nephelometric immunoassays and particle size and shape determinations. The laser beam is used specifically in some nephelometers because of its high intensity; in addition, the coherent nature of laser light makes it ideally suited for nephelometric applications.

In addition, ratio-referencing fluorometers are well suited for nephelometric measurements.

LIMITATIONS OF LIGHT-SCATTERING MEASUREMENTS

Antigen excess and matrix effects are limitations encountered in the use of turbidimeters and nephelometers in measurement of analytes of clinical interest.

Antigen Excess

Antigen-antibody reactions are complex and appear to result in a mixture of aggregate sizes. As the turbidity increases during addition of antigen to antibodies, the signal increases to a maximum value and then decreases. The point at which the decrease begins marks the beginning of the phase of antigen excess; this phenomenon is explained in Chapter 9.

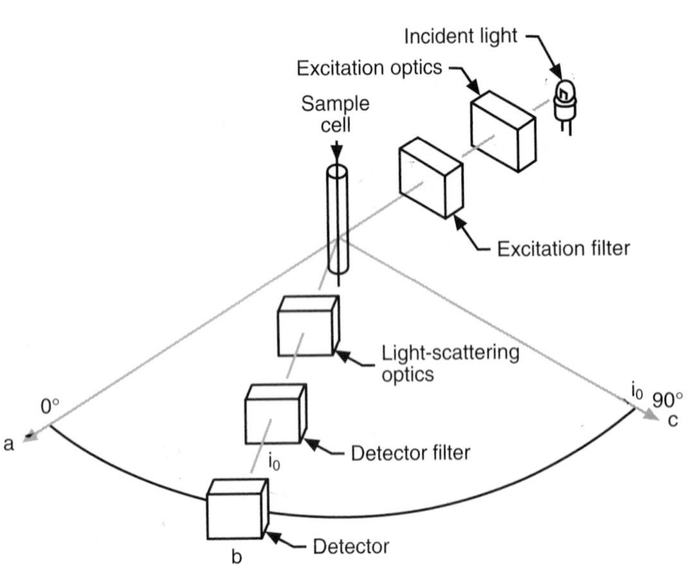

Figure 3-23 Schematic diagram of light-scattering instrumentation showing **A,** the optics position for a turbidimeter; **B,** the optics position for a forward-scattering nephelometer; and **C,** the optics position for a right angle nephelometer.

Consequently, light-scattering methods for quantitation of antigen-antibody reactions must provide a method for detecting antigen excess. The kinetics of immune complex formation measured either by nephelometry or turbidimetry are sufficiently different in the three phases—antibody excess, equivalence, and antigen excess—that computer algorithms have been developed to flag antigen excess automatically.[10,21]

Matrix Effects

Particles, solvent, and all serum macromolecules scatter light. Lipoproteins and chylomicrons in lipemic serum provide the highest background turbidity or nephelometric intensity. With appropriate dilutions, the relative intensity of light scattering from a lipemic sample is less than that of the antiserum blank. However, as the concentration of the antigen in serum decreases and correspondingly less dilute samples are used, the background interference from lipemic samples becomes greater. An effective method for minimizing this background interference is the use of rate measurements, where the initial sample blank is eliminated.

Large particles, such as suspended dust, also cause significant background interference. This background interference is controlled by filtering all buffers and diluted antisera before analysis is attempted.

REFERENCES

1. Blackburn GF, Shah HP, Kenten JH, et al. Electrochemiluminescence development of immunoassays and DNA probe assays for clinical diagnostics. Clin Chem 1991;37:1534-9.
2. DeLuca M, McElroy WD. Bioluminescence and Chemiluminescence, Part B. Methods in Enzymology, vol 133, San Diego:Academic Press, 1986, 649pp.
3. Diamandis E, Christopoulos TK. Europium chelate labels in time-resolved fluorescence immunoassays and DNA hybridization assays. Anal Chem 1990;62:1149A-57A.
4. Epperson PM, Sweedler JV, Billhorn RB et al. Applications of charge transfer devices in spectroscopy. Anal Chem 1988;60:327A-35A.
5. Evenson ME. Spectrophotometric techniques. In: Burtis CA, Ashwood ER, eds. Tietz textbook of clinical chemistry, 3nd ed. Philadelphia:WB Saunders Co, 1999:75-93.
6. Fletcher P, Andrew KN, Calokerinos AC, Forbes S, Worsfold PJ. Analytical applications of flow injection with chemiluminescence detection–a review. Luminescence. 2001;16(1):1-23.
7. Galban J, Andreu Y, Sierra JF, de Marcos S, Castillo JR. Intrinsic fluorescence of enzymes and fluorescence of chemically modified enzymes for analytical purposes: a review. Luminescence. 2001;16(2):199-210.
8. Harma H, Soukka T, Lovgren T: Europium nanoparticles and time-resolved fluorescence for ultrasensitive detection of prostate-specific antigen. Clin Chem 2001;47:561-8.
9. Heiftje GM, Vogelstein EE. : A linear response theory approach to time-resolved fluorometry. In: Wehry EL, ed. Modern fluorescence spectroscopy. New York:Plenum Press, vol 4, 1981:25-50.
10. Hills LP, Tiffany TO. Comparison of turbidimetric and light scattering measurements of immunoglobulins by use of a centrifugal analyzer with absorbance and fluorescence light scattering optics. Clin Chem 1980;26:1459-66.
11. Jolley ME, Stroupe SD, Schwenzer KS, et al. Fluorescence polarization immunoassay. III. An automated system for therapeutic drug determination. Clin Chem 1981;27:1575-9.
12. Masters BR, Kino GS. Charge coupled devices for quantitative Nipkow Disk real-time scanning confocal microscopy. In: Shotton D, ed. Electron light microscopy: The principles and practice of video-enhanced contrast, digital intensified fluorescence, and confocal scanning light microscopy. New York:Wiley-Liss, 1993.
13. Mestre YF, Zamora LL, Calatayud JM. Flow-chemiluminescence: a growing modality of pharmaceutical analysis. Luminescence 2001;16(3):213-35.
14. Patrick CW. Clinical flow cytometry. MLO 2002, 34 (9):10-16.
15. Peterson JI,Vurek GG. Fiber-optic sensors for biomedical applications. Science 1984;224:123-7.
16. Shapiro H M. Practical flow cytometry. 4th ed. Hoboken, NJ: John Wiley & Sons, 2003:576pp.
17. Slavin W. Atomic absorption spectroscopy: The present and future. Anal Chem 1982;54:685A-94A.
18. Soini E, Kojola H. Time-resolved fluorometer for lanthanide chelates: A new generation of nonisotopic immunoassays. Clin Chem 1983;29:65-8.
19. Soukka T, Paukkunen J, Harma H, Lonnberg S, Lindroos H, Lovgren T. Supersensitive time-resolved immunofluorometric assay of free prostate-specific antigen with nanoparticle label technology. Clin Chem 2001;47:1269-78.
20. Soukka T, Antonen K, Harma H, Pelkkikangas AM, Huhtinen P, Lovgren T. Highly sensitive immunoassay of free prostate-specific antigen in serum using europium(III) nanoparticle label technology. Clin Chim Acta 2003; 328:45-58.
21. Sternberg J. A rate nephelometer for measuring specific proteins by immunoprecipitin reactions. Clin Chem 1977;25:1456-64.
22. Stevens JF, Vadgama P. Infrared analysis in clinical chemistry: its use in the laboratory and in non-invasive near patient testing. Ann Clin Biochem 1997;34:215-21.
23. Sweedler JV, Billhorn RB, Epperson PM et al. High performance charge transfer devices. Anal Chem 1988;60:282A-91A.

24. Tiffany TO. Fluorometry, nephelometry, and turbidimetry. In: Burtis CA, Ashwood ER, eds. Tietz textbook of clinical chemistry, 3nd ed. Philadelphia:W.B. Saunders Co., 1999: 94-112.
25. Vignali DA. Multiplexed particle-based flow cytometric assays. J Immunol Methods 2000; 243:243-55.
26. Wieder I. Background rejection in fluorescent immunoassay. In: Knapp W, Holubar K, Wick G, eds. Proceedings of the VIth International Conference on Immunofluorescence. Amsterdam:Elsevier/North-Holland, 1978:67-80.
27. Ziegler MM, Baldwin TO, eds. Bioluminescence and Chemiluminescence, Part C. Methods in Enzymology, vol 305, San Diego:Academic Press, 2000:732pp.

ADDITIONAL READING

General

Harris DC. Quantitative chemical analysis. 6th ed. New York: W.H. Freeman and Company, 2002:1200pp.

Karnik HB. Laboratory instruments in clinical chemistry, principles of. In: Meyers RA, ed. Encyclopedia of analytical chemistry: Applications, theory, and instrumentation. New York: John Wiley & Sons, 2000: 1395-410.

Kricka, LJ. Optical Methods: A Guide to the "-escences." Washington DC; AACC Press, 2003:191pp.

Rooke MA, Mader SL. The Science of spectroscopy. http://www.scienceofspectroscopy.info

Rouessac F, Rouessac A: Chemical analysis: Modern instrumentation methods and techniques. New York: John Wiley & Sons, 2000:300pp.

Ryder A. Light measurement handbook. Newburyport, MA: International Light, 1997:64pp. (see http://www.intl-light.com/handbook/).

Skoog DA, Holler FJ, Nieman TA. Principles of instrumental analysis. 5th ed. New York: Saunders College Publishing, 1998.

Van Dyke K, Van Dyke C, Woodfork K, eds. Luminescence biotechnology: Instruments and applications. Boca Raton,FL: CRC Press, 2001.

Willard HH, Dean JA, Settle FA, Dean J, Merritt, LL. Instrumental methods of analysis. 7th ed. Belmont, CA:Wadsworth Publishing Company, 1988:895pp.

Wolfbeis OS. Fiber-optic chemical sensors and biosensors. Anal Chem 2002;74:2663-78.

Atomic Spectrometry

Bings NH, Bogaerts A, Broekaert JAC. Atomic spectroscopy. Anal Chem 2002;74:2691-2712.

Parson PJ. Atomic spectrometry in clinical chemistry. In: Meyers RA, ed. Encyclopedia of analytical chemistry: Applications, theory, and instrumentation. New York: John Wiley & Sons, 2000:1091-1122.

Chemiluminescence

Case JF, Herring, PJ, Robinson BH, Haddock SHD, Kricka LJ, Stanley PE, Robinson BH (eds). Bioluminescence & chemiluminescence 2000. 1st ed, Teaneck, NJ: World Scientific Pub Co, 2001:540pp.

Colowick SP, M DeLuca (eds). Bioluminescence and chemiluminescence. In: Methods in enzymology, San Diego: Academic Press V57, 1997:653pp.

Garcia-Campana AM, Baeyens WRG (eds). Chemiluminescence in analytical chemistry. New York: Marcel Dekker, 2001:621pp.

Pazzagli M, Roda A, Stanley P. Bioluminescence and chemiluminescence: Perspective for the 21st Century: Proceedings of the 10th International Symposium on Bioluminescence and Chemiluminescence. New York: John Wiley & Sons, 1999:648pp.

Stanley PE, Kricka LJ. Bioluminescence and chemiluminescence: Progress and current applications. Teaneck, NJ: World Scientific Pub Co, 2002:556pp.

Ziegler MM, Baldwin TO (eds). Bioluminescence and chemiluminescence. In: Methods in Enzymology, San Diego: Academic Press 2000, Part C V305, 581pp.

Flow Cytometry

Earley MC, Vogt RF Jr, Shapiro HM, et al. Report from a workshop on multianalyte microsphere assays. Cytometry 2002;50:239-42.

Patrick CW. Clinical flow cytometry. MLO 2002, 34 (9):10-16.

Shapiro H M. Practical flow cytometry. 4th ed. Hoboken, NJ: John Wiley & Sons, 2003:576pp.

Fluorescence

Lakowicz JR, (ed). Principles of fluorescence spectroscopy. 2nd ed. NewYork: Plenum Pub Corp, 1999:725pp.

Oldham PB, McCarroll ME, McGown, LB, Warner IM. Molecular fluorescence, phosphorescence, and chemiluminescence spectrometry Anal Chem 2000;72:197-210R.

Schulman JM, Schulman SG. Phosphorescence, fluorescence, chemiluminescence in clinical chemistry. In: Meyers RA, ed. Encyclopedia of analytical chemistry: Applications, theory, and instrumentation. New York: John Wiley & Sons, 2000:1570-82.

Udenfriend S. Fluorescence assay in biology and medicine. New York:Academic Press, Inc., 1962:517pp.

Infrared Spectroscopy

Ng LM, Simmons R. Infrared spectroscopy in clinical chemistry. In: Meyers RA, ed. Encyclopedia of analytical chemistry: Applications, theory, and instrumentation. New York: John Wiley & Sons, 2000:1375-1394.

Spectrophotometry

Clark RJH, Hester RE, Eds. Biomedical applications of spectroscopy. New York: John Wiley & Sons, 1996:402pp.

Dean JA. Electronic Absorption and luminescence spectroscopy. In: Analytical chemistry handbook. New York: McGraw-Hill Inc, 1995:Section 5.

Gore MG (ed). Spectrophotometry and spectrofluorimetry: a practical approach, 2nd ed. London: Oxford University Press, 2000:368pp.

Upstone SL. Ultraviolet/visible light absorption spectrophotometry in clinical chemistry. In: Meyers RA, ed. Encyclopedia of analytical chemistry: Applications, theory, and instrumentation. New York: John Wiley & Sons, 2000:1699-713.

Turbidity/Nephelometry

Berry GC. Light scattering, classical:size and size distribution characterization. In: Meyers RA, ed. Encyclopedia of analytical chemistry: Applications, theory, and instrumentation. New York: John Wiley & Sons, 2000:5413-47.

Kourti T. Turbidimetry in particle size analysis. In: Meyers RA, ed. Encyclopedia of analytical chemistry: Applications, theory, and instrumentation. New York: John Wiley & Sons, 2000:5549-80.

Mishchenko MI, Travis LD, Lacis AA. Scattering, absorption, and emission of light by small particles. 1st ed, Cambridge: Cambridge University Press, 2002:480pp.

INTERNET SITES

http://ull.chemistry.uakron.edu/analytical/Mol_spec_equip/

CHAPTER 4

Electrochemistry and Chemical Sensors*

Paul D'Orazio, Ph.D., and Mark E. Meyerhoff, Ph.D.

Electrochemical and optical sensors (and associated biosensors) are firmly established in clinical analysis systems. Sensors for measurement of blood gases, electrolytes, and metabolites are particularly well suited for incorporation into automated, point-of-care, and critical-care analyzers (see Chapters 11, 12, and 27 respectively), because of their ease of use, low maintenance, and ability to measure clinically important analytes in undiluted blood.[51] When integrated into chromatographic systems (see Chapter 6), electrochemical detectors provide a very sensitive and selective means to detect a variety of other analytes, such as therapeutic drugs, neurotransmitters, glutathione, and homocysteine. Also, electrochemical detection has been applied successfully for monitoring coagulation reactions, detecting toxic lead in blood samples, and developing novel ultrasensitive immunoassay schemes. When bioelements are integrated with electrodes, the resultant biosensors further expand the analytical capabilities of such devices. In addition, the development and application of "optodes," based on some of the same selective chemistries used in electrochemical devices, provide yet another analytical tool for measuring blood gases and electrolytes.

In this chapter, the fundamental electrochemical principles of potentiometry, voltammetry and/or amperometry, conductance, and coulometry will be summarized and clinical applications presented. Next, optodes and biosensors will be discussed. The chapter concludes with a discussion of in vivo and minimally invasive sensors.

*The authors gratefully acknowledge the original contributions of Drs. Richard A. Durst and Ole Siggard-Andersen on which portions of this chapter are based.

POTENTIOMETRY AND ION-SELECTIVE ELECTRODES

Potentiometry is widely used clinically for the measurement of pH, PCO_2 and electrolytes (Na^+, K^+, Cl^-, Ca^{2+}, Mg^{2+}, Li^+) in whole blood, serum, plasma and urine, and as the basis for some biosensors for metabolites of clinical interest.

Basic Concepts

Potentiometry is the measurement of an electrical potential difference between two electrodes (half-cells) in an electrochemical cell (Figure 4-1) when the cell current is zero (galvanic cell). Such a cell consists of two electrodes (electron or metallic conductors) that are connected by an electrolyte solution (ion conductor). An *electrode*, or *half-cell*, consists of a single metallic conductor that is in contact with an electrolyte solution. The ion conductors can be composed of one or more phases that are either in direct contact with each other or separated by membranes permeable only to specific cations or anions (see Figure 4-1). One of the electrolyte solutions is the unknown or test solution; this solution may be replaced by an appropriate reference solution for calibration purposes. By convention, the cell notation is shown so that the left electrode (M_L) is the reference electrode; the right electrode (M_R) is the *indicator (measuring) electrode* (see later equation 3).[9]

The *electromotive force* (E or EMF) is defined as the maximum difference in potential between the two electrodes (right minus left) obtained when the cell current is zero. The cell potential is measured using a *potentiometer*, of which the common pH meter is a special type. The *direct-reading potentiometer* is a voltmeter that measures the potential across the cell (between the two electrodes); however, to obtain an accurate potential measurement, it is necessary

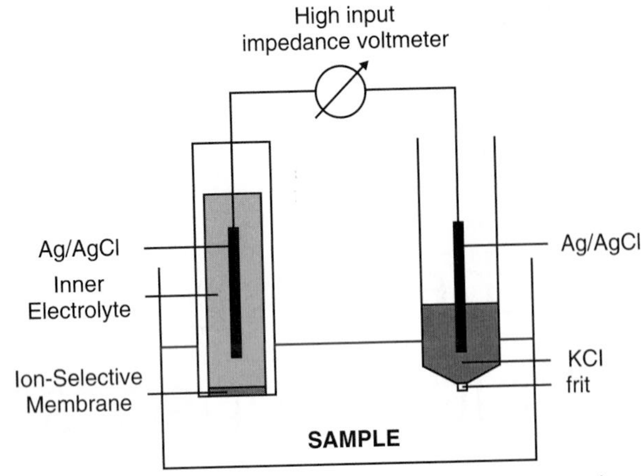

Figure 4-1 Schematic of ion-selective membrane electrode-based potentiometric cell.

that no current flow through the cell. This is accomplished by incorporating a high resistance within the voltmeter (input impedance $>10^{12}\,\Omega$). Modern direct-reading potentiometers are accurate and can be modified to provide direct digital display or printouts.

Within any one conductive phase, the potential is constant as long as the current flow is zero. However, a potential difference arises between two different phases in contact with each other. The overall potential of an electrochemical cell is the sum of all the potential gradients that exist between different phases of the cell. The potential of a single electrode with respect to the surrounding electrolyte and the absolute magnitude of the individual potential gradients between the phases are unknown and cannot be measured. Only the *potential differences* between two electrodes (half-cells) can be measured. The potential gradients can be classified as (1) redox potentials, (2) membrane potentials, or (3) diffusion potentials. Generally, it is possible to devise a cell in such a manner that all the potential gradients except one are constant. This potential can then be related to the activity of a specific ion of interest (e.g., H^+ or Na^+).

Types of Electrodes

Many different types of electrodes are used for potentiometric applications. They include redox, ion-selective membrane (glass and polymer), and PCO_2 electrodes.

Redox Electrodes

Redox potentials are the result of chemical equilibria involving electron transfer reactions:

$$\text{Oxidized form (Ox)} + \text{ne}^- \longleftrightarrow \text{Reduced form (Red)} \quad (1)$$

where n represents the number of electrons involved in the reaction. Any substance that accepts electrons is an *oxidant* (Ox), and any substance that donates electrons is a *reductant* (Red). The two forms, Ox and Red, represent a redox couple (conjugate redox pair). Usually, homogeneous redox processes take place only between two redox couples. In such cases, the electrons are transferred from a reductant (Red_1) to an oxidant (Ox_2). In this process, Red_1 is oxidized to its conjugate Ox_1, whereas Ox_2 is reduced to Red_2:

$$\text{Red}_1 + \text{Ox}_2 \longleftrightarrow \text{Ox}_1 + \text{Red}_2 \quad (2)$$

In an electrochemical cell, electrons may be accepted from or donated to an inert metallic conductor (e.g., platinum). A reduction process tends to charge the electrode positively (remove electrons), and an oxidation process tends to charge the electrode negatively (add electrons). By convention, a heterogeneous redox equilibrium (equation 2) is represented by the cell

$$M_L|\text{Red}_1 - \text{Ox}_1 :: \text{Ox}_2 - \text{Red}_2|M_R \quad (3)$$

A positive potential ($E > 0$) for this cell signifies that the cell reaction proceeds spontaneously from left to right; $E < 0$ signifies that the reaction proceeds from right to left; and $E = 0$ indicates that the two redox couples are at mutual equilibrium.

The *electrode potential* (reduction potential) for a redox couple is defined as the couple's potential measured with respect to the standard hydrogen electrode, which is set equal to zero (see hydrogen electrode later). This potential, by convention, is the electromotive force of a cell, where the standard hydrogen electrode is the reference electrode (left electrode) and the given half-cell is the indicator electrode (right electrode). The reduction potential for a given redox couple is given by the Nernst equation:

$$E = E^\circ - \frac{N}{n} \times \log\frac{a_{\text{Red}}}{a_{\text{Ox}}} = E^\circ - \frac{0.0592V}{n} \times \log\frac{a_{\text{Red}}}{a_{\text{Ox}}} \quad (4)$$

where

E = electrode potential of the half-cell
E° = standard electrode potential when $a_{\text{Red}}/a_{\text{Ox}} = 1$
n = number of electrons involved in the reduction reaction
$N = (R \times T \times \ln 10)/F$ (the Nernst factor if n = 1)
$N = 0.0592\,\text{V}$ if $T = 298.15\,\text{K}$ (25 °C)
$N = 0.0615\,\text{V}$ if $T = 310.15\,\text{K}$ (37 °C)
R = gas constant (= 8.31431 Joules $\times\, K^{-1} \times mol^{-1}$)
T = absolute temperature (unit: K, kelvin)
F = Faraday constant (= 96,487 Coulombs $\times\, mol^{-1}$)
ln 10 = natural logarithm of 10 = 2.303
a = activity
$a_{\text{Red}}/a_{\text{Ox}}$ = product of mass action for the reduction reaction

Redox electrodes currently in use are either (1) inert metal electrodes immersed in solutions containing redox couples or (2) metal electrodes whose metal functions as a member of the redox couple.

Inert Metal Electrodes

Platinum and *gold* are examples of inert metals used to record the redox potential of a redox couple dissolved in an electrolyte solution. The *hydrogen electrode* is a special redox electrode for pH measurement. It consists of a platinum or gold electrode that is electrolytically coated (platinized) with highly porous platinum (platinum black) to catalyze the electrode reaction.

$$H^+ + e^- \longleftrightarrow \frac{1}{2}H_2 \qquad (5)$$

The electrode potential is given by

$$E = E^\circ - N \times \log\frac{(f_{H_2})^{1/2}}{a_{H^+}} \qquad (6)$$

or

$$E = E^\circ - N \times \left[\log(f_{H_2})^{1/2} - \log a_{H^+}\right] \qquad (7)$$

where

$E^\circ = 0$ at all temperatures (by convention)
f_{H_2} = fugacity of hydrogen gas
a_{H^+} = activity of hydrogen ions
$-\log a_{H^+}$ = negative log of the H^+ activity (pa_{H^+} or pH)

When the partial pressure of hydrogen (PH_2) in the solution (and hence f_{H_2}) is maintained constant by bubbling hydrogen through the solution, the potential is a linear function of log a_{H^+} (= −pH). In the *standard hydrogen electrode (SHE),* the electrolyte consists of an aqueous solution of hydrogen chloride with a_{HCl} equal to 1.000 (or c_{HCl} = 1.2 mol/L) in equilibrium with a gas phase and with f_{H_2} equal to 1.000 (or PH_2 = 101.3 kPa = 1 atm). The SHE is also used as a reference electrode.

Metal Electrodes Participating in Redox Reactions

The silver-silver chloride electrode is an example of a metal electrode that participates as a member of a redox couple. The silver-silver chloride electrode consists of a silver wire or rod coated with $AgCl_{(s)}$ that is immersed in a chloride solution of constant activity; this sets the half-cell potential. The Ag/AgCl electrode is itself considered a potentiometric electrode, as its phase boundary potential is governed by an oxidation-reduction electron transfer equilibrium reaction that occurs at the surface of the silver:

$$AgCl_{(solid)} + e^- \longleftrightarrow \overset{\circ}{Ag}_{(solid)} + Cl^- \qquad (8)$$

The Nernst equation for the reference half-cell potential of an Ag/AgCl reference electrode can be written as:

$$E_{Ag/AgCl} = E^0_{Ag/AgCl} + \frac{RT}{nF} \times \ln\frac{a_{AgCl}}{a_{Ag}a_{Cl^-}} \qquad (9)$$

Since AgCl and Ag are both solids, their activities are equal to unity ($a_{AgCl} = a^0_{Ag} = 1$). Therefore, from equation 9, the half-cell potential is controlled by the activity of chloride ion in solution (a_{Cl^-}) contacting the electrode.

The Ag/AgCl electrode is used both as an internal reference element in potentiometric ISEs, and as an external reference electrode half-cell of constant potential, required to complete a potentiometric cell (see Figure 4-1). In both cases, the Ag/AgCl electrode must be in equilibrium with a solution of constant chloride ion activity.

The Ag/AgCl element of the external reference electrode half-cell is in contact with a high-concentration solution of a soluble chloride salt. Saturated potassium chloride is commonly used. A porous membrane or frit is frequently employed to separate the concentrated KCl from the sample solution. The frit serves both as a mechanical barrier to hold the concentrated electrolyte within the electrode and as a diffusional barrier to prevent proteins and other species in the sample from coming into contact with the internal Ag/AgCl element, that could poison and alter its potential. The interface between two dissimilar electrolytes (concentrated KCl/calibrator or sample) occurs within the frit and develops the liquid-liquid junction potential (E_j), a source of error in potentiometric measurements. The difference in liquid-liquid junction potential between calibrator and sample (residual liquid junction potential) is responsible for this error and can be minimized and usually neglected in practice if the compositions of the calibrating solutions are matched as closely as possible to the sample with respect to ionic content and ionic strength. An equitransferant electrolyte at high concentration as the reference electrolyte further helps to minimize the residual liquid junction potential. Potassium chloride at a concentration ≥2 mol/L is preferred. Differences of approximately −2% in the measurement of sodium by ISEs have been demonstrated when the KCl concentration in the reference electrolyte is lowered from 3 to 0.5 mol/L.[24] The magnitude of the residual liquid junction potential may also be estimated by the Henderson equation[82] with sufficient knowledge of ionic activities, ionic charges, and ionic mobilities for each electrolyte on both sides of the junction and the temperature. Using this estimate, a correction to the overall cell potential may be applied.

The presence of erythrocytes in the sample may also affect the magnitude of the residual liquid junction potential in a less predictable manner. For example, erythrocytes in blood of normal hematocrit are estimated to produce approximately 1.8 mmol/L positive error in the measurement of sodium by ISEs when an open, unrestricted liquid-liquid junction is used.[11] This bias may be minimized if a restrictive membrane or frit is used to modify the liquid-liquid junction.

The *calomel electrode* consists of mercury covered by a layer of calomel (Hg_2Cl_2), which is in contact with an electrolyte solution containing Cl^-. Calomel electrodes are frequently used as reference electrodes for pH measurements using glass pH electrodes.

Ion-Selective Electrodes

Membrane potentials are caused by the permeability of certain types of membranes to selected anions or cations. Such membranes are used to fabricate ISEs that selectively interact with a single ionic species. The potential produced at the membrane-sample solution interface is proportional to the logarithm of the ionic activity or concentration of the ion in question. Measurements with ISEs are simple, often rapid, nondestructive, and applicable to a wide range of concentrations.

The ion-selective membrane is the "heart" of an ISE as it controls the selectivity of the electrode. Ion-selective membranes are typically composed of glass, crystalline, or polymeric materials. The chemical composition of the membrane is designed to achieve an optimal permselectivity toward the ion of interest. In practice, other ions exhibit finite interaction with membrane sites and will display some degree of interference for determination of an analyte ion. In clinical practice, if the interference exceeds an acceptable level, a correction is required.

The Nicolsky-Eisenman equation describes the selectivity of an ISE for the ion of interest over interfering ions:

$$E = E^{\circ} + \left(\frac{2.303RT}{z_iF}\right)\log\left(a_i + \sum K_{i/j}a_j^{zi/zj}\right) \quad (10)$$

where

a_i = activity of the ion of interest

a_j = activity of the interfering ion

$K_{i/j}$ = selectivity coefficient for the primary ion over the interfering ion. Low values indicate good selectivity for the analyte "*i*" over the interfering ion "*j*".

z_i = charge of primary ion

z_j = charge of interfering ion

All other terms are identical to those in the Nernst equation (equation 4).

There are various approaches for determining the selectivity of an ISE for a primary ion over an interfering ion.[7,12] A straightforward approach is the *separate solution method,* where the potential of an ISE is determined in solutions of the primary and interfering ions separately but at equal ionic activities. The selectivity coefficient is then calculated as:

$$\log K_{i/j} = \frac{E_j - E_i}{\frac{2.303RT}{nF}} + \left(1 - \frac{z_i}{z_j}\right)\log a_i \quad (11)$$

Most ISEs used in clinical practice have sufficient selectivity and do not require correction for interfering ions. Oesch et al have published required ISE selectivity coefficients for ions commonly measured in clinical chemistry over other ions found in blood.[69] Table 4-1 shows required selectivity coefficients for the measurement of cations of interest in clinical chemistry over potentially interfering cations, assuming an acceptable maximum interference of 1% for the ion of interest.

Glass membrane and polymer membrane electrodes are two types of ISEs that are commonly used in clinical chemistry applications.

TABLE 4-1 Required Selectivities for Cation-Selective ISEs for Whole Blood, Plasma, and Serum Measurements

Primary Ion (i)	Required Selectivity Coefficient ($\log K_{i/j}$) for Interfering Cation (j)					
	H^+	Li^+	Na^+	K^+	Mg^{2+}	Ca^{2+}
H^+	—	−6.5	−8.5	−7.0	−7.7	−7.7
Li^{+*}	2.1	—	−4.3	−2.8	−3.5	−3.6
Na^+	4.4	−0.1	—	−0.6	−1.2	−1.3
K^+	2.8	−1.7	−3.6	—	−2.8	−2.9
Mg^{2+}	8.9	0.1	−3.9	−0.9	—	−2.4
Ca^{2+}	9.3	0.4	−3.6	−0.6	−1.9	—

*Assumes a therapeutic range for Li^+ between 0.7 and 1.5 mmol/L.

The Glass Electrode

Glass membrane electrodes are employed to measure pH and Na^+, and as an internal transducer for PCO_2 sensors. The H^+ response of thin glass membranes was first demonstrated in 1906 by Cremer.[22] In the 1930s, practical application of this phenomenon for measurement of acidity in lemon juice was made possible by the invention of the pH meter by Arnold Beckman.[9] Glass electrode membranes are formulated from melts of silicon and/or aluminum oxide mixed with oxides of alkaline earth or alkali metal cations. By varying the glass composition, electrodes with selectivity for H^+, Na^+, K^+, Li^+, Rb^+, Cs^+, Ag^+, Tl^+ and NH_4^+ have been demonstrated.[29] However, glass electrodes for H^+ and Na^+ are today the only types with sufficient selectivity over interfering ions to allow practical application in clinical chemistry. A typical formulation for H^+ selective glass is: 72% SiO_2; 22% Na_2O; 6% CaO, that has a selectivity order of $H^+ >>> Na^+ > K^+$. This glass membrane has sufficient selectivity for H^+ over Na^+ to allow error free measurements of pH in the range of 7.0 to 8.0 ($[H^+] = 10^{-7}$ to 10^{-8} mol/L) in the presence of >0.1 mol/L Na^+. Glass pH electrodes with selectivity coefficients ($K_{H/Na}$) over Na^+ of 10^{-7} and better have been realized. By altering slightly the formulation of the glass membrane to: 71% SiO_2; 11% Na_2O; 18% Al_2O_3 its selectivity order becomes $H^+ > Na^+ > K^+$. Thus, the preference of the glass membrane for H^+ over Na^+ is greatly reduced, resulting in a practical sensor for Na^+ at pH values typically found in blood.[28]

Polymer Membrane Electrodes

Polymer membrane ISEs are employed for monitoring pH and for measuring electrolytes, including K^+, Na^+, Cl^-, Ca^{2+}, Li^+, Mg^{2+}, and CO_3^{2-} (for total CO_2 measurements). They are the predominant class of potentiometric electrodes used in modern clinical analysis instruments.

The mechanism of response of these ISEs falls into three categories: (1) charged, dissociated ion-exchanger; (2) charged associated carrier, and (3) the neutral ion carrier (ionophore).[6,13] An early charged associated ion-exchanger type ISE for Ca^{2+} was developed and commercialized for clinical application in the 1960s. This electrode was based on the Ca^{2+}-selective ion-exchange/complexation properties of 2-ethylhexyl phosphoric acid dissolved in dioctyl phenyl phosphonate (charged associated carrier).[34] A porous mem-

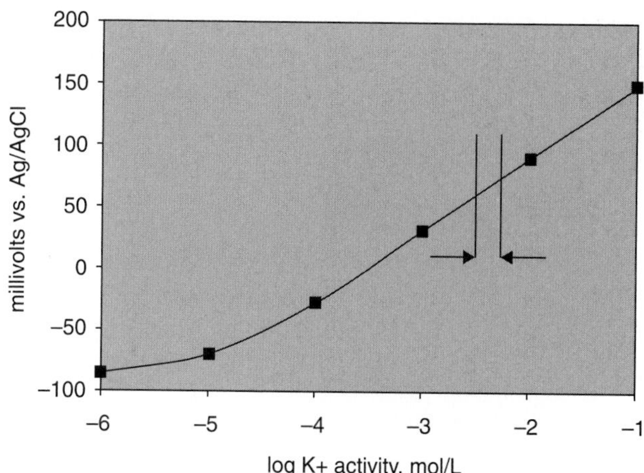

Figure 4-2 Typical EMF response of potassium selective membrane electrode to changes in the activity of potassium in the sample solution. Bracketed interval represents the normal reference interval of potassium concentration in blood. *(From D'Orazio P. In: Clinical chemistry laboratory management and clinical correlations, Lewendrowski K, ed. Philadelphia: Lippincott, Williams and Wilkins, 2002: 455.)*

brane was impregnated with this cocktail and mounted at the end of an electrode body. This type sensor was referred to as the "liquid membrane" ISE. Later a method was devised where these ingredients could be cast into a plasticized poly(vinyl chloride) (PVC) membrane, that was more rugged and convenient to use than its wet liquid predecessor. This same approach is still used today to formulate PVC-based ISEs for clinical use.[66]

A major breakthrough in the development and routine application of PVC type ISEs was the discovery by Simon and co-workers that the neutral antibiotic valinomycin could be incorporated into organic liquid membranes (and later plasticized PVC membranes), resulting in a sensor with high selectivity for K^+ over Na^+ ($K_{K/Na} = 2.5 \times 10^{-4}$).[75] The K^+ ISE based on valinomycin was the first example of a neutral carrier ISE and is extensively used today for the routine measurement of K^+ in blood. Figure 4-2 shows the response of the valinomycin-based K^+ ISE in the presence of physiological levels of Na^+, Ca^{2+}, and Mg^{2+}. The wide linear range of this ISE over three orders of magnitude makes it suitable for the measurement of K^+ in blood and urine. The K^+ range in blood is only a small portion of the electrode linear range and is spanned by a total ΔEMF of about 9 mV. Interference from other cations, seen as deviation from linearity, is not apparent at K^+ activities $>10^{-4}$ mol/L. Other, less selective polymer-based ISEs (e.g., for the measurement of Mg^{2+} and Li^+), are subject to interference from Ca^{2+}/Na^+, and Na^+, respectively, requiring simultaneous determination and correction for the presence of significant levels of interfering ions.[63,77]

Studies regarding the relationship between molecular structure and ionic selectivity have resulted in the development of polymer-based ISEs using a number of naturally occurring and synthetic ionophores, with sufficient selectivity for application in clinical analysis. The chemical structures of several of these neutral ionophores are illustrated in Figure 4-3.

Dissociated anion exchanger-based electrodes employing lipophilic quaternary ammonium salts as active membrane components are also still used commercially for the determination of Cl^- in whole blood, serum, and plasma despite some limitations.[55] Selectivity for this type of ISE is controlled by extraction of the ion into the organic membrane phase and is a function of the lipophilic character of the ion (since, unlike the carriers described above, there is no direct binding interaction between the exchanger site and the anion in the membrane phase). Thus, the selectivity order for Cl^- ISE based on an anion exchanger is fixed as $R^- > ClO_4^- > I^- > NO_3^- > Br^- > Cl^- > F^-$. The application of the Cl^- ion-exchange electrode is therefore limited to samples without significant concentrations of anions more lipophilic than Cl^-. Blood samples containing salicylate or thiocyanate, for example, will produce positive interference for the measurement of Cl^-. Repeated exposure of the electrode to the anticoagulant heparin will lead to loss of electrode sensitivity toward Cl^- because of extraction of the negatively charged heparin into the membrane. Indeed, this extraction process has been used successfully to devise a method to detect heparin levels in blood by potentiometry.[58]

High selectivity for carbonate anion can be achieved using a neutral carrier ionophore possessing trifluoroacetophenone groups doped within a polymeric membrane.[53,83] Such ionophores form negatively charged adducts with carbonate anions, and the resulting electrodes have proven useful in commercial instruments for determination of total carbon dioxide in serum/plasma, after dilution of the blood to a pH value in the range of 8.5 to 9.0, where a significant fraction of total carbon dioxide will exist as carbonate anions.

A typical formulation of a PVC membrane ISE used in clinical instrumentation is:

1 to 3 wt% ionophore
~64 wt% plasticizer
~30 wt% PVC
<1 wt% additives

The plasticizer is crucial in controlling the polarity of the membrane and thus, along with the ionophore, plays a pivotal role in determining the selectivity of the membrane toward the ion of interest. A large lipophilic anion (e.g., tetraphenylborate derivative) is often included as an additive for preparation of cation selective ISE membranes. This anion serves as a counteranion for the cation of interest as it is extracted into the membrane phase forming a positively charged complex with the neutral ionophore. However, it is the ratio of bound to unbound ionophore sites at the membrane surface that determines the magnitude of the phase boundary potential generated by the ISE membrane.[3] Thus, the selective response to the activity of the ion of interest is an interfacial property of the given ISE membrane.

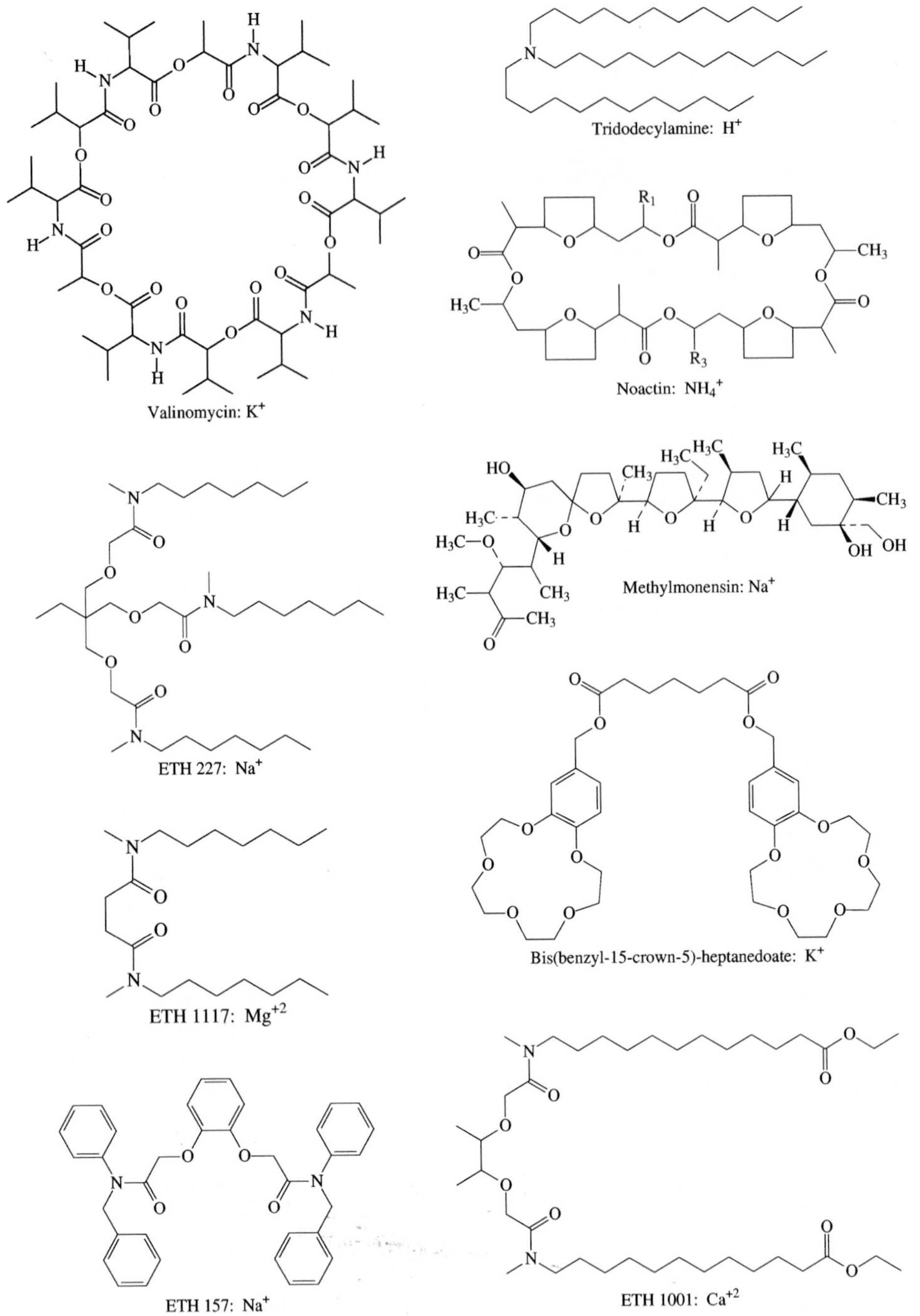

Valinomycin: K^+

Tridodecylamine: H^+

Noactin: NH_4^+

Methylmonensin: Na^+

ETH 227: Na^+

Bis(benzyl-15-crown-5)-heptanedoate: K^+

ETH 1117: Mg^{+2}

ETH 157: Na^+

ETH 1001: Ca^{+2}

Figure 4-3 Structures of common ionophores used to fabricate polymer membrane type ISEs for clinical analysis.

Studies have demonstrated that the ultimate detection limits of polymer membrane type ISEs are controlled in part by the leakage of analyte ions, from the internal solution to the outer surface of the membrane, and into the sample phase in close contact with the membrane.[61] Hence, much lower limits of detection can often be achieved by decreasing the concentration of the primary analyte ion within the internal solution of the electrode. Further, this leakage of analyte ions, coupled with an ion-exchange process at the membrane sample interface when assessing the selectivity of the membrane over other ions, can often yield a measured potentiometric selectivity coefficient that underestimates the true selectivity of the membrane. To determine "unbiased" selectivity coefficients by the separate solution method, the membrane should not be exposed to the analyte ion for extended periods of time, and the concentration of analyte ion in the internal solution should be low.[8]

Electrodes for PCO_2

Electrodes have been developed to measure PCO_2 in body fluids. The first PCO_2 electrode, developed in the 1950s by Stow and Severinghaus, used a glass pH electrode as the

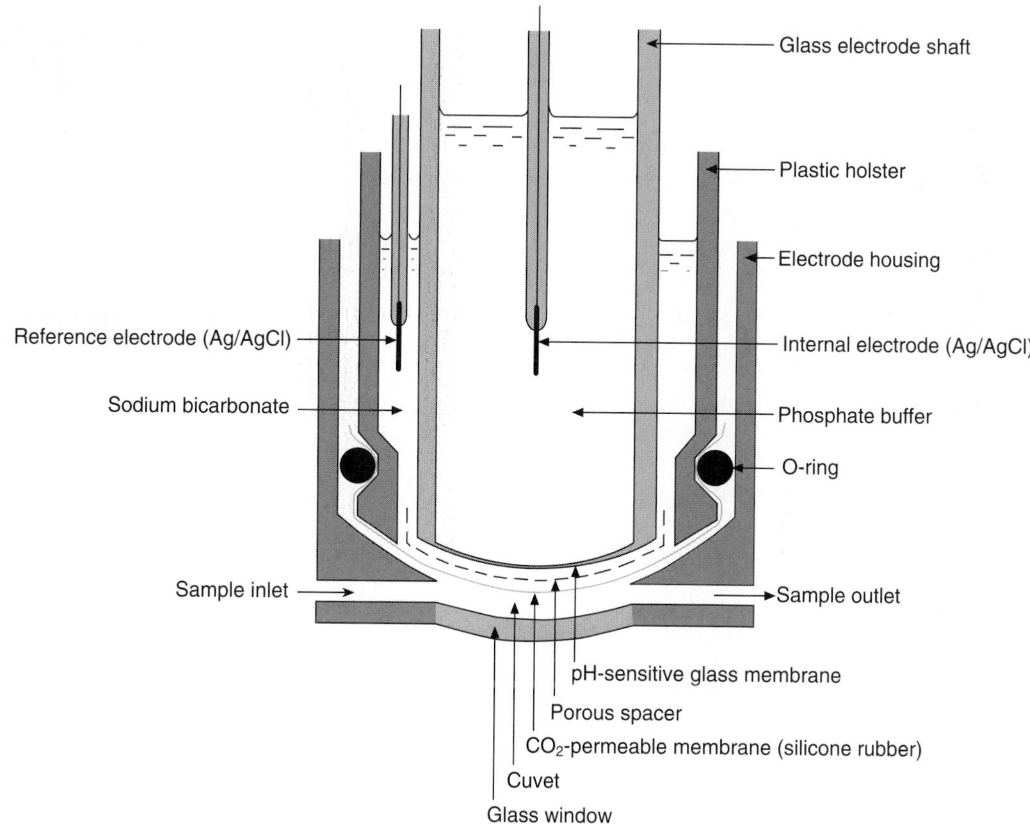

Figure 4-4 Schematic of Severinghaus style PCO_2 sensor used to monitor CO_2 levels in blood samples. *(From Siggard-Andersen O. The acid-base status of the blood. 4th ed. Baltimore: Williams & Wilkins, 1974: 172.)*

internal element in a potentiometric cell for measurement of the partial pressure of carbon dioxide.[4] This important development paved the way for commercial availability of the three-channel blood analyzer (pH, PCO_2, PO_2) to give the complete picture of the oxygenation and acid-base status of blood.

Figure 4-4 shows a diagram of a typical Severinghaus style electrode for PCO_2. A thin membrane (~20 µm), permeable to only to gases and water vapor, is in contact with the sample. Membranes of silicone rubber, Teflon, and other polymeric materials are suitable for this purpose. On the opposite side of the membrane is a thin electrolyte layer consisting of a weak bicarbonate salt (about 5 mmol/L) and a chloride salt. A pH electrode and Ag/AgCl reference electrode are in contact with this solution. The PCO_2 electrode is a self-contained potentiometric cell. Carbon dioxide gas from the sample or calibration matrix diffuses through the membrane and dissolves in the internal electrolyte layer. Carbonic acid is formed and dissociates, shifting the pH of the bicarbonate solution in the internal layer:

$$CO_2 + H_2O \leftrightarrow H_2CO_3 \leftrightarrow H^+ + HCO_3^- \quad (12)$$

and

$$\Delta\log PCO_{2(\text{sample})} \approx \Delta pH_{(\text{internal layer})} \quad (13)$$

The relationship between the sample PCO_2 and the signal generated by the internal pH electrode is logarithmic and governed by the Nernst equation. The electrode may be calibrated using precision gas mixtures or by solutions with stable PCO_2 concentrations. While Severinghaus style electrodes for PCO_2 have gained widespread use in modern blood gas analyzers, the format in which such sensors may be constructed is limited by the size, shape, and ability to fabricate the internal pH sensitive element.

A slightly different potentiometric cell for PCO_2 is shown in Figure 4-5. This cell arrangement uses two PVC type pH selective electrodes in a differential mode. The electrode membranes contain a lipophilic amine type neutral ionophore that exhibits very high selectivity for H^+ (see Figure 4-3). One electrode has an internal layer, which is buffered, while the other is unbuffered, consisting of a low concentration of bicarbonate salt. Carbon dioxide gas from the sample or calibration matrix diffuses across the outer H^+-selective PVC membranes of both sensors. On the unbuffered side, CO_2 diffusion produces a potential shift at the internal interface of the pH responsive membrane proportional to sample PCO_2 concentration. The signal at the electrode with the buffered internal layer is unaffected by CO_2 that diffuses across the membrane. Consequently, one half of the sensor responds to pH alone, while the other half responds to both pH and PCO_2. The signal difference

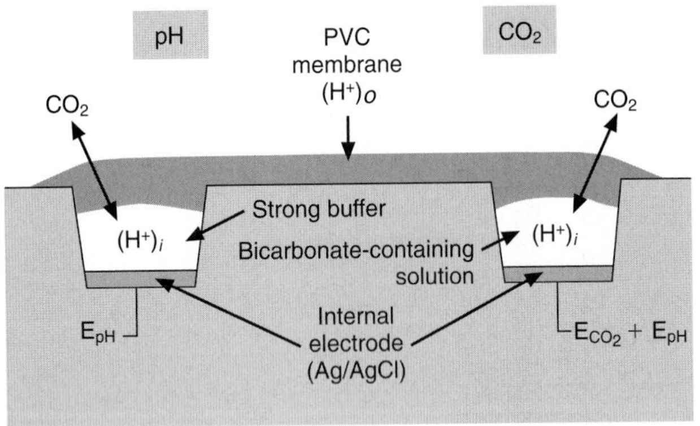

Figure 4-5 Differential planar PCO_2 potentiometric sensor design, based on two identical polymeric membrane pH electrodes, but with different internal reference electrolyte solutions. Both pH sensing membranes are prepared with H^+-selective ionophore.

between the two electrodes cancels any contribution of sample pH to the overall measured cell potential. The differential signal is proportional only to PCO_2. Unlike the traditional Severinghaus style electrode, this differential potentiometric cell PCO_2 sensor has been commercialized in a planar format and is more easily adaptable to mass production in sensor arrays.[14]

Direct Potentiometry by ISE—Units of Measure and Reporting for Clinical Applications

Classical analytical methods such as flame photometry for the measurement of electrolytes provide the total *concentration (c)* of a given ion in the sample, usually expressed in units of millimoles of ion per liter of sample (mmol/L). *Molality (m)* is a measure of the moles of ion per mass of water (mmol/kg) in the sample. Using the sodium ion as an example, the relationship between concentration and molality is given by:

$$c_{Na^+} = m_{Na^+} \times \rho H_2O \tag{14}$$

where ρH_2O is the mass concentration of water in kg/L. For normal blood plasma, the mass concentration of water is approximately 0.93 kg/L, but in specimens with elevated lipids or protein, the value may be as low as 0.8 kg/L. In these specimens, the difference between concentration and molality may be as great as 20%. A significant advantage of direct potentiometry by ISE for the measurement of electrolytes is that the technique is sensitive to molality and is therefore not affected by variations in the concentration of protein or lipids in the sample. Techniques such as flame photometry and other photometric methods requiring sample dilution are affected by the presence of protein and lipids. In these methods, only the water phase of the sample is diluted, producing results lower than molality as a function of the concentration of protein and lipids in the sample. Thus there is a risk for errors, such as a falsely low Na^+ concentration (pseudohyponatremia), in cases of extremely elevated protein and lipid concentrations.[2]

In addition to the difference between molality and concentration, measurement of ions by direct potentiometry provides yet another unit of measurement known as *activity (a)*, the concentration of free, unbound ion in solution. Unlike methods sensitive to ion concentration, ISEs do not sense the presence of complexed or electrostatically "hindered" ions in the sample. The relationship between activity and concentration using, again, sodium ion as an example, is expressed as:

$$a_{Na^+} = \gamma_{Na^+} \times c_{Na^+} \tag{15}$$

where γ is a dimensionless quantity known as the activity coefficient. The activity coefficient is primarily dependent on ionic strength of the sample as described by the Debye-Huckel equation:

$$\log \gamma = -\frac{(A \times z^2 \times I^{1/2})}{1 + B \times a \times I^{1/2}} \tag{16}$$

where A and B are temperature-dependent constants (A = 0.5213 and B = 3.305 in water at 37 °C), a is the ion size parameter for a specific ion, and I is the ionic strength ($I = 0.5\ \Sigma m \times z^2$, where z is the charge number of the ions). Equation 16 shows that a decrease in the activity coefficient occurs with an increase in ionic strength. This effect is more pronounced when the charge *(z)* of the ion is high. Activity coefficients for ions in biological fluids, such as blood and serum, are difficult to calculate with accuracy because of the uncertain contribution of macromolecular ions, such as proteins, to the overall ionic strength. However, assuming that the normal ionic strength of blood plasma is 0.160 mol/kg, estimates of activity coefficients at 37 °C are: Na^+ = 0.75, K^+ = 0.74, and Ca^{2+} = 0.31. Referring to equation 15, activity and concentration will differ greatly in samples of physiological ionic strength, especially for divalent ions.

Physiologically, ionic activity is assumed to be more relevant than concentration when considering chemical equilibria or biological processes. Practically, however, ionic concentration is the more familiar term in clinical practice, forming the basis of reference intervals and medical decision levels for electrolytes. Early in the evolution of ISEs as practical tools in clinical chemistry, it was decided that changing clinical reference intervals to a system based on activity instead of concentration was impractical and carried the risk for clinical misinterpretation. A pragmatic approach for using ISEs in modern analyzers without changing established concentration-based reference intervals is to formulate calibration solutions with ionic strengths and ionic compositions as close as possible to that of normal blood plasma. In this way, the activity coefficient of each ion in the calibrating solutions approximates that in the sample matrix, allowing calibration and measurement of electrolytes in units of concentration instead of activity.[71]

A typical set of solutions for multi-ISE calibration in an analyzer is shown in Table 4-2. Two points are used to calibrate each ISE. The difference in the cell potential generated

TABLE 4-2 Example of Two-Level Calibrating Solutions for Measurement of pH and Electrolytes by Direct Potentiometry*

Analyte	Calibration Point (mmol/L)	Slope Point (mmol/L)	Expected Signal Δ (millivolts)
Na^+	140	110	6.6
K^+	4.0	8.0	18
Ca^{2+}	1.25	2.50	9
Cl^-	100	80	6
pH	7.38 (pH units)	6.84 (pH units)	32.4

*Ionic strength adjusted to 160 mmol/kg with buffer salts and inert electrolytes.

by these two solutions (ΔE) is used to calculate the response slope of the cell (slope = (ΔE/Δlog c) where c is the concentration of ion in each calibrating solution, substituted for activity. The standard electrode potential, E^0, is calculated as the y-intercept. Determination of ion concentration in an unknown sample is then a straightforward solution of the Nickolsky-Eisenman equation (equation 10), after measuring the cell potential generated by the sample.

Calibration of the cell is in units of concentration; however, as mentioned above, direct potentiometry is sensitive to the molality of the ion, which is related to concentration by the water content of the sample (equation 14). The water content of aqueous calibrating solutions shown in Table 4-2 is approximately 0.99 kg/L. The water content of normal blood plasma is ~0.93 kg/L. Molality is 7% greater than concentration in this normal plasma specimen. The direct potentiometric cell will report results approximately 6% greater than the concentration in normal specimens because of this difference in water content between sample and calibrator (0.99/0.93 = 1.06). Direct potentiometry presents an advantage in that the technique is not affected by the presence of protein and lipids in the sample; however, the application of clinical reference intervals based on concentration again poses a risk for confusion and clinical misinterpretation. Most manufacturers of electrolyte measurement systems have overcome this problem in a practical way by following National Committee for Clinical Laboratory Standards (NCCLS) guidelines recommending the use of correlation factors to standardize ISE measurements to units of concentration. These factors may be obtained by standardizing the ISE measurement to certified reference materials based on human serum, with electrolyte values assigned in units of concentration.[42,68,86] The appropriate correlation factors are then applied to sample calculations using algorithms resident in the instrument software.

VOLTAMMETRY/AMPEROMETRY

Voltammetric and amperometric techniques are among the most sensitive and widely applicable of all electroanalytical methods.

Basic Concepts

In contrast to potentiometry, voltammetric and amperometric methods are based on electrolytic electrochemical cells, in which an external voltage is applied to a polarizable working electrode (measured versus a suitable reference electrode: $E_{appl} = E_{work} - E_{ref}$), and the resulting cathodic (for analytical reductions) or anodic (for analytical oxidations) current of the cell is monitored and is proportional to the concentration of analyte present in the test sample. Current only flows if E_{appl} is greater than a certain voltage (decomposition voltage), determined by the thermodynamics for a given redox reaction of interest ($Ox + ne^- \leftrightarrow Red$; defined by the E^0 value for that reaction (standard reduction potential)), and the kinetics for heterogeneous electron transfer at the interface of the working electrode. Often, slow kinetics of electron transfer for the redox reaction on a given inert working electrode (Pt, carbon, gold, etc.) mandates use of a much more negative (for reductions) or positive (for oxidations) E_{appl} than predicted based merely on the E^0 for a given redox reaction. This is called an overpotential (η). Regardless of whether or not an overpotential for electron transfer exists, in voltammetry/amperometry, a specific oxidation or reduction reaction occurs at the surface of the working electrode, and it is the charge transfer at this interface (current flow) that provides the analytical information.

For electrolytic cells that form the basis of voltammetric and amperometric methods:

$$E_{appl} = E_{cell} + \eta - iR_{cell} \tag{17}$$

where E_{cell} is the thermodynamic potential between the working and reference electrode in the absence of an applied external voltage. When the external voltage is greater or less than this equilibrium potential, plus or minus any overpotential (η), then current will flow because of either an oxidation or reduction reaction at the working electrode. A voltammogram is simply the plot of observed current, i, vs. E_{appl} (Figure 4-6). In amperometry (see below), a fixed voltage is applied, and the resulting current is monitored. The amount of current is inversely related to the resistance of the electrolyte solution, and any "apparent" resistance that develops because of the mass transfer of the analyte species to the surface of the working electrode. Because the electrochemical reactions are heterogeneous, occurring only at the surface of the working electrode, the amount of current observed is also highly dependent on the surface area (A) of the working electrode.

When a potential is applied to a working electrode that will oxidize or reduce a species in the solution phase contacting the electrode, the electrochemical reaction causes the concentration of electroactive species to decrease at the

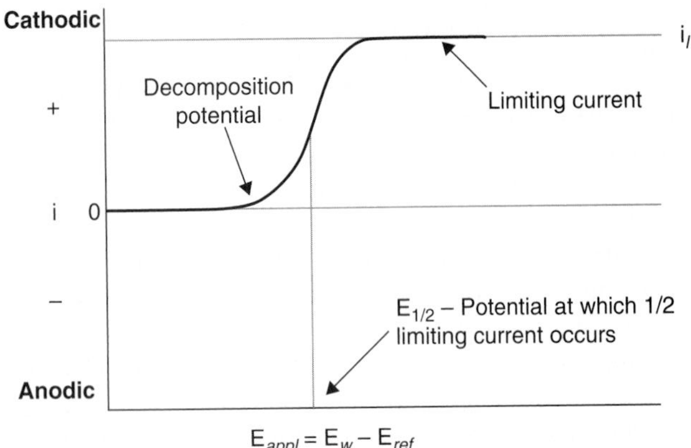

Figure 4-6 Illustration of the current vs. voltage curve (voltammogram) obtained for oxidized species (Ox) being reduced to Red at the surface of working electrode, as the E_{appl} is scanned more negative, and the solution is stirred to yield a steady-state response.

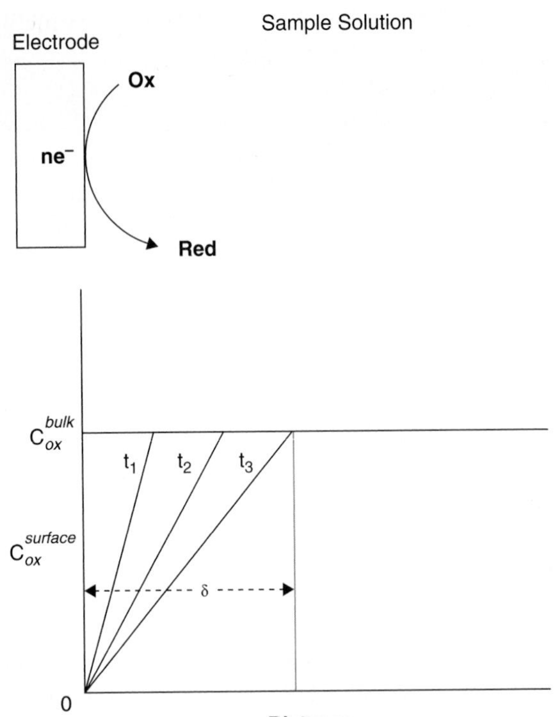

Figure 4-7 Concept of electrochemical reaction increasing the diffusion layer thickness (concentration polarization) of analyte via a reduction (or oxidation) at the surface of the working electrode. As time (t) increases, the diffusion layer thickness grows quickly to a value that is determined by degree of convection in the sample solution.

surface of the electrode (Figure 4-7), a process termed "concentration polarization." This in turn causes a concentration gradient of the analyte species between the bulk sample solution and the surface of the electrode.[32] When the bulk solution is stirred, the diffusion layer of analyte grows out from the surface of the electrode very quickly to a fixed distance controlled by how vigorously the solution is stirred. This diffusion layer is termed the Nernst layer and has a finite thickness (δ) after a relatively short time period (see Figure 4-7) when the solution is moving (convection). Voltammetry carried out in the presence of convection (either by stirring the solution, rotating the electrode, flowing solution by electrode, etc.) is called steady-state voltammetry. When the solution is not moving, the diffusion layer grows further and further with time (i.e., not constant), creating larger and larger δ values with time. This is termed nonsteady state voltammetry and often results in peak currents in i vs. E_{appl} plots for electrolytic cells.

In steady-state voltammetry, when the potential of the working electrode is scanned past a value that will cause an electrochemical reaction, the current will rise rapidly, and then level off to a near constant value, even as E_{appl} changes further. Figure 4-6 illustrates such a wave for a hypothetical reduction of an oxidized species (Ox) via an n electron reduction to a reduced species (Red). When the applied potential is much more negative than required, the current reaches a limiting value (termed the limiting current, i_l). This limiting current is proportional to the concentration of the electroactive species (Ox in this case) as expressed by the following equation:

$$i_l = nFA\left(\frac{D}{\delta}\right)C_{ox} \quad (18)$$

where i is the measured current in amperes, n equals the number of electrons in the electrochemical reaction (reduction in this case), F is Faraday's constant (96,487 coulombs/mol), A is the electrochemical surface area of the working electrode (in cm^2) (assuming a planar electrode geometry), D is the diffusion coefficient (in cm^2/sec) of the electroactive species (Ox in this case), δ is the diffusion layer thickness (in cm), and C is the concentration of the analyte species in mol/cm^3. The D/δ term is often denoted as m_o, the mass transfer coefficient of the Ox species to the surface of the working electrode. Note that equation 18 indicates a linear relationship for limiting current and concentration. The exact same equation applies for detecting reduced species by an oxidation reaction at the working electrode. In this case, by convention, the resulting anodic current is considered a negative current. As shown in Figure 4-6, the potential of the working electrode that corresponds to a current that is exactly one half the limiting current is termed the $E_{1/2}$ value. This value is not dependent on analyte concentration. The $E_{1/2}$ is determined by the thermodynamics (E^0) of the given redox reaction, the solution conditions (e.g., if protons are involved in reaction, then the pH will influence the $E_{1/2}$ value), along with any overpotential caused by slow electron transfer, etc., at a particular working electrode surface. The $E_{1/2}$ values are indicative of a given species undergoing an electrochemical reaction under specified conditions; hence, the $E_{1/2}$ values enable one to distinguish one electroactive species from another in the same sample. If the

$E_{1/2}$ values for various species differ significantly (e.g., >120 mV), then measurements of several limiting currents in a given voltammogram can yield quantitative results for several different species simultaneously.

Electrochemical cells employed to carry out voltammetric or amperometric measurements can involve either a two or three electrode configuration. In the two electrode mode, the external voltage is applied between the working and a reference electrode, and the current monitored. Since the current must also pass through the reference electrode, such current flow can potentially alter the surface concentration of electroactive species that poises the actual half-cell potential of the reference electrode, changing its value by a concentration polarization process. For example, if an Ag/AgCl reference electrode were used in a cell in which a reduction reaction for the analyte occurs at the working electrode, then an oxidation reaction would take place at the surface of the reference electrode:

$$Ag^0 + Cl^- \rightarrow AgCl_{(s)} + 1\,e^- \tag{19}$$

Hence, the activity/concentration of chloride ions near the surface of the electrode would decrease, which would make the potential of the reference electrode more positive than its true equilibrium value based on the actual activity of chloride ion in the reference half-cell since the Nernst equation for this half-cell is:

$$E_{Ag/AgCl} = E^0_{Ag/AgCl} - 0.059\log\left(a^{surface}_{Cl^-}\right) \tag{20}$$

Such concentration polarization of the reference electrode is prevented by maintaining the current density (J; amperes/cm^2) very low at the reference electrode. This is achieved in practice by making sure that the area of the working electrode in the electrochemical cell is much smaller than the surface area of the reference electrode; hence the total current flow will be limited by this much smaller area, and J values for the reference will be very small, as desired, to prevent concentration polarization.

To completely eliminate changes in reference electrode half-cell potentials, a three electrode potentiostat is often employed. In simple terms, the potentiostat applies a voltage to the working electrode, which is measured versus a reference electrode via a zero current potentiometric type measurement, but the current flow is between the working electrode and a third electrode, called the counter electrode. Thus if reduction takes place at the working electrode, oxidation would occur at the counter electrode; but no net reaction would take place at the surface of the reference electrode, since no current flows through this electrode. A potentiostat circuit is relatively simple to construct using modern operational amplifiers.

In voltammetric methods, the E_{appl} is varying via some waveform, to alter the working electrode potential as a function of time and the resulting current measured. The current change occurs at the decomposition potential range, which is hopefully specific for a given analyte. However, the location of the current response as a function of E_{appl} provides information on the nature of the species present (e.g., $E_{1/2}$) along with a concentration-dependent signal. This scan of E_{appl} can be linear (linear sweep voltammetry) or it can have more complex shapes that enable greatly enhanced sensitivity to be achieved for monitoring the concentration of a given electroactive species (e.g., normal pulsed voltammetry, differential pulse voltammetry, square wave voltammetry, etc.).[72] When a dropping mercury electrode (DME) is used, such voltammetric methods are considered polarographic methods of analysis.

Amperometric methods differ from voltammetry in that E_{appl} is fixed, generally at a potential value that occurs in the limiting current plateau region of the voltammogram and simply monitoring the resulting current, which will be proportional to concentration. Amperometry can be more sensitive than common voltammetric methods because background charging currents, which arise from changing the E_{appl} as a function of time in voltammetry, do not exist. Hence, when selectivity can be assured at a given E_{appl} value, amperometry may be preferred to voltammetric methods for more sensitive quantitative measurements.

APPLICATIONS

Molecular oxygen is capable of undergoing several reduction reactions, all with a significant overpotentials at solid electrodes, such as Pt, Au, or Ag. For example, the following reaction:

$$\begin{gathered} O_2 + 2H_2O + 4e^- \rightarrow 4OH^- \\ \left(E^0 = +0.179 \quad vs \quad Ag/AgCl;1\,M\,Cl^-\right) \end{gathered} \tag{21}$$

exhibits an $E_{1/2}$ at around −0.500 V on a Pt electrode (vs. a Ag/AgCl reference electrode), with a limiting current plateau beginning at approx. −0.600 V. This reaction can be used to monitor the partial pressure of oxygen (PO_2) in blood, which is the basis of the widely used Clark style amperometric oxygen sensor (Figure 4-8). This device employs a small area planar platinum electrode as a working electrode (encased in insulating glass or other material), and a Ag/AgCl reference electrode, typically a cylindrical design (Figure 4-8). This two electrode electrolytic cell is placed within a sensor housing, on which a gas permeable membrane (e.g., polypropylene, silicone rubber, Teflon, etc.) is held at the distal end. The inner working platinum electrode is pressed tightly against the gas-permeable membrane to create a thin film of internal electrolyte solution (usually buffer with KCl added). Oxygen in the sample can permeate across the membrane and be reduced in accordance with the above electrochemical reaction. An E_{appl} of −0.650 or −0.700 V vs. Ag/AgCl (within the limiting current regime) to the Pt working electrode will result in an observed current that is proportional to the PO_2 present in the sample (including whole blood). In the absence of any oxygen, the current at this applied voltage under amperometric conditions will be very near zero.

The outer gas-permeable membrane enables the Clark electrode to detect oxygen with very high selectivity over

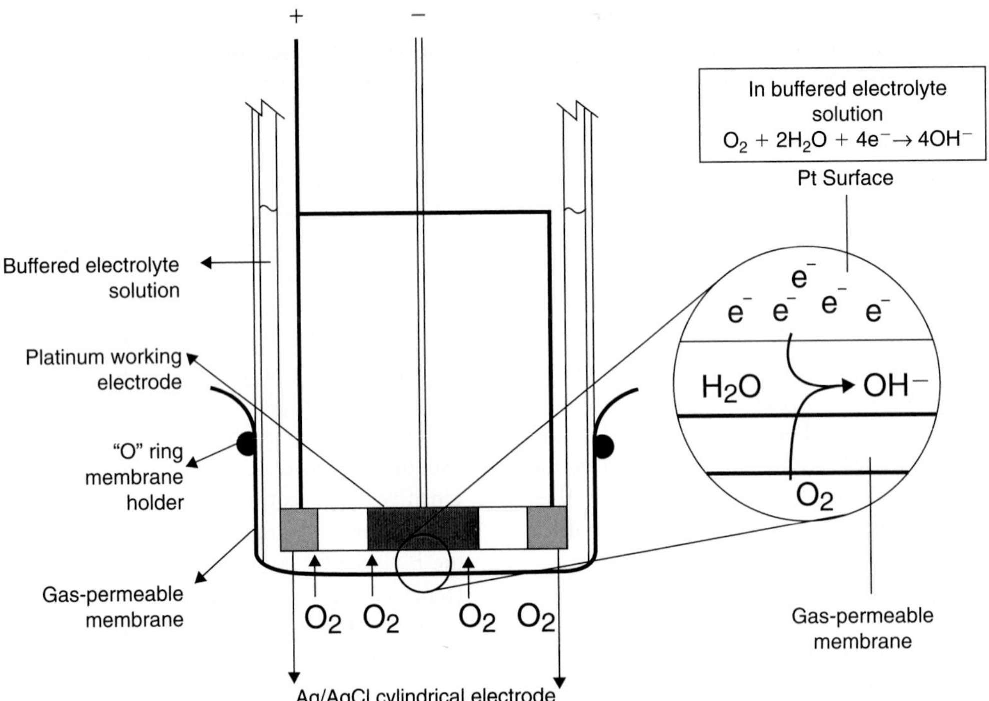

Figure 4-8 Design of Clark style amperometric oxygen sensor used to monitor PO_2 levels in blood.

other easily reduced species that might be present in a given sample (e.g., metal ions, cystine, etc.). Indeed, only other gas species or highly lipophilic organic species can partition into and pass through such gas-permeable membranes. One type of interference in clinical samples can be certain anesthesia gases, such as nitrous oxide, halothane, and isoflurane. These species can also diffuse through the outer membrane of the sensor, be electrochemically reduced at the platinum electrode, and yield a false positive value for the measurement of PO_2.[26] However, optimized gas-permeable membrane materials and appropriate control of the applied potential to the cathode of the sensor have greatly reduced this problem in modern instruments. The outer gas-permeable membranes also help restrict the diffusion of analyte to the inner working electrode; hence the membrane can control the mass transport of analyte (D/δ term in equation 16), such that in the presence or absence of sample convection, mass transport of oxygen to the surface of the platinum working electrode is essentially the same.

The basic design of the Clark amperometric PO_2 sensor can be extended to detect other gas species by altering the applied voltage to the working electrode. For example, it is possible to detect nitric oxide (NO) with high selectivity using a similar gas electrode design in which the platinum is polarized at +0.900 vs. Ag/AgCl to oxidize diffusing NO to nitrate at the platinum anode.[10] Such NO sensors can be used for a variety of biomedically important studies to deduce the amount of NO locally at or near the surface of various NO-producing cells.

Beyond amperometric devices, one specialized method for detecting trace levels of toxic metal ions in clinical samples is anodic stripping voltammetry (ASV). In ASV a carbon working electrode is used (sometimes further coated with a Hg film), and the E_{appl} is first fixed at a very negative E_{appl} voltage so that all metal ions in the solution will be reduced to elemental metals (M^0) within the mercury film and/or on the surface of the carbon. Then the E_{appl} is scanned more positive, and the reduced metals deposited in and/or on the surface of the working electrode are reoxidized, giving a large anodic current peak proportional to the concentration of metal ions in the original sample. The potential at which these peaks are observed indicates which metal is present, and the height of stripping peak current is directly proportional to the concentration of the metal ion in the original sample. Such ASV techniques can be used to detect the total concentration of Pb in whole blood samples, providing a rapid screening method for lead exposure and poisoning.[33]

Another biomedical example of modern voltammetry is a rapid scan cyclic voltammetric technique that has been used to quantify dopamine in brain tissue of freely moving animals.[78] In this application, oxidation of dopamine to a quinone species at an implanted microcarbon electrode (at approximately +0.600 V vs. Ag/AgCl) yields peak currents proportional to dopamine levels. The electrode can be used to measure this neurotransmitter in different regions of the brain or in a fixed location. Often, pharmacological or electrical stimulation can be employed to measure the

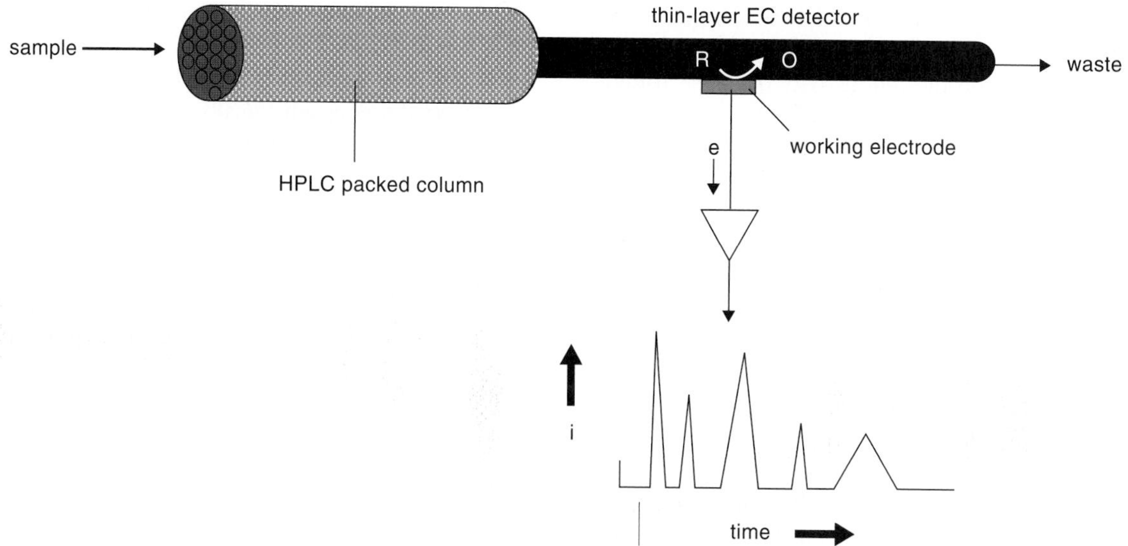

Figure 4-9 Schematic of LC-EC system, with electrochemical detector monitoring the elution of analytes from an HPLC column, by either their oxidation or reduction (shown here as example) at a suitable thin-layer working electrode.

change in local dopamine levels due to such stimulation techniques.

While voltammetric/amperometric techniques can be applied to detect a wide range of species, the selectivity offered for measurements in complex clinical samples—where many species can be electroactive—is rather limited. For example, as stated in the above discussion relevant to the Clark oxygen sensor, in the absence of the gas-permeable membrane, other species that can be reduced at or near the same E_{appl} as oxygen would cause significant interference.

To greatly expand the range of analytes that can be detected with voltammetric/amperometric methods, electrochemical techniques can be used as highly sensitive detectors for modern high performance liquid chromatographic (HPLC) systems (see Chapter 6). In liquid chromatography with electrochemical detection (LC-EC), eluting solutes are detected by flow-through electrodes (usually carbon or mercury) designed to have extremely low dead volumes (Figure 4-9). The electrodes can be operated in amperometric or voltammetric modes (with high scan speeds), and several electrodes can be operated simultaneously in series or in parallel flow arrangements to gain additional selectivity.[48] For example, homocysteine can be measured with (1) the addition of reducing agents to a serum sample to generate free homocysteine, (2) precipitation of proteins in the sample (with trichloroacetic acid), and (3) separation of the serum components on a reversed phase octadecylsilane HPLC column. The eluting homocysteine is detected and measured with online electrochemical detection via homocysteine oxidation to the corresponding mercuric dithiolate complex

$$2\,RSH + Hg \rightarrow Hg(RS)_2 + 2H^+ + 2e^- \qquad (22)$$

using a thin-layer Hg/Au amalgam electrode poised at +0.150 V vs. Ag/AgCl.[81] Integration of the eluting band for homocysteine provides quantitative results, with very high selectivity. Similarly, catechols and catecholamines can also be readily detected in serum by a similar LC-EC method, with the eluted catechols oxidized to quinones at a flow-through carbon working electrode poised at potentials typically >0.200 V vs. Ag/AgCl. Further, a host of therapeutic drugs can also be quantitated in serum or urine via LC-EC methods.

CONDUCTOMETRY

Conductometry is an electrochemical technique used to determine the quantity of an analyte present in a mixture by measurement of its effect on the electrical conductivity of the mixture. It is the measure of the ability of ions in solution to carry current under the influence of a potential difference. In a conductometric cell, potential is applied between two inert metal electrodes. An alternating potential with a frequency between 100 and 3000 Hz is used to prevent polarization of the electrodes. A decrease in solution resistance results in an increase in conductance and more current is passed between the electrodes. The resulting current flow is also alternating. The current is directly proportional to solution conductance. Conductance is considered the inverse of resistance and may be expressed in units of ohm^{-1} (siemens). In clinical analysis, conductometry is frequently used for the measurement of the volume fraction of erythrocytes in whole blood (hematocrit) and as the transduction mechanism for some biosensors.

Erythrocytes act as electrical insulators because of their lipid-based membrane composition. This phenomenon was first used in the 1940s to measure the volume fraction of erythrocytes in whole blood (hematocrit) by conductivity[80] and is used today to measure hematocrit on multianalyte instruments for clinical analysis. The conductivity of whole blood depends not only on the volume fraction and shape of the erythrocytes but also on the conductivity of the surrounding plasma. An increase in the volume fraction of erythrocytes, that are less conductive than the surrounding plasma, leads to a decrease in conductivity shown by the following relationship[95]

$$G_b = \frac{a}{1} + \frac{H}{100-H} \times c \qquad (23)$$

where G_b is the conductivity of whole blood, a is the plasma conductivity, H is the percent of hematocrit and c is a factor for erythrocyte orientation. In practice, plasma conductivity also contains correction factors for Na^+ and K^+ concentrations. These cations are usually measured in conjunction with hematocrit on systems designed for clinical analysis.

Conductivity-based hematocrit measurements have limitations.[88] Abnormal protein levels will change plasma conductivity and interfere with the measurement. Low protein concentrations resulting from dilution of blood with protein-free electrolyte solutions during cardiopulmonary bypass surgery will result in erroneously low hematocrit values by conductivity. Preanalytical variables, such as insufficient mixing of the sample, will also lead to errors.[99] Hemoglobin is the preferred analyte to monitor blood loss and the need for transfusion during trauma and surgery. However, the electrochemical measurement of hematocrit in conjunction with blood gases and electrolytes remains in use mainly because of simplicity and convenience, despite some limitations.

Another clinical application of conductance is for electronic counting of blood cells in suspension. Termed the "Coulter principle," it relies on the fact that the conductivity of blood cells is lower than that of a salt solution used as a suspension medium.[21] The cell suspension is forced to flow through a tiny orifice. Two electrodes are placed on either side of the orifice, and a constant current is established between the electrodes. Each time a cell passes through the orifice, the resistance increases; this causes a spike in the electrical potential difference between the electrodes. The pulses are then amplified and counted.

COULOMETRY

Coulometry measures the electrical charge passing between two electrodes in an electrochemical cell. The amount of charge passing between the electrodes is directly proportional to oxidation or reduction of an electroactive substance at one of the electrodes. The number of coulombs transferred in this process is related to the absolute amount of electroactive substance by Faraday's Law:

$$Q = n \times N \times F \qquad (24)$$

where

Q = is the amount of charge passing through the cell (unit: C = coulomb = ampere · second)

n = the number of electrons transferred in the oxidation or reduction reaction

N = the amount of substance reduced or oxidized in moles

F = Faraday constant (96,487 coulombs/mole)

The measurement of current is related to charge as the amount of charge passed per unit time (ampere = coulomb/second). Coulometry is used in clinical applications for the determination of chloride in serum or plasma and as the mode of transduction in certain types of biosensors.

Commercial coulometric titrators have been developed for determination of chloride. A constant current is applied between a silver wire (anode) and a platinum wire (cathode). At the anode, Ag is oxidized to Ag^+. At the cathode, H^+ is reduced to hydrogen gas. At a constant applied current, the number of coulombs passed between the anode and cathode is directly proportional to time (coulombs = amperes × seconds). Therefore, the absolute number of silver ions produced at the anode may be calculated from the amount of time current passes through it. In the presence of Cl^-, Ag^+ ions formed are precipitated as $AgCl_{(S)}$ and the amount of free Ag^+ in solution is low. When all the Cl^- ions have been complexed, there is a sudden increase in the concentration of Ag^+ in solution. The excess Ag^+ is sensed amperometrically at a second Ag electrode, polarized at negative potential. The excess Ag^+ is reduced to Ag, producing a current. When this current exceeds a certain value, the titration is stopped. The absolute number of Cl^- ions present in the sample is calculated from the time during which the titration with Ag^+ was in progress. Knowing the volumetric amount of serum or plasma sample originally used, it is possible to calculate the concentration of Cl^- in the sample. Coulometric titration is one of the most accurate electrochemical techniques since the method measures the absolute amount of electroactive substance in the sample. Coulometry is considered the gold standard for determination of chloride in serum or plasma. However, the method is subject to interference from anions in the sample with affinity for Ag^+ greater than chloride, such as bromide.[97]

OPTICAL CHEMICAL SENSORS

An "optode" is an optical sensor used in analytical instruments to measure blood gases and electrolytes. Optodes have certain advantages over electrodes, including ease of miniaturization, less noise (no transduction wires), potential long-term stability using ratiometric type measurements at multiple wavelengths,[84] and no need for a separate reference electrode. These advantages promoted the development of optical sensor technology initially for design of intravascular blood gas sensors (see in vivo sensor section below). However, the same basic sensing principles can be used in clinical chemistry instrumentation designed for more classical in vitro measurements on discrete samples. In such systems, light can be brought to and from the sensing site either by optical fibers or simply by appropriate positioning of light sources (light emitting diodes, LEDs), filters, and

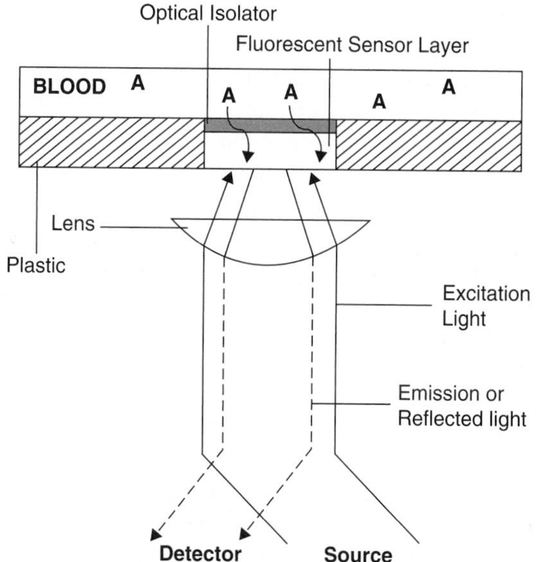

Figure 4-10 General design for in vitro optical sensor designed to detect given analyte in blood sample. Polymer film contains dye that changes spectral properties in proportion to the amount of analyte in the sample phase. Example shown is for sensing film that changes luminescence (fluorescence or phosphorescence).

photodetectors to monitor absorbance (by reflectance), fluorescence, or phosphorescence (Figure 4-10).

Basic Concepts

Optical sensors devised for PO_2 measurements are typically based on the immobilization of certain organic dyes (e.g., pyrene, diphenylphenanthrene, phenanthrene, fluoranthene, etc.) or metal ligand complexes (e.g., ruthenium[II] tris[dipyridine], Pt and Pd metalloporphyrins, etc.) within hydrophobic polymer films (e.g., silicone rubber) in which oxygen is very soluble.[25] The fluorescence or phosphorescence of such species at a given wavelength is often quenched in the presence of paramagnetic species, including molecular oxygen. In the case of embedded fluorescent dyes, the intensity of the emitted fluorescence of such films will decrease in proportion to the PO_2 level of the sample in contact with the polymer film, in accordance with the Stern-Volmer equation for quenching:

$$\frac{I_0}{I_{PO_2}} = 1 + kPO_2 \qquad (25)$$

where

I_0 = fluorescence intensity in the absence of any oxygen
I_{PO_2} = fluorescence intensity at a given PO_2 level
k = quenching constant for the particular fluorophore used

Hence a linear relationship exists between the ratio I_0/I_{PO_2} and the PO_2 in the sample phase. The larger the Stern-Volmer constant, the greater the degree of quenching for the given fluorophore. However, it is important that the quenching constant is in a range that will yield linear Stern-Volmer behavior over the physiologically relevant range of PO_2 in blood. For example, if k is too large, then maximum quenching possible will occur over a range of PO_2 that is less than physiological.

Phosphorescence intensity or phosphorescence lifetime measurements of immobilized metal ligand complexes can also be employed (i.e., binding of oxygen decreases excited state lifetimes). Sensors based on changes in luminescent lifetime have the inherent advantage of being insensitive to perturbations in the optical pathlength and the amount of active dye present in the sensing layer.

Optical pH sensors require immobilization of appropriate pH indicators (e.g., fluorescein, 8-hydroxy-1,2,6-pyrene trisulfonate [HPTS], phenol red, etc.) within thin layers of hydrophilic polymers (e.g., hydrogels), since equilibrium access of protons to the indicator is essential. The absorbance or fluorescence of the protonated or deprotonated form of the species can be used for sensing purposes.[84] One issue with respect to using immobilized indicators for accurate physiological pH measurements is the effect of ionic strength on the pKa of the indicator. Because optical sensors measure the concentration of protonated or deprotonated dye as an indirect measure of hydrogen ion activity, variations in the ionic strength of the physiological sample can influence the accuracy of the pH measurement.

Applications

Optical sensors suitable for the determination of PCO_2 employ optical pH transducers (with immobilized indicators) as inner transducers in an arrangement quite similar to the classical Severinghaus style electrochemical sensor design (see Figure 4-4). The addition of bicarbonate salt within the pH sensing hydrogel layer creates the required electrolyte film layer, which varies in pH depending on the level of PCO_2 in equilibrium with the film. The optical pH sensor is covered by an outer gas-permeable hydrophobic film (e.g., silicone rubber), to prevent proton access, yet allows CO_2 equilibration with the pH-sensing layer. As the PCO_2 level in the sample increases, the pH of the bicarbonate layer decreases, and the corresponding decrease in the concentration of the deprotonated form of the indicator (or increase in the concentration of protonated form) is sensed optically.

Two approaches have been used to sense electrolyte ions optically in physiological samples. One method employs many of the same lipophilic ionophores developed for polymer membrane type ion-selective electrodes (see Figure 4-3).[6,13] These species are doped into very thin hydrophobic polymeric films along with a lipophilic pH indicator. In the case of cation ionophores (e.g., valinomycin for sensing potassium), when cations from the sample are extracted by the ionophore into the thin film, the pH indicator (RH) loses a proton to the sample phase to maintain charge neutrality within the organic film (yielding R^-). This results in a change in the optical absorption or fluorescence spectrum of the polymer layer. If the thickness of the films is kept <10 μm, equilibrium response times on the order of <1 min have been achieved. The main limitation of this design is that the pH of the sample phase also influences the overall extraction equilibrium for ions into the film. Thus either simultaneous and independent measurement of sample pH is required, or buffered dilution and/or pH control of the sample phase is necessary to obtain accurate measurements of electrolytes.

A second methodology used to sense electrolyte ions is to immobilize a cation and/or anion recognition agent within a hydrogel matrix, similar to the pH sensors described above. The recognition agent in this case is not usually lipophilic, and therefore it must be covalently anchored to the hydrogel so that it does not leach into the sample phase. The agent is designed so that selective cation or anion binding alters the absorbance or fluorescence spectrum of the species within the hydrogel. Typically, this is achieved by linking both ion recognition and chromophoric properties within a single organic molecule. Such ion sensors have been employed successfully in at least one commercial blood gas-electrolyte analyzer using an array of sensors of the generic design similar to that illustrated in Figure 4-10.

BIOSENSORS

A biosensor is a specific type of chemical sensor consisting of a biological recognition element and a physico-chemical transducer, often an electrochemical[45,90] or an optical device. The biological element is capable of recognizing the presence and activity and/or concentration of a specific analyte in solution. The recognition may be either a *biocatalytic reaction (enzyme-based biosensor)* or a *binding process (affinity-based biosensor),* when the recognition element is, for example, an antibody, DNA segment, or cell receptor. The interaction of the recognition element with a target analyte results in a measurable change in a solution property locally at the surface of the device, such as formation of a product or consumption of a reactant. The transducer converts the change in solution property into a quantifiable electrical signal. The mode of transduction may be one of several, including electrochemical, optical, and the measurement of mass or heat. The present discussion will be limited to biosensors based on electrochemical and optical modes of transduction since they comprise the majority of biosensors used for clinical applications.

Enzyme-Based Biosensors with Amperometric Detection

Enzyme-based biosensors based on electrochemical transducers, specifically amperometric electrodes, are the most commonly used for clinical analyses and the most frequently cited in the literature.[44] Clark and Lyons developed the first amperometric biosensor; it was used for measuring glucose in blood and was based on immobilizing glucose oxidase on the surface of an amperometric PO_2 sensor.[18] A solution of glucose oxidase was physically entrapped between the gas-permeable membrane of the PO_2 electrode and an outer semipermeable membrane (see Figure 4-11 general design). The outer membrane was of a low molecular weight cut-off to allow substrate (glucose) and oxygen from the sample to pass, but not proteins and other macromolecules. In this way, enzymes could be concentrated at the sensor's surface. The oxidation of glucose, catalyzed by glucose oxidase

$$\text{Glucose} + O_2 \xrightarrow{\text{glucose oxidase}} \text{gluconic acid} + H_2O_2 \quad (26)$$

consumes oxygen near the surface of the sensor. The rate of decrease in PO_2 is a function of the glucose concentration and is monitored by the PO_2 electrode. A steady-state reduced level of oxygen can be achieved at the surface in a

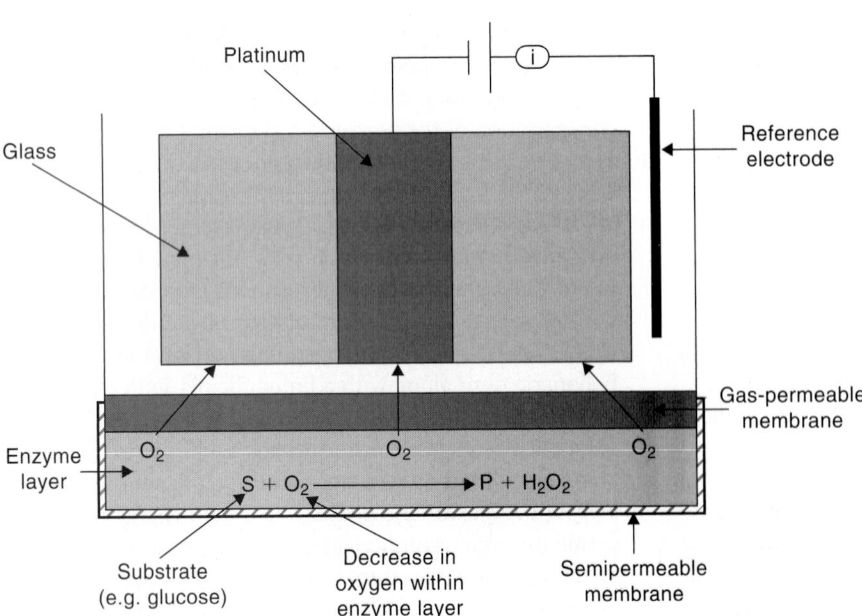

Figure 4-11 Illustration of enzyme electrode prepared using oxidase enzyme immobilized at the surface of amperometric PO_2 sensor. Increase in substrate concentration S reduces the amount of oxygen present at the surface of the sensor.

short period of time, yielding a steady-state current value that decreases as a function of glucose concentration in the sample.

If the polarizing voltage of the PO_2 electrode is reversed, making the platinum electrode positive (anode) relative to the Ag/AgCl reference electrode, and if the gas permeable membrane is replaced with a hydrophilic membrane containing the immobilized enzyme, it is possible to oxidize the H_2O_2 produced by the glucose oxidase:

$$H_2O_2 \rightarrow 2e^- + O_2 + 2H^+ \quad (27)$$

The steady-state current produced is now directly proportional to the concentration of glucose in the sample.

In practice, a sufficiently high voltage (overpotential) must be applied to the platinum anode to drive the oxidation of the hydrogen peroxide. An applied voltage of +0.7 volts or greater (relative to Ag/AgCl) is typically used. Figure 4-12 illustrates this basic hydrogen peroxide detection design, which is suitable for use in devising clinically useful sensors for glucose, but also for a host of other substrates for which there are suitable oxidase enzymes that generate hydrogen peroxide.

Immobilization of enzymes in the early biosensors was a simple entrapment method behind a membrane of low molecular weight cut-off, and this approach is still used in some commercial applications. Many other schemes for enzyme immobilization for biosensor development have been suggested.[41] Most common are cross-linking of the enzyme with an inert protein, such as bovine serum albumin (BSA), using glutaraldehyde, simple adsorption of enzyme to electrode surfaces, or covalent binding of enzymes to insoluble carriers, such as nylon or glass. Another immobilization technique involves bulk modification of an electrode material, mixing enzymes with carbon paste, which serves as both the enzyme immobilization matrix and the electroactive surface.[38]

One of the first biosensor based systems for the measurement of glucose in blood was commercialized by Yellow Springs Instruments, Inc. (YSI), Yellow Springs, Ohio, in 1975 and used the amperometric detection of H_2O_2 as the measurement principle (see Figure 4-12). Dependence of the measured glucose value on the oxygen concentration in the sample was a problem since there is significantly less than the stoichiometric amount of dissolved oxygen in blood to support the glucose oxidase reaction and produce a linear relationship of signal with glucose concentration. This is especially true at high levels of glucose found in samples from diabetic patients (>500 mg/dL). In the case of the YSI system, the sample and calibration solutions are diluted at least 1:10 in buffer (depends on model), which is in equilibrium with atmospheric PO_2, fixing the oxygen concentration in the calibrator and sample at a constant level.

The problem of oxygen limitations of biosensors based on oxidase enzymes has been addressed by designing semipermeable membranes that restrict the diffusion of the primary analyte (substrate) to the enzyme layer, avoiding saturation of the enzyme, and keeping the ratio of oxygen to analyte always in excess of 1. This extends the linearity of response to analyte concentrations substantially higher than the K_m of the enzyme, and reduces the signal dependence on oxygen. Outer track-etched polycarbonate membranes are commonly used,[76] and membranes of poly (vinyl chloride), polyurethanes, and silicone emulsions.[60] Another approach has been to use an oxygen-rich electrode material as a reservoir of oxygen to support the bioreaction. A fluorocarbon (Kel-F oil) has been used to formulate a carbon paste electrode to act both as a source of oxygen and the working electrode.[96]

Electron acceptors other than oxygen can serve as mediators in the glucose oxidase reaction, and completely eliminate any dependence of the amperometric response on oxygen concentration of the sample. The mediator, usually co-immobilized with the enzyme, transports electrons to the

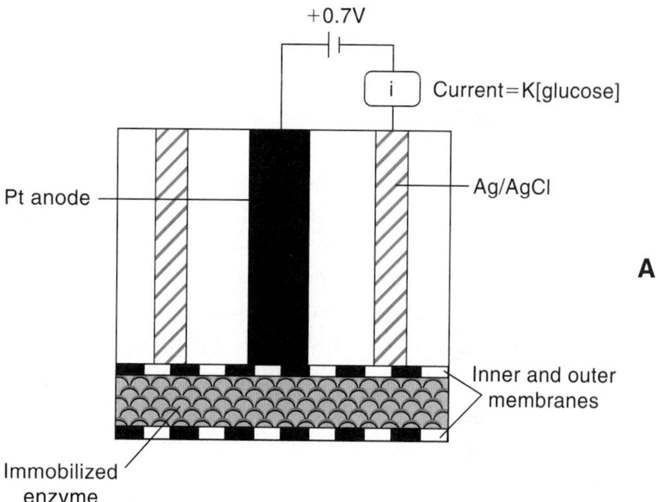

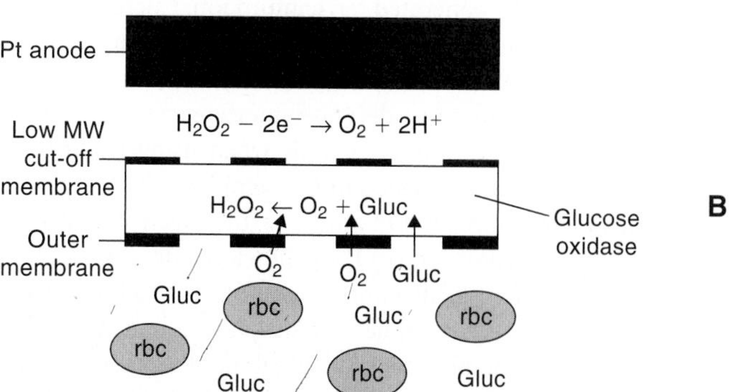

Figure 4-12 Design of amperometric enzyme electrode based on anodic detection of hydrogen peroxide generated from oxidase enzymatic reaction (e.g., glucose oxidase) **(A)**, and expanded view of the sensing surface showing the different membranes and electrochemical process that yield the anodic current proportional to the substrate concentration in the sample **(B)**. *(From Meyerhoff M, New in vitro analytical approaches for clinical chemistry measurements in critical care. Clin Chem 1990;36:1570.)*

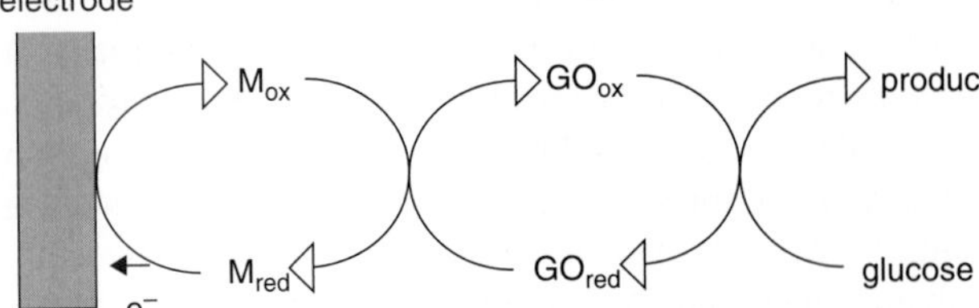

Figure 4-13 Scheme showing the use of electroactive mediator in the design of an amperometric enzyme electrode. The mediator accepts electrons directly from the enzyme, and is oxidized at the surface of the working electrode, creating more oxidized mediator to continue this process. *(From D'Orazio P. In: Lewendrowski, K, ed. Clinical chemistry laboratory management and clinical correlations, Philadelphia: Lippincott, Williams and Wilkins, 2002: 464.)*

anode surface, where it is reoxidized, resulting in a cyclic reaction mechanism (Figure 4-13). Mediators with electron transfer kinetics (little or no overpotential) more favorable than oxygen allow operation of the sensor at lower applied potentials (+0.2 V vs. Ag/AgCl or lower) than is typically used for the oxidation of H_2O_2. This approach not only eliminates dependency of the reaction rate on oxygen, but also serves to reduce the contribution from oxidizable interfering substances (e.g., uric acid, ascorbic acid, acetaminophen, etc.) on the sensor response. Examples of mediators that have been used include quinones and conductive organic salts, such as tetrathiafulvalene-tetracyanoquinodimethane (TTF-TCNQ).[35,74] Ferricyanide and ferrocene derivatives have also been employed,[15] including commercial application in a device for home blood glucose monitoring (ExacTECH™, Abbott-Medisense). In this device, dimethylferrocene is impregnated into a graphite electrode to which glucose oxidase has been immobilized. Reduced glucose oxidase from the enzymatic reaction is reoxidized by the electrochemically generated ferricinium ion. Current is produced during this cycling mechanism, which is proportional to the concentration of glucose in the blood sample.

Another technique to decrease interferences from easily oxidized species in a blood sample when using traditional H_2O_2 electrochemical detection is to employ selectively permeable membranes in proximity to the electrode surface that allow transport of H_2O_2 to the electrode surface, but reject the interfering substances based on size exclusion (see Figure 4-12, *B*). An example is as simple as a low molecular weight cut-off membrane, such as cellulose acetate, used in many commercial amperometric biosensors.[50] Also used are electropolymerized films, such as poly (phenylenediamine), formed in-situ, to reject interfering substances based on size.[30] Another approach employed in a commercial application involves using a second correcting electrode, identical to the working electrode, but without enzyme, sensitive only to the presence of oxidizable interfering substances. The resulting differential signal is proportional to the concentration of analyte.

A novel approach used for the elimination of electroactive interfering substances in a commercially available glucose sensor is to directly "wire" the redox center of the enzyme glucose oxidase to a metallic, amperometric electrode using an osmium (III/IV)-based redox hydrogel.[70] The osmium sites effectively serve as mediators, and can accept electrons directly from the entrapped enzyme, without need for oxygen. This approach allows the operating potential of the electrode to be dramatically lowered to +0.2 V vs. SCE (saturated calomel reference electrode), where currents resulting from electrooxidation of ascorbate, urate, acetaminophen, and L-cysteine are negligible.

Substitution of other oxoreductase enzymes for glucose oxidase allows amperometric biosensors for other substrates of clinical interest to be constructed. Practical sensors with commercial application in critical care analyzers for blood lactate have been realized.[1] Other amperometric biosensors reported include cholesterol, pyruvate, alanine, glutamate, and glutamine. By using the multiple enzyme cascade shown in the reactions below, an amperometric biosensor for creatinine is also possible. Electrochemical oxidation of H_2O_2 is the detection mechanism.

$$\text{Creatinine} + H_2O \xrightarrow{\text{creatinine amidohydrolase}} \text{Creatine} \quad (28)$$

$$\text{Creatine} + H_2O \xrightarrow{\text{creatine amidinohydrolase}} \text{Sarcosine} + \text{Urea} \quad (29)$$

$$\text{Sarcosine} + H_2O + O_2 \xrightarrow{\text{sarcosine oxidase}} \text{Glycine} + \text{formaldehyde} + H_2O_2 \quad (30)$$

This three-enzyme scheme suffers interference from endogenous creatine in the sample, requiring correction. Low concentrations of creatinine found in blood ($\leq 100\,\mu mol/L$) must be measured in the presence of oxidizable interfering substances, sometimes present at higher concentrations than the analyte.[47] Special electroactive layers within the biosensor have been proposed to remove redox-active interfering substances.[85] Since the useful life of the creatinine biosensor based on these reactions requires three enzymes to retain activity, reusable commercial biosensors for creatinine based on this measurement principle typically suffer from a short useful life of only a few days.

Enzyme-Based Biosensors with Potentiometric and Conductometric Detection

Ion selective electrodes can also be used as transducers in potentiometric biosensors. An example is a biosensor for urea (blood urea nitrogen, BUN) based on a polymembrane ISE (vinyl chloride) for ammonium ion (Figure 4-14).[52] The enzyme urease is immobilized at the surface of the ammonium selective ISE based on the antibiotic nonactin (see structure of ionophore in Figure 4-3), and catalyzes the hydrolysis of urea to NH_3 and CO_2.

$$\text{Urea} \xrightarrow{\text{urease}} 2NH_3 + CO_2 \quad (31)$$

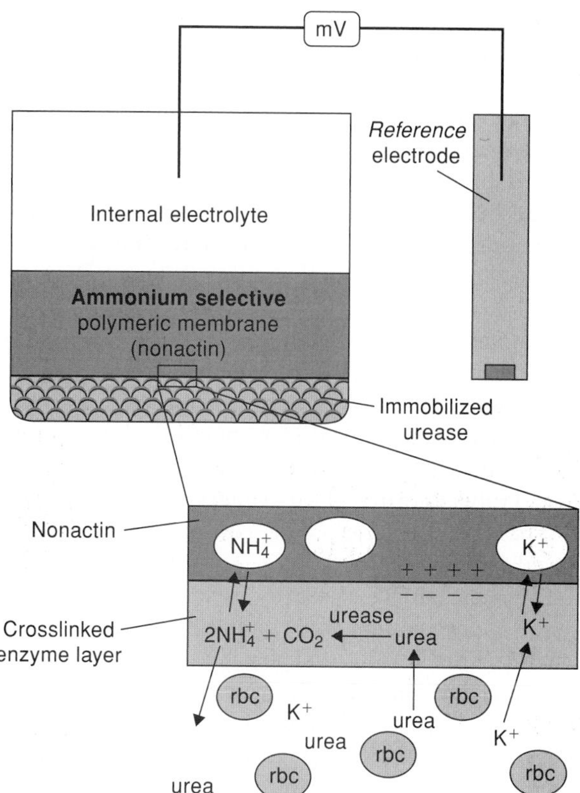

Figure 4-14 Potentiometric enzyme electrode for determination of blood urea, based on urease enzyme immobilized on the surface of an ammonium ion–selective polymeric membrane electrode.

The ammonia produced dissolves to form NH_4^+, which is sensed by the ISE. The signal generated by the NH_4^+ produced is proportional to the logarithm of the concentration of urea in the sample. The response may be either steady state or transient. Typically, correction for background potassium is required, since the nonactin ionophore has limited selectivity for ammonium over potassium ($K_{NH4/K} = 0.1$). Potassium is measured simultaneously with urea and used to correct the output of the urea sensor using the Nicolsky-Eisenman equation.

The above approach for measurement of urea using an enzyme-based potentiometric biosensor assumes that the turnover of urea to ammonium at steady state provides a constant ratio of ammonium ions to urea, independent of concentration. This is rarely the case, especially at higher substrate concentrations, resulting in a nonlinear sensor response. The linearity of the sensor is also limited by the fact that hydrolysis of urea produces a local alkaline pH in the vicinity of the ammonium-sensing membrane, partially converting NH_4^+ to NH_3 (pKa = 9.3). Ammonia (NH_3) is not sensed by the ISE. The degree of nonlinearity may be reduced by placement of a semipermeable membrane between enzyme and sample to restrict diffusion of urea to the immobilized enzyme layer.

A change in solution conductivity has also been used as a transduction mechanism in enzyme-based biosensors. Examples include the measurement of glucose, creatinine, and acetaminophen using interdigitated electrodes.[23] Practical applications of conductometric biosensors are few because of the variable ionic background of clinical samples and the requirement to measure small conductivity changes in media of high ionic strength. A commercial system for the measurement of urea in serum, plasma, and urine is a BUN analyzer (Beckman-Coulter) based on the enzyme urease.[27] Dissolution of the products to NH_4^+ and HCO_3^- produces a change in sample conductivity. The initial rate of change in conductivity is measured to compensate for the background conductivity of the sample. This approach is limited to the measurement of analytes at relatively high concentrations because of small changes in conductivity produced by low levels of analyte.

Enzyme-Based Biosensors with Optical Detection

Optical sensors with immobilized enzymes and indicator dyes have been developed for the measurement of glucose and other substrates of clinical interest.[54] These biosensors are based on optical detection chemistries for pH and oxygen, described earlier in this chapter, and rely on absorbance/reflectance, fluorescence, and luminescence as modes of detection. Enzyme immobilization methods resemble those used to construct electrochemical biosensors, including physical entrapment or encapsulation in a gel matrix, physical adsorption onto substrates, and covalent binding or absorption on an insoluble support. Using an example based on an optode for PO_2, a sensitive indicator is co-immobilized with an oxidase enzyme at the end of a fiber optic probe. The probe is used to monitor fluorescence of the indicator. Quenching of fluorescence of the indicator by O_2 is followed. A decrease in PO_2 resulting from a reaction catalyzed by the enzyme will result in less quenching of the indicator and a fluorescent signal directly proportional to the concentration of substrate. In an example of an optical biosensor probe for glucose, an oxygen, sensitive cationic dye, $Ru(phen)_3^{2+}$, is immobilized along with glucose oxidase on the surface of an optical fiber.[67] A decrease in PO_2 arising from the enzyme-catalyzed oxidation of glucose results in an increase in luminescence intensity of the ruthenium tris(phenanthrene).

Similar optical biosensors have been prepared for many other analytes. For example, a cholesterol optical biosensor has been devised based on fluorescence quenching of an oxygen-sensitive dye that is coupled to consumption of oxygen resulting from the enzyme-catalyzed oxidation of cholesterol by the enzyme cholesterol oxidase.[93] Serum bilirubin has been detected using bilirubin oxidase, co-immobilized with a ruthenium dye, on an optical fiber.[56] The bilirubin sensor was reported to exhibit a lower detection limit of 10 μmol/L, a linear range up to 30 mmol/L, and a typical reproducibility of 3% (CV), certainly adequate for clinical application.

The pH change resulting from enzyme-catalyzed reactions has also been measured optically. The indicator dye fluorescein is often used as a pH-sensitive indicator to construct such sensors. The protonated form of fluorescein does not fluoresce, but the conjugate base strongly fluoresces at 530 nm, when excited at 490 nm. Using glucose oxidase as the enzyme, a pH optode has been employed to follow the formation of gluconic acid.[92] A disadvantage of optical sensors based on pH changes is that they are strongly dependent on the pH and buffer capacity of the sample. Moreover, the working range of the sensor is determined by the pKa of the indicator, 6.8 to 7.2 for fluorescein, depending on ionic strength of the sample matrix. A pH-sensitive indicator may also be used to follow enzymatic reactions producing ammonia (e.g., urease action on urea).

Affinity Sensors

Affinity sensors are a special class of biosensors in which the immobilized biological recognition element is a binding protein, antibody (immunosensors), or oligonucleotide (e.g., DNA, aptamers, etc.) with high binding affinity and high specificity toward a clinically important analyte/partner. Such sensors are being developed as alternatives to conventional binding assays to enhance the speed and convenience of a wide range of assays that would be normally run on sophisticated instruments (e.g., immunoassay analyzers, etc.). Ideally, direct binding of the immobilized species with its target in a clinical sample should yield a sensor signal proportional to the concentration of the analyte. However, "direct" sensing (without use of exogenous labels/tracers) of the binding events at analyte concentrations that would cover the full range for clinical applications is very difficult to achieve. Further, high affinity of such binding reactions, required to achieve optimal sensitivity, also limits the reversibility of such devices (slow reverse rate constant). Indeed, unlike ISEs, oxygen sensors, and many of the enzyme type biosensors described above, affinity sensors based on electrochemical, optical, or other transduction modes are typically single-use devices.[31] For repeated multi-use applications, some type of regeneration step (pH change, etc.) to dissociate the tight binding between the recognition element and target is required.[57]

A host of "direct" sensing affinity sensors have been proposed, based on either electrochemical (including capacitance changes), optical, thermal, mass, and acoustic detection methods.[46,57,62,87] Of these, few have adequate specificity to be used in complex clinical samples, owing to significant signals arising from nonspecific binding. One report, however, suggests that alpha fetoprotein can be detected reliably in serum samples via a quartz crystal microbalance type mass detector, possessing immobilized antialpha-fetoprotein antibodies on the surface of the quartz crystal transducer.[17] Increasing concentrations of analyte in the sample yield increased binding to the surface, changing the mass loaded because of the immunological reaction. Incubation times as low as 20 min are required to achieve results that compare favorably to a conventional radioimmunoassay method for serum samples.

Some success for direct sensing devices has also been achieved in the area of DNA sensors.[46] Generally, in such devices, a segment of DNA complementary to the target strand is immobilized on a suitable transducer. Electrochemical DNA sensors have received considerable attention in this regard, since they can operate in the direct (based on electrochemical oxidation of guanine in target DNA) (see Figure 4-15, *A*) or indirect (with exogenous electrochemical markers/labels, see below and Figure 4-15, *B*) transduction modes. For example, Ozkan et al. demonstrated a relatively simple label-free electrochemical "genosensor" for detecting the presence of factor V Leiden mutations, using capture probes with inosine substituted for guanosine nucleic acids.[73] Probes were developed to bind wild-type and mutant DNA, based on the known base sequences in the regions of the wild and mutant DNA species. These probes were immobilized on the surface of carbon paste working electrodes. After PCR amplification of the sample DNA, a small volume of such samples (10 μL) is incubated for 6 minutes with the probe-modified electrode. Then, after a quick washing step, the presence of the target amplicon bound to the surface can be observed by differential pulse voltammetry using an anodic scan. The presence of a guanine oxidation peak, occurring at +1.00 V vs. Ag/AgCl reference, indicates the presence of the target DNA in the original sample.

Most affinity type sensors that function well for real clinical measurements are usually based on labeled reagents such as enzymes, fluorophores, and electrochemical tags, and hence function more like traditional binding/immunoassays, except that one recognition element is immobilized on the surface of a suitable electrode or other type of transducer.[57,62,87] For example, electrochemical oxygen sensors have been employed to carry out heterogeneous enzyme immunoassays (sandwich or competitive type), using catalase as a labeling enzyme (catalyzes $H_2O_2 \rightarrow 2H^+$ and O_2), and immobilizing capture antibodies on the outer surface of the gas-permeable membrane. After binding equilibration and washing steps, the amount of bound enzyme is detected by adding the substrate and following the increase in current generation, owing to local production of oxygen near the surface of the sensor. Similar, heterogeneous enzyme immunoassays have been developed based on electrode detection of peroxide using oxidase enzyme labels, pH changes using urease as an enzyme label, etc.

DNA detection using electrochemical labeled oligonucleotides, or electrochemical probes that selectively intercalate into hybridized DNA duplexes, represents a growing area of investigation, with several "gene" sensor arrays of this type poised to become commercial products (see Chapter 37). As illustrated in Figure 4-15, *B*, when not using the intrinsic electroactivity of guanine (that requires use of electrode immobilized capture oligo probes with inosine replacing guanosine, see above), detection of hybridization of a target DNA sequence is achieved in either of two ways. In one case,

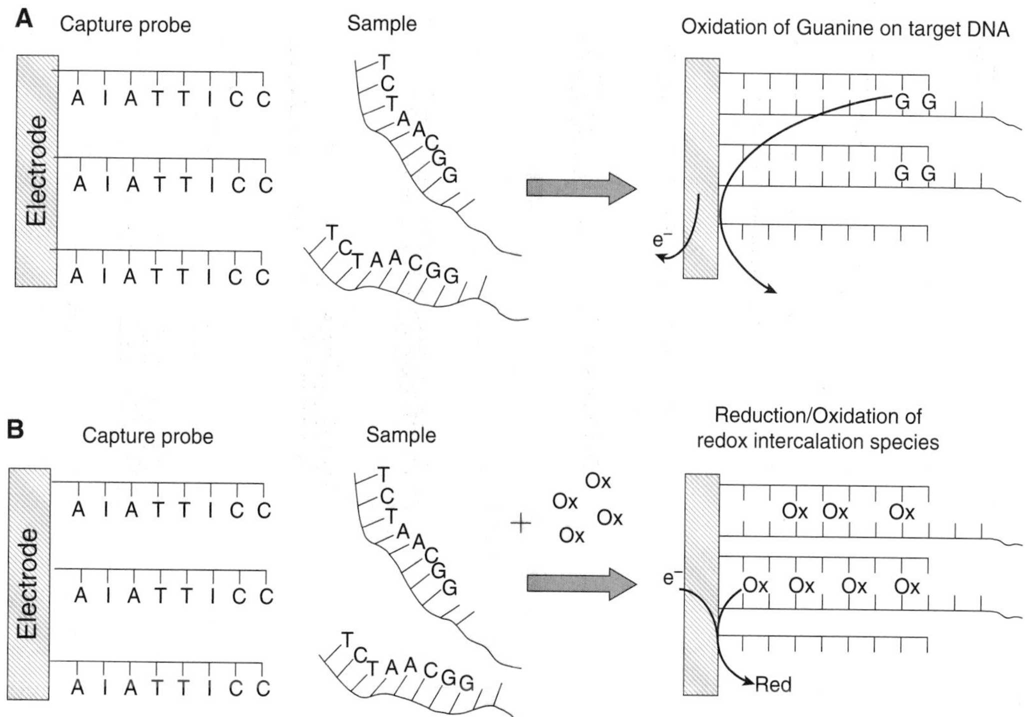

Figure 4-15 Examples of DNA biosensor configurations: **(A)** direct electrooxidation detection of guanosine bases in target DNA after hybridization with immobilized capture probe on electrode surface; **(B)** electrochemical detection of hybridization using exogenous redox species that intercalates into hybridized complex between immobilized capture DNA probe and target DNA.

after allowing the immobilized capture oligo anchored to the electrode surface to bind the target sequence, hybridization is detected by exposing the surface of the electrode to an exogenous electroactive species (Co(III)tris-phenanthroline, ruthenium complexes, etc.) that can interact (intercalate) with the duplex, but not single-stranded DNA. After washing away unbound electroactive species, the presence of hybridization can be readily detected by voltammetry, scanning the potential of the underlying electrode to oxidize or reduce any intercalated electroactive species, with the level of current detected being proportional to the number of duplex DNA species on the surface of the electrode.

A second route involves the detection of target DNA via a sandwich type binding assay, using an electrochemical-labeled oligonucleotide (oligo labeled with ferrocene, osmium(III) trisbipyridine, etc. to bind to another sequence of the targeted DNA different than the capture oligo on the surface of the electrode). Sequential exposure of the electrode to the sample of DNA (usually after amplification via PCR), excess of the labeled reporter oligo, a wash solution, and then electrochemical detection of surface bound label yields the analytical signal. Again, the amount of current monitored is proportional to the number of target DNA species present in the original sample.

The basic advantage of immobilizing affinity reagents on the surface of electrodes and optical sensing devices is somewhat diminished when separate washing steps are required to remove unbound label species. Indeed, true biosensors should yield analytically useful responses in the presence of undiluted physiological samples, without need for discrete incubation and washing steps. One example of an electrochemical-based immunosensor method that partly achieves this goal is a technique termed NEEIA (nonseparation electrochemical enzyme immunoassay).[64] The basic concept is illustrated in Figure 4-16. As indicated, no separation or washing steps are required. The method was used to detect prostate specific antigen (PSA) and hCG at ng/mL levels in undiluted plasma and whole blood.[64]

IN VIVO AND MINIMALLY INVASIVE SENSORS

Progress has been made in the development of miniaturized, implantable electrochemical/optical sensors that can be employed for in vivo, real-time monitoring of clinically important species. Unfortunately, the biological response of the living system toward such sensors (e.g., clotting, etc.) can have a dramatic impact on the analytical accuracy of such indwelling probes,[5,43,59,65] and has thus far prevented their widespread use in clinical practice. Progress is being made, however, to improve the reliability of in vivo measurements, and some commercial products are already on the market for in vivo blood gas and glucose monitoring.

Analytical sensors that can be implanted within human blood vessels or subcutaneously mandate that such sensing

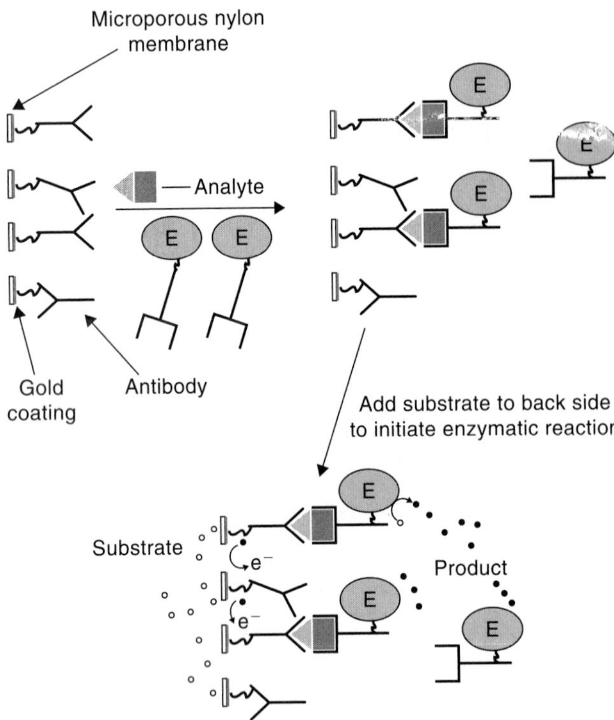

Figure 4-16 Principle of nonseparation electrochemical enzyme immunoassay (NEEIA) concept, configured in sandwich immunoassay mode to detect a given protein analyte. Enzyme label on reporter antibody generates an electroactive product that is detected at surface of porous gold electrode when substrate for enzyme is added to the back side of membrane.

devices have an outside diameter of <0.6 mm. Both electrochemical and optical sensor technologies have been employed to create devices having the required size. These are basically miniaturized versions of the electrochemical and optical sensor devices described above. However, in addition to small size, such devices must exhibit very stable output signals, since reliable calibration of the probes with calibrating solutions is not possible once the probes are inserted in vivo. While so-called in-situ calibration is possible (periodically removing in vitro blood sample to obtain current value of analyte, and update in vivo sensor output to this value), if the frequency of such in situ calibrations is high, the true advantage of having an in vivo probe is greatly diminished.

Continuous in vivo measurement of oxygen saturation (SaO_2) has been achieved with small optical fibers placed into the blood stream via a catheter and then measuring the reflective absorbance of the blood at two or three appropriately selected wavelengths that are based on the absorbance spectra of oxy- and deoxy-Hb.[19] In addition, implantable analytical sensors that provide continuous readings of blood gases (pH/PCO_2/PO_2) when inserted within the radial artery, especially for critically ill patients already fitted with an arterial line, are being developed.[79] Such sensors are usually based on the classical Clark style design in which oxygen is reduced at a microplatinum, silver, or gold working electrode confined (along with Ag/AgCl reference) within a narrow-diameter gas-permeable catheter tube made of a given polymer (see Figure 4-17, *A*), with the resulting current being proportional to the partial pressure of oxygen in the medium surrounding the catheter. Indwelling electrochemical pH and PCO_2 sensors are typically potentiometric devices, based on either polymer membrane pH electrode technology or use of solid-state metal oxide–based pH sensors. Incorporation of lipophilic proton ionophores (e.g., tridodecylamine; see Figure 4-3) within the walls of plastic tubing provides a convenient means to prepare a novel dual-lumen pH/PCO_2 sensing design that has been demonstrated to provide accurate in vivo results in animal experiments.[89]

Miniaturization of electrode designs that enable several sensors to be bundled into a single implantable device, however, remains a significant engineering challenge. Consequently, many of the efforts aimed at developing commercially viable intravascular blood gas sensors for monitoring pH, PCO_2 and PO_2 simultaneously have employed modern optical fiber–based technology alone or in combination with a single electrochemical device. As the outer diameter of available fibers continues to decrease, it is now possible to bundle three or more separate chemically sensitive fibers in a single catheter with an outer diameter <600 μm for implantation within human radial arteries, without dampening the pressure waveform detected by a microelectronic pressure transducer within the arterial line. Absorbance-, fluorescence-, and phosphorescence-based chemistries have all been investigated in the design of sensors with suitable selectivity and calibration stability.[65] Appropriate indicators are usually immobilized on the distal ends of the fibers, although alternate configurations/locations have also been proposed. Most optical oxygen measurements are made with indicators whose luminescence is quenched in the presence of oxygen, whereas pH sensors are prepared by immobilizing pH indicators (e.g., phenol red) in hydrogel type films.[84] Optical sensors for PCO_2 can be easily prepared from the same pH sensors by incorporating bicarbonate salt in the hydrogel layer and then covering this layer with a gas-permeable polymeric film (usually silicone rubber material), as described above in the section on optical sensors.

The Paratrend™ probe is commercially available and is used for the intravascular measurement of blood gases. It was originally developed by Pfizer/Biomedical Sensors and is currently distributed by Diametrics Inc. As shown in Figure 4-17, *B*, this indwelling sensor consists of a novel hybrid design, in which oxygen is sensed electrochemically (catheter form of Clark sensor) while pH and PCO_2 are determined via fiber-based optical fluorescence sensors.[94] While acceptable clinical performance of the Paratrend has been reported, frequent in situ recalibrations have been suggested.[20] A newer version of this product replaces the electrochemical oxygen sensor with an optical fiber design.

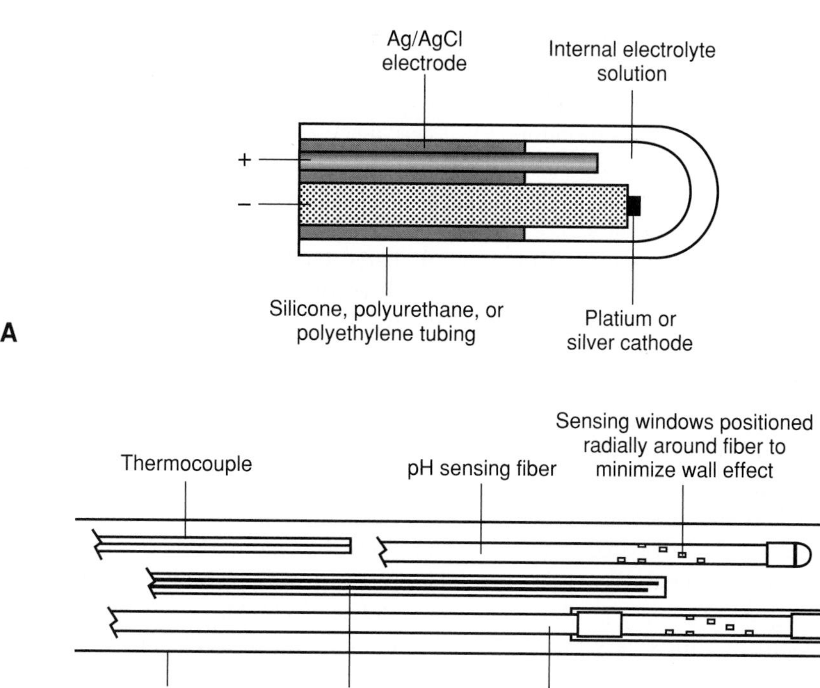

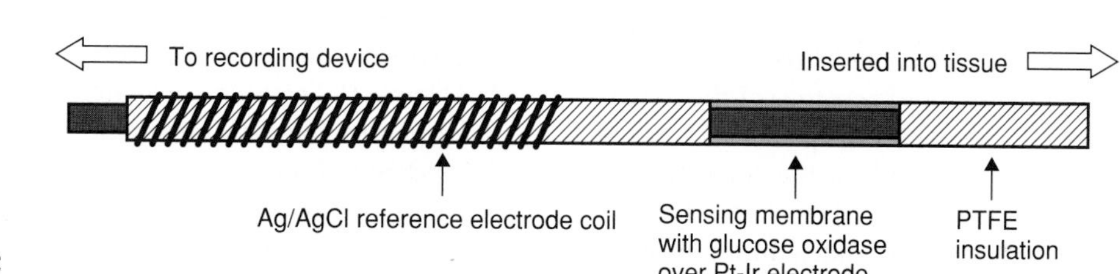

Figure 4-17 Schematics of various implantable electrochemical/optical sensors useful for continuous in vivo monitoring: **(A)** catheter style amperometric oxygen sensor; **(B)** design of Paratrend intravascular combined PO_2, PCO_2, and pH sensor (hybrid electrochemical/optical design); **(C)** needle type electrochemical glucose sensor useful for monitoring glucose subcutaneously to track blood glucose levels continuously.

Another class of in vivo chemical sensor that is now available are glucose sensors designed to help manage diabetic patients, with the ultimate goal of fully automated feedback control of subcutaneous insulin delivery via newly devised, highly portable insulin pumps. Since such sensors need to function within patients outside the hospital setting, and for extended time periods (days, weeks), placement of such devices subcutaneously, rather than intravascularly, is desirable.[49] In addition, sensors are being developed that could be implanted within the vena cava for periods of 1 year. In the case of subcutaneous devices, several studies have now shown that the levels of glucose in interstitial fluid track blood concentrations closely, although there is some time delay in achieving identical values in the two sample environments.[37]

Implantable glucose (and lactate) sensors have been based, almost exclusively, on electrochemical transducers. For example, one such sensor is based on using dual oxygen sensors in a single catheter design for indwelling blood glucose and lactate measurements.[39] One oxygen sensor with immobilized glucose or lactate oxidase provides response to glucose levels (decreasing surface oxygen levels in response to increase in glucose or lactate) while the second matched oxygen sensor, without enzyme, is able to correct for unknown and varying levels of endogenous PO_2. Others have focused on the design of probes with amperometric detection of the hydrogen peroxide (via oxidation) at an underlying iridium/platinum anode similar in operation to those used in vitro in commercial instruments.[98] In such designs, use of outer polymer films to restrict glucose (or lactate) diffusion relative to oxygen is critical to achieve linear electrochemical response to glucose from normal (90 mg/dL) to elevated levels found in diabetic patients (>500 mg/dL). Figure 4-17, *C* illustrates a design in which the needle type probe is constructed by multiple membrane coatings and electrodeposition of the glucose oxidase layer.[16] A design quite similar to this is the only currently FDA-approved sensor that is available for subcutaneous monitoring of glucose.[40] The sensor is actually fabricated on a very narrow planar substrate, rather than on a cylindrical wire–based system. Relatively frequent calibration of the sensor is required via periodic in vitro blood tests, and after explantation, and hence the output of the device is not readable by the patient at this time.

Instead of implanting glucose sensors intravascularly or subcutaneously, an alternative approach employs electrochemical glucose sensors to monitor glucose levels in interstitial fluid brought to the surface of the sensors via an iontophoresis process.[91] Electrical current is passed through the skin to move fluid in a given direction toward the surface of the electrochemical glucose sensors that are based on peroxide detection (see Chapter 25 for additional discussion of this device.)

Current research and development efforts have focused on the use of more biocompatible coatings to reduce the biological response of both intravascular and subcutaneous devices. These efforts are based on the expectation that such developments will be critical to the ultimate success in developing implanted sensors that yield continuous analytical results that match closely with conventional in vitro test methods. One new approach in this direction employs novel nitric oxide (NO) release polymers to coat the surface of intravascular sensors.[36] The potent antiplatelet activity of NO has been shown to greatly reduce the formation of thrombus on the surface of implantable electrochemical oxygen sensing catheters, and yield much more accurate continuous PO_2 values in animal experiments.

REFERENCES

1. Aduen J, Bernstein WK, Khastigir T, Miller J, Kerzner R, Bhatiani A, et al. The use and clinical importance of a substrate specific electrode for rapid determination of blood lactate concentrations. JAMA 1994;272:1678-85.
2. Apple FS, Koch DD, Graves S, Ladenson JH. Relationship between direct potentiometric and flame photometric measurement of sodium in blood. Clin Chem 1982;28:1931-5.
3. Armstrong RD, Lockhart JC, Todd M. The mechanism of transfer of K^+ between aqueous solutions and PVC membranes containing valinomycin. Electrochim Acta 1986;31:591-4.
4. Astrup P, Severinghaus JW. The history of blood gases, acids and bases. Copenhagen:Munksgaard, 1986.
5. Baker DA, Gough DA. Dynamic delay and maximal dynamic error in continuous biosensors. Anal Chem 1996; 68:1292-7.
6. Bakker E, Bühlmann P, Pretsch E. Carrier-based ion-selective electrodes and bulk optodes. 1. general characteristics. Chem Rev 1997;97: 3083-132.
7. Bakker E, Pretsch E, and Bühlmann P. Selectivity of potentiometric ion sensors, Anal Chem 2000;72:1127-33.
8. Bakker E. Determination of improved selectivity coefficients of polymer membrane ion-selective electrodes by conditioning with a discriminated ion. J Electrochem Soc 1996;143:L83-L85.
9. Bates RG. Determination of pH: theory and practice. New York: John Wiley & Sons, 1973.
10. Bedioui F, Villeneuve N. Electrochemical nitric oxide sensors for biological samples-principle, selected examples and applications. Electroanalysis 2003;15:5-18.
11. Bijster P Vader HL, Vink CLJ. Influence of erythrocytes on direct potentiometric determination of sodium and potassium. Ann Clin Biochem 1983;20:116-20.
12. Buck RP, Lindner E. Recommendations for Nomenclature of Ion-Selective Electrodes. Pure Appl Chem 1994;66:2527-36.
13. Bühlmann P, Pretsch E, Bakker E. Carrier-based ion-selective electrodes and bulk optodes. 2. ionophores for poteniometric and optical sensors. Chem Rev 1998;98:1593-687.
14. Burgess B, Martin G. Combined pH and dissolved carbon dioxide gas sensor. US Patent 4,818,361, April 4, 1989.
15. Cass AEG, Davis G, Francis GD, Hill HAO, Aston WJ, Higgins IJ. Ferrocene mediated enzyme electrode for amperometric determination of glucose. Anal Chem 1984;56:667-71.
16. Chen X, Matsumoto N, Hu Y, Wilson GS. Electrochemically mediated electrodeposition/ electropolymerization to yield a glucose microbiosensor with improved characteristics. Anal Chem 2002;74:368-72.
17. Chou SF, Hsu WL, Hwang JM, Chen CY. Determination of alpha-fetoprotein in human serum by a quartz crystal microbalance-based immunosensor. Clin Chem 2002;48:913-8.
18. Clark LC Jr, Lyons C. Electrode systems for continuous monitoring in cardiovascular surgery. Ann NY Acad Sci 1962;102:29-45.
19. Collison, ME, Meyerhoff, ME. Chemical sensors for bedside monitoring of critically ill patients. Anal Chem 1990;62:425A-37A.
20. Coule LW, Truemper EJ, Steinhart CM, Lutin WA. Accuracy and utility of a continuous intra-arterial blood gas monitoring system in pediatric patients. Crit Care Med 2001;29:420-6.
21. Coulter WH. Means for counting particles suspended in a fluid. US Patent 2,656,508, Oct 20, 1953. Washington DC: US Patent Office.
22. Cremer M. Uber die ursahce der elektromotorishcen eigneschaften der gewebe, zugliech ein beitrag zur lehre von den polyphasichen elektrolytketten. Z Biol 1906;47:562-608.

23. Cullen D, Sethi R, Lowe C. A multi-analyte miniature conductance biosensor. Anal Chim Acta 1990;231:33-40.
24. Czaban JD, Cormier AD, Legg KD. Establishing the direct potentiometric normal range for Na/K: residual liquid junction potential and activity coefficient effects. Clin Chem 1982;28:1936-45.
25. Demas JN, DeGraff BA, Coleman PB. Oxygen sensors based on luminescence quenching. Anal Chem 1999;71:793A-800A.
26. Eberhard P, Mindt W. Interferences of anesthetic gases at oxygen sensors. In Birth defects: original article series 1979;XV:65-74.
27. Eckfeldt J, Levine AS, Greiner C, Kershaw M. Urinary urea: are currently available methods adequate for revival of an almost abandoned test? Clin Chem 1982;28:1500-2.
28. Eisenman G, Rudin DO, Casby JU. Glass electrode for measuring sodium ion. Science 1957;126:831-4.
29. Eisenman G. Theory of membrane electrode potentials: An examination of the parameters determining the selectivity of solid and liquid ion exchangers and of neutral ion sequestering molecules. In: Durst RA, ed. Ion-Selective Electrodes, NBS Special Publication 314, Washington DC: US Govt. Printing Office, 1969; 1-56.
30. Emr S, Yacynych A. Use of polymer films in amperometric biosensors. Electroanalysis 1995;7:913-23.
31. Enzer S, Burgess BM, Wyman JS, Hendershot R. Disposable self-calibratable electrode package. US Patent 4,871,439, October 3, 1989.
32. Faulkner LR. Understanding electrochemistry: some distinctive concepts. J Chem Ed 1983;60:262-4.
33. Feldman BJ, Oserioh JD, Hata BH, D'Alessandro A. Determination of lead in blood by square wave anodic stripping voltammetry at a carbon disk ultramicroelectrode. Anal Chem 1994;66:1983-7.
34. Frant MS. Where did ion selective electrodes come from? The story of their development and commercialization. J Chem Ed 1997;74:159-66.
35. Frew J, Hill HA. Electrochemical biosensors. Anal Chem 1987;59:933A-44A.
36. Frost MC, Rudich SM, Zhang H, Marashio MA, Meyerhoff ME. In vivo biocompatibility and analytical performance of intravascular oxygen sensors prepared with improved nitric oxide-releasing silicone rubber coating. Anal Chem 2002;74:5942-7.
37. Gerritsen M, Jansen JA, Lutterman JA. Performance of subcutaneously implanted sensors for continuous monitoring. Netherlands J Med 1999;54:167-79.
38. Gorton L. Carbon paste electrodes modified with enzymes, tissues and cells. Electroanalysis 1995;7:23-45.
39. Gough DA, Lucisano JW, Pius HST. Two dimensional enzyme electrode sensor for glucose. Anal Chem 1985;57:2351-7.
40. Gross TM, Bode BW, Einhorn D, Kayne DM, Reed JH, White NH, Mastrototaro JJ Performance evaluation of the MiniMed Continuous Glucose Monitoring System during patient home use. Diabetes Techno Therap 2000;2:49-56.
41. Guilbault GG. Handbook of immobilized enzymes. New York: Marcel-Dekker, 1984.
42. Gunaratna PC, Koch WF, Paule RC, Cormier AD, D'Orazio P, Greenberg N, et al. Frozen human serum reference material for standardization of sodium and potassium measurements in serum or plasma by ion selective electrode. Clin Chem 1992;38:1459-65.
43. Halbert SA. Intravascular monitoring: problems and promise. Clin Chem 1990;36:1581-4.
44. Heller A. Amperometric biosensors. Curr Opin Biotechnol 1996;7:50-4.
45. Henning TP, Cunningham DD. Biosensors for personal diabetes management. In: Ramsay G, editor. Commercial biosensors: application to clinical, bioprocess, and environmental samples. New York: John Wiley & Sons, 1998:3-46.
46. Homs, MC. DNA sensors. Anal Letters 2002;35:1875-94.
47. Killard AJ, Smyth MR. Creatinine biosensors: principles and design. Trends Biotechnol 2000;18:433-7.
48. Kissinger P. LCEC: The combination of liquid chromatography and electrochemistry. J Chem Ed 1983;60:308-11.
49. Koschchinsky T, Heinemann L. Sensors for glucose monitoring: technical and clinical aspects. Diabetes Metab Res Rev 2001;17:113-23.
50. Kost GJ, Nguyen TH, Tang Z. Whole blood glucose and lactate: trilayer biosensors, drug interference, metabolism and practice guidelines. Arch Pathol Lab Med 2000;124:1128-34.
51. Kost GJ. New whole blood analyzers and their impact on cardiac and critical care. Crit Rev Clin Lab Sci 1993;30:153-202.
52. Kuan SS, Guilbault GG. Ion selective electrodes and biosensors based on ISEs. In: Turner APF, Karube I, Wilson GS, editors. Biosensors, fundamentals and applications. Oxford: Oxford University Press, 1987.
53. Lee HJ, Yoon IJ, Yoo CL, Pyun HJ, Cha GS, Nam H. Potentiometric evaluation of solvent polymeric carbonate-selective membranes based on molecular tweezer-type neutral carriers. Anal Chem 2000;72: 4694-9.
54. Leiner MJP. Luminescence chemical sensors for biomedical applications: scope and limitations. Anal Chim Acta 1991;255:209-22.
55. Lewandowski R, Sokalski T, Hulanicki A. Influence of aspirin on in vitro direct potentiometry of chloride in serum. Clin Chem 1989;35:2146.
56. Li X, Rosenweig Z. A fiber-optic sensor for rapid analysis of bilirubin in serum. Anal Chim Acta 1997;353:263-73.

57. Luppa PB, Sokoll LJ, Chan DW. Immunosensors—principles and applications to clinical chemistry. Clin Chim Acta 2001;314:1-26.
58. Ma SC, Meyerhoff ME, Yang V. Heparin-responsive electrochemical sensor: a preliminary report. Anal Chem 1992;64:694-7.
59. Mahutte CK. On-line arterial blood gas analysis with optodes: current status. Clin Biochem 1998;31:119-30.
60. Maines A, Ashworth D, Vadgama P. Diffusion restricting outer membranes for greatly extending linearity measurements with glucose oxidase enzyme electrodes. Anal Chim Acta 1996;333:223-31.
61. Mathison S, Bakker E. Effect of transmembrane electrolyte diffusion on the detection limit of carrier-based potentiometric ion sensors. Anal Chem 1998;70:303-9.
62. Medyantseva EP, Khaldeeva EV, Budnikov GK. Immunosensors in biology and medicine: analytical capabilities, problems, and prospects. J Anal Chem 2001:56:886-900.
63. Metzger E, Aeschimann R, Egli M, et al. 3,7-Dioxa-azela-amides as ionophores for lithium ion selective liquid membrane electrodes. Helvetica Chim Acta, 1986;69:1821-8.
64. Meyerhoff ME, Duan C, Meusel M. Novel nonseparation sandwich-type electrochemical enzyme immunoassay system for detecting marker proteins in undilute blood. Clin Chem 1995;41:1378-84.
65. Meyerhoff ME: In vivo blood-gas and electrolyte sensors: progress and challenges. Trends Anal Chem 1993; 12:257-66.
66. Moody GJ, Thomas JDR. Selective ion sensitive electrodes. Watford, England: Merrow, 1971.
67. Moreno-Bondi MC, Wolfbeis OS, Leiner MJP, Schaffar BPH. Oxygen optrode for use in a fiber-optic glucose biosensor. Anal Chem 1990;62:2377-80.
68. National Committee for Clinical Laboratory Standards. A designated comparison method for the measurement of ionized calcium in serum; Approved Standard. NCCLS Document C39-A, Wayne PA: NCCLS, 2000.
69. Oesch U, Ammann D, Simon W. Ion-selective membrane electrodes for clinical use. Clin Chem 1986;32:1448-59.
70. Ohara TJ, Rajagopalan R, Heller A. "Wired" enzyme electrodes for amperometric determination of glucose or lactate in the presence of interfering substances. Anal Chem 1994;66:2451-7.
71. Osswald HF, Wuhrmann HR. Calibration standards for multi ion analysis in whole blood samples. In: Lubbers DW, Acker H, Buck RP, et al., eds. Progress in enzyme and ion-selective electrodes. Berlin: Springer-Verlag, 1981;74-8.
72. Osteryoung J. Pulse voltammetry. J Chem Ed 1983;60:296-8.
73. Ozkan D, Erdem A, Kara P, Kerman K, Meric B, Hassmann J, et al. Allele-specific genotype detection of factor V leiden mutation from polymerase chain reaction amplicons based on label-free electrochemical genosensor. Anal Chem 2002:74:5931-6.
74. Pandey PC, Upadhyay S, Upadhyay B. Peroxide biosensors and mediated electrochemical regeneration of redox enzymes. Anal Biochem 1997;252:136-42.
75. Pioda LA, Simon W, Bosshard HR, Curtius CH. Determination of potassium ion concentration in serum using a highly selective liquid-membrane electrode. Clin Chim Acta. 1970; 29:289-93.
76. Reddy SM, Vadgama PM. Membranes to improve amperometric sensor characteristics. In: Kress-Rogers E, editor. Handbook of biosensors and electronic noses. New York: CRC Press, 1997:111-35.
77. Rehak N, Cecco SA, Niemela JE, et al. Linearity and stability of the AVL and Nova magnesium and calcium ion selective electrodes. Clin Chem 1996;42:880-7.
78. Robinson DL, Venton BJ, Helen MLAV, Wightman RM. Detecting sub-second dopamine release with fast-scan voltammetry in freely moving rats. Clin Chem 2003;49:1763-73.
79. Rolfe P. In vivo chemical sensors for intensive-care monitoring. Med Biol Eng Comput 1990:28:B34-B47.
80. Rosenthal RL, Tobias CW. Measurement of the electrical resistance of human blood: use in coagulation studies and cell volume determinations. J Lab Clin Med 1948;33:1110-22.
81. Rubenstein D, Yahashita GT. Determination of homocysteine, penicillamine and their symmetrical and mix disulfides by liquid chromatography with electrochemical detection. Anal Biochem 1989;180:259-63.
82. Salling N, Siggaard-Andersen O. Liquid junction potentials between plasma or erythrolysate and KCl solutions. Scand J Clin Lab Invest 1971;28:33-40.
83. Scott WJ, Chapoteau E, Kumar A. Ion-selective membrane electrode for rapid automated determinations of total carbon dioxide. Clin Chem 1986;312:137-41.
84. Seitz WR. Chemical sensors based on fiber optics. Anal Chem 1984;56:16A-34A.
85. Shin JH, Choi YS, Lee HJ, Choi SH, Ha J, Yoon IJ, et al. A planar amperometric creatinine biosensor employing an insoluble oxidizing agent for removing redox-active interferences. Anal Chem 2001;73:5965-71.
86. Standardization of sodium and potassium ion selective electrode systems to the flame photometric reference method; Approved Standard, 2nd edition. NCCLS Document C29-A2, Wayne, PA: NCCLS, 2000.
87. Stefan RI, van Staden JF, Aboul-Enein HY. Immunosensors in clinical analysis. Fresenius J Anal Chem 2000:366:659-68.
88. Stott RAW, Hortin GL, Wilhite TR, Miller SB, Smith CH, Landt M. Analytical artifacts in hematocrit measurements by whole blood chemistry analyzers. Clin Chem 1995;41:306-11.

89. Telting-Diaz M, Collison ME, Meyerhoff ME. Simplified dual lumen catheter design for simultaneous potentiometric monitoring of carbon dioxide and pH. Anal Chem 1994;66:576-83.
90. Thevenot DR, Toth K, Durst RA, Wilson GS. Electrochemical biosensors: recommended definitions and classifications. Biosen Bioelectron 2001;16:121-31.
91. Tierney MJ, Tamada JA, Potts RO, Jovanovic L, Garg S. Clinical evaluation of the GlucoWatch biographer: a continual, noninvasive glucose monitor for patients with diabetes. Biosens Bioelectron 2001;16:621-9.
92. Trettnak W, Leiner MJP, Wolfbeis OS. Fiber optic glucose sensor with a pH optrode as the transducer. Biosensors 1988;4:15-26.
93. Trettnak W, Wolfbeis OS. A fiber-optic cholesterol biosensor with an oxygen optrode as the transducer. Anal Biochem 1990;184:124-7.
94. Venkatesh B, Clutton-Brock TH, Hendry SP. Continuous measurement of blood gases using a combined electrochemical and spectrophotometric sensor. J Med Eng Technol 1995;18:165-8.
95. Visser KR. Electrical conductivity of stationary and flowing blood at low frequencies. Med Biol Eng Comput 1992;30:636-40.
96. Wang J, Lu F. Oxygen rich oxidase enzyme electrodes for operation in oxygen-free solutions. J Am Chem Soc 1998;120:1048-50.
97. Wenk RE, Lustgarten JA, Pappas NJ, Levy RI, Jackson R. Serum chloride analysis, bromide detection, and the diagnosis of bromism. Am J Clin Path 1976;64:49-57.
98. Yang Q, Atanasov P, Wilkins E. A needle-type sensor for monitoring glucose in whole blood. Biomed Instrum Technol 1997;31:54-62.
99. Zaloga GP, Hill TP, Strickland RA, Kennedy D, Visser M, Ford K, et al. Bedside blood gas and electrolyte monitoring in critically ill patients. Crit Care Med 1989;17:920-5.

ADDITIONAL READING

Astrup P, Severinghaus JW. The history of blood gases, acids and bases. Copenhagen: Munksgaard, 1986.

Bard AJ, Faulkner LR. Electrochemical methods, 2nd ed. New York:John Wiley, 2001.

Cass AEG, Ed. Biosensors, a practical approach. Oxford:Oxford University Press, 1990.

D'Orazio P. Biosensors in clinical chemistry. Clin Chim Acta. 2003; 334:41-69.

Durst RA, Siggaard-Adersen O. Electrochemistry. In: Burtis CA, Ashwood ER eds. Tietz Textbook of Clinical Chemisry 3rd ed. Philadelphia: W B Saunders, 1999:133:49.

Killard AJ, Sequeira M, Diamond D, Smyth MR. Electroanalysis and biosensors in clinical chemistry. In: Meyers RA (ed). Encyclopedia of analytical chemistry. Chichester: John Wiley & Sons, 2000:1257:90.

Kissinger PT, Heineman WR. Laboratory techniques in electroanalytical chemistry, 2nd Ed. New York:Marcel Dekker, 1996.

Koryta, J. Ions, electrodes and membranes. Chichester:John Wiley, 1982.

Su EJ. Bocarsly AB. Electroanalytical chemistry in clinical analysis. In: Meyers RA (ed). Encyclopedia of analytical chemistry. Chichester: John Wiley & Sons, 2000: 1291-9.

Turner APF, Karube I, Wilson GS, Eds. Biosensors-fundamentals and applications. Oxford:Oxford University Press, 1987.

Urban GA. Biosensor design and fabrication. In: Meyers RA (ed). Encyclopedia of analytical chemistry. Chichester: John Wiley & Sons, 2000:1164-80.

Wang J. Analytical Electrochemistry. 2nd ed. New York:Wiley-VCH, 2000.

Young V. Ion-selective electrodes: Fundamentals. In: Meyers RA (ed). Encyclopedia of analytical chemistry. Chichester: John Wiley & Sons, 2000:9878-907.

CHAPTER 5

Electrophoresis*

Raymond Karcher, Ph.D.,
and James P. Landers, Ph.D.

Developments in deoxyribonucleic acid (DNA) testing, improvements in ease of performance through automation, and advantages of speed and miniaturization afforded by the technique of *capillary electrophoresis* (CE) have led to a renaissance and growth of *electrophoresis* as an analytical tool that is widely used in clinical laboratories. These developments and improvements have enabled clinical laboratories to keep pace with higher volumes of testing and introduce more sophisticated technology to meet the demands of modern clinical practice. This chapter will review the principles and practice of the technique and separately discuss conventional, capillary, and microchip electrophoresis. Particular attention is given to newer methods and their promise in fields such as *genomics* and *proteomics.*

BASIC CONCEPTS AND DEFINITIONS

Electrophoresis is a comprehensive term that refers to the migration of charged solutes or particles of any size in a liquid medium under the influence of an electrical field. *Iontophoresis* and *isotachophoresis (ITP)* are similar terms but refer specifically to the migration of small ions. The first electrophoresis method used to study proteins was the free solution or moving boundary method devised by Tiselius in 1937. The Tiselius apparatus was a rectangular, sectional U-tube equipped with sensitive Schlieren optics. It allowed changes in refractive index to be observed as segments of solution with different protein content migrated past. This technique was used in research to measure electrophoretic mobility and to study protein-protein interaction. It was able to resolve the serum proteins into only four component mixtures, with the α_1 fraction incompletely separated from albumin.

Zone electrophoresis refers to the migration of charged molecules, usually in a porous supporting medium like agarose gel film, such that each protein zone is sharply separated from neighboring zones by a protein-free area. Zones are visualized by staining with a protein-specific stain to produce an *electropherogram* that is then scanned and quantified using a densitometer. The support medium can also be handled after drying and kept as a permanent record. This is the most commonly applied technique in clinical chemistry and is used to separate proteins in serum, urine, cerebrospinal fluid (CSF), other physiological fluids, erythrocytes and tissue, and nucleic acids in various tissue cells.

THEORY OF ELECTROPHORESIS

Depending on the kind of charge they carry, ionized solutes move toward either the cathode (negative electrode) or the anode (positive electrode) in an electrophoresis system. For example, positive ions (cations) migrate to the cathode and negative ions (anions) to the anode. An ampholyte (a molecule that is either positively or negatively charged, formerly called a zwitterion) becomes positively charged in a solution more acidic than its isoelectric point (pI)* and migrates toward the cathode. In a more alkaline solution, the ampholyte becomes negatively charged and migrates toward the anode. Because proteins contain many ionizable amino (—NH_2) and carboxyl (—COOH) groups, and the bases in nucleic acids may also be positively or negatively charged, they both behave as ampholytes in solution.

*The authors gratefully acknowledge the original contributions of Drs. Emmanuel Epstein and Kern L. Nuttall on which portions of this chapter are based.

*The isoelectric point of a molecule is the pH at which it has no net charge and will not move in an electrical field.

The rate of migration of ions in an electrical field depends on factors such as the (1) net charge of the molecule, (2) size and shape of the molecule, (3) strength of the electric field, (4) properties of the supporting medium, and (5) temperature of operation. The equation expressing the driving force in such a system is given by

$$F = (X)(Q) = \frac{(\text{EMF})(Q)}{d} \qquad (1)$$

where

F = the force exerted on an ion
X = the current field strength (V/cm) (i.e., voltage drop per unit length of medium)
Q = the net charge on the ion
EMF = the electromotive force (voltage [V] applied)
d = the length of the electrophoretic medium (cm)

The steady acceleration of the migrating ion is counteracted by a resisting force characteristic of the solution in which migration occurs. This force, expressed by Stokes' law, is

$$F' = 6\pi r\eta v \qquad (2)$$

where

F' = the counter force
r = the ionic radius of the solute
η = the viscosity of the buffer solution in which migration is occurring
π = 3.1416
v = the rate of migration of the solute = velocity, length (l) traveled per unit of time (cm/s)

The force F' counteracts the acceleration that would be produced by F if no counter force were present, and the result of the two forces is a constant velocity. Therefore when

$$F = F' \qquad (3)$$

then

$$6\pi r\eta v = (X)(Q) \qquad (4)$$

or

$$\frac{v}{X} = \frac{l \times d}{t \times E} = \frac{Q}{6\pi r\eta} = \mu \qquad (5)$$

where v/X is the rate of migration (cm/s) per unit field strength (E/cm), defined as the electrophoretic mobility. It is expressed by the symbol μ and has the units $cm^2/(V)(s)$.

The electrophoretic mobility is directly proportional to the net charge and inversely proportional to the size of the molecule and the viscosity of the electrophoresis medium. In practice the equation $\mu = cm^2/(V)(s)$ is used to calculate the electrophoretic mobility. Thus if albumin travels 3 cm (l) on a 10-cm (d) long agarose gel and does so in 75 minutes (or 75 × 60 s) at a voltage of 250 V, then

$$\mu = \frac{(3)(10)}{(75)(60)(250)} = 2.7 \times 10^{-5}\ cm^2/(V)(s)$$

Since one mobility unit is defined as $10^{-5}\ cm^2/(V)(s)$, this result is converted to 2.7 mobility units. Mobility may be positive or negative, depending on whether a protein migrates in the same or the opposite direction as the electrophoretic field (defined as extending from the anode to the cathode). In the example just given, electrophoresis was performed at pH 8.6 where proteins have a negative charge; therefore migration occurred from the cathode to the anode, and the mobility would be −2.7 mobility units.

Another factor and potential problem that can affect mobility is *wick flow.* During electrophoresis heat evolved because of the passage of current through a resistive medium can cause evaporation of solvent from the electrophoretic support. This drying effect draws buffer into the support from both buffer compartments. If significant, the flow of buffer from both directions can affect protein migration and hence the calculated mobility.

CONVENTIONAL ELECTROPHORESIS

In this section, instrumentation, general electrophoretic operations, technical and practical considerations, and types of conventional electrophoresis are discussed.

INSTRUMENTATION

Although modern electrophoresis equipment and systems vary considerably in form and degree of automation, the essential components common to all systems (Figure 5-1) include two reservoirs (1), which contain the buffer used in the process a means of delivering current from a power supply via platinum or carbon electrodes (2), which contact the buffer, and a support medium (3) in which separation takes place connecting the two reservoirs. In some systems, wicks (4) may connect the medium to the buffer solution or directly to the electrodes. The entire apparatus is enclosed (5) to minimize evaporation and protect both the system and the operator. The direct current power supply sets the polarity of the electrodes and delivers current to the medium.

Power Supplies

The power supply drives the movement of ionic species in the medium and allows adjustment and control of either the current or the voltage. In more sophisticated units, the power may be controlled as well and conditions may be programmed to change during electrophoresis. Capillary systems use power supplies capable of providing voltages in the kilovolt range.

Current flowing through a resistive medium produces heat:

$$\text{Heat} = (E)(I)(t) \qquad (6)$$

where

E = EMF in volts (V)
I = current in amperes (A)
t = time in seconds (s)

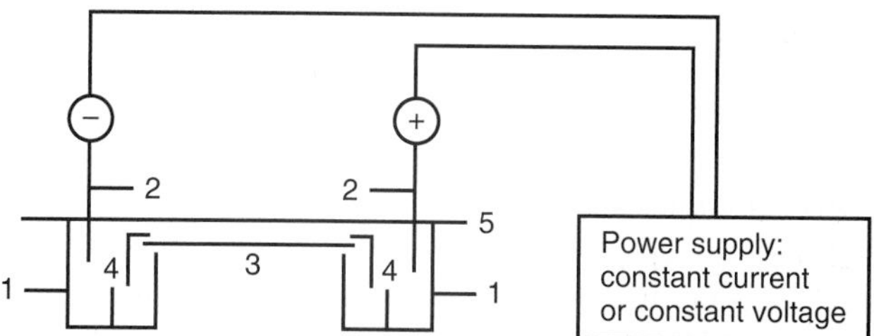

Figure 5-1 A schematic diagram of a typical electrophoresis apparatus showing two buffer boxes with baffle plates (*1*), electrodes (*2*), electrophoretic support (*3*), wicks (*4*), cover (*5*), and power supply.

This heat is released into the medium and increases the thermal agitation of all dissolved ions, and therefore the conductance of the system (decreases the resistance). With constant-voltage power supplies, the resultant rise in current increases both protein migration and evaporation of water from the medium. Any water loss increases the ion concentration and further decreases the resistance (R). Under these circumstances, the current and therefore the migration rate will progressively increase. To minimize these effects, it is best to use a constant-current power supply. According to Ohm's law:

$$E = (I)(R) \tag{7}$$

Therefore if R decreases, the applied EMF also decreases, keeping the current constant. This in turn decreases the heat effect and stabilizes the migration rate.

For *isoelectric focusing* (IEF) (see later section), a power supply that provides constant power is advisable. During electrophoresis, current drops significantly because of lower conductivity as carrier ampholytes focus at their isoelectric points and because of creation of zones of pure water. If a constant-voltage supply is used, frequent voltage adjustments may be necessary. Constant-current power supplies are not customarily used in IEF. *Pulsed-power* or *pulsed-field* techniques (see later section) require a power supply that can periodically change the orientation of the applied field relative to the direction of migration.

Buffers

Buffer ions have a twofold purpose in electrophoresis; they carry the applied current, and they fix the pH at which electrophoresis is carried out. Thus they determine the kind of electrical charge on the solute, the extent of ionization of the solute, and therefore the electrode toward which the solute will migrate. The buffer's ionic strength determines the thickness of the ionic cloud (buffer and nonbuffer ions) surrounding a charged molecule, the rate of its migration, and the sharpness of the electrophoretic zones. With increasing concentration of ions, the ionic cloud increases in size, and the molecule becomes more hindered in its movement. For the separation of serum proteins, the barbital or tris-boric acid-EDTA buffers remain the most popular.

According to Joule's law, power produced when current flows through a resistive medium is dissipated as heat. This heat increases in direct proportion to the resistance but in proportion to the square of the current. The reduction in resistance caused by a high ionic strength buffer therefore leads to increased current and excessive heat. These buffers yield sharper band separations, but the benefits of sharper resolution are diminished by the Joule (heat) effect that leads to denaturation of heat-labile proteins or degradation of other components.

Ionic strength (also denoted by the symbol μ) is computed according to the following

$$\mu = 0.5\sum c_i z_i^2 \tag{8}$$

where

c_i = ion concentration in mol/L

z_i = the charge on the ion

The ionic strength μ of an electrolyte (buffer) composed of monovalent ions is equal to its molarity (mol/L). The ionic strength of a 1 mol/L electrolyte solution with one monovalent and one divalent ion is 3 mol/L, and for a doubly divalent electrolyte, it is 4 mol/L.

A relatively high ionic strength buffer ($\mu = 0.075$, pH 8.6) containing calcium lactate has been used in *high-resolution electrophoresis* to improve the separation of serum proteins into as many as 13 bands, with two or more bands in the α_1, α_2, and β-globulin regions and one or more additional bands seen in various pathological conditions. Because of higher conductivity and the associated heat produced, it is necessary to reduce the temperature of the system to 10 °C to 14 °C. "Submarine" techniques, in which gels are submersed in circulating buffer cooled by an external cooling device or a Peltier plate built into the electrophoresis chamber itself, provide exact temperature control. Effective cooling with less precise temperature control may also be achieved using chambers designed with a sealed compartment of cooled ethylene glycol, which is in contact with the gel during running.

Support Media

The support medium provides the matrix in which protein separation takes place. Various types of support media are used in electrophoresis and range from pure buffer solutions in a capillary to insoluble gels (e.g., sheets, slabs, or columns of starch, agarose, or polyacrylamide), or membranes of cellulose acetate. Gels are cast in a solution of the same buffer to be used in the procedure and may be used in a horizontal or vertical direction. In either case, maximum resolution is achieved if the sample is applied in a very fine starting zone. Separation is based on differences in charge-to-mass ratio of the proteins and, depending on the pore size of the medium, possibly molecular size.

Starch Gel

Starch gel is prepared from partially hydrolyzed native starch, which in raw form does not gel. It is used in starch gel electrophoresis (SGE) to separate macromolecular ions on the basis of both charge-to-mass ratio and molecular size. Applying electrical current compacts proteins on the surface of the gel so that a thin uniform starting zone is produced, giving improved band resolution. However, because proper preparation of gels is relatively difficult and requires considerable skill, this technique is now rarely used in the clinical laboratory.

Cellulose Acetate

Cellulose acetate is a thermoplastic resin made by treating cellulose with acetic anhydride to acetylate the hydroxyl groups. The membranes contain about 80% air space within the interlocking cellulose acetate fibers and come as dry, opaque, brittle films that crack easily. When the film is soaked in buffer, the air spaces fill with liquid and the film becomes pliable. Membrane characteristics depend upon the extent of acetylation, the prewashing procedure used by the manufacturer, the additives used, the pore size, and the thickness of the membrane.

Samples (0.3 to 2.0 µL) are generally applied to cellulose acetate strips (presoaked with buffer) with a twin-wire applicator or the edge of a glass slide, and electrophoresis is carried out for 20 to 60 minutes. Stained membranes may be made transparent (cleared) for densitometry by soaking in a solvent containing 95 parts methanol and 5 parts glacial acetic acid. The cellulose acetate fibers are partially dissolved by the action of this solvent and coalesce to eliminate the original air spaces. Cleared membranes are strong and may be stored as a permanent record, but because of the necessity for presoaking before use and clearing the strips before densitometry, cellulose acetate has largely been replaced by agarose gel in most clinical applications.

Agarose

Agarose is a purified, essentially neutral fraction of agar obtained by separating agarose from agaropectin, a more highly charged fraction caused by acidic sulfate and carboxylic side groups. It is used in agarose gel electrophoresis (AGE) for the separation of serum, urine or CSF proteins, hemoglobin variants, isoenzymes, lipoproteins, and other substances. Because the pore size in agarose gel is large enough for all proteins to pass through unimpeded, separation is based only on the charge-to-mass ratio of the protein. Advantages of agarose gel include its lower affinity for proteins and its native clarity after drying, which permits excellent densitometric examination. It is essentially free of ionizable groups and so exhibits little endosmosis.

Most routine procedures for agarose electrophoresis today are carried out on commercially produced, prepackaged microzone gels, and the sample is applied by means of a thin plastic template with small slots corresponding to sample application points. The template is placed on the agarose surface, and 5- to 7-µL samples are placed on each slot. The serum sample is allowed to diffuse into the agarose for 5 minutes, excess sample is removed by blotting, and the template is removed. An AGE separation for most routine serum applications requires an electrophoresis time of 20 to 30 minutes.

Polyacrylamide Gel

Polyacrylamide is thermostable, transparent, strong, relatively chemically inert, and—depending on concentration—can be made in a wide range of pore sizes. Its average pore size in a typical 7.5% gel is about 5 nm (50 Å), large enough to allow most serum proteins to migrate unimpeded. However, proteins with a molecular radius and/or length that exceed critical limits will be impeded in their migration. Some of these proteins are fibrinogen, β-lipoprotein, α_2-macroglobulin, and γ-globulins. Thus separation is based on both charge-to-mass ratio and molecular size (a phenomenon referred to as molecular sieving), and serum proteins can be resolved into more individual fractions than with agarose gel. Furthermore, these gels are uncharged thus eliminating electroendosmosis, which is discussed later. Because of the potential carcinogenicity of acrylamide, however, appropriate caution must be exercised when handling this material during gel preparation.

Attempts to improve the hydrophilic nature of polyacrylamide have led to the development of mono- and di-substituted monomers, one of which is N-acryloyl-tris(hydroxymethyl)aminomethane or poly NAT™.[4] This material is more hydrophilic than polyacrylamide and its matrix has larger pores, thereby presenting less resistance to the passage of large molecules. It is ideally suited to the separation of DNA fragments up to 20 kilobases (kb) in size using a homogeneous (nonpulsed) electric field. Fragments that differ in size by as little as 2% can be resolved. Gels are submersed in buffer during use, allowing temperatures to be tightly controlled at values between 50 °C and 60 °C. Using elevated temperature results in shorter run times and more reproducible band migration.

Automated Systems

Because of increased volume of testing, primarily for serum proteins, many laboratories are converting to automated systems for electrophoresis. Such a system is the Helena SPIFE 3000, an automated electrophoresis system providing automated reagent application and a variety of gel sizes that permit the analysis of 10 to 100 samples simultaneously. It also features in-line sample application, automated electrophoretic separation and staining of analytes, multiple stain ports, and positive sample identification. Other systems that have partially automated the procedure or incorporated the ability to process multiple gels of different compositions sequentially include the Phast System (Pharmacia, LKB), the HITE Fractoscan (Olympus), the Hydragel-Hydrasys (Sebia), and the High-Performance Gel Electrophoresis (HPGE)-1000 system (LabIntelligence). Most CE systems (see Capillary Electrophoresis section) have autosampling capability for sequentially processing specimens, but the Beckman Coulter capillary zone electrophoresis (CZE) system permits simultaneous processing of seven samples by using multiple capillaries. Newer microchip-based analyzers like the Agilent 2100 Bioanalyzer significantly miniaturize and increase the speed of the process for separating proteins, nucleic acids, or even entire cells. These advances substantially reduce the labor component associated with this technique.

General Operations

General operations performed in conventional electrophoresis include separation, detection and quantification, and a number of "blotting" techniques.

Electrophoretic Separation

When electrophoresis is performed on precast microzone agarose gels, the following steps are typical: (1) the excess buffer is first removed from the support surface by blotting, taking care that bubbles are not present; (2) 5 to 7 μL of sample is applied using a plastic template, allowed to diffuse into the gel, and then blotted to remove the excess (in some systems, samples may be applied with a comb); (3) the gel is placed into the electrode chamber; (4) electrophoresis is performed at specified current, voltage, or power; (5) the gel is rinsed, fixed, and then dried; (6) the gel is stained and redried; (7) the gel is scanned in a densitometer. If isoenzymes are the analyte, substrate-dye solution is incubated on the gel to stain zones before fixing and drying. Alternative procedures would be required if more sophisticated methods described later are used.

Detection and Quantification

Once separated, proteins may be detected either by staining followed by quantification using a densitometer or by direct measurement using an optical detection system.

Staining

If staining is used to visualize the separated proteins, the proteins are usually first fixed by precipitating them in the gel with a chemical agent like acetic acid and methanol. This prevents diffusion of proteins out of the gel when submersed in the stain solution. The amount of dye taken up by the sample is affected by many factors, such as the type of protein and the degree of denaturation of the proteins by the fixing agents.

Table 5-1 lists dyes commonly used in electrophoresis along with suggested wavelengths for quantitation by densitometry. Most commercial methods for serum protein electrophoresis use Amido Black B or members of the Coomassie Brilliant Blue series of dyes for staining. Isoenzymes are typically visualized by incubating the gel in contact with a solution of substrate, which is linked structurally or chemically to a dye before fixing. Silver nitrate and silver diammine stain proteins and polypeptides with sensitivity 10- to 100-fold greater than that of conventional dyes.[45] Selective fixing and staining of protein subclasses also can be achieved by combining a stain molecule with an antiglobulin as is done in immunofixation.

Quantification

Stained zones can be quantified in a *densitometer,* an instrument that measures the absorbance of each fraction as the gel (or other medium) is moved past a photometric optical system and displays an *electropherogram* on a recorder chart or computer display. Microprocessor-containing units automatically integrate the area under each peak and report each as a percent of total or as absolute concentration or activity computed from the total protein or activity of enzyme in the sample.

Reliable densitometric quantitation requires light of an appropriate wavelength, a linear response from the instru-

TABLE 5-1 Suggested Wavelengths for Quantitation of Protein Zones by Direct Densitometry

Separation Type	Stain	Nominal Wavelength (nm)
Serum proteins in general	Amido Black (Naphthol Blue Black)	640
	Coomassie BrilliantBlue G—250 (Brilliant Blue G)	595
	Coomassie BrilliantBlue R—250 (Brilliant Blue R)	560
	Ponceau S	520
Isoenzymes	Nitrotetrazolium Blue	570
Lipoprotein zones	Fat Red 7B (Sudan Red 7B)	540
	Oil Red O	520
	Sudan Black B	600
DNA fragments	Ethidium bromide (fluorescent)	254 (Ex) 590 (Em)
CSF proteins	Silver nitrate	—

ment, and a transparent background in the medium being scanned. The linearity may be tested with a neutral density filter designed with either separated or adjacent areas of linearly increasing density. The densities are permanent and have expected absorbance values. The very small sample sizes used and transparency of agarose gels satisfy the requirement for a clear background. Nevertheless, problems can occur with densitometry because of differences in quantity of stain taken up by individual proteins and differences in protein zone sizes.

Essential features of a densitometer include (1) the ability to scan gels 25 to 100 mm in length; (2) automatic gain control, which adjusts the most intense peak of an electropherogram to full scale; (3) automatic background zeroing, which selects the lowest point in the electropherogram as baseline so that minor peaks are not lost or "cut off"; (4) variable wavelength control over the range of 400 to 700 nm; (5) variable slits to allow adjustment of the beam size; (6) an integrating device with both automatic and manual selection of cut points between peaks; (7) automatic indexing, a feature that advances the electrophoresis strip from one sample channel to the next; and (8) the ability to measure ultraviolet fluorescence.

Desirable features of a densitometer include (1) computerized integration and printout, (2) built-in diagnostics for instrument troubleshooting, (3) a choice of one of several scanning speeds, and (4) ability to measure in the reflectance mode. Models with a separate personal computer for data processing permit storage and reformatting of data, if desired, and reprinting or delayed transmission to a host computer.

DNA analysis requires the ability to scan larger gels, which may contain several dozen bands of different length DNA fragments. Modern automated electrophoresis systems also use larger gels containing 30 or more samples, which are scanned on a new generation of densitometers referred to as "flat bed scanners" or "digital image analyzers."[17] These instruments are capable of scanning and storing digitized light intensity readings from large areas and use ultrasensitive charge coupled device (CCD) detectors having a resolution of up to 1200 dots per inch (21 μm). Sophisticated data processing software permits manipulation of the stored image information to produce conventional scans and computations or more complex outputs, such as overlaying and subtraction of patterns from two different samples. Chemiluminescence has also been used in this way to quantify IgE (Lumi-Phos 530).[54] DNA fragments have been detected by linking with a fluorescent dye label.[27]

Blotting Techniques

In 1975 Edward Southern developed a technique that is widely used to detect fragments of DNA. This technique, known as *Southern blotting*,[20] first requires an electrophoretic separation of DNA or DNA fragments by AGE. Next a strip of nitrocellulose or a nylon membrane is laid over the agarose gel, and the DNAs or DNA fragments are transferred or "blotted" onto it by either capillary, electro-, or vacuum blotting. They are then detected and identified by hybridization with a labeled, complementary nucleic acid probe. This technique is widely used in molecular biology for identifying a particular DNA sequence, determining the presence, position, and number of copies of a gene in a genome, and typing DNA (see Chapters 36 and 37 for further details).

Northern[20] and *Western*[20] blotting techniques, named by analogy to Southern blotting, were subsequently developed to separate and detect ribonucleic acid (RNAs) and proteins, respectively. Northern blotting is carried out identically to Southern blotting except that a labeled RNA probe is used for hybridization. Western blotting is used to separate, detect, and identify one or more proteins in a complex mixture. It involves first separating the individual proteins by polyacrylamide gel and then transferring or "blotting" onto an overlying strip of nitrocellulose or a nylon membrane by electro-blotting. The strip or membrane is then reacted with a reagent that contains an antibody raised against the protein of interest. (See Chapter 9 for further details and applications of this technique.)

TECHNICAL AND PRACTICAL CONSIDERATIONS

In performing electrophoretic separations, a number of technical and practical aspects need to be considered as they affect the process.

Electroendosmosis or Endosmosis

An electrophoretic support medium, such as a gel in contact with water, takes on a negative charge caused by adsorption of hydroxyl ions. These ions are fixed to the surface and are immobile. Positive ions in solution cluster about the fixed negative charge sites, forming an ionic cloud of mostly positive ions and creating what is referred to as the Stern potential. The number of negative ions in the solution increases with increasing distance from the fixed negative charge sites until eventually positive and negative ions are present in equal concentration (Figure 5-2). The potential that exists between the fixed ions and the associated cloud of ions is termed the *electrokinetic potential* or the *zeta potential* (ζ).

When current is applied to such a system, charges attached to the immobile support remain fixed, but the cloud of ions in solution moves to the electrode of opposite polarity. Because ions in solution are highly hydrated, this results in movement of the solvent as well. The movement of solvent and its solutes relative to the fixed support is referred to as *endosmosis,* and it causes preferential movement of water in one direction. Macromolecules in solution that move in the direction opposite this flow may remain immobile or may even be swept back toward the opposite pole if they are insufficiently charged. In media in which endosmosis is strong, such as conventional cellulose acetate and conventional agarose gel, γ-globulins are swept back from the application point. Because the inner surface of a

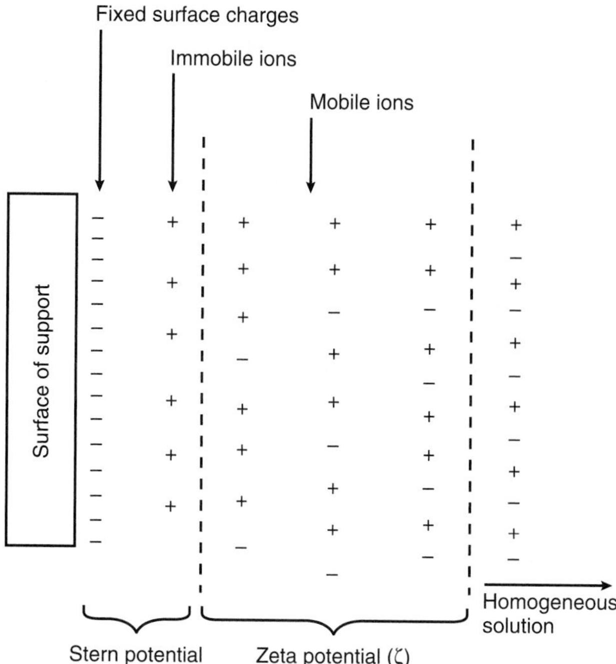

Figure 5-2 Distribution of + and – ions around the surface of an electrophoretic support. Fixed on the surface of the solid is a layer of – ions. (These may be + ions under suitable conditions.) A second layer of + ions is attracted to the surface. These two layers compose the Stern potential. The large, diffuse layer containing mostly + ions is the electrokinetic or zeta (ζ) potential. Extending farther from the surface of the solid is homogeneous solution. The Stern potential plus the zeta potential equals the electrochemical potential, or epsilon (ε) potential.

glass capillary contains many such charged groups, endosmosis is very strong and is actually the primary driving force for migration in CE systems.

Most of the endosmotic effect observed using agarose is caused by the presence of charged groups, such as sulfate or carboxylic acid groups. It is possible to reduce endosmotic effects considerably by removing or chemically modifying these charged groups. Endosmosis can be manipulated similarly in CE to modify the magnitude of the endosmotic effect. In electrophoretic media in which surface charges are minimal (starch gel, purified agarose gel, or polyacrylamide gel), endosmosis is also minimal.

Sampling

To achieve a proper balance between sensitivity and resolution, the amount of serum protein that is applied to an electrophoretic support must be optimum. Albumin is about 10 times more concentrated in serum than the smallest fraction, the α_1-globulins. Therefore the amount of serum applied should prevent overloading with albumin but still be adequate to quantify α_1-globulin. For the separation of serum proteins using polyacrylamide gel electrophoresis (PAGE), 3 µL of serum containing approximately 210 µg of total protein is applied. For alkaline phosphatase isoenzymes, up to 25 µL of a normal serum may be applied (less may be used if activity is greatly increased). Urine specimens require 50- to 100-fold concentration for adequate sensitivity, and CSF may or may not require concentration, depending on the staining approach used.

Discontinuities in Sample Application

Discontinuities in sample application may be caused by dirty applicators in cellulose acetate or inclusion of an air bubble in AGE. In practice, caution must be used in cleaning applicators because they are easily bent. Twin-wire applicators are best cleaned merely by agitating in water followed by gently pressing the applicators against absorbent paper. It is inadvisable to clean wires by manual wiping. The pipette tip should be checked for air bubbles before application of the sample to the agarose gel template.

Unequal Migration Rates

Unequal migration of samples across the width of the gel may be caused by dirty electrodes causing uneven application of the electric field or by uneven wetting of the gel. If wicks are used to connect the gel to a power supply, uneven wetting of the wicks could cause unequal migration or bowing of sample lanes at the gel edges. Gels, which may have been stored too close to heat sources (e.g., in a cabinet over a light fixture), could have partially and unevenly dried areas, contributing to similar problems.

Distorted, Unusual, or Atypical Bands

Distorted protein zones may be caused by bent applicators, incorporation of an air bubble during sample application, overapplication, or inadequate blotting of the sample. Distorted zones may also be caused by excessive drying of the electrophoretic support before or during electrophoresis or by improper tension on a cellulose acetate film, resulting in zones that look "bent over." Irregularities (other than broken zones) in the sample application probably are due to excessively wet cellulose acetate films or agarose gels. Parts of the applied samples may look washed out.

In most cases, unusual bands are artifacts that may be easily recognized. Hemolyzed samples are frequent causes of an increased β-globulin (where free hemoglobin migrates) or an unusual band between the α_2- and β-globulins, the result of a hemoglobin-haptoglobin complex. A band occurring at the starting point of an electropherogram may be fibrinogen. The sample should be verified as being serum before this band is reported as an abnormal protein. The α- and β-lipoproteins may migrate ahead of their normal positions in some samples. Occasionally a split albumin zone is observed in the rare, benign, genetically related condition of *bis*albuminemia. However, a grossly widened albumin zone could be due to albumin-bound medication and not faulty electrophoretic practice.

Atypical bands in an isoenzyme pattern may be the result of binding by an immunoglobulin (a macroenzyme), causing abnormal migration of one or more of the normal isoenzymes. Occasionally an irregular but sharp protein zone is seen at the starting point. Unlike fibrinogen or other proteins that may be seen at about the same point, the artifact lacks the regular, somewhat diffuse appearance that proteins normally show; it is actually denatured protein resulting from a deteriorated serum. Of course when faced with an unusual band anywhere in a serum protein pattern, the possibility that it is a true paraprotein must always be considered. Finally, it is good laboratory practice to include a control serum with each electrophoretic run to evaluate its quality and that of the densitometer.

Buffers

Because buffers used in electrophoresis are good culture media for the growth of microorganisms, they should be refrigerated when not in use. Moreover, a cold buffer is preferred in an electrophoretic run, because it improves resolution and decreases evaporation from the electrophoretic support. Buffer used in a small-volume apparatus should be discarded after each run because of pH changes resulting from the electrolysis of water that accompany electrophoresis. If volumes used are larger than 100 mL, buffer from both reservoirs may be combined, mixed, and reused up to four times.

Staining

In practice, a typical stain solution may be used several times before being replaced. A good rule of thumb is that a stain solution of 100 mL may be used for a combined total of 387 cm^2 (60 in^2) of cellulose acetate or agarose film. The stain solution may be considered faulty if leaching of stained protein zones occurs in the 5% acetic acid wash solution or in the clearing solution (cellulose acetate only). Whenever protein zones appear too lightly stained, the stain or substrate reagent—in the case of isoenzymes—should always be suspected. Stain solution must be stored tightly covered to prevent evaporation.

Types of Electrophoresis

Using different media in different physical formats and a variety of instrumental configurations, several different types of electrophoretic techniques are used for the separation of a diverse range of analytes.

Slab Gel Electrophoresis

Traditional methods, using a rectangular gel regardless of thickness, are referred to collectively by the term *slab gel electrophoresis.* Its main advantage is its ability to simultaneously separate several samples in one run. Starch, agarose, and polyacrylamide media have all been used in this format. It is the primary method used in clinical chemistry laboratories for separation of various classes of serum or CSF proteins and DNA and RNA fragments. Gels (usually agarose) may be cast on a sheet of plastic backing or completely encased within a plastic walled cell, which allows either horizontal or vertical electrophoresis and submersion for cooling, if necessary.

Slab gels may be cast with additives such as (1) ampholytes, which create a pH gradient (see Isoelectric Focusing Electrophoresis), or (2) sodium dodecyl sulfate (SDS), which denatures proteins (see Two-Dimensional [2-D] Electrophoresis). In some applications, a gradient of concentration or denaturant is created in the gel to improve separation.[12] Very thin gradient or nongradient gels have been used to improve the efficiency and speed of separation of DNA fragments.[52,61] In addition to conventional serum proteins, applications include the separation of isoenzymes, lipoproteins, hemoglobins, and fragments of DNA and RNA. One-dimensional separations of the last two often involve the addition of a mixture of known fragment size markers, referred to as a ladder, in one lane to enable size identification of sample fragments.

Disc Electrophoresis

Protein electrophoresis using agarose gel yields only five zones, namely: (1) albumin, (2) α_1-, (3) α_2-, (4) β-, and (5) γ-globulins, although some subfractionation of the α_2- and β-globulins is possible with high resolution gels. *Disc electrophoresis* was developed to improve this situation and derives its name from *discontinuities* in the electrophoretic matrix caused by layers of gel that differ in composition and pore size.[7,40] The pore size in a polyacrylamide or starch gel is controlled by the percent composition of the polyacrylamide or starch and is much smaller than that found in agarose gel. These gels may yield 20 or more fractions and are widely used to study individual proteins in serum, especially genetic variants and isoenzymes.

With PAGE, samples are separated in individual gels prepared in open-ended glass tubes, which form a bridge between two buffer reservoirs. Although precast gel tubes are now commercially available, the original technique involved a three-gel system prepared in situ. A small-pore *separation gel* filled the majority of the tube followed, after gelation, by a thin segment of large-pore *spacer gel* cast on top of the separation gel. Then another thin layer of large-pore monomer solution containing a small amount of serum, about 3 µL, was polymerized above the spacer gel. When electrophoresis begins, all protein ions migrate easily through the large-pore gels (which do not impede movement of most proteins in serum) and stack up on the separation gel in a very thin zone. This process improves resolution and concentrates protein components at the border (or starting zone) so that preconcentration of specimens with low protein content (e.g., CSF) may not be necessary. Separation then takes place in the bottom separation gel with retardation of some proteins caused by the molecular sieve phenomenon. A schematic representation of serum protein electrophoresis by PAGE is shown in Figure 5-3.

Isoelectric Focusing Electrophoresis

IEF separates amphoteric compounds, such as proteins, with increased resolution in a medium possessing a stable pH gradient. The protein becomes "focused" at a point on the gel as it migrates to a zone where the pH of the gel matches

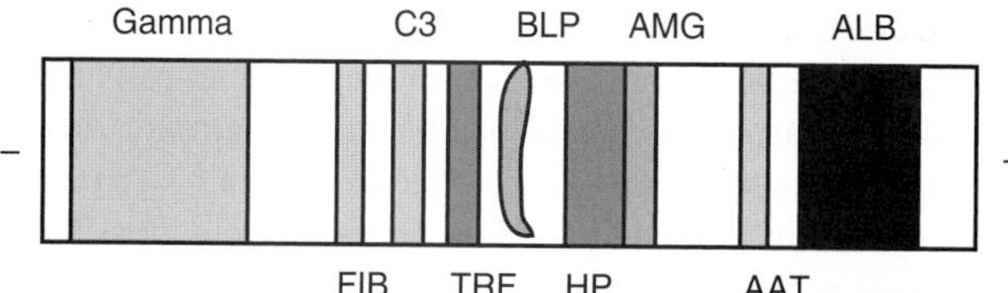

Figure 5-3 A simplified schematic drawing of a protein pattern from the serum of a subject with haptoglobin type 2-1 (separation by PAGE). Some zones contain more than the one protein shown, as demonstrated by immunological techniques. *AAT*, Alpha$_1$-antitrypsin; *ALB*, albumin; *AMG*, alpha$_2$-macroglobulin; *BLP*, beta-lipoprotein; *C3*, complement 3; *FIB*, fibrinogen; *gamma*, gamma-globulin; *HP*, haptoglobin; *TRF*, transferrin.

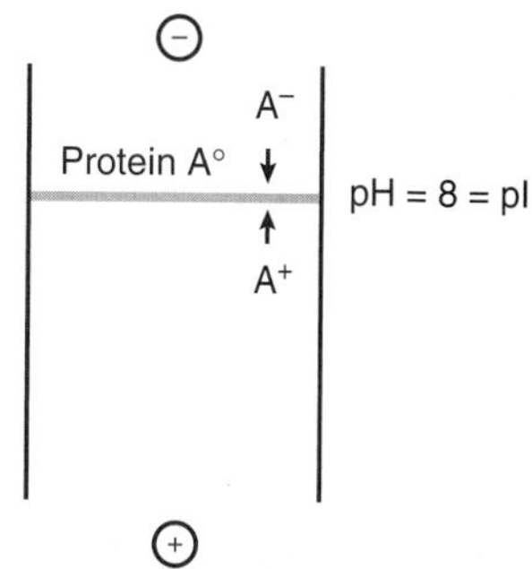

Figure 5-5 After attaining the pH where protein A has a net charge of zero (A°), diffusion toward the cathode bestows a negative charge on A (A⁻), and migration in the electric field forces A⁻ back to A°. Diffusion toward the anode causes A to take on the opposite charge A+, and migration is toward the cathode and to the point where A° exists. IF processes of this kind cause sharp zones to form (i.e., the protein is focused).

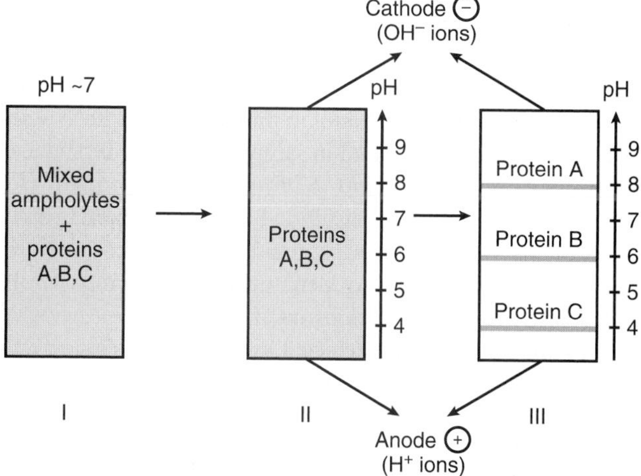

Figure 5-4 Schematic of an IEF procedure. **I,** A homogeneous mixture of carrier ampholytes, pH range 3 to 10, to which proteins A, B, and C with pI 8, 6, and 4, respectively, were added. **II,** Current is applied and the carrier ampholytes rapidly migrate to the pH zones where the net charge is zero (the pI value). **III,** The proteins A, B, and C migrate more slowly to their respective pI zones where migration ceases. The high buffering capacity of the carrier ampholyte creates stable pH zones in which each protein may reach its pI.

the protein's isoelectric point (pI). At this point, the charge of the protein becomes zero and its migration ceases. Figure 5-4 illustrates the procedure and shows the electrophoretic conditions before and after current is applied. The protein zones are very sharp, because the region associated with a given pH is very narrow. Normal diffusion is also counteracted by the acquisition of a charge as a protein varies from its pI position and subsequently migrates back because of electrophoretic forces (Figure 5-5). Proteins that differ in their pI values by only 0.02 pH units have been separated by IEF.

The pH gradient is created with *carrier ampholytes,* a group of amphoteric polyaminocarboxylic acids, which have slight differences in pKa value and molecular weights of 300 to 1000. Mixtures of 50 to 100 different compounds are added to the medium and create a "natural pH gradient" when the individual ampholytes reach their pI values during electrophoresis. They establish narrow buffered zones, with stable but slightly different pHs, through which the slower-moving proteins migrate and stop at their individual pIs.

As Figure 5-4 illustrates, the anode is surrounded by a dilute acid solution and the cathode by a dilute alkaline solution. After focusing, the most negatively charged carrier ampholytes and proteins will be found at the anodal end and the most positively charged near the cathodal end of the electrophoretic matrix. The other carrier ampholytes and proteins focus at intermediate points according to their isoelectric points. Because carrier ampholytes are generally used in relatively high concentrations, a high-voltage power source (up to 2000 V) is necessary (power is in the vicinity of 2 to 50 W, depending on experimental conditions). As a result, the electrophoretic matrix must be cooled. A modification of this technique, in which an immobilized pH gradient (IPG-IEF) is produced in the gel before applying the sample, is reported to improve resolution and reproducibility.[11]

PAGE-IEF is widely used in analytical work as it is essentially free of electroendosmosis. The polyacrylamide gel must have a large enough pore size, however, so that protein migration will not be impeded by molecular sieving effects. In actual practice, impeded migration of some proteins, such as IgM, cannot be prevented. With the availability of endosmosis-free materials, IEF methods have been adapted for agarose, cellulose acetate, and Sephadex electrophoresis. AGE-IEF and cellulose acetate electrophoresis-IEF (CAE-IEF) have the advantages that operating conditions are simple, and that large pore sizes make it unlikely that any proteins will be excluded on the basis of molecular size.[9] Sephadex, like polyacrylamide, provides advantages of separation on the basis of molecular size. IEF has been applied to the separation of alkaline phosphatase isoenzymes and is widely used in neonatal screening programs to test for variant hemoglobins (see Chapter 31).

Isotachophoresis

ITP completely separates smaller ionic substances into adjacent zones that contact one another with no overlap, and all migrate at the same rate. In this technique, no background electrolyte (buffer) is mixed with the sample, so current flow is carried entirely by charged sample ions. An aliquot of a sample is typically placed in a capillary between a leading electrolyte solution that contains faster-migrating ions than any in the sample and a trailing solution containing slower-migrating ions than any in the sample. Once a faster-moving component separates completely from a slower-moving one, any further separation creates a region of depleted charge and increases the resistance and therefore the local voltage in that region. The increased voltage causes the slower component to migrate faster and close the gap, thereby concentrating it and increasing the conductivity of its zone until it matches that of the faster ion. Ultimately, all ions migrate at the rate of the fastest ion in zones that differ in size depending on their original concentrations. Zone size is determined by measuring ultraviolet (UV) absorbance, temperature difference, or conductivity as the sample passes a detector. Applications include the separation of small anions and cations, organic and amino acids, peptides, nucleotides, nucleosides, and proteins.

Pulsed-Field Electrophoresis

In pulsed-field electrophoresis, power is alternately applied to different pairs of electrodes or electrode arrays, so the electrophoretic field is cycled between two directions. The directions can differ spatially by 105° to 180°, and molecules must reorient themselves to the new field direction during each cycle before migration can continue. Because reorientation time depends on molecular size, net migration becomes a function of the frequency of field alteration. This permits separation of very large molecules, such as DNA fragments greater than 50 kb that cannot be resolved by the relatively small pores in agarose or polyacrylamide gels.[39] Fragments of 50 to 400 kb can be resolved using 10 s pulse times, whereas larger fragments up to 7 megabases in size or intact chromosomes require pulse times of several hours for complete resolution. This technique has been applied to typing various strains of bacterial DNA.[15,46]

Two-Dimensional (2-D) Electrophoresis

Two-dimensional (2-D) electrophoresis is extensively used in the field of proteomics to study families of proteins and search for genetic- or disease-based differences or to study the protein content of cells of various types.[29] It has also been applied to the study of human gene mutations[55] and the DNA of various bacteria and tumor cells as a means to earlier diagnosis.[12,44] By combining charge-dependent IEF in the first dimension with molecular weight–dependent electrophoresis in the second, the technique is able to resolve up to 1100 separate protein spots using autoradiographic detection and up to 400 using Coomassie dyes. The first dimension separation is carried out in a large-pore medium, such as agarose gel or large-pore polyacrylamide gel. The second dimension is often polyacrylamide in a linear or gradient format.

The 2-D electrophoresis method of O'Farrell[38] uses PAGE-IEF in 130 × 2.5-mm (internal diameter) tubes for the first dimension and covers a pH range of 3 to 10 units. The anodal compartment is in contact with 10 mmol/L phosphoric acid and the cathodal compartment with 20 mmol/L NaOH. After electrophoresis is complete, the gel is extruded from the tube and placed in contact with a thin, polyacrylamide gradient gel slab that incorporates SDS. At the end of the process, the polypeptides are detected by one of several different methods.

In the O'Farrell method, SDS is used in the second dimension, β-mercaptoethanol in the first. Others have used SDS in both dimensions and in sample preparation. The use of β-mercaptoethanol and SDS denatures proteins to polypeptides by reducing disulfide bonds and depolymerizing proteins. When native proteins, such as enzymes, are desired for further study, nondenaturing sample preparation and electrophoresis conditions must be used.

Separated proteins are detected by use of Coomassie dyes, silver staining, radiography (exposure of photographic film to emissions of isotopically labeled polypeptides), or fluorographic analysis (x-ray film exposed to tritium-labeled polypeptides in the presence of a scintillator). The latter two methods represent the greatest analytical sensitivity, because they are 100 to 1000 times more sensitive than the Coomassie dyes.

Newer developments in this area combine analytical techniques to achieve a 2-D separation by linking, for example, liquid IEF with nonporous silica reverse phase, high performance liquid chromatography (HPLC; see Chapter 6) and detecting intact proteins by electrospray ionization, time of flight, and mass spectrometry[57] (see Chapter 7).

CAPILLARY ELECTROPHORESIS

In CE, the classic techniques of zone electrophoresis, ITP, IEF, and gel electrophoresis are carried out in a small-bore (10- to 100-μm internal diameter) fused silica capillary tube of 20 to 200 cm in length.[36]

Two distinct advantages of the capillary format include the ability to apply much higher voltages than in traditional electrophoresis and the ease of automation. Applications are also more extensive and include separation of low-molecular-weight ions in addition to proteins and other macromolecules. Even uncharged molecules can be separated using CE in the micellar electrokinetic chromatography (MEKC) mode that is discussed later in this section. CE has also proved useful for separations of inorganic ions, amino

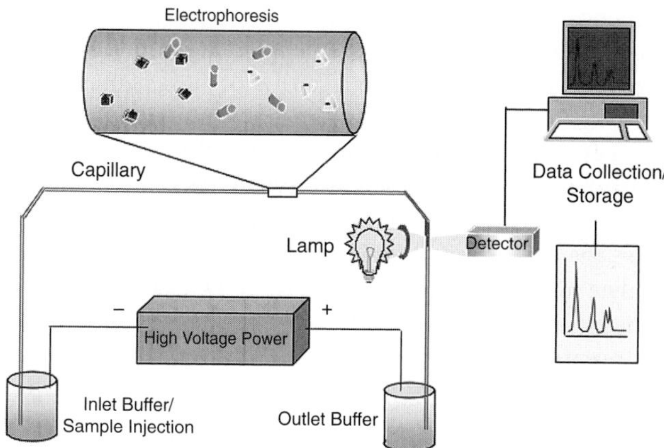

Figure 5-6 A schematic for CE instrumentation.

acids, organic acids, drugs, vitamins, porphyrins, carbohydrates, oligonucleotides, proteins, and DNA fragments.[8,22,51,60]

INSTRUMENTATION

A schematic diagram of a typical CE instrument is shown in Figure 5-6. As indicated, the capillary tube serves as an electrophoretic chamber that is connected to a detector at its terminal end and, via buffer reservoirs, to a high-voltage power supply. Improved heat dissipation permits the application of voltages in the range of 10 to 30 kV, which enhances separation efficiency and reduces separation time in some cases to less than 1 minute. Only a few microliters of the sample are required, with volumes in the picoliter to nanoliter range actually used. This minimizes distortions in the applied field caused by the presence of samples.

In contrast to the cumbersome and time-consuming tasks of conventional electrophoresis, CE is well suited to automation. Samples are easily applied to the capillary, a variety of detector types can be used, and the resulting electropherograms can be analyzed and manipulated in much the same manner as chromatograms. Commercial instruments resemble many HPLC instruments in terms of automated sample loading and data analysis. Traditional serum protein electrophoresis, for example, can be fully automated with CE.

The Capillary Format

The capillary tubes used as separation chambers in CE are most commonly made from fused silica (i.e., pure glass) coated with a thin exterior covering of polyimide to provide strength and flexibility. Although capillaries can be made from other materials, such as polyethylene or Teflon, such capillaries have seen limited use. The polyimide coating is usually removed from a small portion of the capillary towards the terminal end, creating a window for online optical detection. Caution must be taken with capillaries after a detection window has been created since loss of the polyimide coating from the capillary tubing weakens the wall of the tube in these locations. The outer diameter of the capillary tubing typically varies from 180 to 375 μm, the inner diameter from 20 to 180 μm, and the total length from 20 cm up to several meters. Noncylindrical capillary tubing suitable for CE is now available from some commercial providers. For example, rectangular capillaries (Polymicro Technologies, Phoenix) provide a flat surface that is more amenable to optical detection than their curved counterparts.

The main advantage of performing electrophoresis in a narrow-bore capillary comes from efficient heat dissipation. The relatively poor dissipation of Joule heat in traditional electrophoresis limits it to relatively low electric fields. The large surface-to-volume ratio inherent in capillaries, however, allows for more effective heat dissipation and much higher voltages can be applied, often up to 30 kV.[33] An additional advantage gained from using a narrow-bore capillary chamber is that it improves resolution by minimizing band broadening.

Sample Injection

In CE, sample volumes of 1 to 50 nL are loaded into the capillary chamber by one of two primary methods, *hydrodynamic injection* and *electrokinetic (EK) injection.* In practice, to maintain high separation efficiency, the sample plug length is usually less than 2% of the total capillary length. With hydrodynamic injection, an aliquot of a sample is introduced by applying a positive pressure at the inlet vial or alternately vacuum at the outlet vial. The volume of sample loaded is governed by a number of parameters including (but not restricted to) the inner diameter of the capillary, buffer viscosity, applied pressure, temperature, and time. Alternatively, gravity may be used as the source of pressure by raising the inlet vial (or lowering the outlet vial) and allowing "siphoning" to occur for a timed interval.

With EK injection, an aliquot of a sample is introduced by applying a voltage for a timed interval. The magnitude of the voltage is dependent on the analyte and buffer system used but typically involves a field strength 3 to 5 times lower than that used for separation. It is important to note that although hydrodynamic methods introduce a sample representative of the bulk specimen, EK injection favors the preferential movement of more mobile ions into the capillary.

Direct Detection

With CE, separated analytes are detected and measured as they migrate past an optical detector without prior staining. Optical detection is based on classical methods, such as photometric absorbance, refractive index, and fluorescence (see Chapter 3). These techniques miniaturize and simplify the process of measurement by eliminating several of the steps required in conventional gel electrophoresis. Because the amount of protein measured and the measurement path are both very small, however, special conditions are often used to improve sensitivity.

Optical Detection

As with HPLC, ultraviolet-visible photometers are widely used as detectors to monitor CE separations.[42] To interface such online detectors with the capillary, a "detection window" is created towards the outlet end of the capillary tube. The "window" serves as an inline cuvet and is typically formed by burning off the polyimide with a small flame and cleaning the window with ethanol. It is not recommended that the polyimide be removed (by scraping) with a sharp object because this could scratch the surface of the fused silica and interfere with optical detection. Although this configuration allows for high efficiency separation because there is no band broadening caused by component mixing or dead volume, the inner diameter of the capillary tube defines the optical light path (OLP) length of the in-line cuvet. Since absorbance is directly proportional to the length of the cuvet (OLP) used in an optical system (see Chapter 3), the 20 to 100 µm inner diameter limits UV-visible absorbance detection to the 10^{-6} to 10^{-8} M range.

Improving Limits of Detection

A number of approaches have been devised to improve the limit of detection of online CE detectors. These include increasing the length of the OLP, using more sensitive optical techniques, and preconcentrating the sample.

Increased OLP. Capillary tubes modified at the detector window with a "bubble" cell (a glass-blown expansion of the internal diameter of the capillary tube) can expand the OLP by almost an order of magnitude, with a concomitant lowering of the system's limit of detection. Alternatively a "Z" geometry has been developed that increases the OLP via detection down the core of the capillary with lengths up to 1 mm possible.

Sensitive Optical Detectors. More sensitive optical techniques that have been used with CE include fluorescence, refractive index, chemiluminescence, Raman spectrophotometry, and circular dichroism.[51] The most sensitive optical detection method used in CE is laser-induced fluorescence (LIF), which is capable of detection limits in the 10^{-18} to 10^{-21} mol (or better) range. This detection mode is easily accomplished with analytes that are either easily labeled with a fluorescent substrate (e.g., intercalators for double-stranded DNA) or are naturally fluorescent (e.g., proteins or peptides containing tryptophan). CE systems have also been interfaced with mass spectrometers,[48] and electrochemical detection methods[13] have been developed, although such detectors must be isolated electrically from the electrophoretic voltages.

Online Sample Concentration. Another technique used in CE systems to increase their limit of detection is to preconcentrate the sample. One of the simplest methods for sample preconcentration is to induce a "stacking" effect with the sample components, something easily accomplished by exploiting the ionic strength differences between the sample matrix and separation buffer.[5] This results from the fact that sample ions have decreased electrophoretic mobility in a higher conductivity environment. When voltage is applied to the system, sample ions in the sample plug instantaneously accelerate toward the adjacent separation buffer zone. Upon crossing the boundary, the higher conductivity environment induces a decrease in electrophoretic velocity and subsequent "stacking" of the sample components into a smaller buffer zone than the original sample plug. Within a short time, the ionic strength gradient dissipates and the charged analyte molecules begin to move from the "stacked" sample zone toward the cathode. Stacking can be used with either hydrostatic or EK injection and can typically yield a tenfold enhancement in sample concentration and hence sensitivity.

An alternative approach to stacking is a "focusing" that is based on pH differences between the sample plug and separation buffer. This has been shown to be very useful for the analysis of peptides, mainly caused by their relative stability over a wide pH range.[1] By increasing the pH of the sample above that of the net pI of the analytes of interest and flanking the sample plug with low pH separation buffer zones (i.e., an equivalent volume of low pH separation buffer following introduction of the sample plug), the negatively charged peptides are electrophoretically driven toward the anode. Upon entering the lower pH separation buffer, a pH-induced change in their charge state causes a reversal in their electrophoretic mobility, resulting in a "focusing" of the peptides at the interface of the sample (high pH) and low pH buffer plugs (similar to those in isoelectric focusing). After the pH gradient dissipates, the peptides, again positively charged, migrate toward the cathode as a sharp zone. This approach can be applied to a variety of analytes, but is limited to those that can withstand the inherent changes in pH without substantial denaturation and may yield as much as a fivefold enhancement in a system's limit of detection.[50]

Other types of sample concentration enhancement approaches applicable to CE include ITP[56] and those involving concentration on an online solid phase.[43] This latter method shows much promise for both small and large molecules and is covered in detail in the review by Wettstein and Strausbauch.[58]

Indirect Detection

When strong chromophores are lacking in the analyte of interest, absorbance and fluorescence detection can also be used in an indirect mode.[10,26,34] In this mode of detection, a strongly absorbing ion is added to the running electrolyte and monitored at a wavelength that gives a constant, high background absorbance. As solute ions move into their discrete zones during the electrophoretic process, they displace the indirect detection agent through mutual repulsion, and this produces a decrease in the background absorbance as the zone passes through the detector. Reagents with the appropriate fluorescence properties can also be employed in a similar manner. The indirect detection of amino acids by CE has been demonstrated with the potential for use in diagnosis of aminoacidurias.[30] These investigators show the direct extrapolation of this technique to microchip detection where UV detection is difficult, if not impossible.

Technical Considerations

Temperature and surface effects influence the separation capabilities of CE. Artifacts also can arise with CE.

Temperature Effects

In most slab or tube platforms for electrophoresis, moderate electric fields (up to 1000 volts) are used because the Joule heating that accompanies the use of higher field strengths can cause nonuniform temperature gradients, local changes in viscosity, and subsequent zone broadening. CE is distinguished from other forms of electrophoresis by the fact that extraordinarily high fields (30,000 volts) can be used to obtain rapid, high efficiency separations. The problems encountered with noncapillary platforms are prevented because of the effective dissipation of Joule heat by either forced air convection or liquid cooling of the capillary, both of which are possible because of the narrow bore of the capillary. The Joule heat produced is a function of the buffer type, concentration, voltage applied, capillary inner diameter, and length, and can be determined for any given system by generating an *Ohm's law plot,* which allows for easy determination of the maximum voltage that can be used effectively.[32] Although the heat produced by the electrophoretic process can be decreased by reducing the inner diameter of the capillary, the ionic strength of the running buffer, or the applied voltage, the latter is less desirable since resolution is directly proportional to the applied field. Consequently, attempts should be made to alter other parameters before reducing the field.

Surface Effects

As in electrophoresis in general, the flow of liquid (electroosmotic or electroendosmotic flow [EOF]) in CE is a consequence of surface charge on the solid support. In CE it plays a significant role in the separation process. The charge on the inner surface of a fused silica capillary is determined by the ionization state of the silanol groups (SiOH) that populate it. Interaction of positively charged buffer species with the bound surface anions generates a layer of mobile cations that move toward the cathode when voltage is applied. This induces a very strong EOF that carries all analytes in the same direction, regardless of their charge. Separation is then achieved because of differences in the electrophoretic migration rates of the analytes superimposed on this EOF.

Because the driving force of the flow is distributed along the wall of the capillary, the flow profile is nearly flat or plug-like, contrasting the laminar or parabolic flow generated by a pressure-driven system caused by shear forces at the wall. A flat flow profile is beneficial because it does not contribute to the dispersion of solute zones. The magnitude and direction of the EOF can be impacted by the type of electrolyte used, the pH, the ionic strength, the use of additives (e.g., surfactants and organic solvents), and the polarity and magnitude of the applied electric field.

Although advantageous for dissipation of Joule heat, the large surface area-to-volume ratio of the capillary chamber increases the likelihood of analyte adsorption onto the surface of its inner wall. This causes phenomena such as peak tailing and even total and irreversible adsorption of the analyte. Adsorption is typically between cationic solutes and the negatively charged wall of the capillary chamber, primarily through ionic interactions (with silanols), but can also involve hydrophobic interactions (with siloxanes). Because of the numerous charges and hydrophobic regions, significant adsorptive effects have been noted, especially for proteins. In practice, adsorption of substances, whether from the sample or from the buffer, to the inner surface of the capillary can alter migration times and other separation characteristics; unaddressed, the capillary can eventually become fouled. Buffer components, such as surfactants, can often render permanent changes to the inner surface of the capillary (through adsorption) and may warrant dedication of specific capillaries for use with particular surfactants.

To minimize these inner wall effects, capillary chambers are conditioned by chemical treatment, most commonly with base to remove adsorbates and refresh the surface. A typical wash method includes flushing the chamber with 10 to 20 capillary volumes of 0.1 to 1.0 mol/L NaOH, followed by flushing with running electrolyte. To prevent exposing the capillary surface to drastic fluctuations in the pH, conditioning procedures for separations at low pH may be better served by using strong acids (e.g., HNO_3), surfactants (e.g., SDS), or organic solvents, such as acetonitrile or methanol, may also be warranted with certain separations.

Artifacts

Because CE uses online optical detection, artifacts can result in the form of "system peaks." These often originate from the sample or the interfaces between the sample and the separation buffer because any species that absorbs at the detection wavelength will generate a response. This differs from protein slab gel electrophoresis where detection specificity is governed by a protein specific stain. It is not uncommon, for example, for buffer species present in the sample but not in the separation buffer to generate system peaks. However, clinical serum protein electrophoresis provides one example where artifacts are eliminated by CE.

One problem associated with conventional electrophoresis of serum proteins is its proclivity for point-of-application artifacts. These are bands that result from the fact that electrophoretic mobility (e.g., with AGE) is bidirectional from the point of application. Consequently the point of application remains part of the scanned area of interest. The fact that these must be immunotyped to distinguish real monoclonal proteins from artifacts is costly and time consuming.

CE prevents point-of-application artifacts for two reasons. First, the net mobility in CE is the vectorial addition of both protein electrophoretic mobility and the EOF. As a result of this unidirectional movement (toward the detector), the point-of-application remains remote from the detector. Second, unlike AGE where precipitates cannot exit the loading well and enter the gel (thus appearing as a band in the scanned region of the gel), there is no gel matrix in CZE to impede electrophoretic migration since analysis occurs in free solution (i.e., CZE). This was demonstrated by Clarke et al who evaluated a small subset of serum samples containing monoclonal proteins that remained at the point-of-application on agarose gels (and cellulose acetate) but were handled by CZE with ease.[3] These precipitates may be euglobulin or cryoprecipitates and may or may not contain a monoclonal protein; only immunoelectrophoresis or immunofixation can determine the presence of monoclonal proteins.

Modes of Operation

Modes in which CE systems are operated include (1) CZE, (2) MEKC, (3) capillary gel electrophoresis (CGE), (4) capillary IEF, and (5) capillary ITP.

Capillary Zone Electrophoresis

CZE, also called *open-tube* or *free-solution* CE, is the simplest form of CE. It includes *capillary ion electrophoresis,* which refers to the analysis of inorganic ions by CZE, particularly when indirect detection is used. The power of the CZE mode is the ability to resolve charged species electrophoretically without a sieving matrix; this applies to a broad spectrum of analytes ranging from proteins, peptides, and amino acids to small molecules (e.g., drugs) and ions. There is abundant literature denoting the advantages of CZE for serum protein analysis over AGE and even CAE.[18,19,37] Figure 5-7 shows a comparison of the separation of serum proteins by cellulose acetate (CAE), agarose (AGE), and CE. The presence of the classical zones with CE is apparent, albeit in a reversed order, as is the identification of serum protein abnormalities in gamma regions. Retrospective studies have shown CE to be effective for detecting monoclonal proteins, which could then be immunotyped by conventional techniques (IF and IEP).[37] Moreover, one study demonstrated the utility of CE for doing both the serum protein electrophoresis and immunotyping for greater than 1500 serum samples.[19] These and other studies lead to the same conclusions—that CE is more sensitive than AGE for identifying abnormalities.

Micellar Electrokinetic Chromatography

MEKC is a hybrid of electrophoresis and chromatography. MEKC, a mode that is separate and distinct from capillary electrokinetic chromatography (CEC), is an effective electrophoretic technique, because it can be used for the separation of neutral and charged solutes. The separation of neutral species is accomplished by the use of micelles formed in the running buffer, when the concentration of surfactant exceeds the critical micelle concentration (e.g., 8 to 9 mmol/L for SDS). During migration the micelles can interact with analytes in a chromatographic manner through hydrophobic interactions in which analytes are micellized based on their degree of hydrophobicity. With charged micelles (e.g., SDS), analytes can also interact through electrostatic interactions via the charge on the surface of the micelle. For neutral species, only partitioning in and out of the micelle affects the separation.

Capillary Gel Electrophoresis

CGE is directly comparable to traditional slab or tube gel electrophoresis because the separation mechanisms are identical. The size separation is achieved with a suitable polymer, which acts as a molecular sieve or sizing mechanism. As charged analytes migrate through the polymer network, they become hindered to a degree that is governed by their size (larger solutes hindered more than smaller ones). Macromolecules, such as DNA and SDS-saturated proteins, cannot be separated without a gel or some other separation mechanism, because they contain mass-to-charge ratios that do not vary with size. The term "gel" in CGE is a misnomer, primarily because cross-linked "gels," as we know them in slab format, are not routinely used in CE. A more suitable term might be "sieving matrix" or "soluble polymer network," a linear polymeric structure that is soluble, reasonably low viscosity, and capable of self-entangling in a manner that forms

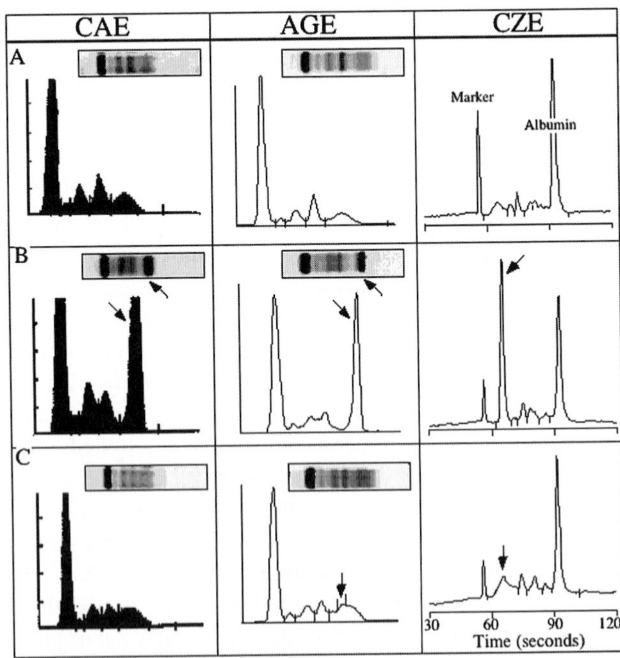

Figure 5-7 Rapid protein electrophoresis of serum protein; comparison with scanning densitometry profiles obtained from CAE and AGE electrophoresis. Panel A—normal serum, Panel B—patient serum containing a large M-protein; Panel C—patient serum containing a small monoclonal protein. The arrows indicate the position of the monoclonal proteins.

pores through which sieving can occur. A variety of polymeric matrices have been defined for both DNA (polyacrylamide and cellulosic materials) and protein analysis (e.g., dextran-base matrices). One of the requirements that often accompanies this type of analysis is to reduce electroosmotic flow. This is accomplished by covalently, adsorptively, or dynamically coating the surface. Cross-linked polyacrylamide has been the main polymer of choice for this but more recently has been supplanted by a host of polymeric matrices that not only provide effective molecular sieving but also adsorptively coat the capillary surface.[23,53] An example of a CGE separation of DNA is provided in a later section.

Capillary Isoelectric Focusing Electrophoresis

cIEF is comparable to tube IEF and is governed by the same principles and procedures. It differs from conventional IEF in that it can be carried out using either a free solution of ampholytes or a precast gel. As expected with a CE mode and unlike conventional IEF, the focused zones migrate past the online detector either during the focusing process or following it. Figure 5-8 shows an example of this where the separation by cIEF is completed in ~15 minutes, circumventing conventional IEF protocols and/or the necessity for other electrophoretic methods (e.g., CAE), both of which are much less time efficient.[14]

Capillary Isotachophoresis

Capillary ITP has essentially the same features as ITP in other formats, except that conditions of pure ITP are usually not achieved. This is not commonly used as a bonafide CE mode, but instead it is more typically used for online sample preconcentration (as described earlier). Most of the time it functions as a preconcentrating step in a mixed mode with CZE, MEKC, or CGE.

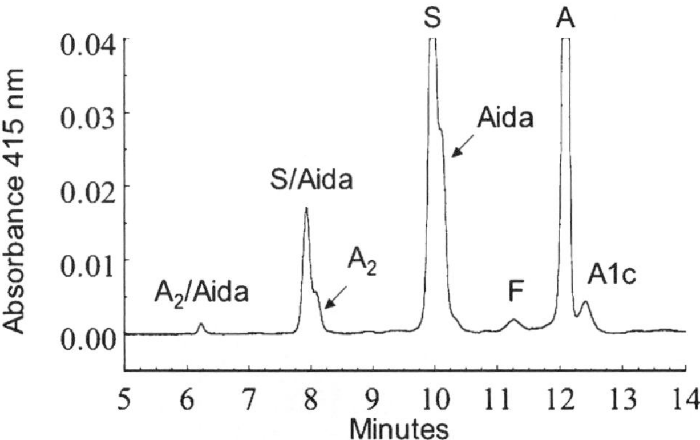

Figure 5-8 CE-based identification of uncommon hemoglobin (Hb) variants by cIEF.[14] Analysis of blood from a patient with Hb S/Aida trait detected the presence of seven different normal and abnormal structural Hb variants, some of which are not detectable by conventional electrophoresis because of a lack of sensitivity or inadequate resolution. The four abnormal variants include Hb S, Aida, S/Aida hybrid, and A_2/Aida. Identifying α-variants of Hb A_2 by cIEF helps discriminate between α- and β-globin gene mutations in samples containing unknown Hb variants. Glycated Hb A (HbA1c) is also apparent in the electropherogram.

MICROCHIP ELECTROPHORESIS

In the past decade, microchip electrophoresis has undergone substantial development, including integrated microchip designs, advanced detection systems, and new applications.[6,24,25,28] In the clinical diagnostic arena, the main analytes of interest for extrapolation to the microchip platform are proteins and DNA.

Among the attributes of microchip electrophoresis separations, the most notable is high speed—normally fourfold to tenfold faster than conventional CE and at least an order of magnitude faster than the slab gel format. Other advantages of microchips include simplicity, capabilities for chip integration of multiple functions, and certainly the potential for automation.

Instrumentation

Although similar in principle, the microchip system differs from its CE counterpart. For example, with the microchip approach, the separation channels, sample injection channels, reservoirs, sample preparation and/or precolumn or postcolumn reactors, and detectors and excitation sources can all be fabricated using photolithographic processes defined by the microelectronics industry, onto the surface of a microchip (see Chapter 10 for additional details on the manufacturing of such devices). Thus a truly multifunctional, "integrated" analytical device embedded in a single monolithic substrate is possible. The classic cross-t design of a single channel microchip involves a short (injection) channel that intersects a longer (separation) channel with a reservoir found at the ends of each of these as shown in Figure 5-9. The setup for LIF detection on a single channel microchip is shown in Figure 5-10.

Comparing volumes, the volume of the separation channel on a microchip is roughly an order of magnitude smaller (low nanoliters) than conventional capillary systems. With their decreased volume requirements (nanoliter to picoliters range), only the electrokinetic sample injection mode is used in microchips, because pressure injection is not easily controlled at these small volumes. In practice, an injection voltage of several hundred volts is applied across the sample and sample waste reservoirs to migrate the sample to the injection cross, which typically represents an injection volume of 50 to 100 pL. A separation voltage (1 to 4 kV) is then applied to the separation channel, which induces separation of the analyte zones before they reach the detection window downstream. It is important to note that, although the sample volume injected is ~100 pL, the actual sample volume necessary (for handling) is ~2 to 4 μL, depending on the reservoir size.

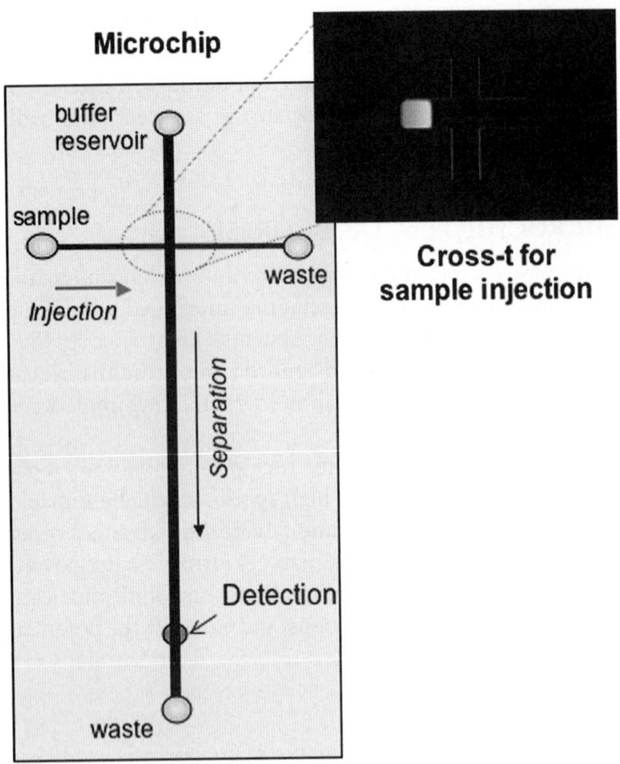

Figure 5-9 Simple cross-t microstructure design on chips used for electrophoretic separation.

Detection with a microchip is primarily through LIF, since this is easily implemented with the planar configuration of the microchip (Figure 5-10). Limits of detection for fluorescein-like fluors have been easily demonstrated at the 10^{-11} M level and pushed as low as 10^{-13} M—a mass detection limit of a few hundred molecules.[35] This allows for detection, for example, of polymerase chain reaction (PCR)-amplified DNA fragments at a level that competes with ^{32}P-autoradiography from Southern blots.[41] Typical microchip separation times are around 50 to 200 seconds.

Fabrication of Microchips

Other than the standard cross-t configurations, electrophoretic microchips are not currently commercially available and tend to be fabricated in the laboratories that use them. They can be constructed from glass (Pyrexlike or soda lime), silicon (as per microelectronic chips), or a variety of plastics, or cast from silicone-like materials (polydimethylsiloxane).[21] The first two of these constitute the vast majority of the electrophoretic devices described in the literature.

Etching the desired structures into a glass wafer surface is done with a buffered solution of hydrofluoric acid, thereby producing a series of U-shaped troughs [typically 70 μm (w) × 20 μm (d)] that interconnect appropriately. Smooth walls are typically achieved, but channels are U-shaped because of both downward and lateral etching by the etch solution. Consequently, features are often designed smaller than they have to be to allow for this type of spreading.

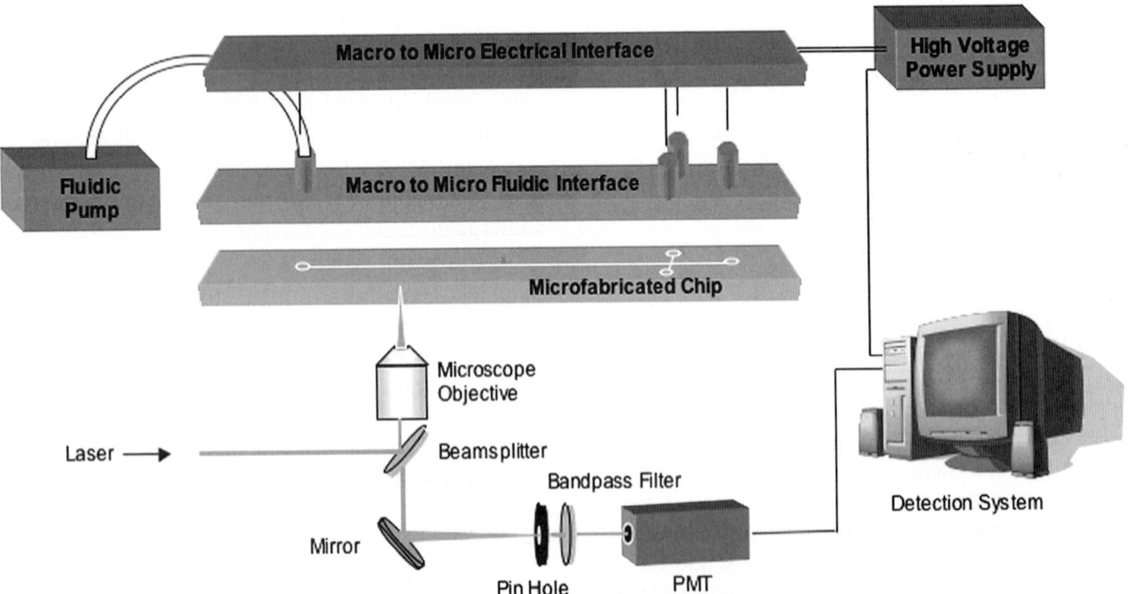

Figure 5-10 Detection system for LIF detection on microchips. Fluidic and electrical interfaces are indirectly fundamental to the detection system. The fluidic interface drives the preparation and flushing of the chip preseparation and postseparation, while the electrical interface drives the electrophoretic separation and controls the flow of fluid through the chip architecture via electrokinetic valving.

Following successful etching, the etched wafer is then bonded to a second piece of glass, into which reservoirs have been drilled, to enclose the chambers and channels of the device.

Molecular Diagnostics Using Microchips

As a result of the ease with which double-stranded (ds)DNA can be made to fluoresce via high affinity dsDNA fluorescent intercalators and the excellent detection sensitivity that results from LIF, DNA separations on microchips have developed more rapidl than protein separations. Consequently, capillary and microchip electrophoresis have emerged as alternatives to traditional slab gel electrophoresis for DNA analysis, this signified by the sequencing of the Human Genome using CE. A variety of polymers have been defined as "polymer networks" or "sieving matrices" effective for molecular sieving and size-based microchip DNA separations, many of which had been previously used in CE.

As described in the CE section, the chemical nature of the microchannel surface is equally important in DNA separations, where the electroosmotic flow has to be minimized or eliminated. For microchip-based electrophoretic DNA analysis, the chip surface must be passivated to reduce EOF. This can be accomplished by covalent modification with polymers like polyacrylamide (PA)[16]; however, the PCR samples must be desalted to achieve optimal resolution and acceptable longevity.[2,49] More attractive alternatives developed for CE involve polymers that have dual functionality, in that they both coat the microchannel surface and act as effective sieving polymers. The polydimethylacrylamide (PDMA) and the cellulosic polymers, hydroxyethyl cellulose and hydroxypropyl cellulose, have been shown to be very effective in this respect.[47]

There has been an almost exponential growth of literature with respect to the application of microchip electrophoresis to the molecular diagnosis of disease based on PCR-amplification of DNA (see Chapter 10).[23] Rudimentary microchip designs have been used to demonstrate the application of this platform in the most simplistic form—detecting the presence of a PCR product of diagnostic significance. This has been demonstrated with a number of applications including the detection of herpes simplex viral DNA in CSF for diagnosis of encephalitis, the detection of gene rearrangements correlative with lymphoproliferative dis-

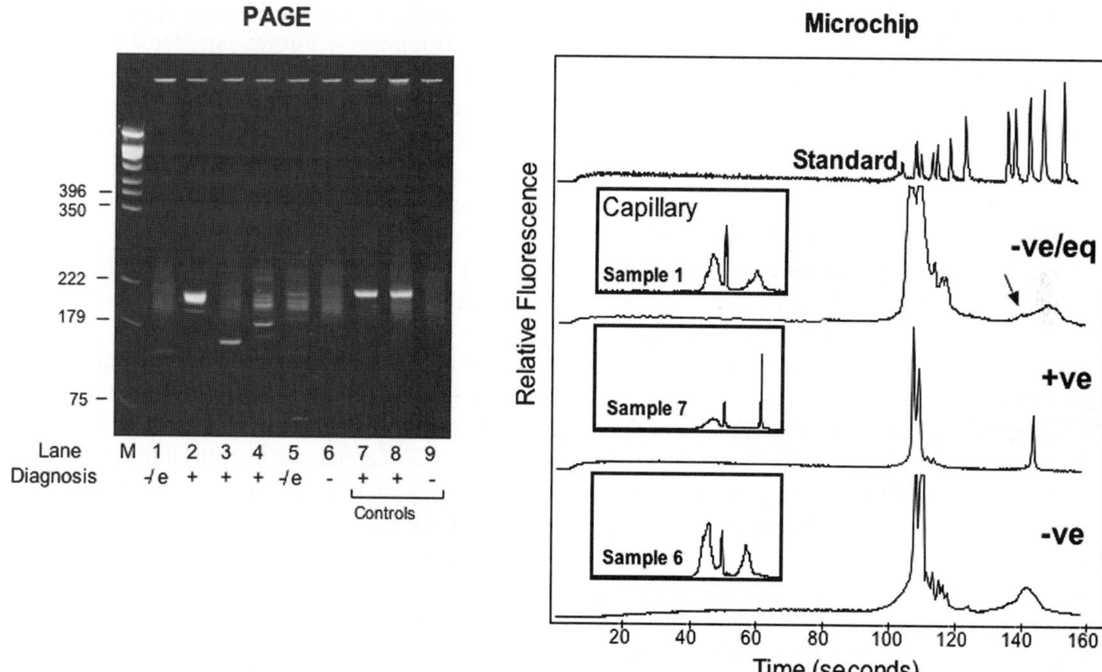

Figure 5-11 Electrophoretic detection of T-cell receptor γ-gene rearrangement products. Left—Slab gel electrophoresis of the amplified products resulting from PCR of nine patient samples. Right—capillary *(inset)* and microchip separations of select samples analyzed by gel electrophoresis on the left. The top profile results from separation of a DNA sizing standard. Sample 6 was consistent with a negative diagnosis for the gene rearrangement; sample 7 was positive as indicated by the dominant peak signifying clonality (peak at 142 seconds); sample 1 was deemed negative and/or equivocal based on the suspicious peak indicated by the arrow. Separation in both systems used hydroxyethylcellulose (HEC) as a polymeric sieving matrix and applied fields of 300 volts/cm and 275 volts/cm, respectively, for the capillary and microchip systems.[31]

orders, polymorphisms in the methylenetetrahydrofolate reductase (MTHFR) gene, the diagnosis of fragile X syndrome, the detection of tetranucleotide repeats associated with hypercholesterolemia, and the diagnosis of muscular dystrophy. More complicated DNA assays have been accomplished on electrophoretic microchips, including single-stranded conformation polymorphism (SSCP) or heteroduplex analysis for the detection of common mutations in the breast cancer susceptibility genes, BRCA1 and BRCA2.[23]

An example of microchip DNA separations applied to diagnosis of lymphoproliferative disorders is shown in Figure 5-11.[31] The high resolution (8%) acrylamide slab gel used for conventional analysis is given on the left for comparison. Because of the short separation length of the electrophoretic chamber (~4 cm) and the use of applied electrical fields comparable to those used in CE, separation on the microchip is complete in 160 seconds (in comparison with 8 hours for the slab gel).

More complicated microchip systems have been developed to address the high throughput requirements of molecular diagnostics laboratories (see Chapters 4, 10, and 37). For example, high throughput genetic typing has been performed on a 96-channel radial capillary array electrophoresis microplate with an unprecedented sample throughput of ~0.6 samples/s.[28,49] This has been extrapolated to a variety of other applications including the genotyping of the marker gene for diagnosis of hereditary hemochromatosis.[59]

REFERENCES

1. Abersold R, Morrison HD. Analysis of dilute peptide samples by capillary zone electrophoresis. J Chromatog 1990;16:79-880.
2. Carrilho E. DNA sequencing by capillary array electrophoresis and microfabricated array systems. Electrophoresis 2000;21:55-65.
3. Clark R, Katzmann JA, Kyle R, Fleisher M, Landers JP. Differential diagnosis of gammopathies by automated capillary electrophoresis: Analysis of serum samples problematic by agarose gel electrophoresis. Electrophoresis 1998;19:2479-84.
4. Chiari M, et al. Towards new formulations for polyacrylamide matrices: N-Acryloylaminoethoxyethanol, a novel monomer combining high hydrophilicity with extreme hydrolytic stability. Electrophoresis 1994;15:177-86.
5. Chien R-L, Burgi DS. Field amplified sample injection in high-performance capillary electrophoresis. J Chromatog 1991;559:141-52.
6. Colyer CL, Mangru SD, Harrison DJ. Microchip-based capillary electrophoresis of human serum proteins. J Chromatog A 1997;781:271-76.
7. Davis BJ. Disc electrophoresis—II. Method and application to human serum proteins. Ann NY Acad Sci 1964;21:404-27.
8. Deyl Z, Tagliaro F, Miksik I. Biomedical applications of capillary electrophoresis. J Chromatog 1994;656: 3-27.
9. Drysdale JW. Isoelectric focusing in polyacrylamide gel. In: Catsimpoolas, ed. Methods of protein separation, Vol 1. New York: Plenum Publishing Corp, 1975.
10. Foret F, Fanali S, Ossicini L. Indirect photometric detection in capillary zone electrophoresis. J Chromatog 1989;470:299-308.
11. Gorg A, Postel W, Gunther S. The current state of two-dimensional electrophoresis with immobilized pH gradients. Electrophoresis 1988;9:531-46.
12. Gurtler V, Barrie HD, Mayall BC. Use of denaturing gradient gel electrophoresis to detect mutation in VS2 of the 16S-23SrDNA spacer amplified from Staphylococcus aureus isolates. Electrophoresis 2001;22:1920-4.
13. Haber C. Electrochemical detection in capillary electrophoresis, In: Landers JP, ed. Handbook of capillary electrophoresis, 2nd Edition. Boca Raton: CRC Press, 1997:425-47.
14. Hempe JM, Vargas A, Craver RD. Clinical analysis of structural hemoglobin variants and Hb A1c by capillary isoelectric focusing. In: Petersen JR, Mohammad AA, eds. Clinical and forensic applications of capillary electrophoresis. Totowa, NJ: Humana Press, 2001: 145-63.
15. Hennekine JA, Kerouanton A, Brisabois A, DeBuyser ML. Discrimination of Staphylococcus aureus biotypes by pulsed-field gel electrophoresis of DNA macrorestriction fragments. J Applied Micro 2003;94: 321-9.
16. Hjerten S. High-performance electrophoresis—Elimination of electroendosmosis and solute adsorption. J Chromatog 1985;347:191-98.
17. Horgan G, Glasbey CA. Uses of digital image analysis in electrophoresis. Electrophoresis 1995;16:298-305.
18. Katzmann JA, Clark R, Namyst-Goldberg C, Sanders L, Kyle RA, Landers JP. Identification of monoclonal proteins by capillary electrophoresis: quantitative comparison with acetate and agarose electrophoresis. Electrophoresis 1997;18:1775-80.
19. Katzmann JA, Clark R, Sanders E, Landers JP, Kyle RA. Prospective study of serum protein capillary zone electrophoresis and immunotyping of monoclonal proteins by immunosubtraction. Am J Clin Pathol 1998;110:503-9.
20. Kendrew J, ed. The Encyclopedia of molecular biology. Oxford: Blackwell Science, 1994.
21. Lacher NS, de Rooij NF, Verpoorte E, Lunte SM. Comparison of the performance characteristics of poly(dimethylsiloxane) and Pyrex microchip electrophoresis devices for peptide separations, J Chromatog A 2003;1004:225-35.
22. Landers JP. Clinical capillary electrophoresis. Clin Chem 1995;41:495-509.

23. Landers JP. Molecular diagnostic analyses using electrophoretic microchips. Anal Chem 2003;75: 2919-27.
24. Liu YJ, Foote RS, Jabobson SC, Ramsey RS, Ramsey JM. Electrophoretic separation of proteins on a microchip with noncovalent postcolumn labeling. Anal Chem 2000;72:4606-13.
25. Harrison DJ, Manz A, Fan Z, Leudi H, Widmer HM. Capillary electrophoresis and sample injection systems integrated on a planar glass chip. Anal Chem 1992;64:1926-32.
26. Marsh DB, Nuttall KL. Methylmalonic acid in clinical urine specimens by capillary zone electrophoresis using indirect photometric detection. J Cap Elec 1995;2:63-7.
27. McGrath SB, Bounpheng M, Torres L, Calavetta M, Scott CB, Rines D, van Orsouw N, Vijg J. High speed, multicolor fluorescent two-dimensional gene scanning. Genomics 2001;78:83-90.
28. Medintz I, Wong WW, Sensabaugh G, Mathies RA. High speed single nucleotide polymorphism typing of a hereditary haemochromatosis mutation with capillary array electrophoresis microplates. Electrophoresis 2000;21:2352-58.
29. Molloy MP. Two-dimensional electrophoresis of membrane proteins using immobilized pH gradients. Anal Biochem 2000;280:1-10(Review).
30. Munro NJ, Finegold DN, Landers JP. Indirect fluorescence detection of amino acids on electrophoretic microchips. Anal Chem 2000;72:2765-73.
31. Munro NJ, Snow K, Kant J, Landers JP. Molecular diagnostics on microfabricated electrophoretic devices: Translating slab gel-based T- and B-cell lymphoproliferative disorder assays from the capillary to the microchip. Clin Chem 1999;45:1906-17.
32. Nelson RJ, Burgi DS. Temperature control in capillary electrophoresis. In: Landers JP, ed. Handbook of capillary electrophoresis. Boca Raton: CRC Press, 1994: 549-62.
33. Nelson RJ, Paulus A, Coehn AS, et al. Use of Peltier thermoelectric devices to control column temperature in high-performance capillary electrophoresis. J Chromatog 1989;80:111-27.
34. Nielen MW. Quantitative aspects of indirect UV detection in capillary zone electrophoresis. J Chromatog 1991;588:321-6.
35. Ocvirk G, Tang T, Harrison DJ. Optimization of confocal epifluorescence microscopy for microchip-based miniaturized total analysis systems. The Analyst 1998;123:1429-34.
36. Oda RP, Bush VJ, Landers JP. Clinical applications of capillary electrophoresis. In: Landers JP, ed. Handbook of capillary electrophoresis, 2nd Edition. Boca Raton: CRC Press, 1997:639-73.
37. Oda RP, Clark RJ, Katzmann JA, Landers JP. Capillary electrophoresis as a clinical tool for the analysis of protein in serum and other body fluids. Electrophoresis 1997;18:1715-23.
38. O'Farrell PH. High resolution two-dimensional electrophoresis of proteins. J Biol Chem 1975;250: 4007-21.
39. O'Reilly MJ, Kinnon C. The technique of pulsed field gel electrophoresis and its impact on molecular immunology. J Immunol Methods 1990;131:1-31.
40. Ornstein L. Disc electrophoresis—I. Background and theory. Ann NY Acad Sci 1964;121:321-49.
41. Pancholi P, Oda RP, Mitchell PS, Persing DA, Landers JP. Clinical diagnostic detection of hepatitis C and herpes simplex viral PCR amplification products by capillary electrophoresis with laser-induced fluorescence. Molec Diagnos 1997;2:27-38.
42. Pentoney Jr SL, Sweedler JV. Optical detection techniques for capillary electrophoresis. In: Landers JP, ed. Handbook of capillary electrophoresis, 2nd Edition. Boca Raton: CRC Press, 1997:379-423.
43. Peri-Okonny UL, Kenndler E, Stubbs RJ, Guzman NA. Characterization of pharmaceutical drugs by a modified nonaqueous capillary electrophoresis—mass spectrometry method. Electrophoresis 2003;24: 139-50.
44. Pohlod-Miller S, Fanning J, Gu P, Crist KA, You M. Detection of genomic alterations in human endometrial cancer by two-dimensional gel electrophoresis. Am J Ob and Gyn 2002;186:855-7.
45. Rabilloud T. A comparison between low background silver diammine and silver nitrate protein stains. Electrophoresis 1992;13:429-39.
46. Saeedi B, Hallgren A, Jonasson J, Nilsson LE, Hanberger H, Isaksson B. Modified pulsed-field gel electrophoresis protocol for typing of enterococci. APMIS 2002;110:869-74.
47. Sanders JC, Breadmore MC, Kwok YC, Horsman KM, Landers JP. Hydroxypropyl cellulose as an adsorptive coating sieving matrix for DNA separations: artificial neural network optimization of polymer and electrolyte conditions for microchip analysis. Anal Chem 2003;75:986-94.
48. Severs JC, Smith RD. Capillary electrophoresis-mass spectrometry. In: Landers JP, ed. Handbook of capillary electrophoresis, 2nd Edition. Boca Raton: CRC Press, 1997:791-826.
49. Shi Y, Simpson PC, Scherer JR, Wexler D, Skibola C, Smith MT, Mathies, RA. Radial capillary array electrophoresis microplate and scanner for high-performance nucleic acid analysis. Anal Chem 1999;71:5354-61.
50. Shihabi ZK. Effects of sample matrix on capillary electrophoretic analysis. In: Landers JP, ed. Handbook of capillary electrophoresis, 2nd Edition. Boca Raton: CRC Press, 1997:457-77.
51. St. Claire RL. Capillary electrophoresis. Anal Chem 1996;68:569R-86R.

52. Szoke M, Sasvari-Szelely M, Guttman A. Ultra-thin-layer agarose gel electrophoresis. I. Effect of the gel concentration and temperature on the separation of DNA fragments. J Chromatog A 1999;830:465-71.
53. Tian H, Brody LB, Mao D, Landers JP. Effective capillary electrophoresis-based heteroduplex analysis through surface coatings and polymers. Anal Chem 2000;72:5483-92.
54. Vesterberg O, Acevedo F, Bayard C. Sensitive quantification of proteins by electrophoresis in gels by use of chemiluminescence. Electrophoresis 1995;16:1390-93.
55. Vijg J, van Orsouw NJ. Two-dimensional gene scanning: exploring human genetic variability. Electrophoresis 1999;20:1239-49.
56. Wainright A, Williams SJ, Ciambrone G, Xue Q, Wei J, Harris D. Sample pre-concentration by isotachophoresis in microfluidic devices. J Chromatog A 2002;979:69-80.
57. Wang H, Kachman MT, Schwaratz DR, Cho KR, Lubman DM. A protein molecular weight map of ES2 clear cell ovarian carcinoma cells using a two-dimensional liquid separations/mass mapping technique. Electrophoresis 2002;23:3618-81.
58. Wettstein PJ, Strausbauch MA. Fraction collection in micro-preparative capillary electrophoresis. In: Landers JP, ed. Handbook of capillary electrophoresis, 2nd Edition. Boca Raton: CRC Press, 1997:841-64.
59. Woolley AT, Sensabaugh GF, Mathies RA. High-speed DNA genotyping using microfabricated capillary array electrophoresis chips. Anal Chem 1997;9:2181-6.
60. Xu Y. Capillary electrophoresis. Anal Chem 1995;67:463R-73R.
61. Zheng J, Odake T, Kitamori T, Sawada T. Miniaturized ultrathin slab gel electrophoresis with thermal lens microscope detection and its application to fast genetic diagnosis. Anal Chem 1999;71:5003-8.

ADDITIONAL READING

Books

Baker DR. Capillary electrophoresis. New York: John Wiley & Sons, 1995.

Gersten D. Gel Electrophoresis of proteins; Essential Techniques Series. New York: John Wiley & Sons, 1996.

Harris DC. Principles of capillary electrophoresis. In: Harris DC. Quantitative chemical analysis. New York: W H Freeman and Company, 2003:654-74.

Jones P, Rickwood D. Gel electrophoresis: Nucleic acids. Essential Techniques Series. New York: John Wiley & Sons, 1995.

Keren DF. High-resolution electrophoresis and immunofixation. Techniques and interpretation. Oxford: Butterworth-Heinemann, 1994.

Landers JP, ed. Handbook of capillary electrophoresis, 2nd edition. Boca Raton: CRC Press, 1997.

Monaco AP. Pulsed field gel electrophoresis: A practical approach. Oxford: Oxford University Press, 1995.

Righetti PG, Hancock W. Capillary Electrophoresis in Analytical Biochemistry. Boca Raton: CRC Press, 1995.

Xu Y. Capillary electrophoresis in clinical chemistry. In: Meyers RA (ed). Encyclopedia of analytical chemistry. Chichester: John Wiley & Sons, 2000:1181-99.

Reviews

Anderson NG, Anderson L. Twenty years of two-dimensional electrophoresis: Past, present and future. (Review) Electrophoresis 1996;17:443-53.

Gebauer P, Bocek P. Recent progress in capillary isotachophoresis. Electrophoresis 2002;23:3858-64.

Guttman A, Ronai Z. Ultrathin-layer gel electrophoresis of biopolymers. (Review) Electrophoresis 2000;21:3952-64.

Holland LA, Leigh AM. Amperometric and voltammetric detection for capillary electrophoresis. Electrophoresis 2002;23:3649-58.

Landers JP. Molecular diagnostics on electrophoretic microchips. Anal Chem 2003;75:2919-28.

Righetti PG, Gelfi C, D'Acunto MR. Recent progress in DNA analysis by capillary electrophoresis. Electrophoresis 2002;23:1361-74.

Shamsi SA. Chiral capillary electrophoresis-mass spectrometry: modes and applications. Electrophoresis 2002;23:4036-51.

Shen Y, Smith RD. Proteomics based on high-efficiency capillary separations. Electrophoresis 2002;23:3106-24.

Shimura K. Recent advances in capillary isoelectric focusing:1997-2001. Electrophoresis 2002;23:3847-57.

Slater GW, Guillouzic S, Gauthier MG, Mercier JF, Kenward M, McCormick LC, Tessier F. Theory of DNA electrophoresis (approximately 1999-2002). Electrophoresis 2002;23:3791-816.

Underberg WJ, Waterval JC. Derivatization trends in capillary electrophoresis: an update. Electrophoresis 2002;23:3922-33.

CHAPTER 6

Chromatography*

M. David Ullman, Ph.D., and Carl A. Burtis, Ph.D.

On March 8, 1903, Mikhail Tswett presented a lecture at the meeting of the Biological Section of the Warsaw Society of Natural Sciences entitled "On a New Category of Adsorption Phenomena and Their Applications to Biochemical Analysis."[7] Later he reported that plant pigments were separated by differential adsorption on a column of calcium carbonate into a number of colored bands.[17] He originated the term "chromatography" to describe this process.

This chapter contains general discussions on basic concepts, separation mechanisms, resolution, specific types of chromatography, and qualitative and quantitative analysis.

BASIC CONCEPTS

Chromatography is a physical process whereby components (solutes) of a sample mixture are separated by their differential distribution between stationary and mobile phases.[6] During this process, the mobile phase carries the sample through a bed, layer, or column containing the stationary phase. As the mobile phase flows past the stationary phase, the solutes may (1) reside only on the stationary phase (no migration); (2) reside only in the mobile phase (migration with the mobile phase); and (3) distribute between the two phases (differential migration). Those solutes with higher affinity for the stationary phase reside in the stationary phase longer than those with less affinity, who therefore reside mostly in the mobile phase. Thus the lower affinity solutes travel faster and separate from solutes having greater affinities for the stationary phase. Strongly bound solutes subsequently are displaced from the stationary phase by changing the physical or chemical nature of the mobile phase. In this chapter, the term *chromatograph* is used as either a verb or a noun. As a verb, it means to separate by chromatography. As a noun, it refers to the assembly of components that are necessary to effect a chromatographic separation.

Planar and column are the two basic forms of chromatography (Figure 6-1). In planar chromatography, the stationary phase is coated on a sheet of paper (paper chromatography) or bound to a solid surface (thin-layer chromatography; TLC). For paper chromatography, the stationary phase is a layer of water or a polar solvent coated onto the paper fibers. In TLC, a thin layer of particles of a material such as silica gel is spread uniformly on a glass plate or a plastic sheet. When the thin layer consists of particles with small diameters (4.5 µm), the technique is known as *high-performance, thin-layer chromatography* (HPTLC).[18]

In column chromatography, the stationary phase may be a pure silica or polymer, or it may be coated onto, or chemically bonded to, support particles. The stationary phase may be "packed" into a tube, or it is coated onto the inner surface of the tube. The technique is termed either gas chromatography (GC) or liquid chromatography (LC), depending on whether the mobile phase is a gas or a liquid. Operationally the instrument used to perform a GC or LC separation is known as either a *gas* or *liquid chromatograph.* When the stationary phase in LC consists of small-diameter particles, the technique is high-performance liquid chromatography (HPLC). When a gas or liquid chromatograph is connected to a mass spectrometer, the combined or "hyphenated" techniques are gas chromatography/mass spectrometry (GC/MS) and liquid chromatography/mass spectrometry (LC/MS), respectively (see Chapter 7).

In analytical GC and LC, the mobile phase, or eluent, exits from the column and passes through a detector or series of detectors that produce a series of electronic signals that are plotted as a function of time, distance, or volume. The resulting graphical display is a chromatogram (Figure 6-2). The retention time or volume is the time or volume when a solute exits the column and passes through the detector. The data represented by the chromatogram are used to help identify

*The authors gratefully acknowledge the original contributions of Dr. Larry D. Bowers on which portions of this chapter are based.

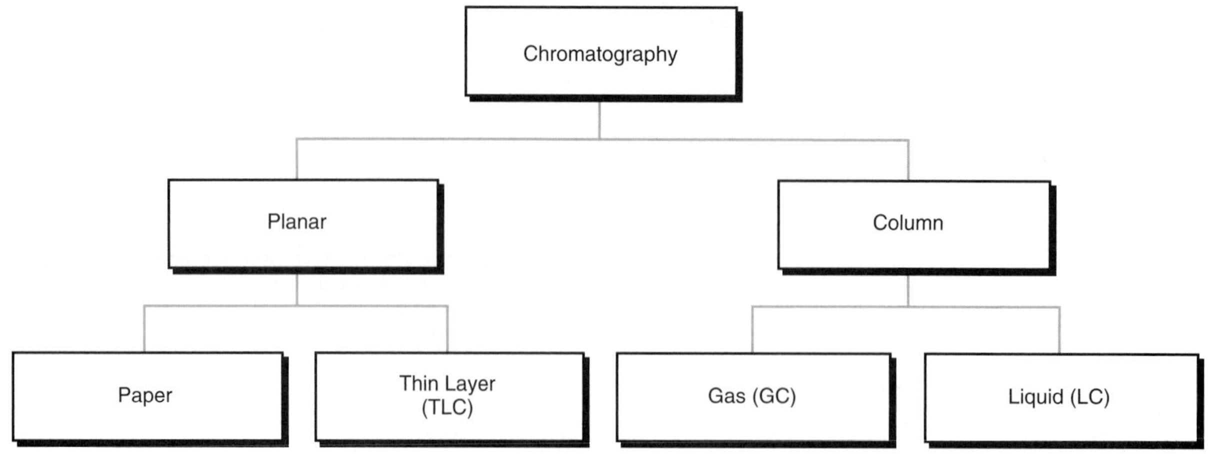

Figure 6-1 Forms of chromatography.

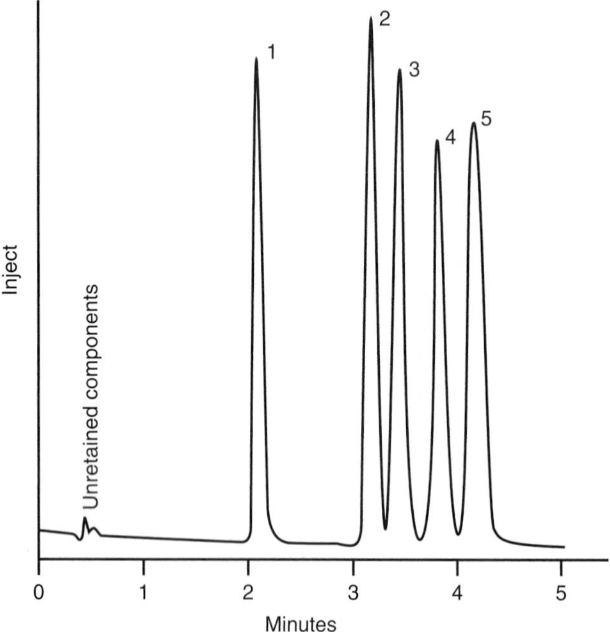

Figure 6-2 Chromatogram from an HPLC reversed-phase separation of tricyclic antidepressants with the use of a UV photometer detector set at 215 nm. Signal is displayed at 0.1 AUFS. *HPLC,* high-performance liquid chromatography; *UV,* ultraviolet; *AUFS,* absorbance units full scale. *(Courtesy Vydac/The Separations Group, Hesperia, Calif.)*

and quantify the solute(s). Because eluting solutes are displayed graphically as a series of peaks, they are frequently referred to as *chromatographic peaks.* These peaks are described in terms of peak width, peak height, and peak area. In planar chromatography, the separated zones are detected by their natural colors or visualized through chemical modification that produces colored "spots" or "bands" that are used qualitatively to identify various analytes or quantify them.

SEPARATION MECHANISMS

Chromatographic separations are classified by the chemical or physical mechanisms used to separate the solutes. These include ion-exchange, partition, adsorption, affinity, and size-exclusion mechanisms. Predominantly, clinical applications use chromatographic separations based on ion-exchange and partition mechanisms.

ION-EXCHANGE CHROMATOGRAPHY

As its name implies, ion-exchange chromatography is based on an exchange of ions between a charged stationary surface and mobile phase of the opposite charge (Figure 6-3). Depending on the conditions, solutes are either cations (positively charged) or anions (negatively charged). They are separated depending on the differences in their ionic charge or the magnitude of their ionic charges. Operationally, the particle surfaces of a plastic resin or silica serve as the stationary phase to which functional groups with fixed cationic or anionic charges are bound. To maintain electrochemical neutrality, an exchangeable ion, termed the *counterion,* is found in close proximity to the fixed charge and solute ions in the mobile phase exchange with the counterions. The solute ions then are eluted selectively by variation of the mobile phase pH, ionic strength, or both.

Cation-exchange particles contain covalently bound, negatively charged functional groups and are used to separate or "exchange" cationic solutes. Examples include strongly acidic

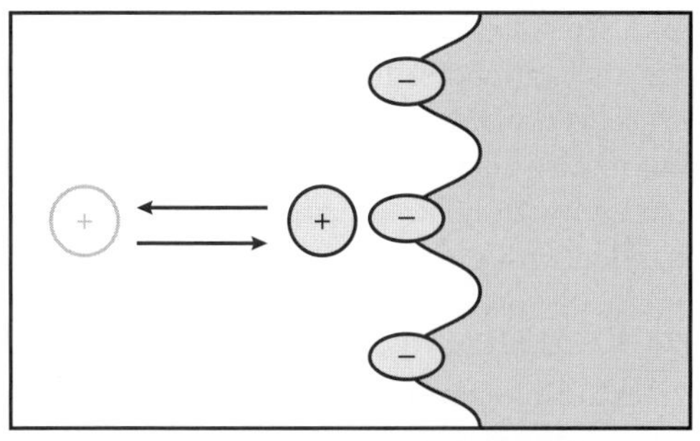

Ion-exchange chromatography

Separation is based on exchange of ions between surface and eluents.

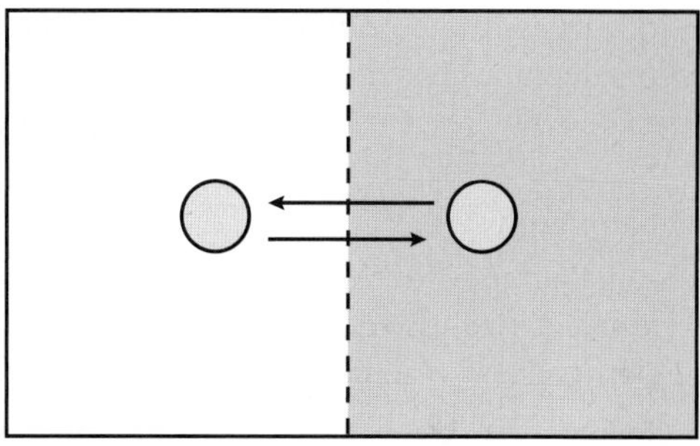

Partition chromatography

Separation is based on solute partitioning between two liquid phases.

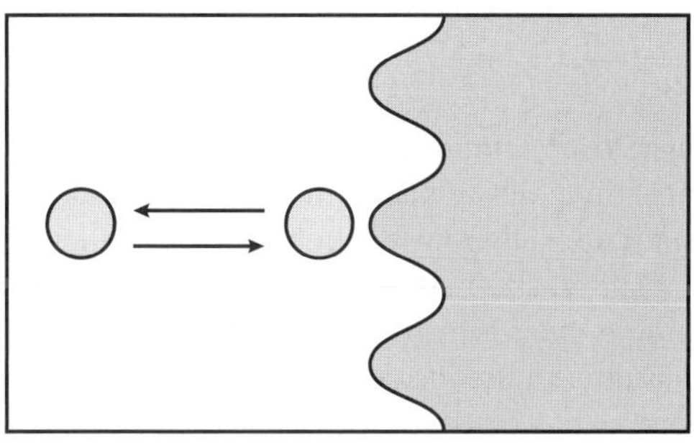

Adsorption chromatography

Separation is due to a series of adsorption/desorption steps.

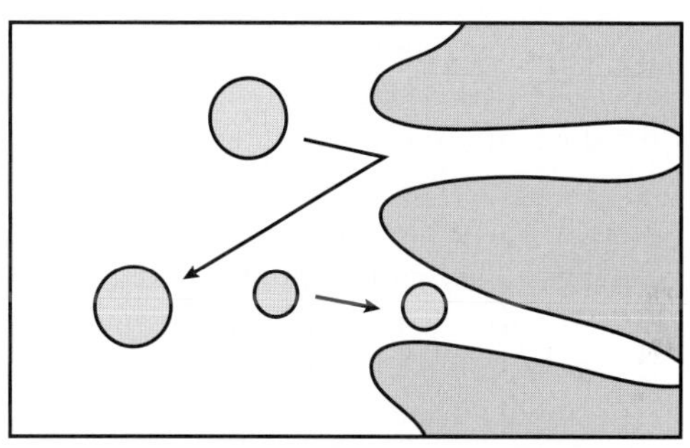

Size-exclusion chromatography

Separation is based on molecular size.

Figure 6-3 Examples of separation mechanisms used in chromatography. *(Courtesy James K. Hardy, Akron, Ohio [http://ull.chemistry.uakron.edu/].)*

groups—such as sulfonate ions, or weakly acidic groups—such as carboxylate ions or carboxymethyl (CM), phosphate (P), sulfomethyl (SM), sulfoethyl (SE), or sulfopropyl (SP) groups. Anion-exchange packings are used to separate anionic solutes. They have strongly basic quaternary amines with positive charges. Examples include triethylaminoethyl groups or weakly basic groups, such as aminoethyl (AE), diethylaminoethyl (DEAE), guanidoethyl (GE), and epichlorohydrin-triethanolamine (ECTEOLA) groups.

Ion-exchange chromatography has many clinical applications, including the separation of amino acids, peptides, proteins, nucleotides, oligonucleotides, and nucleic acids. Another important application of ion-exchange chromatography is the separation and removal of inorganic ions from aqueous mixtures. Thus most water purification units used to prepare deionized water for the laboratory contain "mixed-bed" columns of cation and anion resins (see Chapter 1).

Partition Chromatography

The differential distribution of solutes between two immiscible liquids is the basis for separation by partition chromatography (see Figure 6-3). Operationally, one of the immiscible liquids serves as the stationary phase. To prepare this phase, a thin film of the liquid is adsorbed or chemically bonded onto the surface of support particles or onto the inner wall of a capillary column. Separation is based on differences in the relative solubility of solute molecules between the stationary and mobile phases.

Partition chromatography is categorized as either GLC or liquid-liquid chromatography (LLC). LLC is further categorized as either normal phase or reversed phase. For normal-phase LLC a polar liquid is used as the stationary phase, and a relatively nonpolar solvent or solvent mixture is used as the mobile phase. In reversed-phase partition chromatography, the stationary phase is nonpolar, and the mobile phase is relatively polar.[13]

Ion-suppression and ion-pair chromatography are two forms of reversed-phase chromatography used to separate ionic solutes.

Ion-Suppression Chromatography

With ion-suppression chromatography, the ionic character of a weakly acidic or basic analyte is neutralized or "suppressed" through modification of the mobile phase pH. By neutralizing its ionic group, the solute is less polar and better able to interact with the nonpolar stationary phase. The suppressed analyte thus has the properties of a neutral species and is separated by reversed-phase chromatography.

Ion-Pair Chromatography

In ion-pair chromatography, a counter ion—opposite in charge to that of the analyte—is added to the mobile phase, where it forms ion pairs with ionic analytes, displaces the usual base pairs, and neutralizes the analyte ion(s). These ion pairs then are separated by reversed-phase chromatography. In practice, ion-pair chromatography is particularly useful for separations of therapeutic drugs and their metabolites.

Adsorption Chromatography

The basis of separation by adsorption chromatography is the differences between the adsorption and desorption of solutes at the surface of a solid particle (see Figure 6-3). Electrostatic, hydrogen-bonding, and dispersive interactions are the physical forces that control this type of chromatography. In GC, this mode is used to separate low molecular weight compounds (e.g., methyl, ethyl, and isopropyl alcohols) and compounds that are normally gases at room temperature. It uses particles of support, such as "molecular sieves," alumina, and styrene-divinylbenzene copolymers. In LC, three types of adsorbents are generally used—nonpolar, acid polar, and basic polar. The nonpolar adsorbents include charcoal and polystyrene-divinylbenzene. The main acidic polar adsorbent is silica gel, the surface silanol (SiOH) groups of which adsorb basic substances. Alumina is the main basic adsorbent for retaining acidic substances. Florisil has also been used as a basic adsorbent when catalytic decomposition of the analyte is observed with alumina.

Affinity Chromatography

In affinity chromatography the unique and specific biological interaction of the analyte and ligand is used for the separation (Figure 6-4). The specificity resulting from enzyme-substrate, hormone-receptor, or antigen-antibody interactions has been used in this type of chromatography.

The stationary phase in affinity chromatography is prepared by immobilizing a *ligand* on particles of a support either directly or via a *spacer.* A variety of chromatographic supports have been used, including agarose, cross-linked dextrans, polyacrylamide, cellulose, polystyrene, and controlled-pore glass. Adjustments of pH and ionic strength are required to achieve optimal binding of the analyte to the ligand. If the interaction between analyte and ligand is specific, the analyte may be displaced in a single step by the addition of a substrate or an inhibitor, or by a pH change, an ionic strength change, or addition of a hydrogen bond–breaking agent—such as guanine hydrochloride, urea, or sulfite. The latter group of compounds is also known as *chaotropic agents.*

The power of affinity chromatography lies in its selectivity. In the clinical laboratory, affinity chromatography has been used to separate and prepare larger quantities of proteins and antibodies for further study. Cells with different surface carbohydrate moieties are separated with lectin columns; low-density and very low-density lipoproteins are separated with heparin columns; glycated hemoglobins are separated with phenyl boronate columns.

Size-Exclusion Chromatography

Size-exclusion chromatography, also known as *gel-filtration, gel-permeation, steric-exclusion, molecular-exclusion,* or *molecular-sieve chromatography,* separates solutes on the basis of their molecular sizes (Figure 6-5; see Fig. 6-3). Molecular shape and hydration are also factors in the process.

A variety of materials are used as stationary phases for size-exclusion chromatography, including cross-linked dextran, polyacrylamide, agarose, polystyrene-divinylbenzene, porous glass, and combinations of the above. Beads of these materials are porous with pore sizes that allow small molecules to be temporarily entrapped. Molecules too large to enter the pores remain entirely in the mobile phase and are rapidly eluted from the column. Molecules that are intermediate in size have access to various fractions of the pore volume and elute between the large and small molecules according to the relation:

$$V_r = V_0 + KV_i \quad (1)$$

where V_r is the retention volume, V_0 is the void volume between the particles, K is the fraction of the pore volume accessible to the molecule, and V_i is the volume within the support particles. The retention is limited to one column volume; therefore resolution is limited. For this reason, steric exclusion is used more for preparative than for analytical purposes.

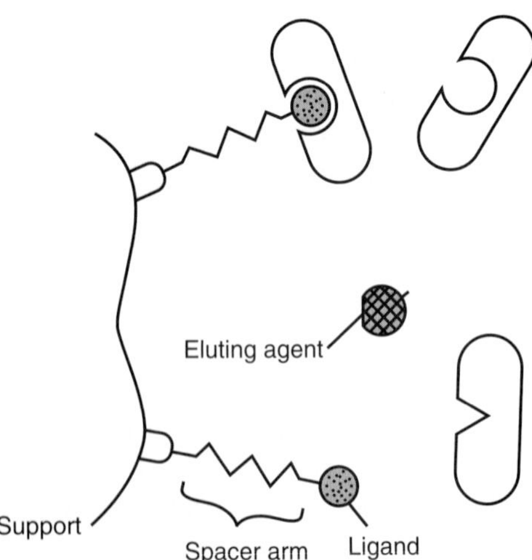

Figure 6-4 Principle of affinity chromatography. The analyte (enzyme, antibody, antigen, tissue receptor, etc.) binds to the support-bound ligand. Subsequently, it is eluted with a general eluent (such as a chaotropic agent), pH change, or biospecific eluent (such as an inhibitor or substrate).

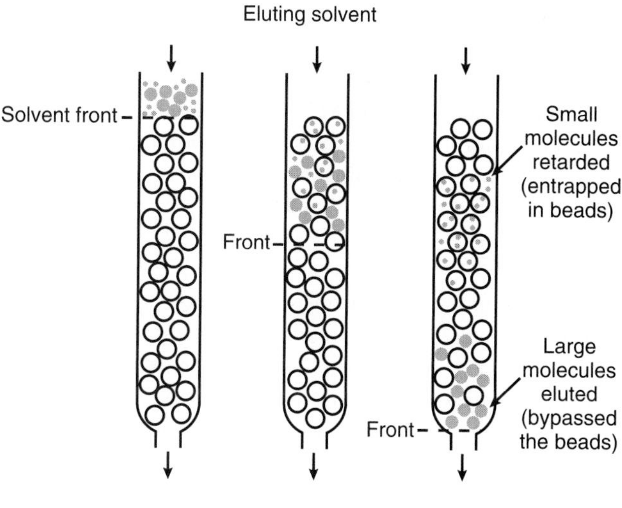

Figure 6-5 Schematic representation of gel-filtration column chromatography. *(Modified from Bennett TP: Graphic biochemistry, vol 1. Chemistry of biological molecules. New York: Macmillan, 1968.)*

RESOLUTION

Resolution (R_s) is a measure of a successful chromatographic separation and requires that two peaks have different elution times for the peak centers and sufficiently narrow bandwidth to eliminate or minimize overlap (Figure 6-6).[3] It is expressed mathematically as follows:

$$R_s = \frac{V_r(B) - V_r(A)}{\left[\frac{w(A) + w(B)}{2}\right]} \quad (2)$$

where

$V_r(A)$ = retention volume for solute A
$V_r(B)$ = retention volume for solute B
$w(A)$ = bandwidth (units of volume) measured at base for solute A
$w(B)$ = bandwidths (units of volume) measured at base for solute B

Resolution also is expressed in terms of time, with $V_r(A)$ and $V_r(B)$ being replaced with retention times $t_r(A)$ and $t_r(B)$, and $w(A)$ and $w(B)$ being expressed in units of time.

Incomplete separation occurs when the calculated value for R_s is less than 0.8, whereas baseline separation is obtained when R_s is greater than 1.25 (Figure 6-7). As demonstrated in Figure 6-8, when R_s is unacceptable for a given separation,

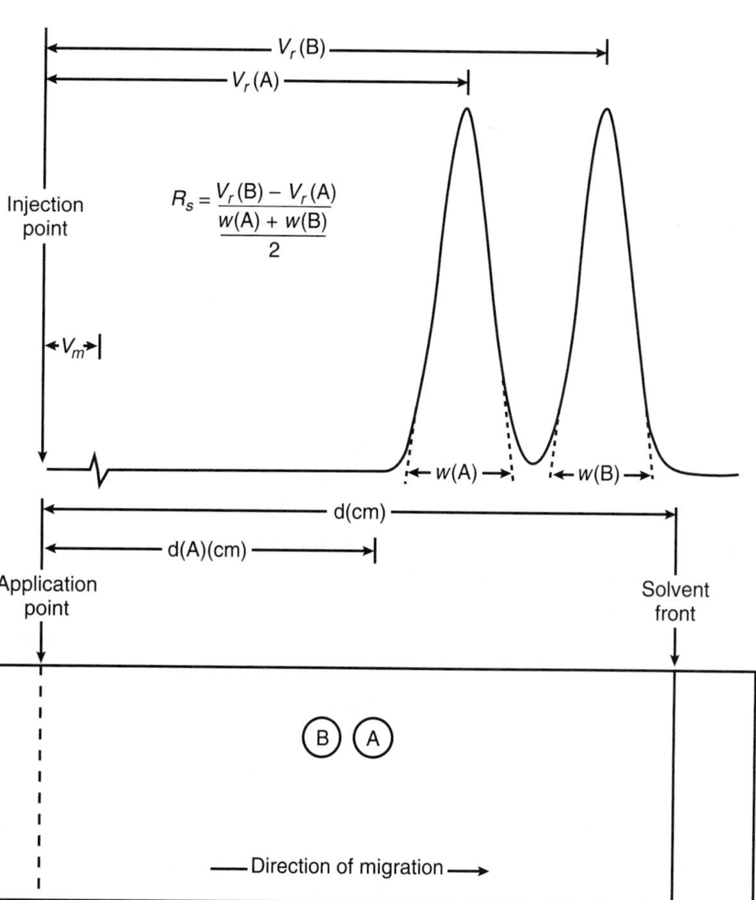

Figure 6-6 Schematic diagram of a chromatogram obtained from a column and open-bed chromatograph (planar). In open-bed chromatography *(bottom)*, strongly retained compounds (B) move more slowly than less strongly retained compounds. In column chromatography *(top)*, compound B is eluted later than compound A, again because of stronger retention. R_s, Resolution; $V_r(A)$, retention volume for solute A; $V_r(B)$, retention volume for solute B; $w(A)$, bandwidth (units of volume) measured at base for solute A; $w(B)$, bandwidth (units of volume) measured at base for solute B; V_m, volume between injector and detectors; $d(A)$, distance traveled by solute A; *A*, solute A; *B*, solute B.

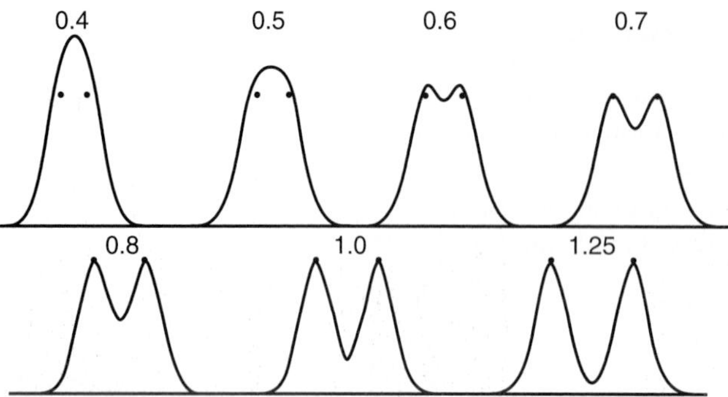

Figure 6-7 Separation of chromatographic peaks present in a 1 : 1 ratio as a function of resolution (R_s). *(From Snyder LR: A rapid approach to selecting the best experimental conditions for high-speed liquid column chromatography. Part I. Estimating initial sample resolution required by a given problem. J Chrom Sci 1972; 10:202.)*

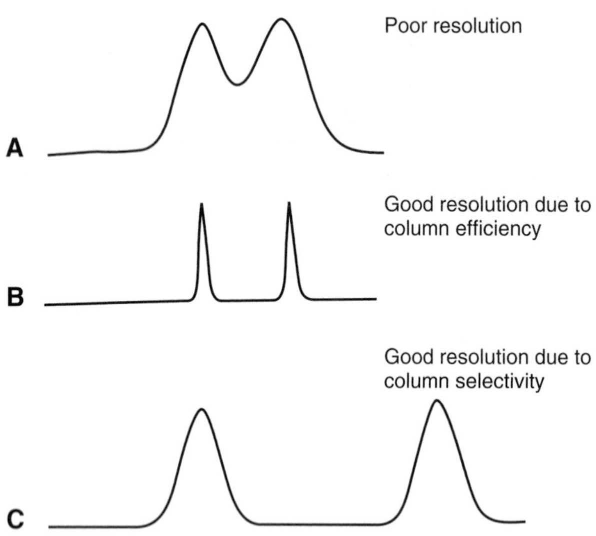

Figure 6-8 Effect of selectivity and efficiency on chromatographic resolution. **A,** Poor resolution. **B,** Good resolution because of column efficiency. **C,** Good resolution because of column selectivity. *(From Johnson EL, Stevenson R: Basic liquid chromatography, Palo Alto, Calif, Varian Associates, 1978.)*

it is improved through a change in (1) the column retention factor *(k')*, (2) column efficiency *(N)*, or (3) column selectivity (α). The retention factor describes the distribution of solutes between stationary and mobile phases. Column efficiency accounts for the ease of physical interaction between solute molecules and column-packing material. Selectivity characterizes the specific chemical affinity between solute molecules and column packing. Thus by rearranging equation (1) and expressing the parameters in terms of retention, efficiency, and selectivity, resolution also is expressed as:

$$R_s = \left(\frac{k'}{k'+1}\right) \times \frac{\sqrt{N}}{4} \times \left(\frac{\alpha - 1}{\alpha}\right) \tag{3}$$

where k' = retention or capacity factor (a thermodynamic term), N = number of theoretical plates (a kinetic term representing column efficiency), and α = selectivity factor (a thermodynamic term).

These factors are varied to affect the degree of resolution of a given separation. However, a practical approach to improve resolution is to adjust first the retention factor to an acceptable value and then improve the efficiency. Finally, if required, the selectivity is changed.

Retention Factor *(k')*

"The retention factor is a measure of the time the sample component resides in the stationary phase relative to the time it resides in the mobile phase."[8] Mathematically, it is the ratio of the adjusted retention volume (v_r) or retention time (t_r) to the void volume (v_0) or hold-up time (t_0) (the time for unretained components to elute from the column).

$$k' = \frac{V_r - V_0}{V_0} = \frac{t_r - t_0}{t_0} \tag{4}$$

The distribution of a solute between the stationary and mobile phases affects the rate at which it migrates through a column or bed. The resultant distribution constant (K_D) is defined as the ratio between the concentrations of the solute molecules in the stationary phase (C_s) relative to those in the mobile phase (C_m):

$$K_D = \frac{C_s}{C_m} \tag{5}$$

Substituting these concentrations with the numbers of molecules (N_s and N_m) per unit volume (V_s and V_m) and rearranging terms, equation (9) becomes:

$$K_D = \left[\frac{N_s}{N_m}\right] \times \left[\frac{V_m}{V_s}\right] = k' \times \beta \tag{6}$$

The ratios N_s/N_m and V_m/V_s are defined as the retention factor, k', and the phase ratio, β, respectively. The retention factor is also a measure of the time a solute molecule spends in the stationary phase relative to the time it spends in the mobile phase and thus is related to the retention time of the solute:

$$k' = \frac{t_r - t_0}{t_0} \tag{7}$$

where t_r is the elution or retention time of retained solute, and t_0 is the elution time of the unretained solutes.

The magnitude of k' is a function of the solute chemical and physical properties, the stationary and mobiles phases, and the column temperature. Also, solute retention is increased by increasing the amount of the stationary phase relative to that of the mobile phase. A large k' is indicative of a slowly moving solute band, which improves the resolution between it and those of other solutes but also results in its broadening. In practice, optimum values of k' are between 2 and 6, although values between 1 and 10 can be used.

In some circumstances, when (1) 10 or more compounds in a sample are of interest, (2) analytes vary widely in their chemical characteristics, or (3) *isocratic* conditions (constant mobile phase composition and column conditions) are employed, a range of k' values may be required to achieve the desired separation or separations. When k' values are high, an extremely long time is required for separation, and detection limits are compromised because of band spreading. This situation (high k' values, long analysis time, and decreased detection limit) is known as the *general elution problem.* In practice, this problem is solved by changing peak retention as a function of time. In TLC, this is accomplished by two-dimensional development; in GC, by programmed changes in column temperature; and in LC, by altering the composition of the mobile phase as a function of time *(gradient elution).*

The retention factor is also used to predict the position in time of a particular compound under the selected conditions of separation. For example, the k' can be used to compare solute retention from one chromatographic system to another because—given the same mobile phase, stationary phase, and stationary phase particle size—it will not differ with flow rate or column diameter and length.

In planar chromatography, all separation activity must occur within the distance traveled by the mobile phase. In TLC, a solute's migration is expressed by its R_f value, which is calculated from the relation:

$$R_f = \frac{\text{distance from application point to solute center}}{\text{distance from application point to solvent front}} \quad (8)$$

Therefore the greater the solute affinity for the stationary phase, the smaller the R_f value. For comparison R_f and k' are related as follows:

$$R_f = \frac{1}{1 + k'} \quad (9)$$

EFFICIENCY *(N)*

Ideally, as a solute moves through a bed or column of the stationary phase, it migrates as a very narrow band. In practice, however, the band broadens as it passes through the column. This is primarily a result of (1) nonuniform flow of the mobile phase as it moves past the stationary phase particles, (2) variability in the physical dimensions of the particles, and (3) diffusion. Using column chromatography as an example, band spreading implies that if identical molecules start as a narrow band in a small volume at the top of the column, they will appear at the column outlet in a larger volume and broader band. Two of the major contributions to band spreading are *eddy diffusion* and *mass transfer* phenomena. Eddy diffusion results when solute molecules traverse different flow paths through the bed of the stationary phase. Some flow paths may be linear, and others are circuitous. Further, the flow paths may be narrower or broader so that molecules in the broader paths travel faster than those in the narrower. Solute molecules distribute randomly into these paths, and those following the more direct and/or wider paths will emerge from the end of the column sooner than those in the more circuitous and/or narrower paths. Thus the solute band is broadened.

Mass transfer processes are composed of (1) mobile phase mass transfer, (2) stagnant mobile phase mass transfer, and (3) stationary phase mass transfer. *Mobile phase mass transfer* is caused by the different mobile phase flow rates for different parts of a single flow path between two stationary phase particles. The mobile phase close to one of the particles moves slowly, and the center of the flow stream (farthest from particles) moves fastest. *Stagnant mobile phase mass transfer* occurs when solute molecules become temporarily delayed in stagnant pools of mobile phase located in pores of the support particles. Here, the solute molecules must reenter the flowing mobile phase through diffusional movement. *Stationary phase mass transfer* occurs when solute molecules diffuse into and within the stationary phase. These molecules must be extricated from the particles and the stagnant pool by diffusional movement. Mass transfer processes are strongly dependent on the characteristics (e.g., particle size, pore size, and particle shape) of the column packing.

Because the equilibria (thermodynamics) are identical for a given solute, band broadening is related to flow dynamics (kinetics). In chromatographic terminology, a bed or column of stationary phase that minimizes the broadening of solute bands is considered "efficient." In column chromatography, a very efficient column is characterized by the appearance of narrow peaks in the chromatogram (see Figure 6-8). Column efficiency is expressed as N, the number of "*theoretical plates.*" Mathematically, N is defined as:

$$N = \left[\frac{V_r(\text{A})}{s(\text{A})}\right]^2 \quad (10)$$

where $V_r(\text{A})$ and $s(\text{A})$ are the retention volume and standard deviation of the peak volume for solute A (see Figure 6-6). The standard deviation of a graphical display, however, is difficult to measure. A more easily measured quantity is used to determine the number of theoretical plates. Tangents are drawn to the ascending and descending curves of the gaussian peak. The distance between the points where the tangents intersect the chromatographic baseline is four standard deviations. Alternatively the width of a gaussian peak at one half its height corresponds to 2.354 standard deviations, and therefore:

$$s(A) = \frac{w_{1/2}(\text{A})}{2.354} \quad (11)$$

Substituting the latter relationship into equation (10), the number of theoretical plates is determined by measuring the width of a peak at half height, $w_{1/2}(\text{A})$, and using the relationship:

$$N = 5.54\left[\frac{V_r(\text{A})}{w_{1/2}(\text{A})}\right]^2 \quad (12)$$

Efficiency is often expressed as the number of theoretical plates per unit length of column (N/L) or the reciprocal

(L/N) of this relationship, which is called the plate height (H) or the *height equivalent of a theoretical plate (HETP)*. Thus:

$$H = \frac{L}{N} \quad (13)$$

where L is the column length. These expressions correspond to "imaginary" physical entities widely used to characterize the relationship of band spreading to column characteristics in chromatographic systems.

In theory a theoretical plate is equivalent to the length of a column necessary to allow one equilibration of the solute to occur between the stationary and the mobile phases. To increase the efficiency of a column, the number of theoretical plates is increased. In practice, this can be accomplished by increasing the length of the column. It should be remembered, however, that, as shown in equation (3), resolution is proportional to the square root of column efficiency. Therefore doubling the column length would only result in a 40% increase in resolution.

Other factors that affect efficiency are characteristics of the stationary support particles, mobile phase viscosity, column temperature, and noncolumn contributions. In general a decrease in (1) mobile phase flow rate, (2) average particle size of the stationary phase, (3) particle size distribution, and (4) volume of sample will increase efficiency. Increases in column length, temperature, and sample viscosity also increase efficiency.

For GC the relationship between the plate height and flow velocity is given by the van Deemter equation:

$$H = \mathrm{A} + \frac{\mathrm{B}}{v} = \mathrm{C}v \quad (14)$$

where v is the flow velocity of the mobile phase, and A, B, and C are constants related to the mechanistic components of dispersion. Eddy diffusion, that is independent of flow velocity, contributes to the A term. The B term arises from diffusion of the analytes along the longitudinal axis of the column and is important only at low-flow velocities. The C term includes contributions from radial diffusion in the mobile phase and diffusion in the stationary phase. Because basic differences in the rates of these processes exist in gases and liquids, the relationship for LC is given by the Knox equation:

$$H = \mathrm{A}v^{1/3} + \frac{\mathrm{B}}{v} + \mathrm{C}v \quad (15)$$

For both GC and LC, the efficiency of a chromatographic system is optimal at intermediate flow velocities. Optimal performance is usually not obtained in practice because of the emphasis on separation speed, which requires the use of greater than optimal flow rates. Theoretical considerations of the thermodynamic and kinetic aspects of chromatography led to the development of HPLC and capillary GC, both of which possess the speed necessary for clinical analyses.

The efficiency of any chromatographic system will be reduced if noncolumn contributions to band spreading are not properly minimized. For example, precolumn and postcolumn tubing, connectors, column fittings, and detector cell must all be of minimum volume.

Selectivity (α)

The *selectivity factor* (α) is a measure of the relative separation between the band centers of two solutes. It is expressed as the ratio of the retention factors of the second eluting solute k'(B) and the first eluting solute k'(A) of the two solutes A and B:

$$\alpha = \frac{k'(\mathrm{B})}{k'(\mathrm{A})} = \frac{[t_r(\mathrm{B}) - t_0]}{[t_r(\mathrm{A}) - t_0]} \quad (16)$$

where t_r (A) and t_r (B) are the elution times of solutes A and B, respectively. By convention the solute with the larger k' is placed in the numerator. Thus the value of α is always 1 or greater. To develop a chromatographic separation, the chosen mechanism should afford a large α value. After the separation mechanism has been chosen, alteration in the magnitude of α is achieved by changing the composition of the mobile phase (e.g., pH, ionic strength, and solvent polarity in LC and HPLC), the column temperature in GC and HPLC, the chemical and physical nature of the column packing or stationary phase, or chemical modification of the solute. When two solutes have identical values for k', α is equal to 1.0, and the solutes are not separated. It is technically feasible, but difficult, to separate two compounds having a α of 1.01; however, it is reasonably easy to separate them if α is 1.05 and easy to separate them if α is 1.10 or greater.

PLANAR CHROMATOGRAPHY

Planar chromatography was developed in the 1950s.[16] With it, solutes are separated on a planar surface of the stationary phase. Paper and TLC are subclassifications of planar chromatography (see Figure 6-1). In paper chromatography, the stationary phase is a layer of water or a polar solvent coated onto the paper fibers.

In TLC a thin layer of sorbent, such as silica gel (usually only 0.2 mm thick), is spread uniformly on a glass plate, plastic sheet, or aluminum foil. Prepared plates are available commercially that are coated with a variety of sorbents (e.g., silica gel, microcellulose, alumina, or cross-linked dextran). The sample is added as a small spot or band near an edge of the plate. The plate then is placed in a closed glass container or tank with the lower edge in, and the sample band just above, the mobile phase (Figure 6-9). The mobile phase then migrates up the plate by capillary action. After the mobile phase travels a desired distance, the plate is removed from the tank and dried. Additional separation is achieved if the plate is developed in a second direction. In addition to this "ascending" technique, thin-layer plates also are developed in a radial mode. After the plate is dry, the separated com-

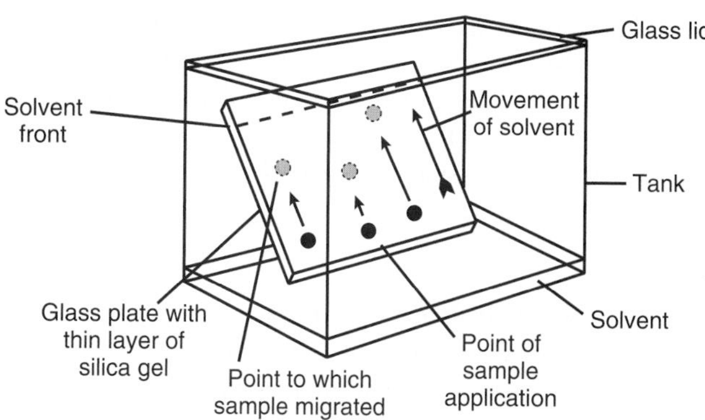

Figure 6-9 Illustration of TLC. The solvent moves up the thin layer of adsorbent by capillary action. *TLC,* Thin-layer chromatography. *(Modified from Bennett TP: Graphic Biochemistry, vol 1. Chemistry of biological molecules, New York: Macmillan, 1968.)*

ponents are located and identified by a variety of procedures, such as ultraviolet (UV) illumination (fluorescence), spraying with specific, color-generating reagents, or autoradiography. Provided the detection method is nondestructive, the appropriate sorbent region can be scraped from the plate and extracted to recover the solute for further study or analysis.

Silica gel continues to be a widely used sorbent for TLC. Other sorbents include inorganic and organic sorbents, such as alumina (neutral and acidic), magnesium silicate, diatomaceous earth (kieselguhr), cellulose, polyamide, and ion-exchange resins.[11] In the 1990s, a range of alkyl-bonded silica TLC plates became commercially available including C_{18}, C_{12}, C_8, C_2, aminopropyl, diphenyl, and cyanopropyl bonded plates.[8] Plates coated with a chiral complexing agent are also available and used for the separation of amino acid enantiomers and similar compounds. The bonded silica plates are used in reversed-phase TLC, which has proven useful for the chromatography of polar compounds. The use of small-diameter, stationary phase particles led to the development of HPTLC. The HPTLC separations are more efficient and reproducible because particles of small diameters are used. Inadequate wetting and solvent evaporation must be controlled carefully. Laser-coded TLC plates are available in which each plate is identified individually to prevent recording and archiving errors.

In practice, the majority of TLC separations are qualitative or semiquantitative (visual comparison) in nature. However, modern computer-controlled densitometers are now available that scan sample and calibrator chromatograms in tracks on HPTLC plates and provide quantitative capabilities.[15] Clinically relevant analytes that have been measured by TLC include amino acids, bile acids, carbohydrates, drugs, lipids, glycolipids, phospholipids, porphyrins, prostaglandins, steroid hormones, purines, pyrimidines, derivatives of nucleic acid, and urinary organic acids. The advantages of TLC include simplicity, rapidity, versatility, ability to process a large number of samples in minimal time, and low cost in terms of reagent and equipment.[11]

COLUMN CHROMATOGRAPHY

In column chromatography, the stationary phase is coated onto or chemically bonded to support particles that are then "packed" into a tube, or the stationary phase is coated onto the inner surface of the tube. GC and LC are subclassifications of column chromatography (see Figure 6-1).

Gas Chromatography

GC was developed by James and Martin in 1952[9] to separate fatty acids. With it a gaseous mobile phase is used to pass a mixture of volatile solutes through a column containing the stationary phase. The mobile phase is typically an inert gas, such as nitrogen, helium, hydrogen, or argon, referred to as the *carrier gas.* Solute separation is based on the relative differences in the solutes' vapor pressures and interactions with the stationary phase. Thus a more volatile solute elutes from the column before a less volatile one. In addition, a solute that selectively interacts with the stationary phase elutes from the column after one with a lesser degree of interaction. The column effluent carries separated solutes to the detector in the order of their elution. Solutes are identified qualitatively by their similar retention times. Peak size (area or height) is proportional to the amount of the solute detected and is used to quantify it.

Gas-solid chromatography (GSC) and gas-liquid partition chromatography (GLC) are variations of GC. In GSC separations occur primarily by differences in absorption at the solid phase surface. In GLC a nonvolatile liquid is coated or chemically bonded onto particles of column packing or directly onto the wall of a capillary column. Separation occurs primarily by differences in solute partitioning between the gaseous mobile phase and the liquid stationary phase.

Instrumentation

The components of a basic gas chromatograph are illustrated in Figure 6-10.

Column Technology

The function of the chromatographic column is to separate the solutes. The main types of columns are packed and capillary. Packed columns are filled with support particles that are used uncoated (GSC) or have been coated or chemically bonded with the stationary phase (GLC). They vary from 1 to 4 mm in internal diameter (ID), from 1 m or more in length, and are fabricated from tubes of glass or stainless steel. Although narrow columns are more efficient, wider columns have increased sample capacities. Fast GC is a type of GC in which high-speed separations are achieved using short lengths of conventional columns. Longer columns are more efficient but require increased carrier gas pressures.

Capillary columns, also known as *wall-coated open tubular columns,* are fabricated by coating the inner wall of a fused-silica tube with a thin film of liquid phase. They vary from 0.1 to 0.5 mm in ID and from 10 to 150 m in length. The ultrapure fused silica capillary tubing is very fragile. To physically strengthen the tubing a thin outside coating of polyimide or aluminum is added; this improves column durability. These modified capillary columns have the structural strength and flexibility necessary to withstand coiling and placement in ovens. Capillary columns are very efficient but have low sample capacities.

In addition to the packed and capillary columns, progress has been made in the development of micro GC columns on silicon chips. These microdevices have great potential for high-speed GC, a miniature GC, and eventually even a pocket GC[5] (see Chapter 10 for a discussion on nanotechnology).

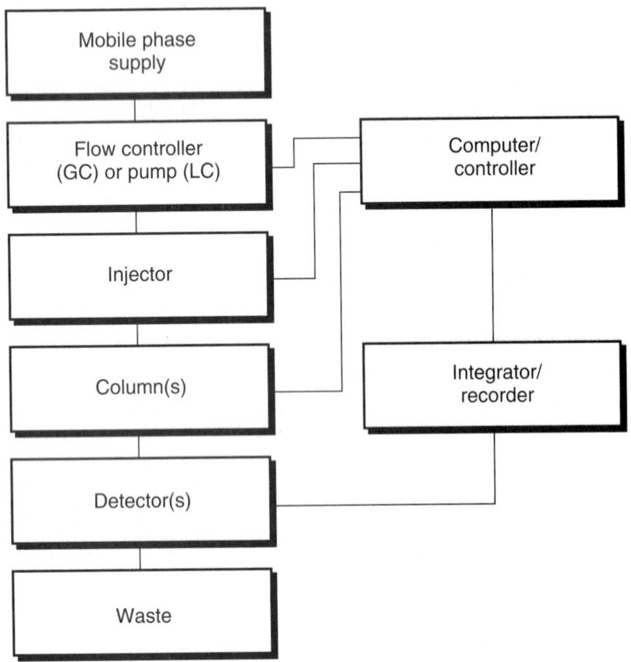

Figure 6-10 Schematic diagram of a gas or liquid chromatograph. *GC,* Gas chromatography; *LC,* liquid chromatography.

A variety of compounds have been used as the stationary phase in GLC. These include methyl silicone polymers, substituted silicone polymers, and silicone polyesters (Table 6-1). These materials are coated or chemically bonded onto the surface of the support particles or onto the walls of the column. Although more expensive, bonded materials are preferable because of their stability.

Carrier Gas Supply and Flow Control

The function of the carrier gas supply and flow control is to provide carrier gas to the chromatographic column and to regulate its flow through the system. Operationally a constant flow of carrier gas is required for column efficiency and reproducible elution times. Systems that provide constant flow rates vary from simple mechanical devices to sophisticated electronic ones. For example, a simple system consisting of a tank of compressed gas, a needle valve to adjust flow, a flow meter, and a pressure gauge is sufficient for many applications. More demanding temperature-programmed operation (discussed later) requires a more sophisticated differential flow controller, such as an electronic pressure control system programmed to regulate the carrier gas flow rate and pressure during a chromatographic run. Such a controller is operated in either a constant-flow or a constant-pressure mode. In the constant-flow mode, the pressure required to maintain a constant flow independent of carrier gas viscosity is calculated. A pressure transducer then measures and maintains the inlet pressure required for the constant flow.

The magnitude of the carrier gas flow rate depends on the type of column. For example, packed columns require a flow rate from 10 to 60 mL/min. Flow rates for capillary columns are much lower (1 to 2 mL/min), and the maintenance of a constant flow rate is even more critical for the efficient operation of these columns.

A number of gases are used as carrier gases, depending on the column and detector. Hydrogen and helium are the carrier gases of choice with capillary columns. Only high-purity hydrogen and helium should be used, however, because carrier-gas impurities (1) harm the column, (2) decrease the performance of some detectors, and (3) adversely affect quantification in trace analysis. For packed columns, the most frequently used carrier gas is nitrogen,

TABLE 6-1 Stationary Phases Commonly Used in Gas Chromatography for Clinical Separations

Composition	Polarity	Similar Phases	Applications
100% dimethyl-polysiloxane	Nonpolar	OV-1, SE-30	Drugs, amino acid derivatives
5% diphenyl—95% dimethyl-polysiloxane	Nonpolar	OV-101, SP-2100	Drugs
50% diphenyl—50% dimethyl-polysiloxane	Intermediate	OV-17	Drugs, steroids, glycols
50% cyanopropylmethyl—50% phenylmethyl-polysiloxane	Intermediate	OV-225	Fatty acid methyl esters, carbohydrate derivatives
Polyethylene glycol	Polar	Carbowax 20 M	Acids, alcohols, glycols, ketones

which is used with flame ionization (FID), electron capture (ECD), or thermal conductivity (TCD) detectors. Helium is used with FIDs and TCDs, and nitrogen-argon-methane mixtures are used with the ECD. Carrier gases should be pure and dry, and the tubing used to connect the gas source to the GC should be uncontaminated. Molecular sieve beds and specialized inline traps have been used to remove or reduce the moisture, hydrocarbon, or oxygen content of the carrier gas.[4]

Injector

The function of an injector is to introduce an aliquot of the sample to be analyzed into the column; this begins the chromatographic process and has to be done with a minimal disruption of the gas flow into the column. In most clinical GC methods, samples are dissolved in nonaqueous liquids introduced into the column via an inline injector. With packed columns, a glass microsyringe is used to inject a 1- to 10-μL aliquot of the dissolved sample through a septum, which serves as the interface between the injector and the chromatographic system. In practice, the syringe needle is inserted through the injector septum and into a heating region. The volatile analytes and the solvent are then "flash-vaporized" and swept into the column by the carrier gas. To ensure rapid and complete solute volatilization, the temperature of the injector is maintained at 30° to 50 °C higher than the column temperature.

Common problems with GC analysis include septum leaks and adsorption of components from the sample onto the septum during injection. In addition, because the septum is heated, decomposition products often form and "bleed" into the column. This results in spurious peaks, termed "ghost" peaks, appearing in the chromatogram. Septum bleed is greater at higher injection-port temperatures. To minimize this problem, a Teflon-coated, low-bleed septum is used. The inner surface of the septum is purged continuously with the carrier gas that is vented before it passes into the column. This approach is especially effective, and most commercial injectors are equipped with continuous-purge capabilities. The septum is a consumable component of the gas chromatograph and should be replaced at least once every 100 injections.

Because of the low sample capacities and carrier-gas flow rates used with capillary columns, split and splitless injection techniques are used to introduce samples into the columns. In the split mode (Figure 6-11), only a small portion of the vaporized sample enters the column, whereas in the splitless mode most of the sample enters the column (Figure 6-12). Operationally the split flow mode is used for samples that contain relatively high concentrations of the target analyte(s); the splitless mode is used for samples that contain relatively low levels of the target analyte(s).

Temperature-programmable injection ports are available and are used in either the split or splitless mode. The sample is injected at a temperature slightly higher than the boiling point of the solvent. Most of the sample components condense on glass or fused silica wool in the injector insert, while the solvent is removed. The injector is then rapidly heated at rates of up to 100 °C/min. The rapid heating vaporizes the analytes, which then move into the column. Very rapid heating is advantageous in that thermally labile compounds are only exposed to high temperatures for a short time. Separation of solvent removal and analyte vaporization allows injection of sample volumes up to hundreds of microliters. This obviously improves analyte detection when the sample matrix is not the limiting factor.

Temperature Control

Operationally, both packed and capillary columns require careful control of the column, injector, and detector temperatures. Control of the column temperature is achieved when the column is placed in an oven or when the column is heated directly by resistive heating.[10] Injector and detector temperatures usually are controlled by electrical resistance

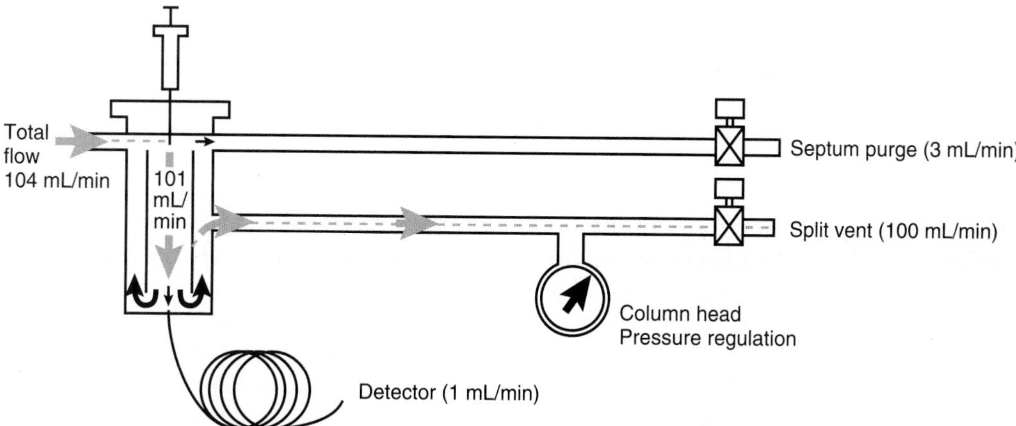

Figure 6-11 Flow diagram of a GC inlet system for split injection. The head pressure and total flow are adjusted to achieve a desired flow rate in the column and a fractional split between the column and the split vent. *GC*, Gas chromatography.

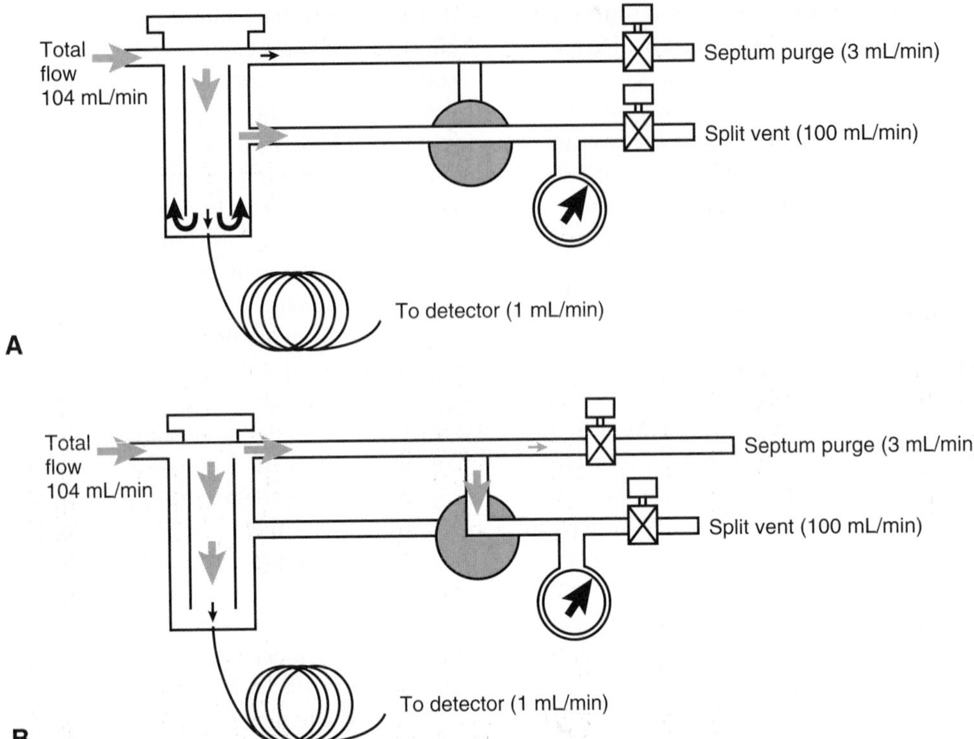

Figure 6-12 Flow diagram of a GC inlet system for splitless injection. Initially the system has most of the flow through the injection liner, with the majority of it directed to the split vent **(A).** When an injection is made, flow is directed through the septum purge line, and all material in the injection liner is transferred into the column **(B).** After 50 to 80 seconds, the flow is again directed through the liner **(A)** to purge any material remaining in the liner through the split vent; meanwhile, a constant flow is maintained through the column. *GC,* Gas chromatography.

heating. Depending on the application, the column temperature is maintained at either a constant preset level (isothermal operation) during the chromatographic run or varied as a function of time (temperature-programmed or temperature-gradient operation).

In practice, temperature-programmed column heating is used for most clinical applications. With temperature programming, the solutes having the lower boiling points elute first, followed by those having higher boiling points. Consequently a complex mixture of solutes with a wide range of boiling points is separated into sharp, distinct chromatographic peaks in less time than with isothermal operation. The temperature is programmed and controlled by a computer and its resident software.

In capillary gas chromatographs, the accurate and precise control of column and injector temperatures is required to obtain optimal performance and accurate results. Temperature control of the column is especially important, particularly in qualitative applications in which the retention times or volumes of eluting peaks are compared with those of authentic standards for identification. A change of only 1 °C causes a 5% change in retention time. In addition, instability of the column temperature adversely affects retention time or volume comparability among instruments or with values in the literature. Temperature gradients in the oven and rapid temperature programming rates also causes variable analyte retention.

The thermal stability of the stationary phase is also important. Because each stationary phase has a range of thermal stability, it is important to control column temperature within the specified range. For the nonpolar phases, the temperature limit is determined by the stability of the polyimide coating. The introduction of aluminum clad columns notably broadens the useable temperature range. Oxidation at higher temperatures limits the operating temperature of intermediate to polar phases.

Before any column is used, it must be "thermally conditioned" by heating the column at various temperatures for different lengths of time. This removes volatile contaminants, including residual monomers, in the polymeric stationary phase. In addition, thermal conditioning of used columns removes accumulated nonvolatile contaminants that cause unstable baselines. To condition a column thermally, it is disconnected from the detector and purged for at

TABLE 6-2 Examples of Detectors Used in Gas Chromatographs

Type of Detector	Principle of Operation	Selectivity	Limit of Detection	Comments
Thermal conductance (TCD)	Measures thermal conductivity change in carrier gas on elution of compounds	Universal	<400 pg propane/mL He	
Flame ionization (FID)	CHNO + heat $\rightarrow$ $CHNO^+ + e^-$; electrons collected for detection	Hydrocarbon	10 to 100 pg CHO	
Thermionic selective (TSD; NPD)	Alkali bead selectively ionizes N- or P-containing compounds	N, P	0.4 to 10 pg N 0.1 to 1.0 pg P	
Electron capture (ECD)	$e^- + R + N_2 \rightarrow Re^- + N_2 + e^-$; excess electrons collected; concentration inversely related	Electronegative groups	0.05 to 1.0 pg Cl^- containing compounds	
Mass spectrometer (MS)	$e^- + ABC \rightarrow A^+ + BC$; monitor mass-to-charge ratio by either scanning or single-ion monitoring (SIM)	Universal (tunable)	1 ng scan 10 pg SIM	Provides structural confirmation; ion ratios constant in SIM
Photoionization (PID)	CHNO + photon $\rightarrow$ $CHNO^+ + e^-$; detect electron	Hydrocarbon	1 to 10 pg CHO	May be improvement on FID
Electrolytic conductivity (Hall)	Postcolumn reaction detector for selective detection of halogen-, S-, or N-containing compounds	Halogen-, S-, and N-containing compounds	0.1 to 1.0 pg Cl 2.0 pg S 4.0 pg N	
Flame photometric (FPD)	P- and S-containing hydrocarbons emit light when burned in FID-type flame; emitted light detected	P- and S-containing compounds	0.9 pg CHP 20 pg CHS	
Fourier transform infrared (FTIR)	Infrared wavelength light absorbed by the compound of interest	Universal (tunable)	1 ng strong infrared absorber	Scanned for structural information or absorbance-measured for quantitation

NPD, Nitrogen-phosphorus detector.

least 5 minutes with pure carrier gas. It is then heated to above 50 °C. The column temperature is then cycled through a normal temperature program three or four times. Alternatively the column can be maintained at the maximum operating temperature for 12 to 24 hours. The thermal conditioning of columns at lower temperatures prolongs the life of the column, but longer conditioning times are required to achieve baseline stability.

Detectors

The purpose of an online detector is to sense and measure the separated analytes as they elute from the column. A variety of sensitive detectors are used with gas chromatographs. These include universal units that detect most analytes and extremely selective devices that detect only specific ones (Table 6-2). Examples include FID, thermionic selective (TSD), ECD, photoionization (PIDs), and TCD. Many other devices have been used as GC detectors, and it has become a common practice to place two or more detectors in a series to enhance analytical specificity and sensitivity.[5] Different types of mass spectrometers are also used as detectors for gas chromatographs (see Chapter 7).

Flame Ionization Detector. The FID is the most commonly used detector for clinical analysis (Figure 6-13). Its advantages include simplicity, reliability, versatility, sensitivity, and ease of operation. During operation the column effluent is mixed with hydrogen and air, and the eluting compounds are burned by a flame. About one molecule in 10,000 produces an organic cation and releases an electron, which is detected by a collector electrode positioned above the

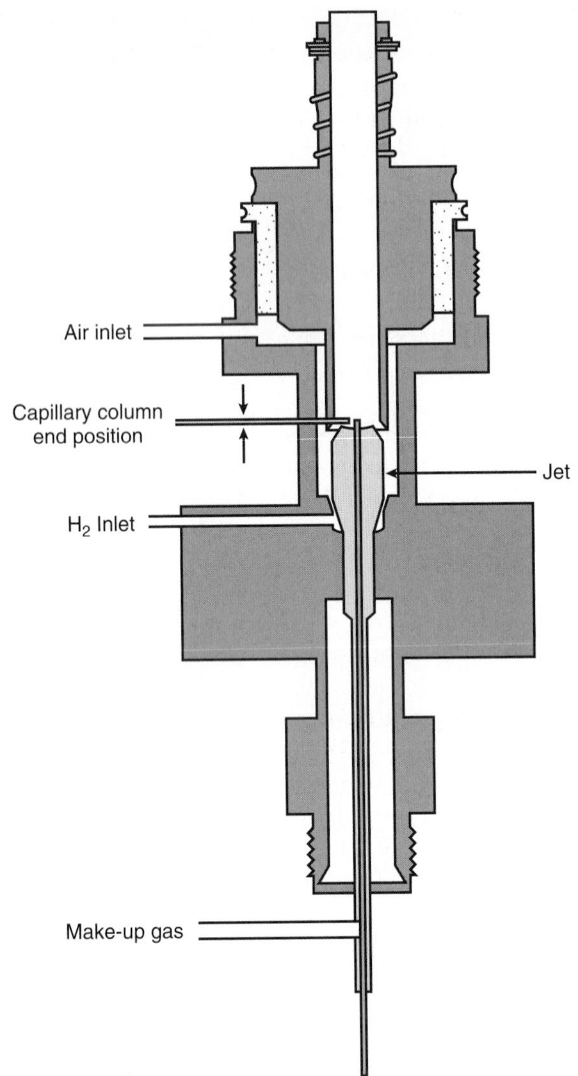

Figure 6-13 Schematic diagram of an FID equipped with make-up gas. *FID,* Flame ionization detector. *(Modified from Hyver KJ: High resolution gas chromatography, 3rd edition, Palo Alto Calif: Hewlitt Packard, 1989.)*

flame. The magnitude of the generated current is related to the mass of carbon material delivered to the detector; after measurement, it is used for detection and quantification of the eluting solutes.

Thermionic Selective Detector. The TSD, also known as the *nitrogen-phosphorus detector (NPD),* is a modification of the FID in which an alkali bead is heated electrically in the area above the jet. In the presence of alkali atoms in the flame, nitrogen-containing compounds give a 15 times greater, and phosphorus-containing compounds a 300 times greater, response.

Electron Capture Detector. The operating principle of the ECD is based on the reaction between electronegative compounds and thermal electrons. The electrons are normally provided from a radioactive source, such as ^{63}Ni or ^{3}H housed in the detector. A collector electrode is pulsed to collect "excess" electrons. This is called the *standing current.* If electronegative species are not present in the detector cell, the nitrogen or argon/methane (95/5) sweep gas removes most of the electrons from the cell. When a compound capable of capturing an electron passes through the cell, some electrons are removed, and a decrease in the standing current is observed. The use of nitrogen or argon/methane is important, because these gases reduce the energy of the electrons via collisions and thus improve the ability of the compounds to "capture" them. It is also important that the gasses be very pure and dry because oxygen and water foul the detector. In some detector designs, the collection pulse rate is varied to maintain a constant amount of current. Then the pulses are counted and used to determine the concentration of electronegative species passing through the cell. The ECD is a concentration-dependent detector. The presence of electronegative constituents, such as fluorine, chlorine, bromine, and iodine, increases the ECD's response. Because not all compounds contain these functional groups, derivatization with reagents containing polychlorinated or polyfluorinated groups to increase detector response is a common practice.

Photoionization Detector. The PID is a variant of the FID. With the PID, however, the energy for ionization is provided by an intense UV lamp rather than by a flame. The PID has a lower limit of detection than the FID because it produces less baseline "noise."

Thermal Conductivity Detector. The TCD is based on the principle that addition of a compound to a gas alters the thermal conductance of the gas. It is used often with capillary GC. The operating principle of the ECD is based on the reaction between electronegative compounds, such as fluorine, chlorine, bromine, and iodine, and thermal electrons. Because not all compounds contain these functional groups, derivatization with reagents containing polychlorinated or polyfluorinated moieties is a common practice used with an ECD.

Different types of mass spectrometers are also used as detectors for gas chromatographs (see Chapter 7).

Computer/Controller

For many years, various digital devices provided both system control and data processing functions for chromatographs (Figure 6-14). The incorporation of computer technology into chromatographic instrumentation resulted in cost-effective, easy-to-operate automated systems with impressive analytical performance. As a process controller, the computer regulates various parameters, such as (1) mobile phase composition and flow rate, (2) column back pressure, (3) column and detector temperatures, (4) sample injection, detector selection and operation, and (5) the various timing steps that command the operation of the system. For data processing, the computer monitors signals generated by the system's detectors and commands the acquisition and storage of data at specified time intervals. The area, or height, of each chromatographic peak is determined from the stored

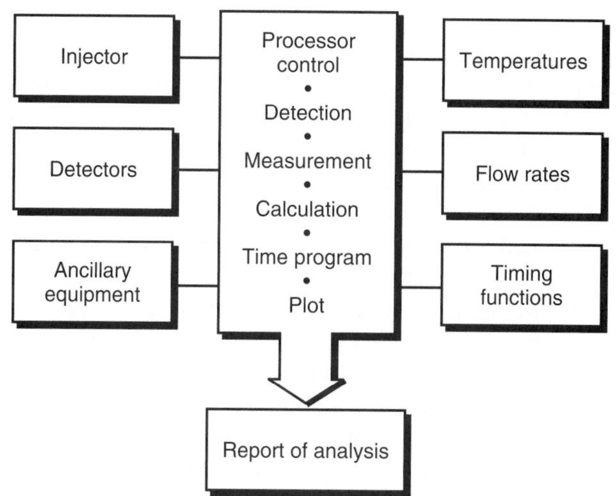

Figure 6-14 Functions of computers in gas and liquid chromatographs.

data and used to compute the analyte concentration represented by each peak. Available algorithms for this computation include those based on calibration curves or conversion factors from internal or external calibration. If desired a complete report can be prepared and printed for each chromatographic run. Alternatively, data are stored to be recalled and reprocessed, with different integration parameters, when desired.

Practical Considerations

Several techniques affect the practical application of GC in the clinical laboratory, including those used to extract and derivatize samples for analysis.

Sample Extraction

For GC analysis, extraction of the analyte from the sample is often necessary. For example, to extract barbiturates from serum, the serum first is acidified to convert the barbiturates into a form soluble in an organic solvent, such as dichloromethane. A volume of this solvent then is shaken vigorously with the acidified serum. When the aqueous and organic layers separate, most of the barbiturates are present in the organic phase, and many interferences, such as proteins, remain in the aqueous phase. Solvent extraction is also frequently used to increase the concentration of an analyte before chromatographic analysis.

Sample Derivatization

Many clinically relevant compounds are nonvolatile, and therefore they are difficult to separate by GC. However, chemical modification or derivatization of such compounds increases their volatility for GC analysis. Chemical reactions used to form these nonpolar derivatives include acylation, silylation, esterification, and oximation. In addition to enhancing solute volatility, derivatization is also used to enhance the specificity and sensitivity of particular separations. For example, the use of a chiral reagent to derivatize amphetamine improves specificity and allows the separation of the D- and L-isomers on a standard GC column. Enhanced ability to detect is also achieved via preparation of pentafluoropropyl derivatives for use with the ECD.

LIQUID CHROMATOGRAPHY

In 1941 Martin and Synge[14] developed *partition chromatography* (also known as *liquid-liquid chromatography*). They demonstrated that monoamino acids and monocarboxylic acids were separated more efficiently by a short column of water-coated silica gel than by any solvent extraction apparatus.

In the late 1960s, emphasis was placed in developing LC as a complementary technique to GLC. In the early 1970s, the evolution and application of chromatographic theory, coupled with the technical improvements and advancements made in instrumentation and separation media, resulted in the development of HPLC and later *capillary gas and liquid chromatography.*[2]

Separation by LC is based on the distribution of the solutes between a liquid mobile phase and a stationary phase. When particles of small diameter are used as the stationary-phase support, the technique is HPLC. Because column efficiency is inversely related to the column packing particle size and pressure drop is related to the square of the particle diameter, relatively high pressures are required to pump liquids through efficient HPLC columns. Consequently the technique has also been referred to as *high-pressure liquid chromatography.* In the clinical laboratory, HPLC is the most widely used form of LC. It has been used for assaying or monitoring many clinically relevant analytes, including amino acids, peptides, proteins, carbohydrates, lipids, nucleic acids and related compounds, vitamins, hormones, metabolites, and drugs such as antiarrhythmics, antibiotics, antiepileptics, analgesics, bronchial smooth muscle relaxants, and tricyclic antidepressants.

Instrumentation

The basic components of a liquid chromatograph are shown in Figure 6-10.[12] With these components, various types of HPLC systems are assembled. These range from single-pump, single-solvent units to versatile, automated systems.

Column Technology

Advances in column technology have improved the selectivity, stability, and reproducibility of LC analytical columns. For example, analytical columns are packed with a variety of stationary phases, providing enormous versatility in the separation process. This section describes (1) column dimensions, (2) particulate column packings, (3) monolithic column packings, and (4) the use of guard columns.

Column Dimensions. Modern column technology has produced columns in different dimensions with the tendency toward smaller internal volumes prevailing for analytical, especially hyphenated, techniques (see Chapter 7).

For use in the clinical laboratory, most analytical HPLC are fabricated from tubes made of 316 stainless steel that have IDs ranging from 0.3 mm to 5 mm and lengths from 50 mm to 250 mm (Table 6-3). Column end fittings, which have zero dead volume and frits to retain the support particles, are used to connect the column to the injector on the inlet end and the detector on the outlet end. Generally, lower detection limits are achieved with columns having smaller IDs. These smaller ID columns are manufactured from narrow bore (approximately 2.1 mm ID) and microbore (approximately 1.0 mm ID) tubes. In addition to providing improved efficiency, columns with smaller IDs use decreased volumes of mobile phase. For example, a 2-mm-ID column requires about fivefold less solvent than a 4.6-mm-ID column (see Table 6-3).

Capillary columns used in LC are constructed by coating the inner wall of a fused-silica tube with a thin film of liquid phase. These columns vary from 0.1 to 0.5 mm in ID and from 10 to 50 cm in length.

Particulate Column Packings. Particulate packings have particle diameters ranging from 1.8 to 10 μm. The packings provide efficient columns with acceptable operating back pressures. Since the back pressure is inversely proportional to the square of the particle diameter, very small mean particle diameter packings require shorter columns to prevent prohibitive back pressures. These types of columns are useful with HPLC/mass spectrometry (HPLC/MS) techniques because of the low solvent volumes required to effect adequate separations. Irregularly shaped or spherical packings that provide lower back pressures are also available.

Types of particulate packings include bonded, polymeric, chiral, and restricted access materials.

Bonded Phase Packings. In this type of packing, the stationary phase is bonded chemically to the surface of silica particles through a silica ester or silicone polymeric linkage. Bonded phase packings (1) are mechanically and chemically stable, (2) have long lifetimes, and (3) provide excellent chromatographic performance. Bonded phase packings are available for ion-exchange and both normal-phase and reversed-phase chromatography. In normal-phase HPLC, the functional groups of the stationary phase are polar relative to those of the mobile phase, which usually consists of nonpolar solvents, such as hexane. Examples of polar functional groups for normal-phase HPLC packings are silanol, amino, and nitrile groups. Reversed-phase HPLC requires a nonpolar stationary phase. The most popular reversed-phase packing is the C18 type, in which octadecylsilane molecules are bonded to silica particles. A column with octadecyl packing is often called an *ODS column* (ODS, octadecyl silica). Reversed-phase column retention and selectivity characteristics are altered via attachment of other groups, such as octyl, phenyl, or cyanopropyl, to the silica.

Polymeric Packings. Graphitized carbon or mixed copolymers are used as polymeric packing (e.g., polystyrene-divinylbenzene) or further derivatized with ion-exchange or C4, C8, or C18 functional groups. Columns filled with these packings feature levels of performance comparable to those of silica-based columns and are stable from pH 2 to 13.

Chiral Packings. Chiral packings are used to separate enantiomers, which are mirror-image forms of the same compound. In the clinical laboratory this type of packing is used to separate and quantify drug enantiomers.

Restricted Access Packings. With this type of packing, the outer surfaces of the support particles are protected by a hydrophilic network. Smaller solutes, such as drugs, pass through the network into the pores, which are coated with hydrophobic stationary phase. Large protein molecules are denied access to the inner core and pass through the column. Columns filled with restricted access packing allow the direct injection of biological samples with high protein concentrations, which bypasses sample preparation and improves analytical accuracy.

In addition to the packings described above, particulate packings (1) with both reversed phase and normal-phase characteristics, (2) compatible with high temperatures (up to 100 °C), or (3) having large pore sizes (e.g., 300 Å) are available commercially.

Monolithic Particulate Column Packings. In recent years, monolithic column packings have been introduced that have some advantages over the classical particulate packings. Monolithic column packings with silica-based or polymer-based monolithic rods have bimodal pore structures with large pores (approximately 2-μm diameter), which create high pore density, and smaller ones (approximately 13-nm diameter), which create a large internal surface area. The high surface area provides good separation, and the high porosity minimizes flow back pressure that allows high flow rates. Thus analysis time is greatly reduced. Further, existing silica-based and polymer-based particle separations are transferred with minimal investment in method development. Also, the lower back pressure appears to provide highly reproducible column characteristics because many of the factors that degrade particulate columns are eliminated (e.g., packing down and channeling). The monolithic rods are encased in inert polytetrafluoroethylene (PTFE) tubing and housed in stainless steel

TABLE 6-3 Types of Columns Used in HPLC

Column Terminology	Column ID (mm)	Optimum Flow Volume
Standard	4.6	1.25 mL/min
	4.0	1.0 mL/min
Narrow bore	3.0	0.6 mL/min
	2.0	200 μL/min
Microbore/capillary	1.0	50 μL/min
	0.5	12 μL/min
	0.3	4 μL/min

HPLC, High-performance liquid chromatography; *ID*, internal diameter.

tubes. The inert tubing eliminates void volumes at the stainless steel tube monolithic rod interface, thus improving resolution. Two additional advantages of these columns are that they can be used with mobile phase flow gradients (e.g., increasing flow rate at the end of a separation), and several columns can be coupled in a series to improve resolution with little increase in flow back pressure. Also, capillary monolithic columns are available.

Guard Columns. To prevent an analytical column from irreversibly adsorbing proteins, with a subsequent reduction in both resolution and column life, a guard column is placed between the injector and analytical column. A guard column is packed with the same or similar stationary phase as the analytical column. It collects particulate matter and any strongly retained components from the sample and thus conserves the life of the analytical column. After a predetermined number of separations, a guard column is routinely replaced.

Solvent Reservoir

Solvents used as the mobile phase are contained in solvent reservoirs. In their simplest forms, the reservoirs are glass bottles or flasks into which "feed lines" to the pump are inserted. To remove particles from solvents, inline filters are placed on the inlets of the feed lines. Sophisticated mobile phase handling systems available commercially contain specially designed bottles with internal, conically shaped bottoms that allow small solvent volumes to be used. These handling systems also feature three or four valve caps that permit the filtration, storage, and delivery of solvents, and a stopcock for vacuum degassing.

Pump

Both constant pressure and constant displacement pumps are used in liquid chromatographs. Constant displacement pumps, however, are used more widely. During its operation the constant displacement pump withdraws (aspirates) the mobile phase from the solvent reservoir and delivers a reproducibly constant flow of it through the chromatographic system. Several different types of pumps are used for this purpose, including the syringe pump single-piston, rapid-refill reciprocating pump; diaphragm pump; and the most widely used dual-piston reciprocating pump.

A dual-piston reciprocating pump uses an asymmetrical cam to drive two pistons into and from two pumping chambers (Figure 6-15). The reciprocating action of the pump, however, creates "pump pulsations" that result from changes in the flow rate. The changes affect the output signals of some detectors, thereby increasing baseline noise that influences the detection limit of the system. Thus most reciprocating pumps use mechanical or electronic pulse dampers and/or multiple heads that operate out of phase to deliver a mobile phase continuously. Another technique uses a significantly more rapid refill stroke than delivery stroke. Reciprocating pumps operate at up to 10,000 psi and generate flow rates from 0.01 mL/min to 20 mL/min or greater, depending on pump head size and configuration.

The HPLC pump is operated in either an isocratic or gradient mode (Figure 6-16). In the isocratic mode, the mobile phase composition remains constant throughout the chromatographic run. This mode is usually used for simpler separations and separations of those compounds with similar structures and/or retention times. An isocratic mobile phase is a single solvent (e.g., methanol) or a prepared mixture of several solvents (e.g., methanol, acetonitrile, and water) delivered from a single solvent reservoir. Alternatively a multisolvent mobile phase can be metered and proportioned from two or more reservoirs. Most HPLC separations are performed under isocratic conditions.

Gradient elution is used for more complex separations.[1] In this mode, mobile phase composition is changed during the run in either a stepwise or continuous fashion. Many different techniques are used to generate gradient profiles. In one technique, two or more pumps are used in parallel. A variety of gradient profiles are generated through programming of the output of each pump. Alternatively the

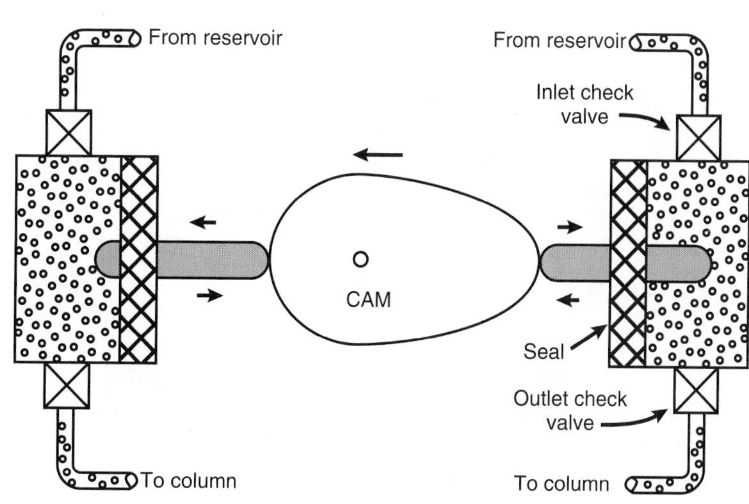

Figure 6-15 Cross-sectional view of a dual-piston reciprocating pump. *(From Walker JQ, Jackson MT Jr, Maynard JB: Chromatographic systems: Maintenance and troubleshooting, 2nd edition, New York: Academic Press, 1977.)*

mobile phase is proportioned on the inlet side of a single pump. For example, up to four solvent reservoirs may be connected via proportioning valves to the inlet check valve of a single pump. The composition of the mobile phase is then varied through programming of the time during which solvent is delivered through each of the proportioning valves.

Injector

To initiate an LC separation, an aliquot of sample (e.g., 0.2 to 50 μL) is first introduced into the column via an injector. The most widely used type of injector is the fixed-loop injector (Figure 6-17). In the fill position, an aliquot of sample is introduced at atmospheric pressure into a stainless steel loop. In the inject mode, the sample loop is rotated into the flowing stream of the mobile phase, and the sample is swept into the chromatographic column. These injectors are precise, function at high pressures, and can be programmed for use in automated systems.

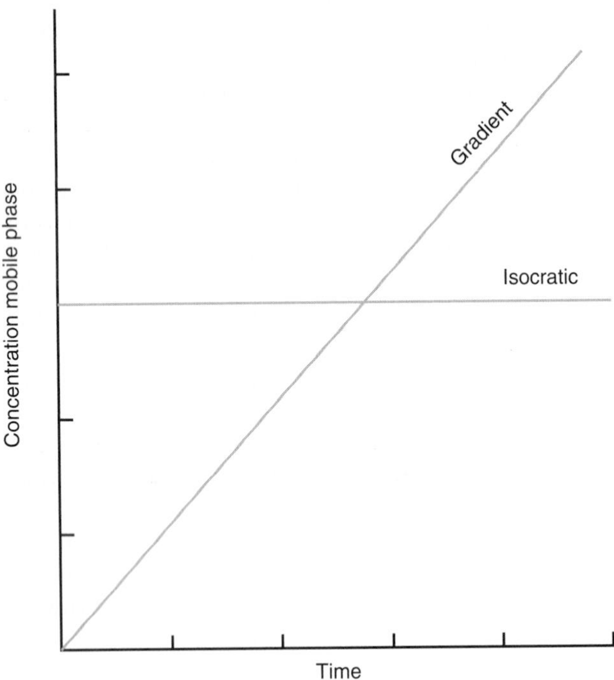

Figure 6-16 Examples of isocratic and gradient elution in LC. *LC,* Liquid chromatography.

Digitally controlled autosamplers that incorporate a loop injector are available commercially. These sophisticated devices are extremely precise and can be programmed for continuous and automated operation. In addition, the sample loop is flushed automatically with the mobile phase between samples to prevent sample carry over. The ability to inject multiple aliquots from a single sample vial or to add reagents from designated vials to derivatize the analyte just before injection are additional features of many autosamplers.

Detectors

Many detectors have been developed for use with liquid chromatographs (Table 6-4). Examples include photometric, spectrophotometric, fluorometric, and electrochemical detectors. A key and integral component of such detectors is the flow cell (Figure 6-18), through which passes the eluate from the chromatographic column. Dissolved analytes are then detected and an electronic signal generated. (Mass spectrometers, which also have been used as LC detectors, are discussed in Chapter 7.)

Photometers and Spectrophotometers. UV and visible photometers measure the radiant energy absorbed by compounds as they elute from the chromatographic column (see Chapter 3). These detectors operate in the radiant energy regions of 190 to 400 nm and 400 to 700 nm, respectively. The devices are versatile and detect many solutes because most organic compounds absorb in the UV region, with a few in the visible region of the electromagnetic spectrum.

Photometers operate as either fixed-wavelength or variable-wavelength detectors. Most fixed-wavelength UV

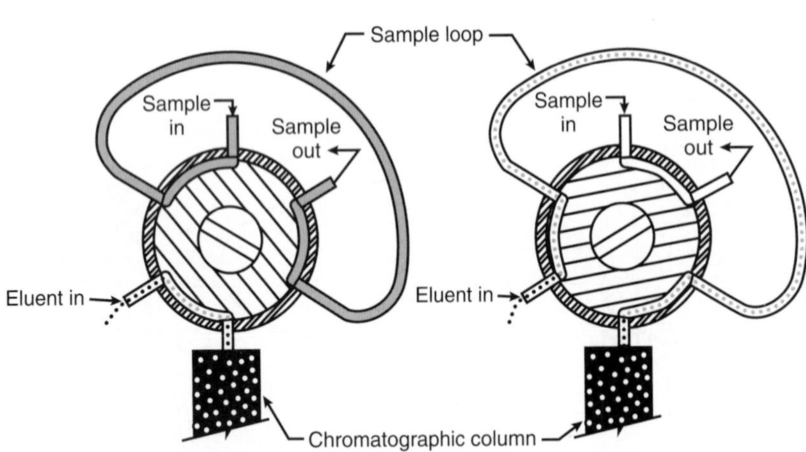

Figure 6-17 Cross-sectional view of a commonly used sample loop injector.

photometers use the intense 254-nm resonance line produced by a mercury arc lamp. This type of detector is extremely sensitive and operates at 0.005 absorbance units full scale (AUFS). To provide the fixed-wavelength detectors with greater flexibility, other less intense resonance lines of the mercury lamp are used. Alternatively a phosphor is placed between the lamp and the flow cell, and the emitted fluorescence resulting from the 254-nm excitation is used as the light source. This latter approach is used in the dual-wavelength photometers that operate at two fixed wavelengths (e.g., 254 nm and 280 nm). The intense 214-nm or 229-nm resonance lines of a zinc or cadmium arc lamp, respectively, also are used for detection at lower wavelengths, where more compounds absorb.

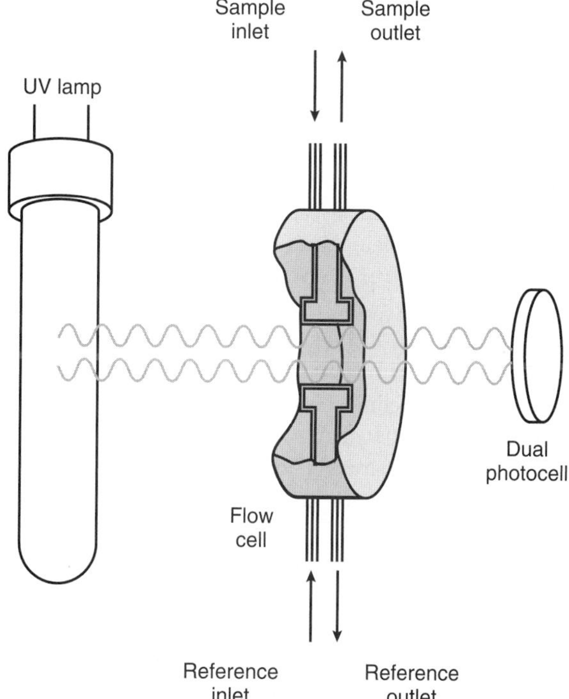

Figure 6-18 Optical schematic of a simple photometer and flow cell. *UV*, Ultraviolet.

The second type of photometer is the variable-wavelength detector. It operates at a wavelength selected from a given wavelength range. Thus the detector is "tuned" to operate at the absorbance maximum for a given analyte or set of analytes, which enhances greatly the applicability and selectivity of the detector (see Fig. 6-2). Another advantage of this detector is its ability to operate at lower wavelengths (e.g., 190 nm). Because more compounds (e.g., cholesterol) absorb at lower wavelengths, this capability enhances the versatility of the detector. At lower wavelengths, however, many solvents absorb UV light and cannot be used as mobile phases. Fortunately, acetonitrile and methanol, two widely used solvents in reversed-phase chromatography, have minimum UV absorptions at 200 nm.

In addition, diode arrays are used as HPLC detectors because they rapidly yield spectral data over the entire wavelength range of 190 to 600 nm in about 10 milliseconds. During operation the diode array detector passes polychromatic light through the detector flow cell. The transmitted light is dispersed by a diffraction grating and then directed to a photodiode array, where the intensity of light at multiple wavelengths in the spectrum is measured. Such detectors have been helpful in the identification of drugs in urine and serum.

Fluorometers. As discussed in Chapter 3, fluorescence occurs when a molecule absorbs light at one wavelength and reemits light at a longer wavelength. Online fluorometers

TABLE 6-4 Examples of Detectors Used in High-Performance Liquid Chromatographs

Type of Detector	Principle of Operation	Range of Application	Detection Limit	Comments
UV photometer (fixed wavelength)	Measures absorbance of UV light	Selective	<1 ng	Analyte must absorb UV light or be derivatized
UV photometer (variable wavelength)	Measures absorbance of UV light	Selective	<1 ng	Detector can be "tuned" to a specific wavelength
Diode array	Measures absorbance of light	Selective	<1 ng	Detector provides complete spectra
Fluorometer	Measures fluorescence	Very selective	pg to ng	Analyte must fluoresce or be derivatized
Refractometer	Measures change in refractive index	Universal	1 μg	
Electrochemical	Electrochemically measures oxidized/reduced analyte	Selective	pg to ng	Detector is useful for catecholamines

UV, Ultraviolet.

are used in liquid chromatographs to detect fluorescing compounds as they elute from the column. In addition, either a precolumn or postcolumn reactor can be used to chemically tag a compound with a fluorescent label for subsequent detection. For example, amino acids or other primary amines often are labeled with either a dansyl or fluorescamine tag and followed by HPLC separation and fluorometric detection. Most fluorometers used with liquid chromatographs are relatively simple in design and extremely selective and sensitive for compounds fluorescing within the detector's operating wavelength range. Deuterium or xenon arc lamps or lasers have been used as light sources in such detectors.

Electrochemical Detectors. In amperometric electrochemical detectors (see Chapter 4), an electroactive analyte enters the flow cell, where it is either oxidized or reduced at an electrode surface under a constant potential. Electroactive compounds of clinical interest conveniently analyzed by HPLC with electrochemical detection include the urinary catecholamines (see Chapter 29). In addition, electrochemically active tags (e.g., bromine) are added to compounds such as unsaturated fatty acids or prostaglandins.

Coulometric detectors are also used. When placed in a series, such detectors are used to detect and quantify co-eluting compounds that differ in their half-wave potentials (the potential at half-signal maximum) by at least 60 mV. These detectors are extremely selective and sensitive, with reasonably wide linear response ranges. They are used in the clinical laboratory for the analysis of metanephrines, vanillymandelic acid, homovanillic acid, and 5-hydroxyindole acetic acid in human urine without extensive sample preparation.

Computer

As with gas chromatographs, the incorporation of computer technology into HPLC instrumentation has resulted in cost-effective, easy-to-operate automated systems with improved analytical performances (see Figure 6-14). In these systems, a computer provides both system control and data processing functions. For details the reader should consult the previous discussion on the use of computers in gas chromatographs.

Practical Considerations

Several techniques affect the practical application of HPLC in the clinical laboratory, including those used to prepare samples and mobile phases.

Sample Preparation

Sample preparation is an important step in chromatographic analysis by HPLC and includes procedures for sample concentration, purification, and derivatization.

Sample Concentration and/or Purification. Concentrating or purifying an analyte in a sample is often necessary before separation and quantification by HPLC. Several liquid extraction and solid phase extraction (SPE) techniques are used for this purpose. The latter has become very popular because solid phase extraction cartridges or 96-well plate SPE formats greatly simplify sample preparation. The cartridges are usually 1- or 3-mL syringe barrels made of polypropylene that contain a stationary phase. The plate format uses smaller quantities of the stationary phase and requires smaller elution volumes. Both the cartridge and plate formats are available with disk designs that have small stationary phase–impregnated disks for use with small sample and elution volumes. Silica-based or polymeric normal-phase, reversed-phase, or ion-exchange (anion, cation, or mixed) stationary phases are available. Monolithic packings are also available. As an aliquot of urine or serum passes through the stationary phase, it retains the analytes. The column is then rinsed with solutions of different pH values or solvent compositions to selectively elute interfering substances. The analytes are then eluted with a different mobile phase. Alternatively, analytes are eluted directly, with unwanted solutes being retained on the cartridge. This approach is popular in the preparation of samples for therapeutic drug monitoring, drugs of abuse testing, and catecholamine analysis. Product manufacturers usually have a compilation of methods and protocols for specific analytes, including those of clinical interest.

Devices are now available for automated online extraction and sample preparation. These consist mainly of robotic arms and mechanisms for highly accurate and precise delivery of solvent volumes. Depending on the instrument, samples may be prepared and analyzed individually or in batches.

Sample Derivatization. For HPLC analyses, many analytes are chemically derivatized before or after chromatographic separation to increase their ability to be detected. For example, in automated amino acid analyzers, eluted amino acids are reacted with ninhydrin in a postcolumn reactor (see Chapter 20). The resulting chromogenic species are then detected with a photometer. Other examples include labeling amino acids or other primary amines with dansyl or fluorescamine tags either before or after the chromatographic step.

Preparation of Mobile Phase. In preparing the mobile phase, dissolved gases in the solvent must be removed or suppressed. The solvent must also be free of particulate matter. When the mobile phase is composed of two or more solvents, the solvents must be adequately mixed.

Solvent Degassing. A common problem in LC is the evolution of dissolved gas bubbles that evolve as the mobile phase passes from the high-pressure (column) side to the ambient-pressure (postcolumn) side of the chromatographic system. These bubbles must be removed or suppressed because they create an unstable electronic signal (noisy baseline) when they pass through a detector. Operationally, vacuum degassing, helium purging, postdetector back pressure, or vacuum membrane degassing are techniques used to prevent this problem.

With vacuum degassing, the mobile phase is stirred in a side-armed flask or mobile phase handling system under reduced pressure. Nonpolar mobile phases require less than 1 minute to degas, but polar mobile phases require several minutes. Prolonged degassing under vacuum should be avoided, however, because it alters the mobile phase composition, especially when volatile solvents are used.

Another degassing technique, helium "sparging," requires a constant, gentle stream of helium bubbled through the solvents in the solvent reservoirs. The relatively insoluble helium extracts the dissolved gases, which then are vented into the atmosphere. Helium degassing is particularly useful with fluorescence detectors because it efficiently removes oxygen that quenches the fluorescence signal. Helium is expensive, however, and is best used with low-vapor-pressure solvents. Nonpolar solvents over time will be removed from the mobile phase mixture by the helium. Placing a drying agent in the helium line (between the helium tank and solvent reservoir) is helpful because it removes any water in the gas. Also, a back-pressure valve can be attached to the outlet of the system's detector, forcing gasses to remain in the solution until they have passed through the detector cell.

Vacuum membrane degassing uses PTFE tubing that is several meters long. As the tubing is permeable to gasses, solvents passing through the tubing are degassed when an external vacuum is applied. The efficiency of degassing is dependent on tubing length and solvent flow rate. Degassing can also be accomplished using Teflon AF tubing, which possesses excellent gas permeability characteristics. Thus degassing chamber internal volumes can be reduced to about 500 uL. In addition, gas-impermeable tubing can be used after the degassing to keep the solvent free of gasses. Vacuum membrane degassing systems can be purchased separately or as an integral part of an HPLC system. This economical form of degassing is satisfactory for most analytical procedures. Other degassing methods include mild heating and ultrasonic vibration of the mobile phase.

Solvent Clarity. Mobile phases should be prepared from HPLC-grade solvents free of particulate matter. Most commercial HPLC solvents are prefiltered. If they are not, however, they should be filtered through a 0.5-μm screen.

Solvent Mixing. During gradient operation, the HPLC solvents that comprise the mobile phase must be mixed adequately, most commonly with either a static or dynamic mixer. Static mixers rely on laminar-flow dynamics, whereas dynamic mixers use magnetic stirrers. Solvent viscosity affects mixing characteristics; inadequate mixing is detected by many UV detectors and may be expressed as an unstable baseline.

Safety

Normal laboratory precautions must be exercised during HPLC operation. The column effluent should be collected in a suitable container and stored appropriately before disposal. The explosive release of pressure in an HPLC system is not a major hazard; liquids compress only slightly and therefore accumulate little energy.

QUALITATIVE AND QUANTITATIVE ANALYSES

Chromatography is basically a separation technique. However it can be used for both qualitative [identifying the analyte(s) of interest] and quantitative analyses.

ANALYTE IDENTIFICATION

The retention time or volume at which an unknown solute elutes from a column or the distance traveled on a plate is often matched to that of a reference compound. The appearance of a solute peak, band, or spot at the same time as that of a reference compound is consistent with the two compounds being the same. The simultaneous appearance does not prove identity, however, because other compounds can have the same retention time as the reference compound.

In planar chromatography, reference compounds are chromatographed with the unknown sample. Tentative identification is made by comparison of the migration distances and detection characteristics of the reference compounds with those of the unknown analytes. If the R_f of the unknown analyte and the R_f of the reference compound do not match, the compounds are judged to be different. If they match, the compounds are presumed to be identical. However, as more than one compound can have the same R_f in a particular chromatographic system, the presumptive identification has to be confirmed by the use of specific spray reagents, antibody complexation, or isolation of the compound followed by chemical and/or instrumental analysis. Software is now available for compound identification by library searching of UV spectra based on corrected R_f values.[15]

With capillary GC and LC columns, it is possible to simultaneously introduce the components of a single injection into two columns made of dissimilar stationary phases. The columns are connected to separate detectors of the same or a different type. Matching the retention properties of a single analyte with a reference compound on two columns of dissimilar phases enhances the chance for correct identification of the analyte. The most reliable analyte identification, however, is provided by a detector that features structural information, such as a mass spectrometer (see Chapter 7).

ANALYTE QUANTIFICATION

The electronic signals from the detector(s) are also used to produce quantitative information. Both external and internal calibrating techniques have been used. With external calibration, reference solutions containing known quantities of analytes are processed in a manner identical to the samples containing the analyte (Figure 6-19). A calibration curve of peak height, peak area, or spot density versus calibrator concentration is constructed and used to calculate the concentration of the analyte in the samples. With internal calibration, also called *internal standardization,* reference solutions of known analyte concentrations are prepared, and a constant amount of a different compound, the internal standard, is added to each reference solution and each

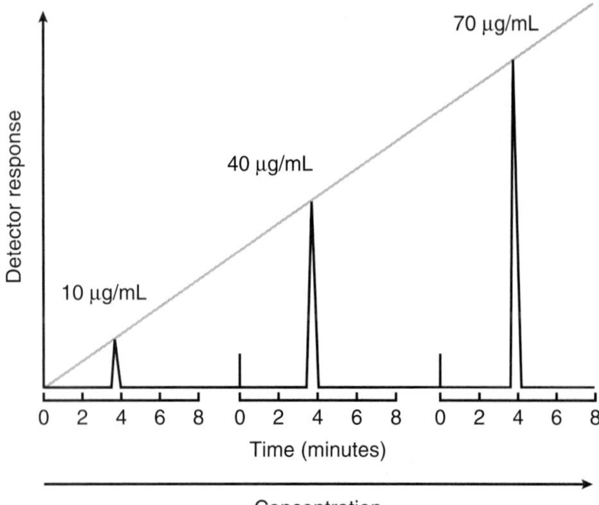

Figure 6-19 The use of external calibrators in the production of a calibration plot. *(From Krull I, Swartz M: Quantitation in method validation. LC-GC 1998; 16:1084-90.)*

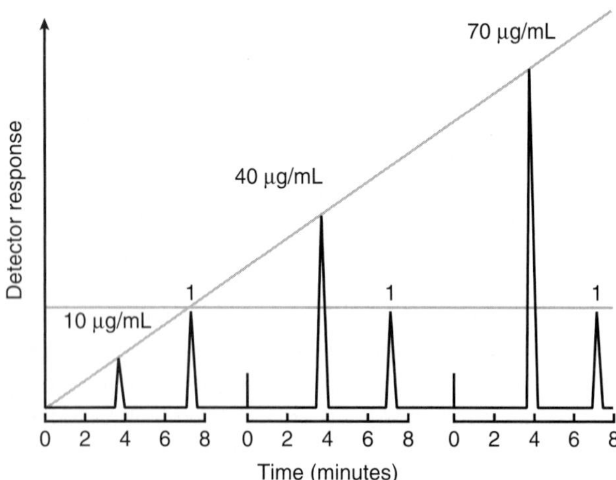

Figure 6-20 The use of internal calibrators in the production of a calibration plot (peak 1 being the internal standard). *(From Krull I, Swartz M: Quantitation in method validation. LC-GC 1998; 16:1084-90.)*

sample (Figure 6-20). By plotting the ratio of the peak height (or area) or spot density of the analyte to the peak height (or area) or spot density of the internal standard versus the concentration of the analyte, a calibration curve that corrects for systematic losses is constructed. This curve is then used to compute the analyte concentration in the samples by interpolation.

REFERENCES

1. Dolan JW, Snyder LR. Gradient Elution Chromatography. In: Meyers, RA (ed). Encyclopedia of analytical chemistry. Chichester: John Wiley & Sons, 2000: 11342-60.
2. Dorsey JG. Liquid Chromatography: Introduction. In: Meyers, RA (ed). Encyclopedia of analytical chemistry. Chichester: John Wiley & Sons, 2000:11231-3.
3. Dorsey JG. Column Theory and Resolution in Liquid Chromatography. In: Meyers, RA (ed). Encyclopedia of analytical chemistry. Chichester: John Wiley & Sons, 2000:11334-42.
4. Eiceman GA. Instrumentation of Gas Chromatography in Clinical Chemistry. In: Meyers, RA (ed). Encyclopedia of analytical chemistry. Chichester: John Wiley & Sons, 2000:10671-9.
5. Eiceman GA, Gardea-Torresdey J, Overton E, Carney K, Dorman F. Gas Chromatography. Anal Chem 2002;74:22771-80.
6. Ettre LS: Nomenclature for chromatography. IUPAC recommendations 1993. Pure & Appl Chem 1993;65:819-72.
7. Ettre LS. M.S. Tswett and the Invention of Chromatography. LC/GC North Amer 2003;21:458-67.
8. Gocan S. Stationary phases for thin-layer chromatography. J Chromatogr Sci 2002;40:538-49.
9. James AT, Martin AJP. Separation and identification of methyl esters of saturated and unsaturated fatty acids from n-pentanoic to n-octadecanoic acids. Analyst 1952;77:915.
10. Jain V, Phillips JB. Fast temperature programming on fused-silica open-tubular capillary columns by direct resistive heating. J Chromatogr Sci 1995;33: 55-9.
11. Jain R, Sherma J. Planar Chromatography in Clinical Chemistry. In: Meyers, RA (ed). Encyclopedia of analytical chemistry. Chichester: John Wiley & Sons, 2000:1583-603.
12. LaCourse WR. Column Liquid Chromatography: Equipment & Instrumentation. Anal Chem 2002;74:2813-32.
13. Lough WJ. Reversed Phase Liquid Chromatography. In: Meyers, RA (ed). Encyclopedia of analytical chemistry. Chichester: John Wiley & Sons, 2000: 11442-50.
14. Martin AJP, Synge RLM. A new form of chromatography employing two liquid phases. I A theory of chromatography. II Applications to the microdetermination of the higher monoamino acids in proteins. Biochem J 1941;35:1358.
15. Sherma J. Planar Chromatography. Anal Chem 2002;74:2653-62.
16. Stahl E. Dunnschicht-chromatographie: Methoden Einflussfactoren und einige. Anwendungsbeispiele Pharmazie 1956;11:63.
17. Tswett M. The macrochemical and microchemical detection of carotin. Ber Deut Botan Geo 1906;24: 385.
18. Zlatkis A, Kaiser RE (eds). HPTLC: High performance thin layer chromatography. New York: Elsevier Science Publishing Co, 1977.

ADDITIONAL READING

Books

General

Ahuja S (ed). Chromatography and separation science (SST). San Diego: Academic Press, 2002: 250pp.

Cazes J, Scott RPW. Chromatography theory. New York: Marcel Dekker, 2002: 496pp.

Millner P. High resolution chromatography: A practical approach. London: Oxford University Press, 1999: 320pp.

Poole C. The Essence of chromatography. Oxford: Elsevier Health Sciences, 2002: 900pp.

Walker JQ, Minneci J (eds). Chromatography fundamentals applications & troubleshooting. Niles IL: Preston Publications 1996.

Gas Chromatography

Grant DW: Capillary gas chromatography. New York: John Wiley & Sons, 1996.

Grob K. Split and splitless injection for quantitative gas chromatography: Concepts, processes, practical guidelines, sources of error, 4th ed. Weinheim, Germany: Vch Verlagsgesellschaft Mbh, 2001; 460pp.

Hinshaw JV. Getting the best results from your gas chromatograph. New York: John Wiley & Sons, 2002: 299pp.

Jennings W, Mittlefehldt E, Stremple PP, Stremple P (eds). Analytical gas chromatography, 2nd ed. San Diego: Academic Press, 1997: 89pp.

McNair HM, Miller JM. Basic gas chromatography. New York; Wiley-Interscience, 1998: 200pp.

Rood D. A practical guide to the care, maintenance, and troubleshooting of capillary gas chromatographic systems, 3rd ed. Weinheim, Germany: Vch Verlagsgesellschaft Mbh, 1999: 344pp.

Sacks RD, Dimandja J-M D, Patterson DG Jr (eds). High speed gas chromatography. New York: John Wiley & Sons, 2001: 400pp.

Scott RPW, Perry JA. Introduction to analytical gas chromatography, 2nd ed. New York: Marcel Dekker, 1998: 397pp.

Liquid Chromatography/ High-Performance Liquid Chromatography

Cunico RL, Gooding KM, Wehr T. Basic HPLC and CE of biomolecules. Hercules, CA: Bay Bioanalytical Laboratory, 1998: 388pp.

Gooding KM, Regnier FE (eds). HPLC of biological macromolecules revised and expanded, 2nd ed. New York: Marcel Dekker, 2002: 792pp.

Neue UD. HPLC Columns: Theory, technology, and practice. Weinheim, Germany: VCH Publishing, 1997: 393pp.

Sadek PC. Troubleshooting HPLC systems: A bench manual. New York: Wiley-Interscience, 1999: 306pp.

Snyder LR, Kirkland JJ, Glajch JL. Practical HPLC method development, 2nd ed. New York: Wiley-Interscience, 1997: 765pp.

Planar Chromatography

Fried B, Sherma J (eds). Practical thin-layer chromatography: A multidisciplinary approach. Boca Raton, FL: CRC Press, 1996: 88pp.

Hahn-Deinstrop E. Applied thin layer chromatography: Best practice and avoidance of mistakes. New York: John Wiley & Sons, 2002: 318pp.

Sherma J: Handbook of thin layer chromatography. 2nd ed, New York: Marcel Dekker Inc, 1996.

Touchstone JC: Practice of thin layer chromatography. 3rd ed, New York: John Wiley & Sons, 1992.

Reviews

Ettre LS. The centenary of the invention of chromatography. J Chromatogr Sci 2003;41:225-6.

Haginaka J. LC packing materials for pharmaceutical and biomedical analysis. Se Pu 2002;20:508-18.

Hooijschuur EW, Kientz CE, Brinkman UA. Analytical separation techniques for the determination of chemical warfare agents. J Chromatogr A 2002;982:177-200.

Kostiainen R, Kotiaho T, Kuuranne T, Auriola S. Liquid chromatography/atmospheric pressure ionization-mass spectrometry in drug metabolism studies. J Mass Spectrom 2003;38:357-72.

McDonald PD. Improving our understanding of reversed-phase separations for the 21st century. Adv Chromatogr 2003;42:323-75.

Sherma J. Planar Chromatography [Review]. Anal Chem 2002;74:2653-62.

Vogeser M. Liquid chromatography-tandem mass spectrometry–application in the clinical laboratory. Clin Chem Lab Med 2003;41:117-26.

CHAPTER 7

Mass Spectrometry*

Thomas Annesley, Ph.D., Alan L. Rockwood, Ph.D., and Nicholas E. Sherman, Ph.D.

Mass spectrometry (MS) is a powerful qualitative and quantitative analytical technique that is used to measure a wide range of clinically relevant analytes. When MS is coupled with either gas or liquid chromatographs, the resultant analyzers have expanded analytical capabilities with widespread clinical applications. In addition, because of its ability to identify and quantify proteins, MS is a key analytical tool that is used in the emerging field of proteomics.

We begin this chapter with a discussion of the basic concepts and definitions of MS followed by discussions of MS instrumentation and clinical applications.

BASIC CONCEPTS AND DEFINITIONS

MS is the branch of science dealing with all aspects of mass spectrometers and the results obtained with them. A *mass spectrometer* is an analytical instrument that first ionizes a target molecule and then separates and measures the mass of a molecule or its fragments. *Mass analysis* is the process by which a mixture of ionic species is identified according to the mass-to-charge *(m/z)* ratios (ions).[88] The analysis is qualitative, quantitative, and extremely useful for determining the elemental composition and structure of both inorganic and organic compounds.

All MS techniques require an ionization step in which an ion is produced from a neutral atom or molecule. In fact development of versatile ionization techniques has led to MS being the excellent analytical tool it is today. In 2002 the Nobel prize was shared by John Fenn and Koichi Tanaka for their development of electrospray[28,29] and laser desorption[49,69,85] ionization, respectively.

Chemical, electron field desorption, laser desorption, photon, plasma desorption, spark, and *thermal* ionization are all used as primary ionization processes. *Secondary ionization* is the term used to describe a process in which ions are ejected from a surface as a result of bombardment by a primary beam of atoms or ions.[88] If low energy or "soft" ionization techniques are used, the mass of the target molecule can be determined. Advances in soft ionization techniques have extended the use of MS to the direct measurement of peptide and protein mass.[3,70] Ionization at higher energy results in more extensive fragmentation of target molecules.

A *mass spectrum* is represented by the relative abundance of each ion plotted as a function of its mass-to-charge *(m/z)* ratio (Figure 7-1). Usually, each ion has a single charge ($z = 1$); thus the *m/z* ratio is equal to the mass. The unfragmented ion of the original molecule is called the *molecular ion.* The ion with the highest abundance in the mass spectrum is assigned a relative value of 100% and is called the *base peak.* By using the relative abundance of each ion fragment, instrument-dependent variability is minimized, and the mass spectrum can be compared to spectra obtained on other instruments. Since the fragmentation at specific bonds can be predicted from their chemical nature, the structure of an analyte can be reconstructed from its mass spectrum. Computer-based libraries of spectra are available to assist in identification of the analyte(s).

When interfaced to a liquid or a gas chromatograph, the mass spectrometer functions as a powerful detector, providing structural information in real time on individual analytes as they elute from a chromatography column. Depending on the operating characteristics of the mass spectrometer and the analyte peak width, several mass spectral scans can be acquired across the peak. The sum of all ions produced is displayed as a function of time to yield a *total ion chromatogram.* The mass spectrometer is considered to be a "universal detector" because all compounds have mass

*The authors gratefully acknowledge the original contributions by Larry D. Bowers on which portions of this chapter are based.

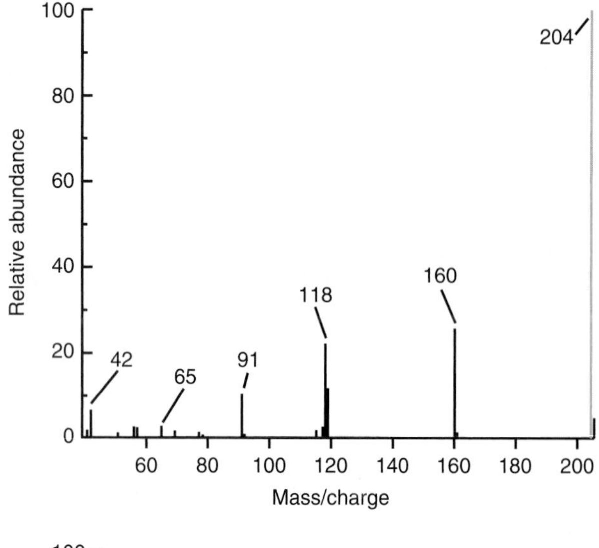

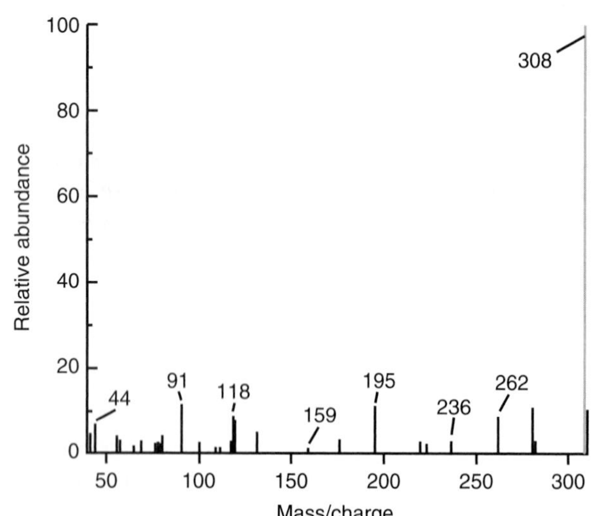

Figure 7-1 Mass spectrum of the pentafluoropropionyl **(A)** and carbethoxyhexafluorobutyryl **(B)** derivatives of d-methamphetamine.

and can, in theory, be detected. The data system can also be programmed to display only preselected ions acquired during the mass spectral scan. The resultant display is called an *extracted ion profile.* Both of these displays have the appearance of a chromatogram with signal intensity plotted as a function of time. Retention times can be measured and peak heights or peak areas can be integrated for use in quantitative analysis.

When only a few analytes are of interest for quantitative analysis and their mass spectrum is known, the mass spectrometer can be programmed to monitor only those ions of interest. This selective detection technique is known as *selected ion monitoring* (SIM). Because SIM focuses on a limited number of ions, more signal can be collected for each selected mass. This increases the signal-to-noise ratio of the analyte and improves the lower limit of detection. In general, however, an unknown is considered identified if the relative abundances of three or four ions agree within ±20% of those from a reference compound.

A distinct advantage of the mass spectrometer is that it can simultaneously differentiate and quantify a compound with a normal abundance of isotope from an analog enriched with a stable isotope (e.g., ^{2}H relative to ^{1}H, ^{13}C relative to ^{12}C, ^{15}N relative to ^{14}N, or ^{18}O relative to ^{16}O). A compound labeled with a stable isotope is used as an internal standard because it behaves nearly identically to the native compound during sample preparation and chromatographic analysis. The internal standard must have a sufficient amount of heavy isotope so that no naturally occurring ^{2}H or ^{13}C contributes significantly to the ion current. For the methamphetamine derivatives shown in Figure 7-2, an internal standard with at least three ^{2}H or ^{13}C atoms is preferred, because at this point the natural abundance of these isotopes is ~0.1% at 3 mass units above the molecular ion [$(M + 3)^+$]. The placement of the stable isotope atoms in the structure is also important. For example, the *m/z* 204 ion for metham-

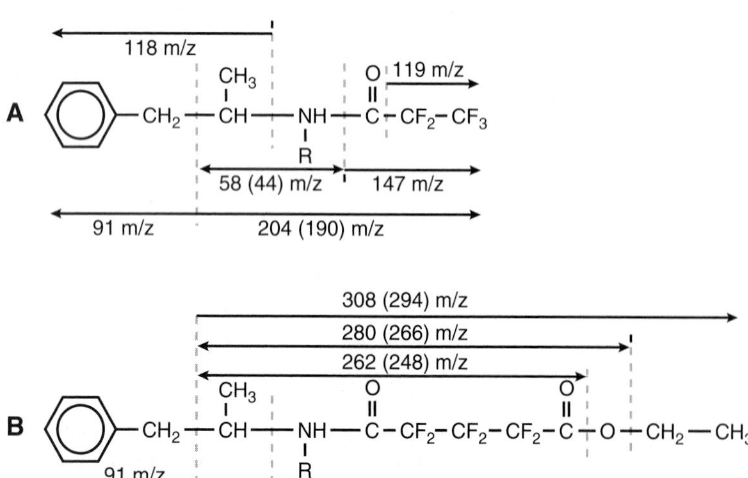

Figure 7-2 Fragmentation patterns for the pentafluoropropionyl **(A)** and carbethoxy-hexafluorobutyryl **(B)** derivatives of methamphetamine (R = CH_3) and amphetamine (R = H; masses in parentheses). Compare the predicted masses with the spectrum shown in Figure 7-1. Note that for the pentafluoropropionyl derivative, only one ion (204, 190 *m/z*) is characteristic of the aliphatic portion of the molecule.

phetamine represents the aliphatic portion of the molecule (loss of the aromatic ring). If five deuterium atoms were present on the aromatic ring of methamphetamine, the pentafluoropropionyl derivatives of both native and isotope-labeled drug would yield the *m/z* 204 ion. Similarly the stable isotope must be located so that it will not exchange with solvent molecules. In general, monitoring ions with higher mass results in lower limits of detection because there are fewer background ions. The ability to quantify a compound relative to an isotopic species of known or fixed concentration is known as *isotope dilution analysis,* and the specific mass spectrometric technique is known as *isotope dilution mass spectrometry* (IDMS). The IDMS technique has been used to develop definitive methods for a number of clinically relevant analytes.

INSTRUMENTATION

A mass spectrometer consists of an ion source, vacuum system, mass analyzer, detector, and computer (Figure 7-3).

Ion Source

Many approaches have been used to form ions, both in high-vacuum and near-atmospheric pressure conditions. *Electron ionization* (EI) and *chemical ionization* (CI) are ionization techniques used when gas phase molecules can be introduced directly into the analyzer from a gas chromatograph. In other analyses, such as high-performance liquid chromatography-mass spectrometry (HPLC-MS), electrospray ionization (ESI), sonic spray ionization (SSI), atmospheric pressure chemical ionization (APCI), and atmospheric pressure photoionization (APPI) interfaces are used as ionization sources.[14,26,33,39] Other ionization techniques include inductively coupled plasma (ICP), matrix-assisted laser desorption ionization (MALDI), atmospheric pressure matrix-assisted laser desorption (AP-MALDI), and fast atom bombardment (FAB).

Electron Ionization

In the EI gas phase molecules are bombarded by electrons emitted from a heated filament and attracted to a collector electrode (Figure 7-4). This process must occur in a vacuum to prevent filament oxidation. A potential difference of 70 eV generates electrons with sufficient energy that a near collision with most organic molecules produces a *radical* cation for EI that is both an ion and a radical.[88] This radical ion then undergos unimolecular rearrangement to produce a cation and a radical:

$$AB^{+\cdot} \rightarrow A^{+} + B^{\cdot}$$

As determined by their chemical stability, the relative proportions of molecular ion and fragment ions are reasonably reproducible. Positive ions are repelled or drawn out of the ionization chamber by an electrical field. The cations are then electrostatically focused and introduced into the mass analyzer.

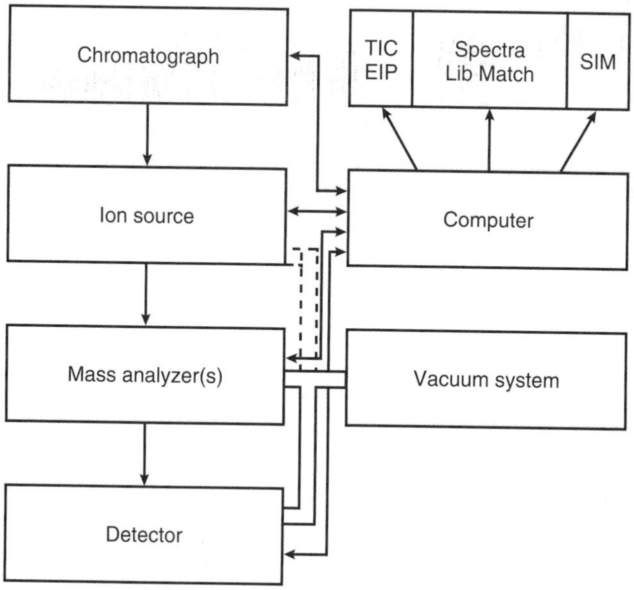

Chromatograph
TIC EIP
Spectra Lib Match
SIM
Ion source
Computer
Mass analyzer(s)
Vacuum system
Detector

Figure 7-3 Block diagram of the components of a chromatograph-mass spectrometer system. The mass analyzer and detector are always under vacuum. The ion source may be under vacuum or under near-atmospheric pressure conditions, depending on the ionization mode. The computer system is an integral part of data acquisition and output.

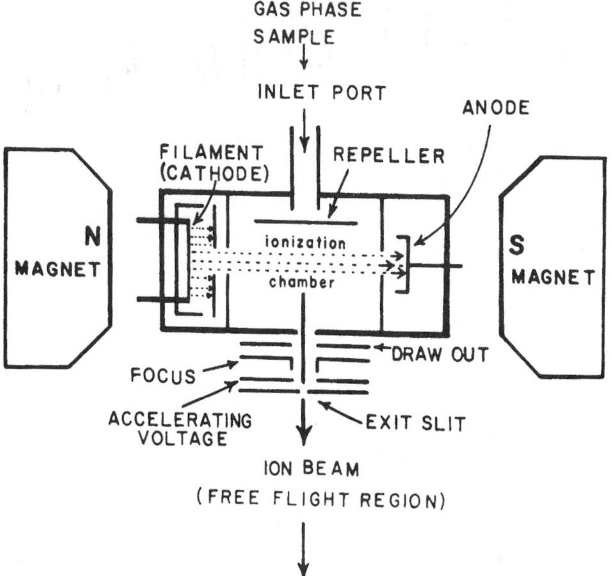

Figure 7-4 Electron impact ion source. The small magnets are used to collimate a dense electron beam, which is drawn from a heated filament placed at a negative potential. The electron beam is positioned in front of a repeller, which is at a slight positive potential compared with the ion source. The repeller sends any positively charged fragment ions toward the opening at the front of the ion source. The accelerating plates strongly attract the positively charged fragment ions.

Chemical Ionization

CI is a "soft" ionization technique in which a proton is transferred to, or abstracted from, a gas phase analyte by a reagent gas molecule. Typical reagent gases are methane, ammonia, isobutane, and water. The reagent gas is bled into a special CI source so the source pressure is increased to about 0.1 torr. An electron beam produces reactive species (such as CH_5^+ for methane). Collisions between the reactive reagent gas and the analyte cause proton and energy transfer. Because the protonated molecule is not highly excited in this process, relatively little fragmentation occurs. This is advantageous for analyte molecular mass determination and for quantification. Negative ion electron capture CI has become popular for quantification of drugs such as benzodiazepines. Negative ion formation occurs when thermalized electrons are captured by an electronegative substituent, such as chlorine or fluorine on the analyte. Thus the number of compounds undergoing negative ionization is small and background signal (noise) is decreased. When applicable, negative ion CI has very low limits of detection. Another use of CI is its application in the quadrupole ion trap (QIT) (discussed later). With a QIT, much lower gas pressures is used because the analyte and the reagent gas are stored for much longer periods of time than in a conventional CI source. This provides a wider range of potential CI reagents. For example, a vial of liquid acetonitrile can be attached to the ion trap and the gas vapor from the solvent used to produce reagent gas ions.

Electrospray Ionization

ESI is a technique in which a sample is ionized at atmospheric pressure before introduction into the mass analyzer.[92,94] The sample, typically an HPLC effluent, is passed through a narrow metal or fused silica capillary to which a 3 to 5 kV charge has been applied (Figure 7-5, *A*). The partial charge separation between the liquid and the capillary results in instability in the liquid that in turn results in the expulsion of a charged droplet series from a Taylor cone, which forms at the tip of the capillary. A coaxial nebulizing gas helps direct the charged droplets toward a counter electrode. The droplets evaporate as they migrate through the atmospheric pressure region, expelling smaller droplets as the charge-to-volume ratio exceeds the Raleigh instability limit. The proton- or ammonium-adduct of the molecule, which may be associated with solvent molecules, is "desolvated" to form "bare" ions, which then pass through a sampling cone and one or more extraction cones (skimmers) before entering the mass analyzer. ESI interfaces are available from all manufacturers of MS detectors, including (1) Agilent Technologies (http://www.agilent.com), (2) Applied Biosystems (http://www.appliedbiosystems.com), (3) Bruker Daltonics (http://www.daltonics.bruker.com), (4) Hitachi (http://www.hitachi.com/), (5) JEOL (http://www.jeol.com/), (6) LECO (http://www.leco.com), (7) Shimadzu (http://www.shimadzu.com), (8) Thermo Finnigan (http://www.thermo.com), (9) Varian (http://www.varianinc.com), and (10) Waters Micromass (http://www.waters.com). JEOL has also introduced a "cold electrospray" interface designed for the analysis of labile compounds.

One unique feature of ESI is the production of multiple charged ions, particularly from peptides and proteins. It is common to observe one charge for every 10 amino acid residues in a protein. For example, because a molecule of mass 20,000 can yield 20 charges, it can be detected at *m/z* 1000 (20,000/20) on a lower resolution and less expensive analyzer. This greatly extends the accessible mass range of such an instrument.

It should be noted that Figure 7-5, being a simplified illustration, shows the probe being directed toward the sampling cone of the mass detector. To enhance performance and minimize contamination of the mass detector, modern hardware configurations have offset the probe and/or the mass detector relative to the sampling cone. This results in the *z-spray* or *orthogonal* configuration employed by instrument manufacturers.

Sonic Spray Ionization

In ESI a high voltage is applied to the capillary. This yields charged droplets that are sprayed from the tip and evaporate to produce ions that enter the MS detector. The size properties of the droplets vary with flow rate, solvent composition, and chemical properties of the compounds being analyzed. An alternate ionization process has been introduced in which coaxial nitrogen gas, traveling at the speed of sound (Mach 1), is used to both create the spray and cause ions to be produced. This technique is known as sonic spray ionization (SSI). As the sonic velocity gas flows over the surface of the mobile phase exiting the capillary, two effects occur. First, droplet fission occurs as a result of shear stress created by the sonic gas flow, yielding fine charged droplets.[36] The charge density of the droplets is then enhanced by application of an external electric field.[35] Second, at sonic velocity, droplet size is at its minimum; this optimizes ionization efficiency. Since neither heating nor high voltage is required in SSI, this technique has been purported to be advantageous when highly polar solvents must be used, or when thermally unstable compounds are analyzed.

Atmospheric Pressure Chemical Ionization

APCI is similar to ESI. It takes place at atmospheric pressure, involves nebulization and desolvation, and uses the same sample and extraction cones as ESI. The major difference lies in the mode of ionization. In APCI no voltage is applied to the inlet capillary. Instead, a separate corona discharge needle,[12] located perpendicular to the capillary, is used to emit a cloud of electrons that ionize compounds after they are converted to the gas phase[37]:

$$CH_3OH + H^+ \rightarrow CH_3OH_2^+$$

$$\text{A (analyte)} + CH_3OH_2^+ \rightarrow AH^+ + CH_3OH$$

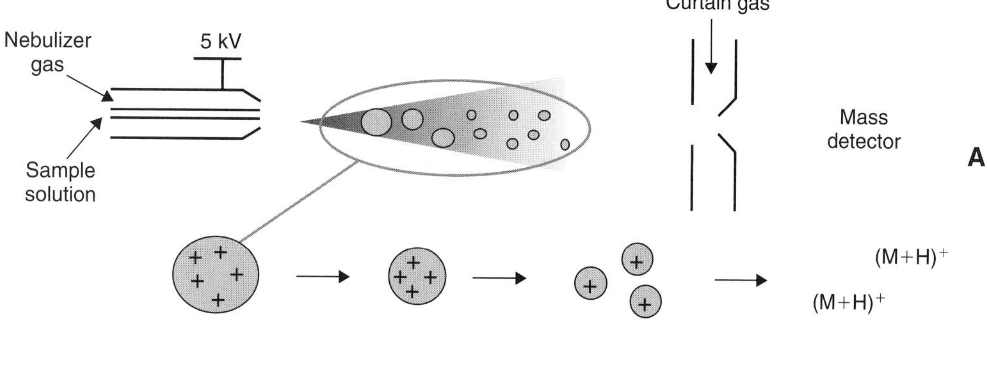

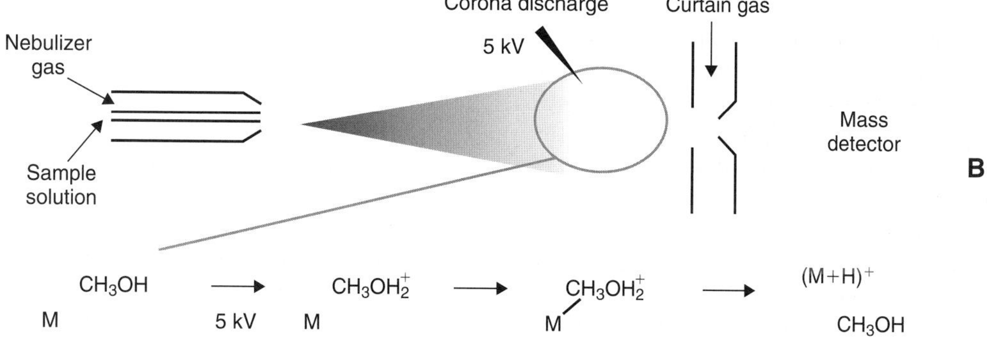

CH3OH M → 5 kV CH3OH2+ M → CH3OH2+ M → (M+H)+ CH3OH

Figure 7-5 Schematics of **(A)** electrospray and **(B)** atmospheric pressure chemical ionization sources. Note the different points where ionization occurs, as described in the text.

or

$$H_2O + H^+ \rightarrow H_3O^+$$

$$\text{A (analyte)} + H_3O^+ \rightarrow AH^+ + H_2O$$

Because eluent molecules (e.g., water, methanol) are present in excess relative to the analytes in the sample, they are predominantly ionized and then act as a reagent gas that reacts secondarily to ionize analyte molecules (Figure 7-5, *B*). Because the products of these secondary reactions may contain clusters of solvent and analyte molecules, either a heated transfer tube or a countercurrent flow of a curtain gas, such as nitrogen, is used to decluster the ions. There is relatively little fragmentation, so much work with APCI has been for quantitative analysis or for tandem MS. As a well-proven interface, APCI sources are available from the major instrument manufacturers (see ESI section above).

Atmospheric Pressure Photoionization

Because of their ionization mechanisms ESI and APCI easily ionize polar compounds, but are less effective at ionizing many nonpolar compounds. APPI is a relatively new ionization technique that provides a complementary approach to ESI or APCI, and which is touted to be more universal across the polarity scale. First introduced by Syagen Technology (http://www.syagen.com), APPI sources are available through several manufacturers, including Agilent, Applied Biosystems, Bruker Daltonics, Thermo Finnigan, and Waters Micromass. The physical configuration of an APPI source is similar to that for APCI, but a photon flux is used instead of a corona discharge needle to generate ions in the gas phase.[74,83,84] The photon source is a krypton discharge lamp with a magnesium fluoride window for transmission of ultraviolet (UV) light, operated at a photon energy of 10 eV. This energy level has been carefully chosen because it is high enough to achieve the ionization potential thresholds for many classes of organic compounds, yet is low enough to be below the ionization thresholds for solvents, such as methanol, acetonitrile and water, and constituents of air. In theory this selective ionization should decrease charge-competition effects, allowing better quantitation and a potential higher dynamic range. The relatively lower ionization energy with APPI also minimizes fragmentation so that molecular ions predominate.[84] In APPI an ionizable dopant, such as toluene or acetone, is often infused coaxially to the nebulizer to provide a source of ions that provide charge or proton transfer to analytes, thus increasing the efficiency of analyte ionization.

Inductively Coupled Plasma

ICP is an atmospheric pressure ionization method. However, unlike most atmospheric pressure ionization methods, which are "soft" (i.e., producing little fragmentation), ICP is the ultimate in "hard" ionization, typically leading to complete atomization of the sample during ionization. Consequently, its primary use is for elemental analysis. In the clinical lab, it is particularly useful for trace metal and heavy metal analysis in tissue or body fluids. ICP is extremely sensitive (e.g., parts per trillion) and is capable of extremely high dynamic ranges. The sample is typically prepared by acid digestion, and the liquid digest is introduced into the ion source via a nebulizer fed by a peristaltic pump. The nebulized sample is transmitted into hot plasma generated at atmospheric pressure by inductively coupling power into the plasma using a high-powered, radio frequency (RF) generator. A small orifice samples the plasma, and ions are transmitted to the mass analyzer through a series of differential pumping stages. The atmospheric sampling apparatus is similar to that of other atmospheric pressure ion sources, such as electrospray, except that the device must withstand the extremely high temperatures generated by the plasma. ICP-MS is comparatively free from most interference. However, some interferences can be extremely troublesome. Most interfering species are small polyatomics formed in the torch via ion-molecule reactions. For example ArO^+ interferes with iron at *m/z* 56. One solution to this problem is the dynamic reaction cell, which consists of a moderate pressure gas placed before the *m/z* analyzer. A reactant gas, such as NH_3, is bled into the reaction cell. The reactant gas reacts with polyatomic interferences and removes them before introduction into the *m/z* analyzer. The dynamic reaction cell is proprietary technology marketed by PE/Sciex (http://www.appliedbiosystems.com; http://www.sciex.com). The Agilent 7500c ICP-MS uses an octopole reaction system to remove the plasma and matrix-based interferences. Other suppliers of ICP-MS instruments include Thermo Finnigan, Thermo Elemental, and Varian.

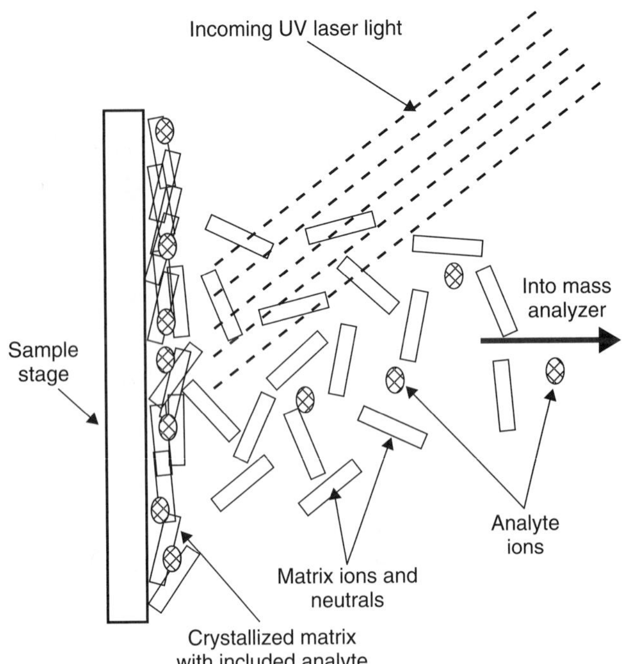

Figure 7-6 A generic view of the process of matrix-assisted laser desorption ionization. Co-crystallized matrix and analyte molecules are irradiated with a UV laser. The laser vaporizes the matrix, producing a plume of matrix ions, analyte ions, and neutrals. Gas-phase ions are directed into a mass analyzer.

Matrix-Assisted Laser Desorption/Ionization

MALDI was originally described in 1987.[43,44] The original work consisted of purely laser desorption/ionization where a sample was placed on a target and, in a combined process, desorbed and ionized so its mass could be measured. Limitations on size and stability of the analyte quickly led to the addition of a matrix to assist in this process. In the current method, the analyte is dissolved in a solution of matrix, a small molecular weight UV-absorbing compound, and this solution is placed on a target that can be introduced into the mass spectrometer. The matrix-to-analyte ratio is generally around 1000 to 1. As the volatile solvents evaporate, the matrix compound crystallizes and incorporates analyte molecules. Figure 7-6 illustrates the use of a UV laser to vaporize small amounts of matrix and analyte into a plume of ions that can be directed into a mass analyzer. MALDI has most classically been coupled with a time of flight (TOF) mass analyzer because it produces discrete, pulsed-ion packets, and because analysis by mass alone generally relies on the resolution and mass accuracy found in the TOF analyzer.

Atmospheric Pressure Matrix-Assisted Laser Desorption/Ionization

The MALDI source has been coupled to other mass analyzers, but these combinations have gained little popularity, generally because the MALDI source is under vacuum and most other sources are at atmosphere, and changing sources is not as straightforward as advertised. In 2000 an ion source was introduced[53] that produces ions in a manner similar to a traditional MALDI ion source but does so at atmospheric pressure (AP-MALDI).[66] The major advantage of this configuration is the ability to switch sources easily while coupling the inherent speed and multiple sample wells of traditional MALDI with mass analyzers capable of easily generating sequence information, such as ion trap or quadrupole TOF systems. The added ability to produce fragmentation overcomes a serious problem in eliminating ambiguous (or no) identifications obtained with protein mass fingerprinting (PMF). One current disadvantage is the poor fragmentation of the singly charged ions produced in the MALDI source, compared with the multiply charged ion produced in an electrospray source. The difference is not great for spectral confirmation but increases dramatically for de novo spectral interpretation. In collaboration with Mass Tech, Inc., AP-MALDI sources have been adapted to the Agilent LC/MSD, Bruker Esquire and Bio-TOF, Thermo Finnigan LCQ, and Waters Micromass Q-Tof instruments.

Surface-Enhanced Laser Desorption/Ionization

A potential change in the area of MALDI involves the development of Surface-Enhanced Laser Desorption Ionization (SELDI).[40,41,64] This technique, developed by Ciphergen Biosystems (http://www.ciphergen.com/), combines affinity purification and MALDI on the target. The most common setup involves producing a MALDI target surface modified with some type of affinity capture property (hydrophobic, ionic, immobilized metal affinity chromatography [IMAC], DNA, antibody, etc). The sample of interest, often in a complex mixture such as serum, is exposed to one or more of these affinity surfaces, and certain analytes will preferentially bind. The surface is washed to remove as much nonspecific binding as possible, and a matrix is added to enhance desorption and/or ionization. The target can then be analyzed by TOF or another method of choice. The interaction can be very specific, such as an antibody, and purify essentially one protein, or it can be specific for a class of compounds, for example, phosphorylated or glycosylated species. The major advantage is low sample loss as purification and analysis occur on the same surface.

Fast Atom Bombardment

Several techniques to produce ions from high molecular weight polymers have been developed. FAB produces ions when a high-velocity beam of atoms impacts the surface of a liquid containing the analyte(s). Protonization is thought to occur when analytes on the surface of vaporized droplets are transferred to the gas state. Since the bombardment occurs in high vacuum, the liquid used (e.g., glycerol) must have a high boiling point. FAB is used to ionize proteins and smaller molecules. Continuous flow FAB[10,11] allows automated sequential introduction of samples. It is often used in conjunction with tandem MS for the diagnosis of short-chain fatty acid acylcarnitine deficiencies from newborn blood spots.

Vacuum System

Ion separation in any of the mass analyzers requires that the ions do not collide with any other molecules during their interaction with the magnetic or electric fields. This requires the use of a vacuum from 10^{-3} to 10^{-9} torr, depending on mass analyzer type. The length of the ion path in the analyzer must be less than the mean free path length, unless collisions play a role in mass analysis. Fourier transform ion cyclotron resonance (FT-ICR), which will be discussed later, requires the lowest pressure (10^{-9} torr), and the QIT tolerates the highest pressure (10^{-3} torr). The mass analyzer is usually maintained at an elevated temperature (150 °C to 250 °C) to prevent gas molecules or organic compounds from adsorbing to the inner surfaces of the vacuum chamber. Routine quality assurance checks for vacuum leaks should include an evaluation of air and water in the mass analyzer.

Efficient high-vacuum pumps generally do not operate well near atmospheric pressure. Thus the vacuum system must have a mechanical vacuum pump to evacuate the system to a pressure where the high-vacuum pumps are effective. Mechanical pumps require routine maintenance, such as ballasting and replacing the pump oil. The diffusion pump is the least expensive and most reliable high-vacuum pump. Turbomolecular pumps and cryopumps are also used on mass analyzers. The high-vacuum pumps also require routine maintenance for optimal operation. A key consideration in construction of the vacuum system is pumping speed. The ability of the pump to maintain the vacuum by removing any gas (or solvent vapor) that enters the system determines the flow rate of gas or liquid that is introduced into the mass spectrometer. In general, higher pump capacities are associated with lower detection limits because noise arising from the gas background is reduced.

Mass Analyzers, Ion Detectors, and Tandem Mass Spectrometers

As mentioned earlier, "mass spectrometry" is a somewhat of a misnomer because mass spectrometers do not measure molecular mass, but rather they measure mass-to-charge ratio (m/z). This fact is fundamental to the physical operating principles of mass spectrometers and consequently impacts all aspects of instrumentation design, operation, and interpretation of results. The conventional definition of m/z creates a problem because it is defined as a dimensionless quantity,[73] which is not consistent with the equations of ion motion in the presence of electric and magnetic fields. These equations require units of mass divided by charge. Therefore in this section a slightly nonstandard definition of m/z will be used in which it has dimensions of mass divided by charge. Under this definition the numerical value of m/z is identical to the usual convention, provided that m is specified in daltons and z is specified in elementary charges. However, in actual calculations of ion motion it is best to convert these quantities to meter/kilogram/second (MKS) units to prevent mixing macroscopic and microscopic units.

The unit of m/z is sometimes referred to as the *Thomson* (Th) in honor of one of the pioneers of MS.[18,23] This notation distinguishes the quantity actually measured by mass spectrometers (m/z) from the quantity somewhat loosely (and incorrectly) associated with MS (mass), which is usually expressed as daltons, Da, or equivalently as unified atomic mass units, u.

General Classes of Mass Spectrometers

Mass spectrometers are broadly classified into two groups, beam-type instruments and trapping-type instruments. In a beam-type instrument, the ions make one pass through the instrument and then strike the detector, where they are destructively detected. The entire process, from the time an ion enters the analyzer until the time it is detected, generally takes microseconds to milliseconds. In a trapping-type analyzer ions are held in a spatially confined region of space by a combination of magnetic, and/or electrostatic, and/or RF electrical fields. The trapping fields are manipulated in ways that allow m/z measurements to be performed. Trapping times may range from a fraction of a second to minutes, though most clinical applications are at the low end of this range. Detection of the ions in a trapping-type instrument may be destructive or nondestructive, depending on the specific type of mass spectrometer used. Additional discussions of mass analyzers, tandem mass spectrometers, and ion detectors are available.[24,80]

Beam-Type Designs

The three main beam-type mass spectrometer designs are quadrupole, magnetic sector, and TOF. It is convenient to categorize beam-type instruments into two broad categories, those that produce a mass spectrum by scanning the *m/z* range over a period of time (quadrupole and magnetic sector) and those that acquire successive instantaneous snapshots of the mass spectrum (TOF). This categorization is not hard and fast. Certain instrument designs can be adapted to either scanning or nonscanning operation. Nevertheless, the categorization is a useful one because it covers the majority of instruments currently available, and because scanning and nonscanning instruments are adapted to different optimal usages.

Quadrupole. Quadrupole mass spectrometers, sometimes known as quadrupole mass filters (QMF), are currently the most widely used mass spectrometers, having displaced magnetic sector mass spectrometers as the standard instrument. Although these instruments lag behind magnetic sector instruments in terms of sensitivity, upper mass range, resolution, and mass accuracy, they offer an attractive and practical mix of features that accounts for their popularity, including ease of use, flexibility, adequate performance for most applications, relatively low cost, noncritical site requirements, and highly developed software systems.

A quadrupole mass spectrometer consists of four parallel electrically conductive rods arranged in a square array (Figure 7-7). The four rods form a long channel through which the ion beam passes. The beam enters near the axis at one end of the array, passes through the array in a direction generally parallel to the axis, and exits the far end of the array. The ion beam entering the quadrupole array may contain a mixture of ions of various *m/z* values, but only ions of a very narrow *m/z* range (typically $\Delta m/z \approx 1$) are successfully transported through the device to reach the detector. Ions outside this narrow range are ejected radially. The $\Delta m/z$ range represents a passband, analogous to the passband of an interference filter in optics (see Chapter 3), which is why quadrupole mass spectrometers are often referred to as "mass filters" rather than "mass spectrometers."

Quadrupole mass spectrometers rely on a superposition of RF and direct current (DC) potentials applied to the quadrupole rods. Considering first the DC component, DC voltages are applied to the electrodes in a quadrupolar pattern. For example, a positive DC potential is applied to electrodes 1 and 3, as indicated in Figure 7-8, and an equivalent negative DC potential is applied to electrodes 2 and 4. The DC potentials are relatively small, of the order of a few volts. Superimposed on the DC potentials are RF potentials, also applied in a quadrupolar fashion. The RF potentials range up to the kilovolt range, and the frequency is of the order of 1 MHz. The frequency is typically fixed, which will be considered the case throughout this discussion, though variable frequency operation is possible.

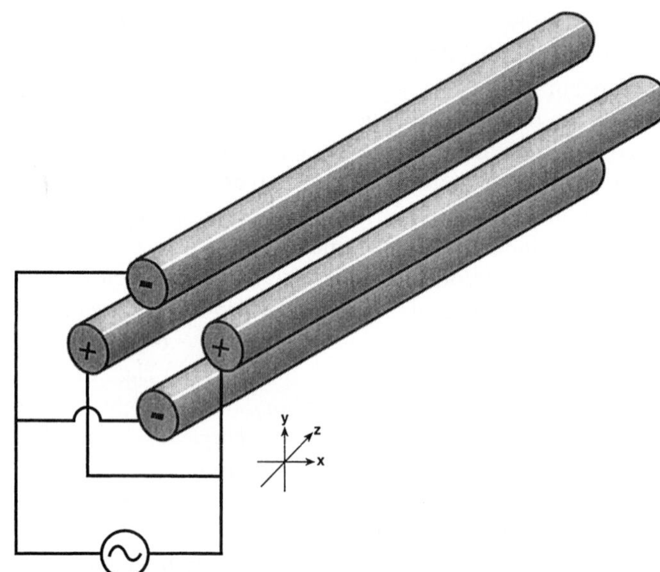

Figure 7-7 Diagram of quadrupole mass filter, including the RF part of the voltages applied to the quadrupole rods.

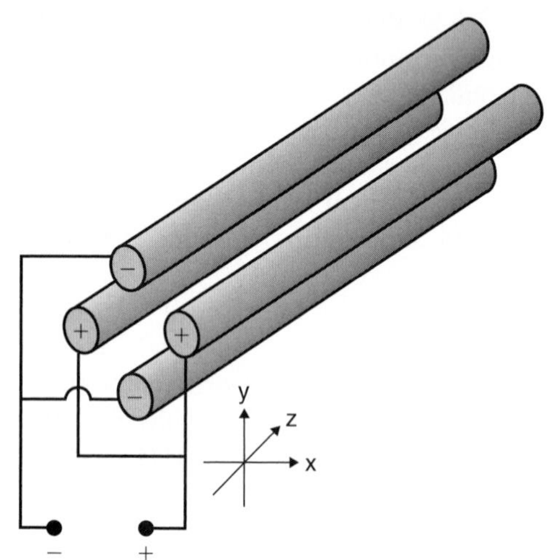

Figure 7-8 DC voltages applied to quadrupole rod assembly.

The device may be operated in either a SIM mode or a scanning mode. In SIM mode, both the DC and RF voltages are fixed. Consequently, both the center of the passband and the width of the passband are fixed. For example, the mass spectrometer may be set to pass ions of *m/z* 363 ± 0.5. Both the center *m/z* and the $\Delta m/z$ can be adjusted by the appropriate choice of DC and RF.

In the scanning mode of operation, the RF and/or DC voltages are continuously varied to scan a range of *m/z* values. As with SIM mode, the $\Delta m/z$ is also determined by the RF and DC voltages. Usually the scan function is designed to maintain a constant $\Delta m/z$ across the full *m/z* range. Thus the resolution increases as *m/z* increases. The value of $\Delta m/z$ is frequently chosen in the range 0.5 to 0.7 to resolve isotopic peaks across the full *m/z* range.

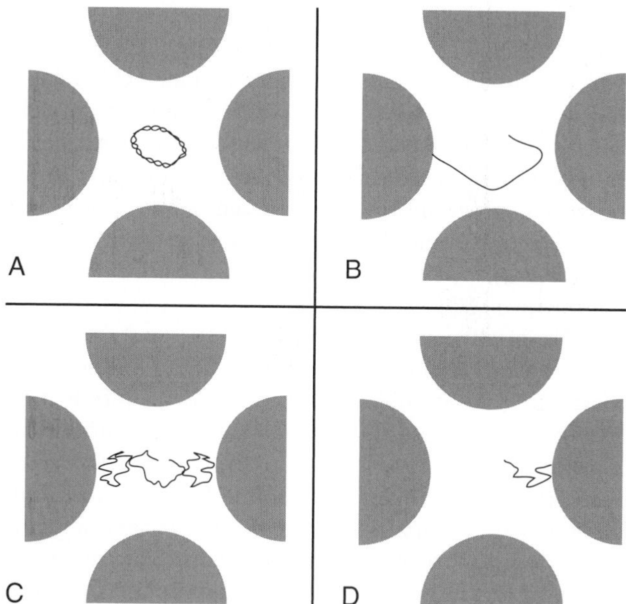

Figure 7-9 Ion trajectories showing confinement and ejection in quadrupole mass filters. **A,** Ion confinement by RF-only field. **B,** Ion ejection by RF-only field. **C,** Ion confinement with a combination of RF and DC fields. **D,** Ion ejection with a combination of RF and DC fields. All trajectories were simulated using Simion.[20]

The physical principles underlying the operation of a quadrupole mass spectrometer require the solving of a complicated differential equation, the Mathieu equation.[22] In operation when an ion is subjected to a quadrupolar RF field, its trajectory can be described qualitatively as a combination of fast and slow oscillatory motions. For descriptive purposes, the fast component will be ignored here and the slow component emphasized, which oscillates about the quadrupolar axis and resembles the motion of a particle in a fictitious harmonic "pseudopotential." The frequency of this oscillation is sometimes called the *secular frequency.*

The "effective force" associated with the pseudopotential points inward toward the quadrupolar axis and is proportional to the distance from the axis. It therefore acts as a confining force, preventing ions from being ejected radially from the quadrupolar assembly. Figure 7-9, *A* shows an example of an ion confined by an RF-only quadrupole. Below a certain *m/z* cutoff frequency (which depends on the frequency and amplitude of the RF field) ions are ejected rather than confined. Figure 7-9, *B* shows an example of an ion ejected by an RF-only quadrupolar field. This establishes the low mass cutoff for the *m/z* pass band. The effective confining force is strongest just above the low *m/z* cutoff, and then decreases asymptotically toward zero at high *m/z.*

The DC part of the quadrupolar potential is independent of *m/z.* Positive ions are attracted toward the negative poles. Negative ions are attracted toward the positive poles. Attraction increases as the distance from the quadrupolar axis increases. Since a quadrupolar DC potential always has both negative and positive poles, the quadrupolar DC potential always contributes to ejection in at least one direction. Whether ejection of an ion of a particular *m/z* actually occurs depends on whether the ejecting force caused by the quadrupolar DC potential overcomes the effective confining force caused by the RF potential. Above a certain *m/z* value the DC part dominates, and ions are ejected radially from the device. This establishes an upper *m/z* limit for ion transmission. Figures 7-9, *C* and *D* show examples of ion trajectories under the influence of combined RF-DC fields, one being confined and the other being ejected. Trajectories in Figure 7-9 were calculated using the Simion ion optics computer program.[20]

A rigorous description of low- and high-mass cutoffs is found in so-called stability diagrams, which graphically describe the lower and upper *m/z* cutoffs of a quadrupole mass spectrometer in terms of parameters related to voltages, frequencies, and *m/z.* An earlier edition of this book presents an example of a stability diagram. However, to fully understand the meaning of the stability diagram, one must delve more deeply into a mathematical description than can be accommodated here.

A large number of manufacturers make numerous quadrupole mass spectrometer models. A few prominent companies among the many in the field include Agilent, Thermo Finnigan, Waters Micromass, and Applied Biosystems/MDS Sciex. Most QMFs are intended primarily for use with separations, such as GC or LC. Nearly any ion source imaginable is marketed with one quadrupole mass spectrometer or another, including EI, ESI, APCI, ICP, and others.

The combination of lower and upper *m/z* limits establishes a passband ($\Delta m/z$), and ultimately a resolution $[(m/z)/(\Delta m/z)]$. Generally quadrupole instruments are limited to a resolution of several thousand, which is sufficient to achieve isotopic resolution for singly charged ions of *m/z* as high as several thousand. However, technical advances have enabled quadrupole mass spectrometers to achieve resolutions exceeding 10,000. The Thermo Finnigan TSQ Quantum Ultra AM is an example of such an instrument. The benefits of high resolution include reduction of interferences. In addition, high resolution, combined with high accuracy electronics, has enabled the measurement of exact masses using quadrupole instruments. Exact mass measurements are useful for confirmation of a chemical formula.

Magnetic Sectors. Because magnetic sector mass spectrometers are rarely used in the clinical laboratory and are rapidly losing popularity among mass spectrometrists generally, they will not be described in detail here. For a good introduction to magnetic sector technology, refer to the previous edition of this book. It should be noted, however, that these classic mass spectrometers are easy to understand (given a basic understanding of physics), are versatile, reliable, highly sensitive, and in their "double focusing" variation are capable of very high *m/z* resolution and mass accuracy. However, they are typically expensive, large, and heavy. In addition, they have the reputation of being difficult to use. Consequently, other instruments have largely displaced magnetic sector mass spectrometers. However, there are two small bench top double focusing magnetic sector mass spectrometers that are potentially interesting to clinical chemists, the LCmate and the GCmate, both from JEOL.

Time of Flight. TOF mass spectrometry (TOF-MS) is a nonscanning technique where a full mass spectrum is acquired as a snapshot rather than sweeping through a sequential series of *m/z* values while sampling the sample. In recent years, TOF mass spectrometers have become very popular. They have a number of advantages, including a nearly unlimited *m/z* range, high acquisition speed, high mass accuracy, moderately high resolution, high sensitivity, and reasonable cost. They are also well adapted to pulsed ionization sources, which is an advantage in some applications, particularly with MALDI and related techniques.

A significant advantage of modern TOF mass spectrometers is that some of them produce exact mass measurements, typically with low parts per million (ppm) accuracy. This allows TOF measurements to confirm the molecular formula of a compound. Unlike magnetic sector instruments, which are also capable of exact mass measurements, exact mass measurements by TOF are practical in routine chromatography experiments and are therefore potentially useful to the clinical chemist.

TOF mass spectrometers are conceptually simple to understand as they are based on the fact that a lighter ion travels faster than a heavier ion, provided that both have the same kinetic energy. Figure 7-10 presents a simplified conceptual diagram of a TOF mass spectrometer. It resembles a long pipe. Ions are created or injected at the source end of the device and are then accelerated by a potential of several kilovolts. They travel down the flight tube and strike the detector at the far end of the flight tube. The time it takes to traverse the tube is known as the flight time, which is related to the mass-to-charge ratio of the ion.

The flight time for an ion of mass m and kinetic energy E to travel a distance L in a region free of electric fields is given by:

$$t = L\left(\frac{m}{2E}\right)^{1/2} \quad (1)$$

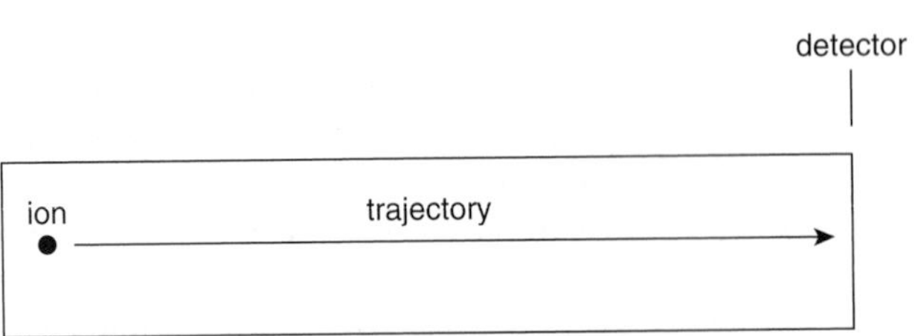

Figure 7-10 Diagram of simplified time of flight mass spectrometer.

A sample calculation for an ion of molecular weight 200 Da (3.32×10^{-25} kg) with a kinetic energy of 10 keV (1.60×10^{-15} J), traveling through a distance of 1 m, yields a flight time of 10.18 microseconds, and an ion of molecular weight 201 takes just 25 nanoseconds longer. To accurately capture such fleeting signals, the data recording system must operate on a ~1 nanosecond time scale. Recent advances in signal processing electronics have made this practical at relatively modest cost, and this has been a major factor in the rise in popularity of TOF-MS.

TOF is inherently a pulsed technique, and it couples readily to pulsed ionization methods, with MALDI being the most common example. A variety of MALDI-TOF mass spectrometers are offered by vendors. Examples include the Waters Micromass MALDI-LR, the Voyager-DE PRO Biospectrometry Workstation from Applied Biosystems (separate from Applied Biosystems/MDS Sciex), and the ultraflex from Bruker Daltonics. MALDI-TOF makes its biggest impact in the area of protein and peptide identification and is presently little used for quantitative analysis because the shot-to-shot variation of signal amplitude makes quantitation difficult.

Unlike many mass spectrometers, which allow the use of several different ionization methods on the same instrument, MALDI-TOF instruments are generally single purpose, being devoted exclusively to MALDI. In practice, EI and ESI methods are also used with TOF mass spectrometers. However, the continuous nature of these sources causes a natural mismatch to TOF-MS, which is a pulsed technique. The traditional way to couple a continuous ion source to a TOF-MS is to dynamically deflect the ion beam past a narrow slit, thus generating a pulsed ion beam at the exit side of the slit.[9] However, this results in low sensitivity as more than 99% of the ion beam is discarded.

To decrease this loss in sensitivity, the beam is injected orthogonal to the axis of the TOF-MS.[21,54,55,78,79] During the injection period the acceleration voltage is turned off. Once the injection region is filled with the traversing beam, the acceleration voltage is suddenly turned on, and the TOF timing cycle starts. The process is cycled repeatedly. The overall duty cycle for this method can be much more than 10%, a vast improvement over the traditional method. For full spectrum sensitivity with continuous ion sources, orthogonal injection TOF mass spectrometers are generally considered the most sensitive of all mass spectrometers. However, for the monitoring of a single *m/z* rather than a full mass spectrum, the use of SIM mode with a quadrupole MS provides superior sensitivity.

The conceptual simplicity of TOF-MS disappears when one considers actual instrumentation design. A good understanding of this issue is important in the selection and use of TOF mass spectrometers because there is a good deal of confusion about the true significance of terms like "linear," "reflectron," "orthogonal acceleration," "delayed extraction," and so forth. This may lead to poor selection and use of instruments.

Resolution is of primary concern. Assumptions underlying equation (1) are that ions all have the same kinetic energy, and that they are never subjected to electric fields. In practice neither assumption holds.

The kinetic energy, E, is imparted to the ion beam primarily via acceleration through an electric field. Each ion starts at a different point in the voltage gradient, and hence each ion acquires a different kinetic energy, resulting in a spread of velocities and flight times as inferred from equation (1). This ultimately leads to a loss of resolution. Early in the development of TOF-MS, Wiley and McLaren[93] showed that proper design of the acceleration field profile produces a compensating effect. In the Wiley-McLaren design, ions starting at the higher end of the potential gradient spend more time in the acceleration region than those starting at the lower end. This extra time compensates for the fact that the higher energy ions spend less time traveling through the field-free region. Wiley-McLaren instruments are classed as "linear" TOF mass spectrometers because ion motion is substantially unidirectional from source to detector.

Thermal motion provides another source of kinetic energy variation. Typical thermal energies are of the order of 0.025 eV, whereas a typical acceleration potential of a TOF mass spectrometer is 5000 V. The direct effect of a variation of 0.025 eV out of 5000 produces negligible effect on equation (1). Instead the resolution degradation is primarily a result of the so-called turnaround time, which occurs during the initial part of the flight time when ions are being accelerated up to full flight energy. Consider two ions with 0.025 eV of kinetic energy. In the acceleration region of the instrument one ion initially travels down the potential gradient (in the direction of the detector), and the other travels up the potential gradient. It takes notable time to turn the trajectory of the second ion around so it is traveling down the potential gradient, and this results in a notable loss of resolution for the instrument, limiting simple TOF mass spectrometers to a resolution of a few hundred.

There are two main approaches to solving the turnaround time problem. One is to extend the flight time of the ions so that the turnaround time is a smaller percentage of the total time, and the second is to inject ions into the instrument in a direction orthogonal to the flight tube of the TOF mass spectrometer. The first approach, extending the flight time, cannot be done by simply lengthening the field-free region. To do so would upset the fine balance inherent in the Wiley-McLaren design. Scaling up the dimension of the complete instrument without a change of basic configuration is also ineffective because the turnaround time increases with the scale of the instrument. What is required is to lengthen the flight path without introducing additional dispersion to the flight time. This is done using a device known as a "reflectron."[60] A reflectron consists of a length of field-free region, followed by an ion reflector. The reflector consists of a potential gradient that acts as an ion mirror. High-energy ions penetrate farther into the mirror and spend greater time in the mirror than low-energy ions. This compensates for the fact that high-energy ions spend less time traversing the field-free region.

Interestingly, reflectrons and Wiley-McLaren designs are similar from the point of view of their ion optics designs. Both use the same electric field profiles but differ in the type of resolution-degrading effect for which they are corrected. Wiley-McLaren designs are corrected for changes in start positions of ions (related to initial ion potential energy), and reflectrons are corrected for changes in the kinetic energy of ions. If a reflectron is added to a Wiley-McLaren section, the total flight time is extended without increasing the turnaround time, and the resolution increases. This is particularly effective if the Wiley-McLaren section is short and the reflectron section is long, because this design approach minimizes turnaround time.

The second approach to solving the turnaround time problem is to inject ions into the instrument in a orthogonal direction to the flight tube of the instrument. This was already discussed in relation to the interfacing of continuous ion sources to TOF mass spectrometers, and it was shown that this method results in an increase in sensitivity. By a fortunate coincidence, the method also produces an increase in resolution. This method relies on the fact that ions injected in a direction nearly perpendicular to the flight tube have a very small velocity component in the direction of the flight tube. Hence, the turnaround time is negligible. This allows even a Wiley-McLaren design to achieve a resolution of several thousand. An example of this approach is the Jaguar mass spectrometer marketed by LECO, which routinely operates at a resolution of 2500. Jaguar is based on an improved Wiley-McLaren design somewhat whimsically referred to as an "inverted perfectron."[67,75] Thus even a linear TOF-MS can be capable of quite good resolution if it is properly designed, and for many applications a reflectron may not be necessary.

Most TOF mass spectrometers used today with continuous-ion sources combine all three resolution-enhancing techniques. They use orthogonal injection into a short Wiley-McLaren stage, followed by a reflectron stage. A well-designed instrument of this type is capable of resolution well in excess of 5000, and resolution exceeding 20,000 has been reported in some cases. The Waters Micromass LCT, the Waters Micromass GCT, the Bruker Daltonics BioTOF II, the Agilent LC/MSD TOF, and the JEOL AccuTOF are typical examples of modern high performance reflectron TOFs interfaced to continuous-ion sources.

The resolution-degrading effects of variable kinetic energy also appear in TOF mass spectrometers using pulsed ion sources, such as MALDI and SELDI. Ion production in MALDI involves ejection of ions from a solid matrix as a result of a laser pulse. Ions are ejected with a distribution of kinetic energies, and this degrades the resolution available in a simple linear MALDI instrument. One technique for increasing resolution is to delay the application of acceleration voltage after application of the ion-forming laser pulse.

This is sometimes referred to as delayed extraction. A second technique is to use a reflectron. More recently, orthogonal introduction of ions has been introduced, in analogy to the orthogonal introduction of ions discussed above. The prOTOF 2000 marketed by Perkin Elmer Sciex is an instrument using orthogonal introduction. The prOTOF 2000 also uses collisional cooling in the interface between ion source and mass analyzer.

The technical features of TOF-MS lead to several operational advantages. TOF-MS is extremely fast. The fundamental repetition rate of most TOF-MS instruments is 5000 spectra/s or greater. This is far too fast for most applications, but signal averaging electronics allow the TOF instrument to be cycled at full speed (greater than or equal to 5000 spectra/s), while storing spectra at a lower rate (1 to 500 spectra/s). The high speed of TOF-MS also allows it to be interfaced to high-speed separations. For example, a TOF-MS capable of storing 100 spectra/s could easily handle chromatographic peak widths of 0.1 second. The Jaguar is an example of a high-speed, LC-capable instrument (100 spectra/s), and the Pegasus, also marketed by LECO, is a high-speed, GC-capable instrument (500 spectra/s).

TOF-MS is not only fast, but it is also a nonscanning technique. Each mass spectrum is an instantaneous snap-shot of the sample composition. This simplifies the use of MS as a chromatographic detector, because it eliminates peak skew. Peak skew is a distortion of mass spectra from scanning instruments when sample composition is dynamically changing. For example, assume that the mass spectrum is being scanned from low to high, and that it is monitoring the elution of a chromatographic peak. On the leading edge of the peak, the intensities at the high-mass end of the mass spectrum will be exaggerated, and on the trailing edge of the chromatograph the intensities of the low-mass end of the mass spectrum are exaggerated. By contrast the spectrum from a TOF-MS is undistorted, regardless of what part of the chromatographic peak is being sampled.

The lack of peak skew and high acquisition speed also facilitate the ability to mathematically deconvolute overlapping chromatograms. This technique attempts to resolve compounds whose chromatographic bands are highly overlapped. It requires that the compounds to be resolved have spectra that are not identical, though spectra can be quite similar. It also requires that the compounds are not perfectly co-eluting, though their chromatograms can be highly overlapped.

Use of deconvolution is advantageous when (1) there are many samples across the chromatographic peak, (2) there is no skewing of the spectra across the chromatographic peak, (3) full mass spectra are used, and (4) the signal-to-noise ratio is high. Of all mass spectrometer technologies available today, TOF-MS best fulfils all these requirements. AMDIS is freely available software for performing this kind of deconvolution,[59] and several instrument vendors also offer proprietary software for performing deconvolution. For example, the Pegasus from LECO, the TEMPUS from Thermo Finnigan, and the GCT from Waters Micromass all have deconvolution software available for their data systems. These deconvolution strategies are especially successful with very high speed GC-MS methods and show great potential for clinical applications as throughput and turnaround time become ever more important.

Another area where TOF-MS has an advantage is in high-mass analysis where its mass range is nearly unlimited. In MALDI-TOF, for example, it is not unusual to detect proteins with molecular weights exceeding 100,000. The ability for high-mass analysis is expected to increase in importance as clinical laboratories embrace proteomic-based diagnostic methods.

Trapping-Mass Spectrometers

In contrast to beam-type designs, these mass spectrometers are based on the trapping of ions to capture and hold ions for an extended amount of time in a small region of space. Trapping times vary from a fraction of a second to minutes. Unlike beam-type instruments, the division between scanning and nonscanning instruments has less meaning for ion-trapping instruments. The main practical difference between scanning and nonscanning instruments relates to peak skew, as discussed in the section on TOF. In terms of producing skewed spectra, trapping devices are more similar to nonscanning instruments, such as TOF (no skew) than to scanning instruments. This is because the sample is captured in an instant and then analyzed at leisure. Because the sample is captured in an instant there is no skewing of the spectra, regardless of whether the *m/z* analysis is performed by a scanning procedure or a nonscanning procedure.

Traditionally, ion traps have been divided into three classes: QIT, which rely on RF fields to provide ion trapping; a linear ion trap, which is closely related to the QIT in its operating principles; and ion cyclotron resonance (ICR) mass spectrometers, which rely on a combination of magnetic fields and electrostatic fields for trapping.

Quadrupole Ion Trap. QITs are primarily used as GC or HPLC detectors. They are relatively compact, inexpensive, and versatile instruments, excellent for exploratory studies, structural characterization, and sample identification. They are also used for quantitative analysis, though quantitative analysis is not the best use for these devices.

The operation of the QIT is based on the same physical principle as the quadrupole mass spectrometer described above. Both devices make use of the ability of RF fields to confine ions. However, the RF field of an ion trap is designed to trap ions in three dimensions rather than to allow the ions to pass through as in a QMF, which confines ions in only two dimensions. This difference has a significant impact on the operation and limitations of the QIT. The physical arrangement of a QIT is different from that of a QMF. If an imaginary axis is drawn through the *y*-axis of the quadrupole rods, and the rods are rotated around the axis, a solid ring with a hyperbolic inner surface results from the *x*-axis pair of rods.

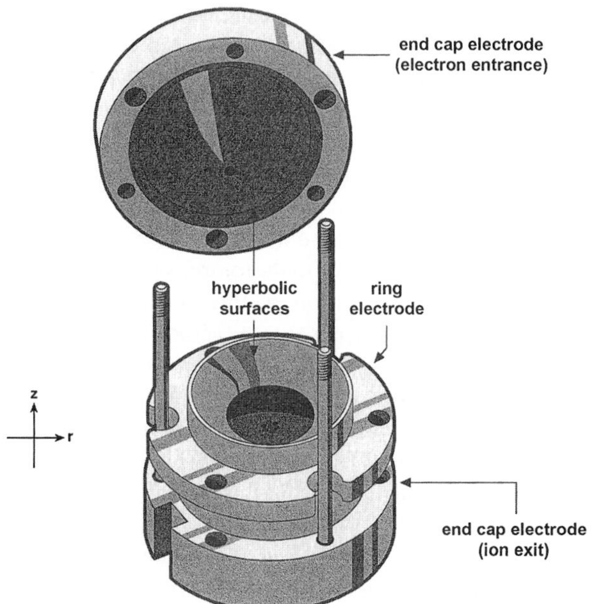

Figure 7-11 Diagram of quadrupole ion trap.

The two y-axis rods form two solid endcaps. The description of the fields within the electrodes must now include a radial component and an axial (between the endcaps) component. This slightly changes the precise conditions required for ion confinement when compared with a QMF, though the qualitative description of ion confinement discussed above is still valid.

A diagram of an ion trap mass spectrometer is given in Figure 7-11. The trap is quite small, of the order of a few centimeters in length. The trapping of ions, by itself, would be little more than an oddity of physics were it not for the fact that ions within the trap can be manipulated in interesting ways (mainly to dissociate them into characteristic fragments) and ejected in a manner to generate a mass spectrum.

Although QITs and QMFs were described at approximately the same time, the QMF initially achieved greater popularity as an analytical device. Two major discoveries changed the usage of the QIT. First, it was found that inclusion in the trap of a higher pressure (10^{-3} torr) of low molecular weight gas improved mass resolution and sensitivity. Second, the development of the mass-selective ejection, or mass-instability scan function, improved QIT scanning. With no DC voltage (i.e., along the x-axis) and a low RF voltage, ions of all m/z are stored in the QIT field. By increasing the RF voltage, ions of increasing m/z become axially unstable and leave the QIT sequentially by m/z. The ions leaving the QIT through one endcap are detected by an external electron multiplier. An additional improvement to the sensitivity of the QIT was the application of an axial modulation waveform to the endcap electrodes. This oscillating voltage improved the efficiency of ion ejection from the trap and improved mass resolution. All of these features and automatic gain control have been incorporated into the Thermo Finnigan PolarisQ GC/MS and the Varian 2000 series GC/MS systems.

In addition to the oscillating voltage mode of operation, the QIT is capable of operation in other modes. For example, the QIT can also be operated in a mass-selective storage mode. This mode of operation is similar to the QMF and involves selecting RF and DC conditions such that only ions of one mass are stored in the QIT at any time.

When interfaced with a gas chromatograph, confinement of all the ions and neutrals emerging from the GC column in the QIT results in two problems. First, the ions in the trap repel each other, disturbing the electrical field generated by the electrodes. This is called *space charge* and results in mass misassignments and a reduced dynamic range. Automatic gain control was introduced to resolve the mass accuracy problem. It monitors the number of ions in the trap in a prescan, then adjusts ionization time for the analytical scan so a targeted number of ions is formed. The dynamic range of QIT nevertheless remains inferior to a QMF, and for many applications, the QMF remains the better instrument for quantitative analysis.

The second problem is that ion-ion or ion-neutral reactions can occur. Reactions (e.g., proton transfer) result in high abundance of protonated molecular ions in the mass spectrum. Thus QIT can be disadvantageous for determining chemical composition in manual spectral interpretation, because the presence of the $(M + 1)^+$ ion tends to confuse the interpretation. Library spectral matching, however, is not affected if the spectral matching algorithm reflects the unique features of the QIT spectrum. An external ionization source with ion injection into the QIT is an alternative solution, because only ions are present in the trap (i.e., neutral analyte molecules that could participate in ion-molecule reactions are not present). The Thermo Finnigan PolarisQ GC/MS is an example of such an instrument.

For ion traps interfaced to HPLC via ESI, external sources are absolutely essential because the electrospray process cannot be carried out inside the trap. The Thermo Finnigan LCQ series ion traps and the Bruker Daltonics Esquire are examples of such instruments.

The storage capabilities of the QIT also change the practical aspects of monitoring selected ions. Because ions do not transiently pass through the QIT, as they do in a QMF, there is no opportunity to focus one ion on the detector and accumulate signal for a specified period of time (dwell time). Instead, the storage capabilities of the QIT can be used to increase the numbers of specific ions in the trap while ejecting unwanted ions. This is known as selected ion storage (SIS). Ions of different mass oscillate radially and axially at a specific frequency, called the *secular frequency,* which depends on the QIT geometry, the RF voltage, and RF frequency. By applying a voltage to the endcap electrodes at the same frequency as the secular frequency, ions of that mass efficiently absorb energy. They also become energetic enough to escape the trapping field. Selective ejection of unwanted ions is achieved by using various combinations of waveforms applied to the endcaps or a combination of waveforms with RF voltage changes on the ring electrode. Basically, any voltage change combination that keeps the ion of interest within its stability envelope while making all other ion trajectories unstable can be used. This diversity, however, makes comparison of SIS techniques difficult. Desired ions stored in the QIT are ejected by using the mass-instability scan function.

The ability to apply customized waveforms to the QIT, together with the fact that ions are trapped and therefore can be subjected to different treatment over a period of time, makes the QIT one of the most versatile of mass spectrometers, rivaled only by the ICR mass spectrometer. This is most strongly evident in tandem mass spectrometry (MS/MS and related techniques), which will be discussed separately. It should be noted here, however, that multiple stage MS/MS experiments (MS/MS/MS . . . , or MS^n) experiments are readily performed in ion traps.

The ability to store ions also has other distinct advantages. Using the mass-selective ejection scan approach, mass resolution on the QIT is inversely proportional to the scan rate. By slowing the scan rate, mass resolution similar to that achieved in sector instruments has been achieved. For example, this technique has been used to determine the charge state of multiply charged protein ions generated by ES ionization. In commercial instruments, higher mass resolution is available over a limited mass range in the Bruker Esquire and Thermo Finnigan LCQ mass spectrometers. Unfortunately, one of the advantages normally conferred by high resolution—exact mass capability—is not fully realized by this technique.

The QIT also shares some advantages with TOF-MS. In particular, ion trap mass spectrometry is known for high sensitivity. Furthermore, sampling is decoupled from scanning, so there is no mass spectral peak skewing in GC-MS and HPLC-MS.

Linear Ion Trap. This is a RF ion trap that is based on a modified linear QMF. Rather than being a pass-through device as in a normal linear QMF, electrostatic fields are applied to the ends to prevent ions from exiting out the ends of the device. Thus being trapped, ions can be manipulated in many of the same ways as in a QIT. An advantage of the linear quadrupole trap is that the trapping field can be turned off at will and the device operated as a normal QMF. Thus a single device combines most of the features of a QIT and QMF and is extremely versatile. Commercial triple quadrupole mass spectrometers are being offered in which the third quadrupole is modified to function as a linear trap. The exploration of the capabilities of the linear ion trap is a very active field of research, and one can expect many new capabilities to be discovered in the next few years. Both Thermo Finnigan and Applied Biosystems/MDS Sciex market linear QIT.

Ion Cyclotron Resonance. The ICR-MS excels in high-resolution and high-mass accuracy measurements. Measurements at resolution exceeding 1 million are not unusual, and sub-ppm mass accuracy is being explored by some investigators. ICR is a trapping technique and shares many of the advantages of RF ion traps; however, there are even more ways to manipulate ions in a ICR-MS than in QIT, and MS^n measurements are easily done with a ICR-MS. Sensitivity of a ICR-MS is generally high. Furthermore, sampling is decoupled from spectral acquisition, so there is no peak skewing in chromatographic experiments, a feature that ICR shares with TOF and QIT.

An ICR-MS is based on the principle that ions immersed in a magnetic field undergo circular motion (cyclotron motion). A typical ICR-MS uses a high-field (3 to 12 tesla) superconducting magnet. Within this field and within a high vacuum is mounted a "cell" typically composed of six metal electrodes, arranged as the faces of a cube. Ions are suspended inside the cell and undergo cyclotron motion, which keeps ions from being lost radially (the radial direction being defined as perpendicular to the magnetic field lines). A low (~1 V) potential is applied to the endcaps to keep ions from leaving the trap axially. Thus the combination of electric and magnetic fields keeps ions confined within the cell.

Each m/z is associated with a specific cyclotron frequency. The relationship is given by:

$$\frac{m}{z} = \frac{B}{2\pi f} \tag{2}$$

where B is the magnetic field strength and f is the frequency. This equation is an approximation to the frequency of an ion's orbital motion in the magnetic field. The frequency is shifted slightly because of the trapping voltage. For presentation purposes, this small shift in frequency is ignored here. This equation is independent of ion kinetic energy, and this fact, combined with the fact that frequency can be measured very precisely, means that very accurate m/z measurements can be performed by an ICR-MS.

The side electrodes of an ICR cell are used for ion detection. The electrodes are used in pairs, with opposite electrodes making a pair. To one pair of electrodes is applied a transient waveform, typically containing a superposition of many frequencies within the tens to hundreds of kHz range. This excites the cyclotron motion of ions in the cell, but only if the waveform contains frequency components matching the cyclotron frequency. Before excitation the diameter of an ion's cyclotron orbit is small, and the phases are random. After excitation the diameter is large. Furthermore the orbital motion of the ions of a given m/z is now synchronized, meaning that ions orbit in phase with each other. This orbital motion induces an electrical signal in the other pair of electrodes. Following the excitation step, the induced signal is amplified electronically and recorded in the data system computer. If there are a variety of ions of different *m/z* present in the cell, the recorded waveform is a complex superposition of many frequencies. A mathematical operation, known as a Fourier transform (FT), is applied to this signal. Each *m/z* value present in the sample produces a peak in the transformed signal. The transformed function is a frequency spectrum of the signal. The frequency of a peak is related to *m/z* according to the preceding equation. Thus the frequency spectrum of ions in the cell is equivalent to the mass spectrum of the sample. The actual mass spectrum is obtained by changing the *x*-axis from frequency to mass using the equation presented above. Because of the frequent use of FT in ICR, the technique is often referred to as FT-ICR or FTMS.

The most notable feature of the process described above is that ions are not destroyed by the detection process. Therefore ions can be further manipulated after detection. The simplest example is the remeasurement of ions (i.e., repeating the excite and/or detect sequence to obtain another mass spectrum of the same group of ions). More complex manipulations include multiple stages of MS/MS. The facts that ions are detected nondestructively and that they are trapped in a region of space mean that very complex sequences of ion manipulations are possible, making FT-ICR instruments the most versatile of all mass spectrometers.

Like the QIT, ionization in the FT-ICR may be performed either internally or externally to the cell. For several reasons, external ionization has become the technique of choice. External ionization allows the use of virtually any ionization method, and commercially available instruments are typically designed as general purpose instruments incorporating interchangeable ion sources. All three major suppliers of FT-ICR instruments (IonSpec, Bruker Daltonics, and Finnigan) offer external sources.

Although having many advantages, ICR-MS has several disadvantages including (1) high instrument cost; (2) very demanding site requirements, both in terms of space and in terms of access restrictions; (3) it uses a high-field superconducting magnet, and its magnetic field introduces safety concerns, such as flying iron objects, and practical concerns, such as the erasing of credit cards and other magnetically encoded strips; (4) cost of operation, care, and maintenance is high because the instruments consume liquid helium, and they must never be allowed to go dry; (5) a highly skilled operator level is necessary to operate it. Consequently, these instruments have yet to make an impact in the clinical lab, though they could well become important in the future if some of their disadvantages are overcome.

Tandem Mass Spectrometers

Tandem mass spectrometry, or mass spectrometry/mass spectrometry (MS/MS), is rapidly becoming an important technique in clinical laboratories where it is mainly used for quantitative analysis of routine samples.[16] However, it is also excellent for structural characterization and compound identification, and is therefore useful for exploratory work, even when a final assay may be based on a different technology, such as an immunoassay. The most important feature of this technique is very high selectivity together with good sensitivity. When coupled with the added selectivity of an HPLC, interferences in a well-designed MS/MS assay (and particularly an HPLC-MS/MS assay) are very low. Because of its low interference rate, low consumable cost (as with most MS methods) and high sample throughput rates, more and more clinical labs are purchasing and using tandem mass spectrometers.

The physical principle of tandem mass spectrometers is best understood by considering beam-type instruments, either a magnetic sector or a quadrupole mass spectrometer. Two mass spectrometers are arranged sequentially, with a "collision cell" placed between the two instruments. The first instrument is used to select ions of a particular *m/z,* called either the "parent ion" or "precursor ion." The parent ion is directed into the collision cell, where ions collide with background gas molecules and are broken into smaller ions. These have been traditionally referred to as "daughter ions" to emphasize the fact that they are derived from the parent ion, though the terminology "product ions" is now preferred by some.[32] The second mass spectrometer acquires the mass spectrum of the daughter ions.

There are a variety of scan functions possible with tandem mass spectrometers. In practice, a product ion scan involves setting the first mass spectrometer, MS1, to select a given *m/z* and scanning through the full mass spectrum of product ions. This scan function is often used for structural characterization. A precursor ion scan reverses this relationship, with the second mass spectrometer, MS2, set to select a specific daughter ion, and MS1 is scanned through the spectrum. The peaks in the parent ion scan tell us which parent ions produce a specific product ion, a capability that is often used to analyze for specific classes of compounds. For example, acylcarnitines are often analyzed by searching for the precursors to the *m/z* 85 product ion. In a constant neutral loss scan, the two mass spectrometers are scanned synchronously, with a constant *m/z* offset between parent and product ion. This scan indicates what ions lose a particular neutral fragment. For example, an offset of 18 *m/z* units would select for ions losing H_2O in the dissociation process. Another scan function is multiple reaction monitoring or MRM. This is not actually a scan function at all but consists of a series of parent/product ion pairs, with the mass spectrometer set to jump through the table of pairs in a cyclical fashion. This is primarily used for quantitative analysis of a few selected target compounds and is a close analogue to SIM monitoring used in GC-MS.

The key to the high selectivity of MS/MS is that it characterizes a compound by two physical properties, parent ion mass and daughter ion mass, rather than a single property. If combined with a chromatographic separation, the retention time is then added to the characterization, and the analytes are characterized by three physical properties. This high selectivity eliminates that vast majority of potential interferences.

As with single-stage mass spectrometers, tandem mass spectrometers can be roughly categorized as beam-type instruments and trapping instruments. The most popular beam-type instrument is the triple quadrupole. In this instrument the first quadrupole (Q1) functions as MS1, and the third quadrupole (Q3) functions as MS2. Between these two quadrupoles is another quadrupole, Q2, which functions as the collision cell. The pressure is raised in Q2 (e.g., greater than 10^{-3} torr) to the point that ions traversing Q2 undergo several collisions, leading to dissociation. Q2 is operated as an "RF-only" quadrupole, ideally passing all ions regardless of *m/z*, although in reality the passband would typically cover a ~10:1 *m/z* range.

Two magnetic sector instruments have also been operated in tandem, with a collision cell placed between the two instruments. These instruments permit high resolution selection of both parent and product ions. However, these instruments are now rarely used as they are expensive and cumbersome to operate. Double focusing mass spectrometers can also be used as tandem mass spectrometers by a technique known as "linked scanning." A product ion scan by linked scanning involves low resolution for MS1 and high resolution for MS2.

Another technological development in tandem mass spectrometry is the combination of two TOF mass spectrometers, TOF/TOF. These instruments have excellent sensitivity and throughput for MALDI-MS/MS and are especially suited for proteomics research. However, these instruments are unable to perform true precursor ion scans or constant neutral loss scans. The Bruker Daltonics ultraflex and Applied Biosystem 4700 proteomics analyzer are examples of this type of instrument. Such instruments have yet to make an impact in clinical chemistry.

So-called hybrid mass spectrometers include a combination of two different types of mass spectrometers in a tandem arrangement. The combination of a magnetic sector mass spectrometer with a quadrupole mass spectrometer was an early instrument of this type. More popular is the combination of a quadrupole for MS1 and a TOF for MS2. As with TOF/TOF, these instruments are presently used mainly for proteomics research but could eventually find applications in the clinical lab. These instruments are unable to perform true precursor ion scans or constant neutral loss scans. Commercial examples of this type of instrument include the qTOF by Waters Micromass and the QSTAR by Applied Biosystems/MDS Sciex.

Trapping mass spectrometers can also be used as tandem mass spectrometers. Unlike beam-type instruments, which are referred to as "tandem in space," trapping mass spectrometers are "tandem in time," meaning that ions are held in one region of space while the parent ion is selected and dissociated and the daughter ion analyzed sequentially in time. The ability to perform tandem mass spectrometry is inherent in the design of trapping mass spectrometers. Generally, little or no additional hardware is required, with tandem capability supplied via a software change. Both QIT and ICR instruments are capable of tandem mass spectrometry. These instruments are capable of multiple stages of mass spectrometry. Thus product ions may be further dissociated to produce another generation of product ions (MS/MS/MS or MS^3). In principle any number of dissociation stages may be performed. This capability finds its greatest use in structural characterization, such as the sequencing of peptides, and is less useful for quantitative analysis. Trapping designs are extremely versatile, but unlike triple quadrupoles they are unable to perform true precursor ion scans or constant neutral loss scans.

DETECTORS

With the exception of an ICR-MS, nearly all mass spectrometers use electron multipliers for ion detection. There are three main classes of electron multipliers: discrete dynode multipliers, continuous dynode electron multipliers (CDEM), also known as channel electron multipliers (CEM), and microchannel plate (MCP) electron multipliers, also known as multichannel plate electron multipliers. Though different in detail, all three work on the same physical principle. An additional detector used in mass spectrometers is the Faraday cup.

Discrete Dynode Multipliers

Figure 7-12 presents a conceptual diagram of the operation of a discrete dynode electron multiplier. When an ion strikes the first dynode, it causes the ejection of one or more electrons ("secondary electrons") from the dynode surface. The electron is accelerated toward the second dynode by a voltage difference of ~100 V. Upon striking the second dynode, this electron causes the ejection of additional electrons, typically 2 or 3 in number. The second group of electrons is then accelerated toward the third dynode, and upon striking the third dynode, causes the ejection of several more electrons. The process is repeated through a chain of dynodes, num-

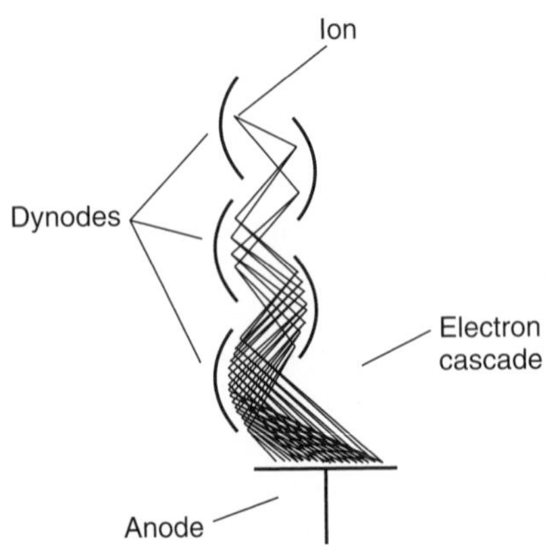

Figure 7-12 Discrete dynode electron multiplier showing dynode structure and generation of electron cascade.

bering between 12 and 24 for most designs. The cascade process typically produces a gain of 10^4 to 10^8, meaning that the generation of one electron at the first dynode produces a pulse of 10^4 to 10^8 electrons at the end of the cascade. The duration of the pulse is very short, typically less than 10 nanoseconds.

Continuous Dynode Electron Multiplier

CDEMs, sometimes called CEMs, work on the same principle as discrete dynode electron multipliers but differ in their physical construction. The set of dynodes of a discrete dynode electron multiplier is replaced by a single continuous surface. Usually the continuous surface takes the form of the inside of a tube, flared at the entrance end. The surface of the tube contains an electrically resistive layer. A voltage gradient is generated down the length of the tube by applying a voltage difference between the entrance and exit ends. The voltage gradient in the CEM takes the place of the discrete voltage drops between the dynodes of the discrete dynode electron multiplier. The resistive layer also serves as the secondary electron emitter. The CDEM is generally fabricated from a specialized glass, and the resistive surface is formed by chemically treating the surface of the glass. DeTech, Burle, and K and M Electronics all market a variety of CDEMs.

Microchannel Plate Electron Multipliers

MCPs operate on the same principle as CDEMs. A microchannel plate is essentially a monolithic array of miniaturized CDEMs fabricated in a single wafer or disk of glass. The disk contains pores extending from the upper surface to the lower surface. These pores are known as channels and perform the same function as the interior of the tube in a CEM, but in contrast to a typical CEM, the entrance ends of the channels are not flared. The channels are typically 3 to 30 micrometers in diameter depending on the design. The length of the channels is set by the thickness of the disk, typically 200 to 1000 micrometers. Microchannel plates can be fabricated in areas measured in cm^2, and because the disk-shaped profile forms a nearly flat stopping surface for ions, they are ideal detectors for TOF mass spectrometers. Burle and Hamamatsu are the major suppliers of these devices.

Faraday Cup

The Faraday cup is a simple electrode that intercepts the ion beam directly. This current is then amplified using electronic amplifiers. Because the Faraday cup measures signal intensity directly, rather than indirectly (as in saturation-prone electron multipliers) it provides an absolute measure of ion current and is also useful when signal levels are too high for electron multiplier–based detection. Some instruments use both electron multiplier– and Faraday cup–based detection to provide for extended dynamic range, a capability that can be especially useful for elemental analysis of trace metals in samples.

Computer and Software

Because of their mass resolution capabilities, scanning functions, ability to automatically switch from positive to negative ionization modes, and speed with which multiple *m/z* signals can be monitored, modern MS instruments generate enormous amounts of raw data. In addition, the use of MS, in such areas as proteomics, biomarker discovery, synthetic combinatorial chemistry, high throughput drug discovery, pharmacogenomics, toxicology, and therapeutic drug monitoring requires that manufacturers provide sophisticated computers and software programs.

In toxicology laboratories one important function of the data system is library searching to assist in compound identification. There are several commercial libraries, including the Wiley Registry of Mass Spectral Data, the NIST Mass Spectral Database, and the Pfleger, Maurer, and Weber drug libraries. In addition, many laboratories generate their own libraries. The quality and quantity of available spectra, the search algorithm, and whether condensed or full spectra are searched are all important in spectral matching. There are several library search algorithms available, the most popular being probability-based matching and the dot product matching approach modified by the NIST. Both approaches provide an assessment of match quality between the observed spectra and the library spectra.

In proteomics and biomarker discovery, complex mass spectra from single proteins, protein mixtures, or protein digests are obtained. Data systems exist that aid in characterization of spectral data to identify such properties as intact protein mass, amino acid subsequences, and post-translational modifications. Fragmentation information can also be compared with peptide databases to identify structural mutations that may be present.

Software programs are also available to locate and identify components in complex chromatographic separations. Deconvolution protocols have been developed that identify and characterize the mass spectra of co-eluting compounds. In some cases two separate sets of chromatographic data can be compared to evaluate similarities or unique differences (e.g., controls versus disease state).

CLINICAL APPLICATIONS

Mass spectrometers coupled with gas and liquid chromatographs (GC-MS and LC-MS) result in versatile analytical instruments that combine the resolving power of the chromatographs with the exquisite specificity and sensitivity of a mass spectrometer. Such instruments are powerful analytical tools that are used by clinical labs to identify and quantify organic analytes. They provide structural and quantitative information in real time on individual analytes as they elute from a chromatographic column. These coupled techniques are very sensitive and only nanogram or picogram quantities of an analyte are required for analysis. Specific applications of these coupled instruments are found in Chapters 33 and 34.

MALDI-TOF mass spectrometers and SELDI and ICP ionization techniques have also enhanced the analytical capabilities of mass spectrometers. In addition, an important application of MS is its use as the primary analytical tool in the rapidly developing and expanding field of proteomics. Also included in this section is a discussion of ion suppression and how it relates to the analytical capabilities of mass spectrometers.

Gas Chromatography-Mass Spectrometry

GC-MS has been used for the analysis of biological compounds for several decades. This technique is used by the U.S. National Institute of Standards and Technology as a definitive method to qualify standard reference materials and to assign certified values to many clinical analytes, including cholesterol, glucose, creatinine, and urea nitrogen (see Chapter 1). One of the most common applications of GC-MS is in drug screening for clinical or forensic purposes (see Chapter 34). Many drugs have relatively small molecular weights and nonpolar and/or volatile properties, which make these compounds particularly suitable for analysis by GC. Electron ionization with full-scan mass detection is the most widely used approach for comprehensive drug screening. Identification of unknown compounds can be achieved by comparison of their full mass spectrum with a mass spectral library or database. Numerous state and federal agencies mandate that only GC-MS be used to confirm the presence of drugs in samples presumptively found to be positive by immunochemical analyses.

GC-MS has many applications beyond drug screening. Numerous xenobiotic compounds can be readily analyzed by GC-MS. Applications for anabolic steroids, pesticides, pollutants, and inborn errors of metabolism have been described.[46,63,81]

One important limitation to GC-MS is the requirement that compounds be sufficiently volatile to allow transfer from the solid phase to the mobile carrier gas and thus elute from the analytical column to the detector. Although many biological compounds are amenable to chromatographic separation with GC, there are a large number of compounds that are too polar or too large in size to be analyzed with this technique.

Liquid Chromatography-Mass Spectrometry

Compared with gas chromatographs, it is more difficult to interface liquid chromatographs with mass spectrometers because the analytes are dissolved in a liquid rather than a gas. As discussed previously, several interface techniques have been developed for coupling a liquid chromatograph to a mass spectrometer, which has allowed HPLC-MS and HPLC-MS/MS to be successfully applied to a wide range of compounds. In theory as long as a compound can be dissolved in a liquid, it can be introduced into an HPLC-MS system. Thus polar and nonpolar analytes and large molecular weight compounds, such as proteins, can be monitored using this technique.

An important area where tandem MS is used clinically is screening and confirmation of genetic disorders and inborn errors of metabolism (see Chapter 55).[17] The ability to analyze multiple compounds in a single analytical run makes this technique an efficient tool for screening purposes. Electrospray tandem MS has become the recognized reference method for carnitine and acylcarnitine analysis to identify organic acidemias and fatty acid oxidation defects.[15,34] It is also becoming more recognized as an excellent tool for the analysis of amino acids. In the case of carnitine and amino acid analysis, these compounds vary widely in their polarity, which creates problems with consistency of response factors. To address this, most procedures employ a butyl ester derivatization of the carboxyl group to force cationic character upon the amino acids and thus yield similar ionization efficiencies for these compounds.[13] Direct flow injection analysis works well for these screens but can have the limitation of a lack of specificity for isobaric amino acids, such as leucine, isoleucine and hydroxyproline, or isobutyrylcarnitine and butyrylcarnitine. In these cases chromatographic separation is required before tandem MS.[13]

Other clinically relevant compounds that are amenable to HPLC-MS analysis include all of the major immunosuppressants, antiretrovirals, homocysteine, biogenic amines, methylmalonic acid, and hemoglobin variants.*

MS is widely used in pharmaceutical development via the process of "high throughput screening." To most efficiently use available resources, research labs synthesize large sets of diverse organic compounds or derivatives of starting core structures. This is often called combinatorial chemistry. The same process of identification is also applied to natural products as pharmaceutical candidates. These vast sets of compounds must be screened for unique structure and evaluated for potential as candidates for further study. This requires high throughput screening of large mixtures or isolates containing many compounds. MS has become the most efficient technique to identify these types of compounds. One example is the use of HPLC-MS to identify new taxanes in botanical extracts as effective anticancer agents.[87]

Important to investigating therapeutic approaches is the recognition of target protein receptors that may be associated with selected diseases. This information can facilitate structure-based approaches to drug design and ideally selective activity toward specific targets. The challenge in drug design has been how to test whether a compound binds to a protein receptor and whether this binding modulates the structure of the receptor. Size exclusion chromatography coupled with MS can be used to help answer these types of questions. After incubating a drug with protein(s), small size

*References 6, 25, 51, 52, 58, 90.

exclusion columns (e.g., Sephadex G25 or Bio-Gel P6) are used to separate free and bound drug. Small unbound molecules diffuse into particle pores and are retained, and larger drug-protein complexes are not retained and elute from the column. The small columns are often placed into a centrifuge and centrifugal force used to speed up the separation. The eluted drug-protein complexes are then analyzed by HPLC-ESI-MS to identify the structural properties of those compounds that effectively bind to the protein target.[82] This process can also be combined with nuclear magnetic resonance (NMR) to investigate bound complexes. NMR chemical shift perturbations can be used to help identify the binding site on a protein and whether this is specific or nonspecific binding.[65] Similar experiments can be performed to evaluate cellular absorption and/or permeability and intestinal cytochrome P4503A4 metabolism using Caco-2 cell monolayers,[19] and inhibition of metabolism with mixtures of hepatic microsomal enzymes, where probe substrates for each enzyme are used to monitor inhibition of multiple enzymes in one assay.[8]

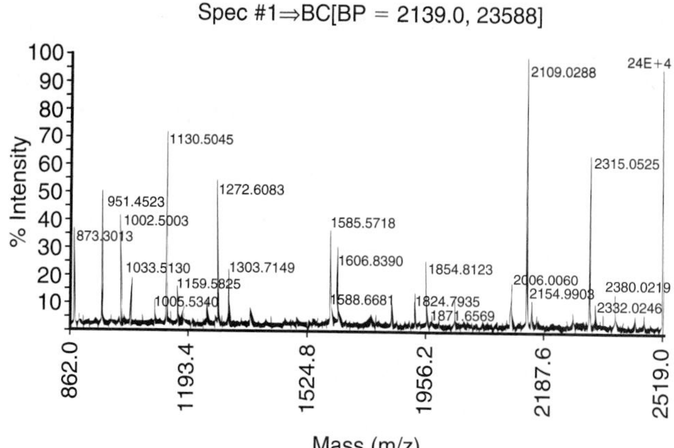

Figure 7-13 An example of a MALDI-TOF spectrum showing peptides generated in a tryptic digest of a spot cored from a 2-D, SDS-PAGE gel. The 16 most abundant *m/z* were submitted to MS-FIT for searching against the nonredundant database. The top result for this search is shown in Table 7-1.

MALDI-TOF Mass Spectrometry

MALDI-TOF has been used to analyze thousands of different classes of compounds. The major considerations for this ionization technique are the ability to co-crystallize with one of the hundreds of matrix molecules available and the ability to form positive or negative ions or a charged adduct that is measured in the mass analyzer. Uses generally fall into one of three broad categories: (1) detection of a particular compound(s), (2) identification of a protein(s), or (3) identification of an organism.

The detection of phosphatidylcholine and its digestion products[71] is a good example of detection of a specific compound and in this case the monitoring of the progress of an enzymatic reaction. These small molecules can be detected as positive ions and readily retain sodium adducts. In addition to simple identification, the authors also monitor progression of the phospholipase digestion. Although MALDI should not be considered quantitative, the use of relative signal-to-noise ratios can be used to monitor the progression of this digestion (or reaction). The main point of small molecule detection by MALDI is that the molecule must co-crystallize with the matrix (and not react), be able to be desorbed back out of the matrix, and form an ion or adduct that can be detected. Although MALDI is simple and fast, other MS and non-MS techniques are often as good or better for small molecule analysis.

MALDI-TOF is often used to determine the identity of proteins through peptide mass fingerprinting (PMF). This technique has been used to identify a large number of 2-D gel spots for the bacterial pathogen *Pseudomonas aeruginosa*.[77] The procedure generally involves in-gel tryptic digestion followed by accurate mass measurement of the peptides. The generated mass list is then compared with theoretical tryptic masses for proteins in a database (Figure 7-13 and Table 7-1). The procedure works best for organisms with complete and annotated genomes. The procedure is very rapid, under 2 minutes per sample, because 100 or greater samples may be automatically processed and deposited on a single MALDI target plate. In the above example,[77] the group rapidly identified a large number of proteins that were expressed differently between laboratory and pathogenic bacteria. In addition, it was found that some proteins were listed as "hypothetical," meaning previously undescribed or confirmed to be expressed, and that theoretical molecular weights and/or isoelectric points (pIs) in some cases were extremely different from those measured in the gel, indicating possible terminal clipping and/or posttranslational modification. These observations are extremely useful in targeting areas of focus given the large amount of data generated by this technique.

The third area that MALDI-TOF is emerging in is identification of organisms, such as bacteria. A method has been described that attempts to identify bacteria by fingerprinting proteins that were extracted using gentle conditions.[91] The basis of this technique is that different bacteria should express unique proteins in the 2 to 20 kDa mass range, allowing classification according to the protein mass fingerprint. Although the other two areas mentioned above are quite mature, this area is still under final development. The major problems[91] are a lack of actual protein mass information for various bacteria and a lack of investigation into different strains of the same bacteria. The protein mass fingerprints must be cataloged for each bacterium and determined to be completely reproducible for a given extraction method. Further, more work will have to be done on changes at the protein level among different strains or isolates of putatively the same bacterium.

TABLE 7-1 Example of Printout of Bacterial Identification Through PMF Using MALDI-TOF. A Generated Mass List Is Compared With Theoretical Tryptic Masses for Proteins in a Database. Match Quality Is Used for Pathogen Identification.

Rank	MOWSE Score	# (%) Masses Matched	Protein MW (Da)/pI	Species	NCBInr.81602 Accession #	Protein Name
1	1.07e + 008	14/16 (87%)	101754.9/9.15	SACCHAROMYCES CEREVISIAE	6321275	(Z72685) ORF YGL163c

1. 14/16 matches (87%). 101754.9 Da, pI = 9.15. Acc. # 6321275. SACCHAROMYCES CEREVISIAE. (Z72685) ORF YGL163c.

m/z Submitted	MH^+ Matched	Delta ppm	Start	End	Peptide Sequence (Click for Fragment Ions)	Modifications
870.4746	870.4797	−5.8732	598	606	(K) GVGGSQPLR(A)	
873.3981	873.3929	5.9793	774	779	(K) DCFIYR(F)	
951.4901	951.4900	0.1050	814	821	(R) LFSSDNLR(Q)	
1002.5385	1002.5373	1.2224	515	522	(K) NFENPILR(G)	
1033.5513	1033.5543	−2.8793	46	55	(K) NTHIPPAAGR(I)	
1130.6349	1130.6322	2.4037	120	128	(R) LSHIQYTLR(R)	
1130.6349	1130.6322	2.4037	514	522	(R) KNFENPILR(G)	
1159.6039	1159.6071	−2.7957	56	67	(R) IATGSDNIVGGR(S)	
1272.6508	1272.6483	1.9865	734	746	(K) AGGCGINLIGANR(L)	
1303.7573	1303.7599	−1.9457	270	280	(K) ILRPHQVEGVR(F)	
1585.7190	1585.7215	−1.5602	446	459	(K) NCNVGLMLADEGHR(L)	
1606.8861	1606.9029	−10.4650	22	35	(R) LVPRPINVQDSVNR(L)	
2138.0756	2138.0704	2.4250	747	765	(R) LILMDPDWNPAADQQALAR(V)	
2315.1093	2315.0951	6.1321	401	423	(K) SSMGGGNTTVSQAIHAWAQAQGR(N)	
2388.0671	2388.0731	−2.5004	293	313	(K) DYLEAEAFNTSSEDPLKSDEK(A)	

SELDI Mass Spectrometry

Currently the area of greatest interest in SELDI analysis is its use for the discovery of biomarkers for disease. An excellent example is biomarker identification in breast cancer.[56] The basic premise is that diagnosis of disease state can be done by monitoring away from the actual site of disease—most often serum, urine, or cerebrospinal fluid. This study follows the basic technique that proteins are affinity purified from the biological fluid, and markers are identified based on a large difference in abundance between control and disease. These markers are not even identified in the early stages of the experiment. The power of the technology is the rapid identification of multiple, potential biomarkers that can be used in concert as a diagnostic tool—highly desirable over many current single biomarker tests.

ICP Mass Spectrometry

As noted earlier in the chapter, ICP-MS is used for the determination of trace elements in many types of samples (see Chapter 35).[5] However, it is known that the toxicity of an element may depend on the organic or inorganic state in which the element is present. In these cases it is more important to ascertain the concentrations of toxic species rather than the total concentration of the element. To extend the utility of this technique, GC and HPLC systems are now being coupled to ICP-MS to separate individual elemental species before ICP-MS analysis.[61]

Proteomics

The past 20 years have seen tremendous progress in genomics, with hundreds of genomes completed or near completion and many now parsed and annotated. However, this information has often failed to provide vast new understanding into cellular function—mainly because of the myriad changes that occur to the proteins produced from the genome throughout the life cycle of a cell. In the mid 1990s, MS came to the forefront of analytical techniques used to study proteins and the term proteomics was coined. Although the definition is still debated, proteomics in the largest sense encompasses knowledge of the structure, function, and expression of all proteins in the biochemical or biological contexts of all organisms.[45] In a more basic and practical sense, proteomics refers to the identification and quantitation of proteins and their posttranslational modifications in a given system or systems. This is a challenging task as every gene has potentially 100 or more distinct, chemical protein isoforms. In addition, many other molecules (metals, lipids, etc.) interact with proteins in a noncovalent fashion. Therefore in a genome, such as human, there may be a repertoire of millions of "proteins" requiring identification and quantitation.

Two foundations are necessary to begin this daunting challenge. The first is the basic sequence expected for each possible protein in a cell (i.e., a completed genome). The second is instrumentation, currently advanced mass spectrometers that identify and quantitate protein isoforms in an automated fashion at very low limits of detection. Both foundations are now essentially in place, and the field of proteomics has leapt forward over the past several years. The goal above is far from complete, however, as considerable advances will have to be made before we truly examine all the proteins in a cell.

Currently, MS is routinely used to accomplish many tasks in proteomics. The most basic task is protein identification. The typical approach is known as the "bottom-up" method, where proteins are separated—either by gel electrophoresis or by solution-based methods—and then digested. The resulting enzymatic fragments are analyzed and used to identify the protein(s) present. This process is time consuming and has many pitfalls. Increasingly, much research has been devoted to analysis of mixtures of proteins. These mixtures can be from cellular compartments, tissue, or immunoprecipitations. Although solving many problems associated with analysis of proteins isolated by gels, this technique suffers one major drawback—complexity. Currently, both instrumentation and analysis software are not sufficiently advanced to easily identify all the proteins in truly complex mixtures. As a result, much emphasis has been placed on separation methods for proteins and/or peptides. Many groups have introduced methods to begin handling this level of complexity. The most popular approaches are subcellular fractionation, multidimensional chromatography, and affinity labeling and/or purification. By combining these approaches, several thousand protein species can routinely be identified. Obviously these numbers are better than "bottom-up" methods from gels, but they still fall far short of those necessary for complete proteomics.

Two last areas that have to be addressed are quantitation and de novo sequencing and/or posttranslational modifications. First, most identified proteins must be quantitated in relation to changes in cell state or cell type. Quantitation in MS for these purposes is relative, (i.e., standard condition to perturbed condition). Current techniques in this area are still in the development phase but generally involve labeling either a subset of peptides (isotope-coded affinity tagging) or all peptides (metabolic labeling). Although some problems exist with the labeling, the greatest—as with identification—involves the sheer complexity of the sample to be analyzed. The second problem is both separate and related. Posttranslational modifications clearly are the major control mechanism in cells. Mass spectrometry is unique as a technique that can both identify and precisely locate a modification. However, the software to automate this process lags far behind the ability to collect the data. What is lacking is software for de novo sequencing, which can interpret a mass spectrum with little or no user intervention, especially in the area of posttranslational modifications. Currently, most modified spectra are manually interpreted by highly skilled mass spectrometrists, adding days or even weeks of analysis time per sample. These two problems, in addition to sample complexity, will have to be solved before proteomics evolves into a mature field.

All of these issues are addressed in numerous papers every month in journals ranging from *Proteomics* to *Clinical Chemistry*. Although an exhaustive listing is impossible, there are several review or opinion references that represent good starting points for exploration into the rapidly changing world of proteomics.*

ANALYTICAL PROBLEM OF ION SUPPRESSION

Ion suppression results from the presence of less volatile compounds that can change the efficiency of droplet formation or droplet evaporation, which in turn affects the amount of charged ion in the gas phase that ultimately reaches the detector.[1,47] Sample matrix, co-eluting compounds, and cross talk can contribute to this effect. Ionization effects can theoretically occur in either the solution phase or the gas phase. For biological extractions, one cause of ion suppression is a change in the spray droplet solution properties caused by the presence of nonvolatile or less volatile solutes.[47] These nonvolatile materials (e.g., salts, ion-pairing agents, endogenous compounds, drugs, and/or metabolites) change the efficiency of droplet formation or droplet evaporation, which in turn affects the amount of charged ion in the gas phase that ultimately reaches the detector. Anions, such as phosphate or borate in buffers, can also neutralize the effective ionization of an analyte.

The presence of ion suppression, or other deleterious effects, can be evaluated via several experimental protocols. One involves comparison of (1) the instrument response for standards (including any internal standards) injected directly in mobile phase and (2) the same amount of compound spiked into preextracted samples.[62] The data for the standard in mobile phase provide a relative 100% response value. The data for the same amount of compound spiked into preextracted samples show the effect of sample matrix on MS response (ion suppression).

A second protocol involves postcolumn continuous infusion of compound into the MS detector.[7,38,68] The instrumental setup includes a syringe pump connected via a tee to the column effluent (Figure 7-14). Because the compound being tested is introduced into the mass detector at a constant rate, a constant electrospray ionization response should

*References 30, 42, 57, 72, 76, 86.

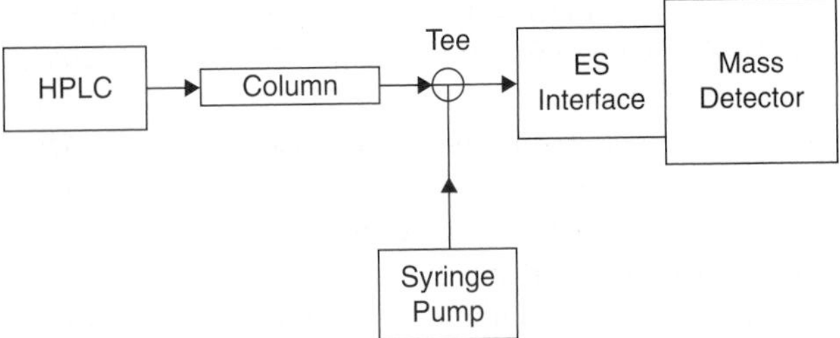

Figure 7-14 Postcolumn infusion system. Mobile phase or specimen extracts are injected into the HPLC system. The analyte being evaluated is continuously infused, postcolumn, and is mixed with the column effluent through a tee before entering the electrospray interface.

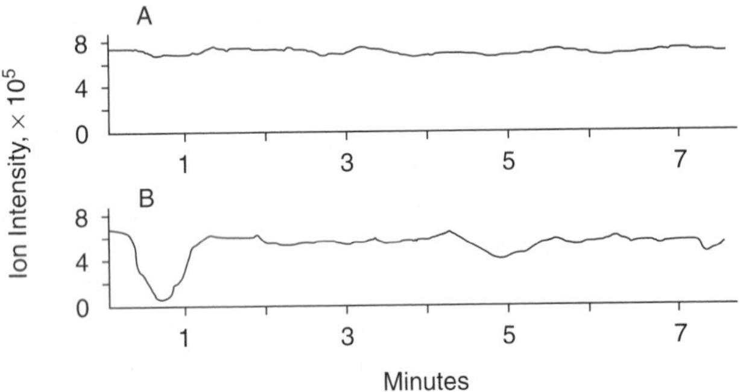

Figure 7-15 Infusion chromatograms for hypothetical analyte. **A,** Mobile phase injection. **B,** Serum liquid-liquid extract injection. These profiles illustrate that ion suppression can be greater than 90%, a recovery time may exist, and that suppression is not limited to the solvent front region. For a comprehensive presentation of these types of effects, the reader is referred to references 7, 38, and 68.

ideally be observed (Figure 7-15, *A*) if no ionization interferences occur when an extract from a biological specimen, such as serum, is injected into the HPLC portion of the instrument. In actuality it is common to see a suppression of the signal at the time point that corresponds to the void volume of the column (Figure 7-15, *B*). The degree of ion suppression and the recovery time to full response can vary from compound to compound[7] and from sample to sample and can also be dependent on the sample preparation method. Since endogenous compounds from the specimen matrix can continue to elute at any time during the chromatographic run, ion suppression is not limited to the column void. The observed degree of ion suppression can also be dependent on the concentration of the analyte being monitored,[89] which relates to the matrix/analyte ratio.

Another potential source of ion suppression is the effect that chromatographic ion-pairing agents may have on signal intensity. For example, trifluoroacetic acid (TFA) has been used in HPLC-UV analyses because it improves peak shape and retention times. Unfortunately, for MS analyses TFA also causes signal suppression and must be considered if this acid is used in the mobile phase. Being a component of the mobile phase this agent will continuously be introduced into the ESI interface, so that signal suppression may be observed throughout the entire chromatographic run.

There are several options that can be used to minimize or correct for ion suppression during HPLC-MS analysis. For ion pairing other weaker acids—such as acetic, formic, or hexafluorobutyric acid—may be successfully substituted for TFA in HPLC-MS analysis. The use of surface tension–lowering modifiers in the ESI source has also been reported to be successful when TFA is used as a mobile phase modifier.[27] The postcolumn addition of acids and solvent carriers to displace TFA from compounds and aid ionization has also been successfully employed. This is a process termed the "TFA fix."[2] It may also be possible to modify the chromatographic conditions so that the compound(s) of interest elute in a region where ion suppression is not observed.[4] Since many HPLC assays include an internal standard, another possibility is to modify chromatographic conditions such that the compound of interest and the internal standard co-elute.[48] The ion suppression for both compounds should be similar if the peaks chromatographically coincide, thus "correcting" for the degree of suppression.

Ion suppression is not limited to just HPLC-MS or ESI interfaces. For MALDI analysis, arginine-containing peptides have been reported to dominate the peptide pattern for protein digests,[50] the extent of which depends on the matrix used. The presence of ionic detergents, such as Triton X-100 and Tween 20, has also been shown to cause signal suppression in MALDI experiments, which can be countered by modifications to the matrix.[31]

REFERENCES

1. Annesley TM. Ion Suppression in mass spectrometry. Clin Chem 2003;49:1041-4.
2. Apffel A, Fischer S, Goldberg G, Goodley PC, Kuhlmann FE. Enhanced sensitivity for peptide mapping with electrospray liquid chromatography-mass spectrometry in the presence of signal suppression due to trifluoroacetic acid-containing mobile phases. J Chromatogr A 1995;712:177-90.
3. Arnott D, Shabanowitz J, Hunt DW. Mass spectrometry of proteins and peptides. Sensitive and accurate mass measurement and sequence analysis. Clin Chem 1993;39:2005-10.
4. Beato BD, Gray DD, Wong P, Hampsch J, Peters S. Ramifications of pump-switching step gradients for bioanalytical LC/MS/MS assays. Current Separations 2000;19:55-8.
5. Beauchemin D. Inductively coupled plasma mass spectrometry. Anal Chem 2002;74:2873-94.
6. Bisse E, Schauber C, Zorn N, Epting T, Eigel A, Van Dorsselaer A, Wieland H, Kister J, Kiger L. Hemoglobin Gorwihl1 [alpha2beta(2)5(A2)Pro → Ala], an electrophoretically silent variant with impaired glycation. Clin Chem 2003;49:137-43.

7. Bonfiglio R, King RC, Olah TV, Merkle K. The effects of sample preparation methods on the variability of the electrospray ionization response for model drug compounds. Rap Comm in Mass Spectrometry 1999;13:1175-85.
8. Bu HZ, Magis L, Knuth K, Teitelbaum P. High-throughput cytochrome P450 (CYP) inhibition screening via cassette probe-dosing strategy. 1. Development of direct injection/on-line guard cartridge extraction/tandem mass spectrometry for the simultaneous detection of CYP probe substrates and their metabolites. Rapid Commun Mass Spectrom 2000;14:1619-24.
9. Cameron AE, Eggers DF Jr. An ion velocitron. Rev Sci Instrum 1948;19:605-7.
10. Caprioli RM, Fan T. Continuous-flow sample probe for fast atom bombardment mass spectrometry. Anal Chem 1986;58:2949-54.
11. Caprioli RM. Continuous-flow fast atom bombardment mass spectrometry. Anal Chem 1990;62:477A-85A.
12. Carroll DI, Dizdic I, Stillwell RN, Haegele KD, Horning EC. Atmospheric pressure ionization mass spectrometry. Corona discharge ion source for use in liquid chromatograph-mass spectrometer-computer analytical system. Anal Chem 1975;47:2369-73.
13. Casetta B, Tagliacozzi D, Shushan B. Development of a method for rapid quantitation of amino acids by liquid chromatography-tandem mass spectrometry (LC-MSMS) in plasma. Clin Chem Lab Med 2000;38:391-401.
14. Cech NB, Enke CG. Practical implications of some recent studies in electrospray ionization fundamentals. Mass Spectrometry Reviews 2001;20:362-87.
15. Chace DH, DiPerna JC, Mitchell BL, Sgroi B, Hofman LF, Naylor EW. Electrospray tandem mass spectrometry for analysis of acylcarnitines in dried postmortem blood specimens collected at autopsy from infants with unexplained cause of death. Clin Chem 2001;47:1166-82.
16. Chace DH. Mass spectrometry-based diagnostics: the upcoming revolution in disease detection has already arrived. Clin Chem 2003;49:1228-9.
17. Chace DH, Kalas TA, Naylor EW. Use of Tandem Mass Spectrometry for Multianalyte Screening of Dried Blood Specimens from Newborns. Clin Chem 2003;49:1797-817.
18. Cooks RG, Rockwood AL. The "Thomson". A suggested unit for mass spectroscopists. Rap Comm in Mass Spectrom 1991;5:93.
19. Crespi CL, Penman BW, Hu M. Development of Caco-2 cells expressing high levels of cDNA-derived cytochrome P4503A4. Pharm Res 1996;13:1635-41.
20. Dahl D. Simion ion optics program version 6.0.
21. Dawson JHJ, Gilhaus M. Orthogonal-acceleration time-of-flight mass spectrometer. Rap Comm Mass Spectrom 1989;3:155-9.
22. Dawson PH. Quadrupole mass spectrometry and its applications. New York: Elsevier Scientific Publishing, 1976:65-78.
23. de Hoffman E, Stroobant V. Mass spectrometry principles and applications, second edition. New York: John Wiley and Sons 2001: Appendix 1, 361.
24. de Hoffman E, Stroobant V. Mass spectrometry principles and applications, second edition. New York: John Wiley and Sons, 2001:63-122 and 132-55.
25. Deters M, Kirchner G, Resch K, Kaever V. Simultaneous quantification of sirolimus, everolimus, tacrolimus and cyclosporine by liquid chromatography-mass spectrometry. Clin Chem Lab Med 2002;40:285-92.
26. Ermer J, Voge, M. Applications of hyphenated LC-MS techniques in pharmaceutical analysis. Biomedical Chromatography 2000;14:373-83.
27. Eshraghi J, Chowdhury SK. Factors affecting the electrospray ionization of effluents containing trifluoroacetic acid for high-performance liquid chromatography/mass spectrometry. Anal Chem 1993;65:3528-33.
28. Fenn JB, Mann M, Meng CK, Wong SF, Whitehouse CM. Electrospray ionization for mass spectrometry of large biomolecules. Science. 1989 Oct 6;246(4926):64-71.
29. Fenn JB. Electrospray Wings for Molecular Elephants (Nobel Lecture). Angew Chem Int Ed Engl. 2003 Aug 25;42(33):3871-94.
30. Figeys D. Novel approaches to map protein interactions. Current Opinion in Biotechnology 2003;14:119-25.
31. Gharahdaghi F, Kirchner M, Fernandez J, Mische SM. Peptide-mass profiles of polyvinylidene difluoride-bound proteins by matrix-assisted laser desorption/ionization time-of-flight mass spectrometry in the presence of nonionic detergents. Anal Biochem 1996;233:94-9.
32. Glish G. To the editor. J Amer Soc Mass Spectrom 1992;2:349.
33. Glish GL, Vachet RW. The basics of mass spectrometry in the twenty-first century. Nature Reviews Drug Discovery 2003;2:140-50.
34. Hardy DT, Preece MA, Green A. Determination of plasma free carnitine by electrospray tandem mass spectrometry. Ann Clin Biochem 2001;38:665-70.
35. Hirabayashi A, de la Mora JF. Charged droplet formation in sonic spray. Int J Mass Spectrometr Ion Processes 1998;175:277-82.
36. Hirabayashi A, Sakairi M, Koizumi H. Sonic spray mass spectrometry. Anal Chem 1995;67:2878-82.
37. Horning EC, Horning MG, Carroll DI, Dzidic I, Stillwell RN. New picogram detection system based on a mass spectrometer with an external ionization source at atmospheric pressure. Anal Chem 1973;45:936-43.

38. Hsieh Y, Chintala M, Mei H, Agans J, Brisson J-M, Ng K, Korfmacher WA. Quantitative screening and matrix effect studies of drug discovery compounds in monkey plasma using fast-gradient liquid chromatography/ tandem mass spectrometry. Rap Comm Mass Spectrometry 2001;15:2481-7.
39. Huang EC, Wachs T, Conboy JJ, Henion JD. Atmospheric pressure ionization mass spectrometry. Anal Chem 1990;62:713A-25A.
40. Hutchens T, Yip T. New desorption strategies for the mass spectrometric analysis of macromolecules. Rapid Commun Mass Spectrom 1993;7:576-80.
41. Issaq H, Veenstra T, Conrads T, Felschow D The SELDI-TOF approach to proteomics. protein profiling and biomarker identification. Biochem Biophys Res Commun 2002;292:587-92.
42. Jeffery DA, Bogyo M. Chemical proteomics and its application to drug discovery. Current Opinion in Biotechnology 2003;14:87-95.
43. Karas M, Hillencamp F. Laser Desorption ionization of proteins with molecular masses exceeding 10,000 daltons. Anal Chem 1988;60:2299-301.
44. Karas M, Bachmann D, Bahr U, Hillenkamp F. Matrix-assisted ultraviolet laser desorption of non-volatile compounds. Int J Mass Spectrom Ion Processes 1987;78:53-68.
45. Kenyon GL, DeMarini DM, Fuchs E, Galas DJ, Kirsch JF, et al. Defining the mandate of proteomics in the post-genomics era: Workshop report. Mol Cell Proteomics 2002;1(10):763-80.
46. Kelley RJ. Diagnosis of Smith-Lemli-Opitz syndrome by gas chromatography/mass spectrometry of 7-dehydrocholesterol in plasma, amniotic fluid, and cultured skin fibroblasts. Clin Chim Acta 1995;236:45-58.
47. King R, Bonfiglio R, Fernandez-Metzler C, Miller-Stein C, Olah T. Mechanistic investigation of ionization suppression in electrospray ionization. J Am Soc Mass Spectrometry 2000;11:942-50.
48. Kitamura R, Matsuoka K, Matsushima E, Kawaguchi Y. Improvement in precision of the liquid chromatographic-electrospray ionization tandem mass spectrometric analysis of 3′-C-ethynylcytidine in rat plasma. J Chromatogr B 2001;754:113-19.
49. Koy C, Mikkat S, Raptakis E, Sutton C, Resch M, Tanaka K, Glocker MO. Matrix-assisted laser desorption/ionization-quadrupole ion trap-time of flight mass spectrometry sequencing resolves structures of unidentified peptides obtained by in-gel tryptic digestion of haptoglobin derivatives from human plasma proteomes. Proteomics. 2003 Jun;3(6):851-8.
50. Krause E, Wenschuh H, Jungblut PR. The dominance of arginine-containing peptides in MALDI-derived tryptic mass fingerprints of proteins. Anal Chem 1999;71:4160-5.
51. Kushnir MM, Komaromy-Miller G, Shushan B, Urry FM, Roberts WL. Analysis of dicarboxylic acids by tandem mass spectrometry. High-throughput quantitative measurement of methylmalonic acid in serum, plasma, and urine. Clin Chem 2001;47:1993-2002.
52. Kushnir MM, Urry FM, Frank EL, Roberts WL. Analysis of catecholamines in urine by positive-ion electrospray tandem mass spectrometry. Clin Chem 2002;48:323-31.
53. Laiko V, Baldwin M, Burlingame A. Atmospheric pressure matrix-assisted laser desorption/ionization mass spectrometry. Anal Chem 2000;72:652-7.
54. Laiko VV, Dodonov AF. Resolution and spectral-line shapes in the reflecting time-of-flight mass spectrometer with orthogonally injected ions. Rap Comm Mass Spectrom 1994;8:720-6.
55. Lazar IM, Lee ED, Rockwood AL, Lee ML. General Considerations for optimizing a capillary electrophoresis-electrospray time-of-flight mass spectrometry system, J Chromatogr A 1998;829:279-88.
56. Li J Zhang Z, Rosenzweig J, Wand Y, Chan D. Proteomics and bioinformatics approaches for identification of serum biomarkers to detect breast cancer. Clin Chem 2002;48:1296-304.
57. Lin D, Tabb DL, Yates JR III. Large-scale protein identification using mass spectrometry. Biochim Biophys Acta 2003;1646:1-10.
58. Magera MJ, Lacey JM, Casetta B, Rinaldo P. Method for the determination of total homocysteine in plasma and urine by stable isotope dilution and electrospray tandem mass spectrometry. Clin Chem 1999;45:1517-22.
59. Mallard WG, Reed J. AMDIS-User Guide, National Institute of Standards and Technology, 1997.
60. Mamyrin BA, Karataev VI, Shmikk DV, Zagulin VA. Mass reflectron. New nonmagnetic time-of-flight high-resolution mass spectrometer. Zh Eksp Teor Fiz 1973;64:82-9.
61. Mandal BK, Ogra Y, Suzuki KT. Speciation of arsenic in human nail and hair from arsenic-affected area by HPLC-inductively coupled argon plasma mass spectrometry. Toxicol Appl Pharmacol 2003;189:73-83.
62. Matuszewski BK, Constanzer ML, Chavez-Eng CM. Matrix effect in quantitative LC/MS/MS analyses of biological fluids. a method for determination of finasteride in human plasma at picogram per milliliter concentrations. Anal Chem 1998;70:882-9.
63. Maurer HH. Role of gas chromatography-mass spectrometry with negative ion chemical ionization in clinical and forensic toxicology, doping control, and biomonitoring. Ther Drug Monitor 2002;24:247-54.
64. Merchant M, Weinberger S. Recent advancements in surface-enhanced laser desorption/ionization-time of flight-mass spectrometry. Electrophoresis 2000;21:1164-77.
65. Moy FJ, Haraki K, Mobilio D, Walker G, Powers R, Tabei K, Tong H, Siegel MM. MS/NMR. a structure-

based approach for discovering protein ligands and for drug design by coupling size exclusion chromatography, and nuclear magnetic resonance spectroscopy. Anal Chem 2001;73:571-81.

66. Moyer S, Cotter R Atmospheric pressure MALDI. Anal Chem 2002;74:469A-76A.
67. Muddiman DC, Rockwood AL, Gao Q, Severs JC, Udseth HR, Smith RD. Application of sequential paired covariance to capillary electrophoresis electrospray ionization time-of-flight mass spectrometry. Unraveling the signal from the noise in the electropherogram. Anal Chem 1995;67:4371-5.
68. Muller C, Schafer, P, Stortzel, M, Vogt, Weinmann, W. Ion suppression effects in liquid chromatography-electrospray-ionization transport-region collision induced dissociation mass spectrometry with different serum extraction methods for systematic toxicological analysis with mass spectral libraries. J Chromatogr B 2002;773:47-52.
69. Nakanishi T, Okamoto N, Tanaka K, Shimizu A. Laser desorption time-of-flight mass spectrometric analysis of transferrin precipitated with antiserum: a unique simple method to identify molecular weight variants. Biol Mass Spectrom. 1994 Apr;23(4):230-3.
70. Opiteck GJ, Lewis KC, Jorgenson JW. Comprehensive on-line LC/LC/MS of proteins. Anal Chem 1997;69:518-24.
71. Petkovic M, Muller J, Muller M, Schiller J, Arnold K, Arnhold J. Application of matrix-assisted laser desorption/ionization time-of-flight mass spectrometry for monitoring the digestion of phosphatidylcholine by pancreatic phospholipase A2. Anal Biochem 2002;308:61-70.
72. Petricoin EF, Liotta LA. Clinical applications of proteomics. J Nutr 2003;133(7 Suppl):2476S-84S.
73. Price P. Standard Definition of Terms Relating to Mass Spectrometry, J Amer Soc Mass Spectrometry 1991;2:336-48.
74. Robb DB, Covey TR, Bruins AP. Atmospheric pressure photoionization. an ionization method for liquid chromatography-mass spectrometry. Anal Chem 2000;72:3653-9.
75. Rockwood AL. An improved time of flight mass spectrometer. Proc 34th Am Soc for Mass Spectrom 1986;Cincinnati, 173-4.
76. Romijn EP, Krijgsveld J, Heck AJR. Recent liquid chromatographic—(tandem) mass spectrometric applications in proteomics. J Chromatogr A 2003;1000:589-608.
77. ShermanNE, Stefansson B, Fox JW, Goldberg JB. Pseudomonas aeruginosa and a proteomic approach to bacterial pathogenesis. Disease Markers 2001;17:285-93.
78. Sin CH, Lee ML. Apparatus and method for trace analysis, US patent no 5,070,240, December 3, 1991.
79. Sin CH, Lee ED, Lee ML. Atmospheric pressure ionization time-of-flight mass spectrometry, Anal Chem 1991;63:2897-900.
80. Siuzdak G. Mass analyzers and ion detectors. In: Siuzdak G, Mass spectrometry for biotechnology. San Diego: Academic Press, 1996:32-55.
81. Stelland, F, ten Brink, HJ, Kok, RM, Jakobs, C. Stable isotope dilution analysis of very long chain fatty acids in plasma, urine, and amniotic fluid by electron capture negative ion mass fragmentography. Clin Chim Acta 1990;192:133-44.
82. Strege M. High-performance liquid chromatographic-electrospray ionization mass spectrometric analyses for the integration of natural products with modern high-throughput screening. J Chromatogr 1999;725:67-78.
83. Syage JA, Evans MD, Hanold KA. Photoionization mass spectrometry. Amer Lab 2000;Issue 12:24-9.
84. Syage JA, Hanning-Lee MA, Hanold KA. A man-portable, photoionization time-of-flight mass spectrometer. Field Anal Chem Toxicol 2000;4:204-15.
85. Tanaka K. The Origin of Macromolecule Ionization by Laser Irradiation (Nobel Lecture). Angew Chem Int Ed Engl. 2003 Aug 25;42(33):3860-70.
86. Tao WA, Aebersold R. Advances in quantitative proteomics via stable isotope tagging and mass spectrometry. Current Opinion in Biotechnology 2003;14:110-18.
87. Theodoritis G, Laskaris G, de Jong CF, Hofte AJP, Verpoorte R. Determination of paclitaxel and related diterpenoids in plant extracts by high-performance liquid chromatography with UV detection in high-performance liquid chromatography-mass spectrometry. J Chromatogr A 1998;802:297-305.
88. Todd JFT. Recommendations for nomenclature and symbolism for mass spectroscopy. IUPAC recommendations 1991. Pure & Appl Chem 1991;63:1541-66.
89. van Hout MWJ, Hoffland CM, Niederlander HAG, de Jong GJ. On-line coupling of solid-phase extraction with mass spectrometry for the analysis of biological samples. II. Determination of clenbuterol in urine using multiple-stage mass spectrometry in an ion-trap spectrometer. Rap Comm Mass Spectrometry 2000;14:2103-11.
90. Villani P, Feroggio M, Gianelli L, Bartoli A, Montagna M, Maserati R, Regazzi MB. Antiretrovirals. simultaneous determination of five protease inhibitors and three nonnucleoside transcriptase inhibitors in human plasma by a rapid high-performance liquid chromatography-mass spectrometry assay. Ther Drug Monitor 2001;23:380-8.
91. Wang Z, Dunlop K, Long R, L, L. Mass spectrometric methods for generation of protein mass database used for bacterial identification. Anal Chem 2002;74:3174-82.

92. Whitehouse CM, Dreyer RN, Yamashita M, Fenn JB. Electrospray interface for liquid chromatographs and mass spectrometers. Anal Chem 1985;57:675-9.
93. Wiley CH, McLaren IH. Time-of-flight mass spectrometer with improved resolution. Rev Sci Instrum 1955;26:1150-7.
94. Yamashita M, Fenn, JB. Electrospray ion source. Another variation on the free-jet theme. J Phys Chem 1984;88:4451-9.

ADDITIONAL READING

Ardrey RE. Liquid chromatography—Mass spectrometry: An introduction. Hoboken NJ: John Wiley and Sons, 2003.

Binz PA, Hochstrasser DF, Appel RD. Mass spectrometry-based proteomics: current status and potential use in clinical chemistry. Clin Chem Lab Med 2003;41:1540-51.

Campbell AM, Heyer lJ. Discovering genomics, proteomics, and bioinformatics. San Francisco:Benjamin/Cummings, 2002.

Cole RB. Electrospray ionization mass spectrometry. Hoboken NJ: John Wiley and Sons, 1997.

Dass C. Principles and practice of biological mass spectrometry. Hoboken NJ: Wiley-Interscience, 2000.

De Hoffman E, Stroobant V. Mass spectrometry: Principles and applications. Hoboken NJ: John Wiley and Sons, 2001.

Fathi M, Corthals G, Hochstrasser D. Mass spectrometry in laboratory medicine. Clin Chem Lab Med 2003;41:1539.

Ferrer I, Thurman, EM. Liquid chromatography/Mass spectrometry, MS/MS and time of flight MS. Cary NC: Oxford University Press, 2003.

Grayson MA. Measuring mass from positive rays to proteins. Philadelphia: Chemical Heritage Press, 2002.

Herbert CG, Johnstone RAW. Mass spectrometry basics. Boca Raton FL: CRC Press, 2002.

Kinter M, Sherman, NE. Protein sequencing and identification using tandem mass spectrometry. Hoboken NJ: Wiley-Interscience, 2000.

Lee MS. LC/MS applications in drug development. Hoboken NJ: John Wiley and Sons, 2002.

Liebler D, ed. Introduction to proteonomics: Tools for the new biology. Totowa NJ: Humana Press, 2002.

McMaster MC, McMaster C. GC/MS: A practical user's guide. Hoboken NJ: John Wiley and Sons, 1998.

Niessen WM, Niessen WMA. Current practice of gas chromatography-Mass spectrometry. New York NY, Marcel Dekker, 2001.

Pramanik BN, Ganguly AK, Gross ML. Applied Electrospray Mass Spectrometry. New York NY, Marcel Dekker, 2002.

Simpson RJ. Proteins and proteomics: A laboratory manual. Woodbury NY: Cold Spring Harbor Laboratory Press, 2002.

Vogeser M. Liquid chromatography-tandem mass spectrometry–application in the clinical laboratory. Clin Chem Lab Med 2003;41:117-26.

Vogeser M, Kyriatsoulis A, Huber E, Kobold U. Candidate reference method for the quantification of circulating 25-hydroxyvitamin D3 by liquid chromatography-tandem mass spectrometry. Clin Chem 2004;50:1415-17.

Willoughby R, Sheehan E, Mitrovich S.: A global view of LC/MS, 2nd ed. Pittsburgh PA: Global View Publishing, 2002.

CHAPTER 8

Principles of Clinical Enzymology*

Renze Bais, Ph.D., and Mauro Panteghini, M.D.

Enzymes are proteins with catalytic properties; clinical enzymology is the application of the science of enzymes to the diagnosis and treatment of disease. The principles of clinical enzymology will be introduced and discussed in this chapter. Individual topics include basic principles, enzyme kinetics, analytical enzymology, and diagnostic enzymology.

BASIC PRINCIPLES

This section begins with a discussion of enzyme nomenclature and is followed with discussions of enzymes as proteins and catalysts.

ENZYME NOMENCLATURE

Historically, individual enzymes were identified using the name of the substrate or group upon which the enzyme acts and then adding the suffix *-ase*. For example, the enzyme hydrolyzing urea was ure*ase*. Later, the type of reaction involved was also identified, as in carbonic anhydrase, D-amino acid oxidase, and succinate dehydrogenase. In addition, some enzymes had been given empirical names such as trypsin, diastase, ptyalin, pepsin, and emulsin.

Because this combination of trivial common names and semisystematic names was found to be inadequate, the International Union of Biochemistry (IUB) appointed an Enzyme Commission (EC) in 1955 to study the problem of enzyme nomenclature. Its subsequent recommendations, with periodic updating, provide a rational and practical basis for identifying all enzymes now known and enzymes that will be discovered in the future (http://www.chem.qmw.ac.uk/iubmb/enzyme/).[9]

With the IUB system, a systematic and trivial name is provided for each enzyme. The systematic name describes the nature of the reaction catalyzed and is associated with a unique numerical code designation. The trivial or practical name, which may be identical to the systematic name but is often a simplification of it, is suitable for everyday use. The unique numerical designation for each enzyme consists of four numbers, separated by periods (e.g., 2.2.8.11). The number is prefixed by the letters *EC*, denoting *Enzyme Commission*. The first number defines the class to which the enzyme belongs. All enzymes are assigned to one of six classes, characterized by the type of reaction they catalyze: (1) oxidoreductases, (2) transferases, (3) hydrolases, (4) lyases, (5) isomerases, and (6) ligases. The next two numbers indicate the subclass and sub-subclass to which the enzyme is assigned. For example, these may differentiate the amino-transferring subclass from the phosphate-transferring category or the ethanol acceptor sub-subclass from that accepting acyl groups. The last number is the specific serial number given to each enzyme within its sub-subclass.

To illustrate how this system is used to name an enzyme, consider the enzyme creatine kinase that catalyzes the reaction:

$$\text{ATP} + \text{creatine} \rightleftharpoons \text{ADP} + \text{creatine phosphate}$$

*The authors gratefully acknowledge the original contributions by Drs. A. Ralph Henderson and Donald W. Moss, upon which portions of this chapter are based.

Its system number is:

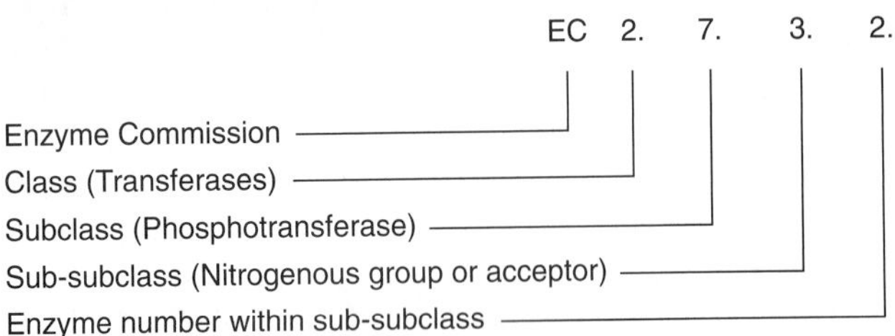

Table 8-1 lists some selected enzymes of clinical interest, identified by trivial, abbreviated, and systematic names and by their code numbers.

Although it is not recommended by the EC, it is a common and convenient practice to use capital letter abbreviations for the names of certain enzymes, such as ALT (formerly GPT) for alanine aminotransferase (EC 2.6.1.2). Other examples are AST for aspartate aminotransferase, LD for lactate dehydrogenase, and CK for creatine kinase (see Table 8-1).

Enzymes as Proteins

Basic Structure

All enzyme molecules possess the primary, secondary, and tertiary structural characteristics of proteins (see Chapter 20). In addition, most enzymes also exhibit the quaternary level of structure. The *primary* structure, the linear sequence of amino acids linked through their α-carboxyl and α-amino groups by peptide bonds, is specific for each type of enzyme molecule. Each polypeptide chain is coiled up into three-dimensional secondary and tertiary levels of structure. *Secondary* structure refers to the conformation of limited segments of the polypeptide chain, namely α-helices, β-pleated sheets, random coils, and β-turns. The arrangement of secondary structural elements and amino acid side chain interactions that define the three-dimensional structure of the folded protein is referred to as its *tertiary* structure. In many cases biological activity, such as the catalytic activity of enzymes, requires two or more folded polypeptide chains (subunits) to associate to form a functional molecule. The arrangement of these subunits defines the *quaternary* structure. The subunits may be copies of the

TABLE 8-1 Enzyme Commission (EC) Numbers, Systematic and Trivial Names, Together With Frequently Adopted Abbreviations of Enzymes of Major Diagnostic Importance

EC Number	Systematic Name	Trivial Name	Abbreviation
1.1.1.27	L-Lactate: NAD^+ oxidoreductase	Lactate dehydrogenase	LD
1.1.1.42	Threo-Ds- isocitrate: $NAD(P)^+$ oxidoreductase (decarboxylating)	Isocitrate dehydrogenase	ICD
1.4.1.3	L-Glutamate: $NAD(P)^+$ oxidoreductase (deaminating)	Glutamate dehydrogenase	GLD
2.3.2.2	(5-Glutamyl)-peptide: amino-acid 5-glutamyltransferase	γ-Glutamyltransferase	GGT
2.6.1.1	L-Aspartate: 2-oxoglutarate aminotransferase	Aspartate aminotransferase (transaminase)	AST
2.6.1.2	L-Alanine: 2-oxoglutarate aminotransferase	Alanine aminotransferase (transaminase)	ALT
2.7.3.2	ATP: creatine *N*-phosphotransferase	Creatine kinase	CK
3.1.1.3	Triacylglycerol acylhydrolase	Lipase	Lip
3.1.1.7	Acetylcholine acetylhydrolase	Acetylcholinesterase, true cholinesterase, cholineesterase I	—
3.1.1.8	Acylcholine acylhydrolase	Pseudocholinesterase, benzoyl cholinesterase, cholineesterase II (serum cholinesterase)	ChE (SChE)
3.1.3.1	Orthophosphoric-monoester phosphohydrolase (alkaline optimum)	Alkaline phosphatase	ALP
3.1.3.2	Orthophosphoric-monoester phosphohydrolase (acid optimum)	Acid phosphatase	ACP
3.1.3.5	5′-Ribonucleotide phosphohydrolase	5′-Nucleotidase	5NT, NTP
3.2.1.1	1,4-α-D-Glucan glucanohydrolase	Amylase	Amy
3.4.2.14		Trypsin	—
4.1.2.13	D-Fructose-1,6-bisphosphate D-glyceraldehyde-3-phosphate-lyase	Aldolase	ALD

same polypeptide chain (homomultimers [e.g., as the MM isoenzyme of creatine kinase, or the H_4 isoenzyme of lactate dehydrogenase]) or they may represent distinct polypeptides (heteromultimers). The biological activity, such as the catalytic activity of enzymes, is often found to be a property of the oligomeric molecule so that activity is usually lost under conditions in which the subunits separate from each other.

The application of physical methods, such as x-ray crystallography and multidimensional nuclear magnetic resonance (NMR) methods, has provided structural insights upon which theories of enzyme mechanisms have been built. Furthermore the tools of molecular biology, such as molecular cloning, have enabled the purification and characterization of enzymes that were previously only available in minute amounts. Molecular biology also enables the manipulation of the amino acid sequence of enzymes, and site-directed mutagenesis (substituting one amino acid residue for another) and deletion mutagenesis (elimination of sections of the primary structure) have allowed the identification of chemical groups that participate in ligand binding and in specific chemical steps during catalysis.

No feature of primary structure, such as repetition of particular amino acid sequences, is common to all enzyme molecules. However, considerable homologies of sequence are found between enzymes that appear to share a common evolutionary origin, such as the proteases trypsin and chymotrypsin, and similarities of sequence are even more marked among the members of a family of isoenzymes. The amino acid sequence in the immediate neighborhood of the active center of the enzyme (discussed later) is often closely similar in enzymes of related function (e.g., the *serine proteases* are so called because they all have this amino acid in the active center).

Enzyme molecules differ in the proportion of secondary-level structures—such as α-helices—they contain, although no enzyme molecule so far studied approaches the large proportion of α-helices found in myoglobin and hemoglobin. The tertiary structures of different types of enzyme molecules are as individually characteristic as their primary structures; nevertheless, some common features can be discerned at this structural level. Enzyme molecules are roughly globular in overall shape, with a preponderance of polar amino acid side chains on the outside of the molecule and nonpolar side chains in the interior. The ionizable residues in contact with the surrounding medium are responsible for many of the properties of the enzyme molecules in a solution, such as their migration in an electric field and their solubility. Covalent disulfide bridges may link different parts of the polypeptide chains in some enzyme molecules, but the three-dimensional structure is mainly stabilized by the large number of hydrophobic interactions that are formed between the nonpolar side chains in the interior of the molecule.

The biological activity of a protein molecule depends generally on the integrity of its structure. Any disruption of the structure is accompanied by a loss of activity, a process known as *denaturation.* If the process of denaturation is minimal, it may be reversed with the recovery of enzyme activity upon removal of the denaturing agent. However, prolonged or severe denaturing conditions result in an irreversible loss of activity. Denaturing conditions include elevated temperatures, extremes of pH, and chemical addition. Heat inactivation of most enzymes takes place at an appreciable rate at room temperature and becomes almost instantaneous in most cases above about 60 °C. The polymerases are an exception and retain activity at temperatures as high as 90 °C. Low temperatures are therefore used to preserve enzyme activity, especially in aqueous solutions, such as serum (see Chapter 21). Extremes of pH also cause unfolding of enzyme molecular structures and, except for a few exceptions, should be avoided when preserving enzyme samples. Addition of chemicals, such as urea and related compounds, disrupts hydrogen bonds and hydrophobic interactions so that exposure of enzymes to strong solutions of these reagents results in inactivation.

Isoenzymes and Other Multiple Forms of Enzymes

Isoenzymes are multiple forms of an enzyme that possess the ability to catalyze the enzyme's characteristic reaction but that differ in structure because they are encoded by distinct structural genes.* These enzyme variants may occur within a single organ or even within a single type of cell. The forms can be distinguished on the basis of differences in various physical properties, such as electrophoretic mobility or resistance to chemical or thermal inactivation. They often have significant quantifiable differences in catalytic properties. However, all the forms of a particular enzyme retain the ability to catalyze its characteristic reaction.

The existence of multiple forms of enzymes in human tissue has important implications in the study of human disease. The presence in different organs of isoenzymes with distinctive properties helps in understanding organ-specific patterns of metabolism, but genetically determined variations in enzyme structure between individuals account for such characteristics as differences in sensitivity to drugs and differences in metabolism, which manifest themselves as hereditary metabolic diseases. For diagnostic enzymology, the existence of multiple forms of enzymes, whether due to genetic or nongenetic causes, may provide opportunities to increase the diagnostic specificity and sensitivity of enzyme assays in body fluid samples.

Like other proteins, enzymes usually elicit the production of antibodies when they are injected into animals of a species other than those in which they originate. Even small structural differences between closely similar molecules, such as the members of a family of isoenzymes, are often sufficient to render them antigenically distinct, allowing antibodies to

*The IUB recommends that the term "isoenzyme" be restricted to forms that originate at the level of the genes that encode the structures of the enzyme proteins in question.[1]

be produced specific to a single type of molecule. The availability of enzyme-specific antisera opens up a wide range of methods in enzyme analysis, some of which—such as immunoassay—do not depend on the catalytic activity of the enzyme molecules. The availability of immunochemical methods has been particularly important in the analysis of isoenzyme mixtures.

Genetic Origins of Enzyme Variants

True isoenzymes are due to the existence of more than one gene locus coding for the structure of the enzyme protein. Many human enzymes (perhaps more than one third) are known to be determined by more than one structural gene locus. The genes at the different loci have undergone differential modifications during the course of evolution so that the enzyme proteins coded by them no longer have identical structures, although they are recognizably similar; in other words, they are isoenzymes. *Multiple-gene loci* have become disseminated throughout a whole species during the course of evolution, so that these genes and their resultant isoenzymes typically are present in all individuals of that species.

The multiple genes that determine a particular group of isoenzymes are not necessarily closely linked on one chromosome; they are often located on different chromosomes. For example, the structural genes that code for human salivary and pancreatic amylases both are located on chromosome 1, whereas the genes that code for mitochondrial and cytoplasmic malate dehydrogenase are carried on chromosomes 7 and 2, respectively. Among the enzymes of clinical importance that exist as isoenzymes because of the presence of multiple gene loci are lactate dehydrogenase, creatine kinase, α-amylase, and some forms of alkaline phosphatase.

A mechanism that results in an enzyme existing in molecular forms that differ from one individual to another is the existence of alternative alleles that are inherited according to Mendelian laws. These give rise to gene products with the same function. The isoenzymes that result from the existence of allelic genes are termed *allozymes.* The proportion of human gene loci subject to allelic variation is considerable, and the probability that individual human beings will differ to some degree in their isoenzyme patterns is correspondingly high.

The number of allelic variants and the frequency with which particular variants occur within the population vary considerably from one enzyme to another. For example, mutations at either of the two principal loci that determine human lactate dehydrogenase are extremely rare, but a high incidence of mutant alleles occurs at the single locus that determines the structure of placental alkaline phosphatase. More than 340 mutations in the glucose-6-phosphate dehydrogenase gene have now been identified on the X chromosome (up-to-date genetic information on this and other enzymes, can be obtained from the Online Mendelian Inheritance in Man (OMIM) database at http://www3.ncbi.nlm.nih.gov/Omim/searchomim.html). Some of these alleles are extremely rare, whereas others occur with appreciable frequency in particular populations or geographical locations. When isoenzymes, due to variation at a single locus, occur with appreciable frequency in a human population, the population is said to be *polymorphic* with respect to the isoenzymes in question.

Another category of multiple molecular forms can arise when enzymes are oligomeric and consist of molecules made up of subunits. The association of different types of subunits in various combinations gives rise to a range of active enzyme molecules. When the subunits are derived from different structural genes, either multiple loci or multiple alleles, the hybrid molecules so formed are called *hybrid isoenzymes.* The ability to form hybrid isoenzymes is evidence of considerable structural similarities between the different subunits. Hybrid isoenzymes can be formed in vitro, but they are also formed in vivo in cells in which the different types of constituent subunits are present in the same subcellular compartment.

The number of different hybrid isoenzymes that can be formed from two nonidentical protomers depends on the number of subunits in the complete enzyme molecule. For a dimeric enzyme, one mixed dimer (hybrid isoenzyme) can be formed. If the enzyme is a tetramer, three heteropolymeric isoenzymes may be formed (Figure 8-1). Examples of

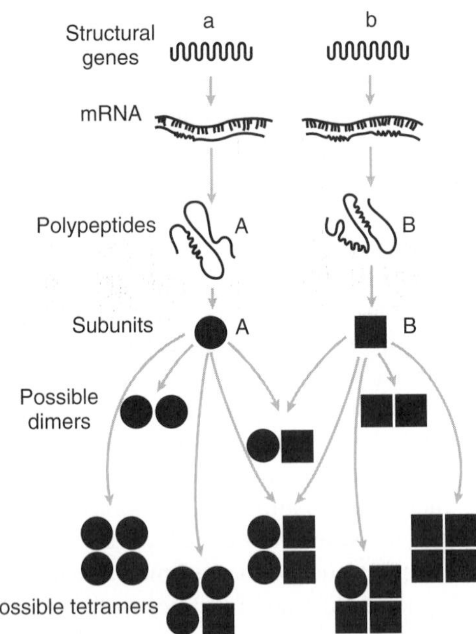

Figure 8-1 Diagram showing the origin of isoenzymes, assuming the existence of two distinct gene loci. When the active enzymes are polymers containing more than one subunit, hybrid isoenzymes consisting of mixtures of different subunits may be formed. One such isoenzyme can be formed in the case of a dimeric enzyme, such as creatine kinase, and three if the enzyme is a tetramer (e.g., lactate dehydrogenase). In both cases, two homopolymeric isoenzymes can also exist. *(From Moss DW. Isoenzyme analysis. London: The Chemical Society, 1979.)*

hybrid isoenzymes are the mixed MB dimer of creatine kinase and the three hybrid isoenzymes, LD-2, LD-3, and LD-4, of lactate dehydrogenase.

Nongenetic Causes of Multiple Forms of Enzymes

Many different types of posttranslational modification of enzyme molecules can give rise to multiple forms that are commonly known as *isoforms* (Figure 8-2). Several of these processes have been shown to cause the heterogeneity of various enzymes, either in living matter or as a result of changes taking place during extraction or storage.

Modification of the residues in the polypeptide chains of enzyme molecules can take place in living cells to give multiple forms. For example, removal of amide groups accounts for some of the heterogeneity of amylase and carbonic anhydrase (these enzymes also each exist as true isoenzymes). Modification can also take place as a result of extraction procedures. Many erythrocyte enzymes, including adenosine deaminase, acid phosphatase, and some forms of phosphoglucomutase, contain sulfhydryl groups that are susceptible to oxidation. In hemolysates, oxidation may be brought about by the action of oxidized glutathione, although in the intact cells, this compound is present in its reduced form. Thus, variant enzyme molecules with altered molecular charge may be generated.

Modifications affecting nonprotein components of enzyme molecules may also lead to molecular heterogeneity. Many enzymes are glycoproteins, and variations in carbohydrate side chains are a common cause of nonhomogeneity of preparations of these enzymes. Some carbohydrate moieties, notably *N*-acetylneuraminic acid (sialic acid), are strongly ionized and consequently have a profound effect on some properties of enzyme molecules. For example, removal of terminal sialic acid groups from human liver and/or bone alkaline phosphatase with neuraminidase greatly reduces the electrophoretic heterogeneity of the enzyme.

Aggregation of enzyme molecules with each other or with nonenzymatic proteins may give rise to multiple forms that can be separated by techniques that depend on differences in molecular size. For example, four catalytically active cholinesterase components with molecular weights ranging from about 80,000 to 340,000 are found in most sera, with the heaviest component, C_4, contributing most of the enzyme activity. Other enzyme forms are also occasionally present, but it appears that the principal serum cholinesterase fractions can be attributed to different states of aggregation of a single monomer.

A specific form of interaction between enzymatic and nonenzymatic proteins is the cause of unusual enzyme components noted when some samples of human plasma are fractionated by electrophoresis or chromatography. These components are due to a combination of apparently normal enzyme or isoenzyme molecules with plasma immunoglobulins. The enzyme-protein complexes ("macrocomplexes")

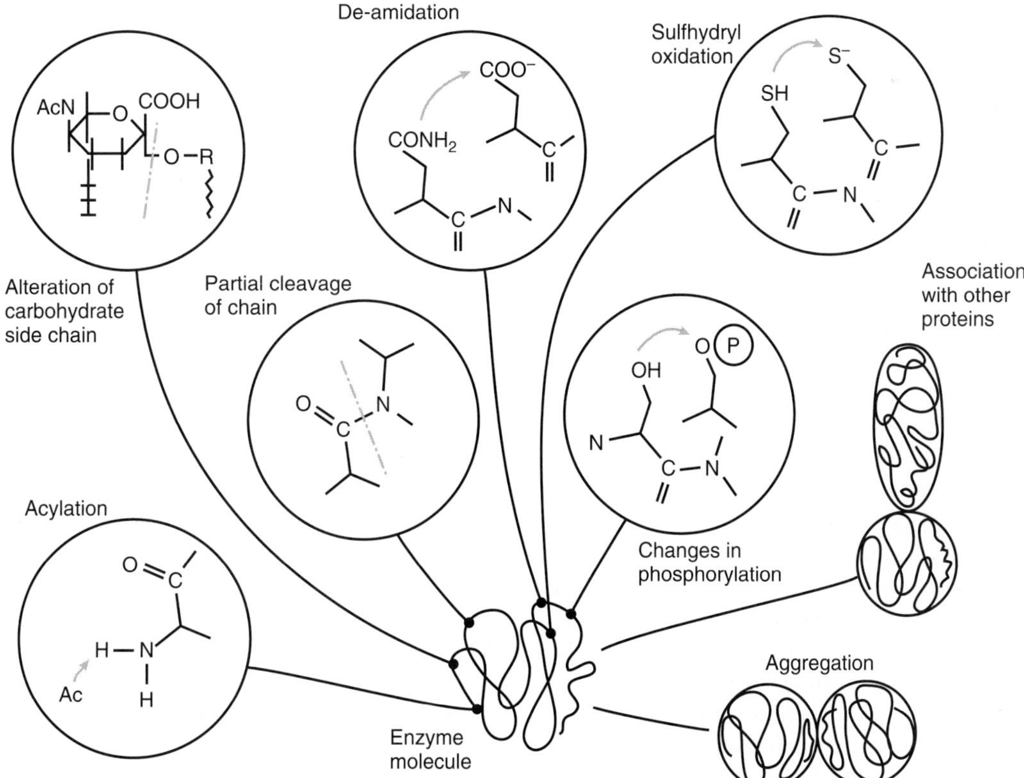

Figure 8-2 Nongenetic modifications that may give rise to multiple forms of enzymes. *(From Moss DW. Isoenzymes. London, Chapman & Hall, 1982.)*

thus formed may themselves be heterogeneous. Since the identification of "macroamylase," the first such enzyme-immunoglobulin complex to be identified, similar complexes have been observed involving lactate dehydrogenase, creatine kinase, alkaline phosphatase (ALP), and other enzymes.

A single polypeptide chain can in theory exist in an infinite number of different conformations. However, one specific conformation generally appears to be the most stable for any given sequence of amino acids, and this conformation is assumed by the chain as it is synthesized within the cell. Thus, the primary structure of the polypeptide chain also determines its three-dimensional secondary and tertiary structures. It is conceivable that in some cases there may be several alternative conformations ("conformers") of a single chain that are of nearly equal stabilities and therefore these alternative forms may coexist. This possibility was first suggested to account for the heterogeneity noted in preparations of the cytoplasmic and mitochondrial isoenzymes of malate dehydrogenase and has also been proposed as an explanation of the multiple electrophoretic zones of erythrocyte acid phosphatase. However, no multiple enzyme forms have been shown unequivocally to be due to conformational isomerism.

Distribution of Isoenzymes and Other Multiple Forms of Enzymes

The existence of multiple gene loci, and the isoenzymes derived from them, has presumably conferred an evolutionary advantage on the species and has thus become part of its normal metabolic pattern. Some of these adaptations are related to the division of function between and within different types of specialized cells and tissues. Thus, the distribution of isoenzymes is not uniform throughout the body, and wide variations in the activity of different isoenzymes are found at the organ, cellular, and subcellular levels. Tissue-specific differences are also found in the distributions of some multiple forms of enzymes that are not due to the existence of multiple gene loci. The tissue-specific distribution of isoenzymes and other multiple forms of enzymes provides the basis for organ-specific diagnosis through isoenzyme measurements.

Certain gene loci may be expressed almost exclusively in a single tissue, perhaps at a particular stage in development. In addition to the two gene loci that determine the two most common subunits of lactate dehydrogenase, a third locus is active only in mature testes. It determines the structure of a third type of subunit, X or C, which makes up a specific isoenzyme, LD-X or LD-C, found only in testes. The isoenzyme of ALP that occurs in the human placenta is the product of a single structural gene locus, which is distinct from the loci that specify the structures of other forms of ALP, and the product of the placental phosphatase locus is normally detectable only in the placenta.

A particularly striking example of the local expression of multiple gene loci is provided by distinct isoenzymes that occur exclusively in specific subcellular organelles. Differences between mitochondrial isoenzymes and their functionally analogous counterparts in the cytoplasm have been demonstrated in several cases (e.g., for aspartate aminotransferase and malate dehydrogenase.)

Changes in Isoenzyme Distribution During Development and Disease

Multiple gene loci and their resultant isoenzymes provide a means for the adaptation of metabolic patterns to the changing needs of different organs and tissues in the course of normal development or in response to environmental change. Pathological conditions may also be associated with alterations in the activities of specific isoenzymes.

The patterns of several sets of isoenzymes change during normal development in tissues from many species. For example, changes in the relative proportions of several isoenzymes are noted during the embryonic development of skeletal muscle. The proportions of the electrophoretically more cathodal isoenzymes, of both LD and CK, progressively increase in this tissue, until approximately the sixth month of intrauterine life, when the pattern resembles that of differentiated muscle. Smaller quantitative changes in isoenzyme distribution may continue to birth and into early postnatal life.

The liver also shows characteristic changes in the patterns of several isoenzymes during embryogenesis. In early fetal development, three aldolase isoenzymes, A, B, and C, together with the various hybrid tetramers, can be detected in extracts of liver. However, at birth as in the adult liver aldolase B is the predominant isoenzyme. Striking changes in the distribution of isoenzymes of alcohol dehydrogenase also occur in human liver during prenatal development.

The changes in isoenzyme patterns during development result from changes in the relative activities of gene loci within developing cells of a particular type (e.g., muscle cells). Other alterations in the balance of isoenzymes within the whole organism may derive from changes in the number or activity of cells that contain large amounts of a characteristic isoenzyme. An example of this is the increased number and activity of the osteoblasts, which are responsible for mineralization of the skeleton between the early postnatal period and the beginning of the third decade of life. The excess of ALP from the active osteoblasts enters the circulation, where its presence can be recognized by its characteristic properties and where it elevates the total serum ALP activity of young people above that of skeletally mature adults. An ALP from the liver also contributes to the total activity of this enzyme in normal plasma, and the amount of this isoenzyme in plasma shows a small, progressive increase with age. The reason for the latter age-dependent change is not known, but it may result from increased synthesis of the isoenzyme by hepatocytes in response to continuing exposure to inducing factors.

Certain diseases, such as the progressive muscular dystrophies, appear to involve a failure of the affected tissues to mature normally or to maintain a normal state. Cancer cells show a progressive loss of the structure and metabolism of the healthy cells from which they arise. Therefore the pattern of isoenzymes of mature, differentiated tissue may be lost or modified if normal differentiation is arrested or reversed, and many examples have been reported of isoenzyme changes accompanying such processes.

The distributions of isoenzymes of aldolase, LD, and CK in the muscles of patients with progressive muscular dystrophy have been found to be similar to those in the earlier stages of development of fetal muscle. The isoenzyme abnormalities in dystrophic muscle have been interpreted as a failure to reach or maintain a normal degree of differentiation. Isoenzyme patterns in regenerating tissues may also show some tendency to approach fetal distributions. This tendency may result from relaxation or modification of control systems in rapidly dividing cells and may account for some of the isoenzyme changes noted (e.g., in muscle in acute polymyositis).

Reemergence of fetal patterns of isoenzyme distribution is also a feature of malignant transformation in many tissues. This phenomenon was first studied extensively in the case of lactate dehydrogenase isoenzymes. Malignant tumors in general show a significant shift in the balance of isoenzymes toward the electrophoretically more cathodal forms, LD-4 and LD-5. The decline in activity of the LD-1 and LD-2 isoenzymes results in patterns that are reminiscent of those occurring in embryonic tissues. Tumors of prostate, cervix, breast, brain, stomach, colon, rectum, bronchus, and lymph nodes are among those that show this transformation. In contrast, comparatively benign gliomas show a relative increase in anionic isoenzymes. A relative increase in the proportion of cathodal isoenzymes of LD has also been observed in tissue adjacent to malignant tumors (e.g., the colon), although the cells in these regions are morphologically normal.

The isoenzyme patterns of aldolase, pyruvate kinase, and hexosaminidase have also been shown to undergo a change toward fetus-like patterns in hepatoma.

In 1968, Fishman and his collaborators reported the identification of an ALP in the serum of a patient with metastatic squamous cell carcinoma of the lung that was biochemically and immunologically identical with the ALP of a normal placenta. The newly discovered isoenzyme was termed the *Regan isoenzyme* after the patient in whom it was discovered. The Regan isoenzyme has been detected in tumor tissues and in sera of patients with many types of malignant disease and in some patients with nonmalignant diseases. An incidence of the isoenzyme of 3% to 15% in sera of cancer patients has been estimated, but this varies with the sensitivity of the methods used for its detection. Other variant forms of ALP have since been discovered in tumor tissues. These variants show many similarities to normal placental ALP but may differ in other properties, such as response to certain inhibitors.

Differences in Properties Between Multiple Forms of Enzymes

The structural differences between the multiple forms of an enzyme give rise to greater or lesser differences in physicochemical properties, such as electrophoretic mobility, resistance to inactivation, and solubility, or in catalytic characteristics, such as the ratio of reaction with substrate analogues or response to inhibitors. Methods of isoenzyme analysis have therefore been designed to investigate a wide range of catalytic and structural properties of enzyme molecules.[7] However, it is usually possible to make only limited deductions about the nature of the underlying structural differences between isoenzymes that are responsible for the dissimilar properties. Equally, the changes in catalytic and other properties that may result from specific structural alterations in enzyme molecules can rarely be predicted from current theoretical knowledge of the relationship between structure and function of proteins.

Techniques of molecular biology, such as gene cloning and sequencing, have revolutionized the investigation of the primary structures of isoenzymes. The differences in primary structures between isoenzymes, whether derived from multiple gene loci or different alleles, are now known in a growing number of cases. Furthermore, many questions have been answered about whether multiple enzyme forms represented true (genetically determined) isoenzymes or arose from posttranslational modification.

Isoenzymes caused by the existence of multiple-gene loci usually differ quantitatively in catalytic properties. These differences may be manifested in such characteristics as molecular activity, K_m values for substrate(s), sensitivity to various inhibitors, and relative rates of activity with substrate analogues (when the specificity of the isoenzymes allows the substrate to be varied), underscoring the biological importance of isoenzymatic variation. In contrast, multiple enzyme forms that arise by such posttranslational modifications as aggregation usually have similar catalytic properties.

Multilocus isoenzymes also usually differ in antigenic specificity, although these differences may be less pronounced among isoenzymes that have emerged relatively recently in evolutionary history and are closely related in structure. Immunological cross-reaction is also not uncommon among multilocus isoenzymes. Multiple enzyme forms caused by postsynthetic modification frequently have common antigenic determinants. Isoenzymes derived from allelic genes (allozymes) are often antigenically similar, even to the extent that they may cross-react with antisera to the common isoenzyme even when a mutation has abolished enzyme activity altogether. The capacity for detecting differences between antigenically similar isoenzyme molecules depends on the extent of monoclonal antibody specificity.

Differences in resistance to denaturation (e.g., by heat or concentrated urea solutions) are commonly found between true isoenzymes, whether these are the products of multiple loci or multiple alleles. Other multiple forms of enzymes often do not differ or differ only slightly in this respect. The most commonly exploited difference between isoenzymes is the difference in net molecular charge that results from the altered amino acid compositions of the molecules; this forms the basis of separation by zone electrophoresis, ion-exchange chromatography, or isoelectric focusing. Separation methods that depend on differences in molecular size, such as gel filtration, do not distinguish between the small differences in size that often exist between true isoenzyme molecules but are important in the detection of multiple forms that involve aggregation or association of enzyme molecules with other proteins.

ENZYMES AS CATALYSTS

A *catalyst* is a substance that increases the rate of a particular chemical reaction without being consumed or permanently altered; enzymes are *protein catalysts* of biological origin. Metabolism is a coordinated series of chemical reactions that occur within a living cell to provide energy and accomplish biosynthesis. The process can be regarded as an integrated series of enzymatic reactions and some diseases as a derangement of the normal pattern of metabolism. Apart from these fundamental considerations, it is the remarkable properties of enzymes that make them such sensitive indicators of pathological change.

Efficiency

Because of their remarkable catalytic activity, a given number of enzyme molecules convert an enormous number of substrate molecules to products within a short time. Therefore, the appearance of increased amounts of enzymes in the blood stream is easily detected, although the amount of enzyme protein released from damaged cells is small compared with the total level of nonenzymatic proteins in blood. Thus a particular enzyme is recognized by its characteristic effect on a given chemical reaction despite the presence of a vast excess of other proteins.

Like other catalysts, an enzyme changes only the rate at which equilibrium is established between reactants and products; it does not alter the equilibrium constant of the reaction. In a reaction in which only one set of products is chemically possible, the catalyst cannot effect any change in the nature of the products. But when several different possible pathways exist, the enzyme directs the reaction along only one pathway.

Specificity and the Active Center

With the exception of enzymes such as proteases, nucleases, and amylases, which act on macromolecular substrates, enzyme molecules are considerably larger than the molecules of their substrates. Consideration of the structure of an enzyme's active site and its relationship to the structures of the enzyme's substrate(s) in its ground and transition states is necessary to understand the rate enhancement and specificity of the chemical reactions performed by the enzyme. The active site of an enzyme will vary between enzymes but in general:[2]

1. The active site of an enzyme is relatively small compared with the total volume of the enzyme molecule because its structure may involve less than 5% of the total amino acids in the molecule.
2. The active sites of enzymes are three-dimensional structures that are formed as a result of the overall tertiary structure of the protein. This results from the amino acids and co-factors in the active site of an enzyme being spatially structured in an exact, three-dimensional relationship with respect to one another and the structure of the substrate molecule.
3. Typically, the attraction between the molecules of the enzyme and its substrate molecules is noncovalent binding. Physical forces used in this type of binding include hydrogen bonding, electrostatic and hydrophobic interactions, and van der Waals forces.
4. Active sites of enzymes typically occur in clefts and crevices in the protein. This excludes bulk solvent and reduces the catalytic activity of the enzyme.
5. The specificity of substrate binding is a function of the exact special arrangement of atoms in the enzyme active site that complements the structure of the substrate molecule.

ENZYME KINETICS

THE ENZYME-SUBSTRATE COMPLEX

Enzymes act through the formation of an enzyme-substrate (*ES*) complex, in which a molecule of substrate is bound to the *active center* of the enzyme molecule. The binding process transforms the substrate molecule to its activated state. The energy required for this transformation is provided by the free energy of binding of *S* to *E*. Therefore activation takes place without the addition of external energy so that the energy barrier to the reaction is lowered and the breakdown to products is accelerated (see Figure 8-3). The ES complex breaks down to give the reaction products (*P*) and free enzyme (*E*):

$$E + S \rightleftarrows ES \longrightarrow P + E \qquad (1)$$

All reactions catalyzed by enzymes are in theory reversible. However, in practice the reaction is usually found to be more rapid in one direction than in the other, so that an equilibrium is reached in which the product of either the forward or the backward reaction predominates, sometimes so markedly that the reaction is virtually irreversible.

If the product of the reaction in one direction is removed as it is formed (e.g., because it is the substrate of a second enzyme present in the reaction mixture), the equilibrium of the first enzymatic process will be displaced so that the reaction will proceed to completion in that direction. Reaction sequences in which the product of one enzyme-catalyzed reaction becomes the substrate of the next enzyme and so on, often through many stages, are characteristic of biologi-

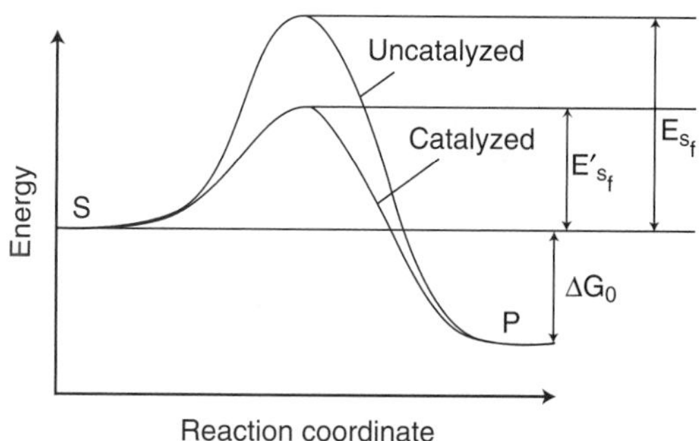

Figure 8-3 Activation energy barrier and reaction course, with and without enzyme catalysis. E_{S_f} is the activation energy for the forward reaction (S → P) in the absence of a catalyst and E'_{S_f} is the activation energy in the presence of a catalyst. ΔG_0 is the change in free energy for the reaction.

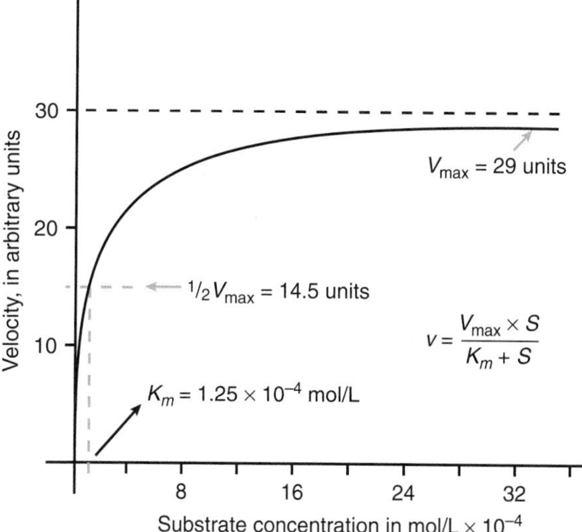

Figure 8-4 Michaelis-Menten curve relating velocity (rate) of an enzyme-catalyzed reaction to substrate concentration. The value of K_m is given by the substrate concentration at which one half of the maximum velocity is obtained.

cal processes. In the lab also, several enzymatic reactions may be linked together to provide a means of measuring the activity of the first enzyme or the concentration of the initial substrate in the chain. For example, the activity of CK is usually measured by a series of linked reactions, and the concentration of glucose is determined by consecutive reactions catalyzed by hexokinase and glucose-6-phosphate dehydrogenase.

When a secondary enzyme-catalyzed reaction, known as an *indicator reaction,* is used to determine the activity of a different enzyme, the primary reaction catalyzed by the enzyme to be determined must be the rate-limiting step. Conditions are chosen to ensure that the rate of reaction catalyzed by the indicator enzyme is directly proportional to the rate of product formation in the first reaction.

Factors Governing the Rate of Enzyme-Catalyzed Reactions

Factors that affect the rate of enzyme-catalyzed reactions include enzyme and substrate concentration, pH, temperature, and the presence of inhibitors, activators, co-enzymes, and prosthetic groups.

Enzyme Concentration

The simplest enzymatically catalyzed reaction for converting substrate S into product P with the intermediate formation of an ES complex, is:

$$E_f + S \underset{k_{-1}}{\overset{k_1}{\rightleftarrows}} ES \xrightarrow{k_2} E_f + P \qquad (2)$$

where

E_f = free enzyme
k_1 = rate constant for the association of the complex
k_{-1} = rate constant for the dissociation of the complex
ES = enzyme-substrate complex
k_2 = rate constant for breakdown of ES to E_f and P
P = product

Michaelis and Menten assumed that equilibrium is attained rapidly among E, S, and ES with the effect of product formation (ES → P) on the concentration of ES being negligible. In addition, the formation of product is written as an irreversible process because there is no product in the solution under initial conditions. Therefore the overall rate of the reaction under otherwise constant conditions is proportional to the concentration of the ES complex.

Provided that an excess of free substrate molecules is present, addition of more enzyme molecules to the reaction system increases the concentration of the ES complex and thus the overall rate of reaction. This accounts for the observation that the rate of reaction is generally proportional to the concentration of enzyme present in the system and is the basis for the quantitative determination of enzymes by measurement of reaction rates. Reaction conditions are selected to ensure that the observed reaction rate is proportional to enzyme concentration over as wide a range as possible.

Substrate Concentration

In addition to explaining the dependence of reaction rate on enzyme concentration under conditions in which excess substrate is present, the formation of an ES complex also accounts for the hyperbolic relationship between reaction velocity and substrate concentration (Figure 8-4). In this section both single-, two-substrate, and consecutive enzyme reactions will be discussed.

Single-Substrate Reactions

If the enzyme concentration is fixed and the substrate concentration is varied, the rate of reaction is first order with respect to substrate concentration and proportional to substrate concentration at low values of the latter. Under these conditions, only a fraction of the enzyme is associated with substrate, and the rate observed reflects the low concentration of the ES complex. At high substrate concentrations, variation in substrate concentration has no effect on rate, and the reaction is zero order with respect to substrate concentration. Under these conditions, all the enzyme is bound to the substrate, and a much higher rate of reaction is obtained. Moreover, because all the enzyme is now present in the form of the complex, no further increase in complex concentration and no further increment in reaction rate are possible. The maximum possible velocity for the reaction has been reached. The significance of substrate-rate curves was first emphasized by Michaelis and Menten, and such curves are referred to as *Michaelis-Menten plots.*

Referring again to equation (2), the overall rate of the reaction (v) is determined by the rate at which product is formed:

$$\text{v} = \frac{d[P]}{dt} = k_2[ES] \qquad (3)$$

The formation of ES will depend on the rate constant k_1 and the availability of enzyme and substrate. If it its assumed the system is in a steady state with the ES complex being formed and broken down at the same rate so that overall $[ES]$ is constant, then the steady state equation is

$$k_1[E][S] = k_{-1}[ES] + k_2[ES] \qquad (4)$$

This equation can be rearranged to

$$[ES] = \frac{k_1[E][S]}{k_{-1} + k_2} \qquad (5)$$

when these rate constants are combined into a single term, the Michaelis constant (K_m) written as

$$K_m = \frac{k_{-1} + k_2}{k_1} \qquad (6)$$

and then substituting this into equation (5) gives

$$[ES] = \frac{[E][S]}{K_m} \qquad (7)$$

Because the amount of ES will be a negligible fraction of the total ([S] >>> [E]), the concentration of free substrate is equated to the total substrate concentration. By substituting equation (3) into equation (7) and eliminating $[ES]$

$$\text{v} = k_2 \times \frac{[E_t] \times [S]}{K_m + [S]} \qquad (8)$$

For a given amount of enzyme, the maximum reaction velocity (V_{max}) is reached when all of the enzyme is saturated with substrate (i.e., $[ES] = [Et]$) and therefore, $V_{max} = k_2 \times [Et]$. Substituting this in equation (6) gives

$$\text{v} = \frac{V_{max}[S]}{K_m + [S]} \qquad (9)$$

A plot of v against $[S]$ gives a section of a rectangular hyperbola (see Figure 8-4), and this is the shape of the curve that is found experimentally for most enzymes. When $[S] = K_m$, manipulation of equation (9) yields $\text{v} = \frac{V_{max}}{2}$, thus K_m is the substrate concentration at which the reaction proceeds at one half of its maximum velocity. In practice, it is now customary to restrict K_m to the experimentally determined substrate concentration at which $v = 0.5\ V_{max}$ and to use the symbol K_s to represent the true ES association constant, where this is known.

Although it is quite simple to set up an experiment to determine the variation of v with $[S]$, the exact value of V_{max} is not easily determined from hyperbolic curves. Furthermore, many enzymes deviate from ideal behavior at high substrate concentrations and indeed may be inhibited by excess substrate, so the calculated value of V_{max} cannot be achieved in practice. In the past it was common practice to transform the Michaelis-Menten equation (9) into one of several reciprocal forms (equations [10] and [11]), and either $1/v$ was plotted against $1/[S]$, or $[S]/v$ was plotted against $[S]$.

$$\frac{1}{\text{v}} = \left(\frac{K_m}{V_{max}} \times \frac{1}{[S]}\right) + \frac{1}{V_{max}} \qquad (10)$$

$$\frac{[S]}{\text{v}} = \left(\frac{1}{V_{max}} \times [S]\right) + \frac{K_m}{V_{max}} \qquad (11)$$

Equation (10), for example, when plotted, results in a *Lineweaver-Burk* plot that gives a straight line with intercepts at $1/V_{max}$ on the ordinate and $-1/K_m$ on the abscissa. For illustrative purposes, the data for Figure 8-4 are recast in Lineweaver-Burk form in Figure 8-5. Regarding inhibition, the Michaelis-Menten curve and its linearized plots are altered in a way that is described later.

It is now routine practice to determine kinetic constants such as K_m and V_{max} using a software package. There are a large number of such packages available that vary from specialized routines for kinetic simulations or for data fitting to general mathematical, statistical, or graphical packages (http://med.umich.edu/biochem/enzresources/software.ttm). Some of these packages are free (public domain, shareware, or free license) or commercially available. An example of the former is the ENCORA 1.2 freeware package available from R.J.W. Slats and colleagues at the Delft University of Technology (http://www.bt.tudelft.nl/), that was developed for an enzymatic kinetic parameter fitting using progressive curve analysis. DynaFit is an example of a commercially available routine (http://www.biokin.com/dynafit) that performs nonlinear least-squares regression of chemical kinetic, enzyme kinetic, or ligand receptor binding data. The data can be either initial reaction velocities in dependence on the concentration of varied species (e.g., inhibitor concentration vs. velocity), or the reaction progress curves (e.g., time vs. absorbance).

The value of K_m has been used to compare the binding of homologous or related substrates to the same enzyme. Also, if measured against the same substrate under defined conditions, the K_m value can be used to compare the properties

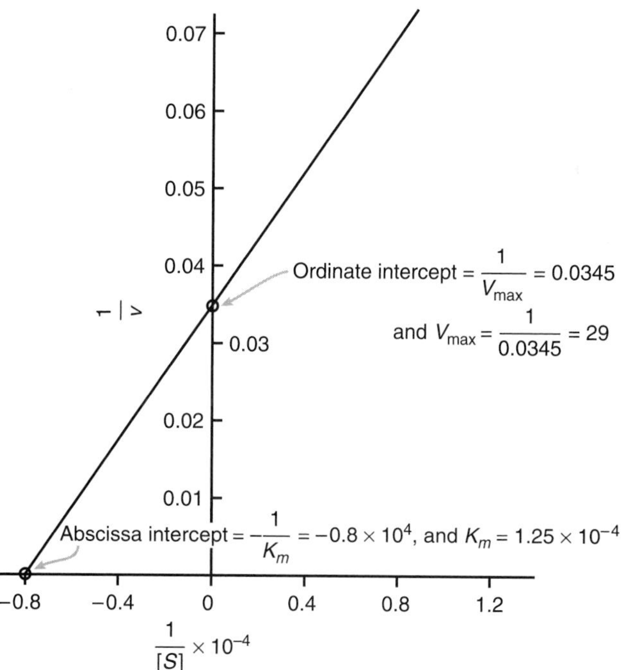

Figure 8-5 Lineweaver-Burk transformation of the curve in Figure 8-4, with $1/v$ plotted on the ordinate (y-axis), and $1/[S]$ on the abscissa (x-axis). The indicated intercepts permit calculation of V_{max} and K_m. The units of v and $[S]$ are those given in Figure 8-4.

of similar enzymes from different sources. Isoenzymes determined by distinct genetic loci typically differ in their K_m, as has been shown (e.g., for the isoenzymes of lactate dehydrogenase.)

When setting up methods of enzyme assay, it is necessary to (1) explore the relationship between reaction velocity and substrate concentration over a wide range, (2) determine K_m, and (3) detect any inhibition at high substrate concentrations. Zero-order kinetics are maintained if the substrate is present in large excess (i.e., concentrations at least 10 and preferably 100 times that of the value of K_m). When $[S] = 10 \times K_m$, v is approximately 91% of the theoretical V_{max}. The K_m values for the majority of enzymes are of the order of 10^{-5} to 10^{-3} mol/L; therefore substrate concentrations are usually chosen to be in the range of 0.001 to 0.10 mol/L. On occasion, the optimal concentrations of substrate cannot be used (e.g., when the substrate has limited solubility or when the concentration of a given substrate inhibits the activity of another enzyme needed in a coupled reaction system).

Two-Substrate Reactions

Most enzymes catalyze reactions with two or more interacting substrates symbolized by the following equation:

$$\underset{S_1}{\text{Substrate 1}} + \underset{S_2}{\text{Substrate 2}} \overset{E}{\rightleftharpoons} \underset{P_1}{\text{Product 1}} + \underset{P_2}{\text{Product 2}} \quad (12)$$

When one of the substrates is water (i.e., when the process is one of hydrolysis), with the reaction taking place in aqueous solution, only a fraction of the total number of water molecules present participates in the reaction. The small change in the concentration of water has no effect on the rate of reaction and these pseudo–one substrate reactions are described by one-substrate kinetics. More generally the concentrations of both substrates may be variable, and both may affect the rate of reaction. Among the bisubstrate reactions important in clinical enzymology are the reactions catalyzed by dehydrogenases, in which the second substrate is a specific coenzyme, such as the oxidized or reduced forms of nicotinamide adenine dinucleotide, (NADH), or nicotinamide adenine dinucleotide phosphate, (NADPH), and the amino-group transfers catalyzed by the aminotransferases.

If a bisubstrate reaction proceeds by way of intermediate ES complexes, so that

$$E + S_1 \rightleftharpoons ES_1 \quad (13)$$

followed by

$$ES_1 + S_2 \rightleftharpoons ES_1S_2 \longrightarrow P_1 + P_2 + E \quad (14)$$

and if S_1 and S_2 combine with separate sites on the enzyme molecule, the rate of reaction is given by

$$v = \frac{V_{max} \times [S_1][S_2]}{[S_1][S_2] + [S_2]K_m^1 + [S_1]K_m^2 + K_s^1 K_m^2} \quad (15)$$

K_m^1 and K_m^2 are the K_m values for the two substrates, and $[S_1]$ and $[S_2]$ are their concentrations. K_s^1 is the equilibrium constant for the reversible reaction between the enzyme and S_1. If the equation is rearranged into the double reciprocal form

$$\frac{1}{v} = \frac{1}{[S_1]}\left(\frac{K_m^1}{V_{max}} + \frac{K_m^2 K_s^1}{[S_2]V_{max}}\right) + \frac{1}{V_{max}}\left(1 + \frac{K_m^2}{[S_2]}\right) \quad (16)$$

a plot of $1/v$ against $1/[S_1]$ gives a straight line, but both the slope of the line and its intercept on the ordinate are affected by $[S_2]$, the concentration of the second substrate (Figure 8-6, *A*). Similarly, a plot of $1/v$ against $1/[S_2]$ is rectilinear but with the slope and intercept dependent on $[S_1]$.

Values of K_m and V_{max} for each substrate are derived from experiments in which the concentration of the first substrate is held constant at saturating levels while the concentration of the second substrate is varied, and vice versa. There is no reason why the K_m values for the two substrates should be the same or even similar (e.g., pyruvate and NADH, the two-substrate pair in the reaction catalyzed by lactate dehydrogenase of beef heart, have K_m values of 2×10^{-5} mol/L and 3×10^{-6} mol/L, respectively).

In some bisubstrate reactions, no ternary complex ES_1S_2 is formed, because the binding of the first substrate is followed by release of the first product before the second substrate is bound and the second product is released. This sequence is described as a *ping-pong bi-bi* type of reaction. It occurs in reactions catalyzed by aminotransferases.

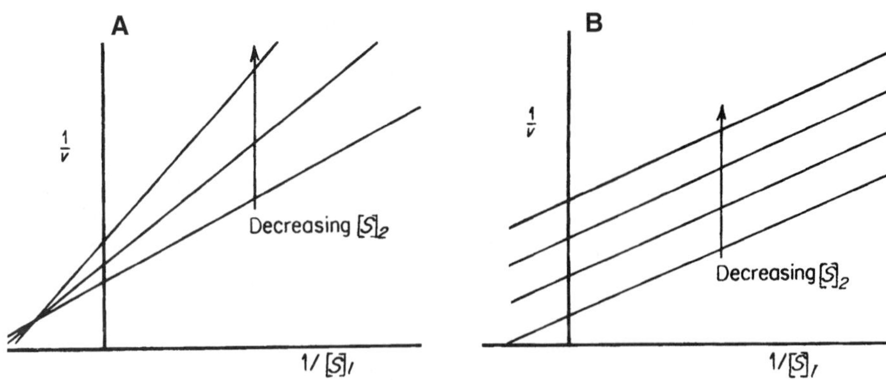

Figure 8-6 Double-reciprocal plots of $1/v$ against $1/[S_1]$ for two-substrate reactions, showing the effect of falling concentration of the second substrate, $[S_2]$. **A,** In a dehydrogenase reaction in which a ternary complex is formed. **B,** In a *ping-pong bi-bi* reaction mechanism (e.g., aminotransferase) in which no ternary complex is formed. *(From Moss DW. Measurement of enzymes. In: Enzymes in cardiology: Diagnosis and research. Hearse DJ, de Leiris J, Eds. New York: John Wiley & Sons Inc, 1979. Reprinted by permission of John Wiley & Sons, Inc.)*

The relationship between reaction velocity and the concentrations of the two substrates in *ping-pong bi-bi* reactions reduces to the form

$$v = \frac{V_{max} \times [S_1][S_2]}{[S_1][S_2] + [S_2]K_m^1 + [S_1]K_m^2} \quad (17)$$

The reciprocals of v and $[S_1]$ are related by the equation

$$\frac{1}{v} = \frac{1}{[S_1]} \times \frac{K_m^1}{V_{max}} + \frac{1}{V_{max}}\left(1 + \frac{K_m^2}{[S_2]}\right) \quad (18)$$

so that a plot of $1/v$ against $1/[S_1]$ is unchanged in slope by variation in $[S_2]$, but the intercept on the ordinate and therefore the value of V_{max} changes as $[S_2]$ is varied (see Figure 8-6, *B*). Similar equations describe the variation of V_{max} with $[S_1]$ when $1/v$ is plotted as a function of $1/[S_2]$.

The selection of reaction conditions for the measurement of enzymatic activity involving two substrates is approached empirically by varying the concentration of the first substrate and keeping the concentration of the second substrate constant until maximum activity is reached. The process is then repeated with the concentration of the first substrate held at the value thus determined, while the concentration of the second substrate is varied.

In practice, the choice of substrate concentrations is limited by such considerations as the solubility of the substrates, the viscosity and high initial absorbance of concentrated solutions, and the relative costs of the reagents. Furthermore, the selection of appropriate substrate concentrations is only one of the factors to be considered in formulating an optimal assay system for the measurement of a specific enzyme activity. Critical choices must also be made with respect to other, frequently interdependent factors that affect reaction rate, such as the concentrations of activators and the nature and pH of the buffer system. The traditional empirical approach to optimization has been replaced by newer techniques of simplex co-optimization and response-surface methodology.[11] As an example, this technique has recently been used to determine optimum conditions for the IFCC-recommended method for amylase.[6]

Consecutive Enzymatic Reactions

As discussed above, an enzymatic reaction is usually found to be more rapid in one direction than the other so that the reaction is virtually irreversible.If the product of the reaction in one direction is removed as it is formed (i.e., because it is the substrate of a second enzyme present in the reaction mixture), the equilibrium of the first enzymatic process is displaced so that the reaction may continue to completion in that direction. Reaction sequences in which the product of one enzyme-catalyzed reaction becomes the substrate of another enzyme, often through many stages, are characteristic of metabolic processes. Analytically, several enzymatic reactions also may be linked together to provide a means of measuring the activity of the first enzyme or the concentration of the initial substrate in the chain. For example, the activity of creatine kinase is usually measured by a series of linked reactions, and glucose can be determined by consecutive reactions catalyzed by hexokinase and glucose-6-phosphate dehydrogenase.

When a linked enzyme assay, known as an *indicator reaction*, is used to determine the activity of a different enzyme, it is essential that the primary reaction be the rate-limiting step. For example, in the determination of aspartate aminotransferase activity, the indicator reaction is the reduction of the oxaloacetate formed in the aminotransferase reaction to malate by malate dehydrogenase and NADH. The activity of the indicator enzyme must be sufficient to ensure the virtually instantaneous removal of the product of the first reaction, to prevent significant reversal of the first reaction. The measured enzyme is typically acting under conditions of saturation with respect to its substrate; however, the concentration of the substrate of the indicator enzyme (i.e., the product of the first reaction) remains in the region of the Michaelis-Menten curve in which v is directly proportional to $[S]$. Therefore the rate of reaction catalyzed by the indicator enzyme is directly proportional to the rate of product formation in the first reaction.

During a lag period that occurs after the start of the first reaction, the concentration of its product reaches a steady state. Because the rate of the second reaction depends on the activity of the indicator enzyme and on the concentration of its substrate (the product of the primary reaction), the duration of the lag period is reduced by increasing the concentration of the indicator enzyme, thus lowering the steady-state concentration of the product of the primary reaction.

The rate of the indicator reaction, v_i, is related to substrate concentration and therefore to the product concentration [P] by the Michaelis-Menten equation

$$v_i = \frac{V_{max}^i \times [P]}{[P] + K_m^i} \qquad (19)$$

in which V_{max}^i and K_m^i are the maximum velocity and K_m of the indicator enzyme, respectively. For the rate of the indicator reaction not to be the rate limiting factor, vi must at least equal the limiting velocity of the primary reaction, vt, which the assay system is expected to measure. Therefore the minimum activity of indicator enzyme needed is given by

$$v_t = \frac{V_{max}^i \times [P]}{[P] + K_m^i} \qquad (20)$$

or rearranged

$$V_{max}^i = v_t\left(1 + \frac{K_m^i}{[P]}\right) \qquad (21)$$

The ratio of activities of the indicator and primary enzymes varies from one assay method to another, depending on (1) the range of activity measured, (2) the K_m of the indicator enzyme, and (3) the lag period that is considered acceptable. Nevertheless the catalytic concentration of the indicator enzyme in the reaction mixture must always be much greater than that of the enzyme being determined.

Effect of pH

The rate of enzyme-catalyzed reactions typically shows a marked dependence on pH (Figure 8-7). Many of the enzymes in blood plasma show maximum activity in vitro in the pH range from 7 to 8. However, activity has been observed at pH values as low as 1.5 (pepsin) and as high as 10.5 (ALP). The optimal pH for a given forward reaction may be different from the optimal pH found for the corresponding reverse reaction. The form of the pH-dependence curve is a result of a number of separate effects including the ionization of the substrate and the extent of dissociation of certain key amino acid side chains in the protein molecule, both at the active center and elsewhere in the molecule. Both pH and ionic environment will also have an effect on the three-dimensional conformation of the protein and

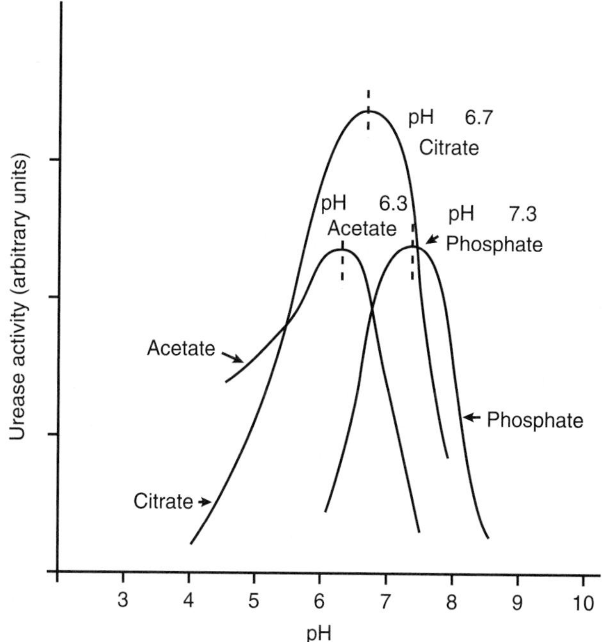

Figure 8-7 The pH activity curves for urease show effect of buffer species on pH optimum. *(Modified from Howell SF, Sumner JB. J Biol Chem 1934;104:619.)*

therefore on enzyme activity to such an extent that enzymes may be irreversibly denatured at extreme values of pH.

The pronounced effects of pH on enzyme reactions emphasize the need to control this variable by means of adequate buffer solutions. Enzyme assays should be carried out at the pH of optimal activity, because the pH-activity curve has its minimum slope near this pH, and a small variation in pH will cause a minimal change in enzyme activity. The buffer system must be capable of counteracting the effect of adding the specimen (e.g., serum itself is a powerful buffer) to the assay system, and the effects of acids or bases formed during the reaction (e.g., formation of fatty acids by the action of lipase). Because buffers have their maximum buffering capacity close to their pK_a values, whenever possible a buffer system should be chosen with a pK_a value within 1 pH unit of the desired pH of the assay (see Chapter 1). Interaction between buffer ions and other components of the assay system (e.g., activating metal ions) may eliminate certain buffers from consideration.

Temperature

The rate of an enzymatic reaction is proportional to its reaction temperature. For most enzymatic reactions, values of Q_{10} (the relative reaction rates at two temperatures differing by 10 °C) vary from 1.7 to 2.5. However, an increase in the rate of the catalyzed reaction is not the only effect of increasing temperature on an enzymatic reaction. In theory, the initial rate of reaction measured instantaneously will increase with a rising temperature. In practice, however, a

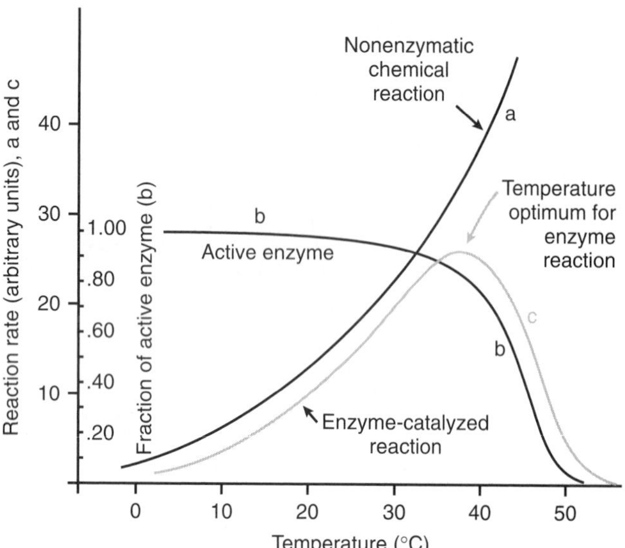

Figure 8-8 Schematic diagram showing effect of temperature on the rate of nonenzyme-catalyzed and enzyme-catalyzed reactions.

finite time is needed to allow the components of the reaction mixture, including the enzyme solution, to reach temperature equilibrium and to permit the formation of a measurable amount of the product. During this period the enzyme is undergoing thermal inactivation and denaturation, a process that has a very large temperature coefficient for most enzymes and thus becomes virtually instantaneous at temperatures of 60 °C to 70 °C. The counteracting effects of the increased rate of the catalyzed reaction and more rapid enzyme inactivation as the temperature increases account for the existence of an apparent *optimal temperature* for enzyme activity (Figure 8-8).

As stated earlier, at some critical temperature, an enzyme will undergo thermal inactivation influenced by a number of factors. These include the presence of substrate and its concentration, the pH, and the nature and ionic strength of the buffer. The presence of other proteins, as in serum samples, may help to stabilize enzymes. Storage of serum samples at low temperatures is necessary to minimize loss of enzyme activity while awaiting analysis, although repeated freezing and thawing should be avoided. However, individual enzymes vary in their stability characteristics, and appropriate storage conditions vary correspondingly. Amylase, for example, is stable at room temperature (22 °C to 25 °C) for 24 hours, whereas acid phosphatase is exceedingly unstable, even when refrigerated, unless kept at a pH below 6.0. ALP exhibits an unusual property: the tendency for the activity of frozen, partially purified preparations of the enzyme to increase after thawing over a period of 24 hours or longer. This effect is shared by reconstituted, lyophilized preparations of the enzyme and affects their use for quality control purposes. A few enzymes are inactivated at refrigerator temperatures; a clinically important example is the liver-type isoenzyme of lactate dehydrogenase, LD-5, which appears to be less stable at lower temperatures. As a result, sera for lactate dehydrogenase determinations should be kept at room temperature and not refrigerated.

Historically, the choice of temperature for the assay of enzymes of clinical importance has been the subject of extensive debate. Currently, the choice of reaction temperature has become a nonissue because most if not all analytical systems operate at 37 °C. In addition, reference methods for several clinically relevant enzymes have now been qualified at 37 °C.[12-17] In practice, accurate temperature control to within ±0.1 °C during the enzymatic reaction is essential. An accurate temperature standard that readily is transferred from one laboratory to another is provided by the gallium melting-point cell.[1] Pure gallium melts at 29.77 °C.

Inhibitors and Activators

The rates of enzymatic reactions are often affected by substances other than the enzyme or substrate. These modifiers may be inhibitors because their presence reduces the reaction rate or activators as they increase the rate of reaction. Activators and inhibitors are usually small molecules (compared with the enzyme itself) or even ions. They vary in specificity from modifiers that exert similar effects on a wide range of different enzymatic reactions at one extreme, to substances that affect only a single reaction. Reagents, such as strong acids or multivalent anions and cations that denature or precipitate proteins, destroy enzyme activity and thus may be regarded as extreme examples of nonspecific enzyme inhibitors. These effects are not usually included in discussions of enzyme inhibition, although they have obvious practical implications in the treatment and storage of specimens in which enzyme activity is to be measured. The activity of some enzymes depends on the presence of particular chemical groups, such as reduced sulfhydryl (–SH) groups, in the active center. Reagents that alter these groups (e.g., oxidants of SH groups) therefore act as general inhibitors of such enzymes.

Some phenomena of enzyme activation or inhibition are caused by interaction between the modifier and a nonenzymatic component of the reaction system, such as the substrate (e.g., Mg^{2+} combining with ATP to form MgATP, the required substrate for the creatine kinase reaction). In most cases, however, the modifier combines with the enzyme itself in a manner analogous to the combination of enzyme and substrate.

Inhibition of Enzyme Activity

Inhibitors are classified into reversible and irreversible types. *Reversible inhibition* implies that the activity of the enzyme is fully restored when the inhibitor is removed from the system in which the enzyme acts by some physical separative process, such as dialysis, gel filtration, or chromatography. An *irreversible inhibitor* combines covalently with the enzyme so that physical methods are ineffective in separating the two. For example, organophosphorus compounds are extremely potent irreversible inhibitors of esterases, including acetylcholinesterase. The enzyme breaks one of the bonds in the inhibitor, but part of the molecule is left bound to the active center of the enzyme, preventing further activity. In some cases, enzymes that have combined with irreversible inhibitors can be reactivated by a chemical reaction that removes the blocking group (e.g., the phosphoryl enzymes formed with organophosphorus compounds can sometimes be reactivated by treatment with oximes or hydroxamic acids).

Reversible Inhibition. Reversible inhibition is characterized by the existence of equilibrium between enzyme, *E*, and inhibitor, *I*:

$$E + I \rightleftarrows EI \tag{22}$$

The equilibrium constant of the reaction, *Ki* (the *inhibitor constant*), is a measure of the affinity of the inhibitor for the enzyme, just as K_m generally reflects the affinity of the enzyme for its substrate.

A *competitive* inhibitor is usually a structural analogue of the substrate that can combine with the free enzyme in such a way that it competes with the normal substrate for binding at the active site. The actual rate of the reaction is strictly dependent on the relative concentrations of substrate and inhibitor. Two equilibriums are therefore possible:

$$E + S \rightleftarrows ES \longrightarrow E + \text{Products}$$

and

$$E + I \rightleftarrows EI$$

The equation that relates the observed reaction velocity to the concentrations of substrate, [*S*], and inhibitor, [*I*], is:

$$v = \frac{V_{max}[S]}{[S] + K_m\left(1 + \frac{[I]}{K_i}\right)} \tag{23}$$

This is the Michaelis-Menten equation, but with K_m modified by a term including the inhibitor concentration and inhibitor constant. V_{max} is unaltered. Therefore, curves of v against [*S*] in the presence and absence of inhibitor reach the same limiting value at high substrate concentrations, but when the inhibitor is present, K_m is apparently greater. Plots of $1/v$ against $1/[S]$ with and without inhibitor cut the ordinate at the same point but have different slopes and intercepts on the abscissa (Figure 8-9).

Competitive inhibition is responsible for the inhibition of some enzymes by excess substrate because of competition between substrate molecules for a single binding site. In two-substrate reactions, high concentrations of the second substrate may compete with the binding of the first substrate. For example, aspartate aminotransferase is inhibited by excess concentrations of the substrate 2-oxoglutarate, and this inhibition is competitive with respect to L-aspartate. Therefore, to maintain a given velocity at high 2-oxoglutarate concentrations, the concentration of L-aspartate has to be increased above the value needed at lower concentrations of 2-oxoglutarate.

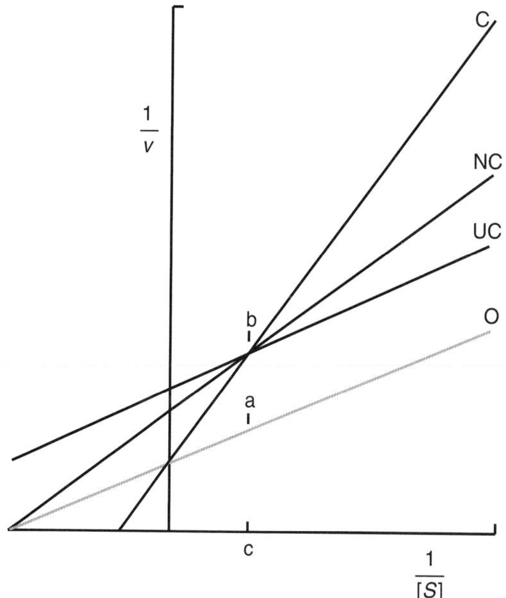

Figure 8-9 Effects of different types of inhibitors on the double-reciprocal plot of $1/v$ against $1/[S]$. Each of the inhibitors has been assumed to reduce the activity of the enzyme by the same amount, represented by the change in $1/v$ from *a* to *b* at a substrate concentration of *c*. *Line O* is the plot for enzyme without inhibitor, *C* with a competitive inhibitor, *NC* with a noncompetitive inhibitor, and *UC* with an uncompetitive inhibitor. *(From Moss DW. Measurement of enzymes. In: Hearse DJ, de Leiris J, Eds. Enzymes in cardiology: Diagnosis and research. New York: John Wiley & Sons Inc, 1979. Reprinted by permission of John Wiley & Sons, Inc.)*

Competitive inhibition also contributes to the reduction of the rate of an enzymatic reaction with time. For example, a rate reduction can occur because increasing concentrations of reaction products tend to drive the reaction backward, if it is freely reversible. A product may itself be an inhibitor of the forward reaction, so even if the reaction is not readily reversible, it proceeds against a rising concentration of inhibitor. A familiar example of "product inhibition" is the release of the competitive inhibitor, inorganic phosphate, by the action of ALP on its substrates. In this case, both organic phosphates and inorganic phosphates bind to the active center of the enzyme with similar affinities (i.e., K_m and K_i are of the same order of magnitude).

Product inhibition is a cause of nonlinearity of reaction progress curves during fixed-time methods of enzyme assay. For example, oxaloacetate produced by the action of aspartate aminotransferase inhibits the enzyme, particularly the mitochondrial isoenzyme. The inhibitory product may be removed as it is formed by a coupled enzymatic reaction: malate dehydrogenase converts the oxaloacetate to malate and at the same time oxidizes NADH to NAD^+.

Competitive inhibition by metal ions can arise when two metal ions compete for the same binding site on the enzyme.

Sodium and lithium are potent inhibitors of pyruvate kinase, for which potassium is an obligatory activator.

A *noncompetitive* inhibitor is usually structurally different from the substrate. It is assumed to bind at a site on the enzyme molecule that is different from the substrate-binding site; thus, there is no competition between inhibitor and substrate, and a ternary enzyme-inhibitor-substrate (ESI) complex forms. Attachment of the inhibitor to the enzyme does not alter the affinity of the enzyme for its substrate (i.e., K_m is unaltered) but the ESI complex does not break down to give products. Since the substrate does not compete with the inhibitor for binding sites on the enzyme molecule, increasing the substrate concentration does not overcome the effect of a noncompetitive inhibitor. Thus V_{max} is reduced in the presence of such an inhibitor, whereas K_m is not altered, as the Lineweaver-Burk plot shows (see Figure 8-9).

In a rather unusual type of reversible inhibition, *uncompetitive* inhibition, parallel lines are obtained when plots of $1/v$ against $1/[S]$ with and without the inhibitor are compared (see Figure 8-9); that is, both K_m and V_{max} are decreased. Uncompetitive inhibition is due to a combination of the inhibitor with the ES complex. It is more common in two-substrate reactions, in which a ternary ESI complex forms after the first substrate has combined with the enzyme.

Irreversible Inhibition. Irreversible inhibitors render the enzyme molecule inactive by covalently and permanently modifying a functional group required for catalysis. An irreversible inhibitor is not in equilibrium with the enzyme. Its effect is progressive with time, becoming complete if the amount of inhibitor present exceeds the total amount of enzyme. The rate of the reaction between enzyme and inhibitor is expressed as the fraction of the enzyme activity that is inhibited in a fixed time by a given concentration of inhibitor. The velocity constant of the reaction of the inhibitor with the enzyme is a measure of the effectiveness of the inhibitor.

When the inhibitor is added to the enzyme in the presence of its substrate, the reaction between the enzyme and inhibitor may be delayed because some of the enzyme molecules are combined with the substrate and are therefore protected from reacting with the inhibitor. However, as the substrate molecules react chemically, the active centers become available and inhibition will eventually become complete even though an excess of substrate may initially have been present. Furthermore, addition of more substrate is ineffective in reversing the inhibition in contrast to its effect on reversible competitive inhibition, which is discussed later.

Irreversible inhibitors have been useful in mapping active sites by covalently modifying different types of functional groups in the enzyme molecule to establish whether such groups are necessary for catalytic activity.

A physiologically important category of irreversible enzyme inhibition is produced by the *antienzymes,* exemplified by various trypsin inhibitors. These are proteins that bind to trypsin irreversibly, nullifying its proteolytic activity. One such inhibitor is present in the α_1-globulin fraction of serum proteins; others are found in soybeans and lima beans. Similar proteolysis inhibitors present in plasma prevent the accumulation of excess thrombin and other coagulation enzymes, thus keeping the coagulation process under control.

Inhibition by Antibodies. The combination of enzyme molecules with specific antibodies often has no effect on catalytic activity, which is retained by the enzyme-antibody complex. However, in some cases, reaction of the enzyme and antibody reduces or even abolishes enzymatic activity. The most probable explanation for this type of inhibition is that the antibody molecule restricts access of the substrate molecules to the active center by steric hindrance or, in extreme cases, completely masks the substrate-binding site. However, it appears that some examples of enzyme inhibition by combination with antibodies are caused by a conformational change induced in the enzyme molecule.

Inhibition of the activity of an enzyme molecule labeled with a hapten (e.g., morphine) as a result of combination with a specific antibody is the basis of homogeneous enzyme immunoassay (EMIT, Syva Corp., Palo Alto, Calif.). See Chapter 9 for further details.

Enzyme Activation

Activators are considered to increase the rates of enzyme-catalyzed reactions by promoting formation of the most active state either of the enzyme itself or of other reactants, such as the substrate. This generalization covers a wide variety of mechanisms of activation.

Many enzymes contain metal ions as an integral part of their structures (e.g., zinc in ALP and carboxypeptidase A). The function of the metal may be to stabilize tertiary and quaternary protein structures. Removal of divalent metal ions by treatment with an appropriate concentration of EDTA solution is accompanied by conformational changes with inactivation of the enzyme. The enzyme can often be reactivated by dialysis against a solution of the appropriate metal ion or simply by adding the ion to the reaction mixture. Reactivation may take some time, because rearrangement of the polypeptide chains into the active conformation is not instantaneous.

When the activator ion is an essential part of the functional enzyme molecule, whether as a purely structural element or with an additional catalytic role, it is usually incorporated quite firmly into the enzyme molecule. Therefore it is not usually necessary to add the activator to reaction mixtures, and excess of the ion may even have an inhibitory effect. However, in some cases the activating ion is attached only weakly or transiently to the enzyme (or its substrate) during catalysis. Enzyme samples may therefore be deficient in the ion so that addition of the ion increases the reaction rate or indeed may be essential for the reaction to take place. For example, all phosphate transfer enzymes (kinases), such as creatine kinase, require the essential presence of Mg^{2+} ions. Other common activating cations are Mn^{2+}, Fe^{2+}, Ca^{2+}, Zn^{2+}, and K^{+}. More rarely, anions may act as activators. Amylase functions at its maximal rate only if Cl^{-} or other monovalent anions, such as Br^{-} or NO_3^{-}, are present. Addition of 5 mmol/L of chloride increases amylase activity almost threefold, at the same time shifting the pH optimum from 6.5 to 7.0. The chloride ion may combine with a positively charged group in the enzyme, changing the ionization constant of a group important in catalysis. However, other anions—such as bromide—are less effective activators of amylase, so some degree of specificity is involved in the process of activation. Some enzymes require the obligate presence of two activating ions. K^{+} and Mg^{2+} are essential for the activity of pyruvate kinase, and both Mg^{2+} and Zn^{2+} are required for ALP activity.

The velocity of the reaction depends on the concentration of a reversible activator in a fashion similar to its dependence on substrate concentration, and an activator constant, K_a, analogous to K_m, can be determined from data relating enzyme activity to increasing activator concentration in the presence of excess substrate. The simplest interpretation of K_a is that it is the dissociation constant of the equilibrium between E and the activator, A. However, this is true only when the combination of enzyme and activator is independent of the reaction between E and S, and the same value for K_a is obtained at all concentrations of the substrate. If the free enzyme and the enzyme-substrate complex have different affinities for the activator, the value for K_a varies with $[S]$.

Apparent activation of an enzyme may be observed whenever a substance that can counteract the presence of some inhibiting agent is added.

Coenzymes and Prosthetic Groups

Coenzymes are usually more complex molecules than activators, although smaller molecules than the enzyme proteins themselves. Some compounds, such as the dinucleotides NAD and NADP, are classified as coenzymes and are specific substrates in two-substrate reactions. Their effect on the rate of reaction follows the Michaelis-Menten pattern of dependence on substrate concentration. The structures of these two coenzymes are identical except for the presence of an additional phosphate group in NADP; nevertheless, individual dehydrogenases, for which these coenzymes are substrates, are predominantly or even absolutely specific for one or the other form.

Coenzymes such as NAD and NADP are bound only momentarily to the enzyme during the course of reaction, as is the case for substrates in general. Therefore no reaction takes place unless the appropriate coenzyme is present in solution (e.g., by adding it to the reaction mixture in the assay of dehydrogenase activity). In contrast to these entirely soluble coenzymes, some coenzymes are more or less permanently bound to the enzyme molecules, where they form part of the active center and undergo cycles of chemical change during the reaction.

The active *holoenzyme* results from the combination of the inactive *apoenzyme* with the *prosthetic group,* as such a bound coenzyme is called. An example of a prosthetic group is pyridoxal phosphate (P-5′-P), a component of AST and ALT. The P-5′-P prosthetic group undergoes a cycle of conversion of the pyridoxal moiety to pyridoxamine and back again during the transfer of an amino group from an amino acid to an oxo-acid. Prosthetic groups, such as activators with a structural role, do not usually have to be added to elicit full catalytic activity of the enzyme unless previous treatment has caused the prosthetic group to be lost from some enzyme molecules. However, both normal and pathological serum samples contain appreciable amounts of apo-aminotransferases, which is converted to the active holoenzymes by a suitable period of incubation with P-5′-P.

A study of the formulas of coenzyme and prosthetic groups shows that many contain structures derived from the vitamins (see Chapter 30). Thus, the nicotinamide portion of NAD and NADP derives from the vitamin niacin, whereas the P-5′-P prosthetic group of the aminotransferases is a derivative of pyridoxine, vitamin B_6. Other derivatives of the B-group vitamins participate in enzymatic reactions.

ANALYTICAL ENZYMOLOGY

Analytically the clinical laboratorian is concerned with measuring the activity or mass in serum or plasma of enzymes that are predominantly intracellular and that are normally present in the serum in low levels only. By measuring changes in the levels of these enzymes in disease, it is possible to infer the location and nature of pathological changes in the tissues of the body.

Measurement of Reaction Rates

The rate of an enzyme-catalyzed reaction is directly proportional to the amount of active enzyme present in the system. Consequently, the determination of the rate of reaction under defined and controlled conditions provides a very sensitive and specific method for the measurement of enzymes in samples such as serum.

Determination of reaction rate involves the kinetic measurement of the amount of change produced in a defined time interval. Both *fixed-time* and *continuous-monitoring* methods are used to measure reaction rates. In the fixed-time method, the amount of change produced by the enzyme is measured after stopping the reaction at the end of a fixed-time interval. In the continuous-monitoring method, the progress of the reaction is monitored continuously. These two methods have different advantages and limitations. To appreciate these, it is necessary to consider the way in which the rate of an enzymatic reaction varies with time.

The progress of conversion of the substrate into products in the presence of an enzyme is monitored by measuring the decreasing concentration of the substrate or the increasing concentration of the products. Measurement of product formation is preferable, as determination of the increase in concentration of a substance above an initially zero or low level is analytically more reliable than measurement of a decline from an initially high level.

At the moment when the enzyme and substrate are mixed, the rate of the reaction is zero. The rate then typically rises rapidly to a maximum value, which remains constant for a period of time (Figure 8-10). During the period of constant reaction rate, the rate depends only on enzyme concentration and is completely independent of substrate concentration. The reaction is said to follow zero-order kinetics, because its rate is proportional to the zero power of the substrate concentration. Ultimately, however, as more substrate is consumed, the reaction rate declines and enters a phase of first-order dependence on substrate concentration. Other factors that contribute to the decline in reaction rate include accumulation of products that may be inhibitory, the growing importance of the reverse reaction, and even enzyme denaturation. Although it is possible to compare the rates of reaction produced by different amounts of an enzyme under first-order conditions, it is obviously easier to standardize such comparisons when the enzyme concentration is the only variable that influences the reaction rate. Therefore, enzyme assays are usually made under conditions that are initially saturating with respect to substrate concentration. The rate of reaction during the zero-order phase is determined by measuring the product formed during a fixed period of incubation where the rate remains constant. This is illustrated in Figure 8-11. Measurement of reaction rates at any portion of curve A gives results that are identical to the true "initial rate." However, curve B deviates from linearity over its entire course, and rates fall off with time. From curve C, correct results are obtained only if the rate is measured along segment II. Incorrect results are

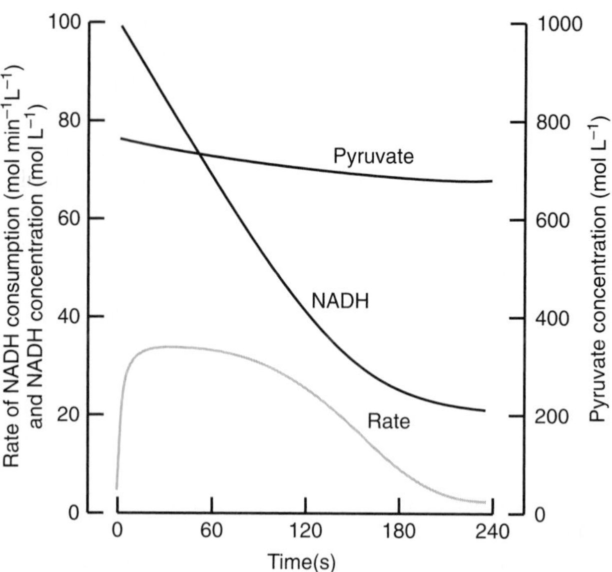

Figure 8-10 Changes in substrate concentrations and rate of reaction during an assay of lactate dehydrogenase activity at 37 °C in phosphate buffer, with pyruvate and NADH as substrates. The reaction is followed by observing the fall in absorbance at 340 nm as NADH is oxidized to NAD^+. The rate of reaction rises rapidly to a maximum value, from which it declines only slightly until about half the NADH has been used up. During this phase of the reaction, the rate is essentially zero order with respect to substrate concentration. At the point at which the rate falls below about 90% of its maximum value, NADH concentration is approximately $10 \times K_m$. The K_m for NADH is of the order of 5×10^{-6} mol/L, whereas for pyruvate it is 9×10^{-5} mol/L. Thus an initial pyruvate concentration approximately 10 times that of NADH is used. (Concentrations are per liter of reaction mixture.) *(From Moss DW. Measurement of enzymes. In: Hearse DJ, de Leiris J, Eds. Enzymes in cardiology: Diagnosis and research. New York: John Wiley & Sons Inc, 1979. Reprinted by permission of John Wiley & Sons, Inc.)*

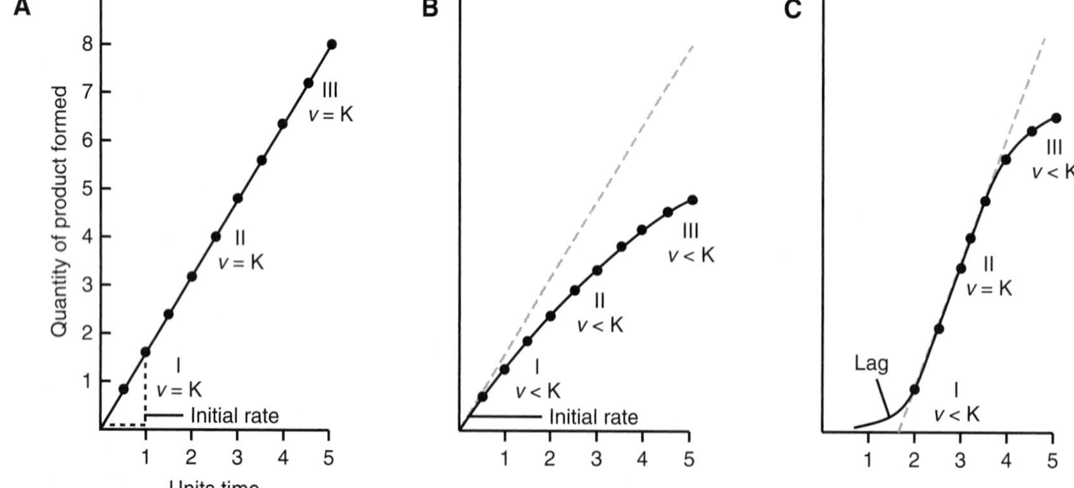

Figure 8-11 Forms of graphs showing change in enzyme reaction rate as a function of time. In **A,** the rate is constant during the entire run, and rates calculated as I, II, and III will be identical to the initial rate. In **B,** the rate falls off continuously; rates calculated at I, II, and III will be different and less than the true initial rate. In **C,** a measurement at II will be representative of the maximum rate, but at I (lag period) and III (substrate depletion), it will be less than at II.

obtained if the rate is measured during the lag phase (I) or during phase III.

Careful selection of reaction conditions, such as the concentrations of substrates and cofactors, improves the reaction progress curves, eliminating lag phases and prolonging the period of linearity, so that fixed-time methods of analysis become feasible. Improvements in optical techniques, leading to more reliable and sensitive measurement of product formation, have also allowed the duration of incubation to be shortened compared with older assays. This has resulted in a corresponding increase in the interval over which enzyme activity is measured. Nevertheless, an upper limit of activity exists in all fixed-time methods, above which progress curves will no longer be linear. In that case the amount of change measured over the fixed-time interval no longer represents true zero-order rate conditions.

The existence of an upper limit of enzyme activity implies that samples with activities above this limit must receive special attention. The upper limit of activity acceptable in the unmodified method must be chosen so that samples with activities below it are presumed with a high degree of certainty to give linear progress curves; on the other hand, if the limit is set too low, many samples will be reanalyzed unnecessarily. Samples that are above the limit should ideally be reassayed by shortening the incubation period until a constant reaction rate is obtained. However, this is difficult or impossible in some automated methods, in which the duration of incubation is fixed by the configuration of the apparatus. It then becomes necessary to dilute the specimen; however, dilution may not always result in a proportionate change in activity.

The initial rate of reaction theoretically increases without limit as enzyme concentration increases, as long as no other factor, such as substrate concentration, becomes limiting. In practice, the reaction rate becomes so rapid at high enzyme activities that it is impossible to measure the initial rate of reaction, even with continuous-monitoring methods. Therefore, an upper limit of activity that is accepted without modification of the assay procedure exists even in continuous-monitoring methods, but this limit is usually much higher than that applicable in corresponding fixed-time methods. Fewer samples therefore require special treatment. Furthermore, continuous monitoring allows identification of the appropriate zero-order portion of the progress curve for each sample and identification of samples that require special treatment. Continuous-monitoring methods therefore possess a decisive advantage in enzyme assay and should be used whenever possible. Enzyme activity can also be measured by noting the time required to consume all of a fixed amount of substrate, but methods of this type have largely been discontinued.

Units for Expressing Enzyme Activity

When enzymes are measured by their catalytic activities, the results of such determinations are expressed in terms of the concentration of the number of activity units present in a convenient volume or mass of specimen. The unit of activity is the measure of the rate at which the reaction proceeds (e.g., the quantity of substrate consumed or product formed in a chosen unit of time). In clinical enzymology, the activity of an enzyme is generally reported in terms of some convenient unit of volume, such as activity per 100 mL or per liter of serum or per 1.0 mL of packed erythrocytes. Because the rate of the reaction depends on experimental parameters, such as pH, type of buffer, temperature, nature of substrate, ionic strength, concentration of activators, and other variables, these parameters must be specified in the definition of the unit.

To standardize how enzyme activities are expressed, the Enzyme Commission of the IUB proposed that the unit of enzyme activity be defined as the quantity of enzyme that catalyzes the reaction of 1 μmol of substrate per minute and that this unit be termed the *international unit* (U). Catalytic concentration is to be expressed in terms of U/L or kU/L, whichever gives the more convenient numerical value. In this chapter, the symbol U is used to denote the international unit. In those instances in which there is some uncertainty about the exact nature of the substrate or when there is difficulty in calculating the number of micromoles reacting (as with macromolecules such as starch, protein, and complex lipids), the unit is to be expressed in terms of the chemical group or residue measured in following the reaction (e.g., glucose units, or amino acid units formed).

The international unit itself may eventually be replaced by the SI unit termed the *katal,* the SI derived unit for catalytic activity (see Chapter 1). It is defined as moles per second. The name katal had been used for this unit for decades, but did not become an official SI derived unit until 1999 with Resolution 12 of the 21st CGPM, on the recommendation of the International Federation of Clinical Chemistry and Laboratory Medicine. Both the International Union of Pure and Applied Chemistry and the IUB now recommend that enzyme activity be expressed in moles per second and that the enzyme concentration be expressed in terms of katals per liter (kat/L).[3] Thus, $1\ U = 10^{-6}\ mol/60\ s = 16.7 \times 10^{-9}\ mol/s$, or $1.0\ nkat/L = 0.06\ U/L$. The formal adoption of the katal is hoped to discourage the use of a non-SI unit called "unit," symbol "U," defined as micromoles per minute. "Units" are more commonly used than the katal in practice at present, but their definition lacks coherence with the SI system.

Measurement of Substrates

The amount of substrate transformed into products during an enzyme-catalyzed reaction can be measured with any appropriate analytical method, such as spectrophotometry, fluorometry, or chemiluminescence. For example, if an enzyme reaction is accompanied by a change in the absorbance characteristics of some component of the assay system, in either the visible or ultraviolet spectrum, it can be photometrically observed while it is proceeding. "Self-indicating" reactions of this type are particularly valuable as they allow continuous monitoring. Important examples of self-indicating reactions are the determination of dehydrogenase activity by monitoring the change in absorbance at 339 (340) nm of the coenzymes NADH or NADPH during oxidation or reduction and the measurement of ALP activity by the generation of the yellow *p*-nitrophenolate ion from the substrate *p*-nitrophenyl phosphate in alkaline solution. These assays are so versatile that coupled reactions are frequently used to provide an observable optical change accompanying a primary reaction in which such a change is not present.

The introduction of prism or diffraction-grating spectrophotometers capable of isolating a narrow beam of monochromatic light in the ultraviolet or visible spectrum and with stable and sensitive photomultipliers as detectors greatly improved the reproducibility of photometric measurements. Consequently, it has become customary to make use of the known molar absorptivity of well-defined reaction products (such as NADH) when calculating changes in their concentrations based on measurements made with spectrophotometers. However, the absorbance and wavelength accuracy of the spectrophotometer should be checked regularly. (See Chapter 3 for details of validating the performance of a spectrophotometer.)

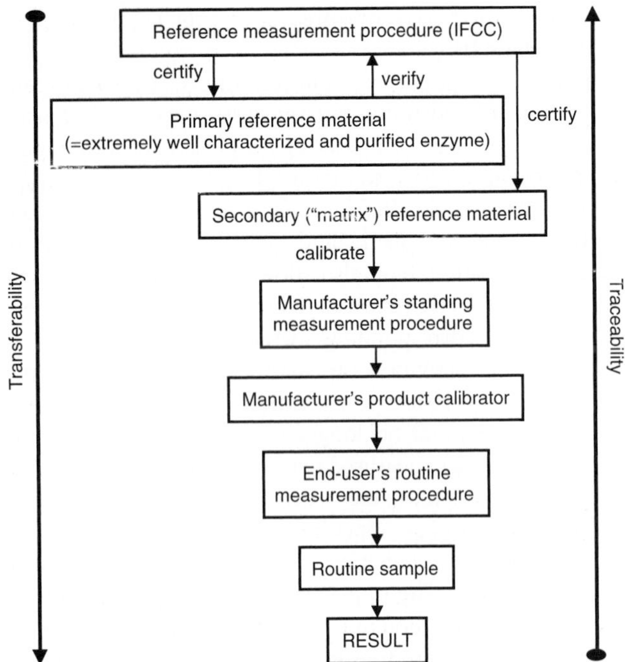

Figure 8-12 The proposed reference system for enzyme measurement showing the traceability of the laboratory result to the reference measurement procedure. *(From Panteghini et al, Clin Chem Lab Med 2001;39:795-800. Reprinted with permission of Walter de Gruyter.)*

Optimization, Standardization, and Quality Control

To measure enzyme activity reliably, all the factors that affect the reaction rate—other than the concentration of active enzyme—must be optimized and rigidly controlled. Furthermore, because the reaction velocity is at or near its maximum under optimal conditions, a larger analytical signal is obtained that can be more accurately and precisely measured than a smaller signal obtained under suboptimal conditions. Much effort has therefore been devoted to determining optimal conditions for measuring the activities of enzymes of clinical importance.

Optimization

Optimization of reaction conditions for enzyme assays has traditionally been carried out by varying a single factor and studying its effect on the reaction rate, then repeating the experiment with a second factor and so on until effects of all the variables have been tested. An optimal combination of variables is selected on the basis of these experiments, and the validity of the chosen conditions is verified. Not only is this approach labor intensive, but it also is not well adapted to situations in which the effects of different variables are interdependent, as is frequently the case in enzyme analysis. This traditional empirical approach to optimization has been replaced by newer techniques of simplex co-optimization and response-surface methodology.[11]

Standardization

Despite considerable effort, the goal of a single universally used procedure to measure the catalytic activity of a given enzyme has not been achieved. Consequently, current enzyme standardization efforts are focused on the development of a system that provides for comparability of test results, independent of the measurement method. To achieve this, a "reference system" based on the concepts of metrological traceability and of hierarchy of analytical methods has been proposed.[10] A reference procedure and certified reference materials are the basis of the metrological traceability chain (Figure 8-12). As part of this hierarchy, reference procedures at 37 °C for the most common enzymes have been developed and a group of reference laboratories are being selected to perform the measurements at an appropriately high metrological level.[12–17]

Reference procedures set standards of precision and accuracy against which the relative performances of methods intended for routine use can be judged. The reference procedure is used to assign a certified value to the reference material. This certified material can then be used by the manufacturers to assign values to commercial calibrators resulting in traceability of the value obtained in the laboratory.

Several studies have demonstrated that enzyme preparations with reproducible properties and purity and having assured stability can be made. These may be from animal sources in which the enzymes closely resemble their human counterparts, although new possibilities have been created by gene-transfer and mass-cell culture techniques ("recombinant" proteins).

For a reference system to be capable of standardizing the results of different assays of a given enzyme activity, some conditions must be satisfied.[8] First, the reference procedure used to assign the value of the reference material and the routine method(s) to be calibrated must have identical specificities for the analyte enzyme (i.e., for the specific isoenzyme or isoform under study). Second, the properties of the calibrator material must be the same as or closely similar to those of the analyte enzyme in its natural matrix, typically serum (i.e., the material must be "commutable" with human serum samples for that particular method).

Quality Control

Despite various difficulties, systematic application of quality control programs is as essential in enzyme analysis as in other forms of clinical analysis if the results obtained are to be useful in diagnosis and treatment.

The application of quality control procedures to ensure that satisfactory analytical performance of enzyme assays is maintained on a day-to-day basis is complicated by the tendency of enzyme preparations to undergo denaturation with loss of activity. This makes it difficult to distinguish between poor analytical performance and denaturation as possible causes of a low result obtained for a control sample introduced into a batch of analyses. Assured stability within a defined usable time span is therefore the prime requirement for enzyme control materials, as it is for enzyme calibrators. However, specifications for the two types of materials can differ in other respects. Because the function of a calibrator is to provide a stated activity under defined assay conditions, it is not necessary for it to show sensitivity to changes in the assay system identical to those of the samples under test; therefore within certain limits, enzymes from various sources can be considered in the search for stability. However, it is the function of a *control* to reveal small variations in reaction conditions, so it must mimic the samples being analyzed. The preparation of enzymes from human sources is not by itself a guarantee of an effective control. For example, human placental ALP is very stable, but it differs significantly in kinetic properties from the liver and bone enzymes that contribute most of the ALP activity of human serum samples; it is therefore not an ideal enzyme for use in control material for the determination of ALP.

Lyophilized and liquid preparations containing various enzymes are available from commercial sources, and these have a useful function in quality control. Serum pools can also be prepared in the laboratory for quality control purposes (with care to exclude any specimens contaminated with hepatitis virus or human immunodeficiency virus), then assayed for enzyme activity and stored in a freezer in small portions for daily use.

Measurement of Enzyme Mass Concentration

A number of immunoassays for human enzymes and isoenzymes measuring protein mass instead of catalytic activity have been described. To develop such assays, purified enzyme protein has to be prepared to act as a calibrator, to be labeled, and to be used to raise the enzyme-specific antibody. These methods determine all molecules with the antigenic determinants necessary for recognition by the antibody so that inactive enzyme molecules that are immunologically unaltered are measured along with active molecules. This has been found to be significant in the determination of some digestive enzymes, such as trypsin, when inactive precursors and inhibitors of catalytic activity are present in plasma. In the majority of cases, however, no degradation or changes of the active enzyme occur in blood so that clinical equivalence of the different measurement approaches (i.e., estimation of catalytic activity and mass concentration) can be obtained.

In practice, however, immunoassays have not been widely used for the determination of total enzyme activities for diagnostic purposes as these assays generally cannot compete in speed, precision, and costs with automated measurement of total catalytic activity. Furthermore, several enzyme activities in serum are due to mixtures of immunologically distinct isoenzymes, so an assay using a single type of antibody usually determines only one of the enzyme forms. However, this disadvantage in the determination of total enzyme activity becomes a marked advantage in the measurement of specific isoenzymes and isoforms, and immunological methods have assumed great importance in isoenzyme analysis for diagnostic purposes.

Enzymes as Analytical Reagents

Enzymes are used as analytical reagents for the measurement of several metabolites and substrates and in immunoassays to detect and quantitate immunological reactions.

Measurement of Metabolites

The use of enzymes as analytical reagents to measure metabolites frequently offers the advantage of great specificity for the substance being determined. This high specificity typically removes the need for preliminary separation or purification stages, so the analysis can be carried out directly on complex mixtures such as serum. Uricase (urate oxidase), urease, and glucose oxidase are examples of highly specific enzymes used in clinically important assays, such as the measurement of uric acid, urea, and glucose in biological fluids. However, high specificity cannot always be achieved in practice, and knowledge of the substrate specificities of reagent enzymes is therefore essential to allow possible interferences with the assay to be anticipated and corrected. Coupled reactions are often used to construct an enzymatic analytical system for determining a particular compound, because they are in measurements of enzyme activity, and the specificity of the coupled reactions may modify the specificity of the overall process. An example of this is the determination of glucose by the hexokinase reaction. Hexokinase converts sugars other than glucose to their 6-phosphate esters. However, the indicator reaction used to monitor this change is catalyzed by glucose-6-phosphate dehydrogenase, an enzyme that is highly specific for its substrate; so the overall process is highly specific for glucose.

In practice, both equilibrium and kinetic (rate) methods have been developed that use enzymes as reagents.

Equilibrium Methods

For most assays used to determine the amount of a substance enzymatically, they are allowed to continue to completion so that all the substrate has been converted into a measurable product. These methods are called *end point* or, more correctly, *equilibrium* methods, because the reaction ceases when equilibrium is reached. Reactions in which the equilibrium point corresponds virtually to complete conversion of the substrate are obviously preferable for this type of analysis. However, unfavorable equilibriums can often be displaced in the desired direction by additional enzymatic or nonenzymatic reactions that convert or "trap" a product of the first reaction (e.g., in measuring lactate with lactate dehydrogenase, the pyruvate formed can be trapped by the addition of hydrazine, with which it forms an irreversible hydrazone.)

Theoretically the time required to transform a fixed quantity, Q, of substrate into products is inversely proportional to the amount of enzyme, $[E]$, present.

$$Q = k_1 + [E] \times t \tag{24}$$

and

$$[E] = \frac{Q}{k_1} \times \frac{1}{t} \tag{25}$$

where k_l is the rate constant and t is the elapsed time. Equilibrium methods may therefore require the use of appreciable amounts of enzyme for each sample to avoid inconveniently long incubation periods. As the substrate concentration falls to low levels toward the end of the reaction, the K_m of the enzyme becomes important in determining the reaction rate. Enzymes with high affinities for their substrates (low K_m values) are therefore most suitable for equilibrium analysis. Equilibrium methods are largely insensitive to minor changes in reaction conditions. It is not necessary to have exactly the same amount of enzyme in each reaction mixture or to maintain the pH or temperature absolutely constant, provided that the variations are not so great that the reaction is not completed within the fixed time allowed.

Kinetic Methods

First- or pseudo–first-order reactions are the most important reactions for the kinetic determination of substrate concentration. For any first-order reaction, the substrate concentration $[S]$ at a given time t after the start of the reaction is given by

$$[S] = [S_0] \times e^{-kt} \tag{26}$$

where $[S_0]$ is the initial substrate concentration, e is the base of the natural log, and k is the rate constant.

The change in substrate concentration $\Delta[S]$ over a fixed-time interval, t_1 to t_2, is related to $[S_0]$ by the equation

$$[S_0] = \frac{-\Delta[S]}{e^{-kt_1} - e^{kt_2}} \tag{27}$$

As this equation indicates, the change in substrate concentration over a fixed time interval is directly proportional to its initial concentration. This is a general property of first-order reactions.

For an enzymatic reaction, first-order kinetics are followed when $[S]$ is small compared with K_m. Thus,

$$v = \frac{V_{max}}{K_m} \times [S] \tag{28}$$

or

$$v = k[S] \tag{29}$$

Thus, the first-order rate constant, k, is equal to $\frac{V_{max}}{K_m}$.

Methods in which some property related to substrate concentration (such as absorbance, fluorescence, chemiluminescence, etc.) is measured at two fixed times during the course of the reaction are known as *two-point* kinetic methods. They are theoretically the most accurate for the enzymatic determination of substrates. However, these methods are technically more demanding than equilibrium methods and all the factors that affect reaction rate, such as pH, temperature, and amount of enzyme, must be kept constant from one assay to the next, as must the timing of the two measurements. These conditions can readily be achieved in automatic analyzers. A reference solution of the analyte (substrate) must be used for calibration. To ensure first-order reaction conditions, the substrate concentration must be low compared to the K_m (i.e., in the order of less than 0.2 $\times K_m$. Enzymes with high K_m values are therefore preferred for kinetic analysis to give a wider usable range of substrate concentration.

Immunoassay

In enzyme immunoassay, enzyme-labeled antibodies or antigens are first allowed to react with ligand, and then an enzyme substrate is subsequently added. ALP, horseradish peroxidase, glucose-6-phosphate dehydrogenase, and β-galactosidase have all been used as enzyme labels. A modification of this methodology is the enzyme-linked immunoabsorbent assay (ELISA) in which one of the reaction components is bound to a solid-phase surface. In this technique, an aliquot of sample is allowed to interact with the solid-phase antibody. After washing, a second antibody labeled with enzyme is added to form an Ab-Ag-Ab-enzyme complex. Excess free enzyme-labeled antibody is then washed away and the substrate is added; the conversion of substrate is proportional to the quantity of antigen. In immunoassays, it is not the specificity of enzymes that is important but their sensitivity.

Analytical Applications of Immobilized Enzymes

The consumption of relatively expensive enzymes, one of the disadvantages of enzymatic analysis, can be reduced by the use of immobilized enzymes that can be reused for several analyses. Immobilized enzymes have been chemically bonded to adsorbents, such as microcrystalline cellulose, diethylaminoethyl (DEAE) cellulose, carboxymethyl cellulose, and agarose. Diazo, triazine, and azide groups are used to join the enzyme protein to the insoluble matrix, forming either particles in contact with the substrate solution or a surface in contact with substrate solution, such as a membrane or a coating on the inner surface of a vessel holding the substrate solution. Among enzymes available in such immobilized form are urease, hexokinase, α-amylase, glucose oxidase, trypsin, and leucine aminopeptidase. Stability to heat and other forms of inactivation is considerably increased compared with enzymes in solution. Immobilized proteolytic enzymes are not subject to autodigestion. However, some properties of the enzyme, such as its K_m or its pH optimum, may be altered.

Techniques such as potentiometry, polarography, and microcalorimetry have been chosen in exploiting the benefits of immobilized enzymes (see Chapter 4). Enzymes incorporated into membranes form part of enzyme electrodes. The surface of an ion-sensitive electrode is coated with a layer of porous gel in which an enzyme has been polymerized. When the electrode is immersed in a solution of the appropriate substrate, the action of the enzyme produces ions to which the electrode is sensitive. For example, an oxygen electrode coated with a layer containing glucose oxidase can be used to determine glucose by the amount of oxygen consumed in the reaction, and urea can be estimated by the combination of a selective ammonium ion–sensitive electrode and a urease membrane.

Measurement of Isoenzymes and Isoforms

A number of analytical techniques have been used to measure isoenzymes or isoforms. They include electrophoresis (see Chapter 5), chromatography (see Chapter 6), chemical inactivation, and differences in catalytic properties, but the most common routine methods are now based on immunochemical methods.

Electrophoresis

Isoelectric focusing (see Chapter 5), has been used successfully to separate isoenzymes that differ in the amount of covalently bound sugar residues, such as sialic acid.

Chromatography

Ion-exchange chromatography makes use of differences in net molecular charge at a given pH to separate isoenzymes. A typical ion-exchange material is DEAE cellulose, in which ionizable DEAE groups are attached to an inert cellulose matrix. Ion-exchange chromatography is not in general as highly resolving of closely similar proteins as is zone electrophoresis, but relatively large amounts of proteins can be separated with good recoveries of enzymatic activity, so the method is of great value in enzyme purification.

Other forms of chromatography that have been applied to fractionation of isoenzyme mixtures include high-performance liquid chromatography (HPLC) and affinity chromatography. The latter makes use of differences between isoenzymes in their affinities for a specific ligand that is attached to an inert insoluble support used as the stationary phase in a chromatography column or in a batch technique.

Chemical Inactivation and Differences in Catalytic Properties

Selective inactivation under controlled conditions has been used in the past in isoenzyme characterization. The method is based on differences in stability that result from small changes in the structure of protein molecules. Elevated temperatures or concentrated solutions of urea or other reagents were used to denature the enzyme. Rates of enzyme inactivation by these agents are critically dependent on the conditions of the experiment, which must therefore be strictly controlled if reliable comparisons between samples are to be made.

Differences in catalytic properties, such as differences in K_m, relative rates of reaction with substrate analogues (when the specificity of the enzyme allows for variation in the structure of the substrate), pH optima, and response to inhibitors, typically exist between isoenzymes that are the products of multiple gene loci. These differences can be made the basis of methods of identification and measurement of particular isoenzymes.

Immunochemical Assays

Immunochemical methods of isoenzyme analysis are particularly applicable to isoenzymes derived from multiple gene loci, because these are usually most clearly antigenically distinct. However, the greater discriminating power of monoclonal antibodies has potentially brought all multiple forms of an enzyme within the scope of immunochemical analysis. Some of these methods make use of catalytic activity of the isoenzymes. For example, residual activity may be measured after reaction with antiserum. Radioimmunoassays, in which isoenzyme labeled with a radioactive tracer competes with unlabeled isoenzyme for antibody-binding sites, have also been applied to isoenzyme measurement. These methods do not depend on the catalytic activity of the isoenzyme being determined. However, with the development of automated immunoassay systems, the most common routine methods for measuring isoenzymes, such as CK-MB, are solid phase enzyme-linked immunosorbent assays (ELISA).

The choice and application of various methods of isoenzyme analysis in clinical enzymology are discussed in Chapter 21 in relation to specific isoenzyme systems.

DIAGNOSTIC ENZYMOLOGY

In general, clinical laboratorians are principally concerned with changes in the activity in the serum or plasma of enzymes that are predominantly intracellular and that are normally present in the serum at low activities only. By measuring changes in the activities of these enzymes in disease, they attempt to infer the location and nature of pathological changes in the tissues of the body. Therefore understanding the factors that affect the rate of release of enzymes from their cells of origin and the rate at which they are cleared from the circulation is necessary so that changes in activity in disease can be interpreted correctly.

FACTORS AFFECTING ENZYME LEVELS IN PLASMA OR SERUM[4,5]

The measured level of activity of an enzyme in blood is the result of the balance between the rate at which it is entering the circulation from its cells of origin and the rate at which it is removed.

Entry of Enzymes into the Blood

The measured levels of an enzyme in blood are the result of the balance between the rate at which it enters the circulation from its cells of origin and the rate at which it is inactivated or removed.

Leakage of Enzymes from Cells

Enzymes are retained within their cells of origin by the plasma membrane surrounding the cell. The plasma membrane is a metabolically active part of the cell, and its integrity depends on the cell's production of ATP. Any process that impairs ATP production, either by depriving the cell of oxidizable substrates or by reducing the efficiency of energy production by restricting the access of oxygen (ischemia or anoxia), promotes deterioration of the cell membrane. The earliest sign of impaired energy metabolism is the efflux of potassium and influx of sodium; water thus accumulates within the cell, causing it to swell. The next and most serious stage is the entry of Ca^{2+}, which stimulates intracellular enzymes, leading to both cell damage and disruption of the cell membrane. Finally, free radicals formed during these processes may cause further damage. The membrane becomes leaky; if cellular injury becomes irreversible, the cell will die, although enzyme loss may also occur without irreversible injury occurring. Small molecules are the first to leak from damaged or dying cells, followed by larger molecules, such as enzymes and other proteins. Cytosolic proteins appear early on in the plasma, followed much later by mitochondrial and membrane-bound enzymes. Ultimately, the contents of the now necrotic cells are discharged.

Because of the very high concentrations of enzymes within the cell—thousands or even tens of thousands of times greater than the concentrations in extracellular fluid—and because extremely small amounts of enzyme can be detected by their catalytic activity, an increase of enzyme activity in the extracellular fluid or plasma is an extremely sensitive indicator of even minor cellular damage, some causes of which are listed in Table 8-2.

Direct attack on the cell membranes by such agents as viruses or organic chemicals also causes enzyme release and

TABLE 8-2 Causes of Cell Damage or Death

Category	Examples
Hypoxia (an extremely common accompaniment of clinical disease)	Loss of blood supply due to narrowing (atheromatous plaques) or blocking (thrombosis) of artery or vein; ischemic-perfusion injury; inadequate oxygenation due to cardiorespiratory failure; loss of oxygen-carrying capacity, CO poisoning, and anemia
Chemicals and drugs (an important cause of cellular damage)	Environmental pollutants—lead, mercury; drugs—use and abuse; alcohol; tobacco
Physical agents	Trauma; extremes of heat and radiation; electrical energy; toxic chemicals
Microbiological agents	Bacteria, viruses, fungi, protozoa, and helminths
Immune mechanisms	Immune disorders can cause tissue damage by a number of mechanisms: 1. Anaphylaxis (causing release of vasoactive amines) 2. Cytotoxicity (causing the target cell to be lysed) 3. Immune complex disease (leading to release of lysosomal enzymes) 4. Cell-mediated hypersensitivity (leading to cytotoxicity)
Genetic defects	Disorders with polygenic inheritance—diabetes mellitus, gout Mendelian disorders—X-linked disorders, autosomal dominant and recessive disorders, disorders with variable modes of transmission
Nutritional disorders	Protein-calorie malnutrition, vitamin deficiencies, mineral deficiencies; obesity and its consequences

Based on the classification of Robbins and colleagues. In: Basic pathology, 3rd ed. Philadelphia: WB Saunders, 1981.

one that is particularly important in the case of the liver. A reduction in the supply of oxygenated blood perfusing any tissue will also promote enzyme release. An example of a clinical condition in which such a reduction occurs is myocardial infarction. The cells of the affected region rapidly begin to deteriorate and die, releasing their enzyme contents to the systemic circulation, which accounts for the rapid rise in serum enzyme activity that is characteristic of this condition. The liver is very sensitive to hypoxia, which results from diminished cardiac output (heart failure). Increased activities of hepatocellular enzymes in the blood accompany a wide variety of conditions, such as congestive heart failure, shock, and hypoxemia.

Skeletal muscles also contribute enzymes to blood. Again, the cause may be poor perfusion, hypothermia, or direct trauma to the muscles (crush injuries). Infection, inflammation (polymyositis), degenerative changes (dystrophies), drugs, and alcohol (alcoholic myopathy) will cause enzyme leakage from myocytes. Enzyme release from muscles and other tissues also occurs as a result of anesthesia.

Efflux of Enzymes from Damaged Cells

Once the conditions for leakage of enzymes from cells have become established, the speed and extent with which the process is reflected in enzyme changes in the blood depend on several factors.

The driving force of enzyme release is the steep concentration gradient of enzyme activity that exists between the interior and the exterior of the cells. The rate of escape of enzyme molecules is presumably controlled to some extent by diffusion; therefore, smaller enzyme molecules might be expected to appear in the extracellular fluid earlier than larger ones. Although this is probably true to some extent, the range of molecular weights covered by enzymes of diagnostic interest is rather narrow, so this factor may be less important.

The way in which released enzyme molecules are transferred from the interstitial fluid to the blood varies from one tissue to another, passing directly through the capillary wall or by lymphatic transfer. Direct transfer probably occurs to a large extent in the liver, which is a highly vascular tissue with many permeable capillaries, although there is some evidence that liver enzymes may also be subject to lymphatic transfer. On the other hand, the capillaries of skeletal muscle are relatively impermeable, and in this tissue it is probable that released enzymes mainly reach the circulatory system by way of drainage from the lymphatic system. Lymph drainage is also important in transporting enzymes released from damaged intestinal and myocardial cells to the circulation although a considerable proportion of myocardial enzymes also reaches the circulation by direct capillary transfer following infarction.

The intracellular location of the leaking enzymes also affects the rates at which they appear in the circulation. As would be expected, the most sensitive indicators of cell damage are the enzymes that are present in the soluble fraction of the cell. Enzymes associated with subcellular structures, such as mitochondria, are less readily released into the circulation. This fact has been used in attempts to distinguish reversible leakage, presumed to reflect damage only to the cell membrane, from necrotic lesions in which the intracellular structures are destroyed.

The relation between tissue injury and the appearance of enzymes in the circulation is most clearly seen in the condition of myocardial infarction, in which a relatively short episode of damage is followed by a rapid transfer of enzymes to the circulatory system. About 24 hours after a myocardial infarction, the pattern of relative activity of various enzymes in the circulatory system closely resembles that in the myocardial tissue. These relationships are less clearly recognized in other conditions, such as chronic liver disease, in which enzyme release is a process that continues for a period of time. The pattern of relative enzyme activities in serum in chronic disease may also become distorted by differential rates of removal of enzymes from the circulation and possibly also by differential changes of rates of enzyme synthesis in the affected tissue.

Some of the small amounts of intracellular enzymes normally present in the plasma can be assumed to result from wear and tear of cells or overflow of enzyme from healthy cells. This contribution of enzymes to the circulating blood may decrease, either as the result of a genetic deficiency of enzyme production (e.g., as is the case for ALP in hypophosphatasia or in individuals homozygous for the "silent" gene for serum cholinesterase), or when enzyme production is depressed as a result of disease (e.g., the production of serum cholinesterase is often depressed in liver disease).

Release of enzymes from damaged or dying cells and changes in the rate of enzyme production constitute the most important mechanisms by which changes in enzyme activity in the serum or plasma are produced. However, other possibilities exist and appear to account for some changes of diagnostic importance. For example, much of the γ-glutamyl transferase activity of liver cells is located on their exterior surfaces. It is possible that ectoenzymes, such as this, may be eluted from the surfaces, especially where there is increased detergent action of the blood through accumulation of bile salts. This process does not involve cell damage in the sense of increased membrane permeability, as evidenced by the lack of correlation between the activities of γ-glutamyl transferase and aminotransferases in serum in liver diseases of different types.

Altered Enzyme Production

The small amounts of intracellular enzymes normally present in plasma are thought to result from turnover of cells or leakage of enzymes from healthy cells. This contribution of enzymes to the circulating blood may decrease either as the result of a genetic deficiency of enzyme production or when enzyme production is depressed as a result of disease. However, cases in which enzyme production is increased are of more general interest in diagnostic enzymology. For example, an increase in the number and activity of the ALP producing osteoblasts of bone is responsible for the increased level of ALP in the serum of normally growing children. Increased osteoblastic activity also accounts for the increased levels of this enzyme in serum in various types of bone disease. Toward the end of normal pregnancy, the placenta constitutes a new source of ALP and contributes its characteristic isoenzyme to the maternal circulation.

The process of enzyme induction also increases enzyme production. An example of such induction is the increased activity of γ-glutamyltransferase in serum, which results from the administration of drugs such as barbiturates or phenytoin, and from the intake of ethanol. Biliary obstruction induces increased synthesis of ALP in the liver.

Clearance of Enzymes

Significant evidence is now available about the way in which enzymes are cleared from circulation. Few enzyme molecules are small enough to pass through the healthy glomerulus of the kidney; therefore urinary excretion is not a major route for elimination of enzymes from circulation. An exception to this is α-amylase; increased concentrations of this enzyme in the blood (e.g., after *acute pancreatitis*) are accompanied by increased excretion in the urine. Evidence now suggests that many enzymes are probably not inactivated in the plasma, but that they are rapidly removed, probably by the reticuloendothelial system, such as the bone marrow, spleen, and liver (Kupffer's cells) or, to a lesser extent, by nearly all cells in the body. The mechanism appears to be by receptor-mediated endocytosis (the process of recognition, specific accumulation, and uptake of protein by specific cell-surface receptors followed by fusion with the lysosomes, digestion of the ingested protein, and recycling of the receptor back to the cell membrane). For example, hepatic Kupffer's cells have been shown to take up several tissue-derived enzymes—such as LD-5, CK-MM, adenylate kinase, cytoplasmic and mitochondrial aspartate aminotransferase, and malate and alcohol dehydrogenases—by receptor-mediated endocytosis, which may have affinity for the lysine residues on these enzymes. The adult isoform of intestinal ALP is a galactosyl-terminal glycoprotein that reacts with a galactosyl-specific receptor on the hepatocyte membrane and undergoes subsequent endocytosis. This process is rapid, accounting for the extremely short plasma half-life of this isoform. However, in hepatic cirrhosis, in which considerable reduction in parenchymal cell mass often occurs, the plasma concentration and half-life of the isoform increase. Other ALP isoenzymes and isoforms are sialoglycoproteins that do not react with the galactosyl receptor and are therefore protected from rapid uptake from blood. Indeed, many examples are now known of excessive sialylation of ALPs, produced by malignant cells, prolonging their plasma half-lives and facilitating their detection. This example illustrates the importance of understanding the processes by which enzymes are cleared from plasma.

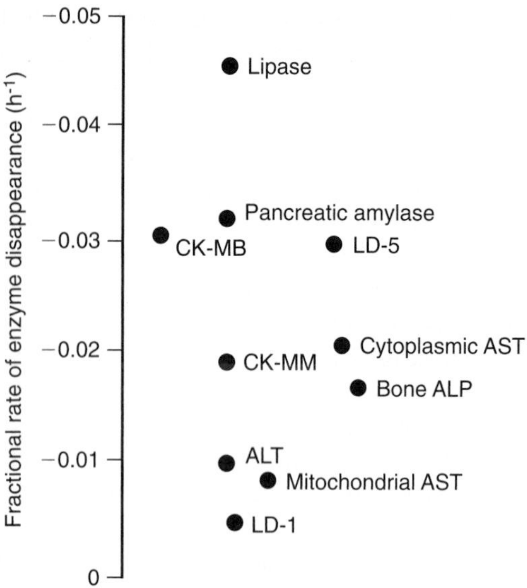

Figure 8-13 Fractional disappearance rates (k_d) from human blood of the most important enzymes.

The half-lives of enzymes in plasma vary from a few hours to several days, but in most cases, with an average half-life ($t_{1/2}$) of 6 to 48 hours. Rates of decay may also be expressed as k_d values—the fractional disappearance rate—and the relationship to $t_{1/2}$ values is:

$$k_d = 2.303\log\frac{2}{t_{1/2}} = \frac{0.693}{t_{1/2}} \qquad (30)$$

Typical disappearance rates from human blood for several clinically relevant enzymes are shown in Figure 8-13.

Selection of Enzyme Tests

The selection of which enzyme to measure in serum for diagnostic or prognostic purposes depends on a number of factors. An important factor is the distribution of enzymes among the various tissues, shown, for example, for aspartate aminotransferase, alanine aminotransferase, and creatine kinase in Figure 8-14. The main enzymes of established clinical value, together with their tissues of origin and their major clinical applications, are listed in Table 8-3 (see also Chapter 21).

The mass of the damaged or malfunctioning organ, together with the enzyme cell/blood gradient, obviously has a profound influence on the resulting elevation of enzyme activity in blood. Thus the gradient of activity of prostatic acid phosphatase between prostate and blood is about $10^3:1$, and the mass of that organ is 20 g. By contrast, the cell and/or blood gradient of alanine aminotransferase in the liver cell is $10^4:1$, and the mass of the liver can exceed 1000 g. Obviously, fewer cells have to be damaged in the liver than in the prostate for the abnormality to be detected by an enzyme elevation in blood. If on the other hand there is total

TABLE 8-3 Distribution of Diagnostically Important Enzymes

Enzyme	Principal Sources of Enzyme in Blood	Principal Clinical Applications
Alanine aminotransferase	Liver, skeletal muscle	Hepatic parenchymal disease
Alkaline phosphatase	Liver, bone, intestinal mucosa, placenta	Bone diseases, hepatobiliary diseases
Amylase	Salivary glands, pancreas	Pancreatic diseases
Aspartate aminotransferase	Liver, skeletal muscle, heart, erythrocytes	Hepatic parenchymal disease, muscle disease
Cholinesterase	Liver	Organophosphorus insecticide poisoning, suxamethonium sensitivity, hepatic parenchymal diseases
Creatine kinase	Skeletal muscle, heart	Muscle diseases, myocardial infarction
Glutamate dehydrogenase	Liver	Hepatic parenchymal diseases
γ-Glutamyltransferase	Liver, kidney	Hepatobiliary diseases
Lactate dehydrogenase	Heart, liver, skeletal muscle, erythrocytes, platelets, lymph nodes	Hemolysis, hepatic parenchymal diseases, myocardial infarction
Lipase	Pancreas	Pancreatic diseases
5′-Nucleotidase	Hepatobiliary tract	Hepatobiliary disease
Trypsin(ogen)	Pancreas	Pancreatic diseases

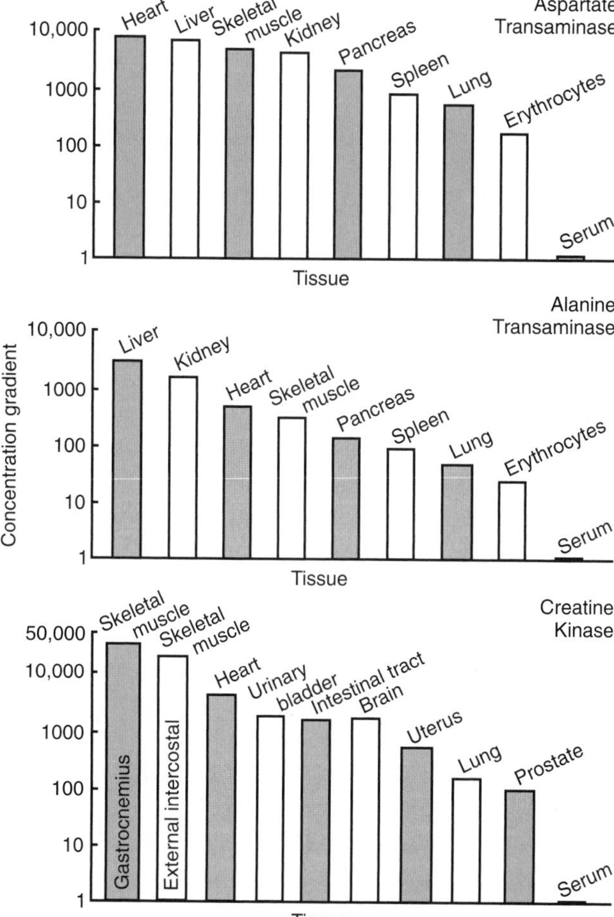

Figure 8-14 The concentration gradients between some human tissues and serum for aspartate transaminase, alanine transaminase, and creatine kinase. The concentration gradient axis is logarithmic.

organ involvement, then clearly the vast number of affected liver cells will markedly elevate blood concentrations of any liver enzyme. It has been estimated that if only 1 liver cell in every 750 is damaged, elevation in the blood level of alanine aminotransferase would be detectable.

Knowledge of the intracellular location of enzymes can assist in determining the nature and severity of a pathological process if suitable enzymes are assayed in the blood. For instance, a mild, reversible viral inflammation of the liver, such as a mild attack of viral hepatitis, is likely to increase only the permeability of the cell membrane and allow cytoplasmic enzymes to leak out into the blood, whereas a severe attack causing cell necrosis also disrupts the mitochondrial membrane, and both cytoplasmic and mitochondrial enzymes are detected in the blood. Finally, in selecting a suitable enzyme to assay in blood for diagnostic purposes, the rate at which its activity disappears from the blood is of significance. As previously indicated, the most commonly assayed enzymes are those with half-lives in the range of 12 hours or greater.

REFERENCES

1. Commission on Biochemical Nomenclature. I. Nomenclature of multiple forms of enzymes. J Biol Chem 1977;252:5939-41.
2. Copeland RA. Enzymes: A Practical Introduction to Structure, Mechanism, and Data Analysis. Basel: V C H Publishers, 1996.
3. IUPAC Commission on Quantities and Units and IFCC Expert Panel on Quantities and Units: Approved Recommendations (1978). Quantities and units in clinical chemistry. Clin Chim Acta 1979;96:157F-83F.
4. Kristensen SR. Mechanisms of cell damage and enzyme release. Dan Med Bull 1994;41:423-33.

5. Kristensen SR, Horder M. Principles of diagnostic enzymology. *In:* Enzyme Tests in Diagnosis. Moss DW, Rosalki SB, Eds. London: Edward Arnold, 1996, pp. 7-24.
6. Lorenz K. Approved recommendation on IFCC methods for the measurement of catalytic concentrations of enzymes. Part 9. IFCC method for amylase. Clin Chem Lab Med 1998;36:185-203.
7. Moss DW. Isoenzyme Analysis. London: The Chemical Society, 1979.
8. Moss DW. Enzyme reference materials: their place in diagnostic enzymology. Ann Biol Clin 1994;52:143-6.
9. Nomenclature Committee, I.E. 1978. Recommendations of the Nomenclature Committee of IUB on the Nomenclature and Classification of Enzymes. New York: Academic Press, 1979.
10. Panteghini M, Ceriotti F, Schumann G, Siekmann L. Establishing a reference system in clinical enzymology. Clin Chem Lab Med 2001;39:795-800.
11. Rautela GS, Snee RD, Miller WK. Response-surface co-optimization of reaction conditions in clinical chemical methods. Clin Chem 1979;25:1954-64.
12. Schumann G, Bonora R, Ceriotti F, Clerc-Renaud P, Ferrero CA, et al. IFCC primary reference procedures for the measurement of catalytic activity concentrations of enzymes at 37°C. Part 2. Reference procedure for the measurement of catalytic concentration of creatine kinase. Clin Chem Lab Med 2002 Jun;40(6):635-42.
13. Schumann G, Bonora R, Ceriotti F, Clerc-Renaud P, Ferrero CA, et al. IFCC primary reference procedures for the measurement of catalytic activity concentrations of enzymes at 37°C. Part 3. Reference procedure for the measurement of catalytic concentration of lactate dehydrogenase. Clin Chem Lab Med 2002;40:643-8.
14. Schumann G, Bonora R, Ceriotti F, Ferard G, Ferrero CA, et al. IFCC primary reference procedures for the measurement of catalytic activity concentrations of enzymes at 37°C. International Federation of Clinical Chemistry and Laboratory Medicine. Part 4. Reference procedure for the measurement of catalytic concentration of alanine aminotransferase. Clin Chem Lab Med 2002;40:718-24.
15. Schumann G, Bonora R, Ceriotti F, Ferard G, Ferrero CA, et al. IFCC primary reference procedures for the measurement of catalytic activity concentrations of enzymes at 37°C. International Federation of Clinical Chemistry and Laboratory Medicine. Part 5. Reference procedure for the measurement of catalytic concentration of aspartate aminotransferase. Clin Chem Lab Med 2002;40:725-33.
16. Schumann G, Bonora R, Ceriotti F, Ferard G, Ferrero CA, et al. IFCC primary reference procedures for the measurement of catalytic activity concentrations of enzymes at 37°C. International Federation of Clinical Chemistry and Laboratory Medicine. Part 6. Reference procedure for the measurement of catalytic concentration of gamma-glutamyltransferase. Clin Chem Lab Med 2002;40:734
17. Siekmann L, Bonora R, Burtis CA, Ceriotti F, Clerc-Renaud P, et al. IIFCC primary reference procedures for the measurement of catalytic activity concentrations of enzymes at 37°C. International Federation of Clinical Chemistry and Laboratory Medicine. Part 7. Certification of four reference materials for the determination of enzymatic activity of gamma-glutamyltransferase, lactate dehydrogenase, alanine aminotransferase and creatine kinase accord. Clin Chem Lab Med 2002;40:739-45.

ADDITIONAL READING

Bergmeyer HU. Methods of enzymatic analysis, 3rd ed. Basel: Verlag Chemie, 1983.

Boyer PD. The enzymes, 3rd ed. San Diego: Academic Press, 1981.

Colowick SP. Kaplan NO. Methods in enzymology. San Diego: Academic Press.

Copeland RA. Enzymes: A practical introduction to structure, mechanism, and data analysis. Basel: V C H Publishers, 1996.

Cornish-Bowden A. Fundamentals of enzyme kinetics, Aldershot UK: Ashgate Publishing Company, 1995.

Dressler D. Enzymes. San Francisco: W H Freeman & Company, 1995.

Enzyme Nomenclature. San Diego: Academic Press, 1992.

Fersht A. Enzyme structure and mechanism. San Francisco: W H Freeman & Company, 1995.

Krebs EG. The Enzymes. Vol. 18. San Diego: Academic Press, 1987.

Marangoni AG. Enzyme kinetics: A modern approach. Hoboken NJ: Wiley-Interscience. 2002:1-248.

Palmer T. Understanding enzymes. Englewood Cliffs, NJ: Prentice Hall, 1995.

Passonneau JV, Lowry OH. Enzymatic analysis: A practical guide. Clifton, NJ: Humana Press, 1993.

Purich DL, Allison RD. Handbook of biochemical kinetics. San Diego: Academic Press. 2000:1-788.

Schomburg D, Stephan D. Enzyme handbook. New York: Springer-Verlag, 1996.

CHAPTER 9

Principles of Immunochemical Techniques*

L.J. Kricka, D.Phil., F.A.C.B., C.Chem., F.R.S.C., F.R.C.Path.

Immunochemical reactions form the basis of a diverse range of sensitive and specific clinical assays. In a typical immunochemical analysis, an antibody is used as a reagent to detect an antigen of interest. The exquisite specificity and the high affinity of antibodies for specific antigens, coupled with the unique ability of antibodies to cross link antigens, allow the identification and quantitation of specific substances by a variety of methods. The principles of the methods most commonly used in the laboratory are discussed in this chapter. This introduction is intended to acquaint the reader with the structure and function of antibodies (immunoglobulins) in relation to their use as reagents in immunoanalyses.

BASIC CONCEPTS

The binding of antibodies and their complementary antigens forms the basis of all immunochemical techniques.

ANTIBODIES

Antibodies are immunoglobulins that are capable of binding specifically to a wide array of natural and synthetic antigens, including proteins, carbohydrates, nucleic acids, lipids, and other molecules. Immunoglobulins consist of five general classes designated as IgG, IgA, IgM, IgD, and IgE. Immunoglobulin G is the most prevalent immunochemical reagent in use. Currently, immunoglobulins A, M, D, and E do not play an important role in immunochemical analysis. A schematic diagram of the IgG molecule is shown in Figure 9-1. IgG is a glycoprotein (MW 158,000) composed of two duplex chains with each set being made up of a heavy (γ) and light (κ and λ) chain joined by disulfide bonds. Interchain disulfide bonds hold the duplex chains together and create a symmetrical molecule. For more information on immunoglobulins, see Chapter 20.

The variable amino acid sequence at the amino terminal end of each chain determines the antigenic specificity of the particular antibody. Each unique amino acid sequence is a product of a single plasma cell line or clone. The normal host response to an immunogen* results in the stimulation of one or two major classes of lymphocytes that are able to divide and produce plasma cells capable of secreting antibodies. Each plasma cell line produces antibodies with a single specificity. A complex antigen is capable of eliciting a multiplicity of antibodies with different specificities that are derived

*The author gratefully acknowledges the original contribution by Dr. Gregory Buffone, upon which portions of this chapter are based.

*An *immunogen* is any chemical substance capable of inducing an immune response. The term immunogen is now used instead of the term *antigen* when referring to materials capable of eliciting antibody formation when injected into a host. The term *antigen* is used for any material capable of reacting with an antibody, without necessarily being capable of inducing antibody formation. For example, egg albumin is an immunogen, because it is capable of inducing formation of antiegg albumin antibody. Because it will react with antimorphine antibodies, morphine is an antigen. However, it is not an immunogen, because it does not induce antibody formation unless first conjugated with a protein.

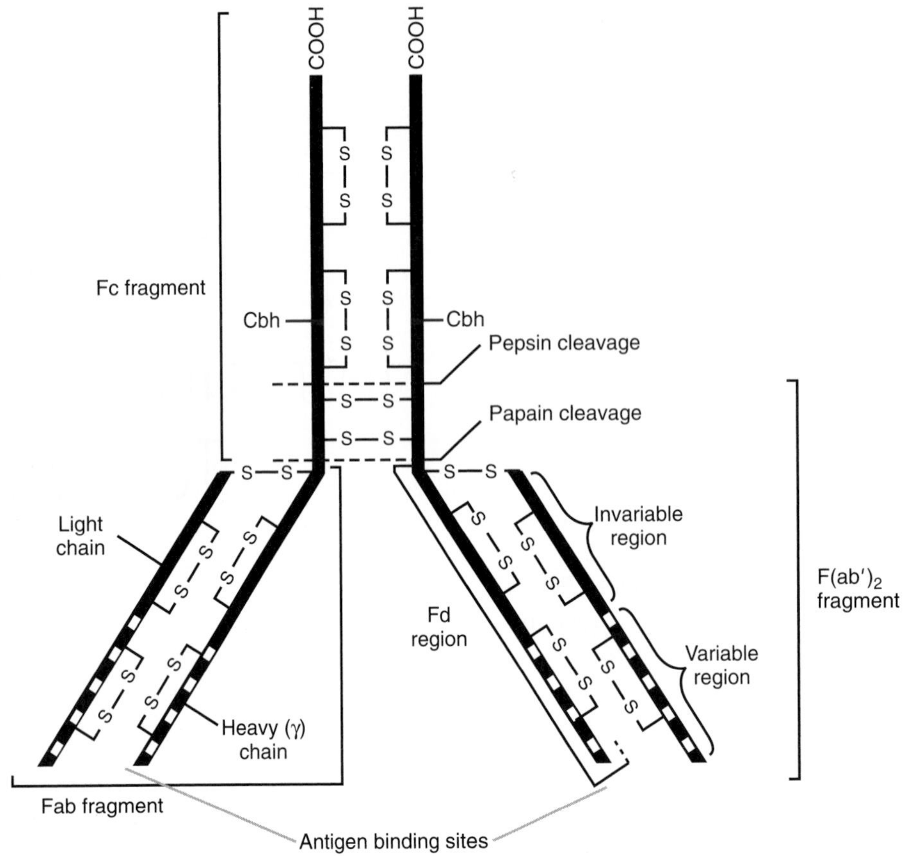

Figure 9-1 Schematic diagram of IgG antibody molecule showing carbohydrate (Cbh), disulfide bonds (—S—S—), and major fragments produced by proteolytic enzyme treatment ($F[ab']_2$, Fc, Fab, Fd).

from different cell lines. Antibodies derived in this manner are termed *polyclonal* and exhibit diverse specificities in their reactivity with the immunogen. Each unique region of the antigen molecule that will bind a complementary antibody is termed an *epitope* (antigenic determinant).

IMMUNOGENS

An *immunogen* is either a protein or a substance coupled to a carrier, usually a protein, that when introduced into a foreign host is capable of inducing the formation of an antibody in the host. The route of introduction of the immunogen is usually, but not always, intradermal. The antibody produced may be either circulating *(humoral)* or tissue bound *(cellular),* as in delayed hypersensitivity reactions or graft host reactions.

A *hapten* is a chemically defined determinant that when conjugated to an immunogenic carrier stimulates the synthesis of antibody specific for the hapten. It is capable of binding an antibody but cannot by itself stimulate an immune response. Natural immunogens are usually more complex than haptens and have several epitopes. Such immunogens are capable of reacting with several antibodies, allowing cross-linking and the formation of large immune complexes. In addition to proteins and polypeptides, lipids (such as the Wasserman antigen and cardiolipin), nucleic acids (e.g., double-stranded deoxyribonucleic acid [dsDNA]), and many other materials function as antigens. Some general properties required for immunogenicity include: (1) areas of structural stability within the molecule, (2) randomness of structure, (3) a minimal molecular weight of 4000 to 5000, (4) ability to be metabolized (a necessary but not sufficient criterion for some classes of antigens), (5) accessibility of a particular immunogenic configuration to the antibody-forming mechanism, and (6) the foreignness of structure to the host. The overall shape and charge of the molecule in most cases have very little influence on the ability to induce antibody formation.

Injection of an immunogen into a host animal induces a series of biological changes leading to markedly increased production of certain serum globulins with specific antibody activity—the immunoglobulins—and to changes in the capability of certain cellular elements to give an immune response. Continued stimulation by an immunogen results in increasing production of immunoglobulins of different types and of different binding characteristics for antigens. In some cases excessive stimulation leads to immunological paralysis in which no antibody response is mounted until a major fraction of the immunogen is cleared from the organism. After the first exposure to an immunogen, a latent period (induction) occurs during which no antibody is present in serum; this period may last from 5 to 10 days. Because antibody formation by sensitized (immunogen coated) cells can be demonstrated in vitro in a period of minutes, the long delay in antibody build up in vivo is caused by the time required for transport of immunogen to the site of antibody production, for transmission of information, and for actual synthesis of the antibody.

The strength or energy of interaction between the antibody and antigen is described by two terms. *Affinity* refers to the thermodynamic quantity defining the energy of interaction of a single antibody-combining site and its corresponding epitope on the antigen. *Avidity* refers to the overall strength of binding of an antibody and an antigen and includes the sum of the binding affinities of all the individual combining sites on the antibody. For example, IgG has two affinity-binding sites, whereas IgM has 10 affinity-binding sites per antibody molecule. Thus affinity is a property of the substance bound (antigen), and avidity is a property of the binder (antibody). For polyclonal antibodies, avidity is difficult to determine primarily because of the diversity of the antibody population.

Polyclonal antiserum is raised in a normal animal host in response to immunogen administration. In contrast, *monoclonal antiserum* is produced in a very different manner and represents the product of a single clone or plasma cell line rather than a heterogeneous mixture of antibodies produced by many cell clones in response to immunization. Monoclonal antibodies are now widely used as reagents in immunoassay techniques.[45,61] The usual method of production of monoclonal antibodies involves fusing sensitized lymphocytes from the spleens or lymph nodes of mice that have been immunized once or more over a 2- to 4-week period with a murine myeloma cell line from tissue culture in the presence of polyethylene glycol (PEG), which promotes cell fusion through an unknown mechanism. The murine myeloma cell line is an immortal B-cell line. The murine myeloma cell lines most commonly used are deficient in the enzyme hypoxanthine guanine phosphoribosyl transferase (HGPRT) and therefore cannot synthesize purine bases from thymidine and hypoxanthine in the presence of aminopterin. Following the fusion, the cells are placed into a selection medium containing hypoxanthine, aminopterin, and thymidine (HAT medium) to grow *fused hybrid cell* lines selectively. The fused hybrid cells can survive in a HAT medium, because the cells combine the immortality of the myeloma cell with the genetic material of the spleen cell necessary for synthesis of HGPRT. The unfused myeloma cells are killed by the HAT medium because they do not have the HGPRT gene and the unfused spleen cells cannot be maintained in the culture. Colonies arising from the fused cells are then screened for antibody production, and cell lines secreting antibody of the desired specificity are cloned in subcultures. In this way, a single clonal line can be isolated that produces an antibody with a specificity for a single antigen epitope and having a single binding energy or affinity.

Because of the unique ability of a monoclonal antibody to react with a single epitope on a multivalent antigen, the majority of monoclonal antibodies will not cross link and precipitate macromolecular antigens. Consequently, monoclonal antibodies have not found broad applicability in traditional precipitin methods. A practical advantage of using monoclonal antibodies is that two different antibody specificities can be used in a single incubation step. A solid phase antibody specific for a unique epitope and another enzyme-labeled or radiolabeled antibody specific for a different epitope can be reacted with an antigen in a single step. This eliminates the two-step sequential addition of an antigen and labeled antibody to the solid phase and one incubation step and one washing step, which would be necessary when using polyclonal antibodies binding to both sites.

Phage display technology provides a new in vitro approach for producing antibodies (single chain Fv fragments, Fab fragments, and whole antibody molecules) that mimics the immune system but does not require B-cell immortalization.[15,92] V genes coding for the heavy and light chain variable domains of immunoglobulin isolated from lymphocytes are amplified by the polymerase chain reaction and ligated into a filamentous bacteriophage vector to form combinatorial libraries of V_H and V_L genes. Individual bacteriophages display copies of a specific antibody on their surface and the phage library can be screened for the antibody of a defined specificity using immobilized antigen ("panning"). Large libraries displaying antibodies formed from greater than 10^{12} different V_H and V_L combinations can be constructed; this provides a rich source of antibodies with binding constants of 10^8 to 10^9 L/mol. Soluble antibody from selected bacteriophages can be secreted from infected bacteria (e.g., *Escherichia coli*) in yields of greater than 500 mg/L.

ANTIGEN ANTIBODY BINDING

Binding Forces

The strength of the binding of an antigen to an antibody depends on several forces acting cooperatively. They include van der Waals-London dipole-dipole interaction, hydrophobic interaction, and ionic coulombic bonding.[43,76]

Van Der Waals-London Dipole-Dipole Interactions

Van der Waals-London binding is caused by the attraction between atoms when they are brought together in close proximity. These interactions are basically electrostatic in nature and are applicable to polarizable, noncharged molecules, whose structure allows the electron cloud around the molecule to be distorted by outside forces in such a way that a transient dipole is produced. Such polarization results in the formation of an instantaneous dipole moment, which in turn induces a dipole moment in adjacent molecules. The induced dipole moment is oriented in an antiparallel fashion with respect to the original dipole moment such that a net attractive force is produced. These forces operate over short distances (4 to 6 nm) and are more significant for larger molecules. Because polarizability varies inversely with temperature, the attractive force is inversely proportional to the temperature.

Hydrophobic Interaction

Hydrophobic interactions result because the association of nonpolar groups is energetically favored in aqueous or other polar solutions. In proteins, hydrophobic interactions serve to bend and fold a molecule in a way that brings nonpolar R groups inside to the less polar interior; polar R groups are oriented outside toward the more polar aqueous environment. Thus hydrophobic bonding forms an interior, hydrophobic protein core, where most hydrophobic side chains can closely associate and weakly bind. Hydrophobic interaction enhances or stabilizes antigen antibody binding but is not necessarily a driving force in such binding.[78]

Coulombic Bonds

Coulombic bonding results from the attraction between charged groups on the antigen and antibody, primarily COO^- and NH_4^+. The attraction between the charged groups is greatest in a medium with a low dielectric constant caused by reduced interaction of the solvent or other solute (salts) with the macromolecular ions. In a medium of high dielectric constant (aqueous solutions containing added salt), a diffuse double layer of charged particles will tend to shield the attraction of the charged species in the reactive sites of the antigen and antibody. This inhibition under certain circumstances can considerably reduce the binding constant for many antigen antibody systems.

Considering these forces, one would predict that changing pH, temperature, and ionic strength of the reaction medium should influence the binding of antigen and antibody. However, given that the lower and upper limit of pH is 6 and 8 and the temperature between 25 °C and 35 °C, these variables have only minimal effect on the rate of association and immune complex formation.[60,80] In fact, extremes in pH (less than 4.0 and greater than 8.0) can cause inhibition of binding or dissociation of already formed antigen antibody complexes. Such extremes ultimately result in some degree of denaturation of the proteins involved. Thus only changes in ionic strength will produce a significant affect on the rate of binding of antigen and antibody. This concept is studied further in the following sections.

Reaction Mechanism

The binding of antigen to antibody is not static but is an equilibrium reaction that proceeds in three phases. The initial reaction (phase 1) of a multivalent antigen (Ag_n) and a bivalent antibody (Ab) occurs very rapidly in comparison with the subsequent growth of the complexes (phase 2) and is depicted by the following equation:

$$Ag_n + Ab \underset{k_{-1}}{\overset{k_1}{\rightleftharpoons}} Ag_nAb \underset{k_{-2}}{\overset{k_2}{\rightleftharpoons}} Ag_aAb_b \quad (1)$$

where $k_1 >>> k_2$, n is the number of epitopes per molecule, and a and b are the numbers of antigen and antibody molecules per complex. Phase 3 of the reaction involves the precipitation of the complex after a critical size is reached. The speed of these reactions depends on electrolyte concentration, pH, and temperature, and on antigen and antibody types and the binding affinity of the antibody. The concentration of NaCl is important, and in most cases normal saline (NaCl, 0.15 mol/L) is used. Higher concentrations of NaCl can lead to smaller amounts of precipitate; this is due not to increased solubility of the antigen antibody complex, but to an equilibrium shift causing a given amount of antigen to combine with smaller amounts of antibody. Decreasing the NaCl concentration can lead to increased precipitation of other proteins. Generally the presence of divalent cations has no effect on precipitation.

It is best to use dilute solutions for determining the influence of such factors as ionic species, ionic strength, pH, and concentration of soluble linear polymers, or for optical analytical methods. Use of dilute solutions slows the growth of the antigen antibody complexes, and a more stable and more homogeneous population of complexes results. Most of the discussions presented in subsequent sections are based on dilute systems and may not pertain to solutions in which reactants are present in much higher concentrations.

Factors Influencing Binding

Factors that influence the strength of binding between an antigen and antibody include the ion species, ionic strength, and polymers.

Ion Species and Ionic Strength Effects

Cationic salts produce an inhibition of the binding of antibody with a cationic hapten.[31] The order of inhibition by various cations is $Cs^+ > Rb^+ > NH_4^+ > K^+ > Na^+ > Li^+$. This order corresponds to the decreasing ionic radius and increasing radius of hydration. Presumably the lesser degree of hydration permits greater interaction of the salt with an anionic group located in the antibody-combining site. Similar results were found for anionic haptens and anionic salts. For example, the order of inhibition of binding for anionic salts is $CNS^- > NO^{-3} > I^- > Br^- > Cl^- > F^-$, which again is in the order of decreasing ionic radius and increasing radius of hydration. If the competition theory as suggested by these experiments is correct, one would expect the degree of inhibition to be a concentration-dependent phenomenon, and indeed the rate of formation of immune complexes is slower in normal saline (NaCl, 0.15 mol/L) than the same reaction carried out in deionized water. Given the above observation, F^- should be the anion of choice for immunochemical reaction buffers. In fact, F^- does provide a modest improvement over Cl^-, but the advantage is so small that laboratories rarely substitute toxic fluoride ion for innocuous chloride ion in buffer solutions. A small but measurable difference in the initial rate of combination of antigen and antibody can be seen for phosphate as compared with tris buffer, presumably owing to the charge difference in the buffer molecules.[74] In general, the most notable differences in reaction rates for the various anionic species evaluated are seen at *t* less than 5 minutes. When the reactions are evaluated at longer times (i.e., *t* greater than 5 minutes), the difference in rate of antigen antibody complex formation is relatively small for different anionic species.[60]

Polymer Effect[54]

In general, the solubility of a protein in the presence of different linear polymers is inversely proportional to the molecular weight of the polymer (i.e., the higher the molecular weight of the polymer, the lower the solubility of the protein). For example, in the presence of Dextran 500, the solubility of α-crystalline < fibrinogen < γ-globulin < albumin <<< tyrosine.[53,54] Laurent thus proposed a steric exclusion mechanism to explain the effect of polymers on protein solubility.[54] Assuming a fixed total volume (V_T) of solvent being occupied by both polymer and protein and defining the volume occupied by polymer as V_E (excluded volume, i.e., volume not accessible to proteins) and the volume occupied by protein as V', then the relation

$$V_T = V' + V_E \tag{2}$$

implies that any increase in V_E caused by an increase in number or size of polymer molecules forces a decrease in V' and an effective increase in the concentration of protein molecules. Hence, as V_E is increased, the *effective* protein concentration is increased, the probability of collision and self-association of protein molecules is increased, and large insoluble aggregates are formed.

Studies by Hellsing[35,36] have provided support for the steric exclusion model and have demonstrated that (1) the *composition* of the immune complex formed is not affected by the presence of a polymer; (2) there is no complex formed between the polymer and the antigen, antibody, or immune complex; (3) the polymer effect is dependent on the molecular weight of both antigen and polymer; (4) and the use of polymer in a reaction mixture can increase the precipitation of immune complex with low-avidity antibody. Addition of polymer to a mixture of antigen and antibody causes a notable increase in the rate of immune complex growth, especially during the early phase of the reaction.[74]

Numerous polymer species have been tested (Box 9-1) for applications in immunochemical methods. The most desirable characteristics of the polymer are high molecular weight, a high degree of linearity (minimal branching), and high aqueous solubility. Most investigators have found PEG 6000 in concentrations of 3 to 5 g/dL to be most useful.

TYPES OF REACTIONS

Types of antigen antibody reactions that are of analytical importance are the precipitin reaction and those at a solid-liquid interface.

The Precipitin Reaction

If the number of antibody-combining sites is notably greater than the antigen-binding sites, ([Ab] >>> [Ag]), then antigen-binding sites are quickly saturated by antibodies before cross-linking can occur, and the formation of small antigen antibody complexes of the composition AgAb results (Figure 9-2, *A*). When an antibody is in moderate excess (i.e., [Ab] greater than [Ag]), the probability of cross-linking of Ag by Ab is more likely and hence large complex formation is favored (see Figure 9-2, *B*). When [Ag] is in great excess, large complexes would be less probable, and the theoretical minimum size of complexes would be Ag_2Ab (see Figure 9-2, *C*). This model describes the results observed when antigens and antibodies are mixed in various concentration ratios. The curve shown in Figure 9-3 is a schematic diagram of the classical precipitin curve. Although the concentration of total antibody is constant, the concentration of free antibody $[Ab]_f$ (i.e., not bound to antigen) and free antigen $[Ag]_f$ varies throughout the range for any given Ag/Ab ratio. A low Ag/Ab ratio exists in *A* of Figure 9-3 (zone of antibody excess). Under these conditions, $[Ab]_f$ exists in solution but $[Ag]_f$ does not. As total antigen increases, the size of the immune complexes increases up to equivalence (see *B*, Figure 9-3) where little or no $[Ab]_f$ or $[Ag]_f$ exists. This is the zone of maximum immune complex size. This equivalence zone does not represent a ratio of exact molar equivalence of reactants but is the optimal combining ratio for cross-linking in the particular system under evaluation. As Ag/Ab increases (see *C*, Figure 9-3), the immune complex size will decrease and $[Ag]_f$ will increase (zone of antigen excess). No $[Ab]_f$ should exist in this area of the curve. However, for a given Ag/Ab ratio, the population of immune complexes formed at equilibrium will be heterogeneous with respect to size and composition.

Reactions at a Solid-Liquid Interface

If the antigen or antibody of interest is bound to a solid phase, such as a cell membrane, or to a synthetic particle (polystyrene or cellulose), the protein will exist in a microenvironment that is different from that of a protein in free solution. The water surrounding the protein is more highly ordered near the surface of the solid phase, and a condition results that is more favorable for van der Waals-London dipole-dipole interaction and coulombic bonding. This situation favors the formation of low- and high-avidity antigen antibody complexes and, hence, can provide lower detection limits for analytical applications. Some studies

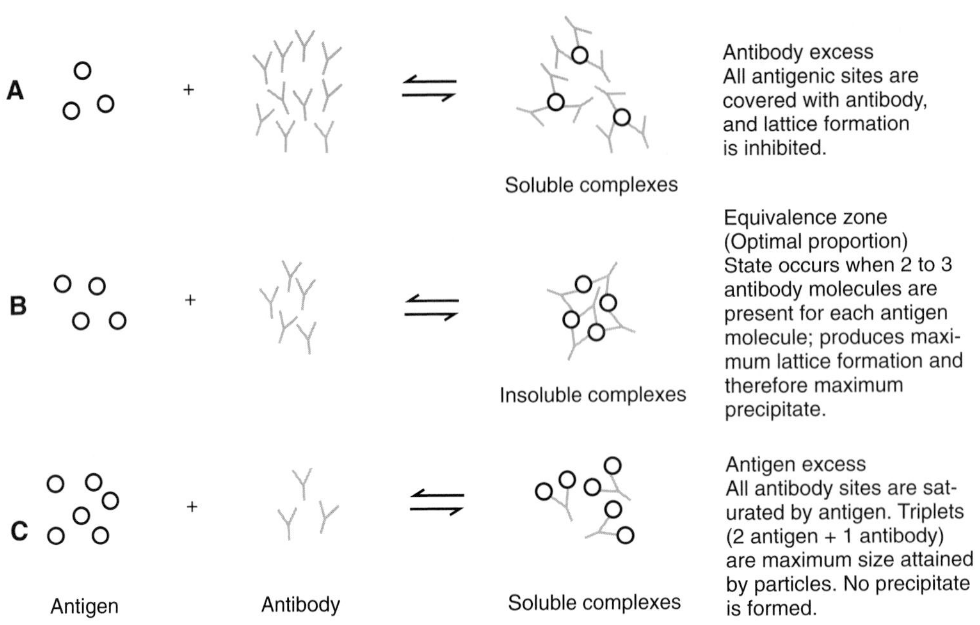

A
Antibody excess
All antigenic sites are covered with antibody, and lattice formation is inhibited.
Soluble complexes

B
Equivalence zone
(Optimal proportion)
State occurs when 2 to 3 antibody molecules are present for each antigen molecule; produces maximum lattice formation and therefore maximum precipitate.
Insoluble complexes

C
Antigen excess
All antibody sites are saturated by antigen. Triplets (2 antigen + 1 antibody) are maximum size attained by particles. No precipitate is formed.
Antigen
Antibody
Soluble complexes

Figure 9-2 Schematic diagram for precipitin reaction.

have shown radiometric solid phase assays to be more sensitive than their counterpart solution assays. In one study using the same antibody pool of antihuman α_1-antitrypsin, the lower limit of detection for the solution method was 20 to 30 ng/mL; for the solid phase method, it was 5 to 10 ng/mL. The difference in the lower limit of detection is most likely a result of additional low-avidity antibody binding during the initial incubation in the solid phase system that does not occur as readily in the liquid phase.

Because of the exquisite specificity and the high affinity of antibodies for specific antigens, thousands of immunoassays have been developed to detect and measure a wide variety of biological analytes. In the next two sections, both qualitative and quantitative immunotechniques are discussed.

QUALITATIVE METHODS

Various types of immunotechniques have been used for qualitative purposes and include passive gel diffusion, immunoelectrophoresis (IEP), and Western and dot blotting.

Passive Gel Diffusion

Many qualitative and quantitative immunochemical methods are performed in a semisolid medium, such as agar or agarose. The primary advantage in using a gelatinous medium is to stabilize the diffusion process with regard to mixing caused by vibration or convection and to allow visualization of precipitin bands for qualitative and quantitative evaluation of the reaction. Antigen antibody ratio, salt concentration, and polymer enhancement have the same influence on the antigen antibody reaction in gels as they have on reactions in solution.

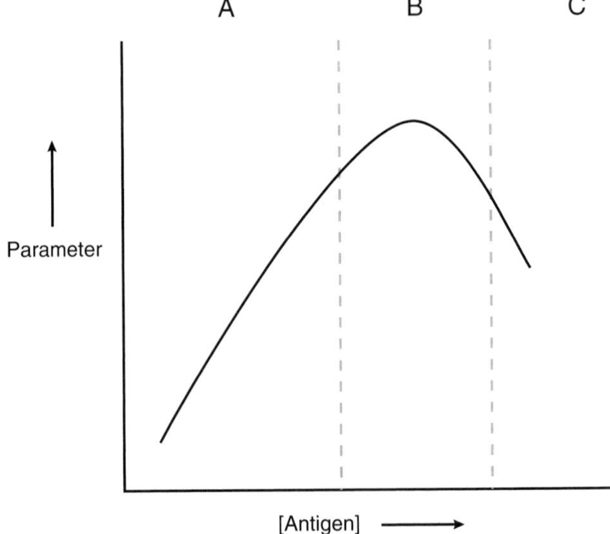

Figure 9-3 Schematic diagram of precipitin curve illustrating zones of antibody excess **(A)**, equivalence **(B)**, and antigen excess **(C)**. The parameter measured may be quantity of protein precipitated, light scattering, or another measurable parameter. Antibody concentration is held constant in this example.

BOX 9-1 Linear Polymers Used to Enhance Antigen Antibody Reaction

Polyethylene glycol (Carbowax)
Polypropylene glycol
Dextran
Polyvinyl alcohol
Modified cellulose
Polyvinyl pyrrolidone

If the matrix does not interact with the molecular species under investigation, passive diffusion of reactants in a semisolid matrix can be described by Fick's equation:

$$\frac{dQ}{dt} = -DA\frac{dC}{dx} \qquad (3)$$

where dQ is the amount of diffusing substance that at time t passes through the area A; dC/dx is the concentration gradient; and D is the diffusion coefficient. The diffusion coefficient, D, is a directly proportional function of temperature; it is also a function inversely proportional to hydrated molecular volume of the diffusing species. The amount of diffusing species transferred from the origin to a distant point (over the migration distance) is dependent on the length of time diffusion is allowed to occur.

The initial concentration of antigen and antibody is critical. Each molecule in the system will achieve a unique concentration gradient with time. When the leading fronts of antigen and antibody diffusion overlap, the reaction will begin, but formation of a precipitin line will not occur until moderate antibody excess is achieved. A precipitin band may form and be dissolved many times by incoming antigen before equilibrium is established, and the position of the precipitin band becomes stable. Because heavier molecules diffuse more slowly, the position of the precipitin band is in part a function of the molecular masses of both antigen and antibody. The precipitin band acts as a specific barrier; neither specific antigen nor antibody can penetrate without being precipitated by the other, but unrelated molecules can cross the band of precipitation freely. However, if both antigen and antibody concentrations are too high, the excessive precipitate formed in the gel can physically block further diffusion of other molecules, including the antigen and antibody of interest, and cause anomalous results.

Basic approaches to passive diffusion include simple diffusion and double diffusion. With simple diffusion, a concentration gradient is established for only a single reactant. *Single immunodiffusion* usually depends on diffusion of an antigen into agar impregnated with antibody. A quantitative technique based on this principle is radial immunodiffusion (RID), which is discussed later. The second approach is double diffusion, in which a concentration gradient is established for both reactants (antigen and antibody).

Double immunodiffusion in two dimensions is a widely used immunotechnique and is known as the Ouchterlony method. It allows direct comparison of two or more test materials and provides a simple and direct method for determining whether the antigens in the test specimens are identical, cross reactive, or nonidentical.

The simplest method uses a standard Petri dish filled with agar in saline (2 to 4 g/dL) to a depth of about 3 mm. Holes are cut in the agar plate with a punch or a sharp cork borer. The plugs of agar are removed by suction, and the bottom of each well is sealed with a drop of agar in saline (1 g/dL) to prevent diffusion under the agar. When the same antigen is in both wells, the lines of precipitation fuse and are continuous—the reaction of identity (Figure 9-4, *A*). When the precipitin bands cross each other, it is a reaction of nonidentity (see Figure 9-4, *B*); if the two antigens are related but not identical, a reaction of partial identity is observed (see Figure 9-4, *C*). Here the cardinal point is that the precipitate serves as a barrier that does not block unrelated diffusing reactants. As shown in Figure 9-4, *D*, when two related antigens, Ag and Ag_1, are in separate wells and the respective antibodies, Ab and Ab_1, are in the third well, an AgAb precipitate forms on one side and blocks further diffusion of Ab from the antibody well. However, on the other side, the Ag_1Ab_1 precipitate does not stop Ab from migrating further and forming an AgAb spur.

Double diffusion can easily be done on a microscale using small glass slides. Only a small sample (1 μL) is required, and the reaction time is markedly decreased from as long as 1 week to 24 hours or less in some cases. Sharp lines are produced because the agar layer is thin, and the area from which the reactants diffuse is minute. Finally the slides can be stained or photographed unstained with an oblique light source illuminating the precipitant bands.

Note that a negative reaction does not necessarily imply absence of antibody or antigen. A negative reaction can result from using amounts of material too small for the detection limit of the method, or the antibody may be nonprecipitating.

Immunoelectrophoresis (IEP)

If several antigens of interest exist in a common solution (e.g., spinal fluid or serum), the various protein species can be separated and identified by IEP. This technique has been used extensively for the study of antigen mixtures, the evaluation of the specificity of antiserum, and the evaluation of human gammopathies.[44]

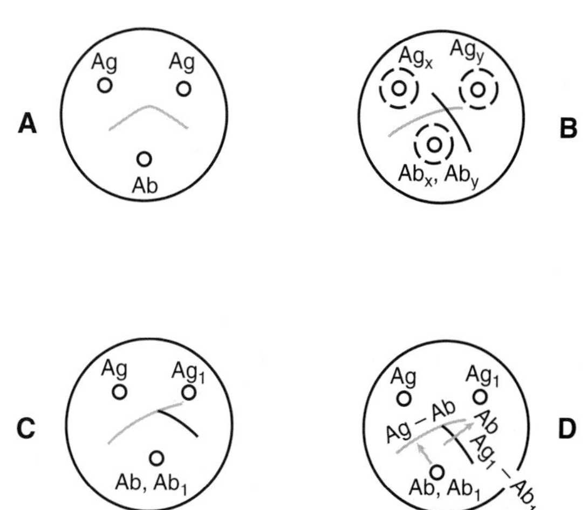

Figure 9-4 Double immunodiffusion in two dimensions by the Ouchterlony technique. **A,** Reaction of identity; **B,** reaction of nonidentity; **C,** reaction of partial identity; **D,** scheme for spur formation. *Ag,* Antigen; *Ab,* antibody.

The procedure is performed using an agarose gel medium poured onto a thin plastic sheet. The sample to be analyzed is placed in a reservoir in the gel, and an electrical field is applied across the gel surface. During electrophoresis, the proteins in the serum are separated according to their electrophoretic mobilities (Figure 9-5). Following electrophoresis, an antiserum against the protein of interest is placed in a trough parallel and adjacent to the electrophoresed sample. Simultaneous diffusion of the antigen from the separated sample and antibody from the trough results in formation of precipitin arcs, whose shape and position are characteristic of the individual separated proteins in the specimen. The pattern is interpreted after overnight development of the precipitate. By comparison with a known control separated on the same plate, tentative identification of individual proteins can be made. In some cases the characteristics of the precipitin arc, such as bowing, brushing at the end of the arc, or thickening, may suggest to the experienced observer the presence of special types of proteins.

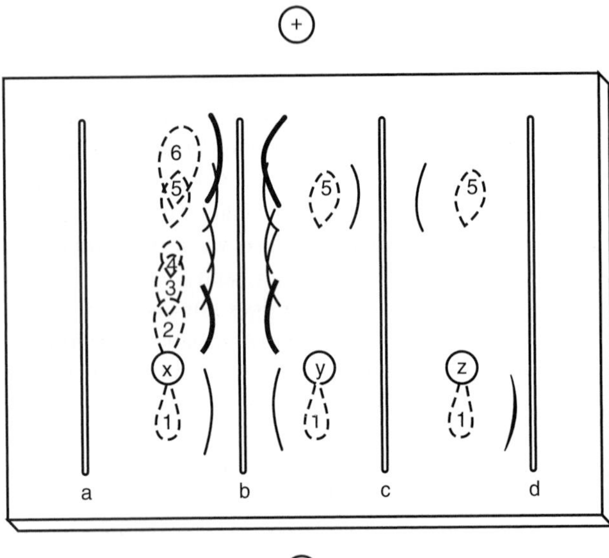

Figure 9-5 Configuration for immunoelectrophoresis. Sample wells are punched in the agar and/or agarose, sample is applied, and electrophoresis is carried out to separate the proteins in the sample. Antiserum is loaded into the troughs and the gel incubated in a moist chamber at 4 °C for 24 to 72 hours. Track *x* represents the shape of the protein zones after electrophoresis; tracks *y* and *z* show the reaction of proteins 5 and 1 with their specific antisera in troughs *C* and *D*. Antiserum against protein 1-6 is present in trough *B*.

In clinical laboratory medicine, this procedure has been applied to the evaluation of human myeloma proteins. However, the method is being replaced by immunofixation (IF) electrophoresis, particularly for the study of protein antigens and their split products, and for evaluation of human myeloma proteins (see later discussion of IF electrophoresis).

Crossed Immunoelectrophoresis (CRIE)

This technique, also known as two-dimensional IEP, is a variation of IEP wherein electrophoresis is also used in the second dimension to drive the antigen into a gel containing antibodies specific for the antigens of interest (Figure 9-6).[19,51] This technique is more sensitive and produces higher resolution than is possible with IEP. As with IEP, the specimen is applied to a cylindrical well cut in an agar medium and is then subjected to electrophoresis in the first dimension, followed by electrophoresis at a 90° angle to the first run through the gel that contains antibodies. Precipitin bands form at the zones of equivalence for each antigen. Precipitation occurs along lateral margins as the antigen advances and results in precipitation "peaks" for each antigen. An example of the application of CRIE is shown in Figure 9-7. A serum specimen treated with two different quantities of trypsin was evaluated for changes in α_1-antitrypsin. Formation of trypsin-antitrypsin complexes results in a second smaller peak cathodal to the native species. The resolution of the peaks in the second dimension may be improved by the use of a linear application of the sample into a rectangular slot instead of a well in the agar. Such application causes the proteins to move from the origin

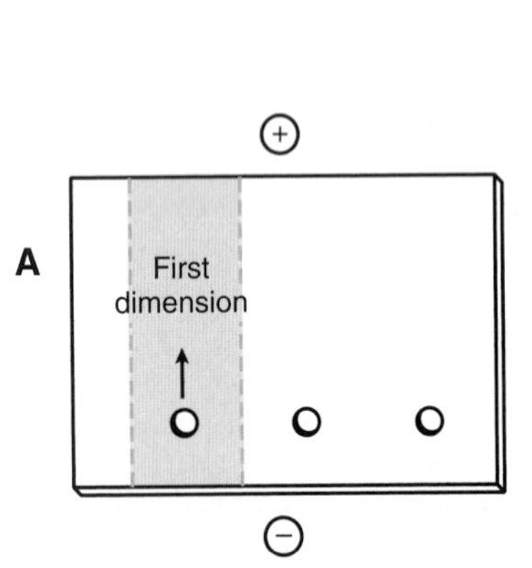

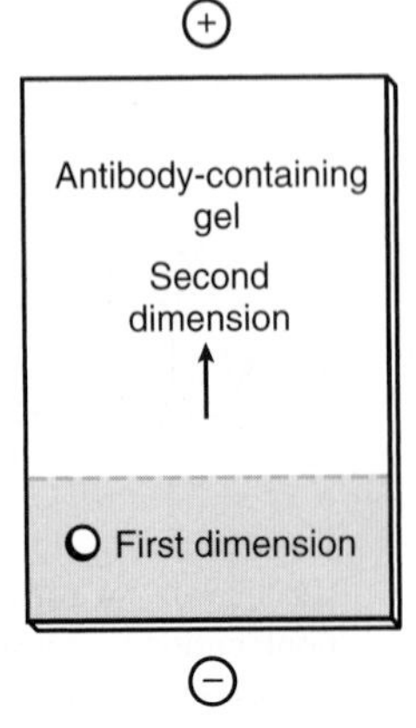

Figure 9-6 Two-dimensional (CRIE) electrophoresis. Diagram **(A)** shows the configuration for the first dimension of CRIE. The segment of the gel denoted by the *dashed lines* in diagram **(A)** is cut out and placed on a second plate. An upper gel containing antibody is added as shown in diagram **(B)**. Electrophoresis is now carried out at 90° relative to the first dimension run.

in relatively narrow bands and not in teardrop-shaped zones. Quantities of individual antigens can be estimated by measuring the peak area of the antigen under the precipitin arc and comparing it with the peak area of a standard antigen preparation.

Counterimmunoelectrophoresis (CIE)

With CIE, two parallel lines of wells are punched in the agar. One row is filled with antigen solution, and the opposing row is filled with antibody solution (Figure 9-8). If the solutions were allowed to passively diffuse over the next 18 to 24 hours, a precipitin line would form between the opposing wells where the antigen reacted with a specific antibody. With CIE, this process is made to occur more rapidly by applying a voltage across the gel so that the antigen and antibody move toward each other at a faster rate. The antigen migrates toward the anode; the antibody moves in the opposite direction as a result of electrophoresis, and a precipitin line is formed where they meet. Qualitative information (i.e., identification of antigen) is provided within 1 to 2 hours. This method has found application in the detection of bacterial antigens in blood, urine, and cerebrospinal fluid.

Immunofixation (IF)

This technique has gained widespread acceptance as an immunochemical method for identifying proteins.[3] As in IEP and CRIE, a first-dimension electrophoresis is performed in agarose gel to separate the proteins in the mixture. Subsequently, antiserum spread directly on the gel causes the protein(s) of interest to precipitate. The immune precipitate is trapped within the gel matrix, and all other nonprecipitated proteins can be removed by washing the gel. The gel may then be stained for identification of the proteins. CRIE is more sensitive than IF in terms of detection limit and also shows better resolution. For instance proteins of closely related or identical electrophoretic mobility can be distinguished better by CRIE, because in IF they will appear as a single band. In practice, IF is technically more efficient than either IEP or CRIE, and it produces patterns that are more easily interpreted. The utility of IF, which is now widely used for the evaluation of myeloma proteins, is illustrated in Figure 9-9.

Western Blotting

The techniques discussed above use a direct evaluation of the immunoprecipitation of the protein(s) in the gel. However, certain media, such as polyacrylamide, do not lend themselves to direct immunoprecipitation, nor is there always sufficient antigen concentration to produce an immunoprecipitate that will be retained in the gel during subsequent processing. Under these circumstances, a technique termed *Western blotting* can be used.[11,26] This technique involves an electrophoresis step followed by transfer of the separated proteins onto an overlying strip of nitrocellulose or a nylon membrane by a process called "electroblotting." Once the proteins are fixed to the membrane they can be detected

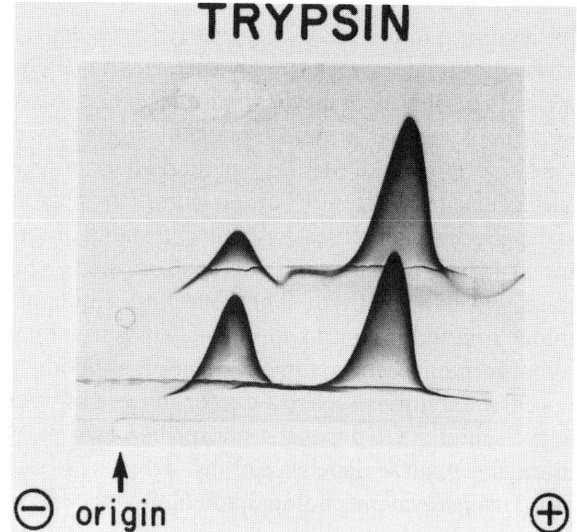

Figure 9-7 A CRIE pattern obtained with two different concentrations of trypsin added to normal serum. The first dimension was carried out from left to right and the second dimension from bottom to top. Two separate gels are shown, with the highest trypsin concentration at the bottom. Antibody against α_1-antitrypsin was present in the second dimension gel. The resulting pattern shows two distinct α_1-antitrypsin species, the free protease inhibitor *(right)* and protease-antiprotease complex *(left)*. This example illustrates the ability of CRIE to evaluate changes in specific protein structure.

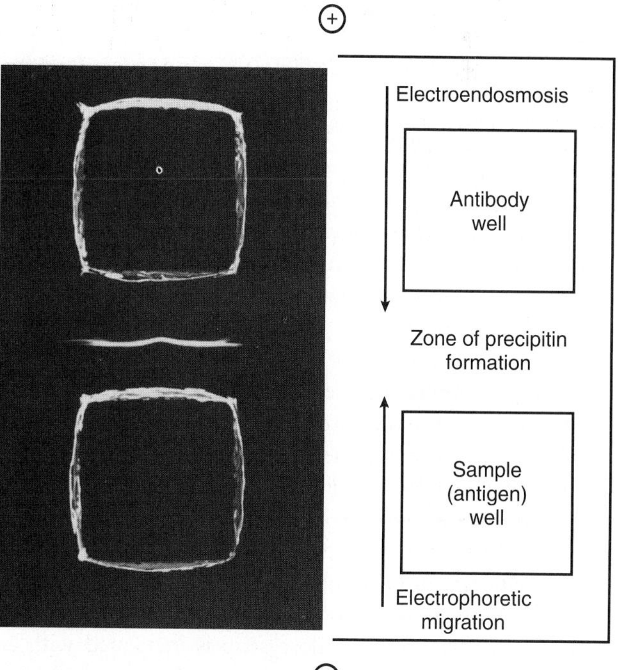

Figure 9-8 CRIE showing positive reaction between anti–*Haemophilus influenzae* B (*upper* well) and a cerebrospinal fluid (CSF) sample containing *H. influenzae* B (*lower* well).

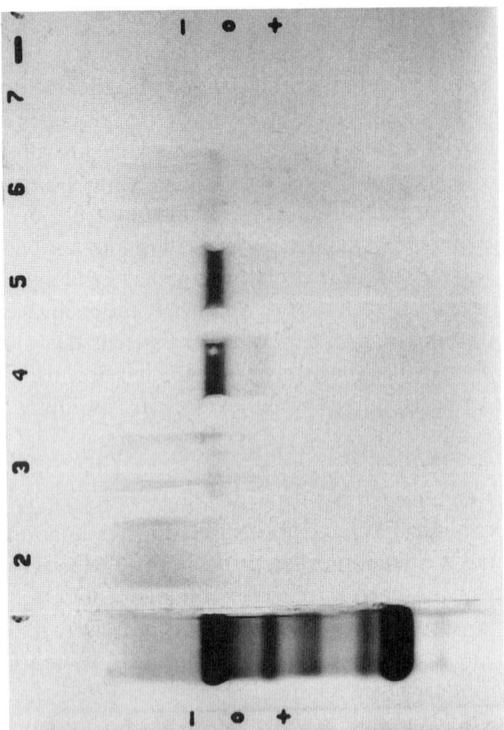

Figure 9-9 IF of a serum containing an IgM kappa paraprotein. Lane 1, serum electrophoresis stained for protein; lane 2, anti-IgG, Fc piece-specific; lane 3, anti-IgA, α-chain specific; lane 4, anti-IgM, μ-chain specific; lane 5, anti-κ light chain; lane 6, anti-λ light chain. *(Courtesy Katherine Bayer, Protein Laboratory, Hospital of the University of Pennsylvania, Philadelphia, Pa.)*

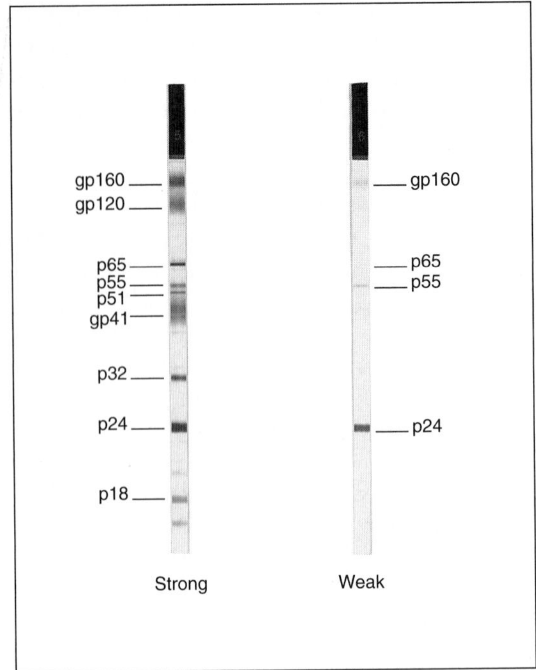

Figure 9-10 Western blot analysis of serum samples strongly positive and weakly positive for HIV-1 antibody. Core proteins (GAG, group-specific antigens) p18, p24, and p55; polymerase (POL) p32, p51, and p65; envelope proteins (ENV) gp41, gp120, and gp160. *(Courtesy Bio-Rad Laboratories Diagnostics Group, Irvine, Calif.)*

using antibodies labeled with probes, such as radioactive isotopes or enzymes. By using such probes, the limits of detection can be 10 to 100 times lower than by using direct immunoprecipitation and staining of proteins. This technique is analogous to *Southern blotting* (electrophoresed DNA blotted onto a membrane), and *Northern blotting* (electrophoresed RNA blotted onto a membrane).

An example of this technique applied to the detection of human immunodeficiency virus type 1 (HIV-1) antibodies is shown in Figure 9-10. HIV-1 antigens are separated according to molecular weight by gel electrophoresis and then transferred to a nitrocellulose membrane by electroblotting. A serum sample is then incubated with a strip of the membrane. HIV-1 antibodies in the sample bind to the viral antigens transferred to the strip as discrete bands. After washing, the strip is incubated with an alkaline phosphatase antihuman immunoglobulin conjugate, which forms a complex with bound HIV-1 antibody. After a further washing step, the nitrocellulose strip is incubated with an alkaline phosphatase substrate solution (5-bromo-4-chloro-3-indolyl phosphate and nitroblue tetrazolium) to reveal bound conjugate as purple bands (where HIV-1 antibody is bound to specific viral antigen fixed in the membrane).

Protein transfer and immobilization following separation by electrophoresis, isoelectric focusing, sodium dodecyl sulfate polyacrylamide electrophoresis (see Chapter 5 for further discussion on these techniques), or other methods provide a powerful tool for the analytical study of proteins present in low concentrations in cell culture or body fluids. When applied to antigen assays, concentrations of antigen as low as 500 ng/mL or 2.5 ng per band in the gel can be detected by this method. The detection limit of the technique can be lowered to approximately 100 pg by using chemiluminescent assays for the labeled antibody (e.g., enhanced chemiluminescence assay for horseradish peroxidase labels, and a 1,2-dioxetane phosphate-based assay for alkaline phosphatase labels) and by detecting the light emission using x-ray or photographic film.[10,48,82]

Dot Blotting

A similar technique that bypasses the electrophoretic separation step is known as *dot blotting*. A protein sample to be analyzed is applied to a membrane surface as a small "dot" and dried. The membrane is then exposed to a labeled antibody specific for the test antigen contained in the dotted protein mixture. After washing, bound labeled antibody is detected with a photometric or chemiluminescent detection system.

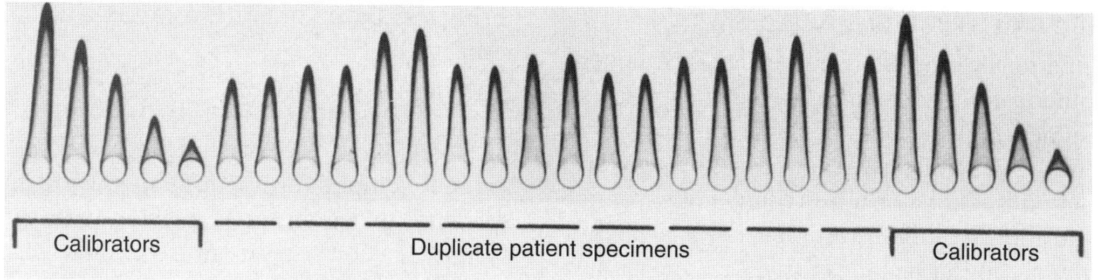

Figure 9-11 Rocket immunoelectrophoresis of human serum albumin. Patient samples were applied in duplicate. Standards were placed at opposite ends of the plate.

QUANTITATIVE METHODS

A number of immunochemical techniques have been used to quantify analytes of clinical interest. They include radial diffusion (RID) and electroimmunoassays, turbidimetric and nephelometric assays, and labeled immunochemical assays.

RADIAL IMMUNODIFFUSION AND ELECTROIMMUNOASSAY

Typically the two most commonly encountered gel-based methods for quantitative immunochemical studies are RID immunoassay and electroimmunoassay ("rocket" technique).

Radial Immunodiffusion Immunoassay

With this technique, a concentration gradient is established for a single reactant, usually the antigen. The antibody is uniformly dispersed in the gel matrix. Antigen is allowed to passively diffuse from a well into the gel until antibody excess exists and immune precipitation occurs; the antigen antibody interaction is manifested by a defined ring of precipitation around the antigen well. The ring diameter will continue to increase until equilibrium is reached. Calibrators are run at the same time as the sample, and a calibration curve of ring area or diameter versus concentration is plotted. The original procedure described by Mancini[59] requires the establishment of equilibrium before measurement of the precipitin ring diameter. Under equilibrium conditions, a linear relationship exists between antigen concentration and the square of the precipitin ring diameter. In addition, the precision of the measurement of the ring diameter is better than if the rings are measured before equilibrium is established. However, quantitative data can also be derived by reading the ring diameter before equilibrium is established.[23] This approach, although less precise, is often more practical for a clinical laboratory if available time for testing is at a premium.

Fick's equation predicts that the rate of diffusion is dependent on antigen size, molecular weight, and concentration. Whereas this is indeed the case for the *rate* of diffusion, the ultimate area of the precipitin ring at equilibrium is independent of these factors and dependent instead on the antigen antibody concentration ratio.[59] Antigen concentrations are calculated in both the preequilibrium and Mancini RID methods[23,59] by plotting the square of the precipitin ring diameter against calibrating antigen concentrations and by interpolating unknowns from this curve. RID can be made more sensitive using PEG to enhance precipitin line formation or by using ^{125}I- or enzyme-labeled reagents.[34,63,71]

Electroimmunoassay

In *electroimmunoassay,* as in RID, a single concentration gradient is established for the antigen, but in this case, an applied voltage is used to drive the antigen from the application well into a homogeneous suspension of antibody in the gel (Figure 9-11).[52] Unlike RID this produces a unidirectional migration of antigen and results in a lower limit of detection for electroimmunoassay methods. The height of the resulting rocket-shaped precipitin line is proportional to the antigen concentration. Quantitation is affected by using calibrators on the same plate along with the unknowns and then estimating the concentrations of unknowns from the heights of the "rockets" obtained. The calibration curve is linear only over a narrow concentration range, so samples may have to be diluted or concentrated as necessary. Electroimmunoassay methods produce the best results with antigens having a strong anodic mobility and intermediate to low molecular weight. Proteins, such as transferrin, C3, or IgG, with low anodal mobility or virtually no net charge at pH 8.6 (the most common pH used for the method) can be modified by carbamoylation or run at a lower pH to make their measurements by electroimmunoassay feasible. One advantage of electroimmunoassay is that more than one antigen can be measured simultaneously if appropriate conditions are chosen. The simultaneous use of more than one antiserum results in superimposed rockets that can be measured separately. Other modifications, such as the use of an intermediate gel that causes precipitation of C3, allow measurement of C3d in human serum and illustrate the exceptional versatility of this method.[9]

In many clinical laboratories, gel-based methods are restricted to qualitative studies. Quantitative data are more commonly obtained by turbidimetric and nephelometric methods, radioimmunoassays, enzyme immunoassays (EIAs), and fluorometric immunoassays.

Turbidimetric and Nephelometric Assays

Turbidimetry and nephelometry are convenient techniques for measuring the rate of formation of immune complexes in vitro. Instrumental principles for these methods are described in Chapter 3. Studies have shown that the reaction between antigen and antibody begins within milliseconds and continues for hours.[31,74] Both turbidimetric and nephelometric immunochemical methods using rate and pseudoequilibrium protocols have been described for proteins, antigens, and haptens. In rate assays, measurements are usually made within the first few minutes of the reaction, because the largest change *(dIs/dt)* in intensity of scattered light *(Is)* with respect to time is obtained during this time interval. For so-called equilibrium assays, it is necessary to wait 30 to 60 minutes so that the *dIs/dt* is small relative to the time required to make the necessary measurements. For the purpose of this discussion, such conditions are referred to as pseudoequilibrium because true equilibrium is not reached within the time allowed for these assays. Measurement of the *rate* of immune complex formation can also be used for quantitative immunochemical studies. Either *dIs/dt* or the time required to reach peak rate can be related to antigen concentration in a manner analogous to any other rate methodology. Rate nephelometric assays have the advantage that blank correction is not required, and that several samples can be assayed in a few minutes instead of the 30 to 60 minutes required for pseudoequilibrium methods.[6,14,38]

The analytical performance of nephelometric or turbidimetric assays can be significantly improved by increasing the reaction rate by addition of water-soluble linear polymers. This allows the use of much lower reactant concentrations and results in a more stable immune complex suspension.[13]

Nephelometric methods in general are more sensitive than turbidimetric assays and have an average lower limit of detection of 0.1 to 10 mg/L for a serum protein. Lower detection limits are obtained in fluids, such as cerebrospinal fluid and urine, because of their lower lipid and protein concentrations, which results in a better signal-to-noise ratio. In addition, for low molecular weight proteins (e.g., myoglobin, MW 17,800), assay detection limits can be lowered using a latex-enhanced procedure based on antibody-coated latex beads.[29]

Nephelometric and turbidimetric assays have also been applied to the measurement of drugs (haptens) using *inhibition techniques.* The reagent is made by attaching the drug of interest to a carrier molecule, such as bovine serum albumin. The hapten-bound albumin then competes with free hapten (drug introduced in sample) for the antihapten antibody. In the presence of free hapten, immune complex formation is decreased, because more antibody sites are saturated; thus light scattering is decreased. The decrease of light scattering is related to the concentration of free hapten. Both kinetic and pseudoequilibrium methods have been described.[17,25] In the absence of free hapten, bound hapten albumin reacts with available antihapten antibody sites to form cross-linked immune complexes with high light-scattering ability.

Labeled Immunochemical Assays

The previously discussed methods rely on evaluating the immune complex formation as an index of antigen antibody reaction. As demonstrated previously in equation (1), the overall reaction occurs in sequential phases, and only the final phase is the formation of the immune complex. However, the initial binding of the antibody and antigen has also been demonstrated to be very useful analytically and has been used with labeled antigens and antibodies to develop many sensitive and specific immunochemical assays. The reaction describing this initial binding and the kinetic constant for the overall reaction are shown in equations (4a) and (4b), respectively:

$$\mathrm{Ab} + \mathrm{Ag} \underset{k_{-1}}{\overset{k_1}{\rightleftharpoons}} \mathrm{AbAg} \tag{4a}$$

$$K = \frac{[\mathrm{AbAg}]}{[\mathrm{Ab}][\mathrm{Ag}]} \tag{4b}$$

where

k_1 = the rate constant for the forward reaction
k_{-1} = the rate constant for the reverse reaction
K = the equilibrium constant for the overall reaction

As would be predicted from the law of mass action, the concentration of Ab, Ag, and AbAg will be dependent on the magnitude of k_1 and k_{-1}. For polyclonal antiserum, the average avidity of the antibody populations will determine K (typically 10^8 to 10^{10} L/mol), and the magnitude of k_1 in comparison with k_{-1} will determine the ultimate limit of detection attainable with a given antibody population.

The original assays used radioactive labels, but concerns about the safe handling and disposal of radioactive reagents and waste have led to the development of alternative nonisotopic labels (Table 9-1).[47,66] In this section, the methodological principles on which these assays are based and the factors that affect their analytical sensitivity are discussed. In addition, specific examples of these assays and the types of labels that are used in them are evaluated. Commercial versions and applications of these assays are discussed in other chapters (see Chapters 3 and 11).

Methodological Principles

To exploit analytically the exquisite specificity and enhanced sensitivity that are possible with immunochemical assays, various methodological principles have been applied in their development. These include competitive and noncompetitive reaction formats and different processing schemes for performing the assays.

Competitive Versus Noncompetitive Reaction Formats

The two major types of reaction formats that are used in immunochemical assays (Figure 9-12) are termed *competi-*

TABLE 9-1 Labels Used for Nonisotopic Immunoassay

Chemiluminescent	Acridinium ester, sulfonyl acridinium ester, isoluminol
Cofactor	Adenosine triphosphate, flavin adenine dinucleotide
Enzyme	Alkaline phosphatase, marine bacterial luciferase, β-galactosidase, firefly luciferase, glucose oxidase, glucose-6-phosphate dehydrogenase, horseradish peroxidase, lysozyme, malate dehydrogenase, microperoxidase, urease, xanthine oxidase
Fluorophore	Europium chelate, fluorescein, phycoerythrin, terbium chelate
Free radical	Nitroxide
Inhibitor	Methotrexate
Metal	Gold sol, selenium sol, silver sol
Particle	Bacteriophage, erythrocyte, latex bead, liposome, quantum dot
Phosphor	Up-converting lanthanide-containing nanoparticle
Polynucleotide	DNA
Substrate	Galactosyl-umbelliferone

Competitive (limited reagent)

Simultaneous

$$\text{Ab} + \text{Ag} + \text{Ag–L} \rightleftharpoons \text{Ab:Ag} + \text{Ab:Ag–L}$$

(free) (bound)

Sequential

$$\text{Step 1 Ab} + \text{Ag} \underset{k_{-1}}{\overset{k_1}{\rightleftharpoons}} \text{Ab:Ag} + \text{Ab}$$

$$\text{Step 2 Ab:Ag} + \text{Ab} + \text{Ag–L} \rightleftharpoons \text{Ab:Ag} + \text{Ab:Ag–L} + \text{Ag–L}$$

Noncompetitive (excess reagent, two-site, sandwich)

$$\text{–Ab} \xrightarrow{+\text{Ag}} \text{– Ab:Ag} \xrightarrow{+\text{Ab–L}} \text{– Ab:Ag:Ab–L}$$

Figure 9-12 Immunoassay designs. *L*, Label.

tive (limited reagent assays) and *noncompetitive* (excess reagent, two-site, or sandwich assays).

Competitive Immunoassays. In a *competitive* immunochemical assay, all reactants are mixed together either *simultaneously* or *sequentially.* In the simultaneous approach, the labeled antigen (Ag*) and unlabeled antigen (Ag) compete for binding to the antibody. In such a system, the avidity of the antibody for both the labeled and unlabeled antigen must be the same. Under these conditions, the probability of the antibody binding the labeled antigen is inversely proportional to the concentration of unlabeled antigen; hence, bound label is inversely proportional to unlabeled antigen concentration.

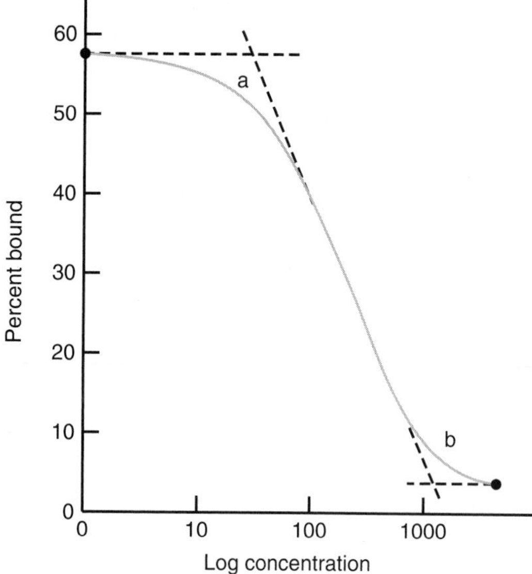

Figure 9-13 A schematic diagram of the dose-response curve for a typical immunoassay. The analytically useful portion of the curve is bracketed by points *a* and *b*.

In a *sequential* competitive assay, unlabeled antigen is first mixed with excess antibody, and binding is allowed to reach equilibrium (see Figure 9-12, step 1). Labeled antigen is then sequentially added (step 2) and allowed to equilibrate. After separation the bound label is determined and used to calculate the unlabeled antigen concentration. Using this two-step method, a larger fraction of the unlabeled antigen can be bound by the antibody than in the simultaneous assay, especially at low antigen concentrations. Consequently, this strategy can provide a twofold to fourfold improvement in the detection limit of a sequential immunoassay compared with that of a simultaneous assay, provided $k_1 >> k_{-1}$. This improvement in detection limit results from an increase in AgAb binding (and thus in a decrease in Ag* binding), which is favored by the sequential addition of Ag and Ag*. If $k_1 >> k_{-1}$, dissociation of AgAb becomes more likely, resulting in an increased competition between Ag* and Ag. A typical immunochemical binding curve is shown in Figure 9-13.

Noncompetitive Immunoassays. In a typical *noncompetitive assay* for an antigen, a capture antibody is first passively adsorbed or covalently bound to the surface of a solid phase. Various sequences in which the capture antibody can be attached are shown in Box 9-2. The simplest involves direct attachment to the solid phase. However, this can lead to some loss of antibody binding capacity because of steric factors or attachment of the antibody via its Fab region. To protect the binding properties of the antibody, more complex sequences have been devised. For example, the solid support can be coated with an antispecies antibody, and then

BOX 9-2 Immobilization Schemes for Preparation of Solid Phase* Antibodies for Use in Immunoassay

■ : AB
■ : Anti-FITC Ab : FITC-AB
■ : Anchor protein-reptavidin : biotin-AB
■ : Antispecies Ab : AB

AB, Capture antibody; *FITC*, fluorescein isothiocyanate.
*Solid phase (tube, bead, microparticle, microwell) is indicated by the *solid boxes*.

the antispecies antibody can be used to immobilize the capture antibody via an antigen antibody reaction.

In the second stage of the assay, the antigen from the sample is allowed to react with the solid phase, capture antibody; other proteins are washed away; and a labeled antibody (conjugate) is added that reacts with the bound antigen through a second and distinct epitope. After washing again, the bound label is determined, and its concentration or activity is directly proportional to the concentration of antigen.

In noncompetitive assays, the capture and labeled antibody can be either polyclonal or monoclonal. If monoclonal antibodies having specificity for distinct epitopes are used, it is possible to incubate the sample and conjugate simultaneously with the capture antibody, thus simplifying the assay protocol.

Noncompetitive immunoassays can be performed in either a simultaneous or sequential mode. However, in the simultaneous mode, a situation can occur in which a high concentration of analyte can saturate both the capture and labeled antibodies. When this occurs, the calibration curve of the assay exhibits a "hook effect" in which the assay response drops off at high analyte concentrations. Under these conditions, the analyte is present in such high concentrations that it reacts simultaneously with the capture antibody and the labeled antibody. This reduces the number of complexes formed and produces a falsely low result. Assays for analytes for which the normal pathological concentration range is very wide (e.g., hCG, AFP) are particularly prone to this problem. Dilutions of a sample are usually reanalyzed to check for this type of analytical interference. The hook effect can be eliminated by adopting a sequential assay format[66] and by ensuring that the concentrations of capture and labeled antibody are sufficiently high to cover analyte concentrations over the entire analytical range of the assay.

Heterogeneous Versus Homogeneous Immunochemical Assays

Immunochemical assays that require a separation of the free from the bound label are termed *heterogeneous*; those that do not are called *homogeneous*.

BOX 9-3 Separation Methods Used in Immunoassays

Adsorption
Charcoal, Florisil, talc

Precipitation
Polymer precipitation: polyethylene glycol
Solvent or salt precipitation: ethanol, dioxane, $(NH_4)_2SO_4$
Protein A or double (second) antibody precipitation

Solid Phase Antibodies
Antibodies or other binding proteins (e.g., protein A, biotin-avidin, and biotin-streptavidin) adsorbed or covalently attached to an insoluble matrix (e.g., plastic beads, inside surface of a plastic tube or microwell, and magnetic beads)

Miscellaneous
Electrophoresis
Gel filtration
Ion exchange
Radial partition

Heterogeneous Assays. Heterogeneous assays implicitly assume that $k_1 >> k_{-1}$ and that a variety of physical separation techniques (Box 9-3) are used to separate the free-label (Ag*) from the bound-labeled antigen (Ag*Ab). The most widely used of these techniques are precipitation and liquid phase and solid phase adsorption.

Precipitation of the bound-labeled antigen (Ag*Ab) from the reaction mixture can be achieved chemically by the addition of a protein-precipitating chemical, such as $(NH_4)_2SO_4$, or immunologically by the addition of a second, "precipitating" antibody. In the latter approach, if the primary antibody was obtained from rabbit antiserum, the precipitating antibody would be contained in a goat or sheep antiserum raised against rabbit globulin. This approach has the advantage that it can be used for practically any assay; however, it has the disadvantage that it usually requires longer assay times and additional processing steps.

In liquid phase adsorption, the free antigen is adsorbed onto particles of activated charcoal or dextran-coated charcoal that are added directly to the reaction mixture. The particles of charcoal and the adsorbed antigen are then removed by allowing them to settle or by centrifugation. The disadvantage of this separation technique is that the time of contact between the adsorbent and the incubation mixture is critical, especially for the more active adsorbents, such as activated charcoal.

Solid phase adsorption is the separation technique that is currently the most popular and widely used in both manual and automated immunoassays (see Chapter 11). In this technique, the binding and competition of the labeled and unlabeled antigens for the binding sites of the antibody occur on the surface of a solid support onto which the capture anti-

TABLE 9-2 Detection Limits for Isotopic and Nonisotopic Immunoassay Labels

Label	Detection Limit in Zeptomoles* (10^{-21} moles)	Method
Alkaline phosphatase	50,000	Photometry
	300	Time-resolved fluorescence
	100	Fluorescence
	10	Enzyme cascade
	1	Chemiluminescence
β-D-galactosidase	5000	Chemiluminescence
	1000	Fluorescence
Europium chelate	10,000	Time-resolved fluorescence
Glucose-6-phosphate dehydrogenase	1000	Chemiluminescence
^{3}H	1,000,000	Scintillation
Horseradish peroxidase	2,000,000	Photometry
	1	Chemiluminescence
^{125}I	1000	Scintillation
Ruthenium (II) tris(bipyridyl)	20†	Electrochemiluminescence

*One zeptomole = 10^{-3} attomoles or 10^{-6} femtomoles.
†Personal communication.

body has been attached by either physical adsorption or covalent bonding. Several different types of solid support have been used, including the inner surface of plastic tubes or wells of microtiter plates and the outer surface of insoluble materials, such as cellulose or magnetic latex beads or particles. With the tubes and microtiter plates, the solid surface containing the attached antibody and bound antigen is washed "in place," and indicator reagents are subsequently added to complete the assay. When beads or particles are used, they are added directly to the reaction mixture and after incubation are removed by centrifugation or magnetic separation. After the supernatant is removed by siphoning or decanting, the beads or particles are washed and indicator reagents subsequently added to complete the assay.

Homogeneous Assays. The development of homogeneous assays that do not require a separation of the bound- and free-labeled antibody or antigen was a major advance in the field of immunochemical analysis. In this type of assay, the activity of the label attached to the antigen is directly modulated by antibody binding, with the magnitude of the modulation being proportional to the concentration of the antigen or antibody being measured. Consequently, in practice it is only necessary to incubate the sample containing the analyte antigen with the labeled antigen and antibody and then directly measure the activity of the label "in place," thus making these assays technically easier and faster. The original homogeneous immunoassay was developed for drug analysis and used a nitroxide spin label and was termed a free radical immunoassay technique.[56] The electron spin resonance spectrum of this label was modulated when the nitroxide-labeled drug was bound by a drug-specific antibody. This procedure was quickly superseded by homogeneous immunoassays that used enzyme labels and could be performed on spectrophotometric analyzers (see subsequent descriptions of enzyme multiplied immunoassay technique (EMIT) and cloned enzyme donor immunoassay [CEDIA]).[37,72]

Analytical Detection Limits

The analytical detection limits of competitive and noncompetitive immunoassays are determined principally by the affinity of the antibody and the detection limit of the label used, respectively.[21,40,41,69] Calculations have indicated that a lower limit of detection of 10 fmol/L (i.e., 600,000 molecules of analyte in a typical sample volume of 100 μL) is possible in a competitive assay using an antibody with an affinity of 10^{12} L/mol.* Table 9-2 illustrates the detection limits for isotopic and nonisotopic labels. A radioactive label, such as ^{125}I, has low specific activity (7.5 million labels necessary for detection of 1 disintegration/s) compared with enzyme labels and chemiluminescent and fluorescent labels. Enzyme labels provide an amplification (each enzyme label produces many detectable product molecules), and the detection limit for an enzyme can be improved by replacing the conventional photometric detection reaction by a chemiluminescent or bioluminescent reaction. The combination of amplification and an ultrasensitive detection reaction makes noncompetitive chemiluminescent EIAs among the most sensitive types of immunoassay. Fluorescent labels also have

*In 1989, Spencer introduced the term "functional sensitivity" and defined it as the lowest concentration of an analyte for which clinically useful results can be reported (Spencer CA. Thyroid profiling for the 1990s: free T4 estimate or sensitive TSH measurement. J Clin Immunoassay 1989; 12:82-9.) This term has become widely adopted and used as one of the measures of the analytical performance of an immunoassay.

high specific activity, and a single high-quantum yield fluorophor can produce 100 million photon/s. In practice, several factors degrade the detection limit of an immunoassay; these include background signal from the detector, assay reagents, and nonspecific binding of the labeled reagent.

Secondary labels, such as biotin, can also be used to introduce amplification into an immunoassay. The binding constant of the biotin-avidin complex is extremely high (10^{15} L/mol); capitalizing on this system allows immunoassay systems to be devised that are even more sensitive than the simple antibody systems. A biotin-avidin system uses a biotin-labeled first antibody. Biotin can be attached to the antibody in relatively high proportion without loss of immunoreactivity by the antibody.[5,32] When an avidin-conjugated label is added, a complex of Ag:Ab-biotin:avidin label is formed. Further amplification can be achieved by a biotin:avidin:biotin linkage, because the binding ratio of biotin:avidin is 4:1. If the label is an enzyme, then large numbers of enzyme molecules in the complete complex provide a large increase of enzymatic activity coupled with the small amount of antigen being determined, and the antigen assay is correspondingly more sensitive. Other strategies to lower the analytical detection limits of immunoassays include the use of streptavidin-thyroglobulin conjugates and macromolecular complexes of multiple-labeled thyroglobulin and streptavidin-thyroglobulin.[19] In these reagents, the thyroglobulin acts as a carrier for multiple labels (e.g., Eu^{3+}), and amplification factors of several thousand are achieved.

Examples of Labeled Immunoassays

In the decade following the pioneering developments of Yalow and Berson,[94] all immunoassays used a radioactive label in a competitive assay format. Since the introduction of enzyme immunochemical assays in the 1970s,[56,72] a vast array of sophisticated immunochemical assays have evolved and have been very widely applied. Specific examples of several of these assays follow; others are briefly described in Box 9-4.

Radioimmunoassay

Radioimmunoassays (RIAs) were developed in the 1960s and used radioactive isotopes of iodine (^{125}I, ^{131}I) and tritium (^{3}H) as labels.[20,94] Radiolabeling of antigen with an isotope can cause changes in reactivity with the antibody. Therefore labeled and unlabeled antigens always need to be evaluated when a competitive assay is used to ensure that the antibody reacts equally with each form. Labeled antibody assays (immunoradiometric assay) have the advantage of not requiring a quantity of purified antigen because the antigen does not have to be labeled. This also obviates potential problems that may be caused by iodination of labile antigens. Antibodies are more stable proteins and are less difficult to label without damaging the protein's function. Combinations of labels (e.g., ^{57}Co and ^{125}I) have been used for simultaneous assays of vitamin B_{12} and folate,[90] lutropin and follitropin, and thyrotropin and free thyroxine. Nonseparation RIAs have also been developed based on the modulation of a tritium label by particles loaded with scintillation molecules and on the modulation of a ^{125}I label by a tungsten particle[81] and have found application in drug discovery assays.

Enzyme Immunoassay

Enzyme immunoassays use the catalytic properties of enzymes to detect and quantify immunological reactions. In practice, enzyme-labeled antibodies or antigens (i.e., conjugates) are first allowed to react with ligands, and enzyme substrates are subsequently added. Measurement of the resultant decrease in substrate concentration or increase in product concentration is then used either to detect or quantitate the antigen antibody reaction. Alkaline phosphatase, horseradish peroxidase, glucose-6-phosphate dehydrogenase, and β-galactosidase enzyme labels predominate in EIA.[27,28] Enzyme-labeled antibody and antigen conjugates are prepared by covalent coupling procedures using bifunctional reagents (e.g., glutaraldehyde, N-succinimidyl 3-[pyridyl] propionate),[4] and recombinant conjugates have been prepared from fused genes and used in research EIAs (e.g., proinsulin-alkaline phosphatase).[58]

Various detection systems have been used to monitor and quantify EIAs. Assays that produce compounds that can be monitored photometrically are very popular, because compact, high-performance photometers are now available that are versatile, reliable, simple to operate, and relatively inexpensive. However, EIAs that use fluorescent- or chemiluminescent-labeled substrates or products are often preferred to photometry-based assays owing to the inherent sensitivity of fluorescent and chemiluminescent measurements (see Chapter 3 and Table 9-2). Immunoassays that incorporate horseradish peroxidase as a label can be assayed by a chemiluminescence using a mixture of luminol, peroxide, and an enhancer such as *p*-iodophenol[82] or by using an acridan derivative.[2] Umbelliferone phosphate is a nonfluorescent substrate that is converted to the highly fluorescent umbelliferone by alkaline phosphatase. This reaction is used to quantify the alkaline phosphatase label.[24] A very sensitive assay for alkaline phosphatase labels uses a chemiluminescent adamantyl 1,2-dioxetane aryl phosphate substrate.[10] The enzyme dephosphorylates the substrate, which decomposes with a concomitant long-lived glow of light (detection limit for alkaline phosphatase using this assay is 1 zeptomole [10^{-21} moles]). Enzyme cascade reactions have also been applied to the detection of enzyme labels in EIA; the principle of a cascade assay for alkaline phosphatase is illustrated in Figure 9-14. The advantage of such an assay is that it combines the amplification properties of two enzymes—the alkaline phosphatase label and the alcohol dehydrogenase in the assay reagent—thus producing a very sensitive assay (see Table 9-2).

BOX 9-4 Examples of Other Nonisotopic Immunoassays*

Bioluminescent Immunoassays[68]

Native or recombinant apoaequorin (from the bioluminescent jellyfish *Aequorea*) is used as the label. It is activated by reaction with coelenterazine, and light emission at 469 nm is triggered by reaction with calcium ions (calcium chloride).

Fluorescence Excitation Transfer Immunoassay[84]

Homogeneous competitive assay in which a fluorophore (donor)-labeled antigen competes with an antigen in the sample for binding sites on an antibody labeled with a fluorescent dye (acceptor). The fluorescence of the donor is quenched when it is bound to the acceptor-labeled antibody.

Immuno-PCR[73]

Heterogeneous immunoassay in which a piece of single- or double-stranded DNA is used as a label for an antibody in a sandwich assay. Bound DNA label is amplified using the polymerase chain reaction (PCR). The amplified DNA product is separated by gel electrophoresis and quantitated by densitometric scanning of an ethidium stained gel.

Luminescent Oxygen Channeling Immunoassay (LOCI)[83]

Homogeneous sandwich immunoassay in which an antigen links an antibody-coated sensitizer dye-loaded particle (250-nm diameter) and an antibody-coated particle (250-nm diameter) loaded with a mixture of a precursor of a chemiluminescent compound and a fluorophore. Irradiation produces singlet oxygen at the surface of the sensitizer dye-loaded particle. This diffuses ("channels") to the other particle held in close proximity by the immunochemical reaction between the antigen and antibodies on the particles. The singlet oxygen reacts with the chemiluminescent compound precursor in the particle to form a chemiluminescent dioxane, which then decomposes to emit light via a fluorophore-sensitized mechanism. No signal is obtained from precursor fluorophore-loaded particles that are not linked via immunological reaction with an antigen.

Phosphor immunoassay[62,95]

Heterogeneous immunoassay in which an upconverting phosphor nanoparticle is used as a label. The nanoparticle (200- to 400-nm diameter) is a crystalline lanthanide oxysulfide. It absorbs two or more photons of infrared light (980 nm) and produces light emission at a shorter wavelength (antiStokes shift). The phosphorescence is not influenced by reaction conditions (e.g., temperature or buffer) and there is no up-converted signal from biological components in the sample (low background). Multiplexing is possible because different types of particle produce different wavelengths of phosphorescence (e.g., yttrium/erbium oxysulfides are green [550 nm] and yttrium/thulium oxysulfide particles are blue [475 nm]).

Quantum Dot Immunoassay[16,33,70]

Heterogeneous immunoassay in which a nanometer-sized (less than 10 nm) semiconductor quantum dot is used as a label. A quantum dot is a highly fluorescent nanocrystal composed of CdSe, CdS, ZnSe, InP, or InAs or a layer of ZnS or CdS on, for example, a CdSe core. Multiplexing is possible with these labels because the emission properties can be modulated by changing the size and composition of the nanocrystal (e.g., CdS emits blue light, InP emits red light).

Solid Phase, Light-Scattering Immunoassay[67]

Indium spheres are coated on glass to measure an antibody binding to an antigen. Binding of antibodies to antigens increases dielectric layer thickness, which produces a greater degree of scatter than in areas where only an antigen is bound. Quantitation is achieved by densitometry.

Surface Effect Immunoassay[77]

An antibody is immobilized on the surface of a waveguide (a quartz, glass, or plastic slide, or a gold- or silver-coated prism), and binding of an antigen is measured directly by total internal reflection fluorescence, surface plasmon resonance, or attenuated total reflection.

*Superscript numbers refer to the references found at the end of this chapter.

Types of enzyme-linked immunoassay include *enzyme-linked immunosorbent assay (ELISA), enzyme multiplied immunoassay technique (EMIT),* and *CEDIA.*

Enzyme-Linked Immunosorbent Assay. ELISA is a heterogeneous EIA technique that is widely used in clinical analyses.[22,86] In this type of assay, one of the reaction components is nonspecifically adsorbed or covalently bound to the surface of a solid phase, such as that of a microtiter well, a magnetic particle, or a plastic bead. This attachment facilitates separation of bound- and free-labeled reactants. In the most common approach to using the ELISA technique, an aliquot of sample or calibrator containing the antigen to be quantitated is added to and allowed to bind with a solid phase antibody. After washing, enzyme-labeled antibody is added and forms a "sandwich complex" of solid phase Ab-Ag-Ab-enzyme. Excess (unbound) antibody is then washed away, and enzyme substrate is added; the enzyme catalytically converts the substrate to product(s), the amount of which is proportional to the quantity of antigen in the sample. Antibodies in a sample can also be quantitated using an ELISA procedure in which antigen instead of antibody is bound to a solid phase, and the second reagent is an enzyme-labeled antibody specific for the analyte antibody. The procedure is otherwise identical to that described earlier for the measurement of antigens. For example, in a microtiter plate format, ELISA assays have been used extensively for detection of antibodies to viruses and parasites in serum or whole blood.[87] In addition, enzyme conjugates coupled

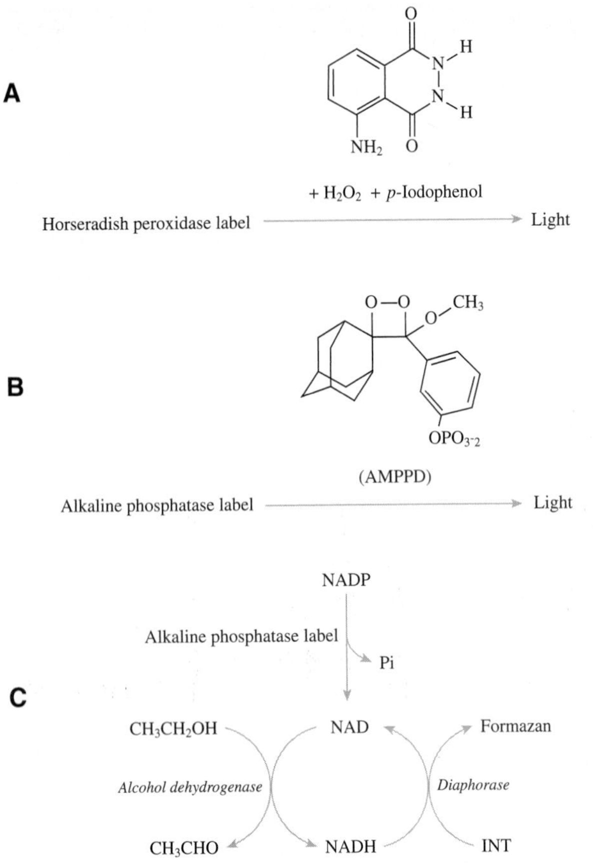

A

NH_2

$+ H_2O_2 + p$-Iodophenol

Horseradish peroxidase label → Light

B

CH_3

OPO_3^{-2}

(AMPPD)

Alkaline phosphatase label → Light

C

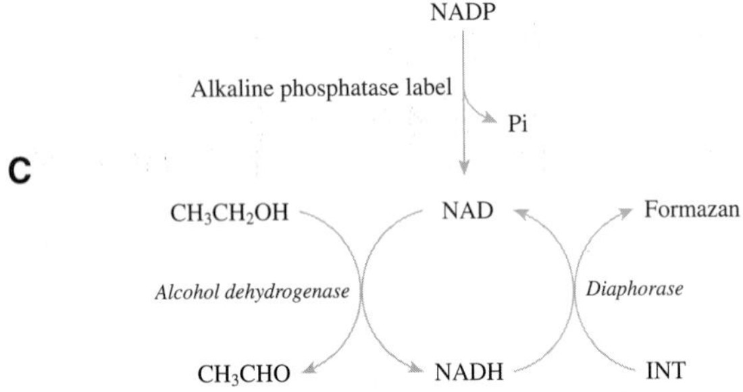

Figure 9-14 Ultrasensitive assays for horseradish peroxidase and alkaline phosphatase labels. **A,** Chemiluminescent assay for horseradish peroxidase label using luminol. **B,** Chemiluminescent assay for an alkaline phosphatase label using AMPPD. **C,** Photometric assay for an alkaline phosphatase label using a cascade detection reaction. *INT, p*-iodonitrotetrazolium violet.

with substrates that produce visible products have been used to develop ELISA type of assays with results that can be interpreted visually. Such assays have been found to be very useful in screening, point-of-care, and home testing applications.

Enzyme Multiplied Immunoassay Technique. EMIT is a homogeneous EIA that is also very widely used in clinical analyses, an illustration of which is shown in Figure 9-15. Because EMIT does not require a separation step, it is simple to perform and has been used to develop a wide variety of drug, hormone, and metabolite assays.[72] Because of their operational simplicity, EMIT type assays are easily automated and are included in the repertoire of many automated clinical and immunoassay analyzers (see Chapter 11). In this technique, antibody against the analyte drug, hormone, or metabolite is added together with substrate to the patient's sample. Binding of the antibody and analyte occurs. An aliquot of the enzyme conjugate of the analyte drug, hormone, or metabolite is then added as a second reagent; the enzyme-analyte conjugate then binds with the excess analyte antibody, forming an antigen antibody complex.

CEDIA

Ab + EA + ED-Ag —(+ Ag)→ Ab:Ag + $(EA{:}ED\text{-}Ag)_4$ *Active enzyme*

↓ No Ag

Ab:Ag-ED + EA *No enzyme activity*

EMIT

Ag-Enzyme + Ab —(+ Ag)→ Ab:Ag + Ag-Enzyme *Active enzyme*

↓ No Ag

Ab:Ag-Enzyme *No enzyme activity*

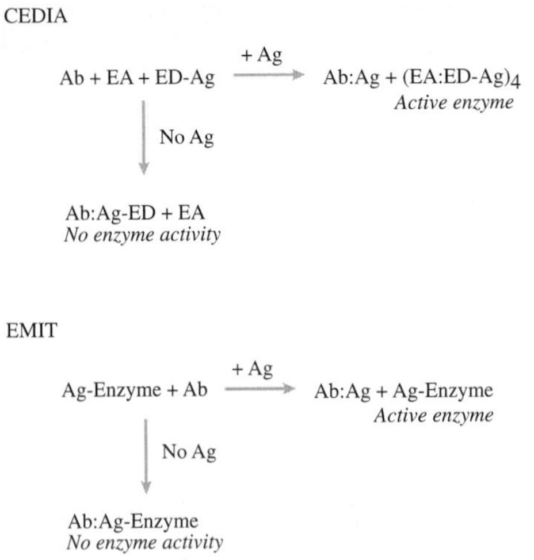

Figure 9-15 CEDIA and EMIT homogeneous immunoassays. *EA,* Enzyme acceptor; *ED,* enzyme donor.

This binding of the analyte antibody with the enzyme analyte conjugate affects enzyme activity by physically blocking access of the substrate to the active site of the enzyme or by changing the conformation of the enzyme molecule and thus altering its activity. To complete the assay, the resultant enzyme activity is measured. The relative change in enzyme activity resulting from the formation of the antigen antibody complex is proportional to the drug, hormone, or metabolite concentration in the patient's sample. Concentration of the analyte is calculated from a calibration curve prepared by analyzing calibrators that contain known quantities of the analyte in question.

Cloned Enzyme Donor Immunoassay. As shown in Figure 9-15, CEDIA is a second type of homogeneous EIA; this assay was the first EIA designed and developed using genetic engineering techniques.[37] Inactive fragments (the enzyme donor and acceptor) of β-galactosidase are prepared by manipulation of the Z gene of the *lac* operon of *E. coli.* These two fragments spontaneously reassemble to form active enzyme even if the enzyme donor is attached to an antigen. However, binding of antibody to the enzyme donor antigen conjugate inhibits reassembly, and no active enzyme is formed. Thus competition between antigen and the enzyme donor antigen conjugate for a fixed amount of antibody in the presence of the enzyme acceptor modulates the measured enzyme activity (high concentrations of antigen produce the least inhibition of enzyme activity; low concentrations produce the greatest inhibition).

Fluoroimmunoassay

Examples of fluorophores that are used as labels in *fluoroimmunoassay* and their properties are listed in Table 9-3.[93] Initially, background fluorescence from drugs, drug metabolites, and protein-bound substances, such as bilirubin, limited the utility of this technique. However, this problem has largely been overcome by the use of rare earth (lanthanide) chelates and background rejection (time-resolved)

TABLE 9-3 Properties of Fluorescent Labels

Fluorophore	Excitation (nm)	Emission (nm)	Fluorescence Quantum Yield*	Lifetime (ns)
Fluorescein isothiocyanate	492	520	0.0-0.85	4.5
Europium (β-naphthoyl trifluoroacetone)	340	590, 613	—	500,000
Lucifer yellow VS	430	540	—	—
Phycobiliprotein	550-620	580-660	0.5-0.98	—
Rhodamine B isothiocyanate	550	585	0.0-0.7	3.0
Umbelliferone	380	450	—	—

*Fluorescence quantum yield: Fraction of molecules that emit a photon.

procedures (see Chapters 3 and 11).[18,19,75] Fluorescent emissions from lanthanide chelates (e.g., europium, terbium, and samarium) are long lived (greater than 1 µs) compared with the typical background fluorescence encountered in biological specimens. In a time-resolved fluoroimmunoassay, a europium chelate label is excited by a pulse of excitation light (0.5 µs), and the long-lived fluorescence emission from the label is measured after a delay (400 to 800 µs). By this time, any short-lived background signal has decayed.

Fluorescent polarization immunoassay is a type of homogeneous fluoroimmunoassay that is widely used to measure drugs and other analytes (Figure 9-16). The polarization of the fluorescence from a fluorescein-antigen conjugate is determined by its rate of rotation during the lifetime of the excited state in solution. A small, rapidly rotating fluorescein antigen conjugate has a low degree of polarization; however, binding to a large antibody molecule slows down the rate of rotation and increases the degree of polarization. Thus binding to antibody modulates polarization, and a homogeneous assay is possible.[42,57,65] Another type of nonseparation fluoroimmunoassay uses a multilayer device to eliminate the necessity for separation of bound and free fractions.[30] The device consists of two agarose layers separated by an opaque layer of iron oxide. A sample is added to the upper (10 µm) layer and diffuses through the iron oxide (10 µm) layer to the thin (1 µm) signal layer that contains antibody:antigen rhodamine complexes. Antigen rhodamine conjugate is displaced from the signal layer by antigen in the sample and diffuses into the upper layer. Residual bound antigen rhodamine conjugate in the signal layer is measured by front-surface fluorometry. Displaced free conjugate does not contribute to the signal, because it is shielded from the fluorescence excitation light by the iron oxide layer. As listed in Box 9-4, many other types of homogeneous fluoroimmunoassays have been described in the literature.[28,47,66,84]

Chemiluminescence Immunoassay

Chemiluminescence is the name given to light emission produced during a chemical reaction (see Chapter 3). Isoluminol and acridinium esters are important examples of chemiluminescent labels used in *chemiluminescent immunoassay.* Oxidation of isoluminol by hydrogen peroxide in the presence of a catalyst, such as microperoxidase, produces a relatively long-lived light emission at 425 nm, and oxidation of an acridinium ester by alkaline hydrogen peroxide in the presence of a detergent (e.g., Triton X-100) produces a rapid flash of light at 429 nm. Acridinium and sulfonyl acridinium esters are high specific activity labels (detection limit for the label is 800 zeptomoles) that can be used to label both antibodies and haptens (Figure 9-17).[1,50,89]

Electrochemiluminescence Immunoassay

Ruthenium (II) tris(bipyridyl) (Figure 9-17, *B*) undergoes an electrochemiluminescent reaction (620 nm) with tripropylamine at an electrode surface, and this chelate is now used as a label in competitive and sandwich *electrochemiluminescence immunoassays.* Using this label, various assays have been developed in a flow cell using magnetic beads as the solid phase. Beads are captured at the electrode surface, and an unbound label is washed out of the cell by a wash buffer. Label bound to the bead undergoes an electrochemiluminescent reaction, and the light emission is measured by an adjacent photomultiplier tube.[7,39]

Simplified Immunoassays

The integration of the technical advances made in molecular immunology with those made in the material and processing sciences has resulted in the development of a number of "simplified" immunoassays for use in physicians' offices or the home (i.e., the so-called point-of-care market). Early efforts were directed toward pregnancy and fertility testing and were based on agglutination and inhibition of agglutination using labeled red blood cells or latex particles in a slide format. Subsequently, sandwich immunoassays have been adapted for similar applications. For example, as listed in the package insert, the ICON II pregnancy test (Beckman Coulter, Fullerton, Calif.) is an operationally simple and sensitive assay for human chorionic gonadotropin (hCG) that detects hCG down to 10 mIU/mL for serum and 20 mIU/mL

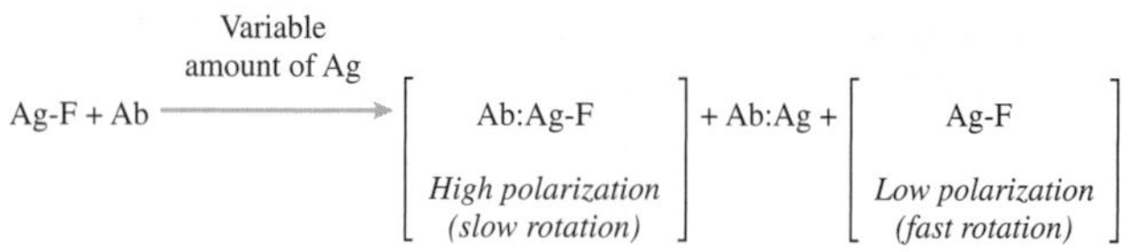

Ag-F + Ab —(Variable amount of Ag)→ [Ab:Ag-F, High polarization (slow rotation)] + Ab:Ag + [Ag-F, Low polarization (fast rotation)]

Figure 9-16 Homogeneous polarization fluoroimmunoassay. *F,* Fluorescein.

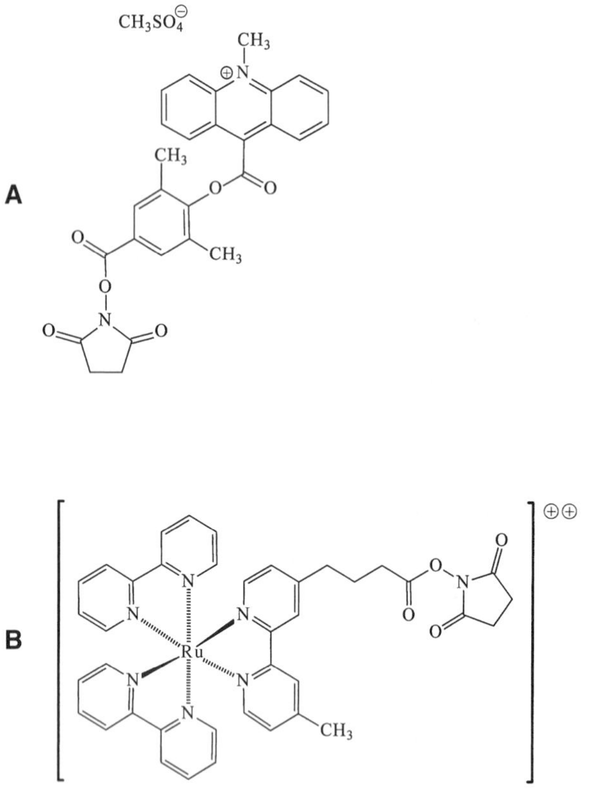

Figure 9-17 Luminescent labels. **A,** Chemiluminescent acridinium ester label. *(From Law S-J, Miller T, Piran U, et al. Novel polysubstituted aryl acridinium esters and their use in immunoassay. J Biolum Chemilum 1989;4:88-98. Reprinted by permission of John Wiley & Sons, Ltd.).* **B,** Electrochemiluminescent ruthenium (II) tris(bipyridyl) NHS ester label.

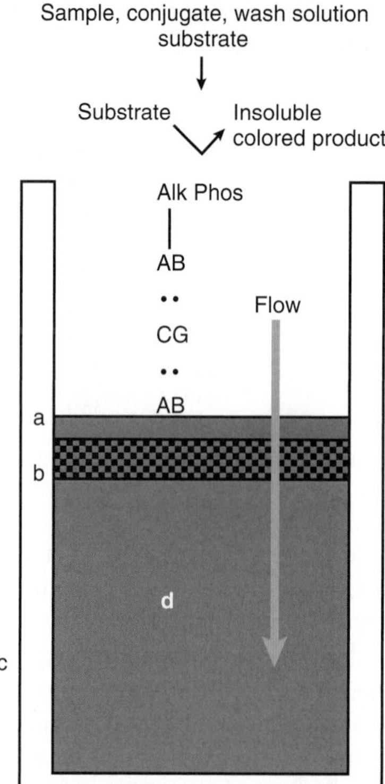

Figure 9-18 ICON immunoassay device (*a,* immobilized antibody membrane; *b,* separating membrane; *c,* container; *d,* adsorbent pad). *hCG,* Human chorionic gonadotropin; *AB,* monoclonal antibody to hCG.

for urine. As shown in Figure 9-18, the ICON II test is a sandwich EIA device that uses a murine monoclonal antibody, which is immobilized onto the surface of a microporous nylon membrane located on top of an adsorbent pad.[85] The pad functions as a capillary pump to draw liquid through the membrane. To perform an analysis, an aliquot of urine is added to the surface of the membrane; hCG is removed as liquid is drawn through it, resulting in the removal of hCG in the sample by its binding to the capture antibody on the membrane. Next, a matched murine monoclonal anti-hCG antibody alkaline phosphatase conjugate is added and allowed to drain into the adsorbent pad. Wash solution is then added, followed by an indoxyl phosphate substrate. Bound conjugate converts this to an insoluble indigo dye, which appears as a discrete blue spot. The second generation of the ICON test includes two additional control zones. An immobilized antialkaline phosphatase zone acts as a procedural control; it binds the alkaline phosphatase conjugate and also appears as a blue spot. A further zone contains an immobilized irrelevant murine monoclonal antibody; this detects the presence of heterophile antibodies in samples, particularly human antimouse antibodies.[8] These mimic antigen and bridge the capture and conjugated mouse antibodies, thus giving what appears to be a positive result.

Newer tests require only the addition of sample, thus simplifying the assay protocol and minimizing possible malfunction resulting from operator error. The TestPack PLUS (Abbott Laboratories, Abbott Park, Ill.) one-step pregnancy test illustrates the general principles of the new devices.[64] It uses a colloidal selenium particle (160-nm diameter) labeled with monoclonal anti-α-hCG antibody, which is red and easily visible. Sample (urine) is applied to the sample well and soaks into a glass-fiber pad containing the conjugate. Any hCG in the urine sample combines with the selenium-labeled antibody, and the mixture migrates along a nitrocellulose track to a region where a line of polyclonal anti-hCG antibody and an orthogonal line of anti-β-hCG:hCG complex has been immobilized. The complex captures unreacted selenium-labeled anti-α-hCG to form a minus sign visible in the viewing window. If hCG is present in the urine sample, then the selenium-labeled anti-α-hCG:hCG complexes bind to the immobilized polyclonal anti-hCG, and a plus sign is formed, denoting a positive result. The remainder of the reaction mixture migrates to the end of the track and reacts with a Quinaldine Red pH indicator in an "end-of-assay" window to signal that the flow in the device has functioned correctly.

A variant of this type of device is the Clearview hCG test (Unipath Diagnostics Inc., Waltham, Mass.). This test uses an absorbent strip that contains blue beads attached to an anti-hCG monoclonal antibody. As urine moves by capillary action through the strip, labeled antibodies are mobilized and move up the test strip, which contains regions of immobilized antibodies loaded with a blue dye. Each strip has separate windows for the positive, negative, and procedural control. If hCG is present at a level of 25 mIU/mL or greater, a blue line becomes visible in the test region window. This region remains clear if the test is negative. A blue line appears in the Reference Region of the result window to show the test is complete and has worked correctly.

Simultaneous multianalyte immunoassays in which two or more analytes are detected in a single assay represent a further means of work simplification in immunoassay. Two different strategies have been developed based on either discrete reaction zones or combinations of different labels. In the Triage panel for drugs of abuse point-of-care test device (Biosite Incorporated, San Diego), simultaneous detection of up to nine drugs is achieved using discrete test zones on a small piece of nylon membrane.[12] Each test zone consists of antibodies for a specific drug immobilized on the membrane surface. This zone captures free gold-drug conjugate from the sample, antidrug antibody, and gold-drug conjugate reaction mixture and appears as a purple band. Combinations of distinguishable labels, such as europium (613 nm, emission lifetime 730 μs) and samarium (643 nm, emission lifetime 50 μs) chelates provide the basis of quantitative simultaneous immunoassays. These two chelates have different fluorescence emission maxima and different fluorescence decay times and thus can be easily distinguished by making measurements at 613 nm, delay time 0.4 ms (europium), and 643 nm, delay time 0.05 ms (samarium). An assay for free and bound prostate-specific antigen and an assay for myoglobin and carbonic anhydrase III are two examples of clinically useful tests combined in this simultaneous assay format.[55,88]

Protein Microarrays

Arrays of hundreds or thousands of micrometer-sized dots of antigens or antibodies immobilized on the surface of a glass or plastic chip are emerging as an important tool in genomic studies and in assessing protein-protein interactions. This format facilitates simultaneous multianalyte immunoassays using, for example, enzyme or fluorophore-labeled conjugates. The arrays are made by printing or spotting 1-nL drops of protein solutions onto a flat surface, such as a glass microscope slide. In a typical sandwich assay, the array on the surface of the slide is incubated with sample and then with conjugate. Bound conjugate is detected using chemiluminescence or fluorescein using a scanning device. The pattern of the signal provides information on the presence and amount of individual analytes in the sample or the reactivity of a single analyte with the range of proteins arrayed on the surface of the slide.[79] (Such devices are discussed in more detail in Chapter 10.)

Interferences in Immunoassays

Immunological assays are prone to interferences, in spite of the use of highly specific antibodies for molecular recognition of the analyte. Falsely low results can occur because of the hook effect at high antigen concentrations (see above). False negative or false positive results are encountered if the sample contains antianimal antibodies. For example, in a two-site sandwich assay for hCG based on mouse antibodies, any human antimouse antibodies (HAMA) present in the specimen will recognize the immobilized mouse capture and mouse conjugate antibodies and form a complex that is indistinguishable from an immobilized capture antibody: hCG:conjugate complex. This leads to a false positive result. A false negative result will be obtained if the HAMA react with either the capture antibody or conjugate to such an extent that specific antibody binding to hCG is prevented. Many different types of circulating antianimal antibodies have been detected (e.g., human antigoat, human antibovine antibodies) and shown to interfere in immunoassays. In practice, this type of interference is minimized by including additives in the immunoassay reagents. Nonimmune serum or IgG from the species used to raise the antibodies has been a popular choice for this purpose.[8,46,49]

OTHER IMMUNOCHEMICAL TECHNIQUES

Other analytical methods of clinical interest that employ antibodies include cytochemical and agglutination assays.

Immunocytochemistry

The use of labeled antibody reagents as specific probes for protein and peptide antigens allows the researcher and pathologist to evaluate single cells for synthetic capability and for specific markers for identification of various cell lines. Immunochemistry in recent years has been rapidly expanded by immunoenzymatic methods, especially with regard to the use of horseradish peroxidase–labeled (immunoperoxidase) assays. Using enzyme labels provides several advantages over fluorescent labels. They permit the use of fixed tissue embedded in paraffin, which provides excellent preservation of cell morphology and eliminates the problem of autofluorescence from tissue. In addition, immunoperoxidase stains are permanent, and only a standard light microscope is necessary to identify labeled features. The immunoperoxidase methods are also applicable to electron microscopy. Several approaches for immunoenzymatic assay have been used, including direct, indirect, peroxidase-antiperoxidase, and enzyme bridge methods.

Agglutination Assays

Agglutination assays have been used for many years for the qualitative and quantitative measurement of antigens and antibodies. In an agglutination method, the visible clumping of particulates, such as cells and latex particles, is used as an indicator of the primary reaction of antigen and antibody. Agglutination methods require stable and uniform particulates, pure antigen, and specific antibody. IgM antibodies are more likely to produce complete agglutination than are IgG antibodies because of the size and valence of the IgM molecule. Therefore when only IgG antibodies are involved, it may be necessary to use chemical enhancement or an antiglobulin agglutination method. As with all immunochemical reactions in which aggregation is the measured end point, the ratio of antigen and antibody is critical. Extremes in antigen or antibody concentration will result in inhibition of aggregation.

An incomplete agglutination reaction is one in which the primary reaction occurs, but no or only minimal aggregation of the particles occurs. Many particles, such as erythrocytes and bacteria in solution, have a net negative charge (zeta potential), which causes mutual repulsion.[91] For successful agglutination, the antigen antibody reaction must overcome this normal resistance. In the case of a weak antigen antibody reaction or one in which only IgG is involved, this mutual repulsion may be sufficient to inhibit agglutination completely or partially. In systems in which incomplete agglutination results, enhancement may be achieved by lowering the ionic strength or by introducing polymeric molecules, such as polymerized albumin (5% to 30%), dextran, polybrene, polyvinylpyrrolidone, or PEG.[91]

Hemagglutination refers to agglutination reactions in which the antigen is located on an erythrocyte. Erythrocytes are not only good passive carriers of antigen, but are also easily coated with foreign proteins and can be easily obtained and stored.

Direct testing of erythrocytes for blood group, Rh, and other antigenic types is used widely in blood banks; specific antisera, such as anti-A, anti-C, and anti-Kell, are used to detect such antigens on the erythrocyte surface.

In *indirect* or *passive* hemagglutination, the erythrocytes are used as a particulate carrier of foreign antigen (and in some tests of antibodies); this technique has wide applications. Other materials available in the form of fine particles, such as bentonite and latex, also have been used as antigen carriers, but they are more difficult to coat, standardize, and store. In a related variation of this technique, known as *hemagglutination inhibition,* the ability of antigens, haptens, or other substances to specifically inhibit hemagglutination of sensitized (coated) cells by antibody is determined.

In general, the agglutination methods are quite sensitive but are not as quantitative as other immunochemical methods discussed thus far. Nonisotopic immunoassays, especially EIAs, are as convenient as agglutination reactions and are therefore replacing agglutination methods in many laboratories.

REFERENCES

1. Adamczyk M, Chen YY, Fishpaugh JR, et al. Linker-mediated modulation of the chemiluminescent signal from N(10)-(3-Sulfopropyl)-N-sulfonylacridinium-9-carboxamide tracers. Bioconj Chem 2000;11:714-24.
2. Akhavan-Tafti H, Sugioka K, Arghavani Z, et al. Lumigen™ PS: Chemiluminescent detection of horseradish peroxidase by enzymatic generation of acridinium esters. Clin Chem 1995;41:1368-9.
3. Alper CA, Johnson AM. Immunofixation electrophoresis: A technique for the study of protein polymorphism. Vox Sang 1969;17:445-52.
4. Avrameas S, Ternynck T, Guesdon JL. Coupling of enzymes to antibodies and antigens. Scand J Immunol 1978;8(Suppl 7):7-23.
5. Bayer EA, Wilcheck M. The use of the avidin-biotin complex as a tool in molecular biology. Methods Biochem Anal 1980;26:2-42.
6. Beck OE, Kaiser PE. Rate nephelometry of human IgE in serum. Clin Chem 1982;28:1349-51.
7. Blackburn GF, Shah HP, Kenten JH, et al. Electrochemiluminescence detection for development of immunoassays and DNA probe assays for clinical diagnostics. Clin Chem 1991;37:1534-9.
8. Boscato LM, Stuart MC. Heterophilic antibodies. A problem for all immunoassays. Clin Chem 1988;34:27-33.
9. Brandshund I, Siersted SE, Teisner B. Double-decker rocket immunoelectrophoresis for direct quantitation of complement split products with C3d specificities in plasma. J Immunol Methods 1981;44:63-71.
10. Bronstein I, Edwards B, Voyta JC. 1,2-Dioxetanes: Novel chemiluminescent enzyme substrates: Applications to immunoassays. J Biolum Chemilum 1989;4:99-111.
11. Brunette WN. Western blotting: Electrophoretic transfer of proteins from sodium dodecyl sulfate-polyacrylamide gels to unmodified nitrocellulose and radiographic detection with antibody and radioiodinated protein A. Anal Biochem 1981;112:195-203.
12. Buechler KF, Moi S, Noar B, et al. Simultaneous detection of seven drugs of abuse by the Triage™ panel for drugs of abuse. Clin Chem 1992;38:1678-4.
13. Buffone GJ, Lewis SA. Advantages of small angle light scattering measurements in immunonephelometry. In: Peeters H, Wright PH, eds. Plasma protein pathology. New York, Pergamon Press, 1979:55-61.
14. Buffone GJ, Savory J, Cross RE, et al. Evaluation of kinetic light scattering as an approach to the measure-

ment of specific proteins with the centrifugal analyzer. I. Methodology. Clin Chem 1975;21:1731-4.
15. Burton DR, Barbas III CF. Human antibodies from combinatorial libraries. Adv Immunol 1994;57: 191-280.
16. Chan WC, Maxwell DJ, Gao X, Bailey RE, Han M Nie S. Luminescent quantum dots for multiplexed biological detection and imaging. Curr Opin Biotechnol 2002;13:40-6.
17. Cheng A, Bray K, Polito A. Nephelometric inhibition assay for gentamicin. Clin Chem 1979;25:1078.
18. Diamandis E. Immunoassays with time resolved fluorescence spectroscopy: Principles and applications. Clin Biochem 1988;21:139-50.
19. Diamandis EP. Multiple labeling and time-resolvable fluorophores. Clin Chem 1991;37:1486-91.
20. Ekins RP. The estimation of thyroxine in human plasma by an electrophoretic technique. Clin Chim Acta 1960;5:453-9.
21. Ekins RP. Current concepts and future developments. In: Collins WP, ed. Alternative Immunoassays. New York; John Wiley & Sons, Inc, 1985:219-37.
22. Engvall E, Perlmann P. Enzyme-linked immunosorbent assay (ELISA). Quantitative assay of immunoglobulin G. Immunochemistry 1971;8:871-4.
23. Fahey JL, McKelvey EM. Quantitative determination of serum immunoglobulins in antibody agar plates. J Immunol 1965;94:84-90.
24. Fiore M, Mitchell J, Doan T, et al. The Abbott IMx™ automated benchtop immunochemistry analyzer system. Clin Chem 1988;34:1726-32.
25. Gauldie J, Bienenstock J. Automated nephelometric analysis of haptens. In: R Ritchie R, ed. Automated Immunoanalysis Vol. 7, Part 1. New York; Marcel Dekker, Inc, 1978:321-33.
26. Gershoni JM, Palade GE. Electrophoretic transfer of proteins from sodium dodecyl–sulfate–polyacrylamide gels to a positively charged membrane filter. Anal Biochem 1982;124:396-405.
27. Giegel JL, Brotherton MM, Cronin P, et al. Radial partition immunoassay. Clin Chem 1982;28: 1894-98.
28. Gosling, JP. A decade of development in immunoassay methodology. Clin Chem 1990;36:1408-27.
29. Grange J, Roch AM, Quash GA. Nephelometric assay of antigens and antibodies with latex particles. J Immunol Methods 1977;18:365-75.
30. Grenner G, Inbar S, Maneghini EW, et al. Multilayer fluorescent immunoassay technique. Clin Chem 1989;35:1865-8.
31. Grossberg AL, Chen CC, Rendina L, et al. Specific cation effects with antibody to a hapten with a positive charge. J Immunol 1962;88:600-03.
32. Guesdon JL, Ternynck T, Avrameas S. The use of avidin-biotin interaction in immunoenzymatic techniques. J Histochem Cytochem 1979;27:1131-9.
33. Han M, Gao X, Su JZ, Nie S. Quantum-dot-tagged microbeads for multiplexed optical coding of biomolecules. Nat Biotechnol 2001;19:631-5.
34. Harrington JL, Fenton JW, Pert H. Polymer-induced precipitation of antigen-antibody complexes: "Precipiplex reactions." Immunochemistry 1971;8:413-21.
35. Hellsing K. Immune reactions in polysaccharide media: Polysaccharide-enhanced precipitation reactions with antigens of various sizes. Biochem J 1969;114:145-9.
36. Hellsing K. Immune reactions in polysaccharide media: I. The effect of dextran on the reaction between ^{125}I-labeled human serum albumin and gamma-G-globulin from rabbit. Acta Chem Scand 1966;20: 1251-62.
37. Henderson DR, Friedman SB, Harris JB, et al. CEDIA, a new homogeneous immunoassay system. Clin Chem 1986;32:1637-41.
38. Hills LP, Tiffany TO. Comparison of turbidimetric and light-scattering measurements of immunoglobulins by use of a centrifugal analyzer with absorbance and fluorescence-light-scattering optics. Clin Chem 1980;26:1459-66.
39. Hoyle NR. The application of electrochemiluminescence to immunoassay-based analyte detection. In: Campbell AK, Kricka LJ, Stanley PE, eds. Bioluminescence and Chemiluminescence. Fundamentals and Applied Aspects. Chichester: Wiley, 1994:28-31.
40. Jackson TM, Ekins RP. Theoretical limitations on immunoassay. Methods Enzymol 1986;74:28-60.
41. Jackson TM, Ekins RP. Theoretical limitations of immunoassay sensitivity: Current practice and potential advantages of fluorescent Eu^{3+} chelates as non-radioisotopic tracers. J Immunol Methods 1986;87:13-20.
42. Jolley ME, Stroupe SD, Wang CJ. Fluorescence polarization immunoassay: I. Monitoring aminoglycoside antibiotics in serum and plasma. Clin Chem 1981;27:1190-7.
43. Kabat EA. Structural Concepts in Immunology and Immunochemistry, 2nd ed. New York: Holt, Rinehart & Winston Inc, 1976.
44. Keren DF. High Resolution Electrophoresis and Immunofixation Techniques. Boston: Butterworth-Heineman, 1994.
45. Kohler G, Milstein C. Continuous cultures of fused cells secreting antibody of predefined specificity. Nature 1975;256:495-7.
46. Kohse KP, Wisser H. Antibodies as a source of analytical errors. J Clin Chem Clin Biochem 1990;28:881-92.
47. Kricka LJ. Ligand-Binder Assays. New York: Marcel Dekker, Inc, 1985.
48. Kricka LJ. Chemiluminescent and bioluminescent techniques. Clin Chem 1991;37:1472-81.
49. Kricka LJ. Human anti-animal antibody interferences in immunological assays. Clin Chem 1999;45:942-56.

50. Krodel E, Boland J, Carey G, et al. Technical challenges in the development of the CIBA Corning ACS:180 benchtop immunoassay system. In: Stanley PE, Kricka LJ, eds. Bioluminescence and chemiluminescence: Current status. Chichester: John Wiley & Sons, 1991:107-10.
51. Laurell CB. Antigen-antibody crossed electrophoresis. Anal Biochem 1965;10:358-61.
52. Laurell CB. Electroimmunoassay. Scand J Clin Lab Invest 1972;29(Suppl 124):21-37.
53. Laurent TC. In: Quintarelei G, ed. The chemical physiology of mucopolysaccharides. Boston: Little, Brown & Co, Inc, 1968:153.
54. Laurent TC. The interaction between polysaccharides and other macromolecules. 5. The solubility of proteins in the presence of dextran. Biochem J 1963;89:253-7.
55. Leinonen J, Lovgren T, Vornanen T, Stenman U-H. Double-label time-resolved immunofluorometric assay of prostate-specific antigen and its complex with alpha1-antichymotrypsin. Clin Chem 1993;39: 2098-103.
56. Leute RK, Ullman EF, Goldstein A, et al. Spin immunoassay technique for determination of morphine. Nature 1972;236:93-4.
57. Li TM, Benovic JL, Burd JF. Serum theophylline determination by fluorescence polarization immunoassay utilizing an umbelliferone derivative as a fluorescent label. Anal Biochem 1981;118:102-7.
58. Lindbladh C, Persson M, Bulow L, et al. The design of a simple competitive ELISA using human proinsulin-alkaline phosphatase conjugates prepared by gene fusion. Biochem Biophys Res Commun 1987;149: 607-14.
59. Mancini G, Carbonara AO, Heremans JF. Immunochemical quantitation of antigens by single radial immunodiffusion. Immunochemistry 1965;2:235-54.
60. Marrack JR, Richards CB. Light scattering studies of the formation of aggregates in mixtures of antigen and antibody. Immunology 1970;20:1019-40.
61. McCormack RT, Ludwig JR, Wolfert RL. Advances in design, generation, and manipulation of monoclonal antibodies. In: Nakamura RM, Kasahara Y, Rechnitz GA, eds. Immunochemical assays and biosensor technology for the 1990s. Washington DC: American Association for Microbiology, 1992:57-82.
62. Niedbala RS, Feindt H, Kardos K, et al. Detection of analytes by immunoassay using up-converting phosphor technology. Anal Biochem 2001;293:22-30.
63. Nygren H, Stenberg M. Diffusion-in-gel enzyme-linked immunosorbent assay (DIG-ELISA): Quantification of antigen by diffusion over an antibody-coated surface. Scand J Clin Lab Invest 1982;42:355-9.
64. Osikowicz G, Beggs M, Brookhart P, et al. One step chromatographic immunoassay for qualitative determination of choriogonadotrophin in urine. Clin Chem 1990;36:1586.
65. Popelka BR, Miller DM, Holen JT, et al. Fluorescence polarization immunoassay: II. Analyzer for rapid, precise measurement of fluorescence polarization with use of disposable cuvettes. Clin Chem 1981;27: 1198-201.
66. Price CP, Newman DJ, eds. Principles and practice of immunoassay. 2nd ed New York: Stockton Press, 1996.
67. Rej R, Keese CR, Giaever I. Direct immunochemical determination of aspartate aminotransferase isoenzymes. Clin Chem 1981;27:1597-601.
68. Rigl CT, Patel MT, Rivera HN, Stults NL, Smith DF. A bioluminescent immunoassay based on the recombinant photoprotein. In: Campbell AK, Kricka LJ, Stanley PE, eds. Bioluminescence and chemiluminescence. Fundamentals and applied aspects. Chichester: Wiley, 1994:345-8.
69. Rodbard D. Data processing for radioimmunoassays: An overview. In: Natelson S, Pesce AJ, Mietz AA, eds. Clinical oImmunochemistry, Vol 3. Washington DC: American Association for Clinical Chemistry, 1978:477-94.
70. Rosenthal SJ. Bar-coding biomolecules with fluorescent nanocrystals. Nat Biotechnol 2001;19:621-22.
71. Rowe DS. Radioactive single radial diffusion: A method for increasing the sensitivity of immunochemical quantitation of proteins in agar gel. Bull WHO 1969;40:613-6.
72. Rubenstein KE, Schneider RS, Ullman EF. "Homogeneous" enzyme immunoassay: New immunochemical technique. Biochem Biophys Res Commun 1972;47:846-51.
73. Sano T, Smith CL, Cantor CR. Immuno-PCR: Very sensitive antigen detection by means of specific antibody-DNA conjugates. Science 1992;258:120-2.
74. Savory J, Buffone GJ, Reich R. Kinetics of the IgG anti-IgG reaction, as evaluated by conventional and stopped-flow nephelometry. Clin Chem 1974;20: 1071-5.
75. Soini E, Kojola J. Time-resolved fluorometer for lanthanide chelates: A new generation of non-isotopic immunoassays. Clin Chem 1983;29:65-8.
76. Steward MW. Immunochemistry. New York: John Wiley & Sons, Inc, 1977:233.
77. Sutherland R, Simpson B, Allman B. Surface effect immunoassay. In: Price CP, Newman DJ, eds. Principles and practice of immunoassay. New York: Stockton Press, 1991:515-42.
78. Tanford C. The Hydrophobic Effect: Formation of micelles and biological membranes. New York: John Wiley & Sons, Inc, 1980.
79. Templin MF, Stoll D, Schrenk M, Traub PC, Vohringer CF, Joos TO. Protein microarray technology. Trends Biotechnol 2002;20:160-6.

80. Tengerdy RP. Reaction kinetic studies of the antigen antibody reaction. J Immunol 1967;99:126-32.
81. Thorell JI. Internal sample attenuator counting (ISAC): A new technique for separating and measuring bound and free activity in radioimmunoassays. Clin Chem 1981;27:1969-73.
82. Thorpe GHG, Kricka LJ. Enhanced chemiluminescent reactions catalyzed by horseradish peroxidase. Methods Enzymol 1986;133:331-5.
83. Ullman EF, Kirakossian H, Singh S, Irvin BR, Irvine JD, Wagner DB. Luminescent oxygen channeling immunoassay (LOCI) for human thyroid stimulating hormone. In: Campbell AK, Kricka LJ, Stanley PE eds. Bioluminescence and chemiluminescence. Fundamentals and applied aspects. Chichester: Wiley, 1994:6-19.
84. Ullman EF, Khana PL. Fluorescence excitation transfer immunoassay (FETI). Methods Enzymol 1981;74: 28-60.
85. Valkirs GE, Barton R. ImmunoConcentration™: A new format for solid-phase immunoassays. Clin Chem 1985;31:1427-31.
86. Van Weeman BK, Schuurs AHWM. Immunoassay using antigen-enzyme conjugates. FEBS Letts 1971;15:232-6.
87. Voller A, Bartlett A, Bidwell DE. Enzyme immunoassays with special reference to ELISA techniques. J Clin Pathol 1978;31:507-19.
88. Vuori J, Rasi S, Takala T, Vaananen K. Dual-label time-resolved fluoroimmunoassay for simultaneous detection of myoglobin and carbonic anhydrase III. Clin Chem 1991;37:2087-92.
89. Weeks I, Campbell AK, Woodhead JS. Two-site immunochemiluminometric assay for human alpha-1 fetoprotein. Clin Chem 1983;29:1480-3.
90. Wians FH Jr, Dev J, Powell MM, et al. Evaluation of simultaneous measurements of lutropin and follitropin with the SimulTropin™ radioimmunoassay kit. Clin Chem 1986;32:887-90.
91. Williams CA, Chase MM, Eds. Methods in immunology and immunochemistry, Vol 3. New York: Academic Press, Inc, 1970:1-125.
92. Winter G, Griffiths AD, Hawkins RE, Hoogenboom HR. Making antibodies by phage display technology. Ann Rev Immunol 1994;12:433-55.
93. Wood P. Heterogeneous fluoroimmunoassay. In: Price CP, Newman DJ, eds. Principles and Practice of Immunoassay. New York: Stockton Press, 1991: 365-92.
94. Yalow RS, Berson SA. Assay of plasma insulin in human subjects by immunological methods. Nature 1959;184:1648-69.
95. Zijlmans HJ, Bonnet J, Burton J, et al. Detection of cell and tissue surface antigens using up-converting phosphors: a new reporter technology. Anal Biochem 1999;267:30-6.

ADDITIONAL READING

Andrey L, Ghindilis AL, Pavlov, AR, Atanassov PB, eds. Immunoassay methods and protocols. Totowa, NJ: Humana Press, 2003.

Crowther JR. ELISA: Theory and practice. Clifton, NJ: Humana Press, 1995.

Deshpande SS. Enzyme immunoassays: From concept to product development. Norwell, MA: Kluwer Academic Publishers; 1996.

Diamandis EP, Christopoulos TK. Immunoassay. San Diego: Academic Press, 1996.

Price CP, Newman DJ, eds. Principles and practice of immunoassay, 2nd ed. New York: Stockton Press, 1996.

Proceedings of the Twenty-Eighth Annual Oak Ridge Conference on Advanced Analytical Concepts for the Clinical Laboratory: Special Topic: Sensitive Detection Systems. Clin Chem 1996;42:1472-1556.

Van Vunakis H, Colowick SP, Langone JJ, Van Vunakis H, eds. Immunochemical techniques (Methods in enzymology, Volume 70, Part A). New York: Academic Press; 1997.

Wild D, ed. The immunoassay handbook, 2nd ed. New York: Stockton Press, 2001.

Wu JT. Quantitative Immunoassay: A practical guide for assay establishment, troubleshooting, and clinical application. Washington D.C: AACC Press, 2000.

CHAPTER 10

Nanotechnology and Microfabrication

Peter Wilding, Ph.D., F.R.C.Path., F.R.S.C., H.C.L.D.(A.B.B.)

On December 29, 1959, at the annual meeting of the American Physical Society, Nobel Laureate Richard Feynman gave his classic talk entitled "There's Plenty of Room at the Bottom" (http://www.zyvex.com/nanotech/feynman.html). In it, he suggested that ordinary machines could build smaller machines that could build still smaller machines, working step by step down toward the molecular level. To quote, "The principles of physics, as far as I can see, do not speak against the possibility of maneuvering things atom by atom."

Norio Taniguchi at the University of Tokyo coined the term "nanotechnology" in 1974 to describe rapidly emerging and converging technologies that are all based upon the scaling down of existing technologies to the next level of miniaturization. In 1981 Eric Drexler defined molecular nanotechnology as a technology based on the ability to build structures to complex, atomic specifications by means of mechanosynthesis and published the first scientific article on the subject entitled "Molecular Engineering: An Approach to the Development of General Capabilities for Molecular Manipulation."[26] Later in 1992, he authored a book entitled *Nanosystems: Molecular Machinery, Manufacturing, and Computation.*[27]

In 2000 the National Science and Technology Council (NSTC) expanded the definition of nanotechnology to:

"nanotechnology involves research and technology development at the atomic, molecular, or macromolecular levels in the dimension range of approximately 1-100 nanometers to provide fundamental understanding of phenomena and materials at the nanoscale and to create and use structures, devices, and systems that have novel properties and functions because of their small and/or intermediate size. The novel and differentiating properties and functions are developed at a critical length scale of matter typically under 100 nm. Nanotechnology research and development includes control at the nanoscale and integration of nanoscale structures into larger material components, systems, and architectures. Within these larger scale assemblies, the control and construction of their structures and components remains at the nanometer scale." (http://www.becon2.nih.gov/nstc_def_nano.htm).

As articulated by Feynman[37] and Drexler[27] and later by many others,[23,88] nanotechnology and miniaturization in general promise many advantages including economy of scale, ease of operation, reliability of instrumentation, and potential for microscale, massive parallel analyses. Consequently, tremendous efforts in terms of scope, diversity, and rate of progress are being invested in developing miniaturized devices.

From the perspective of the clinical laboratory, miniaturization has been a long-term trend in clinical diagnostics instrumentation.[67] For example, capillary electrophoresis instruments (see Chapter 5) and mass spectrometers have been implemented on microchips of silicon, glass, or plastic. In actuality, however, these devices are not manufactured on a nanometer scale but rather on a micrometer scale. Consequently, this chapter will be concerned with microminiaturized devices whose key components (1) are approximately 100 micrometers in size, (2) are employed in analytical measurement, and (3) require special forms of fabrication designed for microdevices. Although this chapter does not attempt to discuss submicron or molecular structures at the nanometer scale, it should be noted that applications discussed later in it require only nanoliter (nL) quantities of a sample or deal with individual cells that may have cell volume in the picoliter (pL) to nL range.

BACKGROUND

Early efforts to reduce the volume requirements of clinical analyzers resulted in the modification of existing technology to use microvolume quantities of a sample. For example, in the 1970s the Chem-1 Analyzer (Technicon Corp, Tarrytown, N.Y.) was modified to perform a single analysis on a sample volume of only 1.0 µL.[13] Before this date, virtually all clinical analyzers used sample or reaction volumes in excess of 50 µL. By the 1980s concerted efforts to develop hand-held devices led to the introduction of the i-STAT system (i-STAT Corp, East Windsor, N.J.; Abbott Diagnostics, Abbott Park, IL.) in 1990; it was one of the first such devices to include microfabricated electrodes and chemical sensors on silicon microchips (Figure 10-1).[33,56] This analyzer featured a functional microsystem employing new fabrication technology that was associated with effective computer-based controls and monitoring capabilities. The use of photolithographic etching technology borrowed from the microelectronics industry illustrated to clinical scientists that microanalytical devices and components could be made in large numbers and be adapted effectively to include chemical components, electrodes, capacitors, and microfluidic features. This illustration by i-STAT laid the basis for numerous other applications to be considered.

Engineering laboratories have been successful in developing miniaturized devices, such as miniature injection valves, actuators, and pumping systems.[11,122,157] Notable efforts with distinct implications for the clinical laboratory community were microdevices for pH measurement fabricated from wafers of silicon.[103,124,130] One of these devices[103] facilitated the measurement of acidic metabolites (e.g., lactic acid) in living cells confined to a flow chamber in silicon. The pH was measured using a light-addressable potentiometric sensor that detects attachment of protons to the chamber surface coated with protonatable silanol and amine groups. Using this device, the changes of metabolism in various forms of cells were monitored. In all of these developments, the exploitation of microfabrication techniques has been essential.

Since these early efforts, the scope of microtechnology has expanded markedly in the early 2000s with developments of applications being driven by the realization of the potential benefit from microtechnology and also from huge investments, particularly to support the science of drug develop-

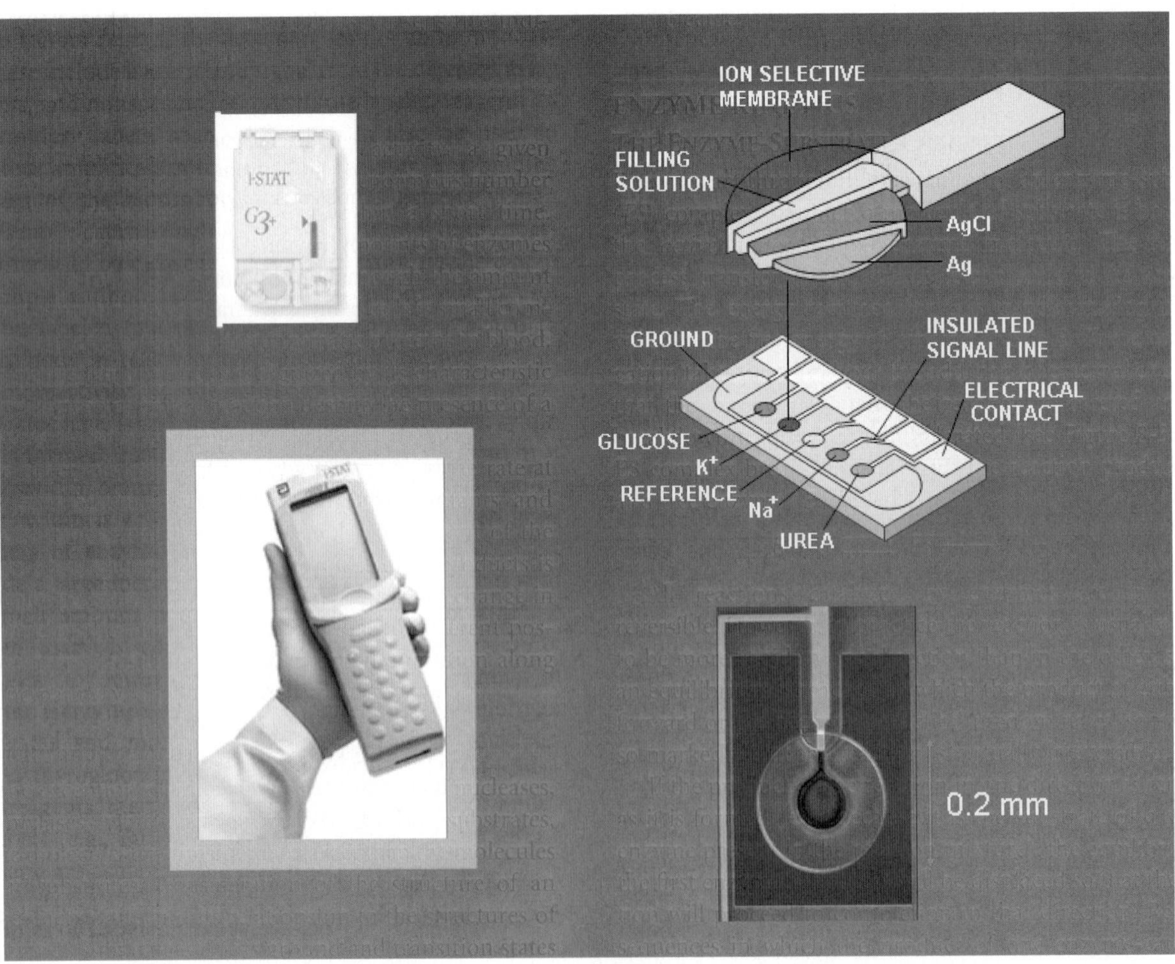

Figure 10-1 The i-STAT system showing a cartridge and the microchip-based electrode assembly. *(Reproduced by permission of i-STAT Corporation, East Windsor, N.J.)*

ment.[65,69,71] Furthermore, hundreds of small companies worldwide have been created to explore and develop applications where the fabrication of microdevices allows for exploitation of new fabricating techniques and the potential benefit of being able to handle and process microsamples.[67] Some of the most notable developments are identified to exemplify the direction of this rapidly developing field. The notable developments are microelectromechanical systems (MEMS), miniaturized total analytical systems (μTAS), microarray type devices for hybridization of deoxyribonucleic acid (DNA) and ribonucleic acid (RNA), microfluidic-based devices for capillary electrophoresis, cell-based assays, and numerous other applications.* However, it is realized that clinical laboratorians require systems, not components, for analytical measurement and so the difficulty facing manufacturers has been to produce microdevices that operate competitively within a microenvironment with macrotechnology or conventional technology. The development of microsystems has therefore been delayed because of the necessity to provide associated components, such as valves and sensors that combine to maintain a microenvironment. An additional requirement, not fully appreciated in the early days of microdevice development, is the necessity for appropriate surface chemistry in microdevices where the impact of an adverse charge or chemical grouping on a surface profoundly modifies the behavior and function of a system. Finally, it is important to realize that microtechnology can be limiting when attempting to adapt conventional methods or procedures.

There are numerous excellent articles, books, editorials, and reviews that cover the topic of microtechnology. A short list of some of the most relevant for a clinically oriented reader is presented in Table 10-1; however, attention is drawn to three reviews published in 2002.[3,111,132] Authors of these reviews have pioneered the development of microtechnology, and their reports highlight the scope and magnitude of development that took place in the prior decade.

*References 23, 57, 88, 126, 129, 146.

FABRICATION AND MATERIALS

Computer chips are categorized by their "minimum feature size"—the dimension of the smallest feature actually constructed in the manufacturing process. The minimum feature size is continually getting smaller to pack more circuitry into the same space. For example, advanced chips in production in 2000 had minimum feature sizes of 180 nm, with chips with a size of 90 nm under development.

The concept of a "minimum feature size" is also important in fabrication of microdevices; its actual dimensions are determined by the choice of fabrication process. As discussed below, conventional photolithography (405 or 436 nm) is generally limited to features of approximately 1 μm. Deep ultraviolet (UV) (230 to 260 nm) lithography has a minimum feature size of 0.3 μm, and x-ray and e-beam can be used to generate features as small as 0.1 μm.

In this section, the techniques used to manufacture, drill, and seal microdevices are discussed.

MANUFACTURING TECHNIQUES

A range of techniques and materials are available for the fabrication of microdevices.[2,66] Photolithography on silicon, glass, and plastic surfaces and molding of polymers are commonly employed processes used to fabricate microdevices. Other processes in use or under investigation include embossing, laser ablation, molding, and atomic force microscopic etching.

Photolithography

Photolithography is the process of transferring geometric shapes on a mask to the surface of a silicon wafer. It involves

TABLE 10-1 Significant Papers in Miniaturization of Relevance to Clinical Analyses

Author(s)	Year	Topic	Ref. #
Manz et al	1993	Early Review	88
Colyer	1997	Clinical Potential of Microchips	23
Kopp et al	1997	Developments in Technology	62
Kricka	1998	Miniaturization of Analytical Systems	67
Ekins & Chu	1999	Microarrays: Origins, and Applications	31
Wilding & Kricka	1999	Micro-microchips: How Small?	145
Medintz et al	2001	Applications of Capillary Electrophoresis	90
Sanders & Manz	2000	Chip-Based Micro-Systems	112
Reyes et al	2002	μ-TAS* Theory and Technology	111
Auroux et al	2002	μ-TAS* Operations and Applications	3
Kricka & Fortina	2002	Microchips: Literature Survey	72
Verpoorte	2002	Microfluidic Chips	132
Lee & Mrksich	2002	Protein Chips: Concept to Practice	75

*μ*TAS*, = Miniaturized total analytical system.

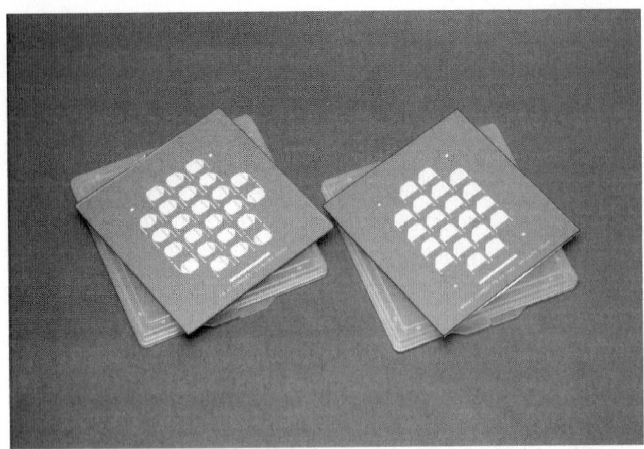

Figure 10-2 Two glass photo masks (approx 125 × 125 mm) showing patterns for multiple PCR devices to be fabricated in silicon.

a series of steps.[2,106] First, a photo mask defining the shapes of the structures to be etched on the silicon wafer is generated from larger drawings that can be accurately duplicated and reduced in size using computer-based programs (Figure 10-2). The silicon wafer is then oxidized to produce a thin surface layer of chemically resistant silicon dioxide that will allow coating with a photo resist material. The wafer is then evenly coated with a polymeric photo resist using a spin-coating procedure and patterned using a photo mask and a UV light source. The photo resist is either a positive resist (photo resist in areas of the wafer exposed to light is rendered soluble) or a negative resist (photo resist in areas of the wafer unexposed to light is rendered soluble). The insoluble polymerized resist remaining on the wafer forms an image of the photo mask on the silicon dioxide surface of the wafer. The wafer is now ready to have the oxide etched away either by a wet or dry etching process.

Wet Etching

Wet etching covers any form of etching where etching is performed by immersing the silicon wafer or glass or plastic surface in a bath of the chemical etchant. The chemical etchants are either isotropic or anisotropic. Isotropic etchants such as hydrofluoric acid (HF) will etch a given material at the same rate whatever direction they are etching in, and are less used because they are difficult to control and etch underneath the protective resist. By contrast, anisotropic etchants will etch at different rates in a given material depending on a number of factors, the most useful one being the crystal structure and orientation. Etching of glass is usually achieved using HF. Microstructures in glass can also be formed by laser ablation techniques.

Figure 10-3 illustrates how the angles of etching can be controlled using an anisotropic etchant. The most widely used anisotropic etchant is potassium hydroxide (KOH). Most etchants will not etch impure silicon at the same rate as pure silicon; this fact can be used to the advantage of the engineer. An example of this would be that if a small part of the silicon substrate is doped with boron, the doped section will not be etched as fast as the normal silicon; if an isotropic etchant is used, the silicon beneath the boron doped area will be etched away. The main disadvantage with using this doping method is that it alters the electrical properties of the silicon so that fabricating and microelectronic devices on the same substrate will be much more difficult.

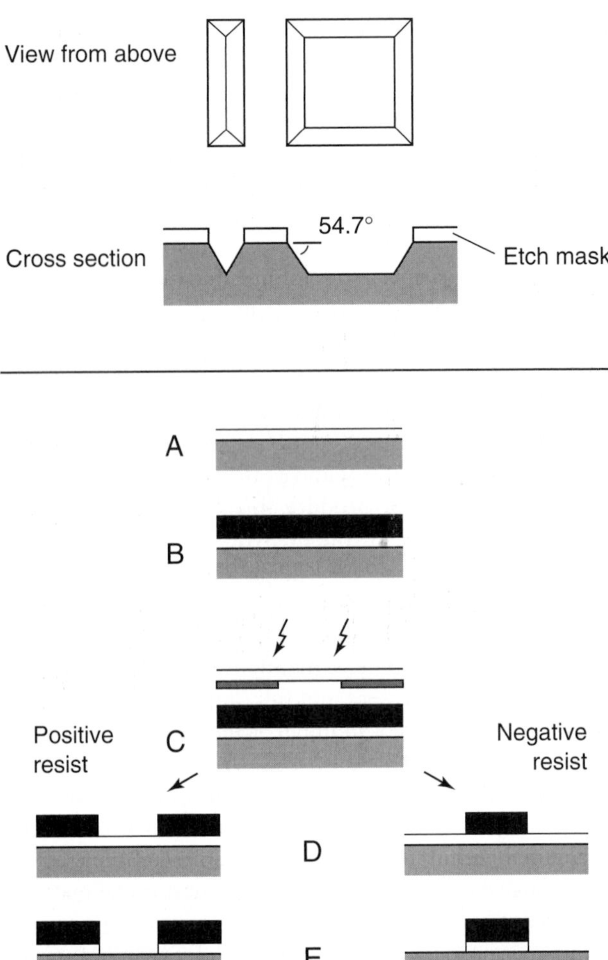

Figure 10-3 Schematic of the etching process used in photolithographic-based fabrication. Upper box: Anisotropic etch of silicone by KOH using silicon nitride mask. Lower box: **A,** Silicon wafer (hashed) with etch mask (white). **B,** Application of photo resist (black) onto etch mask. **C,** Exposure of photo resist through photo mask. **D,** Positive and negative photo resist after development of resist. **E,** Removal of etch mask. **F,** Removal of photo resist, leaving either the pattern present in the photo mask or its opposite patterned into the etch mask.

Dry Etching

This type of etching does not use any chemicals directly on the wafer; instead the most popular method involves accelerating ions toward the wafer to be etched. These ions will etch more in the direction in which they are traveling. This method is called reactive ion etching (RIE). RIE is an anisotropic etching method because the direction of the etching controls the rate of etching (see Figure 10-3). In the final steps, the photo resist and the silicon oxide layers are removed to give the final etched silicon wafer. By using multiple masks and sacrificial layers that permit undercutting to produce movable components, it is possible to fabricate complex multicomponent structures on the surface of a silicon wafer. All of these fabrication steps are performed in a clean room environment, thus permitting the production of sterile devices suitable for in vivo or clinical application.

Molding of Polymeric Materials

The LIGA process was developed at the Institut für Mikrostrukturtechnik (IMT) at the German University of Karlsruhe, in the early eighties under the leadership of W. Ehrfeld. LIGA is an German acronym (Lithographie, Galvanoformung, Abformung) standing for the main steps of the process; it involves deep x-ray lithography,[142] electroforming, and plastic molding. These three steps make it possible to mass produce microcomponents at a low cost.

In practice, the LIGA process provides a way to manufacture a mold for a microstructure. It consists of the following steps. First, a resist-coated substrate is patterned using a mask and a source of synchrotron radiation (oriented x-rays). Secondly, after development, the resist structure is electroplated. This electroforming produces a metal microstructure (a negative replica of the structure), and this is then used as the mold for the final structure. Advantages of the LIGA process are that high aspect ratios are attained (e.g., lateral dimensions of a few μm and vertical dimensions of up to 1000 μm), and the molds can be used to prepare multiple replicas of the structure in a variety of materials (e.g., polyimide, polymethylmethacrylate [PMMA]).[8]

Direct molding using a silicon master and a thermoplastic fluoropolymer (e.g., Hostaflon) at 150 °C and at a pressure of 50 kg/cm^2 has been employed to fabricate channels for performing electrophoresis. The plastic molded part was then clamped between two plates to complete the sealing of the channel. Other methods have also been employed to create microfluidic devices in various polymeric materials.[54] Laser ablation of poly dimethylsiloxane (PDMS) has been used to create elastomeric molds that pattern structures,[48,125] or nickel molds produced from a silicon master pattern device from acrylic polymers[89] or polystyrene.[160] Copolyester microfluidic devices have also been constructed using this principle for use in ultrafiltration of food contaminants and for use in drug screening.[59] Other devices for capillary electrophoresis of DNA samples have been made by compression molding of polycarbonate against a silicon master.[79,83] In some of these devices using polymeric materials, such as polyimides, the molding has been coupled with metallization layers to allow the production of electrodes inside or outside the fluidic channels.[76,91] With all of these structures, there is a need for bonding or sealing processes that allow the formation of channels or chambers.

Incorporation of Electronic Components

Another requirement in certain microchips is the incorporation of electronic components, such as electrodes (see Chapter 4).[138] So-called bioelectronic chips have been constructed that use arrays of platinum electrodes (80 μm in diameter) coated with streptavidin. By modifying the charge applied to the electrodes, molecules such as DNA or RNA are differentially attracted to, or displaced from, the electrode surfaces.[16,42]

DRILLING

Mechanical, ultrasonic, and laser drilling are processes also used to fabricate chambers in microdevices. Laser drilling is particularly suited for drilling very small size holes (e.g., less than 2 μm using a deep UV excimer laser).[5] This type of drilling is of increasing importance for the manufacture of devices used for high throughput systems that are used for ion channel studies on isolated cells in the pharmaceutical industry where exact holes of approximately 1 μm are required.[152] In these situations, the contours of the small holes being created and the surrounding surface area are critical to success, and the demanding criteria are rarely met by silicon with its crystalline structure.

Chambers have also been drilled through glass by means of an electrodischarge process in which the glass is submerged in an alkaline solution (e.g., NaOH) and a needle (30-μm diameter tip) contacting the glass and a negative potential applied (40 volts).[122]

BONDING AND SEALING

Sealing structures to produce liquid-tight enclosures (chambers and channels) is a key step in the fabrication of a microdevice. Several different processes are available depending on the materials employed. However, in nearly all cases some method of surface cleaning is necessary before the bonding process.

Surface Cleaning

One of the most common methods of cleaning surfaces for subsequent sealing is the use of the so-called "piranha clean," which involves emersion in a mixture of H_2SO_4 and H_2O_2 (3:1) followed by washing with deionized water. When this method is unsuitable (e.g., the device contains metal electrodes), then alternative methods—such as treatment of the surfaces with oxygen plasma[141] or laser radiation[143]—have been used.

Anodic Bonding

Pyrex glass has been bonded to silicon using an anodic bonding technique.[1] With it, the thermal expansion coefficients of the two materials are similar thus residual stress after bonding is minimized. Operationally, a mirror-polished, clean flat piece of glass is placed on top of a clean piece of polished silicon and heated to near the annealing point of the glass (180 °C to 500 °C). A negative voltage of 200 to 1000 volts is applied by attaching electrodes to the silicon (anode) and glass (cathode). The DC voltage creates an electric field between the two surfaces and pulls them into contact. This electrostatic attraction arises as follows: glass behaves as an electrolyte at high temperature, and there is a migration of ions (mostly Na^+ from the dissociation of Na_2O) toward the cathode that leaves a residual negative charge on the glass surface adjacent to the silicon surface. The actual bond is believed to be chemical, possibly a thin layer of silicon dioxide. Other materials have also been bonded using this process, including gallium arsenide–glass and silicon-silicon. The latter is achieved by first sputtering a thin layer of Pyrex glass (4 µm thick) onto one of the silicon surfaces.[61] Glass has also been bonded to glass using a simple thermal cycle process[35] or without thermal treatment if rigorous cleaning is used[20] or using a UV curable glue at room temperature.[55]

Eutectic Bonding

This method is used for bonding two silicon surfaces. A thin layer of gold is coated onto the surface of one of the wafers, or a thin sheet of gold-silicon or gold-tin mixture is placed between the two surfaces (a preform). The assembled device is then clamped together and heated in a vacuum chamber above the eutectic temperature for the particular materials (e.g., eutectic temperature for Si/Au is 36 °C). The preform melts and a diffusion process (gold into the silicon surface) leads to the formation of a silicon alloy between the contacted surfaces. As this cools, a bond is formed between the two surfaces.[61]

Other Bonding Methods

Other methods of bonding include direct bonding[127] and clamping.[118] However, most of these methods preclude the treatment of channels or chambers within the device before bonding. Several methods have been employed for bonding polymeric materials. These include pressure between aluminum plates[59] and the use of adhesives or materials modified by UV light.[29]

MICROFLUIDICS

Microfluidics is a key functionality in the success of microdevices. It is defined as a branch of physics and biotechnology that studies the behavior of fluids at the microscale and mesoscale, volumes thousands of times smaller than a common droplet. It also concerns the design of systems in which such small volumes of fluids will be used. For example, the gene chips and labs-on-a-chip are based on the transport of nanoliter or picoliter volumes of fluids through microchannels within a glass or plastic chip.

The success of microfluidics research is seen in the innovative designs of microdevices that have been constructed so that either stable fluid flow or chaotic mixing is achieved depending on the requirement. To ensure adequate mixing, numerous systems have been developed. Some simple systems are based on the positioning of baffles in the flow stream; others achieve the mixing with complex three-dimensional serpentine structures[81,82] or use of closed loop devices.[158] Furthermore, the design of microfluidic devices that facilitate rapid analysis of sequential samples without carryover or the separation of particulate materials (e.g., blood cells or bead preparations) has required meticulous study of flow characteristics. Early studies in 1992 showed that electroosmotic pumping or electrokinesis could be used to control the movement of solutions in microcapillaries.[52,87] Later in 1994, it was demonstrated that using pressure, blood could be pumped through microchannels on a silicon microchip[148] without causing obstruction of the channels. Subsequently the science of microfluidics has expanded greatly to the point where this subject is regarded as a scientific discipline. In many devices, especially those involved with capillary electrophoresis, there is a requirement to accurately meter and mix nL volumes of liquids with great precision followed by transfer of a small aliquot to a detection area.[86] These activities are now characterized in terms of fluid dynamics, and future designs will be based on the understanding of these phenomena. An example of the progress made in such designs is illustrated in Figure 10-4.[46,109] Application of this type of design dramatically diminishes deterioration of sample integrity as it flows through a microchannel.

As the designs of microdevices have developed, there has also been an increasing demand to exploit this technology for high throughput screening, especially within the pharmaceutical industry. In an effort to accommodate this demand, creative designing has been necessary. In Figure 10-5 a microchip is shown that accommodates 96 capillary electrophoresis channels in one device.[117] Other developments have resulted in a device that allows for up to 384 parallel channels on one glass microchip (wafer).[32] However, the problem with such designs is achieving convenient peripheral equipment that allows (1) filling of the multichannel devices; (2) the parallel, or sequential, monitoring of the fluid flow; and (3) the detection and quantitation of the various reactions. As a result, it is important to ensure that a sample injection into microdevices occurs with as much precision and accuracy as the process requires. Ensuring that a sample is injected as a distinct bolus has initiated the design of numerous injection systems that are dictated by the pumping system being used.[41] Electrokinetic pumping (see Chapter 5) tends to employ T-junctions where the fluid flow is controlled by application of differential voltages, and pressure-based systems use rapid injection from syringes operated by pumps.

VALVING SYTEMS

To successfully implement microtechnology systems into the clinical laboratory, where accuracy and precision are

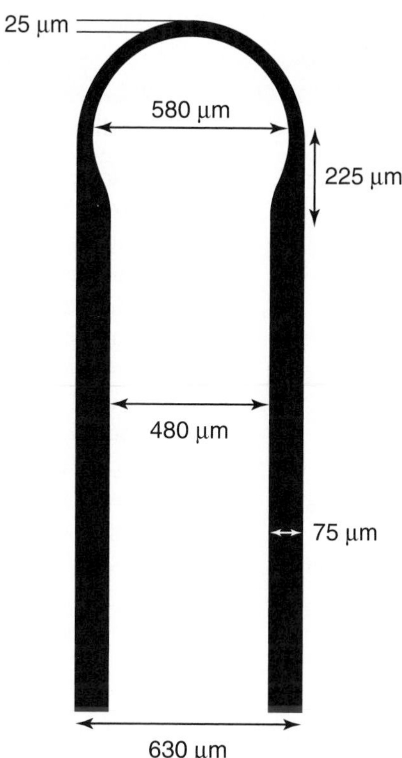

Figure 10-4 Design of an asymmetric turn used in microchip-based capillary electrophoresis system constructed in glass. The design facilitates the maintenance of sample integrity during flow in a microchannel around a curve. The dimensions are indicated on the figure and are taken from the tops of the channels. The channels were filled with black ink for contrast. *(From Ramsey JD, Jacobson SC, Culbertson CT, Ramsey JM. High efficiency, two-dimensional separations of protein digests on microfluidic devices. Anal Chem 2003;75:3758-64.)*

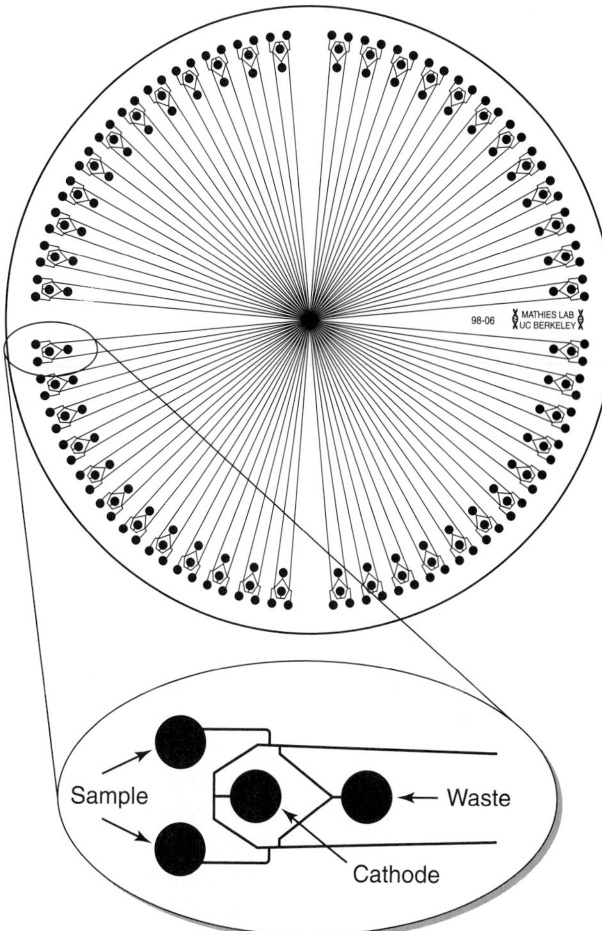

Figure 10-5 Design of a complex microfluidic device for parallel capillary electrophoresis. Figure shows the mask pattern for a 96-channel radial capillary electrophoresis microplate in glass. The separation channels with 200 μm twin-T injectors were masked to 10 μm width and then etched to form 110 μm wide by approximately 50 μm deep channels. The diameter of the reservoir holes is 1.2 mm. The distance from the injector to the detection point is 33 mm. The glass substrate is 10 cm in diameter. *(From Shi Y, Simpson PC, Scherer JR, et al. Radial capillary array electrophoresis microplate and scanner for high-performance nucleic acid analysis. Anal Chem 1999;71:5354-61.)*

mandatory requirements, there is basic requirement in many instances for accurate and precision volume metering of fluids and reagents.[115] In many reported applications on microchips, this requirement has not been included, or the requirement is circumvented by the use of internal standards.

However, to realize a practical and cost-effective system for biomedical applications, a microvalve system that will process human whole blood is essential. To date, most microvalve systems have been microfabricated from silicon,[123] although valves using plastic membranes have also been developed.[159] Chip-based microvalve systems have been classified as either active microvalves (with an actuator) or passive (check) microvalves (without an actuator).[123] The miniaturization of the active microvalve systems is restricted by the size of the actuator.

Actuators used for the active microvalve systems include solenoid plungers,[128] bimetallic actuators,[58] and piezoelectric actuators.[34,120,121] However, numerous other principles have been employed, such as springs,[120] pneumatic pressure,[99] or electrostatic[45] or electromagnetic forces.[155] Other microvalve systems have been developed that employ a variety of principles, including hydrogel bistrips that are activated and deactivated by pH change[156] or a bistable gate valve, actuated by electrolytically generated gas bubbles.[102] However, none of these systems have been widely adopted even though one of them may well provide the basis of future analytical platforms.

The characteristics of the silicon chip–based active and passive microvalve systems have been reviewed.[159] As expected, the sizes of the passive microvalve systems were generally smaller than the active microvalve systems, and the response time of the active microvalve systems ranged from 5 milliseconds to 10 seconds, whereas many of the passive microvalve systems based on electrokinetic forces in

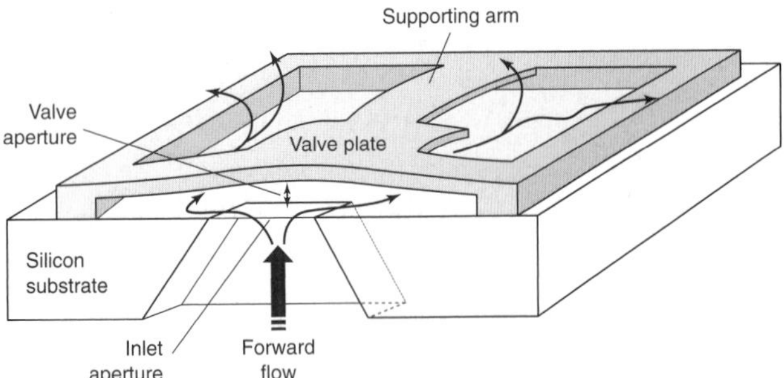

Figure 10-6 Example of a microfluidic valve constructed in silicon (1200 × 1200 μm) with an etched aperture to form the inlet for gas or liquid. The movable valve plate is supported by four polycrystalline-silicon arms, 400 μm long and 200 μm wide, attached to the silicon substrate. *(From: Bien DCS, Mitchell SJN, Gamble HS. Fabrication and characterization of a micromachined passive valve. J Micromech Microeng 2003;13:557-62.)*

TABLE 10-2 General and Medical Applications of Nanotechnology and Microtechnology

General Applications	Medical Applications
Analytical chemistry	Basic research
Biotechnology	Disease discovery
Combinatorial chemistry	Drug development
Electronics	Drug manufacturing
Engineering	Gene expression
Environmental monitoring	Genotyping
Fabrication	Genomics
Fluidics	Medical diagnostics
Materials science	Medical screening
Pharmaceuticals	Nucleic acid analysis
Reactor technology	Proteomics
Robotics	
Waste minimization	

microchannels can operate in microseconds. Silicon chip–based microvalve systems for medical and biomedical applications are still limited, especially a microvalve system that is suitable for whole blood handling. Developing an effective microvalve for use with body fluids and suspensions of particulates (e.g., whole blood) represents a major challenge because passive types of valves based on electrokinesis will not handle these types of fluids. Overcoming this challenge is a vital step toward developing practical totally integrated microfluidic systems for blood analysis. A partly disposable three-way microvalve employing a silicon membrane also has been developed that claims to be suitable for whole blood handling using pneumatic actuation.[99] However, no data on whole blood handling in this valve are yet available. Integrated systems aimed at the clinical market are under development and prototype systems have been reported[17,47,119,149] for a variety of purposes. An example of a microfluidic valve is shown in Figure 10-6.

APPLICATIONS

As previously stated, the scope of applications of nanotechnology and microtechnology in science, industry, and medicine is extremely wide and diverse (Table 10-2). Here we wish to emphasize those applications with relationships or relevance to biomedicine, even though many of the scientists involved in the field work strictly in the disciplines of electroengineering and mechanical engineering, microfluidics, and industrial physics. Examples are drawn from the wide assortment of applications to illustrate the direction and capability of this technology. Some of the applications in different fields employ the same principles or technology—such as microchip-based electrophoresis,[131] microarrays, or thermal cycling—but they are discussed according to their clinical subdiscipline.

Genomics

Microdevices and microtechnological developments have had their greatest impact in the field of genomics, and thousands of papers have been published describing their application in this arena. In essence the involvement covers several main areas, including techniques for DNA and amplification, hybridization arrays, sample preparation, and detection and quantitation of nucleic acids and small polynucleotides (see Chapters 36 and 37).

Early reports by Northrup et al[96] and Wilding, Kricka, and colleagues[17,150] established that DNA amplification using the polymerase chain reaction (PCR) was possible in a microchip. Both groups used elementary microchambers etched in silicon and demonstrated that effective amplification could be achieved. Subsequent reports indicated that this technology, including microfluidics, provided effective, reliable, and precise (CV less than 10%)[150] nucleic acid amplification on a microchip.[73,148] Using elementary microchips, this degree of performance of PCR on a chip was attained with volumes of 10 to 50 μL of PCR reaction mixtures containing target DNA, Taq-polymerase, DNA primers, and the requisite nucleotides that were heated by external thermocyclers. Early efforts were successful, but the reports lacked evidence of the reliability, precision, and sensitivity of amplification, and it soon became apparent that other issues, such as surface chemistry[149] and good heating control,[95,151] had to be resolved before effective systems could be developed. Based on earlier work using glass capillary-based devices and forced air heating,[151] it was assumed that very short cycling times for PCR would be achieved. However, forced air for thermocycling seems an unlikely basis for more complex devices.

Since the early demonstrations of microchip-based PCR, numerous authors have reviewed the topic and forecast the direction that this technology will follow.* The large number of potential applications in the clinical laboratory based on DNA amplification made this an attractive field for commercial reasons. Other reviews† have described the role of microchip-based PCR and reverse transcription PCR (RT-PCR) in DNA sequencing and genetic analysis and the problems of process control and the state of the art.

It was projected in the mid-1990s that chip-based devices would become more complex and incorporate features that would facilitate sample preparation, amplification, and amplicate detection. As a result, the next generation of chip-based devices not only brought complexity but a clear awareness of the limitations and hurdles that microchip-based technologies present. As of 2005, the majority of the benefits of using microchip-based devices for PCR are still perceived, rather than realized. It has been assumed since the first illustration of microchip-based PCR in the early 1990s that features such as low-reagent consumption, low-volume sample requirements, and rapid cycle times would be a consequence of this technology. However, the ability to couple the PCR process with other features such as sample preparation and amplicate detection quickly initiated a drive to the design and construction of integrated devices, that ultimately should provide more convenient and cheaper methods in the many fields in which molecular biology is practiced. The expected economy of scale of manufacturing has yet to be realized, but it is assumed that the pattern will follow that of the electronics industry where millions of microdevices are produced at low cost. This is a realistic projection, because it is likely that the microdevices that ultimately serve the needs of the analyst and researcher will eventually incorporate much of the degree complexity of electronic microchips. Furthermore, because of the relative simplicity of the biological microchips and the roles they will serve, it is probable that the manufacturing processes will be more likely based on plastic than silicon.

Many commercial and academic centers that are exploring this technology have already demonstrated that DNA targets from several biological systems, including the human genome, viruses, and microbes, can be amplified by PCR on miniaturized devices.[4,62,116] Newer developments have been directed toward total systems (Figure 10-7) that incorporate sample preparation, amplification, and detection.[18,60,74,139,140] These developments achieve greater convenience and shorter cycle times for the PCR. Another approach used to achieve faster cycle time has been to use a microfluidic chip that pumps nL quantities of PCR-reaction mixture through a circular channel arranged over three heaters that facilitate denaturation, annealing, and extension during the PCR.[80]

The fields in which the growth of microchip-based genomics have first emerged relate to drug development in the pharmaceutical industry where determination of inhibition or enhancement of nucleotide replication is important. Other early products include devices designed for the defense industry, where the detection and identification of toxic agents is desirable. Another key area is the provision of products that facilitate the parallel operation of PCR on microsamples for the life sciences where production of sufficient amplicate is a requisite for sequencing studies.

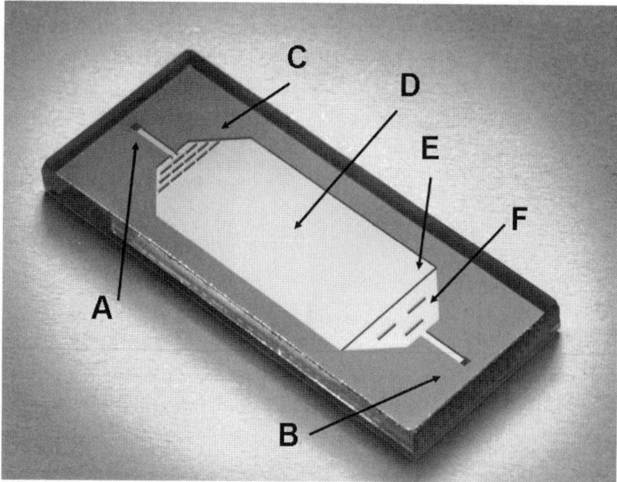

Figure 10-7 Silicon-glass microchip (14×35 mm) for cell isolation and PCR. By flowing 1.0 μL of whole blood into the chamber, WBCs can be isolated on the filter bed. PCR is performed after releasing the cells back into the main microchip chamber. Thermocycling is achieved by external heating. *A,* Entrance port to chip. *B,* Exit port from chip. *C,* Deflectors for forward flow. *D,* Chip chamber that is 80 μm deep and passivated with 2000 angstroms of thermal oxide. *E,* Filter bed having 667 pillars (10×20 μm, 3.3 μm gaps). *F,* Exit baffles.

Hybridization Arrays

Hybridization arrays are now widely used in genomic research (see Chapter 37). Primarily these arrays have been developed to meet the growing demands of pharmaceutical research. However, there are few academic centers today that do not have core facilities to prepare low- and high-density arrays to meet the requirements of academic research studying gene expression.

The basic principle underlying hybridization arrays is the immobilization of a DNA probe onto a planar surface of glass, silicon, or polymer material. The length of the DNA probe may vary greatly depending on the nature or role of the array. Attachment of probes to the surface has become a complex science involving coupling reagents, spacer molecules, and customized surface chemistry. Hybridization generally requires single-stranded DNA as both a probe and a sample. To facilitate detection of successful hybridization, a fluorescent tag is added to the sample. Moreover the density and size of individual spots on any array have varied from less than 10 on a glass slide to over 10,000 per square cm in

*References 9-11, 14, 15, 30, 67, 68, 97, 107, 110, 144.

†References 3, 62, 97, 98, 112, 132, 162.

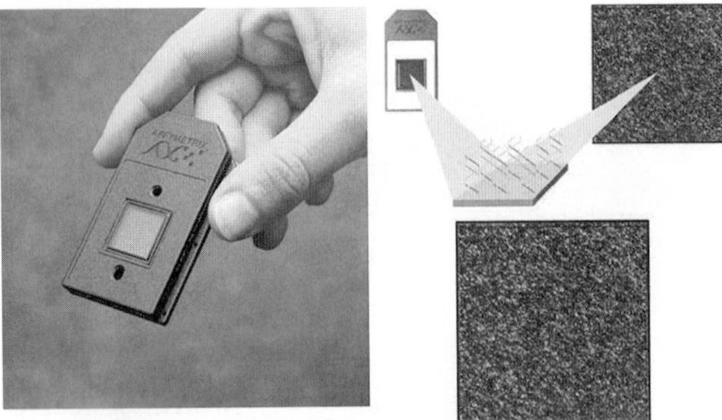

Figure 10-8 Microarray device showing principle and detail of high-density array. *(Courtesy Affymetrix Corp, Palo Alto, Calif.)*

certain commercial products. Methods for creating or manufacturing arrays vary from simple spotting of a DNA probe solution with a micropipette to complex photolithographic techniques, as used by the Affymetrix Corp., that allow for the synthesis of each probe in a spot to create oligonucleotides up to 20 base pairs or more (Figure 10-8).[6,38,39]

The conditions under which the hybridization process takes place have varied from 24 hours in certain static systems to a few minutes in some of the newer devices with microfluidic flow and mixing features. Detection of the hybridization is effected with an array reader that quantitates the level of fluorescence and identifies the location of the spot. When the array is high density, the reader frequently involves confocal microscopy and considerable computing capacity. Because partial hybridization can occur, usually caused by use of an inappropriate length of probe or sample DNA, the fluorescent signal is modified. Therefore the interpretation of high-density array information is complex. In efforts to improve the specificity of hybridization, many techniques have been developed, which include the use of microarrays created on electrodes that facilitate the selection of appropriate targets and the elimination of interfering molecules or other materials. A technique of so-called electronic stringency has been developed to achieve this by the Nanogen Corp.[16,114] Other expanding technologies based on hybridization arrays are those used for gene expression and gene mapping.[30] For this procedure, the assessment of sample quality is required to prevent the inappropriate use of expensive arrays. As a result, convenient microchip-based capillary electrophoresis devices have been developed that facilitate the assessment of DNA and RNA preparations and that are capable of providing a fast and accurate determination of the size and quantity of DNA or RNA fragments. One device (The Agilent 2100, Agilent Technologies, Palo Alto, Calif.) analyzes up to 12 specimens in less than 30 minutes using only 1 μL of a sample[94,101] and incorporates up to 13 internal standards. This device has also been adapted to facilitate testing of protein solutions.

Nucleic Acid Sequencing

The human genome project has been successful in the sequencing of the human genome (see Chapter 36) using conventional technology. However, it is now apparent that advancements made in microtechnology will provide another opportunity for the biologist eager to sequence DNA. Using long capillary channels fabricated in microfluidic devices of glass or silicon, several workers have demonstrated successful sequencing of up to 800 base pairs with a reported accuracy of 99%. The microdevices involved used 16-channel electrophoresis arrays,[82] 40-cm-long microchannels,[63] or a radially conformed 96-channel microcapillary electrophoresis system.[100] Using such systems, a dramatic improvement in the speed of sequencing has been achieved, resulting in parallel sequencing separations of 450 bases in less than 15 minutes.

Drug Detection and Assay

The huge commercial potential for the development of assays for therapeutic drugs or drugs of abuse that employ microsamples and disposable microdevices has yet to be realized. However, it is clear that assays for these compounds will be performed in a convenient manner and will impact the clinical laboratory in the near future. An early report showed that serum theophylline could be measured using immunoassay and capillary chromatography on a microchip.[133] Subsequent work illustrated the successful measurement of imipramine and desipramine in human plasma using capillary electrophoresis– and mass spectrometry–based microchips[25] and drug screening assays for barbiturates and phenobarbital antibodies.[59] The problem with these assays is that no device has yet been produced that meets the requirements of "user friendliness" necessary for the busy clinical laboratory or the rigid specifications demanded for recording quality assurance data.

Protein Chips

It is expected that microdevices that facilitate studies on the existence and classification of protein chips will have a great impact on the emerging field of proteonomics (see Chapter 43). For example, microarrays printed or spotted with proteins have already been developed.[75,85] However, problems were encountered obtaining the prerequisite specificity of binding between the antigens and antibodies. In addition, arrays containing thousands of phage libraries or unique clones have now been constructed using glass, hydrogels, or gold,[28,49] but again problems with identification were encountered. It has been found that some proteins incur structural changes when attached to solid surfaces. These efforts have also demonstrated that "blocking proteins" are useful to diminish nonspecific binding. In addition, new immobilization strategies and techniques are being developed that optimize the binding of the receptor protein (antibody or antigen) to the surface of a chip. As with the DNA array, detection is usually accomplished with fluorescent tags,[84,161] but other methods, including radiolabels or mass spectrometry,[43] have been employed.

Immunoassay for Antibodies and Peptides

One of the earliest efforts of qualitative measurement of a protein (human serum albumin) in a microchip-based device was based on bead agglutination in a microchamber (approximately 10 μL).[147] Subsequently, several quantitative immunoassays have been performed using microchip electrophoretic systems that permit separation and quantitation of free- and bound-labeled antigens in competitive assays (see Chapter 5). Most are carried out in channels micromachined into fused silica substrates. Early work on quantitative assays achieved measurement of cortisol in serum.[64] The assay used cortisol labeled with fluorescein and an argon laser detector at 488 nm and required only 80 μL of a 40× dilution of serum as the sample. Other capillary electrophoresis–based assays for a variety of antibodies have also been developed that include immunoglobulins (IgG, IgA, and IgM), antibovine serum albumin, and antiestradiol.[19]

Isolation of target proteins using immobilized antibodies or proteins on bead or microchannel surfaces has also been successfully demonstrated. Other assays for IgG and IgA using magnetic or polystyrene microbeads in microchip assays have demonstrated that viable alternatives to capillary electrophoresis do exist. In another microchip method, polystyrene beads were introduced into a glass microchannel and then human secretory immunoglobulin A (s-IgA) adsorbed on the microbead surface. This in turn was reacted with colloidal gold conjugated anti-s-IgA antibody and detected by a thermal lens microscope.[113] This system creates an environment that shortens the antigen antibody reaction to less than 10 minutes and has a level of detection of approximately 1 μg/mL, far below the requirements of a clinical assay.

A 2002 variation of a microchip-based immunoassay employs amperometric detection of the redox tracer ferrocene after separation by capillary electrophoresis.[137] A direct assay (noncompetitive) involves (1) mixing the ferrocene-tagged antibody and an antigen analyte, (2) rapid electrophoretic separation of labeled free antibody and the labeled antigen and/or antibody complex, and (3) a downstream anodic detection of the ferrocene tracer at a gold-plated carbon screen-printed electrode detector. The competitive assay integrates precolumn reactions of the labeled antigen and the target antigen with the antibody with electrophoretic separation of the free- and bound-labeled antigens, along with amperometric detection of the redox tag. In this study, the authors state that the use of a redox tracer offers the advantages of simplified protocol, wider linear range, higher stability, and higher separation efficiency compared with an analogous use of enzyme tags. Assays for direct mouse-immunoglobulin G (IgG) and the competitive 3,3′,5-triiodo-L-thyronine (T3) were accomplished within less than 150 and 130 seconds, respectively, and offer minimum detectable concentrations of 2.5, 10, 12 and 1, 10, 6 g/mL, respectively.

The technique of isoelectric focusing has proven to be a useful tool in protein chemistry, and this too has been adapted to the microchip. Using 7-cm-long channels in glass microchips (200 μm wide and 10 μm deep) mixtures of Cy5-labeled peptides can be focused in less than 30 seconds.[53] This same procedure has also been applied to plastic microchips made from PMMA by laser ablation and shown to focus mixtures of peptides labeled with rhodamine green.[53,108] Results for this type of microchannel isoelectric focusing are available in less than 5 minutes compared with traditional techniques that take over 1 hour.

The scope of assays using microchips has also encompassed lipoproteins. Low-density lipoprotein analyses have been performed in an uncoated glass microchannel capillary electrophoresis chip.[14] Analyses using mixtures of lipoproteins isolated from blood have been completed in under 25 seconds. However, no convenient method is yet available for the clinical laboratory.

Enzymology

Several enzyme-based assays have been developed for microdevices but few, if any, are applicable to native biological specimens such as plasma or serum. This is mainly because the bulk of assays developed are carried out in devices employing capillary electrophoresis using electrokinesis as the driving force in the microdevice, which is unsuitable for liquids with high concentrations of ions, proteins, metabolites, or particulates (e.g., cells). However, it is anticipated that future convenient assays will be developed that will facilitate use of biological specimens, such as serum or plasma, using pressure-driven systems in microchips are perfected. The motivation for developing enzyme assays in microdevices has been derived mainly from the necessity to perform assays for multiple enzymes in high throughput screening of compounds that are candidates for therapeutic drugs. For this reason, multiplexed enzyme assays have been developed for groups of kinases and phospholipases using a single-use capillary electrophoresis type of microchips.[153] Also, successful use of microchip-based devices, again using capillary electrophoresis, has been developed for measurement of β-galactosidase, and inhibitory action on this enzyme[51] and acetylcholinesterase.[50] A generic microchip method has also been described that uses enzymatic detection for glucose, ethanol, theophylline, and amino acids.[134] Other microchip-based assays have also been developed for the measurement of protein kinases,[22] leucine aminopeptidase,[164] insulin, and glucose.[135]

Metabolites

Because the bulk of assays in the clinical chemistry laboratory stem from the various metabolites, the potential for microchip-based assays is extremely large. The possibility that multiple assays will be carried out using microsamples with minimal use of reagents has many implications for the clinical laboratory and the diagnostics industry. However, apart from an impressive list of assays available on the i-STAT device, which includes Na, K, chloride, urea nitrogen, creatinine, glucose, lactate, and ionized calcium,[56] the number of assays developed to date is few, and most rely on the use of microchip-based capillary electrophoresis with various forms of detection.

Simultaneous assays for glucose, uric acid, and ascorbic acid have been demonstrated in aqueous solutions of the analytes using a glass microchip system of capillary electrophoresis employing amperometric detection with a silver–silver chloride electrode.[136] Microchip-based capillary electrophoresis technology has also been adapted to measure carnitine and selected acylcarnitines in urine extracts by using mass spectrometry as the detection method.[24] A method using similar technology but with electrodes for detection has been used to measure homocysteine and glutathione in plasma.[104] This method measures homocysteine up to levels of 50 μMol/L, well above the healthy concentrations of 5 to 15 μMol/L.

An assay for uric acid in urine employing a PDMS and/or glass microchip for capillary electrophoresis has also been developed.[36] This device can achieve separation and quantitation of uric acid in less than 30 seconds and a linear response over a range of 0 to 100 μM/L. To facilitate this measurement, dilutions of urine of the order of fiftyfold to seventy-fivefold were required. Other similar devices for the renal markers creatine, creatinine, p-aminohippuric acid, and uric acid in urine,[135] and a microchip-based method for zone electrophoretic analysis of oxalate in urine have been reported.[163]

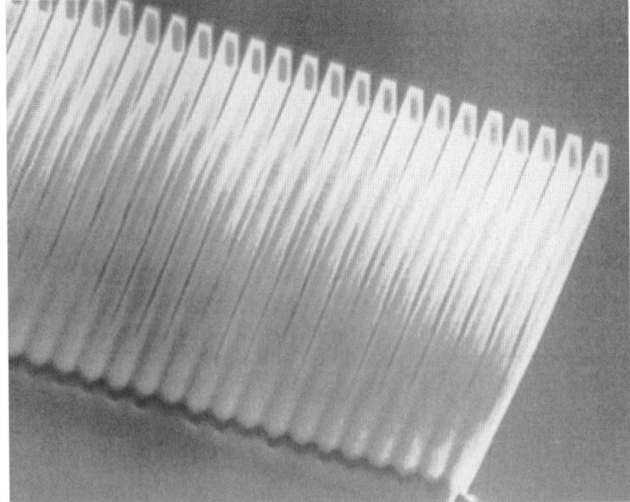

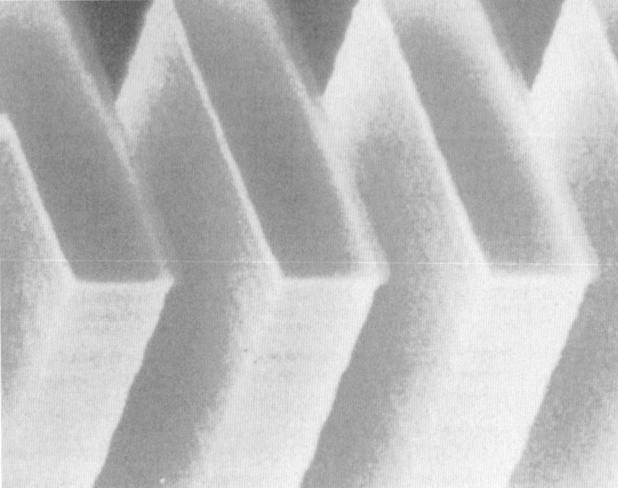

Figure 10-9 Microfiltration device made in silicon by reactive-ion etching. Upper picture shows low magnification of electron micrograph. Each pillar is 90 mm high. Lower picture shows detail of the gaps between filter elements (3.5 mm). Each pillar is 20 mm long and 10 mm wide, which allows easy passage of RBCs but precludes large granulocytes. *(Courtesy Wilding P, Kricka LJ, University of Pennsylvania.)*

Cell Handling and Cell Culture

Using the microenvironment of a microdevice to facilitate cell culture and the study of cellular behavior has resulted in several applications. For example, the incubation process of *E. coli* in a gas-permeable PDMS microfluidic device has been monitored by fluorescence[92]; also screening for agonists and antagonists in cultured cells has been achieved by monitoring calcium flux.[21] In addition, using specifically designed filter systems or electrodes, it was shown that cells could be isolated by size or charge from other populations or surrounding media followed by a variety of treatments, such as immunoattachment, lysis, or DNA and RNA release. For example, the ability to create filter systems with selected pore sizes for isolation of white blood cells (WBCs) has been demonstrated starting with volumes of whole blood less than 5 μL.[40,146] Figure 10-9 illustrates the nature of a microfilter used for this purpose.

Additional applications include the study of red blood cell (RBC) mobility[7] and chemotaxis and locomotion of WBCs in a confined environment.[12]

Other Applications

Other avenues of miniaturization are being pursued that have medical applications. These include the opportunity to manipulate analytes and cells to (1) provide improved methods of reagent and sample transfer; (2) mix aliquots using techniques such as electrokinesis[110]; (3) isolate or separate macromolecules or cells by filtration[146] and electrical charge; (4) ensure electronic stringency[16]; and (5) use nanoparticles to measure biomolecules.[105]

SURFACE CHEMISTRY ISSUES

An early discovery during the development of microchip PCR was the importance of surface chemistry in microchip operation and design.[119,149] This work demonstrated that PCR in silicon microchips was severely inhibited if the surface chemistry was unsuitable. These workers noted that the increase in surface area in microchips, relative to volume, could be twentyfold greater compared with conventional tubes used for PCR. Moreover, if the surface was only partially coated or existed as silicon, silicon nitride, or certain other substances, then it was very difficult to achieve reproducible or adequate amplification. However, successful and reproducible amplification could be achieved if the surface was subjected to coating with a suitable passivating layer (e.g., 2000 angstroms of silicon oxide). Passivation of the silicon surface has also been achieved with polymeric coatings of the microchip channels and chambers[93] or by silanization of glass microchips followed by a coating of polyacrylimide.[74]

Other studies have sought to employ other substrates with fewer problems, but the inherent one of increased surface-to-volume ratio always applies. One of the approaches has been to incorporate substances such as polyethylene glycol (PEG), polyvinylpyrrolidone (PVP), or epoxy compounds that significantly reduce or eliminate binding of analytes or key reagents to surfaces.[44] Others have used silanization followed by coating of the channels or chambers with polymeric compounds.[93] Additionally, microchip-based capillary electrophoresis devices constructed from PDMS and glass have been modified with a three-layer biotin-neutravidin sandwich coating, made of biotinylated IgG, neutravidin, and biotinylated dextran. By replacing biotinylated dextran with any biotinylated reagent, the modified surface can be readily patterned with biochemical probes, such as antibodies.[77,78]

LIMITATIONS OF MICROTECHNOLOGY

The limitations of microtechnology are invariably related to the concentration of the analyte or type of cell under study. If the device is only capable of receiving microliter quantities, then the final signal strength being measured will depend on the inclusion of an amplification process (e.g., PCR) or the ability to detect extremely low levels of analyte concentration or type of cell identification. For example, only 0.5 μL of whole blood are necessary to allow for isolation of 500 WBCs, more than sufficient to provide genomic DNA for mutation detection by PCR. Similarly, submicroliter quantities of protein or DNA solutions provide adequate material for analysis by capillary electrophoresis (see Chapter 5). However, if the aim is to identify and isolate an infected WBC in whole blood that is present at an incidence of only 1 in 10 million, then quantities in excess of 10 mL of whole blood may be required just to encounter 5 cells. This does not provide the ideal situation for a microdevice. Another key limitation, namely the impact of surface chemistry, has been addressed in a previous section.

An application in microchip technology that highlights the limitation of the sole use of microtechnology is the use of a microfabricated filter to enhance the enrichment of fetal cells in a preparation that will be used for genomic studies.[126,154] In this study, the goal was to provide a sample that contains 5 to 50 nucleated red blood cells (n-RBCs) of fetal origin so that chromosomal or genomic studies could be performed. The starting specimen for this isolation and/or enrichment procedure is 20 mL of maternal blood, and so the 5 to 50 fetal n-RBCs are being isolated from a matrix containing approximately 100 billion adult RBCs, 100 million adult WBCs, and 1.4 g of protein. The encouraging data resulting from this work is achieved only because microtechnology is used in combination with preparative steps using conventional technology (cell agglutination and immunoprecipitation with magnetic beads). This example illustrates that successful application of microtechnology in the clinical field will probably result in hybrid systems that exploit both conventional and microtechnology.

THE FUTURE

The future of nanotechnology and microfabrication in the clinical field, particularly where it will impact the clinical laboratory, is difficult to forecast. However, because the necessity to reduce analytical costs is a constant theme there is little doubt that products of this technology will be implemented and used. Moreover, as the demand grows for increased effort at the point of care, coupled with the growing demand to achieve low-cost, high-throughput screening for malignancies and other diseases, it is inevitable that microtechnology will be a developing science for many years. Forecasting which subdisciplines in laboratory medicine will be the first to benefit is more difficult. The advances made in microcapillary electrophoresis, nucleic acid amplification, and the many detection techniques suggest that molecular pathology will benefit first, but that many other subdisciplines will soon follow. The application of nanostructures and the manipulation of molecular architecture to facilitate clinical assays have already commenced with the use of nanosized beads as labels for ligands or antibodies and for the modification of surface chemistry.[70,71] However, it will be necessary for these technologies to surpass current achievements using present day techniques and to compete on an economic basis in the ever demanding world of healthcare.

REFERENCES

1. Albaugh KB, Cade PE, Rasmussen D. Mechanism of anodic bonding of silicon to Pyrex glass. Tech Dig. IEEE Solid-State Sens. Actuator Workshop. Hilton Head, SC, 1988:109-10.
2. Angell JB, Terry SC, Barth PW. Silicon micromechanical devices. Sci Am 1983;248:44-55.
3. Auroux PA, Lossifidis D, Reyes DR, Manz A. Micro total analysis systems. 2. Analytical standard operations and applications. Anal Chem 2002;74:2637-52.
4. Belgrader P, Benett W, Hadley D, Long G, Mariella RJ, Milanovich F, et al. Rapid pathogen detection using a microchip PCR array instrument. Clin Chem 1998;44:2191-4.
5. Bellows G, Kohls JB. Drilling without drills. Am Mach Special Rep 1982;743:173-88.

6. Bowtell DDL. Options available-from start to finish-for obtaining expression data by microarray. Nature Genet 1999;21 (Suppl.):33-7.
7. Brody JP, Han Y, Austin RH, Bitensky M. Deformation and flow of red blood cells in a synthetic lattice: evidence for an active cytoskeleton. Biophys J 1995;68:2224-32.
8. Bryzek J, Peterson K, McCully W. Micromachines on the march. IEEE Spectrum 1994;31:20-31.
9. Burke DT, Burns MA, Mastrangelo C. Microfabrication technologies for integrated nucleic acid analysis. Genome Res 1997;7:189-97.
10. Burns MA, Johnson BN, Brahmasandra SN, Handique K, Webster JR, Krishnan Mea. An integrated nanoliter DNA analysis device. Science 1998;282: 484-7.
11. Burns MA, Mastrangelo CH, Sammarco TS, Man FP, Webster JR, Johnsons BN, et al. Microfabricated structures for integrated DNA analysis. Proc Natl Acad Sci U S A 1996;93:5556-61.
12. Carlson RH, Gabel C, Chan S, Austin RH. Activation and sorting of human white blood cells. J Biomed Devices 1998;1:39-47.
13. Cassaday M, Diebler H, Herron R, Pelavin M, Svenjak D, Vlastelica D. Capsule chemistry technology for high-speed clinical chemistry analysis. Clin Chem 1985;31:1453-6.
14. Ceriotti L, Shibata T, Folmer B, Weiller BH, Roberts MA, de Rooij NF, et al. Low density lipoprotein analysis in microchip capillary electrophoresis systems. Electrophoresis 2002;23:3615-22.
15. Cheng J, Fortina P, Surrey S, Kricka LJ, Wilding P. Microchip-based devices for molecular diagnosis of genetic diseases. Mol Diagn 1996;1:183-200.
16. Cheng J, Sheldon EL, Wu L, Uribe A, Gerrue LO, Carrino J, et al. Preparation and hybridization analysis of DNA/RNA from E.coli on microfabricated bioelectronic chips. Nature Biotechnol 1998;16:541-6.
17. Cheng J, Shoffner MA, Hvichia GE, Kricka LJ, Wilding P. Chip PCR. II. Investigation of different PCR amplification systems in microfabricated silicon glass chips. Nucleic Acids Res 1996;24:380-5.
18. Cheng J, Waters LC, Fortina P, Hvichia G, Jacobson SC, Ramsey JM, et al. Degenerate oligonucleotide primed-polymerase chain reaction and capillary electrophoretic analysis of human DNA on microchip-based devices. Anal Biochem 1998;257:101-6.
19. Cheng SB, Skinner CD, Taylor J, Attiya S, Lee WE, Picelli G, et al. Development of a multichannel microfluidic analysis system employing affinity capillary electrophoresis for immunoassay. Anal Chem 2001;73:1472-9.
20. Chiem N, Lockyear-Schultz L, Andersson P, Skinner C, Harrison DJ. Room temperature bonding of micromachined glass devices for capillary electrophoresis. Sens Actuators B 2000;63:147-52.
21. Chow A, Kopf-Sill A, Nikiforov T, Zhou A, Coffin J, Wada G, et al. Proceedings of Micro Total Analysis Systems 2000. Dordrecht, The Netherlands: Kluwer Academic Publishers, 2000:489-92.
22. Cohen CB, Chin-Dixon E, Jeong S, Nikiforov TT. A microchip-based enzyme assay for protein kinase A. Anal Biochem 1999;273:89-97.
23. Colyer CL, Tang T, Chiem N, Harrison DJ. Clinical potential of microchip capillary electrophoresis systems. Electrophoresis 1997;18:1733-41.
24. Deng Y, Henion J, Li J, Thibault P, Wang C, Harrison DJ. Chip-based capillary electrophoresis/mass spectrometry determination of carnitines in human urine. Anal Chem 2001;73:639-46.
25. Deng Y, Zhang H, Henion J. Chip-based quantitative capillary electrophoresis/mass spectrometry determination of drugs in human plasma. Anal Chem 2001;73:1432-9.
26. Drexler KE. Molecular engineering: An approach to the development of general capabilities for molecular manipulation. Proc Natl Acad Sci USA 1981;78: 5275-8.
27. Drexler KE. Nanosystems: Molecular machinery, manufacturing, and computation. New York: John Wiley & Sons, 1992.
28. deWildt RM. Antibody arrays for high-throughput screening of antibody-antigen interactions. Nature Biotechnol 2000;18:989-94.
29. Duffy DC, Schueller OJA, Brittain ST, Whitesides GM. Rapid prototyping of microfluidic switches in poly(dimethyl siloxane) and their actuation by electroosmotic flow. J Micromech Microeng 1999;9: 211-7.
30. Eggers M, Erlich D. A review of microfabricated devices for gene-based diagnostics. Hematol Pathol 1995;9:1-15.
31. Ekins R, Chu FW. Microarrays: their origins and applications. Trends Biotechnol 1999;17: 217-8.
32. Emrich CA, Tian H, Medintz IL, Mathies RA. Microfabricated 384-lane capillary array electrophoresis bioanalyzer for ultrahigh-throughput genetic analysis. Anal Chem 2002;74:5076-83.
33. Erickson KA, Wilding P. Evaluation of a novel point-of-care system, the i-STAT portable clinical analyzer. Clin Chem 1993;39:283-7.
34. Esahi M. Integrated microflow control systems. Sensors Actuators A 1990;21/23:161-78.
35. Fan ZH, Harrison DJ. Micromachining of capillary electrophoresis injectors and separators on glass chips and evaluation of flow at capillary intersections. Anal Chem 1994;66:177-84.
36. Fanguy JC, Henry CS. The analysis of uric acid in urine using microchip capillary electrophoresis with electrochemical detection. Electrophoresis 2002;23:767-73.

37. Feynman R. There's Plenty of Room at the Bottom. In: Gilbert HD, ed. Miniaturization. New York: Reinhold, 1961: 282-96.
38. Fodor SPA, Rava RP, Huang XC, A.C. P, Holmes CP, Adams CL. Multiplexed biochemical assays with biological chips. Nature Biotechnol 1993;364:555-6.
39. Fodor SPA, Read JL, Pirrung MC, Stryer L, Lu AT, Solas D. Light-directed, spatially addressable parallel chemical synthesis. Science 1991;251:767-73.
40. Fortina P, Cheng J, Kricka LJ, Waters LC, Jacobson SC, Wilding P. DOP-PCR amplification of whole genomic DNA and microchip-based capillary electrophoresis. Methods in Molecular Biology 2001;163:211-9.
41. Fu LM, Yang RJ, Lee GB, Liu HH. Electrokinetic injection techniques in microfluidic chips. Anal Chem 2002;74:5084-91.
42. Gilles PN, Wu DJ, Foster CB, Dillon PJ, Channock SJ. Single nucleotide polymorphic discrimination by an electronic dot blot assay on semi-conductor microchips. Nature Biotechnol 1999;17:365-70.
43. Gilligan JJ, Schuck P, Yergey AL. Mass spectrometry after capture and small volume elution of analyte from a surface plasmon resonance biosensor. Anal Chem 2002;74:2041-7.
44. Giordano BC, Copeland ER, Landers JP. Towards dynamic coating of glass microchip chambers for amplifying DNA via the polymerase chain reaction. Electrophoresis 2001;22:334-40.
45. Goll C, Bacher W, Bustgens B, Maas D, Ruprecht R, Schomburg WK. An electrostatically actuated polymer microvalve equipped with a movable membrane electrode. J Micromech Microeng 1997;7:224-6.
46. Griffiths SK, Nilson RH. Low-dispersion turns and junctions for microchannel systems. Anal Chem 2001;73:272-8.
47. Grover WH, Skelley AM, Liu CN, Lagally ET, Mathies RA. Monolithic membrane valves and diaphragm pumps for practical large-scale integration into glass microfluidic devices. Sensors and Actuators B 2003;89:315-23.
48. Grzybowski BA, Haag R, Bowden N, Whitesides GM. Generation of micrometer sized patterns for micro-analytical applications using a laser direct-write method and microcontact printing. Anal Chem 1998;70:4645-52.
49. Haab BB. Advances in protein microarray technology for protein expression and interaction profiling. Curr Opin Drug Discov Devel 2001 Jan;4(1):116-23.
50. Hadd AG, Jacobson SC, Ramsey JM. Microfluidic Assays of Acetylcholinesterase Inhibitors. Anal Chem 1999;71:5206-12.
51. Hadd AG, Raymond DE, Halliwell JW, Jacobson SC, Ramsey JM. Microchip device for performing enzyme assays. Anal Chem 1997;69:3407-12.
52. Harrison DJ, Manz A, Fan ZH, Ludi H, Widdmer HM. Capillary Electrophoresis and Sample Injection Systems Integrated on a Planar Glass Chip. Anal Chem 1992;64:1926-32.
53. Hofmann O, Che D, Cruickshank KA, Muller UR. Adaptation of capillary isoelectric focusing to microchannels on a glass chip. Anal Chem 1999;71:678-86.
54. Hong JW, Hosokawa K, Fujii T, Seki M, Endo I. Microfabricated polymer chip for capillary gel electrophoresis. Biotechnol Prog 2001;17:958-62.
55. Huang Z, Sanders JC, Dunsmor C, Ahmadzadeh H, Landers JP. A method for UV-bonding in the fabrication of glass electrophoretic microchips. Electrophoresis 2001;22:3924-9.
56. Jacobs E, Vadasdi E, Sarkozi L, Colman N. Analytical evaluation of i-STAT Portable Clinical Analyzer and use by nonlaboratory health-care professionals. Clin Chem 1993;39:1069-74.
57. Jacobson SC, Ramsey JM. Integrated microdevice for DNA restriction fragment analysis. Anal Chem 1996;68:720-3.
58. Jerman H. Electrically-activated micromachined diaphragm valves. Technical Digest IEEE Sensors and Actuators Workshop, 1990:65-9.
59. Jiang Y, Wang PC, Locascio LE, Lee CS. Integrated plastic microfluidic devices with ESI-MS for drug screening and residue analysis. Anal Chem 2001;73:2048-53.
60. Khandurina J, McKnight TE, Jacobson SC, Waters LC, Foote RS, Ramsey JM. Integrated system for rapid PCR-based DNA analysis in microfluidic devices. Anal Chem 2000;72:2995-3000.
61. Ko WH, Suminto JT, Yeh GH. Bonding techniques for microsensors. In: Fung CD, Cheung PW, Ko WH, Fleming DG, eds. Micromachining and micropackaging of transducers. New York: Elsevier Science, 1985:41-61.
62. Kopp MU, Crabtree HJ, Manz A. Developments in technology and applications of microsystems. Curr Opin Chem Biol 1997;1:410-9.
63. Koutny L, Schmalzing D, Salas-Solano O, EI-Difrawy S, Adourian A, Buonocore S, et al. Eight hundred-base sequencing in a microfabricated electrophoretic device. Anal Chem 2000;72:3388-91.
64. Koutny LB, Schmalzing D, Taylor TA, Fuchs M. Microchip electrophoretic immunoassay for serum cortisol. Anal Chem 1996;68:18-22.
65. Kricka LJ, Nozaki O, Wilding P. Micromechanics and nanotechnology: implications and applications in the clinical laboratory. J Intnl Fed Clin Chem 1994;6:52-6.
66. Kricka LJ, Wilding P. Micromachining: A new direction for clinical analyzers. Pure & Appl Chem 1996;68:1831-6.
67. Kricka LJ. Miniaturization of analytical systems. Clin Chem 1998;44:2008-14.

68. Kricka LJ. Nucleic acid detection technologies—labels, strategies, and formats. Clin Chem 1999;45:453-8.
69. Kricka LJ, Fortina, P. Microarray technology and applications: an all-language literature survey including books and patents. Clin Chem 2001;47:1479-82.
70. Kricka LJ. Microchips, microarrays, biochips and nanochips: personal laboratories for the 21st century. Clinica Chimica Acta 2001;307:219-23.
71. Kricka LJ, Fortina P. Nanotechnology and applications: an all-language literature survey including books and patents. Clin Chem 2002;48:662-5.
72. Kricka LJ, Fortina, P. Microchips: an all-language literature survey including books and patents. Clin Chem 2002;48:1620-2.
73. Kricka LJ, Nozaki O, Heyner S, Garside WT, Wilding P. Applications of a microfabricated device for evaluating sperm function. Clin Chem 1993;39:1944-7.
74. Lagally ET, Medintz I, Mathies RA. Single-molecule DNA amplification and analysis in an integrated microfluidic device. Anal Chem 2001;73:565-70.
75. Lee Y-S, Mrksich M. Protein chips: from concept to practice. Trends Biotechnol 2002;20:S14-8.
76. Lichtenberg J, de Rooij NF, Verpoorte E. A microchip electrophoresis system with integrated in-plane electrodes for contactless conductivity detection. Electrophoresis 2002;23:3769-80.
77. Linder V, Verpoorte E, de Rooij NF, Sigrist H, Thormann W. Application of surface biopassivated disposable poly(dimethylsiloxane)/glass chips to a heterogeneous competitive human serum immunoglobulin G immunoassay with incorporated internal standard. Electrophoresis 2002;23:740-9.
78. Linder V, Verpoorte E, Thormann W, de Rooij NF, Sigrist H. Surface biopassivation of replicated poly(dimethylsiloxane) microfluidic channels and application to heterogeneous immunoreaction with on-chip fluorescence detection. Anal Chem 2001;73:4181-9.
79. Liu BF, Ozaki M, Utsumi Y, Hattori T, Terabet S. Chemiluminescence detection for a microchip capillary electrophoresis system fabricated in poly (dimethylsiloxane). Anal Chem 2003;75:36-41.
80. Liu J, Enzelberger M, Quake S. A nanoliter rotary device for polymerase chain reaction. Electrophoresis 2002;23:1531-6.
81. Liu RH, Stremler MA, Sharp KV, Olson MG, Santago JG, Adrian RJ, et al. Passive mixing in a three-dimensional serpentine channel. J Microelectromech Systems 2000;9:190-7.
82. Liu S, Ren H, Gao Q, Roach DJ, Loder RT, Armstrong TM, et al. Automated parallel DNA sequencing on multiple channel microchips. Proc Natl Acad Sci U S A 2000;97:5369-74.
83. Liu Y, Ganser D, Schneider A, Liu R, Grodzinski P, Kroutchinina N. Microfabricated polycarbonate CE devices for DNA analysis. Anal Chem 2001;73:4196-201.
84. Lizardi PM, Huang X, Zhu Z, Bray-Ward P, Thomas DC, Ward DC. Mutation detection and single-molecule counting using isothermal rolling-circle amplification. Nat Genet 1998;19:225-32.
85. MacBeath G, Schreiber SL. Printing proteins as microarrays for high-throughput function determination. Science 2000;289:1760-3.
86. Manica DP, Ewing AG. Prototyping disposable electrophoresis microchips with electrochemical detection using rapid marker masking and laminar flow etching. Electrophoresis 2002;23:3735-43.
87. Manz A, Harrison DJ, Verpoorte EMJ, Fettinger JC, Paulus A, Ludi H, et al. Planar chips technology for miniaturization and integration of separation techniques into monitoring systems. J Chromatog 1992;539:253-8.
88. Manz A, Harrison DJ, Verpoorte EMJ, H.M. W. Planar chips technology for miniaturization of separation systems: A developing perspective in chemical monitoring. In: Brown PR, Grushka E, eds. Advances in chromatography. New York: Marcel Dekker, 1993:1-66.
89. McCormick RM, Nelson RJ, Alonso-Amigo MG, Benvegnu DJ, Hooper HH. Microchannel electrophoretic separations of DNA in injection-molded plastic substrates. Anal Chem 1997;69:2626-30.
90. Medintz IL, Paegel BM, Blazej RG, Emrich CA, Berti L, Scherer JR, et al. High performance genetic analysis using microfabricated capillary array electrophoresis microplates. Electrophoresis 2001;22:3845-56.
91. Metz S, Holzer R, Renaud P. Polyimide-based microfluidic devices. Lab Chip 2001;1:29-34.
92. Monaghan PB, Manz A, Nichols WW. Proceedings of micro total analysis systems 2000. Dordrecht, The Netherlands: Kluwer Academic Publishers, 2000: 111-4.
93. Munro NJ, Huhmer AF, Landers JP. Robust polymeric microchannel coatings for microchip-based analysis of neat PCR products. Anal Chem 2001;73:1784-94.
94. Nachamkin I, Panaro NJ, Li M, Ung H, Yuen PK, Kricka LJ, et al. Agilent 2100 bioanalyzer for restriction fragment length polymorphism analysis of the Campylobacter jejuni flagellin gene. J Clin Microbiol 2001;39:754-7.
95. Northrup MA, Gonzalez C, Hadley D, Hills RF, Landre P, Lehew S, Saiki R, Sninsky JJ, Watson R, Watson R Jr. A MEMS-based miniature DNA analysis system. 8th Int. Conf. Sol.-State Sens. Actuators Eurosens. IX Digest of Technical papers (IEEE Cat. No. 95TH8173). Stockholm: Foundation Sensors & Actuator Technology, 1995:764-7.
96. Northrup MA, Ching MT, White RM, Watson RT. DNA amplification with a microfabricated reaction

chamber. In: IEEE, ed. IEEE International Conference on Solid-State Sensors and Actuators (Transducers '93). New York, 1993.
97. O'Donnell-Maloney MJ, Little DP. Microfabrication and array technologies for DNA sequencing and diagnostics. Gen Anal Biomol Eng 1996;13:151-5.
98. O'Donnell-Maloney MJ, Smith CL, Cantor CR. The development of microfabricated arrays for DNA sequencing and analysis. Trends Biotechnol 1996;14:401-7.
99. Ohori T, Shoji S, Miura K, Yotsumoto A. Partly disposable three-way microvalve for a medical micro total analysis system (JAS). Sensors Actuators A 1998;64:57-62.
100. Paegel BM, Emrich CA, Wedemayer GJ, Scherer JR, Mathies RA. High throughput DNA sequencing with a microfabricated 96-lane capillary array electrophoresis bioprocessor. Proc Natl Acad Sci U S A 2002;99:574-9.
101. Panaro NJ, Yuen PK, Sakazume T, Fortina P, Kricka LJ, Wilding P. Evaluation of DNA fragment sizing and quantification by the agilent 2100 bioanalyzer. Clin Chem 2000;46:1851-3.
102. Papavasaliou A, Pisano A, Liepmann A. High speed and bi-stable electrolysis bubble actuated gate valves. Transducers '01. Munich, Germany, 2001:940-3.
103. Parce JW, Owicki JC, Kercso KM, Sigal GB, Wada HG, Muir VC, et al. Detection of Cell-Affecting Agents with a Silicon Biosensor. Science 1989;246:243-7.
104. Pasas SA, Lacher NA, Davies MI, Lunte SM. Detection of homocysteine by conventional and microchip capillary electrophoresis/electrochemistry. Electrophoresis 2002;23:759-66.
105. Penn SG, He L, Natan MJ. Nanoparticles for bioanalysis. Curr Opin Chem Biol 2003;7:609-15.
106. Petersen KE. Silicon as a mechanical material. Proc IEEE 1982;70:420-56.
107. Peterson KE, McMillam WA, Kovacs GTA, Northrup MA, Christal LA, Pourahmadi F. Towards next generation clinical diagnostic instruments: Scaling and new processing paradigms. J Biomed Devices 1998;1:71-9.
108. Raisi F, Belgrader P, Borkholder DA, Herr AE, Kintz GJ, Pourhamadi F, et al. Microchip isoelectric focusing using a miniature scanning detection system. Electrophoresis 2001;22:2291-5.
109. Ramsey JD, Jacobson SC, Culbertson CT, Ramsey JM. High-efficiency, two dimensional separations of protein digests on microfluidic devices. Anal Chem 2003;75:3758-64.
110. Ramsey JM, Jacobson SC, Knapp MR. Microfabricated chemical measurements systems. Nature Med 1995;1:1093-6.
111. Reyes DR, Lossifidis D, Auroux PA, Manz A. Micro total analysis systems. 1. Introduction, theory, and technology. Anal Chem 2002;74:2623-36.
112. Sanders GHW, Manz A. Chip-based microsystems for genomic and proteomic analysis. Trends in Anal Chem 2000;19:364-78.
113. Sato K, Tokeshi M, Odake T, Kimura H, Ooi T, Nakao M, et al. Integration of an immunosorbent assay system: analysis of secretory human immunoglobulin A on polystyrene beads in a microchip. Anal Chem 2000;72:1144-7.
114. Schena M, Heller RA, Theriault TP, Konrad K, Lachenmeier E, Davis RW. Microarrays: biotechnology's discovery platform for functional genomics. Trends Biotechnol 1998;16:301-6.
115. Schomburg WK, Fahrenberg J, Mass D, Rapp R. Active valves and pumps for microfluidics. J Micromech Microeng 1993;3:216-8.
116. Shalon D, Smith SJ, Brown PO. A DNA microarray system for analyzing complex DNA samples using two-color fluorescent probe hybridization. Genome Res 1996;6:639-45.
117. Shi Y, Simpson PC, Scherer JR, Wexler D, Skibola C, Smith MT, et al. Radial capillary array electrophoresis microplate and scanner for high-performance nucleic acid analysis. Anal Chem 1999;71:5354-61.
118. Shimbo M, Furukawa K, Fukuda K, Tanzawa K. Silicon-to-silicon direct bonding method. J Appl Phys 1986;60:2987-9.
119. Shoffner MA, Cheng J, Hvichia GE, Kricka LJ, Wilding P. Chip PCR. I. Surface passivation of microfabricated silicon-glass chips for PCR. Nucleic Acids Res 1996;24:375-9.
120. Shoji S, Esashi M. Micromachining for chemical sensors. In: Seiyama T, ed. Chemical sensor technology. Tokyo: Kodansha, 1988:179-93.
121. Shoji S, van der Schoot BH, de Rooij NF, Esashi M. Smallest dead volume microvalves for integrated chemical analyzing systems. Tech Dig Transducers 1991;91:1052-5.
122. Shoji S, Esashi M. Microfabrication and microsensors. Appl Biochem Biotechnol 1993;41:21-34.
123. Shoji S, Esashi M. Microflow devices and systems. J Micromech Microeng 1994;4:157-71.
124. Shoji S, Esashi M, Matsuo M. Prototype miniature blood gas analyzer fabricated on a silicon wafer. Sensors Actuators 1988;14:101-7.
125. Slentz BE, Penner NA, Lugowska E, Regnier F. Nanoliter capillary electrochromatography columns based on collocated monolithic support structures molded in poly(dimethyl siloxane). Electrophoresis 2001;22:3736-43.
126. Somprasit C, Marquez-Do DA, Yamanishi D, Simpson JL, Bischoff FZ. A novel approach for enrichment of fetal cells using a microfabricated silicon membrane. Los Angelas: Amer Soc Human Genet, 2003.
127. Stengl R, Ahn K, Gosele U. Bubble-free silicon wafer bonding in a nonclean room environment. Jpn J Appl Phys 1988;60:2364-6.

128. Terry SC, Jerman JH, Angell JB. A, gas chromatographic air analyzer fabricated on a silicon wafer. IEEE Trans Electron Device 1979;26:1880-6.
129. Tracey M, Johnston I, Greenaway R, Davis J, Sutton N, Schulze G, et al. Proceedings of micro total analysis systems 1998. Dordrecht, The Netherlands: Kluwer Academic Publishers, 1998:89-92.
130. van der Schoot B, Bergveld P. An ISFET-based microlitre titrator: integration of a chemical sensor-actuator system. Sensors Actuators 1985;8:11-22.
131. Vandaveer WR, Pasas SA, Martin RS, Lunte SM. Recent developments in amperometric detection for microchip capillary electrophoresis. Electrophoresis 2002;23:3667-77.
132. Verpoorte E. Microfluidic chips for clinical and forensic analysis. Electrophoresis 2002;23:677-712.
133. von Heeren F, Verpoorte E, Manz A, Thormann W. Micellar electrokinetic chromatography separations and analyses of biological samples on a cyclic planar microstructure. Anal Chem 1996;68:2044-53.
134. Wang J. On-chip enzymatic assays. Electrophoresis 2002;23:713-8.
135. Wang J, Chatrathi MP. Microfabricated electrophoresis chip for bioassay of renal markers. Anal Chem 2003;75:525-9.
136. Wang J, Chatrathi MP, Tian B, Polsky R. Microfabricated electrophoresis chips for simultaneous bioassays of glucose, uric acid, ascorbic acid, and acetaminophen. Anal Chem 2000;72:2514-8.
137. Wang J, Ibanez A, Chatrathi MP. Microchip-based amperometric immunoassays using redox tracers. Electrophoresis 2002;23:3744-9.
138. Wang J, Pumera M. Dual conductivity/amperometric detection system for microchip capillary electrophoresis. Anal Chem 2002;74:5919-23.
139. Waters LC, Jacobson SC, Kroutchinina N, Khandurina J, Foote RS, Ramsey JM. Microchip device for cell lysis, multiplex PCR amplification, and electrophoretic sizing. Anal Chem 1998;70:158-62.
140. Waters LC, Jacobson SC, Kroutchinina N, Khandurina J, Foote RS, Ramsey JM. Multiple sample PCR amplification and electrophoretic analysis on a microchip. Anal Chem 1998;70:5172-6.
141. Weinert A, Amirfeiz P, Bengtsson S. Plasma assisted room temperature bonding for MST. Sensors Actuators A 2001;92:214-22.
142. White V, Ghodssi R, Herdey C, Denton DD, McCaughan L. Use of photosensitive polyimide for deep x-ray lithography. Appl Phys Lett 1995;66:2072-3.
143. Wild MJ, Gillner A, Poprawe R. Locally selective bonding of silicon and glass with laser. Sensors Actuators A 2001;93:63-9.
144. Wilding P. Nucleic Acid Amplification in Microchips. In: Cheng JKL, ed. Biochip technology. Philadelphia: Harwood Academic Publishers, 2001:173-84.
145. Wilding P, Kricka LJ. Micro-microchips: just how small can we go? Trends Biotechnol 1999;17:465-8.
146. Wilding P, Kricka LJ, Cheng J, Hvichia G, Shoffner MA, Fortina P. Integrated cell isolation and polymerase chain reaction analysis using silicon microfilter chambers. Anal Biochem 1998;257:95-100.
147. Wilding P, Kricka L, Zemel JN. Methods and apparatus for the detection of an analyte utilizing mesoscale flow systems. US Patent 5,637,469, June 10, 1997.
148. Wilding P, Pfahler J, Bau HH, Zemel JN, Kricka LJ. Manipulation and flow of biological fluids in straight channels micromachined in silicon. Clin Chem 1994;40:43-7.
149. Wilding P, Shoffner MA, Hvichia G, Kricka LJ. Thermal cycling and surface passivation of micromachined devices for PCR. Clin Chem 1995;41:1367-8.
150. Wilding P, Shoffner MA, Kricka LJ. PCR in a silicon microstructure. Clin Chem 1994;40:1815-8.
151. Wittwer CT, Fillmore GC, Garling DJ. Minimizing the time required for DNA amplification by efficient heat transfer to small samples. Anal Biochem 1990;186:328-31.
152. Xu J, Guia A, Rothwarf D, Huang M, Sithiphong K, Ouang J, et al. A benchmark study with sea/chip planar patch-clamp technology. Assay Drug Develop Technol 2003;1:1-10.
153. Xue Q, Wainright A, Gangakhedkar S, Gibbons I. Multiplexed enzyme assays in capillary electrophoretic single-use microfluidic devices. Electrophoresis 2001;22:4000-7.
154. Yamanishi DT, Xu J, Hujsak PG, Yang Z, Wang X-B, Wu L. Enrichment of rare fetal cells from maternal peripheral blood. Expert Rev. Mol. Diagn. 2002;2:303-11.
155. Yanagisawa K, Kuwano H, Tago A. An electromagnetically driven microvalve. Tech Dig Transducers 1993;93:102-5.
156. Yu Q, Bauer JM, Moore JS, Beebe DJ. Responsive biomimetic hydrogel valve for microfluidics. Appl Phys Lett 2001;78:2589-91.
157. Yuen PK, Kricka L, Fortina P, Panaro NJ, Sakazume T, Wilding P. Microchip module for blood sample preparation and nucleic acid amplification reactions. Genome Res 2001;11:405-12.
158. Yuen PK, Li G, Bau Y, Muller UY. Microfluidic devices for fluidic circulation and mixing improve hybridization signal intensity on DNA arrays. Lab Chip 2003;3:46-50.
159. Yuen PK, Kricka LJ, Wilding P. Semi-disposable microvalves for use with microfabricated devices or microchips. J Micromech Microeng 2000;10:401-9.
160. Zhao XM, Xia YN, Whitesides GM. Soft lithographic methods for nanofabrication. J Mater Chem 1997;7:1069-74.

161. Zhu H, Bilgin M, Bangham R, Hall D, Casamayor A, Bertone P, et al. Global analysis of protein activities using proteome chips. Science 2001;293:2101-5.
162. Zlatnova J, Bavykin S, Mirzabekov A. Biological microchips: State-of-the-art. Biophys J 1999;76:A456.
163. Zuborova M, Masar M, Kaniansky D, Johnck M, Stanislawski B. Determination of oxalate in urine by zone electrophoresis on a chip with conductivity detection. Electrophoresis 2002;23:774-81.
164. Zugel SA, Burke BJ, Regnier FE, Lytle FE. Electrophoretically mediated microanalysis of leucine aminopeptidase using two-photon excited fluorescence detection on a microchip. Anal Chem 2000;72:5731-5.

CHAPTER 11

Automation in the Clinical Laboratory*

James C. Boyd, M.D., and
Charles D. Hawker, Ph.D., M.B.A., F.A.C.B.

The term "automation" has been applied in the field of clinical chemistry to describe the use of laboratory instruments and specimen processing equipment to perform clinical laboratory assays with only minimal involvement of the technologist.

The development of automated instruments for the clinical laboratory began in the 1950s at the same time as the demand for tests escalated dramatically. The availability of automated instruments enabled laboratories to process a much larger workload without a comparable increase in staff.[23] The evolution of automation in the clinical laboratory has paralleled that in the manufacturing industry, progressing from fixed automation—whereby an instrument performs a repetitive task by itself—to programmable automation—which allows it to perform a variety of different tasks—to intelligent automation, where individual instruments or systems are able to self-monitor and respond appropriately to changing conditions.

One benefit of automation is a reduction in the variability of results and errors of analysis by eliminating tasks that are repetitive and monotonous for a human and that can lead to boredom or inattention. The improved reproducibility gained by automation has led to a significant improvement in quality of laboratory tests in recent years caused largely by the combination of skillfully designed automated instrumentation with good analytical methods and effective quality assurance programs.[37] In recent years many small laboratories have consolidated into larger, more efficient entities in response to market trends for reducing costs. The pioneering work to automate these merged laboratories has pointed to new avenues in laboratory automation. No longer is automation being used simply to assist the laboratory technologist in performing tests, but it now extends to (1) processing and transporting specimens, (2) loading them into automated analyzers, and (3) assessing the results of the performed tests. Automation of these additional functions is basic to the future prosperity of the clinical laboratory.

In this chapter, we discuss the principles that are applied to automate the individual steps of the analytical process both in individual analyzers and in the integration of automation throughout the clinical laboratory. We provide examples of these principles as implemented in commercially available chemistry, hematology, immunoassay, and nucleic acid systems; point-of-care (POC) analyzers; and automated specimen processing systems.* Definitions of terms used in the automation of clinical chemistry have been published by the International Union of Pure and Applied Chemistry (IUPAC).[48]

HISTORICAL OVERVIEW

Automation of laboratory assays has occurred incrementally over the past 50 years.[13,15] Key to the successful automation of these assays was the incorporation of continuous flow and

*The authors acknowledge the original contributions of Ernest Maclin and D.S. Young upon which portions of this chapter are based.

*Many times throughout this chapter, we refer to various commercially available analyzers. The addresses and web addresses of the companies that offer these analyzers are available on this book's accompanying Evolve site, found at http://evolve.elsevier.com/Tietz/textbook/.

discrete processing steps in the design of automated instruments and systems for use in clinical laboratories. Ancillary developments of note include the development of laboratory information systems, robotics, and the concepts of total and modular automation.

Processes Used in Automation

Types of liquid processing steps used to automate laboratory assays include continuous-flow and discrete processing.

Continuous-Flow Analysis

The development of the continuous-flow analyzer by Leonard Skeggs in the 1950s was a landmark step forward from the manual performance of laboratory analyses.[82,83] Skeggs' pioneering device, eventually marketed as the Technicon AutoAnalyzer, was a single-channel, continuous-flow batch analyzer that provided one result per analyte for each specimen at a rate of 40 to 60 specimens per hour. In continuous-flow systems, the reaction occurred in tubing that served as both flow container and cuvet. Specimens and reagent were combined using a roller pump that pushed them through a fluid manifold designed specifically for each assay. To control reagent and specimen volumes, different internal diameter pump tubing was used. Mixing was achieved by running the reactants through coils. Carryover of one specimen to the next was minimized by injecting air bubbles at regular intervals into the specimen stream. Air bubbles were removed as the reactant stream reached the photometer where absorbance readings were taken. Temperature control, if necessary, was supplied by immersing coils of tubing in temperature-regulated water baths. Timing of the reaction was controlled by the distance the stream traveled in the tubing. Protein-free filtrates of the reaction mixture could be provided using dialyzers. Continuous-flow analyzers remained a mainstay of routine laboratory analysis for more than 20 years. The second and third generations of continuous-flow analyzers—the Technicon SMA 12/60 and the SMAC—were able to provide multiple test results on the same specimen.

Discrete Analysis

Discrete analysis, in contrast with continuous-flow analysis, allows each specimen in a batch its own physical and chemical space, separate from every other specimen. Early discrete analyzers, such as the 1970 vintage robot chemist, mimicked the steps of manual human analysis.[57] Subsequently, many discrete analyzers were developed and are still widely used in clinical laboratories. Centrifugal and random access analyzers are examples of instruments that use discrete processing.

Centrifugal Analyzers

Centrifugal analyzers were invented and developed in the early 1970s by Norman Anderson and his colleagues at the Oak Ridge National Laboratory with funding provided by the U.S. Atomic Energy Commission, National Institute of General Medical Sciences, and National Aeronautics and Space Administration.[5,80] With a centrifugal analyzer, discrete aliquots of specimens and reagents are pipetted into discrete chambers in a rotor. The specimens are subsequently analyzed in parallel by spinning the rotor and using the resultant centrifugal force to simultaneously transfer and mix the aliquots of specimens and reagent(s) into radially located cuvets. The rotary motion is then used to move the cuvets through the optical path of an optical system. Under control of an integrated computer system, multiple absorbance readings are taken from each cuvet and resultant software used to calculate enzyme activity or substrate concentration. Although early centrifugal analyzers analyzed multiple specimens for a single analyte in parallel, the development of technologies to select different optical wavelengths rapidly enabled centrifugal analyzers to perform several analyses in parallel at different wavelengths. Thus the rotor could contain specimens for several different tests at the same time and the appropriate tests on each specimen could be scheduled by keyboard entry or bar coded labels on specimen tubes.

Random-Access Analyzers

Random-access analyzers perform analyses on a batch of specimens sequentially with each specimen analyzed for a different selection of tests. The tests performed in the random-access analyzers are selectable through the use of different containers of liquid reagents, different reagent packs, or different reagent tablets depending on the analyzer. This approach permits measurement of a variable number and variety of analytes in each specimen. Profiles or groups of tests are defined for a specimen at the time the requested tests are entered into the analyzer by means of a keyboard (used in most systems), by instruction from a laboratory information system in conjunction with bar coding on the specimen tube, or by operator selection of appropriate reagent packs. Like centrifugal analyzers, random-access analyzers incorporate computers and are able to take multiple absorbance or reflectance measurements for each assay. In addition, enough self-diagnosis features are programmed into each analyzer's software to allow the technologist operating the instrument to leave the instrument for brief periods of time. This latter feature, termed "walk-away" automation by the manufacturers, offered the first opportunities for a single technologist to operate more than one analyzer at a time.

Most current chemistry and immunoassay analyzers are random-access analyzers. Manufacturers have steadily improved the mechanical reliability of these systems, and provided software that allows technologists to operate the analyzers easily.

Laboratory Information Systems

Integral to the automation of the clinical laboratory was the development of the laboratory information system (LIS) that first appeared in laboratories in the latter part of the

1960s and early 1970s (see Chapter 18). At first these systems served primarily as a way of generating consolidated laboratory result reports. However, LISs quickly evolved into tools to capture all test requests, to manage laboratory work flow, and to improve the quality of laboratory results. Particularly important in the improvement of laboratory quality was the development of direct electronic interfaces between laboratory analyzers and the LIS that supplanted the necessity for manual transcription of results from analyzer to laboratory report. The modern LIS has extensive software for supporting the entire clinical laboratory enterprise (see Chapter 18). In hospital settings, the LIS may also be interfaced to other clinical systems, such as admitting, billing, electronic medical records, and pharmacy.

Robotics

Robotic technology was first applied in the clinical laboratory in the 1980s as an outgrowth of developments in industrial robotic automation, which started a quarter of a century earlier. Microprocessor-controlled robot arms developed in the early 1980s allowed development of robotic laboratory workstations capable of carrying out programmable multistep specimen manipulations. The programmability of these new devices gave them flexibility to be adapted to many different assay and specimen-handling approaches. This new generation of robots was first used in laboratories for automated specimen preparation in chromatographic and spectroscopic assays.

Types of Automation

Types of automation developed for use in the clinical laboratory include total and modular automation.

Total Laboratory Automation

A laboratory constructed by Dr. Masahide Sasaki and his laboratory technologists in the early 1980s at the Kochi Medical School in Nankoku, Japan, provided an early model of total laboratory automation.[77] In Sasaki's laboratory, conveyor belts transported carriers containing patient specimens to various analytical workstations throughout the laboratory, and mobile robots moved the empty carriers back to a central location. When these carriers arrived via the conveyor belt at each workstation, automated pipettors aspirated serum from each tube for the required laboratory assays. At some workstations, one-armed stationary robots performed pre-programmed pipetting and dispensing steps on the patient specimens to accomplish more complex preanalytical processing steps.

Sasaki's laboratory provided the first glimpse of a total laboratory automation system. A total laboratory automation (TLA) system is generally constructed on a large scale and includes some or all of the preanalytical automation functions, such as centrifugation of blood specimens, aspiration of serum from centrifuged tubes into aliquot tubes, decapping of tubes, splitting of specimens into additional aliquot tubes, bar code labeling of aliquot tubes, and sorting of tubes according to predetermined laboratory destinations.[7,8] In addition, a TLA system also includes a transport system, such as a conveyor that delivers tubes to specific automated analyzers that are mechanically interfaced to the system for automated sampling and analysis. TLA systems also often include a tube recapping machine, a delivery location for specimens that are not analyzed on interfaced analyzers, and an automated storage system for specimens for which testing has been completed (for possible repeat tests or additionally ordered tests). TLA will be discussed in depth later in this chapter.

Sasaki's vision of an integrated automated laboratory coupled with the demonstration of successful robotic applications by other groups created much enthusiasm for robotic automation of the laboratory in the early 1990s.[12] For example, enthusiasts touted the ability of robotic systems to improve the quality and reproducibility of testing, while providing shorter test turnaround times, reduced costs of testing, and improved worker safety. Because commercially developed TLA systems were very expensive, all but the largest laboratories were slow to adopt the new technology.

Modular Automation

By the mid-1990s, manufacturers had begun to market modular automation products in which selected modules—such as analyzers, ion-selective electrodes (ISE), and rack lanes or tracks—could be integrated together to meet the requirements of the individual laboratory.[33] Examples of modern modular systems are shown in Table 11-1. Although modular automation was marketed to the laboratory community much more successfully, there was also widespread recognition that automation of the preanalytical steps (particularly sorting, centrifugation, and aliquoting) would yield the greatest labor (and cost) savings. These steps have been focal points for new automation development.

Laboratory Automation Systems

The development of TLA and modular automation required the development of computer systems known as laboratory automation systems (LAS) with extensive software to support these systems in the clinical laboratory. For a more detailed description of the relationships between an LAS, LIS, automation equipment, and laboratory analyzers, the reader is referred to the National Committee for Clinical Laboratory Standards (NCCLS) standard on laboratory automation communications.[61]

INDIVIDUAL STEPS IN THE ANALYTICAL PROCESSES

The individual steps required to complete an analysis are often referred to as "unit operations." They include the following:

1. Specimen acquisition
2. Specimen identification
3. Specimen delivery to laboratory

TABLE 11-1 Examples of Modular Systems with Key Parameters

System Name	Modules	Throughput Range, Results per Hour	Key Common Elements	Module Assembly	Comments
SYNCHRON CX7	Analyzers	825	Sampler and computer	At factory	Combines the CX3 and CX4
MODULAR	D, P, E modules	170-10,000	Rack lanes, loading station, and computer	At factory and in field	Multiple common analytical modules can be used
WorkCell	Analyzers	1650 chemistry and 240 immunochemistry	Track and computer	At factory	Combines the 1650 and Centaur
LX4201	Analyzers	2880	Computer	At factory	Combines two LX20 analyzers
AU5400 Series	Analyzer(s)	3200-6600	Rack transfer lanes and computer	At factory	Combines up to 3 analyzer modules and 2 ISE modules

4. Specimen preparation
5. Specimen loading and aspiration
6. On-analyzer specimen delivery
7. Reagent handling and storage
8. Reagent delivery
9. Chemical reaction phase
10. Measurement approaches
11. Signal processing, data handling, and process control

In this section, we describe these operations individually and intersperse examples of how they have been automated in terms of operational and analytical performance. In most automated systems, these steps are usually performed sequentially, but in some instruments they may be combined and occur in parallel.

Specimen Acquisition

Techniques used to acquire specimens for subsequent analysis in the clinical laboratory are discussed in Chapter 2, but few devices have been developed that automate these techniques. There is, however, ongoing work to develop approaches to automate collection of blood specimens traditionally collected by finger stick or phlebotomy. For example, various new hand-held devices for automated monitoring of blood glucose have been designed to sample blood from sites on the body such as the fingertip, forearm, thigh, and calf (see Chapters 4 and 25). One such device applies a small vacuum, lances the skin, transfers blood onto an electrochemical test strip, and measures glucose.[35]

Additionally, Zivanovic and Davis have evaluated a robotic system for blood sampling that presses a flat-headed probe against the surface of the skin and uses force and/or position profiles to determine the location of a vein.[94] When a needle is inserted, the characteristic force and/or position profile, on puncturing the vein wall, is distinctive enough to implement automatic needle withdrawal to prevent overshoot. The authors plan to develop both an autonomous blood sampling robot and a force-feedback surgical trainer.

Specimen Identification

Typically the identifying link between patient and specimen is made at the patient's bedside, and it is imperative that this connection be maintained throughout the transport of the specimen to the laboratory, its subsequent analysis, and the preparation of a report. Many technologies are available for automatic identification and data collection purposes, including labeling, bar coding, optical character recognition,[11] magnetic stripe and magnetic ink character recognition, voice, radiofrequency identification, touchscreens, light pens, handprint tablets, optical mark readers, and smart cards. Historically, labeling was the technology used for identification purposes. However, bar coding is now the technology of choice.

Labeling

In many laboratory information systems, electronic entry either in the laboratory or at a nursing station of a test order for a uniquely identified patient generates a specimen label bearing a unique laboratory accession number.[11] A record is established that remains incomplete until a result (or set of results) is entered into the computer against the accession number. The unique label is affixed to the specimen collection container when the blood is drawn. Proper alignment of the label on the collection container is critical for subsequent specimen processing when using bar coded labels. Arrival of the specimen in the laboratory is recorded by a manual or computerized log-in procedure. In other systems, the specimen is labeled at the patient's bedside with the patient identification and collection information and enters the laboratory with a requisition form; there it is assigned an accession number as part of the log-in procedure, which may or may not be computer implemented.

After accessioning, specimens undergo the technical handling processes. For those processes requiring physical removal of serum from the original tube, secondary labels bearing essential information from the original label must be affixed to any secondary tubes created. The secondary labels are generated at the time of accessioning by a special, usually computerized device.

For analyzers that do not automatically link specimen identity and aspiration, the sequence of results produced must be linked manually with the sequence of entry of specimens. Some analyzers print out or transmit to a host computer each result or set of results from a specimen, either by position of the specimen in the loading zone or by the accession number programmed to that position.

Figure 11-1 Examples of bar codes used in chemistry analyzers containing the same information. **A,** Code 39. **B,** Code I 2/5. **C,** Code 128B. **D,** Codabar. *(Courtesy Computer Transceiver Systems, Inc.)*

Bar Coding

A major advance in the automation of specimen identification in the clinical laboratory has been the incorporation of bar coding technology into analytical systems.[4,10,85,90,93] In practice, a bar coded label (often generated by the laboratory information system and bearing the specimen accession number) is placed onto the specimen container and is subsequently "read" by one or more bar code readers that have been strategically placed at key positions in the analytical train. The resultant identifying and ancillary information is then transferred to and processed by the system software.

Unequivocal positive identification of a specimen can be achieved in analyzers with bar code readers in less than 2 seconds. Advantages of the use of coded labels that can be automatically scanned and identified by the analyzer include: (1) elimination of work lists for the system, (2) prevention of mix ups in the placement of tubes in the analyzer or during sampling, (3) analysis of specimens in a defined sequence, and (4) absence of possible tube mix up when serum must be transferred into a secondary container.[87] The reader is cautioned, however, that most automation systems require individual container identification instead of relying only on the LIS accession number. The NCCLS automation standards also require unique container identification.[59-63] Since a given patient order could consist of two or more different types of specimen, all bearing the same accession number, the use of unique container identification is the only way to ensure that an automation system delivers the correct type of specimen to the appropriate analyzer or destination. Most manufacturers have incorporated computer software to detect the different symbologies. The bar code detector can "autodiscriminate" or automatically recognize and read codes in one of several common symbologies so that operator intervention is not required. Examples of bar codes that are used in chemistry analyzers are presented in Figure 11-1.

Initiating bar code identification at a patient's bedside ensures greater integrity of the specimen's identity in an analyzer. Systems to transfer information concerning a patient's identity to blood tubes at the patient's bedside have been introduced in some hospitals and several companies are now offering these systems (Becton, Dickinson & Co., Bridge Medical, Inc., Lattice, McKesson, and Systemme INFORMATICA). One difficulty in applying these systems is the necessity to cross traditional administrative boundaries; this can create conflict with established procedures that are beyond the control of the laboratory staff. However, the Food and Drug Administration has issued a proposed rule that would require matching of bar codes on medications and blood products to patient bar code wristbands.[29] Thus, most healthcare facilities are now adopting these systems (and solving their administrative issues), which enable the laboratories to ensure accurate and reliable specimen identification.

Both one- and two-dimensional (2-D) bar coding systems are now available. Of the two, one-dimensional bar codes have been the most widely used in the clinical laboratory.

One-Dimensional Bar Codes

A one-dimensional bar code is defined as "an array of rectangular bars and spaces that are arranged in a predetermined pattern following unambiguous rules to represent elements of data that are referred to as characters.[6]" A bar code is transferred and affixed to an object by a "bar code label," which carries the bar code and, optionally, other human-readable information. "Symbology" is the term used to describe the rules specifying the way the data are encoded into the bars and spaces. The width of the bars and spaces, and the number of each, is determined by a specification for that symbology. Different combinations of the bars and spaces represent different characters. On passing a bar code scanner over the bar code, the light beam from the scanner is absorbed by the dark bars and not reflected; the beam is reflected by the light spaces. A photocell detector in the scanner receives the reflected light and converts the light into an electrical signal that can be digitized. A one-dimensional bar code is "vertically redundant" in that the same information is repeated vertically—the heights of the bars can be truncated without any loss of information. In practice, vertical redundancy allows a symbol with printing defects, such as spots or voids, to be read.

Different types of symbologies are used to encode information into one-dimensional bar code labels.[1,4,66,90] Some are numeric only (Universal Product Code [UPC], European Article Numbering [EAN] system [now also called IAN for International Article Numbering], Interleaved 2 of 5), some are of fixed length (UPC-A is 12 digits, UPC-E is 6 digits, EAN-13 is 13 digits, and EAN-8 is 8 digits), and some have both numbers and alphabetic characters (Code 93, Code 128, and Code 39). Code 128 allows the encoding of all 128 ASCII characters. Standards for symbologies have been developed and the Health Industry Business Communications Council endorses the use of six of them.[44] The NCCLS has published a standard for the use of bar codes to support clinical laboratory automation.[60] This standard recommends that Code 128 replace all other symbologies in laboratory automation systems such as Code 39, Codabar, and Interleaved 2 of 5 by December 31, 2003. The standard also specifies bar code symbol and label placement zones for tubes of various lengths (66 mm, 75 mm, and 100 mm) and specifying the minimum widths of a narrow bar and the quiet zone. (See http://www.taltech.com/TALtech_web/resources/intro_to_bc/bcsymbol.htm for examples).

Two-Dimensional Bar Codes

As its name implies, a 2-D bar code stores information along the height and the length of the symbol and is designed to place a portable database in as little space as possible.[6] The term "matrix code" applies to 2-D codes that code the data based on the position of black spots within a matrix. Each black element is the same dimension and it is the position of the element that codes the data. Moving-beam laser scanners and charge-coupled device (CCD) scanners are used to read 2-D labels. More than 20 different 2-D symbologies have been developed for encoding 2-D labels. They include Codablock, Code 16K, Code 49, Data Matrix, MaxiCode, Portable Data File (PDF) 417, and Softstrip, each of which allows for more information to be encoded into a 2-D label than can be encoded into a one-dimensional bar code label. For example, the PDF 417 allows for between 1000 and 2000 characters to be encoded per symbol, with an information density of between 100 and 340 characters. Few, if any, clinical laboratories are employing 2-D codes because the data that could be contained in those codes, such as patient name, age, sex, collection date and time, specimen type, ordered tests, etc., are widely desired to be human readable. Additionally, the price of 2-D readers is much higher than 1-D bar code scanners.

Identification Errors

Specimen identification and test ordering errors occur frequently in the clinical laboratory and emanate from errors that occur in the specimen collection and accessioning process.[9,73,86] With the 1999 publication of the Institute of Medicine (IOM) report, *To Err is Human: Building a Safer Health System,*[50] there has been increasing scrutiny of identification errors in medical practice. The IOM report urges improved understanding of the causes of errors in the healthcare system and development of approaches using computerized and other "mechanical" support systems to decrease error rates.

Operationally, many opportunities arise in the clinical laboratory for mismatching specimens and results.[37] The risks begin at the bedside and are compounded with every processing step that a specimen undergoes between collection from the patient and analysis by the instrument. The risks are particularly great when hand transcription is invoked for accessioning, labeling and relabeling, and making load lists. An incorrect accession number or one with a transposition of digits, or a load list with transposed accession numbers, may cause test results to be attributed to the wrong patient. An additional hazard exists when specimens must be inserted into certain positions in the loading zone defined for them by a load list. Human misreading of either specimen label or loading list may cause misplacement of specimens, calibrators, or controls. In one study, automatic reading of bar coded labels was found to reduce the error rate from 1 in 300 characters (for human entry) to about 1 in 1 million characters.[66]

SPECIMEN DELIVERY TO LABORATORY

Several methods may be used to deliver specimens to the laboratory, which is often in a location distant from the patient. These include courier service, pneumatic tube systems, electric track vehicles, and mobile robots. In some laboratories, phlebotomists may also bring specimens with them as they return to the laboratory.

Courier Service

Human couriers have been extensively used to transport specimens from collection sites to the laboratory and between laboratories. Although in general reliable, there are problems with courier service. For example, human delivery is a batch process, and couriers usually only service a given pickup point at specified times. Arrangements for stat pickup can be made, but this adds costs to the analytical process and delays the reporting of results. In addition, specimen breakage or loss can occur with manual handling of specimens.

Pneumatic Tube Systems

Pneumatic tube systems provide rapid specimen transportation and are quite reliable when installed as point-to-point services. However, when switching mechanisms are introduced to allow carriers to be sent to various locations, additional mechanical problems may arise and cause carriers to be misrouted. Although pneumatic tubes have been reported to damage specimens because of rapid acceleration or deceleration,[39,70] and have limited carrying capacity, they have been found to be cost effective.[38]

Electric Track Vehicles

Electric track vehicles have a larger carrying capacity than pneumatic tube systems and do not appear to have problems with damaging specimens by acceleration and/or deceleration forces. Some systems maintain the carrier in an upright position by use of a gimbal (a device that permits a body to incline freely in any direction or suspends it so that it will remain level when its support is tipped). Compared with pneumatic tube systems, electric track vehicles usually require a larger station for loading and unloading, and this fact often limits where a station may be placed. If the station is not located directly in the central laboratory, additional staff may be necessary to unload the carts and transport the specimens to their final destination, and the electric track system may not achieve its desired goal of rapid specimen transport.

Mobile Robots

Mobile robots have been used successfully to transport laboratory specimens both within the laboratory[32,47] and outside the central laboratory.[71] Further studies are required to establish the usefulness of mobile robots for specimen transport, but it is already apparent that mobile robot transportation will have many of the same limitations as the human messenger (e.g., batched specimen pickup and time delay in notifying of necessity for pickup). In a busy laboratory setting, however, delivery of specimens to lab benches by a mobile robot can be more frequent than human pickup and has been shown to be cost effective.[17]

SPECIMEN PREPARATION

The clotting of blood in specimen collection tubes, their subsequent centrifugation, and the transfer of serum to secondary tubes require time to complete. When performed manually, it has been known to cause delays in the preparation of a specimen for analysis. Consequently, to eliminate the problems associated with specimen preparation, systems are being developed to automate this process. The following developments are noteworthy.

Use of Whole Blood for Analysis

When an assay system has been designed to analyze whole blood samples, specimen preparation time is essentially eliminated. Automated or semiautomated ion-selective electrodes, which measure ion activity in whole blood rather than ion concentration, have been incorporated into automated systems to provide certain test results within minutes of the drawing of a specimen. This approach is now commonly used for assaying electrolytes and some other common analytes. Another approach involves either manual or automated application of whole blood to dry reagent films and visual or instrumental observation of a quantitative change. This approach is exemplified by the Reflotron Plus.

Automation of Specimen Preparation

Several manufacturers have developed fully automated specimen preparation systems. These systems are described later in the chapter.

SPECIMEN LOADING AND ASPIRATION

In most situations, the specimen presented to an automated analyzer is serum or plasma. Many state-of-the-art analyzers (e.g., CX/LX series, ADVIA 1650 and 2400, Architect c-8000 series, MODULAR, DIMENSION) directly sample serum from primary collection tubes of various sizes. With such analyzers, the collecting tubes most frequently used contain a separator material that forms a barrier between supernatant and cells (see Chapter 2). Some analyzers also sample from a cup or tube that is filled with serum transferred from the original specimen tube.

Evaporation of specimen from cups or tubes in the loading zone has caused analytical errors as great as 50% over 4 hours.[14] Operationally, all cups or tubes containing solution for analysis should be covered until the time the specimen is to be analyzed. Many manufacturers of automated analyzers provide covers for individual cups or for part or the whole of the loading zone to reduce losses caused by evaporation. Cups may be covered by Parafilm or by caps that are placed over the cups and that have crosscuts to permit ready entry of a specimen probe. A type of antievaporative cover that reduces evaporative losses to less than 0.1%/hr has been described.[16]

Also, specimens may undergo thermal or photo degradation. For example. temperature-labile constituents may undergo degradation if held at ambient temperature. Other constituents that are photolabile, such as bilirubin, are destroyed by ultraviolet light. The adverse effects of ambient temperature may be overcome by holding both specimens and calibrators in a refrigerated loading zone. Photo degradation is reduced by the use of semiopaque specimen containers and by protecting specimens from light both in storage and on the analyzer.

The *loading zone* of an analyzer is the area in which specimens are held in the instrument before they are analyzed. The holding area may be in the form of a circular tray, a rack or series of racks, or a serpentine chain of containers into which individual tubes are inserted. When specimens are not identified automatically, they must be presented to the sampling device in the correct sequence as specified by a loading list. The sampling mechanism determines the exact volume of specimen removed from the specimen. For most analyzers, specimens for a second run may be prepared on a separate tray while one run is already in progress. This permits machine operation and human actions to proceed in parallel for optimal efficiency. In some analyzers, specimens may be added continuously by the operator as the specimens become available. A desirable feature of any automated analyzer is the ability to insert new specimens ahead of specimens already in place in the loading zone. This feature allows the timely analysis of specimens with a high medical priority when they are received in the clinical laboratory. When specimen identification is machine read, it is easy for the operator to reposition specimens in the loading zone; however, when specimen identification is tied to a loading list, insertion or repositioning of specimens must be accompanied by revision of the loading list.

Transmission of infectious diseases by automated equipment is a concern in clinical laboratories.[81] The method of transmission by equipment is primarily by means of the splatter of serum or blood during the acquisition of specimens from rapidly moving specimen probes.[27] The use of level sensors, which restrict the penetration of sample probes into specimens and provide smoother motion control, greatly reduces splatter. There is no evidence that aerosols, which may be generated by instrument systems, are a source of transmission of infectious diseases.[28,64] However, there is a potential for contamination when the stoppers of primary containers are "popped" to decant serum into specimen cups.[27] To obviate this hazard and the risk of exposure from broken glass, spillage, and stopper disposal, several firms have developed closed-container sampling systems for use in their automated hematology and chemistry analyzers. One such system is used in the Synchron LX PRO chemistry analyzer. On this analyzer, tubes are positioned under the piercing unit where they are clamped and pierced by a blade. Once the cap has been pierced, the sample probe can easily slide through the cap and withdraws an aliquot of specimen. Closed-container sampling is widely used in hematology analyzers.

On-Analyzer Specimen Delivery

The method of specimen delivery within the analyzer is the major difference between continuous-flow and discrete systems. In continuous-flow systems, the specimen is aspirated through the sample probe into a continuous reagent stream, whereas in discrete analyzers, the specimen is aspirated into the sample probe and then delivered through the same orifice into a reaction cup or other container.

Discrete Pipetting

Positive–liquid-displacement pipettes are used for specimen handling in most discrete automated systems. With them, specimens, calibrators, and controls are delivered by a single pipette to the next stage in the analytical process.

A positive-displacement pipette may be designed for one of two operational modes: (1) to dispense only aspirated specimen into the reaction receptacle or (2) to flush out specimen together with diluent. Both systems use a plastic or glass syringe with a plunger whose tip is usually made of Teflon. When a liquid (e.g., diluent or reagent) is used as displacement medium, liquid-displacement pipettes are capable of highly reproducible measurement of serum. However, when air is the displacement medium, viscous fluids can be measured with less accuracy. This inaccuracy becomes apparent when sera containing large amounts of lipids or proteins are pipetted and the analytical results are compared against aqueous calibrators.

Pipettes may be categorized as fixed-, variable-, or selectable-volume (see Chapter 1). Selectable-volume pipettes allow the selection of a limited number of predetermined volumes. In general, pipettes with selectable volumes are used in systems that allow many different applications, whereas fixed-volume pipettes are usually used for specimens and reagents in instruments dedicated to performing only a small variety of tests.

Inaccuracy and imprecision for delivery of specimens from pipettes should not exceed 1%. Similar performance is desired for reagent delivery. The accuracy of the pipetting must be verified periodically, and such checks are a key factor in assessing the quality of instrument performance (see Chapter 14). The accuracy and reproducibility of pipettes in automated instruments are checked in the same way as they are for pipettes in manual systems (see Chapter 1).

On analyzers with several analytical modules (MODULAR, Architect, AU 5400 series), delivery of specimens from the specimen input area to the various modules is accomplished using either built-in conveyor tracks (MODULAR, AU 5400 series) or robotic handling of specimen carriers (Architect) (Figure 11-2). These devices will be discussed in more detail later.

Carryover

Carryover is defined as the unintended transfer of a quantity of analyte or reagent by an analytical system from one specimen reaction into a subsequent one. Because carryover introduces error into the analytical results from the subsequent reaction, it should be minimized. Details for determining the extent of analyte carryover are described in the NCCLS document EP 10-A2, "Preliminary Evaluation of Quantitative Clinical Laboratory Methods; Approved Guideline Second Edition."[58] More elaborate protocols are required to evaluate the extent of reagent carryover.[52] Most

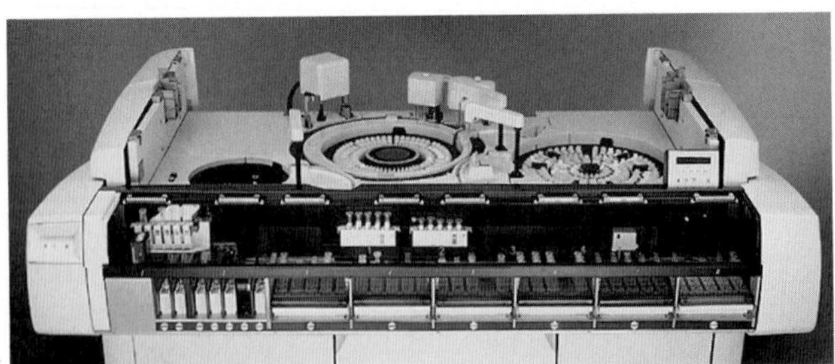

Figure 11-2 A robotic device is used in the Abbott Architect c8000, ci8200, and i2000SR to move racks of specimens from multiple specimen introduction bays located across the front of the analyzer to a bar code reading station *(left)* and to analyzer module sampling areas *(center)*. Covers normally present on this c8000 analyzer have been removed. *(Reproduction of this photograph has been granted with approval of Abbott Laboratories, Inc, all rights reserved by Abbott Laboratories, Inc; www.abbottdiagnostics.com.)*

manufacturers of discrete systems reduce the carryover by setting an adequate flush-to-specimen ratio and by incorporating wash stations for the sample probe. The ratio of flush to specimen may be as much as 4:1 to limit carryover to less than 1%, although recent advances in materials and dispenser velocity control have permitted lower ratios. Appropriate choice of sample probe material, geometry, and surface conditions minimizes imprecision and inaccuracy.

Carryover has been reduced in some systems by flushing the internal and external surfaces of the sample probe with copious amounts of diluent. The outside of the sample probe is wiped in some instruments to prevent transfer of a portion of the previous specimen into the next specimen cup. In discrete systems with disposable reaction vessels and measuring cuvets, carryover is caused by the pipetting system. In instruments with reusable cuvets or flow cells, carryover may arise at every point through which specimens pass sequentially. Disposable sample-probe tips eliminate both the contamination of one specimen by another inside the probe and the carryover of one specimen into the specimen in the next cup. Such an approach is used in the Vitros analyzers, in which a separate disposable tip for each specimen is automatically mounted onto a single, positive-displacement pipette. In these systems, a specimen is partially expelled, and the resultant pendant drop of serum on the tip is touched to the spreading layer of the test slide, where it spreads and subsequently diffuses into the next layer, consisting of a dry reagent matrix. Although the imprecision and inaccuracy of specimen dispensing may be as high as 2%, the volume of fluid that passes to the area exposed to the photometric light beam remains constant, and the resulting final precision is equivalent to 0.2%. Because a new pipette tip is used for each specimen, carryover is totally eliminated.

Reduction of carryover is a more stringent requirement for automated analyzers that perform immunoassays because for some analytes the concentration range in specimens can be as high as 6 decades (as for human chorionic gonadotropin). Some systems use extra steps, such as additional washes, or an additional washing device to reduce carryover to acceptable limits. Because extra steps can reduce overall throughput, additional rinsing functions are initiated (by computer operator selection) only for assays with a large dynamic range.

Reagent Handling and Storage

Most automated systems use liquid reagents stored in plastic or glass containers. For those analyzers in which a working inventory is maintained in the system, the volumes of reagents stored depend on the number of tests to be performed without operator intervention to refill. Whenever possible, manufacturers use single reagents for test procedures, although two or more reagents may be required for some tests. Others (e.g., Vitros and Reflotron Plus) use reagent-impregnated slides and strips, respectively. Still others rely entirely on electrodes to react with specimens (e.g., Bayer RapidLab systems, GEM Premier 3000, Radiometer ABL 700, and i-STAT Portable Clinical Analyzer).

For many analyzers in which specimens are not processed continuously, reagents are stored in laboratory refrigerators and introduced into the instruments as required. In larger systems (e.g., SYNCHRON CX and LX systems, Architect, MODULAR, AND DIMENSION), sections of the reagent storage compartments are maintained at 4 °C to 10 °C. Refrigerated storage for reagents is also provided in most immunoassay systems. Many of the reagents delivered in liquid form by the manufacturers of these systems are stable for 2 to 12 months.

Liquid Reagent Systems

The DIMENSION Clinical Chemistry System, MODULAR, ADVIA 2400, and SYNCHRON series are examples of systems that use liquid reagents. Large volumes of reagents, adequate for operation of the analyzer for hours or days, are stored in the systems. The containers are reservoirs that provide reagents test by test. Reagents with limited stability may be prepared during the analyzer set-up phase and may be stored, during a run, in refrigerated space adjoining the system.

Nonliquid Reagent Systems

No or very little liquid is used in the analytical process on dry reagent systems such as the Vitros and Reflotron Plus. For "color reactions," the Vitros uses a multilayered, 16-mm square slide (Figure 11-3) in which reagents dispersed in emulsions are activated by diffusion of the specimen fluid into the layers. From three to seven layers containing reagents are used for each of the different tests available. The Vitros also uses slides for electrometric assays that incorporate miniature ion-selective electrodes. On these, a reference solution and patient specimen provide fluid that turns the electrodes into electrochemical half-cells (see Chapter 4). Slides of this type that measure sodium, potassium, carbon dioxide, and chloride are currently in use.

The OPUS system has dry reagents impregnated in a coated multilayer film chip encased within a plastic bar coded test module. No external or supplementary reagents are required. A serum or plasma specimen is applied to the test module by the instrument and the fluorescence intensity from the module is measured after an assay-specific time interval.

Systems with Reusable Reagent Capability

Some systems use reagents or antibodies that have been immobilized in a reaction coil or chamber to repetitively carry out a chemical reaction or a separation of an analyte contained in aliquots of successive specimens. Other systems use enzymes immobilized on membranes that are coupled to sensing electrodes. The reaction products are then measured by the sensing device. Only a buffer is required as a diluent and wash solution, and thus the membrane has an extended life of approximately several months. Some

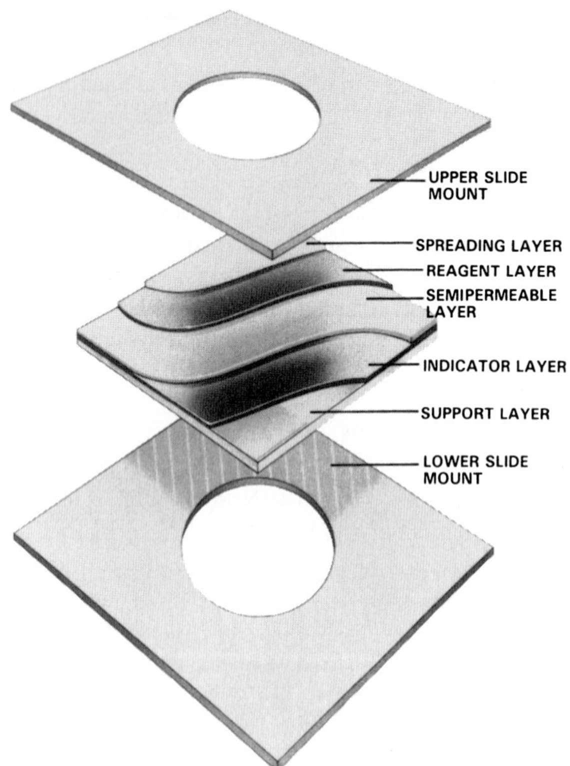

Figure 11-3 A schematic, exploded view of the multilayer dry film reagent used in Vitros analyzers. *(Courtesy Ortho-Clinical Diagnostics.)*

assemblies can be recycled for as many as 7500 tests, resulting in a low cost per test. Application of these systems is found in the 2300 STAT Plus for glucose and lactate assay.

Reagent Identification

Labels on reagent containers include information such as reagent identification, volume of the contents or number of tests for which the contents of the containers can be used, expiration date, and lot number. Provision of much of this information on labels is required by law. Many reagent containers now carry bar codes that contain some or all of this information and the manufacturer is able to retrieve any pertinent information when necessary. Other advantages of using reagent bar codes include: (1) facilitation of inventory management; (2) ability to insert reagent containers in random sequence; (3) ability to automatically dispense a particular volume of liquid reagent. In immunoassay systems, a bar code on a reagent container contains key information about (multiple) calibrators, such as definition of a calibration curve algorithm and values of curve constants that are defined at the time of reagent manufacture. Accompanying calibrator materials provided in their own bar coded tubes at the time of manufacture ensure that calibration functions are properly integrated into the analysis process.

Open Versus Closed Systems

Automated analyzers also are classified as "open" or "closed." In an open analyzer, the operator is able to change the parameters related to an analysis and to prepare "in-house" reagents or use reagents from a variety of suppliers. Such analyzers usually have considerable flexibility and are readily adapted to new methods and analytes. A closed-system analyzer requires the reagent in a unique container or format provided by the manufacturer. In general, liquid reagents for open systems are less expensive than the proprietary components required for closed analyzers. Yet, closed systems have a hidden cost advantage because reconstitution or preparation of the reagents for use does not require a technologist's time. The variability arising from reconstitution of dry reagents can be overcome by the use of predispensed liquid reagents or through the provision of premeasured liquids. The stability of liquid reagents for some open systems is now approaching the longer stability that has characterized many closed systems. Most immunoassay systems are closed, as are most systems that have been developed for POC applications.

Reagent Delivery

Liquid reagents are taken up and delivered to mixing and reaction chambers either by pumps (through tubes) or by positive-displacement syringe devices. In the early continuous-flow systems, such as the SMAC, a peristaltic pump and manifold both delivered fluids and determined the proportion of reagents to specimen. In the SYNCHRON CX series, a stepper motor is used to drive a pump that functions in the same way as the peristaltic pump of the AutoAnalyzer by alternately compressing and releasing a single reagent tube. Syringe devices for both reagent and specimen delivery are common to many automated systems. They are usually positive-displacement devices, and the volumes of reagents they deliver are programmable. Reproducibility of delivered volume is frequently better than ±1% with an accuracy within ±1%. In those analyzers in which more than one reagent is acquired and dispensed by the same syringe, washing or flushing of the probe is essential to prevent reagent carryover that may be deleterious to successive analytical steps in the same assay or to successive and different assays.

Chemical Reaction Phase

As its name implies, the chemical reaction phase occurs when aliquots of specimen and reagents are allowed to chemically react. Concerns related to this operation and the measurement of the reaction are addressed in the design of every automated analyzer. Design issues to be considered include (1) the vessel in which the reaction occurs and the cuvet in which the reaction is monitored, (2) the timing of the reaction(s), (3) the mixing and transport of reactants, and (4) the thermal conditioning of fluids. Separation of bound and unbound fractions is a fifth issue for immunoassay systems, as described in Chapter 9.

Type of Reaction Vessel and Cuvet

In older continuous-flow systems, each specimen passed through the same continuous stream and was subjected to the same analytical reactions as every other specimen and at the same rate. In such systems the reaction occurred in the tube that served as both a flow container and a cuvet.

In discrete systems each specimen in a batch has its own physical and chemical space, separate from every other specimen. Discrete analyzers use (1) individual (disposable or reusable) reaction vessels that are transported through the system after specimen and reagent have been dispensed (Immulite 2000), or (2) a stationary reaction chamber, as in the SYNCHRON CX Series. In some discrete systems, reaction vessels are reused; in others, they are discarded after use. The use of disposable cuvets has simplified automation and eliminated carryover in the cuvets and maintenance of flow cells. Disposable cuvets became possible through the development of superior plastics (notably acrylic and polyvinyl chloride) and manufacturing technology. Large-scale production of cuvets with excellent dimensional tolerances is an essential requirement. The cuvets must be transparent in the spectral range of interest. Disposable components are increasingly used in discrete automated systems.

Reaction vessels are reused in many instruments (e.g., SYNCHRON CX Series, Abbott Architect c8000 series, MODULAR, and the AU 400, AU 640, and AU 5400). The time before reusable cuvet and/or reaction vessels must be replaced depends on their composition (e.g., 1 month for plastic and 2 years for standard glass vessels). Pyrex glass vessels are not replaced unless physically damaged.

The typical cleaning sequence of a reusable cuvet and/or reaction vessel involves aspiration of the reaction mixture out of the cuvet at an in situ wash station. A detergent, alkaline, or acid wash solution is then repeatedly dispensed into and aspirated out of the cuvet. The cuvet is rinsed several times with deionized water and dried by vacuum or pressurized air. Optical clarity is verified automatically in most systems (usually while the cuvets contain the water). If performance is unsatisfactory, the operator is alerted to replace individual cuvets. If the cuvets are not replaced promptly, the system cannot be used for analysis; until they are replaced, the results for the unsatisfactory cuvets will be flagged.

Although the use of reusable cuvets reduces expenditure on consumables and extends walk-away time, it does contribute to instrument complexity and requires that a supply of cleaning liquids be maintained. In Centaur, a supply of individual cuvets is loaded onto the instrument. The number of loaded cuvets ranges from 200 to 1000, permitting walk-away times of approximately 1 to 3 hours.

In the DIMENSION, cuvets of 5-mm path length are manufactured in the instrument by drawing two strips of Surlyn clear plastic around the circumference of a ring mold that contains 100 separate cavities (Figure 11-4). A canister containing sufficient plastic to make 12,000 cuvets is loaded into the instrument. A schematic diagram of the Immulite 2000 analyzer is shown in Figure 11-5. This analyzer is equipped with an automatic tube feeder that accepts polystyrene reaction tubes in bulk, orients them vertically, and delivers them to the bead drop and the pipetting positions. The reaction tube serves as the vessel for all incubations, washes, and signal development. It is discarded automatically after analysis.

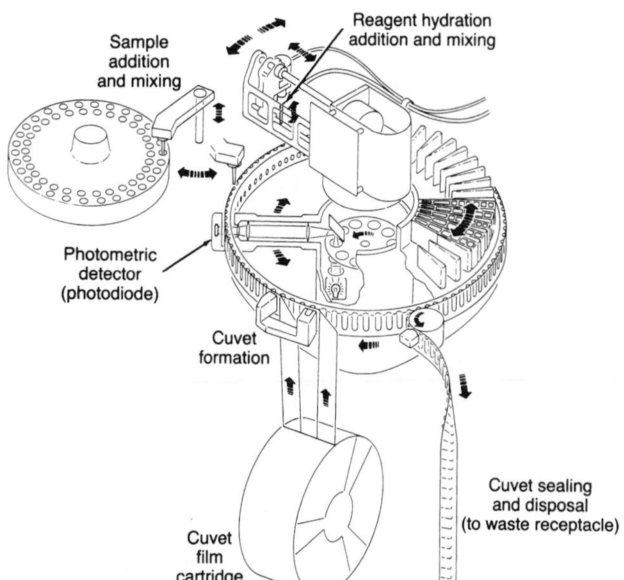

Figure 11-4 Arrangement of key elements of the DIMENSION. Relationships of elements used for in situ cuvet manufacturing are shown. *(Courtesy Dade Behring; www.dadebehring.com.)*

Timing of Reactions

The time allowed for a reaction to occur depends on a variety of factors. In some analyzers reaction time depends on the rate of transport through the system to the measurement station or on timed events of reagent addition (or activation) relative to measurement, or on both. In discrete random-access analyzers specimens and reagents are added to a cuvet in a timed sequence, and absorbance readings are performed at intervals to follow the course of each reaction. Usually, the total read time for a reaction in these systems is constrained to a maximum value defined by the manufacturer but may be programmed for a shorter period.

Mixing of Reactants

Various techniques are used to mix reactants. These include the following: (1) forceful dispensing, (2) magnetic stirring, (3) a rotating paddle, and (4) the use of ultrasonic energy (DIMENSION). Continuous-flow analyzers relied on the tumbling action of the stream flowing through a mixing coil. The dry reagent systems, such as Vitros, Reflotron Plus, Stratus, and OPUS, obviate the necessity for mixing because the serum completely interacts with the dry chemicals as it flows through the matrix of the reaction unit. Regardless of the technique used, mixing is a difficult process to automate.

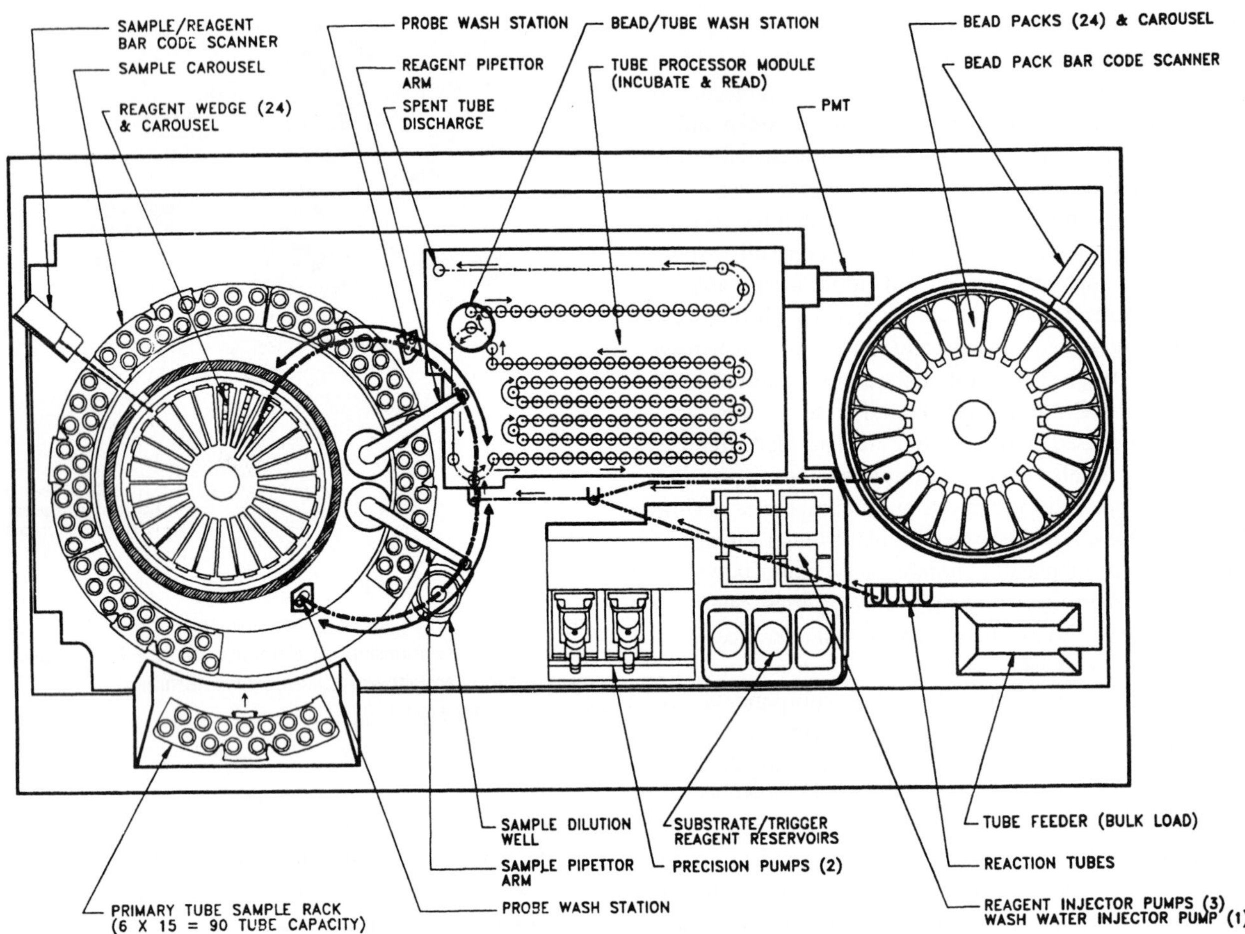

Figure 11-5 A schematic view of the Immulite 2000 analyzer. The relationship of the tube feeder, bead pack carousel, reagent carousel, specimen carousel, tube processor module, and photomultiplier tube (PMT) is shown. *(Courtesy Diagnostic Products Corporation; www.dpcweb.com.)*

Thermal Regulation

Thermal regulation requires the establishment of a controlled-temperature environment in close contact with the reaction container and efficient heat transfer from the environment to the reaction mixture. Air baths, water baths, and contact with a heating or cooling plate (e.g., Peltier device) have been used for thermal regulation in commercial analyzers (mostly at 37 °C).

Measurement Approaches

Automated chemistry analyzers have traditionally relied on photometers and spectrophotometers for measurement of absorbance. Alternative approaches now being incorporated into analyzers include reflectance photometry and fluorometry. Immunoassay systems have used fluorescence (IMX), chemiluminescence (Centaur and Immulite), and electrochemiluminescence (ELECSYS) to enhance sensitivity. Ion-selective electrodes and other electrochemical techniques are also widely used. Principles of these measurement techniques have been discussed previously (see Chapter 4). This section reviews the special features and application of the various approaches to automated analysis.

Photometry

The measurement of absorbance requires three basic components: (1) an optical source, (2) a means of spectral isolation, (3) and a detector (see Chapter 3).

Optical Source

The radiant energy sources used in automated systems include tungsten, quartz halogen, deuterium, mercury, and xenon lamps and lasers. In the quartz-halogen lamp, low-pressure halogen vapor (such as iodine or bromine) is enclosed in a fused silica envelope in which a tungsten filament serves as an incandescent light source. The spectrum produced includes wavelengths from approximately 300 to 700 nm.

Spectral Isolation

In automated systems spectral isolation is commonly achieved with interference filters. Such filters are now quite inexpensive, and only a few are necessary in any one instrument, because only a limited number of wavelengths is required for analysis of a large number of absorbing species. Typical interference filters have peak transmission of 30% to

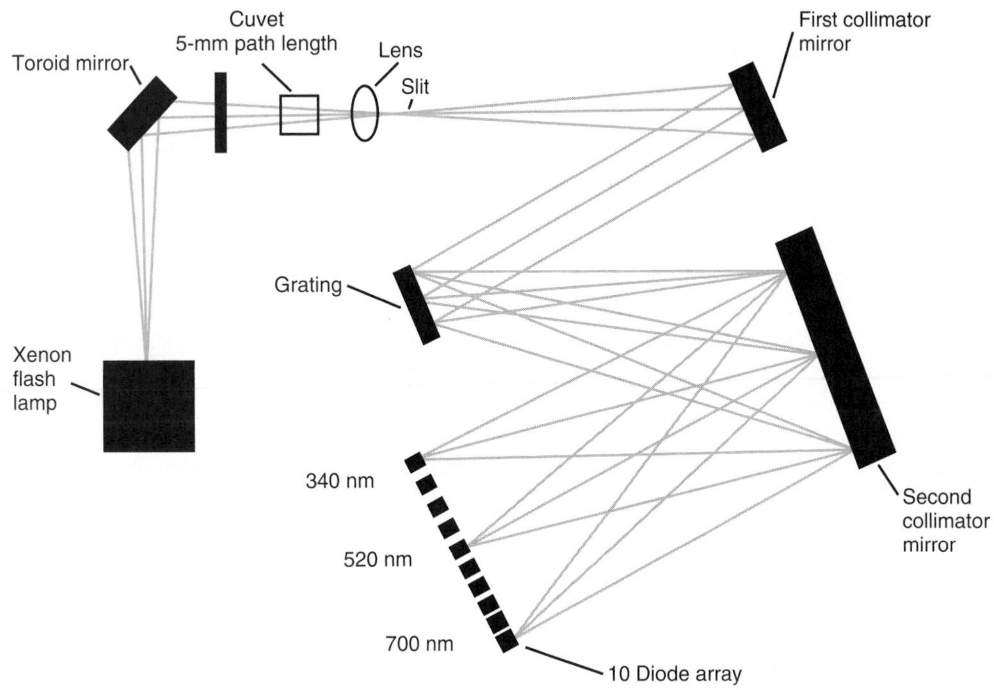

Figure 11-6 Use of a diode array in the SYNCHRON CX7 monochromator reduces requirements for moving parts. For simplicity, ray traces for only three wavelengths are shown. *(Courtesy Beckman Coulter Inc; www.beckmancoulter.com.)*

80% and bandwidths of 5 to 15 nm (see Chapter 3). In several multitest analyzers, filters are mounted in a filter wheel, and the appropriate filter is moved into place under computer control. Monochromators with movable gratings and slits provide a continuous choice of wavelengths. They offer a high amount of flexibility and are especially suited for the development of new assays. However, because relatively few wavelengths are required for analyses in routine analyzers, many manufacturers use a stationary, holographically ruled grating coupled with a stationary photodiode array to isolate the spectrum. These two elements are also coupled with fiberoptic light guides to transfer the passage of light energy through cuvets at locations convenient for mechanization. Use of these passive elements enhances the reliability of a system because no moving parts are required for spectral isolation. Figure 11-6 shows the arrangement of a grating and/or diode array for the SYNCHRON CX Series.

Photometric Detectors

Photodiodes are used as detectors in many automated systems either as individual components or in multiples as an array. Photomultiplier tubes are required in many immunoassay systems to provide adequate sensitivity and fast detector response times for fluorescent and chemiluminescent measurements. Several approaches have been used for the electrooptical integration and packaging in different analyzers. A logarithmic amplifier or microprocessor and/or computer software converts transmittance to absorbance. Low-cost analog-to-digital converters with conversion times of fractions of a millisecond, together with low-cost oscillators with timing accuracy of microseconds, are coupled with high-performance computers to accumulate, store, and process optical signals on a real-time basis. Analyzers that use time sharing of the optical system components tend to be less costly while still providing good performance and reliability. In general an electrooptical package should offer an absorbance range of up to 2.5 absorbance units (*A*) to permit the extended linearity desirable for some reactions. Its photometric detection limit should be 0.001 *A* at 1 *A* and its noise level should not exceed 0.0005 *A* at 1 *A*, to ensure precision adequate for measuring kinetic reactions. The spectral range typically required is from 340 to 650 nm, but lower wavelengths may be necessary for some applications. Spectral isolation does not have to be more exact than is necessary for enzyme determinations. For analytes with broad absorbance peaks, interference filters with a bandpass up to 20 nm are satisfactory.

Proper alignment of cuvets with the light path(s) is equally important in automated and manual photometry; stray energy and internal reflections must be kept to acceptable levels. If the light path is not perpendicular to the cuvet, inaccuracy and imprecision may occur, particularly in kinetic analyses. Stray energy is reduced to 0.2% or less by careful design of the wavelength isolation filters or the monochromator to increase rejection of stray light.

Other Forms of Measurement

Several other optical techniques now are widely used in automated systems. Among these techniques are the following:

(1) reflectance photometry, (2) fluorometry, (3) fluorescence polarization, (4) turbidimetry and nephelometry, (5) chemiluminescence and bioluminescence.

Reflectance Photometry

In reflectance photometry, diffuse reflected light is measured. The reflected light results from illumination, with diffused light, of a reaction mixture in a carrier or from the diffusion of light by a reaction mixture in an illuminated carrier. The intensity of the reflected light from the reagent carrier is compared with that reflected from a reference surface. Intensity of reflected light is not linear with concentration of the analyte, and two algorithms are commonly used to linearize the relation of reflectance to concentration.[89] The electrooptical components used in reflectance photometry are essentially the same as those required for absorbance photometry. Reflectance photometry is used primarily in analyzers using dry, unit-dose reagent systems (e.g., Vitros and Reflotron Plus). In the Vitros, equilibrium measurements and kinetic enzyme measurements are monitored by separate reflectometers, each with a permanent reflectance reference. A Clapper-Williams transformation[89] is used to linearize the relation of reflectance to concentration. Adaptive algorithms define the number of points selected for calculation of enzyme activity to provide, in essence, a variable-time analysis as defined by Pardue.[67]

Fluorometry

Fluorescence is the emission of electromagnetic radiation by a species that has absorbed exciting radiation from an outside source. Intensity of emitted (fluorescent) light is directly proportional to the concentration of the excited species (see Chapter 3).

Fluorometry is widely used for automated immunoassay. It is approximately 1000 times more sensitive than comparable absorbance spectrophotometry, but background interference caused by fluorescence of native serum can create a major problem. This interference is minimized by careful design of the filters used for spectral isolation, by the selection of a fluorophore with an emission spectrum distinct from those of interfering compounds, or by using time- or phase-resolved fluorometry (see Chapter 3).

Different optical arrangements are represented in different manufacturers' equipment. Right-angle fluorescence measurement is one of the most common approaches, with emitted light passing through the emission interference filter to a photomultiplier tube.

Front-Surface Reflectance Fluorometry

Front-surface reflectance fluorometry is used in the Stratus CS analyzer, where light passed through a 360-nm filter is reflected from a dichroic mirror onto the front of the reagent tab on which the reaction of the antigen-conjugated enzyme occurs. The light emitted from the front surface of the tab travels back through the dichroic mirror and to a photomultiplier through an interference filter that selects only 450-nm light. Fluorescence intensity is monitored over a 30-second interval, and the rate of fluorescence development is calculated by the microprocessor. The rate of fluorescence change is then compared with the calibration curve stored in the microprocessor, and the test value is computed.

Polarization Fluorometry

In fluorescence polarization, the radiant energy is in the form of polarized light. Measurement is then made of the change in the degree of polarized light emitted by a fluorescent molecule, as described in Chapter 3. Fluorescence polarization is applied in the Abbott TD_x and AxSYM for homogeneous assays of low molecular weight compounds. Radiant energy in the form of polarized light is alternately pulsed vertically and horizontally to impinge on a reaction mixture containing antibody, specimen, and tracer. Free tracer not bound to antibody depolarizes the emitted light, whereas light emitted from a bound tracer is highly polarized. As a result, in this system, polarization is inversely proportional to concentration. The optical system consists of a 50-W projector bulb, an interference filter, a fixed horizontal polarizer, and a photomultiplier tube. An electrically switched liquid crystal is located between the polarizer and the reaction mixture. Absence or presence of voltage on the crystal changes the orientation of the polarized light. Because variability of path length is immaterial to the analytical principle used, inexpensive borosilicate tubes are satisfactorily used for reaction cells. Use of a liquid crystal instead of mechanical devices to modulate the polarized light significantly improves the reliability of the optical system for this sensitive technique.

Turbidimetry and Nephelometry

These two optical techniques are particularly applicable to methods measuring the precipitate formation in antigen antibody reactions (see Chapter 9). Turbidimetry is used in several chemistry immunoassay systems for therapeutic drug monitoring and specific protein assays. Details of turbidimetry and nephelometry are discussed in Chapter 3.

Nephelometers such as the ARRAY, IMAGE, and BN series are widely used for analysis of serum specific proteins (see Chapter 20). These analyzers direct light to a flow cell and detect forward angle light scattering from different sized immune complexes. Reading the light scattering at a forward angle rather than the classical 90° angle is known to increase the sensitivity of nephelometric assays.[78]

Chemiluminescence and Bioluminescence

Chemiluminescence and bioluminescence differ from fluorometry in that the excitation event is caused by a chemical or electrochemical reaction and not by photoillumination (see Chapter 3). The applications of chemiluminescence and bioluminescence have greatly increased with the development of automated instrumentation and several new reagent systems. Because of their attomole to zeptomole detection limits, chemiluminescence and bioluminescence reactions have been widely used as direct and indicator labels in the development of immunoassays (see Chapter 9). Several of these schemes have been used in new automated immunochemistry analyzers (CENTAUR, Immulite, and ELECSYS).

Electrochemical

A variety of electrochemical methods have been incorporated into automated systems. The most widely used electrochemical approach involves ion-selective electrodes. These electrodes have replaced flame photometry for the determination of sodium and potassium in many analyzers and have lately found direct application in the measurement of other electrolytes and indirect application in the analysis of several other serum constituents. The operating principle of ion-selective electrodes is given in some detail in Chapter 4. The relationship between ion activity and the concentration of ions in the specimens must be established with calibrating solutions, and frequent recalibration must be done to compensate for alterations of electrode response.

Peristaltic pumps are used to move the specimen into chambers containing fixed specimen and reference electrodes. The electrodes must remain in contact with the specimen for a sufficiently long time (from 7 to 45 seconds) to reach steady-state conditions. Response time, therefore, determines throughput of an automated system, and care must be taken to monitor response time and to restore it, when it degrades, by implementing appropriate maintenance procedures. The most common arrangement is to provide electrodes to assay three analytes, typically sodium, potassium, and chloride. Because specimens and calibrators usually flow past a group of electrodes, results for all analytes are reported for most systems. However, ion-selective electrode capability has also been incorporated into automated analyzers as individual channels (SYNCHRON CX series). Integrated three- and four-parameter modules have been incorporated into many small and large random-access systems (e.g., COBAS Integra, MODULAR, Architect c-8000 series, AU 400, AU 640, and AU 5400); this has significantly increased these systems' throughput, because several results are produced in parallel.

Ion-selective electrodes coupled with immobilized enzymes represent an extended application. In such systems, the enzymatic reaction with the analyte involves a product that can be measured electrochemically. An example is the YSI 2300 STAT Plus used to measure glucose in whole blood. In this system, glucose oxidase is immobilized between two membrane layers and catalyzes oxidation of glucose in the fluid, in contact with the membrane, to produce hydrogen peroxide. The hydrogen peroxide in turn is oxidized at a platinum anode. The oxidation results in an electrical current directly proportional to hydrogen peroxide concentration and, therefore, proportional to glucose concentration.

Conductimetry is another electrochemical approach that is used in the SYNCHRON CX series, specifically for the measurement of urea nitrogen. The specimen is introduced into the reaction cup along with a buffered urease solution. With the conversion of urea to ammonium and carbonate ions, the rate of change of conductivity across gold electrodes embedded in the cup is proportional to the concentration of urea nitrogen.

Signal Processing, Data Handling, and Process Control

Computers and computer telecommunications are integral components of the entire analytical and reporting process and control the data input, operation, monitoring, and data reporting functions in automated analyzers. Also, workstations have been used to integrate the operation of one or more laboratory analyzers. Individual analyzers and/or their workstations are electronically interfaced with large central data repositories on laboratory information systems (LIS) and/or laboratory automation systems (LAS) (see Chapter 18).

Computers installed in each analyzer are essential in the acquisition and processing of analytical data. Ancillary internal electronic components include analog-to-digital converters that rapidly (10^{-3} to 10^{-5} seconds) convert analog signals to digital form. Such digitized data are passed to the microprocessor and/or computer that processes the data into useful and meaningful output. Data processing and other computer functions in analyzers depend upon sophisticated software developed by each instrument manufacturer. For example, automation of procedures such as nonisotopic immunoassays and reflectance spectrometry relies on computer algorithms to transform complex, nonlinear standard responses into linear calibration curves. The nature and character of data output can be as varied as output software and hardware allow and as analytical purposes require. Some functions performed by computers incorporated into automated analyzers are listed in Box 11-1.

Other functions of integrated computers include:

1. Computers *command* and *phase* the electromechanical operation of the analyzer, thus ensuring that all functions are performed uniformly, are repeatable, and are in the correct sequence (e.g., transfer of solutions, placement of proper filters, and regulation and change in speed of rotation). Computer control of operational features of automated equipment, calculation of results, and monitoring of operation contribute to the increased reproducibility of results. These combined features, theoretically at least, allow less-skilled operators to operate such systems.
2. Computers *acquire, assess, process,* and *store* operational data from the analyzers. Many computers include built-in test equipment that monitors instrument functions for correct execution and reacts to improper function by recording the site and nature of the malfunction.
3. Computers enable important *communication interactions between the analyzer and the operator.* Alphanumeric displays on monitors or on light-emitting diode arrays provide operator-readable information and signals. The signals may instruct the operator to intervene to replen-

BOX 11-1 Some Signal and Data Processing Functions Performed by Computers of Automated Analyzers

Data Acquisition and Calculation

Acquisition of response signal and signal averaging
Subtraction of blank response
Correction of response of unknown for interferences (e.g., Allen-type corrections)
Linear regression for determining slope
($\Delta A/\Delta t$) of rate reactions; ($\Delta A/\Delta C$) of absorbance/concentration relation; ($\Delta R/\Delta C$) of any response parameter to concentration
Statistics (mean, SD, CV) on patient or control values
Mathematical transformation of nonlinear relations to linear counterpart
Mathematical transformation of results to alternative reporting units

Monitoring

Test for fit of data to linearity criteria for calibration curves or rate reactions
Test of patient result against reference interval criteria
Test of control result against criteria of a quality control standard of performance
Test of moving average of patient results against quality criteria for detecting assay drift

Display

Display of specimens currently being analyzed, tests ordered on each specimen, and expected times of completion
Accumulation of sets of patient results
Collation of results for patient-oriented printout
Provide warning messages to alert operator to instrument malfunction, need for maintenance, or unusual clinical situation
Provide quality control charts for operator review
Provide troubleshooting flowcharts to assist operator

SD, Standard deviation; *CV*, coefficient of variation.

ish reagent supply or to empty waste containers, or they may warn of operating problems that can compromise test results. The message describing the site and type of problem, together with the manufacturer's service manuals, enables quick identification of problems and their prompt correction. Personal computer (PC) operating systems provide detailed and interactive troubleshooting guidance to operators of instruments and visual display of the status of every specimen. Output data tested against preset criteria can be flagged and displayed for the operator's evaluation and assessment. Such information may specify that linearity of a reaction has been exceeded, a reaction is nonlinear, substrate exhaustion has occurred, absorbance of a reagent is too high or too low, or baseline drift is excessive. The computer can also receive commands from the operator through the keyboard or a touch-sensitive screen. These commands may reprogram certain functions of the analyzer (e.g., timing interval for a kinetic reaction and set point of the reaction temperature); enter certain values, such as calibrator concentrations; display stored information in raw or processed form; or define the format of printed output.

4. Integrated computers can in turn *communicate with mainframe computers.* A typical interface implemented in computers is a UART (universal asynchronous receiver and transmitter), which is in turn connected to an RS-232, RS-488, or Ethernet interface to permit interactive communication with other computer systems. The same interface capability permits transmission by modem (modulator-demodulator) over telephone lines. The telephone line may allow the manufacturer's central service department to enhance the ability of the on-site operator to service and repair the analyzer. With a bidirectional interface, it is possible to "download" from the main LIS computer such data as specimen identification, which governs specimen location in the analyzer's loading zone, and to send test results from the analyzer back to the LIS, either in real time or by batch.
5. Computers incorporated into instruments or connected through stand-alone PCs have expanded the capabilities of instrument systems to include those previously available only by connection to the mainframes of LISs. These capabilities include summaries of quality control (production of Shewhart plots), fitting of immunoassay calibration curves using various models (e.g., four parameter log-logistic),[74] and linkage of patient information with specimen identification.

Computer workstations can be used to monitor and integrate the functions of one or more analyzers. Typically, the workstation serves as the point of interaction with the instrument operator, accepts test orders, monitors the testing process, assists with analysis of process quality, and provides facilities for review and verification of test results. The workstation is usually directly interfaced with the LIS host, accepting downloaded test orders, and uploading test results. Most workstations have facilities to display Levy-Jennings quality control charts, to monitor the progress of each test order, and to troubleshoot the analyzers. They may also provide facilities to assist with the review of completed test results. Some workstations have rule-based software, which allows the operator to program rules for autoverification of test results (MODULAR Middleware Software).

INTEGRATED AUTOMATION FOR THE CLINICAL LABORATORY

Significant progress has been made in integrating the individual steps of the analytical process discussed in the previous section into analytical systems. Consequently, advanced analytical systems are now available from multiple vendors for automated chemistry, hematology,[41,69] immunoassay,[18,19,72,91,92] coagulation,[45,88] microbiology, and nucleic acid testing (see Chapter 37),* which provide efficient and cost-effective operation with a minimum of operator input. Because of increased financial pressures to reduce costs, clinical laboratorians are integrating these analytical systems with "front-end" specimen handling and transport systems to "totally" automate their laboratories and are even considering the automation of previously nonautomated areas.

Some manufacturers have also developed stand-alone "front-end" automation systems, which perform tasks such as sorting, centrifugation, decapping, aliquoting, and labeling of aliquot tubes. These systems may require manual transport of the tubes to the analytical areas, but they have automated steps in specimen processing with acceptable returns on investment for the laboratories that have acquired them. Including the total and modular automation systems described above and these stand-alone systems, total worldwide installations of laboratory automation are estimated at well more than 800 systems as of this writing.

The potential economic benefits of large-scale automation of the laboratory are enormous. Carried to the fullest extent, large-scale automation of the laboratory includes an automated specimen processing area where the operations of specimen identification, labeling, scheduling, centrifugation, and sorting of specimens are initiated. After specimen processing, automated specimen conveyor devices transport the sorted specimens to the appropriate workstations in the laboratory, where they are analyzed without human intervention. Rule-based expert system software assists with the review of laboratory results by automatically releasing results that have no associated problems, but drawing any problematic results to the attention of trained medical technologists. All specimens are cataloged after analysis and stored in a central storage facility, available for automated retrieval if necessary. As pointed out previously, particularly important aspects of large-scale automation projects are the approaches used to process and transport specimens and the overall integration of the automated components into a smoothly functioning whole.

We begin this section with discussions of the roles that workstations, instrument clusters, and workcells have in laboratory automation, followed by discussions of specimen transportation, automated specimen processing, automated specimen sorting, and automated specimen storage and retrieval subsystems.

WORKSTATIONS

The task of integrating laboratory automation begins with the laboratory workstation.[12,56] In general, a clinical laboratory workstation is usually devoted to a defined task (e.g., performing chemistry profiles, complete blood counts, hormone testing, polymerase chain reaction testing, and urinalysis) and contains appropriate laboratory instrumentation to carry out that task. Frequently, the workstation in the modern laboratory is defined in terms of the automated analyzer that is being used. Current laboratory instruments and systems are highly developed for stand-alone operation and fit into the workstation concept. Movement of specimens into and out of the workstation is accomplished by manual transport, and the instrument operator activities are largely independent of those at other workstations. On a typical instrument, the instrument operator follows a manufacturer-recommended sequence of calibration, quality control, and daily maintenance activities, and uses the instrument's front-panel functions to introduce specimens for analysis. If the analyzer has a bidirectional interface with a laboratory information system (LIS; see Chapter 18) and bar code reading capabilities, information regarding what assays to run on each specimen is downloaded from the LIS, and the instrument operator simply loads bar code–labeled specimens into the specimen input area. The built-in diagnostics supplied in most modern analyzers (e.g., to detect malfunctions during the assay process, to track usage of reagents, and to notify the operator of out-of-range results) provide enough "intelligence" in the analyzer that the operator is able to "walk away" from the instrument for short periods, confident of its reliable operation. Nevertheless, the operator needs to attend periodically to instrument operation, replenishing reagents, evaluating instrument diagnostic messages, and introducing new specimens into the specimen input tray.

INSTRUMENT CLUSTERS

To reduce labor costs, instrument manufacturers are developing approaches that will allow a single technologist to simultaneously control and monitor the functions of several instruments. Initially, such workstations have been configured with *clusters* of identical instruments, such as Vitros or Architect i2000 analyzers (Figure 11-7). Each cluster of analyzers has its own central control module (typically a PC) with software designed to assist the technologist in monitoring the functions of each analyzer and to aid in the review of laboratory results generated by the cluster. Access to the many front-panel functions of each analyzer is provided by the interface between the analyzer and the central control module. More advanced instrument clusters incorporate both chemistry and immunoassay analyzers (MODULAR and Architect CI series). The development of instrument clusters is possible in large part because the manufacturers have designed sufficient diagnostic capacities into their instruments to enable the autonomous "walk-away" mode of operation discussed previously. Thus the technologist can load specimens onto each instrument in the cluster and then monitor subsequent instrument operation and review the results at the central workstation. By incorporating the activities of what would be *several* workstations in most current laboratories into a *single* integrated workstation, this approach shows promise in saving laboratory manpower.

*References 20, 22, 34, 51, 65, 68, 92.

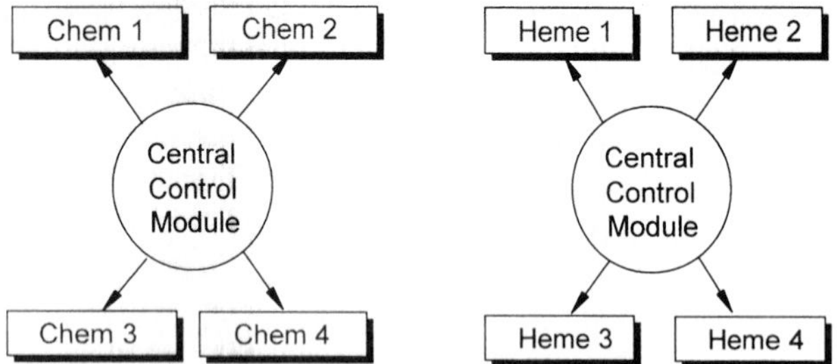

Figure 11-7 Workstations with clusters of like instruments (e.g., chemistry analyzers, Chem 1 through Chem 4, or hematology analyzers, Heme 1 through Heme 4) enable one technologist to operate and monitor the functions of several analyzers simultaneously. The central control module is usually provided by the manufacturer of the analyzers in each cluster. *(From Boyd JC, Felder RA, Savory J. Robotics and the changing face of the clinical laboratory. Clin Chem 1996; 42:1901-10.)*

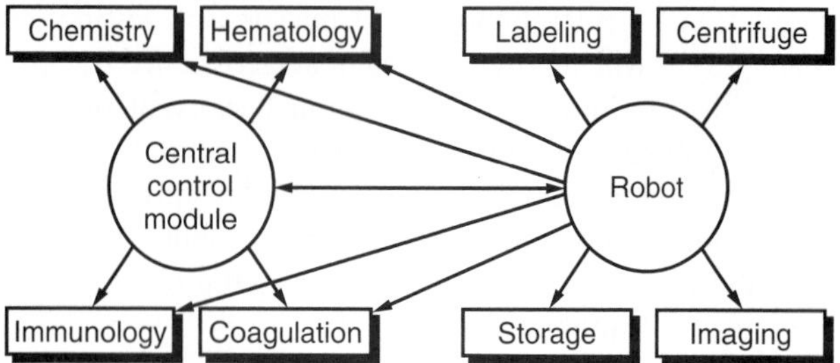

Figure 11-9 Example of a workstation configured with a cluster of unlike instruments and robotic specimen processing that could be useful in remote automated laboratories or in small outpatient laboratories. *(From Boyd JC, Felder RA, Savory J. Robotics and the changing face of the clinical laboratory. Clin Chem 1996; 42:1901-10.)*

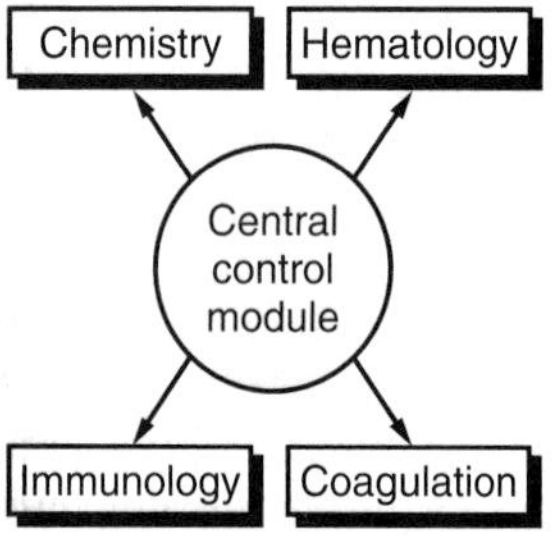

Figure 11-8 A workstation configured with a cluster of unlike instruments theoretically allows one technologist to operate and monitor the functions of several unlike analyzers. The software provided for the central control module is vitally important for successful implementation of such a configuration. Central control modules for this type of instrument cluster are under development by some LIS vendors and independent system integrators. *(From Boyd JC, Felder RA, Savory J. Robotics and the changing face of the clinical laboratory. Clin Chem 1996; 42:1901-10.)*

A possible extension of this concept is the development of clusters of unlike instruments (Figure 11-8) that cross traditional laboratory disciplines. When it is possible for a single technologist to monitor a workstation performing simultaneous testing from several disciplines, further reduction of laboratory manpower is envisioned. Bush[17] used a "chematology laboratory" to describe his joining of routine chemistry and hematology into a single instrument cluster in his laboratory. Interfaces between laboratory instruments in a cluster and the central control module are critical components of such a cluster. Standard interface design that would allow uniform communication of instructions to instruments from the central control module, and reporting of status information and laboratory results from the instruments to the central control module would facilitate the development of hybrid instrument clusters; however, current instrument interface standards do not yet allow for standardized transmission of instrument control instructions, and most laboratory instruments are not designed to accept commands from a remote computer.[53] Thus enhanced communication between different types of laboratory automation is necessary if this extended instrument cluster concept is to be successful (see later, under Development of Standards for Laboratory Automation).

WORKCELLS

Another extension of the instrument cluster concept is to add robotic specimen handling and preparation (Figure 11-9).[54] The robot is used to carry out various specimen preparation steps, including checks of specimen adequacy, centrifugation, aliquoting, labeling, and specimen storage after analysis. The robot is then responsible for introducing specimens into the appropriate analyzer, allowing the technologist to assume a primarily monitoring role. An interface between the central control module and the robot controller (or combining these functions on a single computer) allows the activities of the robotic cluster to be fully coordinated. The ability to carry out serial centrifugation of specimens as described by Godolphin et al[36] and others[25,26] would be ideal at a workstation because it would prevent the time delays introduced by batching of specimens in traditional centrifugation. As is mentioned in a section below on stand-alone specimen processing systems, several vendors are now marketing workcells that combine specimen processing with analytical testing. The Ortho enGen 1 system interfaces the enGen processing system with a Vitros 950AT analyzer. The Olympus OLA4000 workcell integrates an automated specimen processing system with up to two AU series analyzers depending on desired capacity.

AUTOMATED SPECIMEN TRANSPORT

Different approaches have been developed to transport specimens within the laboratory, including mobile robots, conveyor belts, and robotic arms.

Mobile Robots Versus Conveyor Belts

Mobile robots and conveyor belts have been used in the laboratory as aids to transport specimens from one clinical laboratory workstation to another. *Conveyor belt technology* has been applied successfully in industry for carefully defined transportation requirements. However, the difficulty this technology has in handling the large variety of specimen containers found in the clinical laboratory (ranging from microspecimen containers to large urine collection containers) is a disadvantage. To increase the variety of types of specimen containers that can be carried on a conveyor belt system, specimens are placed into specially designed carriers that fit on the conveyor belt line. Known as "pucks" or "racks" (depending on whether they carry individual specimens or groups of specimens), the carriers have receptacles for variously sized tubes. The Beckman Coulter Power Processor system carries specimens individually in disk-shaped pucks, whereas the Roche Diagnostics-Hitachi system carries specimens in racks that hold five tubes. Both of these systems have limitations on the tube sizes they can accommodate. Although some conveyor belt systems are custom manufactured for a facility (Simpliflex), others (Beckman Coulter, Roche Diagnostics-Hitachi, and Flexlink) are sold in modular form, including straight and curved pieces of track of varying lengths, crossover modules, and gating modules that can be assembled in various configurations to match a given laboratory geometry.

Elevator modules are available for some systems that allow pucks or racks to be moved up to ceiling height or under the floor for transport. Elevator modules vary in their ability to keep the specimen in an upright position, an important consideration if the tubes are being transported in an uncapped state. Eggert et al[24] have developed a unique overhead conveyor system for delivery of specimens from a central receiving area to appropriate laboratory workstations. Diamond et al[21] have described the use of conveyor belt technology in carrying out automated analyses in the hematology laboratory. Rothe et al[75] have provided estimates of the cost savings that may be achieved by such an approach.

Transfer of specimens from the conveyor belt to the laboratory workstation has been implemented in various ways. For example, many manufacturers have equipped their laboratory instruments with devices to obtain specimens from conveyor belt systems. The Vitros 950 AT and 250 AT analyzers, Dade Behring Dimension RxL, Abbott Architect, and Bayer ADVIA Centaur are examples of analyzers that can sample directly from open tubes on a conveyor belt track that has been physically attached to the back or side of the analyzer. Diagnostic Products Corp. has a specimen management system (SMS) that can be linked to a single Immulite 2000 or that can form an immunoassay workcell by linking with two Immulite 2000 analyzers. The SMS uses a robot arm to transfer specimens back and forth between racks of specimens that have been loaded into the SMS and the analyzer carousels. Thus racks of specimens have merely to be loaded into the SMS, which then manages the process of loading and unloading both analyzers. The SMS can also be attached to a conveyor system from which the same robot arm can transfer specimens from the conveyor directly into an Immulite 2000 or into empty racks in the immunoassay workcell. The SMS can also return specimens to the conveyor after the test results have been verified, provided there is an empty carrier in the proper position on the conveyor.

In contrast with the limited ability to reconfigure conveyor belt systems and their limited ability to handle different sized specimen containers, *mobile robots* are easily adapted to carry various sizes and shapes of specimen containers, and can be reprogrammed to travel to new (and distant) locations with changes in laboratory geometry. Limitations of mobile robots include their requirement of having to batch specimens, and their difficulty in interfacing mechanically with laboratory analyzers so that specimens are introduced directly from the mobile robot onto the analyzer. In many situations, laboratory personnel are still required to place specimens onto or remove specimens from the mobile robot at each stopping place. Mobile robots have been used to return conveyor belt specimen carrier racks to the central dispatch area and for transport of specimens within and outside the laboratory. In the latter application, mobile robots may be a useful alternative to pneumatic tube delivery systems.

Mobile robots have been equipped with simple (Robocart) or sophisticated (Helpmate) guidance systems. Robots with simple guidance systems follow a predetermined route (such as a line on the floor) to reach their destination, whereas robots with more sophisticated guidance systems are expected to navigate independently through a facility. The costs of the technology, not unexpectedly, vary directly with the degree of sophistication. Sophisticated guidance systems require more built-in sensors to provide enough information about the robot's outside environment to enable independent navigation. A review of commercially available mobile robots has been published.[32]

Robot Arms

The early applications of programmable robotic arms in the clinical laboratory have been reviewed.[30,31] Robotic arms were first used by the pharmaceutical industry to conduct drug dosage studies, and then by clinical laboratories to carry out highly complex clinical assays. Three types of robotic devices are commercially available: cartesian, cylindrical, and articulating (Figure 11-10). Robots, by virtue of their operational flexibility, enable systems to be reconfigured rapidly for new and varying protocols. This enhances versatility and safety, improves precision and productivity, and reduces errors caused by human mismatching of specimen identity. However, misprogramming of the systems can result in repetitive errors with potentially grave medical and legal consequences; thus great care is required to ensure that such errors do not occur.

Cartesian systems are the most common form of robotics in use in laboratories at present. Embodied in programmable pipetting stations, they provide flexible pipetting routines to suit varied protocols. They have been applied

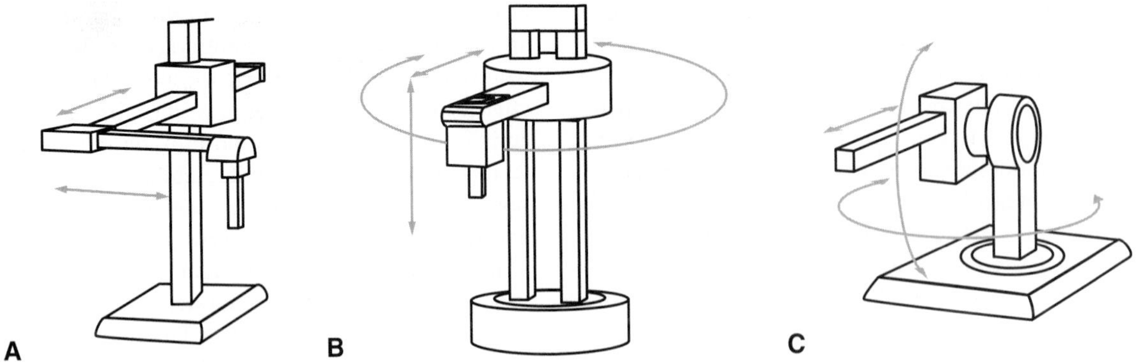

Figure 11-10 Three basic configurations of robotic devices that have application in the clinical laboratory. **A,** Cartesian. **B,** Cylindrical. **C,** Articulating (polar) or jointed. *(Courtesy the Journal of the International Federation of Clinical Chemistry 1992; 4:175.)*

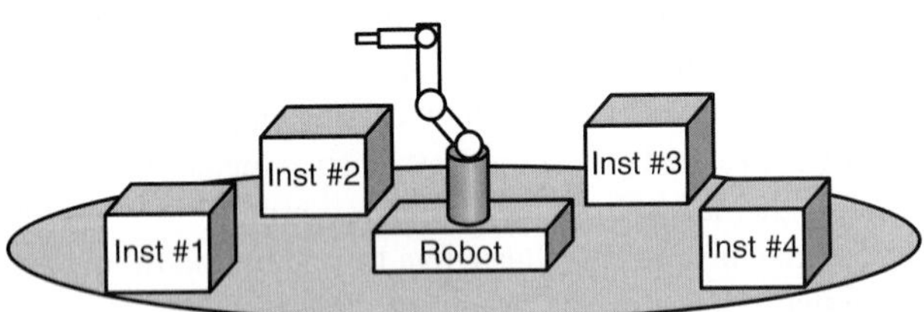

Figure 11-11 Radial arrangement of peripheral equipment around a centrally located robot. Such a workstation requires a circular work space in the laboratory with easy access from all sides. *(From Boyd JC, Felder RA, Savory J. Robotics and the changing face of the clinical laboratory. Clin Chem 1996; 42:1901-10.)*

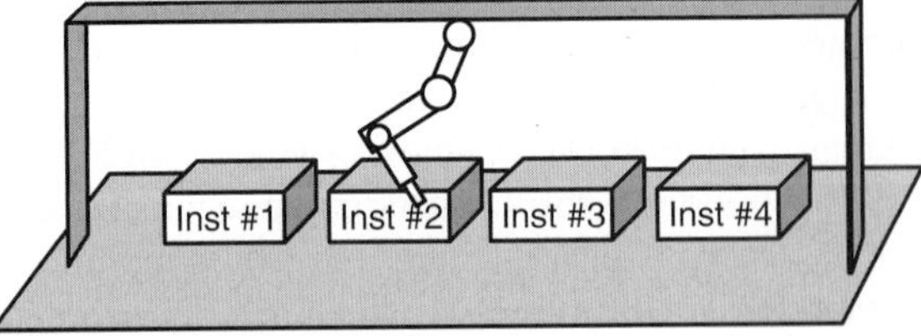

Figure 11-12 Use of a robot on a linear track allows placement of peripheral equipment with which the robot interacts on a rectangular table. This workstation configuration uses a more conventional rectangular space that can be set along a wall. *(From Boyd JC, Felder RA, Savory J. Robotics and the changing face of the clinical laboratory. Clin Chem 1996; 42:1901-10.)*

most often to automating heterogeneous assays. Examples of cartesian systems include Microlab 2000 and 2200, Plato 3000 series, and Tecan. The Integra incorporates a cartesian robot for carrying out all pipetting activities on the analyzer.

Robot arms have varying configurations and degrees of freedom of movement.[30] Two types of arms have been used in clinical laboratories: (1) cylindrical robot arms with interchangeable hands (Zymate); and (2) fully articulated robot arms with wrist and elbow joints (Thermo CRS). When the arm is attached to a stationary base, its range of motion is constrained (Figure 11-11) to a hemispherical or cylindrical space around the robot base (depending on the type of robot). This limit on the range of motion restricts the positions of devices with which the robot interacts to a radial pattern around the robot base. Some robot manufacturers have mounted their robot arms on mobile bases attached to a track (Figure 11-12). The track extends the range of motion of the robot so that instruments and devices with which the robot interacts can be arrayed linearly along a table or bench.

The reproducibility of robot arm motions is in general very good, having a standard deviation of less than 1 mm for positional repeatability.[79] Although high-level programming languages are available for robot arms and are relatively easy to use, it has been difficult to find laboratory personnel who understand the existing robot control programs and can make appropriate modifications to the programs when improvements are made to the assay protocol or when the assay protocol changes with the acquisition of newer analytical devices.

Few of the originally described robot arm applications in North American clinical laboratories remain operational today because there are too few trained personnel to maintain the software. Applications of robot arms in the Kochi Medical School (Nankoku, Japan), by contrast, appear to have enjoyed greater longevity because the technologists working in that laboratory have had appropriate training in programming and maintaining these applications. Because the applications of robotic arms in pharmaceutical laboratories have been highly repetitive procedures with relatively low complexity, competent systems integrators have been able to profitably produce and maintain working pharmaceutical robotic testing systems. Systems integrators have not been eager to develop customized medical robotics systems in U.S. clinical laboratories because of issues related to compliance with Food and Drug Administration regulations for medical devices.

Automated Specimen Processing

Although the manual operations carried out in a specimen processing area have the outward appearance of being simple, considerable complexity underlies these operations. Consequently, specimen processing has been one of the most difficult areas of the clinical laboratory to automate.

Automating the specimen processing area has been approached in various ways using both integrated and modular approaches, which are discussed below. Each specimen passing through a specimen processing area has to undergo a series of operations, beginning with (1) receiving the specimen, (2) inspecting it for appropriateness (labeling, container type, and quantity of specimen), (3) logging onto the laboratory information system, (4) labeling with an accession number, and (5) separating urgent and stat specimens from routine specimens. Also, specimens must be sorted for centrifugation, aliquoting, or otherwise prepared for the appropriate laboratory station. Centrifugation must be performed for the appropriate period of time usually based upon matrix and assays to be performed, and each centrifuged specimen must be inspected for appropriate quality (e.g., noting presence of hemolysis, lipemia, and icterus) and sorted according to its workstation destination. Adding to the difficulty of programming an automated system is the fact that typical clinical laboratories receive diverse specimen containers with all types of specimens to be evaluated (ranging from blood to hair) and have a test repertoire exceeding 2000 different tests.

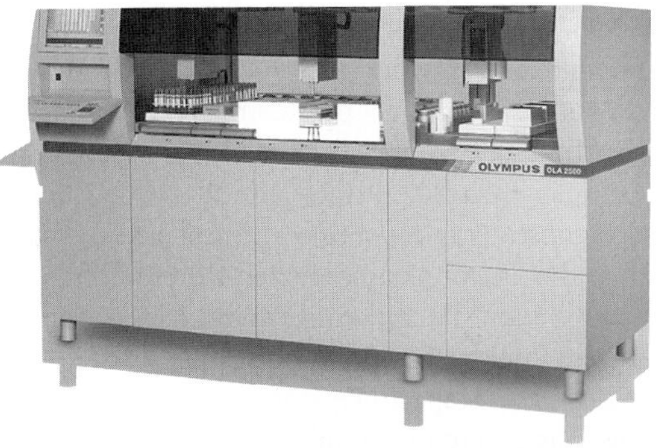

Figure 11-13 The Olympus OLA-2500 Decapper/Sorter/Archiver/Aliquotter has a maximum sorting throughput of 800 tubes per hour and a typical aliquoting throughput of 600 tubes per hour. Olympus also has an OLA-4000 system, which includes centrifugation and can be integrated with up to two Olympus AU-series automated analyzers. *(Courtesy Olympus America, Inc; www.olympusamerica.com.)*

Stand-Alone Specimen Processing Systems

Several manufacturers (AI Scientific, Aloka, Olympus [Figure 11-13], Ortho-Clinical Diagnostics, and Tecan [Figure 11-14]) offer stand-alone or independent specimen processing systems that automate various tasks but do not provide conveyors for transporting specimens between subsystems. All of these systems place processed specimens into racks that must be transported manually to the testing areas, with some exceptions. The system from Olympus can also be directly interfaced to Olympus analyzers and the systems from Ortho-Clinical Diagnostics (which is made by Thermo Electron Corporation) can be directly interfaced to analyzers from different vendors. Some of these stand-alone systems are about the size of a large automated analyzer and others may be a little larger. They may be a good choice for laboratories with daily workloads of 500 to 2500 specimens, laboratories with space limitations, or laboratories that desire an upgrade path and ease of use with different analyzers from different vendors. Some laboratories may choose to use multiples of a stand-alone specimen processing system to automate archiving and preanalytical specimen processing.

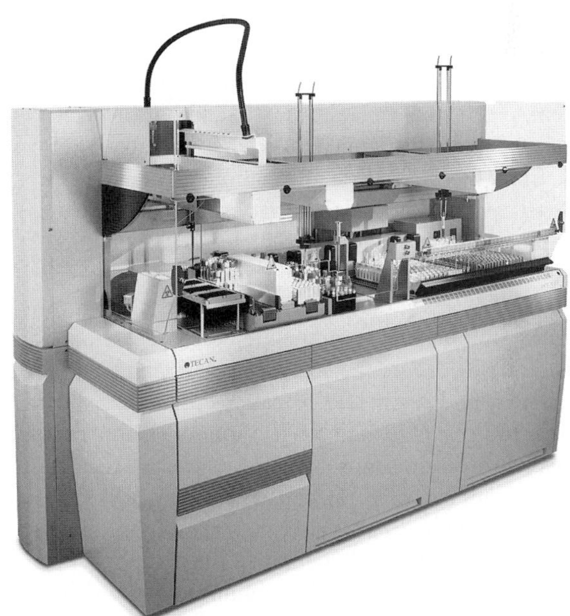

Figure 11-14 The Tecan Genesis FE-500 Workcell performs presorting, specimen volume inspection, centrifugation, decapping, aliquoting, and destination sorting into racks specific to a number of different analyzers with a throughput of up to 500 primary tubes per hour. *(Courtesy Tecan, US, Inc; www.tecan-us.com.)*

Each of these systems has the following capabilities: (1) receiving incoming specimens, (2) sorting, (3) decapping, (4) aliquoting, and (5) bar coded labeling of aliquot specimen containers. All can be interfaced to the laboratory's LIS. In addition, the Ortho-Clinical Diagnostics, Tecan, and one of the two Olympus systems include automated centrifugation. Several of the systems sort into instrument-specific racks for analyzers from a number of different vendors. In addition to sorting for particular analyzers or laboratory sections, some users apply these systems for aliquoting and sorting their reference or "send-out" testing, saving considerable time in locating the original specimens after testing in their own laboratory. The AI Scientific and Aloka systems are not yet marketed in the United States.

Integrated and Modular Automation Systems

Several manufacturers offer integrated or modular automation systems for specimen processing that includes additional functionality (A&T Corp., Bayer, Beckman Coulter, MDS AutoLab Systems, Ortho-Clinical Diagnostics, PVT, Roche Diagnostics, and Thermo Clinical Lab Systems). In addition to the functions described in the preceding section, these systems typically add conveyor transport, interfacing to automated analyzers, more sophisticated process control, and in some cases a specimen storage and retrieval system. All of the systems are of modular design, allowing the customer to choose the functions (e.g., centrifugation, sorting, aliquoting, etc.) to be included. Some of the systems use an open design, which permits interfaces to analyzers from a variety of vendors, whereas other systems are of a closed design and can only be interfaced to the vendor's own or a limited number of analyzers. It should be noted that closed systems typically do not have process control software that is independent of the instruments or system, but rather the automation process control is integrated to work with the vendor's analyzers. This design may make it difficult for the laboratory to change analyzers to another vendor in the future.

To achieve maximum effectiveness of an automation system, process control software should be able to read the specimen's identification (ID) bar code and obtain information from the laboratory's LIS about specimen type and ordered tests. It should then determine the processes the specimen requires—such as centrifugation, decapping, or aliquoting—and the exact route or course of action for each specimen. It should be able to calculate the number of aliquots and the proper volume for each depending on the tests requested, route the specimens to analyzers, recap the specimens, and retain the specimens for automatic recall. The software should be able to monitor analyzers for in-control production status and automatically make decisions if a test is not available. Specimen integrity checking should be automatic; rules-based decisions should monitor specimen quality and make these decisions. Finally, most process control software should include "autoverification," which is validation of analyzer results by making rules-based decisions that flag exceptions for technologist review, and "autoretrieval" of specimens for repeat, reflex, and dilution testing.

Although most of these systems are restricted to handling specific types of specimen containers, they are capable of processing much of the daily workload of a laboratory and have been installed in more than 500 laboratories around the world. Although a few laboratories with daily workloads as low as 600 to 800 specimens tubes have justified these systems because of a shortage of technical help, normally these systems are designed for laboratories with workloads of 1000 to 10,000 specimens per day. In addition to process control software and the ability to be interfaced to the laboratory's LIS, each of these systems incorporates some or all of the following components:

1. *Specimen input area:* A holding area where bar code–labeled specimens are introduced into the system.
2. *Bar code reading stations:* Multiple bar code readers are placed at critical locations in the processing system to track specimens and provide information for their proper routing to various stations in the processing system.
3. *Transport system:* Segments of a conveyor belt line that move specimens to the appropriate location.
4. *High-level sorting or routing device:* A device that separates specimens by type (such as by tube height) or by order code and passes them to the transport system or to a racking system. High-level sorting is often used to separate specimens that require centrifugation, or other processing steps from specimens that do not, or to route specimens into completely different pathways within the total automation system.
5. *Automated centrifuge:* An area of the specimen processor in which specimens requiring centrifugation are removed from the conveyor belt, introduced into a centrifuge that is automatically balanced, centrifuged (either refrigerated or at room temperature), and then removed from the centrifuge and placed back on the transport system.
6. *Level detection and evaluation of specimen adequacy (specimen integrity):* An area in which sensors are used to evaluate the volume of specimen in each specimen container and to look for the presence of hemolysis, lipemia, or icterus.
7. *Decapping station:* An area or device in the automated system in which specimen caps or stoppers are automatically removed and discarded into a waste container.
8. *Recapping station:* An area or device in the automated system in which specimen tubes are automatically recapped with new stoppers or covered with an air-tight closure.
9. *Aliquoter:* Aspirates appropriately sized aliquots from each original specimen container and places them into bar coded secondary specimen containers for sorting and transport to multiple analytical workstations.
10. *Interface to automated analyzer:* a direct physical connection to an automated analyzer that permits the analyzer's sampling probe to aspirate directly from an open specimen container while the container is still on the conveyor, or that may robotically lift the container from the conveyor and place it in the analyzer. Some automation systems only interface to their own brand of analyzers or to a limited number of systems, whereas other automation systems use a so-called open design that complies with the NCCLS standards and permits interfaces to a variety of automated analyzers.
11. *Sorter:* an automated sorting system for sorting of specimens not going to a conveyor-interfaced analyzer or workstation. Such a sorter typically sorts into 30 to 100 different sort groups in racks or carriers. In some systems the racks can be specific to certain analyzers for convenience.

12. *Take-out stations:* Temporary storage areas for specimens before or after analysis. The take-out station may be the same as the sorter described above where specimens are sorted for manual delivery. However, it may also serve as a holding area (stockyard) for specimens awaiting autoverification of results in case a repeat test is required.
13. *Storage and retrieval system.* This unit may serve the same function as the take-out station or stockyard—that of holding specimens after analysis in case a specimen is necessary for a repeat test, but it has one major difference. These units are typically refrigerated and hold many more specimens (several thousand) than the typical take-out station or stockyard. Depending on daily workloads, the laboratory may be able to retain one week's worth of specimens for possible repeat or additional tests. Specimen containers are loaded and retrieved robotically.

Brief descriptions of the integrated (modular) automation systems appear in the following sections.

A&T Corporation

The A&T CliniLog system includes specimen input, bar code reading, high-level sorting or routing, conveyor transporting, centrifugation, decapping, aliquoting, bar code labeling of racks of aliquot specimens, interfacing to chemistry and immunochemistry analyzers, and a terminal stocker. Specimens can be transported in racks of 5 or 10 specimen containers. A&T has approximately 60 installations in hospitals and laboratories in Asian countries and has recently begun marketing in the United States. A&T participates in the Open LA21 Project, an effort involving 10 different companies to develop a modular automation system by following the NCCLS and Japanese standards for laboratory automation. This system allows single specimen transport and has all of the 13 functions listed above.

Bayer Diagnostics

The Bayer Diagnostics ADVIA LabCell and ADVIA WorkCell Modular Automation Systems use circular single tube carriers capable of transporting various size primary tubes and a unique dual conveyor design that allows specimen tubes to bypass intermediate stations to quickly reach other stations in the total system. The capabilities of these systems include specimen input, bar code reading, high-level sorting and/or routing, conveyor transporting, centrifugation, decapping, interfacing to Bayer's chemistry, immunochemistry, hematology, urine analyzers, a take-out station, and archiving capabilities for finding specimens postanalysis. An automated aliquoter is under development. Bayer's ADVIA CentraLink provides a single LIS interface for all automation and analyzers and serves as the consolidated data and quality control (QC) manager. There are more than 73 U.S. installations worldwide with approximately half in the United States as of this writing.

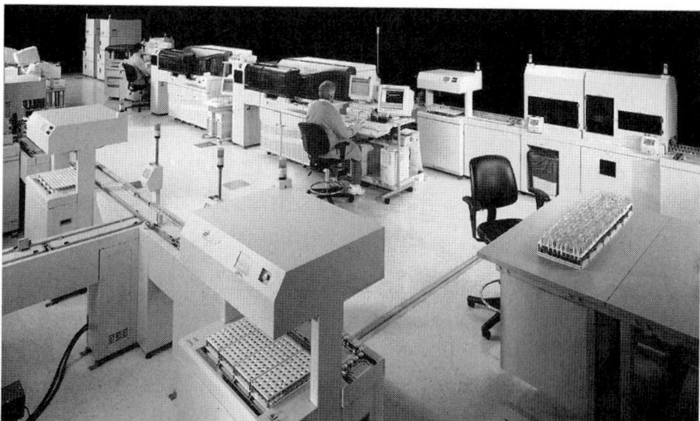

Figure 11-15 Beckman Coulter Power Processor System. This photograph is of an actual system installed in a large hospital laboratory. This system design includes modules for preanalytical processing and analyzers. *(Courtesy Beckman Coulter Inc; www.beckmancoulter.com.)*

Beckman Coulter

The Beckman Coulter Power Processor (formerly the Coulter IDS System) transports specimens in disk-shaped carriers known as "pucks" (Figure 11-15). The system includes specimen input, sorting, centrifugation, decapping, specimen volume detection, aliquoting, bar code labeling of aliquot specimens, interfaces to Synchron LX and other vendors' analyzers, recapping, a downstream sorter or stockyard, and a refrigerated storage system for finished specimens. The pucks cannot be removed from the track. Therefore devices such as the centrifuge or analyzers into which tubes are transferred have an adjacent area of track in which empty pucks are queued to await the return of each tube to a puck. Beckman Coulter has approximately 180 installations of the Power Processor or the IDS system worldwide and offers a full line of systems from entry level to very complex custom systems.

MDS AutoLab

MDS AutoLab generally only builds automation systems in laboratories that are wholly or partly owned by MDS. However, one very large reference laboratory not owned by MDS does have a highly successful AutoLab system, which has been described in publications.[42,43] There are a total of seven MDS installations in the United States and Canada. The AutoLab system uses unique transport carriers that transport individual specimens, but which can be removed from the track and snapped together into blocks of carriers that resemble tube racks for tubes. Capabilities of the MDS AutoLab systems include high-speed specimen input, conveyor transport, decapping, interfacing to chemistry and immunochemistry analyzers from different vendors, recapping, and high-speed sorting.

Ortho-Clinical Diagnostics

Ortho's automation systems are designed and built by Thermo Electron Corp. This arrangement gives customers an option of acquiring the automation system and Ortho's analyzers as a package and having a single source for service. These systems have the following functionalities: specimen input, bar code reading, transporting system, high-level sorting or routing, centrifugation, decapping, aliquoting, interfacing to various chemistry and immunochemistry analyzers, recapping, and an exit-sorting system. Ortho-Clinical Diagnostics has also partnered with Thermo Electron for automated systems outside the United States.

PVT

The capabilities available with PVT's modular automation include specimen input, sorting, automated centrifugation, specimen integrity inspection, decapping, aliquoting, bar code labeling of aliquot specimens, recapping, specimen distribution with cap piercing, and a take-out and sorting station. All PVT systems can accommodate all common container sizes and all specimen types. PVT uses the Hitachi 5-position rack for their single-task modules. The multi-task workstations from the RSD 800 series work with racks from almost any vendor. Their specimen integrity system measures specimen volume and detects clots, hemolysis, icterus, and lipemia. Each PVT module can be purchased independently to meet specific laboratory requirements. PVT has more than 300 installations in Europe and more than 20 installations in the United States.

Roche Diagnostics

Roche Diagnostics' MODULAR *PREANALYTICS* (MPA *Plus*) automation system is manufactured by Hitachi and is based on the Hitachi 5-tube rack. The capabilities of this system include specimen input, centrifugation, decapping, aliquoting, bar code labeling of aliquot tubes, specimen integrity checking, interfacing to Roche and/or Hitachi MODULAR analyzers, recapping, sorting, and a take-out station. Components can be purchased in a customized fashion to meet the requirements of individual laboratories. Roche Diagnostics and Hitachi have approximately 120 installations worldwide.

Thermo Electron Corporation

Thermo Clinical Labsystem's TC Automation system uses single specimen carriers, which can accommodate a variety of container sizes and multiple tube carriers. Their system can also accommodate racks of different sizes or types in their exit sorting system. The system's capabilities include specimen input, bar code reading, high-level sorting or routing, centrifugation, decapping, aliquoting, bar code labeling of aliquot specimens, interfaces to various chemistry and immunochemistry analyzers, and an exit-sorting system. To date, Thermo Electron has 14 installations, which have all been in Europe, but they are now marketing in the United States.

AUTOMATED SPECIMEN SORTING

Several approaches to automated sorting of specimens have been taken including (1) use of a conveyor belt, (2) automated sorting into racks, and (3) stand-alone sorters. Selecting the correct one of these approaches is an extremely important determinant of the overall scheme of automation in any particular laboratory.

Integration with a Conveyor System

Three types of conveyor sorting systems have been used. One type uses a continuous loop in which all specimens follow the loop and go past each workstation or analyzer. Specimens are either sampled directly by the analytical instrument while on the conveyor, or a robot attached to the workstation removes selected specimens from the conveyor for analysis (Figure 11-16). This approach has the advantage that specimen aliquoting is not required because specimens pass by all workstations at which tests are performed. However, the continuous loop also has some drawbacks in that specimen throughput is often limited by the slowest direct sampling analyzer on the loop. One exception is the Bayer ADVIA system, which uses double tracks enabling specimens to bypass stations to get to their correct destinations. It should also be noted that if specimens are removed from their carriers on the line for testing, a system of queuing empty carriers is required to return the tubes to the conveyor.

In a second approach, instead of a continuous loop, some automated processing conveyor systems use a high-level sorting device to sort specimens into groups according to their routing destination in the laboratory, such as for hematology or chemistry tests. Downstream from the sorting device, separated specimens are routed down a dedicated conveyor line (Figure 11-17). This sorting method follows the approach used in most manual specimen processing areas; the extent of specimen transport via conveyor can depend on the activities to be included. For example, these designs may include a centrifuge and aliquoter, interfaced chemistry or immunochemistry analyzers, additional sorting, a take-out station, and even a refrigerated storage and retrieval station at the end of the chemistry line. The

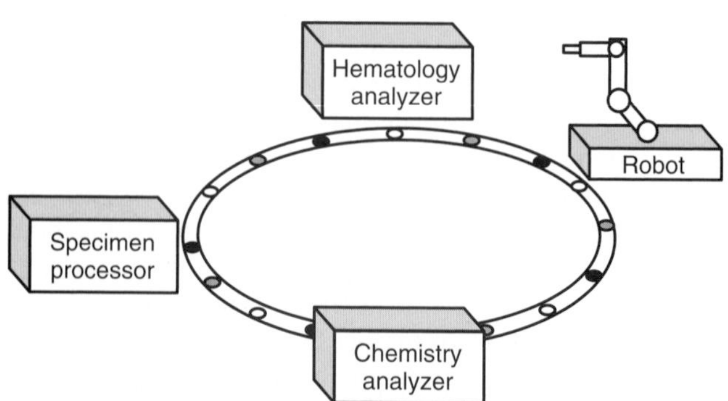

Figure 11-16 Direct sampling from a conveyor track in a loop configuration eliminates the need for separate equipment to sort specimens but may limit the rate of specimen movement on the track to the sampling speed of the slowest workstation. *(From Boyd JC, Felder RA, Savory J. Robotics and the changing face of the clinical laboratory. Clin Chem 1996; 42:1901-10.)*

hematology line may lead directly to hematology and coagulation analyzers and to an automated slide preparation machine.

In the third approach, sorting is integral to the conveyor system and specimens are sorted as they are transported (Figure 11-18). The advantages of this approach are that a dedicated specimen sorting device is not necessary in the specimen processing system, and that with appropriate specimen rerouting, the requirement for specimen aliquots may be avoided. Possible disadvantages of this approach are the expense of multiple bar code reading stations and specimen routing gates and the complexity of the process control software required.

Automated Sorting into Racks

Some systems are designed to sort the specimens into racks for transfer to particular laboratory sections or analyzers as described above. These systems (AI Scientific, Aloka, Olympus, Ortho-Clinical Diagnostics, and Tecan) sort the aliquot and original tubes into racks for manual transport to analyzers or lab sections. In some cases the racks may be specific for a specific analyzer, eliminating additional handling of tubes.

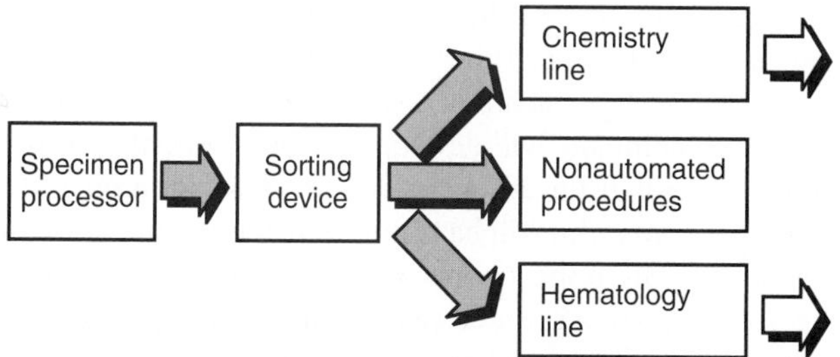

Figure 11-17 Sorting laboratory specimens before introduction to an automated specimen conveyor system simplifies the design and construction of the conveyor. *(From Boyd JC, Felder RA, Savory J. Robotics and the changing face of the clinical laboratory. Clin Chem 1996; 42:1901-10.)*

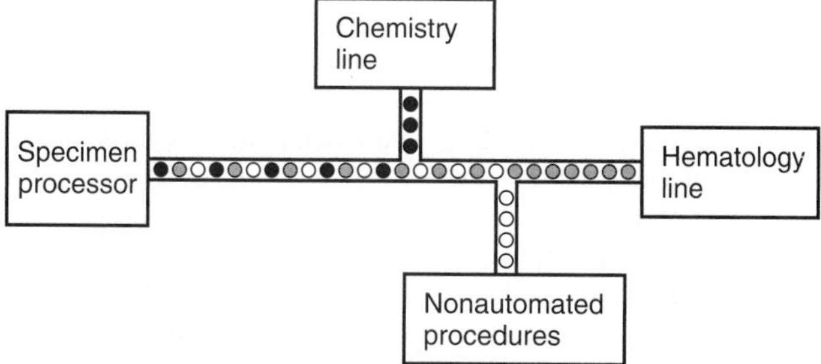

Figure 11-18 Use of the conveyor system to sort specimens dynamically during specimen transport eliminates the requirement for separate equipment to sort specimens, but requires a more sophisticated conveyor system with numerous bar code reading stations and gates to direct the specimens to the appropriate workstation. *(From Boyd JC, Felder RA, Savory J. Robotics and the changing face of the clinical laboratory. Clin Chem 1996; 42:1901-10.)*

Stand-Alone Sorting System

Some systems use a stand-alone sorting system, where specimens are manually loaded and unloaded (MDS AutoLab, Megamation, and Motoman). These systems require manual loading of tubes in racks or carrier devices; in some instances these may be analyzer specific racks or carriers. At speeds of 1000 tubes per hour or greater, tubes can be sorted into as many as 30 to 100 different sort groups. Typically the laboratory determines what each sort group is. The sort group could be all tests for a particular laboratory section, a group of closely related tests performed on the same analyzer or at the same bench, or an individual high-volume test. These systems may be very useful in a setting such as a reference laboratory, which may have many different tests and high volumes, but for which online centrifugation and aliquoting are less important considerations.

Automated Specimen Storage and Retrieval

Automated capability to store and retrieve specimens on demand is an important aspect of automated specimen delivery systems. A few of the integrated systems described above (e.g., Beckman Coulter) offer specimen storage and retrieval modules as options in their systems. These robotic modules store specimens refrigerated in specific locations that are logged into a database maintained by the specimen delivery system. When a user requests a specific specimen to be retrieved, the robot is given commands to retrieve the specimen from the appropriate archived location and to route the specimen to the requested station using the specimen transportation system.

A variety of free-standing refrigerated or frozen systems are also available and have been employed in some clinical laboratories. Biophile has a low temperature (−80 °C, etc.) robotic freezer, which is ideal for vials such as those used in molecular testing. Jouan Robotics has a robotic frozen storage system for microtiter plates. For laboratories with larger daily workloads, SK Daifuku, Diamond Phoenix, and Remstar each have different types of automated storage and retrieval systems that can be installed in either refrigerators or freezers. In these systems, trays or racks of specimens can be stored and retrieved by an operator or by using a robotic system, depending on the degree of automation desired.

PRACTICAL CONSIDERATIONS

In this section we discuss the practical considerations that influence a laboratory's decision to automate part or all of its operations. Included are discussions of evaluating a laboratory's requirements and other problems laboratorians face in integrating and automating their laboratories. The section concludes with a discussion on measuring the impact of automating a laboratory.

Evaluation of Requirements

Any consideration of total or modular laboratory automation should start with an evaluation of requirements.[42] Such an evaluation begins with mapping of the current laboratory work flow from the arrival of patient specimens through completion of testing and reporting of results. Box 11-2 lists potential work-flow steps that should be mapped.

Middleton et al have described work-flow mapping in their discussion of process control and online optimization.[55] They relate the mapping of material (specimen) flows and data flows to process flow and show how such mapping assists the laboratory in determining process steps that are bottlenecks, steps that waste labor, and steps that are prone to errors. Work-flow mapping thus enables the laboratory to better identify what steps should be considered for automation. Although work-flow analysis at the beginning of an automation project may seem time consuming when the steps to be automated appear obvious, the authors believe that the mapping effort is well worth the investment in time and labor.

Some laboratorians use 80% as a "rule of thumb" in guiding decisions about automation. Clinical laboratories have many exceptional tests, specimen containers, and handling situations. Nevertheless, if 80% of the specimen containers and handling situations can be standardized and automated, the laboratory will achieve a dramatic reduction in its labor and costs, which should be sufficient to justify the investment in automation and the planning and evaluation time involved.

Once the laboratory's work flow has been mapped and its requirements have been identified, alternative solutions can be considered. Vendors are then invited to make presentations and to host visits of the laboratory management team to other laboratories where the vendors have successful installations. It is important at this stage to focus on the requirements identified by the work-flow mapping and not allow the vendor to try to sell equipment that may not be necessary.

Not every laboratory automation project has been successful. The authors believe that the poorer than expected results for at least some of those projects were due to inadequate planning and lack of evaluation of requirements. Box 11-3 lists 10 potential reasons why automation fails to meet expectations.

BOX 11-2 Clinical Laboratory Steps for Work-flow Mapping

Unpacking from transport containers
Presorting
Temperature preservation
Order entry
Document management (requisitions, etc.)
Labeling
Sorting
Centrifugation
Labeling of aliquot tubes
Pouring of aliquots
More sorting
Delivery to laboratory sections
More sorting
Preparing work lists
Decapping
Labeling analyzer-specific tubes for specimens
Pouring or pipetting analyzer-specific specimens
Loading tubes on analyzers
Performing tests (steps such as extraction, centrifugation, precipitation, dilution, etc., are not specifically listed)
Unloading analyzers
Recapping
Data manipulations (calculations)
Result review and verification
Reporting of results
Delivery of specimens to archival storage system
Archival storage of specimens
Reflexive testing
Repeat testing, diluting, if necessary
Additional physician-ordered testing
Specimen retrieval for additional or repeat testing
Disposal of expired specimens

PROBLEMS OF INTEGRATION

Building a highly integrated laboratory generates many potential problems. Because it is unlikely that a laboratory will use only the equipment of a single equipment manufacturer, integration of the instruments and robotic devices from different manufacturers is necessary. Decisions must be made concerning which device will be the master controller and which company will develop the software that provides overall control of the automation scheme. In addition, individuals or firms who will be responsible for configuration of the automation to the geometry and production schedule of the laboratory must be recruited and trained. Although industrial automation schemes have been developed to solve

BOX 11-3 Ten Reasons Why Automation Fails to Meet Expectations

- Incomplete understanding of current environment, processes, costs, customer expectations
- Loss in flexibility because of fixed processes and limited throughput
- Unrealistic expectations of system—cost reduction, throughput, return on investment
- Unplanned and poorly developed "workarounds" required to interface automation with manual processes
- Unclear expectations of system functionality
- Overbuilt and unnecessarily complicated system design
- Inadequate technical support
- Credible and realistic impact analysis never conducted
- Hidden costs—labor, supplies, maintenance
- Failure to optimize current processes before automation (never automate a poor process)

Modified from Argent Global Services, Solutions Newsletter, page 4, April 2003, Oklahoma City, Okla.

many of these problems, there is as yet insufficient experience with these approaches in the very different operating environment of a clinical laboratory.

The reader is referred to the NCCLS standard AUTO3-A, which is described in the following and in particular to the Functional Control Model (Section 4.2), which describes the relationships between the LIS, LAS, and various devices. In this model, and throughout the series of NCCLS automation standards, the term LAS represents the computer system that controls the automation system, not the actual automation hardware. Most often, it is the LAS that has the requisite process control software to support automation. The functional control model, which is depicted in Figure 11-19, supports analytical instruments that may be physically attached to the automation system and analyzers that may not be attached but are still interfaced to the LIS. The model does not give dominance to either the LIS or the LAS, but rather allows for essential information flows in either direction to make the most efficient use of the strengths of each system.

Although laboratory automation has the potential to improve laboratory productivity and reduce operational costs,[76] integrated laboratory automation has not always proven to be cost effective. Tatsumi et al[84] have reviewed the Japanese experience with integrated laboratory systems and found that these systems do not always succeed in reducing laboratory costs. With an increasing emphasis on cost-effective laboratory testing in Japan, many hospitals there have replaced total laboratory systems with smaller modular systems that allow rapid and convenient testing and are responsive to the political changes in the Japanese healthcare system.

Device Integration

One objective in developing an integrated laboratory is to link laboratory instruments and devices into an automated system to maximize the number of functions automated.

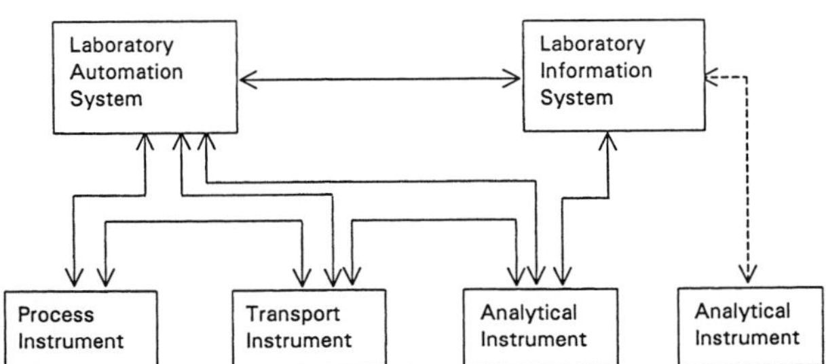

Figure 11-19 Functional control model of NCCLS AUTO3-A standard. The solid lines and arrows depict logical information flows supported by the standard. The dotted line and arrows are logical information flows permitted, but not supported, by the standard. *(National Committee for Clinical Laboratory Standards [NCCLS]. Laboratory automation: Communications with automated clinical laboratory systems, instruments, devices, and information systems, approved standard. NCCLS Document AUTO3-A Wayne PA: NCCLS, 2000. Figure reproduced with permission of NCCLS.)*

Automatic specimen introduction requires the development of mechanical interfaces between each laboratory analyzer and devices such as conveyor belts, mobile robots, or robot arms. Enhancements to electronic interfaces for laboratory instruments are necessary to allow remote computer control of front-panel functions, notification of instrument status information, and coordination of the distribution of specimens between instruments. Most existing LIS interfaces with laboratory analyzers provide only the ability to download accession numbers and the tests requested on each specimen, and to upload the results generated by the analyzer.

Process Controllers and Software

Process controllers provide computer integration of the many decision-making tasks that occur in the daily activity of a laboratory. Consequently, process control software is needed to coordinate the overall activities of the laboratory. To integrate the various devices in the laboratory, communications with a master controller device must be established. In addition, communication is needed between the LIS computer, the LAS computer (that provides process control), the laboratory analyzers, and the specimen conveyor and specimen manipulation devices, such as automated centrifuges, aliquoters, decappers, etc. The distribution of tasks must be carefully specified in developing such a communications network. A possible distribution of tasks is the following:[12]

1. The LAS assumes responsibility for assigning a dispatch priority and schedule to each specimen, providing specimen tracking information to the LIS, rerouting specimens for reanalysis, implementing reflex orders, and troubleshooting, and has final authority in resolving any priority conflicts that arise in specimen handling.
2. The LAS also controls specimen distribution. It monitors all specimen distribution system bar code readers and gates, routes specimens to workstations as required, monitors specimen tracking information, monitors instrument status, alerts an operator of any instrument problems, and notifies instruments of each specimen that has to be sampled.
3. The LIS downloads specimen information to instruments and the LAS, monitors and provides to users all information related to specimen tracking received from the LAS, and receives all completed laboratory test results from each analyzer. Software with user-definable algorithms for automatic reflex testing may reside in either the LAS or the LIS depending on system capabilities and the overall design.

This list of tasks is not necessarily complete but demonstrates the complexity of the software engineering task of integrating automation in a laboratory. Although the functions of the LIS and LAS are often provided on separate computers, they may also be integrated on a single computer. Several manufacturers (e.g., MDS AutoLab, Odysis, and Zymark) have process control software that can manage many functions in an automated laboratory. However, the integration of the LAS functions with the LIS functions remains a formidable project often requiring the development of custom software.

Measuring the Impact of Automation

It is highly recommended that performance metrics be used to assess the performance of automation systems to objectively determine whether the implementation has been successful in meeting the original objectives and to monitor continued improvement. This statement is applicable, whether the automation is a simple mobile delivery robot or a total laboratory automation system with specimen processing and integrated analyzers. Ideally, the metrics should be identified and implemented in advance of implementation of the automation to establish an adequate baseline for comparison. Recommended parameters for measurement include stat and routine turnaround time at median and 90 or 95 percentiles; quality parameters, such as lost specimens, mishandled specimens, mislabeled specimens, misdelivered specimens, and aliquoting or pouring errors; and productivity parameters, such as requisitions or orders processed per employee, billed units reported per employee, etc. Since automation usually improves employee safety, postautomation employee accidents may decrease. Automation also may improve employee job satisfaction and reduce training time, so measures such as employee turnover rates are useful.

DEVELOPMENT OF STANDARDS FOR LABORATORY AUTOMATION

The rate of development of standards continues to influence the speed of technical advancement in the field of laboratory automation. Typical laboratory instruments are interfaced to LIS systems using either the RS 232C serial or 802.3 Ethernet connection standards. The latter may often be set up using Transmission Control Protocol/Internet Protocol (TCP/IP), through local area network (LAN) connections, and may also use an interface engine. The American Society for Testing and Materials (ASTM) standards E1391 and E1384 are the more commonly used communication standards, although the newer NCCLS standard AUTO3-A (see next paragraph) now offers many improvements over ASTM. The commonly used cabling standards employed are IEEE-422 serial or IEEE-488 parallel. Although these electronic standards help to reduce the work involved in development of an interface, each interface with a laboratory device must still be developed individually and tested.

The NCCLS has developed standards to meet the requirements of vendors and users of clinical laboratory automation systems. Five standards have now been published at the approved level dealing with specimen container and specimen carrier[59]; bar codes for specimen container identification[60]; communications with automated clinical laboratory systems, instruments, devices, and information systems[61]; systems operational requirements, characteristics, and information elements[62]; and electromechanical interfaces.[63] The communications standard was developed in collaboration with Health Level Seven (HL7). A new chapter of the HL7 standard (Chapter 13), which appears in HL7 version 2.4[46] and newer versions, was written specifically to address the requirements for laboratory automation communications, which had not been met by the older standards developed by ASTM.[2,3] The NCCLS communications standard[61] includes all of HL7 Chapter 13 plus additional information of value in applying the HL7 communications standard to specific automation requirements. In addition to the new Chapter 13, some changes were also made in Chapters 4 and 7 of the HL7 standard to coordinate with the automation requirements detailed in Chapter 13. Vendors and users of automation are therefore advised to obtain both the HL7 and NCCLS standards.

The NCCLS has an Area Committee on Automation and Informatics, which oversees the above standards and initiates new standards development projects. Current standards development projects include Data Content for Specimen Identification, Protocols to Validate Laboratory Information Systems, and Remote Access to Hospital Diagnostic Devices via the internet. In 2002, ASTM transferred to NCCLS the ownership and copyright of all nine standards in its E31.13 group, including the two standards referenced above. These standards all relate to the clinical laboratory, with some of them simply preceding or overlapping the NCCLS automation standards. NCCLS is now in the process of evaluating which of these standards will be maintained and updated and which may be abandoned.

OTHER AREAS OF AUTOMATION

In addition to the automated devices and processing units that were developed primarily to automate chemistry and immunoassay that are described above, a variety of other instruments and processes have been automated and used in the clinical laboratory. They include urine analyzers, flow cytometers, hematology cell counters, nucleic acid analyzers, microtiter plate systems, point-of-care analyzers, and remotely located systems.

Urine Analyzers

Many of the same analytical principles are used for the quantitation of serum and urine constituents, but it is more difficult to automate testing of urine than serum, because the broad range of concentrations of many urine constituents requires a low limit of detection to measure low concentrations, and expanded linearity to permit measurements of high concentrations without dilution. This requirement, together with the relatively low demand for urine tests compared with that for serum tests, has restricted the development of analyzers designed specifically for urine constituents. Nevertheless, selected urine analyses are performed on the available analyzers in some institutions.[40]

Flow Cytometers

Cytometry refers to the measurement of physical and/or chemical characteristics of cells, or, by extension, of other biological particles. Flow cytometry is a process in which such measurements are made while the cells or particles pass, preferably in single file, through the measuring apparatus in a fluid stream (see Chapter 3). Flow sorting extends flow cytometry by using electrical or mechanical means to divert and collect cells with one or more measured characteristics falling within a range or ranges of values set by the user.

Flow cytometers are used in the clinical laboratory to analyze cells that have been stained with a supravital or fluorescent dye (although unstained cells can also be measured) and travel in suspension one by one past a laser light source. Scattered and emitted light is collected in front of the light source and at right angles, respectively (see Chapter 3). Information derived by measuring *light scatter* when a cell is struck by the laser beam can be used to estimate cell shape, size, cellular granularity, nuclear lobularity, and cell surface structure. Some cell counters classify white cells using the Coulter principle, cell conductivity, and light scattering of unstained cells (e.g., Gen-S, HmX, and MAXM) to differentiate cell types, whereas other cell counters (ADVIA-120) use two flow cytometry channels (one with peroxidase-stained, fixed cells, one with unstained or lysed cells). The Cell-Dyn 4000 uses one flow cytometry channel and aperture resistance to count white blood cells and light scattering from unstained cells measured at four different light-scatter angles to provide a five-part differential analysis. The aperture resistance transducer is also used to provide the red blood cell and platelet counts. The Sysmex XE-2100 uses flow cytometry with light scattering measured at three angles to determine the white cell count and differential. A separate channel provides additional information on the presence of immature white blood cells. This channel uses a hemolytic reagent that selectively protects immature white blood cells that are counted using the Sysmex radiofrequency direct current detection method.

Hematology Cell Counters

Analyzers that perform a complete blood count have been automated using the Coulter principle, cell conductivity, light scatter, and flow cytometry. Individual blood cells are analyzed by application of one or more of these techniques. The *Coulter principle* is based on changes in electrical impedance, which are produced by nonconductive particles suspended in an electrolyte as they pass through a small aperture between electrodes. In the sensing zone of the aperture, the volume of electrolyte displaced by the particle (cell) is measured as a change in voltage that is proportional to the volume of the particle. By carefully controlling the quantity of electrolyte drawn through the aperture, several thousand particles per second are individually counted and sized. An electronic correction is applied if more than one cell passes through the aperture at the same time. Red blood cells, white blood cells, and platelets can be identified by their size. Alternating current in the radiofrequency range short circuits the bipolar lipid layer of the cell membrane, allowing energy to penetrate the cell. Information about intracellular structure, including chemical composition and nuclear volume, can be collected using this technique, known as *cell conductivity.*

Nucleic Acid Analyzers

Automation of the analysis of nucleic acids developed rapidly as an outgrowth of the Human Genome Project.[49] Several manufacturers have developed automation to assist with the isolation of nucleic acids and with analysis of nucleic acids using several amplification schemes. Two common examples of such analyzers are presented below.

The MagNA Pure LC Instrument allows automated isolation and preparation of nucleic acids. The instrument performs up to 32 nucleic acid isolations in 1 to 3 hours from various specimens, which can include blood, blood cells, culture cells, plasma, serum, sputum, stool, broncho-alveolar lavage, plant tissues, or food products.

Specimen identifications are entered at the user terminal or acquired by reading bar codes. All subsequent steps are performed automatically. Nuclease-free disposable reaction tips are used for transfer of specimens and as reaction vials. Separation of nucleic acids is carried out using magnetic beads, washing steps, and elution of nucleic acids from the beads into the cooled specimen cartridge. Used reaction tips are automatically discarded into an attached autoclavable waste bag and liquid waste is pipetted at the end of the run into an appropriate waste container. The device provides increased reproducibility and scalability of purification and reduced risk of cross contamination when compared with standard manual methods. Following nucleic acid purification, the MagNA Pure can transfer the nucleic acid to various container types (programmable by the user) including capillaries, 96-well polymerase chain reaction (PCR) plates, A-rings, or tubes. The instrument can provide pager notification to the user regarding the status of the instrument and the processes.

The LightCycler system combines a thermal cycler platform with a fluorescence detection system. The unique design of this device allows real-time monitoring of amplification cycles and melting temperature curves. Each amplification specimen is placed in a glass capillary with a maximum capacity of 20 μL. The capillary is tightly closed to prevent contamination and is not opened at any time during analysis. The small specimen volume saves reagents, and the high surface-to-volume ratio of the capillary allows very fast heating and cooling. Fluorescence emitted during the PCR process is focused on the tip of the capillary. The instrument uses air for heating and cooling. Given the very low thermal capacity of air and the high surface-to-volume ratio of the capillary, the temperature can be changed very rapidly (about 20 °C per second). Thus thermal cycling can occur at very rapid rates. A typical amplification cycle requires only 30 to 60 seconds, which means that an amplification reaction with 30 cycles is usually completed within 15 to 30 minutes. The amplification products are quantified by fluorescence measurement using a single microvolume fluorimeter. The fluorimeter uses a blue LED that emits light at 470 nm as an excitation source and provides three channels that detect emitted light with wavelengths of 530 nm, 640 nm, and 710 nm.

The LightCycler instrument can use fluorescence-labeled, sequence-specific hybridization probes (oligonucleotides) for the specific detection of amplification products. This detection format permits high-throughput genotyping without the requirement for any post-PCR specimen manipulation. Once suitable oligonucleotides are designed, the genotyping of a specimen is straightforward. The instrument is programmed to amplify the DNA and to perform a subsequent melting curve analysis.

Microtiter Plate Systems

Microtiter plate systems are commonly used in immunoassays and nucleic acid analyses. As used for enzyme-linked immunosorbent assay (ELISA) assays, microtiter plates usually are made of polystyrene and have 48 or 96 wells coated with antibody specific for the antigen of interest. After incubation of serum in the microtiter plate well, the well is washed to remove unbound antigen, and a second antibody with conjugated indicator enzyme is added. After a second incubation period, the well is washed to remove the unbound conjugate. Color is developed by the addition of enzyme substrate and the reaction is terminated at a set time. With the development of automated pipetting stations (e.g., Gilson Model 215, Hamilton Microlab FAME, and Perkin Elmer Multiprobe), the liquid handling steps required for microtiter plate assays have been fully automated to make microtiter plate assays a viable technology for carrying out large numbers of immunoassays. Automated pipetting stations have a cartesian robot with a pipette fixed to the end of a probe that moves about a rectangular space. The probe is capable of moving in the X, Y, and Z axes. Liquids may be aspirated and dispensed in any location within the rectangular space.

Automated Pipetting Stations

Pipetting stations may be used to automate an analytical procedure for which an automated analyzer does not exist or cannot be cost justified. Most pipetting robots are relatively easy to program, rarely malfunction, and can deliver liquids with extreme precision and accuracy. Multiple-channel pipetting robots allow parallel processing of specimens with 8- or 12-channel probes to handle microtiter plates.

POCT Analyzers

Point-of-care testing (POCT) is a rapidly growing component of laboratory testing. It is known by a variety of names, including "near-patient," "decentralized," and "off-site" testing and is discussed in detail in Chapter 12. In addition, technologies incorporated into POCT analyzers are discussed in Chapters 4 and 10 and examples of POCT glucose analyzers are described and discussed in Chapter 25.

Remote Automated Laboratory System

Unmanned satellite laboratories are a possible alternative to a central laboratory facility. To demonstrate the practicality of such an approach, investigators at the University of Virginia have developed remote automated laboratory systems (RALS) designed to automate POCT in hospital intensive care units. The results from the analytical instruments in each RALS are sent to a central monitoring workstation several floors away from the satellite laboratory by a network interface, where results are viewed and either accepted or rejected by a trained medical technologist before being released for clinical use. Error codes built into the analytical instruments are also passed to the main laboratory by the computer network. Technologists in the control center can also shut down the satellite laboratory when necessary, as in the case of instrument failure. Patient information is downloaded from the hospital information system in real time so that users can select their patients and the tests to perform from a list presented on the computer touchscreen.

REFERENCES

1. A Bar Code Primer. Santa Cruz, CA, Worthington Data Solutions, 1996.
2. American Society for Testing and Materials. Transferring information between clinical instruments and computer systems. E1394-91. Philadelphia (http://www.astm.org), ASTM, 1991.
3. American Society for Testing and Materials. Low-level protocol to transfer messages between clinical laboratory instruments and computer systems. E1381-95. Philadelphia (http://www.astm.org), ASTM, 1995.
4. American Society for Testing and Materials. Use of bar codes on specimen tubes in the clinical laboratory. E1466-92. Philadelphia (http://www.astm.org), ASTM, 1992.
5. Anderson NG. Computer interfaced fast analyzers. Science 1969;166:317-24.
6. Bar Code 1 (http://www.adams1.com/pub/russadam), Adams Communications, 1995.
7. Bauer S, Teplitz C. Total laboratory automation: a view of the 21st century. Medical Laboratory Observer 1995;27(7):22-5.
8. Bauer S, Teplitz C. Total laboratory automation: system design. Medical Laboratory Observer 1995;27(9):44-50.
9. Becan-McBride K. Laboratory sampling: does the process affect the outcome? J Intraven Nurs 1999 May-Jun;22:137-42.
10. Bond LW. Consideration of laboratory parameters in design and implementation of automated systems with bar coding. Clin Chem 1990;36:1583-6.

11. Bonini PA, Alpert N, Luzzana M, Rubin MR. Guidelines for the identification and distribution of patient samples in the medical laboratory. Journal of Automatic Chemistry 1994;16:35-32.
12. Boyd JC, Felder RA, Savory J. Robotics and the changing face of the clinical laboratory. Clin Chem 1996;42:1901-10.
13. Boyd J. Robotic laboratory automation. Science 2002;295:517-8.
14. Burtis CA. Factors influencing evaporation from sample cups, and assessment of their effect on analytical error. Clin Chem 1975;21:1907-17.
15. Burtis CA. Converging technologies and their impact on the clinical laboratory. Clin Chem 1996;42:1735-49.
16. Burtis CA, Watson JS. Design and evaluation of an anti-evaporative cover for use with liquid containers. Clin Chem 1992;38:768-75.
17. Bush E. The role of an integrated chematology laboratory. Advance for Administrators of the Laboratory 2001;(2):38-42.
18. Chan DW. Clinical instrumentation (immunoassay analyzers). Anal Chem 1995;67:519R-24R.
19. Chan DW. Immunoassay automation. From concept to system performance. In Kost GJ, ed. Handbook of clinical automation, robotics, and optimization. New York, John Wiley & Sons, 1996:419-41.
20. Cheng J, Fortina P, Surrey S, Kricka LJ, Wilding P. Microchip-based devices for molecular diagnosis of genetic diseases. Molecular Diagnosis 1996;1:183-200.
21. Diamond LW, Nguyen DT, Sheridan BL, Strul M, Bailey K, Bak A. An automated hematology laboratory with computer-controlled robotics. Medinfo 1995;8:620-3.
22. DiDomenico N, Link H, Knobel R, Caratsch T, Weschler W, Loewy ZG, Rosenstraus M. COBAS AMPLICOR & tm: Fully automated RNA and DNA amplification and detection system for routine diagnostic PCR. Clin Chem 1996;42:1915-23.
23. E-Health Insider. New automated lab is one of Europe's largest. 2004: Jan 27. (http://www.e-health-insider.com/news/item.cfm?ID=634).
24. Eggert AA, Bowers KL, Smulka GJ, Emmerich KA, Iwanski AL, Quam FF. An overhead specimen handling system for variable workloads. J Med Syst 1999;23:1-11.
25. Estey CA, Felder RA. Clinical trials of a novel centrifugation method. Axial separation. Clin Chem 1996;42:402-9.
26. Estey CA, Felder RA. Clinical evaluation of serial blood processing at point of care. Clin Chem 1997;43:360-2.
27. Evans MR, Henderson DK, Bennett JE. Potential for laboratory exposures to biohazardous agents found in blood. Am J Public Health 1990;80:423-7.
28. Favero MS, Peterson NJ, Bond WW. Transmission and control of laboratory-acquired hepatitis infection. In Laboratory Safety. Principles and Practices. Washington, DC: American Society for Microbiology, 1986: 49-58.
29. Federal Register, March 14, 200321CFR Parts 201, 606, and 610Bar code label for human drug products and blood. Proposed rule. Vol 68, No 50, 12500-34.
30. Felder RA, Boyd JC, Margrey K, Holman W, Savory J. Robotics in the medical laboratory. Clin Chem 1990;36:1-310.
31. Felder RA, Boyd JC, Margrey KS, Holman W, Roberts J, Savory J. Robots in health care. Anal Chem 1991;63:741A-7A.
32. Felder RA. Automation of preanalytical processing and mobile robotics. In Kost GJ, ed. Handbook of clinical automation, robotics and optimization. New York, John Wiley & Sons, 1996:252-82.
33. Felder R. Modular workcells—modern methods for laboratory automation. Clin Chim Acta 1998;278: 257-67.
34. Findlay JB, Atwood SM, Bergmeyer L, Chemelli J, Christy K, Cummins T, Donish W, Ekeze T, Falvo J, Patterson D, et al. Automated closed-vessel system for in vitro diagnostics based on polymerase chain reaction. Clin Chem 1993;39:1927-33.
35. Fineberg SE, Begenstal RM, Bernstein RM, Laffel LM, Schwartz SL. Use of an automated device for alternative site blood glucose monitoring Diabetes Care 2001;24:1217-20.
36. Godolphin W, Bodtker K, Uyeno D, Goh LO. Automated blood-sample handling in the clinical laboratory. Clin Chem 1990;36:1551-5.
37. Grannis GF, Grumer HD, Lott JA, Edison JA, McCabe WC. Proficiency evaluation of clinical chemistry laboratories. Clin Chem 1972;18:222-36.
38. Green M. Successful alternative to alternate site testing: use of a pneumatic tube system to the central laboratory. Arch Pathol Lab Med 1995;119:943-7.
39. Greendyke RM, Banzhaf JC, Pelysko S, Bauman B. Immunologic studies of blood samples transported by a pneumatic tube system. Am J Clin Pathol 1977;68:508-10.
40. Guder WG, Ceriotti F, Bonini P. Urinalysis–challenges by new medical needs and advanced technologies. Clin Chem Lab Med 1998 Dec;36:907.
41. Gulati GL, Hyun BH, Ashton JK. Advances of the past decade in automated hematology. Am J Clin Pathol 1992;98:S11-6.
42. Hawker CD, Garr SB, Hamilton LT, Penrose JR, Ashwood ER, Weiss RL. Automated transport and sorting system in a large reference laboratory part 1: evaluation of needs and alternatives and development of a plan. Clin Chem 2002;48:1751-60.
43. Hawker CD, Roberts WL, Garr SB, Hamilton LT, Penrose JR, Ashwood ER, Weiss RL. Automated transport and sorting system in a large reference laboratory part 2: implementation of the system and performance measures over three years. Clin Chem 2002;48:1761-7.

44. Health Industry Business Communications Council. Coexistence of bar coding symbologies under the HIBCC standard. Phoenix, AZ: Health Industry Business Communications Council, August 20, 1991.
45. Heins M, Reinauer H. Automation in coagulation testing. J Int Fed Clin Chem 1996;8:117-22.
46. HL7 Standard, Version 2.4, Health Level Seven, Inc., 3300 Washtenaw Ave., Suite 227, Ann Arbor, MI 48104-4261 USA 2000.
47. Howanitz PJ, Sunseri DA, Love LA, Lohr A. Adapting mobile robotic technology to intralaboratory specimen transport. Arch Pathol Lab Med 1996;120:944-50.
48. International Union of Pure and Applied Chemistry. Nomenclature for automated and mechanised analysis (recommendation 1989). Pure and Applied Chemistry 1989;61:1657-64.
49. Jaklevic JM, Garner HR, Miller GA. Instrumentation for the genome project. Annu Rev Biomed Eng 1999;1:649-78.
50. Kohn LT, Corrigan JM, Donaldson M, eds. To Error is Human: Building a Safer Health System. Washington, DC: Institute of Medicine, 1999.
51. Kricka LJ, Wilding P. Micromechanics and nanotechnology. In Kost GJ, ed. Handbook of clinical automation, robotics, and optimization. New York, John Wiley & Sons, 1996:45-77.
52. Krouwer JS, Stewart WN, Schlain B. A multi-factor experimental design for evaluating random-access analyzers. Clin Chem 1988;34:1894-6.
53. Margrey KS, Martinez A, Vaughn DP, Felder RA. A standard clinical instrument interface for robotic applications. Clin Chem 1990;36:1572-5.
54. Markin RS. Recent trends in clinical laboratory automation. Clin Lab Manage Rev 1998;12:176-80.
55. Middleton S, Mountain P, Kemp A. Laboratory automation: a model. Leadersh Health Serv 1993;2:20-4.
56. Moore R, Luczyk K, Wu A. Workstation optimization: needs and steps for implementation. In Kost GJ, ed. Handbook of clinical automation, robotics, and optimization. New York, John Wiley & Sons, 1996:497-514.
57. Morgenstern S, Kessler G, Auerbach J, Flor RV, Klein B. An automated p-nitrophenylphosphate serum alkaline phosphatase procedure for the "Robot Chemist". Clin Chem 1965;11:889-97.
58. National Committee for Clinical Laboratory Standards (NCCLS). Preliminary evaluation of quantitative clinical laboratory methods, approved guideline-second edition. NCCLS document EP10-A2. Wayne, PA:NCCLS, 2002.
59. National Committee for Clinical Laboratory Standards (NCCLS). Laboratory automation: Specimen container/specimen carrier, approved standard. NCCLS Document AUTO1-A Wayne, PA:NCCLS, 1999.
60. National Committee for Clinical Laboratory Standards (NCCLS). Laboratory automation: Bar codes for specimen container identification, approved standard. NCCLS Document AUTO2-A Wayne, PA:NCCLS, 1999.
61. National Committee for Clinical Laboratory Standards (NCCLS). Laboratory automation:. Communications with automated clinical laboratory systems, instruments, devices, and information systems, approved standard. NCCLS Document AUTO3-A Wayne, PA:NCCLS, 2000.
62. National Committee for Clinical Laboratory Standards (NCCLS). Laboratory automation: Systems operational requirements, characteristics, and information elements, approved standard. NCCLS Document AUTO4-A Wayne, PA:NCCLS, 2000.
63. National Committee for Clinical Laboratory Standards (NCCLS). Laboratory automation: Electromechanical interfaces, approved standard. NCCLS Document AUTO5-A Wayne, PA:NCCLS, 2000.
64. Newsom SWB, Matthews J. A microbiology survey of automated biochemical machines. J Clin Pathol 1980;33:566-70.
65. Paegel BM, Blazej RG, Mathies RA. Microfluidic devices for DNA sequencing: sample preparation and electrophoretic analysis. Curr Opin Biotechnol 2003 Feb;14:42-50.
66. Palmer RC. The bar code book. Peterborough, NH: Helmers Publishing, Inc., 1989:3-9.
67. Pardue HL. A comprehensive classification of kinetic methods of analysis used in clinical chemistry. Clin Chem 1977;23:2189-201.
68. Pease AC, Solas D, Sullivan EJ. Light-generated oligonucleotide arrays for rapid DNA sequence analysis. Proc Natl Acad Sci USA 1994;91:5022-6.
69. Pierre RV. Peripheral blood film review. The demise of the eye count leukocyte differential. Clin Lab Med 2002;22:279-97.
70. Pragay DA, Fan P, Brinkley S, Chilcote ME. A computer directed pneumatic tube system: its effects on specimens. Clin Biochem 1980;13:259-61.
71. Prasad P. Effective use of robots as mechanized couriers at Stanford University Hospital. Biomed Instrum Technol 1995;29:398-404.
72. Price CP, Newman DJ, eds. Principles and practice of immunoassay, 2nd ed. New York: Stockton Press, 1997.
73. Renner SW, Howanitz PJ, Bachner P. Wristband identification error reporting in 712 hospitals: a College of American Pathologists' Q-Probes study of quality issues in transfusion practice. Arch Pathol Lab Med 1993;117:573-7.
74. Rodbard D, Bridson W, Rayford PL. Rapid calculation of radioimmunoassay results. J Lab Clin Med 1969;74:770-81.
75. Rothe M, Wingfield S, Barranco P, Charache S. Robotics in the hematology laboratory: an evaluation of the productivity of the Sysmex HS-330. Am J Clin Pathol 1995;103:154-8.

76. Sarkozi L, Simson E, Ramanathan L. The effects of total laboratory automation on the management of a clinical chemistry laboratory: retrospective analysis of 36 years. Clin Chim Acta 2003;329:89-94.
77. Sasaki M. Total laboratory automation in Japan: past, present, and the future. Clin Chim Acta 1998;278: 217-27.
78. Savory J, Buffone G, Reich R. Kinetics of the IgG-anti-IgG reaction, as evaluated by conventional and stopped-flow nephelometry. Clin Chem 1974;20: 1071-5.
79. Schmidt WA, Rollheiser JJ, Stelting KM. The laboratory robotics evolution: a survey of today's robot options. In Strimaitis JR, Hawk GL, eds. Advances in laboratory automation robotics Vol 5. Hopkinton, MA; Zymark Corporation, 1989:479-501.
80. Scott CD, Burtis CA, Johnson WF, Thacker LH, Tiffany TO. A small portable centrifugal fast analyzer system. Clin Chem 1974;20:1003-8.
81. Sewell DL. Laboratory-associated infections and biosafety. Clin Microbiol Rev 1995;8:389-405.
82. Skeggs LT Jr. An automatic method for colorimetric analysis. Am J Clin Pathol 1957;28:311.
83. Skeggs LT Jr. Persistence . . . and prayer: from the artificial kidney to the AutoAnalyzer. Clin Chem 2000;46:1425-36.
84. Tatsumi N, Okuda K, Tsuda I. A new direction in automated laboratory testing in Japan: five years of experience with total laboratory automation system management. Clin Chim Acta 1999;290:93-108.
85. Tilzer LL, Jones RW. Use of bar code labels on collection tubes for specimen management in the clinical laboratory. Arch Pathol Lab Med 1988;112:1200-2.
86. Valenstein PN, Howanitz PJ. Ordering accuracy: a College of American Pathologists Q-Probes study of 577 institutions. Arch Pathol Lab Med 1995;119: 117-22.
87. Van Damme H, Van Velthoven T, Kaelen E, Pelssers E. Fluid elements. A concept for automation of diagnostic tests. Clin Chem 1997;43:369-78.
88. Walenga JM, Fareed J. Automation and quality control in the coagulation laboratory. Clin Lab Med 1994 Dec;14(4):709-28.
89. Walter B. Dry reagent chemistries in clinical analysis. Anal Chem 1983;55:498A-514A.
90. Weilert M, Tilzer LL. Putting bar codes to work for improved patient care. Clin Lab Med 1991;11:227-38.
91. Wheeler MJ. Automated immunoassay analysers. Ann Clin Biochem 2001 May;38(Pt 3):217-29.
92. Winn-Dean ES. Automation of molecular genetics and diagnosis. In Kost GJ, ed. Handbook of clinical automation, robotics, and optimization. New York, John Wiley & Sons, 1996:396-418.
93. Whisler K, Maffetone M, Watt S. Automated system for positive specimen identification and sample handling. Clin Chem 1990;36:1587-8.
94. Zivanovic A, Davies BL. A robotic system for blood sampling. IEEE Trans Inf Technol Biomed 2000;4: 8-14.

ADDITIONAL READING

Chan, DW. Immunoassay automation: An updated guide to systems. San Diego, CA: Academic Press, 1995.
Hall, GM. The age of automation: Technical genius, social dilemma. Westport, CT: Greenwood Publishing Group, 1995.
1996 Health care automation and reimbursement survey report. Gaithersburg, MD: Aspen Publishers, 1996.
Hurst, WJ. Automation in the laboratory. New York: VCH Publishers, 1995.
Kost, GJ. ed. Handbook of clinical automation, robotics, and optimization. New York: John Wiley & Sons, 1996.

CHAPTER 12

Point-of-Care Testing

Christopher P. Price, Ph.D.,
and Andrew St. John, Ph.D., M.A.A.C.B.

Point-of-care testing (POCT) is a rapidly growing component of healthcare services* and is used in many healthcare settings (Box 12-1). They include coronary care units,† intensive care units,[45,96,153] surgical wards,[12,19,34] emergency wards,[40,146] pediatric units,[41,128] and for monitoring both acute[46,52,91] and chronically ill patients.‡ For the purpose of this chapter, POCT is defined as "any test that is performed at the time at which the test result enables a decision to be made and an action taken that leads to an improved health outcome." Other terms used to describe POCT include "bed side,"[107] "near patient,"[28] "physician's office,"[88] "extralaboratory,"[114] "decentralised,"[5] "off site," "ancillary," and "alternative site"[49,106] testing. Reduced turnaround time (TAT) of test results[119] and improved patient management are advantages of this type of testing (Box 12-2).[75]

In the early days of diagnostic testing, tests were undertaken close to the patient—at the point-of-care—integrating information gained from simple tests into the clinician's observation of the patient's current symptoms and previous history (Figure 12-1).[117] With technical progress in the development and availability of sophisticated analyzers and analytical systems, these tests moved away from the patient and were analyzed in a central or core clinical laboratory where all samples were transported for subsequent analysis. Eventually, this resulted in a disconnect in the time between the individual, specimen(s), physician, laboratory, results, and medical decision making process (Figure 12-2). This has led to logistical, management, and analytical problems in laboratory operations and an increase in the TAT of test results from minutes to hours and sometimes even days. With the trend toward miniaturization of components (see Chapters 4 and 10) and their integration into small, self-contained, analytical systems, the means became available of returning to POCT with a goal of reducing TAT of test results and improving patient management (Box 12-2).

The following sections of this chapter will describe the technology available for POCT and the organizational factors that are important when POCT is implemented in a healthcare setting. The chapter concludes with a short discussion of the future of POCT.

*References 10, 27, 48, 61, 65, 76, 80, 93, 103, 117, 129.
†References 4, 6, 58, 86, 135, 136.
‡References 8, 54, 72, 84, 133, 139.

ANALYTICAL AND TECHNOLOGICAL CONSIDERATIONS

The technical advances that have catalyzed the evolution of POCT instruments are the development of a miniature sensor to measure electrolytes, blood gases, and other analytes and the development of dry, stable reagents in disposable unit-dose devices. Although the throughput of tests for these systems is low, the time required to produce the results is usually short. These systems are often small enough to be portable, further enhancing the possibility of "bringing tests to the patient."

Topics to be discussed in this section include (1) instrument requirements, (2) instrument and operator interface design, (3) examples of POCT devices, and (4) the role of informatics. Readers requiring additional information are referred to more comprehensive texts[74,115] or to the vendors of POCT devices.

REQUIREMENTS

All POCT devices should meet the following overall requirements: (1) simple to use, (2) robust in terms of storage and usage, (3) producing results concordant with the central laboratory and consistent with the clinical need,and (4) capable of being safely operated. Additional characteristics and requirements of POCT devices are listed in Box 12-3.

BOX 12-1 Environments Where Point-of-Care Testing Might Be Employed

Primary Care
Home
Community pharmacist
Health centers (general practice, primary care)
Workplace clinic
Physician's office and community clinic
Diagnostic and treatment center
Paramedical support vehicle (ambulance, helicopter, aircraft)

Secondary and Tertiary Care
Emergency room
Admissions unit
Ambulatory diagnostic and treatment center
Operating room
Intensive care unit
Ward
Outpatient clinic

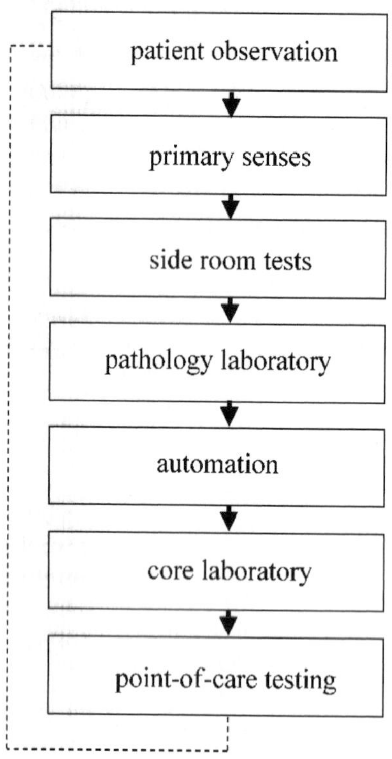

Figure 12-1 The trend in the evolution of diagnostic testing from observation of the patient, through simple testing, to sophisticated testing in the laboratory and back to a more patient-centered approach.

BOX 12-2 Advantages of Point-of-Care Testing

Reduced TAT of test results
Improved patient management
Reduction in the administrative work associated with test requesting
Minimization of delays occurring during sample collection and sample requirement(s)
Reduction in the time delay resulting from the transport of the sample to the testing lab
Reduction in the time delay resulting from having to log in (register) the sample
Reduction in the time delay that results from the entry of a sample into a complex testing facility

BOX 12-3 Characteristics/Requirements of a Point-of-Care Testing Analyzer

First results in a minute or less
Portable instruments with consumable reagent cartridges
A one- or two-step operating protocol
The capability of performing direct specimen analysis on whole blood and urine (nonprocessed samples)
Simple operating procedures that do not require a laboratory-trained operator
Flexible test menus
Quantitative results with accuracy and precision comparable with those of the central laboratory
Built-in/integrated calibration and quality control
Ambient temperature storage for reagents
Results provided as hard copy, stored, and available for transmission
Low instrument cost
Service by exchange
Built-in regulatory record keeping

Modified from Maclin E, Mahoney WC. Point-of-care testing technology. J Clin Ligand Assay 1995;18:21-33.

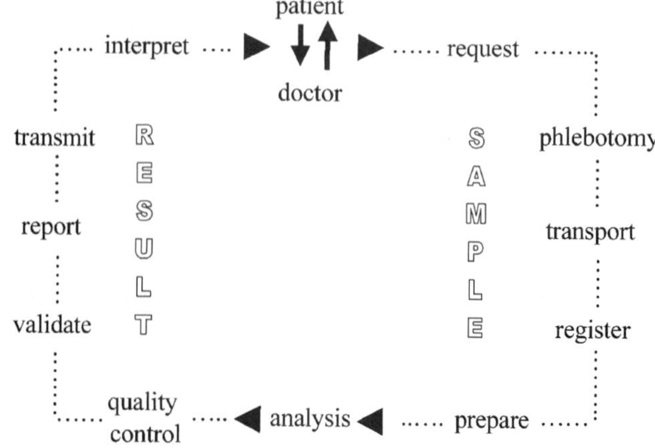

Figure 12-2 A schematic representation of the key steps in requesting, delivering, and using a diagnostic test result.

DESIGN

There is a great diversity of devices being used at point-of-care, ranging from relatively simple dipstick or strip tests to large, bench top, chemistry analyzers (Table 12-1). This breadth of technology encompasses a large range of analytes (Table 12-2), and many of the devices use the same analytical principles, such as enzymatic conversion and antibody recognition, as those found in conventional mainframe laboratory analyzers. The design of individual components or processes to be considered for POCT devices includes (1) operator interface, (2) bar code identification systems, (3) sample delivery devices, (4) reaction cell, (5) sensors, (6) control and communications systems, (7) data management and storage, and (8) manufacturing requirements.

Operator Interface

The operator or user interface is a very important design feature of POCT devices and should require minimal oper-

TABLE 12-1 Classification of Types of Point-of-Care Testing Instruments or Devices

Type of Technology	Analytical Principle	Analytes
Single-use, qualitative or semiquantitative cartridge/strip tests	Reflectance	Urine and blood chemistry
	Lateral-flow or flow-through immunoassays	Infectious disease agents, cardiac markers, hCG
Single-use quantitative cartridge/strip tests with a reader device	Reflectance	Glucose
	Electrochemistry	Glucose
	Reflectance	Blood chemistry
	Light scattering/optical motion	Coagulation
	Lateral-flow, flow-through, or solid phase immunoassays	Cardiac markers, drugs, CRP, allergy, and fertility tests
	Immunoturbidimetry	HbA_{1c}, urine albumin
	Spectrophotometry	Blood chemistry
	Electrochemistry	pH, blood gases, electrolytes, metabolites
Multiple-use quantitative cartridge/bench top devices	Electrochemistry	pH, blood gases, electrolytes, metabolites
	Fluorescence	pH, blood gases, electrolytes, metabolites
	Multiwavelength spectrophotometry	Hemoglobin species, bilirubin
	Time-resolved fluorescence	Cardiac markers, drugs, CRP
	Electrical impedance	Complete blood count

TABLE 12-2 Examples of Single or Multipad Stick Tests

Test	Sample	Chemistry
Acetaminophen	Whole blood	Acyl dehydrogenase
Alanine aminotransferase	Whole blood	Alanine/glutamate
Albumin	Whole blood, urine	Dye binding
Cholesterol	Whole blood	Cholesterol oxidase
Creatinine	Whole Blood, urine	Copper complexation
Glucose	Whole blood	Glucose oxidase
Lactate	Whole blood	Lactate dehydrogenase
Uric acid	Whole blood	Uricase
Alcohol	Urine	Alcohol dehydrogenase
Bilirubin	Urine	2,4-dichloroaniline
Hemoglobin	Urine	Peroxidase activity
Leukocyte esterase	Urine	Pyrrole amino ester hydrolysis
Ketones	Urine	Sodium nitroprusside reaction
Nitrite	Urine	p-Arsanilic acid reaction
pH	Urine	Double indicator principle
Protein	Urine	Protein error of indicators
Specific gravity	Urine	Polyacid pH change
Urobilinogen	Urine	Ehrlich's reaction

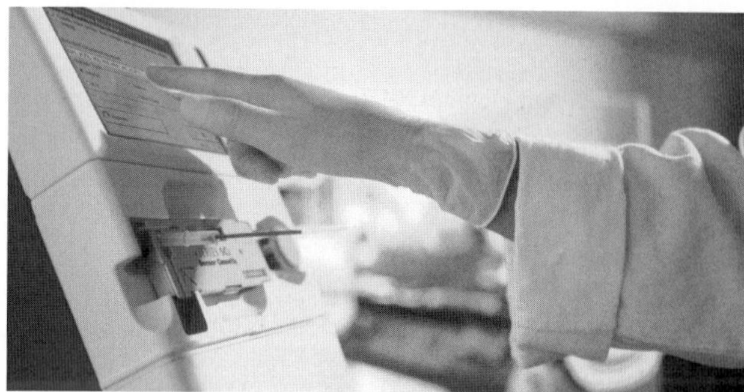

Figure 12-3 Touchscreen of the ABL77 blood gas analyzer. *(Courtesy Radiometer, Copenhagen.)*

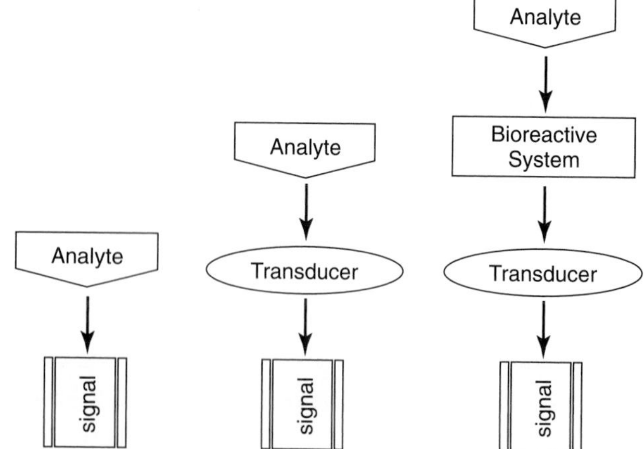

Figure 12-4 Diagram showing the key types of sensor technology used in POCT instruments.

ator interaction, guide the user through the operation, and tolerate minor operator errors. A minimum number of steps should include identifying the operator, patient, and test to be measured. Advances in information technology and consumer electronics have had a major impact on this area, such as the production of inexpensive liquid crystal display (LCD) screens.[89] Other forms of user interface include keypads, bar code readers, and possibly a printer. In some devices, the display is the only means to show the result, and in others it may incorporate a touch screen that is used to control the device (Figure 12-3). An alternative to the touch screen is a membrane type of keypad, but both displays and keypads can lead to significant increases in the size of the device when other user demands require smaller devices.

Bar Code Identification Systems

Many POCT devices incorporate bar code reading systems for a number of purposes. These include (1) identifying the test package to the system, (2) incorporating factory calibration data, and in some cases (3) programming the instrument to process a particular test or group of tests. Some POCT devices use magnetic strips as a way of storing similar information, such as lot-specific calibration data. Other functions of a bar code reader that are of growing importance are to identify both the operator and the patient sample to the system. This will ensure that there is traceability of the person who performed the test, and that the results are linked to the correct patient.

Sample Delivery

Sample access and delivery of the sample to the actual sensing component of the strip, cassette, or cartridge are also key interactions of the user with the device and in some cases, removal of the sample may also require user intervention. Ideally, following the addition of the sample, results should be produced without further intervention.

Reaction Cell

The design of the location where the analytical reaction takes place can be very simple, such as a porous pad, a cell, or a surface within a chamber. However, to simplify the user interface, it is often necessary to design complexity into the reaction chamber. Advances in microfluidics and techniques, such as molding, micromachining, photolithography, and screen printing, have all played a substantial role in the development of POCT devices.[71,78]

Sensors

Much of the focus on POCT devices has been concerned with the advances in sensor design (see Chapter 4).[140] Various sensor designs are illustrated in Figure 12-4. The chemosensor shown in the first column of Figure 12-4 is an example where the analyte has an intrinsic property, such as fluorescence, that enables it to be detected without a recognition element. The chemosensor shown in the second column of Figure 12-4 is a much more common design and is used in many POCT devices. The transducing element might be a chemical indicator or binding molecule that recognizes the analyte to be measured and produces a signal, usually electrical or optical. A biosensor is shown in the third column of Figure 12-4 and is distinguished from a chemosensor by having a biological or biochemical component as the recognition element. Enzymes are the most common biological element used followed by antibodies; transduction can be via an optical or electrical signal.

Control and Communications Systems

These constitute a major component of all POCT devices other than qualitative or semiquantitative strip tests that do not require a reader or measurement device. In even the smallest device, there is a control subsystem that coordinates all the other systems and ensures that all the required processes for an analysis take place in the correct order. Operations that require control include insertion or removal of the strip, cartridge, or cassette; temperature control; sample injection or aspiration; sample detection; mixing; timing of the detection process, such as absorbance measurement; and waste removal. Fluid movement can often be accomplished by mechanical means through pumps or centrifugation, and by fluidic properties, such as surface tension; the latter is often a critical element in the design of the simple strip tests and in microfabricated systems.[71]

Data Management and Storage

There are substantial requirements for data storage for POCT devices and in some cases data management, depending on the size and complexity of the device and testing menu. Data management includes calibration curve data and quality control (QC) limits and patient results. In some systems, data transfer and management takes place when the meter or reader is linked to a small bench top device called a docking station. These and other devices include communication protocols that allow data to be transferred to other data management systems.

Manufacturing of POCT Devices

Since many POCT methods are only used once and then discarded, reproducibility of manufacture is a key requirement so that consistent performance extends across a large number of strips or devices. The manufacturing process includes steps that are taken to ensure that the devices are reproducible (e.g., with respect to fluid movement) and remain stable during transit and storage for the stated period of time (e.g., with respect to calibration and reagent performance.)

EXAMPLES OF POCT DEVICES

POCT devices are classified as (1) in vitro and (2) in vivo, ex vivo, or minimally invasive.

In Vitro Devices

A 2003 survey of POCT analyzers, excluding glucose meters, indicated that the majority of POCT analyzers were in vitro devices and performed their analysis on whole blood, although others used serum, plasma, urine, or saliva samples.[36] The majority of instruments used less than 100 μL of the sample, and there were more than 15 different detection systems used for analytical measurement. The diversity of in vitro POCT technology and the range of analytes make it difficult to devise a simple classification that avoids any overlap between various technologies. For the purposes of highlighting key or novel POCT technologies, the following discussion classifies the various devices largely according to size and complexity: (1) single-use cartridge and/or strip tests, (2) single-use quantitative cartridge and/or strip tests with a monitoring device, and (3) multiple-use cartridge and bench top systems.

Single-Use Qualitative Strip or Cartridge and/or Strip Devices

A wide range of devices fall into this category, including single-pad urine tests (dipsticks) that are read visually; more complex strips that use light reflectance for measurement; and fabricated cassettes or cartridges that incorporate techniques such as immunochromatography[116] and are used as immunosensors.

Dipsticks. Dipsticks are single-pad devices that are relatively simple in construction and are composed of a pad of porous material, such as cellulose, that is impregnated with reagent and then dried.[154]

Complex Strips. More complex pads are composed of several layers, the uppermost of which is a semipermeable membrane that prevents red cells from entering the matrix. Despite their simplicity, critical operator factors include the need to cover the whole pad with the sample. Because the reactions often do not proceed to completion, it is necessary to time the period between placing the sample on the pad and comparing the resulting color to a color chart. In addition, for blood tests it may be necessary to remove all the blood before placing the sample in the reflectance meter; sometimes it is possible to read the color from the underside of the strip. Developments of these single stick devices include two pads for measurement of (1) different concentrations of the same analyte, such as hemoglobin and glucose[150]; (2) both albumin and creatinine (semiquantitative) to provide an albumin-creatinine ratio[120]; and (3) up to 10 different urine analytes using reflectance technology.[82] A chromatographic device has also been developed for the quantitative measurement of cholesterol, which does not require the use of any instrumentation.[1] Table 12-2 lists the tests performed by single or multipad dipsticks and the chemistry used for analysis.

Immunosensors. These devices are biological sensors in which the recognition agent is an antibody that binds to the analyte (see Chapters 4 and 9). Detection of the binding event or signal transducer is usually via an optical mechanism, either reflectance or fluorescence spectrophotometry, for quantification. Most immunosensing devices use reactions that are not reversible, although reversible reactions have now been described, which will facilitate their application in multiple-use cartridges and similar formats in the future.[57] Immunosensors usually use solid phase technologies in conjunction with either flow-through, lateral-flow, or immunochromatography processes. In the flow-through format, a heterogeneous immunoassay takes place in a porous matrix cell that acts as the solid phase, and in lateral flow the separation stage take place as the sample passes along the porous matrix.

A typical immunoassay format in a flow-through device has an antibody covalently coupled to the surface of a porous matrix. When the patient sample is added to the matrix, the analyte of interest binds to the antibody. Addition of a second labeled antibody forms a sandwich and traps the label at the position of the first antibody.[144] If the label is gold sol particles or colored latex, the label is directly visualized or quantified by reflectance spectrophotometry in a separate reader.[3] Another important feature of this type of technology is the incorporation of a built-in quality monitor that indicates positive if all the reagents have been stored and the device operated correctly. In all these different formats,

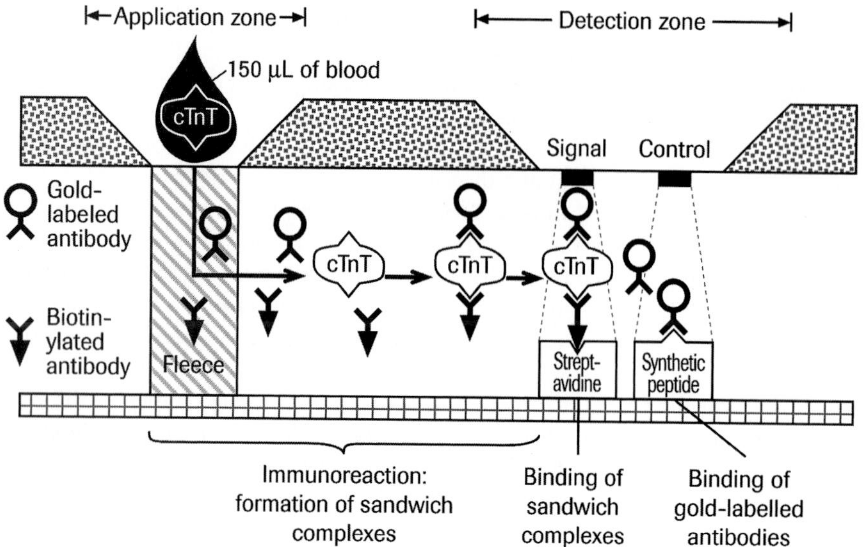

Figure 12-5 Schematic diagram of a lateral flow immunoassay for troponin T. *(Courtesy Roche Diagnostics, Mannheim, Germany.)*

uniform and predictable flow of the sample through or along the solid phase matrix is a major determinant of the reproducibility of the technique. Therefore the choice of matrix and how it interacts with the sample is of particular importance, and advances in the understanding of solid phase and surface chemistry technology have made a major contribution to the development of immunosensors.[131]

The Roche Trop T test strip for the qualitative determination of troponin T is an example of this technology (Figure 12-5). In this device, the blood sample is added and first flows through a glass fiber fleece, that separates the plasma from whole blood. Simultaneously, two monoclonal antihuman cTnT antibodies, one conjugated to biotin and one labeled with gold particles, bind to the troponin T in the sample. The antibody troponin complex then flows in a lateral direction along the cellulose nitrate test strip until it reaches the capture zone, which contains streptavidin bound to a solid phase. The biotin in the antibody troponin complex binds to the streptavidin and immobilizes the complex. The complex is then visualized as a purple band by the gold particles attached to one of the antibodies.[3] The unreacted gold-labeled antibody moves farther down the strip where it is captured by a zone containing a synthetic peptide consisting of the epitope of human cardiac troponin T and is visualized as a separate but similar colored band. The presence of this second band serves as an important quality indicator, because it indicates that the sample has flowed along the test strip, and the device has worked correctly.

A growing application of the strip type of technology for immunoassay is for infectious disease testing and the rapid detection of various infectious antigens and antibodies including *Chlamydia*,[21,62] group A streptococci,[20] *Helicobacter pylori*,[50] infectious mononucleosis,[39] and human immunodeficiency virus.[64,67] These tests commonly use a lateral-flow format for urine, serum, plasma, or whole blood samples in conjunction with analytical techniques, such as enzyme immunoassay and immunochromatography. An alternative

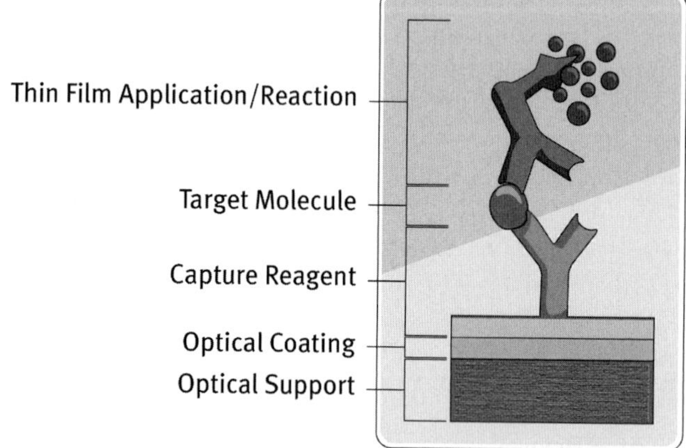

Figure 12-6 Schematic diagram of the principles of an optical immunoassay (OIA®) using thin film detection. *(Courtesy Thermo Electron Corporation, Louisville, CO.)*

approach manufactured by the Point-of-Care and Rapid Diagnostics business unit of the Thermo Electron uses light reflection and thin film amplification in what are termed optical immunoassays. The presence of an infectious disease antigen, such as Streptococcus A, is detected through binding to an antibody coated on a test surface. Light reflected through the antibody film alone produces a gold background that changes to purple when the thickness of the film is increased because of the presence of an antigen (Figure 12-6). The tests include built-in controls and provide results comparable with those provided by conventional microbiological assays but much more rapidly.[44]

Although most single-use devices currently rely upon reflectance or absorbance as the detection mechanism, other techniques of measurement are being investigated including surface plasmon resonance, evanescent wave, fixed-polarized ellipsometry, and diffraction. For example, evanescent wave technology has been used for the measurement of cardiac markers.[94,138]

Single-Use Quantitative Cartridge and Strip Tests with a Monitoring Device

The technologies or devices described in this section differ from those described above in that they include a meter or monitoring device, thereby enabling detection and quantification of the analyte(s). The availability of small, compact detectors is a result of advances in modern electronics and miniaturization. An integral part of many of these instruments is a charge-coupled device (CCD) camera that is a multichannel light detector, similar to a photo multiplier tube in a spectrophotometer, but with a higher signal to noise ratio so that it can detect much lower signals at low levels of light. For example, the Roche Cardiac Reader contains a CCD that can quantitate separate lateral-flow immunoassay strips for measurement of troponin T,[3,26] myoglobin, and D-Dimer. The majority of devices included in this category are used to measure glucose. In addition, many other analytes of clinical interest are measured with such devices.

Glucose Measurement. Clinically, POCT is most frequently used to measure glucose (see Chapter 25). The first glucose test strips were introduced more than 25 years ago, and now many millions of diabetics around the world use these strips in conjunction with a glucose meter to monitor their blood glucose level. These devices are biosensors since they all use an enzyme as the recognition agent, either glucose oxidase (GO), hexokinase (HK), or glucose dehydrogenase (GDH), with photometric (reflectance) or electrochemical detection.[53]

In general, all glucose strips are a form of what is called *thick-film* technology in that the film is composed of several layers each having a specific function. When blood is added to a strip, both water and glucose must pass into the film or analytical layer; for photometric systems erythrocytes must be excluded. These processes are achieved by what is called the separating layer that contains various components including glass fibers fleeces, membranes, and special latex formulations. In photometric systems, a spreading layer is important for the fast homogeneous distribution of the sample, whereas electrochemical strips use capillary fill systems. The support layer is usually a thin plastic material that in the case of reflectance-based strips may also have reflective properties. Additional reflectance properties have been achieved through the inclusion of substances such as titanium oxide, barium sulfate, and zinc oxide.

With systems that measure reflectance, the relationship between reflectance and the glucose concentration is described by the Kubelka-Munk equation:

$$C \alpha \frac{K}{S} = \frac{(1 - R)^2}{2R}$$

where C is the analyte concentration, K is the absorption coefficient, S is the scattering coefficient, and R is the percent of reflectance. In practice, glucose strips are produced in large batches and, after extensive quality assurance procedures, each batch is given a code that is stored in a magnetic strip on the underside of each test strip. This code describes the performance of the batch, including the calibrating relationship between the photometric or electrochemical signal and the concentration of glucose.

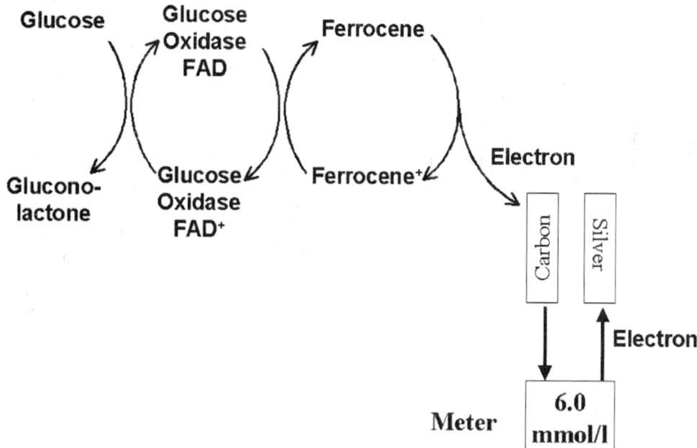

Figure 12-7 Schematic diagram of the reactions taking place in a MediSense electrochemical glucose strip. *(Modified from Henning TP, Cunningham TP. Biosensors for personal diabetes management. In Ramsay G ed, Commercial Biosensors. New York: John Wiley & Sons, 1998:3-46.)*

Since their introduction, there has been a steady stream of innovation in the development of glucose meters with the goal of making the devices smaller and easier to use with less risk of error and reducing interference from other compounds. The latter includes other reduction of substances, oxygen, and hematocrit. A major step in this development process was the use of ferrocene and its derivatives as immobilized mediators in the construction of an electrochemical glucose strip, the principles of which are shown in Figure 12-7.[30] The strip is composed of an Ag-AgCl reference electrode and a carbon-based active electrode, both manufactured using screen printing technology with the ferrocene or its derivatives contained in the printing ink. The sample is placed in the sample observation window and the hydrophilic layer serves to direct the sample over the reagent layer. The conversion of glucose is accompanied by the reduction of ferrocene and the release of electrons. The introduction of electrochemical technology has facilitated the production of smaller meters, nonwipe strips, less need to clean the instrument optics, and more rapid results. Some of these features are now available with photometric glucose meters.

Other Applications. Several immunosensor-based POCT devices have been developed that are capable of measuring a panel of analytes, such as cardiac markers,[4] allergy tests,[56] and fertility tests.[13] In these devices, a mixture of antibodies is immobilized at the origin, and complementary antibodies for the various analytes are immobilized at varying positions along the porous strip. In the case of drugs of abuse, devices are designed such that positive responses are only obtained if the concentration is above a precalibrated cut-off value.[15]

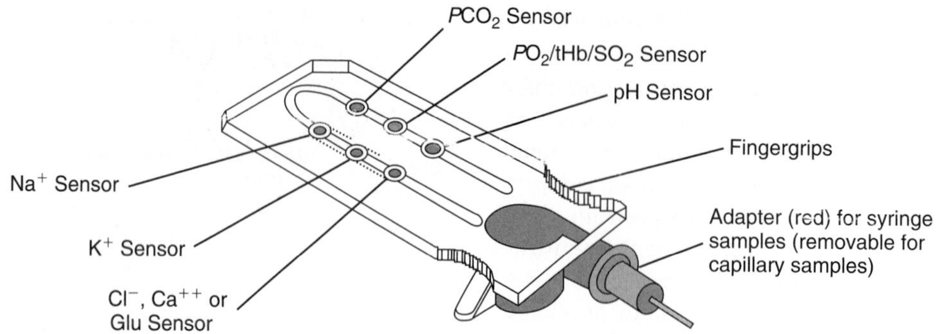

Figure 12-8 Schematic view of the measurement cassette for the Osmetech OPTI Critical Care Analyzer. *(Courtesy Osmetech, Roswell, GA.)*

In contrast to the thick-film technology described above, single-use sensors have also been constructed using *thin-film* technology, the most common commercial example being the i-STAT analyzer (see Chapter 10). This is a hand-held blood gas device, which measures electrolytes, glucose, creatinine, and certain coagulation parameters.[9,38] In thin-film sensors, electrodes are wafer structures constructed with thin metal oxide films using microfabrication techniques directly comparable with those used in the computer industry. The results are small, single-use cartridges containing an array of electrochemical sensors that operate in conjunction with a hand-held analyzer that can be used directly at the bedside.[32] Because the sensor layer is very thin, blood can permeate this layer quickly, and the sensor cartridge can be used immediately after it is unwrapped from its packing. This is an advantage over some thick-film sensors that require an equilibration or wet-up time before they can be used to measure blood samples.

Single-use devices for blood gas and other critical care measurements are also available through optical sensors or optodes[84] (see Chapters 4 and 27). The Osmetech OPTI Critical Care Analyzer (Figure 12-8) and the Radiometer NPT 7 are examples of this type of technology.[11,125] The advantages of optical systems compared with electrochemical transducers include the fact that they do not have to be calibrated to correct for electrode drift, and therefore the sensors are calibrated at the time of manufacture.[83]

A number of single-use, quantitative POCT devices are available that employ a cassette or cartridge design rather than lateral-flow strips. These include the Cholestech LDX system that uses a cassette that separates plasma from red cells after which the plasma reacts with pads of dry reagents for glucose or cholesterol or triglycerides and measurement of the absorbance in a small photometer.[24] Several cassette-based systems have been developed for measurement of hemoglobin, including the HemoCue. In this system, red cells are lysed in a minicuvet hemoglobin converted to methemoglobin and the methemoglobin measured at 570 nm; turbidity is corrected for by an additional measurement at 880 nm.[147]

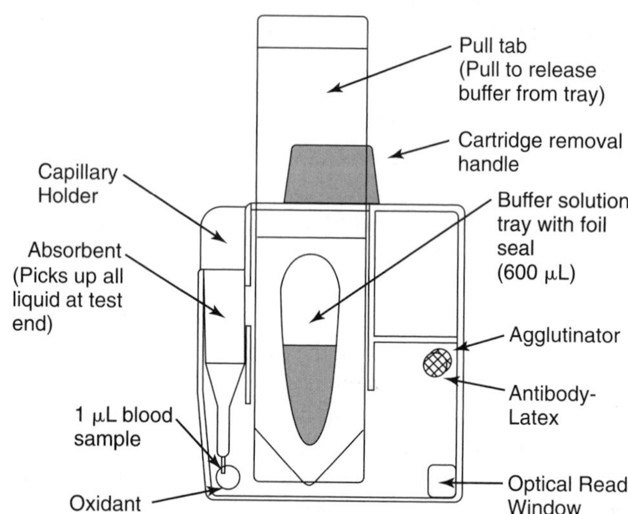

Figure 12-9 A schematic diagram of the Bayer DCA 2000 HbA_{1c} immunoassay cartridge. *(Courtesy Bayer HealthCare, Medfield, MA.)*

The Bayer DCA system is another example of a cartridge design but using a light-scattering immunoassay to measure glycated hemoglobin, together with a photometric assay for total hemoglobin. The cartridge is a relatively complex structure that contains antigen-coated latex particles, antibodies to HbA_{1C} and lysing reagents that are mixed following addition of the sample (Figure 12-9). Measurement takes place when the cartridge is placed into a temperature-controlled reader, and the analytical performance is sufficient for quantitative monitoring of diabetic control.[113] The size of the device allows it to be used in diabetic clinics where it can also be used for measurement of urinary albumin and creatinine.[23,108]

POCT devices for monitoring anticoagulant therapy have also been developed for use in clinics or by the patient at home.[104,105] These devices have been made possible by advances in optical detection techniques and the ability to miniaturize electromechanical devices. For example, early systems used magnets to detect the decrease in sample flow or movement that results from the clotting process, but this required careful timing and a large blood sample. An alternative technology pumps a defined amount of the sample backward and forward through a narrow aperture. Optical sensors monitor the speed at which the sample moves and, as the clot forms, the speed decreases and when a predetermined level is reached, the instrument indicates the time.[2] Yet another approach also uses magnetism in the form of paramagnetic iron oxide particles that are included with the sample and induced to move by an oscillating magnetic field. When a clot is formed, the movement of the particles is restricted; this is detected by an infrared sensor, and the time taken to reach this state is an indication of the clotting time.[104]

Speckle detection technology has also been used to measure prothrombin time (PT), activated partial thromboplastin time (APTT), and activated clotting time (ACT). In this approach, the instrument contains an infrared light source that directs a coherent light beam onto the oscillating sample. The movement of the red cells in the blood results in the refraction of the light to produce an interference or "speckle" pattern that is recorded by the photodetector. This "speckle" pattern changes when the capillary flow slows as the sample clots. The time it takes for this to happen is a measure of the clotting time.[130] Other point-of-care devices that measure aspects of hemostasis and thrombosis include the Thromboelastograph and Sonoclot.[41a,145]

It should be noted that the sizes of some of the single-use, cartridge-based systems are comparable with certain of the bench top, multiple-use devices described later in this chapter. Examples of these analyzers, which are usually used in clinics and physician practices rather than at the bedside, are the Vision,[126] Stratus,[66] and Piccolo[124] devices, all of which incorporate onboard centrifugation. Other small analyzers that are used at point-of-care but require preliminary centrifugation of the sample include the Ortho-Clinical Diagnostics DT60, which uses the same dry-slide technology that is used in the larger, laboratory analyzers.[29]

Multiple-Use Cartridge and Bench Top Systems

Many of the POCT devices in this category are used for critical care testing in locations such as the intensive care unit, surgical suite, and emergency room. Some of these devices use thick-film sensors or electrodes in strips to measure glucose, lactate, and urea and use the same technology described above but differ in that the sensors are designed to be reusable. They are manufactured from thick films of paste and inks using screen printing techniques to produce individual or multiple sensors. In addition to measuring metabolites, these sensors are also used to measure blood gases and electrolytes.[31] The sensors have been incorporated with reagents and calibrators into a single cartridge or pack that is placed in the body of a small- to medium-sized, portable critical care analyzer (Figure 12-10). Each pack will measure a certain number of samples during a certain time period, after which it is a relatively simple procedure to replace. This type of technology is available as the Instrumentation Laboratory GEM Premier,[59] the Radiometer ABL77,[81] and the Bayer Diagnostics Rapidpoint 400.[85]

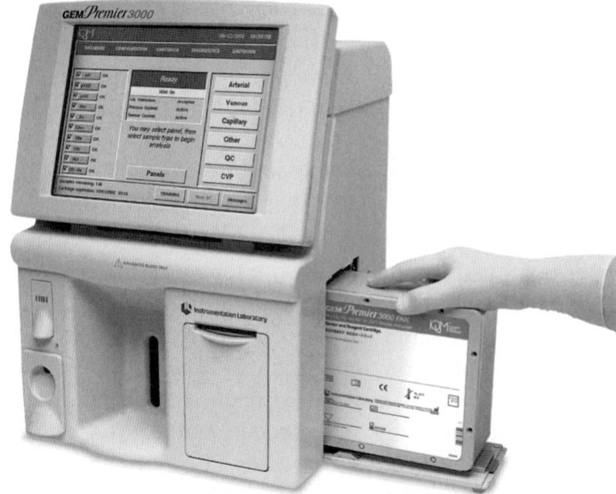

Figure 12-10 The GEM® Premier™ 3000 critical care analyzer. *(Courtesy Instrumentation Laboratory, Lexington, MA.)*

Other key developments for devices include the development of liquid calibration systems that use a combination of aqueous base solutions and conductance measurements to calibrate the pH and PCO_2 electrodes, with oxygen being calibrated with an oxygen-free solution and room air.[92] In addition, automated QC packages are integrated into these analyzers that ensure that QC samples are analyzed at regular intervals. These comprise packs or bottles of QC material that are contained within the instrument and sampled at predetermined intervals with onboard software interpreting the results and generating alerts, if necessary. Such devices can even be remotely monitored and programmed to respond to problems on instruments located long distances from the central laboratory.[55]

Critical care POCT instruments are also available for measuring various hemoglobin species and performing CO-oximetry determinations. The latter relies upon multiwavelength spectrophotometry where light absorption by hemolyzed blood is measured at up to 60 or more wavelengths to determine the concentration of the five hemoglobin species.[14] One manufacturer has recently extended the multiwavelength spectrophotometry to measure bilirubin directly in whole blood.[123]

Bench top devices are also available to perform complete blood counts (CBC) using analytical principles similar to those used in laboratory-based devices.[33,35] In addition, single-use cartridge technology is being developed that will have the capability to offer full white cell differentiation. Immunoassay measurements are also now available in a compact device, for use in clinics and similar locations. The Innotrac Aio! is an example of such a device and uses dry-coated reagents and time-resolved fluorescence for detection.[110] Results are produced in less than 20 minutes, and the assay menu includes C-reactive protein (CRP), human chorionic gonadotropin (hCG), and cardiac markers.[51]

In Vivo, Ex Vivo, or Minimally Invasive Devices

Although the majority of POCT devices are used for in vitro applications, there is a smaller group that is classified as in vivo, ex vivo, or minimally invasive (Table 12-3). In vivo or continuous monitoring applications are those in which the sensing device is inserted into the bloodstream. For many years, this application was confined to blood gases using optical technology,[148] but electrochemical applications also have been developed for both blood gases and glucose.[7] Electrochemical sensors are also used in an ex vivo application for the same parameters, the difference being that the sensors are actually external to the body but in a closed loop of blood that leaves the body and is then returned downstream from the sensing device.[152] The major application for minimally invasive devices is primarily glucose, such as the Gluco Watch Biographer device,[137] but devices for transcutaneous measurement of bilirubin are also now available,[122] although they are only suitable for screening purposes.

TABLE 12-3 Types of Ex Vivo, In Vitro, and Noninvasive Point-of-Care Testing Technology

Type of Technology	Analytical Principle	Analytes
Ex vivo	Optical fluorescence	pH, blood gases
	Electrochemistry	pH, blood gases, electrolytes, glucose
In vivo	Optical fluorescence	pH, blood gases
	Electrochemistry	Subcutaneous glucose
Noninvasive	Electrochemistry/ iontophoresis	Transcutaneous glucose
	Multiwavelength spectrophotometry	Bilirubin

Informatics and POCT

Most analytical devices used in clinical laboratories are directly linked or connected via an electronic interface to a laboratory information system (LIS). In this progression, many different informatic functions (see Chapter 18) are used, including the electronic transfer of data from the analyzers to the LIS and ultimately into a patient's electronic medical record. This provides healthcare professionals with quick, accurate, and appropriate access to the patient's medical history and information.

Considerable effort has been expended to incorporate these informatic processes into POCT devices. However, this has proved extremely difficult (Table 12-4), with early POCT devices lacking the hardware and software to acquire and store data and transfer it to an LIS. Consequently, analytical data were often not captured in a patient's medical record or had to be entered manually into an LIS with a major risk of transcription error. Thus important clinical information may be lost with the additional possibility of costly duplicate testing.[63] Newer POCT devices have addressed this problem by incorporating the prerequisite hardware and software into their design, but linking them to information management systems has proven problematic as each device had its own proprietary interface. The extent of this problem was highlighted by a survey of more than 500 United States hospitals conducted by the Enterprise Corporation for the American Association of Clinical Chemists in 1999 where it was found that only 15% of POCT data was sent to the LIS electronically, 18% entered manually, and 67% never reached the LIS. This lack of "connectivity" was identified as a major barrier to the effective deployment of POCT.[132]

To address the problem of a lack of connectivity in POCT instruments, a group of more than 30 companies involved in the POCT industry created a Connectivity Industry

TABLE 12-4 Informatic Issues With Present-Day Point-of-Care Testing Devices

Principle	Problem with POCT
Patient samples should be positively identified with the system	Strip devices do not carry identification (ID) and meters do not read IDs.
Operator access to the system should be password protected	This is not true of many hand-held meters
A hard copy of the record of the results, positively identified, should be generated	Many meters do not carry printers and results must be manually transcribed
Data should be stored in a local or remote database	This capability is not available on many devices
A log of events and of access should be maintained	This capability is not available on many devices

Modified from Jones R. Informatics and point-of-care testing. In: Price CP, Hicks JM, eds. Point-of-care testing. Washington DC: AACC Press, 1999: 175-95.

Consortium (CIC), that developed a set of seamless—"plug and play"—point-of-care communication standards. Adherence to these connectivity standards ensures that POCT devices meet critical user requirements, such as bidirectionality, device connection commonality, commercial software intraoperability, security, and QC and/or regulatory compliance. The design of the standards was based on (1) the use of a proven architecture and notation, (2) the use of existing standards and architectural patterns wherever possible, (3) a focus on services that would enable software intraoperability and add value to overall functionality, and (4) a reduction in the complexity of device communications.

Description of Connectivity Standards

The CIC connectivity standards are represented simply as the two interfaces between the POCT devices and information systems (Figure 12-11). The device interface passes patient results and QC information between the POCT instrument and devices, such as docking stations, concentrators, terminal servers, and point-of-care data managers. The latter have to be linked to a variety of information systems via the observation reporting interface or electronic data interface, for transmission of ordering information and patient results.

The connectivity standard was approved by the National Committee for Clinical Laboratory Standards (NCCLS) in 2001 as the POCT1-A standard.[100] Essentially, if a POCT device incorporates this standard, it should easily be able to communicate with laboratory and hospital information management systems, allowing exchange of data and information in a standardized format irrespective of vendor, location, or interface.

Benefits of POCT Connectivity

The full informatic benefits of connectivity may be some years away since the standards are only likely to be included in new products. However, pressure from laboratory scientists and users should encourage its adoption just as it helped with the formation of the CIC. At this stage, one of the most important benefits of connectivity will be to facilitate the transfer and capture of patient POCT and quality-related data into permanent medical records.[22] Other destinations for point-of-care data include the bedside monitors and clinical information systems that reside in critical care units. These systems integrate data from various sources, including vital signs and diagnostic results. In conjunction with clinical guidelines and expert systems, they can produce critical care maps used in the management of the critically ill patient.[47] Integration of POCT data with other clinical information is now quite commonly seen in disease management systems supporting the care of patients with chronic diseases, such as diabetes mellitus and hyperlipidemia. In the case of diabetes mellitus, the data manager serves to maintain a record of the blood glucose results and any other observations that the patient wishes to record to bring to the attention of the clinician at the next clinic visit. This record is then used to help patients with the management of their own disease. In the case of hyperlipidemia, the data may be fed into an algorithm together with other observations to calculate a risk score that is then used by the patient and his

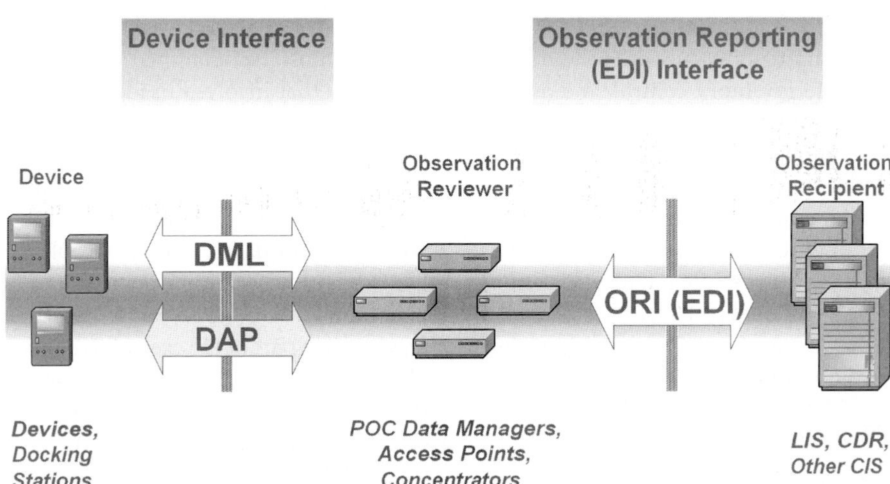

Figure 12-11 Schematic diagram of the interfaces between POCT devices and information systems. *(Modified from National Committee for Clinical Laboratory Standards: Point-of-Care Connectivity; Approved Standard. NCCLS Document POCT1-A. Wayne, PA. National Council for Clinical Laboratory Standards, 2001.)*

or her clinician to identify life style, dietary, and therapy changes, together with the expected outcomes (e.g., reduced risk of cardiovascular disease).

Innovations in the area of POCT quality will also be assisted by being able to easily link devices to networks and to those who are ultimately responsible for the device. Several manufacturers of POCT devices now provide software to allow central laboratories to monitor their instruments in remote locations. Currently, these packages are primarily in the critical care testing area, such as blood gases and related parameters, but with easier access to interfacing, it is likely that this type of software will be available for a wider range of devices. In conjunction with network technology, remote control software not only allows monitoring of the performance of the device but also enables those responsible for the instrument to carry out some service procedures or even shut the instrument down completely if required. Such software can manage a large number of devices that may be geographically dispersed and, by reducing the necessity to physically visit each device, it can result in significant staff savings.[55]

Although the need to have a permanent record of patient data is the most important benefit of connectivity for many laboratory scientists, others might place more emphasis on the requirement for accurate financial accounting of POCT. This would certainly be applicable in those countries where diagnostic testing has to be charged to the patient or their insurer. Easier connectivity of POCT data to accounting or billing systems will help prevent the obvious financial consequences of uncharged testing.

IMPLEMENTATION AND MANAGEMENT CONSIDERATIONS

Implementation, management, and maintenance of a POCT service in a healthcare facility require providing the necessary planning, oversight, and inventory control, and assuring the reliability of the results through adequate training and QC. Consequently a number of factors must be considered including (1) establishing need; (2) organizing and implementing of a coordination committee; (3) establishing a POCT testing policy and accountability; (4) procuring equipment and its evaluation; (5) training and certification of operators, establishing a QC, quality assurance, and audit policy; (6) ensuring documentation; (7) establishing an accreditation and regulation of POCT policy.

Establishment of Need

As with laboratory testing in general, the decision to implement a POCT service requires (1) establishment of need, (2) consideration of the clinical, operational, and economic benefits, and (3) the costs involved.*

BOX 12-4 Assessing the Need for a Point-of-Care Testing Service

Which tests are required?
What is the TAT required?
What clinical question is being asked when requesting this test?
What clinical decision is likely to be made upon receipt of the result?
What action is likely to be taken upon receipt of the result?
What outcome should be expected from the action taken?
Why isn't the laboratory able to deliver the required service?
Will POCT provide the required accuracy and precision of result?
Is there staff available to perform the test?
Are there adequate facilities to perform the test and store the equipment and reagents?
Will you abide by the organizations POCT policy?
Are there operational benefits to this POCT strategy?
Are there economic benefits to this POCT strategy?
Will a change in practice be required to deliver these benefits?
Is it feasible to deliver the changes in practice that might be required?

Addressing the questions listed in Box 12-4 is useful for establishing the requirement for a POCT service. Answering them will help identify the test itself but should also explain why the current service is not meeting the needs of the patient or the clinician. Specifically, establishing the need for a POCT service should identify what benefits are likely to accrue to the patient and/or the healthcare provider by introducing a more rapid service. An economic assessment of the costs of delivering the current service and the costs associated with the POCT service should also be conducted. The benefits must be identified and accounted for in a way similar to that involved in identifying the cost of other elements of the health service. However, it is important in such an exercise to ensure that the costs associated with the benefits are recognized in terms of those that will redirect resources, as against those that may be more associated with an improved quality of care and ultimately quality of life. Some of the costs in the latter cannot be readily leveraged, and therefore resources are required to fund the POCT service. This part of the exercise is extremely useful as it often identifies the changes in practice that are required to release the resources to fund the new service and the potential difficulties associated with achieving such a change.

A risk assessment should also be conducted that will focus primarily on the procedures and processes that have to be put in place to ensure the maintenance of a high quality of service.[73] Issues of concern include (1) robustness of the POCT device, (2) quality of the results produced, (3) competence of the operator of the device, (4) effectiveness of the process for transmission of the results to the caregiver, (5) competence of the caregiver to interpret the results provided,

*References 68, 79, 87, 95, 109, 118.

(6) procedures in place to ensure that an accurate record of the results is kept, (7) identification of what practice changes may have to be made to deliver the benefits that have been identified, (8) how the staff will be retrained if appropriate, and (9) how the changes in practice will be implemented.[69,102,121,127,146]

Organization and Implementation of a Coordination Committee

When organizing and implementing POCT service, it is important to consult with all of the parties involved in delivering such a service. This can be best achieved by establishing a POCT coordinating committee. Such a committee is then charged with managing the whole process of delivering a high quality POCT service. Membership of the committee should include representatives of those who use the service and those that deliver the service, together with a representative of the organization's management team. The users will include physicians, nurses, other healthcare providers, and maybe even a patient. The providers should include at least one representative from the laboratory and those involved in the use of other diagnostic and therapy equipment close to the patient (e.g., respiratory measurement technologists and nurses). Typically a laboratory professional will chair such a committee because it is the laboratory that will provide the necessary backup if there is a service failure; furthermore the laboratory professional will have had training and expertise with the analytical issues that are likely to arise. For many reasons, the committee should report to the medical director. The committee should then designate members who will take the responsibility for overseeing the training and accreditation of all POCT operators and also for QC and quality assurance. The work of the committee should be governed by the organization's policy on POCT.

POCT Policy and Accountability

Implementation of a POCT service requires a POCT policy that establishes all of the procedures required to ensure the delivery of a high quality service, together with the responsibility and accountability of all staff associated with the POCT. This may be (1) part of the organization's total quality management system,[60] (2) part of its clinical governance policy,[42] and (3) required for accreditation purposes.[17,18] The elements of a POCT policy are listed in Box 12-5.

BOX 12-5 Elements of a Point-of-Care Testing Policy

Catalog information—review time
- Approved by
- Original distribution
- Related policies
- Further information
- Policy replaces

Introduction—background
- Definition
- Accreditation of services
- Audit of services

Laboratory services in the organization—location
- Logistics
- Policy on diagnostic testing

Management of POCT—committee and accountability
- Officers
- Committee members
- Terms of reference
- Responsibilities
- Meetings

Equipment and consumable procurement—criteria for procurement
- Process of procurement

Standard operating procedures
- Training and certification of staff—training
- Certification
- Recertification

Quality control and quality assurance—procedures
- Documentation and review

Health and safety procedures
Bibliography

Equipment Procurement and Evaluation

After establishing the requirement, coordination committee, and policy, the next stage in the process is equipment procurement. This involves first identifying candidate POCT equipment having the prerequisite analytical and operational capabilities to meet the clinical requirements of a POCT service. As discussed in Chapter 15, the performance characteristics of these devices are then obtained and compared. These include parameters such as accuracy, precision, TAT, calibration frequency, potential interferants, calibrator and reagent stability, variation in different lot numbers of reagents and calibrators, and QC requirements. In addition, operational requirements made of the operator also have to be identified, and the potential for operator error (including delayed addition of the sample and use of an incorrect sample volume) determined. Independent validation of these analytical and operational characteristics can be obtained from (1) the manufacturer; (2) published evaluations performed by agencies such as the Medical Devices Agency in the United Kingdom; and (3) reports in the peer-reviewed literature. When reviewing performance data, particular attention should be paid to the precision and accuracy of measurement, including the concordance between the results produced by the POCT device and by a routine laboratory method, because patients are likely to be managed using both analytical systems. This concordance may be difficult to assess, and it may be necessary to seek endorsements from current users of the systems and possibly conduct some form of internal trial. Evaluation of analytical performance will be addressed in Chapter 14 and in the NCCLS protocol.[99]

An economic assessment of the equipment, including the cost of consumables and servicing, should also be made. This is likely to be a comparative exercise between the various point-of-care systems under consideration. Any comparison of costs with the laboratory service will only be highlighting the cost per test, which, as stated earlier, will not give an accurate assessment of the cost utility of the system. However, it is helpful at this point to have a good assessment of the relative staff costs associated with different systems because these are likely to be key features in the decision-making process. It is likely that the chosen system will be operated by staff already performing a wide range of duties involving the care of patients, and therefore the amount of time required to operate the device may be critical.

After the comparison data have been obtained, tabulated, and interpreted, a POCT device is selected. It is then recommended that the laboratory professional conduct a short evaluation of the equipment to gain familiarization with the system. This evaluation will help to determine the content of the training routine that will have to be subsequently developed and if troubleshooting of problems is required. Such an evaluation should document the concordance between the results generated with the device and those provided by the laboratory. All of this information should then be recorded in a logbook associated with the equipment. In addition, the organization may wish to undertake some form of safety check, give the device some form of local code, and enter the code into the local equipment register.

Training and Certification

The confidence of the clinician, the caregiver, and the patient in the results generated by a POCT device depends heavily on the robustness of the instrument and the competence of the operator, given that it has already been shown to meet the analytical requirements of the clinical setting. Many of the agencies involved in the regulation of healthcare delivery now require that all personnel associated with the delivery of diagnostic results demonstrate their competence through a process of regulation, and this applies equally to POCT personnel. Typically, those healthcare professionals involved in POCT will not have received training in the use of analytical devices as part of their core professional training but may be called upon to operate a number of complex pieces of equipment.

The elements of a training program are listed in Box 12-6. In practice such a program is tailored to suit the needs of the individual and the organization.[134] These may include formal presentation to groups, or on a one-to-one basis, self-directed learning using agreed documentation or computer-aided learning. For example, several of the current models of blood gas and electrolyte analyzers have onboard computer-aided training modules. Whatever the training strategy employed, it is important to document the satisfactory completion of training and that the individual has been tested and found competent with a combination of questions concerned with understanding and practical demonstration of the skills gained. The latter can be achieved by performing tests on a series of QC materials and repeat testing of samples that have recently been analyzed (parallel testing). Finally the operator should be observed through the whole procedure involved in the POCT on a minimum of three occasions.

BOX 12-6 The Main Elements of a Point-of-Care Testing Training Program

Understanding the context of the test—pathophysiological context
- Clinical requirement for the test
- Action taken on basis of result
- Nature of test and method used

Patient preparation required—relevance of diurnal variation
- Relevance of drug therapy

Sample requirement and specimen collection
Preparation of analytical device—machine and/or consumables
Performance of test
Performance of quality control
Documentation of test result and quality control result
Reporting of test result to appropriate personnel
Interpretation of result and sources of advice
Health and safety issues (e.g., disposal of sample and test device, cleaning of machine and test area)

Competence on a long-term basis is maintained through regular practice of skills and continuing education, and it is important to build these features into any education and training program. Regular review of performance in QC and quality assurance programs will provide a means of overseeing the competence of operators. However, this is not always sufficient, particularly when operators are employed on irregular shifts or may not always be called upon to perform POCT. In this latter situation, it may be necessary to create specific arrangements for individuals to undertake tests on QC material. The error log may also highlight when problems are arising. However, the most important thing is to encourage an open approach to the assessment of competence so that operators themselves seek help if they believe that problems are occurring. Such an open approach should be supported with audit and performance review meetings where problems are aired and developments discussed. The regular assessment of competence should be built into a formal program for recertification that will be a requirement of most accreditation programs.

Quality Control, Quality Assurance, and Audit

QC and quality assurance programs provide a formal means of monitoring the quality of a service (see Chapter 19). The internal QC program is a relatively short-term view and typically compares the current performance with that of the last time the analysis was made. External quality assurance on the other hand takes a longer-term view and in some respects addresses other issues surrounding the quality of the result. Thus quality assurance compares the testing performance of different sites and/or different pieces of equipment or methods.[16,145] An audit is a more retrospective form of analysis of performance and, furthermore, can take a more holistic view of the whole process. However, the foundation to ensuring good quality remains a successful training and certification scheme.

Classically, quantitative internal QC involves the analysis of a sample for which the analyte concentration is known, either because the material has been analyzed on many occasions and the distribution of results documented, or because it has been analyzed independently and the mean and range of results quoted for the method used. The essence of using the internal QC material is to establish the interval of results that is acceptable; the current analytical result is compared with the interval of results deemed to be acceptable (see Chapter 16). The result must then be documented, usually graphically, because it shows the conformity of results and any trends in results that may be occurring. The major aim is to use a means of documentation that ensures that comparative performance is assessed.

There are several challenges to the classical approach with POCT. The first concerns the frequency of testing—should a QC sample be analyzed every time that (1) a sample is analyzed, (2) a new operator uses the system, (3) a new lot number of reagents is used, or (4) the system is recalibrated? There is no consistent agreement on the correct approach, and one probably has to be guided by the reproducibility and overall analytical performance of the system and local circumstances, such as the number and competence of the operators, together with the frequency with which the system is used. For a bench top and/or multitest analyzer, at least one QC sample should be run a minimum of once per shift—three times a day. Some critical care analyzers can be programmed to perform a QC check at intervals set by those responsible for the device.

For single-use POCT disposable devices, the above strategy cannot completely monitor the quality of the test system.[111,151] For example, when conventional QC material is analyzed on a unit-use or single-test POCT system, only that testing unit is monitored. Thus it is impossible to test every unit with control material because by definition these are single-test systems and one cannot analyze both control material and a patient sample with the single unit. Under these circumstances, there is greater dependence placed on the manufacturing reproducibility of the devices to ensure a good quality service. A 2002 NCCLS guideline reports quality management procedures for unit-use testing both from a manufacturer's and a user's perspective.[101]

In the case of the user, some may wish to continue with a QC testing strategy that is similar to that for multiuse devices, namely analyze a minimum of one QC sample per run during each shift. If testing is infrequent, then another approach would be to analyze a QC sample whenever there is a change to the testing system, such as a different batch of testing materials or a different operator.[98] There are also other QC approaches, but many do not test the whole process. For example, the use of a plastic surrogate reflectance pad as a QC sample will only test the performance of the reflectance meter and does not test the process of sample addition, etc. Similarly the same forms of electronic internal QC, used for example with the i-STAT cassette system, also do not test the sampling technique but simply the functionality of the cassette and the docking station.[151]

External quality assurance or proficiency testing is a systematic approach to QC monitoring in which standardized samples are analyzed by one or more laboratories to determine the capability of each participant. In this approach, the operator has no knowledge of the analyte concentration, and therefore it is considered closer to a "real testing situation." The results are transmitted to a central authority, who then prepares a report and returns a copy to each participating laboratory. The report will identify the range of results obtained for the complete group of participants and may be classified according to the different methods used by participants in the scheme. The scheme may encompass both laboratory and POCT users, which gives an opportunity to compare results with laboratory-based methods. In practice, external quality assurance or proficiency testing is used in POCT to determine and document long-term performance and the concordance of results between the POCT service and an organization's central laboratory. It is also possible to operate an external quality assurance scheme within a hospital or organizational setting; such a scheme would typically be run by qualified laboratory personnel. This provides the opportunity to compare the results being reported by both the laboratory and other POCT sites within the same organization. This can be important when patients are managed in several departments—or when machines break down and samples are taken to other sites for testing. When deteriorating or poor performance is identified in one of these schemes, it is important to document the problem, and then provide and document a solution. It may be necessary as part of this exercise to review some of the patient's notes to ensure that incorrect results have not been reported and inappropriate clinical actions taken. In addition, if the solution highlights a vulnerable feature of the process overall or for one particular operator then a process of retraining must be instituted.

An example of data from an external quality assurance scheme for POCT is shown in Figure 12-12. Such schemes are run on a national and international basis, and some Web site schemes are listed in references.[25,141,149]

Maintenance and Inventory Control

The implementation and maintenance of a POCT service require that a supply of devices be maintained at all times and a formal program for doing so employed. The key points in this process are to (1) adhere to the recommended storage conditions, (2) be aware of the stated shelf life of the consumables, and (3) ensure that stocks are released in time for any preanalytical preparation to be accommodated (e.g., thawing). When multiple sites are using the same materials, then a central purchasing, supply and inventory control system should be put in place—not only to gain the benefit from bulk purchasing, but also to ensure that individual systems are not supplied unknowingly with different batches of consumables.

The complexity in the maintenance of reusable devices will vary from system to system, but clear guidelines will be available from the manufacturer and should be adhered to rigorously. Issues that usually require particular vigilance include expiration dates, bio-contamination, electrical safety, maintenance of optics, and inadvertent use of inappropriate consumables.

DOCUMENTATION

The documentation of all aspects of a POCT service has been a major issue for many years, compounded by the fact that often the storage of data in laboratory and hospital information systems has been limited and often inconsistent. Thus it is critically important to keep an accurate record of the test request, the result, and the action taken as an absolute minimum. Some of the issues concerning documentation are now being resolved with the advent of the patient electronic record, electronic requesting, and better connectivity of POCT instrumentation to information systems and the patient record (see earlier discussion). The

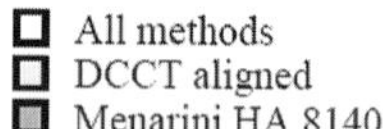

Specimen : 257A	n	Mean	SD	CV(%)
DCCT aligned	228	5.64	0.24	4.3
Bayer DCA 2000	34	5.65	0.14	2.4
BioRad Variant (I)	6	5.43	0.21	3.9
BioRad Variant (II)	34	5.57	0.18	3.2
Menarini HA 8121	9	5.71	0.13	2.3
Menarini HA 8140	53	5.84	0.25	4.3
Menarini HA 8160	15	5.54	0.24	4.3
Primus	9	5.73	0.20	3.6
Roche Integra	20	5.64	0.19	3.3
Tosoh 2.2	17	5.51	0.21	3.8
Tosoh G7	17	5.39	0.13	2.5
Non-aligned by choice	18	5.09	0.45	8.8
Menarini HA 8140	7	5.02	0.14	2.7

no. of laboratories: 100, 80, 60, 40, 20, 0
3.8 4.7 5.6 6.5 7.4

Your result	5.8
Target value (DCCT aligned)	5.64
Your specimen:	
%bias	+2.9
transformed bias	+69
Accuracy Index	69
IFCC reference value	3.91
DCCT comparison value	5.67
ALTM (for information only)	5.61

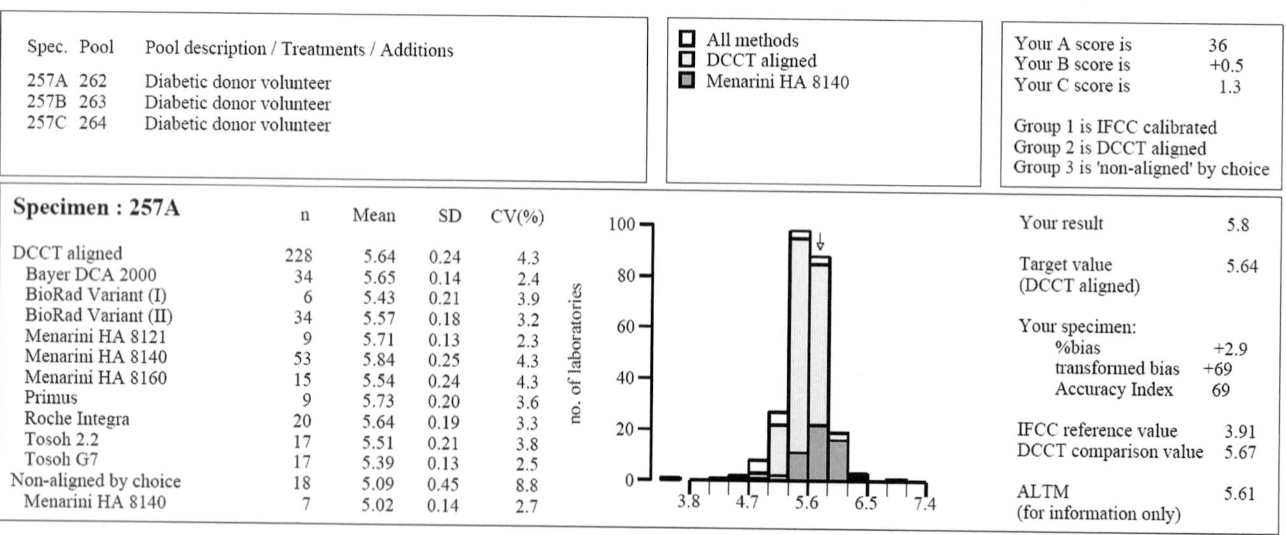

Spec.	Pool	Pool description / Treatments / Additions
257A	262	Diabetic donor volunteer
257B	263	Diabetic donor volunteer
257C	264	Diabetic donor volunteer

Your A score is	36
Your B score is	+0.5
Your C score is	1.3

Group 1 is IFCC calibrated
Group 2 is DCCT aligned
Group 3 is 'non-aligned' by choice

Specimen : 257A	n	Mean	SD	CV(%)
DCCT aligned	228	5.64	0.24	4.3
Bayer DCA 2000	34	5.65	0.14	2.4
BioRad Variant (I)	6	5.43	0.21	3.9
BioRad Variant (II)	34	5.57	0.18	3.2
Menarini HA 8121	9	5.71	0.13	2.3
Menarini HA 8140	53	5.84	0.25	4.3
Menarini HA 8160	15	5.54	0.24	4.3
Primus	9	5.73	0.20	3.6
Roche Integra	20	5.64	0.19	3.3
Tosoh 2.2	17	5.51	0.21	3.8
Tosoh G7	17	5.39	0.13	2.5
Non-aligned by choice	18	5.09	0.45	8.8
Menarini HA 8140	7	5.02	0.14	2.7

no. of laboratories: 100, 80, 60, 40, 20, 0
3.8 4.7 5.6 6.5 7.4

Your result	5.8
Target value (DCCT aligned)	5.64
Your specimen:	
%bias	+2.9
transformed bias	+69
Accuracy Index	69
IFCC reference value	3.91
DCCT comparison value	5.67
ALTM (for information only)	5.61

Figure 12-12 Extract of data from Distribution 257 of the UK NEQAS for Glycated Hemoglobin, May 2003. *(Courtesy Dr. J. Middle, UK NEQAS.)*

documentation should extend from the standard operating procedure(s) for the POCT systems to records of training and certification of operators, internal QC and quality assurance, together with error logs and any corrective action taken.

Accreditation and Regulation of POCT

The features of the organization and management of POCT described above are the same as those for the accreditation of any diagnostic services.[17,18] Accreditation of POCT should be part of the overall accreditation of laboratory medicine services, or indeed as part of the accreditation of the full clinical service, as has been the case in many countries, including the United States and the United Kingdom for a number of years. Thus the Clinical Laboratory Improvement Amendments of 1988 (CLIA) legislation in the United States stipulates that all POCT must meet certain minimum standards.[142,143] In the United States, the Centers for Medicare and Medicaid Services, the Joint Commission on Accreditation of Healthcare Organizations, and the College of American Pathologists are responsible for inspecting sites and each is committed to ensuring compliance with testing regulations for POCT.[37]

FUTURE OF POCT

We believe that the three key drivers for expansion of POCT services in the future will be (1) changes in the way healthcare is provided, (2) patient's needs and expectations, and (3) technological innovation. Currently the trends in the manner that clinical care is being delivered are completely opposite to the way in which diagnostic testing services are moving. For example, although laboratories are being consolidated with emphasis on more efficient and productive testing facilities, patient care is being moved closer to the patient and away from the larger hospital unit (Figure 12-13). This will effectively lead to either an increase in the logistics effort required to support the TATs expected by clinicians and patients, or a dramatic increase in the volume of POCT.

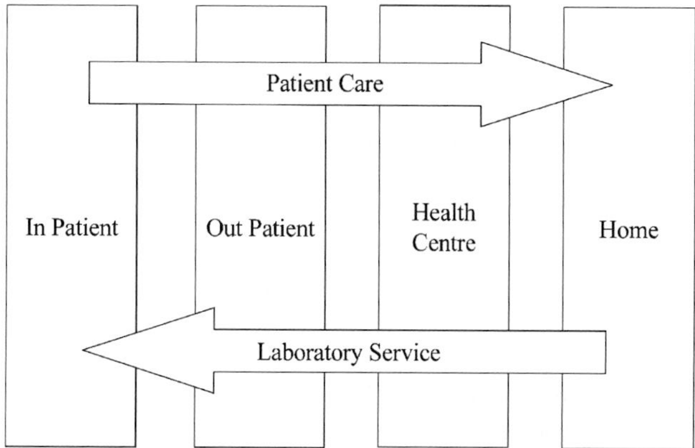

Figure 12-13 Diagram of the trends in healthcare today that include devolution of patient care to the primary care sector while laboratory medicine is consolidating in the "opposite direction."

Patient expectations are increasing and will drive the trend toward more patient-focused style of care with fewer clinic visits, shorter waiting times, and an expectation of better care. POCT has been shown to be capable of shorter "lengths of stay" and in many cases improved health outcomes. As health service decision makers (both purchasers and providers) realize that it is possible to achieve lower "costs per patient episode" with the use of POCT, more of the effort will be put into this testing modality. So what will facilitate this revolution? The answer lies in the new technology—both in terms of the new delivery platforms that are being developed and also in the discovery of new markers.

There are now considerable efforts being made to develop and manufacture miniaturized analytical devices (see Chapters 4 and 10) that will enable faster analytical times to be achieved, with smaller sample requirements. There are now several examples in the field of microfabricated devices that have been shown to meet these aspirations.[77,78] In the future, continued technological advances will result in even smaller devices that can be tailored for a large number of analytes and that are very simple to operate.

Noninvasive testing has promised much, and over the past decade, there is now evidence of some success in this area. The majority of work has been performed on a range of imaging techniques that seek a signature of the molecule of interest (e.g., glucose from among the many signatures of the extracellular and tissue matrix[70,90,97,112]). Alternative approaches have sought to access the extracellular fluid space or to sample the extracellular fluid directly, such as with the Glucowatch.[137]

The three areas of testing that will increase significantly are testing for infectious agents using molecular based techniques, testing for the predisposition to disease, and assessing an individual's response profile toward a new drug. In the case of all three scenarios, the key to having a POCT is the need for early decision making to implement therapy (or life style change), together with the need for patient counseling. There is clearly now the technology available to detect any form of biological entity at the point-of-care, including very rapid analysis of deoxyribonucleic acid (DNA) from saliva samples.[43] However, there are clearly many ethical issues surrounding the analysis for genetic predisposition and tests for certain infectious diseases.

An area of great interest, however, lies in the field of pharmacogenomics (see Chapter 43)—although it is not yet clear whether it will be the proteomic or the genomic markers that will predominate. It is already acknowledged that each person responds to or metabolizes drugs differently. Tailoring drug therapy to achieve an individualized optimal level is preferable—and from the foregoing examples it is clear that to be able to perform that optimization at the time of the clinic visit reduces the need for future clinic visits, improves compliance, and meets with both patient's and caregiver's approval. Individualization of drug therapy has already been shown to be effective for the management of diabetes, anticoagulation status, hypertension, anticonvulsant therapy, azothioprine treatment, Herceptin treatment, and many others, although POCT has not been implemented on a routine basis in many of these clinical conditions.

In closing, it is difficult to predict the role of POCT in self-testing as part of a wellness program. For example, the level of self-testing for cholesterol has not reached the predictions that were made several years ago—and the reasons for this are not entirely clear. If testing for some analytes remains restricted as is the case in some countries today, then it is possible that individuals will seek the tests from a POCT source. Examples include tests for cancers such as prostate, bladder, and colon that have attained a high level of media coverage in recent years.

REFERENCES

1. Allen MP, DeLizza A, Ramel U, Jeong H, Singh P. A non-instrumental quantitative test system and its application for determining cholesterol concentration in whole blood. Clin Chem 1990;36:1591-7.
2. Andrew M, Marzinotto V, Adams M, Cimini C. LaDuca F. Monitoring of oral anticoagulant therapy in pediatric patients using a new microsample PT device. Blood 1995;86(Suppl):863.
3. Antmann EM, Grudzien C, Sachs DB. Evaluation of a rapid bedside assay for detection of serum cardiac troponin T. JAMA 1995;273:1279-82.
4. Apple FS, Christenson RH, Valdes R, Wu AHB, Andriak AJ, Duh SH et al. Simultaneous rapid measurement of whole blood myoglobin, creatine kinase MB, and cardiac troponin I by the Triage Cardiac Panel for detection of myocardial infarction. Clin Chem 1999;273:1279-82.
5. Ashby JP, ed. The Patient and Decentralised Testing. Lancaster, UK: MTP Press Ltd, 1988.
6. Azzazy HM, Christenson RH. Cardiac markers of acute coronary syndromes: is there a case for point-of-care testing? Clin Biochem. 2002;35:13-27.
7. Bailey PL, McJames S, Cluff ML, Wells DT, Orr JA, Westernskow DR. Evaluation in volunteers of the VIA V-ABG automated bedside blood gas, chemistry and haematocrit monitor. J Clin Monit Comput 1998;14:339-46.
8. Belsey R, Baer D, Sewell D. Laboratory test analysis near the patient. JAMA 1986;255:775-86.
9. Bingham D, Kendall J, Clancy M. The portable laboratory: an evaluation of the accuracy and reproducibility of I-STAT. Ann Clin Biochem 1999;36:66-71.
10. Bissell M. Point-of-care testing at the millennium. Crit Care Nurs Q 2001;24:39-43.
11. Boalth N, Wandrup J, Larsson L, Frischauf PA, Lundsgaard FC, Andersen WL, et al. Blood gases and oximetry: calibration-free new dry-chemistry and optical technology for near-patient testing. Clin Chim Acta 2001;307:225-33.
12. Boldt J. Point of care (POC) monitoring in anesthesia and intensive care–an overview of available POC systems. Anasthesiol Intensivmed Notfallmed Schmerzther 2003;38:158-64.
13. Bonnar J, Flynn A, Freundl G, Kirkman R, Royston R, Snowden R. Personal hormone monitoring for contraception. Brit J Fam Planning 1999;24:128-34.
14. Brunelle JA, Degtiarov AM, Moran RF, Race LA. Simultaneous measurement of total hemoglobin and its derivatives in blood using CO-oximeters; Analytical principles; their application in selecting analytical wavelengths and reference methods; a comparison of the results and the choices made. Scand J Clin Lab Invest 1996;56,Suppl 224:47-69.
15. Buechler KF, Moi S, Noar B, McGrath D, Villela J, Clancy M, et al. Simultaneous detection of seven drugs of abuse by the triage panel for drugs of abuse. Clin Chem 1992;38:1678-84.
16. Bullock DG. Quality control and quality assurance. In Price CP, StJohn A, Hicks JH, eds. Point-of-care testing. Washington DC: AACC Press, 2004:137-45.
17. Burnett D. Accreditation and point-of-care testing. Ann Clin Biochem 2000;37:241-3.
18. Burnett D. A practical guide to accreditation in laboratory medicine. ACB Venture Publications, London, 2002:1-314.
19. Calatzis A, Heesen M, Spannagl M. Point-of-care testing of hemostatic alterations in anaesthesia and intensive care. Anaesthesist 2003;52:229-37.
20. Chapin KC, Blake P, Wilson CD. Performance characteristics and utilization of rapid antigen test, DNA probe, and culture for detection of group a streptococci in an acute care clinic. J Clin Microbiol. 2002;40:4207-10.
21. Chernesky M, Jang D, Krepel J, Sellors J, Mahony J. Impact of reference standard sensitivity on accuracy of rapid antigen detection assays and a leukocyte esterase dipstick for diagnosis of Chlamydia trachomatis infection in first-void urine specimens from men. J Clin Microbiol 1999;37:2777-80.
22. Chin HL, Krall MA. Successful implementation of a comprehensive computer-based patient record system in Kaiser Permanente Northwest: strategy and experience. Eff Clin Pract 1998;1:51-60.
23. Claudi T, Cooper JG. Comparison of urinary albumin excretion rate in overnight urine and albumin creatinine ratio in spot urine in diabetic patients in general practice. Scand J Prim Health Care 2001;19:247-8.
24. Cobbaert C, Boerma GJ, Lindemans J. Evaluation of the Cholestech LDX desktop analyzer for cholesterol,

HDL-cholesterol and triglycerides in heparinized venous blood. Eur J Clin Chem & Clin Biochem 1994;32:391-4.

25. College of American Pathologists:www.cap.org (e.g., drugs of abuse testing program).
26. Collinson PO, Gerhardt W, Katus HA, Muller-Bardoff M, Braun S, Schricke U et al. Multicenter evaluation of an immunological rapid test for the detection of Troponin T in whole blood samples. Eur J Clin Chem Clin Biochem 1996;34:591-8.
27. Creed GM. Point-of-care testing in the United Kingdom. Crit Care Nurs Q 2001;24:44-8.
28. Crook M. Handbook of Near-Patient Testing. London: Greenwich Medical Media Limited, 1999: 1-116.
29. Curme HG, Columbus RL, Dappen GM, Elder TW, Fellow WD, Figueras J et al. Multilayer film elements for clinical analysis: General concepts. Clin Chem 1978;24:1335-42.
30. D'Costa EJ, Higgins IJ, Turner AP. Quinoprotein glucose dehydrogenase and its application in an amperometric glucose sensor. Biosensors 1986;2: 71-87.
31. D'Orazio P. Biosensors in clinical chemistry. Clin Chim Acta 2003;334:41-69.
32. Davis G. Microfabricated sensors and the commercial development of the i-Stat® point-of-care system. In Ramsay G, ed. Commercial Biosensors. New York: John Wiley & Sons, 1998:47-76.
33. Despotis GJ, Alsoufiev A, Hogue CW, Zoys TN, Goodnough LT, Santora SA, et al. Comparison of CBC results from a new, on-site hemocytometer to a laboratory-based hemocytometer. Crit Care Med 1996;24:1163-7.
34. Despotis GJ, Joist JH, Goodnough LT. Monitoring of hemostasis in cardiac surgical patients: impact of point-of-care testing on blood loss and transfusion outcomes. Clin Chem 1997;43:1684-96.
35. Despotis GJ, Saleem R, Bigham M, Barnes P. Clinical evaluation of a new point-of-care hemocytometer. Crit Care Med 2000;28:1185-9.
36. ECRI. Point-of-care analyzers, Clinical Laboratory. Healthcare product comparison system, 2003;May: 1-67.
37. Ehrmeyer SS, Laessig RH. Regulation, accreditation and education for point-of-care testing. In: Kost G, ed. Principles and practice of point-of-care testing. Philadelphia: Lippincott Williams and Wilkins, 2002:434-43.
38. Erickson KA, Wilding P. Evaluation of a novel point-of-care system: The i-Stat portable clinical analyzer. Clin Chem 1993;39:283-7.
39. Farhat SE, Finn S, Chua R, Smith B, Simor AE, George P, et al. Rapid detection of infectious mononucleosis-associated heterophile antibodies by a novel immunochromatographic assay and a latex agglutination test. J Clin Microbiol 1993;31: 1597-600.
40. Fermann GJ, Suyama J. Point of care testing in the emergency department. J Emerg Med 2002;22: 393-404.
41. Fiallos MR, Hanhan UA, Orlowski JP. Point-of-care testing. Pediatr Clin North Am 2001;48:589-99.

41a. Forestier F, Belisle S, Contant C, Harel F, Janvier G, Hardy JF. Reproducibility and interchangeability of the Thromboelastograph, Sonoclot and Hemochron activated coagulation time in cardiac surgery. Can J Anaesth 2001;48:902-10.

42. Freedman DB. Clinical governance: implications for point-of-care testing. Ann Clin Biochem 2002;39: 421-3.
43. French DJ, Archard CL, Andersen MT, McDowell DG. Ultra-rapid DNA analysis using HyBeacon probes and direct PCR amplification from saliva. Mol Cell Probes 2002;16:319-26.
44. Fries SM. Diagnosis of group A streptococcal pharyngitis in a private clinic: comparative evaluation of an optical immunoassay method and culture. J Pediatr 1995;126:933-6.
45. Giuliano KK, Perkins S. Implementing a point-of-care testing program in the critical care setting. Clin Leadersh Manag Rev 2002;16:139-47.
46. Halpern MT, Palmer CS, Simpson KN, Chesley FD, Luce BR, Suyderhoud JP, et al. The economic and clinical efficiency of point-of-care testing for critically ill patients: a decision-analysis model. Am J Med Qual 1998;13:3-12.
47. Halpern N. Point of care diagnostics and networks. Crit Care Clin 2000;16:623-39.
48. Halpern NA, Brentjens T. Point of care testing informatics. The critical care-hospital interface. Crit Care Clin 1999;15:577-91.
49. Handorf CR. College of American Pathologists Conference XXVIII on alternate site testing: Introduction. Arch Pathol Lab Med 1995;119:867-71.
50. Harrison JR, Bevan J, Furth EE, Metz DC. AccuStat whole blood fingerstick test for Helicobacter pylori infection: a reliable screening method. J Clin Gastroenterol 1998;27:50-3.
51. Hedberg P, Valkama J, Puukka M. Analytical performance of time-resolved fluorometry-based Innotrac Aio! cardiac marker immunoassays. Scand J Clin Lab Invest 2003;63:55-64.
52. Heslop L, Howard A, Fernando J, Rothfield A, Wallace L. Wireless communications in acute healthcare. J Telemed Telecare 2003;9(4):187-93
53. Henning TP, Cunningham TP. Biosensors for personal diabetes management. In Ramsay G, ed. Commercial Biosensors. New York: John Wiley & Sons, 1998:3-46.
54. Hicks JM, Haeckel R, Price CP, Lewandrowski K, Wu AH. Recommendations and opinions for the use of

point-of-care testing for hospitals and primary care: summary of a 1999 symposium. Clin Chim Acta 2001;303:1-17.
55. Hirst D, St John A. Keeping the spotlight on quality from a distance. Accred Qual Assur 2000;5;9-13.
56. Hobbs FD, Delaney BC, Fitzmaurice DA, Wilson S, Hyde CJ, Thorpe GH, et al. A review of near patient testing in primary care. Health Technol Assess 1997;1:1-230.
57. Hoffman A. Bioconjugates of intelligent polymers and recognition proteins for use in diagnostics and affinity separations. Clin Chem 2000;46:1478-86.
58. Hudson MP, Christenson RH, Newby LK, Kaplan AL, Ohman EM. Cardiac markers: point of care testing. Clin Chim Acta 1999;284:223-37.
59. Jacobs E, Nowakowski M, Colman N. Performance of Gem Premier blood gas/electrolyte analyzer evaluated. Clin Chem 1993;39:189-93.
60. Jacobs E, Hinson KA, Tolnai J, Simson E. Implementation, management and continuous quality improvement of point-of-care testing in an academic health care setting. Clin Chim Acta 2001;307:49-59.
61. Janssen HW, Bookelman H, Dols JL, Gerritzen WE, de Keyzer RH. Point-of-care testing: the views of the working group of the Dutch Association of Clinical Chemistry. Clin Chem Lab Med 1999;37:675-80.
62. Johnson RE, Newhall WJ, Papp JR, Knapp JS, Black CM, Gift TL, et al. Screening tests to detect Chlamydia trachomatis and Neisseria gonorrhoeae infections—2002. MMWR Recomm Rep. 2002;51:1-38;quiz CE1-4.
63. Jones R, St John A. Informatics in point-of-care testing. In: Price CP, St John, A, Hicks JM, eds. Point-of-Care testing. Washington DC: AACC Press, 2004:197-208.
64. Jurgens R, Elliott R. Rapid HIV screening at the point of care: legal and ethical issues. Can HIV AIDS Policy Law Newsl 2000;5:28-33.
65. Kamino N. Coagulation monitoring in point of care testing—A global point of view. Rinsho Byori 2002;50:1035-40.
66. Kamm C, Elser R, Eitel D, Napier J. Evaluation of the Stratus CS® analyzer and three cardiac markers. Clin Chem 1998;44:1457-63.
67. Kassler HIV, Kassler WJ. Advances in HIV testing technology and their potential impact on prevention. AIDS Educ Prev 1997;9(3 Suppl):27-40.
68. Keffer JH. Economic considerations of point-of-care testing. Am J Clin Pathol. 1995;104(4 Suppl 1):S107-10.
69. Kendall J, Reeves B, Clancy M. Point of care testing: randomised, controlled trial of clinical outcome. BMJ 1998;316:1052-7.
70. Khalil OS. Spectroscopic and clinical aspects of noninvasive glucose measurements. Clin Chem 1999;45:165-75.
71. Khandurina J, Guttman A. Bioanalysis in microfluidic devices. J Chromatogr A 2002;943:159-83.
72. Kiechle FL. The impact of continuous glucose monitoring on hospital point-of-care testing programs. Diabetes Technol Ther 2001;3:647-50.
73. Kost GJ. Preventing medical errors in point-of-care testing: security, validation, safeguards, and connectivity. Arch Pathol Lab Med 2001;125:1307-15.
74. Kost GJ, ed. Principles and practice of point-of-care testing. Philadelphia: Lippincott Williams & Wilkins. 2002:1-654.
75. Kost GJ. New whole blood analyzers and their impact on cardiac and critical care. Crit Rev Clin Lab Sci 1993;30:153-202.
76. Kost GJ, ed. Point-of-care testing: pathology patterns. Am J Clin Pathol 1995;104(Supplement):S1-S127.
77. Kricka LJ. Microchips, microarrays, biochips, and nanochips: personal laboratories for the 21st century. Clin Chim Acta 2001;307:219-23.
78. Kricka LJ. Microchips: the hitchhiker's guide to analytical microchips. Washington: AACC Press, 2002:1-94.
79. Lee-Lewandrowski E, Laposata M, Eschenbach K, Camooso C, Nathan DM, Godine JE, et al. Utilization and cost analysis of bedside capillary glucose testing in a large teaching hospital: implications for managing point of care testing. Am J Med 1994;97:222-30.
80. Lee-Lewandrowski E, Lewandrowski K. Point-of-care testing. An overview and a look to the future. Clin Lab Med 2001;21:217-39.
81. Lindemans J, Hoefkens P, van Kessel AL, Bonnay M, Kulpmann WR, van Suijlen JD. Portable blood gas and electrolyte analyzer evaluated in a multiinstitutional study. Clin Chem 1999;45:111-17.
82. Lott JA, Johnson WR, Luke KE. Evaluation of an automated urine chemistry reagent-strip analyzer. J Clin Lab Anal 1995;9:212-17.
83. Lubbers DW. Optical sensors for clinical monitoring. Acta Anaesthesiol Scand 1995;35(Suppl 104):37-54.
84. Lubbers DW, Koster T, Holst GA. O2 flux optode: a new sensing principle to determine the oxygen flux and other gas diffusions. Adv Exp Med Biol 1996;388:59-68.
85. Magny E, Renard MF, Launay JM. Analytical evaluation of Rapidpoint 400 blood gas analyzer. Ann Biol Clin (Paris) 2001;59:622-8.
86. Males RG, Stephenson J, Harris P. Cardiac markers and point-of-care testing: a perfect fit. Crit Care Nurs Q 2001;24:54-61.
87. Marshall DA, O'Brien BJ. Economic evaluation of diagnostic tests. In Price CP and Christenson RH, eds. Evidence-based laboratory medicine; from principles to outcomes. Washington DC: AACC Press, 2003:159-86.
88. Mass D. Consulting to physician office laboratories. In: Snyder JR, Wilkinson DS, eds: Management in laboratory medicine, Third edition. New York: Lippincott, 1998:443-50.
89. McClelland I, Adamson K, Black ND. Information issues in telemedicine systems. J Telemed Telcare 1995;1:7-12.

90. MacKenzie HA, Ashton HS, Spiers S, Shen Y, Freeborn SS, Hannigan J et al. Advances in photoacoustic noninvasive glucose testing. Clin Chem 1999;45: 1587-95.
91. Mikkelsen DJ, James KR, Dohrman DH. Experience with laboratory instrumentation placed in critical care situations over a seven year period. N Z Med J 1987;100:686-8.
92. Mollard J-F. Single phase calibration for blood gas and electrolyte analysis. In D'Orazio P, ed. Preparing for critical care analyses in the 21st century. Proceedings of the 16th International Symposium. Washington: AACC Press, 1996.
93. Mor M, Waisman Y. Point-of-care testing: a critical review. Pediatr Emerg Care 2000;16:45-8.
94. Morgan CL, Newman DJ, Price CP. Immunosensors: technology and opportunities in laboratory medicine. Clin Chem 1996;42:193-209.
95. Muir Gray JA. Evidence-Based Healthcare. How to make health policy and management decisions. Edinburgh: Churchill Livingstone, 1997:1-270.
96. Muller MM, Hackl W, Griesmacher A. Point-of-care-testing—the intensive care laboratory. Anaesthesist 1999;48:3-8.
97. Nadeau RG, Groner W. The role of a new noninvasive imaging technology in the diagnosis of anemia. J Nutr 2001;131:1610S-4S.
98. National Committee for Clinical Laboratory Standards: Point-of-care in vitro diagnostic (IVD) testing: Approved Guideline. NCCLS Document AST2-A. Wayne, PA:National Committee for Clinical Laboratory Standards 1999.
99. National Committee for Clinical Laboratory Standards: Evaluation of precision performance of clinical chemistry devices; Approved Guideline. NCCLS Document EP5-A. Wayne, PA:National Committee for Clinical Laboratory Standards 1999.
100. National Committee for Clinical Laboratory Standards: Point-of-Care Connectivity; Approved Standard. NCCLS Document POCT1-A. Wayne, PA:National Council for Clinical Laboratory Standards 2001.
101. National Committee for Clinical Laboratory Standards: Quality management for Unit-Use testing: Approved Guideline. NCCLS Document EP18-A. Wayne, PA:National Committee for Clinical Laboratory Standards 2002.
102. Nichols JH, Kickler TS, Dyer KL, Humbertson SK, Cooper PC, Maughan WL, Oechsle DG. Clinical outcomes of point-of-care testing in the interventional radiology and invasive cardiology setting. Clin Chem 2000;46:543-50.
103. Nichols JH, Poe SS. Quality assurance, practical management, and outcomes of point-of-care testing: laboratory perspectives, Part I. Clin Lab Manage Rev 1999;13:341-50.
104. Oberhardt BJ, Dermott SC, Taylor M, Alkadi ZY, Abruzzini AF, Gresalfi NJ. Dry reagent technology for rapid convenient measurement of blood coagulation and fibrinolysis. Clin Chem 1991;37:520-6.
105. Oberhardt BJ. Thrombosis and homeostasis testing at the point of care. Am J Clin Pathol 1995;104(4 Suppl 1):S72-8.
106. O'Leary D. Global view of how alternate site testing fits in with medical care. Arch Pathol Lab Med 1995;119:877-80.
107. Oliver G. On Bedside Testing. London: HK Lewis, 1884:1-128.
108. Parsons MP, Newman DJ, Newall RG, Price CP. Validation of a point-of-care assay for the urinary albumin:creatinine ratio. Clin Chem 1999;45:414-17.
109. Parvin CA, Lo SF, Deuser SM, Weaver LG, Lewis LM, Scott MG. Impact of point-of-care testing on patients' length of stay in a large emergency department. Clin Chem 1996;42:711-7.
110. Pettersson K, Katajamaki T, Irjala K, Leppanen V, Majamaa-Volti K, Laitinen P. Time-resolved fluorometry (TRF)-based immunoassay concept for rapid and quantitative determination of biochemical myocardial infarction markers from whole blood, serum and plasma. Luminescence 2000;15:1-9.
111. Phillips DL. Quality systems for unit-use testing devices. Clin Chem 1997;43:893-6.
112. Pickup J, Rolinski O, Birch D. In vivo glucose sensing for diabetes management: progress towards non-invasive monitoring. BMJ 1999;319:1289-92.
113. Pope RM, Apps JM, Page MD, Allen K, Bodansky HJ. A novel device for the rapid in-clinic measurement of haemoglobin A1c. Diabet Med 1993;3:260-3.
114. Price CP. Quality assurance of extra-laboratory analyses. In Marks V, Alberti KGMM, eds. Clinical biochemistry nearer the patient II. London: Bailliere Tindall, 1987:166-78.
115. Price CP, St John A, Hicks JM, eds. Point-of-care testing. Washington DC: AACC Press, 2004:1-488.
116. Price CP, Thorpe GH. Disposable analytical devices for point-of-care testing. In: Price CP, Hicks JM, eds. Point-of-care testing. Washington DC: AACC Press, 1999:19-40.
117. Price CP. Point-of-care testing. BMJ 2001;322:1285-8.
118. Price CP. Medical and economic outcomes of point-of-care testing. Clin Chem Lab Med 2002;40:246-51.
119. Price CP. Point of care testing. Potential for tracking disease management outcomes. Dis Manage Health Outcomes 2002;10:749-61.
120. Pugia MJ, Lott JA, Clark LW, Parker DR, Wallace JF, Willis TW. Comparisons of urine dipsticks with quantitative methods for microalbuminuria. Eur J Clin Chem Clin Biochem 1997;35:693-700.
121. Rink E, Hilton S, Szczepura A, Fletcher J, Sibbald B, Davies C, et al. Impact of introducing near patient testing for standard investigations in general practice. BMJ 1993;307:775-8.
122. Robertson A, Kazmierczak S, Vos P. Improved transcutaneous bilirubinometry: comparison of SpectR$_X$

BiliCheck and Minolta Jaundice Meter JM-102 for estimating total serum bilirubin in a normal newborn population. J Perinatol 2002;22:12-4.
123. Rolinski B, Kuster H, Ugele B, Gruber R, Horn K. Total bilirubin measurement by photometry on a blood gas analyzer: potential for use in neonatal testing at the point of care. Clin Chem 2001;47:1845-7.
124. Schembri CT, Ostoich V, Lingane PJ, Burd TL, Buhl SN. Portable simultaneous multiple analyte whole-blood analyzer for point-of-care testing. Clin Chem 1992;38:1665-70.
125. Schlebusch H, Paffenholz I, Zerbach R, Leinberger R. Analytical performance of a portable critical care analyzer. Clin Chim Acta 2001;307:107-12.
126. Schultz SG, Holen JT, Donohue JP, Francoeur TA. Two-dimensional centrifugation for desktop clinical chemistry. Clin Chem 1985;31:1457-63.
127. Scott MG. Faster is better-it's rarely that simple! Clin Chem 2000;46:441-2.
128. Sirkin A, Jalloh T, Lee L. Selecting an accurate point-of-care testing system: clinical and technical issues and implications in neonatal blood glucose monitoring. J Spec Pediatr Nurs 2002;7:104-12.
129. St-Louis P. Status of point-of-care testing: promise, realities, and possibilities. Clin Biochem 2000;33:427-40.
130. Solomon H, Mullins R, Lyden P, Thompson P, Hudoff S. The diagnostic accuracy of bedside and laboratory coagulation procedures used to monitor the anticoagulation status of patients treated with heparin. Am J Clin Pathol 1998;109:371-8.
131. Spitznagel TM, Clark DS. Surface density and orientation effects on immobilized antibodies and fragments. Biotechnology 1993;11:825-9.
132. Stephens EJ. Developing open standards for point-of-care connectivity. IVD Technology 1999;10:22-5.
133. Stief TW, Fareed J. Point of care: diagnostics in hemostasis—the wrong direction? Clin Appl Thromb Hemost 2003;9:191-5.
134. Storto Poe S, Case-Cromer DL. Nursing strategies for point-of-care testing. In Kost G, ed: Principles and practice in point-of-care testing. Philadelphia: Lippincott Williams and Wilkins, 2002:214-35.
135. Storrow AB, Gibler WB. The role of cardiac markers in the emergency department. Clin Chim Acta 1999;284:187-96.
136. Stubbs P, Collinson PO. Point-of-care testing: a cardiologist's view. Clin Chim Acta 2001;311:57-61.
137. Tamada JA, Garg S, Jovanovic L, Pitzer KR, Fermi S, Potts RO. Noninvasive glucose monitoring: comprehensive clinical results. Cygnus Research team. JAMA 1999;282:1839-44.
138. Tang Z, Louie RF. Kost GJ. Principles and performance of point-of-care testing instruments. In Kost GJ, ed: Principles and practice of point-of-care testing. Philadelphia: Lippincott Williams & Wilkins, 2002:67-92.
139. Terry LM. Point-of-care testing and recognizing and preventing errors. Br J Nurs 2002;11:1036-9.
140. Turner APF. In: Karube I, Wilson GS, eds. Biosensors: Fundamentals and Applications. Oxford: Oxford University Press, 1987:770.
141. United Kingdom National External Quality Assessment Scheme: www.ukneqas.org.uk (e.g., cholesterol testing programme).
142. US Department of Health and Human Services. Medicare, Medicaid and CLIA programs: regulations implementing the Clinical Laboratory Improvement Amendments of 1988 (CLIA). Final rule. Federal Register 1992;57:7002-186.
143. US Department of Health and Human Services. Medicare, Medicaid and CLIA programs: regulations implementing the Clinical Laboratory Improvement Amendments of 1988 (CLIA) and Clinical Laboratory Act program fee collection. Federal Register 1993;58:5215-37.
144. Valkirs GE, Barton R. Immunoconcentration™. A new format for solid-phase immunoassays. Clin Chem 1985;31:1427-31.
145. van den Besselaar AM. Accuracy, precision, and quality control for point-of-care testing of oral anticoagulation. J Thromb Thrombolysis 2001;12:35-40.
146. Van Heyningen C, Watson ID, Morrice AE. Point-of-care testing outcomes in an emergency department. Clin Chem 1999;45:437-8.
147. Von Schenck H, Falkensson M, Lundberg B. Evaluation of HemoCue, a new device for determining hemoglobin. Clin Chem 1986;32:562-9.
148. Wahr JA, Tremper KK. Continuous arterial blood gas monitoring. J Cardio Vasc Anesth 1994;8:342-53.
149. Wales External Quality Assessment Scheme: www.weqas.co.uk (e.g., urinalysis program).
150. Walter B. Dry reagent chemistries. Anal Chem 1983;55:A498-514.
151. Westgard JO. Electronic quality control, the total testing process, and the total quality system. Clin Chim Acta 2001;307:45-8.
152. Widness JA, Kulhavy JC, Johnson KJ, Cress GA, Kromer IJ, Acarregui MJ, Feld RD. Clinical performance of an in-line point-of-care monitor in neonates. Pediatrics 2000;106:497-504.
153. Zaloga GP, Hill TR, Strickland RA, Kennedy D, Visser M, Ford K, Whitley J, Holt G, Booker C. Bedside blood gas and electrolyte monitoring in critically ill patients. Crit Care Med 1989;17:920-5.
154. Zipp A, Hornby WE. Solid phase chemistry: Its principles and application in clinical analyses. Talanta 1984;31:863-77.

SECTION III

Principles of Laboratory Medicine

CHAPTER 13

Introduction to Laboratory Medicine and Evidence-Based Laboratory Medicine

Christopher P. Price, Ph.D., Patrick M.M. Bossuyt, Ph.D., and David E. Bruns, M.D.

This chapter introduces the section "Principles of Laboratory Medicine." In the beginning of the chapter, we consider the meaning of the term "laboratory medicine" and the relationships among clinical chemistry, laboratory medicine, and evidence-based laboratory medicine. The remainder of the chapter focuses on key concepts of evidence-based laboratory medicine and thus provides a transition from the chemical principles presented in the preceding chapters to the more clinical focus of the following six chapters in this section. Key chapter topics are diagnostic accuracy of tests, clinical outcomes studies, economic evaluations of medical tests, systematic reviews of diagnostic tests, clinical practice guidelines, and clinical audit. The principles provide a foundation for the rational and appropriate use of diagnostic tests.

CONCEPTS, DEFINITIONS, AND RELATIONSHIPS

In this section, laboratory medicine and clinical chemistry are defined. The relationships between these two fields of endeavor are discussed.

WHAT IS LABORATORY MEDICINE?

The term "laboratory medicine" refers to the discipline involved in the selection, provision, and interpretation of diagnostic testing that uses primarily samples from patients. The field includes research, administration, and teaching activities and clinical service. Testing in laboratory medicine may be directed at (a) *confirming* a clinical suspicion (which could include *making* a diagnosis), (b) *excluding* a diagnosis, (c) assisting in the *selection, optimization, and monitoring* of treatment, (d) providing a *prognosis*, or (e) *screening* for disease in the absence of clinical signs or symptoms. Testing is also used to establish and monitor the severity of a physiological disturbance.

The field of laboratory medicine includes clinical chemistry and molecular diagnostics and their traditional subdisciplines (such as toxicology and drug monitoring, endocrine and organ-function testing, "biochemical" and "molecular" genetics, etc.) and areas such as microbiology, hematology, hemostasis and thrombosis, blood banking (transfusion medicine), immunology, and identity testing. In some parts of the world, laboratory medicine also encompasses cytology and anatomical pathology (histopathology). The analytical components of these specialties are delivered from central laboratories or through a more distributed type of service (point-of-care testing [POCT]) or both.

Data management and interpretation (including laboratory informatics) are key aspects of the laboratory medicine service, as are activities concerned with maintaining quality (e.g., quality control and proficiency testing, audit, benchmarking, and clinical governance).

Clinical Chemistry and Laboratory Medicine

The ties between clinical chemistry (or clinical biochemistry) and other areas of laboratory medicine have deep roots. Individuals working primarily in the area of clinical chemistry have developed tools and methods that have become part of the fabric of laboratory medicine. Examples include the theory and practice of reference intervals (Chapter 16), the use of both (internal) quality control and proficiency testing (Chapter 19), the introduction of automation in the clinical laboratory (Chapter 11), and concepts of diagnostic testing, which are discussed in this and other sections of the book. From the physician's and the patient's perspective, there is no distinction between the specialties and invariably the repertoire of more than one specialty will be called upon when making a clinical decision (e.g., in the diagnosis and management of renal failure, or in the management of the patient in intensive care).

The boundaries between clinical chemistry and other areas of laboratory medicine are not always distinct. In many institutions, clinical chemists initiate and direct activities, such as laboratory informatics and POCT. In some areas of the world, the term "clinical chemistry" has long been used to include laboratory areas such as hemostasis, thrombosis testing, immunology testing, and parts of hematology that in the United States are not considered to be part of classical clinical chemistry.

Boundaries between and among the parts of the clinical laboratory have blurred further with the increasing emphasis on use of chemical and "molecular" testing. Molecular diagnostics testing has evolved beyond human genetic testing, an area in which clinical chemists have long been active. Now, clinical chemists in "molecular" laboratories contribute their expertise in laboratory medicine to infectious disease testing, cancer diagnostics, and identity testing, activities that were formerly associated almost solely with, respectively, clinical microbiology, hematology, and blood bank laboratories. Successful contribution to these areas requires an understanding of the principles of laboratory medicine and close collaboration with clinical microbiologists, hematologists, and others who have specialized expertise in those areas of laboratory medicine.

The relationship between laboratory medicine and the clinical chemist has evolved further with the advent of "core" laboratories. These laboratories, which provide all high-volume and emergency testing in many hospitals, depend on automation (see Chapter 11), informatics and computers (Chapter 18), and a high level of quality control and quality management (Chapter 19). Clinical chemists, who have long been active in these areas, have assumed increasing responsibility in core laboratories and thus have become more involved in areas such as hematology, coagulation, urinalysis, and even microbiology. Thus a new type of "clinical chemist" has emerged, and again the functions require a broader knowledge of laboratory medicine and greater collaboration with other specialists.

The close associations of clinical chemistry and laboratory medicine have been evident in other public ways. Most journals in the field of clinical chemistry publish papers in all of the areas of laboratory medicine. The subtitle of the journal *Clinical Chemistry* even includes the term "Laboratory Medicine." Moreover, the international association of clinical chemistry societies is now called the International Federation of Clinical Chemistry and Laboratory Medicine.

Clinical Chemistry, Laboratory Medicine, and Evidence-Based Laboratory Medicine

In this chapter, we review the new influences on clinical chemistry and laboratory medicine from the fields of clinical epidemiology and evidence-based medicine (EBM). Clinical epidemiologists have developed study designs to quantify the diagnostic accuracy of the tests developed in laboratory medicine, and study methods to evaluate the effect and value of laboratory testing in healthcare. Practitioners of EBM focus on use of the best available evidence from such well-designed studies in the care of individual patients. EBM rephrases problems in the clinical care of patients as structured clinical questions, looks for the available evidence, evaluates the quality of clinical studies, evaluates the clinical implications of the results, and provides tools to help clinicians optimally use those results in the care of individual patients.

EVIDENCE-BASED MEDICINE—WHAT IS IT?

This brief section contains a definition of EBM and describes its goals and key practices. Following this, evidence-based laboratory medicine will be addressed.

Definition and Goals of Evidence-Based Medicine

Among the definitions proposed for EBM, the foremost probably is "*the conscientious, judicious, and explicit use of the best evidence in making decisions about the care of individual patients.*"[81] The word *judicious* implies use of the skills of experienced clinicians to put the evidence in context, and to recognize patient individuality and preferences.[62] A goal of EBM is "*to incorporate the best evidence from clinical research into clinical decisions.*"[40] The word *best* implies the necessity for critical appraisal. The words *making decisions* indicate why the principles of EBM can, and must, be applied in laboratory medicine as laboratory medicine is one of the fundamental tools used in making decisions in the practice of medicine.

Since the introduction[29] of the term "evidence-based medicine" in 1991 by Gordon Guyatt (initially in an editorial in *ACP Journal Club* and in a supplement to *Annals of Internal Medicine*), volumes have been written on the topic. A PubMed search on January 2, 2005, for the term returned

16,421 articles. The papers address every area of medicine and activities such as disease management.[27] Compared with practitioners in many of these areas, workers in clinical laboratories were late in embracing the activities of EBM, but numerous studies are now influencing the practice of clinical chemistry and laboratory medicine.

The justifications for an evidence-based approach to medicine are founded on the constant requirement for information[72]; the constant addition of new information[63]; the poor quality of access to good information[1]; the decline in up-to-date knowledge and/or expertise with advancing years of an individual clinician's practice[18]; the limited time available to spend with the patient, let alone read the literature[82]; and the variability in individual patients' values and preferences. To this one might add, particularly in relation to laboratory medicine, (1) the limited number and poor quality of studies linking test results to patient benefits,[59] (2) the poor perception of the value of diagnostic tests, (3) the ever-increasing demand for tests, and (4) the disconnected approach to resource allocation (reimbursement) in laboratory medicine, "silo budgeting," which addresses only laboratory costs without consideration of benefit outside the laboratory, thus forcing decisions to save expense in the laboratory with insufficient attention to the needs of patients, their caregivers, and the payers.

The Practice of Evidence-Based Medicine

Guyatt and colleagues[41] summarized the practice of EBM as follows:

> "An evidence-based practitioner must understand the patient's circumstances or predicament; identify knowledge gaps and frame questions to fill those gaps; conduct an efficient literature search; critically appraise the research evidence; and apply that evidence to patient care."

The efficient practice of EBM requires:

- A knowledge of the *clinical process* and conversion of a clinical goal into an answerable question
- Facility to generate and critically appraise information to generate knowledge
- A critically appraised knowledge resource
- Ability to use the knowledge resource
- A means of accessing and delivering the knowledge resource
- A framework of clinical and economic accountability
- A framework of quality management

The identification of a clinical goal provides the foundation of the service provided by the healthcare professional. In the area of laboratory medicine, as described later in this chapter, the goal can be expressed in terms of answering a clinical question; appropriate laboratory investigations help to answer the question.[75] Knowledge of the characteristics of these investigations is needed to decide which test to use, when to use it, and how to interpret the results.

Finding and appraising knowledge that is relevant to the question requires awareness of the information resources available, ready access to them, and an ability to critically appraise the relevance of the available data.

A knowledge resource in the form of systematic reviews (see later in this chapter) should provide the critically reviewed evidence of the efficacy, benefits, limitations, and risks from using a test, intervention, or device. Access has classically been through scientific journals and textbooks, and electronic communication of various sorts (including textbooks and journals) is making access faster and more up to date.

Knowledge on the use of a test or intervention ultimately has to be placed in the context of a clinical and economic accountability framework and ensuring the highest quality and lowest risk to patients. Clinical audit is a key element of meeting this objective.

EVIDENCE-BASED MEDICINE AND LABORATORY MEDICINE

When a patient has symptoms or signs of a health problem, the clinician establishes hypotheses about their etiology. Competing hypotheses must be resolved. After decisions are made about the nature of the condition, the process of care may then involve further decisions depending on the nature of the problem or disease. The services of laboratory medicine are one of the tools at the disposal of the clinician to answer the questions posed by the hypothesis generation and to help make decisions.[79]

The tools provided by laboratory medicine are called *diagnostic* tests, but it must be understood that tests are used far more broadly than in making a diagnosis. As mentioned above and discussed below, they are also used in making a prognosis, excluding a diagnosis, monitoring a treatment or disease process, and screening for disease. Thus the word "diagnostic" is used (often unknowingly) in the formal sense of a diagnostic system, the quotidian example of which is the daily weather forecast.

What Is Evidence-Based Laboratory Medicine?

Evidence-based laboratory medicine is simply the application of principles and techniques of EBM to laboratory medicine. A clinician requesting an investigation has a question and must make a decision. The clinician hopes that the test result will help to answer the question and assist in making the decision. Thus a definition of evidence-based laboratory medicine could be "*the conscientious, judicious, and explicit use of best evidence in the use of laboratory medicine investigations for assisting in decision-making about the care of individual patients.*" It might also be expressed more directly in terms of health outcomes as "*ensuring that the best evidence on testing is made available and the clinician is assisted in using the best evidence to ensure that the best decisions are made about the care of individual patients and lead to increased probability of improved health outcomes.*" As discussed later, outcomes can be clinical, operational, and/or economic.[76]

Types of Diagnostic Questions Addressed in Laboratory Medicine

The decision-making process involves one of four scenarios typified by these questions (Figure 13-1):

- What is the diagnosis?
- Can another diagnosis be ruled out?
- What is this patient's prognosis?
- How is the patient doing?

In the first case, a diagnosis is being sought, with a diagnostic conclusion leading to a decision and some form of action, which often involves an intervention; the intention is that the cascade for diagnostic question through result, decision, and action should lead to an improved outcome. An example of this scenario would be when a test for acetaminophen indicates that there has been ingestion of an excessive amount of drug, and the administration of *N*-acetylcysteine reduces the risk of a fatal outcome. The measurement of acetaminophen in this scenario is referred to as a "rule-in test."

In the second scenario, the test result excludes a diagnosis; this is referred to as a "rule-out test." The actions resulting from excluding a diagnosis will invariably involve the evaluation or creation of another hypothesis. When a patient is admitted with atypical chest pain and acute myocardial infarction is suspected, the measurement of troponin may be used to rule out (or rule in) acute myocardial necrosis.

The third use of an investigation is for prognosis, which may be considered as the assessment of risk, and complements the diagnostic application. For example, the measurement of human immunodeficiency virus (HIV) viral load following initial diagnosis of HIV infection predicts the time interval before immune collapse if the condition is not treated.

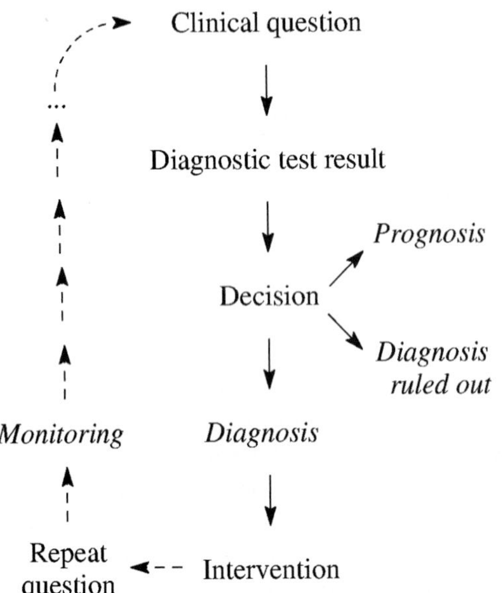

Figure 13-1 Schematic representation of four common decision-making steps in which the result of an investigation is involved.

The fourth broad use of a test result is concerned with patient management. In a patient with a chronic disease, the result may be used to select the type of intervention and assess the effectiveness of an intervention, and the action will be to change or continue the treatment. In women with metastatic breast cancer, the HER-2/*neu* status is used to assess the potential usefulness of Herceptin therapy. In a person with diabetes, hemoglobin (Hb) A_{1c} measurements are used to assess glycemic control and thus the effectiveness of therapy.

These scenarios illustrate the importance of identifying the triad of *question, decision, and action*. Identifying these three components proves to be critical in designing studies of utility or outcomes of testing (see later in this chapter and Chapter 15). They are also important in audit (see below) of the use of investigations both from the point of clinical governance (clinical accountability) and financial governance (controlling the test demand in the context of economic governance). The recognition of this triad has led to the definition of an *appropriate test request* as one in which there is a clear clinical question for which the result will provide an answer, enabling the clinician to make a decision and initiate some form of action leading to a health benefit for the patient.[75]" This benefit could be extended to the health provider and to society as a whole to encompass more directly the potential for economic benefit.

Examples of questions that specify the detail required to accurately qualify the use of a test result are given in Table 13-1. The criteria for a screening test have been established for many years; importantly one of the key criteria is that there must be valid treatment available. The clinical episode involves a series of diagnostic questions with binary responses[16]—a point illustrated in Table 13-1.

Test Results Alone Do Not Produce Clinical Outcomes

In most cases, testing is followed by an appropriate intervention to produce a desired outcome, particularly when the outcome is defined as improved morbidity or mortality. A test result alone may provide reassurance or an understanding of the origin of one's complaint, but usually these good outcomes require an intervention in the form of an explanation of the result in the context of the patient's symptoms. Thus it is difficult to design EBM studies that investigate the utility of the test in isolation. Thus most laboratory medicine research encompasses only test characteristics. This restricted research leads to a poor understanding and appreciation of the contribution that the test result makes to improved outcomes. In relation to certain scenarios it is possible to find valid study data, most particularly when the test result is being used to exclude a diagnosis. Thus in a randomized study of a rapid chest pain evaluation protocol, cardiac markers had a high negative predictive value in patients evaluated with chest pain. Testing led to fewer admissions to the coronary care unit, without adversely affecting morbidity and mortality.[68] Reducing the turn-

TABLE 13-1 Examples of Clinical Questions in Which a Laboratory Assessment May Be of Value, and the Associated Action and Potential Outcome (Benefit)

Test	Question	Result	Possible Action	Possible Outcome
Rule In				
B-type natriuretic peptide (BNP)	Is this breathless patient suffering from heart failure?	450 ng/L	Confirm with cardiac ultrasound, decide to admit and treat	Reduced symptoms, decreased morbidity and mortality
Troponin I (TnI)	Has this patient had a myocardial infarction?	7.2 μg/L	Decide to admit, intensity of care required, and treat	Decreased morbidity and mortality
TSH	Does this child have hypothyroidism?	12.2 mU/L	Treat with thyroxine	Decreased morbidity and mortality
Urine leukocyte esterase (LE) and nitrite	Does this patient have a urinary tract infection?	Positive LE, positive nitrite, or both	Send urine to laboratory for microscopy, culture and sensitivity and treat if positive	Appropriate use of antibiotics, decreased morbidity
Rule Out				
BNP	Is this breathless patient suffering from heart failure?	56 ng/L	Seek alternative diagnosis	Avoid incorrect diagnosis and treatment with its potential for harm
TnI	Has this patient had a myocardial infarction?	<0.1 μg/L	Consider other possible diagnoses and early discharge	Less worry for patient, reduce unnecessary admissions to cardiac care unit
TSH	Does this patient have hypothyroidism?	2.1 mU/L	No further action	Any patient disquiet allayed
Urine LE and nitrite	Does this patient have a urinary tract infection?	Normal dipstick result	Do not send urine to laboratory, look for alternative cause of symptoms	Inappropriate antibiotic treatment avoided, unnecessary laboratory work avoided
Monitoring				
BNP	Is the patient taking the correct dosage of β-blocker?	No change	Review dosage and patient compliance	No change in symptoms, risk of cardiac event, more clinic visits
BNP	Is the patient taking the correct dosage of β-blocker?	Fallen from 216 to 160 ng/L	No change to dosage, encourage patient	Reduced symptoms and risk of cardiac event
HbA_{1c}	Is patient complying with treatment protocol?	10.6% (no change in a year)	Consider changing treatment, closer monitoring of compliance, clinic visits and consultations with diabetes nurse	Persistently high HbA_{1c} carries increased risk of complications; intervention necessary to decrease risk
HbA_{1c}	Is patient complying with treatment protocol?	5.8%	Congratulate patient, maintain treatment regimen	Continued reduced risk of complications

Continued.

TABLE 13-1 Examples of Clinical Questions in Which a Laboratory Assessment May Be of Value, and the Associated Action and Potential Outcome (Benefit)—*Continued*

Test	Question	Result	Possible Action	Possible Outcome
Prognosis				
BNP	Is this patient's heart failure deteriorating?	Increase from 450 to 650 ng/L in last year	Adjust therapy, perhaps advise on palliative care	Poor prognosis
TnI	What is this patient's risk of a further cardiac event?	0.9 μg/L	Consider intervention	Increased risk without intervention
Her-2/*neu*	What is this patient's prognosis?	3+ by immuno-histochemical staining at primary diagnosis	Consider Herceptin treatment	Improvement of poor prognosis by selection of appropriate therapy

around time for blood-gas and electrolyte testing may allow faster discharge from the emergency room,[66] unless other evaluations (such as other laboratory tests or radiological investigations) are rate limiting.[48] Reduced length of stay appeared to be primarily because normal results with the POCTs enabled some patients to be discharged more quickly (i.e., a rule-out decision).[66]

If a result is not received or accessed, it will not contribute to an improved outcome. In a systematic study, Kilpatrick and Holding[50] found when they introduced an electronic transmission of data to the emergency department and admissions unit that a notable number of results were never accessed.

Using the Test Result

In many clinical scenarios, the first criterion for a useful test is that the result leads to a change in the probability of the presence of the target condition. Boyd and Deeks,[11] for example, showed that the (pretest) probability of pulmonary embolism fell from about 0.28 to a posttest probability of 0.041 when the D-dimer test result was less than 500 μg/L. The change in probability does not, in itself, make the decision. The clinician must use this information along with other findings and clinical judgment to make decisions or recommendations about care.

The Clinical Setting of an Outcome Study

The setting of a research study may or may not be the same as that of the individual patient. The evidence from a study may be unreliable when differences exist in age, sex, ethnic origin, lifestyle, prevalence of the disease in the population, or prevalence of comorbidities. Transferability of study results may also be affected by analytical variables, such as patient preparation (effects of fasting, posture, exercise, and biological variation) and method performance (accuracy and precision).

CHARACTERIZATION OF DIAGNOSTIC ACCURACY OF TESTS

When a new test is developed or an old test is applied to a new clinical question, users need information about the extent of agreement of the test's results with the correct diagnoses of patients. For this purpose, researchers design studies in which results from the new test are compared with the results obtained with the reference standard on the same patients. The results of the comparison can be expressed in a number of ways, including sensitivity and specificity, predictive values, likelihood ratios, diagnostic odds ratios, and areas under receiver operating characteristic (ROC) curves (see Chapter 15). We will refer to such studies as diagnostic accuracy studies.

Study Design

In studies of diagnostic accuracy, the results of one test (often referred to as the index test, the test of interest) are compared with those from the reference standard (referred to as the reference test, the best current practice). A "test" can be any method for obtaining additional information on a patient's health status. This includes not only laboratory tests, imaging tests, and function tests but also data from the history and physical examination, and genetic data.

The *reference standard* is the best available method for establishing the presence or absence of the target condition (the suspected condition and/or disease for which the test is to be applied). The reference standard can be a single test, or a combination of methods and techniques, including clinical follow-up of tested patients.

There are several potential threats to the internal and external validity of a study of diagnostic accuracy, of which only the major ones will be addressed in this section. (For more detail and examples, see Chapter 15.) Poor *internal validity* will produce bias, or systematic error, because the estimates do not correspond to what one would have obtained using optimal methods, whereas poor *external validity* limits the generalizability of the findings, as the results of the study, even if unbiased, do not correspond to settings encountered by the decision maker. For example, the results of a study of patients in a tertiary-care medical center may not be generalizable to patients seen in a general practice, and studies done exclusively in older men may not be applicable to women or children.

The ideal study examines a consecutive series of patients, enrolling all consenting patients suspected of the target condition within a specific period. All of these patients then undergo the index test and then the reference test. The term "consecutive" refers to total absence of any form of selection, beyond the a priori definition of the criteria for inclusion and exclusion, and requires explicit efforts to identify and enroll patients qualifying for inclusion.

Alternative designs are possible. Some studies first select patients known to have the target condition, and then contrast the results of these patients with those from a control group. This approach has been used to characterize the performance of tests in settings in which the condition of interest is uncommon as in maternal serum screening testing for detecting Down syndrome in the fetus. It is also used in preliminary studies to assess the potential of a test before embarking on prospective studies of a series of patients. With this design, the selection of the control group is critical. If the control group consists of healthy individuals only, diagnostic accuracy of the test will tend to be overestimated, as has been shown in an analysis that compared the results of such studies with results of studies of consecutive series of patients.[57] (See Chapter 15 for further discussion.)

In the ideal study, the results of all patients tested with the test under evaluation are contrasted with the results of a single reference standard. If fewer than all patients are verified with the reference standard, then *partial verification* exists, and verification bias may occur if the selection of subjects for reference testing is not purely random. For example, if selection is associated with the outcome of the index test, or the strength of prior suspicion, or both, then verification bias is certain. In a typical case, some patients with negative test results (test-negatives) are not verified by the reference standard if this involves a costly or invasive procedure, and these patients are not included in the analysis. This may result in an underestimation of the number of false-negative results.

A different form of verification bias can happen if more than one reference standard is used, and the two reference standards correspond to different manifestations of disease. This study design can produce *differential verification bias.* Suppose test-positive patients are verified with further testing and test-negative patients are verified by clinical follow-up. An example is the verification of suspected appendicitis, with histopathology of the appendix versus natural history as the two forms of the reference standard. A patient is classified as having a false-positive test result if the additional test does not confirm the presence of disease after a positive index test result. Alternatively, a patient is classified as a false-negative if an event compatible with appendicitis is observed during follow-up after a negative test result. Yet these are different definitions of disease because not all patients who have positive test results by the reference standard would have experienced an event during follow-up if they had been left untreated. The use of two reference standards, one pathological and the other based on clinical prognosis, can affect the assessment of diagnostic accuracy. It can also lead to variability among studies that depend on the proportions of patients verified with each of the two standards. For additional discussion, see Chapter 15.

There is a long-standing debate on whether or not clinical data should be provided to those performing or reading the index test, especially when that test has a subjective component. Withholding this information is known as blinding or masking. Some clinical information is often routinely known by the reader of the test, such as when radiologists see the patients on whom they are performing a test, or a pathologist is told the site from which a biopsy is obtained. To try to withhold such information in the context of a study of diagnostic accuracy may create an artificial scenario that has no counterpart in patient care. Thoughtful attention to this question is important in the early phases of designing a study. For most study questions, masking is preferable, because knowledge of the results will tend to increase agreement of the result of the studied (index) test with the reference standard (test).

The severity of disease in the studied patients with the target condition and the range of other conditions in the other patients (controls) can affect the apparent diagnostic accuracy of a test. For example, if a test that is designed to detect early cancer is evaluated in patients with clinically apparent cancer, the test is likely to perform better than when used for persons who do not yet show signs of the condition. This problem has been called "spectrum bias." Similarly, if a test is developed to distinguish patients with the target condition from patients with a similar condition, it may be misleading to use healthy subjects as controls when evaluating the diagnostic accuracy of the test.

THE REPORTING OF STUDIES OF DIAGNOSTIC ACCURACY AND THE ROLE OF THE STARD INITIATIVE

Complete and accurate reporting of studies of diagnostic accuracy should allow the reader to detect the potential for bias in the study and to assess the ability to generalize the results and their applicability to an individual patient or group. Reid, Lachs, and Feinstein[77] documented that most studies of diagnostic accuracy published in leading general medical journals either had poor adherence to standards of clinical epidemiological research or failed to provide information about adherence to those standards.[5] A later study showed similar problems in studies of genetic tests. These reports led to efforts at the journal *Clinical Chemistry* in 1997 to produce a checklist for reporting of studies of diagnostic accuracy.[12] The quality of reporting in that journal increased after introduction of this checklist,[58] though not to an ideal level.[9]

The work of Lijmer et al[57] showing that poor study design and poor reporting are associated with overestimation of the diagnostic accuracy of evaluated tests indicated the necessity to improve the reporting of studies of diagnostic accuracy for all types of tests, not only those in clinical chemistry. An initiative on Standards for Reporting of Diagnostic Accuracy (STARD) was begun at the 1999 meeting of the Cochrane Diagnostic and Screening Test Methods Working Group. The initiative[7] aimed to improve the quality of reporting of diagnostic accuracy studies by following the model of the successful Consolidated Standards of Reporting Trials (CONSORT) initiative for reporting of trials of therapies (see discussion of outcomes studies later in this chapter).

The key components of the STARD document[7] are a checklist of items to be included in reports of studies of diagnostic accuracy and a flow diagram to document the flow of participants in the study. The checklist was developed from an extensive literature search that identified 75 potential items. The list was pared to 25 items (Figure 13-2) in a consensus meeting of researchers, editors, methodologists, and representatives of professional organizations. The flow diagram (Figure 13-3) has the potential to clearly communicate vital information about the *design* of a study—including the method of recruitment and the order of test execution—and about the *flow* of participants.

The final, single-page checklist (Figure 13-2) has been endorsed by numerous journals (such as *Journal of the American Medical Association [JAMA]* and *Annals of Internal Medicine)* and published in many of them, including all the major journals of clinical chemistry and other leading journals including *Radiology*, *British Medical Journal (BMJ)*, and *Lancet.* A separate document explaining the meaning and rationale of each item and briefly summarizing the available evidence was published in *Annals of Internal Medicine* and *Clinical Chemistry.*[8] The STARD group will prepare updates of the STARD document when new evidence on sources of bias or variability becomes available. In the experience of one of the authors of this chapter (DB), use of the checklist has increased the information content of all manuscripts to which it has been applied at *Clinical Chemistry*, and use of the flow diagram has led to correction of errors in many manuscripts.

Use of the STARD initiative is recommended for all reports of studies of diagnostic accuracy. Most if not all of the content of STARD applies to studies of tests used for prognosis, monitoring, or screening.

OUTCOMES STUDIES

Medical and public health interventions are intended to improve the well-being of patients, the population at large, or population segments. For therapeutic interventions, patients are interested, for example, not only if a drug decreases serum cholesterol or blood pressure (risk factors), but more importantly whether it decreases the risk of heart attack, stroke, and cardiovascular death. Similarly, on the diagnostic side of medicine, patients have little interest in knowing the numerical value of their serum cholesterol concentration or blood pressure unless that knowledge will lead to actions that will in some way improve their quality or quantity of life. For example, a test result may identify the need for a life-saving therapeutic intervention for an existing disease or it may lead to a change in lifestyle that will decrease risk of developing a disease. At other times, the test result itself can provide valuable reassurance, as when a genetic test indicates that a family member does not carry a mutation that is present in the family. In still other cases, a laboratory test may provide prognostic information that allows the patient to better plan for the future despite a bad prognosis, or it may provide reassurance that symptoms are not signs of serious disease, thus allowing him or her to better manage the symptoms without fear. The test-related outcomes in these examples range from preventing imminent death to being better able to plan for death.

WHAT ARE OUTCOMES STUDIES?

Outcomes may be defined as results of medical interventions in terms of health or cost. "Patient outcomes" are results that are perceptible to the patient.[3] Outcomes that have been studied commonly include mortality, complication rates (such as the nosocomial infection rate), length of stay in the hospital, waiting times in a clinic, cost of care, and patients' satisfaction with care. In studying and comparing diagnostic tests, other highly desirable "outcomes" are an improved ability to make a correct diagnosis of a treatable condition and an improved ability to exclude a diagnosis or monitor treatment or screen for disease. Test results themselves are not widely considered to be outcomes, but an argument can be made that they should be considered as such when it is certain that real outcomes will change for the better with a superior test. Some tests are increasingly being used as surrogate outcome markers in intervention studies when a strong relationship has been documented between the test result and morbidity or mortality; examples include the use of HbA_{1c} and the urine albumin:creatinine ratio in studies on the management of diabetes mellitus.

Outcomes studies must be distinguished from studies of prognosis. Studies of the prognostic value of a test ask the question, "Can the test be used to predict an outcome?" By contrast, outcomes studies ask questions such as, "Does use of the test improve outcomes?" For example, a study of the former type asks the question, "Does the concentration of a cardiac troponin in serum correlate with the mortality rate after myocardial infarction?" An outcomes study might ask, "Is the mortality rate of patients with suspected myocardial infarction decreased when physicians use troponin testing to guide therapy?" Recent outcomes studies have asked questions such as the following: "Is availability of POCT in the emergency room, compared with testing

Section and Topic	Item #		On page #
TITLE/ABSTRACT/ KEYWORDS	1	Identify the article as a study of diagnostic accuracy (recommend MeSH heading sensitivity and specificity).	
INTRODUCTION	2	State the research questions or study aims, such as estimating diagnostic accuracy or comparing accuracy between tests or across participant groups.	
METHODS		Describe	
Participants	3	The study population: The inclusion and exclusion criteria, setting and locations where the data were collected.	
	4	Participant recruitment: Was recruitment based on presenting symptoms, results from previous tests, or the fact that the participants had received the index tests or the reference standard?	
	5	Participant sampling: Was the study population a consecutive series of participants defined by the selection criteria in items 3 and 4? If not, specify how participants were further selected.	
	6	Data collection: Was data collection planned before the index test and reference standard were performed (prospective study) or after (retrospective study)?	
Test methods	7	The reference standard and its rationale.	
	8	Technical specifications of material and methods involved including how and when measurements were taken, and/or cite references for index tests and reference standard.	
	9	Definition of and rationale for the units, cutoffs and/or categories of the results of the index tests and the reference standard.	
	10	The number, training, and expertise of the persons executing and reading the index tests and the reference standard.	
	11	Whether or not the readers of the index tests and reference standard were blind (masked) to the results of the other test and describe any other clinical information available to the readers.	
Statistical metheds	12	Methods for calculating or comparing measures of diagnostic accuracy, and the statistical methods used to quantify uncertainty (e.g. 95% confidence intervals).	
	13	Methods for calculating test reproducibility, if done.	
RESULTS		Report	
Participants	14	When study was done, including beginning and ending dates of recruitment.	
	15	Clinical and demographic characteristics of the study population (e.g. age, sex, spectrum of presenting symptoms, comorbidity, current treatments, recruitment centers).	
	16	The number of participants satisfying the criteria for inclusion that did or did not undergo the index tests and/or the reference standard; describe why participants failed to receive either test (a flow diagram is strongly recommended).	
Test results	17	Time interval from the index tests to the reference standard, and any treatment adminstered between.	
	18	Distribution of severity of disease (define criteria) in those with the target condition; other diagnoses in participants without the target condition.	
	19	A cross tabulation of the results of the index tests (including indeterminate and missing results) by the results of the reference sandard; for continuous results, the distribution of the test results by the results of the reference standard.	
	20	Any adverse events from performing the index tests or the reference standard.	
Estimates	21	Estimates of diagnostic accuracy and measures of statistical uncertainly (e.g. 95% confidence intervals).	
	22	How indeterminate results, missing responses, and outliers of the index tests were handled.	
	23	Estimates of variability of diagnostic accuracy between subgroups of participants, readers, or centers, if done.	
	24	Estimates of test reproducibility, if done.	
DISCUSSION	25	Discuss the clinical applicability of the study findings.	

Figure 13-2 STARD checklist.

performed in the hospital laboratory, associated with a decreased length of stay for patients in the emergency department?"[48,66,73] and "Does routine testing of elderly patients before cataract surgery decrease postoperative complication rates?"[84]

Many test attributes are amenable to studies of outcomes. Studies can address not only the test availability or non-availability but also such attributes as the methodology used for a measurement, the analytical quality of test performance (e.g., precision), the turnaround time (as for POCT in the emergency department), and the method of reporting of test results (e.g., with or without extensive interpretation of the result).

WHY OUTCOMES STUDIES?

Outcomes studies have taken on considerable importance in medicine. On the therapeutic side of medicine, few drugs can be approved by modern government agencies (or paid for by healthcare organizations or health insurers) without randomized, controlled trials of their safety and effectiveness. Increasingly, diagnostic testing is entering a similar environment in which physicians, governments, commercial health insurers, and patients demand evidence of effectiveness of diagnostic procedures. To appreciate this, one need only recall the enormous interest in controversies about the value of mammography and the effectiveness of measuring prostate-specific antigen in serum. These issues (and many others) hinge on demonstration of improved outcomes.

In the United States, the important Joint Commission on Accreditation of Healthcare Organizations (JCAHO) defines *quality* as increased probability of desired **outcomes** and decreased probability of undesired **outcomes.** If a healthcare organization, or a unit of it, such as the clinical laboratory,

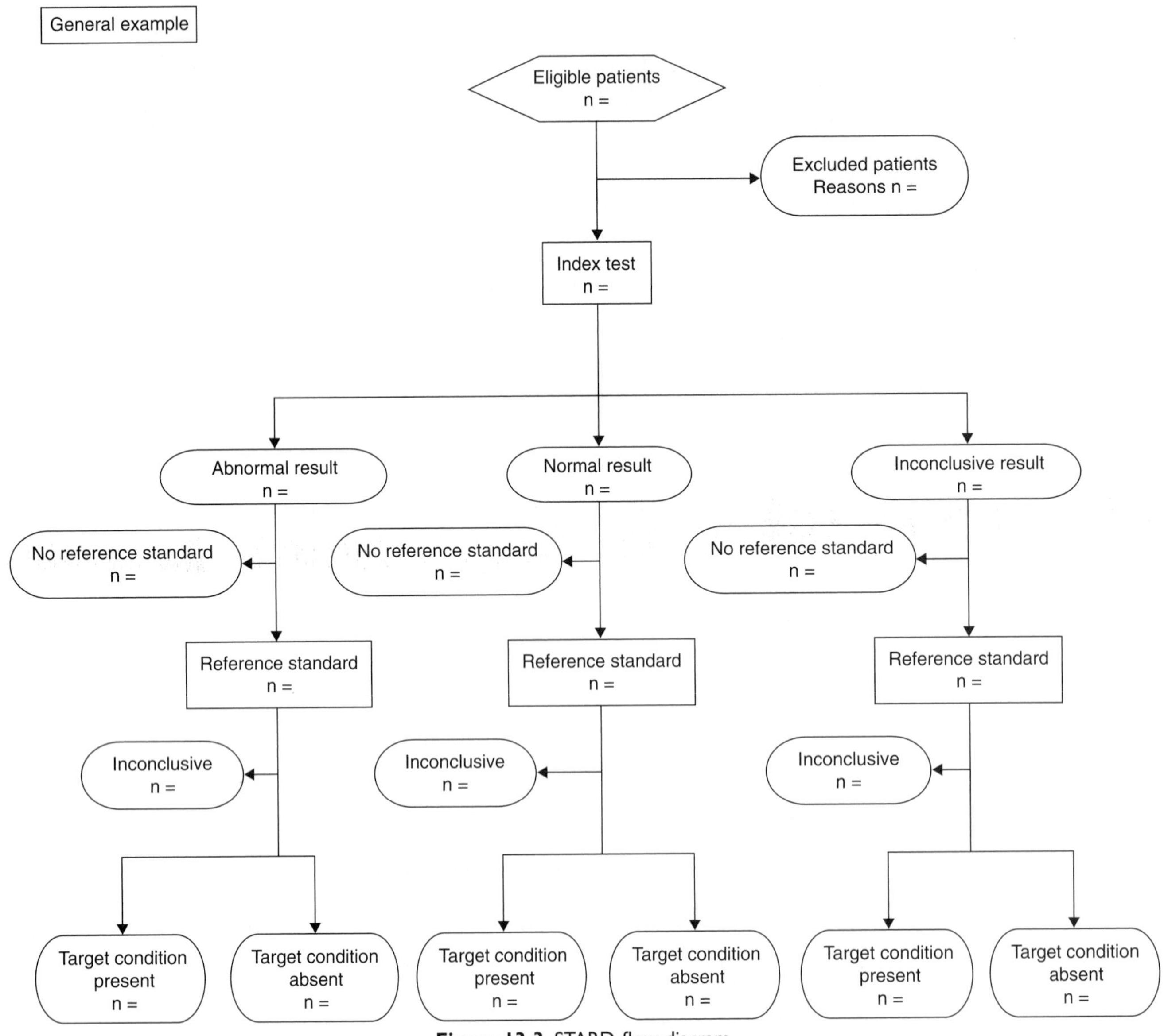

Figure 13-3 STARD flow diagram.

wishes to propose that its quality is high or that it contributes to the quality of the institution, the message is clear.

Design of Studies of Medical Outcomes

The randomized controlled trial (RCT) is the de facto standard for studies of the health effects of medical interventions. In these studies, patients are randomized to receive either a therapy to be tested or an alternative (either a placebo or a conventional treatment), and an outcome is measured. RCTs have been used to evaluate therapeutic interventions, including drugs, radiation therapy, and surgical interventions, among others. The measured outcomes vary from hard evidence, such as mortality and morbidity, to softer evidence, such as patient-reported satisfaction and surrogate end points typified by markers of disease activity (e.g. HbA_{1c} and urine albumin : creatinine ratio as mentioned earlier).

The high impact of RCTs of therapeutic interventions led to scrutiny of their conduct and reporting. An interdisciplinary group (largely clinical epidemiologists and editors of medical journals) developed a guideline known as CONSORT[61] for the conduct of these studies. Although initially designed for trials of therapies, CONSORT provides useful reminders when designing or appraising outcomes studies of tests in clinical chemistry and molecular diagnostics. The key features of the guideline are a checklist (Figure 13-4) of items to include in the report and a flow diagram (Figure 13-5) of patients in the study.

The optimal design of an RCT of a diagnostic test is not always obvious. A classical design is to randomize patients to

Checklist of items to include when reporting a randomized trial

PAPER SECTION And topic	Item	Description	Reported on page #
TITLE & ABSTRACT	1	How participants were allocated to interventions (*e.g.*, "random allocation," "randomized," or "randomly assigned").	
INTRODUCTION Background	2	Scientific background and explanation of rationale.	
METHODS Participants	3	Eligibility criteria for participants and the settings and locations where the data were collected.	
Interventions	4	Precise details of the interventions intended for each group and how and when they were actually administered.	
Objectives	5	Specific objectives and hypotheses.	
Outcomes	6	Clearly defined primary and secondary outcome measures and, when applicable, any methods used to enhance the quality of measurements (*e.g.*, multiple observations, training of assessors).	
Sample size	7	How sample size was determined and, when applicable, explanation of any interim analyses and stopping rules.	
Randomization -- Sequence generation	8	Method used to generate the random allocation sequence, including details of any restriction (*e.g.*, blocking, stratification).	
Randomization -- Allocation concealment	9	Method used to implement the random allocation sequence (*e.g.*, numbered containers of central telephone), clarifying whether the sequence was concealed until interventions were assigned.	
Randomization -- Implementation	10	Who generated the allocation sequence, who enrolled participants, and who assigned participants to their groups.	
Blinding (masking)	11	Whether or not participants, those administering the interventions, and those assessing the outcomes were blinded to group assignment. When relevant, how the success of blinding was evaluated.	

Figure 13-4 CONSORT checklist.

Continued.

Statistical methods	12	Statistical methods used to compare groups for primary outcome(s); methods for additional analyses, such as subgroup analyses and adjusted analyses.	
RESULTS Participant flow	13	Flow of participants through each stage (a diagram is strongly recommended). Specifically, for each group report the numbers of participants randomly assigned, receiving intended treatment, completing the study protocol, and analyzed for the primary outcome. Describe protocol deviations from study as planned, together with reasons.	
Recruitment	14	Dates defining the periods of recruitment and follow-up.	
Baseline data	15	Baseline demographic and clinical characteristics of each group.	
Numbers analyzed	15	Number of participants (denominator) in each group included in each analysis and whether the analysis was by "intention-to-treat." State the results in absolute numbers when feasible (*e.g.*, 10/20, not 50%).	
Outcomes and estimation	17	For each primary and secondary outcome, a summary of results for each group, and the estimated effect size and its precision (*e.g.*, 95% confidence interval).	
Ancillary analyses	18	Address multiplicity by reporting any other analyses performed, including subgroup analyses and adjusted analyses, indicating those pre-specified and those exploratory.	
Adverse events	19	All important adverse events or side effects in each intervention group.	
DISCUSSION Interpretation	20	Interpretation of the results, taking into account study hypotheses, sources of potential bias or imprecision, and the dangers associated with multiplicity of analyses and outcomes.	
Generalizability	21	Generalizability (external validity) of the trial findings.	
Overall evidence	22	General interpretation of the results in the context of current evidence.	

Figure 13-4 *Cont'd*

receive or not receive a test, and then to modify therapy from conventional therapy to a different therapy based on the test result in the tested patients. This approach leads to interpretive problems.[6] For example, if the new therapy is always effective, the tested group will always fare better even if the test is a coin toss, because only the tested group had access to the new therapy. The conclusion that the testing was valuable would thus be wrong. A similar problem occurs if the tested group had merely an increased access to the therapy. (A possible example is the apparent benefit of fecal occult blood testing in decreasing the incidence of colon cancer where the tested group is more likely to undergo colonoscopy and removal of premalignant lesions in the colon. A random selection of patients for colonoscopy might achieve results similar to the results for the group tested for fecal occult blood.) This problem will lead to the erroneous conclusion that the test itself is useful. By contrast, if the new therapy is always worse than the conventional treatment, patients in the tested group will do worse and the test will be judged worse than useless, no matter how accurate it is. Similarly, if the two treatments are equally effective, the outcomes will be the same with or without testing; this scenario will lead to the conclusion that the test is not good, no matter how diagnostically accurate it is. When a truly better therapy becomes available, the test may prove to be valuable, so it is important to not discount the test's potential based on a study with a new therapy that offers no advantage over the old therapy.

Bossuyt and colleagues[6] describe a study design to determine whether ultrasound testing of the fetus can be used to

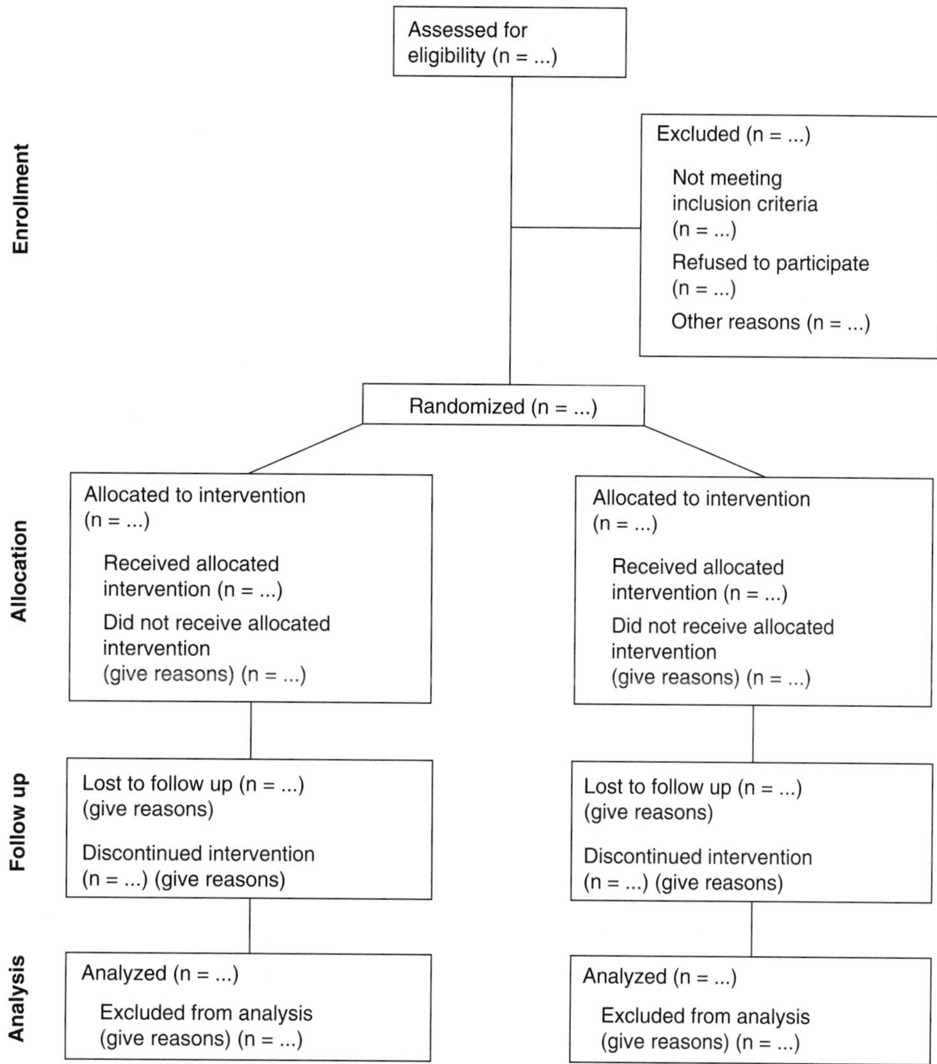

Figure 13-5 CONSORT flow diagram for patients in an RCT.

identify those women with growth-restricted fetuses who can be safely managed at home rather than in the hospital. In a common study design, women with fetuses showing intrauterine growth restriction (IUGR) are randomized to receive Doppler ultrasound. Women with positive test results would be kept in the hospital and those with negative test results would go home. Women in the control arm would stay in the hospital, the usual approach. One can see here that if some women benefit from home care, whereas all other women do equally well with either of the two treatments, home care patients will do better regardless of the intrinsic value of the ultrasound test. Thus patients in the tested arm will fare better, and the testing itself will erroneously be declared a success. By contrast, a proper interpretation would be that the strategy worked well, and a testable hypothesis might be generated from the study that all patients can be sent home without testing.

Alternative designs have been described to address the question of use of ultrasound in women with IUGR.[6] In one design, all patients undergo the new test, but the results are hidden during the trial. Patients are randomized to receive or not receive the new therapy. In this design, the new test should be adopted only if there is an improvement in patient outcome caused by switching to the new therapy, and if that improvement in outcome is associated with the test outcome. For example, the improvement may be larger in the subgroup that had positive test results on ultrasound compared with the subgroup that had negative test results.

An RCT is not always feasible. Alternatives to the RCT include studies that use historical or contemporaneous control patients in whom the intervention was not undertaken. Other studies include patients with and patients without the outcome of interest. These studies are called case-control studies. Uncertainty about the comparability of the controls and the patients in such designs is a threat to the validity of these studies.

Researchers have turned to other methods for exploring the outcomes of testing strategies. To address the multitude of available options when several tests are available, decision analysis has been proposed. These studies rely on a model that links data on diagnostic accuracy with data on health outcomes. Patients with true-positive test results receive the benefits of treatment for the target condition, in contrast with patients who have true-negative test results. On the other hand, those with false-positive test results undergo the risk of the side effects associated with treatment, without the benefits. For an example, see Perrier et al.[74]

SYSTEMATIC REVIEWS OF DIAGNOSTIC TESTS

Systematic reviews are recent additions to the medical literature. In contrast to traditional "narrative" reviews, these reviews aim to answer a precisely defined clinical question and to do so in a way that is transparent and designed to minimize bias. Some of the defining features of systematic reviews are (1) a clear definition of the clinical question to be addressed, (2) an extensive and explicit strategy to find all studies (published or unpublished) that may be eligible for inclusion in the review, (3) criteria by which studies are included and excluded, (4) a mechanism to assess the quality of each study and, in some cases, (5) synthesis of results by use of statistical techniques of meta-analysis. By contrast, traditional reviews are subjective, are rarely well focused on a clinical question, lack explicit criteria for selection of studies to be reviewed, do not indicate criteria to assess the quality of included studies, and rarely can use meta-analysis.

The explicit methodology of systematic reviews suggests that persons skilled in the art of systematic reviewing should be able to reproduce the data of a systematic review, just as researchers in chemistry or biochemistry expect to be able to reproduce published primary studies in their fields. This concept strengthens the credibility of systematic reviews, and workers in the field of EBM generally consider well-conducted systematic reviews of high-quality primary studies to constitute the highest level of evidence on a medical question.

Why Systematic Reviews?

The explosion of research and the vastness of the medical literature are such that no one can read, much less digest, all relevant work. The massive amount of new technology, the poor quality of narrative reviews,[65] and the necessity to provide an accurate digest for practicing clinicians[36] constitute the background to the call for a more systematic review of literature.

Systematic reviews can achieve multiple objectives.[44] They can identify the number, scope, and quality of primary studies by using an extensive search strategy; provide a summary of the diagnostic accuracy of a test; compare the diagnostic accuracies of tests; determine the dependence of reported diagnostic accuracies on quality of study design; identify dependence of diagnostic accuracy on characteristics of the patients or method for the test; and identify areas that require further research and recognize questions that are well answered and for which further studies may not be necessary.

Conducting a Systematic Review

Systematic reviewing is time consuming and requires multiple skills. Usually a team is required, and the team should include at least one person experienced in the science and art. The team must agree on the clinical problem to be tackled and on the scope of the review.

An early step in preparation for performing a systematic review is to identify whether a similar review has been undertaken recently. Among other things, such a search will help to focus the review. The Cochrane Collaboration provides an excellent resource of reviews, but unfortunately few are reviews of diagnostic tests.[95] The Database of Abstracts of Reviews of Effectiveness (DARE),[69] which is run by the Centre for Reviews and Dissemination at the University of York in the United Kingdom, contains reviews of some diagnostic tests. A third resource is the Bayes Library of Diagnostic Studies and Reviews, which is associated with the Cochrane Collaboration[42] (http://www.bice.ch/engl/content_e/bayes_library.htm, accessed March 18, 2004). Other resources include electronic databases, such as PubMed and Embase, and recent clinical practice guidelines, which are likely to cite systematic reviews that were available at the time of the guideline's development (see section on guidelines later in this chapter). Horvath et al[43] list additional sources.

The review team must develop a protocol for the project. A protocol should include,[2,43,49] in addition to a title, background information, composition of the review group, and a timetable:

- The clinical question(s) to be addressed in the review
- Search strategy
- Inclusion and exclusion criteria for selection of studies
- Methodology of and checklists for critical appraisal of studies
- Methodology of data extraction and data extraction forms
- Methodology of study synthesis and summary measures to be used

Description of all of the details is beyond the scope of this chapter and only some highlights will be discussed. Review of the references cited here is recommended before embarking on a systematic review.

The Clinical Question and Criteria for Selection of Studies

Among the steps in conducting a systematic review of a diagnostic test (Box 13-1), the most important is the identification of the clinical question for which the test result is required to give an answer, and thus formulation of the question that forms the basis of the review. Two types of questions can be addressed in a systematic review in diagnostic medicine: one type is related to the diagnostic accuracy of a test, and the other to the clinical value (to patients or to others) of using the test. The questions that arise are similar in structure but require different approaches.

BOX 13-1 Selected Key Steps in a Systematic Review of a Diagnostic Test

Identify the clinical question
Define the inclusion and exclusion criteria
Search the literature
Identify the relevant studies
Select studies against explicit quality criteria
Extract data and assess quality
Analyze and interpret data
Present and summarize findings

Examples:

Type 1 question regarding diagnostic accuracy of a test:

In patients coming to the emergency department with shortness of breath, how well does B-type natriuretic peptide (BNP) or N-terminal pro-BNP predict (identify the presence of) heart failure as assessed by the cardiac ejection fraction measured by echocardiography?

Type 2 question regarding the value of a test in improving patient outcomes (called a phase 4 evaluation of a test by Sackett and Haynes[80]):

In patients admitted to the hospital for treatment of heart failure, how well does use of BNP or N-terminal pro-BNP help as a guide to therapy, improve the ability to treat heart failure as assessed by the rate of subsequent readmission for heart failure?

Note that each question (1) identifies the patient's problem (shortness of breath and the clinical setting [emergency department or hospital]), (2) the test being used (BNP or N-terminal pro-BNP), (3) the reference standard for the diagnosis (ejection fraction as measured by echo) or for the clinical outcome (rate of subsequent readmission), and (4) an outcome (ability to detect the presence of heart failure or ability to treat heart failure).

More complex questions often arise. For example, a type 1 question may involve comparing the diagnostic accuracies of two or more tests, or it may address the improvement in diagnostic accuracy from adding results of a new test to results of an existing test or tests. A complex type 2 question may involve the utility of therapeutic drug testing at the time of a clinic visit to reduce clinic visits by helping to establish optimum drug dosages. In all cases, however, it is usually best that the clinical question be specific and focused on defined clinical scenarios and clinical settings.

The clinical question leads to inclusion and exclusion criteria for studies to be included in the review. These criteria include the patient cohort and setting in which the test is to be used, as well as the outcome measures to be considered. These are all important as both the "patient setting" and the nature of the question affect the diagnostic performance of a test.[75]

Until recently, methodologists interested in systematic reviews have focused on studies of the effects of interventions, especially drugs, on patient outcomes. That work is generally applicable to systematic reviews of diagnostic tests that start with a question of the second type above. The opportunities to use the techniques, however, are limited as it is unusual to find more than one study on any combination of a test and an outcome. We therefore focus on systematic reviews of the diagnostic accuracy of tests and express the hope that the quality of primary studies will continue to improve so that many such systematic reviews will become feasible.

When the questions to be addressed are defined, the review group must agree on the scope of the review. Irwig et al[44] summarized the two main approaches to defining the scope of a systematic review of studies of diagnostic accuracy:

- Restrict the review to studies of high quality directly applicable to the problem of immediate interest to the reviewer.
- Explore the effect of variability in study quality and other characteristics (setting, type of population, disease spectrum, etc.) on estimates of accuracy, using subgroup analysis or modeling.

The second approach is more complex, but allows estimates of such things as the applicability of estimates of diagnostic accuracy to different settings and the effect of study design and inherent patient characteristics (e.g., age, sex, symptoms) on estimates of a test's diagnostic accuracy.

Search Strategy

Searching of the primary literature is usually carried out in three ways: (1) an electronic search of literature databases, (2) hand searching of key journals, and (3) review of the references of key review articles. It is usual to search both Medline and Embase, as the overlap between the two can be as low as 35%.[90] Searching of databases is a detailed exercise and the help of a librarian or information scientist is recommended. An incorrectly structured search can generate a large number of irrelevant references and miss crucial references.[53] Guidance that is tailored to searching for studies of diagnostic accuracy in the published literature is available in Irwig et al.[44]

Additional studies may be found in the "gray" literature that is not indexed by the major databases. These sources include theses, conference proceedings, technical reports, and monographs. Consultation with individuals active in the field may uncover studies in these sources and studies that are being prepared for publication.

Data Extraction and Critical Appraisal of Studies

Identified papers should be read independently by two persons and data extracted according to a template. A checklist of items to extract from primary studies in preparing a systematic review on test accuracy is available online[44] and on this book's accompanying Evolve site, found at http://evolve.elsevier.com/Tietz/textbook/. The STARD checklist[7] can also be used as an additional guide in designing the template.

The quality of studies must be assessed as part of the systematic review. Rating schemes for the quality of primary studies have been concerned mostly with studies of therapeutic interventions. These schemes have focused on the type of study design, with large RCTs routinely considered to have the highest level of quality and other designs given lower ratings. Glasziou et al[37] have pointed out, however, that different types of clinical questions (such as questions related to diagnostic approaches) often require different types of study design. Thus, a randomized trial, though ideal for studies of the effects of interventions, is not the most appropriate design to study whether (their examples) computerized or human reading of cervical smears is better (or to study the natural history of a disease or the cause of a disease, etc.). Moreover, a study may use a good design but suffer from serious drawbacks in other dimensions, such as the number of patients lost to follow-up. Thus adequate grading of the quality of studies must go beyond the categorization of study design.[37]

Summarizing the Data

The characteristics and data from critically appraised studies should be presented in tables. The data should include sensitivities, specificities, and likelihood ratios wherever possible. These can then be summarized in plots that provide an indication of the variation among studies. The summary should also include an assessment of the quality of each study, using an explicit scoring system. A review should also present critical analysis of the data highlighted in the review.

Meta-analysis

It may be possible to undertake a meta-analysis if data are available from a number of similar studies (i.e., asking the same question in the same type of patients and in the same or similar clinical settings). Meta-analyses can explore sources of variability in the results of clinical studies, increase confidence in the data and conclusions, and signal when no further studies are necessary. For guidelines on conduct of meta-analyses of RCTs, see the Quality of Reporting of Meta-analyses (QUORUM) statement at http://www.consort-statement.org/QUOROM.pdf (accessed April 22, 2004).

Although meta-analyses are hampered in diagnostic research by the paucity of high-quality primary studies,[44] the quality of these studies is improving.[58] For descriptions of meta-analytic techniques in diagnostic research, including the summary ROC curve, see papers by Irwig et al[45,46] and Deeks[19] and the book chapter by Boyd and Deeks.[11] Deeks has argued that likelihood ratios provide the most transparent expression of the utility of a test, because they enable the clinician to calculate the posttest probability if the pretest probability is known.[19]

ECONOMIC EVALUATIONS OF DIAGNOSTIC TESTING

Healthcare costs worldwide have surged in recent decades. For example, the United States spent $1.55 trillion dollars on healthcare in 2002, or 14.9% of its gross domestic product (see http://www.cms.hhs.gov/statistics/nhe/historical/t1.asp, accessed March 18, 2004). Although the direct laboratory costs are small in comparison, the tests have a profound influence on medical decisions and therefore total costs.

A Hierarchy of Evidence

A hierarchy of evidence regarding clinical tests[34] begins with assessment of the test's technical performance and proceeds through the study of the test's diagnostic performance to an identification of potential benefits and thus to economic evaluation. The hierarchy has also been expressed as moving up from the efficacy of a test through efficiency to the effectiveness of a test.[60] This hierarchy of evidence can also be seen in the context of the data that are required to make decisions about the implementation of a test.[76] It therefore lies at the heart of the process of policy making and service management.[64] Economic evaluation provides a means of evaluating the comparative costs of alternative care strategies and providing a means of evaluating health outcomes at the highest level in terms of life years gained and social benefit.[26,89]

Methodologies for Economic Evaluations

Health economics is concerned with the *cost* and *consequences* of decisions made about the care of patients. It therefore involves the identification, measurement, and valuation of both the costs and the consequences. The process is complex and is an "inexact science."[67] The approaches to economic evaluation include (1) cost minimization, (2) cost benefit, (3) cost effectiveness, and (4) cost utility analysis (Table 13-2).

Cost minimization can be considered as the simplest approach and provides the least information; it is an evaluation of the costs of alternative approaches that produce the same outcome. In the area of diagnostic testing, it is applicable only to the cost of alternative suppliers of the same test, device, or instrument. It is therefore a technique that is limited to the procurement process where the specifications of the service are already established and the outcomes clearly defined. It might be considered as providing the "cost per test," an often quoted parameter that is not, however, a true economic evaluation because it does not identify an outcome except the provision of a test result.

Cost-benefit analysis determines whether the cost of the benefit exceeds the cost of the intervention and therefore whether the intervention is worthwhile. The value of the consequence or benefit is assessed in monetary terms; this

TABLE 13-2 Approaches to Economic Evaluations

Type of Evaluation	Test Evaluated	Effect or Outcome	Decision Criteria
Cost minimization	Alternative tests or delivery options	Identical outcomes	Least expensive alternative
Cost benefit	Alternative tests or delivery options	Improved effect or outcome	Effect evaluated purely in monetary terms
Cost effectiveness	Alternative tests or delivery options	Common unit of effect but differential effect	Cost per unit of effect (e.g., dollars per life years gained)
Cost utility	Alternative tests or delivery options	Improved effect or outcome	Outcome expressed in terms of survival and quality of life

can be quite challenging, because it may require the analyst to equate a year of life to a monetary amount. There are a number of methods, including the "human capital approach," which assesses the individual's productivity (in terms of earnings), and the "willingness to pay approach," which is more of a modeling approach having determined by questionnaire what individuals are prepared to pay. Cost-benefit evaluation is not widely used, but it might have some value in comparisons of different testing modalities.

Cost-effectiveness analysis looks at the most efficient way of spending a fixed budget and the effects are measured in terms of a natural unit. The ultimate natural unit is the life year, but more practical measures include reduction in the frequency of hypoglycemic episodes, or number of strokes prevented. Surrogate measures with clear relationships to morbidity and mortality have also been used (e.g., change in blood pressure). When assessing an intervention, the number of cases of disease prevented may be used as a measure of benefit, as in the case of alternative approaches to the management of patients with suspected peptic ulcer.[30] In this study, investigative and treatment strategies were compared for outcome measures of costs per ulcer cured and cost per patient treated. The serological testing strategy was found to be more effective than endoscopy by both measures.

Cost-utility analysis includes the quality and the quantity of the health outcome, or in other words looking at the quality of the life years gained. The cost of the intervention is assessed in monetary terms, but the outcomes are expressed in "quality-adjusted life years" (QALYs). Approaches that assess the quality of life include Quality of Wellbeing,[47] Heath Utilities Index,[94] and EuroQol.[51] Cost-utility analysis has seen little use in the study of diagnostic tests probably because of the complexity of the clinical process involving both diagnostic test and treatment necessary to produce a measurable clinical outcome. It has, however, been used to assess the utility of some screening programs.

The inclusion of a quality of life component can affect choices among alternatives. In the Centers for Disease Control and Prevention Diabetes Cost-Effectiveness Study, the lifetime costs and benefits of opportunistic screening for diabetes were compared with those of current practice,[15] with primary outcome measures of life years saved and QALYs. The incremental cost effectiveness was found to be $35,768 per life year gained and $13,376 per QALY, showing that adjustment for quality of life has a major impact on the cost effectiveness. This suggests that in addition to the extension of life through screening there is also a gain in the quality of life that increases the attractiveness of the benefits accruing from screening.

The addition of new technology often increases both cost and benefit. A cost-effectiveness study[33] of screening for colorectal cancer (versus no screening) showed that the "least expensive" strategy was a single sigmoidoscopy at 55 years of age, with an incremental cost-effectiveness ratio of $1200 per life year saved. Alternative strategies gave incremental cost-effectiveness ratios of $21,200, $51,200, and $92,900 with the addition of increasingly complex and frequent screening for fecal occult blood.

When tests increase both the cost and benefit, decisions about their use will depend on factors such as willingness to pay and other political and individual pressures. A figure of $50,000 per QALY has been used in the United States as a reference point, the figure deriving from a decision by the U.S. Congress to approve dialysis treatment for end-stage renal failure.[54] Although providing useful comparative data, there are concerns about the use of tables of cost per QALY.[23]

The underlying issue of economic evaluations is to compare the costs that will be incurred with an estimate of the gain, and for this there are four possible findings and three possible decisions:

- Test more costly but providing greater benefit—possibly introduce depending on overall gain
- Test more costly but providing less benefit—do not introduce test
- Test less costly but providing greater benefit—introduce test
- Test less costly but providing less benefit—possibly introduce test depending on the size of the loss in the benefit and the magnitude of savings (which may be able to produce a demonstrably greater benefit if spent on a different intervention or test).

These options have been expressed graphically in a two-dimensional plot called the "cost- effectiveness plane"[4,70] with cost on one axis and benefit on the perpendicular axis.

Quality of Economic Evaluations

In exactly the same way as for studies on diagnostic performance and for outcomes studies, there is a minimal set of criteria for evaluating an economic study of a diagnostic test. A suggested list of criteria includes[22]:

- Clear definition of economic question including perspective of the evaluation (e.g., perspective of a patient or society or an employer or a health insurance company or a hospital administrator; long-term versus short-term perspective)
- Description of competing alternatives
- Evidence of effectiveness of intervention
- Clear identification and quantification of costs and consequences including incremental analysis
- Appropriate consideration of effects of differential timing of costs and benefits
- Performance of sensitivity analysis (How sensitive are results to changes in assumptions or in input, e.g., cost of drugs or expected benefit in life years?)
- Inclusion of summary measure of efficiency, ensuring that all issues are addressed

Two reviews of economic evaluations of diagnostic tests have shown poor adherence to the criteria outlined above, with only about half of the evaluated papers meeting the criteria.[21,85]

Perspectives of Economic Evaluations

The perspective from which an economic evaluation is performed affects the design, conduct, and results of the evaluation. The perspective may, for example, be that of a patient, a payer (government health agency or health insurance company), or society. The perspective may be long term or short term. The perspective is a practical consideration when attempting to assess the benefit of a particular test or device as part of a more complex clinical protocol. Perspective is also important in relation to many of the routine decisions made about a diagnostic test. The questions below illustrate the importance of perspective:

- What is the cost of the test result produced on analyzer A compared with analyzer B?
- What is the cost of the test result produced by laboratory A compared with laboratory B?
- What is the cost of the test result produced by POCT compared with the laboratory?
- Will provision of rapid testing for the emergency department reduce the length of patients' stays in the department and thus decrease cost for the hospital?
- Will HbA_{1c} testing in a clinic save time for *patients* by providing results at the time of the clinic visit? Will it save money for the patients' *employers* by reducing employees' time away from work for physician appointments? Will it save time for the physician and thus money for the *clinic*? Will it improve care of diabetes (perhaps by facilitating counseling at the time of the clinic visit) for the *patient* as indicated by independent measures of glycemic control? Will it save money for the *health system* by improving glycemic control and thus decreasing hospitalizations? Will it provide benefit for *society* by decreasing society's healthcare costs (for hospitalizations) and increasing patients' functioning and contributions to society?

The first scenario is the type of evaluation made when making a deal, and is a simple procurement exercise. The outcome is the same—the provision of a given test result, to a given standard of accuracy and precision within a given time (the specification). The second question might appear to be the same, but it is not and will undoubtedly have to take into account other issues, namely the logistical issues associated with sample transport or the level of communication support provided by the laboratories. To make a relevant evaluation concerning the value of POCT, it is important to also take into account the implications outside of the laboratory that may result from the delay in sending the sample to another laboratory.

Most economic evaluations of diagnostic tests will have a perspective beyond the bounds of the laboratory if the value of the test is to be appreciated and understood. Unfortunately, many of the early economic data on POCT looked solely at the costs of producing the test result.[56] The studies overlooked the potential value of the key objective of producing the result more quickly so that a decision can be made immediately and a treatment instituted or changed. When a test is proposed to reduce the use of other resources within the hospital (e.g., use of drugs or blood products or other expensive diagnostic technology) the expectation is that the clinical outcome will be unchanged (e.g., the patient is not put at risk by using less blood or the less expensive technology). When provision of a test result may have a longer-term impact, as in management of chronic disease, use of intermediate measures of outcome may be especially important.

Choice of Outcome Measures

Tests are not always evaluated in terms of life years gained. Even for cost-effectiveness and cost-utility studies, surrogate clinical markers and surrogate economic markers may have a place.[91] The use of surrogate markers of clinical outcome requires the existence of a clear, demonstrated relationship between the marker and morbidity and mortality. Even if such a relationship is demonstrated, however, changes in the surrogate do not reliably lead to changes in the associated patient-important outcome.[14] This limits the strength of inferences from such studies.

Many of the questions listed above address issues within the "clinical episode," but the evaluation of the longer-term value or benefit of a diagnostic test is more complex. Long-term costs and benefits, as in management of a chronic condition such as diabetes, may be influenced by other (confounding) factors. The complexity depends on the relationship between test and treatment and also on the compliance of both patient and clinician in use of both the test and the treatment. In diabetes, the measurement of blood glucose and HbA_{1c} is an integral part of management. Although short-term studies have been done,[39] rigorous economic evaluations of the long-term use of these tests are rare. Economic modeling of both the Diabetes Control and Complications Trial (DCCT) and United Kingdom Prospective Diabetes Study (UKPDS) demonstrated the economic benefits of intensive glycemic control[20,38] but did not indicate the value of the testing component. An observational study of the implementation of an intensive glycemic control program demonstrated long-term savings from improved clinical outcomes that reduced clinic visits and hospital admissions and their attendant costs.[97]

Use of Economic Evaluations in Decision Making

The stream of new tests in laboratory medicine requires frequent decisions about whether or not to implement them. Economic evaluations can help in making these decisions. The finite resources for healthcare require use of an objective means of determining how resources are allocated and how the efficiency and effectiveness of service delivery can be improved.

Use of economic evaluations faces several challenges. First, the laboratory medicine budget is usually "controlled" independently of the other costs of healthcare. This is often referred to as "silo budgeting." In practical terms the budget for testing is established independently of the budgets for all of the other services, including budgets for which the contemplated diagnostic test might be able to provide savings. Second, achievement of a favorable outcome (e.g., from a reduction in length of stay or a decrease of admissions to the coronary care unit) is of use from a management standpoint only if the potential savings can be turned into real money (leveraged). Third, the introduction of a new test or testing modality (e.g., POCT) will undoubtedly lead to a change in practice and so the benefits can be achieved only if the change in practice can be implemented. Finally, even if the desired cost savings are achieved, silo budgeting ensures that the savings are seen in a budget different from the laboratory's, and the laboratory budget shows only an increased cost. Fortunately the drawbacks of silo budgeting are being recognized, and a broader view of health economics seems to be developing in some healthcare settings.

Regardless of any problems in introducing them, economic evaluations can provide the objective measure of what can be achieved, and the standard against which the change in practice can be audited after implementation.

CLINICAL PRACTICE GUIDELINES

The patient-centered goals of evidenced-based laboratory medicine cannot be reached by primary studies and systematic reviews alone. The results of these investigations must be turned into action. Increasingly, health systems and professional groups in medicine have turned to the use of clinical practice guidelines as one tool to facilitate implementation of lessons from primary studies and systematic reviews. Important motivations for development of guidelines have been to decrease variability in practice (and improve the use of best practices) and to decrease the (often prolonged) time required for new information to be used for the benefit of patients for prevention of disease.

Although most guidelines have been developed primarily for use by clinicians, publication of guidelines on the Internet, and descriptions of them in articles in the popular press, have led to their use by patients and their families.[13] The development of such guidelines is a challenging new area about which some things are becoming clearer, including the absence of tested guidelines for the development of laboratory-related guidelines. A start in this direction for laboratory medicine has appeared recently.[71]

What Is a Clinical Practice Guideline?

A widely quoted definition of clinical practice guidelines comes from a report of the U.S. Institute of Medicine. "Clinical practice guidelines are systematically developed statements to assist practitioner and patient decisions about appropriate healthcare for specific clinical circumstances."[31] This definition appears broad enough to accommodate the laboratory-related guidelines that are appearing in the literature and on the Internet. Guidelines of various sorts have long addressed issues of concern to laboratorians, such as requirements or goals for accuracy, precision, and turnaround time of tests and considerations about the frequency of repeat tests in the monitoring of patients. In contrast to many earlier pronouncements on such issues, the focus of modern clinical practice guidelines, such as recent ones on laboratory testing in diabetes[83] and liver disease,[24,25] is the patient in the "specific clinical circumstances" referred to in the definition of clinical practice guidelines. The new ingredient in development of these guidelines is the tool kit of EBM and clinical epidemiology, which allow the guidelines to grow in a more transparent way from well-conducted studies and systematic reviews.

A Transparent Process Must Be Used in the Development of Guidelines

In the absence of a transparent process for development of a guideline, the credibility of the product is compromised and can be legitimately questioned. When guidelines are developed by a professional group (such as specialist physicians or laboratory-based practitioners), the recommendations (e.g., to perform a diagnostic procedure in a given setting) may be suspected of promoting the welfare of the professional group. By contrast, when guidelines are prepared under the auspices of payers for healthcare (governments and insurance companies), the recommendations may be seen as cost-control measures. In this setting, a key danger is that the absence of evidence of a benefit from a medical intervention may be interpreted as evidence of absence of benefit.

Steps in the Development of Guidelines

The development of guidelines is best undertaken with a step-by-step plan. One such scheme is shown in Figure 13-6, only selected issues of which will be discussed here. For a more detailed discussion, see Bruns and Oosterhuis[13] or Oosterhuis et al.[71]

Selection and Refinement of a Topic

The critical importance of this first step is analogous to the importance of the corresponding step in development of a systematic review. The scope must not exceed the capabilities (in time, funding, and expertise) of the group, the topic must not be without evidence (or the guideline will lack credibility), and the area must be one requiring attention (or the guideline will have little value and will attract no attention).

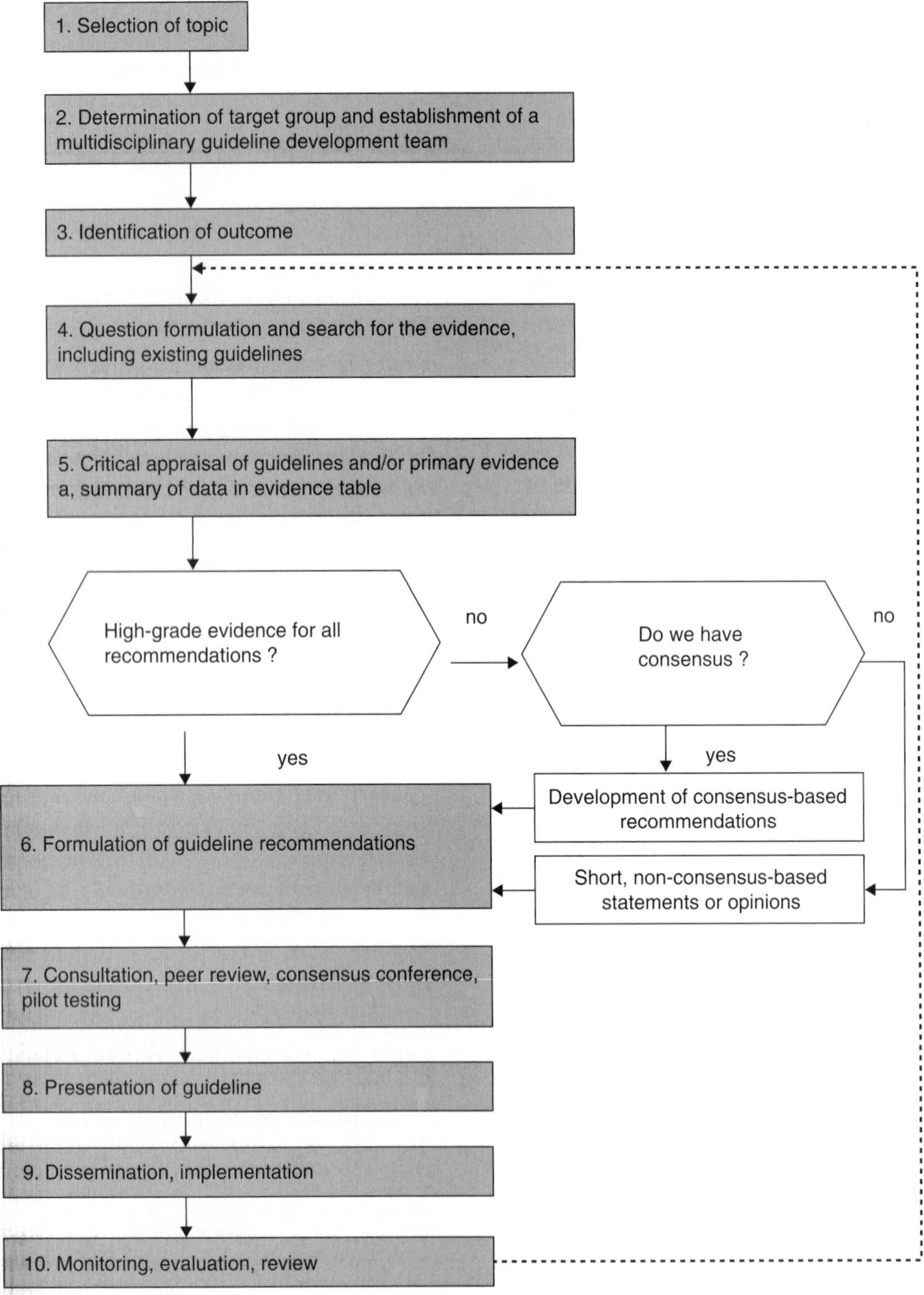

Figure 13-6 Steps in development of a clinical practice guideline. *(Modified from Oosterhuis WP, Bruns DE, Watine J, Sandberg S, Horvath AR. Evidence-based guidelines in laboratory medicine: principles and methods. Clin Chem 2004;50: 806-818.)*

Guidelines can address clinical conditions (such as diabetes and liver disease), symptoms (chest pain), signs (abnormal bleeding), or interventions, whether therapeutic (coronary angioplasty and aspirin) or diagnostic (cardiac markers). The priority for a guideline should be: Is there variation in practice that suggests uncertainty? Is the issue of public health importance, such as in the increasing problem of diabetes and obesity? Is there a perceived necessity for cost reduction?

The critical issues to be addressed must be identified and distinguished from those that may be considered peripheral or simply beyond the scope that can reasonably be included. Ideally, this process involves a multidisciplinary group, with clinicians, laboratory experts, patients, and likely users of the guidelines. The scope will be affected by the staff (if any) and financial support available to the guideline group. The cost is usually underestimated.

Determination of Target Group and Establishment of a Multidisciplinary Guideline Development Team

The intended audience must be identified: Is it nurses, general practice physicians, clinical specialty physicians, laboratory specialists, or patients?

The team should include representatives of all key groups involved in the management of the target condition. In development of guidelines in laboratory medicine, teams ideally include relevant medical specialists, laboratory experts, methodologists (for expertise in statistics, literature search, critical appraisal, and guideline development), and those who deliver services (such as nurse practitioners and patients for guidelines on home monitoring of glucose; laboratory technicians and managers for a guideline that addresses turnaround times for cardiac markers).

As the composition of guideline development groups affects recommendations, with those who perform procedures more likely to recommend their use,[55] potential conflicts of interest of all members must be noted. The role if any of sponsors (commercial or nonprofit) in the guideline development process must be agreed upon and reported. Ideally, staff support is available for arranging meetings and conference calls and assisting with publication and other forms of dissemination (e.g., audioconferences).

A minimum group size of six has been recommended.[88] Making the team larger than 12 to 15 persons can inhibit the airing of each person's views. A recommended tool is the use of subgroups to focus on specific questions, with a steering committee responsible for coordination and the production of the final guideline. Other ways of using subgroups can be envisioned.

Identifying and Assessing the Evidence

When available, well-performed systematic reviews form the most important part of the evidence base for guidelines. Systematic reviews are necessary when there is expected to be variation between studies, sometimes attributable to effects too small to be measured. Where no systematic reviews exist, the group effectively must undertake to produce one. The level of evidence supporting each conclusion in the review will affect the recommendations made in the guidelines.

Translating Evidence into a Guideline and Grading the Strength of Recommendations

The processes for reaching recommendations within an expert group are poorly understood. For clinical practice guidelines, the process may involve balancing of costs and benefits after values are assigned and the strength of evidence is weighed. Conclusive evidence for recommendations is only rarely available. Authors of guidelines thus have an ethical responsibility to make very clear the level of evidence that supports each recommendation.

Various schemes are available for grading the level of evidence, and one of them should be adopted and used explicitly.[13,71] A rather simple one, with a rather typical four levels (A through D), is shown in Table 13-3. More complex schemes are shown in Tables 13-4 and Box 13-2. For a recent and different approach, see the additional readings at the end of this chapter. The level of evidence does not always predict the strength of a recommendation, as recommendations may either follow directly from clinical studies or be extrapolated from the results of the studies. For example, multiple studies supporting use of a drug may have been done well and a competent systematic review may be available, so that the evidence may be graded as high. However if the study was done in adults and the guideline is for children, the strength of the recommendation may be low.[13]

TABLE 13-3 A Scheme for Grading of Strength of Recommendations in Clinical Guidelines

Level	Characteristics
A	Directly based on meta-analysis of RCTs or on at least one RCT
B	Directly based on at least one controlled study without randomization or at least one other type of quasiexperimental study, or extrapolated from RCTs
C	Directly based on nonexperimental studies or extrapolated from RCTs or nonrandomized studies
D	Directly based on expert reports or opinion or experience of authorities, or extrapolated from RCTs, nonrandomized studies, or nonexperimental studies

From Shekelle PG, Woolf SH, Eccles M, Grimshaw J. Clinical guidelines: developing guidelines. BMJ 1999; 318: 593-6.

TABLE 13-4 Categories of Evidence Supporting Guidelines (A-E) and Quality of Evidence on Which Recommendation Is Based (I-IV) as Used by the American Association for the Study of Liver Disease

Category	Explanation
I	Evidence from multiple well-designed randomized controlled clinical trials, each involving a number of patients to be of sufficient statistical power
II	Evidence from at least one large well-designed clinical trial with or without randomization, from cohort or case-controlled analytical studies, or well-designed meta-analysis
III	Evidence based on clinical experience, descriptive studies, or reports of expert committees
IV	Not rated
A	Survival benefit
B	Improved diagnosis
C	Improvement in quality of life
D	Relevant pathophysiological parameters improved
E	Impacts cost of healthcare

From Dufour DR, Lott JA, Nolte FS, Gretch DR, Koff RS, Seeff LB. Diagnosis and monitoring of hepatic injury. II. Recommendations for use of laboratory tests in screening, diagnosis, and monitoring. Clin Chem 2000;46:2050-68.

BOX 13-2 System to Rate the Strength of a Body of Evidence

Quality of Primary Studies and Reviews: Rating the Level of Evidence of Individual Articles:

Ia Meta-analysis or systematic review based on at least several level Ib studies
Ib Diagnostic trial or outcome study of good quality
II Diagnostic trial or outcome study of medium quality, insufficient patients, or other trials (case-control, other designs)
III Descriptive studies, case reports, other studies
IV Statements of committees, opinion of experts etc., review, not systematic

Rating of the Strength of the Evidence Supporting Guideline Recommendations:

A Supported by at least two independent studies of level Ib or one review of level Ia ("it was shown/demonstrated")
B Supported by at least two independent studies of level II ("it is plausible")
C Not supported by sufficient studies of level I or II ("indications"), poorly
D Advice of experts, etc. ("there is no proof")

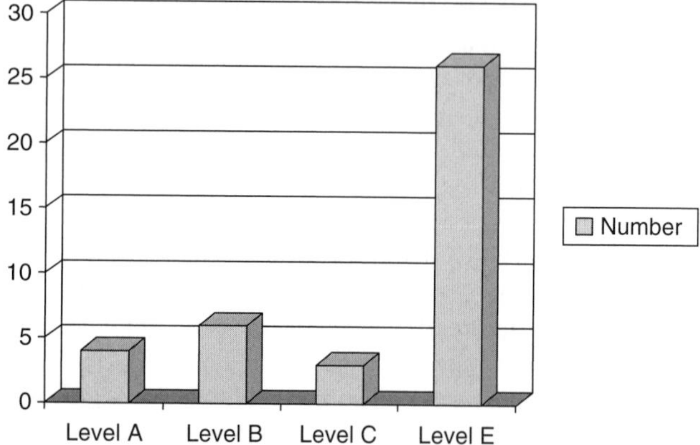

Figure 13-7 Level of evidence for recommendations in NACB guideline for testing in diabetes.[83] *(From Bruns DE, Oosterhuis WP in Price CP, Christenson RH, eds Evidence-Based Laboratory Medicine: from principles to outcomes. AACC Press, 2003.)*

Level A evidence is rare in guidelines on the use of diagnostic tests. The recommendations made in the National Academy of Clinical Biochemistry (NACB) guidelines on laboratory testing in diabetes[83] were graded by the scheme of the American Diabetes Association, a scheme similar to that in Table 13-3 except that level D is referred to as level E. As shown in Figure 13-7, the vast majority of the recommendations were graded only as level E (expert opinion) by the authors of the guidelines, and only three were graded as A. The high proportion of recommendations in the NACB document supported only by expert opinion is far from unique or peculiar to that document or to guidelines for diagnostic tests.

For analytical goal setting or "quality specifications" for analytical methods in guidelines, randomized controlled clinical trials (outcomes studies) are rarely available. As discussed by Bruns and Oosterhuis,[13] a different hierarchy of evidence[32] (Table 13-5) may be useful for grading of such laboratory-related recommendations. The highest level of evidence is evidence related to medical needs. It is conceivable that even statistical modeling of specific clinical decisions could be considered as a subtype of evidence related to medical needs. For example, Klee et al[52] have shown rates of misclassification of cardiac risk as a function of analytical bias of cholesterol assays. Similarly, error rates in insulin dosing can be calculated[10] as a function of imprecision (or bias or both) of home glucose measurements, with increas-

TABLE 13-5 Hierarchy of Criteria for Quality Specifications

Level	Basis
1A	Medical decision making: Use of test in specific clinical situations
1B	Medical decision making: Use of test in medicine generally
2	Guidelines—"experts"
3	Regulators or organizers of external quality assurance schemes
4	Published data on state of the art

From Fraser CG, Petersen PH. Analytical performance characteristics should be judged against objective quality specifications. Clin Chem 1999;45:321-3.

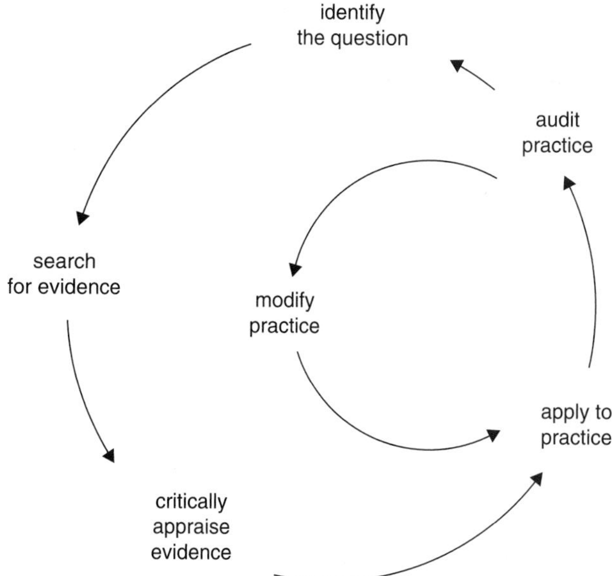

Figure 13-8 The audit cycle. *(From Price CP. Clin Chem 2000;46:1041-50.)*

ing imprecision (or bias) of the glucose assay leading to increasingly frequent errors in the administered dose of insulin. Although such studies do not demonstrate an effect on patient outcomes, they may be a distinct advance over anecdotes, and an expert group can make reasoned recommendations for imprecision based on such data and mathematical modeling when the clinical action follows a well-defined rule.

Level 1B in Table 13-5 refers primarily to the concepts of within-person and among-person biological variation. Levels of optimum, desirable, and minimum performance for both imprecision and bias have been defined[32] based on these concepts. When a test is to be used for monitoring, use of this type of quality specification for imprecision appears appropriate in guidelines. Failure to use this approach is difficult to justify, because data on within-person and among-person biological variation are available for virtually all commonly used tests. The quality specifications relate directly to the ability to use assays for monitoring and the ability to use common reference intervals within a population. These may be considered patient-centered objectives in a broad sense if not in a narrow one.

Obtaining External Review and Updating the Guidelines

Three types of outside examiners can evaluate the guideline[88]:

- Experts in the clinical content area—to assess completeness of literature review and the reasonableness of recommendations
- Experts on systematic reviewing and guideline development—to review the process of guideline development
- Potential users of the guidelines

In addition, journals, sponsoring organizations, and other potential endorsers of the guidelines may undertake formal reviews. Each of these reviews can add value.

As part of the guideline development process, a plan for updating should be developed. The importance of this step is underscored by the finding that one of the most common reasons for nonadherence to guidelines is that the guidelines are outdated.[96] Consistent with that finding, a study[87] of clinical practice guidelines of the Agency for Healthcare Research and Quality showed that about half the guidelines were outdated in 5.8 years (95% confidence interval [CI] 5.0 to 6.6 years). No more than 90% of conclusions were still valid after 3.6 years (CI 2.6 to 4.6 years). These findings suggest that the time interval between completion and review of a guideline should be short.

CLINICAL AUDIT

The term "audit" is associated with a particular connotation in healthcare, namely clinical audit and refers to the review of case histories of patients against the benchmark of current best practice.[86] The clinical audit was proposed as a tool to improve clinical practice and a recent study indicates that it can do so, though the effects are modest.[93] A more general role for audit, however, is that it can be used as part of the wider management exercise of benchmarking of performance with the use of relevant performance indicators against the performance of peers.

Four distinct activities can be considered under the broad umbrella of an audit: (1) solving problems associated with the process or outcome, (2) monitoring workload in the context of controlling demand, (3) monitoring the introduction of a new test and/or changes in practice, and (4) monitoring the adherence with best practices (e.g., with guidelines).

The components of the audit cycle are depicted in Figure 13-8. All of the audit activities are found in the practice of evidence-based laboratory medicine, namely that there is a clinical question for which the test result should provide an answer and that the answer will lead to a decision being made and an action taken, leading to an improved health outcome. There should be evidence to support the use of the test in the setting for which it is being used.

Audit to Help Solve Problems

All audits involve the collection of observational data and comparison against a standard or specification. In many cases a standard does not exist, and maybe not even a specification; then it is important to establish a specification as the first stage of auditing a process. Such a specification may then generate observations, which can lead to the creation of a standard. At the outset it provides the comparative measure against which to judge the performance data collected.

Solving a problem relating to a process may first involve collecting data on aspects of the process that are considered to have an influence on the outcome with the goal of identifying rate-limiting steps. For example, a study of test result turnaround times might collect data on phlebotomy waiting time, quality of patient identification, transport time, sample registration time, quality of sample identification, sample preparation time, analysis time, test result validation time, and result delivery time.

The study of process may extend to the way in which the results are accessed and used. For example, the use of POCT in an emergency department (not in an audit) did not decrease the length of stay despite the fact that the delivery time for the results was much shorter than when results were provided by the laboratory.[48] The authors concluded that the test result was not the rate-limiting step.[48] Murray, in a similar study,[66] did find a reduction in the length of stay and identified a subset of patients in which the POCTs could be used to rule out diagnoses and allow a faster discharge. They noted that in other cases the triage decision was delayed by the need for results from the laboratory.

Monitoring Workload and Demand

The true demand for a test will depend on the number of patients and the spectrum of disease in each case where the test is appropriate. The appropriateness of the test request is a valuable arbiter in situations in which workload or demand for tests is questioned. A portfolio of evidence helps to define the basis for the appropriate use of tests. When conducting an audit of workload for a test it is possible to ask a number of questions, usually by questionnaire that are directly related to the original generation of the evidence upon which the use of the test should be based (guidelines). These include:

- What clinical question is being asked?
- What decision will be aided by the results of the test?
- What action will be taken following the decision?
- What risks are associated with not receiving the result?
- What are the expected outcomes?
- Is there evidence to support the use of the test in this setting?
- And, for tests ordered urgently, why was this test result required urgently?

This approach is likely to identify unnecessary use of tests, misunderstandings about the use of tests, and instances of use of the wrong test. With the advent of electronic requesting and the electronic patient record, it is possible to build this approach into a routine practice.

After receipt of the results from the questionnaire, a number of actions may follow depending on the findings from the survey. They are likely to include (1) feedback of results to the users, (2) reeducation of users, (3) identification of unmet needs and research to satisfy, for example, a need for advice on alternative test, (4) creation of an algorithm or guideline on use of the test, and (5) reaudit in 6 months time to review for change in practice. Any algorithm may be embedded in the electronic requesting package to provide an automatic bar to inappropriate requesting (e.g., to prevent liver function tests from being requested every day).

Monitoring the Introduction of a New Test

In this situation the main objectives of the audit are to ensure (1) that the change in practice that is often consequent upon the introduction of a new test has been effected, and (2) that the outcomes originally predicted are being delivered. The development of any new test should lead to evidence that identifies the way in which the test is going to be used, including:

- Identification of the clinical question(s), patient cohort, clinical setting, etc.
- Identification of preanalytical and analytical requirements for the test
- Identification of any algorithm into which the test might have to be inserted (e.g., use in conjunction with other tests, signs, or symptoms)
- Identification of the decision(s) that is likely to be made on receipt of the result
- Identification of the action(s) likely to be taken on receipt of the result
- Identification of the likely outcome(s)
- Identification of any risks associated with introduction of a new test
- The evidence (and strength of that evidence) that supports the use of the test and the outcomes to be expected
- Identification of any changes in practice (e.g., deletion of another test from the repertoire, move to POCT, and reduction in laboratory workload)

This "summary of use" and portfolio of evidence forms the basis of the "standard operating procedure" for the clinical use of the test, the core of the educational material for users of the service, and the basis for conducting the audit.

Before auditing, the introduction of a new test is obviously important to have ensured that a full program of education of users has been completed and that any other changes in practice have been accommodated in the clinic and/or ward routines. Thus if a test is moving to the point-of-care then there has to have been the necessary training and certification of operators completed.

Monitoring Adherence to Best Practice

This is the scenario that probably best reflects the way in which the "clinical audit" was first envisaged and practiced. Typically, it is based on the review of randomly selected cases from a clinical team with the review undertaken by an independent clinician. This approach is the most likely to identify when a test has not been performed and identifying unnecessary testing. The audit is best performed against some form of benchmark, which may be a local, regional, or national guideline; the existence of a guideline appropriately written (see earlier) will have taken into account the best evidence available and in so doing takes away any bias that may exist between clinical teams.

In recent years registers have been established to track the performance of health institutions and organizations. Typically, such registers are disease specific and will measure outputs at a high level (e.g., morbidity and mortality).[17,28,35] In some cases (e.g., the UK Renal Registry[92]), the data collected are extensive and include laboratory information. This depth of data is extremely helpful to the laboratory specialist because it begins to provide a basis for looking at issues, such as the impact of the analytical performance of certain tests on clinical outcomes.

APPLYING THE PRINCIPLES OF EVIDENCE-BASED LABORATORY MEDICINE IN ROUTINE PRACTICE

It is hopefully clear from the foregoing discussion that the principles of evidence-based laboratory medicine can underpin the way in which laboratory medicine is practiced, from the discovery of a new diagnostic test through to its application in routine patient care. The principles provide the logic on which all of the elements of practice are founded. The tools of evidence-based laboratory medicine provide the means of delivering the highest quality of service in meeting the needs of patients and the healthcare professionals who serve them. The application of evidence-based practice is far more complex in the case of laboratory medicine than in the major area in which such principles have previously been applied, namely the pharmaceutical intervention.

The ways in which the test is used, once its efficacy has been demonstrated, will be embodied in the laboratory handbook which, increasingly, will be electronic, fully searchable in real time, and built into clinical protocols and care pathways. Such a handbook can then be supported by an information resource, again searchable, which will inform the clinician (and the patient) of the strength of evidence to support the use of the test in a specific situation. Use of these resources is practical as shown by Richardson and Burdette, who observed that information resources could be accessed during patient consultations, with each access completed in 4 to 5 seconds.[78]

The demonstration of improved outcomes in addition to providing a validation of the test also provides the data on which to undertake some form of economic analysis. As indicated earlier, this will show where the benefits are generated and what the costs and savings will be—costs to the laboratory medicine budget and savings elsewhere in the health economy. This information will enable a business case to be produced, supporting a reimbursement strategy—the style of which will depend on the type of healthcare system. The real challenge, however, comes in identifying the changes in practice, which will undoubtedly have to be implemented should the test be introduced (e.g., to leverage the benefits from reduction in length of stay, faster optimization of therapy, earlier discharge, and rule-out decisions in primary care).

The evidence base then underpins the activities that ensure the maintenance of a high quality of service: (1) provision of a knowledge resource that summarizes the evidence and its application, (2) use of this resource in education and training of health professionals, and (3) audit to ensure correct implementation and maintenance of good practice.

EBM expects clinicians to turn to primary studies of diagnostic performance and outcomes to guide decision making. However, as has been observed during the course of this chapter, there are few such studies available for diagnostic tests and devices. Furthermore in the case of many tests it will be difficult to undertake such studies as use of the markers has become embedded in routine practice and consensus guidelines. In these cases it will be necessary to depend on a more audit style of evaluation to attempt to validate the use of a test. Although this may appear as a limitation it still embodies many of the principles of evidence-based practice in laboratory medicine; crucially, recognition of the question for which the test result is seeking to provide an answer. Furthermore, the focus on outcomes will certainly help to demonstrate the value of the laboratory medicine service.

REFERENCES

1. Antman EM, Lau J, Kupelnick B, Mosteller F, Chalmers TC. A comparison of results of meta-analyses of randomized control trials and recommendations of clinical experts. Treatments for myocardial infarction. JAMA 1992;268:240-8.
2. Battaglia M, Bucher H, Egger M, et al. (writing committee). The Bayes Library of Diagnostic Studies and Reviews. 2nd Edition Basel: Division of Clinical Epidemiology and Biostatistics, Institute of Social and Preventive Medicine, University of Berne and Basel Institute for Clinical Epidemiology, University of Basel, Switzerland; 2002; pp1-60, available at www.ispm.unibe.ch (accessed on April 22, 2004).
3. Bissel MG. Laboratory Related Measures of Patient Outcomes: an introduction. Washington: AACC Press, 2000:194pp.

4. Black WC. The CE plane: a graphic representation of cost-effectiveness. Med Decis Making 1990;10: 212-4.
5. Bogardus ST Jr, Concato J, Feinstein AR. Clinical epidemiological quality in molecular genetic research: the need for methodological standards. JAMA 1999;281:1919-26.
6. Bossuyt PM, Lijmer JG, Mol BW. Randomised comparisons of medical tests: sometimes invalid, not always efficient. Lancet 2000;356:1844-7.
7. Bossuyt PM, Reitsma JB, Bruns DE, Gatsonis CA, Glasziou PP, Irwig LM, et al. Towards complete and accurate reporting of studies of diagnostic accuracy: the STARD initiative. Standards for Reporting of Diagnostic Accuracy. Clin Chem 2003;49:1-6.
8. Bossuyt PM, Reitsma JB, Bruns DE, Gatsonis CA, Glasziou PP, Irwig LM et al. The STARD statement for reporting studies of diagnostic accuracy: explanation and elaboration. Clin Chem 2003;49:7-18.
9. Bossuyt PM. The quality of reporting in diagnostic test research: getting better, still not optimal. Clin Chem 2004;50:458-6.
10. Boyd JC, Bruns DE. Quality specifications for glucose meters: assessment by simulation modeling of errors in insulin dose. Clin Chem 2001;47:209-14.
11. Boyd JC, Deeks JJ. Analysis and presentation of data. In: Price CP, Christenson RH, eds. Evidence-Based Laboratory Medicine: from principles to outcomes. Washington: AACC Press, 2003:115-36.
12. Bruns DE, Huth EJ, Magid E, Young DS. Toward a checklist for reporting of studies of diagnostic accuracy of medical tests. Clin Chem 2000;46:893-5.
13. Bruns DE, Oosterhuis WP. From evidence to guidelines. In: Price CP, Christenson RH, eds. Evidence-Based Laboratory Medicine: from principles to outcomes. Washington: AACC Press, 2003:187-208.
14. Bucher H, Guyatt G, Cook D, Holbrook A, McAlister F. Surrogate Outcomes. In: Guyatt G, Rennie D. The Users' Guides to the Medical Literature: A Manual for Evidence-Based Clinical Practice. JAMA and Archive Journals, American Medical Association, Chicago, 2002.
15. CDC Diabetes Cost-Effectiveness Study Group, Centers for Disease. The cost-effectiveness of screening for type 2 diabetes. JAMA 1998;280:1757-63.
16. Christenson RH, Duh S-H, Price CP. Identifying the question: the laboratory's role in testing provisional assumptions aimed at improving patient outcomes. In Price CP and Christenson RH (editors). Evidence-Based Laboratory Medicine: from principles to outcomes. AACC Press, Washington, 2003:21-37.
17. Cystic fibrosis Registry of Australia at http://www.cysticfibrosisaustralia.org/dataregistry.shtml (accessed on April 10, 2003)
18. Davis DA, Thomson MA, Oxman AD, Haynes RB. Changing physician performance. A systematic review of the effect of continuing medical education strategies. JAMA 1995;274:700-5.
19. Deeks JJ. Systematic reviews in health care: Systematic reviews of evaluations of diagnostic and screening tests. BMJ 2001;323:157-62.
20. Diabetes Control and Complications Trial Research Group. Lifetime benefits and costs of intensive therapy as practiced in the Diabetes Control and Complications Trial. JAMA 1996;276:1409-15.
21. Drummond MF, Jefferson TO. Guidelines for authors and peer reviewers of economic submissions to the BMJ. The BMJ Economic Evaluation Working Party. BMJ 1996;313:275-83.
22. Drummond MF, O'Brien BJ, Stoddart GL, Torrance GW. Methods for the Valuation of Health Care Programs, 2nd edition. Toronto; Oxford University Press, 1997.
23. Drummond MF, Torrance GW, Mason J. Cost-effectiveness league tables: more harm than good? Soc Sci Med 1993;37:33-40.
24. Dufour DR, Lott JA, Nolte FS, Gretch DR, Koff RS, Seeff LB. Diagnosis and Monitoring of Hepatic Injury. I. Performance characteristics of laboratory tests. Clin Chem 2000;46:2027-49.
25. Dufour DR, Lott JA, Nolte FS, Gretch DR, Koff RS, Seeff LB. Diagnosis and monitoring of hepatic injury. II. Recommendations for use of laboratory tests in screening, diagnosis, and monitoring. Clin Chem 2000;46:2050-68.
26. Eisenberg JM. Clinical economics. A guide to the economic analysis of clinical practices. JAMA 1989;262:2879-86.
27. Ellrodt G, Cook DJ, Lee J, Cho M, Hunt D, Weingarten S. Evidence-based disease management. JAMA. 1997;278:1687-92.
28. European Network of Cancer Registries at http://www.encr.com.fr (accessed on April 10, 2003).
29. Evidence-Based Medicine Working Group. Evidence-based medicine. A new approach to teaching the practice of medicine. JAMA 1992;268:2420-5.
30. Fendrick AM, Chernew ME, Hirth RA, Bloom BS. Alternative management strategies for patients with suspected peptic ulcer disease. Ann Intern Med 1995;123:260-8.
31. Field MJ, Lohr KN, eds. Clinical Practice Guidelines: directions for a new program. Washington, DC: National Academy Press, 1990: p 38.
32. Fraser CG, Petersen PH. Analytical performance characteristics should be judged against objective quality specifications. Clin Chem 1999;45:321-3.
33. Frazier AL, Colditz GA, Fuchs CS, Kuntz KM. Cost-effectiveness of screening for colorectal cancer in the general population. JAMA. 2000;284:1954-61.
34. Fryback DG, Thornbury JR. The efficacy of diagnostic imaging. Med Decis Making 1991;11:88-94.

35. Gaucher Registry at http://www.gaucherregistry.com (accessed on April 10, 2003).
36. Glasziou P, Irwig L, Bain C, Colditz G. Systematic Reviews in Health Care; a practical guide. Cambridge, UK. Cambridge University Press, 2001.
37. Glasziou P, Vanderbroucke J, Chalmers I. Assessing the quality of research. BMJ 2004;328:39-41.
38. Gray A, Raikou R, McGuire A, et al. Cost effectiveness of an intensive blood glucose control policy in patients with type 2 diabetes: economic analysis alongside randomised controlled trail (UKPDS 41). BMJ 2000;320:1373-8.
39. Grieve R, Beech R, Vincent J, Mazurkiewicz J. Near patient testing in diabetes clinics: appraising the costs and outcomes. Health Technol Ass 1999;3:1-74.
40. Guyatt G, Haynes B, Jaeschke R et al. Introduction: the philosophy of evidence-based medicine. In Guyatt G and Rennie D (editors) User's Guide to the Medical Literature. A manual for evidence-based clinical practice. JAMA and Archive Journals, American Medical Association, Chicago, 2002:3-12.
41. Guyatt GH, Haynes RB, Jaeschke RZ, Cook DJ, Green L, Naylor CD, et al. Users' Guides to the Medical Literature: XXV. Evidence-based medicine: principles for applying the Users' Guides to patient care. Evidence-Based Medicine Working Group. JAMA 2000;284:1290-6.
42. Horvath AR, Pewsner D, Egger M. Systematic reviews in laboratory medicine: potentials, principles and pitfalls. In: Price CP, Christenson RH, eds. Evidence-Based Laboratory Medicine: from principles to outcomes. Washington: AACC Press, 2003:137-58.
43. Horvath AR, Pewsner D. Systematic reviews in laboratory medicine: principles, processes and practical considerations. Clin Chim Acta 2004;342:23-39
44. Irwig L, Glasziou P. Cochrane Methods Group on Systematic Review of Screening and Diagnostic Tests: recommended methods. Updated 6 June 1996. http://www.cochrane.org/cochrane/sadtdoc1.htm (Accessed on March 15, 2003)
45. Irwig L, Macaskill P, Glasziou P, Fahey M. Meta-analytic methods for diagnostic test accuracy. J Clin Epidemiol 1995;48:119-30.
46. Irwig L, Tosteson ANA, Gatsonis C, Lau J, Colditz G, Chalmers TC, Mosteller F. Guidelines for meta-analyses evaluating diagnostic tests. Ann Intern Med 1994;120:667-76.
47. Kaplan RM, Anderson JP. A general health policy model: update and applications. Health Serv Res 1988;23:203-35.
48. Kendall J, Reeves B, Clancy M. Point of care testing: randomised, controlled trial of clinical outcome. BMJ 1998;316:1052-7.
49. Khan KS, ter Riet G, Glanville J, Sowden AJ, Kleijnen J., eds. Undertaking Systematic Reviews of Research on Effectiveness. CRD's Guidance for those Carrying Out or Commissioning Reviews. CRD Report No 4 (2nd Edition). NHS Centre for Reviews and Dissemination, University of York: York Publishing Services Ltd, March 2001.
50. Kilpatrick ES, Holding S. Use of computer terminals on wards to access emergency test results; a retrospective audit. BMJ 2001;322:1101-3.
51. Kind P. The EuroQol instrument: an index of health-related quality of life. Quality of Life and Pharmacoeconomics in Clinical Trials. Philadelphia: Lippincott-Raven, 1996:191-201.
52. Klee GG, Schryver PG, Kisabeth RM. Analytic bias specifications based on the analysis of effects on performance of medical guidelines. Scand J Clin Lab Invest 1999;59:509-12.
53. Klovning A, Sandberg S. Searching the literaure and relevant databases. In: Price CP, Christenson RH, eds. Evidence-Based Laboratory Medicine: from principles to outcomes. Washington: AACC Press, 2003:93-114.
54. Laupacis A, Feeny D, Detsky AS, Tugwell PX. How attractive does a new technology have to be to warrant adoption and utilization? Tentative guidelines for using clinical and economic evaluations. CMAJ 1992;146:473-81.
55. Leape LL, Park RE, Kahan JP, Brook RH. Group judgments of appropriateness: the effect of panel composition. Qual Assur Health Care 1992;4:151-9.
56. Lee-Lewandrowski E, Laposata M, Eschenbach K, Camooso C, Nathan DM, Godine JE, Hurxthal K, Goff J, Lewandrowski K. Utilization and cost analysis of bedside capillary glucose testing in a large teaching hospital: implications for managing point of care testing. Am J Med 1994;97:222-30.
57. Lijmer JG, Mol BW, Heisterkamp S, Bonsel GJ, Prins MH, van der Meulen JH, Bossuyt PM. Empirical evidence of design-related bias in studies of diagnostic tests. JAMA 1999;282:1061-6.
58. Lumbreras-Lacarra B, Ramos-Rincón JM, Hernández-Aguado I. Methodology in diagnostic laboratory test research in *Clinical Chemistry* and *Clinical Chemistry and Laboratory Medicine.* Clin Chem 2004;50:530-6.
59. Lundberg GD. The need for an outcomes research agenda for clinical laboratory testing. JAMA 1998;280:565-6.
60. Marshall DA, O'Brien BJ. Economic evaluation of diagnostic tests. In Price CP and Christenson RH (editors). Evidence-Based Laboratory Medicine: from principles to outcomes. AACC Press, Washington, 2003:159-86.
61. Moher D, Schulz KF, Altman DG for the CONSORT group. The CONSORT statement: revised recommendations for improving the quality of reports of parallel group randomized trials 2001. JAMA 2001;285:1987-91. Available at: http://www.consort-statement.org/revisedstatement.htm (accessed on April 22, 2004).

62. Montori V, Guyatt GH. Evidence-based medicine and the diagnostic process. In Price CP and Christenson RH (editors). Evidence-Based Laboratory Medicine: from principles to outcomes. AACC Press, Washington, 2003:1-19.
63. Moore RA. Evidence-based clinical biochemistry. Ann Clin Biochem 1997;34:3-7.
64. Muir Gray JA. Evidence-Based Healthcare: how to make health policy and management decisions. Edinburgh: Churchill Livingstone, 1997:1-270.
65. Mulrow CD. The medical review article: state of the science. Ann Intern Med 1987;106:485-8.
66. Murray RP, Leroux M, Sabga E, et al. Effect of point of care testing on length of stay in an adult emergency department. J Emer Med 1999;17:811-4.
67. Mushlin AI, Ruchlin HS, Callahan MA. Cost effectiveness of diagnostic tests. Lancet 2001;358:1353-5.
68. Ng SM, Krishnaswamy P, Morissey R, Clopton P, Fitzgerald R, Maisel AS. Ninety-minute accelerated critical pathway for chest pain evaluation. Am J Cardiol 2001;88:611-7.
69. NHS Centre for Reviews and Dissemination. http://agatha.york.ac.uk/darehp.htm (accessed on April 22, 2004).
70. O'Brien BJ, Heyland D, Richardson WS, Levine M, Drummond MF. Users' guide to the medical literature. XIII. How to use an article on economic analysis of clinical practice. B. What are the results and will they help me in caring for my patients? Evidence-Based Medicine Working Group. JAMA 1997;277:1802-6.
71. Oosterhuis WP, Bruns DE, Watine J, Sandberg S, Horvath AR. Evidence-based guidelines in laboratory medicine: principles and methods. Clin Chem 2004;50: 806-18.
72. Osheroff JA, Forsythe DE, Buchanan BG, Bankowitz RA, Blumenfeld BH, Miller RA. Physicians' information needs: analysis of questions posed during clinical teaching. Ann Intern Med 1991;114:576-81.
73. Parvin CA, Lo SF, Deuser SM, Weaver LG, Lewis LM, Scott MG. Impact of point-of-care testing on patients' length of stay in a large emergency department. Clin Chem 1996;42:711-7.
74. Perrier A, Nendaz MR, Sarasin FP, Howarth N, Bounameaux H. Cost-effectiveness analysis of diagnostic strategies for suspected pulmonary embolism including helical computed tomography. Am J Respir Crit Care Med 2003;167:39-44.
75. Price CP. Applications of the principles of evidence-based medicine to laboratory medicine. Clin Chim Acta 2003;333:147-54.
76. Price CP. Evidence-based laboratory medicine: supporting decision-making. Clin Chem 2000;46: 1041-50.
77. Reid MC, Lachs MS, Feinstein AR. Use of methodological standards in diagnostic test research. Getting better but still not good. JAMA 1995;274:645-51.
78. Richardson WS, Burdette SD. Practice corner: taking evidence in hand. Evidence-Based Medicine 2003;8:4-5.
79. Sackett DL, Haynes RB, Guyatt GH, Tugwell P. Clinical Epidemiology; a basic science for clinical medicine. Second edition. Little, Brown, Toronto, 1991:1-441.
80. Sackett DL, Haynes RB. The architecture of diagnostic research. BMJ 2002;324:539-41.
81. Sackett DL, Rosenberg WMC, Muir Gray JA, Haynes RB, Richardson WS. Evidence-based medicine: What it is and what it isn't. BMJ 1996;312:71-2.
82. Sackett DL, Straus SE. Finding and applying evidence during clinical rounds: the "evidence cart." JAMA 1998;280:1336-8.
83. Sacks DB, Bruns DE, Goldstein DE, Maclaren NK, McDonald JM, Parrott M. Guidelines and recommendations for laboratory analysis in the diagnosis and management of diabetes mellitus. Clin Chem 2002;48:436-72.
84. Schein OD, Katz J, Bass EB, Tielsch JM, Lubomski LH, Feldman MA, Petty BG, Steinberg EP. The value of routine preoperative medical testing before cataract surgery. Study of Medical Testing for Cataract Surgery. N Engl J Med 2000;342:168-75.
85. Severens JL, van der Wilt GJ. Economic evaluation of diagnostic tests. A review of published studies. Int J Technol Assess Health Care. 1999;15:480-96.
86. Shaw CD. Measuring against clinical standards. Clin Chim Acta 2003;333:115-24.
87. Shekelle PG, Ortiz E, Rhodes S, Morton SC, Eccles MP, Grimshaw JM, Woolf SH. Validity of the Agency for Healthcare Research and Quality clinical practice guidelines: how quickly do guidelines become outdated? JAMA 2001;286:1461-7.
88. Shekelle PG, Woolf SH, Eccles M, Grimshaw J. Clinical guidelines: developing guidelines. BMJ 1999;318: 593-6.
89. Sloan FA. Valuing Health Care. Cambridge, Cambridge University Press, 1995:1-273.
90. Smith BJ, Darzins PJ, Quinn M, Heller RF. Modern methods of searching the medical literature. Med J Aust 1992;157:603-11.
91. StJohn A, Price CP. Measures of outcome. In Price CP and Christenson RH (editors). Evidence-Based Laboratory Medicine: from principles to outcomes. Washington: AACC Press, 2003:55-74.
92. The Renal Association. www.renalreg.com (accessed on April 22, 2004).
93. Thompson O'Brien MA, Oxman AD, David DA, Haynes RB, Freemantle N, Harvey EL. Audit and feedback; effects on professional practice and health care outcomes (Cochrane review). In: The Cochrane Library, issue 4, 2002. Oxford: Update Software.
94. Torrance GW, Furlong W, Feeny D, Boyle M. Multi-attribute preference functions. Health Utilities Index. Pharmacoeconomics. 1995;7:503-20.

95. Update Software. http://www.update-software.com/cochrane/ (accessed on April 22, 2004).
96. van Wijk MA, van der Lei J, Mosseveld M, Bohnen AM, van Bemmel JH. Compliance of general practitioners with a guideline-based decision support system for ordering blood tests. Clin Chem 2002;48:55-60.
97. Wagner EH, Sandhu N, Newton KM, McCulloch DK, Ramsey SD, Grothaus LC. Effect of improved glycemic control on health care costs and utilization. JAMA 2001;285:182-9.

ADDITIONAL READING

Atkins D, Best D, Briss PA, Eccles M, Falck-Ytter Y, Flottorp S et al. (GRADE Working Group). Grading quality of evidence and strength of recommendations. BMJ 2004:1490.

Glasziou P, Vandenbroucke JP, Chalmers I. Assessing the quality of research. BMJ 2004;328:39-41.

CHAPTER 14

Selection and Analytical Evaluation of Methods—With Statistical Techniques

Kristian Linnet, M.D.,
*and James C. Boyd, M.D.**

The introduction of new or revised methods is a common occurrence in the clinical laboratory. Method selection and evaluation are key steps in the process of implementing new methods (Figure 14-1). A new or revised method must be selected carefully, and its performance evaluated thoroughly in the laboratory before being adopted for routine use. The establishment of a new method may also involve an evaluation of the features of the automated analyzer on which the method will be implemented.

Method evaluation in the clinical laboratory is influenced strongly by guidelines. The National Committee for Clinical Laboratory Standards (NCCLS) has published a series of consensus protocols[76-81] for clinical chemistry laboratories and manufacturers to follow when evaluating methods (see the NCCLS website http://nccls.org). The International Organization for Standardization (ISO) has also developed several documents related to method evaluation.[34-43] In addition, meeting laboratory accreditation requirements has become an important aspect in the method selection and/or evaluation process. In recent years, accrediting agencies have placed increased focus on the importance of total quality management and assessment of trueness and precision of laboratory measurements. An accompanying trend has been the emergence of an international nomenclature to standardize the terminology used for characterizing method performance. This chapter presents an overview of considerations in the method selection process, followed by sections on method evaluation and method comparison. The latter two sections focus on graphical and statistical tools that are used to aid in the method evaluation process, provide examples of the application of these tools, and summarize current terminology within the area.

*The authors gratefully acknowledge the original contributions by David D. Koch, Theodore Peters, Jr., Robert O. Kringle, and Mike Bogovich, on which portions of this chapter are based.

METHOD SELECTION

Optimal method selection involves consideration of medical, analytical performance, and practical criteria.

MEDICAL CRITERIA

The selection of appropriate methods for clinical laboratory assays is a vital part of rendering optimal patient care, and advances in patient care are frequently based upon the use of new or improved laboratory tests. Ascertainment of what is necessary clinically from a laboratory test is the first step in selecting a candidate method (Figure 14-1). Key parameters such as desired turnaround time and necessary clinical utility for an assay can often be derived by discussions between laboratorians and clinicians. When introducing new

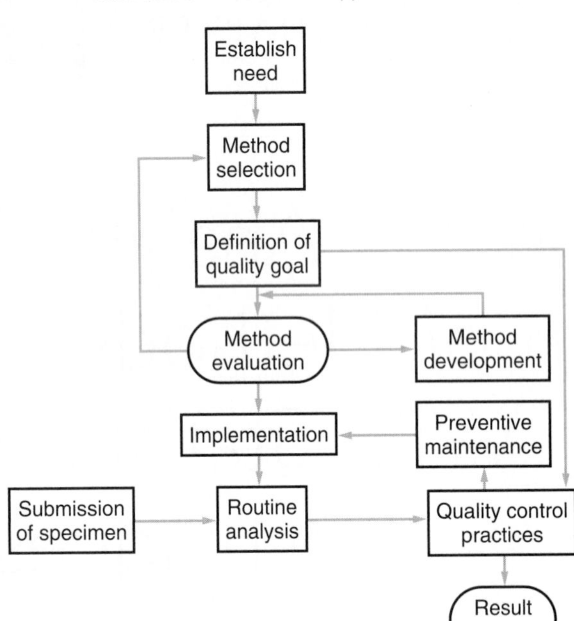

Figure 14-1 A flow diagram that illustrates the process of introducing a new method into routine use. The diagram highlights the key steps of method selection, method evaluation, and quality control.

diagnostic assays, reliable estimates of clinical sensitivity and specificity must be obtained either from the literature or by conducting a clinical outcome study (see Chapter 15). With established analytes, a common scenario is the replacement of an older, labor-intensive method with a new, automated assay that is more economical in daily use. In these situations, consideration must be given to whether the candidate method has sufficient precision, accuracy, analytical measurement range, and freedom from interference to provide clinically useful results.

Analytical Performance Criteria

In evaluation of the performance characteristics of a candidate method, precision, accuracy (trueness), analytical range, detection limit, and analytical specificity are of prime importance. The sections in this chapter on method evaluation and comparison contain a detailed outline of these concepts and their assessment. The estimated performance parameters for a method can then be related to quality goals that ensure acceptable medical use of the test results (see section on Analytical Goals). From a practical point of view, the "ruggedness" of the method in routine use is of importance. Reliable performance when used by different operators and with different batches of reagents over longer time periods is essential.

When a new clinical analyzer is included in the overall evaluation process, various instrumental parameters also require evaluation, including pipetting precision, specimen-to-specimen carryover and reagent-to-reagent carryover, detector imprecision, time to first reportable result, onboard reagent stability, overall throughput, mean time between instrument failures, and mean time to repair. Information on most of these parameters should be available from the instrument manufacturer, and the manufacturer should also be able to furnish information on what user studies to conduct in estimating these parameters for an individual analyzer.

Other Criteria

Various categories of candidate methods may be considered. New methods described in the scientific literature may require "in-house" development. Commercial kit methods, on the other hand, are ready for implementation in the laboratory, often in a "closed" analytical system on a dedicated instrument. When reviewing prospective methods, attention should be given to the following:

1. The principle of the assay, with original references
2. The detailed protocol for performing the test
3. The composition of reagents and reference materials, the quantities provided, and their storage requirements (e.g., space, temperature, light, and humidity restrictions) applicable both before and after opening the original containers
4. The stability of reagents and reference materials (e.g., their shelf life)
5. Technologist time and required skills
6. Possible hazards and appropriate safety precautions according to relevant guidelines and legislation
7. The type, quantity, and disposal of waste generated
8. Specimen requirements (i.e., conditions for collection, specimen volume requirements, the necessity for anticoagulants and preservatives, and necessary storage conditions)
9. The reference interval of the method, including information on how it was derived, typical values obtained in health and disease, and the necessity of determining a reference interval for one's own institution (see Chapter 16 for details on how to generate a reference interval)
10. Instrumental requirements and limitations
11. Cost effectiveness
12. Computer platforms and interfacing to the laboratory information system
13. The availability of technical support, supplies, and service

Other questions concerning placement of the method in the laboratory should be taken into account. Does the laboratory possess the necessary measuring equipment? If not, is there sufficient space for a new instrument? Does the projected workload match with the capacity of a new instrument? Is the test repertoire of a new instrument sufficient? What is the method and frequency of calibration? Is the staffing of the laboratory sufficient for the new technology? If training the entire staff in a new technique is required, is such training worth the possible benefit? How frequently will quality control samples be run, and what materials will be used for quality control? What approach will be used with the method for proficiency testing? What is the estimated cost of performing an assay using the proposed method, including the cost of calibrators, quality control specimens, and technologists' time?

Questions applicable to implementation of new instrumentation in a particular laboratory may also be relevant. Does the instrument on which the method is implemented satisfy local electrical safety guidelines? What are the power, water, drainage, and air-conditioning requirements of the instrument? If the instrument is large, does the floor have sufficient load-bearing capacity?

A qualitative assessment of the above factors is often made, but it is also possible to use a value scale to assign points to the various features of a method weighted according to their relative importance; the latter approach allows a more quantitative selection process. Decisions can then be made regarding the analytical methods that best fit the laboratory's requirements and that have the potential for achieving the necessary analytical quality.

TABLE 14-1 The Four-Parameter Logistic Model Expressed in Three Different Forms

Algebraic Form	Variables*	Parameters†
$y = (a - d)/[1 + (x/c)^b] + d$	(x, y)	a, b, c, d
$R = R_0 + K_c/(1 + \exp[-(a + b\log(C))])$	(C, R)	R_0, K_c, a, b
$y = y_0 + (y_¥ - y_0)(x^d)/(b + x^d)$	(x, y)	$y_0, y_¥, b, d$

*Concentration and instrument response variables shown in parentheses.
†Equivalent letters do not necessarily denote equivalent parameters.

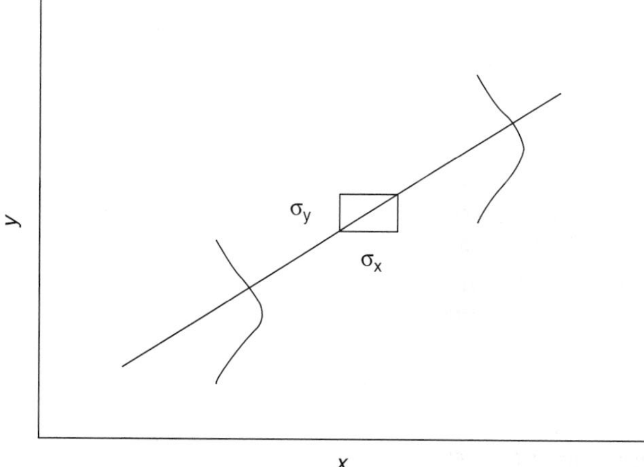

Figure 14-2 Relation between concentration (x) and signal response (y) for a linear calibration curve. The dispersion in signal response (σ_y) is projected onto the x axis giving rise to assay imprecision (σ_x).

BASIC CONCEPTS IN RELATION TO ANALYTICAL METHODS

This section defines the basic concepts used in this chapter (e.g., calibration, accuracy, precision, linearity, limit of detection, and others).

CALIBRATION

The calibration function is the relation between instrument signal (y) and concentration of analyte (x) i.e.,

$$y = f(x)$$

The inverse of this function, also called the measuring function, yields the concentration from response:

$$x = f^{-1}(y)$$

This relationship is established by measurement of samples with known amounts of analyte (calibrators).[14] One may distinguish between solutions of pure chemical standards and samples with known amounts of analyte present in the typical matrix that is to be measured (e.g., human serum). The first situation applies typically to a reference measurement procedure, which is not influenced by matrix effects, and the second case corresponds typically to a field method that often is influenced by matrix components and so preferably is calibrated using the relevant matrix.[90] Calibration functions may be linear or curved, and in the case of immunoassays often of a special form (e.g., modeled by the four-parameter logistic curve).[92] This model (logistic in log x) has been used for both radioimmunoassay and enzyme immunoassay techniques and can be written in several forms as shown (Table 14-1). Nonlinear regression analysis is applied to estimate the relationship, or a logit transformation to a linear form is carried out. An alternative, model-free approach is to estimate a smoothed spline curve, which often is performed for immunoassays. The only requirement is that there should be a monotonic relationship between signal and analyte concentration over the analytical measurement range. Otherwise the possibility of errors occurs (e.g., the hook effect in immunoassays) caused by a decreasing signal response at very high concentrations. If the assumed calibration function does not correctly reflect the true relationship between instrument response and analyte concentration, a systematic error or bias is likely to be associated with the analytical method. A common problem is deviation from linearity in the high concentration range.

The precision of the analytical method depends on the stability of the instrument response for a given amount of analyte. In principle, a random dispersion of instrument signal at a given concentration transforms into dispersion on the measurement scale as schematically shown (Figure 14-2). The detailed statistical aspects of calibration are rather complex,[95,97] but in the following, some approximate rela-

TABLE 14-2 An Overview of Qualitative Terms and Quantitative Measures Related to Method Performance

Qualitative Concept	Quantitative Measure
Trueness Closeness of agreement of mean value with "true value"	**Bias** A measure of the systematic error
Precision Repeatability (within run) Intermediate precision (long term) Reproducibility (interlaboratory)	**Imprecision (SD)** A measure of the dispersion of random errors **Error of Measurement** Comprises both random and systematic influences
Accuracy Closeness of agreement of a single measurement with "true value"	

tions are outlined. If the calibration function is linear, and the imprecision of the signal response is the same over the analytical measurement range, the analytical standard deviation (SD_A) of the method tends to be constant over the analytical measurement range (Figure 14-2). If the imprecision increases proportionally to the signal response level, the analytical SD of the method tends to increase proportionally to the concentration level (x), which means that the *relative* imprecision (coefficient of variation, $[CV] = SD/x$) is constant over the analytical measurement range—supposing that the intercept of the calibration line is zero. In the case of nonlinear calibration curves, the precision often varies over the analytical measurement range, being best at the steepest part of the calibration curve, at least if the imprecision of the signal is the same over the analytical measurement range (see also the Analytical Sensitivity section in this chapter).

In modern automated clinical chemistry instruments, the relation between analyte concentration and signal is often very stable so that calibration is necessary infrequently (e.g., at intervals of several months).[89] Built-in process control mechanisms may help ensure that the relationship remains stable and indicate when recalibration is necessary. In traditional chromatographic analysis (e.g., high-performance liquid chromatography [HPLC]), on the other hand, it is customary to calibrate each analytical series (run), which means that calibration is carried out daily. Aronson et al[2] established a detailed simulation model of the various factors influencing method performance with focus on the calibration function.

TRUENESS AND ACCURACY

Trueness of measurements is defined as closeness of agreement between the average value obtained from a large series of results of measurements and a true value.[21,37] The difference between the average value (strictly, the mathematical expectation) and the true value is the *bias,* which is expressed numerically and so is inversely related to the trueness. Trueness in itself is a qualitative term that can be expressed as, for example, low, medium, or high. From a theoretical point of view, the exact true value is not available, and instead an "accepted reference value" is considered, which is the "true" value that can be determined in practice.[21] Trueness can be evaluated by comparison of measurements by a given (field) method and a reference method. Such an evaluation may be carried out by parallel measurements of a set of patient samples or by measurements of reference materials (see traceability and uncertainty). The ISO has introduced the trueness expression as a replacement for the term "accuracy," which now has gained a slightly different meaning. *Accuracy* is the closeness of the agreement between the result of a measurement and a true concentration of the analyte.[37] Accuracy is thus influenced by both bias and imprecision and in this way reflects the total error. Accuracy, which in itself is a qualitative term, is inversely related to the "uncertainty" of measurement, which can be quantified as described later (Table 14-2).

In relation to trueness, the concepts *recovery, drift,* and *carryover* may also be considered. Recovery is the fraction or percentage increase of concentration that is measured in relation to the amount added. Recovery experiments are typically carried out in the field of drug analysis. One may distinguish between *extraction recovery,* which often is interpreted as the fraction of compound that is carried through an extraction process, and the recovery measured by the entire analytical procedure, in which the addition of an internal standard compensates for losses in the extraction procedure. A recovery close to 100% is a prerequisite for a high degree of trueness, but it does not ensure unbiased results, because possible nonspecificity against matrix components is not detected in a recovery experiment. *Drift* is caused by instrument instability over time, so that calibration becomes biased. Assay *carryover* also must be close to zero to ensure unbiased results. Drift or carryover or both may be conveniently estimated by multifactorial evaluation protocols[52] (see the NCCLS guideline EP10-A2, *Preliminary evaluation of quantitative clinical laboratory methods*).[77]

PRECISION

Precision may be defined as the closeness of agreement between independent results of measurements obtained under stipulated conditions.[21] The degree of precision is usually expressed on the basis of statistical measures of imprecision, such as the SD or CV (CV = SD/x, where x is the measurement concentration), which thus is inversely related to precision. Imprecision of measurements is solely related to the random error of measurements and has no relation to the trueness of measurements.

Precision is specified as follows[21,35]:

Repeatability: closeness of agreement between results of successive measurements carried out under the same conditions (i.e., corresponding to within-run precision).

Reproducibility: closeness of agreement between results of measurements performed under changed conditions of measurements (e.g., time, operators, calibrators, and reagent lots). Two specifications of reproducibility are often used: total or between-run precision in the laboratory, often termed *intermediate precision,* and interlaboratory precision (e.g., as observed in external quality assessment schemes [EQAS]) (see Table 14-2).

The total standard deviation (σ_T) may be split into within-run and between-run components using the principle of analysis of variance components (variance is the squared SD):[97]

$$\sigma_T^2 = \sigma_{\text{Within-run}}^2 + \sigma_{\text{Between-run}}^2$$

It is not always clear in clinical chemistry publications what is meant by "between-run" variation. Some authors use the term to refer to the total variation of an assay, whereas others apply the term between-run variance component as defined above. The distinction between these definitions is important but is not always explicitly stated.

In laboratory studies of analytical variation, it is *estimates* of imprecision that are obtained. The more observations, the more certain are the estimates. Commonly the number 20 is given as a reasonable number of observations (e.g., suggested in the NCCLS guideline on the topic).[76] To estimate both the within-run imprecision and the total imprecision, a common approach is to measure duplicate control samples in a series of runs. For example, one may measure a control in duplicate for more than 20 runs, in which case 20 observations are present with respect to both components. One may here notice that the dispersion of the means (x_m) of the duplicates is given as:

$$\sigma_{xm}^2 = \sigma_{\text{Within-run}}^2/2 + \sigma_{\text{Between-run}}^2$$

From the 20 sets of duplicates, we may derive the within-run SD using the shortcut formula:

$$\text{SD}_{\text{Within-run}}^2 = \sum d_i^2/(2 \times 20)$$

where d_i refers to the difference between the ith set of duplicates. When estimating standard deviations, the concept degrees of freedom (df) is used. In a simple situation, the number of degrees of freedom equals $N - 1$. For N duplicates, the number of degrees of freedom is $N(2 - 1) = N$. Thus both variance components are derived in this way. The advantage of this approach is that the within-run estimate is based on several runs, so that an average estimate is obtained rather than only an estimate for one particular run, if all 20 observations had been obtained in the same run. The described approach is a simple example of a *variance component analysis.* The principle can be extended to more components of variation. For example, in the NCCLS EP5-A guideline a procedure is outlined based on the assumption of two analytical runs per day, in which case within-run, between-run, and between-day components of variance are estimated by a *nested* component of variance analysis approach.[76]

There is nothing definitive about the selected number of 20. Quite generally, the estimate of the imprecision improves the more observations that are available. Exact confidence limits for the standard deviation can be derived from the χ^2 distribution. Estimates of the variance, SD^2, are distributed according to the χ^2-distribution (tabulated in most statistics textbooks): $(N-1)\text{SD}^2/\sigma^2 \sim \chi^2_{(N-1)}$, where $(N-1)$ is the degrees of freedom.[97] Then the two-sided 95% confidence interval (CI) (95% CI) is derived from the relation:

$\Pr(\chi^2_{97.5\%(N-1)} < (N-1)\text{SD}^2/\sigma^2 < \chi^2_{2.5\%(N-1)}) = 0.95$

which yields the 95% CI expression:

$$\text{SD} \times \left((N-1)/\chi^2_{2.5\%(N-1)}\right)^{0.5} < \sigma < \text{SD} \times \left((N-1)/\chi^2_{97.5\%(N-1)}\right)^{0.5}$$

Example

Suppose we have estimated the imprecision to an SD of 5.0 on the basis of $N = 20$ observations. From a table of the χ^2-distribution, we get the 2.5 and 97.5 percentiles:

$$\chi^2_{2.5\%(19)} = 32.9 \text{ and } \chi^2_{97.5\%(19)} = 8.91$$

where 19 in the parenthesis refers to the number of degrees of freedom. Substituting in the equation, we get:

$$5.0 \times (19/32.9)^{0.5} < \sigma < 5.0 \times (19/8.91)^{0.5}$$

or $3.8 < \sigma < 7.3$.

For reasonable values of N, approximate limits can be derived from the normal approximation[45] of the distribution of the SD being based on the expression of the standard error of σ equal to $[\sigma^2/(2(N-1))]^{0.5}$. Using the normal approximation, the interval equals $5 \pm t_{19}[5^2/(2(20-1))]^{0.5}$, which corresponds to $5 \pm 2.093 \times 0.81 = 3.30 - 6.7$. Thus at the sample size of 20, the approximation is not so good because of the asymmetric distribution of the SD. For a sample size of 50, the approximate interval can be calculated to 4.0 to 6.0, which is a somewhat better approximation of the exact interval of 4.2 to 6.25. Quite generally, it is observed that the uncertainty of the estimated SD is considerable at moderate sample sizes. In Table 14-3 factors corresponding to the 95% CI are given as a function of sample size for simple SD estimation according to the χ^2-distribution. These factors provide guidance on the validity of estimated SDs for

TABLE 14-3 Factors Corresponding to 95% CI Limits for an SD. The number of degrees of freedom is N – 1.

N	95% CI Lower	95% CI Upper
20	0.760	1.460
30	0.797	1.346
40	0.819	1.283
50	0.835	1.243
60	0.848	1.217
70	0.857	1.198
80	0.865	1.183
90	0.872	1.171
100	0.878	1.161
150	0.898	1.128
200	0.911	1.109
250	0.919	1.096
300	0.926	1.087

precision. For individual variance components, the relations are more complicated.

Precision Profile

Precision often depends on the concentration of analyte being considered. A presentation of the precision as a function of analyte concentration is the precision profile, which is usually plotted in terms of the SD or the CV as a function of analyte concentration (Figure 14-3, *A-C*). Some typical examples may be considered. First, the SD may be constant (i.e., independent of the concentration), as it often is for analytes with a limited range of values (e.g., electrolytes). When the SD is constant, the CV varies inversely with the concentration (i.e., it is high in the lower part of the range and low in the high range). For analytes with extended ranges (e.g., hormones), the SD frequently increases as the analyte concentration increases. If a proportional relationship exists, the CV is constant. This may often apply approximately over a large part of the analytical measurement range. Actually, this relationship is anticipated for measurement error arising because of imprecise volume dispensing. Often a more complex relationship exists. Not infrequently, the SD is relatively constant in the low range so that the CV increases in the area approaching the detection limit. At intermediate concentrations, the CV may be relatively constant and perhaps decline somewhat at increasing concentrations. A square root relationship may model the relationship in some situations as an intermediate form of relation between the constant and the proportional case. A constant SD in the low range can be modeled by truncating the assumed proportional or square root relationship at higher concentrations. The relationship between the SD and the concentration is of importance when considering the method specifications over the analytical measurement range, and in the context of selecting appropriate statistical methods for method comparison (e.g., whether a difference or relative difference plot should be applied or whether a simple or a weighted regression analysis procedure should be used) (see the sections entitled "Relative Distribution of Differences Plot" and "Regression Analysis" later in this chapter).

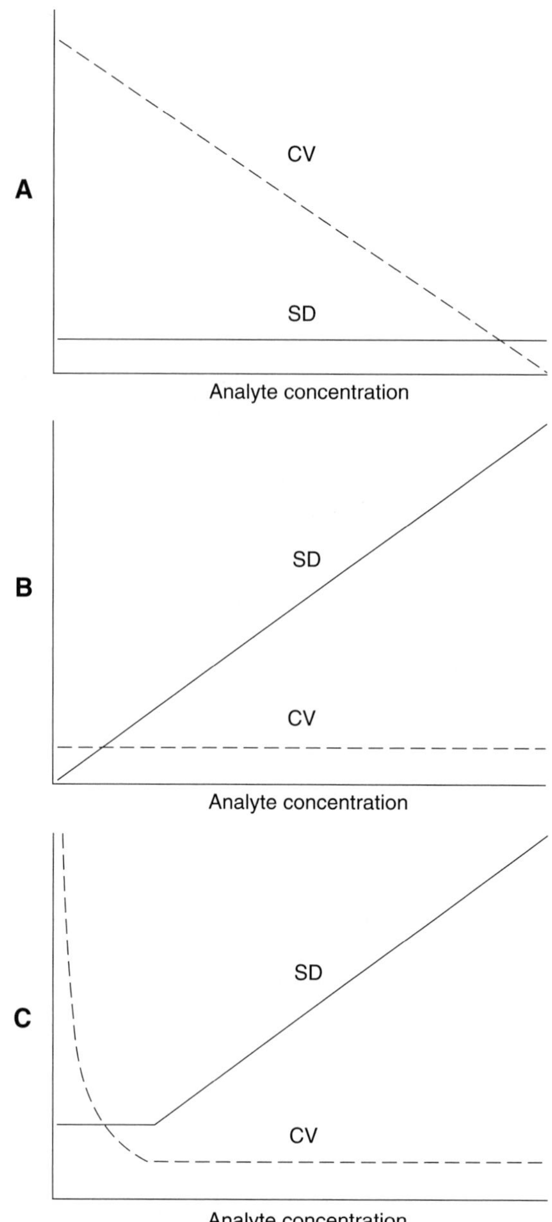

Figure 14-3 Relations between analyte concentration and SD/CV. **A,** The SD is constant so that the CV varies inversely with the analyte concentration. **B,** The CV is constant because of a proportional relationship between concentration and SD. **C,** Illustrates a mixed situation with constant SD in the low range and a proportional relationship in the rest of the analytical measurement range.

LINEARITY

Linearity refers to the relationship between measured and expected values over the analytical measurement range. Linearity may be considered in relation to actual or relative analyte concentrations. In the latter case, a dilution series of a sample may be studied. This is often carried out for immunoassays, in which case it is investigated whether the measured concentration declines as expected according to the dilution factor. Dilution is usually carried out with the appropriate sample matrix (e.g., human serum [individual or pooled serum]).

The evaluation of linearity may be carried out in various ways. A simple, but subjective, approach is to visually assess whether the relationship between measured and expected concentration is linear or not. A more formal evaluation may be carried out on the basis of statistical tests. Various principles may be applied here. When repeated measurements are available at each concentration, the random variation between measurements and the variation around an estimated regression line may be evaluated statistically (by an *F*-test).[31] This approach has been criticized because it only relates the magnitudes of random and systematic error without taking the absolute deviations from linearity into account. For example, if the random variation among the measurements is large, a given deviation from linearity may not be declared statistically significant. On the other hand, if the random measurement variation is small, even a very small deviation from linearity that may be clinically unimportant is declared significant. When significant nonlinearity is found, it may be useful to explore nonlinear alternatives to the linear regression line (i.e., polynomials of higher degrees).[24,51]

Another commonly applied approach for detecting nonlinearity is to assess the residuals of an estimated regression line and test for whether positive and negative deviations are randomly distributed. This can be carried out by a runs test[20] (see regression analysis section). An additional consideration for evaluating dilution curves that should be considered is whether an estimated regression line passes through zero or not. Furthermore, testing for linearity is related to assessment of trueness over the analytical measurement range. The presence of linearity is a prerequisite for a high degree of trueness. A NCCLS guideline suggests procedure(s) for assessment of linearity.[79]

ANALYTICAL MEASUREMENT RANGE

The analytical measurement range (measuring interval, reportable range) is the analyte concentration range over which the measurements are within the declared tolerances for imprecision and bias of the method.[21] In practice, the upper limit is often set by the linearity limit of the instrument response and the lower limit corresponds to the lower limit of quantitation (LoQ—see below). Usually, it is presumed that the specifications of the method apply throughout the analytical measurement range. However, there may also be situations in which different specifications are applied to various segments of the analytical measurement range. One should also be aware of whether the SD or the CV is specified within certain limits over the analytical measurement range (see Precision Profile, p. 358).

LIMIT OF DETECTION

The limit of detection (LoD) is medically important for many analytes, especially hormones. The first generation hormone assay frequently has a high LoD, rendering the low results medically useless. Thyroid stimulating hormone (TSH) is a good example. As the assay methods improved, lowering the LoD, low TSH results could be distinguished from the lower limit of the reference interval, making the test useful for the diagnosis of hyperthyroidism.

Concepts

Conventionally the limit of detection often has been defined as the lowest value that significantly exceeds the measurements of a blank sample. Thus the limit has been estimated on the basis of repeated measurements of a blank sample and reported as the mean plus 2 or 3 SDs of the blank measurements. Some problems exist with this conventional approach, and the ISO has recently recommended a formal procedure for estimation of the LoD that is more complicated.[38,41] Therefore the LoD concept is treated in depth in the present exposition to introduce the suggested concepts. First, the distribution of blank values is often asymmetric, making the application of parametric statistics inappropriate (Figure 14-4, *A*). Second, repeated measurements of a sample with a true concentration exactly equal to the limit of statistical significance for blank measurements will yield a distribution with 50% of values below and 50% exceeding the limit because of random measurement error (Figure 14-4, *A*). Only if the true concentration of the sample is higher than the significance limit can one be sure that a measured value will exceed the limit with a probability higher than 50% (Figure 14-4, *B*). In a statistical sense, one should take into account not only the Type I error (the significance test) but also the Type II error, the error of not detecting the presence of analyte that indeed is present.

Given an asymmetric distribution of blank values and applying a significance level (alpha) of 5% (Figure 14-4, *A*), the most straightforward procedure for estimation of the significance limit is to apply a nonparametric principle based on the ordered values for estimation of the 95th percentile. Having ranked N_B values according to size, the 95 percentile may be estimated as the value of the $(N(95/100) + 0.5)$ ordered observation.[15,70,71] In case of a noninteger value, interpolation is carried out between neighbor values (see example). The limiting percentile (Perc) of the blank distribution, which cuts off the percentage α in the upper tail of the distribution, will in the following be called the limit of blank (LoB)

$$\mathrm{LoB} = \mathrm{Perc}_{100-\alpha}$$

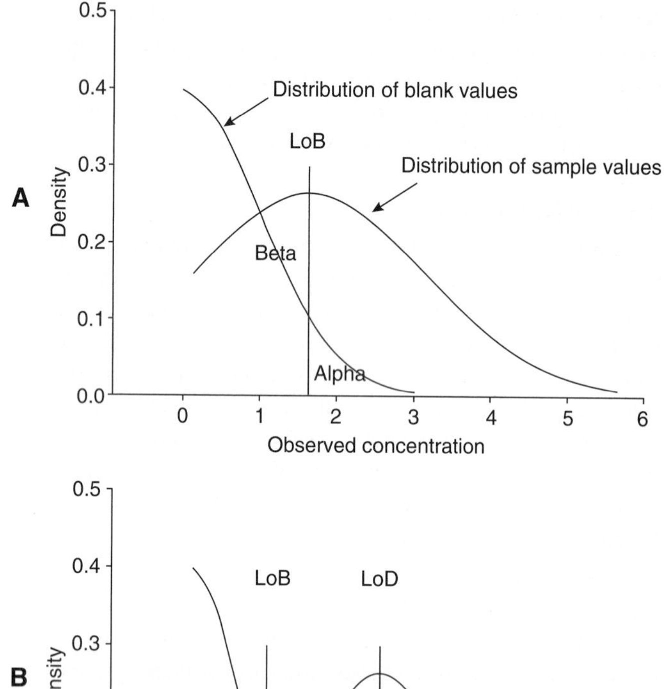

Figure 14-4 Outline of the distribution of blank values, which is truncated at zero, and the distribution of sample values. **A,** When the true sample concentration equals LoB, 50% of the measurements exceed LoB. **B,** At a true sample concentration equal to LoD, (100% – β) (here 95%) of the sample measurements exceed LoB.

To address the Type II error level, one has to consider the minimum sample concentration that provides measured concentration values exceeding LoB with a specified probability. If the Type II error level β is set to 5%, 95% of the measurements should exceed LoB (Figure 14-4, *B*). Usually the sample distribution is Gaussian, and in this case the 5th percentile of the distribution can be estimated from the mean and standard deviation as:

$$x_{mS} - 1.65\,SD_S$$

where x_{mS} and SD_S are the mean and standard deviation of the sample measurements, respectively. Overall, we have:

$$LoD = LoB + 1.65\,SD_S$$

In case the sample distribution is not normal, the 5 percentile of the sample distribution can be estimated nonparametrically in the same way as the LoB. However, parametric estimation is more efficient and should be used when possible.

It is important to realize the exact meaning of the LoD. The LoD expresses a *capability* of the method and should not be used for direct comparison with actually measured sample values. These should be related to the LoB.

Characteristics of Blank and Sample

The blank sample(s) should be as similar as possible to the natural patient samples (e.g., for a drug assay it might be a serum or plasma sample free of drug and not just a buffer solution). To ensure that the measurements are representative, compilation of measurements on a number of blank samples might be preferable. Thus instead of only repeatedly measuring one particular serum sample, a set of 5 to 10 or more blank serum samples would be preferable, because matrix differences exist from sample to sample. For endogenous compounds, it might be samples stripped by the component (e.g., by precipitation using an antibody), by enzymatic degradation, or by adsorption to charcoal. In relation to hormones, blank samples may in some cases be provided from diseased subjects or subjects with suppressed concentrations caused by pharmacological treatment. Concerning tumor markers, samples from nondiseased subjects may be appropriate.

With regard to the sample(s) with low analyte concentration, one may preferably spike a set of serum samples from various patients with the analyte (e.g., a drug), rather than just one serum sample or a serum pool. For endogenous compounds, ideally a set of patient samples with concentrations in the low range might be used. A pooled SD_S estimate can then be derived from repeated measurements of the set of samples (e.g., 10 measurements of each of 10 samples [see the example presented later in this chapter]). Measurements on different days should be carried out, so that SD_S reflects the total analytical variation.

Reporting of Results

In a laboratory, the LoB may be used to decide whether to report patients' results as "detected" or "not detected." Not detected (i.e., a result below LoB) means that the *true* concentration is less than the LoD with 100 – β percent assurance where β is the Type II error level, which often is set to 5%. Thus a result less than LoB should be reported as "less than LoD" and not as "less than LoB" or "zero." A result exceeding LoB (i.e., "detected") means that the true concentration exceeds *zero* with 100 – α percent assurance (where α is the Type I error level), and the reporting could be "greater than zero" or "detected." Results at or exceeding the LoQ (see below) are reported as quantitative results.

A modification of the above-mentioned principles for reporting of results might be considered in case the results are going to be used in scientific studies. Here, unbiased results for groups of subjects being investigated are obtained by reporting the actual measured concentrations irrespective of whether the values are below or above the LoB threshold. Otherwise, biased results may be obtained for the groups.

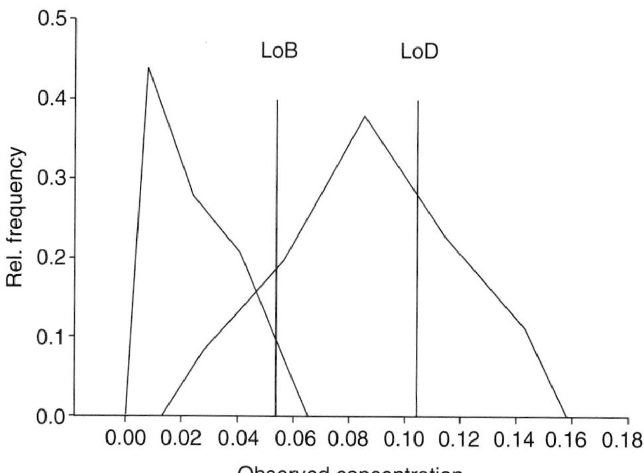

Figure 14-5 Recorded distributions of 100 blank and 100 sample values for the hypothetical hormone example. The estimated LoB (= 95th percentile of the distribution of blank values) and the estimated LoD are indicated. SD_S was derived from the distribution of sample values (actually as a pooled estimate of sets of 10 measurements that are here merged together).

An Example of Estimating the LoD of an Assay

We consider here a hypothetical hormone assay, for which the manufacturer or a research laboratory wants to estimate the LoD. The default values $\alpha = \beta = 5\%$ are used. It is supposed that the manufacturer has 10 samples available from patients lacking the hormone because of disease or pharmacological suppression. Ten measurements of each blank sample are performed on 10 different days to ensure that the total assay variation is reflected. Only nonnegative values are provided by the assay, and the distribution of the 100 blank measurements is skew (Figure 14-5). Thus LoB is estimated nonparametrically as the 95th percentile of the measurement distribution. The 95th percentile corresponds to the 95.5 ordered observation (= 100 × (95/100) + 0.5). The 95 and 96 observations have the values 0.0539 and 0.0548 U/L, respectively. Linear interpolation between the 95 and 96 observations yields an LoB estimate of 0.0544 U/L (= 0.0539 + 0.5 × (0.0548 − 0.0539)).

Samples with low concentrations are obtained from patients. We suppose here that one sample is obtained from each of 10 patients, and that each sample is assayed 10 times (Figure 14-5). A pooled estimate of the SD_S was computed (in this case the square root of the average of the variances—a more general computation procedure is available on this book's accompanying Evolve site, found at http://evolve.elsevier.com/Tietz/textbook/). An estimate of the LoD is then obtained

$$\begin{aligned} \text{LoD} &= \text{LoB} + 1.65\,SD_S = 0.0544 + 1.65 \times 0.0299 \\ &= 0.104\,\text{U/L} \end{aligned}$$

This is a point estimate, and the real LoD may be slightly lower or higher. It is possible to derive a CI as described by Linnet and Kondratovich.[71]

Analytical Sensitivity

The detection limit of a method should not be confused with the so-called analytical sensitivity. Analytical sensitivity is the ability of an analytical method to assess small variations of the concentration of analyte.[14] This is often expressed as the slope of the calibration curve.[21] However, in addition to the slope of the calibration function, the random variation of the calibration function should also be taken into account. In point of fact, the analytical sensitivity depends on the ratio between the SD of the calibration function and the slope. As mentioned previously, the smaller the random variation of the instrument response and the steeper the slope, the higher is the ability to distinguish small differences of analyte concentrations. In reality, analytical sensitivity depends on the precision of the method. Historically the meaning of the term analytical sensitivity has been the subject of much discussion.

Limit of Quantitation

The relative uncertainty of measurements at or just exceeding the LoD may be large, and often a quantitative result is not reported. The lower limit for reporting quantitative results, the limit of quantitation (LoQ), relates to the total error being considered acceptable for an assay. From a precision profile for the assay and an evaluation of the bias in the low range, LoQ may be determined in relation to specifications of the method. For example, a laboratory may specify that the total error (e.g., expressed here as Bias + 2 SD) of an assay is lower than 45% (corresponding to a bias of 15% and a CV of 15%) of the measurement concentration.[14,108] In this case, the LoQ is the lowest assay value at which this specification is fulfilled. LoQ constitutes the lowest limit of the reportable range for quantitative results of an assay.

Analytical Specificity and Interference

The analytical specificity is the ability of an assay procedure to determine specifically the concentration of the target analyte in the presence of potentially interfering substances or factors in the sample matrix (e.g., hyperlipemia, hemolysis, bilirubin, anticoagulants, antibodies, and degradation products). For example, in the context of a drug assay, specificity is of relevance in relation to drug metabolites. The interference from hyperlipemia, hemolysis, and bilirubin is generally concentration dependent, and can be quantitated as a function of the concentration of interfering compound.[29] A detailed protocol for evaluation of interference has been published by NCCLS.[80]

In relation to immunoassays, interference from proteins (usually antibodies) should be recognized. Ismail et al[44] found in a survey comprising more than 5000 TSH results that interference occurred in 0.5% of the samples, leading to incorrect results that in a majority of the cases could have changed the treatment. Rotmensch and Cole[94] described 12 patients in whom a diagnosis of postgestational choriocarcinoma was made based on false-positive test results for human chorionic gonadotropin (hCG). Most of these patients were subjected to unnecessary surgery or chemotherapy. In each case, the false-positive result traced to the presence of heterophilic antibodies that interfered with the immunoassay for hCG. Marks[74] found that almost 10% of immunoassay results from patients with autoimmune disease were erroneous. In many cases, addition of heterophilic antibody blocking reagent or the study of dilution curves or both may help clarify suspected false-positive immunoassay results. Such limitations in the results of immunoassays should be directly communicated to clinicians.

ANALYTICAL GOALS

Setting goals for analytical quality can be based on various principles. A hierarchy has been suggested on the basis of a consensus conference on the subject[86] (Table 14-4). The top level of the hierarchy specifies goals on the basis of the clinical outcome in specific clinical settings, which is a logical principle. For example, one may consider the impact of analytical quality on the error rates of diagnostic or risk classifications.[47,84] A supplementary approach is to study the impact of imprecision and bias on clinical outcome on the basis of a simulation model as described by Boyd and Bruns.[8] For a given analyte, a series of specific clinical settings may then be evaluated, and in principle, the most demanding specification then becomes the goal, at least for a general laboratory serving various clinical applications.

Analytical goals related to biological variation have attracted considerable interest. Originally, focus was on imprecision, and Cotlove et al[13] suggested that the analytical SD (σ_A) should be less than half the intraindividual biological variation, $\sigma_{Within\text{-}B}$. The rationale for this relation is the principle of adding variances. If a subject is undergoing monitoring of an analyte, the random variation from measurement to measurement consists of both analytical and biological components of variation. The total SD for the random variation during monitoring then is determined by the relation

$$\sigma_T^2 = \sigma_{Within\text{-}B}^2 + \sigma_A^2$$

where the biological component includes the preanalytical variation. If σ_A is equal to or less than half the $\sigma_{Within\text{-}B}$ value, σ_T only exceeds $\sigma_{Within\text{-}B}$ by less than 12%. Thus if this relation holds true, analytical imprecision only adds limited random noise in a monitoring situation, and the relationship may be called a *desirable* relation. Alternatively, Fraser et al[27] considered grading of the relationship with additional specifications corresponding to an *optimum* relation ($\sigma_A = 0.25\ \sigma_{Within\text{-}B}$) yielding only 3% additional noise and a *minimum* relation corresponding to 25% additional variation ($\sigma_A = 0.75\ \sigma_{Within\text{-}B}$).[27,28]

In addition to imprecision, goals for bias should also be considered. Gowans et al[30] related the allowable bias to the width of the reference interval, which is determined by the combined within- and between-subject biological variation in addition to the analytical variation. On the basis of considerations concerning the included percentage in an interval in the presence of analytical bias, it was suggested that:

$$\text{Bias} < 0.25\left(\sigma_{Within\text{-}B}^2 + \sigma_{Between\text{-}B}^2\right)^{0.5}$$

where $\sigma_{Between\text{-}B}$ is the between-subject biological standard deviation component.

Thus the bias should *desirably* be less than a fourth of the combined biological standard deviation. One may further extend the suggested relationships to comprise an optimum relation corresponding to a factor 0.125 and a minimum relation with a factor 0.375. Given a normal distribution of reference values, the desirable relationship corresponds to maximum deviations for proportions outside the interval from the expected 2.5% at each side to 1.4% and 4.4%. This gives an overall deviation of 0.8% from the expected total of 5%, corresponding to a relative deviation of 16%, which may be considered acceptable.[28]

Other widely used principles are to relate goals to limits set by regulatory bodies (e.g., Clinical Laboratory Improvements Amendments [CLIA])[104] or professional bodies (e.g., the bias goal of 3% for serum cholesterol [originally 5%]) set by the National Cholesterol Education Program.[75] Table 14-5 provides an overview of analytical goals for important analytes. The goals are given in concentration units using decision levels or critical concentrations (x_c). The decision concentrations are limits of reference or therapeutic intervals or originate from Barnett.[3] Burnett and Westgard[9] have suggested that the analytical CV for a method should not exceed one fourth of CLIA limits so as to include the possibility of

TABLE 14-4 Hierarchy of Procedures for Setting Analytical Quality Specifications for Laboratory Methods

I	Evaluation of the effect of analytical performance on clinical outcomes in specific clinical settings
II	Evaluation of the effect of analytical performance on clinical decisions in general:
	A. Data based on components of biological variation
	B. Data based on analysis of clinicians' opinions
III	Published professional recommendations
	A. From national and international expert bodies
	B. From expert local groups or individuals
IV	Performance goals set by
	A. Regulatory bodies (e.g., CLIA)
	B. Organizers of EQA schemes
V	Goals based on the current state of the art
	A. Data from EQA/proficiency testing scheme
	B. Data from current publications on methodology

unstable method performance and the use of cost-effective quality control procedures. Ricos et al[91] have published a comprehensive listing of data on biological variation with a database that is available on the internet (Ricos et al, Biological Variation Database, www.westgard.com/guest17.htm, accessed August, 2003).

Qualitative Methods

Qualitative methods, which currently are gaining increasing use in the form of point-of-care testing (POCT), are designed to distinguish between results below or above a predefined cut-off value. Notice that the cut-off point should not be confused with the detection limit. These tests are primarily assessed on the basis of their ability to correctly classify results in relation to the cut-off value.

Performance Measures

The probability of classifying a result as positive (exceeding the cutoff), in case the true value indeed exceeds the cutoff, is called the clinical sensitivity. Classifying a result as negative (below the cutoff), in case the true value indeed is below

TABLE 14-5 Analytical Goals

Analyte	Decision Level, x_c	Acceptable Performance, CLIA '88[104]	Precision Goals (Maximum SD)		Fixed-Limit Goals (Maximum Total Error) CLIA '88
			x_c × CLIA/4	Fraser[a]	
Routine Chemistry					
Alanine aminotransferase[b]	50 U/L	20%	2.5	6.1	10
Albumin	3.5 g/dL	10%	0.09	0.06	0.35
Alkaline phosphatase	150 U/L	30%	11	4.8	45
Amylase	100 U/L	30%	7.5	4.8	30
Aspartate aminotransferase[b]	30 U/L	20%	1.5	1.8	6.0
Bicarbonate	20 mmol/L			0.46[c]	
	30 mmol/L			0.69[c]	
Bilirubin, total[b]	1.0 mg/dL	0.4	0.10	0.13	0.40
	20 mg/dL	20%	1.0	2.6	4.0
Blood gas, PCO_2	35 mm Hg	5 mm Hg	1.3	0.84	5.0
	50 mm Hg	5 mm Hg	1.3	1.2	5.0
Blood gas, PO_2	30 mm Hg	3 SD[d]	0.75 SD[d]		3 SD[d]
	80 mm Hg	3 SD	0.75 SD		3 SD
	195 mm Hg	3 SD	0.75 SD		3 SD
Blood gas, pH	7.35	0.04	0.01	0.01[e]	0.04
	7.45	0.04	0.01	0.01[e]	0.04
Calcium, total[b]	7.0 mg/dL	1.0	0.25	0.07	1.0
	10.8 mg/dL	1.0	0.25	0.11	1.0
	13.0 mg/dL	1.0	0.25	0.13	1.0
Chloride[b]	90 mmol/L	5.0%	1.1	0.54	4.5
	110 mmol/L	5.0%	1.4	0.66	5.5
Cholesterol, total[b]	200 mg/dL	10%	5.0	6.0	20
Cholesterol, high-density lipoprotein	35 mg/dL	30%	2.6	1.3	10.5
	65 mg/dL	30%	4.9	2.3	19.5
Creatine kinase[b]	200 U/L	30%	15	23	60
Creatine kinase, MB isoenzyme	13 μg/L	3 SD	0.75 SD	1.2	3 SD
Creatinine	1.0 mg/dL	0.30	0.08	0.02	0.30
	3.0 mg/dL	15%	0.11	0.07	0.45

CLIA, Clinical Laboratory Improvements Amendments.

[a]Goal calculated from one half the intraindividual biological variation data given by Fraser in ref. 28 or as demarcated.

[b]Reference method/material credentialed by the National Reference System for Clinical Laboratories.

[c]Fraser CG. Biological variation in clinical chemistry. An update: Collated data, 1988-1991. Arch Pathol Lab Med 1992;116:916-923.

[d]SD limits are based on peer group data from the Proficiency Testing program used.

[e]Fraser CG. Generation and application of analytical goals in laboratory medicine. Annali dell' Instituto Superiore di Sanita 1991;27:369-376.

Continued.

TABLE 14-5 Analytical Goals—*Continued*

Analyte	Decision Level, x_c	Acceptable Performance, CLIA '88[104]	Precision Goals (Maximum SD)		Fixed-Limit Goals (Maximum Total Error) CLIA '88
			x_c × CLIA/4	Fraser[a]	
Routine Chemistry—Cont'd					
Glucose[b]	50 mg/dL	6.0	1.5	1.7	6.0
	126 mg/dL	10%	3.15	4.2	12.6
	200 mg/dL	10%	5.0	6.6	20
Iron	150 µg/dL	20%	7.5	20	30
Lactate dehydrogenase	300 U/L	20%	15	13	60
Lactate dehydrogenase isoenzymes	100 U/L	30%	7.5	3.8	30
Magnesium	2.0 mg/dL	25%	0.13	0.04	0.50
Phosphate, inorganic	4.5 mg/dL			0.19	
Potassium[b]	3.0 mmol/L	0.50	0.13	0.07	0.50
	6.0 mmol/L	0.50	0.13	0.14	0.50
Protein, total[b]	7.0 g/dL	10%	0.18	0.10	0.70
Sodium[b]	130 mmol/L	4.0	1.0	0.52	4.0
	150 mmol/L	4.0	1.0	0.60	4.0
Triglycerides	160 mg/dL	25%	1	17	40
Urea nitrogen[b]	27.0 mg/dL	9%	0.6	1.7	2.4
Uric acid	6.0 mg/dL	17%	0.25	0.26	1.02
Endocrinology and Related Markers					
11-Deoxycortisol	8.0 µg/L			0.86[f]	
17-OH Progesterone	0.5 µg/L			0.073[c]	
Aldosterone	15 ng/dL			2.2	
	30 ng/dL			4.4	
Androstenedione	260 ng/dL			15	
CA 15-3	25 U/mL			0.73	
CA 125	35 U/mL			2.4	
CA 549	11 U/mL			0.5	
Carcinoembryonic antigen	5 ng/mL			0.23	
Chorionic gonadotropin	25 IU/L	3 SD	0.75 SD		
	10,000 IU/L	3 SD	0.75 SD		
Cortisol	5 µg/dL	25%	0.31	0.53	1.25
	30 µg/dL	25%	1.88	3.15	7.5
C-peptide	37 µg/L			1.7	
Dehydroepiandrosterone sulfate	2000 µg/L			34	
	4500 µg/L			77	
Estradiol	60 ng/L			6.8	
	450 ng/L			51	
Follicle-stimulating hormone	10 U/L			0.51	
	95 U/L			4.8	
Luteinizing hormone	6 U/L			0.44	
	55 U/L			4.0	
Prolactin	15 µg/L			0.53[c]	
	200 µg/L			7.0[c]	
Prostate-specific antigen	2 µg/L			0.14	
T_3 uptake	25%	3 SD	0.75 SD		3 SD

[f]Fraser CG, Peterson PH, Ricos C, Haeckel R. Quality specifications. *In:* Evaluation Methods in Laboratory Medicine. R. Haeckel, Ed. New York, VCH Publishers, 1993, pp. 87-99.

TABLE 14-5 Analytical Goals—*Continued*

Analyte	Decision Level, x_c	Acceptable Performance, CLIA '88[104]	Precision Goals (Maximum SD)		Fixed-Limit Goals (Maximum Total Error) CLIA '88
			$x_c \times$ CLIA/4	Fraser[a]	
Endocrinology and Related Markers—Cont'd					
Testosterone	90 ng/dL			4.0	
	1000 ng/dL			44	
Thyroid-stimulating hormone	0.3 mIU/L	3 SD	0.75 SD	0.030	3 SD
	5.0 mIU/L	3 SD	0.75 SD	0.50	3 SD
Thyroxine, free	0.8 ng/dL	3 SD	0.75 SD	0.023[c]	3 SD
	4.0 ng/dL	3 SD	0.75 SD	0.11[c]	3 SD
Thyroxine, total	3.0 μg/dL	1.0	0.25	0.09	1.0
	13 μg/dL	20%	0.65	0.39	2.6
Transferrin	375 mg/dL			5.6	
Triiodothyronine	80 ng/dL	3 SD	0.75 SD	3.5	3 SD
	200 ng/dL	3 SD	0.75 SD	8.8	3 SD
Toxicology and Therapeutic Drug Monitoring					
Alcohol, blood	0.10 g/dL	25%	0.006		0.025
Carbamazepine	8 mg/L	25%	0.50	0.51[f]	2.0
	12 mg/L	25%	0.75	0.77[f]	3.0
Digoxin	0.8 μg/L	0.20	0.05	0.03[f]	0.20
	2.0 μg/L	20%	0.10	0.08[f]	0.40
Ethosuximide	40 mg/L	20%	2.0	2.0[g]	8.0
	100 mg/L	20%	5.0	4.9[g]	20.0
Gentamicin	10 mg/L	25%	0.6		2.5
Lead, blood	10 μg/dL	4.0	1.0		4.0
	40 μg/dL	4.0	1.0		4.0
Lithium	0.5 mmol/L	0.3	0.08	0.02[f]	0.3
	1.5 mmol/L	20%	0.08	0.06[f]	0.3
Phenobarbital	15 mg/L	20%	0.75	0.33[f]	3.0
	40 mg/L	20%	2.0	0.88[f]	8.0
Phenytoin	10 mg/L	25%	0.6	0.36[f]	2.5
	20 mg/L	25%	1.2	0.72[f]	5.0
Primidone	5 mg/L	25%	0.3	0.56[g]	1.3
	12 mg/L	25%	0.75	1.36[g]	3.0
Procainamide	4 mg/L	25%	0.25		1.0
	20 mg/L	25%	1.25		5.0
Quinidine	7 mg/L	25%	0.45		1.8
Theophylline	10 mg/L	25%	0.63	1.1[f]	2.5
	20 mg/L	25%	1.2	2.2[f]	5.0
Valproate	50 mg/L	25%	3.1	3.2[f]	12.5
	100 mg/L	25%	6.2	6.4[f]	25
Hematology					
Cell identification		90% consensus			
Erythrocyte count	4.5 M/μL	6%	0.07	0.07	0.27
	5.9 M/μL	6%	0.09	0.09	0.35
Fibrinogen	150 mg/dL	20%	7.5	8	30
Hematocrit	35%	6%	0.53%	0.49%	2.1%
	50%	6%	0.75%	0.70%	3.0%

INR, International Normalized Ratio.

[g]Fraser CG. Desirable standards of performance for therapeutic drug monitoring. Clin Chem 1987;33:387-389.

Continued.

TABLE 14-5 Analytical Goals—*Continued*

Analyte	Decision Level, x_c	Acceptable Performance, CLIA '88[104]	Precision Goals (Maximum SD)		Fixed-Limit Goals (Maximum Total Error) CLIA '88
			x_c × CLIA/4	Fraser[a]	
Hematology—Cont'd					
Hemoglobin	12 g/dL	7%	0.21	0.17	0.84
	17 g/dL	7%	0.30	0.24	1.19
Leukocyte count	3.5 k/μL	15%	0.13	0.19	0.52
	11 k/μL	15%	0.41	0.58	1.65
Partial thromboplastin time	40 s	15%	1.5		6.0
Platelet count	50 k/μL	25%	3.12	2.3	12.5
	500 k/μL	25%	31.2	23	125
Prothrombin time	INR 3.6	15%	INR 0.14		INR 0.54
White cell differentiation		3 SD			3 SD
Immunology					
Alpha$_1$- antitrypsin	80 mg/dL	3 SD	0.75 SD		3 SD
Alpha-fetoprotein	10 μg/L	3 SD	0.75 SD		3 SD
Antinuclear antibody		2 Titers or ±	1 Titer		
Antistreptolysin O		2 Titers or ±	1 Titer		
Antihuman immunodeficiency virus		R/N	R/N		
Complement C3	100 mg/dL	3 SD	0.75 SD	2.6	3 SD
Complement C4	20 mg/dL	3 SD	0.75 SD	0.9	3 SD
Hepatitis (HB_sAg, anti-HB_c, HB_eAg)		R/N	R/N		
IgA	400 mg/dL	3 SD	0.75 SD	10	3 SD
IgE	200 IU/mL	3 SD	0.75 SD		3 SD
IgG	500 mg/dL	25%	31	12	125
	2000 mg/dL	25%	125	46	500
IgM	300 mg/dL	3 SD	0.75 SD	9.0	3 SD
Infectious mononucleosis		2 Titers or ±	1 Titer		
Rheumatoid factor		2 Titers or ±	1 Titer		
Rubella		2 Titers or ±	1 Titer		

R/N, Reactive/nonreactive.

the cutoff, is termed the clinical specificity. Determination of clinical sensitivity and specificity is based upon comparison of the test results with a gold standard. The gold standard may be an independent test that measures the same analyte, but it may also be a clinical diagnosis determined by definitive clinical methods (e.g., radiographic testing, follow-up, or outcomes analysis). Determination of these performance measures is covered in Chapter 15. The clinical sensitivity and specificity may be given as a fraction or as a percentage after multiplication by 100. Standard errors of estimates are derived from the binomial distribution.[97] Comparison of the performance of two qualitative tests applied on the same groups of nondiseased and diseased subjects can be performed by McNemar's test.[60]

One approach for determining the recorded performance of a test in terms of clinical sensitivity and specificity is to determine the true concentration of analyte using an independent reference method. The closer the concentration is to the cut-off point, the larger error frequencies are to be expected. Actually the cut-off point is defined in such a way that for samples having a true concentration exactly equal to the cut-off point, 50% of the results will be positive and 50% will be negative.[25] The concentrations above and below the cut-off point at which repeated results are 95% positive or 95% negative, respectively, have been called the "95% interval" for the cut-off point for that method[25] (notice that this is not a CI; Figure 14-6). Thus in an evaluation of a qualitative test, it is important to specify the composition of the samples in detail. Recently a NCCLS guideline on the topic has suggested a protocol for evaluation.[78] Briefly, it is recommended to prepare samples with a concentration equal to the cut-off point and with concentrations 20% below and above the point. Twenty replicate measurements are then carried out at each concentration, and the percentages of positive and neg-

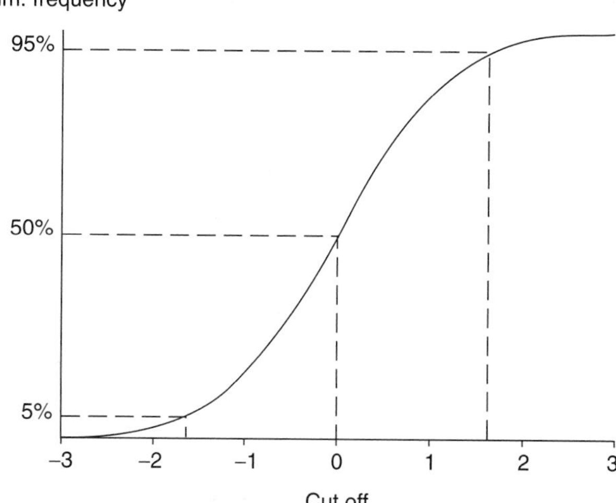

Figure 14-6 Cumulative frequency distribution of positive results. The *x*-axis indicates concentrations standardized to zero at the cut-off point (50% positive results) with unit SD.

ative results are recorded. On the basis of these measurements, it can be judged whether the "95% interval" for the cut-off point is within or outside this interval. In relation to the suggested procedure, one should be aware of the limitations associated with repeated measurements of pools. Measurements of individual patient samples with the specified concentrations are preferable to get a true impression of possible matrix effects.

Agreement Between Qualitative Tests

As outlined above, if the outcome of a qualitative test can be related to a true analyte concentration or a definitive clinical diagnosis, it is relatively straightforward to express the performance in terms of clinical specificity and sensitivity. In the absence of a definitive reference or "gold standard," one should be cautious with regard to judgments on performance. In this situation, it is primarily *agreement* with another test that can be assessed. When considering replacement of an old or expensive routine method with a new or cheap method, it is of interest to know whether similar test results are likely to be obtained. If both methods are imperfect, however, it is not possible to judge which test has the best performance, unless additional testing by a reference procedure is carried out.

In a comparison study, the same individuals are tested by both methods to prevent bias associated with selection of patients. Basically the outcome of the comparison study should be presented in the form of a 2 × 2 table, from which various measures of agreement may be derived (Table 14-6). An obvious measure of agreement is the overall fraction or percentage of the subjects tested that have the same test result (i.e., both results negative or positive)

$$\text{Overall percent agreement} = (a + d)/(a + b + c + d) \times 100\%$$

TABLE 14-6 2 × 2 Table for Assessing Agreement between Two Qualitative Tests

		Test 1	
		+	–
Test 2	+	*a*	*b*
	–	*c*	*d*
Total		*a* + *c*	*b* + *d*

If the agreement differs with respect to diseased and healthy individuals, the overall percent agreement measure becomes dependent on the disease prevalence in the studied group of subjects. This is a common situation, and accordingly it may be desirable to separate this overall agreement measure into agreement concerning negative and positive results:

Percent agreement given test 1 positive: $a/(a + c) \times 100\%$

Percent agreement given test 1 negative: $b/(b + d) \times 100\%$

For example, if there is a high agreement with regard to positive results, the overall agreement will be high when the fraction of diseased subjects is high; but in a screening situation with very low disease prevalence, the overall agreement will mainly depend on agreement with regard to negative results. Standard errors of the estimates can be derived from the binomial distribution.[62,97]

A problem with the above-mentioned simple agreement measures is that they do not take agreement by chance into account. Given independence, the expected proportions observed in the fields of the 2 × 2 table are obtained by multiplication of the fractions of negative and positive results for each test. Concerning agreement, it is the excess agreement beyond chance that is of interest. More sophisticated measures have been introduced to account for this aspect. The most well-known measure is kappa, which is defined generally as the ratio of observed excess agreement beyond chance to the maximum possible excess agreement beyond chance.[26] We have:

$$\text{Kappa} = (I_o - I_e)/(1 - I_e)$$

where I_o is the observed index of agreement and I_e is the expected agreement from chance. Given complete agreement, kappa equals +1. If observed agreement is greater than or equal to chance agreement, kappa is larger than or equal to zero. Observed agreement worse than chance yields a negative kappa value.

Example

Table 14-7 shows a hypothetical example of observed numbers in a 2 × 2 table. The proportion of positive results for Test 1 is 75/(75 + 60) = 0.555 and 80/(80 + 55) = 0.593 for Test 2. Thus by chance we expect the ++ pattern in 0.555 × 0.593 × 135 = 44.44 cases. Analogously, the –– pattern is

TABLE 14-7 2 × 2 Table with Example of Agreement Data for Two Qualitative Tests

		Test 1		
		+	−	**Total**
Test 2	+	60	20	80
	−	15	40	55
Total		75	60	135

expected in $(1 - 0.555) \times (1 - 0.593) \times 135 = 24.45$ cases. The expected overall agreement by chance I_e is $(44.44 + 24.45)/135 = 0.51$. The observed overall agreement is $I_o = (60 + 40)/135 = 0.74$. Thus we have:

$$\text{Kappa} = (0.74 - 0.51)/(1 - 0.51) = 0.47$$

Kappa values greater than 0.75 are generally taken to indicate excellent agreement beyond chance, values from 0.40 to 0.75 are regarded as fair-to-good agreement beyond chance, and finally, values below 0.40 represent poor agreement beyond chance. A standard error for the kappa estimate can be computed.[26] Kappa is related to the intraclass correlation coefficient, which is a widely used measure of interrater reliability for quantitative measurements.[26] The considered agreement measures, percent agreement, and kappa can also be applied to assess the reproducibility of a qualitative test when the test is applied twice in a given context.

Various methodological problems are encountered in studies on qualitative tests. An obvious mistake is to let the result of the test being evaluated contribute to the diagnostic classification of the subjects being tested (circular argument). Another problem is partial as opposed to complete verification. When a new test is compared with an existing, imperfect test a partial verification is sometimes undertaken, in which only discrepant results are subjected to further testing by a perfect test procedure. On this basis, sensitivity and specificity are reported for the new test. This procedure (called discrepant resolution) leads to biased estimates and should not be accepted.[72] The problem is that for cases with agreement, both the existing (imperfect test) and the new test may be wrong. Thus only a measure of agreement should be reported, not specificity and sensitivity values. In the biostatistical literature, various procedures have been suggested to correct for bias caused by imperfect reference tests, but unrealistic assumptions concerning independence of test results are usually put forward.

METHOD COMPARISON

Comparison of measurements by two methods is a frequent task in the laboratory. Preferably, parallel measurements of a set of patient samples should be undertaken. To prevent artificial matrix-induced differences, fresh patient samples are the optimal material. A nearly-even distribution of values over the analytical measurement range is also preferable. In an ordinary laboratory, comparison of two field methods will be the most frequently occurring situation. Less commonly, comparison of a field method with a reference method is undertaken. When comparing two field methods, the focus is on the observed differences. In this situation, it is not possible to establish that one set of the measurements is the correct one and then consider the deviation of the other set of measurements from the presumed correct concentrations. Rather, the question is whether the new method can replace the existing one without a general change in measurement level. To address this question, the dispersion of observed differences between the paired measurements by the methods may be evaluated. To carry out a formal, objective analysis of the data, a statistical procedure with graphics display should be applied. Various approaches exist: (1) a frequency plot or histogram of the distribution of differences with measures of the central tendency and the dispersion (distribution of differences [DoD] plot); (2) a difference (bias) plot, which shows the differences as a function of the average concentration of the measurements (Bland-Altman plot); and (3) a regression analysis. In the following, a general error model is presented, and some typical measurement relationships are considered. Each of the mentioned statistical approaches will be presented in detail with a discussion of their advantages and disadvantages.

BASIC ERROR MODEL

The occurrence of measurement errors is related to the performance characteristics of the assay, primarily bias, imprecision, and specificity as defined above. The overall influence of these factors may be incorporated in an error model.

True Value and Target Value

Taking into account that an analytical method measures analyte concentrations with some uncertainty, one has to distinguish between the measured value (x_i) and the target value ($X_{Targeti}$) of a sample subjected to analysis by a given method. The latter is the average result we would obtain, if the given sample was measured an infinite number of times. The measured value is likely to deviate from the target value by some small "random" amount (ε). For a given sample measured by an analytical method, we have:

$$x_i = X_{\text{Target}i} + \varepsilon_i$$

If the method is a reference method without bias and nonspecificity, the target value equals the true value, i.e.,

$$X_{\text{Target}i} = X_{\text{True}i}$$

Given a field method, some bias or nonspecificity may be present, and the target and true values are likely to differ somewhat. For example, if we measure creatinine with a chromogenic method, which co-determines some other components with creatinine in serum, we will likely obtain a higher target value than when we use a specific isotope-dilution mass spectrometry (ID-MS) reference method (i.e.,

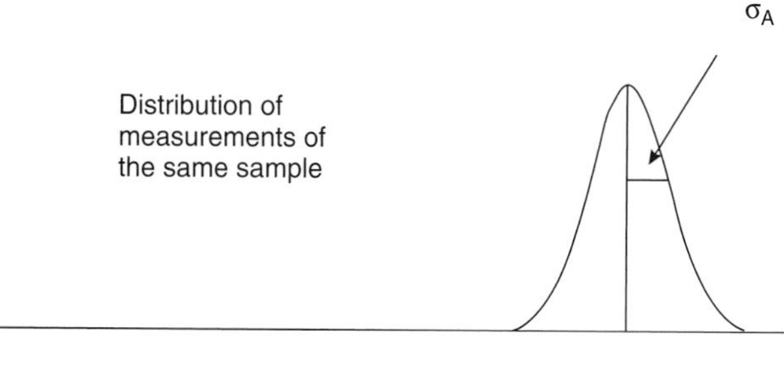

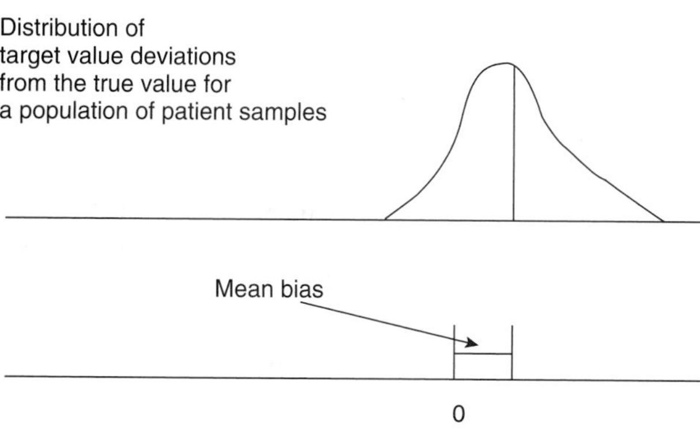

Figure 14-7 Outline of basic error model for measurements by a field method. *Upper part:* The distribution of repeated measurements of the *same* sample, representing a normal distribution around the target value *(vertical line)* of the sample with a dispersion corresponding to the analytical standard deviation, σ_A. *Middle part:* Schematic outline of the dispersion of target value deviations from the respective true values for a population of patient samples. A distribution of an arbitrary form is displayed. The vertical line indicates the mean of the distribution. *Lower part:* The distance from zero to the mean of the target value deviations from the true values represents the mean bias of the method.

the target value of the chromogenic method exceeds the true value determined by repetitive reference method measurements). Thus we have the relation

$$X_{Target i} = X_{True i} + \text{Bias}_i$$

Because the amounts of co-determined substances may vary from sample to sample, the bias is likely to differ somewhat from sample to sample. For a representative set of patient samples, we may describe the biases associated with the individual samples by the central tendency (mean or median) and the dispersion (Figure 14-7). Thus the bias may be split into an average amount: the mean bias, and a random part, random bias.[48,53,55,58] For an individual sample, we have

$$X_{Target i} = X_{True i} + \text{Mean-Bias} + \text{Random-Bias}_i$$

For example, the chromogenic creatinine method may on average determine creatinine values 15% too high, which then constitutes the mean bias. For individual samples, the particular bias may be slightly higher or lower than 15% depending on the actual chromogenic content.

Mean Bias and Random Bias

Taking mean bias and random bias into account, we obtain the following expression for an individual measurement of a given sample by a field method

$$x_i = X_{Target i} + \varepsilon_i = X_{True i} + \text{Mean-Bias} + \text{Random-Bias}_i + \varepsilon_i$$

For such an individual measurement the total error is the deviation of x_i from the true value, i.e.,

$$\text{Total error of } x_i = \text{Mean-Bias} + \text{Random-Bias}_i + \varepsilon_i$$

Thus the total error is composed of a mean bias, a random matrix-related interference component, and finally a random measurement error element. The latter component can be assessed from repeated measurements of the given sample by the method in question and can be expressed as a standard deviation (i.e., the analytical standard deviation as previously described [either within or between runs]). Estimation of the other elements requires parallel measurements between the method in question and a reference method as outlined in detail later.

The exposition above defines the total error in somewhat broader terms than often is seen. A traditional total error expression is[106]

$$\text{Total error} = \text{Bias} + 2\,\text{SD}_A$$

which often is interpreted as the mean bias plus 2 SD_A. If a one-sided statistical perspective is taken, the expression is modified to Bias + 1.65 SD_A, indicating 5% of results being located outside the limit. If a lower percentage is desired, the multiplication factor is increased accordingly, supposing a normal distribution. Interpreting the bias as being identical with the mean bias may lead to an underestimation of the total error.

When the mean bias is considered, one should distinguish between specific (systematic) sample-related interference (e.g., the influence of hemolysis on a photometric assay) in which a clear concentration dependent effect is present and general nonspecificity of the assay. The former can be handled appropriately, either by systematic corrections or by setting limits for allowed degrees of hemolysis.[29]

Random matrix-related interference may take several forms. It may be a regularly occurring additional random error component, perhaps of the same order of magnitude as the analytical error. In this context, it is natural to quantify the error in the form of an SD or CV. The most straightforward procedure is to carry out a method comparison study based on a set of patient samples, where one of the methods is a reference method as outlined later. Often reference methods are not available, and Lawton et al[58] described a multiple method comparison technique based on principal component analysis to quantify random bias components. Applying at least three field methods, it is possible, given certain assumptions concerning independence with regard to interference, to estimate random bias components. Krouwer[53] formally quantified sample-related random effects in a comparison experiment of two cholesterol methods and found that the CV of the sample-related random interference component exceeded the analytical CV. Kringle and Bogovich[48] considered random bias of a Jaffé creatinine method by components of variance analysis and also found random bias to be a pronounced random error component, constituting 80% of the total random error. This relatively high amount should be regarded in light of the limited specificity of the Jaffé creatinine measurement principle.

Another form of random matrix-related interference is more rarely occurring gross errors, which typically are seen in the context of immunoassays and relate to unexpected antibody interactions (see interference section).[44,74,94] Such an error will usually show up as an outlier in method comparison studies. A well-known source is the occurrence of heterophilic antibodies. This is the background for the fact that outliers should be carefully considered and not just discarded from the data analysis procedure. Supplementary studies may help clarify such random matrix-related interferences and may provide specifications for the assay that limit its application in certain contexts (e.g., with regard to samples from certain patient categories).

Mean Bias and Analyte Concentration

When considering mean bias, one should recognize that the mean bias may be a function of the analyte concentration. For example, it may be positive at low concentrations and negative at high concentrations. This may occur in cases in which there is some nonspecificity of the method, yielding values that are generally too high. In the high concentration range, however, nonlinearity in the negative direction may predominate over the positive bias because of nonspecificity. In this case, the recorded mean bias for a set of samples becomes dependent on the distribution of sample values. For an even distribution of sample values over the whole range, the mean bias may be close to zero (see later example concerning the paired *t*-test). For a set of samples with values limited to the lower part of the analytical measurement range, the mean bias may be positive. Finally the recorded mean bias may be negative for sets of samples with only high values.

Blunders or Clerical Errors

Another reason for outliers in method comparison studies and in daily practice is *blunders* or *clerical errors.* In the past, this type of error usually arose in relation to manual transfer of results. Today, this kind of error typically is related to computer errors originating at interfaces between computer systems. Bonini et al[6] concluded on the basis of a literature review that laboratory errors occurred more frequently in the preanalytical or postanalytical phases than in the analytical part. Errors on test order forms or errors related to handling of order forms appear to occur relatively frequently (1% to 5% of recorded cases). In the postanalytical phase, inappropriate interpretation may take place (e.g., in relation to erroneous reference intervals).

METHOD COMPARISON DATA MODEL

We here consider our error model in relation to the method comparison situation. For a given sample measured by two analytical methods, 1 and 2, we have

$$x1_i = X1_{\text{Target}i} + \varepsilon 1_i = X_{\text{True}i} + \text{Mean-Bias1} + \text{Random-Bias1}_i + \varepsilon 1_i$$

$$x2_i = X2_{\text{Target}i} + \varepsilon 2_i = X_{\text{True}i} + \text{Mean-Bias2} + \text{Random-Bias2}_i + \varepsilon 2_i$$

From this general model we may study some typical situations. First, comparison of a field method with a reference method will be treated. Secondly the more frequently occurring situation, the comparison of two field methods, is considered.

Comparison of a Field Method With a Reference Method

We may start supposing that method 1 is a reference method. In this case, the bias components per definition disappear, and we have the following situation:

$$x1_i = X1_{\text{Target}i} + \varepsilon 1_i = X_{\text{True}i} + \varepsilon 1_i$$

$$x2_i = X2_{\text{Target}i} + \varepsilon 2_i = X_{\text{True}i} + \text{Mean-Bias2} + \text{Random-Bias2}_i + \varepsilon 2_i$$

The paired differences become

$$(x2_i - x1_i) = \text{Mean-Bias2} + \text{Random-Bias2}_i + (\varepsilon 2_i - \varepsilon 1_i)$$

We thus have an expression consisting of a constant term (the mean bias of method 2) and two random terms. The random bias term is distributed around the mean bias according to an undefined distribution. The second random term is a difference between two random measurement errors that are independent and commonly, normally distributed. Under these assumptions, the differences between the random measurement errors are also random and normally distributed. However, we remind the reader that the standard deviation for analytical methods often depends on the concentration level as mentioned earlier. For analytes with a wide analytical measurement range (e.g., some hormones), both the random matrix-related interferences and the analytical SDs are likely to depend on the measurement concentration, often in a roughly proportional manner. It may then be more useful to evaluate the *relative* differences: $(x2_i - x1_i)/[(x2_i + x1_i)/2]$ and accordingly express mean and random bias, and analytical error as proportions. An alternative is to partition the total analytical measurement range into segments (e.g., three parts), and consider mean bias, random bias and analytical error separately for these segments. The segments may preferably be divided in relation to important decision concentrations (e.g., in relation to reference interval limits and/or treatment decision concentrations).

Comparison of Two Field Methods

In the comparison of two field methods, the paired differences become:

$$(x2_i - x1_i) = (\text{Mean-Bias2} - \text{Mean-Bias1}) + (\text{Random-Bias2}_i - \text{Random-Bias1}_i) + (\varepsilon 2_i - \varepsilon 1_i)$$

The expression again consists of a constant term, the difference between the two mean biases, and two random terms. The first random term is a difference between two random-bias components that may or may not be independent. If the two field methods are based on the same measurement principle, the random bias terms are likely to be correlated. For example, two chromogenic methods for creatinine are likely to be subject to interference from the same chromogenic compounds present in a given serum sample. On the other hand, a chromogenic and an enzymatic creatinine method are subject to different types of interfering compounds, and the random-bias terms may be relatively independent. In the $\varepsilon 2_i - \varepsilon 1_i$ term, the same relationships as described above are likely to apply. One may notice that the general form of the expressed differences is the same in the two situations. Thus the same general statistical principles actually apply. In the following sections, we will consider the distribution of differences under various circumstances and also consider the measurement relations between method 1 and 2 on the basis of regression analysis.

Preliminary Practical Work in Relation to a Method Comparison Study

When preparing a method comparison study, the analytical methods to be studied should be established in the laboratory according to written protocols and stable in routine performance. Reagents are commonly supplied as ready-made analytical kits, perhaps implemented on a dedicated analytical instrument (open or closed system). The technologists performing the study should be trained in the procedures and associated instrumentation. Further, it is important that an internal quality control system is in place to ensure that the methods being compared are running in the in-control state.

Planning a Method Comparison Study

In the planning phase of a method comparison study, several points require attention, including the number of samples necessary, the distribution of analyte concentrations (preferably uniform over the analytical measurement range), and the representativeness of the samples. To address the latter point, samples from relevant patient categories should be included, so that possible interference phenomena can be discovered. Practical aspects related to storage and treatment of samples (container, etc.) and possible artifacts induced by storage (e.g., freezing of samples) and addition of anticoagulants should be considered. Comparison of measurements should preferably be undertaken over several days (e.g., at least 5 days), so that the comparison of methods does not become dependent on the performance of the methods in one particular analytical run. Finally, ethical aspects (e.g., informed consent from patients whose samples will be used) should be considered in relation to existing legislation.

When considering the comparison protocol, various guidelines may be consulted. The NCCLS Evaluation Protocol (EP) guidelines give advice on various aspects. For example, the NCCLS guideline EP-9A2: *Method Comparison and Bias Estimation Using Patient Samples* suggests measurement of 40 samples in duplicate by each method, when a new method is introduced in the laboratory as a substitute for an established one.[81] Additionally, it is proposed that a vendor of an analytical test system should have made a comparison study based on at least 100 samples measured in duplicate by each method. The principle of a more demanding requirement for vendors appears reasonable. This initial validation should be comprehensive to disclose the performance of the assay system in detail. Then the requirement for the ordinary user may be more modest.

Although these general guidelines on sample size are useful, further aspects are important. Statistical power may be considered as a basis for considering the appropriate sample size as presented under regression analysis. Additionally the probability of detecting rarely occurring interferences showing up as outliers should be taken into account when considering the necessary sample size. Finally, in relation to evaluation of automated methods, special consideration should be given to the sample sequence to evaluate drift, carryover, and nonlinearity (e.g., by a multifactorial design).[52]

Distribution of Differences Plot (DoD plot)

From the end-user viewpoint, it is the differences per se that matter. Thus with regard to the outcome of replacing an established field method with a new one that perhaps is cheaper or more practical, it is important to focus on the distribution of differences between paired measurements by the old and the new method. A graphic display with assessment of the central tendency and the dispersion of the differences in the form of an ordinary histogram or frequency polygon plot is useful. The differences may or may not be normally distributed. Because both analytical error components and random matrix-related interferences may contribute to the differences, the distribution may be irregular and outliers may occur. Further, the random dispersion elements may be dependent on analyte concentration. Therefore a nonparametric approach for interpreting the distribution of differences may generally be preferable as a starting point.

Nonparametric Approach

Both the central tendency (median) and extreme percentiles are of interest when using the nonparametric approach to the distribution of differences. Given a traditional 95% level, the 2.5 and 97.5 percentiles are considered. A 99% or more extreme level may also be selected, and the related percentiles

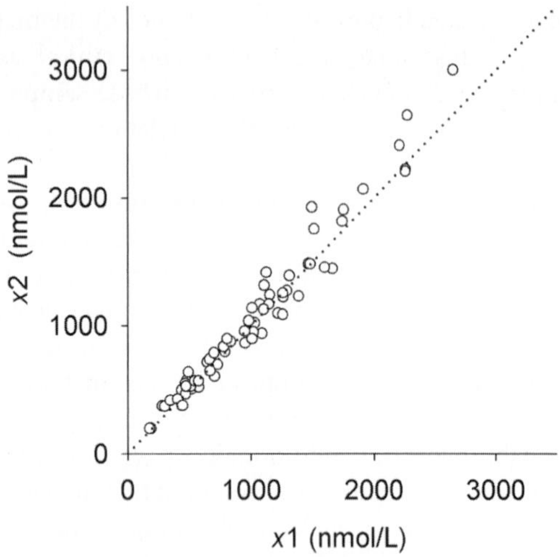

Figure 14-8 A scatter plot of $N = 65$ ($x1, x2$) data points for comparison of two drug assays. The dashed line is the line of identity.

(0.5 and 99.5 or more extreme ones) are then applied for description of method differences. Nonparametric estimation of the 2.5 and 97.5 percentiles requires 2.5 times as many observations as the parametric approach to provide the same precision, which implies that sample sizes cannot be too small.[70] Estimating confidence limits of the percentiles can give an indication of their imprecision. The CIs can be estimated from the ordered observations as described in Chapter 16 in the section on nonparametric estimation of the 95% reference interval. Alternatively a bootstrap procedure, available on the book's accompanying Evolve site, can be applied as described.[70] The advantage of the bootstrap procedure is that standard errors can be derived using smaller sample sizes than by the simple nonparametric approach.

A method comparison example from one of the authors' laboratory is considered (KL). Two in-house developed drug assays for serum concentrations of the antipsychotic drug clozapine are compared. The established assay (method 1) is an HPLC method based on manual liquid-liquid extraction. The new method (method 2) is an HPLC method with an automated on-column extraction step. An initial impression of the relation between $x1$ and $x2$ measurements can be obtained from a scatter plot of the 65 measurement sets ($x1$, $x2$) with the identity line outlined (Figure 14-8). The $x1$ and $x2$ values are displayed in Table 14-17, which is available on the book's accompanying Evolve site. The $x1$ measurements range from 177 to 2650 nmol/L, and the range of $x2$ values is from 200 to 3004 nmol/L (i.e., we have a relatively wide analytical measurement range in the present example). A histogram of the differences ($x2 - x1$) is shown in Figure 14-9. Applying a nonparametric data description, we order the observed differences according to size and derive the median difference as the value of the ($0.5N + 0.5$) ordered observation, here 26 nmol/L. In case the order is a noninteger, interpolation between neighbor-ordered values is carried out. A paired nonparametric test, the Wilcoxon test,[97] showed that the median difference was significantly higher than zero (P less than 0.02). The 2.5 and 97.5 percentiles correspond to the values of the ($0.025N + 0.5$) and the ($0.975N + 0.5$) ordered observations, respectively, as displayed in Table 14-8.[15,70] For a sample size of less than 120, it is not possible to derive CIs for the percentiles by the simple nonparametric procedure. Therefore we also applied the bootstrap procedure to estimate nonparametric percentiles with 90% CIs[70] (Table 14-8) (see the book's accompanying Evolve site). The bootstrap procedure, which is based on computerized random resampling of the observations, provides slightly different percentile estimates as shown in the table. In this way, we obtain an estimation of the size of negative and positive differences with uncertainties. In the present example, there is a considerable range of differences, the 2.5 percentile being −169 nmol/L (90% CI: −214 to −123), and the 97.5 percentile being 356 nmol/L (90% CI: 255 to 457). The relatively large differences should be related to the considerable analytical measurement range for the analyte, and an

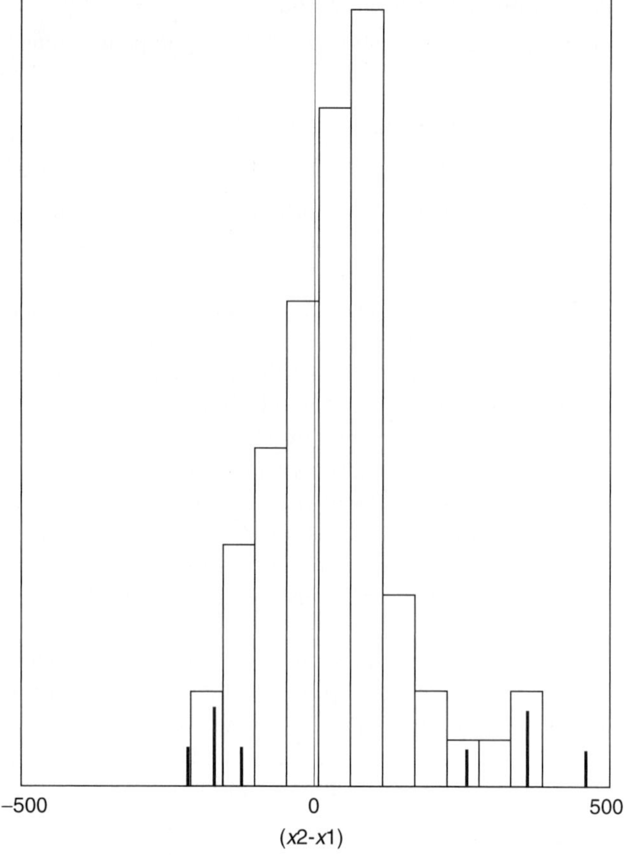

Figure 14-9 DoD plot for comparison of two drug assays: nonparametric analysis. A histogram shows the relative frequency of $N = 65$ differences with demarcated 2.5 and 97.5 percentiles determined nonparametrically. The 90% CIs of the percentiles are shown. These were derived by the bootstrap technique.

TABLE 14-8 Analysis of Distribution of Differences for the Comparison of Drug Assays Example. $N = 65$. The unit is nmol/L.

Total range of $x1$ measurements	177 to 2650		
Total range of $x2$ measurements	200 to 3004		
Total range of differences ($x2 - x1$)	−210.00 to 437.00		
Test for normality of differences (Anderson-Darling test)	$P < 0.01$		
Statistical analysis of differences	Simple nonparametric	Bootstrap	Parametric
Median	26.00 ($P < 0.02$)		
Mean			42.00 ($P < 0.01$)
SD			124.42
Coefficient of skewness			+0.83
Coefficient of kurtosis			+1.27
Outlier test (4 SD)			n.s.
2.5 percentile	−166.00	−169.11	−201.86
97.5 percentile	372.38	355.90	285.86
90% CI for 2.5 percentile		−214.73 to −123.50	−245.24 to −158.47
90% CI for 97.5 percentile		255.03 to 456.77	242.47 to 329.24

evaluation of *relative* differences may in the present example be more relevant (see later in this chapter).

In the presented examples, no evident outliers were present. However, outliers deserve special attention. Unless they are related to obvious method or apparatus malfunction, the discarding of outliers should be considered with caution. Outliers may indicate the presence of large random matrix-related interferences, which may be of major clinical importance (e.g., interference by antibodies or degradation products that only occur rarely). Thus a special investigation of outlying results with reanalysis and exploration of the reasons for the outlying observations should be considered. A statistical evaluation of outliers is available on the book's accompanying Evolve site.

Parametric Approach

If application of a goodness-of-fit test does not disprove that the distribution of differences is normally distributed, a parametric statistical approach may be undertaken. In the presented example, there was a significant deviation from normality as assessed by the Anderson-Darling test[61] (P less than 0.01), and a parametric analysis should in principle not be carried out. However, to demonstrate the procedure, the parametric approach is also carried out (Figure 14-10 and Table 14-8). The mean and standard deviation (SD_{Dif}) of the paired differences ($x2 - x1$) are estimated according to standard procedures. A paired t-test is used to determine whether the mean difference is significantly different from zero or not (P less than 0.01 in this case). The 2.5 and 97.5 percentiles for the differences are estimated as the mean $\pm t_{0.025,(N-1)}$ SD_{Dif}. A standard error for the percentiles (SE_{perc}) may be computed as specified on the book's accompanying Evolve site, and the 90% CI limits are then derived as ± 1.65 SE_{perc} around the

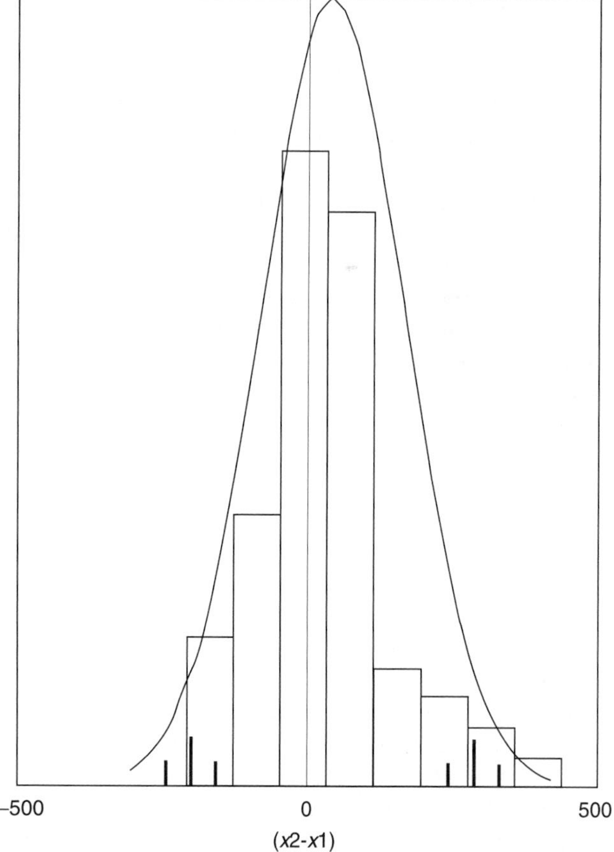

Figure 14-10 DoD plot for comparison of two drug assays: parametric analysis. A histogram shows the relative frequency of $N = 65$ differences with the estimated Gaussian density distribution. Parametrically estimated 2.5 and 97.5 percentiles are shown with 90% CIs.

percentiles (Figure 14-10 and Table 14-8). The parametrically derived 2.5 and 97.5 percentiles (−202 and 286 nmol/L) differ somewhat from the nonparametrically derived percentiles, which in the present context with proven nonnormality may be regarded as the most reliable estimates.

Relative Distribution of Differences Plot (Rel. DoD plot)

In many cases in which there is a wide analytical measurement range (i.e., corresponding to 1 or several decades), the random error components depend on the concentration as previously mentioned. The analytical SDs may be approximately proportional to the concentration over the major part of the analytical measurement range, and this relationship may also apply to the random matrix-related interferences. In the present example, the initial scatter plot of ($x1$, $x2$) values suggests that the random error of the differences increases with the concentration (see Figure 14-8). A formal test for this possible relation is to compute the correlation coefficient between the average concentration and the *absolute* value of the differences. This correlation coefficient, r, is +0.57 (P less than 0.001) and thus confirms the relationship of an increasing scatter with the concentration, which also can be visualized in a scatter plot of the absolute differences against the average concentration (Figure 14-11). A natural next step is then to assess the *relative* differences in relation to the average concentration. The correlation coefficient between the absolute values of the relative differences ($[x2 - x1]/[\{x1 + x2\}/2]$) and the average concentration ($[x1 + x2]/2$) was not significantly different from zero ($r = -0.15$), and a scatter plot also suggests a more homogeneous dispersion (Figure 14-12). In this situation, it is more reasonable to deal with *relative* differences or percentage differences ($[x2 - x1]/[\{x1 + x2\}/2] \times 100\%$). The same nonparametric descriptive measures as used above may be applied for the central tendency and the dispersion (Figure 14-13). The median relative difference amounts to 0.042 or 4.2%, which is significantly

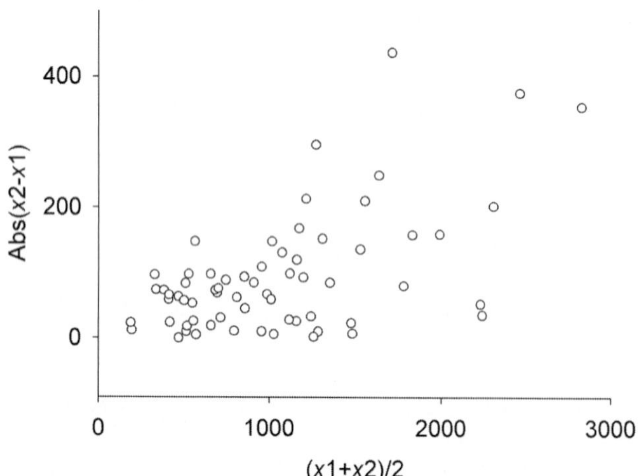

Figure 14-11 Plot of absolute differences (ordinate) against average concentration (abscissa) for the comparison of drug assays example. The scatter increases with the average concentration ($r = +0.57$).

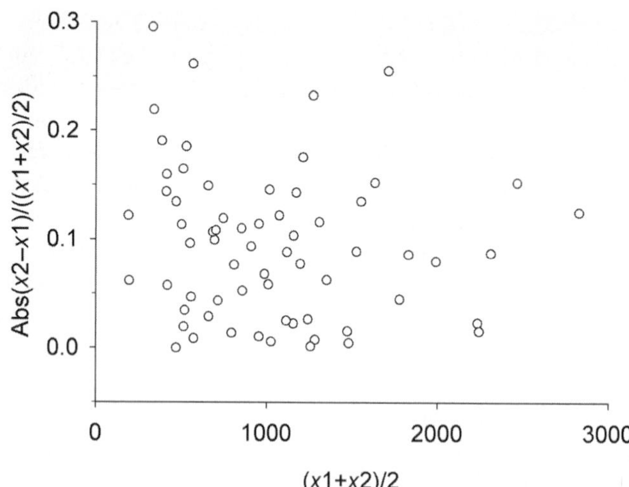

Figure 14-12 Plot of absolute *relative* differences (ordinate) against average concentration (abscissa) for the comparison of drug assays example. The scatter is not significantly correlated with the average concentration ($r = -0.15$, not significant).

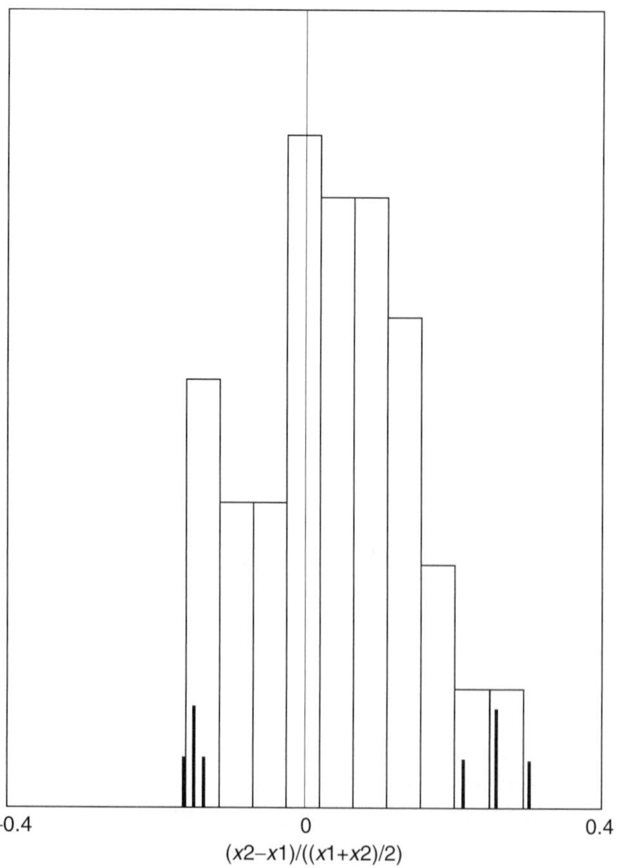

Figure 14-13 Rel. DoD plot for comparison of two drug assays: nonparametric analysis. A histogram shows the relative frequency of relative differences with demarcated 2.5 and 97.5 percentiles determined nonparametrically. The 90% CIs (bootstrap) of the percentiles are shown.

higher than zero (P less than 0.01) (Table 14-9). The 2.5 and 97.5 percentiles are –0.15 and 0.26, respectively. The 90% CIs derived by the bootstrap procedure were –0.16 to –0.14 and 0.21 to 0.30, respectively. Thus from this analysis we may conclude that the 95% interval for percentage differences ranges from about –15% to +26%.

Finally, we may consider a parametric analysis of the relative differences (Figure 14-14 and Table 14-9). A goodness-of-fit test (Anderson-Darling test, P greater than 0.5) showed that the relative differences did not depart significantly from a normal distribution, which in this case supports the parametric approach (Figure 14-15). The parametric 2.5 and 97.5

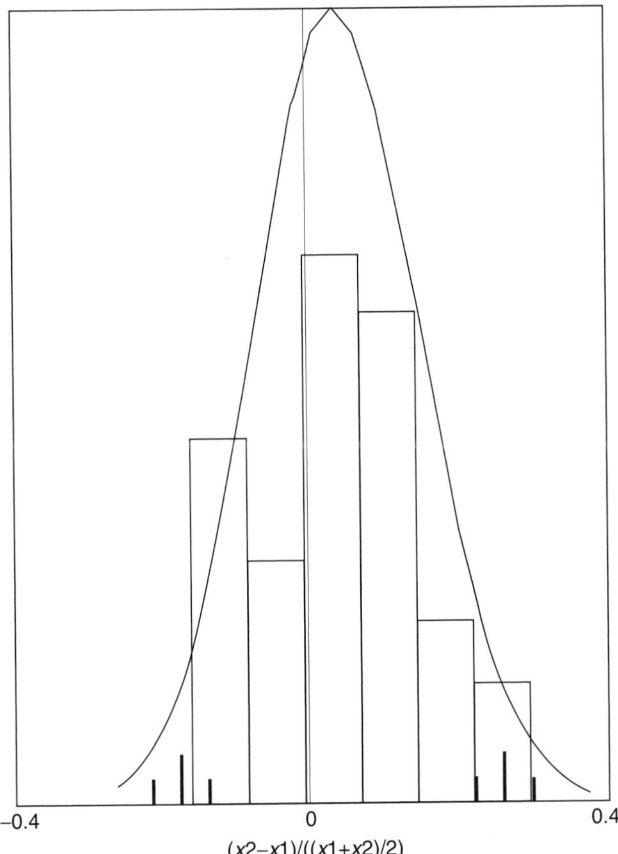

Figure 14-14 Distribution of *relative* differences plot for comparison of two drug assays: parametric analysis. A histogram shows the relative frequency of relative differences with the estimated Gaussian density distribution. Parametrically estimated 2.5 and 97.5 percentiles are shown with 90% CIs.

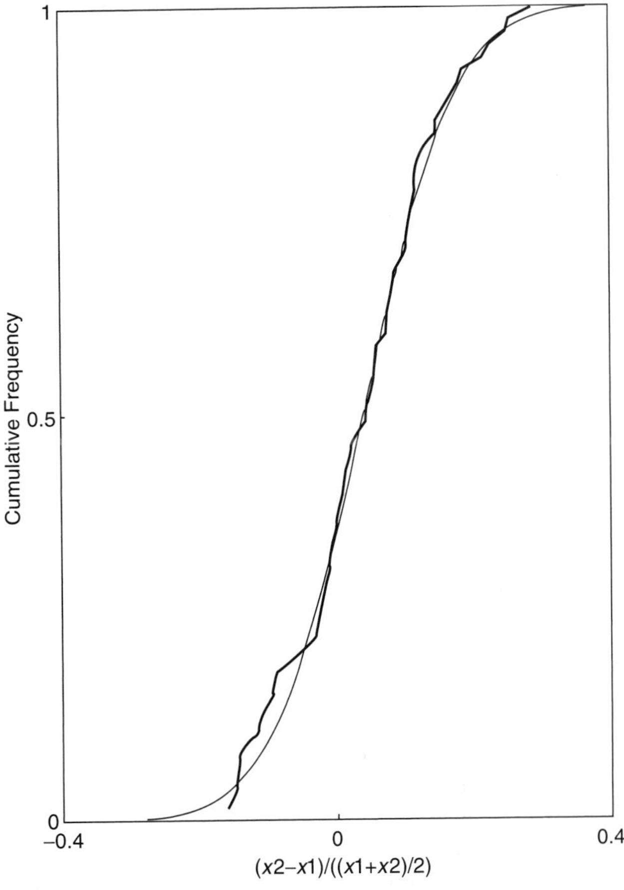

Figure 14-15 Cumulative frequency distribution of relative differences for the comparison of drug assays example. The lighter curve indicates the Gaussian cumulative frequency distribution curve. In accordance with the test for normality, a good agreement is observed.

TABLE 14-9 Analysis of Distribution of *Relative* Differences for the Comparison of Drug Assays Example. $N = 65$

Total range of relative differences	–0.1598 to 0.2953		
Test for normality (Anderson-Darling test)	n.s.		
Statistical analysis	Simple nonparametric	Bootstrap	Parametric
Median	0.0467 ($P < 0.01$)		
Mean			0.0418 ($P < 0.01$)
SD			0.1109
Coefficient of skewness			+0.05
Coefficient of kurtosis			–0.60
Outlier test			n.s.
2.5 percentile	–0.1487	–0.1492	–0.1754
97.5 percentile	0.2607	0.2570	0.2591
90% CI for 2.5 percentile		–0.1627 to –0.1357	–0.2141 to –0.1368
90% CI for 97.5 percentile		0.2135 to 0.3005	0.2204 to 0.2978

percentiles were −0.18 and 0.26, respectively. The mean was 0.042 and the SD of the relative differences was 0.11. Thus we may conclude that there is a mean bias of about 4% and a random error corresponding to a CV of 11%. If we ascribe the random variation equally to the two assays, it corresponds to a random error level of $11\%/\sqrt{2} = 7.8\%$ for each assay. In the present example, this error level was considered acceptable in relation to the clinical use of the assay, and it was decided to replace the manual assay with the new, automated assay.

A modification of the histogram display of differences is a plot suggested by Krouwer and Monty[54] known as the "mountain plot." This is a plot of cumulative frequencies (*cf*%) of differences up to 50% with subsequent subtracted cumulative frequencies (100% − *cf*%). Such a plot shows in principle the same information as a histogram or frequency polygon plot. An advantage may be that the percentiles can be directly read from the plot.

Verification of Distribution of Differences in Relation to Specified Limits

In many situations in which a field method is being considered for implementation, it may be desired primarily to *verify* whether the differences in relation to the existing method are located within given specified limits rather than *estimating* the distribution of differences. For example, one may set limits corresponding to ±15% as clinically acceptable, and desire that the majority, for example, 95% of differences are located within this interval.

By counting, it may be determined whether the expected proportion of results is within the limits (i.e., 95%). One may accept percentages that do not deviate significantly from the supposed percentage at the given sample size derived from the binomial distribution (Table 14-10). For example, if 50 paired measurements have been performed in a method comparison study, and it is observed that 46 of the results (92%) are within the specified limits (e.g., ±15%), the study supports that the achieved goal has been reached, because the lower bound for acceptance is 90%. It is clear that a reasonable number of observations should be obtained for the assessment to have an acceptable power. If very few observations are at hand, the risk is high of falsely concluding that at least 95% of the observations are within the specified limits, in case it is not true (i.e., to commit a Type II error).

TABLE 14-10 Lower Bounds (One-sided 95% CI) of Observed Proportions (%) of Results Being Located Within Specified Limits for Paired Differences That Are in Accordance With the Hypothesis of at Least 95% of Differences Being Within the Limits

N	Observed Proportions
20	85
30	87
40	90
50	90
60	90
70	90
80	91
90	91
100	91
150	92
200	93
250	93
300	93
400	93
500	93
1000	94

Difference (Bland-Altman) Plot

In recent years, the type of difference plot for evaluation of method comparison data suggested by Bland and Altman has become increasingly popular.[4] The procedure was originally introduced for comparison of measurements in clinical medicine, but the procedure has been adopted also in clinical chemistry.[65,85,88] The Bland-Altman plot is usually understood as a plot of the differences against the average results of the methods. Thus the difference plot in this version provides information on the relation between differences and concentration, which is useful to evaluate whether problems exist at certain ranges (e.g., in the high range) caused by nonlinearity of one of the methods. It may also be of interest to observe whether the differences tend to increase proportionally with the concentration, or whether they are independent of concentration. In some situations, particular interest may be directed toward the low concentration region. Information on the relation between differences and concentration is useful in the context of how to adjust for an irregularity (e.g., by changing the method with nonlinearity or by restricting the analytical measurement range). Thus this type of plot may be useful for the laboratory, whereas the DoD plot perhaps may be regarded more as directed toward the end user. The underlying error model outlined above applies also in principle to the difference plot.

The basic version of the difference plot consists of plotting the differences against the average of the measurements. Figure 14-16 shows the plot for the comparison of drug assay data. If one set of the measurements is without random measurement error, one may plot the differences against this value. If errors are present in $x1$, however, an artificial bias is induced by plotting the differences against $x1$.[5] The interval ±2 SD of the differences is often delineated around the mean difference (i.e., corresponding to the mean and the 2.5 and 97.5 percentiles considered in the parametric DoD plot).

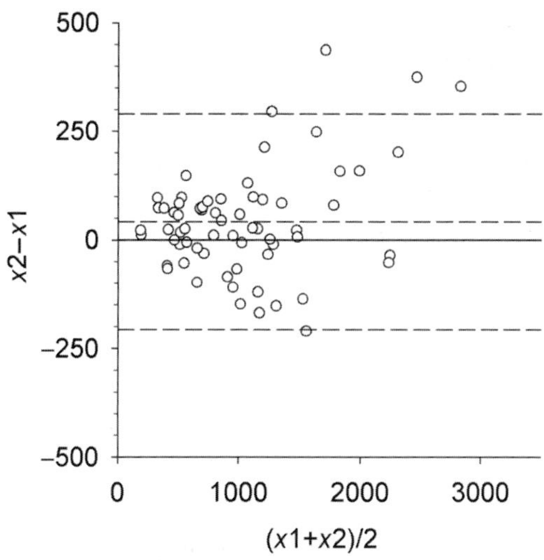

Figure 14-16 Bland-Altman plot of differences for the drug comparison example. The differences are plotted against the average concentration. The mean difference (42 nmol/L) with ±2 SD of differences is shown *(dashed lines).*

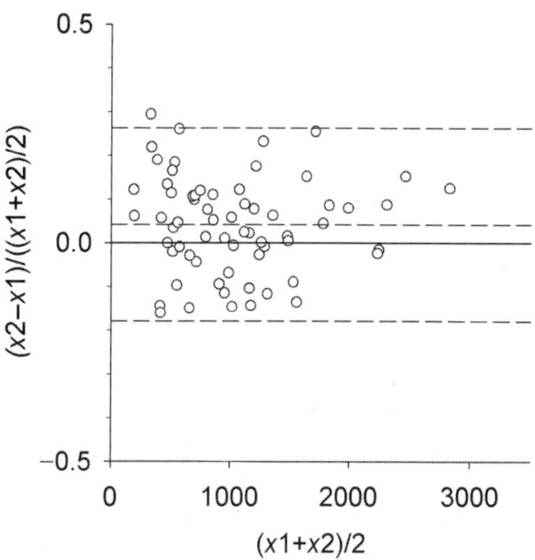

Figure 14-17 Bland-Altman plot of *relative* differences for the drug comparison example. The differences are plotted against the average concentration. The mean relative difference (0.042) with ±2 SD of relative differences is shown *(dashed lines).*

Nonparametric limits may also be considered. The distribution of the differences as measured on the *y*-axis of the coordinate system corresponds to the relations outlined for the DoD plot, which represents a projection of the differences on the *y*-axis. A constant mean bias over the analytical measurement range changes the average concentration away from zero. The presence of random matrix-related interferences increases the width of the distribution. If the mean bias depends on the concentration or if the dispersion varies with the concentration or both, the relations become more complex, and the interval mean ±2 SD of the differences may not fit very well as a 95% interval throughout the analytical measurement range.

In the displayed Bland-Altman plot for the drug assay comparison data, there is a tendency toward increasing scatter with increasing concentration, which is a reflection of the increasing random error with the concentration level considered in detail above. Thus a plot of the relative differences against the average concentration is of relevance (Figure 14-17). Now there is a more homogeneous dispersion of values agreeing with the estimated limits for the dispersion (i.e., the relative mean difference $\pm t_{0.025,(N-1)}$ SD_{RelDif} analogous to the situation with the relative DoD plot considered above).

Focus on *relative* differences in situations with a proportional random error relationship prevents very large differences in the high concentration range from dominating the analysis and making a balanced interpretation difficult. In the low range, the proportional relationship may not necessarily hold true, and sometimes the relative difference plot makes an overcompensation in this region. It is then possible to make a truncation of the proportional relationship at some lower limit, and assume a constant SD for the differences below this limit[66] (i.e., corresponding to the relationship in Figure 14-3, *C*). In the actual example with a slightly negative correlation coefficient between relative differences and average concentration, there is a tendency toward this pattern. An alternative to the relative difference plot is to plot log differences against the average concentration, but this type of plot is more difficult to interpret.

Although it is customary to display the *estimated* limits for the differences (often mean $\pm 2\ SD_{dif}$), one may as an alternative display specification limits considered being reasonable as mentioned for the DoD plot.[85] It may then be assessed whether the observed differences conform to these limits as discussed earlier (see Table 14-10). Application of the difference plot in various specific contexts has been considered.[11,98] It has also been suggested to estimate a regression line for the differences as a function of the average measurement concentration.[101]

A Caution Against Incorrect Interpretation of Paired *t*-Tests in Method Comparison Studies

In association with the difference plot, the paired *t*-test is usually applied as described above.[4] One should here be careful with regard to the interpretation. For example, consider the case shown below, in which method 2 ($x2$) measurements tend to exceed method 1 ($x1$) measurements in the low range and vice versa at high concentrations (Figure 14-18, *A*). This corresponds to a positive mean bias in the low range changing to a negative bias in the high range. In this situation, the overall averages of both sets of measurements are about identical, and the paired *t*-test yields a nonsignificant result, because the average paired difference (i.e., the mean bias) is close to zero (Table 14-11). This does not mean that the measurements are equivalent. Subjecting the data to Deming regression analysis (see the next section) clearly discloses the relation[68] (Figure 14-18, *B*). The results of the regression analysis confirm the existence of both a systematic constant error (intercept different from zero) and a systematic proportional error (slope different from 1). Therefore the statistical significance revealed by the paired *t*-test cannot be used to indicate whether measurements are equivalent or not as also previously pointed out. The paired *t*-test is just a test for the mean bias and does not say anything about the equivalency of the measurements throughout the analytical measurement range.

Regression Analysis

Regression analysis is commonly applied in comparing the results of analytical method comparisons. Typically an experiment is carried out in which a series of paired values is collected when comparing a new method with an established method. This series of paired observations ($x1_i$, $x2_i$) is then used to establish the nature and strength of the relationship between the tests. This discussion outlines various regression models that may be used, provides criteria for when each should be used, outlines approaches for determining how many specimens to use in a given comparison, and provides guidelines for interpreting the results.

Regression analysis has the advantage that it allows the relation between the target values for the two compared methods to be studied over the full analytical measurement range. If the systematic difference between target values (i.e., the mean bias difference between the two methods or the systematic error) is related to the analyte concentration, such a relationship may not be clearly shown when using the previously mentioned types of difference plots. Although nonlinear regression analysis may be applied, the focus is usually on linear regression analysis. In linear regression analysis, it is assumed that the systematic difference between target values can be modeled as a constant systematic difference (intercept deviation from zero) combined with a proportional systematic difference (slope deviation from unity). The intercept may typically represent some average matrix-induced difference, and the proportional difference may be due to a discrepancy with regard to calibration of the methods. In situations with constant SDs of random errors, unweighted regression procedures are used (i.e., ordinary least-squares (OLR) and Deming regression analysis). For cases with SDs that are proportional to the measurement level, the corresponding weighted regression procedures are preferred.

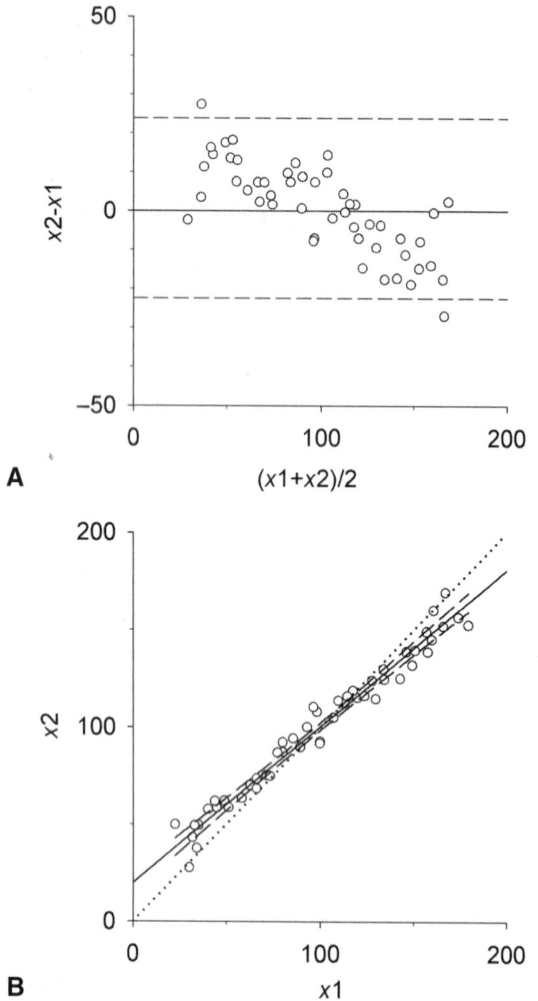

Figure 14-18 Simulated example with positive and negative differences in the low and high range, respectively: **A,** Bland-Altman plot. **B,** An x-y plot with diagonal *(dotted straight line)* and estimated Deming regression line *(solid line)* with 95% confidence curves *(dashed lines)*.

Error Models in Regression Analysis

As outlined previously, we distinguish between the measured value (x_i) and the target value ($X_{Targeti}$) of a sample subjected

TABLE 14-11 Comparison of Paired *t*-test Results and Deming Regression Results for a Simulated Method Comparison Example With Positive Intercept ($a_0 = 20$) and Slope Below Unity ($b = 0.80$). N = 50 ($x1$, $x2$) Measurements

	Paired t-Test	Regression Analysis (Deming)
Mean difference (SEM)	0.78 (1.63)	
t = Mean difference/(SEM)	0.78/1.63 = 0.48 (n.s.)	
Slope (b) (SE(b))		0.80 (0.027)
$t = (b - 1)/\mathrm{SE}(b)$		−7.4 ($P < 0.001$)
Intercept (a_0) (SE(a_0))		20.3 (2.82)
$t = (a_0 - 0)/\mathrm{SE}(a_0)$		7.2 ($P < 0.001$)

to analysis by a given method. In linear regression analysis we assume a linear relationship

$$X2'_{\text{Target}i} = \alpha_0 + \beta X1'_{\text{Target}i}$$

where $X1'_{\text{Target}i}$ and $X2'_{\text{Target}i}$ correspond to the target values without random bias, i.e., we have the relations:

$$X1_{\text{Target}i} = X1'_{\text{Target}i} + \text{Random-Bias}1_i$$
$$X2_{\text{Target}i} = X2'_{\text{Target}i} + \text{Random-Bias}2_i$$

This model is generally useful when the systematic difference between $X1'_{\text{Target}i}$ and $X2'_{\text{Target}i}$ depends on the measured concentration

$$X2'_{\text{Target}i} - X1'_{\text{Target}i} = \alpha_0 + (\beta - 1)X1'_{\text{Target}i}$$

The systematic difference is thus composed of a fixed part and a proportional part.

Because of random matrix-related interferences and analytical error, the individually measured pairs of values ($x1_i$, $x2_i$) will be scattered around the line expressing the relationship between $X1'_{\text{Target}i}$ and $X2'_{\text{Target}i}$. Figure 14-19 outlines schematically how the random distribution of $x1$ and $x2$ values occurs around the regression line. We have:

$$x1_i = X1_{\text{Target}i} + \varepsilon1_i = X1'_{\text{Target}i} + \text{Random-Bias}1_i + \varepsilon1_i$$
$$x2_i = X2_{\text{Target}i} + \varepsilon2_i = X2'_{\text{Target}i} + \text{Random-Bias}2_i + \varepsilon2_i$$

The random error components may be expressed as SDs, and generally we can assume that random bias and analytical components are independent for each analyte yielding the relations

$$\sigma^2_{x1} = \sigma^2_{\text{RB1}} + \sigma^2_{\text{A1}}$$
$$\sigma^2_{x2} = \sigma^2_{\text{RB2}} + \sigma^2_{\text{A2}}$$

The random bias components for method 1 and 2 may not necessarily be independent. They may also not be normally distributed, which is less likely as regards the analytical components. Thus when applying a regression procedure, the explicit assumptions to take into account should be considered. In situations without random bias components of any significance, the relationships simplify to

$$\sigma^2_{x1} = \sigma^2_{\text{A1}}$$
$$\sigma^2_{x2} = \sigma^2_{\text{A2}}$$

In this situation, it can usually be assumed that the error distributions are normal, and the standard deviations may be known from quality control data.

Another methodological problem concerns the question whether the dispersion of the random error components is constant or changes with the analyte concentration as considered previously in the difference plot sections. For most clinical chemical compounds, the analytical SDs vary with the measured concentration, and this relationship may also apply to the random-bias components. In cases with a considerable range (i.e., a decade or more), this phenomenon should also be taken into account when applying a regression analysis. Figure 14-20 schematically shows how the dispersions may increase proportionally with concentration.

Deming Regression Analysis and Ordinary Least-Squares Regression Analysis (OLR) (Constant SDs)

To estimate the relationship between the target values accurately (i.e., a_0 for α_0 and b for β), a regression procedure taking errors in both $x1$ and $x2$ into account is preferable

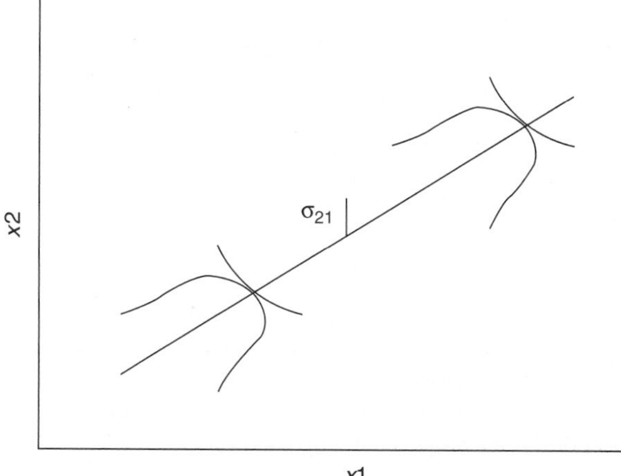

Figure 14-19 Outline of the relation between $x1$ and $x2$ values measured by two methods subject to random errors with constant standard deviations over the analytical measurement range. A linear relationship between the target values ($X1'_{\text{Target}i}$, $X2'_{\text{Target}i}$) is presumed. The $x1_i$ and $x2_i$ values are Gaussian distributed around $X1'_{\text{Target}i}$ and $X2'_{\text{Target}i}$, respectively, as schematically shown. σ_{21} (σ_{yx}) is demarcated.

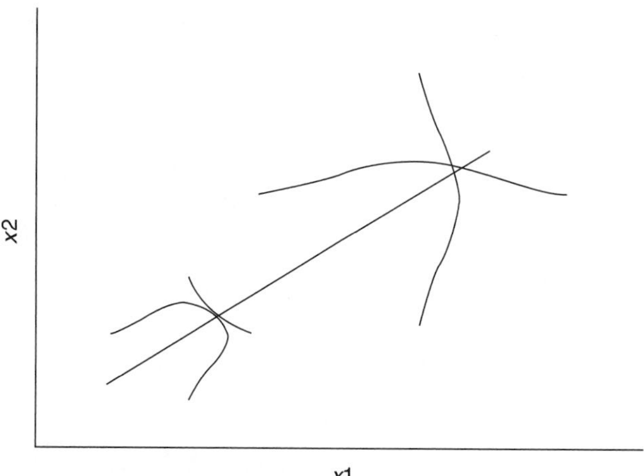

Figure 14-20 Outline of the relation between $x1$ and $x2$ values measured by two methods subject to proportional random errors. A linear relationship between the target values is assumed. The $x1_i$ and $x2_i$ values are Gaussian distributed around $X1'_{\text{Target}i}$ and $X2'_{\text{Target}i}$, respectively, with increasing scatter at higher concentrations as schematically shown.

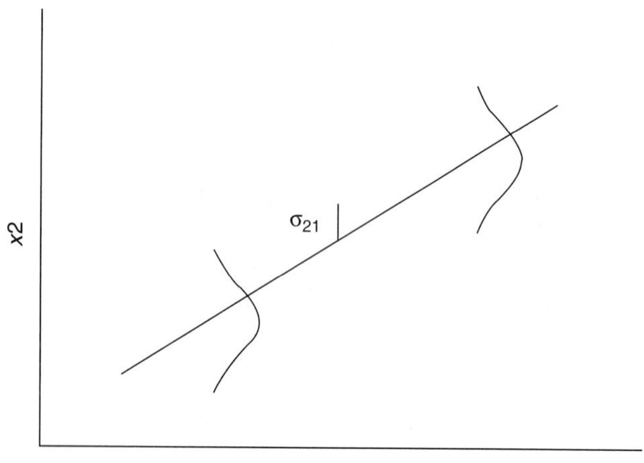

Figure 14-21 The model assumed in ordinary OLR. The $x2$ values are Gaussian distributed around the line with constant standard deviation over the analytical measurement range. The $x1$ values are assumed to be without random error. σ_{21} (σ_{yx}) is shown.

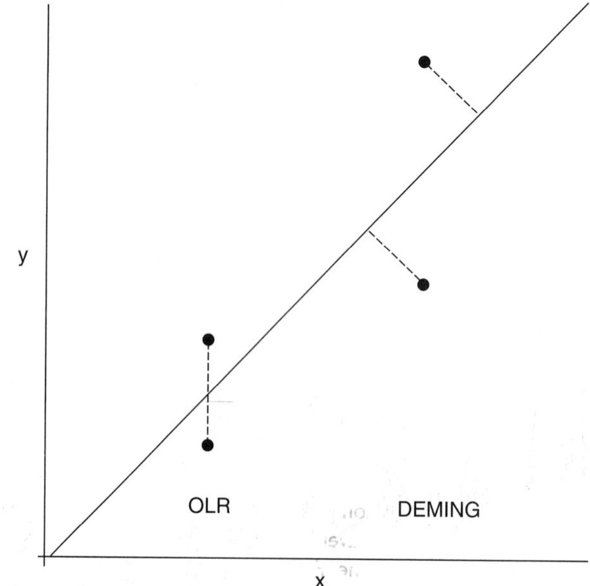

Figure 14-22 In OLR, the sum of squared deviations from the line is minimized in the vertical direction. In Deming regression analysis, the sum of squared deviations is minimized at an angle to the line depending on the random error ratio. Here the symmetric case is displayed with orthogonal deviations. *(From Linnet K. The performance of Deming regression analysis in case of a misspecified analytical error ratio. Clin Chem 1998;44:1024-1031 [Figure 1]).*

(Figures 14-19 and 14-20). In the statistical literature, this type of regression analysis is called errors-in-variables analysis or is referred to as structural or functional relationship models.[46] Various modifications exist, comprising both parametric and nonparametric approaches. In clinical chemistry, a parametric approach described in the following is usually called the Deming method.[12,17] However, the most widely used regression procedure in method comparison studies, OLR, does not take errors in $x1$ into account but is based on the assumption that only the $x2$ measurements are subject to random errors (Figure 14-21). In the Deming procedure, the sum of squared distances from measured sets of values ($x1_i$, $x2_i$) to the regression line is minimized at an angle determined by the ratio between the standard deviations for the random variations of $x1$ and $x2$. It can be theoretically proven that given Gaussian error distributions, this estimation procedure is optimal. In Figure 14-22, the symmetric case is illustrated with a regression slope of 1 and equal standard deviations for the random variations of $x1$ and $x2$, in which case the sum of squared distances is minimized orthogonally in relation to the line. In OLR, the sum of squared distances is minimized in the vertical direction to the line (Figure 14-22). It can be proven theoretically that neglect of the random error in $x1$ induces a downward biased slope estimate

$$\beta' = \beta(\sigma^2_{X1'\text{target}}/(\sigma^2_{X1'\text{target}} + \sigma^2_{x1})) = \beta/\left[1+(\sigma_{x1}/\sigma_{X1'\text{target}})^2\right]$$

where $\sigma_{X1'\text{target}}$ is the standard deviation of $X1'$ target values.[97] According to the formula, the amount of bias depends on the ratio between the standard deviation for the random error in $x1$ and the standard deviation of the $X1'$ target values. In situations with a wide range of $X1'$ target values, this bias may be negligible, and OLR may be used for estimation of slope and intercept despite the assumption of a wrong error model. Figure 14-23 shows the bias as a function of the ratio of the random error standard deviation to the standard deviation of the $X1'$ target value dispersion. For a ratio up to 0.1, the bias is less than 1%. At a ratio of 0.33, the bias amounts to 10%, and then increases further for increasing ratios.

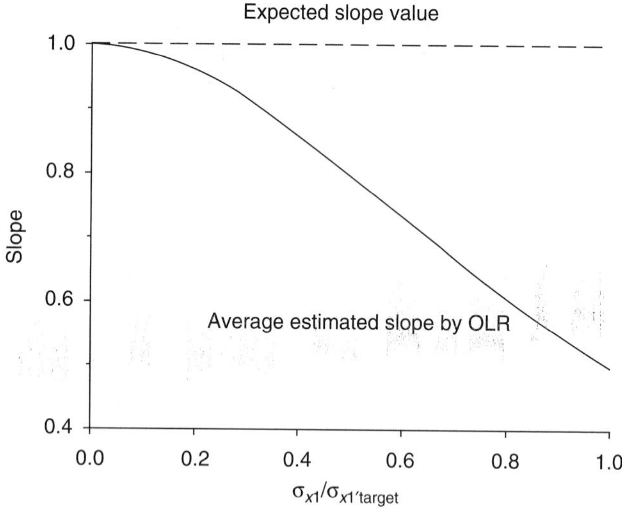

Figure 14-23 Relations between the true (expected) slope value and the average estimated slope by OLR. The bias of the OLR slope estimate increases negatively for increasing ratios of the standard deviation random error in $X1$ to the standard deviation of the $X1$ target value distribution.

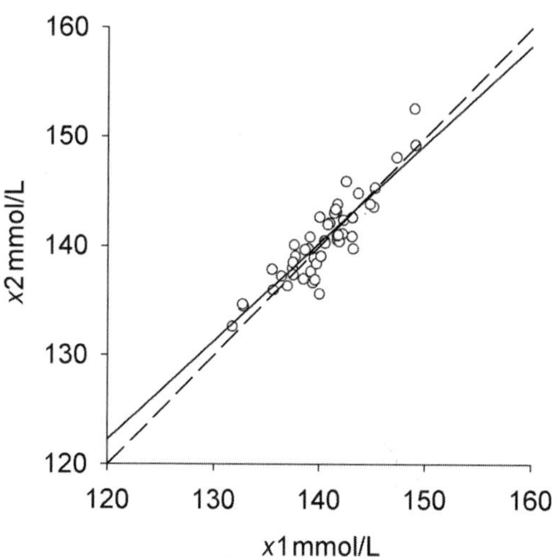

Figure 14-24 Simulated comparison of two sodium methods. The solid line indicates the average estimated OLR line, and the dashed line is the identity line. Even though there is no systematic difference between the two methods, the average OLR line deviates from the identity line corresponding to a downward slope bias of about 10%.

Example

As an illustration of the bias problem associated with application of the OLR procedure, we will study by simulation the comparison of two sodium methods. Fifty paired measurements are simulated. It is assumed that there is no systematic difference between the measurements, and we will expect an average slope estimate of 1.0 for 1000 repeated experiments. The mean value is 140.5 mmol/L corresponding to the mean of a reference interval 136 to 145 mmol/L. The dispersion of the target values was set to 3.8 mmol/L, which corresponds to a range exceeding the reference interval by about 5 mmol/L in each direction, corresponding to inclusion of some pathological samples. The analytical SDs for the methods are presumed constant throughout the analytical measurement range with values of 1.27 mmol/L corresponding to CVs of 0.9% at the mean 140.5 mmol/L. The average estimated regression line for the 1000 repetitions corresponds to the solid line in Figure 14-24, which is tilted downward corresponding to a slope value of 0.90 (i.e., 10% lower than the expected value of 1.0). The slope bias of −10% occurs, because the ratio between the SD of the random error in x to the SD of the dispersion of the target X' values is 0.33.

In the example presented above, the ratio of the analytical SD to the SD of the target value distribution is large because of the tight physiological regulation of electrolyte concentrations, which means that the biological variation is limited. Most other types of analytes exhibit wider distributions, and the ratio of error to target value distribution is smaller. For example, for analytes with a distribution of more than 1 decade and an analytical error corresponding to a CV of 5% at the middle of the analytical measurement range, the OLR slope bias amounts to about −1%.

Whether this is considered a problem may depend on the situation. In the context of assessing the ability to trace analytical methods from regression analysis of paired patient sample measurements, an error of 1% solely because of the applied regression procedure would indeed constitute a problem (see Traceability and Measurement Uncertainty later in this chapter).

Computation Procedures for OLR and Deming Regression

Assuming no errors in $x1$ and a Gaussian error distribution of $x2$ with constant standard deviation throughout the analytical measurement range, OLR is the optimal estimation procedure as proved by Gauss in the eighteenth century. About 50 years later, the first version of the errors-in-variables regression model was outlined by Adcock[1] and later supplemented by Kummel.[57] It should be noted for these parametric procedures that only the error distributions must be normal. The least-squares principle does not presume normality to be applied, but it is optimal under normality conditions, and the nominal Type I errors for the associated statistical tests for slope and intercept hold true under this assumption. The procedures are generally robust toward deviations from normality, but they are sensitive toward outliers because of the squaring principle. Finally the distribution of the target values of $x1$ and $x2$ does not have to be normal. A uniform distribution over the analytical measurement range is generally of advantage, but the distribution may in principle take any form.

It can be proved theoretically that the lines that minimize the sum of squared distances from the line in the two situations can be estimated as described below.[46] In both cases the mean values, the sum of squared deviations, and a sum of cross products should be computed:

$$x1_m = \sum x1_i/N \qquad x2_m = \sum x2_i/N$$

$$u = \sum (x1_i - x1_m)^2 \qquad q = \sum (x2_i - x2_m)^2$$

$$p = \sum (x1_i - x1_m)(x2_i - x2_m)$$

For OLR we have:

$$b = p/u \qquad a_0 = x2_m - bx1_m$$

and so

$$X2'_{\text{Targetest}i} = a_0 + bx1_i$$

$X2'_{\text{Targetest}i}$ refers to the *estimated* $X2'$ target value for a given $x1_i$ according to the regression equation (under the OLR model $x1_i$ and $X1'_{\text{Target}i}$ are identical). In case of duplicate sets of measurements, each $x1_i$ and $x2_i$ represents the mean of individual measurements ($x1 = (x1_{1i} + x1_{2i})/2$ and $x2_i = (x2_{1i} + x2_{2i})/2$).

To compute the slope in Deming regression analysis, the ratio between the standard deviations of the random errors of $x1$ and $x2$ is necessary, i.e.,

$$\lambda = (\sigma^2_{\text{RB1}} + \sigma^2_{\text{A1}})/(\sigma^2_{\text{RB2}} + \sigma^2_{\text{A2}})$$

(assuming independence of the random-bias terms).

Analytical standard deviations can be estimated from duplicate sets of measurements as:

$$SD^2_{A1} = (1/2N)\sum(x1_{2i} - x1_{1i})^2$$
$$SD^2_{A2} = (1/2N)\sum(x2_{2i} - x2_{1i})^2$$

or they may be available from quality control data.

If a specific value for λ is not available and the two field methods that are compared are likely to be associated with random error levels of the same order of magnitude, λ can be set to 1. The Deming procedure is generally relatively insensitive to a misspecification of the λ value.[67] The slope and intercept may now be derived as

$$b = \left[(\lambda q - u) + \left[(u - \lambda q)^2 + 4\lambda p^2\right]^{0.5}\right] \Big/ (2\lambda p)$$
$$a_0 = x2_m - bx1_m$$

and so

$$X2'_{\text{Targetesti}} = a_0 + bX1'_{\text{Targetesti}}$$

For both procedures, we may evaluate the standard deviation of the dispersion in the *vertical* direction around the line (commonly denoted $SD_{y.x}$ and here given as SD_{21}). We have

$$SD_{21} = \left[\sum(x2_i - X2'_{\text{Targetesti}})^2 / (N-2)\right]^{0.5}$$

For the OLR procedure we may further derive the standard errors of the slope and intercept estimate as follows

$$SE(b) = SD_{21}/\sqrt{u} \quad SE(a_0) = SD_{21}\left[1/N + x1^2_m/u\right]^{0.5}$$

For the OLR procedure, given that the assumptions are fulfilled (which they almost never are), these SEs are exact. For the Deming procedure, they apply approximately. More correct formulas have been given[99] or they can be conveniently derived by a computerized method (see later in this chapter). For both OLR and Deming regression analysis, the correct interpretation of SD_{21} is important, but quite often it is misinterpreted (see the next section).

Evaluation of the Random Error Around an Estimated Regression Line

The estimated slope and intercept provide an estimate of the systematic difference or error between two methods over the analytical measurement range. Additionally an estimate of the random error is important. As mentioned above, it is commonplace to consider the dispersion around the line in the vertical direction, which is quantified as $SD_{y.x}$ (here denoted SD_{21}). SD_{21} has originally been introduced in the context of OLR, but it may as well be considered in relation to Deming regression analysis.

Interpreting $SD_{y.x}$ (SD_{21}) With Random Error only in x2

In the model assumed in OLR, we only have random errors associated with $x2$ measurements (see Figure 14-21). This situation occurs infrequently in practice, but it can happen (e.g., when a set of reference materials is available that have been determined repetitively by a reference method), so that in practice there is no random measurement error present. In this case, the scatter around the line solely reflects the random error of $x2$ measurements. If there are no random matrix-related interferences, the random error equals the analytical imprecision, and we have

$$\sigma_{21} = \sigma_{A2}$$

If random matrix-related interferences are present, we have

$$\sigma^2_{21} = \sigma^2_{A2} + \sigma^2_{RB2}$$

where σ_{RB2} is the standard deviation of the random matrix-related effects, which are here supposed to be normally distributed and independent of method imprecision.

Interpreting $SD_{y.x}$ (SD_{21}) With Random Errors in Both x1 and x2

With regard to σ_{21}, we have here without sample-related random effects

$$\sigma^2_{21} = \beta^2\sigma^2_{A1} + \sigma^2_{A2}$$

Thus σ_{21} reflects both the random error in $x1$ (with a rescaling) and in $x2$. Often β is close to unity, and in this case σ^2_{21} becomes approximately the sum of the individual squared standard deviations.[73] This relation holds true for both Deming and OLR analysis. Frequently, OLR is applied in situations associated with random measurement error in both $x1$ and $x2$, and in these situations σ_{21} reflects the errors of both.

The presence of sample-related random interferences in both $x1$ and $x2$ gives the following expression

$$\sigma^2_{21} = \left[\beta^2\sigma^2_{A1} + \sigma^2_{A2}\right] + \left[\beta^2\sigma^2_{RB1} + \sigma^2_{RB2}\right]$$

Thus, the σ_{21} value is influenced by the slope value, the analytical error components σ_{A1} and σ_{A2} (grouped in the first bracket) and σ_{RB1} and σ_{RB2} (grouped in the second bracket). In many cases, the slope is close to unity, in which case we have simple addition of the components. As mentioned earlier, the matrix-related random interferences may not be independent. In this case, simple addition of the components is not correct, because a covariance term should be included. However, in a real case, we can estimate the combined effect corresponding to the bracket term. Information on the analytical components is usually available, either from duplicate sets of measurements or from quality control data. On this basis, the combined random bias term in the second bracket can be derived by subtracting the analytical components from σ_{21}. Overall, it can be judged whether the total random error is acceptable or not. The systematic difference can be adjusted for relatively easily by a rescaling of one of the sets of measurements. However, if the random error term is very large, such a rescaling does not ensure equivalency of measurements with regard to individual samples. Thus it is important to assess both the systematic difference and the random error when deciding whether a new field method can replace an existing one. Figure 14-25 shows the random distributions around the regression lines for simulated

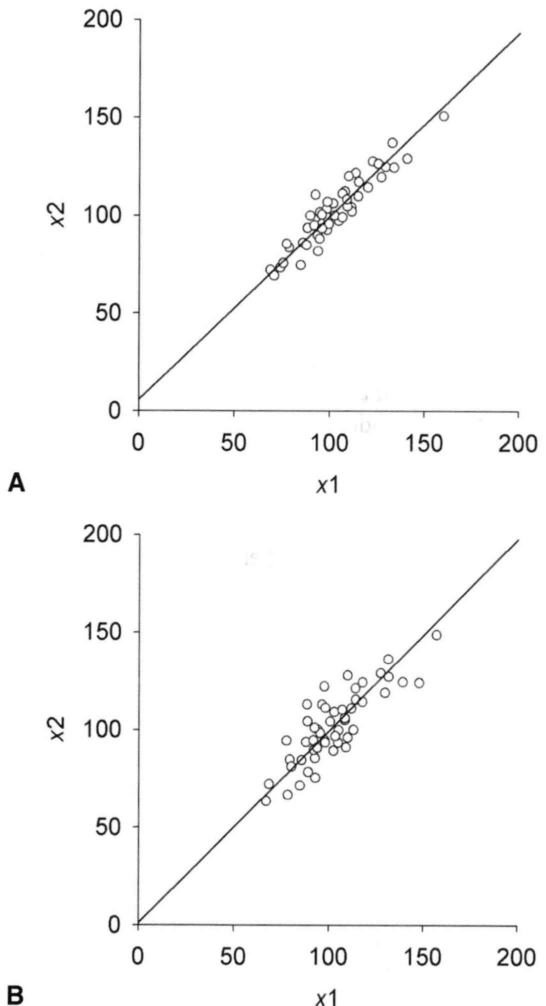

Figure 14-25 Simulated examples that illustrate the effect of sample-related random interferences in a scatter plot with regression analysis. **A,** $x1$ and $x2$ are subject to only analytical errors. **B,** Additional random bias of the same magnitude is present, which results in a wider scatter around the line.

examples with only analytical error (A) and both analytical error and random bias of an equal magnitude (B). In a roughly symmetric situation with a slope close to unity and two field methods of presumed equal specificity and precision, the total random error expressed as SD_{21} may be subdivided into component errors associated with each test by dividing with the square root of two. One may then assess the random error levels in relation to stated goals.

Assessment of Outliers

The principle of minimizing the sum of squared distances from the line makes the described regression procedures sensitive toward outliers, and an assessment of the occurrence of outliers should be carried out routinely. The distance from a suspected outlier to the line is recorded in standard deviation units, and rejection of the outlier is performed if the distance exceeds a predetermined limit (e.g., 3 or 4 standard deviation units). In the case of OLR, the standard deviation unit equals SD_{21}, and the vertical distance is considered. For Deming regression analysis, the unit is the standard deviation of the deviation of the points from the line at an angle determined by the error variance ratio λ. A plot of these deviations, a so-called residuals plot, conveniently illustrates the occurrence of outliers.[64] Figure 14-26, *A* illustrates a Deming regression analysis example with occurrence of an outlier and the associated residuals plot (B), which clearly shows the outlier pattern. In this example, the residuals plot was standardized to unit standard deviation. Using in this example an outlier limit of 4 standard deviation units, the outlier was rejected and a reanalysis was undertaken. In this example, rejection of the outlier changed the slope from 1.14 to 1.03. With regard to outliers, these measurements should not just be rejected automatically, but the reason for their presence should be scrutinized.

The Correlation Coefficient

Having outlined the random error components related to regression analysis, some comments on the correlation coefficient may be appropriate. The ordinary correlation coefficient ρ, also called the Pearson product moment correlation coefficient, is estimated as r from sums of squared deviations for $x1$ and $x2$ values as follows using the same notation as above[97]

$$r = p/[uq]^{0.5}$$

Looking at the theoretical model, ρ is related to the ratio between the standard deviations of the distributions of target values ($\sigma_{X1'\text{target}}$ and $\sigma_{X2'\text{target}}$) and the associated independent total random error components (σ_{x1} and σ_{x2})[7]

$$\rho = \sigma_{X1'\text{target}}\sigma_{X2'\text{target}}/[(\sigma^2_{X1'\text{target}}+\sigma^2_{x1})(\sigma^2_{X2'\text{target}}+\sigma^2_{x2})]^{0.5}$$

The total random error components comprise both imprecision error and sample-related random interferences (i.e., $\sigma^2_{x1} = \sigma^2_{A1} + \sigma^2_{RB1}$ and $\sigma^2_{x2} = \sigma^2_{A2} + \sigma^2_{RB2}$). Thus ρ is a *relative* indicator of the amount of dispersion around the regression line. If the range of values is short, ρ tends to be low and vice versa for a long range of values. For example, consider simulated examples, where the random errors of $x1$ and $x2$ are the same, but the width of the distributions of target values differs (Figure 14-27, *A* and *B*). In (A) the target values are uniformly distributed over the range 1 to 3, and in (B) the range is 1 to 6. The random error SD is presumed constant, and it is in both cases set to 0.15 for both $x1$ and $x2$ corresponding to a CV of 5% at the level 3. Given sets of 50 paired measurements, the correlation coefficient is 0.93 in case (A) and 0.99 in case (B). Further, a single point located outside the range of the rest of the observations exerts a strong influence (Figure 14-27, *C*). In (C) 49 of the observations are distributed within the range 1 to 3 with a single point located apart from the others around the value 6, other factors being equal. The correlation coefficient here takes an intermediate value, 0.97. Thus a single point located away from the rest has a strong influence (a so-called influential point). Notice that it is not an outlying point, just an aberrant point with regard to the range.

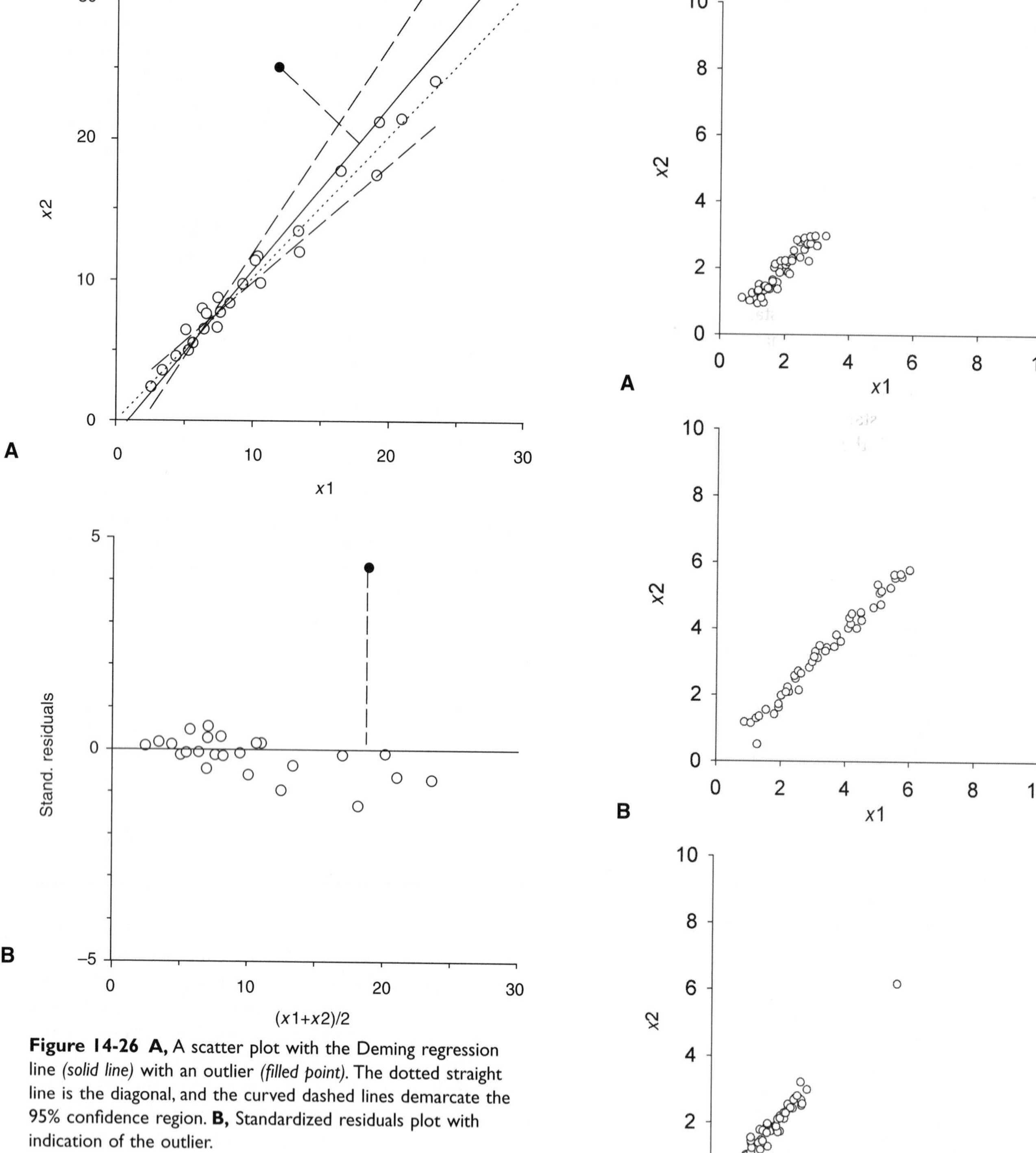

Figure 14-26 **A,** A scatter plot with the Deming regression line *(solid line)* with an outlier *(filled point)*. The dotted straight line is the diagonal, and the curved dashed lines demarcate the 95% confidence region. **B,** Standardized residuals plot with indication of the outlier.

Figure 14-27 Scatter plots illustrating the effect of the range on the value of the correlation coefficient ρ. **A,** The target values are uniformly distributed over the range 1 to 3 with random errors of both *x*1 and *x*2 corresponding to an SD of 5% of the target value at 3 (constant error standard deviations). **B,** The range is extended to 1 to 6 with the same random error levels. The correlation coefficient equals 0.93 in **A** and 0.99 in **B.** In **C** the effect of a single aberrant point is shown. Forty-nine of the target values are distributed over the range 1 to 3 with a single point at 6. The correlation coefficient is 0.97.

Although σ_{21} is the relevant measure for random error in method comparison studies, ρ is still widely used as a supposed measure of agreement between two methods. It should be noted that a systematic difference is not expressed through ρ; thus even though the correlation coefficient is very high, there may be a considerable bias between the measurements of two methods.

Regression Analysis in Case of Proportional Random Errors

As discussed in relation to the precision profile, for analytes with extended ranges (e.g., 1 or several decades), the analytical standard deviation is seldom constant. Rather a proportional relationship may apply. This may also be true for the random bias components. In this situation, the regression procedures described above may still be used, but they are not optimal because the standard errors of slope and intercept become larger than is the case when applying a weighted form of regression analysis. The optimal approaches are weighted forms of regression analysis that take into account the relationship between random error and analyte concentration. Given a proportional relationship, a weighted procedure assigns larger weights to observations in the low range; the low-range observations are more precise than measurements at higher concentrations that are subject to larger random errors. More specifically, weights are applied in the computations that are inversely proportional to the squared standard deviations (variances) that express the random error. In the weighted form of least-squares regression analysis (WLR) the distances from $(x1_i, x2_i)$ to the line in the vertical direction are inversely weighted according to the squared SD_A value at the given concentration level (Figure 14-28).

The following computations are performed

$$x1_{mw} = \sum w_i x1_i / \sum w_i \qquad x2_{mw} = \sum w_i x2_i / \sum w_i$$

$$u_w = \sum w_i (x1_i - x1_{mw})^2 \qquad q_w = \sum w_i (x2_i - x2_{mw})^2$$

$$p_w = \sum w_i (x1_i - x1_{mw})(x2_i - x2_{mw})$$

$$b = p_w / u_w \qquad a_0 = x2_{mw} - b x1_{mw}$$

$$X2'_{\text{Targetesti}} = a_0 + b x1_i$$

The weights (w_i) are inversely proportional to the squared standard deviation of random errors of $x2$ measurements at a given concentration. These standard devations are assumed to be a function $(h(\cdot))$ of $x1$:

$$\sigma_{A2} = k_{A2} h(x1_i) \qquad w_i = [h(x1_i)]^{-2}$$

$$\sigma_{RB2} = k_{RB2} h(x1_i)$$

where k_{A2} and k_{RB2} are proportionality factors and $w_i = [h(x1_i)]^{-2}$.[31,66] Alternatively, weighting might be given as a function of $X2'_{\text{Targetest}}$ determined iteratively, which provides essentially the same results apart from different proportionality constants. For the proportional standard deviation case, which is assumed to hold true in the present context, $w_i = 1/x1_i^2$. The proportionality factor is estimated from the dispersion around the line in the vertical direction

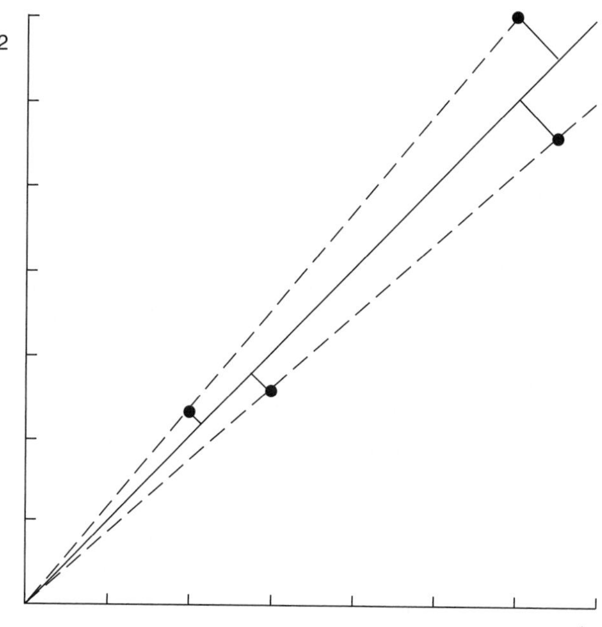

Figure 14-28 Distances from data points to the line in the vertical direction in WLR assuming proportional standard deviations for random errors in $x2$ and no random error in $x1$. *(From Linnet K. Necessary sample size for method comparison studies based on regression analysis. Clin Chem 1999;45:882-94.)*

$$k = \left[\sum (x2_i - X2'_{\text{Targetesti}})^2 w_i / (N-2)\right]^{0.5}$$

The standard errors of slope and intercept are[31,66]

$$SE(b) = k/\sqrt{u_w} \qquad SE(a_0 = k[1/\sum w_i + x_{mw}^2/u_w])^{0.5}$$

The Deming method can also be carried out in a weighted form (e.g., assuming proportional standard deviations). In the weighted modification of the Deming procedure, distances from $(x1_i, x2_i)$ to the line are inversely weighted according to the squared standard deviations at a given concentration (Figure 14-29). The regression procedures are most conveniently performed using dedicated software, which is available on the book's accompanying Evolve site.

For the weighted Deming procedure, the slope and intercept are estimated as[64]

$$b = \left[(\lambda q_w - u_w) + \left[(u_w - \lambda q_w)^2 + 4\lambda p_w^2\right]^{0.5}\right] / 2\lambda p_w$$

$$a_0 = x2_{mw} - b x1_{mw}$$

$$X2'_{\text{Targetesti}} = a_0 + b X1'_{\text{Targetesti}}$$

It is here presumed that the *ratio* between the squared standard deviations for the random error components

$$\lambda = (\sigma_{RB1}^2 + \sigma_{A1}^2)/(\sigma_{RB2}^2 + \sigma_{A2}^2)$$

is constant throughout the analytical measurement range. The standard deviations are functions of the target values

$$\sigma_{A1} = k_{A1}h(X1'_{Targeti}) \text{ and } \sigma_{A2} = k_{A2}h(X2'_{Targeti})$$

$$\sigma_{RB1} = k_{RB1}h(X1'_{Targeti}) \text{ and } \sigma_{RB2} = k_{RB2}h(X2'_{Targeti})$$

Assuming a proportional relationship, the weights w_i $(= 1/[(X1'_{Targetesti} + \lambda X2'_{Targetesti})/(1+\lambda)]^2)$ are obtained by an iterative approach as described.[64,66]

For the weighted Deming procedure, general formulas for standard errors of slope and intercept are complicated, and computerized methods (e.g., jackknife or bootstrap) may be applied in their estimation (available on the book's accompanying Evolve site). Using these computerized approaches, a 95% confidence region around the line may also be estimated (Figure 14-30). The confidence region as outlined here refers to the CIs for estimated $X2'$ target values in relation to given $X1'$ target values and is accordingly not a 95% region for the individual paired observations (i.e., it is not a prediction region). It is observed that the interval is most narrow at a level corresponding to the weighted mean of $x1$ values and widens toward the extremes of the $x1$ range, especially at high concentrations where the random error is largest. For a simplified situation with a slope close to unity and equal CVs for random error components of $x1$ and $x2$, the formulas given under WLR approximately apply.

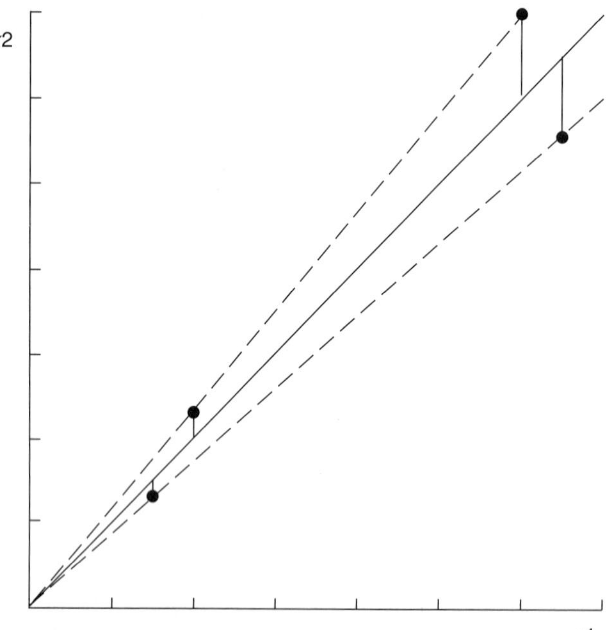

Figure 14-29 Distances from data points to the line in weighted Deming regression assuming proportional random errors in $x1$ and $x2$. The symmetric case is illustrated with equal random errors and a slope of unity yielding orthogonal projections onto the line. *(From Linnet K. Necessary sample size for method comparison studies based on regression analysis. Clin Chem 1999;45:882-94.)*

Determination of the Random Error Around an Estimated Regression Line in Case of Proportional Random Errors

In regression analysis with proportional random errors, we will also consider the dispersion around the line in the vertical direction. SD_{21} is dependent on the measured concentration. Supposing a proportional error relationship and an intercept of the regression line close to zero, SD_{21} can be characterized by a proportionality factor.[31,66]

Relations with Random Error Only in x2

In the model assumed in WLR, we only have random errors associated with $x2$ measurements. If there are no random matrix-related interferences, the random error equals the analytical imprecision, and we have

$$CV_{21} = CV_{A2}$$

If random matrix-related interferences are present, we have

$$CV_{21}^2 = CV_{A2}^2 + CV_{RB2}^2$$

where CV_{RB2} is the coefficient of variation for the random matrix-related effects, which are here supposed to be normally distributed and independent of method imprecision.

Relations with Random Errors in Both x1 and x2

Assuming there are random errors in $x1$ and $x2$ without sample-related random effects, CV_{21} can be determined as follows

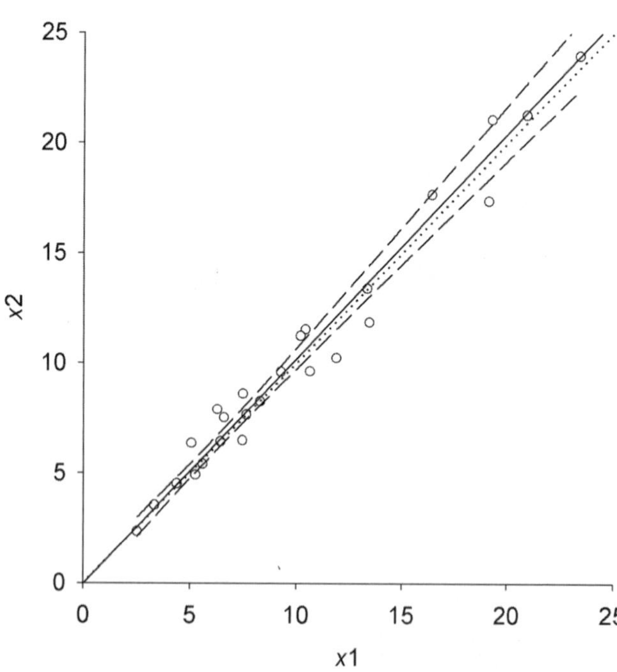

Figure 14-30 An example of application of weighted Deming regression analysis. The solid line is the estimated regression line, and the dotted line is the line of identity. The estimated 95% confidence bands obtained by the jackknife approach are the curved dashed lines.

$$CV_{21}^2 = CV_{A1}^2 + CV_{A2}^2$$

Thus CV_{21} reflects both the random error in $x1$ and in $x2$. In case of proportional errors, there is no rescaling of the $x1$ error contribution. This relation holds true for both weighted Deming and WLR analysis. Frequently, WLR is applied in situations associated with random measurement error in both $x1$ and $x2$, and in these situations CV_{21} reflects the errors of both.

The presence of proportional sample-related random interferences in both $x1$ and $x2$ gives the following expression

$$CV_{21}^2 = [CV_{A1}^2 + CV_{A2}^2] + [CV_{RB1}^2 + CV_{RB2}^2]$$

As mentioned earlier, the matrix-related random interferences may not be independent. In this case, simple addition of the components is not correct, because a covariance term should be included. However, we can estimate the combined effect corresponding to the bracket term, which then strictly refers to the CV of the differences ($CV_{RB2-RB1}^2$). As in the case with constant standard deviations, information on the analytical components is usually available, either from duplicate sets of measurements or from quality control data, and the combined random bias term in the second bracket can then be derived by subtracting the analytical component from CV_{21}. Systematic and random errors can then be determined, and it can be decided whether a new field method can replace an existing one. Figure 14-31 shows an example with proportional random errors around the regression line.

In a situation with proportional random errors, a weighted modification of the correlation coefficient can be computed from sums of squared deviations for $x1$ and $x2$ values as follows

$$r_w = p_w/[u_w q_w]^{0.5}$$

Adjustments for Recalibration

Having estimated a linear relationship between two field methods, one may wish to recalibrate one of the methods in relation to the other (e.g., for method 2 one may make the adjustment)

$$x2_{rec} = (x2 - a_0)/b$$

where $x2_{rec}$ is the recalibrated $x2$ value. The systematic bias is now adjusted between the methods, and it is of interest to study the random error elements. Figures 14-32, *A* and 14-33, *A* show two simulated situations in which $\sigma_{A1} = \sigma_{A2} = 5$ and $\sigma_{RB1} = \sigma_{RB2} = 5$. In Figures 14-32, *A* and 14-33, *A* the slopes are 1.5 and 0.5, respectively. The random error of the differences between the values of method 1 and the recalibrated $x2$ values ($x2_{rec} - x1$) is observed from the displayed recalibration difference plots (Figures 14-32, *B* and 14-33, *B*). It is evident that in the case with a slope of 0.5, the dispersion of the differences is largest. This is due to the rescaling of the $x2$ values, which leads to an associated rescaling of the random error. We have

$$\sigma_{A2rec} = \sigma_{A2}/\beta \text{ and } \sigma_{RB2rec} = \sigma_{RB2}/\beta$$

Thus in the case with a slope value below unity, the random error of the rescaled value is amplified, and vice versa for a

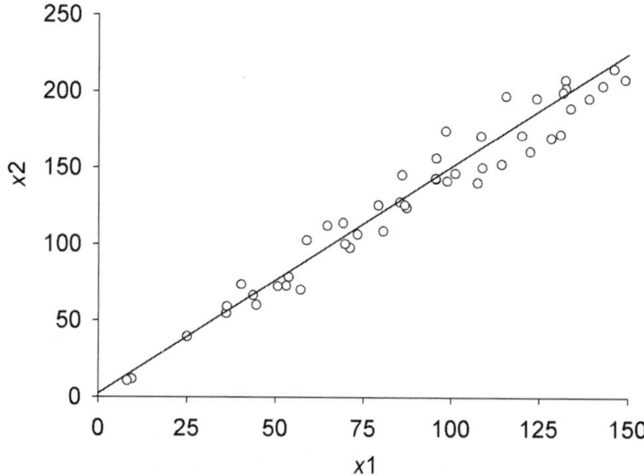

Figure 14-31 An example of proportional random errors around a regression line estimated by the weighted Deming approach.

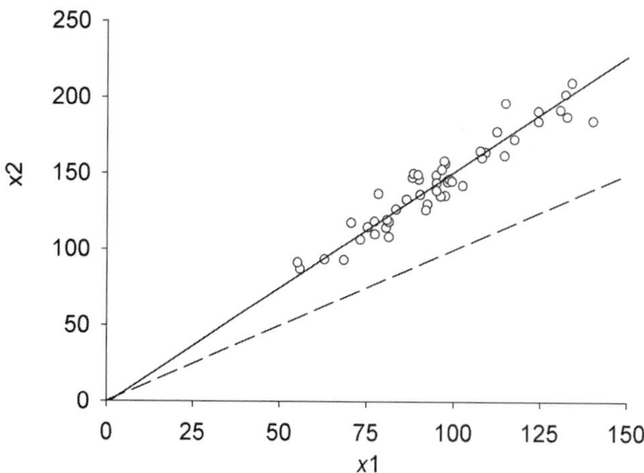

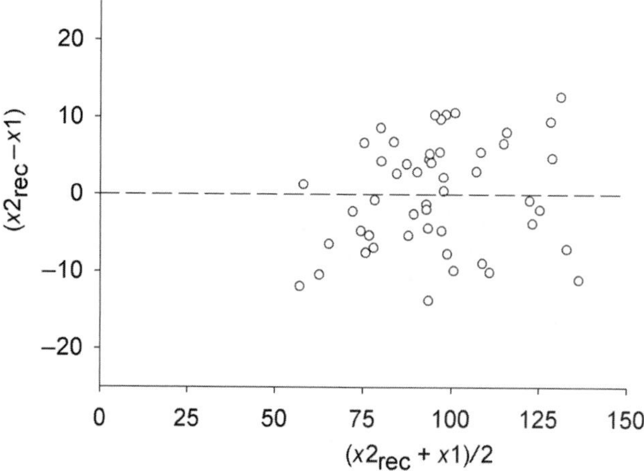

Figure 14-32 *Scatter* plot *(top)* and recalibration difference plot *(bottom)* of ($x2_{rec} - x1$) differences against ($x2_{rec} + x1$)/2 for situations corresponding to one simulation run of $N = 50$ ($x1$, $x2$) sets for the following parameter values: $\alpha_0 = 0$, $\beta = 1.5$, $\sigma_{x1} = 5$, and $\sigma_{x2} = 5$.

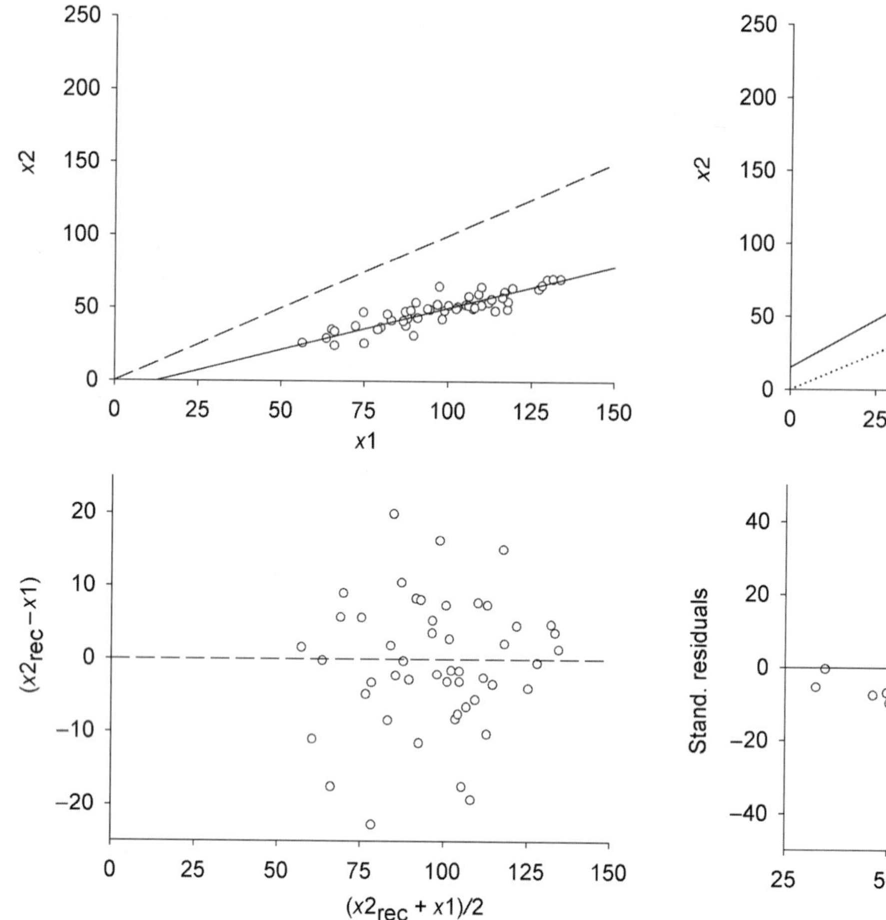

Figure 14-33 Scatter plot *(top)* and recalibration difference plots *(bottom)* of $(x2_{rec} - x1)$ differences against $(x2_{rec} + x1)/2$ for situations corresponding to one simulation run of $N = 50$ $(x1, x2)$ sets for the following parameter values: $\alpha_0 = 0$, $\beta = 0.5$, $\sigma_{x1} = 5$, and $\sigma_{x2} = 5$.

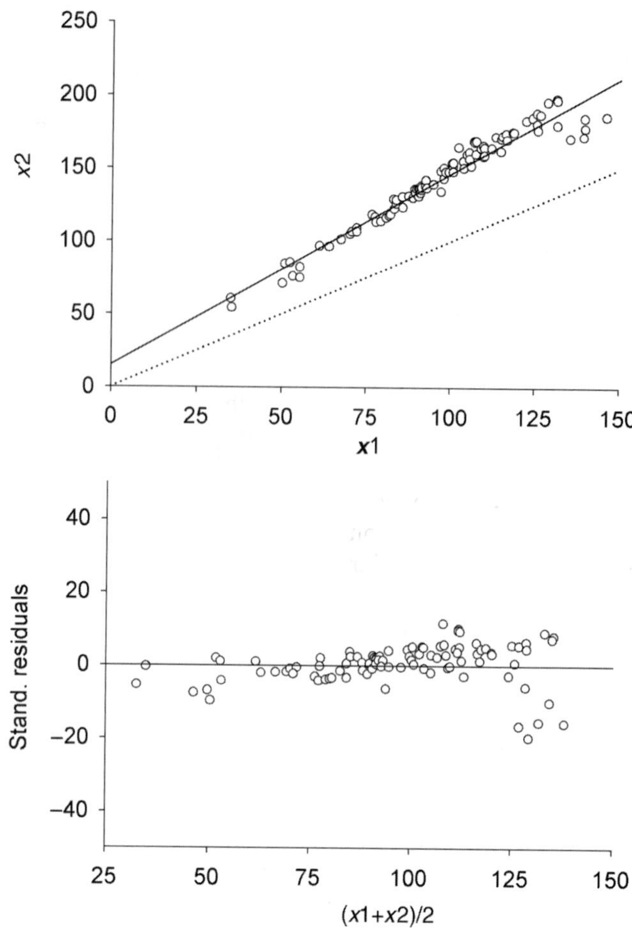

Figure 14-34 *Top,* Scatter plot showing an example of nonlinearity in the form of downward deviating $x2$ values at the upper part of the range. *Bottom,* Plot of residuals showing the effect of nonlinearity. At the upper end of the analytical measurement range, a sequence (run) of negative residuals is present from $x = 150$ to 200.

slope exceeding unity. The overall expression for the random error between the differences of $x1$ and $x2_{rec}$ becomes

$$\sigma_{(x2rec-x1)} = \left[(\sigma_{A2}/\beta)^2 + (\sigma_{RB2}/\beta)^2 + \sigma_{A1}^2 + \sigma_{RB1}^2\right]^{0.5}$$

In a real example, $\sigma_{(x2rec-x1)}$ is estimated from the set of paired differences between rescaled $x2$ values and $x1$ values and may be conveniently displayed in the form of a recalibration difference plot that also serves as a validation of the presumed linear relationship between the original sets of measurements. From the magnitude of the standard deviation of the paired differences, one may then judge whether it is acceptable to interchange measurements between method 1 and the rescaled method 2.

Testing for Linearity

Splitting of the systematic error into a constant and a proportional component depends on the assumption of linearity, which should be tested. A convenient test is a runs test, which in principle assesses whether the negative and positive deviations from the points to the line are randomly distributed over the analytical measurement range.[20] The term *run* here relates to a sequence of deviations with the same sign. Consider for example the situation with a downward trend of $x2$ values at the upper end of the analytical measurement range (Figure 14-34, *A*). The standardized deviations from the line (i.e., the residuals) will then tend to be negative in this area instead of being randomly distributed above and below the line[64] (Figure 14-34, *B*). Given a sufficient number of points, such a sequence will turn out to be statistically significant in a runs test.

Nonparametric Regression Analysis (Passing-Bablok)

The slope and intercept may be estimated by a nonparametric procedure, which is robust to outliers, and requires no assumptions of Gaussian error distributions.[82] Notice, however, that the parametric regression procedures do not presume Gaussian distributions of target values, but only of the error distributions. Furthermore, the jackknife principle used for estimation of standard errors for Deming and weighted Deming procedures is also in principle nonparametric. Thus the main advantage of the nonparametric procedure is its robust performance in the presence of outliers. The method takes measurement errors for both $x1$ and $x2$ into account, but the method presumes that the ratio between analytical standard deviations is related to the slope in a fixed manner

$$\lambda = (SD^2_{RB1} + SD^2_{A1})/(SD^2_{RB2} + SD^2_{A2}) = 1/\beta^2$$

Otherwise, a biased slope estimate is obtained.[66,83] The procedure may be applied both in situations with constant analytical standard deviations and in cases with proportional analytical standard deviations. The method is not as efficient as the corresponding parametric procedures (i.e., Deming and weighted Deming procedures).[66]

Slope and intercept with CIs are provided together with Spearman's rank correlation coefficient. A software program is required for the procedure.

Principle of Computations

The procedure consists of calculating all sets of possible slopes from the set of $N(x1, x2)$ values

$$S_{ij} = (x2_i - x2_j)/(x1_i - x1_j) \text{ for } 1 \le i < j \le N$$

The slope is in principle obtained as a shifted median

$$b = S_{((n+1)/2+K)} \text{ for odd } n$$

$$b = \exp((\log(S_{(n/2+K)}) + \log(S_{(n/2+1+K)}))/2) \text{ for even } n \text{ (geometric mean)}$$

where n is the total number of S_{ij} values, and K is the number of S_{ij} values below −1.

The intercept a_0 is obtained as the median of all $(x2_i - bx1_i)$.

CIs for slope and intercept are derived as described.[82] No standard error is obtained in this purely nonparametric procedure. If the CI for the slope does not include 1, the deviation is statistically significant and analogous for the intercept.

Interpretation of Systematic Differences between Methods Obtained on the Basis of Regression Analysis

A systematic difference between two methods is identified, if the estimated intercept differs significantly from zero, or if the slope deviates significantly from 1. This is decided on the basis of t-tests

$$t = (a_0 - 0)/\text{SE}(a_0)$$

$$t = (b - 1)/\text{SE}(b)$$

SE(a_0) and SE(b) are the standard errors of the estimated intercept a_0 and slope b, respectively. For OLR and WLR, the standard errors are calculated from the formulas presented previously. These formulas also apply approximately for the Deming and weighted Deming procedures. An exact procedure is to apply a computerized resampling principle called the jackknife procedure, which in practice can be carried out using appropriate software[69] (described on the book's accompanying Evolve site).

Having estimated a_0 and b, we have the estimate of the systematic difference between the methods, D_c, at a selected concentration $X1'_{\text{Targetc}}$

$$D_c = X2'_{\text{Targetestc}} - X1'_{\text{Targetc}} = a_0 + (b - 1)X1'_{\text{Targetc}}$$

$X2'_{\text{Targetestc}}$ is the estimated $X2'$ target value at $X1'_c$. Notice that D_c refers to the *systematic* difference (i.e., the difference between target values), and so it is not a total error including random measurement errors.

The standard error of the estimated systematic difference D_c should be considered. For OLR the formula applies

$$\text{SE}(D_c) = \text{SD}_{21}\left[1/N + (X1'_{\text{Targetc}} - x_m)^2/u\right]^{0.5}$$

For WLR we have the analogous formula

$$\text{SE}(D_c) = k_{21}\left[1/\sum w_i + (X1'_{\text{Targetc}} - x_{mw})^2/u_w\right]^{0.5}$$

where $k_{21} = [\Sigma(x2_i - X2'_{\text{Targetest}i})^2 w_i/(N-2)]^{0.5}$. The formulas given above for OLR and WLR apply approximately for Deming and weighted Deming regression, respectively. An exact procedure is to apply the jackknife procedure using a software program.[69] By evaluating the standard error throughout the analytical measurement range, a confidence region for the estimated line can be displayed (see Figure 14-30). It is apparent from the structure of the formulas that the confidence region is narrowest at the center of the range (x_m or x_{mw}). If method comparison is performed to assess the ability to trace, correction of a significant systematic difference D_c will often be performed by recalibration ($x2_{\text{rec}} = (x1 - a_0)/b)$). The associated standard uncertainty is the standard error of D_c (see section on Traceability). Even though the intercept and slope are not significantly different from zero and one, respectively, the combined expression D_c may be significantly different from zero. This may occur in situations in which the intercept and slope deviations are in the same direction.

Example of Application of Regression Analysis (Weighted Deming Analysis)

Application of weighted Deming regression analysis may be illustrated by the comparison of drug assays example (N = 65($x1$, $x2$) measurements). As outlined in detail previously, in this example the random error of the differences increases with the concentration, suggesting that the weighted form of Deming regression analysis is appropriate. Figure 14-35 shows (A) the estimated regression line with 95% confidence bands and (B) a plot of residuals. The nearly homogeneous scatter in the residuals plot supports the assumed proportional random error model and the assumption of linearity. The slope estimate (1.014) is not significantly different from 1 (95% CI: 0.97 to 1.06), and the intercept is not significantly different from zero (95% CI −6.7 to 47.4) (Table 14-12). A runs test for linearity does not contradict the assumption of linearity. The amount of random error is

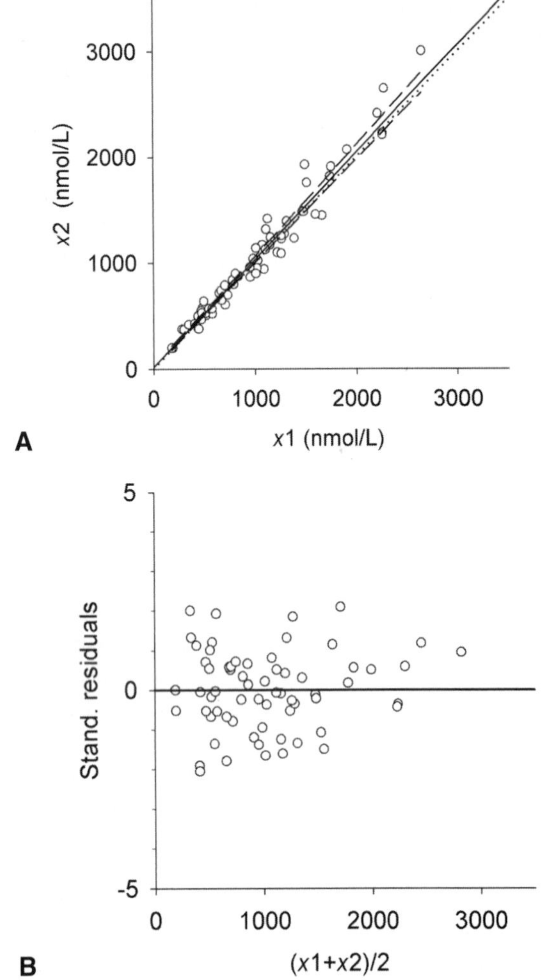

Figure 14-35 An example of weighted Deming regression analysis for the comparison of drug assays. **A,** The solid line is the estimated weighted Deming regression line, the dashed curves indicate the 95% confidence region, and the dotted line is the line of identity. **B,** A plot of residuals standardized to unit standard deviation. The homogeneous scatter supports the assumed proportional error model and the assumption of linearity.

quantified in the form of the SD_{21} proportionality factor equal to 0.11 or 11%. In the present example with a slope close to unity and two field methods with assumed random errors of about the same magnitude we divide the random error by the square root of two and get $CV_{x1} = CV_{x2} = 7.8\%$. In this simple case with a slope of unity, the results correspond to those previously derived in the analysis of the distribution of relative differences. Quality control data in the laboratory have provided CV_As of 6.1% and 7.2% for method 1 and 2, respectively. Thus in this example the random error largely may be attributed to analytical error. The assay principle is for both methods HPLC, which generally is a rather specific measurement principle, and considerable random bias effects are not expected in this case. If one or both of the assays had been immunoassays, the situation might have been different.

In the table, the estimated systematic differences at the limits of the therapeutic interval (300 and 2000 nmol/L) are displayed (24.6 and 48.9 nmol/L, respectively). This corresponds to percentage values of 8.2% and 2.4%, respectively. The estimated standard errors by the jackknife procedure yield the 95% CIs as shown in the table. At the low concentration, the difference is significant (95% CI: 5.7 to 44 nmol/L does not include zero), which is not the case at the high level (95% CI: −19 to 117 nmol/L). Even though the intercept and slope estimates separately are not significantly different from the null hypothesis values of zero and 1, respectively, the combined difference $Delta_c$ is significant at low concentrations in this example. If the difference is considered of medical importance and both methods are to be used simultaneously in the laboratory, a recalibration of one of the methods might be considered.

Estimating Sample Size Necessary for Method Comparison Studies

In the planning phase of a method comparison study, one should consider the size of the medically significant difference or critical difference Δ_c that should be detected at a given concentration $X1'_{Target\,c}$ (see *Analytical Goals*)

TABLE 14-12 Results of Weighted Deming Regression Analysis for the Comparison of Drug Assays Example, $N = 65$ $(x1, x2)$ Measurements

	Estimate	SE	95%-CI
Slope (b)	1.014	0.022	0.97 to 1.06
Intercept (a_0)	20.3	13.5	−6.7 to 47.4
Weighted correlation coefficient	0.98		
SD_{21} proportionality factor	0.11		
Runs test for linearity	n.s.		
$Delta_c = X_2 - X_1$ at $X_c = 300$	24.6	9.5	5.72 to 43.6
$Delta_c = X_2 - X_1$ at $X_c = 2000$	48.9	34.2	−19.3 to 117

(Figure 14-36). One may then derive the requirements for detecting critical sizes of α_0 and slope deviation from unity ($\beta - 1$):

$$\Delta_c = X2'_{\text{Target}c} - X1'_{\text{Target}c} = \alpha_0 + (\beta - 1)X1'_{\text{Target}c}$$

In the following section, statistical power considerations with regard to testing for intercept and slope deviations are presented.

Statistical Power Considerations in Method Comparison Studies

The investigator should consider whether the study design is likely to disclose critical differences of clinical relevance. Important factors in this context are the range of measurements, the SDs of the random errors of the involved methods, and the number of samples. These factors determine the statistical power of a method comparison study (i.e., the ability of the data analysis procedure to verify the presence of a given systematic difference).

Having decided from above what values of α_0 and ($\beta - 1$) should be detected, the next step is to design the method comparison study appropriately. First, a relevant range of values should be included (i.e., covering the range of clinical interest). A uniform distribution of values over the range is preferable and is primarily supposed in the present evaluation. Secondly, we have to consider the random errors of the methods. Two situations should be considered: the presence of constant and variable SDs for random error. The first possibility is mainly of interest given a short range of measured concentrations (e.g., in case of electrolyte methods). Given ranges of more than 1 or more decades, the standard deviations of the random error distributions usually vary with the measured concentration, often in a roughly proportional way.[93] Finally, specific values for the SDs or CVs of the methods should be assigned from available quality control data and assumptions concerning random matrix-related errors. According to the formula presented below and as explained in more detail,[69] we now have the necessary information to plan the comparison study (i.e., to decide on the necessary number of samples).

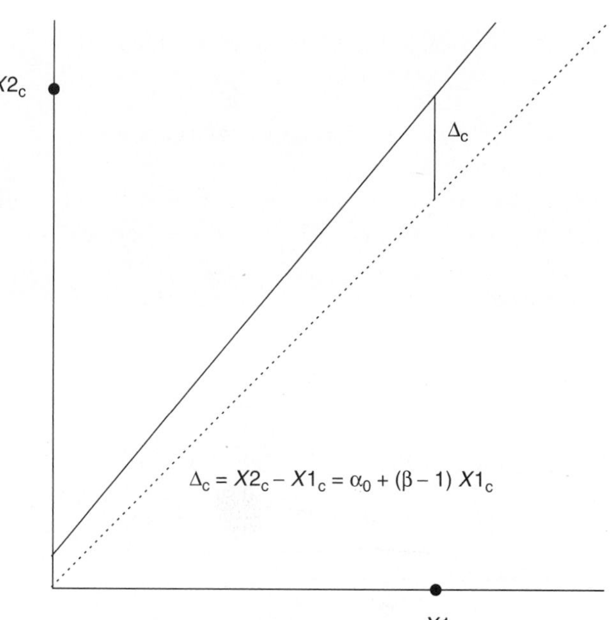

Figure 14-36 Illustration of the systematic difference Δ_c between two methods at a given level $X1_c$ according to the regression line. The difference is a result of a constant systematic difference (intercept deviation from zero) and a proportional systematic difference (slope deviation from unity). The dotted line represents the diagonal $X2 = X1$.

A general, simplified formula for approximating the sample size necessary for detection of a given deviation Δ of slope from unity or intercept from zero is[69]:

$$N = (c/\Delta)^2(t_{p/2} + t_{1-q})^2$$

Δ is the actual difference in slope from unity (or intercept from zero), and c is a constant determining the standard error ($= c/\sqrt{N}$) of the *estimated* difference D corresponding to the true difference Δ. $t_{p/2}$ depends on the significance level p (Type I error) and is 1.96 (asymptotically) for p less than or equal to 5%. t_{1-q} reflects the statistical power $(1 - q)$, which is the probability of verifying a real difference Δ. The complement of statistical power is the Type II error (q), which is the probability of overlooking a real difference Δ. For a traditional power level of 90%, t_{1-q} takes the value 1.28. Finally the sample size is, in principle, inversely related to the squared difference Δ (i.e., if a given difference is halved, the sample size requirement is increased by a factor of four). At small to moderate sample sizes, however, adjustment of the t-value from the asymptotic value and the general impact of approximations disturb this relationship slightly.[69]

The relation between the null hypothesis situation of no difference (difference = 0) and the alternative hypothesis of the presence of a real difference (difference = Δ) is schematically shown in Figure 14-37. The figure outlines the hypothetical situation corresponding to a set of repeated method comparison studies that results in observed differences D that are distributed around the true difference, which is zero under the null hypothesis of no difference and equal to Δ under the alternative hypothesis. The larger the sample size is, the narrower the dispersions of observed differences around the true values are. Thus for a given Δ and Type I error the power increases with the sample size.

The necessary sample sizes for a series of standard method comparison situations in clinical chemistry have been tabulated (Tables 14-13 and 14-14). A Type I error (significance level) of 5% and a power of 90% have been assumed. Table 14-13 concerns the situation with *constant* SDs over the analytical measurement range, and Table 14-14 covers cases with *proportional* SDs.

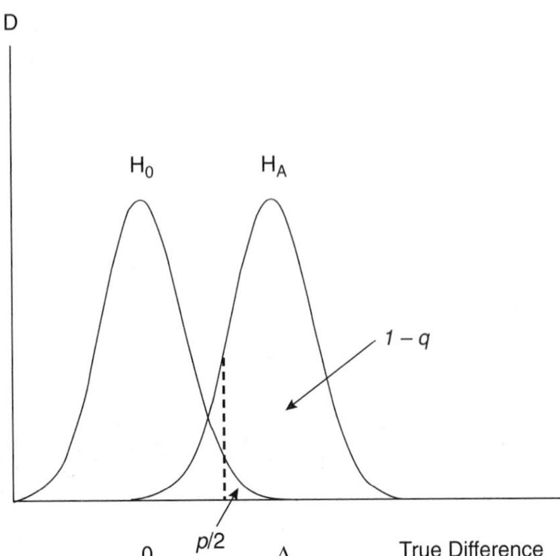

Figure 14-37 Schematic illustration of distributions of differences D under the null hypothesis (H_0) of no real difference and the alternative hypothesis (H_A) of the presence of a real difference Δ. The vertical dotted line indicates the limit of statistical significance. *p* is the Type I error (5%), and 1 − *q* is the power (90%). *(From Linnet K. Necessary sample size for method comparison studies based on regression analysis. Clin Chem 1999;45:882-94.)*

Power in Case of Constant Error Standard Deviations

Table 14-13 covers intervals with ratios from 1.25 to 10 for the maximum value divided by the minimum value (range ratio = maximum value/minimum value). The other entry in the table is the standardized delta value for slope or intercept. As regards the slope, this value refers to the slope deviation from unity measured in analytical coefficient of variation units:

$$\Delta\beta_{st} = (\beta - 1)/CV$$

where CV refers to $[CV_A^2 + CV_{RB}^2]^{0.5}$. Notice that the CVs (expressed as fractions) enter the formula, even though constant SDs are supposed, implying that the CVs are not constant over the analytical measurement range. The CVs in the formula refer to the specific CV value at the middle of the interval of interest (i.e., CV = SD/x_m), where x_m is the mean of the interval for the analytes.[69] It is assumed in the present context that the CV values for method 1 and 2 are identical. CV_A values may be known from quality control data. CV_{RB} values are usually not known. Depending on knowledge about the analytical principles and the likely influence of matrix effects a reasonable value should be assumed. In some situations, a value of zero is reasonable; in other cases a value similar to the CV_A might be assumed.

With regard to the intercept deviation from zero, the standardized delta value is:

$$\Delta\alpha_{0st} = (\alpha_0 - 0)/SD$$

TABLE 14-13 Sample Size Table for Comparison of Methods With *Constant* Standard Deviations for Random Errors Using Deming Regression Analysis*

Necessary sample sizes for test of slope deviation from 1 or intercept deviation from zero by Deming regression analysis given constant error standard deviations: $SD_{x1} = SD_{x2}$ = SD. Uniform *x*1 and *x*2 distributions on intervals with the given range ratio. The range ratio is the maximum value divided by the minimum value of the considered interval.

OLR (given no random error in *x*1) requires half the listed sample sizes.

Type I error: 5%; Power: 90%.

	RANGE RATIOS								
$\Delta\beta_{st} = (\beta - 1)/CV$†	1.25	1.5	2	2.5	3	4	5	8	10
1	5104	1575	567	343	256	182	150	116	108
2	1276	410	152	90	69	48	39	32	27
3	585	185	70	42	32	25	20	16	15
4	325	104	41	27	20	15	13	11	≤10
	RANGE RATIOS								
$\Delta\alpha_{0st} = (\alpha_0 - 0)/SD$	1.25	1.5	2	2.5	3	4	5	8	10
1	5125	1596	588	364	273	196	168	125	120
2	1281	410	152	91	71	52	44	35	32
3	580	187	71	42	33	26	22	17	16
4	330	110	40	27	21	15	13	11	≤10

*From Linnet K. Necessary sample size for method comparison studies based on regression analysis. Clin Chem 1999;45:882-94.

†CV refers to the coefficient of variation for the random error at the middle of the given interval (SD/x_m).

where SD refers to $[SD_A^2 + SD_{RB}^2]^{0.5}$. The standard situations presuppose that the analyte values are uniformly distributed over the intervals of interest. The table has only selected entry values. With regard to standardized deviations that are not covered, an approximate sample size may be obtained by interpolation or extrapolation. At large sample sizes, squared interpolation or extrapolation is reasonable (examples of squared interpolation and extrapolation are given in the example below), but for small sample sizes this relationship is not exactly valid. Concerning the tabulated range ratios, approximate interpolations can also be carried out. Estimation of N given assumptions not covered in the table may be performed on the basis of formulas as described.[69] Moreover, it may be prudent to add additional samples to take nonideal conditions into account (e.g., target value distributions that are not exactly uniform over the given interval) (see later). The tabulated values refer to application of Deming regression analysis assuming equal random errors for both methods. If OLR is applied and there are no random errors associated with the $x1$ values, the required sample sizes are half the tabulated values.

It is apparent from the table that the range of values is very important with regard to the required sample size for detection of a given standardized slope or intercept deviation. For very short ranges characteristic for electrolyte measurement methods, detection of a standardized slope or intercept deviation equal to 1 may require more than 1000 samples. On the other hand, the sample size requirements may be rather modest for analytes with values dispersed over wider ranges. As regards standardized deviations that are not covered, the approximate sample size may be obtained by squared interpolation or extrapolation

Example: Planning a Comparison of Two Potassium Methods (Constant SDs)

We first decide on the critical differences that should be detected. For convenience, we take as a basis the CLIA '88 demand, which amounts to 0.5 mmol/L throughout the analytical measurement range. Notice that CLIA '88 demands relate to the total error in relation to a target value of a quality control sample:

$$\text{Total Error} = \text{systematic error} + 1.65\,SD_A$$

The factor 1.65 corresponds to a total error assuming that 95% of the measurements are within the given limit.

We consider here decision levels of 3 and 6 mmol/L and suppose in the present example that the SD_A is 0.09 mmol/L, which corresponds to a CV_A of 2% at the mean (4.5 mmol/L) of the considered range. In the present example we set the random bias component to zero. Thus the systematic difference that should be detected is:

$$\Delta_c = 0.5\,\text{mmol/L} - 1.65 \times 0.09\,\text{mmol/L} = 0.35\,\text{mmol/L}$$

TABLE 14-14 Sample Size Table for Comparison of Methods With *Proportional* Standard Deviations for Random Errors Using Weighted Deming Regression Analysis*
Necessary sample sizes for test of slope deviation from 1 or intercept deviation from zero by weighted Deming regression analysis given proportional SDs (i.e., constant coefficients of variation): $CV_{x1} = CV_{x2} = CV$. Uniform distributions of $x1$ and $x2$ on intervals with the given range ratio. The range ratio is the maximum value divided by the minimum value of the considered interval.
WLR analysis (given no random error in $x1$) requires approximately half the listed sample sizes.
Type I error: 5%; Power: 90%.

	RANGE RATIOS									
$\Delta\beta_{st} = (\beta - 1)/CV$	**2**	**2.5**	**3**	**4**	**5**	**8**	**10**	**25**	**50**	**100**
1	544	320	226	150	114	75	64	45	37	37
2	144	82	61	40	33	23	20	18	15	15
3	66	42	29	22	17	14	12	≤10	≤10	≤10
4	39	26	19	15	12	≤10	≤10	≤10	≤10	≤10
	RANGE RATIOS									
$\Delta\alpha_{0st} = (\alpha_0 - 0)/(CV \times x_m)$†	**2**	**2.5**	**3**	**4**	**5**	**8**	**10**	**25**	**50**	**100**
1	521	281	180	99	69	34	26	≤10	≤10	≤10
2	130	70	45	28	20	14	11	≤10	≤10	≤10
3	60	32	24	15	12	≤10	≤10	≤10	≤10	≤10
4	35	22	15	≤10	≤10	≤10	≤10	≤10	≤10	≤10

*From Linnet K. Necessary sample size for method comparison studies based on regression analysis. Clin Chem 1999;45:882-94.
†x_m is the midpoint of the actual interval of interest (e.g., x_m equals 6 for the interval [4; 8]), which has a range ratio of 2.

From the general formula:

$$\Delta_c = X2'_{\text{Target}c} - X1'_{\text{Target}c} = \alpha_0 + (\beta - 1)X1'_{\text{Target}c}$$

we obtain at $X1'_{\text{Target}c} = 3\,\text{mmol/L}$:

$$0.35 = 3.35 - 3 = \alpha_0 + (\beta - 1)3$$

This corresponds to a requirement for detecting α_0 equal to ±0.35 mmol/L, if the systematic difference is ascribed to an intercept deviation. Relating the systematic difference to a slope deviation results in a demand of detecting $\beta = 1.12$ (3.35/3) or 0.88. Similarly, at the upper decision level of $X1'_{\text{Target}c} = 6\,\text{mmol/L}$, we have again the limits ±0.35 mmol/L for detection of α_0, but now the demand for detecting a slope deviation has been sharpened to $\beta = 1.06$ (6.35/6) or 0.94.

We may now consider the various factors in the estimation of sample size. The first factor to consider is the analytical measurement range: 3 to 6 mmol/L (i.e., a range ratio of 2). We suppose as mentioned above that both methods have constant SDs corresponding to a CV% of 2% at the middle of the range (i.e., 0.09 mmol/L). We are now able to convert the slope delta value to a standardized value:

$$\Delta\beta_{\text{st}} = (\beta - 1)/\text{CV} = 0.06/0.02 = 3.0$$

Deming regression analysis is performed with a significance level (Type I error) of 5% and a statistical power of 90%. To get the necessary sample size, we consult Table 14-13 and look under a range ratio of 2 and a standardized slope deviation of 3 and find the sample size $N = 70$.

Table 14-13 also covers cases studied by the use of OLR. Under the given assumptions, the approximate sample size requirement for OLR is obtained by dividing the numbers by 2 (i.e., $N = 35$ in this case) (see the accompanying Evolve site). However, a correct statistical analysis based on OLR requires that the $x1$ method is without analytical errors.

For the intercept, we want to detect a deviation of ±0.35 mmol/L, which may be converted to:

$$\Delta\alpha_{0\text{st}} = (\alpha_0 - 0)/\text{SD} = 0.35/0.09 = 3.9$$

According to Table 14-13 the sample size requirement is $N = 40$ for a standardized deviation 4. By squared interpolation, we obtain $N = 42$ $(= 40 \times (4/3.9)^2)$. Thus in this example the sample size requirement with regard to testing for intercept deviation from zero is less demanding than that of testing for a critical slope deviation.

Power in Case of Proportional Error Standard Deviations

Table 14-14 covers application of weighted Deming regression analysis in situations with *proportional* SDs (constant CVs) and includes intervals with range ratios extending from 2 to 100. The standardized slope deviation is here:

$$\Delta\beta_{\text{st}} = (\beta - 1)/\text{CV}$$

and the standardized intercept deviation from zero is:

$$\Delta\alpha_{0\text{st}} = (\alpha_0 - 0)/(\text{CV} \times x_m)$$

CV refers to $[\text{CV}_A^2 + \text{CV}_{RB}^2]^{0.5}$ and should be expressed as a fraction, not a percentage. x_m is the midpoint of the interval of interest. Application of Table 14-14 presupposes that the analytical methods have identical CVs, and that the analyte concentrations are uniformly distributed over the intervals of interest. The CV refers to single or duplicate sets of measurements as appropriate. Approximate sample sizes for application of WLR, assuming CV = 0 for method 1, are derived by division of the sample size values by 2.

With regard to testing slope deviations, the strong impact on sample size of the range of values is apparent. The required number of samples is of the same order of magnitude as for analogous situations with constant SDs. For example, detection of one standardized slope deviation with the given Type I error and power requires more than 500 samples when the range ratio is 2, but only 37 samples for a range ratio of 50 or higher. Below, the sample size requirement is considered for a comparison of two glucose methods with proportional SDs.

Example: Planning a Comparison of Two Glucose Methods (Proportional SDs)

We first decide on the critical differences that should be detected. For convenience, we apply CLIA '88 requirements, which specify that $\Delta = 10\%$ or 60 mg/L at low concentrations. We consider a decision level corresponding to a fasting plasma glucose concentration of 1260 mg/L, which is of relevance for the diagnosis of diabetes. Again we notice that CLIA '88 requirements relate to the total error. Assuming proportional SD_As with a CV_A of 3% for both methods and CV_{RB} equal to zero, we obtain the critical systematic difference as:

$$\Delta_c = 10\% - 1.65 \times 3\% = 5\%$$

We have:

$$\Delta_c = X2'_{\text{Target}c} - X1'_{\text{Target}c} = \alpha_0 + (\beta - 1)X1'_{\text{Target}c}$$

which corresponds to:

$$(0.05 \times 1260) = X2'_{\text{Target}c} - 1260 = \alpha_0 + (\beta - 1) \times 1260$$
$$\text{or } 63 = 1323 - 1260 = \alpha_0 + (\beta - 1) \times 1260$$

This relation translates to a requirement of detecting α_0 equal to ±63 mg/L, if the systematic difference is related to an intercept deviation. Ascribing the systematic difference to a slope deviation requires detecting $\beta = 1.05$ or 0.95.

Let us now consider the conditions: an analytical measurement range of 600 mg/L to 3000 mg/L (i.e., a range ratio of 5); the midpoint of the interval $(x_m) = 1800$ mg/L; and for both methods, proportional SD_As with $\text{CV}_A\text{s} = 0.03$. The regression procedure is weighted Deming regression analysis with a significance level (Type I error) of 5% and a statistical power of 90%.

We standardize the slope deviation:

$$\Delta\beta_{\text{st}} = (\beta - 1)/\text{CV} = 0.05/0.03 = 1.7$$

From the column corresponding to a range ratio of 5 in Table 14-14, we find the required sample size to be between 114 and 33 measurements by each method. Squared interpolation gives $N = 46$ $(= 33 \times (2/1.7)^2)$. For WLR assuming $CV_A = 0$ for method 1, approximately half the number of samples are required ($N = 23$).

Concerning the intercept, we want to detect a deviation of ±63 mg/L, which may be converted to:

$$\Delta\alpha_{0st} = (\alpha_0 - 0)/(CV_A \times x_m) = 63/(0.03 \times 1800) = 1.2$$

From Table 14-14 we obtain $N = 48$ $(= 69 \times (1/1.2)^2)$ (i.e., in this case about the same number as that obtained for testing the critical slope deviation).

Other decision levels might also be considered (e.g., the nonfasting plasma glucose concentration limit of 2000 mg/L). In this proportional error model, the standardized slope deviation to be detected is the same at all decision levels, but the requirement for intercept detection varies with the concentration, so that the most demanding situations occur at low concentrations.

Discussion of Application of Regression Analysis

Most published method evaluations fail to apply regression analysis in a rigorous fashion. This section considers both the use of OLR instead of Deming regression and the use of unweighted analysis in the setting of proportional random errors.

Application of OLR in Case of Random Errors Associated with Both $x1$ and $x2$

OLR is the most widely used regression analysis procedure in method comparison studies. Thus it is important to consider the significance of the lack of consideration of measurement errors in $x1$ as outlined previously (see Figures 14-23 and 14-24). The bias problem concerning the slope is most significant when dealing with narrow measurement ranges (e.g., when comparing electrolyte measurements). It has been recommended that OLR may be applied when the correlation coefficient exceeds 0.975 or 0.99.[81] The correlation coefficient, however, also depends on the random error of $x2$, which has no influence on the bias problem. The bias of the slope estimate has as a consequence that the Type I error for the statistical analysis increases (i.e., the null hypothesis is rejected too frequently). Depending upon the range of test concentrations considered and the amount of random error associated with $x1$, this increase may be several fold higher than the nominal level of 5%. If the range of $X1'$ target values is large (e.g., corresponding to several decades), the problem is negligible.

Application of Unweighted Forms of Regression Analysis in Case of Proportional Random Errors

According to current practice in method comparison studies, it is usual to apply unweighted forms of regression analysis (i.e., OLR and the Deming procedure), even though the SDs vary with the measured concentration, as occurs with a proportional relation (constant CV_A). Thus it is of interest to consider what happens in these situations.[66]

Basically, OLR provides unbiased estimates of slope and intercept, if $x1$ is without random error, irrespective of whether the SD for random error of $x2$ is constant or varies with the measured concentration. In the same way, the Deming procedure provides unbiased estimates of slope and intercept, when the SDs vary, provided that their ratio is constant throughout the analytical measurement range. This aspect is important and means that generally the estimates of slope and intercept are reliable in this frequently encountered situation. However, additional aspects must be considered: the reliability of the associated statistical analysis and the efficiency of the unweighted estimation procedures. The presence of a proportional SD_A for the $x2$ measurements tends to independently increase the Type I error for the test of slope deviation using the OLR procedure, because the standard error of the slope is underestimated. The phenomenon is most pronounced for skew target value distributions, in which cases the Type I error may increase threefold to fourfold, becoming 15% to 20% compared with the nominal level of 5%.[66] For uniform and Gaussian target value distributions, the increase is up to 7.5% and 10%, respectively. Finally the precision of slope and intercept estimations is lower than that of WLR in case of a proportional SD_A for $x2$ measurements. For a range ratio of 10, 2.3 times as many observations are required for estimation of the slope with a given precision compared with the WLR procedure (Table 14-15). For the intercept, the factor is 3.9.

The major problem associated with application of the unweighted Deming analysis in case of proportional SD_As is the suboptimality of the unweighted approach (Table 14-15). For uniform distributions with range ratios from 2 to 100, 1.2 to 3.7 times as many samples are necessary to obtain the same precision of the slope estimate by the unweighted compared with the weighted approach. Thus the larger the range ratio, the more inefficient the unweighted method. If one intends to apply the unweighted Deming procedure in a situation with proportional SD_As, the sample size values of Table 14-14 should be multiplied by the adjustment factors that may be derived from Table 14-15.

In conclusion, planning a method comparison study to achieve a given power for detection of medically notable differences should be considered. In this way, a method comparison study is likely to be conclusive: either the null hypothesis of no difference is accepted, or the presence of a relevant difference is established. Otherwise, a statistically nonsignificant slope deviation from unity or intercept deviation from zero or both may either imply that the null hypothesis is true, or be an example of a Type II error (i.e., an overlooked real difference of medical importance).

Discussion of Method Comparison Approaches

The various approaches outlined above all have their merits and limitations. Much emphasis has been placed on the difference plot, usually in the form suggested by Bland and

Altman.[4] Its advantage is that the differences are in focus and can be considered in detail. The *x-y* plot with a regression analysis line has been criticized for not displaying the differences explicitly, which may constitute a point in favor of the difference plot. On the other hand, when the relation between target values (i.e., the mean bias at a given concentration) changes drastically from plus to minus or vice versa, the *x-y* plot with regression analysis displays the relations accurately. All in all, the use of both a difference plot and an *x-y* plot with the estimated regression line will provide a good outline of both the mean bias as a function of the concentration and the random differences. It is important to get estimates of relevant measures for mean bias and random differences as outlined above. The use of the correlation coefficient should be avoided, because the interpretation is complex, and the value does not express relevant error measures.

MONITORING SERIAL RESULTS

An important aspect in clinical chemistry is monitoring of disease or treatment (e.g., tumor markers in case of cancer or drug concentrations in case of therapeutic drug monitoring). To assess changes in a rational way, the various imprecision components have to be taken into account. Biological within-subject variation ($SD_{within\text{-}B}$), preanalytical variation (SD_{PA}), and analytical variation (SD_A) all have to be recognized. We assume in the following discussion that preanalytical variation is already included in the estimated within-subject variation SD, which often is the case. On this basis, using the principle of adding squared standard deviations (variances) a total SD (SD_T) can be estimated:

$$SD_T^2 = SD_{Within\text{-}B}^2 + SD_A^2$$

The limit for statistically significant changes then is: $k\sqrt{2}$ SD_T, where *k* depends on the desired probability level. Considering a two-sided 5% level, *k* is 1.96. The corresponding one-sided factor is 1.65. If a higher probability level is desired, *k* should be increased.

Limits for statistically significant changes ($Delta_{stat}$) may be related to changes that are considered of medical importance by clinicians (i.e., action limits [$Delta_{med}$]).[96] We will here consider a one-sided situation, where an increase is of importance, and a 5% significance level is selected (i.e., $Delta_{stat} = 1.65\sqrt{2}\ SD_T = 1.65\ SD_{delta}$). Suppose as a starting point that the true change ($Delta_{true}$) for a patient is zero (Figure 14-38, *A*). If $Delta_{stat}$ is less than $Delta_{med}$, the frequency of false-positive alarms will be less than 5%. If, on the other hand, $Delta_{stat}$ exceeds $Delta_{med}$, the frequency of false-positive alarms will exceed 5% (i.e., medical action will be taken too frequently). Figure 14-38, *A* illustrates the situation with $Delta_{stat}$ equal to $Delta_{med}$. We now consider the situation with a true change equal to the medically important change (i.e., $Delta_{true} = Delta_{med}$) (Figure 14-38, *B*), where exactly 50% of the observed changes exceed the medically important limit. If $Delta_{stat}$ is less than or equal to $Delta_{med}$, less than 5% of the patients will exhibit an observed delta value in the opposite direction of the true change (an obviously misleading trend). If the condition is not met, more than 5% will have a misleading change. Finally, in the case in which the true change equals the sum of $Delta_{med}$ and $Delta_{stat}$ (Figure 14-38, *C*) more than 95% of the observed changes exceed the medically important change and appropriate action will be taken for most patients.

The outline presented above illustrates that in the monitoring situation not only the requirement for statistical significance (i.e., the Type I error problem concerning false alarms), but also the Type II error problem or the risk of overlooking changes should be addressed; the latter is an aspect that often is overlooked.[63] Provided that $Delta_{stat}$ is small relative to $Delta_{med}$, both the Type I and II errors can be kept small. On the other hand, if $Delta_{stat}$ equals or exceeds $Delta_{med}$, the relative importance of Type I and II errors may be weighed against each other. If the consequences of overlooking a medically important change are serious, one should keep the Type II error small and accept a relatively large Type I error (i.e., accept the occurrence of false alarms). On the contrary, if overlooking changes only gives rise to minor or transient problems, the priority may be to keep the Type I error small. In addition to the simple evaluation of a shift between two measurements as considered here, sequen-

TABLE 14-15 Comparison of Sample Sizes Providing the Same Precision of Slope and Intercept Estimates by Unweighted and Weighted Deming Regression Analysis in Situations With Proportional Error SDs
Uniform *x*1 and *x*2 distributions are supposed on intervals with the given range ratio.

	RANGE RATIOS						
	2	**3**	**5**	**10**	**25**	**50**	**100**
Sample size for weighted Deming regression analysis	100	100	100	100	100	100	100
Equivalent sample size for unweighted Deming regression analysis for slope testing	116	132	155	230	307	345	370
Equivalent sample size for unweighted Deming regression analysis for intercept testing	116	145	184	389	1067	1960	4650

From Linnet K. Necessary sample size for method comparison studies based on regression analysis. Clin Chem 1999;45:882-94.

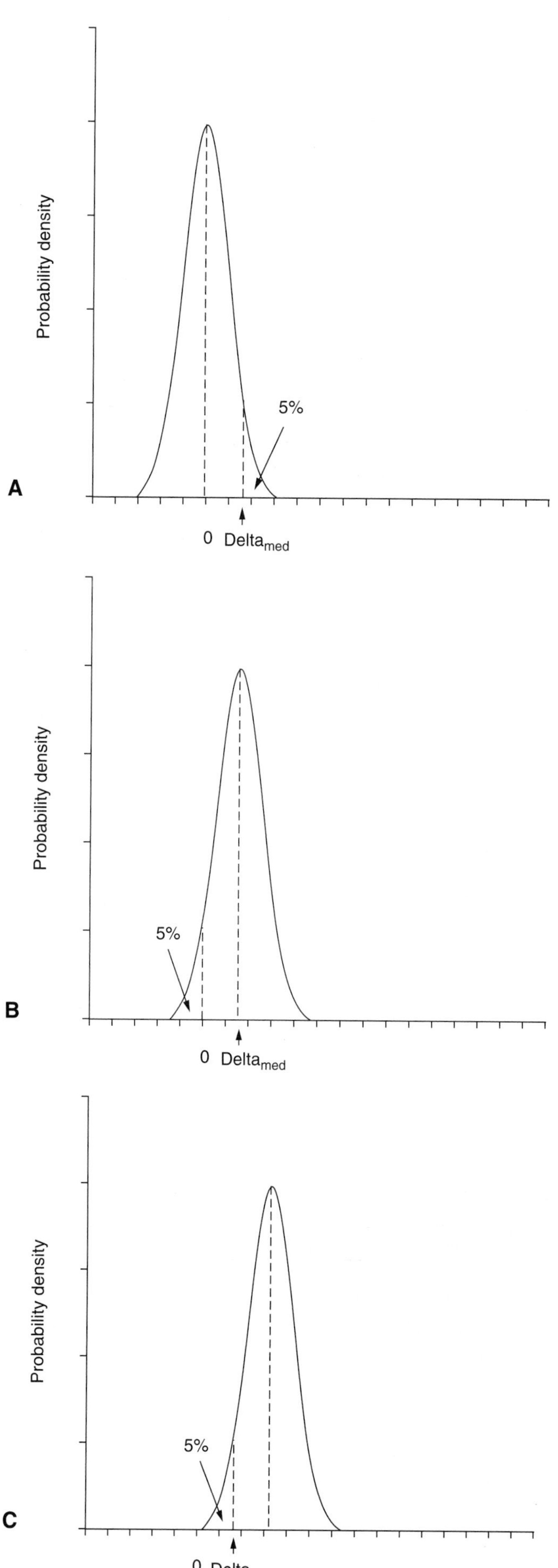

tial results may also be analyzed using more refined time-series models.[32]

TRACEABILITY AND MEASUREMENT UNCERTAINTY

As outlined previously in the error model sections, laboratory results are likely to be influenced by systematic and random errors of various kinds. Obtaining agreement of measurements between laboratories or agreement over time in a given laboratory often can be problematic.

TRACEABILITY

To ensure reasonable agreement between measurements of field methods, the concept of traceability comes into focus. *Traceability* is based on an unbroken chain of comparisons of measurements leading to a known reference value (Figure 14-39). A hierarchical approach for tracing the values of routine clinical chemistry measurements to reference and definitive methods was proposed by Tietz[103] and has been adapted by the ISO. For well-established analytes, a hierarchy of methods exists with *a primary reference procedure* at the top, *secondary reference procedures* at an intermediate level, and finally *routine methods* at the bottom.[10,43,103] A primary reference procedure is a fully understood procedure of highest analytical quality with complete uncertainty budget given in SI units.[21,39] The results of the primary reference method are obtained without reference to a calibrator for the analyte to be measured. The primary reference procedure is used to assign values to *primary calibrators.* Subsequently the primary calibrator is applied in the calibration of secondary reference procedures. Secondary reference procedures are used to measure the analyte concentration in *secondary calibrators,* which typically have the same matrix as the samples that are to be measured by the routine procedures (e.g., human serum). Secondary calibrators are usually of high analytical quality and certified. Using cortisol as an example, the primary measurement procedure may consist of weighing of cortisol and a chemical analysis for impurities. A primary calibrator is then a cortisol preparation with stated mass fraction (purity) (e.g., 0.998 and a 95% CI of ±0.001). The secondary reference measurement procedure is an isotope-dilution gas chromatography-mass spectrometry method. After the secondary calibrator, we have a measurement procedure used for commercial preparation of reagents, calibrators, and analytical kits for routine use in clinical chemistry laboratories. *The selected measurement* procedure is calibrated with a primary or secondary calibrator, and is used for measurement of the quantity in the manufacturer's *working calibrator.* The latter is used to calibrate the company's *standing measurement procedure,* which is a method that has been val-

Figure 14-38 The monitoring situation: **A,** Distribution of observed changes given a true change of zero. **B,** A true change equal to $Delta_{med}$. **C,** A true change of ($Delta_{med}$ + 1.65 SD_{delta}). $Delta_{stat}$ (= 1.65 SD_{delta}) equals $Delta_{med}$ in these examples.

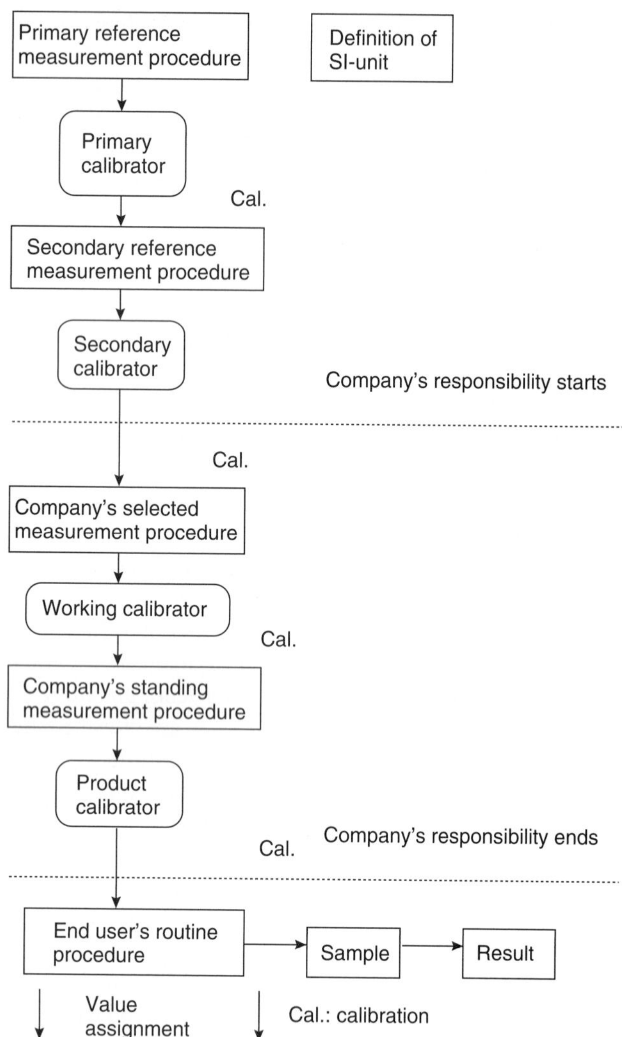

Figure 14-39 The calibration hierarchy from a primary method to a routine method. The uncertainty increases from top to bottom.

idated with regard to analytical specificity. The standing measurement procedure is applied for quantitation of the *product calibrator,* which is the calibrator for the routine method. The uncertainty of the measurement procedures increases from the top level to the bottom. Some recent ISO guidelines (15193 and 15194) address reference methods and reference materials.[39,40]

Only a minority (25 to 30) of clinical chemistry analytes are traceable to SI units (e.g., electrolytes), some metabolites (glucose, creatinine, and uric acid), steroid, and some thyroid hormones.[10,102] With protein hormones, the existence of heterogeneity or microheterogeneity complicates the problem of traceability.[102]

The Uncertainty Concept

To assess errors associated with laboratory results in a systematic way, the *uncertainty* concept has been introduced in laboratory medicine.[23,36] According to the ISO *Guide to the Expression of Uncertainty in Measurement* ("GUM"), *uncertainty* is formally defined as "a parameter associated with the result of a measurement that characterizes the dispersion of the values that could reasonably be attributed to the measurand."[36] In practice, this means that the uncertainty is given as an interval around a reported laboratory result that specifies the location of the true value with a given probability (e.g., 95%). In general the uncertainty of a result, which is traceable to a particular reference, is the uncertainty of that reference together with the overall uncertainty of the traceability chain.[23] Updated information on traceability aspects is available on the website of the *Joint Committee on Traceability in Laboratory Medicine* (www.bipm.org/enus/2_Committees/JCTLM.shtml, Accessed August, 2003).

The Standard Uncertainty (u_{st})

The uncertainty concept is directed toward the end user (clinician) of the result, who is concerned about the total error possible, and who is not particularly interested in the question whether the errors are systematic or random. In the outline of the uncertainty concept it is assumed that any known systematic error components of a measurement method have been corrected, and the specified uncertainty includes the uncertainty associated with correction of the systematic error(s).[36] Although this appears logical, a problem may be that some routine methods have systematic errors dependent on the patient category from which the sample originates. For example, kinetic Jaffé methods for creatinine are subject to positive interference by alpha-keto compounds and to negative interference by bilirubin and its metabolites, which means that the direction of systematic error will be patient dependent and not generally predictable.

In the theory on uncertainty, a distinction between type A and B uncertainties is made. Type A uncertainties are frequency-based estimates of standard deviations (e.g., an SD of the imprecision). Type B uncertainties are uncertainty components for which frequency-based SDs are not available. Instead, the uncertainty is estimated by other approaches or by the opinion of experts. Finally the total uncertainty is derived from a combination of all sources of uncertainty. In this context, it is practical to operate with *standard uncertainties* (u_{st}), which are equivalent to standard deviations. By multiplication of a standard uncertainty with a *coverage factor* (k), the uncertainty corresponding to a specified probability level is derived. For example, multiplication with a coverage factor of two yields a probability level of $\approx$ 95% given a normal distribution. When considering the total uncertainty of an analytical result obtained by a routine method, the preanalytical variation, method imprecision, random matrix-related interferences, and uncertainty related to calibration and bias corrections (traceability) should be taken into account. Expressing the uncertainty components as standard uncertainties, we have the general relation:

$$u_{st} = [u_{PAst}^2 + u_{Ast}^2 + u_{RBst}^2 + u_{Tracst}^2]$$

where the individual components refer to preanalytical, analytical, matrix-related random bias and traceability uncertainty.

Uncertainty can be assessed in various ways, and often a combination of procedures is necessary. In principle, uncertainty can be judged *directly* from measurement comparisons or *indirectly* from an analysis of individual error sources according to the law of error propagation ("error budget"). Measurement comparison may consist of a method comparison study with a reference method based on patient samples according to the principles outlined previously or by measurement of certified matrix reference materials (CRMs).

Example of Direct Assessment of Uncertainty on the Basis of Measurements of a Certified Reference Material

Suppose a CRM is available with a specified value 10.0 mmol/L and a standard uncertainty of 0.2 mmol/L. Ten repeated measurements in independent runs give a mean value of 10.3 mmol/L with SD 0.5 mmol/L. The standard error of the mean is then $0.5/\sqrt{10} = 0.16$ mmol/L. The mean is not significantly different from the assigned value ($t = (10.3 - 10.0)/(0.2^2 + 0.16^2)^{0.5} = 1.17$). The total standard uncertainty with regard to traceability is then $u_{\text{Tracst}} = [0.16^2 + 0.2^2]^{0.5} = 0.26$ mmol/L. If the bias had been significant, one might have considered making a correction to the method, and the standard uncertainty would then be the same at the given level. Thus the measurements of the CRM provide an estimate of the uncertainty related to traceability. The other components have to be estimated separately. Concerning method imprecision, the long-term imprecision (e.g., observed from quality control measurements) should be used rather than the short-term SD observed for the CRM material. We here suppose the long-term SD_A is 0.8 mmol/L. Data on preanalytical variation can be obtained by sampling in duplicates from a series of patients or can be a matter of judgment (type B uncertainty) from literature data or data on similar analytes. We here suppose SD_{PA} equals half the analytical SD (i.e., 0.4 mmol/L). Finally, we lack data on a possible random bias component, which we may choose to ignore in the present example. The standard uncertainty of the results then becomes:

$$u_{\text{st}} = \left[u_{\text{PAst}}^2 + u_{\text{Ast}}^2 + u_{\text{Tracst}}^2\right] = \left[0.4^2 + 0.8^2 + 0.26^2\right]^{0.5}$$
$$= 0.93\ (\text{mmol/L})$$

In this case, the major uncertainty component is the long-term imprecision in the laboratory.

Example of Direct Assessment of Uncertainty on the Basis of a Method Comparison Study with a Reference Method Using Patient Samples

Suppose a set of patient samples has been measured by a field method ($X2$) in parallel with a reference method ($X1$) and that a linear relationship exists between the measurements. We want to assess a possible bias and evaluate the standard uncertainty of the results of the field method on the basis of the regression analysis results and information on the standard uncertainty related to traceability of the reference method results. The imprecision of the reference method is assumed to be 2.5% or as a fraction (used in the following) 0.025 ($= CV_{A1}$), and the component relating to the uncertainty of the traceability chain for the reference method is 0.020 ($= u_{\text{Tracst}}$). Proportional measurement errors are assumed for both methods and a weighted form of Deming regression analysis is applied. The error variance ratio λ is not known exactly, but the reference method is devoid of random bias, so it is assumed that the random error level is about half that of the field method (i.e., λ is set to $1/2^2 = 1/4$). At a decision point ($X1'_{\text{Targetc}}$) (e.g., corresponding to the upper limit of the 95% reference interval), the systematic difference between the methods ($D_c = a_0 + (b-1)\,X1'_{\text{Targetc}}$) is estimated with standard error (see regression section):

$$D_c = X2'_{\text{Targetc}} - X1'_{\text{Targetc}} = 20\,\text{mg/L with SE}(D_c)$$
$$= 1.0\ \text{mg/L}$$

corresponding to a relative SE(D_c) of 0.050 (= (1.0 mg/L)/(20 mg/L)). For OLR analysis ignoring random measurement error with regard to $X1'_{\text{Targetc}}$, SE(D_c) can be computed as outlined in the regression section. For the Deming procedures, the standard error can be conveniently computed by the jackknife procedure (described on the book's accompanying Evolve site). We observe that the difference is highly significant and decide to recalibrate the field method in relation to the reference method using the estimated slope and intercept (i.e., the recalibrated $x2$ values equals $(x2 - a_0)/b$). Having done that, the field method is assumed to have no systematic error in relation to the reference method, but when considering the uncertainty of the results, we have to add the standard uncertainty of the bias correction. The uncertainty related to traceability for the field method is now obtained as the uncertainty inherent to the reference method and the comparison step, i.e.,

$$u_{\text{Tracst}} = \left[0.020^2 + 0.050^2\right]^{0.5} = 0.054$$

We are now further interested in deriving estimates of random error components for the field method from the regression analysis results. Both analytical error and random matrix-related error should be assessed, and it should be recognized that the observed total random error is the result of contributions from both measurement methods. Suppose that CV_{21} of the regression analysis has been calculated to be 0.10 (CV_{21} is analogous to SD_{21} or $SD_{y.x}$ given constant measurement errors over the analytical measurement range [i.e., an expression for the random error in the vertical direction in the x-y plot]). From the regression section, we have:

$$CV_{21}^2 = \left[CV_{A1}^2 + CV_{A2}^2\right] + \left[CV_{RB1}^2 + CV_{RB2}^2\right]$$

By substituting $CV_{A1} = 0.025$, $CV_{RB1} = 0$, and $CV_{21} = 0.10$, we derive

$$CV^2_{A2} + CV^2_{RB2} = 0.009375 \ [CV^2_{A2} + CV^2_{RB2}]^{0.5} = 0.0968$$

Thus the total random error of the field method corresponds to a CV of 0.097. If we had measured samples in duplicate in the method comparison experiment or had available quality control data, we could split the total random error into its components. CV_{A2} is here assumed to be 0.035, which gives a rest of 0.090 corresponding to CV_{RB2}. We may here notice that the assumed error ratio λ of $(½)^2$ is not quite correct. According to our results, λ should be $(0.025/0.0968)^2$. Although the Deming regression principle is rather robust toward misspecified λ values, we could choose to carry out a reanalysis with the more correct λ value, a process that could be iterated. Finally, assuming a value of 0.03 for the preanalytical coefficient of variation, we derive a total standard uncertainty estimate of:

$$u_{st} = [u^2_{PAst} + u^2_{Ast} + u^2_{RBst} + u^2_{Tracst}]$$

$$= [0.03^2 + 0.0968^2 + 0.054^2]^{0.5} = 0.115$$

At the given decision level of 20 mg/L and with a coverage factor of 2, we obtain the 95% uncertainty interval of a single field measurement as:

$$20\,mg/L \pm (2 \times 0.115 \times 20)\,mg/L = 15.4 - 24.6\,mg/L$$

Having estimated the uncertainty as outlined, additional uncertainty sources should be considered. If the comparison was undertaken within a short time period, one might consider adding an additional long-term imprecision component as a variance component to the standard uncertainty expression.

When comparing the two approaches briefly outlined, the latter is the more informative. Using a series of patient samples instead of a pooled sample, individual random bias components are included in the uncertainty estimation, assuming the patient samples are representative. Also, natural patient samples are preferable to a stabilized pool that perhaps is distributed in freeze-dried form that may introduce artifactual errors in some analytical systems. Using a CRM, on the other hand, is more practical and in many situations the only realistic alternative.

With regard to uncertainty estimation from a comparison study of patient samples as outlined above, one should be careful concerning the uncertainty estimation. First, it is important to estimate correctly the standard error of the difference at selected decision points or at points covering the analytical measurement range (i.e., at the lower limit, in the middle part, and at the upper limit). From the expression of the estimated difference ($D_c = a_0 + (b - 1)\ X1'_{Targetc}$), one might at a first glance estimate the standard error (standard uncertainty) by adding (squared) the standard errors of the intercept and slope. However, simple squared addition of standard errors is only correct given independence of estimates (see below). Estimates of intercept and slope in regression analysis are negatively correlated, which implies that simple squared addition of standard errors leads to an overestimation of the total standard uncertainty.[16] Rather, a direct estimation procedure for the standard error should be applied as mentioned above.

A method comparison study based on genuine patient samples represents as mentioned a real assessment of traceability. In Figure 14-39, the focus is on the calibration aspect intended to *mediate* traceability. One should recognize that the matrix of product calibrators for practical reasons often is artificial (e.g., the matrix of a calibrator may be bovine albumin instead of human serum). Many routine methods are matrix sensitive, which implies that calibrators and patient samples are not commutable. To ensure traceability in this situation, the assigned concentration of a calibrator has to be different from the real concentration.

Uncertainty Estimation from External Quality Assessment Schemes

Measurement comparison with reference methods or measurement of CRMs may not be feasible. For example, measurement of newly detected biochemical markers may only be performed in a handful of research laboratories. In this case, collaborative studies or data from EQAS may constitute a source for uncertainty estimations. If the laboratory has performed repeated measurements over a time period, the standard deviation of differences (SD_{dif}) between the measured values and the consensus or assigned values may enter the uncertainty computations. If a significant systematic difference is observed, a correction should be considered. SD_{dif} can be considered as composed of the inherent (short-time) imprecision in the laboratory ($SD_{intralab}$) and a variability component reflecting variations over time of the systematic error (here expressed as SD_{ext}). For example, if an external control material is assayed monthly in duplicate and if the differences between the consensus values and the mean of duplicates are assessed, the following relation applies:

$$SD^2_{dif} = SD^2_{ext} + SD^2_{intralab}/2$$

Taking into account also the preanalytical variation associated with sampling and sample pre-treatment, the total standard uncertainty with traceability stated to the consensus mean is given by:

$$u^2_{st} = SD^2_{PA} + SD^2_{intralab} + SD^2_{ext}$$

In case several laboratories use the same analytical reagent systems, a subgrouping of consensus means is often performed. When considering uncertainty, it should then be distinguished between traceability to the subgroup consensus and the overall consensus mean.

The total dispersion of values for a group of laboratories in an EQAS study for a given method gives an impression of the uncertainty level that can be achieved in practice. From the relation:

$$SD^2_{Total} = SD^2_{intralab} + SD^2_{interlab}$$

it is observed to what extent it is possible for groups of laboratories to conform to a common measurement level. Additional preanalytical uncertainty and uncertainty related to the traceability (bias) of the consensus mean should also be included. This total uncertainty expressed as a standard uncertainty can be used to consider the feasibility of using common decision levels (e.g., internationally agreed diagnostic or treatment limits).

Indirect Evaluation of Uncertainty by Quantification of Individual Error Source Components

On the basis of a detailed quantitative model of the analytical procedure, the standard approach is to assess the standard uncertainties associated with the individual input parameters and combine them according to the law of propagation of uncertainties.[23] The relationship between the combined standard uncertainty $u_c(y)$ of a value y and the uncertainty of the *independent* parameters $x_1, x_2, \ldots x_n$, on which it depends, is:

$$u_c[y(x_1,x_2,\ldots)] = \left[\sum c_i^2 u(x_i)^2\right]^{0.5}$$

where c_i is a sensitivity coefficient (the partial differential of y with respect to x_i). These sensitivity coefficients indicate how the value of y varies with changes in the input parameters x_i. If the variables are not independent, the relationship becomes:

$$u_c[y(x_i,x_k\ldots)] = \left[\sum c_i^2 u(x_i)^2 + \sum c_i c_k u(x_i,x_k)^2\right]^{0.5}$$

where $u(x_i, x_k)$ is the covariance between x_i and x_k, and c_i and c_k are the sensitivity coefficients. The covariance is related to the correlation coefficient ρ_{ik} by:

$$u(x_i,x_k) = u(x_i)u(x_k)\rho_{ik}$$

This is a complex relationship that usually will be difficult to evaluate in practice. In many situations, however, the contributing factors are independent, thus simplifying the picture. Below, some simple examples of combined expressions are shown. The rules are presented in the form of combining SDs or coefficients of variation (CVs) given *independent* input components.

$$q = x + y \qquad SD(q) = \left[SD(x)^2 + SD(y)^2\right]^{0.5}$$

$$q = x - y \qquad SD(q) = \left[SD(x)^2 + SD(y)^2\right]^{0.5}$$

$$q = ax \qquad SD(q) = a\,SD(x) \quad \text{and} \quad CV(q) = CV(x)$$

$$q = x^p \qquad CV(q) = p^{0.5}CV(x)$$

$$q = xy \qquad CV(q) = \left[CV(x)^2 + CV(y)^2\right]^{0.5}$$

$$q = x/y \qquad CV(q) = \left[CV(x)^2 + CV(y)^2\right]^{0.5}$$

The formulas shown may be used, for example, to calculate the combined uncertainty of a calibrator solution from the uncertainties of the reference compound, the weighting, and dilution steps) (see below).

TABLE 14-16 Relations between Standard Deviation and Range for Various Types of Distributions

Normal Distribution	Rectangular Distribution	Triangular Distribution
SD = Half width of 95% interval/ $t_{0.975}(\nu)$ ≈ Half width of 95% interval/2	SD = Half width/$\sqrt{3}$	SD = Half width/$\sqrt{6}$

Some relations between the SD and nonnormal distributions may also be of relevance for uncertainty calculations (type B uncertainties) (Table 14-16). For example, if the uncertainty of a CRM value is given with some percentage, it may be understood as referring to a rectangular probability distribution. In relation to calibration of flasks, the triangular distribution is often assumed.

Example

Briefly, computation of the standard uncertainty of a calibrator solution will be outlined. The concentration C equals the mass M divided by the volume V ($C = M/V$). We will here express the standard uncertainties as relative values and derive the approximate total standard uncertainty by squared addition of the individual contributions. Starting with the mass, the purity is stated on the certificate as 99.4% ± 0.4%. Assuming a rectangular distribution, the relative standard deviation becomes $0.004/\sqrt{3} = 0.0023$. The uncertainty of the weighing process is known in the laboratory to have a CV of 0.1% or 0.0010. Thus the relative standard uncertainty of the mass becomes:

$$u_{Mst} = \left[0.0023^2 + 0.0010^2\right]^{0.5} = 0.0025$$

The certificate of the flask (50 mL at 20 °C) indicates ±0.1 mL as uncertainty. Assuming here a triangular distribution, we derive the standard uncertainty as $0.10\,\text{mL}/\sqrt{6} = 0.0408\,\text{mL}$, which is converted to a relative value of 0.000816. The temperature expansion coefficient is given as 0.020 mL per degree change of temperature. Assuming a variability of 20 ± 4 °C, this contribution amounts to ±0.080 mL. Assuming here a rectangular distribution, we get an SD of $0.080/\sqrt{3}$ mL, or 0.00092 as a relative SD. The repeatability of the volume dispensing process in the laboratory has been assessed to 0.020 mL expressed as an SD, which corresponds to a relative value of 0.00040. The total standard uncertainty of the volume dispensing process becomes:

$$u_{Vst} = \left[0.000816^2 + 0.00092^2 + 0.00040^2\right]^{0.5} = 0.0013$$

The total standard uncertainty of the calibrator solution is:

$$u_{\text{Calst}} = \left[u_{\text{Mst}}^2 + u_{\text{Vst}}^2\right]^{0.5} = 0.0025^2 + 0.0013^2$$
$$= 0.0028 \text{ or } 0.28\%$$

Quite generally, when adding squared CVs, minor contributions can in practice be ignored (e.g., CVs less than a third or quarter of the other components).[23]

The indirect procedure is mainly of relevance for relatively simple procedures. In some situations, a simulation model of a complex analytical method may be established to estimate the combined uncertainty of the method on the basis of the input uncertainties.[2] For closed, automated clinical chemistry procedures it will often not be possible to discern the individual error elements. Further, the correlation aspect is difficult to take into account in practice. In these cases, the direct procedure of measurement comparison is preferable. However, the indirect procedure has been applied in clinical chemistry.[59]

Uncertainty in Relation to the Traditional Systematic and Random Error Classifications

As mentioned above, systematic errors have no place in the uncertainty expression, because it is assumed that they have been corrected, so that it is the uncertainty of the correction procedure that should be taken into account. Otherwise, systematic errors have been added linearly or squared in error propagation models.[87,100] One may further consider that the distinction between systematic effects and random effects may be a matter of the reference frame. For example, a systematic error over time may turn into a random error, because a bias may change over time. Lot to lot reagent effects may be interpreted as either systematic or random errors. When a laboratory changes from an old to a new lot, a shift in measurement level may occur, which initially will be considered as a systematic change. However, over a long time period involving several lots of reagents, the recorded shifts will typically be up and down and be regarded as a long-term random error component. Additionally, a bias in a particular laboratory may be viewed as a random error component, when dealing with a whole group of laboratories, because the individual laboratory biases appear randomly distributed and are quantified as the interlaboratory standard deviation. Thus there are arguments for using the uncertainty concept as outlined above to end up with one overall uncertainty expression directed toward the end user of the laboratory result. Still, as mentioned previously, systematic errors linked to samples from specific patient subcategories may constitute a problem, because a general correction is not possible. A way to quantify this error contribution is to include samples from all patient subgroups in a balanced way in a method comparison study, so that this error type is incorporated in the uncertainty component related to traceability. Another problem with systematic errors is that they often depend on the analyte concentration. Thus if a CRM is measured at a particular concentration, one should consider whether a bias correction is valid only at the given level or generally over the analytical measurement range. Further, the occurrence of outliers caused by rarely occurring interference (e.g., heterophilic antibodies in relation to immunoassays) also constitutes a problem.[56] If the uncertainty estimation is based on parametric statistics (standard uncertainty expanded by a coverage factor), inclusion of gross outliers may increase the standard uncertainty considerably and make the uncertainty specification useless. A solution might here be to omit the outliers in the first hand, compute the 95% uncertainty interval, and then finally add a special note with regard to the probability of occurrence of outliers in the uncertainty specification.

Although it may appear complicated to specify the uncertainty in a detailed manner, a rough estimate may be obtained by adding the squares of CVs corresponding to essential uncertainty elements (e.g., grouped as the factors outside the laboratory) (derived from the traceability chain), the analytical factors inside the laboratory (intermediate precision), and the preanalytical elements.[49] In estimating uncertainty, it is important to include relevant elements, but be careful not to count the same elements twice. It should be recognized that the simple squared addition principle requires independence. Finally, because of the squared addition principle of CVs, minor contributions can in practice be ignored. The application of the uncertainty concept in the field of clinical chemistry is currently subject to some discussion.[50,56]

GUIDELINES, REGULATORY DEMANDS, AND ACCREDITATION

Various guidelines and regulatory demands are of relevance in relation to analytical methods used in clinical chemistry. Examples of the NCCLS guidelines have been referred to in the individual subsections and various ISO documents. Here some general guidelines will be mentioned briefly.

ISO15189 Medical Laboratories—Particular Requirements for Quality and Competence is a universal standard for quality management in medical laboratories that specifies requirements in general terms applicable to all medical laboratory fields.[42] The standard is intended to form the basis for accreditation of medical laboratories. In addition to general laboratory conditions in relation to quality control, the standard focuses on medical competence, interpretation of test results, selection of tests, reference intervals, ethical aspects, and safety. An annex concerns quality management of laboratory computer systems.

Concerning regulatory demands, the CLIA regulations in the United States have exerted a large influence on quality considerations in clinical chemistry[104,105] (see Table 14-5). From a manufacturer's perspective, the Food and Drug Administration (FDA) requirements for validation of new assays are of prime importance in the United States. In Europe, the *IVD-directive* (Directive 98/79 of the European

Community on In-Vitro Diagnostics) is a European legislative regulation directed at in vitro manufacturers.[18] The directive demands that the manufacturer have a quality management system and that products are validated by competent laboratories. It is required that the traceability of values assigned to calibrators or control materials or both must be ensured through available reference measurement procedures and/or available materials of higher order. Explicit statement of the uncertainty of calibrator values is not required, but indirectly the manufacturers have to address the uncertainty of the traceability chain to ensure traceability.

SOFTWARE PACKAGES

Statistical analyses are today usually carried out either in spreadsheets or by statistical programs. Concerning the latter, large general program packages may be applied or smaller programs more or less specialized toward the field of clinical chemistry. Various large general packages are on

BOX 14-1 Abbreviations and Vocabulary

Abbreviations

CI	Confidence interval
CV	Coefficient of variation (= SD/x, where x is the concentration)
CV%	= CV × 100%
CV_A	Analytical coefficient of variation
CV_{RB}	Random bias coefficient of variation
DoD	Distribution of differences (plot)
ISO	International Organization for Standardization
IUPAC	International Union of Pure and Applied Chemistry
OLR	Ordinary least-squares regression analysis
SD	Standard deviation
SD_A	Analytical standard deviation
SD_{RB}	Random bias standard deviation
SEM	Standard error of the mean (= SD/$\sqrt{N}$)
x_m	Mean
x_{mw}	Weighted mean
WLR	Weighted least-squares regression analysis

Vocabulary*

Analyte Compound that is measured.

Bias Difference between the average (strictly the expectation) of the test results and an accepted reference value (ISO 3534-1). Bias is a measure of trueness.[34]

Certified Reference Material (CRM) is a reference material, one or more of whose property values are certified by a technically valid procedure, accompanied by or traceable to a certificate or other documentation that is issued by a certifying body.

Commutability Ability of a material to yield the same results of measurements by a given set of measurement procedures.

Limit of Detection The lowest amount of analyte in a sample that can be detected but not quantified as an exact value. Also called lower limit of detection, minimum detectable concentration (or dose or value).[38]

Matrix All components of a material system, except the analyte.

Measurand The "quantity" that is actually measured (e.g., the concentration of the analyte). For example, if the analyte is glucose, the measurand is the concentration of glucose. For an enzyme, the measurand may be the enzyme *activity* or the *mass concentration* of enzyme.

Measuring interval Closed interval of possible values allowed by a measurement procedure and delimited by the *lower limit of determination* and the *higher limit of determination.* For this interval, the total error of the measurements is within specified limits for the method. Also called the *analytical measurement range.*

Primary measurement standard Standard that is designated or widely acknowledged as having the highest metrological qualities and whose value is accepted without reference to other standards of the same quantity.[40]

Reference material (RM) is a material or substance, one or more properties of which are sufficiently well established to be used for the calibration of a method, or for assigning values to materials.

Quantity The amount of substance (e.g., the concentration of substance).

Random error arises from unpredictable variations of influence quantities. These random effects give rise to variations in repeated observations of the measurand.

Reference measurement procedure Thoroughly investigated measurement procedure shown to yield values having an uncertainty of measurement commensurate with its intended use, especially in assessing the trueness of other measurement procedures for the same quantity and in characterizing reference materials.

Selectivity and/or specificity The degree to which a method responds uniquely to the required analyte.

Systematic error A component of error which, in the course of a number of analyses of the same measurand, remains constant or varies in a predictable way.

Traceability "The property of the result of a measurement or the value of a standard whereby it can be related to stated references, usually national or international standards, through an unbroken chain of comparisons all having stated uncertainties."[34] This is achieved by establishing a chain of calibrations leading to primary national or international standards, ideally (for long-term consistency) the Système Internationale (SI) units of measurement.

Uncertainty A parameter associated with the result of a measurement that characterizes the dispersion of the values that could reasonably be attributed to the measurand, or more briefly: *uncertainty* is a parameter characterizing the range of values within which the value of the quantity being measured is expected to lie.

*A listing of terms of relevance in relation to analytical methods is displayed. Many of the definitions originate from Dybkær[21] with statement of original source where relevant (e.g., ISO document number). Others are from the Eurachem/Citac guideline on uncertainty.[23] In some cases, slight modifications have been performed for sake of simplicity.

the market (e.g., SPSS, SAS, Stata, Systat, Statview, and StatGraphics). Among programs of an intermediate size, one may mention GraphPad (www.graphpad.com) and SPSS SigmaStat. Excel (Microsoft) also contains various statistical routines. The general programs may lack procedures of interest to clinical chemists (e.g., the Deming and Passing-Bablok procedures). Among more or less specialized programs for clinical chemistry, one may mention Analyze-it (www.analyze-it.com), MedCalc (www.medcalc.be), EP-evaluator (D. Rhoads Assoc., www.dgrhoads.com), and a program distributed by one of the authors (KL) CBstat (www.cbstat.com).

REFERENCES

1. Adcock RJ. A problem in least squares. The Analyst 1878;5:53-5.
2. Aronsson T, deVerdier C, Groth T. Factors influencing the quality of analytical methods: A systems analysis, with computer simulation. Clin Chem 1974;20: 738-48.
3. Barnett RN. Medical significance of laboratory results. Am J Clin Pathol 1968;50:671-6.
4. Bland JM, Altman DG. Statistical methods for assessing agreement between two methods of clinical measurement. Lancet 1986;i:307-10.
5. Bland JM, Altman DG. Comparing methods of measurement: why plotting difference against standard method is misleading. Lancet 1995;346: 1085-7.
6. Bonini P, Plebani M, Ceriotti F, Rubboli F. Errors in laboratory medicine. Clin Chem 2002;48:691-8.
7. Bookbinder MJ, Panosian KJ. Using the coefficient of correlation in method-comparison studies. Clin Chem 1987;33:1170-6.
8. Boyd JC, Bruns DE. Quality specifications for glucose meters: assessment by simulation modeling of errors in insulin dose. Clin Chem 2001;47:209-14.
9. Burnett RW, Westgard JO. Selection of measurement and control procedures to satisfy the Health Care Financing Administration requirements and provide cost-effective operation. Arch Pathol Lab Med 1992;116:777-80.
10. Büttner J. Reference materials and reference methods in laboratory medicine: a challenge to international cooperation. Eur J Clin Chem Clin Biochem 1994;32:571-7.
11. Clarke WL, Cox D, Gonder-Frederick LA, Carter W, Pohl SL. Evaluating clinical accuracy of systems for self-monitoring of blood glucose. Diabetes Care 1987;10:622-8.
12. Cornbleet PJ, Gochman N. Incorrect least-squares regression coefficients in method-comparison analysis. Clin Chem 1979;25:432-8.
13. Cotlove E, Harris EK, Williams GZ. Biological and analytic components of variation in long-term studies of serum constituents in normal subjects. III. Physiological and medical implications. Clin Chem 1970;16:1028-32.
14. Currie LA. Nomenclature in evaluation of analytical methods including detection and quantification capabilities (IUPAC Recommendations 1995). Pure & Appl Chem 1995;67:1699-1723.
15. David HA. Order statistics. New York: Wiley 1981: 80-2.
16. Davis RB, Thompson JE, Pardue HL. Characteristics of statistical parameters used to interpret least-squares results. Clin Chem 1978;24:611-20.
17. Deming WE. Statistical adjustment of data. New York: Wiley, 1943:184.
18. Directive 98/79/EC of the European Parliament and of the Council of 27 October on in vitro diagnostic medical devices. Off J Eur Comm 1998(Dec 7);L331: 1-37.
19. Dixon WJ. Processing data for outliers. Biometrics 1953;9:74-89.
20. Draper NR, Smith H. Applied regression analysis. 3. ed. New York: Wiley, 1998:192-8.
21. Dybkær R. Vocabulary for use in measurement procedures and description of reference materials in laboratory medicine. Eur J Clin Chem Clin Biochem 1997;35:141-73.
22. Efron B. An introduction to the bootstrap. London: Chapman and Hall, 1993.
23. Ellison SLR, Rosslein M, Williams A (eds.) Eurachem/ Citac guide: Quantifying uncertainty in analytical measurement. 2. ed. QUAM, 2000:4, 5, 9, 17.
24. Emancipator K, Kroll MH. A quantitative measure of nonlinearity. Clin Chem 1993;39:766-72.
25. European Committee for Clinical Laboratory Standards. Guidelines for the evaluation of diagnostic kits. Part 2. General principles and outline procedures for the evaluation of kits for qualitative tests. Lund, Sweden: ECCLS, 1990.
26. Fleiss JL. Statistical methods for rates and proportions. 2th ed. New York: Wiley, 1981: Chap. 13.
27. Fraser CG, Petersen PH, Libeer JC, Ricos C. Proposals for setting generally applicable quality goals solely based on biology. Ann Clin Biochem 1997;34:8-12.
28. Fraser CG. Biological variation: From principles to practice. Washington, D.C.: AACC press, 2001:50-4, 133-41.
29. Glick MR, Ryder KW. Analytical systems ranked by freedom from interferences. Clin Chem 1987;33:1453-8.
30. Gowans EMS, Petersen PH, Blaabjerg O, Hørder M. Analytical goals for the acceptance of common reference intervals for laboratories throughout a geographical area. Scand J Clin Lab Invest 1988;48:757-64.
31. Hald A. Statistical theory with engineering applications. New York: Wiley, 1952:534-5, 551-7.

32. Harris EK, Boyd J. Statistical bases of reference values in laboratory medicine. New York: Marcel Dekker, 1995:238-50.
33. International Federation of Clinical Chemistry. Approved recommendation (1987) on the theory of reference values. Part 5. Statistical treatment of collected reference values. Determination of reference limits. J Clin Chem Clin Biochem 1987;25:645-56.
34. International Organization for Standardization (ISO). International vocabulary of basic and general terms in metrology (VIM.). Geneva: ISO, 1993.
35. International Organization for Standardization (ISO). Statistics—Vocabulary and symbols—Part 1: Probability and general statistical terms. ISO 3534-1, 1st ed. Geneva: ISO, 1993.
36. International Organization for Standardization (ISO). Guide to the expression of uncertainty in measurement. Geneva: ISO, 1993 (Reprint 1995).
37. International Organization for Standardization (ISO). Accuracy (trueness and precision) of measurement methods and results. ISO 5725—Part 1: General principles and definitions. Geneva: ISO, 1994.
38. International Organization for Standardization (ISO). Capability of detection—Part 1: Terms and definitions (11843-1). Geneva: ISO, 1997.
39. International Organization for Standardization (ISO). In vitro diagnostic devices—Measurement of quantities in samples of biological origin—Presentation of reference measurement procedures (15193). Geneva: ISO, 1999.
40. International Organization for Standardization (ISO). In vitro diagnostic devices—Measurement of quantities in samples of biological origin—Descriptions of reference materials (15194). Geneva: ISO, 1999.
41. International Organization for Standardization (ISO). Capability of detection—Part 2: Methodology in the linear calibration case (11843-2). Geneva: ISO, 2000.
42. International Organization for Standardization (ISO). Medical laboratories—Particular requirements for quality and competence (15189). Geneva: ISO, 2003.
43. International Organization for Standardization (ISO). In vitro diagnostic medical devices—Measurement of quantities in biological samples—metrological traceability of values assigned to calibrators and control materials (17511). Geneva: ISO, 2003.
44. Ismail AAA, Walker PL, Barth JH, Lewandowski KC, Jones R, Burr WA. Wrong biochemistry results: two case reports and observational study in 5310 patients on potentially misleading thyroid-stimulating hormone and gonadotropin immunoassay results. Clin Chem 2002;48:2023-9.
45. Kendall MG, Stuart A. The advanced theory of statistics 4. ed., vol 1. London: C. Griffin & Co., 1977: 258, 352.
46. Kendall MG, Stuart A. The advanced theory of statistics 3. ed., vol 2. London: C. Griffin & Co., 1973: 391-408.
47. Klee G. A conceptual model for establishing tolerance limits for analytical bias and imprecision based on variations in population test distributions. Clin Chim Acta 1997;260:175-88.
48. Kringle RO, Bogavich M. Statistical procedures. In: Burtis CA, Ashwood ER, eds. Tietz textbook of clinical chemistry, 3rd ed. Philadelphia: WB Saunders, 1999:265-309.
49. Kristiansen J. Description of a generally applicable model for the evaluation of uncertainty of measurement in clinical chemistry. Clin Chem Lab Med 2001;39:920-31.
50. Kristiansen J. The Guide to expression of uncertainty in measurement approach for estimating uncertainty: an appraisal. Clin Chem 2003;49:1822-9.
51. Kroll MH, Emancipator K. A theoretical evaluation of linearity. Clin Chem 1993;39:405-13.
52. Krouwer JS. Multifactor protocol designs IV. How multifactor designs estimate the total error by accounting for protocol-specific biases. Clin Chem 1991;37:26-9.
53. Krouwer JS. Estimating total analytical error and its sources. Arch Pathol Lab Med 1992;116:726-31.
54. Krouwer JS, Monti KL. A simple graphical method to evaluate laboratory assays. Eur J Clin Chem Clin Biochem 1996;33:525-7.
55. Krouwer JS. Setting performance goals and evaluating total analytical error for diagnostic assays. Clin Chem 2002;48:919-27.
56. Krouwer JS. Critique of the Guide to the expression of uncertainty in measurement method of estimating and reporting uncertainty in diagnostic assays. Clin Chem 2003;49:1818-21.
57. Kummel CH. Reduction of observation equations which contain more than one observed quantity. The Analyst 1879;6:97-105.
58. Lawton WH, Sylvester EA, Young-Ferraro BJ. Statistical comparison of multiple analytic procedures: application to clinical chemistry. Technometrics 1979;21:397-409.
59. Linko S, Örnemark U, Kessel R, Taylor PDP. Evaluation of uncertainty of measurement in routine clinical chemistry—Application to determination of the substance concentration of calcium and glucose in serum. Clin Chem Lab Med 2002;40:391-8.
60. Linnet K. Assessing diagnostic tests once an optimal cutoff point has been selected. Clin Chem 1986;32:1341-6.
61. Linnet K. Two-stage transformation systems for normalization of reference distributions evaluated. Clin Chem 1987;33:381-6.
62. Linnet K. A review on the methodology for assessing diagnostic tests. Clin Chem 1988;34:1379-86.

63. Linnet K. Choosing quality control systems to detect maximum medically allowable analytical errors. Clin Chem 1989;35:284-8.
64. Linnet K. Estimation of the linear relationship between the measurements of two methods with proportional errors. Stat Med 1990;9:1463-73.
65. Linnet K, Bruunshuus I. HPLC with enzymatic detection as a candidate reference method for serum creatinine. Clin Chem 1991;37:1669-75.
66. Linnet K. Evaluation of regression procedures for methods comparison studies. Clin Chem 1993;39:424-32.
67. Linnet K. The performance of Deming regression analysis in case of a misspecified analytical error ratio. Clin Chem 1998;44:1024-31.
68. Linnet K. Limitations of the paired t-test for evaluation of method comparison data. Clin Chem 1999;45:314-5.
69. Linnet K. Necessary sample size for method comparison studies based on regression analysis. Clin Chem 1999;45:882-94.
70. Linnet K. Nonparametric estimation of reference intervals by simple and bootstrap-based procedures. Clin Chem 2000;46:867-9.
71. Linnet K, Kondratovich M. Partly nonparametric approach for determining the limit of detection. Clin Chem 2004;50:732-40.
72. Lipman HB, Astles JR. Quantifying the bias associated with use of discrepant analysis. Clin Chem 1998;44:108-15.
73. Mandel J. The statistical analysis of experimental data. New York: Wiley, 1964:290-1.
74. Marks V. False-positive immunoassay results: a multicenter survey of erroneous immunoassay results from assays of 74 analytes in 10 donors from 66 laboratories in seven countries. Clin Chem 2002;48: 2008-16.
75. National Cholesterol Education Program. Current status of blood cholesterol measurements in clinical laboratories in the United States: a report from the laboratory Standardization Panel of the National Cholesterol Education Program. Clin Chem 1988;34:193-201.
76. NCCLS. Evaluation of precision performance of clinical chemistry devices; Approved guideline. NCCLS document EP5-A (ISBN 1-56238-368-X). Wayne, PA: NCCLS, 1999;19(No. 2):1-42.
77. NCCLS. Preliminary evaluation of quantitative clinical laboratory methods; Approved Guideline-Second Edition. NCCLS document EP10-A2 (ISBN 1-56238-482-1). Wayne, PA: NCCLS, 2002;22(No. 29):1-56.
78. NCCLS. User protocol for evaluation of qualitative test performance; Approved guideline. NCCLS document EP12-A. NCCLS, Wayne, PA, USA 2002.
79. NCCLS. Evaluation of the linearity of quantitative measurement procedures: A statistical approach; Approved guideline. NCCLS document EP6-A (ISBN 1-56238-498-8). NCCLS, Wayne, PA, USA 2003.
80. NCCLS. Interference testing in clinical chemistry; Approved guideline. NCCLS document NCCLS-EP7-A. NCCLS, Wayne, PA, USA 2002.
81. NCCLS. Method comparison and bias estimation using patient samples; Approved guideline—2. ed. NCCLS document EP9-A2 (ISBN 1-56238-472-4). Wayne, PA: NCCLS, 2002;22(No.19):1-55.
82. Passing H, Bablok W. A new biometrical procedure for testing the equality of measurements from two different analytical methods. J Clin Chem Clin Biochem 1983;21:709-20.
83. Passing H, Bablok W. Comparison of several regression procedures for method comparison studies and determination of sample sizes. J Clin Chem Clin Biochem 1984;22:431-45.
84. Petersen PH, de Verdier C-H, Groth T, Fraser CG, Blaabjerg O, Hørder M. The influence of analytical bias on diagnostic misclassifications. Clin Chim Acta 1997;260:189-206.
85. Petersen PH, Stöckl D, Blaabjerg O, Pedersen B, Birkemose E, Thienpont L, et al. Graphical interpretation of analytical data from comparison of a field method with a reference method by use of difference plots. Clin Chem 1997;43:2039-46.
86. Petersen PH, Fraser CG, Kallner A, Kenny D (eds). Strategies to set global analytical quality specifications in laboratory medicine. Scand J Clin Lab Invest 1999;59(7):475-585.
87. Petersen PH, Stöckl D, Westgard JO, Sandberg S, Linnet K, Thienpont L. Models for combining random and systematic errors. Assumptions and consequences for different models. Clin Chem Lab Med 2001;39:589-95.
88. Pollock MA, Jefferson SG, Kane JW, Lomax K, MacKinnon G, Winnard CB. Method comparison—a different approach. Ann Clin Biochem 1992;29: 556-60.
89. Powers DM. Establishing and maintaining performance claims. Arch Pathol Lab Med 1992;116:718-25.
90. Prichard FE, Day JA, Hardcastle WA, Holcombe DG, Treble RD. Quality in the analytical chemistry laboratory. Chichester, England: Wiley, 1995:136-143, 169.
91. Ricos C, Alvarez V, Cava F, Garcia-Lario JV, Hernandez A, Jimenez CV, Minchinela J, Perich C, Simon M. Current databases on biological variation: pros, cons and progress. Scand J Clin Lab Invest 1999;59: 491-500.
92. Rodbard D, McClean SW. Automated computer analysis for enzyme-multiplied immunological techniques. Clin Chem 1977;23:112-5.
93. Ross JW, Lawson NS. Analytical goals, concentration relationships, and the state of the art for clinical laboratory precision. Arch Pathol Lab Med 1995;119: 495-513.

94. Rotmensch S, Cole LA. False diagnosis and needles therapy of presumed malignant disease in women with false-positive human chorionic gonadotropin concentrations. Lancet 2000;355:712-5.
95. Shukla GK. On the problem of calibration. Technometrics 1972;14:547-53.
96. Skendzel LP, Barnett RN, Platt R. Medically useful criteria for analytic performance of laboratory tests. Am J Clin Pathol 1985;83:200-5.
97. Snedecor GW, Cochran WG. Statistical methods, 8th ed. Ames, IA: Iowa State University Press, 1989:75, 121, 140-2, 170-4, 177, 237-8, 279.
98. Stöckl D. Beyond the myths of difference plots. [Letter] Ann Clin Biochem 1996;36:575-7.
99. Strike PW. Measurement in laboratory medicine. Oxford: Butterworth-Heinemann, 1996, 162-3.
100. Taylor JR. An introduction to error analysis. Oxford: Oxford University Press, 1982.
101. Thienpont LM, Van Nuwenborg JE, Stöckl D. Intrinsic and routine quality of serum total potassium measurement as investigated by split-sample measurement with an ion chromatography candidate reference method. Clin Chem 1998;44:849-57.
102. Thienpont L, Van Uytfanghe K, De Leenheer AP. Reference measurement systems in clinical chemistry. Clin Chim Acta 2002;323:73-87.
103. Tietz NW. A model for a comprehensive measurement system in clinical chemistry. Clin Chem 1979;25:833-9.
104. US Department of Health and Human Services. Medicare, Medicaid, and CLIA programs: Regulations implementing the Clinical Laboratory Improvement Amendments of 1988 (CLIA). Final rule. Fed Regist 1992;57:7002-186.
105. US Department of Health and Human Services. Medicare, Medicaid, and CLIA programs: Laboratory requirements relating to quality systems and certain personnel qualifications. Final rule. Fed Regist 2003;68:3640-714, available at: http://www.phppo.cdc.gov./clia/pdf/CMS-2226-F.pdf (accessed August 2003).
106. Westgard JO, Hunt MR. Use and interpretation of common statistical tests in method-comparison studies. Clin Chem 1973;19:49-57.
107. Wu CFJ. Jackknife, bootstrap and other resampling methods in regression analysis (with discussion). Ann Stat 1986;14:1261-95.
108. Zweig MH, Kroll MH. Linear regression estimation of minimal detectable concentration. Thyrotropin as an example. Arch Pathol Lab Med 1997;121:948-55.

CHAPTER 15

Clinical Evaluation of Methods

Edward K. Shultz, M.D., M.S.,
Constantin Aliferis, M.D., Ph.D.,
and Dominik Aronsky, M.D., Ph.D.

Often it is not clear which procedure offers the best information in a specific setting, which procedure is the most cost effective, or which sequence of procedures offers the most efficient route to the solution of a problem. How does one combine a testing result or testing information with previously obtained information? Addressing these questions, this chapter focuses on how to quantify the diagnostic information content of a test or groups of tests and then on how to compare the results with those of other tests. Finally, the cost effectiveness of a test is discussed in the context of outcomes analysis.

The analytical performance of the methods used for many clinical tests has improved dramatically over the past 4 decades. However, a highly accurate and precise test may provide less clinical information than a different test that is less accurate and less precise. For example, a test for total creatine kinase is often more accurate and precise than one for creatine kinase isoenzymes, yet knowledge of the total enzyme activity is of less value in the diagnosis of cardiac damage. How does one evaluate the information content of a test? What procedure should one use to decide among different tests based on their disease discrimination ability? This chapter discusses these and other nonanalytical aspects of test performance that affect a test's overall medical usefulness.

To demonstrate how the concepts described in this chapter can be practically applied, we present the following example: A urologist questions the performance of the current assay to detect prostatic disease. He suggests replacing the current prostate-specific antigen (PSA) assay with a new one that has a greater ability to detect carcinoma of the prostate. He wishes to use the assay annually on his male patients who are older than 50 years of age to screen for prostatic carcinoma. As can be seen in Table 15-1, it appears that the new assay does offer superior performance in this regard. Of the patients with carcinoma, 88% were detected using the new test (Test A), whereas only 82% were detected using the current test (Test B). When healthy men were tested, 96% were correctly classified as not having prostatic carcinoma using Test A; Test B's performance was slightly better, classifying 99% of the subjects correctly.[15]

SPECTRUM

Before an opinion regarding test superiority can be made, the source of the data in Table 15-1 should be considered. In particular, it is appropriate to examine the populations studied and the criteria used for diagnosis. The *spectrum* concerns the medical characteristics of the patients who are involved in the test evaluation. Important aspects include the duration and severity of the disease state, its specific pathological categorization, and the existence of conditions that may affect test performance. Does the study population contain patients typical of those likely to be tested for the disease in question? If the selection criteria make patients with prostatitis or benign prostatic hypertrophy (BPH) more or less likely in the study population than the population to be tested in routine use, the test's interpretation must be qualified by this information.

In this particular case, the patients with carcinoma were identified (in a study by Chan and associates[15]) as having either symptoms or signs of disease. Advanced disease is associated with increases in the number of symptoms and signs and in PSA values. Thus a greater fraction of those

TABLE 15-1 Correct Prediction of Prostatic Carcinoma by Two Prostate-Specific Antigen Assays

Test	Carcinoma (%)	Healthy Men (%)
A, New test	88	96
B, Old test	82	99

TABLE 15-2 Correct Prediction of Prostatic Carcinoma by Two Tests Using Autopsy Data to Estimate Disease Occurrence

Test	Carcinoma (%)	Nondiseased (%)
A, New test	8	95
B, Old test	4	99

Data from references 11, 18, 24, 33, and 41.

reported in this study would be expected to be over the chosen diagnostic cutoff point than nonsymptomatic individuals undergoing an annual screen. The "normal" subjects (drawn from the same work) were patients without known disease; those with BPH, which is a noncancerous enlargement of the prostate, were intentionally excluded. Because our urologist intends to use the assay on BPH patients, and because BPH is associated with higher PSA values, the percentage quoted in Table 15-1 for predicting the presence of a healthy prostate is inflated.

Problems of spectrum are commonly encountered early on in a test's application. Often, very sick patients with advanced disease are compared with unequivocally normal patients to see if a proposed test has any merit. As more realistic clinical populations are tested, performance typically declines. One would expect to see worse performance than the estimates in Table 15-1 in a screening function. One would see an increase in false-negative results owing to the inclusion of less diseased patients and an increase in false-positive results owing to the presence of BPH in the patients being screened (i.e., in those who are older than 50 years of age).

However, the urologist points out that the problems of spectrum are at least constant for both tests. Although the table estimates are not accurate in his population, the relative difference between Test A and Test B in the study would be expected to extend to other populations. Thus it is still advisable to select Test A.

CLASSIFICATION BIAS

How was the diagnosis of carcinoma or the absence of disease established? This question introduces the concept of *classification bias.* Classification bias occurs when an independent standard is not used to judge the validity of a test. A subtle example that involves both spectrum and classification bias occurs in the well-known study by Light and coworkers[33] of the utility of the ratio of serum lactate dehydrogenase to pleural fluid lactate dehydrogenase. The results appear to document excellent differentiation between effusions and transudates. Unfortunately, when a clinical diagnosis could not be made using the remainder of the clinical information available, the case was excluded from the analysis. For the remaining cases, the test offered excellent discrimination. One would expect that small malignancies, which would be less obvious clinically, would also have a more indeterminate ratio. The lack of a gold standard resulted in an overly optimistic appraisal of the test's ability to discriminate between effusions and transudates. Similarly, assumptions have been made about the existence of disease in nonsymptomatic patients in prostatic disease, because it has been impractical to take biopsies in these individuals. For example, Cooner and associates[17] assumed patients who had negative ultrasound and digital examination results had no prostatic disease. Based on this assumption, they derived estimates of the performance of the PSA assay in detecting disease. Their standard for the establishment of disease absence was the assessment of both biopsy and other test results.

Often, alternative candidates for gold standards exist, and this confounds simple interpretation. For example, when step sections of prostates obtained at autopsy or from patients undergoing radical cystectomy were examined, prostatic carcinoma was found in men at a rate more than 10 times higher than Cooner and associates had estimated.[22,27,29,36,43] The silent fraction of nonsymptomatic control subjects who were called "normal" in Cooner's study clearly were not free of carcinoma. This resulted in a higher estimate of the disease detection capability (sensitivity) of PSA at a specific decision threshold. Other studies have used elevated PSA as a criterion for determining which patients should undergo biopsy. When the test in question is used to determine which patients will have the gold standard test or which ones will be included in the diagnostic set, *test referral bias* occurs. Test referral bias can be shown to erroneously increase the true-positive rate in a study population compared with the clinically relevant population.[46] An estimate of the performance of the assay using autopsy data for an estimate of the frequency of disease expected is found in Table 15-2.

A more subtle issue here is the designation of a true-positive result. Medical professionals have been both frustrated and protected in the past owing to their inability to detect early-stage limited disease; they have been frustrated because earlier detection would often have offered the opportunity to treat disease at a time when a cure is possible, and protected because the temptation to overtreat incidental, clinically insignificant disease did not come into play because of detection limits. This protection is diminishing as

TABLE 15-3 Sensitivity and Specificity of a Test Applied to Healthy and Diseased Populations

	No. of Patients With Positive Test Result	No. of Patients With Negative Test Result	Totals
No. of patients with disease	TP	FN	TP + FN
No. of patients without disease	FP	TN	FP + TN
Totals	TP + FP	FN + TN	TP + FP + TN + FN

TP, True positives (number of diseased patients correctly classified by the test); *FP,* false positives (number of nondiseased patients misclassified by the test); *FN,* false negatives (number of diseased patients misclassified by the test); *TN,* true negatives (number of nondiseased patients correctly classified by the test).

Sensitivity = positivity in disease, expressed as a percent = TP/(TP + FN) × 100

Specificity = absence of a particular disease, expressed as percent = TN/(FP + TN) × 100

Likelihood ratio positive (LR^+) = sensitivity/(1 − specificity)

Likelihood ratio negative (LR^-) = specificity/(1 − sensitivity)

Odds ratio = probability of event/(1 − probability of event)

the sensitivity and specificity of diagnostic tools increase. The desire to detect early disease must now often be tempered by reflection on what is clinically relevant disease.

It would appear that the examination of step sections of patient prostates, although more difficult, might at first seem to be as near an absolute gold standard as possible. However, the great majority of prostatic carcinomas (>99%) are clinically indolent and do not decrease life span or increase morbidity.[24,47] A more reasonable true-positive result should reflect identification of those carcinomas that will progress to cause increased morbidity or mortality if neglected.

In the case of prostatic carcinoma, it has been argued that the size of the carcinoma is the best predictor of morbidity and mortality.[24,47] Minimum tumor sizes from 0.2 to 3 cm^3 have been suggested as worth detecting.[24,47] The Hybritech PSA assay uses 4 µg/L as its cutoff. This can be shown to correspond to an average prostatic carcinoma volume, if present, of approximately 1.3 cm^3.[3,14,48] A tumor of this size would serve as a reasonable cutoff for a gold standard,[56] but it is difficult to size a tumor before complete prostate removal. Using the biopsy as a gold standard is also problematical. Biopsy will detect clinically insignificant disease by chance, but will miss large tumors owing to sampling error. Yet, by its nature, the sampling error of the biopsy is weighted in favor of ignoring small tumors and of detecting large ones. In addition, the number of cancers detected using the biopsy in screening programs is similar to the number of tumors larger than 1.3 cm^3 that were expected. Hence, biopsy is a reasonable substitute for PSA assay. It is adopted as the gold standard for the remainder of this analysis.

Reviewing Table 15-1 after consideration of spectrum and classification bias indicates considerable error in the estimates quoted if they were to be used for annual tests on patient groups consisting largely of BPH patients. A better estimate comes from the data of Chan and colleagues from a comparison of patients with BPH and patients with known prostatic carcinoma.[14,15] The number of carcinoma patients correctly predicted is still an overestimate, because this number includes patients with advanced disease; this would not be the case in the annual screening of the example urologist's patients.

TABLE 15-4 Correct Prediction of Prostatic Carcinoma and Benign Prostatic Hyperplasia (BPH)

Test	Carcinoma (%)	BPH (%)
A, New test	78	58
B, Old test	50	92

SENSITIVITY AND SPECIFICITY

The urologist in the example has assumed that using the test that detects a higher fraction of those with carcinoma is preferable. The *sensitivity* of an assay is the fraction of those with a specified disease that the assay correctly predicts. The *specificity* is the fraction of those without the disease that the assay correctly predicts. Pertinent definitions and formulas for computing sensitivity and specificity are found in Table 15-3. Both sensitivity and specificity are desirable characteristics for a test, but one is typically preferred over the other in different clinical situations.

The data in Table 15-1 have both spectrum problems and bias. The more accurate Table 15-4 can be used to make a decision. However, an illusion has been created here, as is apparent in Figure 15-1. This figure is a dot plot of the performance of a single assay for PSA on patients with BPH and on patients with established carcinoma of the prostate (stages A-D). Note the two dashed lines crossing the graphs that represent diagnostic cutoffs. In fact, Tests A and B in Table 15-4 are not two different assays but rather two decision cutoffs that are applied to the same assay. By moving the decision level to a lower value, the sensitivity has been

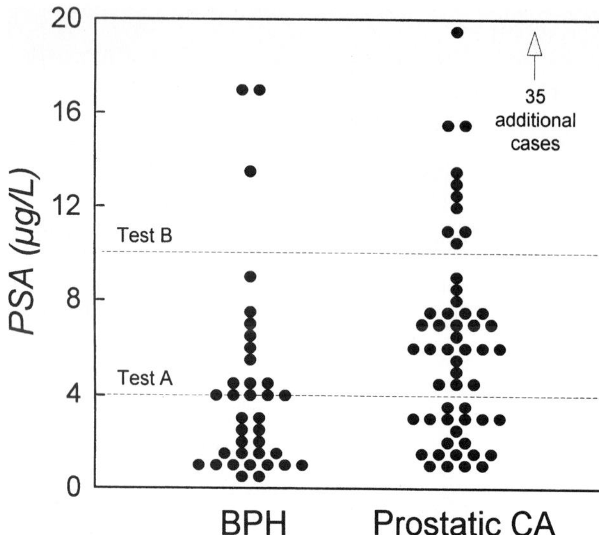

Figure 15-1 Prostate-specific antigen (PSA) levels for patients with benign prostatic hyperplasia (BPH) and known prostatic carcinoma (CA) are shown with two decision-level cutoffs. Tests A and B in Table 15-4 were actually the same test with two different cutoffs.

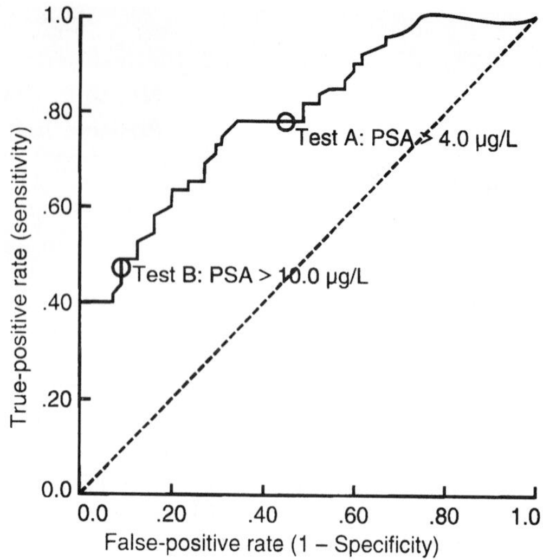

Figure 15-2 Receiver operating characteristic curve of prostate-specific antigen (PSA). Each point on the curves represents a different decision level. The sensitivity (true-positive rate) and 1—the specificity (false-positive rate) can be read for Tests A and B. The true-positive and false-positive rates are demonstrated using 4 and 10 μg/L as decision thresholds.

increased but at the cost of a decrease in specificity. Thus increased true-positive detection was traded for an increase in the number of false-positive results. This tradeoff is not unique to this assay. It occurs in every test performed in medicine. Although it is not often appreciated, it affects the opinions of surgical pathologists and radiologists along with the care provider who performs a physical examination as much as it affects the interpretation of quantitative laboratory results.

RECEIVER OPERATING CHARACTERISTIC CURVES[57]

The dot plot answers quantitative performance questions in only a limited way. One cannot easily estimate sensitivity and specificity for various decision cutoffs using the plot. A graphical technique for displaying the same information called a *receiver operating characteristic* (ROC) curve began to be used during World War II. It was used to examine the sensitivity and specificity associated with the radar detection of enemy aircraft. An ROC curve is generated by plotting sensitivity (y-axis) versus 1 − specificity (x-axis).

For the case at hand, Figure 15-2 shows the ROC curve for PSA using Chan's data.[14] The x-axis plots the fraction of nondiseased patients who were erroneously categorized as positive for a specific decision threshold. This false-positive rate is mathematically the same as 1 − specificity. The y-axis plots the true-positive rate (the sensitivity). A "hidden" third axis is contained in the curve itself: the curve is drawn through points that represent different decision cutoff levels. The whole curve is a graphical display of the performance of the test.

The two Tests A and B from Table 15-4 are displayed as two decision points on the ROC curve. The dotted line extending from the lower left to the upper right represents a test with no discrimination. A curve that is "above" the diagonal line describes performance that is better than random guessing. A curve that extends from the lower left to the upper left and then to the upper right is a perfect test. The area under the curve describes the test's overall performance, although usually we are interested only in the performance in a specific region of the curve.[8] The strength of the ROC graph lies in its provision of a meaningful comparison of different tests. The use in the medical literature of 2 × 2 tables (e.g., Tables 15-1, 15-2, and 15-4) to establish the sensitivity and specificity of a test is a common source of the logical error encouraged in the previous paragraphs. When the initial publication of an assay presents a cutoff for analysis purposes, the assay is often categorized as sensitive or specific based on this cutoff. Yet, as can be seen in the ROC curve, every assay can be as sensitive as desired at some cutoff and as specific as desired at another cutoff.

When comparing two procedures, confusion is avoided by using the ROC curves instead of accepting statements such as "Test A is more sensitive, but Test B is more specific." For example, the usefulness of the prostatic acid phosphatase assay has been compared for years with that of the PSA assay for diagnostic and follow-up purposes. Various claims have been made regarding the relative sensitivity and specificity of the two assays.[18,44]

Figure 15-3 compares the performance of a thymolphthalein acid phosphatase assay with that of the PSA assay for discrimination between BPH and prostatic carcinoma stages A through D. Although each has been claimed to be

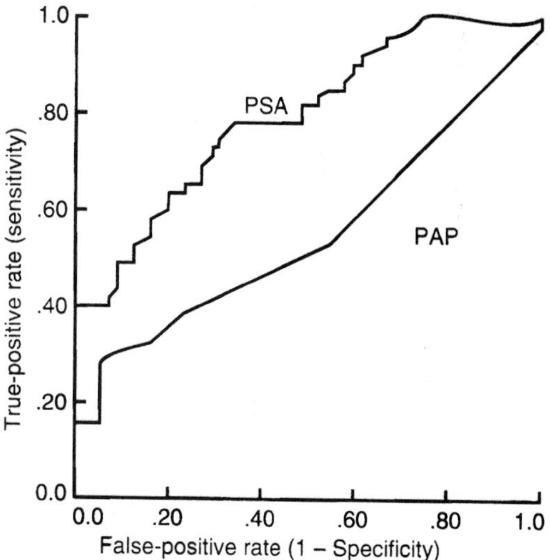

Figure 15-3 Receiver operating characteristic curves of prostatic acid phosphatase (PAP) and prostate-specific antigen (PSA) assays for patients with benign prostatic hyperplasia and prostatic carcinoma. Because the PSA assay curve is above the PAP assay curve at all points, the PSA assay is the better assay for the patients tested.

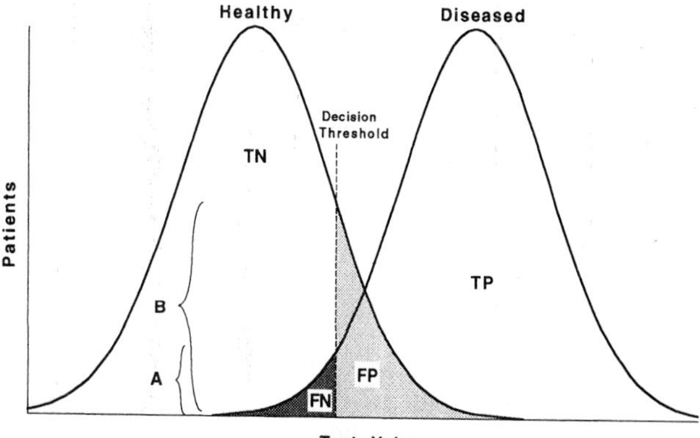

Figure 15-4 Simulated distributions of healthy and diseased populations. Note that the ratio of diseased patients to healthy patients, A to B, is less than 1 and very different at the point of decision (the likelihood ratio) from the ratio of TP to FP, which is much greater than 1. *TP*, True positives; *TN*, true negatives; *FP*, false positives; *FN*, false negatives.

"more sensitive but less specific" than the other by various authors, it is clear from the ROC curves that the authors were choosing different points on the two curves. No matter what level of sensitivity is chosen, the PSA assay offers greater specificity than the acid phosphatase at the same level of sensitivity. This does not mean one should conclude that the PSA assay is always superior. It indicates that for the spectrum of patients used in the assays, the PSA assay offers superior performance compared with that of prostatic acid phosphatase. However, there may be subpopulations in the group tested in which the acid phosphatase assay provides information that the PSA assay misses.

It has been advocated that the area under the ROC curve is a relative measure of a test's performance. A Wilcoxon statistic (or equivalently the Mann-Whitney U-Test) statistically determines which ROC curve has more area under it. Less computationally intensive alternatives, which are no longer necessary, have been described.[8] These methods are particularly helpful when the curves do not intersect. When the ROC curves of two laboratory tests for the same disease intersect, they may offer quite different performances even though the areas under their curves are identical. The performance depends on the region of the curve (i.e., high sensitivity versus high specificity) chosen. Details on how to compare statistically individual points on two curves have been developed elsewhere.[8]

INTERPRETING A TEST

Although the ROC curve improves our capability to judge a test's performance, a result should not be interpreted in isolation. The laboratory scientist must take into account the clinical setting before rendering a specific interpretation. For example, an elevated PSA level in a 35-year-old is not interpreted in the same way as in a 70-year-old because the rate of occurrence of prostatic cancer in 35-year-olds is much lower than in older men.[37] The interpretation is tempered by a knowledge of the prevalence of the disease. The *prevalence* is defined as the frequency of disease in the population examined.[55] For example, using step sectioning of prostate tissue from a random sample of men older than 50 years of age, at least a 25% probability of histological carcinoma can be expected (most of the carcinomas identified will never become clinically important, but they are carcinomas nevertheless).[27,43] Several useful techniques can be applied to combine the prevalence and other previously obtained information with the results of a procedure.

ODDS RATIO

The *odds ratio* is defined as the probability of the presence of a specific disease divided by the probability of its absence. The odds ratio reflects the prevalence of the disease in a population. For example, the probability of the occurrence of a 1.3-cm^3 carcinoma in a 75-year-old man is about 8%. The odds ratio of finding histological carcinoma greater than 1.3 cm^3 in size after sectioning the prostate from the autopsy specimen of a man older than 70 years is thus 0.08/(1 – 0.08), or 1:11.5. Findings from a digital rectal examination, from transrectal ultrasonography, or from both are other data that affect the previous probability of the presence of prostatic disease.

LIKELIHOOD RATIO

The *likelihood ratio* is the probability of the occurrence of a specific result (given that the disease is present) divided by the probability of the same result if the disease were absent (i.e., sensitivity/[1 – specificity]). For a given result, this corresponds to the ratio of the heights A and B of the two curves at the decision point in Figure 15-4.

Note that the areas under each curve in Figure 15-4 are the same. The likelihood ratio does not take disease prevalence or any other prior information into account. To arrive at a realistic probability, one must adjust for the best estimate of the probability of disease before obtaining the test result. Bayes' theorem provides a method for combining the prior probability information.

BAYES' THEOREM

Bayes' theorem provides a method to calculate the probability of a disease after the addition of new information to previously obtained information. These formulas can be incorporated into computer spreadsheets and other computer aids to help in the estimation of updated probabilities. One method, which can be performed without a computer, involves using the odds ratio version of Bayes' theorem. The odds ratio of the occurrence of a disease is calculated before the test result is known; this information is then combined with the results of the test in the form of a likelihood ratio. The final result is again in the form of an odds ratio; this can be converted into a probability, if desired. The advantages of this method are that it is relatively easily memorized and that it requires little mathematical calculation. The odds ratio is useful when it is combined with the likelihood ratio in a more memorable form of Bayes' theorem:

$$\text{Odds ratio after} = \text{Odds ratio before} \times \text{Likelihood ratio}$$

Consider interpretation of a slightly elevated PSA (4.0 to 10.0 μg/L) PSA in BPH. A urologist follows with a transrectal ultrasound examination, which he interprets as giving a positive result. The urologist has performed biopsies on numerous patients similar to this patient and has had many negative results. The urologist finds this perplexing, because both screening tests produced positive results. He or she then requests an estimate of the probability of disease in this patient.

Step 1. *Calculate the odds ratio that carcinoma is present before performing the ultrasound.* Given a PSA of 4.0 to 10.0 μg/L, there is an estimated probability of 12% in a BPH population with biopsy-verifiable disease; thus the probability of no disease is (1 − 0.12) = 0.88. The odds ratio therefore is 0.12/0.88 = 0.14.

Step 2. *Calculate the likelihood ratio of the new information (findings of the transrectal ultrasound).* Screening studies on urology patients report sensitivities of approximately 92% and specificities that range from 30% to 70% (average 50%) for transrectal ultrasound.[13,17,41] The likelihood ratio positive is the sensitivity divided by (1 − specificity), or 0.92/0.50 = 1.8.

Step 3. *Calculate the odds ratio after incorporation of the new information.* The revised odds ratio estimate (the product of Steps 1 and 2) is 0.25.

Step 4. *Convert the odds ratio back into probabilities.* The probability equals the odds ratio divided by (1 + odds ratio), or 0.25/1.25 = 0.2.

Although both tests were positive, the probability of a positive biopsy result is only 20%. If the ultrasound findings had been negative, we would use the inverse of the odds ratio coupled with the likelihood ratio negative. The odds ratio of no disease after the PSA assay, (0.88/0.12) = 7.3, multiplied by the likelihood ratio negative (true-negative rate/false-negative rate = specificity/(1 − sensitivity) = 0.5/0.08 = 6.25) is 43. Converting to probabilities yields 43/(43 + 1) = 98% probability of no disease.

Limitations of Bayes' Theorem

Although Bayes' theorem is widely recommended as an aid to refine the probabilistic estimates of disease, it rests on the assumption of *test independence,* which is often not present. As an extreme example of the possible errors that can occur when nonindependent tests are used, consider testing the PSA level of a BPH patient on 3 consecutive days. Each day, the PSA value is greater than the 4 μg/L cutoff. The likelihood ratio positive of a value greater than 4 μg/L is equal to the sensitivity divided by (1 − specificity), or 0.78/(1 − 0.58) = 1.9. Using the odds ratio form of Bayes' theorem, we would multiply the prior odds (assume 10:90) by the likelihood ratio to obtain the odds after of 0.2, or a probability of 17% after the first test. The odds are 1.9 × 0.2 = 0.38 after the second test, and finally 0.72 after the third test. This gives a 42% probability of disease. Very little new information has been provided by the second and third tests, yet the probability of disease has apparently increased from 17% to 42%. A less obvious and less extreme example would result from the combination of the prostatic acid phosphatase results with the PSA results. Although this combination does provide some new information, an acid phosphatase result is related to the amount of prostatic tissue, much as a PSA result is. In contrast, the ultrasound examination is a different approach to the diagnosis, and the information it yields should be more independent of the PSA assay than information yielded by the acid phosphatase results. The lack of test independence is also a problem when using computerized diagnostic programs that employ a Bayesian approach. The amount of independence among different tests for various diseases must often be estimated and tried using a set of test cases. Techniques are being developed to reduce this problem.

Judging independence is difficult without collecting a large set of clinical data and examining them mathematically. A useful approach is to think about the incorrect results given by each test. If both tests tend to yield incorrect results for the same patients, then the tests are not independent, and thus Bayes' theorem cannot be applied to the combination of their results to correctly estimate the probability of disease. For example, the presence of prostatitis or BPH will result in a large number of false-positive results for both PSA and prostatic acid phosphatase assays. Although the tests are not measuring the same analyte and do provide some independent information, combining their results using Bayes' theorem is not appropriate. On the other hand, if the tests seem intuitively to be independent, then the errors made by assuming independence are not likely to be great.

One should note that test independence is important for accurate probability estimation, but not necessarily for classification. In classification, one has to determine only which disease is the more likely, not its exact probability. Studies have shown that using Bayes' estimation gives quite good diagnostic accuracy even when the tests are not independent. Tests with correlations of up to 0.7 can still be used together to give an idea of the most likely disease.

Combination Testing

Panels of tests are commonly used to increase sensitivity and specificity or when used sequentially to decrease costs. For the practicing laboratorian, the value of panels is limited by the sparse literature on the performance of combinations of tests. The same issue of test independence addressed in the previous section makes it difficult to calculate the performance of panels of tests. In addition, the use of multiple tests can increase the probability of the occurrence of false-positive or false-negative results, depending on how the tests are combined.

Because most reference intervals exclude a fraction of those patients without disease, there is an expected false-positive rate. As multiple tests are added to panels, the probability of false-positive results increases. Efforts to establish multivariate reference intervals that correct for multiple tests and their interrelationships have been made, but the concept has not found widespread acceptance. Although the concept is mathematically quite reasonable, those who have investigated the utility of multivariate reference intervals believe that more work needs to be done before they will be useful.

The gain in test performance to be achieved from combining test results may be illusory. As demonstrated by Table 15-4, by the dot plot in Figure 15-1, and by the ROC curve in Figure 15-2, sensitivity can usually be increased at the expense of decreased specificity. This does not guarantee that the individual test, if the decision threshold were modified to improve sensitivity, would not have comparable performance. For example, consider the data of Chan and associates[14,15] for PSA and prostatic acid phosphatase values in patients with BPH and in those with prostatic disease. Although combining the two individual tests does improve sensitivity, there is a decrease in specificity. Note that using a lower decision threshold for the PSA assay gives comparable sensitivity with improved specificity over the combination. Two observations are important. First, tables can be as misleading for combinations of tests as they can be for single tests. For example, if only the first three rows of Table 15-5 were published, one might conclude that the combination of the two tests offered superior sensitivity. Second, although in this case the two tests do not offer performance that is comparable with that of the single test, in many cases they do. Although it might be assumed that using a single test is to be preferred given equal performance, it is not always the

TABLE 15-5 Performance of Different Test Combinations in Prediction of Prostatic Carcinoma

Test Combination	Sensitivity (%)	Specificity (%)
PSA > 4 μg/L	78	58
PAP > 0.6 U/L	77	25
PSA > 4 μg/L or PAP > 0.6 U/L	92	19
PSA > 1.5 μg/L	91	36

PSA, Prostate-specific antigen; *PAP*, prostatic acid phosphatase.

most cost-effective approach. In this example, the prostatic acid phosphatase assay costs less than the PSA assay. If the combination in row three of Table 15-5 offered performance comparable with that of the PSA assay alone, then using the acid phosphatase assay to exclude some patients and subsequently performing PSA assays on patients with higher PSA values may well be the more economical approach.

A widely held belief[54] is that one should test first with a sensitive test and then follow up the occurrence of positive results with a specific test for best performance. The logic is that if the first test determines which patients are to undergo a second test, then the first test should be the more sensitive of the two to ensure that the disease has not been missed. Somewhat surprisingly, even when the first test determines which patients will undergo a second test, the order in which the tests are performed does not affect the combination of sensitivity and specificity. However, it does affect the overall cost. In the following examples, two hypothetical tests that are independent are used sequentially. It is assumed that fixed decision limits are used for the two tests and that the two tests cost the same. Although the tests are hypothetical, the principles are generally applicable to other sequential testing situations.

Example 1. Often care can be optimized if it can be confirmed that a disease is not present. In this case, if screening Test A yields a positive result, it will be followed by Test B; otherwise, testing stops. If Test B yields a positive result, then the overall interpretation is a positive result. Because A *and* B are necessary for the diagnosis, the specificity is improved; however, the sensitivity decreases compared with the use of Test A alone. As shown in Table 15-6, the average cost of the combination varies with the disease prevalence; however, note that performance of the more *specific* test first results in lower expected costs. This lower cost would be accentuated if the second test were to cost more than the first.

The net effect of the use of the test combination compared with the use of Test A alone has been to decrease our false-positive rate fivefold while decreasing the true-positive rate by 0.8%. Whether this tradeoff is desirable

TABLE 15-6 Combination Test Performance Maximizing Specificity*

	Sensitivity (%)	Specificity (%)	Cost
Test A	80	99	$100
Test B	99	80	$100
A followed by B	79.2	99.8	
Prevalence = 0.2			$117
Prevalence = 0.8			$164
B followed by A	79.2	99.8	
Prevalence = 0.2			$136
Prevalence = 0.8			$183

*Results of Test A *and* Test B must be positive to make a positive diagnosis.

TABLE 15-7 Combination Test Performance Maximizing Sensitivity*

	Sensitivity (%)	Specificity (%)	Cost
Test A	80	99	$100
Test B	99	80	$100
A followed by B	99.8	79.2	
Prevalence = 0.2			$183
Prevalence = 0.8			$136
B followed by A	99.8	79.2	
Prevalence = 0.2			$164
Prevalence = 0.8			$117

*Results of Test A *or* Test B must be positive to make a positive diagnosis.

depends on the implications of missing a diagnosis versus generating false-positive results.

Example 2. Diagnosing a curable disease that has a low-cost therapy often increases the relative worth of sensitivity over specificity. If a first test result is negative, a second test might still be performed to maximize sensitivity. Either of two tests that yields a positive result would be interpreted as a positive finding overall. This is more typically the result of tests that are done simultaneously, but also occurs in sequential testing. In Table 15-7, a negative result on the first test is followed by performance of the second test; otherwise, testing stops. If the result of the second test is negative, then the overall interpretation is negative. The cost of performing tests sequentially with this rule varies with prevalence, as seen in Table 15-7.

Using this rule, the combination sensitivity increases as the specificity decreases. Note that the strategy of using the test with the *lower* specificity first results in lower average cost.

Following the strategy outlined in Table 15-6, the first test's specificity determines the cost of sequential testing. When the strategy is to confirm all the negative results of the first test (see Table 15-7), the first test should be the more sensitive so as to minimize costs. As demonstrated in the two examples presented earlier, the decision rule used preferentially trades off sensitivity at the expense of specificity, or vice versa. Although independent tests have been used in these examples, the conclusions are the same for dependent tests. It should be remembered that it is the interpretive rule and the two tests that determine the overall panel performance and costs; the order of testing does not affect performance but can dramatically affect costs.

Multivariate Data Analysis

Diagnosis using computer-generated probabilities from results of multiple laboratory tests has not received wide use. Use has been limited over time to variation of the same analyte, or simple ratios or combinations of two to five variables, as seen with cardiac enzymes or fetal maturity tests. However, this should change dramatically in the coming years as more computer-based support for diagnosis becomes an expectation. At the far end of the multivariable diagnostic spectrum lie mass-throughput molecular biological assaying techniques (e.g., array technologies,[52] mass spectrometry,[16,34] and serial analysis of gene expression [SAGE[40]]), which provide the ability to rapidly and inexpensively measure gene expression levels, presence of polymorphisms, number of copies of genes, and protein concentrations of thousands of genes and proteins *with a single assay* per patient. These molecular profiling techniques can be used with samples obtained from biopsies or from the patient's serum or other biological fluids, and have opened several possibilities for improved tests for diagnosis and for prognosis of clinical outcome, alone or as a response to treatment.

Techniques for combining multiple tests for diagnostic purposes focus on (1) selecting the best subset of all available diagnostic variables, (2) transforming the variables to facilitate separation between diseases and nondiseases, and (3) selecting the best boundaries around the resultant groupings for optimal categorization. One or more of these techniques may be used. As statistical aids become simpler to use, there is less art and more automated performance of these tasks. However, as with all tools, lack of knowledge of the strengths and limitations of the tools can lead to clinically significant errors.

For 2 to 25 variables, methods such as Fisher's discriminant analysis, quadratic discriminant analysis, and neural networks serve to effectively determine diagnostic combinations.[2] Although they are limited to two variables for clarity, the graphs in Figures 15-5, 15-6, and 15-7 show these different approaches. In Figure 15-5, imagine sitting on the *x*-axis beneath the clouds of diseased and nondiseased above you and trying to pick the best spot for a decision point for Test 1. The curves there show the density of the points above you, and that any point chosen will have a significant tradeoff between false positive and false negatives. An identical

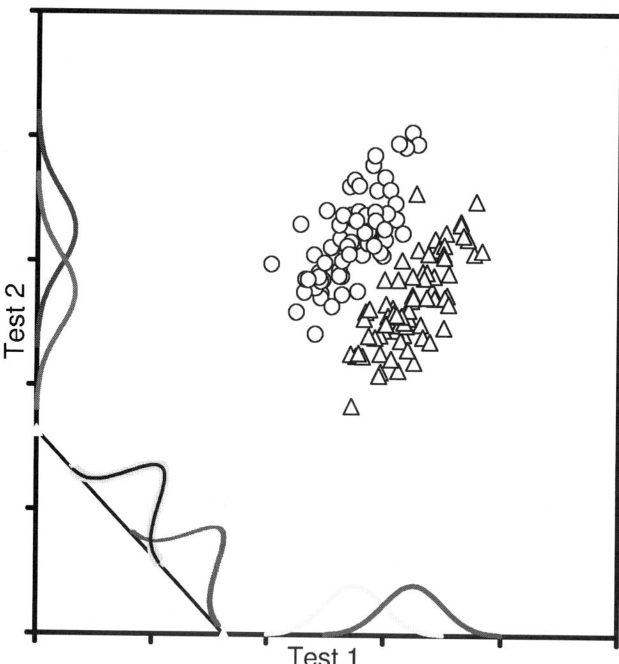

Figure 15-5 Fisher's linear discriminant analysis determines the line, plane, or hyperplane that best separates two populations, based on their mean values and the variance. In the graph, a line bisecting the two curves in the lower left corner provides this "best" discriminator.

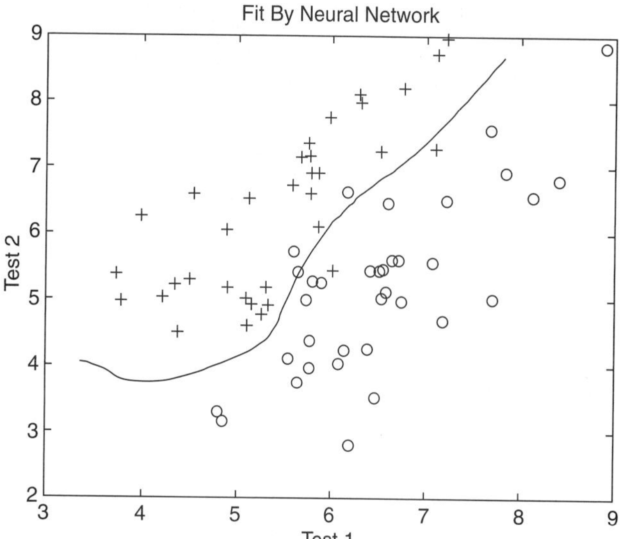

Figure 15-7 Neural networks provide ultimate freedom of discrimination, with the additional danger of "overfitting" a solution. The curved line separating the two populations for this specific set of data may not work well in a subsequent sample since it is custom molded to separate this test set.

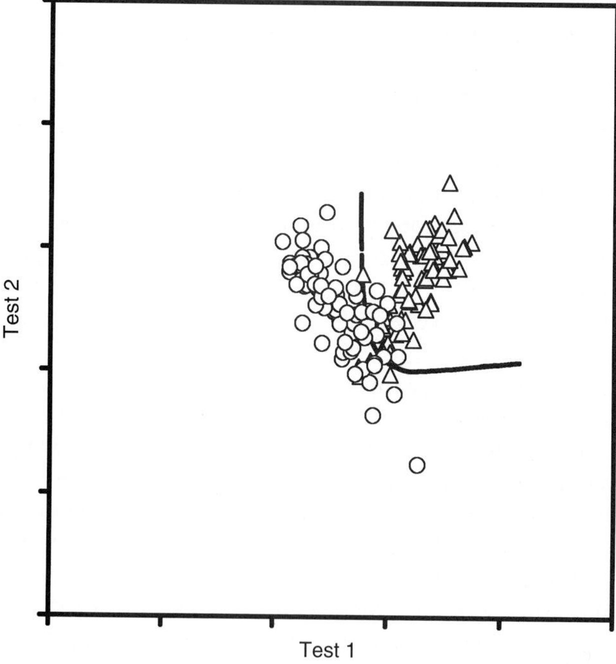

Figure 15-6 Quadratic discriminant analysis removes the constraint of a straight and/or flat plane and allows more molding of the decision boundary than is possible with linear discriminant analysis.

situation is true for Test 2, found on the *y*-axis. In Figure 15-5 we see that Fisher's discriminant analysis is seeking to find a viewing point that "best" separates the diseased and nondiseased. "Best" is defined in this test by finding the location where the difference between the means of the two groups is maximized while the apparent clustering (variance) of the values is minimized. The line found in the bottom left corner provides this viewing point. Here the density curves do not overlap significantly, and we can draw a line at right angles to our viewing point that will optimally separate the two groups of points. When more than two variables are involved, the resultant line becomes a plane (three variables) or hyperplane (more than three).

Fisher's linear discriminant works well when the two sets of data have roughly the same shape, but that is the exception rather than the common case. Where the shapes and orientation are different, quadratic discriminant analysis is preferred. As seen in Figure 15-6, we can provide much better separation using a curved line than we would have been able to with a straight line. You could continue using more and more curves in your lines, or more and more complex transformations. Perhaps the most flexible decision boundaries are derived from neural networks, with a possible solution shown in Figure 15-7. So why not always use neural networks if they're so flexible? The result is shown in Figure 15-8, where another sample from a different set of patients has been classified using the Figure 15-7 decision boundaries. This is an example of "overfitting," where we've derived a solution so specifically tailored to a specific set of data that merely resampling the same test from another set of patients decreases the diagnostic performance observed.

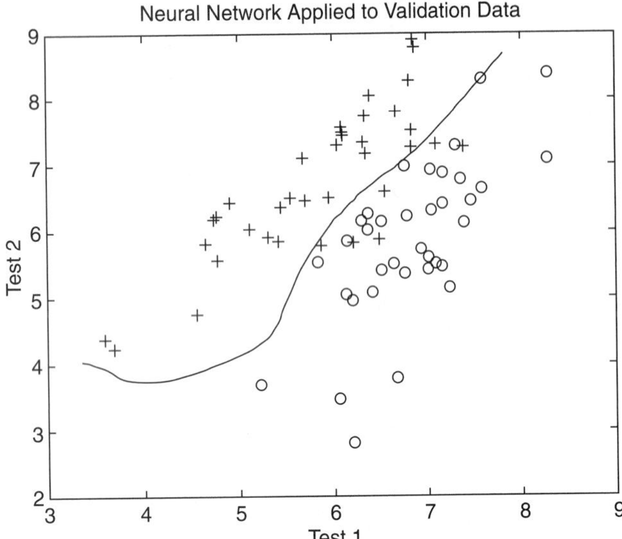

Figure 15-8 The decision boundary derived using a neural net, fit from different data in Figure 15-7, no longer provides optimal separation, although in this case the separation by chance is still good.

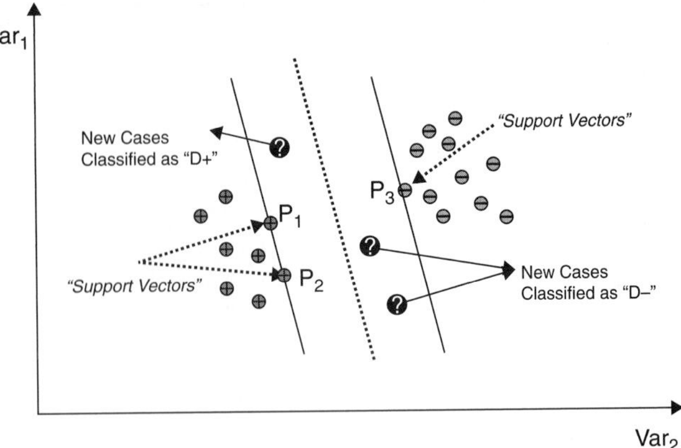

Figure 15-9 A support vector machine (SVM). The patients in the training data are represented by encircled plus and minus signs, while example patients that we have not seen before are represented by encircled question marks. The SVM classifier in this example is the set of the two parallel lines that go through patients P_1, P_2, and P_3, respectively. These two lines specify the "classification margin." Patients P_1, P_2, and P_3 are the "support vectors." Unseen cases are classified according to whether they are closer to the line defined by the disease-positive support vectors P_1, P_3, or to the line parallel to the previous line and the disease-negative support vector P_3.

General procedures for avoiding this are discussed later in the chapter.

Moving from dozens of variables to the thousands of variables found in genomic or proteomic analysis represents a different type of challenge. At least in the current, exploratory stage of examining the diagnostic utility of these profiles, the ratio of *samples to variables* is very small as compared with evaluations of individual tests and traditional panels. In particular, the samples-to-variables ratio is too small to use traditional statistical models (e.g., logistic regression and Fisher's discriminant analysis), because these methods require several patients per estimated model parameter (typically 2 to 10) to function satisfactorily. Genomic and proteomic analyses have a large number of simultaneous variables—in the tens of thousands. In contrast, available data sets of the present and foreseeable future have at most a few hundred patient samples, as is true for most new diagnostic tests. This dilemma is known as "curse of dimensionality" and plagues traditional statistical techniques.

Data Analysis Methods for Very Large Numbers of Variables

Newer data analysis methods overcome the difficulties that small sample-to-variables ratios create for traditional statistical methods. These new methods fall into two major categories: (1) support-vector classification and regression methods, and (2) feature selection and construction techniques. The former are effectively determined by only a small portion of the training data (sample), while the latter select only a small subset of variables such that the available sample is enough for traditional and newer classification techniques.

Support Vector Machines (SVMs)

As with Fisher's linear discriminant analysis, SVMs are classifiers that search for hyperplanes that separate between data points in the data set.[23,42] The separation seeks to maximize the distance between selected (boundary) data points (called the "support vectors") belonging to the different classes (e.g., diseases). Furthermore, nonlinearly separable data are transformed by projection to a higher-dimensional space in which separating hyperplanes can be found. The transformation is achieved through the use of functions ("kernels") such that optimization can be achieved by using only dot products of the original data. Empirical evidence verifies that SVMs are in general very robust to a low sample-to-feature ratio.[12,19,20,26] An intuitive explanation of how SVMs operate and why they have sample requirements much smaller than traditional statistical methods follows.

Consider the example task of classifying patients as having a disease ("D+") or not ("D–") on the basis of real-valued predictive variables *Var1* and *Var2.* Such variables might be for instance gene expression values or protein concentration. For simplicity, the example is in two dimensions but in practice thousands of such dimensions (variables) are used, as discussed earlier in this chapter. Figure 15-9 shows an SVM classifier for this example. First, note that patients in the training data are represented by encircled plus and minus signs, whereas example patients not classified previously are represented by question marks in circles. The SVM classifier in this example is the set of the two parallel lines that go through patients P_1, P_2, and P_3, respectively. These two lines specify the "classification margin." Patients P_1, P_2, and P_3 are the "support vectors" in this example. Unseen cases are classified according to whether they are closer to the line defined by the disease-positive support vectors P_1, P_3, or to the line parallel to the previous line and the disease-negative support vector P_3. A key observation is that the SVM classifier is *fully defined by its support vectors.* In other words, all remaining training cases are not used for classification once support vectors have been identified by the learning algorithm. It follows that since the total number of support vectors is at most the number of available data (i.e., patients), *the available data are always sufficient to fully specify an SVM model.* In contrast, in classical statistical models we do not seek only a means to correctly classify the data but also an estimate of the process that generates our data (the so-called "generative model"); as a result in a classical regression framework we may not have enough data to estimate a model unless the number of training cases is at least as large as the number of free parameters in our model (and in practice the number of such parameters is at least an order of magnitude larger than the number of predictor variables).

So far we established we can specify fully an SVM model even when the number of variables greatly exceeds the number of training samples (e.g., number of variables in the thousands with number of samples in the dozens). But can the classification performance under such conditions be good? We will give here an intuitive explanation why this is indeed the case. First, note that we are interested in good predictive performance for cases previously undiagnosed and sampled independently of the training sample from exactly the same population of patients. In statistical terminology, we say we wish to minimize "i.i.d. generalization error." Hence, as a first step, we need a good method to estimate the generalization error. Statistical sampling theory provides such an unbiased estimator of this generalization error in the form of the *leave-one-out error* (see later in this chapter). It is easy to see that the leave-one-out error is strictly a function of the support vectors (the nonsupport vectors will always be classified correctly). It can be shown easily that the leave-one-out-error has upper bound $s/(2d)$ where s is the number of support vectors and d is the total number of training data instances (patients). Assume for illustrative purposes that in our example three support vectors are selected in all of the leave-one-out splits; in this case the expected generalization error (the error if we were to use the same method on a very large set of data) is at most $3/38 = 7.9\%$. As the number of training instances grows, the generalization classification performance approaches the large sample optimal.

This example and discussion demonstrate that within the framework of SVMs it is possible to build classifiers even when the number of predictors is orders of magnitude larger than the available sample size (something not possible in classical regression-based classifiers); and such classifiers can exhibit very good classification performance.

Feature Selection and Construction

Feature selection is pursued because (1) a decreased set of variables will reduce the computation time from impossible to feasible, (2) feature selection may allow researchers to better understand the domain, (3) collecting a reduced set of predictors may be cheaper, and (4) collecting a reduced set of predictors may be safer (e.g., a blood sample versus a biopsy specimen). Feature selection methods are typically of the *wrapper* or the *filter* variety. Wrapper algorithms perform a search in the space of all possible variable subsets and evaluate each visited subset by applying the classifier for which they intend to optimize the variable selection. Common examples of search strategies are hill climbing (forward, backward, and forward-backward, simulated annealing, branch-and-bound, and genetic algorithms).[32,35] Filter approaches select features on the basis of shape of the data, called its joint distribution. The optimal variable set can be discovered effectively with newer algorithms under mild distributional assumptions[6,49,50] and allows optimal feature selection under those assumptions.

Once a variable subset has been identified, both traditional statistical classifiers and newer methods such as SVMs can be built using only the selected variables. A variant of the variable selection problem is the *feature* (or variable) *construction* problem in which one tries to transform the original variable set into a new set of variables for which building classifiers are easier to compute or fewer samples are required. Examples of such methods include principal components analysis for array gene expression-based diagnosis, and clustering and peak detection as preprocessing to mass spectrometry diagnostic model building.[28]

Clinical Examples

Gene array expression measurements have been used to (1) classify lung cancer patients as having adenocarcinomas or squamous carcinomas,[10] and metastatic cancer or nonmetastatic cancers; and (2) distinguish between normal and cancer samples.[4,5] Classification of adenocarcinoma versus squamous carcinoma[3] was accomplished using array comparative genomic hybridization (CGH) data. Models predictive of prognosis for patients with various stages of lung cancer[9] have been built using gene expression data. Patients with leukemia were classified as having acute myelogenous versus acute lymphocytic leukemia using array gene expression data,[25] while models for predicting clinical outcome of breast cancer have been developed.[51] Models were built to detect early prostate cancer and discriminate it from BPH and normal prostates using mass spectrometry data.[1,40] Mass spectrometry has been used to detect ovarian cancer,[39] to detect malignant cutaneous melanoma,[21] and to detect transitional cell carcinoma of the bladder.[53]

These applications are only a small sample of a large number of molecular-profiling clinical bioinformatics models that apply advanced computational techniques on mass-throughput data to address questions of prevention, diagnosis, treatment selection, and prognosis. A multitude of computational methods not covered here have also been explored in such problems.

Model Validation

In the neural net example above, it was clear that a method that is created and performs well on a training set of data may not perform well when another data sample is encountered. Hence a "validation" (test set) of data is needed to estimate how the classifier would perform in real life.

A variety of procedures are available to assess a model's true expected performance: split sample validation, cross-validation, jackknifing, and bootstrapping.

In split-sample or hold-out validation the data set is split randomly into different subsets: training and test sets. The training set is used for learning, typically estimating the model's parameters; the test set is used to assess the model's expected performance on future sets of data and its ability to generalize. Random case assignment is necessary to obtain representative groups. The split-sample approach works well for large sample data sets and, as long as the number of cases available in each subset is sufficient, will avoid overfitting and generate unbiased estimates.

However, small sample size data sets, in the range of 50 to 200 cases, are more common. With small sample data sets, using all cases for training and then using the same cases for testing is not permissible because biased (overly optimistic) results will be obtained. The cases in the training and test sets are no longer independent of each other. Computer-intensive statistical approaches, such a cross-validation, jackknifing, or bootstrapping are available and are the preferred evaluation methods that overcome some of the limitations inherent to sets with small sample sizes. These procedures are based on resampling theory and have the advantage that all cases can be used for training and testing. In resampling theory the observed data set becomes the underlying population from which samples are drawn repetitively with replacement. The samples are used to estimate parameters of interest.

Cross-validation is used to estimate the generalization error of a model or to compare the performance of different models. K-fold cross-validation divides a data set into k different subsets of equal size n. The validation procedure includes k runs and applies a "round-robin" approach. During each run one of the k subsets is left out and used as the test set while the remaining subsets are used for training the model. Leave-one-out cross-validation is present if k equals the sample size (i.e., each subset includes only one case). The selection between leave-one-out cross-validation and k-fold cross-validation depends on the situation. The former is preferred for continuous error functions, whereas the latter is preferred for determining the number of misclassified cases. A frequent value for k-fold cross-validation is $k = 10$.

Similar to leave-one-out cross-validation, jackknifing also involves omitting one case from the entire subset. However, jackknifing is applied to estimate the bias of a statistic of interest rather than the generalization error.

Bootstrapping involves the repetitive drawing of random samples with replacement from the observed population and computing statistics. A complete bootstrap in an observed population with eight variables would require the calculation of bootstrap statistics for $8^8 = 16,777,216$ samples, quite a computer-intensive process. Therefore bootstrap samples are usually limited to hundreds or thousands of drawings.

The validation procedures based on resampling theory mimic the theoretical process of repetitive sampling from an unobserved population; however, the samples are drawn from an empirically observed population rather than a theoretical, unobserved one. The limitation of resampling procedures is the representativeness of the observed population; unless the observed population is representative, the ability to generalize the model remains biased.

COST EFFECTIVENESS AND OUTCOMES RESEARCH

Optimal use of the laboratory requires examination of both the cost of obtaining the result and the value or quality of the information obtained. Determining the quality of various procedures in medicine has been a subject of increasing interest over the last 2 decades. Some key aspects of value received are the amount of improvement in health care, the extent to which testing is consistent with the wishes and expectations of patients, and the degree to which testing addresses social concerns as embodied in laws and regulations.

The Clinical Laboratory Improvement Act of 1967 (CLIA '67) and the Clinical Laboratory Improvement Amendments of 1988 (CLIA '88) mandate quality control and external quality assurance programs in large part as an effort to address social concerns regarding the quality of testing results. Only indirect measures of the quality of testing in terms of individual or population health benefit are available. The major instruments for measuring the quality of a healthcare intervention, including laboratory testing, are healthcare outcomes. Outcomes can be defined as the state or condition of an individual or population that is a result of antecedent medical care. In an effort to examine these issues and as a result of CLIA '88, the Centers for Disease Control and Prevention initiated the Evaluation of Quality of Laboratory Practices and Standards program, which partners with various groups to investigate the relationship between quality issues in the laboratory (e.g., proficiency testing, quality assurance, and personnel) and their effect on patient outcomes.[11] By tying specific analytical procedures and performance to patient outcome, it may be possible to directly trade off the increase in cost associated with achieving increased precision and accuracy with actual patient benefit. At this point, however, results are very preliminary and few conclusions can be made.

Another approach to quantifying health outcomes is to estimate the cost implications of a true-positive diagnosis and the costs of false-positive, false-negative, and true-negative results. One can calculate a weighted average of cost across all possibilities to determine whether a testing strategy is sensible. The decision threshold can be changed to maximize the benefits or to minimize the costs.[7,38,46,55]

An example of the issues involved can be found in the outcomes analysis of screening for prostate cancer. Prostate screening programs are increasing each year, partially accounting for a 600% increase in radical prostatectomies between 1984 and 1990.[37] For each man who dies each year from prostate cancer, there is a much larger number whose prostate cancer progresses slowly, never causing any morbidity. Screening is expensive and the iatrogenic side effects of surgical treatment for prostate cancer are significant. As a result of these observations, studies have called into question the overall cost effectiveness of prostate screening.

This question is amenable to outcomes analysis. One can examine the dollar costs per life year saved using two strategies. In the first strategy, assume that men age 45 through 75 undergo a screening PSA evaluation. If the screening PSA is greater than 4 µg/L, they are followed up by transrectal ultrasound evaluation and digital examination. If either of the subsequent tests is positive, a biopsy would be performed, and patients with positive biopsies would undergo radical prostatectomy. In the second strategy, there is no screen, and when prostatic carcinoma clinically appears, patients are treated using radiation and hormonal therapy for symptomatic relief. The literature provides the estimated number of life years lost, the patients' normal expected life span, and the expected life span based on the two strategies. Using methods described in more detail elsewhere,[30,45] the cost per life year saved can be computed. The costs of follow-up treatment for surgical side effects (e.g., incontinence and impotence) can be calculated from published frequencies of occurrence. A graphical depiction of the two strategies is shown in Figure 15-10, which is called a decision tree.

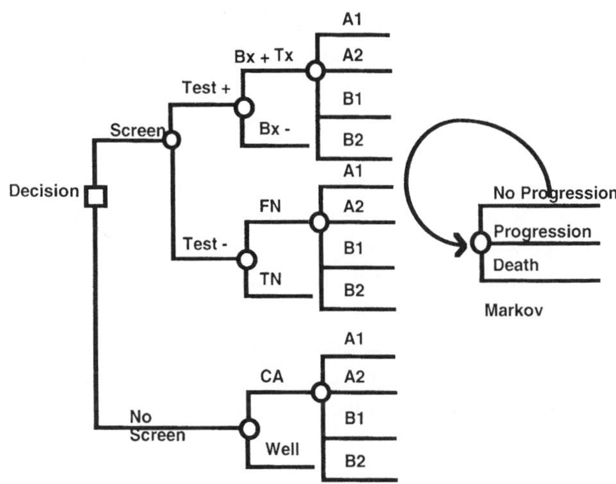

Figure 15-10 The decision tree shows alternative strategies that branch at the *square box*. The *lower* branch assumes no screening, and disease is treated symptomatically as symptoms appear. The *upper* branch evaluates with a screening program, followed by radical prostatectomy for biopsy-positive cases. *A1* through *B2* represent different cancer stages. The Markov model is an algorithm that evaluates costs and life years gained as patients sequentially stay unchanged, progress, or die each year. It repeats for 15 years. *(From Shultz EK. Multivariate receiver operating characteristic curve analysis: Prostate cancer screening as an example. Clin Chem 1995;41:1253.)*

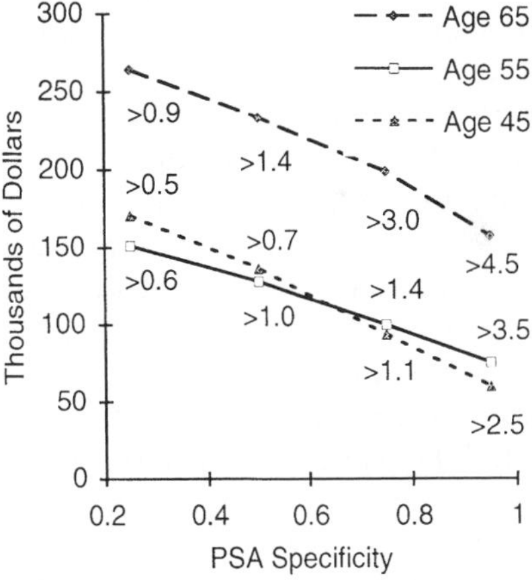

Figure 15-11 Cost per incremental life year in nondiscounted dollars. The decision thresholds on the plot are in micrograms per liter. This is marginal cost per additional life year relative to no screening. In screening, the most cost-effective strategy results from using different decision levels based on the patients' ages. Younger patients have the most to gain from screening, but the overall cost is still high in all groups. *PSA*, Prostate-specific antigen. *(From Shultz EK. Multivariate receiver operating characteristic curve analysis: Prostate cancer screening as an example. Clin Chem 1995;41:1254.)*

Figure 15-11 demonstrates that the overall cost per life year saved decreases with an increasing PSA screening decision threshold. The data for men 75 years of age are not graphed, because it is estimated that there would be a net decrease in life expectancy at all decision levels. The most benefit is achieved for younger men at decision thresholds that are very specific (i.e., have very few false-positive results). The data are limited in not examining all decision thresholds. It would appear likely that using even higher decision thresholds would result in still more cost/life year gains.

But is the program worth it at any decision level? One can estimate the relative worth of the program by comparing the proposed cost per increased life year with those of other programs. After calculating the present-day value of money invested in the future (called "discounting"), the overall cost per life year is higher than is generally spent on other programs, making the use of general prostate screening difficult to justify.[31] Others have proposed quality-adjusted life years (QALY) as a more suitable yardstick. A QALY was developed to try to quantify the relative value of life spent with decreased functionality to a life year with no functional limitation (e.g., how much is a life with chronic incontinence worth compared with a normal life?). However, in the previous analysis, the conclusion would be strengthened if a man found incontinence or impotence less desirable than full health, so use of QALYs is not necessary for the general conclusion.

As new types of procedures, increased test sensitivity, and therapeutic alternatives become increasingly available, the challenge will be to skillfully combine medicine, laboratory expertise, and analytical thinking in the guiding of laboratory practice. Maximizing benefits given a limited set of resources requires a well considered approach to the selective improvement of test accuracy and precision and to the interpretation of test results.

REFERENCES

1. Adam BL, Qu Y, Davis JW, Ward MD, Clements MA, Cazares LH, Semmes OJ, Schellhammer PF Yasui Y, Feng Z, Wright GL Jr. Serum protein fingerprinting coupled with a pattern-matching algorithm distinguishes prostate cancer from benign prostate hyperplasia and healthy men. Cancer Res 2002;62 (13): 3609-14.
2. Agresti A. Categorical data analysis, 2nd ed. New York: Wiley-Interscience, 2002.
3. Aliferis CF, Hardin D, Massion P. Machine learning models for lung cancer classification using array comparative genomic hybridization. Proc AMIA Symp. 2002;7-11.
4. Aliferis CF, Tsamardinos I, Massion P, Statnikov A, Fananapazir N, Hardin D. Machine learning models for classification of lung cancer and selection of genomic markers using array gene expression data. 16th International FLAIRS Conference, St Augustine, Florida, USA, May 2003 (FLAIRS 2003, special track: AI in Medicine) 2003;67-71.
5. Aliferis CF, Tsamardinos I, Massion P, Statnikov A, Hardin D. Why classification models using array gene expression data perform so well: A preliminary investigation of explanatory factors. In: The 2003 International Conference on Mathematics and Engineering Techniques in Medicine and Biological Sciences, 2003;47-53.
6. Aliferis CF, Tsamardinos I, Statnikov, A. HITON: A novel markov blanket algorithm for optimal variable selection. Proc AMIA Symp 2003; {no page numbers, electronically published}
7. Beck JR. The role of new laboratory tests in clinical decision-making. Clin Lab Med. 1982;2:751-77.
8. Beck JR, Shultz EK. The use of relative operating characteristic (ROC) curves in test performance evaluation. Arch Pathol Lab Med 1986;110:13-20.
9. Beer DG, Kardia SL, Huang CC, Giordano TJ, Levin AM, Misek DE, Lin L, Chen G, Gharib TG, Thomas DG, Lizyness ML, Kuick R, Hayasaka S, Taylor JM, Iannettoni MD, Orringer MB, Hanash S. Gene-expression profiles predict survival of patients with lung adenocarcinoma. Nat Med 2002;8(8):816-24.
10. Bhattacharjee A, Richards WG, Staunton J, Li C, Monti S, Vasa P, Ladd C, Beheshti J, Bueno R, Gillette M, Loda M, Weber G, Mark EJ, Lander ES, Wong W, Johnson BE, Golub TR, Sugarbaker DJ, Meyerson M. Classification of human lung carcinomas by mRNA expression profiling reveals distinct adenocarcinoma subclasses. Proc Natl Acad Sci USA 2001;98(24): 13790-5.
11. Boone DJ, Steindel SJ. Conducting outcomes research: past experience and future directions. Clin Chem 1995;41:795-8.
12. Burges CJC. A tutorial on support vector machines for pattern recognition. Data Minining and Knowledge Discovery 1998;2(2):1-47.
13. Catalona WJ, Smith DS, Ratliff TL, Dodds KM, Coplen DE, Yuan JJ, Petros JA, Andriole GL. Measurement of prostate-specific antigen in serum as a screening test for prostate cancer. N Engl J Med. 1991;324:1156-61. Erratum in: N Engl J Med 1991;325:1324.
14. Chan DW. PSA as a marker for prostatic cancer. Lab Manag 1988;35-9.
15. Chan DW, Bruzek DJ, Oesterling JE, Rock RC, Walsh PC. Prostate-specific antigen as a marker for prostatic cancer: A monoclonal and a polyclonal immunoassay compared. Clin Chem 1987;33:1916-20.
16. Chen G, Gharib TG, Huang CC, Thomas DG, Shedden KA, Taylor JM, Kardia SL, Misek DE, Giordano TJ, Iannettoni MD, Orringer MB, Hanash SM, Beer DG. Proteomic analysis of lung adenocarcinoma: identification of a highly expressed set of proteins in tumors. Clin Cancer Res 2002;8(7):2298-305.
17. Cooner WH, Mosley BR, Rutherford CL Jr, Beard JH, Pond HS, Bass RB Jr, Terry WJ. Clinical application of transrectal ultrasonography and prostate specific antigen in the search for prostate cancer. J Urol 1988;139:758-61.
18. Drago JR, Badalament RA, Wientjes MG, Smith JJ, Nesbitt JA, York JP, Ashton JJ, Neff JC. Relative value of prostate-specific antigen and prostatic acid phosphatase in diagnosis and management of adenocarcinoma of prostate: Ohio State University experience. Urology 1989;34:187-92.
19. Duda RO, Hart PE, Stork DG. Pattern classification 2nd ed. New York: Wiley, 2001.
20. Duin RPW. Classifiers in almost empty spaces, International Conference on Pattern Recognition (ICPR'00), Barcelona, Spain, 2000.
21. Ferrar L, Seraglia R, Rossi CR, Bertazzo A, Lise M, et al. Protein profiles in sera of patients with malignant cutaneous melanoma. Rapid Commun Mass Spectrom 2000;14 (13):1149-54.
22. Franks LM. Latent carcinoma of the prostate. J Pathol Bacteriol 1954;68:603-16.

23. Furey TS, Cristianini TS, Duffy N, Bednarski DW, Schummer M, Haussler D. Support vector machine classification and validation of cancer tissue samples using microarray expression data. Bioinformatics 2000;16 (10):906-14.
24. George NJR. Natural history of localized prostatic cancer managed by conservative therapy alone. Lancet 1988;1:494-6.
25. Golub TR, Slonim DK, Tamayo P, Huard C, Gaasenbeek M, Mesirov JP, Coller H, Loh ML, Downing JR, Caligiuri MA, Bloomfield CD, Lander ES. Molecular classification of cancer: class discovery and class prediction by gene expression monitoring, Science 1999;286:531-6.
26. Guyon I, Weston J, Barnhill S, Vapnik V. Gene selection for cancer classification using support vector machines. Machine Learning 2002;46:389-422.
27. Halpert B, Sheehan EE, Schmalhorst WR, Scott R Jr. Carcinoma of the prostate: A survey of 5,000 autopsies. Cancer 1963;16:737-42.
28. Hastings CA, Norton SM, Roy S. New algorithms for processing and peak detection in liquid chromatography/mass spectrometry data. Rapid Commun Mass Spectrom 2002;16 (5):462-7.
29. Kabalin JN, McNeal JE, Price HM, Freiha FS, Stamey TA. Unsuspected adenocarcinoma of the prostate in patients undergoing cystoprostatectomy for other causes: Incidence, histology and morphometric observations. J Urol 1988;141:1091-4.
30. Krahn MD, Mahoney JE, Eckman MH, Trachtenberg J, Pauker SG, Detsky AS. Screening for prostate cancer. A decision analytic view. JAMA 1994;272:773-80.
31. Laupacis A, Feeny D, Detsky AS, Tugwell PX. How attractive does a new technology have to be to warrant adoption and utilization? Tentative guidelines for using clinical and economic evaluations. CMAJ 1992;146:473-81.
32. Li L, Weinberg CR, Darden TA, Pedersen LG. Gene selection for sample classification based on gene expression data: study of sensitivity to choice of parameters of the GA/KNN method. Bioinformatics 2001;17:1131-42.
33. Light Light RW, Macgregor MI, Luchsinger PC, Ball WC Jr. Pleural effusions: the diagnostic separation of transudates and exudates. Ann Intern Med 1972;77:507-13.
34. Lin SM ,Johnson, KF, Eds. Methods of microarray data analysis, Boston: Kluwer Academic Publishers, 2002.
35. Liu H, Motoda H. Feature selection. Boston: Kluwer Academic Publishers, 1998.
36. McNeal JE, Bostwick DG, Kindrachuk RA, Redwine EA, Freiha FS, Stamey TA. Patterns of progression in prostate cancer. Lancet 1986;1:60-3.
37. Parker SL, Tong T, Bolden S, Wingo PA. Cancer statistics, 1996. CA Cancer J Clin. 1996;46(1):5-27.
38. Petersen PH, Horder M. Ways of assessing quality goals for diagnostic tests in clinical situations. Arch Pathol Lab Med 1988;112:435-43.
39. Petricoin EF, Ardekani AM, Hitt BA, Levine PJ, Fusaro VA, Steinberg SM, Mills GB, Simone C, Fishman DA, Kohn EC, Liotta LA. Use of proteomic patterns in serum to identify ovarian cancer. Lancet 2002;359:572-7.
40. Petricoin EF 3rd, Ornstein DK, Paweletz CP, Ardekani A, Hackett PS, Hitt BA, Velassco A, Trucco C, Wiegand L, Wood K, Simone CB, Levine PJ, Linehan WM, Emmert-Buck MR, Steinberg SM, Kohn EC, Liotta LA. Serum proteomic patterns for detection of prostate cancer. J Natl Cancer Inst 2002;94(20):1576-8.
41. Ragde H, Bagley CM, Aldape HC, et al. Screening for prostatic cancer with high-resolution ultrasound. J Endourol 1989;3:115-23.
42. Scholkopf B, Burges CJ, Smola AJ, eds. Advances in kernel methods: support vector learning. Boston:The MIT Press, 1999.
43. Scott R Jr, Mutchnik DL, Laskowski TZ, Schmalhorst WR. Carcinoma of the prostate in elderly men: Incidence, growth characteristics and clinical significance. J Urol 1969;101:602-7.
44. Seamonds B, Yang N, Anderson K, Whitaker B, Shaw LM, Bollinger JR. Evaluation of prostate-specific antigen and prostatic acid phosphatase as prostate cancer markers. Urology 1986;28:472-9.
45. Shultz EK. Multivariate receiver-operating characteristic curve analysis: Prostate cancer screening as an example. Clin Chem 1995;41:1248-55.
46. Sox HC, Blatt MA, Higgins MC, Marton KI, eds. Medical decision making. Stoneham MA: Butterworths, 1988.
47. Stamey TA. Cancer of the prostate: An analysis of some important contributions and dilemmas. Monogr Urol 1983;3:68-92.
48. Stamey TA, Yang N, Hay AR, McNeal JE, Freiha FS, Redwine E. Prostate-specific antigen as a serum marker for adenocarcinoma of the prostate. N Engl J Med 1987;317:909-15.
49. Tsamardinos I, Aliferis CF. Towards principled feature selection: Relevancy, filters and wrappers. Ninth International Workshop on Artificial Intelligence and Statistics, Key West, Florida, USA, 2003.
50. Tsamardinos I, Aliferis CF, Statnikov A. Time and sample efficient discovery of markov blankets and direct causal relations. The Ninth ACM SIGKDD 2003 International Conference on Knowledge Discovery and Data Mining.
51. van't Veer LJ, Dai H, van de Vijver MJ, He YD, Hart AA, et al. Gene expression profiling predicts clinical outcome of breast cancer. Nature 2002;415(6871): 530-6.
52. Velculescu VE, Zhang L, Vogelstein B, Kinzler KW. Serial analysis of gene expression, Science 1995;270, 484-7.

53. Vlahou A, Schellhammer PF, Mendrinos S, Patel K, Kondylis FI, Gong L, Nasim S, Wright Jr GL Jr. Development of a novel proteomic approach for the detection of transitional cell carcinoma of the bladder in urine. Am J Pathol 2001;158(4):1491-502.
54. Watts NB. Medical relevance of laboratory tests: A clinical perspective. Arch Pathol Lab Med 1988;112:379-82.
55. Weinstein MC, Fineberg HV, eds. Clinical decision analysis. Philadelphia: WB Saunders Co, 1980.
56. Whitmore WF Jr. Natural history of low-stage prostatic cancer and the impact of early detection. Urol Clin North Am 1990;17:689-97.
57. Zweig MH, Campbell G. Receiver operating characteristic (ROC) plots: A fundamental evaluation tool in clinical medicine. Clin Chem 1993;39:561-77.

ADDITIONAL READING

Boyd JC. Mathematical tools for demonstrating the clinical usefulness of biochemical markers. Scand J Clin Invest 1997;227:46-63.

National Committee for Clinical Laboratory Standards. Assessment of the Clinical Accuracy of Laboratory Tests Using Receiver Operating Characteristic (ROC) Plots: Approved Guideline. NCCLS Document GP10-A. Wayne PA: NCCLS, 1995 (Reaffirmed 2001).

CHAPTER 16

Establishment and Use of Reference Values

Helge Erik Solberg, M.D., Ph.D.

THE CONCEPT OF REFERENCE VALUES

Medicine is an art and a science in the service of fellow human beings. To improve the health of their patients, physicians (1) collect empirical data, (2) interpret these data using scientific knowledge and professional experience, (3) make decisions concerning diagnoses, (4) recommend preventive measures, and (5) execute therapeutic actions. There is a fundamental limitation in this activity as absolute health does not exist. Health is necessarily a relative concept.[20]

INTERPRETATION BY COMPARISON

To say that health is *relative* implies that the condition of individuals must be related to something. Data collected during the medical interview, clinical examination, and supplementary investigations must be interpreted by *comparison* with reference data. The physician does this when making a diagnosis. If the condition of the patient resembles what is considered typical of a particular disease, the physician may base the diagnosis on this observation (positive diagnosis). This diagnosis is made more likely if observed symptoms and signs do not fit the patterns characterizing a set of alternative diseases (diagnosis by exclusion). Such disease patterns are examples of reference data necessary for the medical interpretation. Also, the different degrees of health have their set of characteristics that serve as reference sources for judging the health of an individual.

The process of medical interpretation by comparison may be more or less formalized. Some diagnoses are recognized by an intuitive assessment based on "clinical experience." Others are based on reasoning using advanced knowledge of normal and pathological anatomy, physiology, and biochemistry and of other relevant areas of medical science. Sometimes, the evaluation is of a qualitative nature; in other cases, it may be quantitative. The decision making may even be computer assisted, using rules based on the laws of probability and statistical techniques or on formalized medical knowledge (expert systems, artificial intelligence).

The interpretation of medical laboratory data is an example of decision making by comparison. We therefore need *reference values* for all tests performed in the clinical laboratory, not only from healthy individuals but from patients with relevant diseases.

Ideally an observed value *in an individual* should be related to *relevant* collections of reference values, such as values from healthy persons, from the undifferentiated hospital population, from persons with typical diseases, and from ambulatory individuals, and previous values from the same subject.[66] A patient's laboratory result simply is not medically useful if appropriate data for comparison are lacking.

NORMAL VALUES—AN OBSOLETE TERM

Historically the term *normal values* was frequently used to refer to medical data used for purpose of comparison. However, the use of the term often leads to confusion because the word "normal" has several different connotations.[48] For example, three medically important but very different meanings of "normal" are given in the following:

1. *Statistical Sense:* Values are often qualified as "normal" if their observed distribution seems to follow closely the theoretical *normal distribution* of statistics (i.e., the Gaussian probability distribution). Somehow this use of "normal" has misled people to believe that the distribution of biological data is symmetrical and bell shaped like the Gaussian distribution. But on closer examination, this is usually found not to be the case. To exorcize the "ghost of Gauss," Elveback and colleagues recommend not using the term *normal limits.*[15] For a similar reason, the term

normal distribution should also be avoided and replaced by the term *Gaussian distribution.*

2. *Epidemiological Sense:* Another meaning of "normal" is illustrated by the following statement: It is "normal" to find that the concentration of triglycerides in serum is between 0.6 and 2.4 mmol/L, whereas it is considered "abnormal" to have a serum triglyceride concentration outside these limits. Here a more exact statement would read as follows: approximately 95% of the values obtained, when measuring the concentration of triglycerides in sera collected from individuals considered to be healthy, is included in the interval 0.6 to 2.4 mmol/L. The obsolete concept of "normal values" partly carried this meaning. Alternative terms for "normal" in this sense are "common," "frequent," "habitual," "usual," and "typical."
3. *Clinical Sense:* The term "normal" is also often used to indicate that values show the absence of certain diseases or the absence of risks for the development of diseases. In this sense, a "normal value" is considered as a sign of health. Better descriptive terms for such values are "healthy," "nonpathological," or "harmless."

Because of the confusion resulting from the different meanings of normal, the term "normal values" is now considered obsolete and should not be used.

To prevent the ambiguities inherent in the term *normal values,* the concept of *reference values* was introduced and implemented in the 1980s.[21,66] At first glance, the substitution of *reference values* for *normal values* appears to be unimportant, but on closer scrutiny this change in nomenclature is an important step toward establishing a scientific basis for clinical interpretation of laboratory data.[71]

Terminology

The International Federation of Clinical Chemistry and Laboratory Medicine (IFCC) recommends the term "reference values" and related terms, such as "reference individual," "reference limit," "reference interval," and "observed values."[34] The definitions given below and the presentation in the following sections of this chapter are in accordance with the IFCC recommendations.*

The definition of *reference values* is based on that of the reference **individual**[34]:

an individual selected for comparison using defined criteria.

As mentioned above, for the interpretation of values obtained from an individual under clinical investigation, we need appropriate comparison values. To provide such values, we must select suitable individuals. The characteristics of the individuals in each group chosen for comparison should be clearly defined. We must specify their age and gender, the conditions for the specimen collection, and whether they should be healthy or have a certain disease. The definition of a reference individual also covers cases in which the individual under clinical investigation is his or her own reference, as discussed in a later section on subject-based reference values.

A **reference value** may then be defined as[34]:

a value obtained by observation or measurement of a particular type of quantity on a reference individual.

If, for example, we measure the concentration of triglycerides in sera collected from a group of reference individuals selected for comparison according to a sufficiently exact set of criteria, the triglyceride results are our reference values.

The **observed value** is defined as[34]:

a value of a particular type of quantity, obtained by observation or measurement and produced to make a medical decision. Observed values can be compared with reference values, reference distributions, reference limits, or reference intervals.

Or rephrased: an observed value is the laboratory result obtained by analysis of a specimen collected from an individual under clinical investigation. Some call such values "test values," but the word "test" in this term is ambiguous (a laboratory test? a statistical test?), and it should be avoided.

The IFCC also defines other terms related to the concept of reference values: reference population, reference sample group, reference distribution, reference limit, and reference interval.[34] Some of these terms are introduced in later sections of this chapter.

Types of Reference Values

In practice it is often necessary or convenient to give a short description associated with the term reference values, such as "health-associated reference values" (close to what was understood by the obsolete term *normal values*). Other examples of such qualifying words are "diabetic," "hospitalized diabetic," and "ambulatory diabetic." These short descriptions prevent the common misunderstanding that reference values are associated only with health.

We may further distinguish between subject-based and population-based reference values. *Subject-based* reference values are previous values from the same individual, obtained when he or she was in a known state of health. *Population-based* reference values are those obtained from a group of well-defined reference individuals and are usually the type of values referred to when the term "reference values" is used without any qualifying words. This chapter deals primarily with population-based values.

The body of this chapter discusses population-based *univariate* reference values and quantities derived from them. If, for example, we produce, treat, and use separate reference values for cholesterol and triglycerides in serum, we have two sets of univariate reference values. The term *multivariate*

*A note on the literature: The Expert Panel on Theory of Reference Values of the IFCC has produced a series of six recommendations on the establishment and use of reference values.[34] A 1989 review by Solberg and Gräsbeck[66] gives in-depth information on this topic.

reference values denotes that results of two or more analytes obtained from the same set of reference individuals are treated in combination. The serum cholesterol and triglyceride values may be used, for example, to define a bivariate reference region. This subject is addressed in a later section.

Requirements

Certain conditions apply for a valid comparison between a patient's laboratory results with reference values[14]:

1. All groups of reference individuals should be clearly defined.
2. The patient examined should sufficiently resemble the reference individuals (in all groups selected for comparison) in all respects other than those under investigation.
3. The conditions under which the specimens were obtained and processed for analysis should be known.
4. All quantities compared should be of the same type.
5. All laboratory results should be produced using adequately standardized methods under sufficient analytical quality control (see Chapters 14 and 19).

To these general requirements one may add others that become necessary when the more advanced techniques for decision making are applied.[71]

6. The stages in the pathogenesis of the diseases that are the objectives for diagnosis should be demarcated.
7. The clinical diagnostic sensitivity and specificity, the prevalence, and the clinical costs of misclassification should be known for all laboratory tests used.

SELECTION OF REFERENCE INDIVIDUALS

A set of *selection criteria* determines which individual should be included in the group of reference individuals.[34,66] Such selection criteria include statements describing the source population, specifications of criteria for health, or the disease of interest.

Often, separate reference values for each sex, different age groups, and other criteria are necessary. Our group of reference individuals may therefore have to be divided into more homogeneous subgroups. For this purpose, we need to specify rules for the division, called stratification or *partitioning criteria.*

It is important to distinguish between selection and partitioning criteria. First, we apply the selection criteria to obtain a group of reference individuals. Thereafter, we may divide this group into subgroups using partitioning criteria. Whether a specific criterion (e.g., gender) is a selection or a partitioning criterion depends on the purpose of the actual project. For example, gender is a selection criterion if reference values from female subjects only are necessary.

Concept of Health in Relation to Reference Values

There is an obvious requirement for health-associated reference values for quantities measured in the clinical chemistry laboratory. But the concept of health[20] is problematical; much confusion may arise if the selection criteria for health are not clearly stated for a specific project.

The World Health Organization has defined health as "a state of complete physical, mental and social well-being and not merely the absence of disease or infirmity." This is an attempt to define *absolute health,* but as such, absolute health is never attained.

Thus in the context of reference values, we need a more modest concept of health. Past experience has taught us that health is a *relative concept.* It is possible to be ill in one respect and well in another; what is considered healthy in a developing country may be judged to be rather unhealthy in Western Europe and North America, and so on.

Furthermore, the diagnosis of health cannot be based solely on excluding pathology. This fact, which has been named the *privative concept of health,* may cause difficulties. If no signs of disease can be demonstrated, uncertainty remains, because such signs might be detected on closer examination. The "feeling" of health is not a reliable criterion because of its subjectivity. In addition, an individual may try to conceal an illness for various reasons (e.g., to qualify for life insurance).

When producing reference values, we should ask ourselves, why do we need these values? How are we going to use them? To what extent does the intended purpose of the project determine how we should identify health? In short, we need a *goal-oriented concept of health.*

Gräsbeck suggested the following **general definition of health,** which summarizes the relative, privative, and goal-oriented aspects discussed previously[20]:

Health is characterized by a minimum of subjective feelings and objective signs of disease, assessed in relation to the social situation of the subject and the purpose of the medical activity, and it is in the absolute sense an unattainable ideal state.

Strategies for Selection of Reference Individuals

Several methods have been suggested for the selection of reference individuals. Table 16-1 shows three pairs of concepts that may be used to describe a sampling scheme. The concepts of each pair are mutually exclusive. For example, the sampling is either direct or indirect. One may, however, combine one concept from several pairs to obtain a more exact description. For example, the selection may be direct, a posteriori, and nonrandom.

The merits and disadvantages of these strategies are described in the following sections. It is not possible to recommend one sampling scheme that is superior in all respects and applicable to all situations. One must choose the optimal approach for a given project and state clearly what has been done.

Direct or Indirect Sampling?

Direct selection of reference individuals (see Table 16-1) is the only method that agrees with the concept of reference

TABLE 16-1 Strategies for Selection of Reference Individuals

Direct	*Individuals* are selected from a parent population using defined criteria.
Indirect	The individuals are not considered, but certain statistical methods are applied to analytical *values* in a laboratory database to obtain estimates with specified characteristics.
A priori*	A direct method (see above) in which individuals are selected for specimen collection and analysis if they fulfill defined inclusion criteria.
A posteriori	A direct method using an already existing database containing both analysis results and information on a large number of individuals. Values of individuals fulfilling defined inclusion criteria are selected.
Random	A process of selection giving each item (individual or test result) an equal chance of being chosen.
Nonrandom	A process of selection giving each item an unequal chance of being chosen.

**Note:* The terms a priori and a posteriori signify in this context "before" and "after" and refer to when inclusion criteria are applied.

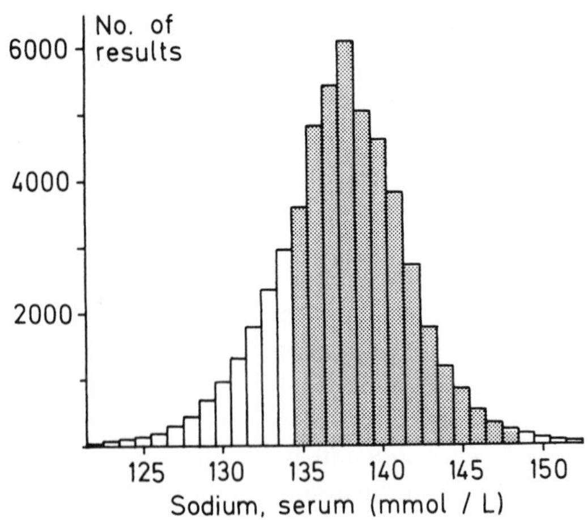

Figure 16-1 Distribution of sodium concentrations in serum obtained in a routine laboratory. The histogram shows the distribution of 53,128 serum sodium concentrations measured in consecutive clinical specimens during a 6-month period in 1982 at Rikshospitalet, Oslo, Norway. The shaded area is within health-associated reference limits as determined by a direct method (193 healthy adults of both sexes).

values as recommended by the IFCC,[34] and it is the basis for the presentation in this chapter. Its only disadvantages are the problems and costs of obtaining a representative group of reference individuals.

These practical problems have led to the search for simpler and less expensive approaches. The *indirect* method has become rather popular.[5,21] It is based on the observation that most analysis results produced in the clinical laboratory seem to be "normal." Figure 16-1 shows one example from the author's laboratory. As can be seen, the values of the serum sodium concentration have a distribution with a preponderant central peak and a shape not too far from that of the Gaussian distribution. The underlying assumption of the indirect method is that this peak is composed mainly of *normal values.* The advocates of the method therefore claim that it is possible to estimate the *normal interval* if we extract the distribution of *normal values* from this part of the distribution. *Normal limits* determined by the indirect method on the basis of the distribution shown in Figure 16-1 would, however, obviously be biased compared with the shown health-associated reference limits. (Note that the term "normal" is here used intentionally to distinguish between the concepts of *normal values* and reference values.)

Several mathematical methods have been used to extract the distribution of *normal values* from routine laboratory data.[5,21]

The indirect method, however, has several important deficiencies. The two major ones are as follows:

1. The estimates of the lower and upper *normal limits* depend heavily on the particular mathematical method used and on its underlying assumptions.
2. The indirect method destroys the scientific basis for obtaining and comparing reference values. The results for each hospital would depend on the characteristics of the hospital's patient group at that particular time. These results would vary not only across hospitals but for the same hospital at different times. The outcome would be a mass of unstable values for each analyte.

Hospital databases may, however, be used for the establishment of reference values that are fully concordant with the IFCC recommendations.[38,64] The requirement is that laboratory data be combined with information stored in clinical databases (i.e., to apply a direct sampling strategy instead of the distribution-based indirect method). Laboratory results are to be used as reference values only if stated clinical criteria are fulfilled. One may define criteria for selecting individuals who have a specified state of health or the disease for which reference data are necessary. Usually certain constraints are also imposed on the use of their laboratory results, such as allowing only one result of each analyte under study from each selected individual. Such reference values have one advantage over those based on direct sampling from other types of populations: hospital-based reference values are ideal for the interpretation of results from hospitalized patients because they are produced under similar conditions.

A Priori or A Posteriori Sampling?

When carefully performed, both a priori and a posteriori sampling (Table 16-1) may result in reliable reference values.

The choice is often a question of practicality. Both require the same set of successive steps, but the order of some of these operations differs depending on the mode of selection, a priori or a posteriori.[21]

The first step in the process of producing reference values for a laboratory test should always be the collection of quantitative information about the sources of biological variation for the analyte studied. A search through relevant literature may give the required information (see Chapter 17).[58,72] If the relevant information cannot be found in the literature, pilot studies may be necessary before the selection of reference individuals is planned in detail.

Serum sodium is an example of a biological analyte that is affected by only a few sources of biological variation. However, the list of factors may be rather long for other analytes, such as serum enzymes, proteins, and hormone.

It is important to distinguish between controllable and noncontrollable sources of biological variation. Some factors may be controlled by the standardization of the procedure for preparation of reference individuals and specimen collection (see a later section of this chapter). Other factors, such as age and gender, may be relevant partitioning criteria. The remaining sources of variation should be considered when defining the criteria for the selection of reference individuals.

The a priori strategy is best suited for smaller studies. Possible reference individuals from the parent population are interviewed and examined clinically and by selected laboratory methods to decide whether they fulfill the defined inclusion criteria. If the decision is positive, specimens for analysis are collected by a standardized procedure (including the necessary preparation of the individuals before the collection).

The a posteriori method is based on the availability of a large collection of data on medically examined individuals and measured quantities. Well-planned studies by centers for health screening or preventive medicine may provide such data. It is important that the data be collected by a strictly standardized and comprehensive protocol concerning the sampling from the parent population, the registration of demographic and clinical data on participating individuals, the preparation for and execution of specimen collection, and the handling and analysis of the specimens. If these requirements are met, values may be selected after application of the defined inclusion criteria to the individuals found in the database. The selection of individuals from large hospital databases (see earlier discussion) is another example of the application of an a posteriori method. In this case, however, the quality of data may be lower than in well-planned population studies.

A study performed in Kristianstad, Sweden,[7] highlights a practical problem often met when selecting reference individuals: the number of subjects fulfilling the inclusion criteria may be too small. In that study, only 17% of the participants were accepted by the criteria used, leaving an insufficient reference sample group. The frequency of exclusion was higher among women and in the older age groups.

There are two possible solutions to this problem:

1. The exclusion criteria may be relaxed. As already discussed, the set of relevant sources of biological variation differs among different analytes. One may define a minimum set of exclusion criteria for a given laboratory test. In the Kristianstad study, the complete group of individuals could probably be used for establishment of reference values (e.g., serum sodium), and most of the individuals would be acceptable for the determination of reference values for several other analytes.[7]
2. Another design of the sampling procedure could reduce the practical problems and costs of obtaining a sufficiently large group of reference individuals. The Kristianstad study showed that 75% of the excluded subjects could have been identified using only a simple questionnaire.[7] In the upper age group, this percentage was even higher. Therefore a preliminary screening of a large number of individuals from the parent population, using a carefully designed autoanamnestic questionnaire, would result in a much smaller sample of individuals to examine clinically and by laboratory methods. If 3000 individuals had been prescreened in Kristianstad, and if only the individuals remaining in the reduced sample were subjected to a closer examination, a group of 240 reference individuals would have been obtained.

The two modifications of the protocol may also be combined.

Random or Nonrandom Sampling?

Ideally, the group of reference individuals should be a random sample of all the individuals fulfilling the defined inclusion criteria in the parent population. Statistical estimation of distribution parameters (and their confidence intervals) and statistical hypothesis testing require this assumption.

For several reasons, most collections of reference values are, in fact, obtained by a nonrandom process.[26] That means that all possible reference individuals in the entire population under study do not have an equal chance of being chosen for inclusion in the usually much smaller sample of individuals studied. A strictly random sampling scheme is in most cases impossible for practical reasons. It would imply the examination of and application of inclusion criteria to the entire population (thousands or millions of persons) and then the random selection (e.g., conduct a raffle) of a subset of individuals from among those accepted.

It is important to realize that we do not obtain a random sample, in the strict sense, if we start by selecting individuals randomly from the entire population and then apply inclusion criteria to sort out the subset of individuals fulfilling these criteria, even though this may be the best approximation we can hope to obtain. Usually the situation is less satisfactory. A sample of reference individuals obtained by selecting among blood donors, persons working in a factory,

BOX 16-1 Examples of Exclusion Criteria for Health-Associated Reference Values*

Diseases

Risk Factors
- Obesity
- Hypertension
- Risks from occupation or environment
- Genetically determined risks

Intake of Pharmacologically Active Agents[36,73]
- Drug treatment for disease or suffering
- Oral contraceptives
- Drug abuse
- Alcohol
- Tobacco

Specific Physiological States
- Pregnancy
- Stress
- Excessive exercise

*The box lists only some major classes of criteria. It should be supplemented with other relevant criteria based on known sources of biological variation (see Chapter 17).[58,72]

or the hospital's staff, or by selection from hospital databases, is definitely not random sampling of the possible reference individuals in the general population.

The conclusions are obvious: (1) we have to use the best reference sample we can possibly get, all practical considerations taken into account; and (2) data should be used and interpreted with due caution, remembering the possible bias introduced by the nonrandomness of the sample selection process.

Selection Criteria and Evaluation of Subjects

The selection of reference individuals consists essentially of applying defined criteria to a group of examined candidate persons.[34] The required characteristics of the reference values determine which criteria should be used in the selection process. Box 16-1 lists some important criteria to consider when the production of health-associated reference values is the aim.

The question of which *diseases* and *risk factors* to consider for exclusion of individuals is difficult (see the discussion on the concept of health earlier in this chapter). The answer lies partly in the intended purpose of establishing reference values; the project must be goal oriented.

The definition of *obesity* is problematical. It might be based on a known or assumed contribution to the risk for development of a specified disease. Scientific data of this type are, however, seldom available for the studied population. Another possibility for establishing obesity is to use upper limits based on weight measurements in different age, gender, and height groups of the general population, using, for example, the national age-, gender-, and height-specific mean weight +20% as the upper limit. National differences are, however, great. Tables of optimum or ideal weights have been published by life insurance companies, and they may be more appropriate for delineation of obesity than this formula.

Similar problems affect the definition of *hypertension* in relation to the establishment of health-associated reference values and exclusion criteria based on *laboratory examinations.* It has been argued that we might be lost in a circular process when we use laboratory tests to assess the health of subjects who are subsequently to be used as healthy control subjects for laboratory tests. But actually there is no difference, in this context, between measuring the height, weight, and blood pressure and performing selected laboratory tests, provided that these laboratory tests are neither those for which we shall produce reference values nor tests that are significantly correlated with them.[20]

It is particularly difficult to define selection criteria when establishing reference values for a geriatric population.[16] In higher age groups it is "normal" to have minor or major diseases and to take drugs. One solution is to collect values at one time and to use the values of survivors after a defined number of years.[20,50]

Usually the clinical evaluation of candidate individuals is based on an anamnestic interview or questionnaire, a physical examination, and supplementary investigations. Anamnestic and examination forms tailored to the requirements of the actual project facilitate the evaluation and document the decisions taken.

Partitioning of the Reference Group

It may also be necessary to define *partitioning criteria* for the subclassification of the set of selected reference individuals into more homogeneous groups (Box 16-2).[34] We shall return in later sections to the question of determining when stratification of the reference sample group is necessary and justified. The number of partitioning criteria should usually be kept as small as possible to obtain sufficient sample sizes to derive valid estimates.

Age and *gender* are the most frequently used criteria for subgrouping because several analytes vary notably among different age and gender groups (see Chapter 17).[16,58,72] Age may be categorized by equal intervals (e.g., by decades) or by intervals that are narrower in the periods of life where greater variation is observed. In some cases it is more convenient to use qualitative age groups, such as postnatal, infancy, childhood, prepubertal, pubertal, adult, premenopausal, menopausal, or geriatric. Height and weight could be used as criteria for categorizing children.

Additional factors are discussed in Chapter 17.[58,72]

SPECIMEN COLLECTION

Several preanalytical factors influence the values of biological quantities, such as the concentration of components in

BOX 16-2 Examples of Partitioning Criteria for Possible Subgrouping of the Reference Group

Age (not necessarily categorized by equal intervals)

Gender

Genetic Factors
Ethnic origin
Blood groups (ABO)
Histocompatibility antigens (HLA)
Genes

Physiological Factors
Stage in menstrual cycle
Stage in pregnancy
Physical condition

Other Factors
Socioeconomic
Environmental
Chronobiological

HLA, Human leukocyte antigen.

blood and in other specimens and the amount excreted in feces, urine, or sweat. This topic is covered elsewhere (see Chapter 17).* In this discussion, we only highlight aspects of special relevance to the generation of reliable reference values.[4,34]

Preanalytical standardization of the preparation of individuals before specimen collection, the procedure of specimen collection itself, and the handling of the specimen before analysis may eliminate or minimize bias or variation from these factors. This reduces biological "noise" that might otherwise conceal important biological "signals" of disease, risk, or treatment effect.

Two Philosophies of Standardization

Preanalytical procedures used before routine analysis of patient specimens and when establishing reference values should be as similar as possible. In general it is much easier to standardize the routines for studies of reference values than those used in the daily clinical setting, especially when collecting specimens in emergency or other unplanned situations. Thus two approaches have been suggested:

1. Only such factors that may be relatively easily controlled in the clinical setting should be part of the standardization when reference values are produced.
2. The rules for preanalytical standardization when producing reference values (Table 16-2) should also serve as ideal standards for the clinical situation. It has been shown that it is possible to apply these rules rather closely in the clinical setting for both hospitalized and ambulatory patients.[66] The same philosophy is the basis for recommendations concerning routine blood specimen collection.*

Either philosophy is, however, concordant with the concept of reference values, provided that the conditions under which reference values are produced are clearly stated.

Standardization Schemes

The magnitudes of preanalytical sources of variation are clearly not equal for different analytes (see Chapter 17).† It could therefore be argued that we should consider only those factors that cause unwanted variation in the biological quantity for which we want to produce reference values. Body posture during specimen collection is, for instance, highly relevant for the establishment of reference values for nondiffusible analytes, such as albumin in serum, but irrelevant for establishment of serum sodium values.[17]

On the other hand, several constituents are routinely analyzed in the same clinical specimen. It would therefore be impractical to devise special systems for every single type of quantity.[66] For that reason, three standardized procedures for blood specimen collection by venipuncture have been recommended[4,21]: (1) collection in the morning from hospitalized patients, (2) collection in the morning from ambulatory patients, and (3) collection in the afternoon from ambulatory patients. Table 16-2 summarizes these procedures.

Such schemes of standardization have to be modified depending on local conditions and necessities and on the intended use of the produced reference values. Published checklists[34,66] may be helpful in the design of a scheme.

A special problem is caused by drugs taken by individuals before specimen collection.[36,73,80] We may distinguish between indispensable and dispensable medication. The latter type of drugs should always be avoided for at least 48 hours. The use of indispensable drugs, such as contraceptive pills or essential medication, may be a criterion for exclusion or partitioning.

In emergency or other unplanned clinical situations, even a partial application of the standardized procedure for collection has been shown to be of great value.[21]

The Necessity for Additional Information

The clinical situation often is different from a controlled research situation; specimens have to be taken during operations, in emergency situations, or when patients are unwilling or unable to follow instructions. Therefore the clinician needs additional information for the interpretation of a patient's values in relation to reference values obtained under fairly standardized conditions.

An *empirical approach*[66] is to produce other sets of reference values, such as postprandial values, postexercise values,

*References 17, 21, 22, 58, 66, 72, 79.

*References 3, 4, 34, 41, 46, 49.
†References 17, 21, 22, 58, 66, 72, 79.

or postpartum values.[21] Such a method, however, is very expensive and does not cover all situations that could possibly arise.

There is another and more general solution to the problem, called the *predictive approach*.[66] Starting from a set of ordinary reference values and using quantitative information on the effect of various factors, such as intake of food, alcohol, and drugs; exercise; stress; or posture, we could estimate "expected reference values" that fit the actual clinical setting (see Chapter 17).[58,72]

More studies of such effects are needed, especially for the combined effect of two or more sources of variation. Is, for example, the combined effect of alcohol and contraceptive drugs on γ-glutamyltransferase activity in serum less than, equal to, or greater than the sum of their individual effects?

ANALYTICAL PROCEDURES AND QUALITY CONTROL

Essential components of the required definition of a set of reference values are specifications concerning (1) the analysis method (including information on equipment, reagents, calibrators, type of raw data, and calculation method), (2) quality control (see Chapter 19), and (3) reliability criteria (see Chapter 14).[21,34]

Specifications should be so carefully described that another investigator can reproduce the study and the user of reference values can evaluate their comparability with values obtained with the methods used for producing the patient's values in a routine laboratory. To ensure comparability between reference values and observed values, the same analytical method should be used.

It is often claimed that the analytical quality should be better when determining reference values than when producing routine values. This may be true for accuracy; all measures should be taken to eliminate bias. The question of imprecision is more difficult because it depends partly on the intended use of the reference values. Increases in analytical random variation result in widening of the reference interval.[21] For some special uses of reference values, the narrower reference interval obtained by a more precise analytical method may be appropriate. However, this is usually not true

TABLE 16-2 Standardization of Preanalytical Factors in the Establishment of Reference Values for Adult Individuals

The Day Before Specimen Collection	
Food	Ordinary intake; last meal before 2200 hr
Alcohol	Maximum of one small bottle of beer (or equivalent of other beverage) taken with a meal
Abstinence	No solid food or tobacco and maximum of one glass of water after 2200 hr
Subjects Lying in Bed; Collection in the Morning	
Rest	Bed rest from 2200 hr until collection; a short visit to the toilet allowed, but minimum of 1 hr before collection
Collection	Between 0700 and 0900 hr (record time); supine position with the arm approximately in the horizontal plane
Ambulatory Subjects; Collection in the Morning	
Rise	1-3 hr before collection (record time)
Transport	Public or car transport for maximum of 45 min; walking a maximum of 500 m (≈ 550 yd) at moderate speed
Rest	Sitting for at least 15 min; arm muscle work not allowed
Collection	Between 0800 and 1000 hr (record time); sitting position with the arm approximately 45° below the horizontal position
Ambulatory Subjects; Collection in the Afternoon	
Breakfast	A light meal in the morning (approximately 310 kcal, 1300 kJ) composed of milk, coffee, or tea (maximum two cups); two open sandwiches with butter, slices of lunch meat/cheese, or marmalade
Activity	No exercise or heavy work
Rest	Sitting at least 15 min; arm muscle work not allowed
Collection	Between 1300 and 1500 hr (record time); minimum of 4 hr after breakfast; otherwise as above
Collection and Handling of Specimen*	
Venipuncture	In the cubital fold; no tourniquet; finger pressure proximal to the site allowed
Difficulties	A new attempt on opposite arm after 15 min rest

Based on Scandinavian recommendations.[4,21]

*Consult Chapter 2 for a discussion of other requirements for the collection and handling of specimens.

for routine clinical use of reference values. The interpretation is simplest if a patient's values and reference values are comparable with regard to analytical imprecision. For the same reason, it is advisable to analyze specimens from reference individuals in several runs to include the between-run components of variation. A safe way to obtain comparability is to include these specimens in routine runs together with the patient's specimens.

STATISTICAL TREATMENT OF REFERENCE VALUES

This section deals with two main topics: the partitioning of reference values into more homogeneous classes and the determination of reference limits and intervals. The subject matter is presented in the order in which data often are treated. Figure 16-2 gives an outline and refers to the corresponding sections in the text. Before the presentation of the methods, some statistical concepts used are briefly discussed (see also Chapter 14). A textbook by Harris and Boyd gives an excellent survey of the statistical bases of reference values in laboratory medicine.[27]

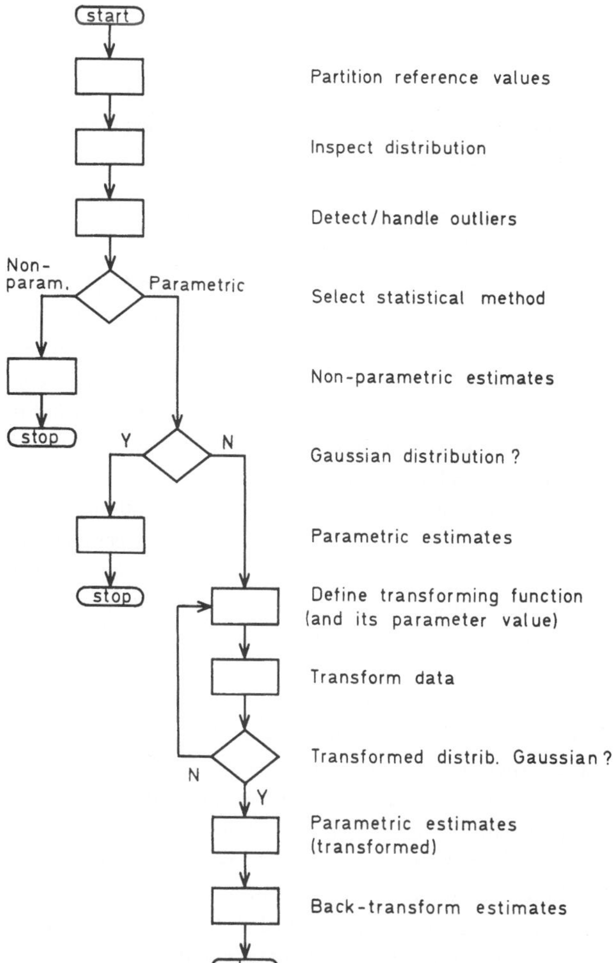

Figure 16-2 The statistical treatment of reference values. The "boxes" in the flow chart refer to sections in the text. NB = Nota bene: The order of the three first actions (partitioning, inspection, and detection and/or handling of outliers) may vary, dependent on the distribution and the statistical methods applied. *Y*, Yes; *N*, no.

STATISTICAL CONCEPTS

The first step in the establishment of reference values is the selection of a group of reference individuals. It is usually not feasible to obtain observations on all possible reference individuals of a certain category of the general population. We therefore hope that the smaller group examined, the *subset* (sometimes called the reference *sample* group), can give us the desired information about the characteristics of the complete *set* of individuals (the reference *population*).[34]

The larger set is often considered *hypothetical* because its characteristics are not observed directly; we know neither the number (the set size) nor the properties of all its individuals. We therefore want to infer from observations made on the subset to the hypothetical set. An obvious requirement is that the individuals in the subset are typical of those in the complete set. Statistical theory usually assumes that the items in the subset are selected at *random* from among those in the set; otherwise, the subset may be biased. If the items are not randomly selected, we can still use statistical techniques, but only with due caution and remembering the possible bias introduced.

There are two main types of *inferences* made from values obtained from the subset (sample group) to the set (total reference population).

1. We can **estimate properties** of the set. A reference limit (a percentile) of a biological quantity, such as the concentration of serum triglycerides, based on subset reference values, is an example of a *point estimate* (a single value). We consider it representative of the property that might have been found if we had observed all possible values in the set. If we examine many randomly selected subsets from the same set, we obtain several estimates with some variation around the "true" value of the set. It is possible to produce an *interval estimate* bounded by limits within which the "true" value is located with a specified confidence: the confidence interval. The *confidence* interval is expressed as a number in the interval 0 to 1, indicating the degree on the scale between "never" and "always." Our reference limit for serum triglycerides could thus be associated by a confidence interval showing its region of uncertainty.

   The "true" (unknown, hypothetical) value of a property of the set is often called a *parameter* and given a lower-case Greek letter symbol. For example, the standard deviation of the population is symbolized by the Greek sigma: σ_x. The corresponding property determined in the subset is named a *statistic* and symbolized by a lower-case Latin letter (e.g., s_x for the standard deviation of the subset).
2. Another inference is to **test hypotheses** regarding properties of the set. We might, for example, state the hypothesis that the distribution of values for serum triglyceride

concentrations is of the Gaussian type (the "null" hypothesis). If the deviations of the subset values from the Gaussian distribution are small, we could ascribe them to variation caused by chance alone. In that case, we should be permitted to use statistical methods based on the Gaussian distribution. However, we must reject the hypothesis if it is unlikely that the observed deviations from the Gaussian distribution are caused by chance alone. *Statistical tests* provide quantitative approaches to these types of decisions: the null hypothesis is rejected if the statistical test shows that the probability of the hypothesis being true is less than a stated *significance level.* The *probability* (p) is a number in the interval of 0 to 1, indicating the degree on the scale between "unlikely" and "certain." If we state a significance level of 0.05 when we test our Gaussian hypothesis for the distribution of serum triglyceride values, we should reject it if the probability obtained by the test is, for example, $p = 0.01$. Then we have to accept the alternative hypothesis that the distribution is nonGaussian. The *power* of a statistical test is the probability of rejection when the "null" hypothesis is false.

In the following sections, we use the term *reference distribution*[34] for the distribution of reference values (x). The two statistics *arithmetic mean* ($\bar{x}$) and *standard deviation* (s_x) are measures of its location and the dispersion of the values in it, respectively. They are defined as

$$\bar{x} = \frac{\sum x}{n}$$

$$s_x = \sqrt{\frac{\sum (x-\bar{x})^2}{n-1}} = \sqrt{\frac{\sum x^2 - \frac{(\sum x)^2}{n}}{n-1}}$$

where x is any of the n reference values in the subset (or a subclass of it). Standard deviations are commonly computed as shown in the second part of the preceding equation. The result may, however, be grossly inaccurate owing to rounding errors introduced by calculators and computers.[61]

The variable x in the preceding formulas denotes a quantity that varies. In our context, it signifies a reference value. If the variable by chance may take any one of a specified set of values, we use the term *variate* (i.e., a random variable). In this section, we consider distributions of single variates (i.e., *univariate* distributions). In a later section, we also discuss the joint distribution of two or more variates (*bivariate* or *multivariate* distributions).

An observed distribution may be presented as a table or graph (histogram) showing the number of observations in small intervals (Figure 16-3, *A*). The number of observations in an interval divided by the total number of observations in the distribution (its size) is an estimator of the probability of finding a value in the corresponding interval of the hypothetical *probability distribution* of the population (assuming random sampling). By consecutive summing of all these ratios, starting with the leftmost interval of the observed distribution, we get an estimate of the hypothetical *cumulative probability distribution* (Figure 16-3, *B*).

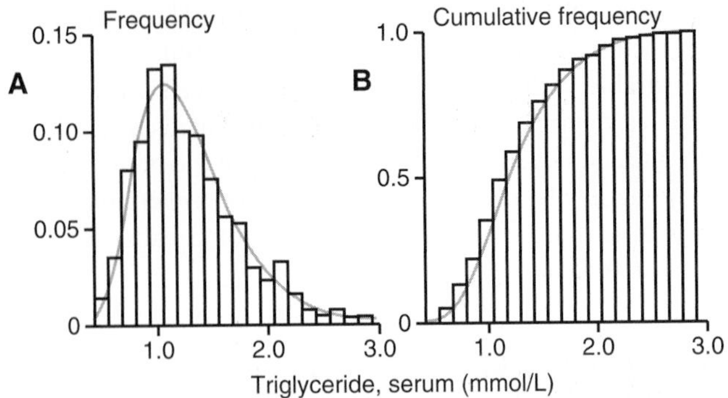

Figure 16-3 Observed and hypothetical distributions of 500 triglycerides values in serum (in mmol/L). **A,** The vertical bars of the left histogram show the number of observations in the interval divided by the total number of observations. The curve is the estimated probability distribution of the population, assuming random sampling and a log-Gaussian distribution. **B,** The cumulated ratios *(bars)* and the estimated cumulative probability distribution *(curve)*. (The data were computer generated for the purpose of illustration.)

Determination of Reference Limits: General Considerations

As mentioned previously, reference values provide a basis for interpretation of laboratory data. In clinical practice, one usually compares a patient's result with the corresponding *reference interval,* which is bounded by a pair of *reference limits.*[34] This interval, which may be defined in different ways, is a useful condensation of the information carried by the total set of reference values.

Three kinds of reference intervals have been suggested: tolerance interval, prediction interval, and interpercentile interval.[34,66] The choice from among these types of intervals may be important for certain well-defined statistical problems, but their numerical differences are negligible when based on at least 100 reference values.

The *interpercentile interval* is simple to estimate, more commonly used, and recommended by the IFCC.[34] This chapter, therefore, focuses on this type of interval. It is defined as an interval bounded by two percentiles of the reference distribution. A *percentile* denotes a value that divides the reference distribution such that a specified percentage of its values have magnitudes less than or equal to the limiting value. For example, if 2.32 mmol/L is the 97.5 percentile of serum triglycerides, 97.5% of the concentration values are equal to or below this value.

It is an arbitrary but common convention to define the reference interval as the *central 95% interval* bounded by the 2.5 and 97.5 percentiles (Figure 16-4) (i.e., 2.5% of the values are cut off in both tails of the reference distribution).[34]

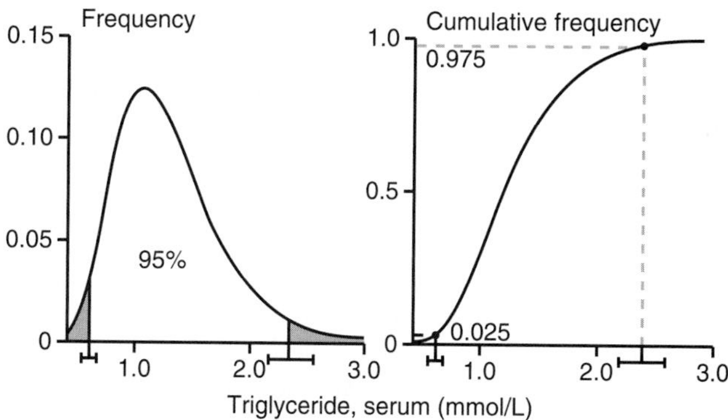

Figure 16-4 Central 95% reference interval. The 2.5 and 97.5 percentiles and their 0.90 confidence intervals of the 500 serum triglyceride concentrations (Figure 16-3), as determined by the parametric method (see text). The curves are the estimated probability distributions.

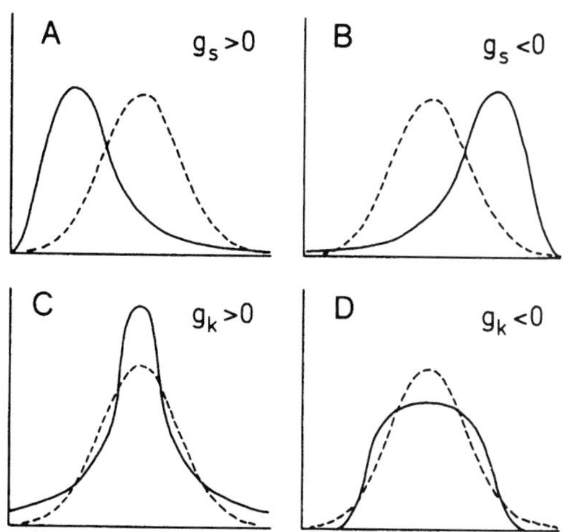

Figure 16-5 Skewness and kurtosis. The two upper figures show asymmetric distributions (**A,** positive skewness; **B,** negative skewness). The two lower figures show distributions with nonGaussian peakedness (**C,** positive kurtosis; **D,** negative kurtosis). The Gaussian distribution *(dashed curve)* is shown in all graphs for comparison. The values of the coefficients of skewness (g_s) and kurtosis (g_k) are also shown.

Another size or an asymmetrical location of the reference interval may be more appropriate in particular cases. To prevent ambiguity, the definition of the interval should always be stated. The estimation of percentiles presented in the following sections is based on the conventional central 95% interval, but the techniques are easily adapted to other locations of the limits.

The percentiles are point estimates of population parameters. Accordingly, they are unbiased estimates only if the subset of values was selected randomly from the population. But, as was discussed earlier, random sampling is often difficult to achieve. The interpercentile interval may always be used, however, as a summary or description of the subset reference distribution.

The precision of a percentile as an estimate of a population value depends on the size of the subset; it is less precise when there are few observations. If the assumption of random sampling is fulfilled, we may determine the *confidence interval* of the percentile (i.e., the limits within which the true percentile is located with a specified degree of confidence) (Figure 16-4). The 0.90 confidence interval of the 97.5 percentile (upper reference limit) for serum triglycerides may, for example, be 2.22 to 2.62 mmol/L. We would expect to find the true percentile in this interval with a confidence of 0.90 if we measured all serum triglyceride concentrations in the total reference population.

The interpercentile interval can be determined by parametric, nonparametric, and "bootstrap" statistical techniques.[27,34]

The *parametric method* for the determination of percentiles and their confidence intervals assumes a certain type of distribution, and it is based on estimates of population parameters, such as the mean and the standard deviation. We are, for example, using a parametric method if we believe that the true distribution is Gaussian and determine the reference limits (percentiles) as the values located 2 standard deviations below and above the mean. Most of the parametric methods are, in fact, based on the Gaussian distribution. If the reference distribution shows another shape, we may use mathematical functions that transform data to approximately Gaussian shape. Some positively skewed distributions (Figure 16-5, *A*) may, for example, be made symmetrical by using logarithms of the data values.

The *nonparametric method* makes no assumptions concerning the type of distribution and does not use estimates of distribution parameters. The percentiles may simply be determined by cutting off the required percentage of values in each tail of the subset reference distribution.

Originally a simple nonparametric method for determination of percentiles was recommended by the IFCC.[34] However, the newer "bootstrap" method[27,57] is currently the best method available for determination of reference limits. The more complex parametric method is seldom necessary, but it will also be presented here owing to its popularity and frequent misapplication. When we compare the results obtained by these methods, we usually find that the estimates of the percentiles are very similar. Detailed descriptions of these methods are given later in this chapter.

Commonly used statistical computer program packages[8,56,67] may aid in the estimation of reference limits, but these packages lack some of the techniques described here. The RefVal program,[65] however, implements these methods completely.

Sample Size

In general the theoretical lower limit of the sample size required for the estimation of the 100α and $100(1-\alpha)$ percentiles is equal to $1/\alpha$. Thus the estimation of the 2.5 percentile requires at least $1/0.025 = 40$ observations. The precision of percentiles increases with an increasing number of observations, as shown by the narrowing of their confidence intervals. A sample size of at least 120 reference values has been recommended.[27,34] However, more values may be necessary if distributions are very skewed.[42]

A Note on Terminology

The terms "reference limits" and "clinical decision limits" should not be confused.[52,71] *Reference limits* are descriptive of the reference distribution: they tell us something about the observed variation of values in the selected subset of reference individuals. Comparison of new values with these limits thus only conveys information about similarity with the given reference values. In contrast, *clinical decision limits* provide optimum separation among clinical categories. The latter limits may be based on analysis of reference values from several groups of individuals (healthy persons and patients with relevant diseases) and can thus be used for the purpose of differential diagnosis.[21,52,68] Here are some examples of terms related to clinical decision limits: diagnostic criterion, prognostic limit, therapeutic value, and toxicity threshold.

The term "reference range" is sometimes used for the IFCC-recommended term "reference interval," but this use should be discouraged because the statistical term *range* denotes the difference (a single value!) between the maximum and minimum values in a distribution.[37]

Partitioning of Reference Values

The best order of the first three actions outlined in Figure 16-2 (partitioning of reference values, inspection of the distribution, and detection and/or elimination of outliers) may in some cases be different from that shown in the figure. For example, it might be more appropriate to eliminate outliers before testing for partitioning. No strict rules for the order of these actions can be given as it depends on data and the statistical methods applied. With this caution in mind, the presentation in this chapter follows Figure 16-2.

The subset of reference individuals and the corresponding reference values may be partitioned according to gender, age, and other characteristics (Box 16-2). The process of partitioning is also called stratification, categorization, or subgrouping, and its results are called partitions, strata, categories, classes, or subgroups. In this chapter, we use the pair of terms *partitioning* (for the process) and *(sub)classes* (for its result).

The aim of partitioning is to provide a better basis for comparison of clinical laboratory results: *class-specific* reference intervals (e.g., age- and gender-specific reference intervals).

Various statistical criteria for partitioning have been suggested.[27,39] For example, an intuitive criterion states that partitioning is necessary if differences between classes are statistically significant (rejection of the "null" hypothesis of equal distributions). The distribution of reference values in the classes may show different locations (mean values vary) or different intraclass variations (standard deviations vary). These differences may be tested by statistical methods, which are not described here. The reader is referred to Chapter 14 and to standard textbooks of parametric[55,59] and nonparametric statistics.[11]

The differences of location or variation, however, may be statistically significant and still too small to justify replacing a single total reference interval with several class-specific intervals. Alternately, statistically nonsignificant differences can lead to situations in which the proportions of each subclass above the upper or below the lower reference limits (without partitioning) are much different from the desired 2.5% on each side. Harris and Boyd[27] therefore suggested criteria based on the ratio between the subclass standard deviations, a normal deviate test of means, and calculation of critical decision values dependent on the sample size.

Lahti and co-workers[39,40] focused on distances between reference limits instead of distances between means, and suggested new distance and proportion criteria for partitioning. Their model also makes it possible to account for unequal subclass prevalences and is applicable to distributions of various types.

Partitioning requires large samples of reference values. If not, the subclass sizes may be too small for reliable estimates of reference intervals.

To solve the subclass size problem, it has been suggested to estimate regression-based reference intervals. Instead of dividing, for example, the total material into several age classes, one may construct continuous age-dependent reference limits and their confidence regions. Simulation studies have shown that this method produces reliable estimates with small sample sizes.[75]

When the intended purpose of the reference interval is to detect individual changes in biochemical status, subject-based reference values may be more appropriate for interpretation than class-specific reference intervals.[24,25,27] We shall return to this problem at the end of this chapter.

In the following sections, we assume that we have a homogeneous reference distribution, either the complete distribution (if partitioning has been shown to be unnecessary) or a subclass distribution (after partitioning).

Inspection of Distribution

It is always advisable to display the reference distribution graphically and to inspect it. A *histogram*, as shown in Figure 16-3, *A*, is easily prepared and is the data display best suited for visual inspection. The examination of the histogram is a safeguard against the misapplication or misinterpretation of statistical methods, and it may give valuable information about data. We should look for the following characteristics of the distribution:

1. Highly deviating values *(outliers)* may represent erroneous values.
2. *Bimodal* or *polymodal* distributions have more than one peak and may indicate that the distribution is nonhomogeneous because of the mixing of two or more distributions. If so, the criteria used to select

reference individuals should be reevaluated, or partitioning of the values according to age, gender, or other relevant factors should be attempted.

3. The shape of the distribution should be noticed. It may be asymmetrical or more or less peaked than the symmetrical and bell-shaped Gaussian distribution (Figure 16-5). The asymmetry most frequently observed with clinical chemistry data is positive *skewness* (Figure 16-5, *A*). A symmetrical distribution with positive *kurtosis* has a high and slim peak and more values in both tails than the Gaussian type of distribution (Figure 16-5, *C*). Conversely, negative kurtosis indicates that the distribution has a broad and flat top with relatively few observations in the tails (Figure 16-5, *D*). Asymmetry and nonGaussian peakedness may be combined.
4. The visual inspection may also provide initial estimates of the location of reference limits that are useful as checks on the validity of computations.

Identification and Handling of Erroneous Values

An *erroneous value* can be traced to a gross deviation from the prescribed procedure for establishment of reference values.[26] Such values may either deviate significantly from the proper reference values (*outliers*) or be hidden in the reference distribution. Only a strict experimental protocol, with adequate controls at each step, can eliminate the latter type of erroneous values.

Visual inspection of a histogram is a reliable method for identification of possible outliers. It is important to keep in mind, however, that values far out in the long tail of a skewed distribution may easily be misinterpreted as outliers. If the distribution is positively skewed, inspection of a histogram displaying the logarithms of the values may aid in the visual identification of outliers.

Some outliers may also be identified by *statistical tests* (see Chapter 14), but no single method is capable of detecting outliers in every situation that may occur. The number of techniques suggested or recommended is, for that reason, very large.[6,27,30] The two main problems encountered are as follows:

1. Many of the tests assume that the type of the true distribution is known before use of the test. Some of these specifically require that the distribution be Gaussian. However, biological distributions are very often nonGaussian, and their types are seldom known in advance. Furthermore, statistical tests of types of distribution are unreliable in the presence of outliers. We then have a difficult dilemma: some tests for outliers assume that the type of distribution is known, but tests for determining the type of distribution require that outliers be absent! As a consequence, it may be difficult to transform the distribution to Gaussian form before the identification of outliers by statistical tests. Some tests are relatively insensitive to departures from Gaussianity. This is the case with Dixon's *range test:* identify the extreme value as an outlier if the difference between the two highest (or lowest) values in the distribution exceeds one third of the range of all values.[27,34,53]
2. Several tests for outliers assume that data contain only a single outlier. The limitation of these tests is obvious. Some tests may detect a specified number of outliers, or they may be run several times, discarding one outlier in each pass of data. The range test, however, usually fails in the presence of several outliers. It is possible to estimate the standard deviation using data remaining after *trimming* of both tails of the distribution by a specified percentage of observations.[27,31] Outliers could be identified by this method as the values lying 3 or 4 standard deviations from the arithmetic mean. The method assumes, however, that the true distribution is Gaussian.

Horn and co-workers[33] have published a novel method in two stages for outlier detection that seems to provide a promising solution to both of the problems mentioned above.

1. Mathematically transform the data to approximate a Gaussian distribution. Horn et al used the Box-Cox transformation,[9] but other transformations that correct for skewness (see below) would probably also work. As mentioned above, it is impossible to achieve exact symmetry by transformation in the presence of outliers, but this does not seem to be critical with Horn's method.
2. Identify (or eliminate) outliers by a criterion based on the central 50% of the distribution, thus reducing the masking effect of several outliers. Compute the interquartile range (*IQR*) between the lower and upper quartiles of the distribution (Q_1 and Q_3, respectively): $IQR = Q_3 - Q_1$. Then identify as outliers data lying outside the two fences $Q_1 - 1.5{*}IQR$ and $Q_3 + 1.5{*}IQR$.

Deviating values identified as possible outliers cannot always be discarded automatically. Values should be included or excluded on a rational basis. Check the records of the dubious values and correct errors. In some cases, deviating values should be rejected because noncorrectable causes have been found, such as previously unrecognized conditions, qualifying individuals for exclusion from the group of reference individuals.

Methods for Determining Reference Values

Nonparametric, parametric, and bootstrap methods are used to determine reference intervals.

Nonparametric Method

This method consists essentially of cutting off a specified percentage of the values from each tail of the reference distribution. Three techniques may be used:

1. The percentiles may be determined *graphically* by plotting the cumulative distribution on ordinary graph paper (Figure 16-4, *B*) or preferably on Gaussian probability paper.

TABLE 16-3 Nonparametric Confidence Intervals of Reference Limits*

Sample Size	Rank Numbers Lower	Rank Numbers Upper	Sample Size	Rank Numbers Lower	Rank Numbers Upper
119-132	1	7	566-574	8	22
133-160	1	8	575-598	9	22
161-187	1	9	599-624	9	23
188-189	2	9	625-631	10	23
190-218	2	10	632-665	10	24
219-248	2	11	666-674	10	25
249-249	2	12	675-698	11	25
250-279	3	12	699-724	11	26
280-307	3	13	725-732	12	26
308-309	4	13	733-765	12	27
310-340	4	14	766-773	12	28
341-363	4	15	774-799	13	28
364-372	5	15	800-822	13	29
373-403	5	16	823-833	14	29
404-417	5	17	834-867	14	30
418-435	6	17	868-871	14	31
436-468	6	18	872-901	15	31
469-470	6	19	902-919	15	32
471-500	7	19	920-935	16	32
501-522	7	20	936-967	16	33
523-533	8	20	968-970	17	33
534-565	8	21	971-1000	17	34

*The table shows the rank numbers of the 0.90 confidence interval of the 2.5 percentile for samples with 119 to 1000 values. To obtain the corresponding rank numbers of the 97.5 percentile, subtract the rank numbers in the table from $(n + 1)$ where n is the sample size.
From IFCC.[34]

2. A *mathematical function* may be fitted to the reference distribution.[27,54,57] The percentiles are then determined using the fitted function.
3. Very simple and reliable methods are based on *rank numbers.*[34,43,53] They also allow nonparametric estimation of the confidence intervals of the percentiles.[53] The method can easily be applied manually or with a spreadsheet program.

The rank-based method as recommended by the IFCC has the following steps:[34]

a. Sort the n reference values in ascending order of magnitude.
b. Rank the values. The minimum value has rank number 1, the next value has rank number 2, and so on until the maximum value, which has rank number n. Consecutive rank numbers should be given to two or more values that are equal ("ties").
c. Compute the rank number of the 100α and $100(1 - \alpha)$ percentiles as $\alpha(n + 1)$ and $(1 - \alpha)(n + 1)$, respectively. Thus the limits of the conventional 95% reference interval have rank numbers equal to $0.025(n + 1)$ and $0.975(n + 1)$.
d. Determine the percentiles by finding the original reference values that correspond to the computed rank numbers, provided that the rank numbers are integers. Otherwise, interpolate between the two limiting values.
e. Finally, determine the confidence interval of each percentile using the binomial distribution.[53] Table 16-3 facilitates this for the 0.90 confidence interval of the 2.5 and 97.5 percentiles. Just enter the table and look up the bounding rank numbers for each percentile.

Table 16-4 shows an example of the nonparametric determination of percentiles using the serum triglyceride values shown in Figure 16-3.

Parametric Method

The parametric method is much more complicated than the simple nonparametric method and requires computer software.[65] The method is presented here under separate headings for testing of type of distribution, transformation of data, and the estimation of percentiles and their confidence intervals.

TABLE 16-4 Nonparametric Determination of Reference Interval*

Sorted and Ranked Serum Triglyceride Values in the Left Tail of the Distribution:

Values:	0.41	0.43	0.45	0.46	0.47	0.49	0.51	0.55	0.55	0.55
Ranks:	1	2	3	4	5	6	7	8	9	10
Values:	0.56	0.58	0.58	0.61	0.62	0.62	0.64	0.64	0.65	0.65
Ranks:	11	12	13	14	15	16	17	18	19	20

Sorted and Ranked Triglyceride Values in the Right Tail of the Distribution:

Values:	2.21	2.22	2.26	2.27	2.27	2.28	2.30	2.31	2.34	2.35
Ranks:	481	482	483	484	485	486	487	488	489	490
Values:	2.48	2.50	2.55	2.62	2.63	2.65	2.72	2.78	2.90	2.91
Ranks:	491	492	493	494	495	496	497	498	499	500

Calculation of Rank Numbers of the Percentiles:

Lower:	0.025(500 + 1) = 12.5
Upper:	0.975(500 + 1) = 488.5

Finding the Original Values Corresponding to These Rank Numbers:

Lower reference limit (2.5 percentile):	0.58
Upper reference limit (97.5 percentile):	2.32 (by interpolation)

Rank Numbers and Values of the 0.90 Confidence Limit of the Lower Reference Limit:

Rank numbers (Table 16-3):	7 and 19
Confidence limits:	0.51 and 0.65

Rank Numbers and Values of the 0.90 Confidence Limit of the Upper Reference Limit:

Rank numbers (Table 16-3):	500 + 1 − 19 = 482
	500 + 1 − 7 = 494
Confidence limits:	2.22 and 2.62

Summary:

Lower reference limit:	0.58 [0.51-0.65] mmol/L
Upper reference limit:	2.32 [2.22-2.62] mmol/L

*The table shows an example using the 500 serum triglyceride concentrations displayed in Figure 16-3. See the text for a description of the nonparametric method. The unit of all concentrations in the table is mmol/L.

Testing Fit to Gaussian Distribution

The parametric method for estimating percentiles assumes that the true distribution is Gaussian. This fact was frequently ignored in the past and caused Elveback[15] to warn against "the ghost of Gauss." Negligence often results in seriously biased estimates of reference limits. If, for example, we compute the mean and standard deviation of the 500 serum triglyceride values displayed in Figure 16-3, and then calculate the reference interval as $\bar{x} \pm 1.960 s_x$, we would find the following limits: 0.4 and 2.2 mmol/L (correct values: 0.6 and 2.3 mmol/L). A highly positively skewed distribution may even result in a negative value for the lower reference limit.

A critical phase in the parametric method is, therefore, to test the goodness-of-fit of the reference distribution to a hypothetical Gaussian distribution. If we must reject the Gaussian hypothesis at a specified significance level, we have two alternatives (Figure 16-2): either we can use the nonparametric method or we can try to apply mathematical transformation of data to approximate the Gaussian distribution. Only when the Gaussian hypothesis is not rejected by the test can we pass directly to parametric estimation of percentiles and their confidence intervals (Figure 16-2).

Goodness-of-fit tests have been reviewed by Mardia.[45] We shall discuss only a few simple tests[63,66] that have proved valuable for our purposes. One can broadly classify these tests into three groups: graphical procedures, coefficient-based tests, and tests that are based on shape differences between the observed and theoretical distributions.

1. *The graphical procedure* consists of plotting the cumulative distribution (Figure 16-3, *B*) on probability paper, which has a nonlinear vertical axis based on the Gaussian distribution. The plot should be close to a straight line if the distribution is Gaussian. It is, however, very diffi-

cult to evaluate visually the deviations from the straight line because of the nonlinearity of the vertical distances in the graph. For that reason, the use of the graphical method is not recommended.

2. *The coefficient-based tests* use statistical measures of skewness and kurtosis (Figure 16-5).[12,34,59,63,66] These measures are computed from the second, third, and fourth subset moments about the mean (m_2, m_3, and m_4, respectively):

$$m_k = \frac{\sum (x-\bar{x})^k}{n} \qquad (k = 2, 3, or\ 4)$$

The subset *coefficient of skewness,* g_s, and its asymptotic standard deviation, s_s (it approaches the true standard deviation as the number of observations increases), are computed by the following formulas:

$$g_s = \frac{m_3}{m_2 \cdot \sqrt{m_2}}$$

$$s_s = \sqrt{\frac{6}{n}}$$

The coefficient g_s is zero for the Gaussian and other symmetrical distributions. The sign of a nonzero coefficient indicates the type of skewness present in the data (Figure 16-5, *A* and *B*).

The subset *coefficient of kurtosis,* g_k, and its asymptotic standard deviation, s_k, are computed as follows:

$$g_k = \frac{m_4}{m_2^2} - 3$$

$$s_k = \sqrt{\frac{24}{n}} = 6 = 2 \cdot \sqrt{\frac{6}{n}}$$

The coefficient g_k is approximately zero for the Gaussian distribution. The sign of a nonzero coefficient indicates the type of kurtosis present in the data (Figure 16-5, *C* and *D*).

The statistical significance of these two coefficients may be found by referring to tables for testing skewness and kurtosis.[59] A rough test is obtained by dividing the coefficient by its standard deviation and then referring to a table of the Gaussian distribution. The latter procedure is only reasonably accurate for sample sizes above 1000 (for g_s) and 2000 (for g_k). Computer programs for calculation and testing of these coefficients are available.[8,29,56,65,67]

Example: The coefficients computed for the serum triglyceride data shown in Figure 16-3 are $g_s = 0.873$ and $g_k = 0.677$. Their critical values for $n = 500$ at the 0.02 level of significance are 0.255 and 0.60, respectively.[59] Both coefficients are thus statistically significant and the Gaussian hypothesis should be rejected (the data were, in fact, approximately log-Gaussian). We arrive at the same conclusion by the approximate tests using the ratio between a coefficient and its asymptotic standard deviation:

$$\frac{g_s}{s_s} = \frac{0.873}{\sqrt{\frac{6}{500}}} = 7.97$$

$$\frac{g_k}{s_k} = \frac{0.677}{\sqrt{\frac{24}{500}}} = 3.09$$

Both coefficients exceed 3 standard deviations. When using a computer program,[65] these probabilities were found: $p < 0.001$ for g_s and $p = 0.011$ for g_k.

3. Three *tests of shape differences* that can be used to evaluate goodness-of-fit are the Kolmogorov-Smirnov test, the Cramer-von Mises test, and the Anderson-Darling test.[34,45,63,66,69] Computer programs for all three tests are available.[65]

Here we focus only on the Anderson-Darling test, which has been recommended by the IFCC.[34] The procedure is as follows[34,63,66,69]:

a. Allow for rounding of data, for example, by adding random "noise":

$$x_i' = x_i + L(r_i - 0.5) \qquad (i = 1, \ldots, n)$$

Here x'_i is the value with random "noise" added, x_i is the original data value, L is the step size of the value scale (least significant digit (e.g., $L = 0.1$ if laboratory results are reported to one decimal place), and r_i is a random number between 0.0 and 1.0.

b. Sort the data values in an ascending order of magnitude.

c. Compute the deviations $v_i = (x'_i - \bar{x})/s_x$, where $\bar{x}$ is the mean and s_x is the standard deviation of the data values.

d. Now find the values w_i of the cumulative Gaussian distribution corresponding to the deviation v_i by using statistical tables or a computerized algorithm.

e. Calculate the test statistic A^2 by this formula:

$$A^2 = -n - \frac{\sum (2i-1) \cdot [\ln(w_i) + \ln(1-w_{n+1-i})]}{n}$$

f. Reject the hypothesis that the data distribution fits the Gaussian distribution at the 0.01 level of significance if the size-adjusted test statistic A^{2*} is greater than 1.092[69]:

$$A^{2*} = A^2 \cdot \left(1 + \frac{4}{n} - \frac{25}{n^2}\right)$$

Transformation of Data: Simple Method

In the previous section it was shown that $\sqrt{x} \pm 1.960 s_x$ of the serum triglyceride data in Figure 16-3 resulted in biased reference limits (too low values), as was to be expected with this positively skewed distribution. However, it is often possible to transform data mathematically to obtain a distribution of transformed values that approximates a Gaussian distribution. With these new values, the 2.5 and 97.5 percentiles are localized at 2 standard deviations on both sides of the mean. The estimates may then be transformed back to the original measurement scale by using the inverse mathematical function.

It is frequently observed that *logarithmically transformed* values, $y = \ln(x)$, of a positively skewed distribution fit the Gaussian distribution rather closely. In other cases, *square roots* of the values, $\sqrt{x}$, result in a better approximation to the Gaussian distribution. This is the basis for the common use of the logarithmic and square root transformations when estimating reference limits. The method is applicable only to positively skewed distributions. The method is easily performed with a spreadsheet program. The procedure is as follows:

1. Test the fit of the distribution of original data to the Gaussian distribution. If the distribution has approximately Gaussian shape, the 2.5 and 97.5 percentiles can be calculated directly as $\bar{x} \pm 1.960s_x$. Otherwise continue with the following steps.
2. Transform data by the logarithmic function $y = \ln(x)$ or by the square root function $y = \sqrt{x}$ and then test the fit to the Gaussian distribution. If the transformed distribution is significantly different from Gaussian shape, try another transformation or estimate the percentiles by the nonparametric method (see earlier in this chapter). Continue with the next step if the transformation to Gaussianity was successful.
3. Compute the mean y and the standard deviation s_y of transformed data. Then estimate the 2.5 and 97.5 percentiles in the transformed data scale as $\bar{y} \pm 1.960s_y$.
4. The final step is reconversion of these percentiles to the original data scale. The inverse functions of the two transformations described here are:

$$\text{Inverse logarithmic function: } x = e^y = \exp(y)$$
$$\text{Inverse square root function: } x = y^2$$

It is also possible to estimate the confidence limits of percentiles determined by the parametric method. The method is presented in a later section.

Example: When using logarithms of the serum triglyceride values of Figure 16-3, we get a distribution very close to Gaussian shape. The mean and standard deviation of transformed data are $\bar{y} = 0.172$ and $s_y = 0.357$, respectively. The transformed 2.5 percentile is $0.172 - 1.960 \times 0.357 = -0.528$. On reconversion to the original data scale we get $\exp(-0.528) = 0.59$. The lower reference limit of serum triglycerides is thus 0.59 mmol/L. Similarly, we find that the upper reference limit is 2.39 mmol/L. These values are in close agreement with those found by the nonparametric method: 0.58 and 2.32 mmol/L (Table 16-4).

Transformation of Data: Two-Stage Method

Because the simple logarithmic and square root transformations often fail to produce the desired Gaussian shape of the distribution, Harris and DeMets[29] introduced the two-stage method: first use a function that transforms the distribution to symmetry (zero coefficient of skewness), and then apply another function that removes any remaining nonGaussian kurtosis. Several mathematical functions may serve the purpose,[27,66] but this chapter presents only the two-stage procedure recommended by the IFCC.[34] This method, which is based on exponential and modulus functions, is implemented in the RefVal computer program.[65] The successive approximations to symmetry and to Gaussian kurtosis (i.e., the iterative determination of the function parameters) are monitored by the coefficient-based tests, whereas the final evaluation has to be done by an independent test (e.g., the Anderson-Darling test; see earlier in this chapter).

The *exponential function* suggested by Manly[44] may correct for both positive or negative skewness:

$$y = \frac{\exp(\gamma \cdot x) - 1}{\gamma} \qquad (\gamma \neq 0)$$
$$y = x \qquad (\gamma = 0)$$

The *modulus function* of John and Draper[35] may remove any nonGaussian kurtosis from a symmetrical distribution:

$$z = sign\left[\frac{(|y|+1)^{\lambda} - 1}{\lambda}\right] \qquad (\lambda \neq 0)$$
$$z = sign[\ln(|y|+1)] \qquad (\lambda = 0)$$

The *sign* in the formulas above is the algebraic sign associated with each input value *y*.

Parametric Estimates of Percentiles and Their Confidence Intervals

General estimates for the 100α and $100(1-\alpha)$ percentiles and their 0.90 confidence intervals can be determined by the following method, provided that data (original or transformed) fit the Gaussian distribution[34]:

The 100α and $100(1-\alpha)$ percentiles are determined as

(mean) $\pm$ c (standard deviation)

where c is the $(1-\alpha)$ standard Gaussian deviate, as can be found in statistical tables. For the 2.5 and 97.5 percentiles, we must find the $(1-0.025) = 0.975$ standard Gaussian deviate: $c = 1.960$.

The 0.90 *confidence intervals* of these percentiles are estimated as[34,66]

$$\text{percentile} \pm 2.81 \cdot \frac{s_y}{\sqrt{n}}$$

where s_y is the standard deviation of the reference values (original or transformed) and n is the number of values. This formula is a special case of a general formula that can be used for confidence intervals of other sizes or for other percentiles.[34,66]

Example: The parametric estimate of the 2.5 percentile of serum triglycerides was determined previously by the logarithmic transformation. The 0.90 confidence limits of the lower percentile are then

$$-0.528 - 2.81 \cdot \frac{0.357}{\sqrt{500}} = -0.573 \qquad \exp(-0.573) = 0.56$$

$$-0.528 + 2.81 \cdot \frac{0.357}{\sqrt{500}} = -0.483 \qquad \exp(-0.483) = 0.62$$

Thus the complete estimate of the 2.5 percentile [and its 0.90 confidence interval] is 0.59 [0.56 – 0.62] mmol/L. The 97.5 percentile is, by the same method, found to be 2.39 [2.29 – 2.50] mmol/L.

Bootstrap Method

Bootstrap-based methods are reliable for estimating reference intervals.[27,43,57] The following version using the rank-based nonparametric method is simple and reliable:

1. Draw, with replacement, random samples of size n from the subset of n reference values. One draws "with replacement" if each value randomly selected from the subset is kept in the subset so that it may participate in the random selection of the next value. The number of resamples should be high (500 is a reasonable number of iterations).
2. For each resample, estimate the upper and lower reference limits (percentiles) by the rank-based nonparametric procedure described previously. Save the two estimates for each iteration.
3. Upon completion of all iterations, use the median of the resample estimates of each of the two reference limits as final estimates.
4. Then estimate the 0.90 confidence interval of each reference limit from the distribution of the percentile estimates.

Among available methods for estimation of reference limits and their confidence intervals, the bootstrap method probably is the most reliable one.[27,43] The location of estimated percentiles is always dependent on the characteristics of the particular subset of reference values. There are only two possible methods to provide percentile estimates that approach population values: using a very large sample or performing repeated sampling from the same parent population. Both methods are obviously expensive. The bootstrap method is a good alternative. Its advantages are: (1) it is economical because it is based upon resampling from a single subset of reference values; (2) it provides robust percentile estimates (with the mentioned single-sample limitation); and (3) the widths of the confidence intervals approach asymptotically those that would have been obtained by repeated sampling from the parent population.[13] A computer is necessary to run the large number of bootstrap iterations.[65]

The bootstrap version described here uses rank-based nonparametric percentile estimates. However, the bootstrap principle may be employed with any kind of estimation, parametric or nonparametric.

PRESENTATION OF AN OBSERVED VALUE IN RELATION TO REFERENCE VALUES

An observed value (patient's value) may be compared with reference values. This comparison is often similar to hypothesis testing, but it is seldom statistical testing in the strict sense. Ideally the patient and the reference individuals should match (i.e., we might state the hypothesis that they were all picked from the same set [population]). Often, however, this is not the case. Thus it is advisable to consider the reference values as the yardstick for a less formal assessment than hypothesis testing.

The clinician should always be supplied with as much information about the reference values as he or she needs for the interpretation. Reference intervals for all laboratory tests may be presented to the physicians in a booklet together with information about the analysis methods, their imprecision, and descriptions of the reference values. The aim must be to present to the physicians enough information for rational clinical judgments.

In addition, a convenient presentation of an observed value in relation to reference values may be a great help for the busy clinician.[14,21,34,62]

The presentation of the observed value together with a *listing of all the reference values* for the corresponding test is a feasible procedure only when few reference values are available. When we have many reference values, it is more convenient to present the *reference distribution* in a table, graphically in the form of a histogram (Figure 16-3, *A*), or by a plot of the cumulative distribution (Figures 16-3, *B* and 16-4, *B*). A very informative presentation of the observed value is to show its location on a graph. This is particularly suited for a computerized display.[21]

A more condensed technique is to present the observed value and the *reference interval* on the same report sheet. The reference intervals may be preprinted on report forms, or the computer system may select the appropriate age- and gender-specific reference interval from a file and print it next to the test result. This type of presentation can be graphical.[21]

It is also possible to compute various *mathematical indices* or to *flag* the results on reports using convenient symbols. When using such presentation methods, the original observed value should also be reported to allow comparison with results of other laboratory tests and metabolic calculations.

An observed value may be classified as "low," "usual," or "high" (three classes), depending on its *location in relation to the reference interval.* On reports, it is convenient to flag unusual results (e.g., by using "L" and "H" for "low" and "high," respectively).[21]

A more detailed division of the value scale has also been advocated.[14] The regions outside the reference interval may be subdivided to indicate how "unusual" the observed value is. The reference interval may also be subclassified. The advantages are doubtful, however, because the shape of the reference distribution is not taken into account.

Another popular method is to express the observed value by a *statistical distance measure.* Such distances are all ratios of the following type:

$$\frac{\text{observed value} - \text{measure of location}}{\text{measure of dispersion}}$$

The well-known *SD unit* or "normal equivalent deviate" is such a measure. It is calculated as the difference between the observed value and the mean of the reference values divided by their standard deviation.[23] Several similar ratios have been suggested,[16] but none has significant advantages over the other. All produce very confusing values if the reference distribution is very skewed. An observed value (e.g., with an SD unit of 2.2) would be above the 97.5 percentile if the reference distribution has a Gaussian shape, but might be well below the upper reference limit of a positively skewed distribution. Mathematical transformation of the reference distribution to the Gaussian shape may solve this problem.[62]

To report the observed value as a *percentile* of the reference distribution provides a very accurate measure of the relation.[14,54] The observed serum triglyceride value 2.4 mmol/L may, for example, be reported as 2.4 mmol/L (98th percentile). Alternatively, we can estimate the probability of finding a value closer to the mean than the observed value, the *index of atypicality*.[2,62]

When observed values of several analytes are reported simultaneously, it is possible to use multivariate analogs of the SD unit and the index of atypicality (see below).[1,2]

ADDITIONAL TOPICS

Transferability of Reference Values

The determination of reliable reference values for each test in the laboratory's repertoire is a major task and is often far beyond the capabilities of the individual laboratory. It would therefore be convenient if reference values generated in another laboratory could be used. This is especially important when ethical considerations limit the number of available individuals (e.g., when producing pediatric reference values). Then, cooperative establishment of reference values may be necessary.

A major prerequisite for transfer of reference values is that the populations be homogeneous (i.e., there should be no major ethnic, social, or environmental differences among them).

However, the problem of analytical transferability remains. The optimal, but usually very unrealistic, situation assumes that the analytical methods, including their calibration and quality assurance, are identical in the laboratories. A more pragmatic approach involves standardization of analytical protocols, common calibration, design of a sufficiently efficient external quality control scheme, and the use of mathematical transfer functions if the results still are not directly comparable.

The parameters of transfer functions may be estimated from the results obtained by analysis of a sufficient number of specimens (preferably human) spanning the relevant range of concentrations in all participating laboratories. Sometimes functions obtained by simple linear regression suffice: using $y = a_0 + a_1x$, the constant term a_0 compensates for systematic shifts among the methods, whereas the coefficient term a_1 adjusts for proportional differences. In other cases, a more elaborate system for transfer of laboratory data is necessary.[70] The mentioned transfer functions account only for analytical bias; however, adjustments for differences in imprecision may also be designed.

Multicenter production of reference values is gaining acceptance, both as a theoretical concept and as a practical approach. A Spanish study[18] introduced a cooperative model, simulating a virtual laboratory for 15 biochemical quantities. A recent project in the Nordic countries (NORIP[51,54a]) was aimed at the production of common reference intervals for 25 analytes.

The verification of transferred reference values or intervals is both important and problematic.[27] The comparison of a locally produced, small subset of values with the large set produced elsewhere using traditional statistical tests often is not appropriate because the underlying statistical assumptions are not fulfilled and because of the unbalanced sample sizes. Alternative methods using nonparametric tests[74] or Monte Carlo sampling[32] have been described.

Multivariate, Population-Based Reference Regions

The topic of the previous sections of this chapter has been univariate population-based reference values and quantities derived from them. Such values do not, however, fit the common clinical situation in which observed values of several different laboratory tests are available for interpretation and decision making. For example, the average number of individual clinical chemistry tests requested on one specimen received in the author's laboratory is 9.7. There are two models for interpretation by comparison in this situation. We can compare each observed value with the corresponding reference values or interval (i.e., we perform *multiple, univariate comparisons*); or we can consider the set of observed values as a single multivariate observation and interpret it as such by a *multivariate comparison.* In this section, the relative merits of these two approaches are discussed, and methods for the latter type of comparison are presented.

The Multivariate Concept

A univariate observation, such as a single laboratory result, may be represented graphically as a point on a line, the axis. The results obtained by two different laboratory tests performed on the same specimen (a bivariate observation) may be displayed as a point in a plane defined by two perpendicular axes. With three results, we have a trivariate observation and a point in a space defined by three perpendicular axes, and so on. We lose the possibility for visualization of a multivariate observation when there are more than three dimensions. Still, we can consider the multivariate observation as a point in a multidimensional hyperspace with as many mutually perpendicular axes as there are results of different tests. The prefix "hyper" signifies, in this context, "more than three dimensions." Such multivariate observations are also

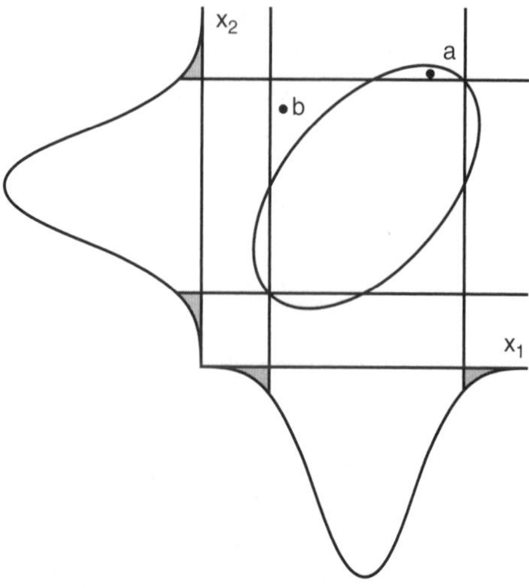

Figure 16-6 Bivariate reference region (*ellipse*) compared with the region defined by the two univariate reference intervals (*box*).

called *patterns* or *profiles.* A multivariate distribution is thus represented by a cluster of points on a plane, in a space, or in a hyperspace, depending on the dimensionality of the observation.[1,60,76] Several statistical methods are based on multivariate methods, and some of them are straightforward extensions of well-known univariate methods.[47]

The Multiple, Univariate Reference Region

The univariate reference interval is bounded by two reference limits on the result axis (Figure 16-4). Figure 16-6 shows that the univariate reference intervals for two laboratory tests describe a square in the plane of the two axes. Similarly, three or more univariate reference intervals define boxes or hyperboxes in the (hyper)space. By multiple, univariate comparison it can be decided whether a multivariate observation point lies inside or outside this square, box, or hyperbox. This method has, however, two very serious deficiencies[78]: an observation may lie outside the limits of the region without being unusual (Figure 16-6, point *a*), or it may be found on the inside and still be a very atypical observation (Figure 16-6, point *b*). If we use the central 95% interval, 5% of the values are by definition expected to be located in the two tails of the univariate reference distribution. But more than 5% of the values would be located outside the square or (hyper)box created by several 95% intervals. To be accurate, $100(1 - 0.95^m)$ percent of multivariate reference values would be excluded by the method of multiple, univariate comparison (m being the number of different tests or the dimensionality). We would, for example, expect to find $100(1 - 0.95^{10}) = 40\%$ of "false positives" when using 10 laboratory tests. This discouraging result has been verified in several multiphasic screening programs. We therefore need a better method.

The Multivariate Reference Region

It is possible to define a common multivariate reference region* based on the joint distribution of the reference values for two or more laboratory tests. This multivariate region is not a right-angled area or hyperbox, but more like an ellipse in the plane (Figure 16-6) or an ellipsoid hyperbody in hyperspace. This region may be a straightforward extension of the univariate 95% interval to the multivariate situation; it may be set to enclose 95% of the central multivariate reference data points. In that case, we would expect to find only 5% "false positives."

The use of multivariate reference regions usually requires the assistance of a computer program, which takes a set of results obtained by several laboratory tests on the same clinical specimen and calculates an index. The interpretation of a multivariate observation in relation to reference values is then the task of comparing the index with a critical value estimated from the reference values. This, obviously, is much simpler than comparing each result with its proper reference interval.

The index is essentially a distance measure, *Mahalanobis' squared distance* (D^2), which expresses the multivariate distance between the observation point and the common mean of the reference values, taking into account the dispersion and correlation of the variables.[1,2,10,47,60] More interpretational guidance may be obtained from this distance by expressing it as a percentile analogous to the percentile presentation of univariate observed values.[10] Also, the index of atypicality has a multivariate counterpart.[1,2]

Mahalanobis' squared distance of an observation is the multivariate analog of the square of the SD unit (d^2) discussed earlier:

$$d^2 = \left(\frac{x-\bar{x}}{s_x}\right)^2 = (x-\bar{x}) \cdot \left(s_x^2\right)^{-1} \cdot (x-\bar{x})$$

The second form of the formula above is given to show the analogy to Mahalanobis' distance, which is defined as follows:

$$D^2 = (\mathbf{x}-\bar{\mathbf{x}})'\mathbf{S}^{-1}(\mathbf{x}-\bar{\mathbf{x}})$$

where $(\mathbf{x} - \bar{\mathbf{x}})'$ and $(\mathbf{x} - \bar{\mathbf{x}})$ are row and column vectors of the differences between each variable and its mean, and $\mathbf{S}^{-1}$ is the inverse matrix of variances and covariances. (According to the notation of matrix algebra, a lower-case boldface letter denotes a vector [an array of numbers]; the symbol for a matrix [a table of numbers] is a boldface capital letter.) The diagonal elements of the matrix $\mathbf{S}$ before inversion are the variances of the measures of the dispersion of individual variables. The covariances are measures of their interrelationship (off-diagonal elements of $\mathbf{S}$). The D^2 for a set of m-dimensional observations follows approximately a χ^2 distribution with m degrees of freedom. The critical value of D^2 for a 95% reference region is thus approximately the (1 –

*References 1, 2, 10, 27, 76, 78.

0.95) fractile of this distribution.[1,2,10] An observed pattern is located outside the multivariate region if its D^2 exceeds the critical value. If we want to report the D^2 as a percentile, we also refer to the same χ^2 distribution.[10]

Although the theory of multivariate reference regions has been known for a long time, surprisingly few applications of it have been reported in the literature. An important report reviews the topic and presents the results of a very careful study on the multivariate 95% region for a 20-test chemistry profile.[10] Some of the findings can be summarized as follows:

1. Sixty-eight percent of the subjects had at least one test result outside univariate reference intervals, which was close to what was theoretically expected: $100(1 - 0.95^{20}) = 64\%$.
2. By contrast, only 5% of the patterns were outside the multivariate reference region (as expected).
3. Transformation to approximately Gaussian shape of the univariate distributions was necessary.
4. A test profile may be distinctly unusual in the multivariate sense even though each individual result is within its proper reference interval (e.g., point B in Figure 16-6).
5. The multivariate reference region could detect minor deviations of multiple analytes.
6. Conversely, it could also be quite insensitive to highly deviating results for a single analyte.
7. The sensitivity could be increased by defining multivariate reference regions for subsets of physiologically related tests.

Subject-Based Reference Values

Figure 16-7 depicts the inherent problem associated with population-based reference values. It shows two hypothetical reference distributions. The one represents the common reference distribution based on single specimens obtained from a group of different reference individuals. It has a true (hypothetical) mean μ and a standard deviation σ. The other distribution is based on several specimens collected over time in a single individual, the *i*th individual. Its hypothetical mean is μ_i and the standard deviation σ_i.

If an observed value is located outside the subject's 2.5 and 97.5 percentiles, the personal or *subject-based reference interval,* the cause may be a change in the biochemical status, suggesting the presence of disease. Figure 16-7 shows that such an observed value may still be within the population-based reference interval. The sensitivity of the latter interval to changes in a subject's biochemical status depends accordingly on the location of the individual's mean μ_i relative to the common mean μ and to the relative magnitudes of the corresponding standard deviations σ_i and σ. A mean μ_i close to μ and a small σ_i relative to σ may conceal the individual's changes entirely within the population-based reference interval.

Harris[24,25] analyzed this topic and found that the ratio R of intraindividual (personal) variation over interindividual (among subjects) variation provides a criterion of the use-

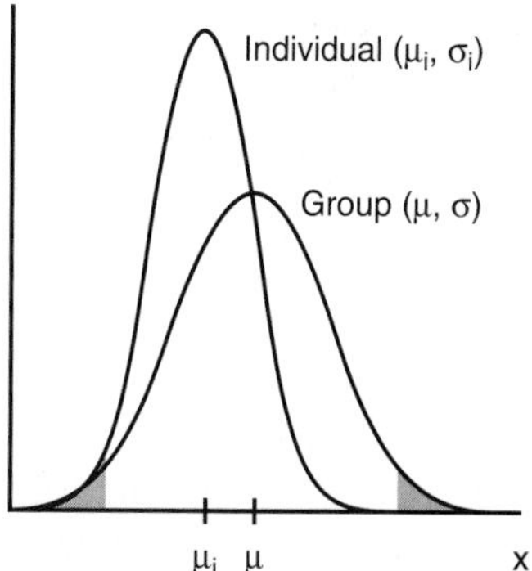

Figure 16-7 Relationship between population-based and subject-based reference distributions and reference intervals. The example is hypothetical, and the two distributions are, for simplicity, Gaussian. *(Modified from Harris EK: Effects of intraindividual and interindividual variation on the appropriate use of normal ranges. Clin Chem 1974; 20:1536.)*

fulness of the population-based reference interval. The population-based reference interval has less than the desired sensitivity to changes in biochemical status if the ratio value is $R \geq 0.6$. This interval is a more trustworthy reference if R is > 1.4, at least for the individual whose standard deviation σ_i is close to the average value. Published data[24,77] usually show that homeostatically tightly controlled quantities, such as serum electrolytes, have high ratio values. The population-based reference intervals of such analytes suffice for clinical use. For example, serum proteins and enzymes have very low ratios because they are not under the same degree of metabolic control. Here, subject-based reference intervals seem more appropriate.

There are two possible solutions to the problem of the clinical insensitivity of population-based reference intervals:

1. We can try to reduce the variation in the reference values by *partitioning* into more homogeneous subclasses, as was discussed in a previous section. But to increase the ratio R, for example, from 0.6 to 1.4 by partitioning, requires that we can obtain the rather dramatic reduction of 37% in the standard deviation.[24] This often is difficult to attain in practice.
2. The other possibility is to use the subject's previous values, obtained when the subject was in a well-defined state of health, as the reference for any future value. The application of *subject-based reference values* becomes more feasible as "health screening" by laboratory tests and as computer storage of results become available to large segments of the general population.

There are two not completely separated classes of models for construction of subject-based reference intervals: statistical and physiological models.[27]

1. Harris has developed several models based on statistical *time series analysis.*[24-28] At the one extreme, we have a stationary or *homeostatic model* suitable for analytes showing relatively fast, random fluctuations around a constant mean (set point). The set point is estimated from past values that are given equal weights. Another

model, the nonstationary *random-walk model,* allows a changing set point over time in healthy subjects. Then, the more recent values are given heavier weights during the estimation of the current set point. Intermediate and more or less complex models exist. Some of these data-following methods are suited for adaptive forecasting in situations in which the time intervals are short (e.g., during hospitalization).[26] They might thus be implemented on a computer as part of a laboratory cumulative reporting system. The reader is referred to papers by Harris for details on statistical time series models.[24-28]

2. It is also possible to construct *physiological models* that use known physiological and biochemical time-dependent relationships. Winkel has developed a time series model for monitoring plasma progesterone in pregnancy using the assumption of a simple exponential growth curve for the size of the placenta.[77]

Dynamic Versus Static Interpretation of Clinical Chemistry Data

The interpretation of observed values by comparison with population-based reference values or intervals is not the only way clinical data may be used. Often, dynamic approaches to data interpretation are more appropriate. Time-dependent variation may provide important information. The time series analysis of consecutive values from the same individual is one example. Other examples are the dynamic analysis of kinetic processes in the organism, such as intermediary metabolism and the exchange of substances between metabolic pools. For example, it is possible to design a model for urea turnover in the body.[19] The model defines the rates of urea input from various sources to the extracellular fluid, the exchange of urea across cell membranes, the urea degradation in the gut, the handling of urea by the kidneys, and so forth. Such a model may facilitate the interpretation of serum urea values with the purpose of detecting hemorrhage or necrosis after major surgery and the evaluation of the magnitude of these complications. Biochemical model building, estimation of model parameters from observed values, and computer simulation of the models may add greatly to our understanding.

REFERENCES

1. Albert A, Harris EK. Multivariate interpretation of clinical laboratory data. New York: Marcel Dekker, 1987.
2. Albert A, Heusghem C. Relating observed values to reference values: The multivariate approach. In: Gräsbeck R, Alström T, eds. Reference values in laboratory medicine. Chichester, England: John Wiley, 1981:289-96.
3. Alström T, Dahl M, Gräsbeck R, et al. Recommendation for collection of skin puncture blood from children with special reference to production of reference values. Scand J Clin Lab Invest 1987;47:199-205.
4. Alström T, Gräsbeck R, Lindblad B, et al. Establishing reference values from adults: Recommendation on procedures for the preparation of individuals collection of blood and handling and storage of specimens. Scand J Clin Lab Invest 1993;53:649-52.
5. Baadenhuijsen H, Smit JC. Indirect estimation of clinical chemical reference intervals from total hospital patient data: Application of a modified *Bhattacharya* procedure. J Clin Chem Clin Biochem 1985;23: 829-39.
6. Barnett V, Lewis T. Outliers in statistical data. Chichester, England: John Wiley, 1994.
7. Berg B, Nilsson JE, Solberg HE, et al. Practical experience in the selection and preparation of reference individuals: Empirical testing of the provisional Scandinavian recommendations. In: Gräsbeck R, Alström T, eds. Reference values in laboratory medicine. Chichester, England: John Wiley, 1981:55-64.
8. BMDP. Cork, Ireland: Statistical Solutions. http://www.statsol.ie/ (Accessed May 2003).
9. Box GEP, Cox DR. Analysis of transformations. J R Stat Soc 1964;B26:211-52.
10. Boyd JC, Lacher DA. The multivariate reference range: An alternative interpretation of multi-test profiles. Clin Chem 1982;28:259-65.
11. Bradley JV. Distribution-free statistical tests. Englewood Cliffs, NJ: Prentice-Hall, 1968.
12. Cramer H. Mathematical methods of statistics. Princeton, NJ: Princeton University Press, 1999.
13. Davison AC, Hinkley DV. Bootstrap methods and their application. Cambridge, UK: Cambridge University Press, 1997:46-52.
14. Dybkær R. Observed value related to reference values. In: Gräsbeck R, Alström T, eds. Reference values in laboratory medicine. Chichester, England: John Wiley, 1981:263-78.
15. Elveback LR, Guillier CL, Keating FR. Health normality and the ghost of Gauss. JAMA 1970;211:69-75.
16. Faulkner WR, Meites S, eds. Geriatric clinical chemistry: Reference values. Washington: AACC Press, 1997.
17. Felding P, Tryding N, Pedersen PH, et al. Effects of posture on concentrations of blood constituents in healthy adults: Practical application of blood specimen collection procedures recommended by the Scandinavian Committee on Reference Values. Scand J Clin Lab Invest 1980;40:615-21.
18. Ferré-Masferrer M, Fuentes-Arderiu X, Alvarez-Funes V, et al. Multicentric reference values: Shared reference limits. Eur J Clin Chem Clin Biochem 1997;35:715-8.
19. Groth T, de Verdier CH. The potential use of biochemical-physiological simulation models in clinical chemistry. Scand J Clin Lab Invest 1979;39:103-10.
20. Gräsbeck R. Health as seen from the laboratory. In: Gräsbeck R, Alström T, eds. Reference values in laboratory medicine. Chichester, England: John Wiley, 1981:17-24.

21. Gräsbeck R, Alström T, eds. Reference values in laboratory medicine: The current state of the art. Chichester, England: John Wiley, 1981.
22. Guder WG, Narayanan S, Wisser H, Zawta B. Samples: From the patient to the laboratory. The impact of preanalytical variables on the quality of laboratory results. 2nd ed. Darmstadt, Germany: GIT Verlag, 2001.
23. Gullick HD, Schauble MK. SD unit system for standardized reporting and interpretation of laboratory data. Am J Clin Pathol 1972;57:517-25.
24. Harris EK. Effects of intra- and interindividual variation on the appropriate use of normal ranges. Clin Chem 1974;20:1535-42.
25. Harris EK. Some theory of reference values: I. Stratified (categorized) normal ranges and a method for following an individual's clinical laboratory values. Clin Chem 1975;21:1457-64.
26. Harris EK. Statistical aspects of reference values in clinical pathology. In: Stefanini M, Benson ES, eds. Progress in clinical pathology. Vol. 7. New York: Grune & Stratton, 1981:45-66.
27. Harris EK, Boyd JC. Statistical bases of reference values in laboratory medicine. New York: Marcel Dekker, 1995.
28. Harris EK, Cooil BK, Shakarji G, et al. On the use of statistical models of within-person variation in long-term studies of healthy individuals. Clin Chem 1980;26:383-91.
29. Harris EK, DeMets DL. Estimation of normal ranges and cumulative proportions by transforming observed distributions to Gaussian form. Clin Chem 1972;18:605-12.
30. Hawkins DM. Identification of outliers. London: Chapman and Hall, 1980.
31. Healy MJR. Outliers in clinical chemistry quality-control schemes. Clin Chem 1979;25:675-7.
32. Holmes EW, Kahn SE Molnar PA, Bermes EW Jr. Verification of reference ranges by using a Monte Carlo sampling technique. Clin Chem 1994;40:2216-22.
33. Horn PS, Feng L, Li Y, Pesce AJ. Effect of outliers and nonhealthy individuals on reference interval estimation. Clin Chem 2001;47:2137-45.
34. International Federation of Clinical Chemistry, Expert Panel on Theory of Reference Values. Approved recommendation on the theory of reference values. Part 1. The concept of reference values. J Clin Chem Clin Biochem 1987;25:337-42; Part 2. Selection of individuals for the production of reference values. J Clin Chem Clin Biochem 1987;25:639-44; Part 3. Preparation of individuals and collection of specimens for the production of reference values. J Clin Chem Clin Biochem 1988;26:593-8; Part 4. Control of analytical variation in the production transfer and application of reference values. Eur J Clin Chem Clin. Biochem 1991;29:531-5; Part 5. Statistical treatment of collected reference values: Determination of reference limits. J Clin Chem Clin Biochem 1987;25:645-56; Part 6. Presentation of observed values related to reference values. J Clin Chem Clin Biochem 1987;25:657-62.
35. John JA, Draper NR. An alternative family of transformations. Applied Statistics 1980;29:190-7.
36. Kallner A, Tryding N. IFCC guidelines to the evaluation of drug effects in clinical chemistry: Based on the IFCC recommendations of the Expert Panel on Drug Effects in Clinical Chemistry. Scand J Clin Lab Invest 1989;49 (Suppl. 195):1-29.
37. Kendall MG, Buckland WR. A dictionary of statistical terms. 5th ed. London: Longman,1990.
38. Kouri T, Kairisto V, Virtanen A, et al. Reference intervals developed from data for hospitalized patients: Computerized method based on combination of laboratory and diagnostic data. Clin Chem 1994;40:2209-15.
39. Lahti A, Petersen PH, Boyd JC, et al. Objective criteria for partitioning Gaussian-distributed reference values into subgroups. Clin Chem 2002;48:338-52.
40. Lahti A, Petersen PH, Boyd JC, Rustad P, Laake P, Helge Erik Solberg HE. Partitioning of Nongaussian-Distributed Biochemical Reference Data into Subgroups Clin Chem 2004;50:891-900.
41. Lindblad B, Alström T, Hansen AB, et al. Recommendation for collection of venous blood from children with special reference to production of reference values. Scand J Clin Lab Invest 1990;50:99-104.
42. Linnet K. Two-stage transformation systems for normalization of reference distributions evaluated. Clin Chem 1987;33:381-6.
43. Linnet K. Nonparametric estimation of reference intervals by simple and bootstrap-based procedures. Clin Chem 2000;46:867-9.
44. Manly BFJ. Exponential data transformations. The Statistician 1976;25:37-42.
45. Mardia KV. Tests of univariate and multivariate normality. In: Krishnaiah PR, ed. Handbook of statistics. Vol. 1. Analysis of variance. Amsterdam: North-Holland Publishing, 1980:279-320.
46. Meites S, Levitt MJ. Skin-puncture and blood-collecting techniques for infants. Clin Chem 1979;25:183-9.
47. Morrison DF. Multivariate statistical methods. 3rd ed. New York: McGraw-Hill, 1990.
48. Murphy EA. The normal and the perils of the sylleptic argument. Perspect Biol Med 1972;15:566-82.
49. National Committee for Clinical Laboratory Standards. Procedures for the collection of diagnostic blood specimens by venipuncture. 4th ed. NCCLS Document H3-A4, 1998; and Procedures and devices for the collection of diagnostic blood specimens by skin puncture. 4th ed. NCCLS Document H4-A4, 1999. Wayne, PA: National Committee for Clinical Laboratory Standards.
50. Nilsson SE, Evrin PE, Tryding N, et al. Biochemical values in persons older than 82 years of age: report

from a population-based study of twins. Scand J Clin Lab Invest 2003;63:1-14.

51. Rustad P, Felding P, eds. Transnational biological reference intervals. Procedures and examples from the Nordic Reference Interval Project 2000. Scand J Clin Lab Invest 2004;64:265-441.
52. Pincus MR. Interpreting laboratory results: Reference values and decision making. In: Henry JB, ed. Clinical diagnosis and management by laboratory methods. 19th ed. Philadelphia: WB Saunders, 1996:74-91.
53. Reed AH, Henry RJ, Mason WB. Influence of statistical method used on the resulting estimate of normal range. Clin Chem 1971;17:275-84.
54. Rossing RG, Hatcher WE. A computer program for estimation of reference percentile values in laboratory data. Comput Progr Biomed 1979;9:69-74.

54a. Rustad P, Felding P. Transnational biological reference intervals. Procedures and examples from the Nordic Reference Interval Project 2000. Scand J Clin Lab Invest 2004;64:265-441.

55. Sachs L. Applied statistics: A handbook of techniques. New York: Springer-Verlag, 1982.
56. SAS System. Cary, NC: SAS Institute. http://www.sas.com/ (Accessed May 2003).
57. Shultz EK, Willard KE, Rich SS, et al. Improved reference-interval estimation. Clin Chem 1985;31:1974-8.
58. Siest G, Henny J, Schiele F, Young DS, eds. Interpretation of clinical laboratory tests: Reference values and their biological variation. Foster City, CA: Biomedical Publications, 1985.
59. Snedecor GW, Cochran WG. Statistical methods. 8th ed. Ames, IA: Iowa State University Press, 1989.
60. Solberg HE. Discriminant analysis. Crit Rev Clin Lab Sci 1978;9:209-42.
61. Solberg HE. Inaccuracies in computer calculation of standard deviation. Anal Chem 1983;55:1611.
62. Solberg HE. Presentation of observed values in relation to reference values. Bull Mol Biol Med 1983;8:21-6.
63. Solberg HE. Statistical treatment of reference values in laboratory medicine: Testing the goodness-of-fit of an observed distribution to the Gaussian distribution. Scand J Clin Lab Invest 1986;46 (Suppl. 184):125-32.
64. Solberg HE. Using a hospitalized population to establish reference intervals: Pros and cons [Editorial]. Clin Chem 1994;40:2205-6.
65. Solberg HE. RefVal: A program implementing the recommendations of the International Federation of Clinical Chemistry on the statistical treatment of reference values. Comput Meth Progr Biomed 1995;48:247-56. (The program is available from the author. Also see Clin Chem Acta 1993;222:19-21.)
66. Solberg HE, Gräsbeck R. Reference values. Adv Clin Chem 1989;27:1-79.
67. SPSS. Chicago, IL: SPSS Inc. http://www.spss.com/ (Accessed May 2003).
68. Statland BE. Clinical decision levels for lab tests. Oradell, NJ: Medical Economics Books, 1987.
69. Stephens MA. EDF statistics for goodness of fit and some comparisons. J Am Stat Assoc 1974;69:730-7.
70. Strike PW, Michaeloudis A, Green AJ. Standardizing clinical laboratory data for the development of transferable computer-based diagnostic programs. Clin Chem 1986;32:22-9.
71. Sunderman FW. Current concepts of "normal values," "reference values," and "discrimination values" in clinical chemistry [Editorial]. Clin Chem 1975;21:1873-7.
72. Tietz NW, ed. Clinical guide to laboratory tests. 3rd ed. Philadelphia: WB Saunders, 1995.
73. Tryding N, Tufvesson C, Sonntag O, eds. Drug effects in clinical chemistry. 7th ed. Stockholm: Apoteksbolaget, 1996. [The references are found in a separate book:] Tryding N, Tufvesson C, eds. References to drug effects in clinical chemistry. Stockholm: Apoteksbolaget, 1996.
74. Van Der Meulen EA, Boogard PJ, Van Sittert NJ. Use of small-sample-based reference limits on a group basis. Clin Chem 1994;40:1698-702.
75. Virtanen A, Kairisto V, Uusipaikka E. Regression-based reference limits: determination of sufficient sample size. Clin Chem 1998;44:2353-8.
76. Winkel P. Patterns and clusters: Multivariate approach for interpreting clinical chemistry results. Clin Chem 1973;19:1329-38.
77. Winkel P. The use of the subject as his own referent. In: Gräsbeck R, Alström T, eds. Reference values in laboratory medicine. Chichester, England: John Wiley, 1981:65-78.
78. Winkel P, Lyngbye J, Jorgensen K. The normal region: A multivariate problem. Scand J Clin Lab Invest 1972;30:339-44.
79. Young DS. Effects of preanalytical variables on clinical laboratory tests. 2nd ed. Washington, DC: AACC Press, 1997.
80. Young DS. Effects of drugs on clinical laboratory tests. 5th ed. Washington, DC: AACC Press, 2000.

CHAPTER 17

Preanalytical Variables and Biological Variation

Donald S. Young, M.B., Ph.D., and Edward W. Bermes, Jr., Ph.D.

The human body is composed of many different compounds and elements; the concentration or activities of these analytes are a reflection of the individual's health or pathophysiological state. However, both preanalytical variables and biological variation affect the concentration or activities of these analytes.[17,30,37]

PREANALYTICAL VARIABLES

Preanalytical variables fall under two categories—those that are controllable and those that are not. Those that can be controlled have short-lived effects. Duration of the other factors is much longer. Standardization of specimen collection practices minimizes the variables that cause changes in test values within one day or from one day to another and thereby reduces the difficulty in interpretation of values (see Chapter 2). However, in many healthcare facilities, standardization is not always possible. Thus one must understand the influences of both controllable and uncontrollable variables on the composition of body fluids.

CONTROLLABLE VARIABLES

Many of the preanalytical variables related to specimen collection that were discussed in Chapter 2 are examples of controllable variables. Others include physiological variables and those associated with diet, lifestyle, stimulants, drugs, herbal preparations, and recreational drug ingestion.

Physiological Variables

Physiological variables that are controllable that affect analytical results include posture, prolonged bed rest, exercise, physical training, circadian variation, and travel.

Posture

In an adult, a change from a lying to an upright position results in a reduction of an individual's blood volume of about 10% (~600 to 700 mL). Because only protein-free fluid passes through the capillaries to the tissue, this change in posture results in the reduction of the plasma volume of the blood and an increase (~8% to 10%) in the plasma protein concentration. Normally the decrease with the change from lying to standing is complete in 10 minutes. However, 30 minutes is required for such a change to occur when one goes from standing to lying.

The typical pressure at the arterial end of a capillary is 24 mm Hg (3.2 kPa) and at the venous end 10 mm Hg (1.3 kPa), although it varies with the distance of the capillary from the heart.[42] Transfer of fluid and solute across a capillary wall depends on a complex interaction of hydrostatic and osmotic pressures of the capillary and interstitial fluids. Fluid moves into the interstitial space at the arteriolar end of the capillary and returns to the capillary at the venular end. A greater volume of fluid leaves the capillary at the arteriolar end than is returned to the venous end. The excess drains into the lymphatic system. When an individual lies down, more fluid returns to the capillaries because the capillary pressure is reduced. The volume of fluid returning to capillaries progressively declines when an individual is recumbent for a long time. Diuresis serves as a mechanism to prevent overloading of the vascular system.

Heart rate and systolic and diastolic blood pressures are greater in the upright than in the recumbent individual. The change in posture from lying to standing increases the secretion of catecholamines, aldosterone, angiotensin II, renin, and antidiuretic hormone. Epinephrine and norepinephrine concentrations in plasma may double within 10 minutes, but there is no change in their urinary excretion. The increase of plasma aldosterone and plasma renin activity is slower, but their concentrations may still double within 1 hour.

Substantial changes also take place with a change from the lying to the sitting position[45] or from standing to a supine or sitting position.[9] The reduction of the extracellular fluid volume with standing reduces the renal blood flow and causes a reduction of the glomerular filtration rate and urine production. The changes are apparent in 1 hour. Lithium, used therapeutically to treat some forms of schizophrenia, responds in the same way as sodium to postural changes. Sodium, potassium, and lithium excretions are reduced in response to increased hormone secretion, but the normal diurnal variation persists. When an individual stands, his urinary pH decreases and excretion of bicarbonate is reduced as hydrogen ions are exchanged for sodium. The excretion of protein is reduced in most individuals with the reduction of the glomerular filtration rate that occurs with standing. Orthostatic proteinuria is a condition in which protein is present when individuals are standing but essentially absent when they are recumbent. This phenomenon is possibly caused by increased glomerular permeability from increased venous pressure. The incidence of orthostatic proteinuria is probably less than 5%.

Normally the alteration of blood volume that takes place with a change from standing to lying is complete in 30 minutes. The decrease with the change from lying to standing is complete in 10 minutes. Changes in concentration of proteins and protein-bound constituents in serum are greater in hypertensive patients than normotensive patients, in individuals with a low plasma protein concentration than in those with a normal concentration, and in the elderly compared with the young. Most of the plasma oncotic pressure is attributable to albumin because of its high concentration, so that protein malnutrition—with its associated reduction of plasma albumin concentration—reduces the retention of the fluid within the capillaries. Conversely the impact of postural changes is less in individuals with abnormally high concentrations of protein, such as those with a monoclonal gammopathy (multiple myeloma).

In general, the concentrations of freely diffusible constituents with molecular weights of less than 5000 Da are unaffected by postural changes. However, a significant increase in potassium (~0.2 to 0.3 mmol/L) occurs after an individual stands for 30 minutes. This increase in K^+ has been attributed to the release of intracellular potassium from muscle. Although postural changes affect urinary sodium excretion, its plasma concentration is only slightly affected.

Changes in the concentration of some major serum constituents with change in posture are listed in Table 17-1.

TABLE 17-1 Change in Concentration of Serum Constituents With Change from Lying to Standing

Constituent	Average Increase (%)
Alanine aminotransferase	7
Albumin	9
Alkaline phosphatase	7
Amylase	6
Aspartate aminotransferase	5
Calcium	3
Cholesterol	7
IgA	7
IgG	7
IgM	5
Thyroxine	11
Triglycerides	6

From Felding P, Tryding N, Hyltoft Petersen P, et al. Effects of posture on concentrations of blood constituents in healthy adults: Practical application of blood specimen collection procedures recommended by the Scandinavian Committee on Reference Values. Scand J Clin Lab Invest 1980;40:615-21.

Prolonged Bed Rest

The plasma and extracellular fluid volumes decrease within a few days of the start of bed rest. Consequently the blood hematocrit may increase by as much as 10% within 4 days. There is usually a slight reduction of total body water.

With prolonged bed rest, fluid retention occurs and plasma protein and albumin concentrations may be decreased by an average of 0.5 and 0.3 g/dL, respectively. The concentrations of protein-bound constituents are also reduced, although mobilization of calcium from bones with an increased free ionized fraction compensates for the reduced protein-bound calcium, so serum total calcium is less affected. Serum aspartate aminotransferase activity is usually slightly less in individuals confined to bed than in those undertaking normal physical activity. Initially and paradoxically, creatine kinase (CK) activity is increased as a result of its release from skeletal muscles, but ultimately, CK activity may be less than in active, healthy individuals. Serum potassium may be reduced by up to 0.5 mmol/L because of reduction of skeletal muscle mass.

Prolonged bed rest is associated with increased urinary nitrogen excretion. Calcium, sodium, potassium, phosphate, and sulfate excretions are increased; hydrogen ion excretion is reduced, presumably caused by decreased metabolism of skeletal muscle.[13] The amplitude of circadian variation of plasma cortisol is reduced by prolonged immobilization, and the urinary excretion of catecholamines may be reduced to one third of the concentration in an active individual. Vanillylmandelic acid excretion is reduced by one fourth after 2 to 3 weeks of bed rest.

When an individual becomes active after a period of bed rest, more than 3 weeks are required before calcium excretion reverts to normal, and another 3 weeks before positive calcium balance is achieved. Several weeks are required before positive nitrogen balance is restored.

Exercise

In considering the effects of exercise the nature and extent of the exercise should be taken into account. Static or isometric exercise, usually of short duration but of high intensity, uses previously stored adenosine triphosphate (ATP) and creatine phosphate whereas more prolonged exercise must use ATP generated by the normal metabolic pathways. The changes in concentrations of analytes as a result of exercise are largely due to shifts of fluid between the intravascular and interstitial compartments, changes in hormone concentrations stimulated by the change in activity and by loss of fluid due to sweating. The physical fitness of an individual may also affect the extent of a change in the concentration of a constituent. Such factors account for the sometimes conflicting reports in the literature. Whether these effects are significant often depends on how long after an exercise activity a specimen was collected.

With *moderate exercise,* the provoked stress response causes an increase in the blood glucose, which stimulates insulin secretion. The arteriovenous difference in glucose concentration is increased by the greater tissue demand for glucose. Plasma pyruvate and lactate are increased by the increased metabolic activity of skeletal muscle. Even mild exercise may increase the plasma lactate twofold. Arterial pH and PCO_2 are reduced by exercise. Reduced renal blood flow causes a slight increase in the serum creatinine concentration. Competition between uric acid and lactate and products of increased tissue catabolism for renal excretion causes the serum urate concentration to increase. Exercise causes a reduction of cellular ATP, which increases cellular permeability. The increased permeability causes slight increases in the serum activities of enzymes originating from skeletal muscle, such as aspartate aminotransferase (AST), lactate dehydrogenase (LD), CK, and aldolase.[51] The increase of enzyme activity tends to be greater in unfit than fit individuals. As little as 5 minutes of walking increases the activity of these enzymes in plasma. Mild exercise produces a slight decrease in the serum cholesterol and triglyceride concentrations that may persist for several days. Those who walk for about 4 hours each week have an average cholesterol concentration 5% lower and high-density lipoprotein (HDL) concentration 3.4% higher than inactive individuals.

In general the effects of *strenuous exercise* are exaggerations of those occurring with mild exercise. Thus hypoglycemia and increased glucose tolerance may occur. The plasma lactate may be increased tenfold. Severe exercise increases the concentration of plasma proteins owing to an influx of protein from interstitial spaces, which occurs after an initial loss of both fluid and protein through the capillaries. The plasma concentrations of glycoproteins, transferrin, and α_2-macroglobulin are typically increased.[23] Fibrinolytic activity is also increased. Strenuous exercise may more than double CK activity, but the activity of enzymes with primarily liver or kidney origins is little changed, although both hepatic and renal blood flow are reduced.

Strenuous exercise for 10 minutes increases plasma renin activity by 400%. Cortisol secretion is stimulated and the normal diurnal variation may be abolished.[12] Urinary free cortisol excretion and the plasma concentrations of cortisol, aldosterone, growth hormone, somatotropin, and prolactin are also increased by exercise. Plasma insulin concentration is decreased by exercise. Strenuous exercise increases both the plasma and urinary concentrations of catecholamines. The changes in hormone concentrations are probably responsible for the increase in leukocyte count to about 25,000 cells/μL that has been observed following strenuous exercise.

The blood pH, oxygen saturation, and venous bicarbonate concentrations are decreased by strenuous exercise. The concentration of triglycerides is reduced briefly by exercise, but the free fatty acid concentration is greatly increased; serum creatinine and urea nitrogen concentrations are also increased. Although the creatinine concentration returns rapidly to normal on the cessation of exercise, the increased urea nitrogen concentration persists for some time. Reversible, benign hematuria and proteinuria occur commonly with exercise and worsen in proportion to the extent of the exercise. These may persist for 3 days following strenuous sports but do not warrant investigation.

Some representative changes in concentration or activity of serum constituents induced by exercise are listed in Table 17-2.

Physical Training

Athletes generally have a higher serum activity of enzymes of skeletal muscular origin at rest than do nonathletes. However, the response of these enzymes to exercise is less in athletes than in other individuals. The reduced release of enzymes from skeletal muscle in well-trained individuals has been attributed to an increase in the number and size of mitochondria allowing the muscle to better metabolize glucose, fatty acids, and ketone bodies. The proportion of CK that is CK-MB is much greater in the trained than untrained individual. Serum concentrations of urea, urate, creatinine, and thyroxine are higher in athletes than in comparable untrained individuals.[55] Urinary excretion of creatinine is also increased. These changes are probably related to the increased muscle mass and a greater turnover of muscle mass in athletes.

The total serum lipid concentration is reduced by physical conditioning; serum cholesterol may be lowered by as much as 25%. HDL cholesterol, however, is increased. Thus the decrease in total cholesterol concentration is mostly due to a reduction in low-density lipoprotein (LDL) cholesterol. The concentration of serum apolipoprotein A-1 increases with training, whereas the concentration of apolipoprotein B decreases. The serum triglyceride concentration may be reduced by up to 20 mg/dL (0.23 mmol/L), but the free fatty acid concentration is higher in fit individuals than others. Loss of body fat is associated with improvement in lipid concentrations. The lactate response to exercise is

TABLE 17-2 Effect of Strenuous Exercise on Selected Serum Constituents*

Constituent Value	% Increase	Constituent Value	% Decrease
Acid phosphatase	11	Albumin	4
Alanine aminotransferase	41	Bilirubin	4
Alkaline phosphatase	3	Iron	11
Aspartate aminotransferase	31	Lactate dehydrogenase	1
Calcium	1	Potassium	8
Chloride	1	Sodium	1
Cholesterol	3	Total lipids	12
Creatinine	17		
Phosphate	12		
Total protein	3		
Urea nitrogen	3		
Uric acid	4		

From Statland BE, Winkel P, Bokelund H. Factors contributing to variation of serum constituents in healthy subjects. In: Siest G, ed. Organisation des laboratoires. Biologie perspective. Paris: L'Expansion Scientifique Francaise, 1975:717-50.
*Changes were determined 15 min after conclusion of 20 min exercise.

reduced in trained athletes compared with untrained individuals. In general the same exercise produces a less marked biochemical response in the fit person than in the unfit person.

Circadian Variation

Many constituents of body fluids exhibit cyclical variations throughout the day.[53] Factors contributing to such variations include posture, activity, food ingestion, stress, daylight or darkness, and sleep or wakefulness. These cyclical variations may be quite large, and therefore the drawing of the specimen must be strictly controlled. For example, the concentration of serum iron may change by as much as 50% from 0800 to 1400, and that of cortisol by a similar amount between 0800 and 1600. Serum potassium has been reported to decline from 5.4 mmol/L at 0800 to 4.3 mmol/L at 1400.[49] The typical total variation of several commonly measured serum constituents over 6 hours is illustrated in Table 17-3. The total variation is listed together with analytical error.

Hormones are secreted in bursts, and this, together with the cyclical variation to which most hormones are subject, may make it very difficult to interpret their serum concentration properly. Corticotropin secretion is influenced by cortisol-like steroids, but it is also affected by posture and by light, darkness, and stress. Its secretion is increased threefold to fivefold from its minimum between afternoon and midnight to its maximum around waking. Cortisol concentrations are greatest around 0600 to 0800 hours and may be twice as high as those observed at midnight.[52]

Maximum renin activity normally occurs early in the morning during sleep; its minimum occurs late in the afternoon. The plasma aldosterone concentration shows a similar pattern. Glomerular filtration rate (GFR) varies inversely with the secretion of renin. GFR is least at the time of maximum renin secretion and 20% greater in the afternoon when renin activity is at a minimum. The excretion of 17-ketosteroids and 17-hydroxycorticosteroids is low at night and reaches a maximum about midafternoon.

There is no circadian variation in the plasma concentrations of follicle-stimulating hormone (FSH) and luteinizing hormone (LH) in men, but a 20% to 40% increase of plasma testosterone occurs during the night. Prolactin is secreted, like other hormones, in multiple bursts; prolactin concentration is greatest during sleep.

The serum thyroid-stimulating hormone (TSH) is at a maximum between 0200 and 0400 and at a minimum between 1800 and 2200. The variation is of the order of 50%. There are also variations in the serum thyroxine concentration, but these appear to be related to the changes in concentration of binding protein brought about by changes in posture. These variations are maximal between 1000 and 1400. Total protein concentration may vary by as much as 10% over 24 hours, but the variation of individual proteins may be even greater.

Growth hormone secretion is greatest shortly after sleep commences. Conversely, basal plasma insulin is higher in the morning than later in the day, and its response to glucose is also greatest in the morning and least about midnight. When a glucose tolerance test is given in the afternoon, higher glucose values occur than when the test is given early in the day. The higher plasma glucose occurs in spite of a greater insulin response, which is nevertheless delayed and less effective.

Urinary excretion of catecholamines and their metabolites is less at night than during the day. The effect is related to activity, because in night workers excretion is less during the day.

The peak urinary excretion of sodium and potassium is about noon, whereas the excretion of calcium and magne-

TABLE 17-3 Total and Analytical Variation for Serum Tests on Specimens Obtained at 0800 and 1400*

Constituent	Mean	Total Variation (%)	Analytical Variation (%)
Sodium (mmol/L)	141	1.9	1.8
Potassium (mmol/L)	4.4	7.1	2.8
Calcium (mg/dL)	10.8	3.2	2.7
Chloride (mmol/L)	102	3.8	3.4
Phosphate (mg/dL)	3.8	10.7	2.4
Urea nitrogen (mg/dL)	14	22.5	2.5
Creatinine (mg/dL)	1.0	14.5	6.3
Uric acid (mg/dL)	5.6	11.5	2.6
Iron (μg/dL)	116	36.6	3.4
Cholesterol (mg/dL)	193	14.8	5.7
Albumin (g/dL)	4.5	5.5	3.9
Total protein (g/dL)	7.3	4.8	1.7
Total lipids (g/L)	5.3	25.0	3.6
Aspartate aminotransferase (U/L)	9	25	6
Alanine aminotransferase (U/L)	6	56	17
Acid phosphatase (U/L)	3	15	8
Alkaline phosphatase (U/L)	63	20	3
Lactate dehydrogenase (U/L)	195	16	12

From Winkel P, Statland BE, Bokelund H. The effects of time of venipuncture on variation of serum constituents. Am J Clin Pathol 1975;64:433-47. Copyright 1975 by the American Society of Clinical Pathologists. Reprinted with permission.
*11 male subjects, age 21-27 years, studied at 0800, 1100, 1400.

sium is greatest during the night. Urinary phosphate excretion is low at night, with the result that serum phosphate is as much as 30% higher at night than during the morning. Urinary volume and creatinine excretion are low during the night. The creatinine clearance may be reduced by up to 10% during the night. Night urine contains excess ammonia and its titratable acidity is high.[50]

Travel

Travel across several time zones affects the normal circadian rhythm. Five days are required to establish a new stable diurnal rhythm after travel across 10 time zones. The changes in laboratory test results are attributable to altered pituitary and adrenal function. Urinary excretion of catecholamines is usually increased for 2 days; serum cortisol is reduced. During a flight, serum glucose and triglyceride concentrations increase, while glucocorticoid secretion is stimulated. During a prolonged flight, fluid and sodium retention occur, but urinary excretion returns to normal after 2 days.[8]

Space travel is associated with a decrease in blood and plasma volumes and is further associated with increases in plasma antidiuretic hormone, atrial natriuretic peptide, growth hormone, cortisol, and corticotropin concentrations. In contrast, the plasma renin activity may be decreased by as much as 50%. Plasma aldosterone may also decrease but to a lesser extent. In spite of the stress of space travel the plasma concentrations of catecholamines are usually unaffected. Plasma and urine calcium concentrations increase during space missions. Plasma sodium concentration decreases while its concentration in the urine increases.

Diet

Diet has considerable influence on the composition of plasma. Studies with synthetic diets have shown that day-to-day changes in the amount of protein are reflected within a few days in the composition of the plasma and in the excretion of end products of protein metabolism.

Four days after the change from a normal diet to a high-protein diet, a doubling of the plasma urea concentration occurs with an increase in its urinary excretion.[6] Serum cholesterol, phosphate, urate, and ammonia concentrations are also increased. A high-protein intake increases both serum and urinary urea and urate. A high-fat diet, in contrast, depletes the nitrogen pool because of the requirement for excretion of ammonium ions to maintain acid-base homeostasis. A high-fat diet increases the serum concentration of triglycerides but also reduces serum urate. Reduction of fat intake reduces serum lactate dehydrogenase activity. The ingestion of very different amounts of cholesterol has little effect on the serum cholesterol concentration; an increase in intake of 50% may only affect the serum concentration by 5 to 10 mg/dL (0.13 to 0.26 mmol/L).[32] Ingestion of monounsaturated fat instead of saturated fat reduces cholesterol and LDL cholesterol concentrations. When polyunsaturated fat is substituted for saturated fat the concentrations of triglycerides and HDL cholesterol are reduced.

When dietary carbohydrates consist mainly of starch or sucrose rather than other sugars, the serum activities of alkaline phosphatase (ALP) and LD are increased. AST activity is also influenced by the type of sugar ingested. The plasma triglyceride concentration is reduced when sucrose intake is decreased. Flatter glucose tolerance curves are observed with a bread diet than when a high-sucrose diet is ingested. A high-carbohydrate diet decreases the serum concentrations of very low-density lipoprotein (VLDL) cholesterol, triglycerides, cholesterol, and protein. Individuals who eat many small meals throughout the day tend to have concentrations of total LDL and HDL cholesterol concentrations that are lower than when the same type and amount of food is eaten in three meals.

In addition to the types of food and drinks ingested, specific food-related situations will also influence plasma composition. They include vegetarianism, obesity, malnutrition, fasting, and starvation.

Food Ingestion

The concentration of certain plasma constituents is affected by the ingestion of a meal, with the time between the ingestion of a meal and the collection of blood affecting the plasma concentrations of many analytes. For example, fasting overnight for 10 to 14 hours noticeably decreases the variability in the concentrations of many analytes and is seen as the optimal time for fasting around which to standardize blood collections. The biggest increases in serum concentrations occurring after a meal are for glucose, iron, total lipids, and ALP. The increase in ALP (mainly intestinal isoenzyme) is greater when a fatty meal is ingested and is influenced by the blood group of the individual and the substrate used for the enzyme assay. In addition, lipemia may affect some analytical methods used to measure serum constituents. Ultracentrifugation or the use of serum blanks can reduce the adverse analytical effects of lipemia.

The effects of a meal may be long lasting. Thus ingestion of a protein-rich meal in the evening may cause increases in the serum urea nitrogen, phosphorus, and urate concentrations that are still apparent 12 hours later. Nevertheless, these changes may be less than the typical intraindividual variability. Large protein meals at lunch or in the evening also increase the serum cholesterol and growth hormone concentrations for at least 1 hour after a meal. The effect of carbohydrate meals on blood composition is less than that of protein meals. No change in the cortisol concentration is noted when breakfast is taken, probably because cortisol completely occupies all cortisol binding sites on its binding protein in the early morning. Glucagon and insulin secretions are stimulated by a protein meal, and insulin is also stimulated by carbohydrate meals.

In response to a meal, the stomach secretes hydrochloric acid, causing a reduction in the plasma chloride concentration. The venous blood from the stomach contains an increased amount of bicarbonate. This condition reflects a mild metabolic alkalosis ("alkaline tide") and an increased PCO_2. The metabolic alkalosis is sufficient to reduce the serum-free ionized calcium by 0.2 mg/dL (0.05 mmol/L). After ingestion of a meal, the liver becomes the prime site for metabolism of the ingested substances. This metabolic activity may impair its secretory capability and thus accounts for the observed increase in postprandial bilirubin concentration, bromsulphalein (BSP) retention, and serum enzyme activity.

The effects of ingestion of a 700-kcal (2.93 MJ) meal on some commonly measured blood constituents are illustrated in Table 17-4. The effects differ with different meals. Thus glucose increase is often greater and phosphate usually decreases after a carbohydrate meal.

The ingestion of one glass of water has been observed to be followed by statistically significant alterations in the concentration of several of the commonly measured test constituents. When 75 g glucose is ingested with water, as in a glucose tolerance test, the concentration of glucose increases. This stimulates the secretion of insulin. Insulin causes the release of sodium from cells and stimulates the transport of potassium into the cells.

Ingestion of Specific Foods and Beverages

Constituents in food and drink will affect the composition of plasma. Bran, serotonin, and caffeine are examples of such constituents.

Bran. Habitual ingestion of bran impedes the absorption of certain compounds, including calcium, cholesterol, and triglycerides from the gastrointestinal tract. The concentration of calcium may be reduced by as much as 0.3 mg/dL (0.08 mmol/L) and that of triglycerides by 20 mg/dL (0.23 mmol/L), especially if triglycerides were high initially. Pectin and dietary fibers reduce the serum apolipoprotein B and cholesterol concentrations.

Serotonin. Many fruits and vegetables that contain 5-hydroxytryptamine (serotonin), such as bananas, cause an increased excretion of 5-hydroxyindoleacetic acid. Avocados impair glucose tolerance by affecting insulin secretion. Onions reduce both the plasma glucose and insulin response to glucose.

Caffeine. Caffeine is contained in many beverages, including coffee, tea, and colas and has considerable effect on the concentration of blood constituents. Caffeine stimulates the adrenal medulla, causing an increased excretion of the catecholamines and their metabolites and a slight increase in the plasma glucose concentration with impairment of glucose tolerance.[3] The adrenal cortex is also affected; plasma cortisol is increased, accompanied by increased excretion of free cortisol, 11-hydroxycorticoids, and 5-hydroxyindoleacetic acid. The effect of caffeine may be so great that the normal diurnal variation of plasma cortisol may be suppressed.

Caffeine has a marked effect on lipid metabolism. Ingestion of two cups of coffee may increase the plasma free fatty acid concentration by as much as 30% and glycerol, total

TABLE 17-4 Influence of a Standard 700-kcal Meal on Serum Constituents

Constituent	Before Meal	2 hr After Meal
Alanine aminotransferase (U/L)	31	33
Albumin (g/dL)	4.5	4.6
Alkaline phosphatase (U/L)	46	46
Aspartate aminotransferase (U/L)	22	28
Bilirubin (mg/dL)	0.7	0.8
Calcium (mg/dL)	9.9	10.0
Cholesterol (mg/dL)	220.0	220.0
Glucose (mg/dL)	71	82*
Lactate dehydrogenase (U/L)	198	198
Phosphate (mg/dL)	3.1	3.6*
Potassium (mmol/L)	3.8	4.0*
Sodium (mmol/L)	140	141
Total protein (g/dL)	7.8	7.9
Urea nitrogen (mg/dL)	16	16
Uric acid (mg/dL)	6.0	6.2

From Steinmetz J, Panek E, Sourieau F, et al. Influence of food intake on biological parameters. In: Siest G, ed. Reference values in human chemistry. Basel: Karger, 1973:193-200.
Results are mean values in 200 healthy individuals.
*Note also that other studies have reported greater increases in the glucose concentration and a reduction of the phosphate and potassium concentrations depending on the type of meal.

lipids, and lipoproteins to a lesser extent. Activation of triglyceride lipase causes the increase in nonesterified fatty acid concentration. Prolonged ingestion of caffeine (e.g., over several weeks) causes a slight reduction of the serum cholesterol concentration but an increase in the serum triglyceride concentration. No differences have been observed between the effects of caffeinated and decaffeinated coffee.

Caffeine is also a potent stimulant of gastric juice, hydrochloric acid, and pepsin secretion. The serum gastrin concentration may be increased by as much as five times after the ingestion of three cups of coffee. Coffee has a diuretic effect and also increases the excretion of erythrocytes and renal tubular cells in the urine. Caffeine increases the absolute amounts of sodium, potassium, calcium, and magnesium in urine—an effect not observed with decaffeinated coffee.

Vegetarianism

In long-standing vegetarians, the concentrations of LDL and VLDL cholesterol are reduced typically by 37% and 12%, respectively, compared with nonvegetarians. The total lipid and phospholipid concentrations are reduced, and the concentrations of cholesterol and triglycerides may be only two thirds of those in people on a mixed diet. Both HDL and LDL cholesterol concentrations are affected. In strict vegetarians the LDL concentration may be 37% less, and the HDL cholesterol concentration 12% less, than in nonvegetarians. The effects are less noted in individuals who have been on a vegetarian diet for only a short time. The lipid concentrations are also less in individuals who eat only a vegetable diet than in those who consume eggs and milk as well. When individuals previously on a mixed diet begin a vegetarian diet, their serum albumin concentration may fall by 10% and their urea concentration by 50%. However, there is little difference in the concentration of protein or of activities of enzymes in the serum of long-standing vegetarians and individuals on a mixed diet.

Urinary pH is usually higher in vegetarians than in meat eaters because of reduced intake of precursors of acid metabolites. The plasma vitamin B_{12} may be reduced in vegetarians to a concentration approaching that observed in deficiency. Vegetarians tend to have a higher serum bilirubin concentration than do meat eaters. An explanation for the low vitamin B_{12} and high bilirubin still has to be established. Differences in the composition of serum of vegetarians and nonvegetarians are listed in Table 17-5.

Malnutrition

In malnutrition, total serum protein, albumin, and β-globulin concentrations are reduced. The increased concentration of γ-globulin does not fully compensate for the decrease in other proteins. The concentrations of complement C3, retinol-binding globulin, transferrin, and prealbumin decrease rapidly with the onset of malnutrition[40] and are measured to define the severity of the condition. The plasma concentrations of lipoproteins are reduced, and serum cholesterol and triglycerides may be only 50% of the concentrations in healthy individuals. In spite of severe malnutrition, glucose concentration is maintained close to that in healthy individuals. However, the concentrations of serum urea nitrogen and creatinine are greatly reduced as a result of decreased skeletal mass, and creatinine clearance is also decreased.

Plasma cortisol concentration is increased because of decreased metabolic clearance. The plasma concentrations of total triiodothyronine (T_3), thyroxine (T_4), and TSH are considerably reduced, with the thyroxine concentration being most affected. This is partly due to reduced concentrations of thyroxine-binding globulin and prealbumin.

Erythrocyte and plasma folate concentrations are reduced in protein-calorie malnutrition, but the serum vitamin B_{12} concentration is unaffected or may even be slightly increased.[33] The plasma concentrations of vitamins A and E are much reduced. Although the blood hemoglobin concentration is reduced, the serum iron concentration is initially little affected by malnutrition.

The activity of most of the commonly measured enzymes is reduced but increases with restoration of good nutrition.

Fasting and Starvation

Withdrawal of most, or all, caloric intake has been used to treat certain cases of obesity. Such withdrawal provokes many metabolic responses. The body attempts to conserve protein at the expense of other sources of energy, such as fat. The blood glucose concentration decreases by as much as 18 mg/dL (1 mmol/L) within the first 3 days of the start of a fast in spite of the body's attempts to maintain glucose production.[36] Insulin secretion is greatly reduced, whereas glucagon secretion may double in an attempt to maintain normal glucose concentration. Lipolysis and hepatic ketogenesis are stimulated. Ketoacids and fatty acids become the principal sources of energy for muscle. This results in an accumulation of organic acids that leads to a metabolic acidosis with reduction of the blood pH, PCO_2, and plasma bicarbonate concentrations. In addition, the concentrations of ketone bodies (acetoacetic acid and β-hydroxybutyric acid), fatty acids, and glycerol in serum rise considerably. Often the blood PO_2 is also reduced. Fasting for 6 days increases the plasma concentrations of cholesterol and triglycerides but causes a decrease in HDL concentration. With more prolonged fasting the concentrations of cholesterol and triglycerides decrease. Amino acids are released from skeletal muscle and the plasma concentration of the branched-chain amino acids may increase by as much as 100% with 1 day of fasting, but the urea concentration decreases.

TABLE 17-5 Comparison of Blood Constituents between Vegetarians and Nonvegetarians

Constituent	Vegetarians	Nonvegetarians
S-Albumin (g/dL)	4.2	4.2
P-Calcium (mg/dL)	9.4	9.7
P-Cholesterol (mg/dL)	213	252
P-HDL cholesterol (mg/dL)	66	66
B-Glucose (mg/dL)	90	101
B-Hemoglobin (g/dL)	13.9	14.3
P-Triglycerides (mg/dL)	106	124
B-Urea nitrogen (mg/dL)	14	16
P-Uric acid (mg/dL)	5.3	5.8

From Gear JS, Mann JI, Thorogood M, et al. Biochemical and haematological variables in vegetarians. BMJ 1980;280:1415.
S, Serum; *P*, plasma; *B*, whole blood.

The breakdown of fat leads to a transient increase in body water. Normally, however, an osmotic diuresis soon reduces the blood volume even though glomerular filtration may be impaired, as demonstrated by increased serum creatinine concentration and reduced creatinine clearance. Hepatic blood supply may also be reduced. BSP retention is increased, and the serum bilirubin rises; the unconjugated bilirubin more than doubles within 48 hours.[1] Increased serum activities of aspartate and alanine aminotransferase and of lactate dehydrogenase are observed. The enzyme changes may be linked more to focal necrosis of the liver than to general circulatory impairment.

In spite of the catabolism of tissue induced by starvation, the serum protein concentration is little affected initially; ultimately, a reduction occurs. However, from the beginning, the catabolism of nucleoproteins causes an increased serum urate. Rise in serum urate is exacerbated by the reduced GFR and the competition for excretion from lactate and ketoacids.

With the onset of starvation, aldosterone secretion increases with the results of increased urinary excretion and decreased plasma concentration of potassium. Magnesium, calcium, and phosphate are affected similarly, although the urinary excretion of phosphate gradually declines. The absolute urinary excretion of ammonia and creatinine increases with prolonged starvation but that of urea decreases.

Plasma growth hormone concentration may rise by as much as 15 times at the start of a fast but may return to normal after 3 days. Reduced energy expenditure is associated with decreased concentrations of thyroid hormones. Free and total triiodothyronine decrease by up to 50% within 3 days of the start of a fast. Free thyroxine concentration is also affected, but to a lesser extent; total thyroxine is little changed. Urinary free cortisol is decreased by fasting, and the plasma cortisol concentration (free and total) shows a slight increase together with loss of the normal diurnal variation.

Early in refeeding, sodium retention occurs as a result of decreased sodium and chloride excretion in the urine.[43] The reduction in potassium excretion takes longer. These events are associated with an even greater secretion of aldosterone than occurs during the period of fasting. The abnormal concentrations of most constituents rapidly revert to normal with refeeding. Nitrogen balance soon becomes positive, especially if the nonprotein calories are mainly from carbohydrate.

Lifestyle

Lifestyle factors that affect the levels of commonly measured analytes include smoking and alcohol ingestion.

Smoking

Smoking, through the action of nicotine, may affect several laboratory tests. The extent of the effect is related to the number of cigarettes smoked and to the amount of smoke inhaled.

Through stimulation of the adrenal medulla, nicotine increases the concentration of epinephrine in the plasma and the urinary excretion of catecholamines and their metabolites.[10] Glucose concentration may be increased by 10 mg/dL (0.56 mmol/L) within 10 minutes of smoking a cigarette. The increase may persist for 1 hour. Plasma lactate is increased, and because the pyruvate concentration is reduced, the lactate-pyruvate ratio is increased. Plasma insulin concentration shows a delayed response to the increased blood glucose, rising about 1 hour after a cigarette is smoked. Typically the plasma glucose concentration is higher in smokers than in nonsmokers, and glucose tolerance is mildly impaired in smokers. The plasma growth hormone concentration is particularly sensitive to smoking. It may increase tenfold within 30 minutes after an individual has smoked a cigarette.

The plasma cholesterol, triglyceride, and LDL cholesterol concentrations are higher (by about 3%, 9.1%, and 1.7%, respectively), as is that of β-lipoprotein, and HDL cholesterol is lower in smokers than in nonsmokers. Free fatty acid concentration tends to be variable, but inhalation during smoking produces an immediate increase of free fatty acids of about 30%. Some of the effects of smoking on serum constituents are listed in Table 17-6.

TABLE 17-6 Reported Increased Concentrations in Serum in Smokers

Constituent	% Change
Albumin	3
Cholesterol	4
Glucose	10
Phospholipids	5
Triglycerides	20
Urea nitrogen	10

From Siest G, Henny J, Schiele F, (eds). Interpretation des examens de laboratoire. Basel: Karger, 1981.

Smoking affects both the adrenal cortex and the medulla; plasma 11-hydroxycorticosteroids may be increased by 75% with heavy smoking. In addition, the plasma cortisol concentration may increase by as much as 40% within 5 minutes of the start of smoking, although the normal diurnal rhythmicity of cortisol is unaffected. Smokers excrete more 5-hydroxyindoleacetic acid than do nonsmokers.

The blood erythrocyte count is increased in smokers. The amount of carboxyhemoglobin may exceed 10% of the total hemoglobin in heavy smokers, and the increased number of cells compensates for impaired ability of the red cells to transport oxygen. The blood PO_2 of the habitual smoker is usually about 5 mm Hg (0.7 kPa) less than in the nonsmoker, whereas the PCO_2 is unaffected. The blood leukocyte concentration is increased by as much as 30% in smokers, but the leukocyte concentration of ascorbic acid is greatly reduced. The lymphocyte count is increased as a proportion of the total leukocyte count.

Fluid retention caused by nicotine causes a mild decrease in the plasma protein concentration but without demonstrable effect on the calcium concentration or on the activity of serum enzymes. The plasma urate concentration is less in smokers than in nonsmokers, probably as a result of lessened intake of food by smokers. Both the serum urea and creatinine concentrations tend to be less in smokers than in nonsmokers.

Nicotine is a potent stimulant of the secretion of gastric juice. Both volume and acid secretion are increased within 1 hour of smoking several cigarettes. In contrast, the bicarbonate concentration and volume of pancreatic juice are reduced.

Smoking affects the body's immune response. For example, serum IgA, IgG, and IgM levels are generally lower in smokers than in nonsmokers, whereas the IgE concentration is higher. Smokers, more often than nonsmokers, may show the presence of antinuclear antibodies and test weakly positive for carcinoembryonic antigen. The sperm count of male smokers is often reduced compared with that in nonsmokers: the number of abnormal forms is greater and sperm motility is less.

The serum vitamin B_{12} concentration is often notably reduced in smokers, and the decrease is in inverse proportion to the serum concentration of thiocyanate.

Alcohol Ingestion

A single moderate dose of alcohol has few effects on laboratory tests. Ingestion of enough alcohol to produce mild inebriation may increase the blood glucose concentration by 20% to 50%. The increase may be even higher in diabetics. More commonly, inhibition of gluconeogenesis occurs and becomes apparent as hypoglycemia and ketonemia and ethanol is metabolized to acetaldehyde and to acetate. Hypoglycemia is most common in children, alcoholics, and the malnourished. Lactate accumulates and competes with urate for excretion in the kidneys so that the serum urate is also increased. Lactate and acetate together decrease the plasma bicarbonate, leading to metabolic acidosis. Marked hypertriglyceridemia after alcohol ingestion is due to a combination of increased triglyceride formation in the liver and impaired removal of chylomicrons and VLDL from the circulation. The effect is most noticeable when alcohol is ingested with a fatty meal. The effect may persist for longer than 12 hours. When moderate amounts of alcohol are ingested for 1 week, the serum triglyceride concentration is increased by more than 20 mg/dL (0.23 mmol/L). Prolonged moderate ingestion of alcohol may increase the HDL cholesterol concentration, which is associated with reduced plasma concentration of cholesterol ester transfer protein (CETP). Phenols in wine with potent antioxidant activity are probably responsible for reducing the oxidation of LDL cholesterol.

Intoxicating amounts of alcohol stimulate the release of cortisol, although the effect is more related to the intoxication than to the alcohol per se. Sympatheticomedullary activity is increased by acute alcohol ingestion but without detectable effect on the plasma epinephrine concentration and only a mild effect on norepinephrine. With intoxication, plasma concentrations of catecholamines are substantially increased. Acute ingestion of alcohol leads to a sharp reduction in the plasma testosterone in men, with an increase in the plasma luteinizing hormone concentration.

Chronic alcohol ingestion affects the activity of many serum enzymes. Gamma-glutamyl transferase (GGT) activity has been extensively studied, and increased activity of the enzyme is used as a marker of persistent drinking. A single acute ingestion of alcohol has been reported to increase the serum activity of the enzyme, a manifestation of hepatic microsomal enzyme induction. Chronic alcoholism is associated with many characteristic biochemical abnormalities, including abnormal pituitary, adrenocortical, and medullary function. Acute alcohol ingestion has been reported to increase the activity of several serum enzymes, including GGT, isocitrate dehydrogenase, and ornithine carbamoyl transferase.[19,21] Alcohol ingestion also has considerable influence on serum HDL cholesterol and total cholesterol concentration.[58] Measurement of carbohydrate-deficient transferrin is becoming increasingly popular as a means of identifying habitual alcohol ingestion. Desialylation of proteins occurs because of inhibition of enzymatic glycosylation in the liver by alcohol. Increased mean cell volume (MCV) has also been used as a marker of habitual alcohol use and may be related to folic acid deficiency or a direct toxic effect of alcohol on red blood cell precursors.

Drug Administration

It is rare for a patient to be hospitalized without receiving medication. For certain medical conditions, more than 10 drugs may be administered at one time. Even many healthy individuals take several drugs regularly, such as vitamins, oral contraceptives, or sleeping tablets. Individuals with chronic diseases often ingest drugs on a continuing basis. Drugs may have both in vivo and in vitro effects on laboratory tests. The in vivo effects arise from the therapeutic intent of drugs, their side effects, and patient idiosyncrasies. Effects on the composition of body fluids are likely to be more apparent when large doses of a drug are administered for a long time than when administration of a single dose occurs on an isolated occasion.

Comprehensive listings of the effects of drugs on laboratory tests have been published.[56,57] Only a few representative effects are discussed here. Many drugs, when administered intramuscularly, cause sufficient muscle irritation to increase amounts of enzyme released into the serum. The activities of CK, aldolase, and the skeletal muscle component of lactate dehydrogenase are increased in the serum. The increased activities may persist for several days after a single injection, and consistently high values may be observed during a course of treatment. *Penicillin* derivatives given intramuscularly are particularly likely to increase the activity of these enzymes, although any drug given intramuscularly appears capable of increasing enzyme activity. Drugs that have been demonstrated to increase serum CK activity after intramuscular injection are listed in Table 17-7. *Opiates,* such as morphine or meperidine, can cause spasm of the sphincter of Oddi. The spasm transmits pressure back to the liver, causing release of liver and pancreatic enzymes into the serum. Increases in aspartate aminotransferase activity may be so large that they may be suggestive of a myocardial infarction.

Oral contraceptives affect many different constituents measured in the clinical laboratory. Tests are affected by both the progestin and estrogen components. The overall effect depends on the proportion and amount of the two components.

Diuretic drugs often cause a mild reduction of the plasma potassium concentration; hyponatremia may be observed. Hypercalcemia may occur with hemoconcentration, but occasionally the free-ionized and the protein-bound fraction is increased. Thiazides cause hyperglycemia and reduce glucose tolerance, especially in diabetics. Thiazides may cause prerenal azotemia with hyperuricemia as a result of decreased renal blood flow and GFR as a result of reduced blood volume. Thiazides, like other diuretics, by causing hemoconcentration increase the plasma concentration of lipids. Many thiazides induce microsomal enzymes and thus affect lipoprotein concentrations.

TABLE 17-7 Drugs Associated With Increased Serum Creatine Kinase Activity After Intramuscular Injection

Ampicillin	Chlorpromazine	Meperidine
Analgesics	Clindamycin	Morphine
Antibiotics	Digoxin	Penicillin
Barbiturates	Diuretics	Phenothiazines
Carbenicillin	Lidocaine	Tubocurarine

The broad range of possible effects of a drug on clinical laboratory tests is exemplified by *phenytoin.* With long-term treatment, many patients have reduced serum calcium and phosphate concentrations and increased activity of ALP. Phenytoin induces the synthesis of bilirubin-conjugating enzymes in the liver. Consequently the serum bilirubin concentration is reduced, serum GGT activity is increased, and urinary glucaric acid excretion is augmented. A few cases of increased serum aminotransferase activity have been reported, together with prolongation of the prothrombin time. Occasionally, cholestatic, cytotoxic, or mixed hepatic injury may occur. The overall incidence of slight alteration of liver function is about 25%.

Phenytoin decreases the urinary excretion of 17-ketosteroids and 17-hydroxycorticosteroids by stimulating the conversion of cortisol to 6-β-hydroxycortisol; it also diminishes serum FSH and the sperm count in semen, and thereby reduces fertility. Phenytoin also lowers the serum thyroxine concentration, probably by competitive displacement of thyroxine from its protein-binding sites; free thyroxine also tends to be low. Serum triiodothyronine is low, probably as a result of stimulated metabolism in the liver, but the concentration of TSH is unaffected by the altered thyroxine metabolism.

Many epileptics receiving anticonvulsants excrete increased amounts of copper and zinc in their urine. Increased serum ceruloplasmin also increases the total serum copper concentration. In 20% to 30% of epileptic children receiving anticonvulsant therapy, erythrocyte aspartate aminotransferase activity is low, indicating a lowered pyridoxal (vitamin B_6) status. In as many as 50% of the adults receiving phenytoin for some time, there will be folate deficiency, manifested by reduced erythrocyte and serum folate concentrations. The mechanism for the deficiency has not yet been established conclusively. In about 10% of adults taking phenytoin, the serum vitamin B_{12} is low.

T-cell function is reduced in many epileptics receiving anticonvulsants, and systemic lupus erythematosus occurs in about 10% of treated individuals. Antinuclear antibodies have been reported in 55%, and low serum IgA and IgG concentrations in 25% of the patients. Other reported biochemical abnormalities include reduced serum concentrations of HDL cholesterol, urate, and urea nitrogen.

Herbal Preparations

Herbal preparations vary greatly in effect and composition. Long-term use of aloe vera, sandalwood, and cascara segrada may cause hematuria and albuminuria. Through their laxative effects, prolonged use of aloe vera, Chinese rhubarb, frangula bark, senna, and buckthorn may lead to hypokalemia provoking hyperaldosteronism. Trailing arbutus may cause hemolytic anemia and liver damage. Green tea has been reported to cause microcytic anemia. Quinine and quinidine have been observed to cause thrombocytopenia. Cayenne *(Capsicum annuum)* increases fibrinolytic activity and induces hypocoagulability. Hyperthyroidism has been caused by bladderwrack. Many herbal preparations affect liver function. Germander has been reported to cause liver cell necrosis, and bishop's weed infrequently causes cholestatic jaundice. Tonka beans can cause reversible liver damage. Comfrey has been associated with one death from liver failure. Bugleweed reduces the plasma concentration of prolactin and reduces the deiodination of thyroxine.

Recreational Drug Ingestion

Amphetamines increase the concentration of free fatty acids. Morphine increases the activity of amylase and lipase, alanine and aspartate aminotransferases, ALP and the serum bilirubin concentration. The concentrations of gastrin, TSH, and prolactin are also increased. In contrast the concentrations of insulin, norepinephrine, pancreatic polypeptide, and neurotensin are decreased. Heroin increases the plasma concentrations of cholesterol, thyroxine, and potassium. PCO_2 is increased but PO_2 is decreased. The plasma albumin concentration is also decreased. Cannabis increases the plasma concentrations of sodium, potassium, urea, chloride, and insulin but decreases those of creatinine, glucose, and urate.

NONCONTROLLABLE VARIABLES

Examples of noncontrollable preanalytical variables include those related to biological, environmental, and long-term cyclical influences and those related to underlying medical conditions.

Biological Influences

There is better agreement between the serum concentrations or activities of several constituents in monozygotic twins than in dizygotic twins.[31] This evidence indicates the importance of genetic constitution in determining the concentration of blood constituents. An influence of heredity has been substantiated on the plasma concentrations of cholesterol, glucose, urea nitrogen, urate, and bilirubin.

An association of blood type with concentration of certain constituents (uric acid, α_1-antitrypsin, cholesterol, and ALP) has been established. In women with blood group O, the blood hemoglobin concentration is generally less than in women with other blood groups. Histocompatibility antigens also have an underlying genetic basis but can be markedly influenced by prior blood transfusions.

The age, sex, and race of the patient influences the results of individual laboratory tests.[41,46] They are discussed individually in various chapters of this book, and reference intervals for various analytes as a function of these biological influences are listed in Chapter 56.

Age

Age has a notable effect on reference intervals; typical changes in serum composition occurring with age are listed

TABLE 17-8 Influence of Age on Mean Concentration of Serum Constituents in Males

	Measured Value	Change Compared With <29 Year Value			
	<29 y	30-39 y	40-49 y	50-59 y	60-69 y
Albumin (g/dL)	4.6	−0.2	−0.3	−0.4	−0.6
Alkaline phosphatase (U/L)	51	−3	−1	1	4
Aspartate aminotransferase (U/L)	41	3	3	1	1
Bilirubin (mg/dL)	0.4	0.1	0	0	0
Calcium (mg/dL)	9.8	−0.1	−0.2	−0.2	−0.3
Cholesterol (mg/dL)	211	29	43	48	36
Creatinine (mg/dL)	11	0	0.1	0.1	0
Glucose (mg/dL)	108	1	6	2	9
Phosphorus (mg/dL)	4.0	−0.1	−0.3	−0.2	−0.2
Total protein (g/dL)	7.6	−0.1	−0.2	−0.2	−0.2
Urea nitrogen (mg/dL)	15	1	1	2	3
Uric acid (mg/dL)	5.9	0	0.2	−0.1	−0.2

From Leonard PJ. The effect of age and sex on biochemical parameters in blood of healthy human subjects. In: Siest G, ed. Reference values in human chemistry. Basel: Karger, 1973:134-40.

in Table 17-8, although the degree of changes differs in various reports. In general, individuals are considered in four groups—the newborn, the older child to puberty, the sexually mature adult, and the elderly adult.

Newborn. The body fluids of the newborn infant reflect both the trauma of birth and the changes related to the infant's adaptation to an independent existence. The composition of the blood is affected by the maturity of the infant at birth. The erythrocyte count and the hemoglobin concentration in the neonate at birth are much higher than those of the adult but within a few days of birth erythrocytes degrade in response to the higher oxygen concentration than that to which the fetus was exposed in utero. In the mature infant, most of the hemoglobin is the adult form, hemoglobin A, whereas in the immature infant, much of the hemoglobin may be the fetal form, hemoglobin F. In both the mature and immature infant, the arterial blood oxygen saturation is very low initially. A metabolic acidosis develops in newborns that results from the accumulation of organic acids, especially lactic acid. The acid-base status, however, reverts to normal within 24 hours.

Within a few minutes of an infant's birth, fluid passes from the blood vessels into the extravascular spaces. This fluid is similar to plasma except that the fluid lost from the intravascular space contains no protein. Consequently the plasma protein concentration increases. The serum activities of several enzymes, including CK, GGT, and AST, are high at birth, but the increase of alanine aminotransferase (ALT) activity is less than that of other enzymes.

In infants, even in the absence of disease, the concentration of bilirubin rises after birth because of the enhanced erythrocyte destruction. Its concentration peaks about the third to fifth day of life. Conjugation of bilirubin is relatively poor in the neonate as a result of immature liver function. The physiological jaundice of the newborn rarely produces serum bilirubin values greater than 5 mg/dL (85 μmol/L). Distinguishing this naturally occurring phenomenon from other conditions that produce neonatal hyperbilirubinemia may be difficult, and the chronological course of the hyperbilirubinemia is important.

The blood glucose concentration is low in newborns because of their small glycogen reserves, although some attribute the low glucose to adrenal immaturity. Blood lipid concentrations are low but reach 80% of the adult values after 2 weeks. The plasma sodium concentration in an infant at birth is slightly higher than in the adult; at 12 hours, it decreases to below the adult value before rising to a value slightly greater than in the adult. The chloride concentration changes similarly, and the changes are largely related to fluid transfer in and out of the blood capillaries. The plasma potassium concentration may be as high as 7 mmol/L at birth, but it falls rapidly thereafter. Plasma calcium is also high initially but falls by as much as 1.4 mg/dL (0.35 mmol/L) during the first day of life.

The plasma urea nitrogen concentration decreases after birth as the infant synthesizes new protein, and the concentration does not begin to rise until tissue catabolism becomes prominent. The plasma amino acid concentration is low as a result of synthesis of tissue protein, although urinary excretion of amino acids may be quite high because of immaturity of the tubular reabsorptive mechanisms. The plasma urate concentration is high at birth, but the high clearance of urate soon reduces the plasma concentration below the adult value.

The serum thyroxine concentration of the healthy newborn, like that in the pregnant woman, is considerably higher than in the nonpregnant adult. After its birth, an infant secretes TSH, which causes a further increase in the serum thyroxine concentration. The physiological hyperthyroidism gradually declines over the first year of life.

Childhood to Puberty. Many changes take place in the composition of body fluids between infancy and puberty. Most of the changes are gradual, and there are rarely abrupt changes to adult concentrations.

The plasma protein concentrations increase after infancy, and adult concentration values are attained by the age of 10. Serum IgG increases slightly out of proportion to the increase in concentration of α_2-globulin. The serum activity of most enzymes decreases during childhood to adult values by puberty or earlier, although the activity of ALT may continue to rise, at least in men, until middle age. Serum ALP activity is high in infancy but decreases during childhood and rises again with growth before puberty. The activity of the enzyme is better correlated with skeletal growth and sexual maturity than with chronological age; it is greatest at the time of maximum osteoblastic activity occurring with bone growth. The activity decreases rapidly after puberty, especially in girls. Total and LDL cholesterol concentrations increase during the rapid growth spurt also.

The serum creatinine concentration increases steadily from infancy to puberty parallel with development of skeletal muscle; until puberty, there is little difference in the concentration between sexes. The serum urate concentration decreases from its high at birth until age 7 to 10 years, at which time it begins to increase, especially in boys, until about age 16 years.

The Adult. Adult values are usually taken as the reference for comparisons with those of the young and elderly. The concentrations of most test constituents remain quite constant between puberty and menopause in women and between puberty and middle age in men.

During the midlife years, serum total protein and albumin concentrations decrease slightly. There may be a slight decrease in the serum calcium concentration in both sexes. In men, the serum phosphate decreases greatly after age 20 years; in women, the phosphate also decreases until menopause, when a sharp increase takes place. The serum ALP begins to rise in women at menopause, so that in elderly women activity of this enzyme may actually be higher than in men. The concentration of glucose in plasma 1 hour after a loading dose rises by 8 mg/dL (0.44 mmol/L) per decade.

Serum urate concentrations peak in men in their twenties and in women during middle age. Urea concentration increases in both sexes in middle age. Age does not affect the serum creatinine concentration in men but does increase the concentration in women. The serum total cholesterol and triglyceride concentrations increase in both men and women at a rate of 2 mg/dL (0.02 mmol/L) per year to a maximum between ages 50 and 60 years. The activity of most enzymes in serum is greater during adolescence than during adult life. This enhanced enzyme activity presumably reflects the greater physical activity of the adolescents.

TABLE 17-9 Changes in Composition of Serum With Menopause

Constituent	% Increase
Alanine aminotransferase	12
Albumin	2
Alkaline phosphatase	25
Apolipoprotein A-1	4
Aspartate aminotransferase	11
Cholesterol	10
Glucose	2
Phosphate	10
Phospholipids	8
Sodium	1.5
Total protein	0.7
Uric acid	10

From Wilding P, Rollason JG, Robinson D. Pattern of change for various biochemical constituents detected in well-population screening. Clin Chim Acta, 1972;41:375-87.

The Elderly Adult. The plasma concentrations of many constituents increase in women after menopause (Table 17-9).[54]

Renal concentrating ability is reduced in the elderly adult, so that creatinine clearance may decline by as much as 50% between the third and ninth decades. This decreased clearance is caused more by a decrease in urinary creatinine excretion as a result of decreased lean body mass than by altered renal function. The tubular maximum capacity for glucose is reduced. The plasma urea concentration rises with age, as does the urinary excretion of protein. The serum median IgG and IgM concentrations are reduced in the elderly although serum IgA concentrations in men increase slightly in the elderly.

Hormone concentrations are also affected by aging. However, changes in concentration are much less pronounced than an endocrine organ's response to stimuli. Triiodothyronine concentration decreases by up to 40% in persons older than 40 years of age. Although thyroxine secretion is reduced, the thyroxine concentration is not changed, because its degradation is also reduced. Yet the plasma parathyroid hormone concentration does decrease with age. Cortisol secretion is reduced, although the serum concentration may not be affected. The reduced secretion leads to a reduction in the urinary excretion of 17-hydroxycorticosteroids. 17-Ketosteroid excretion in the elderly adult is about half that of the younger adult. The secretion and metabolic clearance of aldosterone are decreased, with a reduction of 50% in the plasma concentration. The aldosterone response to sodium restriction is diminished. Basal insulin concentration is unaffected by aging but its response to glucose is reduced. In men, the secretion rate and concentration of testosterone are reduced after age 50 years. In women, the concentration of pituitary gonadotropins, especially FSH, is increased in the blood and urine.

Estrogen secretion in women begins to decrease before menopause and continues at a greater rate after menopause, whereas gonadotropins show a feedback-mediated reciprocal rise. Serum concentrations of estrogens decrease by 70% or more, and urinary excretion of estrogens is decreased comparably. The decreased estrogen secretion may be responsible for the increase of serum cholesterol that occurs up to age 60 in women. Estrogen secretion in men, although always less than in women, declines with age.

Sex

Until puberty, there are few differences in laboratory data between boys and girls. After puberty the characteristic changes in the concentrations of the sex hormones, including prolactin, become apparent. After puberty, the serum activities of ALP, ALT, AST, CK, and aldolase are greater in men than in women. The higher activity of enzymes originating from skeletal muscle in men is related to their greater muscle mass. After menopause, the activity of ALP increases in women until it is higher than in men. Although total LD activity is similar in men and women, the activities of the LD-1 and LD-3 isoenzymes are higher, and LD-2 is less in young women than in men. These differences disappear after the menopause.

The concentrations of albumin, calcium, and magnesium are higher in men than women, but the concentration of γ-globulin is less. Blood hemoglobin concentrations are lower in women; thus, the serum bilirubin concentrations are also slightly lower. The increased turnover of erythrocytes in women leads to their having a higher reticulocyte count than in men. Serum iron is low during a woman's fertile years, and her plasma ferritin may be only one third the concentration in men. The reduced iron concentration in women is attributable to menstrual blood loss. In contrast, the serum copper concentration tends to be higher in women than men. Cholesterol and LDL cholesterol concentrations are typically higher in men than women, whereas the α-lipoprotein, apolipoprotein A-1, and HDL cholesterol concentrations are less. The plasma amino acid concentrations and the concentrations of creatinine, urea, and urate are higher in men than in women. The effect of age on the difference in concentrations of serum constituents between men and women is illustrated in Table 17-10.

Race

Differentiation of the effects of race from those of socioeconomic conditions is often difficult. Nevertheless, the total serum protein concentration is known to be higher in blacks than in whites. This is largely attributable to a much higher γ-globulin, although usually the concentrations of α_1- and β-globulins are also increased. The serum albumin is typically less in blacks than whites. In black men, serum IgG is often 40% higher and serum IgA may be as much as 20% higher than in white men.[7]

The activity of CK and LD is usually much higher in both black men and women than in whites. This effect presumably is related to the amount of skeletal muscle, which tends to be greater in blacks than whites. Because of their greater skeletal development, black children usually have a higher serum ALP at puberty than do white children. Amylase activity in West Indian immigrants to the United Kingdom is typically higher than in native Britons.

Carbohydrate and lipid metabolism differ in blacks and whites.[4] Glucose tolerance is less in blacks, Polynesians,

TABLE 17-10 Influence of Sex on Composition of Serum at Different Ages

Constituent	MALE-FEMALE DIFFERENCE				
	<29 y	30-39 y	40-49 y	50-59 y	60-69 y
Albumin (g/dL)	0.1	0.1	0	0	−0.1
Alkaline phosphatase (U/L)	14	12	−8	2	−1
Aspartate aminotransferase (U/L)	5	8	8	1	−1
Bilirubin (mg/dL)	0.1	0.1	0.1	0.1	0.1
Calcium (mg/dL)	0.1	0.1	0.1	−0.1	−0.2
Cholesterol (mg/dL)	−14	2	6	−16	−34
Creatinine (mg/dL)	0.2	0.2	0.2	0.2	0.1
Glucose (mg/dL)	5	3	6	0	6
Phosphate (mg/dL)	0.1	0.1	0.0	−0.1	−0.2
Total protein (g/dL)	−0.1	−0.1	−0.1	−0.1	−0.2
Urea nitrogen (mg/dL)	3	3	3	2	0
Uric acid (mg/dL)	1.5	1.7	1.7	1.0	0.5

From Leonard PJ. The effect of age and sex on biochemical parameters in blood of healthy human subjects. In: Siest G. Reference values in human chemistry. Basel: Karger, 1973:134-40.
Male values are higher than female except where indicated by a minus sign.

Native Americans, and Inuits than in comparable age- and sex-matched whites. This is substantiated by a plasma glucose 1 hour after glucose challenge that may be as much as 15 to 25 mg/dL (0.8 to 1.4 mmol/L) higher in blacks than whites. After age 40, the serum cholesterol and triglyceride concentrations are consistently higher in both white men and women than in blacks. The lipoprotein (Lp) (a) concentration in blacks may be twice as high as in whites. These may be dietary rather than racial factors, because the concentration of plasma lipids has been shown to be different for the same racial group in different parts of the world. The blood hemoglobin concentration is as much as 10 g/L higher in whites than blacks. Black Americans of both sexes have lower leukocyte counts than white Americans, largely caused by a lower number of granulocytes, but their monocyte count is also less. Some of the indigenous groups of the Pacific (e.g., Maoris of New Zealand) have notably higher mean serum urate concentrations than white populations.

Environmental Factors

Environmental factors that affect laboratory results include altitude, ambient temperature, and place of residence.

Altitude

In individuals living at a high *altitude,* the blood hemoglobin and hematocrit are greatly increased because of reduced atmospheric PO_2.[14] Erythrocyte 2,3-diphosphoglycerate is also increased, and the oxygen dissociation curve is shifted to the right. The increased erythrocyte concentration leads to an increased turnover of nucleoproteins and excretion of urate. The fasting, basal concentration of growth hormone concentration is high in individuals living at a high altitude, but the concentrations of renin and aldosterone are decreased in healthy individuals. Plasma sodium and potassium concentrations are typically unaffected by high altitude although the osmolality is reduced. The serum concentrations of C-reactive protein, transferrin, and β_2-globulin are notably increased with transition to a high altitude. The urinary concentration and clearance are decreased at high altitudes. Complete adaptation to a high altitude takes many weeks whereas adjustment to lower altitudes takes less time.

Ambient Temperature

Ambient temperature affects the composition of body fluids. Acute exposure to heat causes the plasma volume to expand by an influx of interstitial fluid into the intravascular space, and by reduction of glomerular filtration. The plasma protein concentration may decrease by up to 10%. Sweating may cause salt and water loss, but usually there are no changes in the plasma sodium and chloride concentrations. Plasma potassium concentration may decrease by as much as 10% as potassium is taken up by the cells. If sweating is extensive, hemoconcentration rather than hemodilution may occur.

Place of Residence

The geographical location where individuals live may affect the composition of their body fluids. Thus a statistically significant increase in the serum concentrations of cholesterol, triglycerides, and magnesium has been observed in people living in areas with hard water. Trace element concentrations are also affected by locale, for example, in areas where there is much ore smelting, serum concentrations of the trace elements involved may be increased. Carboxyhemoglobin concentrations are higher in areas where there is much heavier automobile traffic than in rural areas (as was true for blood lead in the 1970s in the United States). Individuals who primarily work indoors typically have lower concentrations of 25-hydroxy vitamin D than those who work outdoors, leading to higher serum calcium concentrations and greater urinary excretion of calcium.

Long-Term Cyclical Changes

Long-term cyclical changes also affect laboratory results. Seasonal influences and the menstrual cycle are examples of such changes.

Seasonal Influences

Seasonal influences on the composition of body fluids are small compared with those related to changes in posture or misuse of a tourniquet.[35] Probable factors are dietary changes as different foods come into season and altered physical activity as more or different forms of exercise become feasible. Evaluations of seasonal variation are difficult because they depend on the definition of a season and on the magnitude of temperature change from one season to another. Day-to-day variability in the composition of body fluids is greater in summer than winter. Nevertheless, biological variability is in general only a little greater than analytical variability.

In summer in the northern hemisphere, the blood volume increases in association with the higher temperature. In winter the plasma protein increases by as much as 10%. In contrast, the γ-globulin may increase by as much as 50% in summer. Serum urate concentrations appear to be 5% to 7% higher in summer than in winter. Urea concentrations are also higher in winter than in summer. Serum triglyceride concentrations are up to 10% higher in summer, whereas the serum cholesterol has been reported to be up to 50 mg/dL (1.3 mmol/L) higher in men and 30 mg/dL (0.7 mmol/L) higher in women in winter than in summer. The increased winter cholesterol concentration has been attributed to less physical exercise, greater food intake, and lower amounts of sunshine. However, similar changes in animals suggest that humoral factors may also be involved. Activities of serum enzymes arising from skeletal muscle are higher in summer than in winter, presumably as a result of increased physical activity. The increase of serum lactate dehydrogenase may be as much as 20%.

Calcium metabolism is affected by an individual's exposure to sunlight. Dehydrocholecalciferol in the skin is

TABLE 17-11 Seasonal Effects on Composition of Serum

	CONCENTRATION		
Constituent	**Highest**	**Lowest**	**% Difference Between High and Low**
Alanine aminotransferase	Winter	Spring, summer	5.0
Albumin	Fall	Summer	1.2
Aspartate aminotransferase	Spring	Fall	11.7
Calcium	Fall	Winter	1.0
Creatinine	Summer	Winter	4.7
Glucose	Fall	Spring	1.5
Lactate dehydrogenase	Summer	Winter	1.8
Triglycerides	Spring	Fall	5.4
Urea nitrogen	Fall	Spring, summer	3.2
Uric acid	Summer	Winter	4.3

converted by ultraviolet irradiation to cholecalciferol, which is further metabolized in the liver and kidney to 1,25-dihydroxycholecalciferol. The calcium concentration in serum is increased along with its elimination in urine.[22] Seasonal changes appear to affect other endocrine systems as well. A lower plasma glucose concentration may be observed and glucose tolerance is improved during summer. Serum concentrations of thyroid hormones are generally unaffected but the serum concentration of triiodothyronine is decreased by 20% in summer and its urinary excretion is increased. The excretion of metabolites of adrenal hormones usually is greater in summer than in winter. This could be attributable to greater physical activity.

Exposure to sunshine for a weekend during summer may cause enough photodegradation of bilirubin to reduce the serum concentration by 20%. Protracted exposure to sun during the summer leads to a consistently lower bilirubin concentration than during winter. Some seasonal effects on the composition of body fluids are listed in Table 17-11.

Influence of Menstrual Cycle

The plasma concentrations of many female sex hormones and other hormones are affected by the menstrual cycle (see also Chapters 50 to 53).[58] Thus the plasma corticosterone concentration is as much as 50% higher in the luteal phase than in the follicular phase. The urinary excretion of 17-hydroxycorticosteroids reaches a peak at midcycle. Plasma androstenedione concentration and plasma aldosterone concentration increase from the follicular phase to the luteal phase of the menstrual cycle. On the preovulatory day, the aldosterone concentration may actually be twice that of the early part of the follicular phase. The change in renin activity is almost as great. These changes are usually more pronounced in women who retain fluid before menstruation. Urinary catecholamine excretion increases at midcycle and remains high throughout the luteal phase. These changes within the menstrual cycle make it essential to do repetitive measurements on women at the same time during the cycle.

The plasma cholesterol and triglyceride concentrations tend to be highest at midcycle, corresponding to the time of maximum estrogen secretion. The cyclical variation in cholesterol is not observed with anovulatory cycles. The total protein and albumin concentrations decrease at the time of ovulation but then increase again. The plasma fibrinogen concentration decreases greatly at menstruation. The serum calcium correlates with changes in albumin. Serum phosphate is reduced at the time of menstruation, although the creatinine and urate concentrations are highest at this time and are lowest toward the end of the intermenstrual period.

The plasma iron concentration may be very low with the onset of menstruation; the magnesium concentration is least at this point of the cycle. Plasma sodium and chloride concentrations increase up to the onset of menstruation but may fall by 2 mmol/L with the postmenstrual diuresis.

The plasma ascorbic acid concentration is low at the time of ovulation, whereas that of folate is unaffected by the menstrual cycle. Serum CK activity may be slightly reduced at the time of ovulation, but the activities of other enzymes appear to be unaffected by the menstrual cycle.

Underlying Medical Conditions

Some general clinical conditions have an effect per se on the composition of body fluids. These conditions may exist in addition to the primary complaint that prompted a patient's admission to the hospital. For example, obesity, blindness, fever, shock and trauma, and transfusions and infusions all affect laboratory results.

Obesity

The serum concentrations of cholesterol, triglycerides, and β-lipoproteins are positively correlated with obesity.[47] One study in twins has shown that for an average increase of 7.3% in body mass index there were increases of 2.5% in total cholesterol concentration, 3% in LDL cholesterol concentration, and 18.2% in triglyceride concentration.[9] The increase in the concentration of cholesterol is attributable to LDL cholesterol because the HDL cholesterol is typically reduced. The serum urate concentration is also correlated with body weight, especially in individuals weighing more than 80 kg.[39] Serum LD activity and glucose concentration increase in both sexes with increasing body weight.[47] In men, serum AST, creatinine, total protein, and blood hemoglobin concentration increase with increasing body weight. In women, serum calcium increases with increasing body weight. In both sexes, serum phosphate decreases with increased body mass.

Cortisol production is increased in obese individuals. However, increased metabolism maintains the serum concentration unchanged so that urinary excretion of 17-hydroxycorticosteroids and 17-ketosteroids is increased. Because the growth hormone concentration is reduced in obese individuals, it responds poorly to the normal challenges. Plasma insulin concentration is increased, but glucose tolerance is impaired in the obese (see Chapter 25). Although the serum thyroxine concentration is unaffected by obesity, the serum triiodothyronine correlates significantly with body weight and increases further with overeating. In obese men, the serum testosterone concentration is reduced.

The fasting concentrations of pyruvate, lactate, citrate, and unesterified fatty acids are higher in obese individuals than in those of normal body weight. Serum iron and transferrin concentrations are low.

Gastric juice volume and acid output are increased in obese individuals.

Blindness

With blindness, the normal stimulation of the hypothalamic-pituitary axis is reduced. Consequently, certain features of hypopituitarism and hypoadrenalism may be observed.[5] In some blind individuals, the normal diurnal variation of cortisol may persist; in others it does not. Urinary excretion of 17-ketosteroids and 17-hydroxycorticosteroids is reduced. Plasma sodium and chloride are often low in blind individuals, probably as a result of reduced aldosterone secretion. Plasma glucose may be reduced in blind people, and insulin tolerance is often less. The excretion of urate is reduced. Renal function may be slightly impaired, as evidenced by slight increases in serum creatinine and urea nitrogen.

Negative nitrogen balance may occur in blind people, and the serum protein concentration may be reduced. The serum cholesterol is frequently increased, and bilirubin concentration may also exceed the upper limit of normal. The diurnal variation of serum iron is often lost.

Pregnancy

Many changes in the concentrations of analytes occur during pregnancy and proper interpretation of test results is dependent on knowledge of the duration of pregnancy (see Chapter 54).

Substantial hormonal changes occur during pregnancy including several not normally associated with reproduction. Many of the changes are related to the great increase in blood volume that occurs during pregnancy from about 2600 mL early in pregnancy to 3500 mL at about 35 weeks. This hemodilution reduces the concentration of the plasma proteins. However, the concentration of some transport proteins including ceruloplasmin and thyroxine-binding globulin is increased, resulting in increased concentrations of copper and thyroxine. The concentrations of cholesterol and triglycerides are notably increased. In contrast, pregnancy creates a relative deficiency of iron and ferritin.

Urine volume increases during pregnancy so that it is typically 25% greater in the third trimester than in the non-pregnant woman. The glomerular filtration rate increases by 50% during the third trimester. This results in increased urinary excretion of hydroxyproline and increased creatinine clearance.

Pregnancy triggers many physiological stress reactions and is associated with increased concentrations of acute-phase reactant proteins. The erythrocyte sedimentation rate increases fivefold during pregnancy.

Stress

Physical and mental stress influence the concentrations of many plasma constituents. Anxiety stimulates increased secretion of aldosterone, angiotensin, catecholamines, cortisol, prolactin, renin, somatotropin, TSH, and vasopressin. Plasma concentrations of albumin, cholesterol, fibrinogen, glucose, insulin, and lactate also increase.

Fever

Fever provokes many hormonal responses.[44] Hyperglycemia occurs early and stimulates the secretion of insulin, which improves glucose tolerance; but insulin secretion does not necessarily reduce the blood glucose concentration because increased secretion of growth hormone and glucagon also occurs. Fever appears to reduce the secretion of thyroxine, as do acute illnesses even without fever. In response to increased corticotropin secretion, the plasma cortisol concentration is increased and its normal diurnal variation may be abolished. The urinary excretion of free cortisol, 17-hydroxycorticosteroids, and 17-ketosteroids is increased. As acute fever subsides, or if it lessens but still persists for a prolonged period, the hormone responses diminish.

Glycogenolysis and a negative nitrogen balance occur with the onset of fever. These are prompted by the typically decreased food intake and wasting of skeletal muscle that accompany fever. Although there is usually an increase in the blood volume with fever, the serum concentrations of creatinine and urate are usually increased. Aldosterone secretion is increased with retention of sodium and chloride. Secretion of antidiuretic hormone also contributes to the retention of water by the kidneys. Increased synthesis of protein occurs in the liver, and the plasma concentrations of acute-phase reactants and glycoproteins are increased.

Fever accelerates lipid metabolism. The serum concentrations of cholesterol, nonesterified fatty acids, and the other lipids may decrease initially, but within a few days the free fatty acid concentration may increase. Fever is often associated with a respiratory alkalosis caused by hyperventilation. This pH increase causes a reduction of the plasma phosphate concentration, with an increased excretion of phosphate and other electrolytes.[2] Serum iron and zinc concentrations decline with accumulation of both elements in the liver. The copper concentration increases because of increased production of ceruloplasmin by the liver. Some representative changes in serum composition induced by fever are listed in Table 17-12.

Shock and Trauma

Regardless of the cause of shock or trauma, certain characteristic biochemical changes result.[11] For example, corticotropin secretion is stimulated to produce a threefold to fivefold increase in the serum cortisol concentration. The 17-hydroxycorticosteroid excretion is greatly increased, although the excretion of 17-ketosteroids and metabolites of adrenal androgens may be unaffected. Aldosterone secretion is stimulated. Plasma renin activity is increased, as are the secretions of growth hormone, glucagon, and insulin. Anxiety and stress increase the excretion of catecholamines. The stress of surgery has been shown to reduce the serum triiodothyronine by 50% in patients without thyroid disease.

The general metabolic response to shock includes the normal response to stress with mobilization of lipids, although the serum triglyceride concentration is not usually affected. Following acute myocardial infarction and other cardiac events there tend to be notable decreases in LDL and HDL cholesterols, and apolipoprotein B and A-I concentrations with an increase in the triglyceride concentration. Surgical procedures and intercurrent illnesses produce similar effects. Even minor illnesses, such as colds, can affect lipid concentrations. The concentrations of lipids revert to normal within 1 month of the event. Plasma glucose concentration is increased in response to stress, and glucose tolerance is reduced.

Immediately after an injury, there is loss of fluid to extravascular tissue with a resulting decrease in plasma volume. If the decrease is enough to impair circulation, glomerular filtration is diminished. Diminished renal function leads to the accumulation of urea and other end products of protein metabolism in the circulation. In burned patients, serum total protein concentration falls by as much as 0.8 g/dL because of both loss to extravascular spaces and catabolism of protein. Serum α_1-, α_2-, and γ-globulin concentrations increase, but not enough to compensate for the reduced albumin concentration. The plasma fibrinogen concentration responds dramatically to trauma and may double in 2 to 8 days after surgery. The concentration of C-reactive protein rises at the same time.

The muscle damage associated with the trauma of surgery will increase the serum activity of enzymes originating in skeletal muscle, and this increased activity may persist for several days. Typical alterations in activity of serum enzymes following surgery are illustrated in Table 17-13. Increased tissue catabolism requires increased oxygen consumption and also leads to the production of acid metabolites. Thus blood lactate may increase twofold to threefold. With tissue anoxia and impairment of renal and respiratory function, a metabolic acidosis develops. With tissue destruction, there is increased urinary excretion of the major biochemical components of skeletal muscle.

Transfusion and Infusions

The protein-rich fluid lost from the intravascular space after trauma is replaced with protein-poor fluid from the interstitial spaces. Subsequently, this is replaced by a fluid similar in composition to plasma. Transfusion of whole blood or plasma raises the plasma protein concentration; the amount

TABLE 17-12 Effect of Fever on Composition of Serum

		Concentration After Induction of Fever			
Constituent	**Baseline Value**	**18 h**	**48 h**	**72 h**	**96 h**
Sodium (mmol/L)	141	130	130	132	135
Chloride (mmol/L)	99	91	89	92	94
Potassium (mmol/L)	3.6	3.5	3.0	3.4	3.6
Calcium (mg/dL)	9.7	8.4	8.5	9.0	9.1
Phosphate (mg/dL)	3.3	2.3	3.2	3.2	3.7
Magnesium (mg/dL)	1.85	1.62	1.73	1.78	1.70
Creatinine (mg/dL)	1.10	1.03	1.04	1.00	1.09
Urea nitrogen (mg/dL)	13.4	14.0	15.2	18.5	17.4
Uric acid (mg/dL)	5.0	5.5	5.7	6.2	6.2

From Beisel WR, Goldman RF, Joy RJT. Metabolic balance studies during induced hyperthermia in man. J Appl Physiol 1968;24:1-10.

of increase depends on the amount of blood administered. Serum LD activity, primarily LD-1 and LD-2 isoenzymes, is increased by the breakdown of transfused erythrocytes. Transfusions to replace blood lost because of injury reduce sodium, chloride, and water retention precipitated by the injury. Serum iron and transferrin concentrations are reduced immediately after an injury, but extensive blood transfusions can lead to siderosis and an increased serum iron concentration. Serum potassium may increase with transfusion of stored blood.

Infusions of glucose solutions usually result in a reduction of both the plasma phosphate and potassium concentrations because these compounds are taken up by the erythrocytes. Infusions of solutions of albumin may increase plasma ALP activity if the albumin has been prepared from placentas. Because of the possible influence of infused components on the concentration of circulating constituents, it is inadvisable to collect blood for analysis less than 8 hours after infusion of a fat emulsion or 1 hour after infusion of carbohydrates, amino acids, and protein hydrolysates or electrolytes.

TABLE 17-13 Incidence of Increased Activity of Serum Enzymes and Isoenzymes After Surgery

Enzyme	%
CK	76
CK-2 isoenzyme	6
Aspartate aminotransferase	50
α-Hydroxybutyrate dehydrogenase	28
LD-1 isoenzyme	18
LD-1 ≤ LD-2	10
LD-5 isoenzyme	20

From Krafft J, Fink R, Rosalki SB. Serum enzymes and isoenzymes after surgery. Ann Clin Biochem 1977;14:294-6.
CK, Creatine kinase; *LD,* lactate dehydrogenase.

BIOLOGICAL VARIABILITY*

Data from studies of biological variation may be used to assess the importance of changes in test values within an individual from one occasion to another, determining the appropriateness of reference intervals and, in conjunction with data from analytical variation, establish laboratory analytical goals.[15-17] Application by clinicians of information on biological variability could enhance their ability to precisely identify important changes in test results in their patients.

Overview

Categories of biological variation include (1) within an individual and (2) between individuals. The change of laboratory data around a hemostatic set point from one occasion to another within one person is called within-subject or intraindividual variation (Table 17-14). The difference

*Note: The authors have based much of their discussion of biological variability on CG Fraser's book: Biological variation; From principles to practice. Washington DC: AACC Press, 2–1:1-151. It should be consulted for further details.

TABLE 17-14 Comparison of Intraindividual and Interindividual Variations and Indices of Individuality

Analyte	Intraindividual Variation (%)	Interindividual Variation (%)	Index of Individuality
Alanine aminotransferase	24.3	41.6	0.58
Albumin	3.1	4.2	0.74
Alkaline phosphatase	32.6	39.0	0.84
Bilirubin	25.6	30.5	0.85
Calcium	1.9	2.8	0.68
Chloride	1.2	1.5	0.80
Creatine kinase	22.8	40.0	0.57
Creatinine	4.3	12.9	0.33
Lactate dehydrogenase	6.6	14.7	0.45
Magnesium	3.6	6.4	0.56
Phosphate	8.5	9.4	0.90
Potassium	13.6	13.4	1.02
Protein	2.7	4.0	0.68
Sodium	0.7	1.0	0.70
Urea nitrogen	12.3	18.3	0.67
Uric acid	8.6	17.2	0.50

Reprinted with permission of AACC Press, from Fraser CG, Biological variation: From principles to practice. Washington DC: AACC Press, 2001.

between the set points of different individuals is called interindividual variation. The average intraindividual variability varies greatly for different analytes, even within the same biochemical class of compounds (e.g., 6.1% for total cholesterol, 7.4% for HDL cholesterol, 9.5% for LDL cholesterol, and 22.6% for triglycerides). The major factors influencing the reported intraindividual and interindividual variability are primarily the number of individuals in a study, the standardization (or lack thereof) of patient preparation and specimen collection conditions, the number of measurements per individual, and the homogeneity of the studied population.

Often, biological variability influences clinical decisions. For example, Mogadam et al have shown that intraindividual variability in LDL concentrations led to 10% of subjects moving from high risk for cardiovascular events status to normal or vice versa.[38] Where clinicians rely inappropriately on the upper and lower limits of the reference interval as finite decision points for treatment, this will result in some patients receiving unnecessary treatment and others, who should be candidates for treatment, going untreated and potentially lost to follow-up because their test values suggested that the individuals were healthy.

The test values in a healthy population used to derive a conventional reference interval are subject to the variety of influences including endogenous, exogenous, genetic or ethnic, and laboratory factors discussed above. The statistical approach used to calculate the interval also has considerable influence on the derived reference interval (see Chapter 16). No individual has test results that would span the entire reference interval. Indeed all the results within a healthy individual typically encompass only a small part of most reference intervals. Stratification into more appropriate intervals for subpopulations is sometimes required. The most typical stratifications are based on sex and age. Sinton et al[48] have advocated that separate reference intervals are justified when the difference between the means of the potentially different populations (e.g., men and women or blacks and whites) is greater than 25% of the 95% reference interval of the entire population. An alternative approach to define whether stratification is appropriate is that of Harris and Boyd, which involves calculation of the standard deviations of all of the results from each of the potentially different populations and if the standard deviation of one is more than 1.5 times another stratification is justified.[25]

Inherent in any reported laboratory test results on patients are influences of (1) biological variation, (2) inherent analytical error, (3) preanalytical and postanalytical sources of variation, and (4) possible pathophysiological alterations. When repeated measurements are made over time in one individual, even under standardized conditions, there is a considerable variability in the test results. The variability within the individual is attributable to both analytical and intraindividual factors but the intraindividual (within-subject) variability is typically less than the variability among a group of individuals. This means that when analytical variability is constant, a statistically significant change in the test results in one individual might occur yet all the results could still lie within the reference interval established from the results obtained from many individuals. Many studies have demonstrated remarkable constancy over the years in intraindividual variability. For those analytes that are influenced by the endocrine system, the variation tends to be even less than for those that have no hormonal regulation, especially those that are affected by dietary factors. In general, biological variability is only slightly affected by age[18] or by diseases that do not directly cause abnormal concentrations of a specific analyte.[27,28]

DELTA CHECK

When a patient's clinical condition is generally stable and differences between repeated test results are small, the difference between successive results may be used as a form of quality assurance (see Chapter 19). Most physicians arbitrarily decide when there is a clinically significant difference between repeated measurements of the same analyte. However, it is possible to address the issue more systematically and logically. The *delta check* concept is applied to two successive values regardless of the time interval between them. Delta check values are typically generated in one of two ways: the first is derived from the differences between the collected consecutive values for an analyte in many individuals, which are then plotted in a histogram with the central 95% or 99% of all values used to identify a clinically significant change in values. Delta checks may involve the absolute difference or the percent change between the consecutive numbers. The second approach to establishing the delta relies on a laboratorian's or clinician's best estimate of an appropriate delta to yield a manageable number of flagged results for follow-up. A more refined means of using patient data for assessing statistically significant changes is through rate checks that involve dividing a delta check value by the time interval between successive measurements. Several different delta check methods have been proposed.[34] Delta checks have been based on (1) delta difference: current result – previous result; (2) delta percent change: (current – previous result) × 100%/previous result; (3) rate difference: delta difference/delta time; and (4) rate percent change: delta percent change/delta time (where delta time is the interval between the current and previous specimen collection times). Some laboratory information systems embody delta checks in the reporting of test results but usually in the simplest way, as in delta difference or delta percent change.

In healthy individuals and in stable patients, the delta value between any two results should be small. Acceptable delta values may be calculated within a population of healthy individuals and then averaged, with the average used as a guide to determine whether a difference of possible clinical significance had occurred between serial measurements in patients. An alternative approach is to use the more refined reference change value (RCV), or critical difference, concept.

Calculating Total Variation

To determine what confidence should be placed in a test result it is useful to evaluate the variability of test values. The factors influencing a test value are preanalytical, analytical, and within an individual. As the sources of variation (squares of the standard deviations) are additive, the total variation (SD_T^2) for any one laboratory result is

$$SD_T^2 = SD_P^2 + SD_A^2 + SD_I^2$$

where

SD_P = Standard deviation of preanalytical variation
SD_A = Standard deviation of analytical variation
SD_I = Standard deviation of within individual biological variation

It is possible to substitute the coefficient of variation for the standard deviation in the above equation. If the conditions of patient preparation, sample collection, and sample handling are standardized, preanalytical variation is minimized and the total variation is then determined by the combined influence of the analytical and intraindividual variations, thus:

$$CV_T = \left(CV_A^2 + CV_I^2\right)^{1/2}$$

Reference Change Values

To determine whether the difference between consecutive results for a single analyte in a patient might have clinical significance, Harris and Yasaka developed the concept of *reference change values.*[26] *An RCV,* also known as *critical difference,* is the value that must be exceeded before a change in consecutive test results is statistically significant at a predetermined probability. The concept introduces a scientific approach to an area where clinicians have largely relied on their intuition and experience. Historically, clinicians' impressions of clinically significant differences been results have varied quite markedly. Fraser et al[18] have shown that systematically calculated critical differences for many analytes tend to be less than physicians' assumptions of clinically significant differences.

An RCV takes into account both analytical and within-individual variations that were discussed above. It is calculated using the following equation

$$RVC = 2^{1/2} \times Z \times \left(CV_A^2 + CV_I^2\right)^{1/2}$$

where Z = Z-score (also called standard normal deviate). Z-scores vary with the desired probability for the change. The Z-scores for different probabilities may be derived from statistical tables. For the widely used probability of 95% for clinical laboratory decisions, the Z-score is 1.96. When inserted in the formula above the formula becomes

$$RVC = 2.77 \times \left(CV_A^2 + CV_I^2\right)^{1/2}$$

In practice, a Z-score of 1.96 for a 95% probability is used to identify a significant RCV. A Z-score of 2.58 is used for a 99% probability to ensure an even more significant RCV. The higher the probability used in the calculation the greater the likelihood that all identified changes will be true changes. Yet the greater certainty with the higher probability may make some physicians believe that the change is obvious and that such large RCVs may mask trends in test values. The CV_A used for the calculation should be appropriate for the range of test values, as low analytical variability enhances the likelihood of calculated changes being statistically significant. The probability of change is then largely influenced by intraindividual variation, CV_I. To enhance the utility of the RCV intraindividual, variability should also be minimized with standardization of patient preparation and specimen collection and processing practices. Standardization is more readily achieved in hospital practice, where uniform timing of collections by trained phlebotomists is often possible, than in outpatient practices.

The change in values between successive measurements in a hospitalized patient is generally higher than in the values reported in the literature derived from studies of healthy individuals because of the change in the patient's medical condition and its response to treatment. RCVs are not constant and a significant change is likely to be smaller over the short term than over a longer time span. Thus application of RCVs from healthy individuals derived over a short time will identify an inappropriately large number of apparently significant changes in hospitalized patients. CV_I varies between individuals so that calculations using the mean CV_I also flag a disproportionately large number of significant changes. Table 17-15 shows the effect of using different probabilities of significant changes.

Index of Individuality

Although it would be preferable if the range of values in an individual when healthy could be used as the reference for the same individual when he or she is ill, this is largely impractical. The less specific reference interval derived from many individuals must be used as a guide to determine whether a specific result is abnormal. The *index of individuality* (II) allows a comparison of total within-subject (intraindividual) variation to between-subject (interindividual) variation. It is calculated as the ratio of the total intraindividual variation to interindividual biological variation as

$$II = \frac{\left[CV_A^2 + CV_I^2\right]^{1/2}}{CV_G}$$

where CV_A is the analytical variability, CV_I the intraindividual variability, and CV_G the interindividual variability. In clinical practice for most analytes, CV_A is small in comparison with CV_I or CV_G and can be ignored and the formula for II is thus simplified to

$$II = \frac{CV_I}{CV_G}$$

A low index of individuality indicates that an analyte has marked individuality and a high index indicates that

TABLE 17-15 Significance of Changes in Serial Results: Probability That Changes Between Successive Values Are Significant (%)

Analyte	Units	PROBABILITY					
		60	70	80	90	95	99
Alanine aminotransferase	U/L	3	5	8	13	16	23
Albumin	g/L	<1	1	2	3	4	5
Alkaline phosphatase	U/L	4	9	13	20	26	36
Amylase	U/L	2	5	8	13	16	23
Bilirubin	mmol/L	<1	1	2	3	4	6
Calcium	mmol/L	0.02	0.04	0.06	0.09	0.12	0.17
Chloride	mmol/L	1	2	3	4	5	7
Cholesterol	mmol/L	0.2	0.3	0.5	0.8	1.1	1.5

Reprinted with permission of AACC Press, from Fraser CG, Biological variation: From principles to practice. Washington DC: AACC Press, 2001.

an analyte has little individuality. Examples of indices of individuality for several analytes are listed in Table 17-14. Harris[24] has demonstrated that it is only appropriate to use the reference interval for an analyte to make clinical decisions when CV_I/CV_G is greater than 1.4. When II is less than 0.6, conventional population reference values are of little value and may be misleading. Little variation in test values for an analyte within one person (i.e., a high index of individuality) means that an individual could have considerable changes in laboratory data that might have clinical significance for him or her, yet all these values could fall within the population reference interval. In theory, such analytes are of little use for the diagnosis of disease unless the changes are markedly abnormal but would be better suited for monitoring the progress of a disease or its response to treatment where the differences between consecutive measurements are used to identify a change in a patient's status.

Index of Heterogeneity

The *index of heterogeneity* (IH) provides a means of determining whether the individuals within a population have similar within-individual variation for a given analyte. It is is defined as the ratio of CV of $(SD_A^2 + SD_I^2)^{1/2}$ to $[2/(n-1)]^{1/2}$ where A and I are the analytical and within-subject variations and n is the number of specimens per subject. The higher the index of heterogeneity the greater the intra-individual variation.

Reliability Coefficient

The *reliability coefficient* (R) is the ratio of between-subject variation to total variation. This is another measure of individuality. It is calculated as the between-individual variance divided by the total variation.

$$R = \frac{CV_G^2}{CV_A^2 + CV_I^2 + CV_G^2}$$

The reliability coefficient will always be between 0 and 1. If it approaches 1, this means that there is very little variation of results over time within one individual, indicating that great confidence can be placed in a single result and that repeated measurements are unnecessary.

Quality Specifications for Total Error Allowable

Analytical variations may increase the number of results in a healthy population outside a previously established reference interval. A positive analytical bias increases the number of high values and a negative bias decreases the number below the lower reference limit. It is possible to link the maximum tolerable analytical bias to biological variability.[17] The relationship below is derived on the assumption that the maximum acceptable bias is less than one quarter of the sum of the intraindividual and interindividual variations within a population.

$$\text{Analytical bias} < 0.25 \times \left(CV_I^2 + CV_G^2\right)^{1/2}$$

By substituting different factors in the above formula different targeted analytical biases can be identified. If less analytical bias is deemed to be appropriate (e.g., one fifth of the total biological variation instead of one quarter), 0.20 would be substituted for 0.25. It has been suggested that analytical precision should be less than one half of the mean intraindividual variation ($CV_A = <0.50\ CV_I$). Total error is derived from the sum of imprecision and bias. From the formula above

$$\text{Total allowable analytical error} < 1.65 \times 0.50 \times CV_I + 0.25 \times \left(CV_I^2 + CV_G^2\right)^{1/2}$$

The factor 1.65 is derived from 90% of the distribution of results excluding the highest and lowest 5% of values. Again, substituting different values for 0.50 and 0.25 above allows different goals to be established.

Other formulas have been used to determine quality specifications for bias. Generally, analytical bias should be less than one quarter of interindividual biological variation.

$$B_A < 0.250 \times \left(CV_I^2 + CV_G^2\right)^{1/2}$$

But optimum performance is also defined by substituting 0.125 for 0.250 in the above formula and minimum performance defined by substituting 0.375 for 0.250. When the factor 0.125 is used, 1.8% of values are outside one reference limit and 3.3% outside the other. When 0.375 is used 1.0% values are outside one reference limit and 5.7% outside the other.[17] Fraser has stated that the lower number should be used when desirable performance standards are easily attained and 0.375 should be used when performance goals are not readily attainable with current procedures.[17] Most of the literature has reported total error in terms of the sum of bias plus 1.65 times the precision (TE_A = Bias + 1.65 SD or CV of interindividual variation).

Biological variation has been included in a goal to determine analytical interference.[20] The goal specifies that

$$\text{Interference}\,(\%) < CV_I - (1.96\,CV_A + SE)$$

where SE represents the percentage systematic error (inaccuracy).

Assessment of Mode of Reporting Test Results

The RCV concept is used to determine the most appropriate mode to report several analytes where several possibilities exist. For example, the amount of an analyte in urine could be reported in terms of concentration, absolute amount per unit of time, or the amount relative to that of creatinine. The mode with the smallest relative change value is the most informative. Data on analytical and intraindividual variation together with RCV can pinpoint the most appropriate type of specimen for certain analyses. Howey et al[29] studied random, early morning, and 24-hour urine specimens to determine the most appropriate means to monitor microalbuminuria. The first morning specimen became the preferred specimen because of its smallest within-individual variation, smallest heterogeneity in intraindividual variances, and smallest RCV between consecutive measurements.

Data on biological variability are used to assist in the selection of the most appropriate test in a given situation. For example, creatinine clearance and urine creatinine have less intraindividual variation than serum creatinine so that creatinine clearance is a better choice than serum creatinine for initial assessment of renal function in an individual but the lower RCV for serum creatinine make this test better for monitoring individuals. However, the need for a urine collection reduces the practicality of using clearance in the initial assessment of renal function. Studies to determine whether the GFR calculated from the serum creatinine concentration might enhance the utility of the serum measurement still have to be performed.

REFERENCES

1. Barrett JV. Hyperbilirubinemia of fasting. JAMA 1971;217:1349-53.
2. Beisel WR, Goldman RF, Joy RJT. Metabolic balance studies during induced hyperthermia in man. J Appl Physiol 1968;24:1-10.
3. Bellet S, Roman, L, DeCastro O, et al: Effect of coffee ingestion on catecholamine release. Metabolism, 1969;18:288-91.
4. Benedek TG, Sunder JH. Comparison of serum lipid and uric acid content in white and Negro men. Am J Med Sci 1970;260:331-40.
5. Bodenheimer S, Winter JSD, Faiman C. Diurnal rhythms of serum gonadotropins, testosterone, estradiol and cortisol in blind men. J Clin Endocrinol Metab 1973;37:472-5.
6. Brohult J. Effects of high protein and low protein diets on ornithine carbamoyl transferase activity in human serum (S–OCT). Acta Med Scand 1969;185:357-62.
7. Buckley CE, Dorsey FC. Serum immunoglobulin levels throughout the life-span of healthy men. Ann Intern Med 1971;75:673-82.
8. Carruthers M, Arguelles AE, Mosovich A. Man in transit: Biochemical and physiological changes during intercontinental flights. Lancet 1976;1:977-81.
9. Cooper GR, Smith SJ, Myers GL, Sampson EJ, Magid E. Biological variation in the concentration of serum lipids: sources, meta-analysis, estimation and minimization by relative range measurements. J Int Fed Clin Chem 1995;7;23-8.
10. Cryer PE, Haymond MW, Santiago JV, et al. Norepinephrine and epinephrine release and adrenergic mediation of smoking-associated hemodynamic and metabolic events. NEJM 1976;295:573-7.
11. Cuthbertson DP, Tilstone WJ. Metabolism during the post-injury period. Adv Clin Chem 1969;12:1-55.
12. Davies CTM, Few JD. Effects of exercise on adrenocortical function. J Appl Physiol 1972;35:887-91.
13. Deitrick JE, Whedon GD, Shorr E. Effects of immobilization upon various metabolic and physiologic functions of normal men. Am J Med, 1948;4:3-36.
14. Eaton JW, Brewer GJ, Grover RG. Role of red cell 2,3-diphosphoglycerate in the adaptation of man to altitude. J Lab Clin Med 1969;73:603-9.
15. Fraser CG. Desirable performance standards for clinical chemistry tests. Adv Clin Chem 1983;23;299-339.
16. Fraser CG. Data on biological variation: essential prerequisites for introducing new procedures? Clin Chem 1994;40;1671-3.
17. Fraser CG. Biological Variation: From Principles to Practice. Washington, DC, AACC Press, 2001.
18. Fraser CG, Cummings ST, Wilkinson SP, Neville RG, Knox JDE, Ho O, MacWalker RS. Biological variability of 26 clinical chemistry analytes in elderly people. Clin Chem 1989;5;783-6.
19. Freer DE, Statland BE. The effects of ethanol (0.75 g/kg body weight) on the activities of selected enzymes in sera of healthy adults: 1. Intermediate-term effects. Clin Chem 1977;23:830-4.

20. Fuentes-Arderiu X, Fraser CG. Analytical goals for interference. Ann Clin Biochem 1991;28:393-5.
21. Goldberg DM, Watts C. Serum enzyme changes as evidence of liver reaction to oral alcohol. Gastroenterology 1965;49:256-61.
22. Green AG. Circannual excretory patterns in man. J Clin Pathol 1974;27:932.
23. Haralambie G. Serum glycoproteins and physical exercise. Clin Chim Acta 1974;26:287-91.
24. Harris EK. Statistical aspects of reference values in clinical pathology. Prog Clin Pathol 1981;8;45-66.
25. Harris EK, Boyd JC. On dividing reference data into sub-groups to produce separate reference ranges. Clin Chem 1990;36:265-70.
26. Harris EK, Yasaka T. On the calculation of a "reference change" for comparing two consecutive measurements. Clin Chem 1983;29;25-30.
27. Holzel WGE. Intra-individual variation of analytes in serum of patients with chronic renal failure. Clin Chem 1987;33;670-3.
28. Holzel WGE. Intra-individual variation of analytes in serum in patients with chronic liver diseases. Clin Chem 1987;33:1133-6.
29. Howey JEA, Browning MCK, Fraser CG. Selecting the optimum specimen for assessing slight albuminuria and a strategy for clinical investigation: novel uses of data on biological variation. Clin Chem 1987;33:2034.
30. Irjala KM, Gronroos PE. Preanalytical and analytical factors affecting laboratory results. Ann Med 1998;30:267-72.
31. Jensen J, Blankenhorn DH, Chin HP, et al. Serum lipids and serum uric acid in human twins. J Lipid Res 1965;6:193-204.
32. Keys A, Anderson JT, Mickelsen O, et al. Diet and serum cholesterol in men: Lack of effect of dietary cholesterol. J Nutr 1956;59:39-56.
33. Khalil M, Tanios A, Moghazy M, et al. Serum and red cell folates, and serum vitamin B12 in protein calorie malnutrition. Arch Dis Child 1973;48:366-9.
34. Lancher DA, Connelly DP. Rate and delta checks compared for selected chemistry tests. Clin Chem 1998;34:1966-79.
35. Letellier G, Desjarlais F. Study of seasonal variations for eighteen biochemical parameters over a four-year period. Clin Biochem 1982;15:206-12.
36. Merimee TJ, Fineberg ES. Homeostasis during fasting: II. Hormone substrate differences between men and women. J Clin Endocrinol Metab 1982;37:698-702.
37. Minoia C. Assessment of factors causing pre-analytic variability. Ann Ist Super Sanita. 1995;31:225-32
38. Mogadam M, Ahmed SW, Mensch AH, et al. Within-person fluctuations of serum cholesterol and lipoproteins. Arch Intern Med 1998;150:1645-8.
39. Munan L, Kelly A, PetitClerc C. Association with body weight of selected chemical constituents in blood. Clin Chem 1978;24:772-7.
40. Olusi SO, McFarlane H, Osunkoya BO, et al. Specific protein assays in protein calorie malnutrition. Clin Chim Acta 1975;62:107-16.
41. Pelsers MM, Chapelle JP, Knapen M, et al. Influence of age and sex and day-to-day and within-day biological variation on plasma concentrations of fatty acid-binding protein and myoglobin in healthy subjects. Clin Chem 1999;45:441-3.
42. Pitts RF. Physiology of the kidney and body fluids, 3rd ed. Chicago: Year Book Medical Publishers, 1974.
43. Rapport A, From GLA, Husdan H. Metabolic studies in prolonged fasting: I. Inorganic metabolism and kidney function. Metabolism 1965;14:31-46.
44. Rayfield EJ, Curnow RT, George DT, et al. Impaired carbohydrate metabolism during a mild viral illness. NEJM 1973;289:618-21.
45. Sassard J, Vincent M, Annat G, et al. A kinetic study of plasma renin and aldosterone during changes of posture in man. J Clin Endocrinol Metab 1976;42: 20-7.
46. Sebastian-Gambaro MA, Liron-Hernandez FJ, Fuentes-Arderiu X. Intra- and inter-individual biological variability data bank. Eur J Clin Chem Clin Biochem 1997;35:845-52.
47. Siest G, Henny J, Schiele F, eds. Interpretation des examens de laboratoire. Basel: Karger, 1981.
48. Stinton TJ, Crowley D, Bryant SJ. Reference values of calcium, phosphate, and alkaline phosphatase as derived on the basis of multi-analyzer profiles. Clin Chem 1986;32:76-9.
49. Statland BE, Winkel P, Bokelund H. Factors contributing to intraindividual variation of serum constituents: 1. Within-day variation of serum constituents in healthy subjects. Clin. Chem 1973;19:1374-9.
50. Steinmetz J, Panek E, Sourieau F, et al. Influence of food intake on biological parameters. In: Reference values in human chemistry. Siest G. ed. Basel: Karger, 1973:193-200.
51. Thomson WHS, Sweetin JC, Hamilton IJD. ATP and muscle enzyme efflux after physical exertion. Clin Chim Acta 1975;59:241-5.
52. Weitzman ED. Circadian rhythms and episodic hormone secretion. Ann Rev Med 1976;27:225-43.
53. Wesson LG, Jr. Electrolyte excretion in relation to diurnal cycles of renal function. Medicine 1964;43: 547-92.
54. Wilding P, Rollason JG, Robinson D. Pattern of change for various biochemical constituents detected in well-population screening. Clin Chim Acta 1972;41:375-87.
55. Young DS. Biological variability. In: Brown SS, Mitchell FLDS, Young DS, eds. Chemical diagnosis of disease. Amsterdam: Elsevier Science Publishing Co, 1979:113.
56. Young DS. The effects of frequently prescribed drugs on common laboratory procedures. In: Spittell JA Jr, ed. Practice of medicine. Philadelphia: JB Lippincott Co, 1984:1-21.

57. Young DS. Effects of drugs on clinical laboratory tests, 5th ed. Washington DC: AACC Press, 2001.
58. Young DS. Effects of preanalytical variables on clinical laboratory tests, 2nd ed. Washington DC: AACC Press, 1997.

ADDITIONAL READING

Antonsen S. The estimation of biological and preanalytical variations of inflammation markers. Scand J Clin Lab Invest Suppl 1994;219:55-60.

Dasgupta A. Review of abnormal laboratory test results and toxic effects due to use of herbal medicines. Am J Clin Pathol 2003;120:127-37.

Dugue B, Leppanen E, Grasbeck R. Preanalytical factors and the measurement of cytokines in human subjects. Int J Clin Lab Res 1996;26:99-105.

Faulkner WR, Meites S. Geriatric clinical chemistry, reference values, Washington DC: AACC Press, 1993.

Fraser CG: Biological Variation: From principles to practice. Washington, DC: AACC Press, 2001.

Guder WG, Narayanan S, Wisser H, Zawta B. Samples from the patient to the laboratory, 3rd edition. Weinheim Germany: Wiley-VCH Verlag, 2003.

Hannon R, Eastell R. Preanalytical variability of biochemical markers of bone turnover. Osteoporos Int 2000;11:S30-44.

Kallner A. Preanalytical procedures in the measurement of ionized calcium in serum and plasma. Eur J Clin Chem Clin Biochem 1996;34:53-8.

Keffer JH. Preanalytical considerations in testing thyroid function. Clin Chem 1996;42:125-34.

Narayanan S. Preanalytical aspects of coagulation testing. Haematologica 1995;80:1-6.

Petersen H, Larsen ML, Horder M, Blaabjerg O. Influence of analytical quality and preanalytical variations on measurements of cholesterol in screening programmes. Scand J Clin Lab Invest Suppl 1990;198:66-72.

Soldin SJ, Brugnara C, Wong EC. Pediatric reference ranges, 4rd edition, Washington DC: AACC Press, 2003.

Statland BE, Winkel P. Effects of preanalytical factors on the intraindividual variation of analytes in the blood of healthy subjects: Consideration of preparation of the subject and time of venipuncture. CRC Crit Rev Clin Lab Sci 1977;8:105-44.

Tietz NW (ed). Clinical guide to laboratory tests, 3rd edition. Philadelphia: WB Saunders Co, 1995.

Vesper HW, Demers LM, Eastell R, Garnero P, Kleerekoper M, Robins SP, et al. Assessment and recommendations on factors contributing to preanalytical variability of urinary pyridinoline and deoxypyridinoline. Clin Chem 2002;48:220-35.

Withold W. Monitoring of bone turnover biological, preanalytical and technical criteria in the assessment of biochemical markers. Eur J Clin Chem Clin Biochem 1996;34:785-99.

CHAPTER 18

Clinical Laboratory Informatics*

Kent A. Spackman, M.D., Ph.D.

Many authors have observed that a clinical laboratory produces information as its main product. Information technology plays a key role in the effective management of information, and therefore a certain level of knowledge and skill in information technology and informatics has become essential to clinical laboratory professionals.[2,3,5] *Health informatics* may be defined as the principles and practice of effective information management for health, including the collection, processing, and distribution of health information about individuals and populations. *Clinical laboratory informatics* deals with the total testing process, from the time a clinician perceives a requirement for a test until the time he or she receives and interprets the result of that test. The computer is an important tool for managing this flow of information, but informatics addresses more than just computing; indeed, the most important aspects of informatics often depend on workflow and human factors, rather than on computer hardware or software. Still, a basic understanding of general computing concepts is fundamental to an ability to recognize and solve problems in the effective use of information.

COMPUTING FUNDAMENTALS

This section provides an introduction to informatics concepts, starting with definitions, progressing to hardware descriptions, and finishing with observations regarding the rate of developmental change in computing.

Computer Basics

Any computer system consists of *hardware,* the physical devices connected together forming the computer, and *software,* the set of programs and instructions that tell the hardware what to do. A *program* consists of a set of ordered commands, which the computer hardware can execute in sequence to accomplish a task. *System programs* are designed to support general tasks, such as reading from an input device, displaying on a screen, printing, or allowing a user to log in, and basically making the computer "run." A collection of essential system programs is called the *operating system.* Microsoft Windows and Linux are examples of operating systems. Programs that are designed to do special purpose tasks, such as running a laboratory information system, are called *application programs.* When the program supports interaction with a person (the *user*), it is called a *user application.* Application programs must be compatible with the operating system on which they run. We say the application runs *on top of* the operating system. Upgrades to either the operating system or the application program may introduce incompatibilities, which may or may not be known to the software suppliers, so a new version of either application software or operating system requires testing before the system can be used with confidence. The combination of hardware, operating system, and applications, together with the persons who use them and the processes that they follow, is often called an *information system.* It cannot be overemphasized that the most important determinants of success of an information system are the people and processes, not the hardware and software.

Selecting the hardware correctly is generally a matter of determining or specifying capacity and compatibility with standards. Hardware capacity can usually be simplified to two aspects: size and speed.

*The author gratefully acknowledges the original contribution by Dr. Franklin R. Elevitch, on which portions of this chapter are based.

Size

The smallest quantity of computer information is the *bit,* or binary digit, meaning either a 0 or a 1. Because information represented and stored this way uses such discrete digits, it is called *digital,* in contrast to information represented using essentially unlimited levels of gradation, a representation called *analog.* Putting several bits together in a string results in a series of zeroes and ones; each such combination can be used to represent a different numeral or alphabetic character. By convention, a *byte* consists of eight bits. There are 2^8 or 256 different combinations of bits that can be represented by one byte. Computers can interpret these 256 combinations according to standards such as the American Standard Code for Information Interchange (ASCII). Because ASCII assigns one byte to each typewritten character, a useful rough estimate of the size of a document equates the number of typewritten characters with the number of bytes required to store it. Documents containing special characters or symbols (accents, umlauts, etc.) may be stored using the Unicode standards, which often use more than one byte per character.

Size, in computer terms, uses idiosyncratic units in addition to the bit and byte. Outside the world of computing, the prefixes kilo, mega, giga, and tera ordinarily refer to 10^3, 10^6, 10^9, and 10^{12}, respectively. However, when used with *byte,* they refer instead to 2^{10}, 2^{20}, 2^{30}, and 2^{40}. That is, a kilobyte is not 1000 bytes but 1024 bytes. The reason is that *addresses,* the numbers that refer to the location of digital data, are binary numbers, so a kilobyte is the total number of bytes that can be addressed by a ten bit address, and it carries the kilo prefix because it is the power of 2 closest to 1000. Likewise a megabyte is 1,048,576 bytes because it is the power of 2 closest to 1,000,000, and represents the number of locations addressable by 20 bits.

Prefix	Computer Storage Meaning	Usual Meaning
kilo	$2^{10} = 1024$	10^3
mega	$2^{20} = 1{,}048{,}576$	10^6
giga	$2^{30} = 1{,}073{,}741{,}824$	10^9
tera	$2^{40} = 1{,}099{,}511{,}627{,}776$	10^{12}

Speed

In computer terminology, *speed* has two chief varieties: *clock speed* and *bandwidth.* Clock speeds, which give an indication of how fast a processor runs, have units of Hertz (Hz), or cycles per second. In this case, standard prefix meanings are used, so one megaHertz is 10^6 cycles per second. The simplest computer instructions require one clock cycle to be executed, so a processor with a clock speed of one megaHertz would be able to execute one instruction in one microsecond, and a gigaHertz processor could execute one instruction in a nanosecond. *Bandwidth* refers to the amount of data that can be transmitted per unit time. We might expect it to be measured in bytes per second (or kilobytes, megabytes, gigabytes, and terabytes per second), but curiously it has instead been traditionally measured in mega*bits* per second, with mega meaning 10^6, not 2^{20}.

HARDWARE

As computers have become more integrated, miniaturized, and streamlined, more and more of the internal hardware has become integrated onto a single silicon chip. As a result, it is useful to separately consider the parts of the system that are relatively modular and can be selected by the user, and the parts that are integrated into the "box," which is mainly hidden from the user.

Inside the box, there is a *central processing unit* (CPU), which is where the clock is located that determines processor speed and where the software instructions are executed. The CPU must fetch the instructions from memory. A type of memory that is very fast and located close to the CPU, usually on the same chip, it is called *cache* memory; the ordinary type of memory is called *random access memory* (RAM). Memory should be distinguished from *storage.* Generally speaking, memory can be quickly accessed, for both reading and writing, but its contents disappear when the power is turned off. By contrast, the contents of storage are slower to access and are preserved when the power is off. The exception is *read-only memory* (ROM), which has the speed of RAM but retains its contents without power; but unlike RAM and storage devices, ROM's contents are fixed and cannot be changed.

The CPU and RAM typically are placed on the same *board* or *card,* which is simply a rigid structure into which silicon chips are placed, along with conducting material that allows electrical signals to flow between the chips. A signal-conducting path is called a *bus.* Buses exist between cards, between chips on a card, and within the chips themselves. The width of a bus is simply the number of individual bits (one bit per "wire") that can be transmitted at the same time; the capacity of a bus is determined by its width combined with its clock speed, which isn't necessarily the same speed as the CPU clock speed.

Common storage devices use magnetic media, either as tapes or disks. Disks can be either fixed or removable; early removable magnetic disks were flexible and so were called *floppy disks,* and the name has been retained even though current "floppies" are enclosed in a rigid case. Large capacity magnetic disk storage devices are commonly called *hard drives* because the disks themselves are hard, not flexible, and they have a motor (drive) that spins them. Although floppies are removable from their drives, hard disks are not; if a hard disk is removable, as with some portable laptop machines, both the magnetic disk and its drive are removed as a single enclosed unit.

Magnetic tapes come in a wide variety of sizes and are relatively inexpensive, but they share the characteristic of

TABLE 18-1 Characteristics of Common Storage and Memory Devices

Storage/Memory Device	Typical Storage Capacity in Megabytes	Typical Maximum Data Transfer Rates (Reading) in Megabytes/sec
Cache memory	0.06-0.5	1000-8000
RAM	128-1024	400-2000
Floppy disk	1.44	0.05-0.5
USB flash memory stick	16-512	0.8-1.5
CD-ROM	650-680	2-8
DVD	4700-17,000	1-16
Hard disk	10,000-200,000	5-200
Magnetic tape	1000-500,000	0.5-8

requiring a spool of magnetic-coated material to be wound past a read-write head. As a result, they tend to be relatively slow, and have become relegated to use as storage for routine copies done at periodic intervals *(backups)*.

Optical disks are storage media onto which digital data are written and from which they are read using laser light; these include *compact disks* (CDs) of both read-only (CD-ROM) and read-write (CD-RW) varieties, and *digital versatile disks* (DVDs). Generally slower than magnetic hard drives, they have the advantages of being removable, much faster than magnetic tape, and capable of containing enough storage to be useful for backup and distribution of large quantities of digital data.

Storage and memory devices have a broad range of storage capacity and speed as listed in Table 18-1. The combination of speed and capacity dictates when and where each of these devices is most useful (Figure 18-1).

Any device connected to the computer but not essential for its basic operation can be called a *peripheral device.* Peripherals also may be regarded as those devices connected to the computer via a cable. With the possible exception of the hard drive that contains the operating system, most storage devices can be regarded as peripherals. Other peripherals include printers, scanners, cameras, and other devices for getting data in or moving data out, typically called *input/output* devices or I/O devices.

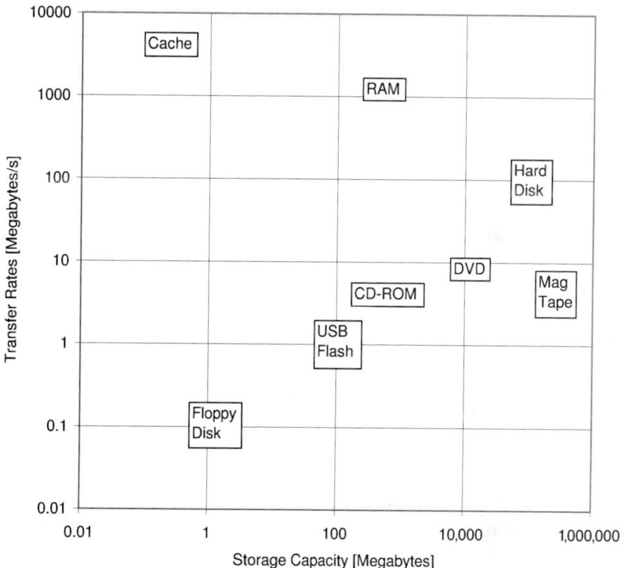

Figure 18-1 Data transfer rate in megabytes/seconds versus storage capacity for selected storage and memory devices.

Rate of Change of Computing Capacity

It could be argued that the field of scientific endeavor that has had the most impact on informatics is computer hardware engineering. Unlike most things in life, the size and expense of computers are rapidly diminishing, and their capacity and speed are rapidly increasing. This dramatic and far-reaching change has been driven primarily by an ever-increasing ability to place large numbers of integrated circuits onto silicon chips. Gordon Moore, one of the founders of the Intel Corp., observed in 1965 that the number of circuits that could be manufactured on a single chip seemed to be doubling approximately every year.[6] This observation has come to be known as "Moore's law" and has been restated and reinterpreted in many ways. For example, some authors have claimed that Moore's law implies that "computer power doubles every 18 months at half the price." Figure 18-2 illustrates the number of transistors on Intel's microprocessors and demonstrates a doubling approximately every 2 years since 1971. This exponential trend toward smaller and more powerful computing devices is seen not just in processors but also in memory, hard disk storage, and communications bandwidth. Although the basic trend continued for approximately 30 years, or 15 doublings, eventually the laws of physics will intervene and the trend will end. Indeed, some authors warn that Moore's law is increasingly an unreliable predictor of future trends.[8] Nevertheless, these changes in power, size, speed, and affordability of computing devices have been nothing short of revolutionary. We can expect this revolution to continue to have a notable impact on healthcare in many ways over the coming years.

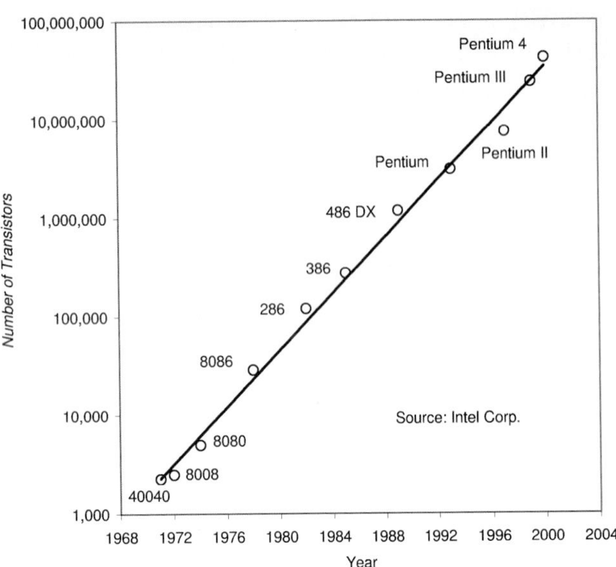

Figure 18-2 Moore's law illustrated: number of transistors per chip doubles every 18 months.

Computer Networks

Communication between computers has become commonplace, and the means of communication is usually some kind of *network.* The basic idea of a network is that a computer can connect to the network and get access, depending on authorization level, to the other computers that have also linked up, and also provide access to itself. Network signals usually travel on electrical or optical cables, although they can also use electromagnetic signals, such as radio waves or infrared light. Networks that connect computers that are all located within a local area, such as one building or perhaps a group of adjacent buildings, are called *local area networks* (LANs). To connect to the network, the computer must have both hardware and software that manages the network connection. The hardware is usually a card, called a *network interface card* (NIC), into which a cable may be connected or, alternatively, to which a wireless transmitter and/or receiver may be connected. A common standard for network hardware is called *ethernet,* which specifies the mechanism for handling the transmission of signals to and/or from the computer's NIC and the transmission medium, such as radio waves, electric pulses in wires, or light pulses in fiberoptic cables. There are also software standards for networking, often called *protocols.* These specify how to divide transmissions into blocks or chunks, how to attach destination addresses, how to signal that a transmission is starting or ending, and so forth. The most widely used set of protocols is called the *Internet protocols,* a nonproprietary suite that includes transmission control protocol (TCP) and Internet protocol (IP), often mentioned together as TCP/IP. These protocols formed the basis for a widely adopted network, called the *Internet,* that grew from what was primarily government and academic use to become virtually ubiquitous. As the Internet grew and became more widely available, additional software protocols were developed for managing the convenient organization and marking of documents that include text, images, and sounds along with the ability to connect from one document to another, even if the other documents are not on the same computer. A document containing such connections is called a *hypertext.* The *hypertext transfer protocol* (HTTP) was specified as a standard for accessing and transmitting hypertext documents that were formatted according to another standard, the *hypertext markup language* (HTML). The set of computers on the Internet that use HTTP to transfer HTML documents is called, collectively, the *Worldwide Web* (WWW). A computer program used for accessing sites or information on a network is termed a *browser.*

Computers may be connected to a LAN but not connected to the Internet. Many businesses, including healthcare organizations, keep their internal networks separate from the wider Internet. An intrainstitutional network is often called an *intranet,* and these are frequently used to connect the institution's information systems.

The phenomenon of the Worldwide Web has resulted in the widespread availability of a vast number of documents and Web pages, easily accessible through search engines such as Google (see www.google.com, accessed May 20, 2004). A search may retrieve a very wide range of quality of documents, ranging from a peer-reviewed journal article to an incoherent rant from a Usenet Newsgroup. Caution is required because the Internet may eliminate, mask, or change the traditional indicators of quality and authoritativeness.

LABORATORY INFORMATION SYSTEMS

Laboratories were the first area of healthcare institutions that adopted computer technology to manage clinical information about the patient. Within the laboratory, chemistry and hematology were the first areas to be supported, followed later by microbiology, blood banking, and anatomical pathology.

One of the first functions supported by laboratory information systems (LISs) was the printing of summary laboratory data for inclusion in the patient's chart. This replaced the labor-intensive and error-prone process of manually writing or typing results on individual slips of paper. Other important intralaboratory functions included assigning accession numbers and tracking specimens and workload. Information system functions have expanded to include virtually every area of laboratory operation.[4]

LIS Modules

Most LISs have different modules that support the natural divisions of the laboratory or groups of those divisions. A *general laboratory module* often supports chemistry and

BOX 18-1 Workflow Steps Necessary to Use a Laboratory Test

Test request	Work list creation
Order entry	Result entry and verification
Collection scheduling	Automated analyzer interface
Label generation	Specimen tracking
Specimen collection	Reflex testing
Specimen transport	Quality assurance
Specimen delivery and accession	Result reporting

hematology, along with immunology, coagulation, urinalysis, and any other parts of the laboratory that tend to perform tests with a fixed numeric result with a reference range. These lab sections and the modules that support them are more likely also to have an automated analyzer to which the LIS is connected via an electronic interface. Laboratory sections that are frequently supported by separate modules include the transfusion service, microbiology, cytopathology, and surgical pathology.

Workflow, Entities, Attributes, and Relationships

To understand the way laboratory information systems work, it is helpful to think about laboratory workflow and the kinds of information required at each step. Box 18-1 lists a set of workflow steps usually followed by a laboratory test.

Different data elements are required at each step in the workflow. The *test request* originates with the ordering physician or provider, and may be hand written, spoken, or entered electronically. *Order entry* signifies the point at which the test request becomes properly specified according to the information system's data structures. At this step, identifiers are required for the patient, the ordering provider, and the test to be performed. Tests must be identified according to the list of tests known to the system, and can sometimes also be modified to include specific timing, pretest preparation, and other variables. *Accession* refers to the point at which a specimen becomes known to the information system, and usually corresponds closely with the delivery of the specimen to the laboratory. A unique accession number is assigned, allowing the information system to track the specimen and correlate it with the order.

Information systems are often described in terms of the *entities* about which they manage information, the *attributes* that describe those entities, and the *relationships* between the entities. This approach to modeling the information is called *entity-relationship modeling* or *E-R modeling.* Patients, providers, specimens, and orders are examples of *entities,* and medical record number, provider identifier, accession number, and order number are all examples of *attributes.* The *relationship* between these entities is represented by a data structure that includes a particular patient identification (ID), provider ID, order ID, and accession number. To design the information system, data analysts often begin by identifying all the *entities* about which we will require information, the *attributes* or data elements that detail the specifics about these entities, and the *relationships* that connect different entities to each other.

Data Standards and Encoding

Whenever information must be shared between two different information systems, a common method of identifying entities must also be shared. The broader the necessity for sharing, the more universal the identifiers have to be. For this reason, numerous standards have been developed to help identify and share information about healthcare information entities such as laboratory tests, images, diagnoses, and procedures.

In the United States, the 1996 HIPAA legislation (the Health Insurance Portability and Accountability Act) resulted in the designation of six required code sets for billing and reimbursement. These are listed in Table 18-2.

The code sets required for billing and reimbursement are capable of representing only a limited amount of information about the health or healthcare of a patient. These limitations are a result of the intended use of the codes (i.e., determining an appropriate dollar figure to attach to a particular procedure or condition). Researchers have evaluated the ability of these code sets to represent the level of detail required for conducting studies of the outcomes of healthcare or enabling computer-based decision support, and have found them to be notably less detailed than required. As a result, a second group of standards was designated by HIPAA as those that support patient medical record information (PMRI). These PMRI standards are not mandated by the government but are recommended for supporting the voluntary movement toward adoption by clinical information systems and healthcare organizations. The most important PMRI standards for clinical laboratories are the Systematized Nomenclature of Medicine—Clinical Terms (SNOMED CT[7]) and Laboratory Logical Observation Identifiers, Names, and Codes (Lab LOINC[9]).

SNOMED CT

SNOMED CT is a clinical terminology, used to code information about health and the care of individuals and populations. At its most basic level, it contains a set of codes, each representing a different concept. For example, "acute appendicitis" is one concept, and "appendicitis" is another concept, and each has its own code. These concept codes are connected to each other in a hierarchy (represented in a data table), with more general concepts such as "appendicitis" located above more specific concepts such as "acute appendicitis." In addition to this hierarchy, concepts are also connected to each other via *attributes* that specify defining characteristics. For example, "appendicitis" may be

TABLE 18-2 U.S. Code Sets for Billing and Reimbursement

Code Set	Purpose
ICD-9-CM vol 1&2: International Classification of Diseases, 9th Edition, Clinical Modification, Volumes 1 and 2	Diseases, injuries, impairments, other health-related problems and their manifestations; causes of injury, disease, impairment, or other health-related problems
ICD-9-CM vol 3: International Classification of Diseases, 9th Edition, Clinical Modification, Volume 3 Procedures	Hospital inpatients: prevention, diagnosis, treatment, management
NDC: National Drug Codes	Retail pharmacies: drugs, biologicals
CDT-2: Code on Dental Procedures and Nomenclature	Dental services
CPT-4: Current Procedural Terminology plus HCPCS: Health Care Financing Administration Common Procedure Coding System	Physician services, physical and occupational therapy services, radiological procedures, clinical laboratory tests, other medical diagnostic procedures, hearing and vision services, transportation services including ambulance
HCPCS	Medical supplies, orthotic and prosthetic devices, durable medical equipment

linked via the attribute *site* to the anatomical concept "appendix."

The scope of SNOMED CT is very broad, encompassing human and veterinary medicine, nursing, dentistry, allied health professions, and population-based health concepts. It includes codes for diagnoses, procedures, findings, drugs, anatomy, organisms, causes of disease, and social aspects of health. Included in SNOMED's procedure hierarchy is a very complete list of laboratory tests and test categories. To provide smooth integration, there is a file that links these SNOMED CT codes to related Lab LOINC codes.

Lab LOINC

Lab LOINC is a set of codes designed to represent laboratory test names. These codes are intended to be used for reporting the values of tests when there is a necessity to provide laboratory test information in electronic form to any information system that does not use the same test identifiers as the originating laboratory information system. This could include transmitting test results from one LIS to another within an institution: (e.g., in providing chemistry results to an anatomical pathology system); or to a more central hospital information system; or beyond to any number of more remote systems. Sharing information in this way requires a common understanding of exactly what test was performed and how it is being reported, and the Lab LOINC codes enable the appropriate level of detail to accomplish this purpose.

The meaning of each code is specified using a six-part name. The six parts are *component* (what is measured), *kind of property* (e.g., concentration versus titer), *time aspect* (single point in time versus timed collection), *system (specimen) type, type of scale* (e.g., quantitative, ordinal, and nominal), and *method*. For example, the LOINC name for a rickettsial antibody titer done on serum by complement fixation and reported as a quantitative number is "Rickettsia sp AB|Titer|PT|Serum|QN|CF," and its code is 5306-6. Table 18-3 lists several LOINC codes, along with a corresponding SNOMED code. The meaning of each part of the LOINC name is illustrated in Figure 18-3.

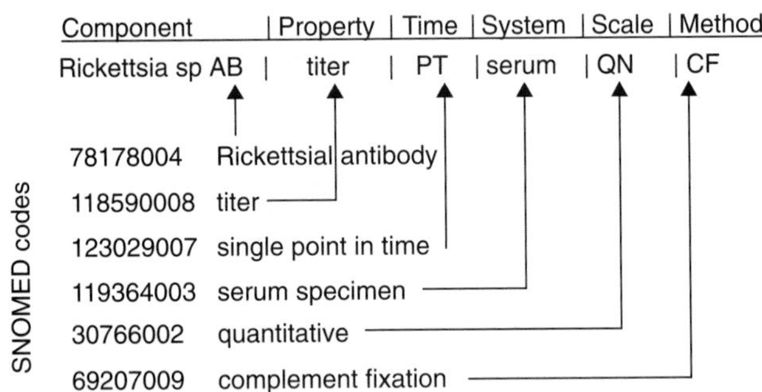

Figure 18-3 Parts of LOINC names, with SNOMED codes.

LOINC-SNOMED Integration

The relationship between the SNOMED hierarchy and the LOINC codes can be illustrated as in Figure 18-3, where more general SNOMED concepts, such as "rickettsial serological test," would be connected to several more specific rickettsial serological tests that would be reported using Lab LOINC codes.

In addition, SNOMED and LOINC are linked through a SNOMED code for each of the LOINC name parts, as illustrated in Figure 18-4. The SNOMED hierarchies for these codes will enable software systems to automatically compute that a complement fixation test for Rickettsia is a subtype of

TABLE 18-3 SNOMED-LOINC Correlation Example

SNOMED Code	LOINC Code	Concept name
17652006		**Serological Test for *Rickettsia rickettsii***
	29705-1	RICKETTSIA RICKETTSII AB|TITR|PT|SER|QN|IF
	29706-9	RICKETTSIA RICKETTSII AB|ACNC|PT|SER|ORD|IF
	29737-4	RICKETTSIA RICKETTSII AB|TITR|PT|SER|QN|
	5307-4	RICKETTSIA RICKETTSII AB.IGG|TITR|PT|SER|QN|IF
	8003-6	RICKETTSIA RICKETTSII AB.IGG|ACNC|PT|SER|QN|
	18430-9	RICKETTSIA RICKETTSII AB.IGM|ACNC|PT|CSF|QN|
	22483-2	RICKETTSIA RICKETTSII AB.IGM|TITR|PT|SER|QN|
	5308-2	RICKETTSIA RICKETTSII AB.IGM|TITR|PT|SER|QN|IF
	8004-4	RICKETTSIA RICKETTSII AB.IGM|ACNC|PT|SER|QN|
117992009		**Rickettsia (Proteus OX19) Antibody Assay**
	21489-0	RICKETTSIA (PROTEUS OX19) AB|TITR|PT|SER|QN|LA
	22468-3	RICKETTSIA (PROTEUS OX19) AB|ACNC|PT|SER|ORD|
	22469-1	RICKETTSIA (PROTEUS OX19) AB|TITR|PT|SER|QN|
	31593-7	RICKETTSIA (PROTEUS OX19) AB|ACNC|PT|SER|QN|
	5303-3	RICKETTSIA (PROTEUS OX19) AB|ACNC|PT|SER|ORD|LA

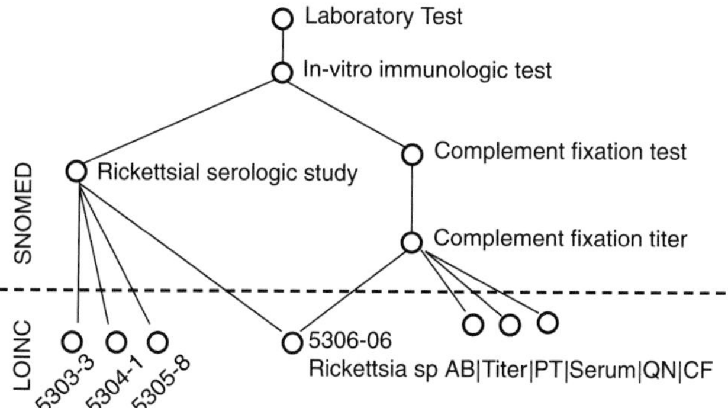

Figure 18-4 LOINC-SNOMED hierarchy integration.

a complement fixation test for a microbial antibody, because the code for Rickettsia species antibody is in the hierarchy for microbial antibodies.

Table 18-3 lists SNOMED codes for rickettsial serologies, along with some of the more specific LOINC codes that are subtypes of these concepts. The LOINC concepts differ based on whether they measure a titer (TITR) or an arbitrary concentration (ACNC); whether they are measuring the antibody in the serum (SER) or another specimen, such as the cerebrospinal fluid (CSF); whether the reported value is quantitative (QN) or ordinal (ORD); and whether the method is specified, such as immunofixation (IF) or latex agglutination (LA). Note that the words "serological test" are intended to mean testing for the antibody to the organism, regardless of the specimen (serum, CSF, or other). Thus in this example the SNOMED code specifies only the "component" part of the LOINC code and leaves the other five LOINC fields unspecified. In Figure 18-4 the SNOMED concept "complement fixation titer" specifies only the SCALE and PROPERTY and leaves the other four LOINC fields unspecified.

Life Cycle of Information Systems

Information systems can be understood as having a life cycle analogous to living organisms. Understanding where a system is in its life cycle can provide insight into the most appropriate steps to be taken to properly manage the system. Major phases in the life cycle of information systems include a definition or specification phase, an acquisition or development phase, an implementation and deployment phase, an operation and maintenance phase, and a disposition phase.

Definition and/or Specification

The earliest phase of an information system cycle, the definition phase involves recognition of and explicit justification of the requirement for the system, including detailed analysis of how information is presently being handled and how the new system would change and improve upon current practices. Success of later phases depends on the care with which the definition and specification are carried out.

Acquisition and/or Development

Although it is possible for a laboratory to develop its own LIS, most healthcare institutions lack the expertise to do this, and when facing a build-or-buy decision they usually come down on the side of "buy." The identification of suitable commercial vendors usually begins with a request for information (RFI), providing basic information about the vendor and its software offerings, followed by a request for proposal (RFP), which asks the vendors to respond to a set of more detailed functional questions designed to assist the laboratory in determining whether, and how well, the vendor's offerings can meet the laboratory's requirements. A convenient source listing vendors is a survey of LIS companies published each fall by *CAP Today* (see www.cap.org, accessed May 20, 2004).

Implementation and Deployment

Once LIS software has been selected, the next step is implementation, a process that usually requires many weeks of concerted effort on the part of both the vendor and the laboratory. The success of an LIS depends directly on how well it is configured to fit the requirements of the laboratory. Transition from a prior information system usually requires extensive training or retraining of laboratory personnel and revision of standard operating procedures. Most implementations also encounter unexpected problems that require additional time and resources.

Most large laboratories will require 12 to 18 months at a minimum, and frequently more, to progress through the first three phases of definition, acquisition, and implementation.

Operation and Maintenance

Once in place, an LIS must be supported and maintained. Software modules and operating systems may have to be upgraded and synchronized. Interfaces to laboratory instruments and communication links with clinical systems also frequently require upgrading and support. Although one might hope that an LIS could evolve gracefully and not require replacement, in practice all information systems inevitably become obsolete, and a new system life cycle begins.

Disposition

Although most of the work to replace an obsolete system involves the definition, acquisition, and implementation of a new system, the disposition of the old system also has to be considered. In particular, data preservation and migration should be carefully evaluated.

Regulatory Issues

In the United States, federal regulations apply to any device, including computers and information systems that directly impact the patient or the process of production of devices and substances that come into contact with the patient. As a result, computer software that is used in the collection, tracking, and processing of blood products is subject to Food and Drug Administration (FDA) preapproval and ongoing inspection. These regulations require careful documentation of the development of the software, and rigorous testing and validation at the time of implementation and again at the time of any upgrade or change.[1]

General LIS applications, outside blood collection or transfusion services, are not subject to FDA regulations, but many laboratories voluntarily subject their LIS to inspection and accreditation. The College of American Pathologists (CAP) inspection and accreditation checklists for laboratory computer software focus on documentation of practices that ensure the safe and reliable operation of the system, such as regular backup of data, validation of system function following software upgrades, and regular testing of the correctness of transmitted or printed laboratory results.

Security and Confidentiality

The administrative simplification provisions of HIPAA were written with the understanding that improvements in safeguards of electronic health information must go hand in hand with increasing detail and sharing of such electronic data. The traditional paper record was inaccessible to all but the individual having possession of the physical record; this created problems when the record was lost, or was necessary at more than one location, but it also provided a natural limit on the accessibility to unauthorized parties. As information becomes available in electronic form, patients have an interest in improved security and confidentiality of their health records.

Security generally refers to the provisions for ensuring that electronic data are prevented from unintentional destruction, loss, alteration, or disclosure. *Confidentiality* refers to the expectation that information about a patient should remain within the patient's control, should be disclosed only to authorized individuals, and should not be used for purposes the patient does not approve.

Achieving a balance between access and security is not simple. In a hospital, numerous individuals have a need to handle patient data; too strict limits on access to data can harm patients by preventing healthcare workers from providing the best care. On the other hand, lax security leaves patients and the institution in danger of harm from unauthorized access to data.

Measures necessary for ensuring security include careful management of access to computer systems, monitoring and tracking access, and judicious application of penalties for violation of security policy. Each user should be required to be identified to the system, and access should depend on a password or other secure mechanism that prevents unauthorized access. Access to patient data, and particularly changes to data, should be automatically logged according to user, date and time, and action taken. These logs are called *audit trails*, an important tool for monitoring system security. When employees inappropriately access patient data for which they have no responsibility, penalties up to and including dismissal should be known and applied when necessary.

PATHOLOGY INFORMATICS RESOURCES

A number of annual meetings are available for laboratory medicine professionals interested in informatics. These include:

- Automated Information Management in the Clinical Laboratory (AIMCL)

- Advancing Pathology Informatics, Imaging, and the Internet (APIII): see apiii.upmc.edu
- Lab InfoTech Summit: see https://www.labinfotech.org/

REFERENCES

1. Brannigan VM. Regulation of clinical laboratory information systems after the 1990 amendments to the Food and Drug Act. Clin Lab Man Rev 1992;6:49-57.
2. Cowan DF, ed. Informatics for the Clinical Laboratory: A Practical Guide. Springer-Verlag New York. 2003.
3. Becich MJ. Information management: moving from test results to clinical information. Clin Leadership Manag Rev 2000;14:296-300.
4. Elevitch FR, Aller RD. The ABCs of LIS: Computerizing your laboratory information system. Chicago: ASCP Press, 1989.
5. Henricks WH, Boyer PJ, Harrison JH, Tuthill JM, Healy JC. Informatics training in pathology residency programs: proposed learning objectives and skill sets for the new millennium. Arch Pathol Lab Med 2003;127:1009-18.
6. Lenzner R. The Reluctant Entrepreneur. *Forbes*, Sept. 11, 1995, p. 162.
7. The Systematized Nomenclature of Medicine, Clinical Terms (SNOMED CT). College of American Pathologists. Northfield IL. 2003.
8. Tuomi, I. The Lives and Death of Moore's Law. *First Monday*, vol 7 no 11, Nov. 2002. See http://www.firstmonday.dk/issues/issue7_11/, accessed on May 20, 2004.
9. Logical Observations, Identifiers, Names and Codes (LOINC). Regenstrief Institute, Indianapolis, IN. 2003.

WORLDWIDE WEB SITES

apiii.upmc.edu—Advancing Pathology Informatics, Imaging, and the Internet
www.aacc.org—American Association for Clinical Chemistry
www.amia.org—American Medical Informatics Association
www.ascp.org—American Society for Clinical Pathology
www.pathologyinformatics.org—Association for Pathology Informatics
www.cdc.gov—Centers for Disease Control and Prevention
www.cap.org—College of American Pathologists
www.nccls.org—National Committee for Clinical Laboratory Standards, Inc.
www.nih.gov—National Institutes of Health, USA
www.nlm.nih.gov—The U.S. National Library of Medicine

CHAPTER 19

Quality Management

James O. Westgard, Ph.D., and George G. Klee, M.D., Ph.D.

The principles of quality management, assurance, and control have become the foundation by which clinical laboratories are managed and operated. This chapter begins with a discussion of the fundamentals of total quality management followed by discussions of (1) total quality management of the clinical laboratory, (2) laboratory error and the Six Sigma process, (3) elements of a quality assurance program, (4) control of preanalytical variables, (5) control of analytical variables, (6) control of analytical quality using stable control materials, (7) control of analytical quality using patient data, (8) external quality assessment and proficiency testing programs, and (9) identifying the sources of analytical errors. We conclude the chapter with a discussion on quality initiatives, including the ISO 9000 certification process.

FUNDAMENTALS OF TOTAL QUALITY MANAGEMENT

Quality systems in healthcare organizations continue to evolve* with numerous sources of information on quality available on the Internet.[26] Public and private pressures to contain costs are now accompanied by pressures to improve quality. The seemingly contradictory pressures for both cost reduction and quality improvement (QI) require that healthcare organizations adopt new systems for managing quality. When faced with these same pressures, other industries implemented "total quality management," or TQM.[101] TQM may also be referred to as total quality control (QC), total quality leadership, continuous quality improvement, or quality management science, or more generally as industrial quality management. TQM provides both a management *philosophy* for organizational development and a management *process* for improving the quality of all aspects of work. Many healthcare organizations have adopted the concepts and principles of TQM.[4]

*References 37, 39, 65, 67, 74, 87, 99, 104, 111.

FUNDAMENTAL CONCEPTS

In this chapter, quality is defined as conformance to the requirements of users or customers. More directly, quality refers to the satisfaction of the needs and expectations of users or customers. The focus on users and customers is important, particularly in service industries such as healthcare. The users of healthcare laboratories are often the nurses and physicians; their customers are the patients and other parties who pay the bills.

Cost must be understood in the context of quality. If quality means conformance to requirements, then "quality costs" must be understood in terms of "costs of conformance" and "costs of nonconformance," as illustrated in Figure 19-1. In industrial terms, costs of conformance are divided into prevention costs and appraisal costs. Costs of nonconformance consist of internal and external failure costs. For a laboratory testing process, calibration is a good example of a cost incurred to prevent problems. Likewise, quality control is a cost for appraising performance, a repeat run is an internal failure cost for poor analytical performance, and repeat requests for tests because of poor analytical quality are an external failure cost.

This understanding of quality and cost leads to a new perspective on the relationship between them. Improvements in quality can lead to reductions in cost. For example, with better analytical quality, a laboratory can eliminate repeat runs and repeat requests for tests. This repeat work is "waste." If quality were improved, waste would be reduced, which in turn would reduce cost. The father of this fundamental concept was the late W. Edwards Deming, who developed and internationally promulgated the idea that quality improvement reduces waste and leads to improved

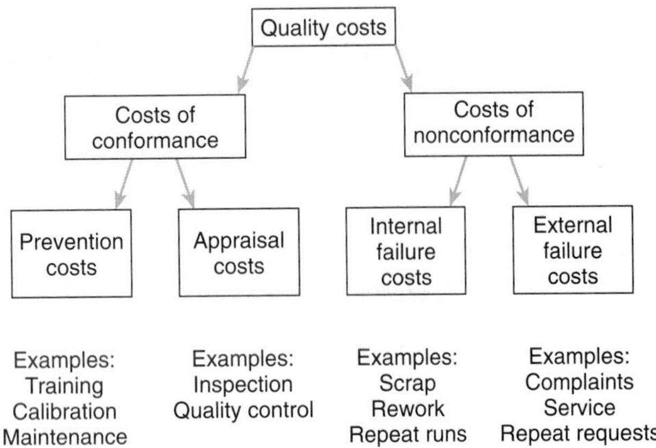

Figure 19-1 The cost of quality in terms of the costs of conformance and the costs of nonconformance to customer requirements. *(From Westgard JO, Barry PL. Cost-effective quality control: Managing the quality and productivity of analytical processes. Washington DC: AACC Press, 1986.)*

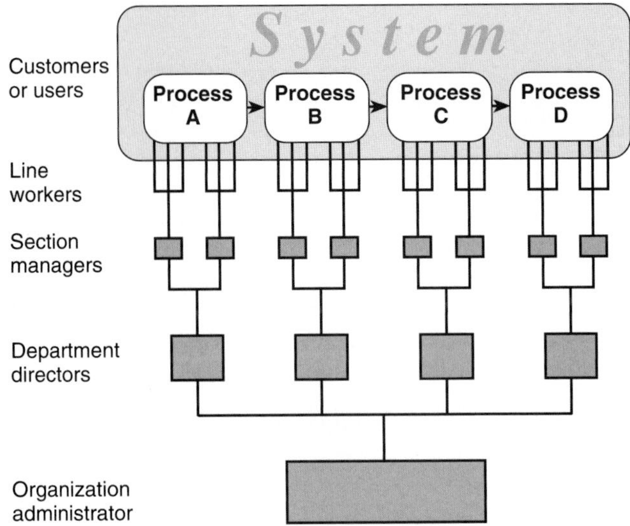

Figure 19-2 TQM view of an organization as a system of processes.

productivity, which in turn reduces costs and provides a competitive advantage.[25] As a result, the organization stays in business and is able to continue providing jobs for its employees.

Fundamental Principles

Quality improvement occurs when problems are eliminated permanently. Problems arise primarily from imperfect processes, not from imperfect people. Industrial experience has shown that 85% of all problems are process problems that are solvable only by managers, with the remaining 15% being problems requiring the action and improvement of performance of individual workers. Thus quality problems are primarily management problems because only management has the power to change work processes.

This emphasis on processes leads to a new view of the organization as a system of processes, as illustrated in Figure 19-2. For example, physicians might view a healthcare organization as a provider of processes for patient examination (A), patient testing (B), patient diagnosis (C), and patient treatment (D). Healthcare administrators might view the activities in terms of processes for admitting patients (A), tracking patient services (B), discharging patients (C), and billing for costs of service (D). Laboratory directors might understand their responsibilities in terms of processes for acquisition of specimens (A), processing of specimens (B), analysis of samples (C), and reporting of test results (D). Laboratory analysts might view their work as processes for acquiring samples (A), analyzing samples (B), performing quality control (C), and releasing patient test results (D). The total system for a healthcare organization involves the interaction of all of these processes and many others.

Given the primary importance of these processes for accomplishing the work of the organization, TQM views the organization as a support structure rather than as a command structure. As a support structure, the most immediate processes required for the delivery of services are those of the frontline employees. Upper management's role is to support the frontline employees and to *empower* them to identify and solve problems in their own work processes.

The importance of empowerment is easily understood if a problem involves processes from two different departments. For example, if a problem occurs that involves the link between process A and process B in Figure 19-2, the traditional management structure requires that the problem be passed up from the line workers to a section manager or supervisor, a department director, and an organization administrator. The administrator then works back through an equal number of intermediaries in the other department. Direct involvement of line workers and their managers should provide more immediate resolution of the problem.

However, such problem solving requires a carefully structured process to ensure that root causes are identified and proposed solutions are verified. Juran's "project-by-project" quality improvement process[42] provides detailed guidelines that have been widely adopted and integrated into current team problem-solving methodology.[3,4,85] The methodology outlines distinct steps for (1) carefully defining the problem, (2) establishing baseline measures of process performance, (3) identifying root causes of the problem, (4) identifying a remedy for the problem, (5) verifying that the remedy actually works, (6) "standardizing" or generalizing the solution for routine implementation of an improved process, and (7) establishing ongoing measures for monitoring and controlling the process.

The quality improvement "project team" provides a new flexible organization unit. A project team is a group of employees appointed by management to solve a specific problem that has been identified by management or staff. The team comprises members from any department and from any level of the organization and includes anyone who

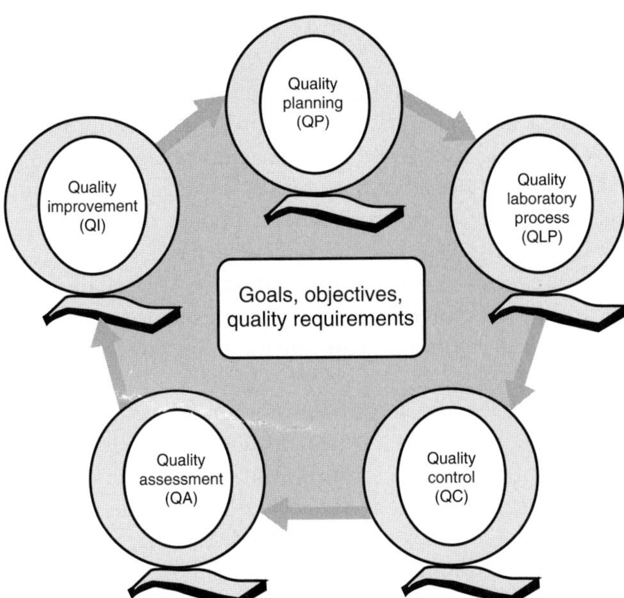

Figure 19-3 TQM framework for managing quality in a healthcare laboratory. *(From Westgard JO, Burnett RW, Bowers GN. Quality management science in clinical chemistry: A dynamic framework for continuous improvement of quality. Clin Chem 1990;36:1712-6.)*

is necessary to understand the problem and identify the solution. Management initiates the project, and the team is empowered and supported to identify the root cause and verify a solution; the management then becomes involved in replanning the process (i.e., planning the implementation of changes in a laboratory process, defining and standardizing the improved process, and establishing appropriate measures for ongoing evaluation and control of the process).[112]

TOTAL QUALITY MANAGEMENT OF THE CLINICAL LABORATORY

The principles and concepts of TQM have been formalized into a quality management process, as illustrated in Figure 19-3. The traditional framework for managing quality in a healthcare laboratory has emphasized the establishment of quality laboratory processes (QLPs), QC, and quality assessment (QA). A QLP includes analytical processes and the general policies, practices, and procedures that define how all aspects of the work get done. QC emphasizes statistical control procedures but also includes nonstatistical check procedures, such as linearity checks, reagent and standard checks, and temperature monitors. QA, as currently applied, is primarily concerned with broader measures and monitors of laboratory performance, such as turnaround time, specimen identification, patient identification, and test utility. Quality "assessment" is the proper name for these activities rather than quality "assurance." Measuring performance does not by itself improve performance and often does not detect problems in time to prevent harmful effects. Quality assurance requires either that causes of problems be identified through QI and eliminated through quality planning (QP) or that QC be able to detect the problems early enough to prevent their consequences.

To provide a fully developed system and framework for managing quality, the QI and QP components must be established.[65,67,111] QI provides a structured problem-solving process for identifying the root cause of a problem and also for identifying a remedy for the problem. QP is necessary to (1) standardize the remedy, (2) establish measures for monitoring performance, (3) ensure that the performance achieved satisfies quality requirements, and (4) document the new QLP. The new process is then implemented through QLP, measured and monitored through QC and QA, improved through QI, and replanned through QP. These five components, working together in a feedback loop, illustrate how continuous QI is accomplished and how quality assurance is built into laboratory processes.

The "five-Q" framework also defines how quality can be managed objectively using the "scientific method" or the *PDCA cycle* (**p**lan, **d**o, **c**heck, **a**ct). QP provides the planning step, QLP establishes standard processes for doing things, QC and QA provide measures for checking how well things are done, and QI provides a mechanism for acting on those measures. The methodology that we naturally apply in scientific experiments should also be the basis for objective management decisions.

Objectivity, however, is dependent on our having quantitative quality requirements for evaluating the performance of existing processes and for planning the performance of new processes.[114] Laboratories must define their service goals and objectives and establish clinical and analytical quality requirements for testing processes. Without such quality goals, there is no objective way to determine whether acceptable quality is being achieved, to identify processes that have to be improved, or to plan or design new processes that ensure that a specified level of quality will be attained.

Quality goals cannot be set on an absolute basis. They vary from laboratory to laboratory, depending on the medical missions of the healthcare facilities and professional interests of the physicians using the laboratory tests. Quality goals must also be considered in relation to cost. A goal of achieving the highest possible quality is not appropriate or practical when costs are being curtailed. In establishing quality goals, it is therefore more realistic to specify the quality that is necessary or adequate for the medical applications of the laboratory test results to be produced.

The balance of this chapter focuses primarily on analytical quality and the procedures by which it is monitored. Goals for analytical quality are established in the same way that they are established for purposes of method evaluation (see Chapter 14). The philosophy is to define an "allowable analytical error" based on "medical usefulness" requirements. A "total error" specification is useful because it will permit the calculation of the sizes of random and systematic errors that have to be detected to maintain performance within the allowable error limit (see Chapters 14 and 17).[71] Medical decision concentrations (i.e., the concentrations at which medical interpretation of laboratory test results is particularly critical) are important in establishing the analytical concentrations at which analytical performance has to be most carefully monitored. Thus analytical goals can be established by specifying the allowable analytical error and the critical medical decision concentration. Method evaluation is only the first step in validating that analytical performance satisfies those goals. Quality control procedures should provide for the continuing verification that those goals are being achieved during routine service.

LABORATORY ERROR AND THE SIX SIGMA PROCESS

A study by the Institute of Medicine has found that more than 1 million preventable injuries and 44,000 to 98,000 preventable deaths occur annually in the United States.[49,53] Further publications have offered suggestions for minimizing medical errors in general.[5,24,53-55,82] The magnitude of laboratory errors and the use of the Six Sigma process in controlling them are discussed in the following sections.

Number of Errors Made in the Clinical Laboratory

In 1989, a study was conducted in which 363 incidents captured by a laboratory's quality assurance program in a hospital were evaluated.[78] Incidents included those in which (1) physicians' orders for laboratory tests were missed or incorrectly interpreted, (2) patients were not properly prepared for testing or were incorrectly identified, (3) specimens were collected in the wrong containers or mislabeled or mishandled, (4) the analysis was incorrect, (5) data were entered improperly, and (6) results were delayed, not available, or incomplete, or they conflicted with clinical expectations.

After evaluation of the data, the authors found no effect on patient care for 233 patients; 78 patients were not harmed, but were subjected to an unnecessary procedure not associated with increased patient risk; and 25 patients were not harmed, but were subjected to an additional risk of inappropriate care. Of the total number, preanalytical mistakes accounted for 218 (45.5%), analytical for 35 (7.3%), and postanalytical, 226 (47.2%). Nonlaboratory personnel were responsible for 28.6% of the mistakes. An average of 37.5 patients per 100,000 treated were placed at increased risk because of mistakes in the testing process.

In a 1997 study, Witte and colleagues investigated the rates of error within the analytical component and found that widely discrepant values were rare, occurring in only 98 of 219,353 analyses.[130] When these results were converted into a standard metric of errors per million episodes, an error rate of 447 ppm was calculated.[5] In another 1997 study, Plebani and Carraro identified 189 mistakes from a total of 40,490 analyses, a relative frequency of 0.47% (4667 ppm). The distribution of mistakes was 68.2% preanalytical (3183 ppm), 13.3 % analytical (620 ppm), and 18.5% postanalytical (863 ppm).[72] Most of the laboratory mistakes did not affect patients' outcomes, but in 37 patients, laboratory mistakes were associated with further inappropriate investigations, thus resulting in an unjustifiable increase in costs. In addition, laboratory mistakes were associated with inappropriate care or inappropriate modification of therapy in 12 patients. The authors concluded that "promotion of quality control and continuous improvement of the total testing process, including preanalytical and postanalytical phases, seems to be a prerequisite for an effective laboratory service."[72]

In a 2002 study of common immunoassays, Ismail and colleagues found only 28 false results from 5310 patients (5273 ppm).[40] However, as a result of incorrect immunoassay results attributable to interference, one patient had 15 consultations, 77 laboratory tests, and an unnecessary pituitary computed tomography scan. The authors stress (1) the necessity for good communication between clinician and laboratory personnel, (2) the importance of the clinical context, and (3) the necessity for use of multiple methods for identifying erroneous test results—a necessity for a rigorous and robust quality system. Heterophilic antibody blocking studies were most effective in identifying interference, but in 21% of patients with false results, dilution studies or alternative assays were necessary to identify the problem. In a similar study, Marks enlisted participation from 74 laboratories from a broad international spectrum of settings and found that 6% of analyses gave false-positive results and, as in the Ismail study, found that use of a heterophilic blocking reagent corrected approximately one third of these.[58] Further evaluation of the data showed no consistent pattern for false results: errors were distributed across donors, laboratories, and systems of analysis. In reviewing the data from these last two studies, Leape suggested setting up a system that would ensure that every result was given a rigorous review before being reported.[53]

In 2002, Bonini and Plebani conducted several MEDLINE studies of laboratory medical errors and found a large heterogeneity in study design and quality and a lack of a shared definition of "laboratory error."[6] However, even with these limitations, they concluded that most such errors occur in the preanalytical phase and suggested that these could be reduced by the implementation of a more rigorous methodology for error detection and classification and the adoption of proper technologies for error reduction. Thus current QA programs that monitor only the analytical phase of the total process have to be expanded to include both the preanalytical (see Chapter 17) and postanalytical phases (www.westgard.com/essay34). By expanded monitoring, the total process would then be managed so as to reduce or eliminate all defects within the process.[72]

Six Sigma Principles and Metrics

Six Sigma[36] is an evolution in quality management that is being widely implemented in business and industry in the new millennium.[76] Six Sigma metrics are being adopted as the universal measure of quality to be applied to their processes and the processes of their suppliers. The principles of Six Sigma go back to Motorola's approach to TQM in the early 1990s and the performance goal that "*6 sigmas or 6 standard deviations of process variation should fit within the tolerance limits for the process*"; hence, the name Six Sigma (http://mu.motorola.com/). For this development, Motorola won the Malcolm Baldridge Quality award in 1988.

Six Sigma provides a more quantitative framework for evaluating process performance and more objective evidence for process improvement. The goal for process performance is illustrated in Figure 19-4, which shows an error distribution of a measurement procedure that fits acceptably within the tolerance specifications or quality requirements for that measurement. Any process can be evaluated in terms of a sigma metric that describes how many sigmas fit within the tolerance limits. The power of the sigma metric comes from having a universal measure of process performance that facilitates benchmarking across industries.

There are two methodologies for assessing process performance in terms of a sigma metric (Figure 19-5). One approach is to measure outcomes by inspection. The other approach is to measure variation and predict process performance. For processes in which poor outcomes can be counted as errors or defects, the defects are expressed as defects per million (DPM), then converted to a sigma metric using a standard table available in any Six Sigma text.[36] At this time, when healthcare outcomes and reducing medical errors are of great interest, Six Sigma provides a general methodology to describe process outcome on the sigma scale.

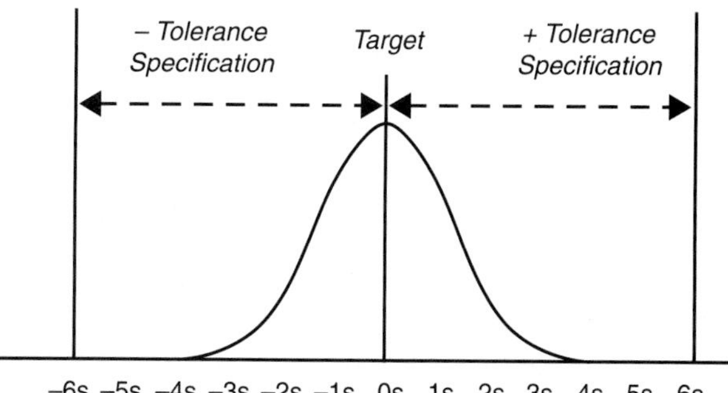

Figure 19-4 Six Sigma goal for process performance "tolerance specification" represents the quality requirement.

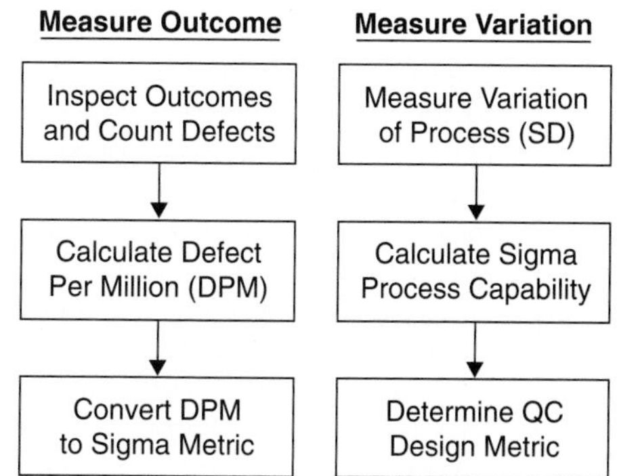

Figure 19-5 Six Sigma methodologies for measuring process performance. Method of measuring process variation is applicable to analytical testing processes.

To illustrate this assessment, consider the well-known problem with a certain brand of tires on a certain brand of sport utility vehicle (SUV) in the United States. A poor outcome, or defect, is defined as a tire blowout that causes an accident. Using data available to the public, there were 2000 accidents in vehicles equipped with these tires, leading to a recall of 6,000,000 tires. The defect rate is then estimated at 333 DPM (2000/6,000,000), or 0.033%, which corresponds to a sigma of 4.9 using a DPM-to-sigma conversion table. For comparison or benchmarking purposes, airline baggage handling has been described as 4.15 sigma performance and airline safety (0.43 deaths per million passenger miles) as better than Six Sigma performance. A defect rate of 0.033% would be considered excellent in any healthcare organization, where error rates from 1% to 5% are often considered acceptable.[5] A 5.0% error rate corresponds to 3.15 sigma performance and a 1.0% error rate corresponds to 3.85 sigma. Six Sigma shows that the goal should be error rates of 0.1% (4.6 sigma) to 0.01% (5.2 sigma) and ultimately 0.001% (5.8 sigma).

The first application describing sigma metrics in a healthcare laboratory was published by Nevalainen[68] in the year 2000. This application focused on preanalytical and postanalytical processes. Order accuracy, for example, was observed to have an error rate of 1.8%, or 18,000 DPM, which corresponds to 3.6 sigma performance. Hematology specimen acceptability showed a 0.38% error rate, or 3800 DPM, which is 4.15 sigma performance. The best performance observed was for the error rate in laboratory reports, which was only 0.0477%, or 477 DPM, or 4.80 sigma performance. The worst performance was therapeutic drug monitoring timing errors of 24.4%, or 244,000 DPM, which is 2.20 sigma performance.

Of the studies discussed in the section above, the error rates computed in DPM can be converted to sigma metrics. For example, for the Ross-Boone study,[78] the computed DPM corresponds to a 3.3 sigma long-term performance. For the Plebani study,[72] a DPM of 620 DPM corresponds to 3.2 sigma long-term performance. In the Ismail study,[40] a DPM of 5273 corresponds to 2.6 sigma long-term performance. On average, this indicates about 3.03 sigma long-term performance.

The application of sigma metrics for assessing analytical performance depends on measuring process variation and determining "process capability" in sigma units.[83,94,103] This approach makes use of the information on precision and accuracy that laboratories acquire initially during method validation studies and have available on a continuing basis from internal and external quality control. An important aspect of this methodology is that the capability, or predictive performance, of the process must be ensured by proper quality control, therefore the ease of assessment comes with the responsibility to design and implement QC procedures that will detect medically important errors.

To apply this methodology, the tolerance limits are taken from performance criteria for external quality assessment programs or regulatory requirements (such as the U.S. Clinical Laboratory Improvement Amendment [CLIA] criteria for acceptable performance in proficiency testing); process variation and bias can be estimated from method validation experiments, peer-comparison data, proficiency testing results, and routine QC data. For laboratory measurements, it is straightforward to calculate the sigma performance of a method from the imprecision: standard deviation (SD) or coefficient of variation (CV) and inaccuracy (bias) observed for a method and the quality requirement (allowable total error, TE_a) for the test [Sigma = $(TE_a - \text{bias})/SD$]. For a cholesterol test with a CLIA criterion of 10.0%, method bias of 1.0%, and method CV of 2.0%, the sigma metric is 4.5 [10.0 – 1.0/2.0]. If the method had a CV of 3.0% and a bias of 3.0% (the maximum allowable figures according to the National Cholesterol Education Program [NCEP] guidelines), the sigma metric is 2.33. Sigma metrics from 6.0 to 3.0 represent the range from "best case" to "worst case." Methods with Six Sigma performance are considered "world class"; methods with sigma performance less than 3 are not considered acceptable for production.

Those conclusions can be readily understood by considering the amount of quality control that is necessary for measurement processes having different performance metrics. Figure 19-6 shows a "power function graph" that describes the probability for rejecting an analytical run on the y-axis versus the size of the systematic error that has to be detected on the x-axis. The bold vertical lines correspond to methods having 3, 4, 5, and 6 sigma performance (left to right). The different lines or power curves correspond to the control rules and number of control measurements given in the key at the right (top to bottom). These different QC procedures have different sensitivities or capabilities for detecting analytical errors. Practical goals are to achieve a probability of error detection of 0.90 (i.e., a 90% chance of detecting the critical-sized systematic error, while keeping the probability of false rejection at 0.05 or less [i.e., 5% or lower chance of false alarms]). That is easy to accomplish for processes with 5 to 6 sigma performance; it requires a more careful selection and increased QC efforts for processes from 4 to 5 sigma; and it becomes very difficult and expensive for processes less than 4 sigma.

Thus the application of Six Sigma principles and metrics is very valuable for all phases of the laboratory testing process. Since the core business of the laboratory is to produce accurate test results, it makes sense to first apply Six Sigma to the analytical processes. That also is the easiest application because there are tolerance limits in the form of acceptability criteria from peer-comparison and proficiency-testing programs, QC data available for estimating method precision, and peer data available for estimating method bias. Laboratories should next expand their efforts to the preanalytical and postanalytical processes, knowing that their core processes are producing the necessary analytical quality.

ELEMENTS OF A QUALITY ASSURANCE PROGRAM

The attainment of quality goals in a clinical laboratory requires a comprehensive quality assurance program. "Quality assurance" is used here to represent practices that are generally recommended for ensuring that desired quality goals are achieved. Quality assurance is a broad spectrum of plans, policies, and procedures that together provide an administrative structure for a laboratory's efforts to achieve quality goals. The term "quality control" is often used to represent those techniques and procedures that monitor performance parameters. Generally, these are quantitative

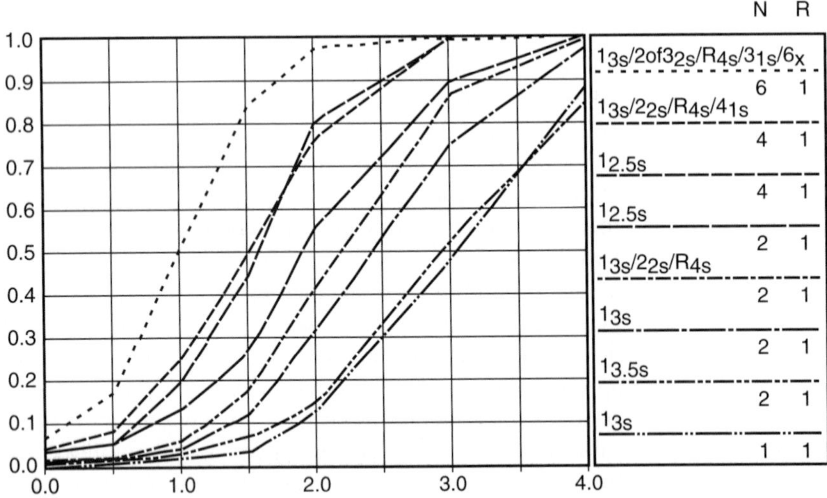

Figure 19-6 Relationship of process performance on the Sigma scale to the performance characteristics of commonly used laboratory QC procedures. Probability for rejection is plotted on the y-axis versus size of systematic error on the x-axis and the Sigma scale on the x-axis. The control rules and number of control measurements are given in the key at the right, where the 8 lines, top to bottom, correspond with the curves on the graph, top to bottom.

techniques that monitor particular sources of errors, estimate the magnitude of the errors, and alert laboratory personnel when there are indications that quality has deteriorated. A quality assurance program involves virtually everything and everybody in the clinical laboratory. An error in any one step during the acquisition, processing, and analysis of a specimen and the reporting of a laboratory test result invalidates the quality of the analysis and causes the laboratory to fall short of its quality goals. There are several essential elements of a quality assurance program.

Commitment

Dedication to quality service must be central and a team effort. Otherwise, quality goals are not likely to be achieved. Quality must be a major consideration in all management decisions because any single decision may compromise other plans and practices for attaining quality goals. A true commitment is required by laboratory directors, managers, and supervisors if the efforts of other laboratory personnel are to be successful.

Facilities and Resources

Laboratories must have the administrative support necessary to provide the quality of services desired. This means having adequate space, equipment, materials, supplies, staffing, supervision, and budgetary resources. These resources provide the basis upon which quality services are developed and maintained.

Technical Competence

High-quality personnel are essential for high-quality services. The educational background and experience of all personnel are important, as is the capability of providing the in-service training that develops and maintains skills. In-service training also is a mechanism for ensuring the competency of laboratory personnel, instilling quality goals, implementing QC procedures, and providing for the continuing development of laboratory personnel, both technically and intellectually.

Technical Procedures

High-quality technical procedures are necessary to provide quality laboratory services. Three groups of procedures are discussed in this chapter:

1. The control of preanalytical conditions or variables, such as test requests, patient preparation, patient identification, specimen acquisition, specimen transport, specimen processing, specimen distribution, preparation of work lists and logs, and maintenance of records (see Chapters 1 and 17).[134]
2. The control of analytical variables, which includes analytical methodology, standardization and calibration procedures, documentation of analytical protocols and procedures, and the monitoring of critical equipment and materials.
3. The monitoring of analytical quality by the use of statistical methods and control charts.

Problem-Solving Mechanism

Although it is a particularly critical element in a quality assurance program, the necessity for a mechanism for problem solving is often underemphasized. Such a mechanism provides the link between the identification of a problem and the implementation of a solution to the problem. It is a "feedback loop" that responds to an error signal by making adjustments to reduce the size of the error or to prevent its recurrence. For problems limited to individual methods or instrument systems, the delegation of responsibility for the systems may provide the corrective mechanism. Specialized trouble-shooting skills need to be developed and improved and preventive maintenance programs instituted. For problems occurring more generally, the in-service training program can be an important part of the mechanism but often requires additional input from a QC specialist or supervisor to initiate the use of this mechanism and to help define its objectives. A different approach to problem solving is the use of quality teams that meet regularly to analyze problems and identify solutions.[85] By involving personnel, quality teams heighten the interest and commitment to quality and also provide a creative feedback mechanism.

The comprehensive nature of quality assurance programs and their missions, goals, and activities have been discussed in greater detail by Eilers.[28] There are also detailed outlines of the elements of cost management for quality assurance[29,44]; detailed recommendations by professional organizations, such as the College of American Pathologists (CAP),[18] the National Committee for Clinical Laboratory Standards (NCCLS),[62-65] and the International Federation of Clinical Chemistry[12-17]; and books devoted to quality assurance practices in clinical laboratories.[23,127]

CONTROL OF PREANALYTICAL VARIABLES

The responsibility for accurate and timely test reports generally lies with the laboratory, but many problems can arise before and after the analysis of the submitted specimens. To monitor and control these errors, it is essential to perform a systems analysis of the laboratory and to identify the types of preanalytical variables.

Systems Analysis

The operation of the clinical laboratory can be viewed as a series of processes, each of which has potential sources of error. Table 19-1 shows the processes that take place from the time of the physician's initial request for a test to the time of the final interpretation of the test result. This "systems analysis" identifies the critical processes for a typical laboratory; however, each laboratory situation is somewhat different, and there may be additional processes and additional sources of error. It is important for each laboratory to perform a

TABLE 19-1 Laboratory Testing Processes and Their Potential Errors

Process	Potential Errors
Test ordering	Inappropriate test Handwriting not legible Wrong patient identification Special requirements not specified Cost or delayed order
Specimen acquisition	Incorrect tube or container Incorrect patient identification Inadequate volume Invalid specimen (e.g., hemolyzed or too dilute) Collected at wrong time Improper transport conditions
Analytical measurement	Instrument not calibrated correctly Specimen mix-up Incorrect volume of specimen Interfering substance present Instrument precision problem
Test reporting	Wrong patient identification Report not posted in chart Report not legible Report delayed Transcription error
Test interpretation	Interfering substances not recognized Specificity of test not understood Precision limitations not recognized Analytical sensitivity not appropriate Previous values not available for comparison

systems analysis of its own laboratory testing system to identify those areas where errors are likely to occur.

Once the processes have been documented, the processes that are most susceptible to error should be identified and should receive the most attention. Many times, the processes that lead to the greatest number of complaints, such as lost specimens or delayed results, are judged to be most important, even though other steps, such as the appropriateness of test selection and the acceptability of a specimen, may be of greater importance for optimal medical care. Guidelines describing procedures for specimen handling are available from organizations such as the NCCLS. Documents by accrediting agencies such as the CAP,[18] Centers for Disease Control and Prevention, and state regulatory agencies are also helpful in this regard.

Types of Preanalytical Variables

It is difficult to establish effective methods for monitoring and controlling preanalytical variables because many of the variables are outside the traditional laboratory areas (see Chapter 17). Monitoring preanalytical variables requires the coordinated effort of many individuals and hospital departments, each of which must recognize the importance of these efforts in maintaining a high quality of service. Accomplishing such monitoring may require support from outside the laboratory, particularly from the institution's clinical practice committee or some similar authority. Variables to consider include the following:

Test Usage and Practice Guidelines

Traditionally, laboratory test utilization has always been monitored or controlled to some degree, but current emphasis on the cost of medical care and government regulation of medical care has increased the importance of this factor. Clinical practice committees may decide that only certain tests are necessary for emergency care and may therefore limit the availability of kind and volume of requests. Peer review audits may lead to the development of other guidelines concerning the appropriate use of diagnostic tests in different clinical situations. Numerous patient care strategies and guidelines are being developed that directly impact laboratory usage.[44] For example, implementation guidelines for the use of bleeding times at the University of Massachusetts Medical Center resulted in a substantial reduction in test requests.[61] Careful monitoring of test requests and their appropriateness is likely to increase in importance, and the laboratory will likely have a role in identifying situations in which test utilization can be optimized and in providing in-service education to effect changes in ordering patterns.

Patient Identification

Correct identification of patients and specimens is a major concern for laboratories. The highest frequency of errors occurs with the use of handwritten labels and request forms. One method for checking identification is to compare identifiers such as the patient's name and his or her unique hospital number. The identification on the specimen label should also correspond with the identification on the requisition form. The use of plastic embossed patient identification cards to imprint the patient's name on test request forms and on blood collection labels can eliminate transcription and identification errors but does not guarantee that the patient name on the labels correctly identifies the donor of the specimen. The integration of bar code technology into the analytical systems that are used by clinical laboratories has significantly reduced identification problems (see Chapter 11).

Turnaround Time

Delayed and lost test requisitions, specimens, and reports have been major problems for laboratories. An essential feature for monitoring the cause of delays is the recording of the actual times of specimen collection, receipt in the laboratory, and reporting of test results. This has been done manually by placing time stamps in key locations such as blood-drawing centers, specimen-processing stations, result-reporting areas, and wards or chart-posting areas. It also has been done more effectively by programming computer systems to automatically document the times of test requests, specimen acquisition, processing, analysis, and reporting.[77] Turnaround time has been monitored like any other QC variable, and limits established to flag "out-of-range" specimens. Lists of delayed specimens also provide a powerful mechanism for detecting lost specimens or reports. Resolution of problems in this area is aided by a systems analysis of the laboratory operations, which would help identify those steps and areas that cause delays and disruptions in service. A good system for monitoring patient, specimen, and information flow may be obtained by integration of the light wand and/or bar code or optical character identification system with a computer that could automatically track each specimen at each of the steps from test request to result posting.

Laboratory Logs

When the serum aliquot tubes arrive in the laboratory, various logging and monitoring systems are necessary. In laboratories without computerized reporting, a request and/or report form generally accompanies the specimens. One should check that the patient name and identification number and the tests requested on the form match the information on the label of the specimen tube. The specimen should be inspected to confirm adequacy of volume and freedom from problems that would interfere with the assay, such as lipemia or hemolysis. The specimens are then stored appropriately, and the identification information and arrival time are recorded in a master log. If the analyses are performed in batches, specimen identification generally is recorded in specific locations on the worksheets using the information on the tube labels. After analysis, the results are recorded on the worksheet, and if both the assay and the individual test results pass the QC criteria, the test results are transferred to the result forms for reporting. However, before reporting the results, a second technologist should verify the adequacy of the QC and should check for transcription errors by comparing the results on the report forms with those on the master log. Specimens that require further analysis because of dilution or assay problems should be indicated either on the master log or on a delayed report log.

Transcription Errors

In laboratories where electronic identification and tracking has not been implemented, a substantial risk of transcription error exists from manual entry of data even with the double checking of results. Computerization will reduce this type of transcription error as such systems have error detection routines programmed into the terminal entry functions, such as check digits, limit checks, test correlation checks, and verification checks with master hospital files (see Chapters 11 and 18).

Patient Preparation

Laboratory tests are affected by many factors, such as recent intake of food, alcohol, or drugs, and by smoking, exercise, stress, sleep, posture during specimen collection, and other variables (see Chapter 17). Proper patient preparation is essential for the test results to be meaningful. Although responsibility for this usually resides with personnel outside the laboratory, the laboratory must define the instructions and procedures for patient preparation and specimen acquisition. These procedures should be included in hospital procedure manuals and should be transmitted to patients in both oral and written instructions. Compliance with these instructions is monitored directly when the laboratory employs its own phlebotomists. Specific inquiry should be made regarding patient preparation before specimens are collected, and efforts should be made to correct noncompliance. For tests in which standardization of the collection is very important (such as for plasma catecholamines), specimens should be collected in a controlled environment, such as a clinical testing unit.

Specimen Collection

The techniques used to acquire a specimen affect many laboratory tests (see Chapter 2).[88] For example, prolonged tourniquet application causes local anoxia to cells and excessive venous back pressure. The anoxia causes small solutes (such as potassium) to leak from cells, and the venous pressure concentrates cells, proteins, and substances bound to proteins (such as calcium). Blood collected from an arm into which an intravenous infusion is running can be diluted or contaminated. Hemolysis during and after collection alters the concentration of any analyte that has a red blood cell/plasma concentration differential. Improper containers and incorrect preservatives greatly affect test results and make them inappropriate. One way to monitor and control this aspect of laboratory processing is to have a specially trained laboratory team assigned to specimen collection. All members of the team should be given explicit instruction in the proper methods of specimen collection. The identification of the person collecting a specimen should be maintained. Individuals who process the specimens should be trained to look for and document collection problems. Physicians should be encouraged to report clinically inconsistent results. Similarly, errors detected by limit checks, delta checks (differences between consecutive results on individual patients), or other algorithms should be recorded. Any collection problems should be reviewed with the individuals collecting the specimens. Pride of workmanship should be encouraged, and quality performance should be rewarded.

Specimen Transport

The stability of specimens during transport from the patient to the laboratory is seldom monitored; however, this aspect may be critical for some tests when performed locally and for most tests when sent to regional centers and commercial laboratories.[63] Most laboratories have recommendations for specimen storage and transport, but many of these are empirical and lack adequate scientific documentation. Even the definition of "stability" is not well agreed upon; some investigators accept changes less than 10%,[50,128] and others relate stability to medically significant changes[80] or a percentage of the established analytical variability.[96]

In controlling specimen transport, the essential feature is the authority to reject specimens that arrive in the laboratory in an obviously unsatisfactory condition (such as a thawed specimen that should have remained frozen). As with other QC procedures, a small number of problems are expected, but if the error rate gets too large, there is a necessity for systems analysis of transport procedures, with resulting modifications. In tests in which stability is a major problem, the design of specific control procedures appropriate for those tests may be necessary.

Specimen Separation and Aliquoting

Separating and aliquoting blood specimens are more directly under the control of the laboratory. The main variables are the centrifuges, the containers used, and the personnel.

Centrifuge Performance

Centrifuges are discussed in Chapter 1. For QC purposes, centrifuges should be monitored by checking the speed, timer, and temperature.

Container Monitoring

Collection tubes, pipettes, stoppers, and aliquot tubes are sources of calcium and trace metal contamination. Also, glass beads or other materials added to blood specimens to aid in the separation of serum from cells may cause contamination. Each lot number of materials used should be tested for contamination by calcium and possibly other elements. Cork stoppers should not be used on specimens intended for calcium determinations because false elevations of 10% to 50% may occur. Some of the plasticizers used in making plastic containers interfere with drug analyses. Also, some plastic materials adsorb trace amounts of some analytes and should not be used for substances in low concentration, such as parathyroid hormone.[41] Because of the intricate relationships between specimen processing and analytical testing, supplies and processing procedures should not be changed without consulting the personnel responsible for the analytical testing (see also Chapter 2).

Personnel Monitoring

As in other areas of the laboratory, the personnel who process the laboratory specimens should be carefully trained and supervised. A written procedure manual should be available in the area. "Fast-track" mechanisms should be established for the processing of emergency specimens. QC mechanisms should monitor both personnel performance and personnel safety. An important part of performance is throughput time, which can be calculated if one records the specimen arrival time and the time when processing is completed. Weekly or monthly summary statistics are an effective method for monitoring processing time. Also, the identification of the technologists should be recorded to facilitate the detection and correction of problems.

In optimizing the efficiency of a specimen-processing laboratory, there is a trade off between the time it takes to record and check parameters and the error rates or inconsistencies of the function. However, these records are necessary for documenting the daily operation and for helping to identify systematic problems.

An elegant system for monitoring manual clerical functions has been developed to detect errors in blood banking records.[92] In this system, known errors are discretely introduced into the system using fictitious patients. The types of errors introduced are chosen to represent errors likely to occur or errors that cause major problems. The fictitious reports are routed to dummy locations and eventually returned to the QC technologist. One can calculate the efficiency of the laboratory error detection program by comparing the number of fictitious errors discovered with the number introduced. This efficiency factor is then used to estimate the actual laboratory error rate based on the number of true errors discovered in the laboratory. The implementation of this scheme requires the cooperation of laboratory personnel and the involvement of a QC specialist. By a combination of paranoia and pride of workmanship, most personnel are more conscientious when they know they are being monitored. Substantial increase in the rate of error detection was observed shortly after this plan was implemented in the blood bank. Public display of individual error rates encourages pride of workmanship.

CONTROL OF ANALYTICAL VARIABLES

Many analytical variables must be controlled carefully to assure accurate measurements by analytical methods. Reliable analytical methods are obtained by a careful process of selection, evaluation, implementation, maintenance, and control (see Chapter 14). Efficient, effective, and uninterrupted laboratory service requires many procedures aimed at preventing the occurrence of problems. Laboratories may experience different problems with the same analytical methods owing to different amounts of effort being allocated to the care and support of those methods.

Certain variables—water quality, calibration of analytical balances, calibration of volumetric glassware and pipettes, stability of electrical power, and the temperature of heating baths, refrigerators, freezers, and centrifuges—should be monitored on a laboratorywide basis because they will affect many of the methods in the laboratory (see Chapter 1). In addition, there will be certain variables that relate more directly to individual analytical methods, and these require that procedures be developed to deal specifically with the characteristics of those methods.

CHOICE OF ANALYTICAL METHODOLOGY

The selection and evaluation of analytical methods are discussed in Chapters 14 and 15. It is important to recognize, however, that the initial evaluation of a method often takes place in a setting somewhat more idealized than the production setting. It is therefore desirable to have a start-up period in the service laboratory before test results are to be reported. This period allows time to (1) discover any additional problems, (2) develop maintenance programs that alleviate those problems, and (3) train a sufficient number of analysts to support the routine service operation.

REFERENCE MATERIALS AND CALIBRATION

The quality of the calibrators and the calibration procedure used are major factors in determining the reliability of the analytical values obtained with a procedure. To appreciate the problems in standardization and calibration, knowledge of the overall structure of an accuracy-based measurement system is necessary. Uriano and Cali[98] and Tietz[97] have defined a hierarchy of analytical methods and reference materials that shows the relationship between reference materials and analytical methods of different quality. Figure 19-7 illustrates how "field methods" are related to "reference methods" by "secondary reference materials" and how reference methods are related to "definitive methods" by "primary reference materials."

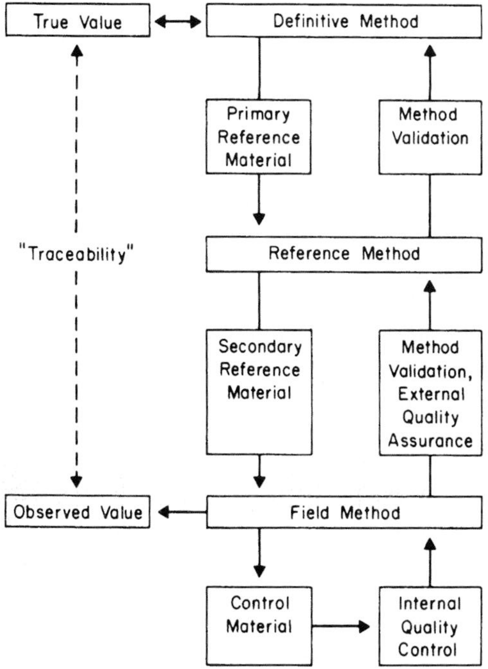

Figure 19-7 Structure of an accuracy-based measurement system showing relationships among reference methods and materials.

The practical meaning of this measurement structure has been discussed by Tietz.[97] The highest quality methods, the *definitive methods,* are to be used to validate reference methods and primary reference materials. The highest quality reference materials, namely *primary reference materials,* should be used in the development and validation of reference methods, the calibration of definitive and reference methods, and the production of secondary reference materials. *Reference methods* should be used to validate field methods. *Secondary reference materials* should be used to provide working calibrators for field methods and to assign values to control materials. *Control materials* are used only to monitor field methods.

Definitions

The following definitions for these materials have been developed by the National Reference System for the Clinical Laboratory (NRSCL)[62]:

Reference material (RM): "A material or substance, one or more whose property values are sufficiently homogeneous and well established to be used for the calibration of an apparatus, the assessment of a measurement method, or for assigning values to materials."

Certified reference material (CRM): "A reference material, accompanied by a certificate, one or more whose property values are certified by a procedure that established its traceability to an accurate realization of the unit in which the property values are expressed, and for which each certified value is accompanied by an uncertainty at a stated level of confidence." For example, standard reference materials from the U.S. National Institute of Standards and Technology (http://www.nist.gov) are considered CRMs.

Calibration material and/or calibrator: "A material (e.g., solution) or a device of known, or assigned quantitative and/or qualitative characteristics (e.g., concentration, activity, intensity, reactivity) used to calibrate, graduate, or adjust a measurement procedure or to compare the response obtained with the response of a test specimen and/or sample."

Control material: "A device, solution, lyophilized preparation, or pool of collected human or animal specimen, or artificially derived material, intended for use in the quality control process."

Use

To illustrate the use of these materials, a field (routine) method would be traceable to a reference method when it has been evaluated against that method or when it has been calibrated with a secondary reference material or calibrator whose value was established by analysis with a reference method. The reference method itself should have been validated against a definitive method and calibrated with a primary reference material or CRM whose value was established by the definitive method. Proper choice of calibrating materials establishes the traceability of the analytical results to the "true value" through the structure of the measurement system (Figure 19-7).[30] Note also that the use of control materials solely for internal quality control does not establish traceability, but use of such materials in external quality assurance may validate field methods against reference methods and thereby may establish traceability. (See Chapter 14 for a discussion of traceability.)

The selection of reference materials is therefore critical in validating the performance of an analytical method (see Chapter 1). CRMs should be used at least in the initial evaluation studies and in establishing the acceptability of calibrators used in routine service. The specific characteristics of calibrators should be documented, along with the number of different concentrations of calibrating solutions and the frequency of their use. These latter choices depend on the characteristics of the analytical method, particularly the stability, reproducibility, and linearity.

Documentation of Analytical Protocols

Step-by-step procedures for performing analytical determinations are critical if the methods are to provide the same results when used by different analysts over a long period of time. Maintaining such consistency requires written protocols or method and procedure manuals. The essential information to be contained in such documents is outlined in Box 19-1. More detailed guidelines are provided in an NCCLS document.[64] Method manuals should be reviewed annually and revised whenever changes occur. Although once a problem because of the time required to retype procedures, the availability of word processors has alleviated this difficulty and permitted rapid revisions whenever changes occur. It is also a good practice to retain outdated procedures in an archival file.

Establishment of Reference Intervals

The details for the establishment of reference values are presented in Chapter 16. An NCCLS document is also available on the topic.[66]

Monitoring Technical Competence

The personal characteristics and techniques of individual analysts may greatly affect certain analytical methods, particularly manual methods. Proper training of laboratory personnel to achieve uniformity in technique is important, as is scheduling sufficient routine service to maintain proper techniques. In training personnel on new analytical methods, it is helpful to have written lists of objectives that outline the critical tasks and knowledge that must be mastered. Having such objectives ensures systematic instruction that covers the critical points. Before performing analyses for clinical use, the technical competence of the personnel should be checked, and practice runs should be performed. Periodic monitoring of competency may be difficult, but incident reports and results from internal and external QC checks will identify specific problems; these problems should be discussed directly with the personnel involved. In-service and continuing education programs will help maintain and improve competence. Employee conferences will also help uncover nontechnical problems that may affect work quality.

BOX 19-1 Outline for a Procedure Manual

A. *Procedure name:* List principal name of procedure first, alternative names next. List commonly used abbreviations.
B. *Clinical significance:* Give a brief explanation of how the test is used in clinical medicine. Include reference intervals for specific diseases and recommended diagnostic and therapeutic action limits.
C. *Principle of method:* Give a brief statement of the principles on which the method is based.
D. *Specimen:* List type of specimens that can be used and recommended volume and minimum volume. Indicate conditions that render the specimen unacceptable, such as hemolysis or lipemia. List patient preparation procedures. Provide instruction for specimen handling before testing.
E. *Reagents and equipment:* Provide a list of reagents in order of their use, including standards. Indicate the names and addresses of suppliers and detailed instructions for preparation, including checks to be performed before use. List equipment used and special precautions required.
F. *Procedure:* This should be a step-by-step description, including calibration and QC procedures. There should be enough detail so that the assay could be performed by a person unfamiliar with the test. The necessary calculations should be included.
G. *Reference values:* List the reference intervals for healthy subjects. Indicate parameters such as age, sex, or race that affect reference values. Include the nature of the population studied, the number of subjects, and the date or reference for the original work.
H. *Comments:* Include any special analytical variables affecting the test, such as pH or temperature. Include effects of commonly used drugs, any dangers or personal hazards in the procedure, and any special safety precautions and procedures.
I. *References:* Give the primary literature references that describe the method or the references upon which the method is based.

Inventory Control of Materials

Stable operation of laboratory methods is critically dependent on the materials used with the methods. Procedures are necessary to inventory materials and initiate orders when supplies are low. These procedures must be tailored to the particular reagents and supplies that are in use. In general, when materials are stable and changes in lot numbers cause problems, large stocks should be maintained, though this may be limited by economic considerations, shelf life, and storage space. Adequate inventory should be maintained to allow time for additional shipment and testing of additional supplies should the current shipment be unsatisfactory. Formal inventory control procedures will help minimize required storage by initiating orders when stock reaches a certain predetermined level. Many companies will ship reagents on a standing order once usage rates are established. In fact, with the arrival of rapid transportation and delivery capabilities, a laboratory is now able to order reagents and supplies and receive them in a very short period of time—a "just-in-time" approach to inventory control.

Input Control of Materials

Along with inventory management, the quality of materials should be monitored when they are received. Interruptions in service can be prevented by testing the adequacy of materials before their introduction for routine use. It is particularly important that patient results from new lots of reagents and calibrators be compared with those obtained with previous lots. New lots of blood-drawing tubes, processing tubes, and the like should receive some parallel or comparison testing before their routine use. In establishing pretesting procedures for monitoring incoming materials, it should be recognized that this kind of testing is costly, both in time and money.

Another part of input control is the proper labeling of reagents and materials. Proper identification should include the name, lot number (particular manufacturing batch), concentration, date received, date prepared, date opened, date of expiration, and recommended storage conditions. In practice, such information is provided by manufacturers via a human-readable bar code.

Monitoring Method Changes

An essential tool for solving analytical problems is a record or log of all changes and problems occurring with a method. These should include the date, time, analyst, and any changes in lots of reagents, materials, or calibrators. All instrument maintenance should be recorded, including all work performed by service personnel from outside the laboratory. The occurrence of control problems should be indicated, along with actions taken to resolve the problems. Periodic review of these logs should lead to implementation of preventive maintenance programs, based on the frequency of occurrence of particular problems.

CONTROL OF ANALYTICAL QUALITY USING STABLE CONTROL MATERIALS AND CONTROL CHARTS

In the routine operation of clinical laboratories worldwide, the performance of analytical methods is routinely monitored by analyzing specimens whose concentrations are known followed by comparing the observed values with the known values. The known values are usually represented by an interval of acceptable values, or upper and lower limits for control (control limits). When the observed values fall within the control limits, the analyst is assured that the analytical method is functioning properly. When the observed values fall outside the control limits, the analyst should be alerted to the possibility of problems in the analytical determination. A number of books are available that discuss the application of QC in the operation of the clinical laboratory.[9,23,107,109,110]

Control Materials

Specimens that are analyzed for QC purposes are called control materials. They are required to be stable, available in aliquots or vials, and amenable to being analyzed periodically over a long time. There should be little vial-to-vial variation so that differences between repeated measurements are attributed to the analytical method alone. The control material should preferably have the same matrix as the test specimens of interest (e.g., a protein matrix may be best when serum is the test material to be analyzed by the analytical method).[59] Materials from human sources have generally been preferred, but because there is some risk of hepatitis infection, bovine materials offer a certain advantage in safety and are more readily available. The concentration of analyte should be in the normal and abnormal ranges, corresponding to concentrations that are critical in the medical interpretation of the test results.

In practice, clinical laboratories are able to purchase materials from one of several companies that manufacture control sera or "control products." These are generally supplied as liquid or lyophilized materials that are reconstituted by adding water or a specific diluent solution. Also available are materials having matrices representing urine, spinal fluid, and whole blood. Liquid control materials are also available and have the potential advantage of eliminating errors caused by reconstitution. However, the matrices of these liquid materials contain other materials that may be a potential source of error with some analytical methods and instruments.

When selecting commercial control materials, there are several other considerations in addition to the matrix of the product. Stability is critical because it is often desirable to purchase a year's supply of one manufacturing lot or batch. Different batches (or lot numbers) of the same material will have different concentrations, which require new estimates of the mean and standard deviation. The size of the aliquots or vials should be convenient for the analytical methods to be monitored. Larger-sized vials are generally less expensive (on a per milliliter basis), but unused materials may eliminate any savings. Two or three different materials should be selected to provide concentrations that monitor performance at different medical decision levels. There may be some advantage in selecting materials from different manufacturers to minimize possible problems with a given manufacturing process. Alternatively, a series of materials designed by one manufacturer to have a certain relationship between concentrations can be used to gain additional information regarding linearity and accuracy.

Control products are purchased as assayed or unassayed materials. Assayed materials come with a list of values for the concentrations that are expected for that material. This list often includes both the mean and standard deviation for several of the common analytical methods and preferably for a reference method used to measure a particular analyte. Because of the work required to determine these values, the assayed materials are in general more expensive. Although the stated assay values are useful in selecting the desired materials, it is advisable to determine the mean and standard deviation in the user's laboratory because this process improves the performance characteristics of statistical control procedures.

General Principles of Control Charts

The most common method of comparing the values observed for control materials with their known values is through the use of control charts. Control charts are simple graphical displays in which the observed values are plotted versus the time when the observations were made.* The known values are represented by an acceptable range of values, as indicated on the chart by lines for upper and lower control limits. When the plotted points fall within the control limits, this is generally interpreted to mean that the method is performing properly. When points fall outside the control limits, problems may be developing.

The control limits are usually calculated from the mean ($\bar{x}$) and standard deviation (s) obtained from repeated measurements on the known specimens by the particular analytical method that is to be controlled. The mean ($\bar{x}$) and standard deviation (s) are calculated from the following equations:

$$\bar{x} = \frac{\sum x_i}{n}$$

$$s = \sqrt{\frac{n\sum_{i=1}^{n} x_i^2 - \sum_{i=1}^{n}(x_i)^2}{n(n-1)}}$$

where x_i is an individual control observation and n is the number of observations in the time period being monitored (see Chapter 14). The initial estimate should be based on measurements obtained over a period of at least 1 month when the method is working properly. These conditions are necessary because the measurements are used to characterize the distribution of values that is expected during stable routine operation of the analytical method.

The initial estimate may not be entirely reliable owing to the low number of data points and possible outliers in the data. The estimates are revised when more data have been accumulated by recording n and the summations of x_i and x_i^2, then using the cumulative totals in the equations above to give cumulative means and standard deviations. The effects of outliers can be minimized by eliminating values exceeding the mean by more than ±3.1 to 3.8 s (where the exact factor depends on the total number of data points: 3.14 for $n = 30$; 3.22, $n = 40$; 3.33, $n = 60$; 3.41, $n = 80$; 3.47, $n = 100$; 3.66, $n = 200$; 3.83, $n = 400$).

It is assumed that error distribution of the analytical method is Gaussian (see Chapter 14). The control limits are set to include most of the control values, usually 95% to 99.7%, which correspond to the mean ±2 or 3 standard deviations. Because it should be a relatively rare occurrence to observe a value in the tails of the distribution (only 1 out of 20 times for 2 s limits and 3 out of 1000 for 3 s limits), such an observation is suspect and suggests that something has happened to the analytical method. Such an occurrence could have caused a shift in the mean (an accuracy problem), which would result in a higher probability for exceeding the limits, or it could have caused an increase in the standard deviation (a precision problem), which would widen the distribution and also result in a higher probability for exceeding the limits.

Figure 19-8, *A* illustrates how the distributions of control values will appear for three different situations: (a) stable performance where only an occasional observation exceeds the control limits; (b) occurrence of a systematic error that shifts the mean of the distribution and causes a much higher expectation or probability of observing control values outside one of the control limits; and (c) occurrence of an increase in random error or imprecision, which widens the distribution and causes a much higher probability of observing a control value outside either of the control limits.

Control charts are used to compare the observed control values with the control limits and to provide a visual display that can be quickly inspected and reviewed. These charts have the concentration or observed value plotted on the *y*-axis versus time of observation on the *x*-axis. It is common practice to plot 1 month's data on a chart, usually only one or two points a day, but the time axis should be chosen to be appropriate for the method being monitored. An example of a control chart is shown in Figure 19-8, *B*, where the control values represent the three situations in Figure 19-8, *A*, with 10 values per situation for a total of 30 values. When the analytical method is operating properly, the control values fall predominantly within the control limits. When there is an accuracy problem, the control values are shifted to one side, and there may be several values in a row falling outside one of the limits. When there is a precision problem, the control values fluctuate much more widely, and there may be values exceeding both the upper and lower control limits.

Interpretation of the control data is guided by certain decision criteria or control rules, which define when an analytical run is judged "in control" (acceptable) or "out of control" (unacceptable). These control rules are given symbols, such as A_L, or n_L, where A is the abbreviation for a statistic n is the number of control observations, and L refers to the control limits. For example, 1_{3s} refers to a control rule where 1 observation exceeding the mean ±3 s control limits is the criterion for rejecting the analytical run.

*Although the discussions in this chapter imply that plots are manually prepared, in actual practice, a wide variety of computer software packages are available for statistically calculating and plotting QA data.

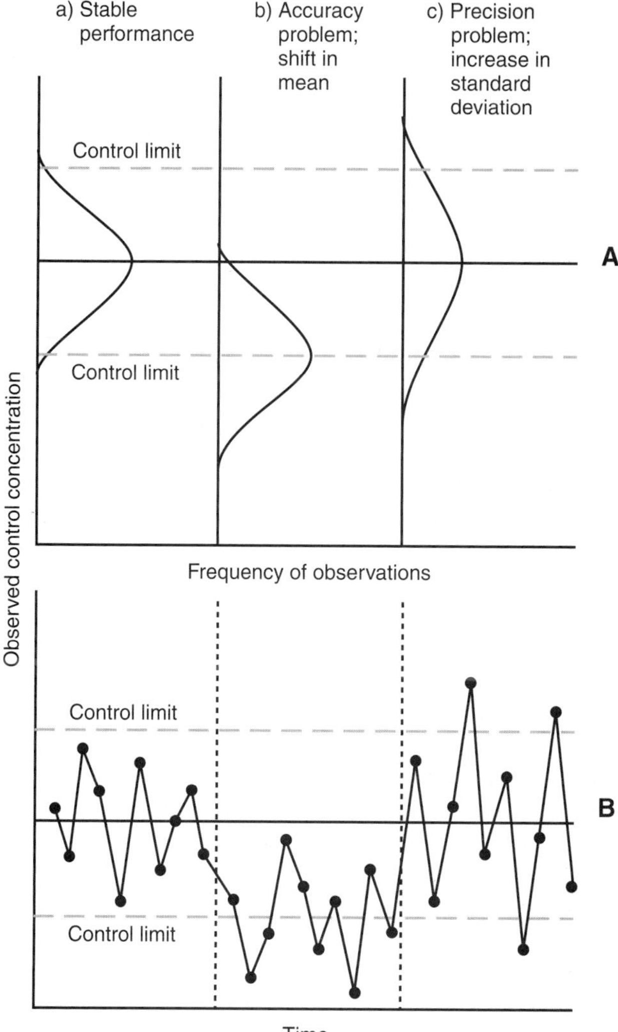

Figure 19-8 Conceptual basis of control charts. **A,** Frequency distributions of control observations for different error conditions. **B,** Display of control values representing those distributions when concentration is plotted versus time on a control chart.

"Analytical run" is used here to refer to that segment of data for which a decision on acceptability is to be made. This is the group of patient results that is to be reported, based on the control results available for inspection at that time.

The total number of control observations available for inspection when a decision is to be made on the acceptability of an analytical run is designated as "*N*." For example, when there is one control observation preceding and one following a group of 10 patient samples whose results are to be reported, there are two control observations in that analytical run.

The different control procedures discussed here have different performance capabilities, depending on the control rules and the number of control observations chosen. These choices should be related to the quality goals set by the laboratory. Many of the procedures in use today have not been chosen for best performance, but rather for ease of use in manual implementation or rule availability in the QC software of instruments and laboratory information systems. Tetrault and Steindel contend that the best set of control rules will vary from method to method.[93] Knowledge of the performance characteristics of control procedures is necessary to select control rules and n's that will detect relevant laboratory problems without causing too many "false alarms" (rejections when there are no analytical problems). Experienced analysts often employ a series of informal rules or judgments to reduce the number of false alarms without knowing their effects on the detection of real problems, or true alarms. There should be some quantitative assessment of these two characteristics, false alarms and true alarms, whenever capabilities of new control procedures are assessed or established control procedures are reviewed.

Performance Characteristics of a Control Procedure

The performance of a control procedure is described by its probability for rejection.[121] Probability refers to the likelihood that an event will occur; in this case, the event is the rejection of an analytical run. Ideally, there should be no rejections of analytical runs when the analytical method is performing properly. Alternatively, when analytical errors occur, the control procedure should provide a rejection signal. This corresponds to having a probability of 0.00 in the first situation and a probability of 1.00 in the second.

The term "probability for false rejection" (p_{fr}) is used to describe the first situation, where there are no analytical errors present except for the inherent imprecision or inherent random error of the analytical method. (There is always some random error associated with an analytical method, even when it is working properly. This is the random error that is estimated by the replication experiment during method evaluation studies.) When only this inherent random error is present, without any additional errors, the probability for false rejection should be zero. The frequency of false rejections is critical, because false rejections are like false alarms. Too many false alarms cause the analyst to disregard the alarm system, even when the alarm is occurring as a result of real errors that should be corrected.

"Probability for error detection" (p_{ed}) is the term used to describe the second case, where there is an analytical error in addition to the inherent or background random error. The probability for error detection should be high (near 1.00) when these errors are large enough to invalidate the quality goals for the analytical method. Unfortunately, this is difficult to achieve because the control procedure is attempting to detect a signal (additional error) in the presence of noise (inherent random error).

These critical performance characteristics—probability for false rejection and probability for error detection—are summarized by graphs of probability for rejection (*y*-axis) versus the size of analytical error (*x*-axis). Graphs such as that shown in Figure 19-9 are called power functions because they describe the statistical power of the control procedure.[119] The different lines on the graph represent different numbers of control observations (e.g., $n = 1, 2$, and 4 for the three lines on this graph). The probability for false rejection is given by the y-intercept, the point where each line intersects the y-axis. For this control procedure with n from 1 to 4, p_{fr} is 0.01 to 0.02, or 1% to 2%. The probability for error detection can be determined for any size error by first locating the size of the error on the x-axis, drawing a line up to intersect the power function curve, drawing a horizontal line from the point of intersection to the y-axis, and reading the probability for rejection from the scale on the y-axis. For this control procedure, p_{ed} is 0.13 for $n = 1$, 0.22 for $n = 2$, and 0.48 for $n = 4$. Thus there is a 13% to 48% chance of detecting an error of this size with this control procedure, depending on the number of control observations used.

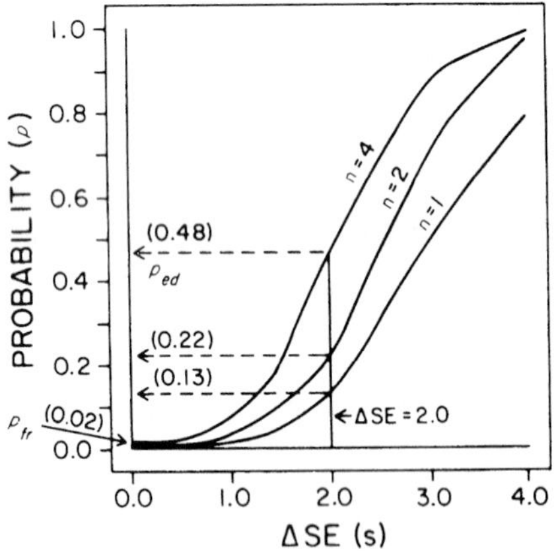

Figure 19-9 Power function graph presenting probability for rejection on the y-axis versus size of error on the x-axis. The different lines represent numbers of control observations, in this case $n = 1, 2$, and 4.

Two power function graphs are necessary, one to describe the performance for random error (RE) and the other for the performance for systematic error. For RE, as shown in Figure 19-10, *A*, the x-axis is labeled ΔRE. A value of 1.0 corresponds with the original standard deviation of the analytical method, a value of 2.0 to a doubling of that standard deviation, 3.0 to a tripling, and so on. For systematic error (SE), the x-axis is labeled ΔSE (see Figure 19-10, *B*). A value of 1.0 s corresponds to a systematic shift equivalent to the size of the standard deviation, a value of 2.0 s to a shift equivalent to two times s, and so on.

Power functions are determined by mathematical calculations or by computer simulation studies, the latter having been used in clinical laboratories to characterize many of the commonly used control procedures.[35,119] Power functions are useful for evaluating the performance capabilities of individual control procedures, for comparing the performance of different control procedures, and for designing new procedures with improved performance characteristics. The best control procedure is the one with the lowest probability for false rejection and the highest probability for detecting those errors that are large enough to invalidate the analytical quality goals for the method.

The sizes of the analytical errors that must be detected if the control procedure is to maintain a specified quality can be determined from a general analytical model for translating quality requirements into laboratory process specifications.[126]

$$TE_a = bias_{meas} + \Delta SE_{cont} s_{meas} + z\Delta RE_{cont} s_{meas}$$

TE_a is the analytical quality requirement expressed as an allowable total error. Minimum total error requirements are

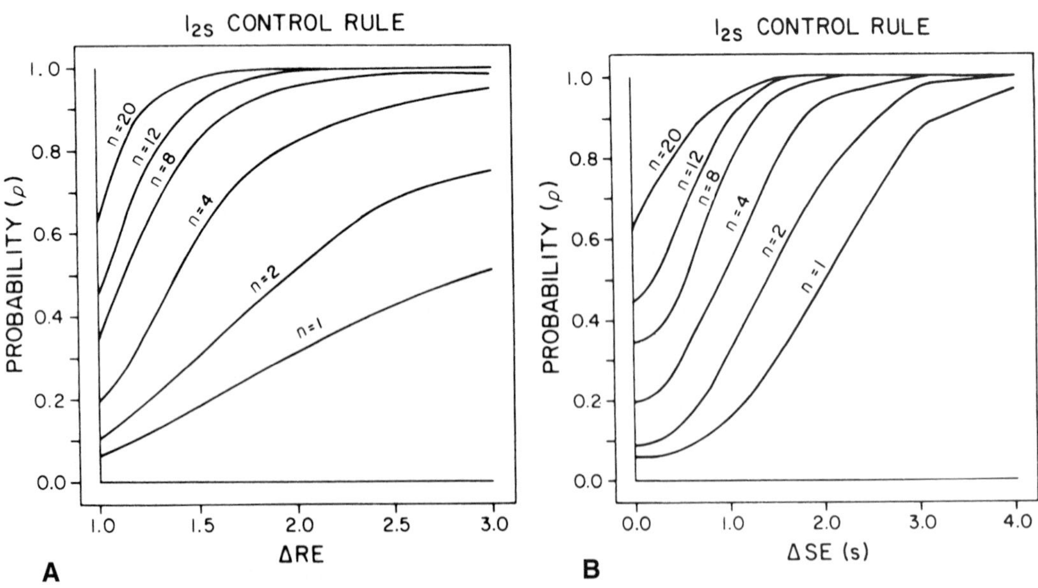

Figure 19-10 Power functions for 1_{2s} control rule. **A,** Random error. **B,** Systematic error. *(From Westgard JO, Groth T. Power functions for statistical control rules. Clin Chem 1979;25:863-9.)*

defined by the CLIA proficiency testing criteria for acceptable performance (see later section). $Bias_{meas}$ is the analytical measurement bias (stable inaccuracy), s_{meas} is the analytical measurement standard deviation (stable imprecision), ΔSE_{cont} is the change in systematic error (unstable inaccuracy) to be detected by the control procedure, ΔRE_{cont} is the change in random error (unstable imprecision) to be detected by the control procedure, and z is related to the chance of exceeding the quality requirement. When z is 1.65, a maximum defect rate of 5% may occur before rejecting an analytical run.

This analytical model is solved for ΔSE_{cont} (by setting ΔRE_{cont} to 1.0) or for ΔRE_{cont} (by setting ΔSE_{cont} to 0.0) to determine the critical sizes of errors that must be detected to maintain performance within the specified quality

$$\Delta SE_{crit} = [(TE_a - |bias_{meas}|)/s_{meas}] - 1.65$$
$$\Delta RE_{crit} = (TE_a - |bias_{meas}|)/1.65 s_{meas}$$

ΔSE_{crit} is the critical systematic error that would shift the distribution enough to cause 5% of the test results to exceed TE_a; ΔRE_{crit} is the critical increase in random error that would widen the distribution enough to cause 5% of the test results to exceed TE_a ($z = 1.65$ for 5% on one side; $z = 1.96$ for 2.5% on each side).

For example, if TE_a were specified as 10 mg/dL at a concentration of 120 mg/dL, and s_{meas} were estimated as 2.0 mg/dL and $bias_{meas}$ as 0.0 mg/dL, ΔSE_{crit} would be 3.4 s, and ΔRE_{crit} is 3.0. This indicates that the control procedure has to be able to detect a systematic shift equivalent to 6.8 mg/dL (3.4 × 2) and a random error equivalent to a standard deviation of 6.0 mg/dL (3.0 × 2).

With knowledge of these values for critical errors and the power functions for a control procedure, it is possible to make a critical assessment of the performance achievable by different statistical control procedures. The quality of the control procedures themselves can be evaluated and related to the quality goals defined for the laboratory.

The relationship between the quality requirement for a test, the imprecision and inaccuracy that are allowable, and the QC that is necessary are shown graphically by a chart of operating specifications (OPSpecs chart).[105] Figure 19-11 shows such a chart that has been prepared for a TE_a of 10%, single and multirules with n's that are commonly used in laboratories, and a p_{ed} of 0.90 or 90% error detection for systematic errors. This OPSpecs chart is derived from the analytical quality planning model shown earlier, setting ΔRE to 1.0, then rearranging as follows:

$$bias_{meas} = TE_a - (\Delta SE_{cont} + 1.65) s_{meas}$$

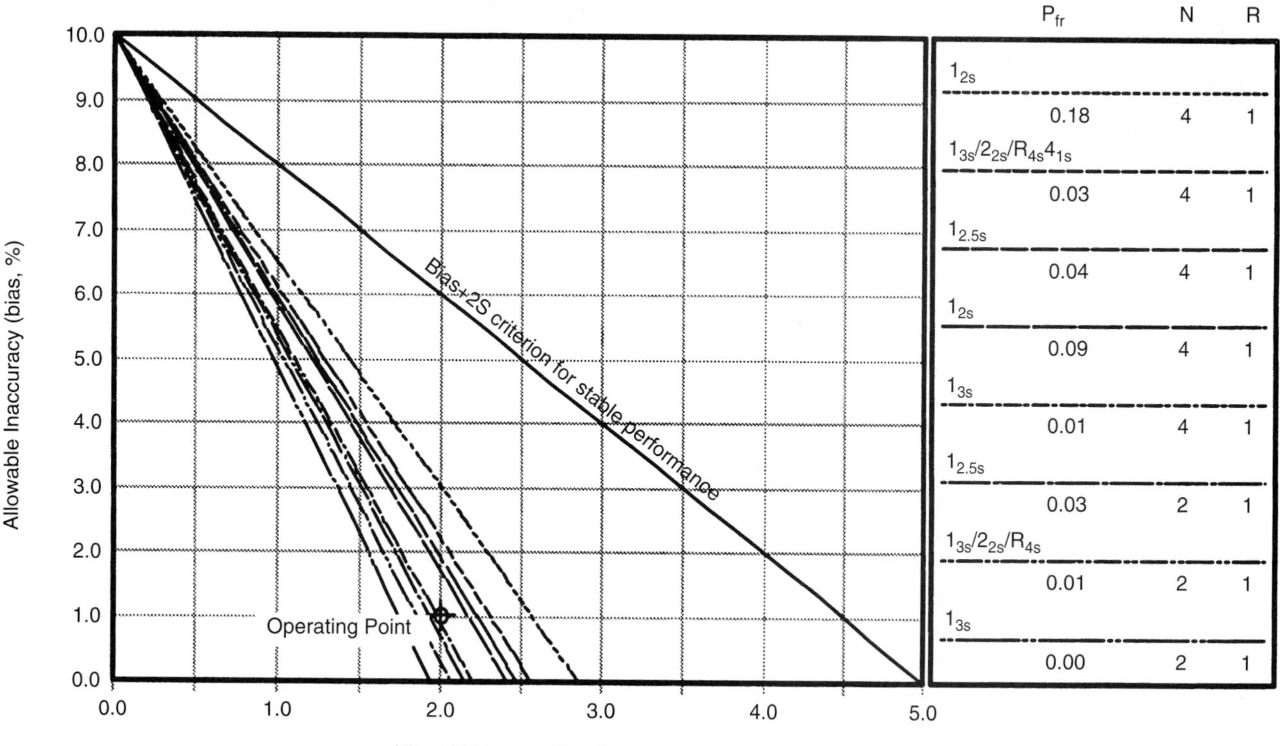

Figure 19-11 Operating specifications chart for an analytical quality requirement of 10% (TE_a) and 90% analytical quality assurance for systematic error. Allowable inaccuracy is plotted on the y-axis versus allowable imprecision on the x-axis.

Notice that this equation has the form of a straight line ($Y = a + bX$), where the y-intercept (a) is TE_a and the slope (b) depends on the sensitivity of the QC procedure. The value for ΔSE_{cont} is obtained from power curves for the control rules and n's of interest and for specified probabilities, such as 90% and 50%.[102] A plot of $bias_{meas}$ versus s_{meas} will describe the allowable limits of imprecision and inaccuracy for different control rules and different numbers of control measurements. A QC procedure can be selected by plotting the observed inaccuracy and imprecision as the method's operating point, then identifying the control rules and n's of the lines above the operating point.

For this example where the observed imprecision is 2.0% and the observed inaccuracy is 1.0%, the four lines above the operating point correspond to the top four QC procedures listed in the key on the right. All four will provide at least 90% detection of critical systematic errors, but their false rejection rates will vary from 0.03 to 0.18, or 3% to 18%. Appropriate choices would be the $1_{2.5s}$ single rule with $n = 4$ or the $1_{3s}/2_{2s}/R_{4s}/4_{1s}$ multirule with $n = 4$ to keep false rejections low.

Step-by-Step Process for Selecting QC Procedures

Laboratories should establish a systematic process for selecting appropriate QC procedures. The necessity for this is illustrated by the statement in the U.S. CLIA regulations[99,100] that "the laboratory must evaluate instrument and reagent stability and operator variance in determining the number, type, and frequency of testing calibration or control materials and establish criteria for acceptability used to monitor test performance during a run of patient specimens." Given that most laboratories must also satisfy certain national proficiency testing requirements, analytical requirements for quality have also been defined by regulatory or professional groups for many of the common tests.

1. Define the analytical quality requirement in the form of an allowable total error (TE_a).

   Use proficiency testing criteria as a practical starting point for defining the minimum quality that must be achieved.
2. Evaluate method performance to obtain estimates of imprecision and inaccuracy.

   Obtain initial estimates from replication and comparison of methods experiments. Obtain ongoing estimates from routine QC and proficiency testing surveys.
3. Obtain power function graphs for the control rules and n's of interest, or OPSpecs charts for the defined TE_a. Power function graphs and OPSpecs charts for commonly used QC procedures with n's of 2, 3, 4, and 6 are available in the scientific literature,[118,119] in workbook format,[106] and also from computer programs (EZ Rules and QC Validator 2.0, Westgard QC, Inc., Madison, Wis.—http://www.westgard.com).
4. Calculate the critical systematic error and draw a vertical line showing its location on the power function graph, or plot the observed imprecision and inaccuracy of your method on the OPSpecs chart for the TE_a of interest.
5. Assess the probabilities for error detection and false rejection.
6. Select control rules and n's that provide 90% detection of the critical systematic error and less than 5% false rejections. For very stable methods, consider 50% error detection if necessary to keep the number of control measurements and false rejections low.
7. Select a total QC strategy to provide an appropriate balance between statistical and nonstatistical QC procedures. With 90% error detection, depend on the statistical QC component and perform the minimal preventive maintenance, instrument function checks, and method validation tests required by good laboratory practice, manufacturers' instructions, and regulatory and accreditation guidelines.

   With 50% to 90% error detection, balance the efforts between statistical and nonstatistical QC procedures; improve method performance by reducing the bias and reducing imprecision.

   With less than 50% error detection, increase the efforts for nonstatistical QC to prevent problems from occurring, improve method performance, or consider replacing the method to achieve better imprecision and inaccuracy and more cost-effective operation of the testing process.
8. Reassess for changes in method performance as necessary. Cost-effective QC depends on doing the right QC to ensure the desired quality is achieved at minimum cost.[110] If method performance improves, less QC will be necessary; if method performance deteriorates, more QC will be necessary. Adjust the QC design as necessary for any changes in method performance.

   Detailed applications based on calculated critical systematic errors have been presented for a multitest chemistry analyzer[48,124]; detailed applications using OPSpecs charts have been presented for automated immunoassays[60]; illustrative examples using OPSpecs charts have also been provided for a variety of tests in chemistry, hematology, coagulation, endocrinology, toxicology, and immunology.[106]

   Manual application of this QC planning process is performed in just a minute using a workbook of OPSpecs charts that cover the range of analytical quality requirements from 1% to 50% and common single and multirules with n's from 2 to 6.[106] Computer support is necessary to use clinical quality requirements stated in the form of a medically important change or a decision interval for test interpretation; clinical requirements are more complicated and require an expanded quality planning model that accounts for additional preanalytical factors, such as within-run biological variation.[122]

With either manual or computer-supported QC planning, laboratories are able to identify appropriate control rules and the minimum number of control measurements that will ensure the desired quality is achieved at the minimum cost. These control rules and n's are usually implemented by setting up a Levey-Jennings control chart or a Westgard multirule chart, and less often by a cumulative sum chart or mean and range charts.

Levey-Jennings Control Chart

Control charts were first introduced into the clinical chemistry laboratory by Levey and Jennings in 1950.[56] They demonstrated how the industrial control procedures developed by Shewhart[86] could be used with the mean and range of duplicate measurements from clinical chemical methods. In an alternate chart, single control values are plotted directly. This "single-value" chart was adopted by most laboratories because data calculations were not required before plotting the control results. Today, this single-value chart is commonly known as a "Levey-Jennings" chart, even though Levey and Jennings recommended plotting the mean and range of replicate measurements.

To use a Levey-Jennings control chart, follow these steps:

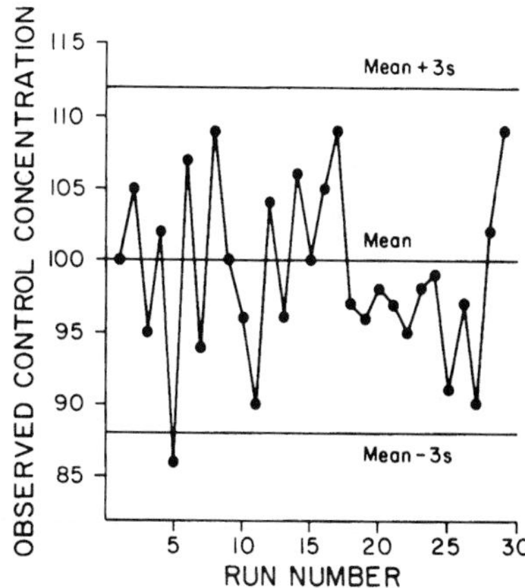

Figure 19-12 Levey-Jennings control chart having control limits set as the mean ±3 *s*. Concentration is plotted on the *y*-axis versus time (run number) on the *x*-axis.

1. Analyze samples of the control material by the analytical method to be controlled on at least 20 different days. Calculate the mean and standard deviation for those results.
2. Construct a control chart either manually on graph paper or electronically using graphical software. Label the *y*-axis "control value" and set the range of concentrations to include the mean ±4 *s*. Draw horizontal lines for the mean and the upper and lower control limits. Set the control limits as the mean ±3 *s* when the number of control observations, *n*, is 2 or greater. When *n* is 1, control limits may be set as the mean ±2 *s*. (See following discussion of performance characteristics.) Label the *x*-axis in terms of time, using day, run number, control observation number, or whatever is most appropriate for recording the relative time of the control observations.
3. Introduce control specimens into each analytical run, record the values, and plot each value on the control chart.
4. When the control values fall within the control limits, interpret the run as being "in control" and report the patient results. When a single control value exceeds the control limits, stop the method; *do not* report patient results. Inspect the method to determine the cause for the errors. Resolve the problem, then repeat the entire run—specimens and control samples. Determine control status for the new run in the same manner.

An example of a Levey-Jennings chart is shown in Figure 19-12, where control limits have been set as the mean ±3 *s*. Power functions for a Levey-Jennings chart having 3 *s* control limits, or a 1_{3s} control rule, are shown in Figure 19-13. The probability for false rejection is seen to be less than 0.05 or 5% even when *n* is very large. The probability for error detection increases as *n* increases, but for an *n* of 2 to 4, the procedure is not very sensitive for either random or systematic errors.

Figure 19-10 shows the power functions for a Levey-Jennings chart having 2 *s* control limits, or the 1_{2s} control rule. Observe that the *y*-intercept increases rapidly as *n* increases. The probabilities for false rejection are as follows: $n = 1$, 0.05; $n = 2$, 0.09; $n = 4$, 0.18; $n = 8$, 0.33; $n = 12$, 0.46; and $n = 20$, 0.64. Because probabilities for false rejection greater than 0.05 or 5% are not desirable, the use of the 1_{2s} rule is limited to the case where $n = 1$.

In practice, the 1_{2s} rule has been widely used with a higher *n*. However, such use causes a false rejection problem that may compromise the usefulness of the control procedure. There is no easy way to tell whether the rejection signal is due to the background random error (false rejection) or whether an additional error has occurred (true rejection). This difficulty has led to a more qualitative interpretation of the control results and often to routine repetition of the control measurements (and sometimes patient sampling) whenever a control value exceeds a 2*s* limit. When the second or repeated control value is observed to be outside the 2 *s* control limits, this provides evidence for a true rejection, and problem-solving procedures should be started.

A similar false rejection problem arises when multichannel instrument systems are controlled using the 1_{2s} rule on each of several channels. For one control material being analyzed by 4, 8, 12, and 20 channels, the chances that the control value on at least one channel exceeds its 2*s* limits are 18%, 33%, 46%, and 64%, respectively. Such a high rate of values exceeding the control limits may cause the same percentage of work to be routinely repeated, obviously compromising the efficiency of the laboratory and increasing its costs.

It is important to recognize the seriousness of the false rejection problem and its relationship to the control limits that are chosen for the Levey-Jennings chart. These false rejections are in effect an inherent property of the control procedure. They occur because of the control limits that have been selected, not because of any problems with the analytical method. Therefore the use of 2*s* control limits cannot be generally recommended. With the use of 3*s* control limits, the false rejection problem is eliminated, but unfortunately error detection is also reduced.

Westgard Multirule Chart

The "multirule" procedure developed by Westgard and associates[113] uses a series of control rules for interpreting control data. The probability for false rejections is kept low by selecting only those rules whose individual probabilities for false rejection are very low (0.01 or less). The probability for error detection is improved by selecting those rules that are particularly sensitive to random and systematic errors. The procedure requires a chart having lines for control limits drawn at the mean ±1 *s*, 2 *s*, and 3 *s*, and is adapted to existing Levey-Jennings charts by the addition of one or two sets of control limits.

The following control rules are used:

Rule	Description
1_{2s}	One control observation exceeding the mean ±2 *s* is used only as a "warning" rule that initiates testing of the control data by the other control rules.
1_{3s}	One control observation exceeding the mean ±3 *s* is a rejection rule that is primarily sensitive to random error.
2_{2s}	Two consecutive control observations exceeding the same mean plus 2 *s* or mean minus 2 *s* limit is a rejection rule that is sensitive to systematic error.
R_{4s}	One observation exceeding the mean plus 2 *s* and another exceeding the mean minus 2 *s* is a rejection rule that is sensitive to random error.
4_{1s}	Four consecutive observations exceeding the mean plus 1 *s* or the mean minus 1 *s* is a rejection rule that is sensitive to systematic error.
$10_{\bar{x}}$	Ten consecutive control observations falling on one side of the mean (above or below, with no other requirement on size of the deviations) is a rejection rule that is sensitive to systematic error.

The use of the multirule procedure is similar to the use of a Levey-Jennings chart, but the data interpretation is more structured. To use the multirule procedure, follow these steps:

1. Analyze samples of the control material by the analytical method to be controlled on at least 20 different days. Two different materials having appropriate concentrations are recommended, but a single material can be used. Calculate the mean and standard deviation for the results for each control material being used.
2. Manually or electronically construct a control chart for each of the control materials being used. The observed concentration or control value should be plotted on the *y*-axis, setting the range of concentrations to include the mean ±4 *s*. Draw horizontal lines for the mean, the mean ±1 *s*, the mean ±2 *s*, and the mean ±3 *s*. It may be desirable to use different colors for these lines, perhaps green, yellow, and red for the 1 *s*, 2 *s*, and 3 *s* limits, respectively. The *x*-axis should be scaled for time, day, or run number, and labeled accordingly.
3. Introduce two control specimens into each analytical run, one for each of the two concentrations when two different materials have been selected. Record the control values and plot each on its respective control chart.
4. When both control observations fall within the 2*s* limits, accept the analytical run and report the patient results. When one of the control observations exceeds a 2*s* limit, hold the patient results. Inspect the control data using the 1_{3s}, 2_{2s}, R_{4s}, and $10_{\bar{x}}$ rules. When any one of these rules indicates the run is out of control, reject the analytical run and do not report the patient results. When all of these rules indicate that the run is in control, accept the analytical run and report the patient results.

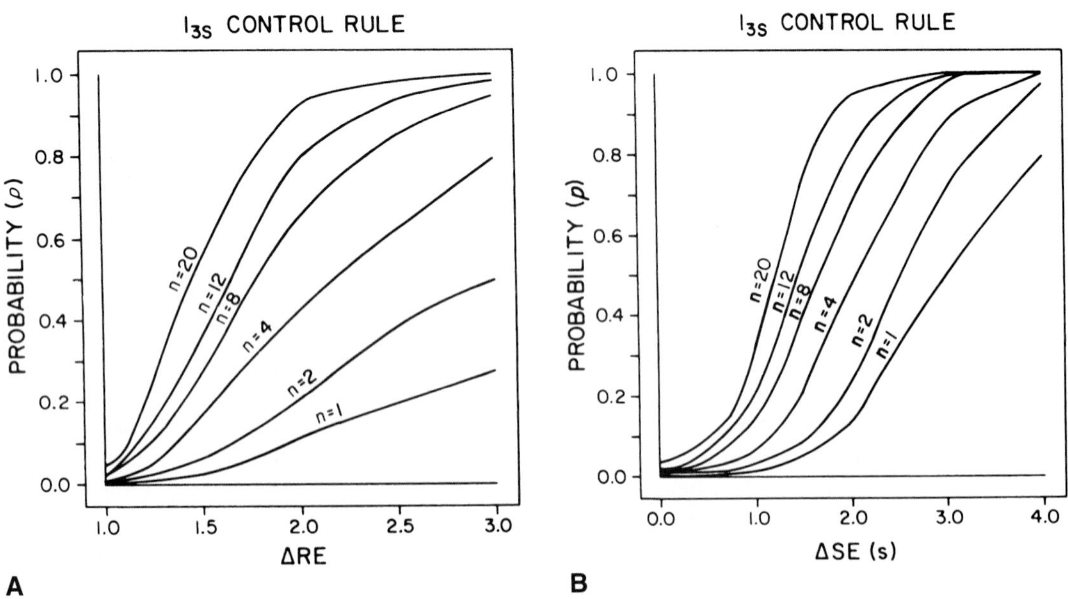

Figure 19-13 Power functions for the 1_{3s} control rule. **A,** Random error. **B,** Systematic error. *(From Westgard JO, Groth T. Power functions for statistical control rules. Clin Chem 1979;25:863-9.)*

5. When a run is out of control, determine the type of error occurring based on the control rule that has been violated. Look for sources of that type of error. Correct the problem, then reanalyze the entire run including both control and patient samples.

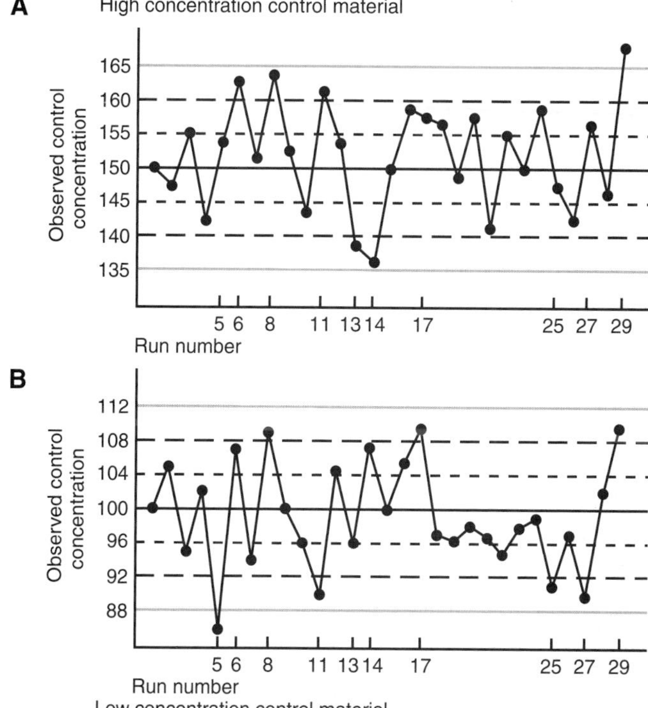

Figure 19-14 Westgard multirule control chart having control limits drawn at the mean ±1 s, 2 s, and 3 s. Concentration is plotted on the *y*-axis versus time (run number) on the *x*-axis. **A,** Chart for high-concentration control material. **B,** Chart for low-concentration control material. *(From Westgard JO, Barry PL, Hunt MR, Groth T. A multi-rule Shewhart chart for quality control in clinical chemistry. Clin Chem 1981;27:493-501.)*

An example application of the multirule procedure is shown in Figure 19-14, where the top chart is for a high-concentration control material and the bottom chart is for a low-concentration material. Table 19-2 summarizes the interpretation of the charted data, providing the run number, the accept and/or reject decision, control rules violated, and the type of error suspected based on the rule violations. It is important to note that the R_{4s} rule is applied only within a run, so that between-run systematic errors are not wrongly interpreted as random errors. However, the rule may be applied "across" materials, meaning that one of the observations can be on the low material and the other on the high material, as long as they are within the same run. On the other hand, note that the 2_{2s}, 4_{1s}, and $10_{\bar{x}}$ rules can be applied across runs and materials. This effectively increases n and improves the error detection capabilities of the procedure.

Power functions for the multirule procedure are shown in Figure 19-15 for n from 2 to 6. The probability for false rejection will be much lower at these n's than for the Levey-Jennings chart having 2*s* control limits. However, the false rejections do increase as n increases, limiting n to a maximum of 4 to 6. For larger n's, it would be necessary to modify the procedure by eliminating the R_{4s} rule, or by replacing this approximate range rule with an exact range rule (see discussion of Shewhart range procedure later in this chapter).

Comparison of the probability for error detection between the multirule procedure and the Levey-Jennings chart having 3*s* limits shows improved error detection for the multirule procedure. The R_{4s} rule improves the detection of random error and the 2_{2s}, 4_{1s}, and $10_{\bar{x}}$ rules improve the detection of systematic error. Elimination of the $10_{\bar{x}}$ rule does not cause much loss in error detection but does considerably reduce the amount of control data that must be inspected; thus the simplification may make the multirule procedure easier to use. The 4_{1s} rule could possibly be elim-

TABLE 19-2 Interpretation of Example Control Data Using the Westgard Multirule Procedure

	Decision on Run		Control Rule Violated					Type of Error	
Run Number	**Accept**	**Reject**	1_{3s}	2_{2s}	R_{4s}	4_{1s}	$10_{\bar{x}}$	**RE**	**SE**
5		×	×					×	
6	×								
8		×		×					×
11		×			×			×	
13	×								
14		×		×					×
17		×				×			×
25	×								
27		×					×		×
29		×	×	×					×

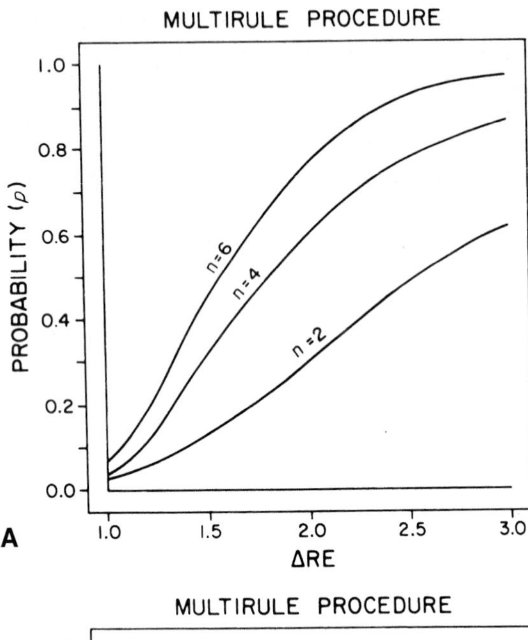

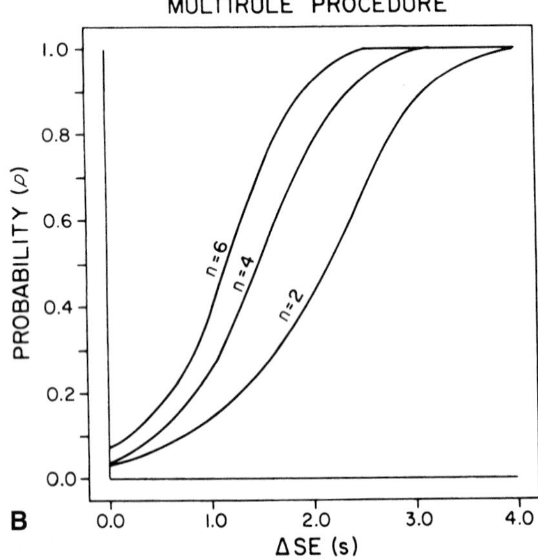

Figure 19-15 Power functions for Westgard multirule control procedure. **A,** Random error. **B,** Systematic error. *(From Westgard JO, Barry PL, Hunt MR, Groth T. A multi-rule Shewhart chart for quality control in clinical chemistry. Clin Chem 1981;27:493-501.)*

inated to further simplify the procedure, but this would be at an appreciable loss in power for detecting systematic errors.

Cumulative Sum (Cusum) Control Chart

The single-value control charts discussed in the previous sections provide a display of the differences between the observed values and the expected mean. Control rules, such as 2_{2s}, 4_{1s}, and $10_{\bar{x}}$ provide one way of determining when these successive differences no longer appear to be random (too many in a row on one side of a limit). A more exact and quantitative method is the cumulative sum control procedure or cusum chart.

TABLE 19-3 Example Cusum Calculations and Tabular Record for V-Mask Cusum Chart (for Control Material with $\bar{x} = 100$, s = 5.0)

Control Observation Number	Control Value	d_i	CS_i
1	110	+10	+10
2	100	0	+10
3	108	+8	+18
4	105	+5	+23
5	105	+5	+28
6	101	+1	+29
7	96	−4	+25
8	105	+5	+30
9	101	+1	+31
10	101	+1	+32
11	111	+11	+43
12	102	+2	+45
13	110	+10	+55
14	107	+7	+62
15	107	+7	+69
16	107	+7	+76

To set up a cusum chart, follow these steps:

1. Analyze the control material by the analytical method to be controlled on at least 20 different days, and calculate the mean and standard deviation of those results. (This is the same as the initial step required for a Levey-Jennings chart or for a multirule chart.)
2. Manually or electronically construct a control chart. Label the *y*-axis "cusum." Draw a horizontal line at the midpoint of the *y*-axis to represent a cusum of zero. Set the range of values above and below to be about 10 times the standard deviation. Label the *x*-axis in terms of time, using day, run number, control observation number, or whatever is most appropriate for recording the relative time of the control observation.
3. Introduce control specimens into each analytical run and record the value obtained.
4. Calculate the difference between the value and the expected mean. Obtain the cusum by adding this difference to the cumulative sum of the previous differences. Plot the cusum on the control chart and inspect the plot.
5. Interpret the charted data by evaluating the slope of the cusum line. A steep slope suggests that a systematic error is present and that the run is out of control.

Example calculations are shown in Table 19-3. These cusum values are plotted versus observation number in Figure 19-16. When control values scatter on both sides of the mean, giving both positive and negative differences, the cusum will alternate in sign, and the plotted values will wander back and forth across the zero line on the control

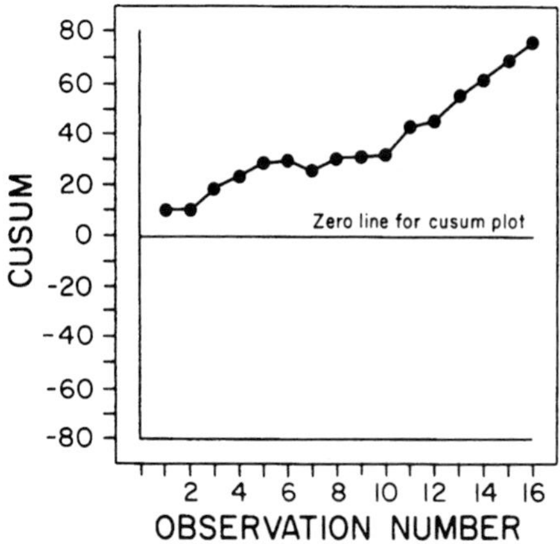

Figure 19-16 V-mask cumulative sum control chart (e.g., data in Table 19-4). The cumulative sum of the differences from the mean is plotted on the *y*-axis versus time (control observation number) on the *x*-axis.

chart. When the control values fall mostly on one side of the mean so that most of the differences have the same sign, the cusum value increases in magnitude, and the plotted values will move away from the zero line of the control chart.

It is more difficult to judge the control status from cusum charts than from Levey-Jennings or multirule charts. The approach that has been used most extensively is to make the judgment based on the slope of the cusum line. In industry, this has often been done by constructing templates having a V-shaped section removed from a rectangular sheet of clear plastic. This V-shaped cutout establishes the angle that is the control limit and gives the technique its name of "V-*mask*" *cusum.* The apex of the V-mask is positioned on the control chart at a specified distance in front of the most recent cusum observation. If all of the plotted values are contained within the angle of the V-mask, the method is judged to be in control. If any of the plotted values fall outside the angle of the V-mask, the method is judged to be out of control. Although this technique for interpreting cusum data is very objective, V-mask overlays have not been very widely used or recommended for clinical laboratories. Instead, interpretation has been based on visual inspection and on judgment of the angle of the cusum line, sometimes aided by use of special graph paper having an underlying pattern of 45° angles (∠∠∠∠∠∠∠.) across the chart. When using this special graph paper, the convention has been to scale the graph so that a change of 2*s* on the *y*-axis is the same distance between two points on the *x*-axis. The 45° angle then represents the slope expected when the observed mean is approximately 2*s* from the expected mean.

An alternative way of interpreting cusum data is to use a numerical limit for the cusum value itself, a technique known as *"decision limit" cusum.* Particular decision limit schemes are characterized by two parameters: *k*, a factor for calculating the threshold, and *h*, a factor for calculating the decision limit or control limit. The cusum calculations do not start until a control value exceeds a certain threshold above (k_u) or below (k_l) the expected mean ($\bar{x}$). Once exceeded, the differences from the threshold are calculated and summed for successive observations to provide the cusum. This process continues until the cusum either exceeds the upper and lower control limits (h_u and h_l) and the method is judged out of control, or until the cusum changes sign, in which case the cusum calculation is stopped and the method judged to be in control. An example of the cusum calculations for the decision limit technique is given in Table 19-4.

TABLE 19-4 Example Cusum Calculations and Tabular Record for Decision Limit Cusum (for Control Material with $\bar{x} = 100$, $s = 5.0$; for Control Chart with $k_u = 105$, $k_l = 95$, $h_u = 13.5$, $h_l = 13.5$)

Control Observation Number	Control Value	d_i	CS_i	Comment
1	110	+5	+5	Start cusum calculation
2	100	−5	0	
3	108	+3	+3	
4	105	0	+3	
5	105	0	+3	
6	101	−4	−1	End cusum calculation
7	96			
8	105			
9	101			
10	101			
11	111	+6	+6	Start cusum calculation
12	102	−3	+3	
13	110	+5	+8	
14	107	+2	+10	
15	107	+2	+12	
16	107	+2	+14	

These example data are plotted in Figure 19-17. One advantage of the decision limit cusum chart is that it has horizontal lines for control limits, permitting the cusum chart to be interpreted in a manner similar to a Levey-Jennings chart. This form of interpretation requires less experience and judgment, thus making possible more consistent interpretation when many analysts use the control procedure. Another advantage of the decision limit technique is that it can be implemented using only tabular operations (without charting), thus making it very easy to program for computerized handling of control data.

Although interpretation is easier and more objective, selecting the threshold and control limits is somewhat difficult. This selection is done with the aid of nomograms,

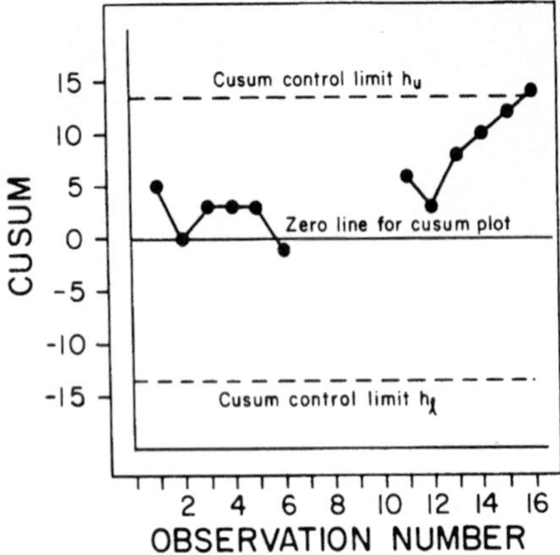

Figure 19-17 Decision limit cumulative sum control chart (e.g., data in Table 19-5). The cumulative sum of the differences from the threshold is plotted on the *y*-axis versus time (control observation number) on the *x*-axis.

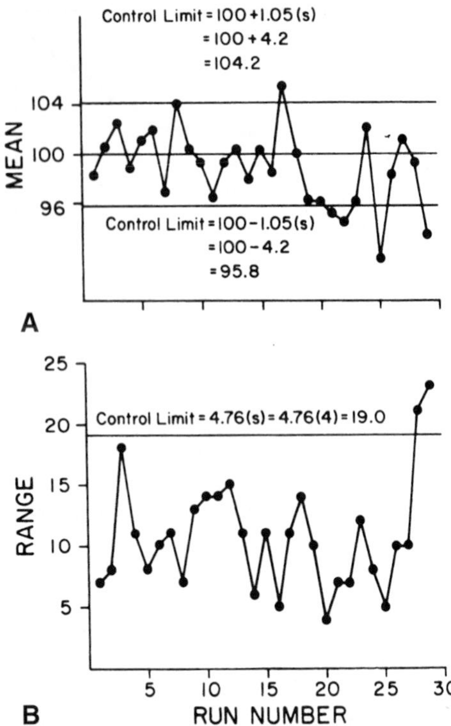

Figure 19-18 Shewhart mean and range control charts. **A,** Mean chart. **B,** Range chart.

which are quite complicated to understand and use, and therefore it is initially perhaps best to use one of the decision limit schemes recommended in the clinical chemistry literature.[120] For manual implementation, set the threshold at the $x \pm 1.0s$ and the control limits at $2.7s$. For computer implementation, set the threshold at the $x \pm 0.5s$ and the control limits at $5.1s$. This latter procedure will be sensitive to smaller errors because of the choice of the lower threshold. However, the charting is not as convenient when performed manually, particularly when the cusum is used in combination with the 1_{3s} control rule to provide better detection of random errors.[120]

When compared with the Levey-Jennings chart with 3*s* limits, the cusum procedure provides better detection of systematic errors but less sensitivity for random errors. Because of the low sensitivity to random errors, cusum should not be used alone, but rather should be included with a Levey-Jennings procedure on a combined chart[120] or used as a separate chart along with a Levey-Jennings chart. Performance is similar to the multirule procedure for low n's, at least as far as detecting systematic errors. However, the multirule procedure is more sensitive to random errors because of the added R_{4s} rule.

Shewhart Mean and Range (or Standard Deviation) Control Charts

Statistical quality control charts were first introduced in industry during the 1930s by Shewhart,[86] who recommended obtaining a group of control measurements, determining the average and standard deviation of the group, then plotting the average on an "*x*-bar" or mean chart and the standard deviation on an *S*-chart. For n's less than 10, the *S*-chart is usually replaced by a "range" or *R*-chart on which is plotted the range, or difference between the highest and lowest observations of the group.

To set up mean and range charts, initial estimates must be obtained for the mean and standard deviation, or the mean and average range, as determined for the control material to be used and the analytical method to be controlled. Control limits for the charts are calculated using appropriate factors (see Table 17-3 in the 3rd edition of this textbook).[123] A group of control measurements is then collected in each analytical run, and the mean and range (or standard deviation) are calculated and plotted. An example set of data is given in Table 19-5 and plotted on the mean and range charts in Figure 19-18.

Implementation by Use of the Z and Chi-Square (χ^2) Tests

Charts for mean, range, and standard deviation are seldom found in clinical laboratories because of the time required for calculating the control statistics. These control procedures are probably practical only when computerized data handling is available. An easy way of implementing these procedures on computers is to employ statistical tests of significance. A *Z*-test can be used to determine whether the mean has changed from its original value, and a χ^2-test can be applied to determine whether the standard deviation has changed from its original value.

The values for *Z* and χ^2 are determined from the following equations:

$$Z_{obs} = \frac{\bar{x}_{obs} - \bar{x}_{exp}}{\frac{s_{exp}}{\sqrt{n}}}$$

$$\chi^2_{obs} = \frac{(s_{obs})^2(n-1)}{(s_{exp})^2}$$

TABLE 19-5 Shewhart Mean and Range Calculations and Tabular Record

	INDIVIDUAL CONTROL MEASUREMENTS						GROUP	
Run	1	2	3	4	5	6	$\bar{x}$	R
1	96	98	101	98	95	102	98.33	7
2	99	100	105	97	100	103	100.67	8
3	101	100	113	95	106	101	102.67	18
4	98	93	96	104	101	102	99.00	11
5	101	103	106	100	99	98	101.17	8
6	95	109	99	103	105	101	102.00	10
7	103	94	92	94	101	98	97.00	11
8	101	105	104	108	103	104	104.17	7
9	96	105	92	105	101	104	100.50	13
10	101	99	93	107	102	95	99.50	14
11	102	88	92	101	99	98	96.67	14
12	92	97	107	95	99	106	99.33	15
13	94	105	96	103	104	100	100.33	11
14	101	96	101	101	95	95	98.17	6
15	107	99	101	96	102	97	100.33	11
16	102	97	98	98	99	97	98.50	5
17	101	112	104	102	107	108	105.67	11
18	97	99	104	96	95	109	100.00	14
19	98	95	101	91	97	96	96.33	10
20	97	96	96	94	96	98	96.17	4
21	98	95	92	99	95	93	95.33	7
22	96	89	95	94	93	94	93.50	7
23	95	100	93	89	98	101	96.00	12
24	96	104	103	102	101	107	102.17	8
25	92	89	94	94	90	90	91.50	5
26	92	101	93	102	102	100	98.33	10
27	100	101	105	101	104	95	101.00	10
28	112	91	97	97	97	102	99.33	21
29	103	102	95	92	80	88	93.33	23

where $\bar{x}_{obs}$ is the mean observed in the analytical run being tested, $\bar{x}_{exp}$ is the mean expected when the method is working properly, n is the number of control measurements in the group, s_{obs} is the standard deviation observed in the analytical run being tested, and s_{exp} is the standard deviation expected when the analytical method is in stable operation. To determine the control status of an analytical run when using the Z-test, the observed Z-value is compared with the critical Z-value for a selected probability for false rejection. The critical values are 1.96, 2.58, and 3.09 for probabilities of false rejection of 0.05, 0.01, and 0.002, respectively. When the observed Z-value is less than the critical Z-value, the run is judged to be in control. When it exceeds the critical Z-value, the run is judged to be out of control.

To determine control status using the χ^2-test, the observed χ^2-value is compared with the critical χ^2-value (see Table 17-3 in the 3rd edition of this textbook).[123] When the observed value is less than the critical value, the run is judged to be in control; when it exceeds the critical value, the run is judged to be out of control.

Alternative Calculations and Applications

Moving averages and moving standard deviations are used in industry and sometimes in clinical laboratories. With these procedures, n is chosen, measurements are collected until n is attained, and then the mean and standard deviation are calculated. With each additional measurement, the oldest measurement is dropped, the newest is added, and new estimates of the mean and standard deviation are obtained after each new control measurement, rather than waiting for new groups of n measurements. Parvin[69] has proposed the use of a multimean rule that combines the means of control values observed in consecutive runs. Similar updated means and standard deviations are obtained from exponential smoothing, a calculation procedure that provides an average that weighs recent observations more heavily than older observations.[118] The "smoothed mean" is sensitive to trends that are just beginning to develop, and therefore it is often referred to as a *trend analysis procedure.* The calculations are too complicated to be implemented manually, but the availability of computers makes these calculations feasible in clinical laboratories.

Power functions for mean (or Z-test), range, and χ^2 (or standard deviation) control procedures, when compared with those for previous control procedures, show higher probabilities for error detection, particularly at larger n's. The probability for false rejection can be set at a suitably low level by proper choice of control limits. Thus these control procedures appear to offer better performance characteristics than single-value control charts because they have higher error detection and lower false rejection as n increases.

The use of mean and standard deviation control procedures (or related procedures) to monitor accuracy and precision is a direct extension of the practices of method evaluation, the mean being used to monitor systematic error and the standard deviation to monitor random error. This relationship helps explain why control procedures having n's from 1 to 4 have relatively low power or error detection capability. Not surprisingly, it is more difficult to estimate precision and accuracy using quality control procedures with n's of 1 to 4 than with method evaluation procedures using n's of 20 to 40. For low ns, all control procedures have relatively low power. As n increases, power will increase, particularly for procedures using mean, range, S-charts, Z-tests, and χ^2-tests, moving averages and moving standard deviations, and trend analysis. Future practices in statistical quality control in clinical laboratories will undoubtedly make greater use of these procedures.

The integration of powerful computer hardware and software into analytical systems has made it practical to use complicated control procedures on a routine basis in clinical laboratories. Calculations on control data, once properly programmed, are performed quickly and without mistakes. Graphical displays can be generated, with color added to aid the interpretation of control data. Specific control rules are programmed to provide "accept" and "reject" signals or printouts. Records are maintained to document instrument changes, preventive maintenance, and control problems. Monthly summary statistics and quality control reports are generated. Many of these features, along with many of the statistical control procedures that have been described, are found in microcomputer quality control programs that are commercially available today.

CONTROL OF ANALYTICAL QUALITY USING PATIENT DATA

QC mechanisms based on patient data provide additional information useful in monitoring the quality of laboratory analyses. These procedures are often time consuming and generally are not sensitive enough to serve as the only means of QC. However, many of the control problems detected with these techniques may not be evident with conventional QC systems. A quality assurance program should make appropriate use of "patient data procedures," and both individual and multiple patient results have been used for QC purposes.

Individual Patient Results

The patient test results are the final product of most laboratory procedures, and the monitoring of these results is the most direct form of QC. Unfortunately, procedures for monitoring results are not very sensitive and have low probabilities for error detection. The most effective procedure is the clinical correlation of test results with other information related to the patient, especially surgical findings, response to therapy, and autopsy data. Less sensitive but easier to implement are comparisons with previous test values and correlation with related test results. The easiest procedure is the comparison of test results with physiological or probabilistic limits.

Clinical Correlation

Operationally, it is impractical for high-volume, core laboratories to correlate all test results with the clinical status of the patients. In general, the clinicians ordering the tests are in a better position to evaluate the appropriateness of test results. However, clinicians often order a test because they are uncertain of the exact clinical status of their patient and base their diagnoses heavily on the laboratory test results. In such cases, it is circular reasoning to correlate clinical diagnoses with laboratory test results. Clinical correlation studies are best done retrospectively when laboratory test results are directly related to other evidence, such as surgical findings. Unfortunately, most laboratory tests do not correlate perfectly with disease states, and one must evaluate multiple cases before determining the diagnostic efficiency of a given test (as discussed further in Chapter 14). In an individual patient, clinical correlation can identify impossible or highly unlikely test results that cannot be flagged in the laboratory, such as a normal serum bilirubin concentration in a highly jaundiced patient. Clinicians should be encouraged to report these discrepancies to the laboratory, and a mechanism should be available to follow up these problems. Also, after using a test for a period of time, many clinicians can detect alterations in test results, and although this is not reliable for documenting problems, informal discussions with clinicians frequently using the test can aid in identifying aspects of laboratory tests that should be further investigated.

A focus on linking laboratory tests to patient care outcomes (see Chapter 13) requires an integrated healthcare system in which all processes are operating properly.[38,131] This integrated system includes the correct assessment of the patient's problem, ordering of the correct tests, accurate and timely analytical performance, correct interpretation of the test results, and implementation of appropriate clinical actions that produce the expected response in the patients. Obviously this complete cycle is subject to numerous variables, which traditionally are outside of the control of the laboratory. However, under managed care there is a strong incentive to ensure that the complete system is working. All patients do not respond the same; therefore the responses of multiple patients with similar disorders must be monitored.

Some examples of this approach are the linkage of adverse outcomes of inappropriate anticoagulation (stroke, myocardial infarct, or death within 6 days) to the measurement of prothrombin times and the linkage of adverse effects of digoxin therapy (death or hospitalization caused by insufficiency, overdose, or drug reaction) with the measurement of digoxin.[129]

Correlation with Other Laboratory Tests

As in clinical correlation, there are a limited number of situations in which a single test result is plausible, but the combination of several test results is impossible or very unlikely. If the tests involved in these comparisons are performed at the same time, one often can identify errors and correct problems before reporting the test results to the clinicians. Even though very few tests have exact clinical relationships and one often must consider statistical percentages rather than the results of a single patient to identify malfunctions, several relationships provide some possibilities for monitoring an individual patient's results, at least for purposes of initiating further review:

1. *Blood typing.* There is a close association between the ABO blood antigens on erythrocytes and isoantibodies found in plasma. Exceptions are found in patients recently transfused with whole blood.
2. *Anion gap.* To maintain electrical neutrality, the sum of the charges of anions in a blood sample must equal the sum of the charges of cations when expressed in molar concentrations. With all units in mmol/L, an anion gap (AG) can be calculated as

$$AG = (Na^+ + K^+) - (Cl^- + HCO_3^-)$$

   Values less than approximately 10 mmol/L or greater than about 20 mmol/L may indicate error. Elevated values may be found in patients with renal failure, diabetic acidosis, cardiac failure, anoxia, and other conditions (see Chapter 46). Low values occur in hypoproteinemia and with intravenous hydration. The capabilities of AG control procedures have been studied by Cembrowski and co-workers,[22] who recommend that the average AG of groups of eight or more patients be used to provide a more sensitive statistical control.
3. *Osmolar gap.* Serum osmolality can be estimated from the concentrations of a few major blood constituents and can also be measured using colligative properties (see Chapter 27).[33] The osmolar gap (OG) is defined as the measured osmolality minus the calculated osmolality or

$$OG = \text{osmolality} - \left[1.86(Na^+) + \frac{\text{glucose}}{18} + \frac{\text{urea}}{2.8} + 9\right]$$

   where osmolality is in mosm/kg, sodium is in mmol/L, and glucose and urea nitrogen are in mg/dL. The factor "9" represents the contribution of other osmotically active substances in plasma, such as K^+, Ca^{2+}, and proteins. Normally this gap is near zero. Alcohol consumption or the ingestion of toxins, such as salicylates or ethylene glycol, causes an increase.[34,132] Alterations of unmeasured electrolytes and dehydration may also increase the gap.
4. *Acid-base balance.* The Henderson-Hasselbalch equation is also used to calculate theoretical bicarbonate and total CO_2 concentrations when pH and PCO_2 are measured. Theoretical and measured results generally agree within 2.0 mmol/L.
5. *Thyroxine-TSH.* Normally, thyroxine sends a negative feedback to the pituitary and reduces the secretion of thyroid stimulating hormone (TSH). Patients with serum thyroxine concentrations above 8.0 μg/dL seldom have elevated concentrations of TSH. Exceptions occur in secondary and tertiary hyperthyroidism.

Intralaboratory Duplicates

Samples can be divided into two aliquots and analyzed, and the duplicates used for control purposes. This is a simple quality control procedure that does not require stable control materials and therefore can be used when stable materials are not available or as a supplemental procedure when stable control materials are available. The differences between duplicates are plotted on a range type of control chart that has limits calculated from the standard deviation of the differences.[110] When the duplicates are obtained from the same method, this range chart monitors only random error and thus is not adequate for ensuring the accuracy of the analytical method. When the duplicates are obtained from two different laboratory methods, then the range chart actually monitors both random and systematic errors but cannot separate the two types of errors. The interpretation becomes more difficult, particularly when there are stable systematic differences or biases between the two analytical methods. Multiplicative factors may be necessary to deal with proportional differences, and additive factors may be necessary to allow for constant differences. Interpretation of observed differences becomes more qualitative; nevertheless, this procedure still provides a useful way of monitoring the consistency of the data being generated by the laboratory.

Delta Checks with Previous Test Results

Certain errors, particularly errors in specimen identification, have been detected by comparing laboratory test results with values obtained on previous specimens from the same patient. The expected variability of test results depends on both the analyte and the time interval between determinations. Ladenson has defined delta check limits based on a 3-day interval in terms of a percentage change from the initial value.[51] His check limits for some common tests are shown in Table 19-6.

In identifying specimen-related errors, it is helpful to examine multiple test parameters, including hematological tests, because differences in a profile of test results often are more obvious and more statistically significant than are changes in individual tests. For example, in a 1979 study, the performance of several delta check methods was evaluated, including two discriminant functions, for detecting mislabeled specimens; a false-positive rate of 5% and an error detection of about 50% for mislabeled specimens were observed.[123]

Limit Checks

A patient's test results should be reviewed to check that they are within the physiological ranges compatible with life. These limit checks are helpful for detecting clerical errors, such as transposed digits or misplaced decimal points. This checking can be combined with warning limit checks for detecting and verifying possible, but infrequently occurring, test results. These warning limits are dependent on test methodology and on the characteristics of the patient population being tested. Table 19-7 shows limits for some common tests.

TABLE 19-6 Recommended Limits for Delta Checks

Test	Delta Check Limit
Albumin	20%
Bilirubin, total	50%
Calcium, total	15%
Creatine kinase	99%
Creatinine	50%
Phosphorus	20%
Potassium	20%
Protein, total	20%
Sodium	5%
Thyroxine	25%
Urea nitrogen	50%
Uric acid	40%

From Ladenson JH. Patients as their own controls: Use of the computer to identify "laboratory error." Clin Chem 1975;21:1648-53.

MULTIPLE PATIENTS

Test Distribution Statistics

Statistics based on distributions of test results from large numbers of patients are useful for detecting systematic errors (shifts and drifts) but are of no value for detecting random errors (increased variability or scatter). They are useful adjuncts to the fundamental control procedures, which use stable control materials, but should not be substituted for them. Patient values include numerous sources of variation—demographical, biological, pathological, and preanalytical (see Chapter 17)[134]—in addition to the analytical variation caused by the analytical method. As a result, individual test values have too much variability to have any utility for QC; however, the mean of multiple test values or groups of patients is more stable and therefore may be useful for control purposes.

The variability of the mean test result from a group of n patients decreases proportionally to the square root of the number of determinations. The variability of the estimated mean is given by the standard error of the mean (SEM), which is equal to the standard deviation of the patient population divided by the square root of n, the number of patient measurements included in the group mean. Consider the following example, where the s of the patient values is 100 units. As n increases to 16, 25, 100, and 400, the SEM becomes 25, 20, 10, and 5 units, respectively. If the s of the analytical method was 10 units, the distribution of patients would be 10 times as large; however, if one considers the mean values of groups of 100 patients, the variability (SEM) of the group mean is approximately equal to the variability

TABLE 19-7 Recommended Ranges for Limit Checks

Test	Low Warning	High Warning
Acid phosphatase* (U/L)	0.1	10
Albumin (g/dL)	1.5	6
Alkaline phosphatase* (U/L)	5	300
Amylase* (U/L)	20	1000
Bilirubin (mg/dL)	0.2	10.0
Calcium (mg/dL)	6.5	13.0
Creatine kinase (U/L)	5	1500
Creatinine (mg/dL)	0.3	7.5
Phosphorus (mg/dL)	1.0	8.0
Potassium (mmol/L)	3.0	6.0
Sodium (mmol/L)	120	150
Urea nitrogen (mg/dL)	3	50
Uric acid (mg/dL)	1.0	12.0

Values are method dependent.

From Whitehurst P, DiSilvio TV, Boyadjian G. Evaluation of discrepancies in patients' results: An aspect of computer-assisted quality control. Clin Chem 1975;21:87-92.

observed on individual observations on stable control materials. For groups of 400 patients, the variability of the mean is half that for individual observations on the stable control material.

Changes in the means of patient populations may be caused by multiple variables (see Chapters 16 and 17). Changes in the demographic and clinical characteristics of the patients, such as the ratio of males to females, the ratio of hospitalized patients to outpatients, or the presence of many specimens from a specialty clinic can alter the mean value. Similarly, changes in preanalytical conditions,[134] such as tourniquet time and specimen storage, alter patient population means and can therefore be monitored by use of patient means. These variables are not monitored by those control procedures employing stable materials; thus the "patient mean procedures" provide additional capabilities and should be used in conjunction with other control procedures.

Statistical Methods for Monitoring Patient Means

The "mean of normals" or "average of normals" (AON) approach calls for establishing limits, usually the limits for reference values, for "trimming" the patient data.[125] Values outside these limits are eliminated from the calculations, thus reducing the response to outliers and subpopulations and also to real errors. An alternative approach has been to use the median as the control statistic, and this may be a more sensitive indicator of change than the mean. More complicated estimates have been recommended to account for hospitalized patients having slightly different test values from those of ambulatory patients. A weighted mean based on the percentage of patients in each category has greater sensitivity for error detection, particularly for measurements of the serum concentration of total protein, albumin, and calcium.

Bull's algorithm has been widely employed for online monitoring of automated hematological cell counters. Bull and colleagues[10] evaluated six statistics for monitoring erythrocyte indices: the sample mean, two moving average means, the mean of a truncated sample, the John's mean, and the median. They assessed the usefulness of these different statistics by mathematically introducing both abrupt bias changes and cyclical time changes. The moving average statistics were found to have superior error detection. The batch size used in calculating the moving average regulates the smoothing of the data. Large batch sizes not only smooth out undesired individual patient effects, but also increase the number of specimens (and time) necessary to detect instrument malfunction. A weighted moving average based on a batch size of 20 specimens was recommended. Cembrowski has developed power function graphs to provide quantitative information of both single-rule and multirule variations of Bull's algorithm.[21,57]

Control statistics based on patient data have been readily implemented in computerized laboratories.[43] However, several authors have shown that these control procedures are not as sensitive as procedures using stable reference material. All of these statistics are designed to detect systematic errors and have virtually no power for detecting random error. The relative sensitivity of these statistics for detection of systematic errors, as compared with stable reference controls, is dependent on three factors: variation of patient test values (and the test statistics derived from them), analytical variation, and the ratio of the number of specimens to the number of controls. Low patient variability, high analytical variability, and a high ratio of specimens to controls favor patient-based QC procedures. Patient test result variability depends not only on the analyte measured, but also on the population being tested. Populations consisting mainly of healthy individuals generally have lower test variability than the populations of medical specialty clinics. A quantitative study of these variables and their effects on the statistical power of procedures using patient means has been performed by Cembrowski and co-workers.[19] Smith and Kroft[89] have further evaluated the performance and relationship of AON and Bull's algorithms and have proposed an exponentially adjusted moving mean whose performance can be optimized for individual applications.

Effect of Analytical Bias on Clinical Decisions

Changes in analytical bias directly shift the distribution of the patient test values. If the elevated values on a test are associated with specific clinical actions, then the shifts in analytical bias can notably alter the number of patients having test values that exceed the action limit.[46] For example, for a serum calcium assay with an action limit of 10.1 mg/dL, an upward bias of 0.2 mg/dL changes the number of patients subjected to further investigation from 6.5% to 15.0%. Similarly, analytical shifts in other critical analytes can cause notable clinical problems, such as false elevations of prostate-specific antigen values triggering prostate ultrasound examinations and biopsies and false elevation of TSH triggering additional thyroid examinations. These small analytical shifts can have major downstream effects on healthcare costs.

Combined Use of Liquid Controls and Moving Averages of Patient Values for Quality Control Monitoring

Distributions of the measured test values have been used to supplement the traditional liquid controls for monitoring analytical bias. These patient specimen measurements generally have much larger variances than liquid controls because they contain biological, pathophysiological, and preanalytical sources of variation in addition to the analytical variation. However, if some of these sources of variation are controlled, averaging techniques often are used to generate tracking parameters, which have variations of the same order of magnitude as liquid controls. Demographic information about specific patients such as age, sex, and medical provider service area have been used to normalize the test values, resulting in smaller variances of the group means for the monitoring parameters. The larger the window size used for

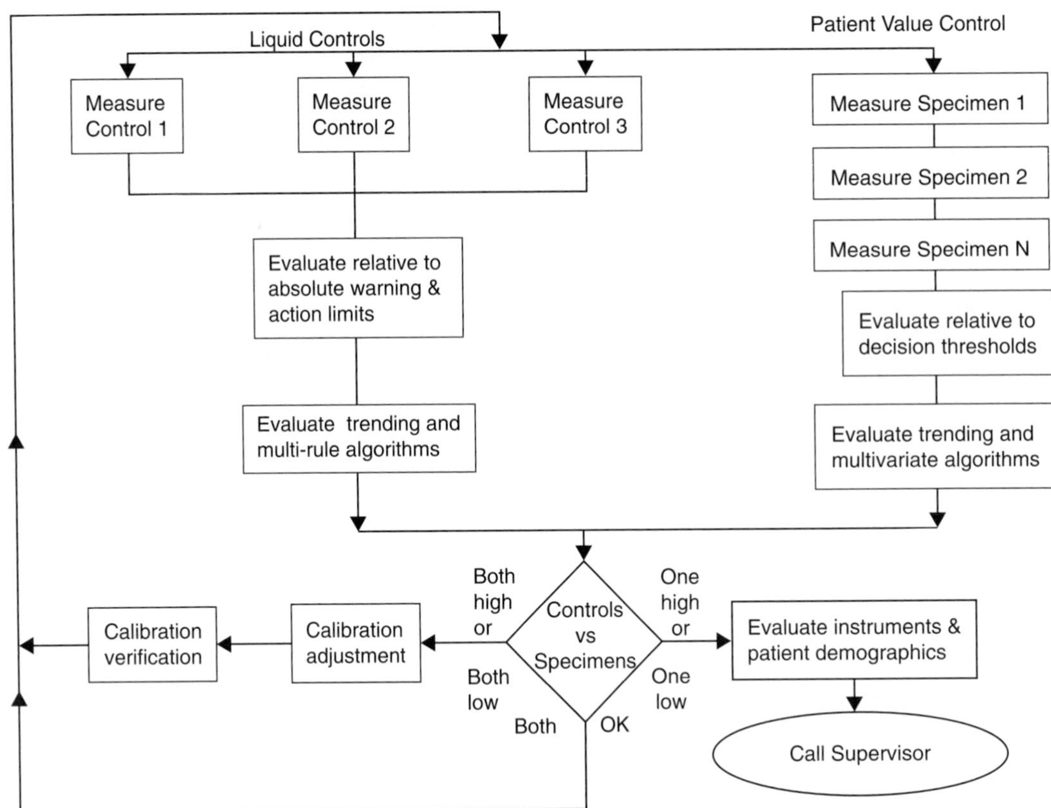

Figure 19-19 Protocol for combining liquid controls and a patient value–derived control.

averaging patient values the smaller the variance. The CV of the group mean decreases approximately proportional to the square root of the number of samples. Various statistical techniques have been used to average the patient values, such as the exponentially adjusted moving mean proposed by Smith and Kroft.[89,90] In general, there is a trade off between decreased variance versus increased time for error detection when larger numbers of patient values are used in these moving averages. For most chemistry tests, window sizes using 50 to 100 sample values often are necessary.[45] An advantage of test value distributions over liquid controls is the inclusion of preanalytical variation caused by specimen collection, transport, and storage. This allows patient value–derived parameters to detect changes in these variables in addition to changes in the analytical testing.

Figure 19-19 illustrates an algorithm for combining liquid controls with a patient value–derived parameter. The same multirule evaluation systems used for liquid controls have been used for tracking the patient value–derived QC statistic. Set points and threshold values are assigned to this derived parameter to optimize the power for error detection for systematic error. Note that the averaging algorithms used to generate these derived parameters average out random errors, so these derived parameters are not useful for detecting random errors. As illustrated in the figure, this combined control protocol is most accurate when both the liquid control and the patient-derived control move in the same direction (both high or both low). When the controls move discordantly, further investigation is necessary to define if the problem is related to instability of the liquid controls, changes in the patient characteristics (such as many sick patients seen at one time), preanalytical test changes, or other causes.

Clinical Correlation Studies

Retrospective correlation studies relating laboratory test results to surgical findings or therapeutic changes in patients are effective mechanisms for long-term QC. Two separate patient populations are necessary to efficiently monitor both false-positive and false-negative laboratory test results. To monitor false-positive results, the records of patients with positive results should be randomly sampled and reviewed for confirmatory evidence of disease. For many laboratory tests, substantial medical follow-up is necessary to confirm or refute test results, and, unfortunately, medical records often do not contain this information. Again, stated diagnoses cannot be used to confirm laboratory test results, since the laboratory test results may have been the primary evidence for the diagnosis. To monitor false-negative results, the records of patients with objective clinical confirmation of the disease should be randomly sampled and reviewed. Examples of objective confirmation are surgical discovery of a tumor, improvement in physical signs and symptoms following pharmacological or surgical therapy, and autopsy findings. It is difficult to obtain unbiased record selection, because test results often alter clinical decisions regarding surgery or therapy. There is less selection bias in autopsy data, but the disease process generally is more advanced in these patients.

EXTERNAL QUALITY ASSESSMENT AND PROFICIENCY TESTING PROGRAMS

All of the control procedures described earlier in the chapter have focused on monitoring a single laboratory. These procedures constitute what is called *internal quality control*[108] to distinguish them from procedures used to compare the performance of different laboratories, the latter being known as *external quality assessment.* The two are complementary activities, internal QC being necessary for the daily monitoring of the precision and accuracy of the analytical method, and external quality assessment being important for maintaining the long-term accuracy of the analytical methods.[15,17]

In practice, internal QC procedures only detect changes in performance between the present operation and the "stable" operation that was characteristic during the baseline period when the analytical method was thought to be operating properly. Although the procedures detect systematic and random errors, the only systematic errors detected are those changes from the original baseline. If the method actually had some undetected systematic errors during the baseline period, those systematic errors would be included in the mean that was used to calculate the control limits for the procedure. Thus only systematic changes from this original mean will be detected by internal QC procedures.

Initial method evaluation studies are essential to ensure that systematic errors are not present before the baseline period and the determination of the mean and the control limits. The accuracy of the method should be initially established by comparison with other analytical methods (and recovery and interference studies) and should continue to be monitored by comparison with other analytical methods. Ongoing comparison-of-methods studies are desirable to ensure that systematic errors do not slowly increase and go undetected by internal QC procedures. These ongoing comparison studies are provided by the external QA programs, which in turn form the basis for proficiency testing programs.

External Quality Assessment

Several external QA programs are available to laboratories, some sponsored by professional societies and others by manufacturers of control materials. The basic operation of these programs involves having all the participating laboratories analyze the same lot of control material, usually daily as part of the internal QC activities. The results are tabulated monthly and sent to the sponsoring group for the data analysis. Summary reports are prepared by the program sponsor and are distributed to all participating laboratories. This reporting takes time for processing all the data from a large number of laboratories; thus the data analysis is not available in real time and is useful only for monthly reviews and periodic problem-solving activities. However, with advances in telecommunications and the arrival of the World Wide Web, real-time external QC is a possibility.

The reports often include extensive data analysis, statistical summaries, and plots. The mean of all results or the mean of results from peer laboratories (those performing the test with similar methods) is taken as the target value and is used for comparison with the individual laboratory's result. Different programs do this in different ways. For example, the statistical significance of any difference between an individual laboratory's observed result and the group mean can be tested by use of the t-test. When the difference is significant, the laboratory is alerted that its results are biased compared with the results of most of the other laboratories. Another approach is to divide the difference by the overall standard deviation of the group, and then to express the difference in terms of the number of standard deviations

$$SDI = \frac{\text{Laboratory Result} - \text{Group Mean}}{\text{Group } s}$$

where SDI is the abbreviation for standard deviation interval or index, and Group s is the standard deviation for the group or a selected subset of the group. Differences greater than 2 or 3 indicate that a laboratory is not in agreement with the rest of the laboratories in the program. These calculations reduce all the test results to the same values, which makes it possible to interpret the data without reference to the exact mean and s for each analytical method. For example, a value of +2.0 has the same meaning for any test, indicating that the value is $2s$ above its target mean.

Additional information about the nature of the systematic error is obtained when there are two different control materials analyzed by each laboratory. For example, the laboratory's observed mean for material A is plotted on the y-axis versus its observed mean for material B on the x-axis; these graphs are called *Youden* plots.[133] Ideally the point for a laboratory should fall at the center of the plot. Points falling away from the center but on the 45° line suggest a proportional analytical error. Points falling away from the center but not on the 45° line suggest either an error that is constant for both materials or an error that occurs with just one material.

The report may also include Levey-Jennings plots of the data, but because this information is not available in real time, it does not effectively serve the purposes of internal QC. Blank control charts that are set up for each analyte and each control material save the laboratory the time that is required when these charts are prepared manually.

The operation of external QA programs is greatly improved by using a PC and appropriate software. Operationally the external comparison is more quickly performed using the PC as a terminal for transmitting data via the

Internet to the central computer. The processing of the data to compare the results from the many different laboratories is then performed and the reports returned to the laboratory. Since the individual control observations are entered into the PC, the control data are then immediately tested by internal control procedures to determine control status. Thus in practice, the PC integrates the internal and external procedures into a more efficient program for QA.

Proficiency Testing and Laboratory Accreditation

Proficiency testing (PT) programs are a type of external quality assessment in which simulated patient specimens made from a common pool are analyzed by the laboratories enrolled in the program. The results are returned to a central facility and evaluated to determine the "quality" of each laboratory's performance. Government and licensing agencies are increasingly using PT as an objective method for accrediting laboratories thereby giving them official authorization to operate.[84]

An example of using PT for such a purpose is the U.S. government's mandate that clinical laboratories be accredited and licensed. Historically, this developed after a series of newspaper articles were published that focused on laboratory quality problems and led to a determined effort by the U.S. government to protect patients' interests and the public welfare.[7,8] In 1988 the U.S. Congress subsequently revised the Clinical Laboratory Improvement Act of 1967 (CLIA '67) and passed the Clinical Laboratory Improvement Amendment (CLIA '88); it mandates PT as a major part of the laboratory accreditation process.[73,100] The implementation rules for this legislation have been evolving, with the final legislative rule being published on January 24, 2003.[99] Additional interpretative guidelines were published by the Centers for Medicare and Medicaid Services (CMS) in January 2004 in the form of the State Operations Manual. Appendix C of that document refers specifically to guidelines for laboratories and laboratory testing services.[1]

The initial CLIA '88 regulations focused primarily on the analytical process. However, it was later stressed that the quality of the "total testing process" must be monitored in addition to the precision and accuracy of the analytical phase.[70,72,78,130] Thus as mentioned earlier in this chapter, current QA programs that monitor only the analytical phase of the total process have to be expanded to include both the preanalytical (see Chapter 17) and postanalytical phases (www.westgard.com/essay34).

CLIA requires all U.S. laboratories to register with the government and to identify the tests they perform. Certain tests are "waived," meaning that any laboratory can perform those tests as long as they follow the manufacturers' directions. There are no other requirements for quality management of those tests. Laboratories that perform "nonwaived" tests are subject to the complete CLIA regulations and must be inspected periodically by the government or by certain professional organizations that are deemed to have standards at least as stringent as the CLIA requirements. Two such organizations are the College of American Pathologists (CAP) and the Joint Commission on Accreditation of Healthcare Organizations (JCAHO). The CLIA implementation rules and interpretative guidelines outline the criteria for acceptable performance in laboratory inspection and accreditation.

The CLIA requirements cover several broad classes: (1) Subpart J. Facility Administration; (2) Subpart K. Quality Systems; (3) Subpart M. Personnel; and (4) Subpart Q. Inspection. The final rule dealt mainly with changes to the subpart on Quality Systems, with particular attention to preanalytical, analytical, and postanalytical systems. It places increased emphasis on having quality systems to monitor preanalytical and postanalytical processes, yet the biggest impact of the final rule is on analytical quality assessment and analytical quality systems.[115]

In general the performance characteristics of PT programs for detecting bias and imprecision are evaluated using methods similar to those listed for assessing internal QC.[52] A commonly used evaluation criterion has been the comparison of PT test results with those of peer groups, considering all values that exceed 2 SD to be "unacceptable." This rule fails to detect many of the laboratories that have poor performance, especially those that have precision problems.[27] The initial CLIA '88 proposal called for the PT of two specimens four times per year, but the final rule expanded this to the study of five samples three times per year so as to improve the capability of detecting "unacceptable" performance. The criterion for PT failure is two of five incorrect results on two of three consecutive PT surveys.

CLIA '88 proposed criteria group laboratory tests into "specialty" and "subspecialty" categories and specify representative tests to be monitored in each category.[70,100] To be totally "successful" in a given category, a laboratory must produce correct results on four out of five specimens for each of the analytes in that category and have an overall score of at least 80% for three consecutive challenges. If there are more than two incorrect results for any analyte, the laboratory is considered "on probation." If a laboratory has two or more incorrect results for any analyte or has an overall score less than 80% on two of three consecutive surveys, it is classified as "suspended" and must cease testing all analytes in that specialty category until it is reinstated.

The CLIA regulations have established fixed limits (either percentages or absolute values from target) for evaluating PT performance. These test categories and limits are shown in Table 19-8. The target values for these analytes will be established by the agencies implementing the PT programs under the federal guideline[100] that states: "Target value means either the mean of all responses after removal of outliers (those responses greater than 3 standard deviations from the original mean) or the mean established by definitive or reference methods acceptable for use in the National Reference System (NRS) for the Clinical Laboratory by the NCCLS. In instances in which definitive or reference methods are not

TABLE 19-8 HCFA/CLIA Proficiency Testing Criteria for Acceptable Performance

Analyte or Test	Acceptable Performance
Routine Chemistry	
Alanine aminotransferase	Target value ± 20%
Albumin	Target value ± 10%
Alkaline phosphatase	Target value ± 30%
Amylase	Target value ± 30%
Aspartate aminotransferase	Target value ± 20%
Bilirubin, total	Target value ± 0.4 mg/dL or ± 20% (greater)
Blood gas PCO_2	Target value ± 55 mm Hg or ± 8% (greater)
Blood gas pH	Target value ± 0.04
Blood gas PO_2	Target value ± 3 SD
Calcium, total	Target value ± 1.0 mg/dL
Chloride	Target value ± 5%
Cholesterol, high-density lipoprotein	Target value ± 30%
Cholesterol, total	Target value ± 10%
Creatine kinase	Target value ± 30%
Creatine kinase isoenzymes	MB elevated (presence or absence) or target value ± 3 SD
Creatinine	Target value ± 0.3 mg/dL or ± 15% (greater)
Glucose	Target value ± 6 mg/dL or ± 10% (greater)
Iron, total	Target value ± 20%
Lactate dehydrogenase (LD)	Target value ± 20%
LD isoenzymes	LD 1/LD 2 positive or negative or target value ± 30%
Magnesium	Target value ± 25%
Potassium	Target value ± 0.5 mmol/L
Sodium	Target value ± 4 mmol/L
Total protein	Target value ± 10%
Triglycerides	Target value ± 25%
Urea nitrogen	Target value ± 2 mg/dL or ± 9% (greater)
Uric acid	Target value ± 17%
Endocrinology	
Cortisol	Target value ± 25%
Free thyroxine	Target value ± 3 SD
Human chorionic gonadotropin	Target value ± 3 SD or positive or negative
T_3 uptake	Target value ± 3 SD
Triiodothyronine	Target value ± 3 SD
Thyroid stimulating hormone	Target value ± 3 SD
Thyroxine	Target value ± 20% or 1.0 µg/dL (greater)
Toxicology	
Alcohol, blood	Target value ± 25%
Blood lead	Target value ± 10% or ± 4 µg/dL (greater)
Carbamazepine	Target value ± 25%
Digoxin	Target value ± 20% or 0.2 ng/mL (greater)
Ethosuximide	Target value ± 20%
Gentamicin	Target value ± 25%
Lithium	Target value ± 0.3 mmol/L or ± 20% (greater)
Phenobarbital	Target value ± 20%
Phenytoin	Target value ± 25%
Primidone	Target value ± 25%
Procainamide (and metabolite)	Target value ± 25%

From the U.S. Department of Health and Human Services: Clinical Laboratory Improvement Amendments of 1988; Final Rules and Notice. 42 CFR Part 493. The Federal Register 1992;57:7188-288.

Continued.

TABLE 19-8 HCFA/CLIA Proficiency Testing Criteria for Acceptable Performance—*Continued*

Analyte or Test	Acceptable Performance
Toxicology—Cont'd	
Quinidine	Target value ± 25%
Theophylline	Target value ± 25%
Tobramycin	Target value ± 25%
Valproic acid	Target value ± 25%
Hematology	
Cell identification	90% or greater consensus on identification
White cell differentiation	Target ± 3 SD based on percentage of different types of white cells
Erythrocyte count	Target ± 6%
Hematocrit	Target ± 6%
Hemoglobin	Target ± 7%
Leukocyte count	Target ± 15%
Platelet count	Target ± 25%
Fibrinogen	Target ± 20%
Partial thromboplastin time	Target ± 15%
Prothrombin time	Target ± 15%
General Immunology	
α_1-antitrypsin	Target value ± 3 SD
α-fetoprotein	Target value ± 3 SD
Antinuclear antibody	Target value ± 2 dilution or positive or negative
Antistreptolysin O	Target value ± 2 dilution or positive or negative
Anti-human immunodeficiency virus	Reactive or nonreactive
Complement C3	Target value ± 3 SD
Complement C4	Target value ± 3 SD
Hepatitis (HBsAg, anti-HBc, HBeAg)	Reactive (positive) or nonreactive (negative)
IgA	Target value ± 3 SD
IgE	Target value ± 3 SD
IgG	Target value ± 25%
IgM	Target value ± 3 SD
Infectious mononucleosis	Target value ± 2 dilution or positive or negative
Rheumatoid factor	Target value ± 2 dilution or positive or negative
Rubella	Target value ± 2 dilution or positive or negative

available, a comparative method may be used. If the method group is less than 20 participants, 'target value' means the overall mean after outlier removal (as defined above) unless acceptable scientific reasons are available to indicate that such an evaluation is not appropriate."

Accepted reference methods do not exist for many of these "controlled analytes," and even when they do exist, the values obtained for PT specimens with some analytical systems may not match those obtained with the reference method owing to differences in matrices and analyte form.[91] The CAP uses peer group mean values as the targets or groups of methods that agree with the definitive method. This target value is termed the definitive method correlated target value (DMCTV). Alternatively, the all-method mean (or median) is used as the target value, but this causes problems if one manufacturer dominates the market, especially if the method used is calibrated differently than the others.

The CLIA '88 regulations specify that the PT specimens should be treated in the same manner as patient specimens and require that the personnel performing the tests sign a statement attesting that they have complied with the regulations. In reality, PT specimens must be treated differently than those from patients, since many are lyophilized or sealed in containers, and reporting of their results requires different forms and is generally not computerized. A study in England showed that "special handling" of PT specimens substantially improved the accuracy of results.[81] A survey of hospital-based laboratories in Pennsylvania showed that the majority of laboratories provided special handling for PT specimens (e.g., running tests in duplicate, reporting the average, and recalibrating methods just before analyzing PT specimens).[20] This "special handling" does not necessarily provide better test results. In a study of proficiency testing problems at a large reference laboratory, it was found that error rates were higher if PT specimens were given special handling than if they were submitted as blind patient specimens. Moreover, it was found that most problems were caused by systematic errors and that the average of replicates did not correct these problems.[32]

A new requirement of the final CLIA regulations is that laboratories must perform method validation studies on all new tests introduced after April 24, 2003. Before this, laboratories that implemented new methods and analytical systems that had been cleared by the Food and Drug Administration (FDA) could simply follow manufacturers' directions for operation and assume that the manufacturer's performance claims were valid. With the issuance of the final rule, the performance of all new tests must be validated in each laboratory to document the reportable range, precision, accuracy, and reference intervals. For some methods, it may also be necessary to determine the detection limit and to test for possible interferences.

Another major change in the final rule was the elimination of an earlier provision that would have required the FDA to review a manufacturer's QC instructions. That was a key provision for allowing laboratories to simply follow a manufacturer's directions. However, with elimination of that provision, laboratories now have more responsibility for establishing effective QC systems that will monitor the complete analytical process, take into account the performance specifications of the method, detect immediate errors, and monitor long-term precision and accuracy.

The most controversial change in the final rule is the introduction of "equivalent QC procedures." CLIA sets a minimum level of QC that must be performed by all laboratories. Typically that requires two levels of controls to be analyzed every 24 hours, or for some tests, one level of control to be analyzed every 8 hours. The new guidelines for "equivalent QC" may allow laboratories to reduce daily QC to weekly or even monthly QC for analytical systems that have built-in procedural controls. The provision is obviously targeted for point-of-care testing (POCT) or near patient testing (NPT) where personnel lack the skills to perform QC and instead rely on instrument checks, most notably electronic checks or electronic QC. In spite of the arguments about the inadequacy of electronic QC,[104] it has become widely accepted in POCT and NPT applications. Although there is at least one example of an analytical system with improved QC technology that requires little or no external QC,[117] most analytical systems have yet to demonstrate the performance that would justify a reduction of daily QC to only weekly or monthly QC.

In the United States, as a result of the personnel standards of CLIA and current staffing shortages, many laboratories have been left without the technical and analytical skills to manage quality effectively. Consequently, in the authors' opinion, the use of statistical QC is declining in many laboratories (www.westgard.com/essay34). Thus QC has come to mean "quality compliance" rather than quality control. The consequences of a regulatory approach to quality have to be carefully assessed relative to other initiatives. Regulation does not appear to be an adequate substitute for professional responsibility for quality.

To summarize this section, PT programs are far from ideal monitors of laboratory performance. In a study of PT survey problems at the Mayo Clinic, more than one half of the errors on surveys were directly related to deficiencies in the surveys (such as invalid specimens and inappropriate evaluation criteria), and only 28% could be linked to specific analytical problems.[47] A novel PT program piloted by the New York State Department of Health involves obtaining aliquots of patient specimens that are routinely processed by the laboratory at the time of its annual inspection.[75] These specimens are reanalyzed in the state's laboratories using reference methods, and the results are compared with those obtained during inspection. This prevents problems such as the presence of unnatural specimens and the clerical errors of foreign forms. Other specimen stability problems and methodological interferences probably continue to exist.

IDENTIFYING THE SOURCES OF ANALYTICAL ERRORS

The control procedures discussed in the previous sections provide a way of alerting the analyst to problems that may cause the quality of analytical performance to fall short of the goals set for the laboratory. However, these control procedures do not identify the sources of the analytical errors and solve the control problems. The following additional procedures are often necessary to identify these sources.

Physical Inspection

When alerted to a control problem, the first step should be to carefully inspect the analytical method, equipment, reagents, and specimens. Does everything look, feel, smell, and sound correct? An inspection may seem to be a very qualitative and subjective technique, but it can be exceedingly useful when performed with checklists developed for specific analytical methods. This inspection should include a review of records documenting changes that occur with the instrument and reagents. Brief instrument function checks are often performed to verify proper system performance and to separate chemical and instrumental sources of errors. An experienced analyst can often spot the problem by making this kind of inspection, whereas inexperienced analysts will be aided by formal checklists.

Relationship of Type and Source of Error

The type of error itself provides a clue about the source of the error. For example, systematic errors are often related to calibration problems (impure calibration materials, improper preparation of calibrating solutions, erroneous set point and assigned values, unstable calibrating solutions, contaminated solutions, inadequate calibration techniques, nonlinear or unstable calibration functions, unstable reagent blanks, and inadequate sample blanks). Random errors are more likely caused by lack of reproducibility in the pipetting of samples and reagents, to the dissolving of reagent tablets and the mixing of sample and reagents, and to the lack of stability of temperature baths, timing regulation, and photometric and other sensors. Individual analytical methods may not be subject to all of these possible sources of error; rather, there may be only a few plausible sources for a particular type of error. Experienced analysts often know what these common sources are for their particular analytical methods and quickly identify the sources once the type of error is known.

Some information about the type of error occurring is obtained by knowing which errors the control procedures respond. As discussed earlier in this chapter, different control rules have different sensitivities to detect random and systematic errors, as illustrated by the multirule control procedure. However, in practice, it is often possible to make a good judgment as to the type of error occurring based on the control procedure that provides the alert. Control procedures that employ patient samples rather than stable control materials can help identify preanalytical sources of errors, such as sample handling and processing. External quality assessment procedures that employ frozen patient samples[79] may provide more extensive information about errors than what is available from internal procedures. The information from all of these procedures is complementary and, when used in combination, provides a more complete assessment of the types of errors occurring and their possible sources.

Method Evaluation Experiments

When the type of error cannot be easily identified and quantified from available control data, it may be necessary to use the experiments employed in method evaluation studies (see Chapter 14). A "comparison-of-methods experiment" may be used to estimate systematic errors when there is another routine method available for measuring the analyte of interest. Interpretation of the results must consider that the observed differences between two methods could be caused by either method and cannot therefore be assigned to the "test" method unless the quality of the "comparison" method is well documented. Recovery, interference, and linearity experiments may be more specific in estimating systematic errors, including the constant or proportional nature of the systematic errors.

To identify sources of random error, a "replication experiment" is designed to estimate the contributions from several different components. For example, when duplicates are analyzed within a run for several different runs, the data are used to determine the components of within-run and between-run variation. This process isolates the errors occurring in different time periods, which in turn may help identify the sources of the random error. Replication experiments of this kind, using analysis of variance statistical techniques, are tailored to particular analytical systems to identify the major factors that contribute to the random error of those analytical methods. The performance of control procedures also depends on the different components of variance, and it is particularly important that the between-run component be kept as small as possible.[116]

Optimization Techniques

More complicated experimental techniques, such as factorial experiments, "simplex" optimization, and "response surface" optimization, have been used to solve complex control problems. Youden[133] described the use of a series of experiments in which several factors could be varied simultaneously, thus reducing the total number of experiments necessary to determine how these factors affect the performance of the analytical method. These "factorial" experiments have been used for testing the "ruggedness" of an analytical method (i.e., its responsiveness to any disturbance in the chosen experimental conditions). A properly optimized method should be rugged—this means that small changes in the analytical conditions should not greatly affect analytical performance. Formal optimization strategies can be employed to decide on those analytical conditions. Simplex optimization techniques have also been applied to optimize clinical chemistry methods. These techniques provide systematic approaches for selecting the analytical conditions that minimize errors and reduce control problems.

QUALITY INITIATIVES

Several organizations have developed and implemented quality initiatives to ensure that clinical laboratories and manufacturers and providers of diagnostic products incorporate the principles of quality management and assurance in their daily operations. Examples include (1) Joint Committee for Traceability in Clinical Laboratories (http://www.bipm.fr/en/committees/jc/jctlm/), (2) International Organization for Standardization (http://www.iso.ch), and (3) National Institute of Standards and Technology (http://www.nist.gov).

Joint Committee for Traceability in Laboratory Medicine (JCTLM)[30]

Many organizations have been involved in developing a traceable accuracy base for analytes of clinical interest (see Chapter 14).[30,95] A driver for current efforts to develop such a base is the European Directive 98/79/EC on in vitro diagnostic medical devices (www.ce-mark.com/ivd.pdf), which requires that: "The traceability of values assigned to calibrators and/or control materials must be assured through available reference measurement procedures and/or available reference materials of a higher order."

In 2002 the JCTLM was created to meet the requirement for a worldwide platform to promote and give guidance on internationally recognized and accepted equivalence of measurements in laboratory medicine and traceability to appropriate measurement standards (www.bipm.org/en/committees/jc/jctlm/). The three principal participants in JCTLM are the International Bureau of Weights and Measures (BIPM), the International Federation for Clinical Chemistry and Laboratory Medicine (IFCC), and the International Laboratory Accreditation Cooperation. Other key participants include producers of certified reference materials (e.g., National Institute for Standards and Technology [NIST] and the Institute for Reference Materials and Measurements [IRMM]). In Vitro Diagnostic (IVD) manufacturers are represented by the Advanced Medical Technology Association (AdvaMed) and the European Diagnostic Manufacturers Association (EDMA); external quality assessment and proficiency testing organizations; standards organizations (e.g., the NCCLS and International Organization for Standardization (ISO)/Technical Committee 212); and regulatory bodies (e.g., FDA, European Union (EU) authorities, and the European Commission).

The JCTLM has created two working groups: (1) JCTLM WG-I, Reference Materials and Reference Procedures and (2) JCTLM WG-II, Reference Laboratory Networks. They are responsible for providing practical support to the worldwide IVD industry in establishing metrological traceability for values assigned to calibrators and/or control materials as required by the forthcoming European Directive on in vitro diagnostics and by comparable regulations in other countries.

International Organization for Standardization

The International Organization for Standardization (ISO) is a worldwide federation of national standards bodies from some 100 countries (http://www.iso.ch), one from each country that is the national body "most representative of standardization in its country." For example, the United States is represented in the ISO by the American National Standards Institute (ANSI). (The national representative for each country can be identified by accessing the ISO homepage—http://www.iso.ch.) The mission of the ISO is to promote the development of standardization and related activities in the world with a view to facilitating the international exchange of goods and services and to developing cooperation in the spheres of intellectual, scientific, technological, and economic activity. The ISO's work results in international agreements, which are published as international standards. The ISO 9000 standards are examples of such standards, and they have been applied on a worldwide basis. The ISO has also organized several technical advisory groups that address quality issues of interest to clinical laboratorians.

ISO 9000

ISO 9000 is a set of four standards for ensuring quality management and quality assurance in manufacturing and service industries. They were first published in 1987 and are used worldwide, with more than 80 countries adopting them as national standards. There have also been two large regional adoptions, the European Committee for Standardization and the Pan American Standards Commission. In brief, ISO 9000 certification is a tangible expression of an organization's commitment to quality that is recognized internationally.

The four ISO 9000 standards are:

ISO 9001 Quality systems—Model for quality assurance in design, development, production, installation, and servicing

ISO 9002 Quality systems—Model for quality assurances in production, installation, and servicing

ISO 9003 Quality systems—Model for quality assurance in final inspection and test

ISO 9004 Quality management and quality system elements—Guidelines

The ISO 9000 standards represent an international consensus on the essential features of a quality system to ensure the effective operation of any business, whether a manufacturer or service provider or other type of organization, whether in the public or private sector. Many major diagnostic companies have received ISO 9000 certification, and in 1996, the Excel Bestview Medical Laboratories of Mississauga, Ontario, Canada became the world's first clinical laboratory to receive ISO 9002 certification.[2] (Note that an organization applies for certification under the section that most closely represents its structure.) Elements of ISO 9002 certification (http://www.revereelectric.com/eleISO.html) include:

Management responsibility—Requires that a quality system be defined, documented, and communicated throughout the organization, and that responsibility for quality be clearly defined. Top management must review the quality system at least once a year to ensure its continuing suitability and effectiveness.

Quality system—Requires that a quality system meeting the requirements of the ISO 9002 standard be established, maintained, and documented as a means of ensuring that product conforms to requirements.

Contract review—Requires review of incoming orders to ensure that requirements are clearly and completely defined, and to ensure the capability exists to meet the requirements.

Document control—Requires establishing and maintaining procedures for controlling documentation through approval, issue, and modification.

Purchasing—Requires purchased product to conform to specified requirements. This is accomplished through vendor assessments, clear and accurate purchasing data, and verification of purchased product where applicable.

Customer-supplied material—Requires procedures for storage and maintenance of customer-supplied product.

Product identification and traceability—Requires procedures for identifying and tracing product if required by the customer.

Process control—Requires procedures to ensure that production processes are carried out under controlled conditions. This includes the documentation, monitoring, and control of suitable process characteristics; use of approved equipment; and workmanship standards.

Inspection and testing—Requires procedures for inspection and testing at receiving, in process, and before shipment.

Inspection, measuring, and test equipment—Requires procedures for selection, control, calibration, and maintenance of measuring and test equipment.

Inspection and test status—Requires evidence to indicate conformance or nonconformance to inspections and tests performed.

Control of nonconforming product—Requires procedures to ensure that product that does not conform to requirements is prevented from unintended use or installation. This includes identification, documentation, evaluation, segregation, and disposition of nonconforming product.

Corrective and preventive action—Requires procedures for the investigation of the cause of nonconformities, actions to eliminate them, and controls to prevent them from recurring.

Handling, storage, packaging, preservation, and delivery—Requires procedures for handling, storing, packaging, preserving, and delivering products to prevent damage or deterioration.

Control of quality records—Requires procedures for identification, collection, indexing, access, filing, storage, maintenance, and disposition of quality records.

Internal quality audits—Requires internal audits by personnel independent of the audited activity to verify whether quality activities comply with requirements and to determine the effectiveness of the quality system.

Training—Requires procedures for identifying training needs and providing training for all personnel to meet them.

Servicing—Requires procedures for performing, verifying, and reporting that the servicing meets specified requirements.

Statistical techniques—Requires procedures, when appropriate, for identifying the necessity for statistical techniques required for establishing, controlling, and verifying process capability.

ISO certification is carried out by accredited organizations known as registrars. Registrars review the organization's quality manual and audit the process to ensure that the system documented in the manual is in place and effective. When an organization receives ISO 9000 certification, benefits are recognized both internally and externally. Internally, it becomes a tool with which to monitor the quality system and to document continuous improvements. In addition, having a documented system ensures consistency, productivity, and effectiveness in all the daily functions of business. Externally, existing and potential customers have confidence knowing that the products or services that they purchase were processed under a controlled and documented system.

ISO Technical Advisory Groups for Laboratory Standards

The ISO also has a number of other activities that relate to quality activities in the clinical laboratory. For example, in response to an NCCLS proposal, the ISO organized in 1995 a Technical Advisory Group (TC 212-Clinical Laboratory Testing and In Vitro Diagnostic Testing Systems). The ISO has delegated responsibility for managing TC 212 to the United States (i.e., ANSI). ANSI in turn has delegated this responsibility to NCCLS. Creation of this technical committee provides a focus for coordination of international standardization in the field of laboratory medicine and in vitro diagnostic test systems. This includes, for example, quality management, preanalytical and postanalytical procedures, analytical performance, laboratory safety, reference systems, and quality assurance. Four working groups for TC 212 have been organized: (1) WG 1—Quality management in the clinical laboratory, (2) WG 2—Reference systems, (3) WG 3—In vitro diagnostic products, and (4) Antimicrobial susceptibility testing. These working groups have produced a number of documents (Table 19-9).

ISO 15189:2003 is an example of an ISO document; it was published by the ISO in 2003 and is based on ISO 9001 :2000 and ISO 17025:1999, the latter being a standard for testing and calibration laboratories.

It identifies specific management requirements, such as laboratory organization and management, a quality management system, document control, review of contracts, evaluation by referral laboratories, external services and supplies, advisory services, resolution of complaints, identification and control of nonconformities, corrective action, preventive action, continual improvement, quality and technical records, internal audit, and management review. Technical requirements cover personnel, accommodation and environmental conditions, laboratory equipment, preexamination procedures, examination procedures, assuring quality of examination procedures, postexamination procedures, and reporting of results. Annexes provide tables that correlate the requirements between ISO 9001:2000 and ISO/IEC 17025:1999. In addition, there are annexes with recommendations for protection of laboratory information systems, ethics in laboratory medicine, and POCT.

Other ISO technical committees that relate to quality in healthcare include (1) TC 48—Laboratory Glassware and Related Apparatus; (2) TC 76—Transfusion, Infusion, and Injection Equipment for Medical Use; (3) TC 176—Quality Management and Quality Assurance; and (4) TC 210—

TABLE 19-9 ISO Standards Relevant to Clinical Laboratories

Number	Title
ISO 15189:2003	Medical laboratories—particular requirements for quality and competence
ISO 15190:2003	Medical laboratories—requirements for safety
ISO 15193:2002	In vitro diagnostic medical devices—measurement of quantities in samples of biological origin—presentation of reference measurement procedures
ISO 15194:2002	In vitro diagnostic medical devices—measurement of quantities in samples of biological origin—description of reference materials
ISO 15195:2003	Laboratory medicine—requirements for reference measurement laboratories
ISO 15197:2003	In vitro diagnostic test systems—Requirements for blood glucose monitoring systems for self-testing in managing diabetes mellitus
ISO 17511:2003	In vitro diagnostic medical devices—measurement of quantities in biological samples—metrological traceability of values assigned to calibrators and control materials
ISO 18153:2003	In vitro diagnostic medical devices—measurement of quantities in biological samples—metrological traceability of values for catalytic concentration of enzymes assigned calibrators and control materials
ISO 19001:2002	In vitro diagnostic medical devices—information supplied by the manufacturer with in vitro diagnostic reagents for staining in biology
Draft Documents	
ISO/DIS 15198	Clinical laboratory medicine—in vitro diagnostic medical devices—validation of manufacturer's recommendations for user quality control
ISO/CD 22869	Technical Report: Medical laboratories—guidance on laboratory implementation of ISO 15189
ISO/CD 22870	Amendment to 15189: Annex D—point-of-care testing (POCT)

Quality Management and Corresponding General Aspects for Medical Devices. The NCCLS also administers the U.S. Technical Advisory Group for ISO/TC 76 on Transfusion, Infusion, and Injection Equipment for Medical Use. ISO/TC 76 is particularly concerned with development of standards for glass containers for blood transfusions, plastic containers for blood collection and transfusion, and blood specimen containers for hematology and biochemistry.

Preparing for ISO Accreditation

In 2002 Burnett compared ISO standards and synthesized an "ideal standard" that becomes a practical guide for laboratories preparing for ISO accreditation.[11] In his comparison, he supplements the original ISO standards and illustrates their application using a fictitious pathology laboratory and hospital (St. Elsewhere's Hospital Trust). In that context, there are many examples of specific forms and policies that would be appropriate for a laboratory. He also provides additional technical information about the quality required for the "intended use" of laboratory tests, which is important if the goal of uniform quality is to be achieved for a patient who moves from place to place and country to country.

Malcolm Baldridge National Quality Award

The Malcolm Baldridge National Quality Award was established by Congress in 1987 to enhance U.S. competitiveness by promoting quality awareness, recognizing quality achievements of U.S. companies, and publicizing successful performance strategies. In conjunction with private industry, the Commerce Department's National Institute of Standards and Technology (http://www.nist.gov) manages the award program. The award is not given for specific products or services. Currently, two awards may be given annually in each of three categories: manufacturing, service, and small business.

Seven areas are evaluated when a company applies for the award: (1) leadership, (2) information and analysis, (3) strategic planning, (4) human resource development and management, (5) process management, (6) business results, and (7) customer focus and satisfaction. Applicants must address a set of examination items within each of these categories. Heavy emphasis is placed on business excellence and quality achievement as demonstrated through quantitative data furnished by applicants. A useful consequence of the award has been the development of worksheets that an organization uses to measure and score its performance against the seven Baldridge criteria.[31] By assessing its quality program against these criteria, an organization verifies the status of its program and identify areas where improvements have to be made.

REFERENCES

1. Appendix C of State Operations Manual. Regulations and Interpretive Guidelines for Laboratories and Laboratory Services. (http://www.cms.gov.clia/appendx.asp).

2. Auxter S. How Excel Bestview became the world's first ISO-registered lab. Clin Lab News 1997;23:1-7.
3. Berry TH. Managing the total quality transformation. St. Louis: McGraw-Hill Book Co, 1991.
4. Berwick DM, Godfrey AB, Roessner J. Curing health care: New strategies for quality improvement. San Francisco: Jossey-Bass Publishers, 1990.
5. Blumenthal D. The Errors of Our Ways. Clin Chem 1997;43:1305. (http://www.clinchem.org/cgi/content/full/43/8/1305).
6. Bonini P, Plebani M, Ceriotti F, Rubboli F. Errors in Laboratory Medicine. Clin Chem 2002;48:691-8. (http://www.clinchem.org/cgi/content/full/48/5/691).
7. Bogdanich W. False Negative: Medical Labs, Trusted and Largely Error-free Are Far from Infallible—Haste, Misuse of Equipment, Specimen Mix-ups Afflict Even Best Labs at Times—Regulation: Weak and Spotty. The Wall Street Journal, February 2, 1987.
8. Bogdanich W. Risk Factor: Inaccuracy in Testing Cholesterol Hampers War on Heart Disease—Some Diagnoses Are Skewed by Glitches Such as Use of Ill-calibrated Lab Gear—Missing the Mark by 100 Percent. The Wall Street Journal, February 3, 1987.
9. Brooks ZC, Plaut D. Quality control—From "Data" to "Decisions": Basic concepts. Washington DC: AACC Press, 2002.
10. Bull BS, Elashoff RM, Heilbron DC, et al. A study of various estimators for the derivation of quality control procedures from patient erythrocyte indices. Am J Clin Pathol 1974;61:473-81.
11. Burnett D. A practical guide to accreditation in laboratory medicine. London: Association of Clinical Biochemists, 2002.
12. Buttner J, Borth R, Boutwell JH, et al. International Federation of Clinical Chemistry provisional recommendation on quality control in clinical chemistry: I. General principles and terminology. Clin Chem 1976;22:532-9.
13. Buttner J, Borth R, Boutwell JH, et al. International Federation of Clinical Chemistry provisional recommendation on quality control in clinical chemistry: II. Assessment of analytical methods for routine use. Clin Chem 1976;22:1922-32.
14. Buttner J, Borth R, Boutwell JH, et al. International Federation of Clinical Chemistry provisional recommendation on quality control in clinical chemistry: III. Calibration and control materials. Clin Chem 1977;23:1784-9.
15. Buttner J, Borth R, Boutwell JH, et al. International Federation of Clinical Chemistry approved recommendation (1983) on quality control in clinical chemistry: V. External quality control. J Clin Chem Clin Biochem 1983;21:885-92.
16. Buttner J, Borth R, Boutwell JH, et al. International Federation of Clinical Chemistry provisional recommendation on quality control in clinical chemistry: VI. Quality requirements from the point of view of health care. Clin Chim Acta 1977;74:F1-9.
17. Buttner J, Borth R, Broughton PMG, et al. International Federation of Clinical Chemistry approved recommendation (1983) on quality control in clinical chemistry: IV. Internal quality control. J Clin Chem Clin Biochem 1983;21:877-84.
18. CAP Standards for Accreditation of Medical Laboratories. Skokie, IL: College of American Pathologists (www.cap.org).
19. Cembrowski GS, Chandler EP, Westgard JO. Assessment of "average of normals" quality control procedures and guidelines for implementation. Am J Clin Pathol 1984;81:492-9.
20. Cembrowski GS, Vanderlinde RE. Survey of special practices associated with College of American Pathologists proficiency testing in the Commonwealth of Pennsylvania. Arch Pathol Lab Med 1988;112:374-6.
21. Cembrowski GS, Westgard JO. Quality control of multichannel hematology analyzers. Am J Clin Pathol 1985;83:337-45.
22. Cembrowski GS, Westgard JO, Iyama–Kurtycz DF. Use of anion gap for the quality control of electrolyte analyzers. Am J Clin Pathol 1983;79:688-96.
23. Cembrowski GS, Carey RN. Laboratory quality management: QC and QA, Chicago: ASCP Press, 1989.
24. Davies HT. Exploring the pathology of quality failings: measuring quality is not the problem–changing it is. J Eval Clin Pract. 2001 May;7(2):243-51.
25. Deming WE. Out of the crisis. Cambridge, MA: Massachusetts Institute of Technology Center for Advanced Study, 1987.
26. DeWoskin RS. Information resources on quality available on the internet. Qual Assur 2003;10:29-65.
27. Ehrmeyer SS, Laessig RH. Ability of the 1_{2s} rule to detect substandard performance in interlaboratory proficiency testing. Clin Chem 1987;33:788-91.
28. Eilers RJ. Quality assurance in health care: Missions, goals, activities. Clin Chem 1975;21:1357-67.
29. Elin RJ. Elements of cost management for quality assurance. Pathologist 1980;34:182-3.
30. Establishing calibration traceability for quantitative assays—CD. Washington DC: AACC Press, 2002.
31. Fischer DC, Simmons BP. The Baldridge workbook for healthcare. New York: Quality Resources Press, 1996.
32. Gambino R, Mallon P, Woodrow G. Managing for total quality in a large laboratory: Some examples. Arch Pathol Lab Med 1991;114:1145-8.
33. Garg AK, Nanji AA. The anion gap and other critical calculations. Diagn Med 1982;5:32-43.
34. Geller RJ, Spyker DA, Herold DA, Bruns DE. Serum osmolal gap and ethanol concentration: a simple and accurate formula. J Toxicol Clin Toxicol 1986;24:77-84.

35. Groth T, Falk H, Westgard JO. An interactive computer simulation program for the design of statistical control procedures in clinical chemistry. Comput Programs Biomed 1981;13:73-86.
36. Harry M, Schroeder R. Six sigma: The breakthrough management strategy revolutionizing the world's top corporations. New York: Currency, 2000.
37. Harteloh PP. Quality systems in health care: A sociotechnical approach. Health Policy. 2003;64: 391-8.
38. Hay ID, Klee GG. Linking medical needs and performance goals: Clinical and laboratory perspectives on thyroid disease. Clin Chem 1993;39:1519-24.
39. Honsa JD, McIntyre DA. ISO 17025: practical benefits of implementing a quality system. J AOAC Int. 2003;86:1038-44.
40. Ismail AAA, Walker PL, Barth JH, Lewandowski KC, Jones R, Burr WA. Wrong biochemistry results: two case reports and observational study in 5310 patients on potentially misleading thyroid-stimulating hormone and gonadotropin immunoassay results. Clin Chem 2002;48:2023-9.
41. Juppner H, Mohr H, Hesch RD. Adsorption of parathyrin: Pitfall for solid phase assays using radiolabelled antibodies? J Clin Chem Clin Biochem 1980;18:585-90.
42. Juran JM, Endres A. Quality improvement for services. Wilton, CT: Juran Institute Inc, 1986.
43. Kazmierczak SC. Laboratory quality control: using patient data to assess analytical performance. Clin Chem Lab Med 2003;41:617-27.
44. Kelly JT. Role of clinical practice guidelines and clinical profiling in facilitating optimal laboratory use. Clin Chem 1995;41:1234-6.
45. Klee GG. Use of patient test values to enhance the quality control of PSA assays. Clin Chem 2003;49:A94.
46. Klee GG. Tolerance limits for short-term analytical bias and analytical imprecision derived from clinical assay specificity. Clin Chem 1993;39:1514-8.
47. Klee GG, Forsman RW. A user's classification of problems identified by Proficiency Testing Surveys. Arch Pathol Lab Med 1988;112:371-3.
48. Koch DD, Oryall JJ, Feldbruegge DH, Dowd DE, Barry PL, Westgard JO. Selection of medically useful QC procedures for individual tests on a multi-test analytical system. Clin Chem 1990;36: 230-3.
49. Kohn KT, Corrigan JM, Donaldson MS. To err is human: building a safer health system Washington DC: National Academy Press, 1993:223pp.
50. Kubasik NP, Ricotta M, Hunter T, et al. Effect of duration and temperature of storage on serum analyte stability: Examination of 14 selected radioimmunoassay procedures. Clin Chem 1982;28:164-5.
51. Ladenson JH. Patients as their own controls: Use of the computer to identify "laboratory error." Clin Chem 1975;21:1648-53.
52. Laessig RH, Ehrmeyer SS. Use of computer modeling to predict the magnitude of intralaboratory error tolerated by proposed CDC interlaboratory proficiency testing performance criteria. Clin Chem 1988;34:1849-53.
53. Leape LL. Striving for Perfection. Clin Chem 2002;48:1871-2. (http://www.clinchem.org/cgi/content/full/48/11/1871).
54. Leape LL, Berwick DM, Bates DW. What practices will most improve safety? Evidence-based medicine meets patient safety. JAMA 2002;288:501-7.
55. Leape LL, Robert E. Gross Lecture. Making health care safe: are we up to it? J Pediatr Surg. 2004;39: 258-66.
56. Levey S, Jennings ER. The use of control charts in the clinical laboratories. Am J Clin Pathol 1950;20:1059-66.
57. Lunetsky ES, Cembrowski GS. Performance characteristics of Bull's multirule algorithm for the quality control of multichannel hematology analyzers. Am J Clin Pathol 1987;33:634-8.
58. Marks V. False-positive immunoassay results: a multicenter survey of erroneous immunoassay results from assays of 74 analytes in 10 donors from 66 laboratories in seven countries. Clin Chem 2002;48:2008-16.
59. Miller WG. Specimen materials, target values and commutability for external quality assessment (proficiency testing) schemes. Clin Chim Acta. 2003;327:25-37.
60. Mugan K, Carlson IH, Westgard JO. Planning QC procedures for immunoassays. J Clin Immunoassay 1994;17:216-22.
61. Nardella A, Farrell M, Pechet L, Synder L. Continuous improvement, quality control, and cost containment in clinical laboratory testing. Arch Pathol Lab Med 1994;118:965-8.
62. National Committee for Clinical Laboratory Standards: Nomenclature and definitions for use in the NRSCL and other NCCLS documents—Third Edition; Proposed Standard, NCCLS Document NRSCL 08-A, Wayne, PA: National Committee for Clinical Laboratory Standards, 1998.
63. National Committee for Clinical Laboratory Standards: Procedures for the handling and transport of diagnostic specimens and etiologic agents—Third Edition; Approved Standard. NCCLS Document H5-A3, Wayne, PA: National Committee for Clinical Laboratory Standards, 1994.
64. National Committee for Clinical Laboratory Standards: Clinical laboratory technical procedure manuals—Fourth Edition; Approved Guideline, NCCLS Document GP02A-A4, Wayne, PA, National Committee for Clinical Laboratory Standards, 2000.

65. National Committee for Clinical Laboratory Standards: A Quality System Model for Health Care; Approved Guideline. HS01-A, Vol 22, Number 13. Wayne, PA: National Committee for Clinical Laboratory Standards, 2002.
66. National Committee for Clinical Laboratory Standards: How to Define and Determine Reference Intervals in the Clinical Laboratory; Approved Guideline, 2nd ed. C28-A2, Vol 20, Number 13. Wayne, PA: National Committee for Clinical Laboratory Standards, 2000.
67. Nevalainen DE. The quality systems approach. Arch Pathol Lab Med 1999;123:566-8.
68. Nevalainen D, Berte L, Kraft C, Leigh E, Morgan T. Evaluating laboratory performance on quality indicators with the six sigma scale. Arch Pathol Lab Med 2000;124:516-9.
69. Parvin CA. Comparing the power of quality-control rules to detect persistent systematic errors. Clin Chem 1992;38:358-63.
70. Peddecord KM, Hammond HC. Clinical laboratory regulation under the Clinical Laboratory Improvement Amendments of 1988: Can it be done? Clin Chem 1990;36:2027-35.
71. Petersen PH, Stockl D, Westgard JO, Sandberg S, Linnet K, Thienpont L. Models for combining random and systematic errors. assumptions and consequences for different models. Clin Chem Lab Med. 2001;39:589-95.
72. Plebani M, Carraro P. Mistakes in a stat laboratory: types and frequency. Clin Chem 1997;43:1348-51. (http://www.clinchem.org/cgi/content/full/43/8/1348).
73. Public Law 100-578. Clinical Laboratory Improvement Amendments of 1988. Stat 42 USC 201. HR 5471, October 31, 1988.
74. Queralto JM. The EC4 quality manual model. Clin Chim Acta. 2001;309:127-36.
75. Rej R, Norton C. External assessment of laboratory cholesterol measurements using patient specimens. Clin Chem 1989;35:1069.
76. Revere L, Black K. Integrating Six Sigma with total quality management: a case example for measuring medication errors. J Healthc Manag. 2003;48: 377-91.
77. Rollo JL, Fauser BA. Computers in Total Quality Management: Statistical process control to expedite stats. Arch Pathol Lab Med 1993;117: 900-5.
78. Ross JW, Boone DJ. Assessing the effect of mistakes in the total testing process on the quality of patient care [Abstract 102]. In Martin L, Wagner W, Essien JDK, eds. 1989 Institute of critical issues in health laboratory practice Minneapolis, MN: DuPont Press, 1991.
79. Ross JW, Miller WG, Myers GL, Praestgaard J. The accuracy of laboratory measurements in clinical chemistry: a study of 11 routine chemistry analytes in the College of American Pathologists Chemistry Survey with fresh frozen serum, definitive methods, and reference methods. Arch Pathol Lab Med 1998;122:587-608.
80. Rossing RG, Foster DM. The stability of clinical chemistry specimens during refrigerated storage for 24 hours. Am J Clin Pathol 1980;73: 91-5.
81. Rowan RM, Laker MF, Albert GMM. The implications of assaying external quality control sera under "special conditions." Ann Clin Biochem 1984;21: 64-8.
82. Samore MH, Evans RS, Lassen A, Gould P, Lloyd J, et al. Surveillance of medical device-related hazards and adverse events in hospitalized patients. JAMA. 2004;291:325-34. (http://www.ncbi.nlm.nih.gov/entrez/query.fcgi?cmd=Retrieve&db=pubmed&dopt=Abstract&list_uids=14734595).
83. Sarewitz SJ. Evaluating laboratory performance with the six sigma scale. Arch Pathol Lab Med. 2000; 124:1748.
84. Savage RA. Proficiency testing and laboratory quality. Lessons from the Ontario Program. Arch Pathol Lab Med 1989;113:983-4.
85. Scholtes PR. The Team Handbook. Joiner Associates Inc, 3800 Regent St, Madison, WI, 1988.
86. Shewhart WA. Economic control of quality of the manufactured product. New York: Van Nostrand, 1931.
87. Siloaho M, Hukkanen K, Kinnunen J. Key elements of the implementation of a quality system in three Finnish clinical laboratories. Clin Chem Lab Med 2001;39:988-96.
88. Slockbower JM, Blumenfeld TA. Collection and handling of laboratory specimens. Philadelphia: JB Lippincott Co, 1983.
89. Smith FA, Kroft SH. Exponentially adjusted moving mean procedure for quality control. An optimized patient sample control procedure. Am J Clin Pathol 1996;105:44-51.
90. Smith FA, Kroft SH. Optimal procedures for detecting analytic bias using patient samples. Am J Clin Pathol 1997;108:254-68.
91. Stewart CE, Koepke JA, Thurrell T. Basic quality assurance practices for clinical laboratories. Philadelphia: JB Lippincott Co, 1987.
92. Taswell HF, Smith AM, Sweatt MA, et al. Quality control in the blood bank: A new approach. Am J Clin Pathol 1974;62:491-5.
93. Tetrault GA, Steindel SJ. Qprobe 94-08. Daily quality control exception practices. Chicago IL: College of American Pathologists, 1994.
94. Tetrault G. Evaluating laboratory performance with the six sigma scale. Arch Pathol Lab Med 2000;124:1748-9.

95. Thienpont LM, Van Uytfanghe K, De Leenheer AP. Reference measurement systems in clinical chemistry. Clin Chim Acta 2002;323:73-87.
96. Thiers RE, Wu GT, Reed AH, et al. Sample stability: A suggested definition and method of determination. Clin Chem 1976;22:176-183.
97. Tietz NW. A model for a comprehensive measurement system in clinical chemistry. Clin Chem 1979;25:833-9.
98. Uriano GA, Cali JP. Role of reference materials and reference methods in the measurement process. In: Validation of the measurement process. DeVoe JR, Ed ACS Symposium Series. Washington DC: American Chemical Society, 1977:140.
99. US Centers for Medicare & Medicaid Services (CMS). Medicare, Medicaid, and CLIA Programs: Laboratory Requirements Relating to Quality Systems and Certain Personnel Qualifications. Final Rule. Fed Regist Jan 24 2003;16:3640-714.
100. US Department of Health and Human Services: Clinical Laboratory Improvement Amendments of 1988; Final Rules and Notice. 42 CFR Part 493. The Federal Register, 57:7188-288, 1992.
101. Warwood S, Antony J. A simple, semi-prescriptive self-assessment model for TQM. Qual Assur 2003;10:67-81.
102. Westgard JO. Assuring analytical quality through process planning and quality control. Arch Pathol Lab Med 1992;116:765-9.
103. Westgard JO. Six sigma quality design and control: Desirable precision and requisite QC for laboratory testing processes. Madison WI: Westgard QC, Inc, 2001.
104. Westgard JO. Electronic quality control, the total testing process, and the total quality control system. Clin Chim Acta 2001;307:45-8.
105. Westgard JO. Charts of operational process specifications ("OPSpecs charts") for assessing the precision, accuracy, and quality control needed to satisfy proficiency testing performance criteria. Clin Chem 1992;38:1226-33.
106. Westgard JO. OPSpecs manual-Expanded edition: Operating specifications for imprecision, inaccuracy, and quality control. Ogunquit ME: Westgard QC, 1996.
107. Westgard JO. Basic planning for quality. Washington DC: AACC Press, 2000.
108. Westgard JO. Internal quality control: planning and implementation strategies. Ann Clin Biochem 2003;40:593-611.
109. Westgard JO. Basic method validation, 2nd ed. Washington DC: AACC Press, 2003.
110. Westgard JO, Barry PL. Cost-Effective quality control: Managing the quality and productivity of analytical processes. Washington DC: AACC Press, 1986.
111. Westgard JO, Barry PL. Total quality control: Evolution of quality management systems. Lab Med 1989;20:377-84.
112. Westgard JO, Barry PL, Tomar RH. Implementing total quality management in health care laboratories. Clin Lab Manage Rev 1991;5:353-70.
113. Westgard JO, Barry PL, Hunt MR, Groth T. A multirule Shewhart chart for quality control in clinical chemistry. Clin Chem 1981;27:493-501.
114. Westgard JO, Burnett RW, Bowers GN. Quality management science in clinical chemistry: A dynamic framework for continuous improvement of quality. Clin Chem 1990;36:1712-6.
115. Westgard JO, Ehrmeyer SS, Darcy TP. CLIA final rules for quality systems: Quality assessment issues and answers. Madison WI: Westgard QC, Inc., 2004.
116. Westgard JO, Falk H, Groth T. Influence of a between-run component of variation, choice of control limits, and shape of error distribution on the performance characteristics of rules for internal quality control. Clin Chem 1979;25:394-400.
117. Westgard JO, Fallon KD, Mansouri S. Validation of iQM active process control technology. Point of Care 2003;2:1-7.
118. Westgard JO, Groth T. Design and evaluation of statistical control procedures: Applications of a computer "QC Simulator" program. Clin Chem 1981;27:1536-45.
119. Westgard JO, Groth T. Power functions for statistical control rules. Clin Chem 1979;25:863-9.
120. Westgard JO, Groth T, Aronsson T, et al. Combined Shewhart-cusum control chart for improved quality control in clinical chemistry. Clin Chem 1977;23:1881-7.
121. Westgard JO, Groth T, Aronsson T, et al. Performance characteristics of rules for internal quality control: Probabilities for false rejection and error detection. Clin Chem 1977;23:1857-67.
122. Westgard JO, Hyltoft-Petersen P, Wiebe DA. Laboratory process specifications for assuring quality in the US National Cholesterol Education Program (NCEP). Clin Chem 1991;37:656-61.
123. Westgard JO, Klee GG. Quality Management. In: Burtis CA, Ashwood ER, eds. Tietz textbook of clinical chemistry, 3rd ed. Philadelphia: WB Saunders, 1999:404.
124. Westgard JO, Oryall JJ, Koch DD. Predicting effects of QC practices on the cost-effective operation of a multitest analytical system. Clin Chem 1990;36: 1760-4.
125. Westgard JO, Smith FA, Mountain PJ, Boss S. Design and assessment of average of normals (AON) patient data algorithms to maximize run lengths for automatic process control. Clin Chem 1996;42:1683-8.
126. Westgard JO, Wiebe DA. Cholesterol operational process specifications for assuring the quality

required by CLIA proficiency testing. Clin Chem 1991;37:1938-44.

127. Westgard JO. Basic QC practices, 2nd ed, Madison WI: Westgard QC Inc, 2002.
128. Wilding P, Zilva JF, Wilde CE. Transport of specimens for clinical chemistry analysis. Ann Clin Biochem 1977;14:301-6.
129. Winkleman JW, Mennemeyer ST. Using patient outcomes to screen for clinical laboratory errors. Clin Lab Manag Rev 1996;10:134-42.
130. Witte DL, VanNess SA, Angstadt DS, Pennell BJ. Errors, mistakes, blunders, outliers, or unacceptable results: how many? Clin Chem 1997;43:1352-6. (http://www.clinchem.org/cgi/content/full/43/8/1352).
131. Wong ET. Improving laboratory testing: Can we get physicians to focus on outcome? Clin Chem 1995;41:1241-7.
132. Wu AH, McKay C, Broussard LA, Hoffman RS, Kwong TC, et al. National academy of clinical biochemistry laboratory medicine practice guidelines: recommendations for the use of laboratory tests to support poisoned patients who present to the emergency department. Clin Chem 2003;49:357-79.
133. Youden WJ. Statistical techniques for collaborative tests. Washington DC: Association of Official Analytical Chemists, 1969.
134. Young DS. Effects of preanalytical variables on clinical laboratory tests, 2nd edition. Washington DC: AACC Press, 1997.

ADDITIONAL READING

CLIA

Westgard JO, Ehrmeyer SS, Darcy TP. CLIA Final Rules for Quality Systems: Quality assessment issues and answers. Madison WI: Westgard QC, Inc., 2004.

Yost, J. Complying with the New CLIA QC Standards 2003. Washington DC: AACC Press, 2003.

ISO 9000

Kimothi SK. The uncertainty of measurements, Milwaukee: ASQ Quality Press, 2002.

Paradis GW. Demystifying ISO 9000. Longman AW, ed., Harlow: UK, 1996.

Peach RW. The ISO 9000 handbook, 3rd ed, New York: Irwin Professional Publishing, 1996.

Seidenfeld A, Christine Glidden C, Henrickson D. Applying ISO 9000 standards to clinical labs: The quest for excellence. CLN 1997; 27:1-10.

Quality Assurance

Brooks ZC. Performance-driven quality control. Washington DC: AACC Press, 2001:1-204.

Brooks ZC, Plaut D. Quality control—From "Data" to "Decisions": Basic concepts. Washington DC: AACC Press, 2002.

Epstein AM. The role of quality measurement in a competitive marketplace. In: Altman S, Reinhardt U, eds. Strategic choices for a changing care system. Chicago: Health Administration Press, 1996:207-34.

Epstein A. Performance reports on quality: Prototypes, problems, and prospects. NEJM 1995;333:57-61.

Montanez JA. Medical device quality assurance manual. Buffalo Grove IL: Interpharm Press, Inc, 1996.

Westgard JO. QC Validator program Version 2.0 with automatic QC selection. Madison WI: Westgard™ QC, Inc. (http://www.westgard.com), 1996.

Westgard JO. OPSpecs manual: Operating specifications for precision, accuracy, and quality control. Madison WI: Westgard™ QC, Inc. (http://www.westgard.com), 1995.

Westgard JO. A method evaluation decision chart (MEDx Chart) for judging method performance. Clin Lab Science 1995;8:277-83.

Westgard JO. Basic planning for quality. Washington DC: AACC Press, 2000.

Westgard JO. Basic method validation, 2nd ed. Washington DC: AACC Press, 2003.

Quality Management

Blumenthal D, Scheck AC, Eds. Improving clinical practice: Total quality management and the physician. San Francisco: Jossey-Bass, 1995.

Deming EW. Out of the crisis. Cambridge: MIT Center for Advanced Engineering Study, 1986.

Deming EW. The new economics for industry, government, education. Cambridge: MIT Center for Advanced Engineering Study, 1995.

Goetsch DL, Davis SB. Introduction to total quality, 2nd ed. New York: Prentice Hall, 1996.

Juran JM. Quality planning and analysis. New York: McGraw-Hill, 1993.

Juran JM. A history of managing for quality. New York: Simon & Schuster Trade, 1995.

National Committee for Clinical Laboratory Standards. Continuous quality improvement: Essential management approaches and their use in proficiency testing; Proposed Guideline GP22-P. Wayne PA: National Committee for Clinical Laboratory Standards, 1997.

National Committee for Clinical Laboratory Standards: A Quality System Model for Health Care; Approved Guideline. HS01-A, Vol 22, Number 13. Wayne PA: National Committee for Clinical Laboratory Standards, 2002.

Six Sigma

Barry R, Murcko AC, Brubaker CE. The six sigma book for healthcare: Improving outcomes by reducing errors. Chicago: Health Administration Press 2002.

Breyfogle FW. Implementing six sigma: Smarter solutions using statistical methods. New York: John Wiley & Sons, 1999.

Chowdhury S. Design for six sigma. Chicago: Dearborn Trade Publishing 2002.
Eckes G. The six sigma revolution—How General Electric and others turned process into profits. New York: John Wiley & Sons, 2001.
Garber C. Six Sigma: Its Role in the Clinical Laboratory. CLN 2004;30:1-10.
George ML. Lean six sigma. New York: McGraw-Hill, 2002.
Pande PS, Newman RP, Cabanagh RR. The six sigma way: Team fieldbook. New York: McGraw-Hill, 2002.
Pyzdek T. The six sigma handbook: A complete guide for greenbelts, blackbelts, & managers at all levels. New York: McGraw-Hill, 2001.

SECTION IV

Analytes

CHAPTER 20

Amino Acids, Peptides, and Proteins*

A. Myron Johnson, M.D.

Amino acids, peptides, and proteins play crucial roles in virtually all biological processes, with amino acids being the basic structural units of proteins. Many genetic mutations result in the incorporation into proteins of amino acids that may alter rates of synthesis, secretion, or metabolism of the proteins and their function. In addition, there are a large number of inherited abnormalities of amino acid metabolism (see Chapter 55).

It is estimated that there are more than 50,000 human proteins, and that the number of distinct proteins within one cell is 3000 to 5000. More than 1400 different proteins can be identified in serum alone. Some proteins are elaborated or circulate only at certain stages of growth or under particular physiological or pathological circumstances. Many proteins are structural elements of cells or organized tissue and can be evaluated only after their separation from the tissue where they reside; others are soluble in intracellular or extracellular fluids. Some soluble proteins that are normally intracellular escape into extracellular and intravascular fluids when cells are damaged; some may be shed into blood or urine in detectable quantities. The variety of proteins is much greater than expected from the number of coding genes because of postsynthetic modifications that may make them selectively functional or degradable. Not only is the number of distinct proteins very large, but also their variations of concentration in health and disease, their distribution in the body, their functions, their compositions, and their structures are seemingly infinite.

*The author gratefully acknowledges the previous contributions of Robert H. Christenson, Hassan M.E. Azzazy, Lawrence M. Silverman, and Elizabeth M. Rohlfs, on which portions of this chapter are based.

This chapter begins with a discussion of amino acids, followed by specific discussions of proteins in plasma and in other fluids and miscellaneous proteins. It concludes with descriptions of analytical techniques used to analyze proteins.

AMINO ACIDS

Amino acids are the basic structural units of proteins. Their measurement in physiological fluids provides important information for fundamental studies and the diagnosis of many pathological and inherited conditions.

BASIC BIOCHEMISTRY

Amino acids are organic compounds containing both an amino group (—NH_2) and a carboxyl group (—COOH). Those occurring in proteins are called α-amino acids and have the empirical formula $RCH(NH_2)COOH$. As shown below, the core of an α-amino acid is the carbon atom next to the carboxylic acid group.

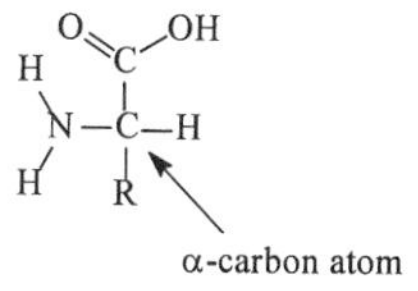

α-carbon atom

With the exception of glycine, all amino acids are asymmetrical, having a hydrogen atom, a carboxyl group, an amino group, and a distinctive R group of a specific chemical structure.

Table 20-1 lists the amino acids that are of importance in protein chemistry. The variety of amino acids provides a large portion of the variability in structure and function of

TABLE 20-1 Amino Acids

Name and Abbreviation	MW	Structure at pH 6–7	Comments
I. Amino Acids Found in Most Proteins			
Hydrophobic Amino Acids; Nonpolar R Groups			
Alanine Ala	89.09	$H_3C-CH(NH_3^{\oplus})-COO^{\ominus}$	Substrate for ALT; least hydrophobic of the group
Leucine Leu	131.17	$(H_3C)_2CH-CH_2-CH(NH_3^{\oplus})-COO^{\ominus}$	Branched-chain R group; essential; ketogenic; metabolism is faulty in maple syrup urine disease
Isoleucine Ile	131.17	$H_3C-CH_2-CH(CH_3)-CH(NH_3^{\oplus})-COO^{\ominus}$	Essential; partly ketogenic; see Leucine above
Valine Val	117.17	$(H_3C)_2CH-CH(NH_3^{\oplus})-COO^{\ominus}$	Essential; partly ketogenic; see Leucine above
Proline Pro	115.13	pyrrolidine ring ($NH_2^{\oplus}$)–$COO^{\ominus}$	Important constituent of connective tissue proteins (e.g., collagen and elastin); some hydroxylated to Hyp during collagen synthesis; destabilizes α-helical and β-structures; contains an α-imino group
Methionine Met	149.21	$H_3C-S-CH_2-CH_2-CH(NH_3^{\oplus})-COO^{\ominus}$	Essential; important in transfer of methyl groups; provides sulfur for other sulfur-containing compounds
Phenylalanine Phe	165.19	$C_6H_5-CH_2-CH(NH_3^{\oplus})-COO^{\ominus}$	Essential; elevated levels in phenylketonuria
Tryptophan Trp	204.22	indole (N)–$CH_2-CH(NH_3^{\oplus})-COO^{\ominus}$	Essential; metabolites found in carcinoid disease; contains indole ring system; precursor of serotonin and melatonin
Hydrophilic Amino Acids; Uncharged Polar Groups			
Glycine Gly	75.07	$H-CH(NH_3^{\oplus})-COO^{\ominus}$	Simplest amino acid; optically inactive; placed in this group because its R group (single H) is unable to affect polarity of the rest of the molecule; used in biosynthesis of purines and porphyrins; used in vitro as a buffer
Serine Ser	105.09	$HO-CH_2-CH(NH_3^{\oplus})-COO^{\ominus}$	Constituent in active center of many enzymes; hydroxyl group can be phosphorylated
Threonine Thr	119.12	$HO(H_3C)CH-CH(NH_3^{\oplus})-COO^{\ominus}$	Essential

ALT, Alanine transaminase.

TABLE 20-1 Amino Acids—*Continued*

Name and Abbreviation	MW	Structure at pH 6–7	Comments
I. Amino Acids Found in Most Proteins—Cont'd			
Hydrophilic Amino Acids; Uncharged Polar Groups—Cont'd			
Cysteine Cys	121.16	$HS-CH_2-CH(NH_3^+)-COO^-$	Sulfhydryl group functional in the activity of many enzymes; is responsible for disulfide bridges in peptides and proteins; cystine is dicysteine, Cys-S-S-Cys; homocysteine has one carbon more than cysteine and forms homocystine (dihomocysteine)
Selenocysteine Secys	168.05	$HSe-CH_2-CH(NH_3^+)-COO^-$	Active form of selenium; found in many enzymes involved in oxidation-reduction reactions
Tyrosine Tyr	181.19	$HO-C_6H_4-CH_2-CH(NH_3^+)-COO^-$	Usually nonessential; intermediate in synthesis of catecholamines, thyroxine, and melanin; functional phenolic group; reacts with Folin's reagent in quantitative protein assay
Glutamine Gln	146.15	$H_2N-C(=O)-CH_2-CH_2-CH(NH_3^+)-COO^-$	Storage form of ammonia in tissue; supplies the amido nitrogen used in purine and pyrimidine biosynthesis
Asparagine Asn	132.12	$H_2N-C(=O)-CH_2-CH(NH_3^+)-COO^-$	Storage form of ammonia in tissues
Hydroxyproline Hyp	131.13	HO-pyrrolidine ring with NH_2^+ and $-COO^-$	Constituent of collagen—the only human protein to contain appreciable amounts; urinary output is used as an indicator of bone matrix metabolism; contains an α-imino group
Dicarboxylic Amino Acids; Acidic R Groups			
Aspartic acid Asp	133.10	$^-OOC-CH_2-CH(NH_3^+)-COO^-$	Cosubstrate with Glu for AST; used in pyrimidine biosynthesis
Glutamic acid Glu	147.13	$^-OOC-CH_2-CH_2-CH(NH_3^+)-COO^-$	Co-substrate with Ala for ALT and with Asp for AST
Basic Amino Acids; Basic R Groups			
Lysine Lys	146.19	$H_3N^+-CH_2-CH_2-CH_2-CH_2-CH(NH_3^+)-COO^-$	Essential; terminal NH_2 called ε-amino
Arginine Arg	174.20	$(H_2N)(H_2N^+)=C-NH-CH_2-CH_2-CH_2-CH(NH_3^+)-COO^-$	Involved in urea synthesis; the basic group is a guanidinium group

AST, Aspartate transaminase.

Continued.

TABLE 20-1 Amino Acids—*Continued*

Name and Abbreviation	MW	Structure at pH 6–7	Comments
I. Amino Acids Found in Most Proteins—Cont'd			
Basic Amino Acids; Basic R Groups—Cont'd			
Histidine His	155.16	$\oplus$HN–(imidazole ring)–N–H, –CH_2–C(H)($NH_3^{\oplus}$)–C(=O)$O^{\ominus}$	The imidazole group of histidine is the most important buffer group in the physiological pH range
II. Miscellaneous Amino Acids			
Thyroxine T_4	776.93	HO–(ring, I, I)–O–(ring, I, I)–CH_2–C(H)($NH_3^{\oplus}$)–C(=O)$O^{\ominus}$	Thyroid hormone
Triiodothyronine T_3	651.01	HO–(ring, I)–O–(ring, I, I)–CH_2–C(H)($NH_3^{\oplus}$)–C(=O)$O^{\ominus}$	Thyroid hormone; more active than T_4
β-Alanine β-Ala	89.09	H_2N–CH_2–CH_2–C(=O)$O^{\ominus}$	Constituent of the vitamin pantothenic acid
Dihydroxyphenylalanine DOPA*	197.18	HO, HO–(ring)–CH_2–C(H)($NH_3^{\oplus}$)–C(=O)$O^{\ominus}$	Intermediate in catecholamine synthesis
γ-Aminobutyric acid GABA*	103.12	$H_3N^{\oplus}$–CH_2–CH_2–CH_2–C(=O)$O^{\ominus}$	Metabolite of Glu; a neurotransmitter
Ornithine Orn*	132.16	$H_3N^{\oplus}$–CH_2–CH_2–CH_2–C(H)($NH_3^{\oplus}$)–C(=O)$O^{\ominus}$	Intermediate in urea synthesis
Citrulline Citr*	175.19	H_2N–C(=O)–NH–CH_2–CH_2–CH_2–C(H)($NH_3^{\oplus}$)–C(=O)$O^{\ominus}$	Intermediate in urea synthesis
Phosphoserine	185.08	HO–P($O^{\ominus}$)($O^{\ominus}$)–O–CH_2–C(H)($NH_3^{\oplus}$)–C(=O)$O^{\ominus}$	In casein and other phosphoproteins
Pyrrolidine carboxylic acid	129.12	O=(pyrrolidine ring, N–H)–C(=O)$O^{\ominus}$	Cyclized form of Glu, rare; used to terminate peptide chains, as at *N*-terminal end of L-chains of γ-globulins
Taurine	125.14	$^{\ominus}$O–S(=O)(=O)–CH_2–CH_2–$NH_3^{\oplus}$	Forms conjugates with bile acids; inhibits nerve impulse transmission
β–Aminoisobutyric β–AIB*	103.12	$H_3N^{\oplus}$–CH_2–C(H)(CH_3)–C(=O)$O^{\ominus}$	Present in urine; a metabolite of pyrimidines

*Abbreviation useful but not official.

peptides and proteins, in which amino acids are combined via *peptide bonds* formed between the α-amino group of one and the α-carboxyl group of the next.

Peptide Bond

A *peptide bond* is formed when the amino group of one amino acid is covalently linked with the carboxyl group of a second amino acid.

$$\underset{\text{First amino acid}}{R_1-CH(NH_2)-COOH} + \underset{\text{Second amino acid}}{HN(H)-CH(R_2)-COOH} \xrightarrow{H_2O} \underset{\text{Dipeptide}}{H_2N-CH(R_1)-\boxed{C(=O)-N(H)}-CH(R_2)-COOH}$$

First amino acid Second amino acid Dipeptide

The peptide bond is described by the structure in the enclosed area. For example, glycine and alanine react to form two different dipeptides, either glycylalanine or alanylglycine.

Acid-Base Properties

Acid-base properties of amino acids depend on the amino and carboxyl groups attached to the α-carbon and on the basic, acidic, or other functional groups represented by R. In the illustration above, the amino acid is shown in an uncharged form. However, in the physiological pH range of 7.37 to 7.47, the carboxyl group is dissociated, and the amino group is protonated to give the following structure:

$$R-CH(\overset{\oplus}{N}H_3)-C(=O)O^{\ominus} \quad \text{or} \quad R-CH(\overset{\oplus}{N}H_3)-COO^{\ominus}$$

This kind of ionized molecule, having coexistent negative and positive charges, is called a *dipolar ion* or *ampholyte.* At low pH, both the amino and carboxyl groups are protonated as $—N^+H_3$ and —COOH, and the amino acid is cationic. As the pH rises, the carboxyl group loses its proton and the ampholyte form appears at about pH 6. At higher pH, the amino $—N^+H_3$ is also deprotonated, and the molecule is anionic. The process is shown for a monoamino acid and monocarboxylic amino acid as follows:

Cation at pH < pI Ampholyte at pH = pI Anion at pH > pI

$$R-CH(\overset{\oplus}{N}H_3)-COOH \underset{K_1}{\overset{OH^{\ominus}}{\rightleftharpoons}} R-CH(\overset{\oplus}{N}H_3)-COO^{\ominus} + H_2O \underset{K_2}{\overset{OH^{\ominus}}{\rightleftharpoons}} R-CH(NH_2)-COO^{\ominus} + 2\,H_2O$$

The dissociation constants, K_1 (ratio of ampholyte to cation) and K_2 (ratio of ampholyte to anion), are usually expressed logarithmically as pK_1 and pK_2, where $pK = -\log K$, in a manner analogous to the notation for pH. A *pK* is the pH at which equal quantities of the protonated (associated) and unprotonated (dissociated) forms are present. The *isoelectric point,* pI, is the pH where the molecules exist in the ampholyte form and have a net charge of 0. The pI of a neutral amino acid can be calculated from the p*K*s of its amino and carboxyl groups ($pI = \frac{1}{2}[pK_1 + pK_2]$). The concept of an ampholyte and its dissociation characteristics is also applicable to proteins as most are negatively charged at physiological pH.

Glycine, with a pK_1 of 2.34 and pK_2 of 9.60, exemplifies the acid-base behavior of amino acids whose R groups have no ionizable constituents. Glycine is sometimes used in vitro to prepare buffers at pH 1.0 to 3.8 or 8.1 to 11.0. The ionization constants in amino acids are given in Table 20-2.

Influence of R Groups

The R groups of individual amino acids are responsible for many of their special properties. Table 20-1 is organized in terms of the differences in R groups, some of which are nonpolar and therefore hydrophobic; others, although uncharged, are polar and hydrophilic. Still others become charged either negatively (the acidic amino acids) or positively (the basic amino acids). R groups may be linear as in valine or cyclical as in proline, small as in glycine or bulky as in tryptophan. Electron density may be low as in aliphatic chains or high as in aromatic rings. This diversity in R group structure and chemistry makes possible several kinds of interaction between the amino acids that are of great importance in determining protein structure and function. Possible interactions among R groups include disulfide bonds, hydrogen bonds, hydrophobic interaction, and steric effects. The disulfide bond (—S—S—) is the only covalent bond, other than the peptide bond, that contributes to polypeptide structure.

The other types of interactions are weaker but are often so numerous that their collective strength is large. Hydrogen bonds result from the sharing of a hydrogen atom between two electronegative atoms (e.g., N or O) that have unbonded electrons. In proteins, groups having a hydrogen atom that can be shared include ═N—H (peptide nitrogen, imidazole, and indole); —OH (serine, threonine, tyrosine, and hydroxyproline); $—NH_2$ and $—N^+H_3$ (arginine, lysine, and α-amino); and —CONH (carbamino). Groups that can accept the sharing of a hydrogen atom include $—COO^-$ (aspartate, glutamate, and α-carboxylate); —S—S— (disulfide); and ═CO (in peptides and ester linkages). Examples of hydrogen bonds linking the ═CO of one peptide bond to the ═NH of another, or the —CO— of one R group to the —OH of another R group.

Hydrophobic interactions result because the association of nonpolar groups (e.g., methyl or phenyl) is energetically favored in aqueous or other polar solutions. In proteins, this association serves to bend and fold a molecule in a way that brings nonpolar R groups inside to the less polar interior; polar R groups are oriented outside toward the more polar aqueous environment.

Some amino acids have R groups that contain charged or ionizable constituents. These constituents have their own

TABLE 20-2 Ionization Constants of Ionizable Groups in Free Amino Acids and in Proteins*

Ionizing Group		Range of pK Values	
		Free Amino Acids	Proteins
Principal carboxyl = pK_1	$-C(=O)O^{\ominus}$	1.7-2.6	3.0-3.2
α-Amino = pK_2	$-\overset{\oplus}{N}H_3$	9.0-10.8	7.6-8.4
Second carboxyls of Glu and Asp	$-C(=O)O^{\ominus}$	3.8-4.3	3.0-4.5
Imidazole nitrogen of His	$\overset{\oplus}{N}H$	6.0	0.6-7.0
Sulfhydryl of Cys	—SH	8.3	9.1-10.8
Phenolic hydroxyl of Tyr	—OH	10.1	9.2-9.8
ε-Amino of Lys	$-\overset{\oplus}{N}H_3$	10.5	9.4-10.6
Guanidinium group of Arg	$-NH-C(NH_2)=\overset{\oplus}{N}H_2$	12.5	11.5-12.6

*Given are the p*K* values for proton-donating charged groups when present in free amino acids and when present in peptide-linked amino acid residues in proteins. The p*K* value for the primary carboxyl varies from 1.71 for Cys to 2.63 for Thr. Similarly, the p*K* for the α-ammonium group varies from 8.95 for Lys to 10.78 for Cys. In protein chains, the proximity of other amino acid residues and charged groups may modify the p*K* for any given ionizable group. The amino acid symbols are those listed in Table 20-1.

p*K*s, which are also shown in Table 20-2. At pH 7, the acidic amino acids, glutamic acid (Glu) and aspartic acid (Asp), have their second carboxyl group fully ionized and are therefore negatively charged in the physiological pH range. Except for histidine, most basic amino acids are positively charged at physiological pH (less than 10% of histidine is positively charged in this range). Charges that reside or develop on R groups are responsible for electrostatic bonding, which may occur in proteins or between a protein and a ligand.

The differing solubilities and acid-base properties of amino acids provide the basis for their separation by electrophoresis, partition chromatography, or ion-exchange chromatography (see Chapters 5 and 6). Differences in the chemical nature of R groups permit, in some cases, their identification or measurement by color reactions. The aromatic amino acids—tyrosine and tryptophan—absorb ultraviolet (UV) light at 280 nm; all amino acids absorb UV radiation at 220 nm. The absorption at 280 nm can be used to estimate the concentration of an individual protein in solution, such as fibrinogen. Aside from the distinctive properties used for analyses, the general and special properties of amino acids are critical to the role they have in determining the structure and function of proteins.

Metabolism

In the healthy state, the primary supply of amino acids for endogenous protein synthesis is provided by dietary proteins. Although most of the amino acids can be formed in vivo, 8 to 10 of the 22 common amino acids cannot be synthesized by most mammals and are therefore considered "essential" constituents of the diet for maintenance of health or growth, or both (see Table 20-1, Comments column). Proteolytic enzymes in the gastrointestinal tract act on ingested proteins, releasing amino acids that are then absorbed from the jejunum into the blood and subsequently become part of the body pool of amino acids. The liver and other tissues draw on this pool for synthesis of plasma and intracellular proteins. The liver and kidneys are also actively involved in interconverting amino acids by transamination and degrading them by deamination. Deamination produces ammonium ions, which are rapidly consumed in the synthesis of urea. Urea in turn is excreted by the kidneys. The major pathways of amino acid metabolism are outlined in Figure 20-1.

Amino acids in blood are filtered through the glomerular membranes but are normally reabsorbed in the renal tubules by saturable transport systems (see Chapter 45). Hence, high blood levels of amino acids may result in significant renal excretion *(aminoaciduria)*. In normal individuals, aminoaciduria is transient and is associated with protein intake in excess of amino acid requirements for repletion of the body pool. The mechanism of reabsorption is not fully understood, although it is known to be an active transport system dependent on membrane-bound carriers and intraluminal Na^+ concentration. Four different transport systems

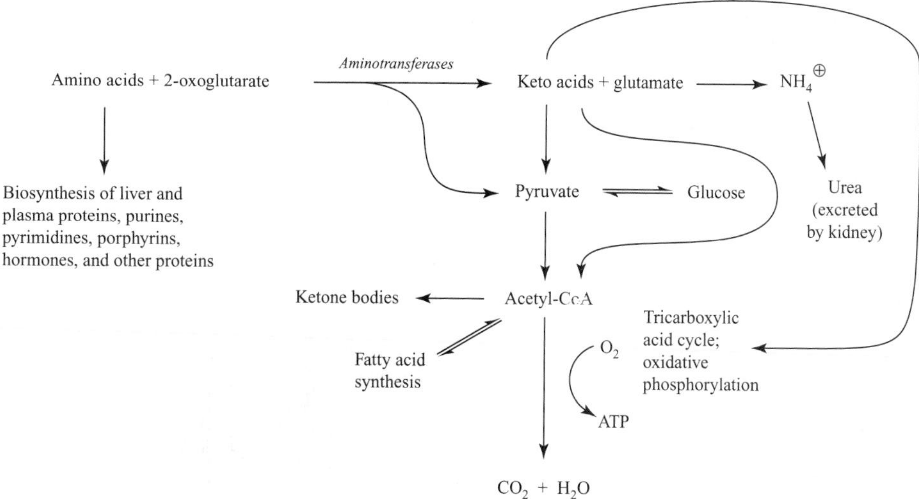

Figure 20-1 A generalized scheme of amino acid metabolism in the liver.

have been identified: one for neutral amino acids; one for basic amino acids; one for proline, hydroxyproline, and glycine; and one for dicarboxylic amino acids. For some amino acids, transport appears to occur by two systems: one of low capacity but of high specificity and the other of high capacity but of low specificity. A few amino acids, such as cystathionine and homocysteine, are not efficiently reabsorbed by renal tubular mechanisms but are cleared by the kidneys and apparently excreted into the urine at the glomerular filtration rate.

Much that is known about renal reabsorption mechanisms has been learned from the study of various forms of aminoaciduria. Three types of aminoaciduria have been identified: (1) *overflow aminoaciduria* occurs when the plasma level of one or more amino acids exceeds the renal threshold (tubular capacity for reabsorption); (2) *renal aminoaciduria* occurs when plasma levels are normal but the renal transport system has a congenital or acquired defect; and (3) *no-threshold aminoaciduria* occurs when excessive amounts of an amino acid, arising from an inherited metabolic block, are present in urine, but plasma levels are essentially normal because all the amino acid is excreted. The no-threshold aminoacidurias, such as homocystinuria, are not due to congenital or acquired kidney defects but solely to saturation of the normal renal tubular reabsorption mechanisms.

Plasma amino acid concentrations are high during the first days of life, especially in premature neonates, but they tend to be low in infants with birth weights low for their gestational age because of placental insufficiency. Maternal values are low in the first half of pregnancy. In adults, increased plasma levels of homocysteine have been linked to increased risk of heart disease (see Chapters 26 and 44).[73]

Plasma amino acid concentrations vary by about 30% during the day; therefore blood specimens should be collected at the same time each day. Values are highest in mid-afternoon and lowest in early morning. This diurnal variation is particularly important when specimens are analyzed for detection of heterozygous states of defective metabolism.

Amino acid excretion in urine varies with maturation of renal tubular function. Premature infants, especially during the first week, have a generalized physiological renal aminoaciduria (see Figure 20-2); even at full term, aminoaciduria is more pronounced than in normal adults. In the urine of normal adults, glycine is usually the dominant fraction, with alanine, serine, glutamine, and—in indulgent meat eaters—histidine and 1-methylhistidine present in smaller quantities. In some normal urine, taurine is prominent; in others, β-aminoisobutyric acid is seen.

Cerebrospinal fluid (CSF) concentrations of most amino acids are lower than those in plasma even though the rate of amino acid transport into the central nervous system is high. The plasma to CSF concentration ratios for individual amino acids vary because of differences in transport systems.

Cells have free amino acid concentrations about 10 times those of plasma. The mechanisms maintaining this tenfold β-aminoisobutyric acid is seen. The mechanisms maintaining the gradient are unknown but may involve the membrane enzyme γ-glutamyl transferase.

Clinical Implications

Aminoacidurias may be primary or secondary. Primary disease is due to an inherited enzyme defect, also called an *inborn error of metabolism.* The defect is located either in the pathway by which a specific amino acid is metabolized or in the specific renal tubular transport system by which the amino acid is reabsorbed. Secondary aminoaciduria is due to disease of an organ, such as the liver, which is an active site of amino acid metabolism, or to generalized renal tubular dysfunction, or to protein-energy malnutrition. Specific inborn errors of metabolism are discussed in more detail in Chapter 55.

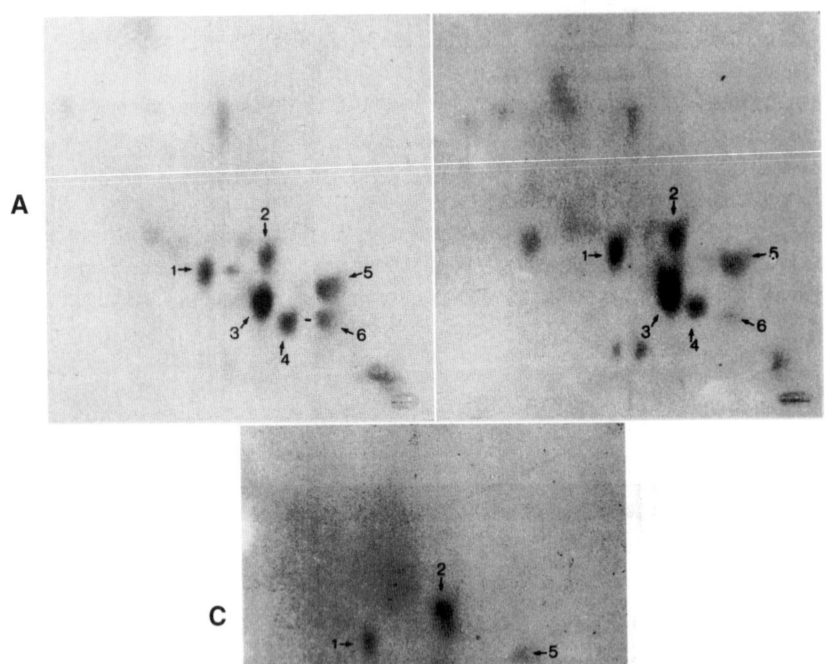

Figure 20-2 Two-dimensional chromatograms of urine showing the variability of amino acid excretion with age. **A,** Neonate. **B,** Infant. **C,** Adult. *1,* Alanine; *2,* serine; *3,* glycine; *4,* glutamine; *5,* histidine; *6,* lysine/ornithine.

Analysis of Amino Acids

Many procedures are available for measuring amino acids in biological samples.[114] In the context of diagnosing pathological disorders, three groups of tests for amino acid analysis are of importance:

1. Screening tests, including thin layer chromatography (TLC), urine color tests, and the Guthrie microbiological test. (Details of these tests are given in a previous edition of this textbook.)[22]
2. Quantitative tests for monitoring treatment or confirming an initial diagnosis. High-performance liquid chromatography (HPLC) and ion-exchange chromatography are widely used for this purpose. Some individual amino acids may also be determined by quantitative chemical methods.
3. Tests that identify an unknown amino acid or metabolite.

Quantitative Tests

Traditionally, amino acids have been quantitatively measured in body fluids using gas chromatography (GC)[129]; liquid chromatography (LC), including HPLC[105] and ion-exchange liquid chromatography[44,65]; and capillary electrophoresis (CE).[50] These techniques are being replaced by tandem mass spectrometry (MS/MS).[17]

Gas Chromatography

Advantages of GC include small sample size, sensitivity, and speed, but a major limitation is the relatively low volatility of amino acids at temperatures conventionally used in this technique (see Chapter 6).[129] However, these compounds can be reacted with derivatizing agents to increase volatility and to enhance their chromatographic and detection characteristics.

Because of the necessity for an initial cleanup step followed by derivatization, GC is not used routinely in the clinical laboratory. However, it is still used for investigation of organic acidurias.

Liquid Chromatography

Because of its excellent sensitivity, high resolution, and relatively short analysis time, ion-exchange liquid chromatography and HPLC have been used to measure amino acids in biological samples (see Chapter 6).[44,65,105] The major advantage of these liquid chromatographic techniques over GC is that the relatively high temperatures necessary for sample volatilization by GC are unnecessary and they avoid the problem of amino acid decomposition at high temperatures.

Only a few amino acids are detected by the UV or visible spectrophotometers, fluorometers, or electrochemical detectors that are routinely used with HPLC analyzers. Consequently, amino acids typically are postcolumn derivatized for analysis by HPLC. The most widely used reagent for this purpose is ninhydrin. A number of colored products are formed, but the major one is presumed to result from deamination and condensation as follows:

Ninhydrin + Amino acid → CO_2 + NH_3 + Hydrindantin + Aldehyde

Ninhydrin + NH_3 + Hydrindantin → Colored product

Most amino acids react with ninhydrin at ambient temperatures to form a blue color that becomes purple on heating. However, proline and hydroxyproline yield yellow compounds that are measured at a different wavelength. Other postcolumn derivatizations use fluorogenic reagents, such as *o*-phthaldialdehyde or fluorescamine. Precolumn derivatization techniques using *o*-phthaldialdehyde, dansyl, phenyl isothiocyanate, or 9-fluorenylmethyl chloroformate derivatives have been used with reversed-phase HPLC. Electrochemical detection has also been coupled with derivatization methods to enhance analytical sensitivity.

Capillary Electrophoresis

In CE, the classic techniques of electrophoresis are performed in small-bore (10 to 100 μm) fused silica capillary tubes of 20 to 200 cm in length (see Chapter 5). It is a very efficient, rapid, sensitive, and versatile analytical technique that is used to analyze a diverse spectrum of analytes ranging from small ions to macromolecular proteins or nucleic acids.[50,62] When coupled with sensitive detectors, it is capable of measuring femtomolar quantities of amino acids.

Tandem Mass Spectrometry

Tandem mass spectrometry (MS/MS) is applicable to the rapid assay of specific analytes in complex biological fluids (see Chapter 7).[13] In practice, it is usually interfaced to a GC[88] or LC.[12] MS/MS has been used to screen neonates[18,19,35,102] for such amino acid metabolic disorders as phenylketonuria (PKU),[20] maple syrup urine disease (MSUD),[16] tyrosinemia,[20] hypermethioninemias,[17] and homocystinuria.[17]

Compared with older methods, MS/MS is a more sensitive technique, offers greater accuracy and precision,[15] has higher clinical specificity and sensitivity, and measures multiple analytes. It has been described as a revolutionary technique for disease detection.[14,82]

PEPTIDES AND PROTEINS

This section begins with a general discussion of the basic biochemistry of peptides and proteins followed by discussions of different proteins. It concludes with a section on the analysis of proteins.

Basic Biochemistry

As discussed earlier, a peptide bond is formed when the α-amino group of one amino acid is linked covalently with the α-carboxyl group of a second amino acid. For example, glycine and alanine can react to form two different dipeptides: either glycylalanine or alanylglycine.

In glycylalanine, alanine is called the *C*-terminal residue of the peptide; glycine is the *N*-terminal residue because its amino group is free. In alanylglycine, the designations are reversed. The *C*- and *N*-terminal designations apply also to polypeptides and proteins. Very short peptide chains are designated as tripeptides, tetrapeptides, or pentapeptides, and so on. Glutathione, for instance, is a tripeptide of glutamine (Glu), cysteine (Cys), and glycine (Gly). The hormones oxytocin and vasopressin are nonapeptides. Chains up to five residues are called *oligopeptides,* and longer chains (6 to 30 residues) are referred to as *polypeptides.* When the number of amino acids exceeds 40 (MW ~ 5000 Da), the chain takes on the physical properties associated with proteins.

The terms *proteose* and *peptone* refer to protein breakdown products of large polypeptides; these differ from true proteins in that they are not coagulated by heat. A wide variety of peptides are formed when proteins are hydrolyzed in the digestive tract or in the laboratory.

The structure of a protein is described at four levels:

1. *Primary structure* refers to the identity and specific order of amino acid residues in the polypeptide chain. This sequence, which depends exclusively on covalent (peptide) bonds, is predetermined by the DNA coding (see Chapter 36); the three-dimensional structure and any special biological properties of the protein follow automatically from this amino acid sequence that folds itself into the most stable structure possible under physiological conditions.
2. *Secondary structure* may be defined as a regular recurring arrangement in space of the primary structure extending along one dimension. The secondary structures of many globular proteins have stretches of α-helix and random coils, all dependent on numerous hydrogen bonds and occasional disulfide covalent bonds.

3. *Tertiary structure* involves the intramolecular folding of the polypeptide chain into a compact three-dimensional structure with a specific shape. This structure is maintained by electrovalent linkages, hydrogen bonds, disulfide bridges, van der Waals forces, and hydrophobic interactions. Hydrophobic interactions are considered to be a major force in maintaining the unique tertiary structure of proteins.
4. *Quaternary structure* refers to the association of several polypeptide chains or subunits into a larger "oligomeric" aggregate unit. This structure depends on the close fit of the polypeptide subunits through interactions at their contact surfaces and with any prosthetic groups.

X-ray diffraction was the primary method used to investigate protein structure in early years. However, other physical, chemical, and biological methods are now used and a number of databases of protein structure have been developed. It is expected that genomics and proteomics (see Chapters 7 and 36) will greatly expand the number of sequenced proteins.

Some proteins contain non–amino acid components known as *prosthetic groups.* Such proteins are often referred to as *conjugated proteins* and are classified according to the nature of their prosthetic groups as metalloproteins, glycoproteins or mucoproteins, phosphoproteins, and so on. Both glycoproteins and mucoproteins have covalently linked carbohydrate prosthetic groups, but the amount of carbohydrate varies—up to 15% in glycoproteins and 15% to 75% in mucoproteins. Many proteins also contain and/or transport ligands, including lipids, hormones, metal ions, and so forth. Conjugated proteins freed of their ligands are called *apoproteins* (e.g., lipoproteins without lipid are called apolipoproteins, and ceruloplasmin without copper is called *apoceruloplasmin*).

Although the soluble globular proteins are especially important in clinical chemistry, thorough investigation of the insoluble, protease-resistant fibrous proteins has revealed many of the basic principles of the three-dimensional structures of proteins. The most familiar fibrous proteins are the α-keratins, which form the principal structural proteins of epidermis, hair, and nails. A molecule of α-keratin is composed of three right-handed α-helix coils supercoiled around each other. Each coil is held together by hydrogen bonding between peptide CO and NH groups of one coil and those of the next or previous coil. The amino acids of these coils include many cysteine residues, which bind the separate α-helices to one another by disulfide bonds aided by hydrogen and electrovalent bonds. This structure gives α-keratins their high tensile strength, flexibility, and elasticity.

Silk contains another type of fibrous protein structure, called a β-*sheet conformation* because of the rippled or pleated structure of these molecules. The polypeptide chains of the extended coils are bound together laterally by disulfide covalent bonds and hydrogen bonds, which connect the peptide bonds of different chains instead of connecting different coils of the same chain as in an α-helix. The β-sheet is strong and inflexible when force is applied parallel to the covalently bonded or long axis, whereas an α-helical structure—such as hair—elongates when tension is applied from an α-helix to a β-sheet structure.

Nearly all proteins of interest in clinical chemistry are soluble globular proteins, such as hemoglobin, enzymes, and most plasma proteins (with the notable exception of fibrinogen). The complex bending and folding of their polypeptide chains are a result of the numerous interactions of their R groups. Globular proteins are compact and have little or no space for water in the interior of the molecule, where most of the hydrophobic R groups are located. On the other hand, most polar R groups are located on the surface of the protein, where they exert a substantial influence on protein solubility, acid-base behavior, and function.

Most globular proteins are fragile, retaining their biological activity within only very limited ranges of temperature and pH, at which their native structural conformations are the most stable. Even short periods of exposure to temperatures of 65 °C to 70 °C or to extremes of pH cause the molecules of protein to "denature," with a concomitant loss of solubility and biological activity. During denaturation, the polypeptide chains of the protein molecules become unfolded or their quaternary structure is lost; their amino acid sequence, however, remains unchanged. After mild denaturation by a change in pH or by the action of agents such as urea, many protein molecules are able to revert spontaneously to their most stable or native globular forms and regain their biological functions when physiological conditions are restored. This is convincing evidence that the amino acid sequence alone determines their normal complex shapes. If, however, a high activation energy barrier exists between the two states, the denatured state does not revert to the native state. Many enzymes, for example, lose their catalytic function irreversibly after denaturation occurs (see Chapter 8).

Many of the properties of proteins are used for their separation, identification, and assay, including the following:

1. ***Molecular size.*** Most proteins are macromolecules having high molecular weights that vary markedly among the proteins. Proteins are separated from smaller molecules by dialysis or ultrafiltration across membranes of specified pore size or by molecular exclusion chromatography (gel filtration). Because of their differing molecular weights, they also are separated by density-gradient ultracentrifugation.
2. ***Differential solubility.*** Loss of solubility is essentially the loss of affinity of the solute for the solvent. The solubility of a protein is affected by the pH, ionic strength, temperature, and dielectric constant of the solvent in which it is placed. Changing the pH of the solvent affects the surface charges of the polar R groups exposed to the solvent; at its pI (net charge zero), a protein in a polar solvent is in its least soluble state because it has the least

affinity for the solvent. Manipulation of ionic strength of the solvent affects the degree of hydration of the protein; in high concentrations, ionic salts compete with protein for water and thus decrease the amount of water available for hydration of the protein molecules. This behavior is the basis of "salting-in" and "salting-out" procedures, the earliest methods for separating and characterizing different proteins and groups of proteins. Raising the temperature affects solubility by decreasing the intramolecular bonding of a protein; loss of secondary and tertiary structure exposes the less polar interior of the protein molecule to the polar medium. Water-miscible neutral organic solvents have dielectric constants that are less than that of water; they suppress the ionization of the surface R groups on the protein and thereby decrease its solubility. Manipulation of solvent character and composition in such ways is often useful in analyses of biological protein-containing fluids.

3. ***Electrical charge.*** The effect of pH to confer, enhance, or change the surface charges on a protein can create, in a mixture of different proteins, various species of different charge-mass ratios, which migrate at different rates in an electrical field; electrophoresis and isoelectric focusing are based on this behavior. Ion-exchange chromatography is based on electrostatic interactions of charged proteins with oppositely charged solid media.
4. ***Adsorption on finely divided inert materials.*** These materials offer a large surface area for interaction with protein. Adsorption of protein on charcoal, a nonpolar substance, presumably occurs by hydrophobic interaction and can be used to separate proteins from a fluid matrix. Adsorption on polar substances such as silica, alumina, or hydroxyapatite depends on ionic interactions or hydrogen bonding; these substances can be used with buffer *elution* in chromatographic separations.
5. ***Specific binding to antibodies, coenzymes, or hormone receptors.*** The unique property of a protein to recognize and bind to complementary antibodies with high specificity is the basis for immunochemical assays (see Chapter 9). Proteins can also be separated by affinity chromatography, in which a ligand attached to a solid medium provides high selectivity (see Chapter 6).

Plasma Proteins

The proteins most amenable to routine laboratory evaluation are those in blood, urine, CSF, amniotic fluid, saliva, feces, and peritoneal or pleural fluids. With few exceptions, the proteins found in all of these are derived from blood plasma. The following discussion is limited to (1) the most abundant *plasma* proteins, (2) changes of their concentrations in the most accessible body fluids, and (3) a few of the analytical techniques used to measure them.

Most plasma proteins, with the exception of immunoglobulins and protein hormones, are synthesized primarily in the liver. They are secreted by the hepatocytes into the spaces of Disse and then move into the bloodstream through the hepatic sinusoids, which open into the central veins of the liver. Plasma proteins circulate in the blood and between the blood and the extracellular tissue spaces; their movement occurs not only by passive diffusion through junctions between capillary endothelial cells but by active transport mechanisms and by pinocytosis and exocytosis. Because of this movement, extravascular fluids normally contain small amounts of many plasma proteins. Differences in molecular size and charge among proteins and the specificity of transport mechanisms account for differences in kind and proportions of individual proteins in different fluids. Disease often alters the amounts of plasma proteins in body fluids in characteristic ways. Most plasma proteins are catabolized in the liver; for some, the signal that marks them for degradation appears to be the loss of part or all of their sialic acid content.

Table 20-3 lists the principal plasma proteins and their half-lives, pI, molecular weights, and preferred method of analysis; the individual proteins are listed in the order of their electrophoretic mobilities in agarose gels at pH 8.6. These proteins are described later in this chapter; other chapters in this book describe many more proteins: enzymes (see Chapter 21); lipoproteins (see Chapter 26); hormones (see Chapter 28); and hemoglobin, fibrinogen, and other coagulation proteins (see Chapter 31). The interim consensus reference intervals for 14 plasma proteins are listed in Table 20-4, pending the publication of more definitive intervals.[28]

Our knowledge of body fluid proteins and their alterations in health and disease has grown rapidly in the past few decades. Some of the alterations have a genetic origin; many more reflect physiological or pathological processes.[59] In many cases, the association of a specific disease with a specific pattern of altered proteins remains empirical, simply because the cause and effect relationships remain unknown. In many instances, laboratory analyses detect and evaluate these variations reliably, but they must always be considered in the context of clinical findings and in terms of all the factors, technical and biological, that may affect the results.

Rates of hepatic synthesis of many plasma proteins are affected by a patient's endocrine status. The effects of some steroid hormones on individual plasma protein levels are given in Table 20-5. The plasma protein levels characteristic of a specific disease may therefore be complicated by the steroid status of a patient and by an inflammatory acute phase reaction. The abnormal steroid status may be the result of an intrinsic hormonal disorder or of treatment with steroid hormones, as in inflammation.

Several of the proteins in Table 20-3 are acute phase reactants (APR) with the concentrations of α_1-antitrypsin (AAT), α_1-acid glycoprotein (AAG), haptoglobin (Hp), ceruloplasmin, C4, C3, procalcitonin (PCT), and serum amyloid A (SAA) increasing in most forms of inflammation; these are called *positive APR.* Others, such as transthyretin

TABLE 20-3 Properties of Selected Plasma Proteins

Electrophoretic Region	Protein	Half-Life	pI	MW (daltons)	Preferred Analysis Method	Comments
	Retinol-binding protein (RBP)	12 hr		21,000	IN, IT, RID	Transports retinol (vitamin A); complexed to TTR
	Transthyretin (TTR)	48 hr	4.7	54,980	IN, IT, RID	Transports thyroid hormones, RBP
	Albumin	15-19 days	4-5.8	66,300	IN, IT, RID, dipstick	A general transport protein; maintains plasma osmotic pressure
α_1	α_1-Antitrypsin (AAT)	4 days	4.8	51,000	IN, IT	Protease inhibitor, especially elastase
	α_1-Acid glycoprotein (AAG, orosomucoid)	5 days	2.7-4	40,000	IN, IT, RID	Function obscure; binds cationic drugs and hormones
	α_1-Fetoprotein (AFP)			69,000	RIA, EIA, fluorescence polarization	Principal fetal protein; albumin analogue
α_2	Haptoglobin (Hp, HAP)	2 days	4.1*	85,000-840,000	IN, IT	Binds hemoglobin; reduced by hemolysis
	α_2-Macroglobulin (AMG)	5 days	5.4	720,000	IN, IT, RID	General proteolytic enzyme inhibitor
	Ceruloplasmin (CER)	4.5 days	4.4	132,000	IN, IT, RID, enzymatic	Oxidant-antioxidant (especially for iron)
β_1	Transferrin (Tf, siderophilin)	7 days	5.7	79,600	IN, IT, RID	Transports iron
	C4			206,000	IN, IT, RID	Complement factor
β_2	C3			180,000	IN, IT, RID	Complement factor
	β_2-Microglobulin (BMG)			11,800	RIA, EIA	Used to test renal tubular function; elevated in

TABLE 20-3 Properties of Selected Plasma Proteins—*Continued*

Electrophoretic Region	Protein	Half-Life	pI	MW (daltons)	Preferred Analysis Method	Comments
						lymphocytosis or lymphocyte breakdown
γ	IgG	24 days	6-7.3	144,000-150,000	IN, IT, immunofixation	Antibody
	IgA	6 days		~160,000	IN, IT, immunofixation	Antibody
	IgM	5 days		900,000	Nephelometry, immunofixation	Antibody
	C-reactive protein (CRP)		6.2	~115,000	RID, RIA, IN, IT, homogeneous enzyme immunoassay	Nonspecific defense against infectious agents; removal of cellular debris

IN, Immunonephelometry; *IT*, immunoturbidimetry; *RID*, radial immunodiffusion; *RIA*, radioimmunoassay.
*For Hp 1-1 phenotype.

TABLE 20-4 Interim Consensus Reference Intervals for 14 Plasma Proteins in Human Serum Referenced to CRM 470

Protein	g/L	mg/dL
α_1-Acid glycoprotein	0.5-1.2	50-120
Albumin	35-52	3500-5200
α_1-Antitrypsin	0.9-2.0	90-200
C3*	0.9-1.8*	90-180*
C4	0.1-0.4	10-40
Ceruloplasmin	0.2-0.6	20-60
C-reactive protein	<5	<0.5
Haptoglobin	0.3-2.0	30-200
IgA	0.7-4.0	70-400
IgG	7-16	700-1600
IgM	0.4-2.3	40-230
Transthyretin (prealbumin)	0.2-0.4	20-40
α_2-Macroglobulin	1.3-3.0	130-300
Transferrin	2.0-3.6	200-360

From Dati F, Schumann G, Thomas L, et al. Consensus of a group of professional societies and diagnostic companies on guidelines for interim reference ranges for 14 proteins in serum based on the standardization against the IFCC/BCR/CAP reference material (CRM 470). Eur J Clin Chem Clin Biochem 1996; 34:517-20.
These values are applicable only to adults between 20 and 60 years of age.
*Values are slightly lower in fresh samples (assayed <8 hr after draw).

TABLE 20-5 Effects of Steroid Hormones on Plasma Protein Concentrations

	Corticoid	Androgen	Estrogen
Prealbumin	+	+	–
Albumin	–	N	–
α_1-Lipoprotein	N	–	++
α_1-Acid glycoprotein	+	+	–
α_1-Antitrypsin	N	+	++
Haptoglobin	+	++	–
Ceruloplasmin	N	N	+++
Transferrin	N	+	+
β-Lipoprotein	++	+	N
IgG	–	N	–

Modified from Whicher JT. Abnormalities of plasma proteins. In: Williams DL, Marks V, editors. Biochemistry in clinical practice. London: William Heinemann, 1983:221-50.
+, Increase; *N*, no change; –, decrease.

(prealbumin), albumin, and transferrin in particular, are *negative APR,* which have levels decreasing with inflammation. Associated disorders include surgery, trauma, myocardial infarction, bacterial infections, and many tumors. Presumably the APR all play a part in the very complex defensive process of inflammation, particularly in complement activation and in control of enzyme activity. The acute phase reaction is a nonspecific reaction to inflammation, comparable with the increase in temperature or leukocyte count, and is not diagnostic for any given disease. Most of the changes are triggered by cytokines released from the site of injury (see Chapter 22).

Plasma levels of the individual acute phase proteins rise at different rates—first, CRP, SAA, and α_1-antichymotrypsin; after the first 12 hours, AAG; after 24 to 48 hours, AAT, Hp, C4, and fibrinogen; and finally C3 and Cp. All reach their maximums within 2 to 5 days following an acute insult and then decrease in the same order as above. Although these changes do not aid in the diagnosis of the cause of inflammation, measurement of those proteins with the largest and earliest rises (e.g., CRP and SAA) can be useful in monitoring the progress of an inflammatory reaction or its response to treatment. In a 2003 study, procalcitonin and SAA levels were found to be more sensitive than CRP for detecting bacterial infection, although SAA levels also rise in most viral infections and are thus less specific.[69]

Individual plasma proteins are discussed in the following sections. They are listed in alphabetical order.

Albumin

The name "albumin" refers to the white precipitate (mostly albumin) formed during the boiling of acidic urine (L. *albus* = white). Normally, albumin is the most abundant plasma protein from midgestation until death, accounting for approximately one half of the plasma protein mass. It is a relatively small protein (molecular mass 66.3 kDa) with a globular conformation, permitting equilibration across the vascular and glomerular basement membranes. Because of this and its high plasma concentration, albumin is a significant component of most extravascular body fluids, including CSF, interstitial fluid, urine, and, during pregnancy, amniotic fluid. Indeed, approximately 60% of the total body albumin is in the extravascular space.[81]

Biochemistry

Albumin has a single polypeptide chain of 580 amino acids, with 17 intrachain S-S bonds aligned in a multiple loop structure. Albumin is one of only a few plasma proteins with no carbohydrate side chains. It is a very stable protein with a high net negative charge at physiological pH and, partly as a result, very high solubility in water. There is one free —SH group at position 34 that reacts completely with thiol compounds, such as cysteine, at physiological pH.[81]

Albumin is synthesized primarily by the hepatic parenchymal cells except in early fetal life, when it is synthesized largely by the yolk sac. The synthetic reserve of the liver is enormous; in nephrotic syndrome, it may be 300% or more of normal. The synthetic rate is controlled primarily by colloidal osmotic pressure (COP) and secondarily by protein intake.[81,92] Synthesis is decreased by inflammatory cytokines,[93] and release (but not synthesis) is decreased by hypokalemia.[92] Catabolism occurs primarily by pinocytosis by all tissue, with lysosomal catabolism of the protein and use of the resulting free amino acids for synthesis of cellular proteins. The rate of pinocytosis is proportional to the local tissue metabolic rate. Small amounts (10% to 20% of the total catabolized) are also lost into the gastrointestinal tract and the glomerular filtrate.[81] Nearly all of the protein in the glomerular filtrate is reabsorbed and catabolized by the proximal renal tubular cells, resulting in a very low concentration in normal excreted urine. The normal plasma half-life of albumin is 15 to 19 days.

Function

The primary function of albumin is generally considered to be the maintenance of COP in both the vascular and extravascular spaces. This is supported teleologically by the fact that its synthesis is regulated primarily by COP. If the plasma albumin level rises or falls, the concentration in extravascular spaces rapidly equilibrates with plasma to compensate for this. As discussed later, most analbuminemic individuals have little or no edema, in part because of this equilibration and in part by increased synthesis of other proteins.

The presence of many charged surface groups plus many specific binding sites, both ionic and hydrophobic, gives albumin the ability to bind and transport a large number of compounds. These include free fatty acids, phospholipids, cholesterol, metallic ions, amino acids, drugs, hormones, and bilirubin, among many others. Albumin is essential for the metabolism and detoxification of many of these, although analbuminemic individuals are significantly affected only by the absence of albumin's lipid and calcium transport properties. High levels of albumin are partially protective against atherosclerosis, probably because of its promotion of cholesterol efflux from fibroblasts and other cells.[41] Albumin binds many hormones, such as triiodothyronine or T_3, but with lower affinity than other proteins (in this case, thyroxine-binding globulin and transthyretin, or prealbumin). It appears to act as a reservoir to ensure that only the physiological amount of free hormone is present, while permitting the rapid release of additional hormone as the free hormone is used or excreted.[81]

Albumin also functions as an amino acid source for peripheral tissue. After ingestion and absorption of amino acid–containing foods, albumin transports them to tissue. In addition, pinocytosed albumin itself can serve as a source of amino acids for tissue. The synthesis of albumin by the liver increases after meals, apparently in an attempt to prevent loss or catabolism of essential amino acids. Complexing by albumin appears to be necessary for the transport of some amino acids across membranes, in particular the transport of tryptophan across the blood-brain barrier.

Other important functions of albumin include the following:

1. Albumin is an important component of plasma antioxidant activity.
2. Albumin acts as a buffer, especially in nonphysiological conditions.
3. The binding of albumin to endothelial membrane-associated glycoproteins increases capillary permeability to small proteins that are important for metabolism in the extravascular space.

4. Albumin inhibits leukotriene and actin production, thus reducing the inflammatory response of platelets and neutrophils.

Clinical Significance

Increased Plasma Levels. Measurably increased levels of albumin are seen only in acute dehydration. As a result, the finding of elevated values has little clinical utility. As noted previously, synthetic rate and intravascular-extravascular shifts usually occur fairly rapidly to stabilize relative osmotic pressures.

Decreased Plasma Levels. Decreased levels of albumin may result from decreased synthesis, increased catabolism (use or loss), or combinations of these. Decreased synthesis may be primary or genetic (as in analbuminemia) or acquired (as in inflammatory processes). Hypoalbuminemia may result in underestimation of the anion gap when evaluating fluid and electrolyte status.[31]

Analbuminemia. Only 20 or so families with inherited analbuminemia have been reported, attesting to the protein's physiological importance.[57] Although affected individuals have plasma albumin levels less than 0.5 g/L (about 1% of normal), they were originally reported to be clinically normal except for mild edema (usually none before the second to fourth decades of life) and altered lipid metabolism. In 1996, the presence of lipodystrophy in women and osteoporosis, hypotension, arcus lipoides corneae, and xanthomatosis in some patients was first reported.[57] In one patient, ankle edema disappeared rapidly with intravenous albumin infusion; however, she developed signs of hypocalcemia during infusions. The infusions did not affect her lipodystrophy. In spite of the lipid abnormalities in affected individuals, there is no increased risk for atherosclerosis. The plasma half-life of infused albumin in affected individuals is 50 to 60 days or approximately three times normal.

Inflammation. Inflammatory disorders, both acute and chronic, are the most common cause of decreased plasma albumin levels. At least four factors are responsible for the decreases: (1) hemodilution; (2) loss into the extravascular space caused by increased vascular permeability; (3) increased consumption by cells locally; and (4) decreased synthesis as the result of direct inhibition by cytokines (see Chapter 22) and by increased COP. This increase in plasma COP results acutely from increased levels of the positive APR; chronically, it results most often from increased levels of immunoglobulins.[81,93]

Hepatic Disease. The liver retains the ability to synthesize even increased amounts of albumin until parenchymal damage or loss is severe, with the loss of 50% to 95% of function. Thus other mechanisms are responsible for the decreased levels seen in most cases of hepatocellular disease.[45] These include, among others, increased immunoglobulin levels, third space loss (extravasation into the extravascular space), and direct inhibition of synthesis by toxins, including alcohol. The inhibitory effect of alcohol is lessened by adequate levels of tryptophan. Albumin levels do not correlate well with severity, prognosis, or level of total hepatic function in either acute hepatitis or cirrhosis.

Urinary Loss. Because albumin is relatively small and globular, relatively large amounts filter into the glomerular urine in spite of its acidic charge at physiological pH. Filtration is increased if acidic groups are blocked (e.g., by glycosylation in patients with diabetes mellitus). Most of the filtered albumin is normally reabsorbed by the proximal tubular cells, but normal excreted urine still contains up to 20 mg albumin/g creatinine, or 20 mg albumin/L urine. Excretion above this amount suggests either increased glomerular filtration (as seen in the nephrotic syndrome), proximal tubular damage, hematuria, or combinations of these. Increased filtration may be seen with "physiological" states, such as physical exercise and fever; therefore urinary albumin should preferably be assayed under controlled conditions and repeated if there is a question.

Although there is still debate about its significance, mildly increased excretion (20 to 300 mg/L) of albumin, so-called *microalbuminuria* (more correctly termed *minimal albuminuria* or *paucialbuminuria*), appears to be a predictor of future development of clinical renal disease in patients with hypertension or diabetes mellitus. It is important to remember that tubular and postrenal causes of albuminuria may also be present in association with these disorders.

Except for hereditary analbuminemia, the lowest levels of plasma albumin are seen in patients with active *nephrotic syndrome*. In this disorder, the glomerular leakage of all proteins is increased, but sieving is usually retained (i.e., small proteins are lost disproportionately). The liver compensates by marked increase in production of many proteins, including albumin. As a result of the sieving and increased production, the concentrations of proteins with high molecular mass, such as α_2-macroglobulin (AMG), larger isotypes of Hp (phenotypes 2-1 and 2-2), and the apolipoproteins are elevated more or less proportionately to the loss of albumin and other small proteins. The resulting electrophoretic pattern is classic, with markedly elevated α_2-globulins (AMG, plus Hp unless Hp 1-1) and lipoproteins, but reductions in most other proteins.

Urinary albumin: α_1-microglobulin and albumin:IgG ratios have been proposed as a means of differentiating among nephropathies and glomerulopathies associated with proteinuria.[52]

Gastrointestinal Loss. Inflammatory disease of the intestinal tract, such as acute viral gastroenteritis, is associated with increased loss of albumin. This is usually of little concern unless the loss is excessive or long lived. However, protein-losing enteropathy may result in losses as great as those seen in the nephrotic syndrome. If protein-losing enteropathy is secondary to lymphangiectasis, larger proteins—especially the immunoglobulins—may be lost in large amounts.

Protein Calorie Malnutrition. Albumin levels have been recommended as a means of detecting and monitoring protein calorie malnutrition, because levels vary directly with adequacy of intake. However, the response of albumin to increased or decreased protein ingestion is relatively slow, in part because of its relatively long half-life (15 to 19 days). Also, as noted previously, the most common cause of low levels is acute or chronic inflammation. Unless inflammation and other causes of increased COP are ruled out, albumin levels do not correlate well with degree of malnutrition.[55]

Edema and Ascites. Edema and ascites rarely are the result of decreased plasma albumin levels per se. Usually they are secondary to increased vascular permeability, which permits the loss of albumin into these spaces. The albumin levels in these fluids vary from very low to higher than those in plasma, the latter in particular with certain forms of ascites.[46] Even with low concentrations, either disorder may be massive enough to contain a substantial portion of the total body albumin.

In patients with edema or ascites associated with low plasma albumin, the effect of albumin infusion is very transient because of rapid equilibration with the extravascular fluid. The only situation in which infusion is usually beneficial is in acute hypovolemic shock; in this case, rapid infusion may result in hypocalcemic tetany, because albumin binds Ca^{2+} with relatively high affinity.

Genetic Aspects

Albumin is coded by a gene on the long arm of chromosome 4, closely linked to the genes for α-fetoprotein (AFP) and vitamin D binding globulin (or Gc globulin), both of which share extensive sequence homology with albumin.[5] Inherited analbuminemia has been reported in a few families. Inheritance is autosomal codominant, with heterozygotes having low normal to reduced levels. Low levels (5% to 10% of normal) are also seen with Alb Hawkes Bay, an electrophoretic variant with a cys → phe substitution at position 177, resulting in abnormal disulfide bonding.[6]

More than 80 additional alleles associated with altered structure but normal concentrations of albumin have been reported. All are inherited in autosomal codominant fashion, with both gene products expressed in approximately equal amounts. Many of the isotypes have altered electrophoretic migration, resulting in so-called *bisalbuminemia.* However, electrophoretic patterns must be interpreted with caution, because bound drugs and metabolites may also change albumin's electrophoretic migration. The common, or wild, type is Alb A; in whites of European descent, the second most frequent variant is Alb B (~1 in 1000 to 10,000 depending on ethnic origin). Alb B has a more cathodal electrophoretic migration because of a glu → lys substitution.

At least two variants are associated with dimer formation, which also results in more cathodal migration. However, they are usually seen as a cathodal blur instead of a distinct, separate band, as is the case with Alb B. The degree of dimer formation and of complexing with other proteins, such as IgA, with these variant albumins varies with storage conditions, pH, and concentration of low molecular weight —SH compounds, such as glutathione; hence the same serum sample may appear different on electrophoresis at different times. Perhaps the most important laboratory consequence of these variants is the formation of complexes with AAT, resulting in apparent deficiency of this protein on electrophoretic patterns. However, quantification of AAT by immunochemical methods is normal.

The function of most albumin isoforms is normal, although some have abnormal binding affinities for thyroxine (T_4). Binding may be increased, as in familial dysalbuminemic hyperthyroxinemia,[116] or decreased.[1] Individuals with familial dysalbuminemic hyperthyroxinemia are euthyroid but have elevated serum T_4 and free T_4 index; the variant albumin comigrates with Alb A. Two glycosylated variants, Alb Redhill and Alb Casebrook, have altered fatty acid binding properties.

Laboratory Considerations

Plasma and Serum. Most clinical laboratories assay albumin in plasma or serum samples by automated dye-binding methods, which rely on a shift in the absorption spectrum of such dyes as bromcresol green (BCG) or purple (BCP) upon binding to proteins. The affinity of these dyes is much higher for albumin than for other proteins, so specificity is increased if only the initial rate of binding is used. Monochromatic methods overestimate albumin in the presence of fibrinogen and heparin (e.g., in heparinized plasma or in "serum" from heparinized patients). This interference can be circumvented by using a bichromatic method.[43] Dye-binding assays also tend to be erroneous if the overall serum protein pattern is abnormal (e.g., in liver disease)—situations in which accurate analysis is most desired. BCP binding assays of albumin in ascitic fluid give spuriously high results.[33] Many other ligands, including drugs and metabolites, bind to albumin but usually do not affect dye-binding assays of serum or plasma significantly unless their concentrations are very high. Because of their simplicity and low cost, dye-binding assays are likely to remain the predominant means for assaying albumin.

The use of densitometric scans of electrophoretic patterns, in association with total protein assays, as a means of quantifying albumin is notoriously inaccurate and is discouraged. The problems relate in part to lateral diffusion of relatively small proteins, including albumin, on support media and to nonlinearity secondary to a lack of saturation of albumin dye-binding sites.

Immunochemical methods, especially automated immunoturbidimetry and immunonephelometry, are more accurate and precise than the methods mentioned previously.

Urine. As previously mentioned, the term *albumin* derives from the white precipitate resulting from boiling acidified urine. The sulfosalicylic acid heat test is still used today to test for albuminuria; however, screening is usually performed by test strips, most of which have lower detection limits of 200 to 300 mg/L. Special strips are now available for detecting microalbuminuria. The immunochemical methods used for serum can assay very low levels of albumin in undiluted urine and are very rapid and precise.

Cerebrospinal Fluid. Immunoturbidimetry and immunonephelometry are also useful for CSF assays.

Reference Intervals

Based on the international protein reference CRM 470, the recommended interim reference interval for albumin in serum of adults 20 to 60 years of age is 35 to 52 g/L (3.5 to 5.2 g/dL).[28] Albumin levels reach adult levels around 20 to 30 weeks of gestation and remain relatively constant until at least 20 years of age. Levels then slowly decrease with age in both sexes. Levels are lower in individuals living in the subtropics and tropics, probably because of higher immunoglobulin levels secondary to infection or parasitic infestation. Levels are very posture dependent, increasing by up to 10% to 15% if the individual is standing.

Alpha$_1$-Acid Glycoprotein (Orosomucoid)

AAG was one of the first plasma glycoproteins to be isolated in the pure state and to be well characterized. Historically, AAG is the major constituent of the seromucoid fraction of plasma, a group of proteins that are precipitated by $HClO_4$ and other strong acids and that are "slimy" on purification ("mucoid" is from Greek *myxa* = slime). The seromucoid fraction has long been of clinical interest because it was one of the first recognized components of the acute phase response.[21]

Biochemistry

AAG contains a high percentage of carbohydrate and a large number of sialic acid residues, giving it a very high net negative charge and high solubility in water. It has a polypeptide chain containing 181 amino acids and a total molecular mass of 40 kDa, of which approximately 45% is carbohydrate (CHO), including 11% to 12% sialic acid. The CHO includes a variable mixture of biantennary, triantennary, and tetraantennary side chains with terminal sialyl residues, resulting in significant microheterogeneity of the intact molecule upon electrophoresis at pH 2.9 or isoelectric focusing. The relative proportions of the different side chains vary with disease states and nutrition, altering their isoelectric points and their reactivity with the lectin concanavalin A. It has also been suggested that changes in glycosylation alter function in vivo.[109]

AAG is synthesized primarily by the hepatic parenchymal cells, but granulocytes and monocytes may also contribute to plasma levels in sepsis. Catabolism is believed to be primarily by removal of desialylated AAG by hepatic asialoglycoprotein receptors. The plasma half-life of intact AAG is ~3 days, whereas that of the desialylated protein is only a few minutes.

Function

Although many functions have been proposed for AAG, its true physiological role still remains unknown. AAG is one of the *lipocalins,* a group of proteins that bind lipophilic substances and share much sequence homology. The lipocalin group also includes retinol-binding protein, β-lactoglobulin, α_{2m}-globulin, α_1-microglobulin (protein HC), bikunin, the chain of complement C8, and inter-α-trypsin inhibitor.[80] AAG has long been known to bind and "inactivate" a large number of basic and lipophilic compounds, including progesterone and related hormones, and the progesterone antagonist RU 486. AAG's binding of progesterone has been proposed to constitute a means of controlling hormonal effects in the fetus. AAG also binds and reduces the bioavailability of many drugs, including propranolol, quinidine, chlorpromazine, cocaine, and benzodiazepines. Most assays for drug levels in plasma or serum assay the total, not just free, drug. If AAG levels are elevated secondary to an acute phase response or corticosteroid therapy, administration of additional drug (and higher blood concentrations) may be necessary to compensate for the increased binding.

Other proposed functions for AAG include down regulation of the immune response, depression of phagocytosis by neutrophils, inhibition of platelet aggregation, inhibition of mitosis, and inhibition of viruses and parasites. In addition, it has been reported to affect collagen fiber formation and to be a cofactor for lipoprotein lipase. It is also essential for maintaining capillary selectivity for passage of albumin and other macromolecules, including in the glomerulus, because of its high negative charge.

Clinical Significance

Various pathological conditions are associated with increased and decreased levels of AAG.

Increased Plasma Levels. Serum AAG increases in inflammation and tissue necrosis and from hormonal effects.

Acute Phase Response. Plasma AAG levels show a threefold to fourfold increase in most conditions associated with inflammation or tissue necrosis, with peak concentrations around 3 to 5 days after the initial insult. AAG may be one of the most reliable indicators of clinical activity of ulcerative colitis.

Hormonal Effects. AAG levels are increased by glucocorticoid hormones, either endogenous (e.g., Cushing's syndrome) or exogenous (as in prednisone or dexamethasone therapy), along with Hp and prealbumin (transthyretin) levels.

Decreased Plasma Levels. Hormonal effects and sieving protein loss are known to decrease AAG levels.

Hormonal Effects. Synthesis and plasma AAG levels are decreased by estrogens.

Sieving Protein Loss. Because of its small molecular size, AAG is lost into the urine in nephrotic syndrome and into gastrointestinal secretions in protein-losing enteropathy.

Genetic Aspects

The presence of different isotypes of the peptide chain of AAG, inherited in autosomal codominant fashion, has long been recognized. There are three genes for AAG in a cluster on chromosome 9q34.3, closely linked to the loci for several other members of the lipocalin family. The originally reported polymorphism (designated *OR*) represented the products of the *ORM1* locus, which accounts for about two thirds of AAG synthesis and most of the isotypic variability. The products of both the *ORM1* and *ORM2* loci can be simultaneously phenotyped by isofocusing of desialylated AAG in immobilized pH gradients containing urea. The variants have no known clinical significance.

Laboratory Considerations

It has been proposed that AAG always be assayed along with haptoglobin when levels of the latter are used to evaluate possible in vitro hemolysis, because hormonal and acute phase effects are similar for the two proteins (see section on Haptoglobin). Although AAG is one of the highest concentration proteins in the α_1-globulin region on routine serum electrophoresis, it does not stain well with protein stains because of its high CHO content. It can be visualized by using periodic acid-Schiff or other carbohydrate stains. AAG can be quantified by all immunochemical methods, including turbidimetry and nephelometry.

Reference Intervals

The proposed interim reference interval for white adolescents and adults is 0.5 to 1.2 g/L (50 to 120 mg/dL), based on CRM 470.[28] Levels at birth are only 20% to 30% of this, but reach approximately adult levels by 6 to 12 months of age.

Alpha$_1$-Antitrypsin

Schultze first described AAT in 1955, later giving it this name because of its inhibition of trypsin. The name "α_1-proteinase inhibitor" was later introduced because of AAT's broad spectrum of inhibition of serine proteases, not just trypsin. Both names are currently used, but AAT is preferred by most clinicians and clinical laboratorians and is used in this chapter.

Biochemistry

AAT has a single polypeptide chain of 394 amino acid residues with three CHO side chains, giving a total molecular mass of ~51 kDa. The active site is contained in a "stressed" reactive loop; on reaction with a serine protease, a small fragment is cleaved, and the remainder of the protein assumes a "relaxed" configuration.[11]

Most if not all plasma AAT is synthesized by the hepatic parenchymal cells, as evidenced by the complete change in phenotype in patients (including those with AAT deficiency) transplanted with livers from individuals with other phenotypes. AAT is an acute phase reactant, with hepatic synthesis and plasma levels rising greatly during inflammatory or necrotic processes. Catabolism occurs by two routes, both primarily in hepatic parenchymal cells: AAT-protease complexes are removed by the serpin-enzyme complex receptors (SEC-R),[79] along with several other serpin-enzyme complexes; in addition, desialylated AAT is removed by asialoglycoprotein receptors. Most proteases complexed with AAT in vivo may be transferred to AMG; the AMG-protease complexes are removed almost immediately by the Kupffer cells of the liver, with a much shorter plasma half-life than AAT-protease complexes.

The normal plasma half-life is 6 to 7 days for the Pi M phenotype; Pi S, and perhaps other variants, has a shorter half-life and secondarily lower plasma levels.

Function

AAT is one of the serpins, or *ser*ine *p*roteinase *in*hibitors, which act as substrates for, then form tetrahedral complexes with the active sites of serine proteases, thus blocking their enzymatic activity. Other members of the serpin superfamily include the proteinase inhibitors α_1-antichymotrypsin, α_2-antiplasmin, antithrombin III, heparin cofactor II, and C1 inhibitor, plus ovalbumin, thyroxine-binding globulin, and other proteins with similar structures but no apparent inhibitory activity. AAT is the second highest concentration proteinase inhibitor in plasma on a mass basis, after AMG; however, AAT has only 7% of the mass of AMG and is by far the highest concentration inhibitor on a molar basis. Its small size allows AAT to pass into all body fluids, whereas AMG is mostly intravascular. AAT inhibits most serine proteases, especially those structurally related to trypsin. It is physiologically most important as an inhibitor of leukocyte elastase, which is released in the process of phagocytosis by polymorphonuclear leukocytes. This enzyme, as its name implies, reacts with elastin in the vascular endothelium and the tracheobronchial tree, in particular. AAT is thus important in the prevention of loss of elastic lung recoil; uninhibited elastase in the bronchial tree can result in the development of emphysema.

AAT may also be a physiologically important inhibitor of leukocyte neutral protease, kallikrein, renin, urokinase, plasmin, and thrombin. It probably does not inhibit leukocyte collagenase (a metalloproteinase), as is often stated; it more likely inhibits a leukocyte protease that activates procollagenase.

Clinical Significance

Increased Plasma Levels. Plasma AAT levels are increased in the acute phase response and with estrogens.

Acute Phase Response. In inflammatory or necrotic processes, serum AAT levels begin to rise after approximately 24 hours and peak at 3 to 4 days if the insult is acute and short lived. Synthesis is stimulated by cytokines, particularly the IL-6 family, and by AAT-elastase complexes taken up via SEC-R. Cytokines induce a broader APR, whereas uptake by the SEC-R induces only AAT synthesis. The acute phase response of AAT probably occurs in an attempt to control the effects of proteases released in areas of inflammation or necrosis. Inflammation of the hepatic parenchymal cells themselves may be associated with increased serum AAT without the other components of the acute phase response.

Estrogens. The synthesis of AAT is stimulated by estrogens; elevated levels are seen particularly during late pregnancy and during estrogen therapy.

Decreased Plasma Levels. Plasma AAT levels are decreased with genetic deficiency, increased use, and urinary or gastrointestinal loss.

Genetic Deficiency. As noted previously, severe genetic deficiency of AAT (Pi Z or null phenotypes) is associated with a very high risk for development of pulmonary emphysema. In affected individuals, emphysema tends to be primarily in the basilar areas (probably because of gravitational vascular pooling), rather than the more typical disease seen in other forms of emphysema. Onset of disease is also much earlier, with changes beginning in the second to fourth decades of life in 90% of Pi ZZ individuals. The primary mechanism for development of emphysema is the degradation of elastin by leukocyte elastase; this process is increased by air pollution and by cigarette smoking because of recruitment and activation of leukocytes in the lung plus the oxidation of methionine 358 in the active site of AAT, rendering it unable to inhibit elastase.[10] The age of onset of symptomatic emphysema and the median age of death are also earlier in individuals who smoke cigarettes. However, there is much variation in the development and progression of disease, even in smokers. Antioxidants may reduce the deleterious effects of smoking, but smoking cessation is by far the better approach.

A deficiency of α_1-antitrypsin is also associated with diseases of the liver, including neonatal cholestasis or "hepatitis," cirrhosis, and hepatocellular carcinoma. Although cirrhosis may be seen at birth, the so-called neonatal hepatitis syndrome is much more common, with varying degrees of hepatocellular damage but particularly with cholestatic jaundice. Neonatal cholestasis was noted in 11% of Pi ZZ infants in Sweden, with another 6% showing biochemical evidence of hepatic disease but no jaundice.[103] This picture is most commonly seen at 3 to 8 weeks of age and usually regresses after a few weeks. Intrahepatic and extrahepatic bile ducts may be very small, probably because of decreased bile flow, even to the point of patients presenting with a picture similar to biliary atresia. It is important to differentiate these two disorders because mortality is high in Pi ZZ infants subjected to major surgery. In most affected infants, the bile ducts dilate to normal size as the inflammatory process regresses and bile flow increases. In Swedish Pi Z adults, 12% of those admitted to hospitals had liver cirrhosis, and a strong correlation was found between Pi Z AAT and primary liver cancer at autopsy.[34]

The cause of hepatic damage in AAT deficiency is probably multifactorial. Liver disease is most commonly seen in patients with variants that are retained within the endoplasmic reticulum of the hepatic parenchymal cells (e.g., Pi Z and Pi M_{malton}). There does not appear to be a familial propensity for development of liver disease in Pi Z individuals, which argues against the likelihood of a second inherited defect. The hypothesis most commonly cited at present is that the accumulation of AAT itself results in the hepatic damage; this is supported by the fact that transgenic mice with multiple copies of the human Pi Z gene develop hepatic disease. In addition, Perlmutter has proposed that upregulation of AAT synthesis, perhaps through uptake of elastase-AAT complexes by the SEC-R, increases the synthesis and accumulation of AAT in affected livers.[79] Reduced rates of catabolism of retained intracellular AAT may also be involved. However, the degree of liver disease does not correlate with the amount of intracellular AAT. Many infants with neonatal cholestasis have very little demonstrable intracellular AAT, and many older children and adults have massive accumulations of AAT but no other hepatic damage. Therefore other factors must be involved.

There is evidence supporting a role for hepatic damage by intravascular proteases in the pathogenesis of neonatal hepatic disease, as reviewed in the previous edition of this textbook.[56] The AAT deposits in the hepatic endoplasmic reticulum do not bind normally to calnexin, one of the chaperones for protein synthesis and release[77]; it is known that proteolytic enzymes reduce the activity of intracellular, membrane-bound proteins involved in metabolic processes. An additional component in congenital and neonatal hepatic disease may be exposure to maternal estrogens, which increase susceptibility to damage from hepatitis viral infections and some toxins.

Several other disorders have been reported in association with AAT deficiency, although many of these may be no more than chance occurrences. However, it appears that the risk for development of systemic vasculitic disease, including Wegener's granulomatosis and Henoch-Schönlein purpura, may be increased in deficient individuals.

Increased Utilization. Secondarily low levels of AAT are seen in the neonatal respiratory distress syndrome, severe neonatal hepatitis, and severe preterminal disease of the pancreas. In nonfatal pancreatitis, levels increase along with those of other APR, and increased levels of complexes with trypsin are probably a better marker for use in either differential diagnosis or prognosis in patients with possible pancreatitis.

Urinary or Gastrointestinal Loss. Because of its small size, AAT diffuses into the glomerular urine and into the gastrointestinal tract; however, AAT is not seen in the excreted urine unless there is damage to the proximal tubular cells or marked overflow proteinuria, as in the nephrotic syndrome. In the latter case, the serum level of AAT may be depressed, especially in the absence of an acute phase reaction. AAT is normally present in the excreted stool, mostly complexed to pancreatic trypsin and elastase. In protein-losing enteropathies, the loss may be greatly increased.

Genetic Aspects

The gene locus for AAT (*PI*, for protease inhibitor) is located on chromosome 14q32.1, just distal to the loci for the immunoglobulin heavy chains and closely linked to the loci for the serpins α_1-antichymotrypsin, protein C inhibitor, and corticosteroid-binding globulin.[9] It is a very polymorphic locus. There are more than 75 distinct genetic variants or isotypes of AAT, designated as Pi (pronounced *pee eye*) plus letters from B to Z in order of decreasing electrophoretic mobility—B being the most anodal variant. Numbers or subscripted place names are used to indicate subtypes (e.g., Pi M1 and Pi M_{malton}), and null for either deleted or non-producing alleles.

Several of the variants are associated with reduced plasma levels, compared with the wild Pi M variant, including the following: Pi P 25%, Pi S 60%, Pi W 80%, Pi Z 15%, and Pi null 0%. Pi Z is most common in northern Europeans, and Pi S is most common in southwestern Europe. Pi Z, clinically the most important deficiency variant, has a lys → glu substitution at position 342, whereas Pi S has a 264 glu → val substitution. There are several known mutations resulting in Pi null, but all are rare. The concentrations and the variants are codominant; therefore an individual with Pi MZ, for example, would normally have a level ~58% of the normal Pi MM level [(100 + 15)/2].

Pi Z, Pi S_{iiyama}, Pi M_{malton}, and Pi M_{duarte} are synthesized by the liver in relatively normal amounts but are only partially secreted, resulting in accumulation within the endoplasmic reticulum of hepatic parenchymal cells and low plasma levels. As a result of a glu → lys substitution in Pi Z, the reactive center loop on one molecule can insert into the β-pleated sheet of a second molecule, resulting in polymerization and retention within the pre-Golgi endoplasmic reticulum. Similar alterations have been shown to be present in Pi S_{iiyama} and Pi M_{malton}.[68] The amino acid substitution and altered molecular folding may also inhibit attachment of CHO side chains, which are necessary for normal secretion by the hepatic parenchymal cells. The retained AAT is seen as "globules" that are eosinophilic and periodic-acid Schiff positive and that react with antibodies to AAT, as shown by immunofluorescence or immunoperoxidase staining of liver sections.

One variant, Pi $M_{pittsburgh}$, has a met → arg substitution at position 358, resulting in a greatly decreased inhibitory activity for elastase but increased activity against several clotting enzymes, including thrombin and kallikrein. Heterozygotes for this variant have a bleeding disorder because of its anticoagulant effects.[96]

Many variants with relatively normal concentrations are apparent on routine clinical electrophoresis; the most common of these are Pi F, Pi X, and Pi V. The low concentration variants should be suspected if the α_1-globulin band appears less intense than normal. As noted in the section on albumin, dimerizing variants of albumin may form complexes with normal AAT variants, resulting in an apparent deficiency of AAT; however, quantification in this case reveals normal levels. If AAT deficiency is suspected by electrophoresis or by quantification, phenotyping may be indicated, particularly if the patient has hepatic or pulmonary disease. Phenotyping is now most often performed by isoelectric focusing in narrow pH range ampholytes (discussed later in this chapter). Genotyping (by deoxyribonucleic acid [DNA] analysis) is also currently in use, particularly for detection of deficiency variants.

Laboratory Considerations

AAT is the major constituent of the α_1-globulin band on routine clinical serum electrophoresis. The two other relatively high concentration α_1-globulins, AAG and α-lipoprotein, do not stain well with peptide stains because of their high contents of CHO and lipid, respectively. Some genetic variants of AAT may be detectable by visual examination of the electrophoresis pattern because of altered mobility or decreased concentration.

There are five to eight AAT bands on either acid gel electrophoresis or isoelectric focusing (pIs approximately 4.2 to 4.9, depending on the genetic phenotype), as shown in Figure 20-3. The microheterogeneity within a single genetic variant results primarily from differences in CHO content and, in the case of the two most cathodal bands, absence of the first five amino acids of the peptide chain.

AAT can be quantified by all immunochemical methods, with immunoturbidimetry and immunonephelometry the most commonly used methods. Because it constitutes about 90% of the serum inhibition of trypsin or elastase activity against small substrates, such as benzoyl-DL-arginine *p*-nitroanilide, it can also be semiquantified by the inhibitory capacity of serum for these enzymes; however, this assay is not specific for AAT.

Leukocyte proteases may be released if serum is allowed to sit on the clot too long after blood drawing. These proteases then form complexes with AAT, altering both electrophoretic mobility and in some cases immunochemical quantification. Bacterial contamination and release of

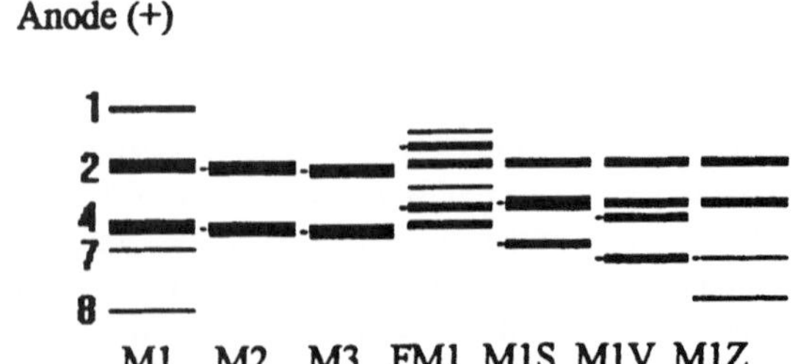

Figure 20-3 Diagrammatic representation of the common variants of α_1-antitrypsin, as demonstrated by isoelectric focusing. The five major bands are shown for M1, but only the 2 and 4 bands for the other variants (with dots to the left of each). Variants F, S, V, and Z are shown in combination with M1 for clarity's sake. If cysteine is added to the samples before focusing, the F-2 and F-4 bands shift to the locations of the faint bands.

bacterial proteases can have a similar effect. Serum should be separated from the retracted clot as soon as possible and stored aseptically at 4 °C (for up to 3 to 4 days) or at −70 °C (for long-term storage).

Reference Intervals

AAT levels remain relatively constant throughout life, from the neonatal period until old age. For adults, the recommended consensus reference interval, based on CRM 470, is 0.9 to 2.0 g/L (90 to 200 mg/dL) for individuals with the Pi MM phenotype,[28] with a median of approximately 1.3 g/L. Levels are slightly higher in women in the childbearing years and in elderly individuals of both sexes. Levels are also higher in inflammatory disorders, malignancy, or trauma, and in women who are pregnant, on estrogen therapy, or taking oral contraceptive pills. Neonates have higher levels, possibly because of maternal estrogen. Individuals with levels below 60 to 70 mg/dL should be phenotyped, especially if they or family members have diseases that may be associated with AAT deficiency.

Alpha$_2$-Macroglobulin

Like the serpins, AMG is a proteinase inhibitor. It is unlike the serpins in many aspects, however. First, it is a very large molecule, with a molecular mass of ~725 kDa. As a result, only very small amounts diffuse out of the plasma space. Second, it acts as a substrate for proteases but does not block their active sites; instead, it "enfolds" the still-active proteases to block access of proteins but not small substrates. Third, it inhibits many different classes of proteinases, including those with serine, cysteine, and metal ions in their proteolytic sites. Fourth, it is structurally related to pregnancy zone protein and to the complement components C3, C4, and C5 rather than to the serpins. Like these proteins, it contains an intrachain thiol ester bond that is necessary for activity and the breaking of which results in a conformational change of the peptide chain.

Biochemistry

A molecule of AMG contains four identical polypeptide chains, present as a pair of dimer subunits. The dimers are covalently linked by disulfide bonds, whereas the pairs are held together by noncovalent bonds. The dimer is the active unit; one molecule of AMG can therefore bind up to two protease molecules. Each monomer contains both the thiol ester mentioned previously and a "bait" site, both of which are essential for inhibitory activity. After the bait site reacts with a protease, the thiol ester is activated and may form covalent bonds with lysine residues on the protease, thus immobilizing it. However, covalent binding is not essential for steric capture and inhibition of proteases.[101]

AMG is synthesized primarily by hepatic parenchymal cells. Catabolism is via two primary routes: once the thiol ester bond is split, AMG—regardless of whether complexed to a protease—is rapidly removed by a hepatic receptor that also acts to remove low-density lipoprotein. Desialylated AMG, like AAT and Cp, is removed by the asialoglycoprotein receptors on hepatocytes. The normal half-life of the intact protein is several days, whereas that of either of these two forms is only a few minutes.

Function

AMG is involved in the primary or secondary ("backup") inhibition of enzymes in the kinin, complement, coagulation, and fibrinolytic pathways. In addition, it acts as a transfer receptor for proteinases complexed to serpins (e.g., elastase-AAT); the AMG-enzyme complexes are then rapidly removed by receptors, as noted earlier.

Oxidation dissociates AMG tetramers into dysfunctional dimers. Thus as is the case for AAT and other serpins, inhibitory activity is reduced or eradicated by increased levels of oxidants (such as those from cigarette smoke or from neutrophils) or decreased levels of physiological antioxidants.

In addition to its critical role as a proteinase inhibitor, AMG transports a large number of small peptides, such as cytokines and growth factors (including insulin and growth hormone), and divalent cations, particularly zinc. Insulin binds covalently to the γ-glutamyl group that is activated from the thiol ester during protease reaction with AMG. Both the native and protease-reacted forms bind cytokines. Binding of these small ligands may be important to prevent diffusional loss or to permit or facilitate cell receptor binding and uptake of them; however, AMG's actual physiological importance as a transport protein is not known.

AMG is also believed to modulate immunological and inflammatory reactions. Complexing of cytokines to protease-reacted AMG reduces cytokine-mediated hepatic production of APR. It, along with AAT, inhibits H_2O_2 release by polymorphonuclear leukocytes; at the same time, it enhances phagocytosis of streptococci and perhaps other organisms.

The physiological importance of AMG is indicated by the fact that no individuals with complete genetic deficiency have been described, whereas total or near-total deficiencies have been described for most other plasma proteins.

Clinical Significance

Increased Plasma Levels. Increased plasma levels of AMG are affected by hormonal effects and age, and seen in the nephrotic syndrome.

Hormonal Effects. Synthesis and plasma levels of AMG are increased by estrogens; women of childbearing age have higher levels than men of the same ages.

Age. Synthesis levels in infants and children are up to three times adult levels, perhaps as a protective mechanism against increased exposure to intestinal proteases in infancy and bacterial or leukocytic proteases during childhood. The high levels may also be responsible in part for the delay in development of clinical signs and symptoms until after puberty in most individuals with either antithrombin III or C1 inhibitor deficiency.

Nephrotic Syndrome. Synthesis levels are increased in the nephrotic syndrome, in part because of volume loss secondary to decreased plasma oncotic osmotic pressure and in part because of increased synthesis of all proteins to compensate for protein loss by the kidneys. The elevated AMG levels partially compensate physiologically for renal loss of lower molecular weight proteinase inhibitors.[58]

Decreased Plasma Levels. Decreased plasma levels of AMG result from various genetic conditions, the acute phase response, pancreatitis, *and* prostatic carcinoma.

Genetic. See Genetic Aspects, later in this chapter.

Acute Phase Response. Synthesis is decreased by IL-1, in parallel with albumin, accounting in part (along with hemodilution) for the mildly decreased levels seen in acute inflammation.

Pancreatitis. In severe attacks of acute pancreatitis, plasma levels of antithrombin III and AMG may be markedly depressed; other inhibitors are normal or increased, and protease-antiprotease complexes are increased. In the peritoneal fluid, all major protease inhibitors are decreased or absent.

Prostatic Carcinoma. Plasma levels of AMG are depressed pretreatment in advanced carcinoma of the prostate and return to normal with successful treatment. AMG binds to prostate-specific antigen (PSA), and levels of the complexes are elevated in plasma during active disease, as is the case for PSA-α_1-antichymotrypsin complexes. In vitro, PSA added to serum has a higher affinity for AMG than for α_1-antichymotrypsin. In vivo, the complexes are probably removed very rapidly by the liver, as are other protease complexes with AMG; usually, free PSA and PSA-α_1-antichymotrypsin are the only forms detected.

Decreased Levels in Extracellular Fluids. Body fluids other than plasma—including extracellular fluid, urine, and CSF—normally contain very low levels of AMG, because of its large molecular size. However, there are several components to the blood-CSF barrier, with a few large pinocytic vesicles transporting proteins up to 1500 Å into the CSF.[67] In some polyneuropathies, the number of these vesicles and the CSF levels of AMG are increased. If there is partial or complete breakdown of the barrier, as in meningitis, or bleeding into the subdural space, levels are also increased. The level of AMG alone, or its relationship to levels of albumin and IgG, may therefore be helpful in differential diagnosis of neurological disorders or of elevated CSF protein. In patients with bacterial meningitis, CSF AMG levels are on average 15 times higher than is the case with nonbacterial meningitis.[87] CSF levels of AMG normally increase with age, suggesting that partial but progressive breakdown of the blood-CSF barrier occurs with aging. Bleeding into the CSF also raises levels in this fluid.

Urinary levels are slightly elevated in the nephrotic syndrome. Levels are higher in malignant ascitic fluid than in nonmalignant ascitic fluid. Increased permeability probably accounts for locally increased levels in areas of inflammation, but IL-6–induced increases in synthesis by monocytes may also contribute.

Genetic Aspects

The gene for AMG is adjacent to the gene for pregnancy zone protein, on chromosome 12p12-13,[70] whereas the gene for its membrane receptor ("low-density lipoprotein–related protein") is at 12q13.1-13.2.[111] As noted previously, no individuals with complete genetic deficiency of AMG have been described. There are known genetic variants, however. Two reported mutations affect either the thiol ester or the bait region. The affected individuals were heterozygous, each having equal amounts of normal and mutant AMG. One patient heterozygous for a variant with either a deletion or a gene arrangement and reduced AMG levels developed chronic lung disease in childhood; reduced inhibition of pulmonary proteases may have played a role in pathogenesis, analogous to the pathophysiology of emphysema in AAT deficiency.

Laboratory Considerations

AMG and Hp together constitute most of the α_2-globulin zone on routine clinical serum electrophoresis. In the newborn period, and in in vivo hemolysis, AMG alone is the major contributor to this zone.

Although the two forms of AMG cannot be distinguished on routine electrophoresis, native AMG migrates slightly cathodal to AMG that has reacted with either proteases or nucleophilic substances that split the thiol ester bond. This characteristic can be used to determine the degree of inactivation that has occurred either in vitro or in vivo (e.g., in pancreatitis); monoclonal antibodies specific for the two forms can also be used in immunoassays for the same purpose. Using the latter assay, normal plasma contains 0.8% to 1.9% of AMG in the complexed form.[54]

AMG levels in urine may be measured to distinguish among causes of proteinuria or hematuria. Elevated levels are seen with intrarenal bleeding from vessel rupture during extracorporeal lithotripsy, and AMG-albumin ratios approximate serum ratios in postrenal bleeding.

Reference Intervals

The interim recommended reference interval for white adults is 1.3 to 3.0 g/L (130 to 300 mg/dL).[28] Levels are approximately twice this in children, with a maximum at 2 to 4 years of age; levels in women are 20% to 30% higher than in men after age 40.

Alpha$_1$-Fetoprotein

Alpha$_1$-fetoprotein (AFP) is a glycoprotein with a single polypeptide chain and approximately 4% carbohydrate. It has a molecular weight of approximately 70 kDa.

Biochemistry and Function

AFP is a major protein in fetal serum, synthesized by the fetal liver and to a lesser extent by the yolk sac and other fetal organs. The maximum level in fetal serum is reached at the end of the first trimester, after which it decreases. The level at birth is approximately 1% of the earlier peak and then decreases with a half-time of about 3 days; after 18 months the level is less than 2 ng/mL. The level in maternal serum peaks at approximately week 30 of gestation. AFP is a fetal albumin analog. In addition, some isoforms bind and inactivate estrogen, presumably protecting the fetus from the high maternal levels of this hormone.

Clinical Significance

Determination of AFP levels in amniotic fluid or maternal serum is used for antenatal screening for certain birth defects and chromosomal abnormalities in the fetus (see Chapter 54). Elevated maternal serum AFP indicates the possibility of a neural tube or open abdominal wall defect in the fetus.[7] The levels may also be elevated with multiple fetuses, low birth weight, fetal demise, and incorrect estimation of gestational age. Trisomy 21 (Down syndrome) and trisomy 18 are associated with low maternal serum AFP levels.[42] AFP is also used as a marker for hepatocellular and germ cell carcinomas. For a discussion of the role of AFP as a tumor marker, see Chapter 23.

Reference Intervals

Newborn	<5 mg/L
>18 mo	<2 µg/L

Beta$_2$-Microglobulin

Beta$_2$-microglobulin (BMG) is a low molecular weight (11.8 kDa) protein found on the cell surfaces of all nucleated cells and shed into the blood, particularly by B lymphocytes and some tumor cells.

Biochemistry

BMG is the light or β-chain of the human leukocyte antigen and consists of a single polypeptide chain with one intrachain disulfide bridge; it does not contain carbohydrate. Its small size allows BMG to pass through the glomerular membrane, but normally less than 1% of the filtered BMG is excreted in the urine; the remainder is reabsorbed and catabolized in the proximal tubules of the kidneys. It has a plasma half-life of only 107 minutes.

Clinical Significance

High plasma levels occur in renal failure, inflammation, and neoplasms, especially those associated with B lymphocytes. BMG assay may be used to test renal tubular function, particularly in kidney transplant recipients in whom rejection of the allograft manifests as diminished tubular function (see Chapter 45). Serial assays of BMG are also useful to monitor B-cell tumors. In acute leukemia and lymphoma with central nervous system (CNS) involvement, the level of BMG is increased in CSF; and in Sjögren's syndrome with lymphoid infiltration of salivary glands, its level rises in saliva.

C-Reactive Protein

Tillet and Francis in 1930 described a substance that is present in the sera of acutely ill patients and that is able to bind the cell wall C-polysaccharide of *Streptococcus pneumoniae* and agglutinate the organisms. In 1941 the substance was shown to be a protein and given the name C-reactive protein (CRP).

Biochemistry

CRP consists of five identical, nonglycosylated polypeptide subunits noncovalently linked to form a disk-shaped cyclical polymer with a molecular weight of ~115 kDa. It contains little or no carbohydrate and is synthesized in the liver.

CRP binds not only the polysaccharides present in many bacteria, fungi, and protozoal parasites but—in the presence of free calcium ions—phosphorylcholine; phosphatidylcholines, such as lecithin; and polyanions, such as nucleic acids. In the absence of calcium ions, CRP also binds polycations, such as histones.

Function

CRP is important in the nonspecific host defense against inflammation, especially infection. In addition, it binds to tissue breakdown products (e.g., from inflammatory processes). The complexes activate the classical complement pathway starting at C1q (see next section), resulting in phagocytosis via C3b receptors. However, CRP complexes bind factor H, a complement inhibitory factor, greatly reducing the activation of late components (C5 to C9) and positive feedback via the alternative pathway (see Complement C3).[74] CRP is catabolized by opsonization, the process by which bacteria are altered in such a manner that they are more readily and more efficiently engulfed by phagocytes. However, whether CRP is catabolized by any other route is not clear. Similar proteins capable of Ca^{2+}-dependent binding to C-polysaccharide occur in fish and birds, and in mammals. Their appearance is similar to CRP on electron microscopy, and they have similar amino acid sequences. No genetic abnormalities have been reported for circulating CRP, although genetic deficiency and DNA variants have been suggested.

Clinical Significance

Acute Phase Response. CRP is one of the most sensitive of the APR with plasma levels rising up to 2000-fold after myocardial infarction, stress, trauma, infection, inflammation, surgery, or neoplastic proliferation. Levels are in general much higher in bacterial than viral infection, although levels greater than 100 mg/L (10 mg/dL) may be seen in uncomplicated influenza and infectious mononucleosis. The increase with inflammation occurs within 6 to 12 hours and peaks at about 48 hours. It is generally proportional to the degree of tissue damage. Because the increase is nonspecific, however, it cannot be interpreted without other clinical information. Umbilical cord blood normally has low CRP concentrations (1 to 35 µg/dL), but in intrauterine (fetal) bacterial infection, levels may be as high as 26 mg/dL.

Determination of CRP is clinically useful for screening for organic disease; for assessing the activity of an inflammatory disease, such as rheumatoid arthritis; for detecting intercurrent infections in systemic lupus erythematosus (SLE), in leukemia, or after surgery (secondary rise in plasma level); for detecting rejection in renal allograft recipients; and for managing neonatal septicemia and meningitis, when collecting specimens for bacteriological investigations may be difficult.

For unknown reasons, the degree of CRP response varies in some diseases that are otherwise apparently similar. For example, the CRP response in SLE and ulcerative colitis, even when there are obvious signs and symptoms of inflammation, is slight in contrast to its frequently large response in rheumatoid arthritis and Crohn's disease.

To summarize, it is very important to remember that CRP levels greater than 5 to 10 mg/L are likely to be associated with clinically significant acute or chronic inflammatory disease (e.g., bacterial infection or malignancy), which should be identified and treated.

Risk of Cardiovascular Disease. Epidemiological studies have demonstrated that increased serum CRP concentrations are positively associated with risk of future coronary events, such as coronary artery disease, cerebrovascular disease, or peripheral arterial disease, and levels may be combined with cholesterol markers in estimating risk[89] (see Chapters 26 and 44). The use of CRP for these purposes requires the use of "high-sensitivity" CRP assays (hs-CRP) having detection limits less than 0.3 mg/L. However, some studies have shown no improvement in risk prediction by adding CRP.[108] It is likely that the increased levels reflect low-grade, chronic intimal inflammation rather than a direct role for CRP in atherogenesis.

Laboratory Considerations

Because CRP is normally present in plasma at a concentration of less than 5 mg/L (50 µg/dL), highly sensitive immunochemical methods are required for its quantification. Current assays include particle-enhanced immunoturbidimetry or nephelometry, immunofluorescence, and immunochemiluminescence. CRP migrates on cellulose acetate or agarose gel electrophoresis anywhere from the slow-γ to mid-β regions, depending upon the calcium ion content of the buffer.

Reference Interval

The reference interval for CRP in adults is 1 < 5 mg/L (500 µg/dL).[28]

Ceruloplasmin

Ceruloplasmin (Cp) is an α_2-globulin that contains approximately 95% of the total copper found in serum. Each molecule of Cp contains six to eight copper atoms, most of which are tightly bound. The high content of copper ions gives Cp a beautiful blue color (L. *caeruleus* = blue). When Cp levels are greatly elevated, as in pregnancy, or the normal yellow pigments of plasma are decreased, as in active rheumatoid arthritis, plasma may have a green tint. Cp can also bind, and perhaps transport, other divalent cations, such as magnesium.

Biochemistry

Ceruloplasmin has a single polypeptide chain with 1046 amino acids and three glucosamine-linked oligosaccharide side chains, with a total carbohydrate content of 8% to 9.5%. The peptide chain and carbohydrate together result in a mean molecular mass of 132 kDa. Cp in serum shows significant size and charge heterogeneity because of differences in glycosylation, the number of copper atoms present, peptide chain variations secondary to alternative DNA splicing, and polymerization. In addition, it is very susceptible to proteolysis, both in vivo and in vitro, by many proteases, including trypsin, plasmin, leukocyte elastase, and a plasma metalloproteinase. This lability accounts for earlier reports of more than one peptide chain.

Ceruloplasmin is synthesized primarily by the hepatic parenchymal cells, with small amounts synthesized by macrophages and lymphocytes. The peptide chain is formed first, then copper is added from an intracellular ATPase (absent in Wilson's disease; see later in this chapter); Cu^+-glutathione complexes may be involved in the transfer. The CHO side chains are subsequently added in the endoplasmic reticulum. Copper appears to be essential for the normal folding of the polypeptide chain and possibly for normal CHO side chain attachment. However, apoCp is synthesized even in the absence of copper or the ATPase; most is degraded intracellularly, but moderate amounts are released into the circulation, where apoCp has a very short half-life.

Sialic acid is slowly removed from circulating Cp by tissue and plasma neuraminidases, resulting in exposure of the penterminal galactose residue on the carbohydrate side chains. Once a critical number of galactose residues are exposed, the protein is rapidly removed by galactose receptors of the hepatic parenchymal cells and catabolized. Markedly increased catabolism by this route may result in deposition of excessive copper in the liver. The normal plasma half-life of intact, holoCp (copper replete) is 4 to 5 days, whereas that of apoCp is a few hours and that of desialylated Cp a few minutes.

Function

The primary physiological role of Cp involves plasma redox reactions. It can function either as an oxidant or an antioxidant depending on other factors, such as the presence of free ferric ions and ferritin binding sites. Acting as a ferroxidase, Cp is vitally important in regulating the ionic state of iron in particular, oxidizing Fe^{2+} to Fe^{3+} (Figure 20-4). It thus permits the incorporation of iron into transferrin without the formation of toxic iron products. Under physiological

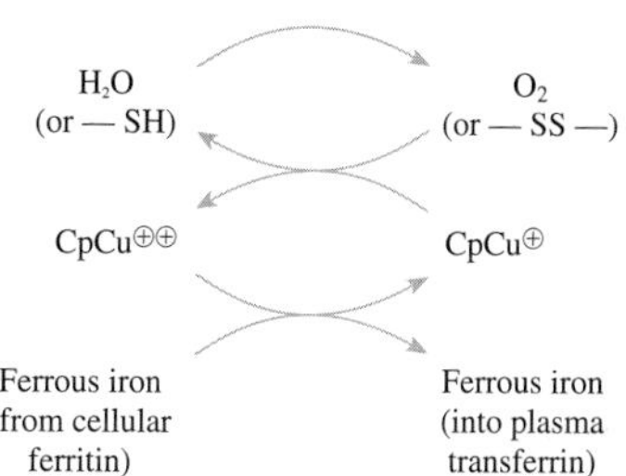

Figure 20-4 Proposed function of ceruloplasmin copper ($CpCu^{2+}$) as a proton (hydrogen ion) recipient from cellular ferrous iron. The resulting oxidation of Fe^{2+} to the ferric state permits its binding and transport by plasma transferrin. $CpCu^{+}$ is oxidized (regenerated to $CpCu^{2+}$) by reaction with oxygen, oxidized thiol groups, or other oxidizing substances. *(Modified from Johnson AM. Ceruloplasmin. In: Ritchie RF, Navolotskaia O, editors. Serum proteins in clinical medicine. Vol. I: Laboratory section. Scarborough, ME: Foundation for Blood Research, 1996:13.01-13.03.)*

conditions, Cp is also important in the control of membrane lipid oxidation—probably by direct oxidation of cations—thus preventing their catalysis of lipid peroxidation. At the same time, in the presence of superoxide (e.g., in inflamed vascular endothelium), Cp is a major contributor to low-density lipoprotein (LDL) oxidation.[37] Its role in oxidation of 6-hydroxydopamine may be important in brain function, perhaps explaining the early neurological symptoms seen in severe genetic deficiency.[36]

Cp may transport small amounts of copper to tissue, which have separate membrane receptors for Cp- and albumin-bound copper. The importance of Cp in transport is debated, however, because turnover of Cp copper is very slow and individuals with genetic deficiency of Cp have no problems related to copper transport (see later in this chapter). Albumin and transcuprein are the major copper transport proteins, especially following absorption from the intestinal tract.

Clinical Significance

Cp is most often measured as a screening test for Wilson's disease. Several other factors, including diet, hormone levels, and other genetic disorders, also influence plasma levels. Immunochemical assays may not distinguish between the active, copper-replete holoCp and apoCp, which is released into the circulation in most of the disorders associated with low total Cp levels. Functional assays might therefore be helpful in clinical circumstances, but they are more difficult to perform and less specific.

Increased Plasma Levels. Cp levels are increased as a result of primary and secondary elevations.

Primary (Genetic) Elevation. EL mice have a Cp gene duplication that results in elevated Cp levels by both immunochemical and copper oxidase methods of assay.[39] Affected mice have an epileptic disorder similar to human complex partial seizures, possibly because of Cp-induced neuronal membrane depolarization. Conversely, rats deficient in copper and Cp have diminished auditory startle responses.[85] There are no published reports of Cp levels in human patients with seizure disorders.

Secondary Elevations. Synthesis of Cp is increased modestly in the APR. The increase occurs relatively slowly, peaking at 4 to 20 days after a single, acute insult. Synthesis is stimulated markedly by estrogens, with moderate increases seen in women taking estrogen-containing medications and larger increases during pregnancy.

Decreased Plasma Levels. Cp levels are decreased as a result of various primary and secondary deficiencies.

Primary (Genetic) Deficiency. Inherited deficiency of Cp has been reported in several families. Clinical findings in homozygous individuals include blepharospasm, retinal degeneration, diabetes mellitus, dementia, and extrapyramidal tract disorders. No patients have shown excessive tissue copper, but all have had increased tissue iron stores and decreased serum iron. This argues strongly for the hypothesis that the primary physiological role of Cp is for maintaining normal iron transport and metabolism. Serum iron levels increase for several hours following infusion of fresh frozen plasma. The clinical picture is similar to that of hereditary hemochromatosis, although CNS effects are greater and no patients to date have shown the arthritis and cardiomyopathy commonly seen in hereditary hemochromatosis.[127,128]

Secondary Deficiency. Low plasma Cp levels caused by a lack of incorporation of Cu^{2+} into the molecule during synthesis are much more common than primary deficiency. Secondary deficiency may be due to dietary Cu^{2+} insufficiency (including malabsorption), inability to release Cu^{2+} from the gastrointestinal epithelium into the circulation, or inability to insert Cu^{2+} into the developing Cp molecule. In all cases, apoCp (noncopper containing) is still synthesized by the hepatic parenchymal cells. However, as mentioned previously, most apoCp is catabolized intracellularly before release into the plasma, and plasma apoCp has a much shorter half-life than does holoCp. Levels may also be low in blood loss or in gastrointestinal or renal protein-losing syndromes.

Dietary Cp deficiency is due to nutritional copper deficiency, with secondarily low levels of Cp, and is associated with neutropenia, thrombocytopenia, low serum iron, and hypochromic, normocytic, or macrocytic anemia unresponsive to iron therapy. The deficiency may be due to inadequate dietary intake, long-term parenteral nutrition without copper supplementation, malabsorption of any cause, penicillamine therapy, or combinations of these. Therapy includes dietary change or copper supplementation, plus treatment of the primary cause of malabsorption if present.

Menkes' disease is an X-linked inherited disorder in which dietary copper is absorbed from the gastrointestinal tract but cannot be transported to the vascular space because of the genetic absence of an intracellular ATPase.[113] Hence, copper is not available to the liver for incorporation into Cp. Affected infants manifest abnormal hair (sparse, brittle, and kinky), growth restriction, and progressive neurological degeneration, with death occurring during the first few years of life if untreated. Subcutaneous injections of copper histidine partially reverse the deleterious effects if started early in life; some residual Menkes' ATPase activity (i.e., incomplete deficiency) may be necessary for this response, however. Patients with deficient gastrointestinal *and* blood-brain barrier transport of copper have also been described; the neurological symptoms in these patients are not reversed by copper therapy.[38] The gene for Menkes' disease is on chromosome Xq13.3-21.2.

Wilson's disease, or hepatolenticular degeneration, differs from dietary deficiency and Menkes' disease in that body copper is markedly increased and is deposited in tissue, including the hepatic parenchymal cells, the brain, and the periphery of the iris (resulting in the characteristic Kayser-Fleischer rings). Copper is absorbed and transported to the liver, but the absence of a hepatocellular P type of ATPase (similar to that missing in Menkes' disease) prevents incorporation of copper into Cp. The gene for this ATPase is on chromosome 13q14.3.[8]

Symptoms in patients with Wilson's disease usually begin in the second or third decade of life, but may be earlier or later. However, mutations that completely destroy gene function may be associated with onset of liver disease as early as 3 years of age. The initial clinical presentation may be hepatic, with presentation similar to acute hepatitis or to chronic active hepatitis; neurological (e.g., clumsiness, dysarthria, ataxia, and tremors); renal (renal tubular acidosis with aminoaciduria); or, less commonly, hematological, with hemolysis secondary to acute release of free copper from tissue and subsequent oxidation of erythrocyte membranes. The hepatic, and possibly CNS, damage may also be secondary to copper-induced oxidative damage to mitochondrial membranes.[99] Hepatic levels of Cp messenger ribonucleic acid (mRNA) are reduced in patients with Wilson's disease, probably secondary to inhibition of transcription by increased intracellular levels of apoCp.[8]

Most patients with Wilson's disease have plasma Cp levels below 0.1 g/L (10 mg/dL), and the mean Cp level in these patients is ~50 mg/L (5 mg/dL). However, some—particularly those with inflammatory diseases or pregnancy—may have low normal levels. Cp levels are low in 10% to 12% of obligate heterozygotes for the Wilson's disease gene and normal in the rest, possibly because of different mutations. Low Cp levels are also seen in other disorders, as noted earlier. Clinical diagnosis of Wilson's disease therefore requires presence of the classical signs of the disease, documentation of copper excess, or both. Slit-lamp examination for Kayser-Fleischer rings, assays of urine copper, and, if these are not diagnostic, liver biopsy for quantitative copper assay may be required for definitive diagnosis. DNA analysis also permits definitive diagnosis in most cases, even in the absence of clinical abnormalities.

Genetic Aspects

There are several genetic variants or isotypes of Cp, but none of these, except for genetic deficiency (see previous discussion in this chapter), has known clinical significance. The most prevalent isotypes are CpA, CpB, and CpC, which are detectable by electrophoresis followed by either immunofixation or functional staining; CpB is the common, or "wild," isotype. The gene encoding Cp is on chromosome 3q25.[126]

Laboratory Considerations

Because of its lability, Cp may lose some or all of its copper either spontaneously or secondary to oxidation during in vitro storage of serum. In addition, fragmentation of the peptide chain by enzymes in normal serum and leukocytes may result in altered reactivity with antibodies. This lability may create problems with calibrators, controls, and quality control materials and with patient samples. Depending on the degree of degradation and the assay method, apparent levels may increase or decrease. Serum or plasma from patient samples should be separated as soon as possible after collection and either assayed promptly or stored under proper conditions (up to 3 days at 4 °C; longer storage at −70 °C).

Ceruloplasmin can be assayed immunochemically or functionally (copper oxidase activity). The latter assays measure only native, copper-containing Cp, whereas the former measure both the intact molecule and, to varying degrees, apoCp and proteolytic fragments.

Reference Intervals

Ceruloplasmin is undetectable before 20 weeks of gestation. Plasma levels then gradually rise by term to 25% to 40% of the normal adult level and by 6 months of age to nearly adult levels (Table 20-6). Levels at birth do not correlate with birth

TABLE 20-6 Plasma Ceruloplasmin Reference Intervals*

Age	Reference Interval (mg/L)	
Cord (term)	50-330	
Birth-4 mo	150-560	
5-6 mo	260-830	
7-36 mo	310-900	
4-12 yr	250-450	
	Male	**Female**
13-19 yr	150-370	220-500
Adults	220-400	250-600 (No OC)
		270-660 (OC; estrogens)
		300-1200 (Pregnant†)

OC, Oral contraceptives.
*Converted to CRM 470 values from multiple references.
†Second and third trimesters; levels increase with increasing gestational age.

weight, and copper supplementation does not increase levels in the first few weeks of life; the low levels are probably secondary to immaturity of the fetal and neonatal liver. The reference interval for neonates is 0.19 to 0.67 g/L.

Serum Cp levels reach a maximum at 2 or 3 years of age, then fall slowly until the adolescent years, when adult levels are reached. Levels are higher in women during their menstrual years (and longer if estrogen replacement therapy is used). There appears to be a genetic influence on synthetic rates; levels within families vary less than do those among families. The recommended interim reference interval for all adults of both sexes, based on CRM 470, is 0.2 to 0.6 g/L (20 to 60 mg/dL).[28]

Haptoglobin

Hp is an α_2-glycoprotein that irreversibly binds hemoglobin (G. *haptein* = to bind).

Biochemistry

Haptoglobin is synthesized by the hepatic parenchymal cells and is composed of four peptide chains linked by disulfide bonds into two pairs, an $(\alpha\beta)_2$ configuration similar to that of hemoglobin. The two chains are synthesized together and then separated by cleavage at an arginine residue. The Hp α-chain exists in two common genetically determined molecular forms, monomeric (α^1) and partially dimeric (α^2; probably the result of incomplete genetic crossover). In addition, one variant has partial triplication. The monomeric Hp α^1-chain has 83 amino acid residues and is partly homologous to kringle 5 of plasminogen; the β-chain, with 245 amino acid residues plus carbohydrate side chains, is related to the serine proteases. The molecular mass of the Hp 1-1 isotype, $(\alpha^1\beta)_2$, is approximately 85 kDa.

During extracellular hemolysis, hemoglobin is released from the erythrocytes, and the hemoglobin tetramers separate into $\alpha\beta$ dimers at the low local concentration of hemoglobin. The free dimers bind almost immediately to free Hp. Each Hp monomer can bind up to two hemoglobin $\alpha\beta$ dimers, the equivalent to one intact hemoglobin molecule; the Hp β-chain binds to hemoglobin α-chains. Hp-hemoglobin complexes are large enough to prevent, or greatly reduce, renal loss of hemoglobin and its iron. The complexes are very rapidly removed by the hepatic Kupffer cells and by macrophages, via CD163 receptors, where the proteins are degraded and the iron and amino acids are reused. Hp is therefore a "suicidal" protein and not strictly a carrier or transport protein. The normal plasma half-life of Hp is approximately 5.5 days.

Function

The primary functions of Hp were initially thought to be the preservation of iron and the prevention of possible damage to the renal tubules by excreted hemoglobin. However, Hp-hemoglobin complexes and free Hp itself also play significant roles in the control of local inflammatory processes:

1. The Hp-hemoglobin complex is a potent peroxidase, capable of hydrolyzing peroxides released during phagocytosis and killing by polymorphonuclear leukocytes at sites of inflammation; complexing of hemoglobin by Hp prevents lipid peroxidation.
2. Hp inhibits cathepsin B released by the phagocytes and binds to and modulates proliferation or activity of lymphocytes, monocytes, and granulocytes, possibly by binding to integrins.
3. Hp is a natural bacteriostatic agent in infection with iron-requiring bacteria, such as *Escherichia coli,* probably by preventing the use of hemoglobin iron by these organisms.
4. Hp synthesis is stimulated by inflammation but not by hemolysis (and depletion of Hp), suggesting teleologically that the role of Hp in local inflammation may be its primary role and function.

Other proposed functions for Hp or the Hp-hemoglobin complex include inhibition of nitric oxide and prostaglandin synthesis, angiogenesis, and control of lymphocyte and neutrophil function. All of these may be relevant to the control of inflammation.

Clinical Significance

Under normal circumstances, approximately 1% of circulating red blood cells are removed from the circulation or destroyed intravascularly each day. An increase to only 2% destruction per day will completely deplete plasma Hp in the absence of a stimulus to production, such as acute inflammation or corticosteroid therapy.

Once Hp is depleted, further hemolysis may be associated with other phenomena. First, hemoglobin may be oxidized to methemoglobin, followed by dissociation of metheme from globin. Metheme is insoluble but can bind to either hemopexin (high affinity) or albumin (low affinity), keeping it in solution. Hemopexin-heme complexes are removed by the reticuloendothelial system (as with Hp-hemoglobin complexes, but more slowly), with subsequent intracellular catabolism of the complex and a decrease in the hemopexin level in plasma.[124] Hemopexin synthesis is relatively unaffected by other factors (such as estrogen) that decrease Hp synthesis, so low values usually reflect fairly severe or prolonged hemolysis. Like Hp, it is a positive (but weak) APR. Disorders with both ineffective hematopoiesis and peripheral or splenic lysis of abnormal cells, including some hemoglobinopathies (e.g., sickle cell disease), are associated with chronic depletion of Hp and hemopexin.[124] Albumin also binds heme, but with lower affinity than hemopexin, to form methemalbumin. Because of the higher affinities of hemoglobin for Hp and of hemopexin for heme, methemalbumin may not be seen until Hp and hemopexin are depleted.

Alternatively, free $\alpha\beta$ dimers may pass through the glomerular filter into the urine. The dimers are normally reabsorbed and catabolized by the proximal tubules and catabolized, with the iron incorporated into cellular ferritin and hemosiderin. Iron may reach toxic levels in the tubular

TABLE 20-7 Correlation of Haptoglobin and α_1-Acid Glycoprotein (Orosomucoid) Changes With Hormonal Effects and Diseases

Haptoglobin	α_1-Acid Glycoprotein	Usual Interpretation
N	*N*	Normal
↑	↑	Acute phase response; corticosteroid or androgen effect
↓	*N*	Hemolysis; hepatocellular disease (with increased red blood cell turnover)
↓	↑	Hemolysis plus acute phase response, corticosteroid therapy, or both
↓	↓	Estrogen effect; hepatocellular disease

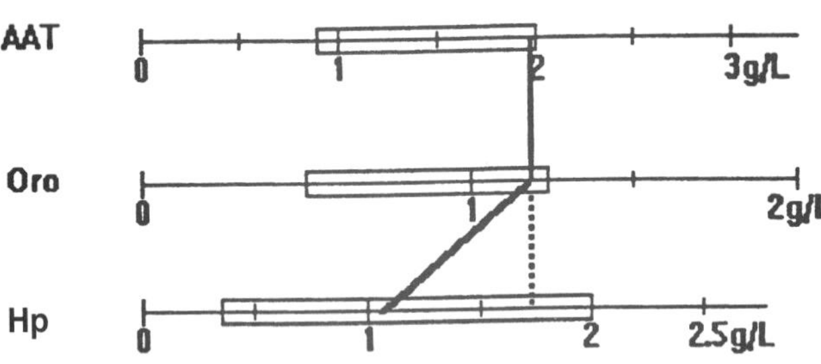

Figure 20-5 Protein profile of α_1-antitrypsin (AAT), α_1-acid glycoprotein (Oro), and haptoglobin (Hp) in a hypothetical individual with in vivo hemolysis. The jagged vertical line connects the concentration values for the proteins.

cells, which may slough into the excreted urine. If the ability of the proximal tubules to reabsorb is exceeded, or if significant damage has occurred, free hemoglobin is seen in the excreted urine. Hemoglobinuria may also be secondary to renal or postrenal bleeding, which must be excluded in the evaluation of hemoglobinuria.

Thus Hp depletion is usually the most sensitive laboratory indicator of hemolysis, followed by hemopexin depletion and finally by the presence of methemalbuminemia, hemoglobinuria, or both. However, Hp levels are influenced by several other factors, as discussed later. It is recommended that Hp always be assayed in association with AAG (orosomucoid), because the other factors—with the exception of protein-losing syndromes—influence the levels of both proteins in parallel (Table 20-7, Figure 20-5). If a patient has a normal Hp level but high AAG level, the possibility of hemolysis plus either corticosteroid therapy or an APR must be considered.

As a result of its role in hemoglobin metabolism, Hp assays are used primarily to screen for, or to follow the course of, hemolytic disorders.

Increased Plasma Levels. Increased levels of Hp are seen in the APR and protein-losing syndromes and associated with corticosteroid effects.

Acute Phase Response. Hp synthesis is increased in the presence of acute inflammatory processes, tissue necrosis, or malignancy. Increased plasma levels are seen approximately 4 to 6 days after the initiation of these processes and take about 2 weeks to fall to normal after the removal of the stimulating factors. Stimulation of synthesis is mediated by cytokines, particularly IL-6.

Protein-Losing Syndromes (in Association with Hp 2-1 or 2-2 Phenotypes). Most protein-losing syndromes, such as the nephrotic syndrome, are associated with sieving loss of plasma proteins, with excretion inversely proportional to the effective diameter of the protein (Stokes radius). There is a concomitant, compensatory increase in synthesis of most if not all proteins synthesized in the liver, including Hp. Hp 1-1 is relatively small and is lost in approximately the same proportion as albumin. However, the 2-1 and 2-2 variants are large; these are retained, and elevated concentrations are usually seen unless hemolysis is also present.

Corticosteroid Effects. Glucocorticoids, such as cortisol (endogenous) and dexamethasone (exogenous), and androgens are associated with increased synthesis of Hp and secondarily elevated plasma levels. Dexamethasone acts, at least in vitro, by enhancing the response of synthesis to interleukins rather than by a direct effect on synthesis.

Decreased Plasma Levels. Decreased levels of Hp are seen with genetic deficiency, hemolytic disease, ineffective erythropoiesis, estrogens, and hepatocellular disease and in neonates.

Genetic Deficiency. Genetic absence (anhaptoglobinemia, or *Hp0*) and hypohaptoglobinemia have been reported in many populations, especially in those of African extraction. However, most reports have been in populations with high rates of hemolytic disease, either genetic (e.g., hemoglobinopathies and glucose-6-phosphatase deficiency) or acquired (e.g., malaria). True *Hp0* (total deficiency) is rare in most if not all populations. More commonly, genetic hypohaptoglobinemia is associated with very low, but phenotypable, levels of Hp probably secondary to altered control of gene transcription rather than a defect in the *Hp* gene itself.

Hemolytic Disease and Ineffective Erythropoiesis. As discussed previously, Hp levels are a sensitive indicator of in vivo hemolysis, as long as other causes of decreased levels are excluded. Splenomegaly and ineffective hematopoiesis are also associated with decreased levels. The latter, with increased hemolysis of red cells and their precursors in the bone marrow space, is seen in megaloblastic anemias (vitamin B_{12} or folate deficiency) and in many hemoglobinopathies.

Estrogens. Either endogenous or exogenous estrogens (e.g., in late pregnancy and in oral contraceptive therapy) result in decreased Hp synthesis and plasma levels.

Hepatocellular Disease. Most forms of acute or chronic hepatocellular disease, including acute viral hepatitis and cirrhosis with jaundice, are associated with decreased levels of Hp, possibly caused in part by altered estrogen metabolism. Increased red cell breakdown secondary to erythrocyte membrane lipid alterations may also play a role, although this has never been documented with turnover studies. In contrast, biliary obstruction is also associated with significant lipid alterations but with increased Hp levels, in the absence of severe hepatocellular disease.

Newborn Period. Hp is absent or present in very low concentration in most newborn infants as a result of hepatic immaturity. In addition, hemopexin levels in newborns are on average one fifth of adult levels. The absence of Hp and hemopexin in the normal fetus may prevent in utero stimulation of the hepatic excretory mechanisms for bilirubin (fetal bilirubin is normally excreted by the placenta and the maternal liver).

Genetic Aspects

The gene encoding Hp is on chromosome 16 at band q22. Both chains are polymorphic, but the α-chain accounts for the commonly recognized isotypes. As mentioned previously, the α-chains exist in different genetically determined sizes, with α^1 the basic monomer. The two common α^1 variants, α^{1F} and α^{1S}, differ only in one amino acid at position 54 (lysine in α^{1F} and glutamic acid in α^{1S}). Of the two, α^{1S} is the more frequent.

The α^2 variants are products of partial gene duplication, probably from unequal crossing over,[98] and are nearly twice the length of the α^1 variants (142 versus 83 amino acid residues). The three possible α^2 products (α^{2FF}, α^{2FS}, and α^{2SS}) have all been described, with α^{2FS} the most common in white populations. Homozygosity for the α^1 alleles results in the phenotype Hp 1-1, with a molecular mass of 85 kDa. Heterozygosity for α^2 and α^1 results in Hp 2-1 (molecular mass of the monomer = 120 kDa), and homozygosity for α^2 in Hp 2-2 (160 kDa). The latter two phenotypes polymerize to form a series of polymers, with molecular masses up to at least 1000 kDa; the Hp 2-2 polymers differ by increments of one $\alpha^2\beta$ dimer (~57.3 kDa). As a result, phenotyping can be performed fairly easily by sieving electrophoresis in starch or polyacrylamide gels (Figure 20-6), usually as Hp-hemoglobin complexes, which can be detected by their peroxidase characteristics. Alternatively, immunofixation can be used after electrophoretic separation. The α-chain subtypes (α^{1S}, α^{1F}, α^{2FF}, α^{2FS}, and α^{2SS}) are detected by isoelectric focusing of reduced, neuraminidase-treated serum or plasma, followed by blotting onto nitrocellulose membranes and immunoperoxidase staining.

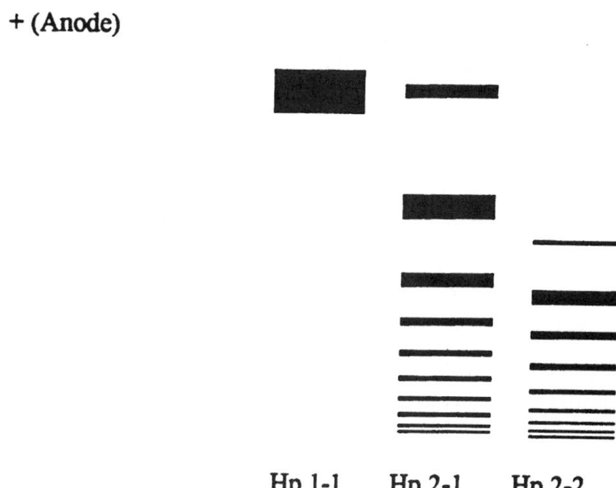

Figure 20-6 The common phenotypes of haptoglobin, as shown by sieving gel electrophoresis of haptoglobin-hemoglobin complexes.

Less common variants include Hp Johnson, in which there is triplication of a portion of the α-chain, and Hp 2-1Mod, a 2-1 phenotype in which there is greatly reduced production in α^2-chains. As mentioned previously, true genetic anhaptoglobinemia (Hp0) is rare; individuals with ring chromosome 16 have terminal deletions of the Hp gene and therefore do have true deficiency. Very low levels on a genetic basis are more commonly caused by decreased transcription, with resulting hypohaptoglobinemia.

The Hp 2-2 phenotype is associated with higher serum iron, ferritin, and transferrin saturation, perhaps because of its preferential uptake by CD163 receptors.[30] Other possible clinical associations of the Hp polymorphism have been reviewed by Langlois and Delanghe.[63]

Laboratory Considerations

Hp and AMG together with Hb-hemoglobin complexes (usually from in vitro hemolysis) migrate more cathodally (Figure 20-6). Traditionally, Hp was measured by assaying peroxidase activity after mixing serum with an excess of free hemoglobin, the so-called hemoglobin binding capacity (BC). On average, [Hp] = [Hp BC] × 1.5; approximately 1 mg hemoglobin is bound by 1.5 mg Hp, depending on the phenotype.

Immunochemical methods are also used for clinical assays because they are rapid and easily automated. Because of the differences in molecular size and corresponding diffusion rates, gel diffusion techniques, such as radial immunodiffusion (RID) require correction for phenotype and are therefore time consuming and inconvenient. Immunoassays in solution, such as nephelometry and turbidimetry, are influenced slightly by size as well, but the differences are relatively insignificant.

Reference Intervals

The recommended interim reference interval for Hp in serum for adults is 0.3 to 2.0 g/L (30 to 200 mg/dL).[28] As noted previously, levels are low to absent in the neonatal period and are low in women who are either pregnant or on exogenous estrogen therapy, including oral contraceptives. For children the reference interval is approximately 0.2 to 1.6 g/L.

Transferrin

Transferrin (originally named *siderophilin*) is the principal plasma transport protein for iron (Fe^{3+}); see Chapter 31.

Biochemistry

Transferrin (Tf) has a molecular weight of approximately 79.6 kDa, including 5.5% carbohydrate. It is a single polypeptide chain, with the carbohydrate moieties in the *C*-terminal domain and two homologous domains, each containing an Fe^{3+} binding site.[110] It is synthesized almost exclusively in the liver, with lesser amounts in the choroid plexus of the brain. Plasma levels are regulated primarily by availability of iron; in iron deficiency, plasma Tf levels rise and, on successful treatment with iron, return to normal. Tf has a half-life of approximately 8 to 10 days. The primary route of catabolism is not known, but some Tf is lost from the body in exfoliated intestinal mucosal cells and other cells. As with albumin, about half of Tf exists outside the vascular compartment in body fluids, such as lymph and CSF.

Tf reversibly binds numerous polycations—iron, copper, zinc, cobalt, and calcium—although only iron appears to have physiological significance. One molecule of Tf binds two ferric ions and an associated anion, usually bicarbonate. There are two binding sites for iron with different affinities; both are strong at physiological pH but decrease with decreasing pH. The iron-Tf complex has an absorbance maximum at 470 nm. Cp is necessary for the oxidation of Fe^{2+} to Fe^{3+} as a preliminary step for binding of Fe^{3+} to Tf.

Function

Iron metabolism is discussed in Chapter 31; thus only a brief discussion of the role of Tf is presented here. Apotransferrin binds iron absorbed from the intestine or released from catabolism of hemoglobin. The iron is then transported to storage sites, such as the liver and reticuloendothelial system, and to sites of synthesis of iron-containing compounds, especially the erythropoietic tissue (for hemoglobin synthesis). However, virtually every cell type has surface receptors for Tf.[64] The receptors have a much higher affinity for Tf-Fe^{3+} than for apotransferrin (Tf without iron). After binding, the Tf-Fe^{+3}-receptor complex is internalized into a caltherin-coated endosome that lowers the internal pH, resulting in release of iron from Tf. The free ferric iron, which is cytotoxic, is reduced and incorporated into ferritin and hemosiderin, for eventual synthesis of compounds, such as hemoglobin, myoglobin, and cytochromes. The receptor-apoTf complex is recycled to the cell surface where the apoTf is released and recycled, making the receptor available again for binding.

Clinical Significance

Increased Plasma Levels. Evaluation of plasma Tf levels is useful in the differential diagnosis of hypochromic microcytic anemia and for monitoring treatment. In iron deficiency, Tf is increased, but the protein is less saturated with iron. On the other hand, if the anemia is due to a failure to incorporate iron into erythrocytes (e.g., with chronic inflammatory disease), the Tf level may be normal or low, but the protein is normally saturated with iron. In iron overload (e.g., hereditary hemochromatosis), Tf concentration is normal, but saturation (normally 30% to 38%) exceeds 55% and may be as great as 100%. Assays of soluble transferrin receptor (sTfR) are useful in differentiating the various causes of microcytic anemia; if tissue iron deficiency is present, the affected cells increase their synthesis of transferrin receptors. Shedding of partial molecules into plasma, in direct proportion to the amount of receptor, is reflected by increased levels of sTfR. Thus levels are high in iron deficiency but normal in other disorders associated with microcytic anemia (e.g., partial α-thalassemia and inflammation). Although assays for sTfR are available, international standardization is needed.

High levels of Tf are also seen in pregnancy and during estrogen administration.

Decreased Plasma Levels. Transferrin is a negative APR; the most common cause of low levels is inflammation or malignancy. Decreased synthesis is seen with chronic liver disease and malnutrition (see Chapter 47). Protein loss, as in the nephrotic syndrome or protein-losing enteropathies, also results in low levels. In hereditary atransferrinemia, a very low level of Tf is accompanied by iron overload but severe hypochromic anemia resistant to iron therapy.

Carbohydrate-Deficient Transferrin (CDT). The glycosylation of transferrin (and of other glycoproteins) may be decreased or absent in certain circumstances. Congenital disorders of glycosylation, or the carbohydrate-deficient glycoprotein syndromes, are increasingly recognized in patients; they may be associated with defects of any of at least 9 genes and result in varying multisystem dysfunction, usually with brain involvement.[53]

CDT is also assayed extensively, especially in Europe, for detection of alcohol abuse. Other proteins, such as α_1-acid glycoprotein, are carbohydrate deficient in this case as well. The "gold standard" for assessment is HPLC, although both capillary electrophoresis and immunoassays are more commonly used in clinical settings. Immunoassays in particular are poorly standardized, both qualitatively and quantitatively; positive tests should be confirmed by an alternative method.[4] Genetic variants of Tf may also complicate interpretation of results.

Genetic Aspects

The gene coding for Tf is on chromosome 3q21-25. At least 22 genetic variants of Tf have been identified (pI 5.5-5.9), with heterozygosity present in up to 25% of some populations. The wild type is Tf C; the most common anodal and cathodal variants are Tf B and Tf C, respectively. The variants all bind iron and have no biological significance except for the rare congenital defect, atransferrinemia. However, they may be misinterpreted as M-components or as CDT.

Laboratory Considerations

Because of the convenience of simultaneous measurement of serum iron and total iron binding capacity (TIBC) and the desirability of knowing percent saturation of Tf (see Chapter 31), Tf is sometimes estimated indirectly from the TIBC value by the following equation:

$$\text{Tf, mg/dL} = 0.70 \times \text{TIBC, } \mu\text{g/dL}$$

or

$$\text{TIBC} = 1.43 \times \text{Tf}$$

This procedure overestimates the Tf concentration by 16% to 20% because it assumes that all plasma iron is bound to Tf. When Tf is more than half saturated (e.g., in hereditary hemochromatosis), some of the iron is bound to other plasma proteins including albumin.

Transferrin is commonly assayed by immunochemical methods, including immunoturbidimetry and immunonephelometry. It migrates in the β_1 region on routine serum electrophoresis; as noted previously, genetic variants may cause problems in interpretation of these patterns.

Reference Intervals

Serum reference intervals based on CRM 470[28] are as follows:

	g/L	mg/dL
Newborn	1.17-2.50	117-250
Adults (20-60 yr)	2.0-3.6	200-360
>60 yr	1.6-3.4	160-340

Transthyretin (Prealbumin) and Retinol-Binding Protein

Transthyretin (prealbumin) and retinol-binding protein (RBP) are transport proteins that migrate together as a 1:1 molecular complex. Transthyretin was originally named prealbumin because of its electrophoretic mobility; it was renamed in 1981 to reflect its binding and transport of both thyroid hormones (thyroxine and triiodothyronine) and RBP.

Biochemistry and Function

Transthyretin (TTR) is a nonglycosylated protein (MW 34.98 kDa) composed of four identical subunits, noncovalently bound to form a hollow core containing the T_3- and T_4-binding sites. It binds and transports approximately 10% of both hormones, with T_3 with higher affinity. (Thyroxine-binding globulin transports approximately 70%, and albumin binds the "overflow" with low affinity.) Because of negative cooperativity, TTR binding of the first hormone molecule decreases the binding affinity of the second, so only one site is normally occupied. TTR is synthesized in the liver and to a lesser extent in the choroid plexus of the CNS.[95] Its synthesis is stimulated by glucocorticosteroid hormones, androgens, and many nonsteroidal antiinflammatory drugs (NSAIDs, including aspirin).

Retinol-binding protein is a small (21 kDa), monomeric transport protein for all *trans* retinol, the physiologically active, alcoholic form of vitamin A.[100] It is synthesized in the liver. Zinc is required for synthesis, and retinol is required for its transportation by the Golgi apparatus.[91] When circulating in the plasma, RBP is in a 1:1 complex with transthyretin, preventing RBP from being filtered by the renal glomeruli and stabilizing the binding of retinol, reducing its release to nontarget cells. Uptake of retinol by target cells is followed by dissociation of the transthyretin-RBP complex and clearance of apoRBP (RBP without retinol) from the circulation by the kidneys. It is reabsorbed by the proximal renal tubular cells and catabolized; the amino acids are then reused.

Clinical Significance

If vitamin A intake is adequate and renal function is normal, levels of TTR and RBP tend to rise and fall synchronistically.

Increased Plasma Levels. Serum RBP increases in chronic renal disease, including diabetic nephropathy.[84] Levels are increased with corticosteroid or NSAID therapy and in Hodgkin's disease.

Decreased Plasma Levels. Decreased levels of RBP are seen primarily with liver disease, protein malnutrition, and the APR. Zinc deficiency is characterized by low serum levels of both RBP and vitamin A.

Transthyretin levels are often used as an indicator of protein status because of its relatively short half-life, a high tryptophan content, a high proportion of essential-to-nonessential amino acids, and small pool size. However, it is a negative APR. Levels fall in inflammation and malignancy and in cirrhosis of the liver and protein-losing diseases of the gut or kidneys. Therefore a sensitive acute phase reactant, such as CRP, should always be assayed along with TTR if levels are to be used to estimate nutritional status. History and physical examination are also important aspects of such evaluations.[55]

Genetic Aspects

The gene coding for TTR is on chromosome 18q. More than 50 genetic variants have been described, a few affecting hormone binding. The substitution of threonine for alanine at codon 109 increases the affinity of transthyretin for thyroxine and is associated with euthyroid *hyper*thyroxinemia. Euthyroid *hypo*thyroxinemia associated with genetic deficiency of thyroxine-binding globulin (TBG) is most commonly seen in males; the gene for TBG is on the X chromosome.

Most TTR variants are associated with extracellular deposition of amyloid fibrils in various tissue. These autosomal dominant hereditary amyloidoses include amyloidotic cardiomyopathy, familial amyloidotic polyneuropathy, and senile systemic amyloidosis. There is phenotypic variability (e.g., variable age of onset), suggesting that other factors may influence pathogenesis of the diseases.

The RBP gene is on chromosome 10q.

Laboratory Considerations

TTR migrates anodal to albumin on routine serum electrophoresis; the presence of a TTR band is considered one marker of good quality electrophoresis. However, levels can be only roughly semiquantified from the intensity of the band. RBP dissociates during electrophoresis and migrates anodal to transferrin, but the band is usually too faint to see. Either protein can be quantified by routine immunochemical methods.

Reference Intervals

The adult reference interval for RBP is 3.0 to 6.0 mg/dL. The RBP level at birth is 1.1 to 3.4 mg/dL and at 6 months increases to 1.8 to 5.0 mg/dL.

The adult reference interval for transthyretin, based on CRM 470, is 20 to 40 mg/dL (0.2 to 0.4 g/L).[28] Levels in healthy neonates are approximately half those found in adults, then increase into puberty, with a larger increase in boys than girls, and decrease in both sexes after age 50.[49]

Other Proteinase Inhibitors

Plasma and other body fluids contain a large number of other proteinase inhibitors in addition to AAT and AMG. A few of the more important ones are presented in Table 20-8.

Complement Proteins

The complement system consists of at least 20 proteins, which can be divided into five groups by function:

1. The *classical pathway,* which includes C1, C4, C2, and C3 (in order of activation)
2. The *alternative pathway,* which includes C3, factors B and D, and properdin
3. The *membrane attack complex,* which includes C5 through C9
4. *Inhibitors* and *inactivators* of the above pathways, including C1 inhibitor, factors H and I, and C4-binding protein, or C4bp
5. *Cellular receptors* for activated or cell-bound components.

The fact that both heat-labile and heat-stable fractions of serum are necessary for the in vitro killing of microorganisms and therefore protection of animals against infection was first recognized in the late 1800s. Ehrlich subsequently named the labile fraction *complement* and the stable fraction *amboceptor,* now known to include primarily the immunoglobulins. Ferrata demonstrated in 1907 that the complement fraction included water-soluble *(pseudoglobulin)* and insoluble *(euglobulin)* components, and Pillemer showed in 1941 that complement contained at least four components. After the development of improved methods for protein purification and characterization in the 1960s, Müller-Eberhard and Nelson, among others, expanded the list to include the nine "classical" components. The current nomenclature was adopted by the World Health Organization (WHO) in 1968.

The classical pathway is activated primarily by the antibody antigen complexes. In 1913, Browning and Mackie showed that cobra venom could trigger serum-mediated lysis of erythrocytes in the absence of an antibody. Pillemer described properdin as a component of the antibody-independent complement pathway in 1954, and proposed the name *properdin pathway.* His work was not accepted until the 1960s, however, when the alternative pathway was

TABLE 20-8 Other Protease Inhibitors

Inhibitor	Molecular Mass (kDa)	Physiological Proteases Inhibited	Diseases Associated With Deficiency
α_1-Antichymotrypsin	68	Cathepsin G; mast cell chymase; prostate-specific antigen*	Hepatic cirrhosis; asthma; emphysema
α_2-Antiplasmin	70	Plasmin	Hemorrhage (increases clot lysis)
Antithrombin III†	65	Thrombin	Thromboembolism
C1 inhibitor†	104	C1r, C1s	Hereditary angioedema
Inter-α-trypsin inhibitor	160	Unknown	None known

*Several inhibitors bind and inactivate prostate-specific antigen (PSA), including α_1-antitrypsin, α_2-macroglobulin, and α_2-antiplasmin. α_1-Antichymotrypsin complexes are usually the predominant ones in serum or plasma, probably because of rapid clearance of the others. Levels of complexed PSA are increased in most patients with prostatic cancer, compared with normal individuals or those with benign prostatic hypertrophy.

†Quantitative and qualitative (functional) deficiencies reported.

shown unequivocally to exist and to be activated by bacterial lipopolysaccharides and cellular proteases or cobra venom. Activation of the classical pathway through C3 also activates the alternative pathway, which then acts to amplify the production of effector molecules.

Any of several mechanisms can activate complement, including continuous and spontaneous "tickover," activation of the classical pathway (e.g., by the antigen antibody complexes or CRP), activation of the alternative pathway, and action of proteases released by leukocytes and other inflammatory cells. The common step involved in all of these is the conversion of C3 to C3b, as shown in Figure 20-7. This figure also demonstrates the sites of action of the inhibitors and inactivators of complement (shown in gray shading), which prevent excessive or continuous depletion of the complement components in addition to controlling complement activity in sites of inflammation.

During activation, many of the complement components are enzymatically cleaved into two fragments, in general a larger fragment plus a smaller fragment that may have activity in chemotaxis, vascular permeability, and the like (see discussion below). The larger fragments are designated by a lowercase *b* and the smaller ones by a lowercase *a*. The larger fragments usually contain a binding site for membranes, immune complexes, and the like, plus in many cases an enzymatic site that can then activate the next component(s). Thus the active cell-bound fragment of C3 is C3b, whereas the anaphylatoxic peptide C3a is released into the surrounding fluid. Inactivated fragments are designated by the letter *i* (e.g., C3bi) or otherwise; for example, the persisting membrane-bound portion of C3b after inactivation is called C3d, and the major fragment after enzymatic cleavage in solution is called C3c. Activated complexes are indicated by a bar over the components (e.g., $\overline{\text{C567}}$).

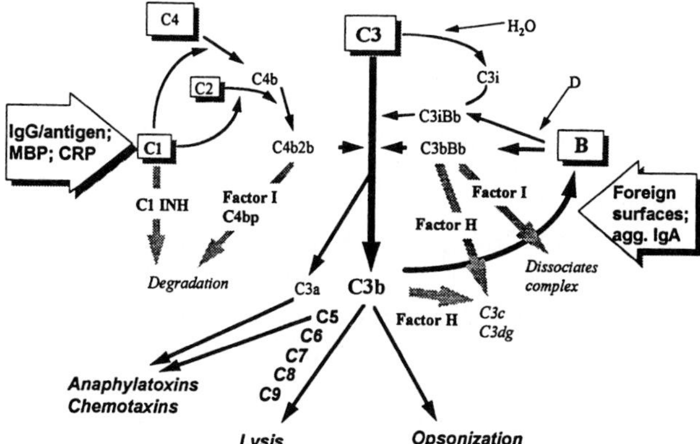

Figure 20-7 Overview of the complement cascades. Activation via the classical pathway is shown on the left and via the alternative pathway on the right. Continuous tickover by hydrolysis of C3 to C3i is shown at the center top. Direct activation of C3 by neutrophil and plasma proteases also may occur. The control mechanisms are shaded. *(Courtesy J.W. Whicher, with modifications.)*

The sequential activation of either the classical or the alternative pathway, with or without complete activation of the membrane-attack complex, produces biological effector molecules that initiate inflammation and facilitate the elimination of the antigens either by lysis (e.g., bacteria) or phagocytosis (e.g., immune complexes). A few of the specific functions of the complement system follow:

1. Some activation fragments, C3a and C5a in particular, act as anaphylatoxins and chemotaxins. Anaphylatoxin activity causes the release of histamine from mast cells, contraction of smooth muscles, and increased vascular permeability. A kinin-like fragment of C2 also increases vascular permeability, as seen in hereditary angioedema. Chemotaxin activity results in migration of phagocytes, such as polymorphonuclear leukocytes and macrophages, into areas of inflammation.
2. Membrane-, immune complex–, or cell-bound C3b acts as an opsonin, resulting in adherence of the substances to which it is bound (e.g., bacteria, viruses, or immune complexes) to specific receptors on phagocytes. They are then ingested and proteolytically destroyed. (The word *opsonin* is derived from a Greek word meaning "preparation of food for ingestion.") This is the primary route of destruction of most foreign agents, including bacteria, yeasts, and viruses, and of complement-mediated hemolysis in human beings.
3. Activation of the membrane-attack complex, through C9, can cause osmotic lysis of cells and viruses. The complete complex appears to be essential primarily for control of *Neisseria* species infections in human beings, because infections with these bacteria are the only significant clinical consequence of genetic deficiencies of the late-acting components.
4. C3d-kallikrein complexes cause the release of polymorphonuclear leukocytes from the bone marrow, increasing their availability.
5. C4b and C3b are important for solubilization of immune complexes (by disrupting lattice formation) and their removal by the reticuloendothelial system.
6. The enzymatic activity of C1s and C2b can activate the clotting, fibrinolytic, and kinin systems and platelets.
7. Interaction with cellular complement receptors is involved in regulation of the antibody response.

Thus complement is one of the major mediators of inflammation. Secondary edema and stasis permit the passage of further antibody, complement, and phagocytes into the extravascular space, aiding in the killing and removal of infectious agents and immune complexes. At the same time, thrombosis as a result of the secondary activation of platelets and the coagulation factors helps to localize infection.

In addition to the inhibitory steps shown in Figure 20-7, complement activity is also controlled by spontaneous hydrolysis of the membrane-binding sites, rapid and spontaneous dissociation of active complexes, and proteolysis by enzymes of the coagulation and fibrinolytic systems and from phagocytic cells.

TABLE 20-9 Clinical Disorders Associated With Inherited Deficiencies of Complement Components

Component	Frequency of Deficiency Gene	Associated Disorders
C1q*	Relatively rare	SLE; DLE; GN
C1r, C1s	Rare	SLE; DLE; infections
C2	≥0.0032	Recurrent infections, vasculitis; SLE, DLE (antinuclear antibody negative); one half of affected individuals are asymptomatic
C3	Rare	Severe and recurrent bacterial infections, especially with encapsulated, pyogenic bacteria (similar to immunoglobulin deficiency)
C4A	0.126	SLE, DLE
C4B	0.132	IgA nephropathy; infections
Combined C4	35% one null, 8-10% two nulls, ~1% three nulls, <0.1% total	Total deficiency: SLE, GN, DLE (many are anti-dsDNA negative but anti-Ro/SSA positive)
C5-C9	Relatively common	Severe or recurrent infections with *Neisseria* sp.
Properdin	Relatively rare	*X*-linked; neisserial infections
Factor D	Rare	Recurrent infections
Factor H or I	Rare	Hypercatabolism of C3 with secondary deficiency; severe and recurrent bacterial infections (as with C3 deficiency); membranoproliferative glomerulonephritis
C1 inhibitor	1/150,000	Hereditary angioedema (autosomal dominant)

Modified from Colten HR, Rosen FS. Complement deficiencies. Annu Rev Immunol 1992;10:809-34.
SLE, Systemic lupus erythematosus (or SLE-like disease); *DLE,* discoid lupus erythematosus; *GN,* glomerulonephritis.
*Both quantitative and qualitative (functional) deficiencies reported.

The clinical importance of the complement system is demonstrated by the disease associations seen in inherited or secondary deficiencies of the various components.[25] Several of the more important of these are listed in Table 20-9. Most of the complement components also demonstrate genetic polymorphism. The genetic aspects of C3 and C4 are discussed in the individual sections following.

The complement components are synthesized primarily by the liver, although small amounts are probably synthesized by monocytes and other cell types.

Complement C3

C3 is the functional link between the classical and alternative pathways of activation and between these pathways and the membrane-attack complex (see Figure 20-7). It is also present in the highest concentration of all the complement components in plasma and acts as a magnification factor. Structurally and genetically, C3 is related to C4, C5, and AMG, all of which contain an internal thiol ester bond that, when activated, can form complexes with membranes and other structures.[104]

Biochemistry

C3 is synthesized as a propolypeptide that is cleaved post-synthetically to two disulfide-linked chains, α (molecular mass, 110 kDa) and β (75 kDa). During the process, an internal thiol ester bond is formed in the α-chain between adjacent glutamic acid and cysteine residues. C3 contains ~3% carbohydrate, added postsynthetically. Most of the plasma C3 is synthesized by the hepatic parenchymal cells, although bacterial endotoxin induces synthesis by monocytes and fibroblasts. Catabolism is primarily by functional activation, followed by hydrolysis.

Activation of either pathway of complement results in the cleavage of C3 to C3b and C3a. The latter is released into the circulation and acts as an anaphylatoxin and a chemotaxin. C3b, with its activated thiol ester, binds to membranes and then activates the subsequent factors in the membrane-attack complex. C3b also acts as an opsonin, binding to receptors on phagocytic cells and resulting in the ingestion of bacteria, viruses, and other foreign particles by these cells.

Function

Low levels of hydrolysis, or tickover, of C3 to C3i occur constantly in plasma. C3i can bind with factor B of the alternative pathway, and the bound factor B may be cleaved by factor D. The resulting C3iBb complex is a weak C3 convertase, resulting in continuous, low-grade activation of C3. Upon activation of the classical pathway, membrane-bound C3b forms similar complexes with factor B; C3bBb is an active C3 convertase. The resulting positive feedback amplifies the complement activity many fold. Fortunately, there are mechanisms that control this; otherwise, C3 may be completely depleted, as seen in hereditary deficiency of factor H or factor I. The control mechanisms include, among others, rapid dissociation of the C3iBb and C3bBb complexes (espe-

TABLE 20-10 Diseases in Which Estimates of Complement Factors May Be Useful for Diagnosis

Disease	Complement Status
Systemic lupus erythematosus	C4 usually low, C3 sometimes low*
Rheumatoid vasculitis	C3 usually low*
Subacute bacterial endocarditis	Both C3* and C4 low
Shunt nephritis	Both C3* and C4 low
Poststreptococcal glomerulonephritis	C3 low,* usually returns to normal in 3 months
Mesangiocapillary glomerulonephritis	C3 low* (persistent), C4 normal
Polymyalgia rheumatica	C3 conversion products found
Mixed cryoglobulinemia	C3 conversion products found
Gram-negative bacteremic shock (early diagnosis)	C3 low,* C4 normal, factor B low
Gram-positive bacteremia	Both C3* and C4 low
Disseminated cytomegalovirus infection	C4 very low, C3* normal or increased

*C3 conversion products are also present.

cially in the presence of factor I), cleavage by proteases, and conversion of C3b to C3c or C3dg by factor H. Conversely, properdin and so-called nephritic factors (autoantibodies) stabilize C3bBb and protect it from the actions of factors H and I.

Clinical Significance

Increased Plasma Levels. Increased levels of C3 are seen with the APR, with biliary obstruction, and with focal glomerulosclerosis.

Acute Phase Response. C3 synthesis is induced by cytokines IL-1, IL-6, and TNFα. Levels rise modestly after trauma or surgery and during inflammatory processes (Table 20-10).

Biliary Obstruction. C3 levels are elevated in biliary obstruction in direct proportion to the level of hyperbilirubinemia.

Focal Glomerulosclerosis. In contrast to nephritic disorders, in which most patients with active disease have low levels of C3 (see later in this chapter), approximately 30% of patients with idiopathic focal glomerulosclerosis have elevated levels, which indicate a favorable prognosis.

Decreased Plasma Levels. Decreased levels of C3 are seen with genetic deficiency, acquired deficiency, and infancy.

Genetic Deficiency. Inherited primary deficiency of C3 is associated with a greatly increased risk for infection, particularly with encapsulated bacteria, similar to the picture seen with the Bruton type of agammaglobulinemia. Deficiency of the inactivators of C3, including factors H and I of the alternative pathway, is associated with severe secondary deficiency of C3 and a similar clinical picture.

Acquired Deficiency. Any cause of increased activation of C3 in vivo is usually associated with decreased plasma or serum concentrations. Disorders include the collagen vascular diseases, such as lupus nephritis, and severe infections. Activation may be through the classical or alternative pathways or both; turnover is increased and extended by the presence of C3 nephritic factor (an autoantibody that protects the alternative pathway's C3bBb convertase from degradation). In addition to increased consumption of C3, acute poststreptococcal glomerulonephritis is associated with decreased synthesis for several weeks after the onset of disease. Sequential levels of C3 may be used to monitor recovery from this disorder. Low levels in patients with systemic lupus nephritis may predict subsequent development of active nephritis, although the correlation is not high. Fulminant septicemia, in particular with *Neisseria meningitidis,* is also associated with activation of both the classical and alternative pathways and secondary hypocomplementemia, whether or not shock develops.

Infancy. Levels in neonates are approximately two thirds of adult levels, which are reached by ~1 year of age.

Genetic Aspects

C3 is coded by a gene on chromosome 19.[123] There are more than 25 known inherited variants demonstrable by prolonged agarose gel electrophoresis of serum or plasma; the most common are C3S and C3F (for "slow" and "fast," respectively). Most are associated with normal concentrations and function; one, C3f, has the same mobility as C3F but is present in approximately 50% of the normal concentration. Genetic deficiency is discussed in the Clinical Significance section above.

Laboratory Considerations

Intact C3 migrates on routine clinical electrophoresis in the β_1 region in ethylenediaminetetraacetic acid (EDTA)-treated plasma and in the β_2 region in the presence of free Ca^{2+}. However, it is a relatively labile protein, with conversion to C3c and C3dg on storage either under suboptimal conditions or for prolonged periods. These fragments migrate more anodally (α_2-β_1). Apparently reduced concentration by electrophoresis is most commonly due to in vitro conversion, not to actual deficiency. Most immunochemical quantification methods measure C3c almost equivalently to intact C3, thus confirming normal concentration.

Electrophoretic variants, including C3F, may be confused with monoclonal immunoglobulins; their identity can be ascertained by immunofixation using specific antiserum.

Activation of C3 has been determined in the past by either immunofixation or two-dimensional, or crossed, immunoelectrophoresis of plasma, with determination of the relative amounts of C3 and C3c.[119] Currently, assays of fragments using antisera to neoantigens (such as those on C3a) are preferred for this determination. For either type of assay, plasma samples must be obtained with precautions to prevent in vitro activation by plasmin, C1s, and leukocyte proteases: The first few milliliters are discarded (or used for other purposes), then whole blood is collected through the same needle into a tube containing EDTA. Centrifugation should be performed as soon as possible and the separated plasma frozen below −40 °C.

Because of differences in immunochemical reactivity of C3 and C3c, reference materials should be completely converted to C3c and stabilized, as is the case for the international reference material CRM 470.[120]

Reference Intervals

C3 levels are low in newborns, then rise and remain relatively constant after the first year of life. The recommended reference interval for adults, based on CRM 470, is 0.9 to 1.8 g/L (90 to 180 mg/dL).[28] Levels are slightly lower in fresh serum (assayed less than 8 hours after drawing).

Complement C4

Although the existence of a fourth component of complement was proposed in 1926, the purification and characterization of C4 did not occur until the 1960s. Müller-Eberhard and Biro originally named it β_{1E}-globulin, but the name C4 was officially adopted in 1968. C4 is enzymatically cleaved by C1s after activation of C1 and is therefore the second component reacting in the classical pathway cascade. C4b, the active fragment, can then bind C2, rendering it susceptible to enzymatic cleavage by C1s. The resulting C4b2b complex is the C3/C5 convertase of the classical pathway.

Biochemistry

C4 has a molecular mass of 206 kDa, including ~4% carbohydrate. Unlike most complement components, it is relatively heat stable. Most synthesis occurs in the hepatic parenchymal cells, although some may be synthesized by monocytes or other tissue. It is originally synthesized as a single chain (proC4) but is enzymatically cleaved at two sites to form three chains, α, β, and γ, held together by disulfide bonds. It has an intramolecular thiol ester bond in the α-chain that, on activation, is the membrane-binding site for "fixation" to membranes, viruses, and immune complexes.[104]

Function

As noted previously, C4b2b is the activating enzyme for C3 and C5 in the classical pathway; C4 is essential for activation of this pathway. However, most individuals with C4 deficiency do not have problems with infection, suggesting that the alternative pathway can compensate for the lack of classical pathway activation in removal of bacterial agents; however, C4 may be critical for clearance of infecting viruses.

C4b2b bound to immune complexes prevents their precipitation and promotes immune complex clearance by the CRa receptor, especially if the C4 is the C4B isotype (see discussion later in this chapter). The binding of C4A to drugs such as procainamide and hydralazine interferes with clearance of immune complexes; this may be important in the etiology of drug-induced lupus syndromes.

C4a, the small fragment released into the circulation on activation of C4, is a weak anaphylatoxin, but its half-life in the circulation is very short.

Clinical Significance

Increased Plasma Levels. C4 levels are modestly increased by the APR (inflammation, trauma, or tissue necrosis; see Table 20-8).

Decreased Plasma Levels. C4 levels are decreased with genetic deficiency, acquired deficiency, and infancy.

Genetic Deficiency. Complete deficiency of C4 is associated with a very high prevalence of autoimmune or collagen vascular disease, particularly SLE, and in a few cases with a propensity for infection. The incidence of isolated deficiency of C4A (see discussion later in this chapter) is markedly increased in patients with SLE as well. It is not yet clear whether these correlations result from decreased clearance of immune complexes or from linkage disequilibrium with immune response genes that predispose to the development of SLE. One extended haplotype is associated with normal C4A levels in clinically normal individuals who nevertheless have anti-DNA antibodies, suggesting that both factors may be required for development of the classical disease. Approximately 20% of individuals with deficiency of IgA also have homozygous deficiency of C4A, as do some with combined IgA and IgG subclass deficiencies, suggesting that the gene for a B-cell maturation factor is linked to C4A.

Acquired Deficiency. Levels of C4 are more commonly depressed because of consumption; > 60% of individuals with SLE and low C4 levels do not have genetic deficiency. Other disorders associated with consumption and low levels include hereditary angioedema (C1 inhibitor deficiency), autoimmune hemolytic anemia, and autoimmune nephritides.

Infancy. C4 levels in newborn infants are approximately 50% to 75% of adult levels.

Genetic Aspects

C4 is coded by two nonallelic loci in the major histocompatibility complex region of chromosome 6p, closely linked to the genes for C2, factor B, and HLA-DR. The close linkage to the immune response genes may account for most of the disease associations reported for C4 variants and deficiency, rather than abnormalities of C4 itself.

The two proteins coded by the C4 loci differ by four amino acids in the binding site region of the α chain and are designated C4A and C4B (note that C4a and C4b refer instead to the cleavage products of C4 activation by C1s). The two have different binding specificities, C4A binding more efficiently with peptides (as in immune complexes) and C4B with hydroxyl groups (e.g., bacterial and erythrocyte membrane polysaccharides). C4d fragments (inactivation products of C4b) of C4A and C4B bound to erythrocyte membranes react with Rodgers and Chido blood grouping antisera, respectively.

Both of the C4 loci are highly polymorphic, with at least 13 known alleles for C4A and at least 21 for C4B, in addition to deletions and nonexpressed genes. Most of the alleles are due to substitutions in the α-chain, although a few variants of the β-chain have also been reported. Either or both loci may be deleted, unexpressed, or duplicated; as a result, a given individual may have zero to four copies of each locus. Both the total C4 level and the ratio of C4A to C4B depend on the number of copies of each locus. Most C4A variants have 25% to 35% of the hemolytic activity of the C4B alleles; one, C4A6, has little if any hemolytic activity and no C5 convertase activity.[32]

Laboratory Considerations

C4 has β_1 electrophoretic mobility, similar to that of transferrin, but is normally not visualized because of its low concentration. It is relatively fragile, especially in the presence of Ca^{2+}, so it is recommended that EDTA or citrated plasma be used for C4 assays when these are considered to be clinically important.

Functional hemolytic assays (CH50) may be used to screen for functional C4 deficiency, although the CH50 must be below 50% for deficiency to be suspected. Most assays are now done by immunochemical methods, especially immunoturbidimetry or nephelometry. Low levels alone cannot differentiate between genetic and acquired deficiency; tests for breakdown products (e.g., C4a des-arginine) or neoantigens may be helpful in detecting increased turnover.[26]

Phenotyping of the C4 proteins is usually performed by electrophoresis of neuraminidase-treated EDTA plasma, followed by immunofixation. Differentiation of overlapping C4A and C4B bands may require the use of a hemolytic gel overlay, which demonstrates primarily the C4B bands. DNA genotyping can also determine the types in most cases but cannot distinguish between synthesizing and nonsynthesizing genes. Some investigators recommend that C4 phenotyping or genotyping be performed routinely in patients with SLE if C4 levels are to be used to monitor disease activity.[117]

Reference Intervals

As with C3, levels are low in neonates but relatively constant after the first year of life. The recommended interim reference interval for adults, based on CRM 470, is 0.1 to 0.4 g/L (10 to 40 mg/dL).[28] The baseline plasma level of C4 in individuals with one or more null genes is lower.[117]

IMMUNOGLOBULINS

Immunoglobulins, or humoral antibodies, recognize the antigens and initiate mechanisms that destroy them (see Chapter 9). The ability to recognize the enormous variety of antigens is accomplished through an unusual degree of structural heterogeneity. For example, a single bacterium has numerous surface antigens; each of these has many determinants or epitopes, and each epitope stimulates production of antibodies to that determinant. This results in marked heterogeneity of the immunoglobulins, illustrated by the diffuse bands seen on electrophoresis, particularly for IgG.

Basic Biochemistry

All immunoglobulin molecules consist of one or more basic units built of two identical heavy (H) chains and two identical light (L) chains. Each of the four chains has a variable and constant region, with the variable region involved in antigen recognition and binding (see Chapter 9, Figure 9-1). The amino acid sequences of the variable regions at the *N*-terminal ends of the four chains determine the antigenic specificity of the particular antibody molecules produced by a single plasma cell or by a "clone" of identical plasma cells. The two antigen-binding sites (Fab) are at the end of each identical light- and heavy-chain pair. The remainder of the molecule, the "constant" part, is the same for every immunoglobulin molecule of a given subclass and carries the effector sites.

Although most plasma proteins are synthesized in the liver, immunoglobulins are synthesized by plasma cells, the progeny of B-lymphocyte stem cells in bone marrow (Table 20-11). More mature B lymphocytes, found mainly in lymph nodes and in blood, develop receptor immunoglobulins on their surface membranes. On encountering the antigen, these B lymphocytes proliferate and develop into plasma cells. These then secrete into the blood specific antibodies capable of binding additional antigen.

B lymphocytes at first have IgM surface receptors (see Table 20-11) and secrete IgM as the first or "primary" response to an antigen. The heavy chains of the IgM surface receptor molecules are then modified in situ to IgG or IgA heavy chains, but the variable regions remain unchanged; as the cells change into plasma cells, a second exposure to the same antigen causes a larger, secondary or anamnestic response of IgG secretion. IgM continues, however, to be synthesized against the antigens confined to the blood, such as erythrocyte surface antigens and tropical parasites.

The effector sites that interact with cells (e.g., IgE with mast cells) and with complement are on the constant (Fc) region of the heavy chains. Variations in the Fc region result in the classes and subclasses into which immunoglobulins are grouped: IgM, IgG (four subclasses), IgA (two subclasses), IgD, and IgE. Their respective heavy chains are called μ, γ, α, δ, and ε. The hinge region between the Fc and Fab portions, which is susceptible to proteolytic cleavage, controls the interaction between the Fab and Fc parts. The

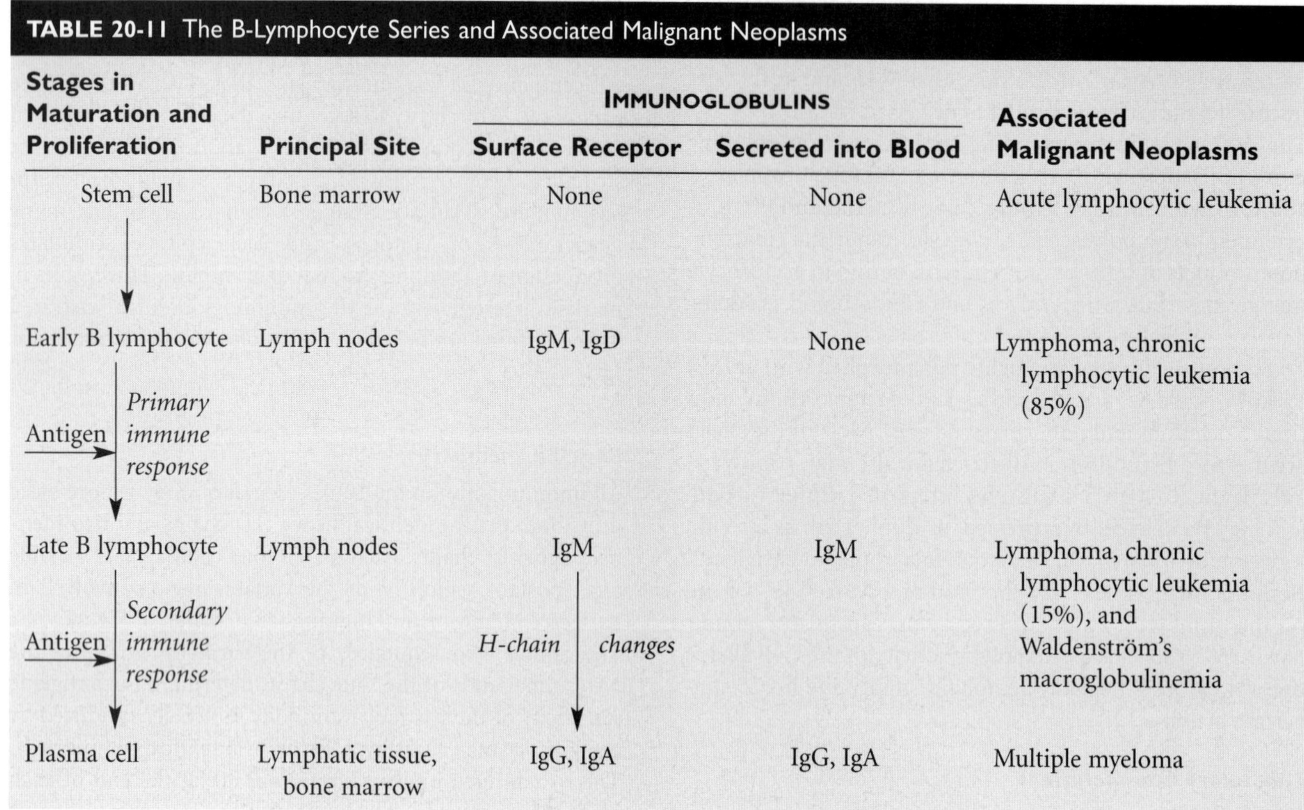

TABLE 20-11 The B-Lymphocyte Series and Associated Malignant Neoplasms

Stages in Maturation and Proliferation	Principal Site	Immunoglobulins: Surface Receptor	Immunoglobulins: Secreted into Blood	Associated Malignant Neoplasms
Stem cell	Bone marrow	None	None	Acute lymphocytic leukemia
↓				
Early B lymphocyte	Lymph nodes	IgM, IgD	None	Lymphoma, chronic lymphocytic leukemia (85%)
Antigen → *Primary immune response* ↓				
Late B lymphocyte	Lymph nodes	IgM	IgM	Lymphoma, chronic lymphocytic leukemia (15%), and Waldenström's macroglobulinemia
Antigen → *Secondary immune response* ↓		*H-chain changes* ↓		
Plasma cell	Lymphatic tissue, bone marrow	IgG, IgA	IgG, IgA	Multiple myeloma

hinge region contains one or more half cystines, which provide the interchain disulfide bridges. The structural variations among immunoglobulin classes also result in differences in function.[86]

Light chains, which are produced independently and in slight excess, are of two types—κ and λ—the constant regions of which have different structures. They occur in all immunoglobulins in the proportion $\kappa:\lambda = 2:1$; the two halves of a given molecule always have the same type. There are four subclasses of λ-chains. The heavy-chain genes are located on chromosome 14; κ light chains are encoded by a gene on chromosome 2, whereas the λ-chain gene is on chromosome 22.

Biochemistry of Individual Immunoglobulins

The individual immunoglobulins G, M, A, D have different biochemical properties.

Immunoglobulin G

Immunoglobulin G (IgG) is the major immunoglobulin produced by plasma cells, making up 70% to 75% of the total immunoglobulins. Of this amount, 65% is extravascular; the remainder is in plasma. IgG antibodies are produced in response to most bacteria and viruses; they bind to and aggregate small, soluble foreign proteins, such as bacterial toxins. IgG consists of two heavy and two light chains (see Chapter 9, Figure 9-1); its molecular weight is 144 to 150 kDa, including less than 3% carbohydrate. On cellulose acetate or agarose gel electrophoresis, IgG migrates broadly in the γ- and slow β-regions as a result of the heterogeneity of the IgG molecules.

Immunoglobulin G has four subclasses, IgG_1, IgG_2, IgG_3, and IgG_4, differing primarily in their hinge regions. In IgG_3, the hinge is extended by up to 15 half cystines, allowing efficient binding to Clq. Both IgG_1 and IgG_3 bind Fc receptors on phagocytic cells, activate killer monocytes (K cells), and cross the placenta by an active transport process dependent on Fc binding. IgG_1 is the principal IgG to cross the placenta and to protect neonates for the first 3 months of postnatal life. The half-life of IgG_1, like those of IgG_2 and IgG_4, is about 22 days, much longer than that of IgG_3 (7 days).

Immunoglobulin M

Immunoglobulin M is the most primitive and least specialized immunoglobulin and is the only immunoglobulin that most neonates normally synthesize. In adult serum, it is the third most abundant immunoglobulin, accounting for 5% to 10% of the total circulating immunoglobulins. IgM as a membrane receptor molecule is monomeric, but most of the serum IgM is a pentamer; each monomer is similar to the IgG molecule shown in Chapter 9, Figure 9-1, except that pentameric IgM also contains a small glycopeptide, the J chain, which is important for polymerization. Plasma cell malignancies may secrete monomeric IgM in addition to, or instead of, pentamers. IgM's high molecular weight (970 kDa; ~10% carbohydrate) prevents its ready passage into extravascular spaces. IgM is not transported across the placenta and is therefore not involved in hemolytic disease of neonates. It is an efficient complement activator, the Fc chains being spaced at the correct distance to match the Clq-binding sites.

Immunoglobulin A

Approximately 10% to 15% of serum immunoglobulin is IgA, which contains 10% carbohydrate, has a molecular weight of 160 kDa, and has a half-life of 6 days. In its monomeric form, its structure is similar to that of IgG, but 10% to 15% of IgA in serum is dimeric, particularly IgA_2, which is more resistant to destruction by some pathogenic bacteria than IgA_1. On electrophoresis, IgA migrates in the β-γ region, anodal to most IgG.

A possibly more important form of IgA is called *secretory* IgA, found in tears, sweat, saliva, milk, colostrum, and gastrointestinal and bronchial secretions. Secretory IgA has a molecular weight of 380 kDa and consists of two molecules of IgA, a secretory component (MW 70 kDa), and a J chain (15.6 kDa). It is synthesized mainly by plasma cells in the mucous membranes of the gut and bronchi and in the ductules of the lactating breast. The secretory component makes secretory IgA more resistant to enzymes, allowing it to protect the mucosa from bacteria and viruses. Its presence in colostrum and milk probably aids in protection of neonates from intestinal infections. IgA can activate complement by the alternative pathway (see Figure 20-7), but the exact role of IgA in serum is not clear.

Immunoglobulin D

Immunoglobulin D accounts for less than 1% of serum immunoglobulins. It is monomeric, contains about 12% carbohydrate, and has a molecular weight of 184 kDa. Its structure is similar to that of IgG. Like IgM, IgD is a surface receptor for the antigen in B lymphocytes, but its primary function is unknown.

Immunoglobulin E

Immunoglobulin E is so rapidly and firmly bound to mast cells that only trace amounts of it are normally present in serum. IgE contains 15% carbohydrate and has a molecular weight of 188 kDa; its structure is similar to that of IgG. IgE binds to mast cells via binding sites on its Fc region. When the antigen (allergen) cross-links two of the attached IgE molecules, the mast cell is stimulated to release histamine and other vasoactive amines that are responsible for the vascular permeability and smooth muscle contraction occurring in such allergic reactions as hay fever, asthma, urticaria, and eczema.

Clinical Significance

Normally, serum contains a heterogeneous, polyclonal mixture of antibodies, which represent multiple "idiotypes" (i.e., the products of many different clones of plasma cells), each producing a single type of immunoglobulin molecule. Benign or malignant proliferation of one such clone produces a high concentration of a single idiotype (a monoclonal antibody), which may appear as a sharp, narrow band on protein electrophoresis. A second, fainter band of free light chains may also be visible. If a few clones proliferate, there may be several sharp bands (e.g., the oligoclonal bands seen in electrophoresis of CSF in demyelinating diseases such as multiple sclerosis, or in serum following successful bone marrow transplantation, or early during a response to such organisms as *Streptococcus pneumoniae*). Disease may therefore be associated with a decrease or an increase in the normal polyclonal immunoglobulins or an increase in one or more monoclonal idiotypes.

Immunoglobulin Deficiency

Immune defense depends on four complex, interactive systems: cell-mediated immunity (T lymphocytes); humoral antibodies (immunoglobulins); the phagocytic system; and the complement system. The last two systems are nonspecific in that they have no immunological memory for the antigen. Only the second and fourth systems are composed of plasma proteins. Immunodeficiency states characterized by recurrent infections may be the result of a defect in any one of these systems or combinations thereof.

An obvious marked reduction or absence of the γ-band on electrophoresis indicates deficiency of IgG antibodies. IgG deficiency may be secondary to protein loss or to acquired failure of synthesis, but may be due to a primary congenital disorder. The causes for various immunoglobulin deficiency disorders are listed in Box 20-1. The diagnosis of a deficiency state is clinically important because replacement therapy with IgG can be provided. Presence of a normal-appearing γ-band on protein electrophoresis does not rule out immunoglobulin deficiency. Some primary deficiencies involve only one or two immunoglobulin classes or subclasses; if the total immunoglobulin level is not greatly affected, the deficiency (e.g., IgA or an IgG subclass) may not be suspected from the electrophoretic pattern. Furthermore, some patients have normal immunoglobulin levels, but the antibodies do not react normally with the antigen.

Infants have transient physiological IgG immunodeficiency, with a nadir at about 3 months of age; either prolonged or severe physiological deficiency may be associated with increased infection rates, especially with encapsulated bacteria. Levels of maternal IgG, transferred across the placenta, rise rapidly in the fetus during the last half of pregnancy but then drop rapidly following birth (Figure 20-8). Two groups of neonates are particularly at risk: premature infants, who start with less maternal IgG, and infants in whom initiation of IgG synthesis is transiently delayed. IgG determinations are invaluable in these cases because levels may become dangerously low if therapy for the infant is not initiated. Rising IgM and normal salivary IgA concentrations at 6 weeks of age suggest a favorable prognosis. Contact of the neonate with environmental antigens normally causes B lymphocytes to begin to multiply and IgM levels to start to rise, followed weeks to months later by IgA and IgG.

BOX 20-1 Causes of Immunoglobulin Deficiency

Secondary Causes (Common)

Defective Synthesis (IgM Falls First, Then IgA, Finally IgG)

- Lymphoid malignancy, multiple myeloma, lymphoma, chronic lymphocytic leukemia
- Toxic reaction (e.g., renal failure, diabetes mellitus)
- Drugs (e.g., phenytoin, penicillamine)
- In neonates only: prematurity, transient delay in initiation of synthesis

Abnormal Loss of Proteins

- Nephrotic syndrome, burns, protein-losing enteropathy

Primary or Inherited Causes (Rare)

Failure of Antibody Production

- Generalized (Severe Pyogenic Infections Occur)
- Infantile X-linked Bruton's type
- Acquired, variable, unclassifiable, occurring at any age
- Selective immunoglobulin deficiency of
- IgA: Most common (1:700), symptomless but those affected tend to suffer allergic or autoimmune disease
- IgG and IgA (IgM increased): recurrent pyogenic infections
- IgA and IgM: Giardiasis common
- IgG: Recurrent Pyogenic Infections
- IgM: Susceptibility to autoimmune disease and to septicemia following splenectomy

Combined Failure of Antibody- and Cell-Mediated Immunity

- Severe combined immunodeficiency. Swiss and sex-linked types, death in infancy from fungal or viral infections
- Associated with thymoma, achondroplasia, or thrombocytopenia and eczema (Wiskott-Aldrich syndrome)

Polyclonal Hyperimmunoglobulinemia

Polyclonal increases in serum immunoglobulins are the normal response to infections. IgG response predominates in autoimmune responses; IgA in skin, gut, respiratory, and renal infections; and IgM in primary viral infections and bloodstream parasites, such as malaria. *Chronic bacterial infections* may cause an increase in serum levels of all immunoglobulins. In such cases, estimations of the individual immunoglobulins seldom provide more information than protein electrophoresis. They are of value, however, in the differential diagnosis of liver disease and of intrauterine infections. In *primary biliary cirrhosis,* the IgM level is greatly increased; in *chronic active hepatitis,* IgG and sometimes IgM are increased; and in *portal cirrhosis,* IgA and sometimes IgG are increased. In *intrauterine infections,* production of IgM by the fetus increases, and the IgM level in umbilical cord blood is increased. Estimations of IgE are used in the management of asthma and other allergic conditions, especially in children.

Monoclonal Immunoglobulins (Paraproteins)

A single clone of plasma cells produces immunoglobulin molecules with identical structure. If the size of the clone increases greatly, the concentration of its particular protein in the patient's serum may produce a narrow, sharply discrete band on electrophoresis. These monoclonal immunoglobulins, termed "*paraproteins,*" may be polymers, monomers, or fragments of immunoglobulin molecules; if fragments, they are usually light chains (Bence Jones proteins) or, rarely, heavy chains or half molecules; both monomers and fragments may polymerize. About 60% of paraproteins are associated with plasma cell malignancies (multiple myeloma or solitary plasmacytoma) and approximately 15% are due to overproduction by B lymphocytes, mainly in lymph nodes (lymphomas, chronic lymphocytic leukemia, Waldenström's macroglobulinemia, or heavy-chain disease). Up to 25% of paraproteins are benign, and many are never discovered.

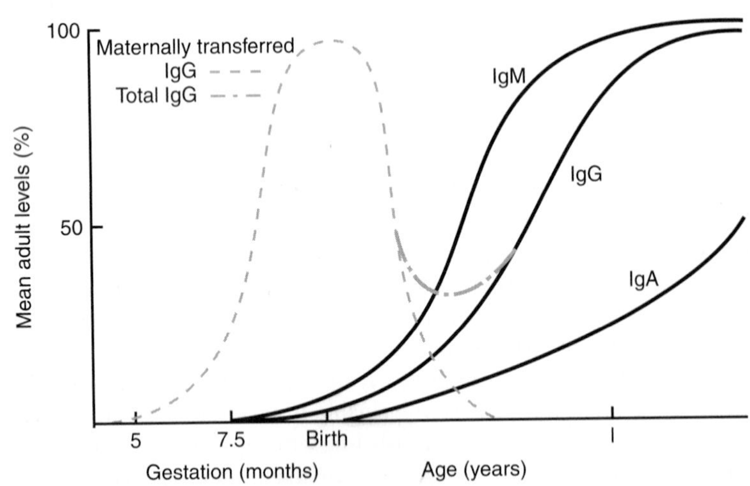

Figure 20-8 Serum immunoglobulin levels as percent of adult levels before birth and for the first year of life.

Should a paraprotein be identified in blood or urine or both, its heavy and light chains should be typed and the concentrations of polyclonal IgG, IgA, and IgM determined. These studies help to confirm whether the band on the electrophoretic pattern is indeed a paraprotein, aid in assessing prognosis, and show whether the polyclonal immunoglobulins are so low that they leave a patient vulnerable to infections. Prognosis is based on the class of the paraprotein found, its concentration at the time of diagnosis, and the rate at which its concentration increases. The concentration at the time of diagnosis usually correlates with the current extent of the disease process. The rate of increase in concentration is indicative of the rate of growth of the neoplasm.

Low-level paraproteins may be clinically benign, with normal bone marrow and bone radiographs. However, the following findings suggest that the condition may eventually become malignant:

1. IgG is greater than 2 g/dL; or either IgA or IgM is greater than 1 g/dL; or the finding of an IgD or IgE paraprotein at any concentration.
2. Immunoglobulin fragments in urine or serum: in urine, usually Bence Jones protein; in serum, occasionally other fragments, such as monomeric IgM or heavy chain fragments.
3. Progressive increase in the concentration of the paraprotein.
4. Low levels of polyclonal immunoglobulins.

The converse of these criteria suggests that the condition is benign or monoclonal gammopathy of unknown significance (MGUS). Even then, patients should be monitored for at least 5 years.

Multiple Myeloma. *Multiple myeloma* is a malignant neoplasm, usually of a single clone of plasma cells although occasionally two or more clones may be involved. The plasma cells most often proliferate diffusely throughout the bone marrow, but occasionally they form a solitary tumor called a *plasmacytoma.* Osteolytic bone lesions are produced, and the other bone marrow cells are reduced so that thrombocytopenia, anemia, and leukopenia develop. At the same time, development of normal clones of plasma cells is inhibited; consequently, synthesis of other immunoglobulins is reduced, and a syndrome of recurrent infections is seen. The incidence of multiple myeloma is low in individuals younger than 60 years but rises rapidly with age. Patients may present with local symptoms of a bone lesion, such as pain or fractures, but more often present with nonspecific symptoms, such as weight loss, anemia, hemorrhage, repeated infections, or renal failure. A normal serum alkaline phosphatase level in a patient with destructive bone lesions is a highly suggestive laboratory finding. Cardinal diagnostic features of the disease are the findings of neoplastic plasma cells in bone marrow aspirate, radiological demonstration of osteolytic lesions, and identification of a paraprotein in serum or urine. All patients who could conceivably have the disease should be screened for paraproteins; fewer than 1% with the disease do not have detectable paraproteins. Table 20-12 lists the paraproteins that may be associated with multiple myeloma and some characteristic findings for them.

Lymphoid Tumors. *Lymphoid tumors,* such as lymphomas or chronic lymphocytic leukemias, arise from less mature stages in B-lymphocyte development; about one in five produce paraproteins, usually of the IgM class.

Waldenström's Macroglobulinemia. If a paraprotein proves to be IgM, the diagnosis is probably *Waldenström's macroglobulinemia,* not multiple myeloma. Waldenström's macroglobulinemia clones arise from the most mature B lymphocytes and invariably produce IgM; in fact, it is the presence of this very high molecular weight protein that produces the salient symptom of the disease—an increase in viscosity of the blood. Bence Jones proteinuria occurs in 80% of these cases, but the condition is much less malignant than multiple myeloma. The lymph nodes and spleen are enlarged, but the lymphoid infiltration is slow growing, and the symptoms are usually treatable by exchange transfusion or plasmapheresis.

Heavy-Chain Disease. Rarely, unusual forms of IgG, IgA, or light chains polymerize and cause a similar syndrome with high blood viscosity. *Heavy-chain diseases* in which the paraprotein consists only of a heavy chain, usually incomplete, are rare conditions associated with lymphoid infiltration. The most common of these is *α-chain disease,* in which the intestine is infiltrated and severe malabsorption may be seen.

Cryoglobulinemia and Amyloid Disease. Both of these disorders are sometimes characterized by paraproteins. A cryoglobulin is a serum protein that precipitates at temperatures lower than normal body temperature. Most cryoglobulins are polyclonal immunoglobulin complexes, but nearly half are monoclonal, usually IgM. For cryoglobulin evaluation, a temperature of 37 °C must be maintained for blood collection and for serum separation and storage to keep the cryoglobulin from precipitating out of the serum. Amyloid disease is characterized by deposits of insoluble fibrillar protein complexes in various tissue; with special staining, the deposits are easily seen in biopsy sections. Some of the deposits contain fragments of light chains, especially from the variable region. Amyloid deposits may also occur in multiple myeloma (see discussion later in this chapter).

Laboratory Considerations

Methodologies

Immunoglobulins are most often quantified by immunoturbidimetry or immunonephelometry.[121] Immunochemical assays of polyclonal immunoglobulins involve determining the concentration of a mixture of protein molecules of different sizes having similar constant regions but different variable regions (idiotypes). Reagent antisera and reference immunoglobulin calibrators used in most immunochemical assays have been generated against normal human sera containing a mixture of immunoglobulin subclasses and idiotypes. However, a monoclonal immunoglobulin has only a few of the determinants with which the antiserum usually reacts, and the antigen excess may be reached at relatively low concentrations. If a paraprotein is suspected or previously identified, the assays should be performed at two or more dilutions to check for this; corrected for dilution, the values should agree within ~10%. Furthermore, if a new batch of antiserum is introduced, the relationship between paraprotein concentration and the calibration curve is likely to change. For these reasons, many laboratories estimate the concentration of paraproteins by electrophoresis and densitometry.

Reference Intervals[28,106]

Reference intervals for IgG and IgM in various human adult populations differ around the world because of different degrees of antigenic stimulation. IgA levels, however, are relatively unaffected by environmental factors. Newborn infants have B lymphocytes with antigen receptors of the IgM type but do not have significant rates of immunoglobulin synthesis. Essentially all of the IgG in neonates has been transferred across the placenta from the mother. Immunoglobulin synthesis is stimulated by environmental antigens, with serum IgM rising fastest after birth (Figure 20-8).

IMMUNOGLOBULIN REFERENCE INTERVALS

Body Fluid	IgG (mg/dL)	IgA (mg/dL)	IgM (mg/dL)	IgD (mg/dL)	IgE (mg/dL)
Serum					
Newborn (4 day)	700-1480	0-2.2	5-30		
20-60 yr	700-1600	70-400	40-230	0-8	0-380
>60 yr	600-1560	90-410	30-360		
CSF	0-5.5	0-0.6	0-1.3		
Saliva	~11				

TABLE 20-12 Monoclonal Immunoglobulins (Paraproteins) in Multiple Myeloma

Plasma Paraprotein	Incidence* (%)	Age of Occurrence* (Mean)	Incidence of Bence Jones Proteinuria (%)	Comments
IgG	50	65	60	Patients more susceptible to immunodeficiency; paraproteins reach highest levels
IgA	25	65	70	Tend to have hypercalcemia and amyloidosis
Bence Jones (free light chains) only	20	56	100	Often renal failure; bone lesions; amyloidosis; poor prognosis
IgD	2	57	100	90% λ type; often have extraosseous lesion, amyloidosis, renal failure; 50% have enlarged lymph nodes, liver, spleen; poor prognosis
IgM	1	—	100	May or may not have hyperviscosity syndrome
IgE	0.1	—	Most	—
Biclonal	1	—	—	—
None detected	<1	—	0	Usually reduction of normal immunoglobulins

*Approximate.

Figure 20-8 shows in graphic form changes in IgA, IgG, and IgM levels in childhood. Readers are cautioned, however, that the data given in the figure and the listing above are only illustrative. Reference intervals change with age and with geographical and methodological differences.

Proteins in Other Body Fluids

In addition to plasma, proteins are found in several other body fluids and tissues, including urine, CSF, amniotic fluid, saliva, and feces.

Urinary Proteins[27,47,52,60]

Biochemistry and Function

The glomeruli act as an ultrafilter for plasma proteins (see Chapter 45). The degree to which individual proteins are normally filtered through the membrane is a function of their molecular size, ionic charge, and plasma concentration. In general, transport of protein molecules through the glomerular membrane progressively diminishes as protein size or negative charge increases. Normally, high molecular weight proteins, such as IgM (MW 970 kDa) appear in glomerular filtrate only in trace amounts. Relatively small yet easily detectable amounts of albumin (66.3 kDa) are passed into the filtrate as a result of its high plasma concentration and relatively low molecular weight. Proteins of MW 15 to 40 kDa filter more readily but in lesser quantities because of their low plasma concentrations.

In addition, the proportions of individual proteins excreted in the urine depend on the extent of their reabsorption by the proximal renal tubules, which is also inversely proportional to molecular size. The reabsorption of low molecular weight proteins involves binding of the protein to specific receptors on the tubule epithelial cells, uptake into the cells by pinocytosis, fusion of uptake vacuoles with lysosomes, and hydrolysis of the protein by lysosomal enzymes, followed by return of the constituent amino acids to the body pool. Very little of the total excreted urinary protein normally consists of small proteins. Only a small amount of protein is excreted normally (20 to 150 mg/dL), and most of it is albumin because of its concentration—it is not completely removed from the filtrate by the tubular cells. The remainder is almost entirely the Tamm-Horsfall protein uromucoid, a constituent of urinary casts, probably secreted by the distal tubules.

Increased permeability of the glomeruli is first signaled by increased amounts of albumin in the urine, and further increase is demonstrated by the appearance in urine of proteins with increasingly higher molecular weights. The appearance of low molecular weight proteins in urine suggests diminished or diminishing tubular reabsorption (e.g., from interstitial inflammation or toxins). (See also Chapter 45.)

Clinical Significance

In addition to hemorrhage, *proteinuria* (increased amounts of protein in urine) occurs with (1) increased glomerular permeability (*glomerular proteinuria*), in which the urinary protein is mainly albumin; (2) defective tubular reabsorption (*tubular proteinuria*), in which the urinary proteins are mainly low molecular weight proteins; (3) increased concentration in the plasma of an abnormal low molecular weight protein, such as immunoglobulin light chains (*overload proteinuria*); and (4) abnormal secretion of protein into the urinary tract (*postrenal proteinuria*). The last two are the least common and here are considered first (see Chapter 45).

Glomerular Proteinuria. This is the most common and serious type of proteinuria. Patients are routinely screened for this disorder by a simple dipstick test for albumin. If the dipstick test result is negative, clinically significant glomerular proteinuria is precluded; if the test result is positive, further investigation, such as a quantitative evaluation of protein excretion, is indicated. Because most of the excreted protein is albumin, glomerular proteinuria is often labeled *albuminuria.* An increase in glomerular permeability occurs in numerous conditions characterized by diffuse injury to the kidneys (see also Chapter 45). In diabetes, vascular permeability increases and albuminuria appears when metabolic regulation is poor, at least in part because of glycosylation and loss of negative charges on the membranes.

Immune complex disease often affects the glomeruli; in nephritis associated with SLE and in most other causes of glomerulonephritis, granular deposits containing immunoglobulins and complement components have been demonstrated on the glomerular membrane. In such progressive diffuse renal diseases, filtration of relatively small proteins, including albumin, is lost first; thus albumin levels in urine increase. As long as molecular sieving determines (by size) which proteins are filtered, the proteinuria is called *selective.* Progressively severe glomerular lesions produce less selective proteinuria until proteins of all sizes pass the glomerulus *(nonselective proteinuria).* Changes in selectivity parallel histological changes on renal biopsy; the earliest changes are seen by electron microscopy. In the final stages of disease, as glomeruli are destroyed or become functionless, proteinuria decreases and renal failure is established. Evaluation of selectivity of the glomerular membrane is thus an aid to differential diagnosis of these diseases and their prognosis.

The protein excretion rate is ordinarily determined from a 24-hour urine collection because random specimens vary considerably in protein concentration. However, a more convenient alternative is to determine, in random samples, the ratio of protein to creatinine (protein-creatinine index). Creatinine concentration is relatively constant in any one subject, and the index correlates well with the 24-hour total excretion of protein. Total protein determination, however, does not discriminate between individual proteins, and when 24-hour excretion or protein-creatinine index values are near normal, estimation of one or two individual representative proteins is preferred. When protein excretion exceeds 1 g/day, the proteinuria is likely to be glomerular. Heavy loss of plasma albumin (>2 g/day) is seen in the nephrotic syndrome, in association with edema. In these cases, selectivity should be assessed by electrophoresis of the urine and comparison of clearance of proteins of differing molecular weights (e.g., IgG-albumin ratio). When selectivity is high (IgG-albumin ratio <0.16), as it often is in children, treatment with corticosteroids is likely to be successful. Effect of treatment can be monitored by measuring excretion rates of total or individual proteins.

Functional or *benign proteinuria* is a form of glomerular proteinuria that is probably due to changes of blood flow through the glomeruli. It is seen with exercise, pyrexia, exposure to cold, congestive heart failure, hypertension, or arteriosclerosis. Protein excretion rates are less than 1 g/day. *Postural* or *orthostatic proteinuria,* associated with the upright position, is also a form of functional proteinuria, but excretion may exceed 1 g/day. Orthostatic proteinuria complicates assessment in otherwise symptomless patients. If transient, it is probably benign; but if chronic or not entirely related to posture, protein excretion rates should be checked at 6-month intervals, preferably by a quantitative test. Persistence of proteinuria suggests underlying renal disease. In normal pregnancy, protein excretion may increase harmlessly to 200 to 300 mg/day. This slight increase is in contrast to the proteinuria of preeclamptic toxemia, a glomerular proteinuria of up to 3 g/day, and to the proteinurias of latent renal disease or of urinary tract infection.

An additional clinical entity, *microalbuminuria,* is recognized as a strong predictor of impending nephropathy in type I diabetic patients (see Chapter 25).

Tubular Proteinuria. This type of proteinuria is characterized by the appearance of low molecular weight proteins in the urine caused by decreased reabsorption by the proximal tubules. It may occur alone but is more commonly associated with glomerular proteinuria. When tubular proteinuria occurs alone, albumin excretion is only slightly increased, but often not enough to give a positive dipstick reaction. More specific tests are required to detect simple tubular proteinuria or to identify it in the presence of glomerular proteinuria. Agarose electrophoresis of urine gives a characteristic pattern—prominent α- and β-bands, a relatively faint albumin band, and sometimes a post-γ-band. Sodium dodecyl sulfate polyacrylamide gel electrophoresis (SDS-PAGE) is even more useful because it separates proteins by molecular size (see Chapter 5) and is used to demonstrate tubular proteinuria in the presence of glomerular proteinuria. The proteins typically excreted in tubular proteinuria (molecular weights in daltons) are β_2-microglobulin (BMG; MW 11,800), lysozyme (MW 14,500), RBP (MW 21,000), α_1-microglobulin (MW 27,000), and AAG (MW 40,000), and various polypeptide hormones and enzymes. A simple way to screen for tubular proteinuria is to measure one of these, such as BMG or lysozyme, quantitatively. The protein-creatinine clearance ratio for the marker protein is a useful index of excretion (e.g., the ratio for lysozyme is increased 100 times in Fanconi syndrome) and is sufficiently reliable for most diagnostic and prognostic purposes.

Acute tubular proteinuria may occur with burns, acute pancreatitis, heavy metal poisoning, or administration of renotoxic drugs and may later resolve completely. *Chronic tubular proteinuria* is usually irreversible. Its etiology may be hereditary, as in Fanconi syndrome, or acquired, as in chronic pyelonephritis or a systemic disease, such as cirrhosis or sarcoidosis. Drugs, such as phenacetin and toxins such as cadmium, also produce tubular damage, which may be severe. In some cases, slight tubular proteinuria may be the only sign of progressive renal damage. Tests for tubular proteinuria are now being used to monitor renal allograft rejection, aminoglycoside and cadmium toxicity, and chronic pyelonephritis; BMG is a favorite marker protein.

Overload Proteinuria. This type of proteinuria includes hemoglobinuria, myoglobinuria, and Bence Jones proteinuria (high plasma concentrations of immunoglobulin light-chain paraproteins, as seen in multiple myeloma). Detection of light chains depends on electrophoretic and immunochemical testing.[40] Hemoglobin or myoglobin can be detected by tests discussed in Chapter 31.

Postrenal Proteinuria. This type of proteinuria refers to protein arising from the urinary tract below the kidneys and is usually due to inflammation or malignancy. It is diagnosed by microscopic evaluation of the urinary sediment for inflammatory cells and malignant cells. The presence of erythrocytes or leukocytes in casts in such a centrifuged urinary sediment is valuable proof that their origin is from the kidneys and is *not* extrarenal.

Laboratory Considerations

Qualitative detection of excess protein in urine is largely based on use of dipstick tests. The reactive portion of the stick is coated with a buffered indicator that develops color in the presence of protein. A typical example is Albustix (Bayer Corporation, Diagnostics Division, Tarrytown, NY), in which bromphenol blue, buffered to pH 3 with citrate, is present mostly in the protonated, yellow form. When protein is added, the affinity of the anionic form of the indicator dye for protein causes a shift of the equilibrium between anionic and protonated forms of the indicator toward formation of the blue anionic species. The intensity of the shade of blue produced is then proportional to the concentration of protein in the specimen. Combur 8 strips (Roche Diagnostics, Inc., Indianapolis, IN) are said to be less subject to drug interferences. Their detection limit is ~7 mg/dL.

Like all dye-binding techniques, the dipstick methods are more sensitive to albumin than to other plasma proteins. They are therefore excellent screening tests for glomerular proteinuria but unsatisfactory for detection of tubular proteinuria or overload proteinuria of the Bence Jones type. Although most tests measure protein in excess of 10 mg/dL, they are only roughly quantitative, and their use should be limited to screening and to rough estimates required before concentrating the specimen for electrophoresis or diluting it for quantitative assay. A first morning urine specimen is preferred because it tends to be concentrated and unaffected by postural factors.

Quantitative assay for total protein or for individual proteins is usually performed on timed collections. Periods of 4, 8, and 12 hours may be appropriate for monitoring a renal transplant recipient or a patient whose acute renal losses of albumin are being compensated with closely regulated replacement therapy. In most cases, however, a 24-hour collection is chosen, both for quantitative total or specific protein assay and for electrophoretic separation. An alternative approach is to measure the protein/creatinine ratios of random specimens.

Quantitative assay of specific proteins is necessary for estimates of glomerular selectivity and for evaluation of tubular proteinuria. Nephelometry and turbidimetry are sufficiently sensitive for most of the analytes (see Chapters 3 and 9). More sensitive immunoassays are required for BMG because of the low levels that are typically excreted. In addition, this protein is susceptible to degradation at low pH, and specimens should be stored at a pH greater than 6.0 during the collection period. In assessment of the nephrotic syndrome, glomerular selectivity is estimated usually by measuring two individual proteins of different molecular size, such as albumin or transferrin plus IgG. A random urine sample and a corresponding serum are collected and analyzed for the two proteins. The ratio of the individual clearances is then calculated

$$\frac{\frac{UV}{P}\text{ for IgG}}{\frac{UV}{P}\text{ for albumin}}$$

where U and P represent the concentration of the compound in urine and plasma and V is the volume of excreted urine per minute. Thus V cancels out and

$$\text{Ratio} = \frac{[\text{serum albumin}] \times [\text{urine IgG}]}{[\text{urine albumin}] \times [\text{serum IgG}]}$$

A value exceeding the upper limit of the reference interval implies loss of selectivity. *Clearance* of individual proteins may also be evaluated by the classical equation

$$\text{Clearance (mL/min)} = \frac{UV}{P}$$

For evaluation of tubular proteinuria, one may use either a 24-hour specimen or a random specimen. In the latter case, the concentrations of both creatinine and the specific protein (e.g., lysozyme) are determined and the protein-creatinine index is calculated as follows:

$$\frac{\text{Lysozyme}}{\text{Creatinine}}\text{ index} = \frac{[\text{lysozyme}]}{[\text{creatinine}]}$$

Reference Intervals

The reference interval for urinary protein is 1 to 14 mg/dL.[106] The excretion rate at rest is 50 to 80 mg/d, but many laboratories indicate the reference value as less than 100 mg/d (less than 150 mg/d in pregnancy). The concentration may reach 300 mg/d in urine of healthy subjects after exercise.

Proteins in Cerebrospinal Fluid[60,115]

CSF circulates around the brain and spinal column. As described in Chapter 2, CSF for testing is normally obtained from the lumbar spinal region.

Biochemistry

CSF is secreted by the choroid plexuses, around the cerebral vessels, and along the walls of the ventricles of the brain. It fills the ventricles and cisternae, bathes the spinal cord, and is reabsorbed into the blood through the arachnoid villi. CSF turnover is rapid, exchanging totally about four times per day. More than 80% of CSF protein content originates from plasma by ultrafiltration and pinocytosis; the remainder is from intrathecal synthesis. The lowest concentration of total protein and the smallest proportion of the larger protein molecules are in the ventricular fluid; as the CSF passes down to the lumbar spine (from which site specimens are usually collected), the protein concentration increases. This difference in concentration at different levels of the CNS is illustrated by the following reference intervals:[106]

TOTAL PROTEIN (mg/dL)	
Ventricular fluid	5-15
Cisternal fluid	15-25
Lumbar fluid	15-45

In CSF from premature and full-term neonates, levels are considerably higher (up to 130 mg/dL); in healthy elderly adults, concentrations up to 60 mg/dL are considered normal.

Because CSF is mainly an ultrafiltrate of plasma, low molecular weight plasma proteins such as prealbumin, albumin, and transferrin normally predominate. No protein with a molecular weight greater than that of IgG is present in sufficient concentration to be visible on electrophoresis. The electrophoretic pattern of normal CSF after concentrating the fluid has two striking features—a prominent prealbumin band and two transferrin bands. The second of the electrophoretic transferrin bands is the τ (tau) protein band, which is produced or transformed intrathecally and, by comparison with plasma transferrin, is deficient in sialic acid content.

Clinical Significance

The blood-CSF barrier is a concept rather than an anatomical structure. The barrier is defined by the many complex factors that govern the distribution of compounds other than water, carbon dioxide, and oxygen between the blood and the extracellular fluid of the brain and its accessory structures. In the present discussion, the term *blood-CSF barrier* is used as a synonym for the capillary endothelium of vessels of the CNS.

Examination of CSF total protein and specific proteins is used primarily to detect either increased permeability of the blood-CSF barrier to plasma proteins or increased intrathecal synthesis of immunoglobulins (Table 20-13).

Increased Permeability. The permeability of the blood-CSF barrier to plasma proteins is increased by high intracranial pressure resulting from a brain tumor, intracerebral hemorrhage, or traumatic injury. In addition, increased permeability to proteins is seen with inflammation associated with bacterial or viral meningitis, encephalitis, or poliomyelitis. Striking elevations of CSF total protein are seen in bacterial meningitis; smaller elevations occur in the other inflammatory diseases and with tumor or hemorrhage. Lumbar CSF protein is increased when the CSF circulation is mechanically obstructed above the puncture site (as by a spinal cord tumor), and plasma proteins equilibrate across the walls of meningeal capillaries into the stagnant CSF. The effect of any of these conditions is that the proportions of specific proteins in CSF increasingly resemble those in serum.

Intrathecal Synthesis. Demonstration of increased *intrathecal synthesis of immunoglobulins,* particularly IgG, has great importance in the diagnosis of demyelinating diseases of the CNS, especially multiple sclerosis.[115] In multiple sclerosis, patchy deterioration of myelin sheaths of axons in the CNS profoundly affects conduction of nerve impulses.

TABLE 20-13 Cerebrospinal Fluid Protein in Various Diseases

Clinical Condition	Appearance and Cells × 10^6/L	Total Protein (mg/dL)
Normal	Clear, colorless; 0-5 lymphocytes	15-45*
Increased admixture of proteins from blood		
Increased capillary permeability:		
Bacterial meningitis	Turbid, opalescent, purulent, usually >500 polymorphs	80-500
Cryptococcal meningitis	Clear or turbid; 50-150 polymorphs or lymphocytes	25-200
Leptospiral meningitis	Clear to slight haze; polymorphs early, then 5-100 lymphocytes	50-100
Viral meningitis	Clear or slight haze, colorless; usually up to 500 lymphocytes	30-100
Encephalitis	Clear or slight haze, colorless; usually up to 500 lymphocytes	15-100
Poliomyelitis	Clear, colorless; up to 500 lymphocytes	10-300
Brain tumor	Usually clear; 0-80 lymphocytes	15-200 (usually normal)
Mechanical obstruction:		
Spinal cord tumor†	Clear, colorless, or yellow	100-2000
Hemorrhage:		
Cerebral hemorrhage	Colorless, yellow, or bloody; blood cells	30-150
Local immunoglobulin production:		
Neurosyphilis	Clear, colorless; 10-100 lymphocytes	50-150
Multiple sclerosis‡	Clear, colorless; 0-10 lymphocytes	25-50
Both increased capillary permeability and local immunoglobulin production:		
Tuberculous meningitis	Colorless, fibrin clot, or slightly turbid; 50-500 lymphocytes	50-300 (occasionally up to 1000)
Brain abscess	Clear or slightly turbid	20-120
After myelography (inflammatory reaction)		Slight increase

*Premature infant: up to 400 mg/dL. Children: 30-100 mg/dL. Old age: up to 60 mg/dL.
†Froin's syndrome: lumbar fluid values are much higher than cisternal fluid values.
‡Similar values may occur in certain other chronic inflammatory conditions of the nervous system.

The cause of demyelination is unknown, and sites of the lesions are unpredictable; resulting symptoms vary widely. B lymphocytes that infiltrate the lesions synthesize IgG and occasionally other immunoglobulins. Because axons of the CNS are in intimate contact with CSF, the immunoglobulins produced in the lesion appear in the CSF.

Laboratory Considerations

Various analytical techniques are used to assess the increased permeability of the blood-CSF barrier to plasma proteins and to detect intrathecal synthesis of immunoglobulins.

Increased Permeability. The degree of permeability of the blood-CSF barrier is evaluated by immunochemical measurements of albumin in CSF and in serum specimens obtained at the same time. (Note that for this purpose, determination of CSF albumin must be made by a quantitative immunochemical method. Electrophoretic separation, although generally informative of increased amounts of specific plasma proteins in the CSF, is not useful for an objective definition of degree of permeability.) Albumin is a particularly suitable indicator protein because it is neither synthesized nor metabolized intrathecally. In CSF that is free of contaminating blood, albumin must necessarily have come from plasma through the blood-CSF barrier.

Using the results of quantitative albumin assays, the following ratio is calculated:

$$\frac{\text{Albumin}_{\text{CSF}}\ (\text{g/dL})}{\text{Albumin}_{\text{serum}}\ (\text{g/dL})}$$

However, because the quotient obtained by dividing 0.015 to 0.045 g/dL for $\text{albumin}_{\text{CSF}}$ by 4.0 to 5.5 g/dL for $\text{albumin}_{\text{serum}}$ would be a very small decimal value, this ratio is renamed the *CSF/serum albumin index* and is arbitrarily calculated as follows (effectively multiplying the ratio by 1000)

$$\frac{\text{CSF}}{\text{serum albumin}}\ \text{index} = \frac{\text{Albumin}_{\text{CSF}}\ (\text{mg/dL})}{\text{Albumin}_{\text{serum}}\ (\text{g/dL})}$$

An index value <9 is considered consistent with an intact barrier. Values of 9 to 14 are interpreted as slight impairment, 14 to 30 as moderate impairment, and >30 as severe impairment.

Intrathecal Synthesis. Determining the protein component of the fatty myelin sheath, *myelin basic protein* (MBP), is a more direct diagnostic approach to assessing diagnosing multiple sclerosis, but such assays have many difficulties because of the fragmentation of MBP in vivo by proteinases and because of the difficulties of making a specific antiserum against MBP. The assay is helpful in assessing the activity of demyelination, MBP levels rising and falling with exacerbation and remission of multiple sclerosis.[122]

Increased intrathecal synthesis of IgG causes an increase in the CSF/serum immunoglobulin concentration ratio and the appearance of oligoclonal immunoglobulin bands on electrophoretic separations of CSF. Investigation of these changes has now become routine when multiple sclerosis is suspected. At least 90% of cases of multiple sclerosis give positive findings, but increased immunoglobulins and oligoclonal immunoglobulins may also be found in some other chronic inflammatory diseases of the CNS, such as chronic meningoencephalitis caused by bacteria, viruses, fungi, or parasites; subacute sclerosing panencephalitis; and Guillain-Barré syndrome. These can be ruled out clinically or by finding a CSF total protein exceeding 100 mg/dL, a CSF leukocyte count greater than 50/µL, or a positive test result for neurosyphilis. The CSF albumin concentration in 70% of cases of multiple sclerosis is within the reference interval.

A complicating factor in testing for intrathecal IgG is that an increase in CSF IgG concentration or in the CSF/serum IgG concentration ratio may occur either because of increased permeability of the blood-CSF barrier, increased local production of IgG, or both. To identify intrathecal production specifically, correction for increased permeability is necessary. Corrections use *CSF and serum* albumin and IgG concentrations in one of several ways:

1. Concentrations *in CSF* of IgG and albumin are measured, and the following ratio is calculated:

   $$\text{Ratio} = \frac{\text{IgG}_{\text{CSF}}\ (\text{mg/dL})}{\text{Albumin}_{\text{CSF}}\ (\text{mg/dL})}$$

   A ratio >0.27 is considered indicative of increased synthesis; in about 70% of cases of multiple sclerosis, the ratio exceeds 0.27.
2. Concentrations *in CSF and serum* of IgG and albumin are measured, and the CSF immunoglobulin index is calculated

   $$\text{Index} = \frac{\text{IgG}_{\text{CSF}}\ (\text{mg/dL}) \times \text{Albumin}_{\text{serum}}\ (\text{g/dL})}{\text{Albumin}_{\text{CSF}}\ (\text{mg/dL}) \times \text{IgG}_{\text{serum}}\ (\text{mg/dL})}$$

   The reference interval for the index is 0.30 to 0.70. Values >0.70 are considered evidence of increased IgG synthesis; in more than 80% of cases of multiple sclerosis, this index exceeds 0.70. This estimator is now the one most often used.
3. Concentrations *in CSF and serum* of IgG and albumin are measured, and the intrathecal rate of IgG synthesis is calculated by an empirical (Tourtellotte's) formula, assessing the increase above normal of IgG in the patient's CSF and deducting from it the amount of leakage through the blood-brain barrier as indicated by excess CSF albumin. The rate of synthesis of IgG in milligrams per day is equal to

$$5\ \text{dL/d}\left[\left\{\text{IgG}_{CSF} - \frac{\text{IgG}_{\text{serum}}}{369}\right\} - \left\{\left(\text{Albumin}_{\text{CSF}} - \frac{\text{Albumin}_{\text{serum}}}{230}\right) \times \frac{0.43\,(\text{IgG}_{\text{serum}})}{\text{Albumin}_{\text{serum}}}\right\}\right]$$

All protein concentrations are expressed in milligrams per deciliter. The first bracketed term represents the difference between IgG found in CSF and the IgG expected if the blood-brain barrier is intact. The second bracketed term represents the same for albumin but is corrected by a ratio, molecular weight of albumin/molecular weight IgG = 0.43, to express the difference in albumin as if it were a difference in IgG, assuming that 1 mol of IgG accompanies every mole of albumin that passes the blood-brain barrier. The term 5 dL/d converts milligrams per deciliter units in the other terms and relates IgG to the average volume of CSF normally formed in 24 hours (~5 dL). The number 369 is the ratio of serum/CSF IgG concentrations in normal subjects; the number 230 is the same ratio but for albumin concentrations. The reference interval for the synthesis rate is −9.9 to +3.3 mg/d. Values exceeding 8 mg/d are found in most cases of multiple sclerosis. This estimator provides no more clinical information than the IgG index; the complex formula merely rearranges the results for serum and CSF IgG and albumin and then factors in several constants.

Reference Intervals[78,106]

The reference interval for albumin in lumbar CSF by RID is 17.7 to 25.1 mg/dL. In normal CSF, IgA, IgD, and IgM are each less than 0.2 mg/dL. Reference intervals for IgG are age related; their means increase from 3.5 mg/dL in the 15- to 20-year-old age group to 5.8 in adults aged 60 years or older. A usual reference interval for CSF IgG in adults is 0.8 to 4.2 mg/dL.

Proteins in Amniotic Fluid, Saliva, Feces, and Peritoneal and Pleural Cavities

Amniotic fluid is analyzed for AFP for detection of open neural tube or abdominal wall defects in the fetus. *Saliva* is tested for secretory IgA in infantile hypogammaglobulinemia and for BMG in Sjögren's syndrome. Assay of *feces* for AAT is sometimes used in the diagnosis of exudative enteropathy, because AAT is not significantly hydrolyzed in the gut. However, intravenous injection of Cr-labeled albumin, followed by measurement of the radioactive label in feces, is a more reliable test.

Pathological accumulations of fluid in the peritoneal and pleural cavities or elsewhere vary greatly in protein content. They may be either ultrafiltrates with low protein concentrations and scant amounts of high molecular weight proteins or fluids with high protein concentrations and significant amounts of large proteins such as immunoglobulins. These fluids are divided arbitrarily according to their protein concentration into *transudates,* with total protein less than 3 g/dL, and *exudates,* with higher total protein concentrations. Transudates ordinarily reflect changes in permeability of filtering membranes, whereas exudates usually result from infection or malignancy; the latter may contain large numbers of leukocytes or malignant cells. Both transudates and exudates usually contain enough protein to allow the biuret method to be used for the determination of total protein.

MISCELLANEOUS PROTEINS

Other proteins of clinical significance that are found in body tissues and fluids include amyloid, heat shock proteins, and other acute phase reactants, such as mannose binding lectin (MBL) and serum amyloid *P* (SAP).

Amyloid[71]

Amyloid (Greek, "resembling starch," because of its staining properties) is a pathological extracellular deposit that appears translucent and structureless. It stains with iodine and various dyes, but its affinity for Congo red is the basis of its definition and identification in biopsy specimens. All types of amyloid bind Congo red, which emits an apple-green fluorescence under polarized light. Under the electron microscope, all types of amyloid share two fibrillar components with characteristic periodicity and a minor rodlike P-component, a glycoprotein that, viewed on end, has the appearance of a pentamer with a hollow core. This component circulates normally in plasma. The fibril deposit consists of a characteristic β-pleated sheet, as determined by x-ray crystallography. It can be extracted from tissue with water but not physiological salt solutions.

Biochemistry

The formation of this insoluble variety of protein, resistant to normal proteolysis due to its β-conformation, is the one characteristic common to all types of amyloid, whatever their composition. Amyloid fibrils may have multiple soluble plasma protein precursors that are either increased in quantity or modified by proteolysis to make them insoluble. The result is a disease group with diverse etiologies, called *amyloidosis.* The deposits can be local or systemic. They exert pressure on vital structures and eventually cause death. No details are known about the local mechanism of formation of these deposits or the determinant for the site of deposition.

Clinical Significance

Clinically, amyloidosis is classified (omitting some rare forms) into five main groups: (1) primary amyloidosis, (2) amyloidosis associated with multiple myeloma, (3) secondary amyloidosis associated with inflammatory or infectious diseases, (4) a form associated with aging, and (5) familial amyloidosis. Increased knowledge of the chemical structure of the deposits has led to a revised classification that takes into consideration the type of amyloid protein present.[61] This classification is used in Table 20-14.

Amyloid Amyloidosis. Primary amyloidosis and amyloidosis associated with multiple myeloma are associated with immunoglobulin light-chain amyloid (AL) amyloidosis. The fibrillar proteins consist of homogeneous immunoglobulin light polypeptide chains mainly of the λ (especially λ_{VI}) type, their amino-terminal variable fragments, or both. AL proteins have a molecular weight of 14-22 kDa and have an affinity for clotting factor X, which may be responsible for the decrease in plasma level of this factor and for associated bleeding. Because they always include the variable part of the immunoglobulin light chain, they differ from one case to

TABLE 20-14 Chemical Classification of the Amyloid Diseases

Clinical Syndrome	Fibril Precursor	Fibril	Common Term	Chemical Description
Primary myeloma with amyloid	Ig L-chain	L-chain or VL fragment	AL	$A_{\lambda(1-n)}$ or $A_{\kappa(1-n)}$
Secondary (inflammation associated)	SAA	AA	AA	$AA_{prototype}$ $AA_{(trp)}$ var*
Localized				
Endocrine			AE	
Thyroid medullary carcinoma[†]	Procalcitonin	Procalcitonin	AE_t	$A_{procalcitonin}$
Pancreatic islet	—	—	AE_i	—
Skin—papular, Macular, nodular	—	—	AD	—
Senile				
Cardiac	Prealbumin	Prealbumin	AS_{c1} AS_{c2}	$A_{prealbumin}$
Brain	—	—	ASb	—
Pancreas	—	—	ASp	—
Familial				
Neuropathic				
Portuguese	Prealbumin	Prealbumin	AF_p	$A_{prealbumin}$ (val30 →met)
Swedish	Prealbumin	Prealbumin	AF_{SW}	$A_{prealbumin}$ (val30 →met)
Israeli	Prealbumin	Prealbumin	AF_{Is}	$A_{prealbumin}$ (thr49 →gly)
Japanese	—	—	AF_j	$A_{prealbumin}$ (val30 →met)
Indiana-Swiss	—	—	$AF_{i\text{-}s}$	$A_{prealbumin}$ (var)
Iowa	—	—	AF_i	—
Cardiomyopathic				
Danish	Prealbumin	Prealbumin	AF_{da}	$A_{prealbumin}$ (var)
Nephropathic				
FMF (North African)	SAA	AA	AF_{FMF}	AA
Irish-American	SAA	AA	AF_{IR}	AA
Urticaria, deafness (England)	—	—	AF_{de}	—
Polish (hypertensive)	—	—	AF_{po}	—
German (renal failure)	—	—	AF_g	—
Vascular				
HCHWA (Iceland)[‡]	Gamma trace[§]	Gamma trace fragment polymer	AF_{HCHWA}	$A_{\lambda\ trace}$

Modified from Buxbaum JN. The amyloid diseases. In: Wyngaarden JB, Smith LH Jr, editors. Cecil Textbook of Medicine. 17th ed. Philadelphia: WB Saunders, 1985:1169.

*This designation is used to denote amino acids that depart from the prototype sequences.

[†]Also found in other APUD (amine precursor uptake and decarboxylation) tumors.

[‡]Hereditary cerebral hemorrhage with amyloidosis.

[§]Gastroenteropancreatic neuroendocrine protein is a hormonelike peptide with no known function found to date in peptidergic central nervous system neurons, the anterior pituitary, and pancreas. Its concentration is high in cerebrospinal fluid.

another. Not all light chains seem capable of precipitation in the β-conformation that constitutes amyloid.

AL amyloidosis is the most common form of these disorders. Bone marrow plasmacytosis and excess plasma cell production of antigenically identical monoclonal light chains are common to primary amyloidosis and multiple myeloma. Thus a clear distinction between these two conditions is not possible chemically. They appear to differ only in the presence or absence of osteolytic lesions. AL deposits may occur in the tongue, heart, lymph nodes, spleen, joints, peripheral nerves, and skin.

Amyloid A Amyloidosis. Secondary amyloidosis is associated with amyloid A (AA) deposits and is called *AA amyloidosis.* In this form, AA proteins (5 to 9 kDa) are the main component and λ-light chains a minor one. AA proteins are amino-terminal fragments of serum amyloid A protein (SAA protein), composed of monomers of 12.5 kDa. It circulates in serum as a polymer of 220 to 235 kDa, most complexed to high-density lipoprotein. SAA is an acute phase protein similar to CRP, increasing rapidly in infections or noninfectious inflammation. AA protein can be distinguished from AL protein by the ability of permanganate to bleach the Congo red staining (AL protein staining is resistant).

AA protein is often deposited in chronic inflammatory diseases such as rheumatoid arthritis (incidence up to 20%) and other inflammatory joint diseases, and in chronic suppurative and granulomatous infections such as tuberculosis and osteomyelitis. Deposits of AA protein are also observed in nonlymphoid tumors such as renal and gastric carcinomas and in Hodgkin's disease. Deposits of AA protein are most often found in the kidneys, liver, and spleen, usually resulting in nephrotic syndrome and hepatosplenomegaly.

Senile Amyloidosis. Senile amyloid protein is found most often in the heart (senile cardiac amyloid), but also in the pancreas and brain. There seems to be an independent pathogenesis for these three forms. Nodular or infiltrative amyloid deposits may also be seen in the skin, lungs, and trachea and may involve endocrine organs such as the pancreas (in long-standing diabetes) or the thyroid (in medullary carcinoma). These forms usually are asymptomatic, except for the cardiac form.

Familial Amyloidosis. Several genetically transmitted forms of amyloid disease have been reported. These have primarily neurological but also renal and vascular symptoms (Table 20-14). The fibrils of the Portuguese and Swedish syndromes and the polyneuropathic amyloid syndrome of Ashkenazic Jews have monomers of 14 kDa that share antigenic determinants and amino acid homology with prealbumin (transthyretin).

Heat Shock Proteins

When exposed to heat shock or other types of stress, a large number of prokaryotic and eukaryotic cells synthesize a small family of proteins that have been termed *heat shock proteins.* These proteins complex with many other proteins, and a wide variety of physiological and molecular functions have been postulated for them. The heat shock proteins function normally as "molecular chaperones" to other proteins. For additional information on heat shock proteins, the reader is referred to reviews[48,94] and textbooks on the subject.[75,112]

Other Acute Phase Reactants

Mannose binding lectin (MBL; also called mannose binding protein) and serum amyloid P (SAP) CRP are acute phase reactants that bind to molecules—sugars or phospholipids—on the surface of infectious agents and products of cell breakdown. Both may act as acute phase reactants, but MBL levels fall during many acute infections. MLB activates C2 and C4 by way of MBL-associated proteases, bypassing C1q. Genetic deficiency or mutations may be associated with increased susceptibility to infection, malignancy, or autoimmune diseases, such as SLE and Sjögren's syndrome.[107] Like CRP, SAP is a pentraxin that, on binding, activates the classical complement pathway. Although its role is not completely known, SAP binds lipopolysaccharides, including those on gram-negative bacteria.[29]

Analysis of Proteins

Methods for the analysis of proteins in body fluids include:

1. Specific quantitative assays of particular proteins by immunochemical methods (see Chapter 9) using specific antisera and measurement of the antigen antibody complexes by nephelometry, turbidimetry, RID, or electroimmuno assay; or, if present in very low concentrations, by RIA, enzyme immunoassay (EIA), fluorescence immunoassay, or chemiluminescence.
2. Detection and identification of proteins by electrophoresis (see Chapter 5).
3. Quantification of total protein in serum, urine, and CSF.
4. Analysis by mass spectrometry, which provides structural and quantitative information (see Chapter 7).

Immunochemical Methods

Most immunochemical methods are applicable to the measurement of any of the proteins in this chapter (see Chapter 9). Because of their speed and ease, nephelometric and turbidimetric methods are most widely used for most serum proteins. These techniques are performed either by measuring the amount of Ag-Ab complex formation (equilibrium methods) or by measuring the rate of complex formation (kinetic methods). The kinetic methods are slightly faster, with measurements completed within ~20 s; however, kinetic assays are somewhat less sensitive because low-affinity antibodies do not have time to react. In addition, many kinetic methods obtain the baseline reading after addition of antiserum, which can reduce the measured signal with high-affinity antibodies.[2] A compromise is often used, with timed measurement before true equilibrium.

Assay Characteristics

Important assay characteristics for immunochemical methods include (1) limit of detection, (2) precision, and (3) turnaround time.

Limit of Detection. Detection limits of approximately 10 μg/mL (10 mg/L) have been attained with routine nephelometric and turbidimetric methods; this limit has been lowered by 10 to 100 fold using antibodies adsorbed onto latex particles. RID methods are able to detect down to a minimum of 10 to 20 μg/mL; the detection limits have been lowered even further by using special "low-level" plates (Calbiochem-Behring Corp., La Jolla, Calif.). Methods using labeled antibodies (e.g., RIA, EIA, chemiluminescence) are very sensitive and can measure levels as low as nanograms per milliliter level.

Precision. With nephelometry and turbidimetry, within-run coefficients of variation (CVs) of less than 5% are usual. RID and EIA have higher within-run and run-to-run CVs, usually in the range of 5% to 15%. RIA, measuring much smaller amounts of protein, generally has within-run CVs of 5% to 10%.

Turnaround Time. Modern nephelometric and turbidimetric methods are fast, giving results within seconds to minutes; however, equilibrium methods take longer to complete. RID requires 24 to 72 hours of incubation, an unacceptable period for stat tests. Depending on the procedure, turnaround time for RIA is usually several hours.

Instrumentation and Equipment

Nephelometric and turbidimetric methods (see Chapter 3) are performed on most current automated analytical systems, although most nephelometric assays are performed on dedicated instruments. RID requires no instrumentation other than pipettes, although some type of illuminated plate reader is advantageous. RIA requires radiation scintillation counters and an automated pipetting station.

Calibration of Immunochemical Methods

The World Health Organization (WHO) has reference preparations for the measurement of complement, immunoglobulins, and a few other proteins, but values are assigned in international units (IU). Two preparations, WHO 6HSP and the United States National Reference Preparation for Specific Human Proteins (USNRP), have values assigned in IU and in some cases mass units for 6 and 13 proteins, respectively. However, conversion factors between mass units and IU differ by as much as 16% between the two preparations.

In 1993 and 1994, the Bureau Commitaire de Référence (BCR) of the European Economic Community, the International Federation of Clinical Chemistry (IFCC), and the College of American Pathologists (CAP) jointly introduced a new reference preparation for serum proteins,[118,120] assigned in IU against WHO materials and in mass units against USNRP for albumin, AMG, complement factors C3 and C4, Cp, Hp, and IgA, IgG, and IgM. Mass values were assigned for AAT (α_1-protease inhibitor), α_1-antichymotrypsin, AAG (orosomucoid), and transferrin against highly purified and thoroughly characterized purified proteins, and for C-reactive protein against WHO 85/506, using the factor 1 IU = 1 mg/dL. In this value assignment, a rigorous transfer protocol was used, and all steps in the preparation were carefully recorded to make it possible to prepare a new lot to be as nearly the same as possible. The material is available from the Institute for Reference Materials and Methods (IRMM; Geel, Belgium) as Certified Reference Material #470 (catalog number *BCR 470*). It is intended for transfer of values to secondary reference materials (e.g., manufacturers' calibrators and controls), not for use as a working calibrator or control.

All manufacturers of immunochemical assays have referenced their individual calibrators and controls against the new material, and national and international quality control studies have shown a marked decrease in interlaboratory variance as a result. Minor differences still exist among manufacturers' assays, however, because of differences in antiserum specificity and in the methods used by the various manufacturers for transfer of values from CRM 470 to working reference materials, including differences in calibration curve fitting and in statistical methods. In most cases, the differences are less than 5%. Tentative international reference intervals for white adults have been established,[28] and the Committee on Plasma Protein Standardization of the IFCC is conducting a large-scale, prospective study to determine reference intervals for several ethnic groups. It is recommended that each laboratory confirm the validity of the values for its own population.

Optimization of Immunonephelometry and Turbidimetry Assays[2]

To minimize complexity and cost, yet retain enough accuracy and precision to meet clinical demands, most commercially available assays for proteins are a compromise In those circumstances in which these are more demanding—for example, for transferring values to a manufacturer's "gold standard" calibrators and controls—signal level should be maximized and all steps in the assay should be performed with as high precision as possible. The criteria for such an assay have been summarized by Blirup-Jensen.[2] Reference laboratories should also use this or similar protocols to maximize accuracy.

In addition, for value transfer, multiple weight-corrected dilutions of the reference (e.g., CRM 470) and the target material should be assayed in multiple runs, with the dilutions of each material calculated to be within the same section of the assay range. If possible, for optimal results, one material should be used as the calibrator and the other as the test sample to avoid the introduction of a third material and increased imprecision.[3]

Specimen Collection and Storage for Immunoassay

Test specimens should be nonhemolyzed, cell-free serum, urine, or CSF. CSF specimens may require centrifugation if cells are present. Serum and CSF samples may be stored at 2 °C to 8 °C for up to 3 days or at −20 °C for longer periods.

Repeated freezing and thawing of specimens may cause deterioration of many proteins and should be avoided. The minimum amount of specimen required is generally 100 μL.

Electrophoretic Techniques

Electrophoresis is used to study and measure the protein content of biological fluids (see Chapter 5). Types include serum protein electrophoresis using either cellulose acetate strip or agarose gel as the separation media, capillary electrophoresis (CE), immunofixation, and "Western blotting."

Serum Protein Electrophoresis

Separation of serum proteins on cellulose acetate or agarose gel is commonly performed on serum to avoid the fibrinogen band in a region in which monoclonal immunoglobulins often migrate. However, some analysts prefer to use plasma to semiquantify the amount of fibrinogen present as evidence of acute inflammation or in vivo fibrinolysis.

The principles of electrophoresis are described in Chapter 5. Figure 20-9 illustrates serum protein electrophoresis separations typical of normal and pathological conditions. In practice, most serum protein electrophoresis is performed using commercial systems that integrate apparatus, materials, and reagents from a single supplier. The standard buffers have low ionic strength (~0.05) and pH ~8.6. The usual sample is 3 to 5 μL, applied with a mechanical device to obtain an even stripe of sample across a track of the medium. Typical parameters for the run are 1.5 mA per 2-cm width of cellulose acetate or 10 mA per 1-cm width of agarose gel, and a run time of 40 to 60 minutes producing a 5 to 6 cm migration distance for albumin. Changes in certain bands are clearly associated with particular disorders, making serum protein electrophoresis a valuable screening method.

Coomassie brilliant blue (CBB) stain is more sensitive than Amido Black or Ponceau S and is widely used. The concentrations of many proteins are too low to be seen as distinct stained bands, or they are overshadowed by proteins of higher concentrations that migrate near them. In addition, some proteins stain poorly because they contain high proportions of lipid (lipoproteins) or carbohydrate (AAG). Densitometry may be used for rough quantification of individual bands and for graphic displays of stained electrophoresis patterns, but visual examination by a trained observer is much preferred.

Special fat stains are needed to visualize lipoproteins that migrate in bands of variable mobility in the fast α_1-region (α_1-lipoprotein), the α_2- or pre-β-region (very low density lipoprotein), and the β_1-region (β-lipoprotein), or remain at the origin (chylomicrons; see also Chapter 26). As mentioned previously, visualization of α_1-acid glycoprotein requires staining for carbohydrate side chains.

In practice, a patient's serum should always be run in parallel with a reference serum for comparison. The following changes may be seen:

1. Intensely stained bands occurring from the α- to the γ-regions in areas not containing normal proteins or free hemoglobin. These suggest monoclonal immunoglobulins (paraproteins).
2. Multiple bands, absent bands, or different mobility of normal bands. These may be due to genetic variants or deficiency, such as AAT in the α_1-region and transferrin or C3 in the β-region.
3. Other causes of altered mobility. Increased mobility of albumin occurs when it is bound to penicillin or salicylates or to greater-than-normal amounts of bilirubin or fatty acids. Mercaptalbumin dimers or complexes with AAT migrate cathodal to monomeric albumin. Decreased mobility of AAT occurs when it binds thiol groups of IgA or Bence Jones protein.
4. Appearance of a band not normally seen. The level of a low-concentration protein may increase to such a level that it becomes visible as a line. For instance, a faint, sharp band may appear between albumin and the α_1-region as a result of a 100-fold increase of AFP with certain tumors. Similarly, a large increase of CRP in a severe APR may generate a faint band in the β- or γ-region (depending on free Ca^{2+} concentration), or an increase of lysozyme in monocytic leukemia may produce a band in the post-γ-region.
5. Changes in relative concentrations. The stained strip should also be observed for changes in relative concentrations of the major plasma proteins. Such changes can suggest the presence of certain pathological conditions:
   a. Decreased albumin and γ-bands in conjunction with an increased α_2-band suggest selective protein loss, such as is displayed in the nephrotic syndrome. Note, however, that the albumin concentration must fall by at least one third of its normal level before its decrease becomes evident on the electrophoretic strip.
   b. An increase in the α_1-band (AAT and AAG) and α_2-band (Hp) suggests an APR. Prealbumin, albumin, and transferrin (α_1) are usually decreased. An increase in only AAT (α_1) may be noted in chronic hepatitis and in APRs accompanied by hemolysis, and in estrogen therapy or pregnancy. In diseases characterized by vasculitis (such as rheumatoid arthritis) or in immune complex diseases, a predominant increase in the α_2-band may be observed.
   c. An increase in the β_1-band (transferrin) suggests iron deficiency (transferrin increase) or high levels of estrogen.
   d. Fusion or bridging of β- and γ-bands suggests an increase in IgA, as seen with cirrhosis, respiratory tract or skin infections, and rheumatoid arthritis.
   e. A diffuse increase in the γ-band suggests a polyclonal γ-globulin increase associated with an immune reaction, chronic inflammatory disease, liver disease, or disseminated neoplasms. Oligoclonal bands are occasionally seen in chronic aggressive hepatitis and

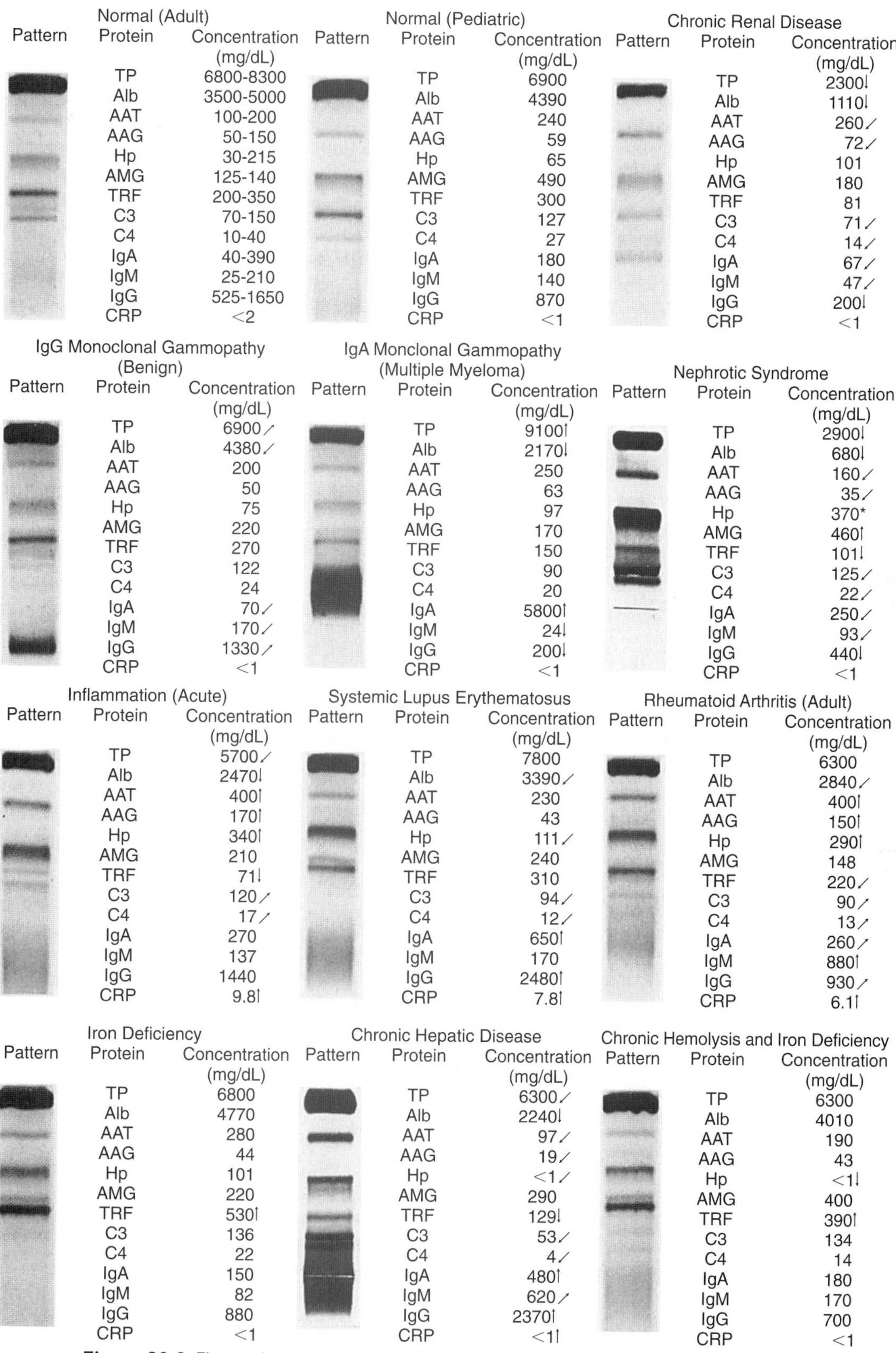

Normal (Adult)

Protein	Concentration (mg/dL)
TP	6800-8300
Alb	3500-5000
AAT	100-200
AAG	50-150
Hp	30-215
AMG	125-140
TRF	200-350
C3	70-150
C4	10-40
IgA	40-390
IgM	25-210
IgG	525-1650
CRP	<2

Normal (Pediatric)

Protein	Concentration (mg/dL)
TP	6900
Alb	4390
AAT	240
AAG	59
Hp	65
AMG	490
TRF	300
C3	127
C4	27
IgA	180
IgM	140
IgG	870
CRP	<1

Chronic Renal Disease

Protein	Concentration (mg/dL)
TP	2300↓
Alb	1110↓
AAT	260↙
AAG	72↙
Hp	101
AMG	180
TRF	81
C3	71↙
C4	14↙
IgA	67↙
IgM	47↙
IgG	200↓
CRP	<1

IgG Monoclonal Gammopathy (Benign)

Protein	Concentration (mg/dL)
TP	6900↗
Alb	4380↙
AAT	200
AAG	50
Hp	75
AMG	220
TRF	270
C3	122
C4	24
IgA	70↙
IgM	170↙
IgG	1330↗
CRP	<1

IgA Monclonal Gammopathy (Multiple Myeloma)

Protein	Concentration (mg/dL)
TP	9100↑
Alb	2170↓
AAT	250
AAG	63
Hp	97
AMG	170
TRF	150
C3	90
C4	20
IgA	5800↑
IgM	24↓
IgG	200↓
CRP	<1

Nephrotic Syndrome

Protein	Concentration (mg/dL)
TP	2900↓
Alb	680↓
AAT	160↙
AAG	35↙
Hp	370*
AMG	460↑
TRF	101↓
C3	125↙
C4	22↙
IgA	250↙
IgM	93↙
IgG	440↓
CRP	<1

Inflammation (Acute)

Protein	Concentration (mg/dL)
TP	5700↙
Alb	2470↓
AAT	400↑
AAG	170↑
Hp	340↑
AMG	210
TRF	71↓
C3	120↗
C4	17↗
IgA	270
IgM	137
IgG	1440
CRP	9.8↑

Systemic Lupus Erythematosus

Protein	Concentration (mg/dL)
TP	7800
Alb	3390↙
AAT	230
AAG	43
Hp	111↙
AMG	240
TRF	310
C3	94↙
C4	12↙
IgA	650↑
IgM	170
IgG	2480↑
CRP	7.8↑

Rheumatoid Arthritis (Adult)

Protein	Concentration (mg/dL)
TP	6300
Alb	2840↙
AAT	400↑
AAG	150↑
Hp	290↑
AMG	148
TRF	220↙
C3	90↗
C4	13↗
IgA	260↗
IgM	880↑
IgG	930↗
CRP	6.1↑

Iron Deficiency

Protein	Concentration (mg/dL)
TP	6800
Alb	4770
AAT	280
AAG	44
Hp	101
AMG	220
TRF	530↑
C3	136
C4	22
IgA	150
IgM	82
IgG	880
CRP	<1

Chronic Hepatic Disease

Protein	Concentration (mg/dL)
TP	6300↙
Alb	2240↓
AAT	97↙
AAG	19↙
Hp	<1↙
AMG	290
TRF	129↓
C3	53↙
C4	4↙
IgA	480↑
IgM	620↗
IgG	2370↑
CRP	<1↑

Chronic Hemolysis and Iron Deficiency

Protein	Concentration (mg/dL)
TP	6300
Alb	4010
AAT	190
AAG	43
Hp	<1↓
AMG	400
TRF	390↑
C3	134
C4	14
IgA	180
IgM	170
IgG	700
CRP	<1

Figure 20-9 Electrophoretic patterns typical of normal and of some pathological conditions (agarose gel). Upward- and downward-pointing arrows indicate increase and decrease from the reference interval, respectively. Right- or left-slanting arrows indicate variation from normal to an increase or from normal to a decrease from the reference interval, respectively. The asterisk indicates Hp 2-2 phenotype.

chronic viral infections, and in some bacterial infections (e.g., pneumococcal pneumonia) or following bone marrow transplantation.

f. Absence or decrease of the γ-band suggests immunodeficiency, either congenital or acquired.

Immunofixation Electrophoresis

Immunofixation electrophoresis (IFE) is gradually replacing immunoelectrophoresis (IEP) for detection of M-components because of its speed and ease of interpretation. Several procedures, including commercial kits, are available for both IFE and IEP. Although these procedures may differ in detail, their principles are similar.

To perform IFE analysis, aliquots of a patient's serum are placed in separate wells in an agarose gel, and their major protein groups separated by electrophoresis. One of these tracks may be treated with a chemical fixative solution to fix all proteins in the agarose and create an electrophoresis reference pattern for the specimen. The other tracks are treated with specific heavy- and light-chain antisera that react with individual immunoglobulins in the specimens, causing them to precipitate (become immunofixed) in the agarose gel. All unreacted proteins are washed out of the gel, which is then stained to visualize the fixed protein bands. By comparing the locations of the stained, immunofixed bands with a band of the same location in the reference pattern, a specific protein may be identified.

Specific antisera may be applied with saturated filter paper or cellulose acetate strips, but many commercial kits use other application methods such as mylar templates that allow direct pipetting of antiserum onto the surface of the gel.

In monoclonal gammopathies, the IFE patterns usually yield a distinct, sharply defined precipitin band with one heavy-chain and one light-chain antiserum. These bands match the location of the particular immunoglobulin in the reference pattern (Figure 20-10). A second, fainter band of free light chains may also be present.

Immunofixation electrophoresis patterns should always be confirmed by quantifying the immunoglobulins (IgG, IgA, IgM) in the specimen. Elevations of specific immunoglobulins should correspond to the more intensely stained bands on the IFE pattern, but if a monoclonal protein is present, the assayed result may be only an approximation because of antigen excess. The unaffected immunoglobulins are often very low in concentration. To determine proper dilutions of the specimen to be used for the various immunoglobulins, it is helpful to perform quantification before IFE is performed.

A comparison of IFE and IEP for two patients with monoclonal gammopathies is shown in Figure 20-10. The principles of IEP are described in Chapters 5 and 9.

Capillary Electrophoresis

CE combines the classic techniques of zone electrophoresis, isotachophoresis, isoelectric focusing, and gel electrophoresis in small-bore (10 to 100 μm), fused silica capillary tubes 20 to 200 cm in length (see Chapter 5). It is a very efficient, rapid, sensitive, and versatile analytical technique that can be used to analyze a diverse spectrum of analytes ranging from small ions to macromolecular proteins or nucleic acids.[62] CE is used for both micropreparative and analytical purposes. One advantage of CE, compared with traditional electrophoretic techniques, is its suitability for automation. However, interpretation of many abnormal samples remains a problem. Commercial systems resemble many high-performance liquid chromatography (HPLC) instruments in terms of automated sample loading and data analysis.

Western Blotting

Western blotting is similar to IFE, except that the separated proteins are blotted onto an overlaying strip of nitrocellulose or a nylon membrane by diffusion or electroblotting. The strip or membrane is then reacted with an antibody raised against the protein of interest and labeled with a radioisotope (e.g., ^{125}I) or enzyme (e.g., horseradish peroxidase). (See Chapter 5 for further details and applications of this technique.)

Determination of Serum Total Protein

In total protein assays, two assumptions are arbitrarily made: (1) All protein molecules are pure polypeptide chains, containing on the average 16% by weight of nitrogen; and (2) each of the several hundred individual proteins present in serum reacts chemically like every other protein. In practice, the first assumption is not true and the second is not always true. Nevertheless, these simplifying assumptions make measurement of total protein a practical, although empirical, procedure.

Specific Methods

Many methods have been developed to measure the total protein content of biological fluids. A number of them are reviewed here.

Biuret Method. The biuret method depends on the presence of peptide bonds, which react with Cu^{2+} ions in alkaline solutions to form a colored product whose absorbance is measured spectrophotometrically at 540 nm. A colored chelate is formed between the Cu^{2+} ion and the carbonyl oxygen and amide nitrogen atoms of the peptide bond. An analogous reaction occurs between cupric ion and the organic compound biuret, hence the name. The reaction occurs with any compound containing at least two H_2N—C—, H_2N—CH_2—, H_2N—CS—, or similar groups covalently linked directly or through a carbon or nitrogen atom. One copper ion is probably linked to six nearby peptide linkages by coordinate bonds. The intensity of the color produced is proportional to the number of peptide bonds that are reacting and therefore to the number of protein molecules present in the reaction system.

Amino acids and dipeptides do not react, but tripeptides, oligopeptides, and polypeptides react to give pink to

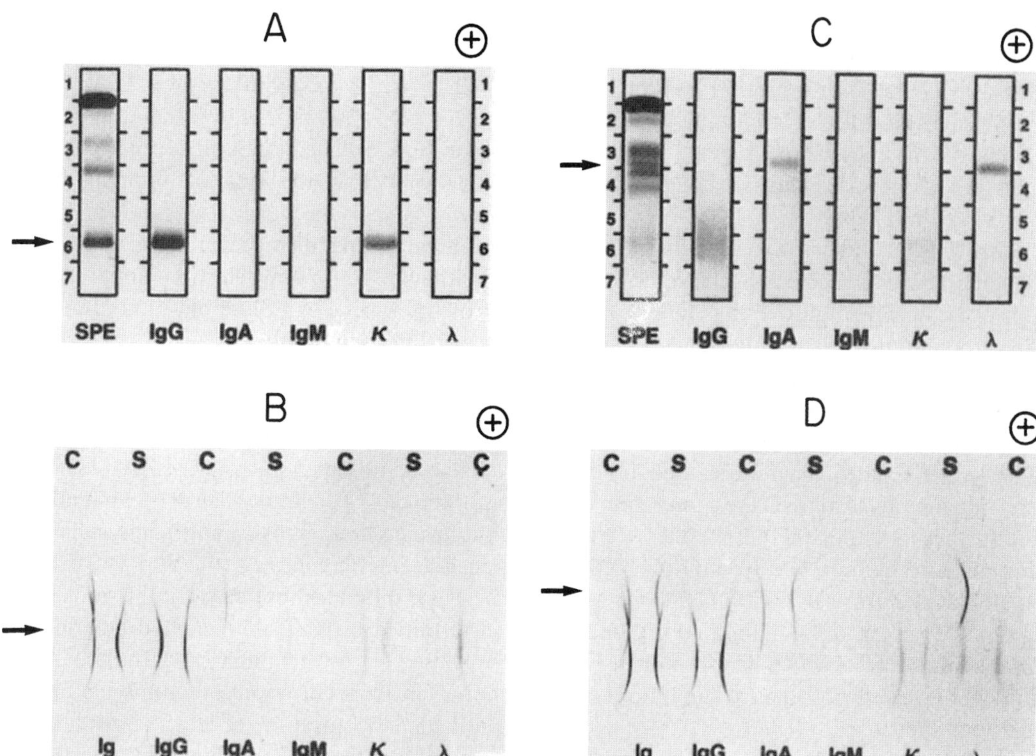

Figure 20-10 Comparison of immunofixation electrophoresis (IFE) and immunoelectrophoresis (IEP) for two patients with monoclonal gammopathies. **A,** Patient specimen with an IgG (kappa, κ) monoclonal protein as identified by IFE. The *arrow* indicates the position of monoclonal protein. After electrophoresis, each track except SPE is reacted with its respective antiserum, then all tracks are stained to visualize the respective protein bands. (SPE: Chemically fixed serum protein electrophoresis; IgG, IgA, IgM, κ, and λ indicate antiserum used on each track.) **B,** Same specimen as in A, with proteins identified by IEP. The *arrow* indicates the position of monoclonal protein. Normal control (C) and patient sera (S) are alternated. After electrophoresis, antiserum is added to each trough as indicated by the labels Ig (polyvalent Ig antiserum), IgG, IgA, IgM, κ, and λ. The antisera react with separated proteins in the specimens to form precipitates in the shape of arcs. The IgG and κ arcs are shorter and thicker than those in the normal control, showing the presence of the IgG (κ) monoclonal protein. The concentrations of IgA, IgM, and λ-light chains are also reduced. **C,** Patient specimen with an IgA (lambda, λ) monoclonal protein identified by IFE procedure as described in A. **D,** Same specimen as in C with proteins identified by IEP as described in B. The abnormal IgA and λ-arcs for the patient specimen indicate an elevated concentration of a monoclonal IgA (λ) protein. All separations were performed using the Beckman-Coulter Paragon system.

reddish-violet products. However, their concentration in serum is so low that they contribute little to the biuret color. Ammonium ions interfere but not at concentrations that can occur in serum. Most biuret methods detect between 1 and 15 mg of protein in the aliquot being measured, an amount present in 15 to 200 µL of a serum containing protein at 7 g/dL. Numerous versions of the biuret method have been reported. All the methods are sufficiently precise for clinical use.

Either serum or plasma may be used for a biuret assay. A fasting specimen is not required but may be desirable to decrease lipemia. Hemolysis should be avoided. Tightly stoppered samples of serum are stable for 1 week or more at room temperature and for 1 month at 2 °C to 4 °C. Specimens that have been frozen and thawed should be thoroughly mixed before assay.

A detailed procedure of a biuret method is available in a previous edition of this textbook.[97]

Direct Photometric Methods. Absorption of ultraviolet (UV) light at 200 to 225 nm and 270 to 290 nm is used to measure the protein content of biological samples. Absorption of UV light at 280 nm depends chiefly on the aromatic rings of tyrosine and tryptophan at pH 8. Accuracy and specificity suffer from an uneven distribution of these amino acids among individual proteins in a mixture and from the presence in body fluids of free tyrosine and tryptophan, uric acid, and bilirubin, which also absorb light near 280 nm. At 200 to 225 nm, peptide bonds are chiefly responsible for UV absorption (70% at A_{205}); specific absorption by proteins at these shorter wavelengths is 10 to 30 times greater than at 280 nm. Interference from free tyrosine and tryptophan is also significant at these short wavelengths, although it can be made negligible for serum by dilution of 1:1000 or 1:2000 in NaCl, 0.15 mol/L. The method has been used for CSF after removal of small interfering molecules by gel filtration. This approach is sensitive and simple but requires the use of an appropriate spectrophotometer and high-quality cuvets having high transmission of light at 220 nm.

Dye-Binding Methods. Dye-binding methods are based on the ability of proteins to bind dyes, such as Coumassie brilliant blue (CBB). The unequal affinities and binding capacities of individual proteins for dyes are a limitation and are complicated further by the inability to define a consistent material for use as a calibrator. The dye-binding method of greatest contemporary interest uses CBB G-250 for assay of total protein in CSF or urine. CBB binds to protonated amine groups of amino acid residues in the polypeptide chain, resulting in decreased absorbance at 465 nm and increased absorbance at 595 nm.

The method is simple, fast, and linear up to 150 mg/dL. Run-to-run CVs with automated analysis are 5.7% at 24 mg/dL and 2.9% at 84 mg/dL. Positive interferences have been noted in urine specimens containing tolbutamide or very high concentrations of urea. Very high concentrations of sodium chloride (NaCl) and hydrogen chloride (HCl), the latter used to preserve specimens, cause very large negative interferences. If the absorbance obtained with albumin is taken as 100%, hemoglobin and transferrin give an absorbance equivalent to that for albumin, but globulins and κ and λ chains are only 60% equivalent.

Folin-Ciocalteu (Lowry) Method. Most proteins contain tyrosine, tryptophan, or both, but each protein contains a unique proportion of them. Albumin, for instance, has only 0.2% tryptophan by weight, whereas the tryptophan content of individual globulins varies between 2% and 3%. These amino acids, either free or in an unfolded polypeptide chain, reduce phosphotungstic-phosphomolybdic acid (Folin-Ciocalteu) reagent to give a blue color. Less chromogenic complexes are formed with histidine and cysteine. This property is more useful for assaying a pure protein whose composition and relative reactivity are known (e.g., fibrinogen) than it is for a mixture of individual proteins with different concentrations and reactivities. However, it has been applied to the assay of total protein (Lowry's method) as an auxiliary to the biuret reaction. In this method, proteins are allowed first to react with Cu^{2+} in alkaline solution to form copper–peptide bond–protein complexes. When the Folin-Ciocalteu reagent is added, the copper-protein complexes join with tyrosine and tryptophan residues in the reduction process. About 75% of the color produced depends on the Cu^{2+} complex; the absorbance of the colored complex is measured at a wavelength between 650 and 750 nm.

The detection limit of the Lowry method (10 to 60 μg/mL) is 100 times lower than the biuret reaction. This lower limit of detection is an advantage for measurement of very low concentrations of protein, and consequently, Lowry's method is widely used in research to measure tissue proteins and purified preparations of enzymes. Despite the desirability of lower detection limits in measuring total protein in urine or CSF, application of the Folin method to these fluids is not wholly satisfactory, because the reagents react nonspecifically with nonprotein compounds, giving a positive error of 3 to 9 mg/dL. Gel filtration can be used to remove interferents from urine or CSF, but this process is time consuming and not always feasible when the specimen volume of CSF is limited. Drugs—such as salicylates, chlorpromazine, tetracyclines, and some sulfa drugs—also give positive interference.

Kjeldahl's Method. Historically, total protein was first determined by Kjeldahl's method, in which acid digestion was used to convert nitrogen in the protein to ammonium ion. The concentration of ammonia nitrogen was then evaluated by titration or nesslerization, a correction was made for nitrogen contributed by nonprotein compounds also present in serum, and the ammonia nitrogen value was multiplied by the factor 6.25 (100%/16%) to express protein nitrogen as total protein. The method was well defined and reproducible but so time consuming and inconvenient that it was impractical for widespread routine use. This method is still used to assign values to reference materials for the biuret method.

Refractometry. Refractometry is a quick alternative to chemical analysis for serum total protein when a rapid estimate is required. Some laboratories find it a convenient way to determine total protein content before serum protein electrophoresis. At protein concentrations less than 3.5 g/dL, refractometric results are likely to be inaccurate. At a level greater than 11.0 g/dL, a valid result is obtained by diluting the serum with equal parts of water followed by reading of the diluted sample. A day-to-day CV of less than 2.0% is acceptable precision.

Nonimmunochemical Turbidimetric and Nephelometric Methods. Precipitation of protein for turbidimetric or nephelometric assays is achieved with sulfosalicylic acid alone, or with sulfosalicylic acid in combination with sodium sulfate or trichloroacetic acid (TCA), or with TCA alone. Precipitation methods for total protein assay depend on formation of a fine precipitate of uniform, insoluble protein particles, which scatter incident light in suspension.

Calibration of Total Protein Methods

Bovine or human albumin is commonly used to calibrate biuret methods. Albumin has been prepared consistently in high purity, it contains only amino acids, its nitrogen content is a constant fraction of its molecular mass, and the number of peptide bonds per molecule is known. Because the peptide bond is the biuret-reacting unit in all proteins and the number of peptide bonds determines the absorbance of the colored product, albumin is a reasonable peptide bond reference material for all the proteins in the mixture.

For the calibration of precipitation and dye-binding methods, the recommendation is usually to use a suitable dilution of a serum (or serum pool) with a normal albumin/globulin ratio, obtained from a healthy subject, and analyzed for total protein with a correctly calibrated and well controlled biuret or Kjeldahl's method. The choice is dictated by the intent to provide in the reference material a mixture of proteins whose precipitation and dye-binding behaviors are similar to those of proteins in the sample to be analyzed. Use of bovine or human serum albumin as calibrators prohibits the use of sulfosalicylic acid because these pure proteins give about 2.5 times the turbidity given by serum globulins. With these pure proteins, TCA is the reagent of choice.

The IRMM is currently preparing a serum-based reference material for serum total protein assays, referenced to highly purified human serum albumin.

Reference Intervals

The total protein concentration of serum obtained from a healthy ambulatory adult is 6.3 to 8.3 g/dL and 6.0 to 7.8 g/dL from an adult at rest. The two general causes of alterations of serum total protein are a change in the volume of plasma water and a change in the concentration of one or more of the specific proteins in the plasma. Decrease in the volume of plasma water *(hemoconcentration)* is reflected as relative hyperproteinemia; concentrations of all the individual plasma proteins are increased. *Hyperproteinemia* is noted in dehydration caused by inadequate water intake or excessive water loss as in severe vomiting, diarrhea, Addison's disease, or diabetic acidosis. *Hemodilution* (increase in plasma water volume) is reflected as relative hypoproteinemia; concentrations of all the individual plasma proteins are decreased. Hemodilution occurs with water intoxication or salt retention syndromes, during massive intravenous infusions, and physiologically when a recumbent position is assumed. A recumbent position decreases total protein concentration by 0.3 to 0.5 g/dL and many individual proteins including albumin by up to 10%.

Of the individual serum proteins, albumin is present in such high concentrations that low levels of this protein alone may cause *hypoproteinemia.* Hypoalbuminemia is very common and has many causes. Mild *hyperproteinemia* may be caused by an increase in the concentration of specific proteins normally present in relatively low concentration, as, for example, increases in APR and polyclonal immunoglobulins as a result of infection. Marked hyperproteinemia may be caused by high levels of the *monoclonal immunoglobulins* produced in multiple myeloma and other malignant paraproteinemias.

Determination of Proteins in Urine

Many methods have been used to measure urinary proteins but none are totally satisfactory. The biuret method applied to acid-precipitated protein or to a concentrate obtained by membrane filtration has the advantage of equal sensitivity to each of the individual proteins in the mixture. Many laboratories, however, find this approach too time consuming for routine use and prefer turbidimetric and dye-binding methods because they are fast and simple. Of the dye-binding methods, pyrogallol red, Ponceau S, and CBB are the most popular. The turbidimetric and dye-binding methods have nonlinear calibration curves and unequal sensitivities for individual proteins. Most underestimate low molecular weight proteins in tubular proteinuria and immunoglobulin light chains in overload proteinuria.

To quantify urinary proteins, a timed collection is usually used. Periods of 4, 8, and 12 hours may be appropriate for monitoring a renal transplant recipient or a patient whose acute renal losses of albumin are being compensated with closely regulated replacement therapy. In most cases, however, a 24-hour collection is chosen, both for quantitative total or specific protein assay and for electrophoretic separation. An alternative approach is to measure the protein-creatinine ratios of random specimens.

Dipstick tests are often used to semiquantitatively measure excess protein in urine. With these tests, the reactive portion of the stick is coated with a buffered indicator that develops color in the presence of protein. Detection limits are approximately 7 mg/dL. Like all dye-binding techniques, the dipstick methods are more sensitive to albumin than to other plasma proteins. They are therefore excellent screening tests for glomerular proteinuria but unsatisfactory for detection of tubular proteinuria or overload proteinuria. Although most tests measure protein in excess of 10 mg/dL, they are only semiquantitative, and their use should be limited to screening and to approximate estimates required before concentrating the specimen for electrophoresis or diluting it for quantitative assay. A first morning urine specimen is preferred because it tends to be concentrated and unaffected by postural factors.

The reference interval for urinary total protein is 1 to 14 mg/dL. The excretion rate at rest is 50 to 80 mg/d, but many laboratories indicate the reference value as less than 100 mg/d (less than 150 mg/d in pregnancy). The concentration may reach 300 mg/d in urine of healthy subjects after exercise.

Determination of Total Protein in Cerebrospinal Fluid

The low levels of protein in CSF limit the methods that are used to measure total protein in it. Turbidimetric methods and versions of the CBB dye-binding method are commonly used for this purpose. The most serious disadvantage of turbidimetric methods is the requirement for 0.2 to 0.5 mL of sample. Coomassie Brilliant Blue (CBB) methods are sensitive enough for use with samples of as little as 25 μL, but they underestimate globulins. Because albumin is the highest concentration protein in CSF, this underestimation may not be serious enough to preclude the use of a CBB method.

Determination of Specific Proteins in Cerebrospinal Fluid

Nephelometry, immunoturbidimetry, electroimmunodiffusion,[23,24] and RID are most often used for measurements of albumin and IgG in cerebrospinal fluid. Apparent absence of IgG may be due to its degradation by proteinases in the specimen. RIA is required for determination of specific proteins present in very low concentrations (e.g., IgM). The reference interval for albumin levels in lumbar CSF by RID is 17.7 to 25.1 mg/dL. IgA, IgD, and IgM, measured by RIA, are each normally less than 0.2 mg/dL. Reference intervals for IgG are age related; their means increase from 3.5 mg/dL in the 15- to 20-year-old group to 5.8 in adults aged 60 or older. The usual reference interval for CSF IgG in adults is 0.8 to 4.2 mg/dL; for total protein, 15 to 45 mg/dL. Total protein levels are considerably higher in neonates, and in healthy elderly adults, concentrations up to 60 mg/dL are considered normal.

Mass Spectrometry

Mass spectrometry is a powerful qualitative and quantitative analytical tool that is used to assess the molecular mass and primary amino acid sequence of peptides and proteins.[13,14] Technical advancements in mass spectrometry have resulted in the development of matrix-assisted laser desorption/ionization (MALDI) and electrospray ionization techniques that allow sequencing and mass determination of picomole quantities of proteins with masses greater than 100 kDa (see Chapter 7). A time-of-flight mass spectrometer is used to detect the small quantities of ions that are produced by MALDI. In this type of spectrometer, ions are accelerated in an electrical field and allowed to drift to a detector. The mass of the ion is calculated from the time it takes to reach the detector. To measure the masses of proteins in a mixture or to produce a peptide map of a proteolytic digest, from 0.5 to 2.0 μL of sample is dried on the tip of the sample probe, which is then introduced into the spectrometer for analysis. With this technique, proteins located on the surfaces of cells are selectively ionized and analyzed.

With electrospray ionization, a fine mist of highly charged particles is produced when a liquid flows from a capillary tube into a strong electrical field (3 to 6 kV). In practice, electrospray ionization sources are often directly coupled with reversed phase HPLC or capillary columns. The ability to couple a liquid chromatograph with an electrospray ionization source and a mass spectrometer allows the online removal of salts and contaminants and the analysis of complex mixtures. Although different from MALDI, electrospray provides similar sensitivity and application to the analysis of large proteins.

Tandem mass spectrometry is a type of mass spectrometry that is applicable to the rapid sequencing of peptides contained in a complex biological mixture. In a tandem mass spectrometer, two or more mass analyzers are connected in tandem. In the first, the targeted compound is selectively ionized and its characteristic ions are separated from others in the mixture. The selected primary ions then collide with molecules of a neutral gas to produce fragments that are separated and identified in the second spectrometer. Using two mass spectrometers in tandem permits the selective and specific analysis of many compounds of various structural classes. The need for a chromatographic step is eliminated because separation and analysis take place simultaneously in the tandem mass spectrometer. Compared with older methods, tandem mass spectrometry offers greater analytical sensitivity, accuracy, and speed.

Because of its ability to identify and quantify proteins, mass spectrometry is a key analytical tool that is used in the emerging field of proteomics (see Chapter 7).[72,83,125] In proteomics, an important task is protein identification.[66] Using mass spectrometry, proteins are separated[51,90] and then digested. The resulting fragments are analyzed by mass spectrometry and used to identify the protein(s) present.[76] This process is complex and several groups are developing instrumentation and analysis software to automatically identify all the "proteins" in truly complex mixtures. Techniques employed include subcellular fractionation, multidimensional chromatography, and affinity labeling and/or purification. By combining these approaches, several thousand protein species are routinely identified.

REFERENCES

1. Barbaree JM, Decker WJ. Studies on a fast-migrating bisalbumin. Biochem Med 1971;5:181-7.
2. Blirup-Jensen S. Protein standardization. III: Method optimization. Clin Chem Lab Med 2001;39:1098-109.
3. Blirup-Jensen S, Johnson AM, Larsen M. Protein standardization. IV: Value transfer. Clin Chem Lab Med 2001; 39:1110-22.
4. Bortolotti F, Tagliaro F, Cittadini F, Gottardo R, Trettene M, Marigo M. Determination of CDT, a marker of chronic alcohol abuse, for driving license issuing: Immunoassay versus capillary electrophoresis. Forensic Sci Int 2002;128:53-8.
5. Braun A, Kofler A, Morawietz S, Cleve H. Sequence and organization of the human vitamin D-binding protein gene. Biochim Biophys Acta 1993;1216: 385-94.
6. Brennan SO, Fellowes AP. Albumin Hawkes Bay: a low level variant caused by loss of a sulphydryl group at position 177. Biochim Biophys Acta 1993;1182: 46-50.
7. Brock DJH, Sutcliffe RG. Alpha-fetoprotein in the antenatal diagnosis of anencephaly and spina bifida. Lancet 1972;2:197-9.
8. Bull PC, Thomas GR, Rommens JM, Forbes JR, Cox DW. The Wilson disease gene is a putative copper

transporting P-type ATPase similar to the Menkes gene. Nat Genet 1993;5:327-37.
9. Byth BC, Billingsley GD, Cox DW. Physical and genetic mapping of the serpin gene cluster at 14q32.1: Allelic association and a unique haplotype associated with alpha-1-antitrypsin deficiency. Am J Hum Genet 1994;55:126-33.
10. Carrell RW. α_1-Antitrypsin: Molecular pathology, leukocytes and tissue damage. J Clin Invest 1986;78:1427-31.
11. Carrell RW, Travis J. α_1-Antitrypsin and the serpins: Variation and counter-variation. Trends Biochem Sci 1985;10:20-4.
12. Casetta B, Tagliacozzi D, Shushan B. Development of a method for rapid quantitation of amino acids by liquid chromatography-tandem mass spectrometry (LC-MSMS) in plasma. Clin Chem Lab Med 2000;38:391-401.
13. Chace DH. Mass spectrometry in the clinical laboratory. Chem Rev 2001;101:445-77.
14. Chace DH. Mass spectrometry-based diagnostics: The upcoming revolution in disease detection has already arrived. Clin Chem 2003;49:1228-9.
15. Chace DH, Adam BW, Smith SJ, Alexander SR, Hillman SL, Hannon WH. Validation of accuracy-based amino acid reference materials in dried-blood spots by tandem mass spectrometry for newborn screening assays. Clin Chem1999;45: 1269-77.
16. Chace DH, Hillman SL, Milllington DS, et al. Rapid diagnosis of maple syrup urine disease in blood spots from newborns by tandem mass spectrometry. Clin Chem 1995;41:62B8.
17. Chace DH, Hillman SL, Milllington DS, et al. Rapid diagnosis of homocystinuria and other hypermethioninemias by tandem mass spectrometry. Clin Chem 1996;42:349B55.
18. Chace DH, Kalas TA, Naylor EW. The application of tandem mass spectrometry to neonatal screening for inherited disorders of intermediary metabolism. Annu Rev Genomics Hum Genet 2002;3:17-45.
19. Chace DH, Kalas TA, Naylor EW. Use of tandem mass spectrometry for multianalyte screening of dried blood specimens from newborns. Clin Chem 2003;49:1797-817.
20. Chace DH, Milllington DS, Terada N, et al. Rapid diagnosis of phenylketonuria by quantitative analysis for phenylalanine and tyrosine in neonatal blood spots by tandem mass spectrometry. Clin Chem 1993;39:66B71.
21. Chandler AM, Neuhaus OW: Synthesis of serum glycoproteins in response to injury. Am J Physiol 1964;206:169-72.
22. Christenson RH, Azzazy ME. Amino acids. In: Burtis CA, Ashwood ER, eds. Tietz textbook of clinical chemistry. Philadelphia: W B Saunders, 1999:444-476.
23. Christenson RH, Russell ME, Gubar KT, Silverman LM, Ebers GD. Oligoclonal banding in cerebrospinal fluid assessed by electrophoresis on agarose after centrifugal sample concentration through a microconcentrator membrane. Clin Chem 1985;31:1734-6.
24. Christenson RH, Russell ME, Hassett BJ. Cerebrospinal fluid: electrophoresis and methods for determining immunoglobulin G compared. Clin Biochem 1989;22:429-32.
25. Colten HR, Rosen FS. Complement deficiencies. Annu Rev Immunol 1992;10:809-34.
26. Cooper NR, Nemerow GR, Mayes JT. Methods to detect and quantitate complement activation. Springer Semin Immunopathol 1983;6:195-212.
27. Cooper EH, Morgan DB. Proteinuria. Specific protein laboratory improvement program. Continuing education monograph. Washington DC: American Association of Clinical Chemistry Press, 1984;1:1-11.
28. Dati F, Schumann G, Thomas L, Aguzzi F, Baudner S, Bienvenu J, et al. Consensus of a group of professional societies and diagnostic companies on guidelines for interim reference ranges for 14 proteins in serum based on the standardization against the IFCC/BCR/CAP reference material (CRM 470). Eur J Clin Chem Clin Biochem 1996;34:517-20.
29. De Haas CJ. New insights into the role of serum amyloid P component, a novel lipopolysaccharide-binding protein. FEMS Immunol Med Microbiol 1999;26:197-202.
30. Delanghe JR, Langlois MR. Haptoglobin polymorphism and body iron stores. Clin Chem Lab Med 2002; 40(3):212-6.
31. Durward A, Mayer A, Skellett S, Taylor D, Hanna S, Tibby SM, Murdoch IA. Hypoalbuminaemia in critically ill children: Incidence, prognosis, and influence on the anion gap. Arch Dis Child 2003; 88(5):419-22.
32. Ebanks R, Jaikaran A, Carroll MC, Anderson MJ, Campbell RD, Isenman DE. A single arginine to tryptophan interchange at β-chain residue 458 of human complement component C4 accounts for the defect in the classical pathway C5 convertase activity of allotype C4A6: Implications for the location of a C5 binding site in C4. J Immunol 1992;148:2803-11.
33. Engel H, Bac DJ, Brouwer R, Blijenberg BG, Lindemans J. Diagnostic analysis of total protein, albumin, white cell count and differential in ascitic fluid. Eur J Clin Chem Clin Biochem 1995;33:239-42.
34. Eriksson S, Carlson J, Velez R. Risk of cirrhosis and primary liver cancer in α_1-antitrypsin deficiency. N Engl J Med 1986;314:736-9.
35. Fearing MK, Levy HL. Expanded newborn screening using tandem mass spectrometry. Adv Pediatr 2003;50:81-111.
36. Floris G, Medda R, Padiglia A, Musci G. The physiopathological significance of ceruloplasmin. A possi-

ble therapeutic approach. Biochem Pharmacol 2000; 60(12):1735-41.
37. Fox PL, Mazumder B, Ehrenwald E, Mukhopadhyay CK. Ceruloplasmin and cardiovascular disease. Free Radic Biol Med 2000; 28(12):1735-44.
38. Fujii T, Okuno T, Ito M, Kaji M, Mutoh K, Mikawa H, et al. Non-Menkes-type copper deficiency with regression, lactic acidosis, and granulocytopenia. Neurology 1991;41:1263-6.
39. Garey CE, Schwarzman AL, Rise ML, Seyfried TN. Ceruloplasmin gene defect associated with epilepsy in EL mice. Nat Genet 1994;6:426-31.
40. Graziani M, Merlini G, Petrini C. Guidelines for the analysis of Bence Jones protein. Clin Chem Lab Med 2003;41:338-46.
41. Ha JS, Ha CE, Chao JT, Petersen CE, Theriault A, Bhagavan NV. Human serum albumin and its structural variants mediate cholesterol efflux from cultured endothelial cells. Biochim Biophys Acta 2003; 1640(2-3):119-28.
42. Haddow JE, Palomaki GE, Knight GJ, Williams JK, Pulkkinen A, Canick JA, et al. Prenatal screening for Down's syndrome with use of maternal serum markers. N Engl J Med. 1992;327:588-93.
43. Hallbach J, Hoffmann GE, Guder WG. Overestimation of albumin in heparinized plasma. Clin Chem 1991;37:566-8.
44. Hara K, Hijikata Y, Hiraoka E, et al. Measurement of urinary amino acids using high-performance liquid chromatography equipped with a strong cation exchange resin pre-column. Ann Clin Biochem 1999;36:202-6.
45. Hedlund JU, Hansson L-O, Ortqvist AB. Hypoalbuminemia in hospitalized patients with community-acquired pneumonia. Arch Intern Med 1995;155:1438-42.
46. Henderson JM, Stein SF, Kutner M, Wiles MB, Ansley JD, Rudman D. Analysis of twenty-three plasma proteins in ascites. The depletion of fibrinogen and plasminogen. Ann Surg 1980;192:738-42.
47. Hofmann W, Rossmuller B, Guder WG, Edel HH. A new strategy for characterizing proteinuria and haematuria from a single pattern of defined proteins in urine. Eur J Clin Chem Clin Biochem 1992;30: 707-12.
48. Hubbard TJP, Sander C. The role of heat-shock and chaperone proteins in protein folding: Possible molecular mechanisms. Protein Engineering 1991;4: 711-7.
49. Ingenbleek Y, Young V. Transthyretin (prealbumin) in health and disease: Nutritional implications. Annu Rev Nutr 1994;14:495-533.
50. Issaq HJ, Chan KC. Separation and detection of amino acids and their enantiomers by capillary electrophoresis: A review. Electrophoresis 1995;16: 467-80.
51. Issaq H, Veenstra T, Conrads T, Felschow D. The SELDI-TOF approach to proteomics, protein profiling and biomarker identification. Biochem Biophys Res Commun 2002;292.587-92.
52. Ivandic M, Hofmann W, Guder WG. Development and evaluation of a urine protein expert system. Clin Chem 1996;42:1214-22, 1996.
53. Jacken J, Matthijs G. Congenital disorders of glycosylation. Annu Rev Genomics Hum Genet 2001;2: 129-51.
54. Jespersen MH, Jensen J, Rasmussen LH, Ejlersen E, Moller-Petersen J, Sperling-Petersen HU. The reference range for complexed α_2-macroglobulin in human plasma: Development of a new enzyme linked immunosorbent assay (ELISA) for quantitation of complexed α_2-macroglobulin. Scand J Clin Lab Invest 1993;53:639-48.
55. Johnson AM. Low levels of plasma proteins: malnutrition or inflammation? Clin Chem Lab Med 1999;37:91-6.
56. Johnson AM, Rohlfs EM, Silverman LH. Proteins. In: Burtis CA, Ashwood ER, editors. Tietz textbook of clinical chemistry, 3rd edition. Philadelphia: WB Saunders, 1999:486-9.
57. Kallee E. Bennhold's analbuminemia: A follow-up study of the first two cases (1953-1992). J Lab Clin Med 1996;127:470-80.
58. Kanfer A. Coagulation factors in nephrotic syndrome. Am J Nephrol 1990;10(Suppl 1):63-8.
59. Killingsworth LM. Plasma protein patterns in health and disease. Crit Rev Clin Lab Sci 1979;11:1-30.
60. Killingsworth LM. Clinical applications of protein determinations in biological fluids other than blood. Clin Chem 1982;28:1093-1103.
61. Kyle RA. Plasma cell disorders. In: Bennett JC, Plum F, editors. Cecil textbook of medicine, 20th edition. Philadelphia: WB Saunders, 1996:958-68.
62. Landers JP. Clinical capillary electrophoresis. Clin Chem 1995;41:495-509.
63. Langlois MR, Delanghe JR. Biological and clinical significance of haptoglobin polymorphism in humans. Clin Chem 1996;42:1589-600.
64. Lash A, Saleem A. Iron metabolism and its regulation. Ann Clin Lab Sci 1995;25:20-30.
65. Le Boucher J, Charret C, CoudrayBLucas C, et al. Amino acid determination in biological fluids by automated ionB exchange chromatography: Performance of Hitachi LB8500A. Clin Chem 1997;43:1421B8.
66. Lin D, Tabb DL, Yates JR III. Large-scale protein identification using mass spectrometry. Biochim Biophys Acta 2003;1646:1-10.
67. Livrea P, Trojano M, Simone IL, Zimatore GB, Pisicchio L, Logroscino G, et al. Heterogeneous models for blood-cerebrospinal fluid barrier permeability to serum proteins in normal and abnormal

cerebrospinal fluid/serum protein concentration gradients. J Neurol Sci 1984;64:245-58.
68. Lomas DA, Elliott PR, Sidhar SK, Foreman RC, Finch JT, Cox DW, et al. α1-Antitrypsin Mmalton (Phe52-deleted) forms loop-sheet polymers in vivo: Evidence for the C sheet mechanism of polymerization. J Biol Chem 1995;270:16864-70.
69. Luzzani A, Polati E, Dorizzi R, Rungatscher A, Pavan R, Merlini A. Comparison of procalcitonin and C-reactive protein as markers of sepsis. Crit Care Med 2003;31(6):1737-41.
70. Matthijs G, Devriendt K, Cassiman JJ, Van den Berghe E, Marynen P. Structure of the human α_2-macroglobulin gene and its promoter. Biochem Biophys Res Commun 1992;184:596-603.
71. Merlini G, Bellotti V, Andreola A, Palladini G, Obici L, Casarini S, et al. Protein aggregation. Clin Chem Lab Med 2001;39:1065-75.
72. Michnick SW. Proteomics in living cells. Drug Discov Today 2004;9:262-7.
73. Miner SES, Evrovski J, Cole DEC. The clinical chemistry and molecular biology of homocysteine metabolism: an update. Clin Biochem 1997;30:189-201.
74. Mold C, Gewurz H, Du Clos TW. Regulation of complement activation by C-reactive protein. Immunopathology 1999; 42(1-3):23-30.
75. Morimoto RI, Tisseres A, Georgopoulos C. The biology of heat shock proteins and molecular chaperones. Cold Spring Harbor, NY: Cold Spring Harbor Laboratory Press, 1994.
76. Nesvizhskii AI, Aebersold R. Analysis, statistical validation and dissemination of large-scale proteomics datasets generated by tandem MS. Drug Discov Today 2004;9:173-81.
77. Ou W-J, Cameron PH, Thomas DY, Bergeron JJM. Association of folding intermediates of glycoproteins with calnexin during protein maturation. Nature 1993;264:771-6.
78. Papadopoulas NM, Costello R, Kay AD, Cutler NR, Rapaport SI. Combined immunochemical and electrophoretic determinations in paired serum and cerebrospinal fluid samples. Clin Chem 1984;30:1814-6.
79. Perlmutter DH. The SEC receptor: A possible link between neonatal hepatitis in α_1-antitrypsin deficiency and Alzheimer's disease. Pediatr Res 1994;36:271-74.
80. Pervaiz S, Brew K. Homology and structure-function correlations between α_1-acid glycoprotein and serum retinol-binding protein and its relatives. FASEB J 1987;1:209-14.
81. Peters T Jr. All about albumin: Serum albumin—biochemistry, genetics, and medical applications. Washington DC: AACC Press, 1996.
82. Petricoin EF, Liotta LA. Mass spectrometry-based diagnostics: The upcoming revolution in disease detection. Clin Chem 2003;49:533-534.
83. Petricoin EF, Liotta LA. Clinical applications of proteomics. J Nutr 2003; 133(7 Suppl):2476S-84S.
84. Pontuch P, Toserova E, Vozar J, Bulas J, Kratochvilova H. Twenty-four hour ambulatory blood pressure, daytime and nighttime urinary albumin and retinol-binding protein excretion in type I diabetic patients. J Diabet Comp 1995;9:234-6.
85. Prohaska JR, Hoffman RG. Auditory startle response is diminished in rats after recovery from perinatal copper deficiency. J Nutr 1996;126:618-27.
86. Pumphrey RSH. Structure and function of immunoglobulin. In: Ward AM, Whicher JT, editors. Immunochemistry in clinical laboratory medicine. Lancaster, UK: MTP Press, 1979:85-98.
87. Rao NR, Pattabiraman TN. Alpha$_2$-macroglobulin, albumin, and chymotrypsin inhibitory capacity in cerebrospinal fluid as indices of blood-cerebrospinal fluid barrier. Biochem Med Metab Biol 1986;36: 317-21.
88. Revelsky IA, Yashin YS, Sobolevsky TG, Revelsky AI, Miller B, Oriedo V. Electron ionization and atmospheric pressure photochemical ionization in gas chromatography-mass spectrometry analysis of amino acids. Eur J Mass Spectrom 2003;9:497-507.
89. Rifai N, Ridker PM. Proposed cardiovascular risk assessment algorithm using high-sensitivity C-reactive protein and lipid screening. Clin Chem 2001;47:28-30.
90. Romijn EP, Krijgsveld J, Heck AJR. Recent liquid chromatographic-(tandem) mass spectrometric applications in proteomics. J Chromatogr A 2003;1000:589-608.
91. Ronne H, Ocklind C, Wiman K, Rask L, Obrink B, Peterson PA. Ligand dependent regulation of intracellular protein transport: effect of vitamin A on the secretion of retinol-binding protein. J Cell Biol 1983;96:907-10.
92. Rothschild MA, Oratz M, Schreiber SS. Albumin synthesis (parts 1 and 2). N Engl J Med,1972;286: 748-821.
93. Ryffel B, Car BD, Woerly G, Weber M, DiPadova F, Kammuller M, et al. Long-term interleukin-6 administration stimulates sustained thrombopoiesis and acute-phase protein synthesis in a small primate—the marmoset. Blood 1994;83:2093-102.
94. Schlesinger MJ. Heat shock proteins: A minireview. J Biol Chem 1990;265:12111-4.
95. Schreiber G, Aldred AR, Jaworowski A, Nilsson C, Achen MG, Segal MB. Thyroxine transport from blood to brain via transthyretin synthesis in choroid plexus. Am J Physiol 1990;258:R338, 1990.
96. Scott CF, Carrell RW, Glaser CB, Kueppers F, Lewis JH, Colman RW. Alpha-1-antitrypsin Pittsburgh: a potent inhibitor of human plasma factor XIa, kallikrein, and factor XIIf. J Clin Invest 1986;77: 631-4.

97. Silverman LM, Christenson RH. Amino acids and proteins. In: Burtis CS, Ashwood ER, editors. Tietz textbook of clinical chemistry. 2nd edition. Philadelphia: W B Saunders, 1993:696-8.
98. Smithies O, Connell GE, Dixon GH. Chromosomal rearrangements and evolution of haptoglobin genes. Nature 1962;196:232-6.
99. Sokol RJ, Twedt D, McKim JM Jr, Devereaux MW, Karrer FM, Kami I, et al. Oxidant injury to hepatic mitochondria in patients with Wilson's disease and Bedlington terriers with copper toxicosis. Gastroenterology 1994;107:1788-98.
100. Soprano DR, Blaner WS. Plasma retinol-binding protein. In: Sporn MB, Roberts AS, Goodman DS, editors. The retinoids, 2nd edition. New York: Raven Press, 1994:257-81.
101. Sottrup-Jensen L. Role of internal thiol esters in the α_2 macroglobulin-proteinase binding mechanism. Ann NY Acad Sci 1994;737:172-87.
102. Sweetman L. Newborn screening by tandem mass spectrometry (MSBMS). Clin Chem 1996;42:345-6.
103. Sveger T. α_1-Antitrypsin deficiency in early childhood. Pediatrics 1978;62:23-5.
104. Tack BF. The β-cys-γ-glu thiolester bond in human C3, C4, and α_2-macroglobulin. Springer Semin Immunopathol 1983;6:259-82.
105. Teerlink T, van Leeuwen PAM, Houdijk A. Plasma amino acids determined by liquid chromatography within 17 minutes. Clin Chem 1994;40:245B9.
106. Tietz NW, editor. Clinical guide to laboratory tests, 3rd edition. Philadelphia: WB Saunders, 1995.
107. Turner MW, Hamvas RM. Mannose-binding lectin: structure, function, genetics and disease associations. Science 2001;29:2370-6.
108. van der Meer IM, de Maat MP, Kiliaan AJ, van der Kuip DA, Hofman A, Witteman JC. The value of C-reactive protein in cardiovascular risk prediction: The Rotterdam Study. Arch Intern Med 2003;163(11):1323-8.
109. van Dijk W, Havenaar EC, Brinkman-van der Linden EC. Alpha 1-acid glycoprotein (orosomucoid): Pathophysiological changes in glycosylation in relation to its function. Glycoconj J 1995; 12(3):227-33.
110. van Eden W, Young DB, editors. Stress proteins in medicine. New York: Marcel Dekker, 1995.
111. van Eijk HG, de Jong G. The physiology of iron, transferrin and ferritin. Biol Trace Elem Res 1992;35:13-24.
112. van Leuven F, Stas L, Raymakers L, Hilliker C. Structure of the human α_2M receptor gene. Ann NY Acad Sci 1994;737:502-3.
113. Vulpe C, Levinson B, Whitney S, Packman S, Gitschier J. Isolation of a candidate gene for Menkes' disease and evidence that it encodes a copper-transporting ATPase. Nat Genet 1993;3:7-13.
114. Walker V, Mills GA. Quantitative methods for amino acid analysis in biological fluids. Ann Clin Biochem 1995;32:28B57.
115. Walsh MJ, Tourtellotte WW.: The cerebrospinal fluid in multiple sclerosis. In: Hallpike JF, Adams CWM, Tourtellotte WW, editors. Multiple sclerosis. London: Chapman & Hall, 1983:275-358.
116. Weiss RE, Sunthornthepvarakul T, Angkeow P, Marcus-Bagley D, Cox N, Alper CA, et al. Linkage of familial dysalbuminemic hyperthyroxinemia to the albumin gene in a large Amish kindred. J Clin Endocrinol Metab 1995;80:116-21.
117. Welch TR, Beischel L, Berry A, Forristal J, West CD. The effect of null C4 alleles on complement function. Clin Immunol Immunopathol 1985;34:316-25.
118. Whicher JT. BCR/IFCC reference material for plasma proteins (CRM 470). Community Bureau of Reference. International Federation of Clinical Chemistry. Clin Biochem 1998;31:459-65.
119. Whicher JT, Higginson J, Riches PG, Radford S. Clinical applications of immunofixation: Detection and quantification of complement activation. J Clin Pathol 1990;33:781-5.
120. Whicher JT, Ritchie RF, Johnson AM, Baudner S, Bienvenu J, Blirup-Jensen S, et al. New international reference preparation for proteins in human serum (RPPHS). Clin Chem 1994;40:934-8.
121. Whicher JT, Warren C, Chambers RE. Immunochemical assays for immunoglobulins. Ann Clin Biochem 1984;21:78-91.
122. Whitaker JN. Indicators of disease activity in MS: studies of myelin basic protein-like materials. Ann NY Acad Sci 1985;436:140-50.
123. Whitehead AS, Solomon E, Chambers S, Bodmer WF, Povey S, Fey G. Assignment of the structural gene for the third component of human complement of chromosome 19. Proc Natl Acad Sci USA 1982;79: 5021-5.
124. Wochner RD, Spilberg I, Iio A, Liem HH, Müller-Eberhard U. Hemopexin metabolism in sickle-cell disease, porphyrias and control subjects: Effects of heme injection. N Engl J Med 1974;290:822-6.
125. Wulfkuhle JD, Paweletz CP, Steeg PS, Petricoin EF 3rd, Liotta L. Proteomic approaches to the diagnosis, treatment, and monitoring of cancer. Adv Exp Med Biol. 2003;532:59-68.
126. Yang F, Naylor SL, Lum JB, Cutshaw S, McCombs JL, Naberhaus KH, et al. Characterization, mapping, and expression of the human ceruloplasmin gene. Proc Natl Acad Sci USA 1986;83:3257-61.
127. Yonekawa M, Okabe T, Asamoto Y, Ohta M. A case of hereditary ceruloplasmin deficiency with iron deposition in the brain associated with chorea, dementia, diabetes mellitas and retinal pigmentation: administration of fresh-frozen human plasma. Eur Neurol 1999; 42(3):157-62.

128. Yoshida K, Furihata K, Takeda S, Nakamura A, Yamamoto K, Morita H, et al. A mutation in the ceruloplasmin gene is associated with systemic hemosiderosis in humans. Nat Genet 1995;9: 267-72.
129. Zumwalt RW: Amino acid analysis by gas chromatography. Boca Raton, FL, CRC Press, 1987.

ADDITIONAL READING

Amino Acids

Cooper C, Packer N, Willims K, eds. Amino Acid Analysis Protocols. Totowa NJ: Humana Press, 2001:1-265.

Cynober LA, ed. Amino acid metabolism in health & nutritional disease. Boca Raton: CRC Press, 1995.

Davies JS. Amino aids, peptides, & proteins. Boca Raton: CRC Press, 1994.

Massey KA, Blakeslee CH, Pitkow, HS. A review of physiological and metabolic effects of essential amino acids. Amino Acids 1998;14:271-300.

Proteins

Allen RC, Budowle B. Gel electrophoresis of proteins and nucleic acids: selected techniques. New York: Walter De Gruyter, 1994.

Copeland RA. Methods for protein analysis: A practical guide in laboratory protocols. London: Chapman & Hall, 1994.

Gersten D. Gel electrophoresis of proteins: Essential techniques. New York: John Wiley & Sons, 1996.

Kellner R. Microcharacterization of proteins. New York: VCH Publishers, 1995.

Keren DF. High-resolution electrophoresis and immunofixation: Techniques and interpretation. 2nd ed. Newton, MA: Butterworth-Heinemann, 1994.

Ritchie R, Navolotskaia O, editors. Serum proteins in clinical medicine. Vol. I: laboratory section. Scarborough, ME: Foundation for Blood Research, 1996.

Ritchie R, Navolotskaia O, editors. Serum proteins in clinical medicine. Vol. II: clinical section. Scarborough, ME: Foundation for Blood Research, 1997.

Rosenberg I. Protein analysis and purification. Cambridge: Birkhauser Boston, 1996.

Westermeier R. Electrophoresis in practice. Part A: Fundamentals and proteins. 2nd. edition. New York: VCH Publishers, 1996.

Proteomics

Kinter M, Sherman NE. Protein sequencing and identification using tandem mass spectrometry. Hoboken NJ: Wiley-Interscience, 2000:1-320.

Liebler DC, ed. Introduction to proteomics: Tools for the new biology. Totowa NJ: Humana Press. 2001:1-198.

Simpson RJ, ed. Proteins and proteomics: A laboratory manual. Cold Spring Harbor NY: Cold Spring Harbor Laboratory, 2002:1-900.

Westermeier R, Naven T. Proteomics in practice: A laboratory manual of proteome analysis. Weinheim Germany: Vch Verlagsgesellschaft Mbh. 2002:1-316.

CHAPTER 21

Enzymes*

Mauro Panteghini, M.D., Renze Bais, Ph.D., and Wouter W. van Solinge, Ph.D.

Measurements of enzymes are used in medicine in two major ways: Enzymes are measured in serum and other bodily fluids to detect injury to a tissue that makes the enzyme. Enzymes are also measured, often within a tissue, to identify abnormalities or absence of the enzyme, which may cause disease. In the first part of this chapter we discuss enzymes as markers of disease, and then describe conditions associated with abnormalities of enzymes in one readily available cell type, the erythrocyte or red blood cell. Many other abnormalities of enzymes exist, of course, and many are described in chapters of this book including Chapters 40 (Inherited Disease), 43 (Pharmacogenetics) and 55 (Inborn Errors of Amino Acid, Organic Acid, and Fastty Acid Metabolism). For descriptions of enzyme abnormalities associated with lysosomal storage disease, and tests for the related enzymes, readers are referred to the Chapter 40 Appendix that is located on this book's accompanying Evolve site, found at http://evolve.elsevier.com/Tietz/textbook/.

Injury to tissue releases cellular substances that can be used as plasma markers of tissue damage. Many of the clinically useful markers of cellular damage are enzymes. Even though various studies have shown that cytoplasmic substances can be lost following reversible cellular injury, clinical findings suggest that enzyme release is highly specific for cell death in some settings.[173] The acute myocardial cell response to ischemia is the most important example: increases of creatine kinase (CK) activity in plasma appear to occur only with myocardial necrosis.[72]

For a substance to serve as a biochemical marker of damage to a specific organ or tissue, it must arise predominantly from the organ or tissue of interest. Highly specific markers have been identified (e.g., cardiac troponin I, which is found only in cardiac myocytes). Some enzymes are predominantly found in the specialized tissue (e.g., lipase in the pancreas), while others, more widely distributed, have tissue-specific isoenzymes or isoforms (e.g., the pancreatic isoenzyme of α-amylase [AMY] or the bone isoform of alkaline phosphatase [ALP]), which can be evaluated to increase tissue and organ specificity.

The timing of the enzyme's diagnostic window is another important aspect to be considered when these markers are used to evaluate acute injuries. According to Noe,[129] the diagnostic window for an injury marker is the interval of time following an episode of injury during which plasma concentrations of the marker are increased and thereby demonstrate the occurrence of the injury. Marker substances that rapidly enter the circulation (i.e., early indicators) tend to have diagnostic windows that begin soon after the onset of the injury. On the contrary, those biomarkers that are slowly released into the circulation and/or slowly cleared from the circulation (i.e., late indicators) generally have diagnostic windows that begin later and last long after the time of injury.[129]

Several enzymes of diagnostic utility are discussed in this chapter. To better clarify their clinical meaning, the individual enzymes are discussed relative to the organ in which they are clinically most important. Overlap occurs for this classification as the same enzyme may be used for investigating disease in several organs.

MUSCLE ENZYMES

Enzymes in this category include CK, lactate dehydrogenase (LD), aldolase (ALD), and glycogen phosphorylase (GP). At the time of this book's writing, the first two are much more commonly measured than are the latter two.

*The authors gratefully acknowledge the original contributions of D.W. Moss, A.R. Henderson, and V.F. Fairbanks upon which portions of this chapter are based.

TABLE 21-1 Approximate Concentrations of Tissue Creatine Kinase (CK) Activity (Expressed as Multiples of CK Activity Concentrations in Serum) and Cytoplasmic Isoenzyme Composition

Tissue	Relative CK Activity	Isoenzymes, %		
		CK-BB	CK-MB	CK-MM
Skeletal muscle (type I, slow twitch, or red fibers)	50,000	<1	3	97
Skeletal muscle (type II, fast twitch, or white fibers)	50,000	<1	1	99
Heart	10,000	<1	22	78
Brain	5000	100	0	0
Smooth muscle:				
Gastrointestinal tract	5000	96	1	3
Urinary bladder	4000	92	6	2

Creatine Kinase

CK (EC 2.7.3.2; adenosine triphosphate : creatine N-phosphotransferase; CK) is a dimeric enzyme (82 kDa) that catalyzes the reversible phosphorylation of creatine (Cr) by adenosine triphosphate (ATP).

Creatine + Adenosine triphosphate ⇌ Phosphocreatine (creatine phosphate) + Adenosine diphosphate

(forward: pH = 9.0; $H^{\oplus}$; CK, Mg_2^+; reverse: pH = 6.7)

Physiologically, when muscle contracts, ATP is converted to adenosine diphosphate (ADP), and CK catalyzes the rephosphorylation of ADP to ATP using creatine phosphate (CrP) as the phosphorylation reservoir.

The optimal pH values for the forward (Cr + ATP → ADP + CrP) and reverse (CrP + ADP ← ATP + Cr) reactions are 9.0 and 6.7, respectively. At neutral pH, CrP has a much higher phosphorylating potential than does ATP; this higher potential favors the reverse reaction, with ATP being formed from CrP. The reverse reaction proceeds two to six times faster than the forward reaction, depending on the reaction conditions.

As is true for all kinases, Mg^{2+} is an obligate activating ion that forms complexes with ATP and ADP. The optimal concentration range for Mg^{2+} is quite narrow, and excess Mg^{2+} is inhibitory. Many metal ions, such as Mn^{2+}, Ca^{2+}, Zn^{2+}, and Cu^{2+}, inhibit enzyme activity, as do iodoacetate and other sulfhydryl-binding reagents. Activity is inhibited by excess ADP and by citrate, fluoride, nitrate, acetate, iodide, bromide, malonate, and L-thyroxine. Urate and cystine are potent inhibitors of the enzyme in serum. Even chloride and sulfate ions inhibit activity, and the concentrations of these ions should be kept low in any enzyme assay system based on the CrP + ADP (reverse) reaction. The enzyme in serum is relatively unstable, activity being lost as a result of sulfhydryl group oxidation at the active site of the enzyme. Activity can be partially restored by incubating the enzyme preparation with sulfhydryl compounds, such as *N*-acetylcysteine, monothioglycerol, dithioerythritol, dithiothreitol (Cleland reagent), and glutathione. The extent of activity recovered by this procedure is inversely proportional to the time delay in adding these reagents after collection of the blood specimen and the type of sulfhydryl reagent. The current agent of choice is *N*-acetylcysteine, used at a final concentration of 20 mmol/L in the assay reagent.

CK activity is greatest in striated muscle and heart tissue, which contain some 2500 and 550 U/g of protein, respectively. Other tissues, such as the brain, the gastrointestinal tract, and the urinary bladder, contain significantly less activity, and the liver and erythrocytes are essentially devoid of activity (Table 21-1).

CK is a dimer composed of two subunits, each with a molecular weight of about 40,000. These subunits (B and M) are the products of loci on chromosomes 14 and 19, respectively. Because the active form of the enzyme is a dimer, only three different pairs of subunits can exist: BB (or CK-1), MB (or CK-2), and MM (or CK-3). The Commission on Biochemical Nomenclature has recommended that isoenzymes be numbered on the basis of their electrophoretic mobility, with the most anodal form receiving the lowest number. Accordingly, the CK isoenzymes are numbered CK-1, CK-2, and CK-3. The distribution of these isoenzymes in the various tissues of humans is shown in Table 21-1. All three of these isoenzyme species are found in the cell in the cytosol or associated with myofibrillar structures. However, there exists a fourth form that differs from the others both immunologically and by electrophoretic mobility. This isoenzyme (CK-Mt) is located between the inner and outer membranes of mitochondria, and it constitutes, in the heart for example, up to 15% of the total CK activity. The gene for CK-Mt is located on chromosome 15.

CK activity may also be found in macromolecular form—the so-called macro-CK. Macro-CK is found, often transiently, in sera of up to 6% of hospitalized patients, but only a small proportion of these have increased CK activities in serum. It exists in two forms, types 1 and 2. Type 1 is a complex of CK, typically CK-BB, and an immunoglobulin, often IgG, but other complexes have been described, such as CK-MM with IgA. Prevalence has been estimated as between 0.8 and 2.3%, but this is dependent on methodology and the population studied. It often occurs in women older than 50. Type 2 is oligomeric CK-Mt, with a reported prevalence of between 0.5 and 2.6%. It is found predominantly in adults who are severely ill with malignancies or liver disease or in children who have notable tissue distress. The appearance of this isoenzyme in serum is usually associated with a poor prognosis. Macro-CK can interfere with the assay of CK-MB by some immunoinhibition methods.

Both M and B subunits have a C-terminal lysine residue, but only the former can be hydrolyzed by the action of carboxypeptidases normally present in blood. Carboxypeptidases B (EC 3.4.17.2) or N (arginine carboxypeptidase; EC 3.4.17.3) sequentially hydrolyze the lysine residues from CK-MM to produce two CK-MM isoforms—CK-MM_2 (one lysine residue removed) and CK-MM_1 (both lysine residues removed). The loss of the positively charged lysine produces a more negatively charged CK molecule with greater anodic mobility. Because CK-MB has only one M subunit, the dimer coded by the M and B genes is named CK-MB_2 and the lysine-hydrolyzed dimer is named CK-MB_1. The assay of the CK isoforms requires special techniques, such as high-voltage electrophoresis (with gel cooling), high-performance liquid chromatography (HPLC), chromatofocusing, or immunoassay.[141]

Serum CK activity is subject to a number of physiological variations. Sex, age, muscle mass, physical activity, and race all interact to affect serum activities.

Clinical Significance

Serum CK activity is greatly elevated in all types of muscular dystrophy. In progressive muscular dystrophy (particularly Duchenne sex-linked muscular dystrophy), enzyme activity in serum is highest in infancy and childhood (7 to 10 years of age) and may be increased long before the disease is clinically apparent. Serum CK activity characteristically falls as patients get older and as the mass of functioning muscle diminishes with the progression of the disease. About 50% to 80% of the asymptomatic female carriers of Duchenne dystrophy show threefold to sixfold increases of CK activity, but values may be normal if specimens are obtained after patients have experienced a period of physical inactivity. Quite high values of CK are noted in viral myositis, polymyositis, and similar muscle diseases. However, in neurogenic muscle diseases, such as myasthenia gravis, multiple sclerosis, poliomyelitis, and parkinsonism, serum enzyme activity is normal. Very high activity is also encountered in malignant hyperthermia, a familial disease characterized by high fever and brought on by administration of inhalation anesthesia (usually halothane) to the affected individual. Apparently, CK-MB replaces part of the CK-MM form in the muscles, resulting in impaired storage of CrP in muscle.

Skeletal muscle that is diseased or damaged (such as by extreme exercise) may contain significant proportions of CK-MB owing to the phenomenon of "fetal reversion," in which fetal patterns of protein synthesis reappear. Thus serum CK-MB isoenzyme may increase in such circumstances. This explanation may also account for the elevated CK-MB values sometimes observed in chronic renal failure (uremic myopathy).

In acute rhabdomyolysis due to crush injuries, with severe muscle destruction, serum CK activities exceeding 200 times the upper reference limit may be found. Serum CK can also be increased by other direct trauma to muscle, including intramuscular injections and surgical interventions. Finally, a number of drugs at pharmacological doses can increase serum CK activities.

The changes of serum CK and its MB isoenzyme following a myocardial infarction are discussed in Chapter 44. Other cardiac conditions have been reported to increase serum CK and CK-MB in serum. These conditions include cardioversion, cardiopulmonary bypass and coronary artery bypass surgery, cardiac transplantation, myocarditis, pericarditis, and pulmonary embolism. Despite improvements in the diagnostic performance and practicality of CK and CK-MB assays, there is no controlled clinical impact trial showing that these tests are effective for decisions to send a patient home or to the appropriate level of care of admission for patients with suspected acute cardiac ischemia, either as one-time or serial tests.[15,182] For diagnosis of acute myocardial infarction, it is now advantageous to use more cardiac-specific nonenzymatic tests, such as cardiac troponin I or T.

Serum CK activity demonstrates an inverse relationship with thyroid activity. About 60% of hypothyroid subjects show an average elevation of CK activity fivefold more than the upper reference limit; elevations of as high as fiftyfold have also been found. The major isoenzyme present is CK-MM, suggesting muscular involvement.

During normal childbirth there is a sixfold elevation in maternal total serum CK activity. Surgical intervention during labor further increases the activity of CK in serum. CK-BB may be elevated in neonates, particularly in brain-damaged or very low birth weight newborns. The presence of CK-BB in blood, usually at low concentrations, may however represent a normal finding in the first days of life.

Methods for the Determination of Creatine Kinase Activity*

Numerous photometric, fluorometric, and coupled enzyme methods have been developed for the assay of CK activity, using either the forward (Cr → CrP) or the reverse (Cr ← CrP) reaction. Analytically the reverse reaction is preferred because it proceeds about six times faster than the forward reaction, although the cost of the starting chemicals, CrP and ADP, is greater than the cost of creatine and ATP.

$$\text{Creatine phosphate} + \text{ADP} \xrightarrow[\text{pH 6.7}]{CK} \text{creatine} + \text{ATP}$$

$$\text{ATP} + \text{glucose} \xrightarrow{HK} \text{glucose-6-phosphate} + \text{ADP}$$

$$\text{Glucose-6-phosphate} + \text{NADP}^{\oplus} \xrightarrow{G6PD} \text{6-phosphogluconate} + \text{NADPH} + \text{H}^{\oplus}$$

CK catalyzes the conversion of CrP to Cr with a concomitant phosphorylation of ADP to ATP.

The ATP produced is measured by hexokinase (HK)/glucose-6-phosphate dehydrogenase (G6PD) coupled reactions that ultimately convert $NADP^+$ to NADPH, which is monitored spectrophotometrically. Oliver first reported this method that Rosalki also described with the improvement of adding AMP to inhibit adenylate kinase (AK) and cysteine to activate CK.[11] Subsequently, Szasz and colleagues optimized the assay by adding *N*-acetylcysteine to activate CK, EDTA to bind Ca^{2+} and to increase the stability of the reaction mixture, and adenosine pentaphosphate (Ap_5A) in addition to AMP to inhibit AK.[11] A reference method based on this previous experience was developed by the International Federation of Clinical Chemistry and Laboratory Medicine (IFCC); it was modified recently to produce a reference procedure for the measurement of CK at 37 °C.[175]

CK activity in serum is relatively unstable and is rapidly lost during storage. The degree of instability varies among specimens. Average stabilities are less than 8 hours at room temperature, 48 hours at 4 °C, and 1 month at −20 °C. CK is susceptible to thermal denaturation; the degree of inactivation corresponds to the degree of temperature increase and is not reversed by addition of sulfhydryl (thiol) reagents. Therefore the serum specimen should be chilled to 4 °C if the serum is not analyzed immediately. It is not necessary to add any thiol agent for storage because the optimized assay formulation, containing EDTA, 2 mmol/L, and *N*-acetylcysteine, 20 mmol/L, reactivates CK in serum to the extent of 99% after it has been stored for 1 week at 4 °C. A slight degree of hemolysis is tolerated because erythrocytes contain no CK activity. However, moderately or severely hemolyzed specimens are unsatisfactory because enzymes and intermediates (AK, ATP, and G6P) liberated from the erythrocytes may affect the lag phase and the side reactions occurring in the assay system.

Reference Intervals

Serum CK activity is influenced by age, sex, race, lean body mass, physical activity, and other less defined genetic differences. The distributions of CK activity are notably skewed toward higher values in reference populations. Men have higher values than women, and blacks have higher values than nonblacks. In Caucasian subjects, the reference interval was found to be 46 to 300 U/L for males and 34 to 180 U/L for females when measured at 37 °C.[8] Experience with the IFCC 37 °C reference procedure has shown reference intervals of 46 to 171 U/L for males and 34 to 145 U/L for females.[180]

Exercise and muscle trauma can increase serum CK. Sustained exercise, such as in well-trained long-distance runners, increases the CK-MB content of skeletal muscle, which may produce abnormal serum CK-MB concentrations.

Methods for the Separation and Quantification of Creatine Kinase Isoenzymes

The techniques most commonly used are electrophoresis and various immunological methods.

Electrophoretic methods for CK isoenzymes use agar, agarose, or cellulose acetate. The isoenzyme bands are visualized by incubating the support with a concentrated CK assay mixture using the reverse reaction. The NADPH formed in this reaction is then detected by observing the bluish-white fluorescence after excitation by long-wave (360 nm) ultraviolet light. NADPH may be quantified by fluorescent densitometry, which is capable of detecting 2 to 10 U/L. Typical examples of results obtained by this technique on a serum sample of a healthy adult and for a patient who has suffered a myocardial infarction 24 hours previously are shown in Figure 21-1, *A*. Alternatively the NADPH can reduce a tetrazolium salt to form a colored formazan. The discriminating power of electrophoresis allows the detection of many abnormal bands, many of which are shown in Figure 21-1, *B*.

In immunoinhibition techniques for measurement of CK-MB, an anti-CK-M subunit antiserum is used to inhibit both M subunits of CK-MM and the single M subunit of CK-MB and thus allow determination of the enzyme activity of the B subunit of CK-MB, the B subunits of CK-BB, macro-CKs, and AK. To determine CK-MB, this technique assumes the absence of CK-BB (and of the other sources of interference mentioned earlier) from the tested serum, a circumstance that does not always occur. In a variation of this technique, the combined activity of the BB isoenzyme, AK, and macro-CKs is determined in a separate reaction and subtracted. The immunoinhibition techniques have been largely supplanted by mass assays of CK-MB.

In contrast with immunoinhibition, which measures the CK-MB isoenzyme by determination of its catalytic activity,

*Methodological details for many of the muscle, liver, pancreatic, and bone methods discussed later in this chapter are found in a prior edition of this textbook (Moss DW, Henderson AR. Clinical enzymology. In: Burtis CA, Ashwood ER eds. Textbook of clinical chemistry, 3rd ed. WB Saunders: Philadelphia, 1999:617-721.)

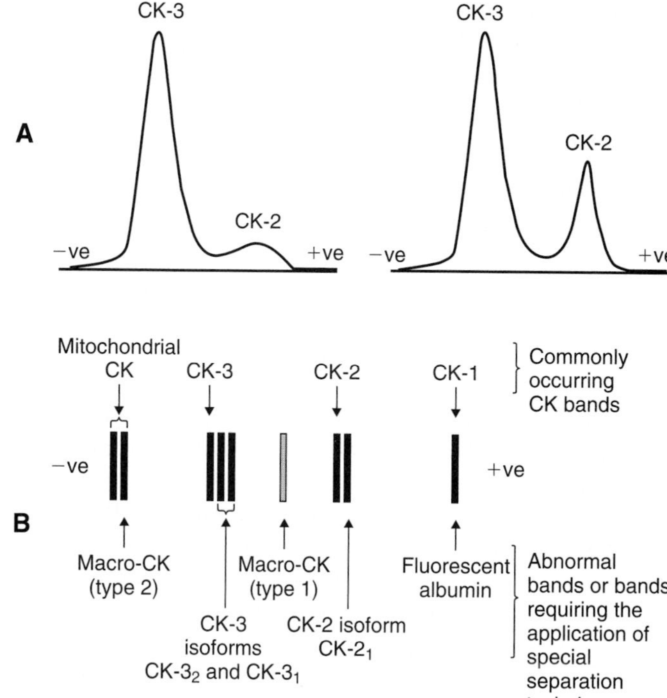

Figure 21-1 **A,** The electrophoretic separation of serum CK isoenzymes from a healthy adult *(left)* and from a patient *(right)* who had a myocardial infarction 24 hours previously. **B,** A diagrammatical representation of the CK isoenzymes (some of which are only seen in disease) and of some of the reported anomalous forms.

immunoassays measure CK-MB mass concentrations. Specific measurements of CK-MB use the "sandwich" technique, in which two antibodies having affinity for different parts of the CK-MB dimer are used. One antibody may be directed against the B-subunit and the other against the M-subunit; an antibody that recognizes only the MB dimer is also used in some assays. The first antibody, which is usually monoclonal, is rendered immobile on a matrix, and the second antibody is conjugated with a label, such as an enzyme or a marker molecule. The sandwich technique ensures that only CK-MB is estimated, because neither CK-MM nor CK-BB reacts with both antibodies. Mass assays are more sensitive than activity-based methods and will detect CK-MB elevations earlier. A number of mass assays, using various labels, are now commercially available and are used for routine and emergency assay of CK-MB. The limit of detection of these systems for CK-MB is usually less than 1 µg/L. The upper reference limit for males is 5.0 µg/L, with values for females being less than the male values, although many laboratories use a single reference limit (male).[136]

Lactate Dehydrogenase

Lactate dehydrogenase (EC 1.1.1.27; L-lactate: NAD^+ oxidoreductase; LD) is a hydrogen transfer enzyme that catalyzes the oxidation of L-lactate to pyruvate with the mediation of NAD^+ as a hydrogen acceptor.

$$\underset{\text{L-Lactate}}{CH_3-CH(OH)-COO^-} + NAD^+ \underset{\text{pH 7.4 to 7.8}}{\overset{\text{Lactate Dehydrogenase, pH 8.8 to 9.8}}{\rightleftharpoons}} \underset{\text{Pyruvate}}{CH_3-C(=O)-COO^-} + NADH + H^+$$

As indicated, the reaction is reversible, and the reaction equilibrium strongly favors the reduction of pyruvate to lactate (P → L)—the "reverse reaction."

The pH optimum for the lactate-to-pyruvate (L → P) reaction is 8.8 to 9.8, and an assay mixture, optimized for LD-1 at 37 °C, contains NAD^+, 9 mmol/L, and L-lactate, 80 mmol/L. For the P → L assay, at 37 °C, the pH optimum is 7.4 to 7.8, NADH 300 µmol/L, and pyruvate 0.85 mmol/L. The optimal pH varies with the predominant isoenzymes in the sample and depends on the temperature and on substrate and buffer concentrations. The specificity of the enzyme extends from L-lactate to various related 2-hydroxyacids and 2-oxo-acids.[107] The catalytic oxidation of 2-hydroxybutyrate, the next higher homologue of lactate, to 2-oxobutyrate is referred to as 2-hydroxybutyrate dehydrogenase (HBD) activity. LD does not act on D-lactate, and only NAD^+ serves as a coenzyme.

The enzyme has a molecular weight of 134,000 and is composed of four peptide chains of two types: M (or A) and H (or B), each under separate genetic control. The structures of LD-M and LD-H are determined by loci on human chromosomes 11 and 12, respectively. The subunit compositions of the five isoenzymes, in order of decreasing anodal mobility in an alkaline medium, are LD-1 (HHHH; H_4); LD-2 (HHHM; H_3M); LD-3 (HHMM; H_2M_2); LD-4 (HMMM; HM_3); and LD-5 (MMMM; M_4). A different, sixth LD isoenzyme, LD-X (also called LD_c), composed of four X (or C) subunits, is present in postpubertal human testes. A seventh LD, called LD-6, has been identified in the sera of severely ill patients.

LD is inhibited by reagents with reactivity against thiol groups, such as mercuric ions and *p*-chloromercuribenzoate, the inhibition being reversed by the addition of cysteine or glutathione. Borate and oxalate inhibit by competing with lactate for its binding site on the enzyme; similarly, oxamate competes with pyruvate for its binding site. Both pyruvate and lactate in excess inhibit enzyme activity, although the effect of pyruvate is greater. Inhibition by either substrate is greater for the H form than for the M form, and substrate inhibition decreases with increase in pH. EDTA inhibits the enzyme perhaps by binding Zn^{2+}; however, the postulated activator role for zinc ions is not fully established.

LD activity is present in all cells of the body and is invariably found only in the cytoplasm of the cell. Enzyme concentrations in various tissues are about 500 times greater than those normally found in serum. Therefore leakage of the enzyme from even a small mass of damaged tissue increases the observed serum activity of LD to a significant extent. Different tissues show different isoenzyme composition. In cardiac muscle, kidneys, and erythrocytes, the electrophoretically faster moving isoenzymes LD-1 and LD-2 predominate, whereas in liver and skeletal muscle, the more cathodal LD-4 and LD-5 isoenzymes predominate—although skeletal muscle damage may also result in anodic LD patterns. Isoenzymes of intermediate mobility account for the LD activity from many sources (e.g., spleen, lungs, lymph nodes, leukocytes, and platelets).

Clinical Significance

Because of its wide distribution in all tissues, serum LD elevations occur in a variety of clinical conditions—including myocardial infarction, hemolysis and disorders of the liver, kidneys, lung, and muscle. A systematic review of the literature concluded that serum LD is relevant in the diagnosis of myocardial infarction, hemolytic anemia, ovarian dysgerminoma, and testicular germ cell tumor.[68] For monitoring purposes, LD is relevant in predicting the survival duration and rate in Hodgkin's disease and non-Hodgkin's lymphoma and in the follow-up of dysgerminoma.

Hemolysis, if sufficiently severe, produces an LD isoenzyme pattern similar to that in myocardial infarction. Megaloblastic anemias, usually resulting from the deficiency of folate or vitamin B_{12}, cause the erythrocyte precursor cell to break down in the bone marrow (ineffective erythropoiesis), resulting in the release of large quantities of LD-1 and LD-2 isoenzymes. Marked elevations of the total LD activity in serum—up to 50 times the upper reference limit—have been observed in the megaloblastic anemias. These elevations rapidly return to normal after appropriate treatment.

Elevations of LD activity are observed in liver disease, but these elevations are not as great as the increases in aminotransferase activity. Elevations are especially high (10 times normal) in toxic hepatitis with jaundice. Slightly lower values are observed in viral hepatitis and in infectious mononucleosis, the latter often associated with elevations of LD-3. LD activity is normal or at most twice the upper reference limit in cirrhosis and obstructive jaundice. Serum LD-5 is often notably elevated in patients with either primary liver disease or liver anoxia secondary to decreased oxygen perfusion.

Patients with malignant disease show increased LD activity in serum; up to 70% of patients with liver metastases and 20% to 60% of patients with other nonhepatic metastases have elevated total LD activity. Notably elevated LD-1 is observed in germ cell tumors (61% of cases), such as teratoma, seminoma of the testis, and dysgerminoma of the ovary. Patients with seminoma have a raised LD-1 in 63% of cases compared with 60% in nonseminoma cases.[206] The percent of patients with increased LD-1 depended on the stage of the disease. LD-1 appeared to be a useful predictor of outcome in patients with testicular germ cell tumors.

In healthy subjects, cerebrospinal fluid (CSF)-LD activity is very much lower than the serum activity, and LD-4 and LD-5 are frequently undetectable. The pattern is also complicated by the possibility of contamination by hemorrhage or the disruption of the blood-brain barrier by disease, which adds LD of systemic origin to the CSF.[34] Additionally, LD isoenzymes may be released from cells that have infiltrated into the CSF. For example, in bacterial meningitis, the resulting granulocytosis produces an elevation of LD-4 and LD-5, whereas viral meningitis produces lymphocytosis, which may create an elevation of LD-1 through LD-3.

Methods for the Determination of Lactate Dehydrogenase Activity

Routine methods for both the forward ($L \rightarrow P$) and reverse ($P \rightarrow L$) reactions are available. However, within the last decade, there has been a significant move from the $P \rightarrow L$ to the $L \rightarrow P$ reaction. An $L \rightarrow P$ continuous-monitoring reference method, optimized for LD-1, has been developed by the IFCC Committee on Enzymes.[13] This method has recently been the basis for developing an IFCC reference procedure for LD at 37 °C.[176]

Serum is the preferred specimen for measuring LD activity. Plasma samples may be contaminated with platelets, which contain high concentrations of LD.[12] Serum should be separated from the clot as soon as possible after the specimen has been obtained. Hemolyzed serum must not be used because erythrocytes contain 150 times more LD activity (particularly LD-1 and LD-2) than serum. The different isoenzymes vary in their sensitivity to cold, LD-4 and LD-5 being especially labile. Activity of LD-4 and LD-5 is lost if the samples are stored at −20 °C. Thus serum specimens should be stored at room temperature, at which no loss of activity occurs for at least 3 days.

Reference Intervals

Values for LD activity in serum vary considerably, depending on the direction of the enzyme reaction and the method used. The reference interval in adult subjects, determined with the IFCC reference procedure at 37 °C, was found to be 125 to 220 U/L.[131] LD reference limits are higher in children (180 to 360 U/L).

Methods for the Separation and Quantification of Lactate Dehydrogenase Isoenzymes

Electrophoretic separation on agarose gels or cellulose acetate membranes is the procedure most commonly used to demonstrate LD isoenzymes.[117] After the isoenzymes have been separated by electrophoresis, a reaction mixture is layered over the separation medium. The mixture (typically D, L-lactate, 500 mmol/L, and NAD^+, 13 mmol/L, often dissolved in a suitable pH 8.0 buffer) is applied as a liquid or in a gel. The NADH generated over the LD zones is detected either by its fluorescence, when excited by long-wave ultraviolet light (365 nm), or by its reduction of a tetrazolium salt to form a colored formazan.

Using an agarose gel technique with fluorometric quantitation of the generated NADH, the following reference intervals for isoenzymes were obtained (expressed as percent of total LD): LD-1, 14% to 26%; LD-2, 29% to 39%; LD-3, 20% to 26%; LD-4, 8% to 16%; and LD-5, 6% to 16%.

Selective chemical inhibition methods have been described to inhibit serum LD-2 through LD-5, thus permitting the assay of LD-1 alone. Chemicals used as inhibitors include 1,6-hexanediol, sodium perchlorate, and guanidine thiocyanate. An immunoprecipitation method using a goat antiserum against purified LD-5 has been used to measure LD-1. This antiserum binds LD isoenzymes LD-2 through LD-5. These bound isoenzymes are precipitated by the addition of a second antibody, leaving only LD-1 in the supernatant.

ALDOLASE

Aldolase (EC 4.1.2.13; D-fructose-1,6-bisdiphosphate D-glyceraldehyde-3-phosphate-lyase; ALD) catalyzes the splitting of D-fructose-1,6-diphosphate to D-glyceraldehyde-3-phosphate (GLAP) and dihydroxyacetone-phosphate (DAP), an important reaction in the glycolytic breakdown of glucose to lactate.

ALD is a tetramer with subunits determined by three separate gene loci. Only two of these loci, those producing A and B subunits, appear to be active simultaneously in most tissues, so the most common isoenzyme pattern consists of various proportions of the components of a five-member set of isoenzymes, of which two members correspond to the A and B homopolymers. The locus that determines the structure of the C subunit is active in brain tissue, as is the A locus, so this tissue contains ALD A and C together with the three corresponding heteropolymers.

Clinical Significance

Serum ALD determinations have been of some clinical interest in primary diseases of skeletal muscle. Some researchers believe that increased ALD activity is useful in distinguishing neuromuscular atrophies from myopathies in combination with the CK/AST ratio.[66] In general, however, measurement of ALD activity in serum does not add information to that available more readily from measurement of other enzymes, such as AST, LD, and especially CK. A recent study, assessing the utility of ALD determination by monitoring patient outcome, showed no clinical benefit when ALD was used in addition to CK in evaluating patients with suspected muscle disease.[62]

Methods for the Measurement of Aldolase Activity

All assay methods are based on the forward ALD-catalyzed reaction. Both photometric fixed-time and continuous-monitoring procedures have been developed. In the analytical approach on which all the commonly used procedures and kits are based, the ALD reaction is coupled with two other enzyme reactions. Triosephosphate isomerase (EC 5.3.1.1) is added to ensure rapid conversion of all GLAP to DAP. Glycerol-3-phosphate dehydrogenase (EC 1.1.1.8) is added to reduce the DAP to glycerol-3-phosphate, with NADH acting as hydrogen donor. The decrease in NADH concentration is then measured.[153]

The ALD activity in serum is quite stable. Activity is unchanged at ambient temperature for up to 48 hours and at 4 °C for several days. Hemolyzed specimens should not be used, and plasma is preferred over serum because of the possible release of platelet enzyme during the clotting process.

Reference Intervals

The reference interval for the activity of ALD in adults is 2.5 to 10 U/L, measured at 37 °C. However, there is a definite sex difference with men having higher values. Serum ALD in the neonate is fourfold the adult activity and in children is twice that of the adult. Adult values are attained by the time the child reaches puberty.[205]

GLYCOGEN PHOSPHORYLASE

Glycogen phosphorylase (EC 2.4.1.1; 1,4-alpha-D-glucan:orthophosphate alpha-D-glucosyltransferase; GP) plays an essential role in the regulation of carbohydrate metabolism by mobilizing glycogen. It catalyzes the first step in glycogenolysis in which glycogen is converted to glucose-1-phosphate. The physiological role of muscle GP is to provide the fuel for the energy supply required for muscle contraction. GP exists in the myocyte in association with glycogen and the sarcoplasmic reticulum, forming a macromolecular complex. The degree of association of GP with this complex depends on the metabolic state of the muscle. With the onset of tissue hypoxia, when glycogen is broken down and disappears, GP becomes soluble and can move from the peri-sarcoplasmic reticulum compartment directly into the extracellular fluid (Figure 21-2).

GP exists as a dimer composed of two identical subunits. Three GP isoenzymes are found in human tissues: GP-LL,

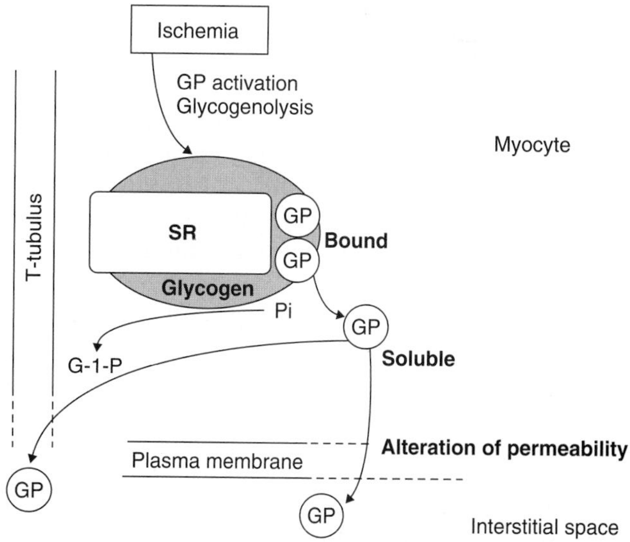

Figure 21-2 Release of glycogen phosphorylase (GP) from damaged muscle. GP and glycogen are tightly associated with the vesicles of sarcoplasmic reticulum (SR) under normal conditions. Ischemic injury is known to favor the conversion of bound GP into soluble GP, giving rise to the efflux of GP into the extracellular fluid. *Pi,* Inorganic phosphate; *G-1-P,* glucose-1-phosphate. *(Modified from Krause EG, Rabitzsch G, Noll F, Mair J, Puschendorf B. Glycogen phosphorylase isoenzyme BB in diagnosis of myocardial ischemic injury and infarction. Mol Cell Biochem 1996;160-1:289-95.)*

GP-MM, and GP-BB. Adult skeletal muscle contains only GP-MM. GP-LL is the predominant isoenzyme in liver and all other human tissues except for heart, skeletal muscle, and brain. GP-BB is the predominant isoenzyme in the human brain. In the heart, the isoenzymes BB and MM are found, but GP-BB is the predominant isoenzyme in the myocardium as well.

Clinical Significance[100]

In preliminary studies, GP-BB was significantly more sensitive than CK and CK-MB for AMI diagnosis during the first 3 to 4 hours after the onset of chest pain. Therefore GP-BB may be an important marker for the early diagnosis of AMI. Similar to other cytoplasmic proteins, such as myoglobin and CK-MB, the time course of GP-BB can be notably influenced by early reperfusion of the infarct-related coronary artery, with a more rapid increase and earlier peak. GP-BB is, however, not a heart-specific protein and its specificity as a marker for myocardial damage is limited.

Methods for the Measurement of Glycogen Phosphorylase Isoenzyme BB

Methods were described for the estimation of GP activity in serum on the enzymic determination of glucose-1-phosphate in a coupled assay system and for the electrophoretic separation of GP isoenzymes.[88] More recently, an immunoenzymometric assay for the measurement of the isoenzyme GP-BB was developed.[157] The upper reference limit of this research assay was 7 µg/L.

LIVER ENZYMES

Enzymes in this category include alanine and aspartate aminotransferases, glutamate dehydrogenase (GLD), ALP, 5′-nucleotidase (NTP), γ-glutamyl transferase (GGT), glutathione S-transferase (GST), and serum cholinesterase (CHE). The aminotransferases and ALP are widely used. They have long been mistakenly called, as a group, "liver function tests." They are not, of course, but the habit persists. GGT is widely available in the United States and on automated analyzers. The others have not been adopted as widely.

AMINOTRANSFERASES

The aminotransferases constitute a group of enzymes that catalyze the interconversion of amino acids to 2-oxo-acids by transfer of amino groups. Aspartate aminotransferase (EC 2.6.1.1; L-aspartate:2-oxoglutarate aminotransferase; AST) and alanine aminotransferase (EC 2.6.1.2; L-alanine:2-oxoglutarate aminotransferase; ALT) are examples of aminotransferases that are of clinical interest.

The 2-oxoglutarate/L-glutamate couple serves as one amino group acceptor and donor pair in all amino-transfer reactions; the specificity of the individual enzymes derives from the particular amino acid that serves as the other donor of an amino group. Thus AST catalyzes the reaction.

$$\underset{\text{L-Aspartate}}{COO^{\ominus}\text{–}CH(NH_2)\text{–}CH_2\text{–}COO^{\ominus}} + \underset{\text{2-Oxoglutarate}}{COO^{\ominus}\text{–}C(=O)\text{–}CH_2\text{–}CH_2\text{–}COO^{\ominus}} \xrightleftharpoons{\text{AST, P-5'-P}} \underset{\text{Oxaloacetate}}{COO^{\ominus}\text{–}C(=O)\text{–}CH_2\text{–}COO^{\ominus}} + \underset{\text{L-Glutamate}}{COO^{\ominus}\text{–}CH(NH_2)\text{–}CH_2\text{–}CH_2\text{–}COO^{\ominus}}$$

ALT catalyzes the analogous reaction.

$$\underset{\text{L-Alanine}}{COO^{\ominus}\text{–}CH(NH_2)\text{–}CH_3} + \underset{\text{2-Oxoglutarate}}{COO^{\ominus}\text{–}C(=O)\text{–}CH_2\text{–}CH_2\text{–}COO^{\ominus}} \xrightleftharpoons{\text{ALT, P-5'-P}} \underset{\text{Pyruvate}}{COO^{\ominus}\text{–}C(=O)\text{–}CH_3} + \underset{\text{L-Glutamate}}{COO^{\ominus}\text{–}CH(NH_2)\text{–}CH_2\text{–}CH_2\text{–}COO^{\ominus}}$$

The reactions are reversible, but the equilibria of the AST and ALT reactions favor formation of aspartate and alanine, respectively.

Pyridoxal-5′-phosphate (P-5′-P) and its amino analogue, pyridoxamine-5′-phosphate, function as coenzymes in the amino-transfer reactions. The P-5′-P is bound to the apoenzyme and serves as a true prosthetic group. The P-5′-P bound to the apoenzyme accepts the amino group from the first substrate, aspartate or alanine, to form enzyme-bound pyridoxamine-5′-phosphate and the first reaction product, oxaloacetate or pyruvate, respectively. The coenzyme in amino form then transfers its amino group to the second substrate, 2-oxoglutarate, to form the second product, glutamate. P-5′-P is thus regenerated.

Both the coenzyme-deficient apoenzymes and the holoenzymes may be present in serum. Therefore, addition of P-5′-P under conditions that allow recombination with the enzymes usually produces an increase in aminotransferase activity. In accordance with the principle that all factors affecting the rate of reaction must be optimized and controlled, IFCC recommends addition of P-5′-P in aminotransferase methods to ensure that all the enzymatic activity is measured.

Transaminases are widely distributed throughout the body. AST is found primarily in the heart, liver, skeletal muscle, and kidney, whereas ALT is found primarily in the liver and kidney, with lesser amounts in heart and skeletal muscle (Table 21-2). ALT is exclusively cytoplasmic; both mitochondrial and cytoplasmic forms of AST are found in cells. These are genetically distinct isoenzymes with a dimeric structure composed of two identical polypeptide subunits of about 400 amino acid residues.[134]

Clinical Significance

Liver disease is the most important cause of increased transaminase activity in serum. In most types of liver disease, ALT activity is higher than that of AST; exceptions may be seen in alcoholic hepatitis, hepatic cirrhosis, and liver neoplasia. In viral hepatitis and other forms of liver disease associated with acute hepatic necrosis, serum AST and ALT

TABLE 21-2 Transaminase Activities in Human Tissues, Relative to Serum as Unity

	AST	ALT
Heart	7800	450
Liver	7100	2850
Skeletal muscle	5000	300
Kidneys	4500	1200
Pancreas	1400	130
Spleen	700	80
Lungs	500	45
Erythrocytes	15	7
Serum	1	1

From King J. Practical Clinical Enzymology. London: D Van Nostrand Co, Ltd, 1965.

concentrations are elevated even before the clinical signs and symptoms of disease (such as jaundice) appear. Activities for both enzymes may reach values as high as 100 times the upper reference limit, although tenfold to fortyfold elevations are most frequently encountered. Peak values of transaminase activity occur between the 7th and 12th days; activities then gradually decrease, reaching normal levels by the 3rd to 5th week if recovery is uneventful. Peak activities bear no relationship to prognosis and may fall with worsening of the patient's condition.

Persistence of increased ALT for more than 6 months after an episode of acute hepatitis is used to diagnose chronic hepatitis. Most patients with chronic hepatitis have maximum ALT less than seven times the upper reference limit. ALT may be persistently normal in 15% to 50% of patients with chronic hepatitis C, but the likelihood of continuously normal ALT decreases with an increasing number of measurements. In patients with acute hepatitis C, ALT should be measured periodically over the next 1 to 2 years to determine if it becomes and stays normal.[45]

The picture in toxic hepatitis is different from that in infectious hepatitis. In acetaminophen-induced hepatic injury, the transaminase peak is more than 85 times the upper reference limit in 90% of cases, a value rarely seen with acute viral hepatitis. Furthermore, AST and ALT activities typically peak early and fall rapidly.[45]

Nonalcoholic steatohepatitis is the most common cause of aminotransferase increases other than viral and alcoholic hepatitis. Increased transaminase concentrations have been observed in extrahepatic cholestasis, with activities tending to be higher the more chronic the obstruction. The aminotransferase activities observed in cirrhosis vary with the status of the cirrhotic process and range from the upper reference limit to four to five times higher, with an AST/ALT ratio greater than 1. The ratio's elevation can reflect the grade of fibrosis in these patients. This appears to be attributable to a reduction of ALT production in a damaged liver. Twofold to fivefold elevations of both enzymes occur in patients with primary or metastatic carcinoma of the liver, with AST usually being higher than ALT, but activities are often normal in the early stages of malignant infiltration of the liver. Slight or moderate elevations of both AST and ALT activities have been observed after administration of various medications, such as nonsteroidal antiinflammatory drugs, antibiotics, antiepileptic drugs, inhibitors of hydroxymethylglutaryl-coenzyme A reductase, or opiates. In patients with increased transaminases, negative viral markers, and a negative history for drugs or alcohol ingestion, the workup should include less common causes of chronic hepatic injury (i.e., hemochromatosis, Wilson's disease, autoimmune hepatitis, primary biliary cirrhosis, sclerosing cholangitis, and α_1-antitrypsin deficiency).[154]

Although serum activities of both AST and ALT become elevated whenever disease processes affect liver cell integrity, ALT is the more liver-specific enzyme. Serum elevations of ALT activity are rarely observed in conditions other than parenchymal liver disease. Moreover, elevations of ALT activity persist longer than do those of AST activity.

After AMI, increased AST activity appears in serum, as might be expected from the high AST concentration in heart muscle. AST activity also is increased in progressive muscular dystrophy and dermatomyositis, reaching concentrations up to eight times normal; they are usually normal in other types of muscle diseases, especially in those of neurogenic origin. If striated muscle is the source of increased AST activity, serum CK will be elevated contemporaneously. Pulmonary emboli can increase AST to two to three times normal, and slight to moderate elevations are noted in celiac sprue, acute pancreatitis, crushed muscle injuries, and hemolytic disease.

Generally, mitochondrial AST (m-AST) activity in serum shows a marked increase in patients with extensive liver cell degeneration and necrosis. Of particular interest is the usefulness of the ratio between m-AST and total AST activities for diagnosing alcoholic hepatitis. The ratio seems to clearly identify the liver-cell "necrotic type" condition (i.e., slight enzyme increase concomitant with relatively high activities of mitochondrial enzymes), typical of alcoholic hepatitis (Figure 21-3).[134]

Several authors have described AST linked to immunoglobulins, or macro-AST. The typical findings are a persistent increase of serum AST activity in an asymptomatic subject, with the absence of any demonstrable pathology in organs rich in AST. The increased AST activity might reflect decreased clearance of the abnormal complex from plasma. Macro-AST has no known clinical relevance. However, identification is important to avoid unnecessary diagnostic procedures in these subjects.[134]

Methods for the Measurement of Transaminase Activity

The assay system for measuring transaminase activity contains two amino acids and two oxo-acids. As there is no convenient method for assaying amino acids, formation or consumption of the oxo-acids is measured. Historically,

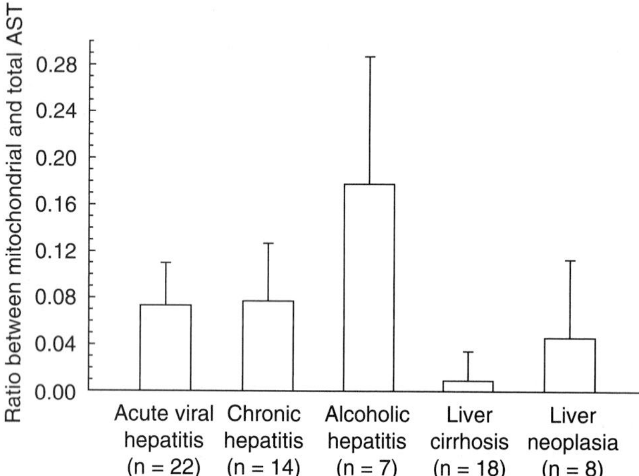

Figure 21-3 The ratio (mean ± SD) of mitochondrial to total AST in hepatic diseases. The difference between alcoholic hepatitis and other hepatic diseases is statistically significant ($p < 0.05$). *(Modified from Panteghini M, Falsetti F, Chiari E, Malchiodi A. Determination of aspartate aminotransferase isoenzymes in hepatic diseases. Lab J Res Lab Med 1983;10:515-9.)*

various photometric substrates (2,4-dinitrophenylhydrazine and various dyes) were coupled to the transaminase reactions. Methods based on these reactions are now considered obsolete. Today, continuous-monitoring methods are used to measure transaminase activity, by coupling the transaminase reactions to specific dehydrogenase reactions. The oxo-acids formed in the transaminase reaction are measured indirectly by enzymatic reduction to the corresponding hydroxy acids, the accompanying change in NADH concentration being monitored spectrophotometrically. Thus oxaloacetate, formed in the AST reaction, is reduced to malate in the presence of malate dehydrogenase (MD).

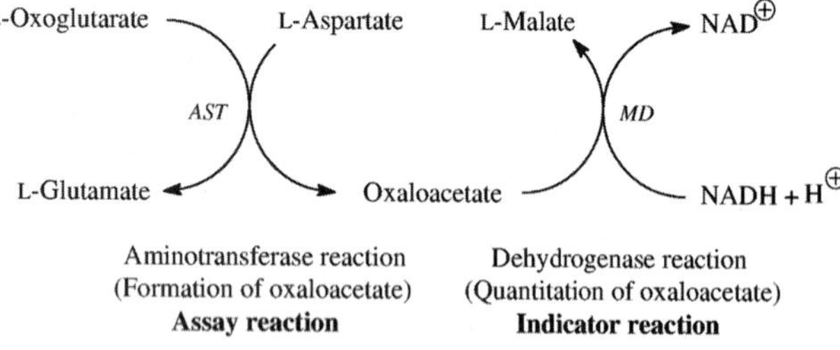

Pyruvate formed in the ALT reaction is reduced to lactate by LD. The substrate, NADH, and the auxiliary enzymes, MD or LD, must be present in sufficient quantity so that the reaction rate is limited only by the amounts of AST and ALT, respectively. As the reactions proceed, NADH is oxidized to NAD^+. The disappearance of NADH is followed by measuring the decrease in absorbance at 340 nm for several minutes, either continuously or at frequent intervals. The change in absorbance per minute (ΔA/min) is proportional to the micromoles of NADH oxidized and in turn to micromoles of substrate transformed per minute. A preliminary incubation period is necessary to ensure that NADH-dependent reduction of endogenous oxo-acids in the sample is completed before adding 2-oxoglutarate to start the transaminase reaction. After a brief lag phase, the change in absorbance (ΔA) is monitored. As already mentioned, supplementation with P-5′-P ensures that all the transaminase activity of the sample is measured.

AST activity in serum is stable for up to 48 hours at 4 °C. Specimens have to be stored frozen if they are to be kept longer. ALT activity should be assayed on the day of sample collection since activity is lost at room temperature, 4 °C, and −25 °C. ALT stability is better maintained at −70 °C. Hemolyzed specimens should not be used.

Standardization[145]

Because of the large numbers of AST and ALT activity measurements performed daily in clinical laboratories throughout the world and because of notable differences when results between laboratories are compared, standardization of transaminase measurements is a priority need for patient care. As discussed in Chapter 8, the reference system approach, based on the concepts of metrological traceability and of hierarchy of analytical measurement procedures, gives clinical laboratories and the medical community universal means of creating and ensuring the comparability of results. In this system, the IFCC reference measurement procedure forms the highest metrological level and thereby constitutes the definition of the respective measurable enzyme quantity. Primary IFCC procedures for the measurement of catalytic activity concentrations of AST and ALT at 37 °C have recently been redesigned and published.[178,179] Values assigned to the manufacturer's product calibrators and measurement results of lower metrological levels, including those in daily routine practice, should be traceable to these top-level reference measurement procedures, thus improving accuracy and comparability of transaminase results. It should be remembered that the concept of the reference system is valid only if the reference procedure and corresponding routine procedures have identical, or at least very similar, specificities for the measured enzyme. Thus it will not be possible to calibrate procedures for aminotransferases that do not incorporate P-5′-P using a procedure that does, such as the IFCC reference procedure, because the ratio of preformed holoenzyme to apoenzyme differs among specimens.

Reference Intervals[180]

When using the new IFCC methods, the AST upper reference limits for adults, calculated as the 97.5 percentile of the reference distribution, are 31 U/L for women and 35 U/L for men, respectively. The corresponding ALT upper reference limits are 34 U/L and 45 U/L.

Methods for the Separation and Quantification of AST Isoenzymes[134]

Several methods have been proposed to quantify AST isoenzymes in human serum. The most commonly used are electrophoresis, selective inhibition, and immunoassays. AST isoenzymes can be separated into an anionic (cytoplasmic AST) and a cationic band (m-AST) by electrophoresis. However, the low concentration of m-AST in normal sera is usually below the limit of detection of this method. Rej described immunoprecipitation assays using antibodies directed against both purified mitochondrial and cytosolic isoenzymes. A similar assay, using anticytoplasmic AST antibody conjugated to sheep erythrocytes, became the basis for a diagnostic kit technique. As a rule, these assays allow direct measurement of low concentrations of the m-AST isoenzyme present in serum. More recently, there have been reports on the selective proteolysis of AST isoenzymes by several proteases. In particular, a homogeneous inhibition assay using proteinase K (EC 3.4.21.14) for selective proteolysis of cytosolic AST was described and made amenable to automation, permitting m-AST to be measured with convenience that approaches that of the total AST assay.[143]

About 5% to 10% of the activity of total AST in serum from healthy individuals is of mitochondrial origin. The upper reference limit for m-AST activity measured at 37 °C is 3.0 U/L.

Glutamate Dehydrogenase

Glutamate dehydrogenase (EC 1.4.1.3; L-glutamate : NAD(P) oxidoreductase, deaminating; GLD) is a mitochondrial enzyme found mainly in the liver, heart muscle, and kidneys, but small amounts occur in other tissue, including brain and skeletal muscle tissue, and in leukocytes.

GLD is a zinc-containing enzyme consisting of six polypeptide chains. The smallest active molecule has a molecular weight of about 350,000 kDa, but larger polymers are also found. The enzyme catalyzes the removal of hydrogen from L-glutamate to form the corresponding ketimino-acid that undergoes spontaneous hydrolysis to 2-oxoglutarate.

$$\text{L-Glutamate} \; (^{-}OOC{-}CH(NH_2){-}CH_2{-}CH_2{-}COO^{-}) + NAD^{+} \xrightleftharpoons{\text{Glutamate Dehydrogenase}} \text{ketimino-acid} \; (^{-}OOC{-}C({=}NH){-}CH_2{-}CH_2{-}COO^{-}) + NADH + H^{+}$$

$$\text{ketimino-acid} + H_2O \xrightarrow{\text{Spontaneous}} \text{2-Oxoglutarate} \; (^{-}OOC{-}C({=}O){-}CH_2{-}CH_2{-}COO^{-}) + NH_3$$

Although NAD^+ is the preferred coenzyme, $NADP^+$ also acts as the hydrogen acceptor. GLD is inhibited by metal ions, such as Ag^+ and Hg^+, by several chelating agents, and by L-thyroxine. The glutamate dehydrogenases of different human tissues may be separated by electrophoresis into several forms, probably resulting from different polymeric states.

Clinical Significance[174]

GLD is increased in serum of patients with hepatocellular damage. Fourfold or fivefold elevations are seen in chronic hepatitis; in cirrhosis, increases are only up to twofold. Very large rises in serum GLD occur in halothane toxicity, and notable increases occur in response to some other hepatotoxic agents.

GLD potentially offers differential diagnostic potential in the investigation of liver disease, particularly when interpreted in conjunction with other enzyme test results. The key to this differential diagnostic potential is to be found in the intraorgan and intracellular distribution of the enzyme. As an exclusively mitochondrial isoenzyme, GLD is released from necrotic cells; therefore, when compared with hepatic disorders with extensive necrosis, release is less in diffuse inflammatory processes, and in these conditions, the release of cytoplasmic enzymes, such as ALT, is quantitatively more pronounced. Together with m-AST, GLD is of value in estimation of the severity of liver cell damage.

GLD is more concentrated in the central areas of the liver lobules than in the periportal zones. This pattern of distribution is the reverse of that of ALT. Pronounced release of GLD is therefore to be expected in conditions in which centrilobular necrosis occurs (e.g., as a result of ischemia or in halothane toxicity).

Methods for the Determination of Glutamate Dehydrogenase Activity

Continuous-monitoring methods have been developed for the determination of GLD using both the forward and reverse reactions. The equilibrium favors the formation of glutamate, and higher reaction rates are observed when 2-oxoglutarate is used as a substrate. Serum is added to a solution of NADH, an ammonium salt, and ADP in buffer at pH 7.5, and the reaction is initiated by the addition of the substrate, 2-oxoglutarate. The rate of decrease in absorbance at 340 nm is measured. The German Society for Clinical Chemistry has published optimum reaction conditions for 37 °C.[42] Oxamate is incorporated into the reaction mixture because this acid inhibits LD activity, avoiding the critical consumption of NADH by this enzyme in serum.

GLD activity in serum is stable at 4 °C for 48 hours and at −20 °C for several weeks.

Reference Intervals

The GLD upper reference limits are 6 U/L (women) and 8 U/L (men), when a method optimized at 37 °C is used.

Alkaline Phosphatase

Alkaline phosphatase (EC 3.1.3.1; orthophosphoric-monoester phosphohydrolase [alkaline optimum]; ALP) cat-

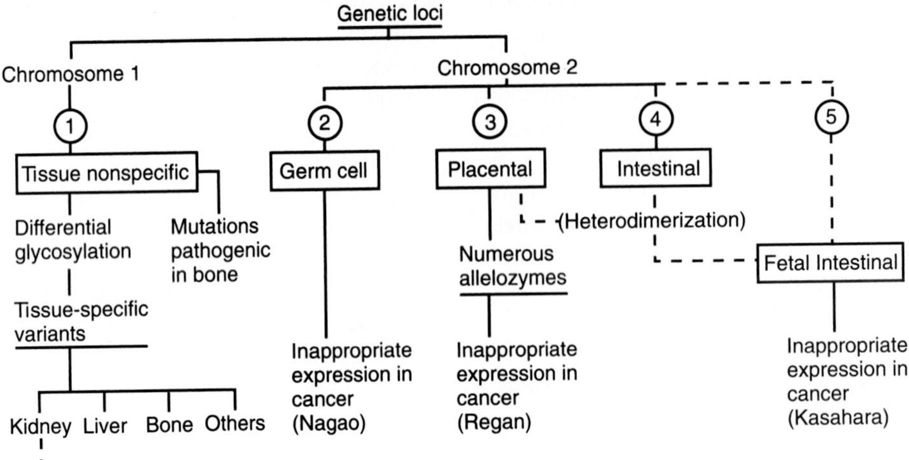

Figure 21-4 Identities, chromosomal assignments, and main physiological and pathological expression of genes encoding human alkaline phosphatases. *Broken lines* show two alternative proposed origins of the fetal intestinal alkaline phosphatase. The sequence of a cDNA is reportedly identical to that of adult intestinal AP. All the isoenzymes and isoforms are glycoproteins, imposing a further level of microheterogeneity. Different processes of cleavage or preservation of the membrane-anchoring domain can generate additional isoforms. *(Modified from Moss DW. Perspectives in alkaline phosphatase research. Clin Chem 1992;38:2486-92.)*

alyzes the alkaline hydrolysis of a large variety of naturally occurring and synthetic substrates.

ALP activity is present in most organs of the body and is especially associated with membranes and cell surfaces located in the mucosa of the small intestine and proximal convoluted tubules of the kidney, in bone (osteoblasts), liver, and placenta. Although the precise metabolic function of the enzyme is not yet understood, it appears that ALP is associated with lipid transport in the intestine and with the calcification process in bone.

ALP exists in multiple forms, some of which are true isoenzymes, encoded at separate genetic loci (Figure 21-4).[120] The bone, liver, and kidney ALP forms share a common primary structure coded for by the same genetic locus, but they differ in carbohydrate content.[118]

Some divalent ions, such as Mg^{2+}, Co^{2+}, and Mn^{2+}, are activators of the enzyme, and Zn^{2+} is a constituent metal ion. The correct ratio of Mg^{2+}/Zn^{2+} ions is necessary to avoid displacement of Mg^{2+} and to obtain optimal activity. Phosphate, borate, oxalate, and cyanide ions are inhibitors of ALP activity. Variations in Mg^{2+} and substrate concentrations change the pH optimum. The type of buffer present (except at low concentrations) affects the rate of enzyme activity. Buffers can be classified as inert (carbonate and barbital), inhibiting (glycine and propylamine), or activating (2-amino-2-methyl-1-propanol [AMP], tris (hydroxymethyl) aminomethane [TRIS], and diethanolamine [DEA]).

The ALP activity present in the sera of healthy adults originates mainly in the liver, with up to half the total activity coming from the skeleton. The respective contributions of these two forms to the total activity are age dependent. A small amount of intestinal ALP may also be present, particularly in the sera of individuals of blood group B or O, i.e., who are secretors of blood group substances. Tissue nonspecific ALP in serum is rapidly denatured at 56 °C but is relatively stable at lower temperatures.

Clinical Significance

Elevations in serum ALP activity commonly originate from one or both of two sources: the liver and bone. Consequently, serum ALP measurements are of particular interest in the investigation of two groups of conditions: hepatobiliary disease and bone disease associated with increased osteoblastic activity (see Bone Enzymes section later in this chapter).

The response of the liver to any form of biliary tree obstruction induces the synthesis of ALP by hepatocytes. Some of the newly formed enzyme enters the circulation to increase the enzyme activity in serum.[121] The elevation tends to be more notable (greater than threefold) in extrahepatic obstruction (e.g., by stone or by cancer of the head of the pancreas) than in intrahepatic obstruction and is greater the more complete the obstruction. Serum enzyme activities may reach 10 to 12 times the upper reference limit and usually return to normal on surgical removal of the obstruction. A similar increase is seen in patients with advanced primary liver cancer or widespread secondary hepatic metastases. Liver diseases that principally affect parenchymal cells, such as infectious hepatitis, typically show only moderately (less than threefold) increased or even normal serum ALP activities (Table 21-3).[139] Increases may also be seen as a consequence of a reaction to drug therapy. Intestinal ALP

TABLE 21-3 Serum Alkaline Phosphatase Activities in Hepatobiliary Diseases

Disorder	No. of Patients	% of Patients With Abnormal ALP	Mean ALP Activity (Multiples of Upper Reference Limit)
Primary and metastatic liver neoplasia	25	92	4.15
Extrahepatic biliary obstruction	19	95	3.98
Acute viral hepatitis	33	79	2.36
Liver cirrhosis	34	76	1.18
Alcoholic hepatitis	33	76	1.13
Chronic hepatitis	14	78	1.03

From Panteghini M. Hepatic alkaline phosphatase isoenzyme: II. Clinical aspects. Giorn It Chim Clin 1990;15:301-8.

isoenzyme, an asialoglycoprotein normally cleared by the hepatic asialoglycoprotein receptors, is often elevated in patients with liver cirrhosis.

An increase of up to two to three times normal has been observed in women in the third trimester of pregnancy, with the additional enzyme being of placental origin. There are also reports of a benign familial elevation in serum ALP activity because of increased concentrations of intestinal ALP.[135] Transient, benign increases in serum ALP may be observed in infants and children, with changes often more than 10 times the upper reference limit. Increases in both the liver and the bone form are seen. These changes seem to reflect a reduction in the removal of ALP from blood caused by transient modifications of enzyme glycosylation.[187]

A result of the application of the techniques of isoenzyme analysis to the characterization of ALP in serum was the discovery that forms of the enzyme essentially identical with the normal placental isoenzyme appear in the sera of some patients with malignant diseases. These carcinoplacental isoenzymes (e.g., Regan isoenzyme) appear to result from the derepression of the placental ALP gene. As described below, the presence of these isoenzymes can be readily detected in serum by their stability at 65 °C. Tumors have also been found to produce ALPs that appear to be modified forms of nonplacental isoenzymes (Kasahara isoenzyme).

Methods for the Determination of Alkaline Phosphatase Activity

Numerous methods have been developed for determining ALP activity. In general, methodological developments have been directed at increasing the speed and sensitivity of the assay by selecting readily hydrolyzed substrates and phosphate-accepting buffers and toward the use of continuous-monitoring methods based on "self-indicating" substrates.

The most popular of the chromogenic or self-indicating substrates for ALP is 4-nitrophenyl phosphate (usually abbreviated 4-NPP or PNPP from the older name, *p*-nitrophenyl phosphate). This ester is colorless, but the final product is yellow at the pH of the reaction:

4-Nitrophenyl phosphate (colorless) + H_2O —(ALP, Mg^{2+}, pH 10.3)→ 4-Nitrophenoxide (colorless, benzenoid form) + phosphate ⇌ (Rearranges at alkaline pH) 4-Nitrophenoxide (yellow, quinonoid form)

The enzyme reaction is continuously monitored by observing the rate of formation of the 4-nitrophenoxide ions. With improvements in the reaction conditions, this reaction forms the basis of current recommended and standard methods of ALP assay. Other self-indicating substrates include phenolphthalein monophosphate, thymolphthalein phosphate, and α-naphthyl phosphate. In the ALP methods discussed, the liberated phosphate group is transferred to water. The rate of phosphatase action is enhanced, however, if certain amino alcohols are used as phosphate-accepting buffers. Among these activators are compounds such as AMP, DEA, TRIS, ethylaminoethanol (EAE), and *N*-methyl-d-glucamine (MEG). Enzyme activity in the presence of optimal concentrations of these buffers is twofold to sixfold greater than in the presence of a nonactivating buffer, such as carbonate.

ALP catalyzes the hydrolysis of 4-NPP, forming phosphate and free 4-nitrophenol (4-NP, PNP), which in dilute acid solutions is colorless. Under alkaline conditions, 4-NP is converted to the 4-nitrophenoxide ion, which has a very intense yellow color. The rate of formation of 4-NP by the action of the enzyme on 4-NPP at 37 °C is then monitored at 405 nm with a recording spectrophotometer. The (provisional) IFCC-recommended method uses 4-NPP as the substrate and AMP as the phosphate-acceptor buffer. It includes Mg^{2+} and Zn^{2+}, optimal concentrations of which are controlled by the addition of Mg^{2+} and Zn^{2+}, and the chelating agent *N*-hydroxyethylethylenediaminetriacetic acid (HEDTA). Although Zn^{2+} ions are present in a total concentration of 1 mmol/L, most are bound to HEDTA, leaving only a small, experimentally determined optimal concentration of free ions. A similar situation exists for Mg^{2+} ions. Thus HEDTA acts as a metal ion buffer, maintaining optimal concentrations of the two ions.[195]

Serum or heparinized plasma, free of hemolysis, should be used. Complexing anticoagulants—such as citrate, oxalate, and EDTA—must be avoided, because they bind cations, such as Mg^{2+} and Zn^{2+}, which are necessary cofactors for ALP activity measurement. Blood transfusion (containing citrate) causes a transient decrease in serum ALP through a similar mechanism. Freshly collected serum samples should be kept at room temperature and assayed as soon as possible but preferably within 4 hours after collection. In sera stored at a refrigerated temperature, ALP activity increases slowly (2%/d). Frozen specimens should be thawed and kept at room temperature for 18 to 24 hours before measurement to achieve full enzyme reactivation.

Reference Intervals[148,197]

ALP activities in serum vary with age. Children show higher ALP activity than healthy adults as a result of the leakage of bone ALP from osteoblasts during bone growth. Using the IFCC procedure at 37 °C, the following reference intervals (central 95 percentiles) have been established:

Sex	Age	Reference Interval
Males-females	4-15 yr	54-369 U/L
Males	20-50 yr	53-128 U/L
	≥60 yr	56-119 U/L
Females	20-50 yr	42-98 U/L
	≥60 yr	53-141 U/L

Activities in growing children are highly variable.

Methods for the Separation and Quantification of Alkaline Phosphatase Isoenzymes

Assays for ALP isoenzymes are needed when: (1) the source of an elevated ALP in serum is not obvious and should be clarified; (2) the main clinical question is concerned with detecting the presence of liver or bone involvement; and (3) in the case of metabolic bone disorders, to ascertain any modifications in the activity of osteoblasts to monitor the disease activity and the effect of appropriate therapies.

Criteria that have been used to differentiate the isoenzymes and other multiple forms of ALP include: (1) electrophoretic mobility; (2) stability to denaturation by heat or chemicals; (3) response to the presence of selected inhibitors; (4) affinity for specific lectins; and (5) immunochemical characteristics.[156]

The same electrophoretic techniques are used for the separation of ALP isoenzymes in serum as for separations of serum proteins. After electrophoresis, ALP zones are made visible by incubating the gel in a solution of buffered substrate (e.g., 1-naphthyl phosphate, to which a chromogenic system, usually represented by a diazonium salt, is added; in the case of electrophoresis on cellulose acetate, the strips are covered with an agar-gel layer containing the staining system). The liver ALP typically moves most rapidly toward the anode. Bone ALP, which typically gives a more diffuse zone than the liver form, has a slightly lower anodal mobility, although the two zones usually overlap to some extent. Intestinal ALP migrates more slowly than the bone enzyme, whereas the placental isoenzyme commonly appears as a discrete band overlying the diffuse bone fraction. An additional band, which is frequently present in the serum of patients with various hepatic diseases, contains a high molecular weight form of ALP but is also strongly negatively charged. Therefore it moves slowly in starch gel or may even fail to enter polyacrylamide gel, but it migrates more anodally than the main liver zone on nonsieving media, such as cellulose acetate. Investigations on this form have revealed that it corresponds to the main liver form attached to the membrane moiety (*membrane particle [fragment] ALP*).[138]

Complexes between ALP and immunoglobulins, or macro-ALP, occur occasionally in serum, giving rise to abnormally migrating bands in the γ-globulin zone; however, these do not provide specific diagnostic information in the present state of knowledge.

Two approaches have been proposed to improve the electrophoretic separation between bone and liver ALPs. Both methods exploit differences in the carbohydrate portions of the two forms of ALP. In one, electrophoresis is carried out in the presence of wheat germ lectin, which retards bone ALP migration more than the liver enzyme migration.[170] In the other, serum is treated briefly (i.e., for 15 min at 37 °C), with neuraminidase to remove part of the terminal sialic acid residues. As the sialic acid residues of bone ALP are more readily attacked than those of liver ALP, the electrophoretic mobility of the bone form is reduced more than that of liver ALP. The improved separation allows quantitative estimates to be made by densitometric scanning (Figure 21-5).[122]

Overnight incubation of the serum sample with neuraminidase also is used to confirm the presence of intestinal ALP. This treatment reduces the anodal mobility of all ALP isoenzymes except that of intestinal origin, which is neuraminidase-resistant because terminal sialic acid residues are not present in the molecule.

Because placental ALP is heat stable, incubation of the serum sample at a temperature as high as 65 °C for 30 minutes provides a convenient test for the presence of this isoenzyme. Other forms of ALP can also be differentiated based on their stability at high temperature. At 56 °C, for example, liver ALP is more stable than the bone ALP. ("Bone burns.") Thus if after 10 minutes at 56 °C, less than 20% of the serum ALP activity remains, the enzyme present is probably largely of bone type. Residual activities of between

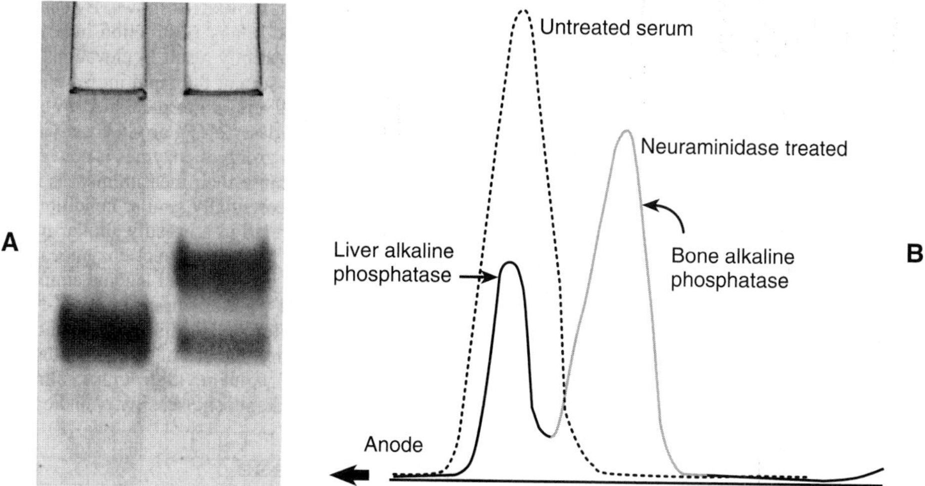

Figure 21-5 A, Polyacrylamide-gel electrophoresis of bone and liver alkaline phosphatases in human serum. *Left,* Mixture of two sera containing, respectively, entirely bone phosphatase and entirely liver phosphatase. *Right,* Mixture of the same two sera after each has been treated with neuraminidase for 10 minutes at 37 °C. The anodal direction is downward. The more anodal zone is liver phosphatase. **B,** Densitometric scans of electrophoretic patterns shown in A. *Broken line,* Scan of mixture of untreated sera; *solid line,* scan of mixture of sera treated briefly with neuraminidase. The anode is to the left. *(From Moss DW, Edwards RK. Improved electrophoretic resolution of bone and liver alkaline phosphatases resulting from partial digestion with neuraminidase. Clin Chim Acta 1984;143:177-82.)*

25% and 55% support electrophoretic evidence that liver ALP is the predominant form. The imprecision of the test reflects difficulties in standardizing the rate of sample heating (related to such things as the type of apparatus used to heat the serum sample, thermal conductivity of the sample container, and the volume of sample in the container during heating), the rate of sample cooling (e.g., in an ice bath), and the fact that the result (as a ratio or percent) includes uncertainties from two measurements. As an alternative to heat fractionation of ALP, measurement of GGT, which is increased in liver disease but not in bone disease, may be a useful rapid tool to distinguish between the two diseases as the explanation for an increased serum ALP. As discussed below, the pattern of increases of serum glutamyl transferase in liver diseases is similar to that for alkaline phosphatase.

The use of wheat germ lectin, binding the *N*-acetylglucosamine residues present in different amounts on individual isoenzymes, has also been the basis of a commercial technique for the selective precipitation and measurement of bone ALP. However, this technique does not provide sufficient accuracy and precision for quantifying the bone fraction.[112]

Immunological methods with polyclonal antisera or monoclonal antibodies provide the best quantitative measurements of intestinal or placental ALPs. Much more difficult is the production of antibodies that selectively react with different products of the tissue-nonspecific ALP gene, including the liver- and bone-derived isoforms, as these antibodies should recognize specific sugar side chains instead of a particular amino acid sequence. Until now, no monoclonal antibodies fully discriminate between liver and bone ALPs. Despite lack of complete specificity, the commercially available immunoassays of bone ALP may offer some advantages, but their value has not been convincingly demonstrated, in part because measurements of total ALP provide the required clinical information in many situations.

5′-NUCLEOTIDASE

5′-Nucleotidase (EC 3.1.3.5; 5′-ribonucleotide phosphohydrolase; NTP) is a phosphatase that acts only on nucleoside-5′-phosphates, such as adenosine-5′-phosphate (AMP) and adenylic acid, releasing inorganic phosphate.

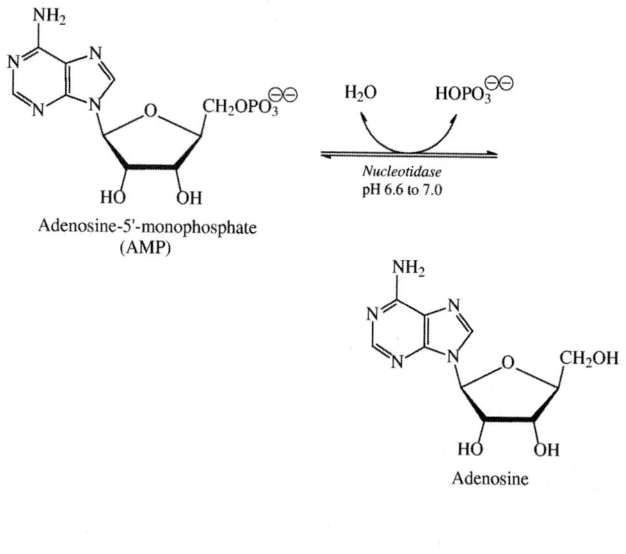

Adenosine-5'-monophosphate (AMP) + H_2O → (*Nucleotidase*, pH 6.6 to 7.0) → Adenosine + $HOPO_3^{2-}$

NTP is a glycoprotein widely distributed throughout the tissues of the body and is principally localized in the cytoplasmic membrane of the cells in which it occurs. Its pH optimum is between 6.6 and 7.0.[188]

Clinical Significance

Despite its ubiquitous distribution, serum NTP activities appear to reflect hepatobiliary disease with considerable specificity. NTP is increased threefold to sixfold in those hepatobiliary diseases in which there is interference with the secretion of the bile. This may be due to extrahepatic causes (a stone or tumor occluding the bile duct), or it may arise from intrahepatic conditions, such as cholestasis caused by chlorpromazine, malignant infiltration of the liver, or biliary cirrhosis. When parenchymal cell damage is predominant, as in infectious hepatitis, serum NTP activity is only moderately elevated.

Assay of NTP activity has been considered of value as an addition to measurement of nonspecific total ALP in patients with suspected hepatobiliary disease, and abnormal NTP activity is routinely interpreted as evidence of a hepatic origin of increased ALP activity in serum. However, approximately half of individuals in whom liver ALP activity is increased in serum may simultaneously show a normal NTP. On the other hand, increased NTP in the serum of patients with normal liver ALP is very often associated with the presence of liver disease. Thus the frequent dissociation of the two enzyme activities supports the utility of determining both (liver) ALP and NTP to increase the diagnostic efficiency for diseases of the liver.[132]

Methods for the Determination of 5′-Nucleotidase Activity

The substrates most generally used in measuring the activity of NTP are AMP or IMP (inosine-5′-phosphate). However, these substrates are organic phosphate esters and thus can be hydrolyzed to an appreciable degree by other nonspecific (alkaline) phosphatases, even at a pH as low as 7.5, which is the pH assumed optimal for NTP activity. Methods for the estimation of NTP in serum must therefore incorporate some means for correcting for the hydrolysis of the substrate by the nonspecific phosphatases.

In a commercially available assay, serum NTP catalyzes the hydrolysis of IMP to yield inosine, which is then converted to hypoxanthine by purine-nucleoside phosphorylase (EC 2.4.2.1). Hypoxanthine is oxidized to urate with xanthine oxidase (EC 1.2.3.2). Two moles of hydrogen peroxide are produced for each mole of hypoxanthine liberated and converted to uric acid. The formation rate of hydrogen peroxide is monitored by a spectrophotometer at 510 nm by the oxidation of a chromogenic system. The effect of ALPs on IMP is inhibited by β-glycerophosphate. This material is substrate for ALP but not for NTP, and by forming substrate complexes with the former enzyme, it reduces the proportion of the total ALP activity that is directed to the hydrolysis of the NTP substrate, IMP.[19]

NTP activity in serum or plasma heparin is stable for at least 4 days at 4 °C and 4 months at −20 °C.

Reference Interval

The reference interval for NTP activity at 37 °C is from 3 to 9 U/L, with no sex-related differences.

GAMMA-GLUTAMYL TRANSFERASE

Peptidases are enzymes that catalyze the hydrolytic cleavage of peptides to form amino acids or smaller peptides. They constitute a broad group of enzymes of varied specificity, and some individual enzymes act as amino acid transferases and catalyze the transfer of amino acids from one peptide to another amino acid or peptide. Gamma-glutamyl transferase (EC 2.3.2.2; γ-glutamyl-peptide:amino acid γ-glutamyltransferase; GGT) catalyzes the transfer of the γ-glutamyl group from peptides and compounds that contain it to some acceptor.[55] The γ-glutamyl acceptor is the substrate itself, some amino acid or peptide, or even water, in which case simple hydrolysis takes place. The enzyme acts only on peptides or peptidelike compounds containing a terminal glutamate residue joined to the remainder of the compound through the terminal (-γ-) carboxyl. Glycylglycine is five times more effective as an acceptor than is either glycine or the tripeptide (gly-gly-gly) but little is known about the optimal properties of the acceptor co-substrate. The peptidase transfer reaction is considerably faster than that of the simple hydrolysis reaction. An example of a reaction catalyzed by the enzyme is:

γ-Glutamyl-*p*-nitroanilide *Substrate (donor)* + Glycylglycine *Acceptor* —(γ-Glutamyltransferase, pH 8.2)→ *p*-Nitroaniline *Donor residue* + γ-Glutamylglycylglycine *Transfer product*

GGT is present (in decreasing order of abundance) in proximal renal tubule, liver, pancreas, and intestine. The enzyme is present in cytoplasm (microsomes), but the larger fraction is located in the cell membrane and may transport amino acids and peptides into the cell across the cell membrane in the form of γ-glutamyl peptides. It may also be involved in some aspects of glutathione metabolism.[214]

GGT activity in serum comes primarily from liver. The enzyme in serum is heterogeneous with respect to both net molecular charge (e.g., shown by electrophoresis) and size. These forms appear to derive from posttranslational modifications of a single type of enzyme molecule rather than to be due to the existence of true isoenzymes. For example, high molecular weight forms may represent the release of cell membrane fragments into the circulation. Despite numerous investigations, clear correlations between patterns of multiple forms and particular diseases cannot be discerned.

Clinical Significance

Even though renal tissue has the highest concentration of GGT, the enzyme present in serum appears to originate primarily from the hepatobiliary system. GGT is a sensitive indicator of the presence of hepatobiliary disease, being elevated in most subjects with liver disease regardless of cause, but its usefulness is limited by the lack of specificity. Like ALP, it is highest in cases of intrahepatic or posthepatic biliary obstruction, reaching activities some 5 to 30 times upper reference limit. High elevations of GGT are also observed in patients with either primary or secondary (metastatic) liver neoplasms; in these conditions, changes may occur earlier and are more pronounced than those with the other liver enzymes are. Moderate elevations (two to five times normal) occur in infectious hepatitis. Patients with chronic hepatitis C infection and high pretreatment serum GGT are unlikely to have a sustained virological response to interferon treatment. Small increases of GGT activity are observed in patients with fatty livers, and similar but transient increases are noted in cases of drug intoxication. In acute and chronic pancreatitis and in some pancreatic malignancies (especially if associated with hepatobiliary obstruction), enzyme activity may be 5 to 15 times the upper reference limit.

Elevated activities of GGT are found in the sera of patients with alcoholic hepatitis and in the majority of sera from people who are heavy drinkers. Increased concentrations of the enzyme are also found in serum of subjects receiving anticonvulsivant drugs such as phenytoin and phenobarbital. Such an increase of GGT activity in serum may reflect induction of new enzyme activity by the action of the alcohol and drugs and/or their toxic effects on microsomal structures in liver cells.

In AMI, GGT activity is usually normal. If there is a rise, it occurs at about the fourth day, reaches a maximum value in another 4 days, and probably implies liver damage secondary to cardiac insufficiency.

Unlike ALP, GGT is not increased in conditions in which osteoblastic activity is increased.

Methods for the Determination of γ-Glutamyltransferase Activity

Early GGT assays used L-γ-glutamyl-*p*-nitroanilide (GGPNA) as the substrate, with glycylglycine serving as the γ-glutamyl residue acceptor. However, GGPNA has limited solubility in the reaction mixture, and it is therefore difficult to obtain saturating substrate concentrations. The *p*-nitroaniline produced in the reaction is determined by its yellow color, which is monitored at 405 nm.

Derivatives of GGPNA are also available and have been used in other methods. In these derivatives, various groups have been introduced into the benzene ring to increase solubility in water. The most useful of these substrates is L-γ-glutamyl-3-carboxy-4-nitroanilide is readily soluble in water and is split by GGT at a rate comparable to that observed with GGPNA. Activities in serum are higher with the carboxyl derivative than with the noncarboxylated substrate, partly because of the higher substrate concentrations attainable with the former.

In the IFCC reference measurement procedure for GGT, L-γ-glutamyl-3-carboxy-4-nitroanilide serves as the substrate, with glycylglycine serving as an acceptor. Buffering is provided by glycylglycine itself. The temperature of reaction is 37 °C and the wavelength of measurement of the reaction product, 5-amino-2-nitrobenzoate, is 410 nm.[177]

GGT is a comparatively stable enzyme in vitro. Activity is stable for at least 1 month at 4 °C and 1 year at −20 °C. Nonhemolyzed serum is the preferred specimen, but EDTA plasma has also been used. Heparin may produce turbidity in the reaction mixture; citrate, oxalate, and fluoride depress GGT activity by 10% to 15%.

Reference Intervals

In adults, the upper reference limit for GGT activity in serum is 38 U/L for females and 55 U/L for males.[180] Reference limits are approximately twofold higher in people of African ancestry. In normal full-term neonates, the GGT activity at birth is approximately six to seven times the adult reference range. The activity then declines, reaching adult values by the age of 5 to 7 months.[33]

Glutathione S-Transferase

Cytosolic glutathione S-transferases (EC 2.5.1.18; GST) are dimeric enzymes that catalyze the nucleophilic addition of glutathione to the electrophilic centers of a wide variety of chemical structures, accomplishing detoxification reactions. In addition, GSTs exert part of the glutathione peroxidase activity and have an important function in intracellular binding and transport of a wide variety of both endogenous and exogenous compounds. The family of human enzymes is divided into four main classes: α, μ, π, and θ.[63]

α-GST is found at high concentrations in the human liver and is released quickly and in large quantities from damaged hepatocytes into the bloodstream.

Clinical Significance

α-GST is an emerging marker for assessing hepatocellular damage. Unlike aminotransferases, which are found predominantly in the periportal hepatocytes, α-GST is evenly distributed across the liver acinus and is therefore released in all types of hepatocyte injury. In liver transplant recipients, α-GST was found more valuable than AST in detecting early rejection episodes postoperatively and less susceptible to the confounding effects of infection.

Methods for the Determination of Glutathione S-Transferase

Several problems have been associated with GST activity measurements. First, normal plasma activity is low and hard to measure. Secondly, GST binds a number of anions, such as bile salts and bilirubin, that inhibit enzyme activity. Immunoassays have been described that allow the precise and specific measurement of α-GST concentrations. At present, the only methodological problem relates to the speed of the assays, which take several hours.

Reference Interval

Using a commercially available enzyme immunoassay for α-GST, the upper reference limit was 11.4 μg/L.[164]

CHOLINESTERASE

Two related enzymes have the ability to hydrolyze acetylcholine. One is acetylcholinesterase (EC 3.1.1.7, acetylcholine acetylhydrolase), which is called true cholinesterase or choline esterase I. True cholinesterase is found in erythrocytes, the lungs and spleen, nerve endings, and the gray matter of the brain. It is responsible for the prompt hydrolysis of acetylcholine released at the nerve endings to mediate transmission of the neural impulse across the synapse. The degradation of acetylcholine is required for the depolarization of the nerve so that it is repolarized in the next conduction event.

The other cholinesterase is acylcholine acylhydrolase (EC 3.1.1.8, acylcholine acylhydrolase, CHE); it is also called pseudocholinesterase, serum cholinesterase, butyrylcholinesterase, or choline esterase II. Although it is found in the liver, pancreas, heart, white matter of the brain, and serum, its biological role is unknown. The assay of this enzyme is clinically useful.

The type of reaction catalyzed by both cholinesterases is:

$$Br^{\ominus}\,(CH_3)_3N^{\oplus}CH_2CH_2OC(=O)CH_3 + H_2O \xrightarrow{\text{Cholinesterase}} CH_3COO^{\ominus} + H^{\oplus} + Br^{\ominus}\,(CH_3)_3N^{\oplus}CH_2CH_2OH$$

Acetylcholine bromide → Acetate + Choline bromide

The two enzymes differ in specificity toward some substrates while behaving similarly toward others. The serum enzyme acts on benzoylcholine but cannot hydrolyze acetyl-β-methylcholine; the red cell enzyme acts on the latter but not on the former. The red cell enzyme splits only choline esters; aryl or alkyl esters are not attacked. The red cell enzyme is inhibited by its substrate, acetylcholine, if present at about 10^{-2} mol/L; the serum enzyme is not inhibited by this substrate.

Both enzymes are inhibited by the alkaloids prostigmine and physostigmine, both of which contain quaternary nitrogen (present in choline) in their structures. These two compounds are typical competitive inhibitors, competing with the choline residue of acetylcholine for its binding site on the enzyme surface. Some organic phosphorus compounds, such as diisopropyl fluorophosphate, irreversibly inhibit both enzymes. The phosphoryl group binds very tightly to the enzyme site at which binding of the acyl group normally occurs, thus preventing attachment of the acetylcholine. Both enzymes are also inhibited by a large variety of other compounds, including morphine, quinine, tertiary amines, phenothiazines, pyrophosphate, bile salts, citrate, fluoride, and borate.

The CHE in normal sera is separated by electrophoresis into 7 to 12 bands, the number depending on the experimental technique used. The forms of CHE differ in molecular size and appear to be aggregates of different numbers of the same basic unit. Of more interest are the atypical (genetic) variants of the enzyme, characterized by diminished activity against acetylcholine and other substrates, which are found in the sera of a small fraction of apparently healthy people.

The gene controlling the synthesis of CHE can exist in many allelic forms. Four of the most common forms are designated as E^u, E^a, E^f, and E^s. These four allelic genes can be combined to form one normal and nine abnormal genotypes. At least 40 other forms exist and another gene locus is recognized (E_2). The normal, most common phenotype is designated as EuEu, or UU (u for *usual*). The gene E^a is referred to as the *atypical* gene; the sera of people homozygous for this gene (E^a E^a = AA) are only weakly active toward most substrates for cholinesterase and demonstrate increased resistance to inhibition of enzyme activity by dibucaine. The E^f gene (f for *fluoride resistant*) also gives rise to a weakly active enzyme but with increased resistance to fluoride inhibition. The E^s gene (s for *silent*) is associated with absence of enzyme or the presence of a protein with minimal or no catalytic activity. The mutations that give rise to the atypical and fluoride-resistant CHE variants involve a change in the structure of the active center. The variant enzymes (allelozymes) are less effective catalysts than the usual form; the affinity of the enzymes for the substrates is reduced (i.e., K_m is increased), and affinity for competitive inhibitors, such as dibucaine or fluoride, is similarly decreased. This gives rise to the characteristic dibucaine- or fluoride-resistant properties of the genetic variants that are exploited in their characterization.

The homozygous forms, AA or FF, are found in 0.3% to 0.5% of the Caucasian population; their incidence among blacks is even lower. Inheritance of increased CHE activity has also been reported in a few families. This is apparently due to increased production of the usual allelozyme.

Clinical Significance[109]

Measurements of CHE activity in serum are used (1) as a test of liver function, (2) as an indicator of possible insecticide poisoning, and (3) for the detection of patients with atypical forms of the enzyme who are at risk of prolonged responses to certain muscle relaxants used in surgical procedures.

Measurement of serum CHE activity can serve as a sensitive indicator of the synthetic capacity of the liver. In the absence of genetic causes or known inhibitors, any decrease in CHE activity reflects impaired synthesis of the enzyme by the liver. A 30% to 50% CHE decrease is observed in acute hepatitis and in chronic hepatitis of long duration. Decreases of 50% to 70% occur in advanced cirrhosis and carcinoma with metastases to the liver. CHE is essentially normal in obstructive jaundice except when the cause is malignant. Serial measurement of CHE has been promoted as an indication of prognosis in patients with liver disease and for monitoring liver function after liver transplantation.

Among the organic phosphorus compounds that inhibit cholinesterase activity are many insecticides, such as parathion, sarin, and tetraethyl pyrophosphate. Workers in agriculture and in organic chemical industries may be subject to poisoning by inhalation of these materials or by contact with them. Obviously, if enough material is absorbed to inactivate all the acetylcholinesterase of nervous tissue, death will result. Both cholinesterases are inhibited, but the activity of the serum enzyme falls more rapidly than does that of the erythrocyte enzyme. A 40% drop in CHE activity occurs before the first symptoms are felt, and a drop of 80% is required before neuromuscular effects become apparent. Near-zero concentrations of enzyme activity require emergency treatment with such enzyme reactivators as pyridine-2-aldoxime. Upon retesting, in 3 to 5 days the CHE activity should increase by 15% to 20% if a significant organophosphate-induced inhibition has previously occurred.

Succinyldicholine (suxamethonium) and mivacurium, drugs used in surgery as muscle relaxants, are hydrolyzed by CHE, and their pharmacological effect normally persists only long enough to meet the needs of the surgical procedure. In patients with low enzyme activities or in those with a weakly active variant, destruction of the drug will not occur rapidly enough, and the patient may enter a period of prolonged paralysis of the respiratory muscles (apnea) requiring mechanical ventilation until the drug effects gradually wear off. Preoperative screening has been advocated to identify patients in whom suxamethonium administration may lead to complications. The degree of drug sensitivity varies with the phenotype of the patient. Total CHE activity is highest in individuals who are homozygous for the usual allele and progressively lower in those who are heterozygous for the usual and a variant allele, those who are homozygous or heterozygous for variant alleles, and those in whom two "silent" alleles are paired and no activity is detected. Subjects who possess one normal allele (i.e., who are heterozygous for the normal and a variant allele) usually produce enough enzyme to protect them against suxamethonium sensitivity, whereas patients with paired variant alleles (either as homozygotes or heterozygotes) show various degrees of sensitivity. The phenotypes most susceptible to apnea after succinylcholine administration are AA, AS, FF, FS, SS, AF, and to some extent UA. Measurements of total CHE activity and determination of the "dibucaine number" and "fluoride number" are needed to characterize CHE variants fully. The latter values indicate the percentage inhibition of enzyme activity toward specified substrates in the presence of standard concentrations of dibucaine or fluoride.

Methods for the Determination of Serum Cholinesterase Activity

Many of the contemporary methods use acylthiocholine esters as substrates. These substrates are hydrolyzed at approximately the same rate as choline esters, and the thiocholine formed can be measured by reaction with chromogenic disulfide agents, such as 5,5′-dithio-bis (2-nitrobenzoate) (DTNB) (Ellman's reagent). The reaction of the thiocholine product with colorless DTNB forms colored 5-MNBA, which is measured spectrophotometrically at 410 nm. The iodide salts of acetylthiocholine, propionylthiocholine, butyrylthiocholine, and succinylthiocholine all have been used as substrates. The reactions for butyrylthiocholine, with DTNB as the chromogen, are:

H_2O → $H^{\oplus}$ (Serum Cholinesterase)

Butyrylthiocholine → Butyrate + Thiocholine

Thiocholine + DTNB (colorless) ⇌ Mixed disulfide + 5-Mercapto-2-nitrobenzoic acid; 5-MNBA (colored)

The clinical question being asked may influence the choice of substrate suitable for measuring the enzyme. Measuring CHE activity using succinyldithiocholine is the method of choice to diagnose succinylcholine sensitivity, purely based on the enzyme activity recorded in serum. This method is, however, well suited for other clinical applications of the test.[116]

Kalow and Genest, using benzoylcholine as a classic substrate, demonstrated the qualitative difference in CHEs. Based on the differences as sensitivity to inhibition by the local anesthetic dibucaine, they developed a simple test to classify the type of CHE as usual, intermediate, or atypical. With 10^{-5} mol/L dibucaine ("dibucaine number"), the usual CHE is inhibited by 80%, but atypical CHE is inhibited by only 20%. Subjects heterozygous for the normal and atypical gene show about 60% inhibition of CHE. To differentiate other genotypes, sodium fluoride can be used as CHE inhibitor.

Serum is the sample of choice. Enzyme activity in serum is stable for several weeks if the specimen is stored under refrigeration, and for several years if stored at −20 °C. Moderate hemolysis does not interfere if separated serum has been centrifuged to remove red blood cell ghosts.

Reference Intervals

Using the succinyldithiocholine/DTNB method at 37 °C, the reference interval for healthy adults with the usual CHE genotype was estimated to be 33 to 76 U/L for women and 40 to 78 U/L for men, respectively. The median activity in individuals with heterozygous genotype was 22 U/L (range 5 to 35 U/L), and for atypical homozygotes 1.5 U/L (range 1 to 4 U/L).[142] A value <23 U/L was approximately five times as likely to occur in a succinyldicholine-sensitive individual as in a normal one.[116] At birth, CHE activity is lower than adult values by about 50%. It increases during the next 3 to 6 years to exceed adult values by about 30%. From the fifth year of life, the activity starts to decrease before stabilizing at the adult value, which is reached at puberty. There is a significant CHE decrease (30%) during pregnancy and early puerperium, explained by hemodilution.

CHE phenotyping, based on the determination of dibucaine (DN) and fluoride (FN) numbers, has been established:

Phenotype	DN Range	FN Range
UU	≥77	≥55
UF	72-76	≥53
UA	48-72	≥44
AF	45-59	<44
FF	64-69	<44
AA	<35	*

*Redundant for AA phenotype attribution.

PANCREATIC ENZYMES

Assays of serum AMY, lipase (LPS), trypsin (TRY), chymotrypsin (CHY), and elastase 1 (E1) are applied to investigation of pancreatic disease. Pancreatic function and pathology are discussed in Chapter 48.

Amylase

α-Amylase (EC 3.2.1.1; 1,4-α-D glucan glucanohydrolase; AMY) is an enzyme of the hydrolase class that catalyzes the hydrolysis of 1,4-α-glucosidic linkages in polysaccharides. Both straight-chain (linear) polyglucans, such as amylose, and branched polyglucans, such as amylopectin and glycogen, are hydrolyzed, but at different rates. In the case of amylose, the enzyme splits the chains at alternate α-1,4-hemiacetal (—C—O—C—) links, forming maltose and some residual glucose; maltose, glucose, and a residue of limit dextrins are formed if branched-chain polyglucans are used as substrate. The enzyme does not attack the α-1,6-linkages at the branch points. AMYs are calcium metalloenzymes, with the calcium absolutely required for functional integrity. However, full activity is displayed only in the presence of various anions—such as chloride, bromide, nitrate, cholate, or monohydrogen phosphate—with chloride and bromide being the most effective activators. AMY in human serum has a moderately sharp pH optimum at 6.9 to 7.0.

AMYs normally occurring in human plasma are small molecules with molecular weights varying from 54,000 to 62,000. The enzyme is thus small enough to pass through the glomeruli of the kidneys, and AMY is the only plasma enzyme normally found in urine. AMY is present in a number of organs and tissues.[215] The greatest concentration is present in the salivary glands, which secrete a potent AMY (S-type) to initiate hydrolysis of starches while the food is still in the mouth and esophagus. The action of the S-AMY, once referred to as *ptyalin,* is terminated by acid in the stomach. In the pancreas, the enzyme (P-type) is synthesized by the acinar cells and then secreted into the intestinal tract by way of the pancreatic duct system. In the intestinal tract, effective action of pancreatic and intestinal AMY is favored by the mildly alkaline conditions in the duodenum. Intestinal maltase then further hydrolyzes maltose to glucose. AMY activity is also found in extracts from semen, testes, ovaries, fallopian tubes, striated muscle, lungs, and adipose tissue. The enzyme is also found in colostrum, tears, and milk. Some tumors of lung and ovary may also contain considerable AMY activity. The enzyme found in urine is derived from the plasma. Ascitic and pleural fluids may contain AMY as a result of the presence of a tumor or pancreatitis.

The enzyme present in normal serum and urine is predominantly of pancreatic (P-AMY) and salivary gland (S-AMY) origin. These isoenzymes are products of two closely linked loci on chromosome 1. AMY isoenzymes also undergo posttranslational modification of deamidation, glycosylation, and deglycosylation to form a number of isoforms. Indeed, nonenzymic deamidation appears to be the mechanism for "aging" that occurs when AMY is sequestered (e.g., pancreatic pseudocysts) or subjected to prolonged in vitro storage. Although P-AMY is not glycosylated, S-AMY may exist in both glycosylated and deglycosylated forms; these isoforms can be separated in both serum and urine using isoelectric focusing or electrophoresis.

Clinical Significance

Blood AMY activity is normally low and constant and greatly increases in acute pancreatitis and salivary gland inflammation. In acute pancreatitis, a rise in serum AMY activity occurs within 5 to 8 hours of symptom onset; activities return to normal by the third or fourth day. A fourfold to sixfold elevation in AMY activity above the upper reference limit is usual, with maximal concentrations attained in 12 to 72 hours. The magnitude of the elevation of serum enzyme activity is not related to the severity of pancreatic involvement; however, the greater the rise, the greater the probability of acute pancreatitis. A portion of the clearance of AMY from the circulation is via renal excretion into the urine, and increased serum activity is reflected in an increase of urinary AMY activity. As compared with serum AMY, urine AMY reaches higher concentrations and persists for longer periods. The clinical specificity of AMY for the diagnosis of acute pancreatitis is, however, low (20% to 60%, depending on the mix of the patient population studied) since increased values are also found in a number of acute intraabdominal disorders and in several extrapancreatic conditions (Table 21-4).

Biliary tract diseases, such as cholecystitis, cause up to fourfold elevations of the serum AMY activity as a result of either primary or secondary pancreatic involvement. Various intraabdominal events can lead to a significant increase in serum AMY activities up to a fourfold elevation and sometimes beyond. Such increases may be due to leakage of the P-AMY from the intestine into the peritoneal cavity and then into the circulation. Peritonitis and acute appendicitis have been reported to produce a slight elevation (up to twofold and threefold) of serum AMY activity. Serum AMY is normal in most patients with ectopic pregnancies, but increases have been seen in advanced cases of ruptured ectopic pregnancy.

In renal insufficiency the serum AMY activity is increased in proportion to the extent of renal impairment (usually, no more than five times the upper reference limit). Hyperamylasemia also occurs in neoplastic diseases. Tumors of the lung and serous and mixed (serous and mucinous) carcinomas of the ovary can produce hyperamylasemia (with an S-type isoenzyme mobility) with elevations as high as 50 times the upper reference limit. Salivary gland lesions caused by infection, irradiation, obstruction, surgery, and tumor have all been reported as producing a significant S-type hyperamylasemia. Postoperative hyperamylasemia occurs in about 20% of all patients subjected to a wide variety of surgical interventions, including extraabdominal procedures. Increases of about four times the upper reference limit are found in as many as 80% of patients with diabetic ketoacidosis. In acute alcoholic intoxication, about 10% of subjects have a threefold elevation. Finally, a wide variety of drugs must always be considered as possible causes of hyperamylasemia.

Macroamylases are sometimes present in sera and may cause hyperamylasemia; these are complexes between ordinary AMY (usually S-type) and IgG or IgA. These macroamylases cannot be filtered through the glomeruli of the kidneys because of their large size (greater than MW 200,000) and are thus retained in the plasma where their presence may increase AMY activity some twofold to eightfold above the upper reference limit. No clinical symptoms are associated with this disorder, but some of these cases have been detected during investigation of abdominal pain.

The lack of specificity of total AMY measurement has led to the interest in the direct measurement of P-AMY instead of total enzyme activity for the differential diagnosis of patients with acute abdominal pain. By applying the best decision limit (i.e., an activity equal to threefold the upper reference limit), the clinical specificity of P-AMY for the diagnosis of acute pancreatitis was greater than 90%.[144] The

TABLE 21-4 Causes of Hyperamylasemia

Pancreatic disease	Pancreatitis, any cause (P-AMY↑)*
	Pancreatic trauma (P-AMY↑)
Intraabdominal diseases other than pancreatitis	Biliary tract disease (P-AMY↑)
	Intestinal obstruction (P-AMY↑)
	Mesenteric infarction (P-AMY↑)
	Perforated peptic ulcer (P-AMY↑)
	Gastritis, duodenitis (P-AMY↑)
	Ruptured aortic aneurysm
	Acute appendicitis
	Peritonitis
	Trauma
Genitourinary disease	Ectopic, ruptured tubal pregnancy (S-AMY↑)
	Salpingitis (S-AMY↑)
	Ovarian malignancy (S-AMY↑)
	Renal insufficiency (Mixed)
Miscellaneous	Salivary gland lesions (S-AMY↑)
	Acute alcoholic abuse (S-AMY↑)
	Diabetic ketoacidosis (S-AMY↑)
	Macroamylasemia (Mixed)
	Septic shock (S-AMY↑)
	Cardiac surgery (S-AMY↑)
	Tumors (usually S-AMY↑)
	Drugs (usually S-AMY↑)

*Predominant isoenzyme type is shown in parentheses: *P-AMY*, pancreatic; *S-AMY*, salivary; *Mixed*, either or both isoenzymes may be present.

sensitivity in late detection of this condition is also notably improved with P-AMY. P-AMY values remain elevated in 80% of patients with uncomplicated pancreatitis 1 week after onset, when only 30% still show increased total AMY activity.[147] This long-standing increase in P-AMY activity in serum also makes redundant the traditional measurement of total AMY in urine, a test performed to achieve a better diagnostic sensitivity in the late phase of pancreatitis.

A decreased P-AMY activity in serum (less than the lower reference limit) identifies with high specificity patients with exocrine pancreatic insufficiency and steatorrhea and can make intubation tests for pancreatic function unnecessary. If, however, P-AMY is normal, a reduced pancreatic function cannot be excluded.[115]

Methods for the Determination of α-Amylase Activity[47]

Historically, saccharogenic, amyloclastic, and chromolytic starch methods were the assays of choice for determining AMY activity. These assays are now completely displaced in favor of ones with well-defined substrates with shorter glucosyl chains. The use of defined AMY substrates and auxiliary and indicator enzymes in the AMY assay has improved the reaction stoichiometry and has led to more controlled and consistent hydrolysis conditions. Substrates used include small oligosaccharides and 4-nitrophenyl (4-NP)-glycoside substrates.

When hydrolyzed by AMY, small oligosaccharides substrates have been found to give better-defined products than do starches. For example, both maltopentaose and maltotetraose show good stability, consistent hydrolysis products, and unambiguous reaction stoichiometry. Several variations of the reaction rate formulation have been devised. For example, the detection of glucose can be achieved by the hexokinase (EC 2.7.1.1) reaction:

$$\text{Maltopentaose} \xrightarrow{\alpha\text{-amylase}} \text{maltotriose} + \text{maltose}$$

$$\text{Maltotriose} + \text{maltose} \xrightarrow{\alpha\text{-glucosidase}} 5\ \text{glucose}$$

$$\text{Glucose} + \text{ATP} \xrightarrow{\text{Hexokinase}} \text{G-6-P} + \text{ADP}$$

$$\text{G-6-P} + \text{NAD}^{\oplus} \xrightarrow{\text{G-6-P dehydrogenase}} \text{6-P-gluconolactone} + \text{NADH} + \text{H}^{\oplus}$$

Maltose generation is detected by the maltose phosphorylase (EC 2.4.1.8) reaction, which avoids interference by the endogenous glucose of the sample.

Maltotetraose has also been used as a substrate in the following reaction scheme:

$$\text{Maltotetraose} \xrightarrow{\alpha\text{-amylase}} 2\ \text{maltose}$$

$$\text{Maltose} + \text{P}_i \xrightarrow{\text{Maltose phosphorylase}} \text{glucose} + \text{glucose-1-P}$$

$$\text{Glucose-1-P} \xrightarrow{\beta\text{-Phosphoglucomutase}} \text{Glucose-6-P}$$

$$\text{G-6-P} + \text{NAD}^{\oplus} \xrightarrow{\text{G-6-P dehydrogenase}} \text{6-P-gluconolactone} + \text{NADH} + \text{H}^{\oplus}$$

With this method, for each bond hydrolyzed by AMY, two molecules of NADH are produced. This holds true only if neither glucose nor maltotriose is produced by the action of AMY. Later work has shown that these products are present in the reaction mixture in significant quantities. Thus the assay underestimates AMY activity.

4-NP-glycoside substrates are prepared by bonding 4-NP to the reducing end of a defined oligosaccharide. If the oligosaccharide is maltoheptaose (G7), the substrate is then 4-NP-G7. AMY splits this substrate to produce free oligosaccharides (G5, G4, and G3) and 4-NP-G2 (9%), 4-NP-G3 (31%), and 4-NP-G4 (60%). P-AMY hydrolyzes the substrate at a greater rate than does S-AMY in the ratio 1.8 : 1:

$$\text{4-NP-(glucose)}_7 \xrightarrow{\alpha\text{-amylase}} \text{4-NP-(glucose)}_{4,3,2} + \text{(glucose)}_{5,4,3}$$

$$\text{4-NP-(glucose)}_{4,3,2} \xrightarrow{\alpha\text{-glucosidase}} \text{4-NP-(glucose)}_4 + \text{x-glucose} + \text{NP}$$

G6, G1, 4-NP-G6, and 4-NP-G5 are not produced in appreciable quantities. In the original assay, the result of the combined hydrolysis by AMY in the specimen and by the reagent α-glucosidase (EC 3.2.1.20; maltase) is that more than 30% of the product is free NP. The free NP is detected by its absorbance at 405 nm. α-Glucosidase does not react with any oligosaccharide containing more than four glucose molecules in the chain; G4 is hydrolyzed only very slowly.[160] Problems arose with the use of the 4-NP-glycoside assay with regard to the poor stability of the reconstituted assay mixture because of the slow hydrolysis of the 4-NP-glycoside by α-glucosidase. This effect has been reduced by covalently linking a "blocking" group, e.g., a 4,6-ethylidene group (ethylidene-protected substrate [EPS]), to the nonreducing end of the molecule. The blocked substrate also shows a different and more advantageous hydrolysis pattern. Thus the ethylidene-4-NP-G7 substrate fragments approximately as 4-NP-G2 (40%), 4-NP-G3 (40%), and 4-NP-G4 (20%). Therefore liberation of 4-NP is increased; however, the reaction rate is reduced in proportion, so these two effects compensate for each other.[90] A novel-type α-glucosidase is available (recombinant enzyme AGH-211 from Toyobo Co., Japan) that completely hydrolyzes nitrophenylated substrates. As a result, the cleavage of one α-glucosidic linkage by AMY results in the release of one molecule of 4-NP. IFCC has optimized this method at 37 °C, deciding to recommend it as a reference measurement procedure for AMY.[98]

An alternative method based on the 2-chloro-*p*-nitrophenol (CNP) indicator uses 2-chloro-*p*-nitrophenyl-α-D-maltotrioside (CNP-G3) as a substrate:

$$10\,\text{CNP} - \text{G3} \xrightarrow{\alpha\text{-amylase}} 9\,\text{CNP} + 1\,\text{CNP} - \text{G2} + 9\,\text{maltotriose} + 1\,\text{glucose}$$

This assay does not require glucosidases and is considered a "direct" assay. Its disadvantages have been stated to include its low substrate conversion rate compared with G4, G5, and G7 assays; the variation in molar absorptivity of CNP associated with changes in pH, temperature, and protein content; and the presence of the activator, potassium thiocyanate, causing allosteric changes to AMY and precluding the use of antibodies for P-AMY determination.[193]

With the exception of heparin, all common anticoagulants inhibit AMY activity because they chelate Ca^{2+}; citrate, EDTA, and oxalate inhibit it by as much as 15%. Therefore, AMY assays should be performed only on serum or heparinized plasma. AMY is quite stable; activity is fully retained during storage for 4 days at room temperature, 2 weeks at +4 °C, 1 year at −25 °C, and 5 years at −75 °C.

Reference Interval

Reference intervals for AMY are method dependent. Using the IFCC recommended method at 37 °C, the serum reference interval was 28 to 100 U/L.[77]

Analytical Methods and Reference Intervals for Amylase Isoenzymes

Methods for AMY isoenzymes based on electrophoresis, ion-exchange chromatography, isoelectric focusing, selective inhibition of the S-AMY by a wheat germ inhibitor, immunoprecipitation by a monoclonal antibody, and immunoinhibition have been introduced. However, only the methods based on the selective isoenzyme inhibition by monoclonal antibodies have shown sufficient precision, reliability, practicability, and analytical speed to allow the introduction of the P-AMY determination in clinical practice.

A double monoclonal antibody assay is commercially available that uses the synergistic action of two immunoinhibitory monoclonal antibodies to S-AMY. After the S-AMY activity is inhibited by the addition of the antibodies, the uninhibited P-AMY activity is measured using EPS-4-NP-G7 as a substrate.[159] The test has been the object of a number of evaluations that have described its characteristics, such as practicability even in emergency conditions, possibility of full automation, and high specificity for P-AMY.[194] False-positive P-AMY results have been reported in subjects with macroamylasemia, in whom the immunoglobulin complexed to AMY forms diminishes or voids the ability of monoclonal antibodies included in the test to efficiently inhibit S-AMY.

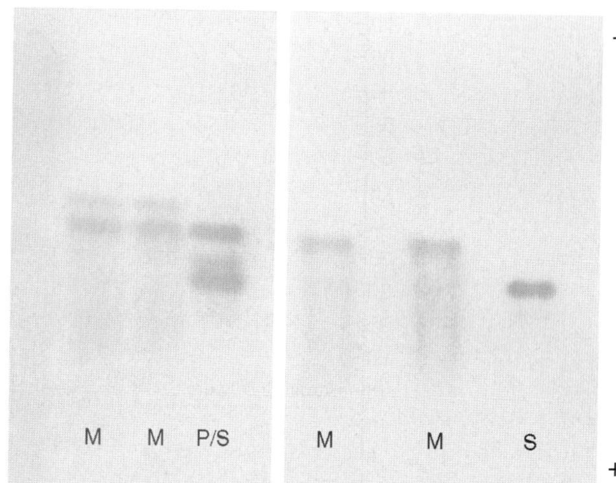

Figure 21-6 Cellulose acetate electrophoresis of amylase isoenzymes. *M*, Macroamylasemia; *P/S*, mixture of two samples containing, respectively, pancreatic juice and saliva; *S*, saliva. The anodal direction is downward.

Upon electrophoresis, macro-AMY usually forms a broad migrating band, clearly different from the homogeneous bands that are produced by AMY isoenzymes present in serum (Figure 21-6). If electrophoretic separation is not available, precipitation of the macrocomplex by a polyethylene glycol (PEG) 6000 solution (240 g/L) represents a good alternative. Residual AMY activity of less than 30% in the supernatant is indicative of macroamylasemia.[201]

In normal adults, P-AMY represents approximately 40% to 50% of the total enzymatic activity in serum. Using the immunoinhibition method at 37 °C, the reference interval for P-AMY activity in sera from adults was 13 to 53 U/L.[77] After birth, serum S-AMY activity increases steadily with age and reaches normal adult values at 2 years of age. Serum P-AMY activity is not demonstrable in most children younger than 6 months, but activity rises slowly thereafter to reach adult levels at 5 years of age, reflecting the postnatal development of exocrine pancreatic function (Figure 21-7).

Lipase

Human lipase (EC 3.1.1.3; triacylglycerol acylhydrolase; LPS) is a single-chain glycoprotein with a molecular weight of 48,000 and an isoelectric point of about 5.8. The LPS gene resides on chromosome 10. LPS concentration in the pancreas is about 5000-fold greater than in other tissues, and the concentration gradient between pancreas and serum is ~20,000-fold.[137] For full catalytic activity and greatest specificity, the presence of bile salts and a cofactor called colipase, which is secreted by the pancreas, is required. Human LPS can also be fully activated in vitro by colipases from other species (e.g., porcine colipase); this property is used in analytical formulations of the LPS assay.[196]

Lipases are defined as enzymes that hydrolyze glycerol esters of long-chain fatty acids. Only the ester bonds at carbons 1 and 3 (α-positions) are attacked, and the products

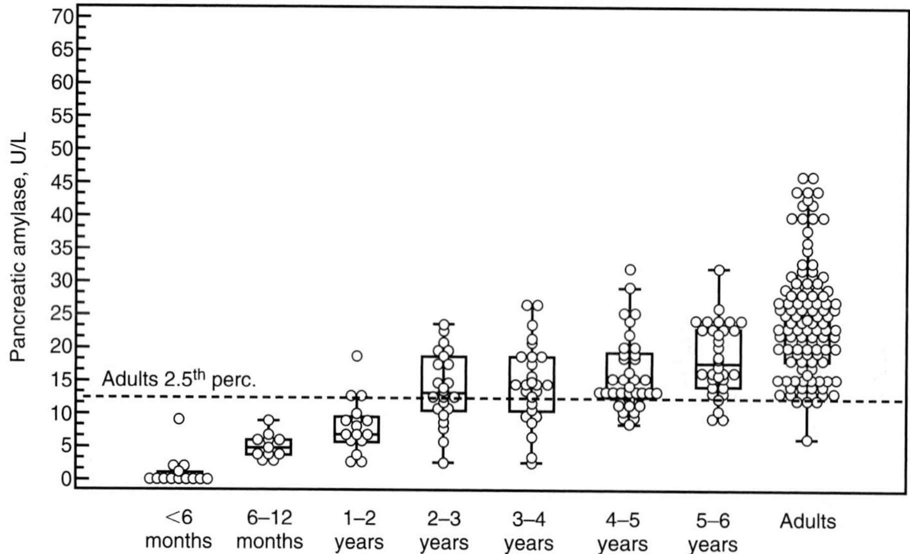

Figure 21-7 Activity values of pancreatic amylase in sera of healthy neonates and children compared with distribution in healthy adults.

of the reaction are 2 mol of fatty acids and 1 mol of 2-acylglycerol (β-monoglyceride) per mole of substrate. The latter is resistant to hydrolysis, probably because of steric hindrance, but it can spontaneously isomerize to the α-form (3-acylglycerol). This isomerization permits the third fatty acid to be split off but at a much slower rate. A scheme for the steps in the complete hydrolysis of a molecule of triglyceride to glycerol and three fatty acids is:

H_2C—OFA(1) / HC—OFA(2) / H_2C—OFA(3) (Triglyceride) —Lipase, H_2O, $OH^{\ominus}$→ H_2C—OH / HC—OFA(2) / H_2C—OFA(3) (α,β-Diglyceride + FA(1)OH (Fatty acid I)) —Lipase, H_2O, $OH^{\ominus}$→ H_2C—OH / HC—OFA(2) / H_2C—OH (β-Monoglyceride + FA(3)OH (Fatty acid III))

—Isomerization→ H_2C—OH / HC—OH / H_2C—OFA(2) (α-Monoglyceride) —Lipase, H_2O, $OH^{\ominus}$→ H_2C—OH / HC—OH / H_2C—OH (Glycerol + FA(2)OH (Fatty acid II))

LPS acts only when the substrate is present in an emulsified form at the interface between water and the substrate. The rate of LPS action depends on the surface area of the dispersed substrate. Bile acids ensure that the surface of the dispersed substrate remains free of other proteins, including lipolytic enzymes, by lining the surface of the insoluble substrate and the aqueous medium. LPS seems to gain access to the substrate surface in the following manner: Colipase attaches to a micelle of bile salts, thus forming a colipase–bile salt complex that reconfigures the structure of colipase with the exposure of a site with high affinity and high specificity for LPS, which therefore attracts LPS and anchors it to the substrate surface, allowing enzyme action to proceed.[140]

Most of the LPS activity found in serum derives from the pancreas, but some is also secreted by the lingual salivary glands and gastric, pulmonary, and intestinal mucosa. LPS is a small enough molecule to be filtered through the glomerulus. It is totally reabsorbed by the renal tubules, and it is not normally detected in urine. Evidence suggests that pancreatic LPS may exist in at least two isoforms, although the exact nature of these is unknown.[137] The complete absence of LPS has been reported. Such congenital absence results in fat malabsorption and severe steatorrhea.

Clinical Significance

LPS measurement on serum is used to diagnose acute pancreatitis. The clinical sensitivity is 80% to 100% depending upon the selected diagnostic cutoff. The clinical specificity is 80% to 100% depending upon the mix of patient population studied. After an attack of acute pancreatitis, serum LPS activity increases within 4 to 8 hours, peaks at about 24 hours, and decreases within 8 to 14 days. Concentrations often remain elevated longer than those of AMY do. Elevations between 2 and 50 times the upper reference limit have been reported. The increase in serum LPS activity is not necessarily proportional to the severity of the attack.[196]

Acute pancreatitis is sometimes difficult to diagnose because it must be differentiated from other acute intraabdominal disorders with similar clinical findings, such as perforated gastric or duodenal ulcer, intestinal obstruction, or mesenteric vascular obstruction. In differential diagnosis, elevation of serum LPS activity greater than 5 times the upper reference limit is a more specific diagnostic finding than increases in serum AMY activity.[146]

Obstruction of the pancreatic duct by a calculus or by carcinoma of the pancreas may increase serum LPS activity, depending on the location of the obstruction and the amount of remaining functioning tissue. In patients with a reduced glomerular filtration rate, the serum LPS activity is increased. Thus care should be exercised in the interpretation of elevated serum LPS values in the presence of renal disease. Finally, investigation of the biliary tract by endoscopic retrograde pancreatography or treatment with opiates (which causes the sphincter of Oddi to contract) may increase serum LPS activity.

Methods for Measuring Lipase Activity

Many LPS methods have been described; they have used both triglyceride and nontriglyceride substrates and titrimetric, turbidimetric, spectrophotometric, fluorometric, and immunological techniques. In general, long-chain triglyceride (and some diglyceride) substrates have demonstrated a correlation of results with the clinical state that is superior to that with methods using other substrates.[95]

In titrimetric methods, LPS catalyzes the hydrolysis of fatty acids from an emulsion of olive oil or oleic acid. The fatty acids liberated are titrated with dilute alkali. Kinetic versions use an automated potentiometric titrator (an instrument commonly referred to as a "pH-stat"). The amount of alkali used is recorded as a function of time and serves as a measure of fatty acid produced during the reaction. This method has been proposed as reference measurement procedure, useful in the evaluation of new LPS methods.[6]

In the turbidimetric method, LPS catalyzes the hydrolysis of fatty acids from an emulsion of oleic acid with a simultaneous decrease in the turbidity of the reaction mixture. Absorbance at 340 nm is read and the Δ*A*/min is taken as a measure of LPS activity. This method requires the use of a LPS calibrator. Turbidities have occasionally been observed to increase rather than to decrease during the reaction period. Such increases have frequently been observed in specimens containing rheumatoid factor. The method linearity (~3 times the upper reference limit) is limited, with many clinical samples needing to be diluted. The upper reference limit at 30 °C was reported to be 150 U/L.

A number of substrates and complex auxiliary and indicator systems are used in spectrophotometric methods. In the Ortho Diagnostics Vitros spectrophotometric reaction rate LPS slide method, the (synthetic) substrate is 1-oleoyl-2,3-diacetylglycerol and the emulsifier dodecylbenzene sulfonate. LPS activity is measured by a complex auxiliary and indicator enzyme system to produce a colored dye detectable at 540 nm. However, the substrate is likely to be more specific for intestinal than pancreatic LPS and may be subject to interference by postheparin lipase and pancreatic carboxylesterase.[191] An upper reference limit of 200 U/L at 30 °C has been reported.

In the enzymatic reaction rate diglyceride assay for LPS, the following sequence of indicator and auxiliary enzymes is used:

$$\text{1,2-Diacylglycerol} + H_2O \xrightarrow[\textit{pH 8.7}]{\textit{Pancreatic lipase, Colipase}} \text{2-monoacylglycerol} + \text{fatty acid}$$

$$\text{2-monoacylglycerol} + H_2O \xrightarrow{\textit{Monoglyceride lipase}} \text{glycerol} + \text{fatty acid}$$

$$\text{Glycerol} + \text{ATP} \xrightarrow{\textit{Glycerol kinase}} \text{L-}\alpha\text{-glycerophospate} + \text{ADP}$$

$$\text{L-}\alpha\text{-glycerophospate} + O_2 \xrightarrow{\textit{L-}\alpha\textit{-glycerophospate kinase}} \text{dihydroxyacetone phosphate} + H_2O_2$$

$$2\,H_2O_2 + \text{4-aminoantipyrine} + \text{TOOS} \xrightarrow{\textit{Peroxidase}} \text{quinonediimine dye (colored)} + 2\,H_2O$$

TOOS is sodium *N*-ethyl-*N*-(2-hydroxyl-3-sulfopropyl)-m-toluidine, and its oxidation produces an intensely colored dye detectable at 550 nm. The suggested upper reference limit is 45 U/L at 37 °C.

A new synthetic substrate (1,2-O-dilauryl-rac-glycero-3-glutaric acid-(4-methyl-resorufin)-ester), consisting of two glycerol ether and one ester bonds, has been proposed. LPS hydrolyze the latter bond in an alkaline medium to an unstable dicarbonic acid ester that spontaneously hydrolyzes to yield glutaric acid and methylresorufin; this is a bluish-purple chromophore with peak absorption at 580 nm.

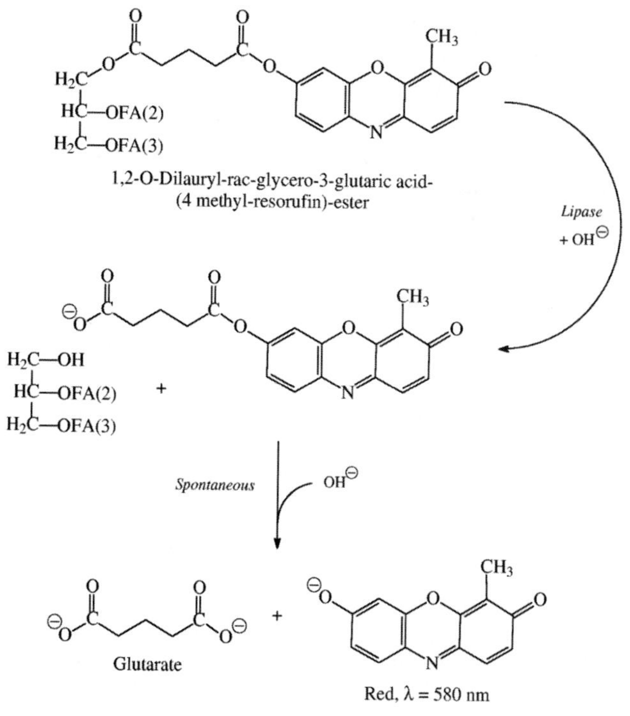

1,2-O-Dilauryl-rac-glycero-3-glutaric acid-(4 methyl-resorufin)-ester

Lipase + $OH^{\ominus}$

Spontaneous $OH^{\ominus}$

Glutarate

Red, λ = 580 nm

The rate of methylresorufin formation is directly proportional to the LPS activity of the sample. The upper reference limit is 38 UL at 37 °C.

LPS activity in serum is stable at room temperature for 1 week; sera may be stored for 3 weeks in the refrigerator and for several years if frozen.

TRYPSIN

Trypsin (EC 3.4.21.4; no systematic name; TRY) is a serine proteinase characterized by the presence at the active site of serine and histidine, both of which participate in the catalytic process. TRY hydrolyzes the peptide bonds formed by the carboxyl groups of lysine or arginine with other amino acids, although esters and amides involving these amino acids are actually split more rapidly than peptide bonds.

The acinar cells of the human pancreas synthesize two different trypsins (1 and 2) in the form of the inactive proenzymes (or zymogens), trypsinogens-1 and -2. These zymogens are stored in zymogen granules and are secreted into the duodenum under the stimulus of either the vagus nerve or the intestinal hormone cholecystokinin-pancreozymin. The two trypsinogens represent approximately 19% of the total protein in pancreatic juice; trypsinogen-1 is present at about fourfold the concentration of trypsinogen-2. In the intestinal tract, the trypsinogens are converted to the active enzyme TRY by the intestinal enzyme enterokinase or by preformed TRY (autocatalysis).[92]

TRY-1 is also described as cationic and TRY-2 as anionic because of their differing electrophoretic mobility; the cationic form predominates and is the better-documented enzyme. TRY-1 and TRY-2 have molecular weights of 25,800 and 22,900 and pI values of 4.6 to 6.5 and greater than 6.5, respectively. TRY-2 differs from TRY-1 in that it rapidly undergoes autolysis at neutral or alkaline pH values and Ca^{2+} does not stabilize it against autolysis. Because the two trypsins show little immunological cross-reactivity, specific immunoassay of each of them is possible.

When trypsinogens are converted to active TRY, a small peptide is cleaved from the *N*-terminal region of trypsinogen (trypsinogen activation peptide or TAP). Determinations of urinary TAP seem to provide useful information on the severity of acute pancreatitis.[48]

Materials such as soybeans, lima beans, and egg whites contain natural TRY inhibitors—small polypeptides such as α_1-antitrypsin (α-1-protease inhibitor) and α_2-macroglobulin—that combine irreversibly with TRY and inactivate it by blocking the active center. Similar nondialyzable TRY inhibitors are present in pancreatic juice, serum, and urine. These inhibitors protect plasma and other proteins against hydrolysis by TRY and other proteases if for some reason any appreciable quantity of the enzyme enters the vascular system. The absence of α_1-antitrypsin is associated with an increased tendency toward panlobular emphysema in early life; this example illustrates the effects of uninhibited proteases on organ function.

Clinical Significance

Trypsin-1 (Cationic Trypsin)[114]

In healthy individuals, free trypsinogen-1 is the major form found in serum. After an attack of acute pancreatitis, serum TRY-1 rises in parallel with serum AMY activity to peak values ranging from 2 to 400 times the upper reference limit. The distribution of the different forms of TRY-1 appears to be related to the type and severity of the acute pancreatitis. Thus in the mildest form of acute pancreatitis, 80% to 99% of the TRY-1 exists as free trypsinogen-1, with smaller proportions existing as bound TRY-1. In the more severe forms, in which mortality ranges from 20% to more than 50%, the proportion of free trypsinogen-1 may be as low as 30% of the total, with appreciable proportions existing as the α_1-antitrypsin- and α_2-macroglobulin-bound TRY-1.[30]

TRY-1 in serum is elevated in chronic renal failure, as is serum AMY. Thus renal failure must be ruled out when interpreting elevated concentrations. In chronic pancreatitis without steatorrhea, plasma concentrations of TRY-1 do not differ from those found in health; when steatorrhea is present, however, fasting concentrations are extremely low.[54] In the relapsing phase of chronic pancreatitis, plasma TRY may be considerably elevated. In carcinoma of the pancreas, TRY concentrations may be high, normal, or even low.

In comparison with P-AMY and LPS measurements, TRY-1 is a more difficult test to perform, requiring several hours to complete. As there is no distinct role of TRY estimation in the routine management of patients with acute pancreatitis, this test is considered of limited clinical value.

In cystic fibrosis, plasma TRY concentrations have been reported to be high in neonates; as the disease progresses, the concentration falls. Dried blood specimens have been suggested for use in screening tests.[60,158]

Trypsin-2 (Anionic Trypsin)

Serum trypsinogen-2 increases more than trypsinogen-1 in acute pancreatitis.[73] Consequently, large amounts of trypsinogen-2 are excreted into urine. Using both quantitative immunofluorimetric assay and qualitative rapid test strips to measure urinary trypsinogen-2, Stenman's group at the University of Helsinki showed high sensitivity and negative predictive value for diagnosis of acute pancreatitis on admission to the hospital. However, the positive predictive value of this test is low.[86]

As noted above, newly formed TRY is inactivated by complexing with α_1-antitrypsin, and assays of this serum complex with TRY-2 have preliminarily shown that this determination can be superior to that of either trypsinogen-2 or AMY in acute pancreatitis.[64] To date, no confirmation of these findings has been published.

Methods for the Determination of Trypsin

Early studies used catalytic assays, but it was soon recognized that other proteolytic enzymes present in serum could also hydrolyze the same substrates. A major advance has been the development of immunoassays to quantify TRY in blood. In the case of TRY-1, immunoassays detect trypsinogen-1, TRY-1, and TRY-1-α_1-antitrypsin complex. They do not detect the TRY-1-α_2-macroglobulin complex, for which different assays are necessary. Free TRY-1 is not usually found in serum; it is always complexed.

Commercial immunoassays are available for measurement of TRY-1. As there is no assay standardization, reference limits are method-dependent.

A rapid (5 minute) urinary trypsinogen-2 test strip is available, which is based on the use of immunochromatography with monoclonal antibodies. At urinary trypsinogen-2 concentrations greater than 50 μg/L, a blue line develops on the strip, and the test is considered positive.

CHYMOTRYPSIN

Chymotrypsin (EC 3.4.21.1; no systematic name; CHY) is also a serine proteinase. It hydrolyzes peptide bonds involving carboxyl groups of Trp, Leu, Tyr, or Phe, with preference for the aromatic residues. The specificity of CHY thus contrasts with that of pepsin, which splits bonds involving amino groups of the aromatic amino acids. CHY also demonstrates hydrolytic activity for other types of bonds in the following order: esters (especially *N*-substituted tyrosine esters) > amide > peptides.[5]

The acinar cells of the human pancreas synthesize two different chymotrypsins (1 and 2, the latter being the major species) in the form of the inactive proenzymes (or zymogens), chymotrypsinogens-1 and -2. These zymogens are stored in granules and are secreted like trypsinogen into the pancreatic duct. In the intestinal tract, the chymotrypsinogens are converted to CHY by the action of TRY. CHY is more resistant than TRY to degradation in the intestine; it is therefore the enzyme of choice for assay in feces.

CHY-1 is also described as anionic and CHY-2 as cationic because of their differing electrophoretic mobility; the cationic form predominates. The molecular weight of both forms is approximately 25,000. There is close immunological similarity between the chymotrypsins and chymotrypsinogens. CHY, like TRY, is bound in plasma by α_1-antitrypsin and α_2-macroglobulin.

Clinical Significance[54]

The major application of the assays that measure CHY activity in stool is in the investigation of chronic pancreatic insufficiency. CHY in feces is often reduced below the lower reference limit in such subjects in whom steatorrhea has developed, but it is not useful in identifying subjects with early pancreatic insufficiency. (See Table 48-15.) CHY measurement in patients with chronic pancreatic insufficiency treated with oral pancreatic enzyme supplements may indicate whether the therapy is adequate or whether increased supplementation is necessary.

Methods for the Determination of Chymotrypsin in Feces

Synthetic substrates are commonly used for this application. A sensitive kinetic assay has been developed that uses succ-ala-ala-pro-phe-4-nitroanilide as a substrate, and made commercially available. Prior treatment of the stool specimen with detergent to release particle-bound CHY is necessary. A cheap device enables a small stool sample to be homogenized, extracted, and centrifuged with minimal inconvenience. The extract is mixed with the substrate, which is hydrolyzed by CHY to produce free 4-nitroanilide, measured photometrically at 405 nm.

CHY activity in stool remains constant at room temperature for up to 7 days.

Reference Interval

The lower reference limit of fecal CHY activity, measured at 37 °C, was found to be 12 U/g stool.[110]

ELASTASE-1

Human elastase-1 (EC 3.4.21.36; no systematic name; E1) is an anionic protease belonging to the family of serine proteases. It is a carboxyendopeptidase that catalyzes hydrolysis of native elastin, the major structural fibrous protein in connective tissue, with a special affinity for the carboxyl group of alanine, valine, and leucine.

Human E1 is synthesized by the acinar cells of the pancreas along with the other digestion enzymes, and is composed of 240 amino acids, with a MW of about 26,000. The enzyme is synthesized as a preproelastase. After processing to proelastase, it is stored in the zymogen granules and later it is activated to elastase by TRY in the duodenum, undergoing minimal degradation during intestinal transit.

Historically, any proteinases that hydrolyze elastin have been named elastases. The genes coding for the elastases are clustered on chromosome 19, and three main types of enzymes are known: (1) pancreatic E1, (2) pancreatic elastase-2 (EC 3.4.21.71), and (3) pancreatic endopeptidase-3 (EC 3.4.21.70), also called cholesterol-binding proteinase.[44]

Clinical Significance[54]

E1 measurement in stool is the most reliable and sensitive noninvasive procedure for the diagnosis of chronic pancreatic insufficiency. However, such a test does not consistently separate mild to moderate insufficiency cases from healthy controls (see Table 48-15). Unlike fecal CHY, E1 provides no information helpful to the therapeutic management of the patient.

Methods for the Determination of Elastase-1 in Feces

An ELISA method in a microplate sandwich format is commercially available to measure E1 mass concentrations in stool samples.

The enzyme has been found to be stable in stool samples for up to 1 week at room temperature.

Reference Interval

The lower reference limit of fecal E1 concentration was found to be 200 μg/g stool.

BONE ENZYMES

Bone enzymes are direct products of active osteoblasts (bone ALP) and osteoclasts (tartrate-resistant acid phosphatase).

Alkaline Phosphatase (Bone Isoform)

Bone, liver, and kidney isoforms of ALP are posttranslational modifications of the same gene product and are identified by their unique carbohydrate content (see Fig. 21-4). They have been described above in the section on liver enzymes. Bone ALP is produced by the osteoblast and has been demonstrated in matrix vesicles deposited as "buds" derived from the cell's membrane. The enzyme is therefore an excellent indicator of global bone formation activity.

Clinical Significance in Bone Disease

Among the bone diseases, the highest concentrations of bone ALP are encountered in Paget's disease (osteitis deformans) as a result of the action of the osteoblastic cells as they try to rebuild bone that is being resorbed by the uncontrolled activity of osteoclasts. Values from 10 to 25 times the upper reference limit are not unusual, and in broad terms the increase reflects the extent of disease. In vitamin D deficiency (osteomalacia and rickets), concentrations two to four times normal may be observed, and these fall slowly to normal on treatment. Primary hyperparathyroidism and secondary hyperparathyroidism are associated with slight to moderate elevations of bone ALP in serum, the existence and degree of elevation reflecting the presence and extent of skeletal involvement. Very high enzyme concentrations are present in patients with osteogenic bone cancer. Concentrations can be slightly increased in osteoporosis, but osteoporotic individuals are not clearly distinguished from age-matched controls. Transient elevations may be found during healing of bone fractures. Physiological bone growth increases bone ALP in serum, and this accounts for the fact that in the sera of growing children, enzyme concentration is 1.5 to 7 times that in healthy adult serum, the maximum being earlier in girls than in boys.

Methods for the Determination of Bone Alkaline Phosphatase

In general, separation of tissue-nonspecific ALP forms (i.e., bone and liver) is difficult because of structural similarity. Bone ALP in serum can be measured by heat inactivation (a poor method), lectin precipitation, and immunochemical and electrophoretic methods (see the section on liver enzymes).

Immunoassays for bone ALP, which measure either enzyme activity or mass, are commercially available; cross-reactivity with liver isoform however, has been established:

Assay	Type	Percentage of Cross-Reactivity
Beckman Tandem-R-Ostase	Mass-based IRMA	12.7-16.5
Beckman Tandem-MP-Ostase	Mass-based ELISA	8.1-16.2
Metra Alkphase-B	Activity-based EIA	5.9-20.0

This general limitation should be borne in mind when interpreting test results.

With the use of immunoassays measuring bone ALP concentrations, the enzyme is said to be stable at −20 °C for 2 years.

Reference Intervals

Using the electrophoretic procedure, the reference interval for bone ALP activity in healthy adults is 10 to 50 U/L.[148] Mean (SD) bone ALP concentrations, determined by immunoassays in healthy adults, were 13 μg/L.[32]

Acid Phosphatase (Tartrate-Resistant)

Under the name of acid phosphatase (EC 3.1.3.2; orthophosphoric-monoester phosphohydrolase [acid optimum]; ACP) are included all phosphatases with optimal activity below a pH of 7.0.

ACP is present in lysosomes, which are organelles present in all cells with the possible exception of erythrocytes. Extra lysosomal ACPs are also present in many cells. The greatest concentrations of ACP activity occur in prostate, bone (osteoclasts), spleen, platelets, and erythrocytes. The lysosomal and prostatic enzymes are strongly inhibited by dextrorotatory tartrate ions, whereas the erythrocyte and bone isoenzymes are not. The majority of the normally low ACP activity of (unhemolyzed) serum is of a tartrate-resistant type (TR-ACP) and probably originates mainly in osteoclasts. Activities of this fraction are increased physiologically in growing children and pathologically in conditions of increased osteolysis and bone remodeling.[119]

At least four ACP-determining genes have been identified and mapped. The erythrocyte ACP gene is located on chromosome 2 and is polymorphic, and a further gene on chromosome 19 encodes the TR-ACP expressed in osteoclasts and other tissue macrophages, such as alveolar macrophages and Kupffer cells (type 5 ACP). Type 5b has been proposed as a specific and sensitive marker of osteoclastic activity. The genes encoding the tartrate-inhibited lysosomal and prostatic ACPs, mapped to chromosomes 11 and 13 respectively, exhibit considerable homology.[123]

The ACPs are unstable, especially at temperatures above 37 °C and at pH above 7.0. Some of the enzyme forms in serum are particularly labile, and more than 30% of the ACP activity may be lost in 3 hours at room temperature. Acidification of the serum specimen to a pH below 6.5 aids in stabilizing the enzyme activity.

Clinical Significance

Slight or moderate elevations in serum TR-ACP activity often occur in Paget's disease, in hyperparathyroidism with skeletal involvement, and in the presence of malignant invasion of the bones by cancers, such as breast cancer in women. Increased concentrations of the osteoclast-derived ACP are also present in serum in osteoclastoma (giant-cell tumor), an osteoclastic neoplasm, and in osteopetrosis (marble bone disease) in which the osteoclasts fail to resorb bone. High concentrations of TR-ACP in serum of these patients reflect increased osteoclastic activity, whether appropriate as in normal bone growth, or damaging as in osteopetrosis. This isoenzyme is therefore a potentially useful marker of conditions with a marked osteolytic component. However, TR-ACP appears to show relatively small dynamic changes in comparison with other markers of bone resorption, e.g., those related to type I collagen metabolism. This may be attributable to the fact that the enzyme is released into the sealed osteoclast microenvironment, rather than directly into circulation.

The only nonbone condition in which elevated activities of TR-ACP are found in serum is Gaucher's disease of spleen, a lysosomal storage disorder. Its source in this disease is the abnormal macrophages in spleen and other tissues, which overexpress this normal macrophage constituent. The hairy cells of hairy-cell leukemia (leukemic reticuloendotheliosis) also express the osteoclast-type ACP, providing a useful histological marker. However, in this condition, the isoenzyme does not enter the plasma in increased amounts.

Although once widely used to detect or monitor carcinoma of the prostate, determination of ACP (tartrate-inhibited) activity in serum is now rarely used for this purpose. It has been replaced by prostate-specific antigen (PSA).

Methods for the Determination of Tartrate-Resistant Acid Phosphatase

Continuous-monitoring methods for assay of TR-ACP activity are based on the principle introduced by Hillmann in which α-naphthol released from its phosphate ester forms a colored product with the stabilized diazonium salt of 2-amino-5-chlorotoluene-1,5-naphthalene disulfonate (Fast Red TR).[9] The introduction of alcohols, such as 1,5-pentanediol, accelerates the reaction and increases sensitivity by acting as phosphate acceptors in transfer reactions. The addition of sodium tartrate inhibits the sensitive isoenzymes (i.e., prostatic and lysosomal ACPs) if they are present in the sample.

Immunological methods based on antibodies raised against TR-ACP have been described. A recently introduced method uses a monoclonal antibody to bind serum TR-ACP in a solid-phase format. After the capture, osteoclastic enzyme is specifically determined by measuring its activity at pH 6.1.

Serum should be immediately separated from erythrocytes and stabilized by the addition of 50 μL of acetic acid (5 mol/L) per milliliter of serum to lower the pH to 5.4, at which the enzyme is stable. Under these conditions, TR-ACP activity is maintained at room temperature for several hours, for up to a week if the serum is refrigerated, and for 4 months if stored at −20 °C. Hemolyzed serum specimens are contaminated with considerable amounts of the erythrocyte tartrate-resistant isoenzyme and should be rejected.

Reference Intervals

In the sera of healthy adults, the reference interval for TR-ACP activity, measured at 37 °C, is 1.5 to 4.5 U/L. Children show higher TR-ACP activities (3.4 to 9.0 U/L).

RED CELL ENZYMES

Erythrocytes perform a variety of functions, the most important being the binding, transport, and delivery of oxygen to all tissues. To do so, they must be capable of passage through microcapillaries, which is achieved by modifications of the erythrocyte's biconcave shape. This is possible because, unlike most other cells in the body, human erythrocytes lose the nucleus and organelles before entering the circulation from the marrow. In addition, remaining RNA in the reticulocyte is lost within the first 2 days in circulation, thereby making further protein synthesis no longer possible.

Normal human red cells survive in the circulation for approximately 120 days, using energy to maintain the electrolyte gradient between plasma and red cell cytoplasm and to keep hemoglobin and the sulfhydryl groups of the red cell enzymes and membrane proteins in the reduced state. Because of the absence of a nucleus and mitochondria, the red cell is incapable of generating energy via the (oxidative) Krebs cycle and depends mainly on the anaerobic conversion of glucose by the Embden-Meyerhof pathway (EMP or direct glycolytic pathway) and the oxidative hexose monophosphate pathway (HMP or pentose phosphate shunt) (Figure 21-8). Numerous red cell enzymes are involved in these pathways, thereby providing the cell with the necessary moles of ATP.

Deficiencies of any of these red cell enzymes may result in impaired ATP generation and consequently loss of function of the erythrocyte. By far the majority of these disorders are hereditary in nature, although acquired deficiencies have been described, mainly in malignant disorders involving the bone marrow. Hereditary enzymatic defects in these pathways disturb the erythrocyte's integrity, shorten its cellular survival, and produce chronic nonspherocytic hemolytic anemia (CNSHA). Deficiencies of some enzymes, however, do not lead to chronic hemolytic anemia, but to acute episodes of severe hemolysis when there is increased oxidative stress on the red cell (as in some types of glucose-6-phosphate dehydrogenase deficiency).

A number of these enzymes are expressed in other tissues as well but cause a notable deficiency predominantly in red blood cells because of the life span of the erythrocyte after the loss of protein synthesis. Once an enzyme is degraded or otherwise becomes nonfunctional, it cannot be replaced by new or other "compensating" proteins because of the lack of nucleus, mitochondria, ribosomes, and other cell organelles in mature red cells. Disorders have been described in the EMP, HMP, Rapoport-Luebering cycle, the glutathione pathway (Figure 21-9), purine-pyrimidine metabolism and methemoglobin reduction.

This section describes the red cell enzymes involved in the metabolic pathways of clinical importance in the human red cell and the disorders associated with defects in these pathways. In addition, diagnostic strategies and pitfalls of laboratory diagnostics for these enzyme deficiencies will be explained. The laboratory methods described have been

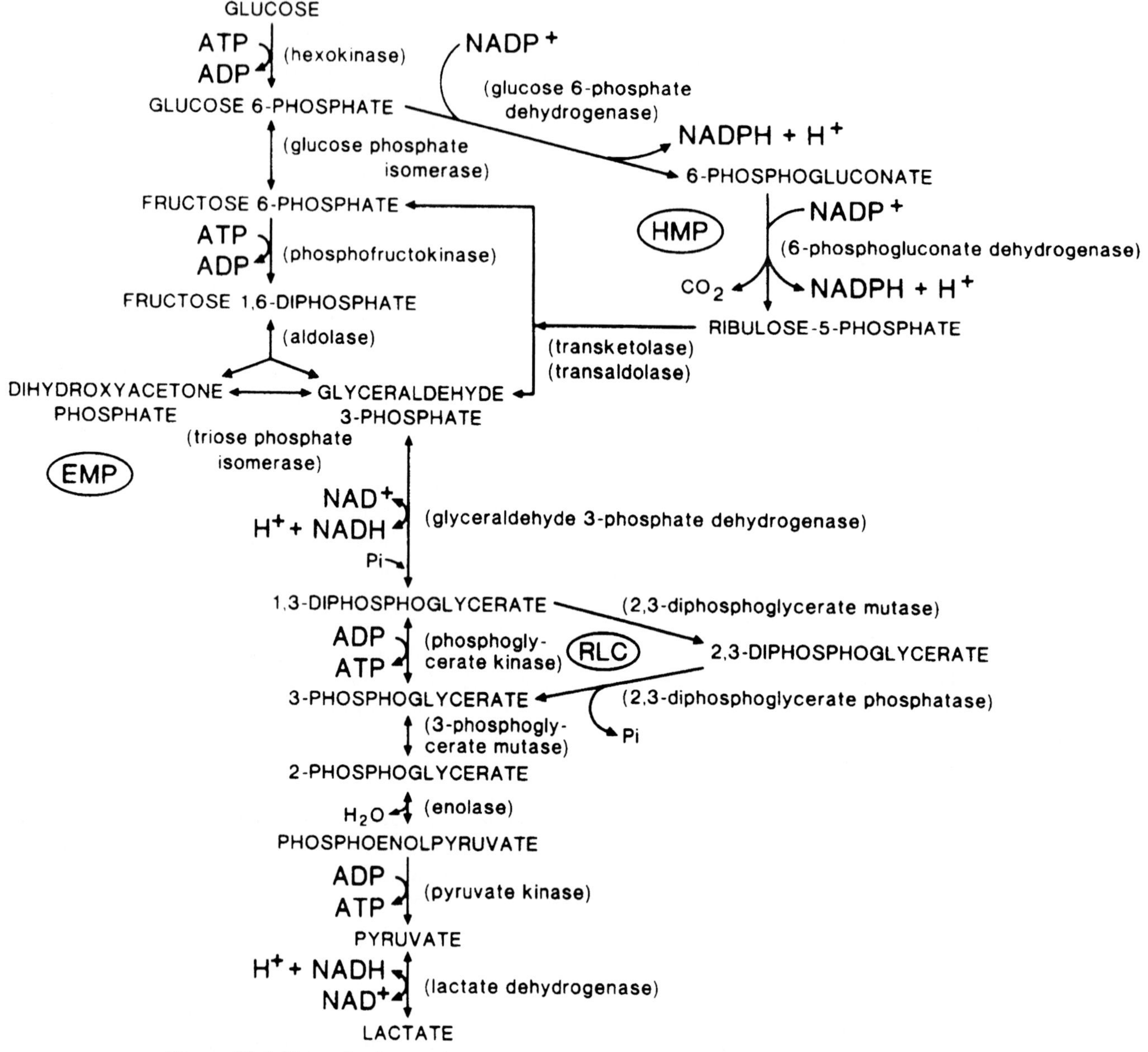

Figure 21-8 Major glycolytic pathways of the erythrocyte. Substrates are in uppercase type, and enzymes are in parentheses. *EMP,* The Embden-Meyerhof pathway; *HMP,* hexose monophosphate pathway or pentose shunt; *RLC,* the Rapoport-Luebering cycle; *ADP,* adenosine diphosphate; *ATP,* adenosine triphosphate; *NAD*$^+$, nicotinamide-adenine dinucleotide; *NADH,* reduced nicotinamide-adenine dinucleotide; *NADP*$^+$, nicotinamide-adenine dinucleotide phosphate; *NADPH,* reduced nicotinamide-adenine dinucleotide phosphate. The step from ribulose-5-phosphate, which is shown as being catalyzed by transketolase and transaldolase, is an abbreviation of this portion of the HMP.

used now for decades and are well documented. During the last few years, however, molecular diagnostics has proven to be an indispensable tool in diagnosing hereditary red cell enzyme deficiencies.

The Embden-Meyerhof Pathway

Glucose is the energy source of the red cell. In the normal situation (without increased "oxidative stress"), 90% of glucose is catabolized anaerobically to pyruvate or lactate by the direct glycolytic pathway or EMP. Although one mole of ATP is used by hexokinase and an additional mole of ATP by phosphofructokinase, the net gain is 2 moles of ATP per mole of glucose, since a total of 4 moles of ATP are formed per mole of glucose by phosphoglycerate kinase and pyruvate kinase. In addition, reducing energy is generated in the form of reduced nicotinamide-adenine dinucleotide (NADH) in the step catalyzed by glyceraldehyde phosphate dehydrogenase. This reducing energy can be used to reduce

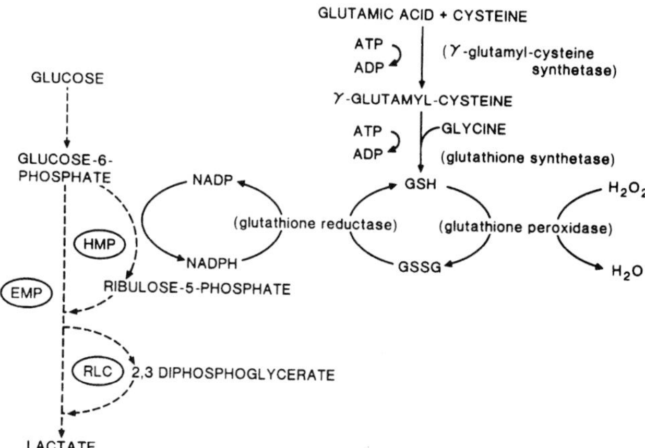

Figure 21-9 Interrelationship of hexose monophosphate and glutathione pathways. *GSH,* Reduced glutathione; *GSSG,* oxidized glutathione.

methemoglobin to hemoglobin by NADH-cytochrome b5 reductase. If this reaction takes place, the end product of the glycolysis is pyruvate. However, if NADH is not reoxidized here, it is used in reducing pyruvate to lactate by lactate dehydrogenase in the last step of the glycolysis.

Although the pathway is reasonably straightforward, it is subjected to a complex mechanism of inhibiting and stimulating factors. Some of the enzymes involved are allosterically stimulated by products of the pathway (such as pyruvate kinase [PK] by fructose diphosphate), while others may serve as strong inhibitors (such as glucose 6-phosphate for hexokinase [HK]).

Hexokinase

Hexokinase (HK; EC 2.7.1.1) catalyzes the phosphorylation of glucose to glucose-6-phosphate (G6P) using ATP as a phosphoryl donor. The activity of HK is significantly higher in reticulocytes compared with mature red cells, where it is very low. The HK reaction is one of two rate-limiting steps in this pathway, the other being the phosphofructokinase reaction.

In mammalian tissues, four isozymes of HK with different enzymatic properties exist, HK-I to III with an M_r of 100,000 kDa and HK-IV (or glucokinase) with an M_r of 50,000 kDa. HK-I to III are considered to have evolved from an ancestral 50 kDa HK by gene duplication and fusion. Consequently, both the *C*- and *N*-terminal halves of HK-I to HK-III show extensive internal sequence similarity, but only in the case of HK-II was catalytic function maintained in both the *C*- and *N*-terminal halves. HK-I and HK-III have further evolved into enzymes with respectively catalytic (*C*-terminal) and regulatory (*N*-terminal) halves.

HK-I is the predominant HK isozyme in tissues that depend strongly on glucose use for their physiological functioning, such as brain, muscle, and erythrocytes. HK-I displays unique regulatory properties in its sensitivity to inhibition by physiological concentrations of the product G6P and, moreover, relief of this inhibition by inorganic phosphate and by high concentrations of glucose.[217] In addition, the enzyme depends on magnesium. HK is a homodimer[3,124] and the recent determination of structures of human and rat HK-I has provided substantial insight into ligand-binding sites and subsequent modes of interaction.[1-3,124,181]

Erythrocytes contain a specific subtype of HK (HK-R),[125] which is encoded by the HK-I gene (*HK1*), localized on chromosome 10q22 and spanning more than 100 kb.[4] The structure of *HK1* is complex: it encompasses 25 exons that, by tissue-specific transcription, generate multiple transcripts by alternative splicing of different 5′ exons.[4] Erythroid-specific transcriptional control results in a unique red blood cell (RBC)–specific mRNA that differs from HK-I mRNA at the 5′ untranslated region (5′-UTR) and at the first 63 nucleotides of the coding region.[126,127,171] Consequently, HK-R lacks the porin-binding domain that mediates HK-I binding to mitochondria.[128]

HK deficiency (OMIM 235700)* is a rare, recessively inherited disease with chronic nonspherocytic hemolytic anemia as the predominant clinical feature. The phenotypic expression of the disease is heterogeneous, as with most glycolytic red cell enzyme deficiencies. The spectrum ranges between severe neonatal hemolysis and death to a fully compensated chronic hemolytic anemia. Patients benefit in general from a splenectomy. Red cell morphology is normal. Since HK activity is dependent on red cell age, reticulocytosis, always present in HK-deficient patients, may obscure enzyme deficiency. Other age-dependent red cell enzymes (e.g., pyruvate kinase and/or G6PD) should be measured simultaneously as an internal control to assess the influence of reticulocyte enzyme activity.

Seventeen families with HK deficiency have been described to date[81] and only three patients have been characterized at the DNA level.[26,27,83,203] One is presumably a splice site mutation, resulting in the skipping of exon 6. In the same patient, a leucine residue at position 529 was mutated into a serine, affecting enzyme stability possibly because of interference with G6P binding.[26,27] The second patient characterized had a homozygous missense mutation in exon 15, leading to substitution of a highly conserved threonine by serine at residue 680 in the enzyme's active site where it interacted with phosphate moieties of ADP, ATP, and inhibitor G6P.[203] The last mutation was lethal and identified in a fetus. A deletion of 9.5 kb of the HK gene, leading

*OMIM stands for Online Mendelian Inheritance in Man. It is a World Wide Web database (http://www.ncbi.nlm.nih.gov/omim) developed under the auspices of the National Center for Biotechnology Information (NCBI). It consists of a catalog of human genes and genetic disorders and contains textual information, pictures, and reference information. It also contains links to NCBI's Entre/database of MEDLINE articles and sequence information. Individual disorders may be found by entering the OMIM numbers into the search engine of the database.

to deletion of exons 5 to 8 of the HK gene was detected, resulting in a null allele.[83]

Glucose Phosphate Isomerase

G6P isomerase (GPI; EC 5.3.1.9) (also known as phosphoglucose isomerase [PGI]), catalyzes the interconversion of G6P and fructose 6-phosphate (F6P), the second step of the EMP. As a result of this reversible reaction, products of the hexose monophosphate pathway can be recycled to G6P. Besides being a housekeeping enzyme of glycolysis, GPI exerts outside the cell cytokine properties and is involved in several extracellular processes.[76] In addition, autoantibodies against GPI seem to be involved in rheumatoid arthritis.[172] GPI is a crucial enzyme, since GPI knockout mice die in the embryological state.[211,212]

Recently, the crystal structure of human GPI was resolved. The enzyme is a multifunctional protein composed of homodimers, each with a molecular mass of 63 kDa. A dimer of GPI is a prerequisite for catalytic activity, because the active site of the enzyme is composed of polypeptide chains from both subunits.[39,162]

The gene encoding GPI is located on chromosome 19q13.1[108] and consists of 18 exons, spanning at least 50 kb, with a cDNA 1.9 kb in length.[218]

GPI deficiency (OMIM 172400) is an autosomal recessive disease and is, after G6PD and PK deficiencies, the third most common red cell enzymopathy. Homozygous or compound heterozygous patients have mild to severe chronic hemolytic anemia, with an enzyme activity less than 25% of normal. Neonatal death, hydrops fetalis, and in some patients neurological symptoms have been reported. Few patients have been described with hemolytic crises after oxidative stress.[70,105,161,213] Usually there is a marked reticulocytosis. Unlike for HK, the GPI activity in reticulocytes is only marginally higher than that of older cells. Heterozygous patients are hematologically normal, with an enzyme activity of 40% to 60%. Red cell morphology is in general without any abnormalities. Patients benefit from a splenectomy. A striking feature of nearly all GPI mutants is that they are thermolabile, while kinetic properties are more or less unaffected. The normal enzyme is very stable.

Around 50 families with GPI deficiency have been described worldwide.[91] In total, 29 mutations are characterized at the molecular level, of which 24 were missense mutations, 3 nonsense, and 2 splice site mutations.[91] Mapping of these mutations in the crystal structure of human GPI gives insight into the molecular mechanisms causing hemolytic anemia in this disorder.[162] Mutations could be placed in three groups: the first affecting the precise structure of the enzyme, the second those that disrupt the dimer interface, and the third those mutants that directly affect the active site.[162]

Phosphofructokinase

Phosphofructokinase (PFK; EC 2.7.1.11) catalyzes the phosphorylation of fructose-6-phosphate by ATP to fructose-1,6-diphosphate. This conversion is rate limiting. The enzyme is a homotetramer or heterotetramer with a molecular mass of around 380 kDa. Three distinct subunits have been identified in humans: PFK-M (muscle), PFK-L (liver), and PFK-P (platelet).[207] In erythrocytes, five isoenzymes can be identified with varying subunit composition (M_4, M_3L_1, M_2L_2, ML_3, and L_4).

The genes for the PFK-M, PFK-L, and PFK-P subunits have been cloned.[46,96,128]

Phosphofructokinase deficiency (OMIM 171850) is a rare autosomal recessively inherited disorder. Since red cells contain both M and L subunits, mutations affecting the genes coding for these subunits will affect enzyme activity. Thus when the PFK deficiency mutation affects only the L subunit, RBCs have only M_4 and are PFK deficient. In such cases, there is a mild hemolytic disorder without myopathy. However, when the M subunit is deficient, muscle PFK is virtually absent together with partial PFK deficiency in RBCs, which will have only L_4. Therefore deficiency of the M subunit causes myopathy and a mild hemolytic disorder.

To date, 15 alleles associated with PFK deficiency have been identified. Missense, nonsense, and a frameshift mutation along with mutations affecting splicing have been characterized in the PFK-M gene.[50]

Patients usually have only a mild, well-compensated hemolytic anemia with an enzyme activity of approximately half normal. The enzyme is relatively unstable in vitro and assays should be carried out, preferably, on fresh blood samples.

Aldolase

Aldolase (fructose-1,6-biphosphate aldolase; EC 4.1.2.13) catalyzes the reversible conversion of fructose-1,6-biphosphate to glyceraldehyde 3-phosphate and dihydroxyacetone phosphate. The enzyme is a tetramer of identical subunits of 40 kDa. Three isoenzymes are identified to date: aldolases A, B, and C. Aldolase A is the isoenzyme that is expressed in the RBC, but also in muscle and brain.

The gene for aldolase A spans 7530 bases and consists of 12 exons. Several transcription-initiation sites were identified along with tissue-specific splicing.[74]

Only three cases of aldolase deficiency have been described.[25,87,89] Beutler et al[25] have described a boy with an unstable enzyme with mental retardation and hemolytic anemia and dysmorphic features. Kishi et al[87] described a patient with severe hemolytic anemia, exacerbated by infection, but none of the features described by Beutler et al. Kishi identified the mutation, leading to a conversion of aspartic acid at position 128 to glycine. Kreuder et al[89] reported on a boy with hemolytic anemia and myopathy caused by aldolase A deficiency. They identified a mutation, causative of an amino acid substitution at position 206 (Glu to Lys).

Aldolase activity is notably influenced by red cell age, thus the activity of this enzyme is increased in patients with hemolytic disease.

Triosephosphate Isomerase

Triosephosphate isomerase (TPI; EC 5.3.1.1) is the enzyme (26.75 kDa) of the anaerobic glycolytic pathway with the highest activity. It catalyzes the interconversion of glyceraldehyde 3-phosphate and dihydroxyacetone phosphate. TPI is a dimer with two identical subunits of 248 amino acids with an eight-stranded barrel structure.[101] There are no isoenzymes known, only three distinct electrophoretic forms due to minor posttranslational modifications.[152,219] In RBCs, TPI is not maturation dependent.

TPI deficiency (OMIM 190450) is a relatively rare autosomal recessive disorder, characterized by hemolytic anemia at onset and severe neuromuscular defects usually at 6 months to 2 years of age. Heterozygotes are clinically normal, but have half normal red cell TPI activity. In the erythrocyte there is a twentyfold to sixtyfold increase in the concentration of dihydroxyacetone phosphate.[169] TPI is transcribed from a single gene, located on chromosome 12p13; the gene spans 3.5 kb and contains seven exons.[31] To date, 14 mutations in the gene encoding TPI have been identified.[165] The most common mutation produces an amino acid substitution at position 104 (glutamate acid to aspartic acid). The other mutations are found only in individual families.

Phosphoglycerate Kinase

Phosphoglycerate kinase (PGK, EC 2.7.2.3) catalyzes the reversible conversion of 1,3-diphosphoglycerate to 3-phosphoglycerate, generating one molecule of ATP.

The reaction catalyzed by PGK can be bypassed by the Rapoport-Luebering shunt (see Figure 21-8), thereby losing the gain of one ATP molecule.

Two isoenzymes PGK-1 and PGK-2 exist, with PGK-1 being ubiquitously expressed in all somatic cells. *PGK-2* is an autosomal gene expressed only in spermatozoa.[106] PGK-1 is a monomeric enzyme of 417 amino acids.[67] The three-dimensional structure of horse muscle PGK (highly homologous with the human enzyme) displays two lobes connected by a hinge, allowing conformational freedom to occur.[16]

The gene encoding PGK-1 is located on the long arm of the X-chromosome (Xq13), making PGK deficiency an X-linked disorder. The gene spans 23 kb and is composed of 11 exons.[36,43,111] Fourteen different mutations in the PGK-1 gene have been described, leading to PGK deficiency (OMIM 311800, for an overview see reference 49). The disease is characterized by hemolytic anemia of varying severity, neurological abnormalities, and muscle disease. However, patients have been described with hemolysis, but without the neurological or muscle symptoms. Thus the expression of the disease can be highly variable.[49] The genotype-phenotype relations of the disorder are still poorly understood.

Pyruvate Kinase

Pyruvate kinase (PK; EC 2.7.1.40) catalyzes the conversion of phosphoenolpyruvate to pyruvate with the concomitant generation of the second molecule of ATP in glycolysis. The activity of PK depends on red cell age. The younger the red cells, the higher the activity.

The enzyme is dependent on K^{2+} and Mg^{2+} or Mg^{2+}.[58] The product of the reaction, pyruvate, is crucial for several metabolic pathways. Because of this important end product, PK is thought to be—together with PFK—the major regulatory enzyme of glycolysis.

PK is active as a homotetramer or heterotetramer, composed of one of four different tissue-specific subunits. The M1 subunit is found in skeletal muscle, heart, and brain. The M2 type is dominant in all tissues in early fetal life, but also in adult tissues including leukocytes and platelets. The L subunit is predominant in the liver, while only the R subunit is found in the erythrocyte. During erythropoiesis, PK-M2 (a homotetramer of M2 subunits) is expressed in normoblasts and reticulocytes. PK-R (a homotetramer of R subunits) increases progressively during erythrocyte maturation, replacing PK-M2. Proteolytic degradation of the 574 amino-acid-long R subunit converts it to the 543 amino-acid-long R′ subunit. This occurs in aging mature erythrocytes, resulting in the preponderance of a PK isoenzyme consisting of a heterotetramer of two R subunits and two R′ subunits in the mature aging red cell.[78-80] Why ultimately no homotetramer of four R′ subunits is formed is unknown.

The red cell enzyme is allosterically regulated by fructose-1,6-diphosphate (FDP). Sigmoid kinetics occur by increasing concentrations of the substrate phosphoenolpyruvate.

The crystal structure of human red cell PK has been elucidated.[67] The enzyme resembles closely the structures of cat and rabbit muscle type PK. The subunit is composed of an *N*-terminal domain, an A-domain containing the active site, a B-domain capable of rotating away from the A-domain generating either the “open” or “closed” conformation, and a C-domain with the binding site for FDP.

The gene encoding both the M1- and M2-type subunits is located on chromosome 15q24-q25, and the respective subunits are formed by alternative splicing.[130,190] The R and L subunits are transcribed from a single gene located on chromosome 1q21, by the use of tissue-specific promoters.[82] The gene consists of 12 exons over 9.5 kb. Exon 1 is specific for the R type, while exon 2 is solely expressed in the L type. Exons 3 to 12 are common to both subtypes.

Pyruvate kinase deficiency (OMIM 266200) is the most common cause of nonspherocytic hemolytic anemia due to defective glycolysis. The allelic frequency is estimated to be around 2%.[22] The consequent lack of sufficient energy, which is required for normal functioning and cellular survival, shortens the life span of the mature PK-deficient erythrocyte. Consequently, PK-deficient patients display a phenotype of nonspherocytic hemolytic anemia albeit with variable clinical severity.[104] The clinical symptoms vary from neonatal death to a well-compensated hemolytic anemia. Patients benefit in general from a splenectomy. Pyruvate kinase deficiency is transmitted as an autosomal recessive disease. To date, more than 130 mutations in *PKLR* have been reported to be associated with pyruvate kinase deficiency (see Figure 21-10; for overview see reference 221). Most (70%) of these mutations are missense mutations affecting conserved residues in structurally and functionally important domains of PK. Splice site mutations, a deletion,

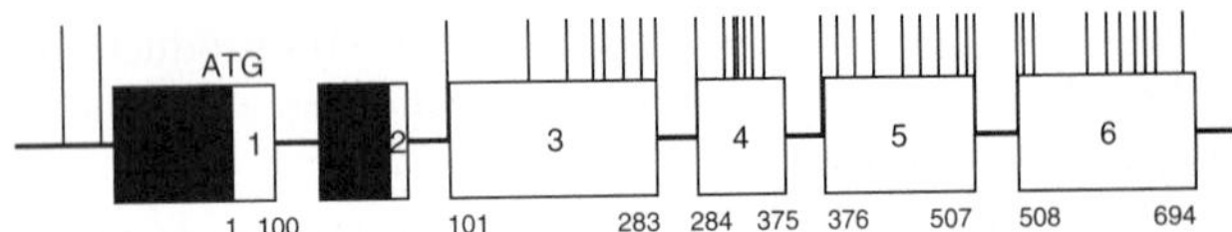

Figure 21-10 Schematic representation (not drawn to scale) of the *PKLR* gene and its erythroid-specific promoter. Exons are numbered and depicted as rectangles, separated by intervening sequences (introns), 5′ and 3′ noncoding sequences are colored black. Nucleotides are numbered according to the erythroid-specific cDNA, the initiator methionine and stop codon (TGA) are indicated. In the figure, the position of each of the more than 130 mutations that have, to date, been described in association with PK deficiency[221] (and our own unpublished observations) is indicated. The horizontal line that encompasses exon 11 indicates the deletion of this exon, as identified on the cDNA level. The figure shows that mutations are encountered throughout the gene, although there tends to be a clustering of mutations toward the 3′-end, in particular in exons 8, 9, and 11.

and point mutations in the red cell–specific promoter have been described. One promoter mutation is of particular interest, as it silences the red cell–specific PK gene completely. This mutation is located in a putative binding domain for an as-yet unidentified trans-acting factor that mediates the effects of factors necessary for regulation of PK gene expression during red cell differentiation and maturation.[204] Because PK activity is related to the age of the red cell, other glycolytic enzymes should be measured simultaneously to assess the influence of reticulocytosis on the enzyme activity.

Modeling the known mutations in the three-dimensional computer model of the tetramer and expressing mutant enzymes in in vitro model systems helps to better understand the genotype-phenotype interactions, since these are still poorly understood in this disorder.[200,202,210]

Lactate Dehydrogenase

Lactate dehydrogenase (LD) catalyzes the conversion of pyruvate to lactate, the last step in the EMP. Deficiency of this enzyme is not associated with hematological disease. LD is described elsewhere.

Hexose Monophosphate Pathway

Normally, approximately 10% of glucose is catabolized through the hexose monophosphate pathway, but this fraction may be markedly increased when there is oxidative stress, as is the case when there is an infection or use of certain drugs. The principal function of the hexose monophosphate pathway is to reduce 2 moles of NADP to NADPH by oxidizing G6P. NADPH is required for a variety of biosynthetic pathways, for the stability of catalase and the regeneration and preservation of the reduced form of glutathione. These processes are crucial in the cell to detoxify hydrogen peroxide and protect the cell from oxidative stress. Since the red cell has no other sources of NADPH, it heavily depends on the prime enzyme of this reaction, glucose 6-phosphate dehydrogenase (G6PD).

Glucose 6-Phosphate Dehydrogenase

Glucose 6-phosphate dehydrogenase (G6PD; EC 1.1.1.49) is expressed in all cells and catalyzes the first step in the hexose monophosphate pathway, the conversion of glucose 6-phosphate to 6-phosphogluconate. This step generates 1 mol of NADPH. The activity of G6PD is higher in reticulocytes than in mature red cells.

The enzyme is a dimer (predominantly) or tetramer (pH dependent) in the active form composed of identical subunits, 515 amino acids long and about 59 kDa.[208] The three-dimensional structure of human G6PD has been elucidated.[7] The monomer is built up by two domains, an N-terminal domain and a large $\beta + \alpha$ domain with an antiparallel nine-stranded sheet. The interface between the two monomers is of crucial importance for proper activity of the enzyme and is located in this second domain.

The gene coding for G6PD is located on the X-chromosome (Xq28), spans 18 kb, and consists of 13 exons. Exon 1 is noncoding. The promoter shares many features common to other housekeeping genes.[103]

G6PD deficiency (OMIM 305900) is the most common enzymopathy, affecting 400 million people worldwide. The disease is X-linked. More than 400 different types of G6PD variants have been described, leading to different enzyme activities associated with a wide range of biochemical and clinical phenotypes. The variants are grouped into five categories according to the level of enzyme activity and clinical phenotype.

The clinical expression of the disease is heterogeneous and five different clinical syndromes can be recognized:

- Drug-induced hemolysis
- Infection-induced hemolysis
- Favism
- Neonatal jaundice (NNJ)
- Chronic nonspherocytic hemolytic anemia (CNSHA)

The majority of G6PD-deficient individuals develop hemolysis only when oxidative stress occurs, as with infections and after ingestion of certain drugs or fava beans. Outside these periods, they are usually asymptomatic. However, G6PD deficiency can also lead to mild to severe chronic hemolysis, exacerbated by oxidative stress. These variants are class I mutants (Table 21-5). Nearly half of the mutations encoding class I G6PD variants directly affect the subunit interface of the G6PD dimer[7] and are located in exons 10 and 11. However, it is not always clear what the exact phenotype of particular mutations will be, since some identical variants might still lead to different phenotypes.[75] The availability of

TABLE 21-5 Classes of Severity of Glucose-6-Phosphate Dehydrogenase (G6PD) Deficiency

Class I	Severe deficiency associated with chronic hemolytic anemia.
Class II	Severe deficiency (<10% residual activity), usually without hemolytic anemia.
Class III	Moderate to mild deficiency (10% to 60% residual activity) (e.g., G6PD A).
Class IV	Very mild or no deficiency (e.g., G6PD A).
Class V	Increased activity (only one such variant has been described, G6PD Hektoen).

the 3-D structure of the human enzyme makes a better understanding of the effect of mutations in G6Pd feasible.

The literature on G6PD and G6PD deficiency is extensive and has been reviewed.[20,99,208]

Transketolase

Transketolase is decreased in thiamin deficiency. Low values of it have also been found in chronic alcoholism.

Rapoport-Luebering Cycle

The Rapoport-Luebering cycle, which is unique to mammalian RBCs, provides the principal physiological means for regulation of the O_2 affinity of hemoglobin.[17,18,198] From the point of view of O_2 transport, one might assert that the Embden-Meyerhof pathway of the RBCs serves principally to generate 2,3-DPG, because quantitatively this substance is the principal glycolytic intermediate of RBCs; the concentration of 2,3-DPG is about equal to the sum of all other glycolytic intermediates. The 2,3-DPG content of RBCs is increased in all anemias; in all but one, the increase is inversely proportional to the hemoglobin concentration.[17] The single exception is PK deficiency, in which 2,3-DPG is increased disproportionately to the hemoglobin deficit as a result of the "bottleneck" at the PK step and of a retrograde accumulation of products of glycolysis. The increase in 2,3-DPG in anemias results in a decrease in O_2 affinity of hemoglobin so that O_2 is more readily transferred to tissues. The O_2 affinity of hemoglobin is also influenced by slight changes in pH of the blood; a corresponding sensitivity to pH exists in the Rapoport-Luebering cycle, which again permits change in 2,3-DPG concentration to fine tune the O_2 affinity of hemoglobin.

Two enzymes involved in the Rapoport-Luebering cycle are diphosphoglyceromutase (2,3-DPG mutase [DPGM]; EC 5.4.2.4) and diphosphoglycerate phosphatase (2,3-DPG phosphatase [DPGP]; EC 3.1.3.13). The same protein molecule is responsible for both DPGM and DPGP activities.[71,167] This multifunctional enzyme regulates the concentration of 2,3-DPG in the erythrocyte and thus is very important in regulating O_2 affinity of hemoglobin. DPGM is a homodimer, with subunits of 258 amino acids (30 kDa).

The single locus for the gene of DPGM is located on chromosome 7q22-34 and is fully expressed only in erythroid tissue during the late stages of differentiation.[209]

DPGM deficiency is a rare autosomal recessive disorder, resulting in reduced synthesis of 2,3-DPG. As a consequence, blood oxygen affinity is increased, accounting for the polycythemia present in affected individuals. Only a few cases have been described. Two mutations in the gene have been identified. One point mutation at nucleotide 413 (Arg89 to Cys) was designated DPGM Creteil I.[168] DPGM Creteil II is a deletion of nucleotide 205, inducing a frameshift and consequently leading to a premature stop codon.[94]

Glutathione Pathway

The sulfhydryl-containing tripeptide reduced glutathione (GSH) protects hemoglobin and other critical RBC proteins from peroxidative injury. In the process of reducing peroxides or oxidized protein sulfhydryl groups, GSH is converted to GSSH (oxidized glutathione). As shown in Figure 21-9, its metabolic pathway includes several enzymes.

Gamma-Glutamylcysteine Synthetase

Gamma-glutamylcysteine synthetase (GCS; EC 6.3.2.2) catalyzes the first step in glutathione biosynthesis in which glutamylcysteine is synthetized using L-glutamate, L-cysteine, and ATP. This amide linking is the rate-limiting step in glutathione synthesis. There is a feedback inhibition by glutathione. The protein is a heterodimer composed of a catalytic heavy chain (GCS_h; 636 amino acids; 73 kDa) and a regulatory light chain (GCS_l; 274 amino acids; 31 kDa).[52,53]

The gene for GCS_h *(GLCLC)* is localized on chromosome 6p12[185] and the gene for GCS_l *(GLCLR)* on chromosome 1p21.[184]

Hereditary GCS deficiency is very rare. Deficiency leads to CNSHA and drug- and infection-induced hemolytic periods. Only 10 patients to date have been described, of which 5 were characterized at the molecular level.[23,59,166] A homozygous 1109A to T (His370Leu) substitution in the GLCLC gene was found,[23] probably resulting in an unstable protein. Another study identified in two related patients a homozygous 473C-to-T substitution resulting in a leucine residue instead of proline at amino acid 158 of GCS_h.[166] Recently, two related patients were reported with a C-to-T missense mutation at nucleotide 379, encoding for a predicted Arg127Cys substitution. Computer modeling indicated the mutation to be localized in a cleft on the protein surface of GCSh.[59]

Glutathione Synthetase

Glutathione synthetase (EC 6.3.2.3; GSH-S) mediates the second step in the synthesis of GSH, by the addition of glycine to the dipeptide γ-glutamylcysteine. The protein is a homodimer of 52 kDa.[51]

The gene for GSH-S is located on chromosome 20q11.2 and contains 12 exons spanning 23 kb.[183-186]

In the few cases that have been described, mild chronic hemolytic anemia is associated with deficiency of GSH-S.[155] The disorder is inherited in an autosomal recessive mode. Such people may also have more severe acute hemolytic crises when exposed to redox substances, such as 8-aminoquinolines or other "oxidant" drugs.

There are two distinct types of GSH-S deficiency, both associated with mild chronic hemolysis; in one type, hemolysis is the only clinical manifestation.[155] In the other, the major clinical features are mental retardation, severe generalized muscle weakness, tremors, incoordination, hemolytic anemia, and metabolic acidosis. This second and much more severe type of GSH-S deficiency is also known as 5-*oxoprolinuria* or *pyroglutamic aciduria.*[186] The difference in severity of these disorders reflects the fact that in the mild form, GSH-S deficiency is confined to the RBCs because in this disorder the GSH-S is unstable. GSH-S activity is present in adequate quantity in young RBCs, but it rapidly declines as the cells age, because the cells are unable to synthesize new molecules of GHS-S. Other cells of the body that have nuclei and ribosomes can compensate for accelerated denaturation of GSH-S by synthesizing more. On the other hand, in the severe systemic form of GSH-S deficiency, all cells of the body have low activities of GSH-S because they cannot form this enzyme in adequate amounts. In both types of GSH-S deficiency, RBCs exhibit notable reduction in GSH concentration.

Several mutations in the gene have been identified recently, associated with the disease. The majority of the mutations are missense, two small deletions and one splice site mutation.[40,41,183]

Glutathione Reductase

Glutathione reductase (EC 1.8.1.7; formerly EC 1.6.4.2; GSR) links the glutathione pathway to the hexose monophosphate pathway through the reversible oxidation and reduction of NADP. Flavin adenine dinucleotide (FAD) is necessary as a cofactor. The enzyme maintains high levels of reduced glutathione in the cell. Two isoforms exist, a mitochondrial and cytoplasmic form, produced by alternative initiation.[85] The molecule is a homodimer, linked by a disulfide bridge. Each subunit (522 amino acids; 56 kDa) is divided into four domains of which domains one and two bind FAD and NADPH, respectively, and domain four forms the interface.[84,192]

The gene encoding GSR is located on chromosome 8p21.1, spans 50 kb, and contains 13 exons.[85]

Glutathione reductase deficiency (OMIM 138300) is an autosomal disease and, except when very severe, is not associated with hemolysis. The disease has been associated with drug-sensitive hemolysis and favism.[97]

Glutathione Peroxidase

Glutathione peroxidase (EC 1.11.1.9; GSH-Px) is active as a homotetrameric enzyme (subunits of 21 kDa) and effects the conversion of hydrogen peroxide to water, thus reducing peroxidative stress to proteins in the cell. Several isoforms exist, but GSH-Px1 is active in the erythrocytes. RBCs also have high catalase (EC 1.11.1.6) activity that converts H_2O_2 to water and O_2; thus GSH-Px is redundant. In fact, deficiencies of either catalase or GSH-Px are without serious consequences for the RBCs because the presence of either of these two enzymes can compensate for deficiency of the other.

Partial deficiencies of GSH-Px have been documented,[56] but a clear cause-effect relationship with hemolysis has not been established. The gene has been assigned to chromosome 3p21.3.[216]

PURINE-PYRIMIDINE METABOLISM

Pyrimidines and purines are the building blocks of DNA and RNA. In addition, they have a role in the formation of coenzymes and active intermediates in carbohydrate and phospholipid metabolism.

Controversy exists concerning the cause and effect relationships between deficiencies of the enzymes adenylate kinase (AK; EC 2.7.4.3) and adenosine triphosphatase (ATPase; EC 3.6.1.3) and hemolytic disease.[61,93] Since the consensus seems to be that there is no association, these enzymes will not be discussed here.

Pyrimidine-5′-Nucleotidase

Pyrimidine-5′-nucleotidases are a group of enzymes dephosphorylating pyrimidine nucleotides to the corresponding nucleosides. The pyrimidine bases diffuse out of the erythrocyte and the phosphates are retained. Pyrimidine phosphates are present on ribosomes of erythroblasts and reticulocytes, but there are normally no pyrimidines in mature RBCs. Two cytoplasmic forms of the enzyme were identified in the erythrocyte, P5′N-1 and P5′N-2. These enzymes are encoded by different genes and have different molecular properties and substrate specificities.[133,189] Since there are no known disorders associated with deficiency of P5′N-2, this enzyme will not be further discussed here.

Pyrimidine-5′-nucleotidase-1 (P5′N-1; uridine 5′ monophosphate hydrolase 1 (UMPH-1); EC 3.1.3.5; MW 34 kDa) is a monomeric unphosphorylated protein and drives the principal mechanism for catabolism of the ribosomal RNA. Enzyme activity is dependent on magnesium ions and has a substrate specificity for UMP, CMP, and dCMP. The tertiary structure is as yet unknown. P5′N-1 is one of the most age-sensitive RBC enzymes, and activity declines rapidly during the first days in circulation to remain stable at a low level in the mature RBC.[24]

The gene encoding P5′N-1 was only very recently identified and maps to chromosome 7p15-p14, spans about 50 kb, and consists of 10 exons. Two pseudogenes were identified on chromosomes 4 and 7. The cDNA of about 1300 base pair (bp) codes for two different proteins, one being 286 amino acids long, the other 297 amino acids.[102] The messenger is alternatively spliced. One mRNA initiates in exon 1 and continues from exon 3, exon 2 being spliced out. The transcript codes for the 286 amino acid protein, being P5′N-1. The longer protein is transcribed from a messenger that initiates from exon 2 and continues through the exons sequentially.[163] The significance of this alternatively spliced messenger is unknown, but the process shows remarkable resemblance to the alternative initiation generating pyruvate kinase mRNA, where it drives tissue specificity (see under pyruvate kinase in this chapter).

P5′N-1 deficiency (OMIM 266120) is a relatively common cause of nonspherocytic hemolytic anemia, and, because of the relatively mild phenotypic expression, many cases might be undetected as yet.[21,65,163] The disease is inherited in an autosomal recessive manner and is the only red cell enzyme deficiency in which red cell morphology is helpful. Prominent and characteristic basophilic stippling is visible in blood films. There usually is an accumulation of high concentrations of pyrimidine nucleotides, mostly uridine triphosphate (UTP) and cytidine triphosphate (CTP), in the red cells.

After the recent identification of the gene, there have been a number of reports describing the mutations that cause P5′N-1 deficiency. To date, 23 patients have been characterized at the molecular level, identifying 14 different mutations. Four are missense, three cause aberrant splicing, two introduce a premature stop codon, and five result in a frameshift.[14,28,102,163] No relationship between the genotype and phenotype could be established.

Adenosine Deaminase

Adenosine deaminase (ADA; EC 3.5.4.4) is the enzyme of the purine metabolism that deaminates adenosine and 2′-deoxyadenosine to inosine and 2′-deoxyinosine, respectively. ADA deficiency, which leads to *severe combined immunodeficiency disease* (SCID), is associated with a decrease in RBC adenosine deaminase activity, without hemolysis. ADA deficiency will not be discussed here.

The abnormality of this enzyme associated with hereditary nonspherocytic hemolytic anemia is an increase in activity in the erythrocyte. This results in the depletion of red cell ATP and hemolysis. Few cases with a thirtyfold to seventyfold increase have been described. It is the only RBC enzymopathy that is inherited as an autosomal dominant disorder. The molecular mechanism of this disorder has not been identified. High levels of normal ADA mRNA were present, suggesting a mutation in an in cis transcriptional regulating element, which could not be identified.*

Methemoglobin Reduction

Hemoglobin can bind oxygen only in the reduced ferrous (Fe^{2+}) state. Consequently, when hemoglobin is oxidized to the ferric (Fe^{3+}) state, the capacity to bind oxygen is lost, which ultimately will lead to pathological consequences. The oxidized state of hemoglobin is called methemoglobin and is normally present at less than 1%. Thus to preserve oxygen-binding capacity, the red cell must keep hemoglobin in the reduced state, a process achieved mainly by the cytochrome b5/cytochrome b5 reductase system, which is NADH-dependent.

NADH-Cytochrome B5 Reductase

Nicotinamide adenine dinucleotide (NADH)-cytochrome b5 reductase (EC 1.6.2.2; cytb5r) uses NADH generated in the reaction in the Embden-Meyerhof pathway by glyceraldehyde 3-phosphate dehydrogenase, to reduce the 12 kDa protein cytochrome b5. Cytochrome b5 in turn reduces methemoglobin to hemoglobin.

The enzyme is present in two different forms. A membrane-bound 300 amino acid form is located mainly in the endoplasmic reticulum and outer mitochondrial membrane.[29,69,149] The membrane form has a role in desaturation and elongation of fatty acids, cholesterol biosynthesis, and drug metabolism.

The second form is a soluble protein of 275 amino acids and is RBC specific.[149] They share an identical hydrophilic *C*-terminal domain, but differ at the *N*-termini. The membrane form has an additional stretch of 25 hydrophobic amino acids.

Both forms of cytb5r are transcribed from the same gene on chromosome 22q 13-qtr spanning 31 kb. It contains 9 exons, but there are two exons[1] (exon 1 and [later discovered] exon 1S).[220] The soluble form is coded by exons 2 through to 9, while the longer membrane bound form is coded for by exon 1 and continues through the exons sequentially.

NADH-cytochrome b5 reductase deficiency (OMIM 250800) is an autosomal recessive disorder, causing hereditary methemoglobinemia. There are three types. In type I, the enzyme is deficient only in erythrocytes. Patients are typically blue and/or gray and cyanotic, but not very sick. Type II is more severe, the enzyme being completely deficient, causing mental retardation and neurological impairment. In type III the enzyme is deficient in all blood cells.

A total of 34 different mutations have been identified associated with cytb5r deficiency to date.[57,150] Sixteen were associated with type I and 16 with type II. These mutations were distributed over all exons, except for exons 1 and 1S.

Detection of Hereditary Red Cell Enzyme Deficiencies

Other than deficiencies of G6PD and possibly PK, RBC enzyme defects are rare; therefore it is not practical to attempt to identify them in laboratories that perform such tests only rarely. Specimens should be shipped by mail to reference laboratories that specialize in performance of these assays. As a rule, whole-blood specimens anticoagulated with EDTA are suitable and the specimens can be shipped at room temperature.[21] Exceptions are assays for phosphorylated sugar intermediates, 2,3-DPG, and nucleotide intermediates, which are unstable in freshly drawn blood and require immediate deproteinization in perchloric acid.[21]

*References 35, 37, 38, 50, 113, 151, 199.

Care must be taken to remove leukocytes and platelets in assays such as for PK, since these cells do contain PK activity, obscuring a deficiency in the red cells.

Other pitfalls in correct diagnosis of glycolytic enzyme deficiencies include the red cell age dependency of enzymes such as PK, HK, and G6PD. The measurement of these enzymes simultaneously can give an idea about red cell age and relative deficiencies. Many patients suffering from severe hemolysis have already received blood transfusions. When this occurs, interpreting results from red cell enzyme assays must be done with great care, since the presence of donor erythrocytes will obscure any deficiencies. In addition, some mutant enzymes display a normal activity in vitro, while in vivo severe hemolysis can occur. More sophisticated assays to measure, for example, heat instability and kinetics have to be used in those cases.

In the last few years, the genes coding for the red cell enzymes have been localized and characterized. This made molecular diagnostics possible, and many causative mutations have been identified. Molecular diagnostics at the DNA and RNA level is very attractive in situations in which the diagnosis of enzyme deficiency is difficult or impossible by activity measurements, such as in transfused patients, as explained above. In addition, prenatal diagnosis is now available. The ability to study the effects of mutations in three-dimentional computer models of the enzymes and the opportunity to express mutant enzymes, will provide a better understanding of the genotype-phenotype relations in these hemolytic disorders.

METHODOLOGY

In this section, methodological principles and reference values are given for several of the methods used to measure red cell enzymes. Methodological details of these methods are given in the Evolve site that accompanies this book at http://evolve.elsevier.com/Tietz/textbook.

Method for the Determination of Glucose-6-Phosphate Dehydrogenase

Principle

Glucose-6-phosphate dehydrogenase (G6PD) catalyzes the oxidation of glucose-6-phosphate to 6-phosphogluconate with a concurrent conversion of $NADP^+$ to NADPH. The activity of G6PD is determined by measurement of the rate of increase of NADPH concentration. Whereas $NADP^+$ is transparent to ultraviolet (UV) light, NADPH strongly absorbs UV light. Therefore the rate of increase in absorbance at 340 nm is the measure of enzyme activity.

Reference Intervals

The reference interval for G6PD in erythrocytes is 8-14 U/g Hb. Values greater than 18 U/g Hb are often encountered in any condition associated with younger than normal RBCs (as in hemolytic anemias not due to G6PD deficiency) but are of no clinical significance.

Method for Screening Erythrocytes for Glucose-6-Phosphate Dehydrogenase Deficiency

In this screening test, $NADP^+$ is reduced to NADPH in both the G6PD and the 6PGD reactions of the hexose monophosphate pathway. If G6PD activity is low, only a small quantity of NADPH is formed. This is reoxidized to $NADP^+$ by glutathione reductase present in RBCs, and no fluorescence is observed. In the presence of adequate amounts of G6PD, the rate of reduction of $NADP^+$ substantially exceeds the rate of oxidation of NADPH by glutathione reductase, and enough NADPH accumulates in RBCs to be demonstrable by its fluorescence.

Method for the Determination of Pyruvate Kinase Activity

Principle

In this assay, the PK reaction is linked with the LD reaction in which NADH is oxidized to NAD^+.

$$\text{Phosphoenolpyruvate} + \text{ADP} \xrightarrow{\text{PK}} \text{pyruvate} + \text{ATP}$$
$$\text{Pyruvate} + \text{NADH} \xrightarrow{\text{LD}} \text{lactate} + \text{NAD}^+ + \text{H}^+$$

Because LD is present in excess, the rate of NADH oxidation is limited by the activity of PK. The reaction rate is measured by the rate of decrease in absorbance at 340 nm. Assays are performed at low substrate concentration with and without the addition of fructose-1,6-diphosphate, because some PK variants associated with hemolysis have atypical reaction kinetics (and thus may exhibit "normal" activity at high substrate concentrations but lower than normal activity at lower substrate concentrations) or may show absence of enhancement by fructose-1,6-diphosphate, the allosteric activator of PK.

Reference Intervals

Reference intervals for pyruvate kinase are:
High substrate 9 to 16 U/g of Hb
Low substrate 1.7 to 6.8 U/g of Hb.

Method for the Determination of Glucose Phosphate Isomerase Activity

Deficiency of glucose phosphate isomerase (GPI) has been associated with chronic hemolytic disease in a few dozen reported cases and may also cause hemolytic disease of the newborn. Although the third most frequently reported enzymopathy causing hemolytic disease, it has been quite rare in our experience.

Principle

GPI catalyzes the interconversion of G6P and F6P:

$$\text{F-6-P} \xleftrightarrow{\text{GPI}} \text{G-6-P}$$
$$\text{NAPH}^+ + \text{G-6-P} \xleftrightarrow{\text{G-6-PD}}$$
$$\text{6-phosphogluconate} + \text{NADPH} + \text{H}^+$$

In this assay, F6P is used as the substrate for GPI. The GPI reaction is linked to the G6PD reaction. The rate of reduction of $NADP^+$, as indicated by the increase in absorbance at 340 nm, is the measure of GPI activity.

Reference Intervals

The reference interval for GPI is 50-70 U/g Hb.

Method for the Determination of Erythrocyte Glutathione Concentration

Erythrocyte GSH concentration is diminished in many people who have defects in the hexose monophosphate or GSH synthesis pathways. The GSH stability test, originally devised to permit identification of people susceptible to hemolysis from primaquine (later shown to be the result of G6PD deficiency), still remains a useful "stress test" of the intactness of these closely linked pathways. Because deficiencies of GSH synthetase and γ-glutamyl cysteine synthetase are rare disorders, it is not practical for clinical laboratories to contemplate assays for these enzymes unless results of the easily performed GSH stability test are abnormal.

Principle

Virtually all of the nonprotein sulfhydryl groups of RBCs are in the form of reduced GSH. 5,5′-Dithiobis(2-nitrobenzoic acid) (DTNB) is a disulfide chromogen that is readily reduced by sulfhydryl compounds to an intensely yellow compound. The absorbance of the reduced chromogen is measured at 412 nm and is directly proportional to the GSH concentration.

Reference Interval

The reference interval for GSH is 5.5-7.5 μmol/g Hb.

Method for Screening for Deficiency of Pyrimidine-5′-Nucleotidase Activity

Principle

Pyrimidine-5′-nucleotidase effects the release of phosphate from cytidine-5′-monophosphate and uridine-5′-monophosphate and thus is an enzyme involved in the catabolism of RNA. RNA is a normal constituent of reticulocytes but not of mature RBCs. In the absence (or notable deficiency) of P-5′-N, RNA persists in RBCs and is manifested by striking basophilic stippling and mild to moderate hemolytic anemia.

Pyrimidine nucleotides, extracted with acid from the RNA remaining in P-5′-N-deficient RBCs, have an absorption peak at 270 nm. This peak is quite distinct from the peak at 257 nm, which is because of purine nucleotides (such as ATP) that are normally present. When P-5′-N is deficient and RNA persists, the P-5′-N deficiency can be inferred by observing a pyrimidine nucleotide peak at 270 nm in an acid extract of RBCs.

Reference Intervals

In normal specimens or in those of any disorder but P-5′-N deficiency, there is an absorbance curve of low amplitude with a peak at about 257 nm, this being caused by the presence of purines, such as ATP and ADP. No peak is seen at 270 nm. In P-5′-N deficiency, a notably higher-amplitude curve is observed, with a peak at 270 nm. The absorbance maximum for normal RBCs is 257 nm, and the observed absorbance value is approximately 0.3/108 RBCs per milliliter. In P-5′-N deficiency, the peak absorbance is at 270 nm, with absorbance values of approximately 0.8/108 RBCs per milliliter having been observed. No interfering substances are known.

Method for the Determination of 2,3-Diphosphoglycerate in Erythrocytes

This enzyme is the predominant glycolytic intermediate of RBCs and has a vital role in modulating the affinity of hemoglobin for O_2.

Principle

The assay of 2,3-DPG is based on an equilibrium system between 3-phosphoglycerate, 2-phosphoglycerate, and PEP when monophosphoglycerate mutase (MPGM) and enolase are present.

$$\text{3-phosphoglycerate} \underset{\text{2,3-DPG}}{\overset{\text{MPGM}}{\rightleftarrows}} 2$$

$$\text{3-phosphoglycerate} \overset{\text{enolase}}{\rightleftarrows} \text{PEP}$$

The addition of 2,3-DPG (in the sample) shifts the equilibrium so that more 2-phosphoglycerate is converted to 3-phosphoglycerate. This in turn results in the conversion of PEP to 2-phosphoglycerate. The rate of decrease in PEP concentration is measured by the decrease in absorbance at 240 nm, which is proportional to the amount of 2,3-DPG in the specimen.

Reference Intervals

The mean (SD) 2,3-DPG is 12.3 (1.87) μmol/g Hb [0.79 (0.12) mol/mol Hb] or 356 (54) μmol/1012 RBCs [356 (54) amol/RBC].

REFERENCES

1. Aleshin AE, Kirby C, Liu X, Bourenkov GP, Bartunik HD, Fromm HJ, et al. Crystal structures of mutant monomeric hexokinase I reveal multiple ADP binding sites and conformational changes relevant to allosteric regulation. J Mol Biol 2000;296:1001-15.
2. Aleshin AE, Zeng C, Bartunik HD, Fromm HJ, Honzatko RB. Regulation of hexokinase I: crystal structure of recombinant human brain hexokinase complexed with glucose and phosphate. J Mol Biol 1998;282:345-57.

3. Aleshin AE, Zeng C, Bourenkov GP, Bartunik HD, Fromm HJ, Honzatko RB. The mechanism of regulation of hexokinase: new insights from the crystal structure of recombinant human brain hexokinase complexed with glucose and glucose-6-phosphate. Structure 1998;6:39-50.
4. Andreoni F, Ruzzo A, Magnani M. Structure of the 5′ region of the human hexokinase type I (HKI) gene and identification of an additional testis-specific HKI mRNA. Biochim Biophys Acta 2000;1493:19-26.
5. Appel W. Chymotrypsin: molecular and catalytic properties. Clin Biochem 1986;19:317-22.
6. Arzoglou P, Goudoula C, Tsantili P, Lessinger JM, Férard G, Mignot V, et al. Transferability of lipase titrimetric assays: deductions from an interlaboratory study. Eur J Clin Chem Lab Med 1994;32:773-7.
7. Au SWN, Gover S, Lam VMS, Adams MJ. Human glucose-6-phosphate dehydrogenase: the crystal structure reveals a structural $NADP^+$ molecule and provides insights into enzyme deficiency. Structure Fold Des 2000;8:293-303.
8. Bais R, Conyers RAJ, Rofe AM, Tormet RI, Geary TD. Creatine kinase reference intervals determined from a multi-centre data pool. Pathology 1988;20: 367-72.
9. Bais R, Edwards JB. An optimized continuous-monitoring procedure for semiautomated determination of serum acid phosphatase activity. Clin Chem 1976;22:25-8.
10. Bais R, Edwards JB. Increased creatine kinase activity associated with haemolysis. Pathology 1980;12: 203-7.
11. Bais R, Edwards JB. Creatine kinase. CRC Crit Rev Clin Lab Sci 1982;16:291-355.
12. Bais R, Edwards JB. Plasma lactate dehydrogenase activity will be increased if detergent and platelets are present. Clin Chem 1977;23:1056-8.
13. Bais R, Philcox M. Approved recommendation on IFCC methods for the measurement of catalytic concentration of enzymes. Part 8. IFCC Method for Lactate Dehydrogenase (l-Lactate: NAD+Oxidoreductase, EC 1.1.1.27). International Federation of Clinical Chemistry (IFCC). Eur J Clin Chem Clin Biochem 1994:32:639-55.
14. Balta G, Gumruk F, Akarsu N, Gurgey A, Altay C. Molecular characterization of Turkish patients with pyrimidine 5′ nucleotidase-I deficiency. Blood 2003;102:1900-3.
15. Balk EM, Ionnidis JP, Salem D, Chew PW, Lau J. Accuracy of biomarkers to diagnose acute cardiac ischemia in the emergency department: a meta-analysis. Ann Emerg Med 2001;37:478-94.
16. Banks RD, Blake CC, Evans PR, Haser R, Rice DW, Hardy GW, et al. Sequence, structure and activity of phosphoglycerate kinase: a possible hinge-bending enzyme. Nature 1979;279:773-7.
17. Bellingham AJ, Huehns ER. Compensatory mechanisms in haemolytic anaemias. Proc R Soc Med 1968;61:1315-16.
18. Benesch RE, Benesch R, Yu CI. The oxygenation of hemoglobin in the presence of 2,3-diphosphoglycerate. Effect of temperature, pH, ionic strength, and hemoglobin concentration. Biochemistry 1969;8:2567-71.
19. Bertrand A, Buret J. A one-step determination of serum 5′-nucleotidase using a centrifugal analyzer. Clin Chim Acta 1982;119:275-84.
20. Beutler E. G6PD deficiency. Blood 1994;84:3613-36.
21. Beutler E. Red cell metabolism: A manual of biochemical procedures. Orlando, FL: Grune & Stratton, 1984.
22. Beutler E, Gelbart T. Estimating the prevalence of pyruvate kinase deficiency from the gene frequency in the general white population. Blood 2000;95: 3585-8.
23. Beutler E, Gelbart T, Kondo T, Matsunaga AT. The molecular basis of a case of gamma-glutamylcysteine synthetase deficiency. Blood 1999;94:2890-4.
24. Beutler E, Hartman G. Age-related red cell enzymes in children with transient erythroblastopenia of childhood and with hemolytic anemia. Pediatr Res 1985;19:44-7.
25. Beutler E, Scott S, Bishop A, Margolis N, Matsumoto F, Kuhl W. Red cell aldolase deficiency and hemolytic anemia: a new syndrome. Trans Assoc Am Physicians 1973;86:154-66.
26. Bianchi M, Crinelli R, Serafini G, Giammarini C, Magnani M. Molecular bases of hexokinase deficiency. Biochim Biophys Acta 1997;1360:211-21.
27. Bianchi M, Magnani M. Hexokinase mutations that produce nonspherocytic hemolytic anemia. Blood Cells Mol Dis 1995;21:2-8.
28. Bianchi P, Fermo E, Alfinito F, Vercellati C, Baserga M, Ferraro F, et al. Molecular characterization of six unrelated Italian patients affected by pyrimidine 5′-nucleotidase deficiency. Br J Haematol 2003;122: 847-51.
29. Borgese N, Pietrini G. Distribution of the integral membrane protein NADH-cytochrome b5 reductase in rat liver cells, studied with a quantitative radioimmunoblotting assay. Biochem J 1986;239:393-403.
30. Brodrick JW, Geokas MC, Largman C, Fassett M, Johnson JH. Molecular forms of immunoreactive pancreatic cationic trypsin in pancreatitis patient sera. Am J Physiol 1979;237:E474-80.
31. Brown JR, Daar IO, Krug JR, Maquat LE. Characterization of the functional gene and several processed pseudogenes in the human triosephosphate isomerase gene family. Mol Cell Biol 1985;5:1694-706.
32. Broyles DL, Nielsen RG, Bussett EM, Lu WD, Mizrahi IA, Nunnelly PA, et al. Analytical and clinical performance characteristics of Tandem-MP Ostase, a new

immunoassay for serum bone alkaline phosphatase. Clin Chem 1998;44:2139-47.
33. Cabrera-Abreu JC, Green A. γ-Glutamyltransferase: value of its measurement in pediatrics. Ann Clin Biochem 2002;39:22-5.
34. Chatterly S, Sun T, Lien Y. Diagnostic value of lactate dehydrogenase isoenzymes in cerebrospinal fluid. J Clin Lab Anal 1991:5:168-74.
35. Chen EH, Tartaglia AP, Mitchell BS. Hereditary overexpression of adenosine deaminase in erythrocytes: evidence for a cis-acting mutation. Am J Hum Genet 1993;53:889-93.
36. Chen SH, Malcolm LA, Yoshida A, Giblett ER. Phosphoglycerate kinase: an X-linked polymorphism in man. Am J Hum Genet 1971;23:87-91.
37. Chottiner EG, Cloft HJ, Tartaglia AP, Mitchell BS. Elevated adenosine deaminase activity and hereditary hemolytic anemia. Evidence for abnormal translational control of protein synthesis. J Clin Invest 1987;79:1001-5.
38. Chottiner EG, Gribbin TE, Ginsburg D, Mitchell BS. Erythrocyte-specific overproduction of adenosine deaminase: molecular genetic studies. Prog Clin Biol Res 1989;319:55-64; discussion 65-8.
39. Cordeiro AT, Godoi PH, Delboni LF, Oliva G, Thiemann OH. Human phosphoglucose isomerase: expression, purification, crystallization and preliminary crystallographic analysis. Acta Crystallogr D Biol Crystallogr 2001;57:592-5.
40. Corrons JL, Alvarez R, Pujades A, Zarza R, Oliva E, Lasheras G, et al. Hereditary non-spherocytic haemolytic anaemia due to red blood cell glutathione synthetase deficiency in four unrelated patients from Spain: clinical and molecular studies. Br J Haematol 2001;112:475-82.
41. Dahl N, Pigg M, Ristoff E, Gali R, Carlsson B, Mannervik B, et al. Missense mutations in the human glutathione synthetase gene result in severe metabolic acidosis, 5-oxoprolinuria, hemolytic anemia and neurological dysfunction. Hum Mol Genet 1997;6: 1147-52.
42. Deutsche Gesellschaft für Klinische Chemie. Proposal of standard methods for the determination of enzyme catalytic concentrations in serum and plasma at 37°C. III. Glutamate dehydrogenase (L-glutamate: $NAD(P)^+$ oxidoreductase (deaminating), EC 1.4.1.3). Eur J Clin Chem Clin Biochem 1992;30:493-502.
43. Deys BF, Grzeschick KH, Grzeschick A, Jaffe ER, Siniscalco M. Human phosphoglycerate kinase and inactivation of the X chromosome. Science 1972;175:1002-3.
44. Dominici R, Franzini C. Fecal elastase-1 as a test for pancreatic function: a review. Clin Chem Lab Med 2002;40:325-32.
45. Dufour DR, Lott JA, Nolte FS, Gretch DR, Koff RS, Seeff LB. Diagnosis and monitoring of hepatic injury. II. Recommendations for use of laboratory tests in screening, diagnosis, and monitoring. Clin Chem 2000;46:2050-68.
46. Eto K, Sakura H, Yasuda K, Hayakawa T, Kawasaki E, Moriuchi R, et al. Cloning of a complete protein-coding sequence of human platelet-type phosphofructokinase isozyme from pancreatic islet. Biochem Biophys Res Commun 1994;198:990-8.
47. Foo AY. Amylase measurement—which method? Ann Clin Biochem 1995;32:239-43.
48. Frossard JL. Trypsin activation peptide (TAP) in acute pancreatitis: from pathophysiology to clinical usefulness. JOP J Pancreas (Online) 2001;2:69-77.
49. Fujii H, Miwa S. Other erythrocyte enzyme deficiencies associated with non-haematological symptoms: phosphoglycerate kinase and phosphofructokinase deficiency. Baillieres Best Pract Res Clin Haematol 2000;13:141-8.
50. Fujii H, Miwa S, Tani K, Fujinami N, Asano H. Overproduction of structurally normal enzyme in man: hereditary haemolytic anaemia with increased red cell adenosine deaminase activity. Br J Haematol 1982;51:427-30.
51. Gali RR, Board PG. Sequencing and expression of a cDNA for human glutathione synthetase. Biochem J 1995;310 (Pt 1):353-8.
52. Gipp JJ, Bailey HH, Mulcahy RT. Cloning and sequencing of the cDNA for the light subunit of human liver gamma-glutamylcysteine synthetase and relative mRNA levels for heavy and light subunits in human normal tissues. Biochem Biophys Res Commun 1995;206:584-9.
53. Gipp JJ, Chang C, Mulcahy RT. Cloning and nucleotide sequence of a full-length cDNA for human liver gamma-glutamylcysteine synthetase. Biochem Biophys Res Commun 1992;185:29-35.
54. Goldberg DM. Proteases in the evaluation of pancreatic function and pancreatic disease. Clin Chim Acta 2000;291:201-21.
55. Goldberg DM. Structural, functional, and clinical aspects of gamma-glutamyltransferase. CRC Crit Rev Clin Lab Sci 1980;12:1-58.
56. Gondo H, Ideguchi H, Hayashi S, Shibuya T. Acute hemolysis in glutathione peroxidase deficiency. Int J Hematol 1992;55:215-18.
57. Grabowska D, Plochocka D, Jablonska-Skwiecinska E, Chelstowska A, Lewandowska I, Staniszewska K, et al. Compound heterozygosity of two missense mutations in the NADH-cytochrome b5 reductase gene of a Polish patient with type I recessive congenital methaemoglobinaemia. Eur J Haematol 2003;70: 404-9.
58. Gupta RK, Oesterling RM. Dual divalent cation requirement for activation of pyruvate kinase; essential roles of both enzyme- and nucleotide-bound metal ions. Biochemistry 1976;15:2881-7.

59. Hamilton D, Wu JH, Alaoui-Jamali M, Batist G. A novel missense mutation in the gamma-glutamylcysteine synthetase catalytic subunit gene causes both decreased enzymatic activity and glutathione production. Blood 2003;102:725-30.
60. Hammond KB, Abman SH, Sokol RJ, Accurso FJ. Efficacy of statewide neonatal screening for cystic fibrosis by assay of trypsinogen concentrations. N Engl J Med 1991;325:769-74.
61. Hanel HK, Cohn J, Harvald B. Adenosine-triphosphatase deficiency in a family with non-spherocytic haemolytic anaemia. Hum Hered 1971;21:313-9.
62. Hawkins RC. Assessment of the utility of aldolase determination in serum by monitoring patient outcomes. Biochim Clin 2001;25:331-5.
63. Hayes PC, Bouchier IAD, Beckett GJ. Glutathione S-transferase in humans in health and disease. Gut 1991;32:813-8.
64. Hedström J, Sainio V, Kemppainen E, Haapiainen R, Kivilaakso E, Schröder T, et al. Serum complex of trypsin 2 and $\alpha_1$antitrypsin as diagnostic and prognostic marker of acute pancreatitis: clinical study in consecutive patients. Br Med J 1996;313:333-7.
65. Hirono A, Forman L, Beutler E. Enzymatic diagnosis in non-spherocytic hemolytic anemia. Medicine (Baltimore) 1988;67:110-7.
66. Hood D, Van Lente F, Estes M. Serum enzyme alterations in chronic muscle disease. A biopsy-based diagnostic assessment. Am J Clin Pathol 1991;95: 402-7.
67. Huang IY, Fujii H, Yoshida A. Structure and function of normal and variant human phosphoglycerate kinase. Hemoglobin 1980;4:601-9.
68. Huijgen HJ, Sanders GT, Koster RW, Vreeken J, Bossuyt PM. The clinical value of lactate dehydrogenase in serum: a quantitative review. Eur J Clin Chem Clin Biochem1997;35:569-75.
69. Hultquist DE, Passon PG. Catalysis of methaemoglobin reduction by erythrocyte cytochrome B5 and cytochrome B5 reductase. Nat New Biol 1971;229:252-4.
70. Hutton JJ, Chilcote RR. Glucose phosphate isomerase deficiency with hereditary nonspherocytic hemolytic anemia. J Pediatr 1974;85:494-7.
71. Ikura K, Sasaki R, Narita H, Sugimoto E, Chiba H. Multifunctional enzyme, bisphosphoglyceromutase/2,3-bisphosphoglycerate phosphatase/phosphoglyceromutase, from human erythrocytes. Evidence for a common active site. Eur J Biochem 1976;66: 515-22.
72. Ishikawa Y, Saffitz JE, Mealman TL, Grace AM, Roberts R. Reversible myocardial ischemic injury is not associated with increased creatine kinase activity in plasma. Clin Chem 1997;43:467-75.
73. Itkonen O, Koivunen E, Hurme M, Alfthan H, Schröder T, Stenman U-H. Time-resolved immunofluorometric assays for trypsinogen-1 and 2 in serum reveal preferential elevation of trypsinogen-2 in pancreatitis. J Lab Clin Med 1990;115:712-18.
74. Izzo P, Costanzo P, Lupo A, Rippa E, Paolella G, Salvatore F. Human aldolase A gene. Structural organization and tissue-specific expression by multiple promoters and alternate mRNA processing. Eur J Biochem 1988;174:569-78.
75. Jablonska-Skwiecinska E, Lewandowska I, Plochocka D, Topczewski J, Zimowski JG, Klopocka J, et al. Several mutations including two novel mutations of the glucose-6-phosphate dehydrogenase gene in Polish G6PD deficient subjects with chronic nonspherocytic hemolytic anemia, acute hemolytic anemia, and favism. Hum Mutat 1999;14:477-84.
76. Jeffery CJ. Moonlighting proteins. Trends Biochem Sci 1999;24:8-11.
77. Junge W, Wortmann W, Wilke B, Waldenström J, Kurrle-Weittenhiller A, Finke J, Klein G. Development and evaluation of assays for the determination of total and pancreatic amylase at 37°C according to the principle recommended by the IFCC. Clin Biochem 2001;34:607-15.
78. Kahn A, Marie J. Pyruvate kinases from human erythrocytes and liver. Methods Enzymol 1982;90: 131-40.
79. Kahn A, Marie J, Boivin P. Pyruvate kinase isozymes in man. II. L type and erythrocyte-type isozymes. Electrofocusing and immunologic studies. Hum Genet 1976;33:35-46.
80. Kahn A, Marie J, Garreau H, Sprengers ED. The genetic system of the L-type pyruvate kinase forms in man. Subunit structure, interrelation and kinetic characteristics of the pyruvate kinase enzymes from erythrocytes and liver. Biochim Biophys Acta 1978;523:59-74.
81. Kanno H. Hexokinase: gene structure and mutations. Baillieres Best Pract Res Clin Haematol 2000;13: 83-8.
82. Kanno H, Fujii H, Miwa S. Structural analysis of human pyruvate kinase L-gene and identification of the promoter activity in erythroid cells. Biochem Biophys Res Commun 1992;188:516-23.
83. Kanno H, Murakami K, Hariyama Y, Ishikawa K, Miwa S, Fujii H. Homozygous intragenic deletion of type I hexokinase gene causes lethal hemolytic anemia of the affected fetus [letter]. Blood 2002;100:1930.
84. Karplus PA, Schulz GE. Refined structure of glutathione reductase at 1.54 A resolution. J Mol Biol 1987;195:701-29.
85. Kelner MJ, Montoya MA. Structural organization of the human glutathione reductase gene: determination of correct cDNA sequence and identification of a mitochondrial leader sequence. Biochem Biophys Res Commun 2000;269:366-8.

86. Kemppainen EA, Hedströ JI, Puolakkainen PA, Sainio VS, Haapiainen RK, Perhoniemi V, et al. Rapid measurement of urinary trypsinogen-2 as a screening test for acute pancreatitis. N Engl J Med 1997;336: 1788-93.
87. Kishi H, Mukai T, Hirono A, Fujii H, Miwa S, Hori K. Human aldolase A deficiency associated with a hemolytic anemia: thermolabile aldolase due to a single base mutation. Proc Natl Acad Sci U S A 1987;84:8623-7.
88. Krause EG, Will H, Böhm M, Wollenberger A. The assay of glycogen phosphorylase in human blood serum and its application to the diagnosis of myocardial infarction. Clin Chim Acta 1975;58: 145-54.
89. Kreuder J, Borkhardt A, Repp R, Pekrun A, Gottsche B, Gottschalk U, et al. Brief report: inherited metabolic myopathy and hemolysis due to a mutation in aldolase A. N Engl J Med 1996;334:1100-4.
90. Kruse-Jarres JD, Kaiser C, Hafkenscheid JCM, Hohenwallner W, Stein W, Bohner J, et al. Evaluation of a new α-amylase assay using 4,6-ethylidene-(G_7)-1-4-nitrophenyl-(G_1)-α-D-maltoheptaoside as substrate. J Clin Chem Clin Biochem 1989;27: 103-13.
91. Kugler W, Lakomek M. Glucose-6-phosphate isomerase deficiency. Baillieres Best Pract Res Clin Haematol 2000;13:89-101.
92. Kylänpää-Bäck ML, Kemppainen E, Puolakkainen P. Trypsin-based laboratory methods and carboxypeptidase activation peptide in acute pancreatitis. JOP J Pancreas (Online) 2002;3:34-48.
93. Lachant NA, Zerez CR, Barredo J, Lee DW, Savely SM, Tanaka KR. Hereditary erythrocyte adenylate kinase deficiency: a defect of multiple phosphotransferases? Blood 1991;77:2774-84.
94. Lemarchandel V, Joulin V, Valentin C, Rosa R, Galacteros F, Rosa J, et al. Compound heterozygosity in a complete erythrocyte bisphosphoglycerate mutase deficiency. Blood 1992;80:2643-9.
95. Lessinger JM, Ferard G. Plasma pancreatic lipase activity: from analytical specificity to clinical efficiency for the diagnosis of acute pancreatitis. Eur J Clin Chem Clin Biochem 1994;32:377-81.
96. Levanon D, Danciger E, Dafni N, Bernstein Y, Elson A, Moens W, et al. The primary structure of human liver type phosphofructokinase and its comparison with other types of PFK. DNA 1989;8:733-43.
97. Loos H, Roos D, Weening R, Houwerzijl J. Familial deficiency of glutathione reductase in human blood cells. Blood 1976;48:53-62.
98. Lorentz K. Approved recommendation on IFCC methods for the measurement of catalytic concentration of enzymes. Part 9. IFCC method for α-amylase (1,4-α-D-glucan 4-glucanohydrolase, EC 3.2.1.1). Clin Chem Lab Med 1998;36:185-203.
99. Luzzatto L, Mehta A. Glucose 6-phosphate dehydrogenase deficiency. In: Scriver C, Beaudet AL, Sly WS, Valle D, eds. The metabolic and molecular basis of inherited disease. 7 ed. New York: McGraw Hill, 1995:3367-98.
100. Mair J, Puschendorf B, Krause EG. Glycogen phosphorylase isoenzyme BB. In: Kaski JC, Holt DW, eds. Myocardial damage. Early detection by novel biochemical markers. Dordrecht, The Netherlands: Kluwer Academic Publishers, 1998:61-71.
101. Mande SC, Mainfroid V, Kalk KH, Goraj K, Martial JA, Hol WG. Crystal structure of recombinant human triosephosphate isomerase at 2.8 A resolution. Triosephosphate isomerase-related human genetic disorders and comparison with the trypanosomal enzyme. Protein Sci 1994;3:810-21.
102. Marinaki AM, Escuredo E, Duley JA, Simmonds HA, Amici A, Naponelli V, et al. Genetic basis of hemolytic anemia caused by pyrimidine 5′ nucleotidase deficiency. Blood 2001;97:3327-32.
103. Martini G, Toniolo D, Vulliamy T, Luzzatto L, Dono R, Viglietto G, et al. Structural analysis of the X-linked gene encoding human glucose 6-phosphate dehydrogenase. EMBO J 1986;5:1849-55.
104. Mattevi A, Valentini G, Rizzi M, Speranza ML, Bolognesi M, Coda A. Crystal structure of Escherichia coli pyruvate kinase type I: molecular basis of the allosteric transition. Structure 1995;3:729-41.
105. Matthay KK, Mentzer WC. Erythrocyte enzymopathies in the newborn. Clin Haematol 1981;10:31-55.
106. McCarrey JR, Thomas K. Human testis-specific PGK gene lacks introns and possesses characteristics of a processed gene. Nature 1987;326:501-5.
107. McComb RB. The measurement of lactate dehydrogenase. In: Homburger HA, ed. Clinical and analytical concepts in enzymology. Skokie, IL: College of American Pathologists, 1983:157-71.
108. McMorris FA, Chen TR, Ricciuti F, Tischfield J, Creagan R, Ruddle F. Chromosome assignments in man of the genes for two hexosephosphate isomerases. Science 1973;179:1129-31.
109. McQueen MJ. Clinical and analytical considerations in the utilization of cholinesterase measurements. Clin Chim Acta 1995;237:91-105.
110. Melzi d'Eril GV, Pollini E, Moratti R, Sprovieri G, Tocchini M, Galeazzi M. Proposed reference values for fecal chymotrypsin as measured photometrically. Clin Chem 1985;31:1088-9.
111. Michelson AM, Markham AF, Orkin SH. Isolation and DNA sequence of a full-length cDNA clone for human X chromosome-encoded phosphoglycerate kinase. Proc Natl Acad Sci U S A 1983;80:472-6.
112. Miura M, Matsuzaki H. Evaluation of a new method for separating bone-type alkaline phosphatase. Ann Clin Biochem 1990;27:501-2.

113. Miwa S, Fujii H, Matsumoto N, Nakatsuji T, Oda S, Asano H, et al. A case of red-cell adenosine deaminase overproduction associated with hereditary hemolytic anemia found in Japan. Am J Hematol 1978;5:107-15.
114. Moller-Petersen J. Clinical evaluation of cathodic trypsin-like immunoreactivity in pancreatic diseases in adults. Scand J Clin Lab Invest 1990;50:463-77.
115. Moller-Petersen J, Pedersen JO, Thorsgaard-Pedersen N, Nyboe Andersen B. Serum cathodic trypsin-like immunoreactivity, pancreatic lipase, and pancreatic isoamylase as diagnostic tests of chronic pancreatitis or pancreatic steatorrhea. Scand J Gastroenterol 1988;23:287-96.
116. Mosca A, Bonora R, Ceriotti F, Franzini C, Lando G, Patrosso MC, et al. Assay using succinyldithiocholine as substrate: the method of choice for the measurement of cholinesterase catalytic activity in serum to diagnose succinylcholine sensitivity. Clin Chem Lab Med 2003;41:317-22.
117. Moses GC, Ross ML, Henderson AR. Ten electrophoretic methods compared with a selected method for quantifying lactate dehydrogenase isoenzymes in serum. Clin Chem 1988;34:1885-90.
118. Moss DW. Alkaline phosphatase isoenzymes. Clin Chem 1982;28:2007-16.
119. Moss DW. Changes in enzyme expression related to differentiation and regulatory factors: the acid phosphatase of osteoclasts and other macrophages. Clin Chim Acta 1992;209:131-8.
120. Moss DW. Perspectives in alkaline phosphatase research. Clin Chem 1992;38:2486-92.
121. Moss DW. Physicochemical and pathophysiological factors in the release of membrane-bound alkaline phosphatase from cells. Clin Chim Acta 1997;257:133-40.
122. Moss DW, Edwards RK. Improved electrophoretic resolution of bone and liver alkaline phosphatases resulting from partial digestion with neuraminidase. Clin Chim Acta 1984;143:177-82.
123. Moss DW, Raymond FD, Wile DB. Clinical and biological aspects of acid phosphatase. CRC Crit Rev Clin Lab Sci 1995;32:431-67.
124. Mulichak AM, Wilson JE, Padmanabhan K, Garavito RM. The structure of mammalian hexokinase-1. Nat Struct Biol 1998;5:555-60.
125. Murakami K, Blei F, Tilton W, Seaman C, Piomelli S. An isozyme of hexokinase specific for the human red blood cell (HK_R). Blood 1990;75:770-5.
126. Murakami K, Kanno H, Miwa S, Piomelli S. Human HK_R isozyme: organization of the hexokinase I gene, the erythroid-specific promoter, and transcription initiation site. Mol Genet Metab 1999;67:118-30.
127. Murakami K, Piomelli S. Identification of the cDNA for human red blood cell-specific hexokinase isozyme [see comments]. Blood 1997;89:762-6.
128. Nakajima H, Noguchi T, Yamasaki T, Kono N, Tanaka T, Tarui S. Cloning of human muscle phosphofructokinase cDNA. FEBS Lett 1987;223:113-16.
129. Noe DA. Tissue injury. In: Noe DA, ed. The logic of laboratory medicine, 2nd ed. Baltimore: Urban & Schwarzenberg, 2001.
130. Noguchi T, Inoue H, Tanaka T. The M_1- and M_2-type isozymes of rat pyruvate kinase are produced from the same gene by alternative RNA splicing. J Biol Chem 1986;261:13807-12.
131. Pagani F, Bonora R, Panteghini M. Reference interval for lactate dehydrogenase catalytic activity in serum measured according to the new IFCC recommendation. Clin Chem Lab Med 2003;41:970-1.
132. Pagani F, Panteghini M. 5′-nucleotidase in the detection of increased activity of the liver form of alkaline phosphatase in serum. Clin Chem 2001;47:2046-8.
133. Paglia DE, Valentine WN, Brockway RA. Identification of thymidine nucleotidase and deoxyribonucleotidase activities among normal isozymes of 5′-nucleotidase in human erythrocytes. Proc Natl Acad Sci U S A 1984;81:588-92.
134. Panteghini M. Aspartate aminotransferase isoenzymes. Clin Biochem 1990;23:311-9.
135. Panteghini M. Benign inherited hyperphosphatasemia of intestinal origin: report of two cases and a brief review of the literature. Clin Chem 1991;37:1449-52.
136. Panteghini M. Diagnostic application of CK-MB mass determination. Clin Chim Acta 1998;272:23-31
137. Panteghini M. Electrophoretic fractionation of pancreatic lipase. Clin Chem 1992;38:1712-6.
138. Panteghini M. Hepatic alkaline phosphatase isoenzyme: I. Biochemical and pathophysiological aspects. Giorn It Chim Clin 1990;15:163-71.
139. Panteghini M. Hepatic alkaline phosphatase isoenzyme: II. Clinical aspects. Giorn It Chim Clin 1990;15:301-8.
140. Panteghini M. Lipase. Clin Chem News 1991;17:6-7.
141. Panteghini M. Serum isoforms of creatine kinase isoenzymes. Clin Biochem 1988;21:211-8.
142. Panteghini M, Bonora R, Pagani F. An alternative approach to the prevention of succinyldicholine-induced apnoea. J Clin Chem Clin Biochem 1988;26:85-90.
143. Panteghini M, Bonora R, Pagani F. Automated measurement of mitochondrial aspartate aminotransferase by selective proteolysis with proteinase K. Clin Chem 1993;39:2199-200.
144. Panteghini M, Ceriotti F, Pagani F, Secchiero S, Zaninotto M, Franzini C for the Italian Society of Clinical Biochemistry and Clinical Molecular Biology (SIBioC) Working Group on Enzymes. Recommendations for the routine use of pancreatic amylase measurement instead of total amylase for the diagnosis

and monitoring of pancreatic pathology. Clin Chem Lab Med 2002;40:97-100.

145. Panteghini M, Ceriotti F, Schumann G, Siekmann L. Establishing a reference system in clinical enzymology. Clin Chem Lab Med 2001;39:795-800.
146. Panteghini M, Pagani F. Clinical evaluation of an algorithm for the interpretation of hyperamylasemia. Arch Pathol Lab Med 1991;115:355-8.
147. Panteghini M, Pagani F. Diagnostic value of measuring pancreatic isoamylase with a double-monoclonal antibody immunoassay in serum of hospitalized hyperamylasemic patients. J Clin Lab Analysis 1990;4:449-52.
148. Panteghini M, Pagani F. Reference intervals for two bone-derived enzyme activities in serum: bone isoenzyme of alkaline phosphatase (ALP) and tartrate-resistant acid phosphatase (TR-ACP). Clin Chem 1989;35:181-1.
149. Passon PG, Hultquist DE. Soluble cytochrome b 5 reductase from human erythrocytes. Biochim Biophys Acta 1972;275:62-73.
150. Percy MJ, Gillespie MJ, Savage G, Hughes AE, McMullin MF, Lappin TR. Familial idiopathic methemoglobinemia revisited: original cases reveal 2 novel mutations in NADH-cytochrome b5 reductase. Blood 2002;100:3447-9.
151. Perignon JL, Hamet M, Buc HA, Cartier PH, Derycke M. Biochemical study of a case of hemolytic anemia with increased (85 fold) red cell adenosine deaminase. Clin Chim Acta 1982;124:205-12.
152. Peters J, Hopkinson DA, Harris H. Genetic and non-genetic variation of triose phosphate isomerase isozymes in human tissues. Ann Hum Genet 1973;36:297-312.
153. Pinto PVC, Kaplan A, Van Dreal PA. Aldolase, II: Spectrophotometric determination using an ultraviolet procedure. Clin Chem 1969;15:349-60.
154. Pratt DS, Kaplan MM. Evaluation of abnormal liver-enzyme results in asymptomatic patients. N Engl J Med 2000;342:1266-71.
155. Prins HK, Oort M, Zurcher C, Beckers T. Congenital nonspherocytic hemolytic anemia, associated with glutathione deficiency of the erythrocytes. Hematologic, biochemical and genetic studies. Blood 1966;27:145-66.
156. Price CP. Multiple forms of human serum alkaline phosphatase: detection and quantitation. Ann Clin Biochem 1993;30:355-72.
157. Rabitzsch G, Mair J, Lechleitner P, Noll F, Hofmann U, Krause EG, et al. Immunoenzymometric assay of human glycogen phosphorylase isoenzyme BB in diagnosis of ischemic myocardial injury. Clin Chem 1995;41:966-78.
158. Ranieri E, Ryall RG, Morris CP, Nelson PV, Carey WF, Pollard AC, Robertson EF. Neonatal screening strategy for cystic fibrosis using immunoreactive trypsinogen and direct gene analysis. Br Med J 1991;302:1237-40.
159. Rauscher E, Gerber M. Pancreatic α-amylase assay employing the synergism of two monoclonal antibodies. Clin Chim Acta 1989;183:41-4.
160. Rauscher E, Neumann U, Schaich E, von Bulow S, Wahlefeld AW. Optimized conditions for determining activity concentration of α-amylase in serum, with 1,4-α-D-4-nitrophenylmaltoheptaoside as substrate. Clin Chem 1985;31:14-9.
161. Ravindranath Y, Paglia DE, Warrier I, Valentine W, Nakatani M, Brockway RA. Glucose phosphate isomerase deficiency as a cause of hydrops fetalis. N Engl J Med 1987;316:258-61.
162. Read J, Pearce J, Li X, Muirhead H, Chirgwin J, Davies C. The crystal structure of human phosphoglucose isomerase at 1.6 A resolution: implications for catalytic mechanism, cytokine activity and haemolytic anaemia. J Mol Biol 2001;309:447-63.
163. Rees DC, Duley JA, Marinaki AM. Pyrimidine 5′ nucleotidase deficiency. Br J Haematol 2003;120:375-83.
164. Rees GW, Trull AK, Doyle S. Evaluation of an enzyme-immunometric assay for serum α-glutathione S-transferase. Ann Clin Biochem 1995;32:575-83.
165. Repiso A, Boren J, Ortega F, Pujades A, Centelles J, Vives-Corrons JL, et al. Triosephosphate isomerase deficiency. genetic, enzymatic and metabolic characterization of a new case from Spain. Haematologica 2002;87:ECR12.
166. Ristoff E, Augustson C, Geissler J, de Rijk T, Carlsson K, Luo JL, et al. A missense mutation in the heavy subunit of gamma-glutamylcysteine synthetase gene causes hemolytic anemia. Blood 2000;95:2193-6.
167. Rosa R, Gaillardon J, Rosa J. Diphosphoglycerate mutase and 2,3-diphosphoglycerate phosphatase activities of red cells: comparative electrophoretic study. Biochem Biophys Res Commun 1973;51:536-42.
168. Rosa R, Prehu MO, Beuzard Y, Rosa J. The first case of a complete deficiency of diphosphoglycerate mutase in human erythrocytes. J Clin Invest 1978;62:907-15.
169. Rosa R, Prehu MO, Calvin MC, Badoual J, Alix D, Girod R. Hereditary triose phosphate isomerase deficiency: seven new homozygous cases. Hum Genet 1985;71:235-40.
170. Rosalki SB, Foo AY. Two new methods for separating and quantifying bone and liver alkaline phosphatase isoenzymes in plasma. Clin Chem 1984;30:1182-6.
171. Ruzzo A, Andreoni F, Magnani M. Structure of the human hexokinase type I gene and nucleotide sequence of the 5′ flanking region. Biochem J 1998;331:607-13.

172. Schaller M, Burton DR, Ditzel HJ. Autoantibodies to GPI in rheumatoid arthritis: linkage between an animal model and human disease. Nat Immunol 2001;2:746-53.
173. Schmidt E, Schmidt FW. Enzyme release. J Clin Chem Clin Biochem 1987;25:525-40.
174. Schmidt ES, Schmidt FW. Glutamate dehydrogenase: biochemical and clinical aspects of an interesting enzyme. Clin Chim Acta 1988;43:43-56.
175. Schumann G, Bonora R, Ceriotti F, Clerc-Renaud P, Ferrero CA, Férard G, et al. IFCC primary reference procedures for the measurement of catalytic activity concentrations of enzymes at 37°C. Part 2. Reference procedure for the measurement of catalytic concentration of creatine kinase. Clin Chem Lab Med 2002;40:635-42.
176. Schumann G, Bonora R, Ceriotti F, Clerc-Renaud P, Ferrero CA, Férard G, et al. IFCC primary reference procedures for the measurement of catalytic activity concentrations of enzymes at 37°C. Part 3. Reference procedure for the measurement of catalytic concentration of lactate dehydrogenase. Clin Chem Lab Med 2002;40:643-8.
177. Schumann G, Bonora R, Ceriotti F, Clerc-Renaud P, Férard G, Ferrero CA, et al. IFCC primary reference procedures for the measurement of catalytic activity concentrations of enzymes at 37°C. Part 6. Reference procedure for the measurement of catalytic concentration of γ-glutamyltransferase. Clin Chem Lab Med 2002;40:734-8.
178. Schumann G, Bonora R, Ceriotti F, Férard G, Ferrero CA, Franck PFH, et al. IFCC primary reference procedures for the measurement of catalytic activity concentrations of enzymes at 37°C. Part 4. Reference procedure for the measurement of catalytic concentration of alanine aminotransferase. Clin Chem Lab Med 2002;40:718-24.
179. Schumann G, Bonora R, Ceriotti F, Férard G, Ferrero CA, Franck PFH, et al. IFCC primary reference procedures for the measurement of catalytic activity concentrations of enzymes at 37°C. Part 5. Reference procedure for the measurement of catalytic concentration of aspartate aminotransferase. Clin Chem Lab Med 2002;40:725-33.
180. Schumann G, Klauke R. New IFCC reference procedures for the determination of catalytic activity concentrations of five enzymes in serum: preliminary upper reference limits obtained in hospitalized subjects. Clin Chim Acta 2003;327:69-79.
181. Sebastian S, Wilson JE, Mulichak A, Garavito RM. Allosteric regulation of type I hexokinase: A site-directed mutational study indicating location of the functional glucose 6-phosphate binding site in the N-terminal half of the enzyme. Arch Biochem Biophys 1999;362:203-10.
182. Selker HP, Zalenski RJ, Antman EM, Aufderheide TP, Bernard SA, Bonow RO, et al. An evaluation of technologies for identifying acute cardiac ischemia in the emergency department: a report from a National Heart Attack Alert Program Working Group. Ann Emerg Med 1997;29:13-87.
183. Shi ZZ, Habib GM, Rhead WJ, Gahl WA, He X, Sazer S, et al. Mutations in the glutathione synthetase gene cause 5-oxoprolinuria. Nat Genet 1996;14:361-5.
184. Sierra-Rivera E, Dasouki M, Summar ML, Krishnamani MR, Meredith M, Rao PN, et al. Assignment of the human gene (GLCLR) that encodes the regulatory subunit of gamma-glutamylcysteine synthetase to chromosome 1p21. Cytogenet Cell Genet 1996;72:252-4.
185. Sierra-Rivera E, Summar ML, Dasouki M, Krishnamani MR, Phillips JA, Freeman ML. Assignment of the gene (GLCLC) that encodes the heavy subunit of gamma-glutamylcysteine synthetase to human chromosome 6. Cytogenet Cell Genet 1995;70:278-9.
186. Spielberg SP, Garrick MD, Corash LM, Butler JD, Tietze F, Rogers L, et al. Biochemical heterogeneity in glutathione synthetase deficiency. J Clin Invest 1978;61:1417-20.
187. Stein P, Rosalki SB, Foo AY, Hjelm M. Transient hyperphosphatasemia of infancy and early childhood: clinical and biochemical features of 21 cases and literature review. Clin Chem 1987;33:313-8.
188. Sunderman FW. The clinical biochemistry of 5′-nucleotidase. Ann Clin Lab Sci 1990;20:123-39.
189. Swallow DM, Aziz I, Hopkinson DA, Miwa S. Analysis of human erythrocyte 5′-nucleotidases in healthy individuals and a patient deficient in pyrimidine 5′-nucleotidase. Ann Hum Genet 1983;47 Pt 1:19-23.
190. Takenaka M, Yamada K, Lu T, Kang R, Tanaka T, Noguchi T. Alternative splicing of the pyruvate kinase M gene in a minigene system. Eur J Biochem 1996;235:366-71.
191. Tetrault GA. Lipase activity in serum measured with Ektachem is often increased in nonpancreatic disorders. Clin Chem 1991;37:447-51.
192. Thieme R, Pai EF, Schirmer RH, Schulz GE. Three-dimensional structure of glutathione reductase at 2 A resolution. J Mol Biol 1981;152:763-82.
193. Tietz NW. Support of the diagnosis of pancreatitis by enzyme tests—old problems, new techniques. Clin Chim Acta 1997:257:85-98.
194. Tietz NW, Burlina A, Gerhardt W, Junge W, Malfertheiner P, Murai T, et al. Multicenter evaluation of a specific pancreatic isoamylase assay based on a double monoclonal-antibody technique. Clin Chem 1988;34:2096-102.
195. Tietz NW, Rinker AD, Shaw LM. IFCC methods for the measurement of catalytic concentration of enzymes. Part 5. IFCC method for alkaline phos-

phatase (orthophosphoric-monoester phosphohydrolase, alkaline optimum, EC 3.1.3.1). J Clin Chem Clin Biochem 1983;21:731-48.
196. Tietz NW, Shuey DF. Lipase in serum—the elusive enzyme: an overview. Clin Chem 1993;38:1000-10.
197. Tietz NW, Shuey DF. Reference intervals for alkaline phosphatase activity determined by the IFCC and AACC reference methods. Clin Chem 1986;32: 1593-4.
198. Torrance J, Jacobs P, Restrepo A, Eschbach J, Lenfant C, Finch CA. Intraerythrocytic adaptation to anemia. N Engl J Med 1970;283:165-9.
199. Valentine WN, Paglia DE, Tartaglia AP, Gilsanz F. Hereditary hemolytic anemia with increased red cell adenosine deaminase (45- to 70-fold) and decreased adenosine triphosphate. Science 1977;195:783-5.
200. Valentini G, Chiarelli LR, Fortin R, Dolzan M, Galizzi A, Abraham DJ, et al. Structure and function of human erythrocyte pyruvate kinase. Molecular basis of nonspherocytic hemolytic anemia. J Biol Chem 2002;17:23807-14.
201. Van Deun A, Cobbaert C, Van Orshoven A, Claeys G, Lissens W. Comparison of some recent methods for the differentiation of elevated serum amylase and the detection of macroamylasaemia. Ann Clin Biochem 1989;26:422-6.
202. van Solinge WW, Kraaijenhagen RJ, Rijksen G, van Wijk R, Stoffer BB, Gajhede M, et al. Molecular modelling of human red blood cell pyruvate kinase: structural implications of a novel G_{1091} to a mutation causing severe nonspherocytic hemolytic anemia. Blood 1997;90:4987-95.
203. van Wijk R, Rijksen G, Huizinga EG, Nieuwenhuis HK, van Solinge WW. HK Utrecht: missense mutation in the active site of human hexokinase associated with hexokinase deficiency and severe nonspherocytic hemolytic anemia. Blood 2003;101:345-7.
204. van Wijk R, van Solinge WW, Nerlov C, Beutler E, Gelbart T, Rijksen G, et al. Disruption of a novel regulatory element in the erythroid-specific promoter of the human PKLR gene causes severe pyruvate kinase deficiency. Blood 2003;101:1596-1602.
205. Visnapuu LA, Karlson LK, Dubinsky EH, Szer IS, Hirsch CA. Pediatric reference ranges for serum aldolase. An J Clin Pathol 1989;91:476-7.
206. Von Eyben FE. A systematic review of lactate dehydrogenase isoenzyme 1 and germ cell tumors. Clin Biochem 2001;34:441-54.
207. Vora S. Isozymes of human phosphofructokinase: biochemical and genetic aspects. Isozymes Curr Top Biol Med Res 1983;11:3-23.
208. Vulliamy TJ, Luzzatto L. Glucose-6-phosphate dehydrogenase deficiency and related disorders. In: Handin RI, Lux SE, IV, P. ST, eds. Blood. Principles and practice of hematology. second ed. Philadelphia: Lippincott Williams & Wilkins, 2003:1921-50.
209. Walker JI, Morgan MJ, Faik P. Structure and organization of the human glucose phosphate isomerase gene (GPI). Genomics 1995;29:261-5.
210. Wang C, Chiarelli LR, Bianchi P, Abraham DJ, Galizzi A, Mattevi A, et al. Human erythrocyte pyruvate kinase: characterization of the recombinant enzyme and a mutant form (R510Q) causing nonspherocytic hemolytic anemia. Blood 2001;98:3113-20.
211. West JD. A genetically defined animal model of anembryonic pregnancy. Hum Reprod 1993;8: 1316-23.
212. West JD, Flockhart JH, Peters J, Ball ST. Death of mouse embryos that lack a functional gene for glucose phosphate isomerase. Genet Res 1990;56: 223-36.
213. Whitelaw AG, Rogers PA, Hopkinson DA, Gordon H, Emerson PM, Darley JH, et al. Congenital haemolytic anaemia resulting from glucose phosphate isomerase deficiency: genetics, clinical picture, and prenatal diagnosis. J Med Genet 1979;16:189-96.
214. Whitfield JB. Gamma glutamyl tranferase. CRC Crit Rev Clin Lab Sci 2001;38:263-355.
215. Whitten RO, Chandler WL, Thomas MGE, Clayson KJ, Fine JS. Survey of α-amylase activity and isoamylases in autopsy tissue. Clin Chem 1988;34:1552-5.
216. Wijnen LM, Monteba-van Heuvel M, Pearson PL, Meera Khan P. Assignment of a gene for glutathione peroxidase (GPX1) to human chromosome 3. Cytogenet Cell Genet 1978;22:232-5.
217. Wilson JE. Hexokinases. Rev Physiol Biochem Pharmacol 1995;126:65-198.
218. Xu W, Lee P, Buetler E. Human glucose phosphate isomerase: exon mapping and gene structure. Genomics 1995;29:732-9.
219. Yuan PM, Talent JM, Gracy RW. Molecular basis for the accumulation of acidic isozymes of triosephosphate isomerase on aging. Mech Ageing Dev 1981;17:151-62.
220. Yubisui T, Miyata T, Iwanaga M, Tamura M, Takeshita M. Complete amino acid sequence of NADH-cytochrome b5 reductase purified from human erythrocytes. J Biochem (Tokyo) 1986;99:407-22.
221. Zanella A, Bianchi P. Red cell pyruvate kinase deficiency: from genetics to clinical manifestations. Baillieres Best Pract Res Clin Haematol 2000;13: 57-81.

CHAPTER 22

Cytokines

*Manuel Santos Rosa, Ph.D., and Anabela Mota Pinto, Ph.D.**

Cytokines are peptides used by cells for intercellular communication and for controlling the inner environment of the cells in which they operate.[30,576] They are produced by cell types that have important roles in the immune response, inflammation, hemopoiesis, healing, and systemic response to injury. Many cytokines are measured by bioassay and immunoassay.[212]

This chapter begins with a background discussion of cytokines followed by discussions of some important cytokines. The chapter concludes with a discussion of the analytical aspects of cytokine measurement.

BACKGROUND INFORMATION

History

The evolution of cytokines as molecules of major biological significance[437] can be divided into four different periods—each is characterized by different technical capacities and scientific purposes.[1,526] For example, initial studies in the 1950s to the 1970s identified a number of cellular protein molecules that had specific functions. Cohen and others[94] first suggested the word "cytokine" to describe these molecules. In the 1970s several cytokines were partially purified and characterized, and specific antibodies against them were produced. The 1980s are considered by many to be the golden age of cytokine research because many individual cytokines were discovered and cloned and specific monoclonal antibodies against them produced. In the 1990s new genetic techniques (e.g., gene knockout and transgenic animals) were developed that led to a better understanding of the biological roles of cytokines and to the production and availability of large amounts of recombinant cytokines for use in therapeutic trials. The development of this deoxyribonucleic acid (DNA) technology has produced evidence for a large number of defined peptides that carry signals for activity, growth, and differentiation of a wide variety of cells.

Initially four groups of molecules were distinguished by either their biological function or by the origin of their scientific discovery.[526] They include (1) lymphocyte-derived proteins (lymphokines and monocyte-derived proteins [monokines]); (2) antiviral interferons (IFNs) and agents; (3) hematopoietic growth factors (colony stimulating factors); and (4) nonhematopoietic growth factors. However, it was quickly found that a redundancy of function occurred both within and between those groups. This led to the view that these molecules act in a network, and their individual functions are often difficult to assess in vivo. Ongoing studies continue to discover and identify additional molecules involved in the communication between cells, and it is now known that we are dealing with a wider and more heterogeneous group of molecules than was once supposed.

Rationale for Measurement

Cytokines are increasingly being measured for clinical applications.[212] Reasons for doing so include:

1. Cytokines are directly implicated in various pathophysiological conditions in humans, and their increased production is responsible for their elevated levels in different body fluids, including blood, synovial fluid, cerebrospinal fluid, amniotic fluid, and bronchoalveolar lavage fluid.
2. Cytokine concentrations reflect the severity of some diseases and are markers of prognosis. This is particularly applicable for infectious diseases (bacterial sepsis and parasitological infections) and immune disorders (autoimmune diseases, such as rheumatoid arthritis[88] and systemic lupus erythematosus, and allergic diseases, such as asthma and skin hypersensitivity).

*The authors gratefully acknowledge the contributions by Drs. Jacques Bienvenu and John Whicher on which portions of this chapter are based.

TABLE 22-1 Cytokines and Their Designations (Abbreviations)

BDNF	Brain-derived neurotrophic factor
CKs	**Chemokines***
CNTF	Ciliary neurotrophic factor
EGF	Epidermal growth factor
Epo	Erythropoietin
FGF	Fibroblast growth factor
FLt3L	Fetal liver tyrosine kinase 3
G-CSF	Granulocyte colony stimulating factor
GM-CSF	Granulocyte-macrophage colony–stimulating factor
IFNα	Interferon α (type I interferon)
IFNβ	Interferon β (type I interferon)
IFNγ	Interferon γ (type II interferon)
IGF	Insulin-like growth factor
IL-1 to IL-18	**Interleukins 1 to 18**
LIF	Leukemia inhibitory factor
M-CSF	Monocyte/macrophage colony stimulating factor
MIF	Migration inhibition factor
NGF	Nerve growth factor
NT-3, NT-4	Neurotrophin-3, neurotrophin-4
OSM	Oncostatin M
PDGF	Platelet-derived growth factor
SCF	Stem cell factor
TGFα	Transforming growth factor α
TGFβ	Transforming growth factor β
TNFα	Tumor necrosis factor α
TNFβ	Tumor necrosis factor β
TPO	Thrombopoietin
VEGF	Vascular endothelial growth factor

*Highlighted cytokines are individually discussed later in the chapter.

3. Clinical trials involving antiinflammatory cytokines or cytokine inhibitors (anticytokines, monoclonal antibodies, and soluble receptors) require the monitoring of cytokines during the course of these treatments.
4. Kits for cytokines quantification are commercially available.

General Characteristics

Many of the more important cytokines are listed in Table 22-1. Most of these have multiple effects as demonstrated by the multiplicity and diversity of effects that they elicit. These effects depend on the responding cell type, biological network, and assay system in use.[472] Also the same molecule produced from different cells may exert a completely different biological action that may be opposite or even unrelated. In fact, the biological activity originally attributed to one cytokine may now be shown to be shared by several different molecules (redundancy), leading to the concept that very few individual cytokines are essential for basic cellular function. For example, knockout animals—lacking a specific cytokine gene—have only subtle abnormalities in their immunoinflammatory reaction. Biological networks are dependent on the influence of one cytokine on the synthesis of other cytokines (positive or negative regulatory mechanisms on cytokine cascades) and on biological activity (enhancing, suppressing, or synergic effects). This leads to modulation mechanisms often connected to the outcome of beneficial or harmful biological effects from a particular pathological event.

The functional modulation of the effect of cytokines requires the presence of cellular and soluble receptors. The expression of these receptors is regulated by specific signals, often dependent on cytokine networks. Transiently produced and of short half-life, cytokines are typically not stored as preformed molecules, and their production is dependent on transient genetic transcriptional activation and short-lived messenger ribonucleic acid (mRNA). Cytokines are rapidly secreted, leading to a brief burst of cytokine release. This burst is very important for cytokines to achieve distant activities, contrasting with the small amount of these molecules necessary for local functions (see later section on interleukin-1).

Biologically, many cytokines have what appears to be an endocrine function, especially when they are released in large quantities. They also exhibit autocrine and paracrine functions because they usually have a short radius of action (Figure 22-1). However, there is an enormous difference between these molecules and the hormones. For example, hormones are produced continuously, although with variation in concentration, and cytokines are usually produced only after the action of an activation signal and for other reasons previously mentioned. In addition, the receptors for cytokines are often of high affinity but are expressed with a low density on cell membranes.

Nomenclature

Cytokines are difficult to define because they encompass different families of molecules with regulatory functions that operate on receptors and are linked only by common biological actions. Here, we define cytokines as low molecular weight proteins (often glycosylated), with a cellular regulatory action, that are produced by different cells and operating preferentially in the immunoinflammatory response. Physiologically, cytokines (1) are produced by and operate on different types of cells, (2) act locally or at a distance, (3) operate in a network, and (4) are repressed or modified by various mechanisms (Figure 22-2).

Classification

Because cytokines were discovered in several different scientific disciplines and are functionally diverse—their classification, like their definition—has been exceedingly difficult.[319] However, they have been classified by their (1) function (Box 22-1),[1,432,436] (2) family group (Box 22-2),[152,421,472,485] and (3) physiochemical structure (Table

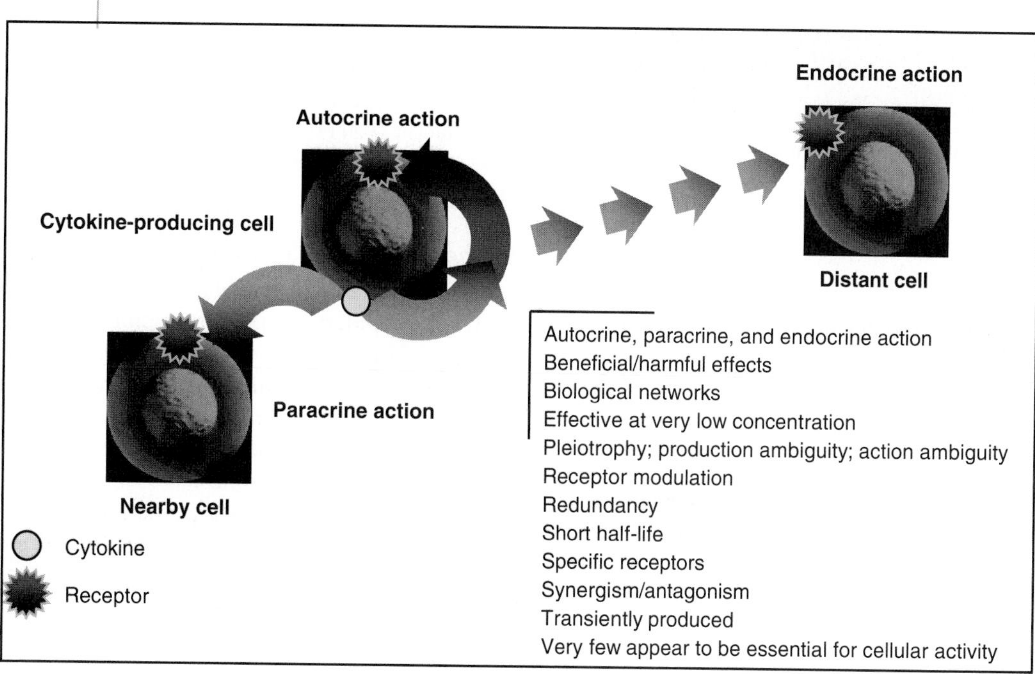

Figure 22-1 Principal functional characteristics of cytokines.

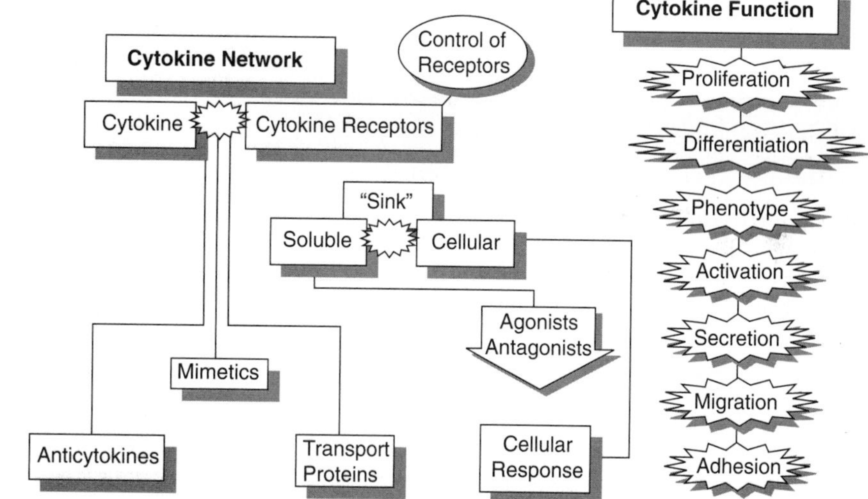

Figure 22-2 Cytokine network and generic function over cells.

22-2).[341,389] Currently, from a practical viewpoint, cytokines are classified as belonging to (1) hemopoietin, (2) interferon, (3) tumor necrosis factor (TNF), or (4) chemokine families.

Biochemistry

Cytokines have very stable structures with the presence of carbohydrates and disulfide bonds imparting solubility, stability, and resistance to cleavage. Despite the lack of amino acid sequence similarity, the limited variation in their overall three-dimensional structure may reflect the evolutionary origins of cytokines. This structural variation has made possible the definition of at least the following four different structural families.[389]

Four-α-Helical Bundles

Molecules having this structure constitute the largest family of cytokines. These molecules have an antiparallel four-α-helical bundle structure (A, B, C, and D helices, A-D and B-C helix pairs). The A-D helix pair frequently represents the region that interacts with the appropriate receptors.

This family includes two subtypes:

1. Short-chain (Sc subtype): interleukin (IL)-2, IL-3, IL-4, IL-5, IL-7, IL-9, IL-13, granulocyte-macrophage colony–stimulating factor (GM-CSF), monocyte/macrophage colony–stimulating factor (M-CSF), stem cell factor (SCF), IFNγ

BOX 22-1 Classification of Cytokines by Function[1]

Cytokines That Mediate Natural Immunity
Type I IFN
TNF
IL-1, IL-6
Chemokines

Cytokines That Regulate Lymphocyte Activation, Growth, and Differentiation
IL-2
IL-4
TGFβ

Cytokines That Regulate Immune-Mediated Inflammation
IFNγ
Lymphotoxin
IL-5, IL-10, IL-12
Migration inhibition factor (MIF)

Cytokines That Stimulate Hematopoiesis
C-Kit ligand
IL-3, IL-7
GM-CSF, M-CSF, G-CSF, other CSFs

BOX 22-2 Elgert's Classification of Cytokines by Family Group[152]

Interleukins: IL-1α, IL-1β, IL-2 to IL-15
Chemokines: IL-8, MCP-1
Interferons: IFNα, IFNβ, IFNγ
Cytotoxic/immunomodulatory/growth factors: TNFβ, TNFα, TGFβ
Colony stimulating factors: G-CSF, GM-CSF, IL-3, IL-7, M-CSF

2. Long-chain (Lc subtype): IL-6, IL-12, Epo, granulocyte colony–stimulating factor (G-CSF), leukemia inhibitory factor (LIF), oncostatin M (OSM), ciliary neurotrophic factor (CNTF), IL-11, GH, IFNα, IFNβ, IL-10

The Sc subtype has a general oblate ellipsoid shape and the Lc subtype an overall elongated cylindrical shape.

Short-Chain α/β Structures

This family has three subfamilies:

1. The epidermal growth factor (EGF) subfamily of cytokines produced as large transmembranar precursor molecules containing at least one EGF domain in the extracellular region. This domain consists of at least two antiparallel β-strands connected to the intervening loops by three disulfide bonds.
2. The chemokine (CK) subfamily of cytokines with a general conformation of an open-face β-sandwich with a C-terminal α-helical segment, divided into three major subgroups based on the amino acid sequence around the conserved cysteine residues.
3. The insulin-related subfamily of cytokines consisting of a conserved set of three disulfide bonds that link three short α-helices.

Long-Chain β-Sheet Structures

This family has three subfamilies:

1. The TNF subfamily of cytokines (TNFα, TNFβ, CD27, and Fas ligand). The members of this subfamily are often cell surface–associated symmetrical homotrimers of which subunits have a conformation of β-jelly rolls. The homotrimer is cone shaped, which may explain the inactivity of isolated monomers and the symmetry of three receptor subunits interacting with the TNF trimer.
2. The IL-1 and the fibroblast growth factor (FGF) subfamilies of cytokines. These molecules adopt a β-trefoil fold, which consists of 12 strands of β-sheet forming six hairpins. They are synthesized with no leader sequence

TABLE 22-2 Classification by Physicochemical Structure of Cytokines and Their Receptors[341,389]

Cytokine	Cytokine Structure	Receptor-Specific Component	Shared Chain
IL-2	6-α-helical short chain	Hemopoietin domain	Common ϖ
IL-4, IL-7, IL-9, IL-13, IL-15	4-α-helical short chain	Hemopoietin domain	Common γ
IL-3, IL-5, GM-CSF	4-α-helical short chain	Hemopoietin domain	Common β
IFNγ	4-α-helical short chain	IFNγR	—
IL-6, IL-11	4-α-helical long chain	Hemopoietin domain	gp130
G-CSF	4α-helical long chain	—	G-CSF-R
TGFβ	β-sheet	Serine/threonine kinase	—
IL-1 α, IL-1β	β-sheet	Ig-like	—
TNFα, TNFβ, CD40L, CD27L, FASL	β-sheet	TNF p75, p55	—
Chemokines	—	Rhodopsin	—

(unlike most other cytokines), and their mechanism of secretion remains unclear.

3. The platelet-derived growth factor (PDGF), transforming growth factor β (TGFβ), and nerve growth factor (NGF) subfamilies of cytokines show β-sheet–rich structures known as cystine knots, which are characterized by an interlocking set of three disulfide bridges and at least four segments of twisted antiparallel β-sheets corresponding to an elongated asymmetric monomer. Usually, each of these growth factors forms a homodimeric complex with a different orientation of the monomers in each type of homodimer.

Mosaic Structures

This family is more heterogeneous than the other three, with diverse members such as heregulins or neuregulins, glial growth factor (GGF), hepatocyte growth factor (HGF), and IL-12.

The heregulins are cell surface proteins with both an EGF and an immunoglobulin (Ig)-like domain on the extracellular side of the molecule; GGF has both an EGF domain and a kringle domain. HGF is a heterodimer with the α-subunit containing four kringle domains (typical of plasminogen) and the β-subunit having homology to serine proteases. IL-12 is a heterodimer with the α-subunit similar to the long-chain, four-α-helical bundle cytokines and the β-subunit overlapping the complementary hemopoietin domain receptor.

Cytokine Receptors

Cytokine receptors represent the functional link between cytokines and target cells and the resultant biological action.

Studies have shown them to be structurally very heterogeneous, and generally confined to five main families of proteins (Table 22-3).

TABLE 22-3 Cytokine Receptor Families and Their Cytokines

Cytokine Receptor Family	Cytokines
Immunoglobulin superfamily	IL-1, M-CSF, C-kit
Class I cytokine receptors (hematopoietin)	IL-2, IL-3, IL-4, IL-5, IL-6, IL-7, IL-9, IL-11, IL-12, IL-13, IL-15, G-CSF, GM-CSF, OSM, LIF, CNTF, growth hormone, prolactin
Class II cytokine receptors (Interferon)	IFNα, IFNβ, IFNγ, IL-10
TNF receptors	TNFa, TNFb, CD40, NGF, FAS
Chemokine receptors	Chemokines

The most important receptors for the immunoinflammatory response are the Class I and Class II receptors; however, the TNF and the chemokine receptors also are biologically important. The Class I and Class II receptors share some characteristics, such as having multiple subunits—one that binds the cytokine and another that mediates signal transduction—with tyrosine phosphorylation of the receptor occurring through the activity of protein tyrosine kinases. The Class I cytokine receptors bind the largest number of cytokines associated with immuno- and hematopoietic systems and are divided into three receptor subfamilies with identical signal-transduction subunits. However, this subunit is shared by different cytokines, explaining the redundancy and antagonism exhibited by some of these molecules. The three subfamilies are the (1) common β-subunit(receptor for GM-CSF, IL-3, and IL-5), (2) common gp130 subunit (receptor for IL-6, IL-11, CNTF, and LIF/OSM), and (3) common γ-subunit (receptor for IL-2, IL-15, as heterotrimers; IL-7, IL-9, and IL-4, as classical two-subunit receptors with a common γ-chain).

Clinical Significance

Because of their diverse biological functions, cytokines have been implicated in a number of pathological conditions, including the inflammatory process and cancer. The clinical significance of individual cytokines is discussed below.

Cytokines and the Inflammatory Process

The immunoinflammatory system is a complex network of cells and humoral elements that includes many cytokines (Figure 22-3). Typically an immunoinflammatory response is triggered by an antigen. The antigen is presented by specialized cells termed antigen-presenting cells (APCs), which present the antigen through either class I or II restrictions of the major histocompatibility complex (MHC). In the case of class I restriction, molecules of antigen are presented to CD8 T lymphocytes. In class II restriction, molecules of antigen are presented to CD4 T lymphocytes (usually referred to as "helpers"). In addition, molecules of antigen can be presented by B lymphocytes (CD19) or can present directly to Tγδ lymphocytes, with a consequent cytotoxic and cytolytical response.[475]

After antigenic presentation to CD4 and CD8 cells, there is a set of effects on other lymphocytes in which the suppressive ability on the proliferation of B lymphocytes is enhanced through CD8 cells. This prevents them from becoming plasma cells and ensures that they produce antibodies. In the case of CD4 (as classical "helpers"), they stimulate B lymphocytes and consequently their conversion into plasma cells and the production of antibodies.

CD4 lymphocytes have two subtypes: T helper (Th)1 and Th2 (Figure 22-4). Th2 is the common CD4 "helper" that "helps" B lymphocytes to be transformed into plasma cells, leading to the production of antibodies. Th1 lymphocytes are implied in a cytotoxic and cytolytical process similar to that developed by CD8 cells, which are not only classical sup-

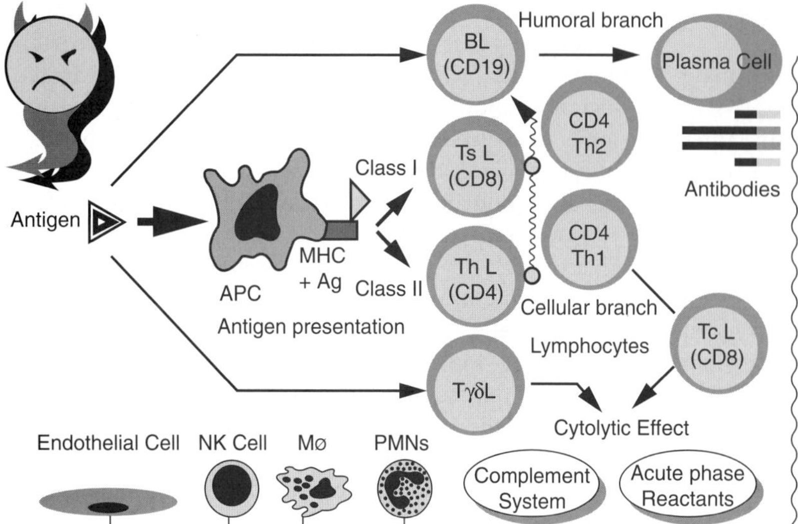

Figure 22-3 Role of cytokines in the immunoinflammatory response.

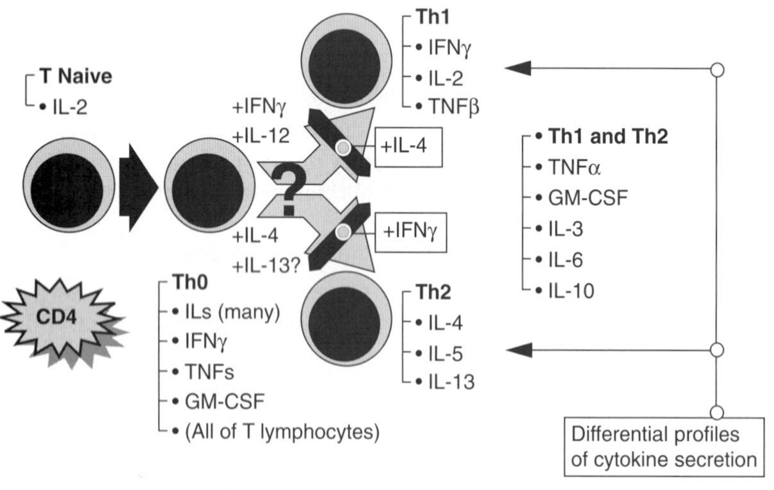

Figure 22-4 Role of cytokines in the polarization of CD4 lymphocytes.

pressors of B lymphocytes but also have cytotoxic ability. Therefore they have an essential role in the cellular polarization, leading to either cytotoxicity or the production of antibodies. The differentiation of Th1 and Th2 cells is based on the local microenvironment of cytokines. Cascades of cytokines are always present during the interactions between antigen-presenting cells and lymphocytes and also in CD4 Th1 and Th2 polarization.

In addition to the lymphocytes, many other cells participate in the immunoinflammatory process, including endothelial cells, natural killer (NK) cells, and macrophages. The complement system and the acute phase proteins are also involved in the amplification of the inflammatory process.

The transformation of CD4 lymphocytes into Th1 or Th2 subtypes is currently thought to be the central stage of the immune response (see Figure 22-4). These cells can polarize into Th1 or Th2 cells according to the cytokines contained in the microenvironment in which the cells are stimulated. For example, in an environment rich in IFNγ and IL-12, there is a Th1 polarization, and in an environment rich in IL-4 (and eventually IL-13), there is Th2 polarization. The kind of cytokine environment reciprocally inhibits the other transformation (i.e., IL-4 blocks the Th1 transformation and IFNγ blocks Th2 transformation).

When CD4 lymphocytes are transformed into Th1 or Th2 subtypes, they produce a characteristic cytokine profile (Figure 22-5) that includes IFNγ, IL-2, and TNFβ for Th1 and IL-4, IL-5, and IL-13 for Th2. TNF, GM-CSF, IL-3, IL-6, and IL-10 are common to both types of cells.

Figure 22-6 represents a general scheme of the development of human CD4 Th1 cells. Typically, there is Th1 polarization when antigenic stimulation is caused by a virus or intracellular bacteria (intracellular pathogen) followed by antigenic presentation from specialized cells such as dendritic cells, with a high production of IFNα and IL-12. The activation of NK cells then creates a high concentration of IFNγ without an increase in levels of IL-4. Thus an environ-

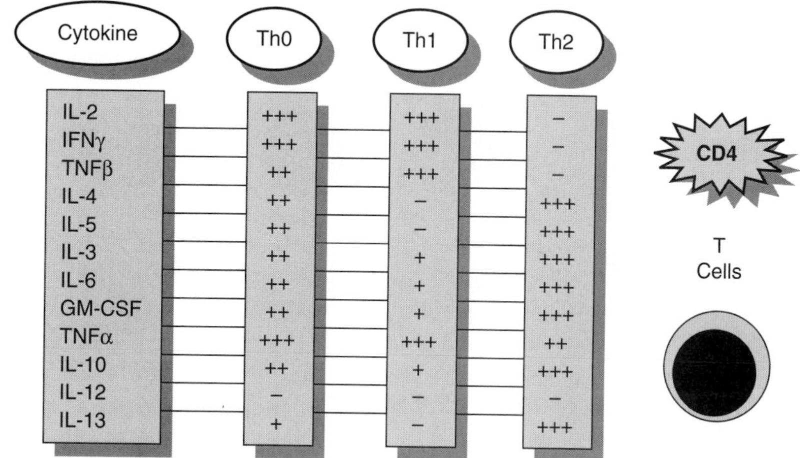

Cytokine	Th0	Th1	Th2
IL-2	+++	+++	–
IFNγ	+++	+++	–
TNFβ	++	+++	–
IL-4	++	–	+++
IL-5	++	–	+++
IL-3	++	+	+++
IL-6	++	+	+++
GM-CSF	++	+	+++
TNFα	+++	+++	++
IL-10	++	+	+++
IL-12	–	–	–
IL-13	+	–	+++

Figure 22-5 Secretion profiles of cytokines from human CD4 T cells. (See Table 22-1 for identification of cytokines.)

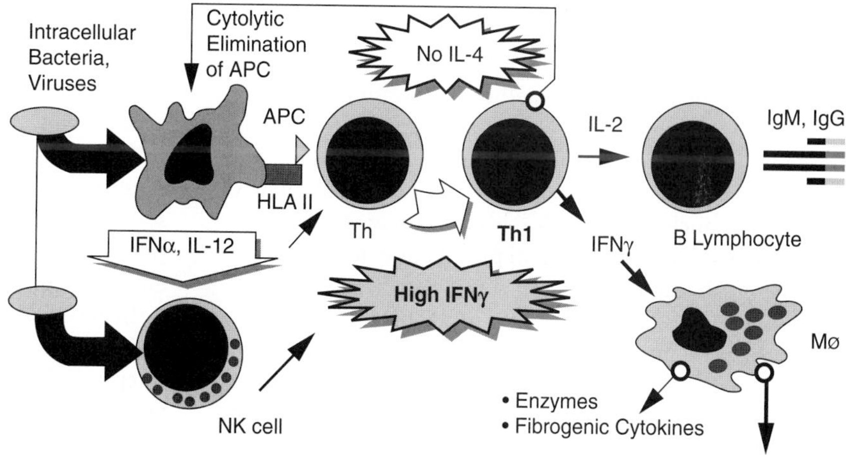

Figure 22-6 Preferential development of human CD4 Th1 cells.

ment rich in IFNγ and poor in IL-4 causes Th1 polarization, which induces a low production of antibodies (usually IgG and IgM). It also causes a cytokine-induced stimulation of phagocytic cells, such as macrophages and polymorphonuclear neutrophils (PMNs) with enzyme and cytokine release boosting the inflammatory reaction. This kind of response is the classic delayed type of hypersensitivity, which is very important for an effective response to intracellular pathogens.[42,316]

Figure 22-7 summarizes the Th2 polarization, which usually occurs because of antigenic stimulation by allergens or extracellular antigens like helminthic (parasite) antigens. This stimulation is associated with a lack of IL-12 and IFNγ production by APCs and the absence of NK activation. However, it is dependent on mast cells and basophils, which are involved in IL-4 synthesis. Thus there is an environment rich in IL-4 (increased by the spontaneous endogenous production of this cytokine) and poor in IFNγ.

An important Th2 cell-specific transcription factor is c-maf, which promotes the differentiation of Th2 cells mainly by an IL-4–dependent mechanism. It remains unclear whether c-maf possesses any IL-4–independent function in regulating the production of Th2 cytokines; c-maf, independent of IL-4, is essential for normal induction of the IL-2 receptor (IL-2R) α (CD25) in developing Th2 cells. The levels of CD25 are remarkably higher in developing Th2 cells than in developing Th1 cells during in vitro differentiation. In addition, timely blockade of IL-2–receptor signaling selectively inhibits the production of Th2 cytokines, but not IFNγ or IL-2. Taken together, they uncover an IL-4–independent and CD25-mediated function of c-maf in promoting the production of Th2 cytokines.[324] Th2 polarization then causes stimulation of B lymphocytes and the production of all classes of Igs (particularly IgE). There is also the stimulation of eosinophils, namely by IL-5, with activation and proliferation of these cells useful against parasitic infections. This kind of response (especially through the high production of IgE) is commonly called the immediate type of hypersensitivity and is associated with atopy.[103,200,264,496]

Cytokines that stimulate the innate immune response are not constitutively expressed but must be induced to function

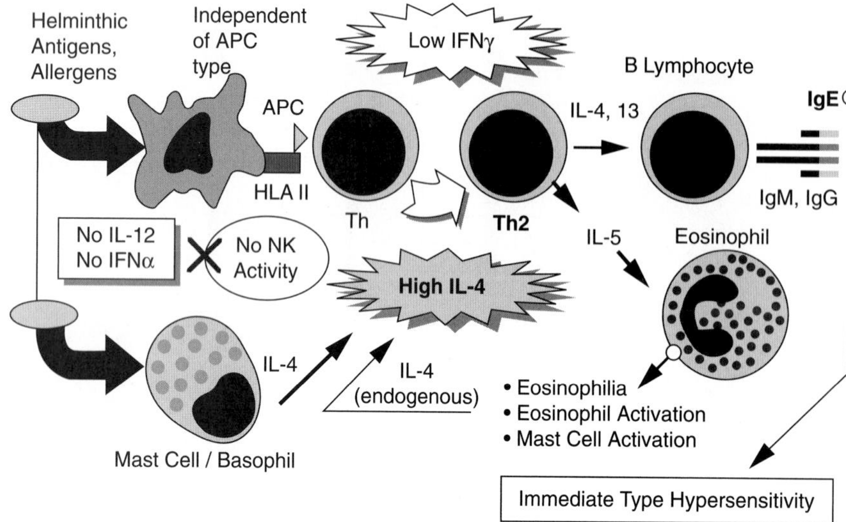

Figure 22-7 Preferential development of human CD4 Th2 cells.

by specific signals that alert the host to invading microorganisms. Toll-like receptors (TLRs) are important signaling receptors in innate host defense with a signal-transduction pathway via a MyD88-dependent pathway, which ultimately involves the nuclear factor-κB (NF-κB) family of transcriptional factors that are involved in proinflammatory cytokine expression. NF-κB serves as a master switch, transactivating various cytokines that are involved in the innate and transition to adaptive immunity: IL-1, IL-6, and IL-8. In addition, TLR4 signal transduction and NF-κB transactivation induces expression of IL-12 p40 and CD80 and CD86, which are co-stimulatory molecules that link innate and adaptive immune responses by activating antigen-specific responses by naive T cells.[414,499] Measurement of the activation of NF-κB may help to predict the outcome of sepsis, for example.[14]

Subsequent findings indicate that cytokines—in part mediators of this "overwhelming" inflammatory reaction, may also stimulate bacterial growth, impair bacterial clearance, and promote the subsequent development of nosocomial infections—may have important implications for the management of the inflammatory syndromes, such as the acute lung injury and/or acute respiratory distress syndrome patient. The interaction between cytokines and bacteria may be an important factor in the development of organ injury and death from severe infections, although numerous host and local factors, including inflammatory cells, profoundly influence the role of a specific cytokine.[130,271,458]

Cytokines regulate activation, differentiation, growth, death, and acquisition of effector functions of various cell types.[246] As a result they are increasingly recognized as important factors in the pathophysiology of chronic heart failure. Inflammatory cytokines may modulate cardiovascular functions by a variety of mechanisms. Cytokines such as TNFα and IL-1β have been shown to depress myocardial contractility. This may be due to the uncoupling of β-adrenergic signaling, an increase in cardiac nitric oxide, or alterations in intracellular calcium homeostasis. TNFα and members of the IL-6 family may also induce structural changes in the failing myocardium, such as cardiomyocyte hypertrophy and interstitial fibrosis. Additionally, TNFα and IL-1β may promote cardiomyocyte apoptosis and activate metalloproteinases and impair the expression of their inhibitors, possibly contributing to cardiac remodeling.[115]

In 2004 Okun and colleagues studied the role of cytokines and growth hormone in the regulation of sleep and narcolepsy. Collectively, proinflammatory cytokines and human growth hormone (HGH), were found to be possibly involved in the development of or the exacerbation of narcolepsy (a disabling neurological sleep disorder characterized by excessive daytime sleepiness and abnormal sleep manifestations). As the role of the immune system in sleep becomes clearer, a better interpretation will be available to assess why narcoleptics have altered cytokine and HGH levels. Future studies should be conducted to fully characterize the sources, patterns, and significance of alterations in patterns of proinflammatory cytokines and HGH in narcolepsy.[397]

Cytokines and Cancer

Cytokines have assumed an increasing importance in cancer biology since the early observations in 1893 of William Coley, who showed that a variety of malignant tumors regressed following infection with certain bacteria. The cytokine revolution of the 1970s led to the supposition that the reasons for this were the release by bacterial endotoxin of tumor inhibitory cytokines, such as the IFNs and TNFs. It is now known that cytokines are involved in the malignant process in a number of ways.

Cancers are a very heterogeneous group of diseases, and the mechanisms of malignant transformation and continuation are very diverse in different tumors; nonetheless, they represent diseases in which intercellular signaling mechanisms have been damaged so as to remove the normal constraints on cellular growth and replication. In many cases, cytokines form part of these control mechanisms or induce other molecules that perform these functions. For example, some proto-oncogenes and oncogenes code for normal or abnormal components of cytokine receptor or signal transduction pathways.

Cytokines may have growth inhibitory properties directly on cancer cells, cause tumor regression because of modification of the host tumor relationship, or enhance antitumor immune effects. They may also act as growth factors for malignant cells, and thus therapeutic strategies to inhibit their action become possible. They may also mediate paraneoplastic effects.

Cytokine-provided survival signals are known to suppress apoptosis through inhibition of mitochondrial pathways that involve Bcl-2 family members. It was also discovered that IFNγ-TNFα synergism, rather than the Fas ligand as currently believed, is responsible for the apoptosis in cancer cell deaths.[307]

In hematopoietic cells, cytokines also regulate death receptor–mediated pathways. Hematopoietic cytokines, such as IL-3 and erythropoietin in normal cells and BCR-ABL oncoprotein in transformed cells, inhibit transcription of tumor necrosis factor–related apoptosis-inducing ligand (TRAIL). The inhibition of TRAIL function is sufficient to partially rescue cytokine-deprived cells from apoptosis. Cytokine and BCR-ABL suppression of TRAIL transcription is mediated through phosphorylation and inhibition of the forkhead FOXO3a transcription factor. BCR-ABL-induced inhibition of TRAIL transcription in hematopoietic cells may provide a novel mechanism for tumorigenicity in chronic myeloid leukemia.[188]

From the perspective of the clinical laboratory, the measurement of cytokines in biological fluids may be useful for monitoring progression of some tumors and for therapeutic monitoring when they are used as anticancer agents.

Regulation of Growth and Differentiation

Because of their growth inhibitory properties, IFNs have assumed great importance in the search for tumor-modifying cytokines. In addition, they can down regulate the expression of cellular proto-oncogenes, such as *myc,* the enzymes associated with DNA replication, and the receptors for growth factors, such as EGF. They may also activate cytotoxic T cells in vivo.

The therapeutic use of IFNα has been evaluated in many clinical trials and it has received approval from the U.S. Food and Drug Administration for use in hairy cell leukemia (HCL), the myeloid leukemias, and a range of solid tumors. It is only in HCL, with median response rates of about 90%, that it is clearly superior to conventional chemotherapy; however, there is considerable interest in including it as a part of multiparameter treatment with chemotherapy, radiotherapy, and surgery for other cancers.

TGFβ blocks the growth-promoting effects of cytokines such as EGF, PDGF, and the FGFs, and many malignant cells both produce and respond to it. A negative autocrine loop thus controls proliferation. In breast cancers, the cells often produce TGF but lose their ability to respond.[55]

IL-6 inhibits the growth of a variety of human cell lines derived from malignant tumors of breast, ovary, and myeloid cells, but it also has a dramatic effect in reducing tumor load in mice transplanted with several murine tumors, an effect that is largely lost if the animals are rendered immune deficient. Conversely, IL-6 is a potent growth factor for plasmacytoma and myeloma cells, and it has been shown that freshly isolated human myeloma cells from patients produced IL-6 in culture, indicating the possibility of an autocrine loop promoting growth in this cancer. Additional evidence also supports a paracrine role for IL-6, with production in myeloma arising not only from the myeloma cells but also from adherent stromal cells in the bone marrow. It is thus of great interest that monoclonal antibodies to IL-6 have shown an effect in retarding tumor growth in early trials.

Cytokines such as IL-6 and TNF also have an important role in regulating estrogen synthesis in peripheral tissue, including normal and malignant breast tissue. The activities of the aromatase, estradiol 17-hydroxysteroid dehydrogenase, and estrone sulfatase enzymes are all increased by IL-6 and TNF. Macrophages and lymphocytes, which invade many breast tumors, are thought to be an important source of factors such as cytokines that can modulate estrogen synthesis in malignant breast tissue.[426]

The incidence of breast cancer is reduced in immunosuppressed women.[426] Because cytokine production is also reduced in immunosuppressed women, this finding supports the concept that cytokines have an important role in breast cancer, possibly acting via stimulation of estrogen synthesis.[426]

Toxicity for Tumor Cells

The TNFs inhibit tumor cell growth by a direct cytotoxic effect, inhibit proliferation, and induce differentiation.[405] The mechanisms are arachidonic acid dependent and may involve the production of oxygen free radicals, which destroy the tumor cell DNA. These molecules have potent antitumor activities in murine models caused by direct inhibition of growth, immunomodulation, and effects on the vascular system. Unfortunately, extensive trials in human malignancies have been very disappointing, largely caused by dose-limiting toxicity when TNF is administered systemically, although isolated limb perfusion and intratumor injection appear promising. TNF can also stimulate growth of some malignant cells.

Modification of Host-Tumor Relationship, Local Spread, and Metastasis

In addition to the effects described previously, TNF also exhibits protumor effects. Transplanted ovarian carcinoma cells in nude mice possess an enhanced ability to invade peritoneal surfaces and metastases following transfection with

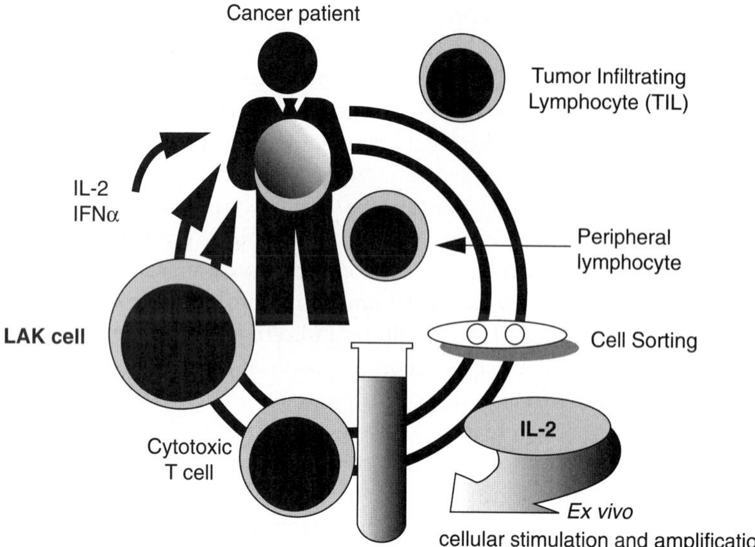

Figure 22-8 Generation of LAK cells in the laboratory.

the human TNFα gene. This suggests more subtle effects (e.g., on the production of adhesion molecules).

Because the control of metastasis is critical to the control of cancer progression, two chemokine receptors and their ligands stand out as likely targets for therapeutics: CCR7/CCL21 for lymph node metastases, and CXCR4/CXCL12 for lung, liver, bone marrow, and brain metastases.[601] It has been reported that the CXC chemokine receptor 4 (CXCR4) and its ligand CXCL12, also known as stromal cell–derived factor 1, or SDF-1, together govern the pattern of breast cancer metastasis.[375,601] In this study, it was suggested that metastatic cancer cells simply use signals that normally control leukocyte transport. Chemokines and their ligands represent one of the more important of these signals because they can be secreted by virtually all types of cells, but in different amounts and combinations. The synthesis of most requires inflammatory signals, whereas a few, such as CXCL12, are molecules of "resting" cells in virtually all organs. Specific combinations of chemokines, chemokine receptors or ligands, and adhesion molecules form a spatial and temporal code that determines which subgroups of human cells migrate and where they migrate.[378]

Immune Response to Tumor

The tumor-suppressor roles of cytokines include many regulatory effects on the immune system. The IFNs enhance the expression of MHC class I antigens on many different normal and malignant types of cells, making them susceptible to killing by cytotoxic T cells.

IL-2 stimulates peripheral blood lymphocytes, rendering a subpopulation of them more cytotoxic for tumor cells. This subpopulation of cells is known as lymphokine-activated killer cells (LAK cells) and probably form part of the NK cell population, which may be responsible for immune surveillance of potentially malignant cells. IL-2 is used therapeutically intravenously or subcutaneously, and in renal cell carcinoma and melanoma gives responses much better than chemotherapy. LAK cells may be stimulated ex vivo using lymphocytes derived from plasmapheresis and reinfused into the patient (Figure 22-8). For still greater specificity, tumor infiltrating lymphocytes (TILs) may be extracted and stimulated. Significant toxicity limits the dose of IL-2.

Tumor infiltrating lymphocytes are very important in immune competence against cancer. A study reported in 2003 demonstrated remarkable differences in the distributions of progression-free survival and overall survival according to the presence or absence of intratumoral T cells.[595] The 5-year overall survival rate was 38.0% among patients with epithelial ovarian cancer whose tumors contained T cells and 4.5% among patients whose tumors contained no T cells in islets. The presence of intratumoral T cells independently correlated with delayed recurrence or delayed death in multivariate analysis and was associated with increased expression of IFN-γ, IL-2, and lymphocyte-attracting chemokines within the tumor. The absence of intratumoral T cells was associated with increased levels of vascular endothelial growth factor.

IL-12 has been shown in animal studies to have potent antitumor and antimetastatic activity, probably by its actions stimulating Th1 cells and inducing IFNγ production.

Cytokines in most cases modulate tumor-specific inhibition dependent on direct lytic activity of cytotoxic CD8 T cells or on polarization of CD4 T cells. But tumor eradication also depends on noncytotoxic CD4 and CD8 lymphocytes releasing high amounts of proinflammatory cytokines that recruit distinct effector leukocytes at the tumor site. This series of events emphasizes the cytokine action in the tumor site upon several distinct cell types and immunoinflammatory mechanisms. However eradication of established tumors involves distinct mechanisms, each endowed with a different curative potential and not only cytokines.[108,486]

Mediation of Paraneoplastic Effects

Many hormonal, neurological, hematological, and other clinical and biochemical disturbances associated with malignant neoplasms (paraneoplastic effects) are considered to be mediated by cytokines. For example, the fever that so often accompanies cancer is mediated by IL-6, IL-1, and TNF and typically occurs in lymphoid malignancies in which these cytokines are released. Anemia may be mediated by TNF, thrombocytosis by IL-6, and cachexia by TNF and IFNγ. Bone reabsorption and hypercalcemia are induced by IL-1.

Cytokines and the Diagnosis of Tumors

A number of situations are emerging in which the measurement of cytokines may provide clinically useful information about prognosis and response to treatment of tumors. For example, great interest has surrounded the role of serum IL-6 measurements in assessing the prognosis in myeloma and in distinguishing it from monoclonal gammopathies of undetermined significance (MGUS). IL-6 levels are elevated in a higher proportion of patients with myeloma and correlate broadly with disease activity, proliferation index, and survival. Patients with MGUS generally have normal or low levels of IL-6, but unfortunately studies have not shown sufficient discrimination to be clinically useful in distinguishing these important conditions. In Hodgkin's disease and non-Hodgkin's lymphoma, there is a correlation between symptoms of fever and malaise (B symptoms) and IL-6 level; raised levels also predict a poorer prognosis. In studies of renal cancer, colorectal cancer, and melanoma, baseline C-reactive protein (CRP) or IL-6 levels have been shown to be related to response to treatment with IL-2, with responders having lower concentrations before therapy and a much greater increase during therapy. Elevated concentrations of the soluble IL-2 receptor (sIL-2R) have been found in a number of malignancies, in particular those of the lymphoid system and the leukemias. In children with acute lymphoid leukemia, raised levels predict relapse and correlate with survival. This is probably also true of adult HCL and T-cell leukemia, suggesting that the use of sIL-2R measurements could have a place in the management of the hematological malignancies. Of the solid tumors, lung cancer has attracted particular attention because raised levels may relate to survival and disease status following treatment, and tend to be higher in small cell lung cancer.

TNF expression or protein production has been demonstrated in many cancer cell lines and biopsies. For example, in ovarian and breast cancers, TNF mRNA or protein has been found in 50% to 70% of the tumors studied. Serum TNF and sTNFR levels are raised in a wide range of malignancies, and their measurement may be useful in follow-up studies.

A high proportion of patients with hematological malignancies have increased levels of the cytokine M-CSF that have been shown to relate to disease type, status, and response to therapy. In addition, elevated levels of this cytokine have been observed in ovarian cancer and have been found to correlate with disease status following treatment. In practice, there is great interest in the use of M-CSF together with CA125 as an index of therapy in this difficult cancer.

A number of the growth factors, such as the IGFs, PDGF, and the TGFs, show raised serum concentrations in various cancers. TGFα is of interest in that it is almost invariably raised in breast cancer irrespective of stage and was higher in the sera of patients with hepatocellular cancer than in normal subjects or those with hepatitis or cirrhosis. This growth factor is excreted in the urine, and urinary levels are often raised in head and neck cancer and may sometimes be useful for monitoring treatment.

INDIVIDUAL CYTOKINES

The structure, function, and clinical significance of many individual cytokines have been extensively studied. In this section, cytokines that are highlighted in Table 22-1 are individually discussed.

INTERLEUKIN-1

Interleukin-1 (IL-1) is a predominantly macrophage-produced interleukin, which mediates the host inflammatory response in innate immunity; two principal forms exist, designated α and β, with apparently identical biological activity. At low concentrations, IL-1 principally acts to mediate local inflammation, causing mononuclear phagocytes and endothelial cells to synthesize leukocyte activating chemokines. At high concentrations, IL-1 enters the blood stream and acts as an endocrine hormone, in some actions resembling TNF by its ability to cause fever, initiate hepatic synthesis of acute phase proteins, and induce cachexia.[138]

Synonyms

IL-1 has also been known as B cell–activating factor, catabolin, endogenous pyrogen, epidermal cell–derived thymocyte activating factor, fibroblast activating factor, hemopoietin-1, hepatocyte stimulating factor (HSF), leukocyte endogenous mediator, lymphocyte activating factor, mononuclear cell factor, osteoclast activating factor, proteolysis inducing factor, and serum amyloid A inducer.

General Characteristics

The IL-1 family has three members: IL-1α, IL-1β, and the IL-1 receptor antagonist (IL-1RA or IL-1γ), all three acting on the same receptors. The structures of the three molecules are related to a limited extent. There is a 20% sequence homology between the two forms of IL-1, which are encoded by two different genes; however, IL-1α and IL-1β are agonists, with IL-1RA being an antagonist having more similarities with IL-1β. The IL-1 family is also related structurally to FGF. Both forms (IL-1α and IL-1β) are stable tetrahedral globular proteins (bowl-like structure)[71] and are processed at the cell membrane or extracellularly to give the mature molecule.[152]

Most of the IL-1 activity in plasma is from IL-1β, IL-1α existing mainly in an intracellular or membrane-associated form.[1,152,437] IL-1 shares many of its functions with TNF, but important differences between IL-1 and TNF exist. For example, IL-1 is in general not toxic, and TNF is a potent cytotoxic effector (see the Biological Actions of TNF section). One of their shared functions is the induction of expression of the vascular cell adhesion molecule (VCAM) by endothelial cells. Studies have indicated that TNF may be more important than IL-1 in induction of VCAM expression at least in the nasal mucosa.[568]

Other general characteristics of IL-1 include:

Molecular Weight

Literature values for the molecular weights of IL-1, IL-1α, and IL-1β vary from 17 to 17.5 kDa.* The molecular weight of the IL-1 receptor core has been reported to be 17 kDa, with three distinct glycosylated forms (18, 22, and 22 kDa).[389]

Cross-Reactivity

The cross-reactivities (amino acid sequence homology between human and mouse) for IL-1 and its receptor include IL-1α (62%), IL-1β (68%), and IL-1RA (77%).[71]

Chromosomal Location

The chromosomal locations of IL-1 and its receptors are 2q12-21 (IL-1α), 2q13-21 (IL-1β), 2q12 (IL-1R type I), and 2q12-22 (IL-1R type II).

Cellular Origin

Activated mononuclear phagocytes are the major cellular sources of IL-1, but almost all nucleated cells are capable of secreting IL-1α and IL-1β after stimulation (Figure 22-9). Also, important sources of IL-1 are classical antigen-presenting cells, including monocytes and macrophages, Langerhans' cells, dendritic cells, B lymphocytes, endothelial cells, T cells, NK cells, astrocytes, keratinocytes, and fibroblasts.[71,152]

*References 1, 71, 152, 341, 389, 421, 436.

Control of Synthesis and Release

Mature forms of IL-1 depend on proteolytic cleavage of precursor forms (prointerleukin-1) into the cytoplasm. Mature molecules and IL-1α precursor are biologically active, but IL-1β precursor is inactive. Activation of this latent form is produced by proteases (such as serine proteases), appropriate proteases from monocytes and/or macrophages, chymase in mast cells, and an aspartate-specific protease called IL-1 converting enzyme (ICE).[341] Normally IL-1 synthesis and secretion occur after cellular stimulation (Box 22-3), but IL-1α is present constitutively in large amounts as a preformed biological response modifier in epithelial cells, such as keratinocytes in the skin, sweat, urine, and amniotic fluid. Damage or stimulation of these cells results in the liberation of enormous amounts of active IL-1.[472] Prointerleukin-1β (pro-IL-1β) is the only known physiological substrate of the ICE. The structural similarities of ICE with a nematode gene, *ced*-3, which initiates a cell death program, suggest that IL-1 could be released from macrophages during apoptosis.[341] Pro-IL-1β has been demonstrated to be a substrate of ICE that is relevant to cell death, and depending on the temporal cellular commitment to apoptosis, mature IL-1β may function as a positive or negative mediator of cell death.[174] However, IL-1β also suppresses apoptosis in CD34 positive bone marrow cells through activation of the IL-1 receptor type I and the subsequent production of endogenous GM-CSF.[444] Following lipopolysaccharide (LPS) stimulation of monocytes, intracellular activity of IL-1 is detected in 30 minutes, extracellular IL-1 activity is detected in 60 minutes, and high levels occur in 3 hours.[152] Urate or silicate

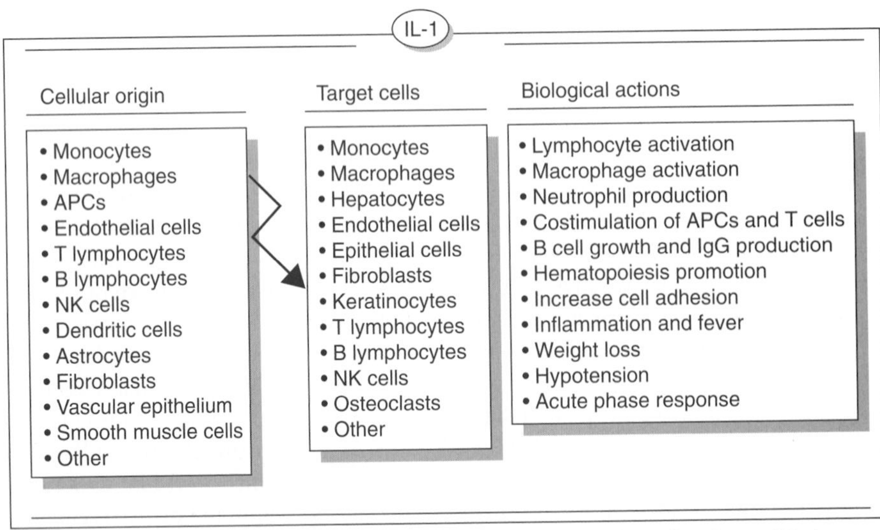

Figure 22-9 Cellular origin, principal target cells, and biological actions of IL-1.

particles and adjuvants, such as aluminum hydroxide, are other external stimuli for cells to produce IL-1. Concerning the regulation of ICE, a cowpox virus inhibitor known as cytokine response modifier A (CRMA) has been described that inhibits the host inflammatory response through the inhibition of ICE.[71] IL-1RA is synthesized by the same cells that secrete IL-1, and an intracellular form has been identified.[71]

Prostaglandins, a class of lipid-derived inflammatory mediators, can also regulate IL-1 expression; for example, IL-1 production by macrophages is enhanced by leukotrienes, but is suppressed by products of the cyclooxygenase pathway, such as prostaglandin (PG) E2 (PGE2). Increased circulating levels of IL-1 are also observed during the luteal phase of the menstrual cycle[268,297,550,556] and during strenuous exercise.

Proteases that activate the precursor forms of IL-1 belong to a class of highly specific cellular proteases termed *caspases*. The number of enzymes in this family of proteases keeps growing, with new members continually being identified and a unified nomenclature being proposed. All caspases share two key features: They require an aspartic acid at the cleavage site, and they are all synthesized as proenzymes that are activated by cleavage at aspartate residues at sites resembling their own targets. This raises the possibility of autoprocessing and transactivation among caspases. This has been shown to be the case for activation of caspase-1 (ICE) by caspase-4, caspase-3 by caspase-1, and caspase-3 and caspase-7 by caspase-10.[347]

IL-4 and IL-10 are inhibitors of IL-1 synthesis, as are glucocorticoids that are produced in response to IL-1, and may represent a feedback mechanism of IL-1 secretion.[437] Multiple stimuli are likely to operate in vivo to promote IL-1β posttranslational processing, such as anion transport inhibitors.[418]

Genetic deletion of IL-1 receptors results in the overproduction of IL-1 mRNA in organs known to produce cytokines during pancreatitis, even when the severity of pancreatitis is lessened. This suggests that a negative feedback loop exists between the IL-1 receptor and IL-1 gene expression.[394]

BOX 22-3 Inducers of IL-1 Synthesis and Secretion[90,152,187,442]

Microbial

- Bacterial endotoxin of gram-negative bacteria—LPS
- Exotoxins, cell walls, muramyl dipeptide (MDP), protein-A
- Yeast cell walls (zymosan)
- Virus-hemagglutinin, double-stranded RNA
- EBV*

Immunoinflammatorial†

- Activated T lymphocytes
- Immune complexes
- Complement C5a
- Leukotrienes
- Platelet activating factor (PAF)
- TNF and IL-6 (their own synthesis and secretion are enhanced by IL-1)
- CRP

Other

- Silica and asbestos particles
- Urate crystals
- Phorbol myristate acetate (PMA)
- UVB radiation (on keratinocytes)

*EBV induces a rapid accumulation of IL-1 and IL-1RA mRNA in neutrophils that was associated with the later appearance of considerable amounts of IL-1α, IL-1β, and IL-RA proteins. The elevated levels of IL-1RA detected for EBV-stimulated neutrophils might be part of a mechanism used by the virus to evade the immune system.

†The cytokine cascade IL-1, TNF, and IL-6 is responsible for many cellular events that are present in acute inflammation, and almost all the inflammatory mediators are enhancers of IL-1 secretion. Also IFNγ and GM-CSF prime cells for IL-1 release after exposure to inducers.

Receptors (IL-1R)

There are two types of IL-1 receptors (Figure 22-10): type I (CDw121a, 80 kDa) and type II (Cw121b, 60 kDa). They are transmembrane glycoproteins and members of the Ig superfamily that bind IL-1α, IL-1β, and IL-1RA. They are profusely distributed on a variety of cell types,[71,152,341] but only type I receptor (IL-1RI) provides intracellular signal. Type II receptor (IL-1RII) acts as an IL-1 regulator (antagonist or decoy receptor). IL-1RI is expressed mainly by T cells, B cells, eosinophils, fibroblasts, endothelial cells, some cells of the nervous system, and muscle cells (25 to 1000 receptors per cell) and IL-1RII by B lymphocytes, activated T lymphocytes, monocytes, neutrophils, eosinophils, placental cells, endothelial cells, fibroblasts, some cells of the nervous system, and megakaryocytes (200 to 8000 receptors per cell).[152,437]

The type I receptor has a large cytoplasmic domain and transmits signals when it binds IL-1; the signaling pathway is not fully known, but shares some components with those

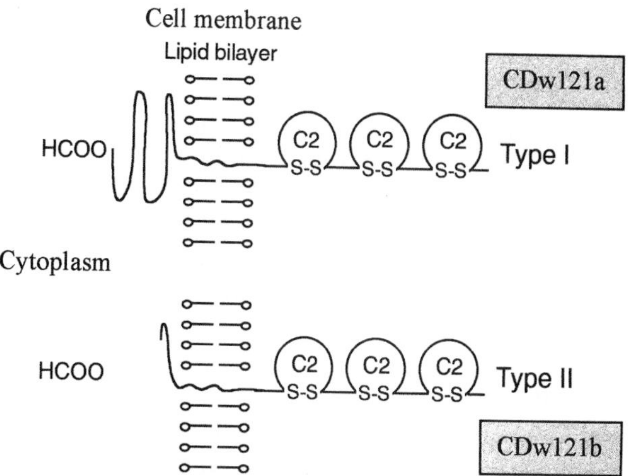

Figure 22-10 Illustrations of the type I and II receptors of IL-1.

used by the IL-18 and TLR families. Binding to as few as five copies of IL-1RI on a cell can be sufficient to produce a response.

A fibroblast may carry several thousand IL-1 receptors; resting T cells express as few as 50, but this number increases after activation. Binding leads to endocytosis of IL-1 together with its receptor.

The biological activity of IL-1 is regulated by IL-1 itself (it enhances synthesis and secretion of IL-1 but suppresses expression of IL-1 receptors); IL-1RII; PGE2, which suppresses IL-1 production and IL-1RA; and TGFβ, which abrogates the immunoinflammatory effects of IL-1. However, the principal functional inhibitor of IL-1 is IL-1RA, acting as a competing molecule for IL-1 receptors. The production of this antagonist is increased by GM-CSF, IL-4, IL-10, and TGFβ. A 1996 study found that IL-1RA is also a common regulatory product of inflammatory macrophages (involved in types 1 and 2 granulomas) and is particularly promoted by CD4 Th1 cytokines, IFNγ, and TNFα.[449] A soluble receptor found in normal human serum has also been described that binds preferentially to IL-1β.[71]

The type II receptor has a small cytoplasmic domain and cannot transduce signals. The extracellular domain of IL-1RII is released in soluble form at sites of local inflammation and into the serum during times of systemic inflammation. This soluble IL-1RII is produced in relatively large amounts, binds IL-1β much more strongly than it binds IL-1α or IL-1RA, and functions as an endogenous inhibitor of IL-1β. Both soluble and cell-associated forms of IL-1RII have therefore been called IL-1 decoy receptors.

Signal Transduction

IL-1 induces hydrolysis of phosphatidylethanolamine (but not other phospholipids), which will release diacylglycerol (DAG) and activate protein kinase C (PKC) without releasing calcium. It has also been reported to activate a G-protein–regulated adenyl cyclase.[71] Association of IL-1 with Janus protein tyrosine kinase signal transducers and activators of transcription (JAK-STAT) signaling has remained unresolved. Tsukada and co-workers have reported an element termed LPS and IL-1–responsive element in the human prointerleukin-1β gene that can be immediately induced by either LPS or IL-1 protein to bind a tyrosine-phosphorylated protein.[539] This LPS and IL-1–induced factor (LIL-factor) is recognized by an antibody raised against the N terminus of STAT1 but not by those specific for either the C terminus of STAT1 or any other gamma interferon activation (GAS)–binding STAT. Moreover, the unique DNA-binding specificity and antigenicity of this factor suggest that LPS, IL-1, and IL-6 may use a common signaling pathway.

Biological Actions

IL-1 plays a central and primary role in the inflammatory response and tissue repair, and weak evidence supports an action of IL-1 as a physiologically important co-stimulator of mature T lymphocyte activation.[1] In a review,[129] Dinarello reports that investigators have studied how production of the different members of the IL-1 family is controlled, the various biological activities of IL-1, the distinct and various functions of the IL-1R family, and the complexity of intracellular signaling. Special attention is paid to IL-1β converting enzyme and programmed cell death (apoptosis). The role of IL-1 in hematopoiesis, leukemia, atherosclerosis, and growth of solid tumors is also discussed.

Systemically, IL-1 exerts a biological effect at the level of a single cell and also has indirect effects (Table 22-4). Its biological activities depend on the quantity of cytokine released.[1] At low concentration, it acts as a mediator of the local immunoinflammatory reaction, inducing a cascade of secondary cytokines in a large number of types of cells (macrophages, endothelial cells, fibroblasts, synovial cells, and keratinocytes), enhancing leukocyte and/or endothelial cell adhesion, and inducing CD4 T-cell proliferation and B-cell growth and differentiation. The latter demonstrates its potential for functional autocrine pathway activation mediated by IL-1α and suggests that the level of expression of IL-1RI may function as a significant control point in physiological IL-1 mediated autocrine pathways.[202] At high concentration, IL-1 diffuses into the blood and subsequently exerts an endocrine action on the brain, liver, adrenals, and other organs; it acts as an endogenous pyrogen, inducing fever, stimulating the synthesis of acute phase proteins, and inducing cachexia. The exact (paracrine) endocrine role of IL-1 on the peripheral immune system, namely on T cells, is not well characterized, but it is known to affect the cell cycle. It regulates IL-2 production (increasing the density and affinity of IL-2 receptors and increasing the production of IL-2). Generally, it seems that every cell, immunoinflammatory or not, is affected by IL-1.[152] The main importance for immunity, however, seems to lie in its ability to enhance the activation of T helper lymphocytes by APCs. IL-1 acts in an autocrine manner to induce or increase expression of various adhesion molecules, IFNγ receptors, and class II MHC proteins on the APC surface and so increase the efficiency with which the APC can bind and activate Th cells.

Dendritic cells are highly effective APCs capable of stimulating the differentiation of naive lymphocytes into effector cells. Specific properties of the dendritic cells determine the quality of immune responses that they initiate. IL-1 and IL-1Ra play a biologically relevant role in the positive and negative regulation of dendritic cell activation. In conjunction with CD40L, IL-1 sends a powerful activation signal to dendritic cells that could be distinguished from other modes of activation. This signal enables the production of proinflammatory cytokines by dendritic cells, and enhances the differentiation of naive T cells into effectors of type 1 cellular immune responses.[573]

IL-1 plays an important role in the pathophysiological responses to infection and inflammation, in part by mediating its own production and that of other proinflammatory cytokines. However, the relative contribution of IL-1α and

TABLE 22-4 Biological Activity of IL-1

Target	Biological Activity
Single Cell Level	
Thymocytes	Proliferation
T lymphocytes	Production of IL-2 and IFN; induction of IL-2 receptors; proliferation, adhesion, inhibition of IL-4 synthesis
Pre-B lymphocytes	Differentiation and expression of IgM
B lymphocytes	Proliferation and antibody production
NK cells	Activation of cytotoxicity
Macrophages	Secretion of IL-1 and prostaglandin (PGE2), chemotaxis, cytotoxicity
PMN neutrophils	Enzyme release; oxidative burst; chemotaxis; production of collagenase
Endothelial cells	Proliferation; synthesis of TNF and IL-6; angiogenesis; prostaglandin synthesis; procoagulant activity; VCAM and E-selectin expression
Epithelial cells	Proliferation; production of collagen, type IV
Keratinocytes	Proliferation; secretion of TNF, IL-6, and GM-CSF
Fibroblasts	Proliferation; secretion of IL-6, collagen, collagenase, and PGE2
Osteoclasts	Bone resorption and calcium release; collagenase synthesis
Chondrocytes	Cartilage breakdown and proteoglycan release; plasminogen activator; prostaglandin and collagenase synthesis
Synovial cells	Proliferation; prostaglandin and collagenase synthesis
Muscle cells	Amino acid oxidation and proteolysis; prostaglandin synthesis
Hepatocytes	Increase in acute phase protein synthesis
Systemic Effects	
Brain	Prostaglandin synthesis; fever; somnolence; anorexia
Adrenals	Induction of ACTH and glucocorticoid production
Blood	Granulocytosis
Bone marrow	Stimulation of hematopoiesis; release of neutrophils into the blood; potentiation of CSFs
Pancreas	Insulin secretion
Body (in general)	Cachexia
Indirect Effects	From cytokine cascades, especially from TNFα and IL-6, through synergy with other cytokines, such as GM-CSF*

From references 1, 90, 152, 349, 457, 528, 568.

*Antigen-presenting cells (APC) can up regulate GM-CSF production through IL-1b and through CD28 triggering by B7 molecules. As GM-CSF itself up regulates B7 expression and IL-1β production by APC, a bidirectional regulatory feedback pathway between APC and T cells seems to modulate GM-CSF production.[229]

IL-1β to the inflammatory response has not been elucidated. This suggests that either IL-1β is not essential for the in vivo systemic response to LPS or that its role can be fulfilled by other cytokines with overlapping activities.[158]

Clinical Significance

IL-1 has been implicated in the pathogenesis of (1) rheumatoid arthritis (RA), (2) septic shock, (3) periodontitis, (4) malignancy, (5) asbestosis, (6) tuberculosis, and (7) human immunodeficiency virus (HIV) infection. Its presence has also been correlated with disease activity or differential diagnosis (synovial fluids, gingival fluids, or even serum). For example, patients with nonallergic bronchial asthma were characterized by increased levels of IL-1β and IL-6 produced by monocytes.[274,368]

IL-1 gene expression is selectively induced in tissue involved in multisystem organ failure during acute pancreatitis, suggesting a role in the pathogenesis of distant organ dysfunction.[394] Acute eosinophilic pneumonia is characterized by locally high levels of IL-5, IL-1RA, and soluble type II IL-1 receptor in the alveolar space.[6] IL-1 has also been found to be associated with inflammatory intestinal diseases, which induce intestinal epithelial cells to produce several cytokines and acute phase proteins (APP) during an inflammatory response. Little is known about the type of IL-1R expressed by intestinal epithelial cells and the effect of cytokines on the expression of these receptors. However, down regulating the expression of the type I IL-1R was suggested as a possible mechanism to limit the effect of IL-1 on intestinal epithelial cell function during the mucosal inflammatory response.[354] Systemic inflammation induces an enhancement of melanoma cell metastasis and growth by IL-1–dependent mechanisms in vivo. In vitro, the mechanism(s) is consistent with IL-1–mediated increase in expression of mannose receptors and production of tumor cell growth factor(s) from the endothelium.[555] Tuberculosis is characterized by a cellular immune response mediated by various cytokines, including IL-1β released by stimulated mononuclear cells. It has been established that IL-1β plays an important role in local and systemic inflammatory response in tuberculosis.[360] In patients with diffuse panbronchiolitis, the relative amounts of IL-1β and IL-1RA or IL-8 may contribute to the neutrophil-mediated chronic airway inflammation.[249] HIV-infected individuals have experienced episodes of localized or systemic bacterial infections caused by gram-negative bacteria associated with the production of proinflammatory cytokines. For example, antiinflammatory cytokines inhibit LPS plus GM-CSF–stimulated HIV expression, and this effect closely correlates with inhibition of IL-1β release and, in particular, with up regulation of endogenous IL-1RA production. Thus the balance between an endogenously produced viral inducer (IL-1β) and an inhibitor (IL-1RA) may represent an important pathway leading to modulation of HIV expression from monocytic cells.[193]

Therapeutic Applications

IL-1 may be useful in protecting patients against lethal doses of radiation and in the stimulation of hematopoiesis. However, the therapeutic application of IL-1 that had generated the greatest interest is the development of anti-IL-1 therapies using either IL-1RA, soluble IL-1R, or other antagonists capable of an antiinflammatory and immunosuppressive effect. Although not very effective, IL-1 has been used in RA and septic shock.[88] Curiously, short-term use of inhibitors of cyclooxygenase (that blunts PGE2-mediated symptoms, such as fever and pain), such as aspirin or ibuprofen, does not decrease IL-1 but results in a "rebound" increase in cytokine-induced cytokine synthesis (IL-1, IL-2, IL-6, TNF, and GM-CSF).[155] Also, anion transport inhibitors—such as tenidap—that suppress cytokine processing independently of the initiating stimulus are attractive candidates as therapeutic regulators of IL-1 production.[418] IL-1 also plays a strategic role in the growth of cancer cells in inflammatory tissue; because IL-1RA is without side effects in humans, studies on intraoperative infusion of IL-1RA during tumor resection may be indicated.[555] The use of IL-1 in humans is associated with dose-limiting toxicity that resembles that of TNFα or IL-2. Activation of neutrophils is thought to contribute to the toxicity caused by these two cytokines but, unlike TNF, IL-1 does not cause neutrophil degranulation in humans, despite its ability to cause neutrophilia and the rapid release of IL-6, IL-8, and nitrite and/or nitrate.[395]

INTERLEUKIN-2

Interleukin-2 (IL-2) is an interleukin produced by T cells in response to antigenic or mitogenic stimulation, acting to regulate the immune response. It (1) stimulates the proliferation of T cells and the synthesis of other T-cell–derived cytokines, (2) stimulates the growth and cytolytic function of NK cells to produce LAK cells, (3) is a growth factor for and stimulates antibody synthesis in B cells, and (4) may promote apoptosis in antigen-activated T cells. IL-2 is used as an anticancer drug in the treatment of a wide variety of solid malignant tumors.[138]

Synonym

IL-2 has also been known as T-cell growth factor (TCGF).

General Characteristics

IL-2 is a globular protein composed of six α-helical regions (A, B, C, D, E, and F) with a disulfide bridge.[71] IL-2 contains variable amounts of carbohydrate in its molecular structure. However, the carbohydrate does not appear to affect the biological function of IL-2.[472] The polypeptide structure of IL-2 consists of 133 amino acid residues with one intramolecular disulfide bridge between residues 58 and 105.[152] Native IL-2 is folded into a globular protein containing two sets of paired parallel α-helices, each sheet oriented at a slight angle to the other. This α-helical folding motif is common to several cytokines, including IL-3, IL-4, IL-5, IL-6, IL-7, GM-CSF, and G-CSF with the WSXWS (tryptophan-serine-X-tryptophan-serine, where X stands for a variable amino acid residue) motif in the amino acid sequence of their receptors.[1]

This cytokine was discovered in the supernatants of T-cell cultures that had been stimulated by antigens or mitogens, such as phytohemagglutinin (PHA). The recognition of IL-2 as a growth and proliferation factor for lymphocytes (namely T cells) made it possible to grow and expand infected T cells for extended periods of time. This allowed the characterization of human T-lymphotropic virus type 1 (HTLV-1) and HIV.[485]

IL-2 represents the most important signal for clonal expansion of T cells. This is achieved by the binding of IL-2 to the high-affinity receptors expressed only by the activated T lymphocytes producing IL-2 (autocrine action) or by nearby activated T or B lymphocytes (paracrine action). Resting T and B cells are limited to the expression of the intermediate affinity receptor. IL-2 does not circulate in the blood at high levels during physiological immune responses and consequently does not act as an endocrine growth factor.[1,152]

Other general characteristics of IL-2 follow:

Molecular Weight

Depending on the degree of glycosylation, literature values for the molecular weight of IL-2 vary from 14 to 23 kDa.[1,71,152,389,472]

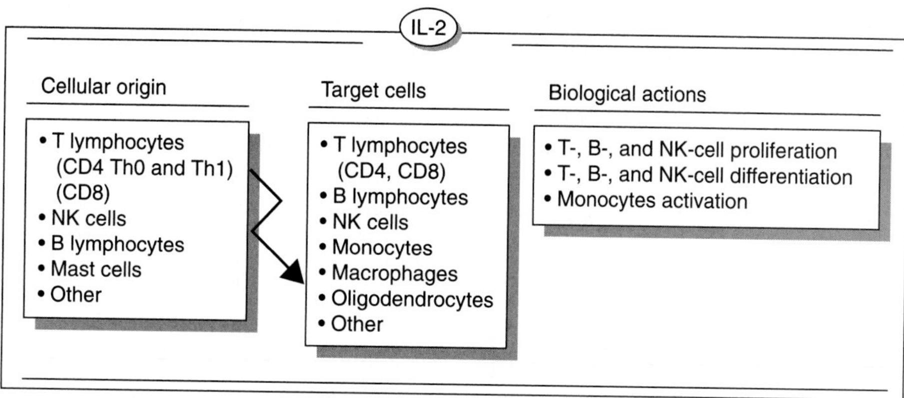

Figure 22-11 Cellular origin, principal target cells, and biological actions of IL-2.

Cross-Reactivity

The cross-reactivity (amino acid sequence homology between human and mouse) for IL-2 is 60%.[71] Human IL-2 is active on mouse lymphocytes, but mouse IL-2 is not active on human lymphocytes.

Chromosomal Location

The chromosomal locations of IL-2 and its receptor are 4q26-27 (IL-2), 10p15-14 (IL-2R α-chain), 22q11.2-12 (IL-2R β-chain), and Xq13 (IL-2R γ-chain).

Cellular Origin

Activated T cells, namely CD4 T cells (Th0 and Th1), and in lesser quantities CD8 lymphocytes and NK cells, all synthesize IL-2 (Figure 22-11). B lymphocytes and mast cells can also produce IL-2.[441,472]

Control of Synthesis and Release

The principal inducers of IL-2 synthesis in vivo are the activators of T lymphocytes. In vitro they include mitogens, phorbol esters, calcium ionophores, and antibodies to cell surface receptors (e.g., CD2, CD3, and CD28).

IL-2 does not exist as a preformed cytokine but is rapidly and transiently synthesized after stimulation, with an early peak of secretion occurring about 4 hours after cellular activation.[1,472] The regulation of IL-2 release is mainly dependent on IL-2 gene expression, which is under inducible control by *cis*-acting regulatory sequences within the IL-2 enhancer. Binding sites have been identified in this region for a nuclear factor of activated T cells (NFAT), NF-κB, AP-1, and octamer proteins. As in other cytokines, a posttranslational control also operates to control the stability of mRNA in the 3′ untranslated region of the IL-2 genetic message.[341] Furthermore, the interaction between APC and lymphocytes is an important regulatory mechanism for IL-2 production and biological activity. Two signals from the APC (interaction of antigen with its specific T-cell receptor [TCR]-CD3 complex and secretion of IL-1) induce both the expression of the gene encoding IL-2 by responding cells and the expression of IL-2 receptors (IL-2R).[152,472] The proliferation rate of activated T cells (one of the principal cellular sources of IL-2) becomes concentration dependent when maximal IL-2R expression occurs. The presence of antigen or mitogen is required for continuous IL-2R expression. Consequently, once antigen or mitogen disappears, IL-2R density declines and cell proliferation drops, followed by a decrease in IL-2 synthesis.[152] It has been demonstrated that individually, IL-2 and TGFβ1 have contrasting effects. For example, TGFβ1 alone down regulates events that are associated with IL-2–mediated signal. When present together, IL-2 and TGFβ1 up regulate activation signals and proliferation of rapidly dividing CD4 T cells.[21] PGE2 inhibits the acquisition of the ability to produce IL-2 and IFNγ by acting directly on naive T cells.[262]

Receptor (IL-2R)

The IL-2 receptors are composed of three noncovalently linked polypeptide chains: α, β, and γ. These chains (or their complex) form the basis for three kinds of IL-2 receptors:

Low-Affinity Receptor

The α-chain (IL-2Rα, CD25), originally called Tac (T activation), is a 55-kDa polypeptide (also named p55) that is a low-affinity receptor ($K_d \cong 10^{-8}$ M). Cells that only express this receptor show detectable biological response to IL-2.[1,152] IL-2Rα is not found on resting T cells, but it is efficiently induced by T-cell activation.[152] A site on the IL-2B α-helix is thought to bind to the p55 receptor.[71]

Intermediate-Affinity Receptor

The β-chain (a polypeptide with 70 to 75 kDa, called p70 or p75, CD122) is a member of the receptor family characterized by the WSXWS motif and is expressed coordinately with the γ-chain (a 64-kDa polypeptide, also a member of the WSXWS family) forming a complex designated IL-2Rαβγ. This is the intermediate-affinity receptor ($K_d \sim 10^{-9}$ M) for IL-2, expressed constitutively by resting T lymphocytes (also by CD8 T cytotoxic cells). It is not expressed by CD4 Th cells,[152] NK cells, macrophages, neutrophils, and other cells causing growth. The β-chain alone binds IL-2 with low affinity, and the γ-chain does not bind IL-2, common γ-chain (p64) together with IL-4R, IL-7R, IL-9R, IL-13R, and IL-15R binds IL-2. Both the β- and γ-chains are required for ligand internalization and signal transduction but not the α-chain.[152] Heterodimers α/γ or α/β form receptors of intermediate affinity.

High-Affinity Receptor

The αβγ-association (IL-2Rαβγ) produces the high-affinity receptor ($K_d \sim 10^{-11}$ M) that is expressed only by activated T (about 2000 binding sites per cell) and B lymphocytes, the latter after stimulation by IL-4 and Ig-receptor binding.[152,341] Also, the control of IL-2 and IL-2Rα-chain production is closely and contemporaneously related, contrasting with the simplicity of β- and γ-chain expression. This is very important because the physiology of cytokines relies on interactions with constitutive and induced receptors.

Although the α-chain is very important (and fundamental for the appearance of high-affinity IL-2R), the γ-chain has a key role based on its molecular pluripresence (found in IL-4, IL-7, IL-9, and IL-15 receptors but possibly not the IL-13 receptor), constitutive expression by lymphoid cells, and genetic defect in the immune response. The latter results in X-linked severe combined immunodeficiency (XSCID) characterized by profoundly diminished cell-mediated and humoral immunity.[152,237,313,341]

As a general rule, resting cells express low- or intermediate-affinity receptors, thereby requiring high levels of IL-2 to have a biological response (as previously stated, the low-affinity receptor is not yet associated with any biological known response to IL-2). On an appropriate stimulus (e.g., antigen-mediated T-cell activation or the IL-2 itself), IL-2Rα is rapidly expressed, thereby reducing the concentration of IL-2 required for cellular growth and proliferation. Nevertheless, IL-2 can also regulate the expression of high-affinity receptors (e.g., IL-2-receptor interactions cause the density of IL-2Rαβγ to diminish).[152] Both IL-2 binding and cellular stimulation can be blocked by antibodies against either α- or β-chains.[1]

Signal Transduction

At least two distinct cytoplasmic regions of the IL-2Rβ-chain are involved in IL-2–mediated cellular signaling: a serine-rich region for induction of *c-myc* and cell proliferation and an acidic region for physical association with *src*-like protein tyrosine kinase (PTK) $p56^{lck}$, activation of $p21^{ras}$, and induction of c-*fos* and c-*jun*.[71]

Many cytokines and growth factors use the JAK-STAT pathway to generate a signal from the cell membrane to the nucleus. While homodimerizing cytokine receptors may transmit a signal via a single form of JAK (i.e., growth hormone receptors), several multicomponent cytokine receptors have been shown to require simultaneous activation of pairs of different JAK kinases (i.e., IFN receptors).[277] In this study, the authors verified the ability of IL-2 to cause tyrosine phosphorylation and activation of JAK1 and JAK3 and demonstrated that IL-2 stimulated JAK3 to a significantly larger extent than JAK1 in human T lymphocytes. Moreover, STAT5 was found to be the dominant STAT transcription factor used by IL-2 in human T cells and specifically required a COOH-terminal region of IL-2Rβ (Ser386-Val525), and STAT5 recruitment was not correlated with activation of IL-2Rγ or JAK3. Several signaling pathways regulate the IL-2 gene, including the NFkB pathway.

Soluble Receptor (sIL-2R)

The measurement of soluble cytokine receptors is generally considered of great importance in the characterization of the immunoinflammatory response. Chronic T-cell stimulation leads to shedding of IL-2Rα. The soluble receptor chains may bind free IL-2, blocking its action on cellular receptors. However, the greater affinity of IL-2Rαβγ compared with shed receptor alone suggests that they do not contribute significantly to immunosuppression. Clinically an increased level of soluble IL-2Rα in a biological fluid, such as serum, is associated with a potent immune response that is often dependent on a strong antigenic stimulation.[1]

Biological Actions

Originally known as a T-cell growth factor, IL-2 is now clearly connected with a variety of cellular actions on T and B lymphocytes, NK cells (Box 22-4), macrophages, monocytes, oligodendrocytes, and fibroblasts.

T Lymphocytes

IL-2 supports growth and proliferation (from the G1 to S phase of the cell cycle) of antigen- or mitogen-primed T lymphocytes and is an important determinant of the magnitude of T-cell–dependent immune responses (IL-2 is the most potent T-cell growth factor and is very important in determining the T-cell functionality).[263] Failure to produce adequate amounts of IL-2 has been described as a cause of antigen-specific T-cell anergy (decreased immunity or lack of immunity to an antigen). However, mice with IL-2 gene knockout appear to have relatively normal immune responses, suggesting that many IL-2 activities may be redundant.[1] This is particularly demonstrable in that other cytokines (e.g., IL-4, IL-6, IL-7, IL-9, and IL-15) can induce similar effects on T and B lymphocytes.[472] The magnitude and duration of the immune response are determined by the interaction of IL-2 with high-affinity IL-2R,[152] which seems to be a good argument for the value of IL-2 in immune responses. Moreover, the kinetic and equilibrium differences between the mouse and human receptor complexes and between IL-2 and IL-15 binding to these receptors clarify the roles of the α- and γ-subunits in the differential response of cells to different cytokines that may be present simultaneously in the environment.[25]

High-dose IL-2 and IL-15 enhance the in vitro priming of naive CD4 T cells for IFNγ but have differential effects on

BOX 22-4 Summary of IL-2 Effects on Lymphocytes*

T Cells
- Growth and proliferation
- Function
- Magnitude and duration of immune response
- Enhanced mobility
- Secretion of IFNγ, TNFα, and TNFβ

CD4 T Cells
- Interaction with B cells, leading to enhanced antibody production
- Interaction with class II MHC molecules on macrophages, leading to IL-1 secretion

CD8 T Cells
- Activation of T cells cytotoxic for tumor cells
- Secretion of IFNγ, leading to macrophage activation and enhanced IL-1 production

B Cells
- Growth and proliferation
- Antibody synthesis
- Immunoglobulin isotype switching IgE production of anergic Th2 cells
- Induces LAK cell capacity
- Modulates human leukocyte antigen expression
- Induces secretion of cytokines

NK Cells
- Proliferation
- Increase cytotoxicity by NK
- Enhanced NK activity
- Induction of LAK activity
- Secretion of TNFα and IFNγ

*References 1, 25, 152, 161, 263, 423, 441, 472.

priming for IL-4.[469] Uncommitted human CD4 CD45RA CD45R0neg* CD25neg CD71neg human leukocyte antigen (HLA)-DRneg T cells can be primed for a Th2 phenotype (see earlier section on inflammation) before they encounter TCR signals and before they are exposed to IL-4. As such, a significant fraction of uncommitted T cells may be primed in vivo for a Th2 phenotype independent of antigen (Ag) and IL-4 if they are exposed to Th1 cell-derived IL-2 and simultaneously interact with accessory cells bearing the natural CD28 ligands B7-1 and B7-2. When stimulated by a specific Ag, such primed Th2 precursor cells may provide a source of IL-4 to promote Th2 immunity.[62] IL-2 and IL-7 reciprocally induce IL-7 and IL-2 receptors on γδ T-cell receptor-positive intraepithelial lymphocytes. The sources of these two cytokines for γδ-T cells were neighboring epithelial cells (IL-7) and αβ-T cells (IL-2 and IL-7).[177]

Paradoxically, however, this cytokine appears equally important in limiting T cell responses and eliminating autoreactive T cells. Prolonged or repeated activation in the presence of IL-2 causes T-cell apoptosis and mutations that inactive IL-2 or its receptor lead to excessive T-cell proliferation and autoimmunity.[114] IL-2 is thus a two-edged sword that initiates immune responses but also limits their intensity and duration.

B Lymphocytes

IL-2 stimulates growth and proliferation of B lymphocytes, leading to antibody synthesis. It does not appear to cause Ig isotype switching.[1] It has been demonstrated that IL-2 restored the helper function of anergic Th2 cells for IgE production by B cells; this effect was greatly enhanced by the addition of IL-4 or IL-13.[161] Also, IL-5 synergizes with Th1 cells to induce B-cell responses to IL-2, which are maintained following T-cell removal.[423] IL-2 induces LAK cell capacity, modulates HLA expression, and induces secretion of other cytokines from different activated cells, like T and B lymphocytes, NK cells, and mononuclear phagocytic cells. This is of particular importance because some cytokines (such as IFNγ) augment NK cell activity, induce the generation of T cytotoxic (Tc) cells, activate macrophages, and modulate the expression of class II MHC molecules.

Other Cells

IL-2 often synergizes with other cytokines (notably IL-12) to induce IFNγ production by NK cells and to increase cytotoxicity by NK and LAK cells.[152] The expression of the receptor for this cytokine on NK cells is, however, continuous in character, but only a very small percentage of these cells have receptors of great affinity.[441] The study of differential use of Janus kinase-signal transducer activator of transcription signaling pathways in the stimulation of human NK cells by IL-2, IL-12, and IFNα has demonstrated a differential phosphorylation and consequent differential activation of both separate and overlapping STAT proteins by IL-2, IL-12, and IFNα. This may provide a molecular basis for the similarities and differences in the actions of these cytokines on NK cells.[591]

The biological actions of IL-2 on other types of cells are less well known, but IL-2 receptor chains have been detected on mononuclear phagocytes. Although they have been known to respond by cytokine synthesis and increase of cell-killing activities, a more specific IL-2 action in this cell population has not been established.[1,472] Mast cells and Langerhans' cells also express IL-2 receptors following activation. Whether IL-2 induces proliferation or alters the activities of these cells is as yet unclear.[472] Investigations reported in 1996 support the concept that a self-directed cytotoxicity against pulmonary fibroblasts is generated during lymphocyte activation with recombinant IL-2.[592]

*CD45R0neg means no expression of CD45R0 (negative). All positive CDs are presented without the plus (+) sign.

Clinical Significance

Excessive production of IL-2 has been reported in pregnancy, multiple sclerosis, sarcoidosis, multiple myeloma, acute rheumatic fever, and chronic rheumatic heart disease.[385,472]

Production of IL-2 is diminished in (1) advanced age, (2) diabetes, (3) RA, and (4) Sjögren's syndrome.[472] Also, reduced synthesis of IL-2 is associated with both acquired immunodeficiency syndrome (AIDS) and SCID.[472] However, 1995 findings support the hypothesis that lymphocytic alveolitis in asymptomatic HIV-positive patients results from IL-2–dependent in situ proliferation of CD8 cytotoxic T cells.[492] Failure to produce either IL-2 or IL-2R is associated with the absence of a T-cell–mediated immune response.[152] Patients with chronic mucocutaneous candidiasis present altered antigen-stimulated IL-2, IL-4, IL-6, and INFγ production, consistent with a predominantly Th2 instead of a Th1 cytokine response.[320] The levels of IL-2 and sIL-2R were found to be lower in some hematological malignancies (Hodgkin's lymphoma and non-Hodgkin's lymphoma).[344]

Down regulation of IL-2 synthesis is associated with the use of immunosuppressive agents, including hydrocortisone, cyclosporin A, Tacrolimus, and cyclophosphamide (see Chapter 33). Also, the immunosuppressive macrolide rapamycin inhibits cytokine-driven proliferation of lymphocytes, acting at a later stage of T lymphocyte activation than the related compound Tacrolimus or cyclosporin A, which block IL-2 transcription. However, the effect of rapamycin on the expression of the IL-2Rα (CD25) is less well documented. Thus rapamycin inhibition of T-cell activation may involve not only IL-2–driven proliferation but also suppression of CD25 up regulation.[582]

Therapeutic Activity

IL-2 was the first cytokine to be used in clinical trials for the treatment of human diseases, especially cancer. This use was based on the discovery that LAK cells (obtained by the stimulation of resting lymphocytes with IL-2) have cytotoxic action against tumor cells while sparing normal cells.[485] IL-2 synergizes with IFNγ and TNFα in a range of antitumor effects but is unique in its ability to mediate activation and expansion of antitumor lymphocytes.[472] However, direct IL-2 therapy (either intravenously or subcutaneously) was only achieved after recombinant IL-2 became available, enabling the use of the large amounts of cytokine required for high-dose therapy in humans (see previous section). These results were limited by the extreme toxicity of IL-2, which affects cardiovascular, respiratory, renal, and hepatic function.[485] The toxic effect of IL-2 depends on the dose and the mode of administration. In the majority of patients, parainfluenza symptoms appear. Most undesirable effects are connected with a multisystemic syndrome of capillary vessel hyperpermeability, leading to increased fluid retention into extravascular spaces, edema, hypotonia, and oliguria.[441] Some of these secondary reactions are in part due to the cytokine cascade effect with production of IFNγ and TNFα.[436] Because of this problem and the relative lack of success with LAK cells, a new regimen of using IL-2 with TIL has been attempted. These cells are 50 to 100 times more potent against homologous tumors than LAK cells. However, despite TIL being found in most human infiltrating ductal breast carcinomas where they should be capable of both in vitro and in vivo activation by IL-2 to produce selective tumor cytolysis, it was observed that the TIL population shows a deficiency in IL-2 and IL-2R expression. This may explain the relative anergic state of native TIL.[100] IL-2R also has been used as a target for IL-2 when coupled with toxins promoting selective cell death.[485] In myelodysplastic syndromes, the in vitro effects of IL-2 suggest the clinical usefulness of this cytokine in a large subgroup of patients, because it may reduce the percentage of blasts and increase clonogenic capacity and cell-mediated cytotoxicity.[99]

Another field of therapeutic interest is the use of IL-2 in immunomodulation, acting as a recovery agent in some immunodeficient conditions, such as that resulting from the administration of immunosuppressive agents.[485] This immunoenhancing capacity in addition has considerable potential for promoting adequate responses to vaccines.[472] As previously mentioned, the use of antibodies against IL-2 or IL-2R subunits can block the activity of this cytokine associated with promising results in the prevention of allograft rejection.[472]

In addition to these uses, IL-2 has been found to be effective in the treatment of patients with disseminate cancer of the kidney and melanoma and in adjuvant therapy of acute myeloid leukemia. Attempts have been made to apply it in the treatment of AIDS and leprosy.[441] The most common areas for IL-2 therapy are renal cell carcinoma,[198] melanoma, and lymphoma.[472,485]

INTERLEUKIN-3

Interleukin-3 (IL-3) is a lymphokine produced by antigen- or mitogen-activated T lymphocytes that stimulate proliferation of hematopoietic and lymphoid stem cells. It is also a colony stimulating factor for all bone marrow progenitor cells.[289] IL-3 supports the growth and differentiation of early hematopoietic and lymphoid stem cells and that of more mature hematopoietic cells, including granulocytes, macrophages, and mast cells.[138]

Synonyms

IL-3 was formerly known as burst promoting activity (BPA), colony forming unit (CFU) stimulating activity, colony stimulating factor (CSF) 2α and 2β, eosinophil-CSF (E-CSF), hematopoietic cell growth factor (HCGF), hemopoietin-2, histamine-producing cell stimulating factor, mast cell growth factor (MCGF) multicolony stimulating factor (M-CSF), multilineage colony stimulating factor, multilineage hemopoietic growth factor, P cell–stimulating factor activity, panspecific hemopoietin, persisting (P) cell–stimulating factor, pluripotential hematopoietic cell stimulating activity, stem cell activating factor, synergistic activity, Thy-1 inducing factor, Thy-1 stimulating activity, and WEHI-3 growth factor. *(Note WEHI is a macrophage-like myelomonocytic leukemia cell line established from inbred BALB/c mice.)*

General Characteristics

IL-3 is a glycoprotein, and glycosylation accounts for most of the heterogeneity of this molecule. Depending on the cleavage position of the precursor polypeptide, there are two mature forms of IL-3: a protein with 134 or 140 amino acid residues.[152] The half-life in the blood is estimated at about 40 minutes. Its structure is a compact globe with four α-helical short chains.

IL-3 stimulates the growth and differentiation of all hematopoietic lineages rather than self-renewal of primitive stem cells.[71,472] Activated T cells secrete IL-3, but its effects are normally restricted to local cellular activation or to nearby sites where T cells migrate (paracrine action).[152]

Other general characteristics of IL-3 include:

Molecular Weight

Depending on the extent of glycosylation, the literature values for the molecular weight of IL-3 vary from 15 to 32 kDa. The following molecular weights have been reported: 15 kDa,[421] 17 kDa,[472] 14 to 30 kDa,[71] 20 to 26 kDa,[152,436,485] and 20 to 32 kDa.[341,389]

Cross-Reactivity

The cross-reactivity (amino acid sequence homology between human and mouse) for IL-3 is 29%.[71] There is no cross-species reactivity.

Chromosomal Location

The chromosomal locations of IL-3 and its receptor are 5q23-31 (IL-3); in this area are located the genes of several hematopoietic growth factors, such as GM-CSF, M-CSF, and the M-CSF receptor (known as the c-*fms* oncogene)[485]; Yp13.3, Xp22.3 (IL-3Rα-chain); and 22 (IL-3Rβ-chain).

Cellular Origin

CD4 T cells of both the Th1 and Th2 subsets are the principal source of IL-3 (Figure 22-12), but NK cells, mast cells, eosinophils, possibly keratinocytes, and thymic epithelium and neuronal cells can also produce this cytokine. GM-CSF and IL-3 are generally thought to be produced in a coordinated fashion by all activated T cells, but studies have indicated that T cells have the potential to display diversity of expression of GM-CSF and IL-3.[167]

Control of Synthesis and Release

IL-3 does not exist in a preformed state, being synthesized after cellular activation. Glucocorticoids and cyclosporin A inhibit IL-3 production by T lymphocytes.[472]

Receptor (IL-3R)

The IL-3 receptor is a heterodimeric structure with high- and low-affinity configurations consisting of two chains (subunits): IL-3Rα (CD123 is a 70 kDa peptide) and IL-3Rβ (150 kDa) signal-transducing subunit, shared with IL-5 and GM-CSF, but does not itself bind any of these cytokines.[71] The α-chain is a member of the hematopoietin receptor superfamily, which includes receptors for IL-2, IL-4, IL-6, IL-7, G-CSF, and GM-CSF and consists of a unique WSXWS-containing subunit.[1,472] IL-3, IL-5, and GM-CSF receptors belong to the cytokine receptor superfamily and are structurally and functionally related; thus these constitute a distinct subfamily.

It has been demonstrated that human IL-3 induces heterodimerization of IL-3Rα- and β-chains and that disulfide linkage of these chains is involved in receptor activation but not high-affinity binding. This may also be applicable to the related GM-CSF and IL-5 receptors.[498] IL-3 down regulates the expression of IL-3 receptor, providing a negative feedback control of its activity.[472] IL-3R is present on progenitor cells, monocytes, pre-B cells, and B cells.[71]

Signal Transduction

Signal transduction requires the presence of the β-chain. IL-3–IL-3R interaction results in rapid phosphorylation of several cellular proteins, including the IL-3Rβ-subunit itself.[71]

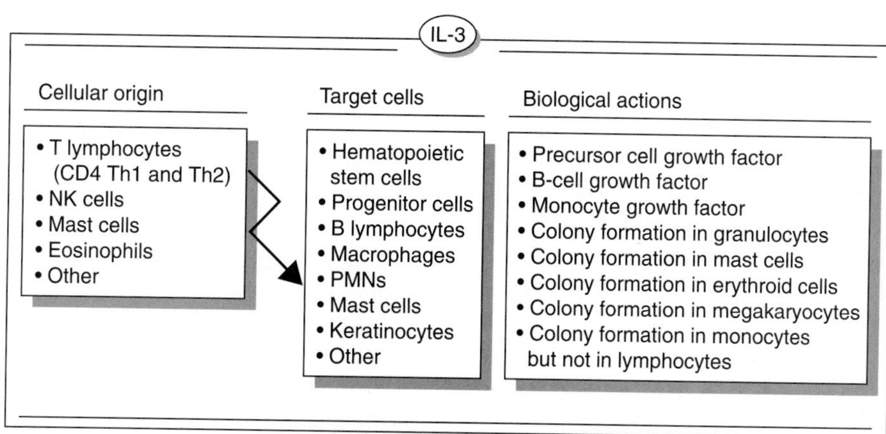

Figure 22-12 Cellular origin, principal target cells, and biological actions of IL-3.

Biological Actions

Effector targets of IL-3 are (1) the pluripotential hematopoietic stem cells and progenitor cells and (2) the other several mature cells, such as B lymphocytes, macrophages, basophils, eosinophils, mast cells, and keratinocytes.[472]

Most functional analyses of IL-3 have been performed in mice and in experimental systems of hematopoiesis. In humans, it has been difficult to establish a role for this molecule. However, many actions attributed to murine IL-3 appear to be performed by human GM-CSF.[1] IL-3 also acts on hematopoietic progenitors, stimulating formation of granulocytes, macrophages, NK cells, erythroid and multipotent precursors, and megakaryocytes, and has biological actions on mast cells, basophils, eosinophils, and macrophages.[341,485] It is thought that IL-3 acts synergistically with IL-1 and IL-6 in the initial phase of erythroid, megakaryocytic, and myelomonocytic development.[436] IL-3 is a broader CSF than more specialized ones, including GM-CSF, G-CSF, and M-CSF. IL-3 seems to cooperate with these factors, providing a very important link between the hematopoietic and immune systems; biological functions of IL-3 are enhanced or depend on the co-stimulation with other cytokines.[71,472] In this manner, the hematopoietic system provides important auxiliary and accessory cells fundamental for an efficient immunoinflammatory reaction.[152] For example, maintenance of local levels of IL-3 is required to (1) increase mast cell in vivo numbers, (2) act as a growth factor for B lymphocytes, and (3) serve as an activator of monocytes.[71,152] Unfortunately, these functions can lead to vascular leak syndrome with extensive hemorrhage, peripheral neuropathy, and reactive erythrophagocytosis as unusual complications of recombinant IL-3 therapy. They suggest a causal mechanism based on the excessive stimulation of macrophages and production of secondary cytokines, such as TNF.[231] The demonstration that T-cell–derived IL-3 induces the production of IL-4 by non-B, non-T cells suggests that IL-3 may amplify the Th2-cytokine response in mice.[291] Also, IL-3 (like IL-4, IL-5, and IL-6), which is mainly produced by Th2 lymphocytes, may possibly regulate the functions of human mast cells in vivo via specific receptors in allergic reactions.[584]

Clinical Significance

Excessive production of IL-3 has been described in several pathological conditions, especially in monocytic or myeloid leukemias and mast cell disorders.[472] However, IL-3 can be measured in blood only after severe immunological stimuli, such as graft-versus-host disease or parasitic infestations. IL-3 may also play an important role in chronic allergic diseases.[152,584]

Therapeutic Applications

IL-3 has been used in clinical trials designed to assess the benefit from hematopoietic stimulation, shortening the duration of cytopenias associated with chemotherapy or irradiation, or following bone marrow transplantation.[472,485] However, the use of IL-3 (GM-CSF or IL-6) to reduce myelosuppression after high-dose chemotherapy appears unlikely to result in stimulation of the growth of the most common solid tumors.[236]

INTERLEUKIN-4

Interleukin-4 (IL-4) is a lymphokine produced by antigen- or mitogen-activated T cells; its principal role is regulation of IgE- and eosinophil-mediated immune reactions. It stimulates switching of B cells for production of IgE. It is a growth and differentiation factor for T cells, particularly Th2 cells; is a growth factor for mast cells; and stimulates the expression of some adhesion molecules on endothelial cells.[138]

Synonyms

IL-4 has been formerly known as B-cell differentiating factor (BCDF), B-cell growth factor I (BCGF-I), B-cell stimulating factor I (BSF-I), MCGF-II, and T-cell growth factor II (TCGF-II).

General Characteristics

IL-4 is a member of the four α-helical short-chain cytokine family. The three-dimensional structure is a compact globe with a predominant hydrophobic core.[71]

IL-4 is a pleiotropic cytokine as demonstrated by the range of cells expressing the IL-4 receptor. IL-4 production is now used as a criterion for classifying CD4 T cells into the Th2 subset. It plays a critical role in IgE- and eosinophil-mediated immunoinflammatory reactions. It is also a growth and differentiation factor for lymphocytes and an antiinflammatory molecule that modulates the biological action of macrophages.[1,436]

Molecular Weight

Depending on the degree of glycosylation, the literature values for the molecular weight of IL-4 vary from 15 to 20 kDa. The following molecular weights have been reported: 18 to 20 kDa,[341,389] 20 kDa (monomer),[1,152,421] 15 kDa (glycoprotein),[472] and 15 to 19 kDa.[71]

Cross-Reactivity

The cross-reactivities (amino acid sequence homology between human and mouse) for different forms of IL-4 include[71,52]:

IL-4 (amino acids 1 to 90 and 129 to 149)—50%

IL-4 (amino acids 91 to 128)—very little

IL-4 is species specific (human IL-4 has no activity on mouse cells and vice versa)

Chromosomal Location

The chromosomal locations of IL-4 and its receptor are 5q23-31 (IL-4), and 16p12.1-11.2 (high-affinity receptor).

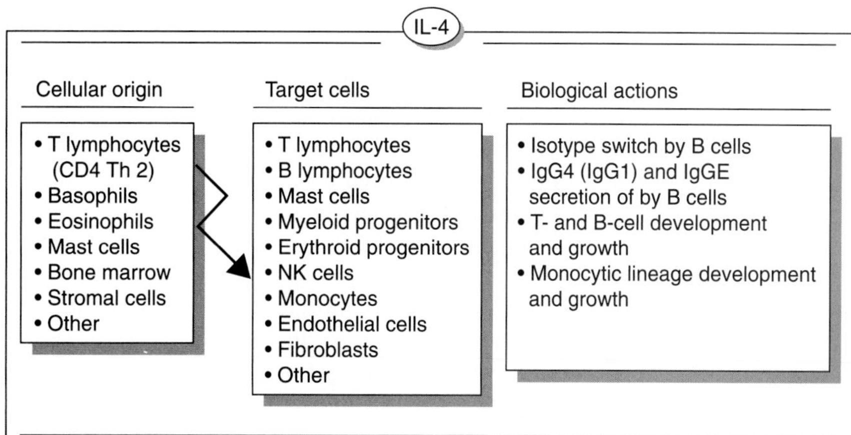

Figure 22-13 Cellular origin, principal target cells, and biological actions of IL-4.

Cellular Origin

IL-4 is synthesized by subtype Th2 of T lymphocytes, basophils, eosinophils, and mast cells and bone marrow stromal cells (Figure 22-13). Some CD8 T cells also produce IL-4.[1,494,584]

Control of Synthesis and Release

IL-4 production depends on T-cell activation or cross-linking of IgE receptors (FcεRI and FcεRII) on mast cells and basophils. In vitro addition of IL-2 or IL-15 to cultures of naive CD4 T cells has differential effects on priming for IL-4. In addition, IL-15 does not restore priming for IL-4, suggesting that IL-2 and IL-15 may have different functional properties during the in vitro differentiation of IL-4–producing cells.[469] It has been suggested that IL-4 synthesis is induced in normal T lymphocytes in the absence of exogenous IL-4 and that CD40L co-stimulation is of fundamental importance in regulation of IL-4 production.[56] This provides a mechanism by which B cells preferentially enhance IL-4 synthesis in T cells at low antigen concentrations.[56] However, it has also been found that CD40-mediated stimulation contributes to lymphocyte proliferation, antibody production, eosinophilia, and mastocytosis during an in vivo Th2 response. IL-4 is not required for T-cell IL-4 production.[333] IL-8 may be an important regulator of CD4 T-cell–derived IL-4, thereby possibly regulating the balance between humoral and cellular T cell-dependent responses.[186] T-cell–derived IL-3 induces the production of IL-4 by non-B, non-T cells to amplify the Th2-cytokine response.[291] No correlation has been found among IL-2-, IL-4-, and IFN-secreting cells, indicating that the production of preponderantly T-cell–derived cytokines is regulated independently.[205]

Production of IL-4 by T cells is induced by mitogens and antigens and suppressed by TGFβ and cyclosporin A. Also, IL-4 expression in T lymphocytes is selectively inhibited by IL-1α and IL-1β; this interaction may represent an important physiological regulator of the balance between proinflammatory cytokines from activated macrophages and antiinflammatory cytokines from T cells.[457] Prednisolone-treated patients show a reduction of the number of cells expressing IL-4.[38] Thiols, usually administered to humans as a mucolytic agent, decrease IL-4 production and IL-4–induced Ig synthesis.[244] Vasoactive intestinal peptide inhibits IL-4 production at a posttranscriptional level. Studies have probed the molecular mechanisms involved in the neuroendocrine regulation of cytokine production.[561] The results support the idea that neuropeptides may participate in the intricate cytokine network controlling local immune responses. Usually IL-4 is a neosynthesized molecule, with the exception of mast cells that contain IL-4 in a preformed state.[472]

Receptor (IL-4R)

The IL-4 receptor is a molecular complex consisting at least of two chains: a high-affinity IL-4 binding chain (p140, α-chain, CD124) and the IL-2R γ-chain also known as the common γ-chain (γc, p64). The high-affinity IL-4 binding chain belongs to the cytokine receptor superfamily and contains the conserved WSXWS motif. The γ-chain is a functional component of the IL-4R and augments IL-4 binding affinity. However, IL-4 does not use or require the common γc of the IL-2R on human endothelial cells to mediate vascular cell adhesion.[465] A soluble form of IL-4R has been found to be a potent IL-4 antagonist.

Monomeric high-affinity IL-4 receptors (CD124) are found on T and B cells, macrophages, mast cells, muscle cells, neuroblasts, stromal cells (brain and bone marrow), myeloid cells, granulocytes, megakaryocytes, hematopoietic progenitor cells, NK cells, fibroblasts, and epithelial and endothelial cells.[152,341] About 300 IL-4 receptors per cell are found on B and T lymphocytes, a number that increases to 100 to 1000 receptors per cell with cell maturation and activation.[71,152]

A second low-affinity IL-4 receptor has also been identified and appears to be coupled to a different signal transduction pathway.[71]

Signal Transduction

IL-4 signaling may involve clustering of the receptor-associated tyrosine kinase and IL-4 binding to the CD124 receptor, resulting in tyrosine phosphorylation of cellular proteins. Activation of tyrosine phosphatase and dephosphorylation of an 80-kDa protein have also been reported. Another signal transduction pathway has been shown to involve breakdown of phosphatidylinositol bisphosphate. This pathway may be coupled to a low-affinity receptor.[1,71] Tyrosine phosphorylation of STAT6 is activated in response to IL-4 and may contribute to various functions, including mitogenesis, CD4 lymphocyte differentiation, and Ig isotype switching, which collectively play a central role in exerting IL-4–mediated biological responses.[480,513]

Biological Actions

The principal functional targets of IL-4 are T cells, B cells, monocytes, endothelial cells, fibroblasts, mast cells, and myeloid and erythroid progenitors. IL-4 (1) induces growth of these cells, (2) promotes class isotype switching in B cells to IgE (keeping up with induced expression of IgE receptors), and (3) augments IgG4 (IgG1 in mouse) production. IL-4 also induces biological responses in other cells, such as NK cells, fibroblasts, and endothelial cells.[341,436]

IL-4 also has the capacity to drive CD4 T-cell differentiation to the Th2 type, thereby blocking Th1 development. This creates a bias in the immune response, with a deleterious effect on the defense capacity against certain biological aggressors, such as intracellular pathogens. Alternately, consequent IgE switching is associated with exacerbated antibody production (especially IgE and IgG classes), immediate hypersensitivity reactions, and defense against helminthic infections (one of the few known physiological functions of the Th2 polarization of CD4 T cells in humans). As a Th2 stimulator, IL-4 inhibits macrophage activation and blocks most of the activating effects of IFNγ, including IL-1, nitric oxide (NO), and PG production. These effects are shared with those of IL-10 (also produced by Th2 cells), resulting in suppression of macrophage-mediated immune reactions. Early IL-4 production after antigen exposure favors the Th2 polarization, further promoting expansion of this T-cell subset because an autocrine growth factor.[1,451] The origin of IL-4 (as a critical element in the induction of Th2 response) during a primary immune response is not yet well defined,[450] although the class I-selected CD4neg CD8neg TCRαβ T cells (double negative CD3 cells) are being proposed as a novel source of this cytokine.[309,310] However, it has been demonstrated that naive human CD4 T cells release low but sufficient levels of IL-4 at priming to support their development into IL-4 producers.[586] IL-4, in the absence of antigen stimulation, induces an anergy-like state in differentiated CD8 Tc1 cells, suppressing IL-2 synthesis and autonomous proliferative pathway but retaining of cytotoxicity and synthesis of other cytokines.[451]

In addition, IL-4 exerts two key regulatory effects in inflammation[472]:

1. It promotes adhesion of lymphocytes (in preference to neutrophils) to endothelial cells, stimulating the expression of adhesion molecules, such as vascular cell adhesion molecule-1 (VCAM-1). IL-4 also induces secretion of CKs by endothelial cells, resulting in an inflammatory response with the attraction of monocytes and eosinophils.[1] Constitutive production of IL-4 itself (also IL-8 and IL-10) by normal peripheral blood eosinophils represents an important role in modulating immune responses in diseases associated with eosinophils and favors Th2 polarization[370,382] amplified by the possibility of enhanced expression of Fcγ RIα by IL-4.[522] The preferential promotion of a lymphocyte's adhesion may hasten the transition from acute neutrophil-dominated to chronic lymphocyte-dominated inflammation. Surprising is the demonstration that the CK growth-regulated oncogene-α (GROα) that induces T lymphocyte chemotaxis* is inhibited by IL-4, IL-10, and IL-13.[245] Alternately, IL-4 may have a protective vascular effect down regulating fibrinogen production.[551]
2. IL-4 induces an antiinflammatory effect by its ability to suppress production of proinflammatory cytokines (IL-1, TNFα, and IL-6) and to favor the release of IL-1RA.[345,360] This antiinflammatory action is evident on activated monocytes and/or macrophages, namely the inhibition of IL-6 production.[132,514] Indeed, not all target cells may be influenced in this way (e.g., IL-4 may be capable of regulating intestinal epithelial cell proliferation without altering the capacity of these cells to function in the inflammatory response by secreting IL-6).[353] IL-4 and IFNγ also synergistically increase total polymeric IgA receptor levels in human intestinal epithelial cells.[126]

Pleiotropic activities of IL-4 include (1) increased class II MHC antigen expression on B cells, (2) enhanced G-CSF–induced proliferation of granulocyte-macrophage precursors, (3) inhibition of LAK cell induction, and (4) synergism with IL-3 and IL-9 in stimulating mast cell and basophil proliferation.[1,152,341,436] IL-4 and IL-13 inhibit bone resorption by suppressing cyclooxygenase-2–dependent PG synthesis in osteoblasts.[400] IL-4 and IL-1β may contribute to the enhanced synthesis of collagen and consequent fibrosis, regulating its production in human skin, liver, and lung fibroblasts.[528]

IL-12 is considered as a counterbalancing cytokine to IL-4 as it cross regulates it.[341] IL-13 has been identified as having

*Chemotaxis is the orientation of a cell along a chemical concentration gradient or movement in the direction of the gradient, either toward (positive chemotaxis) or away from (negative chemotaxis) the greater concentration of the substance, referred to as a chemotactic factor, chemotactin, or chemoattractant. Macrophages, neutrophils, eosinophils, and lymphocytes exhibit chemotaxis in response to a wide variety of substances released at sites of inflammatory reactions, including lymphokines, mediators released by basophils and mast cells, bacterial products, and C5a and other activated complement components.

overlapping biological activities with IL-4, supporting the hypothesis that the two cytokines use a common receptor complex or signal pathway.[124]

Clinical Relevance

IL-4 is the main physiological regulator of allergic reactions (immediate hypersensitivity). As IL-4 boosts immune mechanisms that rely on IgE (that include antigen recognition by mast cells and epidermal Langerhans' cells), excessive production of it is associated with disorders in which these cells are pivotal, such as atopic dermatitis.[472] IL-4 also plays a key role in the contact sensitivity skin reaction.[17] It has been postulated that in atopic patients, IL-4 is the most discriminatory cytokine and that the level of serum IgE has a low predictive value in allergic disease.[157] In this study, because of a lack of correlation between IL-4 and serum IgE, the authors suggest that the measurement of IL-4 in blood mononuclear cells may be of great value in the analysis of allergic responses in atopic donors. Excessive production of IL-4 is associated with T-cell lymphomas (Th2 subtype), also with a corresponding strong expression of the low-affinity receptor for IgE (CD23).[472]

Therapeutic Applications

IL-4 may be useful in the therapy of humoral immunodeficiency.[485] In addition, it has antitumor effects on some solid tumors because it can initiate cytotoxic responses mediated by eosinophils, macrophages, and T lymphocytes, and this activity may be useful in the clinical setting.[341,365,472] Experimental models of vaccination with tumor cells engineered to produce IL-4 have shown that the local release of this cytokine is associated with the development of antitumor immunity that may induce regression of established cancer.[359] IL-4 can also modify integrin expression and adhesive functions of tumor cells in vitro, acting as direct regulators of adhesive mechanisms of tumor cells bearing adequate receptors, thus influencing metastasis.[215]

Anti–IL-4 antibodies could be interesting as a means of correcting the balance between Th1 and Th2 cells in Th2 polarized situations.[341] However, it has been reported that the peripheral blood of allergic individuals contains long-lived allergen-specific B cells that have already switched to IgE production and that are not sensitive to IL-4 and IL-13 treatment. These results may have implications on attempts to use cytokines or cytokine antagonists in therapy of a type I allergy.[133]

In an attempt to develop additional antiviral therapeutic strategies, De Francesco and colleagues have found that HIV-1 p17 matrix protein greatly increased HIV-1 replication in preactivated peripheral blood mononuclear cell cultures obtained from healthy donors.[116] In their studies they have discovered that p17 exerts its biological activity after binding to a specific cellular receptor expressed on activated T-enhancing levels of TNFα and IFNγ released from cells stimulated by IL-2. IL-4 was found to down regulate IFNγ and TNFα, and p17 restored the ability of cells to produce both cytokines. The property of p17 to increase production of proinflammatory cytokines could be a mechanism exploited by the virus to create a more suitable environment for HIV-1 infection and replication.

INTERLEUKIN-5

Interleukin-5 (IL-5) is a lymphokine produced by antigen- or mitogen-activated T cells and by activated mast cells that stimulates the growth and differentiation of eosinophils and activates mature eosinophils to kill helminths. It may act as a cofactor in the growth and differentiation of B cells and may also be involved in increasing synthesis of IgA by mature B cells.[138]

Synonyms

IL-5 was formerly known as BCDF B-cell differentiation factor for IgM (BCDFμ), B-cell growth factor II (BCGF-II), eosinophil colony stimulating factor, eosinophil differentiation factor, IgA-enhancing factor, and T-cell replacing factor (TRF).*

General Characteristics

IL-5 is an antiparallel disulfide-linked homodimer (115 AA). It belongs to the four α-helical short-chain cytokine family with two short β-sheets. The novel dimeric structure is considered unique, containing four helices (A to D) arranged in an up-up-down-down topology. In contrast to other subfamily members, which fold unimolecularly into a single helical bundle, IL-5 forms a pair of helical bundles by the interdigitation of two identical monomers that contribute a D helix to the others' A through C helices.[1,72,127,128,341] The monomer is biologically inactive. It has been predicted that the lack of bioactivity by IL-5 monomer is due to a short loop between helices C and D, which physically prevents unimolecular folding of helix D into a functionally obligate structural motif. By lengthening this loop, an insertional mutant of IL-5 is engineered that is expressed as a monomer with biological activity similar to that of native IL-5. These studies demonstrate that all of the structural features necessary for IL-5 to function are contained within a single helical bundle.[128] Dimerization of this glycoprotein possibly enables enough affinity interaction with the receptor. IL-5 is a cytokine typically produced by the Th2 subset of CD4 T cells and by activated mast cells, having as major activity the stimulation of growth and differentiation of eosinophils and the activation of mature eosinophils.[1,26,71]

Other general characteristics of IL-5 include:

Molecular Weight

Depending on its molecular form, the literature values for the molecular weight of IL-5 vary from 18 to 45 kDa. The following molecular weights have been reported: 24 kDa

*TRF means a factor that could replace T lymphocytes in the stimulation of B lymphocytes to produce antibodies, without MHC restriction and antigen-specific stimulus.

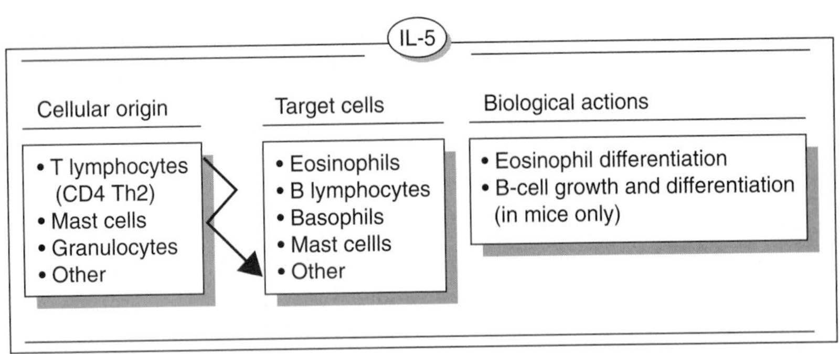

Figure 22-14 Cellular origin, principal target cells, and biological actions of IL-5.

(as a disulfide bonded dimer),[341] 40 kDa homodimeric cytokine,[1,152] 45 kDa,[71,421] 18 kDa,[472] and 40 to 45 kDa.[389]

Cross-Reactivity

The cross-reactivity (amino acid sequence homology between human and mouse) for IL-5 is 71%.[71] There is a significant cross-reactivity in functional assays.

Chromosomal Location

The chromosomal locations of IL-5 and its receptor are 5q23-31 (IL-5) and 3p26 (IL-5R).

Cellular Origin

IL-5 is produced by the activated Th2 subset of CD4 T cells, mast cells, and eosinophils (Figure 22-14).

Control of Synthesis and Release

Parasitic (helminths) and bacterial infections provide a major stimulus for IL-5 secretion by activated T cells (CD4 Th2) and mast cells. It has been demonstrated that naive human CD4 T cells release low but sufficient levels of IL-4 at priming to support its clonal expansion into high IL-4 and/or IL-5 producers.[586] IFNα selectively down regulates IL-5 synthesis by human CD4 T cells.[462] Prednisolone treatment in asthma is associated with reduction in the number of cells expressing mRNA for IL-5.[38] Cyclosporin A reduces the expression and production of IL-5.[235]

Experimental data suggest that activation via the unique sequence combination GATA/CLE0 results in selective expression of the IL-5 gene in response to elevated levels of intracellular cyclic adenosine monophosphate (cAMP).[484]

Receptor (IL-5R)

The IL-5R complex has a specific low-affinity ligand binding chain of 55 kDa (CD125), containing the WSXWS motif, and a nonbinding β-chain (βc) with 150 kDa (common to IL-3R and GM-CSFR); the latter can convert the low-affinity IL-5R into the high-affinity IL-5R and is indispensable for IL-5 signal transduction. Both chains belong to the cytokine receptor superfamily. Soluble forms of IL-5R are produced with unknown significance, unless they modulate IL-5–dependent eosinophilia in humans.* IL-5 receptor is expressed on eosinophils, basophils, and activated murine B cells. These cells display 500 to 1000 low-affinity receptors and 7500 to 10,000 high-affinity receptors per cell.[152] A controversy exists about the expression and biological significance of IL-5R in human B lymphocytes. However, IL-5 can regulate human B cells but only if they have been appropriately stimulated to undergo terminal differentiation.[233]

*References 1, 26, 64, 71, 152, 341, 512.

Signal Transduction

Although not completely elucidated,[71] studies have suggested that JAK2 kinase and an activated isoform of mitogen-activated protein (MAP) kinase, p45, may mediate some of IL-5's effects. This mediation occurs on eosinophils in a manner unique to the activation pathways previously described for other cells.[31,512]

Biological Actions

An important difference between murine and human IL-5 is that murine IL-5 causes B-cell and eosinophil differentiation, while human recombinant IL-5 causes only eosinophil differentiation and regulates IgA isotype selection.[71,152,200]

As in B cells, IL-5 has a very important role in the production of IgA based on a late-acting B-cell differentiation (although IgA synthesis is probably the result of synergistic actions with other cytokines, such as IL-6). However, on B cells, IL-5 (1) can be a co-stimulator for the growth of antigen-activated B cells; (2) may function synergistically with other cytokines, such as IL-2 and IL-4, to stimulate the growth and differentiation of these cells; (3) can induce the expression of IL-2R; (4) can promote IgG and IgM secretion; and (5) can enhance the expression of CD23 and the synthesis of IgE (these two synergistically with IL-4). The general effect of IL-5 on B cells is essential for the proper function of eosinophils during the immune response to infection.[472] In particular, IL-5 plays a critical role in the development of CD5-positive B (B-1) cells.[512]

IL-5 has a recognized effect on eosinophil growth, differentiation, and chemoattraction (inducing the generation of eosinophils from bone marrow precursors, up regulating the expression of CD11b, and activating IgA-induced degranulation).[341,472] Eosinophilia is a uniquely specific phenomenon regulated by IL-5, suggesting specific control for IL-5 gene expression.[257] The activity of IL-5 on eosinophils is complemented by the activities of IL-4 (IgE switching and eosinophil recruitment) and of IL-10 (IgG4 switching), contributing to Th2-mediated allergic reactions.[1,70]

IL-5 also enhances the expression of IL-2R on B cells and stimulates basophils.[341,472] Proeosinophilic and/or proallergic Th2 cytokines, originally described as T lymphocyte products, have been ascribed to mast cells as well, and these cells are probably analogous to T cells in the requirement of co-stimuli for the production of IL-5 protein. Moreover, the rapid kinetics of IgE-mediated IL-5 transcription and protein elaboration are consistent with a primary role for mast cell activation, directly leading to late phase airway eosinophilia.[240]

Clinical Relevance

IL-5 is a key molecule in allergic diseases. For example, the late manifestations of the allergic response in asthmatic patients are associated with eosinophil accumulation in the lung. These granulocytes are implicated in lung damage through release of the eosinophil's major basic protein and neurotoxin.[302,341] The eosinophilia results from T-cell activation (namely CD4 cells),[530] secretion of IL-5, and consequent increase of eosinophil concentration. Compared with patients with adult respiratory distress syndrome, the patients with acute eosinophilic pneumonia had high bronchoalveolar lavage fluid levels of IL-5, IL-1RA, and soluble type II IL-1R but not IL-1β, TNFα, IL-3, or GM-CSF.[6] A 1995 study demonstrated that mononuclear cells from HLA-B8 DR3-positive individuals display a reduction of IL-5 production, suggesting that the IgA synthesis dysregulation (IgA deficiency) observed in HLA-B8 DR3-positive individuals could be due to an impairment of IL-5 production.[324] The expression and production of IL-5 are high in severe atopic dermatitis.[235] Global studies suggest that IL-3, IL-4, IL-5, and IL-6, which are mainly produced by T helper 2 lymphocytes, might regulate the functions of human mast cells in vivo via specific receptors in allergic reactions.[584]

Therapeutic Applications

IL-5 may be useful for the therapy of hypogammaglobulinemia.[485] There is some promise in the clinical setting for treating helminth infections (enhancement of antibody-dependent cell-mediated cytotoxicity; ADCC), as a pivotal molecule in the stimulation of growth and differentiation of eosinophils, and in the activation of mature eosinophils to kill helminths.[152,472] A detailed understanding of IL-5 structure and function is required to develop immunomodulators of IL-5–mediated inflammatory responses (as in asthma and allergic diseases), particularly the A/D helical region of this cytokine.[128]

INTERLEUKIN-6

Interleukin-6 (IL-6) is a lymphokine produced by antigen- or mitogen-activated T cells, fibroblasts, macrophages, and other cells that serves as a differentiation factor for B cells and thymocytes and stimulates immunoglobulin production by B cells; it also induces hepatocytes to synthesize various plasma proteins involved in the acute phase response (APR) and is a cofactor in initiation of the cell cycle in primitive hematopoietic cells in vitro.[138]

Synonyms

IL-6 was formerly known as 26-kDa protein, BCDF, B-cell stimulating factor 2 (BSF-2), cytotoxic T-cell differentiation factor, hepatocyte differentiation factor (HSF), hybridoma/plasmacytoma growth factor, interferon-β2 (IFNβ2), monocyte granulocyte inducer type 2 (MGI-2), and thrombopoietin. The designation of IFNβ-2 is now considered inappropriate, and its use has been discontinued.[1,71,472]

General Characteristics

The molecular configuration of IL-6 is not completely known.[71] However, it is known to belong to the four α-helical long-chain family. It is known to be a pleiotropic cytokine produced by many types of cells (lymphoid and nonlymphoid) and affecting diverse biological areas (regulation of T- and B-cell function, Ig secretion, acute phase inflammatory reactions, and hematopoiesis).[71,421] Like IL-1 and TNFα, IL-6 is a participant in a cytokine cascade that regulates the immunoinflammatory response to infection, assuming a very important role in host defense.[152,472]

Other general characteristics of IL-6 include:

Molecular Weight

The literature values for the molecular weight of IL-6 vary from 20 to 29 kDa. The following molecular weights have been reported: 21 to 26 kDa,[341,389] 26 kDa (homodimer),[1,71,421,436,472] and 20 and 29 kDa.[152]

Cross-Reactivity

The cross-reactivity (amino acid sequence homology between human and mouse) for IL-6 is 42%.[71] Human IL-6 is functional on mouse cells, but murine IL-6 has no activity on human cells.

Chromosomal Location

The chromosomal locations of IL-6 and its receptor are 7p21-14 (IL-6), 1 (IL-6Rα), and 5 and 17 (gp130).

Cellular Origin

IL-6 is secreted by a wide variety of cells, including T and B lymphocytes,* monocytes and/or macrophages, fibroblasts, endothelial cells, epithelial cells, mast cells, neuronal cells, astrocytes, microglia, mesangial cells, osteoblasts, epidermal Langerhans' cells, dendritic cells, and keratinocytes and bone marrow stromal cells (Figure 22-15).†

*Loss of IL-6 secretion is a functional characteristic of human germinal center B lymphocytes. The change from an autocrine to a paracrine IL-6 response may permit a better control of B-cell growth and differentiation during the germinal center reaction.[68]

†References 1, 152, 288, 299, 341, 406.

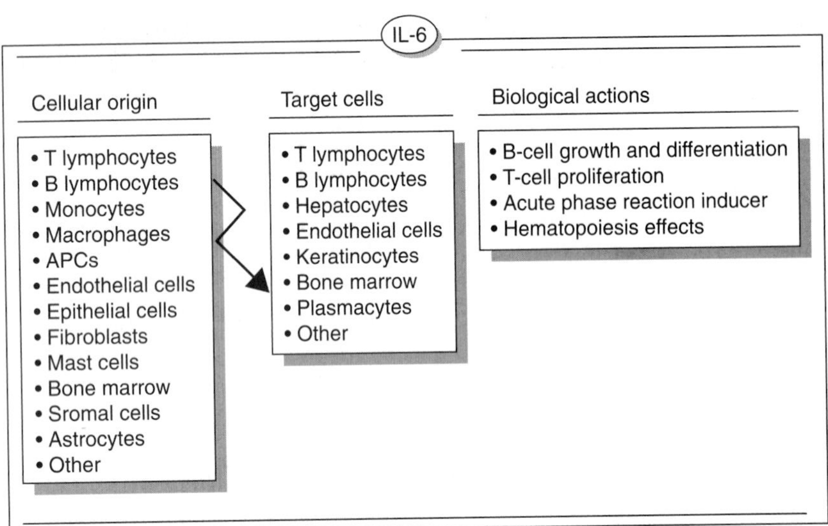

Figure 22-15 Cellular origin, principal target cells, and biological actions of IL-6.

Control of Synthesis and Release

Endotoxins, IL-1 and, to a lesser extent, TNFα are enhancers of IL-6 secretion.[1,152,472] However, studies have demonstrated that unlike TNF, IL-1 does not cause neutrophil degranulation in humans despite its ability to cause neutrophilia and the rapid release of IL-6 and IL-8.[395] Eosinophil major basic protein interacts in a synergistic fashion with IL-1α or TGFβ to augment fibroblast IL-6 type of cytokine production.[443] CD40 ligand triggers IL-6 secretion and related cellular differentiation and primes B cells for responsiveness to IL-10 with a consequent increase of Ig secretion.[543] The subcellular component of type III group B streptococci (GBS) is a potent inducer of IL-6 and may play an important role in tissue inflammation during GBS infection.[546] The complement activation fragment C5a has been shown to induce IL-6 synthesis by peripheral blood mononuclear cells (PBMCs). This may be important in the modulation of IL-6 synthesis in gram-negative bacteremia,[221] particularly because LPS is known to stimulate IL-6 release.

IL-10 and IL-4 inhibit cytokine expression in activated human monocytes, which suggests that IL-4 may inhibit the transcription of the IL-6 gene. IL-10 may inhibit the IL-6 mRNA levels posttranscriptionally, without suppressing promoter activity in human monocytes.[132,514] IL-10 also inhibits the production of IL-6, IL-12, and TNFα.[110] Reduced IL-6 levels in individuals who are exposed to chromate were reported, pointing to its possible role in negative immunomodulation.[490] Also, nitrite (NO^{-2}) induces a decrease of LPS-stimulated IL-1β, IL-6, IL-8, and TNFα release from activated alveolar macrophages.[273]

Receptor (IL-6R)

The IL-6R consists of a noncovalent association of a 60-kDa α-ligand–binding chain subunit (CD126) and a 130-kDa β-signal–transducing subunit (CD130, gp130). The binding protein contains both an Ig domain and a WSXWS motif. The signal transducing subunit does not itself bind IL-6 and also contains both an Ig domain and the WSXWS motif, but it is not specific for IL-6 (shared with IL-11, LIF, and other noninterleukin molecules, such as OSM and CNTF).* IL-6 interacts with the α-ligand–binding chain subunit of IL-6R, initiating interaction with gp130 and its dimerization.[341] However, gp130 transducing receptor cross-linking is sufficient to generate functional IL-6 type responses in hematopoietic, neural, and hepatic cells.[170]

IL-6 receptor has a density of about 50 to 2000 receptors per cell and is expressed on activated B cells (resting B cells do not express the IL-6R but are induced to express it following activation), plasma cells, T cells, monocytes, and many other cells, including epithelial cells, fibroblasts, hepatocytes, and neural cells.[71,152,341] Glucocorticoid-dependent induction of IL-6R expression in human hepatocytes facilitates IL-6 stimulation of amino acid transport, providing the liver with substrate to support key metabolic pathways during catabolic states.[165] Human bronchial epithelial cells constitutively expressed mRNA for IL-6R and IL-1α, and IL-6 itself up regulated IL-6R gene expression; IL-6 might be involved in the regulation of the epithelial functions via an autocrine and a paracrine mechanism.[515] It has also been demonstrated that the IL-11R can serve as a substitute to IL-6R in activating gene expression in target cells that are devoid of the appropriate ligand-binding receptor subunits.[33] Receptors for IL-10 and IL-6 type of cytokines use similar signaling mechanisms for inducing transcription through IL-6 response elements. This demonstrates that the IL-10R, unlike other members of the IFN receptor family, is highly effective in recruiting the signaling pathways of IL-6 type of cytokine receptors.[301] IL-6 has been found to possess three topologically distinct receptor binding sites: site 1 for binding to the subunit-specific chain IL-6Rα and sites 2 and 3 for the interaction with two subunits of the signaling chain

*References 1, 36, 71, 86, 152, 341.

gp130. It may be possible to develop effective IL-6 blocking agents in vivo.[493]

Shed IL-6 receptors (soluble receptors) can also bind IL-6 and signal through the cell-bound gp130 subunit.[1] Because the intracytoplasmic region of the IL-6Rα does not contribute to signaling, soluble forms of the extracytoplasmic domain (sIL-6Rα) potentiate IL-6 bioactivity and induce a cytokine-responsive status in cells expressing gp130 only. This observation, together with the detection of high levels of circulating soluble human IL-6Rα in sera, suggests that the IL-6–sIL-6Rα complex represents an alternative form of the cytokine.[531]

Signal Transduction

IL-6 binds to the IL-6Rα and the IL-6–IL-6Rα complex, which then binds two gp130 molecules to form a gp130 disulfide-linked homodimer, resulting in tyrosine phosphorylation of gp130 and signal transduction. IL-6 has also been shown to induce phosphorylation of the CD40 B-cell receptor.[71,341] Further investigation has revealed that IL-6, but neither IL-4 nor IFNγ, activates the LIL factor. Thus the existence of such a STAT-like factor relates the LPS and IL-1 signaling pathway to other cytokine receptor signaling pathways via the activation of STATs, suggesting that LPS, IL-1, and IL-6 may use a common signaling pathway.[539] IL-6 is the major cytokine-inducing transcription of human CRP during the APR. STAT family members have been shown to be important mediators of the effects of many cytokines—including IL-6, and especially STAT3, which participates in the transcriptional activation of CRP in response to IL-6.[594]

TABLE 22-5 Principal Biological Activities of IL-6*

Target	Action
Immune System	
B cells	Late growth and differentiation factor (increases IgS production)
T cells	Activation and proliferation (increases IL-2R expression)
	Differentiation of Tc cells
Bone marrow	Enhances hematopoiesis
Hepatocytes	Induces acute phase protein synthesis
Brain	
Pituitary	Increases ACTH
Hypothalamus	Rise of temperature
Astrocyte	Increases nerve growth factor production
Kidney	Increases mesangial proliferation
Endothelial cells	Secretion of IL-1 and TNFα
	Increases adherence for lymphocytes
Keratinocytes	Proliferation
	Secretion of IL-1 and TNFα
Human malignant plasma cells	Chemotaxis-inhibitory effect

*References 1, 37, 109, 341, 468, 477, 566.

Biological Actions

IL-6 has multifunctional and pleiotropic effects that are summarized in Table 22-5, but its two most extensively studied effects are on B cells and hepatocytes.[1,341]

IL-6 does not induce production of any other cytokines and has relatively little direct effect on immune cells at physiological concentrations, suggesting that its main immunological function is to potentiate the effect of other cytokines.

B Lymphocytes

In activated B cells, IL-6 acts late in the sequence of antigen- or mitogen-driven B-cell differentiation-promoting growth and facilitates maturation-enhancing Ig secretion (growth factor for plasmacytes). IL-6 and IL-10 from Th2 types of cells may play an important compensatory role in the induction and regulation of mucosal IgA responses.[396] IL-6 can also promote in vitro the growth of somatic cell hybrids (hybridomas) that produce monoclonal antibodies, and it acts as a growth factor for myeloma and/or plasmacytoma and Kaposi's sarcoma cells. Other cytokines (IFNs, TNFα, and TGFβ) and possibly other factors are potent, dominant inhibitors of IL-6–dependent plasmacytoma and/or hybridoma growth in vitro.[468]

Hepatocytes

IL-6 is the principal inducer of the APR, directly acting on hepatocytes to synthesize acute phase proteins, such as CRP, complement components, orosomucoid, haptoglobin, fibrinogen, protease inhibitors, and others. Its effects on the APR involve a complex interaction (namely synergistic actions) with several other cytokines, notably IL-1 and TNF.

T Lymphocytes and Natural Killer (NK) Cells

IL-6 is a co-stimulator of T cells and thymocytes, a differentiation factor for Tc lymphocytes, and a cofactor with other cytokines for the growth of early bone marrow hematopoietic stem cells. IL-10 production is enhanced in human T cells by IL-6 and IL-12.[109] IL-6 augments NK-cell activity (it appears to synergize also with IL-1).

Progenitor and Other Types of Cells

IL-6 synergizes with IL-3 (and probably GM-CSF) to support proliferation of neutrophil, monocyte, eosinophil, and megakaryocyte colonies. Increased mesangial proliferation in the kidney inhibits the growth of fibroblasts and induces class I HLA expression on their cell surfaces.

Endothelial Cells/Chemotaxis

IL-6 acts on endothelial cells to preferentially increase their adherence for lymphocytes (enhanced expression of intercellular adhesion molecule-1 [ICAM-1] and of VCAM-1 and E-selectin). These molecules and the leukocyte integrin LFA-1 all contribute to lymphocyte binding to endothelium activated by IL-6. It is proposed that IL-6 may also be involved in the recruitment of lymphocytes into nonlymphoid tissue.[566]

This cytokine has also been found to have a chemotaxis-inhibitory effect. High levels of IL-6 in the bone marrow microenvironment of patients with multiple myeloma appear to be favorable for the localization of myeloma cells in situ. This capacity to inhibit the chemotaxis of human malignant plasma cells is probably transduced via the signal-transducing receptor component, gp130.[477]

Immunoinflammatory Reactions/Fever

The demonstration that resident epidermal Langerhans' cells and the dendritic cells into which they develop are important sources of IL-6 explains the induction of cutaneous immunoinflammatory responses.[107] Human epidermal keratinocytes are induced to secrete IL-6 and co-stimulate T-lymphocyte proliferation by a CD40-dependent mechanism, amplifying inflammatory processes in the skin.[182] The rapid response in the expression of LIF and IL-6 genes after injury suggests that these cytokines act as trauma factors but with different roles in injured peripheral nerve.[77,295]

In common with IL-1 and TNF, IL-6 has a role as an endogenous pyrogen, inducing fever. It was suggested that central IL-6 is a necessary component of the fever response to both endogenous (IL-1β) and exogenous (LPS) pyrogens in mice and that IL-6 acts downstream from both peripheral and central IL-1β.[80]

Neuroendocrine Axis

IL-6 acts on the pituitary to induce adrenocorticotropic hormone (ACTH) release and directly on the adrenal glands to produce glucocorticoids. It is known that different cytokines that share gp130 as a receptor subunit induce serum amyloid A, and potentiate the induction of IL-6 and the activation of the hypothalamic-pituitary-adrenal axis by IL-1. In particular, LIF, OSM, IL-11, and cardiotrophin-1 potentiate the elevation of serum corticosterone and IL-6 levels induced by IL-1. Furthermore, the potentiation of IL-1–induced serum corticosterone levels is not a consequence of the increased serum IL-6 observed after IL-1 administration. Thus either endogenous IL-6 does not mediate IL-1–induced corticosterone increase, or its role may be fulfilled by other cytokines. This is very important in the understanding of the activation of the hypothalamic-pituitary-adrenal axis and that potentiation of acute phase protein synthesis may represent an important feedback regulatory mechanism of inflammation.[37]

Clinical Relevance

Increased levels in the circulation have been identified following gram-negative bacterial infection and inflammatory reactions. IL-6 is detected in the serum of patients or experimental animals undergoing bacterial sepsis. Studies have indicated that IL-6 protects against virulent infection and suggest that the protective effect may be at least partially mediated through neutrophils.[1,111,436] IL-6 in these conditions is one of the more easily measured cytokines in the blood. Also, LPS responsiveness of proinflammatory cytokines (IL-1β, IL-6, IL-8, and TNFα) in whole blood from people with high and low levels of high-density lipoproteins is different, presumably of importance in inflammation and atherogenesis.[151] By secretion of pro-inflammatory cytokines, mast cells assist in the recruitment of monocytes and T lymphocytes into the vascular tissue, thereby promoting monocyte and/or macrophage-derived, cholesteryl-containing ester foam cell formation. Mast cells facilitate foam cell formation by promoting native and oxidized low-density lipoproptein (Ox-LDL) uptake by macrophages. Mast cell–derived cytokines and growth factors and tryptase might activate proliferation of vascular smooth muscle and fibroblasts, allowing the development of the obstructive lesions observed in human atherosclerosis.[270]

Balanced production of cytokines by alveolar macrophages may be very important for inflammatory outcome. During acute complications of lung transplantation, it has been shown that alveolar Ms display an early activation with oversecretion of IL-6, which is involved in tissue injury, counterbalanced by a late activation in which TGFβ predominates, mediating tissue repair.[337]

IL-6, produced by macrophages in the periprosthetic membranes surrounding joint replacements, has been implicated as a causal agent in osteolysis and prosthetic loosening and, when produced by T cells from the femoral head of patients with rapidly destructive coxopathy, has also been related with this pathological condition.[51,516] Further studies suggest that secretion of IL-6 by osteoblasts is crucial for stimulation of bone resorption not only by parathyroid hormone, but also by parathyroid hormone–related protein, vasoactive intestinal peptide, and β-adrenergic agonists, such as isoproterenol.[199]

Because IL-6 is an autocrine growth factor for many types of cells, its hyperproduction has been associated with a variety of malignancies, including plasmacytoma, multiple myeloma, uterine cervical carcinoma, and Kaposi's sarcoma.[1,472] A consensus regarding myeloma cell growth factor responsiveness and the ability to produce autocrine IL-6 has not yet been obtained; however it is thought to be caused by the heterogeneity observed; between cell lines and in clinical disease.[574] A central role for STAT3 has been suggested in IL-6–induced regulation of growth and differentiation in M1 leukemia cells, which determines the cellular decision from cell growth to differentiation in M1 cells.[383]

Considering the role of IL-6 in inflammation and immune response, and its known association with increased levels of MyD116 and GADD 34 mRNAs (genes involved in the prevention of apoptotic death of cells), pathological effects of herpes simplex virus can result because of a combination of direct viropathic effects and immunological reactions to viral antigens, namely a selective activation of IL-6 expression.[251]

Reviews emphasize the presumed activities of IL-6 in normal skin; in some diseases with cutaneous involvement in the pathogenesis of both local and systemic inflammation, including surgical ones, tumor development, autoimmune diseases, infectious diseases, and others.*

Therapeutic Applications

IL-6 may be useful to support neutrophil and megakaryocyte growth in patients treated with high doses of chemotherapy. However, alterations in platelet function in patients receiving IL-6 as cytokine therapy have been reported.[398] In experimental conditions, IL-6 altered platelet function as measured by reactivity to thrombin, even though effective at promoting platelet production.[415] Also, patients infected with HTLV-1 have been reported to respond to IL-6.[485] IL-6 reduces myocardial damage in mice with viral myocarditis, probably through the modification of immune responses together with reduction in viral replication. However, early activation of immune responses and attenuation of viral replication appear most significant, as reflected in the limited time window during which IL-6 is effective in myocarditis.[252]

Strategies designed to interfere with either autocrine or paracrine growth-promoting effects of IL-6 in malignancies may be useful.[472]

INTERLEUKIN-7

Interleukin-7 (IL-7) is an interleukin produced by epithelial and mesangial stromal cells, which serves as a differentiation factor for B cells in the early stages of their development and also supports the growth of some thymocytes and T lymphocytes.[138]

*References 153, 163, 300, 305, 386, 406, 433, 518, 527.

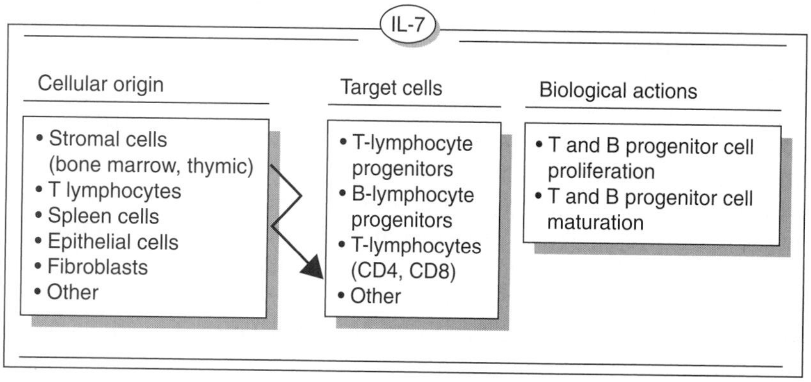

Synonyms

IL-7 was formerly known as lymphopoietin 1 (LP-1), B-cell growth factor, and pre–B-cell growth factor.

General Characteristics

The three-dimensional structure of IL-7 is not known, but it is a member of the four α-helical short-chain cytokine family (152AA). It stimulates early B- and T-lymphocyte growth and the proliferation and differentiation of mature T cells, which are produced by stromal marrow and thymus cells.[71,421,432] IL-7 can be classified as a CSF.[152]

Other general characteristics of IL-7 include:

Molecular Weight

The literature values for the molecular weight of IL-7 vary from 20 to 28 kDa. The following molecular weights have been reported: 25 kDa (monomer),[1,152,341,389,421] 20 to 28 kDa,[71,436] and 22 to 28 kDa.[472]

Cross-Reactivity

The cross-reactivity (amino acid sequence homology between human and mouse) for IL-7 is 60%.[71] Cross-species reactivity also has been observed and verified.

Chromosomal Location

The chromosomal locations of IL-7 and its receptor are 8q12-13 (IL-7) and 5p13 (IL-7R).

Cellular Origin

IL-7 is produced by bone marrow and thymic stromal cells, T lymphocytes, spleen cells, epithelial cells, and fibroblasts (Figure 22-16).[71,177,421,432]

Control of Synthesis and Release

Stromal cells from a variety of lymphoid and nonlymphoid tissues constitutively produce low levels of IL-7. This production is not affected by the lectins and mitogens that normally influence the synthesis of other growth factors.[472]

IL-7

Cellular origin	Target cells	Biological actions
• Stromal cells (bone marrow, thymic) • T lymphocytes • Spleen cells • Epithelial cells • Fibroblasts • Other	• T-lymphocyte progenitors • B-lymphocyte progenitors • T-lymphocytes (CD4, CD8) • Other	• T and B progenitor cell proliferation • T and B progenitor cell maturation

Figure 22-16 Cellular origin, principal target cells, and biological actions of IL-7.

Receptor (IL-7R)

The IR-7 receptor belongs to the hematopoietic receptor family, which includes the receptors for IL-2, IL-4, IL-6, IL-11, and GM-CSF.[341,472] It is a complex structure consisting of an IL-7 binding chain (α-chain, CD127) and the IL-2R γ-chain (γc). The CD127 contains the WSXWS motif, but it is unclear whether it should be included as a member of the cytokine receptor superfamily. The IL-7R γ-chain is a functional component enhancing IL-7 binding (shared with IL-4R, IL-9R, IL-13R, and IL-15R). This chain may explain the described high- and low-affinity binding sites. A soluble form of IL-7R has also been identified that originates by alternative splicing of the IL-7 gene.[71]

IL-7R is expressed on bone marrow lymphoid precursors, pro-B cells, thymocytes, mature T cells, and monocytes.[71,152] Data from a 1993 study suggest that heparin may act as a carrier for IL-7, blocking its interaction with target cells and protecting it from degradation during transit.[92]

Signal Transduction

IL-7 stimulates tyrosine phosphorylation of cellular proteins and tyrosine kinase–dependent activation of phosphatidyl-inositol-specific phospholipase C.[71] IL-7 has been observed to induce a rapid and dose-dependent tyrosine phosphorylation of JAK1 and JAK3 and concomitantly the tyrosine phosphorylation and DNA-binding activity of multiple STAT proteins. The STAT proteins used by IL-7 were identical to those induced by IL-2 and could be identified as various STAT5 isoforms. Moreover, the induction of both JAK1 and JAK3, and STAT5 activity strongly correlated with the growth-promoting effects of IL-7, suggests that this signal transduction mechanism may play a key role in IL-7–induced proliferation.[172]

Biological Actions

IL-7 promotes the growth of B- and T-cell progenitors (probably at the same level of development as IL-3 or GM-CSF) and proliferation of mature T cells (CD4 and CD8). It also facilitates the differentiation of both T-cell progenitors and Tc cells but not of B cells. It can stimulate T cells to proliferate even with a suboptimum concentration of IL-2.[1,71,341,436,485] IL-7 increases production of IL-2 and expression of IL-2R in T lymphocytes and stimulates the generation of LAK activity.[472] It also appears to promote TCR gene rearrangement among pre-T cells, namely D-J β rearrangement.[152,538] It induces secretion of IL-1α, IL-1β, IL-6, and TNFα by monocytes and tumoricidal activity in these cells.[341,485] IL-1 and TGFβ can block the stimulatory effects of IL-7.[472] IFNα and IFNβ have been found to be potent inhibitors of IL-7–induced growth of early B lineage cells and have no effect on cell growth induced by IL-2, IL-3, IL-4, or autogenous factors. The combination of IL-7 and these IFNs induces bcl-2 down regulation and cell death by apoptosis. This may explain this inhibition factor, which maintains the balanced production of normal B lineage cells.[562] Another demonstration of a selective induction of CD23 expression on activated human T cells cultured in the presence of IL-7 indicates that this cytokine has an important role in the regulatory network of the immune response.[75] IL-2 and IL-7 reciprocally induce IL-7 and IL-2 receptors on γδ T-cell intraepithelial lymphocytes with subsequent activation. The sources of these two cytokines were neighboring epithelial cells (IL-7) and αβ T cells (IL-2 and IL-7), respectively.[177] IL-7R is indispensable for normal lymphocyte development, and the IL-7R α chain not only causes progenitors to proliferate, but also has a distinct activity in inducing differentiation. Thus the signals that mediate a differentiative function of the IL-7R in B lymphopoiesis are specific and distinct from those causing proliferation.[97]

Clinical Relevance

IL-7 is known to regulate HIV-1 replication in naturally infected peripheral blood mononuclear cells (PBMCs).[488] From asymptomatic, chronically infected donors, IL-7–induced virus replication and increased proviral DNA levels in these cells are probably independent of the stimulation of IL-1β, IL-6, or TNFα production by PBMCs.

Therapeutic Applications

IL-7 may be useful in tumor therapy because of its ability to enhance the generation of Tc lymphocytes and LAK cells, even in the absence of IL-2.[341] Because of its capacity to stimulate lymphopoiesis, IL-7 may also be helpful for the therapy of some immunodeficiencies or to accelerate recovery following bone marrow transplantation.[472,485] IL-7 is also able to induce the proliferation of pro-B cells and CD4 and CD8 T cells and to enhance cytotoxicity of Tc and NK cells, indicating its possible therapeutic applications by enhancement of the immune system (tumors and infections). Its significant cross-species reactivity allows exogenous administration of human rIL-7, which protects mice against acute parasite challenge. This protection results from the stimulation of IFNγ production and augments the CD8 T-cell–mediated cytotoxic response.[260]

INTERLEUKIN-8

Interleukin-8 (IL-8) is a chemokine produced by monocytes, endothelial cells, and other cells that acts as a chemotactic and activator for neutrophils and may play a role in the extravasation of neutrophils in inflammation.[138] (For additional information, see later section on chemokines.)

INTERLEUKIN-9

Interleukin-9 (IL-9) is a cytokine produced by T cells and macrophages that acts as a growth factor for some T-cell populations and bone marrow–mast cell progenitors.[138]

Synonyms

IL-9 was formerly known as human p40, mouse IL-9 as p40, mast cell growth-enhancing activity, and T-cell growth factor III (TCGF-III).

General Characteristics

The three-dimensional structure of IL-9 is not known. However, it is known to be a glycoprotein of the four α-helical short-chain family (126AA). Similar to IL-2, it is a T-cell–derived T-lymphocyte growth factor with no effect on resting cells.

Other general characteristics of IL-9 include:

Molecular Weight

The literature values for the molecular weight of IL-9 vary from 14 to 40 kDa. The following molecular weights have been reported: 14 kDa,[341] 40 kDa,[421,485] 30 to 40 kDa,[1,152] 20 kDa,[436] and 32 to 39 kDa.[71,389,472]

Cross-Reactivity

The cross-reactivity (amino acid sequence homology between human and mouse) for IL-9 is 55%.[71] Mouse IL-9 has activity on human cells, but human IL-9 is inactive on mouse cells.

Chromosomal Location

The chromosomal location of IL-9 is 5q23-31, 5q31.1(IL-9).[71] The chromosomal location of its receptor is unknown.

Cellular Origin

IL-9 is produced by some activated T cells (mainly by activated CD4 Th2 lymphocytes for which it represents an autocrine growth factor) and Hodgkin's lymphoma cells (Figure 22-17).[71,341]

Control of Synthesis and Release

The mechanisms for controlling the synthesis and release of IL-9 are currently unknown.

Receptor (IL-9R)

This is a single-chain receptor, which is a heavily glycosylated protein of 64 kDa, associated with the IL-2R γ-chain. Both membrane-bound and soluble forms of the IL-9R exist. It is expressed on T helper clones, macrophages, some T-cell tumors, and mast cell lines.[71,341]

Signal Transduction

IL-9 causes tyrosine phosphorylation of proteins but not of MAP kinase.[71] It has also been demonstrated that JAK1 was constitutively associated with the IL-9 receptor. Activated STAT complexes induced by IL-9 have been found to contain STAT1, STAT3, and STAT5 transcription factors. Moreover, sequence homologies between human IL-9R tyrosine 116 and tyrosines of other receptors activating STAT3 and STAT5 have been observed. Collectively, these data indicate that a single tyrosine of the IL-9 receptor required for activation of three different STAT proteins is necessary for distinct activities of this cytokine, including proliferative responses.[125]

Biological Actions

IL-9 is a T-cell growth factor that acts in synergy with other cytokines (with IL-2, it causes proliferation of T cells and with IL-4, it promotes IgE and IgG synthesis by plasmacytes).[341] However, it supports the growth of some Th2 T-cell clones in the absence of IL-2 or IL-4. It has also been found to enhance the proliferative action of IL-3 on mast cell progenitors, to augment basophil proliferation and erythroid colony formation, and to stimulate the proliferation of megakaryoblastic leukemia cells.[71,432,485]

Clinical Relevance

IL-9 can support cell proliferation in the absence of an antigen or APC. Overproduction of it may lead to T-cell tumors, particularly of Th2 lymphocytes. In certain lymphomas, such as Hodgkin's lymphoma, it may act as an autocrine signal for cellular proliferation.[341,472] IL-9 may play a role in the development of acute myeloblastic leukemia by stimulating leukemic cells to enter the S-phase rather than preventing cell death. In addition, IL-9 acts synergistically with stem cell factor for recruiting quiescent leukemic cells in the cell cycle.[312]

IL-9 is a member of the Th2 cytokine family and has been implicated as an essential factor in determining mucosal immunity and susceptibility to atopic asthma. It has also been found in association with severe asthma and to cause airway hyperresponsiveness.[29,57,597]

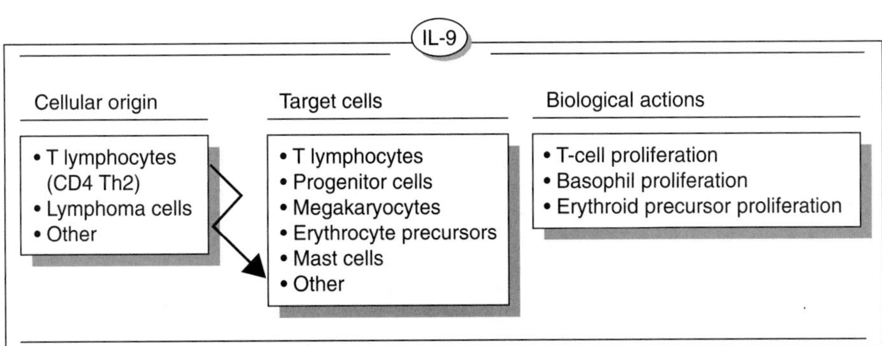

Figure 22-17 Cellular origin, principal target cells, and biological actions of IL-9.

Therapeutic Applications

Currently, there are no therapeutic applications of IL-9.

INTERLEUKIN-10

Interleukin-10 (IL-10) is a cytokine produced by activated macrophages, certain lymphocytes, and other cells that decreases both innate and T-cell–mediated immune inflammation; it inhibits the production of cytokines by activated T cells, plays a role in B-cell activation, inhibits production of IFNγ, and blocks antigen presentation and macrophage formation of IL-1, IL-6, and TNF.[138]

Synonyms

IL-10 was formerly known as B-cell–derived T-cell growth factor, cytokine synthesis inhibitory factor (CSIF), MCGF, and thymocyte growth-promoting factor.*

General Characteristics

IL-10 is a member of the four α-helical cytokine family and probably functions as a homodimer (160AA).[1] However, its three-dimensional structure is not yet known. It is a pleiotropic Th2 CD4 lymphocyte cytokine (also Th1 in humans) with the capacity to inhibit cell-mediated responses but also to enhance some specific aspects of the immune reaction. This gives it unique immunoregulatory properties.

This cytokine has been shown to have a 70% identity with an open reading frame (BCRF1) of the Epstein-Barr virus (EBV) genome. It and the protein encoded by BCRF1 (vIL-10) have some common activities, such as suppression of IFN production and macrophage activation.[71] This homology raises the possibility that EBV has captured and processed the human gene as a means of inhibiting antiviral immunity. EBV infection can cause immune suppression, which is probably dependent on an IL-10–like viral peptide.[472] vIL-10 shares with IL-10 predominantly inhibitory effects, such as macrophage deactivation conducing to a local immunosuppressive effect, which is particularly important in tumor biology and treatment.[43]

Other general characteristics of IL-10 include:

Molecular Weight

The literature values for the molecular weight of IL-10 vary from 17 to 40 kDa. The following molecular weights have been reported: 17 to 21 kDa,[341,389] 18 to 20 kDa,[1] 40 kDa,[421] 18 kDa,[152,436,472] and 35 to 40 kDa.[71]

Cross-Reactivity

The cross-reactivity (amino acid sequence homology between human and mouse) for IL-10 is 72%.[71] Human IL-10 is active on mouse cells, but murine IL-10 is inactive on human cells.

Chromosomal Location

The chromosomal locations of IL-10 and its receptor are 1 (IL-10) and 11 (IL-10R).

Cellular Origin

IL-10 is produced by Th0 and Th2 subsets of CD4 T lymphocytes (Figure 22-18). Data suggest that IL-10 can also be produced by activated B cells, some Th1 cells, CD8 T cells, activated macrophages, and other cells, such as eosinophils, dendritic cells, and keratinocytes.[1,71,152,341,383]

Control of Synthesis and Release

IL-10 production is enhanced in human T cells by IL-12 and IL-6 and in monocytes by TNFα. These findings suggest that IL-10 production by human T cells and monocytes is differentially regulated. IL-10 inhibits the production of IL-6, IL-12, and TNFα, which may indicate a potential mechanism of negative feedback regulation of the immune response.[110,499] IL-12 induces differentiation of Th1 cells, primarily through its ability to prime T cells for high IFNγ production, which in turn is an inhibitor of IL-10 production. Besides the presence of IL-12 during the first several days of in vitro clonal expansion of polyclonally stimulated human

*The same name is more consistently attributed to IL-3 and IL-4 (MCGF-II).

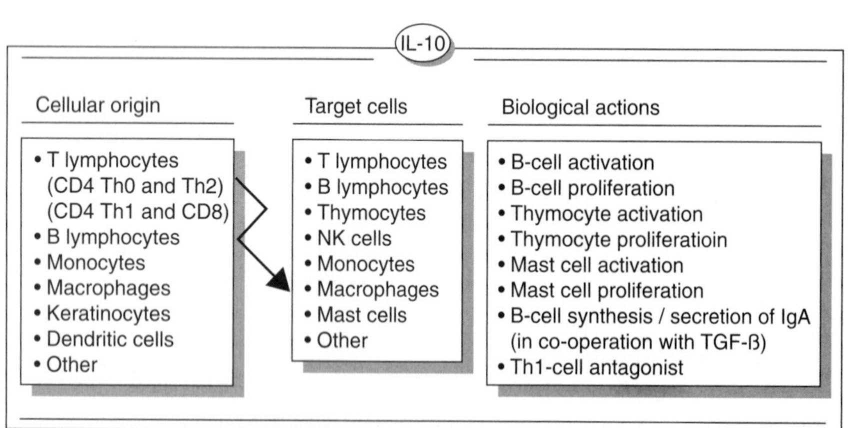

Figure 22-18 Cellular origin, principal target cells, and biological actions of IL-10.

peripheral blood, CD4 and CD8 T cells induce stable priming for high IL-10 production, but IL-4 almost completely suppresses this priming for IL-10 production.[185] Recombinant IFNβ blocks proliferation but enhances IL-10 secretion by activated human T cells.[435] Activation of human monocytes by LPS results in an initial burst of inflammatory cytokines, such as TNFα, that is followed by the secretion of anti-inflammatory mediators, such as IL-10. The regulation of IL-10 expression is more complex than that of TNFα.[358] Vasoactive intestinal peptide (VIP), a neuropeptide present in the peptidergic innervation of lymphoid organs and expressed in thymocytes and peripheral lymphocytes, has the capacity to modulate cytokine expression in T lymphocytes. VIP and the structurally related neuropeptide PACAP-38 inhibit IL-10 production by spleen cells or thymocytes.[348] Proopiomelanocortin peptides may be able to up regulate the production of IL-10 in monocytes and thereby contribute to immunosuppression.[46] Triggering of the CD23 molecule at the surface of human macrophages induces the generation of IL-10 through a cAMP-dependent mechanism. Concomitantly, this generation of IL-10 is down regulated by NO. This generation is also produced after triggering of the CD23 antigen. Collectively, these data indicate that human macrophages produce IL-10 after triggering of the CD23 molecule and that this production can regulate the inflammatory state of these cells.[148]

Receptor (IL-10R)

IL-10R is a single-chain receptor. IL-10R belongs to the class II cytokine receptor family that also includes the IFN receptors (IFNγ and IFNαβ receptors). The extracellular region consists of two homologous fibronectin type III domains that are without the WSXWS motif characteristic of class I cytokine receptors. It is expressed on B cells, thymocytes, and other cellular lines such as mast cells and macrophages. Human IL-10R mRNA is restricted mostly to hematopoietic cells and cell lines.[71]

Signal Transduction

Signal transduction by IL-10 is still unknown but likely to involve the JAK family of kinases.[71] The signal transduction cascades initiated by IL-10 ligation to its cognate receptor seem to rapidly and transiently stimulate phosphatidylinositol 3-kinase activity associated with the p85 subunit of the enzyme. IL-10 also activates p70 S6 kinase that is inhibited by the immunosuppressive drug rapamycin.[104]

Receptors for IL-10 and IL-6 cytokines appear to use similar signaling mechanisms for inducing transcription through IL-6 response elements. The cytoplasmic domain of the IL-10R contains two motifs that have been identified in the signal-transducing receptor subunits for IL-6 and known to be required for activating STAT3 and inducing transcription through IL-6–responsive elements. To determine whether the IL-10R has signaling functions similar to IL-6R in cells normally expressing these receptors, leukocytes of the B-, T-, and NK-cell lineages have been treated with either cytokine. Data demonstrate that the IL-10R, unlike other members of the IFN receptor family, is highly effective in recruiting the signaling pathways of IL-6 type of cytokine receptors.[301]

Biological Actions

IL-10 causes the inhibition of general proinflammatory cytokine synthesis, APC function, and cell-mediated immunity and induces the terminal differentiation of B cells into plasmacytes, which results in production of antibodies. Consequently, it has important effects on T and B lymphocytes, NK cells, monocytes and/or macrophages, and mast cells.[341,436] It is characterized by a paradoxical duality of function (negative and/or positive; Box 22-5).

This cytokine is a pleiotropic cytokine that can suppress cytokine expression by NK cells and Th1 lymphocytes, thus down regulating cell-mediated immunity and stimulating humoral responses.[596] Resulting T-cell anergy may then play an important role in the induction and maintenance of antigen-specific T-cell tolerance.[201] IL-10 is also capable of down regulating the release of IL-6 and PGE2. Endogenously synthesized IL-10 limits the immune complex–induced secretion of proinflammatory cytokines TNFα and IL-1β.[41] The antiinflammatory properties of IL-4, IL-10, IL-13, and TGFβ are associated with their ability to repress the production of proinflammatory cytokines and to favor the release of interleukin I receptor anatagonist (IIRA). Inhibition by IL-10 of proinflammatory cytokine release (IL-2 and IFNγ by Th1 cells) appears to occur at the level of gene

BOX 22-5 Duality of IL-10 Function

Negative Actions

- Inhibition of cytokine synthesis by activated Th1 and NK cells (indirect effect, mediated by a primary action on macrophages [Ms])
- Inhibition of cytokine secretion (IL-1, TNFα, IL-12, chemokines, GM-CSF, and G-CSF) by mononuclear cells
- Inhibition of IFNγ-induced production of reactive oxygen radicals and NO by macrophages
- Down regulation of MHC class II expression and of co-stimulators, such as B7, on Ms (inhibition of the accessory functions of Ms in T-cell activation)
- Antiimmunoinflammatory activity caused by down regulation of Th1 T cells, Ms, and NK cells

Positive Actions

- Chemoattractant for diverse cell types
- Synergizes with IL-2 and IL-7 in the proliferation of thymocytes and T cells
- Synergizes with other cytokines to stimulate proliferation of B cells, thymocytes, and MCs
- Stimulates B lymphocytes (together with TGFβ, causes IgA production, induces B-cell proliferation, and may be a switching factor for the production of IgG4)

transcription for TNFα and both transcriptionally and post-transcriptionally for IL-1β.[315] However, IL-10 is unable to induce IL1-RA by itself or to amplify the LPS-induced production by PMNs. It is able to increase its release when TNFα is the triggering signal.[345] The action of IL-10 as a potent inhibitor of TNFα expression and release from alveolar macrophages and peripheral blood monocytes may have an important role in the cytokine network of local immune response similar to its pulmonary one.[13] Despite IL-1α and TNFα release by alveolar macrophages, IL-6 release can only be suppressed to some extent by a combination of IL-4 and IL-10 (inhibiting the transcription rate of the IL-6 gene).[132,599] It has been suggested that the down regulation of fibrinogen biosynthesis by IL-4, IL-10, and IL-13 represents a protective vascular effect.[551]

Alternately, it is known that IL-10 has both stimulatory and inhibitory effects on diverse types of cells, including co-stimulation of T-cell proliferation (particularly Th2 cells), chemoattraction of CD8 T cells, and stimulation of LAK cell activity.[43] Also, osteoclast-like cells demonstrated an up regulation of NO production and inducible NO synthase mRNA by IL-8 and IL-10.[504]

Clinical Relevance

IL-10 has not been implicated in virus-induced diseases, but the mimicry of IL-10 by EBV is a method for pathogens to interfere with host defense mechanisms. This interference can have possible important pathological consequences.[472] IL-10, in addition to down regulating the cellular immune response to HIV-1, may also play a role in TNFα-mediated activation of HIV-1 replication.[164] During the acute phase of Kawasaki disease, levels of IL-10 are markedly elevated. This increase in serum IL-10 levels may contribute to the up regulation of humoral immunity and to the down regulation of acute inflammation.[275] An imbalance of Th-cell populations leads to the secretion of mostly IL-4 and IL-10 at the start of infection. The concomitant down regulation of IFNγ secretion reversed the host's resistance to *Trypanosoma cruzi.*[27] IL-10 has been shown to exert an inhibitory effect on cell-mediated immunity with a contribution to parasite Ag-induced T-cell hyporesponsiveness observed in patients with chronic *Schistosoma haematobium* infection.[276] It has also been demonstrated that diminished IL-10 production in asthma permits the unopposed synthesis of proinflammatory cytokines, thereby contributing to the development and severity of asthma.[60] Increased IL-10 serum levels in patients with solid tumors may have important implications for future investigations, immunological monitoring, and therapeutic intervention on neoplastic patients and suggests a mechanism for tumor cells escaping from immune surveillance.[168]

Polymorphisms in cytokine genes can influence immune responses, inflammation, and tissue injury and may affect the outcome of hematopoietic stem cell transplantation. Among recipients of hematopoietic cells from an HLA-identical sibling, the IL-10-592A allele seems to be a marker of a favorable outcome after transplantation. Despite advances in supportive care, severe grade III or IV graft-versus-host disease (GVHD) remains a serious complication of transplantation and contributes to transplantation-related mortality. High level of IL-10 production by recipients' cells during the early posttransplantation period mitigates the intensity of the alloimmune response and GVHD-induced inflammation, thereby reducing the clinical manifestations of GVHD and associated mortality. Knowledge of the IL-10 promoter-region genotypes, and possibly of polymorphisms in other immune regulatory genes, could be incorporated into the pretransplantation risk-assessment process and serve as a guide for the planning of treatment. The use of alternative approaches, such as nonablative conditioning regimens, might reduce morbidity and mortality in selected high-risk patients. Further insight into the mechanism underlying the association between the IL-10 promoter-region genotype and GVHD could prompt new strategies for modulating the intensity of the alloimmune response and reducing the toxicity of GVHD.[322]

Therapeutic Applications

Being a modulator of cytotoxic cell activity (macrophages, NK cells, and Th1 cells), IL-10 may be able to ameliorate clinical situations characterized by a hyperinflammatory reaction, such as septic shock. Its capacity to inhibit the production of IFNγ (namely by Th1 cells) is also of interest in various clinical situations, particularly those in which it is important to suppress delayed types of hypersensitivity responses (DTHR) without affecting antibody production.

IL-10 is also an efficient inhibitor of tumor metastasis in experimental models in vivo at doses that do not have toxic effects on normal cells. Histological characterization after IL-10 treatment has confirmed the absence of CD8 and CD4 T cells and macrophages at the sites of tumor growth; however, abundant NK cells were localized at these sites.[596] Human IL-10 differs from its EBV homologue viral IL-10 (vIL-10), because it can stimulate the acquisition of an effective, specific, and long-lived antitumor immune response in murine models and can reverse the local immunosuppressive effects of vIL-10. This indicates a potential role for IL-10 administration in the biological therapy of cancer and suggests a broader interpretation of IL-10 biology.[43]

Interleukin-11

Interleukin-11 (IL-11) is a cytokine produced by bone marrow stromal cells that stimulates megakaryocyte proliferation and B-cell differentiation.[138]

Synonym

IL-11 was formerly known as adipogenesis inhibitory factor.

General Characteristics

IL-11 belongs to the four α-helical long-chain cytokine family (179AA). Information is incomplete about its three-dimensional structure. It is known to be a bone marrow stromal cell–derived cytokine involved in lymphopoiesis and hematopoiesis.[71,485]

Other general characteristics of IL-11 include:

Molecular Weight

The literature values for the molecular weight of IL-11 vary from 19 to 23 kDa. The following molecular weights have been reported: 20 kDa,[1,152] 23 kDa,[71,421,436] and 19 to 21 kDa.[389]

Cross-Reactivity

The cross-reactivity (amino acid sequence homology between human and mouse) for IL-11Rα is 84%.[71,384] Human IL-11 is active on mouse cells.

Chromosomal Location

The chromosomal locations of IL-11 and its receptor are 19q13.3-13.4 (IL-11) and 9p13 (IL-11Rα-chain).

Cellular Origin

IL-11 is produced by bone marrow stromal cells, trophoblast cells, glial cells, and IL-1–stimulated fibroblasts (Figure 22-19).[1,71,152,377]

Control of Synthesis and Release

Synthesis of IL-11 is induced by IL-1 and TGFβ in stromal cells and fibroblasts; cytokines that inhibit its production remain to be defined. In addition, IFNα has been found to down regulate IL-1–induced IL-11 in human bone marrow stromal cultures.[7]

Receptor (IL-11R)

The high-affinity receptor for IL-11 is composed of two subunits, IL-11 receptor α-chain (IL-11Rα) and gp130, the common subunit of the IL-6, CNTF, LIF, and OSM receptors. The IL-11 receptor-specific α chain shares homologies with the α chain of the CNTF and IL-6 receptors, confirming evolutionary conservation at the level of gene organization among the hematopoietic cytokine receptor family.[85]

The IL-11Rα has the requirement of either the human or mouse gp130 molecule for signaling because the human IL-11Rα-chain is able to form a functional receptor complex in association with murine gp130 or human gp130. This complex results in high-affinity IL-11–binding sites and IL-11–dependent cellular proliferation.[384] The functional receptor complexes assembled in response to IL-6, IL-11, LIF, OSM, and CNTF all involve the signal transducer gp130. IL-6 and IL-11 induce homodimerization of gp130, and LIF, OSM, and CNTF heterodimerize gp130 with other gp130-related β subunits. IL-6, IL-11, and CNTF also require a specificity-determining α-subunit not directly involved in signaling. Studies have established that stromal and/or osteoblastic cells are targets for the actions of all the members of the cytokine subfamily that share the gp130 signal transducer; this suggests that different receptor repertoires may be expressed at different stages of differentiation of this lineage.[36]

Signal Transduction

IL-11 intracellular signaling travels through cytoplasmic kinases of the Janus family. How JAKs accomplish the multiple functions of IL-11 has not been determined and only a few associated downstream proteins have been identified, in particular the evidence for the IL-11–induced association of protein phosphatase (PP2A), P13K, and Yes to JAK2. This novel finding of JAK2 and/or PP2A binding and release may have relevance to many serine and/or threonine-regulated mechanisms, such as P13K, STAT, and mitogen-activated protein kinase (MAPK) activation. These associations support a model of JAK2 as a protein kinase docking protein of IL-11 signal transduction, which may be applicable to other gp130 and JAK signal transduction systems.[176] IL-11R can also serve as a substitute IL-6R in activating gene expression in target cells that are devoid of the appropriate ligand-binding receptor subunits.[33]

Biological Actions

The biological activities of IL-11 are not fully characterized, but they are similar to those of IL-6, LIF, and OSM.[485] For example, IL-11 (1) stimulates the development of diverse hematopoietic cell lineages from bone marrow precursors (especially of early hematopoiesis), including monocytes and/or macrophages and megakaryocytes; (2) is a growth factor for plasmacytes, hematopoietic multipotential cells,

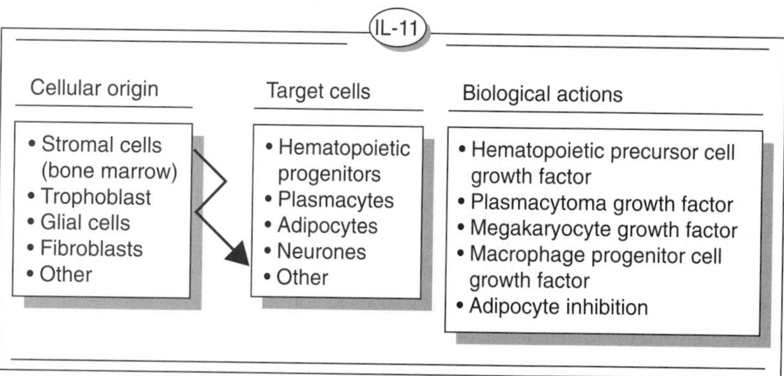

Figure 22-19 Cellular origin, principal target cells, and biological actions of IL-11.

and committed megakaryocytic and macrophage progenitor cells; and (3) inhibits adipogenesis in mouse preadipocytes. It is also involved in the production of APP and has been reported to increase the number of antibody-forming B cells in response to an antigen.[7,71,485] However, when compared with IL-6, IL-11 and LIF induced only minimal stimulation on production of APP by human primary hepatocytes. Thus circulating levels of IL-11 or LIF do not contribute significantly to the production of APR in vivo, and they do not seem to account for the difference in APR response between systemic lupus erythematosus and other inflammatory rheumatic diseases.[181] It has been shown that IL-6, IL-11, and to a lesser extent LIF in rat hepatocytes are potential mediators of metallothionein synthesis in inflammation.[102]

Cerebral expression of IL-11 by glial cells is important because IL-11 has been shown to have effects on neuronal electrophysiology, has overlapping functions with the neuroactive cytokine IL-6, and is part of the gp130-associated neuropoietic family of cytokines.[377]

Clinical Relevance

IL-11 is expressed in leukemic myeloid cells, and their proliferation is regulated by this cytokine, which acts synergistically.[311]

Therapeutic Applications

As a stimulator of megakaryopoiesis, IL-12 may be of therapeutic benefit in patients with platelet deficiencies.[1] Ex vivo expansion with stem cell factor and IL-11 augments both short-term recovery posttransplant and the ability to transplant bone marrow serially.[219]

INTERLEUKIN-12

Interleukin-12 (IL-12) is a heterodimeric cytokine produced by phagocytic cells, B cells, and other antigen-presenting types of cells. It is a potent inducer of cytokine production, causes T and NK cells to secrete IFN-γ, is a growth factor for preactivated T and NK cells, and enhances cytotoxic activity in $CD8^+$ T cells and NK cells. It also has a role in the generation of T helper type 1 cells and in the differentiation of cytotoxic T lymphocytes.[138]

Synonyms

IL-12 was formerly known as cytotoxic lymphocyte maturation factor (CLMF), natural killer cell stimulatory factor (NKSF), and T-cell stimulatory factor.

General Characteristics

Information is incomplete concerning the three-dimensional structure of IL-12. However, it is known to be a heterodimeric four α-helical short-chain cytokine (196AA/306AA) that stimulates T- and NK-cell function.[71,341,421] It consists of two covalently linked polypeptide chains, one of 35 kDa (p35, IL-12α) and the other of 40 kDa (p40, IL-12β). The p35 chain has a four α-helix structure, similar to that of many other cytokines, but the p40 chain of IL-12 is homologous to the IL-6R, containing an Ig domain and a WSXWS motif. Thus, IL-12 appears to be composed of one cytokine-like polypeptide and one receptor-like polypeptide.[1]

Other general characteristics of IL-12 include:

Molecular Weight

Depending on its molecular form, the literature values for the molecular weight of IL-12 vary from 24 to 70 kDa. The following molecular weights have been reported: 24 to 33 kDa (p35) and 34 to 44 kDa (p40),[341] 70 kDa,[1,152,421] 35 (p35) and 40 (p40) kDa,[389,421] and 30 to 33 kDa (p35) and 35 to 44 kDa (p40).[71]

Cross-Reactivity

The cross-reactivities (amino acid sequence homology between human and mouse) for molecular forms of IL-12 include IL-12 p35 (60%) and IL-12 p40 (70%).[71] Human IL-12 is inactive on mouse cells, and murine IL-12 is active on human cells.

Chromosomal Location

The chromosomal locations of the molecular forms of IL-12 are 3p12-3q13.2 (IL-12α) and 5q31-33 (IL-12β).

Cellular Origin

The p35 subunit of IL-12 is produced by T and B cells, NK cells, neutrophils, monocytes, and macrophages (at least in the mouse). The p40 subunit is produced mainly by B lymphocytes, activated monocytes, and dendritic cells (including epidermal Langerhans' cells). Consequently the principal sources of IL-12 are B cells and monocytes and/or macrophages (Figure 22-20).* In the brain, microglia-like cells are the primary producers of the p40 transcripts. In contrast, the IL-12 p35 gene is constitutively expressed in the brain at a very low level.[409]

IL-12 is the only cytokine acting as a regulator of the effector phase of cell-mediated immune reactions that is not produced by T cells. However, the IL-12 receptor is restrictedly expressed by T lymphocytes and NK cells.

Control of Synthesis and Release

It has been suggested that IL-12 is up regulated as part of the early cytokine response of mononuclear phagocytes to infectious agents and that the cellular events associated with phagocytosis are themselves a potent signal for IL-12 production. IL-12 released by infected macrophages can further up regulate pathogen-specific CD4 T-cell effector function.[179] IL-12 expression is regulated by NO, which may exert an autoregulatory and paracrine control of IL-12 gene expression.[448] IL-10 inhibits the production of IL-6, IL-12, and TNFα, probably indicating a potential mechanism of negative feedback regulation of the immune response, as

*References 152, 216, 253, 341, 448, 536, 590.

Figure 22-20 Cellular origin, principal target cells, and biological actions of IL-12.

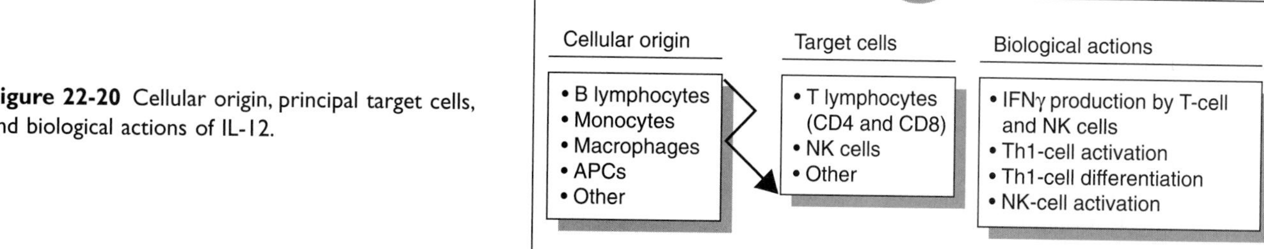

IL-12 or IL-6 can induce the expression of IL-10 by PHA-stimulated T cells.[110] The gp120 glycoprotein of HIV is an inducer of IL-12 expression in monocytes and/or macrophages, and IFNγ is an essential cofactor for IL-12 secretion, especially in differentiated macrophages.[159] The production of IL-12 is stimulated by bacteria, bacterial products, and intracellular parasites and enhanced by priming with GM-CSF and IFNγ. It is inhibited by IL-10.[536] Bioactive IL-12 (p70) is composed of the two subunits (p35, which is only secreted as part of the p70 dimer, and p40, which can also be secreted by itself). The two subunits are encoded by separate genes, and to what extent the expression of each of the subunits contributes to the regulation of IL-12 production is being investigated. Results indicate that in LPS-stimulated whole blood and purified monocytes, p70 and p40 production are enhanced by IFNγ and inhibited by IL-10 and IL-4. However, IFNγ and IL-10 had stronger effects on p70 production than on p40 production, and IL-4 affected p40 production more strongly. Concomitantly, in all experimental conditions tested, p40 production greatly exceeded p70 production, suggesting that p35 expression was limiting. Analysis of p35 and p40 mRNA expression by polymerase chain reaction (PCR) confirmed this belief. Resting purified monocytes expressed neither p40 nor p35 mRNA. The effects of IFNγ, IL-10, and IL-4 on the p35 mRNA expression in LPS-stimulated purified monocytes were similar to the effects of these cytokines on p70 protein production, and the p40 mRNA expression corresponded to p40 protein production. These results imply that production of the two IL-12 subunits is differently regulated for each subunit, mainly at the level of mRNA expression, and that the level of bioactive IL-12 production in monocytes in response to LPS and cytokines is determined by the level of p35 expression.[489] IFNγ, which is up regulated during infection, acted in synergy with other stimuli on IL-12 synthesis, suggesting an amplification loop for IL-12 production, whereas IL-4, IL-10, IL-13, and TGFβ were inhibitory. The existence of a broad range of stimuli from a wide variety of pathogenic organisms underscores the fundamental importance of IL-12 in host defense.[487]

Receptor (IL-12R)

IL-12R is a single-chain receptor expressed only on T cells and NK cells (structurally similar to the G-CSF receptor). One component of the IL-12 receptor complex shows it to be related to gp130.[71] To date, a large number of receptors for IL-12 have been found but only on PBMC following activation with PHA or IL-2. Studies have found that the expression of IL-12R on a human γδ T-cell line responds to IL-12 with enhanced cytolytic activity and increased expression of cytolytic effector molecules granzyme B and perforin.[281]

Signal Transduction

STAT4 has been found to be essential for mediating responses to IL-12 in T lymphocytes and NK cells and regulating the differentiation of both Th1 and Th2 cells.[256,525] IL-12 activates STAT4, STAT1α, and STAT3, and induces complexes containing STAT4 only, STAT4 with STAT1α, STAT3 with STAT1α, or STAT1α only in preactivated primary NK cells. STAT1α activation by IL-12 is correlated with increased phosphorylation of serine but not tyrosine. IL-2 induced tyrosine phosphorylation of JAK1 and JAK3, with IL-12 inducing phosphorylation of JAK2 and TYK2 in both preactivated primary NK and NK3.3 cells. Differential phosphorylation and consequent differential activation of both separate and overlapping STAT proteins by IL-2, IL-12, and IFNα may provide a molecular basis for the similarities and differences in the actions of these cytokines on NK cells.[281,591]

Biological Actions

The major biological activity of IL-12 is on T and NK cells where it increases cytokine production, proliferation, and cytotoxicity. Its production occurs several hours after exposure to infectious agents, which induces a rapid production of IFNγ by NK and later by T cells. Thus IFNγ potentiates APC functions important in clearing infectious agents (phagocytosis, oxidative burst, and production of NO) and increases further production of IL-12. IL-12 has been clearly demonstrated to be important in the generation of CD4 and CD8 type of Th1 cells both in vivo and in vitro. IL-12 also primes naive T cells for concomitant high IFNγ and IL-10 production, whereas IL-4 is required for IL-4 priming, thus suggesting that these corresponding genes and possibly others are independently regulated. IL-12 is therefore involved in the skewing of cytokine production toward a type 1 T response. It is now becoming clear that IL-12 acts as both a proinflammatory cytokine and an immunomodulator and therefore bridges the innate and antigen-specific adaptive immune responses to intracellular bacterial, fungal, and protozoan pathogens.[185,536,579]

IL-12 has been called "the jump starter of cell-mediated immunity," indicating that IL-12 acts early in infection as a switch driving CD4 T cells (with IFNγ) to a cellular Th1 response.[152]

It is likely that IL-12 plays a pivotal role in the host defense against intracellular pathogens.[183] For example, it (1) promotes cell-mediated immunity by polarizing Th types of cytokine responses (causing DTHR), (2) enhances the lytic activity of NK and/or LAK cells, (3) augments specific Tc responses, (4) induces the production of IFNγ, and (5) suppresses the development of Th2 types of cytokine responses and humoral immunity, particularly IgGl and IgE responses. Thus IL-12 selectively promotes differentiation of Th1 lymphocytes and potentiates cell-mediated immunity while suppressing Th2-dependent functions, such as the production of IL-4, IL-10, and IgE antibodies.

Studies have documented that the immunoregulatory functions of IL-12 may play a role in promoting endogenous protective responses during infections or contribute to pathological conditions resulting from unregulated cytokine expression. Pathogen induction of IL-12 elicits IFNγ production by NK cells, contributing to early defense during certain bacterial, parasitic, and viral infections. IL-12 also facilitates the development of Th1 lymphocytes required for late protection against bacteria, parasites, and fungi. During viral infections, however, there appear to be mechanisms independent of IL-12 for inducing protective T-cell responses. In contrast, negative regulation of IL-12 during acute infections can be a key event in the establishment of chronic infection and protection against harmful excessive cellular immune response.[50]

IL-12 is a multifunctional cytokine capable of inhibiting neovascularization.[473] Because the human IFNγ-inducible protein 10 (IP-10) can also inhibit neovascularization, IP-10—induced by IL-12 through the intermediate cytokine IFNγ—was tested to determine if it might be a mediator of IL-12 angiogenesis inhibition. Murine IL-12–induced murine IP-10 expression in mouse splenocytes and human IFNγ-induced human IP-10 expression in purified human endothelial cells suggest that IL-12 can induce IP-10 expression in certain cells. These results document the important role of IP-10 as a mediator of angiogenesis inhibition by IL-12 and raise the possibility that IP-10 may also contribute to the antitumor effect of IL-12.[485]

Cytotoxic activity of both NK cells and Tc lymphocytes is enhanced by IL-12 (it acts synergistically with IL-2 to induce IFNγ synthesis by these cells and is considered as the most potent NK-cell stimulator known). This cytotoxic enhancement occurs in parallel with depression of IgE production and reduction of IL-4 secretion (IL-12 and IL-4 cross regulate one another's activities). IL-12 effects are only seen early, whereas IL-4 effects are maintained. Studies have suggested a molecular basis for these temporal differences of IL-12 and IL-4 on Th1 and Th2 responses.[341,541] These differences are dependent on the specific characteristics of T-cell receptor functions: on Th1 lymphocytes, the IL-4R and the IL-12R remain expressed and functional, whereas on Th2 lymphocytes, IL-12R functional defects were identified following commitment to the Th2 lineage.

CD40-CD40L interaction synergizes with IL-12 in selectively enhancing IFNγ production by T cells. Both CD4 and CD8 T cells were able to produce IFNγ in the presence of helper signals from IL-12 and CD40, although CD8 T cells were less active. CD40-CD40L interaction also up regulates IL-12 production.[416] CD8 Tc lymphocytes are important mediators for resistance to infections and malignant diseases, and IL-12 function in the generation of important human antiviral CD8 T-cell responses also has been demonstrated by augmented IFNγ production during Tc generation.[45]

It has been suggested that CD4 human thymocytes have the potential to develop into cells producing the Th2 cytokines IL-4 and IL-5, whereas the ability to produce both Th1 cytokines and IL-10 is acquired only after priming with IL-12.[364] In the absence of APC, IL-12 and TNFα both demonstrate an inhibitory effect on the proliferation of CD8 Tc lymphocyte clones, whereas IL-10 enhances the proliferation. IL-12–induced inhibition of CD8 Tc clones is not mediated by the endogenous production of TNFα by these clones. The strong inhibitory effect of IL-12 and TNFα does not result in apoptosis, and these cytokines do not alter the cytotoxicity of CD8 Tc clones. When CD4 T-cell clones were tested in the absence of APC, no substantial change in IL-2–dependent proliferation caused by IL-10, IL-12, and TNFα could be measured. Because these effects on established Tc clones are in contrast to the effects of IL-10, IL-12, and TNFα during the induction phase of immune responses, a dichotomy of immunomodulatory cytokines, such as IL-10, IL-12, and TNFα, early and late in the immune response has been suggested.[547]

Clinical Relevance

IL-12 may be a marker of Th1-mediated pathological conditions, such as autoimmune type 1 diabetes mellitus.[341] Th1 cells are critically involved in several pathological conditions, such as contact hypersensitivity, and it has been suggested that IL-12 may play a dominant role in vivo in the induction of this pathology.[438] The relative increase in IL-12 mRNA in chronic atopic dermatitis skin lesions suggests a possible role for IL-12 producing cells in modulating chronic inflammation.[207] The verification that higher mRNA expression of the regulated IL-12 p40 subunit, but not IL-10, was present in sarcoid lung cells, with elevated levels of p40 protein found in sarcoid bronchoalveolar lavage fluid, and that sarcoid alveolar macrophages produce greater amounts of IL-12 than normal alveolar macrophages favors the hypothesis that sarcoidosis is a Th1-mediated pathological condition driven by chronic, dysregulated production of IL-12 at sites of disease.[367]

Defective IL-12 production is associated with increased susceptibility to infection (e.g., familial disseminated *Mycobacterium avium* complex infection, *T. cruzi* infection, and human visceral leishmaniasis), a finding that supports the critical role of this cytokine in host defense and in the regulation of the cellular immune response.[23,175,230] The loss of immune function following infection with HIV may result from altered production of immunoregulatory cytokines, such as IL-10 and IL-12. It was suggested that monocytes from HIV-positive individuals secrete decreased amounts of IL-12, which may lead to the development of Th2 type of responses characterized by high IL-10 secretion and immune dysfunction.[109,110]

As previously discussed, IL-12 is considered to be a key factor for the induction of IFNγ, a cytokine essential for the lethal effects of endotoxin. Administration of a lethal or sublethal dose of live *Escherichia coli* to baboons results in the release of the nonfunctional subunit of IL-12, p40, and biologically active heterodimeric IL-12, p70. This finding is contrary to what might be expected if IFNγ were solely induced by IL-12. Lethally challenged baboons generated threefold more IFNγ at 6 hours than those receiving a sublethal dose. Moreover, higher levels of IFNγ were associated with lower p40 to p70 ratios, suggesting that in agreement with observations, in vitro IFNγ may have preferentially up regulated the release of p70 over p40. These data show that IL-12 is released in experimental septic shock in nonhuman primates and suggest that IL-10 and IFNγ are involved in the regulation of this release. Furthermore, this study indicates that the systemic release of IL-12 might be essential, but is not likely sufficient, to promote lethal production of IFNγ in sepsis.[243] IL-12 and PGE2 are two opposite immunomodulators: IL-12 enhances IFNγ production by activated CD4 T cells, whereas PGE2 inhibits the secretion of this cytokine. The relative contributions of these factors shift in time owing to different production kinetics, from a dominant IL-12 effect to a mixed IL-12/PGE2 effect; this may be largely determinant to T-cell activation and therefore lead to immunological dysfunction.[217]

IL-12 is also a critical cytokine regulating NK and T-cell function, and it has been suggested that reduced expression and production of IL-12 from activated umbilical cord blood may contribute to the immaturity in its cellular immunity and may explain decreased GVHD following umbilical cord blood stem-cell transplantation.[308]

Therapeutic Applications

IL-12 has been shown to exert striking therapeutic effects at nontoxic doses in mouse tumor models and in mouse models of a variety of infectious diseases and airway inflammation. In mouse tumor models, the therapeutic effects of IL-12 have been shown to result from its immunoenhancing activity, which requires both T cells and IFNγ. In some models, administration of IL-12 can result in antiangiogenic effects, which may also contribute to its antitumor activity. Tumor cell–induced angiogenesis is an essential requirement for the growth of solid neoplasms. The mechanism of antitumor action of IL-12 may depend not only on the immunostimulatory activity of this cytokine, but also on its effect on tumor cell–induced angiogenesis (IFNγ being a mediator of the antiangiogenic effect of IL-12).

IL-12 should be considered a potential candidate for the treatment of angiogenesis-dependent malignancies. Enhanced antitumor effects may be achieved by administering IL-12 in combination with certain other cytokines or with radiotherapy or chemotherapy. Additionally, IL-12 has been shown to be more efficacious than IL-2 in several murine tumor models, and toxicology studies suggest that it may have a substantially better therapeutic index. Also, the long serum half-life of IL-12 relative to other cytokines will allow more flexibility in dosing schedules. The striking therapeutic effects of IL-12 in these preclinical models have led to the initiation of clinical trials to evaluate the potential therapeutic activity of IL-12 in human cancer patients and in patients with HIV infection or with chronic hepatitis B or C virus infections.[183,184,339] Despite considerable advancement in anticancer therapy, minimal residual disease is still a major problem in the clinical management of cancer, including lymphoma. Experimental studies suggest that cytokines, such as IL-12, may have the potential to mediate antitumor effects against residual lymphoma without compromising lymphohematopoietic recovery.[552] IL-12 promotes specific and long-lasting antitumor immunity mediated by T cells in a variety of murine tumor models. It also synergizes with B7.1, a co-stimulatory molecule involved in the activation of T lymphocytes (CD80) to induce proliferation and cytokine production by both human and murine T cells in vitro. These activities support the potential clinical utility of combined gene therapy using IL-12 and B7.1-engineered autologous cells (tumor or fibroblasts) as a vaccine to elicit specific antitumor immunity.[600] IL-12 in combination with IL-2 enhanced the autologous antimelanoma Tc lymphocyte response, whereas B7.1 antigen expression on tumor cells did not increase antimelanoma Tc generation. This method represents a novel strategy to enhance the efficacy of recombinant anticancer vaccines and could be used to design more appropriate genetically modified tumor vaccines.[121,429]

Because of its multiple effects on immunoinflammatory response, recombinant IL-12 has been shown to have therapeutic activity in a variety of mouse tumor and infectious disease models and is being evaluated in clinical trials in human cancer patients. IL-12 also appears to play a role in the genesis of some forms of immunopathology, including endotoxin-induced shock and some autoimmune diseases associated with aberrant Th1 activity. Therefore IL-12 antagonists may also have therapeutic potential in the treatment of autoimmune disorders. In addition, intraocular injection of IL-12 significantly inhibited the development of endotoxin-induced intraocular inflammation, suggesting that IL-

12 can have an immunoregulatory function in some forms of inflammatory disease.[577]

IL-12 may also be potentially useful for adoptive immunotherapy, especially in immunosuppressed patients (caused by cancer or HIV infection) with decreased NK function and T-cell cytotoxicity.[1,341,472] Under appropriate conditions, IL-12 has therapeutic efficacy for promoting defense against a variety of pathogens and for use as a vaccine adjuvant to enhance beneficial Th1 over detrimental Th2 lymphocyte responses and provides new tools for the development of treatment and adjuvant strategies to potentiate beneficial or inhibit detrimental endogenous immune responses.[50]

INTERLEUKIN-13

Interleukin-13 (IL-13) is a cytokine produced by activated T lymphocytes that has structural and functional similarities to IL-4; it inhibits inflammatory cytokine production by LPS in human peripheral blood monocytes and may be involved in promoting B-cell division.[138]

Synonyms

IL-13 has been formerly known as NC30 (human complementary DNA [cDNA]) and P600 (mouse cDNA clone).

General Characteristics

IL-13 belongs to the four α-helical short-chain cytokine family (112AA). The structural homology between IL-13 and IL-4 and the juxtaposition of their encoding genes on chromosome 5 are probably related to a process of gene duplication. It is a highly pleiotropic cytokine produced by Th2 cells (such as IL-4), inhibiting macrophage responses.[71,341]

Other general characteristics of IL-13 include:

Molecular Weight

Depending on the degree of glycosylation, the literature values for the molecular weight of IL-13 vary from 9 to 17 kDa. The following molecular weights have been reported: 9 to 17 kDa,[341] 12 kDa,[335] 10 kDa,[389,436] and 12.4 kDa,[152] 9 kDa, and 17 kDa (glycosylated form).[71]

Cross-Reactivity

The cross-reactivity (amino acid sequence homology between human and mouse) for IL-13 is 58%.[71] There is a significant cross-species reactivity. Human and mouse IL-13 have no known activity on mouse B cells.

Chromosomal Location

The chromosomal location of IL-13 is 5q23-31.

Cellular Origin

Previously, IL-13 was considered to be predominantly produced by activated T cells, namely Th2 CD4 lymphocytes. Now it is known that CD4 T-cell clones belonging to Th0, Th1-like, and Th2-like subsets produce IL-13 following antigen-specific or polyclonal activation (Figure 22-21). In addition, EBV-transformed B-cell lines express IL-13 mRNA and produce small amounts of IL-13 protein.[120] IL-13 is also known to be produced by activated human CD4 and CD8 CD45R0 memory T cells and CD4 and CD8 CD45RA naive T cells. Collectively, it appears that IL-13 is also produced by peripheral blood T cells that also produce IL-4, but not IFNγ, and by naive CD45RA T cells. These observations, together with the long-lasting production of IL-13, suggest that IL-13 may have IL-4–like functions in situations in which T-cell–derived IL-4 is still absent or its production has already been down regulated.[248,548]

The production of IL-13 by basophils has been demonstrated to be localized in basophilic granules. Kinetic studies have demonstrated detectable IL-13 release at 3 hours, which steadily increased up to 24 hours. This is significantly different from the kinetics of basophil histamine and IL-4 release and suggests that basophils, in addition to secreting mediators, can represent an important source of proallergic cytokines.[318] Actual findings point to the fact that bone marrow–derived mucosal-like mast cells constitutively expressed IL-13, whereas bone marrow–derived connective tissue–like mast cells demonstrated IL-13 transcription only after Fcε activation or the addition of exogenous IL-3. A similar pattern of expression of IL-10 by these mast cells was also evident and matches that of IL-4 previously reported, suggesting that mucosal mast cells may have a constitutive

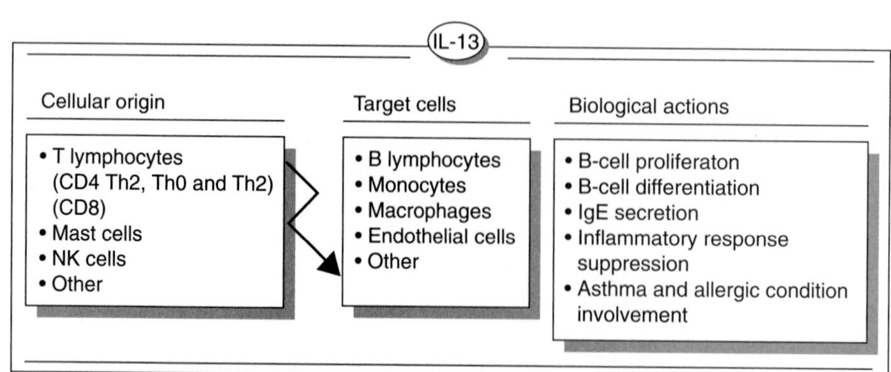

Figure 22-21 Cellular origin, principal target cells, and biological actions of IL-13.

repertoire of Th2 cytokines with potential antiinflammatory activity. Connective tissue MCs may not be this repetitive. However, production of such cytokines can be induced in the connective tissue mast cells and other cell types of the immune response by the addition of IL-3.[346]

Control of Synthesis and Release

Expression of IL-13 mRNA and production of IL-13 protein by peripheral blood T cells and T-cell clones are rapidly induced and are relatively long lasting, whereas IL-4 production by these cells is transient. In addition, IL-13 mRNA expression is induced by modes of activation that failed to induce IL-4 mRNA expression.[120] Because the primed T cells involved in IL-4 and IL-13 production contain higher levels of nuclear factor–activated T cells, preformed (NFATp), capable of binding to P elements of the IL-4 and IL-13 promoters, than do freshly isolated T cells, the NFAT-binding P elements are attractive candidates to mediate the coordinate expression of these two cytokine genes.[135] IL-13 production in all types of cells is enhanced by cyclosporin A. In contrast to IL-13, IL-4 production requires co-stimulation through CD3 and was inhibited by cyclosporin A. The unusual regulation and relative abundance of IL-13 make it an important candidate to be controlled tightly by dose and type of TCR ligands. Cyclosporin A is used widely to inhibit T-cell function, and the finding that IL-13 production is enhanced instead of diminished in the presence of cyclosporin A may explain the Th2-inducing effects of this immunosuppressor in vivo.[548]

Receptor (IL-13R)

The IL-13 receptor may share a subunit with IL-4R but not in the ligand-binding component. IL-13 lacks the T-cell–activating properties of IL-4 that are related to the fact that T cells fail to bind radiolabeled IL-13 and do not express the IL-13–specific receptor component.[120] The overlapping activities of IL-13 and IL-4 are probably due to the existence of common receptor components. Two proteins have been described as constituents of the IL-4R (a high-affinity IL-4 binding chain (p140, α-chain, CD124) and the IL-2R γ-chain also known as the common γ-chain (γc), but neither of these proteins binds IL-13. The IL-13 binding protein (IL-13R) has two consensus patterns characteristic of the hematopoietic cytokine receptor family and a short cytoplasmic tail. It shows homology with the IL-5 receptor, and to a lesser extent with the prolactin receptor.[74] The receptor for IL-4 and IL-13 was described as a shared heteromultimeric complex in which the common γc subunit was essential for activity. Endothelial cells bind both cytokines with high affinity, and it has been demonstrated that they express IL-4Rα but do not express the γc of the IL-2R. Therefore it is probable that the subunit structure of the functional receptors for IL-4 and IL-13 on human endothelial cells do not use or require the common γc of the IL-2R.[465]

IL-13R is expressed on endothelial cells and probably on the same cells expressing IL-4R or IL-5R.

Signal Transduction

IL-13 shares many biological activities with IL-4 and may share a common component required for signal transduction.[120] Compared with IL-4, IL-13 induces a similar alteration of the cytokine cascade and arachidonic acid metabolism, supporting the hypothesis that the two cytokines use a common receptor complex or signal pathway.[124] IL-13 activates STAT6 in B cells but not JAK3. This leads to the conclusion that γc is essential for activation of JAK3 and STAT6 in the signal transduction pathway of IL-4 in human B cells and that IL-13 does not use γc but activates STAT6 through an alternative pathway that is not impaired in B cells of XSCID patients.[237] However, IL-4 and IL-13 differentially regulate epithelial chloride secretion, which indicates that although postreceptor signaling events induced by IL-13 and IL-4 may be similar, endpoint function is cytokine specific.[560,603]

Biological Actions

IL-13 is a regulator of B cells and monocyte activity. On B cells, IL-13 functions as a co-stimulatory signal (together with a B-cell receptor or CD40), increasing B-cell proliferation and CD23 expression. In the presence of IL-13, interaction between CD40 and CD40L induces isotype switching to IgE synthesis (as occurs with IL-4). IL-13 can also inhibit monocyte and/or macrophage responses, suppressing the production of IL-1α, IL-1β, IL-6, IL-8, and TNFα (this action is shared by IL-4 and IL-10). IL-13 synergizes with IL-2 on NK cells to produce IFNγ. IL-13 has also been shown to prolong survival of human monocytes and increase surface expression of MHC class II and CD23.[71,341] IL-13 is a cytokine secreted by activated T lymphocytes and shares some, but not all, of its biological activities with IL-4. This includes inhibition of monocyte and macrophage activation, stimulation of human B cells, and induction of growth and differentiation of mouse bone marrow cells in vitro.[74,303]

IL-13 lacks the T-cell–activating properties of IL-4, relying instead on differences in expression and biological activities of these two cytokines on T cells with possible consequences for their relative roles in the immune system response.[120] IL-13 is described as a cytokine with Th2-like actions.[207] IL-13 and IL-4 exert similar, nonadditive effects on endothelial cells, inducing VCAM-1 expression and subsequent transmigration of eosinophils.[465] Experimental data indicate that exogenous rIL-13 induces extramedullary hematopoiesis in mice and suggest that endogenous IL-13 may contribute to replenishment of effector cells during strong Th2 responses.[303] IL-13 has also been found to induce the expression and release of the IL-1 decoy receptor (type II) in human neutrophils along with the production of the IL-1RA. Human rIL-13 induces cellular morphological changes in neutrophils that are typical of activated cells, increases tyrosine phosphorylation of several neutrophil proteins, and induces the synthesis of several neutrophil proteins but has no significant effect on phagocytosis and

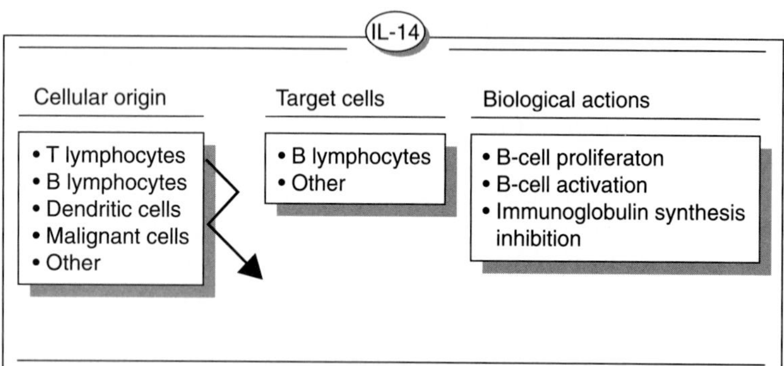

Figure 22-22 Cellular origin, principal target cells, and biological actions of IL-14.

apoptosis. Collectively, these results demonstrate that IL-13 is a modulator of several human neutrophil functions.[189] For example, IL-13 has been identified as a powerful regulatory tool for the inhibition of NO synthesis in human cells, which may be pathophysiologically relevant in NO-related inflammatory processes.[460] IL-13 suppresses the bone-resorbing activity stimulated by IL-1α by suppressing cyclooxygenase-dependent PG synthesis in osteoblasts.[400]

Clinical Relevance

Laboratory data have shown that acute atopic dermatitis skin lesions are associated with an increased expression of IL-13 mRNA.[207] IL-4 and IL-13 down regulate both the increase of fibrinogen secretion induced by IL-6 and fibrinogen mRNA levels, probably protecting vessel walls from monocyte injuries leading to atherosclerosis.[551] IL-13 may also exhibit a negative regulatory effect on neoplastic B cells in contrast with that observed in normal B cells and could be an important factor in the pathogenesis of chronic lymphocytic leukemia by preventing the death of monoclonal B cells.[83] IL-13 gene expression has been detected in the epithelial compartment of the nasal mucosa of 18 of 19 perennial allergic rhinitis patients but was undetected in normal volunteers and chronic infectious rhinitis patients, pointing to its intervention in local allergic reactions.[413]

Therapeutic Applications

IL-13 may have a role as an inhibitor of monocyte inflammatory cytokines (for example, induced by LPS) and thus may be useful as a therapeutic agent in septic shock. The peripheral blood of allergic individuals contains long-lived allergen-specific B cells that have already switched to IgE production and that are not sensitive to IL-4 and IL-13 treatment. This information may have implications for attempts to use cytokines or cytokine antagonists in therapy of type I allergy.[133]

Interleukin-14

Interleukin-14 (IL-14) is a cytokine produced by T lymphocytes and malignant B lymphocytes; it induces B-cell proliferation and inhibits Ig secretion.[138]

Synonym

IL-14 was formerly known as high molecular weight B-cell growth factor (HMW-BCGF).

General Characteristics

IL-14 is unrelated to any other cytokines but shares homology with complement factor Bb.[71] It is a B-cell growth factor produced by T cells (483AA).

Other general characteristics of IL-14 include:

Molecular Weight

The literature values for the molecular weight of IL-14 vary from 50 to 60 kDa. The following molecular weights have been reported: 50 to 60 kDa,[341] 53 kDa,[152,436] and 60 kDa.[71]

Cross-Reactivity

There are no reports of cross-activity of murine IL-14.

Chromosomal Location

The chromosomal location of IL-14 is unknown.

Cellular Origin

IL-14 is produced by activated T, B, follicular dendritic, and malignant cells (Figure 22-22).[71,152,341]

Control of Synthesis and Release

Mechanisms for controlling the synthesis and release of IL-14 are currently unknown.

Receptor (IL-14R)

A single type of receptor was detected on B cells; IL-14 causes up regulation of its receptor on these cells. IL-14R also binds complement fragment Bb.[71]

Signal Transduction

IL-14 causes increases in intracellular cAMP, DAG, and calcium.[71]

Biological Actions

IL-14 enhances the proliferation of activated B cells and may play a role in the development of B-cell memory. The

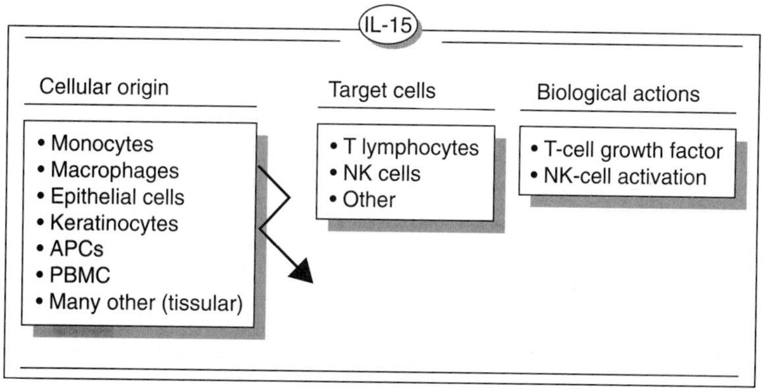

Figure 22-23 Cellular origin, principal target cells, and biological actions of IL-15.

presence of IL-14 in germinal center T cells and follicular dendritic cells suggests that during a secondary immune response, naive B cells migrating through the lymph node encounter antigen, become activated, express IL-14R, and consequently bind IL-14. This results in increased bcl-2 expression, which prevents apoptosis and permits B-cell memory development.[341] Despite the proliferative action on B cells, inhibition of Ig secretion is produced by IL-14.[71,152,341,432] IL-14, like IL-13 and TGFβ, is considered to be a down regulatory cytokine.[131]

Clinical Relevance

Hyperproduction of IL-14 together with IL-6 and IL-10 has been reported in patients with systemic lupus erythematosus.[341]

Therapeutic Applications

In a variety of malignant conditions, lymphoma or leukemia cells are able to proliferate with an IL-14 stimulus, implicating this cytokine in their expansion and survival. IL-14 down regulation or inhibition may also prove useful.[341]

INTERLEUKIN-15

Interleukin-15 (IL-15) is a cytokine released by mononuclear phagocytes and some tissue cells in response to events triggering innate immunity, such as viral infection; its primary function appears to be promotion of NK-cell proliferation.[197]

General Characteristics

The three-dimensional structure of IL-15 is a four α-helical bundle similar to IL-2 (four α-helical short-chain cytokine, 114AA). IL-15 has biological characteristics similar to those of IL-2, acting mainly on the proliferation of T cells. The discovery of IL-15 may explain the perplexing observation that IL-2–deficient mice have surprisingly conserved immune responses.[71,152]

Other general characteristics of IL-15 include:

Molecular Weight

The literature values for the molecular weight of IL-15 vary from 14 to 15 kDa. The following molecular weights have been reported: 14 to 15 kDa,[71,341] 12.9 kDa,[436] and 14 kDa.[152]

Cross-Reactivity

Human IL-15 is active on murine T cells.

Chromosomal Location

The chromosomal location of IL-15 is unknown. The chromosomal location of IL-15 is 4q31.

Cellular Origin

IL-15 is produced by multiple cellular and tissue sources (blood mononuclear cells, placenta, skeletal muscle, kidney, lung, liver, heart, bone marrow stromal cells, keratinocytes, Langerhans' cells, and other tissue-specific dendritic cells) and particularly by epithelial cells and monocytes (Figure 22-23).[53,71,152,373]

Control of Synthesis and Release

Optimal induction of IL-15 in murine macrophages requires both priming (IFNγ) and triggering (LPS, mycobacteria, or *Toxoplasma gondii*) stimuli. When compared with IL-12 mRNA synthesis by the same macrophages, IL-15 mRNA production was more resistant to inhibition by the down regulatory cytokines IL-14, IL-13, and TGFβ. Moreover, IL-10, which is inhibitory for most other monokines, increased levels of the IL-15 mRNA found after stimulation. Thus IL-15 is a product of the macrophage-monocyte lineage that is up regulated on activation. IL-15 could thus play an important role in the initiation of immune responses by microbial agents.[131] Ultraviolet B radiation (UVB) up regulates the expression of IL-15 in human skin, suggesting a new mechanism by which UVB can promote Ag-independent T-cell responses via elaboration of IL-15.[366]

Receptor (IL-15R)

IL-2R β- and γ-chains are both required for binding IL-15 and for signal transduction; the α-chain is not required.[71,152,191] Like IL-2, IL-15 causes the release of sIL-2Rα from PHA-activated human PBMCs in a concentration and time-dependent manner. This effect of IL-15 is largely direct and independent of IL-2. Blocking of the IL-2Rβ-chain prevents the release of sIL-2Rα by IL-15 but not by IL-2. IL-7, another cytokine using the γ-chain of the IL-2R, drives the release of sIL-2Rα as well. Several clinical conditions are associated with abnormal serum sIL-2Rα levels and are monitored by the measurement of sIL-2Rα. The reason for sIL-2Rα release is not fully understood. In one study, IL-15, like IL-2, was shown to be a potent inducer of sIL-2Rα release in vitro.[534] Comparing the interactions of IL-2 and IL-15 with the IL-2Rβ and IL-2Rγ-chain subunits, it has been suggested that the existence of a human IL-15Rα subunit and physical evidence of this molecule has been obtained.[191] This indicates that IL-15 creates a less stable bridge between the IL-2Rβ and IL-2Rγ-chains than does IL-2.[118] IL-2 and IL-15 share many biological activities as a consequence of their use of the β- and γ-chains of the IL-2R. However, each cytokine binds to a specific receptor α-chain: IL-2 with low affinity and IL-15 with high affinity. IL-15, like IL-2, is also thought to up regulate expression of IL-2Rα on human T and B cells, but rapidly down regulate IL-15 high-affinity binding sites that represent IL-15Rα. This leads to a decreased responsiveness to IL-15 as measured by induction of JAK3 tyrosine phosphorylation. These results suggest a mechanism by which IL-15 may cooperate with IL-2 at the initiation of an immune response and enhance subsequent IL-2 responsiveness during T-cell expansion.[292] A murine IL-15–specific α-subunit has been identified, cloned, and shown to be structurally related to IL-2Rα. However, the murine IL-15Rα alone binds IL-15 with a 1000-fold higher affinity than that seen with IL-2Rα and IL-2. These studies have been extended into the human system with the isolation of three differentially spliced human IL-15Rα variants that are all capable of high-affinity binding of IL-15. The cytoplasmic domain of IL-15Rα, like that of IL-2Rα, is dispensable for mitogenic signaling, suggesting that the primary role of the α-chains is to confer high-affinity binding. At high concentrations, IL-15, like IL-2, is able to signal through a complex of IL-2Rβ and γ in the absence of the α subunit. The distribution and expression of the IL-15Rα are much wider than those of the IL-2Rα, suggesting a broader range of cellular targets for IL-15.[10]

Biological Actions

IL-15 has been shown to stimulate T-lymphocyte proliferation (especially Tc cells) and to facilitate their generation.[392] The similarity of IL-15 to IL-2 is also evident from its ability to enhance LAK activity and from the inhibition of IL-15 responses by anti–IL-2Rβ-chain antibody.[341] However, IL-15 has only some IL-2 functions, perhaps dependent on differences between the two cytokine receptors (presence of a unique IL-15 binding protein associated with the IL-2Rβ subunit). Unlike IL-2, IL-15 is produced by monocytes and/or macrophages and not by lymphocytes.[53,341]

NK-cell proliferation could not be initiated with rIL-15 as the sole co-stimulatory cytokine. However, NK-cell proliferation was initiated with rIL-15. Either rIL-10 or rIL-12, cytokines also produced by monocytes and other APCs are implicated in innate immune responses. These results support the notion that NK-cell proliferation occurs at different phases of the immune response, with the particular cytokine milieu influencing the repertoire of NK-cell–secreted cytokines, and that IL-15 may be a physiologically relevant ligand for NK-cell differentiation in vivo.[373,564] IL-2 and IL-15 may have different functional properties during the in vitro differentiation of IL-4–producing cells. The role of IL-15 in priming for IFNγ is not as important as that of IL-2, leaving this cytokine as the preponderant controller of Th1 differentiation in physiological situations. Finally, IL-15 has been shown to increase proliferation of activated CD4 T-cell blasts but not of naive CD4 T cells. Moreover, cultures containing both IL-2 and IL-15 show greater proliferation than either cytokine alone, suggesting an additive effect between these cytokines.[469]

IL-15 promotes cytokine production by human Th cells by (1) inducing IL-5 synthesis; (2) having a role at the site of allergic inflammation; and (3) having a role in the recruitment and activation of eosinophils by inducing Th2 cytokine production by T cells.[371] IL-15 has other activities, including chemotactic properties and inducing uropod formation on T lymphoblasts to which ICAM-3 is redistributed, representing a potent T-lymphocyte chemoattractant. Other adhesion molecules, such as ICAM-1, ICAM-2, CD43, and CD44, are also redistributed to the uropod, although in a smaller proportion of the cells. The effect of IL-15 was dose dependent and specifically inhibited by a monoclonal antibody (mAb) against this cytokine. Blocking experiments with anti–IL-2Rβ-chain mAb showed an inhibitory effect on IL-15–mediated redistribution of ICAM-3, whereas no effect was observed in the presence of anti–IL-2Rα-chain mAb. The M16, N9 uropod induced by IL-15 is enriched in many different adhesion receptors and, being well exposed to the external milieu, is likely to modulate the adhesive properties of lymphocytes.[355,390] In addition, because IL-15 is produced by keratinocytes, Langerhans' cells, and other tissue-specific dendritic cells, it may be important in attracting and activating antigen-specific Th1 T cells.[53]

It has been suggested that IL-15 derived from infected macrophages may contribute to the early activation of γδ T cells during salmonellosis.

Clinical Relevance

IL-15 and IL-2 induce expression of cell-surface IL-2Rα (CD25) on freshly isolated human PBMCs in the absence of other exogenous stimuli. They also stimulate the release of sIL-2Rα. On stimulation with rIL-15, more than 80% of all NK cells express CD25, and more CD8 lymphocytes are positive for CD25 compared with stimulation by rIL-2. These results may be clinically relevant because several diseases are associated with high serum levels of sIL-2Rα, which may be due not only to IL-2 but also to IL-15 stimulation.[533] UVB-induced down regulation of keratinocyte IL-15 production may contribute to the relative state of immunosuppression induced by sun exposure.[53] Experimental findings demonstrate that IL-15 triggers the growth of leukemic B cells through IL-2R system subunits, pointing to the role of this cytokine in regulating the neoplastic proliferation in chronic lymphoproliferative disorders.[535] Synovial fluids from RA patients were found to contain chemotactic activity, which was attributable in part to the presence of IL-15. Moreover, in a murine model, injection of rIL-15 was found to induce a local tissue inflammatory infiltrate consisting of mostly T lymphocytes. Synovial fluid T lymphocytes proliferate in response to IL-15, demonstrating that continued responsiveness to IL-15 is a feature of T cells after entry into the synovial compartment. These data suggest that IL-15 can recruit and activate T lymphocytes in the synovial membrane, thereby contributing to RA pathogenesis.[355] A defect in IL-15 signaling may contribute to the XSCID in humans, resulting from mutations in the receptor common γ-chain.[191]

Therapeutic Applications

IL-2 and IL-15, which uses the β- and γ-chains of the IL-2R, have been found in melanoma cells and anti–IL-15 mAbs to inhibit HLA class I expression in these cells. Therefore these cytokines may modify the behavior of both stromal and neoplastic cells inside a tumor. These data may have important implications for our understanding of tumor–host interactions and in future strategies of immunotherapy.[22] When compared with IL-2, which enhances both spontaneous and antigen-induced lymphocyte proliferative responses, IL-15 rarely increases spontaneous lymphocyte proliferation. Thus IL-15 may help to correct the impaired proliferative response of CD4 lymphocytes from HIV-1–infected persons without the mitogenic effect of IL-2, which also may induce HIV-1 expression.[411]

INTERLEUKIN-16

Interleukin 16 (IL-16) is a proinflammatory cytokine that is chemotactic for CD4+ T lymphocytes, monocytes, and eosinophils.[78]

Synonym

IL-16 was formerly known as lymphocyte chemoattractant factor (LCF).

General Characteristics

IL-16 has a tetrameric structure that appears to be an absolute requirement for biological activity. The amino acid structure predicts six β-sheets, of which the β2-sheet contains a sequence probably important in the autoaggregation of monomers (130AA). The 15 hydrophilic C-terminal amino acids are thought to be important in IL-16 binding to its receptor. There is no direct evidence that the secreted molecule is glycosylated. A protein of 80 kDa has been identified on both human and murine lymphocytes using various antibodies directed against the 14-kDa secreted protein. Biological activity suggests that IL-16 is a proinflammatory and immunomodulatory cytokine.[79]

Other general characteristics of IL-16 include:

Molecular Weight

Depending on its molecular form, the literature values for the molecular weight of IL-16 vary from 14 to 80 kDa. The following molecular weights have been reported: 14 to 17 kDa, 56 kDa (homotetramer), and 80 kDa (precursor).[79]

Cross-Reactivity

The cross-reactivity (amino acid sequence homology between human and mouse) for IL-16 is more than 85%.[79] Murine IL-16 has chemoattractant bioactivity for human CD4 T cells, and this activity is inhibited by antihuman IL-16 mAb.[79]

Chromosomal Location

The chromosomal location of IL-16 is 15q26.1. No similarities to other cytokine genes have been found, and the chromosomal location is not proximal to that of any other cytokines.[79]

Cellular Origin

IL-16 synthesis has been demonstrated in CD8 lymphocytes (Figure 22-24).[336] CD4 and CD8 T cells constitutively express mRNA for IL-16; however, fully assembled bioactive tetrameric cytokine is preformed only in CD8 T cells. CD8 T cells contain constitutively synthesized and stored IL-16 in bioactive form. It is unclear whether IL-16 is synthesized

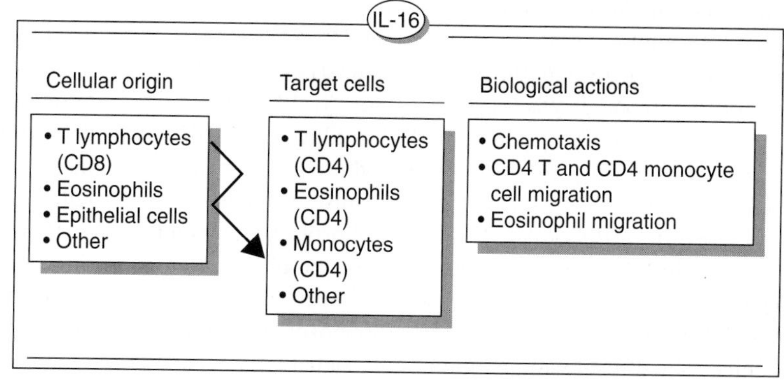

Figure 22-24 Cellular origin, principal target cells, and biological actions of IL-16.

and released from classic Tc or other CD8 T subsets, but the immunosuppressive effect is more consistent with a suppressive T-cell origin. CD4 T lymphocytes contain IL-16 mRNA and the 80-kDa precursor but no preformed bioactive cytokine. Following mitogen, antigen, or CD3 stimulation, CD4 T cells release bioactive IL-16. Eosinophils and airway epithelial cells are sources of bioactive IL-16, and brain, thymus, spleen, whole blood leukocytes, and pancreas express IL-16 mRNA.[79,321]

Control of Synthesis and Release

Serotonin induces secretion of IL-16 from CD8 but not from CD4 T cells. This induction does not require *de novo* protein synthesis. Serotonin, via serotonin type 2 receptors, may promote the recruitment of CD4 T lymphocytes into an inflammatory focus.[298] IL-16 is released in response to an antigen, mitogen, histamine, or serotonin. Histamine induces secretion of IL-16 by interaction with H2-type histamine receptors on CD8 cells, and serotonin induces secretion by interaction with S2-type receptors. The mechanism of IL-16 secretion is unknown; however, the intracellular 80-kDa molecule suggests the necessity of protein processing, resembling IL-1 (which also lacks leader sequences) that is secreted after processing and formation of pore complexes.[79]

Receptor (IL-16R)

The CD4 molecule is thought to be the IL-16 receptor[407] because it serves as a receptor for the secreted form of IL-16, and IL-16 binding to CD4 induces signal transduction, which affects the activation state of the cell.[336] The binding region on CD4 appears to be distant from the MHC and HIV-1 gp120 binding regions and related with the CDR3 region near the OKT4 binding domain. The use of CD4 as the receptor for IL-16 implies that CD4, in addition to being an accessory molecule in APC/T-cell binding, has functions as a chemoattractant and growth factor receptor. The tetramerization of CD4 seems to be indispensable for IL-16 binding (also in a tetrameric complex), whereas gp120 can bind to single CD4 molecules.[79]

Signal Transduction

The interaction between IL-16 and its receptor CD4 leads to an increase in intracytoplasmic calcium and inositol triphosphate. Recombinant IL-16 induces rapid translocation of PKC from the cytosol to the membrane in CD4 cells, including normal blood T cells, suggesting a role for PKC in CD4-mediated migratory responses.[408] The binding of IL-16 to CD4 results in activation of p56(lck), whose adaptor function is essential for the chemotactic response. Subsequently, increases in intracellular Ca^{2+} and phosphatidylinositol 1,4,5-triphosphate occur, as does translocation of PKC from cytosol to membrane.[105] IL-16 induces rises in intracellular Ca^{2+} and inositol triphosphate and autophosphorylation of p56lck. The transmission of a migratory signal is associated with the SH2- and SH3-mediated recruitment of other signaling molecules and not with lck kinase activity. The requirement for the SH2 and SH3 recruitment domains for other intracellular proteins suggests that they provide the link to the cytoskeleton for the motile response. Phosphoinositide 3-kinase, phospholipase Cγ, and PKC are also implicated in IL-16–induced motile response. There are similarities in the signal transduction pathways and cellular functions induced by IL-16 and HIV-1 gp120, although it is not known if IL-16 induces other biological activities that have been attributed to gp120, such as cytokine synthesis and arachidonate metabolism in monocytes.[79]

Biological Actions

The principal known action of IL-16 is its chemoattractant activity for CD4 lymphocytes and for CD4 eosinophils and monocytes.[79,321] The chemoattractant activity for activated and resting T cells is both chemokinetic and chemotactic. For eosinophils and monocytes, this is mostly a chemotactic activity. IL-16 is a competence growth factor for CD4 lymphocytes, inducing a G0 to G1 cell-cycle change but not cell division. IL-16 induces the expression of high-affinity IL-2R on these cells but not the synthesis of IL-2. IL-16 provides a functional role for the existence of CD4 receptor on non-T cells (besides chemoattraction, it increases adhesion of eosinophils to matrix proteins and induces IFNγ-independent HLA-DR expression on monocytes).[79,408] IL-16 is chemotactic for CD4 T cells and induces functional IL-2 receptors in CD4 T cells. The investigation of the potential regulatory effects of IL-16 on CD3/TCR-mediated lymphocyte activation indicates that this proinflammatory state is associated with subsequent transient inhibition of responsiveness via the CD3/TCR complex.[105] IL-16 is a natural CD4 ligand that suppresses T-cell proliferation in a dose-dependent manner. The unresponsiveness induced by rIL-16 is distinct from that of other CD4 ligands in that CD4 and IL-2R expression are unaffected. The failure of rIL-2 to restore proliferation suggests that the decrease in T-cell responsiveness induced by rIL-16 may result from an interruption in the IL-2R–signaling mechanism. These experiments may help explain how CD4 delivers both activating and inhibitory signals and provides a rationale for the role of IL-16 in the regulation of immune responses.[523] CD4 plays an important regulatory role in T-cell activation by switching from augmentation of antigen-specific responses in the presence of APCs, to antigen-independent inflammatory responses following dimerization by anti-CD4 antibodies or tetramerization by IL-16. This cytokine could contribute in part to a general recruitment of T cells during an inflammatory process and render the responsive lymphocytes temporarily less susceptible to antigen stimulation.

IL-16 has also been described as a suppressor of HIV infectivity, inhibiting HIV-1 replication in infected PBMCs. Pretreatment of CD4 lymphoid cells with rIL-16 repressed HIV-1 promoter activity up to sixtyfold. This effect of IL-16 requires sequences contained within the core enhancer but is not due simply to the down regulation of transcription factors binding to this element.[79,336] In patients undergoing hepatic resection, both IL-6 and IL-16 are suggested to induce hepatic regeneration and the production of APP in the liver.[478] IL-16 produced by eosinophils could contribute to enhancing the recruitment of additional populations of CD4 lymphocytes and eosinophils into sites of allergic inflammation.[321]

Clinical Relevance

IL-16 is thought to play a role in allergic inflammation.[321] Accumulation of CD4-activated lymphocytes in the airways of asthmatics is generally attributed to the presence of chemoattractant cytokines, namely IL-16 and MIP1α.[106] Most studies have focused on asthma and granulomatous diseases because IL-16 represents about 80% of the CD4 lymphocyte chemoattractant activity found in bronchoalveolar lavage from patients with asthma. Mast cell histamine might induce the secretion of IL-16 after an allergenic challenge. In granulomatous inflammatory responses, the production of histamine and serotonin by mast cells induces the secretion of IL-16 and consequent intervention of CD4 T cells. IL-16 has been found in sarcoid granuloma and in granulomas of infective origin, particularly *Mycobacterium tuberculosis.*[79]

Therapeutic Applications

IL-16 inhibitors may prove useful in suppressing the proinflammatory effects of IL-16. The capacity of this cytokine to inhibit HIV infection and simultaneously prime CD4 lymphocytes for IL-2–induced proliferation suggests a complementary role in the treatment of HIV infection.[79]

INTERLEUKIN-17

Interleukin-17 (IL-17) is a prototype member of a new cytokine family secreted by activated $CD4^+$ and $CD8^+$ T lymphocytes. It is classified as proinflammatory cytokine, because it induces many mediators of inflammation that are involved in the proliferation, maturation, and chemotaxis of neutrophils.[581]

Synonyms

Two T-cell–derived molecules termed cytotoxic T lymphocyte-associated antigen 8 (CTLA 8) and herpesvirus saimiri gene 13 (HVS13) were proposed as novel cytokines that bind to a novel cytokine receptor named IL-17, vIL-17, and IL-17R, respectively.[587] Analysis of the cDNA-encoding murine IL-17 (cytotoxic T lymphocyte–associated antigen 8) predicted a secreted protein sharing 57% amino acid identity with the protein predicted from ORF13, an open reading frame of a T lymphotropic virus, HVS.[169]

General Characteristics

Human IL-17 has been described as a glycoprotein of 155 amino acids secreted as a homodimer by activated memory CD4 T cells.[169] Like IL-10 and BCRF1, IL-17 and ORF13 suggest a virus-captured gene with possible functional activity. Both glycosylated and nonglycosylated forms of the homodimeric IL-17 molecule are secreted yet are not related to the functional activity of this cytokine.[65]

Human IL-17

A cDNA encoding human IL-17 (hIL-17) has been cloned from a CD4 T-cell library.[588] The predicted 155–amino acid sequence contains an N-terminal signal peptide and exhibits 72% amino acid identity with HVS13 and 63% with murine CTLA-8. High levels of hIL-17 were induced from primary peripheral blood $CD4^+$ T cells on stimulation. When expressed in CV1/EBNA cells, recombinant hIL-17 was secreted in both glycosylated and nonglycosylated forms. An hIL-17 Fc fusion protein and supernatants from cells transfected with hIL-17 induced IL-6 and IL-8 production and enhanced the surface expression of the ICAM-1 in human fibroblasts.[588]

Mouse IL-17

Mouse IL-17 is a cytokine preferentially expressed by αβ TCR CD4neg CD8neg T cells. It represents a novel molecule, originally designated murine CTLA-8, and later described as a cDNA isolated from an activated T-cell hybridoma produced by fusing a mouse cytotoxic T-cell clone and a rat T lymphoma. This cDNA, which contains mRNA instability sequences characteristic of many cytokines, encodes a putative secreted protein that is homologous to the ORF13 gene of herpesvirus saimiri. The human homologue to this molecule has been identified as the proinflammatory cytokine IL-17. The cDNA encoding mouse IL-17 from a cDNA library, generated from αβ TCR CD4neg CD8neg thymocytes, shares 87.3% amino acid identity to the previously described murine CTLA-8. Comparison of murine CTLA-8 with the cDNA isolated from activated rat splenocytes revealed that murine CTLA-8 is the rat homologue of IL-17. Mouse IL-17 mRNA is specifically expressed by activated αβ TCR CD4neg CD8neg T cells, a small subset with a potentially important role in immune regulation. Mouse, rat, and human IL-17 can induce IL-6 secretion in mouse stromal cells, indicating that all homologues can recognize the mouse receptor.[272]

Other general characteristics of IL-17 include:

Cross-Reactivity

Human IL-17 cross-reacts with mouse cells.[272]

Chromosomal Location

The chromosomal location of IL-17 is 2q31.[65]

Cellular Origin

IL-17 is produced by activated memory CD4 T cells (Figure 22-25).[169] This represents a rather restricted set of T lymphocytes that contrasts with the ubiquitous expression of IL-17 receptor.[65]

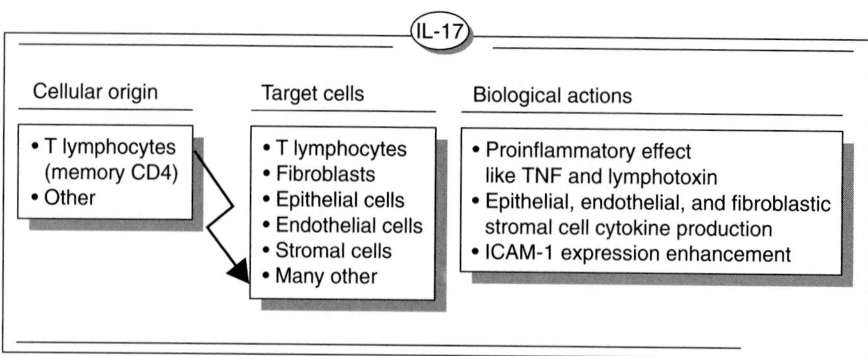

Figure 22-25 Cellular origin, principal target cells, and biological actions of IL-17.

Control of Synthesis and Release

Under normal conditions, the IL-17 gene is induced to synthesize cytokine from activated memory CD4 of T lymphocytes. Whether IL-17 itself has a role in IL-17 production and what kind of stimuli will be able to activate IL-17 synthesis remain to be elucidated.[65]

Receptor (IL-17R)

IL-17R is unrelated to previously identified cytokine receptor families. A recombinant soluble receptor inhibits T-cell proliferation and IL-2 production induced by mitogens and anti-TCR monoclonal antibodies.[587] It has been suggested that a large variety of cells can express IL-17R, including fibroblasts; epithelial; and endothelial cells.

Signal Transduction

Murine IL-17 stimulates the activity of the transcriptional factor NF-κB, which is known to regulate a number of gene products involved in cell activation and growth control, raising the possibility that some of IL-17 activities may be mediated by a common intracellular event.[65,587]

Biological Actions

Recombinant HVS13 and CTLA-8 stimulate transcriptional factor NF-κB activity and IL-6 secretion in fibroblasts and co-stimulate T-cell proliferation.[587] IL-17 and the product of its viral counterpart—ORF13—stimulate epithelial, endothelial, and fibroblastic cells to secrete cytokines such as IL-6, IL-8, and G-CSF, and PGE2. Furthermore, when cultured in the presence of IL-17, fibroblasts can sustain the proliferation of CD34 hematopoietic progenitors and their preferential maturation into neutrophils. These observations suggest that IL-17 may constitute an early initiator of the T-cell–dependent inflammatory reaction and be an element of the cytokine network that bridges the immune system to hematopoiesis. TNFα and IFNγ have been found to have additive effects on the IL-17–induced secretion of IL-6; neither IL-17 nor TNFα induces release of GM-CSF. However, the combination of IL-17 plus TNFα is effective in this event.[65,169] Knowing that IL-17 induces the production of other cytokines (IL-6, IL-8, and G-CSF) from fibroblasts, endothelial cells, and epithelial cells, the release of PGE2 enhances the expression of ICAM-1. Considering that these molecules have very different activities, a single cytokine can have a broad set of not entirely predictable effects, which may have the potential of counterbalancing each other.[66]

INTERLEUKIN-18

Interleukin-18 (IL-18) is structurally similar to IL-1 and functionally similar to IL-12. It increases the cytotoxic activity of NK cells and cytotoxic T lymphocytes and may play a role both as a neuroimmunomodulator and in the induction of mucosal immunity.[49]

Synonym

IL-18 was formerly known as IFNγ-inducing factor (ICIF).

General Characteristics

The amino acid sequence determined from the human IL-18 from normal human liver cDNA clones indicates a 193–amino acid precursor peptide with 65% homology with that of murine IL-18. The amino acid sequence of IL-18 also includes an IL-1 signature-like sequence. IL-18 possesses potent biological activities, including the induction of IFNγ production by spleen cells and the enhancement of NK-cell cytotoxicity.[544]

Other general characteristics of IL-18 include:

Molecular Weight

The molecular weight of IL-18 is though to be ~18 kDa.[112]

Cross-Reactivity

The cross-reactivity (amino acid sequence homology between human and mouse) for IL-18 is 65%.[544]

Chromosomal Location

The chromosomal location of IL-18 is unknown.

Cellular Origin

Human IL-18 is produced primarily by liver cells (Figure 22-26).[544]

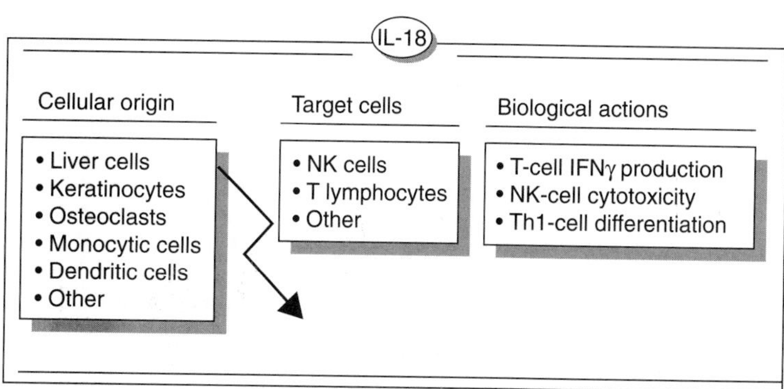

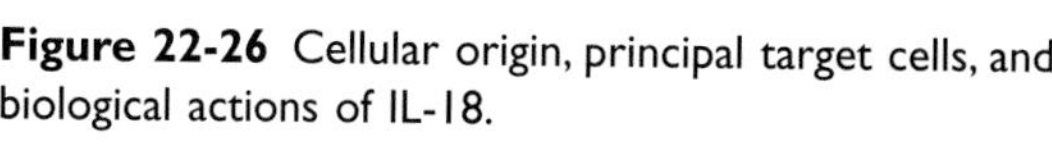
Figure 22-26 Cellular origin, principal target cells, and biological actions of IL-18.

Biological Actions

IL-18 augments NK-cell activity in cultures of human PBMCs similar to that of the structurally unrelated cytokine IL-12. In addition, it has been found to enhance the production of IFNγ and GM-CSF while decreasing the production of IL-10 by mitogen-stimulated PBMCs but had no effect on IL-4 production by concanavalin A–stimulated PBMC. IL-18 enhances T-cell proliferation apparently through an IL-2–dependent pathway. It also enhances Th1 cytokine production in vitro and exhibits synergism when combined with IL-12 in terms of enhanced IFNγ production but not IL-2 and GM-CSF production.[362,544]

IL-18 selectively enhances the FasL-mediated* cytotoxicity of cloned murine Th1 cells but not Th0 or Th2 cells. Anti-IFNγ antibody does not block the IL-18–induced cytotoxicity of Th1 cells, nor does IFNα, IFNγ, or TNFα augment the cytotoxic activity of Th1, thus indicating that this enhanced cytotoxicity of Th1 cells was mediated by IL-18. In addition, IL-12 has been found to also enhance the FasL-mediated cytotoxicity of Th1 cells, suggesting that Th1 cells possess receptors for both cytokines, although these cytokines can act via different pathways. Data indicate that IL-18 might play a potential role in immunoregulation or in inflammation by augmenting the functional activity of FasL on Th1 cells.[112]

INTERFERONS

Interferons (IFNs) are a family of glycoproteins that exert virus-nonspecific but host-specific antiviral activity by inducing the transcription of cellular genes coding for antiviral proteins that selectively inhibit the synthesis of viral RNA and proteins. The name of IFNs derives from the common property *to interfere with the viral infection of cells.* They represent the most important element of natural immune defenses against viral infection.[152,472]

IFNs also have immunoregulatory functions (inhibition of B-cell activation and antibody production enhancement of T-cell activity, and enhancement of NK cell cytotoxic activity) and can inhibit the growth of nonviral intracellular parasites. Production of interferon can be stimulated by viral infection, especially by the presence of double-stranded RNA, by intracellular parasites (chlamydiae and rickettsiae), by protozoa *(Toxoplasma),* and by bacteria (streptococci and staphylococci) and bacterial products (endotoxins). Interferons have been divided into three distinct types (α, β, and γ) associated with specific producer cells and functions, but all animal cells are able to produce interferons, and certain producer cells (leukocytes and fibroblasts) produce more than one type (both IFNα and IFNβ).[138]

IFNα and IFNβ show little structural similarity (30% homologous at the amino acid level), but they share a common receptor, have similar functions, and both genes are located on chromosome 9. There are at least 24 structurally related subtypes of IFNα,* each encoded by a separate gene with 95% homology, and only one IFNβ gene in humans and mice (the so-called IFNβ2 is now demonstrated to be IL-6). Collectively, they are known as type I IFNs and acid-stable (pH2) IFNs. IFNγ has a different receptor and partially different functionality. It is known as type II IFN and acid-labile IFN.[1,71,436,485]

All IFNs have antiviral capacity and immunomodulatory and antiproliferative effects on both normal and tumor cells. Consequently, they have been used in the treatment of several pathologies, ranging from viral infection (e.g., common cold and viral hepatitis) and intracellular parasitosis to malignancies (e.g., leukemia, lymphoma, and melanoma). Generally, IFNs enhance the effectiveness of the cellular immune response, but their use in anticancer therapy is based on the antiproliferative effect of IFNs. This duality of increased synthesis of several proteins, such as other cytokines, MHC molecules, β2-microglobulin, carcinoembryonic antigen, enzymes, and decreased synthesis of several other proteins followed by decreased expression of the *myc* and *ras* oncogenes, is characteristic of IFNs.[485]

*Fas ligand (FasL), expressed on activated T cells, plays a central role in regulating the immune response by inducing apoptosis in activated lymphocytes through binding to its receptor, Fas.

*Some investigators now subdivide the IFNα family into the IFN I and IFN II (also known as IFNθ) groups on the basis of the number of amino acids (166 or 165 amino acids for IFNαI and 172 amino acids for IFNαII) and the respective sequences within the family.[1,71]

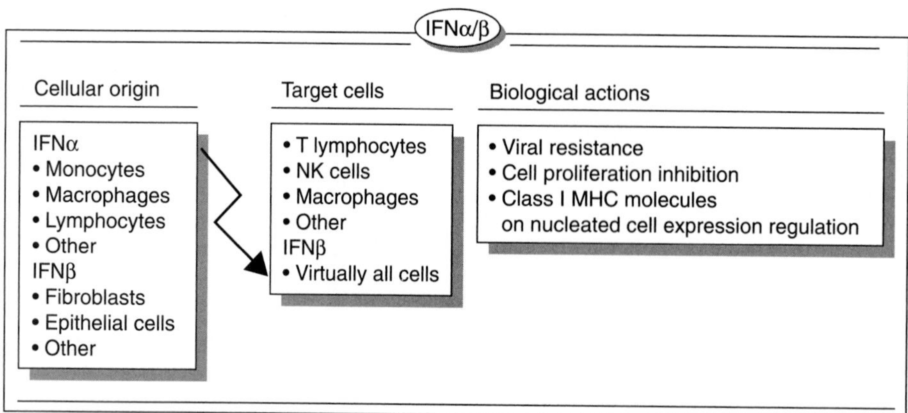

Figure 22-27 Cellular origin, principal target cells, and biological actions of IFNα and IFNβ.

IFNα and IFNβ

Interferonα (IFNα) is the major interferon produced by virus-induced leukocyte cultures; the primary producer cells are null lymphocytes, and the major activities are antiviral activity and activation of NK cells. It is used in the experimental treatment of hairy cell leukemia and other selected neoplasias.[138]

Interferonβ (IFNβ) is the major interferon produced by double-stranded RNA-induced fibroblast cultures; the primary producer cells are fibroblasts, epithelial cells, and macrophages, and the major activity is antiviral activity.[138]

Synonyms

IFNα was formerly known as acid-stable IFN, B-cell IFN, buffy coat IFN, leukocyte-derived IFN, lymphoblast IFN, Namalwa IFN, and type I IFN. IFNβ was formerly known as acid-stable IFN, fibroblast-derived IFN, IFNβ1, and type I IFN.

General Characteristics

IFNβ is glycosylated, but the majority of human IFNα type I molecules are not. The three-dimensional structure of either molecule is yet to be fully elucidated, but there may be a similarity between the two. IFNβ has five helices (three parallel to each other and two antiparallel to the other three), and the general structure is a variant of the α-helix bundle but with a new chain-folding topology common to all type I IFNs.[71,436]

Other general characteristics of IFNα and IFNβ include:

Molecular Weight. The literature values for the molecular weight of IFNα vary from 16 to 27.5 kDa. The following molecular weights have been reported: 18 kDa,[1] 20 kDa,[421] 16 kDa,[436] 19 to 26 kDa (monomer),[472] 16 to 27 kDa,[71] and 16 to 27.5 kDa.[389] The literature values for the molecular weight of IFNβ vary from 15 to 32 kDa. The following molecular weights have been reported: 20 kDa (monomer),[1,71,421,472] 27 kDa,[436] and 22 to 23 kDa.[389]

Cross-Reactivity. The cross-reactivities (amino acid sequence homology between human and mouse) of IFNs are IFNα (40%) and IFNβ (48%). IFNs are more species specific and preferential in their biological activities than most other cytokines.

Chromosomal Location. The chromosomal locations of α and β IFN and their receptors are 9p22 (IFNα), 9p22 (IFNβ), and 21q22.1 (IFNαBR, shared with IFNβ).

Cellular Origin. IFNα is produced by monocytes, macrophages, lymphocytes, and cellular lines such as Namalwa and KG1 (Figure 22-27). IFNβ is produced by fibroblasts and epithelial cells. However, many other cells can also produce these cytokines, including hematopoietic cells for IFNα.[71,152,341,436]

Monocytes differentiate into macrophages during cell culture and lose their ability to produce IFNα when challenged with HIV-1. However, these cells remain capable of producing IFNα in response to other stimuli, suggesting that as monocytes differentiate into macrophages, they selectively lose their ability to produce IFNα through the double-stranded RNA (dsRNA)–independent mechanism.[173]

Control of Synthesis and Release

Viral infection is the most potent signal that elicits type I IFN production. Both IFNα and IFNβ are also secreted during immune responses to antigens (antigen-activated T cells stimulate mononuclear phagocytes to synthesize type I IFNs).[1] IFNα production is increased if the cellular source is previously exposed to either IFNα or IFNβ. IFNβ synthesis is enhanced by bacterial endotoxins, TNFα, and IL-1.[472] Data suggest that there are dsRNA-dependent and dsRNA-independent mechanisms for the induction of IFNα production.[173] Glucocorticoids regulate IFNα production (inhibition) but fail to elicit this activity from acquired immunodeficiency syndrome (AIDS)–glucocorticoid resistant monocytes.[393]

IFNα and IFNβ Receptors

The receptors for IFNα and IFNβ are shared and consist of a single-chain polypeptide (CD118) that is homologous to the type II IFN. Two types of receptors have been cloned.

The first specifically binds IFNαB (IFNα8, a variety of IFNα) and is known as the IFNαB receptor. The second binds both IFNα and IFNβ and is called the IFNα/β receptor. The IFNαβR is a member of the class II cytokine receptor family, which also includes the IFNγR, IL-10R, and tissue factor. The IFNα/βR is also a class II cytokine receptor and contains at least two components that interact with type I IFNs. It is not known if these two receptors are expressed independently on the cell surface or are associated with each other in an IFN receptor complex. The receptors are present on most types of cells. A soluble form of the IFNα/βR has been identified in human serum and urine.[1,71,152,335]

Signal Transduction

Receptor signaling results in phosphorylation and activation of PTK, TYK2, and JAK1 but not KAK2. Although IFNα activates STAT1α and STAT5, STAT1α is predominantly activated. Differential phosphorylation and consequent differential activation of both separate and overlapping STAT proteins by IL-2, IL-12, and IFNα may provide a molecular basis for the similarities and differences in the actions of these cytokines on NK cells. IFNα has also been shown to activate PLC-A2 releasing arachidonic acid and DAG. The IFNα/βR is physically associated with JAK1.[71,591]

Biological Actions

Antiviral action was the first biological property of IFNα and IFNβ to be described. However, type I IFNs also (1) inhibit cell proliferation; (2) induce MHC class I expression on cell surfaces (representing cellular targeting for the immune system); (3) increase the cytolytic activity of NK cells, macrophages, and Tc lymphocytes; and (4) improve ADCC.[1,71,472,485] This results in the enhancement of particular host-nonspecific responses against intracellular pathogens, tumor cells, and graft cells. Inhibition of viral replication is based on the induced synthesis of a number of enzymes that interfere with replication of viral RNA or DNA. This antiviral action is primarily paracrine (a virally infected cell secretes type I IFNs [typically IFNβ] to protect neighboring cells not yet infected, thus limiting the area of infection and the extent of cellular damage). IFNβ is a physiological inhibitor of normal cell growth, and IFNα is an antiproliferative molecule for certain tumors as will be discussed later. Inhibition of cell growth and proliferation may result from the induction of the same enzymes that inhibit viral replication and possibly other ones that prevent synthesis of essential amino acids. Inhibition may also result from the inhibitory effect in the production of hematopoietic growth factors that originate in the bone marrow microenvironment.[8] MHC class I expression is increased by type I IFNs in parallel to a profound inhibition of class II expression. This MHC modulation boosts the effector phase of CD8 T cells (Tc response), preventing the activation of class II–restricted CD4 T cells.[1,472] Several activities are probably involved in the antiinflammatory effects mediated by IFNβ, including complex immunoregulatory effects on endothelial cells with differential modulatory effects on various cell surface markers.[363] The effects of IFNβ on T-cell functions in vitro are centered on the inhibition of T-cell proliferation and T-cell–dependent Ig secretion in a dose-dependent manner. IFNβ does not inhibit up regulation of CD40L on activated T cells but blocks induction of CD25 on stimulated T and B lymphocytes. Secretion of IFNγ, TNFα, and IL-13 is inhibited by the addition of IFNβ, whereas IL-4 secretion is unaffected. IFNβ also enhances secretion of IL-2 and of IL-10.[345] Moreover, the influence of IFNα on CD4 T cells is very important through cytokine synthesis and Th1/Th2 polarization. IFNα also markedly inhibits IL-5 production and stimulates production of IL-10 in activated CD4 T cells. This effect might enhance the negative-feedback mechanism ascribed to IL-10, which limits inflammatory reactions and contributes to CD4 polarization.[8,379,462] Most T cells derived in the presence of IFNα produce IFNγ but no or only limited amounts of IL-4 and IL-5 (Th1 or Th0 cells). IFNα also shifts the TCR Vβ repertoire of specific T-cell lines.[410] However, neither IFNγ nor IFNα alone can induce Th1 polarization.[571] IFNα also induces a variety of central actions (e.g., fever, anorexia, slow wave sleep, and depression). The cellular mechanism by which this cytokine affects neuronal activity appears to be the suppression of the N-methyl-D-aspartate (NMDA) responses through its action on opioid receptors and the production of free radicals, such as hydroxyl radicals and NO, caused by the neuron-glial cell interactions.[261] Systemic administration of human IFNα stimulates the pituitary-adrenal axis in humans, but the exact mechanism still remains to be established. However, circulating IL-6 increases, resulting in activation of the pituitary-adrenal axis.[479]

Clinical Relevance

IFNα is an antiviral cytokine detected in plasma of HIV-infected patients during acute viremia and during late-stage disease.[173] It is known to inhibit expression of GM-CSF in adherent cells of human long-term bone marrow cultures stimulated with IL-1, TNFα, or endotoxin. These results indicate a regulatory role for IFNα in the bone marrow microenvironment possibly involved in the myelosuppressive effect of IFNα therapy on viral infections.[194] Both hyperthyroidism and hypothyroidism have been reported during prolonged recombinant human IFNα therapy. These changes in thyroid hormone metabolism are possibly mediated in part by IL-6.[98] Undetectable IFNα serum levels in a patient with atopic dermatitis with normal IL-4 and increased IFNγ suggest the role of IFNα in the pathogenesis of atopic dermatitis.[134]

Therapeutic Applications

Type I IFNs have clinical application in the treatment of viral infections, especially infections characterized by a tendency toward a chronic state (such as hepatitis B and C). Also, IFNs have potential as adjuvants in the treatment of HIV infection. Their antitumor effects are significant (especially

IFNα) in leukemia, lymphoma, multiple myeloma, melanoma, renal cell carcinoma, and Kaposi's sarcoma. Side effects include flulike syndrome, fever, myalgias, rashes, thrombocytopenia, and neutropenia.[472,485]

Some therapeutic results have been encouraging: Treatment with IFNα of a posttransplant lymphoproliferative disorder led to dramatic clinical, radiographic, and histological improvement probably directly related to the inhibition of Th2 CD4 lymphocytes.[160] IFNα modulates the development of allergen-specific T cells in vitro, which suggests that it may represent a useful tool for novel immunotherapeutic approaches in allergic disorders.[410] Also a growing body of evidence indicates that IFNα has a major place in the long-term treatment of idiopathic hypereosinophilic syndrome, especially in cases resistant to conventional treatment.[340] Results from clinical trials have indicated that recombinant IFNβ is a promising drug for the treatment of multiple sclerosis, although this treatment decreases TNFα and increases IL-6, which could potentially counteract its beneficial immunomodulatory effects[63,435]; it has been suggested that IFNβ gene transfection by the use of liposome coupled with a monoclonal Ab might become a useful technique for gene therapy of malignant glioma.[557] However, a phase II trial of IL-2 and IFNα in the treatment of metastatic colorectal carcinoma has shown that the toxicity and short duration of response without survival benefit do not support the routine use of this therapeutic modality for this type of tumor.[82]

IFNγ

Interferonγ (IFNγ) is the major interferon produced by immunologically stimulated (by mitogens or antigens) lymphocyte cultures; the primary producer cells are T lymphocytes, and the major activity is immunoregulation. IFNγ has been implicated in aberrant expression of class II histocompatibility antigens by tissue cells (such as thyroid cells) that do not normally express them, leading to autoimmune disease.[138]

Synonyms

IFNγ was formerly known as immune IFN, macrophage activating factor, T-cell IFN, and type II IFN.

General Characteristics

IFNγ is a homodimer (native IFNγ is a monomeric glycoprotein, but the active moiety is a dimer, which interacts with α- and β-receptors causing their aggregation and subsequent activation) formed by antiparallel association of two subunits. Each subunit has six α-helices held together by short nonhelical sequences. There are no β-sheets. The subunits have a flattened elliptical shape, whereas the overall structure of the dimer is globular.[71]

IFNγ was originally described as an antiviral molecule but is a pleiotropic cytokine influencing the growth, differentiation, and function of T cells, B cells, NK cells, macrophages, and other types of cells, such as endothelial cells and fibroblasts. It is involved in the regulation of almost all phases of the immunoinflammatory responses. Because IFNγRs are expressed on almost all types of cells, this cytokine directly mediates a vast biological spectrum.[472] However, it has low antiviral and antiproliferative activity but potentiates the antiviral and antitumor effects of IFNα and IFNβ.[71,341]

IFNγ binds with high affinity to heparin sulfate and heparin molecules through its carboxyl-terminal domain. In vivo, IFNγ is eliminated from the blood stream with a half-life of 1.1 minutes, caused by binding to heparin sulfate. Unbound IFNγ is cleaved rapidly at the carboxyl-terminal side, a process that inactivates the cytokine. When bound to heparin, the plasma clearance of IFNγ is greatly decreased (half-life ≅99 minutes), and the cytokine activity is increased by as much as 600%. These data demonstrate that the blood clearance of IFNγ is a nonreceptor-mediated process and that in vivo the local concentration of heparin sulfate and/or heparin-like molecules regulates the activity of this cytokine.[330]

Other general characteristics of IFNγ include:

Molecular Weight. Depending on its molecular form and extent of glycosylation, the literature values for the molecular weight of IFNγ vary from 20 to 70 kDa. The following molecular weights have been reported: 20 to 25 kDa (dimer),[341,389,472] 21 to 24 kDa subunits (the size variation is due to variable degrees of glycosylation, but each subunit contains an identical 18 kDa polypeptide),[1] 45 kDa (normally dimerized),[421] 40 to 70 kDa,[436] 20 and 25 kDa forms (these two glycosylated forms are caused by the post-translational modification of a 17 kDa polypeptide, but the extent of glycosylation is variable and not necessary to the biological activity),[152] 20 or 25 kDa (corresponding to different species of monomeric human IFNγ, which differ only in the degree and sites of glycosylation), and 40 to 70 kDa (caused by dimerization and some multimerization).[71]

Cross-Reactivity. The cross-reactivity (amino acid sequence homology between human and mouse) of IFNγ is 40%.[71] It has no significant cross-species activity.

Chromosomal Location. The chromosomal location of IFNγ and its receptor are 12q24.1, 6q12-q22, and 21q22 (AF-1).

Cellular Origin. IFNγ is synthesized by activated T cells (CD4 Th0, CD4 Th1, and CD8) and NK cells (Figure 22-28).*

Control of Synthesis and Release

IFNγ is produced by CD4 Th1 cells following antigen activation.[380] Transcription is directly initiated after antigen activation and is enhanced by IL-2, IL-12, and IL-15. Depending on the type of antigenic stimulus, Th1 CD4 T cells and CD8 T cells are the main producers of IFNγ. CD40/CD40L interaction synergizes with IL-12 in selectively enhancing IFNγ production through purified anti-CD3-stimulated T cells. Both CD4 and CD8 T cells are able to produce IFNγ in the

*References 1, 19, 71, 152, 341, 472.

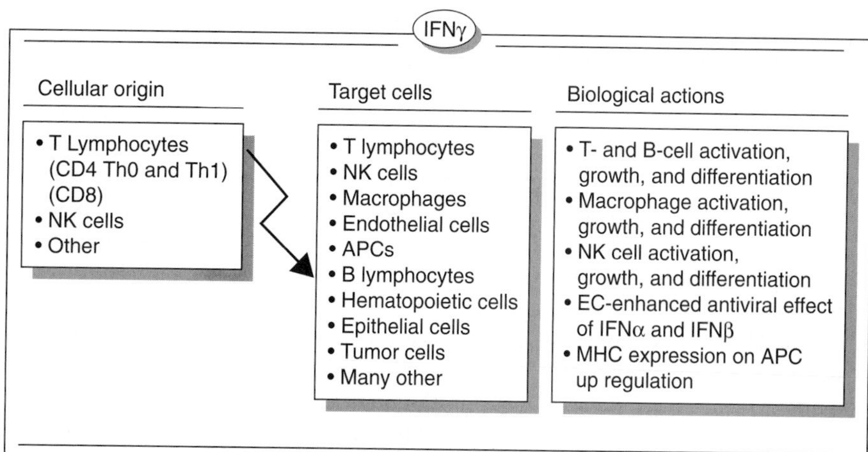

Figure 22-28 Cellular origin, principal target cells, and biological actions of IFNγ.

presence of helper signals from IL-12 and CD40, although CD8 T cells are less active.[416] Th1 cells can be the primary producers of IFNγ when exposed to antigens, but on appropriate stimulation, NK cells are potent producers; when exposed to IL-1, IL-2, and IL-12, they become the primary source of IFNγ.[1,152,185,341,469] IL-12 is a very critical factor for skewing the immune response toward a Th1 of cytokine profile (high IFNγ and low IL-4) and is thought to be a key factor for the induction of IFNγ synthesis.[216,242] IL-18 has been found to enhance the production of IFNγ. When T cells were exposed to a combination of IL-18 and IL-12, a synergistic effect was observed in the production of IFNγ.[362,544] The bacillus Calmette-Guerin may exert part of its antitumor action on melanoma through the induction of IFNγ, which can be greatly enhanced through the concomitant addition of IL-2 or GM-CSF.[178] Bacterial DNA induces NK cells to produce IFNγ in vivo and is associated with an increase in LPS-induced TNFα and IL-6 release.[101]

PGE2 inhibits the secretion of IFNγ, and the net IFNγ production of CD4 T cells is largely determined by the ratio of IL-12 and PGE2 at the point of T-cell activation.[217] Retinoic acid inhibits IFNγ synthesis when the CD28 co-stimulatory pathway is activated in addition to the TCR/CD3 pathway, suggesting that it blocks some step in the CD28 pathway.[73] Cyclosporin A inhibits IFNγ production by preventing the activation of key promoter sites, in particular, the binding of NFAT.[72]

Receptor (IFNγR)

All human cells are thought to have the IFNγ receptor; it is a complex of a high-affinity IFNγ binding chain (CD119) and a second accessory protein required for signal transduction. This specific receptor is different from, but structurally related to, the receptor used by IFNγ and IFNβ. The IFNγ binding subunit is a single-chain transmembrane glycoprotein. Although the receptor binds IFNγ with high affinity, signal transduction requires a species-specific accessory protein, which associates with the extracellular domain of the receptor. The accessory subunit has been called accessory factor 1 (AF-1) and the IFNγ receptor β-chain (being CD119 the α-chain). It is a type I membrane-spanning glycoprotein and a member of the class II cytokine receptor family. The IFNγR is also a member of the class II cytokine receptor family, characterized by an extracellular region of about 200 amino acids but no WSXWS motif characteristic of class I cytokine receptors.

The IFNγR is expressed on a wide variety of hematopoietic cells, including T cells, B cells, macrophages, PMNs, and platelets. It is not expressed by erythrocytes. The receptor is also on many somatic cells, such as epithelial and endothelial cells, and on many tumor cells. The receptor density ranges from 200 to 10,000 per cell. Membrane-bound IFNγ is rapidly internalized and degraded at 37 °C.[1,71,152]

Signal Transduction

IFNγ induces receptor dimerization and internalization, but its receptor-mediated ligand internalization is not sufficient to induce a biological response.[39] Signal transduction is mediated by phosphorylation and activation of JAK1 and JAK2 PTKs and involves phosphorylation of the receptor. The IFNγ and IFNα/β receptors share common signal transduction components, including p91, which binds directly to the GAS response element after translocation to the nucleus.[71] With the use of chimeric receptors involving the IFNγR complex as a model system, it has been demonstrated that JAK2 activation is not an absolute requirement for IFNγ signaling because other members of the JAK family can functionally substitute for JAK2.[285] STAT1 transcription factor is activated by IFNγ, synthesized, and released on stimulation of T-lymphocyte populations. There is evidence that Th1 cells lack the IFNγR chain necessary for activation of STAT1.[190]

Biological Actions

IFNγ shares many biological actions with type I IFN (it has antiviral activity and antiproliferative effect). As IFNγ enhances the antiviral activity of IFNα and IFNβ in a synergistic fashion, production of IFNγ by specific T cells is an important pathway by which the immune system is able to enhance the nonspecific protection against intracellular infection.[472] However, IFNγ has several properties that are especially attributed to this cytokine.*

Macrophage and Lymphocyte Functionality. IFNγ is a powerful activator of macrophage functionality (NO, superoxide, TNFα, IL-1 production, and Fc receptors increase) and has a very important role in cellular cytotoxicity, providing the means by which T lymphocytes activate macrophages. The diverse effects of IFNγ converge to promote Th1 polarization and macrophage inflammatory reactions, while suppressing Th2 and eosinophil-dependent responses; it thus has an essential role in the destruction of intracellular pathogens. However, in the differentiation of CD4 cells to a Th1 phenotype, the role for IFNγ is controversial. With optimal TCR stimulation and co-stimulation, endogenous IFNγ, without IL-12, is sufficient to elicit Th1 cells via an autocrine mechanism. With suboptimal stimulation, exogenous rIFNγ or rIL-12 is required for Th1 development, and optimal development of the Th1 phenotype is mediated by the synergistic actions of both cytokines. Human peripheral blood T cells that are stimulated through the TCR and expanded with IL-2 are unresponsive to IFNγ. This nonresponsiveness occurs because of a lack of expression of the AF-1 of the IFNγR, while at the same time maintaining IFNγR CD119 expression. Expression of the AF-1 can be restored by secondary TCR ligation or phorbol myristate acetate (PMA) treatment. Therefore as T cells progress from primary TCR activation through IL-2–dependent proliferation, followed by secondary TCR stimulation, their responsiveness to IFNγ varies, and this may affect their ability to participate in an ongoing immune response.

Major Histocompatibility Complex Class I and II Expression. INFγ is the principal enhancer of MHC class I expression on many different types of cells. In contrast to type I IFN, it is also an inducer of MHC class II expression in APCs (mast cells included) and lymphocytes, promoting the activation of class II–restricted CD4 T cells. These cells are an important target for IFNγ, leading to the differentiation of the Th1 subset and inhibiting the proliferation of Th2 cells.

Antigen Presentation. Both IFNγ and IL-10 are thought to suppress antigen presentation by Langerhans' cells for Th1 cells by suppressing their CD80 (B7-1) expression. The inhibitory effect of IFNγ on CD80 expression on Langerhans' cells appears to be partially mediated through the suppression of GM-CSF production by keratinocytes.

Cellular Adhesion. The previously discussed effects of IFNγ on CD4 cells are complemented by its enhancement of adhesion and morphological alterations on cells that facilitate lymphocyte extravasation to tissue and the expression of CD54 adhesion molecules (ICAM-1) fundamental in binding effector lymphocytes to target cells. Treatment with TNFα plus IFNγ causes PECAM-1 to decrease or disappear from endothelial cells' intercellular contacts. This phenomenon is accompanied by a reduction of leukocyte migration through endothelial cell monolayers. On the basis of several observations, it has been suggested that a primary role for IFNγ is to promote intercellular adhesion between the leukocytes in an effector focus, promoting its ability to block pathogen migration. Monocytes stimulated with exogenous IFNγ lose their capacity to bind to fibronectin, which coincides with the down regulation of surface α5 integrin expression. Although IFNγ-treated monocytes also show a decreased ability to adhere to laminin, no alteration of β2 integrin expression is detectable, thus suggesting a modification of the functional state of surface β2 integrins. Furthermore, when stimulated with TGF1, IFNγ-pretreated monocytes reacquire the ability to bind to fibronectin and laminin. Conversely, IFNγ reduces adhesiveness to fibronectin and laminin of monocytes initially stimulated with TGFβ1. These in vitro adhesive-deadhesive responses of monocytes to TGFβ1 and IFNγ modulation may reflect mononuclear phagocyte motility within sites of inflammation.

T-Cell Cytotoxicity and Acute Phase Response. The maturation of CD8 Tc lymphocytes is dependent on IFNγ, which acts synergistically with other cytokines (e.g., with TNFα).[84] As an inducer of cellular cytotoxicity, IFNγ is a less potent activator than TNF, up regulating the respiratory burst of neutrophils, but much more potent than type I IFNs, stimulating the activity of NK cells. IFNγ also augments the APR, increasing the production of IL-1 and TNF. IFNγ can be an important regulatory cytokine in chronic inflammatory sites, and its purported antiinflammatory effects may be explained by significant suppression on the induction of IL-1β gene expression in macrophages.

Immunoglobulin Production. IFNγ produced by T and NK cells after CpG DNA stimulation contributes to the B-cell secretion of IL-6 and the subsequent Ig production.* However, IFNγ inhibits IgM secretion, which is triggered by a different bacterial product, LPS. Thus in contrast to its antagonistic interaction with LPS, IFNγ causes a dose-dependent increase in the level of IgM secretion induced by CpG DNA. Like IgM secretion, B-cell secretion of IL-6 more than doubles after the addition of exogenous IFNγ.[589]

Other Activities. IFNγ causes a concentration-dependent decrease in steady-state lipoprotein receptor-related protein (LRP) mRNA expression and gene transcription rate. When TGFβ1 is added 24 hours before IFNγ, the extent of LRP down regulation is reduced. This suggests

*References 1, 16, 32, 35, 61, 89, 149, 154, 232, 241, 332, 341, 404, 440, 454, 471, 472, 485, 497, 549, 578.

*The dinucleotide CpG is significantly under-represented in vertebrate DNA and is usually methylated. In contrast, CpG dinucleotides are generally present at the expected frequency in bacterial DNA and are unmethylated. These unmethylated CpG motifs induce B cells to secrete IL-6 and IgM and can induce NK and CD4 T cells to produce the immunoregulatory IFNγ.

TABLE 22-6 Principal Cellular Actions of IFNγ[1,341,436,472,485]

Cell Type	Biological Effects
Many cells*	Enhanced MHC class I expression (antigen recognition by CD8 Tc cells)
APCs	Enhanced MHC class II expression (antigen recognition by CD4 cells)
Stem cells	Inhibition of hematopoiesis
B cells	Growth and differentiation (late-acting agent);† inhibition of proliferation‡
T cells	Differentiation and activation (synergizes with IL-2); inhibition of proliferation†
Monocytes	Differentiation into macrophages
Møs	Effector activation (together with TNFα)
Neutrophils	Activation, adhesion to endothelium
NK cells	Activation (synergizes with IL-2)
Endothelial cells	Activation, enhanced MHC expression
Tumor cells	Enhanced susceptibility to Tc and NK cells (synergizes with TNFα)

*Do not normally express IFNγ.
†Synergistically with other B-cell stimulating factors.
‡Dependent on its capacity to inhibit protein synthesis.

that the balance between IFNγ and TGFβ1 may be critical in determining LRP expression at sites of infection and inflammation. The results from LRP being a major receptor for multiple ligands, including chylomicrons and very low-density lipoprotein remnants, bacterial toxins, viruses, proteinases, lipoprotein lipase, and activated α_2-macroglobulin. In contrast to Th2 cell–associated cytokines, IFNγ does not affect PGE2 production and cyclooxygenase activity.

Experimental data support the hypothesis that IFNγ is antifibrogenic; this may be a consequence of cytokine therapy. Some of the most important classical cellular actions of IFNγ are summarized in Table 22-6.

Clinical Relevance

Humans with deficient IFNγ response show several immunological defects, such as increased susceptibility to infections with intracellular pathogens. Impaired IFNγ production has been demonstrated in human pathological conditions, namely chronic mucocutaneous candidiasis[320] and systemic lupus erythematosus.[206]

Increased IFNγ production is associated with food-sensitive atopic dermatitis,[482] Crohn's disease (local mucosal synthesis),[180] RA synovial tissue (suggesting a role for this cytokine in the ongoing immunological reaction of the inflamed joint),[136] and poor antibody-mediated immunity in hypovitaminosis A. IFNγ in relatively small amounts can limit Th2 cell growth and interfere with the B-cell stimulatory functions of Th2 cell cytokines.[73]

IFNγ has also been found to be associated with immunodeficiency after allogeneic bone marrow transplantation,[287] the pathophysiology of aplastic anemia,[470] and atherogenesis.[481]

Detection in carcinoma tissue of IFNγ mRNA that leads to the induction of the HLA-DR antigen on adjacent normal cells may be an indicator of a host's immune response to carcinoma. This in vivo observation might be clinically applicable to the prediction of patients' immune responsiveness to carcinomas.[350]

Therapeutic Applications

Based on a broad spectrum of activity, IFNγ is of great pharmaceutical interest with a wide variety of clinical expectancy, including antiviral, antiproliferative, and immunomodulatory effects.[279] However, the thermodynamic stability of recombinant IFNγ is low, limiting its clinical application. New research has indicated that the insertion of additional new disulfide bonds will enhance the thermodynamic stability and protect the protein against proteolytic degradation, resulting in better pharmaceutical characteristics.[203]

As a macrophage activator, IFNγ is responsible in part for the increased ability of this cell to kill intracellular pathogens and tumor cells. However, IFNγ only partly activates mononuclear phagocytes to kill tumor cells, a function that probably requires the action of second signals, such as TNF.[1] To be an important stimulus for the TNF, IL-1, and IL-6 cytokine cascade, it antagonizes the bone-resorbing effects of these cytokines, which may be important for the treatment of RA.[472] As an inhibitor of cell growth and proliferation, IFNγ has been used to treat malignancies; however, its immunotherapeutic effect gives mixed results.[152]

Some investigators believe that the most important therapeutic application of IFNγ will be to revert or maintain a Th1 preferential response basically necessary for diverse successful defense reactions (e.g., against intracellular pathogens—namely parasites and virus—and tumor cells). IFNγ has also been shown to be a suppressor of β-amyloid precursor protein promoter activity and is the first cytokine reported to possess such down regulating effects. Attenuating β-amyloid precursor protein gene expression may have relevance in diseases such as Alzheimer's disease, in which this protein has been implicated in neuropathological processes.[439]

Using retrovirus-mediated somatic gene transfer techniques to produce IFNγ from human peripheral blood CD34 hematopoietic progenitor cells, IFNγ was found to activate monocytes that may be specifically suited to cellular therapy requiring homing to sites of inflammation where their antimicrobicidal, cytotoxic, and APC functions play an important role in host defense against foreign pathogens.[4]

At least theoretically, IFNγ and also IL-12 and IL-18, either alone or in combination, have therapeutic potential for inhibiting the synthesis of IgE.[264]

Tumor Necrosis Factors

Tumor necrosis factors (TNF) are lymphokines that exist in either an α or β form; they are capable of causing in vivo hemorrhagic necrosis of certain tumor cells, but not affecting normal cells. They also have been used as experimental anticancer agents but can also induce shock when bacterial endotoxins cause their release. TNFα contains 157 amino acids and is produced by macrophages, eosinophils, and NK cells. TNFβ is a lymphotoxin and contains 171 amino acids.[138]

Synonyms

TNFα was formerly known as cachectin, cytotoxin, cytotoxic factor, differentiation-inducing factor, hemorrhagic factor, macrophage cytotoxic factor, macrophage cytotoxin, and necrosin. TNFβ was formerly known as cytotoxin, differentiation-inducing factor, and lymphotoxin (LT). Although TNFβ and LT are considered synonyms, some authors prefer the restricted equivalence of TNF to TNFα, and consider LT to be a different related cytokine.[1,71]

LTα and TNFβ have been found to be structurally similar and biologically indistinguishable. LTβ is a type II integral membrane-bound protein of 33 kDa that forms a heteromeric complex with LT on the cell surface without a known function.[71]

General Characteristics

TNFα and TNFβ are closely related proteins and may have arisen by ancestral duplication of a common gene.[472]

TNFα is expressed as a type II membrane protein attached by a signal anchor transmembrane domain and is processed intracellularly by an enzyme called ADAM-17 (a disintegrin and metalloprotease domain17; also referred to as TACE [TNF-alpha converting enzyme] and TACA [TNF-alpha converting activity]). It is synthesized as a nonglycosylated protein of approximately 25 kDa whose orientation is reversed (its amino terminus is intracellular, and its carboxy terminus is extracellular). After its synthesis, latent pro-TNFα (a 26 kDa protein) is deposited on the cell surface of monocytes and other cells. ADAM-17 cleaves pro-TNFa, releasing an active, soluble 17 kDa form. Other proteolytic functions of ADAMs include shedding of members of the family of TNF receptors and other cell-surface cytokines, adhesion molecules, and growth factors and receptors that are involved in inflammation, cell proliferation, and cell death.[474] The 17 kDa membrane fragment, including the carboxy terminus, is proteolytically cleaved by a matrix metalloproteinase from the plasma membrane of the mononuclear phagocytes and assembled into a stable 51 kDa to 52 kDa biologically active homotrimer (secreted form).[1,71,152]

Secreted TNF assumes a triangular pyramidal shape with each side of the pyramid being formed by a different monomeric subunit. This pyramidal shape is characterized by an edge-to-face association of the antiparallel sandwich structure of the wedge-shaped monomers. The receptor binding sites are at the base of the pyramid, allowing simultaneous binding to more than one receptor. The tertiary structure is very similar to the so-called "jelly roll" motif of some plant and animal virus capsids.[1,71]

TNFβ is also a homotrimer cytokine and shares approximately 30% to 35% sequence homology with TNFα. It binds to the same receptors, contains one or two N-linked oligosaccharides (accounting for the variability in molecular weights), and is a truly secretory protein with a normal signal peptide and without a membrane-spanning region.[1,71,152]

TNFβ also exists in membrane form when bound by a transmembrane protein (LTβ), resulting in a cell-surface complex that mediates the effects of TNFβ on other cells. Both proteins belong to a general family that includes CD40L, CD30L, and CD29L.[1,341]

In general, the quantities of TNFβ synthesized are much less than those of TNFα. Consequently, TNFβ is not easily detected in the circulation and is usually considered a locally acting paracrine factor and not a mediator of systemic injury. Like TNFα, it has many biological functions, from stimulation of fibroblasts and killing of tumor cells to modulation of immunoinflammatory responses. However, TNFα is a potent paracrine and endocrine mediator of immunoinflammatory reactions. It is also known to regulate growth and differentiation of a wide variety of types of cells and to be cytotoxic (especially in combination with IFNγ) for many transformed cells. In vivo it promotes necrosis of murine sarcomas.[1,71]

TNFα and TNFβ also are thought to have unique and critical roles both in the development of the immune system and in immune responses to specific pathogens.[71,472]

Other general characteristics of TNFs include:

Molecular Weight

Depending on their molecular form, the molecular weights of TNFs vary from 17 to 70 kDa. The following molecular weights have been reported for TNFα: 17 kDa,[152,341,389,421,472] 35 kDa (trimer),[436] and 52 kDa (trimer).[71] The following have been reported for TNFβ: 25 kDa,[71,341] 21 to 24 kDa (lymphotoxin),[1] 17 kDa,[421] 60 to 70 kDa (trimer),[436] 20 kDa,[472] and 24 kDa.[152]

Cross-Reactivity

The cross-reactivities (amino acid sequence homology between human and mouse) for different TNFs are TNFα (79%) and TNFβ (74%).[71] There is a significant cross-species reactivity. However, human TNF binds to the mouse p55 receptor but not to the mouse p75 receptor. Mouse TNF binds to both human receptors.

Chromosomal Location

The chromosomal location of both TNFα and TNFβ is 6p21.3. Genes lie within the class III region of the MHC. The location of TNFα, TNFβ, and LTβ within the MHC region gives the possibility that these proteins may be implicated in

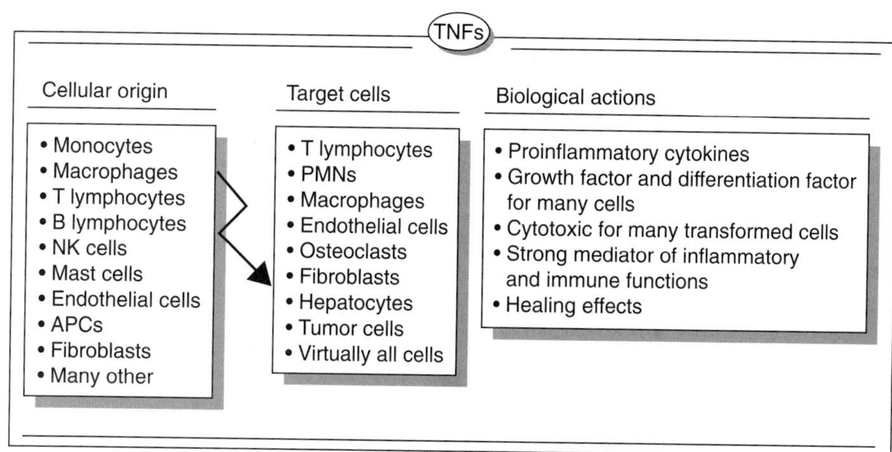

Figure 22-29 Cellular origin, principal target cells, and biological actions of TNFs.

some MHC-linked genetic effects.[341] The chromosomal locations of their receptors are 12p13 (type I receptor) and 1p36-p32 (type II receptor).

Cellular Origin

TNFα is produced primarily by activated monocytes and/or macrophages and, to a lesser extent, by many other types of cells, such as activated T cells (Th1 cells), B cells, NK cells, mast cells, endothelial cells, fibroblasts, keratinocytes, microglia, astrocytes, Kupffer's cells, smooth muscle cells, synovial lining cells, and basophils (Figure 22-29).*

Unlike TNFα, cellular sources of TNFβ are few, mostly activated T and B cells, NK cells, and astrocytes.† TNFα is produced by 0.7% to 20% of PBMCs. The primary sources of this cytokine are CD14 monocytes and/or macrophages. A significant positive correlation is found in the frequency of cells secreting IL-6, IL-10, and TNFα ex vivo, suggesting that the release of such cytokines is coordinately regulated.[205]

Control of Synthesis and Release

TNFα is released in response to bacteria (endotoxins and LPS), viruses, protozoa, cytokines (GM-CSF, IL-1, IL-2, IFNγ, and TNFα itself), immune complexes, complement component C5a, neuropeptide substance P, and reactive oxygen intermediates. Unlike TNFα, sources of preformed TNFβ have not been identified.[341,472]

Production of TNFα is inhibited by IL-10, TGFβ, cyclosporin A, PGE2, dexamethasone, ibuprofen, methylprednisolone, and pentoxifylline. Adenosine agonists inhibit TNFα production in macrophages and monocytes, but the mechanism for doing this is unknown. Nitrite exposure of LPS-stimulated alveolar macrophages resulted in a functional impairment of TNFα production. Endurance also down regulates ex vivo TNFα production.‡ An additional biological role for C3a and C3a desArg is its regulation of TNFα and IL-1β synthesis. C3a desArg may enhance cytokine synthesis by adherent monocytes at local inflammatory sites, while inhibiting the systemic synthesis of proinflammatory cytokines by circulating cells.[511]

Up regulation of TNFα production is activated by NO, reactive oxygen intermediates, nonsteroidal antiinflammatory drugs, and hypoxia.[122,196,211,537] The increased cytokine production during hypoxia may be due to decreased PGE2 synthesis. PGE1 suppresses T-cell adhesion to endothelial cells by selectively inhibiting TNFα-induced up regulation of ICAM-1 on these cells.[211,569]

The α-subunit of the heterotrimeric G protein, Gz, can regulate production of TNFα, modulating the stimulatory pathways for induction of this cytokine synthesis in mast cells.[34]

A20 (a zinc finger protein—a product of a cytokine-induced primary response gene) has been found to specifically inhibit signal transduction pathways induced by TNF and IL-1, suggesting that it functions as a negative regulator of the cytokine response.[238]

Postranscriptional regulation may be accomplished by controlling the rate of precursor mRNA splicing of TNFβ and message stability of both TNFα and TNFβ.[341]

Receptor (TNFsR)

Two different TNF receptors of 55 and 75 kDa, each encoded by a separate gene, bind both TNFα and TNFβ. Although all types of cells, including both TNF-sensitive and TNF-resistant cells, express TNFsRs (with few exceptions, such as erythrocytes and resting T cells), the type I (TNFR-1, type B, p55, CD120a) receptor is expressed on many different types of cells, and the type II (TNFR-2, type A, p75, CD120b) receptor is expressed predominantly on hematopoietic cells.[1,71,341,472] Both receptors contain four cys-rich repeats in the extracellular domain. The two receptors are members of the nerve growth factor receptor (NGFR)/TNFsR superfamily and are less than 25% identical. (They have similar homology to each other and to other members of the

*References 1, 11, 71, 152, 341, 420, 432, 472, 485.
†References 1, 152, 299, 341, 421, 432, 436, 472.
‡References 1, 3, 34, 48, 273, 427, 453, 472, 540.

superfamily.) There is also no significant homology between the intracellular domains of the two TNFαs receptors, indicating different signaling mechanisms. Receptor density ranges from 2000 to 3000 binding sites per cell, and the amount of cell lysis is proportional to the number of TNF molecules bound to susceptible cells. The affinity of TNFs for these receptors is unusually low for a cytokine (k_d of 5×10^{-10} mol for type II receptor and 1×10^{-9} mol for type I); however, TNF is synthesized in very large quantities and can easily saturate its receptors.[1,71,152] Each of these receptors has a large cytoplasmic domain and can transmit signals through the NF-κB pathway that give rise to most of the immunological effects of TNFα.

The role of TNFR-1 and TNFR-2 in mediating the capacity of TNFs to stimulate NGF production in fibroblasts has been investigated, indicating that TNFR-1 alone mediates the TNF's activity to stimulate NGF production in fibroblasts.[210] The role of the two TNFRs in discriminating TNFα and LTα (TNFβ) effects has been studied. Data suggest that LTα is less potent than TNF because of its lower ability to properly trigger the p55 TNFR and because of its lack of signaling through the p75 TNFR.[357] In addition, whereas the p75 TNFR can both directly propagate TNF signals and "pass" TNF to the p55 TNFR, it attenuates LTα and may serve as a decoy receptor for this cytokine.[356]

In general, TNFR-1 is the principal mediator of TNFα activity, with TNFR-2 serving an auxiliary role. Moreover, unlike TNFR-2, the cytoplasmic portion of TNFR-1 includes an 80–amino acid sequence known as the death domain, which is also found in the Fas protein. Receptor expression is modulated by vitamin D3, IL-1, IL-2, GM-CSF, and TNF itself.[341]

Activated cells shed their TNF receptors and soluble forms of both the human p55 and p75 receptors; they have been found in serum of cancer patients and in urine. They may act as competitive inhibitors of the cell surface receptors.[1,71,267,341] These are soluble receptors, as many cytokines and soluble cytokine receptors are generated by limited proteolysis of membrane-bound precursors. A TNFα protease inhibitor and other protease inhibitors have also been found to have the ability to modulate shedding.[374]

Signal Transduction

Receptor cross-linking by the TNF trimer is important for signal transduction. TNFs activate a sphingomyelinase, resulting in release of ceramide from sphingomyelin, which in turn activates a Mg^{2+}-dependent protein kinase. These include the three types of mitogen-activated protein kinase (extracellular signal-regulated kinase [ERK], jun amino-terminal kinase [JNK/p54], and p38) and a β-casein kinase. TNF-induced sphingomyelinase activity is secondary to the generation of DAG produced by a phosphorylcholine-specific phospholipase C (PC-PLC). Activation of phospholipase D and phospholipase A2 (PLA2) by TNFs has also been described. There is some evidence for G protein coupling of the TNFsRs to PLA2. Type I and type II receptors probably activate different cellular responses, and they may be coupled to distinct signal transduction pathways.[39,71,341,455]

Biological Actions

TNFs are mediators of both specific and nonspecific biological responses and an important link between immune and inflammatory reactions. Unfortunately, TNFs represent a two-edged sword in that severe catabolic effects (cachexia), tissue damage, and death can result from excessive uncontrolled production of these cytokines.[341,436,472,485]

TNFs were first known for their capacity to cause tumor necrosis in vitro, and they may also be the mediator of the occasional antitumor cytotoxicity observed after serious gram-negative infections. TNFα is the principal mediator of the host response to LPS of gram-negative bacteria and may play a role in multiple biological activities (antiviral, antiparasitic, lipolytic, glycogenolytic, and osteoclastic), some of them synergistically with IFNγ and IL-1.[1,152,436] TNFs also have widespread effects in inflammation and healing and are involved in granuloma formation, tissue necrosis, and fibrosis in many organ systems and, when produced in excess, vascular shock.[13,421,436]

TNFα is primarily responsible for a laboratory phenomenon known as the localized hemorrhagic "Shwartzman" reaction in which repeated injection of LPS into a solid tissue leads to hemorrhagic infarction. This occurs because LPS-induced TNFα secretion by macrophages can stimulate endothelial cells to release PGs, IL-6, and other mediators that cause coagulation, clotting, and obstruction of local blood supply.

TNFα, together with IFNγ, is also a powerful modulator of immune responses, mediating the induction of adhesion molecules, other cytokines (IL-1 and IL-6), and the activation of phagocytes. It is also a growth factor for fibroblasts and a major inducer of the acute phase response. TNFα influences the behavior of a wide variety of types of cells, and many of the activities of TNFα are shared with IL-1. In general, IL-1 is not toxic, and TNFα is a potent cytotoxic effector.

TNFβ manifests a wide range of similar parallel activities (inflammatory and antitumor immunity) affecting not only lymphocytes and neutrophils but also bone (resorption), endothelium (ability to enhance adhesion molecule expression), and neuronal cells.[341,436] However, several differences between TNFβ and TNFα are recognized, and the effect of TNFβ on endothelial cell growth is of particular interest. TNFβ appears to exert antiangiogenic effects on tumor blood vascular endothelial cells, with resulting hemorrhagic necrosis. In contrast, in wound healing, angiogenic effects such as those exerted by TNFα are thought to occur.[192,472]

The biological actions of TNFs are concentration dependent.[1] At low concentrations (approximately 1×10^{-9} mol/L), they act locally as paracrine and autocrine regulators of immunoinflammation—being rapidly released or secreted at sites of injury or infection. TNFα primes both neutrophils and endothelial cells for adhesion and directs further the migration of leukocytes via chemotactic effects. TNFα-mediated proliferation of fibroblasts and endothelial cells is an important element of wound healing. In many of these activities, the effects of TNFα are amplified by IL-1, which acts synergistically with TNFα.[1,432,472] At high concentrations, TNFs (namely TNFα) act as an endocrine hormone with notorious systemic effects.

At low concentrations, the principal biological actions of TNFs locally include[1,152,432]:

1. Expression of adhesion molecules on endothelial cells (accumulation of leukocytes at local sites of inflammation, which is probably the physiologically most important local effect of TNFs)
2. Activation of inflammatory leukocytes to fight against microorganisms or tumor cells (especially potent for neutrophils, but also for eosinophils and mononuclear phagocytes)
3. Stimulation of cytokine synthesis (IL-1, IL-6, TNFα itself, CKs) by mononuclear phagocytes and other types of cells
4. Interferon-like protective effect against viruses

These effects of TNFs are critical for inflammatory responses to microbes and tumors. If inadequate quantities of TNFs are present, an organism may fail to suppress the infection. TNFβ is especially considered as a paracrine-type factor. It is cytostatic and cytotoxic for some tumor cell lines and causes necrosis of certain tumors in vivo. TNFβ also influences the function of B cells, T cells, connective tissue cells, and hematopoietic cells.

At moderate concentrations, TNFα enters the blood stream where it can act as an endocrine factor. The principal systemic actions of TNFs include[1,152]:

1. Acting as an endogenous pyrogen (shared with IL-1) and mediated by increased synthesis of PGs
2. Stimulation of secretion by mononuclear phagocytes and endothelial cells of IL-1 and IL-6 into the circulation
3. Increased synthesis of APPs by liver cells together with IL-1 and IL-6 (the spectrum of hepatocyte proteins induced by TNF is identical to that induced by IL-1 but differs from that induced by IL-6: IL-6 → fibrinogen, IL-1/TNF → serum amyloid protein)
4. Activation of the coagulation system
5. Suppression of bone marrow stem cell division
6. Cachexia, produced largely by TNF-induced appetite suppression; with IL-1, may also contribute to the cachectic state accompanying certain chronic diseases, such as tuberculosis and cancer

Because of activities similar to IL-1, TNFα is also considered an inflammatory cytokine. T-cell–derived IFNγ induces LPS-activated macrophages to make more TNFα. In fact, IFNγ enhances many of the effects of TNFα.

High quantities of TNFs are produced during gram-negative bacterial sepsis (serum concentration can exceed 10^{-7} mol/L), being a critical mediator in the complex cytokine network of septic shock (Figure 22-30). Several specific actions of TNFs may contribute to their lethal effects at extremely high concentrations[1]:

1. Reduction of tissue perfusion by depressing myocardial contractility (induction of nitric oxide synthase, producing NO, which inhibits myocardial contractility)
2. Reduction of blood pressure and tissue perfusion by relaxing vascular smooth muscle tone
3. Intravascular thrombosis (combination of endothelial and mononuclear phagocyte alterations, which promote coagulation, and activation of neutrophils—disseminated intravascular coagulation)
4. Severe metabolic disturbances, such as fall in blood glucose concentrations to levels that are incompatible with life

Many of the biological actions of TNF are augmented by IFNγ as previously mentioned (in some cells explained by IFNγ-stimulated increases in TNF receptor numbers). The

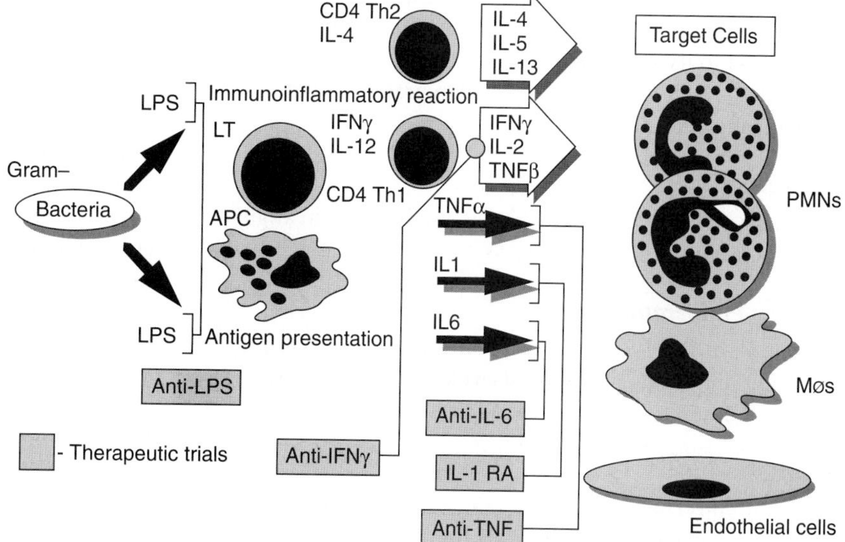

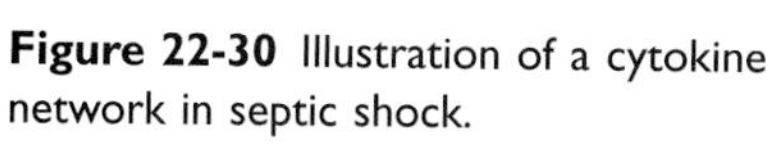
Figure 22-30 Illustration of a cytokine network in septic shock.

full significance of this interaction is not clear, but activated T cells often secrete TNF and IFNγ coordinately. Coordinate secretion of these two cytokines may provide a means of locally enhancing the actions of TNF without requiring concentrations that produce systemic toxicity.[225,351]

In addition, TNFs also have a number of other effects including (1) apoptosis, (2) adhesion and cellular trafficking, (3) angiogenesis, (4) myocyte proliferation, (5) fibrosis, (6) phagocytosis, (7) cytokine production and/or cellular activation, (8) leukocyte/macrophages function, (9) inflammation, and (10) tumor control.

Apoptosis

TNFα can induce apoptosis in many normal and transformed types of cells.[239] For example, activation of TNF receptors by TNFα or other members of the TNF superfamily causes an aggregation of receptors, which leads to the recruitment of various adaptor proteins that activate downstream kinases and proteases, including caspases. Mitochondria are important targets for TNF-initiated death signals. The subsequent release from mitochondria of reactive oxygen species, such as superoxide anion and cytochrome *c* oxidase and other factors that induce apoptosis, plays a pivotal part in TNF-induced cell death.[529]

TNFα and IL-1α also induce mannose receptors and apoptosis in glomerular mesangial but not in endothelial cells.[326] TNFα does not induce necrosis or apoptosis in EBV-positive or EBV-negative cell lines, regardless of the culture conditions of the cells or the presence or absence of cytokines.[408]

Adhesion and Cellular Trafficking

TNFα and IFNγ collectively and synergistically promote the inhibition of PECAM-1 (CD31) synthesis and leukocyte transmigration in endothelial cells, and human ICAM-1 expression can be up regulated by IFNγ or TNFα. Regulation of PECAM-1 expression on endothelial cells may modulate leukocyte trafficking, angiogenesis, and vascular permeability.[241,440,497] TNFα and IL-1 stimulate endothelial cell expression of CD54 (ICAM-1) and CD106 (VCAM-1). In addition to its ability to activate endothelial cell adhesion molecules, TNFα can induce directed migration of lymphocytes through collagen pads.[119,250]

Angiogenesis

TNFα is a pleiotropic cytokine that is also involved in angiogenesis and immunoregulation.[294]

Myocyte Proliferation

Activation of the TNFα p55 receptor induces myocyte proliferation and modulates agonist-evoked calcium transients in cultured human tracheal smooth muscle cells.[9]

Fibrosis

TNFα inhibits collagen synthesis and at high concentrations stimulates collagenase synthesis in fibroblasts.[553] Moreover, TNFα inhibits adherence and phagocytosis of collagen. These effects are mediated by a reduction in the strength of α2β1 integrin binding to collagen, possibly through tyrosine kinases in focal adhesions. At low concentrations of TNFα (10 ng/mL) that are found in the periphery of chronic inflammatory lesions, it has been suggested that inhibition of the collagen phagocytic pathway may contribute to fibrosis.[87]

Phagocytosis

Experimental data suggest that upregulation of complement receptor (CR3) and CR3-mediated phagocytosis are mechanisms by which TNFα and IFNγ stimulate nonphagocytic, nonbactericidal macrophage precursors to kill intracellular bacterial pathogens.[144]

Cytokine Production/Cellular Activation

TNFα and IFNγ mediate the induction of other cytokines (IL-1 and IL-6) and the activation of phagocytes.[472] It has been suggested that particle-induced expression of MIP-2 and cytokine-induced neutrophil chemoattractant CKs in the rat lung are mediated at least in part by production of TNFα.[145] TNF is involved in control of monocyte-mediated regulation of cytokine production by T cells. Preincubation of monocytes with rTNF enhanced their ability to induce IFNγ production, and TNF synthesis inhibitors decreased this induction. However, Th2 cells are stimulated in the relative absence of monocyte co-stimulatory signal(s), probably IL-6.[301] Concerning pain responsivity, TNFα produces dose-dependent hyperalgesia mediated via the induced release of IL-1β.[565]

Leukocytes/Macrophages Function

TNFα renders human neutrophils responsive to PF-4, a member of the CK superfamily. Over a broad range of concentrations, PF-4 by itself is unable to induce functional changes in PMN. However, neutrophils preincubated or coincubated with physiologically relevant concentrations of TNFα responded to PF-4 by the selective mobilization of the secondary granule marker lactoferrin but not of the primary granule marker elastase.[419] Stimulation of macrophages with IFNγ or TNFα shuts off the suppressive effect played by PGE2, which can explain how macrophage tumoricidal activity may be induced and maintained even in the presence of higher levels of PGE2.[598] The regulation of CD4 expression on macrophages and its role in immune cell interactions remain obscure. Experimental results show that LPS, TNFα, and IL-1β selectively down regulate CD4 expression in primary human macrophages and that decreased CD4 expression induced by LPS results from endogenous secretion of TNFα and IL-1β from the macrophages.[213]

Inflammation

TNF-stimulated gene 6 (TSG-6), encoding a 35 kDa secretory glycoprotein (TSG-6), is induced in fibroblasts, chondrocytes, synovial cells, and mononuclear cells by the proinflammatory cytokines TNFα and IL-1. TSG-6 protein forms a stable complex with components of the serine protease inhibitor inter-α-inhibitor. The antiinflammatory effect of the TNF/IL-1–inducible TSG-6 protein, along with its ability to inhibit protease action (especially plasmin activity), suggests that TSG-6 production during inflammation is part of a negative feedback loop operating through the protease network.[458] IL-10 and IL-4 synergize with TNFα to induce IL-1RA production by human neutrophils and to favor an antiinflammatory condition.[345]

Tumor Control

The antitumor effects of TNFα are based on several distinct activities, including (1) direct cytotoxic effect on tumor cells but not on normal cells, (2) modification of the vasculature in such a manner that migration of lymphocytes into tumors is enhanced, and (3) stimulation of the immune response by activating cells that mediate antitumor immunity.[472]

Clinical Relevance

TNFs have been found to have clinical relevance in the disorders discussed below.

Infection/Septic Shock

TNFα is classically associated with septic shock and diverse infectious pathological conditions. It is involved in the development of a protective immune response in tuberculosis.[341] Measurable serum TNFα levels have been detected in 10.5% of children with pulmonary tuberculosis, all of whom belonged to the group with active disease.[28] Results suggest a protective role for TNFα in respiratory syncytial virus infection.[388] In patients with chronic hepatitis C during treatment with IFNα, elevated production of TNFα by PBMCs may be due to host response to the virus.[278] In HIV infection, TNFs and IL-6 stimulate viral replication.[15,436]

Autoimmune Diseases

TNFβ is considered to be an important mediator in a number of T-lymphocyte–mediated autoimmune diseases, such as type 1 diabetes.[472] Also, TNFs seem to play a pivotal role in certain autoimmune diseases, such as in the pathogenesis of RA, because transgenic mice constitutively overexpress TNF inflammatory arthritis but no systemic lupus erythematosus–like lesions. These findings in animals and humans suggest that the ambient level of TNF might have a hitherto underappreciated capacity to control the form in which autoimmunity is expressed as a specific syndrome or disease.[171]

Inflammatory/Allergic Diseases

TNFα is released by many inflammatory cells, including mast cells and eosinophils, and promotes mediator and cytokine secretion, adhesion molecule expression, and granulocyte migration. Consequently, TNFα is considered an important effector molecule and a pivotal mediator[57] in the pathogenesis of allergic respiratory reactions and in the acute stages of RA, being implicated in the cartilage damage.[76,88,286] Soluble receptors for TNF (sTNFR) are present at elevated concentrations in the synovial fluid of patients with RA. They are presumably released by cells of the synovial membrane, including the monocyte-derived synovial macrophages. Cytokines from the synovium, including IL-1 and TNFα, may stimulate sTNFR release. These observations help to explain why elevated levels of sTNFR in synovial fluid coexist with enhanced expression of cell-surface TNFR on synovial macrophages in RA.[52,247] DNA profiles (immunoprints) have been generated for patients suffering from early-onset pauciarticular chronic arthritis. The TNFα allele is not found in linkage disequilibrium with HLA-DRB1 and may be present on either chromosome 6. Thus a novel susceptibility factor probably within the TNFα/TNFβ gene region has been identified via linkage with the TNFα microsatellite allele.[156] Excessive synthesis and release of proinflammatory cytokines following trauma have been correlated with poor outcome in injured patients. TNFα appears to play a pivotal role as a trigger for the induction of systemic inflammation. Two naturally occurring inhibitors of TNFα, sTNFRs p55 and p75, have been characterized. Injured patients revealed increased plasma levels of both sTNFRs compared with healthy volunteers. Patients with severe injury revealed higher levels of sTNFRs on the day of admission than patients with minor trauma.[267]

Endometriosis

TNFα concentrations have been reported higher in the peritoneal fluid of women with endometriosis than in the peritoneal fluid of those without.[294] The mean concentration of IL-1β and TNFα has been found to be much higher in macrophage-conditioned media of patients with endometriosis without significant changes in peritoneal fluid.[269]

Cerebral Ischemia

Early increases in TNFα, IL-6, and IL-1β levels following transient cerebral ischemia suggest that regionally selective increases in cytokines may be involved in the pathophysiological changes in the hippocampus and striatum following transient cerebral ischemia.[452]

Acute Pancreatitis

As with sepsis, there is evidence that TNFα in particular may play a central role in acute pancreatitis and mediate the systemic sequelae of the disease. Analytical data have provided evidence that TNFα is a major contributor to the morbidity and mortality from acute pancreatitis.[227]

Nephropathies

Plasma levels of cytokines were measured in subjects hospitalized with nephropathia epidemica. Concentrations of TNFα, IL-6, and IL-10 were increased in all of these patients at admission. TNFα concentrations were still increased 1 week after onset of disease; levels of IL-6 and IL-10 normalized. Serum levels of the two soluble TNF receptors p55 and p75 correlated with levels of the cytokine, indicating that receptor binding may be the reason for lack of bioactivity in vitro.[323]

Neurological Disorders

Two cytokines, TNFα and IFNγ, are involved in the progression of neurological disorders, such as multiple sclerosis and AIDS dementia complex, with an emphasis on cytokine effects on glial cells.[38]

Alcoholic Liver Disease

Increased serum and/or tissue TNF levels have been observed in alcoholic liver disease (see Chapter 47), and TNF has been postulated to play a role in ethanol-induced liver injury. It appears that both TNF and ethanol are capable of increasing manganese superoxide dismutase activity, presumably via enhanced oxidative stress.[417]

Transplant Rejection

TNFα has been implicated in the pathogenesis of both acute and chronic transplant rejection. Levels of this cytokine are known to vary in a normal population, leading to speculation that high responders may be at greater risk of rejection. Particular TNF region polymorphic markers have been associated with increased TNFα levels and a biallelic polymorphism has been identified in the TNFα promoter, which may contribute significantly to the interindividual variation in healthy persons. There is evidence for a new association between a polymorphic locus in the TNF gene region and increased production of TNFα in heart transplant recipients. No association was demonstrated for the promoter region polymorphism.[541]

Therapeutic Applications

Clinical trials have revealed that diseases that are related directly to excessive TNF production, such as septic shock, GVHD, and lupus nephritis, may be amenable to treatment either with anti-TNFα antibodies or with antiinflammatory agents that reduce TNF production, such as cyclosporin A and steroids.[343,472]

Neutralizing TNF in patients with RA by means of soluble TNF receptors or anti-TNF monoclonal antibodies has proven to be a powerful means of controlling disease activity. For example, the combination of neutralizing TNF with methotrexate has been found to improve the symptoms and signs of inflammation, physical function, and the quality of life and prevents radiographic evidence of progressive joint damage in a majority of patients with RA who have no response to methotrexate alone. Studies are in progress to obtain additional information regarding long-term safety of TNF blockade and its effects on disease progression as it was already evaluated with Crohn's disease.*

Infection/Septic Shock

A recombinant, soluble fusion protein that is a dimer of an extracellular portion of the human TNF receptor and the Fc portion of IgG1 (TNFR:Fc) binds and neutralizes TNFα and prevents death in animal models of bacteremia and endotoxemia. In patients with septic shock, treatment with the TNFR:Fc fusion protein does not reduce mortality, and higher doses appear to be associated with increased mortality.[166]

Inflammatory Diseases/Trauma

Anti-TNF therapies may have potential use in inflammatory arthritis. A review study of cytokine expression and regulation in rheumatoid joints has culminated in demonstrating that TNFα blockade markedly ameliorates arthritis. This defines an important therapeutic target for RA.[162] Experimental investigations have shown that a decrease in TNFα level or the inhibition of its activity is accompanied by reduced brain damage, affecting the development of cerebral edema and neurological dysfunction and hippocampal cell loss after closed head injury. These findings emphasize the role that TNFα plays in the inflammatory response following trauma.[483]

Tumors

TNFα has been shown to have limited success in the chemotherapy of some tumors, including melanomas (alone, or in combination with IFNγ), and it does not appear very promising for the treatment of human cancer. This is thought to be because of the observation that its toxicity in vivo precludes the administration of sufficient doses required to obtain blood levels high enough to cause cell death.[341,485] TNFα is one of the cytokines administered in immunotherapy of advanced neoplastic disease. Its action is exerted through immune endocrine and central nervous systems, and it might be possible that some side effects of human recombinant TNFα administration are connected with the decreasing cortisol level.[602] Because TNFα induces changes in integrin expression and adhesive properties, it can regulate adhesive mechanisms of tumor cells bearing adequate receptors, thus influencing lung-metastasis formation.[215]

CHEMOKINES

Chemokines (CKs) are a group of low molecular weight cytokines that are identified on the basis of their ability to induce chemotaxis or chemokinesis in leukocytes (or in particular populations of leukocytes); in inflammation, the group is now divided into four subgroups on the basis of genetic, structural, and functional criteria. They function as regulators of the immune system and may also play roles in the circulatory and central nervous systems.[138]

CKs were discovered in the late 1980s as a result of advancements made in molecular biological techniques used to identify proteins. More than 50 have been identified but

*References 18, 24, 171, 266, 314, 325, 505, 529, 593.

their biological functions are not always known.[461] They are, however, thought to play key roles in the processes of inflammation and leukocyte migration, lymphocyte trafficking, and immune activation that precedes the wound healing process.[304,372,583]

General Characteristics

Chemokines is a condensation of the term "chemoattractant cytokines." Former names include (1) intercrines, (2) PF-4 superfamily of cytokines, or (3) SIS cytokines. CKs are now defined as a superfamily of low molecular weight proteins (8 to 10 kDa), regulating the motility and orientation of leukocytes. They are (1) proinflammatory mediators, (2) potent immunomodulators (lymphocyte activation and diversification), (3) biological modifiers of erythrocyte function, and (4) angiogenic factors. Their functional role indicates that CKs play a very important function as pathogenic mediators in several pathological conditions, including asthma, allergic diseases, infection, cancer, RA, sarcoidosis, pulmonary fibrosis, and atherosclerosis. In addition, they may also serve as targets for molecular mimicry in microbial invasion.

Classification

CKs are grouped into a CK superfamily that is further divided into four families (CXC, CC, C, and CX_3C) according to their amino acid sequence around one conserved motif that includes four cysteines (Box 22-6).* These four families also correlate with separate gene clusters (in humans, the CXC family is located on chromosome 4q12-21, the CC on 17q11-32, C on 1, and CX_3C on 16q13). The classical members of these families are summarized in Table 22-7. The respective acronyms, main function, and new nomenclature are listed in Table 22-8 and Figure 22-31. Despite the large size of this superfamily, there are elements (like the NAP-4 and P500) that are not easily integrable inside the previously described families, because they lack some cysteines in the classical four-cysteine conformation.

As indicated in Table 22-8, most of CXC CKs are attractants for PMNs (neutrophils, eosinophils, and basophils) but not for monocytes. Most of the ELR-CXC molecules are potent neutrophil chemoattractants and share the CXC CK

*References 1, 228, 293, 304, 372, 436, 461, 485, 542, 583.

BOX 22-6 Chemokine Families

CXC (also known as α family): Contains one amino acid (X) between the first two cysteines
- CXC subfamilies (according to the sequence of amino terminal region)
- ELR-CXC (glutamic acid-leucine-arginine-cysteine-amino acid X-cysteine)
- No ELR preceding CXC

CC (also called β family): Absence of one amino acid between the first two cysteines

C (also called γ family): Lack of the first and third cysteines (one instead of two cysteines in their N-terminus)

CX_3C (also called δ family): Novel arrangement of cysteine residues (CysXaaXaaXaaCys), followed by an extended mucinlike stalk, a transmembrane domain, and an intracellular domain

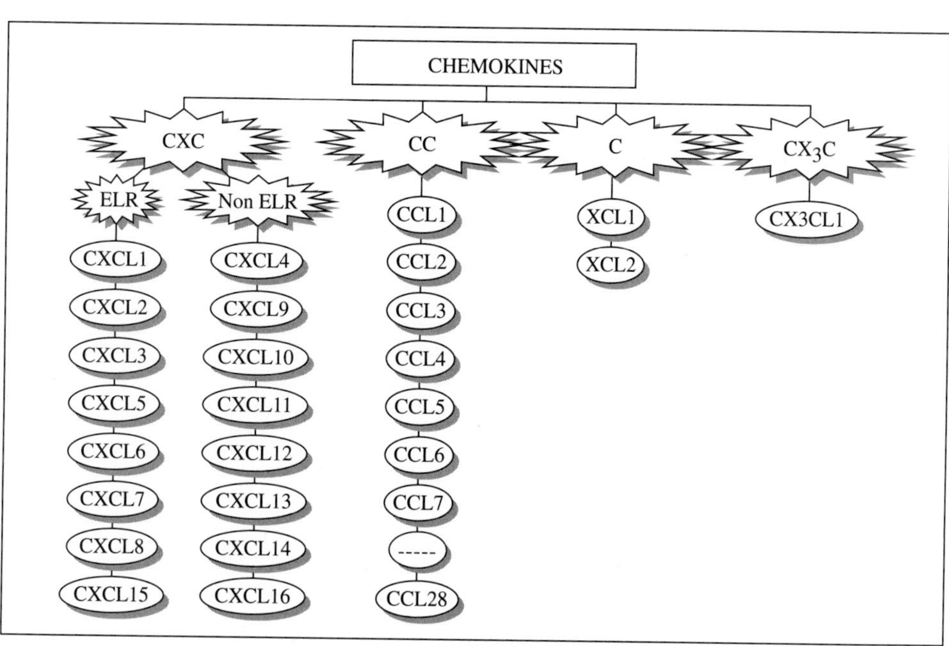

Figure 22-31 Chemokine families (see Box 22-6 for definitions).

TABLE 22-7 Classical Members of Chemokine Families*

Chemokine	Cellular Origin	Cellular Targets	Cellular Receptors
CXC Family: ELR Group			
ENA-78 (CXCL5)	Epithelial lung cells Endothelial cells Fibroblast ECRF3 Platelets	Neutrophils	CXCR2
GCP-2 (CXCL6)	Osteosarcoma cells Kidney tumors	Granulocytes Neutrophils	CXCR1, CXCR2
GROα/MGSA (CXCL1 GROβ CXCL2 GROγ CXCL3)	Monocytes/macrophages Melanoma cells Epithelial cells Endothelial cells	Neutrophils Lymphocytes Monocytes Melanoma cells	CXCR, CXCR2 IL-8RA DARC ECRF3
IL-8 (CXCL8)	Many cells Monocytes/macrophages Lymphocytes Epithelial cells Fibroblasts	Neutrophils Basophils Eosinophils T lymphocytes B lymphocytes	CXCR1, CXCR2
NAP-2 (CXCL7)	Platelets	Neutrophils Basophils Eosinophils Fibroblasts NK cells	CXCR2
SDF-1 (CXCL12)	Stromal cells Bone marrow Liver	T cells/monocytes Pre-B cells	CXCR4
CXC Family: NonELR Group			
MIG (CXCL9)	Macrophages IFNγ-activated monocytes	TIL Monocytes	CXCR3
IP-10 (CXCL10)	Monocytes Fibroblasts Endothelial cells Keratinocytes	Monocytes Endothelial cells NK cells T lymphocytes	CXCR3
PF-4 (CXCL4)	Platelets Megakaryocytes	Fibroblasts Platelets Mast cells Basophils Endothelial cells Megakaryocytes	
CC Family			
Eotaxin (CCL11)	Endothelial cells Macrophages Lung cells Intestinal cells	Eosinophils	CCR3

TABLE 22-7 Classical Members of Chemokine Families*—Continued

Chemokine	Cellular Origin	Cellular Targets	Cellular Receptors
CC Family—Cont'd			
I-309 (CCL1)	T lymphocytes Mast cells	Monocytes/macrophages Neutrophils/basophils Microglial cells	CCR8
MCP-1 (CCL2)	Many cells Monocytes/macrophages Lymphocytes Endothelial cells Epithelial cells	Monocytes T lymphocytes Basophils/eosinophils NK cells Many cells	CCR2
MCP-2 (CCL8)	Monocytes/macrophages Fibroblasts Osteosarcoma cells	T lymphocytes Monocytes Basophils/eosinophils NK cells	CCR3, CCR5
MCP-3 (CCL7)	Fibroblasts Platelets Osteosarcoma cells Monocytes/mast cells	Monocytes/neutrophils T lymphocytes Basophils/eosinophils NK cells	CCR1, CCR2, CCR3
MIP-1α (CCL3)	Many cells T and B lymphocytes Monocytes/macrophages Neutrophils/eosinophils Langerhans' cells Astrocytes	T lymphocytes Monocytes/neutrophils Basophils/eosinophils NK cells Myeloid stem cells Keratinocytes	CCR1, CCR5
MIP-1β (CCL4)	Monocytes/macrophages T and B lymphocytes Fibroblasts	Monocytes T lymphocytes Basophils	CCR5
RANTES (CCL5)	T lymphocytes Monocytes Fibroblasts Platelets Endothelial cells Epithelial cells	Monocytes T lymphocytes Neutrophils Basophils/eosinophils NK cells Mast cells	CCR1, CCR3, CCR5
HCC-1 (CCL14)	Liver cells Spleen cells Bone marrow cells	Monocytes CD34 myeloid cells	CCR1, CCR5
C Family			
SCM-1α (XCL1)	T lymphocytes Thymocytes	T lymphocytes	Specific XCR1
SCM-1β (XCL2)	T lymphocytes Spleen cells		XCR1
CX_3C Family			
Fractalkine (CX_3CL1)	Endothelial cells Many cells	Leukocytes Many cells	CX_3CR1

*References 3, 140, 271, 280, 376, 428, 461, 466, 526, 545, 558.

TABLE 22-8 New Nomenclature and Principal Acronyms of Chemokines[140,372]

New Name	Original Name	Receptors	Function
CXC Chemokines			
CXCL1	GROα	CXCR2, CXCR	Inflammatory
CXCL2	GROβ	CXCR2	Inflammatory
CXCL3	GROγ	CXCR2	Inflammatory
CXCL4	PF-4	Unknown	
CXCL5	ENA-78	CXCR2	Inflammatory
CXCL6	GCP-2	CXCR1, CXCR2	Inflammatory
CXCL7	NAP-2	CXCR2	Inflammatory
CXCL8	IL-8	CXCR1, CXCR2	Inflammatory
CXCL9	MIG	CXCR3	Dual function
CXCL10	IP-10	CXCR3	Dual function
CXCL11	I-TAC	CXCR3	Dual function
CXCL12	SDF-1 a/b	CXCR4	Homeostatic
CXCL13	BCA-1	CXCR5	Homeostatic
CXCL14	BRAK	Unknown	
CXCL16	—	CXCR6	Dual function
CC Chemokines			
CCL1	I-309	CCR8	Dual function
CCL2	MCP-1	CCR2	Inflammatory
CCL3	MIP-1α	CCR1, CCR5	Inflammatory
CCL3L1	LD78β	CCR1, CCR5	
CCL4	MIP-1β	CCR5	Inflammatory
CCL5	RANTES	CCR1, CCR3, CCR5	Inflammatory
CCL6	Unknown	Unknown	
CCL7	MCP-3	CCR1, CCR2, CCR3	Inflammatory
CCL8	MCP-2	CCR3, CCR5	Inflammatory
CCL9/CCL10	Unknown	CCR1	
CCL11	Eotaxin	CCR3	Inflammatory
CCL12	Unknown	CCR2	
CCL13	MCP-4	CCR2, CCR3	Inflammatory
CCL14	HCC-1	CCR1, CCR5	Inflammatory
CCL15	HCC-2/Lkn-1/MIP-1β	CCR1, CCR	Inflammatory
CCL16	HCC-4/LEC/LCC-1	CCR1, CCR2	
CCL17	TARC	CCR4	Dual function
CCL18	DC-CK1	Unknown	Homeostatic
CCL19	MIP-3β/ELC	CCR7	Homeostatic
CCL20	MIP-3α/LARC	CCR6	Dual function
CCL21	6Ckine/SLC	CCR7	Homeostatic
CCL22	MDC	CCR4	Dual function
CCL23	MPIF-1/CKb8	CCR1	
CCL24	Eotaxin-2	CCR3	Inflammatory
CCL25	TECK	CCR9	Dual function
CCL26	Eotaxin-3	CCR3	Inflammatory
CCL27	CTACK	CCR10	Inflammatory
CCL28	MEC	CCR3, CCR10	Inflammatory

TABLE 22-8 New Nomenclature and Principal Acronyms of Chemokines[140,372]—Continued

New Name	Original Name	Receptors	Function
C Chemokines			
XCL1	Lymphotactin/SCM-1α	XCR1	Inflammatory
XCL2	SCM-1β	XCR1	
CX3C Chemokines			
CX3CL1	Fractalkine	CX3CR1	Inflammatory

BCA-1, B-cell–attracting chemokine 1; *CTACK,* cutaneous T-cell–attracting chemokine; *DC-CK1,* dendritic cell–derived CC chemokine 1; *ELC,* EBL-1-ligand chemokine; *ENA-78,* epithelial cell–derived neutrophil attractant 78; *GCP,* granulocyte chemotactic protein; *GRO,* growth-related oncogene; *HCC,* hemofiltrate CC chemokine; *IL,* interleukin; *IP-10,* interferon-inducible protein 10; *I-TAC,* interferon-inducible T-cell alpha chemoattractant; *LARC,* liver- and activation-regulated chemokine; *LCC-1,* liver-specific CC chemokine-1; *LEC,* liver-expressed chemokine; *Lkn-1,* leukotactin; *MCP,* monocyte chemoattractant protein; *MDC,* macrophage-derived chemokine; *MEC,* mammary-enriched chemokine; *MIG,* monokine induced by interferon γ; *MIP,* macrophage inflammatory protein; *MPIF,* myeloid progenitor inhibitory factor; *NAP,* neutrophil activating peptide; *PF-4,* platelet factor 4; *RANTES,* "regulated on activation, normally T-cell expressed and secreted"; *SCM-1α/β,* single C motif-1 α/β; *SDF,* stromal cell–derived factor; *SLC,* secondary lymphoid tissue chemokine; *TARC,* thymus- and activation-regulated chemokine; *TECK,* thymus-expressed chemokine.

receptor. In contrast, those without the ELR motif show different chemotactic functional capacities and do not seem to link themselves to the same receptor. CC CKs attract mononuclear cells (monocytes and lymphocytes) but not neutrophils. C CKs attract specific kinds of leukocytes (lymphocytes) but not neutrophils and monocytes. Exceptions to these general rules include CXC CKs IL-8, IP-10, and melanoma growth stimulatory protein (MGSA), which are chemotactic to T cells, and CC CKs MCP-1, MCP-3, RANTES gene, and MIP-1α, which are chemotactic to basophils.[461,545]

Functionally, CKs are categorized as "homeostatic" or "inflammatory." Homeostatic CKs are produced and secreted constitutively and are generally involved in lymphocyte trafficking and immune surveillance. Inflammatory CKs are only produced by cells during infection or following a proinflammatory stimulus; they prompt the migration of leukocytes to an injured or infected site and can also activate cells to raise an immune response.[304,583]

In general, the CKs are remarkably diverse, in terms of both individual proteins and their production by blood and tissue cells, and some cannot be assigned unambiguously to either one of the two functional categories. These are referred to as "dual-function" CKs and generally participate in immune defense functions, such as those that are up regulated under inflammatory conditions and target noneffector leukocytes, including precursor and resting mature leukocytes, at sites of leukocyte development and immune surveillance. Many dual-function CKs are highly selective for lymphocytes and have a role in T-cell development in the thymus and in T-cell recruitment to inflammatory sites. In contrast to homeostatic and dual-function CKs, inflammatory CKs have broad receptor selectivities.[372]

Molecular Structure

The three-dimensional structures have been elucidated for many CXC and CC CKs. As expected from the high degree of sequence identity of these molecules, the structures of all the monomers are very similar. However, the quaternary structures of the CXC and CC CKs are distinct and the dimer interface is formed by a totally different group of residues. The three-dimensional conformation is globular for IL-8 (CXC CK) and elongated and cylindrical for MIP-1β (CC CK). PF-4 (a CXC CK) is a tetramer composed of a dimer of IL-8–type dimers. The differences in the quaternary structure provide an explanation for the lack of receptor cross-binding between CXC and CC CKs.[545] However, although dimerization and aggregation is often observed, the CKs function as monomers, and the critical receptor-binding regions are in the NH2-terminal 20 residues of the protein.[91,195]

Biological Function

CKs have many important biological functions, several of which are summarized below.

Inflammation

Chemoattractant properties are the major biological effect of CKs. Their receptors are G protein–coupled receptors that form a family of structurally and functionally related proteins. CKs are induced in cells and tissue in response to proinflammatory cytokines. They are produced by a large diversity of cells (Figure 22-32). The CK superfamily, with the exception of RANTES, β-TG, HCC-1, and PF-4, is not expressed in resting cells but is rapidly induced in response to various inflammatory and mitogenic stimuli. Probably all CKs have some activities that are unique and many that are

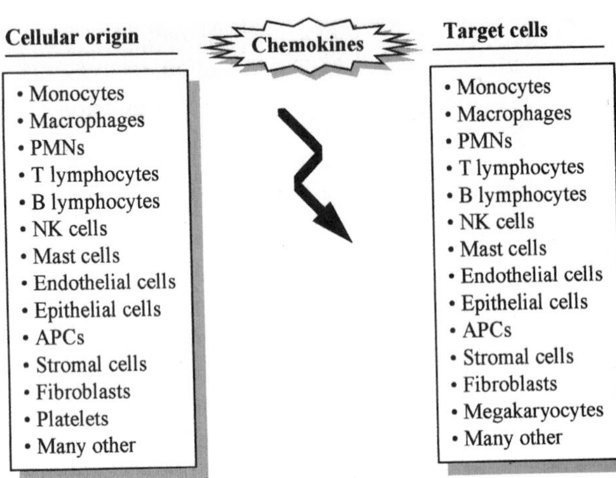

Figure 22-32 Cellular origin and principal target cells of chemokines.

overlapping that include (1) cellular migration, (2) calcium mobilization, (3) cellular adhesion, and (4) signal transduction. In addition, CKs are implicated as major participants in (1) acute and chronic inflammatory reactions, (2) inhibition of hematopoiesis, (3) modulation of angiogenesis, and (4) fibroplasia. They act on T lymphocytes, presumably influencing the recruitment of immunocompetent cells to immunoinflammatory sites. Although there is no evidence that CKs play a role in the induction of immune reactions, they promote the effector limb of immunity. CKs may also contribute to the normal homing and distribution of leukocytes. Although CKs obviously have major differentiative effects on the functions of target cells, the possibility that they act as co-stimulants of cell growth is also being studied. Finally, CKs are attractive targets for the development of new therapeutic agents. For example, inhibition of their activities may be an effective antiinflammatory strategy; promoting their activity might enhance wound healing and tissue repair.[519,572]

Chemokines in Leukocyte Trafficking

CKs are thought to be centrally involved in leukocyte trafficking and not limited to attraction of monocytes by the CC family and neutrophils by the CXC family.[399] Other functions of the CKs include expression of adhesion molecules, especially for the lymphocytes in both the migratory response and maturation and proliferation.[461] The selective chemoattractant qualities shown by CKs explain the directed migration of each kind of leukocyte or even of subtypes of these cells (as T and B lymphocytes, perhaps even Th1 and Th2). Several studies have shown that CC CKs attract T lymphocytes and that CD45R0, memory-phenotype cells are considered to be the main responders. The results, however, have often been contradictory, and the role of lymphocyte activation and proliferation is still unclear. The CC CKs MCP-2, MCP-3, RANTES, MIP-1α, MIP-1β, and MCP-1 induce significant, dose-dependent transendothelial chemotaxis of CD3 T lymphocytes. In contrast, the CXC CKs IL-8 and IP-10 fail to induce transendothelial chemotaxis of CD3 T lymphocytes or T-lymphocyte subsets. RANTES, MIP-1α, and MIP-1β induce significant transendothelial chemotaxis of CD4, CD8, and CD45R0 T-lymphocyte subsets. Phenotyping of mononuclear cells that underwent transendothelial migration to MCP-2, MCP-3, RANTES, or MIP-1α shows both monocytes and activated (CD26 high) memory-type (CD45R0) T cells. Both CD4 and CD8 T lymphocytes were recruited but not NK cells or many B cells. In fact, MCP-2 was the only CC CK tested that attracted a substancial number of naive type (CD45RA) T lymphocytes. In the absence of endothelium, IL-8 but not IP-10 promoted modest but significant chemotaxis of CD3 T cells.[329,447]

CKs also play a role in leukocyte trafficking during ovarian function. For example, CKs are expressed and leukocytes accumulate within the ovulatory follicle and the corpus luteum. Hormonal and embryonic regulation of CKs are thought to be responsible.[137,532]

For CKs to act in vivo, they require a solid phase in which normal conditions of blood flow would be unable to wash away the chemoattractant gradient. In this manner, CKs secreted by each cell trafficking through a vessel are sequestered and maintained by stable components of the extracellular matrix, such as proteoglycans.[461] This model of CK action in leukocyte migration is summarized in Figure 22-33.

Hematopoietic Function

Several CKs have marked activity in hematopoietic precursor cell cycling regulation and differentiation, MSGA/GRO acts as a growth factor, and IL-8 is a potent angiogenic factor (possibly shared by other ELR-CXC CKs). Although this pro-hematopoietic capacity is important, some are suppressive (such as IP-10 and MIP-1α), inhibiting the action of growth factors in hematopoietic cells.[16] However, PF-4 presents the most fascinating spectrum of biological activities, including inhibition of tumor growth, megakaryopoiesis, reversal of immunosuppression, and bactericidal capacity. Curiously, MIP-1α and MIP-1β, despite their structural similarities, show diverging signaling capacities. Depending on the MIP-1 subtype and its NH2-terminal processing, one or more of the CC CK receptors CCR1, CCR2, CCR3, and CCR5 are recognized.[142] Since both human MIP-1α subtypes (LD78α and LD78β) and MIP-1β signal through CCR5, the major co-receptor for M-tropic HIV-1 strains, these CKs are capable of inhibiting HIV-1 infection in susceptible cells.[361]

Proliferation of B-Cell Progenitors

SDF-1 stimulates proliferation of B-cell progenitors in vitro and is constitutively expressed in bone marrow–derived stromal cells.[381]

Leukocyte Activation/Inflammation

The biological role of PF-4 in the regulation of neutrophil function is different from that of IL-8 and other CKs. It

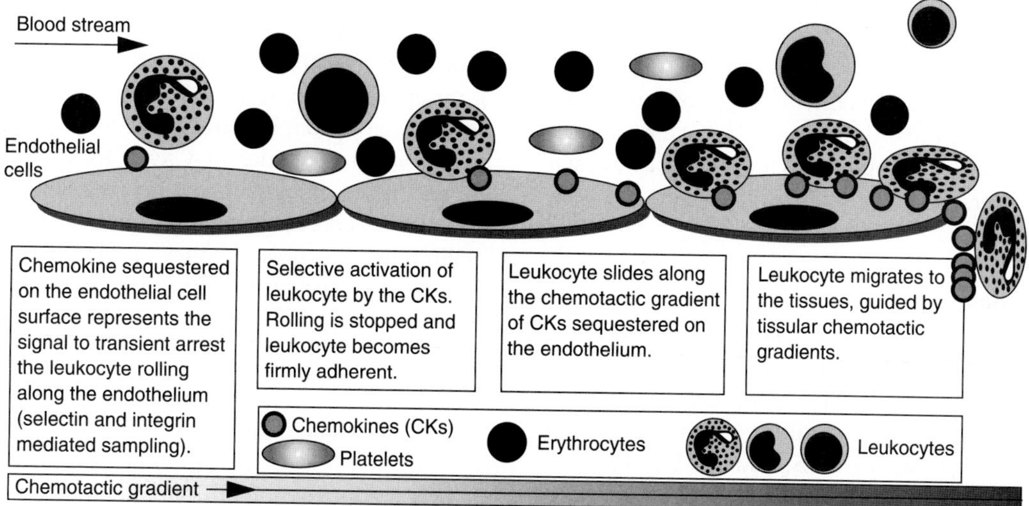

Figure 22-33 Function of chemokines in leukocyte migration.

is limited to the selective mobilization of the secondary granule marker lactoferrin but not of the primary granule marker elastase from neutrophils treated with TNFα.[419] The β-CK family contains members that stimulate basophils and eosinophils to secrete proinflammatory substances, such as histamine or eosinophil cationic protein. MCAF/MCP-1, MCP-2, MCP-3, RANTES, and MIP-1α all attract and stimulate basophils; MCP-1 and MCP-3 are the most potent. RANTES, MCP-3, and to a lesser degree MIP-1α are chemotactic factors and activators of eosinophils. These substances may have particular importance as mediators of allergic inflammation, particularly the late phase component of the allergic response.[254] It is surprising that RANTES, MCP-1, MCP-2, MCP-3, MIP-1α, and MIP-1β have no effect on mast cell activation, showing evidence for the differences between human mast cells and basophils regarding cytokine-dependent activation.[209]

During organogenesis, immunosurveillance, and inflammation, CKs selectively recruit leukocytes by activating seven transmembrane-spanning receptors. It has been suggested that an important component of this process is the formation of a haptotactic gradient by immobilization of CKs on cell surface glycosaminoglycans (GAGs). Each tissue produces specific repertoires of GAGs, some of which are known to bind and regulate CK activity. Several lines of evidence point to the importance of one particular GAG, heparan sulfate (HS), in promoting CK activity.[331,425]

Lymphocyte Recruitment and Activation

The β-CKs, MIP-1α, and MIP-1β; RANTES; and MCP-1 have been found in vitro capable of directly co-stimulating purified human T-cell and human T-cell clone proliferation and IL-2 production in the presence of anti-CD3 but not phorbol esters. CK treatment of human T cells in vitro increases the level of cell surface CD25 and soluble CD25. In addition, these CKs enhance both antigen and alloantigen-specific T cells and T-cell clone proliferation. This activity was further augmented in the presence of the CD28 ligand, B7-1. Together, these results suggest that CKs not only play an important role in lymphocyte recruitment to inflammatory sites, but also participate in T-cell activation.[520] CD8 T-lymphocyte accumulation is strongly enhanced by MIP-1α, and RANTES may have a physiological role in T-lymphocyte recirculation.[521] RANTES is a CK whose gene is expressed immediately after stimulation of several types of cells but up regulated late (3 to 5 days) after activation in normal T lymphocytes. This is dependent on two cis-acting elements in the human RANTES promoter that act in T lymphocytes. One is activated within the first 24 hours after T-cell activation, and the second site is up regulated later, between days 3 and 5. These data provide an explanation for the immediate early expression of RANTES in some types of cells and identify apparently novel factors contributing to late RANTES transcription in T cells.[403] MIG is a CK of the CXC subfamily that is inducible in macrophages and in other cells in response to IFNγ. Human MIG induces the transient elevation of [Ca^{2+}] in TIL and human peripheral activated lymphocytes. No responses have been seen in human neutrophils, monocytes, or transformed lymphoblastoid cell lines. It was concluded that human MIG plays a role in T-cell trafficking and perhaps in other aspects of the physiology of activated T cells.[317] Evidence indicates that MCP-1, MCP-2, and MCP-3 are active on NK cells.[491]

Lymphocyte trafficking through internal organs is thought to be controlled by rather general, tissue-nonspecific, "inflammatory" adhesion molecules and CK receptors, unlike lymphocyte homing to epithelial surfaces. The so-called homing subsets of effector and memory T cells with distinct tissue tropism have been identified: the integrin and

CK receptor CCR9 target T cells to the small intestinal mucosa. By contrast, skin-homing T cells display selectin ligands in combination with CCR4 and/or CCR10. It remains to be determined whether T cells expressing skin-homing markers are exclusively homing to skin or also to other tissue. Distinct homing subsets for other organs, such as the lung, liver, brain, or kidney, have not yet been reported.[147]

Platelet Activation

Tethering of the monocytes by P-selection is required for their activation by RANTES. This suggests that activated platelets regulate CK secretion by monocytes in inflammatory lesions.[575] Platelets express mRNAs for the following CKs: CTAP-III, ENA-78, RANTES, and MCP-3. Platelets also express mRNAs for IL-8RA and a novel CK receptor CCR4. These results suggest that CKs may not only play an important role in platelet activation, but also influence the nature of the leukocyte infiltrate to sites of inflammation and infection.[424]

Immune Response

Induction of oral tolerance was prevented by the administration of anti-MCP-1. These results indicate that CKs play an important role in the induction of oral tolerance.[258] There is evidence that both CXC and CC CKs are integral components of antibacterial host defense. Specifically, in vitro studies indicate that CXC CKs (IL-8 and MIP-2) and the CC CK MIP-1α augment the ability of PMNs and alveolar macrophages, respectively, to phagocytose and kill *E. coli.* In addition, the intratracheal instillation of *Klebsiella pneumoniae* in mice results in time-dependent production of MIP-2 and MIP-1α. Inhibition of MIP-2 bioactivity in vivo results in decreases in lung PMN influx, impaired bacterial clearance, and early mortality.[495]

MIP-1α, MIP-1β, RANTES, and ATAC are not only chemoattractants but also co-activators of macrophages, so together with IFNγ they constitute a group of cytokines that act together as a functional unit, which is used by NK cells in the innate phase and in the antigen-specific phase of the immune defense, thus bridging the two components of a Th1 immune reaction.[139] T cells express a large variety of CK receptors and respond to an impressive number of CKs. In most cases, regulation of CK receptor expression depends upon the phenotype and consequent functional properties of the T cells (namely Th1 and Th2 phenotypes).[445,583]

Angiogenic Activity

The CXC CK family displays disparate angiogenic activity, depending on the presence or absence of the ELR motif (a NH2-terminal motif previously found to be important in ligand/receptor interactions). CXC CKs containing the ELR motif, such as IL-8, are potent angiogenic factors, inducing both in vitro endothelial chemotaxis and in vivo corneal neovascularization. In contrast, CXC CKs lacking the ELR motif (PF-4, IP-10, and MIG) not only fail to induce significant in vitro endothelial cell chemotaxis or in vivo corneal neovascularization, but are found to be potent angiostatic factors in the presence of CXC CKs containing the ELR motif. These findings support the idea that the net biological balance in the magnitude of expression of angiogenic and angiostatic CXC CKs at either the site of wound repair or during tumorigenesis may be important in the regulation of net angiogenesis.[44,446,500,502]

Cell Adhesion

The CKs RANTES, MCP-1, and to a lesser extent MIP-1α, MIP-1β, and IL-8 are able to induce uropod formation and ICAM-3 redistribution in T lymphoblasts adhered to ICAM-1 or VCAM-1. A similar CK-mediated effect has been observed during T cells binding to the binding sites for the integrins VLA-4 and VLA-5. The uropod structure concentrates the ICAM-3 adhesion molecule (a ligand for LFA-1) and emerges to the outer milieu from the area of contact between lymphocyte and protein ligands. In addition, this study demonstrates that other adhesion molecules, such as ICAM-1, CD43, and CD44, also redistribute to the lymphocyte uropod upon RANTES stimulation, whereas a wide number of other cell-surface receptors do not redistribute. CKs display a selective effect among different T-cell subsets; MIP-1β had more potent action on CD8 T cells and TIL, whereas RANTES and MIP-1α targeted selectively CD4 T cells. These results demonstrate that uropod formation and adhesion receptor redistribution are novel functions mediated by CKs. This phenomenon may represent a mechanism that significantly contributes to the recruitment of circulating leukocytes to inflammatory foci.[123]

The molecular basis of cancer metastasis suggests that metastatic cancer cells simply use signals that normally control leukocyte transport focused on CKs and there is some evidence to support that CXC CK receptor 4 (CXCR4) and its ligand CXC CK ligand 12 (CXCL12) together govern the pattern of breast cancer metastasis.[378]

Clinical Relevance

CKs have important roles in a large diversity of human pathological conditions, namely in HIV infection; transplant rejection; rheumatic, allergic, and autoimmune diseases; cancer; atherosclerosis; and general immunoinflammatory processes (systemic or related with central nervous system), and are expected as promising targets for new molecular therapies.*

*References 54, 59, 69, 214, 222, 226, 265, 282, 327, 328, 376, 378, 500, 506, 510, 554, 558.

AIDS/HIV Infection

CKs are promising molecules for therapy in AIDS.[524] This hypothesis is based on two observations: (1) increased levels of MIP-1α, MIP-1β, and RANTES in long-term nonprogressors (individuals who do not show evidence of disease from HIV, even a long time after being infected) and (2) the observation that CCR5 plays a critical role in HIV capacity to infect CD4 cells. In addition, MIP-1α and MIP-1β are induced in human monocyte cultures following infection with the HIV-1. Induction depends on productive viral infection: Not only does the kinetics of MIP-1 peptide induction closely follow that of viral replication, but monocyte cultures inoculated with heat-inactivated virus or infected in the presence of 3′-azido-3′-deoxythymidine (AZT) failed to produce these β-CK peptides.[464] The RANTES is a T-cell–expressed, proinflammatory CK that has been implicated as a suppressive agent of HIV replication.[12,387] However, some investigators have argued against the CKs being clinically relevant for AIDS therapy.[93,141,456]

Several CK receptors have been implicated in HIV entry in various experimental systems, with CCR5 being the most important mediator of R5 HIV entry because of its role in transmission early in the disease. CCR5 is now a highly validated target for the treatment of HIV-1 infection. In vitro, cells cannot become infected with certain strains of HIV-1, designated R5-tropic, if they do not express CCR5 in conjunction with the primary receptor CD4. Natural and synthetic ligands for CCR5, such as RANTES, AOP-RANTES, MIP-1α, MIP-1β, Met-RANTES, andLD78β (MIP-1α isoform), protect against R5 virus infection in vitro. This extends to in vivo where it has been observed that individuals with high levels of MIP-1β have decreased risk of HIV progression.[265]

Transplant Rejection/Kidney Pathological Conditions

CKs are thought to play a role in directing inflammatory cells to graft sites and initiate rejection.[434] For example, in murine allogeneic skin grafts, two general patterns of CK gene expression have been observed. In the first, CK genes—including MIP-1α, MIP-1β, JE, and KC—are observed at peak levels 3 days posttransplant. In the second pattern, CKs such as RANTES and IP-10 are expressed at high levels 3 to 4 days before rejection of the allografts is complete. These two patterns of chemoattractant cytokine gene expression may be representative of the early inflammatory and the late T-cell–mediated phases of the allograft rejection process, respectively.[284] CKs are also involved in mediating renal pathological conditions and proteinuria. IL-8, RANTES, and MCP have been extensively studied in the kidney.[572]

Allergic Diseases

Both CXC and CC CKs have been found to be expressed in pulmonary-derived mast cells, suggesting an important contribution to leukocyte responses in the allergic airway.[334,399] This CK expression contrasts with the previously mentioned observation that RANTES, MCP-1, MCP-2, MCP-3, MIP-1α, and MIP-1β have no action on mast cell activation.[209]

Studies in both animals and humans have demonstrated a positive correlation between the inflammatory state of the airways and the severity of airway hyperreactivity. However, because the type and etiology of this inflammation and the extent and consequences of the inflammatory process vary between different diseases exhibiting airway hyperreactivity, the direct contribution of individual types of cells or CKs to airway hyperreactivity requires further investigation.[54]

Autoimmune Diseases

Production in the central nervous system of MIP-1α plays an important role in directing the chemoattraction of mononuclear inflammatory cells in the T-cell–mediated experimental autoimmune encephalomyelitis.[259]

Persons with type 1 diabetes have increased peripheral blood mononuclear cell expression of CK receptors CXCR4 (naive T cells), CCR5 and CXCR3 (Th1-associated), CCR3 and CCR4 (Th2-associated) and serum CK levels of MCP-1, MIP-1α, MIP-1β, and RANTES. A reduced expression of the Th1-associated CK receptors CCR5 and CXCR3 in type 1 diabetes patients and a genetic association involving a single-base polymorphism in CCR2 has been suggested.[20]

Rheumatic Diseases

MIP-1β has been identified as a unique CK that is increased in the synovial fluid from osteoarthritic patients but not in the synovial fluid of RA patients. This observation indicates that MIP-1β may play a role in the ingress of monocytes into the osteoarthritic joint.[283]

In addition, several studies have emphasized the role and therapeutic approaches of CKs and CK receptors in RA and inflamed synovia.[328,412,508,517]

Hemolytic Diseases/Transfusion

PF-4, β-thromboglobulin, and RANTES are released from platelets during storage and accumulated over time in the platelet concentrates. These CKs might play a causative role in nonhemolytic transfusion reactions because of their inflammatory potential, but the clinical effects of the transfusion of platelet concentrates with high CK contents are still being investigated.[67]

Inflammatory Processes[204]

MCP-1 and RANTES are thought to contribute to the recruitment and activation of leukocytes in mucosa from patients with inflammatory bowel disease, suggesting that these CKs play a role in the pathogenesis of mucosal inflammation. Furthermore, the expression of the MCP-1 gene in vessel-associated cells may indicate its involvement in mechanisms regulating the adhesion of blood monocytes to endothelial cells.[352] Eotaxin and CCR-3 may be host factors highly specialized for eosinophil recruitment in inflammation and may be good targets for the development of selective drugs for inflammatory diseases in which eosinophils contribute to pathogenesis, such as asthma.[280,428]

Chemokine Receptors (CKRs)

Several kinds of structures able to receive functional signals of CK are known. The most important ones can be formed into the following categories: (1) specific receptors, (2) shared receptors, (3) promiscuous receptors, (4) virally encoded receptors, and (5) orphan receptors.[461,545]

The attempt to define CK receptors has been based primarily on four different methods: direct binding, signal transduction, molecular cloning, and structure function. All of these have advantages and handicaps related to the intrinsic methodology, but the complexity of receptor characterization derives also from the biological model, including the number of CKs simultaneously used (for example, CC, CKR-1 binds MIP-1α, RANTES, MIP-1β, and MCP-1 and has been reported as an MIP-1α/RANTES receptor).[526] Among the CKRs, the IL-8 receptors were the first to be studied at the molecular level. Now, several CK receptors have been cloned and characterized and all found to be members of the G-protein coupled receptor superfamily (GPCR). Rhodopsin is the typical GPCR, although other molecules exist, namely calcitonin-like, metabotropic, pheromone-like, and cAMP-like. Using gene mapping studies, receptors with the highest sequence similarity have been found to be closely linked on human chromosomes. This close genetic association suggests a functional relationship as well.[431] These receptors are integral membrane glycoproteins with a structure composed of seven helices snaking through the cell membrane with the N-terminus on the extracellular face. CKRs are coupled to regulatory GTP-binding proteins, leading to signal transduction.[545]

Specific Receptors

Specific receptors bind only one CK. In practice, it is difficult to define the specificity of a receptor for CKs.[3] However, some of them, such as the IL-8 receptor A (IL-8RA) and the MCP-1 receptor (MCP-1R), have been found to be specific.

Shared Receptors

Shared receptors are defined as able to bind more than one CK; this concept is only valid inside each CK family. For example CCL20, alternatively named liver and activation-regulated CK (LARC), macrophage inflammatory protein-3α (MIP-3α) or Exodus-1, is the only CK known to interact with CC CK receptor 6 (CCR6), a property shared with the antimicrobial β-defensins. The ligand-receptor pair CCL20-CCR6 is responsible for the chemoattraction of immature dendritic cells, effector/memory T cells, and B cells and plays a role at skin and mucosal surfaces under homeostatic and inflammatory conditions and in pathological conditions, including cancer and RA.[467]

CXC Chemokine Receptors (CXC CKRs or CXCRs). The CXC CKs have been found to have six human receptors: CXCR1, CXCR2, CXCR3, CXCR4, CXCR5, and CXCR6.*

CC Chemokine Receptors (CC CKRs, or CCRs). The CC CKs have at least 10 receptors: CCR1, CCR2, CCR3, CCR4, CCR5, CCR6, CCR7, CCR8, CCR9, and CCR10.† CC CKs do not bind to the CXC receptors because the three-dimensional structure of the ligand differs in a region between the two families and by a modification of the amino terminus. This suggests a two-site model for receptor activation and for selectivity between CC and CXC CKs, with an initial receptor contact provided by the main body of the CK and activation provided by the amino terminal region.[570] The different cellular expression of CC CKRs enables selective biological actions (e.g., monocyte responses to MCP-3 that could be mediated by both CCR2 and CCR1), whereas eosinophil responses to MCP-3 could be mediated by CCR1.[96]

Promiscuous Receptors

By definition, promiscuous receptors bind several CKs outside their family (CXC or CC). The most important is the Duffy antigen receptor complex (DARC), or Duffy antigen receptor for CKs, that is present on several cellular types, especially on erythrocytes (thus it also has been called erythrocyte CK receptor). In a 1995 study, Szabo and coworkers[507] suggest that the promiscuous nature of DARC is limited because C and non–ELR-CXC CKs do not bind to it. This also occurs inside the CC family with MIP-1α and MIP-1β, contrasting with RANTES and MCP-1, that bind to the Duffy antigen.[3,223] This demonstrates that the ELR motif is not crucial for CK binding to DARC. The presence of this receptor must be seen mostly as a regulatory mechanism of the CK's biological function with a clear "sink" role and a "drain" capacity clearing excess CK from the circulation‡ and maintaining the sensitivity of blood leukocytes to CK gradient generated by local inflammatory foci but also allowing the action of CK on cells without other more specific receptors (such as IL-8RA and IL-8RB). It is curious, for instance, that lymphocytes appear to vary the level of DARC expression according to their state of activation and differentiation.[293,461] DARC is also a receptor for the malaria parasite *Plasmodium vivax* but the parasite ligand has no similarity to the CKs.[1,341] However, the lack of DARC expression

*References 3, 223, 229, 376, 338, 401, 476, 545, 558, 570.

†References 95, 141, 220, 296, 338, 369, 376, 401, 402, 422, 430, 456, 545, 558.

‡Although the normal circulating levels of IL-8 are in the picomole range, they can be as high as 8 nmol/L in sera of patients with sepsis or acute respiratory distress syndrome, implying the "drain" of surplus IL-8 molecules.

(Duffy-negative phenotype) has not yet been correlated with any kind of disease susceptibility, but only with the advantage to individuals exposed to *P. vivax.*

DARC is mapped in human chromosome 1q21-25 and is expressed in human erythrocytes and on endothelial cells lining postcapillary venules, brain, kidney, spleen, lungs, and thymus. The expression of DARC by subsets of endothelial cells and neurons in discrete anatomical sites in the brain suggests that this enigmatic receptor may have multiple roles in normal and pathological physiology. Conservation of this promiscuous CK-binding activity is evident from the similarity in nucleotide sequence of DARC homologues from multiple species and the high-affinity binding of human CKs to murine and avian erythrocytes. The hierarchical expression of DARC in neurons in the cerebellum suggests that CKs may play an important role in the modulation of neuronal activity by glial cells.[223,224]

The platelet activating factor receptor as a GPCR (rhodopsin family) is possibly also a promiscuous receptor for CKs. The same can be considered for the chemoattractant receptors, complement 5 anaphylatoxin receptor, and FPR/FMLPR (N-formyl peptide receptor).

Virally Encoded Receptors

Virally encoded receptors (homologues of the native CK receptors) represent the possible subversion of these receptors by viruses and the two known to date are of shared type. The first is the human cytomegalovirus open reading frame US28; it is a CC-shared receptor (it binds MIP-1α, MIP-1β, MCP-1, and RANTES). The second is the Herpesvirus saimiri (HVS) ECRF3; it is a CXC-shared receptor (it is activated by the same CKs that bind to IL-8 RB but with different capacity; for IL-8 RB, the hierarchy is IL-8 greater than GROα = NAP-2, and for ECRF3 is GROα greater than NAP-2 greater than IL-8). The biological significance of these receptors is not well understood and is the subject of intensive research. It is already clear that a few microorganisms use the plasticity of genomes to immunomodulate the host defense. ECRF3 is functionally active (in contrast with US28, which lacks a known signaling activity), and it may sensitize HVS-infected T lymphocytes (without IL-8 RB) to CXC CKs as a way to establish cytosolic ideal conditions for replication.[3] This may be very important in clinical practice, mainly for immunocompromised hosts.[218,338]

Orphan Receptors

Several DNAs have been cloned that have homology to the already known members of the CK-receptor family, although they have not yet shown functional significance. The principal orphan receptors are CMK-BRL-1 (CK β-receptor-like-1), BLR-1/MDR-15 (Burkitt's lymphoma receptor-1/monocyte-derived receptor-15), V28, and EBI1.[545]

Functional Signaling

The biological effects of CKs are mediated by complex components requiring seven transmembrane, G-protein-linked receptors on the surface of target cells. The complexities of interactions between CKs and cytoplasmic components of target cells are summarized in Figure 22-34.[461]

Experimental research regarding the types of G proteins coupled to CC CKRs suggests that MCP-1 and RANTES receptors are promiscuously coupled to multiple G proteins in IL-2-activated NK-cell membranes and that this coupling is different from MIP-1α receptors, which seem to be coupled to G(s), G(o), and G(z) but not to G(i).[5] The CCR1 and CCR2 can reconstitute ligand-induced accumulation of inositol phosphates with PLC β2 in a pertussis toxin-sensitive manner, presumably through Gβγ released from the G(i) proteins.[563] However, these receptors demonstrate different specificity in coupling to the α subunits of the G(q) class. The results suggest that some of the CC CK receptors, unlike the CXC CK receptors, discriminate against Gα16, a hematopoietic-specific Gα subunit. The intriguing specificity in coupling of the G(q) class of G proteins implies

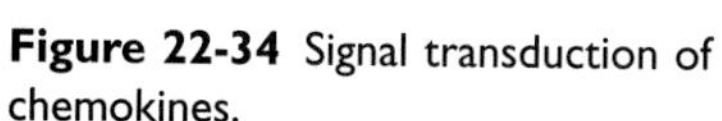

Figure 22-34 Signal transduction of chemokines.

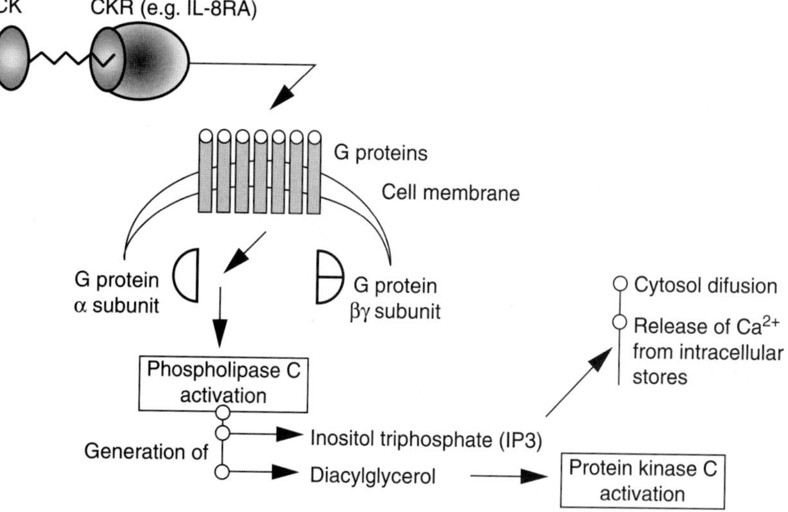

that the CKs may be involved in some distinct functions in vivo.[290]

Regulation of Chemokine Activity

The control of CK activity probably depends on several mechanisms, such as the presence of a clearance receptor in red blood cells, such as DARC, and anti-CK antibodies in the circulation.[461] Also the genetic expression of some CKs (such as IL-8) seems to be tightly regulated, leading to a short half-life of mRNA expression.[341] Oxidized low-density lipoprotein (LDL) has been found to greatly potentiate the expression of the KC (murine equivalent to GROα) CK gene in LPS-stimulated macrophages, whereas levels of IP-10 mRNA are altered in the opposite fashion. These effects on KC gene transcription are in marked contrast to previous reports demonstrating inhibitory effects of oxidized LDL on LPS-induced M CK expression. Thus extensively oxidized LDL acts on the transcriptional control process in macrophages in both a positive and negative fashion on separate members of the same gene family.[208] These experimental data indicate a large diversity of influences controlling CK production and interaction with receptors. Moreover, because CKs are important mediators of immunoinflammatory reactions and they belong to a complex cascade of events in part dependent on inflammatory cytokines.

MEASUREMENTS OF CYTOKINES

The basic goal for the clinical determination of cytokines is the measurement of their physiological and physiopathological concentrations. Thus the definition of physiological concentration is very important in defining the actual biological functions of cytokines. Again, cytokines are different from hormones, which normally act in a distant anatomical region from the site where they are produced (of course, systemic levels will represent a good approach for the physiological concentration of hormones). Cytokines frequently act on the same cell that produced them (autocrine action) or in neighboring cells (paracrine action), leaving the systemic concentration (endocrine action) as a very distant reflection of biological action. Considering present knowledge, only the on-site determination (at the cell membrane or in the intracellular compartment) will be physiologically relevant[2,255,585] except in the case of cytokines, such as IL-1 and IL-6, that have endocrine functions.[2] However, circulating cytokine concentrations may still act as simple disease markers in conditions such as cancer and inflammation. In practice, even in the systemic compartment, it is necessary to study several cytokines (IL-2, IFNγ, IL-4, IL-10, and IL-13) using not only enzyme-linked immunosorbent assay (ELISA) but also PCR techniques.[157]

Requirements

To study local concentrations of cytokines, it is necessary to define the (1) secreted concentration of the cytokine per cell per time unit, (2) number of secretory vesicles fusing with the plasma membrane per time unit, (3) distribution of fusing vesicles on cell surface (normally not evenly spaced), (4) size of secretory vesicles, (5) concentration of cytokines in secretory vesicles, (6) liberation of vesicle contents (normal versus propulsion), and (7) superficial diffusion (over cell membranes) coefficient and time.[255]

In addition, many physiological factors affect the circulating levels of cytokines and their measurement (Figure 22-35). For example, cytokines usually act in a paracrine and autocrine mode by binding to their receptors; only a few cytokines have endocrine actions. In addition, although the circulating levels of cytokines can be high (e.g., IL-6 can reach blood concentrations up to 20,000 pg/mL in severe bacterial infections), their normal circulating levels are typically very low (e.g., a few pg/mL). Thus methods used to

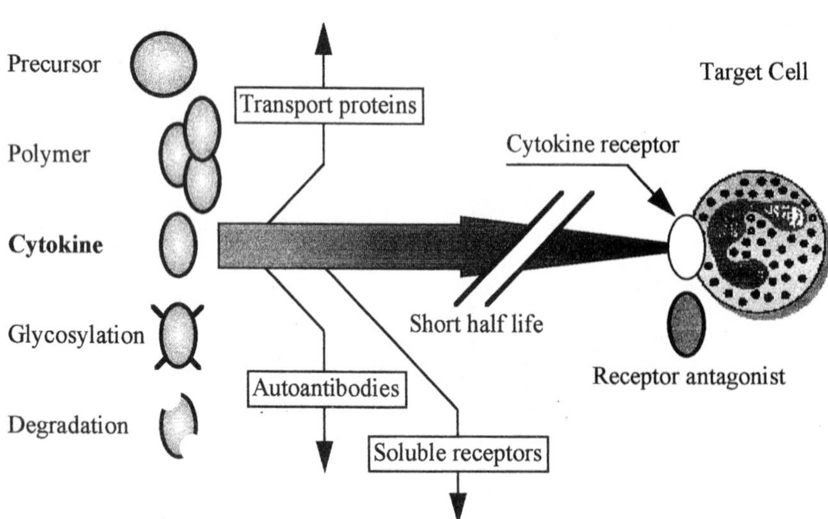

Figure 22-35 Factors influencing the measurement of cytokines.

measure them must have a wide dynamic range and a low limit of detection. The molecular forms of cytokines are very diverse (monomers and polymers), and some are synthesized as precursors (e.g., the 31-kDa precursor of IL-1α is converted by proteolysis to the mature 17-kDa form of IL-1α). Cytokines can also be degraded by proteases, which are produced during the inflammatory process.

Many cytokine inhibitors have been described. Among them, soluble receptors or autoantibodies (with affinity constant sometimes being as high as 10^{-11} mol/L) can influence cytokine assays. Nonspecific inhibitors are represented by plasma proteins, which bind cytokines (e.g., α_2-macroglobulin and IL-6). The presence of such inhibitors can contribute to inaccurate results. The half-lifes of cytokines are also very short (generally a few minutes), which explains the very rapid plasma peaks of these molecules. Furthermore, in some instances, a circadian rhythm has been reported (IL-6 and RA) and intraindividual variation is very high (Figure 22-36).

Sample Collection and Storage

In the measurement of cytokines in body fluids, samples must be collected and stored in the proper manner. The main problems encountered in the collection process include: (1) cytokines can continue to be produced after sample collection by the various cells present in the biological fluid; (2) collection tubes can become contaminated by microorganisms, which are a potent stimulus of cytokine production; (3) cytokines can be degraded in the collection container; and (4) cytokines can bind to cell receptors during storage.

For bioassays, serum collected in pyrogen-free tubes is required. After rapid centrifugation, freezing of the plasma (or serum) at −80 °C is recommended for storage. Freezing-thawing cycles must be prevented.

For immunoassays in biological fluids, ethylenediaminetetraacetic acid (EDTA) plasma is the most suitable sample, because tubes containing heparin are often contaminated by endotoxin, and cytokine release may occur during coagulation. Some investigators recommend the addition of protease inhibitors (Trasylol).

For intracellular cytokine detection by flow cytometry, PBMCs are often used, but to have a more specific analysis, it may be necessary to use cells from other biological fluids (e.g., synovial fluid, cerebrospinal fluid, and bronchoalveolar lavage fluid) or to separate cells according to functional characteristics or expression of membrane antigens (e.g., CD3, CD4, CD8, and CD56).

In practice, all analyses for cytokines must be performed within a narrow interval of time (not more than 5 hours) after sample collection to prevent cellular interactions and possible cytokine release. Blood samples must be collected with endotoxin-free heparin. The same is true for immunoassays dealing with cytokine production by blood cells.

Principles of Cytokine Assays

Bioassay and immunoassay are the analytical techniques of choice to measure cytokines.[463] However, newer instrumental techniques are also beginning to be used to measure cytokines and CKs. These techniques are used to quantify their (1) concentration and activity in biological fluids, (2) production by whole blood cells,[40] (3) concentration of receptors, and (4) intracellular levels.

Bioassays

Historically the functions of cytokines have been elucidated first with bioassays preceding immunoassays for cytokine quantification. The bioassay of a given cytokine is based on its bioactivity in a defined biological model, normally based on a certain cell line. Various approaches have been reported: (1) proliferation tests—induction of cell growth (e.g., B9 cell line for IL-6); (2) tests for cytotoxicity—TNFα on WEHI 164

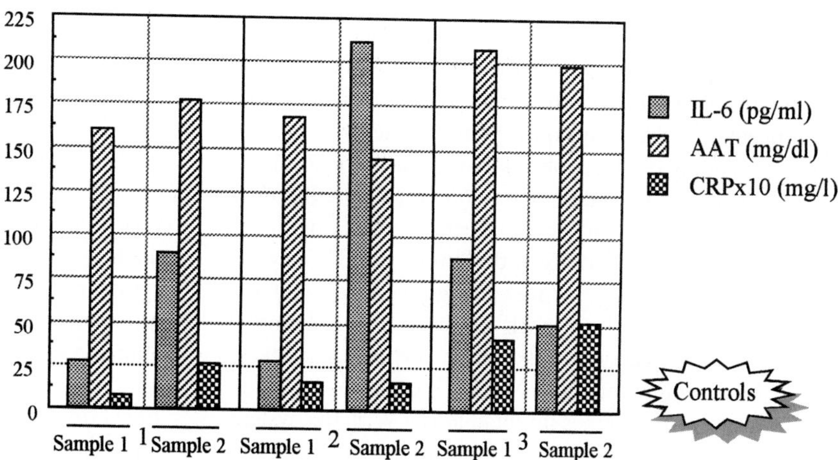

Figure 22-36 Intraindividual variation of IL-6, α_1-antitrypsin (AAT), and C-reactive protein. Data obtained from the analysis of peripheral blood samples obtained from three healthy volunteers. Sample 1 was obtained from each volunteer with sample 2 obtained 2 weeks later.

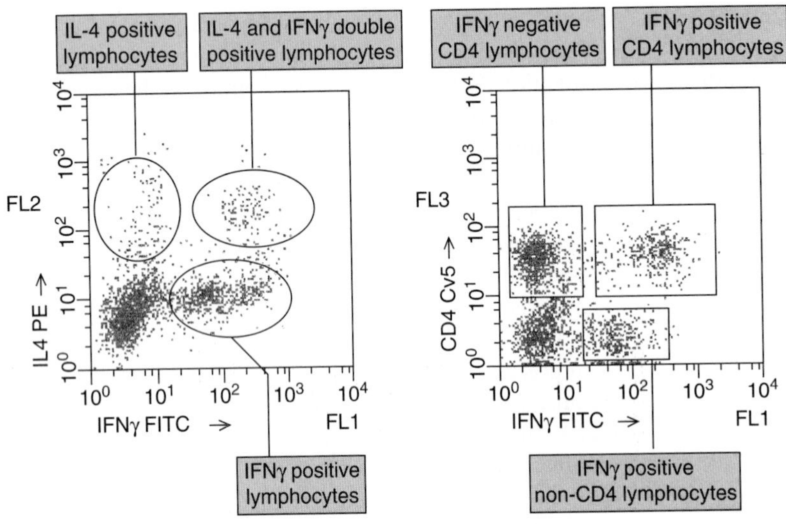

Figure 22-37 Flow cytometric analysis of IL-4 and IFNγ.

cell line, and (3) tests for chemotactic activity—migration of cells in a Boyden chamber or in agarose (e.g., IL-8).

The major drawback of these techniques is their lack of specificity, poor precision (CV = 15% to 100%), and long analysis time (1 to 4 days). Their main advantages are that they measure biologically active molecules and detect as little as 0.1 pg/mL.

A standard method for the quantitation of cytokines is to perform a bioassay in which aliquots of samples are compared with known concentrations of a cytokine in supporting the proliferation of a cytokine-dependent cell line. In most instances, however, these cell lines are dependent on the cytokine not only for proliferation, but also for survival.[58]

Immunoassays

Currently, immunoassay is the practical method of choice for measuring cytokines and their receptors. As cytokines are proteins, specific antibodies can be raised against recombinant cytokines and have also been measured as an indicator of cytokine presence.[146] The general characteristics of cytokine immunoassays are comparable with the classical immunoassays, with monoclonal, oligoclonal, or polyclonal antibodies all being used (see Chapter 9). The most popular formats are immunoradiometric assay (IRMA) and ELISA, which use a first monoclonal antibody for the capture and a second antibody labeled with a radioisotope or an enzyme.

Typically, ELISA assays only measure one cytokine at a time. Depending on the application, this may be a disadvantage, because it may be desirable to measure more than one cytokine. This disadvantage has been overcome with the development and appearance of the "multiplexed" analytical systems that are capable of measuring several cytokines at once.[117,150] An example of such a system is the Luminex 100/xMAP analytical system (Luminex Corp., Austin, Texas); http://www.luminexcorp.com), which is capable of measuring more than 70 cytokines simultaneously. With this system, molecular reactions take place on the surface microspheres. For each reaction in an xMAP profile, thousands of molecules are attached to the surface of internally color-coded microspheres. The assigned color code identifies the reaction throughout the test. Instrumentally the analyzer integrates laser optics, fluidics, a controller, advanced digital signal processing, and a bar code reader into a single compact unit. Other systems incorporate microchip, immunoassay, and flow cytometry to measure cytokines,[81,459,509,559,567] cytokine antibodies,[146,567] or cytokine genes.[113,391]

The main disadvantage of immunoassays is that they measure total cytokine, which contains both functional and nonfunctional levels.[342] Cross-reactivity with the precursors or degradation products of the cytokine is frequently observed. The detection limit (about 1 to 10 pg/mL) of immunoassays is higher than bioassays. A 1995 study reported a lack of comparability between the different kits for IL-2, IL-6, IL-8, and TNFα.[306] The major advantages of immunoassays are their excellent analytical performance and their ability to be automated.

The comparative characteristics of bioassays and immunoassays when applied to cytokine measurements in biological fluids are listed in Table 22-9.[47]

Instrumental Techniques

Instrumental techniques such as capillary electrophoresis, high-performance liquid chromatography,[503] flow cytometry, and multiplexing techniques have been used to measure cytokines or their receptors, antibodies, or genes. For example, flow cytometry has been found useful in measuring intracellular cytokines in less than 2 hours. This gives very useful information about the frequency and cell-surface phenotype of individual cytokine-producing cells. Flow cytometry allows the rapid analysis of sufficiently large numbers of cells previously treated with fixative and permeabilizing agents. Three- to four-color analysis (FL1, FL2, FL3, and FL4) is advised to undertake concomitant cellular identification using antigenic markers (e.g., FL1-IFNγ, FL2-CD3, and FL3-CD4 gives the identification of CD4 T lymphocytes with intracellular IFNγ) as shown in Figure 22-37.

TABLE 22-9 Comparative Characteristics of Bioassays and Immunoassays*

	Bioassays	Immunoassays
Limit of detection	<1 pg/mL	1-10 pg/mL†
Specificity	Low	High
Precision	CV ≅ 15%-100%	CV ≅ 5%-10%
Assay range	Narrow	Wide
Assay time	1-4 days	A few hours
Calibration	Difficult	Simple
Clinical significance	Biological active molecule	Antigenic presence

*Cytokine measurements in biological fluids.
†New high-sensitivity kits allow detection of 0.1 to 1 pg/mL.

In practice,[463] the main problems experienced by flow cytometric assays are (1) the necessity for a negative control to define the cutoff level (normally the upper limit of the negative control) between positive and negative fluorescent cells; (2) the background induced by autofluorescence (frequently important in bronchoalveolar lavage cells); (3) the nonsuitability of automatic gating of cells; and (4) the complexity of quantifying the number of cytokine molecules inside each cell.

REFERENCES

1. Abbas AK, Lichtman AH, Pober JS. Cellular and molecular immunology, 2nd ed. Philadelphia: WB Saunders, 1994.
2. Agouridakis P, Kyriakou D, Alexandrakis MG. The predictive role of serum and bronchoalveolar lavage cytokines and adhesion molecules for acute respiratory distress syndrome development and outcome. Respir Res 2002;3:25.
3. Ahuja SK, Gao JL, Murphy PM. Chemokine receptors and molecular mimicry. Immunol Today 1994;15:281-7.
4. Ahuja SS, Brown MR, Fleisher TA, et al. Autocrine activation of hemopoietic progenitor-derived myelo-monocytic cells by IFN-γ gene transfer. J Immunol 1996;156:4345-3.
5. Al Aoukaty A, Schall TJ, Maghazachi AA. Differential coupling of CC chemokine receptors to multiple heterotrimeric G proteins in human interleukin-2-activated natural killer cells. Blood 1996;87:4255-60.
6. Allen JN, Liao Z, Wewers MD, et al. Detection of IL-5 and IL-1 receptor antagonist in bronchoalveolar lavage fluid in acute eosinophilic pneumonia. J Allergy Clin Immunol 1996;97:1366-74.
7. Aman MJ, Bug G, Aulitzky WE, et al. Inhibition of interleukin-11 by interferon-α in human bone marrow stromal cells. Exp Hematol 1996;24:863-7.
8. Aman MJ, Tretter T, Eisenbeis I, et al. Interferon-α stimulates production of interleukin-10 in activated CD4+ T cells and monocytes. Blood 1996;87:4731-6.
9. Amrani Y, Panettieri RA Jr, Frossard N, Bronner C. Activation of the TNFα-p55 receptor induces myocyte proliferation and modulates agonist-evoked calcium transients in cultured human tracheal smooth muscle cells. Am J Respir Cell Mol Biol 1996;15:55-63.
10. Anderson DM, Kumaki S, Ahdieh M, et al. Functional characterization of the human interleukin-15 receptor α chain and close linkage of IL15RA and IL2RA genes. J Biol Chem 1995;270:29862-9.
11. Anderson WH, Davidson TM, Broide DH. Mast cell TNF mRNA expression in nasal mucosa demonstrated by in situ hybridization: a comparison of mast cell detection methods. J Immunol Methods 1995;189:145-55.
12. Appay V, Rowland-Jones SL. RANTES: a versatile and controversial chemokine. Trends Immunol 2001;22:83-7.
13. Armstrong L, Jordan N, Millar A. Interleukin 10 (IL-10) regulation of tumour necrosis factor α (TNF-α) from human alveolar macrophages and peripheral blood monocytes. Thorax 1996;51:143-9.
14. Arnalich F, Garcia-Palomero E, López J, et al. Predictive value of nuclear factor kb activity and plasma cytokine levels in patients with sepsis. Infect Immunity 2000;68:1942-5.
15. Arnalich F, López J, Codoceo R, et al. Relationship of plasma leptin to plasma cytokines and human survival in sepsis and septic shock. J Infect Dis 1999;180:908-11.
16. Aronica SM, Mantel C, Gonin R, et al. Interferon-inducible protein 10 and macrophage inflammatory protein-1 alpha inhibit growth factor stimulation of Raf-1 kinase activity and protein synthesis in a human growth factor-dependent hematopoietic cell line. J Biol Chem 1995;270:21998-2007.
17. Asherson GL, Dieli F, Sireci G, Salerno A. Role of IL-4 in delayed type hypersensitivity. Clin Exp Immunol 1996;103:1-4.
18. Ashton RW, Daniels CE, Ryu JH. Thrombolytic therapy in patients with submassive pulmonary embolism. N Engl J Med 2003;348:357.
19. Assenmacher M, Scheffold A, Schmitz J, et al. Specific expression of surface interferon-gamma on interferon-gamma producing T cells from mouse and man. Eur J Immunol 1996;26:263-7.
20. Atkinson MA, Wilson SB. Fatal attraction: chemokines and type 1 diabetes. J Clin Invest 2002;110:1611-3.
21. Ayoub IA, Yang TJ. Growth regulatory effects of transforming growth factor-β 1 and interleukin-2 on IL-2 dependent CD4+ T lymphoblastoid cell line. Immunol Invest 1996;25:129-51.

22. Azzarone B, Pottin-Clemenceau C, et al. Are interleukin-2 and interleukin-15 tumor promoting factors for human non-hematopoietic cells? Eur Cytokine Netw 1996;7:27-36.
23. Bacellar O, Brodskyn C, Guerreiro J, et al. Interleukin-12 restores interferon-gamma production and cytotoxic responses in visceral leishmaniasis. J Infect Dis 1996;173:1515-8.
24. Baert F, Norman M, Vermeire S, et al. Influence of Immunogenicity on the Long-Term Efficacy of Infliximab in Crohn's Diseas. N Engl J Med 2003;348: 601-8.
25. Balasubramanian S, Chernov-Rogan T, Davis AM, et al. Ligand binding kinetics of IL-2 and IL-15 to heteromers formed by extracellular domains of the three IL-2 receptor subunits. Int Immunol 1995; 7:1839-49.
26. Banks M, Graber P, Proudfoot AE, et al. Soluble interleukin-5 receptor α-chain binding assays: use for screening and analysis of interleukin-5 mutants. Anal Biochem 1995;230:321-8.
27. Barbosa-de-Oliveira LC, Curotto-de-Lafaille MA, Collet-de-Araujo-Lima GM, et al. Antigen-specific IL-4- and IL-10-secreting $CD4^+$ lymphocytes increase in vivo susceptibility to Trypanosoma cruzi infection. Cell Immunol 1996;170:41-53.
28. Barlan IB, Basaran MM, Bakir M, et al. Serum TNF-α, sCD8 and sIL-2R levels in childhood tuberculosis. Infection 1995;23:237-9.
29. Barnes PJ, Lim S. Inhibitory cytokines in asthma. Mol Med Today 1998 Oct;452-8.
30. Barrett KE. Cytokines: sources, receptors, and signaling. Bailliers Clin Gastroenterol 1996;10:1-15.
31. Bates ME, Bertics PJ, Busse WW. IL-5 activates a 45-kilodalton mitogen-activated protein (MAP) kinase and Jak-2 tyrosine kinase in human eosinophils. J Immunol 1996;156:711-8.
32. Batten P, Yacoub MH, Rose ML. Effect of human cytokines (IFN-γ, TNF-γ, IL-1 β, IL-4) on porcine endothelial cells: induction of MHC and adhesion molecules and functional significance of these changes. Immunology 1996;87:127-33.
33. Baumann H, Wang Y, Morella KK, et al. Complex of the soluble IL-11 receptor and IL-11 acts as IL-6-type cytokine in hepatic and nonhepatic cells. J Immunol 1996;157:284-90.
34. Baumgartner RA, Hirasawa N, Ozawa K, et al. Enhancement of TNF-α synthesis by overexpression of G α z in a mast cell line. J Immunol 1996;157:1625-9.
35. Bauvois B, Van-Weyenbergh J, Rouillard D, Wietzerbin J. TGF-β1-stimulated adhesion of human mononuclear phagocytes to fibronectin and laminin is abolished by IFN-γ: Dependence on α 5 β 1 and β 2 integrins. Exp Cell Res 1996;222:209-17.
36. Bellido T, Stahl N, Farruggella TJ, et al. Detection of receptors for interleukin-6, interleukin-11, leukemia inhibitory factor, oncostatin M, and ciliary neurotrophic factor in bone marrow stromal/ osteoblastic cells. J Clin Invest 1996;97:431-7.
37. Benigni F, Fantuzzi G, Sacco S, et al. Six different cytokines that share GP130 as a receptor subunit, induce serum amyloid A and potentiate the induction of interleukin-6 and the activation of the hypothalamus-pituitary-adrenal axis by interleukin-1. Blood 1996;87:1851-4.
38. Bentley AM, Hamid Q, Robinson DS, et al. Prednisolone treatment in asthma. Reduction in the numbers of eosinophils, T cells, tryptase-only positive mast cells, and modulation of IL-4, IL-5, and interferon-gamma cytokine gene expression within the bronchial mucosa. Am J Respir Crit Care Med 1996;153:551-6.
39. Benveniste EN, Benos DJ. TNF-α- and IFN-γ-mediated signal transduction pathways: effects on glial cell gene expression and function. FASEB J 1995;9:1577-84.
40. Benyoucef S, Hober D, Shen L, et al. TNF-α production by whole blood from HIV-1 infected patients. Pathol Biol Paris 1996;44:393-6.
41. Berger S, Ballo H, Stutte HJ. Immune complex-induced interleukin-6, interleukin-10 and prostaglandin secretion by human monocytes: a network of pro- and anti-inflammatory cytokines dependent on the antigen:antibody ratio. Eur J Immunol 1996;26:1297-301.
42. Berguer R, Braco CN, Bowyer M, et al. Major surgery suppresses maximal production of helper T-Cell type 1 cytokines without potentiating the release of helper T-Cell type 2 cytokines. Arch Surg 1999;134:540-4.
43. Berman RM, Suzuki T, Tahara H, et al. Systemic administration of cellular IL-10 induces an effective, specific, and long-lived immune response against established tumors in mice. J Immunol 1996;157: 231-8.
44. Bernardini G, Ribatti D, Spinetti G, et al. Analysis of the role of chemokines in angiogenesis. J Immunol Methods 2003;273:83-101.
45. Bhardwaj N, Seder RA, Reddy A, Feldman MV. IL-12 in conjunction with dendritic cells enhances antiviral $CD8^+$ CTL responses in vitro. J Clin Invest 1996;98:715-22.
46. Bhardwaj RS, Schwarz A, Becher E, et al. Pro-opiomelanocortin-derived peptides induce IL-10 production in human monocytes. J Immunol 1996;156:2517-21.
47. Bienvenu J. Exploration of cytokines in inflammation in biological fluids. C R Seances Soc Biol Fil 1995;189:545-55.
48. Bienvenu J, Doche C, Gutowski MC, et al. Production of proinflammatory cytokines and cytokines involved in the TH1/TH2 balance is modulated by pentoxifylline. J Cardiovasc Pharmacol 1995;25:S80-4.

49. Biet F, Locht C, Kremer L. Immunoregulatory functions of interleukin 18 and its role in defense against bacterial pathogens. J Mol Med 2002;80: 147-62. Epub 2001 Dec 08.
50. Biron CA, Gazzinelli RT. Effects of IL-12 on immune responses to microbial infections: A key mediator in regulating disease outcome. Curr Opin Immunol 1995;7:485-96.
51. Blaine TA, Rosier RN, Puzas JE, et al. Increased levels of tumor necrosis factor-α and interleukin-6 protein and messenger RNA in human peripheral blood monocytes due to titanium particles. J Bone Joint Surg Am 1996;78:1181-92.
52. Blaschke S, Koziolek M, Scjwarz A, et al. Proinflammatory role of Fractalkine (CX3CL1) in rheumatoid arthritis. J Rheumatol 2003:30:1918-27.
53. Blauvelt A, Asada H, Klaus V, et al. Interleukin-15 mRNA is expressed by human keratinocytes Langerhans cells, and blood-derived dendritic cells and is down-regulated by ultraviolet B radiation. J Invest Dermatol 1996;106:1047-52.
54. Blease K, Lukacs NW, Hogaboam CM, Kundel SL. Chemokines and their role in airway hyper-reactivity. Respir Res 2000;1:54-61.
55. Blobe GC, Schiemann WP, Lodish HF. Role of transforming growth factor β in human disease. N Engl J Med 2000;342:1350-8.
56. Blotta MH, Marshall JD, DeKruyff RH, Umetsu DT. Cross-linking of the CD40 ligand on human CD4+ T lymphocytes generates a costimulatory signal that up-regulates IL-4 synthesis. J Immunol 1996;156: 3133-40.
57. Bochner BS, Busse WW. Advances in mechanisms of allergy topics being presented. J Allergy Clin Immunol 2004;113:868-75.
58. Boise LH, McShan CL, Thompson CB. Introduction of the cell survival gene bcl-xL improves the viability of CTLL-2 cells without affecting their IL-2 proliferative response. Implications for the development of bioassays. J Immunol Methods 1996;191:143-8.
59. Boisvert WA. Modulation of atherogenesis by chemokines. Trends Cardiovasc Med 2004;14:161-5.
60. Borish L, Aarons A, Rumbyrt J, et al. Interleukin-10 regulation in normal subjects and patients with asthma. J Allergy Clin Immunol 1996;97:1288-96.
61. Bradley LM, Dalton DK, Croft M. A direct role for IFN-γ in regulation of Th1 cell development. J Immunol 1996;157:1350-8.
62. Brinkmann V, Kinzel B, Kristofic C. TCR-independent activation of human CD4+ 45RO-T cells by anti-CD28 plus IL-2: Induction of clonal expansion and priming for a Th2 phenotype. J Immunol 1996;156:4100-6.
63. Brod SA, Marshall GD Jr, Henninger EM, et al. Interferon-β 1b treatment decreases tumor necrosis factor-α and increases interleukin-6 production in multiple sclerosis. Neurology 1996;46:1633-8.
64. Brown PM, Tagari P, Rowan KR, et al. Epitope-labeled soluble human interleukin-5 (IL-5) receptors. Affinity cross-link labeling, IL-5 binding, and biological activity. J Biol Chem 1995;270:29236-43.
65. Broxmeyer HE. Is interleukin-17, an inducible cytokine that stimulates production of other cytokines, merely a redundant player in a sea of other biomolecules? J Exp Med 1996;183:2411-5.
66. Broxmeyer HE, Cooper S, Hague N, et al. Human chemokines: enhancement of specific activity and effects in vitro on normal and leukemic progenitors and a factor-dependent cell line and in vivo in mice. Ann Hematol 1995;71:235-46.
67. Bubel S, Wilhelm D, Entelmann M, et al. Chemokines in stored platelet concentrates. Transfusion 1996;36:445-9.
68. Burdin N, Galibert L, Garrone P, et al. Inability to produce IL-6 is a functional feature of human germinal center B lymphocytes. J Immunol 1996;156: 4107-13.
69. Burke-Gaffney A, Brooks AVS, Bogle RG. Regulation of chemokine expression in atherosclerosis. Vascular Pharmacy 2002;38:283-92.
70. Busse WW, Lemanske RF. Asthma. New Engl J Med 2001;344:350-62.
71. Callard R, Gearing A. The cytokine factsbook. Orlando: Academic Press, 2001.
72. Campbell PM, Pimm J, Ramassar V, Halloran PF. Identification of a calcium-inducible, cyclosporine sensitive element in the IFN-γ promoter that is a potential NFAT binding site. Transplantation 1996;61:933-9.
73. Cantorna MT, Nashold FE, Chun TY, Hayes CE. Vitamin A down-regulation of IFN-γ synthesis in cloned mouse Th1 lymphocytes depends on the CD28 costimulatory pathway. J Immunol 1996;156:2674-9.
74. Caput D, Laurent P, Kaghad M, et al. Cloning and characterization of a specific interleukin IL-13 binding protein structurally related to the IL-5 receptor α chain. J Biol Chem 1996;271:16921-6.
75. Carini C, Fratazzi C. CD23 expression in activated human T cells is enhanced by interleukin-7. Int Arch Allergy Immunol 1996;110:23-30.
76. Casale TB, Costa JJ, Galli SJ. TNF α is important in human lung allergic reactions. Am J Respir Cell Mol Biol 1996;15:35-44.
77. Catania RA, Schwacha MG, Cioffi WG, et al. Does uninjured skin release proinflammatory cytokines following trauma and hemorrhage? Arch Surg 1999;134:368-74.
78. Center DM, Cruikshank WW. Modulation of lymphocyte migration by human lymphokines. I. Identification and characterization of chemoattractant

activity for lymphocytes from mitogen-stimulated mononuclear cells. J Immunol 1982;128:2563-8.

79. Center DM, Kornfeld H, Cruikshank WW. Interleukin-16 and its function as a CD4 ligand. Immuno Today 1996;17:476-81.
80. Chai Z, Gatti S, Toniatti C, et al. Interleukin (IL)-6 gene expression in the central nervous system is necessary for fever response to lipopolysaccharide or IL-1 β: a study on IL-6-deficient mice. J Exp Med 1996;183:311-6.
81. Chan SD, Luedke G, Valer M, Buhlmann C, Preckel T. Cytometric analysis of protein expression and apoptosis in human primary cells with a novel microfluidic chip-based system. Cytometry 2003;55A(2):119-25.
82. Chang AE, Cameron MJ, Sondak VK, et al. A phase II trial of interleukin-2 and interferon-α in the treatment of metastatic colorectal carcinoma. J Immunother Emphasis Tumor Immunol 1995;18:253-62.
83. Chaouchi N, Wallon C, Goujard C, et al. Interleukin-13 inhibits interleukin-2-induced proliferation and protects chronic lymphocytic leukemia B cells from in vitro apoptosis. Blood 1996;87:1022-9.
84. Chavarria A, Alcocer-Varela J. Is damage in central nervous system due to inflammation? Autoimmunity Rev 2004;3:251-60.
85. Cherel M, Sorel M, Apiou F, et al. The human interleukin-11 receptor α gene (IL11RA): genomic organization and chromosome mapping. Genomics 1996;32:49-53.
86. Chevalier S, Fourcin M, Robledo O, et al. Interleukin-6 family of cytokines induced activation of different functional sites expressed by gp130 transducing protein. J Biol Chem 1996;271:14764-72.
87. Chou DH, Lee W, McCulloch CA. TNF-α inactivation of collagen receptors: Implications for fibroblast function and fibrosis. J Immunol 1996;156:4354-62.
88. Choy EHS, Panayi GS. Cytokine pathways and joint inflammation in rheumatoid arthritis. New Engl J Med 2001;344:907-16.
89. Chujor CS, Klein L, Lam C. Selective inhibition of interleukin-1 β gene expression in activated RAW 264.7 macrophages by interferon-gamma. Eur J Immunol 1996;26:1253-9.
90. Chung JH, Youn SH, Koh WS, et al. Ultraviolet B irradiation-enhanced interleukin (IL)-6 production and mRNA expression are mediated by IL-1 α in cultured human keratinocytes. J Invest Dermatol 1996;106:715-20.
91. Clark-Lewis I, Kim KS, Rajarathnam K, et al. Structure-activity relationships of chemokines. J Leukoc Biol 1995;57:703-11.
92. Clarke D, Katoh O, Gibbs RV, et al. Interaction of interleukin 7 (IL-7) with glycosaminoglycans and its biological relevance. Cytokine 1995;7:325-30.
93. Cohen J. AIDS conference. Chemokines share center stage with drug therapies [news]. Science 1996;273:302-3.
94. Cohen S, Pick E, Oppenheim JJ, Eds Biology of the Lymphokines. New York, Academic Press, 1979.
95. Combadiere C, Ahuja SK, Tiffany HL, Murphy PM. Cloning and functional expression of CC CKR5, a human monocyte CC chemokine receptor selective for MIP-1(α), MIP-1(β), and RANTES. J Leukoc Biol 1996;60:147-52.
96. Combadiere C, Ahuja SK, Van-Damme J, et al. Monocyte chemoattractant protein-3 is a functional ligand for CC chemokine receptors 1 and 2B. J Biol Chem 1995;270:29671-5.
97. Corcoran AE, Smart FM, Cowling RJ, et al. The interleukin-7 receptor chain transmits distinct signals for proliferation and differentiation during B lymphopoiesis. EMBO J 1996;15:1924-32.
98. Corssmit EP, Heyligenberg R, Endert E, et al. Acute effects of interferon-α administration on thyroid hormone metabolism in healthy men. J Clin Endocrinol Metab 1996;80:3140-4.
99. Cortelezzi A, Sarina B, Cattaneo C, et al. In vitro effects of IL-2 on NK-activity, clonogenic potential, blast cell proliferation and cytokine release of MDS bone marrow patients. Leukemia 1996;10:1181-9.
100. Coventry BJ, Weeks SC, Heckford SE, et al. Lack of IL-2 cytokine expression despite Il-2 messenger RNA transcription in tumor-infiltrating lymphocytes in primary human breast carcinoma: selective expression of early activation markers. J Immunol 1996;156:3486-92.
101. Cowdery JS, Chace JH, Yi AK, Krieg AM. Bacterial DNA induces NK cells to produce IFN-γ in vivo and increases the toxicity of lipopolysaccharides. J Immunol 1996;156:4570-5.
102. Coyle P, Philcox JC, Rofe AM. Metallothionein induction in cultured rat hepatocytes by arthritic rat serum, activated macrophages, interleukin-6, interleukin-11 and leukaemia inhibitory factor. Inflamm Res 1996;44:475-81.
103. Coyne CB, Vanhook MK, Gambling TM. Regulation of airway tight junctions by proinflammatory cytokines. Molecular Biology of the Cell 2002;13;3218-34.
104. Crawley JB, Williams LM, Mander T, et al. Interleukin-10 stimulation of phosphatidylinositol 3-kinase and p70 S6 kinase is required for the proliferative but not the antiinflammatory effects of the cytokine. J Biol Chem 1996;271:16357-62.
105. Cruikshank WW, Lim K, Theodore AC, et al. IL-16 inhibition of CD3-dependent lymphocyte activation and proliferation. J Immunol 1996;157:5240-8.
106. Cruikshank WW, Long A, Tarpy RE, et al. Early identification of interleukin-16 (lymphocyte chemoattractant factor) and macrophage inflamma-

tory protein 1 α (MIP1 α) in bronchoalveolar lavage fluid of antigen-challenged asthmatics. Am J Respir Cell Mol Biol 1995;13:738-47.
107. Cumberbatch M, Dearman RJ, Kimber I. Constitutive and inducible expression of interleukin-6 by Langerhans cells and lymph node dendritic cells. Immunology 1996;87:513-8.
108. Curcio C, Di Carlo E, Clynes R, et al. Nonredundant roles of antibody, cytokines, and perforin in the eradication of established Her-2/neu carcinomas. J Clin Invest 2003;111:1161-70.
109. Daftarian PM, Diaz-Mitoma F, Creery WD, et al. Dysregulated production of interleukin-10 (IL-10) and IL-12 by peripheral blood lymphocytes from human immunodeficiency virus-infected individuals is associated with altered proliferative responses to recall antigens. Clin Diagn Lab Immunol 1995;2:712-8.
110. Daftarian PM, Kumar A, Kryworuchko M, Diaz-Mitoma F. IL-10 production is enhanced in human T cells by IL-12 and IL-6 and in monocytes by tumor necrosis factor-α. J Immunol 1996;157:12-20.
111. Dalrymple SA, Slattery R, Aud DM, et al. Interleukin-6 is required for a protective immune response to systemic *Escherichia coli* infection. Infect Immun 1996;64:3231-5.
112. Dao T, Ohashi K, Kayano T, et al. Interferon-gamma-inducing factor, a novel cytokine, enhances Fas ligand-mediated cytotoxicity of murine T helper 1 cells. Cell Immunol 1996;173:230-5.
113. Dasu MR, Hawkins HK, Barrow RE, Xue H, Herndon DN. Gene expression profiles from hypertrophic scar fibroblasts before and after IL-6 stimulation. J Pathol 2004;202:476-85.
114. Davidson A, Diamond B. Autoimmune diseases. New Engl J Med 2001;345:340-50.
115. Damås JK, Gullestad L, Aukrust P. Cytokines as new treatment targets in chronic heart failure. Curr Control Trials Cardiovasc Med 2001;2:271-7.
116. De Francesco MA, Baronio M, Fiorentini S, et al. HIV-1 matrix protein p17 increases the production of proinflammatory cytokines and counteracts IL-4 activity by binding to a cellular receptor. Proc Natl Acad Sci USA 2002;99:9972-7.
117. de Jager W, te Velthuis H, Prakken BJ, Kuis W, Rijkers GT. Simultaneous detection of 15 human cytokines in a single sample of stimulated peripheral blood mononuclear cells. Clin Diagn Lab Immunol 2003;10:133-9.
118. de Jong JL, Farner NL, Widmer MB, et al. Interaction of IL-15 with the shared IL-2 receptor β and gamma c subunits. The IL-15/β/gamma c receptor-ligand complex is less stable than the IL-2/β/gamma c receptor-ligand complex. J Immunol 1996;156:1339-48.
119. de Jong AL, Green DM, Trial JA, Birdsall HH. Focal effects of mononuclear leukocyte transendothelial migration: TNF-α production by migrating monocytes promotes subsequent migration of lymphocytes. J Leukoc Biol 1996;60:129-36.
120. de Waal-Malefyt R, Abrams JS, Zurawski SM, et al. Differential regulation of IL-13 and IL-4 production by human $CD8^+$ and $CD4^+$ Th0, Th1 and Th2 T cell clones and EBV-transformed B cells. Int Immunol 1995;7:1405-16.
121. de Wit D, Flemming CL, Harris JD, et al. IL-12 stimulation but not B7 expression increases melanoma killing by patient cytotoxic T lymphocytes (CTL). Clin Exp Immunol 1996;105:353-9.
122. Deakin AM, Payne AN, Whittle BJ, Moncada S. The modulation of IL-6 and TNF-α release by nitric oxide following stimulation of J774 cells with LPS and IFN-γ. Cytokine 1995;7:408-16.
123. del Pozo MA, Sanchez-Mateos P, Nieto M, Sanchez-Madrid F. Chemokines regulate cellular polarization and adhesion receptor redistribution during lymphocyte interaction with endothelium and extracellular matrix. Involvement of cAMP signaling pathway. J Cell Biol 1995;131:495-508.
124. Deleuran B, Iversen L, Deleuran M, et al. Interleukin 13 suppresses cytokine production and stimulates the production of 15-HETE in PBMC. A comparison between IL-4 and IL-13. Cytokine 1995;7:319-24.
125. Demoulin JB, Uyttenhove C, Van Roost E, et al. A single tyrosine of the interleukin-9 (IL-9) receptor is required for STAT activation, antiapoptotic activity, and growth regulation by IL-9. Mol Cell Biol 1996;16:4710-6.
126. Denning GM. IL-4 and IFN-γ synergistically increase total polymeric IgA receptor levels in human intestinal epithelial cells. Role of protein tyrosine kinases. J Immunol 1996;156:4807-14.
127. Dickason RR, Huston DP. Creation of a biologically active interleukin-5 monomer. Nature 1996;379:652-5.
128. Dickason RR, Huston MM, Huston DP. Delineation of IL-5 domains predicted to engage the IL-5 receptor complex. J Immunol 1996;156:1030-7.
129. Dinarello CA. Biologic basis for interleukin-1 in disease. Blood 1996;87:2095-147.
130. Dinarello CA, Abraham E. Does blocking cytokines in sepsis work? Am J Respir Crit Care Med 2002;166:1155-6.
131. Doherty TM, Seder RA, Sher A. Induction and regulation of IL-15 expression in murine macrophages. J Immunol 1996;156:735-41.
132. Dokter WHA, Koopmans SB, Vellenga E. Effects of IL-10 and IL-4 on LPS-induced transcription factors (AP-1, NF-IL6 and NF-kappa B) which are involved in IL-6 regulation. Leukemia 1996;10:1308-16.
133. Dolecek C, Steinberger P, Susani M, et al. Effects of IL-4 and IL-13 on total and allergen specific IgE production by cultured PBMC from allergic patients determined with recombinant pollen allergens. Clin Exp Allergy 1995;25:879-89.

134. Dolen JG, Mathur A. Undetectable interferon-α serum levels in a patient with atopic dermatitis. J Interferon Cytokine Res 1995;15:973-5.
135. Dolganov G, Bort S, Lovett M, et al. Coexpression of the interleukin-13 and interleukin-4 genes correlates with their physical linkage in the cytokine gene cluster on human chromosome 5q23-31. Blood 1996;87:3316-26.
136. Dolhain RJ, ter Haar NT, Hoefakker S, et al. Increased expression of interferon (IFN)-gamma together with IFN-γ receptor in the rheumatoid synovial membrane compared with synovium of patients with osteoarthritis. Br J Rheumatol 1996;35:24-32.
137. Dominguez F, Pellicer A, Simon C. The chemokine connection: Hormonal and embryonic regulation at the human maternal-embryonic interface—A review. Placenta 2003;24:S48-55.
138. Dorland WA. Dorland's illustrated medical dictionary, 30th Edition. Philadelphia: W B Saunders, 2003.
139. Dorner BG, Scheffold A, Rolph MS. MIP-1α, MIP-1β, RANTES, and ATAC/lymphotactin function together with IFN-γ as type 1 cytokines. Proc Natl Acad Sci USA 2002;99:6181-6.
140. Douglas MR, Morrison KE, Salmon M, Buckley CD. Why does inflammation persist: a dominant role for the stromal microenvironment? Expert Reviews in Mol Med 2002, 9/12, 1-18.
141. Dragic T, Litwin V, Allaway GP, et al. HIV-1 entry into CD4+ cells is mediated by the chemokine receptor CC-CKR-5 [see comments]. Nature 1996;381:667-73.
142. Dragic T. An overview of the determinants of CCR5 and CXCR4 co-receptor function. J Gen Virol 2001;82:1807-14
143. Drenth JP, Van Uum SH, Van Deuren M, et al. Endurance run increases circulating IL-6 and IL-1ra but down-regulates ex vivo TNF-α and IL-1 β production. J Appl Physiol 1995;79:1497-503.
144. Drevets DA, Leenen PJ, Campbell PA. Complement receptor type 3 mediates phagocytosis and killing of Listeria monocytogenes by a TNF-α- and IFN-α-stimulated macrophage precursor hybrid. Cell Immunol 1996;169:1-6.
145. Driscoll KE, Hassenbein DG, Carter JM, et al. TNF α and increased chemokine expression in rat lung after particle exposure. Toxicol Lett 1995;82-83:483-9.
146. Du W, Xu Z, Ma X, Song L, Schneider EM. Biochip as a potential platform of serological interferon alpha2b antibody assay. J Biotechnol 2003;106:87-100.
147. Dudda JC, Martin SF. Tissue targeting of T cells by DCs and microenvironments. Trends Immunol 2004;25:417-21.
148. Dugas N, Vouldoukis I, Becherel P, et al. Triggering of CD23b antigen by anti-CD23 monoclonal antibodies induces interleukin-10 production by human macrophages. Eur J Immunol 1996;26:1394-8.
149. Dunger A, Cunningham JM, Delaney CA, et al. Tumor necrosis factor-α and interferon-gamma inhibit insulin secretion and cause DNA damage in unweaned-rat islets. Extent of nitric oxide involvement. Diabetes 1996;45:183-9.
150. Earley MC, Vogt RF Jr, Shapiro HM, Mandy FF, Kellar KL, et al. Report from a workshop on multianalyte microsphere assays. Cytometry 2002;50:239-42.
151. Eggesbo JB, Hjermann I, Hostmark AT, Kierulf P. LPS induced release of IL-1 β, IL-6, IL-8 and TNF-α in EDTA or heparin anticoagulated whole blood from persons with high or low levels of serum HDL. Cytokine 1996;8:152-60.
152. Elgert KD. Immunology: Understanding the immune system. New York: Wiley-Liss, 1996.
153. Ellstrom M, Bengtsson A, Tylman M, et al. Evaluation of tissue trauma after laparoscopic and abdominal hysterectomy: measurements of neutrophil activation and release of interleukin-6, cortisol, and C-reactive protein. J Am Coll Surg 1996;182:423-30.
154. Endo T, Ogushi F, Sone S. LPS-dependent cyclooxygenase-2 induction in human monocytes is down-regulated by IL-13, but not by IFN-γ. J Immunol 1996;156:2240-6.
155. Endres S, Whitaker RE, Ghorbani R, et al. Oral aspirin and ibuprofen increase cytokine-induced synthesis of IL-1 β and of tumour necrosis factor-α ex vivo. Immunology 1996;87:264-70.
156. Epplen C, Rumpf H, Albert E, et al. Immunoprinting excludes many potential susceptibility genes as predisposing to early onset pauciarticular juvenile chronic arthritis except HLA class II and TNF. Eur J Immunogenet 1995;22:311-22.
157. Esnault S, Benbernou N, Lavaud F, et al. Differential spontaneous expression of mRNA for IL-4, IL-10, IL-13, IL-2 and interferon-gamma (IFN-γ) in peripheral blood mononuclear cells (PBMC) from atopic patients. Clin Exp Immunol 1996;103:111-8.
158. Fantuzzi G, Zheng H, Faggioni R. Effect of endotoxin in IL-1 β-deficient mice. J Immunol 1996;157:291-6.
159. Fantuzzi L, Gessani S, Borghi P, et al. Induction of interleukin-12 (IL-12) by recombinant glycoprotein gp120 of human immunodeficiency virus type 1 in human monocytes/macrophages: Requirement of gamma interferon for IL-12 secretion. J Virol 1996;70:4121-4.
160. Faro A, Kurland G, Michaels MG, et al. Interferon-α affects the immune response in post-transplant lymphoproliferative disorder. Am J Respir Crit Care Med 1996;153:1442-7.
161. Fasler S, Aversa G, Terr A, et al. Peptide-induced anergy in allergen-specific human Th2 cells results in lack of cytokine production and B cell help for IgE synthesis. Reversal by IL-2, not by IL-4 or IL-13. J Immunol 1995;155:4199-206.

162. Feldmann M, Brennan FM, Elliott MJ, et al. TNF α is an effective therapeutic target for rheumatoid arthritis. Ann N Y Acad Sci 1995;766:272-8.
163. Fiebich BL, Biber K, Gyufko K, et al. Adenosine A2b receptors mediate an increase in interleukin (IL)-6 mRNA and IL-6 protein synthesis in human astroglioma cells. J Neurochem1996;66:1426-31.
164. Finnegan A, Roebuck KA, Nakai BE, et al. IL-10 cooperates with TNF-α to activate HIV-1 from latently and acutely infected cells of monocyte/macrophage lineage. J Immunol 1996;156:841-51.
165. Fischer CP, Bode BP, Takahashi K, et al. Glucocorticoid-dependent induction of interleukin-6 receptor expression in human hepatocytes facilitates interleukin-6 stimulation of amino acid transport. Ann Surg 1996;223:610-18, [discussion] 618-9.
166. Fisher CJ, Agosti JM Jr, Opal SM, et al. Treatment of septic shock with the tumor necrosis factor receptor: Fc fusion protein. The Soluble TNF Receptor Sepsis Study Group. N Engl J Med1996;334:1697-702.
167. Fitzpatrick DR, Kelso A. Dissociated expression of granulocyte-macrophage CSF and IL-3 in short-term T cell clones from normal mice. J Immunol 1995;155:5140-50.
168. Fortis C, Foppoli M, Gianotti L, et al. Increased interleukin-10 serum levels in patients with solid tumours. Cancer Lett 1996;104:1-5.
169. Fossiez F, Djossou O, Chomarat P, et al. T cell interleukin-17 induces stromal cells to produce proinflammatory and hematopoietic cytokines [see comments]. J Exp Med 1996;183:2593-603.
170. Fourcin M, Chevalier S, Guillet C, et al. gp130 transducing receptor cross-linking is sufficient to induce interleukin-6 type responses. J Biol Chem 1996;271:11756-60.
171. Fox DA. Cytokine Blockade as a New Strategy to Treat Rheumatoid Arthritis-Inhibition of Tumor Necrosis Factor. Arch Intern Med. 2000;160:437-44.
172. Foxwell BM, Beadling C, Guschin D, et al. Interleukin-7 can induce the activation of Jak 1, Jak 3 and STAT 5 proteins in murine T cells. Eur J Immunol 1995;25:3041-6.
173. Francis ML, Fan XS, Meltzer MS. Loss ability to produce IFN-α in response to HIV-1 as monocytes differentiate into macrophages. Induction through a mechanism independent of double-stranded RNA. J Immunol 1996;156:2481-7.
174. Friedlander RM, Gagliardini V, Rotello RJ, Yuan J. Functional role of interleukin 1 β (IL-1 β) in IL-1 β-converting enzyme-mediated apoptosis. J Exp Med 1996;184:717-24.
175. Frucht DM, Holland SM. Defective monocyte costimulation for IFN-γ production in familial disseminated Mycobacterium avium complex infection: abnormal IL-12 regulation. J Immunol 1996;157:411-6.
176. Fuhrer DK, Yang YC. Complex formation of JAK2 with PP2A, P13K, and Yes in response to the hematopoietic cytokine interleukin-11. Biochem Biophys Res Commun 1996;224:289-96.
177. Fujihashi K, Kawabata S, Hiroi T, et al. Interleukin 2 (IL-2) and interleukin 7 (IL-7) reciprocally induce IL-7 and IL-2 receptors on gamma delta T-cell receptor-positive intraepithelial lymphocytes. Proc Natl Acad Sci USA 1996;93:3613-8.
178. Fujimoto T, O'Donnell MA, Szilvasi A, et al. Bacillus Calmette-Guerin plus interleukin-2 and/or granulocyte/macrophage colony stimulating factor enhances immunocompetent cell production of interferon-gamma, which inhibits B16F10 melanoma cell growth in vitro. Cancer Immunol Immunother 1996;42:280-4.
179. Fulton SA, Johnsen JM, Wolf SF, et al. Interleukin-12 production by human monocytes infected with Mycobacterium tuberculosis: role of phagocytosis. Infect Immun 1996;64:2523-31.
180. Fuss IJ, Neurath M, Boirivant M, et al. Disparate CD4[+] lamina propria (LP) lymphokine secretion profiles in inflammatory bowel disease. Crohn's disease LP cells manifest increased secretion of IFN-γ, whereas ulcerative colitis LP cells manifest increased secretion of IL-5. J Immunol 1996;157:1261-70.
181. Gabay C, Singwe M, Genin B, et al. Circulating levels of IL-11 and leukaemia inhibitory factor (LIF) do not significantly participate in the production of acute-phase proteins by the liver. Clin Exp Immunol 1996;105:260-5.
182. Gaspari AA, Sempowski GD, Chess P, et al. Human epidermal keratinocytes are induced to secrete interleukin-6 and co-stimulate T lymphocyte proliferation by a CD40-dependent mechanism. Eur J Immunol 1996;26:1371-7.
183. Gately MK, Brunda MJ. [The potential of interleukin-12 for use in cancer therapy]. Gan To Kagaku Ryoho 1996;23:961-71.
184. Gately MK, Gubler U, Brunda MJ, et al. Interleukin-12: a cytokine with therapeutic potential in oncology and infectious diseases. Ther Immunol 1994;1:187-96.
185. Gerosa F, Paganin C, Peritt D, et al. Interleukin-12 primes human CD4 and CD8 T cell clones for high production of both interferon-gamma and interleukin-10. J Exp Med 1996;183:2559-69.
186. Gesser B, Lund M, Lohse N, et al. IL-8 induces T cell chemotaxis, suppresses IL-4, and up-regulates IL-8 production by CD4[+] T cells. J Leukoc Biol 1996;59:407-11.
187. Gewurz H, Zhang XH, Lint TF. Structure and functions of the pentraxins. Curr Opin Immunol 1995;7:54-64.
188. Ghaffari S, Jagani, Kitidis C, et al. Cytokines and BCR-ABL mediate suppression of TRAIL-induced

apoptosis through inhibition of forkhead FOXO3a transcription factor. PANS 2003;100:6523-8.
189. Girard D, Paquin R, Naccache PH, Beaulieu AD. Effects of interleukin-13 on human neutrophil functions. J Leukoc Biol 1996;59:412-9.
190. Girdlestone J, Wing M. Autocrine activation by interferon-gamma of STAT factors following T cell activation. Eur J Immunol 1996;26:704-9.
191. Giri JG, Anderson DM, Kumaki S, et al. Il-15, a novel T cell growth factor that shares activities and receptor components with Il-2. J Leukoc Biol 1995;57:763-6.
192. Glaser R, Kiecolt-Glaser JK, Marucha PT, et al. Stress-related changes in proinflammatory cytokine production in wounds. Arch Gen Psychiatry 1999;56:450-6.
193. Goletti D, Kinter AL, Hardy EC, et al. Modulation of endogenous IL-1 β and IL-1 receptor antagonist results in opposing effects on HIV expression in chronically infected monocytic cells. J Immuno 1996;56:3501-8.
194. Gollner G, Aman MJ, Steffens HP, et al. Interferon-α (IFN-α) inhibits granulocyte-macrophage colony stimulating factor (GM-CSF) expression at the post-transcriptional level in murine bone marrow stromal cells. Br J Haematol 1995;91:8-14.
195. Gong JH, Uguccioni M, Dewald B, et al. RANTES and MCP-3 antagonists bind multiple chemokine receptors. J Biol Chem 1996;271:10521-7.
196. Gossart S, Cambon C, Orfila C, et al. Reactive oxygen intermediates as regulators of TNF-α production in rat lung inflammation induced by silica. J Immuno 1996;156:1540-8.
197. Grabstein KH, Eisenman J, Shanebeck K, Rauch C, Srinivasan S, et al. Cloning of a T cell growth factor that interacts with the beta chain of the interleukin-2 receptor. Science 1994;264:965-8.
198. Gratama JW, Schmitz PI, Goey SH, et al. Modulation of immune parameters in patients with metastatic renal-cell cancer receiving combination immunotherapy (IL-2, IFN α and autologous IL-2-activated lymphocytes). Int J Cancer 1996;65:152-60.
199. Greenfield EM, Horowitz MC, Lavish SA. Stimulation by parathyroid hormone of interleukin-6 and leukemia inhibitory factor expression in osteoblasts is an immediate-early gene response induced by cAMP signal transduction. J Biol Chem 1996;271:10984-9.
200. Greenfeder S, Umland SP, Cuss FM, et al. Th2 cytokines and asthmaThe role of interleukin-5 in allergic eosinophilic disease. Respir Res 2001;2:71-9.
201. Groux H, Bigler M, de Vries JE, Roncarolo MG. Interleukin-10 induces a long-term antigen-specific anergic state in human $CD4^+$ T cells [see comments]. J Exp Med 1996;184:19-29.
202. Groves RW, Rauschmayr T, Nakamura K, et al. Inflammatory and hyperproliferative skin disease in mice that express elevated levels of the IL-1 receptor (type I) on epidermal keratinocytes. Evidence that IL-1-inducible secondary cytokines produced by keratinocytes in vivo can cause skin disease. J Clin Invest 1996;98:336-44.
203. Gunther G, Fechteler T, Villmann C, et al. Computer-aided modeling of structure stabilizing disulfide bonds in recombinant human interferon-gamma. Pharm Acta Helv 1996;71:37-44.
204. Gura T. Chemokines take center stage in inflammatory ills [news]. Science 1996;272:954-6.
205. Hagiwara E, Abbasi F, Mor G, et al. Phenotype and frequency of cells secreting IL-2, IL-4, IL-6, IL-10, IFN and TNF-α in human peripheral blood. Cytokine 1995;7:815-22.
206. Hagiwara E, Gourley MF, Lee S, Klinman DK. Disease severity in patients with systemic lupus erythematosus correlates with an increased ratio of interleukin-10: interferon-gamma-secreting cells in the peripheral blood. Arthritis Rheum 1996;39:379-85.
207. Hamid Q, Naseer T, Minshall EM, et al. In vivo expression of IL-12 and IL-13 in atopic dermatitis. J Allergy Clin Immuno 1996;98:225-31.
208. Hamilton TA, Major JA. Oxidized LDL potentiates LPS-induced transcription of the chemokine KC gene. J Leukoc Biol 1996;59:940-7.
209. Hartmann K, Beiglbock F, Czarnetzki BM, Zuberbier T. Effect of CC chemokines on mediator release from human skin mast cells and basophils. Int Arch Allergy Immuno 1995;108:224-30.
210. Hattori A, Hayashi K, Kohno M. Tumor necrosis factor (TNF) stimulates the production of nerve growth factor in fibroblasts via the 55-kDa type 1 TNF receptor. FEBS Lett 1996;379:157-60.
211. Hempel SL, Monick MM, Hunninghake GW. Effect of hypoxia on release of IL-1 and TNF by human alveolar macrophages. Am J Respir Cell Mol Biol 1996;14:170-6.
212. Heney D, Whitcher JT. Factors affecting the measurement of cytokines in biological fluids: Implications for their clinical measurement. Ann Clin Biochem 1995;32:358-68.
213. Herbein G, Doyle AG, Montaner LJ, Gordon S. Lipopolysaccharide (LPS) down-regulates CD4 expression in primary human macrophages through induction of endogenous tumour necrosis factor (TNF) and IL-1 β. Clin Exp Immuno 1995;102:430-7.
214. Heredia A, Davis C, Amoroso A, et al. Induction of G1 cycle arrest in T lymphocytes results in increased extracellular levels of β-chemokines: A strategy to inhibit R5 HIV-1. Proc Natl Acad Sci USA 2003;100:4179-84.
215. Herzberg F, Schoning M, Schirner M, et al. IL-4 and TNF-α induce changes in integrin expression and adhesive properties and decrease the lung-colonizing potential of HT-29 colon carcinoma cells. Clin Exp Metastasis 1996;14:165-75.

216. Heufler C, Koch F, Stanzl U, et al. Interleukin-12 is produced by dendritic cells and mediates T helper 1 development as well as interferon-gamma production by T helper 1 cells. Eur J Immuno 1996;26:659-68.
217. Hilkens CM, Snijders A, Vermeulen H, et al. Accessory cell-derived IL-12 and prostaglandin E2 determine the IFN-γ level of activated human $CD4^+$ T cells. J Immuno 1996;156:1722-7.
218. Holst PJ, Rosenkilde MM. Microbiological exploitation of the chemokine system. Microbes and Infection 2003;5:179-87.
219. Holyoake TL, Freshney MG, McNair L, et al. Ex vivo expansion with stem cell factor and interleukin-11 augments both short-term recovery posttransplant and the ability to serially transplant marrow. Blood 1996;87:4589-95.
220. Hoogewerf A, Black D, Proudfoot AE, et al. Molecular cloning of murine CC CKR-4 and high affinity binding of chemokines to murine and human CC CKR-4. Biochem Biophys Res Commun 1996;218:337-43.
221. Hopken U, Mohr M, Struber A, et al. Inhibition of interleukin-6 synthesis in an animal model of septic shock by anti-C5a monoclonal antibodies. Eur J Immuno 1996;26:1103-9.
222. Horuk R. Development and evaluation of pharmacological agents targeting chemokine receptors. Methods 2003;29:369-75.
223. Horuk R. The interleukin-8-receptor family: from chemokines to malaria. Immuno Today 1994;15: 169-74.
224. Horuk R, Martin A, Hesselgesser J, et al. The Duffy antigen receptor for chemokines: structural analysis and expression in the brain. J Leukoc Biol 1996;59:29-38.
225. Hotchkiss RS, Karl IE. The pathophysiology of treatment of sepis. N Engl J Med 2003;248:138-50.
226. Houshman P, Zlotnik A. Therapeutic applications in the chemokine superfamily. Curr Opin Chem Biol 2003;7:457-60.
227. Hughes CB, Gaber LW, Mohey-el-Din AB, et al. Inhibition of TNF α improves survival in an experimental model of acute pancreatitis. Am Surg 1996;62:8-13.
228. Huising MO, Stet RJM, Kruiswijk CP, et al. Molecular evolution of CXC chemokines: extant CXC chemokines originate from the CNS. Trends Immunol 2003;24:206-12.
229. Huising MO, Stet RJM, Kruiswijk CP, et al. Response to shields: molecular evolution of CXC chemokines and receptors. Trends Immunol 2003;24:256-7.
230. Hunter CA, Slifer T, Araujo F. Interleukin-12-mediated resistance to Trypanosoma cruzi is dependent on tumor necrosis factor α and gamma interferon. Infect Immun 1996;64:2381-6.
231. Hurwitz N, Probst A, Zufferey G, et al. Fatal vascular leak syndrome with extensive hemorrhage, peripheral neuropathy and reactive erythrophagocytosis: an unusual complication of recombinant IL-3 therapy. Leuk Lymphoma 1996;20:337-40.
232. Hussaini IM, LaMarre J, Lysiak JJ, et al. Transcriptional regulation of LDL receptor-related protein by IFN-γ and the antagonistic activity of TGF-β(1) in the RAW 264.7 macrophage-like cell line. J Leukoc Biol 1996;59:733-9.
233. Huston MM, Moore JP, Mettes HJ, et al. Human B cells express IL-5 receptor messenger ribonucleic acid and respond to IL-5 with enhanced IgM production after mitogenic stimulation with Moraxella catarrhalis. J Immuno 1996;156:1392-401.
234. Hwang ES, White IA, Cheng Ho I. An IL-4-independent and CD25-mediated function of c-maf in promoting the production of Th2 cytokines. Proc Natl Acad Sci USA 2002;99:13026-30.
235. Ishii E, Yamamoto S, Sakai R, et al. Production of interleukin-5 and the suppressive effect of cyclosporin A in childhood severe atopic dermatitis. J Pediatr 1996;128:152-5.
236. Izquierdo MA, Degen D, Myers L, et al. Effects of the hematopoietic growth factors GM-CSF, IL-3, and IL-6 on human tumor colony-forming units taken directly from patients. Ann Oncol 1995;6:927-32.
237. Izuhara K, Heike T, Otsuka T, et al. Signal transduction pathway of interleukin-4 and interleukin-13 in human B cells derived from X-linked severe combined immunodeficiency patients. J Biol Chem 1996;271:619-22.
238. Jaattela M, Mouritzen H, Elling F, Bastholm L. A20 zinc finger protein inhibits TNF and IL-1 signaling. J Immuno 1996;156:1166-73.
239. Jacobsen FW, Veiby OP, Stokke T, Jacobsen SE. TNF-α bidirectionally modulates the viability of primitive murine hematopoietic progenitor cells in vitro. J Immuno 1996;157:1193-9.
240. Jaffe JS, Glaum MC, Raible DG, et al. Human lung mast cell IL-5 gene and protein expression: temporal analysis of upregulation following IgE-mediated activation. Am J Respir Cell Mol Biol 1995;13: 665-75.
241. Jahnke A, Johnson JP. Intercellular adhesion molecule 1 (ICAM-1) is synergistically activated by TNF-α and IFN-γ responsive sites. Immunobiology 1995;193: 305-14.
242. Jansen PM, de Jong IW, Hart M, et al. Release of leukemia inhibitory factor in primate sepsis. Analysis of the role of TNF-α. J Immuno 1996;156:4401-7.
243. Jansen PM, van der Pouw-Kraan TC, de Jong IW, et al. Release of interleukin-12 in experimental *Escherichia coli* septic shock in baboons: Relation to plasma levels of interleukin-10 and interferon-gamma. Blood 1996;87:5144-51.

244. Jeannin P, Delneste Y, Lecoanet-Henchoz S, et al. Thiols decrease human interleukin (IL) 4 production and IL-4-induced immunoglobulin synthesis. J Exp Med 1995;182:1785-92.
245. Jinquan T, Frydenberg J, Mukaida N, et al. Recombinant human growth-regulated oncogene-α (GRO) induces T lymphocyte chemotaxis. A process regulated via IL-8 receptors by IFN-γ, TNF-α, IL-4, IL-10, and IL-13. J Immuno 1995;155:5359-68.
246. Jones BM. Changes in cytokine production in healthy subjects practicing Guolin Qigong: a pilot study. BMC Complementary and Alternative Medicine 2001;1:8.
247. Joyce DA, Steer JH. Tumor necrosis factor α and interleukin-1 α stimulate late shedding of p75 TNF receptors but not p55 TNF receptors from human monocytes. J Interferon Cytokine Res 1995;15:947-54.
248. Jung T, Wijdenes J, Neumann C, et al. Interleukin-13 is produced by activated human CD45RA$^+$ and CD45RO$^+$ T cells: modulation by interleukin-4 and interleukin-12. Eur J Immuno 1996;26:571-7.
249. Kadota J, Matsubara Y, Ishimatsu Y, et al. Significance of IL-1β and IL-1 receptor antagonist (IL-1Ra) in bronchoalveolar lavage fluid (BALF) in patients with diffuse panbronchiolitis (DPB). Clin Exp Immuno 1996;103:461-6.
250. Kallmann BA, Hummel V, Lindenlaub T, et al. Cytokine-induced modulation of cellular adhesion to human cerebral endothelial cells is mediated by soluble vascular cell adhesion molecule-1. Brain 2000;123:687-97.
251. Kanangat S, Babu JS, Knipe DM, Rouse BT. HSV-1-mediated modulation of cytokine gene expression in a permissive cell line: Selective upregulation of IL-6 gene expression. Virology 1996;219:295-300.
252. Kanda T, McManus JE, Nagai R, et al. Modification of viral myocarditis in mice by interleukin-6. Circ Res 1996;78:848-56.
253. Kang K, Kubin M, Cooper KD, et al. IL-12 synthesis by human Langerhans cells. J Immuno 1996;156:1402-7.
254. Kaplan AP, Kuna P, Reddigar SR. Chemokines and the allergic response. Exp Dermatol 19959;4:260-5.
255. Kaplan D. Autocrine secretion and the physiological concentration of cytokines. Immuno Today 1996;17:303-4.
256. Kaplan MH, Sun YL, Hoey T, Grusby MJ. Impaired IL-12 responses and enhanced development of Th2 cells in Stat4-deficient mice. Nature 1996;382: 174-7.
257. Karlen S, D'Ercole M, Sanderson CJ. Two pathways can activate the interleukin-5 gene and induce binding to the conserved lymphokine element 0. Blood 1996;88:211-21.
258. Karpus WJ, Lukacs NW. The role of chemokines in oral tolerance. Abrogation of nonresponsiveness by treatment with antimonocyte chemotactic protein-1. Ann NY Acad Sci 1996;778:133-44.
259. Karpus WJ, Lukacs NW, McRae BL, et al. An important role for the chemokine macrophage inflammatory protein-1 α in the pathogenesis of the T cell-mediated autoimmune disease, experimental autoimmune encephalomyelitis. J Immuno 1995;155:5003-10.
260. Kasper LH, Matsuura T, Khan IA. IL-7 stimulates protective immunity in mice against the intracellular pathogen, Toxoplasma gondii. J Immuno 1995;155:4798-804.
261. Katafuchi T, Take S, Hori T. Roles of cytokines in the neural-immune interactions: Modulation of NMDA responses by IFN-α. Neurobiology Bp 1995;3:319-27.
262. Katamura K, Shintaku N, Yamauchi Y, et al. Prostaglandin E2 at priming of naive CD4$^+$ T cells inhibits acquisition of ability to produce IFN-γ and IL-2, but not IL-4 and IL-5. J Immuno 1995;155:4604-12.
263. Katsikis PD, Cohen SB, Londei M, Feldmann M. Are CD4$^+$ Th1 cells pro-inflammatory or anti-inflammatory? The ratio of IL-10 to IFN-γ or IL-2 determines their function. Int Immuno 1995;7: 1287-94.
264. Kay AB. Allergy and Allergic Diseases. N Engl J Med 2001;344:30-7.
265. Kazmierski W, Bifulco N, Yang H, et al. Recent progress in discovery of small-molecule CCR5 chemokine receptor ligands as HIV-1 inhibitors. Bioorganic Medicinal Chem 2003;11:2663-76.
266. Keane J, Gershon S, Wise RP, et al. Tuberculosis associated with infliximab, a tumor necrosis factor α-neutralizing agent. N Engl J Med 2001;345: 1098-104.
267. Keel M, Bonaccio M, Steckholzer U, et al. [Increased plasma level of Type I (p55) and Type II (p75) TNF-receptors following trauma]. Swiss Surg 1995;5: 241-4.
268. Keelan JA, Blumenstein M, Helliwel RJA, et al. Cytokines, Prostaglandins and Parturition—A Review. Placenta 2003;17;S33-S46.
269. Keenan JA, Chen TT, Chadwell NL, et al. IL-1 β, TNF-α, and IL-2 in peritoneal fluid and macrophage-conditioned media of women with endometriosis. Am J Reprod Immuno 1995;34:381-5.
270. Kelley JL, Chi DS, Abou-Auda W, et al. The molecular role of mast cells in atherosclerotic cardiovascular disease. Mol Med Today 2000 Aug;6:304-8.
271. Kelner GS, Zlotnik A. A cytokine production profile of early thymocytes and the characterization of a new class of chemokine. J Leukoc Biol 1995;57:778-81.
272. Kennedy J, Rossi DL, Zurawski SM, et al. Mouse IL-17: A cytokine preferentially expressed by α β TCR$^+$ CD4-CD8-T cells. J Interferon Cytokine Res 1996;16:611-7.

273. Kienast K, Knorst M, Muller-Quernheim J, Ferlinz R. Modulation of IL-1 β, IL-6, IL-8, TNF-α, and TGF-β secretions by alveolar macrophages under NO_2 exposure. Lung 1996;174:57-67.
274. Kilby JM, Eron JJ. Novel therapies based on mechanisms of HIV-1 cell entry. N Engl J Med 2003;348:2228-38.
275. Kim DS, Lee HK, Noh GW, et al. Increased serum interleukin-10 level in Kawasaki disease. Yonsei Med J 1996;37:125-30.
276. King CL, Medhat A, Malhotra I, et al. Cytokine control of parasite-specific anergy in human urinary schistosomiasis. IL-10 modulates lymphocyte reactivity. J Immuno 1996;156:4715-21.
277. Kirken RA, Rui H, Malabarba MG, et al. Activation of JAK3, but not JAK1, is critical for IL-2-induced proliferation and STAT5 recruitment by a COOH-terminal region of the IL-2 receptor β-chain. Cytokine 1995;7:689-700.
278. Kishihara Y, Hayashi J, Yoshimura E, et al. IL-1 β and TNF-α produced by peripheral blood mononuclear cells before and during interferon therapy in patients with chronic hepatitis C. Dig Dis Sci 1996;41:315-21.
279. Kishimoto K, Sandner S, Imitola J et al. Th1 cytokines, programmed cell death, and alloreactive T cell clone size in transplant tolerance. J Clin Invest 2002;109:1471-9.
280. Kitaura M, Nakajima T, Imai T, et al. Molecular cloning of human eotaxin, an eosinophil-selective CC chemokine, and identification of a specific eosinophil eotaxin receptor, CC chemokine receptor 3. J Biol Chem 1996;271:7725-30.
281. Klein JL, Fickenscher H, Holliday JE, et al. Herpesvirus saimiri immortalized gamma delta T cell line activated by IL-12. J Immuno 1996;156:2754-60.
282. Klein RS, Rubin JB. Immune and nervous system CXCL12 and CXCR4: parallel roles in patterning and plasticity. Trends Immunol 2004;25:306-14.
283. Koch AE, Kunkel SL, Shah MR, et al. Macrophage inflammatory protein-1 β: A C-C chemokine in osteoarthritis. Clin Immuno Immunopathol 1995;77:307-14.
284. Kondo T, Novick AC, Toma H, Fairchild RL. Induction of chemokine gene expression during allogeneic skin graft rejection. Transplantation 1996;l61:1750-7.
285. Kotenko SV, Izotova LS, Pollack BP, et al. Other kinases can substitute for Jak2 in signal transduction by interferon-gamma. J Biol Chem 1996;271:17174-82.
286. Kowanko IC, Ferrante A. Adhesion and TNF priming in neutrophil-mediated cartilage damage. Clin Immuno Immunopathol 1996;79:36-42.
287. Krenger W, Falzarano G, Delmonte J Jr, et al. Interferon-gamma suppresses T-cell proliferation to mitogen via the nitric oxide pathway during experimental acute graft-versus-host disease. Blood 1996;88:1113-21.
288. Kruger-Krasagakes S, Moller A, Kolde G, et al. Production of interleukin-6 by human mast cells and basophilic cells. J Invest Dermatol 1996;106:75-9.
289. Kruger M, Van Gool S, Peng XH, et al. Production of granulocyte-macrophage colony-stimulating factor by T cells is regulated by B7 and IL-1β. Immunology 1196;88:49-54.
290. Kuang Y, Wu Y, Jiang H, Wu D. Selective G protein coupling by C-C chemokine receptors. J Biol Chem 1996;271:3975-8.
291. Kullberg MC, Berzofsky JA, Jankovic DL, et al. T cell-derived IL-3 induces the production of IL-4 by non-B, non-T cells to amplify the Th2-cytokine response to a non-parasite antigen in Schistosoma mansoni-infected mice. J Immuno 1996;156:1482-9.
292. Kumaki S, Armitage R, Ahdieh M, et al. Interleukin-15 up-regulates interleukin-2 receptor α chain but down-regulates its own high-affinity binding sites on human T and B cells. Eur J Immuno 1996;26:1235-9.
293. Kunkel SL, Strieter RM, Lindley IJ, Westwick J. Chemokines: new ligands, receptors and activities. Immuno Today 1995;16:559-61.
294. Kupker W, Felberbaum R, Bauer O, Diedrich K. [Significance of tumor necrosis factor α (TNF-α) in endometriosis]. Geburtshilfe Frauenheilkd 1996;56:239-42.
295. Kurek JB, Austin L, Cheema SS, et al. Up-regulation of leukaemia inhibitory factor and interleukin-6 in transected sciatic nerve and muscle following denervation. Neuromuscul Disord 1996;6:105-14.
296. Kurihara T, Bravo R. Cloning and functional expression of mCCR2, a murine receptor for the C-C chemokines JE and FIC. J Biol Chem 1996;271: 11603-7.
297. Kutteh WH, Franklin RD. Quantification of immunoglobulins and cytokines in human cervical mucus during each trimester of pregnancy. Am J Obstet Gynecol 2001;184:865-74.
298. Laberge S, Cruikshank WW, Beer DJ, Center DM. Secretion of IL-16 (lymphocyte chemoattractant factor) from serotonin-stimulated $CD8^+$ T cells in vitro. J Immuno 1996;156:310-5.
299. Lafortune L, Nalbantoglu J, Antel JP. Expression of tumor necrosis factor α (TNF α) and interleukin 6 (IL-6) mRNA in adult human astrocytes: comparison with adult microglia and fetal astrocytes. J Neuropathol Exp Neurol 1996;55:515-21.
300. Lagneaux L, Delforge A, Snoeck R, et al. Human cytomegalovirus increases constitutive production of interleukin-6 and leukemia inhibitory factor by bone marrow stromal cells. Blood 1996;87:59-66.
301. Lai CF, Ripperger J, Morella KK, et al. Receptors for interleukin (IL)-10 and IL-6-type cytokines use similar signaling mechanisms for inducing transcription through IL-6 response elements. J Biol Chem 1996;271:13968-75.

302. Lai CK, Ho AS, Chan CH, et al. Interleukin-5 messenger RNA expression in peripheral blood CD4+ cells in asthma. J Allergy Clin Immuno 1996;97: 1320-8.
303. Lai YH, Heslan JM, Poppema S, et al. Continuous administration of IL-13 to mice induces extramedullary hemopoiesis and monocytosis. J Immuno 1996;156:3166-73.
304. Laing KJ, Secombes CJ. Chemokines. Developmental and Comparative Immunology 2004;28:443-60.
305. Law K, Weiden M, Harkin T, et al. Increased release of interleukin-1 β, interleukin-6, and tumor necrosis factor-α by bronchoalveolar cells lavaged from involved sites in pulmonary tuberculosis. Am J Respir Crit Care Med 1996;153:799-804.
306. Ledur A, Fitting C, David B, et al. Variable estimates of cytokine levels produced by commercial ELISA kits: results using international cytokine standards. J Immuno Methods 1995;186:171-9.
307. Lee MS. Cytokine synergism in apoptosis: Its role in diabetes and cancer. J Bioch Mol Biol 2002;35:54-60.
308. Lee SM, Suen Y, Chang L, et al. Decreased interleukin-12 (IL-12) from activated cord versus adult peripheral blood mononuclear cells and upregulation of interferon-gamma, natural killer, and lymphokine-activated killer activity by IL-12 in cord blood mononuclear cells. Blood 1996;88:945-54.
309. Leite de Moraes MC, Dy M. MHC class I-selected CD4-CD8-TCR α β+ T cells: an important source of IL-4. Braz J Med Biol Res 1995;28:903-5.
310. Leite de Moraes MC, Herbelin A, Machavoine F, et al. MHC class I-selected CD4-CD8-TCR-α β+ T cells are a potential source of IL-4 during primary immune response. J Immuno 1995;155:4544-50.
311. Lemoli RM, Fogli M, Fortuna A, et al. Interleukin-11 (IL-11) acts as a synergistic factor for the proliferation of human myeloid leukaemic cells. Br J Haematol 1995;91:319-26.
312. Lemoli RM, Fortuna A, Tafuri A, et al. Interleukin-9 stimulates the proliferation of human myeloid leukemic cells. Blood 1996;87:3852-9.
313. Leonard WJ. The molecular basis of X-linked severe combined immunodeficiency: defective cytokine receptor signaling. Annu Rev Med 1996;47:229-39.
314. Leonardi CL, Powers JL, Matheson RT, et al. Etanercept as monotherapy in patients with psoriasis. N Engl J Med 2003;349:2014-22.
315. Levitz SM, Tabuni A, Nong SH, Golenbock DT. Effects of interleukin-10 on human peripheral blood mononuclear cell responses to Cryptococcus neoformans, Candida albicans, and lipopolysaccharide. Infect Immun 1996;64:945-51.
316. Lew W, Bowcock AM, Krueger JG. Psoriasis vulgaris: cutaneous lymphoid tissue supports T-cell activation and 'Type 1' inflammatory gene expression. Trends Immunol 2004;25:295-305.
317. Liao F, Rabin RL, Yannelly JR, et al. Human Mig chemokine: Biological and functional characterization. J Exp Med 1995;182:1301-14.
318. Li H Sim, TC Alam R. IL-13 released by and localized in human basophils. J Immuno 1996;156:4833-8.
319. Liles WC, Van Voorhis WC. Review: Nomenclature and biologic significance of cytokines involved in inflammation and host immune response. J Infect Dis 1995;172:1573-80.
320. Lilic D, Cant AJ, Abinun M, et al. Chronic mucocutaneous candidiasis. I. Altered antigen-stimulated IL-2, IL-4, IL-6 and interferon-gamma (IFN-γ) production. Clin Exp Immuno 1996;105:205-12.
321. Lim KG, Wan HC, Bozza PT, et al. Human eosinophils elaborate the lymphocyte chemoattractants. IL-16 (lymphocyte chemoattractant factor) and RANTES. J Immuno 1996;156:2566-70.
322. Lin M-T, Storer B, Martin PJ, et al. Relation of an interleukin-10 promoter polymorphism to graft-versus-host disease and survival after hematopoietic-cell transplantation. N Engl J Med 2003;349:2201-10.
323. Linderholm M, Ahlm C, Settergren B, et al. Elevated plasma levels of tumor necrosis factor (TNF)-α, soluble TNF receptors, interleukin (IL)-6, and IL-10 in patients with hemorrhagic fever with renal syndrome. J Infect Dis 1996;173:38-43.
324. Lio, D D'Anna, C Gervasi, F et al. In vitro impairment of interleukin-5 production in HLA-B8, DR3-positive individuals implications for immunoglobulin A synthesis dysfunction. Hum Immuno 1995;44:170-4.
325. Lipsky PE, van der Heijde DMFM, St. Clair EW, et al. Infliximab and methotrexate in the treatment of rheumatoid arthritis. N Engl J Med 2000;343:1594-602.
326. Liu ZH, Striker GE, Stetler-Stevenson M, et al. TNF-α and IL-1 α induce mannose receptors and apoptosis in glomerular mesangial but not endothelial cells. Am J Physiol 1996;270:C1595-C1601.
327. Liu Q-H, Williams DA, McManus C, et al. HIV-1 gp120 and chemokines activate ion channels in primary macrophages through CCR5 and CXCR4 stimulation. Proc Natl Acad Sci USA 2000;97:4832-7.
328. Loetscher P, Moser B. Homing chemokines in rheumatoid arthritis. Arthritis Res 2002;4:233-6.
329. Loetscher P, Seitz M, Baggiolini M, Moser B. Interleukin-2 regulates CC chemokine receptor expression and chemotactic responsiveness in T lymphocytes [see comments]. J Exp Med 1996;184:569-77.
330. Lortat-Jacob H, Baltzer F, Grimaud JA. Heparin decreases the blood clearance of interferon-gamma and increases its activity by limiting the processing of its carboxyl-terminal sequence. J Biol Chem 1996;271:16139-43.
331. Lortat-Jacob H, Grosdidier A, Imberty A. Structural diversity of heparan sulfate binding domains in

chemokines. Proc Natl Acad Sci USA 2002;97: 1229-34.

332. Love KS, Lakshmanan RR, Butterfield JH, Fox CC. IFN-γ-stimulated enhancement of MHC class II antigen expression by the human mast cell line HMC-1. Cell Immuno 1996;170:85-90.

333. Lu P, Urban JF, Zhou XD, et al. CD40-mediated stimulation contributes to lymphocyte proliferation, antibody production, eosinophilia, and mastocytosis during an in vivo type 2 response, but is not required for T cell IL-4 production. J Immuno 1996;156:3327-33.

334. Lukacs NW, Strieter RM, Chensue SW, Kunkel SL. Activation and regulation of chemokines in allergic airway inflammation. J Leukoc Biol 1996;59:13-7.

335. Lutfalla G, Holland SJ, Cinato E, et al. Mutant U5A cells are complemented by an interferon-α β receptor subunit generated by alternative processing of a new member of a cytokine receptor gene cluster. EMBO J 1995;14:5100-8.

336. Maciaszek JW, Parada NA, Cruikshank WW, et al. IL-16 represses HIV-1 promoter activity. J Immuno 1997;158:5-8.

337. Magnan A, Mege JL, Escallier JC, et al. Balance between alveolar macrophage IL-6 and TGF-β in lung-transplant recipients. Marseille and Montreal Lung Transplantation Group. Am J Respir Crit Care Med 1996;153:1431-6.

338. Mahalingam S, Friedland JS, Heise MT, et al. Chemokines and viruses: friends or foes? Trends Microbiol 2003;11:383-91.

339. Majewski S, Marczak M, Szmurlo A, et al. Interleukin-12 inhibits angiogenesis induced by human tumor cell lines in vivo. J Invest Dermatol 1996;106:1114-8.

340. Malbrain ML, Van den Bergh H, Zachee P. Further evidence for the clonal nature of the idiopathic hypereosinophilic syndrome: complete haematological and cytogenetic remission induced by interferon-α in a case with a unique chromosomal abnormality. Br J Haematol 1996;92:176-83.

341. Male D, Cooke A, Owen M, Trowsdale J, Champion B. Advanced Immunology. St. Louis: CV Mosby, 1996.

342. Malone D, Napolitano LM, Genuit T, Bochicchio GV, Kole K, Scalea TM. Total cytokine immunoassay: a more accurate method of cytokine measurement? J Trauma 2001;50:821-5.

343. Mandi Y, Farkas G, Ocsovszky I. Effects of pentoxifyllin and PentaglobinO on TNF and IL-6 production in septic patients. Acta Microbiol Immuno Hung 1995;42:301-8.

344. Mantovani G, Maccio A, Lai P, et al. Membrane-bound/soluble IL-2 receptor (IL-2R) and levels of IL-1 α, IL-2, and IL-6 in the serum and in the PBMC culture supernatants from 17 patients with hematological malignancies. Cell Biophys 1995;27: 1-14.

345. Marie C, Pitton C, Fitting C, Cavaillon JM. IL-10 and IL-4 synergize with TNF-α to induce IL-1ra production by human neutrophils. Cytokine 1996;8: 147-51.

346. Marietta EV, Chen Y, Weis JH. Modulation of expression of the anti-inflammatory cytokines interleukin-13 and interleukin-10 by interleukin-3. Eur J Immuno 1996;26:49-56.

347. Martins LM, Earnshaw WC. Apoptosis: alive and kicking in 1997. Cell Biol 1997;20:111-4.

348. Martinez C, Delgado M, Gomariz RP, Ganea, D. Vasoactive intestinal peptide and pituitary adenylate cyclase-activating polypeptide-38 inhibit IL-10 production in murine T lymphocytes. J Immuno 1996;156:4128-36.

349. Masamune A, Igarashi Y, Hakomori S. Regulatory role of ceramide in interleukin (IL)-1 β-induced E-selectin expression in human umbilical vein endothelial cells. Ceramide enhances IL-1 β action, but is not sufficient for E-selectin expression. J Biol Chem 1996;271:9368-75.

350. Matsushita K, Takenouchi T, Kobayashi S, et al. HLA-DR antigen expression in colorectal carcinomas: influence of expression by IFN-γ in situ and its association with tumour progression. Br J Cancer 1996;73:644-8.

351. Mayer K, Gokorsch S, Fegbeutel C, et al. Parenteral nutrition with fish oil modulates cytokine response in septic patients. AJRCCM 2003;167:1321-8. Epub 2003 Feb 25.

352. Mazzucchelli L, Hauser C, Zgraggen K, et al. Differential in situ expression of the genes encoding the chemokines MCP-1 and RANTES in human inflammatory bowel disease. J Pathol 1996;178:201-6.

353. McGee DW, Vitkus SJ. IL-4 enhances IEC-6 intestinal epithelial cell proliferation yet has no effect on IL-6 secretion. Clin Exp Immuno 1996;105:274-7.

354. McGee DW, Vitkus SJ, Lee P. The effect of cytokine stimulation on IL-1 receptor mRNA expression by intestinal epithelial cells. Cell Immuno 1996;168: 276-80.

355. McInnes IB, al-Mughales J, Field M, et al. The role of interleukin-15 in T-cell migration and activation in rheumatoid arthritis. Nat Med 1996;2:175-82.

356. Medvedev AE, Espevik T, Ranges G, Sundan A. Distinct roles of the two tumor necrosis factor (TNF) receptors in modulating TNF and lymphotoxin α effects. J Biol Chem 1996;271:9778-84.

357. Medvedev AE, Laegreid A, Sundan A, Espevik T. A non-competitive P55 TNF receptor antibody enhances the specific activity of lymphotoxin-α. Scand J Immuno 1996;43:439-48.

358. Meisel C, Vogt K, Platzer C, et al. Differential regulation of monocytic tumor necrosis factor-α and interleukin-10 expression. Eur J Immuno 1996;26: 1580-6.

359. Melani C, Sule-Suso J, Arienti F, et al. A human melanoma cell line transduced with an interleukin-4 gene by a retroviral vector releases biologically active IL-4 and maintains the original tumor antigenic phenotype. Hum Gene Ther 1995;6:1427-36.
360. Mendez-Samperio P, Hernandez-Garay M, Badillo-Flores A, Nunez-Vazquez A. Down-modulation of mycobacterial-induced IL-1 β production in human mononuclear cells by IL-4. Clin Exp Immuno 1996;104:374-9.
361. Menten P, Wuyts A, Van Damme J. Macrophage inflammatory protein-1. Cytokine & Growth Factor Reviews 2002;13:455-81.
362. Micallef MJ, Ohtsuki T, Kohno K, et al. Interferon-gamma-inducing factor enhances T helper 1 cytokine production by stimulated human T cells: synergism with interleukin-12 for interferon-gamma production. Eur J Immuno 1996;26:1647-51.
363. Miller A, Lanir N, Shapiro S, et al. Immunoregulatory effects of interferon-β and interacting cytokines on human vascular endothelial cells. Implications for multiple sclerosis autoimmune diseases. J NeuroImmuno 1996;64:151-61.
364. Mingari MC, Maggi E, Cambiaggi A, et al. Development in vitro of human CD4[+] thymocytes into functionally mature Th2 cells. Exogenous interleukin-12 is required for priming thymocytes to produce both Th1 cytokines and interleukin-10. Eur J Immuno 1996;26:1083-7.
365. Missol E, Sochanik A, Szala S. Introduction of murine IL-4 gene into B16(F10) melanoma tumors by direct gene transfer with DNA-liposome complexes. Cancer Lett 1995;97:189-93.
366. Mohamadzadeh M, Takashima A, Dougherty I, et al. Ultraviolet B radiation up-regulates the expression of IL-15 in human skin. J Immuno 1995;155:4492-6.
367. Moller DR, Forman JD, Liu MC, et al. Enhanced expression of IL-12 associated with Th1 cytokine profiles in active pulmonary sarcoidosis. J Immuno 1996;156:4952-60.
368. Moniuszko T, Rutkowski R, Chyrek-Borowska S. [Production of selected cytokines by monocytes (IL-1β, IL-6) and lymphocytes (IL-2, IL-4) in peripheral blood of patients with nonallergic bronchial asthma treated with Broncho-Vaxom]. Pneumonol Alergol Pol 1995;63 Suppl 2:66-70.
369. Monteclaro FS, Charo IF. The amino-terminal extracellular domain of the MCP-1 receptor, but not the RANTES/MIP-1α receptor, confers chemokine selectivity. Evidence for a two-step mechanism for MCP-1 receptor activation. J Biol Chem 1996;271: 19084-92.
370. Moqbel R, Ying S, Barkans J, et al. Identification of messenger RNA for IL-4 in human eosinophils with granule localization and release of the translated product. J Immuno 1995;155:4939-47.
371. Mori A, Suko M, Kaminuma O, et al. IL-15 promotes cytokine production of human T helper cells. J Immuno 1996;156:2400-5.
372. Moser B, Wolf M, Walz A, Loetscher P. Chemokines: multiple levels of leukocyte migration control. Trends Immunol 2004;25:75-84.
373. Mrozek E, Anderson P, Caligiuri MA. Role of interleukin-15 in the development of human CD56[+] natural killer cells from CD34[+] hematopoietic progenitor cells. Blood 1996;87:2632-40.
374. Mullberg J, Durie FH, Otten-Evans C, et al. A metalloprotease inhibitor blocks shedding of the IL-6 receptor and the p60 TNF receptor. J Immuno 1995;155:5198-205.
375. Muller A, Homey B, Soto H, Ge N, Catron D, et al. Involvement of chemokine receptors in breast cancer metastasis. Nature 2001;410:50-6.
376. Murakami T, Cardones AR, Hwang ST. Chemokine receptors and melanoma metastasis. J Dermatol Sci 2004;36:71-8.
377. Murphy GM, Jr Bitting L, Majewska A, et al. Expression of interleukin-11 and its encoding mRNA by glioblastoma cells. Neurosci Lett 1995;196: 153-6.
378. Murphy PM. Chemokines and the molecular basis of cancer metastasis. N Engl J Med 2001;345: 833-5.
379. Musselman DL, Lawson DH, Gumnick JF, et al. Paroxetine for the prevention of depression induced by high-dose interferon alfa. N Engl J Med 2001;344:961-6.
380. Mytar B, Woloszyn M, Ruggiero I, et al. Monocyte-mediated regulation of antigen-driven IFN gamma production by T cells. The role of endogenously produced TNF. Immuno Invest 1995;24:897-906.
381. Nagasawa T, Hirota S, Tachibana K, et al. Defects of B-cell lymphopoiesis and bone-marrow myelopoiesis in mice lacking the CXC chemokine PBSF/SDF-1. Nature 1996;382:635-8.
382. Nakajima H, Gleich GJ, Kita H. Constitutive production of IL-4 and IL-10 and stimulated production of IL-8 by normal peripheral blood eosinophils. J Immuno 1996;156:4859-66.
383. Nakajima K, Yamanaka Y, Nakae K et al. A central role for Stat3 in IL-6-induced regulation of growth and differentiation in M1 leukemia cells. EMBO J 1996;15:3651-8.
384. Nandurkar HH, Hilton DJ, Nathan P, et al. The human IL-11 receptor requires gp130 for signalling: demonstration by molecular cloning of the receptor. Oncogene 1996;12:585-93.
385. Narin N, Kutukculer N, Ozyurek R, et al. Lymphocyte subsets and plasma IL-1 α, IL-2, and TNF-α concentrations in acute rheumatic fever and chronic rheumatic heart disease. Clin Immuno Immunopathol 1995;77:172-6.

386. Navikas V, Matusevicius D, Soderstrom M, et al. Increased interleukin-6 mRNA expression in blood and cerebrospinal fluid mononuclear cells in multiple sclerosis. J NeuroImmuno 1996;64:63-9.
387. Nelson PJ, Ortiz BD, Pattison JM, Krensky AM. Identification of a novel regulatory region critical for expression of the RANTES chemokine in activated T lymphocytes. J Immuno 1996;157:1139-48.
388. Neuzil KM, Tang YW, Graham BS. Protective Role of TNF-α in respiratory syncytial virus infection in vitro and in vivo. Am J Med Sci 1996;311:201-4.
389. Nicola NA. Guidebook to Cytokines and Their Receptors. Oxford: Oxford University Press, 1995.
390. Nieto M, del Pozo MA, Sanchez-Madrid F. Interleukin-15 induces adhesion receptor redistribution in T lymphocytes. Eur J Immuno 1996;26:1302-7.
391. Niiya M, Niiya K, Kiguchi T, Shibakura M, Asaumi N, Shinagawa K, Ishimaru F, Kiura K, Ikeda K, Ueoka H, Tanimoto M. Induction of TNF-alpha, uPA, IL-8 and MCP-1 by doxorubicin in human lung carcinoma cells. Cancer Chemother Pharmacol 2003;52:391-8. Epub 2003 Aug 08.
392. Nishimura H, Hiromatsu K, Kobayashi N, et al. IL-15 is a novel growth factor for murine gamma delta T cells induced by Salmonella infection. J Immuno 1996;156:663-9.
393. Norbiato G, Bevilacqua M, Vago T, Clerici M. Glucocorticoids and interferon-α in the acquired immunodeficiency syndrome. J Clin Endocrinol Metab 1996;81:2601-6.
394. Norman JG, Fink GW, Sexton C, Carter G. Transgenic animals demonstrate a role for the IL-1 receptor in regulating IL-1β gene expression at steady-state and during the systemic stress induced by acute pancreatitis. J Surg Res 1996;63:231-6.
395. Ogilvie AC, Hack CE, Wagstaff J, et al. IL-1 β does not cause neutrophil degranulation but does lead to IL-6, IL-8, and nitrite/nitrate release when used in patients with cancer. J Immuno 1996;156:389-94.
396. Okahashi N, Yamamoto M, Vancott JL, et al. Oral immunization of interleukin-4 (IL-4) knockout mice with a recombinant Salmonella strain or cholera toxin reveals that $CD4^+$ Th2 cells producing IL-6 and IL-10 are associated with mucosal immunoglobulin A responses. Infect Immun 1996;64:1516-25.
397. Okun ML, Giese S, Lin L et al. Exploring the cytokine and endocrine involvement in narcolepsy. Brain, Behavior, and Immunity 2004;18:326-332.
398. Oleksowicz L, Puszkin E, Mrowiec Z, et al. Alterations in platelet function in patients receiving interleukin-6 as cytokine therapy. Cancer Invest 1996;14:307-16.
399. Ono SJ, Nakamura T, Miyazaki D, et al. Chemokines: Roles in leukocyte development, trafficking, and effector function. J Allergy Clin Immunol 2003;111:1185-99.
400. Onoe Y, Miyaura C, Kaminakayashiki T, et al. IL-13 and IL-4 inhibit bone resorption by suppressing cyclooxygenase-2-dependent prostaglandin synthesis in osteoblasts. J Immuno 1996;156:758-64.
401. Onuffer JJ, Horuk R. Chemokines, chemokine receptors and small-molecule antagonists: recent developments. Trends Pharmacol Sci 2002;23:459-467.
402. Oppermann M. Chemokine receptor CCR5: insights into structure, function, and regulation. Cell Singalling 2004;16:1201-10.
403. Ortiz BD, Krensky AM, Nelson PJ. Kinetics of transcription factors regulating the RANTES chemokine gene reveal a developmental switch in nuclear events during T-lymphocyte maturation. Mol Cell Biol 1996;16:202-10.
404. Ozawa H, Aiba S, Nakagawa-Tagami H. Interferon-gamma and interleukin-10 inhibit antigen presentation by Langerhans cells for T helper type 1 cells by suppressing their CD80 (B7-1) expression. Eur J Immuno 1996;26:648-52.
405. Pan G, O'Rourke K, Chinnaiyan AM, et al. The receptor for the cytotoxic ligand TRAIL. Science 1997;276:111-3.
406. Paquet P, Pierard GE. Interleukin-6 and the skin. Int Arch Allergy Immuno 1996;109:308-17.
407. Parada NA, Cruikshank WW, Danis HL, et al. IL-16- and other CD4 ligand-induced migration is dependent upon protein kinase C. Cell Immuno 1996;168:100-6.
408. Park E, Kalunta CI, Nguyen TT, et al. TNF-α inhibits anti-IgM-mediated apoptosis in Ramos cells. Exp Cell Res 1996;226:1-10.
409. Park JH, Shin SH. Induction of IL-12 gene expression in the brain in septic shock. Biochem Biophys Res Commun 1996;224:391-6.
410. Parronchi P, Mohapatra S, Sampognaro S, et al. Effects of interferon-α on cytokine profile, T cell receptor repertoire and peptide reactivity of human allergen-specific T cells. Eur J Immuno 1996;26: 697-703.
411. Patki AH, Quinones-Mateu ME, Dorazio D, et al. Activation of antigen-induced lymphocyte proliferation by interleukin-15 without the mitogenic effect of interleukin-2 that may induce human immunodeficiency virus-1 expression. J Clin Invest 1996;98:616-21.
412. Patterson AM, Schmutz C, Davis S, et al. Differential binding of chemokines to macrophages and neutrophils in the human inflamed synovium. Arthritis Res 2002;4:209-14.
413. Pawankar RU, Okuda M, Hasegawa S, et al. Interleukin-13 expression in the nasal mucosa of perennial allergic rhinitis. Am J Respir Crit Care Med 1995;152:2059-67.
414. Peck OM, Williams DL, Breuel KF, et al. Differential regulation of cytokine and chemokine production in

lipopolysaccharide-induced tolerance and priming. Cytokine 2004;26:202-8.
415. Peng J, Friese P, Wolf RF, et al. Relative reactivity of platelets from thrombopoietin- and interleukin-6-treated dogs. Blood 1996;87:4158-63.
416. Peng X, Kasran A, Warmerdam PA, et al. Accessory signaling by CD40 for T cell activation: induction of Th1 and Th2 cytokines and synergy with interleukin-12 for interferon-gamma production. Eur J Immuno 1996;26:1621-7.
417. Perera CS, St Clair DK, McClain CJ. Differential regulation of manganese superoxide dismutase activity by alcohol and TNF in human hepatoma cells. Arch Biochem Biophys 1995;323:471-6.
418. Perregaux DG, Svensson L, Gabel CA. Tenidap and other anion transport inhibitors disrupt cytolytic T lymphocyte-mediated IL-1 β post-translational processing. J Immuno 1996;157:57-64.
419. Peterson F, Ludwig A, Flad HD, Brandt E. TNF-α renders human neutrophils responsive to platelet factor 4. Comparison of PF-4 and IL-8 reveals different activity profiles of the two chemokines. J Immuno 1996;156:1954-62.
420. Pettipher ER, Salter ED. Resident joint tissues, rather than infiltrating neutrophils and monocytes, are the predominant sources of TNF-α in zymosan-induced arthritis. Cytokine 1996;8:130-3.
421. Playfair JHL. Immunology at a Glance. 6th ed. New York: Blackwell Science, 1996.
422. Post TW, Bozic CR, Rothenberg ME, et al. Molecular characterization of two murine eosinophil β chemokine receptors. J Immuno 1995;155: 5299-305.
423. Poudrier J, Owens T. Th1 and Th2 help for B cells: differential capacity for induction of autonomous responsiveness to IL-2. Int Immuno 1995;7:1021-7.
424. Power CA, Clemetson JM, Clemetson KJ, Wells TN. Chemokine and chemokine receptor mRNA expression in human platelets. Cytokine 1995;7:479-82.
425. Proudffot AEI, Handel TM, Johnson Z, et al. Glycosaminoglycan binding and oligomerization are essential for the in vivo activity of certain chemokines. Proc Natl Acad Sci USA 2003;100: 1885-90.
426. Purohit A, Newman SP, Reed MJ. The role of cytokines in regulating estrogen synthesis: implications for the etiology of breast cancer. Breast Cancer Res 2002;4:65-9.
427. Qiu H, Pan J, Zhao Y. [The role of TNFα, IL-1 β and MIP-1 α in LPS-induced organ injury]. Chung Hua I Hsueh Tsa Chih 1996;76:254-7.
428. Rankin SM, Conroy DM, Williams TJ. Eotaxin and eosinophil recruitment: implications for human disease. Mol Med Today 2000 Jan;6:20-7.
429. Rao JB, Chamberlain RS, Bronte V, et al. IL-12 is an effective adjuvant to recombinant vaccinia virus-based tumor vaccines: enhancement by simultaneous B7-1 expression. J Immuno 1996;156:3357-65.
430. Raport CJ, Gosling J, Schweickart VL, et al. Molecular cloning and functional characterization of a novel human CC chemokine receptor (CCR5) for RANTES, MIP-1β, and MIP-1α. J Biol Chem 1996;271:17161-6.
431. Raport CJ, Schweickart VL, Chantry D, et al. New members of the chemokine receptor gene family. J Leukoc Biol 1996;59:18-23.
432. Reeves G, Todd I. Lecture Notes on Immunology. 3rd ed. New York: Blackwell Science, 1996.
433. Reichner JS, Mulligan JA, Palla ME, et al. Interleukin-6 production by rat hepatocellular carcinoma cells is associated with metastatic potential but not with tumorigenicity. Arch Surg 1996;131:360-5.
434. Reinders MEJ, Laning JC, Paul LC, Briscoe DM. The role of chemokines in transplant immunology. Transplant Rev 2003 Apr;17(2):87-95.
435. Rep MH, Hintzen RQ, Polman CH, van Lier RA. Recombinant interferon-β blocks proliferation but enhances interleukin-10 secretion by activated human T-cells. J NeuroImmuno 1996;67:111-8.
436. Revillard JP. Immunologie, 2nd ed. Paris: De Boeck & Larcier SA, 1995.
437. Rich AR, Lewis MR. Mechanisms of allergy in tuberculosis. Proc Soc Exp Biol Med 1928, 25:296-8.
438. Riemann H, Schwarz A, Grabbe S, et al. Neutralization of IL-12 in vivo prevents induction of contact hypersensitivity and induces hapten-specific tolerance. J Immuno 1996;156:1799-1803.
439. Ringheim GE, Szcepanik AM, Burgher KL, et al. Transcriptional inhibition of the β-amyloid precursor protein by interferon-gamma. Biochem Biophys Res Commun 1996;224:246-51.
440. Rival Y, Del-Maschio A, Rabiet MJ, et al. Inhibition of platelet endothelial cell adhesion molecule-1 synthesis and leukocyte transmigration in endothelial cells by the combined action of TNF-α and IFN-γ. J Immuno 1996;157:1233-41.
441. Robak T. [Biological properties and therapeutic use of interleukin 2 (IL-2)]. Postepy Hig Med Dosw 1995;49:367-93.
442. Roberge CJ, Poubelle PE, Beaulieu AD, et al. The IL-1 and IL-1 receptor antagonist (IL-1Ra) response of human neutrophils to EBV stimulation. Preponderance of IL-Ra detection. J Immuno 1996;156:4884-91.
443. Rochester CL, Ackerman SJ, Zheng T, Elias JA. Eosinophil-fibroblast interactions. Granule major basic protein interacts with IL-1 and transforming growth factor-β in the stimulation of lung fibroblast IL-6-type cytokine production. J Immuno 1996;156:4449-56.
444. Rodriguez C, Lacasse C, Hoang T. Interleukin-1 β suppresses apoptosis in CD34 positive bone marrow cells through activation of the type I IL-1 receptor. J Cell Physiol 1996;166:387-96.

445. Romagnani P, Annunziato F, Piccinni M-P, et al. Cytokines and chemokines in T lymphopoiesis and T-cell effector function. Immunol Today 2000;21: 415-7.
446. Romagnani P, Lasagni L, Annunziato F, et al. CXC chemokines: the regulatory link between inflammation and angiogenesis. Trends Immunol 2004;25: 202-9.
447. Roth SJ, Carr MW, Springer TA. C-C chemokines, but not the C-X-C chemokines interleukin-8 and interferon-gamma inducible protein-10, stimulate transendothelial chemotaxis of T lymphocytes. Eur J Immuno 1995;25:3482-8.
448. Rothe H, Hartmann B, Geerlings P, Kolb H. Interleukin-12 gene-expression of macrophages is regulated by nitric oxide. Biochem Biophys Res Commun 1996;224:159-63.
449. Ruth JH, Bienkowski M, Warmington KS, et al. IL-1 receptor antagonist (IL-1ra) expression, function, and cytokine-mediated regulation during mycobacterial and schistosomal antigen-elicited granuloma formation. J Immuno 1996;156:2503-9.
450. Sabin EA, Pearce EJ. Early IL-4 production by non-CD4$^+$ cells at the site of antigen deposition predicts the development of a T helper 2 cell response to Schistosoma mansoni eggs. J Immuno 1995;155: 4844-53.
451. Sad S, Mosmann TR. Interleukin (IL) 4, in the absence of antigen stimulation, induces an anergy-like state in differentiated CD8$^+$ TC1 cells: loss of IL-2 synthesis and autonomous proliferation but retention of cytotoxicity and synthesis of other cytokines. J Exp Med 1995;182:1505-15.
452. Saito K, Suyama K, Nishida K, et al. Early increases in TNF-α, IL-6 and IL-1 β levels following transient cerebral ischemia in gerbil brain. Neurosci Lett 1996;206:149-52.
453. Sajjadi FG, Takabayashi K, Foster AC, et al. Inhibition of TNF-α expression by adenosine: role of A3 adenosine receptors. J Immuno 1996;156:3435-42.
454. Sakatsume M, Finbloom DS. Modulation of the expression of the IFN-γ receptor β-chain controls responsiveness to IFN-γ in human peripheral blood T cells. J Immuno 1996;156:4160-6.
455. Saklatvala J, Davis W, Guesdon F. Interleukin 1 (IL1) and tumour necrosis factor (TNF) signal transduction. Philos Trans R Soc Lond B Biol Sci 1996;351:151-7.
456. Samson M, Libert F, Doranz BJ, et al. Resistance to HIV-1 infection in caucasian individuals bearing mutant alleles of the CCR-5 chemokine receptor gene [see comments]. Nature 1996;382:722-5.
457. Sandborg CI, Imfeld KL, Zaldivar F Jr, et al. IL-4 expression in human T cells is selectively inhibited by IL-1 α and IL-1 β. J Immuno 1995;155: 5206-12.
458. Santos CC, Zhang H, Slutsky AS. From bench to bedside: bacterial growth and cytokines. Critical Care 2002;6:4-6.
459. Sato K, Yamanaka M, Takahashi H, Tokeshi M, Kimura H, Kitamori T. Microchip-based immunoassay system with branching multichannels for simultaneous determination of interferon-gamma. Electrophoresis 2002;23:734-9.
460. Saura M, Martinez-Dalmau R, Minty A, et al. Interleukin-13 inhibits inducible nitric oxide synthase expression in human mesangial cells. Biochem J 1996;313(Pt 2):641-6.
461. Schall TJ, Bacon KB. Chemokines, leucocyte trafficking, and inflammation. Curr Opion Immunolog 1994;6:865-73.
462. Schandene L, Del Prete GF, Cogan E, et al. Recombinant interferon-α selectively inhibits the production of interleukin-5 by human CD4$^+$ T cells. J Clin Invest 1996;97:309-15.
463. Schauer U, Jung T, Krug N, Frew A. Measurement of intracellular cytokines. Immuno Today 1996;17: 305-6.
464. Schmidtmayerova H, Nottet HS, Nuovo G, et al. Human immunodeficiency virus type 1 infection alters chemokine β peptide expression in human monocytes: implications for recruitment of leukocytes into brain and lymph nodes. Proc Natl Acad Sci USA 1996;93:700-4.
465. Schnyder B, Lugli S, Feng N, et al. Interleukin-4 (IL-4) and IL-13 bind to a shared heterodimeric complex on endothelial cells mediating vascular cell adhesion molecule-1 induction in the absence of the common gamma chain. Blood 1996;87:4286-95.
466. Schulz-Knappe P, Magert HJ, Dewald B, et al. HCC-1, a novel chemokine from human plasma. J Exp Med 1996;183:295-9.
467. Schutyser E, Struyf S, Van Damme J. The CC chemokine CCL20 and its receptor CCR6. Cytok Growth Factor Rev 2003;14:406-26.
468. Schwabe M, Cox GW, Bosco MC, et al. Multiple cytokines inhibit interleukin-6-dependent murine hybridoma/plasmacytoma proliferation. Cell Immuno 1996;168:117-21.
469. Seder RA. High-dose IL-2 and IL-15 enhance the in vitro priming of naive CD4$^+$ T cells for IFN-γ but have differential effects on priming for IL-4. J Immuno 1996;156:2413-22.
470. Selleri C, Maciejewski JP, Sato T, Young NS. Interferon-gamma constitutively expressed in the stromal microenvironment of human marrow cultures mediates potent hematopoietic inhibition. Blood 1996;87:4149-57.
471. Sempowski GD, Derdak S, Phipps RP. Interleukin-4 and interferon-gamma discordantly regulate collagen biosynthesis by functionally distinct lung fibroblast subsets. J Cell Physiol 1996;167:290-6.

472. Seymour GJ, Savage NW, Walsh LJ. Immunology: An Introduction for the Health Sciences. New York: McGraw-Hill, 1995.
473. Sgadari C, Angiolillo AL, Tosato G. Inhibition of angiogenesis by interleukin-12 is mediated by the interferon-inducible protein 10. Blood 1996;87: 3877-82.
474. Shapiro SD, Owen CA. ADAM-33 Surfaces as an Asthma Gene. N Engl J Med 2002;347:936-8.
475. Sherwood ER, Toliver-Kinsky T. Mechanisms of the inflammatory response. Best Pract Res Clin Anaesthesiol 2004;18:385-405.
476. Shields DC. Molecular evolution of CXC chemokines and receptors. Trends Immunol 2003;24:355.
477. Shibayama H, Tagawa S, Hattori H, et al. Interleukin-6 inhibits the chemotaxis of human malignant plasma cell lines. Br J Haematol 1996;93:534-41.
478. Shimada M, Matsumata T, Taketomi A, et al. The role of interleukin-6, interleukin-16, tumor necrosis factor-α and endotoxin in hepatic resection. Hepato-gastroenterology 1995;42:691-7.
479. Shimizu H, Ohtani K, Sato N, et al. Increase in serum interleukin-6, plasma ACTH and serum cortisol levels after systemic interferon-α administration. Endocr J 1995;42:551-6.
480. Shimoda K, van Deursen J, Sangster MY, et al. Lack of IL-4-induced Th2 response and IgE class switching in mice with disrupted Stat6 gene. Nature 1996;380: 630-3.
481. Shin WS, Hong YH, Peng HB, et al. Nitric oxide attenuates vascular smooth muscle cell activation by interferon-gamma. The role of constitutive NF-kappa B activity. J Biol Chem 1996;271: 11317-24.
482. Shinbara M, Kondo N, Agata H, et al. Interferon-gamma and interleukin-4 production of ovalbumin-stimulated lymphocytes in egg-sensitive children. Ann Allergy Asthma Immuno 1996;77:60-6.
483. Shohami E, Bass R, Wallach D, et al. Inhibition of tumor necrosis factor α (TNFα) activity in rat brain is associated with cerebroprotection after closed head injury. J Cereb Blood Flow Metab 1996;16: 378-84.
484. Siegel MD, Zhang DH, Ray P, Ray A. Activation of the interleukin-5 promoter by cAMP in murine EL-4 cells requires the GATA-3 and CLE0 elements. J Biol Chem 1995;270:24548-55.
485. Sigal LH, Ron Y. Immunology and Inflammation: Basic Mechanisms and Clinical Consequences. New York: McGraw-Hill, 1994.
486. Signore A, Capriotti G, Scopinaro F, et al. Radiolabelled lymphokines and growth factors for in vivo imaging of inflammation, infection and cancer. Trends Immunol 2004;24:395-402.
487. Skeen MJ, Miller MA, Shinnick TM, Ziegler HK. Regulation of murine macrophage IL-12 production. Activation of macrophages in vivo, restimulation in vitro, and modulation by other cytokines. J Immuno 1996;156:1196-206.
488. mithgall MD, Wong JG, Critchett KE, Haffar OK. IL-7 up-regulates HIV-1 replication in naturally infected peripheral blood mononuclear ells. J Immuno 1996;156:2324-30.
489. Snidjers A, Hilkens CM, van der Pouw-Kraan TC, et al. Regulation of bioactive IL-12 production in lipopolysaccharide-stimulated human monocytes is determined by the expression of the p35 subunit. J Immuno 1996;156:1207-12.
490. Snyder CA, Udasin I, Waterman SJ, et al. Reduced IL-6 levels among individuals in Hudson County, New Jersey, an area contaminated with chromium. Arch Environ Health 1996;51:26-8.
491. Sozzani S, Locati M, Zhou M, et al. Receptors, signal transduction, and spectrum of action of monocyte chemotactic protein-1 and related chemokines. J Leukoc Biol 1995;57:788-94.
492. Spain BA, Soliman DM, Sidner RA, Twigg HL. Enhanced proliferation and IL-2 secretion by lung lymphocytes from HIV-infected subjects. Am J Physiol 1995;269(4 Pt 1):L498-L506.
493. Sporeno E, Savino R, Ciapponi L, et al. Human interleukin-6 receptor super-antagonists with high potency and wide spectrum on multiple myeloma cells. Blood 1996;87:4510-9.
494. tanciu LA, Shute J, Holgate ST, Djukanovic R. Production of IL-8 and IL-4 by positively and negatively selected $CD4^+$ and $CD8^+$ human T cells following a four-step cell separation method including magnetic cell sorting (MACS). J Immuno Methods 1996;189:107-15.
495. Standiford TJ, Kunkel SL, Greenberger MJ, et al. Expression and regulation of chemokines in bacterial pneumonia. J Leukoc Biol 1996;59:24-8.
496. Steinke JW, Borish L. Th2 cytokines and asthma Interleukin-4: its role in the pathogenesis of asthma, and targeting it for asthma treatment with interleukin-4 receptor antagonists. Respir Res 2001;2: 66-70.
497. Stewart RJ, Kashxur TS., Marsden PA. Vascular endothelial platelet endothelial adhesion molecule-1 (PECAM-1) expression is decreased by TNF-α and IFN-γ. Evidence for cytokine-induced destabilization of messenger ribonucleic acid transcripts in bovine endothelial cells. J Immuno 1996;156:1221-8.
498. Stomski FC, Sun Q, Bagley CJ, et al. Human interleukin-3 (IL-3) induces disulfide-linked IL-3 receptor α- and β-chain heterodimerization, which is required for receptor activation but not high-affinity binding. Mol Cell Biol 1996;16:3035-46.
499. Strieter RM, Belperio JA, Keane MP. Cytokines in innate host defense in the lung. J Clin Invest 2002;109:699-705.

500. Strieter RM, Belperio JA, Phillips RJ, Keane MP. CXC chemokines in angiogenesis of cancer. Semin Cancer Biol 2004;14:195-200.
501. Strieter RM, Polverini PJ, Arenberg DA, Kunkel SL. The role of CXC chemokines as regulators of angiogenesis. Shock 1995;4:155-60.
502. Strieter RM, Polverini PJ, Arenberg DA, et al. Role of C-X-C chemokines as regulators of angiogenesis in lung cancer. J Leukoc Biol 1995;57:752-62.
503. Sullivan CM, Smith DM, Matsui NM, et al. Identification of constitutive and gamma-interferon- and interleukin 4-regulated proteins in the human renal carcinoma cell line ACHN. Cancer Res 1997;57: 1137-43.
504. Sunyer T, Rothe L, Jiang X, et al. Proinflammatory agents, IL-8 and IL-10, upregulate inducible nitric oxide synthase expression and nitric oxide production in avian osteoclast-like cells. J Cell Biochem 1996;60:469-83.
505. Svensson Å, Möller H, Björkner B. Rheumatoid arthritis, gold therapy, contact allergy and blood cytokines. BMC Dermatology 2002;2:1-5.
506. Szabo I, Chen X-h, Xin L, et al. Heterologous desensitization of opioid receptors by chemokines inhibits chemotaxis and enhances the perception of pain. Proc Natl Acad Sci USA 2002;99:10276-81.
507. Szabo MC, Soo KS, Zlotnik A, Shall T. J Chemokine class differences in binding to the Duffy antigen-erythrocyte chemokine receptor. J Biol Chem 1995;270:25348-51.
508. Szekanecz Z, Kim J, Koch AE. Chemokines and chemokine receptors in rheumatoid arthritis. Semin Immunol 2003;15:15-21.
509. Szodoray P, Alex P, Dandapani V, Nakken B, Pesina J, et al. Apoptotic effect of rituximab on peripheral blood B cells in rheumatoid arthritis. Scand J Immunol 2004;60:209-18.
510. Szekanecz Z, Koch AE. Therapeutic inhibition of leukocite recruitment in inflammatory diseases. Curr Opin Pharmacol 2004;4:423-8.
511. Takabayashi T, Vannier E, Clark BD, et al. A new biologic role for C3a and C3a desArg: regulation of TNF-α and IL-1 β synthesis. J Immuno 1996;156:3455-60.
512. Takatsu K. [Structure and function of IL-5 receptor]. Yakugaku Zasshi 1995;115:570-83.
513. Takeda K, Tanaka T, Shi W, et al. Essential role of Stat6 in IL-4 signalling. Nature 1996;380:627-30.
514. Takeshita S, Gage JR, Kishimoto T, et al. Differential regulation of IL-6 gene transcription and expression by IL-4 and IL-10 in human monocytic cell lines. J Immuno 1996;156:2591-8.
515. Takizawa H, Ohtoshi T, Yamashita N, et al. Interleukin 6-receptor expression on human bronchial epithelial cells: regulation by IL-1 and IL-6. Am J Physiol 1996;270(3 Pt 1):L346-L352.
516. Tamai M, Sagawa K, Kawabata R, et al. Production of IL-6 by T cells from the femoral head of patients with rapidly destructive coxopathy (RDC). Clin Exp Immuno 1996;103:506-13.
517. Tamamura H, Fujisawa M, Hiramatsu K, et al. Identification of a CXCR4 antagonist, a T140 analog, as an 3 anti-rheumatoid arthritis agent. FEBS Letters 2004;569:99-104.
518. Tang GJ, Kuo CD, Yen TC, et al. Perioperative plasma concentrations of tumor necrosis factor-α and interleukin-6 in infected patients. Crit Care Med 1996;24:423-8.
519. Taub DD, Oppenheim JJ. Chemokines, inflammation and the immune system. Ther Immuno 1994;1: 229-46.
520. Taub DD, Turcovski-Corrales SM, Key ML, et al. Chemokines and T lymphocyte activation: I. chemokines costimulate human T lymphocyte activation in vitro. J Immuno 1996;156:2095-103.
521. Tedla N, Palladinetti P, Kelly M, et al. Chemokines and T lymphocyte recruitment to lymph nodes in HIV infection. Am J Pathol 1996;148:1367-73.
522. Terada N, Konno A, Terada Y, et al. IL-4 upregulates Fc epsilon RI α-chain messenger RNA in eosinophils. J Allergy Clin Immuno 1995;96(6 Pt 2):1161-9.
523. Theodore AC, Center DM, Nicoll J, et al. CD4 ligand IL-16 inhibits the mixed lymphocyte reaction. J Immuno 1996;157:1958-64.
524. Theodorou I, Capolable C, Combadiere C, Debre P. Genetic control of HIV disease. Trends Microbiol 2003;11:392-7.
525. Thierfelder WE, van Deursen JM, Yamamoto K, et al. Requirement for Stat4 in interleukin-12-mediated responses of natural killer and T cells. Nature 1996;382:171-4.
526. Thompson AW, Lotze MT. The Cytokine Handbook. 4th ed. Orlando: Academic Press, 2003.
527. Thuma PE, Weiss G, Herold M, Gordeuk, VR. Serum neopterin, interleukin-4, and interleukin-6 concentrations in cerebral malaria patients and the effect of iron chelation therapy. Am J Trop Med Hyg 1996;54:164-8.
528. Tiggelman AM, Boers W, Linthorst C, et al. Collagen synthesis by human liver (myo)fibroblasts in culture: evidence for a regulatory role of IL-1 β, IL-4, TGF β and IFN gamma. J Hepatol 1995;23:307-17.
529. Tilg H, Dielhl AM. Cytokines in alcoholic and non-alcoholic steatohepatitis. New Engl J Med 2000;343:1467-76.
530. Till S, Li B, Durham S, Humbert M, et al. Secretion of the eosinophil-active cytokines interleukin-5, granulocyte/macrophage colony-stimulating factor and interleukin-3 by bronchoalveolar lavage $CD4^+$ and $CD8^+$ T cell lines in atopic asthmatics, and atopic and non-atopic controls. Eur J Immuno 1995;25: 2727-31.

531. Toniatti C, Cabibbo A, Sporena E, et al. Engineering human interleukin-6 to obtain variants with strongly enhanced bioactivity. EMBO J 1996;15:2726-37.
532. Tpownson DH, Liptak AR. Chemokines in the corpus luteum: implications of leukocyte chemotaxis. Reprod Biol Endocrinol 2003;1:94.
533. Treiber-Held S, Stewart DM, Barraclough HA, et al. Release of sIL-2R α from and activation of native human peripheral blood mononuclear cells by recombinant IL-15. Clin Immuno Immunopathol 1996;80:67-75.
534. Treiber-Held S, Stewart DM, Kurman CC, Nelson DL. IL-15 induces the release of soluble IL-2Rα from human peripheral blood mononuclear cells. Clin Immuno Immunopathol 1996;79:71-8.
535. Trentin L, Cerutti A, Zambello R, et al. Interleukin-15 promotes the growth of leukemic cells of patients with B-cell chronic lymphoproliferative disorders. Blood 1996;87:3327-35.
536. Trinchieri G, Gerosa F. Immunoregulation by interleukin-12. J Leukoc Biol 1996;59:505-11.
537. Tsuboi I, Tanaka H, Nakao M, et al. Nonsteroidal anti-inflammatory drugs differentially regulate cytokine production in human lymphocytes: up-regulation of TNF, IFN-γ and IL-2, in contrast to down-regulation of IL-6 production. Cytokine 1995; 7:372-9.
538. Tsuda S, Rieke S, Hashimoto Y, et al. IL-7 supports D-J but not V-DJ rearrangement of TCR-β gene in fetal liver progenitor cells. J Immuno 1996;156:3233-42.
539. Tsukada J, Waterman WR, Koyama Y, et al. A novel STAT-like factor mediates lipopolysaccharide, interleukin 1 (IL-1), and IL-6 signaling and recognizes a gamma interferon activation site-like element in the IL1B gene. Mol Cell Biol 1996;16:2183-94.
540. Tuncer AM, Hicsonmez G, Gumruk F, et al. Serum TNF-α, gamma-INF, G-CSF levels in neutropenic children with acute leukemia treated with short-course, high-dose methylprednisolone. Leuk Res 1996;20:265-9.
541. Turner DM, Grant SC, Lamb WR, et al. A genetic marker of high TNF-α production in heart transplant recipients. Transplantation 1995;60:1113-7.
542. Umehara H, Bloom ET, Okazaki T, et al. Fractalkine and vascular injury. Trends Immunol 2001;22: 602-7.
543. Urashima M, Chauhan D, Hatziyanni M, et al. CD40 ligand triggers interleukin-6 mediated B cell differentiation. Leuk Res 1996;20:507-15.
544. Ushio S, Namba M, Okura T, et al. Cloning of the cDNA for human IFN-γ-inducing factor, expression in *Escherichia coli,* and studies on the biologic activities of the protein. J Immuno 1996;156:4274-9.
545. Vaddi K, Keller M, Newton RC. The chemokine facts book. Orlando: Academic Press, 1997.
546. Vallejo JG, Baker CJ, Edwards MS. Interleukin-6 production by human neonatal monocytes stimulated by type III group B streptococci. J Infect Dis 1996;174:332-7.
547. van Bergen CA, Smit WM, van Sluijters DA, et al. Interleukin-10, interleukin-12, and tumor necrosis factor-α differentially influence the proliferation of human $CD8^+$ and $CD4^+$ T-cell clones. Ann Hematol 1996;72:245-52.
548. van der Pouw Kraan TC, Boeije LC, Troon JT, et al. Human IL-13 production is negatively influenced by CD3 engagement. Enhancement of IL-13 production by cyclosporin A. J Immuno 1996;156:1818-23.
549. Vanky F, Hising C, Sjowall K, et al. Interferon-gamma and tumor necrosis factor-α treatment of ex vivo human carcinoma cells potentiates their interaction with allogeneic lymphocytes. J Interferon Cytokine Res 1996;16:201-7.
550. van Nieuwenhoven ALV, Bouman A, Moes H, et al. Endotoxin-induced cytokine production of monocytes of third-trimester pregnant women compared with women in the follicular phase of the menstrual cycle. Am J Obstet Gynecol 2003;188:1073-7.
551. Vasse M, Paysant I, Soria J, et al. Down-regulation of fibrinogen biosynthesis by IL-4, IL-10 and IL-13. Br J Haematol 1996;93:955-61.
552. Verbik DJ, Stinson WW, Brunda MJ, et al. In vivo therapeutic effects of interleukin-12 against highly metastatic residual lymphoma. Clin Exp Metastasis 1996;14:219-29.
553. Verrecchia F, Mauviel A. TGF-β and TNF-α: antagonistic cytokines controlling type I collagen gene expression. Cellular Signalling 2004;16:873-80.
554. Vicari AP, Treilleux I, Lebecque S. Regulation of the trafficking of tumour-infiltrating dendritic cells by chemokines. Semin Cancer Biol 2004;14:161-9.
555. Vidal-Vanaclocha F, Alvarez A, Asumendi A, et al. Interleukin 1 (IL-1)-dependent melanoma hepatic metasasis in vivo, increased endothelial adherence by IL-1-induced mannose receptors and growth factor production in vitro. J Natl Cancer Inst 1996;88: 198-205.
556. Viganò P, Mangioni S, Pompei F, Chiodo I. Maternal-conceptus cross talk. A review. Placenta 2003;24:S56-S61.
557. Wakabayashi T, Mizuno M, Yoshida J [The effectiveness of interferon-β against glioma cells and its augmentation of growth inhibitory effect by transfection of its gene]. Hum Cell 1995;8:95-8.
558. Wallace GR, Curnow SJ, Wloka K, et al. The role of chemokines and their receptors in ocular disease. Progress in Retinal and Eye Research 2003;23:435-48.
559. Wang CC, Huang RP, Sommer M, Lisoukov H, Huang R, et al. Array-based multiplexed screening and quantitation of human cytokines and chemokines. J Proteome Res 2002;1:337-43.

560. Wang I-M, Lin H, Goldman SJ, Kobayahi M. STAT-1 is activated by IL-4 and IL-13 in multiple cell types. Mol Immunol 2004;41:873-84.
561. Wang HY, Xin Z, Tang H, Ganea D. Vasoactive intestinal peptide inhibits IL-4 production in murine T cells by a post-transcriptional mechanism. J Immuno 1996;156:3243-53.
562. Wang J, Lin Q, Langston H, Cooper MD. Resident bone marrow macrophages produce type 1 interferons that can selectively inhibit interleukin-7-driven growth of B lineage cells. Immunity 1995;3:475-84.
563. Ward SG. Do phosphoinositide 3-kinases direct lymphocyte navigation? Trends Immunol 2004;25:68-73.
564. Warren HS, Kinnear BF, Kastelein RL, Lanier LL. Analysis of the costimulatory role of IL-2 and IL-15 in initiating proliferation of resting (CD56dim) human NK cells. J Immuno 1996;156:3254-9.
565. Watkins LR, Goehler LE, Relton J, et al. Mechanisms of tumor necrosis factor-α (TNF-α) hyperalgesia. Brain Res 1995;692:244-50.
566. Watson C, Whittaker S, Smith N, et al. IL-6 acts on endothelial cells to preferentially increase their adherence for lymphocytes. Clin Exp Immuno 1996;105:112-9.
567. Waukau J, Jailwala P, Wang Y, Khoo HJ, Ghosh S, Wang X, Hessner MJ. The design of a gene chip for functional immunological studies on a high-quality control platform. Ann N Y Acad Sci 2003;1005:284-7.
568. Weinberger MS, Davidson TM, Broide DH. Differential expression of vascular cell adhesion molecule mRNA and protein in nasal mucosa in response to IL-1 or tumor necrosis factor. J Allergy Clin Immuno 1996;97:662-71.
569. Weiss JM, Pilarski KA, Weyl A, et al. Prostaglandin E1 inhibits TNF α-induced T-cell adhesion to endothelial cells by selective down-modulation of ICAM-1 expression on endothelial cells. Exp Dermatol 1995;4:302-7.
570. Wells TN, Power CA, Lusti-Narasimhan M, et al. Selectivity and antagonism of chemokine receptors. J Leukoc Biol 1996;59:53-60.
571. Wenner CA, Guler ML, Macatonia SE, et al. Roles of IFN-γ and IFN-α in IL-12-induced T helper cell-1 development. J Immuno 1996;156:1442-7.
572. Wenzel UO, Abboud HE. Chemokines and renal disease. Am J Kidney Dis 1995;26:982-94.
573. Wesa A, Galy A. Increased production of proinflammatory cytokines and enhanced T cell responses after activation of human dendritic cells with IL-1 and CD40 ligand. BMC Immunology 2002;3:1-11.
574. Westendorf JJ, Ahmann GJ, Greipp PR, et al. Establishment and characterization of three myeloma cell lines that demonstrate variable cytokine responses and abilities to produce autocrine interleukin-6. Leukemia 1996;10:866-76.
575. Weyrich AS, Elstad MR, McEver RP, et al. Activated platelets signal chemokine synthesis by human monocytes. J Clin Invest 1996;97:1525-34.
576. Whicher JT, Evans SW. Cytokines in Disease. Clin Chem 1990;37:1269-81.
577. Whitcup SM, Rizzo LV, Lai JC, et al. IL-12 inhibits endotoxin-induced inflammation in the eye. Eur J Immuno 1996;26:995-9.
578. Wilson RA, Coulson PS, Betts C, et al. Impaired immunity and altered pulmonary responses in mice with a disrupted interferon-gamma receptor gene exposed to the irradiated Schistosoma mansoni vaccine. Immunology 1996;87:275-82.
579. Windhagen A, Anderson DE, Carrizosa A, et al. IL-12 induces human T cells secreting IL-10 with IFN-γ. J Immuno 1996;157:1127-31.
580. Wisniewski HG, Hua JC, Poppers DM, et al. TNF/IL-1-inducible protein TSG-6 potentiates plasmin inhibition by inter-α-inhibitor and exerts a strong anti-inflammatory effect in vivo. J Immuno 1996;156:1609-15.
581. Witowski, Ksiazek, Jorres A. Interleukin-17: A mediator of inflammatory responses. CMLS Cell Mol Life Sci 2004;61:567-79.
582. Woerly G, Brooks N, Ryffel B. Effect of rapamycin on the expression of the IL-2 receptor (CD25). Clin Exp Immuno 1996;103:322-7.
583. Wong MM, Fish EN. Chemokines: attractive mediators of the immune response. Semin/621Immunol 2003;15:5-14.
584. Yanagida M, Fukamachi H, Ohgami K, et al. Effects of T-helper 2-type cytokines, interleukin-3 (IL-3), IL-4, IL-5, and IL-6 on the survival of cultured human mast cells. Blood 1995;86:3705-14.
585. Yáñez-Mó M, Lara-Pezzi E, Selgas R, et al. Peritoneal Dialysis and Epithelial-to-Mesenchymal Transition of Mesothelial Cells. N Engl J Med 2003;348:403-13.
586. Yang LP, Byun DG, Demeure CE, et al. Default development of cloned human naive CD4 T cells into interleukin-4- and interleukin-5-producing effector cells. Eur J Immuno 1995;25:3517-20.
587. Yao Z, Fanslow WC, Seldin MF, et al. Herpesvirus Saimiri encodes a new cytokine, IL-17, which binds to a novel cytokine receptor. Immunity 1995;3:811-21.
588. Yao Z, Painter SL, Fanslow WC, et al. Human IL-17: a novel cytokine derived from T cells. J Immuno 1995;155:5483-6.
589. Yi AK, Chace JH, Cowdery JS, Krieg AM. IFN-γ promotes IL-6 and IgM secretion in response to CpG motifs in bacterial DNA and oligodeoxynucleotides. J Immuno 1996;156:558-64.
590. Yoshimoto T, Kojima K, Funakoshi T, et al. Molecular cloning and characterization of murine IL-12 genes. J Immuno 1996;156:1082-8.

591. Yu CR, Lin JX, Fink DW, et al. Differential utilization of Janus kinase-signal transducer activator of transcription signaling pathways in the stimulation of human natural killer cells by IL-2, IL-12, and IFN-α. J Immuno 1996;157:126-37.
592. Zambello R, Trentin L, Enthammer C, et al. Lysis of pulmonary fibroblasts by lymphokine (IL-2)-activated killer cells—a mechanism affecting the human lung microenvironment? Clin Exp Immuno 105:383-388, 1996.
593. Zganiacz A, Santosuosso M, Wang J, et al. TNF-α is a critical negative regulator of type 1 immune activation during intracellular bacterial infection. J Clin Invest 2004;113:401-413.
594. Zhang D, Sun M, Samols D, Kushner I. STAT3 participates in transcriptional activation of the C-reactive protein gene by interleukin-6. J Biol Chem 1996;271:9503-9.
595. Zhang L, Conejo-Garcia JR, Katsaros D, et al. Intratumoral T cells, recurrence, and survival in epithelial ovarian cancer. N Engl J Med 2003;348: 3203-13.
596. Zheng LM, Ojcius DM, Garaud F, et al. Interleukin-10 inhibits tumor metastasis through an NK cell-dependent mechanism. J Exp Med 1996;184: 579-84.
597. Zhou Y, McLane M, Levitt RC Th2 cytokines and asthma Interleukin-9 as a therapeutic target for asthma. Respir Res 2001;2:80-4.
598. Zicari A, Lipari M, Di Renzo L, et al. Stimulation of macrophages with IFN gamma or TNF α shuts off the suppressive effect played by PGE2. Int J Immunopharmacol 1995;17:779-86.
599. Zissel G, Schlaak J, Schlaak M, Muller-Quernheim J. Regulation of cytokine release by alveolar macrophages treated with interleukin-4, interleukin-10, or transforming growth factor β. Eur Cytokine Netw 1996;7:59-66.
600. Zitvogel L, Robbins PD, Storkus WJ, et al. Interleukin-12 and B7.1 co-stimulation cooperate in the induction of effective antitumor immunity and therapy of established tumors. Eur J Immuno 1996;26:1335-41.
601. Zlotnik A. Chemokines in neoplastic progression. Semin Cancer Biol 2004;14:181-5.
602. Zubelewicz B, Braczkowski R, Romanowski W, Grzeszczak W. [Influence of treatment using recombinant tumor necrosis factor (hrec TNF α) on circadian rhythm of cortisol secretion in patients with advanced neoplastic disease]. Pol Arch Med Wewn 1995;94:506-11.
603. Zund G, Madara JL, Dzus AL, et al. Interleukin-4 and interleukin-13 differentially regulate epithelial chloride secretion. J Biol Chem 1996;271:7460-4.

ADDITIONAL READING

Balkwill RF. Cytokines: A practical approach, 3rd ed. Oxford: Oxford University Press, 2000.

Kunkel SL. The role of cytokines in the inflammatory response. Farmington CT: S Karger AG, 1996.

Oppenheim JJ, Feldmann M, Durum SK. Cytokine reference: A compendium of cytokines and other mediators of host defense. San Diego: Academic Press, 2000.

Thompson AW. The cytokine handbook, 4th ed. San Diego: Academic Press, 2003.

CHAPTER 23

Tumor Markers

Daniel W. Chan, Ph.D., D.A.B.C.C., F.A.C.B., Ronald A. Booth, Ph.D., and Eleftherios P. Diamandis, M.D., Ph.D.

A tumor marker is a substance produced by a tumor or by the host in response to a tumor that is used to differentiate a tumor from normal tissue or to determine the presence of a tumor based on measurements in the blood or secretions. Such substances are found in cells, tissue, or body fluids and are measured qualitatively or quantitatively by chemical, immunological, or molecular biological methods.[199]

Morphologically, cancer tissue has been recognized by pathologists as resembling fetal tissue more than normal adult differentiated tissue. Tumors are graded according to their degree of differentiation as being (1) well differentiated, (2) poorly differentiated, or (3) anaplastic (without form). Tumor markers are the biochemical or immunological counterparts of the differentiation state of the tumor. In general, some tumor markers represent reexpression of substances produced normally by embryogenically closely related tissue (Table 23-1).

Some tumor markers are specific for one type of cancer, and others are seen in several cancer types. Many of the well-known markers are seen in noncancerous conditions and cancer. Consequently, these tumor markers are not diagnostic for cancer. However, it is thought that the blood levels of tumor markers reflect tumor activity and volume.

Clinically an ideal tumor marker should be both specific for a given type of cancer and sensitive enough to detect small tumors for early diagnosis or during screening. Unfortunately, few markers are specific for a single individual tumor (tumor-specific markers); most are found with different tumors of the same tissue type (tumor-associated markers). They are present in higher quantities in cancer tissue or in blood from cancer patients than in benign tumors or in the blood of normal subjects. In practice, tumor markers are most useful in evaluating the progression of disease status after the initial therapy and monitoring subsequent treatment modalities.[14,15]

This chapter begins with general discussions on (1) cancer, (2) the historical background of tumor markers, (3) their clinical applications, (4) how their utility is evaluated, (5) clinical guidelines for their use, and (6) how they are measured. Several clinically relevant tumor markers from each of these categories are then discussed in detail. These are grouped under the general categories of enzymes, hormones, oncofetal antigens, carbohydrate markers, blood group antigens, proteins, receptors, or genes. More detailed information on tumor markers is found in a 2002 textbook on the subject.[59]

CANCER

In 2004 the estimated number of new cancer cases excluding skin cancer was 1.37 million. Prostate cancer was the leader, followed by cancer of the breast, lung, colon-rectum, and bladder.[31] Together, diseases of the heart and malignant neoplasms account for 52% of all deaths in the United States. Despite heart disease still being the leading cause (699,697 deaths in 2001), malignant neoplasms are a close second (553,251 deaths) and they are projected to surpass heart disease in approximately 10 years.[10] Even in the face of an enormous research effort, the overall mortality rate of cancer has not changed significantly over the past 40 years. However, the trend of cancer mortality varies with individual types of cancer. Significant decreases (greater than 15%) in mortality have been observed in Hodgkin's disease and cancer of the cervix, stomach, and uterus. Alternately, significant increases in mortality (greater than 15%) have occurred in lung cancer, melanoma, multiple myeloma, and non-Hodgkin's lymphoma.[95] These trends support the conclusion that early detection and more effective treatment combined with prevention (e.g., decreasing smoking and improving diet) could greatly reduce the mortality rate of cancer in the future.

TABLE 23-1 "Levels" of Expression of Oncodevelopmental Markers

	Production of Tumor Markers by Various Tissues			
Marker	**Normal Producing**	**Embryogenically Closely Related**	**Distantly Related**	**Unrelated**
CEA	Colon	Stomach, liver, pancreas	Lung, breast	Lymphoma
AFP	Liver, yolk sac	Colon, stomach, pancreas	Lung	
hCG	Placenta	Germinal tumors	Liver	Epidermal lung
Serotonin	Enteroendocrine carcinoid	Adrenal	Oat cell, lung	Epidermal lung

Modified from Sell S. Cancer markers. In: Moossa AR Schempff SC, Robson MC, eds. Comprehensive textbook of oncology, 2nd ed, Vol. 1. Baltimore: Williams & Wilkins, 1991: 225-38.
CEA, Carcinoembryonic antigen; *AFP*, alpha fetoprotein; *hCG*, human chorionic gonadotropin.

A simple definition of cancer is "a relatively autonomous growth of tissue."[175] Understanding the cause of autonomous growth would clearly facilitate the search for a cure. A *carcinogen* is an agent that causes cancer. A carcinogen may be physical (e.g., radiation), chemical (e.g., a polycyclic hydrocarbon), or biological (e.g., a virus). Exposure to such an agent may cause cancer either by producing direct genotoxic effects on deoxyribonucleic acid (DNA) (e.g., as with radiation) or by increasing cell proliferation (e.g., by a hormone), or both (e.g., through the use of tobacco).

Advances in molecular genetics have provided a better understanding of the genesis of human cancer. The proliferation of normal cells is thought to be regulated by growth-promoting *oncogenes* and counterbalanced by growth-constraining *tumor suppressor genes.* The development of cancer appears to involve the activation or the altered expression of oncogenes[1] or the loss or inactivation of a tumor suppressor gene.[246] A pathway to cancer development has been published.[66]

Early detection of cancer offers the best chance for cure. The goal is to diagnose cancer when a tumor is still small enough to be completely removed surgically. Unfortunately, most cancers do not produce symptoms until the tumors are either too large to be removed surgically or until cancerous cells have already spread to other tissue (metastasized).

Although other modes of therapy, such as administration of chemical toxins or irradiation, are often effective in destroying most tumor cells, they are usually not curative. The few residual viable tumor cells are able to proliferate, develop resistance to further therapy, and eventually kill the patient.

HISTORICAL BACKGROUND

The first tumor marker reported was the Bence Jones protein. Since its discovery in 1847 by precipitation of a protein in acidified boiled urine,[17] the measurement of Bence Jones protein has been a diagnostic test for multiple myeloma (a tumor of plasma cells). More than 100 years after its discovery, the Nobel Prize–winning studies of Porter and of Edelman and Poulik identified the Bence Jones protein as the monoclonal light chain of immunoglobulin secreted by tumor plasma cells. Monoclonal paraproteins appear as sharp bands in the globulin area in electrophoretic patterns of serum. Diagnosis of multiple myeloma is often made based on this finding or on the presence of an elevated level of "monoclonal" immunoglobulin in the serum.[213]

A brief history of tumor markers is shown in Table 23-2.[197] The first period of tumor marker history was the era of the Bence Jones protein. The second era, from 1928 to 1963, included the discovery of hormones, enzymes, isoenzymes, and proteins and their application to the diagnosis of cancer and the beginnings of the chromosomal analysis of tumors. Occasionally, such markers were useful in the diagnosis of individual tumors, but the general application of tumor markers for monitoring cancer patients did not start until the third era with the discovery of alpha fetoprotein (AFP) in 1963[2] and carcinoembryonic antigen (CEA) in 1965.[80] The production of such markers during fetal development and in tumors led to the use of the term *oncodevelopmental markers.*[71]

The fourth era started in 1975 with the development of monoclonal antibodies and their subsequent use to detect oncofetal antigens and antigens derived from tumor cell lines. Examples are carbohydrate antigens such as CA 125, CA 15-3, and CA 27.29. Advances in molecular genetics using molecular probes and monoclonal antibodies to detect chromosome or protein alterations, including the study of oncogenes, suppressor genes, and genes involved in DNA repair,[115] have led to the rapid understanding and use of tumor markers at the molecular level. These markers are becoming increasingly useful at the cellular level. For example, mutated *ras* oncogene can be detected in sloughed cellular DNA in fecal material and thus can be used to diagnose colon cancer.[204] Discovery of the breast cancer susceptibility genes, *BRCA 1* and *BRCA 2,*[144,251] has led to the possibility of screening for familial breast cancer in high-risk individuals.[174]

As we begin the twenty-first century, new technologies are being applied to the discovery of tumor markers and their

TABLE 23-2 A Brief History of Tumor Markers

Year	Author	Marker
1846	H. Bence Jones	Bence Jones protein
1928	W.H. Brown	Ectopic hormone syndrome
1930	B. Zondek	hCG
1932	H. Cushing	ACTH
1949	K. Oh-Uti	Deletions of blood group antigens
1959	C. Markert	Isoenzymes
1963	G.I. Abelev	AFP
1965	P. Gold and S. Freeman	CEA
1969	R. Heubner and G. Todaro	Oncogenes
1975	H. Kohler and G. Milstein	Monoclonal antibodies
1980	G. Cooper, R. Weinberg, and M. Bishop	Oncogene probes and transfection
1985	H. Harris, R. Sager, and A. Knudson	Suppressor gene
2001	Multiple investigations	Genomics and proteomics using microarrays, mass spectrometry, neural networks, multiparametric analysis

Modified from Sell S. Cancer markers. In: Moossa AR, Schempff SC, Robson MC, eds. Comprehensive textbook of oncology, 2nd ed, Vol. 1. Baltimore: Williams & Wilkins, 1991: 225-38.
hCG, Human chorionic gonadotropin; *ACTH,* adrenocorticotropic hormone; *AFP,* alpha fetoprotein; *CEA,* carcinoembryonic antigen.

clinical applications. Notable among these discoveries are the introduction of genomics and proteomics technologies[162] such as the measurement of complementary DNA (cDNA) protein and the tissue microarrays and the use of mass spectrometry as a diagnostic and discovery tool. Furthermore, the advent of bioinformatic techniques, including neural networks, logistic regression, and other algorithms, is facilitating the use of multiparametric analysis for cancer diagnosis, prognosis, and prediction of therapy.[263]

CLINICAL APPLICATIONS

The potential uses of tumor markers are summarized in Table 23-3. In general, tumor markers may be used for diagnosis, prognosis, and monitoring the effects of therapy and as targets for localization and therapy.[199] Ideally a tumor marker should be produced by the tumor cells and be detectable in body fluids. It should not be present in healthy people or in benign conditions. Therefore it could be used for screening for the presence of cancer in asymptomatic individuals in a general population. Most tumor markers are present in normal, benign, and cancer tissues and are not specific enough to be used for screening cancer. However, if the incidence of cancer is high among certain populations, screening could be feasible. An example is the use of AFP in the screening of hepatocellular carcinoma in China and Alaska.[141] Prostate-specific antigen (PSA) has been used in conjunction with digital rectal examination for early detection of prostate cancer. Because of the elevation of serum PSA in benign prostatic hyperplasia (BPH), PSA velocity and free PSA have been used to improve the detection of prostate cancer.[167]

The clinical staging of cancer is aided by quantitation of the marker (i.e., the serum level of the marker reflects tumor burden). The marker value at the time of diagnosis may be used as a prognostic indicator for disease progression and patient survival. This is possible for an individual patient, but different levels of markers produced by different tumors do not usually allow one to determine the prognosis of a tumor from the initial level. However, after successful initial treatment, such as surgery, the marker value should decrease. The rate of the decrease can be predicted by using the half-life of the marker. For example, the half-life of PSA is 2 to 3 days, that of human chorionic gonadotropin (hCG) is 12 to 20 hours, and that of AFP is 5 days. If the half-life after treatment is longer than the expected half-life, then the treatment has not been successful in removing the tumor. The magnitude of marker reduction may, however, reflect the degree of success of the treatment or the extent of disease involvement.

Detecting cancer recurrence may be helpful to initiate early treatment or change therapy. Ultrasensitive PSA assays allow earlier detection of prostate cancer after radical prostatectomy. The breast cancer marker CA 27.29 has been shown to detect recurrent disease before any clinical evidence in breast cancer patients receiving adjuvant chemotherapy.[39]

Most tumor marker values correlate with the effectiveness of treatment and responses to therapy. In breast cancer, the concentration of markers, such as CA 15-3 or CA 27.29, changes with the treatment and the clinical outcome of the patient. Marker values usually increase with progressive disease, decrease with remission, and do not change significantly with stable disease. The tumor marker kinetics in the monitoring of cancer may be more complicated. The marker values in response to treatment may show an initial delay before demonstrating the expected pattern of change.[110]

In addition, antibodies to tumor markers labeled with a radioactive tag are used to localize the tumor masses (radioimmunoscintigraphy)[52] or to provide direction for labeled antibodies to attack the tumor site. Examples are the use of radiolabeled antibodies to CEA to localize colon tumors and the application of labeled antibodies against ferritin to target hepatocellular carcinoma. This approach is

TABLE 23-3 Current Applications of Tumor Markers and Their Limitations

Application	Current Usefulness	Comments
Screening for cancer	Limited	1. For screening, you must have a marker that is elevated at early disease stages, when the disease is localized and potentially curable. Most circulating cancer markers (with the exception of PSA) are elevated notably in the late stages of disease. Thus diagnostic sensitivity is usually low for early-stage disease. 2. With the exception of PSA, most cancer markers are not specific for a particular tissue and elevations may be due to diseases of other tissue, including benign and inflammatory diseases. Thus diagnostic specificity may be low, leading to many false positives. In screening, there is a necessity for a definitive diagnostic method that will separate true positives from false positives. If this procedure is invasive (e.g., surgery) and/or expensive, patients will not accept it. 3. Screening, even if effective for early cancer diagnosis, must demonstrate benefit to the screened population in terms of survival or other clinical endpoints.
Diagnosing cancer	Limited	Same as above. Low diagnostic sensitivity and specificity. However, for selected subgroups of high-risk patients, in whom the chance of cancer is high (high prevalence), tumor marker analysis may not aid the clinician in ordering more elaborate testing (e.g., imaging techniques or laparoscopic investigations).
Evaluating cancer prognosis	Limited	Most cancer markers have prognostic value but their accuracy is not good enough to warrant specific therapeutic interventions. For example, higher preoperative levels of PSA are associated with capsular penetration, high Gleason score, positive surgical margins, and positive lymph node status, but the decision to treat with two different modalities (e.g., radical prostatectomy versus nonsurgical approaches) cannot be made based on tumor marker data alone. Same applies to many other cancers.
Prediction of therapeutic response	Important	Despite the importance of using biomarkers in predicting response to specific therapies, very few known markers have such predictive power. These include the steroid hormone receptors for predicting response to antiestrogens and Her-2/neu amplification for predicting response to Herceptin in breast cancer patients. We must have more predictive markers to individualize therapy and maximize clinical response.
Tumor staging	Limited	Same as for prognosis. The data are not good enough for accurate staging unless the value is reflecting tumor volume.
Detecting tumor recurrence or remission	Controversial	Despite the importance of using biomarkers to detect cancer relapse, current markers are limited by the following: (a) Lead time is short (weeks to a few months) and does not significantly affect outcome, even if therapy is instituted earlier; (b) Therapies for treating recurrent disease are not effective at present; (c) In certain groups of patients, biomarkers are not produced and do not detect relapses; (d) Sometimes biomarkers provide misleading information (e.g., clinical relapses occur without biomarker elevation, or biomarker is elevated nonspecifically, without progressive disease, leading to either overtreatment or discontinuation of a current and successful treatment protocol).
Localizing tumor and directing radiotherapeutic agents	Limited	Only a few biomarkers are available for this application and success is limited at present

TABLE 23-3 Current Applications of Tumor Markers and Their Limitations—*Continued*

Application	Current Usefulness	Comments
Monitoring the effectiveness of cancer therapy	Important	For patients with advanced disease, who are treated with various modalities, it is important to know if therapy works. In this regard, biomarkers usually provide information that is readily interpretable and more economical, more sensitive, and safer than radiological or invasive procedures. For certain cancers, this may facilitate increased enrollment of patients into therapeutic clinical trials.

Modified from Diamandis EP. Tumor markers: Past, present, and future. In: Diamandis EP, Fritsche HA, Lilja H, Chan DW, Schwartz MK. Tumor markers: Physiology, pathobiology, technology, and clinical application. Washington DC: AACC Press, 2002:5.

also used for treatment by allowing the antibody to bind to the tumor marker epitopes and kill the tumor cell with the dose of radioactivity.[245]

EVALUATING CLINICAL UTILITY

To evaluate the clinical usefulness of a tumor marker, it is necessary to establish reference values, calculate predictive values, evaluate the distribution of marker values, and determine the role of the values in disease management.

REFERENCE VALUES

Reference values of a tumor marker are obtained from a healthy population, preferably with age- and sex-matched individuals.[26] The determination of reference values is time-consuming and requires a large healthy population ($n \geq 120$ subjects). Statistical analysis using the mean ± 2 standard deviation (SD) for a population with a gaussian (normal) distribution is a frequently used method. For a nongaussian distribution, the percentile method is a simple approach and often used (for further discussion of reference values, see Chapter 16).

The reference values determined using healthy subjects in this fashion are applicable to analytes with physiologically well-defined concentrations. For testing with relatively specific applications, such as the use of tumor markers in the diagnosis and management of cancer, a decision level may be more appropriate than the upper limit of the normal population. In most cases, using benign patients as the nondisease group is more appropriate than using a healthy population. The decision level can be determined using a predictive value model.

PREDICTIVE VALUE MODEL

The predictive value model includes the clinical sensitivity, specificity, and predictive value of a test. By varying the decision level, clinical sensitivity and specificity will change in opposite directions. An optimal decision level can be selected based on the strategies outlined in Chapter 15.

A useful approach to evaluating multiple tests for the same analyte or multiple markers for the same type of cancer

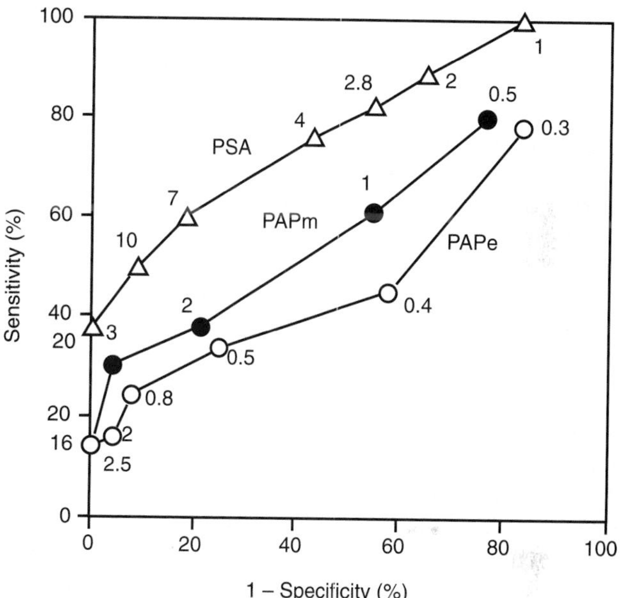

Figure 23-1 ROC curves for PSA, prostatic acid phosphatase by monoclonal immunoassay (M-PAP), and enzymatic prostatic acid phosphatase (E-PAP). The data for all 128 patients with prostatic disease are plotted, with several quantitative decision levels (as indicated in the figure) for each assay. Units are µg/L for M-PAP and PSA, and U/L for E-PAP. *(From Rock RC, Chan DW, Bruzek DJ, et al. Evaluation of a monoclonal immunoradiometric assay for prostate-specific antigen. Clin Chem 1987; 33:2257-61.)*

is the *receiver operating characteristic* (ROC) curve (see Silver and co-workers).[207] The ROC curve can be constructed by plotting sensitivity versus 1 minus specificity or the true-positive rate versus the false-positive rate. The advantage of the ROC curve is the display of performance over the entire range of decision levels. One can pinpoint the decision level where the optimal sensitivity and specificity can be achieved. By superimposing the ROC curves of several markers, the most predictive marker can be selected. Examples are shown in Figures 23-1 and 23-2. The preparation of an ROC curve has been discussed in detail by Zweig and Robertson[266] and in Chapter 15.

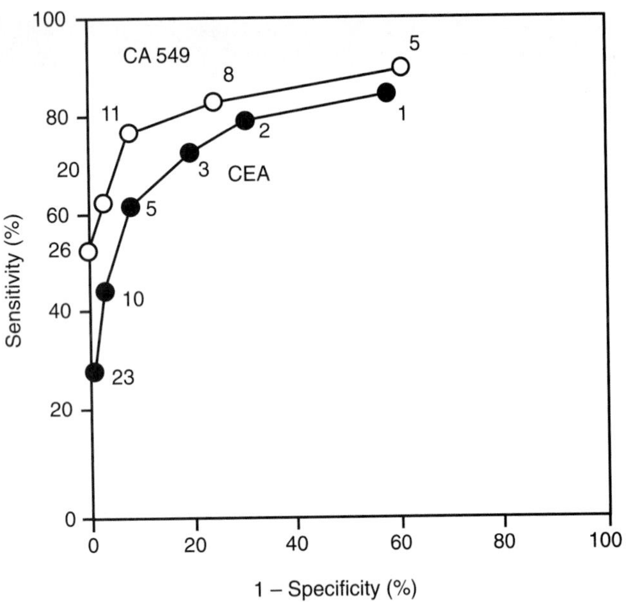

Figure 23-2 ROC for CA 549 (kU/L) and CEA (μg/L). The sensitivity, specificity, and efficiency are based on the decision level of CA 549 (11 kU/L) and CEA (5 μg/L). The data include patients with breast cancer and benign breast diseases (331 for CA 549, and 322 for CEA). The decision values are indicated on the curve. *(From Chan DW, Beveridge RA, Bruzek DJ, et al. Monitoring breast cancer with CA 549. Clin Chem 1988; 34:2000-4.)*

Distribution of Marker Values

Application of the predictive value model is difficult for analytes that are not diagnostic for a single disease. Levels of most, if not all, tumor markers are elevated in more than one disease condition. When using the predictive value model, it is necessary to select a population that includes groups with and without disease. What patients should be included in these two groups? The decision should be based on the specific clinical questions asked. If the question concerns the diagnostic sensitivity of CEA for active colorectal carcinoma, the disease group should include only those patients with active colorectal carcinoma. Selection of the nondisease group is more challenging. Should healthy individuals and those with benign conditions be included? If so, how many benign condition groups should be included? Should the patients in remission be included as well, because they do not have active diseases? The values calculated for sensitivity and specificity greatly depend on the types of groups included and on the number of patients in each group (see Chapter 15 for a discussion on the effect of spectrum on sensitivity and specificity).

The distribution of tumor marker values is usually shown as the percentage of patients with elevated values as determined using various cut-off values in the healthy, benign, and cancerous groups. International staging criteria should be used to classify cancer patients. Diagnosis should be based on pathological findings. The groups are selected from past experiences of similar markers. In breast cancer, for example (Table 23-4), normal women are used as the healthy population for comparison. The nonmalignant or benign groups are selected to include people with the most likely causes of marker elevation: benign liver and breast diseases and pregnancy. The nonbreast metastatic cancer groups are selected to show the specificity of the marker using endometrial, colon, lung, prostate, and ovarian carcinoma.

Grouping all breast cancer patients into a single category is not satisfactory because most markers are elevated in active breast cancer. The adjuvant group consists of patients who had no metastasis, underwent mastectomy and treatment with adjuvant chemotherapy, and have no evidence of disease. The marker value is not expected to be elevated. The metastasis group includes patients in complete remission, in partial remission, or with progressive breast cancer accompanied by local or distant metastases. The progressive breast cancer group should have the highest percentage of elevated marker values. The partial remission group should have an intermediate percentage of elevated marker values. The complete remission group should have the lowest percentage of elevated marker values.

Disease Management

Most tumor markers are used to monitor treatment and progression of cancer. The selection of patient groups is important to illustrate the usefulness of the marker in various clinical settings. Markers may be used to determine the success of the initial treatment (e.g., surgery or radiation), detect the recurrence of cancer, and monitor the effectiveness of the treatment modality.

To determine the success of surgery, an elevated marker level before surgery should fall after a successful operation. The extent of the decrease in the marker value depends on the pretreatment tumor involvement.

With the recurrence of cancer after a successful initial treatment, the marker value may not fall within the normal half-life. It may fall to a steady level that is higher than normal, or it may fall within the reference interval of healthy individuals. A subsequent rise in the marker value suggests recurrence of the cancer. An example of breast cancer is shown in Figure 23-3.

To monitor the effectiveness of cancer therapy, the marker value should increase with the progression of cancer, decrease with the regression of cancer, and not change in the presence of stable disease. When evaluating candidate markers, all the events related to the progression, stability, and regression of disease can be grouped; whether the marker value changes in the predicted direction in all these situations can be evaluated next.[38]

The Working Group on Tumor Marker Criteria of the International Society for Oncodevelopmental Biology and Medicine has published the following criteria for the interpretation of changes in tumor marker values[26]:

"If no therapy is given, at least a linear increase in three

TABLE 23-4 Distribution of CA 549 Values

Diagnosis	Number (and %) of Patients With CA 549 Values (kU/L)						
	No. of Patients	**0-8**	**>8**	**>11**	**>15**	**>20**	**>25**
Normal women	100	85 (85)	15 (15)	5 (5)	0 (0)	0 (0)	0 (0)
Nonmalignant							
Benign liver	42	19 (45)	23 (55)	11 (26)	3 (7)	0 (0)	0 (0)
Benign breast	69	63 (91)	6 (9)	1 (1)	1 (1)	0 (0)	0 (0)
Pregnancy	30	26 (87)	4 (13)	0 (0)	0 (0)	0 (0)	0 (0)
Nonbreast Metastatic Cancer							
Endometrial	8	7 (88)	1 (12)	1 (12)	1 (12)	1 (12)	0 (0)
Colon	41	25 (61)	16 (39)	7 (17)	3 (7)	1 (2)	1 (2)
Lung	40	22 (55)	18 (45)	13 (33)	11 (28)	6 (15)	6 (15)
Prostate	30	13 (43)	17 (57)	12 (40)	5 (17)	5 (17)	3 (10)
Ovarian	60	22 (37)	38 (63)	30 (50)	21 (35)	15 (25)	10 (17)
Breast Cancer							
Adjuvant	88	61 (69)	27 (31)	10 (11)	6 (9)	4 (5)	0 (0)
Metastatic							
Complete remission	16	11 (69)	5 (31)	3 (19)	1 (6)	1 (6)	1 (6)
Partial remission	52	12 (23)	40 (77)	33 (63)	27 (52)	22 (42)	16 (31)
No response (progressive)							
Local	12	5 (42)	7 (58)	5 (42)	3 (25)	2 (17)	2 (17)
Metastasis	94	7 (7)	87 (93)	83 (88)	79 (84)	73 (78)	69 (73)

From Chan DW, Beveridge RA, Bruzek DJ, et al. Monitoring breast cancer with CA 549. Clin Chem 1988; 34:2000-4.

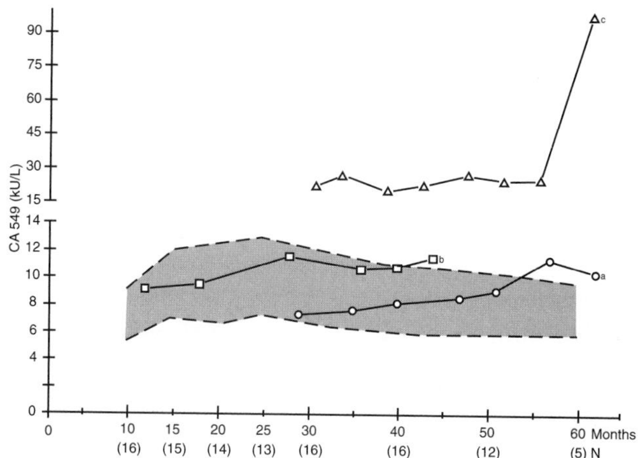

Figure 23-3 Monitoring the clinical sources of adjuvant breast cancer patients ($n = 19$). Mean *(bottom line of the shaded area)* and mean +2 SD *(top line)* of CA 549 values for 16 patients. *Open circles,* Patient A; *open squares,* patient B; *open triangles,* patient C; *N,* number of samples. *(From Chan DW, Beveridge RA, Bruzek DJ, et al. Monitoring breast cancer with CA 549. Clin Chem 1988;34:2000-4.)*

consecutive samples (i.e., two time intervals) on a log scale should be registered to establish a recurrence. Usual intervals could be three months but are clinically determined. After a first increase, next samples should be taken after 2 to 4 weeks, irrespective of the absolute level."

If therapy is given, the changes in marker values should reflect the clinical progression of the disease. "Progressive disease is defined by an increase in the marker level of at least 25%. Sampling should be repeated within 2 to 4 weeks for additional evidence. . . . The sampling interval during therapy may depend on the type of tumor and should be related to clinical follow-up." A decrease in marker value of at least 50% is indicative of partial remission "with the concept that tumor load is related to the changes in serum tumor marker levels." The working group also provided a general opinion that "a complete remission cannot be determined by marker levels, but if tumor marker levels are elevated, the clinical decision of complete remission based on conventional methods should be considered incorrect unless an explanation for the presence of the elevated level is given."

CLINICAL GUIDELINES

The diagnosis and staging of cancer involve a number of tools, including physical examination, imaging, and laboratory studies. Application of these tools has resulted in a number of tumor markers that are used for screening, diagnosis, staging, and prognosis, and for directing treatment modalities. However, not all tumor markers are appropriate for all uses, and not all cancers have established tumor markers. Therefore each type of cancer and each tumor marker must be properly evaluated for use, and clinicians must be educated to the proper use of the tumor markers to conserve resources.

A number of international groups have released guidelines on the selection and use of tumor markers in the clinic. These groups include the National Academy of Clinical Biochemistry (NACB), the European Group on Tumor Markers (EGTM), the American Cancer Society (ACS), the American Society for Clinical Oncology (ASCO), and others.[230] All of these groups are composed of experts in the areas being assessed, and a number of criteria are used to form the recommendations, including the level of evidence for the tumor marker (level I to V, with level I being a high-powered prospective trial) and the tumor marker utility grading system (TMUGS).[59] Table 23-5 summarizes the recommendations of a number of these groups.

ANALYTICAL METHODOLOGY

Tumor markers are measured by a variety of analytical techniques including enzyme assay (Chapters 8 and 21); immunoassay (Chapter 9); receptor assay and instrumental techniques such as chromatography (Chapter 6); electrophoresis (Chapter 5); mass spectrometry interfaced with either liquid or gas chromatographs (Chapter 7) and microarrays. Details of these techniques are found in the indicated chapters. Here we expand on the use of mass spectrometry and microarrays for the assay of protein and genetic tumor markers.

MASS SPECTROMETRY

Mass spectrometry for small molecules has been used in the clinical laboratory for more than 40 years. However, recent

TABLE 23-5 Summary of Key Guideline Recommendations

Cancer Type	NACB	ASCO	ACS	EGTM
Breast	ER and PR on all cancers. CA 15-3/CA 27.29 for monitoring advanced disease	Routine use of CA 15-3 or CA 27.29 alone *not* recommended Increasing CA 15-3 or CA 27.29 may be used to suggest treatment failure. Routine use of CEA not recommended. ER and PR determined for primary lesions. Steroid hormone receptors to be used to select patients for endocrine therapy. HER-2/neu (c-ErbB-2) overexpression or amplification may be used to select patients for Herceptin (trastuzumab) therapy	None	Steroid receptors in tissue predicting response to hormone therapy CEA and one MUC1-gene-related protein in serum for prognosis, follow-up, and monitoring of therapy HER-2/neu in tissue for predicting response to Herceptin (trastuzumab) in patients with advanced disease
Ovarian	CA 125 as a diagnostic aid and for monitoring therapy	None	None	CA 125 as an aid in diagnosis, for monitoring treatment, and early prediction of recurrence
Prostate	PSA with DRE. %fPSA when PSA is between 4-10 ng/mL and DRE is negative	Guidelines under development for metastatic disease	PSA and DRE for screening and detection	tPSA with DRE for screening (studies), case finding, or prognosis.

TABLE 23-5 Summary of Key Guideline Recommendations—*Continued*

Cancer Type	NACB	ASCO	ACS	EGTM
				tPSA in follow-up and monitoring of therapy if additional means of therapy can be offered in case of rising tPSA. %fPSA for differential diagnosis when tPSA is between 4-10 ng/mL and DRE is negative
Germ cell	AFP, hCG, LD for detecting and monitoring testicular tumors. AFP is diagnostic for NSGCT	None	None	AFP, hCG, LD, and PLAP* for case finding, staging, prognosis, follow-up, and monitoring of therapy. AFP is diagnostic for NSGCT
Colon	CEA for monitoring therapy	CEA for prognosis, detecting recurrence, and monitoring therapy	None	CEA for case-finding, prognosis, follow-up, and monitoring for therapy
Neuroendocrine	Urinary catecholamines, VMA, HVA as indicators for pheochromocytoma and neuroblastoma. Calcitonin for medullary thyroid carcinoma	None	None	None
Myeloma	Serum protein electrophoresis for M spike	None	None	None
Lung	None	None	None	NSE in differential diagnosis. CYFRA 21-1, CEA, and/or NSA for follow-up and monitoring of therapy

Modified from Diamandis EP. Tumor markers: Past, present, and future. In: Diamandis EP, Fritsche HA, Lilja H, Chan DW, Schwartz MK. Tumor markers: Physiology, pathobiology, technology, and clinical application. Washington DC: AACC Press, 2002:57

NACB, National Academy of Clinical Biochemistry; *ASCO,* American Society of Clinical Oncology; *ACS,* American Cancer Society; *EGTM,* European Group on Tumor Markers; *tPSA,* total PSA; *fPSA,* free PSA; *NSGCT,* nonseminomatous germ cell tumors.

"None" indicates that the relevant group has not yet considered this type of cancer.

Placental alkaline phosphatase (PLAP) is for monitoring of seminomas in nonsmokers only.

developments have allowed for the mass spectrometric identification of high molecular weight compounds, including proteins and nucleic acids. The new ionization technologies were recognized by the Nobel Prize in chemistry in 2002. These advances triggered investigations toward using the technology for either cancer diagnosis or prognosis or for discovering new cancer biomarkers. In one approach, serum or other fluids from cancer patients or controls are treated with various absorbing surfaces, such as ion-exchange, hydrophobic, or metal-binding chips. After washing out excess proteins, the chips are subjected to mass spectrometric analysis by using the so-called MALDI method (matrix-assisted laser desorption ionization) or SELDI (surface-enhanced laser desorption ionization)-TOF (time-of-flight mass spectrometry). This analysis generates a number of peaks of various M-Z (mass to charge) ratios. By comparing these proteomic patterns with patterns obtained from samples from normal individuals, and by using sophisticated bioinformatic and computational tools, it is possible to identify patterns that are only associated with cancer. This technology has now been investigated for diagnosis of ovarian[171,178,264] prostate,[3,172] bladder, and many other cancers.[186] The technology has been reviewed.[162,173,219] The diagnostic sensitivities and specificities of this technology are impressive and surpass those achieved by using current cancer biomarkers.[3,171,172] However, this method has not as yet been prospectively evaluated but clinical trials are now in progress. Also, a number of shortcomings of this technology have been identified.[56-58]

The same technology and principles are also being used to identify novel cancer biomarkers.[125,178,186,264] To date, a number of molecules have been identified, including apolipoprotein A1, transthyretin fragment, interalpha-trypsin inhibitor, haptoglobin-alpha subunit, and vitamin D–binding protein. These molecules are present in serum at concentrations much higher than levels of traditional cancer biomarkers. The clinical evaluation of these proteins as candidate biomarkers is still under investigation.

MICROARRAYS

A microarray is a microchip of silicon that contains a large number of elements ("spots") in a two-dimensional array (see Chapter 10). To each of these spots is attached different molecules of immobilized short oligonucleotides (e.g., the Affymetrix chips), cDNAs of various genes, proteins, antibodies, etc.[129,152,193] It is possible to immobilize up to 20,000 to 40,000 elements on such chips and, consequently, genome-wide analysis at both the messenger ribonucleic acid (mRNA) and protein levels is now possible. Applications of microarrays include quantitative assessment of gene expression, detection of mutations and polymorphisms (such as single nucleotide polymorphisms), DNA sequencing, and study of protein expression and protein-protein interactions. For some applications, the method has been semiautomated.

These devices have been used to discover new candidate biomarkers. For example, Welsh and colleagues used microarray analysis of gene expression profiles of normal and cancerous tissues and identified highly overexpressed genes in ovarian and other cancers.[247,248] These overexpressed genes were then to be evaluated further with more quantitative techniques, such as reverse-transcriptase polymerase-chain reaction, to confirm the overexpression. The identification of an overexpressed gene can be followed by development of assays to measure the protein and then evaluate it as a serological or tissue biomarker.[247] Some successes of this process have recently been reported (e.g., the identification of osteopontin and HE4 as ovarian cancer biomarkers).

Another application of microarrays is in the classification of cancers based on their gene expression profiles. There are now numerous examples of subclassifying breast, ovarian, prostate, brain, hematological, and other cancers using this technology.[109,170] Especially for breast cancer, it has recently been realized that tissue microarray analysis may stratify patients according to prognosis.[239,240] These analyses aid in the selection of adjuvant therapy. Van de Vijver et al have shown that a relatively small number of genes (about 70) can be used to classify patients in high- and low-risk groups. As of June 2003, this method has been applied clinically to select breast cancer patients for adjuvant chemotherapy.

The application of microarrays for cancer classification and prognosis and for discovering new cancer biomarkers is relatively new. This method has the potential to revolutionize cancer prognosis and prediction of therapy by using dedicated chips. Further standardization is necessary.

ENZYMES

Enzymes were one of the first groups of tumor markers identified. Their elevated activities were used to indicate the presence of cancer.[83] Measurement of enzymes was relatively easy using spectrophotometric determination of enzymatic activities. With the introduction of radioimmunoassay (RIA) in the late 1950s, the mass of an enzyme could be measured as a protein antigen instead of its catalytic activity.

With few exceptions, an increase in the activity or mass of an enzyme or isoenzyme is not specific or sensitive enough to be used for identifying the type of cancer or the specific organ involvement. An exception is PSA. PSA has mild protease activity and amino acid sequence homology with serine protease of the kallikrein family.[46,54] It is expressed by normal, benign, hyperplastic, and cancerous prostate glands and minimally by other tissue.[23] Until the application of PSA as a marker for prostate cancer, tumor enzymes had lost most[83,196] of their popularity for use as cancer markers. Enzymes were used historically as tumor markers before the discovery of oncofetal antigens and the advent of monoclonal antibodies.[195] The abnormalities of enzymes as a marker for cancer are either the expression of the fetal form of the enzyme (isozyme) or the ectopic production of enzymes.

Enzymes are present in much higher concentrations inside the cell. Enzymes are released into the systemic

TABLE 23-6 Enzymes as Tumor Markers

Enzyme	Assay	Type of Cancer
Alcohol dehydrogenase	Act	Liver
Aldolase	Act	Liver
Alkaline phosphatase	Act	Bone, liver, leukemia, sarcoma
Alkaline phosphatase-placental	Act	Ovarian, lung, trophoblastic, gastrointestinal, seminoma, Hodgkin's
Amylase	Act	Pancreatic, various
Aryl sulfatase B	Act	Colon, breast
Creatine kinase-BB	Act	Prostate, lung (small cell), breast, colon, ovarian
Esterase	Act	Breast
Galactosyltransferase	Act	Colon, bladder, gastrointestinal, various
γ-Glutamyltransferase	Act	Liver
Hexokinase	Act	Liver
Lactate dehydrogenase	Act	Liver, lymphomas, leukemia, various
Leucine aminopeptidase	Act	Pancreatic, liver
Neuron-specific enolase	RIA	Lung (small cell), neuroblastoma, carcinoid, melanoma, pheochromocytoma, pancreatic
5′-Nucleotidase	Act	Liver
Prostatic acid phosphatase	Act/IMA	Prostate
PSA	IMA	Prostate
Pyruvate kinase	Act	Liver, various
Ribonuclease	Act	Various (ovarian, lung, large bowel)
Sialytransferase	Act	Breast, colon, lung
Terminal deoxytransferase	Act	Leukemia
Thymidine kinase	RIA/Act	Various, leukemia, lymphomas, lung (small cell)

Act, Activity; *RIA*, radioimmunoassay; *IMA*, immunometric assay.

circulation as the result of tumor necrosis or of the change of the membrane permeability of the cancer cells. Increased enzyme levels are also observed in the blockage of pancreatic or biliary ducts and in renal insufficiency. The intracellular location of the enzyme may also determine the rate of the release. By the time enzymes are released into the systemic circulation, the metastasis of tumors may have occurred. Most enzymes are not unique for a specific organ. Therefore enzymes are most suitable as nonspecific tumor markers. Elevated enzyme levels may signal the presence of malignancy.

Isoenzymes and multiple forms of enzymes may provide additional organ specificity. Table 23-6 summarizes various enzymes, their associated types of malignancy, and the assays used to measure their activity (Act) or their mass concentration (RIA or immunometric assay). Enzymes are traditionally measured by their activities. With the introduction of antibody techniques, some enzymes, such as PSA, are measured as protein antigens rather than by their enzyme activity.

Alkaline Phosphatase

Alkaline phosphatase may arise from liver, bone, or placenta. The alkaline phosphatase in the sera of normal adults comes primarily from the liver or biliary tract. Elevated levels of alkaline phosphatase are seen in primary or secondary liver cancer. Its level may be helpful in evaluating metastatic cancer with bone or liver involvement. Greatest elevations are seen in patients with osteoblastic lesions, such as in prostatic cancer with bone metastases. Minimum elevations are seen in patients with osteolytic lesions, such as breast cancer with bone metastases.[70,229]

In liver metastases, the serum alkaline phosphatase level shows a better correlation with the extent of liver involvement than those of other liver tests. To differentiate the origin of elevated alkaline phosphatase levels, tests of other liver enzymes may be performed, such as that for 5′-nucleotidase or γ-glutamyltransferase. Determination of alkaline phosphatase isoenzymes may provide additional specificity. The liver isoenzyme is thermally more stable than the bone isoenzyme (see Chapter 21 for a more detailed discussion). Other malignancies, such as leukemia, sarcoma, and lymphoma complicated with hepatic infiltration, may also show elevated alkaline phosphatase levels.

Placental alkaline phosphatase (PALP) is synthesized by the trophoblast and is elevated in sera of pregnant women. PALP was first identified as the Regan isoenzyme in 1968 by Fishman and colleagues[71] and was recognized as one of the first oncodevelopmental markers along with AFP and CEA. It is elevated in a variety of malignancies, including ovarian, lung, trophoblastic, and gastrointestinal cancers; seminoma; and Hodgkin's disease.

Creatine Kinase

Creatine kinase (CK) catalyzes the phosphorylation of creatine by adenosine triphosphate. CK is a dimer consisting of two subunits, M (muscle) and B (brain). There are three isoenzymes, CK1 (BB), CK2 (MB), and CK3 (MM). CK1 is present in the brain, prostate gland, gastrointestinal tract, lung, bladder, uterus, and placenta. Cardiac muscle has the highest concentration of CK2 (≅ 20%). CK3 is present in skeletal and cardiac muscles.

Elevated levels of CK1 have been demonstrated in prostate cancer and small cell carcinoma of the lung. Although it is also elevated in other malignancies, such as those of the breast, colon, ovary, and stomach, the clinical usefulness of CK1 as a tumor marker requires further investigation.[196] CK isoenzymes have been included in a prostate cancer panel, "ProstAsure."[12,221]

Lactate Dehydrogenase

Lactate dehydrogenase (LD) is an enzyme in the glycolytic pathway and is released as the result of cell damage. The elevation of LD in malignancy is rather nonspecific. It has been demonstrated in a variety of cancers—including liver, non-Hodgkin's lymphoma, acute leukemia, nonseminomatous germ cell testicular cancer, seminoma, neuroblastoma, and other carcinomas, such as breast, colon, stomach, and lung cancer. The serum LD level has been shown to correlate with tumor mass in solid tumors and provides a prognostic indicator for disease progression. Its value in the monitoring of therapy is rather limited. The isoenzymes only provide marginal specificity for organ involvement. For example, the elevation of the LD5 isoenzyme is associated with liver metastases. The elevation of LD5 in the spinal fluid may be an early indication of central nervous system metastases.[196]

Neuron-Specific Enolase

Enolase is a glycolytic enzyme also known as phosphopyruvate hydratase. *Neuron-specific enolase* (NSE) is the form of enolase found in neuronal tissue and in the cells of the diffuse neuroendocrine system and the amine precursor uptake, and decarboxylation (APUD) tissue. NSE is found in tumors associated with the neuroendocrine origin, including small cell lung cancer (SCLC), neuroblastoma, pheochromocytoma, carcinoid, medullary carcinoma of the thyroid, melanoma, and pancreatic endocrine tumors.

Serum NSE level may be measured by RIA. The upper reference limit is 12.5 μg/mL. In patients with SCLC, the sensitivity is reported to be 80%. The specificity is at least 80% to 90%. The NSE level appears to correlate with stages and provides a useful prognosis for disease progression. The value of NSE in detecting disease relapse has not been proven. Although the findings are mixed, NSE also appears to be useful in monitoring chemotherapy and correlates with disease state. The immunostaining of NSE may also provide differential diagnosis between SCLC and other histological carcinoma types.

Among children with advanced neuroblastoma, more than 90% have been reported to have elevated serum levels of NSE. High levels of NSE are associated with poor prognosis. The levels seem to correlate with the stage of the disease. Monitoring therapy using serum NSE is controversial, particularly with respect to the issue of specificity. However, elevated levels of NSE in children with stage IV neuroblastoma were associated with a poorer outcome.[260]

Prostatic Acid Phosphatase

The acid phosphatases include all phosphatases that hydrolyze phosphate esters with an optimum pH of less than 7.0. They are present in the lysozymes of the secretory epithelial cells. Although acid phosphatase is produced primarily by the prostate gland, it is also found in erythrocytes, platelets, leukocytes, bone marrow, bone, liver, spleen, kidney, and intestine.

Prostatic acid phosphatase (PAP), with an optimum pH of 5 to 6, is very labile at a pH of greater than 7.0 and a temperature greater than 37 °C. It can be distinguished from other acid phosphatases by using tartrate, which strongly inhibits the prostatic form. Another approach is to select substrates that are more specific for PAP. Two substrates commonly used are thymolphthalein monophosphate and β-naphthol phosphate. These two substrates are hydrolyzed by PAP much more quickly than by the other acid phosphatases. Thymolphthalein monophosphate appears to be more specific. Acid phosphatase was first used as a tumor marker in 1938 by Gutman and colleagues.[83] PAP was measured first by its enzymatic activity, then using counterimmunoelectrophoresis, and subsequently, in the late 1970s, by RIA. Its use was proposed as a screening tool for prostate cancer. It has been used to help stage prostate cancer, to correlate with the prognosis of the disease, and to monitor therapy. Elevated serum PAP may be seen in malignant conditions, such as osteogenic sarcoma, multiple myeloma, and bone metastases of other cancers. It may also be elevated in some benign conditions, such as BPH, osteoporosis, and hyperparathyroidism.

The clinical use of PAP has been replaced by PSA. PAP is not as sensitive as PSA for screening or for detection of early cancer. The clinical use of PAP is restricted to confirmation of metastatic prostate cancer and staging of prostate cancer.[6,30] It is less likely to be elevated in BPH than is PSA. Currently the method of choice for PAP is the measurement of its enzymatic activity.

Kallikreins

Kallikreins are a subgroup of the serine protease enzyme family, three of which have been assigned a specific biological role.

Biochemistry

The human kallikrein (hK) gene locus spans a region of approximately 300 kb of chromosome 19q13.4, which contains 15 tandemly localized kallikrein genes (*KLK1* to *KLK15*) with no intervention from other genes. This is the largest cluster of serine proteases within the human genome. The members of the kallikrein family are identified by a number of similar features.[61] They all have a nearly identical genetic structure (5′ untranslated region, intron-exon size and organization), and the catalytic triad of serine proteases is conserved by all members, with the histidine always occurring near the end of the second exon, the aspartate in the middle of the third exon, and the serine residue at the beginning of the fifth exon. All kallikreins are produced as prepropeptides with a 17 to 20 amino acid signal sequence and a 4 to 9 amino acid activation peptide. They also contain 10 to 12 conserved cysteines that form five to six disulfide bonds. Finally, most if not all genes are under steroid hormone control.

Kallikreins are expressed in a wide variety of tissue including prostate, breast, ovary, and testis.[252] For example, KLK3 (PSA) is highly expressed in prostate and is discussed in detail later in the chapter. KLK3 also has minor expression in breast, thyroid, salivary glands, lung, and trachea, and KLK11 and KLK12 are highly expressed in more than 10 tissues, with minor expression in at least four others.

Only three of the 15 kallikreins have been assigned a specific biological role. The major biological role of hK1 is the release of lysyl-bradykinin (kallidin) from low molecular weight kininogen; however it has been implicated in the processing of peptide hormones, including proinsulin, low-density lipoprotein (LDL), prorenin, the precursor of atrial natriuretic peptide, and vasoactive intestinal peptide. The role of hK2 has only recently been investigated. Seminal plasma hK2 cleaves seminogelin I and II, but at different sites than hK3 (PSA). Furthermore, a role for hK2 in the regulation of growth factors through the proteolysis of insulin-like growth factor binding protein 3 (IGFBP-3) has been suggested. hK3, also known as PSA, is not only found in prostate tissue (discussed below), but is found in relatively high concentration in nipple aspirate fluid, breast cyst fluid, breast milk, amniotic fluid, and tumor extracts.[23] Its presence in these fluids and tissue suggests a biological function in breast and a possible role in fetal development; however no specific function in these tissue has been identified to date.

Clinical Applications

The role of kallikreins as tumor markers is rather varied; a number of kallikreins have been associated with hormonal malignancies (prostate, breast, testicular, and ovarian cancers). The roles of hK3 (PSA) and hK2 are discussed in detail below. hK6 has been used as a serum marker for diagnosis, prognosis, and monitoring of ovarian cancer,[60] and as a cytosolic marker for prognosis of breast cancer. Serum hK5, hK6, hK10 and hK11 have also been used for diagnosis and monitoring of ovarian cancer[112,137,253,254] and high concentration of cytosolic hK10 in ovarian tumor and breast cells is a poor prognostic marker.[135,136] Kallikrein gene expression is associated with both positive and negative prognosis in various cancers, including prostate, ovarian, and breast cancers. For a review see reference 61.

Analytical Methodology

Reverse transcription-polymerase chain reaction (RT-PCR), northern and western blotting, and immunoassays have been used for detection of kallerin mRNA and protein in tissue extracts of ovarian, breast, testicular, and prostate tumors. Immunohistochemical techniques have been used for the detection of KLK7 in ovarian tumors and KLK10 in ovarian and testicular tumors. The serum levels of KLK3 (PSA) and KLK11 are evaluated by immunoassay.

PROSTATE-SPECIFIC ANTIGEN

PSA is one of the most promising tumor markers of this decade. It is one of the few organ-specific tumor markers. Prostate cancer is the leading cancer in older men. When detected early (organ confined), it is potentially curable by radical prostatectomy. Therefore early detection is important. The role of PSA in prostate cancer has been reviewed.[35,43,54,166]

PSA was discovered by Hara and colleagues in 1971.[89] They called this seminal plasma protein *γ-seminoprotein.* Li and Beling isolated the same protein from seminal plasma and called it "protein E1" because it has a slow β-mobility in electrophoresis and a molecular weight (MW) of 31,000. In 1978 Sensabaugh characterized this glycoprotein with isoelectric points between 6.5 and 8.0 and called it "p30." In 1979 Wang and co-workers purified a protein from prostatic tissue and called it *prostate-specific antigen.* PSA is found in normal, benign, hyperplastic, and malignant prostatic tissues. γ-seminoprotein, p30, and PSA are biochemically very similar.

Biochemistry

PSA is a single-chain glycoprotein that is 7% carbohydrate. It has 237 amino acid residues and four carbohydrate side chains with linkages at amino acid 45 (asparagine), 69 (serine), 70 (threonine), and 71 (serine). The N-terminal amino acid is isoleucine, and the C-terminal residue is proline. Its MW is 28,430,[16] and it has isoelectric points from 6.8 to 7.2 because of its various isoforms. The three-dimensional structure and the antigenic domain of PSA have been characterized.[46]

The complete gene encoding PSA has been sequenced and located on chromosome 19.[59,134] It is similar to the kallikrein-1 gene with 82% homology. Functionally, PSA is a serine protease of the kallikrein family. It is produced exclusively by the epithelial cells of the acini and ducts of the prostate gland. PSA is secreted into the lumina of the prostatic duct. In the seminal fluid, PSA cleaves a seminal vesicle–specific protein into several low molecular weight proteins as part of the process of liquefaction of the seminal coagulum. Therefore PSA possesses chymotrypsin-like and trypsin-like activity. Autodigestion of PSA has been reported at three possible locations—*LYS* 148, *LYS* 185, and *ARG* 85. The addition of protease inhibitors may be important to prevent the autohydrolysis of PSA in solution.[46]

Molecular Forms of Prostate-Specific Antigen

PSA exists in two major forms in blood circulation. The majority of PSA is complexed with protease inhibitor α_1-antichymotrypsin (ACT) (MW 100,000) or with α_2-macroglobulin (AMG) and a minor component of free PSA (MW 28,430). Most immunoassays measure both free and ACT-complexed PSA but not AMG-PSA.[126,226] In human seminal fluid, PSA could be fractionated into five isoforms. PSA-A and PSA-B are active, intact enzymes capable of forming complexation with ACT. PSA-C, PSA-D, and PSA-E are nicked forms with disulfide bonds cleaved; they possess low or no enzymatic activities.[262] The inactive forms of free PSA are composed of three distinct molecular forms—bPSA, pPSA, and iPSA. bPSA in tissue is relatively localized in the transition zone of the prostate and contributes to fPSA in BPH serum. pPSA is localized in the peripheral zone of the prostate and contributes to fPSA in cancer serum.[146,212]

Physiological Properties

The metabolic clearance rate of PSA follows a two-compartment model with initial half-lives of 1.2 and 0.75 hours for free PSA and total PSA and subsequent half-lives of 22 and 33 hours.[168] Because of this relatively long half-life, 2 to 3 weeks may be necessary for the serum PSA to return to baseline levels after certain procedures, including transrectal biopsy, transrectal ultrasonography, transurethral resection of the prostate, and radical prostatectomy. Prostatitis and acute urinary retention can also elevate PSA concentration. Although the digital rectal examination has no clinically important effects on serum PSA levels in most patients, in some it may lead to a twofold elevation.

There appears to be significant physiological variation of serum PSA levels (up to 30%). Serum PSA has been reported to be decreased by 18% after the patient has been hospitalized for 24 hours. The reason for this reduction is not known. It may be that patients become sedentary (e.g., remain in the supine position) or suspend sexual activity. It is perhaps a good practice to collect serum samples from ambulatory patients.

Nonprostatic PSA

Originally, it was thought that PSA was solely expressed in prostate tissue. However, it was later found that PSA also is expressed in numerous tissues, most notably hormonally regulated tissue. It should not be surprising that PSA is expressed in these tissues as its promoter contains three androgen response elements and can be activated by androgens, progestins, and glucocorticoids. The presence of PSA in breast tissue is related to progesterone and estrogen receptor positivity and correlates with a favorable prognosis[256,257] but surprisingly, with resistance to tamoxifen therapy.[72] PSA positivity was found to be significantly associated with smaller tumors, steroid receptor positivity, low cellularity, diploid tumors, low S-phase fraction, less advanced disease, and longer survival. PSA has also been measured in nipple aspirate fluid (NAF) as a possible tool for breast cancer risk assessment.[191] Women with no risk factors had relatively high NAF PSA, and women with breast cancer had overall lower NAF PSA measurements.

Clinical Applications

PSA is an extremely useful tumor marker for prostate cancer. It is used to detect and stage the cancer and to monitor treatment of prostate cancer. It is also thought to be involved in tumor progression.

Early Detection of Prostate Cancer

PSA testing by itself is not effective in the screening or detection of early prostate cancer because PSA is specific for prostatic tissue but not for prostatic cancer. BPH is a common disease in men 50 years of age and older. Studies have shown that the PSA values in patients with BPH are similar yet statistically different from those associated with early prostatic cancer (i.e., those of patients with organ-confined cancer).[157] Unfortunately the overlap of PSA values between these two groups is so extensive that selecting an optimum cut-off value of PSA, either 4 or 10 µg/L, is almost impossible. The use of serum PSA together with digital rectal examination and followed by transrectal ultrasonography provides more accurate and sensitive diagnosis than digital examination alone.[35]

The clinical sensitivity of PSA is 78% at a cut-off value of 4.0 µg/L. By lowering the cut-off value to 2.8 µg/L, sensitivity increases to 92%, whereas specificity decreases from 33% to 23%. Raising the cut-off value to 8 µg/L improves the specificity to 90%.[40] Using ROC analysis (see Figure 23-1), PSA is a better predictor than PAP for the diagnosis of prostatic cancer.[184]

To improve the ability of PSA testing to detect early prostate cancer, several approaches have been suggested. One approach is to use age-adjusted reference intervals: 0 to 2.5 µg/L for men ages 40 to 49 years, 0 to 3.5 µg/L for 50 to 59 years, 0 to 4.5 µg/L for 60 to 69 years, and 0 to 6.5 µg/L for 70 to 79 years. By lowering the upper limit of the reference interval, more cancer will be detected in younger men for whom a potential cure by radical prostatectomy is most beneficial.[158] Another approach is to use PSA density (i.e., divide PSA concentration by the prostatic volume as determined by transrectal ultrasonography).[18] Patients with PSA between 4 and 10 µg/L, a negative digital rectal examination result, and elevated PSA density have increased risk for prostate cancer. The third approach is using PSA velocity—the rate of PSA increase as a function of time. By establishing a baseline level of PSA in each patient, the rate of increase of PSA is then calculated. The increase of PSA in health, BPH, and prostatic cancer appears to be different, with the highest rate (greater than 0.75 µg/L/yr) observed in patients with prostate cancer.[33] The specificity improved to 90% for BPH, and sensitivity is 72% for prostate cancer. A 1996 study of free PSA velocity found that percent free PSA is the earliest serum marker for predicting subsequent diagnosis of prostate cancer.[169]

The percent free PSA has been used to improve the sensitivity and specificity in detecting prostate cancer, particularly for patients in the diagnostic "gray" zone of PSA between 4 and 10 µg/L or 2 and 20 µg/L.[34,164] ProPSA (pPSA) has been reported to improve over fPSA in the detection of prostate cancer with total PSA in the 2.5 to 4.0 ng/mL range.[212] Complexed (cPSA) showed improved specificity over total PSA for prostate cancer detection in a multicenter clinical trial.[163]

In addition to the approaches described above, a number of algorithms using PSA and other analytes have been developed to increase the sensitivity of prostate cancer detection. They include logistic regression and artificial neural networks.

Logistic Regression. Logistic regression (LR) is a technique for making predictions when the dependent variable is a dichotomy (either the patient has cancer or does not), and the independent variables (PSA, f/T-PSA, age, etc.) are continuous and/or discrete. This technique is used to determine which variables (analytes) have the greatest predictive value in determining cancer risk, from which probability curves are generated. Finne et al used 758 men from a group of over 10,000 screened patients (200 confirmed prostate cancer and 558 controls) with total PSA between 4 and 20 µg/L to develop nomograms using total PSA, f/T-PSA, digital rectal examination, and prostate volume for determination of cancer probability.[69] The technique gave improved clinical sensitivity and specificity for cancer detection over total PSA and f/T-PSA and should reduce the number of biopsies performed and increase the detection rate of prostate cancer.

Artificial Neural Networks. Artificial neural networks are computer-based multiparameter techniques inspired by biological neurons, which operate as nonlinear summing devices. These networks have been applied to prostate cancer in determining which patients should undergo biopsy.[51,181,227,228] Unlike LR, neural networks must be trained, in much the same way that biological neural networks must be trained, to correctly categorize patients. The training involves selection of various inputs (total PSA, f/T-PSA, prostate volume, etc.) with known outcomes. Therefore selection of the correct training data set is extremely important. This technique can increase the sensitivity and specificity and the positive and negative predictive value obtained from prostate cancer screening; however care must be taken in training and validation of the neural network. An example is the ProstAsure Index.

The ProstAsure index, developed by Zhang, Stamey, and Chan,[12,221] was designed to increase the sensitivity and specificity of cancer detection, while maintaining a reasonable false positive detection rate. The index is derived from several values, including age, total PSA, creatine kinase isoenzymes, and prostatic acid phosphatase, which are input into a neural network–derived, nonlinear algorithmic procedure. The results are in the form of four zones (zones 1 to 4) based on an ascending probability of cancer. Patients in either zone 3 or 4 should be considered for biopsy. The algorithm performed well when compared with the free-total PSA ratio and had a sensitivity of 93%, with a specificity and apparent positive predictive value of 81% and 61%, respectively, compared with 80%, 74%, and 49%, respectively, for free-total PSA at the 15% threshold. At the 19% free-total PSA threshold, the sensitivity was increased to 93%, but the specificity and PPV decreased to 59% and 48%, respectively. However, the study by Babaian et al was on a limited number of patients and only tested its usefulness in the PSA range of less than or equal to 4 µg/L, not the 4 to 10 µg/L where the free-total PSA ratio is used.

Staging of Prostate Cancer

PSA has been found to correlate with clinical stages of prostate cancer.[222] Higher PSA levels and higher percentages of patients with elevated PSA concentrations are associated with advanced stages. However, PSA testing is not sufficiently reliable to determine stages on an individual basis.

PSA has also been found to correlate with pathological stages of tumor extension and metastases. Advanced pathological stages are associated with higher PSA levels in the serum. Patients with organ-confined disease seldom have a PSA level greater than 50 µg/L, suggesting that patients with these elevated levels are most likely to have extracapsular tumor extension. Because significant overlap occurs in PSA values among stages, PSA cannot be used to determine the pathological stage in a given individual. Therefore, PSA by itself should not be used to decide whether a patient has prostate cancer confined to the organ and therefore is a likely candidate for radical prostatectomy. The level of PSA can serve as a guide and is more useful in evaluating the presence of metastases. Patients with PSA levels less than 20 µg/L rarely have bone metastases. Studies have shown that PSA could replace the radionuclide bone scan in newly diagnosed untreated prostate cancer patients who have a low serum PSA concentration (less than 10 µg/L) and do not have symptoms relating to the skeletal system.[156]

Monitoring Treatment

The greatest clinical use of PSA is in the monitoring of definitive treatment of prostate cancer. This treatment includes radical prostatectomy, radiation therapy, and antiandrogen therapy. PSA has also been suggested to play a role in tumor progression.[55]

Radical Prostatectomy. This surgery removes all prostatic tissue. Because PSA is produced almost exclusively by the prostatic tissue, after radical prostatectomy the PSA level should fall below the detection limit of the assay. This may require 2 to 3 weeks owing to the 2- to 3-day half-life of PSA. If the half-life is longer than normal, it must be assumed that residual tumor is present.[157,222] For example, Walsh and

TABLE 23-7 Prostate-Specific Antigen and Tumor Status in 297 Men Followed 1 to 13 Years After Radical Prostatectomy

	POSTOPERATIVE PSA LEVEL			
		>0.5 µg/L		
Pathological Stage	**<0.5 µg/L NED***	**NED**	**Recurrence†**	**(%)**
Organ confined	169	8	3	6
Capsular penetration	51	3	10	20
Seminal vesicle involvement	9	10	9	68
Positive lymph nodes	4	15	6	84
Total	233	36	28	

From Walsh PC, Oesterling JE, Epstein JI, et al. The value of prostate-specific antigen in the management of localized prostate cancer. In: Murphy G, Khoury S eds. Therapeutic progress in urological cancer. New York: Alan R Liss Inc, 1989:27-33.
*No evidence of disease.
†Local recurrence and/or metastatic disease.

co-workers[244] reported a long-term study of 297 men who were followed for 1 to 13 years after radical prostatectomy (Table 23-7). For the 180 patients with organ-confined cancer, only 11 (6%) showed elevated PSA levels (greater than 0.5 µg/L). Three of these patients had documented recurrence, whereas the other eight had no evidence of cancer. The frequency of elevated PSA levels increased with advancing pathological stage. Of the entire group, 12% had elevated PSA levels without evidence of recurrence. These patients most likely had residual disease. All patients with the recurrence of cancer had elevated PSA levels.

It is recommended that measurement of PSA be done every 3 months during the first year following surgery, every 4 months in the second year, and every 6 months thereafter. The clinical threshold of an elevated PSA varies with each institution and ranges from 0.1 to 0.3 µg/L. The clinical threshold will be affected by the test's analytical sensitivity and biological variation of serum PSA. In any case, an increasing PSA level after radical prostatectomy is a strong indication of disease recurrence. The time between PSA concentration elevation and clinical recurrence is between 1 and 5 years.

Radiation Therapy. The role of PSA in the monitoring of patients after definitive radiation therapy is less well defined as compared with that after radical prostatectomy. The majority of patients show an initial decrease of PSA level after radiation therapy. PSA is better than digital rectal examination for detecting residual cancer after radiation therapy.[202]

Antiandrogen Therapy. Antiandrogen therapy includes bilateral orchiectomy and treatment with luteinizing hormone-releasing hormone analogues, diethylstilbestrol, and flutamide. PSA testing is useful for predicting prognosis and monitoring treatment response to this type of therapy in patients with stage D2 prostate cancer. The level of PSA is inversely proportional to the survival time and increases with cancer progression, decreases in remission, and remains unchanged in stable disease. PSA could replace the radionuclide bone scan for monitoring patients with advanced disease.[47]

Androgen deprivation therapy may have a direct effect on the PSA level that is independent of the antitumor effect. The production of PSA may be under the influence of hormones such as dihydrotestosterone. Thus the PSA levels in patients who receive antiandrogen therapy may have a different meaning than they do in patients receiving other types of therapies.[156]

Tumor Progression

PSA has also been suggested to play a role in tumor progression.[55] PSA digests extracellular matrix proteins laminin and fibronectin that may promote metastasis. PSA also digests IGFBP-3, increasing the local concentration of insulin-like growth factors, which also may promote tumor growth.

Analytical Methodology

Both traditional and ultrasensitive assays are available for measuring PSA.

Traditional Assays

Immunoassays are used to measure PSA and are commercially available. Most of them use nonisotopic labels, such as enzyme, fluorescence, or chemiluminescence. The majority of these assays are automated on an immunoassay system. Different assays and even the same assay with different lots of reagent may produce different results. The reasons for such differences are due to changes in assay calibration, production lot variation, assay reaction time, reagent matrices, assay sensitivity, and imprecision. Antibodies react with different PSA epitopes; therefore, some antibodies react dissimilarly with the various molecular forms of PSA. Assays are classified as equimolar if they bind to free and cPSA equally and nonequimolar if they bind to free or cPSA differently. Examples of equimolar assays are the ACCESS

Hybritech PSA assay (Beckman Coulter, Brea, Calif.) and the TOSOH NexIA immunometric assay (which uses the same antibodies as the Access assay). The World Health Organization, the International Federation of Clinical Chemistry, and the National Committee for Clinical Laboratory Standards have developed two international preparations to facilitate the effort to standardize PSA assays: 100% free PSA (code 96/686) and 90% PSA-ACT complex and 10% free PSA (code 96/700).[44]

Ultrasensitive Assays

Ultrasensitive PSA is the term used for assays with detection limits of 0.01 to 0.001 μg/L, which are significantly less than that of traditional PSA assays.[68] The major use for ultrasensitive PSA is detection of residual prostate cancer after prostatectomy. After radical prostatectomy, circulating levels of PSA are extremely low; 80% have a PSA lower than 0.01 μg/L, and 20% have a PSA below 0.001 μg/L.[53,241,255] A postprostatectomy increase in PSA is associated with disease recurrence. Routine PSA methods cannot detect an increase in PSA until it reaches about 0.1 μg/L; however ultrasensitive methods can detect an increase long before traditional methods (1 to 2 years). This provides the opportunity for earlier treatment and an increased likelihood of a cure.

Ultrasensitive methods are also useful in measuring PSA in women, since normal PSA levels in women are less than or equal to 0.01 μg/L. An increased PSA in women is seen during pregnancy and in breast cancer patients.[24]

Human Glandular Kallikrein 2

Human kallikrein 2 (hK2) and PSA (human kallikrein 3) are serine proteases that share 80% identity in protein sequence[192] and are almost exclusively found in prostatic epithelium.

Biochemistry

Similar to PSA, hK2 concentrations are 100,000-fold higher in seminal fluid than in serum.[131] hK2 has the ability to form complexes with endogenous antiproteases. One important inhibitor is the protein-C-inhibitor (PCI) that is the major ligand complexed to hK2 in seminal fluid, but in vitro, hK2 also forms complexes with alpha$_2$-antiplasmin, alpha$_2$-macroglobulin, ACT, antithrombin III, C1-inactivator, and plasminogen activator inhibitor-1.[145] Gel filtration studies on a relatively low number of samples have suggested that hK2 mainly occurs in a free, noncomplexed form hK2 in serum, where only a minor proportion (5% to 20%) may be complexed with protease inhibitors. In vitro, recombinant hK2 activates proPSA into mature, catalytic active form.

Clinical Applications

Immunohistochemical studies demonstrated that tissue expression of hK2 showed intense staining in high-grade cancers and lymph node metastases, whereas it showed weaker staining for low-grade cancers and BPH.[50] Serum hK2 alone or hK2*total PSA/free PSA has been shown to be a significantly better predictor of pT2a/b-PCa than tPSA.[85] Recker et al confirmed the improvement in staging accuracy, noting that hK2 was the only serum analyte that significantly discriminated pT2a/b from greater than or equal to pT3a-PCa. Moreover, hK2 discriminated aggressive Grade 3 from less aggressive Grade 1 and Grade 2 PCa.[179]

Analytical Methodology

Currently, there are two major hK2 immunoassays. Hease and colleagues found notable differences in values measured by the two immunoassays for hK2 for identical patient samples.[86] Calibration of the two assays by use of a common, ek-rhK2-based calibrator revealed a substantial gain in agreement between the assays.

The Urokinase-Plasminogen Activator System

The urokinase-plasminogen activator system consists of three main components, urokinase-plasminogen activator (uPA, a 53 kDa serine protease), the uPA membrane-bound receptor (uPAR), and the uPA inhibitors, PAI-1 and PAI-2.[5,63,182,185]

Biochemistry

uPA is produced as a single inactive polypeptide, which is activated by cleavage between lysine 158 and isoleucine 159. The cleavage is catalyzed by a number of proteases, including cathepsins B and L and hK2. The active form of uPA consists of an A-chain, which interacts with its cell-surface receptor, uPAR, and a catalytically active B-chain. The most thoroughly characterized activity of uPA is the conversion of plasminogen to active plasmin, which degrades extracellular matrix (ECM) components and activates matrix metalloproteinases (MMPs), and that further degrade the ECM, and activate and release specific growth factors (fibroblast growth factor [FGF]2 and transforming growth factor [TGF]-β). The activity of uPA is controlled in vivo by two inhibitor molecules, PAI-1 and PAI-2. PAI-1 and PAI-2 not only act to inhibit uPA but also have a number of other functions, including angiogenesis, cell adhesion and migration, and inhibition of apoptosis.

Clinical Applications

uPA has been used as a prognostic marker in breast cancer and a number of other cancers.

Breast Cancer

uPA was the first protease implicated in metastasis evaluated for prognostic value in humans. At least 20 independent groups have demonstrated that breast cancer patients with high activity of uPA in their primary tumors have a worse disease-free pattern than those patients with low uPA activity.[62] The prognostic impact of uPA appears to be independent of other traditionally used markers, such as axillary node status, tumor size, grade, and estrogen receptor (ER) status. In most studies, uPA is a more potent predictor of overall survival than tumor size, grade, or ER status, and equally powerful as nodal status. The patients who benefit most from uPA measurement are those who are newly diagnosed with histologically negative local nodes. The long-term survival of this group is 70% to 80% with local therapy alone, and no further benefit is gained from adjuvant chemotherapy. uPA may be able to detect the small number of patients most at risk for recurrent disease and spare other cured patients from unnecessary chemotherapy.

PAI-1 has also been associated with progression of breast cancer. Paradoxically, high levels of PAI-1 correlate with more aggressive disease. This appears to be because of the involvement of PAI-1 in angiogenesis and inhibition of apoptosis as opposed to inhibition of uPA. Recently a prospective study[101] of 674 node-negative breast cancer patients demonstrated that women with high levels of uPA and/or PAI-1 had a notably shorter disease-free period than those with low levels of both proteins. The level 1 evidence for the prognostic use of uPA and PAI-1 should allow these markers to enter routine use in breast cancer evaluation. Recently, reviews and metaanalysis studies suggested that uPA and PAI-1 are ready to be used as prognostic markers of breast cancer at the clinic.[90,130,261]

Other Cancers

uPA has also demonstrated its usefulness as a prognostic marker in colorectal cancer. In one study,[62] uPA was found to be a marker of disease outcome in patients with tumor invasion but negative node status (Dukes' B stage). High levels of uPA were also found to correlate with aggressive disease in both gastric and esophageal cancers. Preliminary studies have implicated uPA as a prognostic marker in ovarian, renal, hepatocellular, pancreatic, gliomas, urinary, bladder, adenocarcinoma of the lung, and cervical cancer. Thus uPA may function as a general prognostic marker in cancer.

Analytical Methodology

The original assay developed for uPA measured its catalytic activity. This assay has been replaced by enzyme-linked immunosorbent assay (ELISA) and a number of research and commercially available kits have been developed for detection of uPA and PAI-1. uPA and PAI-1 can be determined in serum and, more frequently, in tissue extracts. Since a proportion of uPA is bound to its receptor, the addition of Triton X-100 is required for full extraction of uPA, which is necessary to gain maximal prognostic information. Generally, increased levels of uPA and/or PAI-1 indicate poor prognosis. A uPA level below 3 ng/mg total tissue and PAI-1 below 14 ng/mg total tissue have a notably better prognosis.[101] Most studies showing a prognostic value for uPA have used ELISA for detection; however some were done using immunohistochemistry. Immunohistochemical detection is easier, and requires less tissue; however interpretation is subjective and only semiquantitative.

CATHEPSINS

The cathepsins are lysosomal proteases and cathepsin B, D, and L have been investigated for their role in tumor development and progression.

Biochemistry

Like other proteases, cathepsins are synthesized as high molecular weight precursors that require processing for activation. Cathepsin B (CB) is a thiol-dependent protease normally found in lysosomes, and is activated by cathepsin D (CD) and matrix metalloproteinases. Activated CB can in turn activate uPA and specific metalloproteinases. Cathepsin L (CL) is similar in specificity to that of CB; however, it has little activity toward small molecular substrates. Cathepsin D, like CB, is a lysosomal protease; however, CD belongs to the aspartyl group of proteases.

The expression and localization of CB appears to be altered in tumors relative to normal tissue. In tumor tissue, CB can be associated with the plasma membrane or secreted. Increased expression has been demonstrated in breast, colorectal, gastric, lung, and prostate tumors, carcinomas, gliomas, melanomas, and osteoclastomas, suggesting a link with tumor development and/or progression.[116] Altered localization of CB has also been seen in various tumor tissue, such as colon carcinomas, thyroid cancers, gliomas, and breast epithelial tumors. This altered expression and localization is thought to be involved in tissue invasion through ECM degradation and growth promotion. The ECM degradation occurs through activation of CB and other proteases, such as MMPs and uPA. In addition to ECM degradation, CB releases growth factors: basic fibroblast growth factor (bFGF), insulin-like growth factor-1 (IGF-1), epidermal growth factor (EGF), and TGF-β associated with the ECM.

Stromal cells were originally thought to be passive bystanders in tumor development; however, evidence suggests an active role. Increased expression of ECM proteases, including CB, has been demonstrated in stromal cells at the border between tumor cells and normal tissue. Expression of both CB and CD is up regulated by various growth factors (bFGF, EGF, IGF-1) and direct contact with tumor cells. This suggests that as tumor cells invade the stroma, the stromal cells are induced to participate directly in matrix degradation.[116] Therefore detection of CB in stromal cells and tumor cells may have prognostic value.

Clinical Applications

A limited number of studies have associated high levels of CB in multiple tumor types with aggressive disease. All, with one exception, are retrospective studies with low numbers of patients. In the one large study (n = 1500 patients), CB was shown to be an independent prognostic marker for both relapse-free and overall survival in breast cancer patients; however, it is not as good a marker as uPA.

The majority of data relating to the prognostic value of CD is in relation to breast cancer[183]; however, its usefulness in squamous cell carcinoma (SCC) of the head and neck, hepatocellular carcinoma, and gastric adenocarcinoma has been investigated in limited studies. For breast cancer, a 1999 report containing 2810 patients confirmed the prognostic value of CD.[73] The authors, using an RIA to detect cytoplasmic CD in tumor tissue, showed that tumors with high CD had a notably poorer relapse-free survival than did those with low CD levels.

In contrast to RIA detection of CD in tissue extracts, immunohistochemical detection has led to conflicting results. Some investigators have reported significant association between immunohistochemically determined CD and a poor outcome, and others found no relationship. Possible reasons include differences in antibody specificity, different scoring systems to quantify CD staining levels, different cut-off points for discriminating high from low values, and different types of tissue: fresh versus formalin-fixed and paraffin-embedded.[59] Therefore the prognostic usefulness of CD in SCC and other malignancies needs further study to determine the utility of CD as an independent marker.

The use of CL as a prognostic indicator has been best studied in breast cancer. Most studies measured CL from tumor extracts and correlated high levels of CL with a decrease in relapse-free survival. CL appears to be an independent prognostic marker in both node-negative and node-positive breast cancer, especially when combined with other prognostic markers such as CB, CD, node status, and steroid hormone receptor status.

Analytical Methodology

The initial assays for detection of CB used chromogenic substrates containing an Arg-Arg sequence and 2-naphthylamide and 7-amino-4-methylcoumarin as chromophores. These early assays lacked specificity and were likely to have suffered from interference by endogenous inhibitors (e.g., cystatins and stefins). CB and CL are now measured by ELISA; however to date no comparison has been made with the older CB methods. Immunohistochemistry has also been used to detect CB in tissue; however no detailed evaluations have been conducted.

The majority of studies correlating CD with tumor progression and prognosis have used an immunoradiometric assay that detects both the proforms and mature forms of CD. This assay can be used to measure CD in tissue extract generated for detection of steroid hormone receptors. CD has also been measured by western blot, by immunohistochemistry, and by activity.

Matrix Metalloproteinases

Matrix metalloproteinases (MMP) are a family of 23 structurally related zinc-dependent endopeptidases capable of degrading components of the ECM.[159,216]

Biochemistry

Most MMPs are secreted as a zymogen, and activation involves removal of a 10 kDa amino-terminal domain. Once in the active form, their proteolytic activity is inhibited by tissue inhibitors known as tissue inhibitors of metalloproteinases (TIMPs). The MMPs have been functionally grouped into four subgroups, based on their ECM specificity: collagenases, gelatinases, stromelysins, and membrane MMPs.

Clinical Applications

MMPs are involved in a number of functions including tissue remodeling and wound repair; however, they have also been associated with tumor growth, invasion, and metastasis.[242] Direct evidence for the role of MMPs in the development and progression of tumors has been provided by mouse knockout studies in which mice lacking various MMPs showed reduced tumorigenesis and progression. Conversely, increased expression is associated with tumor aggressiveness and poor prognosis. Increased expression of MMP-2 and MMP-9 is associated with accelerated tumor progression in oral carcinoma, lung adenocarcinoma, and bladder, ovarian, and papillary thyroid carcinoma. Similarly, increased staining of MMP-3 and MMP-9 is seen in high-grade versus low-grade endometrial sarcoma. In esophageal carcinoma, MMP-7 expression correlates with tumor aggressiveness.

MMPs also act as predictors of recurrence or metastatic risk. High preoperative serum levels of MMP-2 or MMP-3 are predictive of recurrence in patients with advanced urothelial carcinoma. Furthermore, high levels of MMP-2 in ovarian tumor cells can predict tumor recurrence. The expression of certain MMPs is predictive of metastatic risk. For example, expression of MMP-1 is associated with lymph node metastasis in cervical and peritoneal metastasis in gastric cancer. MMP inhibition may be a therapeutic strategy for cancer.[159]

Analytical Methodology

Gelatin zymography is a technique commonly used to detect MMPs, such as MMP-2 and MMP-9. Zymography is an electrophoretic technique used to identify proteolytic activity in enzymes separated by sodium dodecyl sulfate polyacrylamide gel electrophoresis under nonreducing conditions. The SDS is removed, allowing the MMPs to refold and subsequently digest gelatin at the position of the separated protein. This technique, although tedious, has the advantage of specifically detecting the active form of the protease. MMPs are also detected in tissue sections by immunohistochemistry using specific antibodies, and in tissue extracts and serum by immunoassay.

Tumor-Associated Trypsin Inhibitor

Tumor-associated trypsin inhibitor (TATI) is a 6 kDa trypsin inhibitor that was first identified from the urine of an ovarian cancer patient.

Biochemistry

TATI is identical to the previously identified pancreatic secretory trypsin inhibitor (PSTI), which is also known as the Kazal inhibitor. TATI is strongly expressed by pancreatic acinar cells together with trypsinogen. It is secreted into the pancreatic juice where it constitutes 0.1% to 0.8% of the total protein. It is expressed at lower concentrations in other healthy tissue, such as the gastrointestinal and urogenital tracts, the gallbladder, biliary tract, kidney, lung, liver, and breast. TATI also acts as an acute phase reactant and is induced under strong inflammatory conditions, as would be expected as its promoter contains an IL-6 response element. TATI function in vivo is thought to protect against autodigestion of body tissue by trypsinogen secreted by the pancreas and other tissue. TATI is rapidly cleared from the circulation by the kidneys with a half-life of approximately 6 minutes. Therefore patients with renal disease can have extremely high serum levels of TATI (greater than 1000 μg/L).

Clinical Applications

Although pancreatitis, severe injury, and inflammation can all increase its levels, TATI can still function as a relatively good tumor marker for various cancers. In most cancers, the increase in TATI is due to tumor production; however, inflammation associated with tissue destruction contributes to the overall TATI increase. Serum and urine concentrations correlate well, but because of greater variation in urine, serum is preferred.

Increases in both serum and urine TATI are common in ovarian cancer. In mucinous ovarian cancers, approximately 45% of patients have increased TATI in stage I, and 90% to 100% have increases by stage IV.[225] Fifty-five percent to 60% of patients with late stage endometrial cancer have increased serum TATI; however, only 20% show an increase in early stages. TATI is increased in cervical cancer, but squamous cell carcinoma antigen (SCCA) and CEA are better markers.

TATI is also useful in gastrointestinal and urological cancers. As may be expected due to its pancreatic production, TATI is a useful marker for pancreatic cancer and is increased in 75% to 90% of patients. In gastric cancer, TATI is increased in 40% to 65% of patients and high preoperative values correlate with a poor prognosis. Patients with hepatocellular (60% to 80%) or biliary tract cancer (75% to 100%) show an increase in TATI. The clinical sensitivity of TATI in hepatocellular cancer is similar to that of AFP and is useful in AFP-negative cancers. Colorectal cancers also increase TATI, with approximately 34% to 74% of patients showing an increase. However, CEA is a better marker of disease. In bladder cancer, TATI has been shown to be more useful than other serum markers and is a strong prognostic indicator. In renal cell carcinoma, TATI is a more sensitive marker than CEA, CA 15-3, CA 125, and CA 19-9, and is useful in monitoring disease progression and after surgery.

Analytical Methodology

TATI in either serum or urine is routinely measured by radioimmunoassay. However, other detection methods have been developed that are used mainly for research purposes. The reference interval for TATI is 3 to 21 μg/L in serum, and is method dependent, as a method employing monoclonal antibodies gives a slightly lower reference interval (3.1 to 16 μg/L). Urine concentration is more variable, with a reference interval of 7 to 51 μg/L.

TELOMERASE

Telomeres are specialized structures at the termini of eukaryotic chromosomes.

Biochemistry

Telomeres are composed of hexanucleotide repeats (TTAGGG) that signal the end of a chromosome and inhibit the DNA repair mechanism from joining the ends of chromosomes together. They also appear to function as a mitotic clock, which records the replicative history and sets a finite life span for normal somatic cells. During each replication, cycle telomeric DNA is lost because of the inability of the replication machinery to overcome the loss of terminal RNA primers. However, expression of functional telomerase is a mechanism to overcome telomeric DNA loss in germline cells and stem cells. Telomerase is a ribonucleoprotein reverse transcriptase that elongates telomere ends using a segment of its own RNA as a template. Two main components are required for telomerase activity: human telomerase RNA (hTR), which contains the template for reverse transcription, and human telomerase reverse transcriptase (hTERT), which consists of the enzyme's catalytic subunit.

Telomerase is normally active during embryogenesis, but is repressed in most somatic cells before or shortly after birth. Germline cells, activated lymphocytes, and other immortal cells show no shortening of telomere length and possess telomerase activity. Thus tumor cells should also show telomerase activity that can act as a specific marker of transformation.

Clinical Applications

Telomerase activity has been detected in more than 80% of cancers, including lung, breast, pancreatic, bladder, and many other cancers; however, it does not seem to be necessary for cancer development.[96] Its activity does, however, correlate with tumor progression and prognosis.

The detection of telomerase activity or hTERT mRNA in excretion, secretion, brushings, and washings has been evaluated. In pancreatic secretion samples, which contain freshly exfoliated cells, detection of telomerase activity was encouraging for cancer detection. Telomerase activity was also found to be useful in distinguishing between adenoma and carcinoma in intraductal papillary-mucinous tumors, which can sometimes be difficult to diagnose. In bronchial brushing samples, the clinical sensitivity of cancer detection is below 70% and false-positive results are commonly encountered because of contamination with lymphocytes, which contain measurable telomerase activity. The measurement of telomerase is also expected to become a useful marker in cervical cancer, since most cervical cancers express telomerase. In cancers such as non–small cell lung cancer, gastric cancer and neuroblastoma, and adenocarcinomas of the stomach and colon telomerase activity is up regulated during tumor progression and is useful in the evaluation of malignant grading and patient prognosis.

Analytical Methodology

The TRAP (telomeric repeat amplification protocol) assay is a widely used method for detection of telomerase activity. This technique measures the telomerase activity present in cell extracts. Briefly, cellular extract containing telomerase activity is incubated with a telomeric substrate (a short strand of DNA onto which the telomerase will attach the telomeric repeats) followed by polymerase chain reaction (PCR) amplification of the elongated telomere. Detection of the PCR product is by a number of methods, including gel electrophoresis, radiometric detection, ELISA, and real-time PCR detection.[188]

HORMONES

Hormones have been recognized as tumor markers for more than 50 years. The introduction of specific RIA methods for a particular hormone that has very little cross-reactivity with similar hormones made it possible to monitor the treatment of cancer patients.[244]

With the introduction and use of monoclonal antibodies, the measurement of hormones is now accurate and precise. The production of hormones in cancer involves two separate routes. First, the endocrine tissue that normally produces it can produce excess amounts of a hormone. Second, a hormone may be produced at a distant site by a non-endocrine tissue that normally does not produce the hormone. The latter condition is called *ectopic syndrome.* For example, the production of adrenocorticotropic hormone (ACTH) is normotopic by the pituitary and is ectopic by the small cell of the lung. Consequently, elevation of a given hormone is not diagnostic of a specific tumor, because a hormone may be produced by a variety of cancers.

Multiple endocrine neoplasia (MEN) syndromes (MEN-1, MEN-2A, and MEN-2B) are familial disorders inherited in an autosomal dominant fashion that are manifested by tumors arising from amine precursor uptake and decarboxylase (APUD) neuroendocrine tissues. These tissue synthesize a number of polypeptide hormones, such as ACTH, calcitonin, gastrin, glucagon, insulin, melanocyte-stimulating hormone, secretin, and vasoactive intestinal polypeptide. The frequency of hormone production correlates with the degree of embryological relationship of the cancer origin to other tissues in the APUD system. MEN-1 has been mapped to the long arm of chromosome 11 (11q13). Medullary thyroid carcinoma (MTC) that is part of MEN-2 has been mapped to chromosome 10.[211] Examples of hormones that are used as tumor markers are listed in Table 23-8. ACTH, calcitonin, and hCG are discussed in more detail below.

TABLE 23-8 Hormones as Tumor Markers

Hormone	Type of Cancer
ACTH	Cushing's syndrome, lung (small cell)
Antidiuretic hormone	Lung (small cell), adrenal cortex, pancreatic, duodenal
Bombesin	Lung (small cell)
Calcitonin	Medullary thyroid
Gastrin	Glucagonoma
Growth hormone	Pituitary adenoma, renal, lung
hCG	Embryonal, choriocarcinoma, testicular (nonseminomas)
Human placental lactogen	Trophoblastic, gonads, lung, breast
Neurophysins	Lung (small-cell)
Parathyroid hormone	Liver, renal, breast, lung, various
Prolactin	Pituitary adenoma, renal, lung
Vasoactive intestinal peptide	Pancreas, bronchogenic, pheochromocytoma, neuroblastoma

Adrenocorticotropic Hormone

ACTH is a polypeptide hormone with 39 amino acids and an MW of 4500 that is produced by the corticotropic cells of the anterior pituitary gland (see Chapter 50). In 1928 a patient was described having a small cell carcinoma of the lung who had the signs and symptoms of what is now known to be cortisol excess.[28] A small number of these carcinomas can produce pro-ACTH, the precursor to ACTH. This precursor has an MW of 22,000, a 5% bioactivity, and most of the immunoactivity of ACTH. Traditional RIA measures both the precursor and the hormone. One immunometric assay in use is specific for ACTH.

Elevated serum levels of ACTH could be the result of pituitary or ectopic production. A high level of ACTH (greater than 200 ng/L) is suggestive of ectopic origin. Failure of the dexamethasone suppression test is also indicative of ectopic production. About half of the ectopic production of ACTH is a result of small cell carcinoma of the lung. Other conditions that elevate ACTH levels have been reported, including pancreatic, breast, gastric, and colon cancer, and benign conditions, such as chronic obstructive pulmonary disease, mental depression, obesity, hypertension, diabetes mellitus, and stress. The value of ACTH in the monitoring of therapy is still unknown.[14]

Calcitonin

Calcitonin is a polypeptide with 32 amino acids, has an MW of about 3400, and is produced by the C cells of the thyroid.[11] Normally, calcitonin is secreted in response to increased serum calcium. It inhibits the release of calcium from bone and thus lowers the serum calcium level. The serum half-life is about 12 minutes. The level in healthy individuals is less than 0.1 μg/L. An elevated level is usually associated with medullary carcinoma of the thyroid.

Calcitonin is most useful in the detection of familial medullary carcinoma of the thyroid, an autosomal dominant disorder. Asymptomatic family members of the affected patients benefit from screening with computed tomography because basal levels are increased in such people. Provocative testing with intravenous administration of calcium and pentagastrin also produces increased calcitonin levels. Microscopic or occult malignancy has been detected in patients having a negative radioisotopic scan and normal thyroid glands on physical examination.

Calcitonin levels appear to correlate with such indicators of extent of disease as tumor volume and tumor involvement in local and distant metastases. Calcitonin is useful for monitoring treatment and detecting the recurrence of disease.

Calcitonin levels are also elevated in some patients with carcinoid and cancer of the lung, breast, kidney, and liver. The usefulness of calcitonin as a tumor marker in these malignancies has not been proven. Calcitonin elevation has been reported in other nonmalignant conditions, such as pulmonary disease, pancreatitis, hyperparathyroidism, pernicious anemia, Paget's disease of bone, and pregnancy.

Human Chorionic Gonadotropin

Elevated human chorionic gonadotropin (hCG) levels are seen in pregnancy, trophoblastic diseases, and germ cell tumors. It is a useful tumor marker for tumors of the placenta (trophoblastic tumors) and some tumors of the testes. It is also useful for diagnosing and monitoring pregnancy (see Chapter 54 for a discussion of hCG and pregnancy).

Biochemistry

hCG is a glycoprotein secreted by the syncytiotrophoblastic cells of the normal placenta. hCG consists of two dissimilar α- and β-subunits. The α-subunit is common to several other hormones: luteinizing hormone (LH), follicle-stimulating hormone (FSH), and thyroid-stimulating hormone (TSH). The β-subunit is unique to hCG, and the 28 to 30 amino acids comprising the carboxyl terminal are antigenically distinct. hCG has an MW of 45,000.[238] The upper reference limit in men and nonpregnant women is 5.0 IU/L.

The production of subunits of hCG is under separate genetic control. In early pregnancy, the free β-subunit is produced together with intact (a whole molecule of) hCG. In late pregnancy, the free α-subunit predominates. Differential production of the subunits has been observed in cancer patients. However, the number of patients who produce only the free subunit is very small. Most cancer patients produce both free β-subunits and intact molecules.

Clinical Applications

hCG is elevated in nearly all patients with trophoblastic tumors (greater than 1 million IU/L), in 70% of those with nonseminomatous testicular tumors, and less frequently in those with seminoma. Lower percentages of elevation have been reported in cases of melanoma and carcinoma of the breast, gastrointestinal tract, lung, and ovary, and in benign conditions, such as cirrhosis, duodenal ulcer, and inflammatory bowel disease.

Also, hCG is useful in identifying patients with trophoblastic tumors and, together with AFP, in detecting nonseminomatous testicular tumors. Levels of hCG correlate with the tumor volume and disease prognosis. The presence of hCG in seminoma may indicate the presence of choriocarcinoma. Because hCG does not cross the blood-brain barrier, the normal cerebrospinal fluid–to-serum ratio is 1:60. Higher levels in cerebrospinal fluid may indicate metastases to the brain. Furthermore, the response to therapy for patients with central nervous system metastasis may be indicated by monitoring the hCG level.

hCG is most useful for monitoring the treatment and the progression of trophoblastic disease.[20] Levels of hCG correlate with tumor volume. A patient with an initial hCG level of greater than 400,000 IU/L is considered at high risk for treatment failure. After surgical removal of the tumor, hCG level is expected to decline. The normal half-life of serum hCG is about 12 to 20 hours. Slowly decreasing or persistent levels of hCG may indicate the presence of residual disease. During chemotherapy, weekly hCG measurement is recommended. After remission is achieved, yearly hCG measurement is recommended to detect relapse. The detection limit of the assay is important, because any residual hCG activity may indicate the presence of a tumor. Specificity for the β-subunit of hCG is also a factor because low levels of cross-reactivity with LH or FSH can cause false-positive results.

Analytical Methodology

The measurement of serum hCG improved greatly in the 1970s. The assay specificity improved by using an antibody to the β-subunit of hCG that had little cross-reactivity with other glycoprotein hormones, LH, FSH, and TSH. Currently, most hCG assays use an immunometric ("sandwich") format. The hCG assay measures the intact (whole) molecule when an antibody for the α-subunit and an antibody for the β-subunit are used in the immunometric format. This type of assay does not measure free α- or β-subunits because free subunits cannot form a sandwich with both antibodies. The total β-hCG assay measures both the intact hCG and free β-subunits. As a tumor marker, a total β-hCG assay may be preferred, because cancer patients produce notable amounts of free β-subunit. None of the commercially available hCG assays have been approved by the Food and Drug Administration (FDA) for use as a tumor marker assay.

ONCOFETAL ANTIGENS

Oncofetal antigens are proteins produced during fetal life. These proteins are present in high concentration in the sera

TABLE 23-9 Oncofetal Antigens as Tumor Markers

Name	Nature	Type of Cancer
AFP	Glycoprotein, 70 kDa, 4% CHO	Hepatocellular, germ cell (nonseminoma)
β-Oncofetal antigen	80 kDa	Colon
Carcinofetal ferritin	Glycoprotein, 600 kDa	Liver
CEA	Glycoprotein, 22 kDa, 50% CHO	Colorectal, gastrointestinal, pancreatic, lung, breast
Pancreatic oncofetal	Glycoprotein, 40 kDa	Pancreatic
Squamous cell antigen	Glycoprotein, 44-48 kDa	Cervical, lung, skin, head and neck (squamous)
Tennessee antigen	Glycoprotein, 100 kDa	Colon, gastrointestinal, bladder
Tissue polypeptide antigen	Cytokeratins 8, 18, 19	Various (breast, colorectal, ovarian, bladder)

CHO, Carbohydrate.

of fetuses and decrease to low levels or disappear after birth. In cancer patients, these proteins reappear. The production of these proteins demonstrates that certain genes are reactivated as the result of the malignant transformation of cells.

The discovery of the oncofetal antigens AFP and CEA in the 1960s revolutionized the modern era of tumor markers. AFP was first found in the sera of mice with liver cancer[2] and later[234] in sera of humans with hepatocellular carcinoma. CEA was discovered in 1965 by Gold and Freeman and was known initially as the Gold "antigen."[80] Oncofetal antigens that have been used as tumor markers, including AFP and CEA, are listed in Table 23-9.

Alpha Fetoprotein

AFP is a marker for hepatocellular and germ cell (nonseminoma) carcinoma.[232]

Biochemistry

AFP is a glycoprotein with a molecular mass of 70 kDa. It consists of a single polypeptide chain and is 4% carbohydrate. AFP is synthesized in large quantities during embryonic development by the fetal yolk sac and liver. It is one of the major proteins in the fetal circulation, but its maximum concentration is about 10% that of albumin. AFP is closely related both genetically and structurally to albumin, having extensive homologies in amino acid sequence. The genes coding for both proteins have been localized to chromosome 4q. As albumin synthesis increases during later fetal development, AFP concentrations in fetal serum begin to decline. They finally reach the trace concentrations found in normal adults 18 months after birth.

For tumor-derived AFP, the composition of carbohydrate on AFP depends on the activity of saccharide transferase in the tumor cells. Differences in carbohydrate side chains on AFP may be determined by the binding of AFP to lectins, such as concanavalin A (Con A) and lens culinaris (LCA). Molecular variants of AFP can be separated into the liver type and the yolk sac type; they differ from each other in their carbohydrate moiety. The yolk sac type of AFP contains an additional sugar, N-acetylglycosamine; this blocks the Con A binding site on the AFP. Therefore the yolk sac type of AFP shows a high percentage (50% to 70%) of Con A nonreactive (CNR) fraction, whereas the liver type, which lacks this additional sugar, shows a low CNR fraction (10% to 20%).[42] LCA binds to the fucosylated form of the first core N-acetylglucose, which is present in both liver and yolk sac types of tumor-derived AFP but not in AFP generated by benign liver diseases.

Clinical Applications

The serum AFP level is less than 10 μg/L in healthy adults.[41] During pregnancy, maternal AFP levels increase from 12 weeks of gestation to a peak of about 500 μg/L during the third trimester. The fetal AFP reaches a peak of 2 g/L at 14 weeks and then declines to about 70 mg/L at term. The use of AFP for detecting fetuses with neural tube defects is discussed in Chapter 54. In addition to pregnancy, elevated levels of serum AFP are also associated with benign liver conditions, such as hepatitis and cirrhosis. Most patients with these benign diseases (95%) have AFP levels lower than 200 μg/L.

Except in the pregnant patient, AFP levels greater than 1000 μg/L are indicative of cancer. At these levels of AFP, about half of hepatocellular carcinomas may be detected. However, because the serum level of AFP correlates with the size of the tumor,[108] detection of hepatocellular carcinoma is more useful at the earlier stages, when the tumor is small enough to be resectable (less than 5 cm) than when the tumor is large. To detect small tumors, the cut-off level for AFP has to be set at a low level; a cut-off point of 10 to 20 μg/L has been recommended. However, at this level, hepatitis and cirrhosis must be considered as possible causes of elevation.

Screening for hepatocellular carcinoma has been attempted in high-incidence areas, such as Africa, China, Taiwan, Japan, and Alaska.[141] Initial large-scale screening in China using less sensitive techniques (e.g., agglutination and immunodiffusion, which have cut-off values of 400 to 1000 μg/L) was able to detect notable numbers of new cases of this type of cancer. More sensitive immunoassay methods having cut-off values of 10 to 20 μg/L and ultrasonography have been used in Taiwan and Japan with better success in detecting hepatocellular carcinoma at earlier stages.

AFP is also useful for determining prognosis and in the monitoring of therapy for hepatocellular carcinoma.[108] The level of AFP is a prognostic indicator of survival. Elevated AFP levels (greater than 10 μg/L) and serum bilirubin levels of greater than 2 mg/dL are associated with shorter survival time.

The AFP level is a good indicator for monitoring therapy and the change in clinical status. Elevated AFP levels after surgery may indicate incomplete removal of the tumor or the presence of metastasis. Falling or rising AFP levels after therapy may determine the success or failure of the treatment regimen. A notable increase of AFP levels in patients considered free of metastatic tumor may indicate the development of metastasis.

AFP and hCG combined are useful in classifying and staging germ cell tumors. Germ cell tumors may be predominantly of one type of cell or may be a mixture of seminoma, yolk sac, choriocarcinomatous elements (embryonal carcinoma), or teratoma.[13] AFP is elevated in yolk sac tumors, whereas hCG is elevated in choriocarcinoma. Both are elevated in embryonal carcinoma. In seminomas, AFP is not elevated, whereas hCG is elevated in 10% to 30% of patients who have syncytiotrophoblastic cells in the tumor. Neither marker is elevated in teratoma. One or both of the markers are elevated in about 90% of patients with nonseminomatous testicular tumor. Elevations were found in fewer than 20% of patients with stage I disease, 50% to 80% with stage II disease, and 90% to 100% with stage III disease. These markers correlate with tumor volume and the prognosis of disease.

The combined use of both markers is also useful in monitoring patients with germ cell tumors: Elevation of either marker indicates recurrence of disease or development of metastasis. The success of chemotherapy can be assessed by calculating the decrease of the levels of both markers using the half-lives of AFP (5 days) and hCG (12 to 20 hours).

Analytical Methodology

Serum AFP can be determined by immunometric assay using either a radioactive or enzyme label (see Chapter 54). Automated immunoassay systems to measure AFP using these techniques are available. The detection limit of AFP immunoassay is about 1 to 2 μg/L.

Carcinoembryonic Antigen

CEA is a marker for colorectal, gastrointestinal, lung, and breast carcinoma. CEA was discovered by Gold and Freeman in 1965.[80] Rabbits were immunized with extracts of human colon cancer tissue, and the resultant antisera were absorbed with extracts of normal human colon. Some antisera reacted with the tumor extracts but not with the extracts of normal tissue. The antigen, which was also found in embryonic tissue, was named *carcinoembryonic antigen.*

Biochemistry

CEA is a glycoprotein with a molecular mass of 150 to 300 kDa; it contains 45% to 55% carbohydrate. It is a single polypeptide chain consisting of 641 amino acids, with lysine in the N-terminal position. The heterogeneity of CEA can be demonstrated by using isoelectric focusing to separate the variants.

CEA consists of a large family of related cell-surface glycoproteins. The CEA proteins are encoded by about 10 genes located on chromosome 19. Up to 36 different glycoproteins have been identified in the CEA family. The major proteins are CEA and nonspecific cross-reacting antigen (NCA).[99] The domain structure of CEA, NCA 50, and the heavy chain of the immunoglobulin IgG are very similar. Thus CEA is part of the immunoglobulin gene "superfamily."

Clinical Applications

The CEA level is elevated in a variety of cancers, such as colorectal (70%), lung (45%), gastric (50%), breast (40%), pancreatic (55%), ovarian (25%), and uterine (40%) carcinoma. Because of the elevations associated with benign disease (i.e., false-positive results) and the number of tumors that do not produce CEA (i.e., false-negative results), CEA testing should not be used for screening.[206]

CEA testing may be useful as an adjunct to clinical staging. Persistently elevated levels that are 5 to 10 times the upper reference limit strongly suggest the presence of colon cancer but may be associated with other cancers. In colon cancer, CEA levels correlate with the stage of the disease. CEA levels are elevated in 28% of patients with Dukes' stage A colorectal cancer and in 45% of those with stage B. The pretreatment CEA level is prognostic of the development of metastasis. A high level of CEA is associated with a greater likelihood of developing metastasis. Evidence suggests that CEA is a cellular adhesion molecule that may potentiate invasion and metastasis.[99]

After successful initial therapy, CEA levels decline. During remission, CEA levels are stable. Rising CEA values may indicate recurrence of disease. The lead time from CEA elevation to clinical recurrence is about 5 months. A repeat laparotomy can be performed to confirm the relapse, which is detected in 90% of cases. In the monitoring of metastatic colon cancer, CEA is useful in following patients throughout therapy and the clinical course of the disease.

CEA is also useful in monitoring breast, lung, gastric, and pancreatic carcinoma. In breast cancer, elevated CEA is associated with metastatic disease. Early or localized breast cancer does not show CEA elevation. CEA is most useful in monitoring metastatic breast cancer during therapy and for detecting the development of bone or lung metastasis. For breast cancer, CEA is being replaced by other more specific markers, such as CA 15-3. In lung cancer, CEA determination is helpful in diagnosing non–small cell lung carcinoma (greater than 65% of patients have elevated CEA) and in monitoring lung cancer.

Analytical Methodology

As with AFP, most assays use the immunometric format for the determination of serum CEA. Polyclonal or monoclonal antibodies, or a combination of both types, have been used in CEA immunoassays.

In the healthy population, the upper limit of CEA is about 3 μg/L for nonsmokers and 5 μg/L for smokers. Because the level of CEA measured is method dependent, values should always be compared using the same method. When changing methods, all patients being monitored should be tested in parallel using both the old and new methods. CEA level is elevated in some patients having benign conditions, such as cirrhosis (45%), pulmonary emphysema (30%), rectal polyps (5%), benign breast disease (15%), and ulcerative colitis (15%).

CYTOKERATINS

The cytokeratins are a large group of approximately 20 proteins that make up the cytoskeletal intermediate filaments of epithelial cells and cells of epithelial origin. The cytokeratins can be grossly divided into two groups, type 1 being smaller and acidic and type 2 being larger and neutral to basic. The clinically useful members of this family are tissue polypeptide antigen (TPA), tissue polypeptide-specific antigen (TPS), and cytokeratin 19 fragments (CYFRA 21-1).

Tissue Polypeptide Antigen

The discovery of TPA preceded that of AFP and CEA, but TPA is not a specific tumor marker.[22] It was later found that TPA could be identified by antibodies that react with cytokeratins 8, 18, and 19. TPA is produced by both normal and cancerous cells. Elevated serum levels of TPA are related to the proliferation activity and turnover of cells, allowing it to be used as a proliferation marker.[155] In pregnancy, TPA increases throughout gestation. After pregnancy, the level returns to normal after 5 days. TPA is also elevated in inflammatory diseases and in cancer; thus it is not useful for diagnosis. In the monitoring of metastatic diseases, TPA is useful when combined with CEA and CA 15-3 in breast cancer, with CEA and CA 19-9 in colon cancer, and with CA 125 in ovarian cancer. TPA may be helpful in the differentiation of cholangiocarcinomas (in which TPA level is elevated) from hepatocellular carcinoma (in which TPA level is not elevated).

Tissue Polypeptide-Specific Antigen

TPS is actually an antigenic site on the TPA complex that is specifically recognized by the M3 monoclonal antibody. This epitope has been proposed as a specific marker of cell proliferation, and is detectable in serum using a specific radioimmunoassay. TPS appears to correlate with proliferation activity of lung tumors, irrespective of histology and tumor volume, with increasing TPS levels in increasing stages.[29] Elevated levels of TPS correlate with a poorer outcome as assessed by univariate analysis.

Cytokeratin 19 Fragments

CYFRA 21-1 is elevated in all types of lung cancer, although it is most sensitive for non–small cell lung cancer and SCC. Levels of CYFRA 21-1 positively correlate with increasing stage and are useful in monitoring of disease course, and in postsurgical follow-up. In one study of non–small cell lung cancer patients, CYFRA 21-1 was shown to independently correlate with decreased survival, nodal status, and tumor stage, confirming its utility as a lung tumor marker.[176]

Squamous Cell Carcinoma Antigen

As its name implies, SCCA is useful in monitoring a wide variety of SCCs.

Biochemistry

SCCA is a glycoprotein previously referred to as "tumor-associated antigen 4." Subfractions of SCCA have been separated by isoelectric focusing into neutral and acidic fractions. The molecular weights range from 42,000 to 48,000. Both malignant and nonmalignant squamous cells have been shown to contain the neutral fraction, whereas the acidic fraction is found mainly in malignant cells. The acidic fraction is the one released into the blood circulation. The expression of SCCA appears to correlate with the grade of differentiation of SCCs.[107]

Clinical Applications

SCCA is elevated in a variety of SCCs, including those of the cervix, lung, skin, head, neck, digestive tract, ovaries, and urogenital tract. In general, the level of SCCA is proportional to the advancing stages of cancer. Screening is not effective, since only a small percentage of patients with early stages of cancer show elevated SCCA values. High pretreatment SCCA values appear to be associated with a poor prognosis. SCCA is useful in detecting the recurrence of cancer and in the monitoring of treatment and disease progression.[107]

Analytical Methodology

SCC antigen is measured using immunoradiometric assay or the microparticle enzyme immunoassay on the IMx analyzer (Abbott Diagnostics, Chicago). Healthy, nonpregnant women have SCC antigen values below 1.5 μg/L. Serum SCC antigen levels may be elevated (greater than 1.5 μg/L) in certain benign conditions, including pulmonary infection, skin disease, renal failure, and liver disease. It is also present in saliva, sweat, and respiratory secretions. Because of this, masks should be worn by laboratory personnel when analyzing SCC antigen.

TABLE 23-10 Mucin Tumor Markers

Name	Antigen and Source	Antibody	Type of Cancer
CA 125	Glycoprotein, >200 kDa, OVCA 433	OC 125	Ovarian, endometrial
Episialin			
CA 15-3	Glycoprotein, 400 kDa, membrane-enriched BrCa	DF3 and 115D8	Breast, ovarian
CA 549	High-MW glycoprotein	BC4E549, BC4N154	Breast, ovarian
CA 27.29	High-MW glycoprotein	B27.29	Breast
MCA	350-kDa glycoprotein	b-12	Breast, ovarian
DU-PAN-2	Mucin, 1000-kDa peptide epitope	DU-PAN-2	Pancreatic, ovarian, gastrointestinal, lung

MW, Molecular weight.

TABLE 23-11 Blood Group Antigen-Related Cancer Markers

Name	Antigen and Source	Antibody	Type of Cancer
CA 19-9	Sialylated Le^{xa}, SW-1116 colon CA	19-9	Pancreatic, gastrointestinal, hepatic
CA 19-5	Le^{a} and sialylated Le^{ag}	19-5	Gastrointestinal, pancreatic, ovarian
CA 50	Sialylated Le^{a} and afucosyl form	C50	Pancreatic, gastrointestinal, colon
CA 72-4	Sialylated Tn	B27.3, cc49	Ovarian, breast, gastrointestinal, colon
CA 242	Sialylated CHO	C242	Gastrointestinal, pancreatic

CARBOHYDRATE MARKERS

Carbohydrate-related tumor markers either are (1) antigens on the tumor cell surface or (2) secreted by the tumor cells.[87,88,198] Monoclonal antibodies have been developed against these antigens. These markers have been found to be clinically useful as tumor markers and tend to be more specific than naturally secreted markers, such as enzymes and hormones. Biochemically, they are high molecular weight mucins (Table 23-10) or blood group antigens (Table 23-11).

CA 15-3, CA 549, and CA 27.29 assays detect a high molecular weight glycoprotein mucin expressed by the mammary epithelium, known as *episialin.* The circulating episialin antigen is a heterogeneous molecule. CA 15-3, CA 549, and CA 27.29 assays detect similar yet different epitopes on the episialin. The main differences are the antibodies used for detection. They are used as markers for breast carcinoma.

CA 15-3

CA 15-3 is a marker for breast carcinoma.

Biochemistry

CA 15-3 is detected by a murine monoclonal antibody (MAb) DF3 produced against a membrane-enriched extract of a human breast cancer metastatic to liver. Another monoclonal antibody, 115D8, was developed against human milk fat globule membrane. The circulating DF3-reactive antigen is a heterogeneous molecule with a molecular mass of 300 to 450 kDa. The gene for this molecule is located on chromosome 1q. cDNA cloning indicates that the DF3 peptide core consists of a highly conserved 60-bp tandem repeat sequence. The polymorphism of the antigen is the result of different numbers of repeats in the peptide core. The DF3 antibody recognizes the epitope within this 20 amino acid–repeating sequence of the peptide core. The recognition of the epitope is also affected by glycation.[93]

Clinical Applications

In healthy subjects, the upper limit of CA 15-3 concentration is 25 kU/L. At this level, 5.5% of 1050 normal subjects, 23% of patients with primary breast cancer, and 69% of those with metastatic breast cancer show elevated CA 15-3 levels.[93] Elevated CA 15-3 levels are also found in other malignancies, including pancreatic (80%), lung (71%), breast (69%), ovarian (64%), colorectal (63%), and liver (28%) cancer. It is also reported to be elevated in benign diseases, although with less frequency (e.g., in benign liver [42%] and benign breast diseases [16%]).

CA 15-3 should not be used to diagnose primary breast cancer, because the incidence of elevation (23%) is fairly low. CA 15-3 is most useful in monitoring therapy and disease progression in metastatic breast cancer patients. A significant change must be at least 25% and correlates with disease progression in 90% of patients, with its regression in 78%. No change correlates with disease stability in 60%. CA 15-3 could replace CEA in metastatic breast cancer owing to its sensitivity and specificity.

Analytical Methodology

Two antibodies are used in immunoassays. The MAb 115D8 is attached to a solid support, whereas MAb DF3 is labeled.

CA 549

CA 549 is a marker for breast carcinoma.

Biochemistry

CA 549 is an acidic glycoprotein with an isoelectric point of pH 5.2. By sodium dodecyl sulfate/polyacrylamide gel electrophoresis under reducing conditions, CA 549 can be separated into two species with molecular masses of 400 and 512 kDa. One monoclonal antibody, a murine IgG_1 termed *BC4E 549,* was raised by immunizing mice with partially purified membrane preparations from T417 human breast tumor cell line. The other antibody, *BC4N 154* (a murine IgM), was developed against human milk fat globule membranes.[27]

Clinical Application

In a population of healthy women, 95% of the population has CA 549 values below 11 kU/L. Pregnancy and benign breast disease show minimum elevation. Some patients with benign liver disease show a slight elevation (see Table 23-4). CA 549 has been shown to be elevated in a variety of non-breast metastatic carcinomas, including ovarian (50%), prostate (40%), and lung (33%) carcinomas.

Similar to CA 15-3, CA 549 is not useful in detecting early breast carcinoma, because the proportion of patients with elevated CA 549 levels is low. Using ROC analysis, CA 549 is better than CEA at identifying active breast cancer (see Figure 23-2).[37] CA 549 is useful in detecting recurrence of breast cancer in patients after initial therapy followed by adjuvant therapy. An increasing CA 549 value after an initial decrease or stabilization indicates the development of metastases (see Figure 23-3). In the monitoring of advanced breast cancer patients, CA 549 correlates with disease progression and regression and helps detect metastases.[37,38]

CA 27.29

CA 27.29 is a marker for breast carcinoma.

Biochemistry

CA 27.29 is detected by a monoclonal antibody, B27.29, that is produced against an antigen in ascites of patients with metastatic breast carcinoma. The minimum epitope to which B27.29 reacts is the 8 amino acid sequence (SAPDTRPA) within the 20 amino acid tandem repeating sequence of the mucin core. The reactive sequence of the B27.29 overlaps with the sequence of DF3 used in the CA 15-3 assay. In inhibition studies using labeled MAb, B27.29 effectively competes with DF3 for binding to both CA 27.29 and CA 15-3 antigens.[180]

Clinical Applications

CA 27.29 has been approved by the FDA for clinical use in the detection of recurrent breast cancer in patients with stage II or stage III disease. In a multicenter study over a 2-year period monitoring 166 breast cancer patients, 26 patients developed recurrent disease. When two consecutive CA 27.29 antigen test results above 37.7 kU/L (99th percentile) were considered positive, the CA 27.29 assay had a sensitivity of 57.7%, specificity of 97.9%, positive predictive value of 83.3%, and negative predictive value of 92.6% for the detection of recurrent breast cancer. The performance appeared to be better than that of CA 15-3 in detecting patients with recurrent breast cancer.[39] In a group of metastatic breast cancer patients, CA 27.29 and CA15.3 showed similar clinical performances.[49]

Analytical Methodology

CA 27.29 is measured using a solid-phase competitive immunoassay. A prediluted sample is added to a polystyrene tube coated with B27.29 antigen and incubated with the ^{125}I-labeled murine antibody for B27.29. A calibration curve is constructed using five calibrators from 0 to 200 kU/L.

Mucinlike Carcinoma-Associated Antigen

Mucinlike carcinoma-associated antigen (MCA) is a marker for breast carcinoma.[25]

Biochemistry

MCA was identified on the surface of a breast carcinoma cell line by the monoclonal antibody b-12. MCA is a glycoprotein with a molecular mass of 350 kDa. The epitopes on this molecule are also recognized by DF3 and 115D8 antibodies of the CA 15-3 assay.

Clinical Applications

In a study of 100 healthy women, the upper reference limit for MCA was found to be 14 kU/L. MCA levels increase throughout pregnancy. In contrast, CA 15-3 only increases slightly during pregnancy. MCA level is elevated in 60% of metastatic breast cancer patients. However, elevated levels are also found in ovarian, cervical, endometrial, and prostate carcinoma. Minimum elevation is observed in benign breast disease. MCA levels correlate with CA 15-3 levels but not with CEA levels. In the monitoring of metastatic breast cancer patients, changes in MCA levels parallel those of CA 15-3 levels.

CA 125

CA 125 is a marker for ovarian cancer.[201]

Biochemistry

CA 125 is a high molecular mass (greater than 200 kDa) glycoprotein recognized by the monoclonal antibody OC 125. It contains 24% carbohydrate and is expressed by epithelial ovarian tumors and other pathological and normal tissues of müllerian duct origin. The physiological function is unknown.

Bast and associates developed the MAb OC 125 using a cell line (OVCA 433) from a patient with a serous papillary cystadenocarcinoma of the ovary.[113] The OC 125 clone was selected for its reactivity with the OVCA 433 cell line and for its lack of reactivity with a B-lymphocyte line from the same patient.

Clinical Applications

In a healthy population, the upper limit of CA 125 level is 35 kU/L. CA 125 is elevated in nonovarian carcinoma, including endometrial, pancreatic, lung, breast, and colorectal and other gastrointestinal tumors. CA 125 is useful for determining the prognosis of endometrial carcinoma. It is also elevated in women in the follicular phase of the menstrual cycle and in benign conditions such as cirrhosis, hepatitis, endometriosis, pericarditis, and early pregnancy. CA 125 may be useful in the evaluation of the disease status in patients with advanced endometriosis but is not useful in screening for ovarian cancer in asymptomatic populations.[100] It cannot be used to differentiate ovarian cancer from other malignancies.

In ovarian carcinoma, CA 125 is elevated in 50% of patients with stage I disease, 90% with stage II, and more than 90% with stages III and IV. The level of CA 125 correlates with tumor size and staging. CA 125 is also useful in differentiating benign from malignant disease in patients with palpable ovarian masses. This differentiation is important because surgical intervention for malignant ovarian masses is far more extensive than that for the benign masses. Einhorn and colleagues studied 100 patients undergoing diagnostic laparotomy for palpable adnexal masses; of these, 23 were found to have a malignancy.[64] Using 35 kU/L as the cut-off value, the predictive values for malignant disease were 78% sensitivity, 95% specificity, 82% positive predictive value, and 91% negative predictive value. Tumor differentiation does not affect the CA 125 level.

A preoperative CA 125 level of less than 65 kU/L is associated with a significantly greater 5-year survival rate (42%) than is a level greater than 65 kU/L (5%). Postoperative CA 125 levels and the rate of decline are also predictors of survival. The half-life of CA 125 is normally 4.8 days. A group of patients with a CA 125 half-life of 22 days responded poorly to chemotherapy as compared with another group with a CA 125 half-life of 9 days.

CA 125 is useful in detecting residual disease in cancer patients following initial therapy. The sensitivity of CA 125 for detecting tumors before repeat laparotomy is 50%, and the specificity is 96%. After chemotherapy, the CA 125 level provides an indication of disease prognosis. A decrease in the CA 125 level by a factor of 10 after the first cycle of chemotherapy is indicative of improvement. Persistent elevation of CA 125 levels after three cycles of chemotherapy indicates a poor prognosis.

In the detection of recurrent metastasis, use of CA 125 level as an indicator is about 75% accurate. The lead time from CA 125 elevation to clinically detectable recurrence is about 3 to 4 months. CA 125 correlates with disease progression or regression in 80% to 90% of cases.[100]

Analytical Methodology

An immunoradiometric assay for CA 125 was first developed and manufactured by Centocor, Inc, now Fujirebio Diagnostics. A second generation assay (CA 125II) uses a monoclonal antibody, M11, as the capture and OC 125 as the conjugate. This assay has been approved by the FDA for the quantitative measurement of CA 125 in serum of women with primary epithelial invasive ovarian cancer.

OTHER OVARIAN CANCER BIOMARKERS

A number of other potential ovarian cancer biomarkers have been discovered by using microarray technologies and other methods. The role of kallikreins as potential ovarian cancer biomarkers has already been described.* Some of the newly discovered biomarkers include mesothelin, HE4 protein, prostasin, osteopontin, and other carbohydrate antigens that were found to be elevated in a small proportion of ovarian cancers (e.g., CA 19-9, CA 15-3, etc.).[94,147,237] There is now a general trend for combining multiple biomarkers, including CA 125, to increase the sensitivity of detecting ovarian cancer, especially in screening settings.[97,142] Others have proposed the rate of increase of CA 125 as an effective screening tool.[209] The combined use of serum markers along with transvaginal ultrasonography generally increases the sensitivity in ovarian cancer screening programs but compromises specificity. The use of biochemical markers as panels in ovarian cancer screening is still under investigation.

DU-PAN-2

DU-PAN-2 is a marker for pancreatic cancer.[143]

Biochemistry

The epitope recognized by the antibody DU-PAN-2 is a mucin. Its molecular mass is between 100 and 500 kDa, and it is 80% carbohydrate. cDNA for the core protein has been cloned and sequenced, and the predicted amino acid sequence reveals a protein of 126 kDa containing 1295 amino acid residues with 42 tandem repeats. DU-PAN-2 antigen is found mainly in the glandular epithelia of the pancreatic and biliary systems and in the breast and bronchial ducts. A lower level of expression is found in cells of the salivary glands, stomach, colon, and intestine.[143]

Clinical Applications

Serum DU-PAN-2 levels are elevated in patients with pancreatic (54% to 61%), biliary tract (44% to 47%), and

*References 60, 112, 136, 137, 253, 254.

hepatocellular (44%) carcinomas. Comparative studies between DU-PAN-2 and CA 19-9 levels in pancreatic cancer show similar elevations in 70% to 80% of patients. The correlation of patient values for DU-PAN-2 and CA 19-9 was good except in patients who are Le^{a-b-} and therefore do not express CA 19-9.

Analytical Methodology

An RIA assay was developed by Metzgar and co-workers,[143] and an immunoenzymetric assay was developed by Kyowa Medex (Tokyo). The serum concentration of DU-PAN-2 in a healthy population is less than 100 kU/L. The cut-off level used to differentiate the presence of cancer from health is 300 or 400 kU/L.

BLOOD GROUP ANTIGENS

Blood group carbohydrates identified by monoclonal antibodies that have been used as markers of cancers are listed in Table 23-11. These include CA 19-9 (sialylated Le^{xa}), CA 50 (sialylated Le^{x-1}, afucosyl forms), CA 72-4 (sialyl Tn), and CA 242 (sialylated carbohydrate coexpressed with CA 50).

CA 19-9

CA 19-9 is a marker for both colorectal and pancreatic carcinoma.[120] CA 19-9 has been approved by the FDA for the quantitative measurement in serum and as an aid in monitoring pancreatic cancer patients.

Biochemistry

This carbohydrate antigen is a glycolipid—specifically, sialylated lacto-*N*-fucopenteose II ganglioside, that is a sialylated derivative of the Le^a blood group antigen and is denoted as Le^{xa}.The expression of the antigen requires the Lewis gene product, 1,4-fucosyl transferase. CA 19-9 is synthesized by normal human pancreatic and biliary ductular cells and by gastric, colon, endometrial, and salivary epithelia. In serum, it exists as a mucin, a high molecular mass (200 to 1000 kDa) glycoprotein complex. Patients who are genotypically Le^{a-b-} (about 5%) do not express CA 19-9. The monoclonal antibody against CA 19-9 was developed from a human colon carcinoma cell line, SW-1116.[117]

Clinical Applications

When using the Centocor CA 19-9 assay, the upper reference limit is 37 kU/L. Of 1500 healthy blood bank donors tested, 99% had CA 19-9 values below this limit. Elevated levels (greater than 37 kU/L) were seen in patients with pancreatic (80%), hepatobiliary (67%), gastric (40% to 50%), hepatocellular (30% to 50%), colorectal (30%), and breast (15%) cancer. Some patients (10% to 20%) with pancreatitis and other benign gastrointestinal diseases have elevated levels up to 120 kU/L. CA 19-9 levels correlate with pancreatic cancer staging. With the cut-off of 37 kU/L, 67% of patients with resectable and 87% of those with unresectable pancreatic cancer have elevated values. By raising the cut-off to 1000 kU/L, 35% of patients with unresectable tumors and only 5% of those with resectable tumors have elevated CA 19-9 values. CA 19-9 is useful in monitoring pancreatic and colorectal cancer. Elevated levels can indicate recurrence 1 to 7 months before detected by radiographs or clinical findings.[224] Unfortunately, early detection of relapse may not be useful because of the lack of effective therapy for pancreatic cancer.

Analytical Methodology

Several companies have produced CA 19-9 immunoassays. Typically, the CA 19-9 antibody is used both as the capture and the signal antibody.

CA 50

CA 50 is a marker for pancreatic and colorectal carcinoma.[87]

Biochemistry

CA 50 is a monoclonal antibody developed against the human colon adenocarcinoma cell line COLO 205. The CA 50 antibody recognizes an epitope on two carbohydrate moieties, sialosylfucosyllactotetraose (sialylated Le^a) and sialosyllactotetraose (sialylated Le^a lacking fucose). This antigen exists as a glycoprotein in serum and also as gangliosides in tissue. The sialylated Le^a is the predominant form of CA 50 in epithelial carcinoma and is also recognized by CA 19-9.

Clinical Applications

Elevated CA 50 levels have been reported in benign diseases of the pancreas (12% to 46%), biliary tract (35% to 38%), and liver (22% to 59%). In pancreatic cancer, 80% to 97% of patients have elevated levels. In colon cancer, elevated levels were reported in Dukes' A (19% to 43%), B (30% to 59%), C (53% to 73%), and D (53% to 73%) stages. In digestive tract carcinoma, elevated levels were seen in esophageal (41% to 71%), gastric (41% to 78%), biliary (58% to 70%), and hepatocellular (14% to 78%) cancer. Other malignancies were reported to have lower percentages of elevation, including breast, lung, renal, prostate, bladder, and ovarian cancer. Similar performances and good correlations were reported between CA 50 and CA 19-9 values.

Analytical Methodology

The original inhibition test has been replaced by an immunoradiometric assay and a time-resolved fluorescent immunoassay (the DELFIA method developed by Pharmacia, Uppsala, Sweden). The cut-off values for healthy subjects vary from 14 to 20 kU/L, depending on the method.

CA 72-4

CA 72-4 is a marker for carcinomas of the gastrointestinal tract and of the ovary.[194]

Biochemistry

B72.3 is a monoclonal antibody developed from the membrane-enriched fraction of breast carcinoma in a patient with liver metastasis. The B72.3 reactive antigen was purified and called TAG-72 (tumor-associated glycoprotein). Further purification of TAG-72 from LS-174T human colon carcinoma xenograft produced a new generation of monoclonal antibodies with higher affinity. These antibodies, denoted "cc" for "colon carcinoma," were used in subsequent studies.

Clinical Applications

A cut-off of 6 kU/L is used in the CA 72-4 assay. The following percentages of elevation were observed: in health, 3.5%; in benign gastrointestinal diseases, 6.7%; in gastrointestinal carcinoma, 40%; in lung cancer, 36%; and in ovarian cancer, 24%. A poor clinical correlation between CEA and CA 72-4 levels was found in gastric cancer. CEA and CA 72-4 values may be complementary. The plasma clearance of TAG-72 was studied by measuring serial TAG-72 values in patients with primary carcinoma of breast and with gastric, colorectal, and ovarian cancer. After removal of the tumor, the average time required for the level to decrease to 4 kU/L was 23.3 days. This suggests that TAG-72 may be useful in detecting residual tumor in these cancer patients.

Analytical Methodology

CA 72-4 is measured using an immunoradiometric assay (IRMA). It uses two monoclonal antibodies that were developed at the National Cancer Institute. B72.3 is the conjugate, whereas cc49 is the capture antibody. This IRMA is manufactured by Fujirebio Diagnostics.

CA 242

CA 242 is a marker for pancreatic and colorectal cancer.[119]

Biochemistry

CA 242 is a monoclonal antibody developed from a human colorectal carcinoma cell line, COLO 205. The antigenic determinant is a sialylated carbohydrate. CA 242 recognizes the epitopes of CA 50 and CA 19-9. CA 242 is found in the apical border of ductal cells of the human pancreas and in the epithelial and goblet cells of the colonic mucosa.

Clinical Applications

Using a cut-off value of 20 kU/L, elevated CA 242 values were found in 5% to 33% of patients with benign colon, gastric, hepatic, pancreatic, and biliary tract diseases; in 68% to 79% of patients with malignant pancreatic cancer; in 55% to 85% of patients with colorectal cancer; and in 44% of patients with gastric cancer. The correlation coefficients (R^2) of CA 242, CA 50, and CA 19-9 values in patients with colorectal, liver, pancreatic, and biliary tract disease ranged from 0.81 to 0.95. CA 242 and CEA appeared to have higher percentages of elevation in colorectal cancer than did CA 50 and CA 19-9. CA 242 seems to be less efficient than CA 19-9 or CA 50 in the detection of pancreatic cancer; however, this may depend on the cut-off value.

Analytical Methodology

An immunometric assay uses CA 50 antibody as the capture antibody and the CA 242 antibody as the conjugate. A fluoroimmunoassay for CA 242 is available as a DELFIA assay. The upper reference limit is 20 kU/L.

PROTEINS

Several proteins having tumor marker potential are listed in Table 23-12. Included in this group of tumor markers are proteins that are not enzymes, hormones, or high in carbohydrate content. Additional research is required to assess the clinical usefulness of most of these markers.

IMMUNOGLOBULIN

Monoclonal immunoglobulin has been used as a marker for multiple myeloma for more than 100 years.[17] Monoclonal paraproteins appear as sharp bands in the globulin area of the serum electrophoretic patterns. More than 95% of

TABLE 23-12 Proteins as Tumor Markers

Name	Nature	Type of Cancer
β_2-Microglobulin	11 kDa	Multiple myeloma, B-cell lymphoma, chronic lymphocytic leukemia, Waldenström's macroglobulinemia
C-peptide	3.6 kDa	Insulinoma
Ferritin	450-kDa iron-binding protein	Liver, lung, breast, leukemia
Immunoglobulin	160-900 kDa, 3%-12% CHO	Multiple myeloma, lymphomas
Melanoma-associated antigen	90-240 kDa	Melanoma
Pancreas-associated antigen	100 kDa, 20% CHO	Pancreatic, stomach
Pregnancy-specific protein 1	10 kDa, 30% CHO	Trophoblastic, germ cell
Prothrombin precursor	Des-r-carboxy prothrombin	Hepatocellular
Tumor-associated trypsin inhibitor	6-kDa polypeptide	Lung, gastrointestinal, ovarian

patients with multiple myeloma have such an electrophoretic pattern. Appearance of nonmalignant monoclonal immunoglobulins increases with age, reaching 5% in patients older than 75 years. These nonmalignant monoclonal bands are usually lower in concentration than malignant bands and not associated with Bence Jones protein. Bence Jones protein is a free monoclonal immunoglobulin light chain in the urine. The level of monoclonal immunoglobulin at initial diagnosis is a prognostic indicator of disease progression.[213] During treatment, the serum concentration of urinary Bence Jones protein may reflect the success of therapy. Lower levels are associated with more favorable outcome. The electrophoretic patterns of serum paraproteins are discussed in Chapter 20.

BLADDER CANCER MARKERS

It is estimated that 600,000 Americans are currently affected by bladder cancer, and almost 54,000 new cases will be reported each year. The symptoms range from intermittent hematuria to voiding problems or dysuria. The most common type of cell seen is transitional cell carcinoma (TCC), and the most frequent symptom is hematuria. Bladder cancer is staged pathologically and treated on the basis of the extent of tumor invasion. Carcinoma in situ (stage Tis) and superficial bladder cancers (stages Ta and T1) occur on the epithelial lining and do not invade the muscle layer. Stage Ta tumors are confined to the mucosa, and stage T1 tumors superficially invade the lamina propria. Stage T2 tumors extend into the muscle layer and T3 tumors invade beyond the muscle layer. Stage T4 tumors have metastasized to local nodes or distant organs.

Urinary Bladder Tumor Markers

Detection of bladder cancer is through either cystoscopy or cytology of shed cells, or by detection of noncellular markers, such as NMP22, complement factor-H (CFH), fibronectin, immunocyt, and bladder tumor associated (BTA) analytes voided in urine.[76,205] Tumor antigens present in urine are the easiest to analyze; however they cannot be used as the sole mechanism for tumor detection. They should be used in a complementary manner with cystoscopy and cytology. NMP22, in a series of 300 patients with hematuria, using a cut-off of 10 U/mL, detected 100% of the bladder cancer cases, with a specificity of 85%.[265] In another study, NMP22 and fibronectin were found to have superior sensitivity to that of cytology; however NMP22 and cytology have the highest specificity.[65] Calreticulin has also been suggested as a marker for bladder cancer and its diagnostic accuracy evaluated.[104]

A fluorescence in situ hybridization (FISH) technique, UroVysion, uses fluorescently labeled probes to detect aneuploidy of chromosomes 3, 7, and 17, and deletion of the 9p21 locus that contains the tumor suppressor p16, which is the most common alteration seen in urothelial carcinoma. Table 23-13 compares cytology with that of UroVysion for the detection of bladder cancer.[190]

Nuclear Matrix Protein (NMP22)

Nuclear matrix proteins (NMPs) make up the internal structure of the nucleus. Their function has been associated with regulating key reactions in the nucleus, such as DNA replication and RNA synthesis. The NMPs released by the cancer cell may be different from the normal cell. Furthermore, different types of cells may have different NMPs. Soluble NMPs could be detected in the sera of cancer patients in higher concentrations than the sera from normal subjects.[165] In a multicenter follow-up study (125 cystoscopies) of 90 patients with 33 pathologically confirmed TCC of the urinary tract, 70% of the 33 recurrences had urinary NMP greater than 10 U/mL. Of the patients with NMP less than 10 U/mL, 86% had no malignancy at subsequent cystoscopy.[215]

An ELISA for the measurement of an NMP called nuclear mitotic apparatus protein in urine sample has been approved by the U.S. FDA for the management of patients with TCC of the urinary tract. The test is called NMP22 and is manufactured by Matritech, Inc. (Newton, Mass.)

Bladder Tumor Associated Analytes

A qualitative test for BTA analytes in urine, termed the BTA stat. test, has been developed. BTA analytes are high molecular weight polypeptides composed of complexes of basement membrane proteins. The presence of BTA analytes in urine is thought to involve either invasion of the basement membrane by tumor, production by the tumor itself, or a combination of these, which may be linked with the body's immune response. If BTA analytes are present in a significant level, they will combine with latex particles to produce an agglutination reaction, which produces a visible color change on the

TABLE 23-13 Comparison of Cytology Sensitivity With UroVysion Sensitivity for the Detection of Bladder Cancer by Stage

	UroVysion (percent)	Cytology (percent)
Stage		
Ta, Grade 1-2	62	23
Ta, Grade 3	83	33
T1, Grade 2	100	100
T1, Grade 3	75	50
T2	100	33
Tis	100	33
Grade		
1	55	18
2	78	44
3	94	41

From Sarosdy, M.F., Schellhammer, P., Bokinsky, G., et al. Clinical evaluation of a multi-target fluorescent in situ hybridization assay for detection of bladder cancer. *J Urol* 2002;168:1950-4.

BTA stat. test strip. A multicenter trial compared the BTA stat. test with voided urine cytology studies in 499 patients undergoing surveillance cystoscopy for recurrent bladder cancer. The BTA stat. test identified 40% of patients with positive cystoscopy results, and cytology detected 17%. A positive test may provide a higher degree of suspicion for recurrence.[189] A quantitative test in ELISA format, BTA TRAK, is also available.

Heat Shock Proteins

Heat shock proteins (HSPs) are a conserved group of proteins that were first identified by their ability to be induced by heat and other stressors. Numerous functions have been associated with HSPs, most notably as chaperones to stabilize cellular proteins during periods of unfavorable conditions. HSPs associate with many cellular components, including signal transduction proteins (kinases and phosphatases), steroid receptors, and components of the apoptotic machinery. The ability of HSPs to interact with various cellular components and protect them from stressors, coupled with the fact that increased expression is seen in a number of tumors, suggests that they may play a role in tumorigenicity. Increased expression of HSP27 is seen in breast cancer, endometrial cancer, and leukemia. HSP70 is increased in breast cancer, endometrial cancer, osteosarcoma, and renal cell tumors. High expression of HSP27 and HSP70 in breast, endometrial, or gastric cancer is correlated with metastasis, poor prognosis, and resistance to chemotherapy.[78] HSP60 and HSP90 are also overexpressed in breast and lung cancers, leukemias, and Hodgkin's disease.

S-100 Proteins

The S-100 proteins are a group of at least 19 related calcium binding proteins. They all contain two high affinity and selective EF-hand calcium binding domains. Their physiological role is uncertain; however some members have been associated with cancer progression, namely S-100A4, S-100A2, S-100A6, and S-100β.[139] S-100A4 is normally expressed in selected immune cells, with faint expression in keratinocytes, melanocytes, and Langerhans' cells. It is not expressed in breast, colon, thyroid, lung, kidney or pancreas. The expression of S-100A4 in breast cancer, esophageal-squamous carcinoma, and gastric cancers correlates with a worse outcome and more aggressive disease, and was shown to be an independent marker of prognosis in multivariate analysis. The lack of expression in normal tissue and its expression in cancer tissue make it an excellent candidate for routine histological use as a cancer marker.

S-100β is routinely used as a diagnostic histological marker of melanoma and melanoma metastases. Recently the measurement of serum levels of S-100β has been investigated for monitoring disease recurrence. In the absence of melanoma, serum S-100β levels are normally undetectable; however with recurrent disease S-100β levels rise. Using an immunoassay (LIA-mat Sangtec 100; Byk-Sangtec Diagnostics, Germany) a cut-off of 0.12 μg/L has been suggested[77] that gives a sensitivity and specificity of 0.29 and 0.93, respectively, with a diagnostic accuracy of 0.84. S-100β is a more sensitive and specific marker for recurrent melanoma and is able to detect recurrence earlier than either LD or alkaline phosphatase (traditional markers of melanoma recurrence).

Autoantibodies

Autoantibodies are antibodies that specifically recognize self-antigens, or proteins. They are normally thought of in the context of autoimmune disease; however autoantibodies have been used for the detection and monitoring of cancer.[59] The event that triggers the development of autoantibodies can either be an infection that through molecular mimicry breaks self-tolerance in a susceptible individual or the inappropriate expression of a self-antigen, such as a cancer antigen. Various cancers produce either proteins or antigens that are recognized by the immune system and are targets for the development of autoantibodies. The detection and monitoring of cancer by the use of circulating tumor markers mainly consist of the detection proteins or antigens that are not normally present in the circulation or when a notable change in the level of these antigens occurs. A number of cancers express new antigens (abnormally glycosylated MUC1, detected by CA 15.3) or overexpress existing antigens, such as HER-2/neu, and autoantibodies that recognize these tumor antigens can also be detected.

Healthy individuals normally either do not have autoantibodies or have them at a very low titer, and a change or rise can signify the development of cancer or another disease state. A number of cancer antigens have been investigated for their ability to induce detectable autoantibodies, including p53, MUC1, c-myc, and c-erbB-2. For example, accumulation of mutant p53 proteins within tumor cells may lead to the development of autoantibodies. Nine percent to 48% of primary breast cancer patients have detectable anti-p53 antibodies, as do 11% to 64% of lung cancer patients.[59] Anti-p53 antibodies have also been detected in hepatocellular, bladder, colorectal, gastric, and other cancers.[7-9]

Many cancers are heterogeneous, and do not consistently express tumor markers. It is clear that no single tumor marker will detect all cancers. Therefore the detection of multiple antigens should increase the sensitivity of detection. This is also the case with autoantibody detection. Using a single autoantibody the detection of primary breast cancer was between 35% and 47%; however using four autoantibodies (p53, MUC1, c-myc, and c-erbB-2) the sensitivity can be increased to 82%.[59]

Autoantibodies are also useful in prognosis and monitoring of disease. Elevated levels of autoantibodies to p53 are associated with a poor prognosis, independent of the tumor-related antigens.[59] This may be due to the fact that expression of the tumor antigen at a distant and/or abnormal site triggers an immune response. The titer of the autoantibodies also tends to follow the amount of tumor antigen, which can provide information about tumor volume. In addition, the concentration of autoantibodies decreases in relation to the antigen load, but will quickly rise again in recurrent disease because of a secondary immune response when the antigen is re-introduced (recurrent disease). The use of autoantibodies with the greatest potential is for the early detection of cancer, since a small amount of the antigen has the ability to generate a vigorous humoral immune response; however more research is necessary before autoantibodies will be part of the standard tests ordered.

THYROGLOBULIN AND ANTIBODIES

Biochemistry

Thyroglobulin (Tg) is produced by the thyroid gland as the precursor to thyroid hormone (see Chapter 52).

Clinical Applications

The main use of Tg measurement is as a tumor marker for patients with a diagnosis of differentiated thyroid cancer. Approximately two thirds of these patients have an elevated preoperative Tg level. An elevated preoperative level of Tg confirms the tumor's ability to secrete Tg and validates the use of postoperative measurement of Tg to monitor for tumor recurrence. Postoperatively, the most sensitive method to detect residual tumor or metastasis is after TSH stimulation. In well-differentiated tumors, a tenfold increase in Tg levels is seen after TSH stimulation.[217] Poorly differentiated tumors, that do not concentrate iodide, may display a blunted response to TSH stimulation.

Antithyroglobulin antibodies can also be used to monitor residual disease and/or recurrence. Serial anti-Tg measurements may be an independent prognostic indicator of therapy, because an increase in anti-Tg antibodies may suggest recurrence of the tumor.[218]

Analytical Methodology

IMA and RIA are the two main methods used for the measurement of Tg. The IMA assays have the advantage of having a shorter incubation time and are automatable; however, they suffer from greater interferences. The main interferants in both assays are antithyroglobulin antibodies, which cause an underestimation of Tg levels in the IMA. Antithyroglobulin antibodies can either be measured directly in all patients or if both IMA and RIA are used to measure Tg, a discordant result suggests the presence of anti-thyroglobulin antibodies.

CHROMOGRANINS

Chromogranins are a family of proteins that are major components of the secretory granules of most neuroendocrine cells.

Biochemistry

The granin family consists of three members, chromogranin A (CgA), B (CgB), and secretogranin II, III, IV, and V.[67] Chromogranins are found in neuroendocrine cells throughout the body, including the neuronal cells of the central and peripheral nervous systems. Intracellularly located chromogranins have been suggested to play a role in the regulation of secretory granules. In addition, the secreted chromogranins can be proteolytically processed to form bioactive peptides. Chromogranin A has been the most studied of the chromogranins, has been shown to be widely expressed by neuroendocrine tissue, and is co-secreted by neuroendocrine cells along with peptide hormones and neuropeptides. This wide distribution and co-secretion make it an excellent histochemical and plasma marker of neuroendocrine tumors.

Clinical Applications

Both CgA and CgB are useful in detecting various neuroendocrine tumors including carcinoid tumors, pheochromocytoma, and neuroblastoma. In most cases CgA is produced at higher levels than CgB; however in some cases, CgB is positive when CgA is negative, therefore both should be measured where possible. In the case of carcinoid tumors, the foregut and mid-gut tumors are normally functional tumors producing serotonin. CgA is as specific for detection of both foregut and midgut carcinoid tumors as the serotonin metabolite 5-hydroxyindoleacetic acid (5-HIAA), and is the preferred marker in hindgut tumors, which commonly are non-functional.[59] Although the nonfunctional tumors have lost the ability to secrete serotonin, they retain the ability to secrete chromogranins. For detection of pheochromocytomas, CgA is at least as sensitive and specific as plasma catecholamines or urinary metanephrins.[21]

Analytical Methodology

Currently, CgA is measured by immunoassay. Depending on the assay, polyclonal or monoclonal antibodies are used. Care must be taken in choosing an assay since CgA and the other chromogranins are heavily processed after release, which may render them nondetectable by the assay and produce false-negative results. Therefore an assay that recognizes both the intact and processed molecule may be desirable.

RECEPTORS AND OTHER MARKERS

Other tumor markers—including catecholamines, polyamines, lipid-associated sialic acid, and receptors—have been used clinically with various degrees of success (Table 23-14). Receptors are probably the most successful of this group of markers. The catecholamines and their metabolites are discussed in Chapter 29.

ESTROGEN AND PROGESTERONE RECEPTORS

Estrogen and progesterone receptors are used in breast cancer as indicators for hormonal therapy.[250] Patients with positive estrogen and progesterone receptors tend to respond to hormonal treatment. Those with negative receptors will be treated using other therapies, such as chemotherapy.

TABLE 23-14 Other Tumor Markers

Name	Nature	Type of Cancer
Estrogen and progesterone receptors	(Tissue)	Breast
Catecholamine metabolites	(Urine) VMA, HVA, metanephrines	Neuroblastoma, pheochromocytoma
Hydroxyproline	(Urine)	Bone metastasis (breast), multiple myeloma
Lipid-associated sialic acid	Sialic acid bound to lipid	Gastrointestinal, lung, rheumatoid
Polyamine	(CSF)	Brain
	(Urine)	Various

VMA, Vanillylmandelic acid; *HVA*, homovanillic acid; *CSF*, cerebrospinal fluid.

Hormone receptors also serve as prognostic factors in breast cancer. Patients with positive receptor levels tend to survive longer.

Biochemistry

Estrogen receptors (ER) and progesterone receptors (PR) are members of the nuclear steroid hormone receptor family, and are involved in hormone directed transcriptional activation. The general structure of nuclear steroid hormone receptors, including ER and PR, consists of a large N-terminal domain containing transcriptional activation domains, a DNA-binding domain, a hinge region, and the hormone-binding domain at the C-terminus. Both the ER and PR are present in a large protein complex, and upon hormone binding, some members of the complex dissociate and the receptors bind to their respective response elements, and activate transcription.

Estrogen and progesterone each have at least two separate receptors. Estrogen has ERα and ERβ, which are transcribed from separate genes. ERα and ERβ show 96% and 58% homology in their DNA- and hormone-binding domains, respectively, with a more divergent sequence in the N-terminal region.[118] Two forms of PR, PR-A and PR-B, also exist and are both transcribed from the same gene. PR-A lacks the first 165 amino acids of PR-B.

The ERs and PRs are found in target tissue cells, such as in the uterus, pituitary gland, hypothalamus, and breast, and appear to be involved in tumor development and progression. Furthermore, ER and PR status correlate with both prognosis and treatment response, therefore measuring the levels of ER and PR is clinically useful.

Clinical Applications

Measurement of ER levels in breast tumor tissue is useful as both a prognostic indicator and in determining the probability of hormonal therapy. Of patients with carcinoma of the breast, 60% have tumors that are ER positive. ER-positive tumors are 7 to 8 times more likely to respond to endocrine therapy, such as tamoxifen, toremifene, and droloxifene. Furthermore, the U.S. National Cancer Institute Consensus Statement suggests that all breast cancer patients who have positive ER findings should undergo hormonal treatment regardless of their age, menopausal status, nodal status, or tumor size. Ninety-five percent of the patients with ER-negative tumors fail to respond. The greater the ER content of the tumor, the higher the response rate to endocrine therapy. Approximately one third of women with metastatic breast carcinoma obtain an objective remission following various types of endocrine therapy directed at lowering their estrogen levels. Such therapy includes oophorectomy, hypophysectomy, and adrenalectomy (ablative therapy), and administration of antiestrogens and androgens (additive therapy). As a prognostic indicator, ER positivity suggests a better 5-year outcome; however after 5 years, ER-negative tumors have a better prognosis.[59]

Occasionally, a tumor is defined as ER negative, but the patient responds to endocrine therapy (false-negative results yielded in an ER assay). The following are explanations of false-negative results:

1. Incorrect handling and storage of tissue sample that may degrade the thermolabile receptor proteins. During the collection, the specimen must always be kept cold and transported on ice to its storage in a freezer at −70 °C.
2. Inadvertent biopsy of neighboring nonmalignant tissue.
3. Low protein concentration in the assayed sample.
4. High levels of endogenous estrogens that saturate receptor sites and render them undetectable when standard methodology is used.

False-positive results of ER assays (ER-positive tumor but no response to endocrine therapy) are more common than are false-negative results. The most frequent explanation is heterogeneity of tumor with biopsy of a site that is not representative of the other tumor deposits. In addition to this problem, evidence exists that some tumor cells have receptor defects distal to the initial binding step (e.g., variant cells are able to bind steroid in the cytoplasm but not transport the receptor to the nucleus).

In 1996 ERβ was identified as a second ER; it is thought to modulate the activity of ER (now renamed ERα). When bound to hormone, ERα and ERβ signal differently at the activator protein-1 (AP-1) site: ERα activates transcription, and ERβ represses transcription.[161] This ability may have implications as to which isoform of ER is measured, and may affect its prognostic use. Duffy's group reported that the level of ERβ expression between breast carcinoma and breast fibroadenoma tissue was greatly decreased in breast carcinoma tissue, and the expression of ERα was not.[59] They also showed that the routinely used ELISA method for quantitation of ER predominantly detects ERα. The fact that ERβ seems to attenuate ERα signaling coupled with the fact that levels of ERβ are inversely proportional to PR and ERα levels suggests a possible mechanism for ER-positive tumors that do not respond to hormonal treatment.[59]

PR assay is a useful adjunct to the assay of ERs. Because PR synthesis appears to be dependent on estrogen action, measurement of PR activity provides confirmation that all the steps of estrogen action are intact. Indeed, metastatic breast cancer patients with both ER- and PR-positive tumors have a response rate of 75% to endocrine therapy, whereas those with ER-positive and PR-negative tumors have a 40% response rate. In addition, only 25% of ER-negative/PR-positive patients respond to endocrine therapy, whereas fewer than 5% of ER-negative/PR-negative patients respond. The percentage of positive specimens is greater in postmenopausal women than in those who are premenopausal.

Analytical Methodology

Titration assays, enzyme immunoassays,[98,102] and immunocytochemical assays[36,150,187] are used to measure steroid hormone receptors.

The classic quantitative biochemical method for assaying steroid receptors in tumor tissue specimens is the *multiple-point dextran-coated charcoal (DCC) titration* assay. However, in comparison with the classic DCC assays, enzyme immunoassays are preferred as they cost less and are simpler, require less time, and can be performed using less tissue than DCC titration assays.

With immunocytochemical assays, monoclonal antibodies are used to detect steroid receptor proteins in frozen tissue sections, paraffin-imbedded tissue, fine-needle aspirates, and malignant effusions using immunocytochemical techniques. These methods are useful in evaluating very small lesions when adequate tissue is not available for performing the conventional DCC method or when tissues have been fixed or imbedded. In these procedures, the primary monoclonal antibody is incubated with a thin section of tissue mounted on a microscope slide. Localization and visualization of receptor material are subsequently accomplished by an indirect immunoperoxidase technique. Specimens having staining in at least 20% of the malignant cells are usually considered receptor positive. Immunocytochemical assays are not influenced by the presence of estrogens, antiestrogens, or steroid-binding proteins. In addition, immunocytochemical methods make it possible to study receptor content specifically in malignant cells.

Androgen Receptor

Androgens, namely testosterone and dihydrotestosterone (DHT), are involved in growth and maintenance of the prostate gland. Testosterone and DHT exert their effect through the androgen receptor (AR), a classical nuclear steroid hormone receptor. The AR activates the transcription of genes containing androgen response elements, and thereby modulates prostate growth and development. The role of the AR in development and progression of prostate cancer is suggested by the fact that antiandrogen therapy is highly but transiently effective, and anti-androgen therapy can stimulate prostate cancer cells, as seen in antiandrogen withdrawal syndrome.

Two polymorphic repeats have been identified, a CAG and a GGN repeat, that correlate with prostate cancer development. Shorter CAG repeats are associated with greater cancer risk and increased prostate cancer aggressiveness. Also, mutations have been found that cause inappropriate activation of the AR by estrogens, progestins, glucocorticoids, and antiandrogens that promote prostate cancer cell growth, suggesting that these mutations play a role in cancer progression and development of resistant tumors.

Hepatocyte Growth Factor Receptor (c-Met)

The hepatocyte growth factor (HGF) receptor, also known as c-Met, is a proto-oncogene tyrosine kinase receptor predominantly expressed on healthy epithelial cells. The natural ligand for c-Met is hepatocyte growth factor/scatter factor (HGF/SF) and upon activation by its ligand induces a wide array of cellular responses, including proliferation, survival, angiogenesis, wound healing, scattering, motility, invasion, and branching morphogenesis. c-Met was originally identified as a fusion gene between the TRP locus and the c-Met locus in a human osteogenic sarcoma cell line treated with a chemical carcinogen. This fusion produced a constitutively active receptor that activates downstream proliferation, survival, and migration pathways.

The involvement of c-Met in the progression of cancer has been investigated in numerous types of tumors. The overexpression of c-Met in prostate, colorectal, breast, malignant melanoma, hepatocellular, and uterine cervix cancer is associated with increased stage, metastatic potential, and a poor prognosis. Increased mRNA copy number of c-Met in colorectal cancer has been correlated with the depth of invasion.[233] In addition, its increased expression in breast cancer tumors correlates with a shortened survival time and is an independent prognostic marker from HER-2, EGFR, and hormone receptor status.[236] Overall, both inappropriate expression and overexpression of c-Met appear to be involved in metastases and invasion and correlate with a worse clinical outcome. Considering the potential role that c-Met plays in cancer progression and metastases, it is being studied as a potential target for drug therapy by various investigators.

Epidermal Growth Factor Receptor

The epidermal growth factor receptor (EGFR) is a prototype of a family of tyrosine kinase receptors. The natural ligands for the EGFR are epidermal growth factor (EGF) and transforming growth factor (TGF)-α. In cancerous tissue, these growth factors can promote growth both in a paracrine and autocrine fashion. In an analysis of more than 200 studies completed between 1985 and 2000, it was determined that the overexpression of EGFR had prognostic value in a number of cancers.[151] The EGFR was found to be a strong prognostic indicator in head and neck, ovarian, cervical, bladder, and esophageal cancers. Patients with elevated EGFR levels showed reduced overall survival in 70% of studies. In breast, colorectal, gastric, and endometrial cancers, EGFR was found to be a moderate prognostic indicator, with 52% of studies showing reduced survival when elevated levels of EGFR are observed. The fact that EGFR is implicated in the progression of various tumor types, it represents a potential point of intervention and treatment for these cancers. A number of compounds have been developed that inhibit EGFR signaling by blocking ligand binding or inhibition of tyrosine kinase activity.

GENETIC MARKERS

Cancerous growth is an inheritable characteristic of cells and is thought to be the outcome of genetic changes.[214] Multiple genetic alterations may be necessary for the transformation of a cell from a normal state to a cancerous one and, finally, for metastatic spread. Therefore, the evaluation of chromosomal changes may fill the gap left by the traditional serum biochemical markers in establishing cancer risk and screening for cancer (see Chapters 36 and 37).

Two classes of genes are implicated in the development of cancer: oncogenes (cell activation genes—Table 23-14) and suppressor genes (genes involved in the recognition and repair of damaged DNA—Table 23-15).[79,246] *Oncogenes* are derived from proto-oncogenes that may be activated by dominant mutations, such as point mutations, insertions, deletions, translocations, or inversions. Most oncogenes code for proteins that function at some stage of activation of cells for proliferation, and their activation leads to cell division. Most oncogenes are associated with hematological malignancies, such as leukemia and, to a lesser extent, solid tumors. The other class of tumor genes, the *suppressor genes,* has been isolated from mostly solid tumors. The oncogenicity of suppressor genes is derived from the loss of the gene rather than their activation as with oncogenes. Deletion or monosomy may lead to the loss of tumor suppressor genes. The major tumor suppressor gene, p53, functions to repair damaged DNA by apoptosis (programmed cell death). Repair is mediated by activation of the production of p21, which blocks the cell cycle in late G_1 to allow repair to take place.[105] The loss of function of this gene caused by loss or mutation may result in the inability of the DNA repair process and lead to the development of tumorigenesis.

It is expected that the knowledge of the sequence of the Human Genome and the identification of all genes will allow the determination of which genes are differentially or aberrantly expressed in cancer, and the role of mutations or rearrangements of these genes in the development and progression of cancer (see Chapter 39). For example, the identification of single nucleotide polymorphisms and other genetic differences between individuals may allow the development of models for predicting individual predisposition to cancer and the deployment of effective prevention strategies, such as frequent surveillance, chemoprevention, nutritional and lifestyle modification, etc.

ONCOGENES

Proto-oncogenes are normal cellular genes related to tumor virus genes. Activation of proto-oncogenes is found to be associated with cancer. These genes code for products that are involved in normal cellular processes, such as growth factor signaling pathways. Overexpression of the oncogene will lead to abnormal cell growth, resulting in malignancy. Of the more than 40 proto-oncogenes recognized, only a few have been shown to be useful tumor markers[199] (see Table 23-15).

TABLE 23-15 Some Oncogenes Found in Human Tumors

Oncogene	Function	Product	Type of Cancer
N-*ras* mutation	Signal transduction	Guanine diphosphate (GDP)/ guanine triphosphate (GTP) binding protein	Acute myeloid leukemia, neuroblastoma
K-*ras* mutation	Signal transduction	GDP/GTP binding protein	Leukemia, lymphoma
c-*myc* translocation	Transcription regulation	Binds to DNA	B- and T-cell lymphoma, small cell lung carcinoma
c-*erb* B-2 amplification	Growth factor receptor	Tyrosine kinase	Breast, ovarian, gastrointestinal
c-*abl*/*bcr* translocation	Signal transduction	Tyrosine kinase	Chronic myelocytic leukemia
N-*myc* amplification	Transcription regulation	Binds to DNA	Neuroendocrine
bcl-2	Blocks apoptosis	Mitochondrial membrane protein	Leukemia, lymphoma

ras Genes

The *ras* genes were first identified as being responsible for the tumorigenic properties of the Harvey (H-*ras*) and Kirsten (K-*ras*) sarcoma viruses, which produce tumors in animals, and provided the first evidence that cellular counterparts in human cells might be involved in development of human tumors. The proteins coded for by the *ras* genes are located at the inner face of the plasma membrane. They bind to guanine nucleotides and function as molecular switches that regulate mitogenic signals from growth factors to the nucleus via signal transduction pathways.[48] *Ras* proteins are activated in association with protein–tyrosine kinase receptors and are required for growth-factor proliferation or differentiation of a number of cell types.[132] N-*ras* is found on the short arm of human chromosome 1. Changes in N-*ras* appear to be the critical step in carcinogenesis. The mutated N-*ras* gene is found in neuroblastomas and acute myeloid leukemia. Mutated K-*ras* is present in 95% of pancreatic cancers, 40% of colon cancer, and 30% of lung and bladder cancers, and in lower percentages in other tumors.[48] A single point mutation at the twelfth K-*ras* codon changes the coded amino acid from glycine to valine in the p21 protein. This mutation is by far the most frequently found in cancers. K-*ras* mutations appear to correlate with poor prognosis and shorter disease-free survival in patients with adenocarcinoma of the lung and endometrial carcinoma. However, overall, the presence of *ras* mutations has little practical application to determination of prognosis. Activated *ras* is detected by expression of the *ras* gene product, p21, in cancer tissue. By immunohistochemistry, the *ras* product is found not only in about 40% of colon cancers, but also in colon polyps believed to be premalignant. A higher relative intensity of staining for p21-*ras* may discriminate malignant from normal tissues or benign lesions in breast, pancreas, stomach, lung, uterus, or thyroid tissues.[82] The level of expression in tissue appears to correlate with the stage or grade of the tumor, but p21-*ras* may also be seen in some normal tissue, and other studies show no significant difference between benign and malignant tumors. The use of p21 as a tumor marker in tissue or serum is not well established. Mutations of *ras* oncogenes have been detected in the DNA in the stools of 9 of 15 patients with curable colorectal tumors.[204]

c-*myc* Gene

The c-*myc* gene is the proto-oncogene of avian myelocytoma virus. It binds to DNA and is involved in transcription regulation. The gene product, p62, is located in the nucleus of transformed cells, and levels of c-*myc* correlate with the rate of cell division. The c-*myc* protein is essential for DNA replication and enhances mRNA transcription. Activation of the c-*myc* gene is associated with B- and T-cell lymphoma, sarcomas, and endotheliomas.[203] In leukemias and lymphomas, increased c-*myc* expression may be due to amplification or chromosomal translocation of the gene. In acute T-cell leukemias, there is an (8:14) (q24:q11) translocation that results in activation of the gene, and activation of the gene is associated with a poor prognosis. A decrease in expression of c-*myc* after initiation of chemotherapy suggests a favorable response. Overexpression of p62 may be seen in 70% to 100% of primary breast cancers using immunohistochemistry, and the intensity of staining is greater with the increasing stage of the tumor. Amplification in lung carcinomas and gliomas correlates with clinical aggressiveness. There may be a fivefold to fortyfold higher expression of c-*myc* in colon cancers when compared with normal mucosa, but the level of expression does not correlate with progression. A similar relationship has been found for cervical, gastric, liver, and other cancers. Serum levels of c-*myc* have been used to detect recurrence but not to differentiate cancer and benign conditions.

Her-2/*neu*

The HER-2/*neu* gene (also known as c-erbB-2) is named for its association with neural tumors (*neu*).

Biochemistry

The HER-2/*neu* gene is a 185 kDa transmembrane protein expressed on epithelial cells, and belongs to the EGF family of tyrosine kinase receptors. The EGF family includes four members, the EGF receptor (EGFR; also known as ErbB1/HER-1), ErbB2/HER-2/*neu*, Erb3/HER-3, and ErbB4/HER-4. The EGF family of receptors have the same overall structure consisting of an extracellular ligand-binding domain (ECD), a single transmembrane domain, and an intracellular tyrosine kinase domain. The extracellular domain can undergo proteolytic cleavage by metalloproteases, releasing the ECD (known as p105) into the blood, which can be detected. All are involved in cell proliferation, differentiation, and survival. HER-2/*neu* is normally expressed on the epithelia of numerous organs, including lung, bladder, pancreas, breast, and prostate, and has been found to be elevated in cancer cells.

Clinical Applications

Amplification of HER-2/*neu* is found in breast, ovarian, and gastrointestinal tumors. In breast cancer, it appears to be as useful a prognostic indicator of overall survival as tumor size or ER and PR expression, but not as good as the number of lymph nodes involved in metastases.[210] Elevated serum HER-2/*neu* antigen levels have been shown to correlate with decreased response to hormone therapy of breast cancer.[122] Of the three oncogenes—HER-2/*neu, ras,* and c-*myc*—HER-2/*neu* has the strongest prognostic value in breast cancer.

Serum levels of p105 are most useful in breast cancer with some use in ovarian cancer patients.[59,133] p105 levels in breast cancer correlate with a worse prognosis and a shorter disease-free state. Elevated HER-2/*neu* levels also correlate with larger tumor size, lymph node positivity, and high grading score. HER-2/*neu* serum levels are not only to be used for prognosis, but may be used to guide treatment. One study of 719 breast cancer patients showed that elevated levels of

HER-2/*neu* in patients with ER-positive cancers showed significantly worse clinical benefit from hormonal therapies.[128] Furthermore, the study showed a trend toward improved outcome with aromatase inhibitors for patients with elevated serum HER-2/*neu*. Serum levels of HER-2/*neu* are also useful in monitoring breast cancer patients because the HER-2/*neu* levels decrease in response to treatment. Herceptin treatment is now administered only to those breast cancer patients who have HER-2/*neu* amplification.

In ovarian cancer, elevated p105 correlates with increased aggressiveness of the tumor, more advanced clinical stage, and poor clinical outcome. HER-2/*neu* is not useful in combination with CA 125 or alone in distinguishing between benign and malignant ovarian tumors, but it may be useful in identifying a subset of high-risk patients.[59]

Analytical Methodology

Immunohistochemistry has been used to detect increased levels of the HER-2/*neu* protein in cancer cells.[59] FISH has been used for detection of HER-2/*neu* gene amplification. Immunohistochemistry is a relatively simple procedure and can be done in most labs, but suffers from interanalyst variation. FISH is less analyst dependent, but only detects increases in gene copy number. Detection of the ECD of HER-2/*neu* (p105) in serum is by ELISA and automated immunoassay. Both assays use the same monoclonal antibodies recognizing different epitopes of the ECD, which does not cross-react with any other member of the EGF family. Importantly, there is no interference from the therapeutic monoclonal antibody, Herceptin, with either assay.[133] The ELISA has a lower detection limit of 3.4 ng/mL and an upper limit of 36 ng/mL, and the automated immunoassay has a linear range from 0.1 to 250 ng/mL. The upper limit of normal for both assays has been set at 15 ng/mL.

bcl-2

The product of the *bcl*-2 oncogene is a novel 239 amino acid, 25 kDa integral membrane protein that localizes primarily to the mitochondrial membranes and to other cellular membranes. This protein is known to inhibit apoptosis (programmed cell death) and contribute to survival of cancer cells, especially lymphoma and leukemic cells.[140] The *bcl*-2 proto-oncogene was identified in follicular lymphomas wherein a 14:18 translocation results in formation of a *bcl*-2-immunoglobulin heavy-chain fusion gene. Activation of the *bcl*-2 gene through the immunoglobulin promoter results in production of high levels of *bcl*-2 protein. The protein is normally expressed on cells that have a long life span (e.g., neurons) and on the proliferative cells in rapidly renewing cell lineages, such as basal epithelial cells. The *bcl*-2 oncogene is highly expressed in a variety of hematological malignancies, including lymphomas, myelomas, and chronic leukemias (malignancies characterized by prolonged cell survival). In the normal colon, *bcl*-2 positive cells are restricted to basal epithelial cells, whereas in dysplastic polyps and carcinomas, many positive cells may be found in parabasal and superficial regions.[208,214] Abnormal expression of the *bcl*-2 gene appears to be an early event in colorectal carcinogenesis. In addition, overexpression of the *bcl*-2 gene is associated with development of resistance to cytotoxic cancer chemotherapy in a variety of tumors, including epithelial tumors and lymphomas. Thus detection of the *bcl*-2-gene product in tumors is an indication of progression. Future studies may determine its usefulness for predicting resistance to chemotherapy.

BCR-ABL

Chronic myelogenous leukemia (CML) is a myeloproliferative disorder resulting from the clonal expansion of a transformed multipotent hematopoietic stem cell. In approximately 90% of CML patients, the transforming event is the formation of the Philadelphia chromosome, a balanced translocation between chromosomes 9 and 22 [t(9;22)(q34;q11)] creating the BCR-ABL fusion gene. The protein derived from this fusion is a constitutively active cytoplasmic tyrosine kinase that activates a number of signaling pathways leading to growth and inhibition of apoptosis.

Detection of the BCR-ABL is useful in diagnosis of CML and in directing treatment, since there are a number of strategies that target either the BCR-ABL gene by antisense oligonucleotides or the BCR-ABL kinase domain by the tyrosine kinase inhibitor STI571. BCR-ABL detection, by RT-PCR, is also useful in monitoring minimal residual disease in patients who have undergone bone marrow transplantation. In the subset of acute lymphoblastic leukemia patients that harbor the Philadelphia chromosome, a positive RT-PCR for the BCR-ABL gene carries a much higher risk of relapse compared with a negative result. In CML patients after bone marrow transplantation, positive RT-PCR results at 6 to 12 months were associated with a twenty-sixfold elevated risk of relapse, and a positive result at 3 months was not predictive of risk.[177] Also, the amount of BCR-ABL transcript per μg of RNA correlated with risk of relapse; less than 1% of patients with a decreasing level of BCR-ABL mRNA or less than 50 transcripts per μg of RNA relapsed, and 72% of patients with greater than 50 transcripts per μg of RNA relapsed.[127]

RET

The RET tyrosine kinase receptor is involved in kidney morphogenesis, maturation of the peripheral nervous system, and differentiation of spermatogonia. The RET receptor exists in a multimeric complex that includes one of four glycosyl-phosphatidylinositol (GPI)-linked co-receptors (GFRα 1, 2, 3, and 4). The complex responds to four ligands: glial-derived neurotrophic factor (GDNF), neurturin (NTN), persephin (PSP), and artemin. Activation of RET appears to be through dimerization and transphosphorylation of the receptor that recruits numerous signaling molecules. RET, like other tyrosine kinase receptors, activates

TABLE 23-16 Tumor Suppressor Genes: Chromosomal Location and Tumor Types

Chromosome Region	Tumor Type	Gene
3p	Kidney	VHL mutation
5q21	Colorectal	APC mutation
9p21	Bladder, glioblastoma, melanoma	p16 (cdkn2) mutation
11p13	Wilms tumor	*WT1* mutation
11p15	Wilms, breast, hepatoblastoma, rhabdomyosarcoma, bladder	Loss of heterozygosity
13q	Breast	*BRCA2*, RB1
13q14	Retinoblastoma, osteosarcoma, small cell lung	RB1 mutation
16q	Breast	P16 E-cadherin mutation
17q	Neurofibromatosis 1, melanoma, breast	*BRCA1* mutation
17p13	Breast, colorectal, lung, liver, renal cell, bladder, sarcomas	p53 mutation
18q21	Colorectal	DCC mutation
22q	Neurofibromatosis 2, meningioma	NF2 mutation

Other genes indicated by loss of heterozygosity include 1p, 8p, 9q, 10q, and others.

downstream growth pathways, and with uncontrolled signaling cancer can result.

Inappropriate activation of RET has been extensively studied in (1) papillary thyroid cancer, (2) multiple endocrine neoplasia type 2 (MEN2), and (3) familial medullary thyroid carcinoma (FMTC). In each the mechanism of activation of RET is through unregulated dimerization and transphosphorylation of the RET receptor.[4] In the case of papillary thyroid cancer a genetic event creates a fusion between the RET tyrosine kinase domain and a dimerization domain that can be donated by a number of genes. In MEN2A and FMTC point mutations of the extracellular domain induce disulfide linkages between receptors, thus inducing dimerization. In MEN2B, a point mutation in the kinase domain appears to alter the substrate specificity of the tyrosine kinase and presumably leads to inappropriate activation of downstream growth pathways.

Tumor Suppressor Genes

Several suppressor genes associated with human cancer are listed in Table 23-16. Historically, evidence for tumor suppressor genes was derived from the study of hybrid cells of normal and malignant cells that behaved normally.[91,223] It was concluded that normal cells contained a gene that suppressed the expression of malignancy.[92] Reversion to malignancy occurred when the cultured cells lost normal chromosomes. The study of suppressor genes may provide a clue as to the development of cancer from normal cell status to benign and cancerous status and to metastasis. The development of colon cancer requires multiple steps that involve several mutations. The loss of a chromosome 5 gene leads to an increase in cell growth. Early adenoma is associated with the loss of methyl groups on the DNA strand. With the *ras* gene mutation and the loss of the DCC gene on chromosome 18, adenoma advances to the late stage. Carcinoma is found with the loss of the p53 gene on chromosome 17. Finally, metastasis occurs with other chromosome losses.[66] The clinical usefulness of detection of mutations in tumor suppressor genes lies not only in the diagnosis and prognosis of cancer, but also in the prediction of susceptibility when the mutation is carried in the germline, such as with the breast cancer genes *BRCA1* and *BRCA2*.

Retinoblastoma Gene

Retinoblastoma (RB) is a rare tumor of children that occurs both in families and sporadically. The work of Knudson on the familial-specific incidence of RB led to the two-hit hypothesis.[114,115] He reasoned that in the inherited form of the tumor, one mutation was present in the germline and all cells of the body, the other mutational event occurring somatically in one of the cells of the developing retina. In the sporadic form, both mutations occur somatically in the same developing retinoblast, a relatively rare event. The two-hit hypothesis has served as a model for other tumor suppressor genes. The RB gene has been localized to chromosome 13q by loss of a chromosomal banding region in peripheral blood lymphocytes of patients with the familial form and by loss of heterozygosity studies in both RBs and some osteosarcomas. However, most tumors do not have gross deletions but point mutations or small insertions and deletions that result in premature truncation of the protein product.[79] The protein product of the RB gene is a nuclear phosphoprotein with a molecular mass of about 105 kDa (p105-RB).[121] This protein binds to a product of a DNA tumor virus, including the E1A protein of murine tumor virus and the E7 protein of human papillomavirus. When p105-RB is hypophosphorylated, it complexes with transcription factors such as E2F and blocks transcription of genes in S-phase cells. E2F dimerizes with a DP protein and regulates the transcription of several genes involved in DNA synthesis. Inactivation or loss of p105-RB deregulates DNA syntheses and increases cellular proliferation. Thus RB is a tumor suppressor gene, as it suppresses DNA synthesis. Detection of mutations in RB is useful in determining the susceptibility of an individual to development of RB in the familial form, but it is not used as a tumor marker.

p53 Gene

Of particular interest is the p53 gene[106,138] that lies on chromosome 17q. The native or wild type of p53 is believed to control cell division by regulating entry into the S phase.[105] This controlling effect of p53 protein may be lost by deletion of the gene or production of a competing mutant protein. Seventy-five percent to eighty percent of colon carcinomas show deletion in one p53 allele and a point mutation in the other allele; thus, no wild type of p53 protein is expressed in these tumors. Allelic deletion of p53 occurs only rarely in adenomas (10%), suggesting that p53 inactivation may be a relatively late event in colon carcinogenesis. In addition, up to 70% of breast cancers also have deleted p53. Mutations in p53 produce proteins that inactivate the wild type of p53 protein and allow cells to move through the cell cycle and contribute to the autonomous growth of cancer. A number of different mutations of p53 have been found in human cancers.[124] Most point mutations are localized in four regions of the protein (amino acid residues 117-142, 171-181, 134-158, and 270-286); three "hot spots" affect residues 175, 248, and 273.[124] In addition, selective guanine to thymine mutations are found at codon 249 in human hepatocellular carcinomas taken from patients in high-incidence areas of Africa and Asia[160] associated with aflatoxin exposure. Mutations at codons 245 and 258 are found in Li-Fraumeni syndrome, a rare autosomal dominant syndrome characterized by diverse neoplasms at many different sites in the body.[220]

Monoclonal antibodies to mutated p53 proteins have been developed. The wild type of p53 is normally present in very small amounts that are not detected by immunohistochemistry, whereas the mutant protein accumulates to easily detectable levels. Overexpression of the mutant proteins has been detected in up to 70% of primary colorectal cancers. Overexpression of p53 in breast cancers is associated with poor prognosis, but this association is not as strong as the association with c-*erb*B-2.[153] Up to 75% of small cell lung carcinomas appear to overexpress a mutant (missense mutation) protein. Finally, circulating antibodies to mutant p53 proteins have been found in sera from patients with breast and lung cancer and B-cell lymphomas. This antibody response may be useful in this subset of patients for monitoring for relapse.[138]

p21 *(WAF1)*

The wild type of p53 protein activates transcription of a number of genes, including the *WAF1/CIP1* gene. The p21 protein product of the p21^{WAF1} gene binds to and inhibits the cyclin-dependent protein kinases (cdk) that are active in the G_1 phase of the cell cycle. The cell-cycle arrest function of p53 in response to DNA damage is mediated by p21. Monoclonal antibodies to the p21 protein are now available and are being used to determine if expression of p21 in tumors may be clinically useful.

APC

One of the first events in the putative steps of progression of precursor lesions to colon cancer is loss of the adenomatous polyposis coli (APC) gene in premalignant polyps.[66] The APC gene encodes a 300-kDa protein that may be truncated in cancer cells. The normal function of the APC gene product is not known, but it interacts with proteins, such as α- and β-catenin, involved in cell-cell interactions in epithelial cells. This gene is mutated in hereditary colorectal cancer syndromes, polyposis, and nonpolyposis types. In the polyposis types, hundreds and even thousands or more benign tumors (polyps) arise before the development of cancer. In the nonpolyposis types, very few polyps are seen, but the elevated risk of cancer is essentially similar. The APC gene was detected by an interstitial deletion on chromosome 5q in a patient with hundreds of polyps.[123] Greater than 80% of individuals with hereditary colorectal cancer have germline mutations in one of the APC alleles, including gross deletions or localized mutations. The hereditary forms of colorectal cancer are relatively uncommon, but somatic mutations appear to be of great importance in the development of nonhereditary colorectal cancers. More than 70% of colorectal tumors, regardless of size or histology, have a specific mutation in one of the two APC alleles, and mutation may also be found in other types of tumors, including breast, esophageal, and brain tumors. The usefulness of the loss of the APC protein for diagnosis and prognosis is now under study.

Neurofibromatosis Type 1

Neurofibromatosis type 1 (NF1), or von Recklinghausen disease, is a dominantly inherited syndrome manifested mainly by proliferation of cells from the neural crest resulting in multiple neurofibromas, cafe au lait spots, and Lisch nodules of the iris.[200] Mutations in the *NF1* gene have been found in about 20% of NF1 patients.[243] The *NF1* gene has been localized to the pericentromeric region of chromosome 17q, band 11. It is a large gene coding for a p300 protein, called neurofibromin. This protein has a high degree of similarity to GTPase-activating proteins.[249] Although the exact mechanism of action of the protein is not known, it appears likely that loss or inactivation of neurofibromin function leads to alterations in signal transduction pathways regulated by small *ras*-like G proteins resulting in continuous "on" signals for cell activation. Inactivating mutations of *NF1* have also been found in colorectal cancer, melanoma, and neuroblastoma.

WT1

The Wilms tumor suppressor gene, *WT1*, is located on chromosome 11p13. It codes for a 45-kDa protein that appears to function in transcriptional regulation by suppressing the expression of growth-inducing genes, such as early growth response, insulin-like growth factor-2, and platelet-derived growth factor A chain genes.[84] Other chromosomal changes in Wilms tumors indicate that mutations of *WT1* may be only one step in the process of carcinogenesis. Thus identification and understanding of one tumor suppressor gene in a given cancer may only provide a part of the information eventually required to understand the carcinogenic process.

nm23

The nm23 gene was found overexpressed in a nonmetastatic murine melanoma cell line but present in low levels in a highly metastatic cell line. The nm23 gene product appears to be elevated in metastatic breast, colon, and prostatic cancer and is now being evaluated as a new marker for metastases.[75]

BRCA1 and *BRCA2*

A subset of breast cancer patients have been shown to have an inherited predisposition to developing breast and ovarian cancer that is inherited as an autosomal dominant trait.[111] Two genetic loci have been identified: *BRCA1* on chromosome 17q and *BRCA2,* which localizes to 13q12-13.[144,251] *BRCA1* encodes for an 1863 amino acid protein that may act as a transcription factor. The ability to detect mutations in *BRCA1* and *BRCA2* in somatic cells permits the identification of individuals in breast cancer families who carry the mutated gene. It is estimated that as many as 1 in 200 women in the United States may have a germline mutation in the *BRCA1* gene. This has created an ethical dilemma for physicians, patients and their families, and insurance companies and health maintenance organizations as it is now possible to predict with reasonable certainty that an individual who carries a mutation in one of these genes will develop breast and/or ovarian cancer. What should be done if an otherwise healthy individual is shown to carry a *BRCA* gene mutation? Carriers of a *BRCA1* gene mutation have an 85% risk of developing breast cancer and a 45% risk of developing ovarian cancer by the age of 85.[74] Should such patients have preventive mastectomy or ovariectomy? Should insurance companies and health care maintenance organizations have higher rates for carriers? It has always been a goal of cancer research to be able to identify individuals at risk. Now that this is possible, we must develop a policy of how to deal with the information (e.g., see Harper[91] or Petty and Killeen[174]). Although detection of the mutation is not useful as a tumor marker per se, with further understanding of how the mutated gene products act, it may be possible to understand the molecular events for development of some breast and ovarian cancers.

Deleted in Colorectal Carcinoma

The deleted in colorectal carcinoma (DCC) gene encodes for a membrane protein of the immunoglobulin superfamily. The exact function of DCC has yet to be elucidated. However, studies have suggested a role in axonal development as a component of the Netrin-1 receptor, and others have suggested a role in promoting apoptosis.[81] In colon cancer, DCC is thought to act as a tumor suppressor, thus, deletion or reduced expression correlates with increasing stage and a poorer prognosis.[154] Conversely, loss of DCC expression in gastric cancer was associated with a better prognosis and higher tumor cell differentiation.[154] More work is necessary to determine the exact role of DCC in both colon cancer and other gastric cancers.

PTEN

The PTEN tumor suppressor gene is mutated in numerous cancers, and is probably underestimated in its importance in tumor formation and progression.[231] PTEN functions as a phosphatase that negatively regulates phosphoinositide 3-kinase (PI 3-K) signaling by dephosphorylating the D3 position of phosphatidylinositol (3,4,5)-triphosphate [PtdIns(3,4,5)P_3]. PI 3-kinase and its product PtdIns(3,4,5)P_3 are involved in activation of signaling pathways leading to inhibition of apoptosis, cell migration, cell size, and chemotaxis. Mutation or inactivation of PTEN allows uncontrolled activation of the downstream pathways, which contribute to tumorigenesis.

Germline mutations in PTEN cause the (1) Cowden, (2) Lhermitte-Duclos, (3) Bannayan-Zonana, and (4) Proteus autosomal-dominant syndromes that are all characterized by development of hamartomas and an increased likelihood of tumor development along with other growth-related symptoms. In general, PTEN mutation and/or loss of expression is associated with a more advanced stage, and is a poor prognostic indicator in various cancers, including breast, hepatocellular, endometrial, and cervical.

Single Nucleotide Polymorphisms

Two of the goals of the Human Genome Project are to identify all the approximate 30,000 genes in human DNA and determine the sequences of the 3 billion chemical base pairs that make up human DNA. A by-product of the sequencing effort was the identification of a very large number of single nucleotide polymorphisms (SNPs, single nucleotides that differ between individuals, and these differences are inherited). It has been estimated that one SNP can be found every approximately 1000 bases of genomic sequence. Most of these SNPs are present in introns and only a relatively small number (approximately 60,000 out of the 2,000,000 SNPs) are within exons. It was also identified that groups of SNPs (called haplotypes) are inherited together in a block. It has been hypothesized that it may be possible to correlate SNP composition (e.g., various haplotypes) with disease predisposition. Until now, very few SNPs or haplotypes have been associated consistently with human cancers. Many scientists are currently investigating SNPs and are attempting to correlate them with various diseases. Large numbers of SNPs can now be identified by using either microarrays or mass spectroscopy. The hope is to identify characteristic SNPs or haplotypes that can be used for diagnostic purposes or for determining future risk (predisposition) for developing certain diseases.

MISCELLANEOUS MARKERS

Markers of Angiogenesis

Angiogenesis, the formation of blood vessels, is a highly regulated and ordered process; however in tumor tissue, this process is rather disordered. The development of tumors is thought to involve the inactivation of tumor suppressor genes and/or the uncontrolled activation of oncogenes. Subsequently, another step in the progression toward malignancy has been identified and has been referred to as the "angiogenic switch."[19,32] The first phase of tumor development is an avascular phase, with a lesion size of 1 to 2 mm. At this point the tumor is in a vascular steady state. The vascular state occurs next where there is rapid and unregulated angiogenesis. The architecture of the newly developing vasculature is very distinct from that of normal vasculature. It is irregularly shaped, dilated and can have dead ends, with irregular blood flow patterns, that makes tumors relatively easy to identify histologically. In normal tissue, there is a balance between proangiogenic signals (VEGF, FGF, PDGFB, EGF, Ets-1, and LPA) and antiangiogenic signals (thrombospondin-1, angiostatin, endostatin, canstatin, and tumstatin). It is believed that in tumors there is an increase in proangiogenic signals. Therefore the measurement of proangiogenic markers may provide prognostic information related to tumor status.

Increases in blood vascular endothelial growth factor (VEGF) and soluble Tie-2 receptor (sTie2) both correlate with the development of metastases, with VEGF being the most powerful predictor of outcome.[45] Ets-1, a transcription factor that activates a number of angiogenic genes, also may serve as a prognostic indicator of uterine cervical cancers. Thrombospondin-1 (TSP-1), an antiangiogenic marker, has been found to be a positive prognostic marker in ductal carcinoma of the breast. Other markers of angiogenesis are being considered as prognostic markers in cancer have been reviewed.[19]

Cell-Free Nucleic Acids

Circulating DNA and RNA has been recognized since the 1970s, but it was not until the late 1980s that the neoplastic characteristics of the DNA were recognized.[103] Circulating DNA and RNA have been proposed as a marker for certain types of cancer. To use circulating DNA as a cancer marker, there must be a mechanism to differentiate normal DNA from neoplastic DNA. This is achieved by detecting mutations in the circulating DNA that are present in the cancer cells (e.g., *ras* mutations that occur in various cancers), by microsatellite analysis of the circulating DNA, or by detection of common cancer-causing chromosomal translocations. Epigenetic alterations of circulating DNA, such as altered methylation patterns, can also be detected. Although this technology is relatively new, over the next decade detection of circulating DNA will join a growing number of clinically useful markers; however a number of questions must still be answered, such as the source of cell-free DNA, and what forms of the DNA and RNA exist. In the future this technology may have the ability to provide a more global picture of the abnormalities present in the patient.

Circulating Cancer Cells

Circulating cancer cells may indicate the presence of cancer (for diagnostic purposes) or cancer dissemination (for prognosis and monitoring therapy). It is generally very difficult to detect rare cancer cells in the circulation. However, the advent of the PCR and the identification of genes that are specifically expressed in certain tissue (normal and cancerous) have allowed for the highly sensitive detection of cancer cells in the circulation.[148,149] Others have used flow-cytometric technology with magnetic separation of cancer cells to achieve the same goal.[235]

Currently, this technology is still under evaluation. However, it is well established that patients with more advanced cancer are more frequently positive for circulating cancer cells and the amount of cancer cells has prognostic significance. PSA and prostate-specific membrane antigen have been used successfully for detection of prostatic cancer cells in the circulation. Zehentner et al. used mammoglobin and other related genes for breast cancer.[259] Despite many limitations of this technology (mainly sample preparation variability and quantification), it may be feasible in the future to identify very rare cancer cells in the circulation for the purpose of diagnosis, prognosis, and monitoring of therapy.[258]

REFERENCES

1. Aaronson SA. Growth factors and cancer. Science 1991;254:1146-53.
2. Abelev GI, Perova SD, Khramkova NI, et al. Production of embryonal α-globulins by transplantable mouse hepatomas. Transplantation 1963;1:174-8.
3. Adam B-L, Qu Y, Davies JW, et al. Serum protein fingerprinting coupled with a pattern-matching algorithm distinguishes prostate cancer from benign prostate hyperplasia and healthy men. Cancer Res 2002;62:3609-14.
4. Alberti L, Carniti C, Miranda C, et al. RET and NTRK1 proto-oncogenes in human diseases. J Cell Physiol 2003;195:168-86.
5. Andreasen PA, Kjoller L, Christensen L, et al. The Urokinase-type plasminogen activator system in cancer metastasis: a review. Int J Cancer 1997;72: 1-22.
6. Andriole GL, Catalona WJ. The diagnosis and treatment of prostate cancer. Ann Rev Med 1991;42: 9-15.
7. Angelopoulou K, Diamandis EP, Sutherland DJ, et al. Prevalence of serum antibodies against the p53

tumor suppressor gene protein in various cancers. Int J Cancer 1994;58:480-87.

8. Angelopoulou K, Rosen B, Stratis M, et al. Circulating antibodies against p53 protein in patients with ovarian carcinoma. Correlation with clinico-pathologic features and survival. Cancer 1996;78: 146-52.
9. Angelopoulou K, Stratis M, Diamandis EP. Humoral immune response against p53 protein in patients with colorectal carcinoma. Int J Cancer 1997; 70:46-51.
10. Arias E, Smith BL. Deaths: Preliminary data for 2001. Natl Vital Stat Rep 2003;51:1-48.
11. Austin LA, Heath H. Calcitonin. Physiology and pathophysiology. NEJM 1981;304:269-78.
12. Babaian RJ, Fritsche HA, Zhang Z, et al. Evaluation of ProstAsure index in the detection of prostate cancer: a preliminary report. Urology 1998;51:132-36.
13. Bartlett NL, Freiha FS, Torti FM. Serum markers in germ cell neoplasms. Hematol Oncol Clin North Am 1991;5:1245-60.
14. Bates SE. Clinical applications of serum tumor markers. Ann Intern Med 1991;115:623-38.
15. Bates SE, Longo DL. Use of serum tumor markers in cancer diagnosis and management. Semin Oncol 1987;14:102-38.
16. Belanger A, van Halbeek H, Graves HDB, et al. Molecular mass and carbohydrate structure of prostate specific antigen: Studies for establishment of an international PSA standard. Prostate 1995;27: 187-97.
17. Bence-Jones H. Papers on chemical pathology. Lecture III. Lancet 1847;ii:269-72.
18. Benson MC, Whang IS, Pantuck A, et al. Prostate specific antigen density: A means of distinguishing benign prostatic hypertrophy and prostate cancer. J Urol 1992;147:815-16.
19. Bergers G, Benjamin LE. Tumorigenesis and the angiogenic switch Nat. Rev Cancer 2002;3:401-10.
20. Berkowitz RS, Goldstein DP. Gestational trophoblastic disease. In: Mossa AR, Schimpff SC, Robson MC, eds. Comprehensive textbook of oncology. Baltimore: Williams & Wilkins, 1991:1046-51.
21. Bernini GP, Moretti A, Ferdeghini M, et al. A new human chromogranin "A" immunoradiometric assay for the diagnosis of neuroendocrine tumours. Br J Cancer 2001;84:636-42.
22. Bjorklund B, Bjorklund V. Antigenicity of pooled human malignant and normal tissues by cyto-immunologic techniques: Presence of an insoluble heat labile tumor antigen. Arch Allergy 1957;10: 153-84.
23. Black MH, Diamandis EP. The diagnostic and prognostic utility of prostate-specific antigen for diseases of the breast. Breast Cancer Res Treat 2000;59:1-14.
24. Black MH, Giai M, Ponzone R, et al. Serum total and free prostate-specific antigen for breast cancer diagnosis in women. Clin Cancer Res 2000;6:467-73.
25. Bombardieri E, Gion M. Mucin-like cancer associated antigen (MCA) as available circulating tumor marker for breast cancer. In: Sell S, ed. Serological cancer markers. Totowa NJ: Humana Press, 1992:341-54.
26. Bonfrer JMG. Working group on tumor marker criteria (WGTMC). Tumour Biol 1990:11:287-88.
27. Bray KR, Koda JE, Gaur PK. Serum levels and biochemical characteristics of cancer associated antigen (CA) 549, a circulating breast cancer marker. Cancer Res 1987;47:5853-60.
28. Brown WH. A case of pluriglandular syndrome. Lancet 1928;ii:1022-24.
29. Buccheri G, Ferrigno D. Lung tumor markers of cytokeratin origin: an overview. Lung Cancer 2001;34:S65-S69.
30. Bunting PS. Is there still a role for prostatic acid phosphatase? CSCC Position Statement. Canadian Society of Clinical Chemists. Clin Biochem 1999;32:591-94.
31. Cancer Facts and Figures 2004. American Cancer Society, 2004:1-60.
32. Carmeliet P. Angiogenesis in health and disease. Nat Med 2003;9:653-60.
33. Carter HB, Pearson JD, Metter EJ, et al. Longitudinal evaluation of prostate specific antigen levels in men with and without prostate disease. JAMA 1992;267:2215-20.
34. Catalona WJ, Partin AW, Slawin KM, et al. Use of the percentage of free prostate-specific antigen to enhance differentiation of prostate cancer from benign prostatic disease: a prospective multicenter clinical trial. JAMA 1998;297:1542-47.
35. Catalona WJ, Smith DS, Ratliff TL, et al. Measurement of prostate specific antigen in serum as a screening test for prostate cancer. N Engl J Med 1991;324:1156-61.
36. Cavaliere A, Bucciarelli E, Sidoni A, Bianchi G, Pietropaoli N, et al. Estrogen and progesterone receptors in breast cancer: Comparison between enzyme immunoassay and computer-assisted image analysis of immunocytochemical assay. Cytometry 1996;26:204-08.
37. Chan DW, Beveridge RA, Bhargava A, et al. Breast cancer marker CA549: A multicenter study. AJCP 1994;101:465-70.
38. Chan DW, Beveridge RA, Bruzek DJ, et al. Monitoring breast cancer with CA 549. Clin Chem 1988;34:2000-04.
39. Chan DW, Beveridge RA, Muss H, et al. Use of TRUQUANT BR RIA for early detection of breast cancer recurrence in patients with stage II and stage III disease. J Clin Oncol 1997;15:2322-28.
40. Chan DW, Bruzek DJ, Oesterling JE, et al. Prostatic-specific antigen as a marker for prostatic cancer:

A monoclonal and a polyclonal immunoassay compared. Clin Chem 1987;33:1916-20.
41. Chan DW, Kelsten M, Rock R, Bruzek D. Evaluation of a monoclonal immunoenzymometric assay for alpha-fetoprotein. Clin Chem 1986;32:1318-22.
42. Chan DW, Maio YC. Affinity chromatographic separation of alpha-fetoprotein variants: Development of a minicolumn procedure and application to cancer patients. Clin Chem 1986;32:2143-46.
43. Chan DW, Sokoll LJ. Prostate-specific antigen: Advances and challenges. (Editorial). Clin Chem 1999;45:755-56.
44. Chan DW, Sokoll LJ. WHO first international standards for prostate-specific antigen: The beginning of the end for assay discrepancies? (Editorial). Clin Chem 2000;46:1291-92.
45. Chin KF, Greenman J, Reusch P, et al. Vascular endothelial growth factor and soluble Tie-2 receptor in colorectal cancer: associations with disease recurrence. Eur J Surg Oncol 2003;29:497-505.
46. Chu TM. Prostate Specific Antigen. In: Sell S, ed. Serological cancer markers. Totowa NJ: Humana Press, 1992:99-115.
47. Chybrowski FM, Keller JJL, Bergstralh EJ, Oesterling JE. Predicting radionuclide bone scan findings in patients with newly diagnosed. Untreated prostate cancer: Prostate specific antigen is superior to all other clinical parameters. J Urol 1991;145: 313-18.
48. Clark GJ, Der CJ. Ras proto-oncogene activation in human malignancy. In: Garret G, Sell S, eds. Cellular cancer markers. Totowa NJ: Humana Press, 1995: 17-52.
49. Correale M, Abbate I, Gargano G, et al. Analytical and clinical evaluation of a new tumor marker in breast cancer: CA 27.29. Int J Biol Markers 1992;7: 43-46.
50. Darson MF, Pacelli A, Roche P, et al. Human glandular kallikrein 2 expression in prostate adenocarcinoma and lymph node metastases. Urology 1999; 53:939.
51. Dayhoff JE, DeLeo JM. Artificial neural networks: opening the black box. Cancer 2001;91:1615-35.
52. De Bie SH, Ferreira TC, Pauwels EKJ, Cleton FJ. Immunoscintigraphy for cancer detection: "A thousand ills require a thousand cures." J Cancer Res Clin Oncol 1992;118:1-15.
53. Diamandis EP. Clinical application of ultrasensitive prostate-specific antigen assays. J Natl Cancer Inst 1997;89:1077-78.
54. Diamandis EP. Prostate-specific antigen: Its usefulness in clinical medicine. Trends Endocrinol Metal 1998; 8:310-16.
55. Diamandis EP. Prostate-specific antigen: a cancer fighter and a valuable messenger? Clin Chem 2000; 46:896-900.
56. Diamandis EP. Proteomic patterns in serum and identification of ovarian cancer. Lancet 2002; 360:170.
57. Diamandis EP. Proteomic patterns in biological fluids: Do they represent the future of cancer diagnostics? Clin Chem 2003;49:1271-78.
58. Diamandis EP. Serum proteomic patterns for detection of prostate cancer. J Natl Cancer Inst 2003; 95:489-90.
59. Diamandis EP, Fritsche HA, Lilja H, Chan DW, Schwartz MK, eds. Tumor markers: Physiology, pathobiology, technology and clinical applications. Washington DC: AACC Press, 2002.
60. Diamandis EP, Scorilas A, Fracchioli S, et al. Human kallikrein 6 (hK6): a new potential serum biomarker for diagnosis and prognosis of ovarian carcinoma. J Clin Oncol 2003;21:1035-43.
61. Diamandis EP, Yousef GM. Human tissue kallikreins: a family of new cancer biomarkers. Clin Chem 2002; 48:1198-205.
62. Duffy MJ, Maguire TM, McDermott EW, et al. Urokinase plasminogen activator: a prognostic marker in multiple types of cancer. J Surg Oncol 1999;1:130-35.
63. Duggan C, Maguire T, McDermott E, et al. Urokinase plasminogen activator and urokinase plasminogen activator receptor in breast cancer. Int J Cancer 1995; 29:597-600.
64. Einhorn N, Bast RC Jr, Knapp RC, et al. Preoperative evaluation of serum CA 125 levels in patients with primary epithelial ovarian cancer. Obstet Gynecol 1986;67:414-16.
65. Eissa S, Swellam M, Sadek M, et al. Comparative evaluation of the nuclear matrix protein, fibronectin, urinary bladder cancer antigen and voided urine cytology in the detection of bladder tumors. J Urol 2002;168:465-69.
66. Fearon ER, Vogelstein B. A genetic model for colorectal tumorigenesis. Cell 1990;61:759-67.
67. Feldman SA, Eiden LE. The chromogranins: their roles in secretion from neuroendocrine cells and as markers for neuroendocrine neoplasia. Endocr Pathol 2003;14:3-23.
68. Ferguson RA, Yu H, Kalyvas M, et al. Ultrasensitive detection of prostate-specific antigen by a time-resolved immunofluorometric assay and the Immulite immunochemiluminescent third-generation assay: potential applications in prostate and breast cancers. Clin Chem 1996;42:675-84.
69. Finne P, Auvinen A, Aro J, et al. Estimation of prostate cancer risk on the basis of total and free prostate-specific antigen, prostate volume and digital rectal examination. Eur Urol 2002;41(6):619-26.
70. Fishman WH, Inglis NR, Stolbach LL, Krant MJ. A serum alkaline phosphatase isoenzyme of human neoplastic cell origin. Cancer Res 1968;28:150-54.

71. Fishman WH, Sell S. Onco-developmental gene expression: A preview. In: Fishman WH, Sell S, eds. Onco-Developmental gene expression. New York: Academic Press Inc, 1976.
72. Foekens JA, Diamandis EP, Yu H, et al. Expression of prostate-specific antigen (PSA) correlates with poor response to tamoxifen therapy in recurrent breast cancer. Br J Cancer 1999;79:888-94.
73. Foekens JA, Look MP, Bolt-de Vries J. Cathepsin-D in primary breast cancer: prognostic evaluation involving 2810 patients. Br J Cancer 1999;79: 300-07.
74. Ford D, Easton DF, Bishop DT, et al. Risks of cancer in BRCA1-mutation carriers. Breast Cancer Linkage Consortium. Lancet 1994;343:692-95.
75. Freije JM, MacDonald NJ, Steeg PS. Differential gene expression in tumor metastasis: Nm23. Curr Top Microbiol Immunol 1996;213:215-32.
76. Friedrich MG, Hellstern A, Hautmann SH, et al. Non-invasive urine tests in diagnosis and as prognostic markers for urinary bladder carcinoma. Comparison of the BTAstat and NMP 22 tests with immunocytology using monoclonal antibodies against Lewis X and 486p3/12. Urologe A 2003; 42:523-30.
77. Garbe C, Leiter U, Ellwanger U. Diagnostic value and prognostic significance of protein S-100beta, melanoma-inhibitory activity, and tyrosinase/ MART-1 reverse transcription-polymerase chain reaction in the follow-up of high-risk melanoma patients. Cancer 2003;97:1737-45.
78. Garrido C, Gurbuxani S, Ravagnan L. Heat shock proteins: endogenous modulators of apoptotic cell death. Biochem Biophys Res Commun 2001;286: 433-42.
79. Goddard AD, Balakier H, Clanton M, et al. Infrequent genomic rearrangement and normal expression of the putative RB1 gene in retinoblastoma tumors. Mol Cell Biol 1988;8:2082-91.
80. Gold P, Freeman SO. Demonstration of tumor specific antigens in human colonic carcinomata by immunological tolerance and absorption techniques. J Exp Med 1965;121:439-62.
81. Graziano F, Cascinu S, Staccioli MP, et al. Potential role and chronology of abnormal expression of the Deleted in Colon Cancer (DCC) and the p53 proteins in the development of gastric cancer. BMC Cancer 2001;1:9.
82. Gulbis B, Galand P. Immunodetection of the p21-ras products in human normal and preneoplastic tissues and solid tumors: A review. Hum Pathol 1993; 24:1271-85.
83. Gutman EB, Sproul EE, Gutman AB. Significance of increased phosphatase activity of bone at the site of osteoplastic metastases secondary to carcinoma of the prostate gland. Am J Cancer 1938;28:485-95.
84. Haber DA, Sohn RL, Buckler AJ, et al. Alternative splicing and genomic structure of the Wilms' tumor gene WT1. PNAS USA 1991;88:9618-22.
85. Haese A, Graefen M, Steuber T, et al. Human glandular kallikrein 2 levels in serum for discrimination of pathologically organ-confined from locally-advanced prostate cancer in total PSA-levels below 10 ng/ml. Prostate 2001;49:101.
86. Haese A, Vaisanen V, Finlay JA, et al. Standardization of two immunoassays for human glandular kallikrein 2. Clin Chem 2003;9:601-10.
87. Haglund C, Kuusela P, Roberts P, Jalanko H. CA 50. In: Sell S, ed. Serological cancer markers. Totowa, NJ: Humana Press, 1992:375-86.
88. Hakomori S-I. Tumor associated carbohydrate markers. In: Sell S, ed. Serological cancer markers. Totowa NJ: Humana Press, 1992:207-32.
89. Hara M, Koyanagi Y, Inoue T, Fukuyana T. Some physico-chemical characteristics of gammaseminoprotein: An antigenic component specific for human seminal plasma. Jpn J Leg Med 1971;25:322-24.
90. Harbeck N, Schmitt M, Kates RE, et al. Clinical utility of Urokinase-type plasminogen activator and plasminogen activator inhibitor-1 determination in primary breast cancer tissue for individualized therapy concepts. Clin Breast Cancer 2002;3: 196-200.
91. Harper PS. Research samples from families with genetic diseases. A proposed code of conduct. Br Med J 1993;306:1391-93.
92. Harris H. The analysis of malignancy by cell fusion: The position in 1988. Cancer Res 1988;48:3302-18.
93. Hayes DF, Tondini C, Kufe DW. Clinical applications of CA 15-3. In: Sell S, ed. Serological cancer markers. Totowa, NJ: Humana Press, 1992:281-307.
94. Hellstrom I, Raycraft J, Hayden-Ledbetter M, et al. The HE4 (WFDC2) protein is a biomarker for ovarian carcinoma. Cancer Res 2003;63:3695-700.
95. Henderson BE, Ross RK, Pike MC. Toward the primary prevention of cancer. Science 1991; 254:1131-38.
96. Hiyama E, Hiyama K. Telomerase as tumor marker. Cancer Lett 2003;94:221-33.
97. Hodgall EV, Hodgall CK, Tingulstad S, et al. Predictive values of serum tumour markers tetranectin, OVX1, CASA and CA125 in patients with a pelvic mass. Int J Cancer 2000;89:519-23.
98. Holmes FA, Fritsche HA, Loewy JW, Geitner AM, Sutton RC, et al. Measurement of estrogen and progesterone receptors in human breast tumors: Enzyme immunoassay versus binding assay. J Clin Oncol 1990;8:1025-35.
99. Hostetter RB, Augustus LB, Mankarious R, et al. Carcinoembryonic antigen as a selective enhancer of colorectal cancer metastasis. J Natl Cancer Inst 1990;82:380-85.

100. Jacobs I, Bast RC. The CA 125 tumor-associated antigen: A review of the literature. Hum Reprod 1989;4:1-12.
101. Janicke F, Prechtl A, Thomssen C. Randomized adjuvant chemotherapy trial in high-risk, lymph node-negative breast cancer patients identified by urokinase-type plasminogen activator and plasminogen activator inhibitor type 1. J Natl Cancer Inst 2001;93:913-20.
102. Jarque F, Lluch A, Vizcarra E, Munoz M, Alberola V, Garca-Conde J. Quantitative monoclonal antibody determination of estrogen and progesterone receptors in human breast cancer: Correlation with the radioligand method. Oncology 1994;51:435-39.
103. Johnson PJ, Lo YM. Plasma nucleic acids in the diagnosis and management of malignant disease. Clin Chem 2002;48:1186-93.
104. Kageyama S, Isono T, Iwaki H, Wakabayashi Y, Okada Y, et al. Identification by proteomic analysis of calreticulin as a marker for bladder cancer and evaluation of the diagnostic accuracy of its detection in urine. Clin Chem 2004;50:857-66.
105. Kastan MB, Canman CE, Leonard CJ. P53, cell cycle control and apoptosis: Implications for cancer. Cancer and Metastasis Rev 1995;14:3-15.
106. Kastan MB, Onyekwere O, Sidransky D, Vogelstein B, Craig RW. Participation of p53 protein in the cellular response to DNA damage. Cancer Res 1991;51: 6304-11.
107. Kato H. Squamous cell carcinoma antigen. In: Sell S, ed. Serological cancer markers. Totowa NJ: Humana Press, 1992:437-51.
108. Kelsten ML, Chan DW, Bruzek DJ, Rock RC. Monitoring hepatocellular carcinoma by using a monoclonal immunoenzymometric assay for alpha-fetoprotein. Clin Chem 1988;34:76-81.
109. Khan J, Simon R, Bittner M, et al. Gene expression profiling of alveolar rhabdomyosarcoma with cDNA microarrays. Cancer Res 1998;58:5009-13.
110. Kiang DT, Greenberg LJ, Kennedy BJ. Tumor marker kinetics in the monitoring of breast cancer. Cancer 1990;65:193-99.
111. King MC, Rowell S, Love SM. Inherited breast and ovarian cancer. JAMA 1993;269:1975-80.
112. Kishi T, Grass L, Soosaipillai A. Human kallikrein 8, a novel biomarker for ovarian carcinoma. Cancer R 2003;63:2771-74.
113. KlugTL, Bast RC, Niloff JM, et al. Monoclonal antibody immunoradiometric assay for an antigenic determinant (CA 125) associated with human epithelial ovarian carcinomas. Cancer Res 1984; 44:1048-53.
114. Knudson AG Jr. Mutation and cancer: statistical study of retinoblastoma. PNAS USA 1971;68:820-26.
115. Knudson AG Jr. Hereditary cancer, oncogenes, and anti-oncogenes. Cancer Res 1985;45:1437-81.
116. Koblinski JE, Ahram M, Sloane BF. Unraveling the role of proteases in cancer. Clin Chim Acta 2000; 291(2):113-35.
117. Koprowski HZ, Steplewski K, Mitchell M, et al. Colorectal carcinoma antigens detected by somatic hybridoma antibodies. Cell Genet 1979;5:957-72.
118. Kuiper GG, Enmark E, Pelto-Huikko M. Gustafsson JA. Cloning of a novel receptor expressed in rat prostate and ovary. PNAS U S A; 93:5925-30.
119. Kuusela P, Haglund C, Jalanko H, Roberts PJ. CA 242. In: Sell S, ed. Serological cancer markers. Totowa, NJ: Humana Press, 1992:429-35.
120. Lamerz R. CA19-9: GICA (gastrointestinal cancer antigen). In: Sell S, ed. Serological cancer markers. Totowa, NJ: Humana Press, 1992:309-39.
121. Lee W-H, Shew JY, Hong RD, et al. The retinoblastoma susceptibility gene encodes a nuclear phosphoprotein associated with DNA binding activity. Nature 1987;329:642-44.
122. Leitzel K, Teramoto Y, Konard K, et al. Elevated serum c-erb B-2 antigen levels and decreased response to hormone of breast cancer. J Clin Oncol 1995;13:1129-35.
123. Leppert M, Dobbs M, Scrambler P, et al. The gene for familial polyposis coli maps to the long arm of chromosome 5. Science 1987;238:1411-13.
124. Levine AJ, Momand J, Finlay CA. The p53 tumour suppressor gene. Nature 19991;351:453-56.
125. Li JL, Zhang Z, Rosenzweig J, et al. Proteomics and bioinformatics approaches for identification of serum biomarkers to detect breast cancer. Clin Chem 2002; 48:1296-304.
126. Lilja H, Christensson A, Dahlen U, et al. Prostate specific antigen in human serum occurs predominantly in complex with alpha-1-antichymotrypsin. Clin Chem 1991;37:1618-25.
127. Lin F, van Rhee F, Goldman JM, et al. Kinetics of increasing BCR-ABL transcript numbers in chronic myeloid leukemia patients who relapse after bone marrow transplantation. Blood 1996; 7:4473-78.
128. Lipton A, Ali SM, Leitzel K, et al. Elevated serum Her-2/neu level predicts decreased response to hormone therapy in metastatic breast cancer. J Clin Oncol 2002;20:1467-72.
129. Liotta LA, Espina V, Mehta AI, et al. Protein microarrays: meeting analytical challenges for clinical applications. Cancer Cell 2003;3:317-25.
130. Look M, van Putten W, Duffy M, et al. Pooled analysis of prognostic impact of uPA and PAI-1 in breast cancer patients. Thromb Haemost 2003; 90:538-48.
131. Lovgren J, Valtonen-Andre C, Marsal K, et al. Measurement of prostate-specific antigen and human glandular kallikrein 2 in different body fluids. J Androl 1999;20:348.

132. Lowe PN, Skinner RH. Regulation of RAS signal transduction in normal and transformed cells. Cellular Signaling 1994;6:109-23.
133. Luftner D, Luke C, Possinger K. Serum HER-2/neu in the management of breast cancer patients. Clin Biochem 2003;36:233-40.
134. Lundwall A, Lilja H. Molecular cloning of human prostate specific antigen cDNA. FEBS Lett 1987; 214:317-22.
135. Luo LY, Diamandis EP, Look MP, et al. Higher expression of human kallikrein 10 in breast cancer tissue predicts tamoxifen resistance. Br J Cancer 2002; 86:1790-96.
136. Luo LY, Katsaros D, Scorilas A, et al. Prognostic value of human kallikrein 10 expression in epithelial ovarian carcinoma. Clin Cancer Res 2001;7: 2372-79.
137. Luo LY, Katsaros D, Scorilas A, et al. The serum concentration of human kallikrein 10 represents a novel biomarker for ovarian cancer diagnosis and prognosis. Cancer Res 2003;63:807-11.
138. Marks JR, Davidoff AM, Iglehart JD. p53 in human cancer. In: Sell S, ed. Serological cancer markers. Totowa NJ: Humana Press, 1992:77-110.
139. Mazzucchelli L. Protein S100A4: too long overlooked by pathologists? Am J Pathol 2002;60:7-13.
140. McDonnell TJ, Marin MC, Hsu B, et al. The bcl-2 oncogene: apoptosis and neoplasia. Radiation Res 1993;136:307-12.
141. McMahon BJ, London T. Workshop on screening for hepatocellular carcinoma. J Natl Cancer Inst 1991; 83:916-19.
142. Menon U, Jacobs IJ. Ovarian cancer screening in the general population: current status. Int J Gynecol Cancer 2001;11:3-6.
143. Metzgar RS, Sawabu N, Hollingsworth MA. DU-PAN-2: A clinically useful mucin marker of differentiation of pancreatic and other ductal cells and their tumors. In: Sell S, ed. Serological cancer markers. Totowa, NJ: Humana Press, 1992:355-74.
144. Miki Y, Swensen J, Shattuck-Eidens D, et al. A strong candidate for the breast and ovarian cancer susceptibility gene BRCA 1. Science 1994;266:66-71.
145. Mikolajczyk SD, Millar LS, Kumar A, et al. Prostatic human kallikrein 2 inactivates and complexes with plasminogen activator inhibitor-1. Int J Cancer 1999; 81:438.
146. Mikolajczyk SD, Miller LS, Wang TJ, et al. "BPSA" a specific molecular form of free prostate specific antigen is found predominantly in the transition zone of patients with nodular benign prostatic hyperplasia. Urology 2000;5:41-5.
147. Mills GB, Bast RC Jr, Srivastava S. Future for ovarian cancer screening: Novel markers from emerging technologies of transcriptional profiling and proteomics. J Natl Cancer Inst 2001;19:1437-39.
148. Moreno JG, Croce CM, Fischer R, et al. Detection of hematogenous micrometastasis in patients with prostate cancer. Cancer Res 1992;52:6110-12.
149. Moreno JG, Gomella LG. Circulating prostate cancer cells detected by reverse transcription-polymerase chain reaction (TR-PCR): What do they mean? Cancer Control 1998;5:507-12.
150. Nichols GE, Frierson HF, Boyd JC, Hanigan MH. Automated immunohistochemical assay for estrogen receptor status in breast cancer using monoclonal antibody CC4-5 on the Ventana ES. Am J Clin Pathol 1996;106:332-38.
151. Nicholson RI, Gee JM, Harper ME. EGFR and cancer prognosis. Euro J Cancer 2001;37:S9-S15.
152. Nishizuka S, Chen ST, Gwadry FG, et al. Diagnostic markers that distinguish colon and ovarian adenocarcinomas: identification by genomic, proteomic and tissue array profiling. Cancer Res 2003;63:5243-50.
153. Noguchi M, Mizukami Y, Kinoshita K, et al. c-erbB-2, ras p21, and c-myc expression in breast carcinoma: prognostic value and correlation with clinicopathologic and biologic variables. Int J Oncol 1994;4: 255-60.
154. O'Boyle K. The role of the Deleted Colon Cancer (DCC) gene in colorectal and gastric cancer. Cancer Invest 2003;12:484-85.
155. Oehr P, Luthgens ML, Liu Q. Tissue polypeptide antigen and specific TPA. In: Sell S, ed. Serological cancer markers. Totowa NJ: Humana Press, 1992: 193-206.
156. Oesterling JE. Prostate specific antigen: A critical assessment of the most useful tumor marker for adenocarcinoma of the prostate. J Urol 1991;145:907-23.
157. Oesterling JE, Chan DW, Epstein JI, et al. Prostate specific antigen in the preoperative and postoperative evaluation of localized prostatic cancer treated with radical prostatectomy. J Urol 1988;139:766-72.
158. Oesterling JE, Jacobsen SJ, Chute GG, et al. Serum prostate specific antigen in a community based population of healthy men: Establishment of age-specific reference ranges. JAMA 1993;270:860-64.
159. Overall CM, Lopez-Otin C. Strategies for MMP inhibition in cancer: innovations for the post-trial era. Nat Rev Cancer 2002;2:657-72.
160. Ozturk M, et al. p53 mutation in hepatocellular carcinoma after aflatoxin exposure. Lancet 1991; 338:1356-59.
161. Paech K, Webb P, Kuiper GG, et al. Differential ligand activation of estrogen receptors ERalpha and ERbeta at AP1 sites. Science 1997;277:1508-10.
162. Palmer-Toy D, Kuzdzal S, Chan DW. Proteomic approaches to tumor marker discovery. In: Diamandis EP, Fritsche HA, Lilja H, Chan DW, Schwartz MK, eds. Tumor markers: Physiology, pathobiology, technology and clinical applications. Washington DC: AACC Press, 2002:391-400.

163. Partin AW, Brawer MK, Bartsch G, et al: Complexed prostate specific antigen improves specificity for prostate cancer detection: Results of a prospective multicenter clinical trial. J Urology 2003;170: 1787-91.
164. Partin AW, Catalona WJ, Southwick PC, et al. Analysis of percent free prostate specific antigen (PSA) for prostate cancer detection: Influence of total PSA, prostate volume and age. Urology 1996;48:55-61.
165. Partin AW, Getzenberg RH, Carmichael MJ, et al. Nuclear matrix protein patterns in human benign prostatic hyperplasia and prostate cancer. Cancer Res 1993;53:744-49.
166. Partin AW, Hanks GE, Klein EA, et al. Prostate-specific antigen as a marker of disease activity in prostate cancer. Oncology (Hunting) 2002;16:1024-38.
167. Partin AW, Oesterling JE. The clinical usefulness of percentage free-PSA. Urology 1996;48:1-3.
168. Partin AW, Piantadosi S, Subong ENP, et al. Clearance rate of serum free and total PSA following radical retropubic prostatectomy. Prostate Supp 1996;7: 35-39.
169. Pearson JD, Uderer AA, Metter EJ, et al. Longitudinal analysis of serial measurements of free and total PSA among men with and without prostatic cancer. Urology 1996;48:4-9.
170. Perou CM, Sorlie T, Eisen MB, et al. Molecular portraits of human breast tumours. Nature 2000; 406:747-52.
171. Petricoin III EF, Ardekani AM, Hitt BA, et al. Use of proteomic patterns in serum to identify ovarian cancer. Lancet 2002;359:572-72.
172. Petricoin III EF, Ornstein DK, Paweletz CP, et al. Serum proteomic patterns for detection of prostate cancer. J Natl Cancer Inst 2002;94:1576-78.
173. Petricoin EF, Zoon KC, Kohn EC, et al. Clinical proteomics: Translating benchside promise into bedside reality. Nature Rev Drug Discov 2002;1: 683-95.
174. Petty EM, Killeen AA. BRCA 1 mutation testing: Controversies and challenges. Clin Chem 1997; 43:6-8.
175. Pitot HC. The language of oncology. In: Pilot HC. Fundamentals of oncology. New York: Marcel Dekker Inc, 1978:16.
176. Pujol JL, Boher JM, Grenier J. Cyfra 21-1, neuron specific enolase and prognosis of non-small cell lung cancer: prospective study in 621 patients. Lung Cancer 2001;31:221-31.
177. Radich JP, Gehly G, Gooley T, et al. Polymerase chain reaction detection of the BCR-ABL fusion transcript after allogeneic marrow transplantation for chronic myeloid leukemia: results and implications in 346 patients. Blood 1995;5:2632-38.
178. Rai AJ, Zhang Z, Rosenzweig J, Shih I-M, Pham T, Fung E, Sokoll LJ, Chan DW. Proteomic approaches to tumor marker discovery: Identification of biomarkers for ovarian cancer. Arch Pathol Lab Med 2002;26:1581-26.
179. Recker F, Kwiatkowski MK, Piironen T, et al. Human glandular kallikrein as a tool to improve discrimination of poorly differentiated and non-organ-confined prostate cancer compared with prostate-specific antigen. Urology 2000;55:481.
180. Reddish MA, Helbrecht N, Almeida AF, et al. Epitope mapping of Mab within the peptide core of the malignant breast carcinoma associated mucin antigen coded for by the human MUC 1 gene. J Tumor Marker Oncol 1992;7:19-27.
181. Remzi M, Anagnostou T, Ravery V, et al. An artificial neural network to predict the outcome of repeat prostate biopsies. Urology 2003;62:456-60.
182. Reuning U, Sperl S, Kopitz C, et al. Urokinase-type plasminogen activator (uPA) and its receptor (uPAR): development of antagonists of uPA/uPAR interaction and their effects in vitro and in vivo. Curr Pharm Des 2003;9:1529-43.
183. Rochefort H, Garcia M, Glondu M, et al. Cathespin D in breast cancer: mechanisms and clinical applications, a 1999 overview. Clin Chim Acta 2000; 291:157-70.
184. Rock RC, Chan DW, Bruzek DJ, et al: Evaluation of a monoclonal immunoradiometric assay for prostate-specific antigen. Clin Chem 1987;33:2257-61.
185. Rosenberg S. The Urokinase-type plasminogen activator system in cancer and other pathological conditions: introduction and perspective. Curr Pharm Des 2003;9:4.
186. Rosty C, Christa L, Kuzdzal S, Baldwin WM, Zahurak ML, et al. Identification of hepatocarcinoma-intestine-pancreas/pancreatitis-associated Protein I as a biomarker for pancreatic ductal adenocarcinoma by protein biochip technology. Cancer Research 2002; 62:1868-75.
187. Saccani Jotti G, Johnston SR, Salter J, Detre S, Dowsett M. Comparison of new immunohistochemical assay for estrogen receptor in paraffin wax embedded breast carcinoma tissue with quantitative enzyme immunoassay. J Clin Pathol 1994;47:900-5.
188. Saldanha SN, Andrews LG, Tollefsbol TO. Analysis of telomerase activity and detection of its catalytic subunit, hTERT. Anal Biochem 2003;315:1-21.
189. Sarosdy MF, DeVere White RW, Soloway MS, et al. Results of a multicenter trial using the BTA test to monitor for and diagnose recurrent bladder cancer. J Urol 1995;154:379-84.
190. Sarosdy MF, Schellhammer P, Bokinsky G, et al. Clinical evaluation of a multi-target fluorescent in situ hybridization assay for detection of bladder cancer. J Urol 2002;168:1950-54.
191. Sauter ER, Daly M, Linahan D, et al. Prostate-specific antigen levels in nipple aspirate fluid correlate with

breast cancer risk. Cancer Epidemiol Biomarkers Prev 1996;5:967-70.
192. Schedlich LJ, Bennetts BH, Morris BJ. Primary structure of a human glandular kallikrein gene. DNA 1987;6:429.
193. Schena M, Shalon D, Davis RW, et al. Quantitative monitoring of gene expression patterns with a complementary DNA microarray. Science 1995;270: 467-70.
194. Schlom J, Colcher D, Milenic DE, et al. TAG-72 as a tumor marker In: Sell S, ed. Serological cancer markers. Totowa NJ: Humana Press, 1992: 387-416.
195. Schwartz MK. Laboratory aids to diagnosis-enzymes. Cancer 1976;37:542-48.
196. Schwartz MK. Enzyme tests in cancer. Clin Lab Med 1982;2:479-91.
197. Sell S. Cancer markers of the 1990s. Clin Lab Med 1990;10:27-31.
198. Sell S. Cancer-associated carbohydrates identified by monoclonal antibodies. Hum Pathol 1991;21: 1003-19.
199. Sell S. Cancer markers. In: Moossa AR, Schempff SC, Robson MC eds. Comprehensive textbook of oncology, 2nd ed. Vol. 1. Baltimore: Williams & Wilkins, 1991:225-38.
200. Shen MH, Harper PS, Upadhyaya M. Molecular genetics of neurofibromatosis type 1 (NF1). J Med Genet 1996;33:2-17.
201. Shih IM, Sokoll LJ, Chan DW. Ovarian cancer. In: Diamandis EP, Fritsche HA, Lilja H, Chan DW, Schwartz MK, eds. Tumor markers: Physiology, pathobiology, technology and clinical applications. Washington, DC: AACC Press, 2002:239-52.
202. Shipley WU. Radiation therapy. J Urol 1992;147: 929-30.
203. Shuin T. C-myc as a tumor marker for primary human cancers. In: Sell S, ed. Serological cancer markers. Totowa, NJ: Humana Press, 1992:53-76.
204. Sidransky D, Tokino T, Hamilton SR, et al. Identification of ras oncogene mutations in the stool of patients with curable colorectal tumors. Science 1992; 256:102-5.
205. Siemens DR, Morales A, Johnston B, et al. A comparative analysis of rapid urine tests for the diagnosis of upper urinary tract malignancy. Can J Urol 2003; 10:1754-58.
206. Sikorska HM, Fuks A, Gold P. Carcinoembryonic antigen. In: Sell S, ed. Serological cancer markers. Totowa, NJ: Humana Press, 1992:47-97.
207. Silver HKB, Archibald B-L, Raga J, Coldman AJ. Relative operating characteristic analysis and group modeling for tumor markers: Comparison of CA 15.3, carcinoembryonic antigen, and mucin-like carcinoma-associated antigen in breast carcinoma. Cancer Res 1991;51:1904-09.
208. Sinicrope FA, Ruan SB, Cleary KR, et al. bcl-2 and p53 oncoprotein expression during colorectal tumorigenesis. Cancer Res 1995;55:237-41.
209. Skates SJ, Menon U, MacDonald N, et al. Calculation of the risk of ovarian cancer from serial CA-125 values for preclinical detection in postmenopausal women. J Clin Oncol 2003;21:206-10.
210. Slamon DJ, Godolphin W, Jones LA, et al. Studies of the HER-2/neu proto-oncogene in human breast and ovarian cancer. Science 1989;244:707-9.
211. Sokoll LJ, Chan DW. Malignancy-Associated endocrine disorders. In: Jialal I, Winter WE, Chan DW, eds. Handbook of diagnostic endocrinology. Washington, DC: AACC Press, 1999:215-44.
212. Sokoll LJ, Chan DW, Mikolajczyk SD, et al: Proenzyme PSA for the early detection of prostate dancer in the 2.5-4.0 ng/mL total PSA range: Preliminary analysis. Urology 2003;1:274-76.
213. Soloman A. Homogeneous (monoclonal) immunoglobulins in cancer. Am J Med 1977;63:169-81.
214. Solomon E, Borrow J, Goddard AD. Chromosome aberrations and cancer. Science 1991;254:1153-60.
215. Soloway MS, Briggman JV, Carpinito GA, et al. Use of a new tumor marker, Urinary NMP22, in the detection of occult or rapidly recurring transitional cell carcinoma of the urinary tract following surgical treatment. J Urol 1996;156:363-67.
216. Somerville RPT, Oblander SA, Apte SS. Matrix metalloproteinases: old dogs with new tricks. Genome Biol 2003;4:216.
217. Spencer CA, LoPresti JS, Fatemi S, et al. Detection of residual and recurrent differentiated thyroid carcinoma by serum thyroglobulin measurement. Thyroid 1999;9:435-41.
218. Spencer CA, Wang C, Fatemi S, et al. Serum thyroglobulin autoantibodies: Prevalence, influence on serum thyroglobulin measurement and prognostic significance in patients with differentiated thyroid carcinoma. J Clin Endocrinol Metab 1998;83: 1121-27.
219. Srinivas PR, Srivastava S, Hannah S, Wright GL Jr. Proteomics in early detection of cancer. Clin Chem 2001;47:1901-11.
220. Srivastava S, Zou Z, Pirollo K, et al. Germ line transmission of a mutated p53 gene in a cancer-prone family with Li-Fraumeni syndrome. Nature 1990; 348:747-49.
221. Stamey TA, Barnhill SD, Zhang Z, et al. Effectiveness of ProstAsure in detecting prostate cancer and benign prostatic hyperplasia in men age 50 or older. J Urol 1996;155:436A.
222. Stamey TA, Yang N, Hay AR, et al. Prostatic-specific antigen as a serum marker for adenocarcinoma of the prostate. N Engl J Med 1987;317:909-16.
223. Stanbridge EJ, Cavenee WK. Heritable cancer and tumor suppressor genes: A tentative connection. In:

Weinberg RS, ed. Oncogenes and the molecular origins of cancer. Cold Spring Harbor, MA: Cold Spring Harbor Lab Press, 1989.
224. Steinberg W. The clinical utility of the CA 19-9 tumor-associated antigen. Am J Gastroenterol 1990; 85:350-55.
225. Stenman UH. Tumor-associated trypsin inhibitor. Clin Chem 2002;8:1206-09.
226. Stenman UH, Leinonen J, Alfthan H. A complex between prostate specific antigen and alpha-1-antichymotrypsin is the major form of prostate specific antigen in serum of patients with prostatic cancer. Assay of the complex improves clinical sensitivity for cancer. Cancer Res 1991;51:222-26.
227. Stephan C, Cammann H, Semjonow A, et al. Multicenter evaluation of an artificial neural network to increase the prostate cancer detection rate and reduce unnecessary biopsies. Clin Chem 2002; 48:1279-87.
228. Stephan C, Jung K, Cammann H, et al. An artificial neural network considerably improves the diagnostic power of percent free prostate-specific antigen in prostate cancer diagnosis: results of a 5-year investigation. Int J Cancer 2002;99:466-73.
229. Stigbrand T, Wahren B. Alkaline phosphatase as tumor markers. In: Sell S, ed. Serological cancer markers. Totowa NJ: Humana Press, 1992:135-49.
230. Sturgeon C. Practice guidelines for tumor marker use in the clinic. Clin Chem 2002;48:1151-59.
231. Sulis ML, Parsons R. PTEN: from pathology to biology. Trends Cell Biol 2003;13:478-83.
232. Taketa K. Alpha-fetoprotein in the 1990s. In: Sell S, ed. Serological cancer markers. Totowa, NJ: Humana Press, 1992:31-46.
233. Takeuchi H, Bilchik A, Saha S, et al. c-MET expression level in primary colon cancer: a predictor of tumor invasion and lymph node metastases. Clin Cancer Res 2003;9:1480-88.
234. Tatarinov Y. New data on the embryo-specific antigenic components of human blood serum. Vopr Med Khim 1964;10:584-88.
235. Tibbe AG, de Grooth BG, Greve J, et al. Cell analysis system based on compact disk technology. Cytometry 2002;47:173-82.
236. Tolgay Ocal I, Dolled-Filhart M, D'Aquila TG, et al. Tissue microarray-based studies of patients with lymph node negative breast carcinoma show that met expression is associated with worse outcome but is not correlated with epidermal growth factor family receptors. Cancer 2003;97:1841-48.
237. Uban N, McIntosh MW, Andersen M, et al. Ovarian cancer screening. Hematol Oncol Clin North Am 2003;17:989-1005.
238. Vaitukaitis JL. Human chorionic gonadotropin: A hormone secreted for many reasons. N Engl J Med 1979;301:324-26.
239. van de Vijver MJ, He YD, van't Veer LJ, et al. A gene-expression signature as a predictor of survival in breast cancer. N Engl J Med 2002;347:1999-2009.
240. van't Veer LJ, Dai H, van de Vijver MJ, et al. Gene expression profiling predicts clinical outcome of breast cancer. Nature 2002;415:530-36.
241. Vassilikos EJ, Yu H, Trachtenberg J, et al. Relapse and cure rates of prostate cancer patients after radical prostatectomy and 5 years of follow-up. Clin Biochem 2000;33:115-23.
242. Vihinen P, Kahari VM. Matrix metalloproteinases in cancer: prognostic markers and therapeutic targets. Int J Cancer 2002;99:157-66.
243. Viskochil D, White R, Cawthon RL. The neurofibromatosis type 1 gene. Annu Rev Neurosci 1993; 16:183-202.
244. Walsh PC, Oesterling JE, Epstein JI, et al. The value of prostate-specific antigen in the management of localized prostate cancer. In: Murphy G, Khoury S, eds. Therapeutic progress in urological cancer. New York: Alan R Liss Inc, 1989:27-33.
245. Wawrzynczak EJ. Systemic immunotoxin therapy of cancer: Advances and prospects. Br J Cancer 1991; 64:624-30.
246. Weinberg RA. Tumor suppressor genes. Science 1991; 254:1138-46.
247. Welsh JB, Sapinoso LM, Kern SG, et al. Large-scale delineation of secreted protein biomarkers overexpressed in cancer tissue and serum. PNAS USA 2003;100:3410-15.
248. Welsh JB, Zarrinkar PP, Sapinoso LM, et al. Analysis of gene expression profiles in normal and neoplastic ovarian tissue samples identifies candidate molecular markers of epithelial ovarian cancer. PNAS USA 2001;98:1176-81.
249. Wigler MH. GAPs in understanding Ras. Nature 1990;346:696-99.
250. Wittliff KL, Pasic R, Bland KI. Steroid and peptide hormone receptors identified in breast tissue. In: Kirby KI, Copeland EM, eds. The breast. Philadelphia: WB Saunders Co, 1990:900-36.
251. Wooster R, Neuhausen SL, Mangion J, et al. Localization of a breast cancer susceptibility gene, BRCA 2, to chromosome 13q12-13. Science 1994;265:2088-90.
252. Yousef GM, Diamandis EP. The new human tissue kallikrein gene family: structure, function, and association to disease. Endocr Rev 2001;2:184-204.
253. Yousef GM, Polymeris ME, Grass L, et al. Human kallikrein 5: a potential novel serum biomarker for breast and ovarian cancer. Cancer Res 2003;63: 3958-65.
254. Yousef GM, Polymeris ME, Yacoub GM, et al. Parallel overexpression of seven kallikrein genes in ovarian cancer. Cancer Res 2003;63:2223-27.
255. Yu H, Diamandis EP, Wong PY. Detection of prostate cancer relapse with prostate specific antigen monitor-

ing at levels of 0.001 to 0.1 microg/L. J Urol 1997; 157:913-20.
256. Yu H, Giai M, Diamandis EP, et al. Prostate-specific antigen is a new favorable prognostic indicator for women with breast cancer. Cancer Res 1995;55: 2104-10.
257. Yu H, Levesque MA, Clark GM, et al. Prognostic value of prostate-specific antigen for worm with breast cancer: a large United States cohort study. Clin Cancer Res 1998;4:1489-97.
258. Zehentner BK. Detection of disseminated tumor cells: strategies and diagnostic implications. Expert Rev Mol Diagn 2002;2:41-8.
259. Zehentner BK, Dillon DC, Jiang Y, et al. Application of a multigene reverse transcription-PCR assay for detection of mammaglobin and complementary transcribed genes in breast cancer lymph nodes. Clin Chem 2002;48:1225-31.
260. Zeltzer PM, Marangos PJ, Evans AE, Schneider SL. Serum neuron-specific enolase in children with neuroblastoma. Cancer 1986;57:1230-34.
261. Zemzoum I, Kates RE, Ross JS, et al. Invasion factors uPA/PAI-1 and HER2 status provide independent and complementary information on patient outcome in node-negative breast cancer. J Clin Oncol 2003;21:1022-28.
262. Zhang WM, Leinonen J, Kalkkinen N, et al. Purification and characterization of different molecular forms of prostate specific antigen in human seminal fluid. Clin Chem 1995;41:1567-73.
263. Zhang Z. Combining multiple biomarkers in clinical diagnostics—A review of methods and issues. In: Diamandis EP, Fritsche HA, Lilja H, Chan DW, Schwartz MK, eds. Tumor markers: Physiology, pathobiology, technology and clinical applications. Washington DC: AACC Press, 2002:133-39.
264. Zhang Z, Bast RC, Yu Y, Li J, Sokoll LJ, Rai AJ, et al. Three biomarkers identified from serum proteomic analysis for the detection of early state ovarian cancer. Cancer Res 2004;64:5882-90.
265. Zippe C, Pandrangi L, Agarwal A. NMP22 is a sensitive, cost-effective test in patients at risk for bladder cancer. J Urol 1999;161:62-5.
266. Zweig MH, Robertson EA. Clinical validation of immunoassay: A well-designed approach to a clinical study. In: Chan DW, ed. Immunoassay: A practical guide. San Diego: Academic Press Inc, 1987:97-128.

ADDITIONAL READING

Diamandis EP, Fritsche HA, Lilja H, Chan DW, Schwartz MK, eds. Tumor markers: Physiology, pathobiology, technology and clinical applications. Washington DC: AACC Press, 2002.

Garrett G, Sell S, eds. Cellular cancer markers. Totowa, NJ: The Humana Press, 1995.

Hanausek M, Walaszek Z, eds. Tumor Marker Protocols (Methods in Molecular Medicine, Vol 14). Totowa, NJ: Humana Press, 1998.

NCCN Clinical Practice Guidelines in Oncology. National Comprehensive Cancer Network. Jenkintown, PA 2004, www.nccn.org (accessed November 19, 2004)

Pannall P, Kotasek D. Cancer & clinical biochemistry. London: ACB Venture Publications, 1997.

CHAPTER 24

Kidney Function Tests

Edmund Lamb, Ph.D., David J. Newman, Ph.D., and Christopher P. Price, Ph.D.

Quantitation of overall function of the kidneys is based on the assumption that all functioning nephrons are performing normally and that a decline in renal function is due to loss of functioning nephrons quantitatively related to the loss. Thus in nearly all types of diffuse renal disease, impaired function of the kidneys is attributed to a diminished number of functioning nephrons rather than to compromised function of individual nephrons. Because glomerular filtration is the initiating phase of all nephron functions, quantitative or qualitative assessment of filtration—or some variable that bears a constant relationship to it—generally provides the most useful indices for physicians to assess the severity and progress of kidney damage.

Specific defects in particular functions of the nephrons can also be identified and evaluated. For example, assessment of the maximum concentrating capacity of the kidneys gives an estimate of antidiuretic hormone (ADH)–controlled reabsorption of solute-free water in the distal portion of the tubule. Pinpoint defects, caused by genetically determined deficiencies of specific tubular transport systems or ion channels and giving rise to characteristic biochemical disorders, are considered in Chapter 45.

This chapter will describe chemical tests that have proved the most practical and useful for screening for and diagnosing impaired kidney function and for monitoring the course and management of progressive chronic kidney disease (CKD). In general, either plasma or serum is used for most of these tests: the term plasma is mainly used throughout this chapter. This chapter provides an overview of contemporary methodology with reference intervals, the clinical utility of the tests, and the changes that are observed in disease.

CREATININE

Creatinine is the cyclic anhydride of creatine that is produced as the final product of decomposition of phosphocreatine. It is excreted in the urine; measurements of excretion rates are used as diagnostic indicators of kidney function.

BIOCHEMISTRY AND PHYSIOLOGY

Creatine is synthesized in the kidneys, liver, and pancreas by two enzymatically mediated reactions. In the first, transamidation of arginine and glycine forms guanidinoacetic acid; in the second, methylation of guanidinoacetic acid occurs with S-adenosylmethionine as the methyl donor. Creatine is then transported in blood to other organs, such as muscle and brain, where it is phosphorylated to phosphocreatine, a high-energy compound.

Creatine —(Creatine kinase; ATP → ADP)→ Phosphocreatine

Creatine —(Spontaneous; $-H_2O$)→ Creatinine

Phosphocreatine —(Spontaneous; $-P_i$)→ Creatinine

Interconversion of phosphocreatine and creatine is a particular feature of the metabolic processes of muscle contraction. A proportion of the free creatine in muscle (thought to be between 1% and 2%/day) spontaneously and irreversibly converts to its anhydride waste product, creatinine. Thus the amount of creatinine produced each day is fairly constant and is related to the muscle mass (and body weight). In health, the concentration of creatinine in the bloodstream is also fairly constant, although diet may influence the value, depending on the individual's meat intake.[97] Creatinine (MW 113 Da) is present in all body fluids and secretions and is freely filtered by the glomerulus. Although it is not reabsorbed to any great extent by the renal tubules, there is a small but significant tubular secretion. Creatinine production also decreases as the circulating level of creatinine increases; several mechanisms for this have been proposed, including feedback inhibition of production of creatine, reconversion of creatinine to creatine, and conversion to other metabolites.[25,79,88]

Clinical Significance

The clinical utility of creatinine measurement is discussed later in this chapter.

Analytical Methodology

Plasma creatinine is measured as a test of kidney function; both chemical and enzymatic methods are used to measure it.[45,164,205] Most laboratories use adaptations of the same assay for measurements in both plasma and urine.

Chemical Methods: the Jaffe Reaction

Most chemical methods for measuring creatinine are primarily based on the reaction with alkaline picrate. In this reaction, first described by Jaffe in 1886, creatinine reacts with picrate ion in an alkaline medium to yield an orange-red complex. Despite considerable literature on the subject, the reaction mechanism and the structure of the product remain unclear.[228]

The Jaffe reaction is not specific for creatinine. Many compounds have been reported to produce a Jaffelike chromogen, including protein,[35] glucose, ascorbic acid, ketone bodies,[232] pyruvate, guanidine, blood-substitute products,[3] and cephalosporins[213] and the reader is referred to several comprehensive reviews.[28,205] The degree of interference from these compounds is dependent on the specific reaction conditions chosen. The effect of ketones and ketoacids is probably of the greatest significance clinically, although the effect is very method dependent. Thus reports on acetoacetate interference vary from a negligible increase to an increase of 3.5 mg/dL (310 μmol/L) in the apparent creatinine concentration at an acetoacetate concentration of 8 mmol/L. Bilirubin is a negative interferant with the Jaffe reaction. The addition of buffering ions, such as borate and phosphate, together with surfactant, has been used to minimize the effects of this interference. A popular technique in this context has been the addition of ferricyanide ("O'Leary method"), which oxidizes bilirubin to biliverdin, hence reducing its interference.[115,154] Noncreatinine chromogens do not generally contribute to measured urinary creatinine concentration.

Several approaches have been used in an attempt to improve the general specificity of the Jaffe reaction. These have included absorption, and subsequent elution, of creatinine into hydrated aluminum silicate (Fuller's earth, Lloyd's reagent), acid blanking, the use of ion-exchange resins[233] or solvent extraction, and oxidation of interferants with compounds such as cerium sulfate; generally these modifications have not proved practical.

The greatest success in terms of common usage and specificity has come from the use of a kinetic measurement approach in combination with careful choice of reactant concentrations. Although manual methods have traditionally been equilibrium methods, with 10 to 15 minutes allowed for color development at room temperature, kinetic assays were developed in a quest both for specificity and for faster and automated analyses. Early studies of interferences in the kinetic methods identified two kinds of noncreatinine chromogens, those whose rates of adduct formation were very rapid in the first 20 seconds after mixing reagent and sample (e.g., acetoacetate) and those whose rates did not become rapid until 80 to 100 s after mixing (e.g., protein). The "window" between 20 and 80 s therefore was a period in which the rate signal being observed could be attributed predominantly to the creatinine-picrate reaction (some investigators found 60 s as the upper limit of this window). Thus improvement of specificity in the kinetic assays was achieved by selecting times for rate measurements 20 to 80 s after initiation of the reaction (mixing). This approach has been implemented on various automated instruments, and kinetic assays are now the most widely used approach to creatinine measurement. An extensive literature exists on the choice of reactant concentrations and reading interval and on the choice of wavelength and reaction temperature. Brief comments include:

Picrate concentration. The Jaffe reaction is pseudo first order with respect to picrate up to 30 mmol/L, with the majority of methods employing a concentration between 3 and 16 mmol/L. At concentrations above 6 mmol/L, the rate of color development becomes nonlinear, so a two-point fixed interval rather than a multiple-data-point approach is required.

Hydroxide concentration. The initial rate of reaction is pseudo first order with respect to hydroxide concentrations above 0.5 mmol/L; however, at 500 mmol/L there is an increased degradation of the Jaffe complex. Furthermore, at hydroxide concentrations above 200 mmol/L, the blank absorbance increases significantly.

Wavelength. Although the absorbance maximum of the Jaffe reaction is between 490 and 500 nm, improved method linearity and reduced blank values have been reported at other wavelengths, the choice varying with hydroxide concentration.

Temperature. The rate of Jaffe complex formation and the absorptivity of the complex are temperature dependent, measurable differences being observed even between 25 °C and 37 °C. Consequently, temperature control is an important component of assay reproducibility.

Other chemical approaches to the measurement of creatinine have been tried. These include (1) reaction with

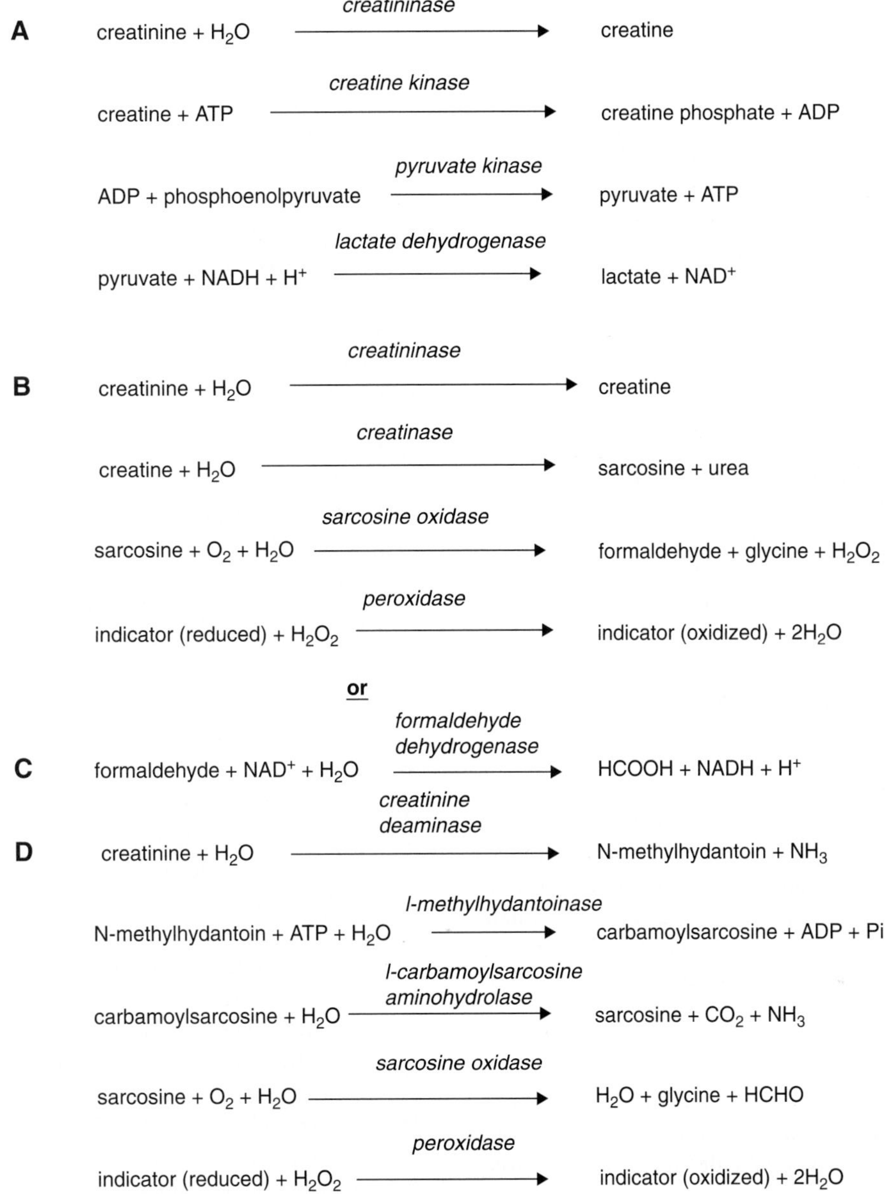

Figure 24-1 Determination of creatinine using a variety of enzymatic methods. For further details, see text.

1,4-naphthoquinone-2-sulfonate; (2) use of *o*-nitrobenzaldehyde to convert creatinine to methylguanidine and its reaction with α-naphthol and sodium hypochlorite under alkaline conditions,[226] and (3) reaction with 3,5-dinitrobenzoic acid.[158] None of these reactions are widely used in clinical laboratories.

Enzymatic Methods

Enzymes from a number of metabolic pathways have been investigated for the enzymatic measurement of creatinine. All of the methods involve a multistep approach leading to a photometric equilibrium (Figure 24-1). There are primarily three approaches, described below.[69,70,216,229]

Creatininase

The enzyme creatininase (EC 3.5.2.10; creatinine amidohydrolase) catalyzes the conversion of creatinine to creatine. The creatine is then detected with a series of enzyme-mediated reactions involving creatine kinase, pyruvate kinase, and lactate dehydrogenase, with monitoring of the decrease in absorbance at 340 nm (Figure 24-1, *A*). Initiating the reaction with creatininase allows for the removal of endogenous creatine and pyruvate in a preincubation reaction. The kinetics of the reaction are poor, and a 30-minute incubation is required to allow the reaction to reach equilibrium. This shortcoming can be overcome by a kinetic approach but with a further reduction in sensitivity. The approach has not been popular, partly because of poor sensitivity, poor precision, and the relatively high cost of reagents.[229]

Creatininase and Creatinase

An alternative, more popular, approach has used the enzyme creatinase (EC 3.5.3.3; creatine amidinohydrolase), which yields sarcosine and urea, the former being measured with further enzyme-mediated steps using sarcosine oxidase (EC 1.5.3.1; yielding glycine, formaldehyde, and hydrogen peroxide) and peroxidase (Figure 24-1, *B*).[69] The hydrogen peroxide has been detected with a variety of methods. Care must be taken to watch for interference (e.g., by bilirubin) in the final reaction sequence. This problem has been approached with the addition of potassium ferricyanide (with limited success) or bilirubin oxidase. The potential interference caused by ascorbic acid can be overcome by the inclusion of ascorbate oxidase. The influence of endogenous intermediate creatine and urea can be overcome by a preincubation step, initiating the reaction with creatininase. This system has been incorporated in a point-of-care testing device using polarographic detection.[184] An alternative detection system involves measurement of the reduction of nicotinamide adenine dinucleotide (NAD) by formaldehyde in the presence of formaldehyde dehydrogenase (Figure 24-1, *C*).[210]

Creatinine Deaminase

Creatinine deaminase (EC 3.5.4.21; creatinine iminohydrolase) catalyzes the conversion of creatinine to N-methylhydantoin and ammonia.[216] Early methods concentrated on the detection of ammonia using either glutamate dehydrogenase or the Berthelot reaction.[134] An alternative approach involves the enzyme N-methylhydantoin amidohydrolase (Figure 24-1, *D*).[70]

Dry Chemistry Systems

A number of multilayer dry reagent methods have been described for the measurement of creatinine using enzyme-mediated reactions. An early "two-slide" approach employed creatinine deaminase, with the ammonia diffusing through a semipermeable and optically opaque layer to react with bromophenol blue to give an increase in absorbance at 600 nm. A second multilayer film lacking the enzyme was used to quantitate endogenous ammonia, enabling blank correction.[212] A later single-slide method used the creatininase-creatinase reaction sequence[136]: lidocaine metabolites have been reported to interfere with this method.[197] The creatinine deaminase system described above has also been used and adapted for use as a point-of-care testing device (Figure 24-1, *D*).[83] In all cases, the color produced in the film is quantitated by reflectance.

A dry chemistry system has also been described in which a nonenzymatic approach was used, based on the reaction with 3,5-dinitrobenzoic acid.[207]

Other Methods

A definitive method employing isotope-dilution mass spectrometry (MS) has been described.[235] A candidate reference method for creatinine linked to this definitive method uses isocratic ion-exchange high-performance liquid chromatography (HPLC) with ultraviolet (UV) detection at 234 nm.[4] A reagent-free midinfrared method for urinary creatinine measurement has been described.[198]

Quality Issues with Creatinine Methods

Different methods for assaying plasma creatinine have varying degrees of accuracy and imprecision. With the advent of automated kinetic analysis, within-laboratory, between-day imprecision of approximately 3.0% can be expected at pathological concentrations, with slightly inferior performance within the reference interval.[22] This is still outside desirable performance standards defined in terms of biological variation.[205] Additionally, accuracy remains a major issue. Reference intervals for creatinine clearance and clearance calculated from one of several formulas (see below) will clearly vary depending on the accuracy of the creatinine measurement used in their calculation. The more a method overestimates "true" creatinine, the greater will be the underestimation of the glomerular filtration rate (GFR), and vice versa. As a result of reaction with noncreatinine chromogens, end-point Jaffe methods were typically judged to overestimate true plasma creatinine concentration by approximately 20% at physiological concentrations. Consequently, kinetic, enzymatic, and chromatographic methods can produce creatinine measurements approximately 20% lower than early Jaffe methods. However, since this could result in a relative overestimation of GFR (for example when measuring or calculating clearance), many reagent and instrument manufacturers have calibrated their assays to produce higher plasma creatinine results. As a consequence, many commercially available creatinine methods continue to demonstrate an approximately 20% positive bias compared with HPLC or isotope-dilution MS methods, particularly at concentrations within the reference intervals.[21,35,124] This calibration is not standardized, leading to variation between laboratories. Indeed, a College of American Pathologists survey reports that systematic differences in the calibration of plasma creatinine assays account for 85% of the observed differences between laboratories.[182] Proficiency studies demonstrate that although between-laboratory coefficients of variation (CVs) of <3% are achievable within method groups, overall between-laboratory agreement across methods is much poorer.[35,124] Systematic variation between laboratories of 0.2 to 0.4 mg/dL (18 to 36 μmol/L) is common.[92,124,146] Further, interlaboratory and within-laboratory agreement deteriorates as plasma creatinine concentration nears the reference interval: the exponential relationship between plasma creatinine and GFR means that imprecision at lower creatinine concentrations contributes to greater error in GFR estimation than at higher creatinine concentrations.

Clearly, standardization of creatinine measurement is crucial to the ability to accurately diagnose, stage, and manage CKD. Further, it is a prerequisite to the meaningful interpretation of epidemiological studies to facilitate health-care planning.[92] Not surprisingly, there have been calls for the use of an international standard to be used when calibrating plasma creatinine assays.[146] Although undoubtedly desirable, there remain practical barriers to implementation. Matrix problems have been identified when lyophilized preparations with isotope-dilution MS-authenticated creatinine concentrations have been used.[35,124] It is clear that serum- or protein-based human material must be used to calibrate creatinine assays, particularly Jaffe-based ones, but this introduces its own inherent problems, such as differing reactivities of the noncreatinine chromogens in the different Jaffe variations. Further, realignment with an authenticated standard will produce results significantly lower than those to which clinicians are accustomed. This will impact not only on the plasma reference interval, but also on the results of calculated and measured clearance estimates, which will therefore require their own realignment.

Reference Intervals

In summary, the methodology for the measurement of creatinine is complex by virtue of the number of variants of the Jaffe reaction and the innovations attempted using enzymatic procedures to overcome the limitations of the former. Although the enzymatic methods are more expensive, they are used in dry chemistry systems (with their lower reagent requirement) including some point-of-care testing devices. Kinetic Jaffe approaches predominate in wet chemistry analytical systems. Any laboratorian assessing a new creatinine method (e.g., as part of an analyzer purchase) should review the data for that method on interference caused by bilirubin, protein, glucose, and ketones and/or ketoacids. Bilirubin will also be particularly important in enzymatic procedures that generate hydrogen peroxide. Despite criticism of the Jaffe methods, there is invariably a good correlation between them and enzymatic procedures, with the differences likely to be due as much to calibration as to interference.

Given the discussion above, reference intervals for plasma creatinine are clearly method dependent.* Typically, reference intervals for plasma creatinine, measured by Jaffe methods, are 0.9 to 1.3 mg/dL (80 to 115 µmol/L) in men and 0.6 to 1.1 mg/dL (53 to 97 µmol/L) in women.[222] Plasma creatinine concentration in patients with untreated end-stage renal disease (ESRD) may exceed 11 mg/dL (1000 µmol/L). Reference intervals for plasma creatinine are also listed in Chapter 56.

Urinary creatinine excretion is higher in men (14 to 26 mg/kg/day, 124 to 230 µmol/kg/day) than in women (11 to 20 mg/kg/day, 97 to 177 µmol/kg/day). Creatinine excretion decreases with age; typically, for a 70-kg man, creatinine excretion will decline from approximately 1640 to 1030 mg/day (14.5 to 9.1 mmol/day) with advancing age from 30 to 80 years.[164] Measurement of urinary creatinine excretion can be a useful indication of the completeness of a timed urine collection.

*References 73, 202, 203, 209, 239, 241.

UREA

Catabolism of proteins and nucleic acids results in the formation of urea and ammonia—the so-called nonprotein nitrogenous compounds.

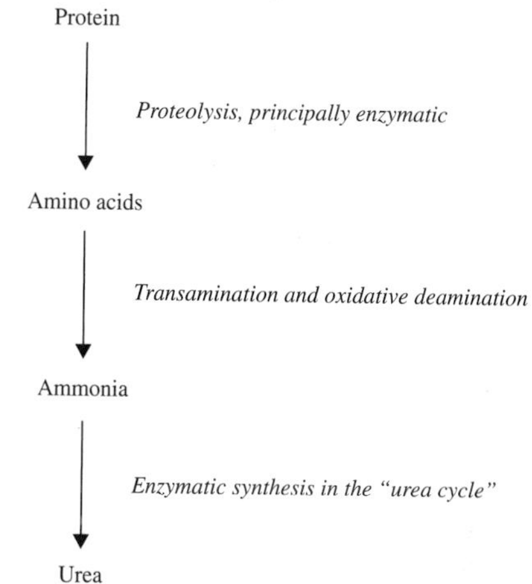

Biochemistry and Physiology

Urea ($CO[NH_2]_2$) is the major nitrogen-containing metabolic product of protein catabolism in humans, accounting for more than 75% of the nonprotein nitrogen eventually excreted. The biosynthesis of urea from amino nitrogen-derived ammonia is carried out exclusively by hepatic enzymes of the urea cycle. During the process of protein catabolism, amino acid nitrogen is converted to urea in the liver by the action of the so-called urea cycle enzymes (Figure 24-2).

More than 90% of urea is excreted through the kidneys, with losses through the gastrointestinal tract and skin accounting for most of the remaining minor fraction. Consequently, kidney disease is associated with accumulation of urea in blood. An increase in plasma urea concentration characterizes the uremic (azotemic) state. Urea is neither actively reabsorbed nor secreted by the tubules but is filtered freely by the glomeruli. In a normal kidney, 40% to 70% of the highly diffusible urea moves passively out of the renal tubule and into the interstitium, ultimately to reenter plasma. The back diffusion of urea is also dependent on urine flow rate, with less entering the interstitium in high-flow states (e.g., pregnancy) and vice versa. Consequently, urea clearance generally underestimates GFR. In stage 5 CKD, the osmotic diuresis in the remaining functional nephrons limits the back diffusion of urea so that urea clearance approaches inulin clearance. Measurement of blood and plasma urea has been used for many years as an indicator of kidney function. However, it is generally accepted that creatinine measurement provides better information in this respect. Plasma and urinary urea measurement may still provide useful clinical information in particular circum-

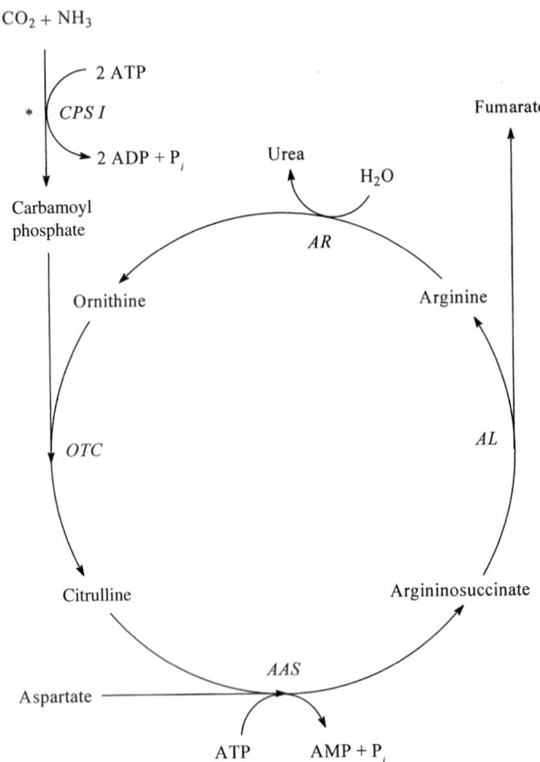

Figure 24-2 The urea cycle pathway. *CPS I*, Carbamyl phosphate synthetase I; *N-acetylglutamate as positive allosteric effector; *OTC*, ornithine transcarbamylase; *AAS*, argininosuccinate synthetase; *AL*, argininosuccinate lyase; *AR*, arginase; *ADP*, adenosine diphosphate, *ATP*, adenosine triphosphate, P_i, inorganic phosphate.

stances, and the measurement of urea in dialysis fluids is widely used in assessing the adequacy of renal replacement therapy (see Chapter 45).

Clinical Significance

A number of extrarenal factors influence the circulating urea concentration, limiting its value as a test of kidney function. For example, plasma urea concentration is increased by a high-protein diet, increased protein catabolism, reabsorption of blood proteins after gastrointestinal hemorrhage, treatment with cortisol or its synthetic analogues, dehydration, and with decreased perfusion of the kidneys (e.g., heart failure). In the above prerenal situations, the plasma creatinine concentration may be normal. In obstructive postrenal conditions (e.g., malignancy, nephrolithiasis, and prostatism), both plasma creatinine and urea concentrations will be increased, although in these situations there is often a greater increase in plasma urea than creatinine because of the increased back diffusion. These considerations give rise to the principal clinical utility of plasma urea, which lies in its measurement in conjunction with that of plasma creatinine and subsequent calculation of the urea nitrogen/creatinine ratio. This can be used as a crude discriminator between prerenal and postrenal azotemia. For a normal individual on a normal diet, the reference interval for the ratio is between 12 and 20 mg urea/mg creatinine (49 and 81 mol urea/mol creatinine). Significantly lower ratios usually denote acute tubular necrosis, low protein intake, starvation, or severe liver disease (decreased urea synthesis). Increased plasma urea with *normal* creatinine concentrations giving rise to high ratios may be seen with any of the prerenal states described above. High ratios associated with *elevated* creatinine concentrations may denote either postrenal obstruction or prerenal azotemia superimposed on kidney disease.

Urea clearance is a poor indicator of GFR, as its production rate is dependent on several nonrenal factors, including diet and the activity of the urea cycle enzymes. A high-protein diet causes significant increases in urinary urea excretion. In addition, the variable amount of back diffusion will influence both plasma and urinary urea concentration.[110] The measurement of urinary urea has little place in clinical diagnosis and management; however, it does provide a crude index of overall nitrogen balance and may be used as a guide to replacement in patients receiving parenteral nutrition. On an average protein diet, urinary excretion expressed as urea nitrogen is 12 to 20 g/day.

Although *blood urea nitrogen* (BUN) continues to be used for ordering the plasma urea nitrogen test, this terminology is incorrect and obsolete, because blood is rarely analyzed for urea. The long-established habit of reporting and expressing results of a urea assay in units of urea nitrogen appears to be strongly entrenched in the United States, although the SI system recommends use of urea, expressed in mmol/L. Thus it behooves students of clinical chemistry to have in mind the conversion factors for urea to urea nitrogen. Because 60 g (1 g molecular weight) of urea contains 28 g (2 g atomic weight) of nitrogen, the factor is 0.467 for converting urea mass units to those of urea nitrogen, and 2.14 for converting urea nitrogen mass units to those of urea. The factor for converting urea nitrogen in mg/dL to urea in mmol/L is 0.357.

Analytical Methodology

Chemical and enzymatic methods are the two principal approaches that have been used to quantify urea in body fluids.

Chemical Methods

Most chemical methods for urea are based on the Fearon reaction in which diacetyl condenses with urea to form the chromogen diazine, which absorbs strongly at 540 nm.

$$(H_2N)_2C{=}O + H_3C{-}CO{-}CO{-}CH_3 \xrightarrow[\text{heat}]{H^{\oplus}} \text{Diazine} + 2\,H_2O$$

Urea Diacetyl Diazine

Because diacetyl is unstable, it is usually generated in the reaction system from diacetyl monoxime and acid. Although once widely used, the method has largely been superseded by enzymatic approaches. For a more detailed description of direct urea measurement, the reader is referred to a review by Taylor and Vadgama.[217]

Enzymatic Methods

Enzymatic methods for the measurement of urea are based on preliminary hydrolysis of urea with urease (urea amidohydrolase, EC 3.5.1.5; main source jack bean meal) to generate ammonium ion, which is then quantified. This approach has been used in end-point, kinetic, conductimetric, and dry chemistry systems.[217]

$$(H_2N)_2C{=}O + 2\,H_2O \xrightarrow{\text{Urease}} 2\,NH_4^{\oplus} + CO_3^{\ominus\ominus}$$

Urea

Spectrophotometric approaches to ammonium quantitation include the *Berthelot reaction* and the *enzymatic assay* with glutamate dehydrogenase [L-glutamate: NAD(P) oxidoreductase (deaminating), EC 1.4.1.3].[188] This latter approach has been accepted as a reference method[189] and adapted to a range of analytical platforms.

$$NH_4^{\oplus} + \text{2-Oxoglutarate} \xrightarrow[\text{NADH} + H^{\oplus} \;\rightarrow\; NAD^{\oplus}]{\text{Glutamate dehydrogenase}} \text{Glutamate} + H_2O$$

For plasma assays, the reaction system is usually formulated with urease so that the addition of sample containing urea starts the reaction. A decrease in absorbance resulting from the glutamate dehydrogenase reaction is monitored at 340 nm. In another example of a coupled-enzyme assay system for urea, ammonia produced from urea by urease then reacts with glutamate and adenosine triphosphate (ATP) in the presence of glutamine synthetase (EC 6.3.1.2). Adenosine diphosphate (ADP) produced in this second enzymatic reaction is then quantitated in a third and fourth step using pyruvate kinase (EC 2.7.1.40) and pyruvate oxidase (EC 1.2.3.3), respectively, thus generating peroxide. In the final step, peroxide reacts with phenol and 4-aminophenazone, catalyzed by peroxidase (EC 1.11.1.7), to yield a quinone-monoamine dye that can be quantitated spectrophotometrically.[127]

Methods for the measurement of urea using dry chemistry systems have been described using the urease approach and a range of detection methods.[170,204] Urea has also been measured using a conductimetric method in which a sample and a urease-containing reagent are incubated in a conductivity cell with the rate of change of the conductivity being monitored as the urea is converted to an ionic species. In a potentiometric approach an ammonium ion-selective electrode is employed and the urease is immobilized on a membrane.[183] This principle has been applied in the NOVA 12 (NOVA Biomedical, Waltham, Mass.),[82] i-STAT (i-STAT Abbott Diagnostics, Chicago),[141] and AVL OMNI (Roche Diagnostics Ltd., Lewes, East Sussex, UK) analytical systems. A similar approach has been used to enable real-time monitoring of dialysis efficiency.[74] Alternative enzymatic approaches to the measurement of urea have more recently been described. Morishita et al[143] have described a system incorporating leucine dehydrogenase (EC 1.4.1.9), in addition to urease, which eliminates interference from endogenous ammonium.

The specificity of all of the methods is good, particularly for the urease-glutamate dehydrogenase procedure; however, endogenous ammonia interference must be expected when the protocol employs the sample to initiate the reaction. This may be relevant in aged samples, in some urines, and in particular metabolic disorders. Typically, within-run CVs of less than 3.0% with between-day values of less than 4.0% are achievable in the concentration range of 14 to 20 mg/dL (5 to 7 mmol/L). Given the high intrinsic biological variation of plasma urea, this is well within desired standards of analytical performance.[217]

Other Methods

An improved isotope-dilution MS method for plasma urea measurement has recently been proposed as a reference method.[113] As discussed above, laboratory urea measurements using standard enzymatic techniques are generally of an acceptable quality for most clinical purposes. New approaches to urea measurement are generally targeted at novel clinical applications, including point-of-care testing. For example, Eddy and Arnold[58] have developed a near-infrared spectroscopy technique for measuring urea in hemodialysis fluids. This would facilitate noninvasive monitoring of dialysis efficacy in real time. A novel enzymatic assay described by Naslund et al,[145] using luminometric detection, demonstrates sensitivity, which would make the method suitable for in vivo monitoring studies using microdialysis techniques.

Reference Intervals

The reference interval for plasma urea nitrogen in healthy adults is 6 to 20 mg/dL (2.1 to 7.1 mmol/L expressed as urea).[221] In adults more than 60 years of age, the reference interval is 8 to 23 mg/dL (2.9 to 8.2 mmol/L). Plasma concentrations tend to be slightly lower in children and in pregnancy and slightly higher in males than in females. Plasma urea concentrations in a patient with untreated ESRD typically reach 108 to 135 mg/dL (40.0 to 50.0 mmol/L).

URIC ACID

Biochemistry and Physiology

In humans, uric acid (2,6,8-trihydroxypurine) is the major product of the catabolism of the purine nucleosides adenosine and guanosine (Figure 24-3). Purines from catabolism of dietary nucleic acid are converted to uric acid directly. The bulk of purines excreted as uric acid arise from degradation of endogenous nucleic acids. The daily synthesis rate of uric acid is approximately 400 mg; dietary sources contribute

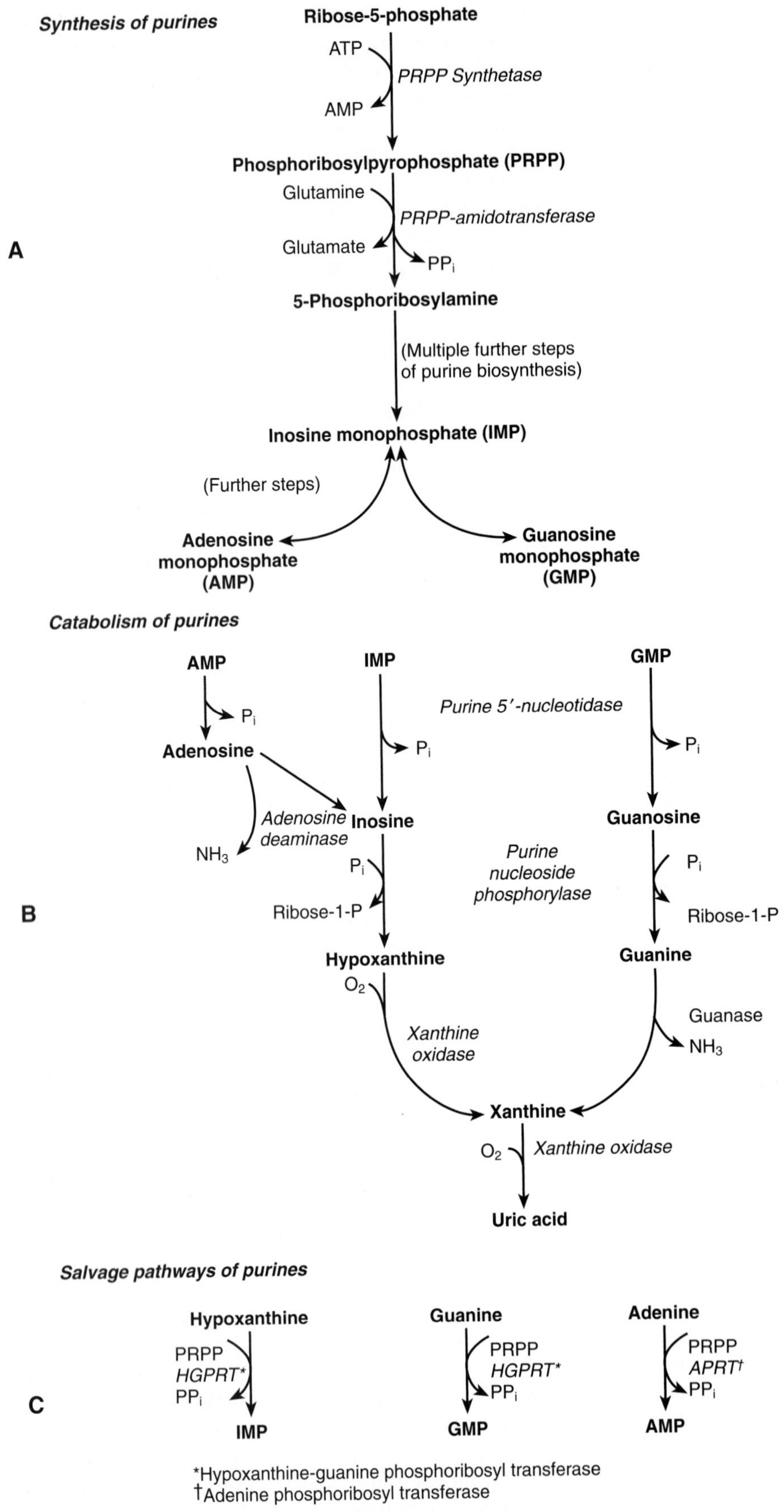

Synthesis of purines

A

Ribose-5-phosphate

ATP

AMP

PRPP Synthetase

Phosphoribosylpyrophosphate (PRPP)

Glutamine

Glutamate

PRPP-amidotransferase

PP_i

5-Phosphoribosylamine

(Multiple further steps of purine biosynthesis)

Inosine monophosphate (IMP)

(Further steps)

Adenosine monophosphate (AMP)

Guanosine monophosphate (GMP)

Catabolism of purines

B

AMP **IMP** **GMP**

P_i

Purine 5′-nucleotidase

Adenosine

P_i

P_i

Adenosine deaminase

NH_3

Inosine

Guanosine

P_i

Ribose-1-P

Purine nucleoside phosphorylase

P_i

Ribose-1-P

Hypoxanthine

Guanine

O_2

Xanthine oxidase

Guanase

NH_3

Xanthine

O_2

Xanthine oxidase

Uric acid

Salvage pathways of purines

C

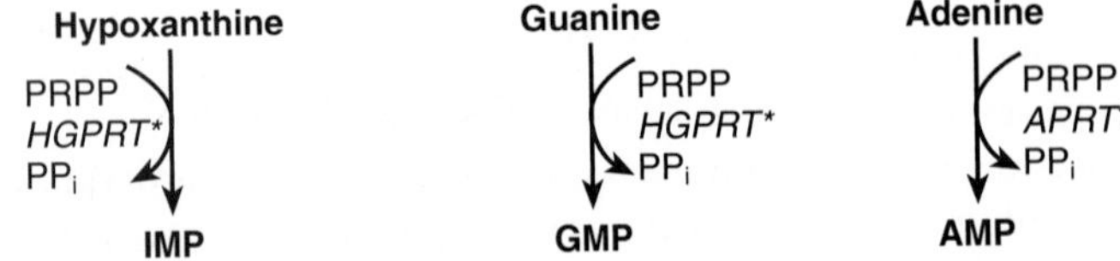

*Hypoxanthine-guanine phosphoribosyl transferase
†Adenine phosphoribosyl transferase

Figure 24-3 Metabolism of purines: **A,** synthesis; **B,** catabolism; and **C,** salvage pathways.

another 300 mg. In men consuming a purine-free diet, the total body pool of exchangeable urate is estimated at 1200 mg; in women it is estimated to be 600 mg. By contrast, patients with gouty arthritis and tissue deposition of urate may have urate pools as large as 18,000 to 30,000 mg.

Overproduction of uric acid may result from increased synthesis of purine precursors. Synthesis and metabolism of the major precursors are illustrated in outline in Figure 24-3. Formation of 5′-phosphoribosylamine is the second enzymatic step in the synthetic pathway (Figure 24-3, *A*); it is the first irreversibly committed step in purine biosynthesis. The intracellular concentration of the substrate phosphoribosylpyrophosphate (PRPP) regulates de novo purine synthesis. The enzyme PRPP-amidotransferase is controlled through feedback inhibition by the purine nucleotides that are the final products of the biosynthetic pathway. The first purine nucleotide formed by ring closure is inosine monophosphate (IMP); adenosine and guanosine monophosphates are derived from IMP through enzymatically mediated interconversions. Adenine and guanine nucleotides may then be used as precursors for the corresponding nucleosides that are the building blocks of deoxyribonucleic acid (DNA) and ribonucleic acid (RNA), or, when further phosphorylated, these nucleotides become carriers of high-energy bonds in the form of ATP and guanosine triphosphate (GTP).

Catabolism of the nucleotides (Figure 24-3, *B*) begins with removal of their ribose-linked phosphate, a process catalyzed by purine 5′-nucleotidase. Removal of the ribose moiety of inosine and guanosine by the action of purine-nucleoside phosphorylase forms hypoxanthine and guanine, both of which are converted to xanthine. Xanthine is converted to uric acid through the action of xanthine oxidase.

Reutilization of the major purine bases adenine, hypoxanthine, and guanine, is achieved through "salvage" pathways (Figure 24-3, *C*), in which phosphoribosylation of the free bases causes resynthesis of the respective nucleotide monophosphates. Adenine is converted to adenosine monophosphate (AMP) through the action of adenine phosphoribosyl transferase (APRT), hypoxanthine, and guanine to their monophosphates through hypoxanthine-guanine phosphoribosyl transferase (HGPRT). The HGPRT pathway is quantitatively more important than the APRT pathway.[236]

Lower primates and mammals other than humans carry purine metabolism one step further with the formation of allantoin from uric acid, a step mediated by uricase ([urate: oxygen] oxidoreductase, EC 1.7.3.3). In humans, approximately 75% of uric acid excreted is lost in the urine; most of the remainder is secreted into the gastrointestinal tract, where it is degraded to allantoin and other compounds by bacterial enzymes.

Renal handling of uric acid is complex and involves four sequential steps: (1) glomerular filtration of virtually all the uric acid in capillary plasma entering the glomerulus; (2) reabsorption in the proximal convoluted tubule of about 98% to 100% of filtered uric acid; (3) subsequent secretion of uric acid into the lumen in the distal portion of the proximal tubule; and (4) further reabsorption in the distal tubule. The net urinary excretion of uric acid is 6% to 12% of the amount filtered.

The physicochemical properties of uric acid are important in considering uric acid concentrations in the circulation, in tissue, and in the kidneys. The first pK_a of uric acid is 5.57; above this pH, uric acid exists chiefly as urate ion, which is more soluble than uric acid.[236] At a urine pH below 5.75, uric acid is the predominant form.

Clinical Significance

More than 20 inherited disorders of purine metabolism giving rise to both hypouricemias and hyperuricemias have been recognized to date. Most are very rare and the diagnosis requires support from a specialist purine laboratory. Symptoms that should raise suspicion include kidney failure or stones in a child or young adult; "gravel" in an infant's diaper; unexplained neurological problems in an infant, child, or adolescent; and gout presenting in a man or woman less than 30 years old.

Hyperuricemia

Hyperuricemia is most commonly defined by plasma uric acid concentrations greater than 7.0 mg/dL (0.42 mmol/L) in men or greater than 6.0 mg/dL (0.36 mmol/L) in women. The major causes of hyperuricemia are summarized in Box 24-1. Asymptomatic hyperuricemia is frequently detected through biochemical screening; long-term follow-up of asymptomatic hyperuricemic patients is undertaken because many are at risk for kidney disease that may develop as a result of hyperuricemia and hyperuricuria; few of these patients ever develop the clinical syndrome of gout.[196]

Measurement of plasma uric acid is predominantly used in the investigation of gout, either as a result of a primary hyperuricemia or caused by other conditions or treatments that give rise to secondary hyperuricemias. It is also used in the diagnosis and monitoring of pregnancy-induced hypertension (preeclamptic toxemia).

Gout occurs when monosodium urate precipitates from supersaturated body fluids; the deposits of urate are responsible for the clinical signs and symptoms. Gouty arthritis may be associated with urate crystals in joint fluid and with deposits of crystals (tophi) in tissue surrounding the joint. The deposits may occur in other soft tissue as well, and wherever they occur they elicit an intense inflammatory response consisting of polymorphonuclear leukocytes and macrophages. The big toe (first metatarsophalangeal) joint is the classic site for gout. Gout is a condition characterized by occasional attacks and long periods of remission: it is important to appreciate that the plasma uric acid concentration is often normal during an acute attack. Kidney disease associated with hyperuricemia may take one or more of several forms: (1) gouty nephropathy with urate deposi-

BOX 24-1 Etiology of Hyperuricemia

Increased Formation

Primary

- Idiopathic
- Inherited metabolic disorders

Secondary

- Excess dietary purine intake
- Increased nucleic acid turnover (e.g., leukemia, myeloma, radiotherapy, chemotherapy, trauma)
- Psoriasis
- Altered ATP metabolism
- Tissue hypoxia
- Preeclampsia
- Alcohol

Decreased Excretion

Primary (idiopathic)

Secondary

- Acute or chronic kidney disease
- Increased renal reabsorption
- Reduced secretion
- Lead poisoning
- Preeclampsia
- Organic acids (e.g., lactate and acetoacetate)
- Salicylate (low doses)
- Thiazide diuretics
- Trisomy 21 (Down syndrome)

tion in renal parenchyma, (2) acute intratubular deposition of urate crystals, and (3) urate nephrolithiasis.[34]

Gout is classified as either primary or secondary. *Primary gout* is associated with "essential" hyperuricemia, which has a polygenic basis. In greater than 99% of cases, the cause is uncertain but is probably due to a combination of metabolic overproduction of purines (25% of patients have increased PRPP-amidotransferase activity), decreased renal excretion (80% of patients show decreased renal tubular secretion of uric acid), and increased dietary intake. Very rarely, primary gout is attributable to inherited defects of enzymes in the pathways of purine metabolism. The *Lesch-Nyhan syndrome* is characterized by complete deficiency of HGPRT (EC 2.4.2.8), the major enzyme of the purine salvage pathways. This X-linked genetic disorder is manifested clinically by mental retardation, abnormal muscle movements, and behavioral problems (self-mutilation and pathological aggressiveness). Patients may present in the first weeks of life with symptoms of crystalluria, acute kidney failure, and gout. Hyperuricemia, hyperuricuria, and markedly decreased activities of HGPRT in erythrocytes, fibroblasts, and other cells are present. Intracellular concentrations of PRPP and rates of purine synthesis are increased. Neurological symptoms of this syndrome may be related to decreased availability of purines to the developing brain, which has limited capacity for de novo purine synthesis and therefore relies on the purine salvage pathways to supply it with most of the purine nucleotides it requires. DNA technology has been applied to prenatal diagnosis in the first trimester using chorionic biopsy material. HGPRT assays on cultured fibroblasts obtained by amniocentesis may be used in the second trimester. Partial deficiency of HGPRT (severe X-linked gout) presents in adolescence or early adulthood as early gout, kidney failure, or nephrolithiasis. Increased concentrations of intracellular PRPP production with consequent increased uric acid concentrations can also occur owing to mutations in PRPP synthetase (EC 2.7.6.1.) (phosphoribosyl pyrophosphate synthetase superactivity), which is also inherited as an X-linked recessive trait. An autosomal dominant familial juvenile hyperuricemic nephropathy has also been recognized. Glucose-6-phosphatase deficiency also leads to hyperuricemia as a result of both overproduction and underexcretion of uric acid.

Secondary gout is a result of hyperuricemia attributable to several identifiable causes. Renal retention of uric acid may occur in acute or chronic kidney disease of any type or as a consequence of administration of drugs; diuretics, in particular, are implicated in the latter instance. Organic acidemia caused by increased acetoacetic acid in diabetic ketoacidosis or by lactic acidosis may interfere with tubular secretion of urate. Increased nucleic acid turnover and a consequent increase in catabolism of purines may be encountered in rapid proliferation of tumor cells and in massive destruction of tumor cells on therapy with certain chemotherapeutic agents.

Management of an acute attack of gout generally involves the use of nonsteroidal antiinflammatory drugs (NSAIDs). Patients should be advised to avoid foods that have a high purine content (e.g., liver, kidneys, red meat, and sardines) and drugs that affect urate excretion (thiazide diuretics and salicylates). Specific pharmacological interventions include the use of uricosuric drugs (e.g., probenecid and sulfinpyrazone), which enhance renal excretion of uric acid by blocking the carriers in the tubular cells that mediate reabsorption, or the xanthine oxidase inhibitor allopurinol. Measurement of urinary uric acid excretion is an aid in selecting appropriate treatment in this context. Patients excreting less than 600 mg/day (3.6 mmol/day) of uric acid are candidates for treatment with uricosuric drugs, which are contraindicated in patients with urate stones or kidney failure. Conversely, patients excreting more than 600 mg/day (3.6 mmol/day) are candidates for treatment with allopurinol. The NSAIDs azapropazone and tiaprofenic acid have a uricosuric effect and so have a place in both the long-term and acute management of gout.[201]

Kidney Stones.[56,87] About one in five patients with clinical gout also has urinary tract uric acid stones. Although plasma and urinary uric acid should be measured in stone formers, many uric acid stone formers do not demonstrate either hyperuricuria or hyperuricemia. However, this may reflect the use of reference intervals derived in a purine-rich, westernized society.[190] The etiology of uric acid stone formation also involves the passage of a persistently acid urine with loss of the postprandial alkaline tide.[34] Undissociated uric acid (pK_a 5.57) is relatively insoluble, whereas urate at pH 7.0 is greater than 10 times more soluble. Thus in patients with urinary pH persistently less than 6.0, normal urinary concentrations of uric acid will produce supersaturation. Measurement of urinary pH throughout the day can be useful.[190] Pure uric acid stones account for approximately 8% of all urinary tract stones and, unlike many of the calcium-containing stones, are radiolucent. Allopurinol is the mainstay of treatment of uric acid stones. Hyperuricuria is also a risk factor for calcium stone formation (see Chapter 45). Consequently, attempts to increase urinary pH with potassium alkali salts may be counterproductive as a result of increased calcium stone formation.

Preeclamptic Toxemia. This condition is associated with increasing plasma uric acid concentration, probably caused by uteroplacental tissue breakdown and decreased kidney perfusion.[62] Plasma urate measurement can be used as an indicator of the severity of preeclampsia. Redman et al[175] noted that concentrations in excess of 6.0 mg/dL (0.36 mmol/L) at 32 weeks gestation are associated with a high perinatal mortality rate.

Hypouricemia

Hypouricemia, often defined as plasma urate concentrations less than 2.0 mg/dL (0.12 mmol/L), is much less common than hyperuricemia. It may be secondary to any one of a number of underlying conditions. Severe hepatocellular disease with reduced purine synthesis or xanthine oxidase activity is one possibility. Another is defective renal tubular reabsorption of uric acid. Defective reabsorption may be congenital, as in generalized Fanconi's syndrome, or acquired. The reabsorption defect may be acquired acutely because of injection of radiopaque contrast media or chronically because of exposure to toxic agents. Overtreatment of hyperuricemia with allopurinol or uricosuric drugs and cancer chemotherapy with 6-mercaptopurine or azathioprine (inhibitors of de novo purine synthesis) may also cause hypouricemia. Very rarely, hypouricemia may occur as a result of an inherited metabolic defect. Hypouricemia in combination with xanthinuria is rarely encountered and suggests a deficiency of xanthine oxidase, either in isolation or as part of combined molybdenum cofactor deficiency (sulfite oxidase/xanthine oxidase deficiency). Purine nucleoside phosphorylase (EC 2.4.2.1) deficiency and other inherited defects have also been described. For further discussion of these, and the primary hyperuricemias, the reader is referred to specialist textbooks.[199]

Analytical Methodology

Phosphotungstic acid (PTA), uricase, and HPLC-based methods have been described for measuring uric acid.[169]

Phosphotungstic Acid Methods

These methods are based on the development of a blue reaction (tungsten blue) as PTA is reduced by urate in an alkaline medium; the color is read by spectrophotometry at wavelengths of 650 to 700 nm. PTA methods are subject to many interferences, and efforts to modify them have had little success in improving their specificity. The reader is referred to a review for a more detailed analysis.[169]

Uricase Methods

Uricase methods are more specific than PTA approaches. Uricase ([urate:oxygen] oxidoreductase; EC 1.7.3.3; main sources *Aspergillus flavus, Candida utilis, Bacillus fastidiosus,* and hog liver) is used either as a single step or as the initial step to oxidize uric acid. Uricase methods became feasible and popular as a result of the availability of high-quality, low-cost preparations of the bacterial enzyme. Preliminary precipitation of protein is not required. Generally, only guanine, xanthine, and a few other structural analogues of uric acid act as alternative substrates, and then only at concentrations improbable in biological fluids. Uricase methods have replaced PTA methods in most current instrumentation.

Uricase acts on uric acid to produce allantoin, hydrogen peroxide, and carbon dioxide.

$$\text{Urate} + O_2 \xrightarrow{\text{Uricase}} \text{Allantoin} + H_2O_2 + CO_2$$

The reaction can be observed in either the kinetic or the equilibrium mode. The *Bacillus fastidiosus* enzyme has the highest Michaelis constant (1.0×10^{-4} mol/L) and the hog liver has the lowest (1.7×10^{-5} mol/L), the choice of enzyme influencing the incubation period required to reach equilibrium and the conditions for a pseudo first-order kinetic approach. The decrease of absorbance as urate is converted may be monitored by a spectrophotometer at 293 nm and this forms the basis of a proposed reference procedure.[55] However, at this wavelength, most of the absorbance is due to plasma proteins. Therefore there is a high signal-noise ratio, which can compromise the precision of the method. A high quality spectrophotometer with narrow bandpass is required and this is rarely satisfied with automated analyzers.

Most current enzymatic assays for uric acid in plasma involve a peroxidase system coupled with one of a number of oxygen acceptors to produce a chromogen.[106,238] For example, one popular method measures hydrogen peroxide with the aid of horseradish peroxidase (donor:hydrogen-peroxide oxidoreductase; EC 1.11.1.7) and an oxygen acceptor to yield a chromogen in the visible spectrum.[68] Its popularity is probably due to the use of less expensive enzymes and greater analytical sensitivity. The most common oxygen acceptor used is 4-aminophenazone together with phenol or a substituted phenol. The benefit of using substituted phenols is the enhanced molar absorptivity: phenol ≈ 5.5×10^3 L · mol/cm, tribromo-phenol ≈ 23.6×10^3 L · mol/cm, and tribromo-3-hydroxybenzoic acid ≈ 30.0×10^3 L · mol/cm. Alternative oxygen acceptors include 3-methyl-1-benzothiazoline hydrazone (MBTH), 2,2′-azino-di-(3-ethyl-benzothiazoline)-6-sulfonate (ABTS), and *o*-dianisidine.

Although many combinations of oxygen acceptor and phenol have been described, the choice should be guided by minimization of interference and sufficient absorbance to ensure good precision. The use of a substituted phenol yielding a highly absorbing product helps to reduce the potential interference by reducing the sample volume requirement. The major interferants to minimize are ascorbic acid and bilirubin. In general it is necessary to employ ascorbate oxidase (L-ascorbate:oxygen oxidoreductase; EC 1.10.3.3) in uric acid methodology.[125] Use of aminophenazone with a substituted phenol or the addition of ferrocyanide[68,93] have been used to minimize bilirubin interference. Alternatively, use of the oxygen acceptor azure-D2 (3,7-diamino-5-pheno-thiazine (thionine) derivative), which can be monitored at 600 nm, reduces the spectral but not the chemical[243] interference caused by hyperbilirubinemia.[121] It has also been shown that unknown metabolites in plasma of patients with kidney failure, thought to be phenolic compounds, will interfere by competing with the reagent phenol, giving a low recovery of urate.[100] The interference can be overcome by using a phenolic derivative, thereby generating a higher absorbing product and reducing the sample volume.

Dry Chemistry Systems

Devices that use uricase in a dry reagent format to measure uric acid have also been described. For example, a multilayer film system employs uricase and peroxidase separated by a semipermeable membrane from a leuco dye that is oxidized to form a colored product.[105] A cellulose matrix pad system employs uricase, peroxidase, and MBTH as oxygen acceptor; the system employs a diluted plasma sample, which helps to reduce interferences, although ascorbic acid was shown to be a significant interferant.[107] A third system incorporates separation of plasma from red cells and uricase, peroxidase, and a substituted phenol to measure uric acid.[225] All three systems employ a reflectance meter system to facilitate accurate and precise quantitation of the color change.

Electrochemical and biosensor systems have also been described for the measurement of uric acid. In all cases uricase is employed, being linked in examples to an oxygen electrode[138] and to Teflon on the photomultiplier tube of a luminometer.[80]

HPLC Methods

HPLC methods using ion-exchange or reversed-phase columns have been used to separate and quantify uric acid. The column effluent is monitored at 293 nm to detect the eluting uric acid. HPLC methods are specific and fast, mobile phases are simple, and the retention time for uric acid is less than 6 minutes, reasonable conditions that recommend these methods for reference use.[94] A proposed definitive method for the assay of uric acid in plasma uses isotope-dilution MS.[60]

Reference Intervals

Although many methods for the quantitation of uric acid are described in the literature, the most popular methods today employ the uricase-mediated reaction; however, the specificity of this reaction may be compromised by the choice of detector reaction, owing to either an interfering enzyme or a molecule that competes in the final color generation step. Today reactions that generate a visible end product are preferred because of the higher color yield; however, care should be taken that interference caused by ascorbate, bilirubin, and unspecified interferants in plasma from patients with kidney failure is minimized.

Using an enzymatic method, the reference interval for uric acid has been reported to be 3.5 to 7.2 mg/dL (0.208 to 0.428 mmol/L) for males and 2.6 to 6.0 mg/dL (0.155 to 0.357 mmol/L) for females.[221] The concentration of plasma uric acid increases gradually with age, rising about 10% between the ages of 20 and 60 years. There is a rise in women after menopause, reaching concentrations similar to those in men. During pregnancy, plasma uric acid concentrations fall during the first trimester and until about 24 weeks of gestation, when concentrations begin to rise and eventually exceed nonpregnant concentrations.[36,130] Using an enzymatic assay, reference intervals at 32, 36, and 38 weeks of gestation have been reported as 1.9 to 5.5 mg/dL (0.110 to 0.322 mmol/L), 2.0 to 5.8 mg/dL (0.120 to 0.344 mmol/L), and 2.7 to 6.5 mg/dL (0.157 to 0.381 mmol/L), respectively.[130]

An alternative approach to the interpretation of plasma uric acid concentrations is to consider the degree of hyperuricemia in relation to the risk of developing gout; men with plasma uric acid concentrations exceeding 9.0 mg/dL (0.540 mmol/L) are approximately 150 times more likely to have coexisting gouty arthritis than are men with uric acid concentrations less than 6.0 mg/dL (0.360 mmol/L).[221]

Urinary uric acid excretion in individuals on a diet containing purines is 250 to 750 mg/day (1.5 to 4.5 mmol/day). Excretion may decrease by 20% to 25% on a purine-free diet to less than 400 mg/day.

SCREEENING FOR KIDNEY DISEASE

Urinalysis

Examination of the urine is often the first step in the assessment of a patient suspected of having, or confirmed to have, deterioration in kidney function. In the laboratory, urine is examined visually, chemically, and microscopically. New instrumental techniques are also being used to examine urine.

Visual Examination

The appearance (color and odor) of urine itself can be helpful, a darkening from the pale normal straw color indicating a more concentrated urine or the presence of another pigment. Hemoglobin and myoglobin can give a pink-red-brown coloration, depending on the concentration. Turbidity in a fresh sample may indicate infection but may also be due to fat particles in a patient with nephrotic syndrome. Excessive foaming of urine when shaken suggests proteinuria. Urine is often chemically evaluated with the help of dipstick tests, which are available for a variety of analytes or microscopically examined.

Dipstick Testing

Many tests of renal significance have been adapted for use on strips of cellulose or pads of cellulose on strips of plastic that have been coated or impregnated with reagents for the analyte in question.[148] This type of analytical test is known as a dipstick test. A dipstick may contain reagents for just one test per stick or reagents for multiple tests on a single stick. For example, up to 10 constituents are now measured on a single dipstick. With this type of test, the different methods detect substances that overflow into the urine, such as glucose, ketones, bilirubin diglucuronate, and urobilinogen, in which changes in the concentration reflect a change in another organ system in the body. These dipstick tests also detect changes in constituents that are more directly linked to alterations brought about by some pathological condition affecting the kidney or urinary tract. Urine samples for dipstick testing should be collected in sterile containers and dipstick testing performed on the fresh urine. Dipsticks should be used only if they have been stored properly desiccated, because they can deteriorate in a matter of hours. Examples of the method principles and comments on the performance of tests pertinent to the assessment of kidney function are given below. In 2003 Clarke and Palmer-Toy[41] have reviewed the literature on outcomes achieved with dipstick urinalysis.

Total Protein

The dipstick test for total protein includes a cellulose test pad impregnated with tetrabromphenol blue and a citrate pH 3 buffer. The reaction is based on the "protein error of indicators" phenomenon in which certain chemical indicators demonstrate one color in the presence of protein and another in its absence. Thus tetrabromphenol blue is green in the presence of protein at pH 3 but yellow in its absence. The color is read after exactly 60 s and the test has a lower detection limit of 150 to 300 mg/L, depending on the type and proportions of protein present. The reagent is most sensitive to albumin and less sensitive to globulins, Bence Jones protein, mucoproteins, and hemoglobin.

Proteinuria is a common finding in patients with kidney disease, and the use of a dipstick assay is an important screening test in any patient suspected of having renal disease. Among patients with suspected or proven CKD, including reflux nephropathy and early glomerulonephritis, and those with hypertension or previously detected asymptomatic hematuria, annual urinalysis for proteinuria is accepted as a useful way of identifying patients at risk of progressive kidney disease. The test has also been used in a number of screening programs in schoolchildren.[140,249] Although these studies have indicated an incidence of about 0.1%, there has been no systematic follow-up of patients to ascertain whether the appearance of protein in the urine is an early predictor of kidney disease.[144] There is currently no proven role for dipstick protein urinalysis in screening of unselected populations.[146,244] Whether it will prove useful in identifying patients at risk of CKD in selected high-risk populations, for instance some ethnic minority populations, remains uncertain. Dipstick testing for proteinuria is inadequate for the detection of CKD among patients with diabetes, who should undergo annual testing for microalbuminuria (see below).

Protein excretion displays considerable biological variability, and may be increased by upright posture, exercise, fever, heart failure, and kidney disease. Because standard urine dipsticks rely on estimation of protein concentration, that in turn depends on hydration or how concentrated the urine sample is; these tests can only give a rough indication of the presence or absence of pathological proteinuria. The specificity of urinalysis protein dipsticks for the detection of proteinuria is approximately 85%[12] and misclassification errors are common. Therefore positive dipstick tests should be confirmed in the laboratory by measuring either the protein/creatinine or albumin/creatinine ratio on an early morning or random urine sample (Figure 24-4). A creatinine test pad (using the peroxidase-like activity of transition metal creatinine complexes) has been added to some strip systems to enable a ratio of protein (or albumin) to creatinine to be reported to reduce the intraindividual variation seen with random urine collections.[150]

Albumin

Dipstick methods are available for the more specific detection of albumin (and also myoglobin and some low molecular weight proteins). Both color-generating and immunological methods for albumin have been described for use with urine samples, the former based on binding of Bis (3′,3″-diiodo-4′,4″-hydroxy-5′,5″-dinitrophenyl)-3,4,5,6-tetrabromosulfonephthalein (DIDNTB) at pH 1.5.[174] The use of the color-generating albumin assay is intended to reduce the variation in reporting of small increases in protein excretion.[174]

Hemoglobin

The presence of hemoglobin in the urine may be due to glomerular, tubulointerstitial, or postrenal disease, although the latter two causes are the more common. The presence of blood in the urine can be detected by the use of a phase contrast microscope to determine the presence of red cells in the urine sediment or by use of a dipstick test. The chemical detection of hemoglobin in urine depends on the peroxidase activity of the protein, employing a peroxide substrate and an oxygen acceptor.[148]

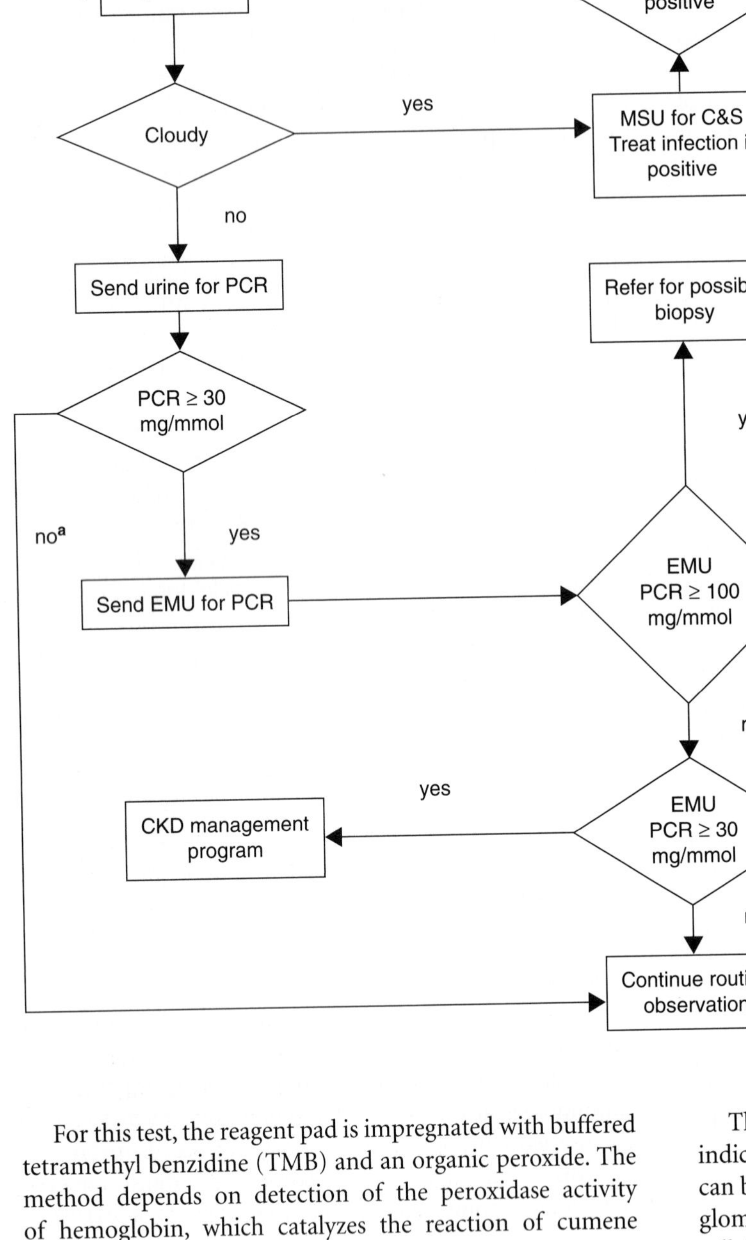

Figure 24-4 Suggested protocol for the further investigation of a positive (trace or above) dipstick or quantitative protein test. Dipstick testing devices show few false-negative results but many false-positive results; positive results should therefore be confirmed using laboratory testing on at least two further occasions. Patients with two or more positive (greater than or equal to 30 mg total protein or albumin/mmole creatinine) tests on early morning samples 1 to 2 weeks apart should be diagnosed as having persistent proteinuria. (The possibility of postural proteinuria should be excluded by the examination of an EMU.) Albumin/creatinine ratio (ACR) measurement can be substituted for the total protein/creatinine ratio. *C&S,* Culture and sensitivity; *CKD,* chronic kidney disease; *EMU,* early morning urine; *MSU,* mid-stream urine; *PCR,* protein/creatinine ratio.
[a]In the absence of a systemic disease, such as diabetes or hypertension, a borderline elevation in total protein or albumin excretion (3 to 30 mg/mmole), without hematuria or a rise in plasma creatinine, a serious primary renal pathology is unlikely. In a diabetic patient, lesser degrees of proteinuria may be significant and should elicit appropriate investigation and management (see "Urinary Albumin and Microalbuminuria Screening" section). *(Algorithm courtesy Dr. R. Burden, Nottingham City Hospital, Nottingham, UK.)*

For this test, the reagent pad is impregnated with buffered tetramethyl benzidine (TMB) and an organic peroxide. The method depends on detection of the peroxidase activity of hemoglobin, which catalyzes the reaction of cumene hydroperoxide and TMB. The color change varies from orange through pale to dark green, and red cells or free hemoglobin are detected together with myoglobin. Again the color of the reagent pad should be compared with a color chart after exactly 60 s. Two reagent pads are employed for the low hemoglobin concentration; if intact red cells are present, the low-concentration pad will have a speckled appearance, with a solid color indicating hemolyzed red cells. The detection limit for free hemoglobin is 150 to 600 μg/L or 5 to 20 intact red cells/μL. The test is equally sensitive to hemoglobin and to myoglobin. Water must not be used as a negative control with this test caused by the matrix requirements of the assay, and will give a false-positive result.

The presence of free hemoglobin or red cells in the urine indicates the presence of renal or bladder disease. Hematuria can be present in a number of kidney diseases, including (1) glomerular nephritis, (2) polycystic kidney disease, (3) sickle cell disease, (4) vasculitis, and (5) several infections. A spectrum of urological diseases may also give rise to hematuria, including bladder, prostate, and pelvic and/or ureteral malignancy, kidney stones, trauma, bladder damage, and ureteral stricture.

Glucose

For glucose measurements, the reagent pad is impregnated with glucose oxidase, peroxidase, potassium iodide, and a blue dye. The reaction employs glucose oxidase and peroxidase to produce hydrogen peroxide, which is subsequently reduced with a concurrent oxidation of potassium iodide to release iodine. The free iodine blends with the background color to produce a variety of colors from green to dark brown. The lower limit of detection for this method is 72 to 127 mg/dL (4.0 to 7.0 mmol/L) with an upper limit of 2018 mg/dL (111 mmol/L). The color change should be read exactly 30 s after sample addition.

Leukocytes

The dipstick test for leukocytes uses an absorbent cellulose pad impregnated with a buffered mixture of derivatized pyrrole amino acid ester and diazonium salt. Granulocytic leukocytes contain esterases that catalyze the hydrolysis of the derivatized pyrrole amino acid ester to liberate 3-hydroxy-5-phenylpyrrole. This pyrrole then reacts with a diazonium salt to produce a purple product. The color of the reagent pad is then compared with the color chart exactly 2 minutes after sample addition. The test is claimed to have a detection limit of 5 to 15 cells/μL in urine and the darkest color block is equivalent to 500 cells/μL or greater. A decrease on the true test result may occur in samples with an elevated glucose concentration, a high specific gravity, or the presence of cephaloxin, cephalothin, tetracycline, or high concentrations of oxalic acid.

Nitrite

To measure nitrite, the reagent pad is impregnated with *p*-arsanilic acid and tetrahydro-benzo(h)quinolin-3-ol. The reaction is based on arsanilic acid in the presence of nitrite converting to a diazonium salt, which couples with the quinolol to produce a pink color. The color should be read exactly 60 s after the sample addition and the detection limit of the test is 61 to 103 μg/dL (13 to 22 μmol/L) nitrite in urine with a normal specific gravity. The test is less sensitive with urine having a high specific gravity. At urine ascorbic acid concentrations above 24.7 mg/dL (1.4 mmol/L) a false-negative result may occur at low nitrite concentrations (81 μg/dL [13 μmol/L] or less). The test will only measure nitrite and is claimed to detect populations of bacteria at an amount of 10^5/mL or more.

The presence of leukocyte esterase is indicative of pyuria. The detection of nitrite is indicative of the presence of bacteria that degrade nitrate excreted in the urine. The combination of the two tests is valuable in patients with urinary tract infection. The absence of both constituents is a valuable test to "rule out" urinary tract infection, thereby reducing the number of samples sent to the laboratory for further tests. The nitrite test may be less helpful in young children in whom the urine remains in the bladder for less time, thereby limiting the time for nitrite production.

Specific Gravity

The test device for specific gravity consists of an absorbent cellulose pad impregnated with bromthymol blue, polymethylvinyl ether and/or maleic anhydride, and sodium hydroxide. The test depends on the apparent pK_a change of the pretreated polyelectrolyte in relation to ionic strength; the hydrogen ions released are detected by the pH indicator. The color changes from a dark blue at a low specific gravity (1.000) to yellow-green at a specific gravity of 1.030. The test is claimed to correlate within 0.005 of refractive index– and hydrometer-derived values; a value of 0.005 can be added to adjust for pH effects above 6.5. In a machine-readable form of the assay (Clinitek System, Bayer Diagnostics, Elkhart, Ind.), automatic adjustment for pH is made (using the data from the pH pad). It is important that the test be read exactly at the time stated (typically 45 s after sample addition). The specific gravity can provide an indication of the concentration of urine; care must be taken with interpretation depending on the method principle because those that detect ionic species will underestimate the specific gravity in the presence of glucose and so forth. Urine collected after intravenous administration of iodine-containing radiopaque compounds for radiological studies may give extraordinarily high values. Glucose and protein may also contribute substantial increments to the density of urine, and semiquantitative determination of these substances is necessary for valid interpretation or correction of urine specific gravity measurements. Diabetic patients with uncontrolled hyperglycemia and glucosuria may have high urine specific gravity even when the normal renal concentrating function is seriously impaired.

pH

To measure the pH of a sample, the test pad is impregnated with indicators—one example being a mixture of methyl red and bromthymol blue. Methyl red in a diluted form is red at pH values below 4.2 and yellow at values above 6.2. Bromthymol blue is yellow at pH values below 6.0 and blue at values above 7.6. At pHs within these values, the indicators give shades of orange and green, respectively. Thus the reagent blocks are evaluated at exactly 60 s and compared with a color chart where the lowest pH block at 5.0 is orange in color and the highest at 8.5 is blue. It is important to recognize that the pH of urine alters with standing and the color of the reagent blocks with time also; therefore careful adherence to the recommended procedure is important. The measurement of urine pH can be helpful in the assessment of patients with renal tubular acidosis and in stone formers, although evaluation using a pH electrode may be more informative.

Microscopic Examination of Urine

Microscopic examination of the sediment obtained from the centrifugation of a fresh urine sample will show the presence of a few cells (erythrocytes, leukocytes, and cells derived from the kidney and urinary tract), casts (composed predominantly of Tamm-Horsfall glycoprotein [THG]), and possibly fat or pigmented particles. An increase in red cells or casts implies hematuria, possibly caused by glomerular disease; white cells or casts imply the presence of white cells in the tubules. Inflammation of the upper urinary tract may result in polymorphonuclear leukocytes and various types of casts, and in lower urinary tract inflammation the casts will not be present. In acute glomerulonephritis, hematuria may lead to coloration of the urine and the presence of large numbers of red cells and white cells; as the duration of the disease increases, the amount of sediment diminishes.[67]

New Instrumental Techniques

Flow cytometry and flow imaging systems have been developed for the characterization of erythrocytes in the differential diagnosis of hematuria, together with a means of improving the recognition of other particulate material in urine. This form of analysis is now used to both discriminate between and quantify the particulate matter in a defined volume of urine, bringing the added benefit of better standardization of the technique.[157] Thus the flow imaging method can identify red blood cells, white blood cells, white blood cell clumps, hyaline casts, pathological casts, squamous epithelial cells, nonsquamous epithelial cells, yeast, crystals, and sperm. These fully automated systems have the potential to replace urinary microscopy,[247] because they offer better discriminatory power and quantitation while also offering closer agreement between laboratories. The principles of flow cytometry are described in Chapter 3. A flow imaging analyzer such as the Iris iQ200 analyzes unspun urine by aspirating sample through a flow cell positioned in a microscope. A digital camera containing a 1.3 megapixel charge coupled device (CCD) is used to capture the images, and neural network–based particle image recognition software is used to identify and count the particles present from 500, 884 × 680 micrometer fields with 0.68 resolution. The number of particles for the volume scanned is then calculated. The flow image analysis has been shown to be more accurate than the flow cytometric approach while also helping to save valuable technologist time by reducing the number of manual microscopic examinations required.[108,109]

Proton nuclear magnetic resonance (NMR) has also been investigated as a means of characterizing low molecular weight molecules.[147] Metabolic profiles have been generated and, using sophisticated computer analysis, distinctive patterns of molecules have been associated with damage to specific parts of the nephron. It is expected that this technique can be used to identify individual molecules for which selective assays can then be developed.[147]

QUANTITATIVE ASSESSMENT OF GLOMERULAR PERMEABILITY: PROTEINURIA

Clinical Significance

Higher molecular weight proteins are retained within the circulation by the glomerular filter, and lower molecular weight proteins are freely filtered and reabsorbed and catabolized within the tubular cells. Clinically, the appearance of significant amounts of protein in the urine suggests renal disease. Commonly, proteinuria is classified as either tubular or glomerular depending on the pattern of proteinuria observed. A third category, overflow proteinuria, is also recognized in which filtration of excessive amounts of low molecular weight protein exceeds the tubular capacity for reabsorption. Examples of the latter include Bence Jones proteinuria and myoglobinuria. Proteinuria is a potent risk marker for progressive kidney disease, and reduction of protein excretion is a therapeutic target. These aspects are considered further in Chapter 45. This section will consider the analytical approach and rationale used in the quantitation of urinary proteins, with emphasis on total protein and albumin measurement.

Sample Collection for Total Protein and Albumin Measurement

There has been extensive discussion in the literature about the appropriate urine sample to use for the investigation of protein excretion. It is generally recognized that a 24-hour sample is the definitive means of demonstrating the presence of proteinuria. However, overnight, first void in the morning (early morning urine [EMU]), second void in the morning, or random sample collections have also been used. Since creatinine excretion in the urine is fairly constant throughout the 24-hour period, measurement of protein/creatinine (or albumin/creatinine) ratios allows correction for variations in urinary concentration.[16,112] Several authors have recommended the use of the protein/creatinine ratio based on the good correlation that has been demonstrated with the 24-hour collection[40,77,187] and at least equivalent power as a predictor of the rate of loss of GFR in nondiabetic nephropathy.[187] Ginsberg et al studied this in detail and showed that there was little variation in the ratio during the daytime, indicating that the first void and either of the two subsequent collections can give a reliable indication of the 24-hour urine protein excretion. Newman et al[150] demonstrated a significant reduction in the intraindividual variation in the protein/creatinine ratio compared with the protein excretion in random urines collected throughout the day (a mean reduction to 38.6% from 96.5%). They found a similar experience with albumin excretion (52.1% from 80.0%).[150] The ratio to osmolality to correct for dilution effects associated with changes in the water excreted during the day has also been reported and that to specific gravity.[150] Saudan et al[192] found positive and negative predictive values of 95% and 90%, respectively, for the use of the protein/creatinine ratio for detecting proteinuria as defined by a 24-hour collection in hypertensive pregnant women. Dyson[57] found positive and negative predictive values of 81% and 96% in kidney transplant patients, suggesting that the random urine protein/creatinine ratio was a useful screening test for proteinuria. Claudi and Cooper[42] made similar observations on the use of the albumin/creatinine ratio in diabetic patients.

Although the reference point remains the accurately timed 24-hour specimen, it is widely accepted that this is a difficult procedure to control effectively; studies have shown that more than 25% of samples have to be discarded because an incomplete collection is suspected. In practice, for screening purposes, spot urine protein/creatinine ratios (or albumin/creatinine ratios) have been used to rule out the necessity for 24-hour collections.[146] An EMU sample is preferred since it correlates well with 24-hour protein excretion and is required to exclude the diagnosis of orthostatic (postural) proteinuria.[146] However, a random urine sample is acceptable if no early morning sample is available. If required, daily protein excretion (in mg/24 hours) can be roughly estimated by multiplying the protein/creatinine ratio (measured in mg/mmole) by a factor of 10 since, although daily excretion of creatinine depends on muscle mass, an average figure of 10 mmol creatinine per day can be assumed.[112] In practice, it is accepted that the use of this number will lead to overestimation of daily protein excretion among patients with low muscle mass and underestimation among patients with high muscle mass; in addition, there may be racial variation in creatinine excretion even after adjustment for muscle mass.[135]

A suitable protocol for the further investigation of patients found to have proteinuria at screening is given in Figure 24-4.

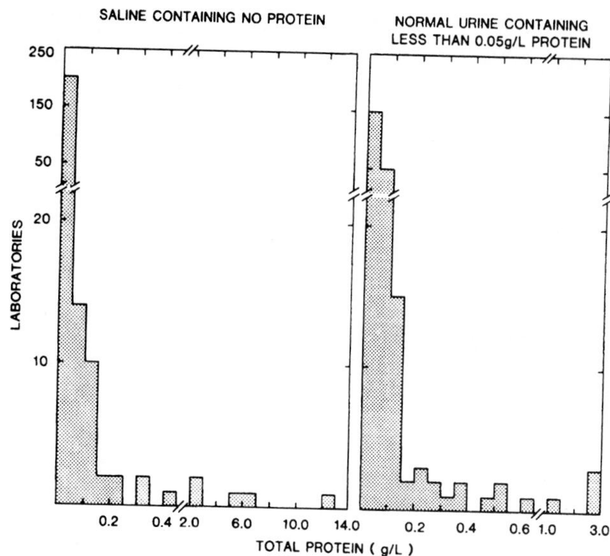

Figure 24-5 Frequency distribution of quantitative results combined with returns of "nil," "zero," or "not detected" for distributions of salt solution and normal urine. Quality control of total protein measurement demonstrates the widespread variation in results achieved using different methods. *(From Chambers RE, Bullock DG, Whicher JT. Urinary total protein estimation: Fact or fiction? Nephron 1989;53:33. Reproduced with permission of S. Karger AG, Basel, Switzerland.)*

Measurement of Total Protein

There are numerous methods used for the measurement of protein in urine (see Chapter 20). They include (1) the original Lowry method,[133] (2) turbidimetry after mixing with trichloroacetic or sulfosalicylic acid,[153] (3) turbidimetry with benzethonium chloride (benzyl dimethyl {2-[2-(*p*-1,1,3,3-tetramethyl butylphenoxy)ethoxy]ethyl} ammonium chloride,[137] (4) dye binding with Coomassie Brilliant Blue,[242] and (5) dye binding with pyrogallol red molybdate.[38]

Concerns about variation in the response to different proteins have led to many variants of the methods being published; this, together with the necessity for automation, resulted in the benzethonium chloride and dye-binding methods becoming the most popular in the United Kingdom.[38] The analytical range of the turbidimetric assays has been of concern, with the equivalent to an "antigen excess" equivalence point being apparent with high protein concentrations giving a lower signal; this can be overcome by monitoring the early period of turbidity formation. The turbidimetric methods and the dye-binding methods do not give equal analytical specificity and sensitivity for all proteins; this may be of particular importance in the detection of light chains, when an immunochemical method is more appropriate. The reactivity of chemical methods to some of the globulins can be enhanced by the inclusion of sodium dodecyl sulfate (SDS) in the reagent.[242] External quality assessment programs have highlighted significant variation between methods (Figure 24-5).[37]

The normal urinary total protein excretion is less than 150 mg/24 hr. The proteins excreted are made up of mostly albumin (50% to 60%) and some smaller proteins, together with proteins secreted by the tubules, of which Tamm-Horsfall glycoprotein (THG) is one. The normal concentrations of proteins found in urine are listed in Table 24-1.

Measurement of Individual Proteins

Immunoassay is the preferred method for the accurate and sensitive quantitation of individual proteins (see Chapter 9). Chromatographic and electrophoretic (including capillary electrophoresis) techniques (see Chapters 5 and 6) provide a semiquantitative or qualitative measurement of many of the proteins appearing in the urine and estimations of a panel or pattern of proteins that are not as easily available with the individual assays. The immunoassay techniques include (1) immunodiffusion immunoassay, (2) electroimmunoassay, (3) light-scattering assays with particle enhancement, and (4) labeled immunometric assays (see Chapter 9). However, immunodiffusion and electroimmunoassays require concentration of the urine to detect the low concentrations of protein present, and immunometric assays might require dilution of the sample. The most common approach today for the quantitation of individual urine proteins employs a light-scattering immunoassay, with either turbidimetric or nephelometric detection of immunoaggregate formation.[219,220]

The choice of the type of assay to be used for such measurements depends on the expected concentration of the protein to be measured. For example, in the case of albumin, the assay chosen must be precise at the upper limit of the reference interval (for maximal clinical effectiveness), while also being able to ensure that antigen excess does not occur at high pathological concentrations. In practice, this cannot be achieved in a direct aggregation assay, where the antibody-created particles are aggregated in the presence of

TABLE 24-1 Characteristics of the Major Urinary Proteins

Protein	M_r (kDa)	Free Plasma Concentration (g/L)	Diameter (nm)	pI	Glomerular Sieving Coefficient	Filtered Load (mg/L)†	Urinary Concentration (mg/L)	% Reabsorbed
IgG	150	10	5.5	7.3	0.0001	1	0.1	99
Albumin	66	40	3.5	4.7	0.0002	8	5	99
α_1-microglobulin	31	0.025	2.9	4.5	~0.3	7.5	5	99
Retinol-binding protein	22	0.025	2.1	4.5	~0.7	17.5	0.1	99
Cystatin C	12.8	0.01	—	9.2	~0.7	0.7	0.1	99
β_2-microglobulin	11.8	0.015	1.6	5.6	0.7	1.1	0.1	99
Total protein	—	70	—	—	NA*	700	<150	NA*

M_r, Molecular mass.
*Not applicable because of tubular secretion of proteins, e.g., THG, which form ~ 50% of urinary total proteins in health.
†Concentration in the glomerular filtrate.

antigen. Consequently, in this situation, it is better to use a method in which a reagent antigen (in this case, albumin) is coupled to particles. In this instance, the sample antigen inhibits the immunoaggregate formation between antigen-labeled particles and antibody in solution (an immunoinhibition assay). At high sample antigen concentrations, the signal falls to a minimum and then plateaus. Thus "antigen excess" is not a problem, as a dilution has to be performed when this minimum is reached. This method is the preferred approach for the measurement of albumin in urine, where decreased selectivity can lead to a very high albumin excretion rate. The problem does not arise with other proteins, either because the plasma concentration is lower or because the size of the protein inhibits its ready loss into the urine even when permeability increases. More detailed descriptions of light-scattering immunoassays are given in Chapters 9 and 20.

With appropriate sample dilution, the light-scattering immunoassays will provide precise results within an interval of 0.1 mg/L to 20 g/L. Choice of an immunoinhibition assay will ensure that the antigen excess does not lead to an erroneously reported result (see Chapter 9), although sample dilution will be required to give an accurate result at high protein concentration. Values for imprecision of less than ±5% within run and ±8% between runs are attainable over a concentration range of 0.1 mg/L to 20 g/L with the appropriate choice of reaction conditions.

Urinary Albumin and Microalbuminuria Screening

In general, proteinuria reflects albuminuria. Albumin is readily measured by quantitative immunoassay methods capable of detecting urine albumin at low concentrations, and several groups have demonstrated that urinary total protein measurement can be replaced by that of urine albumin.[11,152] This may provide a more specific and sensitive measure of changes in glomerular permeability and is consistent with current national guidelines.[146] However, it should also be noted that changes in albumin excretion may reflect overall changes in vascular permeability and therefore may not indicate an explicit deterioration in renal function.[81]

Dry chemistry systems have also been developed for the quantitation of albumin in urine.[119] For example, in one such device the urine albumin flows laterally along a porous matrix through an area containing gold particle–labeled antibodies to albumin. In the presence of albumin, these antibody molecules are neutralized and pass through a portion of the matrix containing immobilized albumin to a detection zone, where they appear as a pink coloration.[119] The excess labeled antibody is captured by the immobilized albumin. Another device produces a semiquantitative result by diffusing the sample into a gel containing gold sol particle–labeled antibody, the diameter of the ring being proportional to the concentration of the antigen being measured.[116] In another approach for use at the point of care an immunoturbidimetric assay for albumin has been developed in a cassette device with a second reagent encompassing a colorimetric creatinine assay in the same cassette device, enabling semiquantitative reporting of the albumin/creatinine ratio.[159] Photometric assays for both albumin and creatinine have been incorporated in a dual pad dipstick with the reactions being monitored using a reflectance meter.[160]

Microalbuminuria is defined as an increase in urinary excretion of albumin above the reference interval for healthy nondiabetic subjects but at a concentration that is not generally detectable by crude clinical tests, such as dipsticks designed to measure total protein.[52] With improved methodology, these low concentrations of albumin can now be measured, and microalbuminuria is now considered a clinically important indicator of deteriorating renal function in diabetic subjects. For example, it is now accepted by both European and U.S. diabetes societies that regular screening of urinary albumin excretion is valuable in monitoring both type 1 and type 2 diabetes.* This came as a consequence of the availability of effective treatments, validated in large multinational trials, along with detailed cost-benefit analyses in the vanguard of evidence-based medicine. The U.S. Agency for Health Research and Quality has recently reviewed the literature on increased albumin excretion and risk of renal disease and deteriorating mortality and found that the preponderance of evidence showed that increased albuminuria was associated with an increased risk of renal disease and cardiovascular mortality.[2]

Because of the large numbers of clinical studies that have been performed, there are now well-established guidelines for microalbuminuria screening (Figure 24-6).[5,18,24,206] The diagnosis of microalbuminuria requires the demonstration of increased albumin excretion (either increased albumin/creatinine ratio or increased albumin excretion rate) in at least two out of three urine samples collected in the absence of infection or an acute metabolic crisis. Establishing the diagnosis has both prognostic and management implications in the care of patients with diabetes mellitus. Tight control of diabetes should be achieved before investigating patients for microalbuminuria and patients should not be screened during intercurrent illness. Screening should commence 5 years after diagnosis in patients with type 1 diabetes mellitus and at diagnosis in patients with type 2 diabetes without proteinuria. Screening for microalbuminuria is not indicated in patients with established proteinuria. All other patients with diabetes mellitus should be screened on an annual basis up to the age of 75 years. An early morning (preferred) midstream urine sample should be sent to the laboratory for albumin estimation. An albumin/creatinine ratio less than 23 mg/g (less than 2.5 mg/mmol) in a male or 32 mg/g (less than 3.5 mg/mmol) in a female requires no further investigation until the patient's next annual review. Patients demonstrating albumin/creatinine ratios above, or equal to this cutoff should have urine samples sent to the laboratory on two further occasions (ideally within 1 month) for albumin estimation. Patients demonstrating increased albumin/creatinine ratios in one or both of these further samples have microalbuminuria. It is important to consider other causes of increased albumin excretion, especially in the case of type 1 diabetes present for less than 5 years. These can include nondiabetic renal disease, menstrual contamination, vaginal discharge, uncontrolled hypertension, urinary tract infection, uncontrolled diabetes, heart failure, intercurrent illness, and strenuous exercise. Occasionally, it may be desirable to confirm the diagnosis by measuring the albumin excretion rate in a timed overnight collection; increased albumin excretion in an overnight collection is defined as an overnight albumin excretion rate greater than 20 μg/min.

Once microalbuminuria has been established, an angiotensin converting enzyme (ACE) inhibitor should be prescribed because this class of antihypertensive agent has distinct antiproteinuria effects above and beyond the effects on blood pressure. Several major trials have shown ACE inhibitors to be effective in reducing not just proteinuria but also the rate of fall in GFR when used in both microalbuminuric and proteinuric diabetes. It has even been suggested that ACE inhibitors should be prescribed for normotensive microalbuminuric diabetes, as the definition of normotension as currently used may not reflect the actual intraglomerular pressure, and a lower cutoff should be used in such a high-risk group as diabetics.

It has been suggested that the identification of diabetic patients at risk of developing nephropathy should be attempted earlier than the microalbuminuric stage, when it may already be too late to prevent the development of nephropathy. The use of tubular markers (see below) has been proposed, but as yet none have been shown to provide any more sensitive indications of damage. Considerable work has been undertaken to look for genetic linkages with the development of nephropathy in diabetics. This work has included studies of polymorphisms of the ACE and insulin genes, but as yet no clear relationship has been demonstrated.[194] Other markers of basement membrane damage have also been used to investigate diabetic nephropathy, including urinary excretion of laminin, collagen IV, and fibronectin.[96,172,193] Laminin and collagen IV excretion were found to give no added benefit, but there has been some evidence that urinary fibronectin and metalloproteinase concentrations are elevated before albumin excretion increases.

Bence Jones Proteinuria

The presence of light chains (Bence Jones proteins, 22 kDa) in the urine is an important indication of the presence of myeloma and, in approximately 20% of cases, may occur in the absence of a paraprotein band in the serum (see Chapter 23).[14] The pathological significance of these proteins is considered in more detail in Chapter 45. Although a variety of tests have been used for the detection of Bence Jones protein, including the classic heat test and the Bradshaw test, electrophoresis supplemented by immunofixation is the most reliable approach.[14,237] It is worth noting that the more sensitive systems are capable of detecting low concentrations of protein occasionally associated with benign proliferation of B cells.[14] Quantitation of Bence Jones protein excretion may be required when monitoring patients with light chain–only myeloma. Although imperfect, this is best achieved by electrophoresis and densitometry.[14]

Myoglobinuria

Myoglobin is a small (17.8 kDa), heme-containing protein normally catabolized by endocytosis and proteolysis in the proximal tubule following glomerular filtration. Typically only 0.01% to 5.0% of filtered protein appears in the urine. However, following rhabdomyolysis large amounts of myoglobin are released into the plasma, saturating the tubular

*References 5, 18, 71, 103, 142, 206.

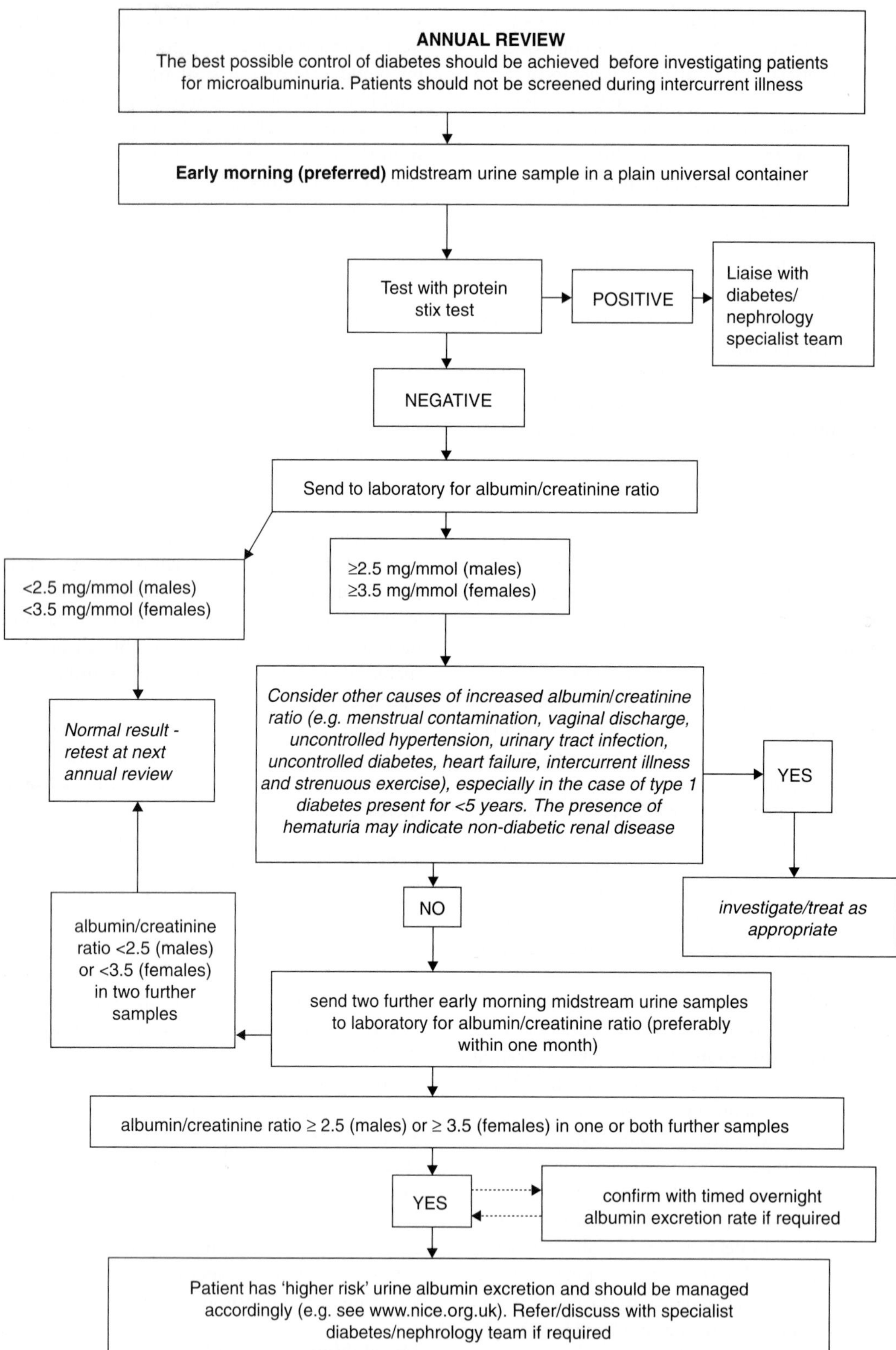

Figure 24-6 Screening for microalbuminuria in diabetes mellitus. Patients demonstrating "higher risk" urine albumin excretion should be managed accordingly. See "Diabetic Renal Disease: Prevention and Early Management" March 2002, available at www.nice.org.uk.

reabsorptive mechanism. This results in the appearance of increased quantities of myoglobin in the urine (which may color the urine red-brown). Further, myoglobin is directly toxic to the renal tubules and can cause acute tubular necrosis with acute renal failure.[251] Myoglobin will give a positive reaction with hemoglobin dipstick tests, and basic methods of detection relied on this principle following removal of hemoglobin (e.g., by ammonium sulfate precipitation), although false-negative and false-positive results are common.[15] Urinary myoglobin is more appropriately measured by immunochemical means, although preconcentration of urine may be required.[132] However, for most purposes evidence that rhabdomyolysis has occurred is better provided by an increase in plasma creatine kinase activity not attributable to a cardiac source. Urinary myoglobin measurement provides no additional prognostic or diagnostic information in this setting.[15]

Tubular Proteinuria

The integrity of the renal tubule can be assessed indirectly through measurement of functional change and detection of tissue damage. The most common approach has been the measurement of urinary concentrations of low molecular weight proteins using immunoassay technology.[17,219] These are freely filtered at the glomerulus and then reabsorbed and catabolized within the proximal tubule. Consequently the appearance of increased quantities of these proteins in the urine reflects failure of the tubular reabsorptive mechanisms. The most commonly measured proteins are retinol binding protein (RBP) and α_1-microglobulin (see Chapters 30 and 20, respectively). Although the excretion of β_2-microglobulin has been extensively studied, it is an impractical marker because of its instability in urine at a pH of less than 6. α_1-microglobulin (Mr 31 kDa) is also referred to as protein HC because of its human complex-forming capacity with IgA. It is synthesized by the liver and the free form is readily filtered at the glomerulus.[234] RBP (Mr 22 kDa) is also synthesized by the liver and is found in the plasma as a complex with prealbumin; the protein is the carrier protein for vitamin A. For the identification of tubular damage, urinary RBP may be more sensitive than α_1-microglobulin, but the higher concentration and excellent stability of the latter in human urine ex vivo facilitate its use as a marker of tubular damage in clinical studies.[104,161] THG, located in the thick ascending limb of the loop of Henle,[91] has also been used as a marker of more distal tubular damage.[163]

Lysozyme is an enzyme that occurs in neutrophilic granulocytes, monocytes, and macrophages, and several organs of the body, including the spleen, kidney, and gastrointestinal tract. It is freely filtered by the kidney and absorbed by the proximal tubules. Thus lysozymuria is seen in conditions associated with both tubular damage and increased endogenous synthesis. Urinary lysozyme is measured by a variety of methods, including catalytic activity and immunoassay; its primary clinical application has been in the monitoring of patients with monocytic leukemia.[156] The reference interval for the excretion of lysozyme in healthy adults is reported to be 1.3 to 3.6 mg/day.[221]

Tubular damage results in the release of intracellular components into the urinary tract, and the measurement of these components reflects the functional integrity of the tubule. A large number of enzymes have been measured in urine.[240] The enzyme *N*-acetyl-β-D-glucosaminidase (NAG) is stable in urine and has been widely used as a marker of tubular integrity. One method for the assay of NAG employs the substrate 4-methylumbelliferyl-N-acetyl-β-D-glucosaminide with a fluorometric measurement of the methylumbelliferone released by the enzyme.[165] Alternative substrates generating products capable of being detected in the visible spectrum have also been described.[250] The measurement of NAG has been undertaken in a variety of diseases associated with renal injury, including hypertension, drug nephrotoxicity, and diabetic nephropathy, as well as transplantation.[171] However, although it is a sensitive marker of kidney damage, it has not generally been shown to provide any unique benefit over other markers of tubular proteinuria. Bazzi et al[13] has demonstrated that urinary NAG could be used to predict progression to renal failure in patients with idiopathic membranous nephropathy. Measurement of α- and π-glutathione-S-transferase (EC 2.5.1.18) isoenzymes has been proposed to discriminate between proximal and distal tubular damage, respectively,[114] but the role of these markers in clinical practice has yet to be established.

Other markers are also available for monitoring the breakdown of the basement membrane components, including collagen breakdown products[96,246] and laminin fragments.[172] However, at present, few of these markers have found a place in the clinical laboratory.

Characterization of Proteinuria

As glomerular damage increases, the permeability of the membrane decreases, with an increasing proportion of higher molecular weight proteins appearing in the urine. The relative clearance of a number of proteins has been measured to assess the selectivity of the membrane and provide an assessment of glomerular damage. The *protein selectivity index* is discussed in the third edition of this textbook, but is generally considered to be of limited value.[33] A commercial semiautomated sodium dodecyl sulfate–agarose gel electrophoresis system (Hydragel, Sebia, France) has been introduced for qualitative analysis of urinary proteins. This separates proteins on the basis of their molecular size, enabling visualization of glomerular, tubular, and mixed patterns of proteinuria. This approach has also been used for the detection and quantitation of Bence Jones proteinuria.[126] Panels of protein measurements, including albumin, α_1-microglobulin, IgG, and α_2-macroglobulin, have been employed in the differential diagnosis of prerenal and postrenal disease.[89] This general strategy was extended with the inclusion of dipstick tests for hematuria, leukocyturia, and proteinuria in the development of an expert system achieving a concordance of 98% with clinical diagnosis.[95]

ASSESSMENT OF KIDNEY FUNCTION: ESTIMATION OF GLOMERULAR FILTRATION RATE

The GFR is widely accepted as the best overall measure of kidney function, enabling a statement of the complex functions of the kidney in a single numerical expression.[146] A decrease in GFR precedes kidney failure in all forms of progressive disease. Different pathological kidney conditions can progress to ESRD and dialysis dependency at rates varying from weeks to several decades.[32,111,178] The symptoms accompanying progressive kidney disease (see Chapter 45) and their correlation with falling GFR will be influenced by this rate of progression. Measuring GFR in established disease is useful in targeting treatment, monitoring progression, and predicting the point at which renal replacement therapy will be required. It is also used as a guide to dosage of renally excreted drugs to prevent potential drug toxicity. A number of methods are used to measure the GFR; most involve the kidneys' ability to clear either an exogenous or endogenous marker. Improving methodology and the discovery of new markers of GFR and glomerular or tubular damage will continue to provide important contributions to the early diagnosis of renal disease.

THE CONCEPT OF CLEARANCE

Most of the clinical laboratory information used to assess kidney function is derived from or related to measurement of the clearance of some substance by the kidneys. The renal clearance of a substance is defined as "the volume of plasma from which the substance is completely cleared by the kidneys per unit of time.[131,224] Provided a substance *S* is in stable concentration in the plasma; is physiologically inert; freely filtered at the glomerulus; and neither secreted, reabsorbed, synthesized, nor metabolized by the kidney, then the amount of that substance filtered at the glomerulus is equal to the amount excreted in the urine (i.e., the amount of *S* entering the kidney must exactly equal the amount leaving it). The amount of *S* filtered at the glomerulus = GFR multiplied by plasma *S* concentration: GFR × PS. The amount of *S* excreted equals the urine *S* concentration (US) multiplied by the urinary flow rate (V, volume excreted per unit time).

Since filtered *S* = excreted *S*, then

$$\text{GFR} \times P_S = U_S \times V \tag{1}$$

or

$$\text{GFR} = \frac{(U_S \times V)}{P_S} \tag{2}$$

where GFR = *clearance* in units of milliliters of plasma cleared of a substance per minute

U_S = urinary concentration of the substance

V = volumetric flow rate of urine in milliliters per minute

P_S = plasma concentration of the substance

The term $(U_S \times V)/P_S$ is defined as the clearance of substance *S* and is an accurate estimate of GFR providing the aforementioned criteria are satisfied. Inulin satisfies these criteria and has long been regarded as the most accurate (gold standard) estimate of GFR (see below).

Kidney size and GFR are roughly proportional to body size. It is conventional therefore to adjust clearance estimates to a standard body surface area (BSA) of $1.73\,\text{m}^2$, according to the formula devised by Du Bois and Du Bois in 1916[53]:

$$\text{BSA} = \text{weight (kg)}^{0.425} \times \text{height (cm)}^{0.725} \times 7.1 \times 10^{-3} \tag{3}$$

MARKERS USED

A variety of exogenous (radioisotopic and nonradioisotopic) and endogenous markers have been used to estimate clearance (Table 24-2). Measurement of clearance may require accurate measurements of both plasma and urinary concentrations of the marker used plus a reliable urine collection. For a reliable plasma measurement, the substance must have reached a steady-state concentration and not be rapidly changing. For a reliable urine collection, the urine flow must be adequate (several mL/min), the collection period of long enough duration, and complete bladder emptying achieved; these requirements are problematic.

Exogenous Markers of Glomerular Filtration Rate

The use of exogenous markers to measure GFR is recommended for the monitoring of slowly progressing nephropathies, such as that associated with diabetes. Exogenous markers are also used to determine a GFR that is used to set a benchmark against which to monitor deterioration in GFR using an endogenous marker, such as creatinine. Measurement of GFR using an exogenous molecule does enable smaller deteriorations in renal function to be observed even when the imprecision in measurement is taken into account.

Both radioisotopic labeled and nonradioisotopic markers are used as exogenous markers. They are administered as a constant infusion or as a single bolus.

Radioisotopic Markers

Radiopharmaceuticals that have been used include (1) ^{51}Cr-EDTA,[7,8,19,30,39] (2) ^{99m}Tc-diethylenetriaminepentaacetic acid (DTPA), and (3) ^{125}I-iothalamate. ^{51}Cr-EDTA is preferred to ^{99m}Tc-DTPA and ^{125}I-iothalamate since its clearance is considered to be closest to that of inulin.[20,30] ^{99m}Tc-DTPA has the advantage that it can also be used for gamma camera imaging. ^{125}I-iothalamate is no longer approved for intravascular use in some countries.[20] GFR measurements may be based on either the urinary or plasma clearance of the marker. To ensure accuracy when measuring GFR using urinary clearance methods it is essential that (1) renal

TABLE 24-2 Markers of Glomerular Filtration Rate: Hierarchical Arrangement

Hierarchy	Marker	Advantages	Disadvantages
Gold standard	Inulin (sinistrin) continuous infusion urinary clearance method	Gold standard	Exogenous Time consuming[61] Requires a timed urine collection Poor specificity of analysis Extrarenal clearance = 0.083 mL/min/kg
Silver standard	Inulin (sinistrin) single bolus plasma clearance method		Exogenous Time consuming[61] Poor specificity of analysis Extrarenal clearance = 0.083 mL/min/kg
	^{51}Cr-EDTA	Radioisotopic (simple measurement) Close correlation with inulin clearance[30]	Exogenous Radioisotopic (risks of ionizing radiation) Time consuming[177] Extrarenal clearance = 0.079 mL/min/kg ^{51}Cr less readily available than ^{99m}technetium (Tc)
	^{99m}Tc-DTPA	Radioisotopic (simple measurement) Can be used for gamma camera imaging	Exogenous Radioisotopic (risks of ionizing radiation) Time consuming[59,177] Protein binding
	^{125}I-iothalamate	Radioisotopic (simple measurement)	Exogenous Radioisotopic (risks of ionizing radiation) Not available in all countries Reports of allergic reactions
	Iohexol	Nonradioisotopic	Exogenous Extrarenal clearance[76,118] = 0.087 mL/min/kg Reports of allergic reactions
Bronze standard	Creatinine	Endogenous Inexpensive Can be used to generate GFR from formula (e.g., MDRD)	Poor sensitivity and specificity
	Cystatin C	Not secreted/reabsorbed Constitutively expressed More sensitive and specific than creatinine	Influence of thyroid function[49,72,101]
Of uncertain clinical use	Creatinine clearance	Endogenous Inexpensive	Requires a timed urine collection Inaccurate
	Urea	Endogenous Inexpensive	Poor sensitivity and specificity
	Retinol-binding protein (RBP)	Endogenous Not secreted/reabsorbed	Nonrenal influences on production rate
	α_1-microglobulin	Endogenous Not secreted/reabsorbed	Nonrenal influences on production rate Less freely filtered than RBP

tubular secretion or reabsorption does not contribute to the elimination of the compound, (2) plasma protein binding of the radiopharmaceutical is negligible, and (3) patients completely empty their bladder. ^{99m}Tc-DTPA has been associated with problems of plasma protein binding of the tracer, but more recent formulations have minimized this problem.[20] Plasma clearance of a radionuclide measures GFR reliably only if nonrenal clearance routes are negligible. For research purposes in patients with low (less than 30 mL/min) GFR and in patients with ascites or edema, measurement is best performed using a urinary clearance method.[20] From a clinical management perspective, in the majority of patients, either urinary or plasma clearance approaches are acceptable.

Nonradiosotopic Markers

Nonradioactive compounds used to measure GFR include inulin and iohexol.[59]

Inulin Clearance. The fructose polymer inulin (molecular mass approximately 5 kDa) satisfies the criteria as an ideal marker of GFR. Inulin clearance using a constant infusion urinary clearance approach has long been regarded as the gold standard measure of GFR. Acceptable single bolus plasma clearance approaches have also been evaluated.[227] However, lack of availability of simple laboratory methods of measurement remains an impediment to universal usage. Early methods for the measurement of inulin were based on the hydrolysis of inulin with concentrated sulfuric acid and condensation with anthrone to give a green product that could be read at 620 nm. Later methods were based on the enzyme inulinase (EC 3.2.17), which converts inulin to fructose; the fructose can then be determined with the aid of sorbitol dehydrogenase (EC 1.1.1.14) according to the following reaction sequence[211]:

$$\text{Inulin} \xrightarrow{\text{Inulinase}} \text{Fructose} + \text{NADH} \xrightarrow[\text{Dehydrogenase}]{\text{Sorbitol}} \text{Sorbital} + \text{NAD}$$

The amount of inulin present is determined from the reduction of nicotinamide-adenine dinucleotide, reduced form (NADH) measured as a decrease in absorbance at 340 nm. The method is calibrated with either inulin or fructose; endogenous fructose in each sample is measured by incubation with an inactivated inulinase reagent. Urine samples require predilution (typically 1 in 40) before analysis. A typical between-run imprecision of less than ±2% for plasma and less than ±4% for urine can be obtained with an automated assay.

An alternative method for detecting the fructose produced involves the use of fructokinase (EC 2.7.1.4), phosphoglucose isomerase, and glucose-6-phosphate dehydrogenase (EC 1.1.1.49), measuring in this case the nicotinamide-adenine dinucleotide phosphate, reduced form (NADPH) produced.[167,209]

Iohexol Clearance. The clearance of the nonradioactive x-ray contrast agent iohexol has been proposed as a simpler alternative to inulin clearance.[6,118] In one method, plasma iohexol is measured by HPLC with reversed-phase separation and UV detection, following prior deproteinization with perchloric acid.[118] Analytical imprecision is less than ±3% intraassay and ±5% interassay. Rapid, inexpensive capillary electrophoresis iohexol measurement techniques have also been described.[102,180] Single bolus plasma clearance of iohexol demonstrates excellent agreement with constant infusion urinary inulin clearance.[76] Biological variability in patients with kidney disease using this technique is approximately 6%.[75] Iohexol clearance appears to provide a suitable method of GFR measurement in the setting of diabetic nephropathy.[90] The nonradioisotopic and stable nature of iohexol enables analysis of samples to be delayed and common reference centers to be used for multinational studies. An outpatient procedure based on filter paper blood spots has been described.[51]

Administration

Both constant infusion and single bolus injection methods are used to administer an exogenous marker. In the constant infusion technique, the fasting subject is required to drink 500 mL of water 1 hour before the study begins, after which he or she is required to take 200 mL every half hour until the end of the study. The subject remains supine throughout the study. An intravenous loading dose of the marker selected is then followed by a constant infusion of a given quantity of marker per minute for 3 hours. After equilibration for 1 hour, blood is taken and urine samples are collected at hourly intervals for 3 hours. This technique can be used with any of the exogenous markers, the dosage being all that will vary between molecules. For example, for inulin, an intravenous loading dose of 2.3 g would be followed by a constant infusion of 18.1 mg/min for 3 hours.

Single bolus plasma clearance methods[98] have obvious practical advantages compared with the complex continuous infusion methods. A single dose of the marker (e.g., inulin, 70 mg/kg; iohexol, 5 mL, Omnipaque 300 mg iodine/mL [Nycomed AS, Oslo, Norway]; or ^{51}Cr-EDTA, 50 to 100 μCi) is injected and venous blood samples are then collected at timed intervals (e.g., typically 120, 180, and 240 minutes after the start of the injection for ^{51}Cr-EDTA). The GFR is calculated using knowledge of the amount of marker injected and the decrease in marker concentration (activity) as a function of time. The elimination of the marker is described by a two-compartment model: this comprises an initial equilibration or distribution phase while the marker mixes between the vascular and extravascular space while also being cleared from the plasma by the kidney. The distribution phase can last between 2 and 8 hours, depending on the size of the subject, the distribution volume of the molecule (e.g., longer in edematous patients), and the GFR of the subject (the lower the GFR, the longer the distribution phase). This gives rise to a biexponential clearance curve (Figure 24-7). However, GFR is normally calculated using single-exponential analysis by plotting log marker concentration against time. The half-life is calculated from the slope (k) and the volume of distribution (C_0) of the marker just after injection.

$$\text{GFR} = k \times C_0 \quad (4)$$

Because this model ignores the distribution phase, GFR is overestimated. Various corrections are used to adjust for this (e.g., those proposed by Chantler and Barrett[39] and Brochner-Mortensen[29]). For further details see Blake et al.[19]

Endogenous Markers of Glomerular Filtration Rate

Although the clearance of infused exogenous markers is generally considered an accurate assessment of GFR, to date these procedures have been considered too costly and cumbersome for routine use, particularly where the GFR is

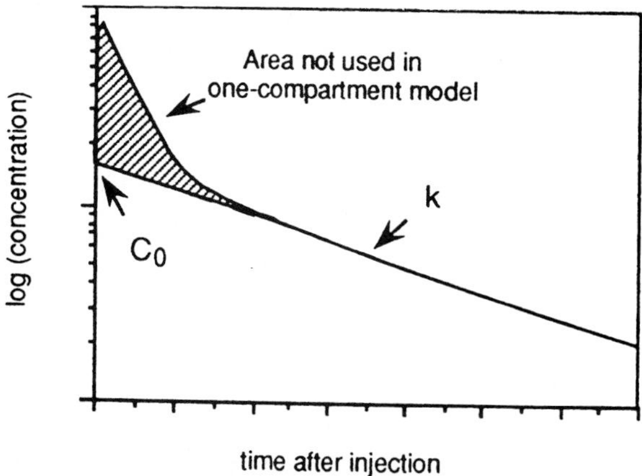

Figure 24-7 Semilog plot used in a single compartmental analysis of the plasma disappearance curve of a GFR marker. In this simplified representation of contrast agent elimination, the distribution phase *(hatched area)* is neglected, which leads to underestimation of the true area under the curve.

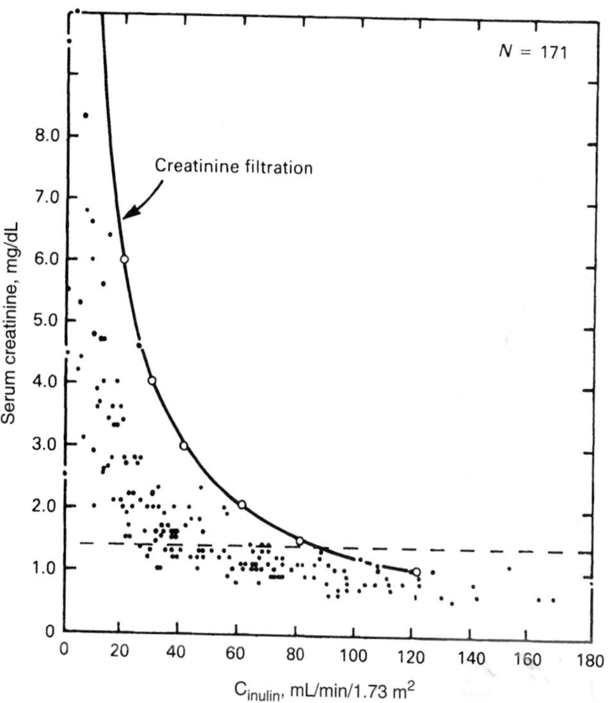

Figure 24-8 The relationship between serum creatinine concentration and GFR, measured as the clearance of inulin, in 171 patients with glomerular disease. The hypothetical relationship between GFR and serum creatinine is shown as a *continuous line,* assuming that only filtration of creatinine takes place. The *dashed horizontal line* represents the upper limit of a normal serum creatinine (1.4 mg/dL). Because of creatinine secretion and/or a creatinine deficit through gut excretion, the serum creatinine consistently overestimates the GFR. *(From Shemesh O, Golbetz H, Kriss JP, Myers BD. Limitations of creatinine as a filtration marker in glomerulopathic patients. Kidney Int 1985;28:830.)*

assessed on a regular basis (e.g., where patients are receiving nephrotoxic drugs). Creatinine and certain low molecular weight proteins such as cystatin C have been used as endogenous markers of GFR. The use of urea in this context is of limited value[214] and will not be discussed further. Endogenous markers obviate the necessity for injection and require only a single blood sample, simplifying the procedure for the patient, clinician, and laboratory.

Creatinine Concentration

The most widely used endogenous marker of GFR is creatinine, expressed either as its plasma concentration or its renal clearance. The use of creatinine as a marker of GFR was developed in 1926 by Rehberg,[176] who used exogenously administered creatinine. This led to the work of Popper and Mandel,[166] who in 1937 developed the use of endogenous creatinine clearance.

Creatinine (molecular mass 113 Da) is freely filtered at the glomerulus and its concentration is inversely related to GFR. As a GFR marker, it is convenient and cheap to measure but is affected by age, sex, exercise, certain drugs (e.g., cimetidine,[223] trimethoprim), muscle mass, nutritional status, and meat intake.[164,205] Further, a small (but significant) and variable proportion of the creatinine appearing in the urine is derived from tubular secretion. Typically, 7% to 10% is due to tubular secretion,[139] but this is increased in the presence of renal insufficiency. As previously discussed, significant analytical interferences continue to be a problem.[117,205] Perhaps most importantly, plasma creatinine remains within the reference interval until significant renal function has been lost (Figure 24-8).[164] Since plasma creatinine is derived from creatine and phosphocreatine breakdown in muscle, the reference interval encompasses the range of muscle mass observed in the population. This contributes to the insensitivity of creatinine as a marker of diminished GFR. Additionally, in patients with CKD, extrarenal clearance of creatinine further blunts the anticipated increase in plasma creatinine in response to falling GFR.[146] Consequently, plasma creatinine measurement will not detect patients with stage 2 CKD (GFR 60 to 89 mL/min/1.73 m^2) and will also fail to identify many patients with stage 3 CKD (GFR 30 to 59 mL/min/1.73 m^2). Thus although an elevated plasma creatinine concentration does generally equate with impaired kidney function, a normal plasma creatinine does not necessarily equate with normal kidney function. Because of all these limitations, it is recommended that plasma creatinine measurement alone is not used to assess kidney function.[146]

Creatinine Clearance

Because creatinine is endogenously produced and released into body fluids at a constant rate, its clearance has been measured as an indicator of GFR.[164] A protocol for the conduct of the creatinine clearance test may be found in the third edition of this textbook.

Utility. Historically, creatinine clearance has been seen as more sensitive for detection of renal dysfunction than measuring plasma creatinine. However, it requires a timed urine collection, which introduces its own inaccuracies,[78,162,179] is inconvenient, and is unpleasant. In adults the intraindividual day-to-day CV for repeated measures of creatinine clearance exceeds 25%.[31] Although tubular secretion undermines the theoretical value of creatinine as a marker of GFR, in the context of creatinine clearance this has previously been offset to some extent by the use of nonspecific methods to measure plasma creatinine, which lead to an overestimation of plasma concentration. Nevertheless, creatinine clearance usually equals or exceeds inulin GFR in adults by a factor of 10% to 40% at clearances above 80 mL/min. However, as GFR falls, plasma creatinine rises disproportionately and the creatinine clearance can reach nearly twice that of inulin.[230] Tubular reabsorption of creatinine has also been reported at low GFRs but may represent diffusion of creatinine through gap junctions between tubular cells or directly through the tubular epithelial cells, down a concentration gradient.[164] Whatever the mechanism, this further devalues the use of creatinine clearance. Hence, at best creatinine clearance can only provide a crude index of GFR.

Calculated Clearance. The mathematical relationship between plasma creatinine and GFR can be improved by correcting for the confounding variables that make that relationship nonlinear. More than 25 different formulas have been derived that estimate GFR using plasma creatinine corrected for some or all of gender, body size, race, and age.[146] These may produce a better estimate of GFR than serum creatinine alone. Indeed the National Kidney Foundation of the United States[146] has recommended that such estimates should be used in preference to serum creatinine, and that either the Cockcroft and Gault or Modification of Diet in Renal Disease (MDRD) formula should be used in adults. The Schwartz[195] and Counahan-Barratt[48] formulas are recommended for use in children.

The Cockcroft and Gault[43] formula is one of the earliest, and perhaps most widely used, of these formulas. The authors measured creatinine clearance in more than 200 patients and used regression analysis to enable prediction of creatinine clearance from the serum creatinine concentration, taking age and patient weight into consideration:

$$\text{Creatinine clearance (mL/min)} = \frac{[(140 - \text{age(years)}) \times \text{weight (kg)}]}{72 \times \text{plasma creatinine (mg/dL)}}$$

or

$$\text{Creatinine clearance (mL/min)} = \frac{[(140 - \text{age(years)}) \times \text{weight (kg)}]}{0.814 \times \text{plasma creatinine } (\mu\text{mol/L})}$$

It should be noted that the formula predicts creatinine clearance, not GFR, and that the results are not corrected for BSA. The formula has become embedded in the medical literature and practice (e.g., aminoglycoside dosage charts have been based upon this estimate of GFR).[191] However, some studies have suggested that it diverges widely from true measures of GFR in certain clinical situations.[164,181] There are also theoretical objections to its use. It was derived among a population only 4% of whom were female: an arbitrary correction factor of 0.85 was recommended for females.[43] A relatively nonspecific Jaffe method was used for measuring plasma creatinine; transferability of data to enzymatic creatinine methods, for example, may not be appropriate. Nevertheless, when compared against exogenous clearance marker methods, subsequent experience has generally shown that the formula produces more accurate and precise estimates of GFR than measured creatinine clearance.[47,122,146,230] An example of the agreement between predicted creatinine clearance and GFR can be seen in Figure 24-9.[47]

In 1999 Levey et al[128] proposed a formula that also included plasma urea and albumin concentrations and race

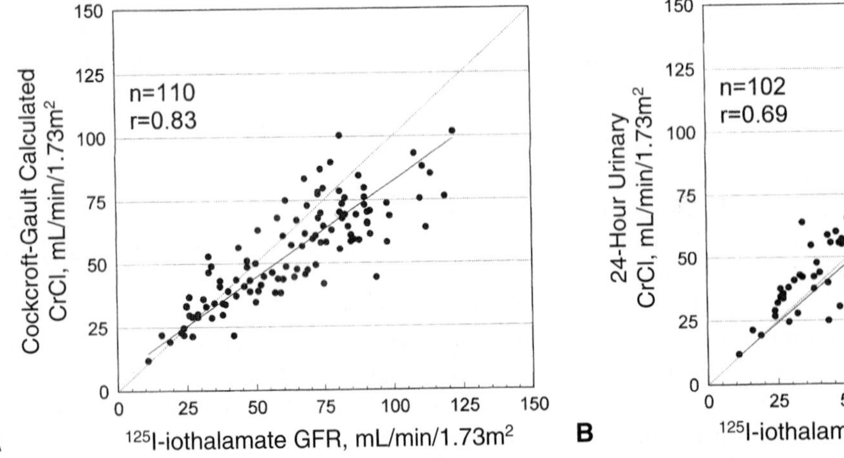

Figure 24-9 Relationship between GFR measured using ^{125}I-iothalamate clearance and estimates of creatinine clearance (CrCl) obtained using the **(A)** Cockcroft and Gault equation and **(B)** measured creatinine clearance. *(From Coresh J, Toto RD, Kirk KA, Whelton PK, Massry S, Jones C, et al. Creatinine clearance as a measure of GFR in screenees for the African-American study of kidney disease and hypertension pilot study. Am J Kidney Dis 1998;32:32-42.)*

as covariables. The formula was developed in 1628 predominantly middle-aged patients enrolled in the MDRD study, which is a study of chronic renal insufficiency, and hence is commonly known as the MDRD formula. Plasma urea was found to be an independent predictor of GFR, probably reflecting the differing renal handling of urea and creatinine by the kidney, and also to improve the strength of relationship between creatinine and GFR, possibly by correcting for the effects of catabolism on plasma creatinine. In addition to urea, they also observed that albumin was an independent predictor of GFR, probably reflecting the known relationship between protein intake and renal function.

$$\begin{aligned}\text{GFR}\left(\text{mL/min/1.73 m}^2\right) &= 170\\ &\times [\text{plasma creatinine (mg/dL)}]^{-0.999}\\ &\times [\text{age}]^{-0.176}\\ &\times [\text{plasma urea nitrogen (mg/dL)}]^{-0.170}\\ &\times [\text{plasma albumin (g/dL)}]^{0.318}\\ &\times [0.762 \text{ if patient is female}]\\ &\times [1.180 \text{ if patient is black}].\end{aligned}$$

or

$$\begin{aligned}\text{GFR}\left(\text{mL/min/1.73 m}^2\right) &= 170\\ &\times [\text{plasma creatinine } (\mu\text{mol/L}) \times 0.011312]^{-0.999}\\ &\times [\text{age}]^{-0.176}\\ &\times [\text{plasma urea (mmol/L)} \times 2.801]^{-0.170}\\ &\times [\text{plasma albumin (g/L)} \times 0.1]^{+0.318}\\ &\times [0.762 \text{ if patient is female}]\\ &\times [1.180 \text{ if patient is black}]\end{aligned}$$

These workers have subsequently also published, in abstract form, an abbreviated version of this formula, which does not require albumin or urea.[129]

$$\begin{aligned}\text{GFR}\left(\text{mL/min/1.73 m}^2\right) &= 186\\ &\times [\text{plasma creatinine (mg/dL)}]^{-1.154}\\ &\times [\text{age}]^{-0.203}\\ &\times [0.742 \text{ if patient is female}]\\ &\times [1.210 \text{ if patient is black}]\end{aligned}$$

or

$$\begin{aligned}\text{GFR}\left(\text{mL/min/1.73 m}^2\right) &= 186\\ &\times [\text{plasma creatinine } (\mu\text{mol/L}) \times 0.011312]^{-1.154}\\ &\times [\text{age}]^{-0.203}\\ &\times [0.742 \text{ if patient is female}]\\ &\times [1.210 \text{ if patient is black}]\end{aligned}$$

They observed that the MDRD equation provided more accurate assessment of GFR than either the Cockcroft and Gault equation or measured creatinine clearance. The MDRD formula has several advantages: (1) it was developed and validated in a large population, (2) it was developed with a population that included both European-Americans and African-Americans, (3) it does not require patient weight, (4) it was validated against an iothalamate clearance estimate of GFR, and (5) the reported GFR is corrected for BSA. However, the MDRD calculations are more complex than the Cockcroft and Gault equation (e.g., some laboratory data systems are unable to compute power calculations) and there has to date been only limited evaluation of this formula, particularly in certain patient groups (e.g., Asians with kidney disease).

Plasma creatinine is an imperfect marker of GFR and therefore it is not altogether surprising that formulas based predominantly upon it are imperfect. Their use cannot circumvent the very significant spectral interferences affecting plasma creatinine measurement (i.e., hemolysis, icterus, and lipemia) and the formulas are unsuitable for use in patients with acute renal failure, in whom plasma creatinine concentrations are changing rapidly. Additionally, the formulas are critically susceptible to variations in creatinine assay calibration and specificity.[46,245] Notwithstanding the MDRD formula is thought to improve the estimation of GFR compared with plasma creatinine alone.

Low Molecular Weight Proteins

A number of proteins with molecular weights of less than 30 kDa are mostly cleared from the circulation by renal filtration and can be considered to be relatively freely filtered at the glomerular filtration barrier. These include α_2-microglobulin, RBP, α_1-microglobulin, β-trace protein,[173] and cystatin C. These proteins are filtered at the glomerulus, then reabsorbed (and metabolized) in the proximal tubule or excreted into the urine, and thus they are entirely eliminated from the circulation. Therefore they have the potential to meet the criteria for use as a marker of GFR. However, apart from cystatin C, all the other proteins have been shown to have plasma concentrations that are influenced by other, nonrenal factors, such as inflammation (α_2-microglobulin) and liver disease (RBP, α_1-microglobulin).[9] The relationship between the circulating concentrations of these proteins shows the same curvilinear form as plasma creatinine, but very recently several groups have demonstrated that cystatin C measurement may offer a more sensitive and specific means of monitoring changes in GFR than plasma creatinine.[64,84,120,151]

Cystatin C

Cystatin C is a low molecular weight (12.8 kDa) protein synthesized by all nucleated cells whose physiological role is that of a cysteine protease inhibitor.[149] With regard to renal function, its most important attributes are its small size and high isoelectric point (pI = 9.2), which enable it to be more freely filtered than the above-mentioned proteins at the glomerulus.[84] The gene has been sequenced, and the promoter region has been identified as of the housekeeping type, with no known regulatory elements. Consequently the production rate of cystatin C has always been considered to be constant,[1] although several publications suggest an influence of thyroid hormone.[49,72,101] Plasma concentrations of cystatin C appear to be unaffected by muscle mass, diet, or gender.[120] There are no known extrarenal routes of elimination, with clearance from the circulation only by glomerular filtration.[84,99,218]

Cystatin C has been measured by immunodiffusion or rocket electroimmunoassay, but the methods are too insensitive, and any form of labeled immunometric assay is too cumbersome and time consuming for the response time required. The most practical approaches described are to use a latex particle–enhanced turbidimetric or nephelometric immunoassay. An intraassay precision of less than ±3% can be expected at the upper limit of the reference interval (~1.00 mg/L), with less than ±4% for the between-day value.[64,120,151,208] Further, cystatin C measurement appears unaffected by the spectral interferences affecting creatinine assays.[208]

There are a number of reports documenting the correlation between plasma cystatin C and creatinine (as a reciprocal), and GFR as assessed by ^{51}Cr-EDTA clearance or using a number of alternative exogenous markers. The correlations vary between 0.32 and 0.88 for cystatin C and 0.25 and 0.89 in the case of creatinine. In almost all of the cases the correlation with cystatin C is superior to that with creatinine.[168] Kyhse-Andersen et al[120] first demonstrated, using receiver operator analysis, the superiority of cystatin C measurement compared with creatinine for the detection of kidney disease (Figure 24-10) and this has been confirmed by a 2002 meta-analysis.[50] A 2002 summary receiver operator curve analysis of all of the studies at the time of publication showed an area under the curve of 0.95 for cystatin C and 0.91 for creatinine ($p = 0.003$).[123] Perhaps more critically, Newman et al found that, in a group of patients with a range of GFRs, the cystatin C concentration increased sooner than creatinine as GFR declined; cystatin C concentration started to increase as GFR fell below about 80 mL/min/1.73 m^2 compared with about 40 mL/min/1.73 m^2 for serum creatinine.[151] Cystatin C is therefore especially useful when trying to detect mild to moderate impairment of kidney function.[26,44]

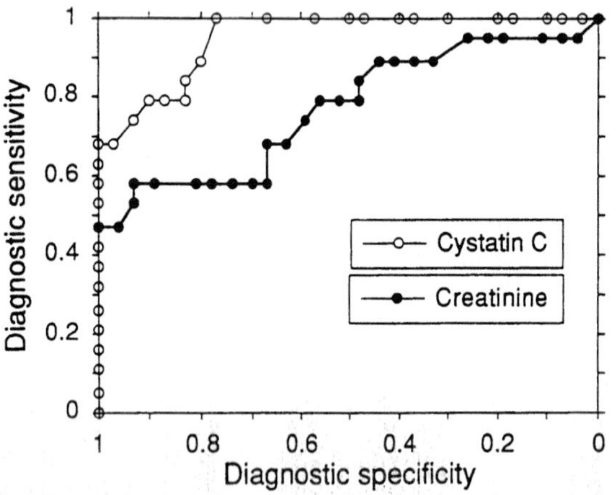

Figure 24-10 Receiver operating characteristic (ROC) curves comparing creatinine and cystatin C in the assessment of GFR. Nonparametric ROC plots were constructed to assess the diagnostic accuracy of serum concentrations of cystatin C and creatinine in distinguishing between normal and reduced GFR (less than 80 mL/min per 1.73 m^2) in 51 patients with various renal conditions. *(From Kyhse-Andersen J, Schmidt C, Nordin G, et al. Serum cystatin C, determined by a rapid, automated particle-enhanced turbidimetric method, is a better marker than serum creatinine for glomerular filtration rate. Clin Chem 1994;40:1921-6.)*

Glomerular Filtration Rate at the Extremes of Age

As discussed previously in this chapter, current markers of GFR are imperfect and the limitations of these tests are accentuated in both pediatric and older populations. At birth, plasma creatinine concentrations approximate those of the maternal circulation. Plasma creatinine concentrations fall rapidly during the neonatal period, with slower falls being observed in premature infants.[186] Plasma creatinine concentrations are lower in infants than in adults, despite their lower GFR, reflecting the lower muscle mass (decreased creatinine production rate). In the setting of pediatric intensive care medicine, the usefulness of plasma creatinine may be further limited by analytical interferences caused by high concentrations of bilirubin and competition with creatinine for tubular secretion by commonly used antibiotics (e.g., trimethoprim and cimetidine). By contrast, plasma cystatin C concentrations in infants appear to more closely reflect GFR, being increased in the first 3 months of life and then falling to approximate adult concentrations by age 1 year (Figure 24-11).[23,65] Further, the diagnostic accuracy of cystatin C for reduced GFR is superior to that of creatinine in children.[86,248]

Plasma creatinine concentrations in healthy older people are not dissimilar to those in younger people, except in nonagenarians and centenarians, despite the decrease in GFR that occurs, on average, with aging.[222] Possible reasons for this include reduced muscle mass and poorer nutrition. Whatever the reason, the same concentration of plasma creatinine may indicate very different degrees of kidney function in younger and older people, and a normal plasma creatinine concentration does not exclude significant renal impairment. The effects of this may be marked and are commonly not appreciated. For example, for a 70-kg man with a plasma creatinine of 1.4 mg/dL (120 μmol/L), the Cockcroft and Gault formula predicts GFRs of 81 and 44 mL/min at age 30 and 80 years, respectively. In two large primary care studies,[54,215] Cockcroft and Gault estimated that GFRs less than 50 mL/min were common in patients with normal plasma creatinine. This was most pronounced in older age groups (e.g., discordance between normal serum creatinine and reduced GFR was observed in 47% of patients aged greater than or equal to 70 years, compared with 1.2% of patients aged 40 to 59 years,[54] and the clinical sensitivity of plasma creatinine for detecting severely reduced GFR [less than 30 mL/min/1.73 m^2] was only 46%).[215] As observed in children, plasma cystatin C, however, does appear to reflect the age-related decline in kidney function[63,231] and appears to be more sensitive than plasma creatinine for detection of reduced GFR.[66,155]

RECOMMENDATIONS AND REFERENCE INTERVALS

The measurement of the urinary clearance of inulin, after continuous infusion, is considered the primary or reference method for the determination of GFR. However, because the necessary plasma and urine assays for inulin often are not practical in clinical laboratories, plasma creatinine or creatinine clearance has almost universally been used for assessment of GFR. With increasing recognition of the importance of early detection and management of CKD, the requirement for more accurate assessment of GFR is being emphasized.[146] Consequently creatinine clearance is no longer considered acceptable as a measure of GFR and plasma creatinine measurements should not be reported in isolation but should be used to generate formulaic estimations of GFR.[146]

In practice, there may be little to choose between the Cockcroft and Gault formula and the more recently described MDRD equation,[22,27,85] and which is chosen will be

TABLE 24-3 Glomerular Filtration Rate: Reference Values

Study	Method	Age (yr)	GFR* (mean [range]) or Mean ± SD (mL/min/1.73 m²)	n
Slack and Wilson[200]	Inulin (constant infusion)	20-29		47
		20	118 (90-146)	
		25	115 (88-142)	
		30-39		28
		30	112 (86-138)	
		35	109 (84-134)	
		40-49		30
		40	106 (82-130)	
		45	104 (80-128)	
		50-59		26
		50	101 (78-124)	
		55	99 (75-123)	
		60	96 (73-119)	4
Prescott et al[167]	Inulin (constant infusion)	30 ± 5	100 ± 19	9
		26 ± 8	88 ± 12	10
Prescott et al[167]	Inulin (single injection)	27 ± 6	104 ± 14	27
		27 ± 3	102 ± 20	8
		26 ± 8	95 ± 12	10
Askergren et al[8]	^{51}Cr-EDTA (single injection)	20-63	103 ± 15	26
		20-63	112 ± 13	15
Bäck et al[10]	Iohexol (single injection)	20-50	100 (78-122)	23
		51-65	83 (58-108)	20
		66-80	72 (52-92)	8
Arvidsson and Hedman[6]	Iohexol (constant infusion) triplicate determinations	19-30	116 ± 10	12
		19-30	117 ± 9	12
		19-30	110 ± 12	12
Rowe et al[185] Males only	Creatinine clearance	17-24	112 (93-131)	10
		25-34	112 (78-146)	73
		35-44	106 (74-138)	122
		45-54	101 (74-129)	152
		55-64	97 (69-122)	94
		65-74	89 (61-114)	68
		75-84	78 (52-102)	29
Sokoll et al[202] Females only	Creatinine clearance	40-49	94 (65-123)	56
		50-59	84 (58-110)	79
		60-69	80 (50-111)	82
		70-79	76 (46-105)	56
		80+	66 (48-85)	6

*All values have been rounded up or down to the nearest whole number.

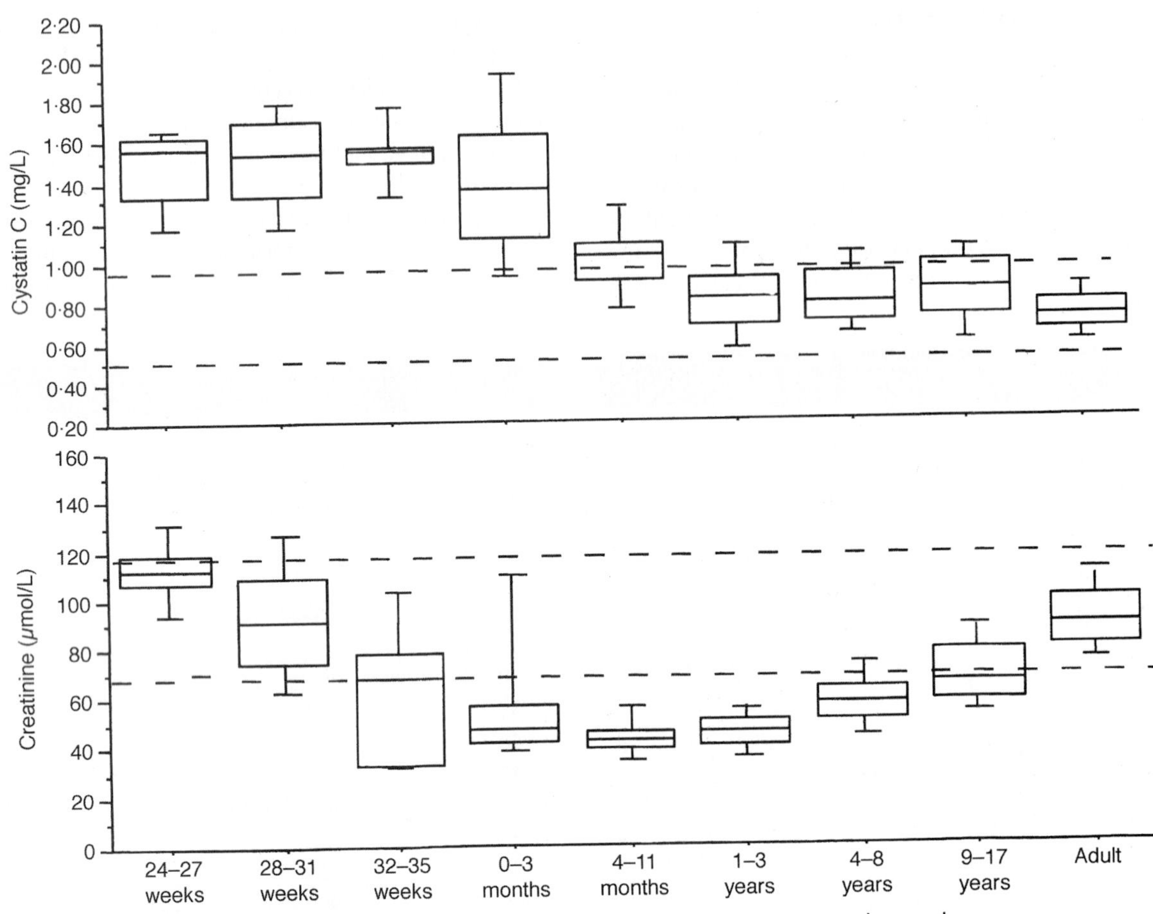

Figure 24-11 Age-related changes in cystatin C and creatinine superimposed upon the reference interval (horizontal dashed lines). Box and Whisker plot; the box represents 25th to 75th percentile with a horizontal line at the median; the whiskers extend to the highest and lowest values. *(From Newman DJ. Cystatin C. Ann Clin Biochem 2002;39:89-104.)*

influenced by local factors (e.g., interfaces between laboratory and clinical data systems). The susceptibility of these formulas to creatinine assay calibration variations must be recognized and, in this sense, the use of cystatin C, which can be reliably and simply measured on a single blood sample with no requirement for anthropomorphic adjustment, may be advantageous. The success of alternative markers such as cystatin C will depend on understanding the benefit of the superior diagnostic efficacy and improved clinical and economic outcomes in relation to the greater cost of the assay when compared with the Jaffe creatinine methods. However, although all of these markers are an improvement over plasma creatinine and creatinine clearance estimation, they are all only approximate measures of true GFR. Obviously, research into new and more accurate methods of estimating GFR is still required. Table 24-3 provides some reference data for GFR using a variety of methods.

REFERENCES

1. Abrahamson M, Grubb A, Olafsson I, Lundwall A. Molecular cloning and sequence analysis of cDNA coding for the precursor of the human cysteine proteinase inhibitor cystatin C. FEBS Letters 1987;216:229-33.
2. Agency for Healthcare Research and Quality. Evidence Report/Technology Assessment No. 84, Use of glycated hemoglobin and microalbuminuria in the monitoring of diabetes mellitus. 2003. Available at www.ahrq.gov
3. Ali ACY, Mihas CC, Campbell JA. Interferences of o-raffinose cross-linked hemoglobin in three methods for serum creatinine. Clin Chem 1997;43:1738-43.
4. Ambrose RT, Ketchum DF, Smith JW. Creatinine determined by "high performance" liquid chromatography. Clin Chem 1983;29:256-9.
5. Anaokar M. Should we screen for microalbuminuria? Med Interf (Sept) 1996;33-55.
6. Arvidsson A, Hedman A. Plasma and renal clearance of iohexol: A study on the reproducibility of a method for the glomerular filtration rate. Scand J Clin Lab Invest 1990;50:757-6.
7. Askergren A, Brandt R, Gullquist R, Silk B, Strandell T. Studies on kidney function in subjects exposed to

organic solvents: IV. Effect on 51-Cr-EDTA clearance. Acta Med Scand 1981;210:373-6.

8. Askergren A, Brandt R, Gullquist R, Silk B, Strandell T. The effect of fluid deprivation, antidiuretic hormone and forced fluid intake on ^{51}Cr-EDTA clearance. Acta Med Scand 1981;210:377-80.
9. Ayatse JOJ, Kwan JTC. Relative sensitivity of serum and urinary retinol binding protein and α_1-microglobulin in the assessment of renal function. Ann Clin Biochem 1991;28:514-6.
10. Back S-E, Ljungberg B, Nilsson-Ehle I, Borga O, Nilsson-Ehle P. Age dependence of renal function: Clearance of iohexol and *p*-amino hippurate in healthy males. Scand J Clin Lab Invest 1989;641-6.
11. Ballantyne FC, Gibbon J, O'Reilly D. Urine albumin should replace total protein for the assessment of glomerular proteinuria. Ann Clin Biochem 1993; 30:101-3.
12. Barratt A, Craig J, Cumming R, Irwig L, Salkeld G. A feasibility study of the early detection and treatment of renal disease by mass screening. University of Sydney, 1999.
13. Bazzi C, Petrini C, Rizza V, Arrigo G, Napodano P, Paparella M, et al. Urinary *N*-acetyl-β-D-glucosaminidase excretion as a marker of tubular cell dysfunction and a predictor of outcome in primary glomerulonephritis. Nephrol Dial Transplant 2002;17:1890-6.
14. Beetham R. Detection of Bence Jones protein in practice. Ann Clin Biochem 2000;37:563-70.
15. Beetham R. Biochemical investigation of suspected rhabdomyolysis. Ann Clin Biochem 2000;37:581-7.
16. Beetham R, Cattell WR. Proteinuria: Pathophysiology, significance and recommendations in clinical practice. Ann Clin Biochem 1993;30:425-34.
17. Beetham R, Dawnay A, Landon J, Cattell WR. A radioimmunoassay for retinol-binding protein in serum and urine. Clin Chem 1985;31:1364-7.
18. Bennett PH, Haffner S, Kasiske BL, Keane WF, Mogensen CE, Parving HH, et al. Screening and management of microalbuminuria in patients with diabetes mellitus: Recommendations to the scientific advisory board of the National Kidney Foundation from an Ad Hoc Committee of the Council on Diabetes Mellitus of the National Kidney Foundation. Am J Kidney Dis 1995;25:107-12.
19. Blake GM, Roe D, Lazarus CR. Long-term precision of glomerular filtration rate measurements using ^{51}Cr-EDTA plasma clearance. Nuclear Medicine Communications 1997;18:776-84.
20. Blaufox MD, Aurell M, Bubeck B, Fommei E, Piepsz A, Russell C et al. Report of radionuclides in nephrourology committee on renal clearance. J Nucl Med 1996;37:1883-90.
21. Blijenberg BG, Brouwer HJ. The accuracy of creatinine methods based on the Jaffe reaction: a questionable matter. Eur J Clin Chem Clin Biochem 1994;32: 909-13.
22. Blijenberg BG, Brouwer HJ, Kuller TJ, Leeneman R, van Leeuwen CJM. Improvements in creatinine methodology: a critical assessment. Eur J Clin Chem Clin Biochem 1994;32:529-37.
23. Bokenkamp A, Domanetzi M, Zinck R, Schumann G, Byrd D, Brodehl J. Cystatin C—a new marker of glomerular filtration rate in children independent of age and height. Pediatrics 1998;101:875-81.
24. Borch-Johnson K, Wenzel H, Viberti, GC, Mogensen CE. Is screening for microalbuminuria worthwhile in patients with insulin dependent diabetes? BMJ 1993; 306:1722-5.
25. Borsook H, Dubnoff JW. The hydrolysis of phosphocreatine and the origin of urinary creatinine. J Biol Chem 1947;168:493-510.
26. Bostom AG, Dworkin LD. Cystatin C measurement: improved detection of mild decrements in glomerular filtration rate versus creatinine-based estimates. Am J Kidney Dis 2000;36:205-7.
27. Bostom AG, Kronenberg F, Ritz E. Predictive performance of renal function equations for patients with chronic kidney disease and normal serum creatinine levels. J Am Soc Nephrol 2002;13:2140-4.
28. Bowers LD. Kinetic serum creatinine assays: 1. The role of various factors in determining specificity. Clin Chem 1980;26:551-4.
29. Brochner-Mortensen J. A simple method for the determination of glomerular filtration rate. Scand J Clin Lab Invest 1972;30:271-4.
30. Brochner-Mortensen J, Giese J, Rossing N. Renal inulin clearance versus total plasma clearance of ^{51}Cr-EDTA. Scand J Clin Lab Invest 1969;23:301-5.
31. Brochner-Mortensen J, Rodbro P. Selection of routine method for determination of glomerular filtration rate in adults. Scand J Clin Lab Invest 1976;36: 35-43.
32. Bruzzi I, Benigni A, Remuzzi G. Role of increased glomerular protein traffic in the progression of renal failure. Kidney Int 1997;62(Suppl):S29-S31.
33. Cameron JS. The patient with proteinuria and/or haematuria. In: Oxford Textbook of Clinical Nephrology 2nd Edition on CD Rom. Davison AM, Cameron JS, Grunfeld J-P, Kerr DN, Ritz E, Winearls CG, Eds. Oxford: Oxford University Press, 1998, Software Copyright Optimedia 1998. Section 3.4.
34. Cameron JS, Simmonds HA. Uric acid, gout and the kidney. J Clin Pathol 1981;34:1245-54.
35. Carobene A, Ferrero C, Ceriotti F, Modenese A, Besozzi M, et al. Creatinine measurement proficiency testing: assignment of matrix-adjusted ID GC-MS target values. Clin Chem 1997;43:1342-7.
36. Carter J, Child A. Serum uric acid levels in normal pregnancy. Aust NZ J Obstet Gynaecol 1989;29: 313-4.

37. Chambers RE, Bullock DG, Whicher JT. Urinary total protein estimation: Fact or fiction? Nephron 1989;53: 33-6.
38. Chambers RE, Bullock DG, Whicher JT. External quality assessment of total urinary protein estimation in the United Kingdom. Ann Clin Biochem 1991;28: 467-73.
39. Chantler C, Barrett TM. Estimation of glomerular filtration rate from plasma clearance of ^{51}chromium edetic acid. Arch Dis Child 1972;47:613-7.
40. Chitalia VC, Kothari J, Wells EJ, Livesey JH, Robson RA, Searle M, et al. Cost-benefit analysis and prediction of 24-hour proteinuria from the spot urine protein-creatinine ratio. Clin Nephrol 2000;55: 436-47.
41. Clarke W, Palmer-Toy DE. Outcomes—based evaluation of dipstick urinalysis. In Nichols JH (editor): Point-of-Care Testing; performance improvement and evidence-based outcomes. New York: Marcel Dekker, 2003:293-323.
42. Claudi T, Cooper JG. Comparison of urinary albumin excretion rate in overnight urine and albumin creatinine ratio in spot urine in diabetic patients in general practice. Scan J Prim Health Care 2001;19:247-8.
43. Cockcroft D, Gault MK. Prediction of creatinine clearance from serum creatinine. Nephron 1976; 16:31-41.
44. Coll E, Botey A, Alvarez L, Poch E, Quinto L, Saurina A et al. Serum cystatin C as a new marker for noninvasive estimation of glomerular filtration rate and as a marker for early renal impairment. Am J Kidney Dis 2000;36:29-34.
45. Cook JGH. Factors influencing the assay of creatinine. Ann Clin Biochem 1975;12:219-32.
46. Coresh J, Astor BC, McQuillan G, Kusek J, Greene T, van-Lente F, et al. Calibration and random variation of the serum creatinine assay as critical elements of using equations to estimate glomerular filtration rate. Am J Kidney Dis 2002;39:920-9.
47. Coresh J, Toto RD, Kirk KA, Whelton PK, Massry S, Jones C, et al. Creatinine clearance as a measure of GFR in screenees for the African-American study of kidney disease and hypertension pilot study. Am J Kidney Dis 1998;32:32-42.
48. Counahan R, Chantler C, Ghazali S, Kirkwood B, Rose F, Barratt TM. Estimation of glomerular filtration rate from plasma creatinine concentration in children. Arch Dis Child 1976;51:875-8.
49. den Hollander JG, Wulkan RW, Mantel MJ, Berghout A. Is cystatin C a marker of glomerular filtration rate in thyroid dysfunction? Clin Chem 2003;49:1558-9.
50. Dharnidharka VR, Kwon C, Stevens G. Serum cystatin C is superior to serum creatinine as a marker of kidney function: a meta-analysis. Am J Kidney Dis 2002;40:221-6.
51. D'Mello L, Niculescu I, Carr E, Barron J, Kwan JTC, Newman DJ. Development of an outpatient GFR procedure suitable for epidemiological investigations. Abstract presented at; The Renal Association, London, UK, Autumn 2001. Available at: http://www.renal.org
52. Dorland's Illustrated Medical Dictionary. 28th ed. Philadelphia: WB Saunders, 1994.
53. DuBois D, Dubois EF. A formula to estimate the approximate surface area if height and weight be known. Arch Intern Med 1916;17:863-70.
54. Duncan L, Heathcote J, Djurdjev O, Levin A. Screening for renal disease using serum creatinine: who are we missing? Nephrol Dial Trans 2001;16:1042-6.
55. Duncan P, Gochman N, Cooper T, Smith E, Bayse D. A candidate reference method for uric acid in serum: I. Optimization and evaluation. Clin Chem 1982;28: 284-90.
56. Dussol B, Berland Y. Urinary kidney stone inhibitors: Where are we? Nephrol Dial Transplant 1996;11:1222-4.
57. Dyson EH, Will EJ, Davison AM, O'Malley AH, Shepherd HT, Jones RG. Use of the urinary protein creatinine index to assess proteinuria in renal transplant patients. Nephrol Dial Transplant 1992;7:450-2.
58. Eddy CV, Arnold MA. Near-infrared spectroscopy for measuring urea in hemodialysis fluids. Clin Chem 2001;47:1279-86.
59. Effersoe H, Rosenkilde P, Groth S, et al. Measurement of renal function with iohexol: A comparison of iohexol, 99mTc-DTPA and 51Cr-EDTA clearance. Invest Radiol 1990;25:778-82.
60. Ellerbe P, Cohen A, Welch MJ, White E. Determination of serum uric acid by isotope dilution mass spectrometry as a new candidate reference method. Anal Chem 1990;62:2173-7.
61. Estelberger W, Petek W, Zitta S, Mauric A, Hom S, Holzer H, et al. Determination of the glomerular filtration rate by identification of sinistrin kinetics. Eur J Clin Chem Clin Biochem 1995;33:201-9.
62. Fay RA. Uric acid in pregnancy and preeclampsia: an alternative hypothesis. Aust NZ J Obstet Gynaecol 1990;30:141-2.
63. Finney H, Bates CJ, Price CP. Plasma cystatin C determinations in healthy elderly population. Arch Gerontol Geriatr 1999;29:75-94.
64. Finney H, Newman DJ, Gruber W, Merle P, Price CP. Initial evaluation of cystatin C measurement by particle enhanced immunonephelometry on the Behring nephelometer systems (BNA, BNII). Clin Chem 1997;43:1016-22.
65. Finney H, Newman DJ, Price CP. Adult reference ranges for cystatin C, creatinine and predicted creatinine clearance. Ann Clin Biochem 2000;37:49-59.
66. Fliser D, Ritz E. Serum cystatin C concentration as a marker of renal dysfunction in the elderly. Am J Kidney Dis 2001;37:79-83.

67. Fogazzi GB. Urinalysis and microscopy. In: Cameron JS, Davison AM, Grunfeld J.-P, Kerr D, Ritz E, eds. Oxford Text Book of Clinical Nephrology, vol 1. Oxford: Oxford University Press, 1992:16.
68. Fossati P, Prencipe L, Berti G. Use of 3,5-dichloro-2-hydroxybenzenesulfonic acid/4-amino-phenazone chromogenic system in direct enzymic assay of uric acid in serum and urine. Clin Chem 1980;26:227-31.
69. Fossati P, Prencipe L, Berti G. Enzymatic creatinine assay: A new colorimetric method based on hydrogen peroxide measurement. Clin Chem 1983;29:1494-6.
70. Fossati P, Ponti M, Passoni G, Tarenghi G, Melzi d'Eril GV, Prencipe L. A step forward in enzymatic measurement of creatinine. Clin Chem 1994;40: 130-7.
71. Freedman BI, Iskander SS, Appel RG. The link between hypertension and nephrosclerosis. Am J Kidney Dis 1995;25:207-21.
72. Fricker M, Wiesli P, Brandle M, Schwegler B, Schmid C. Impact of thyroid dysfunction on serum cystatin C. Kidney Int 2003;63:1944-7.
73. Gardner MD, Scott R. Age- and sex-related reference ranges for eight plasma constituents derived from randomly selected adults in a Scottish new town. J Clin Pathol 1980;33:380-5.
74. Garred LJ, Canaud B, Bosc JY, Tetta C. Urea rebound and delivered K_t/V determination with a continuous urea sensor. Nephrol Dial Transplant 1997;12:535-42.
75. Gaspari F, Perico N, Matalone M, Signorini O, Azzollini N, Mister M, et al. Precision of plasma clearance of iohexol for estimation of GFR in patients with renal disease. J Am Soc Nephrol 1998;9:310-13.
76. Gaspari F, Perico N, Ruggenenti P, Mosconi L, Amuchastegui CS, Guerini E, et al. Plasma clearance of nonradioactive iohexol as a measure of glomerular filtration rate. J Am Soc Nephrol 1995;6:257-63.
77. Ginsberg JM, Chang BS, Matarese RA, Garella S. Use of single voided urine samples to estimate quantitative proteinuria. New Engl J Med 1983;309:1543-6.
78. Goldberg TH, Finkelstein MS. Difficulties in estimating the glomerular filtration rate in the elderly. Arch Intern Med 1987;147:1430-3.
79. Goldman R. Creatinine excretion in renal failure. Proc Soc Exp Biol Med 1954;85:446-50.
80. Gorus F, Schram E. Chemiluminescent assay of uric acid. Arch Int Physiol Biochem 1977;85:981-2.
81. Gosling P. Microalbuminuria: a sensitive indicator of non-renal disease? Ann Clin Biochem 1995;32: 439-41.
82. Gourmelin Y, Gouget B, Truchaud A. Electrode measurement of glucose and urea in undiluted samples. Clin Chem 1990;36:1646-9.
83. Gray MR, Phillips E, Young DM, Price CP. Evaluation of a rapid specific ward based assay for creatinine in blood. Clin Nephrol 1995;43:169-73.
84. Grubb A. Diagnostic value of analysis of cystatin C and protein HC in biological fluids. Clin Nephrol 1992;38(Suppl 1):S20-S27.
85. Harmoinen A, Lehtimaki T, Korpela M, Turjanmaa V, Saha H. Diagnostic accuracies of plasma creatinine, cystatin C, and glomerular filtration rate calculated by the Cockcroft-Gault and Levey (MDRD) formulas. Clin Chem 2003;49:1223-5.
86. Helin I, Axenram M, Grubb A. Serum cystatin C as a determinant of glomerular filtration rate in children. Clinical Nephrology 1998;49:221-5.
87. Henderson MJ. Renal stone disease: Investigative aspects. Arch Dis Child 1993;68:160-2.
88. Heymsfield SB, Arteaga C, McManus C, Smith J, Moffitt S. Measurement of muscle mass in humans: Validity of the 24-hour urinary creatinine method. Am J Clin Nutr 1983;37:478-94.
89. Hofmann W, Regenbogen C, Edel H, Guder WG. Diagnostic strategies in urinalysis. Kidney Int 1994;46:S111-S114.
90. Houlihan C, Jenkins M, Osicka T, Scott A, Parkin D, Jerums G. A comparison of the plasma disappearance of iohexol and 99mTc-DTPA for the measurement of glomerular filtration rate (GFR) in diabetes. Aust N Z J Med 1999;29:693-700.
91. Hoyer JR, Sisson SP, Vernier RL. Tamm-Horsfall glycoprotein: ultrastructural immunoperoxidase localization in rat kidney. Lab Invest 1979;41:168-73.
92. Hsu CY, Chertow GM, Curhan GC. Methodological issues in studying the epidemiology of mild to moderate chronic renal insufficiency. Kidney Int 2002;61: 1567-76.
93. Hullin DA, McGrane MTG. Effect of bilirubin on uricase-peroxidase coupled reactions. Implications for urate measurement in clinical samples and external quality assessment schemes. Ann Clin Biochem 1991;28:98-100.
94. Ingebretsen OC, Borgen J, Farstad M. Uric acid determination: Reversed-phase liquid chromatography with ultraviolet detection compared with kinetic and equilibrium adaptations of the uricase method. Clin Chem 1982;28:496-8.
95. Ivandic M, Hofmann W, Guder WG. Development and evaluation of a urine protein expert system. Clin Chem 1996;42:1214-22.
96. Jackle-Meyer I, Szukics B, Neubauer K, Metze V, Petzoldt R, Stolte H. Extracellular matrix proteins as early markers in diabetic nephropathy. Eur J Clin Chem Clin Biochem 1995;33:211-9.
97. Jacobsen FK, Christensen CK, Mogensen CE, Heilskov NSC. Evaluation of kidney function after meals. Lancet 1980;1:319.
98. Jacobson L. A method for the calculation of renal clearance based upon a single plasma sample. Clin Physiol 1983;3:297-305.
99. Jacobsson B, Lignelid H, Bergerheim US. Transthyretin and cystatin C are catabolized in proxi-

mal tubular epithelial cells and the proteins are not useful as markers for renal cell carcinomas. Histopathology 1995;26:559-64.

100. James DR, Price CP. Interference in colorimetric reactions for measuring hydrogen peroxide. Ann Clin Biochem 1984;21:398-404.
101. Jayagopal V, Keevil BG, Atkin SL, Jennings PE, Kilpatrick ES. Paradoxical changes in cystatin C and serum creatinine in patients with hypo- and hyperthyroidism. Clin Chem 2003;49:680-1.
102. Jenkins MA, Houlihan C, Ratnaike S, Jerums G, Des Parkin J. Measurement of iohexol by capillary electrophoresis: minimizing practical problems encountered. Ann Clin Biochem 2000;37:529-36.
103. Jensen JS, Borch-Johnsen K, Jensen G, Feldt-Rasmussen B. Microalbuminuria reflects a generalized transvascular albumin leakiness in clinically healthy subjects. Clin Sci 1995;88:629-33.
104. Jung K, Pergande M, Priem F, Becker S, Klotzek S. Rapid screening of low molecular mass proteinuria: Evaluation of the first immunochemical test strip for the detection of α_1-microglobulin in urine. Eur J Clin Chem Clin Biochem 1993;31:683-7.
105. Kadinger CL, O'Kell RT. Clinical evaluation of Eastman Kodak's Ektachem 400 analyzer. Clin Chem 1983;29:498-501.
106. Kageyama N. A direct colorimetric determination of uric acid in serum and urine with uricase-catalase system. Clin Chim Acta 1971;31:421-6.
107. Karmen A, Lent R. Clinical chemistry testing with the Ames SERALYZER dry reagent system. J Clin Lab Auto 1982;2:284-90.
108. Kasdan HL, Ashe M, Chapoulaud E, Dougherty WM, Halby S, Tindel JR. Comparison of pathological cast analytical performance and flagging of automated urine sediment analyzers: a new flow imaging system versus flow cytometry. Clin Chem 2003;49:A160.
109. Kasdan HL, Chapoulaud E, Dougherty WM, Halby S, Tindel JR. Comparison of automated urine particle analysis methods: a new flow imaging system versus flow cytometry. Clin Chem 2002;48:A5.
110. Kassirer JP. Clinical evaluation of kidney function: Glomerular function. N Engl J Med 1971;285: 385-9.
111. Keane WF, Brenner BM, Parving H-H, eds. Progression of renal disease. Kidney Int 1994;45(Suppl):S1-S180.
112. Keane WF, Eknoyan G. Proteinuria, albuminuria, risk, assessment, detection, elimination (PARADE): a position paper of the National Kidney Foundation. Am J kidney Dis 1999;33:1004-10.
113. Kessler A, Siekmann L. Measurement of urea in human serum by isotope dilution mass spectrometry: a reference procedure. Clin Chem 1999;45:1523-9.
114. Kharbanda R, Lauder J, Thomson D, Gouldesbrough DR, Harrison DJ. Heterogeneity of glutathione S-transferase isoenzyme expression in renal disease. Nephrol Dial Transplant 1991;6:695-700.
115. Knapp ML, Mayne PD. Development of an automated kinetic Jaffe method designed to minimize bilirubin interference in plasma creatinine assays. Clin Chim Acta 1987;168:239-46.
116. Kouri T, Solakivi T, Harmoinen A. Performance of NycoCard AlbuminTM; and Micral-TestTM; rapid methods for detecting microalbuminuria. Eur J Clin Chem Clin Biochem 1994;32:419-23.
117. Kroll MH, Elin RJ. Interference with clinical laboratory analyses. Clin Chem 1994;40:1996-2005.
118. Krutzen E, Back SE, Nilsson-Ehlr I, Nilsson-Ehle P. Plasma clearance of a new contrast agent, iohexol: A method for the assessment of glomerular filtration rate. J Lab Clin Med 1984;104:955-61.
119. Kutter D, Thoma J, Kremer A, Hansen S, Carol R. Screening for oligoalbuminuria by means of Micral-TestTM;: II. A new immunological test strip. Eur J Clin Chem Clin Biochem 1995;33:243-5.
120. Kyhse-Andersen J, Schmidt C, Nordin G, Andersson B, Nilsson-Ehle P, Lindstrom V, et al. Serum cystatin C, determined by a rapid, automated particle-enhanced turbidimetric method, is a better marker than serum creatinine for glomerular filtration rate. Clin Chem 1994;40:1921-6.
121. Lamb EJ, Price CP. Use of azure-D2 for the measurement of uric acid in serum. Eur J Clin Chem Clin Biochem 1995;33:595-601.
122. Lamb EJ, Webb MC, Simpson DE, Coakley AJ, Newman DJ, O'Riordan SE. Estimation of glomerular filtration rate in older patients with chronic renal insufficiency: is the Modification of Diet in Renal Disease formula an improvement? J Am Geriatrics Soc 2003;51:1012-7.
123. Laterza OF, Price CP, Scott MG. Cystatin C: an improved estimator of glomerular filtration rate? Clin Chem 2002;48:699-707.
124. Lawson N, Lang T, Broughton A, Prinsloo P, Turner C, Marenah C. Creatinine assays: time for action? Ann Clin Biochem 2002;39:599-602.
125. Leary NO, Pembroke A, Duggan PF. Adapting the uricase/peroxidase procedure for plasma urate to reduce interference due to haemolysis, icterus or lipaemia. Ann Clin Biochem 1992;29:85-9.
126. Le Bricon T, Erlich D, Bengoufa D, Dussaucy M, Garnier JP, Bousquet B. Sodium dodecyl sulfate-agarose gel electrophoresis of urinary proteins: application to multiple myeloma. Clin Chem 1998;44: 1191-7.
127. Lespinas F, Dupuy G, Revol F, Aubry C. Enzyme urea assay: A new colorimetric method based on hydrogen peroxide measurement. Clin Chem 1989;35: 654-8.
128. Levey AS, Bosch JP, Lewis JB, Greene T, Rogers N, Roth D. A more accurate method to estimate

glomerular filtration rate from serum creatinine. Ann Intern Med 1999;130:461-70.

129. Levey AS, Greene T, Kusek JW. A simplified equation to predict glomerular filtration rate from serum creatinine. J Am Soc Nephrol 2000;11:A0828.
130. Lind T, Godfrey KA, Otun H. Changes in serum uric acid concentrations during normal pregnancy. Br J Obstet Gynaecol 1984;91:128-32.
131. Lote CJ. Essential anatomy of the kidney. In: Lote CJ, ed. Principles of Renal Physiology, 3rd ed. London: Chapman and Hall, 1994:21-9.
132. Loun B, Copeland KR, Sedor FA. Ultrafiltration discrepancies in recovery of myoglobin from urine. Clin Chem 1996;42:965-9.
133. Lowry OH, Rosebrough NJ, Farr AL. Protein measurement with the Folin phenol reagent. J Biol Chem 1951;193:265-75.
134. Mathies JC. Adaptation of the Berthelot color reaction for the determination of urea nitrogen in serum and urine to an Ultramicro System. Clin Chem 1964;10:366-75.
135. Mattix HJ, Hsu CY, Shaykevich S, Curhan G. Use of the albumin/creatinine ratio to detect microalbuminuria: implications of sex and race. J Am Soc Nephrol 2002;13:1034-9.
136. Mauck JC, Mauck L, Novros J, Norton GE. Development of a single-slide KODAK EKTACHEM thin film assay for serum and urine creatinine [Abstract]. Clin Chem 1986;32:1197-8.
137. McDowell TL. Benzethonium chloride method for proteins adapted to centrifugal analysis. Clin Chem 1985;31:864-6.
138. Meites S, Thompson C, Roach RW. Two ultramicroscale methods for plasma uric acid analysis with uricase. Clin Chem 1974;20:790-3.
139. Miller BF, Winkler AW. The renal excretion of endogenous creatinine in man: Comparison with exogenous creatinine and inulin. J Clin Invest 1938;17:31-40.
140. Miller PF, Speirs NI, Aparicio SR, Lendon M, Savage JM, Postlethwaite RJ, et al. Long term prognosis of recurrent haematuria. Arch Dis Child 1985;60:420-5.
141. Mockel T, Morrison D, Yatscoff R. Evaluation of the i-STAT™ system: a portable chemistry analyser for the measurement of sodium, potassium, chloride, urea, glucose, and hematocrit. Clin Biochem 1995;28:187-92.
142. Mogensen CE, Vestbo E, Poulson PL, Christiansen C, Damsgaard EM, Eiskjaer H, et al. Microalbuminuria and potential confounders. Diabetes Care 1995;18:572-81.
143. Morishita Y, Nakane K, Fukatsu T, Nakashima N, Tsuji K, Soya Y, et al. Kinetic assay of serum and urine for urea with use of urease and leucine dehydrogenase. Clin Chem 1997;43:1932-6.
144. Murakami M. Screening for proteinuria and hematuria in school children: Methods and results. Acta Paediatr Jpn 1990;32:682-9.
145. Naslund B, Stahle L, Lundin A, Anderstam B, Arner P, Bergstrom J. Luminometric single step urea assay using ATP-hydrolyzing urease. Clin Chem 1998;44:1964-73.
146. National Kidney Foundation-K/DOQI. Clinical practice guidelines for chronic kidney disease: evaluation, classification, and stratification. Am J Kidney Dis 2002;39(suppl 1):S1-266.
147. Neild GH, Foxall PJD, Lindon JC, Holmes EC, Nicholson JK. Uroscopy in the 21st century: High-field NMR spectroscopy. Nephrol Dial Transplant 1997;12:404-17.
148. Newall RG, ed. Clinical Urinalysis. Stoke Poges, United Kingdom, Miles Ltd., Ames Division, 1990:133-40.
149. Newman DJ. Cystatin C. Ann Clin Biochem 2002;39:89-104.
150. Newman DJ, Pugia MJ, Lott JA, Wallace JF, Hiar AM. Urinary protein and albumin excretion corrected by creatinine and specific gravity. Clin Chim Acta 2000;294:139-55.
151. Newman DJ, Thakkar H, Edwards RG, Wilkie M, White T, Grubb AO, et al. Serum cystatin C measured by automated immunoassay: A more sensitive marker of changes in GFR than serum creatinine. Kidney Int 1995;47:312-8.
152. Newman DJ, Thakkar H, Medcalf EA, Gray MR, Price CP. Use of urine albumin measurement as a replacement for total protein. Clin Nephrol 1995;43:104-9.
153. Nishi HH, Elin RJ. Three turbidimetric methods for determining total protein compared. Clin Chem 1985;31:1377-80.
154. O'Leary N, Pembroke A, Duggan PF. A simplified procedure for eliminating the negative interference of bilirubin in the Jaffe reaction for creatinine. Clin Chem 1992;38:1749-51.
155. O'Riordan SE, Webb MC, Stowe HJ, Simpson DE, Kandarpa M, Coakley AJ, et al. Cystatin C improves the detection of mild renal dysfunction in older patients. Ann Clin Biochem 2003;40:648-55.
156. Ota H, Yasuma A. Lysozyme activity in hematologic and non-hematologic disorders with special reference to reactive monocytosis associated with chronic infections and inflammatory reactions. Tohoku J Exp Med 1974;114:15-26.
157. Ottiger C, Huber AR. Quantitative urine particle analysis: integrative approach for the optimal combination of automation with UF-100 and microscopic review with KOVA cell chamber. Clin Chem 2003;49:617-23.
158. Parekh AC, Sims C. Serum creatinine assay by use of 3,5 dinitrobenzoates: a critique. Clin Chem 1977;23:2066-71.

159. Parsons MP, Newman DJ, Newall RG, Price CP. Validation of a point-of-care assay for the urinary albumin:creatinine ratio. Clin Chem 1999;45:414-7.
160. Parsons M, Newman DJ, Pugia M, Newall RG, Price CP. Performance of a reagent strip device for quantitation of the urine albumin:creatinine ratio in a point of care setting. Clin Nephrol 1999;51:220-7.
161. Payn MM, Webb MC, Lawrence D, Lamb EJ. α_1-microglobulin is stable in human urine ex vivo. Clin Chem 2002;48:1136-8.
162. Payne RB. Creatinine clearance: A redundant clinical investigation. Ann Clin Biochem 1986;26:243-50.
163. Pergande M, Jung K, Precht S, Fels LM, Herbort C, Stolte H. Changed excretion of urinary proteins and enzymes by chronic exposure to lead. Nephrol Dial Transplant 1994;9:613-8.
164. Perrone RD, Madias NE, Levey AS. Serum creatinine as an index of renal function: New insights into old concepts. Clin Chem 1992;38:1933-53.
165. Pocsi I, Taylor SA, Richardson AC, Aamlid KH, Smith BV, Price RG. "VRA-GlcNAc": Novel substrate for N-acetyl-β-D-glucosaminidase applied to assay of this enzyme in urine. Clin Chem 1990;36:1884-8.
166. Popper H, Mandel E. Filtrations and Reabsorptions Leitung in der Nierenpathologie. Erg Inn Med Kinder 1937;53:685-95.
167. Prescott LF, Freestone S, McAuslane JAN. Reassessment of the single intravenous injection method with inulin for measurement of the glomerular filtration rate in man. Clin Sci 1991;80:167-76.
168. Price CP, Finney H. Developments in the assessment of glomerular filtration rate. Clin Chim Acta 2000; 297:55-66.
169. Price CP, James DR. Analytical reviews in clinical biochemistry: The measurement of urate. Ann Clin Biochem 1988;25:484-98.
170. Price CP, Koller PU. A multicentre study of the new Reflotron™; system for the measurement of urea, glucose, triacylglycerols, cholesterol, gamma-glutamyltransferase and haemoglobin. Eur J Clin Chem Clin Biochem 1988;26:233-50.
171. Price RG. The role of NAG (N-acetyl-β-D-glucosaminidase) in the diagnosis of kidney disease including the monitoring of nephrotoxicity. Clin Nephrol 1992;38:S14-9.
172. Price RG, Taylor SA, Crutchen E. Assay of laminin fragments in the assessment of renal disease. Kidney Int 1994;47:S25-8.
173. Priem F, Althaus H, Birnbaum M, Sinha P, Conradt HS, Jung K. β-trace protein in serum: a new marker of glomerular filtration rate in the creatinine-blind range. Clin Chem 1999;45:567-8.
174. Pugia MJ, Lott JA, Clark LW, Parker DR, Wallace JF, Willis TW. Comparison of urine dipsticks with quantitative methods for microalbuminuria. Eur J Clin Chem Clin Biochem 1997;35:693-700.
175. Redman CWG, Beilin LJ, Bonnar J, Wilkinson RH. Plasma urate measurements in predicting fetal death in hypertensive pregnancy. Lancet 1976;1:1370-3.
176. Rehberg PB. Studies on kidney function: II. The excretion of urea and chloride analyzed according to a modified filtration reabsorption theory. Biochem J 1926;20:461-82.
177. Rehling M, Moller ML, Thram-Drup B, Lund JO, Trad-Jensen J. Simultaneous measurement of renal clearance and plasma clearance of ^{99}mTc-labelled diethylene triaminepenta-acetate, ^{51}Cr-labelled ethylene diamine tetra-acetate and inulin in man. Clin Sci 1984;66:613-9.
178. Remuzzi G, Ruggenenti P, Benigni A. Understanding the nature of renal disease progression. Kidney Int 1997;51:2-15.
179. Ricos C, Jimenez CV, Hernandez A, Simon M, Perich C, Alvarez V, et al. Biological variation in urine samples used for analyte measurements. Clin Chem 1994;40:472-7.
180. Rocco MV, Buckalew VM, Jr, Moore LC, Shihabi ZK. Capillary electrophoresis for the determination of glomerular filtration rate using nonradioactive iohexol. Am J Kidney Dis 1996;28:173-7.
181. Rolin HA, Hall PM, Wei R. Inaccuracy of estimated creatinine clearance for prediction of iothalamate glomerular filtration rate. Am J Kidney Dis 1984; 9:48-54.
182. Ross JW, Miller WG, Myers GL, Praestgaard J. The accuracy of laboratory measurements in clinical chemistry: a study of 11 routine chemistry analytes in the College of American Pathologists Chemistry Survey with fresh frozen serum, definitive methods, and reference methods. Arch Pathol Lab Med 1998; 122:587-608.
183. Rovida E, Mosca A, Dossi G. Serum and whole blood urea determination by the use of a microprocessor controlled differential pH analyzer. Eur J Clin Chem Clin Biochem 1981;19:820.
184. Rowe DJ, Omar H, Barratt SL, Biggs P. An evaluation of blood creatinine measurement by creatinase on the NOVA M7 blood gas analyser. Clin Chim Acta 2001; 307:23-5.
185. Rowe JW, Andres R, Tobin JD, Norris AH, Shock NW. The effect of age on creatinine clearance in men: A cross-sectional and longitudinal study. J Gerontol 1976;31:155-63.
186. Rudd PT, Hughes EA, Placzek MM, Hodes DT. Reference ranges for plasma creatinine during the first month of life. Arch Dis Child 1983;58:212-5.
187. Ruggenenti P, Gaspari F, Perna A, Remuzzi G. Cross-sectional longitudinal study of spot morning urine protein:creatinine ratio, 24-hour urine protein excretion rate, glomerular filtration rate, and end stage renal failure in chronic renal disease in patients without diabetes. BMJ 1998;316:504-9.

188. Sampson EJ, Baird MA. Chemical inhibition used in a kinetic urease/glutamate dehydrogenase method for urea in serum. Clin Chem 1979;25:1721-9.
189. Sampson EJ, Baird MA, Burtis CA, Smith EM, Witte DL, Bayse DD. A coupled-enzyme equilibrium method for measuring urea in serum: optimization and evaluation of the AACC Study Group on urea candidate reference method. Clin Chem 1980;26: 816-26.
190. Samuell CT, Kasidas GP. Biochemical investigations in renal stone formers. Ann Clin Biochem 1995;32: 112-22.
191. Sarrubi FA, Hull JH. Amikacin serum concentrations: prediction of levels and dosage guidelines. Ann Intern Med 1978;89:612-8.
192. Saudan PJ, Brown MA, Farrell T, Shaw L. Improved methods of assessing proteinuria in hypertensive pregnancy. Brit J Obstet Gynaecol 1997;104:1159-64.
193. Scherberich JE, Wolf G. Disintegration and recovery of kidney membrane proteins: Consequences of acute and chronic renal failure. Kidney Int 1994;47(Suppl): S52-S57.
194. Schmidt S, Ritz E. The role of angiotensin in converting enzyme gene polymorphism in renal diseases. Curr Opin Nephrol Hyperten 1996;5:552-5.
195. Schwartz GJ, Gauthier B. A simple estimate of glomerular filtration rate in adolescent boys. J Pediatr 1985;106:522-6.
196. Scott JT. Asymptomatic hyperuricaemia. BMJ 1987; 294:987-8.
197. Sena SF, Syed D, Romeo R, Krzymowski GA, McComb RB. Lidocaine metabolite and creatinine measurements in the Ektachem 700: steps to minimize its impact on patient care. Clin Chem 1988; 34:2144-8.
198. Shaw RA, Low-Ying S, Leroux M, Mantsch HH. Toward reagent-free clinical analysis: quantitation of urine urea, creatinine, and total protein from the mid-infrared spectra of dried urine films. Clin Chem 2000;46:1493-5.
199. Simmonds HA. Purine and pyrimidine disorders. In: Holton JB, ed. The Inherited Metabolic Diseases. Philadelphia: Churchill Livingstone, 1994:297-350.
200. Slack TK, Wilson DM. Normal renal function: C_{IN} and C_{PAH} in healthy donors before and after nephrectomy. Mayo Clin Proc 1976;51:296-300.
201. Snaith ML. Gout, hyperuricaemia, and crystal arthritis. BMJ 1995;310:521-4.
202. Sokoll LJ, Russell RM, Sadowski JA, Morrow FD. Establishment of creatinine clearance: Reference values in older women. Clin Chem 1994;40:2276-81.
203. Soldin SJ, Hicks JM, eds. Pediatric Reference Ranges, Washington: AACC Press, 1995.
204. Spayd RW, Bruschi B, Burdick BA, Dappen GH, Eikenberry JN, Esders TW, et al. Multilayer-film elements for clinical analysis: Application to representative chemical determinations. Clin Chem 1978;24: 1343-50.
205. Spencer K. Analytical reviews in clinical biochemistry: The estimation of creatinine. Ann Clin Biochem 1986;23:1-25.
206. Stephenson JM, Kenny S, Stevens LK, Fuller JH, Lee E. Proteinuria and mortality in diabetes: The WHO Multinational Study of Vascular Disease in Diabetes. Diab Med 1995;12:149-55.
207. Stevens JF, Tsang W, Newall RG. Measurement of bilirubin, cholesterol, and creatinine in serum and plasma, by solid phase reflectance spectroscopy. J Clin Pathol 1983;36:598-601.
208. Stowe H, Lawrence D, Newman D, Lamb EJ. Analytical performance of a particle-enhanced nephelometric immunoassay (PENIA) for serum cystatin C using rate analysis. Clin Chem 2001;47:1482-5.
209. Sugita O, Tomiyama Y, Matsuto T, Okada M, Gejyo F, Arakawa M, et al. A new enzymatic method for the determination of inulin. Ann Clin Biochem 1995;32:561-5.
210. Sugita O, Uchiyama K, Yamada T, Sato T, Okada M, Takeuchi K. Reference values of serum and urine creatinine, and of creatinine clearance, by a new enzymatic method. Ann Clin Biochem 1992;29: 523-8.
211. Summerfield AL, Hortin GL, Smith CH, Wilhite TR, Landt M. Automated enzymatic analysis for inulin. Clin Chem 1993;39:2333-7.
212. Sundberg MW, Becker RW, Esders TW, Figueras J, Goodhue CT. An enzymatic creatinine assay and a direct ammonia assay in coated thin films. Clin Chem 1983;29:645-9.
213. Swain RR, Biggs SL. Positive interference with the Jaffe reaction by cephalosporin antibiotics. Clin Chem 1977;23:1340-2.
214. Swan SK. The search continues—an ideal marker of GFR. Clin Chem 1997;43:913-4.
215. Swedko PJ, Clark HD, Paramsothy K, Akbari A. Serum creatinine is an inadequate screening test for renal failure in elderly patients. Arch Intern Med 2003;163:356-60.
216. Tabata M, Kidneyo T, Totani M. Automated assay of creatinine in serum as simplified by the use of immobilised enzymes, creatinine deaminase and glutamate dehydrogenase. Anal Biochem 1983;134:44-9.
217. Taylor AJ, Vadgama P. Analytical reviews in clinical biochemistry: the estimation of urea. Ann Clin Biochem 1992;29:245-64.
218. Tenstad O, Roald AB, Grubb A, Aukland K. Renal handling of radiolabelled human cystatin C in the rat. Scand J Clin Lab Invest 1996;56:409-14.
219. Thakkar H, Cornelius J, Dronfield DM, Medcalf EA, Newman DJ, Price CP. Development of a rapid latex enhanced turbidimetric assay for retinol binding protein. Ann Clin Biochem 1991;28:407-11.

220. Thakkar H, Newman DJ, Holownia P, Davey CL, Wang CC, Lloyd J. Development and validation of a particle enhanced turbidimetric inhibition assay for urine albumin on the Du Pont aca analyser. Clin Chem 1997;43:109-13.
221. Tietz NW, ed. Clinical Guide to Laboratory Tests. 3rd ed. Philadelphia: WB Saunders Co, 1995.
222. Tietz NW, Shuey DF, Wekstein DR. Laboratory values in fit aging individuals—sexagenarians through centenarians. Clin Chem 1992;38:1167-85.
223. Van Acker BA, Koomen GC, Koopman MG, de Waart DR, Arisz L. Creatinine clearance during cimetidine administration for measurement of glomerular filtration rate. Lancet 1992;340:1326-9.
224. Vander AJ, ed. Renal Physiology, 5th ed. New York: McGraw-Hill, 1995:37.
225. van der Slik W, Leinberger R. Results of a multicentre study for the measurement of uric acid, aspartate aminotransferase and alanine aminotransferase using Reflotron.™ Eur J Clin Chem Clin Biochem 1992;17: 67-73.
226. Van Pilsum JF, Martin RP, Kito E. Determination of creatine, creatinine, arginine, guanidinoacetic acid, guanidine and methyl-guanidine in biological fluids. J Biol Chem 1956;222:225-6.
227. Van Rossum LK, Mathot RAA, Cransberg K, Vulto AG. Optimal sampling strategies to assess inulin clearance in children by the inulin single-injection method. Clin Chem 2003;49:1170-9.
228. Vasiliades J. Reaction of alkaline sodium picrate with creatinine: 1. Kinetics and mechanism of formation of the non creatinine picric acid complex. Clin Chem 1976;22:1664-71.
229. Wahlefeld AW, Siedel J. Creatine and creatinine. In: Methods of Enzymatic Analysis, vol 8. 3rd ed. Weinheim, 1985:488-90.
230. Walser M. Assessing renal function from creatinine measurements in adults with chronic renal failure. Am J Kidney Dis 1998;32:23-31.
231. Wasen E, Suominen P, Isoaho R, Matilla K, Virtanen A, Kivela SL, et al. Serum cystatin C as a marker of kidney function in an elderly population. Clin Chem 2002;48:1138-40.
232. Watkins PJ. The effect of ketone bodies on the determination of creatinine. Clin Chim Acta 1967;18:191-6.
233. Weatherburn MW, Trotman RBB, Jackson SH. Specific method for serum creatinine determination based on ion exchange chromatography and an automated alkaline picrate reaction: A proposed reference method. Clin Biochem 1978;11:159-66.
234. Weber MH, Verwiebe R. α_1-microglobulin (protein HC): features of a promising indicator of proximal tubular dysfunction. Eur J Clin Chem Clin Biochem 1992;30:683-91.
235. Welch MJ, Cohen A, Hertz HS, Ng KJ, Schaffer R, Van der Lijn P. Determination of serum creatinine by isotope dilution mass spectrometry as a candidate definitive method. Anal Chem 1986;58:1681-5.
236. Whelton A, Watson AJ, Rock RC. Nitrogen metabolites and renal function. In: Burtis CA, Ashwood ER, eds. Tietz Textbook of Clinical Chemistry, 2nd ed. Philadelphia, WB Saunders, 1993:1513-75.
237. Whicher JT, Calvin J, Riches P, Warren C. The laboratory investigation of paraproteinaemia. Ann Clin Biochem 1987;24:119-32.
238. White RM, Cross RE, Savory J. Enzyme coupled measurement of uric acid in serum with a centrifugal analyser. Clin Chem 1977;23:1538-40.
239. Whitehead TP, Robinson D, Hale AC, Bailey AR. Clinical Chemistry and Haematology: Adult Reference Ranges. London: BUPA Medical Research and Development, 1994.
240. Whiting PH, Price RG. Importance of early detection of renal dysfunction: value of markers of early renal disease and damage. CPD Clin Biochem 2001;3:3-8.
241. Wilding P, Rollason JG, Robinson D. Patterns of change for various biochemical constituents detected in well population screening. Clin Chim Acta 1972; 41:375-87.
242. Wimsatt DK, Lott JA. Improved measurement of urinary total protein (including light-chain proteins) with a Coomassie Brilliant Blue G 250-sodium dodecyl sulfate reagent. Clin Chem 1987;33: 2100-6.
243. Witte DL, Brown LF, Feld RD. Effects of bilirubin on detection of hydrogen peroxide by use of peroxidase. Clin Chem 1978;24:1778-82.
244. Woolhandler S, Pels RJ, Bor DH, Himmelstein DU, Lawrence RS. Dipstick urinalysis screening of asymptomatic adults for urinary tract disorders. I. Hematuria and proteinuria. JAMA 1989;262:1214-9.
245. Wuyts B, Bernard D, Van Den Noortgate N, Van De Walle J, Van Vlem B, De Smet R, et al. Reevaluation of formulas for predicting creatinine clearance in adults and children, using compensated creatinine methods. Clin Chem 2003;49:1011-4.
246. Yagame M, Suzuki D, Jinde K, Saotome N, Sato H, Noguchi M, et al. Significance of urinary type IV collagen in patients with diabetic nephropathy using a highly sensitive one-step sandwich enzyme immunoassay. J Clin Lab Anal 1997;11:110-6.
247. Yasmi Y, Tatsumi N, Park K. Urinary sediment analysed by flow cytometry. Cytometry 1995;22: 75-9.
248. Ylinen EA, Ala-Houhala M, Harmoinen APT, Knip M. Cystatin C as a marker for glomerular filtration rate in pediatric patients. Pediatr Nephrol 1999;13: 506-9.
249. Yoshikawa N, Uehara S, Yamana K, Ikeuchi H, Hiraumi M, Matsuo T, et al. Clinicopathological correlations of persistent asymptomatic proteinuria in children. Nephron 1980;25:127-33.

250. Yuen CT, Price RG, Chattagoon L, Richardson AC, Praill PFG. Colorimetric assays for *N*-acetyl-β-D-glucosaminidase and β-D-galactosidase in human urine using newly developed ν-nitrostyryl substrates. Clin Chim Acta 1982;124:195-204.
251. Zager RA. Rhabdomyolysis and myohemoglobinuric acute renal failure. Kidney Int 1996;49:314-26.

ADDITIONAL READING

Periodicals

1. Kidney International http://www.blackwellpublishing.com (Accessed 8th November 2004)
2. Nephrology, Dialysis and Transplantation http://www.ndt.oupjournals.org (Accessed 8th November 2004)
3. Journal of the American Society of Nephrology http://www.jasn.org (Accessed 8th November 2004)
4. American Journal of Kidney Diseases http://www2.ajkd.org (Accessed 8th November 2004)
5. Clinical Chemistry http://www.clinchem.org (Accessed 8th November 2004)
6. Annals of Clinical Biochemistry http://www.acb.org.uk/annalsindex.htm (Accessed 8th November 2004)

Useful Internet Sites

1. American Society of Nephrology http://www.asn-online.org (Accessed 8th November 2004).
2. International Society for Nephrology http://www.isn-online.org (Accessed 8th November 2004).
3. United Kingdom Renal Association http://www.renal.org (Accessed 8th November 2004).
4. National Kidney Foundation (USA) http://www.kidney.org (Accessed 8th November 2004).
5. Hypertension, Dialysis & Clinical Nephrology http://www.hdcn.com (Accessed 8th November 2004).
6. British Renal Society http://www.britishrenal.org (Accessed 8th November 2004).
7. United Kingdom Renal Registry http://www.renalreg.com (Accessed 8th November 2004).

Reviews

Blaufox MD, Aurell M, Bubeck B, Fommei E, Piepsz A, Russell C et al. Report of radionuclides in nephrourology committee on renal clearance. J Nuclear Medicine 1996;37:1883-90.

Hsu CY, Chertow GM, Curhan GC. Methodological issues in studying the epidemiology of mild to moderate chronic renal insufficiency. Kidney Int 2002;61: 1567-76.

Lamb EJ, O'Riordan SE, Delaney MP. Ageing and the kidney: pathology, assessment and management. Clin Chim Acta 2003;334:25-40.

Laterza OF, Price CP, Scott MG. Cystatin C: an improved estimator of glomerular filtration rate? Clin Chem 2002;48:699-707.

National Kidney Foundation-K/DOQI. Clinical practice guidelines for chronic kidney disease: evaluation, classification, and stratification. Am J Kidney Dis 2002; 39(suppl 1):S1-266.

Perrone RD, Madias NE, Levey AS. Serum creatinine as an index of renal function: New insights into old concepts. Clin Chem 1992;38:1933-53.

Price CP, Finney H. Developments in the assessment of glomerular filtration rate. Clin Chim Acta 2000;297: 55-66.

Price CP, James DR. Analytical reviews in clinical biochemistry: The measurement of urate. Ann Clin Biochem 1988;25:484-98.

Simmonds HA. Purine and pyrimidine disorders. In: Holton JB (ed) The Inherited Metabolic Diseases. Churchill Livingstone 1994: Chapter 6, p 297-350.

Spencer K. Analytical reviews in clinical biochemistry: The estimation of creatinine. Ann Clin Biochem 1986;23: 1-25.

Taylor AJ, Vadgama P. Analytical reviews in clinical biochemistry: the estimation of urea. Ann Clin Biochem 1992;29:245-64.

CHAPTER 25

Carbohydrates*

David B. Sacks, M.B., Ch.B., F.R.C.Path.

Carbohydrates, including sugar and starch, are widely distributed in plants and animals. They perform multiple functions, ranging from being structural components of deoxyribonucleic acid (DNA) and ribonucleic acid (RNA) (*ribose* and *deoxyribose* sugars) to serving as sources of energy (*glucose*). Glucose is derived from the breakdown of carbohydrates in the diet (grains, starchy vegetables, and legumes) and in body stores (glycogen), and by endogenous synthesis from protein or the glycerol moiety of triglycerides. When energy intake exceeds expenditure, the excess is converted to fat and glycogen for storage in adipose tissue and liver or muscle, respectively. When energy expenditure exceeds calorie intake, endogenous glucose formation occurs from the breakdown of carbohydrate stores and from noncarbohydrate sources (e.g., amino acids, lactate, and glycerol).

The glucose concentration in the blood is maintained within a fairly narrow range under diverse conditions (feeding, fasting, or severe exercise) by hormones, such as insulin, glucagon, or epinephrine.

Measurement of glucose is one of the most commonly performed procedures in hospital chemistry laboratories. The most frequently encountered disorder of carbohydrate metabolism is high blood glucose caused by diabetes mellitus, which affects approximately 8% of the U.S. adult population. The incidence of hypoglycemia (low blood glucose) is unknown, but, excluding patients who use exogenous insulin to control blood glucose, it is low.

CHEMISTRY OF CARBOHYDRATES

Carbohydrates are aldehyde or ketone derivatives of polyhydroxy (more than one –OH group) alcohols, or compounds that yield these derivatives on hydrolysis. The term *carbohydrate* refers to hydrates of carbon and is derived from the observation that the empirical formulas for these compounds contain approximately one molecule of water per carbon atom. Thus glucose, $C_6H_{12}O_6$, and lactose, $C_{12}H_{22}O_{11}$, can be written as $C_6(H_2O)_6$ and $C_{12}(H_2O)_{11}$, respectively. These compounds are not hydrates in the usual chemical sense, however, and noncarbohydrate compounds, such as lactic acid, $CH_3CH(OH)COOH$ or $C_3(H_2O)_3$, can have similar empirical formulas.

MONOSACCHARIDES

Monosaccharides, or simple sugars, consist of a single polyhydroxy aldehyde or ketone unit and cannot be hydrolyzed to a simpler form. The backbone is made up of a number of carbon atoms. Sugars containing three, four, five, six, and seven carbon atoms are known as *trioses, tetroses, pentoses, hexoses,* and *heptoses,* respectively. One of the carbon atoms is double bonded to an oxygen atom to form a carbonyl group. An *aldehyde* has the carbonyl group at the end of the carbon chain, whereas if the carbonyl group is at any other position, a *ketone* is formed (Figure 25-1). The simplest carbohydrate is glycol aldehyde, the aldehyde derivative of ethylene glycol. The aldehyde and ketone derivatives of glycerol are, respectively, glyceraldehyde and dihydroxyacetone (see Figure 25-1). Monosaccharides are termed *aldose* or *ketose,* according to the position of the carbonyl group (Figure 25-2).

Compounds that are identical in composition and differ only in spatial configuration are called *stereoisomers.* The carbon atoms in the unbranched chain are numbered, as shown by the numbers at the left of the formula for D-glucose (see Figure 25-2). The designation D or L refers to the position of the hydroxyl group on the carbon atom adjacent to the last (bottom) CH_2OH group. In general, the designation of D and L *for a sugar molecule refers to the stereoisomeric forms of the highest-numbered asymmetrical*

*The author gratefully acknowledges the original contributions by Drs. Wendell T. Caraway and Nelson B. Watts on which portions of this chapter are based.

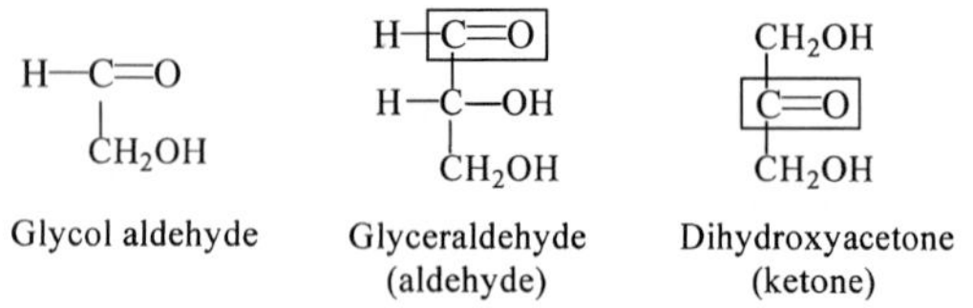

Glycol aldehyde	Glyceraldehyde (aldehyde)	Dihydroxyacetone (ketone)
H—C=O	H—C=O	CH₂OH
CH₂OH	H—C—OH	C=O
	CH₂OH	CH₂OH

Figure 25-1 Two- and three-carbon carbohydrates.

	D-Glucose (Aldose)	L-Glucose (Aldose)	D-Fructose (Ketose)	D-Galactose (Aldose)
1	H—C=O	H—C=O	CH₂OH	H—C=O
2	H—C—OH	HO—C—H	C=O	H—C—OH
3	HO—C—H	H—C—OH	HO—C—H	HO—C—H
4	H—C—OH	HO—C—H	H—C—OH	HO—C—H
5	H—C—OH	HO—C—H	H—C—OH	H—C—OH
6	CH₂OH	CH₂OH	CH₂OH	CH₂OH

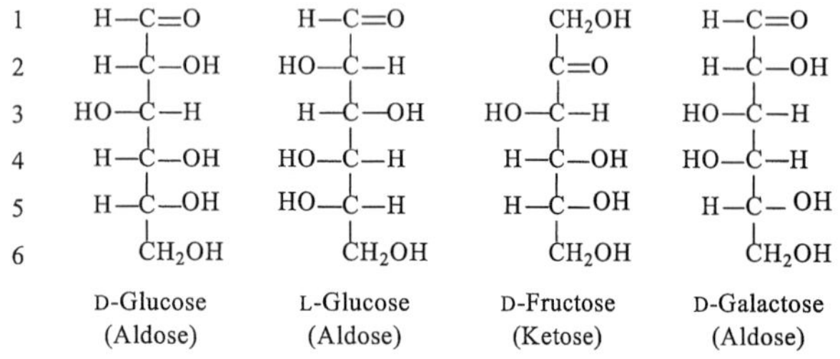

Figure 25-2 Typical six-carbon sugars.

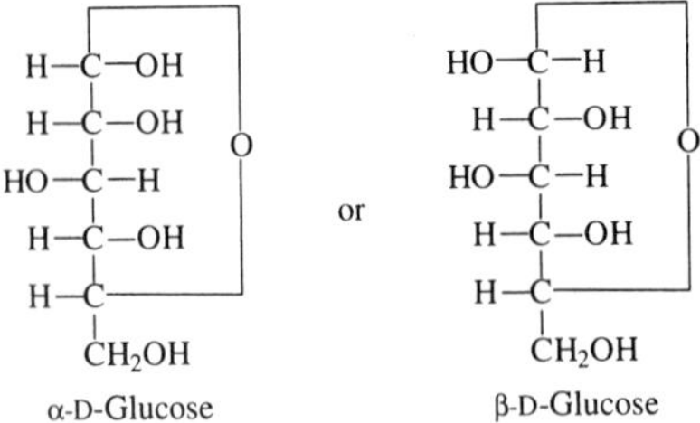

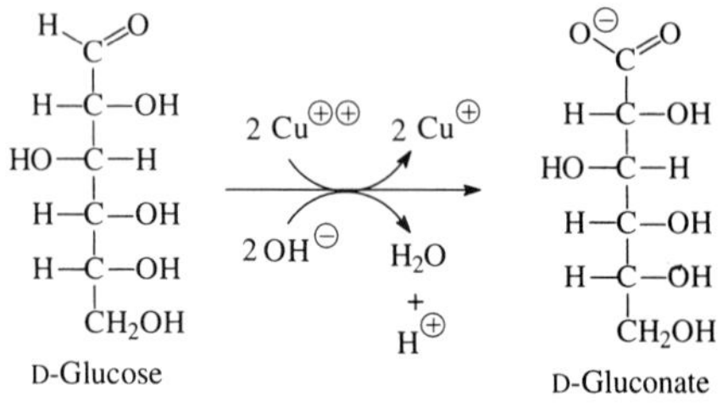

Figure 25-3 Structure of D-glucose (hemiacetal form).

D-Glucose $\xrightarrow[2\,OH^{-}\;\rightarrow\;H_2O\,+\,H^{+}]{2\,Cu^{2+}\;\rightarrow\;2\,Cu^{+}}$ D-Gluconate

*carbon atom.** By convention, the D-sugars are written with the hydroxyl group on the right and the L-sugars are written with the hydroxyl group on the left (see Figure 25-2). *Most sugars in the human body are of the D-configuration.* A number of different structures exist, depending on the relative positions of the hydroxyl groups on the carbon atoms.

The formula for glucose can be written in the form of either aldehyde or enol, a short-lived reactive species. Shift to the enol anion is favored in alkaline solution:

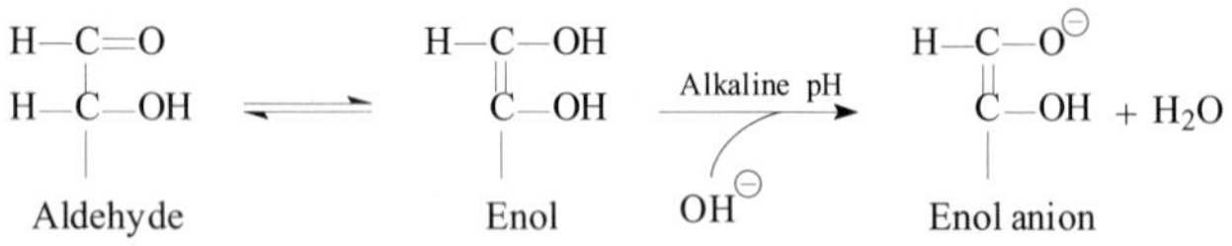

Aldehyde (H—C=O / H—C—OH) ⇌ Enol (H—C—OH / C—OH) $\xrightarrow[OH^{-}]{\text{Alkaline pH}}$ Enol anion (H—C—O⁻ / C—OH) + H_2O

The presence of a double bond and a negative charge in the enol anion makes glucose an active reducing substance that can be oxidized by relatively mild oxidizing agents, such as cupric (Cu^{2+}) and ferric (Fe^{3+}) ions. Glucose in hot alkaline solution readily reduces cupric ions to cuprous ions, and the carbonyl carbon is oxidized to carboxylic acid. The color change can be used as a presumptive indication for the presence of glucose, and for many years blood and urine glucose were measured this way. Other sugars can reduce cupric ions in alkaline solution.

*Although the D and L designations are retained in this chapter, readers should be aware that in the Cahn-Ingold-Prelog system, a series of sequence rules determines configurations. In this new system, the symbols R and S are used to designate configurations instead of D and L. For further information, readers are referred to March J. Advances in organic chemistry: Reactions, mechanisms, and structure, 4th ed. New York: John Wiley & Sons, 1992: 109-111.

Aldehyde and alcohol groups can react to form hemiacetals. In the case of glucose, the aldehyde group reacts with the hydroxyl group on carbon 5 (Figure 25-3). Note that this ring structure contains an additional asymmetric carbon atom and can exist in two stereoisomeric forms. By convention, the form with the hydroxyl group on the right of the first carbon atom is called *α-D-glucose* and the form with the hydroxyl group on the left is called *β-D-glucose.* The common anhydrous crystalline glucose is in the α-D-form. The β-D-form is obtained by crystallization from acetic acid. The two forms differ with respect to optical rotation of polarized light. The specific rotation—$[\alpha]_D^{25}$—for the α-D-form is +113° and for the β-D-form is +19.7°. As a result of mutarotation, either form in aqueous solution gives rise to an equilibrium mixture that has a specific rotation of +52.5°. The equilibrium established at room temperature is such that about 36% of the glucose exists in the α-form and 64% in the β-form; only a trace remains in the free aldehyde form. The enzyme glucose oxidase reacts only with β-D-glucose. For this reason, calibrating solutions to be used in glucose oxidase methods for glucose determinations should be permitted to stand at least 2 hours to obtain equilibrium comparable with that in the test samples to be analyzed.

From the ring structures shown in Figure 25-3, it is not apparent why the aldehyde group should react with the distant hydroxyl group on carbon 5. The spatial arrangement of the atoms is better represented by a symmetrical ring structure, depicted by the Haworth formula, in which glucose is considered as having the same basic structure as pyran (Figure 25-4). In this formula, the plane of the ring is considered to be perpendicular to the plane of the paper, with the heavy lines pointing toward the reader. *Hydroxyl groups in position 1 are then below the plane (α-configuration)* or *above the plane (β-configuration).* A six-member ring sugar, containing five carbons and one oxygen, is a deriva-

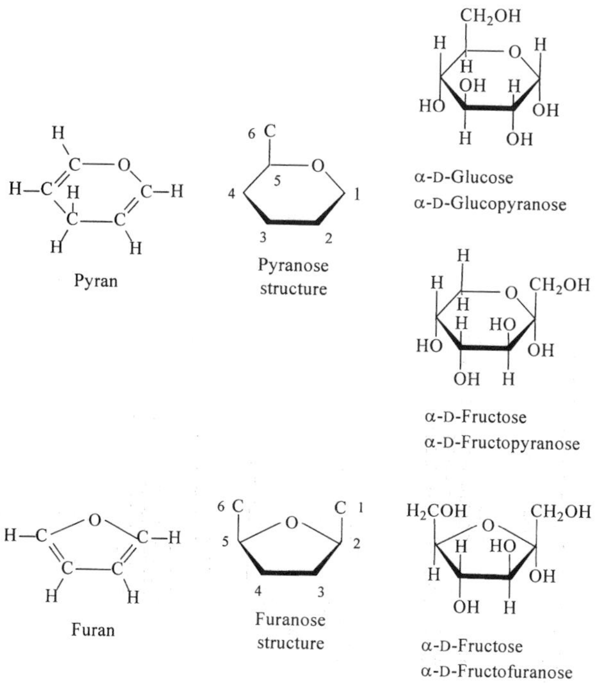

Pyran

Pyranose structure

α-D-Glucose
α-D-Glucopyranose

α-D-Fructose
α-D-Fructopyranose

Furan

Furanose structure

α-D-Fructose
α-D-Fructofuranose

Figure 25-4 The Haworth formula for sugars.

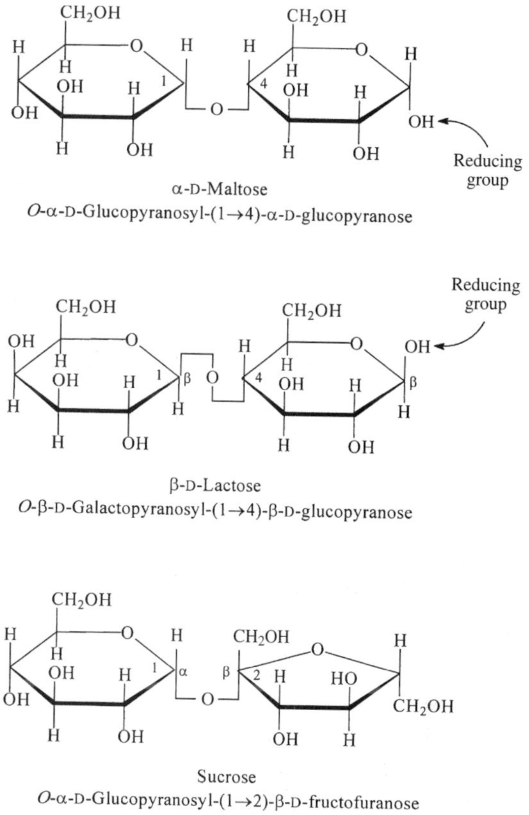

α-D-Maltose
O-α-D-Glucopyranosyl-(1→4)-α-D-glucopyranose

β-D-Lactose
O-β-D-Galactopyranosyl-(1→4)-β-D-glucopyranose

Sucrose
O-α-D-Glucopyranosyl-(1→2)-β-D-fructofuranose

Figure 25-5 Structural formulas of disaccharides.

tive of pyran and is called a *pyranose.* When linkage occurs with formation of a five-member ring, containing four carbons and one oxygen, the sugar has the same basic structure as furan and is called a *furanose.* Representative formulas are shown in Figure 25-4. Fructose is shown in two cyclical forms. Fructopyranose is the configuration of the free sugar, and fructofuranose occurs whenever fructose exists in combination in disaccharides and polysaccharides, as in sucrose and inulin.

DISACCHARIDES

Two monosaccharides join covalently by an *O-glycosidic bond,* with the loss of a molecule of water, to form a disaccharide. The chemical bond between the sugars always involves the aldehyde or ketone group of one monosaccharide joined to an alcohol group (e.g., maltose) or to an aldehyde or ketone group (e.g., sucrose) of the other monosaccharide. The most common disaccharides are

Maltose = glucose + glucose
Lactose = glucose + galactose
Sucrose = glucose + fructose

There are several conventions that are followed in the nomenclature of disaccharides (Figure 25-5). The compound is written with the nonreducing end to the left. An *O* precedes the name of the first (left) monosaccharide, emphasizing that the linkage occurs by an oxygen atom. The configuration of the anomeric (carbonyl) carbon is designated α or β. Five- (furanosyl) and six- (pyranosyl) membered rings are distinguished and the carbon atoms joined by the glycosidic bond are identified. Because sucrose has no reducing end, it can be written as *O*-α-D-glucopyranosyl-(1 → 2)-β-D-fructofuranose or *O*-β-D-fructofuranosyl-(2 → 1)-α-D-glucopyranose. If the linkage between two monosaccharides is between the aldehyde or ketone group of one molecule and a hydroxyl group of another molecule (as in maltose and lactose), one potentially free ketone or aldehyde group remains on the second monosaccharide. Consequently, the second glucose residue can be oxidized (thus the disaccharide is a reducing sugar) and is capable of existing in α- or β-pyranose forms. The reducing power, however, is only approximately 40% of the reducing power of the two single monosaccharides added together, primarily because one of the reducing groups is not available. On the other hand, if the linkage between two monosaccharides involves the aldehyde or ketone groups of both molecules (as in sucrose), a nonreducing sugar results because no free aldehyde or ketone group remains.

POLYSACCHARIDES

The linkage of multiple monosaccharide units results in the formation of polysaccharides. The major storage carbohydrates are *starch* in plants and *glycogen* in animals, both of which form granules inside cells. The suffix *an* attached to a name of a monosaccharide indicates the main type of sugar present in the polysaccharide. Starch and glycogen, for example, are *glucosans,* because they are composed of a series of glucose molecules. Inulin, a polysaccharide found in the tubers of certain plants, consists largely of fructose units and is known as a *fructosan.*

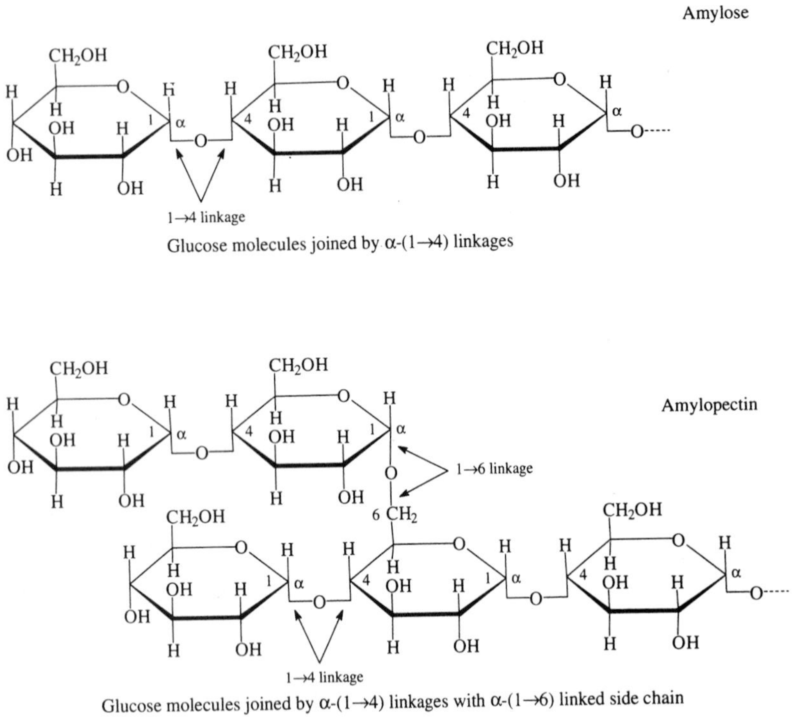

Amylose

1→4 linkage

Glucose molecules joined by α-(1→4) linkages

Amylopectin

1→6 linkage

1→4 linkage

Glucose molecules joined by α-(1→4) linkages with α-(1→6) linked side chain

Figure 25-6 Structures of the polysaccharides amylose and amylopectin.

Nearly all starches consist of a mixture of two kinds of glucosans called *amyloses* and *amylopectins.* The relative proportions of these two glucosans in a starch vary from approximately 20% amylose and 80% amylopectin in wheat, potato, and ordinary corn starch to nearly 100% amylopectin in the starch of waxy corn. On the other hand, a few corn starches are known to contain as much as 75% amylose. Both amylose and amylopectin consist of glucose residues, but their structures exhibit one significant difference. Amylose consists of one long unbranched chain of glucose units linked together by α-1,4-linkages with only the terminal aldehyde group free (Figure 25-6). In amylopectin, most of the units are similarly connected with α-1,4-links, but there are also α-1,6-glycosidic bonds every 24 to 30 residues, producing side chains (see Figure 25-6). Amylopectin contains up to 1 million glucose residues. The structure of glycogen is similar to that of amylopectin, but branching is more extensive in glycogen and occurs every 8 to 12 glucose residues. These branches enhance the solubility of glycogen and allow the glucose residues to be mobilized more readily. Glycogen is most abundant in liver and also is found in skeletal muscle. The most favorable conformation for α-1,4-linked polymers of D-glucose, such as starch or glycogen, is a tightly coiled helical structure.

The difference in structure between amylose and amylopectin is important when selecting the appropriate starch substrate for amylase determinations (see Chapter 21). The rate of hydrolysis is affected by structural differences in the starch. α-Amylase from the pancreas hydrolyzes internal α-1,4-glycosidic linkages. This hydrolysis results initially in the production of some maltose and a mixture of dextrins, which are subsequently hydrolyzed to maltose. The β-1,6-linkages are not attacked by α-amylase, and relatively large molecules of so-called residual (limit) dextrins are left after the action of the enzyme on amylopectin. Iodine gives a deep blue color with amylose and a red to violet color with amylopectin. These characteristic colors disappear when the respective glucosans are hydrolyzed to smaller units, such as dextrins and maltose. This disappearance of the starch-iodine color is used in some older methods for amylase determination.

Dextrins are the products of partial hydrolysis of starch. They are a complex mixture of molecules of different sizes. Those formed from amylose are unbranched chains, whereas amylopectins produce branched chains of glucose molecules. Erythrodextrins are larger branched dextrins that turn a reddish color on complexing iodine.

Cellulose, an important structural polysaccharide in plants, is an unbranched polymer of glucose residues joined by β-1,4-linkages. The β-configuration facilitates the formation of long straight chains, producing fibers of high tensile strength. The β-1,4-linkages are not hydrolyzed by α-amylases. Because humans do not have *cellulases,* they are unable to digest vegetable fiber.

Chitin, the principal component of the exoskeleton of arthropods (insects and crustacea), consists of *N*-acetyl-D-glucosamine residues in a β-1,4-linkage. The only chemical difference from cellulose is that the substituent at C-2 is an acetylated amino group instead of a hydroxyl group.

GLYCOPROTEINS

Glycosylation is the most frequent enzymatic modification of proteins. Many integral membrane proteins have oligosaccharides covalently attached to the extracellular region,

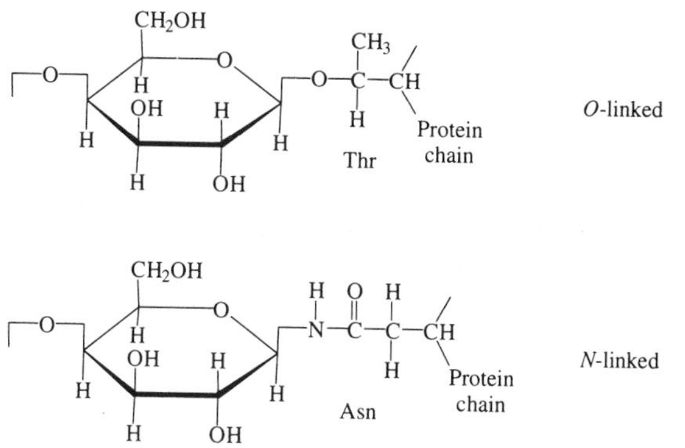

Figure 25-7 Glycosidic linkages between oligosaccharides and protein.

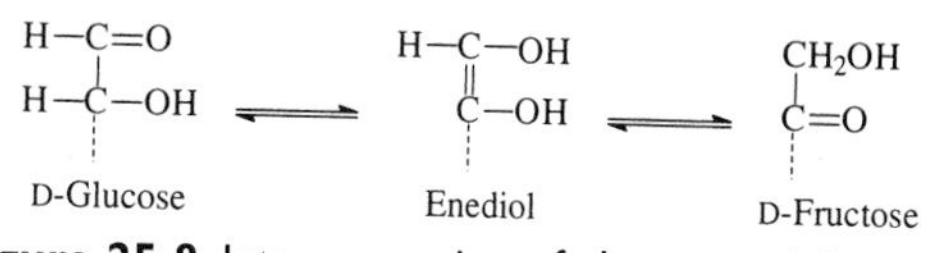

Figure 25-8 Interconversion of glucose and fructose.

forming *glycoproteins.* In addition, most proteins that are secreted, such as antibodies, hormones, and coagulation factors, are glycoproteins. The number of attached carbohydrates varies among proteins and constitutes 1% to 70% of the weight of the glycoprotein. The oligosaccharides are attached either by *O*-glycosidic linkages to the side-chain oxygen of serine and/or threonine residues or by *N*-glycosidic linkages to the side-chain nitrogen of asparagine residues (Figure 25-7).

One of the biological functions of the carbohydrate chains is to regulate the lifespan of proteins. For example, removal of sialic acid residues from the end of oligosaccharide chains on erythrocytes results in the disappearance of the red blood cells from the circulation. Carbohydrates have also been implicated in cell-cell recognition, and in secretion and targeting of proteins to specific subcellular domains. Recently, defects in protein glycosylation have been linked to several forms of congenital muscular dystrophy that are associated with brain abnormalities.[183]

METABOLISM OF CARBOHYDRATES

Carbohydrate metabolism provides glucose, the primary energy source for the human body. After digestion of carbohydrates and absorption of glucose, blood glucose concentration is controlled by the action of several hormones. Glucose can be synthesized de novo or stored in the tissue as glycogen.

Digestion and Absorption

Ingested starch and glycogen are partially digested by the action of salivary amylase in the mouth to form intermediate dextrins and maltose (see also Chapter 48). The acid pH of the stomach inhibits amylase activity, but the alkaline pancreatic secretions increase the pH in the small intestine, allowing pancreatic amylase to complete digestion to oligosaccharides, preponderantly maltose. Maltose, along with any ingested lactose and sucrose, is hydrolyzed by the appropriate disaccharidase (*maltase, lactase,* or *sucrase*) from the intestinal mucosa to glucose, galactose, and fructose.

These monosaccharides are absorbed across the wall of the duodenum and ileum by an active, energy-requiring, carrier-mediated transfer process. The rate of absorption for glucose and galactose is several times greater than for similar molecules absorbed by passive diffusion (e.g., xylose). Some conversion of fructose to glucose may occur during the process of absorption, and the interconversion can be visualized in terms of the enediol form common to both (Figure 25-8). Fructose is absorbed more slowly than glucose and galactose by a carrier-mediated process different from the glucose and galactose transport mechanisms. The monosaccharides are then transported by the portal vein to the liver.

Intermediary Metabolism

The metabolism of hexoses proceeds according to the body's requirements. This results in (1) energy production by conversion to carbon dioxide and water, (2) storage as glycogen in the liver or triglyceride in adipose tissue, or (3) conversion to keto acids, amino acids, or protein.

Some steps in the intermediary metabolism of glycogen and hexoses are shown in Figure 25-9. Each step is enzymatically catalyzed. In some cases, different enzymes are responsible for the forward and reverse reactions. For example, the initial phosphorylation of glucose is mediated by glucokinase, but the reverse reaction depends on glucose-6-phosphatase.

Various inborn errors of metabolism (Table 25-1) result from deficiencies or absence of some of the enzymes listed in Figure 25-9. Some of these are discussed later in the chapter. The relationship of carbohydrate metabolism to the production of lactate, ketone bodies, and triglycerides is also depicted in Figure 25-9. The pentose phosphate pathway, also known as the *hexose monophosphate shunt,* is an alternative pathway for glucose metabolism that generates the reduced form of nicotinamide-adenine dinucleotide phosphate (NADPH), which is used in maintaining the integrity of red blood cell membranes, in lipid and steroid biosynthesis, in hydroxylation reactions, and in other anabolic reactions. The complete picture of intermediary metabolism of carbohydrates is rather complex and interwoven with the metabolism of lipids and amino acids. For details, readers should consult a biochemistry textbook.

Regulation of Blood Glucose Concentration

The concentration of glucose in the blood is regulated by a complex interplay of multiple pathways, modulated by a number of hormones. *Glycogenesis* is the conversion of glucose to glycogen. The reverse process, namely the break-

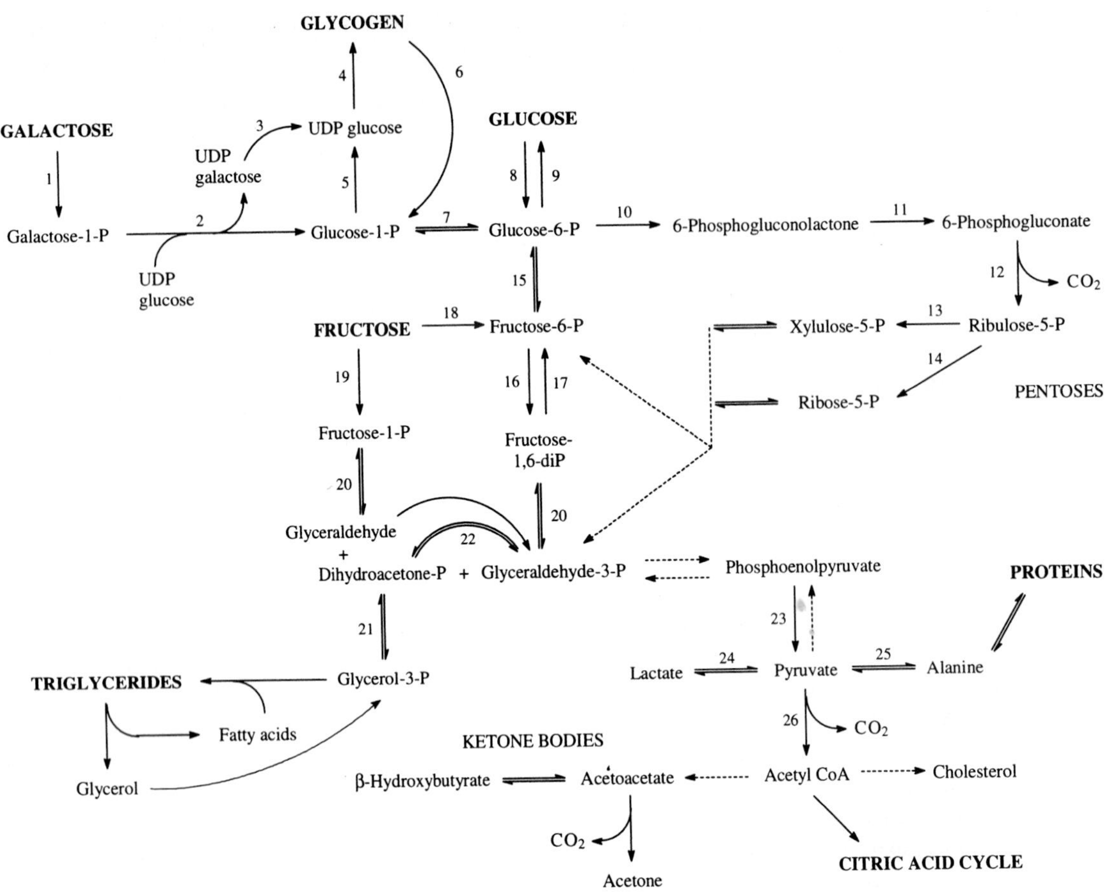

Figure 25-9 Major steps in the intermediary metabolism of carbohydrates. Numbers shown refer to specific enzymes. (---------), Multistep pathway; (———), single-step pathway.

1. Galactokinase
2. Galactose-1-P-uridyl transferase
3. UDP-galactose-4-epimerase
4. Glycogen synthetase (plus branching enzyme)
5. UDP-glucose pyrophosphorylase
6. Glycogen phosphorylase
7. Phosphoglucomutase
8. Glucokinase (and hexokinase)
9. Glucose-6-phosphatase
10. Glucose-6-phosphate dehydrogenase
11. 6-Phosphogluconolactonase
12. 6-Phosphogluconate dehydrogenase
13. Ribulose 5-P-epimerase
14. Ribose 5-P-isomerase
15. Phosphohexose isomerase
16. Phosphofructokinase
17. Fructose-1,6-diphosphatase
18. Hexokinase (extrahepatic)
19. Fructokinase
20. Aldolase
21. Glycerol phosphate dehydrogenase
22. Triose-P-isomerase
23. Pyruvate kinase
24. Lactate dehydrogenase
25. Alanine aminotransferase
26. Pyruvate dehydrogenase

TABLE 25-1 Inborn Errors of Carbohydrate Metabolism

Enzyme Deficiency	Disease State
Glucose-6-phosphatase (9)*	Type I GSD (von Gierke's disease)
Muscle phosphorylase	Type V GSD (McArdle's disease)
Liver phosphorylase	Type VI GSD (Hers' disease)
Galactose-1-phosphate-uridyl transferase (2)	Galactosemia
Galactokinase (1)	Galactosemia
Uridine diphosphate-galactose-4-epimerase (3)	Galactosemia
Fructokinase (19)	Essential fructosuria
Fructose-1-phosphate aldolase (20)	Hereditary fructose intolerance
Pyruvate kinase (23)	Hemolytic anemia
Glucose-6-phosphate dehydrogenase (10)	Hemolytic disease

GSD, Glycogen storage disease.
*Numbers in parentheses refer to enzymes in Figure 25-9.

down of glycogen to glucose and other intermediate products, is termed *glycogenolysis.* The formation of glucose from noncarbohydrate sources, such as amino acids, glycerol, or lactate, is termed *gluconeogenesis.* The conversion of glucose or other hexoses into lactate or pyruvate is called *glycolysis.* Further oxidation to carbon dioxide and water occurs through the Krebs (citric acid) cycle and the mitochondrial electron transport chain coupled to oxidative phosphorylation, generating energy in the form of adenosine triphosphate (ATP). Oxidation of glucose to carbon dioxide and water also occurs through the hexose monophosphate shunt pathway, which produces NADPH.

Hormones That Regulate Blood Glucose Concentration

During a brief fast, a precipitous decline in the concentration of blood glucose is prevented by breakdown of glycogen stored in the liver and synthesis of glucose in the liver. Some glucose is derived from gluconeogenesis in the kidneys.[100] These organs contain glucose-6-phosphatase, which is necessary to convert glucose-6-phosphate (derived from either gluconeogenesis or glycogenolysis) to glucose. Skeletal muscle lacks this enzyme, and muscle glycogen therefore cannot contribute directly to blood glucose. With more prolonged fasting (longer than 42 hours), gluconeogenesis accounts for essentially all of the glucose production. In contrast, after a meal, the absorbed glucose is converted to glycogen (for storage in the liver and skeletal muscle) or fat (for storage in adipose tissue). Despite large fluctuations in the supply and demand of carbohydrates, the concentration of glucose in the blood is normally maintained within a narrow range by hormones that modulate the movement of glucose into and out of the circulation. These include insulin, which decreases blood glucose, and the counter-regulatory hormones (glucagon, epinephrine, cortisol, and growth hormone), which increase blood glucose concentrations (Figure 25-10).[100] Normal glucose disposal depends on: (1) the ability of the pancreas to secrete insulin, (2) the ability of insulin to promote uptake of glucose into peripheral tissue, and (3) the ability of insulin to suppress hepatic glucose production. The major insulin target organs are liver, skeletal muscle, and adipose tissue. These organs exhibit some differences in their responses to insulin. For example, the hormone stimulates glucose uptake through a specific glucose transporter—GLUT4—in muscle and fat cells, but not liver cells.

Insulin

Insulin is a protein hormone produced by the β-cells of the islets of Langerhans in the pancreas. Insulin was the first protein hormone to be sequenced, the first substance to be measured by radioimmunoassay (RIA), and the first compound produced by recombinant DNA technology for practical use. It is an anabolic hormone that stimulates the uptake of glucose into fat and muscle, promotes the conversion of glucose to glycogen or fat for storage, inhibits glucose production by the liver, stimulates protein synthesis, and inhibits protein breakdown.

Chemistry. Human insulin (MW 5808) consists of 51 amino acids in two chains (A and B) joined by two disulfide bridges, with a third disulfide bridge within the A chain. The amino acid sequence of human insulin differs slightly from insulin of other species, but the carboxyl terminal region of the B chain (B23 to B26), which appears crucial for the biological actions of insulin, is highly conserved among species. Insulin from most animals is immunologically and biologically similar to human insulin, and in the past patients were treated with insulin purified from beef or pig pancreas. The most commonly used forms now are recombinant human insulins.

Synthesis. Preproinsulin, a protein of about 100 amino acids (MW 12,000), is formed by ribosomes in the rough endoplasmic reticulum of the pancreatic β-cells (Figure 25-

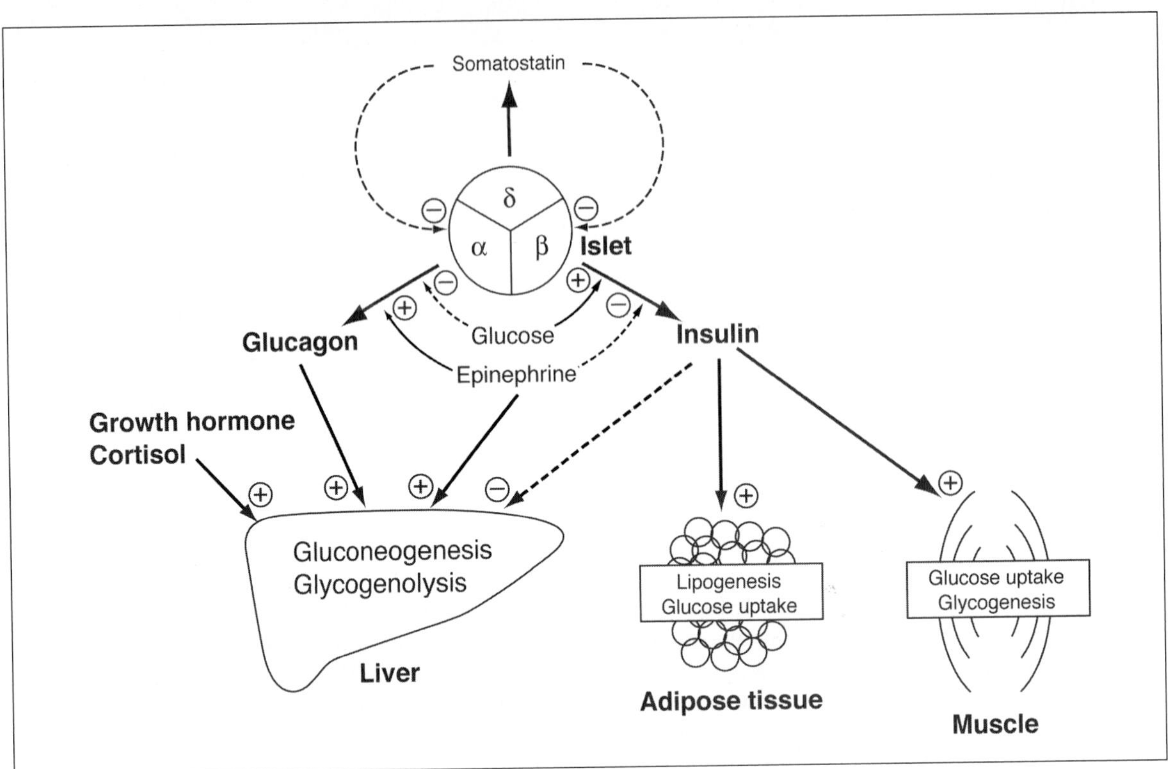

Figure 25-10 Hormonal regulation of blood glucose. Key: +, stimulation; –, inhibition. Cortisol, growth hormone, and epinephrine also antagonize the effect of insulin.

11). Preproinsulin is not detectable in the circulation under normal conditions because it is rapidly converted by cleaving enzymes to proinsulin (MW 9000), an 86–amino acid polypeptide. This is stored in secretory granules in the Golgi complex of the β-cells, where *proteolytic cleavage to insulin and connecting peptide (C-peptide) occurs.*[210] Cleavage of proinsulin is catalyzed by two Ca^{2+}-regulated endopeptidases, prohormone convertases 1 and 2 (PC1 and PC2).[232] PC1 (sometimes designated PC3) hydrolyzes the molecule on the *C*-terminal end of Arg-31 and Arg-32 (at the BC junction) to yield split 32, 33 proinsulin (Figure 25-12). PC2 cleaves proinsulin on the *C*-terminal side of dibasic residues Lys-64 and Arg-65 (at the AC junction) to generate split 65, 66 proinsulin. Each enzymatic hydrolysis is rapidly followed by the removal of two newly exposed *C*-terminal basic amino acids by carboxypeptidase-H to produce insulin and C-peptide. The split proinsulin intermediates are rarely detected in patient samples because of the relatively high quantity of carboxypeptidase-H. This enzyme produces the more commonly observed proinsulin intermediates, des 31, 32 proinsulin and des 64, 65 proinsulin (see Figure 25-12). Most proinsulin processing is sequential. Intact proinsulin is initially hydrolyzed by PC1 and carboxypeptidase-H. The resultant des 31, 32 proinsulin is converted by PC2 and carboxypeptidase-H to insulin and C-peptide. Less than 10% of proinsulin is metabolized via des 64, 65 proinsulin, which is present in negligible amounts in humans. Des 31, 32 proinsulin is the major proinsulin conversion intermediate.[260] Glucose regulates biosynthesis of both proinsulin and PC1, but has no effect on PC2 and carboxypeptidase-H. At the cell membrane, insulin and C-peptide are released into the portal circulation in equimolar amounts. In addition, small amounts of proinsulin and intermediate cleavage forms enter the circulation.

Release. Glucose, amino acids, pancreatic and gastrointestinal hormones (e.g., glucagon, gastrin, secretin, pancreozymin, and gastrointestinal polypeptide), and some medications (e.g., sulfonylureas and β-adrenergic agonists) stimulate insulin secretion. Insulin release is inhibited by hypoglycemia, somatostatin (produced in the pancreatic δ-cells), and various drugs (e.g., α-adrenergic agonists, β-adrenergic blockers, diazoxide, phenytoin, phenothiazines, and nicotinic acid).[219] In healthy individuals, insulin is secreted in a pulsatile fashion, with glucose and insulin the main signals in the feedback loop. Glucose elicits the release of insulin from the pancreas in two phases. The first phase begins 1 to 2 minutes after intravenous injection of glucose and ends within 10 minutes. This phase, illustrated by the sharp spike in Figure 25-13, *A*, represents the rapid release of stored insulin. The second phase, beginning at the point where the first phase ends, depends on continuing insulin synthesis and release and lasts until normoglycemia has been restored, usually within 60 to 120 minutes. With progressive failure of β-cell function, the first-phase insulin response to

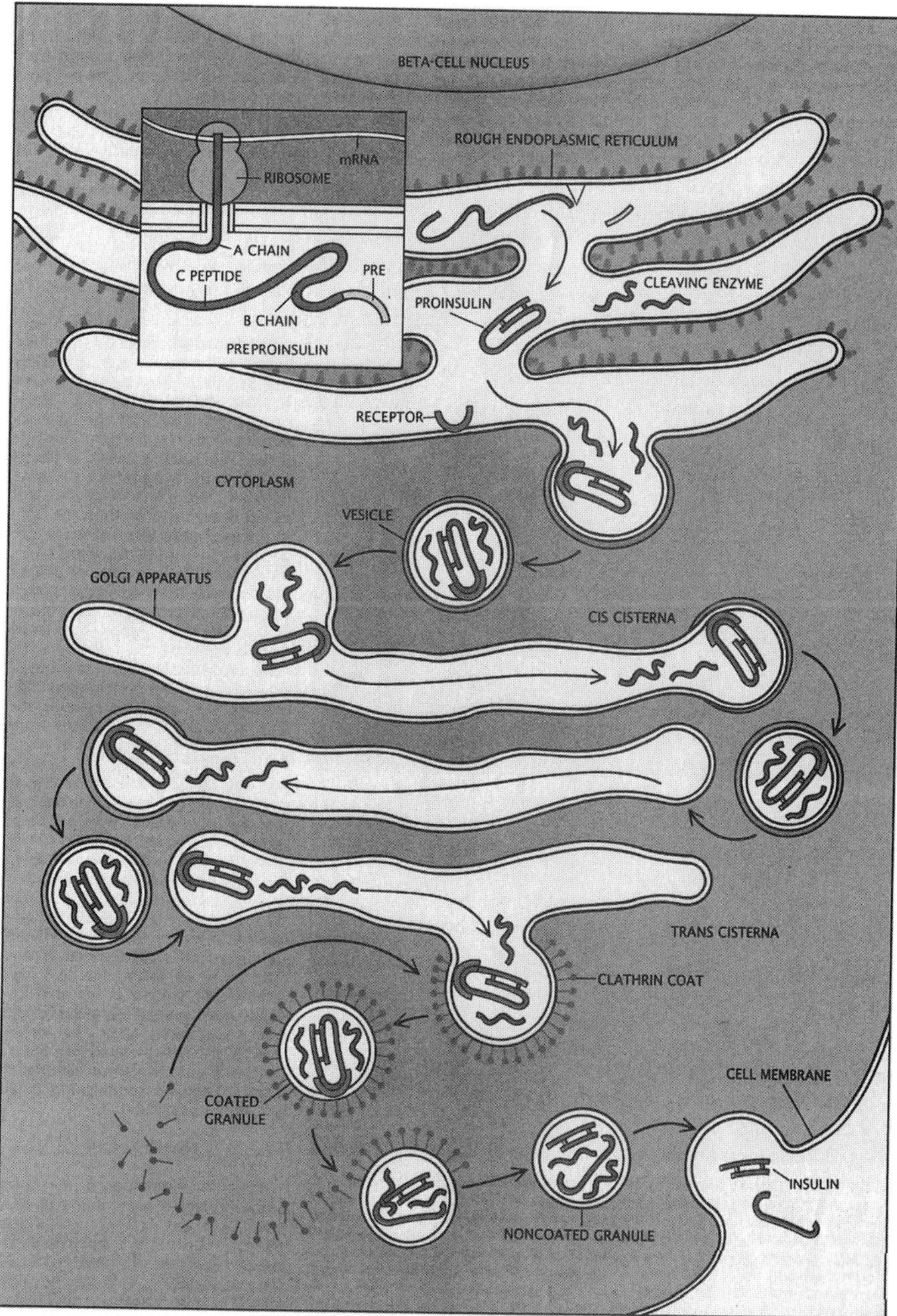

Figure 25-11 Insulin synthesis and release from the pancreatic β-cell. *(From Orci L, Vassalli J-D, Perrelet A. The insulin factory. Sci Am 1988; 259:85-94.)*

glucose is lost, but other stimuli such as glucagon or amino acids may be able to elicit this response. Although the second-phase insulin response is preserved in most patients with type 2 diabetes mellitus, both the first-phase response (see Figure 25-13, *B*) and the normal pulsatile insulin secretion[209] are lost. In contrast, patients with type 1 diabetes mellitus exhibit minimal or no insulin response (see Figure 25-13, *C*).

Degradation. On the first pass through the portal circulation, approximately 50% of the insulin is extracted by the liver, where it is degraded. Because the amount extracted is variable, plasma insulin concentrations may not accurately reflect the rate of insulin secretion. Additional insulin degradation occurs in the kidneys. Insulin is filtered through the glomeruli, reabsorbed, and degraded in the proximal tubule. The basal insulin secretory rate is about 1 U/hr, with total daily secretion of about 40 U. The half-life of insulin in the circulation is between 4 and 5 minutes.

Proinsulin. Proinsulin, which has relatively low biological activity (approximately 10% of insulin potency), is the major storage form of insulin.[236] Normally, only small amounts (about 3% of the amount of insulin, on a molar basis) of proinsulin enter the circulation. However, the hepatic clearance rate for proinsulin is only 25% of that for insulin and the half-life of proinsulin is ~30 minutes. Therefore in the fasting state, circulating proinsulin concentrations are approximately 10% to 15% of insulin concentrations.

C-Peptide. Proinsulin is cleaved to a 31–amino acid connecting (C) peptide (MW 3600) and insulin (see Figure 25-12). C-peptide is devoid of biological activity but appears necessary to ensure the correct structure of insulin.[122] Although insulin and C-peptide are secreted into the portal circulation in equimolar amounts, fasting C-peptide concentrations are fivefold to tenfold higher than those of insulin owing to the longer half-life of C-peptide (about 35 minutes). The liver does not extract C-peptide, which is removed from the circulation by the kidneys and degraded, with a fraction excreted unchanged in the urine.

Antibodies to Insulin. Antibodies to insulin develop in almost all patients who are treated with exogenous insulin.[235] These antibodies are usually present at low titer and produce no adverse effects. On rare occasions (usually in patients with type 2 diabetes) high titers of insulin antibodies may

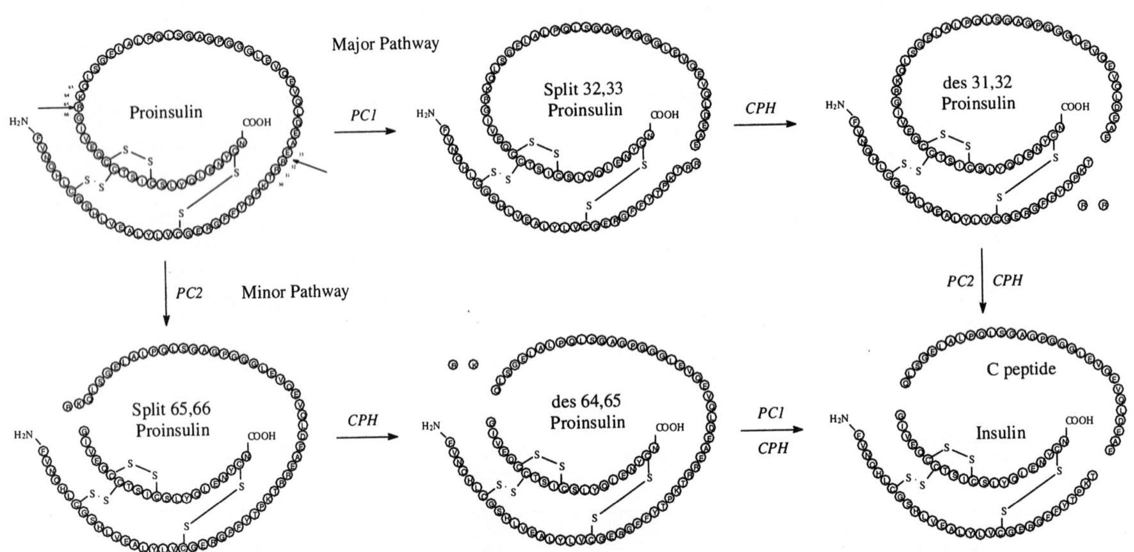

Figure 25-12 Processing of proinsulin. The enzymes prohormone convertase 1 and 2 (PC1 and PC2) act on proinsulin to form the appropriate split proinsulins. Carboxypeptidase-H (CPH) removes the two exposed basic amino acid residues *(circles)*.

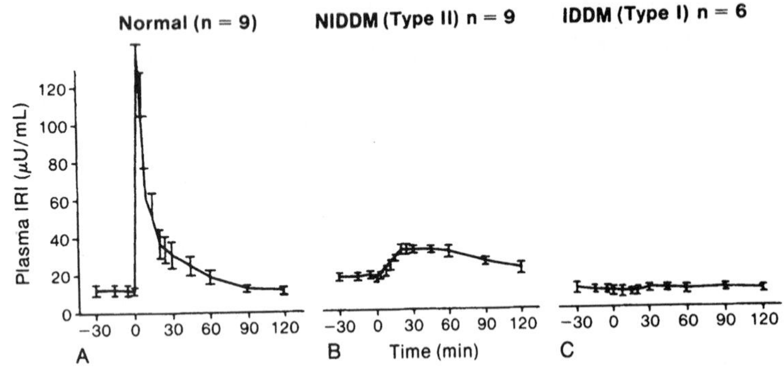

Figure 25-13 Response of plasma insulin to glucose stimulation. A 20-g glucose pulse is given intravenously at time 0. **A,** Healthy subjects. **B,** Patients with type 2 diabetes mellitus (NIDDM). **C,** Patients with type 1 diabetes mellitus (IDDM). *IRI,* Immunoreactive insulin. Values before time 0 represent baseline. *(From Pfeifer MA, Halter JB, Porte D Jr. Insulin secretion in diabetes mellitus. Am J Med 1981; 70:579-88.)*

cause insulin resistance. Improvement in the purity of animal insulins and the widespread use of human insulin have reduced, but not eliminated, antibody production. Antibodies to insulin rarely develop in patients who have not received exogenous insulin.

Although rare, patients with antibodies to the insulin receptor have also been described.[91] On binding the receptor, these antibodies act as either antagonists, producing hyperglycemia (e.g., in patients with acanthosis nigricans), or agonists, resulting in hypoglycemia.

The Mechanism of Insulin Action. Although the metabolic effects produced by insulin are well known, the molecular mechanism of insulin action remains incompletely understood.[233,244] It is generally accepted that the initial event is the binding of insulin to specific receptors in the plasma membrane (Figure 25-14). The human insulin receptor, which is well characterized, is a heterotetramer, comprising two α- and two β-subunits. The α-subunit (MW 135,000) is located on the outer surface of the plasma membrane and contains the site where insulin binds. The β-subunit (MW 95,000) extends intracellularly through the plasma membrane and contains an intrinsic tyrosine kinase. Binding of insulin to the α-subunits induces a conformational change in the receptor, resulting in activation of the tyrosine kinase that catalyzes the phosphorylation of tyrosine residues on several proteins. One of the major substrates for this tyrosine kinase is the receptor itself.

In addition to phosphorylating itself, the insulin receptor catalyzes the tyrosine phosphorylation of a number of specific intracellular proteins (see Figure 25-14). These include the four members of the family of insulin-receptor substrate (IRS) proteins (termed IRS-1, IRS-2, IRS-3, and IRS-4), Shc, and Gab-1. The phosphorylated tyrosines on these target proteins act as docking sites for selected intracellular signal transducer proteins.[290] Most of these transducer proteins contain one or more Src homology 2 (SH2) domains. The SH2 domain is a sequence of approximately 100 amino acids that recognizes phosphotyrosine.[218] Sequence differences in the SH2 domain dictate the specificity of binding. SH2-containing proteins depicted in Figure 25-14 include those labeled phosphatidylinositol 3′-kinase (PI3K) and growth factor receptor-bound protein 2 (Grb2), which mediate downstream signal transduction events. Like other growth factors, insulin stimulates the mitogen-activated protein (MAP) kinase cascade via ras. In addition, phosphatidylinositol 3′-kinase activates atypical protein kinase C (aPKC) via Akt. The latter enzymes regulate glucose transport by modulating translocation of GLUT4 (the insulin-sensitive glucose transporter) to the plasma membrane. Akt also phosphorylates and inactivates GSK-3, thereby enhancing glycogen synthesis. Some of these events are listed in Figure 25-14. The pathways are elaborate, and although several components have been identified, there remain considerable gaps in our knowledge and understanding. Recent studies have clarified a fundamental concept, that the insulin-mediated signaling events are highly redundant. For example, when two key insulin-signaling molecules, IRS-1 and GLUT4, were knocked out in transgenic mouse experiments, the resulting animals had minor metabolic defects rather than overt diabetes.[233] Similarly, mice with knockout of insulin receptors from skeletal muscle or liver do not develop diabetes.

Glucose Transport. The transport of glucose into cells is modulated by two families of proteins.[29] The intestinal sodium/glucose co-transporter promotes the uptake of glucose and galactose from the lumen of the small bowel and their reabsorption from the urine in the kidney. The transporter uses the electrochemical sodium gradient to transport glucose against its concentration gradient. Members of the second family of glucose carriers are called *facilitative glucose transporters* (GLUT) (Table 25-2). These transporters are designated GLUT1 to GLUT7, based on the order in which they were identified. GLUT1 is widely expressed and provides many cells with their basal glucose requirement.

TABLE 25-2 Facilitative Human Glucose Transporters

Name	Tissue	Function
GLUT1 (erythrocyte)	Wide distribution, especially brain, kidney, colon, and fetal tissues	Basal glucose transport
GLUT2 (liver)	Liver, β-cells of pancreas, small intestine, and kidney	Non–rate-limiting glucose transport
GLUT3 (brain)	Wide distribution, especially neurons, placenta, and testis	Glucose transport in neurons
GLUT4 (muscle)	Skeletal muscle, cardiac muscle, and adipose tissue	Insulin-stimulated glucose transport
GLUT5 (small intestine)	Small intestine, kidney, skeletal muscle, brain, and adipose tissue	Transports fructose (not glucose)
GLUT6	—	Pseudogene that is nonfunctional
GLUT7 (microsomal)	Liver	Release of glucose from endoplasmic reticulum

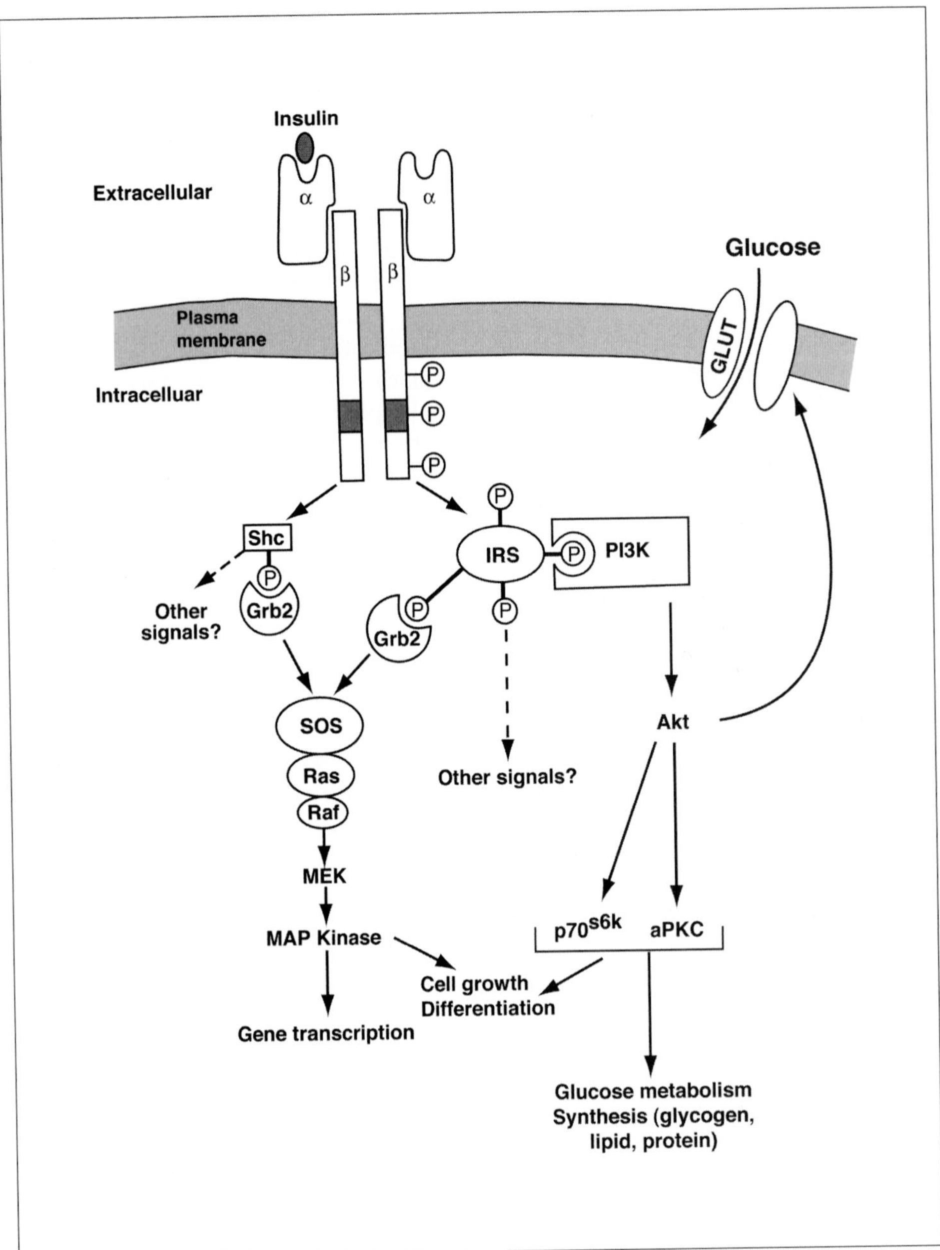

Figure 25-14 Mechanism of insulin action. Binding of insulin to the extracellular α-subunit of the insulin receptor induces autophosphorylation of the β-subunit of the receptor and phosphorylation of selected intracellular proteins, such as Shc and the IRS family. These latter phosphoproteins interact with other targets, thereby activating phosphorylation cascades, which result in glucose uptake (in adipose tissue and skeletal muscle), glucose metabolism, synthesis (of glycogen, lipid, and proteins), enhanced gene expression, cell growth, and differentiation. *p,* protein phosphorylation; *aPKC,* atypical protein kinase C. See text for details.

GLUT1 in the blood-brain barrier and GLUT3 in neuronal cells provide the constant high concentrations of glucose required by the brain. GLUT2 is expressed in hepatocytes, β-cells of the pancreas, and basolateral membranes of intestinal and renal epithelial cells. It is a low-affinity, high-capacity transport system to allow non–rate-limiting movement of glucose into and out of these cells. GLUT4 catalyzes the rate-limiting step for glucose uptake and metabolism in skeletal muscle, the major organ of glucose consumption. When circulating insulin concentrations are low, most of the GLUT4 is localized in intracellular compartments and is inactive. After eating, the pancreas releases insulin, which stimulates the translocation of GLUT4 to the plasma membrane, thereby promoting glucose uptake into skeletal muscle and fat. Insulin-stimulated glucose transport into skeletal muscle is defective in type 2 diabetes mellitus, but the mechanism has not been established. GLUT6 is a pseudogene that is not expressed at the protein level. GLUT7 allows the diffusion of free glucose out of the endoplasmic reticulum of gluconeogenic tissue.

Insulin-Like Growth Factors

Insulin-like growth factors I and II (IGF I and II) are polypeptides structurally related to insulin.[161] These hormones (previously referred to as *nonsuppressible insulin-like activity* or *somatomedin*) exhibit metabolic and growth-promoting effects similar to those of insulin. IGF I (previously somatomedin C) is one of the major regulators of cell growth and differentiation, but the physiological role of IGF II is not known. Synthesis of IGF I depends on growth hormone and occurs predominantly in the liver. In addition, many other cells produce IGF I that does not enter the circulation but acts locally. Circulating IGF concentrations are approximately 1000-fold higher than insulin concentrations, and the hormone is kept inactive by binding to a family of at least six specific binding proteins.[135] These proteins regulate IGF by protecting the ligands in the circulation and delivering them to their target tissue. In contrast to insulin, which is unbound in the circulation, less than 10% of total serum IGF I is free. The biological actions of IGF are exerted through specific IGF receptors or the insulin receptor. The IGF I receptor is closely related to the insulin receptor in structure and biochemical properties. In contrast, the IGF II receptor is quite different; it lacks tyrosine kinase activity and its physiological relevance is not understood. The IGF I receptor has a high affinity for both IGF I and IGF II, but a low affinity for insulin. The IGF II receptor has high, low, and no affinity for IGF II, IGF I, and insulin, respectively. The insulin receptor binds insulin with high affinity and IGF I and II with low affinity.

The significance of IGFs in normal carbohydrate metabolism is not known. Exogenous administration produces hypoglycemia, whereas a deficiency of IGF I results in dwarfism (pygmies and Laron dwarfs). IGFs, particularly IGF II, may be produced in excess by extrapancreatic neoplasms, and patients may have fasting hypoglycemia.[70] The high concentrations of both IGF II protein in the blood and IGF II messenger RNA (mRNA) in tumor extracts has led to the proposal that IGF II is the humoral mediator of nonislet cell tumor-induced hypoglycemia.[257] Measurement of plasma IGF I concentration may be useful in evaluating growth hormone deficiency and excess and in monitoring responses to nutritional support.

Counterregulatory Hormones

Several hormones have actions opposite to those of insulin. These counterregulatory hormones are catabolic and increase hepatic glucose production initially by enhancing the breakdown of glycogen to glucose (glycogenolysis) and later by stimulating the synthesis of glucose (gluconeogenesis).[99,100] The initial response (within minutes) to low blood glucose is an increase in glucose production, stimulated by glucagon and epinephrine. With time (3 to 4 hours), growth hormone and cortisol increase glucose mobilization and decrease glucose use (see Figure 25-10). Evidence also suggests glucose production by the liver as an inverse function of ambient glucose concentration, independent of hormonal factors *(glucose autoregulation)*. The role of other hormones or neurotransmitters is not clear but appears relatively unimportant. The multiple counterregulatory hormones exhibit both redundancy and hierarchy. Glucagon is the most important, and epinephrine becomes critical when glucagon is deficient. The other factors have lesser roles. These hormones, briefly described here, are discussed further in Chapters 29 and 48.

Glucagon. Glucagon is a 29–amino acid polypeptide secreted by the α-cells of the pancreas. The major target organ for glucagon is the liver, where it binds to specific receptors and increases both intracellular adenosine-5′-monophosphate and calcium. Glucagon stimulates the production of glucose in the liver by glycogenolysis and gluconeogenesis.[168] In addition, glucagon enhances ketogenesis in the liver. A minor target organ for glucagon is adipose tissue, where the hormone increases lipolysis. Glucagon secretion is regulated primarily by plasma glucose concentrations, low and high plasma glucose being stimulatory and inhibitory, respectively. Long-standing diabetes mellitus impairs the glucagon response to hypoglycemia, resulting in an increased incidence of hypoglycemic episodes. Stress, exercise, and amino acids induce glucagon release. Insulin inhibits glucagon release from the pancreas and decreases glucagon gene expression, thereby attenuating its biosynthesis. Increased glucagon concentrations, secondary to insulin deficiency, are believed to contribute to the hyperglycemia and ketosis of diabetes.

Proglucagon is also produced in the distal gut by L-cells, which process it into glucagon, glucagon-like peptide I, and glucagon-like peptide II. Food ingestion stimulates release of glucagon-like peptide I, which acts on the β-cell of the pancreas to stimulate insulin gene transcription and potentiate glucose-induced insulin secretion.

Epinephrine. Epinephrine, a catecholamine secreted by the adrenal medulla, stimulates glucose production (glycogenolysis) and decreases glucose use, thereby increasing blood glucose concentrations. It also stimulates glucagon secretion and inhibits insulin secretion by the pancreas (see Figure 25-10). Epinephrine appears to have *a key role in glucose counterregulation when glucagon secretion is impaired* (e.g., in type 1 diabetes mellitus). Physical or emotional stress increases epinephrine production, releasing glucose for energy. Tumors of the adrenal medulla, known as *pheochromocytomas,* secrete excess epinephrine or norepinephrine and produce moderate hyperglycemia as long as glycogen stores are available in the liver.

Growth Hormone. Growth hormone is a polypeptide secreted by the anterior pituitary gland. It stimulates gluconeogenesis, enhances lipolysis, and antagonizes insulin-stimulated glucose uptake.

Cortisol. Cortisol, secreted by the adrenal cortex in response to adrenocorticotropic hormone (ACTH), stimulates gluconeogenesis and increases the breakdown of protein and fat. Patients with Cushing's syndrome have *increased cortisol* owing to a tumor or hyperplasia of the adrenal cortex and may become hyperglycemic. In contrast, people with Addison's disease have *adrenocortical insufficiency* because of destruction or atrophy of the adrenal cortex and may exhibit hypoglycemia.

Other Hormones Influencing Glucose Metabolism

Thyroxine. Thyroxine, secreted by the thyroid gland, is not directly involved in glucose homeostasis but stimulates glycogenolysis and increases the rate of both gastric emptying and intestinal glucose absorption. These factors may produce glucose intolerance in thyrotoxic individuals, but patients usually have a fasting plasma glucose concentration in the reference interval.

Somatostatin. Somatostatin, also called growth hormone–inhibiting hormone, is a 14–amino-acid peptide found in the gastrointestinal tract, the hypothalamus, and the δ-cells of the pancreatic islets. Although somatostatin does not appear to have a direct effect on carbohydrate metabolism, it inhibits the release of growth hormone from the pituitary. In addition, *somatostatin inhibits secretion of glucagon and insulin by the pancreas,* thus modulating the reciprocal relationship between these two hormones.

BOX 25-1 Clinical Utility of Insulin, Proinsulin, C-Peptide, and Glucagon Assays

Insulin
Evaluation of fasting hypoglycemia
Evaluation of the polycystic ovary syndrome
Classification of diabetes mellitus
Predict diabetes mellitus
Assessment of β-cell activity
Select optimal therapy for diabetes
Investigation of insulin resistance
Predict the development of coronary artery disease

Proinsulin
Diagnosis of β-cell tumors
Familial hyperproinsulinemia
Cross-reactivity of insulin assays

C-Peptide
Evaluation of fasting hypoglycemia
  β-cell tumors
  Factitious
Classification of diabetes mellitus
Assessment of β-cell activity
Obtain insurance coverage for insulin pump
Monitoring therapy
  Pancreatectomy
  Transplant (pancreas-islet cell)

Glucagon
Diagnosis of α-cell tumors

Clinical Utility of Measuring Insulin, Proinsulin, C-Peptide, and Glucagon

Box 25-1 lists the clinical conditions in which hormones that regulate glucose, namely insulin, proinsulin, C-peptide, and glucagon, have been measured. Although there is interest in the possible clinical value of measurement of the concentrations of insulin and its precursors, the assays are useful primarily for research purposes. There is no role for routine testing for insulin, proinsulin, or C-peptide in patients with diabetes mellitus.[241] It must be emphasized that the diagnostic criteria for diabetes mellitus do not include measurements of hormones, which remain predominantly research tools.

Insulin

The primary clinical application of insulin measurement is in the evaluation of patients with fasting hypoglycemia (discussed in more detail later in this chapter). Insulin determination has also been proposed to be of value in selecting the optimal initial therapy for patients with type 2 diabetes mellitus. In theory, the lower the pretreatment insulin concentration, the more appropriate might be insulin or an insulin secretagogue as the treatment of choice. Although intellectually appealing, there is no evidence that knowledge of the insulin concentration leads to more efficacious treatment. Evidence indicates that increased concentrations of insulin in nondiabetic individuals predict the development of coronary artery disease.[113] Nevertheless, it is not clear that the increased insulin is responsible for the risk of coronary disease, and the clinical value is questionable.[241] An emerging use for insulin assays is in the evaluation and management of patients with the polycystic ovary syndrome.[241] Women with this condition have insulin resistance and abnormal carbohydrate metabolism that may respond to oral hypoglycemic agents. Although a few investigators have recommended measuring insulin along with glucose during an oral glucose tolerance test as an aid to the early diagnosis of diabetes mellitus, this approach is not recommended.[241]

Proinsulin

High proinsulin concentrations are usually noted in patients with benign or malignant β-cell tumors of the pancreas. Most patients with β-cell tumors have increased insulin, C-peptide, and proinsulin concentrations, but occasionally only proinsulin is increased[98] because the tumors have defective conversion of proinsulin to insulin. Despite its low biological activity, proinsulin production may be adequate to produce hypoglycemia. In addition, a rare form of familial hyperproinsulinemia, produced by impaired conversion to insulin, has been described. Measurement of proinsulin can be useful to determine the extent of proinsulin-like material that cross-reacts in an insulin assay. Patients with type 2 diabetes have increased proportions of proinsulin and proinsulin conversion intermediates,[167] high concentrations of which are associated with cardiovascular risk factors.[197] Even relatively mild hyperglycemia produces hyperproinsulinemia, with values greater than 40% of insulin concentration in type 2 diabetes.[167] Similarly, women with gestational diabetes mellitus (GDM) have notably higher concentrations of proinsulin and split 32, 33 proinsulin than pregnant normoglycemic control subjects. An increased ratio of proinsulin-like molecules to insulin-like molecules at screening may be a better predictor of GDM than age, obesity, or hyperglycemia.[266] Increased proinsulin concentrations may also be detected in patients with chronic renal failure, cirrhosis, or hyperthyroidism.

Accurate measurement of proinsulin has been difficult for several reasons: the blood concentrations are low; antibody production is difficult; most antisera cross-react with insulin and C-peptide, which are present in much higher concentrations; the assays measure intermediate cleavage forms of proinsulin; and reference preparations of pure proinsulin are not readily available. However, a more sensitive nonequilibrium RIA method for measuring proinsulin was developed by adsorbing the initial antiserum with biosynthetic human C-peptide coupled to agarose to eliminate cross-reactivity with C-peptide.[39,120] An enzyme-linked immunosorbent assay (ELISA) has been described that employs an antibody to C-peptide as the coating antibody and antiinsulin antibody for detection.[101] The detection limit is 0.25 pmol/L.[156]

C-Peptide

Measurement of C-peptide has a number of advantages over insulin measurement. Because hepatic metabolism is negligible, C-peptide concentrations are better indicators of β-cell function than is peripheral insulin concentration.[222] Furthermore, C-peptide assays do not measure exogenous insulin and do not cross-react with insulin antibodies, which interfere with the insulin immunoassay.

Fasting Hypoglycemia. The primary indication for measuring C-peptide is for the evaluation of fasting hypoglycemia. Some patients with insulin-producing β-cell tumors, particularly if hyperinsulinism is intermittent, may exhibit increased C-peptide concentrations with normal insulin concentrations. When hypoglycemia is due to surreptitious insulin injection, *insulin* concentrations will be high but C-peptide values will be low[129]; this occurs because C-peptide is not found in commercial insulin preparations and exogenous insulin suppresses β-cell function.

Insulin Secretion. Basal or stimulated (by glucagon or glucose) C-peptide concentrations can provide an estimate of a patient's insulin secretory capacity and rate. For example, diabetic patients with C-peptide concentrations greater than 1.8 μg/L (1.8 ng/mL) after stimulation with glucagon behave clinically like patients with type 2 diabetes, and those with low peak C-peptide values (less than 0.5 μg/L) behave like patients with type 1 diabetes.[123] In rare cases this strategy may be helpful before discontinuation of insulin treatment (e.g., in an obese adolescent). Urinary and fasting serum C-peptide concentrations also appear to be of some value in differentiating patients with type 1 diabetes from those with type 2 diabetes.[147] In addition, patients who have type 1 diabetes but who have no C-peptide response are usually more labile than those with some residual β-cell function. Despite these observations, C-peptide measurement has a negligible role in the routine management of patients with diabetes. A new indication for C-peptide analysis is the recent requirement that Medicare patients in the United States have low C-peptide concentrations to be eligible for coverage of insulin pumps.[241]

Monitoring Therapy. Measurement of C-peptide can be used to monitor patients' response to pancreatic surgery. C-peptide should be undetectable after a radical pancreatectomy and should increase after a successful pancreas or islet cell transplant.

Measurements of urine C-peptide are useful when a continuous assessment of β-cell function is desired or frequent blood sampling is not practical. The 24-hour urine C-peptide content (in the absence of renal failure, which produces increased levels) correlates well with fasting serum C-peptide concentration or with the sum of C-peptide concentrations in sequential specimens after a glucose load. However, the fraction of secreted C-peptide that is excreted in the urine exhibits high intersubject and intrasubject variability, limiting the value of urine C-peptide as a measure of insulin secretion.[275]

Glucagon

Very high concentrations of glucagon are seen in patients with α-cell tumors of the pancreas called glucagonomas. Patients with this tumor frequently have weight loss, necrolytic migratory erythema, diabetes mellitus, stomatitis, and diarrhea.[289] The skin lesions often occur first and are frequently overlooked. Most tumors have metastasized when finally diagnosed. Low glucagon concentrations are associated with chronic pancreatitis and long-term sulfonylurea therapy.

Methods for the Measurement of Specific Hormones

Details of the following methods for specific hormones are found in the Evolve site that accompanies this book at http://evolve.elsevier.com/Tietz/textbook/.

Insulin

Although insulin has been assayed for more than 40 years, there is no highly accurate, precise, and reliable procedure available to measure the amount of insulin in a patient sample. Many insulin assays are commercially available.[61] The techniques most widely used in the United States are immunochemical.[235] Bioassays, although of greater physiological relevance because they measure biological activity, are labor intensive and not widely used. A stable isotope dilution mass spectrometry assay, which was described recently, yields lower values than immunoassays.[154]

Patients treated with exogenous insulin may develop circulating antiinsulin antibodies, which compete with antibodies in the RIA. The endogenous antibodies and their bound insulin can be precipitated from serum with polyethylene glycol (PEG), and the free insulin measured by RIA. The total insulin can be determined by eluting antibody-bound insulin with hydrochloric acid (HCl), precipitating the antibody with PEG, and performing RIA. The bound insulin is the difference between total and free insulin. Unless a patient's insulin requirements change dramatically, total insulin concentrations are usually constant in patients with type 1 diabetes, and repeated assays are not necessary.

Principle. In a typical RIA procedure for measuring insulin, ^{125}I-labeled insulin competes with insulin in a patient sample for binding to an insulin-specific antibody immobilized on the walls of a polypropylene tube. The supernatant is decanted, and the bound ^{125}I determined in a gamma counter. The amount of insulin in the sample is established by comparison with a calibration curve obtained by plotting on logit-log graph paper the percent of total radioactivity bound (B/T%) against the concentration of the calibrators. Various commercial kits for insulin measurement are now available.

Comments. General comments on the measurement of insulin include:

1. The term *immunoreactive insulin* is used in reference to assays that may recognize, in addition to insulin, substrates that share antigenic epitopes with insulin. Examples include proinsulin, proinsulin conversion intermediates, and insulin derivatives, produced by glycation or dimerization.
2. Various insulin preparations, including human insulin, are used as insulin calibrators. For ease of comparison of results among laboratories, the insulin calibrator is expressed in terms of international units (IU). One international unit of insulin is equal to approximately 43 μg of the World Health Organization (WHO) first International Reference Preparation (1st IRP) Code 66/304 (National Institute of Biological Standards and Control, South Mimms, Potters Bar, Hertfordshire, United Kingdom), which is 100% human insulin.
3. *Antisera raised against insulin show some cross-reactivity with proinsulin but not with C-peptide.* Specificity is not a problem in healthy individuals because the low proinsulin concentrations do not appreciably affect the absolute values of insulin. In certain situations (e.g., islet cell tumors and diabetic individuals), proinsulin is present at higher concentrations and direct assay of plasma may falsely overestimate the true insulin concentration. Because proinsulin has very low activity, incorrect conclusions regarding the availability of biologically active insulin may be reached in patients with diabetes. The magnitude of the error depends on the concentration of proinsulin and the extent of cross-reactivity of the antiserum with proinsulin. Monoclonal antibody-based assays that are specific for insulin and do not measure proinsulin,[272] although theoretically advantageous, are not superior to nonspecific assays.[235]
4. A stable isotope dilution assay using mass spectrometry to measure insulin, proinsulin, and C-peptide has been developed.[154] The difference in mass among the three analytes allows specific measurement of each protein. Comparison of patient samples revealed that most, but not all, results were higher by immunoassay than mass spectrometry.[154] Thus immunoassays may overestimate insulin, particularly at low concentrations. The high protein concentration in the serum requires extraction of proteins (e.g., by immunoaffinity) and purification by high-performance liquid chromatography (HPLC) before quantification by mass spectrometry. This method is not suitable for routine laboratory analysis.
5. The American Diabetes Association (ADA) appointed a task force to standardize the insulin assay.[235] Evaluation of unknown samples by 17 different laboratories revealed a wide range in insulin values, with interlaboratory variation of up to threefold.[235] Large differences were observed even among laboratories using the same assays. Use of a common calibrator did not improve agreement among laboratories. Assay coefficients of variation (CVs) ranged from less than 2% to greater than 30%, with ELISAs exhibiting the lowest imprecision. Certain characteristics of some assays, including commercial kits, were unacceptable. The task force judged available proficiency and certification programs for insulin to be inadequate, and recommended the establishment of a central laboratory to provide certification for insulin assays. Complete interlaboratory standardization was deemed to be neither practical nor universally acceptable. The ADA recommendations for analysis of insulin[235] are as follows:
   a. Each laboratory should carefully evaluate its insulin assay to ensure acceptable assay performance.
   b. Each laboratory should compare the performance of its assay with others using common calibrators and unknown samples.
   c. Because assay performance may change with time or with new reagents or equipment, performance characteristics must be remeasured periodically.
6. Acceptance criteria for an insulin assay are less than 15% interassay CV. Minimum detectable concentration of insulin, as calculated from the calibration curve, should be 1 μIU/mL with the overnight procedure or 3 μIU/mL with the same-day procedure. In addition, recovery and linearity should be 100 ± 15%, and the in-house insulin calibrator should be within 5% of the gold standard. No gold standard was specified.
7. Patient samples with high values should be diluted with the zero calibrator.
8. The presence of antibodies to insulin results in spuriously increased or decreased (depending on the method used) insulin values.

Reference Intervals. Reference intervals vary among assays and each laboratory should establish its own reference intervals. After an overnight fast, insulin concentrations in healthy, normal, nonobese people range from 2 to 25 μIU/mL (12 to 150 pmol/L).* More specific assays that have minimal cross-reactivity with proinsulin reveal a fasting plasma insulin concentration of less than 9 μIU/mL (60 pmol/L). Concentrations up to 200 μIU/mL can be reached during a glucose tolerance test. Representative values for insulin concentrations after glucose are shown in Figure 25-13. Fasting insulin values are higher in obese, nondiabetic people and lower in trained athletes.

Insulin Antibodies

Assays for insulin antibodies fall into three categories: (1) quantitative radioimmunoelectrophoresis, which measures the binding of IgG antibody to radiolabeled insulin by rocket immunoelectrophoresis into anti–IgG-containing agarose; (2) RIAs with separation of bound and free insulin by precipitation with PEG or a second antibody; and (3) solid phase immobilization of insulin to test tubes or Sepharose. These are discussed in more detail in Reeves.[230]

Proinsulin

Principle. Accurate measurement of proinsulin has been difficult for several reasons: the blood concentrations are low; antibody production is difficult; most antisera cross-react with insulin and C-peptide, which are present in much higher concentrations; the assays measure intermediate cleavage forms of proinsulin; and reference preparations of pure proinsulin were not readily available.[285] Therefore few accurate data are available in the literature on plasma proinsulin. These problems have, to a large extent, been overcome by the availability of biosynthetic proinsulin, which has allowed the production of monoclonal antibodies to proinsulin[79,260] and provided reliable proinsulin calibrators and reference preparations. An International Reference Preparation for human proinsulin (code 84/611) is available from the National Institute of Biological Standards and Controls (Potters Bar, United Kingdom). Earlier assays may have overestimated proinsulin concentrations.[211]

Reference Intervals. Reference intervals for proinsulin are highly dependent on the method of analysis, the degree of cross-reactivity of the antisera, and the purity of proinsulin calibrators. Each laboratory should establish its own reference intervals.

Reference intervals in healthy, fasting individuals reported in the literature range from 1.1 to 6.9 pmol/L to 2.1 to 12.6 pmol/L (see Reference 130 and references therein).

*The conversion factor of 6.0 used to convert μIU/mL (or mIU/L) of insulin to pmol/L is based on a MW of insulin of 5807.58 and a specific activity of 30 IU/mg.

C-Peptide

Principle. C-peptide undergoes minimal liver metabolism and, in contrast to proinsulin assays, assays are not affected by antiinsulin antibodies. However, various methodological problems produce large between-method variation. These difficulties include variable specificity among different antisera, variable cross-reactivity with proinsulin, and the type of C-peptide preparation used as a calibrator. A comparison, in the clinically relevant range, using four commercial kits and four commercial C-peptide antisera yielded values ranging from 0.54 to 1.06 nmol/L on the same sample. Furthermore, a tyrosine residue must be incorporated onto the C-peptide to enable labeling with ^{125}I. Several immunometric methods have been described for the measurement of C-peptide, and a number of kits are commercially available.[61]

Reference Intervals. Each laboratory should establish its own reference interval for C-peptide. Fasting serum concentrations of C-peptide in healthy people range from 0.78 to 1.89 ng/mL (0.25 to 0.6 nmol/L). After stimulation with glucose or glucagon, values range from 2.73 to 5.64 ng/mL (0.9 to 1.87 nmol/L), three to five times the prestimulation value. Urinary C-peptide is usually in the range of 74 ± 26 μg/L (25 ± 8.8 μmol/L). C-peptide is excreted primarily by the kidney and concentrations in the serum are increased in renal disease.

Glucagon

Principle. A competitive RIA is available for measuring glucagon (Diagnostic Products Corp.). ^{125}I-labeled glucagon competes with glucagon in the patient specimen for binding to the polyclonal glucagon antibody. Bound glucagon is separated from free glucagon by use of PEG and a second antibody. Bound radioactivity for the patient specimen is compared with that of glucagon calibrators. The calibrator values are assigned at the manufacturer using the WHO glucagon international standard (69/194).

Reference Intervals. Fasting plasma concentrations of glucagon vary from 70 to 180 ng/L (20 to 52 pmol/L). Values up to 500 times the upper reference limit may be found in patients with autonomously secreting α-cell neoplasms.

DIABETES MELLITUS

Diabetes mellitus is a group of metabolic disorders of carbohydrate metabolism in which glucose is underused, producing hyperglycemia. Some patients may experience acute life-threatening hyperglycemic episodes, such as ketoacidosis or hyperosmolar coma. As the disease progresses, patients are at increased risk for the development of specific complications, including *retinopathy* leading to blindness, *nephropathy* leading to renal failure, *neuropathy* (nerve damage), and *atherosclerosis.*[200,258] The last may result in stroke, gangrene, and coronary artery disease.

The prevalence of diabetes is unknown. The most recent published information in the United States is from the

Centers for Disease Control and Prevention (CDC), which estimated a prevalence in 2001 of 7.9% in adults.[192] This is equivalent to 16.7 million people. Because at least 30% of all prevalent cases are undiagnosed,[117] the total number may have been almost 22 million. Note that in 1987, the prevalence of diagnosed diabetes was 6.8 million.[225] This large increase in diabetes has been observed globally. The prevalence of diabetes in adults worldwide was estimated to be 4.0% in 1995 and anticipated to rise to 5.4% by the year 2025.[153] The prediction is that in 2025 there will be 300 million adults with diabetes, greater than 75% of whom will live in developing countries. These statistics have led to diabetes being described as "one of the main threats to human health in the twenty-first century."[303] The prevalence of diabetes mellitus increases with age, and approximately half of all cases occur in people older than 55 years. In the United States, ~20% of the population older than 65 years have diabetes.[117] There is racial predilection, and by the age of 65, 33%, 25%, and 17% of Hispanics, blacks, and whites, respectively, in the United States have diabetes mellitus. In 2002 diabetes mellitus was estimated to be responsible for $132 billion in healthcare expenditures in the United States.[125] The direct costs were $92 billion, with 50% of that incurred by those older than 65 years. An estimated 186,000 deaths annually are attributable to diabetes.[125] In fact, American women are twice as likely to die from diabetes mellitus as from breast cancer. Approximately one in five American healthcare dollars spent in 2002 was for people with diabetes mellitus.

CLASSIFICATION

Diabetes was initially diagnosed by the oral glucose tolerance test (OGTT). Values greater than two standard deviations above the mean of the value found in a selected population of healthy volunteers without a family history of diabetes mellitus were accepted as diagnostic. This criterion led to the identification of large numbers of asymptomatic people with abnormally high 1- to 2-hour postload glucose values, but normal fasting blood glucose. They were presumed to have early or mild diabetes mellitus. In 1975 it was estimated that more than half the population older than 60 years was abnormal. Follow-up of these people indicated that most of them with lesser degrees of glucose intolerance did not manifest definite evidence of diabetes mellitus in the next 10 years, and a large percentage returned to normal glucose tolerance.

Most populations have plasma glucose values that exhibit a unimodal, log-normal distribution (i.e., a distribution curve that is skewed to the high end but becomes bell shaped on a logarithmic axis). Ethnic groups with a high prevalence of diabetes, such as the Pima Indians and Nauruans, exhibit bimodal blood glucose distributions.[92] Optimal distinction between normal and diabetic individuals in these groups occurs at a fasting glucose around 140 mg/dL and glucose concentrations greater than 200 mg/dL 2 hours after an oral glucose load. Furthermore the specific microvascular complications of diabetes were believed to be rare in patients with fasting or 2-hour postprandial glucose concentrations less than 140 or 200 mg/dL, respectively. These observations were the basis for the criteria proposed in 1979 by a workgroup of the National Diabetes Data Group[203] and later endorsed by the WHO Committee on Diabetes. Lower cutpoints are used currently.

The 1979 classification scheme recognized two major forms of diabetes: type I (insulin-dependent) diabetes mellitus (IDDM) and type II (non–insulin-dependent) diabetes mellitus (NIDDM).[203] The terms juvenile-onset and adult-onset diabetes were abolished. To base the classification on etiology rather than treatment, the ADA established a workgroup in 1995 to reexamine the classification and diagnosis of diabetes mellitus. The revised classification, published in 1997,[7] eliminates the terms insulin-dependent diabetes mellitus and non–insulin-dependent diabetes mellitus, which are now termed type 1 and type 2 diabetes, respectively (Box 25-2). Furthermore the categories of previous abnormality of glucose tolerance and potential abnormality of glucose tolerance have been eliminated.

Type 1 Diabetes Mellitus (Formerly Insulin-Dependent Diabetes Mellitus [IDDM], Type I, or Juvenile-Onset Diabetes)

Approximately 5% to 10% of all cases of diabetes mellitus are in this category. Patients usually have abrupt onset of symptoms (e.g., polyuria, polydipsia, and rapid weight loss). Patients have insulinopenia (a deficiency of insulin) caused by loss of pancreatic islet β-cells and are dependent on insulin to sustain life and prevent ketosis. Most patients have antibodies that identify an autoimmune process (see later discussion); some patients have no evidence of autoimmunity and are classified as type 1 idiopathic. The peak incidence is in childhood and adolescence. Approximately 75% acquire the disease before age 30 years, but the onset in the remainder may occur at any age. Age at presentation is not a criterion for classification.

BOX 25-2 Classification of Diabetes Mellitus and Other Categories of Glucose Intolerance

Type 1 diabetes
- A. Immune mediated
- B. Idiopathic

Type 2 diabetes
Other specific types of diabetes
GDM
IGT
IFG

From the American Diabetes Association. Report of the expert committee on the diagnosis and classification of diabetes mellitus. Diabetes Care 1997; 20:1183-1201.

Type 2 Diabetes Mellitus (Formerly Non-Insulin-Dependent Diabetes Mellitus [NIDDM], Type II, or Adult-Onset Diabetes

This group comprises approximately 90% of all cases of diabetes. Patients have minimal symptoms, are not prone to ketosis, and *are not dependent on insulin* to prevent ketonuria. *Insulin concentrations may be normal, decreased, or increased,* and most people with this form of diabetes have impaired insulin action. *Obesity* is commonly associated and weight loss alone usually improves the hyperglycemia. However, many individuals with type 2 diabetes may require dietary manipulation, an oral hypoglycemic agent, or insulin to control hyperglycemia. Most patients acquire the disease after age 40, but it may occur in younger people. Type 2 diabetes in children and adolescents is an emerging, significant problem.[10,303] Among children in Japan, type 2 diabetes is now more common than type 1.[303]

Other Specific Types of Diabetes Mellitus

This subclass includes uncommon patients in whom hyperglycemia is due to a specific underlying disorder, such as genetic defects of β-cell function; genetic defects in insulin action; disease of the exocrine pancreas; endocrinopathies (e.g., Cushing's disease, acromegaly, and glucagonoma); the administration of hormones or drugs known to induce β-cell dysfunction (e.g., dilantin and pentamidine) or impair insulin action (e.g., glucocorticoids, thiazides, and β-adrenergics); infections; uncommon forms of immune-mediated diabetes; or other genetic conditions (e.g., Down syndrome, Klinefelter syndrome and porphyria; see American Diabetes Association[7] for a detailed list). This was formerly termed *secondary diabetes.*

Impaired Glucose Tolerance (IGT)

Impaired glucose tolerance is diagnosed in people who have fasting blood glucose concentrations less than those required for a diagnosis of diabetes mellitus, but have a plasma glucose response during the OGTT between normal and diabetic states. An OGTT is required to assign a patient to this class. Development of overt diabetes occurs at a rate of 1% to 5% per year, but a large proportion spontaneously revert to normal glucose tolerance. Microvascular disease is quite rare in this group and patients usually do not experience the renal or retinal complications of diabetes. Patients have an increased prevalence of atherosclerosis and mortality from cardiovascular disease.[76]

Impaired Fasting Glucose (IFG)

This new category is analogous to IGT, but is diagnosed by a *fasting* glucose value between that of normal and diabetic individuals. It is a metabolic stage between normal glucose homeostasis and diabetes. As with IGT, persons with IFG are at increased risk for the development of diabetes and cardiovascular disease. IFG and IGT are not clinical entities, but rather risk factors for diabetes and cardiovascular disease.

Gestational Diabetes Mellitus

This is carbohydrate intolerance of variable severity *with onset or first recognition during pregnancy*[187] (i.e., diabetic women who become pregnant are not included in this category). Estimates of the frequency of abnormal glucose tolerance during pregnancy range from 1% to 14%, depending on the population studied and the diagnostic tests employed.[153] In the United States, GDM occurs in 6% to 8% of pregnancies. Women with GDM are at increased risk for the subsequent development of diabetes mellitus, which develops in 6% to 62% of these women.[213] The risk is particularly high in women who have marked hyperglycemia during or soon after pregnancy, women who are obese, and women whose GDM was diagnosed before 24 weeks of gestation.[157] At 6 to 12 weeks postpartum, all patients who had GDM should be evaluated for diabetes and, if diabetes is not present, reevaluated for diabetes at least every 3 years.[12]

PATHOGENESIS OF TYPE 1 DIABETES MELLITUS

Type 1 diabetes mellitus results from a cellular-mediated autoimmune destruction of the insulin-secreting cells of pancreatic β-cells.[19,118] In the vast majority of patients, the destruction is mediated by T cells. This is termed type 1A or immune-mediated diabetes (Box 25-2). The α-, δ-, and other islet cells are preserved. The islet cells have a chronic mononuclear cell infiltrate, called *insulitis.* The autoimmune process leading to type 1 diabetes begins months or years before the clinical presentation, and an 80% to 90% reduction in the volume of the β-cells is required to induce symptomatic type 1 diabetes. The rate of islet cell destruction is variable and is usually more rapid in children than in adults.

Antibodies

The most practical markers of β-cell autoimmunity are circulating antibodies, which can be detected in the serum years before the onset of hyperglycemia. The best characterized antibodies are[19,118,241]

1. *Islet cell cytoplasmic antibodies* (ICAs) react with a sialoglycoconjugate antigen present in the cytoplasm of all endocrine cells of the pancreatic islets. These antibodies are detected in the serum of 0.5% of normal subjects and 75% to 85% of patients with newly diagnosed type 1 diabetes. The antibodies are detected by immunofluorescence microscopy on frozen sections of human pancreatic tails. Results are compared with a standard serum of the Immunology of Diabetes Workgroup[190] and are expressed in Juvenile Diabetes Foundation (JDF) units. Although not universal, many laboratories use 10 JDF units on two separate occasions or a single result of greater than or equal to 20 JDF units as significant titers. The ICA assay is labor intensive and difficult to standardize. Few clinical laboratories are likely to implement this assay, which has marked interlaboratory variability in sensitivity and specificity.[241]

2. *Insulin autoantibodies* (IAAs) are present in more than 90% of children who develop type 1 diabetes before age 5, but in fewer than 40% of individuals developing diabetes after age 12. Their frequency in healthy people is similar to that of ICA. A radioisotopic method that calculates the displaceable insulin radioligand binding after the addition of excess nonradiolabeled insulin is recommended for IAA. Results are positive when concentrations exceed the mean +2 (or 3) standard deviations (SD) of healthy controls. An important caveat is that insulin antibodies develop after insulin therapy, even in those persons who use human insulin.
3. *Antibodies to the 65-kD isoform of glutamic acid decarboxylase* (GAD_{65})[21] have been found up to 10 years before the onset of clinical type 1 diabetes and are present in ~60% of patients with newly diagnosed diabetes. GAD_{65} antibodies may be used to identify patients with apparent type 2 diabetes who will subsequently progress to type 1 diabetes. Several different assay formats have been used for the measurement of anti-GAD_{65} antibodies, including enzymatic immunoprecipitation assay, radiobinding assay, ELISA, immunofluorescence, and Western blotting.[252] The considerable variability among laboratories has been significantly reduced by the Second International GADAb Workshop.[252] A monoclonal antibody, MICA 3, was suggested as a reference standard. A dual micromethod and RIA performed with ^{3}H-labeled human recombinant GAD_{65} in a rabbit reticulocyte expression system is used by many laboratories. Methods for measurement of GAD_{65} are now commercially available.
4. *Insulinoma-associated antigens* (IA-2A and IA-2βA), directed against two tyrosine phosphatases, have been detected in more than 50% of newly diagnosed type 1 diabetes patients. A widely used method to measure IA-2A uses ^{35}S-labeled recombinant IA-2 in a dual micromethod and RIA. The concurrent analysis of IA-2 and GAD_{65} in a single assay has been reported.[242]

Although antibodies to bovine serum albumin have been reported in patients with newly diagnosed type 1 diabetes,[146] this model is contentious, and conflicting data exist.[18,20]

The CDC is working with the Immunology of Diabetes Society to develop the Diabetes Autoantibody Standardization Program. Because of the difficulty in obtaining adequate patient samples, it is not yet clear whether this program will become generally available.

Autoantibody markers of immune destruction are present in 85% to 90% of individuals with immune-mediated diabetes when fasting hyperglycemia is initially detected.[7] Approximately 10% to 12% of white adult patients who have the type 2 diabetes phenotype also have islet cell autoantibodies, particularly to GAD_{65}. This condition has been termed latent autoimmune diabetes of adulthood (LADA).[224] Up to 1% to 2% of healthy individuals have a single autoantibody and are at low risk of developing immune-mediated diabetes. Because the prevalence of immune-mediated diabetes is low (~0.3% in the general population), the positive predictive value of a single autoantibody will be low. The presence of multiple islet autoantibodies (IAA, GAD_{65}, and IA-2A and/or IA-2βA) is associated with a greater than 90% risk of immune-mediated diabetes. However, no acceptable therapy has been documented to prevent the clinical onset of diabetes in islet cell autoantibody-positive individuals.[19] New strategies for treatment of type 1 diabetes that are being developed focus on immunosuppressive therapy to attenuate the autoimmune response, replacement of insulin-producing β-cells by transplantation, or restoration of insulin with gene therapy.[102,207] Recently, hyperglycemia in diabetic mice was completely reversed by gene therapy that induced the development of β-cells of the pancreas in the liver.[160] Although type 1 diabetes can be prevented in animal models,[38] the possible role of immune intervention in humans remains unresolved.

Genetics

Susceptibility to type 1 diabetes is inherited,[276] but the mode of inheritance is complex and has not been defined. It is a multigenic trait, and the major locus is the major histocompatibility complex on chromosome 6. At least 11 other loci on 9 chromosomes also contribute, with the regulatory region of the insulin gene on chromosome 11p15 being an important locus. The concordance rate between identical twins is approximately 30%, and approximately 95% of whites with type 1 diabetes express either HLA-DR3 or HLA-DR4 histocompatibility antigens. However, up to 40% of the nondiabetic population also express these alleles. In contrast, the HLA-DQB1*0602 allele significantly decreases the risk of type 1 diabetes. HLA typing can indicate absolute risk of diabetes.[241] The risk of a sibling developing diabetes is 1%, 5%, and 10% to 20% if the number of haplotypes shared is none, one, and two, respectively. However, only 10% of patients with type 1 diabetes have an affected first-degree relative. The multiplicity of independent chromosomal regions associated with a predisposition to type 1 diabetes suggests that other susceptibility genes will be identified. Routine measurement of genetic markers is not of value at this time for the diagnosis or management of patients with type 1 diabetes.[241]

Environment

Reports describe that environmental factors are involved in initiating diabetes. Viruses, such as rubella, mumps, and coxsackievirus B, have been implicated.[136] Other environmental factors that have been suggested include chemicals and cow's milk. It seems likely that autoimmunity to β-cells is initiated by a viral protein (that shares amino acid sequence with a β-cell protein) or some other environmental insult. Genetic susceptibility and other host factors (e.g., HLA type) determine the progression of the β-cell destruction.

Pathogenesis of Type 2 Diabetes Mellitus

There are at least two major identifiable pathological defects in patients with type 2 diabetes.[77,144,243] One is a decreased ability of insulin to act on the peripheral tissue. This is called *insulin resistance* and is thought by many to be the primary underlying pathological process. The other is *β-cell dysfunction,* which is an inability of the pancreas to produce sufficient insulin to compensate for the insulin resistance. Thus there is a relative deficiency of insulin early in the disease and absolute insulin deficiency late in the disease. The debate over whether type 2 diabetes is primarily due to a defect in β-cell secretion, peripheral resistance to insulin, or both has been raging for decades. However, there are data to support the concept that insulin resistance is the primary defect, preceding the derangement in insulin secretion and clinical diabetes by as much as 20 years.[144,243] Despite the lack of consensus, it is clear that type 2 diabetes mellitus is an extremely heterogeneous disease and no single cause is adequate to explain the progression from normal glucose tolerance to diabetes. The fundamental molecular defects in insulin resistance and insulin secretion result from a combination of environmental and genetic factors.

Loss of β-Cell Function

The increased β-cell demand induced by insulin resistance is ultimately associated with a progressive loss of β-cell function that is necessary for the development of fasting hyperglycemia. The major defect is a *loss of glucose-induced insulin release* (see Figure 25-13), which is termed *selective glucose unresponsiveness.* Hyperglycemia appears to render the β-cells increasingly unresponsive to glucose (called *glucotoxicity*), and the level of dysfunction correlates with both the glucose concentration and duration of hyperglycemia. Restoration of euglycemia rapidly resolves the defect. Increased free fatty acids in serum have also been implicated in β-cell failure.[30] Other insulin secretory abnormalities in type 2 diabetes include disruption of the normal pulsatile release of insulin and an increased ratio of plasma proinsulin to insulin.[167] More recently, evidence obtained from knockout mice reveals that insulin resistance in the β-cells may contribute to alterations in insulin secretion as occur in type 2 diabetes.[162]

Insulin Resistance

Insulin resistance is defined as *a decreased biological response to normal concentrations of circulating insulin*[90] and is found in both obese, nondiabetic individuals and patients with type 2 diabetes. The underlying pathophysiological defects(s) has (have) not been identified, but insulin resistance is usually attributed to a defect in insulin action. Measurement of insulin resistance in a routine clinical setting is difficult and surrogate measures, namely fasting insulin concentration or the euglycemic insulin clamp,[8] are used to provide an indirect assessment of insulin function. There is a broad clinical spectrum of insulin resistance, ranging from euglycemia (with marked increase in endogenous insulin) to hyperglycemia despite large doses of exogenous insulin.

The insulin resistance syndrome (also known as syndrome X or the metabolic syndrome) is a constellation of associated clinical and laboratory findings, consisting of insulin resistance, hyperinsulinemia, obesity, dyslipidemia (high triglyceride and low HDL cholesterol), and hypertension.[228] The metabolic syndrome is diagnosed if an individual has three or more of the following criteria[87]:

- Abdominal obesity: waist circumference greater than 35 inches (women) or 40 inches (men)
- Triglycerides greater than 150 mg/dL
- HDL cholesterol less than 50 mg/dL (women) or less than 40 mg/dL (men)
- Blood pressure greater than or equal to 130/85 mm Hg
- Fasting plasma glucose (FPG) greater than or equal to 110 mg/dL

Individuals with this syndrome are at increased risk for cardiovascular disease. Several rare clinical syndromes are also associated with insulin resistance. The prototype is the type A insulin resistance syndrome, which is characterized by hyperinsulinemia, acanthosis nigricans, and ovarian hyperandrogenism.

Environment

Environmental factors, such as diet and exercise, are important determinants in the pathogenesis of type 2 diabetes. There is convincing evidence linking obesity to the development of type 2 diabetes, but the association is complex. Although 60% to 80% of patients with type 2 diabetes are obese, diabetes develops in fewer than 15% of obese individuals. In contrast, virtually all obese subjects, even those with normal carbohydrate tolerance, have hyperinsulinemia and are insulin resistant. Other factors, such as family history of type 2 diabetes (genetic predisposition), the duration of obesity, and the distribution of fat are important. Nevertheless, the rising prevalence of diabetes is believed to be a consequence of the increase in obesity (defined as a body mass index greater than or equal to 30 kg/m^2), which was reported to be 20.9% in U.S. adults in 2001.[192] Evaluation of 84,941 healthy women after 16 years in the Nurses' Health Study revealed that obesity was the most important predictor of type 2 diabetes.[131] Compared with women with a body mass index of less than 23, the relative risks of developing diabetes were 38.8 and 20.1 with body mass indexes of greater than or equal to 35 and 30 to 34.9, respectively. Importantly, intervention can delay or prevent the onset of type 2 diabetes. Two randomized studies documented that life-style changes (weight reduction and exercise) in individuals with IGT reduced the incidence of type 2 diabetes.[158,279] Although the weight loss was modest (5% to 7%), the rate of progression to type 2 diabetes was reduced by 58% in both studies.

Interestingly, there is an inverse relationship between the degree of physical activity and the prevalence of type 2 diabetes. For every 500-kcal increase in daily energy expenditure, there is a 6% decrease in the age-adjusted risk of type 2 diabetes. This effect is independent of both body weight and a parental history of diabetes. The mechanism of the protective effect of exercise is thought to be an increased sensitivity to insulin in skeletal muscle and adipose tissue.

Diabetogenes

It is widely acknowledged that genetic factors contribute to the development of type 2 diabetes.[144] For example, the concordance rate for type 2 diabetes in identical twins approaches 100%. Type 2 diabetes is 10 times more likely to occur in an obese person with a diabetic parent than an equally obese person without a diabetic family history. However, the mode of inheritance is unknown, and type 2 diabetes has been described as a "geneticist's nightmare."[204] Many less common diseases (e.g., cystic fibrosis or Duchenne muscular dystrophy) are caused by mutations at a single locus. More common diseases, such as diabetes mellitus, schizophrenia, atherosclerosis, hypertension, and osteoporosis, are not inherited according to simple mendelian rules. These conditions are genetically more complex, and multiple genetic factors interact with exogenous influences (such as environmental factors) to produce the phenotype.

Multiple factors complicate the search for diabetogenes in type 2 diabetes.[243] A variety of approaches have produced several genes that are associated with type 2 diabetes. However, despite considerable investigative effort to identify the genetic basis of type 2 diabetes mellitus (more than 60 candidate genes have been examined), *genetic defects identified to date account for fewer than 5% of patients with type 2 diabetes.* Therefore the gene or genes causing the common forms of type 2 diabetes remain unknown. The known genes can be conveniently separated into those involved in insulin secretion, those participating in insulin action, and those regulating body weight.

Candidate Insulin Secretion Genes

These include genes that are expressed in β-cells, such as amylin, glucagon-like peptide-1 receptor, glucokinase regulatory protein, and islet-1 protein. The greatest success in the search for diabetogenes has been in maturity-onset diabetes of the young (MODY), a rare group of disorders characterized by nonketotic diabetes.[30,241] The clinical spectrum of MODY is broad, ranging from asymptomatic hyperglycemia to an acute presentation. There are several different types of MODY, which result from mutations in the genes that encode glucokinase (an enzyme that phosphorylates glucose in the β-cell) or several transcription factors. These can be diagnosed by molecular diagnostic testing. Although MODY is not a form of type 2 diabetes, the interest in the genetics of MODY is in the hope that insight will be obtained into type 2 diabetes.

Candidate Insulin-Resistance Genes

Numerous mutations of the insulin receptor have been identified.[90] Many patients with these defects have extreme insulin resistance, but these mutations are exceptionally rare and are usually found in only one patient or a single family. Mutations of substrates for the insulin receptor that cause diabetes are not known. Few mutations have been described in other potential candidate genes, including those coding for GLUT4 and glycogen synthase. The sequencing of the human genome has enabled whole-genome screens to identify chromosomal regions linked with type 2 diabetes in families.[3] Genetic variation in the gene encoding calpain-10 appears to increase diabetes susceptibility in selected populations.

Candidate Body Weight Gene

A gene that is expressed only in adipose tissue (*ob*) has been cloned and its protein product, leptin, has been proposed to be a vital signaling factor regulating body weight homeostasis and energy balance.[114] Leptin is synthesized in adipose tissue and binds to specific receptors in the hypothalamus, regulating appetite and energy intake.[93,179] Plasma leptin concentrations are increased in diabetic mice, and both food ingestion and insulin administration increase leptin mRNA in fasted rats. This latter finding suggests that insulin may be an important mediator of the effects of food intake on *ob* expression, thus providing a possible genetic link between obesity and type 2 diabetes. The mouse *diabetes (db)* gene and rat *fatty (fa)* gene, both of which have a diabetes phenotype, have been shown to be identical to the *ob* gene.[60] However, caution should be exercised in interpreting these findings, because extrapolation from animal studies to human disease is often not straightforward and obesity, like diabetes mellitus, is unlikely to have a monogenic basis. Although certain strains of genetically obese mice have leptin deficiency and lose weight when leptin is replaced, most obese humans have increased leptin concentrations.[179]

Other Factors

Amylin (also called *islet amyloid polypeptide* [IAPP]) is a 37–amino-acid peptide, which is stored in the β-cells of the pancreas and is co-secreted with insulin in response to food ingestion.[126,239] It is the major component of the amyloid deposits in the pancreatic islets in more than 90% of patients with type 2 diabetes.[66] Whether amylin deposition contributes to the pathogenesis or is a consequence of type 2 diabetes remains contentious. In addition, the biological effects of amylin are not clearly defined and are controversial. Intravenous infusions of amylin are reported to increase blood lactate and glucose concentrations, decrease glucose uptake, and produce insulin resistance.[94] However, other investigators failed to observe an acute effect of amylin on blood glucose concentrations.[42] In most studies, the metabolic sequelae of amylin occur at supraphysiological concentrations, suggesting that the effects are pharmacological.[263] Excess amylin is believed by some to contribute to insulin resistance and glucose intolerance in type 2 diabetes, but these patients exhibit variable plasma amylin concentrations. Amylin appears to help regulate glucose metabolism by delaying gastric emptying and suppressing glucagon production. Amylin deficiency may occur in insulinopenic type 2 patients and patients with type 1 diabetes. Several trials of amylin analogues, such as pramlintide, are being conducted. At the present time, there is no clinical value in measuring amylin.[241]

BOX 25-3 Criteria for the Diagnosis of Diabetes Mellitus

Diabetes Mellitus

Any one of the following is diagnostic:*

1. Classic symptoms of diabetes and casual† plasma glucose concentration ≥200 mg/dL (11.1 mmol/L)
2. Fasting‡ plasma glucose ≥126 mg/dL (7 mmol/L)
3. 2-hour postload plasma glucose concentration ≥200 mg/dL during the OGTT (11.1 mmol/L)

Impaired Fasting Glucose

Fasting plasma glucose between 110 and 125 mg/dL (6.1 and 7.0 mmol/L)§

Impaired Glucose Tolerance

Two criteria must be met:

1. Fasting plasma glucose <126 mg/dL (7 mmol/L)
2. 2-hour OGTT plasma glucose concentration is between 140 and 199 mg/dL (7.8 and 11.1 mmol/L)

From the American Diabetes Association. Report of the expert committee on the diagnosis and classification of diabetes mellitus. Diabetes Care 1997; 20:1183-1201.

OGTT, Oral glucose tolerance test.

*If positive, confirm by repeat testing on a subsequent day.

†Regardless of the time of the preceding meal.

‡No caloric intake for at least 8 hr.

§In 2003, the ADA recommended a lower limit for the IFG interval of 100 mg/dL (5.6 mmol/L).

Note: Whole-blood glucose concentrations are approximately 10% to 12% lower than plasma concentrations.

New strategies to elucidate the pathogenesis of diabetes have been adopted recently. The expression of integral components of insulin signaling or secretion has been manipulated in transgenic or knockout mice. These approaches have begun to yield some insight.[28] In addition, DNA microarray technology has been applied to identify differences in gene expression patterns in selected tissues between normal, obese, and diabetic mice.[196,301] Similar endeavors are being adopted to discover new proteins as substrates with therapeutic potential. These techniques may identify novel analytes for diagnosis and targets for the development of new therapeutic agents.

DIAGNOSIS

The diagnosis of diabetes mellitus depends solely on the *demonstration of hyperglycemia* (Box 25-3). For type 1 diabetes, the diagnosis is usually easy because hyperglycemia appears abruptly, is severe, and is accompanied by serious metabolic derangements. Diagnosis of type 2 diabetes may be difficult because the hyperglycemia is often not severe enough for the patient to notice symptoms of diabetes. Nevertheless, the risk of complications makes it important to identify people with the disease.

The diagnostic criteria previously recommended were (1) classic symptoms of diabetes with unequivocal increase of plasma glucose, (2) FPG greater than or equal to 140 mg/dL on more than one occasion, or (3) a 2-hour and one other postload glucose concentration greater than or equal to 200 mg/dL during an OGTT.[203] These criteria were widely adopted but are imperfect. The OGTT is more sensitive than fasting glucose early in the course of type 2 diabetes, resulting in a lack of equivalence between the fasting and 2-hour glucose values. Virtually all persons with an FPG concentration greater than or equal to 140 mg/dL have a 2-hour glucose greater than or equal to 200 mg/dL in an OGTT. In contrast, in persons without previously identified diabetes, a fasting glucose greater than or equal to 140 mg/dL is present in only 25% of those who have a 2-hour glucose greater than or equal to 200 mg/dL. To address these and other discrepancies, the diagnostic criteria were revised in 1997 (see Box 25-3).[7,240] The major modification is that the diagnostic threshold for fasting glucose has been lowered from 140 to 126 mg/dL (7 mmol/L) to better identify individuals at risk of retinopathy and nephropathy. The lower cutoff should result in earlier diagnosis of diabetes, with consequent earlier therapeutic intervention.[240]

Fasting Plasma Glucose Concentrations

FPG concentrations exceeding 126 mg/dL (7 mmol/L) on more than one occasion are diagnostic of diabetes mellitus (see Box 25-3). The diagnosis of most cases of diabetes mellitus can be established with this criterion. However, some investigators believe that hyperglycemia may be a relatively late development in the course of type 2 diabetes, delaying the diagnosis and underestimating the prevalence of diabetes mellitus in the population.[271] Complications of diabetes, such as retinopathy, proteinuria, and neuromuscular disease, are present in approximately 30% of patients at clinical diagnosis of type 2 diabetes, and the onset of type 2 diabetes probably occurs at least 4 to 7 years before clinical diagnosis. Screening of high-risk individuals for diabetes is now recommended.[7,112] Fasting glucose should be measured in all asymptomatic people at age 45 (or younger in subjects at increased risk), with follow-up testing every 3 years (see discussion later in this chapter). However, there is no published evidence that treatment based on screening is efficacious.

Oral Glucose Tolerance Test

Serial measurement of plasma glucose before and after a specific amount of glucose given orally should provide a standard method to evaluate individuals and establish values for healthy and diseased subjects. Although more sensitive than FPG determinations, glucose tolerance testing is affected by a large number of factors that result in *poor reproducibility* (Box 25-4).[4] Moreover, approximately 20% of OGTTs fall into the nondiagnostic category (e.g., only one blood sample exhibits increased glucose concentration). Unless results are grossly abnormal initially, *the OGTT should be performed on two separate occasions* before the results are considered abnormal.

BOX 25-4 Factors Other Than Diabetes That May Influence the Oral Glucose Tolerance Test

Patient Preparation
Duration of fast
Prior carbohydrate intake
Medications (e.g., thiazides, oral contraceptives, and corticosteroids)
Trauma
Intercurrent illness
Age
Activity
Weight

Administration of Glucose
Form of glucose (anhydrous or monohydrate)
Quantity of glucose ingested
Volume in which administered
Rate of ingestion

During the Test
Posture
Anxiety
Caffeine
Smoking
Activity
Time of day

The following conditions should be met for performing an OGTT: discontinue, when possible, medications known to affect glucose tolerance; perform in the morning after 3 days of unrestricted diet (containing at least 150 g of carbohydrate per day) and activity; and perform the test after a 10- to 16-hour fast only in ambulatory subjects (bed rest impairs glucose tolerance), who should remain seated during the test without smoking cigarettes. Glucose tolerance testing should not be performed on hospital, acutely ill, or inactive patients. The test should begin between 7 AM and 9 AM. Plasma glucose should be measured fasting, then every 30 minutes for 2 hours after an oral glucose load. For nonpregnant adults, the recommended load is 75 g, which may not be a maximum stimulus[203]; for children, 1.75 g/kg, up to a 75-g maximum is given. The glucose should be dissolved in 300 mL of water, and ingested over 5 minutes. A commercial, more palatable form of glucose may be ingested, but whether the anhydrous or monohydrate form of glucose should be used is still in question.[291]

An OGTT is rarely necessary for the diagnosis of diabetes mellitus and is not recommended by the ADA for routine clinical use. It continues to be recommended in a limited fashion by the WHO[1,241] and its use remains contentious. The sensitivity of FPG concentrations is lower than the OGTT for diagnosing diabetes, and some authors claim that the OGTT better identifies patients at risk for developing complications of diabetes. An FPG value less than 100 mg/dL or a random glucose concentration less than 140 mg/dL is sufficient to rule out the diagnosis of diabetes mellitus. An OGTT is indicated in the following situations:

1. Diagnosis of GDM (discussed later).
2. Diagnosis of IGT. This remains controversial. Individuals with IGT have increased risk of cardiovascular disease, but many of them do not have IFG by ADA criteria.[241]
3. Evaluation of a patient with unexplained nephropathy, neuropathy, or retinopathy, with random glucose concentration less than 140 mg/dL. Abnormal results in this setting do not necessarily denote a cause-and-effect relationship, and other diseases must be ruled out.
4. Population studies for epidemiological data.

Intravenous Glucose Tolerance Test

Poor absorption of orally administered glucose may result in a "flat" tolerance curve. Some patients are unable to tolerate a large oral carbohydrate load or may have altered gastric physiology (e.g., after gastric resection). In these patients, an intravenous glucose tolerance test may be performed to eliminate factors related to the rate of glucose absorption. In addition, measurement of the first-phase insulin response can identify the subgroup of individuals with increased concentrations of multiple autoantibodies who are at greatest risk of progression to type 1 diabetes.[34]

Preparation of patients is the same as for the OGTT. The dose of glucose is 0.5 g/kg of body weight (maximum 35 g), given as a 25-g/dL solution. The dose is administered intravenously over 3 minutes ± 15 seconds, and blood is collected every 10 minutes after the midinjection time for 1 hour. A single forearm vein cannula may be used for infusion and sampling, but it should be flushed with saline after the glucose is infused and dead space should be cleared with several volumes of blood before each sample is drawn. If insulin assays are performed, a specimen is also obtained 5 minutes after the start of the injection. Blood glucose concentrations decrease in an exponential manner, and the rate of glucose disappearance can be calculated from the formula $K = 70/t_{1/2}$, where $t_{1/2}$ is the number of minutes required for the blood glucose value to decrease to one half of the 10-minute value, and K is the rate of disappearance of blood glucose, expressed as percent per minute. The glucose values are plotted on the log scale of semilog paper versus time on the abscissa. The best-fitting straight line is drawn through the points, and the time (in minutes) for the glucose concentration to decrease 50% ($t_{1/2}$) is read. In healthy individuals, K usually exceeds 1.5%; values less than 1.0% are considered diagnostic of diabetes. A poor correlation is found between the results of intravenous and oral glucose tolerance tests.[96] Like oral glucose tolerance, intravenous glucose tolerance deteriorates with age.

In the formula $K = 70/t_{1/2}$, the value of 70 is derived from the logarithmic nature of the decrease in glucose concentration with time. The concentration of glucose at 10 minutes will be twice that of the value obtained from the plot $t_{1/2}$. Using natural logarithms, the rate of decrease in glucose concentration, expressed as percent per minute (K), is given by

$$K = 100(\ln 2 - \ln 1)/t_{1/2} = 69.3/t_{1/2} \cong 70/t_{1/2}$$

The main indication for the intravenous glucose tolerance test is in clinical research to evaluate the first-phase insulin response to glucose (see Figure 25-13).[35] The test is performed as described earlier, but samples are drawn as follows:

Two baseline samples 5 minutes apart (the latter immediately before infusion) and samples 1, 3, 5, and 10 minutes after the end of the glucose infusion. The first-phase insulin release is usually measured by the sum of the insulin concentrations 1 and 3 minutes after the glucose bolus. Alternatively, the 0- to 10-minute incremental insulin area may be used. Like the OGTT, the intravenous glucose tolerance test has poor reproducibility.

Gestational Diabetes Mellitus

Normal pregnancy is associated with increased insulin resistance, especially in the late second and third trimesters. Euglycemia is maintained by increased insulin secretion, with GDM developing in those women who fail to augment insulin sufficiently. Risk factors for GDM include a family history of diabetes in a first-degree relative, obesity, advanced maternal age, glycosuria, and selected adverse outcomes in a previous pregnancy (e.g., stillbirth or macrosomia). The recommendations for screening and diagnosis were formulated in 1984 at the Second International Workshop-Conference on Gestational Diabetes Mellitus[264] and refined at the Third and Fourth International Workshop-Conferences in 1990 and 1998,[187] respectively. Based on the last workshop-conference, the ADA modified their recommendations for laboratory diagnosis of GDM by adopting 5% to 10% lower glucose values.[9] Their guidelines are as follows:

1. Low-risk patients require no testing. Low-risk status is limited to women meeting all of the following:
   - Age less than 25 years
   - Weight normal before pregnancy
   - Member of an ethnic group with a low prevalence of GDM
   - No known diabetes in first-degree relatives
   - No history of abnormal glucose tolerance
   - No history of poor obstetric outcome
2. Average-risk patients (all patients who fall between low and high risk) should be tested at 24 to 28 weeks of gestation (see below for testing strategy).
3. High-risk patients should undergo immediate testing. They are defined as having any of the following:
   - Marked obesity
   - Personal history of GDM
   - Glycosuria
   - Strong family history of diabetes

The first step in laboratory testing is identical to that for diagnosing diabetes in a nonpregnant individual (i.e., an FPG greater than or equal to 126 mg/dL (7 mmol/L) or casual plasma glucose greater than or equal to 200 mg/dL (11.1 mmol/L) (see Box 25-3). However, in the absence of that degree of hyperglycemia, average- and high-risk patients receive a glucose challenge test following one of two methods (Table 25-3):

1. One step: Perform either a 100-g or 75-g OGTT. This one-step approach may be cost-effective in high-risk patients or populations (e.g., some Native-American groups).
   - The 100-g OGTT is the most commonly used standard test supported by outcome data.
   - Alternatively, a 75-g OGTT can be performed, but it is not as well validated as the 100-g test, and cutoffs are arbitrary. In the 75-g test, diagnostic criteria for plasma glucose concentrations are the same as for the 100-g test, except that there is no 3-hour measurement (Table 25-3).
2. Two step (Table 25-3): The first step is a 50-g oral glucose load (the patient does not need to be fasting), followed by a plasma glucose determination at 1 hour. A plasma glucose value greater than or equal to 140 mg/dL (7.7 mmol/L) indicates the necessity for definitive testing. Approximately 15% of patients have a 1-hour venous plasma glucose concentration of 140 mg/dL (7.7 mmol/L)

TABLE 25-3 Screening and Diagnosis of Gestational Diabetes Mellitus

Screening

1. Perform between 24 and 28 wk of gestation on all average- and high-risk pregnant women not identified as having glucose intolerance.
2. Give 50 g oral glucose load without regard to time of day or time of last meal.
3. Measure venous plasma glucose at 1 hr.
4. If glucose is ≥140 mg/dL,* perform glucose tolerance test.

Diagnosis

1. Perform in the morning after a 8–14-hr fast.
2. Measure fasting venous plasma glucose.
3. Give 75 or 100 g of glucose orally.
4. Measure plasma glucose hourly for 3 hr (or 2 hr if 75 g of glucose given)
5. At least two values must meet or exceed the following:

	100-g load	75-g load
Fasting	95 mg/dL	95 mg/dL
1 hr	180 mg/dL	180 mg/dL
2 hr	155 mg/dL	155 mg/dL
3 hr	140 mg/dL	—

6. If results are normal in a clinically suspect situation, repeat during the third trimester.

*Some experts recommend a cutoff of 130 mg/dL.

or greater and require a full diagnostic glucose tolerance test. That subgroup includes ~80% of all women with GDM. Some experts have recommended a value of greater than or equal to 130 mg/dL. This cutoff will increase the sensitivity for GDM to greater than 90%, but will include ~25% of all pregnant women. The second and definitive test is one of the two OGTTs described above.

The criteria for diagnosis are different from those for nonpregnant patients (see Table 25-3).[214] There remains a lack of consensus regarding the use of the 100-g versus 75-g OGTT for the definitive diagnosis of GDM. Although the 75-g OGTT appears practical and acceptable, there are more data with the 100-g OGTT. Moreover, appropriate diagnostic thresholds remain in dispute.[187]

Although usually asymptomatic and not life threatening to the mother, GDM is associated with an increased incidence of neonatal mortality and morbidity, including hypocalcemia, hypoglycemia, and macrosomia.[157,187] The maternal hyperglycemia causes the fetus to secrete more insulin, resulting in stimulation of fetal growth and macrosomia. Recognition is important because therapy can reduce the perinatal morbidity and mortality.[201] Maternal complications include a high rate of cesarean delivery and hypertension. In addition, mothers with GDM are at a significantly increased risk of subsequent diabetes, predominantly type 2. The cumulative incidence of type 2 diabetes varies among populations, ranging from ~40% to 70%.[152] It rises markedly in the first 5 years and reaches a plateau after 10 years.

Distinct from GDM is pregnancy in a patient with preexisting diabetes (~19,000 per annum in the United States). This is associated with an increased incidence of congenital malformations, but meticulous glycemic control during the first 8 weeks of pregnancy can significantly decrease the risk of congenital malformations.[155] Tight control results in an increased incidence of maternal hypoglycemia, which is teratogenic in animals but does not cause malformations in humans.[189]

Women with GDM should be evaluated at the first postpartum visit (at least 6 weeks after delivery) for diabetes by standard criteria (see Box 25-3). If glucose values are normal, glycemia should be reassessed at least every 3 years.

Chronic Complications of Diabetes Mellitus

Pathogenesis

Patients with both type 1 and type 2 diabetes are at high risk for the development of chronic complications.[43,200] Diabetes-specific microvascular pathology in the retina, renal glomerulus, and peripheral nerve produces retinopathy, nephropathy, and neuropathy. As a result of these microvascular complications, diabetes is the most frequent cause of new cases of blindness in the industrialized world in persons between 25 and 74 years and the leading cause of end-stage renal disease.[15] Diabetes is also associated with a marked increase in atherosclerotic macrovascular disease involving cardiac, cerebral, and peripheral large vessels. The consequence is that patients with diabetes have a high rate of myocardial infarction (the major cause of mortality in diabetes), stroke, and limb amputation. Prospective clinical studies document a strong relationship between hyperglycemia and the development of microvascular complications.[72,280] Both hyperglycemia and insulin resistance appear to be important in the pathogenesis of macrovascular complications.[43,105,280]

Progress has been made in our understanding of the molecular mechanisms underlying the derangements produced by hyperglycemia.[43,258] Four main hypotheses have been proposed to explain how hyperglycemia causes the neural and vascular pathology. These are: increased aldose reductase (or polyol pathway) flux; enhanced formation of advanced glycation end products (AGE); activation of protein kinase C; and increased hexosamine pathway flux. Inhibitors of each of these have been shown to ameliorate diabetes-induced abnormalities in cell culture and animal models.[43] The overproduction of superoxide by the mitochondrial electron transport chain integrates these four apparently disparate mechanisms. Clinical trials are underway using novel therapies specifically directed at the signaling molecules (such as protein kinase C) or employing antioxidants to neutralize the effects of the oxidants.

Effect of Intensive Therapy

Type 1 Diabetes

Although it had been theorized for many years that better glycemic control would decrease rates of long-term complications of diabetes mellitus, it was not until the publication of the Diabetes Control and Complications Trial (DCCT) in 1993[72] that this hypothesis was verified. The DCCT was a multicenter, randomized trial that compared the effects of intensive and conventional insulin therapy on the development and progression of complications in 1441 patients with type 1 diabetes. During the study period, which averaged 6.5 years, intensively managed patients maintained significantly lower mean blood glucose concentrations. Compared with conventional therapy, intensive therapy reduced the risk of retinopathy, nephropathy, and neuropathy by 40% to 75%.[72] Intensive therapy delayed the onset and slowed the progression of these three complications, regardless of age, gender, or duration of diabetes. The absolute risks of retinopathy and nephropathy were proportional to the mean glycated hemoglobin (GHb) (discussed later in the chapter). Although intensive therapy also reduced the development of hypercholesterolemia, major cardiovascular and peripheral vascular disease were not significantly decreased. This landmark study has had a significant impact on therapeutic goals and comprehension of the pathogenesis of complications of diabetes.

At the conclusion of the DCCT, 95% of the participants enrolled in the long-term follow-up study, termed the Epidemiology of Diabetes Interventions and Complications (EDIC). Five years after the end of the DCCT, there was no difference in metabolic control (assessed by GHb measurements) between the former conventional and intensively treated groups. Nevertheless, the further progression of retinopathy was ~70% lower in the former intensive group, demonstrating that the beneficial effects of intensive treatment persisted for at least several years beyond the period of strictest intervention.[74]

Type 2 Diabetes

The role of hyperglycemia in the development of complications in individuals with type 2 diabetes was established in the United Kingdom Prospective Diabetes Study (UKPDS).[280] The UKPDS was a major randomized, multicenter clinical study that included 5102 patients with newly diagnosed type 2 diabetes who were followed for an average of 10 years. Analogous to the findings of the DCCT, the UKPDS demonstrated in patients with type 2 diabetes that intensive treatment diminishes by ~10% to 40% the development of microvascular complications.[280] Although intensive treatment decreased the rate of occurrence of macrovascular complications, the reduction was not statistically significant. An important caveat of both the DCCT and UKPDS was that intensive therapy produced a threefold increase in the incidence of severe hypoglycemia.[72,280]

Role of the Clinical Laboratory in Diabetes Mellitus

The clinical laboratory has a vital role in both the diagnosis and management of diabetes mellitus. Some of the important parameters assayed are outlined in Table 25-4. In 2002 the National Academy of Clinical Biochemistry (referred to as the NACB) published evidence-based guidelines for laboratory analysis in diabetes mellitus.[241] The guidelines were reviewed by the Professional Practice Committee of the ADA and were consistent in those areas where the ADA also published recommendations. Specific recommendations for laboratory testing based on published data or derived from expert consensus are presented.[241] A brief overview is presented here.

Diagnosis

Preclinical (Screening)

Type 1 Diabetes. Evidence from animal studies suggests that immune intervention therapy before the appearance of clinical symptoms can delay or prevent type 1 diabetes. Several large clinical trials are underway to assess a variety of therapeutic strategies designed to delay or prevent the

TABLE 25-4 Role of the Laboratory in Diabetes Mellitus

Diagnosis	
Preclinical (Screening)	**Clinical**

Immunological markers
  ICA
  IAA
  GAD antibodies
  Protein tyrosine phosphatase antibodies (IA-2)
Genetic markers (e.g., HLA)
Insulin secretion
  Fasting
  Pulses
  In response to a glucose challenge
Blood glucose
	Blood glucose
	OGTT
	Ketones (urine and blood)
	Other (e.g., insulin, C-peptide, and stimulation tests)

Management	
Acute	**Chronic**

Glucose
  Blood
  Urine
Ketones
  Blood
  Urine
Acid-base status (pH, bicarbonate)
Lactate
Other abnormalities related to cellular dehydration or therapy (e.g., potassium, sodium, phosphate, and osmolality)
	Glucose
	  Blood (fasting-random)
	  Urine
	Glycated proteins
	  GHb
	  Fructosamine
	Urinary protein
	  UAE ("microalbuminuria")
	  Proteinuria
	Evaluation of complications (e.g., creatinine, cholesterol, and triglycerides)
	Evaluation of pancreas transplant (C-peptide, insulin)

onset of type 1 diabetes.[118] The Diabetes Prevention Trial-Type 1 (DPT-1) screened 84,228 relatives of patients with diabetes for islet cell antibodies.[80] Half of the 339 individuals deemed to be at high (greater than 50%) risk for disease were randomly assigned to low-dose insulin therapy. Unfortunately, insulin injections failed to delay the development of type 1 diabetes.[80] Results of the oral arm of the trial have not been reported yet. Despite the negative results, the ADA encourages screening of first-degree relatives of patients with type 1 diabetes by measuring immune-related markers (autoantibodies), provided that individuals who have positive screening results are referred to defined research studies,[13] several of which are underway.[241] Until effective intervention therapy becomes available and cost-effective screening strategies are developed for young children, screening for antibodies is not recommended.[241] Some experts have proposed that testing for islet cell autoantibodies may be useful in the following situations: (1) to identify a subset of adults initially thought to have type 2 diabetes but who have islet cell autoantibody markers of type 1 diabetes and progress to insulin dependency; (2) to screen nondiabetic family members who wish to donate a kidney or part of their pancreas for transplantation; (3) to screen women with GDM to identify those at high risk of progression to type 1 diabetes; and (4) to distinguish type 1 from type 2 diabetes in children to institute insulin therapy at the time of diagnosis.[241] There is wide variability in clinical practice regarding the use of islet-cell autoantibodies. Proponents argue that the results of autoantibody assays are clinically useful, whereas others point to a lack of evidence. Although some clinicians, particularly those who treat pediatric patients, use autoantibody assays, clinical studies are necessary to provide outcome data to validate the clinical use of autoantibody assays.

Screening by determining HLA type is not currently warranted, except in research studies.[241] A decrease in glucose-stimulated insulin secretion is the first functional abnormality in both type 1 and type 2 diabetes. Nevertheless, tests of insulin secretion are not currently recommended for routine clinical use.

Type 2 Diabetes. Screening of asymptomatic individuals for type 2 diabetes has been the subject of much controversy.[112] The ADA, which previously did not support screening, now advocates screening in all asymptomatic individuals over the age of 45 years.[14,86] Screening should be performed, particularly in overweight individuals, by FPG in a healthcare setting. If results are less than 110 mg/dL (6.1 mmol/L), testing should be repeated at 3-year intervals.[241] Testing may be considered at a younger age or be carried out more frequently in individuals at increased risk of diabetes (e.g., family history or a member of certain ethnic groups).[14] The rising incidence of type 2 diabetes in adolescents has led to the recommendation for screening overweight youths with any two of the following risk factors: (1) they have a family history of type 2 diabetes in first- and second-degree relatives; (2) they belong to a certain race and/or ethnic group; or (3) they have signs of insulin resistance.[14,241] Testing should be done every 2 years starting at 10 years of age. Rationales for screening are that at least 33% of individuals with type 2 diabetes are undiagnosed, complications are often present by the time of diagnosis, and treatment delays the onset of complications.[112] Notwithstanding these recommendations, there is no evidence that treatment based on screening has value.

Clinical

The laboratory diagnosis of diabetes is made exclusively by the demonstration of hyperglycemia. Other assays, such as the OGTT, contribute to the classification and characterization. Although other tests (e.g., C-peptide and insulin analysis) have been proposed to assist in the diagnosis and classification of the disease, these do not at present have a role outside of research studies.[241]

Management

Acute

In diabetic ketoacidosis, hyperosmolar nonketotic coma, and hypoglycemia, the clinical laboratory has an essential role in both diagnosis and monitoring of therapy. Several analytes are frequently measured to guide clinicians in treatment regimens to restore euglycemia and correct other metabolic disturbances. The metabolic abnormalities of these conditions are beyond the scope of this book, and interested readers are referred to a standard textbook of medicine. The NACB guidelines also provide information on the tests that are used.

Chronic

The DCCT[72] and UKPDS[280] studies documented a correlation between blood glucose concentrations and the development of long-term complications of diabetes. Measurement of glucose and glycated proteins provides an index of short- and long-term glycemic control, respectively (see section on glycated proteins later in the chapter). The detection and monitoring of complications are achieved by assaying urea, creatinine, urinary albumin excretion, and serum lipids. The success of newer therapies, such as islet cell or pancreas transplantation, can be monitored by measuring serum C-peptide or insulin concentrations.

HYPOGLYCEMIA

Hypoglycemia is a blood glucose concentration below the fasting value, but it is difficult to define a specific limit.[255] The most widely suggested cutoff is 50 mg/dL, but some authors suggest 60 mg/dL.[45] A transient decline may occur 1.5 to 2 hours after a meal, and it is not uncommon for a plasma glucose concentration as low as 40 mg/dL to be observed 2 hours after ingestion of an oral glucose load. Similarly, extremely low fasting blood glucose values may occasionally be noted without symptoms or evidence of underlying disease.

Symptoms of hypoglycemia vary among individuals and none is specific. Epinephrine produces the classic signs and symptoms of hypoglycemia, namely trembling, sweating, nausea, rapid pulse, lightheadedness, hunger, and epigastric discomfort. These autonomic (neurogenic) symptoms are nonspecific and may also be noted in other conditions, such as hyperthyroidism, pheochromocytoma, or even anxiety. Although controversial, it has been proposed that a rapid decrease in blood glucose may trigger the symptoms even though the blood glucose itself may not reach hypoglycemic values, whereas gradual onset of hypoglycemia may not produce symptoms.[78]

The brain cannot store or produce glucose and in resting adults the central nervous system (CNS) consumes approximately 50% of the glucose used by the body.[100] Very low concentrations of plasma glucose (less than 20 or 30 mg/dL) cause severe CNS dysfunction. During prolonged fasting or hypoglycemia, ketones may be used as an energy source. The broad spectrum of symptoms and signs of CNS dysfunction ranges from headache, confusion, blurred vision, and dizziness to seizures, loss of consciousness, and even death; these symptoms are known as *neuroglycopenia.* Restoration of plasma glucose usually produces a prompt recovery, but *irreversible damage may occur.*

The age of onset of hypoglycemia is a convenient way to classify the disorder (Box 25-5), but it should be borne in mind that some overlap occurs among the various groups. For example, some glycogen storage disorders may present in the third decade of life, and hormone deficiencies occur in childhood.

BOX 25-5 Causes of Hypoglycemia

Neonates
Small for gestational age-prematurity
Respiratory distress syndrome
Maternal diabetes mellitus
Toxemia of pregnancy
Other (e.g., cold stress, polycythemia)

Infants
Ketotic hypoglycemia
Congenital enzyme defects
Glycogen storage disease
Deficiency of gluconeogenic enzymes
Galactosemia
Hereditary fructose intolerance
Leucine hypersensitivity
Endogenous hyperinsulinism
Reye's syndrome
Idiopathic

Adults
Medications (insulin, oral hypoglycemic agents)
Toxins (alcohol, hypoglycins)
Severe hepatic dysfunction
Deficiency of hormones (e.g., glucocorticoids, growth hormone)
Insulin-producing pancreatic tumors (insulinoma)
Insulin antibodies
Nonpancreatic neoplasms
Septicemia
Chronic renal failure
Reactive

Hypoglycemia in Neonates and Infants

Neonatal blood glucose concentrations are much lower than adult (mean ≈35 mg/dL) and decline shortly after birth when liver glycogen stores are depleted. Glucose concentrations as low as 30 mg/dL in a term infant and 20 mg/dL in a premature infant may occur without clinical evidence of hypoglycemia. The more common causes of hypoglycemia in the neonatal period include prematurity, maternal diabetes, GDM, and maternal eclampsia (see Box 25-5; for review, see Haymond).[119] These are usually transient. Hypoglycemia with onset in early infancy is usually less transitory and may be due to inborn errors of metabolism or ketotic hypoglycemia, and usually develops after fasting or a febrile illness.

Fasting Hypoglycemia in Adults

Hypoglycemia may result from a *decreased* rate of hepatic glucose production or an increased rate of glucose use. Symptoms suggestive of hypoglycemia are fairly common, but hypoglycemic disorders are rare. However, true hypoglycemia usually indicates serious underlying disease and may be life threatening. A precise threshold for establishing hypoglycemia is not always possible, and values as low as 30 mg/dL may be encountered in healthy premenopausal women after a 72-hour fast.[186] Symptoms usually begin at plasma glucose concentrations below 55 mg/dL, and impairment of cerebral function begins when glucose is less than 50 mg/dL.

The *classic diagnostic test is the 72-hour fast,* which should be conducted in a hospital.[255] During the fast, the patient should be allowed a liberal intake of calorie-free and caffeine-free fluids. All nonessential medications should be discontinued and patients should be active when awake. Samples should be drawn for analysis of plasma glucose, insulin, C-peptide, and proinsulin every 6 hours. When plasma glucose concentration is less than or equal to 60 mg/dL, analysis should be performed every 1 to 2 hours. The fast should be concluded when plasma glucose concentration falls to less than or equal to 45 mg/dL and the patient exhibits signs or symptoms of hypoglycemia. If this does not occur, the fast should be terminated after 72 hours. At the conclusion of the fast, draw blood for glucose, insulin, C-peptide, proinsulin, β-hydroxybutyrate, and sulfonylurea analysis. Then inject 1 mg of glucagon intravenously and measure plasma glucose concentration at 10, 20, and 30 minutes. This concludes the protocol and the patient can be fed. When a deficiency is suspected, plasma cortisol, growth hormone, or glucagon should be measured at the beginning and end of the fast. A gender difference is observed in plasma glucose concentrations during prolonged fasting, with women exhibiting significantly lower concentrations than men. Low plasma glucose alone is not sufficient to establish the diagnosis, and the absence of signs or symptoms of hypoglycemia during the fast excludes the diagnosis of a hypoglycemic disorder.

More than 100 causes of hypoglycemia have been reported. Some of the more common conditions to be considered are listed in Box 25-5. Drugs are the most prevalent cause,[254] and a wide variety, including propranolol, salicylates, and disopyramide, can produce hypoglycemia. Oral hypoglycemic agents, which have a long half-life (35 hours for chlorpropamide), are the most frequent cause of drug-induced hypoglycemia. Sulfonylureas stimulate secretion of insulin, proinsulin, and C-peptide, and may mimic an insulinoma. Differentiation is made by demonstrating the drug in blood or urine. Surreptitious administration of insulin can be detected by finding low C-peptide concentrations with increased insulin concentrations.

Ethanol produces hypoglycemia by inhibiting gluconeogenesis, and this is aggravated by malnutrition (low glycogen stores) in patients with chronic alcoholism. The decreased glucose production in *hepatic failure* (e.g., viral hepatitis, toxins) caused by impaired gluconeogenesis or glycogen storage may result in hypoglycemia. Because this requires dysfunction of more than 80% of the liver, evidence of liver disease is invariably present. Deficiency of *growth hormone* (especially with coexistent ACTH deficiency), glucocorticoids, thyroid hormone, or glucagon may also produce hypoglycemia. Although a deficiency of glucocorticoids (e.g., Addison's disease) is most consistently associated with hypoglycemia, most glucocorticoid-deficient adults are not hypoglycemic. Hormonal deficiency causes hypoglycemia in children more frequently than in adults.

Demonstration of a low plasma glucose concentration in the presence of an abnormally high plasma insulin value is highly suggestive of an insulin-producing *pancreatic islet cell tumor.*[89] Because insulin concentrations exhibit a wide range in normal people, absolute hyperinsulinemia occurs in fewer than 50% of patients with insulinomas. Serum insulin concentrations inappropriately high for concurrent plasma glucose have been proposed to increase diagnostic accuracy. A plasma glucose concentration less than 30 mg/dL with a plasma insulin concentration exceeding 15 μIU/mL, insulin/glucose ratio greater than 0.3, or amended insulin/glucose ratio may be used. However, these ratios have unacceptably low sensitivity. C-peptide concentrations greater than or equal to 0.2 nmol/L at the end of a fast when plasma glucose was less than or equal to 50 mg/dL correctly identified all insulinoma patients. Provocative tests (glucagons,[163] tolbutamide,[256] calcium,[145] or suppression tests [infusion of insulin and measuring C-peptide]), although strongly recommended in the past, are generally not necessary. Intraarterial calcium stimulation with right hepatic vein sampling for insulin gradients appears to be a sensitive preoperative test for localizing insulinoma.[82]

Spontaneous production of *antibodies to insulin* may produce hypoglycemia (these antibodies are distinct from those elicited by insulin therapy and the antibodies detected in certain patients with type 1 diabetes). Antiinsulin antibodies causing hypoglycemia have been reported in Graves' disease, multiple myeloma, systemic lupus erythematosus, and rheumatoid arthritis. Patients exhibit postprandial hyperglycemia and fasting hypoglycemia. Laboratory analysis demonstrates low plasma C-peptide and high plasma insulin concentrations. It is important to test for antibodies to insulin because these may interfere with insulin immunoassays.

Nonpancreatic neoplasms that cause hypoglycemia are often extremely large mesenchymal neoplasms that appear to overuse glucose but may also have an inhibitory effect on glucose mobilization. Tumors of epithelial origin may cause hypoglycemia, frequently by producing IGF II.[70,257]

Hypoglycemia caused by *septicemia* should be relatively easy to diagnose.[188] The mechanism is not well defined, but depleted glycogen stores, impaired gluconeogenesis, and increased peripheral use of glucose may all be contributing factors. Glucose tolerance is commonly depressed in renal disease, and hypoglycemia may occur in end-stage *renal failure.*

Some of the conditions producing fasting hypoglycemia are readily apparent, but others require a lengthy diagnostic workup. Once hypoglycemia is demonstrated, specific tests should be performed to establish the underlying cause. The *OGTT is not an appropriate study for evaluating a patient suspected of having hypoglycemia.*

Postprandial Hypoglycemia

A group of disorders may produce hypoglycemia in the postprandial (fed) state.[124] These include drugs, antibodies to insulin or the insulin receptor, and inborn errors (e.g., fructose-1,6-diphosphatase deficiency). Also included is *reactive hypoglycemia* (also referred to as functional hypoglycemia), which has been the subject of much debate.[45] Many commentaries and editorials have been published regarding the existence of reactive hypoglycemia (Hofeldt[124] and references listed therein). The general consensus is that there is no scientific evidence that supports the existence of "functional hypoglycemia." It has been proposed that for individuals with vague symptoms after food ingestion the preferred terminology should be *idiopathic reactive hypoglycemia*[124] or *idiopathic postprandial syndrome.*[255]

At the Third International Symposium on Hypoglycemia,[169] reactive hypoglycemia was defined as a *clinical disorder in which the patient has postprandial symptoms suggesting hypoglycemia that occur in everyday life and are accompanied by a blood glucose concentration less than 45 to 50 mg/dL as determined by a specific glucose measurement on arterialized venous or capillary blood, respectively.* Patients complain of autonomic symptoms occurring approximately 1 to 3 hours after eating and seem to obtain relief, lasting 30 to 45 minutes, by food intake. These symptoms are rarely due to low blood glucose concentrations (e.g., diabetes mellitus, gastrointestinal dysfunction, or hormonal deficiency states). Most of these individuals have postprandial autonomic symptoms without neuroglycopenia in the postprandial state. Some experts in the field state that there are no true hypoglycemic disorders characterized solely by autonomic symptoms.[255] A 5- or 6-hour glucose tolerance test was the standard procedure to establish the presence of postprandial hypoglycemia, but has been discredited.[45] The test is not reproducible in any particular individual, and low values for plasma glucose may be noted in the absence of symptoms, whereas symptoms may occur with normal glucose concentrations.[56] In addition, patients who have low blood glucose concentrations with autonomic symptoms 3 or 4 hours after an oral glucose load may have identical symptoms with normal blood glucose values after a mixed meal.[56] This may be partly due to anxiety provoked by the stressful environment during the glucose tolerance test. Demonstration of increased plasma epinephrine concentrations at the glucose nadir during an OGTT was reported to differentiate patients with reactive hypoglycemia,[53] but the patients studied were identified on the basis of autonomic symptoms and signs, and only 25% demonstrated hypoglycemia. The *OGTT should not be used in the diagnosis of reactive hypoglycemia.*

Postprandial hypoglycemia is infrequent and the demonstration of hypoglycemia during spontaneously occurring symptomatic episodes is necessary to establish the diagnosis.[215] If this is not possible, a 5-hour meal tolerance test[56] (which simulates the composition of a normal diet) or a "hyperglucidic" (high glucose) breakfast test[45] has been proposed.

A diagnosis of hypoglycemia has also been used to explain a wide variety of disorders that appear unrelated to blood glucose abnormalities.[51] These nonspecific symptoms include fatigue, muscle spasms, palpitations, numbness, tingling, pain, sweating, mental dullness, sleepiness, weakness, and fainting. Behavior abnormalities, poor school performance, and delinquency have been incorrectly attributed to low blood glucose concentrations. The widespread use of the insensitive and nonspecific 5-hour glucose tolerance test caused overdiagnosis of hypoglycemia and led the ADA to publish a statement to discourage the inappropriate use of the OGTT for the diagnosis of hypoglycemia.[261] Lay publications[273] have supported this recommendation, but it is still important for the medical community to reassure such patients that low blood glucose is not the cause of their symptoms and to deal with specific abnormalities that might underlie patients' complaints or problems. A diagnosis of hypoglycemia should not be made unless a patient meets the criteria of *Whipple's triad of low blood glucose concentration with typical symptoms alleviated by glucose administration.* Demonstration of a normal plasma glucose concentration when the subject exhibits symptoms excludes the possibility of a hypoglycemic disorder.

Hypoglycemia in Diabetes Mellitus

Hypoglycemia occurs frequently in both type 1 diabetes and type 2 diabetes.[68,99] Patients using insulin experience approximately one to two episodes of symptomatic hypoglycemia per week, and severe hypoglycemia (i.e., requiring assistance from others or associated with loss of consciousness) affects about 10% of this population per year. In patients practicing intensive insulin therapy (e.g., multiple injections or continuous subcutaneous insulin infusion), these figures are increased twofold to sixfold. The chief adverse event associated with intensive therapy in the DCCT was a threefold increase in the incidence of severe hypoglycemia.[72] Similarly, hypoglycemia occurs in patients with type 2 diabetes (caused by oral hypoglycemic agents or insulin), but is less frequent than in type 1 diabetes. Two pathophysiological mechanisms contribute to hypoglycemia in patients with diabetes.

Defective Glucose Counterregulation

Counterregulatory responses become impaired in type 1 diabetes patients,[68] increasing the risk of hypoglycemia. The response of glucagon to hypoglycemia is impaired by an unknown mechanism early in the course of type 1 diabetes. Epinephrine secretory response to hypoglycemia becomes deficient later in the course of the disease. These defects are selective because other stimuli continue to elicit glucagon and epinephrine secretion. Glucose counterregulation does not appear to be notably defective in patients with type 2 diabetes.

Hypoglycemia Unawareness

Up to 50% of patients with long-standing (more than 30 years) type 1 diabetes do not experience neurogenic warning symptoms and are prone to more severe hypoglycemia. The mechanism is thought to be associated with a decreased epinephrine response to hypoglycemia. Intensively treated patients with type 1 diabetes require lower plasma glucose concentrations to elicit symptoms of hypoglycemia. Some authors have claimed that human insulin results in an increased incidence of hypoglycemia unawareness, but analysis of 45 studies revealed no significant differences in hypoglycemic episodes between insulin species.[234]

Tolbutamide Tolerance Test

Tolbutamide, 1-butyl-3-(*p*-tolylsulfonyl)urea *(Orinase)*, stimulates the normal pancreas to produce insulin. The response of the pancreas to intravenous tolbutamide can be used in the investigation of fasting hypoglycemia. Blood specimens are obtained for glucose and insulin before intravenous injection of 1 g of a water-soluble form of tolbutamide and at 2, 15, 30, 60, 90, and 120 minutes afterward. Normal people have a decrease in plasma glucose concentration to about 50% of the fasting value by 30 minutes, with a return to baseline at 120 minutes. Patients with fasting hypoglycemia exhibit a lower glucose nadir, with hypoglycemia persisting up to 2 hours. The insulin response

TABLE 25-5 Methods of Glucose Analysis in 5409 Laboratories*

Method	Number†	Percent of Total	Mean (mg/dL)	CV (%)
Hexokinase				
Photometric (visible)	207	4	155.1	2.8
Photometric (ultraviolet)	2668	49	154.2	2.4
Glucose Oxidase				
Photometric	1351	25		
Automated (1327)†			154.4	2.6
Manual (24)			158.3	4.5
Oxygen electrode	1148	21	157.5	2.2
Glucose Dehydrogenase	35	1	154.17	2.5

CV, Coefficient of variation for all results by all methods of the indicated method-type from all manufacturers. It may include a component of variation attributable to differences in calibrators and to matrix effects.
*Results are based on 2003 CAP Survey, Set C-A, Specimen C-11 (Copyright, 2003 College of American Pathologists; data used with permission). See text for discussion of methods.
†"Number" and numbers in parentheses indicate how many laboratories use the indicated method-type.

provides further diagnostic information. The peak insulin concentration at 2 minutes is normally less than 150 μIU/mL. This value is increased in patients with islet cell tumors, and the elevated insulin concentration at 60 minutes is reported to be the most reliable discriminator.[36] In various conditions—such as liver disease, malnutrition, or renal insufficiency—plasma glucose responses to tolbutamide are indistinguishable from those seen with islet cell tumors, *but only patients with insulinoma exhibit exaggerated plasma insulin concentrations.*

The test has also been proposed for the diagnosis of diabetes mellitus. If the blood glucose concentration at 20 minutes is between 80% and 84% of the fasting value, the patient is said to have a 50% probability of having diabetes. In some severe cases, the response is even less because the pancreas is unable to secrete adequate amounts of insulin. However, *this test has no role in the diagnosis of diabetes.* Patients must be carefully observed for hypoglycemic reactions, and the test terminated, if necessary, by intravenous administration of glucose. This test is potentially dangerous and should not be performed in people with moderate or severe fasting hypoglycemia. The tolbutamide test should not be administered if the plasma glucose concentration is less than 60 mg/dL immediately before the test.

DETERMINATION OF GLUCOSE IN BODY FLUIDS

Many analytical procedures are used to measure blood glucose concentrations. In the past, analyses were often performed with relatively nonspecific methods that resulted in falsely increased values. Almost all commonly used techniques are now enzymatic (e.g., hexokinase or glucose oxidase), and older methods, such as photometric or oxidation-reduction techniques, are rarely used. The glucose assays most widely used in the United States may be determined by inspecting quality control surveys conducted by the College of American Pathologists (CAP). Results from 5409 laboratories reported in a survey conducted in 2003 are displayed in Table 25-5. These data show that automated hexokinase methods are used in half of the participating laboratories. The extensive use of the hexokinase method is a reflection of the procedures adopted by the manufacturers of automated equipment. Glucose oxidase is the only other method that is widely used. The most significant change in the past 20 years is the disappearance of the *o*-toluidine method, which was used in the SMA 12/60 Autoanalyzer. It must be emphasized that these data apply only to this CAP survey and are weighted to laboratories participating either on a voluntary basis or in compliance with state regulatory agencies. Many kits are commercially available for measuring glucose and are widely used, especially in smaller laboratories. Furthermore, testing performed in physicians' offices is not included. Reference to CAP surveys demonstrates that all the methods exhibit a CV less than 5% for glucose values on lyophilized serum, with automated methods having CVs less than or equal to 2.6%.

Methods for the determination of glucose in blood have been reviewed,[48] and 10 glucose methods have been evaluated and compared with a generally accepted hexokinase reference method.[217]

Specimen Collection and Storage

In individuals with a normal hematocrit, fasting whole-blood glucose concentration is approximately 10% to 12% lower than plasma glucose. Although the glucose concentrations in the water phase of red blood cells and plasma are similar (the erythrocyte plasma membrane is freely permeable to glucose), the water content of plasma (93%) is approximately 11% higher than that of whole blood. In most clinical laboratories, plasma or serum is used for most glucose determinations; methods for self-monitoring of glucose use whole blood samples but may measure the glucose concentration in the plasma phase. During fasting, capillary blood glucose concentration is only 2 to 5 mg/dL higher than that of venous blood. After a glucose load, however, capillary blood glucose concentrations are 20 to 70 mg/dL ([mean ~ 30 mg/dL], equivalent to 20% to 25%) higher than concurrently drawn venous blood samples.[166]

Glycolysis decreases serum glucose by approximately 5% to 7% in 1 hour (5 to 10 mg/dL) in normal uncentrifuged coagulated blood at room temperature.[54,287] The rate of in vitro glycolysis is higher in the presence of leukocytosis or bacterial contamination. Other workers have observed a decrease of only 1.9 mg/dL/hr when blood was drawn into sterile Vacutainer-brand tubes.[247] This negligible decrease can be attributed in part to prevention of bacterial contamination and to lower ambient temperatures. In separated, nonhemolyzed sterile serum, the glucose concentration is generally stable as long as 8 hours at 25 °C and up to 72 hours at 4 °C; variable stability is observed with longer storage periods.[40] Plasma, removed from the cells after moderate centrifugation, contains leukocytes that also metabolize glucose—although cell-free sterile plasma has no glycolytic activity.

Glycolysis can be inhibited and glucose stabilized for as long as 3 days at room temperature by adding sodium fluoride (NaF), or less commonly, sodium iodoacetate to the specimen.[78] Fluoride ions prevent glycolysis by inhibiting enolase, an enzyme that requires Mg^{2+}. The inhibition is due to the formation of an ionic complex consisting of Mg^{2+}, inorganic phosphate, and fluoride ions; this complex interferes with the interaction of enzyme and substrate. Fluoride is also a weak anticoagulant because it binds calcium; however, clotting may occur after several hours, and it is therefore advisable to use a *combined fluoride-oxalate mixture,* such as 2 mg of potassium oxalate ($K_2C_2O_4$) and 2 mg of NaF/mL of blood, to prevent late clotting. Other anticoagulants (e.g., EDTA, citrate, or heparin) can also be used. Fluoride ions in high concentration inhibit the activity of urease and certain other enzymes; consequently the specimens are unsuitable for determination of urea in procedures that require urease and for direct assay of some serum enzymes. $K_2C_2O_4$ causes a loss of cell water, thereby diluting the plasma. Samples collected in these tubes should therefore not be used for measurement of other analytes. Although fluoride maintains long-term blood glucose stability, the rate of decline in the first hour after sample collection is not altered.[54] It is probably not necessary in routine analysis to use a fluoride-containing tube if plasma is separated from cells or if glucose is measured within 60 minutes of blood collection. However, inhibitors of glycolysis are necessary in patients with greatly increased leukocyte counts because differences of up to 65 mg/dL have been observed between glucose values with and without glycolytic inhibitors after 1 to 2 hours of contact with the blood cells.

Cerebrospinal fluid (CSF) may be contaminated with bacteria or other cells and should be analyzed for glucose immediately. If a delay in measurement is unavoidable, the sample should be centrifuged and stored at 4 °C or −20 °C.

In 24-hour collections of urine, glucose may be preserved by adding 5 mL of glacial acetic acid to the container before starting the collection. The final pH of the urine is usually between 4 and 5, which inhibits bacterial activity. Other preservatives that have been proposed include 5 g of sodium benzoate per 24-hour specimen or chlorhexidine and 0.1% sodium nitrate (NaN_3) with 0.01% benzethonium chloride. These may be inadequate, and urine should be stored at 4 °C during collection. Urine samples may lose as much as 40% of their glucose after 24 hours at room temperature.[173]

Methods

Hexokinase and glucose oxidase are the two main types of methods used to measure glucose in body fluids. Other methods are found on the Evolve site that accompanies this book.

Hexokinase Methods

Glucose is phosphorylated by ATP in the presence of hexokinase and Mg^{2+}. The glucose-6-phosphate formed is oxidized by glucose-6-phosphate dehydrogenase (G6PD) to 6-phosphogluconate in the presence of nicotinamide-adenine dinucleotide phosphate (NADP+). The amount of NADPH produced is directly proportional to the amount of glucose in the sample and is measured by absorbance at 340 nm. G6PD derived from yeast is used in the assay with $NADP^+$ as the cofactor. The oxidized form of nicotinamide-adenine dinucleotide (NAD^+) is the cofactor if bacterial (*Leuconostoc mesenteroides*) G6PD is used, and the NADH produced is also measured at 340 nm.

$$\text{Glucose} + \text{ATP} \xrightleftharpoons{\textit{Hexokinase}} \text{Glucose-6-phosphate} + \text{ADP}$$

$$\text{Glucose-6-phosphate} \xrightarrow[\text{NADP}^{\oplus}\ (\text{or NAD}^{\oplus}) \;\rightarrow\; \text{NADPH} + \text{H}^{\oplus}\ (\text{or NADH})]{\textit{G-6-PD}} \text{6-Phosphogluconate}$$

A generally accepted reference method based on this principle has been developed and validated.[206] Serum or plasma is deproteinated by adding solutions of barium hydroxide ($Ba[OH]_2$) and zinc sulfate ($ZnSO_4$). The clear supernatant is mixed with a reagent containing ATP, NAD^+, hexokinase, and G6PD, incubated at 25 °C until the reaction is complete, and NADH measured. Calibrators and blanks are carried through the entire procedure, including the deproteination step. Detailed specifications are given for the equipment, materials, and reagents, including tests of enzyme reagent adequacy.

Although highly accurate and precise, the reference method is too exacting and time consuming for routine use in a clinical laboratory. An alternative approach is to apply the reaction directly to serum or plasma and use a specimen blank to correct for interfering substances that absorb at 340 nm.[205] Because almost all methods are automated and rely on commercially prepared reagents supplied in lyophilized form, only a general discussion of the procedure is presented here.

Either serum or plasma may be used. NaF, with an anticoagulant such as EDTA, heparin, oxalate, or citrate, may be used. Hemolyzed specimens containing more than 0.5 g hemoglobin/dL are unsatisfactory because phosphate esters and enzymes released from red blood cells interfere with the assay. Other sources of interference include drugs, bilirubin, and lipemia (triglyceride greater than or equal to 500 mg/dL causes a positive interference). A sample blank is therefore recommended for lipemic and icteric samples. This blank is prepared by adding 10 μL of sample to isotonic saline or buffer instead of reagent. The absorbance of this mixture, read against water at 340 nm, is subtracted. Although fructose interferes in the assay, normal fasting serum has low fructose concentrations. After ingestion of sucrose 2 g/kg of body weight, serum fructose concentration increases up to 8 to 10 mg/dL within 1 hour and persists for 2 hours. Solutions administered during glucose tolerance testing should therefore not contain any fructose.

Absorbances of sample or calibrator reaction mixtures are measured after the reactions have continued to completion (equilibrium reaction). Although glucose concentrations may be calculated directly, based on the molar absorptivity of NADPH or NADH, inclusion of a set of calibrators is recommended to detect possible deterioration of enzymes, ATP, $NADP^+$, or NAD^+, all of which are unstable. Reagents may also contain substances that react with the coenzymes. Presence of these substances can be evaluated by measuring the increase in absorbance observed in a reagent blank. Reagents are unsuitable for use if the absorbance at 340 nm exceeds 0.35, using water as the blank. The highest calibrator provides a check on the linearity of response and the adequacy of the enzyme reagent. The procedure is linear from 0 to 500 mg/dL. Glucose concentrations that exceed 500 mg/dL should be diluted with isotonic saline and reassayed.

Hexokinase procedures in which indicator reactions produce colored products are also available, enabling absorbance to be measured in the visible range.[299] An oxidation-reduction system containing phenazine methosulfate (PMS) and a substituted tetrazolium compound, 2-(*p*-iodophenyl)-3-*p*-nitrophenyl-5-phenyltetrazolium chloride (INT), is reacted with NADPH formed in the reaction. The reduced INT is colored with maximum absorbance at 520 nm. The PMS-INT color developer must be refrigerated when not in use and must be protected from exposure to light to retard autoreduction.

Glucose Oxidase Methods

The enzyme glucose oxidase catalyzes the oxidation of glucose to gluconic acid and hydrogen peroxide (H_2O_2):

$$\text{Glucose} + 2H_2O + O_2 \xrightarrow{\text{Glucose Oxidase}} \text{Gluconic acid} + 2H_2O_2$$

Addition of the enzyme peroxidase and a chromogenic oxygen acceptor, such as *o*-dianisidine, results in the formation of a colored compound that can be measured:

$$\underset{\text{(Colorless)}}{\text{o-Dianisidine}} + H_2O_2 \xrightarrow{\text{Peroxidase}} \underset{\text{(Colored)}}{\text{Oxidized } o\text{-Dianisidine}} + H_2O_2$$

Glucose oxidase is highly specific for β-D-*glucose*. As noted earlier, 36% and 64% of glucose in solution are in the α- and β-forms, respectively. Complete reaction of glucose therefore requires mutarotation of the α- to β-form. Some commercial preparations of glucose oxidase contain an enzyme—mutarotase—that accelerates this reaction. Otherwise, extended incubation time allows spontaneous conversion.

The second step, involving peroxidase, *is much less specific than the glucose oxidase reaction.* Various substances, such as uric acid, ascorbic acid, bilirubin, hemoglobin, tetracycline, and glutathione, inhibit the reaction (presumably by competing with the chromogen for H_2O_2), producing lower values. Incorporation of potassium ferrocyanide significantly decreases interference by bilirubin. Most interfering substances can be eliminated by use of a Somogyi filtrate (see the discussion under oxidation reduction methods on the Evolve site that accompanies this book at http://evolve.elsevier.com/Tietz/textbook). Acid filtrates cannot be used because peroxides, which cause falsely elevated results, may be released. Most modern methods omit the preparation of protein-free filtrates to make the procedure faster and simpler. Some glucose oxidase preparations contain catalase as a contaminant; catalase activity decomposes peroxide and decreases the final color obtained. Calibrators and unknowns should be analyzed simultaneously under conditions in which the rate of oxidation is proportional to glucose concentration.

In some methods, the final mixture is acidified slightly to stop the reaction, and the intensity of the yellow chromophore is measured at 400 nm. In stronger acid solution, the color becomes pink, with maximum absorbance at 540 nm, and both sensitivity and stability are improved. Other approaches to measurement of the H_2O_2 produced include the peroxide-mediated oxidative coupling of 3-methyl-2-benzothiazolinone hydrazone (MBTH) with *N,N*-dimethyl-aniline (DMA) catalyzed by peroxidase[106] or the oxidative coupling of *p*-aminophenazone (PAP) to phenol.[278] Both procedures have been automated. The

MBTH-DMA and PAP procedures are not affected by high concentrations of creatinine, uric acid, or hemoglobin and are performed directly on serum. The chromogen 2-amino-4-hydroxybenzenesulfonic acid produces a yellow color in the presence of peroxidase and H_2O_2.[231] Additional components are not required to produce the color and the assay can be performed on as little as 2 μL of serum.

Glucose oxidase methods are *suitable for measuring glucose in CSF.* Urine contains high concentrations of substances that interfere with the peroxidase reaction (such as uric acid), producing falsely low results. The glucose oxidase method should therefore *not be used for urine.* A method in which the urine is first pretreated with an ion-exchange resin to remove interfering substances has been described.

Modified Glucose Oxidase Methods

Some instruments use a polarographic oxygen electrode that measures the rate of oxygen consumption after the sample is added to a solution containing glucose oxidase.[143] Because this measurement involves only the first reaction shown earlier, *interferences encountered in the peroxidase step are eliminated.* To prevent formation of oxygen from H_2O_2 by catalase present in some preparations of glucose oxidase, H_2O_2 is removed by two additional reactions:

$$H_2O_2 + C_2H_5OH \xrightarrow{\text{Catalase}} CH_3CHO + 2H_2O$$

$$H_2O_2 + 2H^+ + 2I^- \xrightarrow{\text{Molybdate}} I_2 + 2H_2O$$

The latter reaction is effective even when catalase activity has diminished on storage of reagents. The procedure can be applied directly to *urine, serum, plasma,* or *CSF.* However, this approach cannot be used for the *determination of glucose in whole blood* because blood cells consume oxygen.

In the YSI Model 23A (Yellow Springs Instrument Co., Yellow Springs, Ohio), glucose oxidase is immobilized in a thin layer of resinous material sandwiched between two membranes. When a buffered sample is introduced, glucose diffuses through the first polycarbonate membrane and reacts with the enzyme to produce H_2O_2. This diffuses through the second, smaller pore cellulose acetate membrane and is oxidized at a platinum anode. The current generated is directly proportional to the glucose concentration in the diluted sample.

$$H_2O_2 \rightarrow 2H^+ + O_2 + 2e^-$$

The circuit is completed at a silver cathode, where oxygen is reduced to water.

$$4H^+ + O_2 + 4e^- \rightarrow 2H_2O$$

Any H_2O_2 diffusing back into the sample chamber is destroyed by catalase to prevent interference with the analysis. Determinations may be performed on 25 μL of *plasma, serum,* or *whole blood.* Good precision and correlation with an oxygen consumption rate analyzer have been reported.[59]

The Vitros system (Ortho-Clinical Diagnostics, Raritan, NJ) makes use of dry multilayer films for chemical analyses.[69] Glucose is measured by a glucose oxidase procedure. A 10-μL sample of *serum, plasma, urine, or CSF* is placed on a porous film on top of the layer containing the reagents. Glucose diffuses through the film and reacts with the reagents to produce a colored end product or dye. The intensity of this dye is measured through a lower transparent film by reflectance spectrophotometry. Advantages of this system include small sample size, no liquid reagents, and improved stability on storage.

Glucose Dehydrogenase Methods

The enzyme glucose dehydrogenase (β-D-glucose : NAD oxidoreductase, EC 1.1.1.47) catalyzes the oxidation of glucose to gluconolactone. Mutarotase is added to shorten the time necessary to reach equilibrium. The amount of NADH generated is proportional to the glucose concentration:

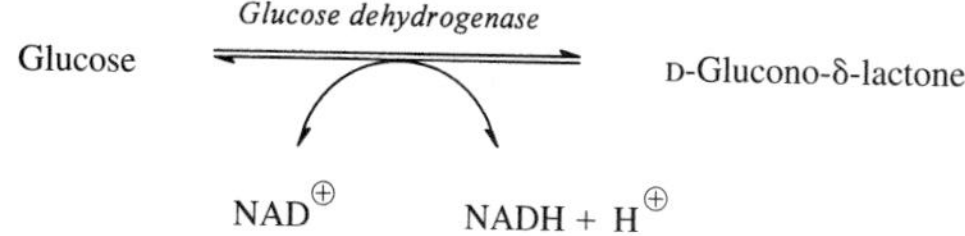

Glucose dehydrogenase for this assay is isolated from *Bacillus cereus.* The reaction appears to be highly specific for glucose, shows no interference from common anticoagulants and substances normally found in serum, and provides results in close agreement with hexokinase procedures. Methods have been adapted to continuous-flow analyzers,[49] including the use of immobilized enzyme,[265] and to a centrifugal analyzer.[176]

REFERENCE INTERVALS

Although glucose can be assayed by several different analytical procedures, reference intervals do not vary significantly among methods. The following values should apply to virtually all currently used glucose assays.

	Sample Fasting Glucose (mg/dL)
Plasma/serum	
Adults	74-106 (4.5-5.9 mmol/L)
Children	60-100 (3.5-5.6 mmol/L)
Premature neonates	20-60 (1.1-3.3 mmol/L)
Term neonates	30-60 (1.7-3.3 mmol/L)
Whole blood	65-95 (3.5-5.3 mmol/L)
CSF	40-70 (2.2-3.9 mmol/L) (60% of plasma value)
Urine	
24 hr	1-15 mg/dL (0.1-0.8 mmol/L)

Note that the ADA criteria,[7] not the reference interval, are used for the diagnosis of diabetes. Moreover, the threshold for diagnosis of hypoglycemia is variable and is considerably less than the lower limit of the reference interval. There is no sex difference. *Plasma glucose values increase with age from the third to the sixth decade:* fasting, approximately 2 mg/dL per decade; postprandial, 4 mg/dL per decade; and after a glucose challenge, 8 to 13 mg/dL per decade.[212] Fasting plasma glucose does not increase significantly after age 60, but glucose concentrations after a glucose challenge are substantially higher in older individuals.[75] Evidence of an association of increasing insulin resistance with age is inconsistent.[137,241]

CSF glucose concentrations should be approximately 60% of the plasma concentrations and *must always be compared with concurrently measured plasma glucose* for adequate clinical interpretation.

Measurement of Glucose in Urine

Examination of urine for glucose is rapid, inexpensive, and noninvasive and can be used to screen large numbers of samples. The older screening tests detect sugars that reduce copper, producing a color.[128] These react with reducing substances other than glucose (Box 25-6). Qualitative, semiquantitative, and quantitative methods are available for measuring glucose in urine and have essentially replaced the nonspecific tests in adults. *Note:* A reducing sugar method, rather than an enzymatic method specific for glucose, must be used when screening neonates and infants for inborn errors of metabolism that result in the appearance of reducing sugars other than glucose (e.g., galactose or fructose) in the urine.

Qualitative Method

In one such method (details of which are found on the Evolve site that accompanies this book), using "Benedict's" reagent (cupric ion complexed to citrate in alkaline solution), reducing substances convert cupric to cuprous ions, forming yellow cuprous hydroxide or red cuprous oxide.

Semiquantitative Methods

Convenient paper test strips are commercially available from a number of manufacturers (Clinistix and Diastix, Bayer Corp., and Chemstrip µG, Roche Diagnostics, Indianapolis).

BOX 25-6 Reducing Substances in Urine

Fructose	Ketone bodies
Lactose	Sulfanilamide
Galactose	Oxalic acid
Maltose	Hippuric acid
Arabinose	Homogentisic acid
Xylose	Glucuronic acid
Ribose	Formaldehyde
Uric acid	Isoniazid
Ascorbic acid	Salicylates
Creatinine	Cinchophen
Cysteine	Salicyluric acid
Glucose	

All strips use the *glucose-specific enzyme glucose oxidase in a chromogenic assay.* For example, Clinistix has filter paper impregnated with glucose oxidase, peroxidase, and the dye *o*-tolidine. Other dyes, such as tetramethylbenzidine (TMB), can be used. The test end of the strip is moistened with freshly voided urine and examined after 10 seconds. A blue color develops if glucose is present at a concentration of 100 mg/dL or greater. Results are read by comparing the test color with a standard color chart. Automated urinalysis systems capable of analyzing 300 strips per hour are commercially available. The test is more sensitive for glucose than the copper reduction test (Clinitest), which has a detection limit of 250 mg/dL. Despite these claims, evaluation of dipsticks reveals high imprecision at low urine glucose concentrations.[95] Clinitest was reported to detect glucose only when it was above 1 g/L, and only Chemstrip µG could differentiate urine glucose at 300 mg/L (upper limit of reference interval) from 600 mg/L.[26] The sensitivity of the strip has been adjusted to take into account the presence of enzyme inhibitors normally present in urine. Thus a positive test result is obtained with lower concentrations of glucose in water than in urine. For the same reason, misleading high results may be obtained with very dilute specimens.

False-positive results may be produced by contamination of urine with H_2O_2 or a strong oxidizing agent, such as hypochlorite (bleach). Exposure of dipsticks to air gives false-positive readings after 7 days.[63] False-negative results may occur with large quantities of reducing substances, such as ketones, ascorbic acid, and salicylates. In one study of 2000 urine specimens, 11 false-negative enzyme paper tests were encountered. Among the inhibitors identified were ascorbic acid, dipyrone, and meralluride sodium (Mercuhydrin). Several antibiotics contain ascorbic acid as a preservative, which is excreted essentially unchanged. For routine examinations, a negative result by the strip test is usually interpreted to mean that the urine specimen is negative for glucose.

Other strip tests (Keto-Diastix, Bayer Corp., and Chemstrip µGK, Roche Diagnostics) are designed for the semiquantitative estimation of both glucose and ketone bodies. The glucose portion of the strip uses the glucose oxidase–peroxidase method. The hydrogen peroxide produced oxidizes iodide to iodine, yielding various intensities of brown that correspond to the concentration of glucose in the urine. The detection limit is 100 mg/dL. The Diastix and Chemstrip glucose tests are reported to be less inhibited by ascorbic acid than Clinistix.

Quantitative Methods

Applications of various procedures for quantitative determination of glucose in urine were discussed earlier in this chapter under Determination of Glucose in Body Fluids. The hexokinase or glucose dehydrogenase procedures are recommended for greatest accuracy and specificity. Glucose oxidase procedures that depend only on the consumption of oxygen or the production of H_2O_2 are also reliable. Glucose oxidase procedures that include the H_2O_2-peroxidase reaction are not acceptable.

SELF-MONITORING OF BLOOD GLUCOSE

Diabetic patients, especially those who need insulin therapy, require careful monitoring to maintain control of blood glucose. This has become particularly important with the results of the DCCT[72] and the recommendation that patients use intensive insulin therapy regimens to achieve nearly normal glycemia. These regimens include multiple daily insulin injections, insulin pumps, and continuous subcutaneous insulin injections. Estimating blood glucose concentrations by monitoring urine glucose concentrations, a simple and convenient method, is undesirable for the following reasons:

1. The renal threshold (the blood glucose concentration above which glucose appears in the urine) averages 160 to 180 mg/dL but varies widely among individuals. It may increase in long-standing diabetes or with age and may be lower in pregnancy or childhood. A decreased threshold (± 100 mg/dL) is known as *renal glycosuria.*
2. Monitoring of urine glucose concentrations lacks sensitivity and specificity. For example, one study demonstrated that patients with plasma glucose concentrations between 150 and 199 mg/dL exhibited normal urine test results 75% of the time. Furthermore, 9% of patients with plasma glucose concentrations below 149 mg/dL had glycosuria.[194]
3. A negative test result does not distinguish between hypoglycemia, euglycemia, and moderate hyperglycemia.
4. Urine testing is not accurate.
5. Other factors influence testing (e.g., fluid intake, urine concentration, ingestion of salicylates or ascorbic acid, and urinary tract infections).

Testing urine for glucose is therefore not adequate for monitoring patients on insulin therapy.[6] Although some evidence suggests that it may be effective for monitoring type 2 diabetes,[2] the ADA states that limitations of urine testing make blood glucose measurements the preferred method of assessing glycemic control.[108]

Glucose Meters

Portable meters for measurement of blood glucose concentrations are used in three major settings: (a) in acute and chronic care facilities (at the patient's bedside and in clinics or hospitals); (b) in physicians' offices; and (c) by patients at home, work, and school. The last, self-monitoring of blood glucose (SMBG), used by approximately 1 million diabetic patients, is performed in the United States at least once a day by 40% and 26% of individuals with type 1 and 2 diabetes, respectively.[241] The worldwide market for SMBG is \$2.7 billion per year, with annual growth estimated at 10% to 12%.[241]

Patients measure their own blood glucose concentration and modify their insulin dose based on this glucose value. It is impractical for patients themselves to perform glucose determinations by the methods described earlier, but a large number of simple test strips that are available permit rapid and reasonably accurate measurements on a drop of whole blood.[65] These use the same methodology as described earlier for glucose analysis—predominantly glucose oxidase or hexokinase—but some strips contain glucose dehydrogenase. In many strips, a dye is colored by the glucose oxidase-peroxidase chromogenic reaction. The reagents are combined in dry form on a small surface area of a test strip, and the colors that develop may be evaluated visually by comparison with a color chart (rarely used any more) or quantified in a specially designed meter. *Visual reading with a color chart is not accurate enough* for most clinical circumstances. At least 25 different blood glucose meters are commercially available and these vary in size, weight, calibration method, and other features. These are reviewed annually in the ADA's Buyer's Guide to Diabetes Products.[11]

To perform the measurement, a sample of blood (usually from a fingerstick, but anticoagulated whole blood collected in EDTA or heparin may be used) is placed on the test pad, which is attached to a plastic support. The test strip is then inserted into the meter. (In some devices, the strip is inserted in the meter before applying the sample.) After a fixed period of time, the result appears on a digital display screen. The meters use reflectance photometry or electrochemistry to measure the rate of the reaction or the final concentration of the products. Reflectance photometry measures the amount of light reflected from a test pad containing reagent. In electrochemical systems, the enzymatic reaction in an electrode incorporated on the test strip produces a flow of electrons. The current, which is directly proportional to the amount of glucose in the sample, is converted to a digital readout. There is large variability among meters as to the test time (15 to 120 seconds) and the claimed reading range (40 to 400 mg/dL to 0 to 600 mg/dL). Calibration is automatic on some devices, whereas others use lot-specific code chips or strips. All manufacturers supply control solutions. Strict adherence to the instructions is necessary to obtain accurate results. Some meters have a porous membrane that separates erythrocytes, and analysis is performed on the resultant plasma. *Whole blood glucose concentrations are approximately 10% to 15% lower than plasma or serum concentrations, but meters can be calibrated to report plasma glucose values, even when the sample is whole blood.* An International Federation of Clinical Chemistry (IFCC) working group recently recommended that glucose meters be harmonized to report the concentration of glucose in plasma, irrespective of the sample type or technology.[47]

Analytical Goals

Multiple analytical goals have been proposed for the performance of glucose meters. The rationale for these is not always clear. In 1987 the ADA recommended a goal of total error (in the hands of users) of less than 10% at glucose concentrations of 30 to 400 mg/dL 100% of the time.[5] The recommendation was modified in response to the significant reduction in complications by tight glucose control in the DCCT. The revised performance goal, published in 1996,[6] is for analytical error to be less than 5%. No published studies of glucose meters have achieved this goal. The Clinical Laboratory Improvement Amendment (CLIA) 88 goal is less stringent than that of the ADA; results with meters should be within 10% of target values or within 6 mg/dL, whichever is larger. The National Committee for Clinical Laboratory Standards (NCCLS) recommendations[202] are that results should fall within 20% of laboratory-measured glucose concentrations when greater than 75 mg/dL and within 15 mg/dL of laboratory glucose if the glucose concentration is less than or equal to 75 mg/dL.

A different method was proposed by Clarke,[62] who developed an error grid that attempts to define clinically important errors by identifying fairly broad target ranges. In addition, a novel approach using simulation modeling revealed that meters that achieve both a CV and a bias less than 5% rarely lead to major errors in insulin dose.[41] The lack of consensus on quality goals for glucose meters reflects the absence of agreed-upon objective criteria. Using biological variation criteria, a goal for total error (including both bias and imprecision) of less than or equal to 7.9% has been proposed.[241] However, additional studies are necessary to accurately define this goal.

Performance of Glucose Meters

The most common errors in SMBG, such as proper application, timing, and removal of excess blood, have been eliminated by advances in technology. Additional innovations that reduce operator error include systems that abort testing if the sample volume is inadequate, built-in programs that simplify quality control, and memory that allows the instrument to store up to several hundred glucose readings that can be downloaded into a computer.

Several factors affect the accuracy and reproducibility of SMBG. These include: (a) user variability—up to 50% of the values may vary more than 20% from the reference values[65]; (b) hematocrit—the presence of anemia (false increase) or polycythemia (false depression) may result in up to 30% variability; and (c) defective reagent strips or instrument malfunction (rare). Other variables include changes in altitude, environmental temperature, or humidity; hypotension; hypoxia; and high triglyceride concentrations. In addition, *these assays are unreliable at very high and very low glucose concentrations* (less than 60 and greater than 500 mg/dL). Because dehydration, a common feature of diabetic ketoacidosis, greatly increases blood viscosity, inaccurately low blood glucose results may be obtained. Several drugs interfere, but not with all meters.[269] Another important factor is the lack of correlation among meters, even from a single manufacturer, caused by different assay methods and architecture. In fact, results from two meters of the same brand have been observed to differ substantially.[270] The analytical performance characteristics of several meters have been published.[140,283] Patient factors are also important, particularly adequate training. Recurrent education at clinic visits and comparison of SMBG with concurrent laboratory glucose analysis improved the accuracy of patients' blood glucose readings.[142] In addition, it is important to evaluate the patient's technique at regular intervals.

The performance of different meters varies widely. Although current meters, as predicted, exhibit performance superior to prior generations of meters,[288] imprecision remains high. Under carefully controlled conditions in which all assays were performed by a single medical technologist, ~50% of analyses met the ADA criterion of less than 5% deviation from reference values.[288] Performance of older meters was substantially worse. Note that the performance of glucose meters achieved by medical technologists is better than that achieved by patients. Another study that evaluated meter performance in 226 hospitals by split samples analyzed simultaneously on meters and laboratory glucose analyzers revealed that 45.6%, 25%, and 14% differed from each other by greater than 10%, greater than 15%, and greater than 20%, respectively.[208] Recent comparison with laboratory values of almost 22,000 measurements of capillary glucose by patients using meters revealed no significant improvement in meter performance between 1989 and 1999.[37]

Indications and Frequency of SMBG

The indications and frequency of self-monitoring vary among patients. *SMBG should be performed by all patients treated with insulin.* The role of SMBG in patients with type 2 diabetes has not been defined.[241] A consensus statement by the ADA[65] recommended the following specific indications for SMBG: (1) patients undergoing intensive insulin treatment programs (in this group, glucose should be measured at least four times a day to achieve glycemic control); (2) preventing and detecting hypoglycemia, especially in people who are asymptomatic or unable to recognize the early warning signs; (3) avoidance of severe hyperglycemia, particularly in situations of increased risk (e.g., medications that alter insulin secretion or action, intercurrent illness, and elderly people); (4) adjusting pharmacological therapy in response to changes in life-style, such as exercise or altering food intake; and (5) determining the necessity for initiating insulin therapy in GDM. *SMBG must not be used to diagnose diabetes mellitus,* and its role in screening remains uncertain.[241]

SMBG should be performed at least four times per day in patients with type 1 diabetes. Monitoring less frequently than four times a day results in a deterioration of glycemic control.[6,199,248] Published studies reveal that self-monitoring is performed by patients much less frequently than recommended: at least once a day by 39% of patients taking insulin and 5% to 6% of those treated with oral agents or diet alone.[116] Moreover, 29% and 65% of patients treated with insulin and oral agents, respectively, monitored their blood glucose less than once per month. However, no evaluation has been performed to verify that four times a day is ideal or whether some other frequency or timing (e.g., postprandial testing) would improve glycemic control. The optimum frequency of SMBG for patients with type 2 diabetes is unknown. Published evidence shows no correlation between the frequency of SMBG in type 2 diabetes and glycemic control.[67,88,116] There is no known role for SMBG in patients with type 2 diabetes who are treated with diet alone.

MINIMALLY INVASIVE MONITORING OF BLOOD GLUCOSE

Fewer than 10% of patients with diabetes routinely perform SMBG because it is painful and inconvenient. Since the 1960s, attempts have been made to develop a painless method for monitoring blood glucose concentrations. Three general approaches have been used, namely implanted sensors, minimally invasive monitoring, and noninvasive monitoring.

Implanted Sensors

Several implanted biosensors have been developed and evaluated in both animals and humans (see Chapter 4). Detection systems are based on enzymes, electrodes, or fluorescence.[149,221] The most widely studied method is an electrochemical sensor that uses glucose oxidase.[295] This sensor can be implanted intravenously or subcutaneously. Intravenous implantation in dogs for up to 3 months has demonstrated the feasibility of this approach.[111] Alternatives to enzymes are being developed, including artificial glucose "receptors." Less success has been achieved with subcutaneous implants. Implantation of a needle type of sensor into the subcutaneous tissue induces a host of inflammatory responses that alters the sensitivity of the device. Microdialysis with hollow fibers or ultrafiltration with biologically inert material can decrease this problem.

Minimally Invasive Glucose Monitoring

The concept underlying these methods is that the concentration of glucose in the interstitial fluid correlates with blood glucose concentration. The principle of the Food and Drug Administration (FDA)–approved Gluco Watch (Cygnus) is the application of a low-level electric current on the skin. This induces movement by electroosmosis of glucose across the skin where it is measured by a glucose oxidase detector.[97,268] Glucose concentrations in transdermal fluid and plasma are highly correlated. The clearest application of the Gluco Watch, which is designed to measure glucose three times per hour for up to 12 hours, appears to be in the detection of unsuspected hypoglycemia. Calibration with reference plasma glucose is required. Initial clinical studies reveal reasonable correlation of the Gluco Watch with SMBG.[97,268] The device has not been rigorously tested in a home setting nor in children, but is likely to stimulate enhanced efforts to bring other technologies into clinical use.

Noninvasive Glucose Monitoring

Noninvasive in vivo monitoring of glucose is an area of active investigation. Near-infrared spectroscopic devices measure either the absorption or reflection of light from subcutaneous tissue. Although glucose has a specific absorption at 1035 nm, many substances interfere. A computer, individually calibrated, screens out interfering information to obtain the glucose result. Similar limitations have prevented successful use of light scattering. Photoacoustic spectroscopy, which uses pulsed infrared light, is a newer technique that shows some promise.

KETONE BODIES

The development of ketosis requires changes in both adipose tissue and the liver. *The primary substrates for ketone body formation are free fatty acids* from adipose stores. Normally, long-chain fatty acids are taken up by the liver, reesterified to triglycerides, and stored in the liver or incorporated in very-low-density lipoproteins and returned to the plasma. In contrast to other tissue, the brain cannot use free fatty acids for energy. When glucose is unavailable, ketone bodies supply the vast majority of the brain's energy. After a 3-day fast, ketone bodies provide 30% to 40% of the body's energy requirements.[165] In uncontrolled diabetes, the low insulin concentrations result in increased lipolysis and decreased reesterification, thereby increasing plasma free fatty acids. In addition, the increased glucagon : insulin ratio enhances fatty acid oxidation in the liver. Increased counterregulatory hormones also augment lipolysis and ketogenesis in fat and liver, respectively. Thus increased hepatic ketone production and decreased peripheral tissue metabolism lead to acetoacetate accumulation in the blood. A small fraction undergoes spontaneous decarboxylation to form acetone, but the majority is converted to β-hydroxybutyrate.

Acetoacetate ⇌ β-Hydroxybutyrate (β-Hydroxybutyrate dehydrogenase (in liver); $NADH + H^{+}$ → NAD^{+})

Acetoacetate + H^{+} → Acetone + CO_2 (Spontaneous)

The relative proportions in which the three ketone bodies are present in blood vary depending on the redox state of the cell. In healthy people, β-hydroxybutyrate and acetoacetate—which are present at approximately equimolar concentrations[165,223,293]—constitute virtually all the serum ketones. Acetone is a minor component. In severe diabetes, the ratio of β-hydroxybutyrate to acetoacetate may increase to 6:1 owing to the presence of a large concentration of NADH, which favors β-hydroxybutyrate production.

None of the commonly used methods for the detection and determination of ketone bodies in serum or urine reacts with all three ketone bodies. Gerhardt's ferric chloride test reacts with acetoacetate only. Tests using nitroprusside are at least 10 times more sensitive to acetoacetate than to acetone, and give no reaction at all with β-hydroxybutyrate.

The fact that *most of the tests for ketosis essentially detect or measure acetoacetate only* may produce a paradoxical situation. When a patient initially presents in ketoacidosis, the test results for ketones may be only weakly positive. With therapy, *β-hydroxybutyrate is converted to acetoacetate and the ketosis appears to worsen.*

Traditional tests for β-hydroxybutyrate are indirect; they require brief boiling of the urine to remove acetone and acetoacetate by evaporation (acetoacetate first breaks down spontaneously to acetone), followed by gentle oxidation of β-hydroxybutyrate to acetoacetate and acetone with peroxide, ferric ions, or dichromate. The acetoacetate thus formed may be detected with Gerhardt's test or one of the procedures using nitroprusside.

Specific determination of β-hydroxybutyrate in urine is not considered to be a routine procedure. A paper strip for semiquantitative measurement of β-hydroxybutyrate in serum and urine has been described[115] but has not gained general acceptance. More recently, quantitative enzymatic assays for β-hydroxybutyrate that can be performed directly on blood or serum became commercially available. Originally available commercially as a bench-top analyzer (KetoSite; GDS Diagnostics, Elkhart, Ind.), hand-held devices are also available now (Precision Xtra; MediSense, Boston, and BioScanner Ketone; Polymer Technology Systems, Indianapolis).[50]

Clinical Significance

Excessive formation of ketone bodies results in increased blood concentrations (*ketonemia*) and increased excretion in the urine (*ketonuria*). This process is observed in conditions associated with decreased availability of carbohydrates (such as starvation or frequent vomiting) or decreased use of carbohydrates (such as diabetes mellitus, glycogen storage disease [von Gierke's disease], and alkalosis). The popular high-fat, low-carbohydrate diets are ketogenic and increase ketone bodies in the circulation. Diabetes mellitus and alcohol consumption are the most common causes of ketoacidosis in adults. (Hyperglycemia is not usually present in the latter condition.) Ingestion of isopropyl alcohol and salicylate poisoning can also produce ketoacidosis. Urine ketone test results are positive in ~30% of first morning void specimens from pregnant women. Semiquantitative determination of ketone bodies in blood is more accurate than determination of these compounds in urine in the treatment of diabetic ketoacidosis. Although not always excreted in proportion to blood ketone concentrations, because of convenience, urine ketones are widely used for monitoring control in patients with type 1 diabetes. The ADA states that *urine ketone testing is an important part of monitoring by patients with diabetes*, particularly those with type 1 diabetes, pregnancy with preexisting diabetes, and GDM.[108] Patients with type 1 diabetes should test for ketones during acute illness or stress, with consistent increase in blood glucose (greater than 300 mg/dL), during pregnancy, or when symptoms of ketoacidosis are present.[108] Measurement of ketones in urine and blood is widely used in patients with diabetes for both diagnosis and monitoring of diabetic ketoacidosis.[241]

Determination of Ketone Bodies in Body Fluids

Although quantitative determination of individual ketone bodies is possible, these methods are not used as routine tests. The semiquantitative Acetest and Ketostix (Ames Co.) are frequently used but are insensitive to β-hydroxybutyrate.[274] It is important to bear in mind, therefore, that a *negative nitroprusside test result does not rule out ketoacidosis.* (Note: Details of the following tests are found on the Evolve site that accompanies this book.)

Detection of Ketone Bodies by Acetest

The Acetest tablets contain a mixture of glycine, sodium nitroprusside, disodium phosphate, and lactose. Acetoacetate or acetone (to a lesser extent) in the presence of glycine forms a lavender-purple complex with nitroprusside. β-hydroxybutyrate does not react with nitroprusside. The disodium phosphate provides an optimum pH for the reaction, and lactose enhances the color.[138]

Detection of Ketone Bodies by Ketostix

Ketostix is a modification of the nitroprusside test in which a reagent strip is used instead of a tablet. The Ketostix test gives a positive reaction within 15 seconds with a specimen containing at least 50 mg of acetoacetate per L. The accompanying color chart gives readings for ketone concentrations of 50, 150, 400, 800, and 1600 mg/L. Acetone also reacts, but the test is less sensitive to it.

Determination of β-Hydroxybutyrate

A 1995 short report on patients with diabetic ketoacidosis indicated that β-hydroxybutyrate correlated better than acetoacetate with changes in acid-base status.[282]

In this test, β-hydroxybutyrate in the presence of NAD^+ is converted by β-hydroxybutyrate dehydrogenase to acetoacetate, producing NADH. Diaphorase catalyzes the reduction of nitroblue tetrazolium (NBT) by NADH to produce a purple compound and its absorbance is read in a special meter that provides a digital readout.

$$\beta\text{-Hydroxybutyrate} \xrightleftharpoons[\text{NAD}^{\oplus} \;\to\; \text{NADH} + \text{H}^{\oplus}]{\beta\text{-Hydroxybutyrate dehydrogenase}} \text{Acetoacetate}$$

$$\text{NADH} + \text{NBT} \xrightleftharpoons{\textit{Diaphorase}} \text{NAD}^{\oplus} + \text{Reduced NBT}$$

Determination of Ketone Bodies in Urine

Acetest and Ketostix are also suitable for detecting ketone bodies in urine. The sensitivity and specificity of the tests are the same as outlined for serum.

Reference Interval

Serum β-hydroxybutyrate values range from 0.02 to 0.27 mmol/L (0.21 to 2.81 mg/dL) in healthy people after an overnight fast. Ketone bodies in the blood can reach 2 mmol/L with prolonged exercise.[165] Patients with diabetic ketoacidosis usually have β-hydroxybutyrate concentrations greater than 2 mmol/L (20 mg/dL).

LACTATE AND PYRUVATE

Lactic acid, an intermediate in carbohydrate metabolism (see Figure 25-9), is derived predominantly from white skeletal muscle, brain, skin, renal medulla, and erythrocytes. The blood lactate concentration depends on the rate of production in these tissues and the rate of metabolism in the liver and kidneys. Approximately 65% of total basal lactate production is used by the liver, particularly in gluconeogenesis. The *Cori cycle* is the conversion of glucose to lactate in the periphery and reconversion of lactate to glucose in the liver. Extrahepatic removal of lactate is by oxidation in red skeletal muscle and the renal cortex. A moderate increase in lactate production results in increased hepatic lactate clearance, but uptake by the liver is saturable when concentrations exceed 2 mmol/L. For example, during strenuous exercise, lactate concentrations may increase significantly, from an average concentration of about 0.9 to more than 20 mmol/L within 10 seconds. There is no uniformly accepted concentration for the diagnosis of lactic acidosis, but lactate concentrations exceeding 5 mmol/L and pH less than 7.25 indicate significant lactic acidosis.

Under certain conditions, the ratio of lactate to pyruvate is an indicator of redox status. By rearranging the equation for the equilibrium constant for the reaction catalyzed by lactate dehydrogenase (EC 1.1.1.27), it can be seen that the ratio of lactate to pyruvate is proportional to the ratio of NADH to NAD^+.

Clinical Significance

Pyruvate is metabolized by four enzyme systems, namely alanine aminotransferase, pyruvate carboxylase (the major regulatory enzyme in gluconeogenesis), lactate dehydrogenase, and pyruvate dehydrogenase (see Figure 25-9). The last is a complex of enzymes that decarboxylate pyruvate in the presence of oxygen to acetyl coenzyme A (CoA), allowing entry into the citric acid cycle. Measurement of pyruvate is useful in the evaluation of patients with inborn errors of metabolism who have increased serum lactate concentrations. A lactate:pyruvate ratio less than 25 suggests a defect in gluconeogenesis, whereas an increased ratio (greater than or equal to 35) indicates reduced intracellular conditions found in hypoxia. Inborn errors associated with an increased lactate:pyruvate ratio include pyruvate carboxylase deficiency and defects in oxidative phosphorylation.[237] A high lactate:pyruvate ratio appears to be a sensitive test for detecting mitochondrial muscle toxicity of zidovudine therapy.[55] Pyruvate is also measured in clinical studies evaluating reperfusion after myocardial ischemia. Patients with Alzheimer's disease were reported to have higher CSF pyruvate concentrations than control subjects, and the concentrations correlate with the severity of the dementia.[216]

Lactic acidosis occurs in two clinical settings: (1) type A (hypoxic), associated with *decreased tissue oxygenation,* such as shock, hypovolemia, and left ventricular failure; and (2) type B (metabolic), associated with *disease* (e.g., diabetes mellitus, neoplasia, liver disease), *drugs and/or toxins* (e.g., ethanol, methanol, and salicylates), or *inborn errors of metabolism* (e.g., methylmalonic aciduria, propionic acidemia, and fatty acid oxidation defects). Lactic acidosis is not uncommon and occurs in approximately 1% of hospital admissions. It has a mortality rate greater than 60%, which approaches 100% if hypotension is also present. Type A is much more common.

The mechanism of type B lactic acidosis is not known but is speculated to be a primary defect in mitochondrial function with impaired oxygen use. This leads to reduced stores of ATP and NAD^+, with accumulation of NADH and H^+. In the presence of decreased liver perfusion or liver disease, lactate removal from the blood is reduced, thereby aggravating the lactic acidosis.

An uncommon but often undiagnosed cause of lactic acidosis is D-lactic acidosis.[284] It was thought that D-lactate was not produced in human metabolism, but normal individuals have a large capacity to metabolize D-lactate.[284] Moreover, absorption and accumulation of D-lactate from abnormal intestinal bacteria may cause systemic acidosis. This occurs after jejunoileal bypass surgery and manifests as altered mental status (from mild drowsiness to coma) with increased blood concentrations of D-lactate. Virtually all the commonly used laboratory assays for lactate use L-lactate dehydrogenase, which does not detect D-lactate. D-Lactate can be measured by gas-liquid chromatography or, more easily, using a specific D-lactate dehydrogenase (Sigma) from *Lactobacillus leichmanni.*[175] The enzyme assay can be readily automated.

Lactate in CSF normally parallels blood levels, but not in children.[134] With biochemical alterations in the CNS, however, CSF lactate values change independently of blood values. Increased CSF concentrations are noted in cerebrovascular accidents, intracranial hemorrhage, bacterial meningitis, epilepsy, inborn errors of the electron transport chain, and other CNS disorders. In aseptic (viral) meningitis, lactate concentrations in CSF are not usually increased; hence, CSF lactate has been used to help discriminate between viral and bacterial meningitis,[22] but the clinical utility has been questioned. In a few children with inherited metabolic diseases, CSF lactate concentrations may be increased despite a plasma lactate in the reference interval.[134]

Methods for Measuring Lactate and Pyruvate in Body Fluids

(Note: Details of the following tests are found on the Evolve site that accompanies this book.)

Determination of Lactate in Whole Blood[17,172,174,181]

Principle

Lactate is oxidized to pyruvate by lactate dehydrogenase in the presence of NAD^+. The NADH formed in this reaction is measured by a spectrophotometer at 340 nm and serves as a measure of the lactate concentration.

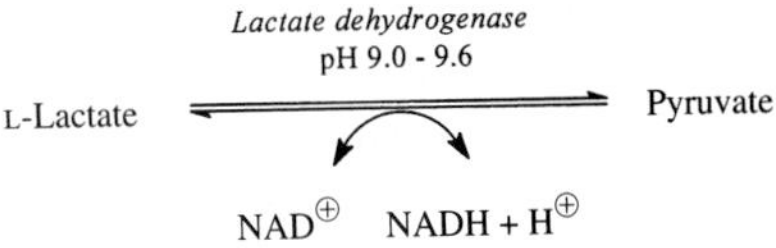

The equilibrium of the reaction normally lies far to the left. However, by using a pH of 9.0 to 9.6, an excess of NAD^+, and trapping the reaction product pyruvate with hydrazine, the equilibrium can be shifted to the right. Pyruvate can also be removed by reacting it with L-glutamate in the presence of alanine aminotransferase. Use of tris (hydroxymethyl)-aminomethane (TRIS) buffer results in more rapid completion of a side reaction between NAD^+ and hydrazine and prevents the "creeping" of blank values observed when glycine buffer is used.[172]

Because of its high specificity and simplicity, the enzymatic method is the method of choice for measuring lactate, although other methods may also be used (e.g., gas chromatography[246] and photometry).

The Vitros analyzer (Ortho-Clinical Diagnostics, Raritan, N.J.) uses an assay in which lactic acid is oxidized to pyruvate by lactate oxidase. The H_2O_2 generated oxidizes a chromogen system, and the absorbance of the resulting dye complex, measured by a spectrophotometer at 540 nm, is directly proportional to the lactate concentration in the specimen. Each mole of lactate oxidized produces 0.5 mol of dye complex.

$$\text{L-Lactate} + O_2 \xrightarrow{\text{Lactate Oxidase}} \text{Pyruvate} + H_2O_2$$

$$2H_2O_2 + \text{4-aminoantipyrine} + \text{1,7-dihydronaphthalene} \xrightarrow{\text{Peroxidase}} \text{red dye}$$

Reference Intervals

The reference intervals for lactate are:

Specimen	LACTATE mmol/L	LACTATE mg/dL
Venous Blood		
At rest	0.5-1.3	5-12
In hospital	0.9-1.7	8-15
Arterial Blood		
At rest	0.36-0.75	3-7
In hospital	0.36-1.25	3-11

Patients in the hospital exhibit a wider range. Lactic acidosis occurs with blood lactate concentrations exceeding 5 mmol/L (45 mg/dL). Severe exercise dramatically increases lactate concentrations, and even movement of leg muscles by patients at bed rest may result in significant increases. Plasma values are about 7% higher than those in whole blood, although differences depend on the procedure used. CSF values are usually similar to blood concentrations, but may change independently in CNS disorders. Age-related reference intervals for CSF lactate (and lactate: pyruvate ratios) have been established in children.[33] The upper limit of the reference interval (90th percentile) for CSF lactate in children in hospital from birth to 15½ years varied continuously from 1.78 to 1.88 mmol/L (16 to 17 mg/dL).[33] Normal 24-hour urine output of lactate is 5.5 to 22 mmol/day.

Determination of Pyruvate in Whole Blood

Principle

The reaction involved in the determination of pyruvate is essentially the reverse of the reaction used in the lactate procedure.

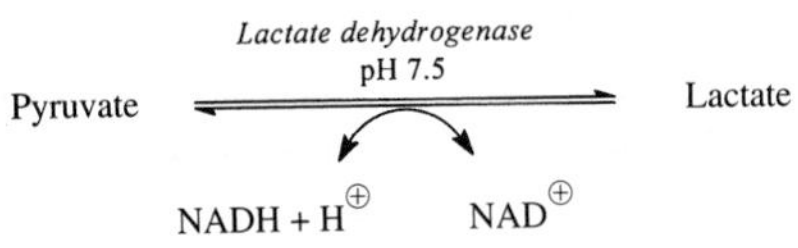

At about pH 7.5, the equilibrium constant strongly favors the reaction to the right. The method is very specific, and 2-oxoglutarate, oxaloacetate, acetoacetate, and β-hydroxybutyrate do not interfere as with colorimetric methods.

Reference Intervals

Fasting venous blood, drawn with a patient at rest, has a pyruvate concentration of 0.03 to 0.10 mmol/L (0.3 to 0.9 mg/dL). Arterial blood contains 0.02 to 0.08 mmol/L (0.2 to 0.7 mg/dL). Values for CSF are 0.06 to 0.19 mmol/L (0.5 to 1.7 mg/dL).[226] Age-related reference intervals in CSF have been established in children.[33] Urine output of pyruvate is normally 1 mmol/day or less. There are few clinical indications for measurement of blood pyruvate concentrations.

GLYCATED PROTEINS

Measurement of glycated proteins, primarily GHb, is effective in monitoring long-term glucose control in people with diabetes mellitus. It provides a retrospective index of the integrated plasma glucose values over an extended period of time and is not subject to the wide fluctuations observed when assaying blood glucose concentrations. GHb concentrations therefore are a valuable and widely used adjunct to blood glucose determinations for monitoring of long-term glycemic control. In addition, GHb is a measure of the risk for the development of complications of diabetes.

Glycated Hemoglobin*

Glycation is the nonenzymatic addition of a sugar residue to amino groups of proteins. Human adult hemoglobin (Hb) usually consists of Hb A (97% of the total), Hb A_2 (2.5%), and Hb F (0.5%). Hb A is made up of four polypeptide chains, two α- and two β-chains. Chromatographic analysis of Hb A identifies several minor hemoglobins, namely Hb A_{1a}, Hb A_{1b}, and Hb A_{1c},which are collectively referred to as Hb A_1, *fast hemoglobins* (because they migrate more rapidly than Hb A in an electrical field), *glycohemoglobins,* or *glycated hemoglobins* (Table 25-6). The Joint Commission on Biochemical Nomenclature of the International Union of Pure and Applied Chemistry recommends the term *neoglycoprotein* for such derivatives and the term *glycation* to describe this process. Therefore although *glycosylated* and *glucosylated* have been widely used in the literature, the term *glycated* is preferred. Hb A_{1c} is formed by the condensation of glucose with the *N*-terminal valine residue of each β-chain of Hb A to form an unstable Schiff base (aldimine, pre-Hb A_{1c}; Figure 25-15). The Schiff base may either dissociate or undergo an Amadori rearrangement to form a stable

*The terms glycated hemoglobin, glycohemoglobin, "glycosylated" (which should not be used as it refers to proteins in which carbohydrates have been attached enzymatically) hemoglobin, Hb A_1, and Hb A_{1c}, have all been used to refer to hemoglobin that has been modified by the nonenzymatic addition of glucose residues. However, these terms are not interchangeable. Glycated hemoglobins comprise Hb A_1 and other hemoglobin-glucose adducts, whereas Hb A_1 is made up of Hb A_{1a}, Hb A_{1b}, and Hb A_{1c}. To eliminate this confusing nomenclature, the term "A1c test" has been suggested. As described in the text, most of the clinical outcome data that are available for the effects of metabolic control on complications (at least for the DCCT and UKPDS) used assay methods that quantified HbA_{1c}. In this chapter, the term glycated hemoglobin includes all forms of glycated hemoglobin.

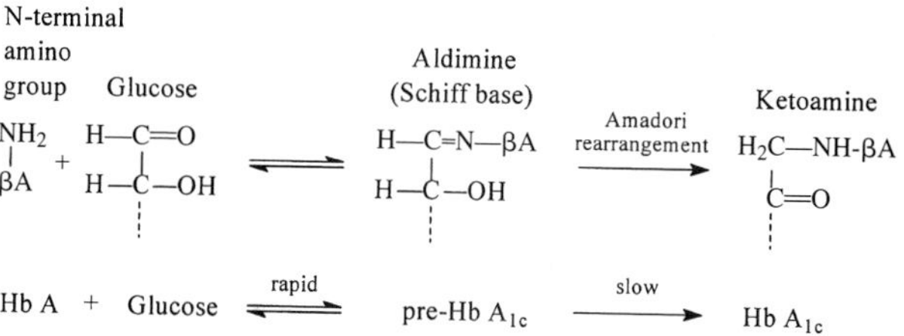

Figure 25-15 Formation of hemoglobin A_{1c}.

ketoamine, Hb A_{1c}. Hb A_{1a1} and Hb A_{1a2}, which make up Hb A_{1a}, have fructose-1,6-diphosphate and glucose-6-phosphate, respectively, attached to the amino terminal of the β-chain (Table 25-6). The structure of Hb A_{1b}, identified by mass spectrometry, contains pyruvic acid linked to the amino terminal valine of the β-chain, probably by a ketamine or enamine bond. *Hb A_{1c} is the major fraction,* constituting approximately 80% of Hb A_1.

Glycation may also occur at sites other than the end of the β-chain, such as lysine residues, or the α-chain. These GHbs, referred to as glycated Hb A_0 or total glycated hemoglobin (Table 25-6), cannot be separated from nonglycated hemoglobin by methods based on charge, but are measured by boronate affinity chromatography.

Formation of GHb is essentially irreversible, and the concentration in the blood depends on both the lifespan of the red blood cell (average 120 days) and the blood glucose concentration. Because the rate of formation of GHb is directly proportional to the concentration of glucose in the blood, *the GHb concentration represents the integrated values for glucose over the preceding 6 to 8 weeks.* This provides an additional criterion for assessing glucose control because GHb values are free of day-to-day glucose fluctuations and are unaffected by recent exercise or food ingestion. It is important to realize that the contribution of the plasma glucose concentration to GHb depends on the time interval, with more recent values providing a larger contribution than earlier values. The

TABLE 25-6 Nomenclature of Selected Hemoglobins

Name	Component(s)
Hb A	Constitutes ~97% adult hemoglobin
Hb A_0	Synonymous with Hb A
Hb A_{1a1}	Hb A with fructose-1,6-diphosphate attached to the *N*-terminal of the β-chain
Hb A_{1a2}	Hb A with glucose-6-phosphate attached to the *N*-terminal of the β-chain
Hb A_{1a}	Comprises Hb A_{1a1} and Hb A_{1a2}
Hb A_{1b}	Hb A with pyruvic acid attached to the *N*-terminal of the β-chain
Hb A_{1c}	Hb A with glucose attached to the *N*-terminal valine of the β-chain
pre-Hb A_{1c}	Unstable Schiff base (aldimine); a labile intermediary component in the formation of Hb A_{1c}
Hb A_1	Consists of Hb A_{1a}, Hb A_{1b}, and Hb A_{1c}
Total glycated hemoglobin*	Consists of Hb A_{1c} and other hemoglobin-carbohydrate adducts

Hb, Hemoglobin
*Also termed "glycated hemoglobin" or "glycohemoglobin"

plasma glucose in the preceding 1 month determines 50% of the Hb A_{1c}, whereas days 60 to 120 determine only 25%.[267] After a sudden alteration in blood glucose concentrations, the rate of change of Hb A_{1c} is rapid during the initial 2 months, followed by a more gradual change approaching steady state 3 months later. The half-time is 35 days.

The interpretation of GHb depends on the red blood cells having a normal lifespan. Patients with hemolytic disease or other conditions with shortened red blood cell survival exhibit a substantial reduction in GHb.[46] Similarly, individuals with recent significant blood loss have falsely low values owing to a higher fraction of young erythrocytes. GHb concentrations can still be used to monitor these patients, but values must be compared with previous values from the same patient, not published reference intervals. High GHb concentrations have been reported in iron deficiency anemia, probably because of the high proportion of old erythrocytes. The effect of hemoglobin variants (such as Hb F, Hb S, and Hb C) depends on the specific method of analysis (discussed later).[46] Depending on the particular hemoglobinopathy and assay method, results may be spuriously increased or decreased. Another source of error in selected methods is *carbamylated hemoglobin.* This is formed by attachment of urea and is present in large amounts in renal failure, which is common in diabetic patients.

Labile intermediates (pre-Hb A_{1c}, Schiff base) may be included in measurements of Hb A_{1c}, especially in the common electrophoretic and ion-exchange methods,[195] and produce misleadingly high results. The *labile fraction changes rapidly with acute changes in blood glucose concentration and thus is not an indicator of long-term glycemic control.* Pre-Hb A_{1c} amounts to 5% to 8% of total Hb A_1 in healthy individuals and ranges from 8% to 30% in patients with diabetes, depending on the degree of control of blood glucose concentration at or near the time of blood sampling.[133] If the analytical method measures both fractions, the labile pre-Hb A_{1c} should first be removed to prevent falsely increased results. In the absence of glucose, pre-Hb A_{1c} reverts to glucose and Hb A (see Figure 25-15). This provides the basis for some procedures to eliminate the labile fraction by incubating washed red blood cells in saline. In some boronate methods, the assay conditions favor rapid dissociation of the Schiff base.

Clinical Utility

GHb has been firmly established as an index of long-term blood glucose concentrations and as a measure of the risk for the development of complications in patients with diabetes mellitus.[107] GHb was a cornerstone of the DCCT.[72] (To prevent assay variability [see section on assay standardization later in this chapter], all GHb assays in the DCCT were done in a central laboratory that measured Hb A_{1c} by HPLC.) The DCCT documented that there is a direct relationship between blood glucose concentrations (assessed by Hb A_{1c}) and the risk of complications.[72] The absolute risks of retinopathy and nephropathy were directly proportional to the mean Hb A_{1c}. The risk of retinopathy increased continuously with increasing Hb A_{1c}, and a single measure of Hb A_{1c} predicted the progression of retinopathy 4 years later. In fact, subsequent analysis revealed that the mean Hb A_{1c} was the dominant predictor of retinopathy progression, and a 10% lower Hb A_{1c} concentration was associated with a 45% lower risk.[73] The risk of microvascular complications varies continuously with Hb A_{1c} and there is not an Hb A_{1c} concentration below which the risk is eliminated.

Analogous correlations between Hb A_{1c} and complications were observed in patients with type 2 diabetes in the UKPDS trial.[280] To ensure that Hb A_{1c} results in the UKPDS were comparable with the DCCT, the same ion-exchange HPLC method was used. The mean Hb A_{1c} values for the intensively treated and conventional groups were 7.0% and 7.9%, respectively.[280] Despite the apparently small difference in Hb A_{1c}, microvascular complications were reduced by ~25%. Each 1% reduction in Hb A_{1c} (e.g., from 8% to 7%) was associated with risk reductions of 37% for microvascular disease, 21% for deaths related to diabetes, and 14% for myocardial infarction.[280] Importantly, in patients without diabetes, Hb A_{1c} is directly related to cardiovascular disease. In the European Prospective Investigation into Cancer and Nutrition [EPIC-Norfolk], an increase of 1% in Hb A_{1c} was associated with a 28% increase in the risk of death.[150] Based on the DCCT and UKPDS, the ADA recommends that a primary treatment goal in adults with diabetes should be "near-normal" glycemia with Hb A_{1c} less than 7%.[15] The American College of Endocrinology and the International Diabetes Federation recommend a Hb A_{1c} target of 6.5%. The more frequent use of this test in the management of patients is reflected in the increased number of laboratories participating in College of American Pathologists (CAP) GHb surveys. In 1985, 1990, and 2003 there were approximately 300, 707, and 2008 laboratories, respectively, enrolled in the GHb surveys.

Methods for the Determination of Glycated Hemoglobins

There are more than 30 different methods for the determination of GHbs. These methods separate hemoglobin from GHb using techniques based on *charge differences* (ion-exchange chromatography, HPLC, electrophoresis, and isoelectric focusing), *structural differences* (affinity chromatography and immunoassay), or *chemical analysis* (photometry and spectrophotometry).[109] Regardless of the method, the result is expressed as a percentage of total hemoglobin. Analysis by chemical techniques is rarely used and is not addressed further here. (Interested readers are referred to earlier editions of this book.) The selection of method by a laboratory is influenced by several factors, including sample volume, patient population, and cost. It is advisable to consult clinicians in this process. The ADA recommends that laboratories should use only GHb assays that are

TABLE 25-7 Methods of Glycated Hemoglobin Analysis[a]

Method	Component	YEAR: 1995 (n = 1947)[b]				2003 (n = 2008)			
		Number[c]	% of Total	Mean (%)[d]	CV (%)[d]	Number[c]	% of Total	Mean (%)[de]	CV (%)[d]
Charge	**Reported**								
Ion exchange			15				42		
	Hb A_{1c}	279		4.9-5.7	4.4-13.8	844		4.9-5.2	1.9-4.9
	Hb A_1	22		6.5	15.2	—			
Electrophoresis			12				<1		
	Hb A_{1c}	138		4.9	16.5	8		N/A[f]	N/A
	Hb A_1	99		6.4-7.8	9.6-12.7	—			
Structure									
Affinity			66				1.5		
	Hb A_{1c}	642		6.5	8.1	21		5.3	3.8
	Total GHb	638		5.9-7.9	6.9-9.3	9		N/A	N/A
Immunoassay			7				56		
	Hb A_{1c}	129		5.7	3.5	1135		5.1-5.7	3.4-7.6

CV, Coefficient of variation; *Hb,* hemoglobin; *GHb,* glycated hemoglobin.
[a]Results are based on 1995 CAP Survey, Set EC-B, Specimen GH-03 and 2003 CAP Survey, Set GH2-A, Specimen GH2-02 (Copyright, 1995 and 2003 College of American Pathologists; data used with permission). See text for discussion of methods.
[b]n is the number of laboratories that participated in the survey.
[c]Indicates how many laboratories use the indicated method.
[d]Where more than one value is listed, the data vary among commercial assays. The range is presented.
[e]The NGSP value in 2003 was 5.2%.
[f]Number of participants was too low to permit statistical analysis.

certified by the National Glycohemoglobin Standardization Program (now known as the NGSP) as traceable to the DCCT reference.[15,241]

The GHb assays most widely used in the United States are depicted in Table 25-7. These data are based on results from 1947 laboratories participating in a 1995 quality control survey and 2008 laboratories participating in a 2003 quality control survey conducted by the CAP. The results demonstrate that in 2003 virtually all laboratories used immunoassay or ion-exchange chromatography. Hb A_{1c} was measured by more than 99% of laboratories (Table 25-7). Total GHb and Hb A_1 measurements had virtually disappeared. These results reflect significant changes from the methods used in 1995 when affinity chromatography was the most common analytical method (Table 25-7). Also, only 60% of laboratories reported Hb A_{1c} in 1995. In addition, the variation among mean values—both between and within methods—and imprecision were substantially lower in 2003. It should be borne in mind that these data refer only to these CAP surveys and are weighted to laboratories that participate. All of the methods described are commercially available from several different manufacturers. Moreover, differences in means among methods may reflect calibration and other differences in addition to inherent differences between methods.

Ion-Exchange Minicolumns

Ion-exchange chromatography separates hemoglobin variants on the basis of charge. The cation exchange resin (negatively charged), packed in a disposable minicolumn, has an affinity for hemoglobin, which is positively charged. The patient's sample is hemolyzed and an aliquot of the hemolysate is applied to the column. A buffer is applied and the eluent collected. The ionic strength and pH of the eluent buffer are selected so that GHbs are less positively charged than Hb A, do not bind as well to the negatively charged resin, and are therefore eluted first. The GHbs—A_{1a} + A_{1b} + A_{1c}, expressed collectively as Hb A_1—are measured in a spectrophotometer. A second buffer of different ionic strength can be added to the column to elute the more positively charged main hemoglobin fraction. This is read in the spectrophotometer and GHb is expressed as a percentage of total hemoglobin. Alternatively, only the Hb A_1 is eluted and a separate dilution of the original hemolysate is made, against which the Hb A_1 is compared. Numerous commercial modifications have been developed. Simple agitation of resins with hemolysates (batch technique) to adsorb Hb A has also been described. In this approach, the supernatant solution containing the Hb A_1 fraction is removed by filtration or centrifugation. Methods that separate Hb A_{1a+b} from Hb A_{1c} by using two different buffers have also been described.[180] Most of the current commercial ion-exchange methods use HPLC.

In all ion-exchange column methods, it is important to *control the temperature of the reagents and columns* to obtain accurate and reproducible results. This is best done by thermostatting the columns. Alternatively, a temperature correction factor can be applied if the room temperature differs from the specified optimum. In addition, rigid control of pH and ionic strength must be maintained. Sample storage conditions are also important.

The labile pre-Hb A_1 fractions elute with the stable ketoamine and produce spuriously high values unless destroyed by pretreatment of the red blood cells. Spuriously increased values are also obtained when the charge on hemoglobin is altered by the attachment of noncarbohydrate moieties, which may co-chromatograph with GHbs, as in uremia (carbamylated hemoglobin), alcoholism, lead poisoning, or chronic treatment with large doses of aspirin (acetylated hemoglobin). Hemoglobin variants or chemically modified hemoglobin that elute separately from Hb A and Hb A_{1c} have little effect on Hb A_{1c} measurements. If the modified hemoglobin (or its glycated derivative) cannot be separated from Hb A or Hb A_{1c}, spuriously increased or reduced results will be obtained.[46] A variant that elutes with Hb A_{1c} will yield a gross overestimation of Hb A_{1c}, and a variant that co-elutes with Hb A will underestimate Hb A_{1c}. Note that a single variant may falsely increase or decrease Hb A_{1c}, depending on the method used.[46]

High-Performance Liquid Chromatography

Hb A_{1c} and other hemoglobin fractions can be separated by HPLC, which employs cation-exchange chromatography.[71] Several fully automated systems are commercially available. Assays require only 5 µL of whole blood, and fingerstick samples can be collected in a capillary tube for analysis. Anticoagulated blood is diluted with a hemolysis reagent containing borate. Samples are incubated at 37 °C for 30 minutes to remove Schiff base and inserted in the autosampler. (Some instruments have a shorter preincubation step, and others [e.g., Tosoh A_{1c}2.2], separate labile A_{1c} chromatographically, eliminating the step to remove the Schiff base.)[103] A step gradient using three phosphate buffers of increasing ionic strength is passed through the column. Detection is performed at both 415 and 690 nm, and results are quantified by integrating the area under the peaks. Analysis time is as short as 3 to 5 minutes. All HPLC methods had CVs less than 3.5% in a 2003 CAP survey. Hb A_{1c} by HPLC was used for analysis of all patient samples in the DCCT[71] and UKPDS.

Electrophoresis

Agar gel electrophoresis on whole-blood hemolysates at pH 6.3 provides good resolution of Hb A and Hb A_1.[185] The gel contains negatively charged moieties that interact with the hemoglobin. After 25 to 35 minutes, the GHb separates on the cathodic side of Hb A. Quantification is performed by scanning densitometry at 415 nm. Results generally agree well with those obtained by HPLC or column chromatography, but are less precise.[185] Minor variations in pH, ionic strength, or temperature have little effect on results. Hb F migrates to the same region as Hb A_1 and causes a falsely increased Hb A_1 value, but Hb S and Hb C do not. The labile form should be removed before assaying.

Isoelectric Focusing

The hemoglobin variants separate on isoelectric focusing on the basis of their migration in gel containing a pH gradient.[262] Ampholines in the pH range of 6 to 8 establish the gradient in 1-mm-thick acrylamide gel slabs. As many as 35 samples per gel slab can be individually applied to filter paper tabs. On completion of isoelectric focusing, the gels are fixed and then scanned on a high-resolution integrating microdensitometer. Hb A_{1c} is adequately resolved from Hb A_{1a}, A_{1b}, S, and F. Results showed close agreement with other methods. The equipment is expensive and is not widely used in the United States, but is more popular in Europe.

Immunoassay

Assays for Hb A_{1c} have been developed using antibodies raised against the Amadori product of glucose (ketoamine linkage) plus the first few (four to eight) amino acids at the *N*-terminal end of the β-chain of hemoglobin.[85,139] A widely used assay measures Hb A_{1c} in whole blood by inhibition of latex agglutination. The agglutinator, a synthetic polymer containing multiple copies of the immunoreactive portion of Hb A_{1c}, binds the anti-Hb A_{1c} monoclonal antibody that is attached to latex beads. This agglutination produces light scattering, measured as an increase in absorbance. Hb A_{1c} in the patient's sample competes for the antibody on the latex, inhibiting agglutination, thereby decreasing light scattering. Enzyme immunoassays using monoclonal antibodies are commercially available and most exhibit low imprecision (see Table 25-7). These assays have been shown to correlate well with HPLC. The antibodies do not recognize labile intermediates or other GHbs (such as Hb A_{1a} or Hb A_{1b}) because both the ketoamine with glucose and the specific amino acid sequences are required for binding. Similarly, other hemoglobin variants, such as Hb F, Hb A_2, Hb S, and carbamylated hemoglobin are not detected.[46] The procedure has been adapted for capillary blood samples using a bench-top analyzer with reagent cartridges designed for use in physicians' office laboratories.

Affinity Chromatography

Affinity gel columns are used to separate GHb, which binds to the column, from the nonglycated fraction. *m*-Aminophenylboronic acid is immobilized by cross-linking to beaded agarose or another matrix (e.g., glass fiber). The boronic acid reacts with the *cis*-diol groups of glucose bound to hemoglobin to form a reversible five-member ring complex, thus selectively holding the GHb on the column (Figure 25-16). The nonglycated hemoglobin does not bind. Sorbitol is then added to elute the GHb. Absorbance of the bound and nonbound fractions, measured at 415 nm, is used to calculate the percentage of GHb.

A commercial assay is performed on an automated analyzer that uses a soluble reagent consisting of dihydroxyboronate coupled to high molecular weight polyacrylic acid.[294] GHb binds to the boronate. The polyanionic-glycated hemoglobin affinity complex attaches by electro-

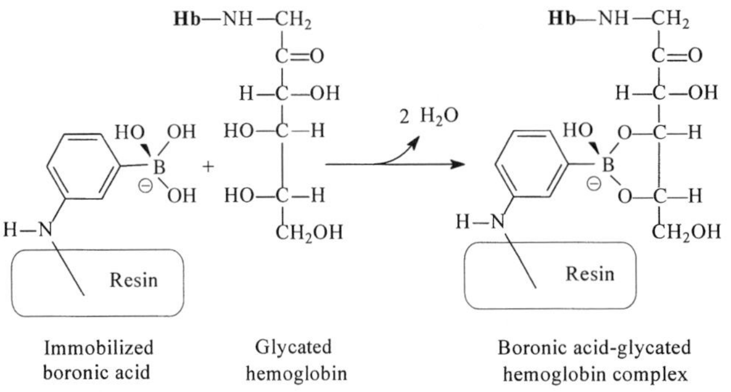

Figure 25-16 Reaction of GHb with immobilized boronic acid.

static interactions to the cationic surface of the solid phase matrix (ion capture). Nonglycated hemoglobin does not bind and is removed in a wash step. GHb is quantified by measuring the quenching by hemoglobin of the fluorescence of an added fluorophore, 4-methyl-umbelliferone. Total hemoglobin is determined by fluorescence quenching of a second sample containing sorbitol. The sorbitol competes for boronate binding sites, and both nonglycated and GHb contribute to inhibition of the quenching. The fluorescence measurements are converted to glycated and total hemoglobin concentrations from separate stored calibration curves.

The major advantages of affinity chromatography are as follows: There is no interference from nonglycated hemoglobins and negligible interference from the labile intermediate form of Hb A_{1c}. It is unaffected by variations in temperature and has reasonably good precision. Hemoglobin variants such as Hb F, Hb S, or Hb C produce little effect. Affinity methods measure total GHb. This includes components other than Hb A_{1c} because the assay detects ketoamine structures on lysine and valine residues on both α- and β-chains of hemoglobin.

Although the method detects all GHbs, several commercially available systems are calibrated to also report an Hb A_{1c} standardized value. The latter are derived from an equation obtained from correlation between total GHb and Hb A_{1c} analysis by HPLC.[294] A linear relationship has been demonstrated, and standardized Hb A_{1c} values are thus comparable with the values obtained by methods specific for Hb A_{1c}. Columns and reagents are readily available from a number of manufacturers, several of whom have automated the procedure.

Removal of Labile Glycated Hemoglobin from Red Blood Cells

The concentration of the labile form of Hb A_{1c} (Schiff base) fluctuates rapidly in response to acute changes in plasma glucose concentrations and should be removed before analysis by charge-based assays. This may be accomplished by incubating red blood cells in saline[110] or in buffer solutions at pH 5 to 6,[27] or by dialysis or ultrafiltration of hemolysates. Most kits for column assays contain reagents to remove this labile component.

Assay Standardization

Clinical laboratories measure GHb with diverse assays that use multiple methods and quantify different components. The DCCT results accentuated the need for accurate GHb measurement and provided a strong impetus for standardization of GHb assays. At the end of the DCCT, it was noted that the absence of both a reference method and a single GHb standard had generated confusion.[245] Interlaboratory comparisons were not possible, and even a single quality-control sample analyzed by a single method exhibited CVs as high as 16.5%. Similar large variability among laboratories was observed in Europe.[104] Committees were established under the auspices of the American Association for Clinical Chemistry and the International Federation of Clinical Chemistry and Laboratory Medicine (IFCC) to standardize GHb assays.

The NGSP (http://web.missouri.edu/~diabetes/ngsp.html) was implemented in 1996 to calibrate GHb results to DCCT-equivalent values. Employing a network of reference laboratories, the NGSP interacts with manufacturers of GHb methods to help them calibrate their methods and trace the values to the DCCT.[171] Manufacturers apply for certification by performing precision testing following NCCLS EP5-A guidelines and report results in DCCT-equivalent hemoglobin A_{1c} values. This calibration effort has markedly improved harmonization of results and reduced imprecision.[171] Results obtained using NGSP-certified assays can be compared with the results of the DCCT and UKPDS, allowing alignment to clinical outcomes data. The ADA recommends that clinical laboratories use only assays certified by the NGSP and participate in proficiency testing offered by the CAP. The CAP-GH2 survey uses pooled whole blood specimens at three GHb concentrations. Target values are assigned by the NGSP network. Thus individual laboratories can directly compare their GHb results with those of the DCCT.

A different approach was adopted by the IFCC. In 1995 a working group was established to devise a reference system for standardization based on Hb A_{1c}. The IFCC group developed a mixture of purified Hb A_{1c} and Hb A_0 as primary reference material.[159] Two candidate reference methods, namely electrospray ionization mass spectrometry (ESI-MS) and capillary electrophoresis, were proposed.[159] These specifically measure the glycated *N*-terminal valine of the β-chain of hemoglobin. Analysis is performed by digesting the hemoglobin molecule with endoproteinase Glu-C, which cleaves the β-chain between Glu-6 and Glu-7, releasing the *N*-terminal hexapeptide. The glycated and nonglycated hexapeptides are separated and quantified by HPLC-ESI-MS or by HPLC-capillary electrophoresis.[159] Hb A_{1c} is measured as the ratio between glycated and nonglycated *N*-terminal hexapeptides. Comparisons between the IFCC and NGSP reference methods (and other reference systems, including others from Japan and Sweden) are under investigation.

Initial analysis indicates a close and stable relationship. However, the Hb A_{1c} results obtained using IFCC reference methods are 1.5% to 2% lower than those of the NGSP (and lower than other reference systems). The difference is probably due to measurement of glycated components other than Hb A_{1c} by the HPLC used by the NGSP. International harmonization would allow worldwide alignment of GHb results with patient outcomes in DCCT and UKPDS. If the IFCC reference method exhibits long-term stability and has a robust relationship with the NGSP, the IFCC method may eventually become the reference method for the NGSP. Consultations among clinicians and laboratorians have been initiated to reach an international consensus on how to reconcile the different Hb A_{1c} values between the standardization programs, with the ultimate goal of enhancing patient care.

Specimen Collection and Storage

Patients need not be fasting. Venous blood should be collected in tubes containing EDTA, oxalate, or fluoride. Sample stability depends on the assay method.[241] Whole blood may be stored at 4 °C for up to 1 week. Above 4 °C, Hb A_{1a+b} increases in a time- and temperature-dependent manner, but Hb A_{1c} is only slightly affected.[259] Storage of samples at −20 °C is not recommended. For most methods, whole blood samples stored at −70 °C are stable for at least 18 months.[83] Heparinized samples should be assayed within 2 days and may not be suitable for some methods of analysis (e.g., electrophoresis).

Reference Intervals

Values for GHbs are expressed as a percentage of total blood hemoglobin. One of three major GHb species, namely Hb A_1, Hb A_{1c}, or total GHb, is usually measured. In the United States, the vast majority of laboratories now measure Hb A_{1c}. Reference intervals vary, depending on the GHb component measured and whether the labile fraction is included in the assay. A consensus, based on several studies of apparently healthy subjects, suggests the following reference intervals:

	Mean (%)	Interval (%)
Hb A_1 (A_{1a+b+c})	6.5	5.0-8.0
Hb A_{1c} only (DCCT-equivalent)	4.5	4.0-6.0
Total glycated Hb ($A_1 + A_0$)	5.5	4.5-7.0

The effects of age on reference intervals are controversial.[241] Some studies show age-related increases (~0.1% per decade after age 30), and other reports show no increase.[151,292] Results are not affected by acute illness. Intraindividual variability is minimal.[238] In patients with poorly controlled diabetes mellitus, values may extend to twice the upper limit of the reference interval or more but rarely exceed 15%. Values greater than 15% should prompt further studies to determine the possible presence of variant hemoglobin.[46] Note that ADA target values derived from DCCT and UKPDS, not the reference values, are used to evaluate metabolic control in patients.

There is no specific value of Hb A_{1c} below which the risk of diabetic complications is eliminated completely. The ADA states that the goal of treatment should be to maintain Hb A_{1c} less than 7%.[15] (Some organizations recommend an Hb A_{1c} target of less than 6.5%.) These values are applicable only if the assay method is certified as traceable to the DCCT reference. Each laboratory should establish its own nondiabetic reference interval. Assay precision is important because each 1% change in Hb A_{1c} represents an approximate 35 mg/dL change in average blood glucose.

There is no consensus on optimum frequency of testing. The ADA recommends that *GHb should be routinely monitored at least every 6 months in patients meeting treatment goals (and who have stable glycemic control).*[15] These recommendations are for patients with either type 1 or type 2 diabetes. In certain clinical situations, such as diabetic pregnancy, when patients are not meeting treatment goals, or a major change in therapy, more frequent monitoring (e.g., every 3 months) may provide useful information.

FRUCTOSAMINE

Clinical Significance

In selected patients with diabetes mellitus (e.g., GDM or change in therapy), there may be a need for assays that are more sensitive than GHb to shorter-term alterations in average blood glucose levels. Nonenzymatic attachment of glucose to amino groups of proteins other than hemoglobin (e.g., serum proteins, membrane proteins, and lens crystallins) to form ketoamines also occurs. Because serum proteins turn over more rapidly than erythrocytes (the circulating half-life for albumin is about 20 days), *the concentration of glycated serum albumin reflects glucose control over a period of 2 to 3 weeks.* Therefore evidence of both deterioration of control and improvement with therapy is evident earlier than with GHb.

Fructosamine is the generic name for plasma protein ketoamines (for reviews, see Armbruster[16] and Hill et al[121]). The name refers to the structure of the ketoamine rearrangement product formed by the interaction of glucose with the ε-amino group on lysine residues of albumin. Analogous to GHb, measurement of fructosamine may be used as an index of the average concentration of blood glucose over an extended period of time.

Because all glycated serum proteins are fructosamines and albumin is the most abundant serum protein, measurement of fructosamine is thought to be largely a measure of glycated albumin, but this has been questioned by some investigators.[250] Although the fructosamine assay can be automated and is cheaper and faster than GHb, *there is a lack of consensus on its clinical utility.* For example, evaluation of 65 studies led the authors to conclude that fructosamine determination is not a reliable test and has not been evaluated sufficiently for routine clinical use.[296] In contrast, a review of essentially the same data concluded that fructosamine could provide information useful in the management of diabetes.[16] Early work using the original assay, introduced in 1983,[23,141] indicated that fructosamine concentrations were significantly higher in diabetic individuals than in healthy subjects. Over the succeeding decade, the assay underwent numerous modifications because several artifacts were identified that rendered the data from the first-generation fructosamine assay difficult to interpret. These include an apparent lack of specificity for glycated proteins (up to 60% of the value was due to nonfructosamine reducing substances), lack of standardization among laboratories, difficulty in calibrating the assay, and interference by urates and hyperlipidemia.[31] Substantial modifications produced second-generation assays that contain uricase and higher detergent concentrations and are calibrated with glycated lysine.[251] In addition, an industry standard was adopted. These improvements resulted in average fructosamine values in nondiabetics that are approximately 10% of those obtained with the first-generation assay. Some clinical evidence suggests that fructosamine may be useful in the elderly[52] and in pregnancy.[148] The potential role of the second-generation fructosamine assay in providing rapid, reliable, inexpensive, and technically easy monitoring of glycemic control requires evaluation. The clinical value of fructosamine has not been firmly established, and there is no convincing evidence that relates its concentration to the chronic complications of diabetes.[241]

As fructosamine determination monitors short-term glycemic changes different from GHb, it may have a role in conjunction with GHb rather than instead of it. In addition, fructosamine may be useful in patients with hemoglobin variants, such as Hb S or Hb C, that are associated with decreased erythrocyte lifespan where GHb is of little value. Gross changes in protein concentration and half-life may have large effects on the proportion of protein that is glycated. Thus fructosamine results may be invalid in patients with nephrotic syndrome, cirrhosis of the liver, or dysproteinemias, or after rapid changes in acute phase reactants. Initial reports indicated that, in the absence of significant alterations in serum protein concentrations, fructosamine results were independent of protein concentrations.[24] However, this observation has been questioned by other investigators who recommend that fructosamine values be corrected for protein concentrations. This issue remains to be resolved. It is generally accepted that the test should not be performed when serum albumin is less than 30 g/L. Although it was initially postulated that the fructosamine assay would replace the OGTT, *there is no role for the fructosamine assay in the diagnosis of diabetes mellitus.* The second-generation fructosamine assay has been reported to have a sensitivity and specificity of close to 80% in screening patients for GDM[132] but this study requires verification.

Determination of Fructosamine

Methods for measuring glycated proteins include (1) affinity chromatography using immobilized phenylboronic acid (similar to the GHb assay)[300]; (2) HPLC of glycated lysine residues after hydrolysis of the glycated proteins[249]; (3) a photometric procedure in which mild acid hydrolysis releases 5-hydroxymethylfurfural—proteins are precipitated with trichloroacetic acid and the supernatant is reacted with 2-thiobarbituric acid[81]; and (4) other procedures using phenylhydrazine and ε-*N*-(2-furoylmethyl)-L-lysine (furosine). None of these assays is popular because they are not suitable for routine clinical laboratories. The development of monoclonal antibodies to glycated albumin,[64] although theoretically advantageous, has not yet resulted in the widespread availability of commercial glycated albumin assays. It should be noted that prolonged storage at ultra-low temperatures (−96 °C) prevents in vitro glycation of serum proteins.[25]

An alternative method for the measurement of fructosamine is a modification[170,251] of the original method of Johnson and colleagues,[141] details of which are included in the Evolve site that accompanies this book. This method is conducted under alkaline conditions and results in fructosamine undergoing an Amadori rearrangement and the resultant compounds having reducing activity that can be differentiated from other reducing substances. In the presence of carbonate buffer, fructosamine rearranges to the eneaminol form, which reduces NBT to a formazan (Figure 25-17). The absorbance at 530 nm is measured at two time points and the absorbance change is proportional to the fructosamine concentration. A 10-minute preincubation is necessary to allow fast-reacting interfering reducing substances to react. It is unnecessary to remove endogenous glucose from patients' samples because a pH greater than 11 is required for glucose to reduce NBT. The assay is easily automated and has excellent between-batch analytical precision. Hemoglobin (greater than 100 mg/dL) and bilirubin (greater than 4 mg/dL) interfere; therefore moderate to grossly hemolyzed and icteric samples should not be used. Ascorbic acid concentrations greater than 5 mg/dL may cause negative interference. Kits are commercially available

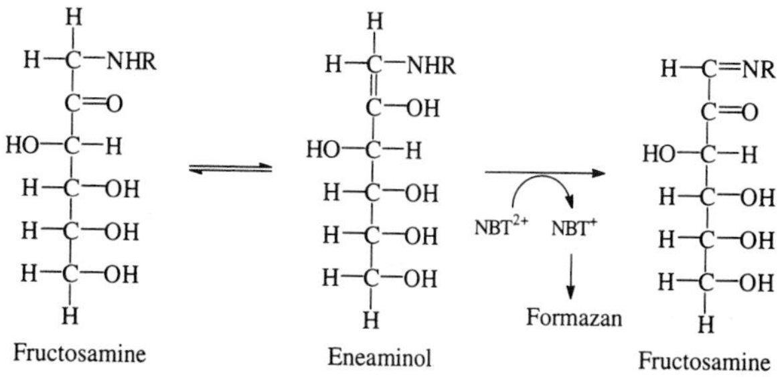

Fructosamine ⇌ Eneaminol → (NBT^{2+} → NBT^{+} → Formazan) Fructosamine

Figure 25-17 Reaction of fructosamine with NBT.

(Roche Diagnostics, Indianapolis). An assay that measures fructosamine by oxidizing the ketoamine bond using ketoamine oxidase, with the release of H_2O_2 that is quantified by a photometric reaction, is available (Randox, Oceanside, Calif.). An FDA-approved device using a hand-held meter for home use by adults excluding pregnant women and children (InCharge, LXN Corp., San Diego) has been discontinued.

Reference Intervals

Values in a nondiabetic population range from 205 to 285 µmol/L. The reference interval corrected for albumin is 191 to 265 µmol/L.

Advanced Glycation End Products

The molecular mechanism by which hyperglycemia produces toxic effects is unknown, but glycation of tissue proteins may be important. Nonenzymatic attachment of glucose to long-lived proteins, such as collagen or DNA, produces stable Amadori early-glycated products. These undergo a series of additional rearrangements, dehydration, and fragmentation reactions, resulting in stable *advanced glycation end products* (AGE). The amounts of these products do not return to normal when hyperglycemia is corrected, and they accumulate continuously over the lifespan of the protein. Hyperglycemia accelerates the formation of protein-bound AGE, and patients with diabetes mellitus thus have more AGE than healthy subjects. Through effects on the functional properties of protein and extracellular matrix, AGE may contribute to the microvascular and macrovascular complications of diabetes mellitus.[44,281] Moreover, an inhibitor of AGE formation, aminoguanidine, has been shown to prevent several of the complications of diabetes in experimental animal models and is undergoing clinical trials in patients.

Several assays for AGE have been developed. An early method, AGE-dependent relative *fluorescence,* suffered from spurious contributions to total fluorescence by non-AGE protein adducts, such as glucose- or lipid-derived oxidation products, that have similar fluorescence spectra. A *radioreceptor assay,* based on the presence of AGE receptors on the surface of a macrophage-like tumor cell line, that was capable of quantifying AGE on both circulating (albumin) and tissue proteins was developed.[227] *Antibodies* were also raised against AGE–keyhole limpet hemocyanin[198] and AGE-bovine serum albumin.[127] These antibodies react with several AGE-proteins. A competitive ELISA using polyclonal anti-AGE antibody was developed to measure hemoglobin-AGE.[178] Using this assay, a linear correlation was demonstrated between Hb A_{1c} and hemoglobin-AGE. In healthy people, hemoglobin-AGE accounts for 0.4% of circulating hemoglobin, with significantly higher values in patients with diabetes mellitus. After an acute change in glycemia, hemoglobin-AGE levels change, but the rate of alteration is 23% slower than that of Hb A_{1c}.[297] Thus hemoglobin-AGE provides a measure of diabetic control longer than that indicated by GHb, reflecting blood glucose concentrations over a greater proportion of the life of red blood cells. It remains to be established whether knowledge of hemoglobin-AGE values offers clinical benefit.

URINARY ALBUMIN EXCRETION

Clinical Significance

Patients with diabetes mellitus are at high risk of suffering renal damage. End-stage renal disease requiring dialysis or transplantation develops in approximately one third of patients with type 1 diabetes,[229] and diabetes is the most common cause of end-stage renal disease in the United States and Europe.[193] Although nephropathy is less common in patients with type 2 diabetes, approximately 60% of all cases of diabetic nephropathy occur in these patients because of the higher incidence of this form of diabetes. Early detection of diabetic nephropathy relies on tests of urinary excretion of albumin. Persistent proteinuria detectable by routine screening tests (equivalent to a urinary albumin excretion [UAE] rate greater than or equal to 200 µg/min) indicates overt diabetic nephropathy. This is usually associated with long-standing disease and is unusual less than 5 years after the onset of type 1 diabetes. Once diabetic nephropathy occurs, renal function deteriorates rapidly and renal insufficiency evolves. Treatment at this stage can retard the rate of progression but not stop or reverse the renal damage. Preceding this stage is a period of increased UAE not detected by routine methods. This range of 20 to 200 µg/min (or 30 to 300 mg/24 hr) of increased UAE defines *microalbuminuria.* Note that it is not defined in terms of urinary albumin concentration, although the albumin:creatinine ratio can be used as a substitute for albumin measurements in a time collection of urine as described below. The term *microalbuminuria,* although generally accepted, is misleading. It implies a small version of the albumin molecule rather than an excretion rate of albumin greater than normal but less than that detectable by routine methods. A more accurate term would be *paucialbuminuria,* but the term microalbuminuria is well entrenched and is unlikely to be superseded.

The presence of increased UAE denotes an increase in the transcapillary escape rate of albumin and is therefore a marker of microvascular disease. Persistent UAE greater than 20 µg/min represents a twentyfold greater risk for the development of clinically overt renal disease in patients with type 1 and type 2 diabetes. Prospective studies have demonstrated that increased UAE precedes and is highly predictive of diabetic nephropathy, end-stage renal disease, cardiovascular mortality, and total mortality in patients with diabetes mellitus.[191,193] The DCCT and UKPDS showed that intensive diabetes therapy can significantly reduce the risk of development of increased UAE and overt nephropathy in people with diabetes.[72,280] In addition, increased UAE identifies a group of nondiabetic subjects at increased risk of coronary artery disease.[101,164] Interventions, such as control of blood glucose concentrations and blood pressure, particularly with angiotensin converting enzyme (ACE) inhibitors, slow the rate of decline in renal function.[193]

METHODS FOR MEASURING URINARY ALBUMIN EXCRETION

There is no consensus about how a urine sample should be collected for measuring UAE. Variations in urine flow rate in a person may be corrected by expressing albumin as a ratio to creatinine (i.e., albumin : creatinine). *UAE is increased by physiological factors* (e.g., exercise, posture, and diuresis) and the method of urine collection must be standardized. Samples should not be collected after exertion, in the presence of urinary tract infection, during acute illness, immediately after surgery, or after an acute fluid load. All the following urine samples are currently acceptable: (1) 24-hour collection; (2) overnight (8 to 12 hours, timed) collection; (3) 1- to 2-hour timed collection (in laboratory or clinic); or (4) first morning sample for simultaneous albumin and creatinine measurement. Only results for timed specimens can be reported as mg albumin excreted per hour, but the albumin : creatinine ratio is more practical and convenient for the patient and is the recommended method.[15] A first morning void sample is best because it has a lower within-person variation for the albumin : creatinine ratio than a random urine sample.[241] *At least three separate specimens, collected on different days, should be assayed* because of the high intraindividual variation (CV of 30% to 50%) and diurnal variation (50% to 100% higher during the day). Urine should be stored at 4 °C after collection. Alternatively, 2 mL of 50 g/L sodium azide can be added per 500 mL of urine, but preservatives are not recommended for some assays. Bacterial contamination and glucose have no effect. Specimens are stable for 2 weeks at 4 °C and for at least 5 months at −80 °C. Albumin concentration decreased by 0.27% at −20 °C.[177] Freezing samples has been reported to decrease albumin,[84] but mixing immediately before assay eliminates this effect.

Semiquantitative Assays

A number of semiquantitative assays for screening for increased UAE are available. These test strips, most of which are optimized to read "positive" at a predetermined albumin concentration, have been recommended for screening programs. In view of the wide variability in UAE, it must be borne in mind that a "normal" value does not rule out renal disease. *Because these assays measure albumin concentration, dilute urine may yield a false-negative test result.* Refrigerated urine samples should be allowed to reach at least 10 °C before analysis. Albu Screen and Albu Sure (Cambridge Life Sciences, Cambridge, United Kingdom) detect urinary albumin concentrations exceeding 20 and 30 mg/L, respectively. The assay is a latex agglutination inhibition test. Briefly, one drop of urine is mixed with one drop of goat anti-human albumin, the titer of which is adjusted so that all the antibody-binding sites are occupied at urinary albumin concentrations of 30 mg/L or greater. Excess albumin-binding sites are detected by adding one drop of albumin-coated latex microspheres and rocking for 2 minutes. Albumin concentrations less than 20 mg/L produce agglutination. Micro-bumintest (Bayer Corp., Tarrytown, N.Y.) uses bromophenol blue in an alkaline matrix to detect albumin concentrations exceeding 40 mg/L. The assay sensitivity for increased urinary albumin as measured by quantitative assays is approximately 95%, but because other proteins are also detected, the specificity is approximately 80%.

Micral (Roche Diagnostics, Indianapolis) uses a monoclonal antialbumin IgG complexed to β-galactosidase. The albumin in the urine binds to the antibody-enzyme conjugate in the test strip. Excess conjugate is retained in a separation zone containing immobilized albumin, and only albumin bound to the antibody-enzyme immunocomplex diffuses to the reaction zone. Here it reacts with a buffered substrate (chlorophenol red galactoside) to produce a red color when the β-galactosidase hydrolyzes galactose. The test strip is dipped into the urine for 5 seconds and the intensity of the color after 5 minutes is proportional to the urinary albumin concentration. Direct visual comparison is made with printed color blocks—yellow, light brown, medium brown, brick red, and burgundy representing 0, 10, 20, 50, and 100 mg/L, respectively. No interference is observed with drugs, glucose, urea, or other proteins. Comparison with a reference method demonstrates a sensitivity and specificity for albumin concentrations greater than 20 mg/L (not for microalbuminuria defined by UAE rate) of approximately 100% and 91%, respectively.[182] The *time that the stick is in contact with the urine and the time of reading are critical.* A modification (Micral II) uses a gold-labeled, instead of an enzyme-labeled, antibody. This enhances the stability, allowing the strip to be read any time from 1 to at least 60 minutes. Urine samples with albumin concentrations greater than 100 to 300 mg/L may be diluted and reassayed. The assigned concentration of the color block is multiplied by the dilution factor to obtain the concentration in the sample. These semiquantitative assays have been *recommended for screening only.* However, published studies reveal sensitivities for detection of increased UAE from 67% to 91%.[241] These low sensitivities limit the value of semiquantitative tests even for screening, and further studies are necessary before the dipstick tests can be recommended as replacements for the quantitative tests.[241]

Quantitative Assays

All the sensitive, specific assays for urine albumin use immunochemistry with antibodies to human albumin. Four methodologies are available: RIA, ELISA, radial immunodiffusion, and immunoturbidimetry.[184] Each method has advantages and disadvantages, and the choice depends on local experience and technical support. In general, the *methods have similar imprecisions, detection limits, and ranges.* A comparison of these methodologies has been performed.[286] Although dye-binding[253] and protein-precipitation[220] assays have been described, these are insensitive and nonspecific and should not be used.

Radial Immunodiffusion

Radial immunodiffusion has not gained wide acceptance because it requires long incubation and a high level of technical skill and cannot be automated. The antibody is incorporated into an agar gel. Aliquots of samples and calibrators are added to wells and allowed to diffuse into the agar. The antigen-antibody complexes precipitate at equilibrium, and after staining, the distance of migration is measured.

Radioimmunoassay

Standard RIA methods have been described[298] with ^{125}I-labeled albumin and antialbumin antiserum, but reagents are radioactive and have a short shelf life. Commercial kits are available.

Enzyme-Linked Immunosorbent Assay

Both competitive and "sandwich" ELISAs are available.[58,277] Although the competitive ELISA is faster because it uses only one incubation with an antibody, it is reported to be less sensitive and exhibits large imprecision. ELISA can be performed on a microplate reader, allowing semiautomation. In the sandwich assay, the primary antibody (antialbumin antiserum) is fixed on the plastic plate, which is then washed. Samples, controls, and calibrators are added, and the complexes detected and quantified by a second antibody conjugated to an enzyme label.

An ELISA method is described in the Evolve site that accompanies this book.

Immunoturbidimetry

Albumin in the urine sample forms an insoluble complex with antibodies to human albumin. PEG accelerates complex formation. The turbidity caused by the complexes is measured by a spectrophotometer at 340 nm and is a measure of albumin concentration. The background absorbance of the initial urine sample is subtracted automatically. This method is simple and less expensive than RIA, and rapid analysis of large numbers of samples is possible. The assays may be performed as either kinetic or equilibrium reactions. Kits are commer-cially available for use on automated analyzers (Roche Diagnostics).

An immunoturbidimetric method for urinary albumin is described in the Evolve site that accompanies this book.

Reference Intervals

URINARY ALBUMIN EXCRETION

	μg/min	mg/24 hr	Corrected (mg/g Urine Creatinine)
Normal	<20	<30	<30
Increased UAE	20-200	30-300	30-300
Clinical albuminuria*	>200	>300	>300

*Also termed "overt nephropathy."

The ADA position statement[15] recommends initial UAE measurement in type 1 diabetes patients who have had diabetes more than or equal to 5 years and in all type 2 diabetic patients. Because of the difficulty in dating the onset of type 2 diabetes, screening should commence at diagnosis. Analysis should be performed annually in all patients who have a negative screening result. Screening may be performed with a semiquantitative assay. If the screening result is positive, UAE should be evaluated by a quantitative assay. Diagnosis requires the demonstration of increased UAE in at least two of three tests measured within a 6-month period.

If the confirmatory test result is positive, treatment with an ACE inhibitor or angiotensin-receptor blocker should be initiated. ACE inhibitors delay the progression to overt nephropathy, and the National Kidney Foundation recommends their use in both normotensive and hypertensive type 1 and 2 diabetic patients.[32] The role of monitoring UAE in patients on ACE inhibitor therapy is less clear, although many experts recommend continued surveillance.[15] Untreated, the UAE would increase 10% to 30% per year, whereas the albumin : creatinine ratio in patients on ACE inhibitors should stabilize or decrease by up to 50%.

INBORN ERRORS OF CARBOHYDRATE METABOLISM

Deficiency or absence of an enzyme that participates in carbohydrate metabolism may result in accumulation of monosaccharides, which can be measured in the urine (see Table 25-1 and Figure 25-9). Most of these conditions are inherited as autosomal recessive traits. Sugars frequently appear in the urine as a result of excessive consumption without underlying disease.

DISORDERS OF GALACTOSE METABOLISM

Galactose is derived from milk in the diet. It resembles glucose in structure, but the hydroxyl group on the fourth carbon has a different spatial arrangement (see Figure 25-2). A deficiency of any of the enzymes that participate in the conversion of galactose to glucose results in *galactosemia.*

Galactose-1-Phosphate Uridyl Transferase Deficiency

Infants with this deficiency fail to thrive on milk because half of the milk sugar, lactose, is galactose. Within a few days of milk ingestion, neonates manifest vomiting and diarrhea. Failure to thrive, liver disease, cataracts, and mental retardation develop later. Hypoglycemia may occasionally develop. The diagnosis should be considered when *the urine demonstrates the presence of a reducing substance that does not react in a glucose oxidase test.* Early detection and treatment (withholding galactose from the diet) are necessary to prevent irreversible changes. Because other reducing sugars may give similar results, galactose should be identified by paper chromatography (discussed later). Diagnosis is suggested by detecting galactose and galactose-1-phosphate in blood and confirmed by directly assaying red blood cell transferase activity. A spot test is also available.

Uridine Diphosphate Galactose-4-Epimerase Deficiency

This extremely rare disorder exhibits clinical findings similar to transferase deficiency.

Galactokinase Deficiency

This is a milder condition manifested predominantly by cataracts caused by galactitol deposits in the lens. The diagnosis is confirmed by demonstrating normal transferase activity and no galactokinase in red blood cells.

Disorders of Fructose Metabolism

Fructose may appear in the urine after eating fruits, honey, and syrups, but has no significance in these circumstances. Three disorders of fructose metabolism, inherited as autosomal recessive traits, produce fructosuria.

Essential Fructosuria

This rare and harmless defect is due to a lack of *fructokinase.*

Hereditary Fructose Intolerance

A *deficiency of fructose-1-phosphate aldolase* produces this rare disorder with hypoglycemia and liver failure. Fructose ingestion inhibits glycogenolysis and gluconeogenesis, producing hypoglycemia. Early detection is important because this condition responds to a diet devoid of sucrose and fructose.

Hereditary Fructose-1,6-Diphosphatase Deficiency

Patients with this deficiency have episodes of apnea and hyperventilation and hypoglycemia, ketosis, and lactic acidosis caused by severe impairment of gluconeogenesis. Diagnosis is by demonstrating the enzyme defect in liver biopsy specimens.

Disorders of Pentose Metabolism

Alimentary Pentosuria

Pentoses may be present in the urine after eating large quantities of fruits such as cherries, plums, or prunes.

Essential Pentosuria

This is a harmless inborn error caused by a *deficiency of L-xylulose reductase,* an enzyme involved in the glucuronic acid pathway.

Other Urinary Sugars

Lactose is sometimes detected in the urine of women during lactation and occasionally toward the end of pregnancy. Patients with *lactase deficiency,* a common disorder caused by a congenital or acquired deficiency of intestinal lactase, exhibit abdominal pain, diarrhea, and lactose in the urine.

Maltose has rarely been detected in the urine of some patients.

Many *reducing substances* other than sugars may be found in urine (Box 25-6). Ascorbic acid (vitamin C) may be ingested in large quantities or may be present in antibiotic preparations administered intravenously. In either case, excess concentrations usually appear in the urine and contribute significantly to the total reducing substances present.

Methods for Measuring Individual Sugars

Qualitative Tests for Glucose

Techniques for separating and identifying sugars have included fermentation, optical rotation, osazone formation with phenylhydrazine, specific chemical tests, and paper or thin-layer chromatography. The availability of glucose oxidase test strips, specific for glucose, has greatly simplified the differentiation of glucose from other reducing substances. For practical purposes, the *urinary sugars of clinical interest are glucose and galactose.* Urine from infants and children should be tested routinely by both the glucose oxidase and copper reduction tests to identify individuals with inborn errors of metabolism. Reducing substances other than glucose should be further identified by chromatographic procedures.

Qualitative Tests for Urinary Sugars Other Than Glucose

Fructose (Selivanoff's Test)

Hot HCl converts fructose to hydroxymethyl furfural (HMF), which links with *resorcinol* to produce a red compound. To make the reagent, dissolve 50 mg of resorcinol in 33 mL of concentrated HCl and dilute to 100 mL with water. Add 0.5 mL of urine to 5 mL of reagent in a test tube and bring to a boil. Fructose produces a red reaction within 30 seconds. The test is sensitive to 100 mg fructose per dL, provided there is no excess glucose. A 2-g/dL solution of glucose produces about the same color as 100 mg/dL of fructose after 30 seconds of boiling. A solution of fructose (0.5 g/dL) should be used as a control. With high concentrations of fructose, a red precipitate forms.

Pentoses (Bial's Test)

By heating with HCl, pentoses are converted to furfural, which reacts with orcinol to form green compounds. Dissolve 300 mg of orcinol in 100 mL of concentrated HCl and add 0.25 mL of ferric chloride solution (10 g/dL). Glucose, if present in the urine, should be removed by fermentation with yeast. Add 0.5 mL of urine to 5 mL of reagent in a test tube and bring to a boil. Pentoses produce a green reaction. The detection limit of the test is 100 mg pentose per dL. A solution of xylose (0.5 g/dL) should be used as a control. Glucuronates produce a similar color if the boiling is prolonged. As with Selivanoff's reagent, fructose produces a red reaction.

Identification of Urinary Sugars by Paper Chromatography

Sugars can be separated by ascending or descending chromatography on paper and located after color development with dinitrosalicylic acid. The variable rates of migration depend on the solubility of the sugars in the particular solvent system. Presumptive identification is made by comparison of the migration (R_f) value of the unknown with those of reference compounds. One procedure may be performed conveniently in a 6 × 18-inch Pyrex jar with a tightly fitting cover.

This method for identifying urinary sugars by paper chromatography is described in the Evolve site that accompanies this book.

Identification of Urinary Sugars by Thin-Layer Chromatography

Identification of urine sugars can also be made by using thin-layer chromatographic techniques as described by Young and Jackson.[302] When frequent chromatographic separations are necessary, this method is preferred over paper chromatography because of the shorter time required. If such studies are performed infrequently, paper chromatography is simple, is adequate for most separations, and requires little actual working time.

GLYCOGEN STORAGE DISEASE

Glycogen, although present in most tissue, is stored principally in the liver and skeletal muscle. During fasting, liver glycogen is converted to glucose to provide energy for the whole body. In contrast, skeletal muscle lacks glucose-6-phosphatase, and muscle glycogen can be used only locally for energy. *Glycogen storage disease* is a generic name encompassing at least 10 rare inherited disorders of glycogen storage in tissue (Table 25-1). The different forms of glycogen storage disease are categorized by numerical type in the chronological sequence in which these defects were identified. Each form is due to a deficiency of a specific enzyme in glycogen metabolism, producing either a quantitative or qualitative defect of glycogen storage. Because the liver and skeletal muscle have the highest rates of glycogen metabolism, these are the structures most affected. The liver forms (types I, III, IV, and VI) are marked by *hepatomegaly* (caused by increased liver glycogen stores) and *hypoglycemia* (caused by the inability to convert glycogen to glucose). The hypoglycemia is manifested by autonomic clinical symptoms (sweating, shakiness, and lightheaded feeling), growth retardation, and laboratory findings of decreased insulin and increased glucagon concentrations in the blood. The muscle forms (types II, IIIA, V, and VII), in contrast, have mild symptoms that *usually appear in young adulthood during strenuous exercise* owing to the inability to provide energy for muscle contraction. Other muscle disorders may exhibit similar symptoms but can be readily differentiated by evaluating glycogen stores. The specific diagnosis of each type is made directly by *demonstrating the enzyme defect in tissue.* A very brief overview is provided here; for a more detailed description, readers should consult Chen and Burchell.[57]

Type I (Glucose-6-Phosphatase Deficiency)

Type I is the most common and severe form (also called *von Gierke's disease*), and patients have accumulation of glycogen of normal chemical structure in the liver. The disease is characterized by massive hepatomegaly, growth retardation, fasting hypoglycemia, increased lactic acid concentrations in the blood (caused by excessive glycolysis), hyperuricemia (caused by competitive inhibition by lactate of renal tubular urate secretion and increased uric acid production), and hypertriglyceridemia (increased lipolysis caused by decreased glucose). Glucagon and epinephrine do not produce hyperglycemia but result in increased lactate concentrations. The failure of blood glucose to increase in response to galactose administration (oral or intravenous) is diagnostic. Galactose is normally converted to glucose (see Figure 25-9), but in these patients glucose-6-phosphate cannot be hydrolyzed to glucose. Treatment includes partaking of frequent meals and nasogastric feeding at night to maintain blood glucose concentrations. Glucose-6-phosphatase activity can be assayed in a liver biopsy. A variant of the disease, type IB, has been identified as a defect in the glucose-6-phosphatase transport system. Other forms include a defect in microsomal phosphate or pyrophosphate transport (type IC) and a defect in microsomal glucose transport (type ID).

Individuals with type I glycogen storage disease (von Gierke's) exhibit decreased availability of liver glycogen demonstrated by a decreased or absent blood glucose response to epinephrine administration. An assay based on this phenomenon is known as the "epinephrine tolerance test." With it an intramuscular injection of 1 mL of a 1/1000 (1-g/L) solution of epinephrine hydrochloride is given, and blood samples are taken at 30, 45, 60, 90, and 120 minutes. Normal people increase blood glucose by 35 to 45 mg/dL in 40 to 60 minutes, with a return to the fasting concentration by 2 hours. The test is rarely used because the diagnosis of von Gierke's disease is made by a failure to increase blood glucose in response to galactose administration, with confirmation by direct assay of glucose-6-phosphatase activity.

TYPE II (ACID α-GLUCOSIDASE DEFICIENCY)

Type II affects predominantly the heart and skeletal muscle, producing muscle weakness and cardiomegaly. Liver function is normal and patients do not have hypoglycemia. Two forms are identified: (1) infantile (*Pompe disease*), which presents in the first few months of life with symptoms of weakness and respiratory difficulties and usually evolves to death caused by cardiac failure within 1 year; and (2) a juvenile form that is milder and may present in the second or third decade of life with difficulty in walking. The diagnosis is made by measuring α-glucosidase activity in muscle, liver, or leukocytes.

TYPE III (AMYLO-1,6-GLUCOSIDASE DEFICIENCY)

Deficiency of glycogen debranching enzyme results in storage of an abnormal form of glycogen (limit dextrinosis). Both the liver and muscle are usually affected (type IIIA), producing hepatomegaly and muscle weakness. Approximately 15% of patients have only liver involvement, without apparent muscle disease (type IIIB). Clinical and biochemical features resemble those of type I disease. Differentiation from type I is by a hyperglycemic response to galactose, lower concentrations of urate and lactate in the blood, and elevated serum transaminase and creatine kinase activities. Enzyme deficiency can be demonstrated in muscle or liver and occasionally in erythrocytes.

TYPE IV (BRANCHING ENZYME DEFICIENCY)

Type IV is an extremely rare disorder manifested by production of an abnormal form of unbranched glycogen in all tissue. Patients exhibit hepatosplenomegaly with ascites and liver failure. Abnormal glycogen can be identified in the tissue and muscles; leukocytes or cultured fibroblasts can be used to demonstrate the enzyme deficiency.

TYPE V (MUSCLE PHOSPHORYLASE DEFICIENCY)

Type V, also called *McArdle's disease,* usually presents in the second or third decade with muscle cramps after exercise. Moderate exercise can be sustained, and patients have a "second wind," when symptoms disappear if exercise is continued. Increased plasma creatine kinase activities at rest, the failure of ischemic exercise to increase serum lactate concentrations while producing an exaggerated increase in ammonia, myoglobinuria, and diminished activity of muscle phosphorylase establish the diagnosis. Patients respond to oral glucose administration or injections of glucagon.

TYPE VI (LIVER PHOSPHORYLASE OR PHOSPHORYLASE KINASE DEFICIENCY)

Type VI is a heterogeneous group of diseases arising from a deficiency of liver phosphorylase or one of the subunits of phosphorylase kinase. It is a rare and relatively benign disorder manifested as hepatomegaly caused by increased deposits of normal glycogen in the liver. Diagnosis is made by measuring enzyme activity in the liver or in red or white blood cells.

TYPE VII (MUSCLE PHOSPHOFRUCTOKINASE DEFICIENCY)

Patients with this rare type have deposits of abnormal glycogen in muscle. Exercise intolerance, unresponsiveness to glucose administration, and hemolysis (caused by decreased glycolysis in erythrocytes) are noted clinically, producing hyperbilirubinemia, pigmenturia, and reticulocytosis. The specific enzyme defect can be demonstrated.

REFERENCES

1. Alberti KG, Zimmet PZ. Definition, diagnosis and classification of diabetes mellitus and its complications. Part 1: diagnosis and classification of diabetes mellitus provisional report of a WHO consultation. Diabet Med 1998;15:539-53.
2. Allen BT, DeLong ER, Feussner JR. Impact of glucose self-monitoring on non–insulin-treated patients with type II diabetes mellitus. Randomized controlled trial comparing blood and urine testing. Diabetes Care 1990;13:1044-50.
3. Almind K, Doria A, Kahn CR. Putting the genes for type II diabetes on the map. Nat Med 2001;7:277-9.
4. American Diabetes Association. Standardization of the oral glucose tolerance test. Report of the Committee on Statistics of the American Diabetes Association June 14, 1968. Diabetes 1969;18: 299-307.
5. American Diabetes Association. Consensus statement on self-monitoring of blood glucose. Diabetes Care 1987;10:93-9.
6. American Diabetes Association. Self-monitoring of blood glucose. Diabetes Care 1996;19 (Supp 1):S62-6.
7. American Diabetes Association. Report of the Expert Committee on the Diagnosis and Classification of Diabetes Mellitus. Diabetes Care 1997;20:1183-97.
8. American Diabetes Association. Consensus Development Conference on Insulin Resistance. 5-6 November 1997. Diabetes Care 1998;21:310-4.
9. American Diabetes Association. Gestational diabetes mellitus. Diabetes Care 2000;23:S77-9.
10. American Diabetes Association. Type 2 diabetes in children and adolescents. Diabetes Care 2000;23: 381-9.
11. American Diabetes Association. Diabetes Forecast—Resource Guide 2001. 2001;54.
12. American Diabetes Association. Gestational diabetes mellitus. Diabetes Care 2003;26 Suppl 1:S103-5.
13. American Diabetes Association. Prevention of type 1 diabetes mellitus. Diabetes Care 2003;26 Suppl 1:S140.
14. American Diabetes Association. Screening for type 2 diabetes. Diabetes Care 2003;26 Suppl 1:S21-4.
15. American Diabetes Association. Standards of medical care for patients with diabetes mellitus. Diabetes Care 2003;26 Suppl 1:S33-50.

16. Armbruster DA. Fructosamine: structure, analysis, and clinical usefulness. Clin Chem 1987;33:2153-63.
17. Astles R, Williams CP, Sedor F. Stability of plasma lactate in vitro in the presence of antiglycolytic agents. Clin Chem 1994;40:1327-30.
18. Atkinson MA, Bowman MA, Kao KJ, Campbell L, Dush PJ, Shah SC, et al. Lack of immune responsiveness to bovine serum albumin in insulin-dependent diabetes. N Engl J Med 1993;329:1853-8.
19. Atkinson MA, Eisenbarth GS. Type 1 diabetes: new perspectives on disease pathogenesis and treatment. Lancet 2001;358:221-9.
20. Atkinson MA, Maclaren NK. The pathogenesis of insulin-dependent diabetes mellitus. N Engl J Med 1994;331:1428-36.
21. Baekkeskov S, Aanstoot HJ, Christgau S, Reetz A, Solimena M, Cascalho M, et al. Identification of the 64K autoantigen in insulin-dependent diabetes as the GABA-synthesizing enzyme glutamic acid decarboxylase [published erratum appears in Nature 1990 Oct 25;347(6295):782]. Nature 1990;347:151-6.
22. Bailey EM, Domenico P, Cunha BA. Bacterial or viral meningitis? Measuring lactate in CSF can help you know quickly. Postgrad Med 1990;88:217-9.
23. Baker J, Metcalf P, Tatnell M, Lever M, Johnson R. Quality assessment of determinations of serum fructosamine in 33 clinical chemistry laboratories. Clin Chem 1986;32:2133-6.
24. Baker JR, O'Connor JP, Metcalf PA, Lawson MR, Johnson RN. Clinical usefulness of estimation of serum fructosamine concentration as a screening test for diabetes mellitus. BMJ (Clin Res Ed) 1983;287:863-7.
25. Balland M, Schiele F, Henny J. Effect of a 6-month storage on human serum fructosamine concentration. Clin Chim Acta 1994;230:105-7.
26. Bandi ZL, Myers JL, Bee DE, James GP. Evaluation of determination of glucose in urine with some commercially available dipsticks and tablets. Clin Chem 1982;28:2110-5.
27. Bannon P. Effect of pH on the elimination of the labile fraction of glycosylated hemoglobin. Clin Chem 1982;28:2183.
28. Baudry A, Leroux L, Jackerott M, Joshi RL. Genetic manipulation of insulin signaling, action and secretion in mice. Insights into glucose homeostasis and pathogenesis of type 2 diabetes. EMBO reports 2002;3:323-8.
29. Bell GI, Burant CF, Takeda J, Gould GW. Structure and function of mammalian facilitative sugar transporters. J Biol Chem 1993;268:19161-4.
30. Bell GI, Polonsky KS. Diabetes mellitus and genetically programmed defects in beta-cell function. Nature 2001;414:788-91.
31. Benjamin RJ, Sacks DB. Glycated protein update: implications of recent studies, including the diabetes control and complications trial. Clin Chem 1994;40:683-7.
32. Bennett PH, Haffner S, Kasiske BL, Keane WF, Mogensen CE, Parving HH, et al. Screening and management of microalbuminuria in patients with diabetes mellitus: recommendations to the Scientific Advisory Board of the National Kidney Foundation from an ad hoc committee of the Council on Diabetes Mellitus of the National Kidney Foundation. Am J Kidney Dis 1995;25:107-12.
33. Benoist JF, Alberti C, Leclercq S, Rigal O, Jean-Louis R, Ogier de Baulny H, et al. Cerebrospinal fluid lactate and pyruvate concentrations and their ratio in children: age-related reference intervals. Clin Chem 2003;49:487-94.
34. Bingley PJ, Bonifacio E, Ziegler AG, Schatz DA, Atkinson MA, Eisenbarth GS. Proposed guidelines on screening for risk of type 1 diabetes. Diabetes Care 2001;24:398.
35. Bingley PJ, Colman P, Eisenbarth GS, Jackson RA, McCulloch DK, Riley WJ, et al. Standardization of IVGTT to predict IDDM. Diabetes Care 1992;15:1313-6.
36. Boehm TM, Lebovitz HE. Statistical analysis of glucose and insulin responses to intravenous tolbutamide: Evaluation of hypoglycemic and hyperinsulinemic states. Diabetes Care 1979;2:479-90.
37. Bohme P, Floriot M, Sirveaux MA, Durain D, Ziegler O, Drouin P, et al. Evolution of analytical performance in portable glucose meters in the last decade. Diabetes Care 2003;26:1170-5.
38. Bowman MA, Leiter EH, Atkinson MA. Prevention of diabetes in the NOD mouse: implications for therapeutic intervention in human disease. Immunol Today 1994;15:115-20.
39. Bowsher RR, Wolny JD, Frank BH. A rapid and sensitive radioimmunoassay for the measurement of proinsulin in human serum. Diabetes 1992;41:1084-90.
40. Boyanton BL, Jr., Blick KE. Stability studies of twenty-four analytes in human plasma and serum. Clin Chem 2002;48:2242-7.
41. Boyd JC, Bruns DE. Quality specifications for glucose meters: assessment by simulation modeling of errors in insulin dose. Clin Chem 2001;47:209-14.
42. Bretherton-Watt D, Gilbey SG, Ghatei MA, Beacham J, Bloom SR. Failure to establish islet amyloid polypeptide (amylin) as a circulating beta cell inhibiting hormone in man. Diabetologia 1990;33:115-7.
43. Brownlee M. Biochemistry and molecular cell biology of diabetic complications. Nature 2001;414:813-20.
44. Brownlee M, Cerami A, Vlassara H. Advanced glycosylation end products in tissue and the biochemical basis of diabetic complications. N Engl J Med 1988;318:1315-21.

45. Brun JF, Fedou C, Mercier J. Postprandial reactive hypoglycemia. Diabetes Metab 2000;26:337-51.
46. Bry L, Chen PC, Sacks DB. Effects of hemoglobin variants and chemically modified derivatives on assays for glycohemoglobin [Review]. Clin Chem 2001;47:153-63.
47. Burnett RW, D'Orazio P, Fogh-Andersen N, Kuwa K, Kulpmann WR, Larsson L, et al. IFCC recommendation on reporting results for blood glucose. Clin Chim Acta 2001;307:205-9.
48. Burrin JM, Price CP. Measurement of blood glucose. Ann Clin Biochem 1985;22 (Pt 4):327-42.
49. Bush JL, Campbell J, Sanderson JA. Performance of a glucose procedure based on the glucose dehydrogenase reaction on Technicon continuous flow equipment. Clin Chem 1981;27:1050.
50. Byrne HA, Tieszen KL, Hollis S, Dornan TL, New JP. Evaluation of an electrochemical sensor for measuring blood ketones. Diabetes Care 2000;23:500-3.
51. Cahill GF, Jr., Soeldner JS. A non-editorial on non-hypoglycemia. N Engl J Med 1974;291:905-6.
52. Cefalu WT, Ettinger WH, Bell-Farrow AD, Rushing JT. Serum fructosamine as a screening test for diabetes in the elderly: a pilot study. J Am Geriatr Soc 1993;41:1090-4.
53. Chalew SA, McLaughlin JV, Mersey JH, Adams AJ, Cornblath M, Kowarski AA. The use of the plasma epinephrine response in the diagnosis of idiopathic postprandial syndrome. JAMA 1984;251:612-5.
54. Chan AY, Swaminathan R, Cockram CS. Effectiveness of sodium fluoride as a preservative of glucose in blood. Clin Chem 1989;35:315-7.
55. Chariot P, Monnet I, Mouchet M, Rohr M, Lefaucheur JP, Dubreuil-Lemaire ML, et al. Determination of the blood lactate: pyruvate ratio as a noninvasive test for the diagnosis of zidovudine myopathy. Arthritis Rheum 1994;37:583-6.
56. Charles MA, Hofeldt F, Shackelford A, Waldeck N, Dodson LE, Jr., Bunker D, et al. Comparison of oral glucose tolerance tests and mixed meals in patients with apparent idiopathic postabsorptive hypoglycemia: absence of hypoglycemia after meals. Diabetes 1981;30:465-70.
57. Chen Y-T, Burchell A. Glycogen storage diseases. In: Scriver AL, Beaudet AL, Sly WS, Valle D, eds. The Metabolic and Molecular Bases of Inherited Disease. 7th ed. New York: McGraw-Hill, 1995:935-65.
58. Chesham J, Anderton SW, Kingdon CF. Rapid, competitive enzymoimmunoassay for albumin in urine. Clin Chem 1986;32:669-71.
59. Chua KS, Tan IK. Plasma glucose measurement with the Yellow Springs Glucose Analyzer. Clin Chem 1978;24:150-2.
60. Chua SC, Jr., Chung WK, Wu-Peng XS, Zhang Y, Liu SM, Tartaglia L, et al. Phenotypes of mouse diabetes and rat fatty due to mutations in the OB (leptin) receptor. Science 1996;271:994-6.
61. Clark PM. Assays for insulin, proinsulin(s) and C-peptide. Ann Clin Biochem 1999;36 (Pt 5):541-64.
62. Clarke WL, Cox D, Gonder-Frederick LA, Carter W, Pohl SL. Evaluating clinical accuracy of systems for self-monitoring of blood glucose. Diabetes Care 1987;10:622-8.
63. Cohen HT, Spiegel DM. Air-exposed urine dipsticks give false-positive results for glucose and false-negative results for blood. Am J Clin Pathol 1991;96:398-400.
64. Cohen MP, Hud E. Production and characterization of monoclonal antibodies against human glycoalbumin. J Immunol Methods 1989;117:121-9.
65. Consensus statement on self-monitoring of blood glucose. Diabetes Care 1996;19 (Suppl 1):S62-6.
66. Cooper GJ. Amylin compared with calcitonin gene-related peptide: structure, biology, and relevance to metabolic disease. Endocr Rev 1994;15:163-201.
67. Coster S, Gulliford MC, Seed PT, Powrie JK, Swaminathan R. Self-monitoring in Type 2 diabetes mellitus: a meta-analysis. Diabet Med 2000;17:755-61.
68. Cryer PE, Fisher JN, Shamoon H. Hypoglycemia. Diabetes Care 1994;17:734-55.
69. Curme HG, Columbus RL, Dappen GM, Eder TW, Fellows WD, Figueras J, et al. Multilayer film elements for clinical analysis: general concepts. Clin Chem 1978;24:1335-42.
70. Daughaday WH. The possible autocrine/paracrine and endocrine roles of insulin-like growth factors of human tumors. Endocrinology 1990;127:1-4.
71. DCCT. Feasibility of centralized measurements of glycated hemoglobin in the Diabetes Control and Complications Trial: a multicenter study. Clin Chem 1987;33:2267-71.
72. DCCT. The effect of intensive treatment of diabetes on the development and progression of long-term complications in insulin-dependent diabetes mellitus. N Engl J Med 1993;329:977-86.
73. DCCT. The relationship of glycemic exposure (HbA1c) to the risk of development and progression of retinopathy in the diabetes control and complications trial. Diabetes 1995;44:968-83.
74. DCCT. Effect of intensive therapy on the microvascular complications of type 1 diabetes mellitus. The Diabetes Control and Complications Trial Research Group. JAMA 2002;287:2563-9.
75. DECODE. Consequences of the new diagnostic criteria for diabetes in older men and women. DECODE Study (Diabetes Epidemiology: Collaborative Analysis of Diagnostic Criteria in Europe). Diabetes Care 1999;22:1667-71.
76. DECODE Study Group. Is the current definition for diabetes relevant to mortality risk from all causes and

cardiovascular and noncardiovascular diseases? Diabetes Care 2003;26:688-96.
77. DeFronzo RA, Bonadonna RC, Ferrannini E. Pathogenesis of NIDDM. A balanced overview. Diabetes Care 1992;15:318-68.
78. DeFronzo RA, Hendler R, Christensen N. Stimulation of counterregulatory hormonal responses in diabetic man by a fall in glucose concentration. Diabetes 1980;29:125-31.
79. Dhahir FJ, Cook DB, Self CH. Amplified enzyme-linked immunoassay of human proinsulin in serum (detection limit: 0.1 pmol/L). Clin Chem 1992;38:227-32.
80. Diabetes Prevention Trial—Type 1 Study Group. Effects of insulin in relatives of patients with type 1 diabetes mellitus. N Engl J Med 2002;346: 1685-91.
81. Dolhofer R, Wieland OH. Increased glycosylation of serum albumin in diabetes mellitus. Diabetes 1980;29:417-22.
82. Doppman JL, Chang R, Fraker DL, Norton JA, Alexander HR, Miller DL, et al. Localization of insulinomas to regions of the pancreas by intra-arterial stimulation with calcium. Ann Intern Med 1995;123:269-73.
83. Duck SC, Lee M, D'Alessio D. 24-42 month stability of internal blood standards for glycated hemoglobin analysis. Diabetes Res Clin Pract 1990;9:195-9.
84. Elving LD, Bakkeren JA, Jansen MJ, de Kat Angelino CM, de Nobel E, van Munster PJ. Screening for microalbuminuria in patients with diabetes mellitus: frozen storage of urine samples decreases their albumin content. Clin Chem 1989;35:308-10.
85. Engbaek F, Christensen SE, Jespersen B. Enzyme immunoassay of hemoglobin A1c: analytical characteristics and clinical performance for patients with diabetes mellitus, with and without uremia. Clin Chem 1989;35:93-7.
86. Engelgau MM, Narayan KM, Herman WH. Screening for type 2 diabetes. Diabetes Care 2000;23:1563-80.
87. Expert Panel. Executive Summary of the Third Report of the National Cholesterol Education Program (NCEP) Expert Panel on Detection, Evaluation, and Treatment of High Blood Cholesterol in Adults (Adult Treatment Panel III). JAMA 2001;285:2486-97.
88. Faas A, Schellevis FG, Van Eijk JT. The efficacy of self-monitoring of blood glucose in NIDDM subjects. A criteria-based literature review. Diabetes Care 1997;20:1482-6.
89. Fajans SS, Vinik AI. Insulin-producing islet cell tumors. Endocrinol Metab Clin North Am 1989;18:45-74.
90. Flier JS. Lilly Lecture: syndromes of insulin resistance. From patient to gene and back again. Diabetes 1992;41:1207-19.
91. Flier JS, Kahn CR, Roth J, Bar RS. Antibodies that impair insulin receptor binding in an unusual diabetic syndrome with severe insulin resistance. Science 1975;190:63-5.
92. Flock EV, Bennett PH, Savage PJ, Webner CJ, Howard BV, Rushforth NB, et al. Bimodality of glycosylated hemoglobin distribution in Pima Indians: relationship to fasting hyperglycemia. Diabetes 1979;28: 984-9.
93. Friedman JM, Halaas JL. Leptin and the regulation of body weight in mammals. Nature 1998;395:763-70.
94. Frontoni S, Choi SB, Banduch D, Rossetti L. In vivo insulin resistance induced by amylin primarily through inhibition of insulin-stimulated glycogen synthesis in skeletal muscle. Diabetes 1991;40:568-73.
95. Froom P, Bieganiec B, Ehrenrich Z, Barak M. Stability of common analytes in urine refrigerated for 24 h before automated analysis by test strips. Clin Chem 2000;46:1384-6.
96. Ganda OP, Day JL, Soeldner JS, Connon JJ, Gleason RE. Reproducibility and comparative analysis of repeated intravenous and oral glucose tolerance tests. Diabetes 1978;27:715-25.
97. Garg SK, Potts RO, Ackerman NR, Fermi SJ, Tamada JA, Chase HP. Correlation of fingerstick blood glucose measurements with GlucoWatch biographer glucose results in young subjects with type 1 diabetes. Diabetes Care 1999;22:1708-14.
98. Gerbitz KD, Spelsberg F. Pancreatic B-cell peptides as parameters for diagnosis and localisation of hormone secreting tumours. J Clin Chem Clin Biochem 1985;23:377-80.
99. Gerich JE. Lilly lecture 1988. Glucose counterregulation and its impact on diabetes mellitus. Diabetes 1988;37:1608-17.
100. Gerich JE. Physiology of glucose homeostasis. Diabetes Obes Metab 2000;2:345-50.
101. Gerstein HC, Mann JF, Yi Q, Zinman B, Dinneen SF, Hoogwerf B, et al. Albuminuria and risk of cardiovascular events, death, and heart failure in diabetic and nondiabetic individuals. JAMA 2001;286:421-6.
102. Giannoukakis N, Rudert WA, Robbins PD, Trucco M. Targeting autoimmune diabetes with gene therapy. Diabetes 1999;48:2107-21.
103. Gibb I, Parnham A, Fonfrede M, Lecock F. Multicenter evaluation of Tosoh glycohemoglobin analyzer. Clin Chem 1999;45:1833-41.
104. Gillery P, Labbe D, Dumont G, Vassault A. Glycohemoglobin assays evaluated in a large-scale quality-control survey. Clin Chem 1995;41:1644-8.
105. Ginsberg HN. Insulin resistance and cardiovascular disease. J Clin Invest 2000;106:453-8.
106. Gochman N, Schmitz JM. Application of a new peroxide indicator reaction to the specific, automated determination of glucose with glucose oxidase. Clin Chem 1972;18:943-50.

107. Goldstein DE, Little RR, Lorenz RA, Malone JI, Nathan D, Peterson CM, Sacks DB. Diabetes Care 2004;27:1761-73.
108. Goldstein DE, Little RR, Lorenz RA, Malone JI, Nathan DM, Peterson CM. Tests of glycemia in diabetes. Diabetes Care 2003;26 Suppl 1:S106-8.
109. Goldstein DE, Little RR, Wiedmeyer H-M, England JD, Rohlfing CG. Glycated haemoglobin estimation in the 1990s: A review of assay methods and clinical interpretation. In: Marshall SM, Home PD, eds. The Diabetes Annual. New York: Elsevier Science B. V., 1994:193-212.
110. Goldstein DE, Peth SB, England JD, Hess RL, Da Costa J. Effects of acute changes in blood glucose on HbA1c. Diabetes 1980;29:623-8.
111. Gough DA, Armour JC. Development of the implantable glucose sensor. What are the prospects and why is it taking so long? Diabetes 1995;44: 1005-9.
112. Greenberg RA, Sacks DB. Screening for diabetes: is it warranted? Clin Chim Acta 2002;315:61-9.
113. Grundy SM. Hypertriglyceridemia, insulin resistance, and the metabolic syndrome. Am J Cardiol 1999;83:25F-9F.
114. Halaas JL, Gajiwala KS, Maffei M, Cohen SL, Chait BT, Rabinowitz D, et al. Weight-reducing effects of the plasma protein encoded by the obese gene. Science 1995;269:543-6.
115. Harano Y, Kosugi K, Hyosu T, Suzuki M, Hidaka H, Kashiwagi A, et al. Ketone bodies as markers for type 1 (insulin-dependent) diabetes and their value in the monitoring of diabetic control. Diabetologia 1984;26:343-8.
116. Harris MI. Frequency of blood glucose monitoring in relation to glycemic control in patients with type 2 diabetes. Diabetes Care 2001;24:979-82.
117. Harris MI, Flegal KM, Cowie CC, Eberhardt MS, Goldstein DE, Little RR, et al. Prevalence of diabetes, impaired fasting glucose, and impaired glucose tolerance in U.S. adults. The Third National Health and Nutrition Examination Survey, 1988-1994. Diabetes Care 1998;21:518-24.
118. Harrison LC. Risk assessment, prediction and prevention of type 1 diabetes. Pediatric Diabetes 2001;2: 71-82.
119. Haymond MW. Hypoglycemia in infants and children. Endocrinol Metab Clin North Am 1989; 18:211-52.
120. Heding LG. Specific and direct radioimmunoassay for human proinsulin in serum. Diabetologia 1977;13:467-74.
121. Hill RP, Hindle EJ, Howey JE, Lemon M, Lloyd DR. Recommendations for adopting standard conditions and analytical procedures in the measurement of serum fructosamine concentration. Ann Clin Biochem 1990;27 (Pt 5):413-24.
122. Hoekstra JB, van Rijn HJ, Erkelens DW, Thijssen JH. C-peptide. Diabetes Care 1982;5:438-46.
123. Hoekstra JB, Van Rijn HJ, Thijssen JH, Erkelens DW. C-peptide reactivity as a measure of insulin dependency in obese diabetic patients treated with insulin. Diabetes Care 1982;5:585-91.
124. Hofeldt FD. Reactive hypoglycemia. Endocrinol Metab Clin North Am 1989;18:185-201.
125. Hogan P, Dall T, Nikolov P. Economic costs of diabetes in the US in 2002. Diabetes Care 2003;26:917-32.
126. Hoppener JW, Ahren B, Lips CJ. Islet amyloid and type 2 diabetes mellitus. N Engl J Med 2000;343: 411-9.
127. Horiuchi S, Araki N, Morino Y. Immunochemical approach to characterize advanced glycation end products of the Maillard reaction. Evidence for the presence of a common structure. J Biol Chem 1991;266:7329-32.
128. Horrocks RH, Manning GB. Partition chromatography on paper: Identification of reducing substances in urine. Lancet 1949;1:1042-5.
129. Horwitz DL, Kuzuya H, Rubenstein AH. Circulating serum C-peptide. A brief review of diagnostic implications. N Engl J Med 1976;295:207-9.
130. Houssa P, Dinesen B, Deberg M, Frank BH, Van Schravendijk C, Sodoyez-Goffaux F, et al. First direct assay for intact human proinsulin. Clin Chem 1998;44:1514-9.
131. Hu FB, Manson JE, Stampfer MJ, Colditz G, Liu S, Solomon CG, et al. Diet, lifestyle, and the risk of type 2 diabetes mellitus in women. N Engl J Med 2001;345:790-7.
132. Hughes PF, Agarwal M, Newman P, Morrison J. An evaluation of fructosamine estimation in screening for gestational diabetes mellitus. Diabet Med 1995;12:708-12.
133. Huisman W, Kuijken JP, Tan-Tjiong HL, Duurkoop EP, Leijnse B. Unstable glycosylated hemoglobin in patients with diabetes mellitus. Clin Chim Acta 1982;118:303-9.
134. Hutchesson A, Preece MA, Gray G, Green A. Measurement of lactate in cerebrospinal fluid in investigation of inherited metabolic disease. Clin Chem 1997;43:158-61.
135. Hwa V, Oh Y, Rosenfeld RG. The insulin-like growth factor-binding protein (IGFBP) superfamily. Endocr Rev 1999;20:761-87.
136. Hyoty H, Taylor KW. The role of viruses in human diabetes. Diabetologia 2002;45:1353-61.
137. Imbeault P, Prins JB, Stolic M, Russell AW, O'Moore-Sullivan T, Despres JP, et al. Aging per se does not influence glucose homeostasis: in vivo and in vitro evidence. Diabetes Care 2003;26:480-4.
138. James RC, Chase GR. Evaluation of some commonly used semiquantitative methods for urinary glucose and ketone determinations. Diabetes 1974;23:474-9.

139. John WG, Gray MR, Bates DL, Beacham JL. Enzyme immunoassay—a new technique for estimating hemoglobin A1c. Clin Chem 1993;39:663-6.
140. Johnson RN, Baker JR. Error detection and measurement in glucose monitors. Clin Chim Acta 2001;307:61-7.
141. Johnson RN, Metcalf PA, Baker JR. Fructosamine: a new approach to the estimation of serum glycosylprotein. An index of diabetic control. Clin Chim Acta 1983;127:87-95.
142. Kabadi UM, O'Connell KM, Johnson J, Kabadi M. The effect of recurrent practice at home on the acceptability of capillary blood glucose readings. Accuracy of self blood glucose testing. Diabetes Care 1994;17:1110-23.
143. Kadish AH. A new and rapid method for the determination of glucose by measurement of rate of oxygen consumption. Clin Chem 1968;14:116-31.
144. Kahn CR. Banting Lecture. Insulin action, diabetogenes, and the cause of type II diabetes. Diabetes 1994;43:1066-84.
145. Kaplan EL, Rubenstein AH, Evans R, Lee CH, Klementschitsch P. Calcium infusion: a new provocative test for insulinomas. Ann Surg 1979;190:501-7.
146. Karjalainen J, Martin JM, Knip M, Ilonen J, Robinson BH, Savilahti E, et al. A bovine albumin peptide as a possible trigger of insulin-dependent diabetes mellitus. N Engl J Med 1992;327:302-7.
147. Katzeff HL, Savage PJ, Barclay-White B, Nagulesparan M, Bennett PH. C-peptide measurement in the differentiation of type 1 (insulin-dependent) and type 2 (non–insulin-dependent) diabetes mellitus. Diabetologia 1985;28:264-8.
148. Kennedy DM, Johnson AB, Hill PG. A comparison of automated fructosamine and HbA1c methods for monitoring diabetes in pregnancy. Ann Clin Biochem 1998;35 (Pt 2):283-9.
149. Khalil OS. Spectroscopic and clinical aspects of noninvasive glucose measurements. Clin Chem 1999;45:165-77.
150. Khaw KT, Wareham N, Luben R, Bingham S, Oakes S, Welch A, et al. Glycated haemoglobin, diabetes, and mortality in men in Norfolk cohort of European prospective investigation of cancer and nutrition (EPIC-Norfolk). BMJ 2001;322:15-8.
151. Kilpatrick ES, Dominiczak MH, Small M. The effects of ageing on glycation and the interpretation of glycaemic control in Type 2 diabetes. QJ Med 1996; 89:307-12.
152. Kim C, Newton KM, Knopp RH. Gestational diabetes and the incidence of type 2 diabetes: a systematic review. Diabetes Care 2002;25:1862-8.
153. King H, Aubert RE, Herman WH. Global burden of diabetes, 1995-2025: prevalence, numerical estimates, and projections. Diabetes Care 1998;21: 1414-31.
154. Kippen AD, Cerini F, Vadas L, Stocklin R, Vu L, Offord RE, et al. Development of an isotope dilution assay for precise determination of insulin, C-peptide, and proinsulin levels in non-diabetic and type II diabetic individuals with comparison to immunoassay. J Biol Chem 1997;272:12513-22.
155. Kitzmiller JL, Gavin LA, Gin GD, Jovanovic-Peterson L, Main EK, Zigrang WD. Preconception care of diabetes. Glycemic control prevents congenital anomalies. JAMA 1991;265:731-6.
156. Kjems LL, Roder ME, Dinesen B, Hartling SG, Jorgensen PN, Binder C. Highly sensitive enzyme immunoassay of proinsulin immunoreactivity with use of two monoclonal antibodies. Clin Chem 1993;39:2146-50.
157. Kjos SL, Buchanan TA. Gestational diabetes mellitus. N Engl J Med 1999;341:1749-56.
158. Knowler WC, Barrett-Connor E, Fowler SE, Hamman RF, Lachin JM, Walker EA, et al. Reduction in the incidence of type 2 diabetes with lifestyle intervention or metformin. N Engl J Med 2002;346:393-403.
159. Kobold U, Jeppsson JO, Dulffer T, Finke A, Hoelzel W, Miedema K. Candidate reference methods for hemoglobin A1c based on peptide mapping. Clin Chem 1997;43:1944-51.
160. Kojima H, Fujimiya M, Matsumura K, Younan P, Imaeda H, Maeda M, et al. NeuroD-betacellulin gene therapy induces islet neogenesis in the liver and reverses diabetes in mice. Nat Med 2003;9:596-603.
161. Kolaczynski JW, Caro JF. Insulin-like growth factor-1 therapy in diabetes: physiologic basis, clinical benefits, and risks. Ann Intern Med 1994;120:47-55.
162. Kulkarni RN, Bruning JC, Winnay JN, Postic C, Magnuson MA, Kahn CR. Tissue-specific knockout of the insulin receptor in pancreatic beta cells creates an insulin secretory defect similar to that in type 2 diabetes. Cell 1999;96:329-39.
163. Kumar D, Mehtalia SD, Miller LV. Diagnostic use of glucagon-induced insulin response. Studies in patients with insulinoma or other hypoglycemic conditions. Ann Intern Med 1974;80:697-701.
164. Kuusisto J, Mykkanen L, Pyorala K, Laakso M. Hyperinsulinemic microalbuminuria. A new risk indicator for coronary heart disease. Circulation 1995;91:831-7.
165. Laffel L. Ketone bodies: a review of physiology, pathophysiology and application of monitoring to diabetes. Diabetes Metab Res Rev 1999;15: 412-26.
166. Larsson-Cohn U. Differences between capillary and venous blood glucose during oral glucose tolerance tests. Scand J Clin Lab Invest 1976;36:805-8.
167. Leahy JL. Natural history of beta-cell dysfunction in NIDDM. Diabetes Care 1990;13:992-1010.
168. Lefebvre PJ. Glucagon and its family revisited. Diabetes Care 1995;18:715-30.

169. Lefebvre PJ, Andreani D, Marks V. Statement on "post-prandial" or reactive hypoglycemia. Hypoglycemia, Serono Symposium: Raven Press, 1987:79.
170. Lin MJ, Hoke C, Ettinger B, Coyne RV. Technical performance evaluation of BM/Hitachi 747-200 serum fructosamine assay. Clin Chem 1996;42:244-8.
171. Little RR, Rohlfing CL, Wiedmeyer HM, Myers GL, Sacks DB, Goldstein DE. The national glycohemoglobin standardization program: a five-year progress report. Clin Chem 2001;47:1985-92.
172. Livesley B, Atkinson L. Letter: Accurate quantitative estimation of lactate in whole blood. Clin Chem 1974;20:1478.
173. Lott JA, Turner K. Evaluation of Trinder's glucose oxidase method for measuring glucose in serum and urine. Clin Chem 1975;21:1754-60.
174. Lubran M. Measurement of lactic and pyruvic acid in biological fluids. In: Sunderman FW, Sunderman FW, Jr., eds. Laboratory Diagnosis of Endocrine Diseases. St. Louis: Warren H. Green, 1971:401-8.
175. Ludvigsen CW, Thurn JR, Pierpont GL, Eckfeldt JH. Kinetic enzymic assay for D(-)-lactate, with use of a centrifugal analyzer. Clin Chem 1983;29:1823-5.
176. Lutz RA, Fluckiger J. Kinetic determination of glucose with the GEMSAEC (ENI) centrifugal analyzer by the glucose dehydrogenase reaction, and comparison with two commonly used procedures. Clin Chem 1975;21:1372-7.
177. MacNeil ML, Mueller PW, Caudill SP, Steinberg KK. Considerations when measuring urinary albumin: precision, substances that may interfere, and conditions for sample storage. Clin Chem 1991;37:2120-3.
178. Makita Z, Vlassara H, Rayfield E, Cartwright K, Friedman E, Rodby R, et al. Hemoglobin-AGE: a circulating marker of advanced glycosylation. Science 1992;258:651-3.
179. Mantzoros CS. The role of leptin in human obesity and disease: a review of current evidence. Ann Intern Med 1999;130:671-80.
180. Maquart FX, Gillery P, Bernard JF, Mante JP, Borel JP. A method for specifically measuring haemoglobin AIC with a disposable commercial ion-exchange column. Clin Chim Acta 1980;108:329-32.
181. Marbach EP, Weil MH. Rapid enzymatic measurement of blood lactate and pyruvate. Use and significance of metaphosphoric acid as a common precipitant. Clin Chem 1967;13:314-25.
182. Marshall SM, Shearing PA, Alberti KG. Micral-test strips evaluated for screening for albuminuria. Clin Chem 1992;38:588-91.
183. Martin-Rendon E, Blake DJ. Protein glycosylation in disease: new insights into the congenital muscular dystrophies. Trends Pharmacol Sci 2003;24:178-83.
184. Medcalf E, Newman DJ, Gorman EG. Rapid latex-enhanced turbidimetric assay for urine albumin. Ann Clin Biochem 1988;25 (Suppl):1645-55.
185. Menard L, Dempsey ME, Blankstein LA, Aleyassine H, Wacks M, Soeldner JS. Quantitative determination of glycosylated hemoglobin A1 by agar gel electrophoresis. Clin Chem 1980;26:1598-602.
186. Merimee TJ, Tyson JE. Stabilization of plasma glucose during fasting; Normal variations in two separate studies. N Engl J Med 1974;291:1275-8.
187. Metzger BE, Coustan DR. Summary and recommendations of the Fourth International Workshop-Conference on Gestational Diabetes Mellitus. The Organizing Committee. Diabetes Care 1998;21: B161-7.
188. Miller SI, Wallace RJ, Jr., Musher DM, Septimus EJ, Kohl S, Baughn RE. Hypoglycemia as a manifestation of sepsis. Am J Med 1980;68:649-54.
189. Mills JL, Knopp RH, Simpson JL, Jovanovic-Peterson L, Metzger BE, Holmes LB, et al. Lack of relation of increased malformation rates in infants of diabetic mothers to glycemic control during organogenesis. N Engl J Med 1988;318:671-6.
190. Mire-Sluis AR, Gaines Das R, Lernmark A. The World Health Organization International Collaborative Study for islet cell antibodies. Diabetologia 2000;43:1282-92.
191. Mogensen CE. Microalbuminuria, blood pressure and diabetic renal disease: origin and development of ideas. Diabetologia 1999;42:263-85.
192. Mokdad AH, Ford ES, Bowman BA, Dietz WH, Vinicor F, Bales VS, et al. Prevalence of obesity, diabetes, and obesity-related health risk factors, 2001. JAMA 2003;289:76-9.
193. Molitch ME, DeFronzo RA, Franz MJ, Keane WF, Mogensen CE, Parving HH. Diabetic nephropathy. Diabetes Care 2003;26 Suppl 1:S94-8.
194. Morris LR, McGee JA, Kitabchi AE. Correlation between plasma and urine glucose in diabetes. Ann Intern Med 1981;94:469-71.
195. Mullins RE, Austin GE. Sensitivity of isoelectric focusing, ion exchange, and affinity chromatography to labile glycated hemoglobin. Clin Chem 1986;32:1460-3.
196. Nadler ST, Stoehr JP, Schueler KL, Tanimoto G, Yandell BS, Attie AD. The expression of adipogenic genes is decreased in obesity and diabetes mellitus. Proc Natl Acad Sci U S A 2000;97:11371-6.
197. Nagi DK, Hendra TJ, Ryle AJ, Cooper TM, Temple RC, Clark PM, et al. The relationships of concentrations of insulin, intact proinsulin and 32-33 split proinsulin with cardiovascular risk factors in type 2 (non–insulin-dependent) diabetic subjects. Diabetologia 1990;33:532-7.
198. Nakayama H, Taneda S, Kuwajima S, Aoki S, Kuroda Y, Misawa K, et al. Production and characterization of antibodies to advanced glycation products on proteins. Biochem Biophys Res Commun 1989;162: 740-5.

199. Nathan D. The importance of intensive supervision in determining the efficacy of insulin pump therapy. Diabetes Care 1983;6:295-7.
200. Nathan DM. Long-term complications of diabetes mellitus. N Engl J Med 1993;328:1676-85.
201. Naylor CD, Sermer M, Chen E, Sykora K. Cesarean delivery in relation to birth weight and gestational glucose tolerance: pathophysiology or practice style? Toronto Trihospital Gestational Diabetes Investigators. JAMA 1996;275:1165-70.
202. NCCLS. Point-of-Care Blood Testing in Acute and Chronic Care Facilities; Approved Guideline—Second Edition. NCCLS document C30-A2. Wayne, Pennsylvania: NCCLS, 2002.
203. NDDG. Classification and diagnosis of diabetes mellitus and other categories of glucose intolerance. National Diabetes Data Group. Diabetes 1979;28: 1039-57.
204. Neel JV. Diabetes mellitus: A geneticist's nightmare. In: Creutzfeldt W, Kobberling J, Neel JV, eds. The Genetics of Diabetes. New York: Springer Verlag, 1976:1-11.
205. Neese JW. Glucose, direct hexokinase method: Selected methods. Clin Chem 1982;9:241-8.
206. Neese JW, Duncan P, Bayse D. Development and Evaluation of a Hexokinase/Glucose-6-Phosphate Dehydrogenase Procedure for Use as a National Glucose Reference Method. HEW Publication No. (CDC) 77-8330. Atlanta: Centers for Disease Control, 1976.
207. Notkins AL. Immunologic and genetic factors in type 1 diabetes. J Biol Chem 2002;277: 43545-8.
208. Novis DA, Jones BA. Interinstitutional comparison of bedside blood glucose monitoring program characteristics, accuracy performance, and quality control documentation: a College of American Pathologists Q-Probes study of bedside blood glucose monitoring performed in 226 small hospitals. Arch Pathol Lab Med 1998;122:495-502.
209. O'Rahilly S, Turner RC, Matthews DR. Impaired pulsatile secretion of insulin in relatives of patients with non–insulin-dependent diabetes. N Engl J Med 1988;318:1225-30.
210. Orci L, Vassalli JD, Perrelet A. The insulin factory. Sci Am 1988;259:85-94.
211. Ostrega D, Polonsky K, Nagi D, Yudkin J, Cox LJ, Clark PM, et al. Measurement of proinsulin and intermediates. Validation of immunoassay methods by high-performance liquid chromatography. Diabetes 1995;44:437-40.
212. O'Sullivan JB. Age gradient in blood glucose levels. Magnitude and clinical implications. Diabetes 1974;23:713-5.
213. O'Sullivan JB. Diabetes mellitus after GDM. Diabetes 1991;40 Suppl 2:131-5.
214. O'Sullivan JB, Mahan CM. Criteria for the oral glucose tolerance test in pregnancy. Diabetes 1964;13:278-85.
215. Palardy J, Havrankova J, Lepage R, Matte R, Belanger R, D'Amour P, et al. Blood glucose measurements during symptomatic episodes in patients with suspected postprandial hypoglycemia. N Engl J Med 1989;321:1421-5.
216. Parnetti L, Gaiti A, Polidori MC, Brunetti M, Palumbo B, Chionne F, et al. Increased cerebrospinal fluid pyruvate levels in Alzheimer's disease. Neurosci Lett 1995;199:231-3.
217. Passey RB, Gillum RL, Fuller JB, Urry FM, Giles ML. Evaluation and comparison of 10 glucose methods and the reference method recommended in the proposed product class standard (1974). Clin Chem 1977;23:131-9.
218. Pawson T. Protein modules and signaling networks. Nature 1995;373:573-80.
219. Pfeifer MA, Halter JB, Porte D, Jr. Insulin secretion in diabetes mellitus. Am J Med 1981;70:579-88.
220. Phillipou G, James SK, Seaborn CJ, Phillips PJ. Screening for microalbuminuria by use of a rapid, low-cost colorimetric assay. Clin Chem 1989;35: 456-8.
221. Pickup J, Rolinski O, Birch D. In vivo glucose sensing for diabetes management: progress towards non–invasive monitoring [interview by Judy Jones]. BMJ 1999;319:1289-92.
222. Polonsky K, Frank B, Pugh W, Addis A, Karrison T, Meier P, et al. The limitations to and valid use of C-peptide as a marker of the secretion of insulin. Diabetes 1986;35:379-86.
223. Porter WH, Yao HH, Karounos DG. Laboratory and clinical evaluation of assays for beta-hydroxybutyrate. Am J Clin Pathol 1997;107:353-8.
224. Pozzilli P, Di Mario U. Autoimmune diabetes not requiring insulin at diagnosis (Latent Autoimmune Diabetes of the Adult): Definition, characterization, and potential prevention. Diabetes Care 2001;24:1460-7.
225. Prevalence incidence of diabetes mellitus–United States 1980-1987. From the Centers for Disease Control. JAMA 1990;264:3126.
226. Pryce JD, Gant PW, Sau KJ. Normal concentrations of lactate, glucose, and protein in cerebrospinal fluid, and the diagnostic implications of abnormal concentrations. Clin Chem 1970;16:562-5.
227. Radoff S, Makita Z, Vlassara H. Radioreceptor assay for advanced glycosylation end products. Diabetes 1991;40:1731-8.
228. Reaven GM. Banting lecture 1988. Role of insulin resistance in human disease. Diabetes 1988;37: 1595-607.
229. Reddi AS, Camerini-Davalos RA. Diabetic nephropathy. An update. Arch Intern Med 1990;150:31-43.

230. Reeves WG. Insulin antibody determination: theoretical and practical considerations. Diabetologia 1983;24:399-403.
231. Reljic R, Ries M, Anic N, Ries B. New chromogen for assay of glucose in serum. Clin Chem 1992;38:522-5.
232. Rhodes CJ, Alarcon C. What beta-cell defect could lead to hyperproinsulinemia in NIDDM? Some clues from recent advances made in understanding the proinsulin-processing mechanism. Diabetes 1994;43:511-7.
233. Rhodes CJ, White MF. Molecular insights into insulin action and secretion. Eur J Clin Invest 2002;32 Suppl 3:3-13.
234. Richter B, Neises G. 'Human' insulin versus animal insulin in people with diabetes mellitus. Cochrane Database Syst Rev 2002:CD003816.
235. Robbins DC, Andersen L, Bowsher R, Chance R, Dinesen B, Frank B, et al. Report of the American Diabetes Association's Task Force on standardization of the insulin assay. Diabetes 1996;45:242-56.
236. Robbins DC, Tager HS, Rubenstein AH. Biologic and clinical importance of proinsulin. N Engl J Med 1984;310:1165-75.
237. Robinson BH. Lactic acidemia (disorders of pyruvate carboxylase, pyruvate dehydrogenase). In: Shriver CR, Beaudet WS, Sly WS, Valle D, eds. The Metabolic and Molecular Bases of Inherited Disease, 7th ed. New York: McGraw-Hill, 1995:1479-99.
238. Rohlfing C, Wiedmeyer HM, Little R, Grotz VL, Tennill A, England J, et al. Biological variation of glycohemoglobin. Clin Chem 2002;48:1116-8.
239. Sacks DB. Amylin–a glucoregulatory hormone involved in the pathogenesis of diabetes mellitus? Clin Chem 1996;42:494-5.
240. Sacks DB. Implications of the revised criteria for diagnosis and classification of diabetes mellitus. Clin Chem 1997;43:2230-2.
241. Sacks DB, Bruns DE, Goldstein DE, Maclaren NK, McDonald JM, Parrott M. Guidelines and recommendations for laboratory analysis in the diagnosis and management of diabetes mellitus. Clin Chem 2002;48:436-72.
242. Sacks DB, Lernmark A. Molecular manipulation of autoantibody testing in type 1 diabetes: two for one. Clin Chem 2001;47:803-4.
243. Sacks DB, McDonald JM. The pathogenesis of type II diabetes mellitus. A polygenic disease. Am J Clin Pathol 1996;105:149-56.
244. Saltiel AR, Kahn CR. Insulin signaling and the regulation of glucose and lipid metabolism. Nature 2001;414:799-806.
245. Santiago JV. Lessons from the Diabetes Control and Complications Trial. Diabetes 1993;42:1549-54.
246. Savory J, Kaplan A. A gas chromatographic method for the determination of lactic acid in blood. Clin Chem 1966;12:559-69.
247. Sazama K, Robertson EA, Chesler RA. Is antiglycolysis required for routine glucose analysis? Clin Chem 1979;25:2038-9.
248. Schiffrin A, Belmonte M. Multiple daily self-glucose monitoring: its essential role in long-term glucose control in insulin-dependent diabetic patients treated with pump and multiple subcutaneous injections. Diabetes Care 1982;5:479-84.
249. Schleicher E, Wieland OH. Specific quantitation by HPLC of protein (lysine) bound glucose in human serum albumin and other glycosylated proteins. J Clin Chem Clin Biochem 1981;19:81-7.
250. Schleicher ED, Mayer R, Wagner EM, Gerbitz KD. Is serum fructosamine assay specific for determination of glycated serum protein? Clin Chem 1988;34:320-3.
251. Schleicher ED, Vogt BW. Standardization of serum fructosamine assays. Clin Chem 1990;36:136-9.
252. Schmidli RS, Colman PG, Bonifacio E. Disease sensitivity and specificity of 52 assays for glutamic acid decarboxylase antibodies. The Second International GADAB Workshop. Diabetes 1995;44:636-40.
253. Schosinsky KH, Vargas M, Luz Esquivel A, Chavarria MA. Simple spectrophotometric determination of urinary albumin by dye-binding with use of bromphenol blue. Clin Chem 1987;33:223-6.
254. Seltzer HS. Drug-induced hypoglycemia. A review of 1418 cases. Endocrinol Metab Clin North Am 1989;18:163-83.
255. Service FJ. Hypoglycemic disorders. N Engl J Med 1995;332:1144-52.
256. Service FJ, Dale AJ, Elveback LR, Jiang NS. Insulinoma: clinical and diagnostic features of 60 consecutive cases. Mayo Clin Proc 1976;51:417-29.
257. Shapiro ET, Bell GI, Polonsky KS, Rubenstein AH, Kew MC, Tager HS. Tumor hypoglycemia: relationship to high molecular weight insulin-like growth factor-II. J Clin Invest 1990;85:1672-9.
258. Sheetz MJ, King GL. Molecular understanding of hyperglycemia's adverse effects for diabetic complications. Jama 2002;288:2579-88.
259. Simon M, Hoover JD. Effect of sample instability on glycohemoglobin (HbA1) measured by cation-exchange chromatography. Clin Chem 1982;28:195-8.
260. Sobey WJ, Beer SF, Carrington CA, Clark PM, Frank BH, Gray IP, et al. Sensitive and specific two-site immunoradiometric assays for human insulin, proinsulin, 65-66 split and 32-33 split proinsulins. Biochem J 1989;260:535-41.
261. Special report. Statement on hypoglycemia. Diabetes 1973;22:137.
262. Spicer KM, Allen RC, Buse MG. A simplified assay of hemoglobin AIc in diabetic patients by use of isoelectric focusing and quantitative microdensitometry. Diabetes 1978;27:384-8.
263. Steiner DF, Ohagi S, Nagamatsu S, Bell GI, Nishi M. Is islet amyloid polypeptide a significant factor in

pathogenesis or pathophysiology of diabetes? Diabetes 1991;40:305-9.
264. Summary and recommendations of the Second International Workshop-Conference on gestational diabetes mellitus. Diabetes 1985;34 Suppl 2: 123-6.
265. Sundaram PV, Blumenberg B, Hinsch W. Routine glucose determination in serum by use of an immobilized glucose dehydrogenase nylon-tube reactor. Clin Chem 1979;25:1436-9.
266. Swinn RA, Wareham NJ, Gregory R, Curling V, Clark PM, Dalton KJ, et al. Excessive secretion of insulin precursors characterizes and predicts gestational diabetes. Diabetes 1995;44:911-5.
267. Tahara Y, Shima K. Kinetics of HbA1c, glycated albumin, and fructosamine and analysis of their weight functions against preceding plasma glucose level. Diabetes Care 1995;18:440-7.
268. Tamada JA, Garg S, Jovanovic L, Pitzer KR, Fermi S, Potts RO. Noninvasive glucose monitoring: comprehensive clinical results. Cygnus Research Team. JAMA 1999;282:1839-44.
269. Tang Z, Du X, Louie RF, Kost GJ. Effects of drugs on glucose measurements with handheld glucose meters and a portable glucose analyzer. Am J Clin Pathol 2000;113:75-86.
270. Tate PF, Clements CA, Walters JE. Accuracy of home blood glucose monitors. Diabetes Care 1992;15: 536-8.
271. Taylor R, Zimmet P. Limitation of fasting plasma glucose for the diagnosis of diabetes mellitus. Diabetes Care 1981;4:556-8.
272. Temple RC, Carrington CA, Luzio SD, Owens DR, Schneider AE, Sobey WJ, et al. Insulin deficiency in non–insulin-dependent diabetes. Lancet 1989;1: 293-5.
273. The fad disease. Hypoglycemia is being diagnosed too often. Time April 7, 1980:71.
274. Thomas GH, Howell RR. Selected Screening Tests for Genetic Metabolic Diseases. Chicago: Year Book Medical Publishers, 1973.
275. Tillil H, Shapiro ET, Given BD, Rue P, Rubenstein AH, Galloway JA, et al. Reevaluation of urine C-peptide as measure of insulin secretion. Diabetes 1988;37:1195-201.
276. Todd JA. Genetic analysis of type 1 diabetes using whole genome approaches. Proc Natl Acad Sci U S A 1995;92:8560-5.
277. Townsend JC. A competitive immunoenzymometric assay for albumin in urine. Clin Chem 1986;32: 1372-4.
278. Trinder P. Determination of glucose in blood using glucose oxidase with an alternative oxygen acceptor. Ann Clin Biochem 1969;6:24-7.
279. Tuomilehto J, Lindstrom J, Eriksson JG, Valle TT, Hamalainen H, Ilanne-Parikka P, et al. Prevention of type 2 diabetes mellitus by changes in lifestyle among subjects with impaired glucose tolerance. N Engl J Med 2001;344:1343-50.
280. U.K. Prospective Diabetes Study (UKPDS) Group. Intensive blood-glucose control with sulphonylureas or insulin compared with conventional treatment and risk of complications in patients with type 2 diabetes (UKPDS 33). UK Prospective Diabetes Study (UKPDS) Group. Lancet 1998;352:837-53.
281. Ulrich P, Cerami A. Protein glycation, diabetes, and aging. Recent Prog Horm Res 2001;56:1-21.
282. Umpierrez GE, Watts NB, Phillips LS. Clinical utility of beta-hydroxybutyrate determined by reflectance meter in the management of diabetic ketoacidosis. Diabetes Care 1995;18:137-8.
283. Urdang M, Ansede-Luna G, Muller B, Newson R, Lacy-Pettit A, O'Shea D. An independent pilot study into the accuracy and reliability of home blood glucose monitors. Lancet 1999;353:1065-6.
284. Uribarri J, Oh MS, Carroll HJ. D-lactic acidosis. A review of clinical presentation, biochemical features, and pathophysiologic mechanisms. Medicine (Baltimore) 1998;77:73-82.
285. Ward WK, Paquette TL, Frank BH, Porte D, Jr. A sensitive radioimmunoassay for human proinsulin, with sequential use of antisera to C-peptide and insulin. Clin Chem 1986;32:728-33.
286. Watts GF, Bennett JE, Rowe DJ, Morris RW, Gatling W, Shaw KM, et al. Assessment of immunochemical methods for determining low concentrations of albumin in urine. Clin Chem 1986;32: 1544-8.
287. Weissman M, Klein B. Evaluation of glucose determinations in untreated serum samples. Clin Chem 1958;4:420-2.
288. Weitgasser R, Gappmayer B, Pichler M. Newer portable glucose meters–analytical improvement compared with previous generation devices? Clin Chem 1999;45:1821-5.
289. Wermers RA, Fatourechi V, Wynne AG, Kvols LK, Lloyd RV. The glucagonoma syndrome. Clinical and pathologic features in 21 patients. Medicine (Baltimore) 1996;75:53-63.
290. White MF, Kahn CR. The insulin signaling system. J Biol Chem 1994;269:1-4.
291. Wiener K. What is 75g of glucose? Ann Clin Biochem 1990;27 (Pt 4):283-4.
292. Wiener K, Roberts NB. Age does not influence levels of HbA1c in normal subject. QJ Med 1999;92: 169-73.
293. Wiggam MI, O'Kane MJ, Harper R, Atkinson AB, Hadden DR, Trimble ER, et al. Treatment of diabetic ketoacidosis using normalization of blood 3-hydroxybutyrate concentration as the endpoint of emergency management. A randomized controlled study. Diabetes Care 1997;20:1347-52.

294. Wilson DH, Bogacz JP, Forsythe CM, Turk PJ, Lane TL, Gates RC, et al. Fully automated assay of glycohemoglobin with the Abbott IMx analyzer: novel approaches for separation and detection. Clin Chem 1993;39:2090-7.
295. Wilson GS, Zhang Y, Reach G, Moatti-Sirat D, Poitout V, Thevenot DR, et al. Progress toward the development of an implantable sensor for glucose. Clin Chem 1992;38:1613-7.
296. Windeler J, Kobberling J. The fructosamine assay in diagnosis and control of diabetes mellitus scientific evidence for its clinical usefulness? J Clin Chem Clin Biochem 1990;28:129-38.
297. Wolffenbuttel BH, Giordano D, Founds HW, Bucala R. Long-term assessment of glucose control by haemoglobin-AGE measurement. Lancet 1996;347:513-5.
298. Woo J, Floyd M, Cannon DC, Kahan B. Radioimmunoassay for urinary albumin. Clin Chem 1978;24:1464-7.
299. Wright WR, Rainwater JC, Tolle LD. Glucose assay systems: evaluation of a colorimetric hexokinase procedure. Clin Chem 1971;17:1010-5.
300. Yatscoff RW, Tevaarwerk GJ, MacDonald JC. Quantification of nonenzymically glycated albumin and total serum protein by affinity chromatography. Clin Chem 1984;30:446-9.
301. Yechoor VK, Patti ME, Saccone R, Kahn CR. Coordinated patterns of gene expression for substrate and energy metabolism in skeletal muscle of diabetic mice. Proc Natl Acad Sci U S A 2002;99:10587-92.
302. Young DS, Jackson AJ. Thin-layer chromatography of urinary carbohydrates. A comparative evaluation of procedures. Clin Chem 1970;16:954-9.
303. Zimmet P, Alberti KG, Shaw J. Global and societal implications of the diabetes epidemic. Nature 2001;414:782-7.

ADDITIONAL READING

American Diabetes Association. American Diabetes Association complete guide to diabetes: The ultimate home reference from the diabetes experts, 3rd ed. New York: McGraw-Hill/Contemporary Distributed Products, 2002: 517pp.

Dominiczak MH, Baynes JW. Diabetes Mellitus. Special Issue. CCLM 2003:41:1103-278.

International Organization for Standardization (ISO). Document ISO 15197, In vitro diagnostic test systems—Requirements for blood-glucose monitoring systems for self-testing in managing diabetes mellitus. Geneva Switzerland: International Organization for Standardization, 2003.

National Committee for Clinical Laboratory Standards. Point-of-Care Blood Glucose Testing in Acute and Chronic Care Facilities, Approved Standard C30-A2. 2nd ed. Wayne PA: National Committee for Clinical Laboratory Standards, 2002.

National Committee for Clinical Laboratory Standards. Harmonization of Glycohemoglobin Measurements; Approved Guideline, Approved Standard C44-A. Wayne PA: National Committee for Clinical Laboratory Standards, 2003.

CHAPTER 26

Lipids, Lipoproteins, Apolipoproteins, and Other Cardiovascular Risk Factors*

Nader Rifai, Ph.D.,
and G. Russell Warnick, M.S., M.B.A.

Lipids are ubiquitous in the body tissue and have an important role in virtually all aspects of life—serving as hormones or hormone precursors, aiding in digestion, providing energy storage and metabolic fuels, acting as functional and structural components in cell membranes, and forming insulation to allow nerve conduction or to prevent heat loss. In this chapter we have categorized lipids into basic lipids, lipoproteins, and apolipoproteins. We discuss the basic biochemistry, clinical significance, and analytical considerations of each.

BASIC BIOCHEMISTRY

For many years, much attention has been focused on certain lipids and the lipoproteins that transport them in the circulation, mainly because of their strong association with coronary heart disease (CHD). Therefore the use of the term *lipids* in clinical chemistry and laboratory medicine has become virtually synonymous with lipoprotein metabolism and atherosclerosis, a cause of CHD. Much of this association has been recognized through the conduct of large national and international collaborative analytical, epidemiological, and clinical studies. In the early 1980s, findings from the Coronary Primary Prevention Trial demonstrated that a decrease in plasma cholesterol concentration results in a reduction in the incidence of CHD. Since that time, several secondary prevention trials using diet or drugs to lower blood cholesterol have also demonstrated a reduction in cardiovascular death and atherosclerotic clinical events. Based on these trials and other evidence, the National Heart, Lung, and Blood Institute established the National Cholesterol Education Program (NCEP) to increase public awareness about cholesterol; devise strategies for diagnosis and treatment of hypercholesterolemia in adults, children, and adolescents; and improve the laboratory measurement of lipids. The European Atherosclerosis Society and other individual countries have also established similar programs to address these issues.

Basic Lipids

The term *lipid* applies to a class of compounds that are soluble in organic solvents and nearly insoluble in water. Chemically, lipids are either compounds that yield fatty acids on hydrolysis or complex alcohols that combine with fatty acids to form esters. Some lipids are more complex, containing nonlipid groups, such as sialic, phosphoryl, amino,

*The authors gratefully acknowledge the contribution by Drs. John Albers and Paul Bachorik on which portions of this chapter are based. Additional portions have been adapted from Rifai N, Kwiterovich PO Jr. Disorders of lipid and lipoprotein metabolism in children and adolescents. In Soldin SJ, Rifai N, Hick JMB eds. Biochemical basis of pediatric diseases, 3rd ed. Washington DC: AACC Press, 1998.

BOX 26-1 Classification of Clinically Important Lipids

Sterol Derivatives
- Cholesterol and cholesteryl esters
- Steroid hormones
- Bile acids
- Vitamin D

Fatty Acids
- Short chain (2-4 carbon atoms)
- Medium chain (6-10 carbon atoms)
- Long chain (12-26 carbon atoms)
- Prostaglandins

Glycerol Esters
- Tri-, di-, and monoglycerides (acylglycerols)
- Phosphoglycerides

Sphingosine Derivatives
- Sphingomyelin
- Glycosphingolipids

Terpenes (Isoprene Polymers)
- Vitamin A
- Vitamin E
- Vitamin K

or sulfate groups. The presence of these groups gives them the property (amphipathic) of having an affinity for both water and organic solvents, which is important in the formation of membranes. Lipids have been broadly subdivided into five groups based on their chemical structure (Box 26-1).

Cholesterol

Although every living organism has been found to contain sterols, cholesterol is found almost exclusively in animals, in which it is also the main sterol. Virtually all cells and body fluids contain some cholesterol. Like other sterols, cholesterol is a solid alcohol of high molecular weight and possesses the tetracyclic perhydrocyclopentanophenanthrene skeleton. The molecule contains 27 carbon atoms, numbered as shown in Figure 26-1. Knowledge of this sterane skeleton and numbering system is important not only to clinical laboratorians but to practicing clinicians because cholesterol is the initial starting point in many metabolic pathways. These include vitamin D synthesis (see Chapter 49), steroid hormone synthesis (see Chapter 51), and bile acid metabolism. Because the enzymes modifying the sterane ring or its radicals in each metabolic pathway are known by both their site and type of reaction (e.g., 21-hydroxylase in cortisol synthesis), the diagnosis of many disease states consequently depends on isolating the site of enzyme dysfunction (e.g., 21-hydroxylase deficiency in adrenogenital syndrome).

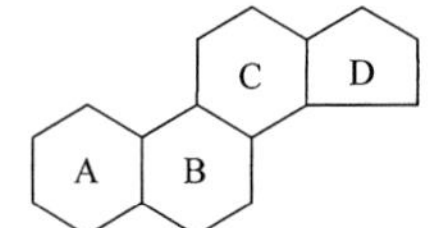

Perhydrocyclopentanophenanthrene (sterane) skeleton

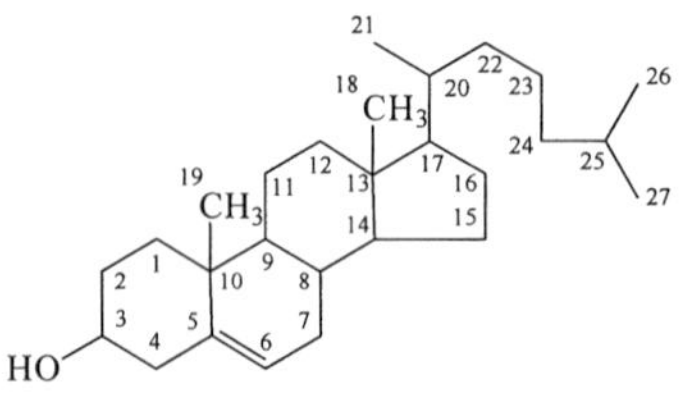

Cholesterol

Figure 26-1 Structure of cholesterol.

Cholesterol Absorption

Cholesterol is presented to the intestinal wall from three sources: the diet, bile and intestinal secretions, and cells. Animal products—especially meat, egg yolk, seafood, and whole-fat dairy products—provide the bulk of dietary cholesterol. Although cholesterol intake varies considerably according to the dietary intake of animal products, the average American diet is estimated to contain approximately 300 to 450 mg of cholesterol per day. A similar amount of cholesterol is present in the gut from biliary secretion and the turnover of mucosal cells. Practically all cholesterol in the intestine is present in the unesterified (free) form. Esterified cholesterol in the diet is rapidly hydrolyzed in the intestine to free cholesterol and free fatty acids by cholesterol esterases secreted from the pancreas and small intestine.

To be absorbed, unesterified cholesterol must first be solubilized. This occurs through the formation of mixed micelles that contain unesterified cholesterol, fatty acids, monoglycerides (derived from triglycerides), phospholipids (lysolecithin), and conjugated bile acids. Formation of mixed micelles aids cholesterol absorption by both solubilizing the cholesterol and facilitating its transport to the surface of the luminal cell, where it is absorbed. Because of their amphipathic properties, the bile acids act as detergents and are the most important factor affecting micelle formation. In the absence of bile acids, digestion and absorption of both cholesterol and triglyceride are severely impaired. The quantity of dietary cholesterol that can be absorbed appears to depend on the amount that can be solubilized by micelles. On the average, 30% to 60% of dietary and intestinal cholesterol is absorbed daily. With increments in dietary cholesterol, additional cholesterol is absorbed to a maximum of approximately 1 g/day when oral intake reaches 3 g/day. The ability of cholesterol to form micelles is also influenced by the quantity of dietary fat but not its degree of saturation. Increased amounts of fat in the diet result in expansion of mixed micelles, which in turn allows for more cholesterol to be solubilized and absorbed. Most cholesterol absorption occurs in the small intestine (middle and terminal ileum), and as absorption of fat and cholesterol occurs in the small intestine, the micelles break up, thus reducing further cholesterol absorption.

In addition to animal cholesterol, approximately 200 to 300 mg of plant sterols are ingested daily. The most common plant sterol is β-sitosterol. Plant sterols differ from cholesterol only by small variations on the sterol side chain. Despite their close similarity to cholesterol, plant sterols are poorly absorbed. When plant sterols are administered in amounts of 5 to 15 g/day, they significantly inhibit the absorption of cholesterol. Although the mechanism for reducing cholesterol absorption has not been determined, plant sterols have been used therapeutically in patients with elevated plasma cholesterol levels.

After its absorption into the intestinal mucosal cell, cholesterol, together with triglycerides, phospholipids, and a number of specific apoproteins, is assembled into a large lipoprotein called the *chylomicron* (see later section on lipoprotein metabolism, exogenous pathway). One apoprotein component known as apolipoprotein (apo) B-48 is vital to the formation of chylomicrons, and in people with a rare deficiency of apo B-48 synthesis, chylomicron formation, and consequently cholesterol and fat absorption, is severely impaired. Chylomicrons enter the lymphatics, which empty into the thoracic duct and eventually enter the systemic venous circulation at the junction of the left subclavian vein and left internal jugular vein.

Cholesterol Synthesis

Of the total cholesterol synthesized daily, about 300 to 1000 mg is derived from dietary intake. Cholesterol is also synthesized endogenously by the liver and other tissue from simple molecules, particularly acetate. Knowledge of the endogenous cholesterol synthetic pathway has assumed great significance in the past decade because agents have been sought to suppress or decrease endogenous cholesterol synthesis. The necessity for clinical medicine to understand the fundamental biochemistry of this pathway was underscored by the triparanol disaster of 1960. Triparanol is a drug that inhibits the final step in the endogenous cholesterol synthetic path (conversion of desmosterol to cholesterol), but does not inhibit the rate-limiting enzyme of cholesterol synthesis, 3-hydroxy-3-methylglutaryl-CoA (HMG-CoA) reductase (Figure 26-2). When triparanol was used to treat hypercholesterolemia, the drug caused tissue accumulation of desmosterol, resulting in the development of cataracts, alopecia, and atherosclerosis in treated patients. Drugs such as atorvastatin, lovastatin, mevastatin, pravastatin, and simvastatin selectively suppress the rate-limiting enzyme HMG-CoA reductase, and thereby lower serum cholesterol levels significantly without the accumulation of water-insoluble intermediates of cholesterol synthesis, such as desmosterol.

Although essentially all cells have the capacity to synthesize cholesterol from acetyl-CoA, almost 90% of synthesis occurs in the liver and gut; peripheral cells and other organs depend on cholesterol delivery from the circulation. Cholesterol biosynthesis is best conceptualized as occurring in three stages (Figures 26-2 through 26-4). In the first stage, acetyl-CoA, a key metabolic intermediate derived from carbohydrates, amino acids, and fatty acids, forms the six-carbon thioester HMG-CoA. In the second stage, HMG-CoA is reduced to mevalonate, then decarboxylated to five-carbon isoprene units. These isoprene units are condensed to form first a 10-carbon (geranyl pyrophosphate) and then a 15-carbon intermediate (farnesyl pyrophosphate). Two of these C_{15} molecules combine to produce the final product of the second stage—squalene, a 30-carbon acyclic hydrocarbon. The second stage is important because it contains the step involving the microsomal enzyme HMG-CoA reductase, which is the rate-limiting enzyme in cholesterol biosynthesis. The enzyme that forms farnesyl pyrophosphate, geranyl transferase, is an important second site of regulation in cholesterol synthesis, and inhibition at this level permits the formation of physiologically important intermediate isoprenoids in the absence of cholesterol synthesis. The third and final stage of synthesis occurs in the endoplasmic reticulum, with many of the intermediate products being bound to a specific carrier protein. Squalene, after an initial oxidation, undergoes cyclization to form the 4-ring, 30-carbon intermediate, lanosterol. In a series of oxidation-decarboxylation reactions, a number of side chains are removed from the pentanophenanthrene structure to form the 27-carbon molecule of cholesterol.

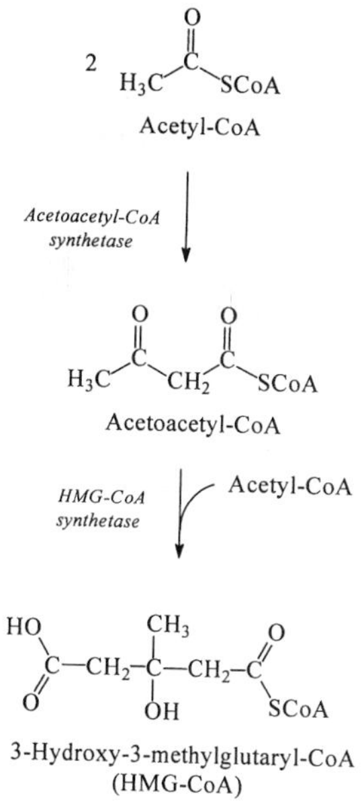

2 Acetyl-CoA

Acetoacetyl-CoA synthetase

Acetoacetyl-CoA

HMG-CoA synthetase ← Acetyl-CoA

3-Hydroxy-3-methylglutaryl-CoA (HMG-CoA)

Figure 26-2 Cholesterol biosynthesis (stage I).

Cholesterol Esterification

Once synthesized, cholesterol is released into the circulation in the form of lipoprotein, primarily very low-density lipoprotein (VLDL; see later section on lipoprotein metab-

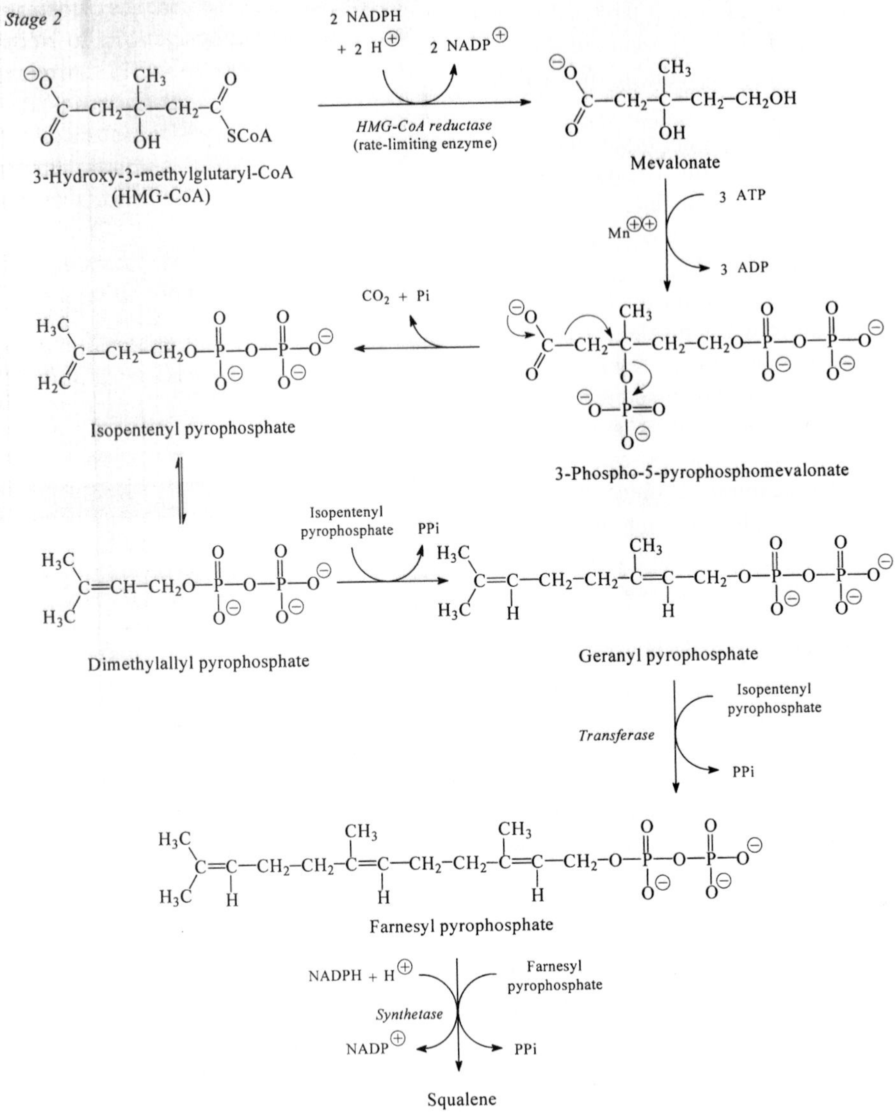

Figure 26-3 Cholesterol biosynthesis (stage 2).

olism, endogenous pathway). The major apoprotein found in VLDL is apo B-100, a protein related to apo B-48, which is found in chylomicrons. Esterification is important because it serves to enhance the lipid-carrying capacity of the lipoprotein in plasma and prevent intracellular toxicity by free cholesterol. The reaction is catalyzed by lecithin-cholesterol acyltransferase (LCAT) in the plasma and acyl-cholesterol acyltransferase (ACAT) within the cell. The intracellular ACAT pathway is the major pathway in the liver, intestine, adrenal cortex, and probably in the arterial wall. This is an energy-requiring pathway, and the initial reaction (Figure 26-5) involves activation of a fatty acid with thio coenzyme A (Co ASH) to form an acyl-CoA, which in turn reacts with cholesterol to form an ester. The LCAT reaction does not require CoASH and results from fatty acid transfer from the second carbon position of lecithin to cholesterol (see Figure 26-5). Cholesteryl esters account for about 70% of the cholesterol in plasma, and LCAT is responsible for the formation of virtually all of this cholesteryl ester. LCAT is synthesized in the liver, released into the circulation, and primarily activated by apo A-I (see later section on apolipoproteins).

Plasma LCAT activity may have some significance analytically because the enzyme continues to esterify plasma cholesterol even after the blood sample is drawn and stored at room temperature. If it is necessary to distinguish between esterified and unesterified cholesterol, analysis should be carried out as soon as possible, or the samples should be cooled to at least 4 °C or frozen, preferably at −70 °C or lower.

Cholesterol Catabolism

Once lipoprotein cholesterol enters the cell, the cholesteryl esters are hydrolyzed by lysosomal acid lipase. The lack or malfunction of this enzyme results in intracellular accumulation of cholesterol esters and produces a clinical disorder known as *cholesteryl ester storage disease.*

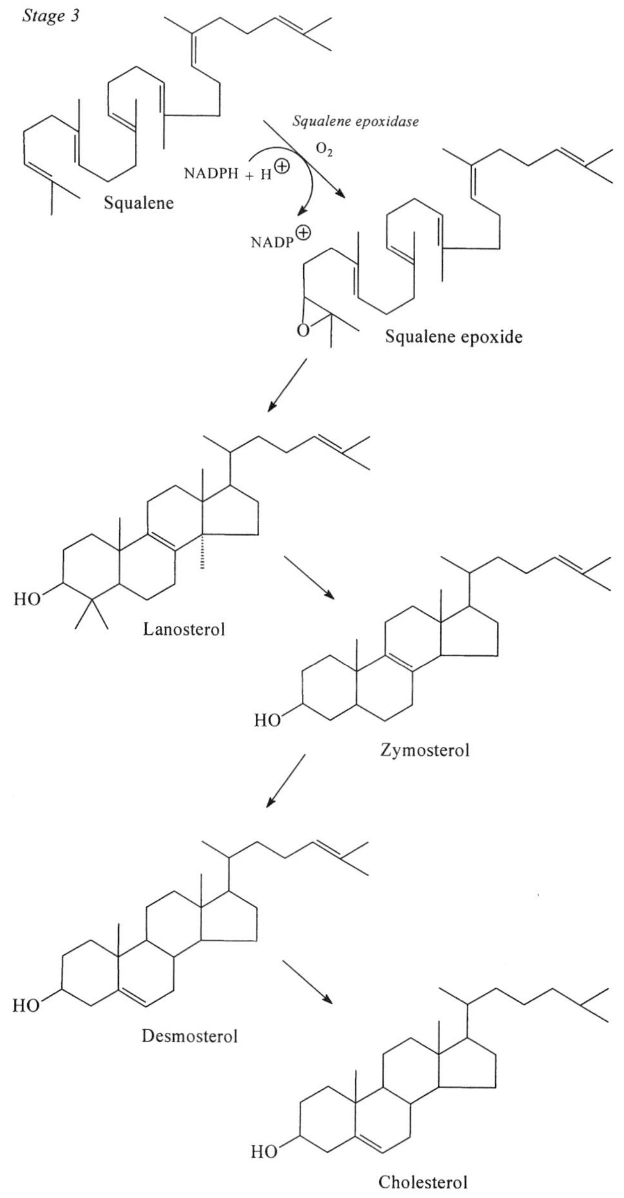

Stage 3

Squalene

Squalene epoxidase

O_2

NADPH + $H^{\oplus}$

$NADP^{\oplus}$

Squalene epoxide

Lanosterol

Zymosterol

Desmosterol

Cholesterol

Figure 26-4 Cholesterol biosynthesis (stage 3).

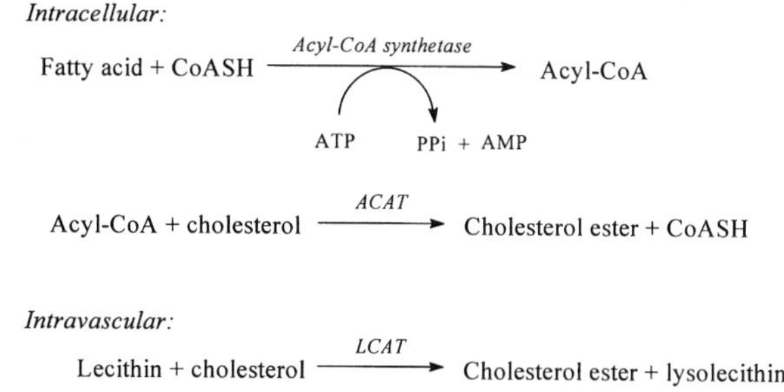

Figure 26-5 Intracellular and intravascular esterification of cholesterol mediated by ACAT and LCAT, respectively.

Cholesterol reaching the liver is either secreted unchanged into bile or metabolized to bile acids. Approximately one third of the daily production of cholesterol, or about 400 mg/day, is converted into bile acids (Figure 26-6). The conversion of cholesterol to cholic and chenodeoxycholic acids, the major bile acids in humans, involves the shortening of the cholesterol side chain and hydroxylation of the sterol nucleus. The first step, which is also the rate-limiting step, is the hydroxylation of the 7-position of the sterol nucleus, catalyzed by the enzyme 7α-hydroxylase (see Figure 26-6). The bile acids are then conjugated with either glycine or taurine and enter the bile canaliculi. After reaching the small intestine, the conjugated bile acids play an active part in cholesterol and fat absorption, as discussed previously. Some of the bile acids are deconjugated and converted by bacteria in the intestine to secondary bile acids. Cholic acid is converted to deoxycholic acid, and chenodeoxycholic acid is metabolized to lithocholic acid. About 90% of the bile acids, except lithocholic, are reabsorbed in the lower third of the ileum and returned to the liver by the portal vein, thus completing the enterohepatic circulation (see also Chapter 47).

A significant amount of cholesterol is also excreted directly into the biliary system, where it is solubilized to form mixed micelles with bile acids and phospholipids. If the amount of cholesterol in bile exceeds the capacity of these solubilizing agents, however, excess cholesterol can precipitate, forming cholesterol gallstones. In westernized societies, approximately 80% of all gallstones are cholesterol-containing stones.

Fatty Acids

The fatty acids are one of the simpler molecular forms of lipids. They are generically indicated by the chemical formula RCOOH, where "R" stands for an alkyl chain. Fatty acid chain lengths vary and are commonly classified according to the number of carbon atoms present. Three somewhat arbitrarily defined groups of fatty acids are those containing 2 to 4 carbon atoms (short chain), 6 to 10 carbon atoms (medium chain), and 12 to 26 carbon atoms (long chain). Those of importance in human nutrition and metabolism are of the long-chain class containing an even number of carbon atoms.

Fatty acids are further classified according to their degree of saturation. Saturated fatty acids have no double bonds between carbon atoms, monounsaturated fatty acids contain one double bond, and polyunsaturated fatty acids contain more than one double bond (Figure 26-7). The double bonds in polyunsaturated fatty acids of both animal and plant origin are usually 3 carbon atoms apart. Some oils from marine fish living in deep, cold waters (e.g., salmon) possess numerous (up to 6) unsaturated bonds and are usually more than 20 carbon atoms long. These oils can be easily oxidated because of their high degree of unsaturation.

The labeling of the carbon atoms in fatty acids can be either from the carboxyl terminal (Δ-numbering system) or from the methyl terminal (η- or ω-numbering system;

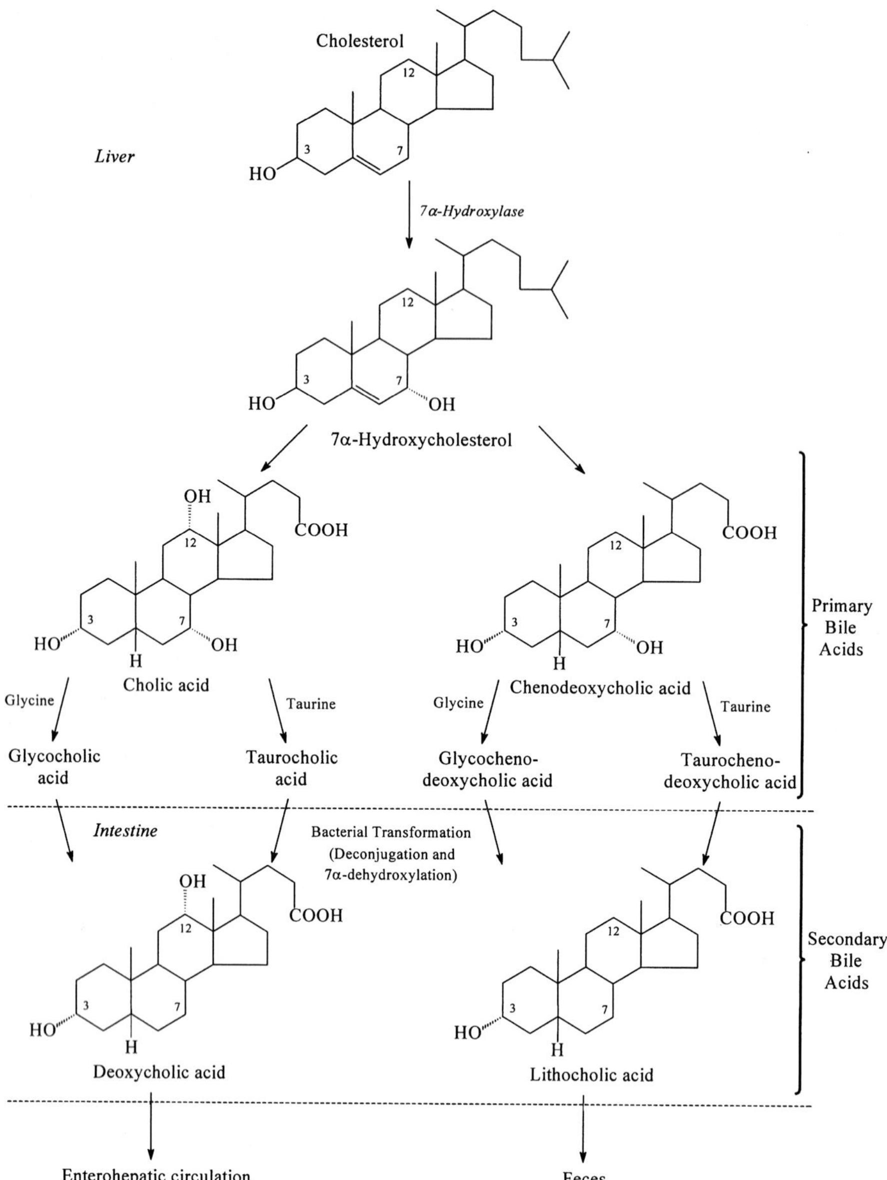

Figure 26-6 Bile acid synthesis.

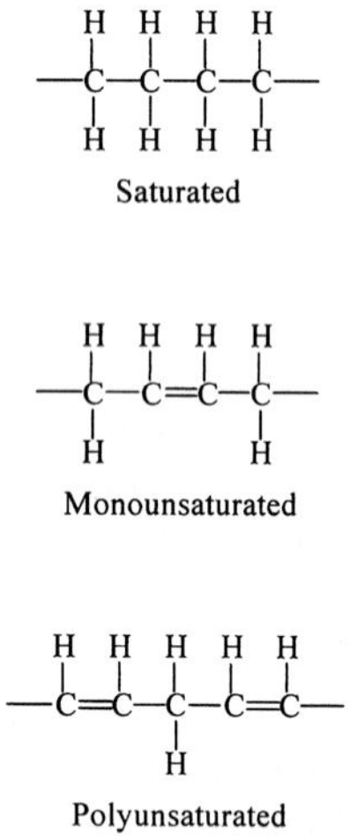

Saturated

Monounsaturated

Polyunsaturated

Figure 26-7 Saturated and unsaturated fatty acids.

Table 26-1). In addition, the carbon atoms may be labeled with Greek symbols, with α being adjacent to the carboxyl group and ω being farthest away. In the Δ-system, fatty acids are abbreviated according to the number of carbon atoms, the number of double bonds, and the position(s) of double bond(s). For example, linoleic acid, which contains 18 carbons and two unsaturated bonds between carbons 9 and 10 and between carbons 12 and 13, could be written as $C_{18}:2^{9,12}$. Using the η- or ω-system, linoleic acid would be abbreviated to $C_{18}:2n-6$, where only the first carbon forming the unsaturated pair is written. The *Geneva* or *systematic* classification is a third system of nomenclature (Table 26-1).

In saturated fatty acids, the chain is extended and flexible (i.e., the carbon atoms rotate freely around the longitudinal axis). Unsaturated fatty acids, however, have fixed 30° bends

TABLE 26-1 Fatty Acids Commonly Found in Human Tissue

Common Name	Systematic Name	Δ-Numbering	η-(ω) Numbering
Lauric	Dodecanoic	12:0	12:0
Myristic	Tetradecanoic	14:0	14:0
Palmitic	Hexadecanoic	16:0	16:0
Palmitoleic	9-Hexadecenoic	$16:1^{9}$	16:1n-7
Stearic	Octadecanoic	18:0	18:0
Oleic	9-Octadecenoic	$18:1^{9}$	18:1n-9
Linoleic*	9,12-Octadecadienoic	$18:2^{9,12}$	18:2n-6
Linolenic*	9,12,15-Octadecatrienoic	$18:3^{9,12,15}$	18:3n-3
Arachidic	Eicosanoic	20:0	20:0
Arachidonic	5,8,11,14-Eicosatetraenoic	$20:4^{5,8,11,14}$	20:4n-6

*Essential fatty acids.

in their chains at each double bond. Depending on the plane in which this bend occurs, either the *cis* or *trans* isomer is produced. In mammals, all naturally occurring unsaturated fatty acids are of the *cis* variety. *Trans* fatty acids result from catalytic hydrogenation, a process used to "harden" fats in the manufacture of certain foods, such as margarine. Most fats in the human body are derived from the diet, which on the average contains up to 40% fat, 90% of which is triglyceride. In addition, humans can synthesize most fatty acids, including saturated, monounsaturated, and some polyunsaturated fats. However, some fatty acids cannot be synthesized. One such fatty acid is linoleic acid ($C_{18}:2^{9,12}$), which is found only in plants. Because it is vital for health and growth and development, it is termed an *essential fatty acid*. Linoleic acid is converted to arachidonic acid, which has an important role in prostaglandin synthesis and perhaps in myelinization of the central nervous system.

The fatty acid carboxyl group has a pK_a of approximately 4.8; thus free fatty acid molecules in both plasma and intracellular fluid (pH of 7.4 and 7.0, respectively) exist in an ionized form. Much of the fatty acid in plasma exists as either esters with cholesterol or glycerol or is transported as a fatty acid–albumin complex or fatty acid–prealbumin complex. One molecule of albumin can carry as many as 20 molecules of fatty acid. The normal level of free fatty acids in human blood is 0.30 to 1.10 mmol/L, or about 8 to 31 mg/dL of plasma. The flux of free fatty acids through the plasma is very large and quite sensitive to physiological energy demands (exercise and physical work), the level of blood glucose, and psychological stresses that cause liberation of epinephrine.

Fatty Acid Catabolism

Long-chain fatty acids are oxidized in the mitochondria and produce energy by a series of reactions that operate in a repetitive manner to shorten the fatty acid chain by two carbon atoms at a time from the —COOH terminal of the molecule, a process known as β-oxidation. For example, 1 mole of C_{16} fatty acid is converted to 8 moles of acetyl-CoA. Acetyl-CoA does not normally accumulate in the cell but is enzymatically condensed with oxaloacetate, derived largely from carbohydrate metabolism (Figure 26-8), to give citrate, which is a major component of the tricarboxylic acid cycle (Krebs cycle). The Krebs cycle serves as a common pathway for the final oxidation of nearly all food material, whether derived from carbohydrate, fat, or protein. It is important to bear in mind that the smooth operation of the Krebs cycle depends on the availability of sufficient oxaloacetate to serve as an acceptor for acetyl-CoA.

The complete oxidation of a single fatty acid molecule produces a large quantity of energy. For example, the complete oxidation of 1 mole of palmitic acid to carbon dioxide and water produces 16 moles of CO_2, 16 moles of H_2O, and 129 moles of adenosine triphosphate (ATP), or 2340 Cal.* Thus the standard free energy for oxidation of palmitic acid is 2340 Cal, whereas the free energy liberated by hydrolysis of 129 moles of ATP is 940 Cal, indicating that the efficiency of energy conservation in fatty acid oxidation is approximately 40% under standard conditions.

By means of suitable enzyme reactions, the chemical energy stored in fatty acids can be released for metabolic processes or stored in the form of high-energy compounds, such as ATP. Triglycerides that contain three fatty acid molecules, therefore, are an efficient storage form for metabolic energy. The amount of energy produced by metabolizing 1 mole of palmitic acid (16 carbon atoms) is approximately twice that produced by metabolizing an equivalent amount (2.5 mol) of glucose (6 carbon atoms per molecule). Carbohydrate storage requires water for hydration; triglyceride storage does not. In addition to their high intrinsic energy content, triglycerides have a low density (<1 g/mL) and, because of their hydrophobic nature and peripheral distribution in the body, provide excellent insulation.

*The unit used in discussing the energy value of food is the Calorie (Cal), equal to 1000 calories or 1 kilocalorie (kcal). In the SI system, the unit of energy is the joule (J), and 1 calorie = 4.1868 J.

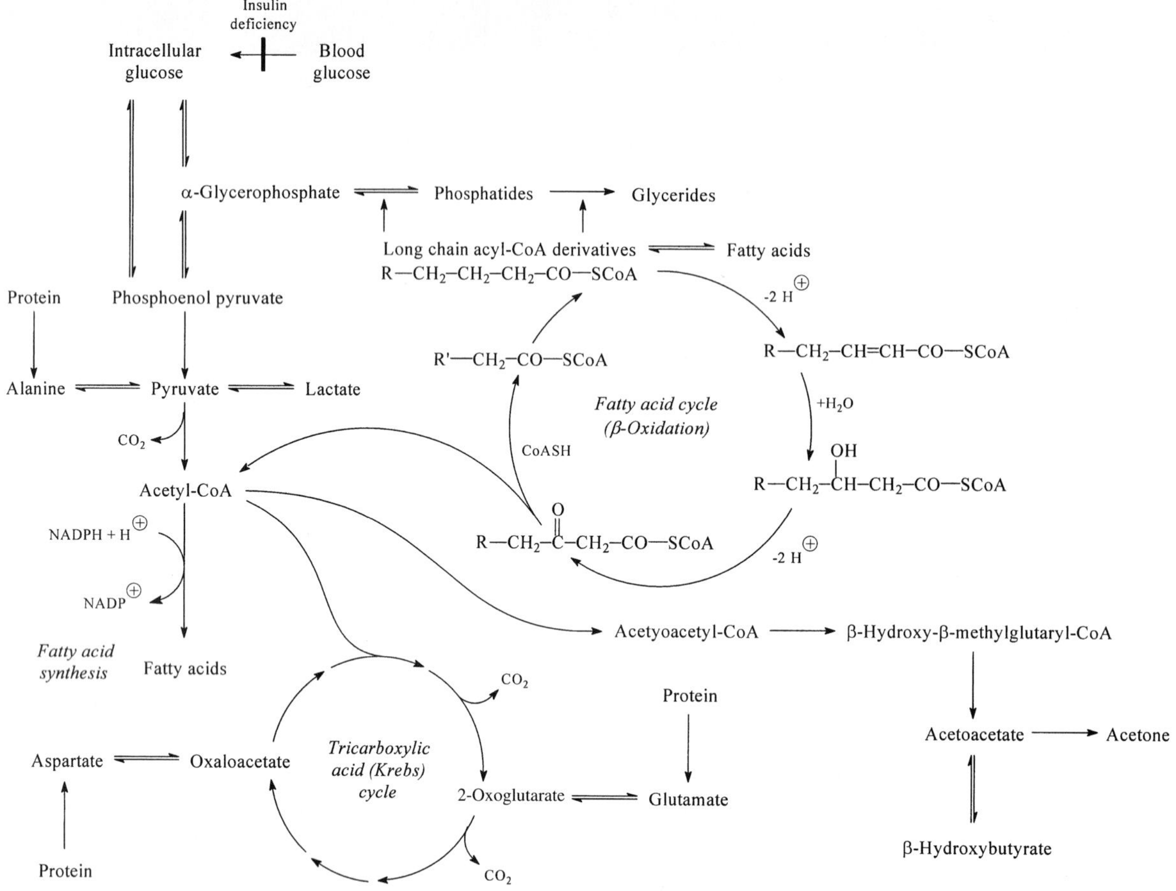

Figure 26-8 Metabolic relations among intermediates of carbohydrate, fat, and protein metabolism. Note that acetyl-CoA is produced from both carbohydrate and fat. The glucogenic amino acids, derived from protein metabolism, enter glycolytic paths as α-keto acids. Ketogenic amino acids enter as acetyl-CoA.

Ketone Formation

During prolonged starvation or when carbohydrate metabolism is severely impaired, as in uncontrolled diabetes mellitus (see Chapter 25), the formation of acetyl-CoA exceeds the supply of oxaloacetate. The abundance of acetyl-CoA results from excessive mobilization of fatty acids from adipose tissue and excessive degradation of the fatty acids by β-oxidation in the liver. The resulting acetyl-CoA excess is diverted to an alternative pathway in the mitochondria and forms acetoacetic acid, β-hydroxybutyric acid, and acetone—three compounds known collectively as *ketone bodies* (Figure 26-9). The presence of ketone bodies is a frequent finding in severe, uncontrolled diabetes mellitus.

As shown in Figure 26-9, the first product, acetoacetyl-CoA, condenses in the mitochondria with a third molecule of acetyl-CoA to yield HMG-CoA. This pool of HMG-CoA is distinct from that in the cytosol that is an intermediate in cholesterol synthesis. The HMG-CoA produced in the mitochondria is then cleaved enzymatically to yield acetoacetate and acetyl-CoA. Some of the acetoacetate formed in liver cells is usually reduced to β-hydroxybutyrate. Because acetoacetate is unstable, a further portion decomposes to form carbon dioxide and acetone, the third ketone body found in severe, untreated diabetes mellitus. Ketosis, therefore, develops from excessive production of acetyl-CoA because the body attempts to obtain necessary energy from stored fat in the absence of an adequate supply of carbohydrate metabolites (see Chapter 25).

Inadequate incorporation of acetyl-CoA into the Krebs cycle may be further aggravated by inhibition of the oxaloacetate-generating enzyme system by excess accumulation of palmitic-CoA and other long-chain fatty acid–CoA derivatives in the liver. Skeletal muscle and heart (and brain in prolonged fasting) use ketone bodies by resynthesizing their CoA derivatives of the acids and subsequently oxidizing them for the production of energy. Although liver cells are largely responsible for converting fatty acids, they cannot metabolize acetoacetate, because liver lacks 3-ketoacid CoA transferase, the enzyme required for transferring CoA from succinyl-CoA.

The entire process of ketosis reversed by restoring an adequate level of carbohydrate metabolism. In starvation, restoration consists of adequate carbohydrate ingestion; in diabetes mellitus, ketosis can be reversed by insulin administration, which permits circulating blood glucose to be taken up by the cells. With production of oxaloacetate, the

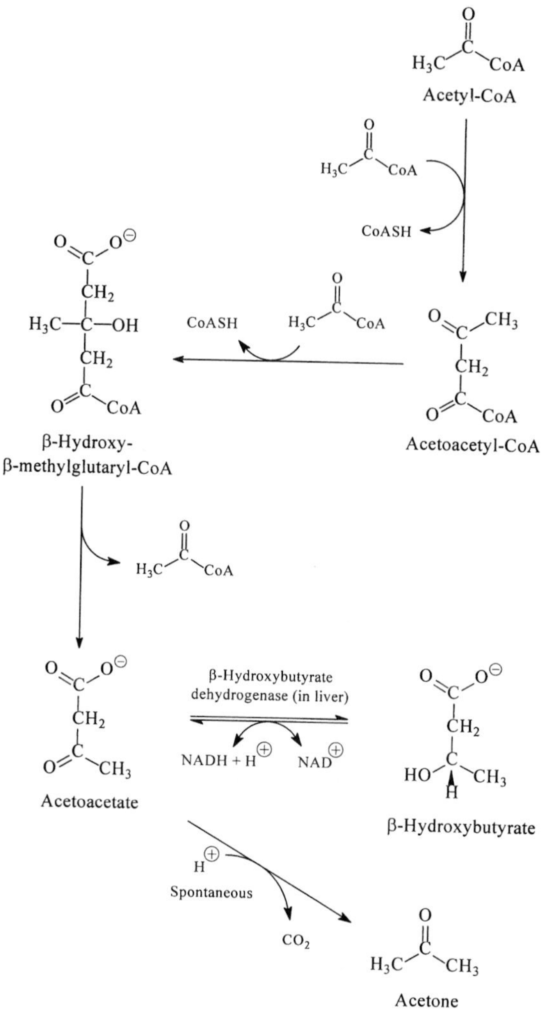

Figure 26-9 Formation of ketone bodies.

acceptor of acetyl-CoA, normal metabolism is restored, and the release of fatty acids from adipose tissue slows and is finally reversed. A graphic view of these metabolic reactions is outlined in Figure 26-8, which shows the interrelationship between carbohydrate, fatty acid, and protein metabolism.

Prostaglandins

Prostaglandins and related compounds are derivatives of fatty acids, primarily arachidonate. The group consists of prostaglandins, thromboxanes, some hydroperoxy- and hydroxy–fatty acid derivatives, and leukotrienes. Although their full physiological role is not completely known, they exert diverse biological actions. They are extremely potent, producing physiological actions at concentrations as low as 1 μg/L.

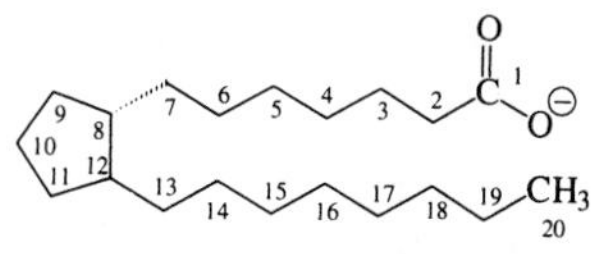

The prostaglandins are a series of C_{20} unsaturated fatty acids containing a cyclopentane ring; the parent fatty acid has been given the trivial name *prostanoic acid.* The seven-carbon chain linked to C-8 of prostanoic acid (R_1) projects below the plane of the ring, whereas the eight-carbon chain attached to C-12 (R_2) projects above the ring.

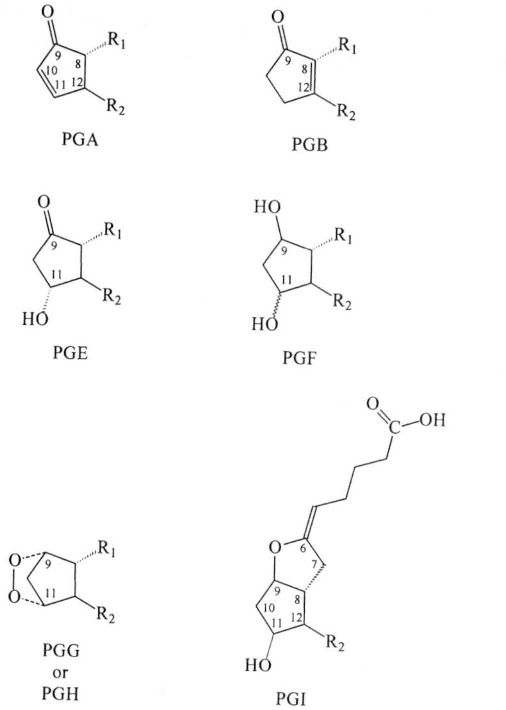

Figure 26-10 Major prostaglandin classes (series). R_1 and R_2 are prostaglandin side chains.

By convention, prostaglandins are abbreviated *PG,* with the class designated by a capital letter (A, B, E, F, G, H, and I), followed by a number and then in some cases a Greek letter (Figure 26-10). With the exception of PGG and PGH, which have the same ring structure (cyclopentane endoperoxide), the letters refer to different ring structures. PGA and PGB have keto groups at C-9, with the A series having a double bond between C-10 and C-11 and the B series having a double bond between C-8 and C-12. PGE also has a C-9 keto bond but a hydroxyl group at C-11. The F series has hydroxyl groups at both C-9 and C-11. The difference between PGG and PGH, which have identical ring structures, occurs in the side chain at C-15 in R_2; the G series has a peroxide group, whereas the H series has a hydroxyl group. The I series has a double-ring formation, C-9 of the cyclopentane ring being linked to C-6 of the side chain by an oxygen molecule to form a second five-sided ring (see Figure 26-10). The endoperoxide PGs (G and H series) are intermediates in the formation of other PGs, such as the A, B, E, F, and I series.

The number after the capital letter is usually written as a subscript and is used to designate the number of unsaturated bonds in the PG side chains and not within the ring structure itself. In PGE_1, for example, a double bond exists between C-13 and C-14; in the 2 series (PGE_2), a double bond exists between C-13 and C-14 and between C-5 and

TABLE 26-2 Naturally Occurring Prostaglandins (PG)

Primary PG	Other PG
PGE_1	PGA_1
$PGF_{1\alpha}$	PGA_2
PGE_2	19α-$OHPGA_1$
$PGF_{2\alpha}$	19α-$OHPGA_2$
PGG_2	PGB_1
PGH_2	PGB_2
PGI_2	19α-$OHPGB_2$
Thromboxane A_2	PGE_3
Thromboxane B_2	$PGF_{3\alpha}$

C-6; and in the 3 series (PGE_3), an additional double bond occurs between C-17 and C-18. The 2 series is most common. The bond between C-13 and C-14 is always *trans*, whereas those between C-5 and C-6 and between C-17 and C-18 are always *cis*. At C-15, all naturally occurring prostaglandins have a hydroxyl group that projects below the plane of the ring. The use of the Greek letter (α or β) applies only to the F series and refers to the hydroxyl group found at C-9. In the α-series, the hydroxyl group projects below the ring plane in the same direction as the C-11 hydroxyl group, whereas the β-series denotes that the hydroxyl at C-9 is above the plane of the ring. Sixteen naturally occurring prostaglandins have been described (Table 26-2), but only seven, along with two thromboxanes, are commonly found throughout the body. These are termed the *primary prostaglandins*.

Although prostaglandins appear hormonelike in action, they are different from hormones in that (1) they are synthesized at the site of action and (2) they are made in almost all tissue. Linoleic acid ($C_{18}:2^{9,12}$) is the precursor of two of the three 20-carbon fatty acids that form prostaglandins; linolenic acid ($C_{18}:2^{9,12,15}$) is the other precursor. Both of these fatty acids are considered essential because they cannot be synthesized in the body and therefore must be present in the diet (see Chapter 48). The three C_{20} fatty acids subsequently formed are $C_{20}:3^{5,8,11}$ (eicosatrienoic acid), $C_{20}:4^{5,8,11,14}$ (eicosatetraenoic or arachidonic acid), and $C_{20}:5^{8,11,14,17}$(eicosatrienoic acid). These three fatty acids form the PG_1, PG_2, and PG_3 series, respectively.

Once formed, prostaglandins exert very short-lived effects and are rapidly catabolized (their half-life is expressed in seconds). Inactivation of prostaglandin appears to be mediated by two enzymes, 15 α-hydroxy-prostaglandin dehydrogenase and Δ^{13}-prostaglandin reductase. Prostaglandins are not stored; instead, the precursor C_{20} fatty acids are present in tissue attached to the C-2 (see later section in this chapter on glycerol esters) of phosphoglycerides. When necessary, the C_{20} precursor is hydrolyzed by phospholipase A_2, which is specific for the C-2 atom of the phosphoglyceride. The release of the C_{20} fatty acid appears

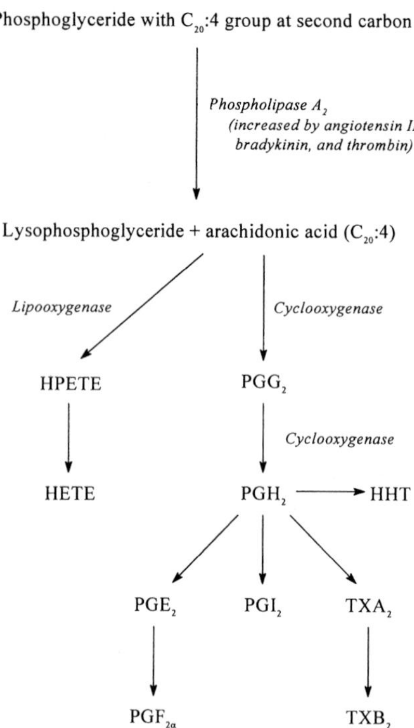

Figure 26-11 Synthesis of prostaglandins from arachidonic precursor. *PG,* Prostaglandin; *TX,* thromboxane; *HPETE, HETE, HHT,* 12-l-hydroxy-5,8,10-heptadecatrienoic acid.

to be the rate-limiting step in prostaglandin synthesis and is stimulated by the effect of bradykinin, thrombins, or angiotensin II.

Although it is probable that all prostaglandins follow a similar synthetic pathway, $C_{20}:4$ (arachidonic acid) has been the most intensively studied and is used to illustrate the pathway (Figure 26-11). Once released, arachidonic acid follows one of two pathways. The lipoxygenase route produces 12-L-hydroperoxy-5,8,10,14 eicosatetraenoic acid (HPETE); HPETE spontaneously decomposes to 12-L-hydroxy-5,8,10,14 eicosatetraenoic acid (HETE). The alternative pathway is mediated by cyclooxygenase (COX) to produce the endoperoxides PGG_2 and PGH_2. The latter can be degraded to 12-L-hydroxy-5,8,10-heptadecatrienoic acid. What controls the entry into a specific pathway remains speculative; however, it is known that nonsteroidal antiinflammatory drugs ([NSAIDs]: aspirin, ibuprofen, and indomethacin) inhibit the COXs, thereby decreasing prostaglandin synthesis. Two isoforms of COX are known, COX-1 and COX-2. COX-1 levels are in general rather constant in cells, whereas COX-2 is synthesized in response to inflammation. Certain drugs that inhibit both COXs have nephrotoxic and ulcerogenic side effects. Therefore newer NSAIDs are being tested to preferentially inhibit COX-2 to reduce side effects while maintaining the desirable antiinflammatory therapy.

Prostaglandin I_2, or prostacyclin, is derived from arachidonic acid (see Figure 26-11) in the vascular endothelium. It has a powerful vasodilatory action, especially on the coro-

Thromboxane A_2 (TXA_2)

Thromboxane B_2 (TXB_2)

Figure 26-12 Structures of thromboxanes.

TABLE 26-3 Prostaglandin-Mediated Effects

Site of Action	Physiological Response
Arterial smooth muscle	Alters blood pressure
Uterine muscle	Induces labor, therapeutic abortion
Lower gastrointestinal tract	Increases motility
Bronchial smooth muscle	Bronchospasm
Platelets	Increases coagulability
Capillaries	Increases permeability
Stomach	Enhances gastric acid secretion
Adipose tissue	Inhibits triglyceride lipolysis

nary arteries, and is also responsible for inhibiting platelet aggregation. Thromboxane A_2 is synthesized from arachidonic acid but is also produced by platelets. It has the opposite effect of prostacyclin (i.e., it stimulates the contraction of arterial smooth muscle and enhances platelet aggregation). It has a very short half-life, about 30 seconds, and is rapidly converted to its inactive metabolite, thromboxane B_2. The thromboxanes are slightly different from the other prostaglandins in that they contain six-sided rings of five carbon atoms and one oxygen atom (Figure 26-12). Table 26-3 lists some of the reported functions of the various prostaglandins. With increasing knowledge of the physiological role of the prostaglandins, it is likely that discrete disorders of prostaglandin metabolism will be discovered and that prostaglandins, prostaglandin analogues, or prostaglandin antagonists will be used in clinical practice.

Glycerol Esters (Acylglycerols)

Virtually all the complex lipids are fatty acid derivatives, and in most cases they are covalently linked to an alcohol. One of the most common alcohols found in human metabolism is glycerol, a three-carbon molecule containing three hydroxyl groups.

```
       H
       |
α   H—C—OH
       |
β   H—C—OH
       |
α'  H—C—OH
       |
       H
```

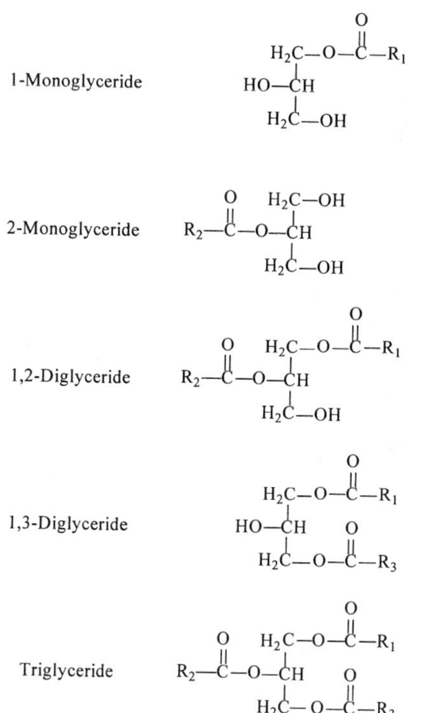

Figure 26-13 Structure and classification of glycerol esters (acylglycerols). R_1, R_2, and R_3 are fatty acid(s) of varying chain length.

The two terminal carbon atoms in the molecule are chemically equivalent and are designated α and α′. The center carbon is labeled β. A common alternative labeling system uses the numeral 1 for the α-carbon, 2 for the β-carbon, and 3 for the α′-carbon.

The class of acylglycerol (glyceride) is determined by the number of fatty acyl groups present; one fatty acid, monoacylglycerols (monoglycerides); two fatty acids, diacylglycerols (diglycerides); three fatty acids, triacylglycerols (triglycerides). In a monoacylglycerol, the fatty acid may be linked to any of the three carbon atoms. By convention, the number system is used to indicate the carbon position (e.g., 1-monoglyceride indicates a fatty acid attachment to the α-carbon). This numbering system applies to all acylglycerols, including the phosphoglycerides, as shown later. Diglycerides are either 1,2- or 1,3-diglycerides (Figure 26-13).

In human nutrition, triglycerides are the most prevalent glycerol esters encountered and constitute 95% of tissue storage fat and are the predominant form of glyceryl ester found in plasma. The fatty acid residues found in monoglycerides, diglycerides, or triglycerides vary considerably and usually include combinations of the long-chain fatty acids, shown in Table 26-1. Triglycerides from plants (e.g., corn, sunflower seed, and safflower oils) tend to have large amounts of C_{18}:2 or linoleic residues and are liquid at room temperature. Triglycerides from animals, especially ruminants, tend to have C_{12}:0 through C_{18}:0 fatty acid residues (saturated fats) and are solids at room temperature. Some plant triglycerides, such as coconut oil, are highly saturated and may be solid at room temperature.

Triglycerides are digested in the duodenum and proximal ileum. Through the action of pancreatic and intestinal lipases and in the presence of bile acids, they are hydrolyzed to glycerol, monoglycerides, and fatty acids. After absorption, triglycerides are resynthesized in the intestinal epithelial cells and combined with cholesterol and apo B-48 to form chylomicrons. Chylomicrons are then secreted to the lymphatic system, travel through the thoracic duct, and eventually reach the bloodstream through the jugular vein.

Another major class of glycerol esters consists of those containing phosphoric acid at the third (α') carbon atom; these esters are called phosphoglycerides (Figure 26-14). In their simplest form, the A group is an H atom and the molecule is therefore a diacylphosphoglyceride. Usually, however, the A is an alcohol-derived group, such as choline, serine, inositol, or ethanolamine (see Figure 26-14). If A is choline, the molecule is referred to as *phosphatidylcholine;* if it is ethanolamine, it will be referred to as *phosphatidylethanolamine,* etc. Phosphatidylcholines have also been collectively referred to as the *lecithins,* whereas phosphatidylethanolamine, phosphatidylserine, and phosphatidylinositol have been called the cephalins. As the fatty acid residues (R_1 and R_2 in Figure 26-14) vary, several different lecithins and cephalins are formed. These phosphoglycerides are named according to the fatty acid acyl ester attached at C-1 and C-2 of the glycerol. The saturated fatty acid attaches to the C-1, whereas (poly)unsaturated fatty acid attaches primarily at C-2. Phosphatidylcholine is the precursor of the potent lipid mediator, platelet-activating factor.

In inner mitochondrial membranes, more complex phosphoglycerides known as *cardiolipins* can be found. They are derived from two phosphoglyceride molecules joined by a glycerol bridge.

Sphingolipids

Sphingolipids are a fourth class of lipids found in humans and are derived from the amino alcohol sphingosine (Figure 26-15). This dihydric 18-carbon alcohol contains an amino group at C-17. A fatty acid containing 18 or more carbon atoms can be bound to the amino group through an amide

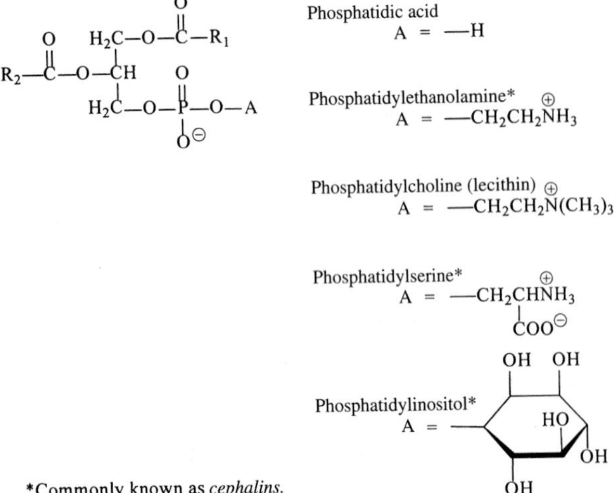

Figure 26-14 Structures of phosphoglycerides and common alcohol groups associated with them. R_1 and R_2 are fatty acid(s) of varying carbon atom lengths.

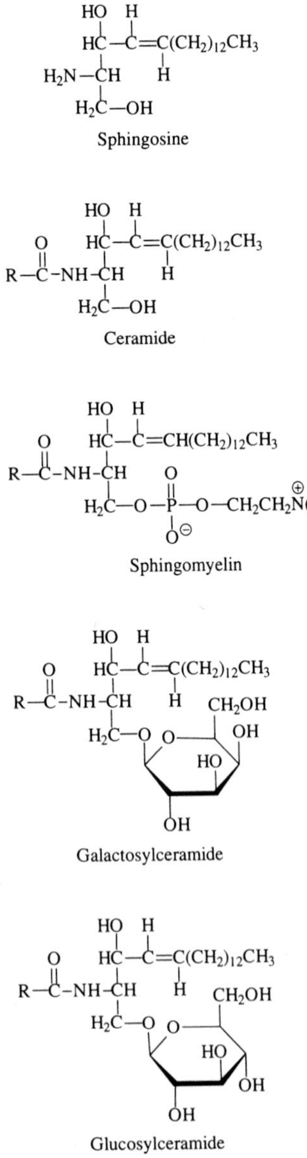

Sphingosine

Ceramide

Sphingomyelin

Galactosylceramide

Glucosylceramide

Figure 26-15 Structures of sphingolipids.

linkage to form *ceramide.* This is the intermediary step in the formation of three important sphingolipids: sphingomyelin, galactosylceramide, and glucosylceramide (see Figure 26-15). The sugar-containing ceramides can have a sulfate group attached (usually to the 2-position of the galactose residue) to form the sulfatides. The glycosyl ceramides can also have additional monosaccharide moieties (such as galactose, *N*-acetylgalactosamine, and *N*-acetylneuraminic acid) to form complex globosides and gangliosides. These complex sphingolipids form the major lipids of cell membranes and the central nervous system. Gangliosides are particularly prevalent in the gray matter of the brain, whereas membrane glycosphingolipids have a major role in cellular interactions, growth, and development, and have been a source of blood group and tumor antigens.

Terpenes

Terpenes are polymers of the five-carbon isoprene unit and include vitamins A, E, and K (see Chapter 30) and the dolichols, which play an important role in protein glycation.

LIPOPROTEINS

Lipids synthesized in the liver and the intestine have to be transported to the various tissues to accomplish their metabolic functions. Because of their insolubility, they are transported in the plasma in macromolecular complexes called lipoproteins. Lipoproteins are spherical particles with nonpolar lipids (triglycerides and cholesterol esters) in their core and more polar lipids (phospholipids and free cholesterol) oriented near the surface. They also contain one or more specific proteins, called apolipoproteins, that are located on their surfaces (Figure 26-16).[255] The association of the core lipids with the phospholipid and protein coat is noncovalent, occurring primarily through hydrogen bonding and van der Waals forces. This binding of lipid to protein is loose

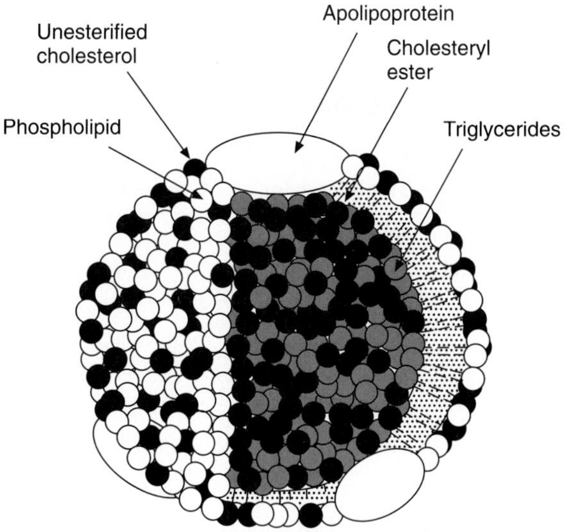

Figure 26-16 Structure of a typical lipoprotein particle.

enough to allow the ready exchange of lipids among the plasma lipoproteins and between cell membranes and lipoprotein, yet strong enough to allow the various classes and subclasses of lipoprotein to be isolated by a variety of analytical techniques.

Lipoproteins have different physical and chemical properties (Table 26-4) as they contain different proportions of lipids and proteins (Table 26-5). Historically, lipoproteins have been categorized based on differences in their hydrated densities as determined by ultracentrifugation. These categories include (1) chylomicrons, (2) VLDL, (3) intermediate-density lipoprotein (IDL), (4) low-density lipoprotein (LDL), (5) high-density lipoprotein (HDL), and (6) lipoprotein(a) [Lp(a)]. HDL is further divided by density into two subpopulations, HDL_2 and HDL_3. As discussed later in this chapter, the two subfractions of HDL seem to differ in their metabolic roles and clinical significance. Lp(a) is a distinct class of lipoprotein (see Table 26-4) that is structurally related to LDL, because both lipoprotein classes possess one molecule of apo B-100 per particle and have similar lipid compositions.[71,173] However, unlike LDL, Lp(a) contains a carbohydrate-rich protein [apo(a)] that is covalently bound to the apo B-100 through a disulfide linkage. The available evidence suggest that Lp(a) contains one molecule of apo(a) and one molecule of apo B-100 per Lp(a) particle. Apo(a) is the unique protein component of Lp(a) and exhibits a significant sequence homology with plasminogen and a high degree of variation in polypeptide chain length. Apo(a) is composed of a serine protease domain and a kringle-containing domain (Figure 26-17). Unlike plasminogen, however, Lp(a) is not activated to form an active protease. The kringle that is contiguous with the protease domain, kringle 5, shares 85% amino acid homology with plasminogen kringle 5, whereas the kringle 4 domain has 78% to 88% amino acid homology with kringle 4 of plasminogen. Apo(a) contains 10 distinct classes of kringle 4–like domains that differ from each other in amino acid sequence. Kringle 4 type 1 and kringle 4 types 3 to 10 are present as a single copy on apo(a) particles. In contrast, kringle 4 type 2 is present in variable number of repeats (3 to >40) and therefore is primarily responsible for the size heterogeneity of apo(a) and consequently of Lp(a) (see Figure 26-17).[150,312]

In the fasting state, most plasma triglycerides are present in VLDL. In the nonfasting state, chylomicrons appear transiently and contribute significantly to the total plasma triglyceride level. LDL carries about 70% of total plasma cholesterol but very little triglyceride (see Table 26-5). HDL contains about 20% to 30% of plasma cholesterol.

Lipoproteins also are separated by electrophoresis on agarose, cellulose acetate, and paper, and polyacrylamide gels.[214] At a pH of 8.6, HDL migrates with the α-globulins, LDL with the β-globulins, and VLDL and Lp(a) between the α- and β-globulins, in the pre-β-globulins region. IDL forms a broad band between β- and pre-β-globulins. Chylomicrons remain at the point of application. The lipoproteins have been referred to by their electrophoretic locations pre-β-lipoprotein, VLDL; β-lipoprotein, LDL; and α-lipoprotein, HDL.

APOLIPOPROTEINS

Apolipoproteins are the protein components of lipoprotein. The characteristics and main known functions of the major apolipoproteins are summarized in Table 26-6.[167,255] Each class of lipoprotein has a variety of apolipoproteins in differing proportions, with the exception of LDL, which contains only apo B-100. Apo A-I is the major protein in HDL. Apo C-I, C-II, C-III, and E are present in various proportions in all lipoproteins except LDL. Apolipoproteins collectively have three major physiological functions. They are involved in (1) activating important enzymes in the lipoprotein metabolic pathways, (2) maintaining the structural integrity of the lipoprotein complex, and (3) facilitating the uptake of lipoprotein into cells through their recognition by specific cell surface receptors.[167]

Apolipoprotein A

Apolipoprotein A-I and apo A-II constitute about 90% of total HDL protein. The ratio of apo A-I to A-II in HDL is about 3:1.[31] In addition to being an important structural

TABLE 26-4 Characteristics of Human Plasma Lipoproteins

Variable	Chylomicron	VLDL	IDL	LDL	HDL	Lp(a)
Density (g/mL)	<0.95	0.95-1.006	1.006-1.019	1.019-1.063	1.063-1.210	1.040-1.130
Electrophoretic mobility	Origin	Prebeta	Between beta and prebeta	Beta	Alpha	Prebeta
Molecular weight (Da)	$0.4\text{-}30 \times 10^9$	$5\text{-}10 \times 10^6$	$3.9\text{-}4.8 \times 10^6$	2.75×10^6	$1.8\text{-}3.6 \times 10^5$	$2.9\text{-}3.7 \times 10^6$
Diameter (nm)	>70	26-70	22-24	19-23	4-10	26-30
Lipid-lipoprotein ratio	99:1	90:10	85:15	80:20	50:50	75:26-64:36
Major lipids	Exogenous triglycerides	Endogenous triglycerides	Endogenous triglycerides, cholesteryl esters	Cholesteryl esters	Phospholipids	Cholesteryl esters, Phospholipids
Major proteins	A-I	B-100	B-100	B-100	A-I	(a)
	B-48	C-I	E	—	A-II	B-100
	C-I	C-II	—	—	—	—
	C-II	C-III	—	—	—	—
	C-III	E	—	—	—	—

VLDL, Very low-density lipoproteins; *IDL,* intermediate-density lipoproteins; *LDL,* low-density lipoproteins; *HDL,* high-density lipoproteins; *Lp(a),* lipoprotein(a).

TABLE 26-5 Chemical Composition (%) of Normal Human Plasma Lipoproteins

		Surface Components		Core Lipids	
	Cholesterol	Phospholipids	Apolipoproteins	Triglycerides	Cholesteryl Esters
Chylomicrons	2	7	2	86	3
VLDL	7	18	8	55	12
IDL	9	19	19	23	29
LDL	8	22	22	6	42
HDL_2	5	33	40	5	17
HDL_3	4	25	55	3	13

From Havel RJ, Kane JP. Introduction: Structure and metabolism of plasma lipoproteins. In Scriver CR, Beaudet AL, Sly WS, Valle D Eds. The metabolic and molecular bases of inherited diseases. 7th ed. Vol II. New York: McGraw-Hill, 1995:1841-50. Reproduced with permission of The McGraw-Hill Companies.

VLDL, Very low-density lipoprotein; *IDL,* intermediate-density lipoprotein; *LDL,* low-density lipoprotein; *HDL,* high-density lipoprotein.

Surface components and core lipids given as percentage of dry mass.

component of HDL, apo A-I is a cofactor for LCAT, the enzyme responsible for forming cholesteryl esters in plasma. Some evidence suggests that apo A-II may inhibit LCAT and activate hepatic triglyceride lipase. Apo A-IV is a component of newly secreted chylomicrons, but is not a major constituent of chylomicron remnants, VLDL, LDL, and HDL. The primary function of apo A-IV is currently unknown, but it has been shown to activate LCAT in vitro,[45] and available data suggest it plays a role in the transport of cholesterol from peripheral tissue to the liver.

Apolipoprotein B

Apolipoprotein B exists in two forms: apo B-100 and apo B-48.[167] The two proteins are known to be translation products of a single structural gene. Apo B-100, a single polypeptide of more than 4500 amino acids, is the full-length translation product of the apo B gene. In humans, apo B-100 is made in the liver and secreted into plasma as part of VLDL. Apo B-100 is the major apolipoprotein of LDL, the end product of VLDL catabolism. Each VLDL particle contains one molecule of apo B-100. In the fasting state, most of the apo B in plasma is apo B-100. Unlike the other apolipoproteins, however, apo B-100 cannot move from one lipoprotein particle to another, and VLDL apo B-100 remains with the lipoprotein as it is catabolized to LDL. Apo B-48 contains 2152 amino acids and is identical to the amino-terminal portion of apo B-100. Apo B-48 results from the posttranscriptional modification of internal apo B-100 messenger ribonucleic acid (mRNA), in which a single base substitution produces a stop codon corresponding to residue 2153 of apo B-100. Apo B-48 is made in the intestine and is the major apo B component of chylomicrons. Both apo B-100 and apo B-48 play important roles in the secretion of VLDL and chylomicrons, respectively. Apo B-100 is recognized by the LDL receptor in hepatic and peripheral tissues and allows the LDL receptor-mediated internalization of LDL[34] (see later sections on lipoprotein metabolism, endogenous and exogenous pathways).

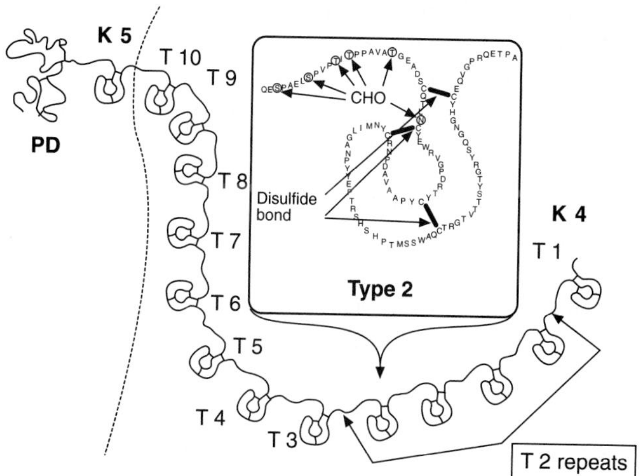

Figure 26-17 Structure of lipoprotein(a).

Apolipoprotein C

Apolipoproteins C-I, C-II, and C-III are associated with all lipoproteins except LDL. Apo C-I, the smallest of the C apolipoproteins, has been reported to activate LCAT in vitro. Apo C-II plays an important role in the metabolism of triglyceride-rich lipoprotein (VLDL and chylomicrons)

TABLE 26-6 Classification and Properties of Major Human Plasma Apolipoproteins

Apolipoprotein	Molecular Weight (Da)	Chromosomal Location	Function	Lipoprotein Carrier(s)
Apo A-I	29,016	11	Cofactor LCAT	Chylomicron, HDL
Apo A-II	17,414	1	Not known	HDL
Apo A-IV	44,465	11	Activates LCAT	Chylomicron, HDL
Apo B-100	512,723	2	Secretion of triglyceride from liver binding protein to LDL receptor	VLDL, IDL, LDL
Apo B-48	240,800	2	Secretion of triglyceride from intestine	Chylomicron
Apo C-I	6630	19	Activates LCAT	Chylomicron, VLDL, HDL
Apo C-II	8900	19	Cofactor LPL	Chylomicron, VLDL, HDL
Apo C-III	8800	11	Inhibits apo C-II activation of LPL	Chylomicron, VLDL, HDL
Apo E	34,145	19	Facilitates uptake of chylomicron remnant and IDL	Chylomicron, VLDL, HDL
Apo(a)	187,000-662,000	6	Unknown	Lp(a)

VLDL, Very low-density lipoproteins; *IDL*, intermediate-density lipoproteins; *LDL*, low-density lipoproteins; *HDL*, high-density lipoproteins; *Lp(a)*, lipoprotein(a); *LCAT*, lecithin cholesterol acyltransferase; *LPL*, lipoprotein lipase.

by activating lipoprotein lipase (LPL), an enzyme that hydrolyzes lipoprotein triglycerides. Because of differences in sialic acid content, apo C-III exists in at least three polymorphic forms.[36] The precise metabolic function of apo C-III is unknown, but it may inhibit LPL and activate LCAT, and therefore may regulate the activities of these enzymes.

Apolipoprotein E

Apolipoprotein E is a 34-kDa plasma glycoprotein that is found primarily in chylomicrons, VLDL, HDL, and chylomicron and VLDL remnants. Removal of apo E–bearing lipoproteins is mediated by several different cellular receptors that recognize a cluster of positively charged amino acids in a specific region of apo E. Apo E plays a central role in the metabolism of chylomicrons and VLDL remnants. It regulates and facilitates lipoprotein uptake in the liver through (1) interaction of chylomicron remnants with chylomicron remnant receptors, and (2) binding of VLDL remnants to the LDL (B, E) receptor.[167]

There are three common apo E isoforms, designated E_2, E_3, and E_4, that were initially distinguished by isoelectric-focusing electrophoresis.[329] These isoforms have amino acid substitutions at residues 112 and 158.[234] Apo E_2 has cysteine residues in both positions and apo E_4 has arginine residues in both positions, whereas apo E_3 has cysteine and arginine at positions 112 and 158, respectively. Apo E_2 exhibits reduced binding affinity for the B and/or E remnant receptor compared with apo E_3, which can lead to an accumulation of apo E–containing lipoprotein in the circulation, whereas apo E_4–containing lipoproteins are cleared more rapidly than those containing apo E_3. These isoforms are coded for by the three alleles of the apo E gene, ε2, ε3, and ε4. The ε3 allele is most frequent, although the relative proportions of the three alleles vary among populations.[59,61,62] These apo E alleles have been shown to contribute significantly to the variability of LDL cholesterol and apo B-100 levels within populations.[272] Individuals with at least one ε2 allele tend to have lower levels of apo B-100 and LDL cholesterol than do those who are homozygous for the ε3 allele, whereas individuals with at least one ε4 allele tend to have higher levels of those analytes, possibly because of the higher affinity of apo E_4 for the LDL receptor, with consequent interference with LDL clearance from the circulation. Also, variation at the apo E locus may explain some of the differences observed in plasma lipid and lipoprotein between individual responses to dietary and drug therapy.[220]

Lipoprotein Metabolism

The pathways of lipoprotein metabolism are complex.[34,103,255] They include exogenous and endogenous pathways based on whether they carry lipids of dietary or hepatic origin (Figures 26-18 and 26-19) and other pathways such as the

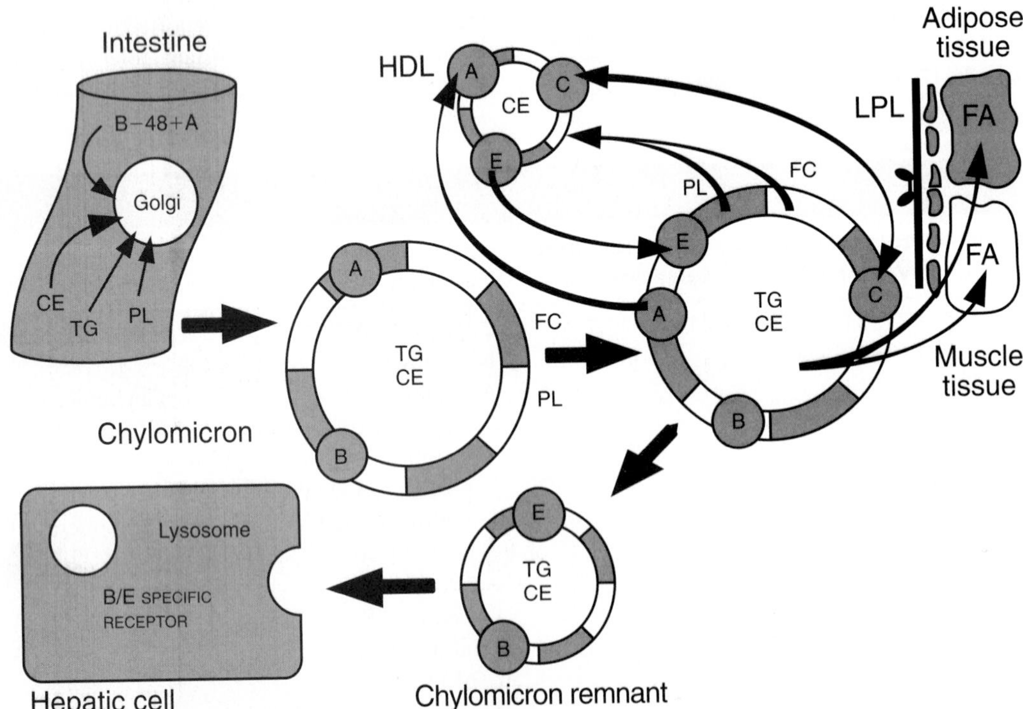

Figure 26-18 Exogenous lipoprotein metabolism pathway. *TG*, Triglyceride; *CE*, cholesterol ester; *FC*, free cholesterol; *PL*, phospholipids; *HDL*, high-density lipoproteins; *FA*, fatty acid; *LPL*, lipoprotein lipase; *B*, apolipoprotein B-48; *A*, apolipoprotein A-I; *C*, apolipoprotein C-II; *E*, apolipoprotein E. *(From Rifai N. Lipoproteins and apolipoproteins: Composition, metabolism, and association with coronary heart disease. Arch Pathol Lab Med 1986;110:694-701. Copyright 1986, American Medical Association.)*

intracellular LDL receptor pathway (Figure 26-20) and the HDL reverse cholesterol transport pathway (Figure 26-21). Although these pathways are viewed as functionally distinct, they have overlapping points that provide sites at which dietary lipid intake can influence the synthesis and catabolism of endogenous lipids.

Exogenous Pathway

Nascent chylomicrons are assembled from dietary triglycerides and cholesterol in the enterocytes and packaged in secretory vesicles in the Golgi apparatus. These particles are then transported by exocytosis into the extracellular space and introduced into circulation through the intestinal villi. The lipid content of nascent chylomicrons consists mainly of triglycerides (90% by mass), whereas the protein components include apo B-48 and the A apolipoproteins (2% by mass).[97] Shortly after entering the circulation, these particles acquire the C apolipoproteins and apo E from circulating HDL (see Figure 26-18). Apo C-II, now present on the surface of chylomicrons, activates the LPL attached to the luminal surface of endothelial cells, which rapidly hydrolyzes the triglycerides to free fatty acids. The fatty acids are associated with albumin and can either be taken up by muscle cells as an energy source or into adipose cells for storage. Simultaneously, some of the phospholipids and the apo A apolipoproteins are transferred from the chylomicron particle onto HDL. The newly formed particle, the chylomicron remnant, contains 80% to 90% of the triglyceride content of the original chylomicron. Because of the presence of apo B-48 and apo E on its surface, the chylomicron remnant can be recognized by specific hepatic remnant receptors and internalized by endocytosis. The components of the particle are then hydrolyzed in the lysosomes. The cholesterol released can form bile acids, be incorporated into newly synthesized lipoprotein, or be stored as cholesteryl ester. Furthermore, the cholesterol from these remnants can down regulate HMG-CoA reductase, the rate-limiting enzyme of cholesterol biosynthesis (see earlier section on cholesterol synthesis).

Endogenous Pathway

Hepatocytes have the ability to synthesize triglycerides from carbohydrates and fatty acids. In addition, when dietary cholesterol acquired from the receptor-mediated uptake of chylomicron remnants is insufficient, hepatocytes also synthesize their own cholesterol by increasing the activity of HMG-CoA reductase. The endogenously made triglycerides and cholesterol are packaged in secretory vesicles in the

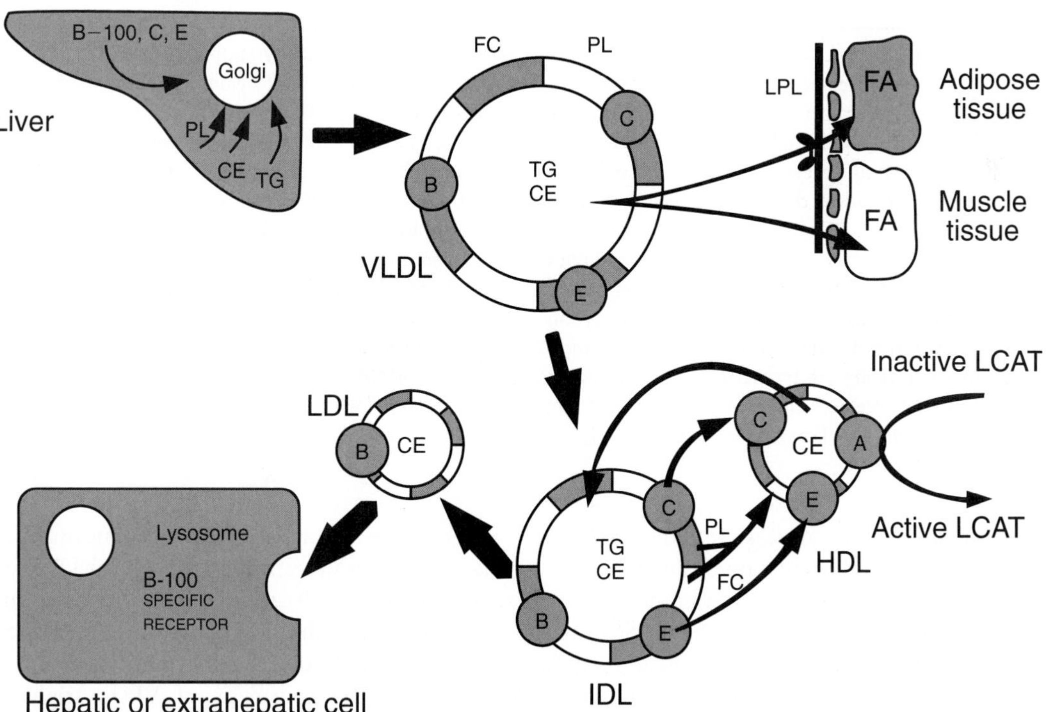

Figure 26-19 Endogenous lipoprotein metabolism pathway. *TG,* Triglyceride; *CE,* cholesterol ester; *FC,* free cholesterol; *PL,* phospholipids; *HDL,* high-density lipoproteins; *LDL,* low-density lipoproteins; *IDL,* intermediate-density lipoproteins; *VLDL,* very low-density lipoproteins; *FA,* fatty acid; *LPL,* lipoprotein lipase; *LCAT,* lecithin cholesterol acyltransferase; *B,* apolipoprotein B-100; *A,* apolipoprotein A-I; *C,* apolipoprotein C-II; *E,* apolipoprotein E. *(From Rifai N. Lipoproteins and apolipoproteins: Composition, metabolism, and association with coronary heart disease. Arch Pathol Lab Med 1986;110:694-701. Copyright 1986, American Medical Association.)*

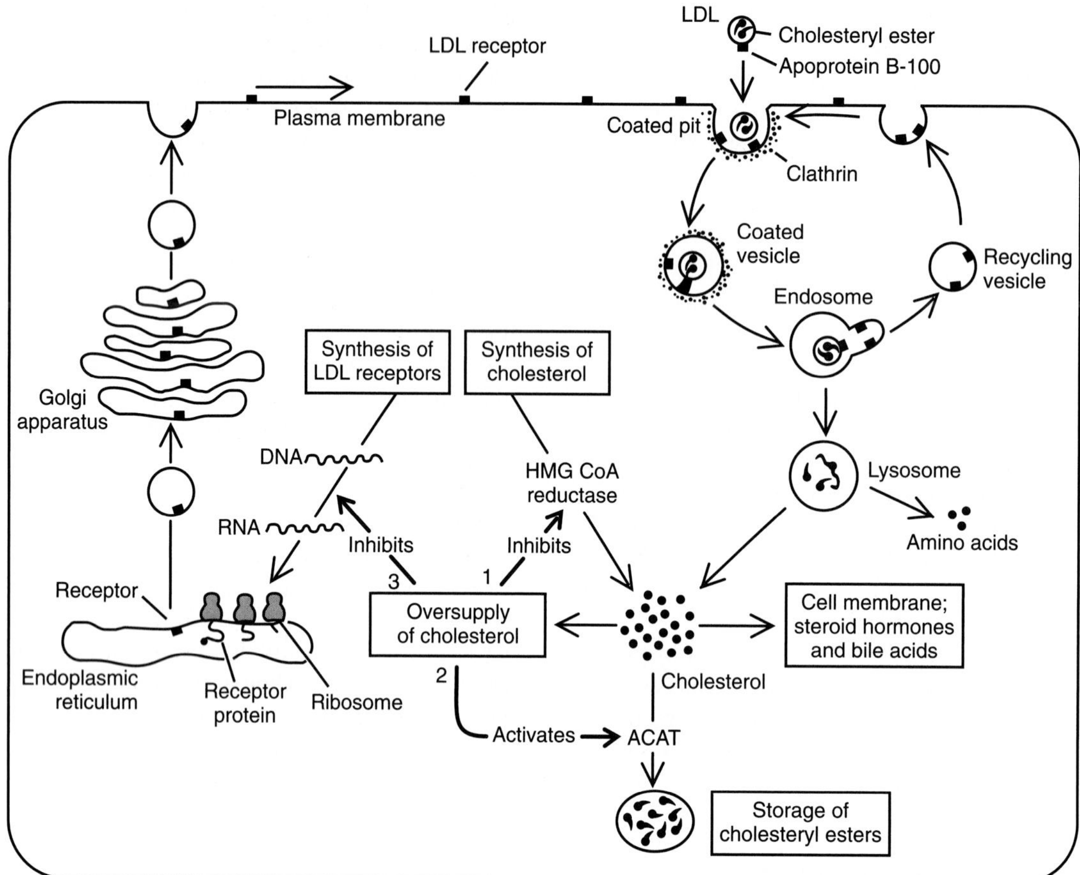

Figure 26-20 Low-density lipoprotein receptor pathway. *LDL,* Low-density lipoproteins; *ACAT,* acyl-CoA cholesterol acyltransferase; *HMG-CoA reductase,* 3-hydroxy-3-methylglutaryl coenzyme A reductase. Because of the presence of apolipoprotein B-100 on its surface, the LDL particle is recognized by a specific receptor in a coated pit and taken into the cell in a coated vesicle *(top right).* Coated vesicles fuse together to form an endosome. The acidic environment of the endosome causes the LDL particle to dissociate from the receptors, which return to the cell surface. The LDL particles are taken to a lysosome, where apolipoprotein B-100 is broken down into amino acids and cholesterol ester is converted to free cholesterol for cellular requirements. The cellular cholesterol level is self-regulated. Oversupply of cholesterol will lead to (1) decreased rate of cholesterol synthesis by inhibiting HMG-CoA reductase, (2) increased storage of cholesteryl esters by activating ACAT, and (3) inhibition of manufacture of new LDL receptors by suppressing the transcription of the receptor gene into mRNA. *(From Brown MS, Goldstein JL. How LDL receptors influence cholesterol and atherosclerosis. Sci Am 1984;251:58-66. Copyright 1984 by Scientific American, Inc. All rights reserved.)*

Golgi apparatus, transported by exocytosis into the extracellular space, and introduced into circulation through the fenestrae of the hepatic sinusoidal endothelium in the form of nascent VLDL (see Figure 26-19). This triglyceride-rich particle (55% by mass) contains apo B-100, apo E, and small amounts of C apolipoproteins on its surface. Additional C apolipoproteins are transferred after secretion from circulating HDL. As in the case of chylomicron metabolism, apo C-II present on the surface of VLDL activates LPL on endothelial cells, which leads to the hydrolysis of VLDL triglycerides and the release of free fatty acids. It is important to note, however, that the rate of hydrolysis of VLDL triglyceride is significantly lower than that of chylomicron triglyceride. The average residence time of VLDL triglyceride is 15 to 60 minutes, compared with the 5 to 10 minutes of chylomicron triglyceride.[111] This difference may be attributed to the fact that VLDL particles are smaller and bind to fewer LPL molecules than chylomicrons.

During the hydrolysis of VLDL triglycerides, the C apolipoproteins are transferred back to HDL. VLDL particles are thus converted to VLDL remnants, some of which are taken up by the liver and the rest converted to smaller, denser particles called IDL. Large IDL particles, which also have several molecules of apo E, bind the hepatic remnant receptors and are removed from circulation. In humans, about 50% of IDL is removed by hepatocytes.

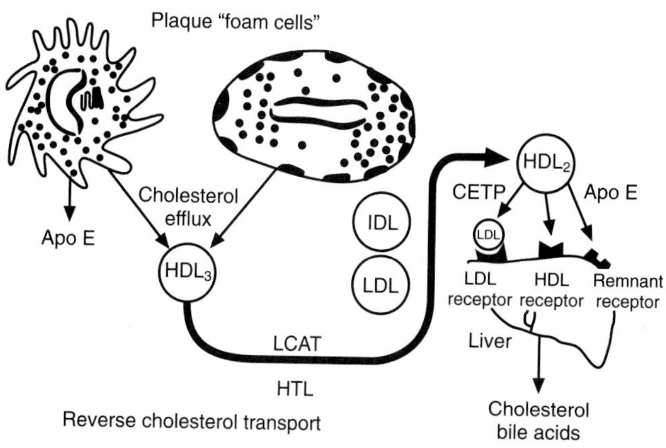

Figure 26-21 Reverse cholesterol transport pathway. *HDL,* High-density lipoproteins; *LDL,* low-density lipoproteins; *IDL,* intermediate-density lipoproteins; *HTL,* hepatic lipoprotein lipase; *LCAT,* lecithin cholesterol acyltransferase; *CETP,* cholesteryl ester transfer protein; *apo E,* apolipoprotein E. Cholesterol is removed from macrophages and other arterial wall cells by an HDL-mediated process. The LCAT esterifies the cholesterol content of HDL to prevent it from reentering the cells. Cholesterol esters are delivered to the liver by one of three pathways: (1) cholesterol esters are transferred from HDL to LDL by CETP and enter the liver through the specific LDL receptor pathway; (2) cholesterol esters are selectively taken from HDL by HDL receptors and HDL particles are returned to circulation for further transport; or (3) HDL have accumulated apo E and therefore the particles can enter the liver through remnant receptors. *(From Gwynne JT. High density lipoprotein cholesterol levels as a marker of reverse cholesterol transport. Am J Cardiol 1989;64:10G-17G. Copyright 1989, with permission from Excerpta Medica Inc.)*

Surface materials from IDL, including some phospholipids, free cholesterol, and apolipoproteins, are transferred to HDL, or form HDL de novo in the circulation. Cholesteryl esters are transferred from HDL to LDL. The net result of the coupled lipolysis and the cholesteryl esters exchange reaction is the replacement of much of the triglyceride core of the original VLDL with cholesteryl esters. IDL undergoes a further hydrolysis in which most of the remaining triglycerides are removed and all apolipoproteins except B-100 are transferred to other lipoproteins. This process ends with ultimate formation of LDL.

Low-Density Lipoprotein Receptor Pathway

The mechanism by which LDL is removed from circulation is well understood. Specific receptors present in coated pits on plasma membranes recognize and bind apo B-100 of LDL (see Figures 26-19 and 26-20). The LDL particles are internalized in coated vesicles, which then fuse to form an endosome. Because of the acidic milieu of the endosome, LDL dissociates from the receptor, which returns to the cell surface for reuse, whereas LDL migrates to the lysosome. Once the LDL is delivered to the lysosome, apo B-100 is degraded to small peptides and amino acids. Cholesterol esters are also hydrolyzed, with the cholesterol then available for the synthesis of cell membranes, steroid hormones in tissue that make them, and bile acids in hepatocytes. Cells have the ability to regulate their cholesterol content. Oversupply of free cholesterol leads to (1) decreased rate of endogenous cholesterol synthesis by inhibiting the rate-limiting enzyme HMG-CoA reductase; (2) increased formation of cholesteryl esters, which is catalyzed by ACAT; and (3) inhibition of the synthesis of new LDL receptors by suppressing the transcription of the receptor gene. The inhibition of HMG-CoA reductase and suppression of the LDL receptor may occur through the interaction of the cholesterol derivative, hydroxycholesterol, with the regulatory portions of the respective genes. Compared with VLDL and chylomicrons, LDL has a relatively long residence time in the circulation, about 3 days.[111]

LDL are also taken up by extrahepatic tissue through scavenger receptors or non–receptor-mediated pinocytosis. The non–receptor-mediated uptake becomes important as plasma LDL concentrations increase, as in familial hypercholesterolemia (FH). Nonreceptor-mediated uptake is not saturable and not regulated. Scavenger receptors are unregulated as well and recognize LDL that has been modified in various ways. They are found in macrophages and other cells. Macrophages that become engorged with cholesteryl esters are called "foam cells," and are considered the earliest components of the atherosclerotic lesion. Two thirds of LDL is normally removed by LDL receptors and the remainder by the scavenger cell system.

High-Density Lipoprotein Reverse Cholesterol Transfer Pathway

High-density lipoproteins are secreted from the liver or intestine as disk-shaped nascent particles that consist primarily of phospholipids and apo A-I. Through the extracellular addition of surface components of triglyceride-rich particles, such as phospholipids, cholesterol, and certain apolipoproteins, nascent HDL is converted to spherical particles. Free cholesterol from cell membranes is also transferred to the nascent HDL (see Figure 26-21). Cholesterol is esterified by the action of LCAT in the presence of its cofactor apo A-I. The size of the HDL particle depends strongly on the amount of accumulated cholesteryl esters and the activity of LCAT. Lysolecithin, a byproduct of this reaction (see previous discussion), is then removed from circulation after binding with albumin. HDL cholesteryl esters are delivered to the liver by one of the following mechanisms: (1) cholesteryl esters are selectively taken up from HDL, probably by the hepatic HDL receptors, and HDL particles are returned to circulation for further transport; (2) cholesteryl esters are transferred from HDL to apo B-100–containing lipoprotein, a process mediated by cholesterol ester transfer protein, then taken up by the liver through receptors for these lipoprotein; or (3) HDL apo E can be recognized by the hepatic remnant receptors.[103] These processes constitute the reverse cholesterol transport mechanism, by which cellular and lipoprotein cholesterol is delivered back to the liver for reuse or disposal.

Although LDL are the major products resulting from the catabolism of VLDL, some conversion of HDL subfractions also occurs during this process. The surface materials from triglyceride-rich particles that have been transferred to the small circulating HDL_3 are subsequently esterified by LCAT, as described earlier, to create the larger cholesteryl ester–rich HDL_2. It has been shown that in vitro HDL_2 is converted back to HDL_3 in the presence of hepatic LPL.[225] HDL_2 contains twice as many cholesterol molecules per unit of apolipoproteins as does HDL_3.

Reference Lipid, Lipoprotein Cholesterol, and Apolipoprotein Concentrations

At birth, the typical plasma cholesterol concentration is about 66 mg/dL,* equally distributed among LDL and HDL with a very small amount in VLDL. Triglyceride concentration is only about 36 mg/dL.[260†] Cord blood apo A-I, apo B-100, and Lp(a) showed mean concentrations of about 80, 33, and 4 mg/dL, respectively.[257,258] Lipid, lipoprotein cholesterol, and apolipoprotein concentrations rise sharply during the first few months of life, with LDL becoming the major carrier of plasma cholesterol, and then remain relatively unchanged until puberty. A profile consisting of a total cholesterol of about 155 mg/dL, LDL cholesterol of 90 mg/dL, HDL cholesterol of 53 mg/dL, triglycerides of 55 mg/dL, apo B-100 of 86 mg/dL, and apo A-I about 130 mg/dL is typical for a normal prepubertal subject. After puberty, there is an increase in triglycerides, LDL cholesterol, and apo B-100 in both sexes and a decrease in HDL cholesterol and apo A-I in men. Lipid concentrations continue to increase throughout adult life, with total and LDL cholesterol and apo B-100 being higher in men than in women up to age 55.[35] Thereafter, women who are not receiving estrogen supplementation have higher total and LDL cholesterol and apo B-100 than their age-matched male counterparts.[104] In contrast to the other lipids, lipoproteins, and apolipoproteins, Lp(a) concentration increases slowly and gradually to reach Lp(a) adult values after the third year of life.[258]

Plasma lipid and lipoprotein concentrations in male and female subjects are presented in Tables 26-7 through 26-10. These reference intervals have been developed using the Lipid Research Clinics (LRC) population. Although reference intervals for apo A-I and B-100 from the Framingham Heart Study using the approved World Health Organization/International Federation of Clinical Chemistry and Laboratory Medicine (IFCC) calibrators have been published,[54,55] distributions of these two proteins that better reflect the North American population have only recently

*To convert mg/dL of cholesterol to mmol/L, multiply by 0.0259.
†To covert milligrams per deciliter of triglyceride to millimoles per liter multiply by 0.0113.

TABLE 26-7 Population Distributions for Total Cholesterol (mg/dL)

Male

Age (yr)	Percentiles 5	10	25	50	75	90	95
0-4	114			155			203
5-9	125	131	141	153	168	183	189
10-14	124	132	144	161	173	191	204
15-19	118	123	135	152	168	183	191
20-24	118	126	142	159	179	197	212
25-29	130	137	154	176	199	223	234
30-34	142	152	161	190	213	237	258
35-39	147	157	176	195	222	248	267
40-44	150	161	179	204	229	251	260
45-49	163	171	188	210	234	255	275
50-54	156	168	189	211	234	262	274
55-59	161	172	188	214	236	260	280
60-64	163	170	191	215	237	262	287
65-69	166	174	192	213	250	275	288
70+	144	160	185	214	236	253	265

Female

Age (yr)	Percentiles 5	10	25	50	75	90	95
0-4	112			156			200
5-9	131	135	150	164	177	189	197
10-14	125	131	142	159	171	191	205
15-19	119	126	140	157	176	198	208
20-24	121	132	147	165	186	220	237
25-29	130	142	158	178	198	217	231
30-34	133	141	158	178	197	215	227
35-39	139	149	165	186	209	233	249
40-44	146	156	172	193	220	241	259
45-49	148	162	182	204	213	256	268
50-54	163	171	188	214	240	267	281
55-59	167	182	201	229	251	270	294
60-64	172	186	207	226	251	282	300
65-69	167	179	212	233	259	282	291
70+	173	181	196	226	249	268	280

From Lipid Research Clinics Program Epidemiology Committee: Plasma lipid distributions in selected North American population: The Lipid Research Clinics Program Prevalence Study. Circulation 1979;60:427-39; and Lipid Metabolism Branch, Division of Heart, Lung, and Blood Institute: The Lipid Research Clinics Population Studies Data Book. Vol. I: The Prevalence Study. NIH Publication No. 80-1527. Bethesda, MD: National Institutes of Health, 1980.
To convert to mmol/L, multiply by 0.0259.

TABLE 26-8 Population Distributions for Triglycerides (mg/dL)

	Male Percentiles								Female Percentiles						
Age (yr)	5	10	25	50	75	90	95	Age (yr)	5	10	25	50	75	90	95
0-4	29			56			99	0-4	34			64			112
5-9	28	34	39	48	58	70	85	5-9	32	37	45	57	74	103	126
10-14	33	37	46	58	74	94	111	10-14	39	44	53	68	85	104	120
15-19	38	43	53	68	88	125	143	15-19	36	40	52	64	85	112	126
20-24	44	50	61	78	107	146	165	20-24	37	42	60	80	104	135	168
25-29	45	51	67	88	120	141	204	25-29	42	45	57	76	104	137	159
30-34	46	57	76	102	142	214	253	30-34	40	45	55	73	104	140	163
35-39	52	58	80	109	167	250	316	35-39	40	47	61	83	115	170	205
40-44	56	69	89	123	174	252	318	40-44	45	51	66	88	116	161	191
45-49	56	65	88	119	165	218	279	45-49	44	55	71	94	139	180	223
50-54	63	75	94	128	178	244	313	50-54	53	58	75	103	144	190	223
55-59	60	70	85	117	167	210	261	55-59	59	65	80	111	163	229	279
60-64	56	65	84	111	150	193	240	60-64	57	66	78	105	143	210	256
65-69	54	61	78	108	164	227	256	65-69	56	64	86	118	158	221	260
70+	63	71	87	115	152	202	239	70+	60	68	83	110	141	189	289

From Lipid Research Clinics Program Epidemiology Committee: Plasma lipid distributions in selected North American population: The Lipid Research Clinics Program Prevalence Study. Circulation 1979;60:427-39; and Lipid Metabolism Branch, Division of Heart, Lung, and Blood Institute: The Lipid Research Clinics Population Studies Data Book. Vol. I: The Prevalence Study. NIH Publication No. 80-1527. Bethesda, MD: National Institutes of Health, 1980.

To convert to mmol/L, multiply by 0.0113.

TABLE 26-9 Population Distributions for Low-Density Lipoprotein Cholesterol (mg/dL)

	Male Percentiles								Female Percentiles						
Age (yr)	5	10	25	50	75	90	95	Age (yr)	5	10	25	50	75	90	95
5-9	63	69	80	90	103	117	129	5-9	68	73	88	98	115	125	140
10-14	64	73	82	94	109	123	133	10-14	68	73	81	94	110	126	136
15-19	62	68	80	93	109	123	130	15-19	59	73	78	93	110	129	137
20-24	66	73	85	101	118	138	147	20-24	57	65	82	102	118	141	159
25-29	70	75	96	116	138	157	165	25-29	71	75	90	108	126	148	164
30-34	78	88	107	124	144	166	185	30-34	70	77	91	109	129	146	156
35-39	81	92	110	131	154	176	189	35-39	75	81	96	116	139	161	172
40-44	87	98	115	135	157	173	186	40-44	74	84	104	122	146	165	174
45-49	97	106	120	140	163	185	202	45-49	79	89	105	127	150	173	186
50-54	89	102	118	143	162	185	197	50-54	88	94	111	134	160	186	201
55-59	88	103	123	145	168	191	203	55-59	89	97	120	145	168	199	210
60-64	83	107	121	143	165	188	210	60-64	100	105	126	149	168	191	224
65-69	98	104	125	146	170	199	210	65-69	92	99	125	151	184	205	221
70+	88	100	119	142	164	182	186	70+	96	108	126	147	170	189	206

From Lipid Research Clinics Program Epidemiology Committee: Plasma lipid distributions in selected North American population: The Lipid Research Clinics Program Prevalence Study. Circulation 1979;60:427-39.

To convert to mmol/L, multiply by 0.0259.

TABLE 26-10 Population Distributions for High-Density Lipoprotein Cholesterol (mg/dL)

	Male Percentiles								Female Percentiles						
Age (yr)	5	10	25	50	75	90	95	Age (yr)	5	10	25	50	75	90	95
5-9	38	43	49	55	64	70	75	5-9	36	38	48	52	60	67	73
10-14	37	40	46	55	61	71	74	10-14	37	40	45	52	58	64	70
15-19	30	34	39	46	52	59	63	15-19	35	38	43	51	61	68	74
20-24	30	32	38	45	51	57	63	20-24	33	37	44	51	62	72	79
25-29	31	32	37	44	50	58	63	25-29	37	39	47	55	63	74	83
30-34	28	32	38	45	52	59	63	30-34	36	40	46	55	64	73	77
35-39	29	31	36	43	49	58	62	35-39	34	38	44	53	64	75	82
40-44	27	31	36	43	51	60	67	40-44	34	39	48	56	65	79	88
45-49	30	33	38	45	52	60	64	45-49	34	41	47	58	68	82	87
50-54	28	31	36	44	51	58	63	50-54	37	41	50	62	71	84	92
55-59	28	31	38	46	55	64	71	55-59	37	41	50	60	73	85	91
60-64	30	34	41	49	61	69	74	60-64	38	44	51	61	75	87	92
65-69	30	33	39	49	52	74	75	65-69	35	38	49	62	73	85	96
70+	31	33	40	48	56	70	75	70+	33	38	45	60	71	82	92

From Lipid Research Clinics Program Epidemiology Committee: Plasma lipid distributions in selected North American population: The Lipid Research Clinics Program Prevalence Study. Circulation 1979;60:427-39.
To convert to mmol/L, multiply by 0.0259.

become available from the National Health and Nutrition Examination Survey III (NHANES-III) (Tables 26-11 and 26-12).[17] Since NHANES has been designed to reflect the U.S. population, data for the distribution of these proteins in the main American ethnic groups are available (Table 26-13). The availability of such information will enable the development of cut points for clinical decision. For example, for apo B-100, cut points similar to those recommended for LDL-C can be developed; the apo B-100 values, which correspond to desirable, borderline high risk, high risk, and very high risk, are 88, 115, 132, and 152 mg/dL and apo A-I values, which correspond to low and high, are 114 and 154 mg/dL.[17] Until Lp(a) measurement is standardized, the development of appropriate reference intervals is not possible.[172]

CLINICAL SIGNIFICANCE

The clinical significance of lipids is primarily associated with coronary heart disease (CHD) and various lipoprotein disorders.

Association with Coronary Heart Disease

Increased cholesterol is a factor in the cause of atherosclerotic diseases (see also Chapter 44). As early as 1910, Windaus described cholesterol in the lesions of diseased arteries. Subsequently, many studies have confirmed that free and esterified cholesterol accumulates in the aorta, coronary arteries, and cerebral vessels, and that the rate of accumulation varies among individuals. The association between serum cholesterol and atherosclerosis in humans was first suggested in 1938, when Muller and Thanhauser each demonstrated familial aggregation of hypercholesterolemia and CHD.[196,302] Further studies showed that when the total cholesterol concentration is high, the incidence and prevalence of CHD are also high.[93]

The relationship between cholesterol and atherosclerotic coronary disease is curvilinear.[102] According to the Multiple Risk Factor Intervention Trial (MRFIT), if a risk ratio of 1.0 is arbitrarily assigned at a cholesterol value of 200 mg/dL, the risk ratio increases to 2.0 at 250 mg/dL and to 4.0 at 300 mg/dL (Figure 26-22). Pathological studies have helped to explain this curvilinear relationship. When 60% of the surface of coronary arteries is covered with plaque, one enters a critical phase in which an increased serum cholesterol concentration will markedly increase coronary disease risk. The results of the LRC-Coronary Primary Prevention Trial (CPPT) showed that the use of the 95th percentile to define hypercholesterolemia is inappropriate. Data from this and other studies suggest that risk increases as cholesterol levels increase; at concentrations of 200 to 240 mg/dL, the risk begins to accelerate at a greater magnitude. On average, each 1% reduction in cholesterol (2 to 3 mg/dL) results in a ~2% reduction in CHD incidence, a relationship of considerable clinical and public health significance.[72] In addition, the Cholesterol-Lowering Atherosclerosis Study (CLAS) demonstrated the benefit of cholesterol lowering even in people with normal or moderately increased cholesterol concentrations (185 to 240 mg/dL) and those with established disease.[26]

Many epidemiological and clinical studies have shown that both increased LDL cholesterol and decreased HDL cholesterol are associated with an increased risk of CHD.[41] Some studies have demonstrated that a reduction in LDL cholesterol is correlated with regression in the atherosclerotic lesion.[32] Various investigations also demonstrated that

TABLE 26-11 Serum Apo A-I Concentrations in Persons Ages ≥ 4 Years by Sex and Age: Means and Selected Percentiles, U.S., 1988-91

	Apo A-I* mg/dL								
			PERCENTILES						
Age, Years	Mean [SEM]†	SD	5th	10th	25th	50th	75th	90th	95th
Males‡									
4-5	135 [2]	19	109	112	122	132	149	159	172
6-11	142	20	111	117	126	141	150	168	177
12-19	129	19	99	106	116	128	141	153	165
≥20	136	22	106	111	121	133	147	164	176
20-29	135	21	105	112	121	132	145	164	173
30-39	135	20	105	111	122	132	145	161	173
40-49	136 [2]	25	103	108	119	133	149	164	178
50-59	136 [2]	21	107	111	121	134	147	167	173
60-69	140 [2]	23	111	116	123	136	153	172	184
≥70	138	23	109	114	122	134	150	167	180
Females‡									
4-5	131	18	104	111	118	130	140	155	163
6-11	136	17	110	117	125	135	145	157	166
12-19	136	23	105	111	120	132	146	165	180
≥20	151	27	113	120	132	147	166	186	202
20-29	148 [2]	30	111	117	128	143	164	185	209
30-39	145	24	110	115	126	143	160	173	189
40-49	149 [2]	24	115	122	134	145	165	181	195
50-59	156 [2]	29	117	123	134	152	173	199	211
60-69	157 [2]	28	120	125	138	154	171	191	205
≥70	155 [2]	26	118	124	137	153	171	189	199

Modified from Bachorik PS, Lovejoy KL, Carroll MD, Johnson CL. Apolipoprotein B and AI distributions in the United States, 1988-1991: results of the National Health and Nutrition Examination Survey III (NHANES III). Clin Chem 1997;43:2364-78.
*Combined data for total population, including all three ethnic groups.
†All SEMs were 1 mg/dL unless otherwise indicated.
‡Estimates based on 400 to 800 subjects in each age and sex subgroup.

the small, dense LDL subfractions correlated better with CHD risk than the large, less dense LDL subfractions.[14,39] Initially, a National Institutes of Health consensus conference on triglyceride and CHD failed to establish increased fasting triglyceride concentration as an independent risk factor.[211] However, the National Cholesterol Education Program (NCEP) and the Adult Treatment Panel III (ATPIII) reports[77,203] have given triglycerides more prominence in CHD risk prediction (see section on diagnosis of lipoprotein disorders later in this chapter). Furthermore, fat tolerance and the ability to rapidly catabolize ingested triglycerides are reported to correlate well with one of the known atherogenic risk indicators, HDL_2 cholesterol.[224] The degree of hypertriglyceridemia appearing after a meal controls the extent to which the basal HDL_2 is converted by hepatic lipase, at least in vitro, to HDL_3. It has also been postulated that chylomicron remnants and IDL, the products of the breakdown of triglyceride-rich lipoprotein, are important in atherogenesis.[337] They may promote atherosclerosis when their concentrations in plasma are high or their presence in circulation is prolonged. A scavenger cell receptor for chylomicron remnants that would provide a mechanism for entry of chylomicron cholesterol in the arterial wall has been identified.

In the early 1970s, Alaupovic suggested that apolipoproteins should also be considered when evaluating the contribution of lipids and lipoproteins to the development of atherosclerotic disease.[2] Several studies demonstrated that in people with CHD, changes in the serum concentrations of apo A-I and apo B-100 are similar to those for HDL and LDL, respectively. Apo B-100 values were increased and apo A-I values were decreased in people with CHD compared with those without disease. In most studies, apo A-I and apo B-100 were somewhat better discriminators of people with CHD than the cholesterol concentration of the corresponding lipoprotein,[145,166] at least in univariate analyses. Further-

TABLE 26-12 Serum Apo B-100 Concentrations in Persons Ages ≥ 4 Years by Sex and Age: Means and Selected Percentiles, U.S., 1988-91

			Apo B-100,* mg/dL						
			Percentiles						
Age, Years	Mean [SEM]†	SD	5th	10th	25th	50th	75th	90th	95th
Males‡									
4-5	79	14	58	0.62	69	79	89	98	103
6-11	79	16	56	0.61	69	76	89	99	105
12-19	78	17	55	0.58	67	75	85	98	110
≥20	107	25	66	0.74	89	106	122	138	150
20-29	91	22	59	0.66	76	88	103	117	130
30-39	106	24	63	0.73	89	107	122	136	143
40-49	112 [2]	24	71	0.82	97	111	126	140	152
50-59	116 [2]	26	75	0.84	98	116	133	149	160
60-69	117 [2]	23	81	0.89	101	116	133	148	156
≥70	110	24	73	0.81	95	109	123	142	152
Females‡									
4-5	82	14	58	0.64	72	82	91	99	104
6-11	82	17	57	0.61	70	81	90	101	113
12-19	81	20	53	0.58	67	79	92	104	119
≥20	103	28	66	0.71	83	99	119	140	153
20-29	91	23	63	0.67	74	86	102	119	132
30-39	93	23	59	0.68	76	89	107	123	132
40-49	99	21	70	0.75	84	96	114	129	136
50-59	116 [2]	29	75	0.84	96	114	133	156	168
60-69	119 [2]	31	75	0.82	98	118	135	156	173
≥70	118	28	79	0.84	98	116	135	152	168

Modified from Bachorik PS, Lovejoy KL, Carroll MD, Johnson CL. Apolipoprotein B and AI distributions in the United States, 1988-1991: results of the National Health and Nutrition Examination Survey III (NHANES III). Clin Chem 1997;43:2364-78.

*Combined data for total population, including all three ethnic groups.

†All SEMs were 1 mg/dL unless otherwise indicated.

‡Estimates based on 400 to 800 subjects in each age and sex subgroup.

more, these two apolipoproteins were shown to correlate better with the degree of coronary stenosis than LDL and HDL cholesterol.[200] It has also been shown that only 14.5% of patients with myocardial infarction younger than the age of 60 years have LDL cholesterol above the 95th percentile. In contrast, 35% of these patients have apo B-100 above the 95th percentile.[284] The measurement of apo B-100 provides information regarding the number of apo B-100–containing particles. If the concentration of LDL cholesterol is normal or slightly increased but apo B-100 is greatly increased, it is likely that the number of the small, more atherogenic and dense, LDL particles is high. Increased serum apo B-100 and decreased apo A-I concentrations were also found in children of parents with premature atherosclerotic disease.[83] These findings suggest that apolipoproteins may be good predictors of the possibility of future CHD. The Familial Atherosclerosis Treatment Study (FATS) demonstrated that the treatment of men, younger than 62 years of age with documented CHD, with-lipid-lowering agents on the basis of their apo B-100 concentration (>the 95th percentile, 125 mg/dL) alone is beneficial. A reduction in apo B-100 concentration in these patients caused a reversal of angiographically demonstrable coronary atherosclerosis and reduced the incidence of clinical events.[32] Data from the Air Force/Texas Coronary Atherosclerosis Prevention Study have shown apo B-100 to be the single most significant and consistent lipid measurement to predict future risk of coronary events.[98] The apo B-100/A-I ratio was a better discriminator of risk than the LDL-C/HDL-C ratio. Data from this study also suggested that the mechanism of the benefit associated with lovastatin-mediated changes in LDL-C and HDL-C may be, in part, a function of the changes in apo B-100 and apo A-I. Findings from the Quebec Cardiovascular Study also showed apo B-100 to be a more powerful independent predictor of CHD than LDL-C.[151] The association of CHD risk with Lp(a) and apo E concentra-

TABLE 26-13 Age-Adjusted* Mean Apo A-I and Apo B Concentrations in Persons Ages ≥ 4 Years by Sex and Age Group, U.S., 1988-1991

	Mean (SEM)† CONC., mg/dL					
	Apo A-I			Apo B		
Age, Years	White	Black	Mexican-American	White	Black	Mexican-American
Males						
All	134	145	135 (2)	99	96	101
4-11	140 (2)	145	139 (2)	79	79	79
12-19	127	139 (2)	131 (3)	78	78	79
≥20	135	146	135 (2)	106	102	109
Females						
All	146	151	144 (2)	97	96	98
4-11	133	142 (2)	132	82	82	81
12-19	122 (2)	144 (2)	140 (4)	80	82	83
≥20	151	154	147 (2)	103	101	105

Modified from Bachorik PS, Lovejoy KL, Carroll MD, Johnson CL. Apolipoprotein B and AI distributions in the United States, 1988-1991: results of the National Health and Nutrition Examination Survey III (NHANES III). Clin Chem 1997;43:2364-78.
*Age-adjusted by the direct method to the 1980 U.S. census population.
†All SEMs were 1 mg/dL unless otherwise indicated.

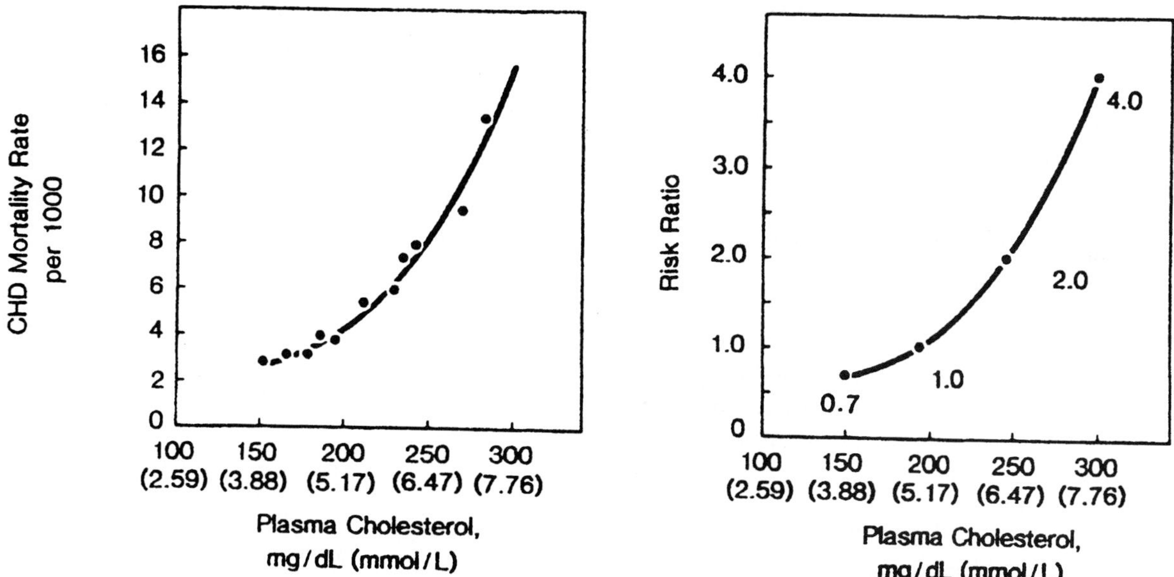

Figure 26-22 Relationship between cholesterol concentration and coronary heart disease mortality expressed by yearly rate per 1000 and risk ratios (Multiple Risk Factor Intervention Trial [MRFIT] participants). *(From Grundy SM. Cholesterol and coronary heart disease: A new era. JAMA 1986;256:2849-55. Copyright 1986, American Medical Association.)*

tions and the various apo E phenotypes is presented later in this chapter.

Although CHD is manifested clinically in the fourth decade of life, evidence clearly indicates that atherosclerosis, its major cause, is a process that begins early in life and progresses silently for decades. Autopsies performed on young American soldiers killed in action in Korea[74] and Vietnam[185] revealed atherosclerotic lesions. Coronary artery lesions were also found in aortas beginning at the age of 3 years[289] and in coronaries starting at the age of 10 years in the International Atherosclerosis Project.[294] In the Pathobiological Determinants of Atherosclerosis in Youth (PDAY) study, intimal lesions appeared in all the examined aortas and more than half of the right coronary arteries of the youngest age group (15 to 19 years) and increased in prevalence and extent with age through the oldest age group (30 to 34 years).[293] This study also demonstrated that some regions of the arteries were lesion prone and others were lesion resistant and the propensity to develop raised or advanced lesions differed among right coronary artery, abdominal aorta, and thoracic aorta. Findings from the Bogalusa Heart Study[328] indicated a correlation between systolic blood pressure, higher total and LDL cholesterol, and lower HDL cholesterol concentrations and the degree of coronary and aortic atherosclerosis in children and adolescents.[24] In the PDAY study, postmortem cholesterol and thiocyanate concentrations predicted the extent of coronary and aortic atherosclerosis, respectively, in autopsies of those aged 14 to 34.[332] Therefore, a direct relation between determinant risk factors and the extent of atherosclerotic lesions in youth seems to exist. Furthermore, children in countries with an increased incidence of CHD were reported to have higher cholesterol concentrations than children of countries with low incidence.[139] About 5% of American children, 5 to 18 years of age, have cholesterol concentrations above 200 mg/dL. In addition, findings from the Muscatine, Bogalusa, and Princeton School District studies have demonstrated that serum cholesterol and lipoprotein cholesterol concentrations cluster in families and display a moderate degree of longitudinal tracking.[134,154,155,328] Thus in those people who have high total and lipoprotein cholesterol concentrations, the levels tend to remain high as they get older. This suggests that the identification and treatment of children who may be at high risk for development of CHD offer the possibility of preventing or delaying the development of this disease.

Disorders of Lipoprotein Metabolism

Dyslipoproteinemia is diagnosed in most patients using plasma lipid and lipoprotein cholesterol concentrations. Dyslipoproteinemias have previously been defined in terms of arbitrarily defined cut points for lipids and lipoprotein, but are now based on the relationship between lipoprotein levels and the risk for CHD (see discussion later in this chapter).

Primary Versus Secondary Hyperlipoproteinemia

On diagnosing hyperlipidemia in a given patient, the hyperlipidemic status should be evaluated to determine whether it is a primary lipoprotein disorder or secondary to any of a variety of metabolic diseases. The diagnosis of primary hyperlipidemia is made after secondary causes have been ruled out. The causes of secondary hyperlipoproteinemia are listed in Table 26-14. The most commonly seen secondary causes in the first year of life are glycogen storage disease and congenital biliary atresia. Hypothyroidism, nephrotic syndrome, and diabetes mellitus are more prevalent later in childhood. Exogenous factors, such as dietary and alcohol intake, oral contraceptives, diabetes mellitus, and pharmacological agents (e.g., steroids, isotretinoin [Accutane], and β-blockers), are the main secondary causes of hyperlipidemia in adults.[125,147]

TABLE 26-14 Causes of Secondary Hyperlipidemia and Dyslipoproteinemia

Disorder	Cause
Exogenous	Drugs: corticosteroids, isotretinoin (Accutane), thiazides, anticonvulsants, β blockers, anabolic steroids, certain oral contraceptives
	Alcohol
	Obesity
Endocrine and metabolic	Acute intermittent porphyria
	Diabetes mellitus
	Hypopituitarism
	Hypothyroidism
	Lipodystrophy
	Pregnancy
Storage disease	Cystine storage disease
	Gaucher's disease
	Glycogen storage disease
	Juvenile Tay-Sachs disease
	Niemann-Pick disease
	Tay-Sachs disease
Renal	Chronic renal failure
	Hemolytic-uremic syndrome
	Nephrotic syndrome
Hepatic	Benign recurrent intrahepatic cholestasis
	Congenital biliary atresia
Acute and transient	Burns
	Hepatitis
	Acute trauma (surgery)
	Myocardial infarction
	Bacterial and viral infections
Others	Anorexia nervosa
	Starvation
	Idiopathic hypercalcemia
	Klinefelter's syndrome
	Progeria (Hutchinson-Gilford syndrome)
	Systemic lupus erythematosus
	Werner's syndrome

Familial Dyslipoproteinemias

Historically, lipoprotein phenotypes reflecting lipoprotein metabolic disorders were classified according to Fredrickson and co-workers. However, these disorders are more rationally approached based on the four metabolic pathways discussed previously (see Figures 26-18 through 26-21). Defects in these pathways, leading to hyperlipidemia, may be related to (1) increased production of lipoproteins, (2) abnormal intravascular processing (e.g., enzymatic hydrolysis of triglyceride), and (3) defective cellular uptake of lipoproteins. Finally, a significant decrease in production or an increase in removal of lipoproteins can lead to a marked reduction in lipid and lipoprotein concentrations.

Deficiency in Lipoprotein Lipase Activity

This disorder is characterized by marked hyperchylomicronemia and a corresponding hypertriglyceridemia (triglyceride as high as 10,000 mg/dL).[36] As discussed previously, LPL is essential for the hydrolysis of triglyceride and the conversion of chylomicrons to chylomicron remnants. The massive accumulation of chylomicrons in the circulation indicates the inability to catabolize dietary fat. The concentration of VLDL cholesterol is usually normal and the concentrations of HDL cholesterol and LDL cholesterol are low (type I pattern). Furthermore, the concentration of apo C-II, the activator of LPL, is normal.

This disorder is usually expressed in childhood. In a review of 43 cases, 35 were manifested before the age of 10.[159,160] It appears that those patients with low to absent LPL activity in all tissue present with symptoms of the disease at an early age (classic form), whereas those with deficiency in LPL activity in only one tissue become symptomatic later in life (variant forms). This disease is usually detected after recurrent episodes of severe abdominal pain and repeated attacks of pancreatitis. Eruptive xanthomas and lipemia retinalis are usually present when plasma triglyceride concentrations exceed 2000 and 4000 mg/dL, respectively.[36] The acuteness of the symptoms is directly proportional to the degree of hyperchylomicronemia. It is important to note that patients with this disorder *do not* appear to be predisposed to atherosclerotic disease.

The diagnosis is made by the determination of LPL activity in postheparin plasma. The intravenously administered heparin binds LPL, causing its dissociation from heparan sulfate, present on the surface of endothelial cells, and subsequent release to plasma.[117] This autosomal recessive disorder is extremely rare (one per million individuals). More than 40 insertions and deletions in the LPL gene that lead to absent or truncated LPL protein with defective catalytic activity have been described.[36]

Deficiency in Apolipoprotein C-II

Deficient or defective apo C-II, the required activator for LPL, reduces the activity of this enzyme, impairs chylomicron catabolism, and increases plasma triglycerides (500 to 10,000 mg/dL). Those affected by this disorder have less than 10% of the normal concentration of apo C-II, the minimum amount necessary for normal LPL activity.[122] Total cholesterol tends to vary considerably (150 to 890 mg/dL) in these patients, but HDL and LDL cholesterol concentrations are below the 5th percentile. Furthermore, plasma apo A-I, A-II, and B-100 concentrations are decreased, whereas apo C-III and E concentrations are increased.

Although the clinical symptoms are similar to those seen in patients with LPL deficiency, they are usually milder and expressed at a later age. The predominant symptom is usually recurrent abdominal pain caused by attacks of pancreatitis. Eruptive xanthomas and lipemia retinalis are not usually seen in these patients. As with LPL deficiency, patients with apo C-II deficiency are not predisposed to atherosclerosis.

The diagnosis is made by the documentation of low LPL activity in postheparin plasma in the absence of added apo C-II. Normal enzymatic activity is restored by the addition of normal apo C-II to the assay mixture. In another approach, the absence of apo C-II can be recognized using an immunoassay for apo C-II. However, the latter approach may not distinguish between normal subjects and those with normal levels of a nonfunctional form of apo C-II. The defective apo C-II disorder is inherited in an autosomal recessive mode, but at a lower frequency than LPL deficiency. More than 10 structural defects in the apo C-II gene that lead to the absence of apo C-II or the production of a defective apo C-II molecule have been described.[36] Subjects heterozygous for a defective apo C-II gene have normal lipid and lipoprotein profiles, because a sufficient amount of normal apo C-II is usually present to activate LPL.

Familial Combined Hyperlipidemia

About 10% to 15% of patients with premature CHD actually have familial combined hyperlipidemia (FCHL).[90] This disorder is recognized as a distinct phenotype by studying family members of survivors of myocardial infarction. Patients with FCHL can have increased plasma concentrations of total and LDL cholesterol (type IIa), or triglyceride (type IV), or both (type IIb). In all cases, apo B-100 concentrations are increased. The presentation of lipoprotein patterns can vary in an individual with time. Furthermore, patients with hypertriglyceridemia with normal partners tend to have offspring with hypercholesterolemia, and vice versa.[102]

FCHL appears to result from the overproduction of VLDL and apo B-100. Kinetic studies have shown that the rate of flux of apo B-100 from VLDL in FCHL is approximately twice that of normal subjects.[44,58] This causes apo B-100 to be increased (more than 125 mg/dL) even in subjects with normal LDL cholesterol. Because of the decreased lipid-to-protein ratio in these patients, both VLDL and LDL particles tend to be small and dense. When increased, LDL cholesterol is about 190 mg/dL, but is lower than that seen in heterozygous familial hypercholesterolemia. Triglyceride levels are usually between 200 and 400 mg/dL, but can be significantly higher. The concentration of HDL cholesterol is usually mildly depressed, particularly in the presence of hypertriglyceridemia. Xanthomas and other clinical symptoms of hyperlipidemia, other than atherosclerosis, are not very common in these patients. The association of FCHL with CHD incidence is high. In addition to the increased IDL in these patients, the presence of high concentrations of small, dense LDL and low concentrations of HDL cholesterol might explain their increased risk.

Although the mutation(s) responsible for FCHL remain unknown, this disorder is associated with a major gene, apparently interacting with other genes, and has a prevalence of 1 in 100 persons. Although the expression of FCHL is delayed until adolescence, young children from families with premature CHD can present with increased cholesterol or triglyceride, or both.[147]

Hyperapobetalipoproteinemia

This disorder is characterized by increased LDL-apo B-100 concentrations with normal or moderately increased concentrations of LDL cholesterol.[148,282] The ratio of LDL cholesterol to apo B-100 is therefore reduced in these patients ($\leq$1.2).[148] Total cholesterol and triglyceride may be normal but are usually increased, and HDL cholesterol and apo A-I are decreased. This disorder appears to be caused by an overproduction of VLDL and apo B-100 in the liver, which leads to the formation of the atherogenic small and dense LDL.[148] The exact mode of inheritance and prevalence of this disorder remain unclear. However, about one third of children of a parent with premature CHD or hyperapobetalipoproteinemia will have this disorder.[283] Features common to hyperapobetalipoproteinemia have also been reported to occur in patients with FCHL, suggesting metabolic and genetic associations between the two disorders.

Familial Hypertriglyceridemia

The production of large VLDL with abnormally high triglyceride content appears to be responsible for familial hypertriglyceridemia (FHTG).[129] The actual number of VLDL particles produced by the liver, however, is not increased. The cholesterol content of VLDL is also increased, but plasma LDL cholesterol and apo B-100 concentrations are normal. This finding suggests that the conversion of VLDL to LDL is not increased in these patients. Furthermore, plasma HDL cholesterol in FHTG is often dramatically decreased, probably secondary to the hypertriglyceridemia.

The cause of the overproduction of VLDL triglyceride is unknown. The administration of estrogen and corticosteroids aggravates hypertriglyceridemia in these patients and can sometimes lead to acute pancreatitis. The diagnosis of FHTG requires study of other family members to differentiate this disorder from FCHL. This disorder appears to be inherited in an autosomal dominant pattern with a delayed expression and an estimated frequency in the population at about 1:500 persons. About one in five children born to affected parents manifest the phenotype early in life.[87]

Type V Hyperlipoproteinemia

This disorder is characterized by an increase in both chylomicrons and VLDL. Although the exact cause for this disorder is not known, it may be due to an increased production or a decreased removal of VLDL, or to a combination of both. The activity of LPL in these patients is either normal or low, and the plasma concentration of apo C-II is normal.[147]

Although this disorder is not usually expressed in childhood, several affected preadolescents have been described.[147] Clinical presentations in adult patients include eruptive xanthomas, lipemia retinalis, pancreatitis, and abnormal glucose tolerance with hyperinsulinism.[36] Premature atherosclerotic complications are not as commonly seen as with FH. This heterogeneous syndrome appears to be inherited in an autosomal dominant mode, but its genetic basis is yet to be elucidated.

Dysbetalipoproteinemia (Type III)

This disorder is caused by a primary genetic defect in the removal of remnants of both intestinal chylomicrons and hepatic VLDL.[167] As indicated earlier, apo E present on the surface of lipoprotein remnants interacts with specific hepatic receptors and facilitates the removal of these particles from the circulation. Patients with dysbetalipoproteinemia are homozygous for a mutant form of apo E (apo E_2) that cannot efficiently bind the specific hepatic receptors, leading to the accumulation of lipoprotein remnants and a cholesterol-enriched lipoprotein of density <1.006 g/mL, commonly referred to as β-VLDL or floating β-lipoprotein, in plasma. This variant form of apo E is the result of a single amino acid substitution of cysteine for the normally occurring arginine at amino acid residue 158.[329]

The disease is characterized in part by increased plasma cholesterol and triglycerides, and the concentrations of the two lipids are about the same when expressed in milligrams per deciliter. β-VLDL present in type III has been shown to contain both apo B-100 and B-48, and is therefore related to triglyceride-rich lipoprotein remnants of both hepatic and intestinal origins. Both LDL and HDL cholesterol are lower than normal in these patients.[167]

This disorder has a late onset; it rarely manifests itself in childhood.[260] The most distinctive clinical presentation of dyslipoproteinemia is the presence of palmar xanthomas, the yellow deposits that occur in the creases of the palms.[132] Tuberous and tuberoeruptive xanthomas also occur but are not unique to this syndrome. Premature atherosclerosis develops in 30% to more than 50% of these patients, particularly in the lower extremities.[295,315]

Apolipoprotein E_2 occurs in about 1% of the population in North America, and homozygotic subjects for this isoform exhibit β-VLDL. However, overt type III hyperlipoproteinemia occurs in only one to two persons per thousand in the general population (LRC prevalence study), indicating that the occurrence of the defective alleles is necessary but not sufficient to produce clinical type III hyperlipoproteinemia.[310] The development of overt hyperlipoproteinemia in these patients is modulated by genetic, hormonal, or environmental factors—such as hypothyroidism, glucose intolerance, decreased estrogen levels after menopause, obesity, and diet—that may lead to decreased LDL receptor activity, increased VLDL production, or increased plasma cholesterol ester transfer protein. Other rare forms of mutant apo E that cause type III hyperlipoproteinemia have also been described. Because of the familial nature of this disorder and the predisposition of the patients to hyperlipoproteinemia and premature atherosclerotic disease, family members should be evaluated. The determination of the apo E phenotype or genotype may serve to better characterize family members who may be more susceptible to the development of this disorder.

Familial Hypercholesterolemia

Familial hypercholesterolemia (FH) is caused by a primary genetic defect in the LDL receptor gene. As discussed earlier, this cell surface receptor is responsible for the recognition and removal of LDL from circulation. The defects seen in patients with FH include reduced LDL binding because of defective or absent LDL receptors. In another variant of this disorder, the person may make defective LDL receptors that bind LDL normally but that cannot efficiently internalize the LDL particles.[34] FH is characterized clinically by increased plasma LDL cholesterol concentration; cholesterol deposition in skin, tendons, and arteries; and autosomal dominant transmission that is expressed in a heterozygous or homozygous mode. Heterozygous FH is one of the most commonly seen genetic metabolic disorders, with an incidence of 1 in 500 persons in the United States. The prevalence of homozygous FH is about one in a million persons. The mean plasma LDL cholesterol in children and adult heterozygotes is usually two to three times that of normal people of similar age, whereas the mean plasma LDL cholesterol of homozygotes is four to six times that of normal subjects.[89] Although the number of LDL particles is increased in these patients, their lipid composition and lipid-to-protein ratio are usually normal.[94] Apolipoprotein B-100, the main protein in LDL, is increased in proportion to LDL cholesterol. Triglyceride concentration is either normal or slightly increased, and HDL cholesterol concentration is slightly decreased in both heterozygotes and homozygotes.

Hypercholesterolemia is present at birth in most FH patients and persists throughout life. In heterozygotes, xanthomas appear toward the end of the second decade and clinical manifestations of atherosclerotic disease appear during the fourth decade.[275] In homozygotes, the unique yellow-orange cutaneous xanthomas develop by the age of 4, if they are not already present at birth.[132] Tendon xanthomas and atherosclerotic complications begin during childhood. Death from myocardial infarction invariably occurs in homozygotes before the end of the third decade.[125,147]

Although increased plasma LDL cholesterol is indicative of the heterozygous form of FH, it is not sufficient to make the diagnosis. Other more complex laboratory tests, such as the demonstration of decreased LDL receptor activity or the confirmation of a mutation in the LDL receptor gene, are necessary to confirm the presence of this disease.[89] However, in routine practice, clinical information—such as the presence of tendon xanthomas, the detection of a child with hypercholesterolemia in the patient's immediate family, and the documentation of autosomal dominant transmission—is sufficient evidence of FH. The diagnosis of homozygous FH is simpler. Patients present at a very early age with symptoms of distinct cutaneous xanthomas, juvenile atherosclerosis, and marked hypercholesterolemia (500 to 1200 mg/dL).

More than 150 different mutations in the LDL receptor gene have been shown to significantly disrupt the normal process of LDL removal from circulation.[89,114] Heterozygotes possess one normal and one mutant allele at the LDL receptor locus and therefore can remove LDL at about half the normal rate. In contrast, homozygotes or compound heterozygotes have two of the mutant alleles and hence are unable to bind or remove LDL particles.

Familial Defective Apolipoprotein B-100

This disorder results from a mutation in the apo B-100 gene rather than the LDL receptor, resulting in a single substitution of glutamine for arginine at residue 3500 of apo B-100. This substitution reduces the positive charge of apo B-100 and decreases the affinity of LDL for the LDL receptor.[286] Plasma LDL cholesterol in heterozygotes can either be normal or moderately or greatly increased because of inadequate removal of LDL particles by LDL receptors.[313] Those with increased LDL cholesterol have an incidence of CHD comparable with that in those with FH. Triglyceride and HDL cholesterol concentrations are not affected. It is very difficult to differentiate clinically between these patients and those with heterozygous FH. However, because the management of patients with the two disorders is similar, the distinction is not clinically important.[129] The frequency of this mutation is 1:500 to 1:600 hypercholesterolemic persons in populations of European descent,[305] but the mutation is very rare in non-European populations.

Familial Hypoalphalipoproteinemia

This disorder is characterized by normal plasma lipids and LDL cholesterol and reduced HDL cholesterol, below the 5th percentile.[260,270] Although patients with this disorder are clinically normal, they have a high incidence of CHD.[303] The molecular basis of familial hypoalphalipoproteinemia is unknown. This disorder is the result of either the decreased biosynthesis or the increased catabolism of HDL or apo A-I.[31] Although the mode of transmission is not certain, in some kindreds familial hypoalphalipoproteinemia is inherited as an autosomal dominant trait.

Defects in the Synthesis of Apolipoprotein A-I

In homozygous familial hypoalphalipoproteinemia, only traces of HDL cholesterol are found in plasma, and apo A-I is undetectable.[31,147] These patients have corneal clouding and are at increased risk for development of premature CHD. Heterozygotes exhibit no clinical signs but have about half the normal concentrations of HDL cholesterol and apo A-I. Mutations—such as a rearrangement at the apolipoprotein gene locus that inactivates both apo A-I and C-III, a deletion of the entire locus, or an insertion in the apo A-I gene—lead to decreased synthesis and low concentrations of apo A-I.[130,147,215] The frequency of recessive genes associated with low HDL cholesterol levels is approximately 10% in the general population.[31]

Defects in Catabolism of Apolipoprotein A-I (Tangier Disease)

Tangier disease, so named because it was first observed in patients from Tangier Island, is characterized by (1) severely reduced plasma HDL concentration, (2) abnormal HDL composition, and (3) accumulation of cholesteryl esters in many tissues throughout the body.[12,271,274] Kinetic studies have demonstrated that increased catabolism of HDL, rather than a defect in biosynthesis, is the cause of Tangier disease.[271] Because plasma HDL concentration is very low, the detailed characterization of this lipoprotein has been difficult to accomplish. Tangier disease is caused by mutations in the *ABC1* (ATP-binding cassette) gene on chromosome 9q31 and appears to be inherited in an autosomal dominant fashion. Plasma cholesterol is decreased to about 70 mg/dL in homozygotes and to about 160 mg/dL in heterozygotes. Triglyceride concentrations vary depending on the diet.[12] In homozygotes, plasma HDL cholesterol and apo A-I concentrations are almost zero, and apo A-II is present at less than 10% of its normal concentration in apo B-100–containing lipoprotein.[13] Heterozygotes are characterized by half-normal concentrations of HDL cholesterol, apo A-I, and apo A-II.

The clinical symptoms of Tangier disease result from the deposition of cholesteryl esters in various tissue in the body. The three major clinical signs are the hyperplastic orange tonsils, splenomegaly, and peripheral neuropathy. Other clinical signs that may be seen include hepatomegaly and corneal opacities. The severely reduced HDL cholesterol and enlarged orange tonsils are pathognomonic.[12,147] Current evidence suggests that these patients have an increased incidence of CHD. Heterozygotes exhibit no clinical manifestations and can be identified only biochemically. Although the incidence of Tangier disease in children is very low, patients as young as 3 years have been identified.[147]

Diagnosis of Lipoprotein Disorders

On the basis of findings from studies such as the MRFIT and the LRC-CPPT discussed previously,[102,163,164] hypercholesterolemia in adults is now defined in terms of CHD risk. The National Institutes of Health ATP of the NCEP[203] has issued its third report for the detection, evaluation, and treatment of hypercholesterolemia (ATP III).[59] The ATP III built on earlier reports and expanded the indications for intensive cholesterol lowering. In ATP I, strategies for primary prevention of CHD in subjects with LDL-C ≥160 mg/dL or 130 to 159 mg/dL and multiple risk factors (2+) were addressed. ATP II added new features; for subjects with existing CHD, a lower LDL-C goal of ≤100 mg/dL was established and the HDL cholesterol value was given more prominence. ATP III called for intensive LDL-C lowering in several other groups of patients. In this section, only a brief description of ATP III will be presented. Those interested in more detailed information should refer to the executive summary[59] or the complete report (http://www.nhlbi.nih.gov/guidelines/cholesterol/index.htm).

TABLE 26-15 ATP III Classification of LDL, Total, and HDL Cholesterol (mg/dL)*

LDL cholesterol	<100	Optimum
	100-129	Near or above optimum
	130-159	Borderline high
	160-189	High
	≥190	Very high
Total cholesterol	<200	Desirable
	200-239	Borderline high
	≥240	High
HDL cholesterol	<40	Low
	≥60	High

Modified from executive summary of the third report of the National Cholesterol Education Program (NCEP) Expert Panel on Detection, Evaluation, and Treatment of High Blood Cholesterol in Adults (Adult Treatment Panel III). JAMA 2001;285:2486-97.

*ATP indicates Adult Treatment Panel; *LDL,* low-density lipoprotein; *HDL,* high-density lipoprotein.

For the primary prevention of CHD, adults age 20 or older should have their fasting lipoprotein profile (total cholesterol, triglycerides, HDL-C, and LDL-C) measured once every 5 years. If a fasting sample is not available, then only total cholesterol and HDL-C should be considered. In this instance if total cholesterol is ≥200 mg/dL or HDL-C is ≤40 mg/dL, then a fasting lipoprotein profile is required. The cut points recommended for classification by ATP III are presented in Table 26-15.[63] In addition to LDL-C, other risk determinants, presented in Box 26-2, are used to assess risk and determine goals and modalities of LDL-C lowering therapy. The highest category of risk consists of those with CHD or CHD-risk equivalents (other forms of atherosclerotic disease, such as peripheral arterial disease, abdominal aortic aneurysm, and symptomatic carotid artery disease, diabetes, or multiple risk factors that confer a 10-year risk for CHD >20%, as estimated by the Framingham risk score) (Table 26-16). The Framingham risk score is calculated for a particular individual using an algorithm that includes age, gender, total cholesterol, HDL-C, history of hypertension and treatment of hypertension, and cigarette smoking. Individuals in this category carry a risk of a major coronary event of >20%/10 years. The second category of risk includes individuals with multiple risk factors (2+) in whom 10-year risk is ≤20%. The third category consists of subjects having 0 to 1 risk factors in whom 10-year risk is ≤10%.

TABLE 26-16 Categories of Risk for LDL Cholesterol Goals

Risk Category	LDL Goal (mg/dL)
CHD and CHD risk equivalents	<100
Multiple (2+) risk factors*	<130
0-1 risk factor	<160

Modified from executive summary of the third report of the National Cholesterol Education Program (NCEP) Expert Panel on Detection, Evaluation, and Treatment of High Blood Cholesterol in Adults (Adult Treatment Panel III). JAMA 2001;285:2486-97.
*Refer to Box 26-2 for list of risk factors. CHD indicates coronary heart disease.

BOX 26-2 Major Risk Factors (Exclusive of LDL Cholesterol)

- Cigarette smoking
- Hypertension (blood pressure ≥140/90 mm Hg or on antihypertensive medication)
- Low HDL cholesterol (<40 mg/dL)*
- Family history of premature CHD (CHD in male first-degree relative <55 years; CHD in female first-degree relative <65 years)
- Age (men ≥45 years; women ≥55 years)

Modified from executive summary of the third report of the National Cholesterol Education Program (NCEP) Expert Panel on Detection, Evaluation, and Treatment of High Blood Cholesterol in Adults (Adult Treatment Panel III). JAMA 2001;285:2486-97.
LDL, Low-density lipoprotein; *HDL,* high-density lipoprotein.
*HDL cholesterol ≥60 mg/dL counts as a "negative" risk factor; its presence removes one risk factor from the total count.

TABLE 26-17 Clinical Identification of the Metabolic Syndrome

Risk Factor	Defining Level
• Abdominal obesity (waist circumference)	
Men	>102 cm (>40 in)
Women	>88 cm (>35 in)
• Triglycerides	≥150 mg/dL
• High-density lipoprotein cholesterol	
Men	<40 mg/dL
Women	<50 mg/dL
• Blood pressure	≥130/≥85 mm Hg
• Fasting glucose	≥110 mg/dL

Modified from executive summary of the third report of the National Cholesterol Education Program (NCEP) Expert Panel on Detection, Evaluation, and Treatment of High Blood Cholesterol in Adults (Adult Treatment Panel III). JAMA 2001;285:2486-97.
HDL, High-density lipoprotein cholesterol.

TABLE 26-18 NCEP Classification of Total and Low-Density Lipoprotein (LDL) Cholesterol in Children and Adolescents*

Category	Total Cholesterol	LDL Cholesterol
Desirable	<170	<110
Borderline	170-199	110-120
High	≥200	≥130

*All values are in mg/dL; to convert to mmol/L, multiply by 0.0259.

Although the primary target of risk-reduction therapy is LDL-C, the ATP III recognized the metabolic syndrome, a constellation of several risk factors (increased triglycerides, decreased HDL-C, obesity, hypertension, and insulin resistance), as a secondary target of therapy. By definition, those with three or more of these risk factors are considered to have the metabolic syndrome.[77] The specific criteria for the clinical identification of the metabolic syndrome are listed in Table 26-17.

The NCEP/Expert Panel on Blood Cholesterol Levels in Children and Adolescents[244] and the American Academy of Pediatrics[7,8] defined "high cholesterol" as concentrations more than the 95th percentile for total and LDL cholesterol in children and adolescents from families with hypercholesterolemia or premature vascular disease (see Table 26-18). "Borderline" total and LDL cholesterol concentrations are defined as values between the 75th and 95th percentiles. The NCEP panel referred to total and LDL cholesterol values below the 75th percentile as "desirable." Low HDL cholesterol was also defined as a concentration below 35 mg/dL. Children tend to have higher HDL cholesterol concentrations than adults. Therefore it is important to determine both LDL and HDL cholesterol concentrations before classifying the child as hypercholesterolemic. Unlike the criteria for the risk-based cholesterol classification system used in adults, the guidelines for children and adolescents were based on consensus rather than directly on the association with coronary disease, because children as a group have very little disease. When such data become available, different cutoffs may be suggested for the pediatric population.

As discussed earlier, cholesterol screening is currently recommended for all adults in the United States. However, for children such a screening program remains highly controversial. According to the NCEP[243] and the American Academy of Pediatrics,[7,8] only children over the age of 2 should be screened for hypercholesterolemia when they have a parent with hypercholesterolemia (>240 mg/dL) or a positive family history (mother, father, uncle, aunt, or grandparent) with early documented CHD (at 55 years or less), myocardial infarction, angina pectoris, peripheral vascular disease, cerebrovascular disease, or sudden cardiac death. Several studies, however, have demonstrated the weakness of

TABLE 26-19 Current Fat Intake in American Adults, Children, and Adolescents and the American Heart Association Step-One and Step-Two Diets

Nutrients	Current Intake			
	Adults	**Children and Adolescents**	**Step-One**	**Step-Two**
Total fat				
Percent of total calories	35%-36%	36%	<30%	<30%
Saturated fat	14%	15%	<10%	7%
Polyunsaturated fat	6%	16%	10%	10%
Monounsaturated fat	13%-14%	15%	10%-15%	10%-15%
Cholesterol (mg/day)	300-400	400-500	<300	<200

Modified from National Cholesterol Education Program, Lipid Metabolism Branch, Division of Heart, Lung, and Blood Institute: The Report of the Expert Panel on Blood Cholesterol Levels in Children and Adolescents. Bethesda, MD: National Institutes of Health, 1991.

this selective approach to screening and have advocated general screening for children.* The Bogalusa Heart Study found that by using the selective screening approach, only 50% of white children and 20% of black children with high LDL cholesterol concentration (>95th percentile) were detected. Furthermore, it has been shown that self-reported cholesterol values in the parents are an ineffective means of identifying children with high cholesterol.[245] More than 90% of children with total cholesterol greater than the 75th or 95th percentile were missed when physicians relied on cholesterol values reported by the parents. General screening, however, is expensive and time consuming and its effectiveness is limited by the fact that a significant number of children with high cholesterol concentrations will *not* remain hypercholesterolemic as adults.[155,239] Universal screening for those older than 16 has also been suggested on the basis of a finding that up to 66% of adolescents with increased LDL cholesterol are missed in a selective screening protocol.[261] When past adolescence, men usually start receiving routine health examinations about the age of 40, and although women visit their physicians earlier, it is because of gynecological needs. Those adolescents with increased LDL cholesterol who are missed in the selective screening process may not be identified until 2 decades later. At that time, the atherosclerotic process may be advanced and the dietary approach may not be sufficiently effective. Another possible yet unpopular approach is to do no screening at all. A prudent low-fat diet, such as the one outlined by the American Heart Association (AHA), can be recommended for all children (Table 26-19).[7,8] Such an approach will not create anxiety, labeling, or overzealous treatment; however, it will miss completely those children with significant hypercholesterolemia most at risk for adult CHD.

Management of Lipoprotein Disorders

Dietary and drug therapies are the cornerstones of the treatment of lipid disorders, such as hypercholesterolemia and hypertriglyceridemia.

*References 67, 68, 85, 101, 245, 261.

TABLE 26-20 Nutrient Composition of the Therapeutic Life-Style Changes (TLC) Diet

Nutrient	Recommended Intake
Saturated fat	<7% of total calories
Polyunsaturated fat	Up to 10% of total calories
Monounsaturated fat	Up to 20% of total calories
Total fat	25%-35% of total calories
Carbohydrate	50%-60% of total calories
Fiber	20-30 g/day
Protein	Approximately 15% of total calories
Cholesterol	<200 mg/day
Total calories	Balance energy intake and expenditure to maintain desirable body weight/ prevent weight gain

Modified from executive summary of the third report of the National Cholesterol Education Program (NCEP) Expert Panel on Detection, Evaluation, and Treatment of High Blood Cholesterol in Adults (Adult Treatment Panel III). JAMA 2001;285:2486-97.

Management of Hypercholesterolemia

According to ATP III, the clinical prevention of CHD is founded on a public health approach and entails a reduction in saturated fat and cholesterol intake (Table 26-20), increased physical activity, and weight control. Although this therapeutic life-style approach offers the opportunity for reducing the morbidity and mortality of CHD in the entire American population, more intensified preventive measures for higher-risk individuals are indicated.[77] The primary goal is to reduce one's long-term (>10 years) and short-term risk (<10 years), and the target LDL-C value depends on the person's absolute risk (Table 26-21). Certainly a more aggressive approach is recommended for those who have already suffered a coronary event or those with established

TABLE 26-21 LDL Cholesterol Goals and Cut Points for Therapeutic Life-Style Changes (TLC) and Drug Therapy in Different Risk Categories

Risk Category	LDL Goal (mg/dL)	LDL Level at Which to Initiate Therapeutic Life Style Changes (mg/dL)	LDL Level at Which to Consider Drug Therapy (mg/dL)
CHD or CHD risk equivalents (10-year risk >20%)	<100	≥100	≥130 (100-129: drug optional)
2+ Risk factors (10-year risk ≤ 20%)	<130	≥130	10-year risk 10%-20%: ≥130 10-year risk <10%: ≥160
0-1 Risk factor (10-year risk <10%)	<160	≥160	≥190 (160-189: LDL-lowering drug optional)

Modified from executive summary of the third report of the National Cholesterol Education Program (NCEP) Expert Panel on Detection, Evaluation, and Treatment of High Blood Cholesterol in Adults (Adult Treatment Panel III). JAMA 2001;285:2486-97.
LDL, Low-density lipoprotein; *CHD,* coronary heart disease.

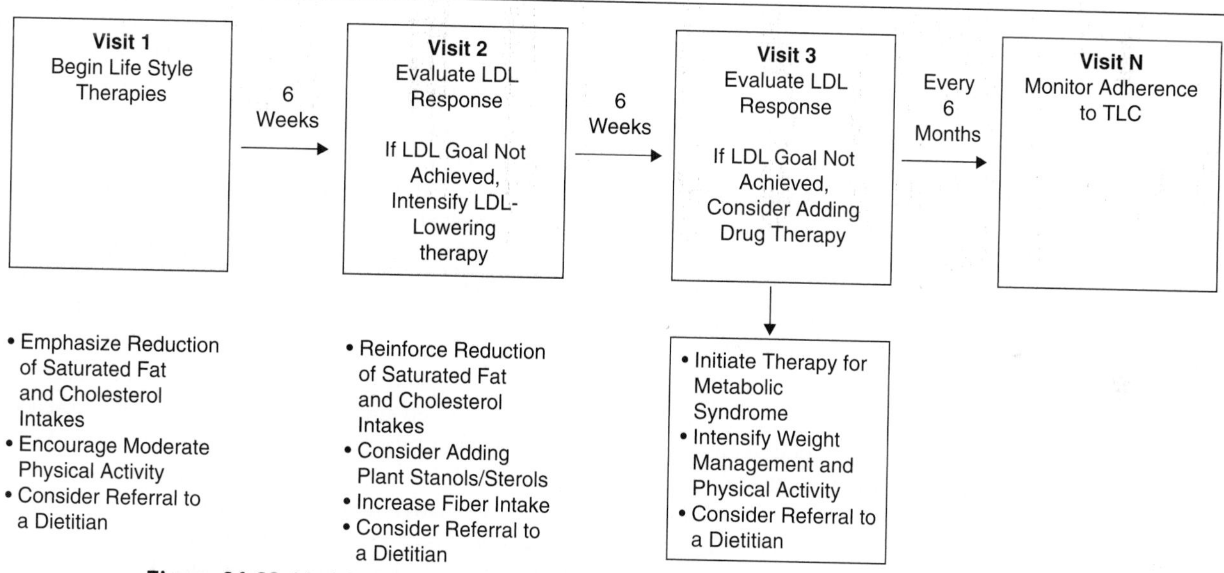

Figure 26-23 Model of steps in therapeutic life-style change. *LDL,* Low-density lipoprotein. *(Modified from Executive summary of the third report of the Expert Panel on Blood Cholesterol Levels in Children and Adolescents, National Cholesterol Education Program. Lipid Metabolism Branch, Division of Heart, Lung, and Blood Institute. NIH Publication No. 01-3670. U.S. Department of Health and Human Services, Public Health Service, National Institutes of Health. Bethesda MD: National Institutes of Health, 2003.)*

CHD or CHD equivalents. Specific models for therapeutic life-style changes and drug therapy in the primary prevention of CHD have been recommended by ATP III (Figures 26-23 and 26-24). As for the management of patients with metabolic syndrome, a combination approach of weight reduction, increased physical activity, and appropriate control of lipid levels is recommended.

A wide variety of pharmacological agents for cholesterol lowering in adults are available,[273] including (1) bile acid–binding resins (cholestyramine and colestipol), (2) niacin, (3) gemfibrozil, (4) probucol, and (5) HMG-CoA reductase inhibitors (e.g., atorvastatin, fluvastatin, lovastatin, pravastatin, and simvastatin) with the latter group having been found to reduce LDL cholesterol by as much as 40%. Some of these drugs are better tolerated by individual patients than others, and all but probucol have demonstrated long-term safety and ability both to increase HDL cholesterol (5% to 20% depending on the drug) and to decrease CHD risk. In certain circumstances, the drugs have been used individually or in combination. For further

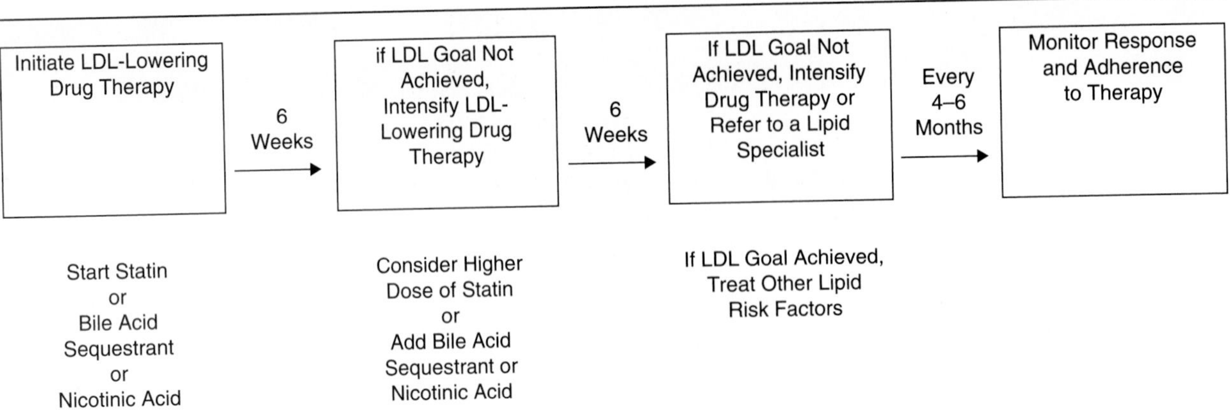

Figure 26-24 Progression of drug therapy in primary prevention. *LDL,* Low-density lipoprotein.

information regarding this subject, the reader is referred to reviews by Gotto.[95,96]

To lower serum cholesterol concentration in children and adolescents, the NCEP adopted a strategy that combines two complementary approaches: a population approach and an individualized approach.[244]

Population Approach

American children and adolescents have relatively high cholesterol concentrations and a high intake of saturated fatty acids and cholesterol (see Table 26-19).[244] The population approach attempts to lower the mean cholesterol concentration in the United States by instituting population-wide modifications in nutrient intake and eating habits. The AHA Step-One diet is recommended (see Table 26-19). Even a modest decrease in mean cholesterol concentration in children and adolescents, if carried into adulthood, could conceivably have a significant impact on lowering the incidence of CHD. The panel did not recommend any dietary changes for infants from birth to 2 years of age. Toddlers ages 2 and 3 should start making the transition to the recommended eating pattern. The NCEP also directed recommendations to schools, health professionals, government agencies, the food industry, and mass media to help influence and modify the eating habits of children and adolescents.

Individualized Approach

The individualized approach aims to lower cholesterol concentrations of children older than 2 years and adolescents who were identified by the selective screening process and the risk assessment protocol (Figure 26-25).[244] Those with an average LDL cholesterol concentration between 110 and 129 mg/dL should be placed on the AHA Step-One diet, counseled about other heart disease risk factors, and reevaluated after 1 year. Those with an average LDL cholesterol concentration more than 130 mg/dL should also be placed on the AHA Step-One diet, evaluated for secondary causes, and their family members screened. If after 3 months of initiating dietary therapy, the LDL cholesterol concentration remains greater than 130 mg/dL, the patient should be placed on the AHA Step-Two diet, which entails further reduction of the saturated fatty acid and cholesterol intake (see Table 26-19). Drug therapy was recommended by the NCEP in children age 10 and older if after careful adherence to dietary therapy (6 months to 1 year) the LDL cholesterol concentration remains more than 190 mg/dL. However, the action level is lower (160 mg/dL) for patients who have a positive family history of premature CHD, or those with two or more other risk factors. Only bile acid–binding resins (cholestyramine and colestipol), which act by binding bile acids in the intestinal lumen, are recommended by the panel for use in children and adolescents. The efficacy, side effects, or safety of other cholesterol-lowering drugs have not been established in children and adolescents, and therefore their use is discouraged in this patient population.

Most FH homozygotes are resistant to drug therapy. Several alternative treatments that have been used are (1) plasmapheresis every 2 weeks, (2) partial ileal bypass or portacaval shunt to lower total and LDL cholesterol in these patients, and (3) liver transplantation, using livers from donors with functional LDL receptors. Five FH homozygote patients have already received liver transplants. Although LDL cholesterol has been normalized after surgery, this treatment has many side effects and the patients must receive immunosuppressive therapy indefinitely. A direct gene therapy in which a normal LDL gene is inserted in the patient's hepatocytes might prove to be a viable treatment option for these patients[89,125] but such an approach is not available at present.

Management of Hypertriglyceridemia

Since recent evidence-based findings have shown triglycerides to be an independent risk factor for CHD in both men and women, more emphasis on the measurement of this marker and management of those with increased triglycerides is seen in ATP III compared with earlier reports.[77]

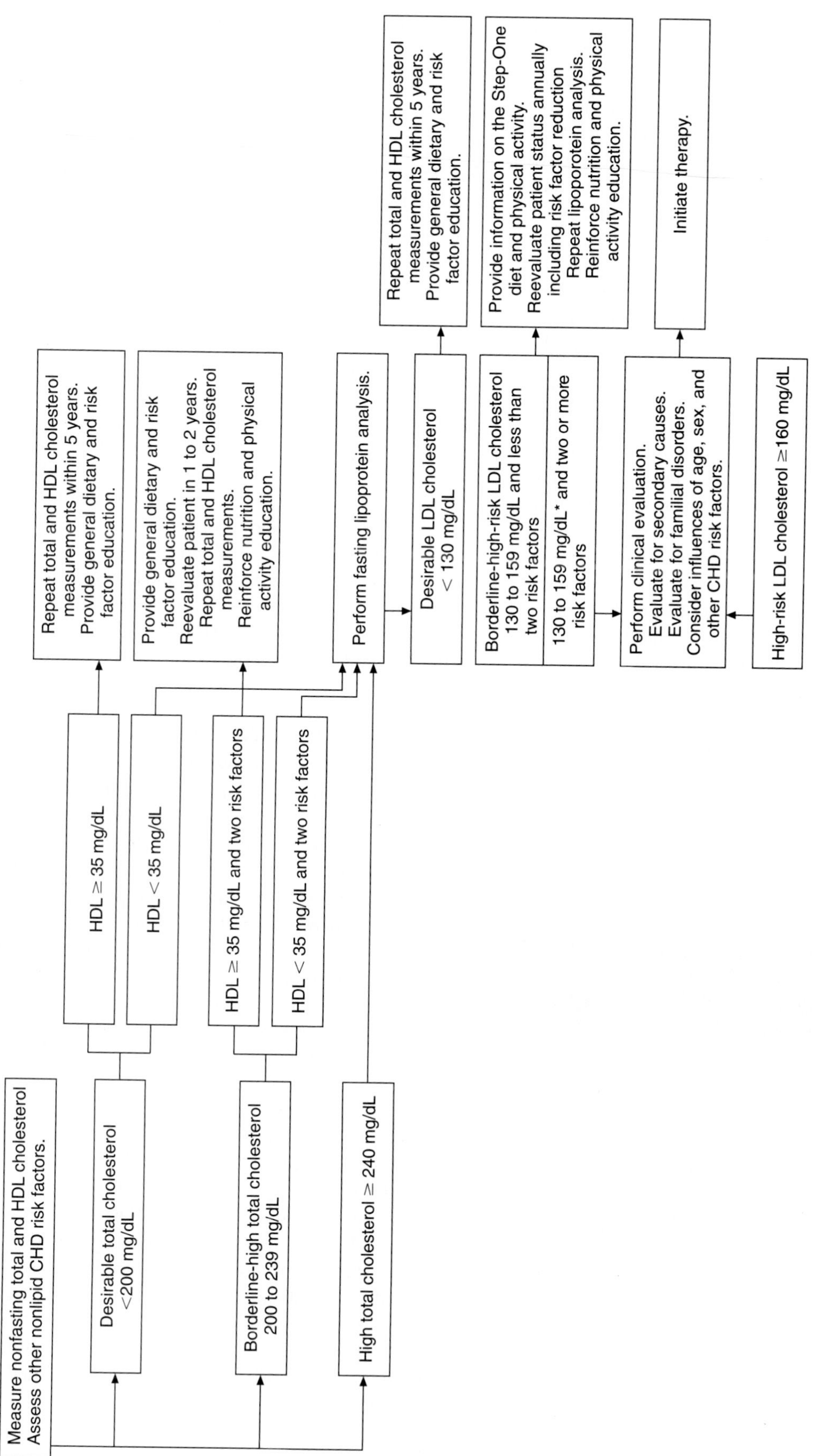

Figure 26-25 Risk assessment flowchart as recommended by the National Cholesterol Education Program Expert Panel on Blood Cholesterol Levels in Children and Adolescents. *(From The Report of the Expert Panel on Blood Cholesterol Levels in Children and Adolescents, National Cholesterol Education Program. Lipid Metabolism Branch, Division of Heart, Lung, and Blood Institute. NIH Publication No. 91-2732. U.S. Department of Health and Human Services, Public Health Service, National Institutes of Health. Bethesda MD: National Institutes of Health, 1991.)*

Furthermore the definition of a *normal* triglyceride level was changed from <200 to <150 mg/dL; values of 150 to 199 mg/dL are considered borderline high, 200 to 499 mg/dL high, and values ≥500 mg/dL very high. In the general population, several factors are associated with increased triglyceride concentrations, including obesity, cigarette smoking, physical inactivity, excess alcohol intake, and several diseases (e.g., type 2 diabetes and chronic renal failure), drugs (e.g., corticosteroids, estrogens, and retinoids), and genetic disorders (e.g., FCHL and FHTG). In clinical practice, hypertriglyceridemia is often associated with the metabolic syndrome. Triglyceride-rich lipoproteins or remnant lipoproteins are currently recognized to be atherogenic. In practice, VLDL cholesterol is used as a measure of these atherogenic lipoproteins. Therefore the ATP III suggested the addition of non-HDL cholesterol (total cholesterol-HDL cholesterol) as an indicator for all atherogenic lipoproteins (mainly LDL and VLDL).[77] The non-HDL-C is used as a secondary target of therapy in persons with triglycerides ≥200 mg/dL. The goal for non-HDL cholesterol in those with increased triglycerides is 30 mg/dL above that set for LDL cholesterol. The treatment of hypertriglyceridemia depends on the cause of the increase and severity. Those with triglycerides <200 mg/dL are treated with weight reduction and increased physical activity; for those at 200 to 499 mg/dL drug therapy is also considered (fibrate, nicotinic acid, and niacin). In the latter group, the non-HDL-C goal becomes a secondary target of therapy (Table 26-22). Those with triglycerides >500 mg/dL are usually at increased risk of pancreatitis and treated with low-fat diets (≤15% of calorie intake), weight reduction, increased physical activity, and triglyceride-lowering drugs.

TABLE 26-22 Comparison of LDL Cholesterol and Non-HDL Cholesterol Goals for Three Risk Categories

Risk Category	LDL Goal (mg/dL)	Non-HDL Goal (mg/dL)
CHD and CHD risk equivalent (10-year risk for CHD >20%	<100	<130
Multiple (2+) risk factors and 10-year risk ≤ 20%	<130	<160
0-1 Risk factor	<160	<190

Modified from executive summary of the third report of the National Cholesterol Education Program (NCEP) Expert Panel on Detection, Evaluation, and Treatment of High Blood Cholesterol in Adults (Adult Treatment Panel III). JAMA 2001;285:2486-97.

LDL, Low-density lipoprotein; *HDL*, high-density lipoprotein; *CHD*, coronary heart disease.

Although nicotinic acid and niacin are usually the drugs of choice, a combination therapy such as gemfibrozil and resins or gemfibrozil and an HMG-CoA reductase inhibitor can also be used.[273]

MEASUREMENT OF LIPIDS, LIPOPROTEINS, AND APOLIPOPROTEINS

The lipoproteins and their lipid and apolipoprotein constituents have become increasingly important in characterizing the risk of cardiovascular diseases and in the diagnosis and management of disorders of lipoprotein metabolism. In recent decades, our knowledge of such disorders has evolved from an essentially descriptive association between elevated plasma lipids and increased risk for premature cardiovascular disease morbidity and mortality to a much broader understanding of the underlying biochemistry, physiology, and genetic interactions. An area of remarkable advance has been in understanding the contribution of the lipoproteins in the development and progression of arterial lesions. Advances have also been made in the analytical techniques and methods for measuring lipids, lipoproteins, and apolipoproteins. In this section, we begin with a brief historical perspective on the development of the measurement technology followed by more detailed discussion of the pertinent methods.

Historical Perspective and Background

The causal relationship between increased plasma concentrations of LDL and the risk of CHD and the efficacy of LDL lowering to reduce risk was widely acknowledged by the mid-1980s*; Awareness of the importance of intervention emphasized the necessity for uniform means of defining hyperlipidemia and CHD risk. Previous practice had been to use arbitrarily defined cutoffs based on prevailing lipid and lipoprotein concentrations, either in the general population or in local populations of "normal patients." Because of the relative nonspecificity of the early chemical methods for cholesterol measurement, and the different kinds of methods then in use, significant biases existed between values obtained in different laboratories, and it was not uncommon for "normal" reference intervals to be laboratory specific. Quantitation of the relationships between total or LDL cholesterol concentration and risk for CHD, the demonstration of the efficacy of treatment, and the development of reference methods and Centers for Disease Control and Prevention (CDC) standardization programs for lipids and lipoproteins,[198] however, made possible the use of risk-related cut-off points (see Tables 26-15 and 26-18). This led to the necessity for uniform definitions of hyperlipidemia based on commonly accepted risk-based lipid and lipoprotein cutoffs and the availability of accurate lipid and lipoprotein measurements.

*References 26, 30, 83, 163, 164, 169.

Formation of Expert Panels

To address the issues discussed previously in this chapter, the NCEP convened expert panels to consider various aspects of diagnosis and treatment of hypercholesterolemia[77,203,244] and develop guidelines for reliable lipid and lipoprotein measurements.[237,238] Two separate laboratory panels considered issues related to blood lipid and lipoprotein measurement. The first, the NCEP Laboratory Standardization Panel, was concerned with the measurement of total cholesterol,[237] and the second, the NCEP Working Group on Lipoprotein Measurement, addressed the measurement of triglycerides, HDL cholesterol, and LDL cholesterol.[238] The recommendations of both panels include extensive reviews of lipid and lipoprotein methodology, and the interested reader is referred to the original reports for details.[237,238] Here we summarize the principal considerations and recommendations for clinical lipid and lipoprotein measurements.

Basic Issues

In developing recommendations for lipid and lipoprotein measurement, the NCEP panels considered several basic issues.

First, in most of the large-scale clinical and epidemiological studies that established the (1) relationships between lipids, lipoproteins, (2) risk for CHD, and (3) efficacy of cholesterol lowering, the measurements were made in standardized laboratories in which the accuracy of the measurements was traceable to CDC reference methods. This included studies such as the National Diet Heart Study in the 1960s, the various LRC program studies (early 1970s to 1990), Specialized Centers of Research in Atherosclerosis (early 1970s to present), and several NHANES studies conducted between 1960 and 1994.[198]

Second, the various methods used in laboratory or nonlaboratory settings should be capable of similar accuracy (i.e., the reliability of the measurements should be independent of how, where, or by whom they are made). Ideally, it should be possible to consider all lipid measurements made in the United States (and eventually globally) as if they had been made in a single laboratory. This premise does *not* require that all laboratories use the same methods; it requires only that all methods be capable of giving values equivalent to those on which the relationships between lipids, lipoproteins, and the risk for CHD were established.

Third, as new methods are developed, particularly those that may be more accurate and precise for the various lipoproteins or lipoprotein subfractions, the particular lipoprotein included in the measurement should be specified. This is to ensure that new methods could be linked to those that were used to establish the known lipoprotein-CHD risk relationships.

To achieve these aims, development of reference methods was required as accuracy targets for lipid and lipoprotein measurements and guidelines were established for analytical performance.

Analytical Challenges

Plasma lipoproteins, as macromolecular complexes that vary considerably in size, composition, and function, present considerable analytical challenge (see Table 26-4). For clinical purposes, lipoprotein concentrations have been traditionally expressed in terms of their cholesterol content, because they carry virtually all of the cholesterol that circulates in the plasma. This simplifies the methods used to measure lipoproteins because the lipoprotein fractions of interest have only to be separated from each other; the other plasma proteins do not have to be removed.

Analytically, cholesterol can be accurately and precisely measured with appropriate chemical or biochemical methods. Triglycerides, and the lipoprotein themselves, however, are not unique chemical entities. Triglycerides consist of three of many possible fatty acyl groups covalently attached to a glycerol backbone through ester linkages (see Figure 26-13).

Fatty acyl groups vary in chain length and degree of saturation, leading to a mixture of triglycerides of somewhat different molecular weights. Consequently, triglyceride methods usually measure the glycerol backbone, and triglyceride concentration is then stated only in terms of molar concentration. In the United States, however, lipids have been traditionally expressed in terms of mass concentration (milligrams per deciliter), which is an approximation requiring an assumption about the average molecular weights of the triglyceride mixture. Because palmitate, stearate, and oleate are the major fatty acids in plasma triglycerides and have similar molecular weights, the conversion between molar and mass concentration usually assumes an average triglyceride molecular weight of 885 Da, the molecular weight of tri-oleyl glycerol (olein).

The situation is even more complicated for LDL and HDL. For example, LDL consists of a population of particles varying in size and lipid composition, each containing apo B-100 as essentially the only apolipoprotein component. Thus LDL has neither a unique molecular weight nor consistent cholesterol composition. Similarly, HDL consists of two major subclasses, HDL_2 and HDL_3, differing in both their lipid and apolipoprotein compositions, and each subclass can be further separated into a number of individual subpopulations.[255] Because of these characteristics, the exact concentration and composition of a fraction identified as LDL or HDL vary depending on how the fraction is isolated. Once isolated, however, the cholesterol content can be measured accurately. A major consideration, therefore, was to define the lipoproteins in a uniform way to afford a common basis for standardization and the assessment of accuracy without inhibiting the development of new methods or necessitating the use of the same methods in all laboratories.

Analytical Approach

For more than 20 years, the CDC had maintained reference methods for cholesterol, triglycerides, and HDL cholesterol and had operated standardization programs[198] targeted for the research laboratories. In addition, these reference methods have been used to establish the accuracy of lipid and lipoprotein measurements in a number of population studies, including the LRC prevalence and CPPT studies,[163,164] several NHANES studies conducted by the National Center for Health Statistics since the 1960s,[124] and others. From these studies, cut points for the risk characterization in patients were derived. Consequently, and because the standardization programs were already accepted as authoritative by the general laboratory and research communities, the NCEP laboratory panels recommended the CDC reference methods as the basis for defining "accuracy" in the context of recommendations for reliable lipid and lipoprotein measurements.

Using this approach had several advantages. First, it established the same basis for accuracy that had been used in developing the relationships between lipid and lipoprotein concentration and CHD, and second, it provided a reference point by which the accuracy of existing or newly developed methods could be assessed.

Lipids and Lipoproteins

Various technologies have been used to measure plasma lipids and lipoproteins and lipoprotein subfractions, including enzymatic, immunochemical, and chemical precipitation reagents, and physical methods, such as ultracentrifugation, electrophoresis, column chromatography, and others. Such methods have been reviewed extensively.[18,256] As mentioned earlier, however, the cholesterol content of any particular lipoprotein class can vary somewhat from individual to individual. Moreover, although different methods of lipoprotein separation may produce similar lipoprotein fractions, they usually do not produce identical fractions, giving rise to systematic biases between methods that purport to measure the same component. The present discussion focuses primarily on methods and procedures commonly used in clinical practice for lipid and lipoprotein measurements.

Reference Methods

Reference methods are the "gold standards" or accuracy targets that have been developed for the more common analytes, such as cholesterol, triglycerides, LDL, and HDL cholesterol.[197] The reference method for cholesterol is fully validated and credentialed through the National Reference System for the Clinical Laboratory. The other methods, although not formally credentialed, have been accepted by consensus.

Cholesterol

The CDC reference method for cholesterol[56,64,72] is based on a chemical method devised by Abell et al. In the CDC version of this method,[72] a 0.5-mL aliquot of serum is treated with 5.0 mL of alcoholic KOH (0.36 mol/L) to hydrolyze the cholesteryl esters. Total cholesterol is then extracted from the mixture with 10 mL of hexane for 15 minutes. An aliquot of the extract is dried in vacuo, and the dry residue is treated with 3.2 mL of a mixture of acetic acid, acetic anhydride, and sulfuric acid (Liebermann-Burchard reagent) for color development. After 30 minutes, absorbance is read at 620 nm using pure cholesterol as the calibrator. This method is operated according to a strict protocol requiring replicate measurements in multiple analytical runs. The method exhibits an approximate 1.6% positive bias compared with isotope dilution mass spectrometry, which, considered to be the definitive method for cholesterol, was developed and applied by the National Institute of Standards and Technology.[72] Cholesterol is expressed either in terms of molar (millimoles per liter) or mass (milligrams per deciliter) concentration. Molar concentration is converted to mass concentration using the following equation:

$$mg/dL = mmol/L \times 38.7 \quad (1)$$

The reference method, demonstrated to be readily transferable to other laboratories,[56] has been widely adopted by other reference laboratories and diagnostic manufacturers as the accuracy target and the basis for calibration in cholesterol measurements.

Triglycerides

In the CDC reference method for triglycerides,[197,198,238] the triglycerides are first extracted quantitatively with chloroform to remove water-soluble interfering substances, such as glucose and glycerol, from the serum. The extract is treated with silicic acid to remove phospholipids, and the triglycerides in the extract are subjected to alkaline hydrolysis to produce unesterified fatty acids and glycerol. The glycerol produced is oxidized to produce formaldehyde, which is then reacted with chromotropic acid for color development. The absorbance of the chromogen in the reaction mixture is measured at 570 nm.

$$\text{Triglycerides} + \text{KOH} \rightarrow \text{fatty acids} + \text{glycerol} \quad (2)$$

$$\text{Glycerol} + \text{periodate} \rightarrow \text{formic acid} + \text{formaldehyde} \quad (3)$$

$$\text{Formaldehyde} + \text{chromotropic acid} \rightarrow \text{chromogen} \quad (4)$$

The results are expressed either in terms of molar concentration (millimoles per liter) or mass concentration (milligrams per deciliter). The following equation is used to convert mmol/dL to mg/dL:

$$mg/dL = mmol/L \times 88.5 \quad (5)$$

The equation assumes an average molecular weight of 885 g/mole (triolein) for plasma triglycerides. In addition, because of the preliminary extraction and adsorption steps, the CDC reference method measures only the glycerides, and does *not* include free glycerol, the so-called triglyceride blank.

Because this assay is so complex, sensitive, and tedious, it has not been readily transferred to other laboratories. As an expedient to facilitate standardization of triglyceride measurements, a designated comparison method (DCM) has been developed by the Cholesterol Reference Method Laboratory Network, involving similar extraction steps followed by more robust enzymatic quantitation of the triglyceride-derived glycerol.[81] This DCM, established in other reference laboratories, is expected to become the secondary accuracy target for triglycerides.

High-Density Lipoprotein Cholesterol

Both a reference method and a designated comparison method have been developed to measure HDL cholesterol.

Reference Method. Because HDL consists of several populations of particles that vary somewhat in their cholesterol content, HDL is commonly defined in terms of the method used to prepare the HDL-containing fraction. The CDC reference method[104,197] uses a combination of ultracentrifugation and polyanion precipitation to prepare the HDL-containing fraction. The cholesterol in this fraction is then quantitated using the CDC reference method for cholesterol. The method is as follows: VLDL and chylomicrons, if present, are first removed by ultracentrifugation of an accurately measured volume of serum for 18 hours at 105,000 × *g*. Under these conditions, VLDL and any chylomicrons accumulate as a floating layer at the top of the ultracentrifuge tube (d = 1.006 g/mL). A tube-slicing technique is used to remove the VLDL fraction.[104,197] The infranatant, which contains IDL, LDL, Lp(a), HDL, and the other serum proteins, is recovered quantitatively. The apo B-100–containing lipoproteins in this fraction are then precipitated with heparin sulfate (1.3 mg/mL) and $MnCl_2$ (0.046 mol/L). The precipitate is removed by centrifugation,[104,197] and cholesterol in the clear supernatant is measured. HDL cholesterol is expressed either in molar or mass concentration; molar concentration is converted to mass concentration using equation (1).

Heparin-$MnCl_2$ was selected as the precipitation reagent primarily for historical reasons because it was the method most commonly used in early studies to establish the relationship between HDL cholesterol concentration and the risk for CHD. The ultracentrifugation step was included to prevent interference with sedimentation of the apo B-100–containing lipoproteins by the lighter triglyceride-rich lipoproteins, VLDL, and chylomicrons.

Designated Comparison Method. Only a few laboratories have an ultracentrifuge and the experience required to reliably perform the CDC reference method for HDL cholesterol. Furthermore, ultracentrifugation is expensive and necessitates obtaining an impractically large specimen volume, typically 5.0 mL. As an practical alternative, the Cholesterol Reference Method Laboratory Network (CRMLN) laboratories developed and validated a modified dextran sulfate (50,000 Da) procedure as a DCM to provide results approximately equivalent to those of the CDC RM but avoiding ultracentrifugation.[135] The $MgCl_2$ concentration in the precipitant reagent was decreased slightly from that used in the previously published primary method to increase the HDL cholesterol values slightly, achieving closer agreement with the CDC reference method.

Low-Density Lipoprotein Cholesterol

The CDC has also defined a reference method for LDL cholesterol based on the same techniques described above for HDL cholesterol.[197] After ultracentrifugation to remove the VLDL and any chylomicrons present, the bottom fraction (d > 1.006) is subjected to precipitation by heparin and manganese as described previously. After measurement of cholesterol in the d > 1.006 fraction and in the heparin-Mn^{2+} supernatant solution, LDL cholesterol is calculated by difference. It should be noted that the LDL fraction as measured by this reference method is a so-called "broad-cut" fraction including any IDL and Lp(a).

Application of the Reference Methods to Standardization

Background

Early efforts in the mid1980s to achieve general standardization of methods used by clinical laboratories began with a fairly traditional approach with secondary reference materials provided to the laboratory community. The reference materials consisted of lyophilized serum pools with target values assigned based on replicate measurements using the reference methods. However, problems were recognized with this approach, primarily from the confounding effects of matrix changes in the reference materials.[191] In practice, conventional reference materials prepared from pooled serum, often deteriorated, sometimes spiked with artificial analytes, and subjected to freezing and freeze drying, did not assay like fresh patient specimens with most routine methods. In several notable cases diagnostic manufacturers used the secondary reference materials to assign presumably reliable targets to their calibrators, but subsequently found that results on patient specimens became quite inaccurate. The problem was compounded by national proficiency testing programs, which in an attempt to improve accuracy began reporting reference method target values with similarly prepared survey materials. Laboratories were adjusting calibration to achieve apparent accuracy on the survey materials; however, in some instances results on actual patient specimens were made inaccurate.

Recognition of these problems focused attention on the issues of "analyte" and "matrix" effects in reference materials.[191] Common procedures used in preparing secondary reference materials were inducing changes in the analytes themselves and in the other constituents and fluids surrounding the analytes that made their analyses no longer comparable with measurements in authentic fresh patient specimens. After considerable study and deliberation, the conclusion was reached that the only universally reliable means of transferring accuracy from the reference methods to diagnostic manufacturers and individual laboratories was through direct comparison studies on fresh, representative patient specimens.[327] As a consequence, the CDC and other groups cooperated to organize a network of reference laboratories providing the reference methods and fresh sample comparison studies.

The Cholesterol Reference Method Laboratory Network

Because the CDC standardization laboratory maintaining the reference methods did not have the capacity to perform all of the necessary comparison studies directly, it was obvious that the reference laboratory capability would have to be expanded to accommodate the needs of the industry and laboratory community. To this end, the CDC and a number of other interested laboratories cooperated to establish the CRMLN. Each participating network laboratory underwent stringent protocols to transfer the CDC reference methods and to maintain comparability with the CDC. In turn the network laboratories performed comparison studies using fresh patient sera with the diagnostic manufacturers and with individual laboratories. Throughout the 1990s the network was large and quite active to accommodate the demands of comparison studies. As standardization has steadily improved in subsequent years, the level of activity has declined and the number of domestic U.S. network laboratories has decreased. However, at the same time the network laboratory program has expanded to include more international laboratories.

In 2004 the CRMLN included four experienced U.S. laboratories and seven international partner laboratories in Canada, Europe, Asia, and South America (Boxes 26-3 and 26-4). The network offers protocols, based on National Committee on Clinical Laboratory Standards guidelines,[209] whereby diagnostic manufacturers ensure accuracy by completing comparison studies with the reference method.[199] A system qualifies for certification by demonstrating agreement within specified limits for total, HDL, and LDL cholesterol and for triglycerides. Based on comparison results, calibrator set points are adjusted if necessary to bring performance into agreement with the reference methods. Diagnostic manufacturers and distributors and instrument partners are encouraged to certify their systems at least every 2 years and to ensure that every production lot is calibrated to maintain accuracy consistent with the accuracy targets, which can be accomplished by ongoing participation in the CDC and/or CRMLN program. The CDC website (http://www.cdc.gov/nceh/dls/crmln/crmln.htm) provides details of the program, protocols for comparison studies, contact information for the CDC and/or CRMLN, and a listing of the commercial methods that have qualified for certification.

Clinical laboratories can promote standardization by encouraging their kit suppliers to participate in the CRMLN comparison process. In addition, individual laboratories can also make arrangements with a CRMLN laboratory to participate in an abbreviated certification protocol for total cholesterol and complete comparison studies for the other analytes, especially useful in the case of new or modified systems. The CRMLN program is supported by modest user fees.

BOX 26-3 U.S. National Reference Method Laboratory Network Participating Laboratories

State Laboratory of Hygiene
University of Wisconsin
Center for Health Sciences
465 Henry Mall
Madison, WI 53706
David Hassemer, M.S.
hassemer@mail.slh.wisc.edu
(608) 265-1100 (×102) Phone
(608) 265-1114 Fax

Wadsworth Center for Laboratories and Research
New York State Department of Health
Empire State Plaza
Albany, NY 12201
Robert Rej, Ph.D.
clinchem@wadsworth.org
(518) 474-5101 Phone
(518) 474-9145 Fax

Northwest Lipid Research Laboratories
Core Laboratory
2121 N. 35th Street
Seattle, WA 98103
Santica Marcovina, Ph.D.
smm@u.washington.edu
(206) 685-3331 Phone
(206) 685-3279 Fax

Pacific Biometrics Research Foundation
220 West Harrison Street
Seattle, WA 98119
Elizabeth Teng Leary, Ph.D.
etl@pacbio.com
(206) 298-0068 (×208) Phone
(206) 298-9838 Fax

Routine Methods

Reference methods are complex, time consuming, at least partially manual, and require a high level of expertise for reliable operation. Consequently, simpler and more practical methods have evolved for routine clinical use.

Cholesterol

Enzymatic methods for cholesterol measurement are precise, accurate when calibrated appropriately, and easily adapted for use on modern analyzers. Commercially available cholesterol reagents commonly combine all of the enzymes and other required components into a single photometric reagent. The reagent usually is mixed with a 3- to 10-μL aliquot of serum or plasma, incubated under controlled

BOX 26-4 Cholesterol Reference Method Laboratory Network Participating Laboratories (International)

University Medical Center Rotterdam
Lipid Reference Laboratory
3015 GD Rotterdam, The Netherlands
Jan Lindemans, Ph.D.
lindemans@ckcl.azr.nl
31-10-463 4509 Phone
31-10 436 7894 Fax

Institute of Biochemistry
Department of Pathological Biochemistry
Glasgow Royal Infirmary
4th Floor Alexandra Parade
Glasgow G31 2ER, Scotland
Chris J. Packard, Ph.D.
44-141-221-4979 (or 4322) Phone
44-141-553-2558 Fax

H. S. Raffaele
Laboratorio Analisi Cliniche
Via Olgettina 60
20132 Milano, Italy
Ferruccio Ceriotti, M.D.
Ferruccio.ceriotti@.hsr.it
39-2-2643-2315 (or 2313) Phone
39-2-2643-2640 Fax

Osaka Medical Center for Health Science and Promotion
Lipid Reference Laboratory
3 Nakamichi 1-chome
Higashinari-ku
Osaka 537-0025, Japan
Masakazu Nakamura, Ph.D.
xnakamura@kenkoukagaku.jp
81-6-6973-5582 Phone
81-6-6973-3574 Fax

Canadian External Quality Assessment Laboratory
307-2083 Alma Street
Vancouver
British Columbia V6R 4N6, Canada
David W. Seccombe, M.D., Ph.D.
dseccombe@ceqal.com
(604) 222-1355 Phone
(604) 222-1373 Fax

Fundacíon Bioquímica Argentina
Laboratorio de Referencia y Estandarización en Bioquímica Clínica (LARESBIC)
Calle 6 N° 1344
La Plata 1900
Argentina
Daniel Mazziotta, M.D.
dmpeec@netverk.com.ar
54-221-4231150 Phone
54-221-4232021 Fax

Beijing Institute of Geriatrics
Beijing Hospital
1 Dahua Road, Post Code 100730
Beijing
P.R. China
Wenxiang Chen, M.D., M.Sc.
chenwenxiang@263.net
86-10-6513-0302 Phone
86-10-6513-2969 Fax

conditions for color development, and absorbance measured in the visible portion of the spectrum, generally at about 500 nm. The reagents typically use a bacterial cholesteryl ester hydrolase to cleave cholesteryl esters.

$$\text{Cholesteryl ester} + H_2O \xrightarrow{\text{Cholesteryl ester hydrolase}} \text{cholesterol} + \text{fatty acid} \quad (6)$$

The 3-OH group of cholesterol is then oxidized to a ketone in an oxygen-requiring reaction catalyzed by cholesterol oxidase,

$$\text{Cholesterol} + O_2 \xrightarrow{\text{Cholesterol oxidase}} \text{cholest-4-en-3-one} + H_2O_2 \quad (7)$$

H_2O_2, one of the reaction products, is measured in a peroxidase catalyzed reaction that forms a colored dye.

$$H_2O_2 + \text{phenol} + \text{4-aminoantipyrine} \xrightarrow{\text{Peroxidase}} \text{quinoneimine dye} + 2\,H_2O \quad (8)$$

These methods are subject to interference from other colored compounds or those that compete with the oxidation reaction, such as bilirubin, ascorbic acid, and hemoglobin. Assays are usually linear up to about 600 or 700 mg/dL. Reagents have been refined by adding substances such as bilirubin oxidase and dual wavelength readings to minimize the effects of hemolysis, and interference from bilirubin is generally not an issue now in concentrations below 5 mg/dL.[18,64,201] Enzymatic reagents are not entirely specific for cholesterol, because β-hydroxy sterols and plant sterols (e.g., β-sitosterol) can also react. In human serum or plasma, however, this is not a major problem because these interfering sterols are generally at very low concentrations.

In practice, reagent formulations vary from manufacturer to manufacturer. In most cases, the reagent from a particular manufacturer will have been optimized for use with one or several specific instruments and calibration materials, usually those sold by that manufacturer. In the past few years, most manufacturers have been supplying calibration materials with assigned values that are traceable to the CDC reference method, which has helped reduce interlaboratory variation. Thus cholesterol methods are best thought of as "measurement systems" composed of reagent, calibrator (cholesterol standard), and instrument. When a reagent-calibrator-instrument system from a single manufacturer is used, cholesterol measurements within a laboratory usually are accurate within 1% to 3% of reference values, and such systems are routinely operated with coefficients of variation of 1.5% to 2.5%. In some cases, however, a reagent from one manufacturer might be used with an instrument from another. In this instance, the responsibility is on the user rather than the manufacturer to ensure that reagent and sample volumes, time and temperature of incubation, and the calibration produce precise and accurate measurements. Although the cholesterol oxidase reagent described previously in this chapter is by far the most common, reagents have been developed using a cholesterol dehydrogenase sequence, which may have advantages in some instances.[131] In addition, highly sensitive enzymatic methods have been described for specialized applications.[137] Free or unesterified cholesterol can be readily quantified by deleting the cholesterol esterase from the reagent.

Triglycerides

Triglycerides also are now commonly measured with enzyme reagents directly in plasma or serum. Reagents combining all the required enzymes, cofactors, and buffers are available from various manufacturers, and as for cholesterol, such reagents are optimized for use with particular instrument-calibrator systems. Several different enzyme sequences have been used. In all of the methods, the first step is the lipase-catalyzed hydrolysis of triglycerides to glycerol and fatty acids.

$$\text{Triglyceride} + 3\,H_2O \xrightarrow{\text{Lipase}} \text{glycerol} + 3\text{ fatty acids} \quad (9)$$

Glycerol is then phosphorylated in an ATP-requiring reaction catalyzed by glycerokinase.

$$\text{Glycerol} + \text{ATP} \xrightarrow{\text{Glycerokinase}} \text{glycerophosphate} + \text{adenosine diphosphate (ADP)} \quad (10)$$

In the most commonly used methods, glycerophosphate is oxidized to dihydroxyacetone and H_2O_2 in a glycerophosphate oxidase-catalyzed reaction,

$$\text{Glycerophosphate} + O_2 \xrightarrow{\text{Glycerophosphate oxidase}} \text{dihydroxyacetone} + H_2O_2 \quad (11)$$

and the H_2O_2 formed in the reaction is measured as described in reaction (8).

Alternatively, glycerophosphate is measured in a reduced form of nicotinamide-adenine dinucleotide (NADH)-producing reaction and the NADH measured by a spectrophotometer set at 340 nm or in a diaphorase-catalyzed reaction to form a reaction product whose absorbance is measured at 500 nm.

$$\text{Glycerophosphate} + \text{nicotinamide-adenine dinucleotide (NAD)} \xrightarrow{\text{Glycerophosphate dehydrogenase}} \text{dihydroxyacetone phosphate} + \text{NADH} + H^+ \quad (12)$$

$$\text{NADH} + \text{tetrazolium dye} \xrightarrow{\text{Diaphorase}} \text{formazan} + \text{NAD}^+ \quad (13)$$

Other methods measure the ADP produced in reaction (10), as shown in equations (14) and (15):

$$\text{ADP} + \text{phosphoenol pyruvate} \xrightarrow{\text{Pyruvate kinase}} \text{ATP} + \text{pyruvate} \quad (14)$$

$$\text{Pyruvate} + \text{NADH} + H^+ \xrightarrow{\text{Lactate dehydrogenase}} \text{lactate} + \text{NAD}^+ \quad (15)$$

The loss of NADH is measured by a photometer at 340 nm.

Enzymatic triglyceride methods are fairly specific in that they do not detect glucose or phospholipids. They are linear in the concentration range up to about 700 mg/dL, and when automated are operated with coefficients of variation in the range of approximately 2% to 3%. The methods are usually calibrated with reference solutions of pure glycerol or with serum-based secondary calibrators. However, because all of these methods measure the glycerol component, any free glycerol in the sample contributes to the apparent amount of triglyceride. Thus assessment of bias in triglyceride measurements is not as straightforward as for cholesterol because the CDC reference method includes only the triglyceride-derived glycerol. With routine methods, the decision must be made whether to correct for free glycerol by using a method that corrects for the free glycerol blank.

Triglyceride Blanks (Correction for Endogenous Glycerol). Glycerol concentrations in freshly collected serum or plasma are usually in the range of about 1 mg/dL, contributing about 5 to 10 mg/dL to the apparent triglyceride concentration. Because this small amount is medically insignificant, the triglyceride blank is usually ignored. However, blanks can be higher in samples with increased triglyceride concentrations and from patients with conditions such as diabetes or those receiving total parenteral nutrition, but even those conditions would generally not substantially affect the interpretation. However, blanks can be increased by fiftyfold to 100-fold in the rare disorder hyperglycerolemia, which results from a deficiency of glycerokinase.[182] In this case, apparent triglyceride concentrations is extremely and artifactually high unless a triglyceride blank is analyzed.

Although triglyceride blanks can in most cases be ignored in clinical measurements, they can dramatically affect conclusions about method accuracy, important in calibration or in standardization of triglyceride measurements.[52] For example, participation in the CDC standardization program requires use of a blanking method, several of which are commercially available. Triglyceride blanking usually requires a separate analysis of glycerol, expressed in terms of equivalent triglyceride concentration, and the measured blank value is subtracted from the total triglyceride measurement.[321] Free glycerol is measured enzymatically using reactions such as shown in equations (10) and (11), using a reagent that is identical to the triglyceride reagent but lacking lipase, an approach designated two-cuvette blanking. Such a reagent has been available from the Bayer Corporation (Tarrytown, N.Y.). In an alternative two-step approach in a single cuvette, any free glycerol in the sample is consumed to produce a colorless product in a preliminary reaction before a lipase enzyme is added to cleave and measure the triglyceride-derived glycerol. Such a reagent is available from Roche Diagnostics (Indianapolis), but can be used only with analyzers capable of adding reagents sequentially.

Triglyceride blanking by either of these approaches can add considerably to the time and cost of triglyceride analysis. Another more practical alternative for routine practice, designated calibration blanking and used by some manufacturers, involves adjusting calibrator set points to compensate for the average amount of free glycerol in specimens. This is accomplished through a comparison study on actual patient specimens versus the reference method or an accurate equivalent. The calibration blanking approach will underestimate the blank in a few specimens but will give a better and reasonably reliable estimation for most specimens.

An ad hoc panel convened to consider the necessity for glycerol blanking in routine practice recommended blank corrections for specimens from inpatients but not outpatients because of the increased likelihood of free glycerol increases in the former.[52] In practice, however, blanking is usually practiced only by research laboratories and those supporting lipid clinics, particularly to facilitate participation in the CDC standardization program.

Phospholipids

Quantitative measurement of phospholipids is rare in routine clinical practice but more common in research (e.g., in studies of dietary influences). The choline-containing phospholipids lecithin, lysolecithin, and sphingomyelin, which account for at least 95% of total phospholipids in serum, are readily measured by an enzymatic reaction sequence using phospholipase D, choline-oxidase, and horseradish peroxidase.[183,299] Kit methods with this enzymatic sequence are available commercially. Before the availability of enzymatic reagents, the common quantitative method involved extraction and acid digestion with analysis of the total lipid-bound phosphorus.[22]

High-Density Lipoprotein Cholesterol

Under current recommendations for characterizing the cardiovascular disease risk in patients, measurement of the two major cholesterol-carrying lipoproteins, HDL and LDL, are most important. Characterization of the beta-VLDL characteristic of the uncommon type III or dysbetalipoproteinemia may be appropriate in a few patients. Measurement of lipoprotein subclasses including IDL or remnant lipoproteins is useful in research and can be helpful in some cases in managing patients.

HDL is classically defined in terms of its density range (1.063 to 1.21 g/mL) obtained by ultracentrifugation, which has been used as the standard by which the accuracy of other HDL methods is judged. However, the density range of Lp(a) (1.04 to 1.08 g/mL) overlaps that of HDL (see Table 26-4), so in patients with high Lp(a) concentrations ultracentrifugation at 1.063 g/mL would overestimate the true HDL concentration. As a consequence, the reference method, described previously, uses precipitation to separate HDL, similar to the approach commonly used for routine determinations.[326]

Precipitation Methods. HDL cholesterol has been most commonly measured (Box 26-5) in the supernatant solution after the precipitation of the apo B-100–containing lipoprotein directly from plasma or serum using agents such as polyanions in the presence of divalent cations.[104] The apo B-100–containing lipoproteins include VLDL, IDL, Lp(a), LDL, and, when present, chylomicrons (see Table 26-4). As indicated earlier, LDL and HDL are the largest contributors to total cholesterol in normal people, with LDL accounting for about two thirds and HDL for about one third of the total cholesterol. On average, IDL and Lp(a) each account for only about 2 to 3 mg/dL of the total cholesterol, although their concentrations can be considerably higher in some individuals.

BOX 26-5 Methods for HDL Separation/Quantification

Precipitation (1st generation)
- Heparin-Mn^{2+}
  - 0.46 mmol/L (LRC method)[78]
  - 0.92 mmol/L (recommended for EDTA plasma)[140]
- Dextran Sulfate (50 kDa) Mg^{2+}[221] (AACC Selected Method and DCM)
- Phosphotungstate-Mg^{2+}[136]

Facilitated Separation (2nd generation)
- Magnetic with/dextran sulfate-Mg^{2+}[143]

Homogeneous (3rd generation)
- Antibody four-reagent method[140] (International Reagents Corp)
- Polyethylene glycol modified enzymes w/cyclodextrin[146] (Kyowa Medex)
- Synthetic polymer/detergent[144] (Daiichi)
- Antibodies[153] (Wako)
- Catalase[154] (Denka Seiken)

Polyanions react with positively charged groups on lipoproteins; their action is facilitated in the presence of divalent cations, which interact with negatively charged groups, causing aggregation and a cloudy precipitate. Precipitation is usually complete within 10 to 15 minutes at room temperature; at 2 °C to 4 °C a 30-minute incubation period is preferred. The precipitate is then sedimented by centrifugation typically for 45,000 *g*-min (i.e., the equivalent of 1500×*g* for 30 minutes). Centrifugation at higher *g* forces, e.g., 10,000×*g* accelerates sedimentation and can actually improve complete precipitation of apo-B–containing particles. HDL cholesterol is then measured in the clear supernatant.

Several polyanion-divalent cation combinations have been used. Initially, heparin sulfate with $MnCl_2$ was adopted by the National Institutes of Health (NIH) and became common in research laboratories, which provided the rationale for employing this combination in the CDC RM. With the transition to enzymatic cholesterol assay methods, residual Mn^{2+} was found to interfere, giving artifactually high results. Techniques were devised to reduce this interference but necessitated additional manipulations, making them inconvenient for routine use. One approach was to add the chelator ethylenediaminetetraacetic acid (EDTA) to the cholesterol reagent to complex residual manganate.[290] Another was to add carbonate in a second precipitation step to precipitate excess Mn^{2+} from the heparin-Mn^{2+} supernatant.[20] Most laboratories avoided these tedious approaches, adopting methods using other precipitants to prevent interference by Mn^{2+} altogether. In time, variations of dextran sulfate or phosphotungstate with Mg^{2+} became most common.[323,238] A method using dextran sulfate with a molecular weight of 50 kDa was validated as a selected method and became the most common precipitation reagent in the United States.

There are several key issues in applying precipitation reagents to measure HDL cholesterol. First, the precipitability of lipoproteins with polyanions and divalent cations depends on the lipid and protein compositions of the molecules.[37] The greater the compositional differences, the more easily the lipoproteins are separated. Thus apo B-100–containing lipoproteins are more easily separated from HDL than they are from each other, and it is for this reason that precipitation methods have been more widely and successfully used for HDL analysis than for LDL or VLDL measurement.

Second, the various precipitants differ in their abilities to precipitate apo B-100–containing lipoprotein completely while leaving most species of HDL in solution,[18,238] resulting in the potential for biases between precipitation methods. With modern reagent-instrument-calibrator systems, conditions are generally optimized to produce values that closely approximate and are traceable to reference method values. But method-to-method biases are observed; however, they appear to be decreasing with experience, although significant discrepancies may be observed on individual specimens.

Third, the precipitation methods can be inaccurate under certain conditions. For example, precipitation of apo B-100–containing lipoprotein can be incomplete in samples with high concentrations of triglyceride-rich lipoproteins. The lipoprotein precipitate should be tightly packed after centrifugation, and the HDL-containing supernatant should be optically clear. Any turbidity at all indicates inadequate sedimentation of the apo B-100–containing lipoprotein, and even a small amount of unsedimented precipitate can produce a significant error in the HDL cholesterol measurement. Samples with high triglyceride concentrations (generally those above 400 mg/dL) frequently produce turbid supernatants because the triglycerides can reduce the density of the lipoprotein-precipitating reagent complex to the point that some of the complex remains unsedimented. In cases of extremely high triglyceride concentrations, some of the precipitate may even form a floating layer over a clear or turbid supernatant, in addition to the usual precipitate at the bottom of the centrifuge tube.

There are several ways to address this problem in hypertriglyceridemic specimens. First, the sample can be ultracentrifuged and the triglyceride-rich lipoprotein removed before precipitation as described for the reference method. Second, a sample with a turbid supernatant can sometimes be cleared by centrifuging for a longer time or at higher *g*-forces.[322] Third, the sample can be diluted to reduce the concentration of triglyceride-rich lipoproteins before the precipitant is added. In general, a dilution greater than twofold should not be used because higher dilutions can cause large dilution errors. This is a particular concern because hypertriglyceridemic patients tend to have low HDL cholesterol levels. A fourth approach is to pass the turbid supernatant through a 0.45-μm filter to remove the unsedimented precipitate before measuring cholesterol in the filtrate.[322]

Finally, matrix effects can influence the results. Matrix effects can arise from the nature of the sample itself or from the addition of anticoagulants or preservatives.[191] For example, HDL cholesterol measurements can be inaccurate, and usually are more variable when obtained from lyophilized samples than from fresh or frozen sera.

Additives including anticoagulants such as citrate and fluoride can have large osmotic effects that cause water to shift from the cells to the plasma. This dilutes the lipoprotein by 10% or more and produces erroneously low values. EDTA, traditionally the preferred anticoagulant for lipoprotein measurements, causes a slight dilution, but has been used because it also inhibits certain oxidative and other changes that can affect some lipoprotein or apolipoprotein measurements. Lipid and lipoprotein concentrations in EDTA plasma tend to be about 3% lower than in serum, an effect that may not be readily noticeable in HDL cholesterol measurements. EDTA, however, complexes some of the Mn^{2+} in the heparin-Mn^{2+} method, and it has been found necessary to use a higher concentration of $MnCl_2$ (0.092 mol/L, final concentration in the reaction system) when the procedure is used with EDTA plasma than with serum (0.046 mol/L).[16,322] Heparin, by virtue of its high molecular weight and when present in concentrations used for anticoagulation, has no measurable effect on lipid or lipoprotein concentration, and does not affect HDL cholesterol measurements.

Second Generation Methods. A second generation dextran sulfate method (Box 26-5) reduces the interference associated with increased triglycerides (POLYMEDCO, Cortlandt Manor, N.Y.). With it, the dextran sulfate precipitant is complexed with magnetic particles, allowing the lipoprotein-precipitant-magnetic particle complex to be removed rapidly by placing the reaction vessel on a magnetic disk. HDL cholesterol is then measured in the usual way. The method can also be adapted for use in an automated clinical chemistry analyzer, allowing the supernatant to be analyzed without the necessity for removing it from the sedimented complex. The method was reported to have a bias of about 4% to 7% in the concentration range 30 to 50 mg/dL compared with ultracentrifugation combined with polyanion precipitation using a conventional dextran sulfate–Mg^{2+} method, and a coefficient of variation (CV) under 4%, similar to the usual dextran sulfate–Mg^{2+} method.[108,206]

Homogeneous Assays. A major breakthrough in HDL assays was reported in 1994,[128] with the introduction of the first of a series of so-called "homogeneous" immunoassay methods for lipoproteins (Box 26-5). Compared with the earlier precipitation methods requiring manual pretreatment steps, the homogeneous methods substantially improve workflow in the modern clinical laboratory, making sample handling as simple as placing a bar-coded specimen tube on the automated analyzer. Elimination of the manual steps provides cost savings with generally higher reagent costs offset by decreased labor costs. The fully automated methods also improve precision through more consistent pipetting of smaller specimen volumes and precise temperature control and reaction timing, which facilitate achieving the NCEP analytical performance goals. Evaluation studies have typically demonstrated substantially better precision, with CVs about half those of conventional pretreatment methods.

The first homogeneous assay for HDL cholesterol required four successive reagent additions (International Reagents Corp., Kobe, Japan). The first reagent contained polyethylene glycol, which causes aggregation of the apo B-100–containing chylomicrons, VLDL, and LDL. The second reagent protected or blocked the aggregated lipoproteins with antibodies to apo B-100 and apo C. The cholesterol reaction enzymes (cholesterol esterase, cholesterol oxidase, and peroxidase) were added in the third reagent, which acted upon only the unprotected HDL cholesterol. The fourth reagent stopped the color reaction and solubilized the aggregates with guanidine salts, clearing the reaction mixture for measurement of color. This breakthrough method, even though not suited for all analyzers because of the multiple reagent additions, was capable of full automation, paving the way for subsequent, two-reagent homogeneous methods.

In 1995, a second homogeneous method became available (Kyowa Medex Co., Tokyo[297]; Roche Diagnostics, Indianapolis) that used sulfated alpha-cyclodextrins together with Mg^{2+} to selectively block but not precipitate chylomicrons and VLDL, providing selectivity without the necessity for precipitation. Secondly, covalently linked polyethylene glycol molecules enhanced the specificities of the enzymes cholesterol esterase and cholesterol oxidase toward the cholesterol in HDL. Polyethylene glycol having an MW of 6000 Da is thought to optimize the specificities at concentrations lower than those used previously to precipitate lipoproteins, implying that the modified enzymes were able to distinguish the lipoprotein classes based on their size and/or charge. The result was a fully automated homogeneous assay with only two reagent additions that is applicable for use with many of the common chemistry analyzers. The original kit included the second enzyme-containing reagent in lyophilized form, necessitating reconstitution, but a modification introduced in mid1998 included both reagents in liquid form.[104] A third modification decreased the Mg^{2+} concentration, apparently to reduce carryover in pipetting.

A synthetic polymer together with a polyanion to block the non-HDL lipoproteins is used in a third homogeneous assay (Daiichi Pure Chemicals Co., Tokyo /Genzyme Corp., Cambridge, Mass.).[107,162,206] A detergent is then added that exposes only cholesterol in HDL to the enzymes, giving specificity for HDL-C. This method also requires two reagent additions, the first with the polyanion and polymer-blocking agents and the second with detergent, enzymes, and substrates. A subsequent modification provided both reagents in liquid form with other changes to improve specificity and decrease potential interference.[105,144,334] A third modification without Mg^{2+} has been reported.[63,121]

A fourth homogeneous assay is based on immunoinhibition and includes two reagents (Wako Pure Chemicals Industry, Osaka, Japan).[156,184,219] The first reagent contains an antibody to human apo B-100 that reacts with the apo B-100–containing lipoproteins, chylomicrons, VLDL, and LDL, blocking their reaction with the enzymes that are added in the second reagent. The current formulation includes both reagents in liquid form.

A fifth homogeneous method (Denka Seiken Co., Niigata, Japan/Polymedco Inc., Cortlandt Manor, N.Y./Randox Laboratories Limited, Crumlin, UK) allows cholesterol esterase and oxidase to react with lipoproteins other than HDL, generating peroxidase, which, in turn, is scavenged by the enzyme catalase.[205,219] An inhibitor of catalase and a surfactant in a second reagent specifically react with HDL cholesterol, producing color through the usual peroxidase sequence.

At least one instrument application for each of the homogeneous assays discussed previously in this chapter has qualified for certification by the CRMLN, implying at least the capability to achieve agreement with the RM. However, conditions and especially calibration may be different on various instrument applications and many have not been evaluated. Thus certification for the reagents cannot be considered universally applicable to all distributor versions, instrument applications, and lots. Similarly, published evaluation studies have confirmed that the methods can be accurate but may not be so in every commercial application.[198] Laboratories choosing to adopt homogeneous assay applications that have not been certified by the CRMLN are encouraged to confirm that their particular systems are accurate. In addition, several more recent evaluations have noted that some homogeneous reagents may lack specificity or ruggedness, especially on specimens with unusual lipoprotein composition.[326]

Specificity and Interference. The accuracy of measuring HDL cholesterol in each individual specimen is a function not only of bias or overall inaccuracy related to calibration, but also of the ruggedness of the assays, their specificity for HDL cholesterol, and absence of interference by other lipoproteins and constituents of the specimen matrix. Laboratories supporting research studies and lipid clinics with a high proportion of atypical specimens must be especially concerned about this issue. The CRMLN certification studies and many published evaluation studies, assessing accuracy, include only samples from relatively normal subjects. Most studies did not determine performance in samples from patients with extreme hyperlipidemias, such as type III or other conditions, such as liver and kidney disease, which often result in unusual lipoproteins with atypical separation characteristics. Only a few studies have included such extreme specimens and have raised questions about the specificity of the homogeneous reagents.[91,113,142,280,319]

Most studies of interference have been fairly traditional and relatively modest.[11,108,119,144,205] Evaluations indicate that triglycerides below 900 mg/dL do not generally interfere with any of the methods and some methods are reportedly free of interference to nearly 2000 mg/dL. Hemoglobin below 2 g/L and bilirubin below 10 mg/dL do not interfere appreciably with any of the homogeneous methods.

Considerations in Choosing an High-Density Lipoprotein Method. Laboratories have had to consider the alternatives in deciding whether to replace a conventional pretreatment method with a homogeneous reagent: improved efficiency on the one hand versus occasional discrepant results on the other. Routine clinical laboratories tend to choose the fully automated methods, often because of unavoidable pressures to improve efficiency. Laboratories performing research and supporting lipid clinics, on the other hand, often choose to retain a conventional precipitation method. An important factor in the latter choice is that a laboratory supporting long-term studies cannot tolerate the potential changes and shifts in results that have occurred because of the frequent modifications in the homogeneous reagents.

Low-Density Lipoprotein Cholesterol

Methods for LDL cholesterol generally quantitate a so-called "broad-cut fraction" including not only the primary LDL species in the 1.019 to 1.063 kg/L density range, but also IDL, density 1.006 to 1.019 kg/L, and Lp(a).[208] Therefore the usual convention based on the following formula is an approximation accepted for convenience:

$$\text{Total cholesterol (chol)} = \text{VLDL chol} + \text{LDL chol} + \text{HDL chol} \quad (16)$$

LDL cholesterol can be measured using both indirect and direct methods, and either approach has been used in major studies that established the relationship between LDL cholesterol concentration and the risk for CHD.

Indirect Methods. Indirect methods for measuring LDL cholesterol are based on measuring a number of lipid-related analytes followed by their use in calculating the LDL cholesterol content of a specimen. This includes the use of the Friedewald equation and the beta-quantification method.

The Friedewald Equation. In the most widely used indirect method (Box 26-6), cholesterol, triglyceride, and HDL cholesterol are measured and LDL cholesterol is calculated from the primary measurements using the empirical equation of Friedewald and colleagues[84]

$$[\text{LDL chol}] = [\text{Total chol}] - [\text{HDL chol}] - [\text{Triglyceride}]/5 \quad (17)$$

where all concentrations are given in milligrams per deciliter (triglyceride/2.22 is used when LDL cholesterol is expressed in millimoles per liter). The factor [triglyceride]/5 is an estimate of VLDL cholesterol concentration, and is based on the average ratio of triglyceride to cholesterol in VLDL.

BOX 26-6 Methods for LDL Separation/Quantification

Beta-quantification
- Ultracentrifugation at density 1.006 Kg/L to float VLDL
- Precipitation with polyanion/cation for HDL
- LDL calculated as density >1.006 – HDL
- Most commonly used by specialty lipid laboratories

Calculation using Friedewald formula
- [LDL chol] = [Total chol] – [HDL chol] – [Triglyceride]/5
- Originally proposed for epidemiology studies
- Became the most common method in routine clinical labs

Homogeneous Reagents
- LDL solubilization (Kyowa Medex)
- LDL protected/deprotected by surfactants (Daiichi)
- LDL protected/catalase (Wako)
- Non-HDL catalase/LDL azide (Denka Seiken)
- LDL protected by Calixarene/cholesterol dehydrogenase (International Reagents Corp)

Several investigators have evaluated the accuracy of LDL cholesterol estimated with equation (17). For example, DeLong and colleagues recommended the use of the expression 0.16 × [triglyceride] as a better estimate of VLDL cholesterol, and consequently, the factor [triglyceride]/6 is used in a few laboratories.[65] Other factors have been suggested for particular populations,[238] but no single factor was accurate under all circumstances. However, when the original factor [triglyceride]/5 was compared with a combined ultracentrifugation-polyanion precipitation method in about 5000 samples, the errors in LDL cholesterol estimated with equation (17) were found to be symmetrically distributed about zero.[324] On balance, the NCEP recommended the use of the original factor [triglyceride/5] for estimating LDL cholesterol with equation (17).[238]

In practice, the Friedewald calculation is reasonably accurate, but there are several well known circumstances under which the Friedewald equation cannot be used. First, calculation is precluded in samples that have triglyceride concentrations above 400 mg/dL or in those that contain great amounts of chylomicrons (nonfasting specimen). At high triglyceride concentrations, the factor [triglyceride]/5 as an estimate of VLDL cholesterol concentration is not appropriate because such samples can also contain chylomicrons, chylomicron remnants, or VLDL remnants, all of which have higher triglyceride/cholesterol ratios. Under these circumstances, the use of the factor [triglyceride]/5 would overestimate VLDL cholesterol and therefore underestimate LDL cholesterol. The Friedewald equation has been found to be most accurate in samples with triglyceride levels below 200 mg/dL,[324] but the error becomes unacceptably large (i.e., >10%) at triglyceride concentrations greater than 400 mg/dL.

The opposite error can occur if the Friedewald equation is used in patients with type III hyperlipoproteinemia. Type III hyperlipoproteinemia is characterized in part by the presence of β-VLDL, not normally present in the blood. Biochemically, β-VLDL occurs in the VLDL, density range, but is much richer in cholesterol than normal VLDL with a ratio of triglyceride/cholesterol on the order of 3:1. Application of the factor [triglyceride]/5 in type IIIs would underestimate VLDL cholesterol and in turn overestimate LDL cholesterol. Thus a patient with type III hyperlipoproteinemia may appear to have an artifactually high LDL cholesterol concentration.

Fortunately, both of these conditions are uncommon. The 95th percentile for fasting plasma triglycerides in the United States is below 300 mg/dL, indicating that only a small percentage of specimens will exceed the 400 mg/dL cutoff. Plasma from fasting subjects does not normally contain chylomicrons, and even if present, chylomicrons can be observed visually as a floating "cream" layer in samples that have been allowed to stand undisturbed at 4 °C overnight. Finally the prevalence of type III hyperlipoproteinemia is only about 1 to 2 per 1000 persons in the general population.[153] Thus the Friedewald calculation will be reasonably reliable in the majority of patients.

Beta-Quantification (Ultracentrifugation-Polyanion Precipitation). This method is the precursor to the HDL and LDL reference methods and is often used in samples for which the Friedewald equation is inappropriate. It follows the procedure used in the LRC Program and combines preparative ultracentrifugation and polyanion precipitation.[104] To use the assay, an accurately measured aliquot of plasma is first ultracentrifuged at 105,000×g for 18 hours at 10 °C to a density of 1.006 g/mL (plasma density). Under these conditions, VLDL and, if present, chylomicrons and β-VLDL, accumulate in a floating layer, with the infranatant containing primarily LDL and HDL (Figure 26-26) plus any IDL and Lp(a) that may be present. The floating layer, removed with the aid of a tube slicer, is sometimes analyzed as a check on recovery and may be saved for electrophoretic analysis. The infranatant solution is remixed, reconstituted to known volume, and its cholesterol content measured. HDL cholesterol is usually measured in a separate aliquot of plasma, but when necessary, an aliquot of the d 1.006 g/mL infranatant can be treated to remove the apo B-100–containing lipoproteins [IDL, LDL, and Lp(a)], and the HDL cholesterol then measured in the clear supernatant. VLDL and LDL cholesterol are calculated as follows:

$$[\text{VLDL chol}] = [\text{Total chol}] - [\text{d} > 1.006\ \text{g/mL chol}] \quad (18)$$

$$[\text{LDL chol}] = [\text{d} > 1.006\ \text{g/mL chol}] - [\text{HDL chol}] \quad (19)$$

LDL cholesterol measured in this way is unaffected by the presence of either chylomicrons or other triglyceride-rich lipoproteins, or by β-VLDL. VLDL cholesterol is usually calculated from equation (18) rather than measured directly in the ultracentrifugal supernatant because it can be difficult to recover this fraction quantitatively, particularly when triglyceride concentrations are high.

Lipoproteins Included in the "LDL Cholesterol" Measurement. From the preceding discussion, it is obvious that in both methods, the term "LDL cholesterol" includes the contributions of cholesterol in the IDL and Lp(a) fractions and that in the core LDL. Although IDL and Lp(a) cholesterol usually contribute only a few milligrams per deciliter to the "total LDL cholesterol" measurement, their contributions can be significant in patients with high IDL or Lp(a) concentrations. For example, assuming that cholesterol (i.e., sterol nucleus) constitutes about 30% of the mass of Lp(a), it can be calculated that the Lp(a) cholesterol concentration would contribute about 12 mg/dL, or about 12%, to the LDL cholesterol measurement in a patient with an Lp(a) concentration of 40 mg/dL and an apparent LDL cholesterol concentration of 100 mg/dL. It has been suggested that a more specific measure of LDL cholesterol could be obtained by correcting the measured LDL cholesterol value for the contribution of Lp(a) cholesterol,[126,267] and a similar argument might be made for IDL. Increased concentrations of both IDL and Lp(a) appear to be related to the increased risk for CHD [see later section on Lp(a)], however, and although such corrections might increase the specificity of the methods for LDL cholesterol, per se, they might also give

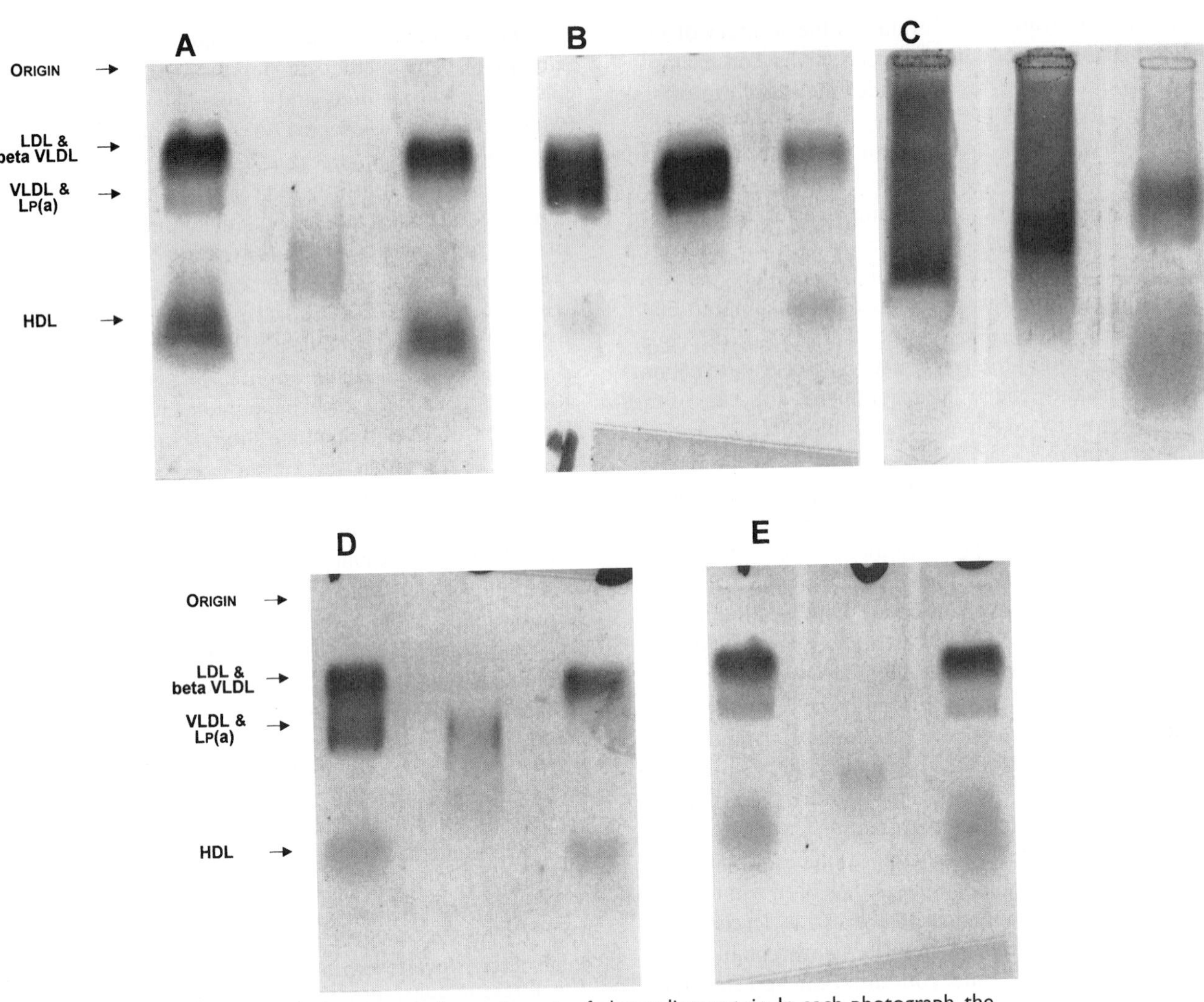

Figure 26-26 Agarose gel electrophoresis of plasma lipoprotein. In each photograph, the samples were applied in the following order, reading left to right: unfractionated plasma, ultracentrifugal density 1.006 g/mL supernatant solution, ultracentrifugal infranatant solution. **A,** Pattern seen in normal samples and samples with high LDL cholesterol concentrations. **B,** Type III hyperlipoproteinemia pattern. **C,** Severe hypertriglyceridemia, triglyceride = 3840 mg/dL. Note chylomicrons at origin. **D,** Pattern observed in samples with moderately elevated triglyceride, triglyceride = 281 mg/dL, LDL cholesterol = 145 mg/dL. Note absence of chylomicrons. **E,** Pattern observed in patients with high concentrations of Lp(a). Note presence of Lp(a) found in infranatant solution. This sample had an Lp(a) concentration of 77 mg/dL. *LDL,* Low-density lipoprotein; *VLDL,* very low-density lipoprotein; Lp(a), lipoprotein(a); *HDL,* high-density lipoprotein.

LDL cholesterol values that underestimate cardiovascular risk because they exclude some of the atherogenic lipoproteins. Moreover, this might occur more frequently with patients with CHD or who are at risk for CHD based on their "LDL cholesterol" concentrations. Consequently, the NCEP Working Group on LDL cholesterol measurement suggested that LDL cholesterol values should *not* be corrected for the contribution of other atherogenic lipoproteins, and also recommended that further research be conducted to establish the individual contributions of IDL, Lp(a), and LDL cholesterol to the CHD risk as reflected in current LDL cholesterol measurements that include all three lipoprotein classes. The most recent guidelines from the NCEP expand on this concept by introducing the term "non-HDL cholesterol," which includes all of the apo B-100–containing atherogenic lipoproteins including not only Lp(a) and IDL but also VLDL cholesterol.[77]

Diagnosis of the Type III Lipoprotein Pattern. The ratio of VLDL cholesterol to plasma triglyceride, expressed in terms of mass, is 0.2 or lower in normal samples and in those from patients with lipoprotein disorders other than type III hyperlipidemia. In type III hyperlipoproteinemia, the ratio is 0.3 or higher because of the presence of β-VLDL, and the elevated ratio can persist even after treatment.

In addition, β-VLDL can also be observed directly by subjecting the VLDL fraction to agarose gel electrophoresis, where it migrates electrophoretically with LDL rather than VLDL (see Figure 26-26). The combination of a VLDL cholesterol/plasma triglyceride ratio of 0.3 or higher and the observation of β-VLDL in the ultracentrifugal supernatant establishes the type III lipoprotein pattern.

Direct Methods. Selective precipitation and homogeneous immunoassay methods have been used to measure LDL cholesterol directly.

Selective Precipitation. Several direct methods have been used for LDL cholesterol measurement that are based on selective precipitation with polyvinyl sulfate or heparin at low pH.[123,165,195] LDL cholesterol is then calculated as the difference between total cholesterol and that in the supernatant, or in another variation, directly in the LDL precipitate. It is not clear whether atherogenic lipoproteins other than LDL itself are also detected, and these methods might be expected to be subject to similar sources of error as those encountered with precipitation methods for HDL separation. A more specific method used a mixture of polyclonal antibodies to apo A-I and apo E linked to a resin to bind VLDL, IDL, and HDL, with LDL cholesterol measured in a filtrate by the usual methods. The method was reasonably precise and in good agreement with ultracentrifugation-polyanion precipitation.[109,123,186,230] The reagent was in commercial distribution for several years but, requiring a separate pretreatment step, was eventually superseded by a new class of direct homogeneous reagents patterned after the homogeneous reagents for HDL cholesterol.

Homogeneous Assays. Following the approach similar to those used with the homogeneous methods for HDL cholesterol,[326] homogeneous assays have been developed to measure LDL cholesterol. For example, five homogeneous LDL methods are commercially available (Box 26-6) and differ by containing different detergents and other chemicals, which allow specific blocking or solubilization of lipoprotein classes to achieve specificity for LDL cholesterol. All suppliers offer kits with two reagents, readily adaptable to most clinical chemistry analyzers.

Sugiuchi and colleagues developed the first homogeneous method for measuring LDL cholesterol[296]; the reagent is distributed by Kyowa Medex, Tokyo and Roche Diagnostics, Indianapolis. With this method, LDL is directly measured by suppressing the other lipoproteins (the other four methods suppress LDL first and react with other lipoproteins before determining LDL cholesterol). The method is formulated in two reagents. The first has $MgCl_2$, dye, buffer (pH 6.75), and the α-cyclodextrin sulfate,[297] which has a highly concentrated negative charge to mask cholesterol in chylomicrons and VLDL in the presence of magnesium ions.[296] The second reagent includes the enzymes cholesterol oxidase and cholesterol esterase, peroxidase, dye, buffer (pH 6.75), and a polyoxyethylene-polyoxypropylene polyether (POE-POP) to block cholesterol, especially in HDL.[296,297] The molecular mass of the POP in the POE-POP molecule and the hydrophobicity index determine selectivity to LDL; 3850 Da was demonstrated to be optimum.[297]

A second method also is formulated in two reagent variations (Daiichi Pure Chemicals Co., Tokyo; Genzyme Diagnostics, Cambridge, Mass.). The first reagent contains ascorbic acid oxidase, 4-aminoantipyrine, peroxidase, cholesterol oxidase, cholesterol esterase, buffer (pH 6.3), and a detergent, which solubilizes all non-LDL lipoproteins, allowing reaction of their cholesterol with the esterase and oxidase enzymes, forming a colorless product. The second reagent contains N,N-bis-(4-sulfobutyl)-m-toluidine Na_2 (DSBmT), buffer (pH 6.3), and a detergent to specifically release LDL cholesterol. The resulting hydrogen peroxide reacts with N,N′-bis-(4-sulfobutyl)-M-toluidine disodium salt to generate a colored product.

A third method (Wako Chemicals, Osaka, Japan) includes a reagent with Good's buffer (pH 6.8), (N-(2-hydroxy-3-sulfopropyl)-3,5-dimethoxyaniline, sodium salt), cholesterol esterase, cholesterol oxidase, catalase, polyanions, and amphoteric surfactants, the latter selectively protecting LDL from enzymatic reaction. The non-LDL cholesterol reacts with esterase and oxidase, producing hydrogen peroxide, which is consumed by catalase. The second reagent includes Good's buffer (pH 7.0), 4-aminoantipyrene, peroxidase, sodium azide, and a de-protecting reagent, which removes the protecting agent from LDL, enabling the specific reaction of cholesterol esterase and cholesterol oxidase with its cholesterol, producing hydrogen peroxide and a blue color complex.[75,189]

Non-LDL cholesterol is removed in a fourth method (Denka Seiken, Niigata, Japan/Polymedco Inc., Cortlandt Manor, N.Y.) via a selective reaction with cholesterol oxidase and cholesterol esterase with the resulting peroxide byproduct eliminated by reaction with catalase (CAT). In this two reagent method, the first reagent contains $MgCl_2$, cholesterol esterase, cholesterol oxidase, catalase, and N-(2-hydroxy-3-sulfopropyl)-3,5-dimethoxyaniline sodium salt, Emulgen 66 (polyoxyethylene compound; Kao), and Emulgen 90, both nonionic surfactants, in Good's buffer (PIPES; 100 mmol/L; pH 7.0). Its second reagent contains peroxidase, 4-aminoantipyrine, sodium azide (to inhibit the catalase), and Triton X-100 in Good's buffer. The hydrophilic/lipophilic balance of the detergents is chosen to obtain appropriate selectivity to the lipoproteins.[218]

In a fifth method (International Reagents Corp., Kokusai-Kobe, Japan), its first reagent contains the detergent calixarene that converts LDL to a soluble complex. Cholesterol esters of HDL-C and VLDL-C are preferentially hydrolyzed by a cholesterol esterase (chromobacterium), cholesterol oxidase, and hydrazine, which divert the accessible cholesterol to cholestenone hydrazone. A second reagent with deoxycholate breaks up the LDL-calixarene complex, allowing LDL-C to react with the esterase, a dehydrogenase, and β-NAD to yield cholestenone and ß-NADH, the latter measured by a spectrophotometer.

Analytical Performance of LDL Methods. Evaluations of the LDL homogeneous assays indicate that CVs are gen-

TABLE 26-23 Analytical Performance of Homogeneous LDL-C Assays

	Imprecision (CVs)	Dynamic range (mg/L)	Recovery (%)			Accuracy	
			LDL	VLDL	IDL	bias (%)	bias (mg/L)
Kyowa	0.7-3.1	2-4100	97-105	16	52-64	0.8-11.2	−60 to −80
Daiichi	<3.1	4-10,000	87	19	31-47	3.9-5.1	−48 to −80
Wako	≤1.2	10-3000	—	—	—	0.4	−15
Denka	<1.8	70-5500	95	10	31	—	—
IRC	≤0.6	?-4000	—	—	—	—	—

erally <3% and consistently within the NCEP performance target of <4% CV (Table 26-23). By contrast, CVs for the Friedewald calculation have been estimated to approximate 4% in expert laboratories and as high as 12% in routine clinical laboratories, estimated from proficiency surveys.[208]

With regard to accuracy, all of the homogeneous assays have qualified for certification through the CRMLN program, suggesting agreement with the reference methods at least in relatively normal specimens. Nevertheless, as indicated previously for HDL cholesterol methods, there are many instrument applications and not all have been evaluated for bias. Factors such as lot-to-lot differences, unique calibrations by distributors, different calibrations from country to country, and reformulations of reagents might affect actual biases.[326] In a 2002 study, four homogeneous assays were compared with the LDL RM; unacceptable total error was found and the authors recommended caution in adopting the methods.[192]

In addition to overall accuracy, primarily a function of calibration, methods should be specific for the LDL-C fraction; this is of particular concern considering the heterogeneity of the lipoproteins. Published studies suggest that the homogeneous assays interact unequally with the different components of the "broad-cut LDL": LDL subclasses, IDL, Lp(a), and Lp-X.* A 2002 study of two homogenous reagents using isolated lipoprotein fractions confirmed the lack of specificity for VLDL and LDL subclasses.[309] The two homogeneous methods included about 20% of isolated VLDL. Also the reagents missed about 30% of IDL and up to 50% of the isolated LDL fractions, especially the important smaller and more atherogenic subclasses. The inclusion of some VLDL will offset the loss of LDL fractions, so the lack of specificity may not be obvious in relatively normal specimens. However, the lack of specificity for lipoprotein subclasses and differences among reagents may make the measured results for each individual different depending on the particular lipoprotein profile and the reagent. Obviously the homogeneous LDL cholesterol assays have to be more rigorously evaluated in other than normal specimens before they can be recommended with confidence.

Conventional interference studies have demonstrated that the methods are not subject to significant interference from bilirubin and hemoglobin. However, higher levels of triglycerides have been shown to interfere, increasing apparent LDL cholesterol values, not surprising considering the reported lack of specificity for VLDL.[118,204,218] Alternately the sulfated α-cyclodextrin used in the Sugiuchi assay to block VLDL cholesterol appeared to cause underestimation of the LDL cholesterol.[75,207,296]

A major potential advantage of the homogeneous methods over the Friedewald calculation is the ability to use nonfasting specimens, convenient in managing patients. Results, judged by mean differences between paired fasting and nonfasting specimens, were promising, but patient classification was poorer with nonfasting specimens.[207,218,335] Lipoprotein composition is affected by recent diet; changes have been observed even with the more robust ultracentrifugation method. However, the changes in vivo are small and the convenience of being able to use nonfasting specimens may offset minor effects on accuracy. Nevertheless, until the use of nonfasting specimens is validated by more comprehensive studies, laboratories are encouraged to specify fasting.

Other Considerations in Adopting a Homogeneous LDL Method. Clinical laboratories are faced with the decision whether to implement the fully automated homogeneous methods for LDL cholesterol, either replacing or supplementing the traditional Friedewald calculation. The considerations are certainly not as compelling for the homogeneous LDL methods as for HDL. Even given the technical disadvantages of the Friedewald method: (1) the necessity for fasting, (2) the poor precision from the cumulative variations in the three underlying measurements, and (3) the well-known limitations in certain patients, it is firmly entrenched in routine practice and will likely be displaced only if the homogeneous methods can demonstrate clear advantages, for example, substantially better analytical performance or overall improved cost effectiveness in characterizing or monitoring patients, advantages that have yet to be shown. A 2002 review suggests that the homogeneous assays can only be recommended to supplement calculation for those patients with elevated triglycerides or other conditions precluding calculation.[208]

*References 75, 78, 118, 218, 259, 266, 296.

Oxidized LDL

In 1983 Brown and Goldstein reported that circulating LDL must undergo some structural modification before it becomes fully proatherogenic.[33] Patients who completely lack LDL receptors accumulate large amounts of cholesterol in their macrophages and form foam cells. The receptors, which recognize the modified LDL, were termed "the scavenger receptors."[88] Currently, several modifications that enhance the uptake of LDL by macrophages in vitro have been described, such as glycation, self-aggregation, immune complex formation, hydrolysis, and oxidation, with the latter receiving the greatest attention.[291]

LDL is oxidized in microdomains in the arterial wall where it is sequestered by proteoglycans and other extracellular matrix constituents and protected from plasma antioxidants. This process is a free-radical–driven lipid peroxidation chain reaction that is initiated by the free radical attacking the double bond associated with PUFA, leading to the generation of malonedialdehyde and 4-hydroxynonenal.[1] These intermediate compounds then bind to apo B-100, giving it an increased net negative charge and rendering it unrecognizable by native LDL receptors.

Oxidized LDL (oxLDL) has several proatherogenic properties including the rapid uptake by macrophages to form foam cells, chemoattraction for circulating monocytes, promotion of the differentiation of monocytes into tissue macrophages, and inhibition of the motility of resident macrophages.[291] It is also cytotoxic to several types of cells and immunogenic. Laboratory, clinical, and epidemiological studies have shown that this oxidation does also occur in vivo. Extracted LDL from human atherosclerotic lesions was shown to be oxidatively modified; circulating anti-oxLDL antibodies were detected in serum, with the titers correlating with progression of atherosclerotic lesions; and the use of various antioxidants (vitamin E and probucol among others) delayed the progression of atherosclerotic lesions.

A commercial enzyme-linked immunosorbent assay (ELISA) method for the determination of oxLDL is currently available (Mercodia).[115] However, at the present time the clinical relevance of oxLDL has not been established and therefore its routine measurement is not recommended.

Total Lipoproteins and Lipoprotein Subclasses

Several approaches have been used to quantitate all of the lipoproteins, and in some cases lipoprotein subclasses, in a single procedure. Nuclear magnetic resonance (NMR) spectroscopy is one of the more efficient methods,[221,222] detecting lipoprotein-associated fatty acyl methyl and methylene groups. The signals from subfractions of VLDL, LDL, and HDL can be resolved mathematically with values reported in terms of lipoprotein cholesterol concentrations based on assumptions about the average cholesterol compositions of the various classes of lipoproteins. A sample can be analyzed quickly using a small volume of serum by the method, which can be automated. A disadvantage of NMR is the inability to distinguish Lp(a) from LDL particles of the same size. Furthermore, the requirement for expensive specialized equipment and expertise limits application.

Density gradient ultracentrifugation is used to measure lipoprotein subclasses; it is performed in a vertical rotor with measurement of cholesterol continuously in the fractions eluted from the gradient.[47-49,53,276] Mathematical curve resolution derives the component lipoprotein profiles and allows calculation of their cholesterol concentrations. The method can determine concentrations of VLDL, IDL, LDL, Lp(a), and HDL cholesterol. LDL cholesterol subclasses can be expressed separately or combined to give a measurement similar to that provided by the Friedewald equation or beta-quantification. A disadvantage is that the procedure is technically demanding and requires instrumentation not usually available in clinical laboratories.

Lipoproteins have also been fractionated by gradient gel electrophoresis with several commercial applications. The electropherogram is scanned densitometrically and the areas under the various lipoprotein peaks are integrated and converted to equivalent lipoprotein cholesterol concentrations using assumed average cholesterol compositions for the lipoprotein. Resolution of the lipoprotein classes is better with gradient gel electrophoresis than with conventional agarose electrophoresis, but electrophoretic quantitation of lipoproteins in unfractionated samples has not gained wide acceptance because of the inherent limitations of such methods,[15,33] including the incomplete resolution of VLDL and LDL, the comigration of β-VLDL with LDL and Lp(a) with VLDL, differences in staining intensity of the lipoproteins, and other methodological challenges. The use of gradient gel electrophoresis for quantitative measurements has been useful in research but not widely used in routine practice.

None of the lipoprotein methods described in this section has been used widely enough to have been validated in independent studies to the same extent as have been the Friedewald and beta-quantification methods. In most cases, the identities of the lipoprotein contributing to the "LDL cholesterol" measurement have not been adequately established. Further evaluations should better define the relationships between these new methods and current reference and routine methods.

Intermediate-Density (Remnant) Lipoproteins

Remnant lipoproteins include the lipolytic products of catabolism of the triglyceride-rich lipoproteins, VLDL and chylomicrons, occurring in the VLDL and LDL ranges. A traditionally defined fraction at the lighter end of the LDL density range, the IDL portion comprises the 1.006 to 1.019 g/mL fraction, which is obtained by sequential ultracentrifugation for quantitation, generally in terms of cholesterol content.

Clinically, remnant lipoproteins have been shown to be predictive of the CHD risk.[110] A method for measuring a remnant fraction designated RLP cholesterol for remnant-like particles (RLP) has become commercially available, using specific antibodies to separate a fraction of lipoprotein remnants. This fraction seems to be particularly indicative of conditions conferring increased CHD risk.[157,187]

Desktop Analyzer Methods

Portable analyzers, also called "desktop analyzers," "physician's office analyzers," or "point-of-care (POC) analyzers," have been developed for use in nonlaboratory settings (see Chapters 4, 10, and 11). Several such devices are capable of measuring cholesterol and most also quantify triglycerides and HDL cholesterol, with calculation of LDL cholesterol, in a few microliters of whole blood, serum, or plasma within a few minutes.

Sources of Variation in Lipid and Lipoprotein Measurements

Lipid and lipoprotein concentrations vary within individuals when measured on several occasions over time. The sources of variation can be broadly categorized as analytical and physiological. Analytical variations are inherent in the measurements themselves and arise from variations in sample collection procedures, volume measurements, instrument function, reagent formulations, uncertainties in the assignment of values to calibration materials, and other such factors. Normal physiological variation occurs independently of analytical error and reflects the actual changes in concentration that occur through the course of normal, day-to-day living. Such variations result from factors such as change in posture, which causes the redistribution of water between the vascular and nonvascular space, thereby changing the concentrations of nondiffusible plasma components.[19,190] Recent food intake produces transient increases in plasma triglycerides of 50% or more and decreases of up to 10% or 15% in LDL and HDL cholesterol depending on the fat content of the meal.[50,51,331] The shifts result from changes in the lipid composition of the lipoproteins that occur as chylomicrons are metabolized. Seasonal changes have also been observed, probably resulting from changes in dietary and exercise patterns throughout the year.[38,92] Normal physiological variations tend to occur in both directions, causing the lipid or lipoprotein concentration to vary somewhat about a mean value for a particular patient. Other kinds of physiological conditions cause changes from the patient's usual steady-state concentrations, for example, acute illness or stress, pregnancy, dietary changes that result in weight loss or gain, changes in saturated fat intake, or the effects of treatment with lipid-lowering medications. In these cases the changes tend to be in one direction, and they are not considered normal physiological fluctuations. Lipoprotein concentrations eventually return to the original steady-state levels when the patient recovers, or a new steady-state level is achieved.

Because normal physiological variations occur, it is difficult to evaluate a patient based on a single measurement because it applies only to the current sample. It is more appropriate to consider the patient's usual range of concentrations, or his or her average steady-state concentration. This distinction is more than academic because it is the basis of a twofold goal of lipid and lipoprotein measurement. From the laboratory's standpoint, the aim is to provide accurate measurements in the particular sample being measured. For this reason, the laboratory is primarily concerned with minimizing analytical error. From the physician's standpoint, however, the goal is to establish the patient's usual range of concentration for purposes of diagnosis and judging the effects of treatment. This aim is affected primarily by physiological variation because physiological variation contributes the larger proportion of the specimen-to-specimen variation observed in serial samples from the same patient. Some sources of physiological variation, such as posture during blood sampling, can be controlled and other factors that cannot be controlled, such as pregnancy, have to be considered in interpreting laboratory results.

Analytical Variation

Table 26-24 illustrates the current overall variation of lipid and lipoprotein measurements in about 4500 laboratories participating in a large, ongoing proficiency survey in 2003. The laboratories used a variety of methods and instruments. For total cholesterol measured with all methods in all laboratories, the average bias was in the range of −0.5% to −2.7% and the CVs were about 3.5%. These numbers represent the total of within- and among-laboratory components of variation, and suggest that reliable cholesterol measurements can be provided by most clinical laboratories. Similarly, the average bias for HDL cholesterol ranged from −3.9% to +4.4%, with overall CVs of about 6%. These results are remarkable because at HDL cholesterol concentrations above 42 mg/dL, they conform to current NCEP recommendations for acceptable HDL cholesterol measurements in single laboratories,[238] and for total cholesterol they meet NCEP criteria for acceptable measurements in single laboratories.[237]

The overall CVs are slightly higher for triglycerides, probably because of the contribution of triglyceride blanks and the inherent greater variability in triglyceride methods, but the bias has improved considerably in recent years. The performance in the calculated LDL cholesterol values is encouraging and reflects the improvement in the reliability of the primary measurements. Data are also now available for the measured LDL cholesterol. Both the overall CV and bias for the measured LDL cholesterol are inferior to those of the calculated values.

Physiological Variation

The normal physiological component of variation is calculated from the total variation of measurements in serial specimens from the same patients, after adjusting for analytical variation.[27,106,127,177,194] Such estimates differ somewhat from study to study, but after an extensive review of the literature,[237,238] the NCEP panels concerned with lipid and lipoprotein measurement assumed average physiological

TABLE 26-24 Analytical Variation of Lipid and Lipoprotein Measurements

Analyte	LP01	LP02	LP03	LP04	LP05
Cholesterol					
Number of laboratories	4580	4623	4607	4608	4587
Mean (mg/dL)	266.7	179.6	(119.7)	152.9	195.4
CV (%)	3.7	3.4	3.5	3.5	3.7
CDC value	274.2	180.5	120.6	154.8	197.2
% Bias*	−2.7	−0.5	−0.5	−1.2	−0.9
Triglyceride†					
Number of laboratories	4499	4529	4522	4516	4512
Mean (mg/dL)	233.4	92.7	92.5	84.9	106.1
CV (%)	5.3	7.1	8.0	7.0	7.6
CDC value	239.3	93.3	91.3	85.7	102.5
% Bias	−2.5	−0.67	+1.37	−0.9	+3.5
HDL Cholesterol‡					
Number of laboratories	4115	4106	4097	4100	4093
Mean (mg/dL)	56.0	44.8	44.7	34.7	51.5
CV (%)	7.4	5.2	5.2	6.1	5.0
CDC value	58.3	43.2	42.8	33.4	50.5
% Bias	−3.9	+3.7	+4.4	+3.9	+2.0
LDL Cholesterol (Calculated)§					
Number of laboratories	2834	2842	2839	2830	2826
Mean (mg/dL)	163.8	116.0	116.4	101.1	122.4
CV (%)	6.6	5.8	5.9	5.6	6.5
CDC value	168.0	118.6	119.5	104.3	126.2
% Bias	−2.5	−2.2	−2.6	−3.1	−3.0
LDL Cholesterol (Measured)					
Number of laboratories	1104	1115	1116	1109	1104
Mean (mg/dL)	157.8	102.7	103.1	86.4	110.2
CV (%)	9.5	10.5	10.2	12.5	9.9
CDC value	150.3	111.1	110.8	97.9	117.3
% Bias	+5.0	−7.6	−6.9	−11.7	−6.1

Data from College of American Pathologists Comprehensive Chemistry Survey, Northfield, IL, 2003.
CV, Coefficient of variation; *CDC*, Centers for Disease Control and Prevention; *HDL*, high-density lipoprotein; *LDL*, low-density lipoprotein.
*Bias calculated as: (Laboratory mean—CDC value/CDC value) × 100
†Blanked and unblanked combined.
‡Combined data for all methods are not provided by College of American Pathologists. Data shown are for all methods using phosphotungstate-Mg^{2+} and enzymatic cholesterol measurement.
§Friedewald equation using [triglyceride/5] as an estimate of very low-density lipoprotein cholesterol concentration.

CVs (Table 26-25). A wide variety of factors contribute to the physiological variations (Table 26-26). The physiological variations observed for cholesterol, HDL cholesterol, and LDL cholesterol are similar. Physiological variation for triglyceride is considerably higher because fasting triglyceride concentrations can vary widely within an individual. Coefficients of analytical variation in a well-controlled laboratory are considerably smaller, generally about 2% to 3% for cholesterol and triglycerides, and 4% to 5% for LDL and HDL cholesterol. It can be calculated that, on average, physiological variations contribute about 70% to 98% of the overall variance of lipid and lipoprotein concentrations in people sampled on several occasions (see Table 26-25). For this reason, a patient's usual lipid or lipoprotein concentration cannot be reliably established from a single measurement. NCEP guidelines recommend that for cholesterol, the average of measurements in two serial samples obtained at least 1 week apart be used; two to three serial specimens are recommended if feasible for triglyceride and HDL and LDL cholesterol.[238]

TABLE 26-25 Physiological Variation of Lipid and Lipoprotein Concentrations in Serial Specimens from the Same Individuals

Component	Physiological Variation (% CV)	Percentage of Variance Contributed by Physiological Variation*
Total cholesterol	6.5	91%
Triglyceride	23.7	98%
HDL cholesterol	7.5	69%
LDL cholesterol	8.2	81%

CV, Coefficient of variation; *HDL*, high-density lipoprotein; *LDL*, low-density lipoprotein.
*Assuming the following analytical CVs: total cholesterol, 2%; triglyceride, 3%; HDL cholesterol, 5%; LDL cholesterol, 4%.

NCEP Recommendations for Lipid and Lipoprotein Measurements

The following information has been summarized from the NCEP recommendations for lipid and lipoprotein measurement.[237,238]

1. *Database linkage.* Laboratories that provide lipid and lipoprotein measurements should maintain linkage with the existing epidemiological databases relating lipid and lipoprotein concentration to the risk for CHD. Because these databases have been established largely based on CDC standardized methods, the methods used for cholesterol, triglycerides, HDL cholesterol, and LDL cholesterol should give results equivalent to those used to establish those databases. Accordingly, CDC reference methods for cholesterol, triglycerides, and HDL cholesterol serve as the basis for judging the accuracy of other methods.
2. *Reference methods.* Reference methods should provide serum equivalent values.
3. *Routine methods.* In most cases, lipid and lipoprotein measurements can be made using specimens of either serum or plasma. Measurements in EDTA plasma can be converted to serum-equivalent values using the following equation:

$$\text{Equivalent serum value} = \text{Plasma value} \times 1.03 \quad (20)$$

4. *Cholesterol measurements.* In practice, either a fasting or nonfasting sample is used for cholesterol measurements. Triglycerides, HDL cholesterol, and LDL cholesterol measurements should preferably be made in samples collected after a 12-hour fast. As a convenience to the patient, such measurements are made after a 9-hour fast without introducing unduly large errors into the measurements.
5. *Blood samples.* Blood samples should be standardized to be taken in the seated position whenever possible. If this is not feasible, the patient should be sampled in the same position on each occasion.
6. *Specimen storage.* Serum or plasma should be removed from cells within 3 hours of venipuncture. Specimens can be stored for up to 3 days at 4 °C; up to several weeks at −20 °C in a nonself-defrosting freezer; and at −70 °C or lower for longer periods.
7. *Serial samples.* Using the mean of several serial measurements for clinical decisions averages out the effects of physiological and analytical variation. Measurements should therefore be made in at least two serial samples collected at least 1 week apart with the values averaged. Three serial samples are preferred for triglycerides, HDL cholesterol, and LDL cholesterol measurements, but two serial specimens can be used if necessary.
8. *Glycerol blanking.* The NCEP Working Group on Lipoprotein Measurement endorses the following recommendations, adapted from the Lipids and Lipoproteins Division of the American Association for Clinical Chemistry:
   - All laboratories should offer a glycerol-blanked triglyceride analysis, even though it may be performed only when requested. Any specimen with triglycerides >200 mg/dL (2.26 mmol/L) should be glycerol blanked using a "reflex" ordering system.
   - Reports from the laboratory should clearly state whether the triglyceride analysis was glycerol blanked (e.g., designated as "Blanked Triglyceride" or "Unblanked Triglyceride"). Physicians need to be educated as to how the inclusion of a glycerol blank may alter the meaning of the results.
   - Glycerol blanking of triglyceride measurements must be done in laboratories participating in the CDC Lipoprotein Standardization Program and is recommended for laboratories that specialize in assessment of lipid status, have large populations of hyperlipidemic subjects, or participate in clinical or basic research.
   - Glycerol blanking of triglyceride analyses does not have to be routinely conducted on outpatient samples unless economically feasible. However, because of the potential for higher glycerol concentrations in hospital inpatient specimens, all inpatient specimens should be routinely glycerol blanked.
9. *Goals for analytical performance.* The NCEP goals for analytical performance differ slightly from CDC standardization criteria because NCEP goals are stated in terms of total error, which reflects both bias and imprecision,[238] whereas CDC standardization criteria consider each separately. NCEP recommendations for total error are shown in Table 26-27.

These guidelines were established after considering levels of accuracy and imprecision that are achievable in well-controlled research and clinical laboratories.[238] A laboratory can approximate its conformance to the total error recommendations using the following equation:

$$\text{Total error} = \%\,\text{Bias} + 1.96\,(\text{CVa}) \quad (21)$$

TABLE 26-26 Representative Preanalytical Sources of Variation (Including Biological)

	TC	HDL-C	TG	LDL-C
Intraindividual biological variation of healthy individuals (coefficient of variation)	6.5%	7.5%	23.7%	8.2%
Sampling				
Nonfasting	NC	–	++	–
Prolonged total fasting	++	–	+	+
Posture from standing to:				
Supine	–	—	—	—
Sitting	–	–	–	–
Anticoagulants from serum:				
Plasma	–	–	–	–
Behavioral				
Diet				
Saturated fatty acids (palmitic acid)	+	NC	+	+
Monounsaturated fatty acids	–	NC	–	–
Polyunsaturated fatty acids	—	–	NC	—
Cholesterol intake	+	NC	NC	+
Fish oil	NC	NC	–	NC
Obesity	+	–	++	+
Smoking	+	–	++	+
Exercise (strenuous)	–	+	–	–
Alcohol intake	+	+	++	–
Clinical Sources				
Myocardial infarction				
24 hr	NC	NC	NC	NC
6 wk	–	–	NC	–
Stroke	–	NC	NC	–
Hypertension diuretics	+	–	++	+
Nephrosis	++	NC	++	++
Diabetes (insulin resistance)	+	–	++	++
Infections	–	–	++	–
Pregnancy > second trimester	+	NC	++	+
Transplantation				
Cyclosporine	++	–	+	++
Prednisone	+	–	++	+

From Cooper GR, Myers GL, Smith SJ, Schlant RC. Blood lipid measurements: Variation and practical utility. JAMA 1992; 267:1652-60. Copyright 1992, American Medical Association.

TC, Total cholesterol; *HDL-C,* high-density lipoprotein cholesterol; *TG,* triglycerides; *LDL-C,* low-density lipoprotein cholesterol; +, minimal to moderate increase; ++, moderate to high increase; –, minimal to moderate decrease; —, moderate to high decrease; *NC,* essentially no change or trend.

where % bias is the mean laboratory difference between the measured value for a serum control pool and the reference value for the pool, and CVa is the overall analytical CV for the pool, including within and among run variations, and calculated as:

$$\frac{\text{Standard deviation}}{\text{Laboratory mean}} \times 100 \qquad (22)$$

Bias should be calculated as the difference from reference values rather than from manufacturers' stated values when these differ.

The individual biases and CVs shown in Table 26-27 should be viewed as examples of conditions under which the total error criteria can be met. A laboratory with less bias can tolerate slightly greater imprecision without exceeding the total error criteria. Conversely, imprecision must be lower if

TABLE 26-27 National Cholesterol Education Program Recommendations for Analytical Performance of Lipid and Lipoprotein Measurements

	Total Error (%)	Consistent With	
		Bias (%)	CV (%)
Cholesterol	8.9	≤±3	≤3
Triglycerides	≤15	≤±5	≤5
HDL cholesterol	≤13	≤±5	≤4
LDL cholesterol	≤12	≤±4	≤4

CV, Coefficient of variation; *HDL,* high-density lipoprotein; *LDL,* low-density lipoprotein.

TABLE 26-28 CDC Standardization Criteria for Lipid and Lipoprotein Measurement

	Bias*†(%)	CV†(%)
Cholesterol	≤±3	≤3
Triglyceride	≤±5	≤5
HDL cholesterol‡	≤±5	≤4

CV, Coefficient of variation; *CDC,* Centers for Disease Control and Prevention; *HDL,* high-density lipoprotein.
*With respect to reference values.
†Maximum allowable.
‡CVs shown apply at HDL cholesterol concentrations greater than 40 mg/dL. At lower concentrations, the precision criteria are based on standard deviation. Acceptable standard deviation is 2.0 mg/dL by July, 1997 and 1.7 mg/dL by 1998.

bias increases. For example, a laboratory operating with a bias of 3% and a CV of 3% for cholesterol would have a total error of 3% + (1.96 × 3%), or 8.9%. If, however, bias is only 1%, the CV could be as high as 4% without exceeding the criteria for total error [1% + (1.96 × 4%) = 8.8%]. (In practice, many laboratories can achieve total errors under 6%, assuming a bias of 2% and CV of 2%.)

It is important to note that the NCEP panels considered that the physician usually does not distinguish between lipid and lipoprotein measurements on the basis of the methodology used to make the measurements. For this reason, the NCEP guidelines do not distinguish between measurements made in the laboratory or those made in alternative settings with desktop analyzers or other methods.

As mentioned previously, CDC standardization criteria consider bias and imprecision separately. For this reason, each of the two criteria must be met to achieve standardization. Current CDC standardization criteria are shown in Table 26-28.

The NCEP guidelines as summarized previously are directed primarily to laboratories and users of the laboratory measurements. The reader is referred to the original reports for more extensive discussions of these issues.[237,238] The NCEP panels have also made a number of other recommendations to improve lipid and lipoprotein measurements, only several of which are mentioned here. First, it was recommended that manufacturers of calibration materials, control pools, and analytical systems calibrate their materials and methods to provide RM equivalent values. Many manufacturers are now doing this, which probably accounts for the relatively small interlaboratory biases for total and HDL cholesterol, as reflected in Table 26-24.

Lipoprotein Separation Procedures

Several methods for separating lipoprotein fractions for subsequent analysis are included in the Evolve site that accompanies this book at http://evolve.com/Tietz/textbook.

APOLIPOPROTEINS

Apolipoproteins are measured by a wide variety of immunoassays, including radioimmunoassay (RIA), ELISA, radial immunodiffusion (RID), immunoturbidimetric assay, and immunonephelometric assay. The concentration of a particular apolipoprotein usually determines the immunotechnique used for its measurement.

Apolipoproteins A-I and B-100

Immunoturbidimetry and immunonephelometry are widely used to measure apo A-I and apo B-100, which are present at relatively high concentrations. According to the College of American Pathologists Proficiency Testing Survey, all clinical laboratories in the United States that are involved in the measurement of apo A-I and apo B-100 use one of these two approaches.[47] Alternatively, more sensitive techniques, such as ELISA and RIA, are perhaps more suitable for those apolipoproteins present at much lower concentrations, such as apo C-I and apo C-II. Additional information about the various analytical techniques used in the determination of apolipoprotein concentrations is provided later.

The following paragraphs discuss some unique analytical issues that pertain to apolipoprotein testing.[149]

Presence of a Given Apolipoprotein on Different Lipoproteins

Apolipoprotein B-100, for example, is present on LDL, IDL, VLDL, and Lp(a) particles, which vary significantly in size and composition. To determine the concentration of total apo B-100 concentration correctly, the anti–apo B-100 antibody used must be able to recognize apo B-100 present on the various lipoprotein classes equally and display similar kinetic patterns with all of them.[263]

"Masking" Phenomenon

Unlike other plasma proteins, such as transferrin and prealbumin, apolipoproteins circulate in the bloodstream as part of the lipoprotein complex. As discussed earlier, lipoprotein particles are heterogenous spheres consisting of lipids and apolipoproteins. The antigenic sites of these proteins are often covered by lipids.[265,292] To have a maximal antigen-antibody interaction, these epitopes must be unmasked. Nonionic detergents such as Tween 20 or Tween 80 are usually added to the assay buffer to disrupt the lipoprotein particles and make all antigenic sites on the apolipoproteins accessible to the antibodies.[195,214]

Suitable Antibodies (Polyclonal Versus Monoclonal)

Polyclonal antibodies are widely used in clinical laboratories for the measurement of plasma protein concentrations. However, immunoassays are often sensitive to the nature of the antibody used.[292] The development of polyclonal antibodies is affected by several factors, such as the purity and dose of the antigen used, the species of host animal, and the immunization procedure. Monoclonal antibodies are viewed as a viable alternative to alleviate these problems. However, the expression of particular epitopes varies with the lipoprotein particles and among individuals; in addition, the apolipoproteins themselves are polymorphic in nature. Therefore the use of a single monoclonal antibody might not detect a particular variant. If a monoclonal antibody is used in the determination of an apolipoprotein, it should be directed to an epitope that is expressed on all polymorphic forms of that particular apoprotein. Furthermore, the epitope should be equally reactive to the antibodies regardless of which lipoprotein class contains it. Alternatively a mixture of monoclonal antibodies directed at different epitopes of the apolipoprotein may also be used. Such mixtures are referred to as "panmonoclonal" antibodies.

Availability of Primary Calibrators

In general, to standardize a particular protein, a purified form of that protein is used as a primary calibrator (see Chapter 20). The purified preparation must, however, express the same immunoreactivity as the native protein. Unfortunately, once removed from its natural milieu, apo B-100 is insoluble in aqueous buffers.[161] This phenomenon is attributed to the very hydrophobic nature of apo B-100. An LDL preparation with density of 1.030 to 1.050 g/mL, often referred to as "narrow-cut" LDL, is generally used as the primary standard for apo B-100. The protein concentration of the purified preparation is determined by amino acid analysis. In contrast, freshly purified apo A-I is soluble in aqueous buffers and is suitable as a primary standard.

As indicated earlier, several immunotechniques are used for the quantification of apo A-I and apo B-100. These techniques are affected differently by the analytical issues discussed previously. RIA and ELISA, for example, are normally used for the determination of analytes present at these very low concentrations (nanograms per milliliter). Therefore large dilutions (up to 40,000-fold) are required when these techniques are applied to apo A-I or apo B-100 measurement, which can result in a substantial analytical error. In addition, these assays are relatively time consuming and not easily automated, and RIA requires the use of isotopes. However, these techniques permit the use of monoclonal or polyclonal antibodies and primary or secondary calibrators, and are less affected by the matrix of the specimen, thus permitting the determination of protein concentration in the presence of lipemia. RID is a slow technique. For example, it takes up to 3 days for VLDL to complete migration through the gel. It is also less precise than automated assays and yields lower apo B-100 values than those obtained by other techniques,[57,263] possibly in part because of the relative selectivity of RID for smaller apo B–containing particles. Either polyclonal or monoclonal antisera may be used with RID.[149] Immunoturbidimetric and immunonephelometric assays are fully automated, highly precise, and can use polyclonal or multiple monoclonal antibodies. However, they can be affected by the background turbidity of the specimen (e.g., in samples with high triglyceride concentrations). The addition of detergents to the assay buffers reduces the nonspecific light scattering, which has helped to diminish this problem.

Considerable effort has been expended over the past decade by national and international organizations in overcoming the problems of apo A-I and B-100 standardization.[57] The lack of internationally available secondary serum reference materials had been a major stumbling block in the standardization of these apolipoproteins. The Committee on Apolipoproteins of the IFCC embarked on an ambitious international collaborative study aimed at developing secondary serum reference materials that can be used, without fear of matrix interaction, as master calibrators for all current commercial assays.[171] This program has been successfully completed.[174,175] A lyophilized serum preparation for apo A-I, designated SP1-01, and a liquid-stabilized serum preparation for apo B-100, designated SP3-07, have been approved as international reference reagents by the World Health Organization (WHO). An apo A-I value of 150 mg/dL was assigned to SP1-01 by a highly standardized RIA calibrated with purified apo A-I for which the mass value had been determined by amino acid analysis.[174] An accuracy-based apo B-100 value of 122 mg/dL was assigned to SP3-07 using a nephelometric method that was calibrated with freshly isolated LDL for which the apo B-100 mass value was determined by a standardized sodium dodecyl sulfate–Lowry protein procedure.[175]

The WHO and the IFCC have appointed the CDC to be the repository for the WHO-IFCC First International Reference Reagents for Apolipoproteins A-I and B-100. Dr. Santica Marcovina of Northwest Lipid Research Laboratories (NWLRL) in Seattle, who is the former Chair of the IFCC Apolipoprotein Working Group, conducts the standardization and distribution program for manufacturers of instruments and reagents using an IFCC calibration protocol. This protocol involves establishing the linearity of dose response, the parallelism of the kinetic responses of standards and calibration sera, and the equality of the intercepts for the reference materials and an analysis of fresh-frozen sera. NWLRL can be contacted for standardization services and the distribution of apolipoprotein reference materials. These reference reagents are also available for reference laboratories in countries where standardized commercial methods are not readily available. It has been shown that through the use of these international reference materials, the analytical performance of apo A-I and apo B-100 measurement, in terms of accuracy and precision, is superior to that of HDL and LDL cholesterol.[174,175] This effort has demonstrated that the use of certified reference materials can significantly reduce the bias of apo A-I and apo B-100 measurements by different immunotechniques. However, an external quality assurance program using fresh or fresh-frozen samples and WHO-IFCC–based value assignments is indispensable in monitoring the performance of clinical chemistry laboratories and manufacturers to ensure that accurate apolipoprotein measurements are made. The NWLRL conducts a quarterly standardization program or Reference Lipoprotein Analysis Basic Survey that provides the accuracy base for cholesterol, triglyceride, HDL, and LDL cholesterol, and apo A-I and apo B-100. To minimize matrix effects, the survey uses fresh human serum and leads to certification of traceability to the National Reference System for cholesterol and to the WHO-IFCC International Reference Reagents for apo A-I and apo B-100.

Apolipoprotein measurements have been shown to further aid in the detection of the CHD risk and the diagnosis of hyperlipoproteinemia. For example, the measurement of apo B-100 provides a reliable clinical tool to identify subjects with an increased risk for CHD who may not be readily identified by the conventional cholesterol or lipoprotein cholesterol measurements (e.g., subjects with a borderline elevation of LDL cholesterol, or subjects with hypertriglyceridemia without an LDL cholesterol elevation). In addition, apo B-100 measurements can assess whether lipid-lowering drugs are effective in lowering the number of atherogenic apo B–containing lipoproteins. However, for apolipoprotein measurements to be used in routine clinical practice, clinically meaningful cut-off values for clinical decision making need to be established, and more information regarding their clinical utility is needed. The use of cut-off values for apo A-I and apo B-100 similar to those recommended by the NCEP for HDL and LDL cholesterol, respectively, has been suggested.[54,55] An apo A-I concentration of <120 mg/dL may be associated with an increased risk of CHD, whereas apo A-I ≥160 mg/dL may be protective. The apo B-100 cut points of 100 and 120 mg/dL approximately correspond to the LDL cholesterol cut points of 130 and 160 mg/dL, which fall at approximately the 50th and 75th percentiles, respectively. Therefore Sniderman and Cianflone have suggested that apo B-100 values greater than the 75th percentile should be regarded as high risk, and a value greater than the 50th percentile as moderate risk.[284]

Lipoprotein(a)

The structural heterogeneity of Lp(a) as a consequence of the apo(a) size heterogeneity has important implications for the accurate measurement of Lp(a) in human plasma.[10,172,173,179,180] Repeated antigenic determinants are present in variable numbers in different Lp(a) particles, and the immunoreactivity of the antibodies directed to these repeated epitopes can vary as a function of apo(a) size. As a consequence, immunoassays using polyclonal antibodies or monoclonal antibodies specifically directed to kringle 4 type 2 epitopes will tend to underestimate apo(a) concentration in samples with apo(a) of smaller size than the apo(a) present in the assay calibrator, and overestimate the apo(a) concentration in samples with larger apo(a). A detailed evaluation of the effect of apo(a) size heterogeneity on the measurement of Lp(a) has been reported.[173] Monoclonal antibody–based assays have the theoretical advantage that the antibodies can be immunochemically characterized and preselected on the basis of their specificity to single epitopes (e.g., those not located in kringle 4 type 2 domain). However, the characterization of monoclonal antibodies is a rather complex procedure, and none of the monoclonal antibodies currently used in commercially available assays has been characterized in terms of epitope specificity. An additional disadvantage of monoclonal antibodies is that they cannot be easily used in immunoassays that require the precipitation of the antigen-antibody complex.

Turbidimetric, nephelometric, radiometric, and enzymatic methods are currently used for Lp(a) measurement. Most of these assays, except the enzyme immunoassays (ELISA), are based on the use of polyclonal antibodies from various animal species. Commercially available, direct-binding, sandwich type ELISAs are usually based on the use of a combination of monoclonal and polyclonal antibodies. One approach takes advantage of the presence of both apo(a) and apo B in Lp(a) particles. In this approach, Lp(a) particles are "captured" using a polyclonal or monoclonal antibody to apo(a), and an enzyme-conjugated antibody to apo B-100 used as the detection antibody. An ELISA method based on this approach has been described and is commercially available.[298] In another approach, both the capture and detection antibodies are specific for apo(a). At present, it is not clear which approach would be better with respect to estimating the risk for CHD or stroke because the pathogenic mechanisms involved have not yet been elucidated. Thus it is not known whether the risk is associated simply with an increased number of Lp(a) particles in the circulation (as measured using an anti–apo B antibody) or also related to the presence of particular size polyforms [as might be detected more readily with anti-apo(a) detection antibodies]. It is likely that both factors influence the risk.

Historically, Lp(a) concentrations have been reported in terms of total Lp(a) particle mass,[3] or alternatively in terms of Lp(a) protein.[172] If the aim is to provide Lp(a) values that are independent of apo(a) size, it is recommended that the Lp(a) assay use antibodies directed to an apo(a) domain other than kringle 4 type 2, or to the apo B-100 component of Lp(a). This would allow the values to be expressed in nanomoles per liter.[4] Panmonoclonal mixtures of antibodies to kringle 4 type 2 may be preferred if particular sizes of polyforms contribute to the risk.

At present, Lp(a) measurements are not standardized, and most of the Lp(a) assays have not been evaluated for their apo(a) size sensitivity. As a result, Lp(a) values reported in clinical studies are difficult to compare. Despite this, a value of about 30 mg/dL of total Lp(a) particle mass has traditionally been used as a cutoff above which elevated levels of Lp(a) are associated with an increased risk of CHD. Lp(a) concentrations can also be expressed in terms of particle number, the mass of apo(a), apo B-100, or Lp(a) cholesterol. Which approach will best predict the risk for CHD has yet to be determined. At present, Lp(a) values are most commonly expressed in terms of total Lp(a) mass, but this should be confirmed with the laboratory making the measurements. In view of the current lack of RMs or standardization procedures for Lp(a), it is difficult to define precise cutoffs that can be used to make clinical decisions. Although less than ideal, one approach would be to establish a reference interval for each assay, and report individual results in terms of percentile values within these intervals. In whites, patients with Lp(a) values above the 80th percentile can be considered at an increased risk for coronary atherosclerosis. However, because Lp(a) values can vary among ethnic groups, reference values need to be population based. Furthermore, such cutoffs may also have to be racially specific. For example, African Americans in general have significantly higher Lp(a) concentrations than whites,[181] but do not manifest a higher incidence of CHD. An IFCC committee, along lines similar to the apo A-I and B-100 committee, has developed reference materials to be used with all commercially available Lp(a) methods.[300,301] As expected, the use of a common calibrator led to harmonization of Lp(a) results but not total standardization.[176] Only when appropriate antibodies are used can standardization be achieved.

Virtually all retrospective case-control studies in whites have reported a strong association between increased Lp(a) and the risk of CHD. In contrast, prospective studies have provided contradictory results, with four of them finding an association between high Lp(a) concentrations and CHD and three not finding any association. Interestingly, the few clinical studies in which Lp(a) was evaluated as a CHD risk factor in African Americans suggest that elevated Lp(a) is not as important a risk factor in this group.

Several studies have suggested that apo(a) size isoforms may be related to a high prevalence of CHD (see earlier discussion). The procedure with the highest resolution and sensitivity for determination of apo(a) phenotypes involves separation of apo(a) on agarose gel electrophoresis, immunoblotting with a specific antibody, and detection with ^{125}I-labeled protein A.[181] This approach identifies at least 34 apo(a) polymorphs. It can be used to express apo(a) size in terms of kringle number, and is consistent with observations on the size variation of the apo(a) gene obtained by pulsed-field gel electrophoresis and genomic blotting.[178]

Apolipoprotein E

As discussed earlier, homozygosity for apo E_2 is characteristic of type III familial hyperlipoproteinemia. Homozygosity for apo E_2 is a necessary but not sufficient condition for expression of the type III hyperlipoproteinemia; a second gene defect or condition appears to be required to cause the characteristic hyperlipidemia. Heterozygosity for some rare apo E mutants may also be associated with type III hyperlipoproteinemia.[311] The study of apo E variants has assumed greater importance in the last few years because of the association between the apo E_4 allele and Alzheimer's disease and dementia.[279] How apo E_4 is related to these disorders is unknown.

Traditionally the determination of apo E isoforms was assessed by isoelectric focusing (IEF) techniques that permit identification of charge variations of the different isoforms. In the early studies, IEF was performed on VLDL that had been extracted to remove the lipids. The separated proteins were then stained for protein.[325] This approach is not used as frequently today because it requires a relatively large volume of plasma and the expensive and time-consuming step of ultracentrifugation to isolate VLDL. Apo E phenotypes are now assessed by IEF of a small volume of plasma followed by immunoblotting with specific antibodies to apo E. This approach can be applied in the clinical laboratory and is well adapted to large-scale population studies. However, it is important that the samples are analyzed fresh, or if stored, that they are kept at −70 °C before analysis to minimize the introduction of artifacts. Misclassification can occur because of posttranslational modifications or nonenzymatic glycation of apo E, the presence of rare variants that have the same charge as the common isoforms, overlooked faint apo E_4 bands, and false-positive apo E_2 bands. The interpretation of the patterns requires significant experience in the use of the technique.

The availability of techniques based on the polymerase chain reaction (PCR) permits an analysis of the variation in the nucleotide sequence of the apo E gene (Figure 26-27). One approach for apo E genotyping uses oligonucleotides to amplify apo E gene sequences containing amino acid positions 112 and 158; the amplified products are digested with *Hha*I and subjected to electrophoresis on polyacrylamide gels.[112] Alternatively, allele-specific oligonucleotide (ASO) primers can be used to specifically amplify E_2, E_3, and E_4 polymorphic sequences of the apo E gene.[99,330] Another approach, the amplification refractory mutation system (ARMS), is based on the strictness of the PCR primer for the 3′ end mismatch and is simple, rapid, and nonisotopic. The reagent costs for the ARMS assay are, however, higher than for the restriction isotyping assay. The single-strand conformation polymorphism (SSCP) method has also been used for apo E genotyping.[73] It can detect unknown apo E mutations but is not very convenient because it requires radiolabeled primers. Because restriction isotyping is rapid, requiring only 1 hour to digest the PCR product and several hours for electrophoresis, and does not require radioactive reagents, it may be the most practical method for apo E genotyping in the diagnostic clinical laboratory. Good-quality deoxyribonucleic acid (DNA) ensures proper amplification and prevents the presence of artifactual bands. Because of potential errors in interpretation or unpreventable artifacts in the apo E phenotype method, apo E genotyping is more reliable for determining the common apo E alleles and would be the method of choice if DNA or whole blood is available. However, most apo E genotyping methods do not detect rare mutations. Discrepancies of 5% to 20% between the results of phenotyping and genotyping have been reported.

OTHER CARDIAC RISK FACTORS

Despite the strong association of lipid concentrations with a CHD risk, it has been long recognized that half of all myocardial infarctions occur among individuals without overt hyperlipidemia. In the Women's Health Study (WHS), for example, 77% of future cardiovascular events occurred among those with LDL cholesterol concentrations <160 mg/dL, and 46% occurred among those with LDL cholesterol <130 mg/dL.[253] Furthermore, in a 2003 study analysis of more than 120,000 patients, approximately 20% of all coronary events occurred in the absence of any of the major classical risk factors: hyperlipidemia, hypertension, diabetes, and smoking.[133] Another large study showed that 85% to 95% of participants with CHD had at least one conventional risk factor, but so too did those participants without CHD, despite follow-up for as long as 30 years.[100] These observations raise the question whether only traditional risk factors are adequate to identify all individuals at an increased risk of CHD.

A wide variety of nonlipid biochemical markers have been suggested in an effort to better identify those individuals at an increased CHD risk, including markers of fibrinolytic and hemostatic function (tissue type plasminogen activator antigen, plasminogen activator inhibitor-1, fibrinogen, von Willebrand, D-dimer, thrombin-antithrombin III complex, and factors V, VII, and VIII), homocysteine, and markers of inflammation (high-sensitivity C-reactive protein (hsCRP), serum amyloid A, interleukins, adhesion molecules, heat shock proteins, and matrix metalloproteases). Clinically the use of most of these markers in screening is of limited value for one or more of the following reasons:

1. Lack of standardization among available methods (e.g., fibrinogen)
2. Inconsistent findings from prospective epidemiological studies regarding their ability to independently predict a future CHD risk (see discussion on homocysteine later in this chapter)
3. Inability to significantly improve prognostic value when added to traditional lipid screening or existing global risk prediction algorithms, such as the Framingham risk score (e.g., tissue type plasminogen activator)

In this section, hsCRP and homocysteine are discussed in more detail.

HIGH-SENSITIVITY C-REACTIVE PROTEIN

Tillet and Francis in 1930 described a substance that was present in the sera of acutely ill patients and able to bind the cell wall C-polysaccharide of *Streptococcus pneumoniae* and agglutinate the organisms. In 1941 the substance was shown to be a protein and given the name *C-reactive protein (CRP).*

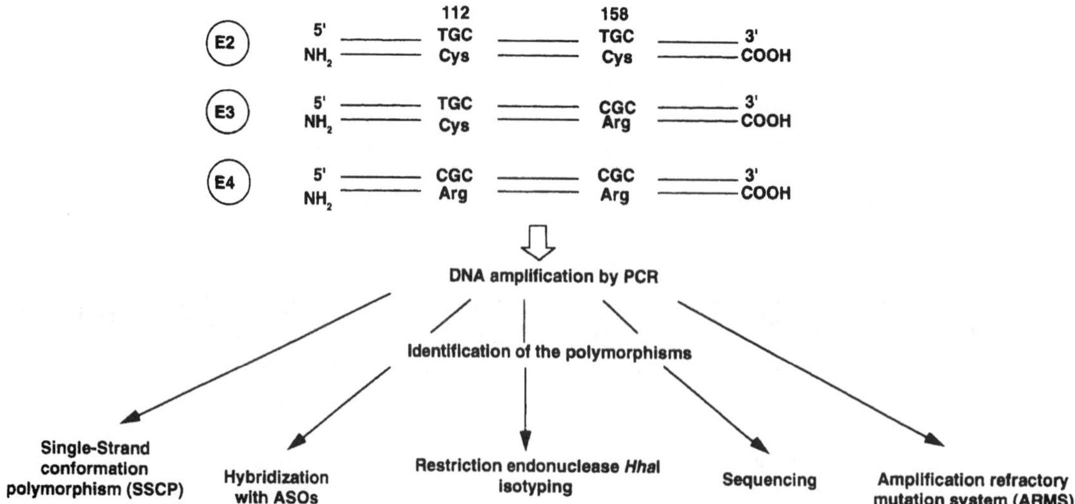

Figure 26-27 Different methods for investigating apolipoprotein E polymorphism at the genomic level. *PCR,* polymerase chain reaction; *ASO,* allele-specific oligonucleotide. *(From Siest G, Pillot T, Regis-Bailly A, et al. Apolipoprotein E: An important gene and protein to follow in laboratory medicine. Clin Chem 1995;41:1068-86.)*

CRP was subsequently shown to be an acute phase reactant and important in the nonspecific host defense against inflammation, especially infection (see Chapter 20) and is routinely monitored as an indication of infection and autoimmune diseases using methods having detector limits of 3 to 8 mg/L.

Chronic inflammation is an important component in the development and progression of atherosclerosis, and numerous epidemiological studies have demonstrated that increased serum CRP concentrations are positively associated with a risk of future coronary events, such as coronary artery disease, cerebrovascular disease, or peripheral arterial disease.[140,247-249] It has also been shown to be predictive of future events in patients with acute coronary syndromes and in patients with stable angina and coronary artery stents.[264]

The use of CRP for these purposes requires the use of hsCPR assays having detection limits less than 0.3 mg/L.[264] A number of automated immunoturbidimetric and immunonephelometric assays are commercially available and capable of sensitive and precise measurements at low concentrations of CRP. The analytical performance of nine of these assays has been evaluated.[264]

In this section, we summarize the basic biochemistry, clinical significance, and analytical considerations of the measurement of hsCRP. Additional information is presented in Chapter 20.

Biochemistry

CRP consists of five identical, nonglycosylated polypeptide subunits noncovalently linked to form a disk-shaped cyclic polymer with a molecular weight of ~115 kDa. It contains little or no carbohydrate and is synthesized in the liver. Its production is controlled by interleukin-6 and it binds to polysaccharides present in many bacteria, fungi, and protozoal parasites and polycations, such as histones.

Clinical Significance

Of the markers mentioned previously in this chapter, only hsCRP has fulfilled the required criteria for a novel marker of CHD risk, and national guidelines for its measurement in the primary prevention of CHD have recently been issued jointly by the American Heart Association (AHA) and the CDC (AHA/CDC).[226] Here we discuss the roles of hsCPR in CHD, the metabolic syndrome, diabetes, and hypertension, and its possible role in atherogenesis. We conclude with a discussion of possible preventive measures in those individuals with increased levels of hsCRP. A comprehensive review on this subject has been published.[23]

Cardiovascular Disease

Prospective epidemiological studies have consistently shown that a single hsCRP measurement is a strong predictor of myocardial infarction,[140,146,249,253] stroke,[146,249,253] peripheral vascular disease,[248,254] and sudden cardiac death[5] in individuals without a history of heart disease. The association between hsCRP and future CHD reflects the current understanding of vascular biology because it is known that chronic inflammation plays a pivotal role in atherogenesis. This association has been observed in the United States and Europe, in the middle aged and elderly, and in high- and usual-risk populations.[5,140,146] The association is apparent even in studies with follow-up periods up to 20 years, as seen in the Honolulu Heart Study.[60] In a direct comparison of traditional and novel biochemical markers of CHD risk, hsCRP was the strongest predictor of future coronary events.[249]

In general, those individuals with baseline hsCRP values in the top quartile of the sample distribution are 2 to 3 times more likely to experience a future vascular event than those in the bottom quartile. The association between hsCRP and future vascular events is linear and is independent of age, smoking, hypertension, dyslipidemia, and diabetes. For example, 8-year follow-up data from the Physicians' Health Study and the WHS showed that after adjustment for traditional risk factors, there was an increase in a future cardiovascular risk of 26% for men and 33% in women for each quintile increase in baseline hsCRP.[249]

Although most of the available data on hsCRP and incident CHD have been derived from nested case-control studies, event-free survival data from large cohorts have been published[250,253] thus enabling the estimation of absolute risks rather than relative risks of disease. Data from the WHS showed hsCRP to be a stronger predictor of the risk than LDL cholesterol (Figure 26-28) and demonstrated that event-free survival was poorest for persons with increases in both LDL cholesterol and hsCRP, and the best survival was observed for those with low values of both measures.[253] Event-free survival was significantly worse for those with high hsCRP and low LDL cholesterol as compared with those with high LDL cholesterol and low hsCRP (Figure 26-29).

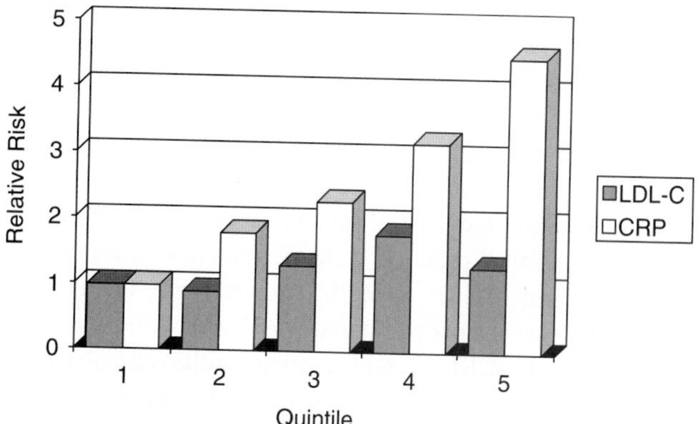

Figure 26-28 Head-to-head comparison of LDL cholesterol and hsCRP in their ability to predict future vascular events. *LDL,* Low-density lipoprotein cholesterol; *hsCRP,* high-sensitivity C-reactive protein. *(From Ridker PM, Rifai N, Rose L, Buring JE, Cook NR. Comparison of C-reactive protein and low-density lipoprotein cholesterol levels in the prediction of first cardiovascular events. N Engl J Med 2002;347:1557-65.)*

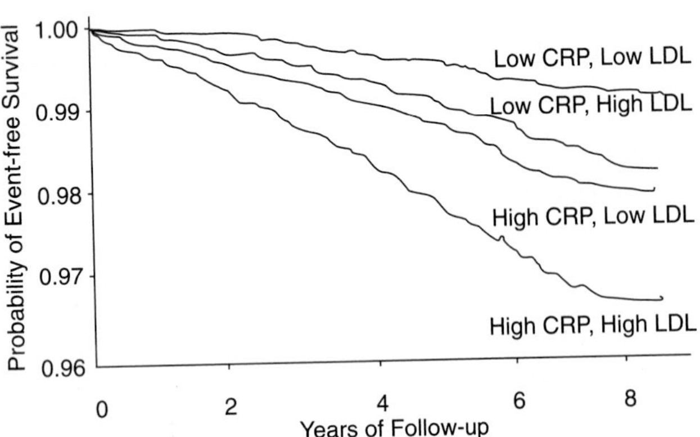

Figure 26-29 Cardiovascular event-free survival according to baseline levels of hsCRP and LDL cholesterol. *(From Ridker PM, Rifai N, Rose L, Buring JE, Cook NR. Comparison of C-reactive protein and low-density lipoprotein cholesterol levels in the prediction of first cardiovascular events. N Engl J Med 2002;347:1557-65.)*

Since hsCRP values minimally correlate with lipid concentrations and lipid parameters account for <3% to 5% of the variance in hsCRP measurement, the measurement of hsCRP does not replace but instead complements the evaluation of lipids and other classical CHD risk factors in primary prevention settings.[6,250,253] Data from the WHS demonstrated that hsCRP adds prognostic information not only at all levels of the risk defined by current LDL cut points of the NCEP but also at all levels of the risk specified by the Framingham risk score algorithm.[253]

Metabolic Syndrome, Diabetes, and Hypertension

Studies have demonstrated a significant association between hsCRP and the future risk of metabolic syndrome,[285] diabetes, and hypertension, conditions that confer an increased cardiovascular risk. The hsCRP values are positively correlated not only with components of the metabolic syndrome that are commonly assessed in clinical practice, such as increased triglycerides, reduced HDL cholesterol, obesity, high blood pressure, and high fasting glucose, but also with other components that are not easily captured in such settings, such as fasting insulin, microalbuminuria, and impaired fibrinolysis.[232] Data from the WHS showed that hsCRP measurement improves the cardiovascular risk prediction beyond that of the metabolic syndrome status as assessed in clinical practice[246]; those women with metabolic syndrome and hsCRP >3 mg/L were at twice the risk of future coronary events compared with those with metabolic syndrome and hsCRP <3 mg/L. Similar results were observed in the West of Scotland Coronary Prevention Study (WOSCOPS).[268]

Increased hsCRP concentrations have also been implicated in the development of type 2 diabetes mellitus. Prospective studies have found strong, graded relationships between hsCRP and incident diabetes, which in many instances persisted after adjustment for body mass index and other covariates.[233] In WOSCOPS, the top quintile of hsCRP was associated with a threefold risk of incident diabetes over a 5-year period compared with the lowest quintile[82] and in the WHS, the top quartile of hsCRP was associated with a fourfold risk during 4 years of follow-up compared with the lowest quartile.[233] These data support the hypothesis that inflammation, atherothrombosis, and diabetes are tightly interrelated disorders of the innate immune system.

Accumulating data also suggest a link between blood pressure and vascular inflammation, perhaps mediated by angiotensin II.[161] For example, angiotensin II infusion activates nuclear factor κB and leads to increased interleukin-6 expression in human vascular smooth muscle cells.[143] Moreover, cross-sectional studies demonstrate graded linear relationships between interleukin-6 and intercellular adhesion molecule-1 and both systolic and diastolic blood pressure.[43] The relationship between blood pressure, hsCRP, and incident cardiovascular events was assessed in the WHS.[25] Despite their strong correlation, hsCRP and blood pressure were independent determinants of future cardiovascular events during an 8-year follow-up period, and hsCRP retained incremental prognostic value at all levels of blood pressure. Compared with women with blood pressures of less than 120/75 mm Hg and hsCRP values of <3 mg/L, those with blood pressures of 160/95 mm Hg and hsCRP values of ≥3 mg/L were more than 8 times as likely to experience a future cardiovascular event. The hsCRP also predicts incident hypertension itself. In the same cohort, after adjustment for multiple potential confounders, those women in the highest quintile of hsCRP were at a 50% higher risk of developing hypertension compared with those in the lowest quintile.[277] Moreover, high hsCRP concentration was associated with an increased risk of incident hypertension at all baseline blood pressures and among individuals without traditional CHD risk factors. On the basis of these data, it has been hypothesized that hsCRP may play a critical role in the development of hypertension. Whether or not blood pressure reduction leads to reduced hsCRP values is uncertain and is being tested in an ongoing clinical trial.

Possible Role of CRP in Atherogenesis

It is not clear at present whether CRP is a marker that reflects systemic or vascular inflammation or is an actual participant in atherogenesis. However, findings from pathological and in vitro studies are increasingly supporting the latter. Recent reports have shown CRP to enhance expression of local endothelial cell surface adhesion molecules,[223] monocyte chemoattractant protein-1,[223] endothelin-1,[314] and endothelial plasminogen activator inhibitor-1[69]; reduce endothelial nitric oxide bioactivity[314]; increase the induction of tissue factor in monocytes[202] and LDL uptake by macrophages[338]; and co-localize with the complement membrane attack complex within atherosclerotic lesions.[304] In addition, it has been demonstrated that the expression of human CRP in CRP-transgenic mice directly enhances intravascular thrombosis in both arterial injury and photochemical injury models of endothelial disruption.[304]

Role in Disease Intervention

Although many behavioral and pharmacological interventions known to reduce the risk of clinical cardiovascular events have been linked to lower hsCRP values, it is not definitely known at present whether the lowering of hsCRP will necessarily lead to a reduction in vascular events. For example, a reduction not only in hsCRP but also in several proinflammatory cytokines and adhesion molecules was seen in obese premenopausal women assigned to a weight-loss program as compared with women in the control group.[336] Whether these effects translate into a reduced risk of subsequent cardiovascular events has not yet been elucidated.

Although no specific drugs are known to lower hsCRP concentrations, several pharmacological agents have demonstrated cardioprotective ability, such as aspirin and statins, with the latter being able to reduce hsCRP values. In the Physicians' Health Study, a large primary prevention trial, the reduction in the risk of future myocardial infarction associated with assignment to aspirin was 56% among those with baseline hsCRP concentrations in the highest quartile and declined proportionately with hsCRP values such that there was a reduction of only 14% among those in the lowest quartile, suggesting that aspirin may prevent ischemic events through antiinflammatory and antiplatelet effects.[247] The effect of aspirin on lowering hsCRP concentrations is uncertain at present.

The ability of statins to lower hsCRP was first described for pravastatin using data accumulated in the Cholesterol and Recurrent Events (CARE) trial.[251,252] These data were initially highly controversial because they suggested that statins have both lipid-lowering and antiinflammatory effects. However, confirmatory work rapidly showed the effect of statins on hsCRP to be a consistent and important class effect. Studies of atorvastatin, cerivastatin, lovastatin, pravastatin, and simvastatin have shown that, on average, median hsCRP concentrations decline 15% to 25% as early as 6 weeks after initiation of therapy.[21] Importantly the magnitude of LDL cholesterol reduction caused by statin therapy is minimally correlated with the magnitude of hsCRP reduction.[21]

Data from two large 5-year randomized trials suggest that the cardiovascular risk reduction attributable to statin therapy may be most marked for those with increased hsCRP concentrations at baseline. In the CARE trial, the proportion of recurrent events prevented by pravastatin was 54% among persons with increased hsCRP values but only 25% among persons with lower hsCRP values, even though baseline lipid concentrations were nearly identical in those with and without evidence of inflammation.[252] Similarly, in the Texas Air Force Coronary Atherosclerosis Prevention Study, lovastatin therapy was associated with a 42% reduction in first cardiovascular events among participants with low LDL cholesterol concentrations (<149 mg/dL) but high hsCRP values (>1.6 mg/L).[250] As a result of these provocative findings, JUPITER—a clinical trial specifically designed to test the efficacy of statins in reducing clinical cardiovascular events among persons with the high hsCRP/low LDL phenotype, who comprise an estimated 25% of the U.S. population—has recently been launched.

Analytical Considerations

As discussed in Chapter 20, historically, CRP has been measured in clinical laboratories to monitor active infection. Although such assays are automated and reproducible, they have a lower detection limit of 3 to 8 mg/L and thus are not sensitive enough to detect the low-end variations required for prediction of the vascular risk. Therefore high-sensitivity methods had to be developed for this clinical application. Of various techniques used by investigators and manufacturers to improve the sensitivity of CRP assays, the most successful approach has been to amplify the light-scattering properties of the antigen-antibody complex by covalently coupling latex particles to a specific antibody, a procedure that is easily automated using standard laboratory instrumentation. More than 30 types of hsCRP assays, most of which use this approach, are now commercially available.[158] In a study of nine such assays, all achieved a lowest detection limit of ≤0.3 mg/L, and five had within-laboratory analytical imprecision of <10% (i.e., reproducibilities >90%).[264] However, hsCRP assays from different laboratories show significant discrepancies in reported results, underscoring the need for additional standardization.[264]

Standardization

Agreement among hsCRP methodologies is essential because an individual patient's result will be interpreted within the context of nationally established cut points. A standardization program led by the CDC has been initiated to address this issue.[136] Phase I, which has been completed, had identified a suitable common calibrator. The European Community Bureau of Reference Certified Reference Material 470 (CRM 470) Phase II, which is ongoing, will verify whether the use of this standard leads to a harmonization of patients' results.

Biological Variability of CRP

Despite being an acute phase reactant, hsCRP exhibits a relatively low degree of intraindividual variability in clinically stable patients. In a study of such patients, the use of two independent measurements of hsCRP taken 90 days apart enabled the classification of 90% of participants into the exact or immediately adjacent biomarker tertile, a percentage comparable with that observed for cholesterol (Figure 26-30).[158,217] Furthermore, the age-adjusted correlation between two hsCRP measurements from blood samples drawn 5 years apart was 0.6, a value comparable with that of cholesterol and other lipid parameters.[251] Other groups of investigators reported a 3-year, age-adjusted reliability coefficient of 0.52.[141] Although findings from this epidemiological study of initially healthy middle-aged men suggest that three independent measurements be taken to maximize the biomarker's predictive ability,[141] whether serial assessment of hsCRP provides incremental clinical benefit is uncertain. Provided that a value of <10 mg/L is obtained, the AHA/CDC panel recommends the use of two hsCRP measures taken 2 or more weeks apart, with the average value used to estimate the vascular risk.[226] Since they may reflect subclinical infection, hsCRP values >10 mg/L should initially be disregarded and the test repeated when the patient has stabilized. Furthermore, since hsCRP values are unaffected by food intake and exhibit almost no circadian variation,[188,217] measurements can be made without regard for fasting status or time of day.

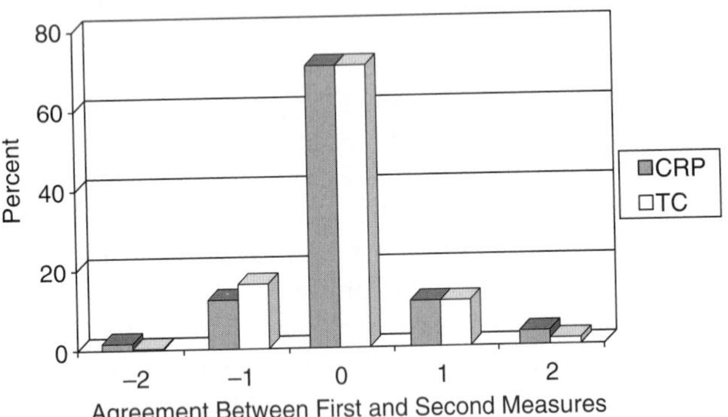

Figure 26-30 Within-person variability: comparison of hsCRP with total cholesterol (Ledue and Rifai 2003). *(From Ledue TB, Rifai N. Preanalytic and analytic sources of variations in C-reactive protein measurement: implications for cardiovascular disease risk assessment. Clin Chem 2003;49:1258-71.)*

Reference Values

Data from several large U.S. and European cohorts indicate that the distribution of circulating hsCRP concentrations appears comparable among men and women not using postmenopausal hormone replacement therapy (HRT),[120,262] with the 50th percentile for both genders being about 1.5 mg/L (Table 26-29). hsCRP concentrations are higher in women who use oral HRT than in women who do not,[253] which suggests that the increased hsCRP may be at least partly responsible for the increased risk of thrombotic events associated with oral HRT use observed in randomized trials, such as the WHS.[170]

Information on the distribution of hsCRP concentrations in nonwhite populations is sparse. In the nationally representative NHANES dataset, there were no significant differences in the distributions of hsCRP concentrations among white, African-American, and Mexican-American men[79] (Table 26-30). Moreover, a comparable hsCRP distribution was seen in Japanese men.[333] Although additional studies on

TABLE 26-29 Population Distributions of CRP, mg/L

	PERCENTILE						
Population	**5th**	**10th**	**25th**	**50th**	**75th**	**90th**	**95th**
American women†	0.2	0.3	0.6	1.5	3.5	6.6	9.1
American men	0.3	0.4	0.8	1.5	3.2	6.1	8.6
European women†	0.3	0.4	0.9	1.7	3.4	6.2	8.8
European men	0.3	0.6	0.8	1.6	3.3	6.5	8.6

Data from Rifai N, Ridker PM. Population distributions of C-reactive protein in apparently healthy men and women in the United States: implication for clinical interpretation. Clin Chem 2003;49:666-9; Imhof A, Frohlich M, et al. Distributions of C-reactive protein measured by high-sensitivity assays in apparently healthy men and women from different populations in Europe. Clin Chem 2003;49:669-72.
†Only women not taking hormone replacement therapy

TABLE 26-30 Distributions of CRP (mg/L) Among Men

	PERCENTILE						
	5th	**10th**	**25th**	**50th**	**75th**	**90th**	**95th**
White American	0.2	0.4	0.7	1.6	3.4	6.7	12.3
African American	0.1	0.2	0.7	1.7	3.9	8.2	13.2
Mexican American	0.2	0.4	0.6	1.6	3.2	6.3	9.8
Japanese	—	<0.3	0.4	1.6	3.5	7.8	—

Data from Ford ES, Giles WH, et al. Population distribution of high-sensitivity C-reactive protein among US men: findings from National Health and Nutrition Examination Survey 1999-2000. Clin Chem 2003;49:686-90; Yamada S, Gotoh T, et al. Distribution of serum C-reactive protein and its association with atherosclerotic risk factors in a Japanese population: Jichi Medical School Cohort Study. Am J Epidemiol 2001;153:1183-90.

the distribution and prognostic ability of CRP in nonwhite populations are clearly necessary, existing data is insufficient to support the exclusion of any racial or ethnic group from current guidelines for CRP testing.

Most studies have reported only a modest relationship between age (range, 18 to 88 years) and serum hsCRP concentrations.[120,262] In the WHS, for example, median hsCRP concentrations for individuals aged 45 to 54, 55 to 64, 65 to 74, and 75 years or older were 1.31, 1.89, 1.99, and 1.52 mg/L, respectively.[262]

Reference values of less than 1, 1 to 3, and greater than 3 mg/L, which correspond to approximate tertiles of the CRP distribution in healthy adults, are recommended for classification of individuals into low-, moderate-, and high-cardiovascular risk groups in primary prevention settings by the AHA/CDC panel.[226] Because of the prognostic additive effect of hsCRP to the lipid screen, an algorithm combining hsCRP and LDL cholesterol using the NCEP cut points has been proposed (Figure 26-31).[262] According to the AHA/CDC recommendation, hsCRP should be part of the global risk assessment of CHD in the primary prevention setting, and individuals with moderate risk as determined by the Framingham risk score will benefit the most from its measurement.[226]

Homocysteine

Many disorders are associated with increased levels of total homocysteine.[241] In this section, the basic biochemistry, clinical significance, and measurement of total homocysteine (tHcy) are summarized.

Basic Biochemistry

Homocysteine is a sulfur-containing amino acid with each molecule of homocysteine containing one atom of sulfur. It is formed during the metabolism of methionine and requires folic acid as a cofactor (see Figure 26-32). At low concentrations, homocysteine is either anabolized back to methionine in a cycle that involves tetrahydrofolate or catabolized to cysteine by enzymes that require vitamin B as a cofactor. Consequently a deficiency of folic acid or vitamins B_6 and B_{12} can result in increased levels of homocysteine (see Chapter 30).[138,269] Homocysteine does not normally accumulate in plasma because it is very unstable in aqueous solution and, when present in excess, undergoes oxidation to homocystine.

Clinical Significance

Numerous studies have suggested an association between elevated levels of circulating homocysteine and various vascular and cardiovascular disorders.* In addition, tHcy levels also are related to birth defects,[236] pregnancy complications,[318] psychiatric disorders,[213] and mental impairment in the elderly.[281] Clinically the measurement of tHcy is considered important (1) to diagnose homocystinuria, (2) to identify individuals with or at a risk of developing

*References 29, 66, 116, 193, 216, 228, 242.

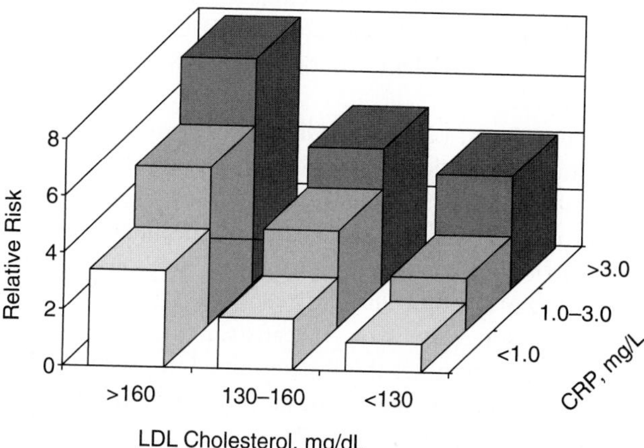

Figure 26-31 Algorithm for risk assessment of CHD risk employing CRP and LDL cholesterol. *(From Rifai N, Ridker PM. Population distributions of C-reactive protein in apparently healthy men and women in the United States: implication for clinical interpretation. Clin Chem 2003;49:666-9.)*

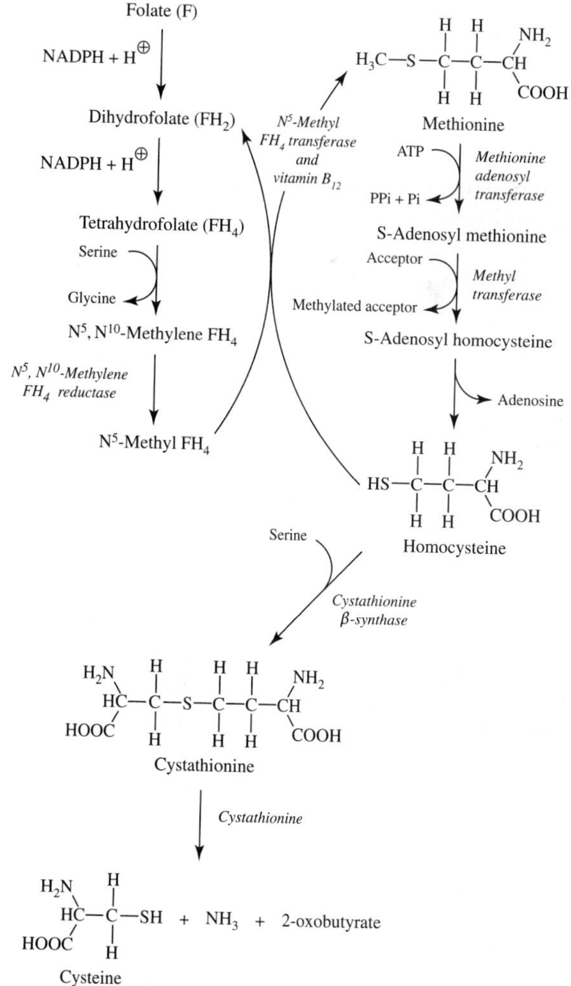

Figure 26-32 Biochemical pathways of the conversion of methionine to homocysteine and cysteine.

cobalamin or folate deficiency, and (3) to assess tHcy as a risk factor for cardiovascular disease (CVD) and other disorders.[40,46,241,320]

Although numerous studies have demonstrated a causal relationship between tHcy and CVD, there is still controversy about the clinical significance of this relationship as (1) the MTHFR 677C→T polymorphism is a strong risk factor for increased tHcy but not for CVD; (2) there is an apparent discrepancy between prospective and retrospective case-control studies; and (3) there is a lack of data from controlled clinical trials.[241]

Because of this concern over the clinical significance of the causal relationship between tHcy and CVD[28,152,168,239,288] Refsum and colleagues developed the following recommendations[241]:

- Measurement of tHcy in the general population to screen for CVD risk is not recommended.
- In young CVD patients (<40 years), tHcy should be measured to exclude homocystinuria.
- In patients with CVD or persons with a high risk of CVD events, a high tHcy concentration should be used as a prognostic factor for CVD events and mortality.
- CVD patients with tHcy >15 µmol/L belong to a high-risk group; it is especially important for them to follow a healthy life-style and to receive optimal treatments for known causal risk factors.
- Increased tHcy combined with low vitamin concentrations should be handled as a potential vitamin deficiency. Other causes of increased tHcy should be considered.

Measurement of Total Homocysteine

Physiologically, homocysteine exists in reduced, oxidized, and protein-bound forms.[193] Methods for tHcy were first introduced in the mid1980s that resolved the problems related to the presence of multiple unstable Hcy species in plasma by converting all Hcy species into the reduced form, HcyH, which is measured as an indication of tHcy content.[235,240,287] Consequently, modern methods require pretreatment of plasma or serum specimens with a reducing agent, such as dithioerythritol, dithiothreitol, mercaptoethanol, tributyl phosphine, and tris(2-carboxyl-ethyl) phosphine that converts all Hcy species into the reduced form, HcyH, which is measured as an indication of tHcy content.

Modern tHcy methods include enzyme immunoassays and chromatographic-based methods.[231,306,308] In practice, immunoassays[80] are most often used for routine purposes (e.g., fluorescence polarization immunoassay [FPIA] as run on Abbott's IMx and AxSYM platforms).[227,278] Chromatographic assays include amino acid analysis; high-performance liquid chromatography (HPLC) with ultraviolet, fluorescence, or electrochemical detection[9,76,307,308,316]; capillary electrophoresis with fluorescence detection; gas chromatography-mass spectrometry (GC-MS); and liquid chromatography with tandem MS (MS-MS).[42,70,231,308]

The different tHcy methods give comparable results[210,229,306] but there is a necessity for standardization of the tHcy assay.[306] A certified reference material is not currently available, but an IFCC working group is preparing such reference materials.

To obtain accurate results, it is recommended that specimens be refrigerated and quickly centrifuged.[193] If specimens are allowed to stand at room temperature, glycolysis can double homocysteine levels. Addition of fluoride or specific S-adenosylhomocysteine hydrolase inhibitors will prevent problems caused by glycolysis.[193] The short-term and long-term variability of plasma homocysteine measurements has been discussed.[86]

Reference intervals for fasting homocysteine levels have been reported to be 13 to 18 µmol/L for serum[212,308] and 10 to 15 µmol/L for plasma.[62] The reference interval for total homocysteine in pediatric patients has been reported to be 3.7 to 10.3 µmol/L.[317]

REFERENCES

1. Abuja PM, Esterbauer H. Simulation of lipid peroxidation in low-density lipoprotein by a basic "skeleton" of reactions. Chem Res Toxicol 1995;8: 753-63.
2. Alaupovic P. Apolipoproteins and lipoprotein. Atherosclerosis 1971;13:141-6.
3. Albers JJ, Hazzard WR. Immunochemical quantification of human plasma Lp(a) lipoprotein. Lipids 1974;9:15-26.
4. Albers JJ, Marcovina SM. Lipoprotein(a) quantification: comparison of methods and strategies for standardization. Curr Opin Lipidol 1994;5:417-21.
5. Albert CM, Ma J, et al. Prospective study of C-reactive protein, homocysteine, and plasma lipid levels as predictors of sudden cardiac death. Circulation 2002;105:2595-9.
6. Albert MA, Danielson E, et al. Effect of statin therapy on C-reactive protein levels: the pravastatin inflammation/CRP evaluation (PRINCE): a randomized trial and cohort study. JAMA 2001;286: 64-70.
7. American Academy of Pediatrics Committee on Nutrition: Indication for cholesterol testing in children. Pediatrics 1989;83:141-2.
8. American Academy of Pediatrics Committee on Nutrition: Prudent life-style for children: dietary fat and cholesterol. Pediatrics 1986;78:521-5.
9. Andersson A, Isaksson A, Brattstrom L, et al. Homocysteine and other thiols determined in plasma by HPLC and thio-specific postcolumn derivatization. Clin Chem 1993;39:1590-7.
10. Ariyo AA, Thach C, Tracy R. Lp(a) lipoprotein, vascular disease, and mortality in the elderly. N Engl J Med 2003;349:2108-15.
11. Arranz-Pena ML, Tasende-Mata J, Martin-Gil FJ. Comparison of two homogeneous assays with a pre-

cipitation method and an ultracentrifugation method for the measurement of HDL-cholesterol. Clin Chem 1998;44:2499-505.

12. Assmann G, Eckardstein A, Brewer HB, Jr. Familial Analphaliproteinemia: Tangier Disease. In: Scriver CR, Beaudet AL, Valle D, Sly WS, Childs B, Kinzler KW, Vogelstein B, eds. The Metabolic and Molecular Bases of Inherited Diseases, Vol. II. 8th ed. New York: McGraw-Hill, 2001:2937-81.
13. Assmann G, Herbert PN, Fredrickson DS, Forte T. Isolation and characterization of an abnormal high density lipoprotein in Tangier Disease. J Clin Invest 1977;60:242-52.
14. Austin MA, Breslow JL, Hennekens CH, Buring JE, Willett WC, Krauss RM. Low-density lipoprotein subclass patterns and risk of myocardial infarction. JAMA 1988;260:1917-21.
15. Bachorik PS. Electrophoresis in the determination of plasma lipoprotein patterns. In: Lewis L, Opplt JJ, eds. CRC Handbook of electrophoresis, Vol. II. Boca Raton: CRC Press, 1980:7.
16. Bachorik PS, Albers JJ. Precipitation methods for quantification of lipoproteins. Methods Enzymol 1986;129:78-100.
17. Bachorik PS, Lovejoy KL, Carroll MD, Johnson CL. Apolipoprotein B and AI distributions in the United States, 1988-1991: results of the National Health and Nutrition Examination Survey III (NHANES III). Clin Chem 1997;43:2364-78.
18. Bachorik PS, Rifkind BM, Kwiterovich PO. Lipids and dyslipoproteinemia. In: Henry JB, ed. Clinical Diagnosis and Management by Laboratory Methods, Vol. 19th ed. Philadelphia: W.B. Saunders, 1996: 208-36.
19. Bachorik PS, Walker R, Brownell KD, Stunkard AJ, Kwiterovich PO. Determination of high density lipoprotein-cholesterol in stored human plasma. J Lipid Res 1980;21:608-16.
20. Bachorik PS, Walker RE, Virgil DG. High-density-lipoprotein cholesterol in heparin-MnCl2 supernates determined with the Dow enzymic method after precipitation of Mn2+ with HCO3. Clin Chem 1984;30:839-42.
21 Balk EM, Lau J, et al. Effects of statins on nonlipid serum markers associated with cardiovascular disease: a systematic review. Ann Intern Med 2003;139: 670-82.
22. Bartlett GR. Phosphorus assay in column chromatography. J Biol Chem 1959;234:466.
23. Benzaquen LR, Yu H, et al. High sensitivity C-reactive protein: an emerging role in cardiovascular risk assessment. Crit Rev Clin Lab Sci 2002;39:459-97.
24. Berenson GS, Wattigney WA, Tracy RE, Newman WP, 3rd, Srinivasan SR, Webber LS, et al. Atherosclerosis of the aorta and coronary arteries and cardiovascular risk factors in persons aged 6 to 30 years and studied at necropsy (The Bogalusa Heart Study). Am J Cardiol 1992;70:851-8.
25. Blake GJ, Rifai N, et al. Blood pressure, C-reactive protein, and risk of future cardiovascular events. Circulation 2003;108:2993-9.
26. Blankenhorn DH, Nessim SA, Johnson RL, Sanmarco ME, Azen SP, Cashin-Hemphill L. Beneficial effects of combined colestipol-niacin therapy on coronary atherosclerosis and coronary venous bypass grafts. JAMA 1987;257:3233-40.
27. Bookstein L, Gidding SS, Donovan M, Smith FA. Day-to-day variability of serum cholesterol, triglyceride, and high-density lipoprotein cholesterol levels. Impact on the assessment of risk according to the National Cholesterol Education Program guidelines. Arch Intern Med 1990;150:1653-7.
28. Booth GL, Wang EE. Preventive health care, 2000 update: screening and management of hyperhomocysteinemia for the prevention of coronary artery disease events. The Canadian Task Force on Preventive Health Care. Canad Med Assoc J 2000;163:21-9.
29. Boushey CJ, Beresford SAA, Omenn GS, et al. A quantitative assessment of plasma homocysteine as a risk factor for vascular disease: Probable benefits of increasing folic acid intakes. JAMA 1995;274:1049-57.
30. Brensike JF, Levy RI, Kelsey SF, Passamani ER, Richardson JM, Loh IK, et al. Effects of therapy with cholestyramine on progression of coronary arteriosclerosis: results of the NHLBI Type II Coronary Intervention Study. Circulation 1984;69:313-24.
31. Breslow JL. Familial disorders of high-density lipoprotein metabolism. In: Scriver CR, Beaudet AL, Sly WS, Valle D, eds. The Metabolic and Molecular Bases of Inherited Diseases, Vol. II. 7th ed. New York: McGraw-Hill, 1995:2031-52.
32. Brown G, Albers JJ, Fisher LD, Schaefer SM, Lin JT, Kaplan C, et al. Regression of coronary artery disease as a result of intensive lipid-lowering therapy in men with high levels of apolipoprotein B. N Engl J Med 1990;323:1289-98.
33. Brown MS, Goldstein JL. Lipoprotein metabolism in the macrophage: implications for cholesterol deposition in atherosclerosis. Annu Rev Biochem 1983;52:223-61.
34. Brown MS, Goldstein JL. A receptor-mediated pathway for cholesterol homeostasis. Science 1986;232:34-47.
35. Brown SA, Hutchinson R, Morrisett J, Boerwinkle E, Davis CE, Gotto AM, Jr., Patsch W. Plasma lipid, lipoprotein cholesterol, and apoprotein distributions in selected US communities. The Atherosclerosis Risk in Communities (ARIC) Study. Arterioscler Thromb 1993;13:1139-58.
36. Brunzell JD, Deeb SS. Familial Lipoprotein Lipase Deficiency, Apo C-II Deficiency, And Hepatic Lipase Deficiency. In: Scriver CR, Beaudet AL, Sly WS, Valle

D, eds. The Metabolic Basis of Inherited Diseases, Vol. 8th ed. New York: McGraw-Hill, 2001: 2789-819.
37. Burstein M, Legmann P. Lipoprotein precipitation. Monogr Atheroscler 1982;11:1-131.
38. Buxtorf JC, Baudet MF, Martin C, Richard JL, Jacotot B. Seasonal variations of serum lipids and apoproteins. Ann Nutr Metab 1988;32:68-74.
39. Campos H, Blijlevens E, McNamara JR, Ordovas JM, Posner BM, Wilson PW, et al. LDL particle size distribution. Results from the Framingham Offspring Study. Arterioscler Thromb 1992;12:1410-9.
40. Carmel R, Jacobsen DW. Homocysteine in health and disease 2001:501 Cambridge University Press, Cambridge, UK.
41. Castelli WP, Doyle JT, Gordon T, Hames CG, Hjortland MC, Hulley SB, et al. HDL cholesterol and other lipids in coronary heart disease. The cooperative lipoprotein phenotyping study. Circulation 1977;55:767-72.
42. Chace DH, Hillman SL, Milllington DS, et al. Rapid diagnosis of homocystinuria and other hypermethioninemias by tandem mass spectrometry. Clin Chem 1996;42:349-55.
43. Chae CU, Lee RT, et al. Blood pressure and inflammation in apparently healthy men. Hypertension 2001;38:399-403.
44. Chait A, Albers JJ, Brunzell JD. Very low density lipoprotein overproduction in genetic forms of hypertriglyceridaemia. Eur J Clin Invest 1980;10: 17-22.
45. Chen CH, Albers JJ. Activation of lecithin: cholesterol acyltransferase by apolipoproteins E-2, E-3, and A-IV isolated from human plasma. Biochim Biophys Acta 1985;836:279-85.
46. Christen WG, Ajani UA, Glynn RJ, Hennekens CH. Blood levels of homocysteine and increased risks of cardiovascular disease: causal or casual?. Arch Intern Med 2000;160:422-34.
47. Chung BH, Segrest JP, Cone JT, Pfau J, Geer JC, Duncan LA. High resolution plasma lipoprotein cholesterol profiles by a rapid, high volume semi-automated method. J Lipid Res 1981;22:1003-14.
48. Chung BH, Segrest JP, Ray MJ, Brunzell JD, Hokanson JE, Krauss RM, et al. Single vertical spin density gradient ultracentrifugation. Methods Enzymol 1986;128:181-209.
49. Chung BH, Wilkinson T, Geer JC, Segrest JP. Preparative and quantitative isolation of plasma lipoproteins: rapid, single discontinuous density gradient ultracentrifugation in a vertical rotor. J Lipid Res 1980;21:284-91.
50. Cohn JS, McNamara JR, Cohn SD, Ordovas JM, Schaefer EJ. Postprandial plasma lipoprotein changes in human subjects of different ages. J Lipid Res 1988;29:469-79.
51. Cohn JS, McNamara JR, Schaefer EJ. Lipoprotein cholesterol concentrations in the plasma of human subjects as measured in the fed and fasted states. Clin Chem 1988;34:2456-9.
52. Cole TG. Glycerol blanking in triglyceride assays: is it necessary? Clin Chem 1990;36:1267-8.
53. Cone JT, Segrest JP, Chung BH, Ragland JB, Sabesin SM, Glasscock A. Computerized rapid high resolution quantitative analysis of plasma lipoproteins based upon single vertical spin centrifugation. J Lipid Res 1982;23:923-35.
54. Contois J, McNamara JR, Lammi-Keefe C, Wilson PW, Massov T, Schaefer EJ. Reference intervals for plasma apolipoprotein A-1 determined with a standardized commercial immunoturbidimetric assay: results from the Framingham Offspring Study. Clin Chem 1996;42:507-14.
55. Contois JH, McNamara JR, Lammi-Keefe CJ, Wilson PW, Massov T, Schaefer EJ. Reference intervals for plasma apolipoprotein B determined with a standardized commercial immunoturbidimetric assay: results from the Framingham Offspring Study. Clin Chem 1996;42:515-23.
56. Cooper GR, Smith SJ, Duncan IW, Mather A, Fellows WD, Foley T, et al. Interlaboratory testing of the transferability of a candidate reference method for total cholesterol in serum. Clin Chem 1986;32: 921-9.
57. Cooper GR, Smith SJ, Wiebe DA, Kuchmak M, Hannon WH. International survey of apolipoproteins A1 and B measurements (1983-1984). Clin Chem 1985;31:223-8.
58. Cortner JA, Coates PM, Bennett MJ, Cryer DR, Le NA. Familial combined hyperlipidaemia: use of stable isotopes to demonstrate overproduction of very low-density lipoprotein apolipoprotein B by the liver. J Inherit Metab Dis 1991;14:915-22.
59. Couderc R, Mahieux F, Bailleul S, Fenelon G, Mary R, Fermanian J. Prevalence of apolipoprotein E phenotypes in ischemic cerebrovascular disease. A case-control study. Stroke 1993;24:661-4.
60. Curb J D, Abbott RD, et al. C-reactive protein and the future risk of thromboembolic stroke in healthy men. Circulation 2003;107:2016-20.
61. Dallongeville J, Lussier-Cacan S, Davignon J. Modulation of plasma triglyceride levels by apoE phenotype: a meta-analysis. J Lipid Res 1992;33: 447-54.
62. Davignon J, Gregg RE, Sing CF. Apolipoprotein E polymorphism and atherosclerosis. Arteriosclerosis 1988;8:1-21.
63. de Keijzer MH, Elbers D, Baadenhuijsen H, Demacker PN. Evaluation of five different high-density lipoprotein cholesterol assays: the most precise are not the most accurate. Ann Clin Biochem 1999;36(Pt 2): 168-75.

64. Deacon AC, Dawson PJ. Enzymic assay of total cholesterol involving chemical or enzymic hydrolysis–a comparison of methods. Clin Chem 1979;25: 976-84.
65. DeLong DM, DeLong ER, Wood PD, Lippel K, Rifkind BM. A comparison of methods for the estimation of plasma low- and very low-density lipoprotein cholesterol. The Lipid Research Clinics Prevalence Study. JAMA 1986;256:2372-7.
66. den Heijer M, Koster T, Blom HJ, et al. Hyperhomocysteinemia as a risk factor for deep-vein thrombosis. N Engl J Med 1996;334:759-62.
67. Dennison BA, Kikuchi DA, Srinivasan SR, Webber LS, Berenson GS. Parental history of cardiovascular disease as an indication for screening for lipoprotein abnormalities in children. J Pediatr 1989;115: 186-94.
68. Dennison BA, Kikuchi DA, Srinivasan SR, Webber LS, Berenson GS. Serum total cholesterol screening for the detection of elevated low-density lipoprotein in children and adolescents: the Bogalusa Heart Study. Pediatrics 1990;85:472-9.
69. Devaraj S, Xu DY, et al. C-reactive protein increases plasminogen activator inhibitor-1 expression and activity in human aortic endothelial cells: implications for the metabolic syndrome and atherothrombosis. Circulation 2003;107:398-404.
70. Ducros V, Demuth K, Sauvant MP, Quillard M, Causse E, Candito M, et al. Methods for homocysteine analysis and biological relevance of the results. J Chromatogr B Anal Technol Biomed Life Sci 2002;781:207-6.
71. Durrington PN. Lipoprotein (a). Baillieres Clin Endocrinol Metab 1995;9:773-95.
72. Ellerbe P, Myers GL, Cooper GR, Hertz HS, Sniegoski LT, Welch MJ, White Et. A comparison of results for cholesterol in human serum obtained by the Reference Method and by the Definitive Method of the National Reference System for cholesterol. Clin Chem 1990;36:370-5.
73. Emi M, Wu LL, Robertson MA, Myers RL, Hegele RA, Williams RR, et al. Genotyping and sequence analysis of apolipoprotein E isoforms. Genomics 1988;3:373-9.
74. Enos WF, Holmes RH, Beyer J. Landmark article, July 18, 1953: Coronary disease among United States soldiers killed in action in Korea. Preliminary report. By William F. Enos, Robert H. Holmes and James Beyer. JAMA 1986;256:2859-62.
75. Esteban-Salan M, Guimon-Bardesi A, de La Viuda-Unzueta JM, Azcarate-Ania MN, Pascual-Usandizaga P, Amoroto-Del-Rio E. Analytical and clinical evaluation of two homogeneous assays for LDL-cholesterol in hyperlipidemic patients. Clin Chem 2000;46:1121-31.
76. Evrovski J, Callaghan M, Cole DEC. Determination of homocysteine by HPLC with pulsed integrated amperometry. Clin Chem 1995;41:757-8.
77. Executive Summary of The Third Report of The National Cholesterol Education Program (NCEP) Expert Panel on Detection, Evaluation, And Treatment of High Blood Cholesterol In Adults (Adult Treatment Panel III). JAMA 2001;285:2486-97.
78. Fei H, Maeda S, Kirii H, Fujigaki S, Maekawa N, Fujii H, et al. Evaluation of two different homogeneous assays for LDL-cholesterol in lipoprotein-X-positive serum. Clin Chem 2000;46:1351-6.
79. Ford ES, Giles WH, et al. Population distribution of high-sensitivity C-reactive protein among US men: findings from National Health and Nutrition Examination Survey 1999-2000. Clin Chem 2003;49: 686-90.
80. Frantzen F, Faaren AL, Alfheim I, Nordhei AK. Enzyme conversion immunoassay for determining total homocysteine in plasma or serum. Clin Chem 1998;44:311-6.
81. Franzin M, Ferro C, Ceriotti F, Carobene A, Martini R, Guerra E. Optimization of a designated comparison method (DCM) for triglycerides measurement. Clin Chem Lab Med 1999;37:S260.
82. Freeman DJ, Norrie J, et al. C-reactive protein is an independent predictor of risk for the development of diabetes in the West of Scotland Coronary Prevention Study. Diabetes 2002;1:1596-600.
83. Freedman DS, Srinivasan SR, Shear CL, Franklin FA, Webber LS, Berenson GS. The relation of apolipoproteins A-I and B in children to parental myocardial infarction. N Engl J Med 1986;315:721-6.
84. Friedewald WT, Levy RI, Fredrickson DS. Estimation of the concentration of low-density lipoprotein cholesterol in plasma, without use of the preparative ultracentrifuge. Clin Chem 1972;18:499-502.
85. Garcia RE, Moodie DS. Routine cholesterol surveillance in childhood. Pediatrics 1989;84:751-5.
86. Garg UT, Zheng Z-J, Folsom AR, et al. Short-term and long-term variability of plasma homocysteine measurement. Clin Chem 43;43:141-5.
87. Glueck CJ, Mellies MJ, Srivastava L, Knowles HC, Jr., Fallat RW, Tsang RC, et al. Insulin, obesity, and triglyceride interrelationships in sixteen children with familial hypertriglyceridemia. Pediatr Res 1977;11: 13-9.
88. Goldstein JL, Ho YK, Basu SK, Brown MS. Binding site on macrophages that mediates uptake and degradation of acetylated low density lipoprotein, producing massive cholesterol deposition. Proc Natl Acad Sci U S A 1979;76:333-7.
89. Goldstein JL, Hobbs HH, Brown MS. Familial Hypercholesterolemia. In: Scriver CR, Beaudet AL, Sly WS, Valle D, eds. The Metabolic and Molecular Bases of Inherited Diseases, Vol. 8th ed. New York: McGraw-Hill, 2001:2863-914.

90. Goldstein JL, Schrott HG, Hazzard WR, Bierman EL, Motulsky AG. Hyperlipidemia in coronary heart disease. II. Genetic analysis of lipid levels in 176 families and delineation of a new inherited disorder, combined hyperlipidemia. J Clin Invest 1973;52: 1544-68.
91. Gomez F, Camps J, Simo JM, Ferre N, Joven J. Agreement study of methods based on the elimination principle for the measurement of LDL- and HDL-cholesterol compared with ultracentrifugation in patients with liver cirrhosis. Clin Chem 2000;46:1188-91.
92. Gordon DJ, Trost DC, Hyde J, Whaley FS, Hannan PJ, Jacobs DR, Jr., Ekelund LG. Seasonal cholesterol cycles: the Lipid Research Clinics Coronary Primary Prevention Trial placebo group. Circulation 1987;76:1224-31.
93. Gordon T, Kannel WB, Castelli WP, Dawber TR. Lipoproteins, cardiovascular disease, and death. The Framingham study. Arch Intern Med 1981;141: 1128-31.
94. Gotto AM, Brown WV, Levy RI, Birnbaumer ME, Fredrickson DS. Evidence for the identity of the major apoprotein in low density and very low density lipoproteins in normal subjects and patients with familial hyperlipoproteinemia. J Clin Invest 1972;51:1486-94.
95. Gotto AM, Jr. Management of dyslipidemia. Am J Med 2002;112 Suppl 8A:10S-8S.
96. Gotto AM, Jr. Treating hypercholesterolemia: looking forward. Clin Cardiol 2003;26:I21-8.
97. Gotto AM, Jr., Pownall HJ, Havel RJ. Introduction to the plasma lipoproteins. Methods Enzymol 1986;128:3-41.
98. Gotto AM, Jr., Whitney E, Stein EA, Shapiro DR, Clearfield M, Weis S, et al. Relation between baseline and on-treatment lipid parameters and first acute major coronary events in the Air Force/Texas Coronary Atherosclerosis Prevention Study (AFCAPS/TexCAPS). Circulation 2000;101: 477-84.
99. Green EK, Bain SC, Day PJ, Barnett AH, Charleson F, Jones AF, Walker MR. Detection of human apolipoprotein E3, E2, and E4 genotypes by an allele-specific oligonucleotide-primed polymerase chain reaction assay: development and validation. Clin Chem 1991;37:1263-8.
100. Greenland P, Knoll MD, et al. Major risk factors as antecedents of fatal and nonfatal coronary heart disease events. JAMA 2003;290:891-7.
101. Griffin TC, Christoffel KK, Binns HJ, McGuire PA. Family history evaluation as a predictive screen for childhood hypercholesterolemia. Pediatric Practice Research Group. Pediatrics 1989;84:365-73.
102. Grundy SM. Cholesterol and coronary heart disease. A new era. JAMA 1986;256:2849-58.
103. Gwynne JT. High-density lipoprotein cholesterol levels as a marker of reverse cholesterol transport. Am J Cardiol 1989;64:10G-7G.
104. Hainline AJ, Karon J, Lippel K. Manual of Laboratory Operations. Bethesda: U.S. Department of Health and Human Services, 1982.
105. Halloran P, Roetering H, Pisani T, van den Berg B, Cobbaert C. Reference standardization and analytical performance of a liquid homogeneous high-density lipoprotein cholesterol method compared with chemical precipitation method. Arch Pathol Lab Med 1999;123:317-26.
106. Harris EK, Kanofsky P, Shakarji G, Cotlove E. Biological and analytic components of variation in long-term studies of serum constituents in normal subjects. II. Estimating biological components of variation. Clin Chem 1970;16:1022-7.
107. Harris N, Galpachian V, Thomas J, Iannotti E, Law T, Rifai N. Three generations of high-density lipoprotein cholesterol assays compared with ultracentrifugation/dextran sulfate-Mg2+ method. Clin Chem 1997;43:816-23.
108. Harris N, Galpchian V, Rifai N. Three routine methods for measuring high-density lipoprotein cholesterol compared with the Reference Method. Clin Chem 1996;42:738-43.
109. Harris N, Neufeld EJ, Newburger JW, Ticho B, Baker A, Ginsburg GS, et al. Analytical performance and clinical utility of a direct LDL-cholesterol assay in a hyperlipidemic pediatric population. Clin Chem 1996;42:1182-8.
110. Havel RJ. Determination and clinical significance of triglyceride-rich lipoprotein remnants. In: Rifai N, Warnick GR, Dominiczak M, eds. Handbook of lipoprotein testing, Vol. Washington DC: AACC Press, 2000:565-80.
111. Havel RJ, Kane JP. Introduction: Structure and metabolism of plasma lipoproteins. In: Scriver CR, Beaudet AL, Sly WS, Valle D, eds. The Metabolic and Molecular Bases of Inherited Diseases, Vol. 8th ed. New York: McGraw-Hill, 2001:2705-16.
112. Hixson JE, Vernier DT. Restriction isotyping of human apolipoprotein E by gene amplification and cleavage with HhaI. J Lipid Res 1990;31:545-8.
113. Hoang MP, Hirany SV, Parupia J, Devaraj S, Jialal I. Comparison of 2 homogeneous high-density lipoprotein cholesterol assays. Arch Pathol Lab Med 1998;122:1005-9.
114. Hobbs HH, Leitersdorf E, Goldstein JL, Brown MS, Russell DW. Multiple crm-mutations in familial hypercholesterolemia. Evidence for 13 alleles, including four deletions. J Clin Invest 1988;81: 909-17.
115. Holvoet P, Vanhaecke J, Janssens S, Van de Werf F, Collen D. Oxidized LDL and malondialdehyde-modified LDL in patients with acute coronary

syndromes and stable coronary artery disease. Circulation 1998;98:1487-94.

116. Homocysteine Syudies Collaboration. Homocysteine and risk of ischemic heart disease and stroke: a meta-analysis. JAMA 2002;288:2015-22.

117. Hoogewerf AJ, Cisar LA, Evans DC, Bensadoun A. Effect of chlorate on the sulfation of lipoprotein lipase and heparan sulfate proteoglycans. Sulfation of heparan sulfate proteoglycans affects lipoprotein lipase degradation. J Biol Chem 1991;266:16564-71.

118. Horiuchi Y, Takanohashi K, Oikawa S, Numabe A, Hishinuma A, Ieiri T. Measurement of serum low density lipoprotein-cholesterol in patients with hypertriglycemia. Electrophoresis 2000;21:293-6.

119. Hubbard RS, Hirany SV, Devaraj S, Martin L, Parupia J, Jialal I. Evaluation of a rapid homogeneous method for direct measurement of high-density lipoprotein cholesterol. Am J Clin Pathol 1998;110:495-502.

120. Imhof A, Frohlich M, et al. Distributions of C-reactive protein measured by high-sensitivity assays in apparently healthy men and women from different populations in Europe. Clin Chem 2003;49: 669-72.

121. Izawa S, Okada M, Matsui H, Horita Y. A new direct method for measuring HDL-cholesterol which does not produce any biased values. J Med Pharm Sci 1997;37:1385-8.

122. Jackson RL, Tajima S, Yamamura T, Yokoyama S, Yamamoto A. Comparison of apolipoprotein C-II-deficient triacylglycerol-rich lipoproteins and trioleoylglycerol/phosphatidylcholine-stabilized particles as substrates for lipoprotein lipase. Biochim Biophys Acta 1986;875:211-19.

123. Jialal I, Hirany SV, Devaraj S, Sherwood TA. Comparison of an immunoprecipitation method for direct measurement of LDL-cholesterol with beta-quantification (ultracentrifugation). Am J Clin Pathol 1995;104:76-81.

124. Johnson CL, Rifkind BM, Sempos CT, Carroll MD, Bachorik PS, Briefel RR, et al. Declining serum total cholesterol levels among US adults. The National Health and Nutrition Examination Surveys. JAMA 1993;269:3002-8.

125. Joint statement for physicians by the Committee on Atherosclerosis and Hypertension in Childhood of the Council on Cardiovascular Disease in the Young and the Nutrition Committee, American Heart Association: Diagnosis and treatment of primary hyperlipidemia in childhood. Circulation 1986;74:1181-A.

126. Jurgens G, Koltringer P. Lipoprotein(a) in ischemic cerebrovascular disease: a new approach to the assessment of risk for stroke. Neurology 1987;37: 513-15.

127. Kafonek SD, Derby CA, Bachorik PS. Biological variability of lipoproteins and apolipoproteins in patients referred to a lipid clinic. Clin Chem 1992;38:864-72.

128. Kakuyama T, Kimura S, Hasiguchi Y. Fully automated determination of HDL-cholesterol from human serum with Hitachi 911. Clin Chem 1994;40:A1104.

129. Kane JP, Havel RJ. Disorders of the biogenesis and secretion of lipoproteins containing the B apolipoproteins. In: Scriver CR, Beaudet AL, Sly WS, Valle D, eds. The Metabolic and Molecular Bases of Inherited Diseases, Vol. 8th ed. New York: McGraw-Hill, 2001:pp. 2717-52.

130. Karathanasis SK, Ferris E, Haddad IA. DNA inversion within the apolipoproteins AI/CIII/AIV-encoding gene cluster of certain patients with premature atherosclerosis. Proc Natl Acad Sci U S A 1987;84: 7198-202.

131. Kayamori Y, Hatsuyama H, Tsujioka T, Nasu M, Katayama Y. Endpoint colorimetric method for assaying total cholesterol in serum with cholesterol dehydrogenase. Clin Chem 1999;45:2158-63.

132. Khachadurian AK, Uthman SM. Experiences with the homozygous cases of familial hypercholesterolemia. A report of 52 patients. Nutr Metab 1973;15:132-40.

133. Khot U N, Khot MB, et al. Prevalence of conventional risk factors in patients with coronary heart disease. JAMA 2003;290:898-904.

134. Khoury P, Morrison JA, Kelly K, Mellies M, Horvitz R, Glueck CJ. Clustering and interrelationships of coronary heart disease risk factors in schoolchildren, ages 6-19. Am J Epidemiol 1980;112:524-38.

135. Kimberly MM, Leary ET, Cole TG, Waymack PP. Selection, validation, standardization, and performance of a designated comparison method for HDL-cholesterol for use in the cholesterol reference method laboratory network. Clin Chem 1999;45:1803-12.

136. Kimberly M M, Vesper HW, et al. Standardization of immunoassays for measurement of high-sensitivity C-reactive protein (hsCRP). Phase I: Evaluation of secondary reference materials. Clin Chem 2003;49:611-16.

137. Kishi K, Ochiai K, Ohta Y, Uemura Y, Kanatani K, Nakajima K, Nakamura M. Highly sensitive cholesterol assay with enzymatic cycling applied to measurement of remnant lipoprotein-cholesterol in serum. Clin Chem 2002;48:737-41.

138. Klee GG. Cobalamin and folate evaluation; measurement of methylmalonic acid and homocysteine vs vitamin B12 and folate. Clin Chem 2000;46:1277-83.

139. Knuiman JT, Hermus RJ, Hautvast JG. Serum total and high density lipoprotein (HDL) cholesterol concentrations in rural and urban boys from 16 countries. Atherosclerosis 1980;36:529-37.

140. Köenig W, Sund M, et al. C-Reactive protein, a sensitive marker of inflammation, predicts future risk of coronary heart disease in initially healthy middle-

aged men: results from the MONICA (Monitoring Trends and Determinants in Cardiovascular Disease) Augsburg Cohort Study, 1984 to 1992. Circulation 1999;99:237-42.

141. Koenig W, Sund M, et al. Refinement of the association of serum C-reactive protein concentration and coronary heart disease risk by correction for within-subject variation over time: the MONICA Augsburg studies, 1984 and 1987. Am J Epidemiol 2003;158:357-64.
142. Kondo A, Muranaka Y, Ohta I, Kanno T. Dynamic reaction in a homogeneous HDL-cholesterol assay visualized by electron microscopy. Clin Chem 1999;45:1974-80.
143. Kranzhofer R, J Schmidt et al. Angiotensin induces inflammatory activation of human vascular smooth muscle cells. Arterioscler Thromb Vasc Biol 1999;19:1623-9.
144. Kubono K, Sakurabayashi I, Nawa T, Tsukada Y. Immunoglobulin interference in the homogeneous HDL cholesterol methods. Clin Chem 2000;46:A98.
145. Kukita H, Hiwada K, Kokubu T. Serum apolipoprotein A-I, A-II and B levels and their discriminative values in relatives of patients with coronary artery disease. Atherosclerosis 1984;51:261-7.
146. Kuller L H, Tracy RP, et al. Relation of C-reactive protein and coronary heart disease in the MRFIT nested case-control study. Multiple Risk Factor Intervention Trial. Am J Epidemiol 1996;44:537-47.
147. Kwiterovich PO, Jr. Diagnosis and management of familial dyslipoproteinemia in children and adolescents. Pediatr Clin North Am 1990;37:1489-523.
148. Kwiterovich PO, Jr. HyperapoB: a pleiotropic phenotype characterized by dense low-density lipoproteins and associated with coronary artery disease. Clin Chem 1988;34:B71-7.
149. Labeur C, Shepherd J, Rosseneu M. Immunological assays of apolipoproteins in plasma: methods and instrumentation. Clin Chem 1990;36:591-7.
150. Lackner C, Cohen JC, Hobbs HH. Molecular definition of the extreme size polymorphism in apolipoprotein(a). Hum Mol Genet 1993;2:933-40.
151. Lamarche B, Tchernof A, Mauriege P, Cantin B, Dagenais GR, Lupien PJ, Despres JP. Fasting insulin and apolipoprotein B levels and low-density lipoprotein particle size as risk factors for ischemic heart disease. JAMA 1998;279:1955-61.
152. Langman LJ, Cole DE. Homocysteine: cholesterol of the 90s?. Clin Chim Acta 1999;286:63-80.
153. LaRosa JC, Chambless LE, Criqui MH, Frantz ID, Glueck CJ, Heiss G, Morrison JA. Patterns of dyslipoproteinemia in selected North American populations. The Lipid Research Clinics Program Prevalence Study. Circulation 1986;73:I12-29.
154. Laskarzewski P, Morrison JA, deGroot I, Kelly KA, Mellies MJ, Khoury P, Glueck CJ. Lipid and lipoprotein tracking in 108 children over a four-year period. Pediatrics 1979;64:584-91.
155. Lauer RM, Clarke WR. Use of cholesterol measurements in childhood for the prediction of adult hypercholesterolemia. The Muscatine Study. JAMA 1990;264:3034-8.
156. Lawlor J, Pelczar D, Sane R, Siek G. Performance characteristic of the RDI homogeneous HDL cholesterol assay. Clin Chem 1998;44:A79.
157. Leary ET, Wang T, Baker DJ, Cilla DD, Zhong J, Warnick GR, et al. Evaluation of an immunoseparation method for quantitative measurement of remnant-like particle-cholesterol in serum and plasma. Clin Chem 1998;44:2490-8.
158. Ledue T B, Rifai N. Preanalytic and analytic sources of variations in C-reactive protein measurement: implications for cardiovascular disease risk assessment. Clin Chem 2003;49:1258-71.
159. Lee J, Lauer RM, Clarke WR. Lipoproteins in the progeny of young men with coronary artery disease: children with increased risk. Pediatrics 1986;78:330-7.
160. Lees RS, Wilson DE, Schonfeld G, Fleet S. The familial dyslipoproteinemias. Prog Med Genet 1973;9:237-90.
161. Libby P. Current concepts of the pathogenesis of the acute coronary syndromes. Circulation 2001;104:365-72.
162. Lin MJ, Hoke C, Ettinger B. Evaluation of homogeneous high-density lipoprotein cholesterol assay on a BM/Hitachi 747-200 analyzer. Clin Chem 1998;44:1050-2.
163. Lipid Research Clinics Coronary Primary Prevention Trial results. I. Reduction in incidence of coronary heart disease. JAMA 1984;251:351-64.
164. Lipid Research Clinics Coronary Primary Prevention Trial results. II. The relationship of reduction in incidence of coronary heart disease to cholesterol lowering. JAMA 1984;251:365-74.
165. Lippi U, Graziani MS, Manzato F, Schinella M. Procedure for effective separation of high-density lipoproteins in normal serum and hypertriglyceridemic samples. Clin Biochem 1987;20:313-15.
166. Maciejko JJ, Holmes DR, Kottke BA, Zinsmeister AR, Dinh DM, Mao SJ. Apolipoprotein A-I as a marker of angiographically assessed coronary-artery disease. N Engl J Med 1983;309:385-9.
167. Mahley RW, Innerarity TL, Rall SC, Jr., Weisgraber KH. Plasma lipoproteins: apolipoprotein structure and function. J Lipid Res 1984;25:1277-94.
168. Malinow MR, Bostom AG, Krauss RM. Homocyst(e)ine, diet, and cardiovascular diseases: a statement for healthcare professionals from the Nutrition Committee, American Heart Association. Circulation 1999;99:178-82.
169. Manninen V, Elo MO, Frick MH, Haapa K, Heinonen OP, Heinsalmi P, et al. Lipid alterations and decline in

the incidence of coronary heart disease in the Helsinki Heart Study. JAMA 1988;260:641-51.

170. Manson JE, Hsia J, et al. Estrogen plus progestin and the risk of coronary heart disease. N Engl J Med 2003;49:523-34.
171. Marcovina SM, Albers JJ. Apolipoprotein assays: standardization and quality control. Scand J Clin Lab Invest Suppl 1990;198:58-65.
172. Marcovina SM, Albers JJ. Lipoprotein Lp(a) quantification: Comparison of methods and strategies for standardization. Curr Opin Lipidol 1994:417-21.
173. Marcovina SM, Albers JJ, Gabel B, Koschinsky ML, Gaur VP. Effect of the number of apolipoprotein(a) kringle 4 domains on immunochemical measurements of lipoprotein(a). Clin Chem 1995;41: 246-55.
174. Marcovina SM, Albers JJ, Henderson LO, Hannon WH. International Federation of Clinical Chemistry standardization project for measurements of apolipoproteins A-I and B. III. Comparability of apolipoprotein A-I values by use of international reference material. Clin Chem 1993;39:773-81.
175. Marcovina SM, Albers JJ, Kennedy H, Mei JV, Henderson LO, Hannon WH. International Federation of Clinical Chemistry standardization project for measurements of apolipoproteins A-I and B. IV. Comparability of apolipoprotein B values by use of International Reference Material. Clin Chem 1994;40:586-92.
176. Marcovina SM, Albers JJ, Scanu AM, Kennedy H, Giaculli F, Berg K, et al. Use of a reference material proposed by the International Federation of Clinical Chemistry and Laboratory Medicine to evaluate analytical methods for the determination of plasma lipoprotein(a). Clin Chem 2000;46:1956-67.
177. Marcovina SM, Gaur VP, Albers JJ. Biological variability of cholesterol, triglyceride, low- and high-density lipoprotein cholesterol, lipoprotein(a), and apolipoproteins A-I and B. Clin Chem 1994;40: 574-8.
178. Marcovina SM, Hobbs HH, Albers JJ. Relation between number of apolipoprotein(a) kringle 4 repeats and mobility of isoforms in agarose gel: basis for a standardized isoform nomenclature. Clin Chem 1996;42:436-9.
179. Marcovina SM, Koschinsky ML, Albers JJ, Skarlatos S. Report of the National Heart, Lung, and Blood Institute Workshop on Lipoprotein(a) and Cardiovascular Disease: Recent Advances and Future Directions. Clin Chem 2003; 49:1785-96.
180. Marcovina SM, Morrisett JD. Structure and metabolism of lipoprotein (a). Curr Opin Lipidol 1995;6:136-45.
181. Marcovina SM, Zhang ZH, Gaur VP, Albers JJ. Identification of 34 apolipoprotein(a) isoforms: differential expression of apolipoprotein(a) alleles between American blacks and whites. Biochem Biophys Res Commun 1993;191:1192-6.
182. McCabe ERB. disorders of glycerol metabolism. In: Scriver CR, Beaudet AL, Sly WS, Valle D, eds. The Metabolic and Molecular Bases of Inherited Diseases, Vol. 7th ed. New York: McGraw-Hill, 1995:1631-52.
183. McGowan MW, Artiss JD, Zak B. A procedure for the determination of high-density lipoprotein choline-containing phospholipids. J Clin Chem Clin Biochem 1982;20:807-12.
184. McMillan TA, Warnick GR. Interlaboratory proficiency survey of cholesterol and high-density lipoprotein cholesterol measurement. Clin Chem 1988;34:1629-32.
185. McNamara JJ, Molot MA, Stremple JF, Cutting RT. Coronary artery disease in combat casualties in Vietnam. JAMA 1971;216:1185-7.
186. McNamara JR, Cole TG, Contois JH, Ferguson CA, Ordovas JM, Schaefer EJ. Immunoseparation method for measuring low-density lipoprotein cholesterol directly from serum evaluated. Clin Chem 1995;41:232-40.
187. McNamara JR, Shah PK, Nakajima K, Cupples LA, Wilson PWF, Ordovas JM, Schaefer EJ. Remnant lipoprotein cholesterol and triglyceride reference ranges from the Framingham Heart Study. Clin Chem 1998;44:1224-32.
188. Meier-Ewert HK, Ridker PM, et al. Absence of diurnal variation of C-reactive protein concentrations in healthy human subjects. Clin Chem 2001;47: 426-30.
189. Miki Y. A Homogeneous assay for the selective measurement of LDL-cholesterol in serum. Enzymatic selective protection method. Clin Lab 1999;45: 398-401.
190. Miller M, Bachorik PS, Cloey TA. Normal variation of plasma lipoproteins: postural effects on plasma concentrations of lipids, lipoproteins, and apolipoproteins. Clin Chem 1992;38:569-74.
191. Miller WG. Matrix effects in the measurement and standardization of Lipids and Lipoproteins. In: Rifai N, Warnick GR, Dominiczak M, eds. Handbook of lipoprotein testing, Vol. Washington DC: AACC Press, 2000:695-716.
192. Miller WG, Waymack PP, Anderson FP, Ethridge SF, Jayne EC. Performance of four homogeneous direct methods for LDL-cholesterol. Clin Chem 2002;48:489-98.
193. Miner SES, Evrovski J, Cole DEC. The clinical chemistry and molecular biology of homocysteine metabolism: An update. Clin Biochem 1997;30: 189-201.
194. Mogadam M, Ahmed SW, Mensch AH, Godwin ID. Within-person fluctuations of serum cholesterol and lipoproteins. Arch Intern Med 1990;150: 1645-8.

195. Mulder K, van Leeuwen C, Schouten JA, van Gent CM, Snel MT, Lahey J, van der Voort HA. An evaluation of three commercial methods for the determination of LDL-cholesterol. Clin Chim Acta 1984;143:29-35.
196. Muller C. Xanthomata, hypercholesterolemia, angina pectoris. Acta Med Scand 1938:75.
197. Myers GL, Cooper GR, L.O. H, Hassemer DJ, Kimberly MM. Standardization of lipid and lipoprotein measurement. In: Rifai N, Warnick GR, Dominiczak M, eds. Handbook of lipoprotein testing, Vol. Washington DC: AACC Press., 2000:717-48.
198. Myers GL, Cooper GR, Winn CL, Smith SJ. The Centers for Disease Control-National Heart, Lung and Blood Institute Lipid Standardization Program. An approach to accurate and precise lipid measurements. Clin Lab Med 1989;9:105-35.
199. Myers GL, Kimberly MM, Waymack PP, Smith SJ, Cooper GR, Sampson EJ. A reference method laboratory network for cholesterol: a model for standardization and improvement of clinical laboratory measurements. Clin Chem 2000;46:1762-72.
200. Naito HK. The association of serum lipids, lipoproteins, and apolipoproteins with coronary artery disease assessed by coronary arteriography. Ann N Y Acad Sci 1985;454:230-8.
201. Naito HK, David JA. Laboratory considerations: determination of cholesterol, triglyceride, phospholipid, and other lipids in blood and tissues. Lab Res Methods Biol Med 1984;10:1-76.
202. Nakagomi A, Freedman SB, et al. Interferon-gamma and lipopolysaccharide potentiate monocyte tissue factor induction by C-reactive protein: relationship with age, sex, and hormone replacement treatment. Circulation 2000;101:1785-91.
203. National Cholesterol Education Program. Second Report of the Expert Panel on Detection, Evaluation, and Treatment of High Blood Cholesterol in Adults (Adult Treatment Panel II). Circulation 1994;89: 1333-445.
204. Nauck M, Graziani MS, Bruton D, Cobbaert C, Cole TG, Lefevre F, et al. Analytical and clinical performance of a detergent-based homogeneous LDL-cholesterol assay: a multicenter evaluation. Clin Chem 2000;46:506-14.
205. Nauck M, Marz W, Jarausch J, Cobbaert C, Sagers A, Bernard D, et al. Multicenter evaluation of a homogeneous assay for HDL-cholesterol without sample pretreatment. Clin Chem 1997;43:1622-9.
206. Nauck M, Marz W, Wieland H. New immunoseparation-based homogeneous assay for HDL-cholesterol compared with three homogeneous and two heterogeneous methods for HDL-cholesterol. Clin Chem 1998;44:1443-51.
207. Nauck M, Rifai N. Analytical performance and clinical efficacy of three routine procedures for LDL cholesterol measurement compared with the ultracentrifugation-dextran sulfate-Mg(2+) method. Clin Chim Acta 2000;294:77-92.
208. Nauck M, Warnick GR, Rifai N. Methods for measurement of LDL-cholesterol: a critical assessment of direct measurement by homogeneous assays versus calculation. Clin Chem 2002;48:236-54.
209. National Committee for Clinical Laboratory Standards (NCCLS). Method comparison and bias estimation using patient samples, approved guideline. NCCLS document EP-9A 1995.
210. Nexo E, Engbaek F, Ueland PM, Westby C, O'Gorman P, et al. Evaluation of novel assays in clinical chemistry: quantification of plasma total homocysteine. Clin Chem 2000;46:1150-6.
211. NIH Consensus conference. Triglyceride, high-density lipoprotein, and coronary heart disease. NIH Consensus Development Panel on Triglyceride, High-Density Lipoprotein, and Coronary Heart Disease. JAMA 1993;269:505-10.
212. Nilsson K, Gustafson L, Faldt R, et al. Plasma homocysteine in relation to serum cobalamin and blood folate in a psychogeriatric population. Eur J Clin Invest 1994;24:600-6.
213. Nilsson K, Gustafson L, Faldt R, Andersson A, Brattstrom L, Lindgren A, et al. Hyperhomocysteinaemia—a common finding in a psychogeriatric population. Eur J Clin Invest 1996;26:853-9.
214. Noble RP. Electrophoretic separation of plasma lipoproteins in agarose gel. J Lipid Res 1968;9: 693-700.
215. Norum RA, Lakier JB, Goldstein S, Angel A, Goldberg RB, Block WD, et al. Familial deficiency of apolipoproteins A-I and C-III and precocious coronary-artery disease. N Engl J Med 1982;306: 1513-19.
216. Nygard O, Vollset SE, Refsum H, et al. Total plasma homocysteine and cardiovascular risk profile. JAMA 1995;274:1526-33.
217. Ockene IS, Matthews CE, et al. (2001). Variability and classification accuracy of serial high-sensitivity C-reactive protein measurements in healthy adults. Clin Chem 2001;47:444-50.
218. Okada M, Matsui H, Ito Y, Fujiwara A, Inano K. Low-density lipoprotein cholesterol can be chemically measured: a new superior method. J Lab Clin Med 1998;132:195-201.
219. Okamoto Y, Tanaka S, Nakano H. Direct measurement of HDL cholesterol preferable to precipitation method. Clin Chem 1995;41:1784.
220. Ordovas JM, Lopez-Miranda J, Perez-Jimenez F, Rodriguez C, Park JS, Cole T, Schaefer EJ. Effect of apolipoprotein E and A-IV phenotypes on the low density lipoprotein response to HMG CoA reductase inhibitor therapy. Atherosclerosis 1995;113: 157-66.

221. Otvos JD, Jeyarajah EJ, Bennett DW. Quantification of plasma lipoproteins by proton nuclear magnetic resonance spectroscopy. Clin Chem 1991;37: 377-86.
222. Otvos JD, Jeyarajah EJ, Bennett DW, Krauss RM. Development of a proton nuclear magnetic resonance spectroscopic method for determining plasma lipoprotein concentrations and subspecies distributions from a single, rapid measurement. Clin Chem 1992;38:1632-8.
223. Pasceri V, Cheng JS, et al. Modulation of C-reactive protein-mediated monocyte chemoattractant protein-1 induction in human endothelial cells by anti-atherosclerosis drugs. Circulation 2001;103: 2531-4.
224. Patsch JR, Patsch W. Exercise, high density lipoproteins, and fat tolerance. Compr Ther 1984;10: 29-37.
225. Patsch JR, Prasad S, Gotto AM, Jr., Bengtsson-Olivecrona G. Postprandial lipemia. A key for the conversion of high density lipoprotein2 into high density lipoprotein3 by hepatic lipase. J Clin Invest 1984;74:2017-23.
226. Pearson T A, Mensah GA, et al. Markers of inflammation and cardiovascular disease: application to clinical and public health practice: A statement for healthcare professionals from the Centers for Disease Control and Prevention and the American Heart Association. Circulation 2003;107: 499-511.
227. Pernet P, Lasnier E, Vaubourdolle M. Evaluation of the AxSYM homocysteine assay and comparison with the IMx homocysteine assay. Clin Chem 2000;46:1440-1.
228. Perry IJ, Refsum H, Morris RW, et al. Prospective study of serum total homocysteine concentration and risk of stroke in middle-aged British men. Lancet 1995;346:1395-8.
229. Pfeiffer CM, Huff DL, Smith SJ, Miller DT, Gunter EW. Comparison of plasma total homocysteine measurements in 14 laboratories: an international study. Clin Chem 1999;45:1261-8.
230. Pisani T, Gebski CP, Leary ET, Warnick GR, Ollington JF. Accurate direct determination of low-density lipoprotein cholesterol using an immunoseparation reagent and enzymatic cholesterol assay. Arch Pathol Lab Med 1995;119:1127-35.
231. Powers HJ, Moat SJ. Developments in the measurement of plasma total homocysteine. Curr Opin Clin Nutr Metab Care 2000;3:391-7.
232. Pradhan AD, Cook NR, et al. C-reactive protein is independently associated with fasting insulin in nondiabetic women. Arterioscler Thromb Vasc Biol 2003;3:650-5.
233. Pradhan AD, Manson JE, et al. C-reactive protein, interleukin 6, and risk of developing type 2 diabetes mellitus. JAMA 2001;286:327-34.
234. Rall SC, Jr., Weisgraber KH, Mahley RW. Human apolipoprotein E. The complete amino acid sequence. J Biol Chem 1982;257:4171-8.
235. Rasmussen K, Møller J. Total homocysteine determination in clinical practice. Ann Clin Biochem 2000;37:627-48.
236. Ray JG, Laskin CA. Folic acid and homocyst(e)ine metabolic defects and the risk of placental abruption, pre-eclampsia and spontaneous pregnancy loss: a systematic review. Placenta 1999;20:519-29.
237. Recommendations for Improving Cholesterol Measurement: A Report from the Laboratory Standardization Panel of the National Cholesterol Education Program., Vol. Bethesda: NIH Publication, 1990: 90-2964.
238. Recommendations on Lipoprotein Measurement: From the Working Group on Lipoprotein Measurement. National Cholesterol Education Program, Vol. Bethesda: NIH/NHLBI NIH Publication, 1995: 95-3044.
239. Refsum H, Fiskerstrand T, Guttormsen AB, Ueland PM. Assessment of homocysteine status. J Inherit Metab Dis 1997;20:286-94.
240. Refsum H, Helland S, Ueland PM. Radioenzymic determination of homocysteine in plasma and urine. Clin Chem 1985;31:624-8.
241. Refsum H, Smith AD, Ueland PM, Nexo E, Clarke R, et al. Facts and recommendations about total homocysteine determinations: an expert opinion. Clin Chem 2004:50:3-32.
242. Refsum H, Ueland PM, Nygård O, Vollset SE. Homocysteine and cardiovascular disease. Annu Rev Med 1998;49:31-62.
243. Relationship of atherosclerosis in young men to serum lipoprotein cholesterol concentrations and smoking. A preliminary report from the Pathobiological Determinants of Atherosclerosis in Youth (PDAY) Research Group. JAMA 1990;264: 3018-24.
244. Report of the Expert Panel on Blood Cholesterol Levels in Children and Adolescents. In: Services. USDoHaH, ed. National Cholesterol Education Program, Vol. Bethesda: NIH Publication, 1991: 91-2732.
245. Resnicow K, Cross D. Are parents' self-reported total cholesterol levels useful in identifying children with hyperlipidemia? An examination of current guidelines. Pediatrics 1993;92:347-53.
246. Ridker PM, Buring JE, et al. C-reactive protein, the metabolic syndrome, and risk of incident cardiovascular events: an 8-year follow-up of 14719 initially healthy American women. Circulation 2003;107: 391-7.
247. Ridker PM, Cushman M, et al. Inflammation, aspirin, and the risk of cardiovascular disease in apparently healthy men. N Engl J Med 1997;336:973-9.

248. Ridker PM, Cushman M, et al. Plasma concentration of C-reactive protein and risk of developing peripheral vascular disease. Circulation 1998;97:425-8.
249. Ridker PM, Hennekens CH, et al. C-reactive protein and other markers of inflammation in the prediction of cardiovascular disease in women. N Engl J Med 2000;342:836-43.
250. Ridker, PM, Rifai N, et al. Measurement of C-reactive protein for the targeting of statin therapy in the primary prevention of acute coronary events. N Engl J Med 2001;344:1959-65.
251. Ridker PM, Rifai N, et al. Long-term effects of pravastatin on plasma concentration of C-reactive protein. The Cholesterol and Recurrent Events (CARE) Investigators. Circulation 1999;100: 230-5.
252. Ridker PM, Rifai N, et al. Inflammation, pravastatin, and the risk of coronary events after myocardial infarction in patients with average cholesterol levels. Cholesterol and Recurrent Events (CARE) Investigators. Circulation 1998;98:839-44.
253. Ridker PM, Rifai N, et al. Comparison of C-reactive protein and low-density lipoprotein cholesterol levels in the prediction of first cardiovascular events. N Engl J Med 2002;347:1557-65.
254. Ridker PM, Stampfer MJ, et al. Novel risk factors for systemic atherosclerosis: a comparison of C-reactive protein, fibrinogen, homocysteine, lipoprotein(a), and standard cholesterol screening as predictors of peripheral arterial disease. JAMA 2001;285:2481-5.
255. Rifai N. Lipoproteins and apolipoproteins. Composition, metabolism, and association with coronary heart disease. Arch Pathol Lab Med 1986;110: 694-701.
256. Rifai N, Dominiczak M, Warnick GR. Handbook of Lipoprotein Testing. Washington: AACC Press, 1997.
257. Rifai N, Heiss G. Gender and race differences in cord blood lipoprotein. Circulation 1988;II:481.
258. Rifai N, Heiss G, Doetch K. Cord blood Lp (a) at birth, in blacks and whites. Atherosclerosis 1992: 123-9.
259. Rifai N, Iannotti E, DeAngelis K, Law T. Analytical and clinical performance of a homogeneous enzymatic LDL-cholesterol assay compared with the ultracentrifugation-dextran sulfate-Mg2+ method. Clin Chem 1998;44:1242-50.
260. Rifai N, Kwiterovich PO, Jr. Disorders of lipid and lipoprotein metabolism in children and adolescents. In: Soldin SJ, Rifai N, Hicks JMB, eds. Biochemical Bases of Inherited Disease, Vol. Washington: AACC Press, 1995:541.
261. Rifai N, Neufeld E, Ahlstrom P, Rimm E, D'Angelo L, Hicks JM. Failure of current guidelines for cholesterol screening in urban African-American adolescents. Pediatrics 1996;98:383-8.
262. Rifai N, Ridker PM. Population distributions of C-reactive protein in apparently healthy men and women in the United States: implication for clinical interpretation. Clin Chem 2003;49:666-9.
263. Rifai N, Silverman LM. Immunoturbidimetric techniques for quantifying apolipoproteins CII and CIII. Clin Chem 1986;32:1969-72.
264. Roberts WL, Moulton L, et al. Evaluation of nine automated high-sensitivity C-reactive protein methods: implications for clinical and epidemiological applications. Part 2. Clin Chem 2001;47:418-25.
265. Rosseneu M, Vercaemst R, Steinberg KK, Cooper GR. Some considerations of methodology and standardization of apolipoprotein B immunoassays. Clin Chem 1983;29:427-33.
266. Sakaue T, Hirano T, Yoshino G, Sakai K, Takeuchi H, Adachi M. Reactions of direct LDL-cholesterol assays with pure LDL fraction and IDL: comparison of three homogeneous methods. Clin Chim Acta 2000;295:97-106.
267. Sandkamp M, Funke H, Schulte H, Kohler E, Assmann G. Lipoprotein(a) is an independent risk factor for myocardial infarction at a young age. Clin Chem 1990;36:20-3.
268. Sattar N, Gaw A, et al. Metabolic syndrome with and without C-reactive protein as a predictor of coronary heart disease and diabetes in the West of Scotland Coronary Prevention Study. Circulation 2003;108:414-19.
269. Savage DG, Lindenbaum J, Stabler SP, Allen RH. Sensitivity of serum methylmalonic acid and total homocysteine determinations for diagnosing cobalamin and folate deficiencies. Am J Med 1994;96:239-46.
270. Schaefer EJ. Clinical, biochemical, and genetic features in familial disorders of high density lipoprotein deficiency. Arteriosclerosis 1984;4:303-22.
271. Schaefer EJ, Blum CB, Levy RI, Jenkins LL, Alaupovic P, Foster DM, Brewer HB, Jr. Metabolism of high-density lipoprotein apolipoproteins in Tangier disease. N Engl J Med 1978;299:905-10.
272. Schaefer EJ, Lamon-Fava S, Johnson S, Ordovas JM, Schaefer MM, Castelli WP, Wilson PW. Effects of gender and menopausal status on the association of apolipoprotein E phenotype with plasma lipoprotein levels. Results from the Framingham Offspring Study. Arterioscler Thromb 1994;14:1105-13.
273. Schaefer EJ, McNamara JR. Overview of the diagnosis and treatment of lipid disorders. In: Rifai N, Dominiczak M, Warnick GR, eds. Handbook of Lipoprotein Testing, Vol. Washington: AACC Press., 1997:25.
274. Schmitz G, Assmann G, Robenek H, Brennhausen B. Tangier disease: a disorder of intracellular membrane traffic. Proc Natl Acad Sci U S A 1985;82:6305-9.
275. Schrott HG, Goldstein JL, Hazzard WR. Familial hypercholesterolemia in a large kindred: Evidence for a monogenic mechanism. Ann Intern Med 1971: 711-20.

276. Segrest JP, Chung BH, Cone JT, Hughes TA. Coronary heart disease risk. Assessment by plasma lipoprotein profiles. Ala J Med Sci 1983;20:76-83.
277. Sesso HD, Buring JE, et al. (2003). C-reactive protein and the risk of developing hypertension. JAMA 2003;290:2945-51.
278. Shipchandler MT, Moore EG. Rapid, fully automated measurement of plasma homocyst(e)ine with the Abbott IMx analyzer. Clin Chem 1995;41:991-4.
279. Siest G, Pillot T, Regis-Bailly A, Leininger-Muller B, Steinmetz J, Galteau MM, Visvikis S. Apolipoprotein E: an important gene and protein to follow in laboratory medicine. Clin Chem 1995;41:1068-86.
280. Simo JM, Castellano I, Ferre N, Joven J, Camps J. Evaluation of a homogeneous assay for high-density lipoprotein cholesterol: limitations in patients with cardiovascular, renal, and hepatic disorders. Clin Chem 1998;44:1233-41.
281. Smith AD. Homocysteine, B vitamins, and cognitive deficit in the elderly [Editorial]. Am J Clin Nutr 2002;75:785-6.
282. Sniderman A, Shapiro S, Marpole D, Skinner B, Teng B, Kwiterovich PO, Jr. Association of coronary atherosclerosis with hyperapobetalipoproteinemia [increased protein but normal cholesterol levels in human plasma low density (beta) lipoproteins]. Proc Natl Acad Sci U S A 1980;77:604-8.
283. Sniderman A, Teng B, Genest J, Cianflone K, Wacholder S, Kwiterovich P, Jr. Familial aggregation and early expression of hyperapobetalipoproteinemia. Am J Cardiol 1985;55:291-5.
284. Sniderman AD, Silberberg J. Is it time to measure apolipoprotein B? Arteriosclerosis 1990;10:665-7.
285. SoRelle R. Metabolic syndrome a major predictor of heart disease. Circulation. 2004;109:e9010-1.
286. Soria LF, Ludwig EH, Clarke HR, Vega GL, Grundy SM, McCarthy BJ. Association between a specific apolipoprotein B mutation and familial defective apolipoprotein B-100. Proc Natl Acad Sci U S A 1989;86:587-91.
287. Stabler SP, Marcell PD, Podell ER, Allen RH. Quantitation of total homocysteine, total cysteine, and methionine in normal serum and urine using capillary gas chromatography-mass spectrometry. Anal Biochem 1987;162:185-96.
288. Stanger O, Herrmann W, Pietrzik K, Fowler B, Geisel J, Dierkes J, et al. D. A. CH.-Liga Homocystein (German, Austrian, and Swiss Homocysteine Society) consensus paper on the rational clinical use of homocysteine, folic acid, and B vitamins in cardiovascular and thrombotic diseases: guidelines and recommendations. J Kardiol 2003;10:190-9.
289. Stary HC. The sequence of cell and matrix changes in atherosclerotic lesions of coronary arteries in the first forty years of life. Eur Heart J 1990;11 Suppl E: 3-19.
290. Steele BW, Koehler DF, Azar MM, Blaszkowski TP, Kuba K, Dempsey ME. Enzymatic determinations of cholesterol in high-density-lipoprotein fractions prepared by a precipitation technique. Clin Chem 1976;22:98-101.
291. Steinberg D, Witztum JL. Is the oxidative modification hypothesis relevant to human atherosclerosis? Do the antioxidant trials conducted to date refute the hypothesis? Circulation 2002;105:2107-11.
292. Steinberg KK, Cooper GR, Graiser SR, Rosseneu M. Some considerations of methodology and standardization of apolipoprotein A-I immunoassays. Clin Chem 1983;29:415-26.
293. Strong JP, Malcom GT, McMahan CA, Tracy RE, Newman WP, 3rd, Herderick EE, Cornhill JF. Prevalence and extent of atherosclerosis in adolescents and young adults: implications for prevention from the Pathobiological Determinants of Atherosclerosis in Youth Study. JAMA 1999;281:727-35.
294. Strong JP, McGill HC, Jr. The pediatric aspects of atherosclerosis. J Atheroscler Res 1969;9:251-65.
295. Stuyt PM, Van 't Laar A. Clinical features of type III hyperlipoproteinaemia. Neth J Med 1983;26: 104-11.
296. Sugiuchi H, Irie T, Uji Y, Ueno T, Chaen T, Uekama K, Okabe H. Homogeneous assay for measuring low-density lipoprotein cholesterol in serum with triblock copolymer and alpha-cyclodextrin sulfate. Clin Chem 1998;44:522-31.
297. Sugiuchi H, Uji Y, Okabe H, Irie T, Uekama K, Kayahara N, Miyauchi K. Direct measurement of high-density lipoprotein cholesterol in serum with polyethylene glycol-modified enzymes and sulfated alpha-cyclodextrin. Clin Chem 1995;41:717-23.
298. Taddei-Peters WC, Butman BT, Jones GR, Venetta TM, Macomber PF, Ransom JH. Quantification of lipoprotein(a) particles containing various apolipoprotein(a) isoforms by a monoclonal anti-apo(a) capture antibody and a polyclonal anti-apolipoprotein B detection antibody sandwich enzyme immunoassay. Clin Chem 1993;39:1382-9.
299. Takayama M, Itoh S, Nagasaki T, Tanimizu I. A new enzymatic method for determination of serum choline-containing phospholipids. Clin Chim Acta 1977;79:93-8.
300. Tate JR, Berg K, Couderc R, Dati F, Kostner GM, Marcovina SM, et al. International Federation of Clinical Chemistry and Laboratory Medicine (IFCC) Standardization Project for the Measurement of Lipoprotein(a). Phase 2: selection and properties of a proposed secondary reference material for lipoprotein(a). Clin Chem Lab Med 1999;37:949-58
301. Tate JR, Rifai N, Berg K, Couderc R, Dati F, Kostner GM, et al. International Federation of Clinical Chemistry standardization project for the measurement of lipoprotein(a). Phase I. Evaluation of the

analytical performance of lipoprotein(a) assay systems and commercial calibrators. Clin Chem 1998;44:1629-40.

302. Thanhauser SJ, Magendantz H. The different clinical groups of xanthomatous diseases: A clinical physiological study of 22 cases. Ann Intern Med 1938;11: 1662-746.
303. Third JL, Montag J, Flynn M, Freidel J, Laskarzewski P, Glueck CJ. Primary and familial hypoalphalipoproteinemia. Metabolism 1984;33:136-46.
304. Torzewski J, Torzewski M, et al. C-reactive protein frequently colocalizes with the terminal complement complex in the intima of early atherosclerotic lesions of human coronary arteries. Arterioscler Thromb Vasc Biol 1998;18:1386-92.
305. Tybjaerg-Hansen A, Gallagher J, Vincent J, Houlston R, Talmud P, Dunning AM, et al. Familial defective apolipoprotein B-100: detection in the United Kingdom and Scandinavia, and clinical characteristics of ten cases. Atherosclerosis 1990;80:235-42.
306. Ubbink JB. Assay methods for the measurement of total homocyst(e)ine in plasma. Semin Thromb Hemost 2000;26:233-41.
307. Ubbink JB, Vermaak WJH, Bissbort S. Rapid high-performance chromatographic assay for total homocysteine levels in human serum. J Chromatogr 1991;565:441-6.
308. Ueland PM, Refsum H, Stabler SP, et al. Total homocysteine in plasma or serum: Methods and clinical applications. Clin Chem 1993;39:1764-79.
309. Usui S, Kakuuchi H, Okamoto M, Mizukami Y, Okazaki M. Differential reactivity of two homogeneous LDL-cholesterol methods to LDL and VLDL subfractions, as demonstrated by ultracentrifugation and HPLC. Clin Chem 2002;48:1946-54.
310. Utermann G. Genetic polymorphism of apolipoprotein E: Impact on plasma lipoprotein metabolism. In: Crepaldi G, Tiengo A, Baggio G, eds. Diabetes, Obesity and Hyperlipidemias: III, Vol. Amsterdam, 1985:1-30.
311. Utermann G, Hees M, Steinmetz A. Polymorphism of apolipoprotein E and occurence of dysbetalipoproteinemia in man. Nature 1977:604-7.
312. van der Hoek YY, Wittekoek ME, Beisiegel U, Kastelein JJ, Koschinsky ML. The apolipoprotein(a) kringle IV repeats which differ from the major repeat kringle are present in variably-sized isoforms. Hum Mol Genet 1993;2:361-6.
313. Vega GL, Grundy SM. In vivo evidence for reduced binding of low density lipoproteins to receptors as a cause of primary moderate hypercholesterolemia. J Clin Invest 1986;78:1410-14.
314. Verma S, Li SH, et al. Endothelin antagonism and interleukin-6 inhibition attenuate the proatherogenic effects of C-reactive protein. Circulation 2002;105:1890-6.
315. Vermeer BJ, van Gent CM, Goslings B, Polano MK. Xanthomatosis and other clinical findings in patients with elevated levels of very low density lipoproteins. Br J Dermatol 1979;100:657-66.
316. Vester B, Rasmussen K. High performance liquid chromatography method for rapid and accurate determination of homocysteine in plasma and serum. Eur J Clin Chem Clin Biochem 1991;29:549-54.
317. Vilaseca MA, Moyano D, Ferrer I, Artuch R. Total homocysteine in pediatric patients. Clin Chem 1997;43:690-1.
318. Vollset SE, Refsum H, Irgens LM, Emblem BM, Tverdal A, Gjessing HK, et al. Plasma total homocysteine, pregnancy complications, and adverse outcomes: the Hordaland Homocysteine Study. Am J Clin Nutr 2000;71:962-8.
319. Wagner AM, Sanchez-Quesada JL, Perez A, Rigla M, Cortes M, Blanco-Vaca F, Ordonez-Llanos J. Inaccuracy of calculated LDL-cholesterol in type 2 diabetes: consequences for patient risk classification and therapeutic decisions. Clin Chem 2000;46:1830-2.
320. Wald DS, Law M, Morris JK. Homocysteine and cardiovascular disease: evidence on causality from a meta-analysis. BMJ 2002;325:1202-8.
321. Warnick GR. Enzymatic methods for quantification of lipoprotein lipids. Methods Enzymol 1986;129:101-23.
322. Warnick GR, Albers JJ. A comprehensive evaluation of the heparin-manganese precipitation procedure for estimating high density lipoprotein cholesterol. J Lipid Res 1978;19:65-76.
323. Warnick GR, Benderson J, Albers JJ. Dextran sulfate-$Mg2^+$ precipitation procedure for quantitation of high-density-lipoprotein cholesterol. Clin Chem 1982;28:1379-88.
324. Warnick GR, Knopp RH, Fitzpatrick V, Branson L. Estimating low-density lipoprotein cholesterol by the Friedewald equation is adequate for classifying patients on the basis of nationally recommended cutpoints. Clin Chem 1990;36:15-19.
325. Warnick GR, Mayfield C, Albers JJ, Hazzard WR. Gel isoelectric focusing method for specific diagnosis of familial hyperlipoproteinemia type 3. Clin Chem 1979;25:279-84.
326. Warnick GR, Nauck M, Rifai N. Evolution of methods for measurement of HDL-cholesterol: from ultracentrifugation to homogeneous assays. Clin Chem 2001;47:1579-96.
327. Warnick GR, Spain M, Kloepfer H, Volke TM. Standardization of a commercial (Boehringer Mannheim diagnostics) enzymic method for cholesterol. Clin Chem 1989;35:409-13.
328. Webber LS, Srinivasan SR, Wattigney WA, Berenson GS. Tracking of serum lipids and lipoproteins from childhood to adulthood. The Bogalusa Heart Study. Am J Epidemiol 1991;133:884-99.

329. Weisgraber KH, Innerarity TL, Mahley RW. Abnormal lipoprotein receptor-binding activity of the human E apoprotein due to cysteine-arginine interchange at a single site. J Biol Chem 1982;257: 2518-21.
330. Weisgraber KH, Newhouse YM, Mahley RW. Apolipoprotein E genotyping using the polymerase chain reaction and allele-specific oligonucleotide probes. Biochem Biophys Res Commun 1988;157:1212-17.
331. Wilder LB, Bachorik PS, Finney CA, Moy TF, Becker DM. The effect of fasting status on the determination of low-density and high-density lipoprotein cholesterol. Am J Med 1995;99:374-7.
332. Wissler RW. New insights into the pathogenesis of atherosclerosis as revealed by PDAY. Pathobiological Determinants of Atherosclerosis in Youth. Atherosclerosis 1994;108 Suppl:S3-S20.
333. Yamada S, Gotoh T, et al. Distribution of serum C-reactive protein and its association with atherosclerotic risk factors in a Japanese population: Jichi Medical School Cohort Study. Am J Epidemiol 2001;153:1183-90.
334. Yamamoto A, Nakamura M, Hino K, Saito K, Manabe M. Development of a new homogeneous method for serum HDL-C. Clin Chem 2000;46:A98.
335. Yu HH, Markowitz R, De Ferranti SD, Neufeld EJ, Farrow G, Bernstein HH, Rifai N. Direct measurement of LDL-C in children: performance of two surfactant-based methods in a general pediatric population. Clin Biochem 2000;33:89-95.
336. Ziccardi P, Nappo F, et al. Reduction of inflammatory cytokine concentrations and improvement of endothelial functions in obese women after weight loss over one year. Circulation 2002;105:804-9.
337. Zilversmit DB. Atherogenesis: a postprandial phenomenon. Circulation 1979;60:473-85.
338. Zwaka TP, Hombach V, et al. C-reactive protein-mediated low density lipoprotein uptake by macrophages: implications for atherosclerosis. Circulation 2001;103:1194-7.

ADDITIONAL READING

Assmann G. HDL deficiency and atherosclerosis. Norwell MA: Kluwer Academic Publishers, 1996.

Bradley WA, Gianturco SH, Segrest JP, Abelson JN, Simon MI, eds. Methods in enzymology: Plasma lipoproteins: Quantitation. Vol 263, Part C. San Diego: Academic Press, 1995.

Jaross W, Dude H, Hanefeld M. Advances in lipoprotein and atherosclerosis research, diagnostics, and treatment. Proceedings of the 8th International Dresden Lipid Symposium. New York: VHC Publishers, 1995.

Milio FR, Loffredo WM, Neidig HA. Qualitative testing for lipids: REAC 447. Palmyra PA: Chemical Education Resources, 1994.

Rifai N, Dominiczak M, Warnick GR, eds. Handbook of lipoprotein testing, 2nd. Washington DC: AACC Press, 2000.

Robins SJ. Management of lipid disorders: A basis and guide for therapy. New York: Igaku-Shoin Medical Publishers, 1997.

Sebedia JL, Perkins EG. New trends in lipid and lipoproteins analysis. Champaign IL: AOCS Press, 1995.

Vance DE, Vance JE. Biochemistry of lipids, lipoproteins, and membranes. New York: Elsevier Science, 1996.

CHAPTER 27

Electrolytes and Blood Gases

Mitchell G. Scott, Ph.D., Vicky A. LeGrys, D.A., M.T.(A.S.C.P.), C.L.S.(N.C.A.) and James Stacey Klutts, M.D., Ph.D.

Maintenance of water homeostasis is paramount to life for all organisms. In mammals, the maintenance of osmotic pressure and water distribution in the various body fluid compartments is primarily a function of the four major electrolytes, Na^+, K^+, Cl^-, and HCO_3^-. In addition to water homeostasis, these electrolytes play an important role in the maintenance of pH, proper heart and muscle function, oxidation-reduction reactions, and as cofactors for enzymes. Indeed, there are almost no metabolic processes that are not dependent on or affected by electrolytes. Abnormal concentrations of electrolytes may be either the cause or the consequence of a variety of disorders. Thus determination of electrolytes is one of the most important functions of the clinical laboratory. Interpretation of abnormal osmolality and acid-base values requires specific knowledge of the electrolytes. Because of their physiological and clinical interrelationship, this chapter discusses determination of electrolytes, osmolality, acid-base status, and blood oxygenation.

ELECTROLYTES

Electrolytes are classified as either *anions,* negatively charged ions that move toward an anode, or *cations,* positively charged ions that move toward a cathode. Physiological electrolytes include Na^+, K^+, Ca^{2+}, Mg^{2+}, Cl^-, HCO_3^-, $H_2PO_4^-$, HPO_4^{2-}, and SO_4^{2-} and some organic anions, such as lactate. Although amino acids and proteins in solution also carry an electrical charge, they are usually considered separately from electrolytes. Hydrogen ion (H^+) concentration is routinely measured as pH, but its concentration is so low relative to other ions (10^{-9} versus 10^{-3} mol/L) in body fluids that it is not considered an electrolyte per se. The major electrolytes (Na^+, K^+, Cl^-, HCO_3^-) occur primarily as free ions, whereas significant amounts (>40%) of Ca^{2+}, Mg^{2+}, and trace elements are bound by proteins, such as albumin.

Determination of body fluid concentrations of the four major electrolytes (Na^+, K^+, Cl^-, and HCO_3^-) is commonly referred to as an "electrolyte profile." Other electrolytes that have special functions in particular contexts are discussed elsewhere: Ca^{2+}, magnesium, and phosphates in Chapter 49; iron in Chapter 31; trace elements in Chapter 30; and amino acids in Chapter 20.

SPECIMENS FOR ELECTROLYTE DETERMINATIONS

Serum and *plasma,* obtained from blood collected by venipuncture into an evacuated tube, are the usual specimens analyzed for Na^+, K^+, Cl^-, and HCO_3^-. Capillary blood, collected in either microsample tubes, capillary tubes, or applied directly from a finger stick to some point-of-care devices, is also a common sample analyzed. Heparinized whole blood arterial or venous specimens obtained for blood gas and pH determinations may also be used with direct ion-selective electrodes (ISEs). Differences of values between serum and plasma and between arterial and venous samples have been documented for these electrolytes (see Tables 2-3 and 2-4), but only the differences between serum and plasma K^+ can be considered clinically significant. Heparin, either the lithium or ammonium salt, is required if plasma or whole blood is assayed. Use of plasma or whole blood has the advantage of shortening turnaround time, because it is not necessary to wait for the blood to clot.[81] Furthermore, plasma or whole blood has a distinct advantage in determining K^+ concentrations, which are invariably higher in serum depending on platelet count.[42,80]

Specimen tubes should be centrifuged unopened, and the serum or plasma separated promptly. Grossly lipemic blood can be a source of analytical error with some methods (see later section on Electrolyte Exclusion Effect), making ultracentrifugation of serum or plasma before analysis necessary for lipemic samples. Hemolysis causes erroneously high K^+ results and this problem is often undetected when analyzing whole blood. In addition, unhemolyzed specimens that are not promptly processed may have increased K^+ concentrations because of K^+ leakage from red blood cells when whole blood is stored at 4 °C. These concerns and others regarding specimen collection and handling are addressed in the following pages with respect to individual analytes.

Urine collection for Na^+, K^+, or Cl^- assay should be made without the addition of preservatives. Feces and aspirates and drainages from different portions of the gastrointestinal tract may also be submitted for electrolyte analysis. Collection and analysis of sweat are described later in this chapter.

SODIUM

Sodium is the major cation of extracellular fluid. Because it represents approximately 90% of the ~154 mmol of inorganic cations per liter of plasma, Na^+ is responsible for almost one half the osmotic strength of plasma. It therefore plays a central role in maintaining the normal distribution of water and the osmotic pressure in the extracellular fluid compartment. The normal daily diet contains 8 to 15 g (130 to 260 mmol) of NaCl, which is nearly completely absorbed from the gastrointestinal tract. The body requires only 1 to 2 mmol/day, and the excess is excreted by the kidneys, which are the ultimate regulators of the amount of Na^+ (and thus water) in the body.

Sodium is freely filtered by the glomeruli. Seventy to 80% of the filtered Na^+ load is then actively reabsorbed in the proximal tubules, with Cl^- and water passively following in an isoosmotic and electrically neutral manner. Another 20% to 25% is reabsorbed in the loop of Henle along with Cl^- and more water. In the distal tubules, interaction of the adrenal hormone aldosterone with the coupled Na^+-K^+ and Na^+-H^+ exchange systems directly results in the reabsorption of Na^+, and indirectly of Cl^-, from the remaining 5% to 10% of the filtered load. It is the regulation of this latter fraction of filtered Na^+ that primarily determines the amount of Na^+ excreted in the urine. These processes are discussed in detail in Chapter 45.

Specimens

Serum, heparinized plasma, whole blood, sweat, urine, feces, or gastrointestinal fluids may be assayed for Na^+. Timed collections of urine, feces, or gastrointestinal fluids are preferred to allow comparison of values with reference intervals and to determine rates of electrolyte loss. Serum, plasma, and urine may be stored at 2 °C to 4 °C or frozen. Erythrocytes contain only one tenth of the Na^+ present in plasma, so hemolysis does not cause significant errors in serum or plasma Na^+ values. Lipemic samples should be ultracentrifuged and the infranatant analyzed unless a direct ISE is used.

Fecal and gastrointestinal fluid specimens require preparation before assay. Only liquid stools justify the trouble of analysis, because it is only when liquid feces occur that losses of electrolytes are significant. Immediately after collection, liquid stool specimens should be clarified of particulate matter by filtration through gauze or filter paper and by centrifugation. Because the risk of bacterial contamination of the automated instrument sampling systems is high with fecal samples, special cleaning and flushing procedures should follow analysis. Another difficulty with these specimens is their unpredictable concentration, which may necessitate a number of different dilutions to bring the concentration within the analytical range of the method. If not analyzed immediately, fecal and gastrointestinal fluids should be stored frozen to prevent microbial growth.

Determination of Sodium in Body Fluids

Sodium may be determined by atomic absorption spectrophotometry (AAS), flame emission spectrophotometry (FES), electrochemically with an Na^+-ISE, or spectrophotometrically. Of these methods, ISE methods are by far the most common. Excellent accuracy and coefficients of variation of less than 1.5% are readily achieved with modern equipment, reliable calibrators, and a good quality assurance program. Because sodium and potassium are routinely assayed together, methods for their analysis are described together later in this chapter.

Reference Intervals[65,101]

The interval for *serum* Na^+ is 136 to 145 mmol/L from infancy throughout life in one reference[101] and 135 to 145 mmol/L in another.[65] The interval for premature newborns at 48 hours is 128 to 148 mmol/L, and the value for umbilical cord blood from full-term newborns is ~127 mmol/L.

Urinary sodium excretion varies with dietary intake, but for people on an average diet containing 8 to 15 g/day, an interval of 40 to 220 mmol/day is typical.[101] There is a large diurnal variation in Na^+ excretion, with the rate of Na^+ excretion during the night being only 20% of the peak rate during the day. The Na^+ concentration of cerebrospinal fluid is 136 to 150 mmol/L. Mean fecal Na^+ excretion (for eight healthy subjects) has been reported as 7.8 ± 2.0 mmol/day (standard error) in one study,[19] and less than 10 mmol/day in another.[101]

POTASSIUM

Potassium is the major intracellular cation. In tissue cells, its average concentration is 150 mmol/L, and in erythrocytes, the concentration is 105 mmol/L (~23 times its concentration in plasma). High intracellular concentrations are maintained by the Na^+, K^+ adenosine triphosphate (ATP)ase pump, which is fueled by oxidative energy and continually transports K^+ into the cell against the concentration gradient. This pump is a critical factor in maintaining and adjusting the ionic gradients on which nerve impulse transmission and contractility of cardiac and skeletal muscle depend. Diffusion of K^+ out of the cell into the plasma exceeds pump-mediated K^+ uptake whenever pump activity is decreased because of (1) depletion of metabolic substrates, such as glucose, for ATP production; (2) competition for ATP between the pump and other energy-consuming activities of the cell; or (3) when cellular metabolism is slowed (as occurs with refrigeration). The importance of these considerations on sample integrity for analysis of K^+ is discussed later in this chapter.

The body requirement for K^+ is satisfied by a dietary intake of 50 to 150 mmol/day. Potassium absorbed from the gastrointestinal tract is rapidly distributed, with a small amount taken up by cells and most excreted by the kidneys. Potassium filtered through the glomeruli is almost completely reabsorbed in the proximal tubules and is then secreted in the distal tubules in exchange for Na^+ under the influence of aldosterone. Aldosterone enhances K^+ secretion and Na^+ reabsorption in the distal tubules by an Na^+-K^+ exchange mechanism. The kidneys respond almost immediately to K^+ loading with an increase in K^+ output, so that urine collected during or after a period of high intake may have a K^+ concentration as high as 100 mmol/L. In contrast, the tubular response to conserve K^+ in instances of depletion is very slow in the initial stages, with the normal kidney continuing to excrete K^+ at a rate of 20 to 30 mmol/day. Unlike the prompt response of the tubules to conserve Na^+ in deficit states, it can take up to 1 week for the tubules to reduce K^+ excretion to 5 to 10 mmol/day.

Factors that regulate distal tubular secretion of K^+ are intake of Na^+ and K^+, plasma concentration of mineralocorticoids, and acid-base balance. Because renal conservation mechanisms are slow to respond, K^+ depletion can be an early consequence of restricted K^+ intake or losses of K^+ by extrarenal routes. Diminished glomerular filtration rate is typical of renal failure, and the consequent decrease in distal tubular flow rate is an important factor in the retention of K^+ seen in chronic renal failure. Renal tubular acidosis and metabolic and respiratory acidoses and alkaloses also affect renal regulation of K^+ excretion. These topics are discussed in much greater detail in Chapters 45 and 46.

Specimens

Comments made earlier on specimens for Na^+ analysis are generally applicable to those for K^+ analysis. However, some additional points must be considered.

Potassium concentrations in plasma and whole blood are 0.1 to 0.7 mmol/L lower than those in serum and stated reference intervals for serum K^+ are 0.2 to 0.5 mmol/L higher than those for plasma K^+. The extent of this difference depends, however, on the platelet count, because the additional K^+ in serum is primarily a result of platelet rupture during coagulation.[42,48,80] This variability in the amount of additional K^+ in serum makes plasma the specimen of choice and emphasizes the necessity of noting on reports whether serum or plasma was assayed and using the appropriate reference intervals.

Specimens for determining K^+ concentrations in serum or plasma must be collected by methods that minimize hemolysis, because release of K^+ from as few as 0.5% of the erythrocytes can increase K^+ values by 0.5 mmol/L. An increase in K^+ of 0.6% has been estimated for every 10 mg/dL of plasma hemoglobin (Hb) caused by hemolysis.[16] Thus slight hemolysis (~50 mg Hb/dL) can be expected to raise K^+ values ~3%, marked hemolysis (~200 mg Hb/dL) 12%, and gross hemolysis (>500 mg Hb/dL) as much as 30%. Therefore it is imperative that any visible hemolysis be noted with reported K^+ values and include a comment that results are falsely elevated. If K^+ concentrations are determined by ISE on whole blood specimens using a blood gas instrument or a point-of-care device, increases in actual K^+ concentrations caused by hemolysis may be easily overlooked. Whenever hemolysis is suspected, a portion of the specimen should be centrifuged and visually inspected.

Clinically significant preanalytical errors can occur in K^+ determinations if blood samples are not processed expediently.[41] As mentioned earlier, maintenance of the intracellular-extracellular K^+ gradient depends on the activity of the energy-dependent Na^+,K^+ ATPase. If a whole blood specimen is chilled before separation, glycolysis is inhibited and the energy-dependent Na^+,K^+ ATPase cannot maintain this gradient and increases in plasma K^+ will occur as a result of K^+ leakage from erythrocytes and other cells. The increase of K^+ in serum is of the order of 0.2 mmol/L in 1.5 hours at 25 °C, whereas at 4 °C, the increase is considerably greater, and has been reported to be as much as a 2-mmol/L increase after 4 hours at 4 °C.[84]

The opposite effect, namely a falsely decreased K^+ value, is initially observed if an unseparated sample is stored at 37 °C because glycolysis occurs and K^+ shifts intracellularly. Even at room temperature, leukocytosis can initially cause falsely decreased K^+ concentrations. The extent of this decrease depends on leukocyte count, temperature, and glucose concentrations, but has been reported to be as much as 0.7 mmol/L at 37 °C.[58] This effect is, however, biphasic. Initially, plasma K^+ decreases as a result of glycolysis, but after the glucose substrate is exhausted K^+ will leak from cells.[3] When the leukocyte count is greater than 100,000/µL and hypokalemia is already a characteristic of the disease (as in acute myeloid leukemia), glycolysis at room temperature may cause the K^+ deficit to seem greater than it actually is. Taking together the effects of glycolysis causing an initial intracellular shift of K^+ followed by K^+ leakage from cells because of glucose exhaustion or inhibition of glycolysis by refrigeration, the recommendation for the most reliable K^+ determinations is to collect blood with heparin to maintain it between 25 °C and 37 °C, and to separate the plasma within minutes by high-speed centrifugation without cooling. However, in practical terms, separation within 1 hour when samples are maintained at room temperature is unlikely to introduce great error in the majority of instances.

Finally, skeletal muscle activity causes K^+ efflux from muscle cells into plasma and can cause a marked elevation in plasma K^+ values. One particular, but common, example occurs when an upper arm tourniquet is not released before beginning to draw blood after a patient clenches his fist repeatedly. The plasma K^+ values can artifactually increase as much as 2 mmol/L because of the muscle activity.[31]

Determination of Potassium in Body Fluids

Like sodium, potassium may be determined by spectrophotometry, AAS, FES, or electrochemically with a K^+-ISE. The ISE method is currently the most common by far. In the physiological range, it should be possible with modern equipment and good quality assurance to achieve coefficients of variation of less than 2% for plasma. Details are described later in this chapter along with the methods for Na^+.

Reference Intervals[65,101]

Reported reference intervals for the serum of adults vary from 3.5 to 5.1 and 3.5 to 5.0 mmol/L, and 3.7 to 5.9 for newborns. For plasma, frequently cited intervals are 3.5 to 4.5 and 3.4 to 4.8 mmol/L for adults. Cerebrospinal fluid concentrations are ~70% of plasma.[106] Urinary excretion of K^+ varies with dietary intake, but a typical range observed in an average diet is 25 to 125 mmol/day. Gastric juice contains K^+ at ~10 mmol/L. Fecal excretion has been reported as 18.2 ± 2.5 mmol/day in one instance[19] and ~5 mmol/day in another.[101] In severe diarrhea, gastrointestinal loss may be as much as 60 mmol/day.

Methods for the Determination of Sodium and Potassium

Although AAS, FES, or spectrophotometric methods may be used for Na^+ and K^+ analysis, most laboratories now use ISE methods. Of approximately 5400 laboratories reporting College of American Pathologists (CAP) proficiency data for Na^+ and K^+, >99% were using ISE methods in 2003.[22] The principles of each of these approaches (which are discussed in detail in Chapters 3 and 4) are the same whether the instrumentation is dedicated or integrated into a multichannel system.

Flame Emission Spectrophotometry

Reference methods using flame photometry for serum have been proposed for both sodium and potassium.[78] Although at one time the most common method for Na^+ and K^+ analysis, FES is no longer a common laboratory method. Advances in electrochemistry combined with the high amount of maintenance and safety procedures for FES have essentially led to the demise of this method for electrolyte analysis.

Principle. Samples are diluted in a diluent containing known amounts of lithium (or cesium, if lithium itself is being measured) and aspirated into a propane-air flame. Sodium, potassium, lithium, and cesium ions, when excited, emit spectra with sharp, bright lines at 589, 768, 671, and 852 nm, respectively. Light emitted from the thermally excited ions is directed through separate interference filters to corresponding photodetectors. The Li^+ or Cs^+ emission signal is used as an internal standard (usually 15 mmol/L) against which the Na^+ and K^+ signals are compared. The system is calibrated relative to low and high concentrations of each analyte, and the relation of signal to concentration is defined by a microprocessor (see also Chapter 3). Details about reagents, procedures, and laboratory safety issues for flame photometry can be found in the third edition of this text (pp. 1059-1060).[18]

Ion-Selective Electrodes[66,68]

Analyzers fitted with ISEs usually contain Na^+ electrodes with glass membranes and K^+ electrodes with liquid ion-exchange membranes that incorporate valinomycin. (Typical electrodes and the principles of potentiometry are described in detail in Chapter 4.) Simply stated, potentiometry is the determination of change in electromotive force (E, potential) in a circuit between a measurement electrode (the ISE) and a reference electrode, as the selected ion interacts with the membrane of the ISE. In instrument applications, the measuring system is calibrated by introduction of calibrator solutions containing defined amounts of Na^+ and K^+. The potentials of the calibrators are determined, and the $\Delta E/\Delta$ log concentration is stored in microprocessor memory as a factor for calculating unknown concentration when E of the unknown is measured. Frequent calibration, initiated either by the user or by automated, microprocessor-controlled uptake of sample from a reservoir of calibrator, is characteristic of most systems. Some instruments are designed to measure Na^+ and K^+ in whole blood, particularly point-of-care testing (POCT) devices and newer blood gas analyzers.

Two types of ISE methods must be distinguished. In the *indirect ISE methods,* the sample is introduced into the measurement chamber after mixing with a rather large volume of diluent. Examples include the Beckman Coulter Synchron CX and LX systems, the Roche Diagnostic Hitachi Modular systems, and the Olympus Diagnostics AU systems. Indirect methods were developed earlier in the history of ISE technology when dilution was necessary to present a small sample in a volume large enough to adequately cover a large electrode and to minimize the concentration of protein at the electrode surface. In the *direct ISE methods,* the sample is presented to the electrodes without dilution. This approach became possible with the miniaturization of electrodes. Examples of direct ISEs include those on blood gas analyzers, such as the Radiometer ABL series, the Instrumentation Laboratories GEM series, and the Bayer Diagnostics Rapid Lab series. Single-use, thin-film ISEs for Na^+, K^+, and Cl^- are unique applications of a direct ISE method that are used by the Ortho Diagnostic's Vitros analyzers.[23] In 2003, of the 5400 laboratories reporting CAP proficiency sample results for Na^+ and K^+, ~two thirds used indirect ISEs and one third used direct ISE methods.[22] Important differences in direct and indirect methods that can cause significant differences in analytical results are discussed in the later section on the electrolyte exclusion effect.

Errors observed in the use of ISEs fall into three categories. First are errors caused by lack of selectivity. For instance, many Cl^- electrodes lack selectivity against other halide ions. Second are errors introduced by repeated protein coating of the ion-sensitive membrane, or by contamination of the membrane or salt bridge by ions that compete or react with the selected ion and thus alter electrode response. These necessitate periodic changes of the membrane as part of routine maintenance. Finally, the "electrolyte exclusion effect," which applies only to indirect methods and is caused by the solvent-displacing effect of lipid and protein in the sample, results in falsely decreased values[5] (see the section on the electrolyte exclusion effect later in this chapter).

Spectrophotometric Methods

Spectrophotometric methods fall into three categories: those based on enzyme activation, those that detect the spectral shift produced when either Na^+ or K^+ binds to a macrocyclic chromophore, and fluorescent sensors. Both approaches have been applied to smaller automated instruments. However, the high cost of reagents for these methods and the fact that few problems exist with ISE methods has resulted in small "niche" use of these methods, primarily in some smaller instruments used in physicians' offices or clinics.

Kinetic spectrophotometric assays for Na^+ are based on activation of the enzyme β-galactosidase by Na^+ to hydrolyze *o*-nitrophenyl-β-D-galactopyranoside (ONPG).[9,85] The rate of production of *o*-nitrophenol (the chromophore) is measured at 420 nm.

CH₂OH, OH, H, OH, H, H, H, OH, O, N=O — *o*-Nitrophenyl-β-D-galactopyranoside $\xrightarrow[\beta\text{-Galactosidase}]{Na^{\oplus}}$ Galactose + *o*-Nitrophenol (λ_{max} = 420 nm)

K^+-specific enzyme activation assays are illustrated by methods using tryptophanase,[53] one of a number of K^+-enhanced enzymes.[8] Accuracy and precision of the method have been reported to compare favorably with those achieved with flame photometry.[47] Bilirubin and hemoglobin and other cations are said to have little effect as interferants, but lipemic samples could not be analyzed.[47]

Macrocyclic ionophores are molecules whose atoms are organized to form a cavity into which metal ions fit and bind with high affinity. Such compounds are also called *polycyclic ethers, crown ethers, cryptands,* or *cryptahemispherands.* Different macrocyclics can be made with cavities tailored to fit the ionic radii of different elements. When chromogenic properties are imparted to these ionophores, spectral shifts occur when the cation is bound. The specificity of many of these ionophores is clearly sufficient for clinical purposes.[55]

One proprietary chromogenic ionophore, *ChromoLyte,* a trinitroanilino-cryptahemispherand, is selective for Na^+ and has been used in some instruments (Bayer Diagnostics, Tarrytown, N.Y.), whereas others are used on smaller, physician's office type of instruments, such as the Abbott Vision (Abbott Laboratories) or Bayer Seralyzer (Bayer Diagnostics, Elkhart, Ind.). These methods give results comparable with methods using ISEs.[55] Potassium can be measured with the same method but using an ionophore with a different cavity size.[55] In fact, an early clinical application of the macrocyclic ionophore principle is the valinomycin ISE for K^+ (see Chapter 4). The Reflotron analyzer (Roche Diagnostics) uses valinomycin in conjunction with a pH indicator to determine serum K^+ concentration. If the cyclic compound has a high binding constant for K^+ and the properties of a chromophore, the process of binding K^+ causes a spectral shift as the molecular structure or ionic form (or both) of the chromophore adjusts to the presence of K^+ in the cavity. Although unsuitable for urine because NH_4^+ is an interferant, results for K^+ in the serum appear to correlate well with those of flame photometric and direct and indirect ISE methods.[96] Finally, fluorescent sensor molecules whose fluorescence is altered by specific binding of electrolytes is the principle of measurement in the OPTI critical care analyzer for POCT from Osmetech, Inc.

ELECTROLYTE EXCLUSION EFFECT[5]

The electrolyte exclusion effect is the exclusion of electrolytes from the fraction of the total plasma volume that is occupied by solids. The volume of total solids (primarily protein and lipid) in an aliquot of plasma is approximately 7% so that ~93% of plasma volume is actually water. The main electrolytes (Na^+, K^+, Cl^-, HCO_3^-) are essentially confined to the water phase. When a fixed volume of total plasma (e.g., 10 μL) is pipetted for dilution before flame photometry or indirect ISE analysis, only 9.3 μL of plasma water containing the electrolytes is actually added to the diluent. Thus a concentration of Na^+ determined by flame photometry or indirect ISE to be 145 mmol/L is the concentration in the total plasma volume, *not* in the plasma water volume. In fact, if the plasma contains 93% water, the concentration of Na^+ in plasma water is $145 \times (100/93)$, or 156 mmol/L. This negative "error" in plasma electrolyte analysis has been recognized for many years.[4] Even though it is the electrolyte concentration in plasma water that is physiological, it is tacitly assumed that the volume fraction of water in plasma is sufficiently constant that this difference could be ignored. In fact, all electrolyte reference intervals are based on this assumption and actually reflect concentrations in total plasma volume and not in the water volume. Indeed, virtually all concentrations measured in the clinical chemistry laboratory are related to the total sample volume rather than to the water volume. This electrolyte exclusion effect becomes problematic when pathophysiological condi-

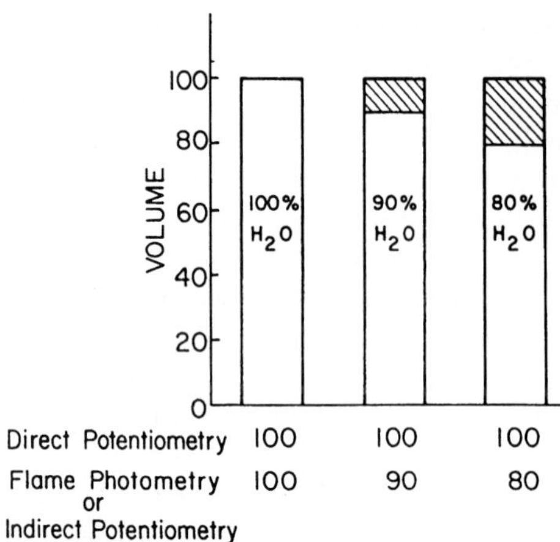

Figure 27-1 Predicted influence of water content on sodium measurements for a 100 mmol/L NaCl solution by direct ion-selective electrode (ISE versus flame emission photometry or indirect ISE). *Hatched areas* represent nonaqueous volumes, which could consist of lipids, proteins, or even a slurry of latex or sand particles. *(From Apple FS, Koch DD, Graves S, Ladenson JH. Relationship between direct-potentiometric and flame-photometric measurement of sodium in blood. Clin Chem 1982;28:1931-5.)*

TABLE 27-1 Methods Measuring the Concentration in the Whole Sample Volume and Thus Subject to Electrolyte Exclusion Effect

Method	Analytes
Flame photometry	Na^+, K^+, Li^+
Atomic absorption spectrometry	Ca^{2+}, Mg^{2+}, and others
Amperometry/coulometry	Cl^-
Indirect potentiometry	Na^+, K^+, Ca^{2+}, Cl^-

tions are present that alter the plasma water volume, such as hyperlipidemia or hyperproteinemia. In these settings, falsely low electrolyte values are obtained whenever samples are diluted before analysis, as in flame photometry or indirect ISE[5] (Figure 27-1).

Indirect ISE methods dilute the sample in a diluent of fixed high ionic strength so that for Na^+, the activity coefficient approaches a value of 1. Under these circumstances, the measurement of activity, a (where $a = \gamma \times$ concentration, and γ is the activity coefficient), is tantamount to measurement of concentration. Flame photometry measures emission of a specific ion after dilution in solutions of high reference ion concentration so that specific emission is also tantamount to the measurement of concentration of the specific ion in total plasma volume. It is the dilution of total plasma volume and the assumption that plasma water volume is constant that render both indirect ISE and flame photometry methods equally subject to the electrolyte exclusion effect. In certain settings, such as ketoacidosis with severe hyperlipidemia[38] or multiple myeloma with severe hyperproteinemia,[57] the negative exclusion effect may be so large that laboratory results lead clinicians to believe that electrolyte concentrations are normal or low when, in fact, the concentration in the water phase may be high or normal, respectively.

The direct ISE methods still determine the concentration relative to activity but do not require sample dilution. Because there is no dilution, activity is directly proportional to the concentration in the water phase, not the concentration in the total volume. To make results from direct ISEs equivalent to flame photometry and indirect ISEs, most direct ISE methods operate in what is commonly referred to as the "flame mode." In this mode, the directly measured concentration in plasma water is multiplied by the average water volume fraction of plasma (0.93). Although the latter may vary widely, as long as the activity of the specific ion is constant, the concentration of the ion in the water phase becomes *independent* of the relative proportions of water and total solids if the ion is not bound by proteins, as is the case for Ca^{2+}. Therefore direct ISE methods are free of the electrolyte exclusion effects, and the values determined by direct ISE methods—even in the flame mode—are directly proportional to activity in the water phase and define electrolyte concentrations in a more physiological and physicochemical sense.

Most clinical chemists and physicians have reached a conclusion that direct ISE methods for electrolyte analysis are the methods of choice. They base their conclusion on the fact that great changes in plasma lipid, protein, and other solids can be expected in relatively common clinical conditions and in therapies such as parenteral alimentation with lipid emulsions. They emphasize further that even in the absence of great changes in the volume fraction of solids, results by direct methods most realistically reflect clinical status and are therefore more effectively used in diagnosis and management. However, it is clear that results from direct methods will continue to be converted to total plasma volume concentrations by use of the "flame mode," and indeed this is the recommendation of the National Committee for Clinical Laboratory Standards (NCCLS).[78] This is also a good recommendation since two thirds of laboratories still use indirect ISE methods[22] and since some reviewers mistakenly believe that modern clinical laboratories are no longer subject to this cause of falsely decreased electrolyte values.[15] Tables 27-1 and 27-2 summarize methods that are and are not subject to the electrolyte exclusion effects, respectively.

The most common causes of the electrolyte exclusion effect leading to pseudohyponatremia or pseudohypokalemia are hyperlipidemia[25] and hyperproteinemia.[58] In severe hypoproteinemia, the effect works in reverse, resulting in a falsely high (2% to 4%) Na^+ or K^+ value. Several approaches have been proposed to improve the physiological accuracy of electrolyte values determined by methods

TABLE 27-2 Methods Measuring the Activity, Molality, or Concentration in the Water Phase and Thus Not Subject to Electrolyte Exclusion Effect

Method	Analytes
ISEs with *undiluted* sample	H^+ (pH), Na^+, K^+, Ca^{2+}, Cl^-, Li^+
Gas electrodes	CO_2 (PCO_2), O_2 (PO_2) HCO_3^- (calculated from pH and PCO_2)
Freezing point depression	H_2O (osmolality)

subject to the electrolyte exclusion effect. For lipemic samples, centrifugation at 100,000 ×*g* and analysis of the chylomicron-poor infranatant is the most common approach.[4] When triglyceride concentrations are less than 1500 mg/dL the error is less than 3%, and it is less than 5% for triglyceride concentrations less than 2500 mg/dL.

In situations in which both lipid and protein content are altered, presenting plasma electrolyte values along with concurrent estimates of plasma water has been suggested. One approach to estimate plasma water is Waugh's empirical equation[107]:

$$\text{Plasma water [g/dL]} = 99.1 - 0.73(P_s) - 1.03(L_s)$$

where P_s is serum total protein and L_s is serum total lipid, both in grams per deciliter. Determination of plasma water by an osmometry-based method[4] is also possible, but cumbersome. A simple, though time-consuming, estimate of serum water can be done by gravimetry. A measured aliquot of serum is weighed, evaporated to dryness, and reweighed, the decrement in weight being the measure of the water fraction. In a practical sense, however, these steps are seldom done, and it is paramount that clinical chemists be aware of the electrolyte exclusion effect and be able to invoke special procedures in these cases to mitigate these errors. Alternatively, the best solution is to use a direct ISE method.

CHLORIDE

Chloride is the major extracellular anion, with median plasma and interstitial fluid concentrations of ~103 mmol/L. This represents by far the largest fraction of the total inorganic anion concentration of ~154 mmol/L. Together, sodium and chloride represent the majority of the osmotically active constituents of plasma. Therefore chloride is significantly involved in the maintenance of water distribution, osmotic pressure, and anion-cation balance in the extracellular fluid (ECF). In contrast to its high ECF concentrations, the concentration of Cl^- in the intracellular fluid of erythrocytes is 45 to 54 mmol/L, and in the intracellular fluid of most other tissue cells it is only ~1 mmol/L. In both gastric and small and large intestinal secretions, Cl^- is the most abundant anion.

Chloride ions in food are almost completely absorbed from the intestinal tract. They are filtered from plasma at the glomeruli and passively reabsorbed, along with Na^+, in the proximal tubules. In the thick ascending limb of the loop of Henle, Cl^- is actively reabsorbed by the chloride pump, whose action promotes passive reabsorption of Na^+. Loop diuretics such as furosemide and ethacrynic acid inhibit the chloride pump. Surplus Cl^- is excreted in the urine and is also lost in the sweat, especially in hot environments.

Methods for Determination of Chloride in Body Fluids

Chloride may be determined by mercurimetric titration, spectrophotometry, coulometric-amperometric titration, or, most commonly today, ISE.

Specimens

Chloride is most often measured in serum or plasma, urine, and sweat. Cl^- is quite stable in serum and plasma. Even gross hemolysis does not significantly alter serum or plasma Cl^- concentration because the erythrocyte concentration of Cl^- is approximately half of that in plasma. Because very little Cl^- is protein bound, changes in posture, stasis, or use of tourniquets also have little effect on its plasma concentration. Measurement of Cl^- lost in gastric aspirates or intestinal drainages is an adjunct to parenteral replacement therapy. Fecal Cl^- determination may be useful for the diagnosis of congenital hypochloremic alkalosis with hyperchloridorrhea (increased excretion of Cl^- in stool). In this condition, the concentration of Cl^- in feces may reach 180 mmol/L, with almost no Cl^- being found in urine.

Mercurimetric Titration

One of the earliest methods for determining Cl^- in biological fluids is mentioned here for historical purposes.[92] A protein-free filtrate of specimen is titrated with mercuric nitrate solution in the presence of diphenylcarbazone as an indicator. Free Hg^{2+} combines with Cl^- to form soluble but essentially nonionized mercuric chloride:

$$2Cl^- + Hg(NO_3)_2 \rightarrow HgCl_2 + 2NO_3^-$$

Excess Hg^{2+} reacts with diphenylcarbazone to form a blue-violet color complex. A more detailed description can be found in the first edition of this textbook (pp. 1184-1185).[100]

Spectrophotometric Methods

Spectrophotometric methods based on the reaction of Cl^- with mercuric thiocyanate used to be common on many automated analyzers. The principle is illustrated in the following equations:

$$Hg(SCN)_2 + 2Cl^- \rightarrow HgCl_2 + 2SCN^-$$

$$3(SCN)^- + Fe^{3+} \rightarrow Fe(SCN)_3$$

Chloride ions react with undissociated mercuric thiocyanate to form undissociated mercuric chloride and free thiocyanate ions. The thiocyanate ions react with ferric ion (Fe^{3+}) to form the highly colored, reddish complex of ferric thiocyanate with an absorption peak at 480 nm. Perchloric acid increases the intensity of the red color. High concentrations of globulins in the serum interfere in these methods because turbidity develops. This reaction is also very temperature sensitive.

Mercurimetric automated methods applied to high-volume testing presented the problem of disposal of reagent waste containing a significant amount of toxic mercury. The mercuric thiocyanate and nitrate methods constituted about 3% of the laboratories reporting Cl^- results in a 1996 CAP survey report but none of ~5400 laboratories used these methods according to a 2003 CAP report.[22] The ferric perchlorate method eliminates the mercurial reagent entirely.[59] Ferric perchlorate and Cl^- react in dilute perchloric acid to form a color complex with absorption maxima at 344 and 562 nm. The absorbance-concentration relationship is linear, and the reaction is more specific for Cl^- than many other spectrophotometric methods. However, this method is also no longer reported as being used in a 2003 CAP survey.[22]

Coulometric-Amperometric Titration

The reactions in coulometric-amperometric determinations of Cl^- depend on the generation of Ag^+ from a silver electrode at a constant rate and on the reaction of Ag^+ with Cl^- in the sample to form insoluble silver chloride[24]:

$$Ag^+ + Cl^- \rightarrow AgCl$$

After the stoichiometric point is reached, excess Ag^+ in the mixture triggers shutdown of the Ag^+ generation system. A timing device records the elapsed time between the start and stop of the Ag^+ generation. (A more detailed description of this principle can be found in Chapter 4.) Because the time interval is proportional to the amount of Cl^- present in the sample, the concentration of Cl^- can be calculated:

$$\text{Chloride (mmol/L)} = \frac{\text{time}_{\text{undnown}} - \text{time}_{\text{blank}}}{\text{time}_{\text{calibrator}} - \text{time}_{\text{blank}}} \times C_{\text{calibrator}}$$

where $C_{calibrator}$ is the concentration of calibrator.

Applications of the coulometric-amperometric principle (often called a Cotlove chloridometer[24]) are the most precise methods for measuring Cl^- over the entire range of concentrations displayed in body fluids. CAP surveys from 1996 showed coefficients of variation of ±1.3% to 1.5% ($n = 42$) for the Beckman ASTRA method and less than ±2.2% for the Corning Titrator (Chiron Diagnostics) over the concentration range of 102 to 119 mmol/L. Calibrator concentrations should, however, be chosen to correlate with the concentration range of unknowns. The method is subject to interferences by other halide ions, by CN^- and SCN^- ions, by sulfhydryl groups, and by heavy metal contamination. Because samples are prediluted before analysis, these methods are also subject to the electrolyte exclusion effect. Maintenance of the systems is crucial to proper operation; electrodes and reaction vials or chambers must be kept scrupulously clean and the proper shape and size of the Ag^+-generating electrodes must be maintained. Only 12 of 5400 laboratories reported in the 2003 CAP survey reported Cl^- results using coulometry.[22] However, some laboratories still maintain these instruments as backups and for sweat analysis.

Ion-Selective Electrode Methods

Solvent polymeric membranes that incorporate quaternary ammonium salt anion-exchangers, such as tri-*n*-octylpropylammonium chloride decanol, are used to construct Cl^--selective electrodes in clinical analyzers.[83] Although by far the most common method for measuring Cl^- in clinical laboratories, these electrodes have been described to suffer from membrane instability and lot-to-lot inconsistency in selectivity to other anions.[83,104] Anions that tend to be problematic are other halides and organic anions, such as SCN^-, which can be particularly problematic because of their ability to solubilize in the polymeric organic membrane of these electrodes.

Approximately 68% of 5394 laboratories reporting in a 2003 CAP proficiency test survey for Cl^- used indirect ISE methodology.[22] Instruments using the indirect ISE method for Cl^- on serum or plasma include the Dade Behring Dimension Series, the Roche Diagnostics Hitachi Modular System, the Beckman Coulter Synchron series, the Abbott Aeroset, and the Olympus AU series of analyzers. In 2003, 1646 of 5394 laboratories (32%) participating in a CAP proficiency survey used direct ISEs, and most of those were the Ortho Diagnostics Vitros series of dry slide analyzers, and blood gas analyzers with direct ISEs.

Reference Intervals[65,101]

Reported reference intervals for Cl^- in the serum or plasma range from 98 to 107 mmol/L to 100 to 108 mmol/L. For neonates, the upper limit of the interval extends to 110 mmol/L. The serum values vary little during the day. The spinal fluid Cl^- concentrations are ~15% higher than in the serum.[106] Urinary excretion of Cl^- varies with dietary intake, but an interval of 110 to 250 mmol/day is typical. Fecal excretion of Cl^- (for eight healthy subjects) has been reported as 3.2 ± 0.7 mmol/day (SEM)[19] and elsewhere as ~2 mmol/day.[101]

BICARBONATE (TOTAL CARBON DIOXIDE)

Total carbon dioxide is used here to describe the quantity that is measured most often in automated analyzers by acidification of a serum or plasma sample and measurement of the carbon dioxide released by the process, or by alkalinization and measurement of total bicarbonate. Under certain conditions of collection and specimen handling, total carbon dioxide values determined in this manner may be almost identical with values for the calculated concentration of total carbon dioxide obtained in blood gas analysis (see later section in this chapter on blood gas methods). The pathophysiology of bicarbonate in acid-base disorders is discussed in detail in Chapter 46.

Specimens

Either serum or heparinized plasma may be assayed. The usual specimen is venous blood drawn into an evacuated tube, although capillary blood taken in microtubes or capillary tubes may also be presented for analysis. Given a specimen in a vacuum-draw tube, the concentration of total CO_2 is most accurately determined when the assay is done immediately after opening the tube and as promptly as possible after collection and centrifugation of the blood in the unopened tube. Ambient air contains far less CO_2 than does plasma, and gaseous dissolved CO_2 will escape from the specimen into the air, with a consequent decrease in the CO_2 value of up to 6 mmol/L in the course of 1 hour.[102] In practical terms, the logistics of high-volume processing and automated analysis of specimens almost ensures that most CO_2 measurements are done on specimens that have lost some dissolved gaseous CO_2, simply because preservation of anaerobic conditions is not practical between the time plasma is placed on an instrument and the time it is sampled. Thus the term "bicarbonate" may actually be preferable to "total CO_2." On the other hand, it is probable that the result of a stat specimen, which is rapidly processed and promptly analyzed, has a much smaller error.

Methods for Determination of Serum or Plasma Total Carbon Dioxide

One of the earliest methods for determining total CO_2 was the *manometric method* for total CO_2 content, using the Natelson microgasometer. This has been supplanted in clinical laboratories by automated methods. This method is described in some detail in an earlier edition of this text.[100]

The first step in automated methods is acidification or alkalinization of the sample. Acidifying the sample converts the various forms of CO_2 in plasma to gaseous CO_2 by dilution with an acid buffer. Alkalinizing the sample converts all CO_2 and carbonic acid to HCO_3^-.[43] The oldest automated methods were those used in *continuous-flow systems* in which the gaseous CO_2 diffused across a silicone membrane into a recipient solution buffered at pH 9.2 and containing the pH indicator phenolphthalein. The change in color over the baseline was determined by a photometer and is proportional to the amount of CO_2 released from the sample. These methods suffered from considerable baseline drift. Also, frequent reagent preparation and recalibration were necessary to keep the method in control. Air lines that supplied bubbles to the sample and reagent streams in these methods were fitted with a CO_2-absorbing trap, which had a short effective life. This method, although a mainstay of the 1960s and 1970s, is not used today.

Methods for total CO_2 measurement in today's automated instruments are either electrode based or enzymatic. In indirect electrode-based methods, such as the Beckman Coulter Synchron and Dade Behring Dimension series of analyzers, the released gaseous CO_2 after acidification is determined by a PCO_2 electrode (discussed in Chapter 4) in the reaction chamber of the CO_2 module. About 47% of 5211 laboratories reporting CAP data used an indirect ISE method in 2003.[22] These methods tend to be linear between ~5 and ~45 mmol/L. *Direct ISE methodology* for total CO_2 is not common on automated analyzers, with only 3% of laboratories from the 2003 CAP using this approach. Direct methods have had some problems with specificity. For instance, one direct total CO_2 electrode reacts almost equivalently with nitrate.[29]

An *enzymatic method* for CO_2 is illustrated by the methods used in the Abbott Aeroset, Bayer Advia, Roche Diagnostics Hitachi Modular, and most Ortho Diagnostics Virtos analyzers. The specimen is first alkalinized to convert all CO_2 and carbonic acid to HCO_3^-. The enzymatic reactions are as follows:

$$\text{Phosphoenolpyruvate} + HCO_3^- \xrightarrow{\text{Phosphoenolpyruvate carboxylase}} \text{Oxaloacetate} + P_i$$

$$\text{Oxaloacetate} + NADH + H^+ \xrightleftharpoons{\text{Malate dehydrogenase}} \text{Malate} + NAD^+$$

Decrease in absorbance of NADH at 340 nm is proportional to the total CO_2 content.

In 2003, these enzymatic methods are used by about 50% of all laboratories reporting total CO_2 values on CAP surveys.[22]

Reference Intervals[65,101]

Reference intervals generally are instrument dependent, and manufacturers' manuals should be consulted in specific cases. The following are reference intervals published in a compendium.[101]

Anaerobic Samples	mmol/L
Whole blood, venous	22-26
Whole blood, arterial	24-29
Plasma/serum, venous	23-29
Plasma, capillary	
Premature, 1 wk	14-27
Newborn	13-22
Infant, child	20-28
Adult	22-29
Adult, >60 yr	23-31
Cord blood	14-22

PLASMA AND URINE OSMOLALITY

Determination of plasma and urine osmolality can be useful in the assessment of electrolyte and acid-base disorders. Comparison of plasma and urine osmolalities can determine the appropriateness and status of water regulation by the kidneys in settings of severe electrolyte disturbances, as might occur in diabetes insipidus or the syndrome of inappropriate antidiuretic hormone (SIADH) (see Chapters 45 and 50). The major osmotic substances in normal plasma are Na^+, Cl^-, glucose, and urea; thus expected plasma osmolality can be calculated from the following empirical equation:

$$\begin{aligned} \text{mOsmol/kg} &= 1.86\,(\text{Na}^+\,[\text{mmol/L}]) \\ &\quad + \text{glucose}\,[\text{mmol/L}] \\ &\quad + \text{urea}\,[\text{mmol/L}] \\ &\quad + 9 \end{aligned}$$

or

$$\begin{aligned} \text{mOsmol/kg} &= 1.86\,(\text{Na}^+\,[\text{mmol/L}]) \\ &\quad + \text{glucose}\,[\text{mg/dL}]/18 \\ &\quad + \text{urea N}\,[\text{mg/dL}]/2.8 \\ &\quad + 9 \end{aligned}$$

The 9 mOsmol/kg added to the above equation represents the contribution of other osmotically active substances in plasma, such as K^+, Ca^{2+}, and proteins, and 1.86 is two times the osmotic coefficient of Na^+, reflecting the contributions of both Na^+ and Cl^-. The reference interval for plasma osmolality is 275 to 300 mOsmol/kg. Comparison of measured osmolality with calculated osmolality can help identify the presence of an "osmolal gap," which can be important in determining the presence of exogenous osmotic substances. Comparison of calculated and measured osmolalities can also confirm or rule out suspected pseudohyponatremia caused by the previously discussed electrolyte exclusion effect.

Principles of Osmotic Pressure and Osmosis

Osmometry is a technique for measuring the concentration of solute particles that contribute to the osmotic pressure of a solution. Osmotic pressure governs the movement of solvent (water in biological systems) across membranes that separate two solutions. Different membranes vary in pore size and thus in their ability to select molecules of different size and shape. Examples of biologically important selective membranes are those enclosing the glomerular and capillary vessels that are permeable to water and to essentially all *small* molecules and ions, but not to large protein molecules. Differences in the concentrations of osmotically active molecules that cannot cross a membrane cause those molecules that can cross the membrane to move to establish an osmotic equilibrium. This movement of solute and permeable ions exerts what is known as osmotic pressure.

As an example, consider an aqueous solution of sucrose placed within a sac made up of a membrane permeable only to water, with an open vertical glass tube (a crude manometer) attached to the sac. If the sac is placed into a beaker of distilled water, water will move from the beaker across the membrane into the sucrose solution. The pressure of this solvent movement will cause the sucrose solution to rise some distance up the tube. At equilibrium, the gravitational pressure of the column of solution in the tube equals the osmotic pressure and prevents further net movement of water from the beaker. The height of the rise of the sucrose solution in the manometer tube is a measure of the *osmotic pressure* of the sucrose solution. This is the pressure that would have to be exerted on the sucrose side of the membrane to prevent the flow of water across the membrane.

Osmosis[105] is the process that constitutes the movement of solvent across a membrane in response to differences in osmotic pressure across the two sides of the membrane. Water migrates across the membrane toward the side containing more concentrated solute.

If the sucrose solution in the aforementioned membrane sac were replaced with a sodium chloride solution of the same molarity, the solution in the manometer would reach equilibrium at a point almost twice as high as that observed with sucrose because sodium chloride dissociates into two ions per molecule. If ion activity is unrestricted, the sodium chloride solution would have twice as many osmotically active particles (osmoles) for the same molecular concentration as the sucrose solution. In reality, the number of active particles is less than this (0.93 for NaCl), as explained later in this chapter. The total number of individual (solute) particles present in a solution per given mass of solvent, regardless of their molecular nature (i.e., nonelectrolyte, ion, or colloid), determines the total osmotic pressure of the solution. In blood plasma, for example, nonelectrolytes such as glucose and urea and even proteins contribute to the osmotic pressure of this body fluid.

Colligative Properties

In addition to increasing osmotic pressure when the solute is added to the solvent, the *vapor pressure* of the solution is *lowered* below that of the pure solvent. As a result of the change in vapor pressure, the *boiling point* of the solution is *raised* above that of the pure solvent, and the *freezing point* of the solution is *lowered* below that of the pure solvent.

These four properties of solutions—(1) increased osmotic pressure, (2) lowered vapor pressure, (3) increased boiling point, and (4) decreased freezing point—are called *colligative properties.* They all are directly related to the total number of solute particles per mass of solvent. For instance, a 1-molal solution in water boils at a temperature 0.52 °C higher and freezes at a temperature 1.858 °C lower than pure water. The vapor pressure of this solution is 0.3 mm Hg lower than the vapor pressure of pure water, which is 23.8 mm Hg at 25 °C. The osmotic pressure of the same solution is increased from zero to 17,000 mm Hg (22.4 atmospheres). The term *osmolality* expresses concentrations relative to *mass* of the solvent (1 osmolal solution is defined to contain 1 Osmol/kg H_2O), whereas the term *osmolarity* expresses concentrations per volume of solution (1 osmolar solution is defined to contain 1 osmol/L solution). Osmolality (Osmol/kg H_2O) is a thermodynamically more exact expression because solution concentrations expressed on a weight basis are temperature independent, whereas those based on volume will vary with temperature. Although the term "osmolarity" is often used in medical literature, osmolality is what the clinical laboratory measures and is a more informative term.

An electrolyte in solution dissociates into two (in the case of NaCl) or three (in the case of $CaCl_2$) particles, and therefore the colligative effects of such solutions are multiplied by the number of dissociated ions formed per molecule. However, because of incomplete electrolyte dissociation and associations between the solute and solvent molecules, many solutions do not behave in the ideal case, and a 1-molal solution may give an osmotic pressure lower than theoretically expected. The osmotic activity coefficient is a factor used to correct for the deviation from the "ideal" behavior of the system:

$$\text{Osmolality} = \text{osmol/kg H}_2\text{O} = \phi n C$$

where

ϕ = osmotic coefficient

n = number of particles into which each molecule in the solution potentially dissociates

C = molality in mol/kg H_2O.

A table of osmotic coefficients of most solutes of biological interest has been compiled.[110]

Glucose and ethanol have osmotic coefficients of 1.00, whereas the ϕ for sodium chloride is 0.93 at the concentrations found in serum—thus the derivation of $1.86 \times Na^+$ (mmol) in the formula to calculate plasma osmolality (NaCl potentially contributes 2 osmotically active particles times $0.93 = 1.86$). The total osmolality or osmotic pressure of a solution is equal to the sum of the osmotic pressures or osmolalities of all solute species present. The electrolytes Na^+, Cl^-, and HCO_3^-, which are present in relatively high concentration, make the greatest contribution to serum osmolality. Nonelectrolytes such as glucose and urea, which are present normally at lower molal concentrations, contribute less, and serum proteins contribute less than 0.5% of the total serum osmolality because even the most abundant protein is present at millimolar concentrations.

Theoretically, any of the four colligative properties (vapor pressure, boiling point, freezing point, or osmotic pressure) could be used as a basis for the measurement of osmolality. However, the freezing point depression is most commonly used in clinical laboratories because of its simplicity. Furthermore, freezing point depression is independent of changes in ambient temperature, unlike vapor pressure. (The vapor pressure of water is 17.5 mm Hg at 20 °C, 23.8 mm Hg at 25 °C, and 47.1 mm Hg at 37 °C.)

Freezing Point Depression Osmometer

The instrument used is a freezing point depression osmometer[1], but it is often referred to simply as an osmometer. The components of a freezing point depression osmometer (Figure 27-2) are as follows:

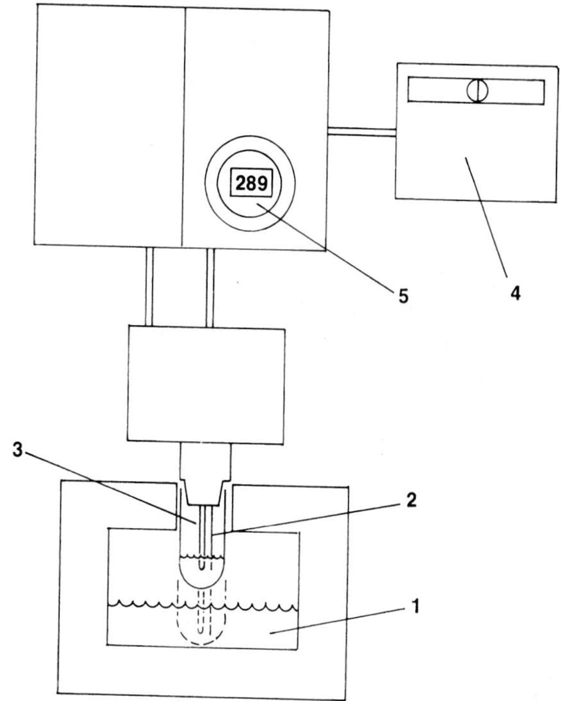

Figure 27-2 Block diagram of a freezing point depression osmometer. *1*, Cooling fluid; *2*, stirring rod; *3*, thermistor; *4*, galvanometer; *5*, potentiometer with direct readout. The test tube is shown above the liquid in the cooling bath *(solid line)* and inside the cooling liquid *(dashed line)*.

1. A thermostatically controlled cooling bath or block maintained at −7 °C.
2. A rapid stir mechanism to initiate ("seed") freezing of the sample.
3. A thermistor probe connected to a circuit to measure the temperature of the sample. (The thermistor is a glass bead attached to a metal stem whose resistance varies rapidly and predictably with temperature.)
4. A galvanometer that displays the freezing curve and that is used as a guide when the measuring potentiometer is used.
5. A measuring potentiometer (variable resistor) is used to null the current in the circuit.

In most instruments, components 4 and 5 are replaced by a light-emitting diode (LED) display that indicates the time course of the freezing curve and the final result.

During analysis, the following steps occur. The sample, in which the thermistor probe and stirring wire are centered, is lowered into the bath and, with gentle stirring, is super cooled to a temperature several degrees below its freezing point (−7 °C). When the galvanometer (or LED display) indicates that sufficient super cooling has occurred, the sample is raised to a point above the liquid in the cooling bath, and the wire stirrer is changed from a gentle rate of stir to a momentary vigorous amplitude, which initiates freezing of the super-cooled solution. This freezing is only to the slush stage, with about 2% to 3% of the solvent solidifying. The released heat of fusion initially warms the solution and then the temperature plateaus and remains stationary, indicating the equilibrium temperature at which both freezing and thawing of the solution are occurring. At the end of the equilibrium temperature plateau, the galvanometer again indicates decreasing temperature as the sample freezes further toward a complete solid.

An example of the calculation to obtain osmolality is: if the observed freezing point is −0.53 °C, then

$$\text{mOsmol/kg } H_2O = \frac{-0.53}{-1.86} \times 1000 = 285$$

where −1.86 °C is the molal freezing point depression of pure water.

Day-to-day precision of ±2 mOsmol/kg H_2O should be obtainable by today's osmometers. More than 98% of the laboratories in the 2003 CAP surveys use freezing point depression osmometers, with the automated instrument from Advanced Instruments (Norwood, Mass.) being the most common.[22]

Vapor Pressure Osmometer

Another type of osmometer is the vapor pressure osmometer. In reality, osmolality measurement in these instruments is not related directly to a change in vapor pressure (in millimeters of mercury), but to the decrease in the *dew point temperature* of the pure solvent (water) caused by the decrease in vapor pressure of the solvent by the solutes. In this instrument, temperature is measured by means of a thermocouple, which is a device consisting of two dissimilar metals joined so that a voltage difference generated between the points of contact (junctions) is a measure of the temperature difference between the points.

In clinical laboratories, the vapor pressure osmolality technique has been reported to be less precise than the freezing point depression method.[69] For serum samples, the coefficients of variation obtained for the vapor pressure osmometer are about twice those obtained for the freezing point depression osmometer. The lesser degree of precision is related to the lower slope of dew point decrease compared with freezing point decrease (i.e., 0.303 °C versus 1.86 °C per osmol/kg H_2O).

An important clinical difference between the vapor pressure technique and the freezing point depression osmometer is the failure of the former to include in its measurement of total osmolality any volatile solutes present in the serum. Substances such as ethanol, methanol, and isopropanol are volatile, and thus escape from the solution and increase the vapor pressure instead of lowering the vapor pressure of the solvent (water). This makes use of vapor pressure osmometers impractical for identifying osmolal gaps in acid-base disturbances (see Chapter 46). Thus use of this type of osmometer cannot be recommended for most clinical laboratories.

Colloid Osmotic Pressure

Because of their large molecular weight, proteins contribute only about 1 mOsmol/kg H_2O to the total serum osmolality measured by freezing point depression. Occasionally, one may be asked to determine the contribution of macromolecules to the serum osmolality. Colloid osmotic pressure (COP) is a direct measure of the contribution of macromolecules (primarily proteins) to the serum osmolality. It is used primarily in the assessment of pulmonary edema or other abnormalities of water balance and serum protein concentrations.[73] However, its utility has been questioned[32] and the method is seldom used. Previous editions of this textbook describe the principles of a COP osmometer.[18,102]

SWEAT TESTING

The analysis of sweat for increased electrolyte concentration is used to confirm the diagnosis of cystic fibrosis (CF). CF is recognized as a syndrome with a wide spectrum of clinical presentations associated with a defect in the cystic fibrosis transmembrane conductance regulator protein (CFTR), a protein that normally regulates electrolyte transport across epithelial membranes. (For a more detailed discussion of CF, see Chapter 40.) Several hundred mutations of CFTR have been identified. Although mutational analysis is available, it is not informative in all cases, and the sweat test remains the standard for diagnostic testing.[89]

The United States Cystic Fibrosis Foundation (CFF) states that the diagnosis of CF is based on the following criteria[89]:

1. The presence of one or more characteristic phenotypic features
2. *Or* a history of CF in a sibling
3. *Plus* laboratory evidence of a CFTR abnormality as documented by elevated sweat chloride concentrations or identification of two CF mutations or in vivo demonstration of characteristic abnormalities in ion transport across the nasal epithelium

To provide appropriate care for CF patients and genetic counseling to their families, it is important that the diagnosis of CF be made accurately and promptly. In the United States, 70% of all CF patients are diagnosed by age 1. However, 8% of patients are diagnosed later than age 10, and more and more patients are being diagnosed as adults.[28] In addition to variable clinical presentation, the diagnosis of CF can be complicated by erroneous sweat-testing results. Unreliable methods, technical errors, and errors in interpretation can all lead to false results.[30,60,88] In an effort to standardize testing, the National Committee for Clinical Laboratory Standards (NCCLS) developed the guidelines document C34-A2: "Sweat Testing: Sample Collection and Quantitative Analysis."[79] The NCCLS document has been adopted by the CFF for use in its accredited care centers.[26] To encourage acceptable performance of the sweat test, the CAP Laboratory Accreditation Program has incorporated sweat collection and analysis into the Special Chemistry checklist.

TABLE 27-3 Methods of Sweat Analysis

Methods	Frequency
Chloride methods (N = 574)	
Chloridometer	199 (34.7%)
Direct skin electrode	197 (34.3%)
ISEs	59 (10.3%)
Manual titration	46 (8.0%)
Test patch	17 (3.0%)
Other	36 (6.3%)
Conductivity (N = 325)	
Wescor Sweat-Chek	206 (63.4%)
Advanced Instruments	60 (18.5%)
Other	59 (18.1%)
Sodium methods (N = 77)	
Flame photometer	41 (53.2%)
ISEs	29 (37.7%)
Other	7 (9.1%)
Osmolality (N = 64)	
Vapor pressure osmometer	47 (73.4%)
Freezing point depression osmometer	17 (26.6%)

From LeGrys VL, Burnett RW. Current status of sweat testing in North America. Arch Pathol Lab Med 1994;118:865-7. Copyright 1994, American Medical Association.
ISE, Ion-selective electrode.

The sweat test occurs in three phases: sweat stimulation by pilocarpine iontophoresis; collection of the sweat onto gauze, filter paper, coil, patch, or capillary tube; and qualitative or quantitative analysis of sweat chloride, sodium, conductivity, or osmolality. A survey of 753 laboratories (Table 27-3) performing sweat testing revealed that 47% analyze chloride, 46% analyze conductivity, and less than 7% analyze sodium or osmolality.[62]

Qualitative Screening Tests

Screening tests may or may not measure the amount of sweat collected and may report a result as positive, negative, or borderline, or give an actual concentration of sweat analytes. Patients having a positive or borderline screening result should have quantitative sweat testing. The use of reliable screening tests may have a role in smaller hospital laboratories where testing frequency does not lend itself to the maintenance of proficiency with quantitative analytical techniques. The CFF forbids accredited CF care centers from using screening sweat tests but rather requires those centers to perform quantitative analysis of sweat chloride.[26] Examples of qualitative screening sweat tests currently in use are the Wescor Sweat-Chek and Nanoduct conductivity analyzers (Wescor, Logan, Utah), the Advanced Instruments conductivity analyzer (Advanced Instruments), the Orion skin electrode for chloride (Orion Research, Cambridge, Mass.), the CF Indicator System chloride patch (Polychrome Medical, Brooklyn, Minn.) and sweat osmolality measurements. The Nanoduct instrument (Wescor) combines pilocarpine iontophoresis with a disposable conductivity cell. Although there are a variety of systems in use for sweat testing, several of the methods have documented problems, making them inappropriate for clinical use. For example, the Orion Skin Measuring System and older conductivity analyzers using unheated collection cups are not recommended as diagnostic procedures because problems have been reported with sample evaporation and condensation and the ability to quantify sweat samples adequately.[30,103,108]

The CFF has approved the Wescor Macroduct Sweat-Chek for screening at clinical sites, such as community hospitals, using the criteria that a patient having a sweat conductivity ≥50 mmol/L should be referred to an accredited CF care center for a quantitative sweat chloride test.[27] Wescor's recommended decision level is higher than that of the CFF, which can lead to confusion between the laboratory and physician as to the appropriate decision level.[14,63,111] The CFF medical advisory committee, in setting the decision limit at 50 mmol/L, did so cautiously, realizing that the goal of screening tests is to tolerate some false-positive results and minimize or prevent false-negative results. Situations with false-positive test results are resolved on further testing, but it would be unacceptable to miss a CF patient. When evaluating sweat conductivity results, it should be noted that values from sweat conductivity methods are approximately 15 mmol/L higher than sweat chloride concentration. The difference is most likely caused by the presence of unmeasured anions, such as lactate and bicarbonate.[44] Because of this difference, laboratories must be clear in reporting that the screening test result represents conductivity, not chloride, and must include appropriate sweat conductivity reference intervals. Confusion, anxiety, and the potential for misdiagnosis arise in patients and their families when a sweat conductivity is mistakenly evaluated using sweat chloride reference intervals. Sixty-eight percent of laboratories performing sweat conductivity had errors in result reporting that included using inappropriate decision levels, reporting conductivity as chloride, and using conductivity as a diagnostic, not screening test.[62]

Quantitative Confirmatory Tests

According to the NCCLS C34-A2 document,[79] a quantitative sweat test consists of collecting sweat into gauze, filter paper, or Macroduct coils; evaluating the amount collected either in weight (milligrams) or volume (microliters) and then measuring the sweat chloride concentration. Chloride provides the greatest discrimination in diagnosis compared with sodium, and is the preferred analyte.[40] For diagnostic purposes, the CFF requires laboratories to perform a quantitative analysis of sweat chloride following the techniques described in the NCCLS document C34-A2.[26,79] Chloride concentration can be determined by either coulometric titration using a chloridometer or manual titration using mercuric nitrate. If a laboratory chooses to quantitate sweat chloride using an automated analyzer that employs an ISE, these methods must be systematically validated for accuracy, precision, and, particularly, the lower limit of the analytical measurement range. Instrumentation used for measuring sweat chloride concentration should be able to detect as low as 10 mmol/L on unadulterated sweat. Analysts should not attempt to boost the analytical sensitivity by adding extraneous chloride standard to patients' specimens.

Reference Intervals for Sweat Chloride

In the context of clinically significant findings, a sweat chloride >60 mmol/L is consistent with CF; concentrations between 40 and 60 mmol/L are considered borderline, and values <40 mmol/L are in general considered normal.[89] The functional upper limit for sweat chloride is 160 mmol/L.[79] Sweat chloride concentrations greater than 160 mmol/L are not physiologically possible and can represent specimen contamination or analytical error.[93] The chloride concentration should be interpreted in the context of the patient's clinical presentation, family history, and age. Some mutations of the CF gene are associated with borderline or normal sweat chloride concentrations.[89]

According to the CFF disease registry, 1.7% of CF patients had sweat chloride concentrations less than 60 mmol/L (mean of 45.1 mmol/L) and 0.5% had sweat chloride concentrations ≤40 mmol/L. These patients were diagnosed with CF on the basis of genotyping, nasal transepithelial potential difference studies, and clinical presentation.[28]

Decision Limits for Sweat Conductivity

There is a lack of consensus on the appropriate decision limit for sweat conductivity. The CFF states that a patient with a sweat conductivity ≥50 mmol/L should be referred for a confirmatory sweat chloride test, and Wescor recommends that conductivity values up to 60 mmol/L can be considered normal, and concentrations >80 mmol/L are positive for CF.[27,111]

Sweat Stimulation and Collection

Localized sweating is produced by iontophoresis of the cholinergic drug pilocarpine nitrate into an area of the skin. Iontophoresis uses a small electric current to deliver pilocarpine into the sweat glands from the positive electrode, and an electrolyte solution at the negative electrode completes the circuit. The current source should be battery powered and regularly inspected according to hospital guidelines by qualified personnel for voltage leak and current control.[79] After iontophoresis, sweat is collected onto preweighed gauze pads or filter paper or into Macroduct coils, using techniques to minimize evaporation and contamination. The Occupational Safety and Health Administration (OSHA) does not list sweat as a potentially infectious material unless it is visibly contaminated with blood.[82] However, laboratory personnel should practice the same universal precautions they would use with any other body fluid.

Because of transient increases in sweat electrolytes shortly after birth, patients should be at least 48 hours old before a sweat test is performed.[79] The patient should be physiologically and nutritionally stable, well hydrated, free of acute illness, and not receiving mineralocorticoids. The inner flexor surface of the forearm is the preferred site for sweat testing. Either the right or left arm is acceptable. If the arms are unavailable, sweat testing can be performed on the patient's upper leg. Never allow the current to cross the patient's chest. The skin should be free of cuts, rashes, and inflammation so as to prevent contamination of the sweat sample with serous fluid. For example, sweat testing should never be performed over an area of eczema.[14] The sweat test can be performed on a patient receiving intravenous fluid, as long as good contact between the skin and the electrode is possible, collection techniques do not interfere with venous flow, and the intravenous fluids do not contaminate the collection area. Iontophoresis should not be performed on a patient receiving oxygen by an open delivery system. Often such patients can temporarily receive oxygen by way of a face mask or nasal cannula, permitting sweat testing.

If sweat is collected onto gauze or filter paper, the electrodes are usually made of copper and are slightly smaller than the stimulation and collection area. Reagents include United States Pharmacopeia (USP) grade 0.2% to 0.5% pilocarpine nitrate solution, a dilute electrolyte solution, and type I distilled water. The composition of the electrolyte solution should be selected to prevent contamination with the sweat sample. A supply of gauze pads, low in electrolyte content, is necessary for cleansing and drying the skin. Before collection, the gauze or filter paper used for sweat collection should be placed into a weighing vial with a secure sealing lid, and the vial should be labeled and weighed using an analytical balance. To minimize contamination, the collection gauze or filter paper and the preweighed vial containing them should never be handled directly. The analyst should always use forceps or powder-free gloves. For a detailed procedure for stimulation and collection, refer to NCCLS document C34-A2.[79]

Alternatively, for sweat stimulation, the electrodes and current source can be integrated as in the Wescor Macroduct system, which uses gel reagents containing pilocarpine. The battery-powered iontophoresis system delivers a current of 1.5 mA for 5 minutes. Type I distilled water and gauze pads or tissues are necessary for cleaning the skin. Using this stimulation system, sweat is collected into a disposable microbore tubing coil collector. After sufficient sweat has been collected, it is transferred from the coil into a sealable microsample cup. When using the Macroduct collection system, the analyst should not touch or otherwise contaminate the concave collecting surface. For specific procedures using the Macroduct collection system, refer to the manufacturer's instructions.

To standardize and simplify the collection process, it is recommended that the size of the electrodes, reagent pads, and collection material be approximately the same. For example, using a 2 × 2-inch gauze or filter paper collection pad, the electrodes should be slightly smaller, about 1.5 × 1.5 inches, and the area of stimulation, represented by the size of reagent pads, should be the same size as the collection pads, 2 × 2 inches. When using the Wescor Macroduct stimulation system and Pilogel, sweat should be collected into the coils designed with the system.

Critical Issues Associated With Sweat Collection

The analyst must address several important issues when collecting sweat. These include adequate patient education, using appropriate stimulation and collection systems, preventing evaporation and contamination, collecting a sufficient sample, and minimizing skin reactions.

Patient Education

Sweat testing is one of the few clinical chemistry tests involving direct patient contact. Patients often have questions about the sweat test that their physicians may not have answered. Patient educational materials on sweat testing have been produced by the CFF in English and Spanish and include both written and video material.

Appropriate Stimulation and Collection Systems

Sweat should be collected in association with compatible stimulation equipment and not be hybridized. For example, laboratories using Wescor Pilogel iontophoresis should collect sweat only into the Macroduct coils and not onto gauze or filter paper.[79] Hybridizing the Wescor Pilogel iontophoresis system with gauze or filter paper collection can dramatically alter the minimum collection volume or weight required to ensure adequate sweat gland stimulation and affect the validity of the sweat electrolyte determination.

Evaporation and Contamination

Testing procedures should minimize the opportunity for evaporation and contamination of the sweat sample. Detailed instructions on minimizing evaporation and contamination can be found in the NCCLS sweat testing document.[79]

Specimen Weight and Collection Time

To have a valid sweat testing result, determination of and adherence to a minimum sweat weight or volume are critical. The requirement for a minimum amount is physiological, to ensure an appropriate sweat rate and sweat electrolyte concentration. It is independent of the instrumentation used to measure sweat electrolytes. Unfortunately, this is poorly understood, leading to false-positive and false-negative sweat test results, which have a significant implication for patient care. Sweat electrolyte concentration is related to sweat rate. At low sweat rates, sweat electrolyte concentration decreases and the opportunity for sample evaporation is increased.[39,79] To ensure a valid result, the average sweat rate should exceed $1\,g/m^2/min$. The minimum acceptable volume or weight depends on the size of the electrode and stimulation area, the type and size of collecting devices, and the length of time the sweat is collected.[79] If a laboratory deviates from standard parameters, the minimum acceptable sweat volume or weight will change. The stimulation and/or collection requirement applies to each site independently, so insufficient samples must not be pooled for analysis.

Applying the acceptable rate to the parameters described in the NCCLS document, the minimum acceptable sample for analysis from a single site using 2 × 2-inch gauze or filter paper for stimulation and collection is 75 mg of sweat collected within 30 minutes. Using the Macroduct system, the electrodes and stimulation area are smaller, and the minimum acceptable sample is 15 μL collected within 30 minutes. Sweat should be collected for only 30 minutes. If the collection time exceeds 30 minutes, the requirement for the amount of sweat necessary to ensure adequate stimulation would have to be increased. Extending the collection time can allow additional opportunity for sweat evaporation and practically does not significantly increase the sweat yield.[60]

Sufficient Sample Collection

Acquiring the minimum sample should not be a problem if the laboratorian follows both the procedure in the NCCLS document and the manufacturer's recommendations. On average, the percentage of insufficient samples should not exceed 5% for patients more than 3 months old.[26] The average amount of sweat collected on 2 × 2-inch gauze pads at one CF center is 282 mg and in Macroduct coils is 65 μL.[44,64] Insufficient sweat samples can be due to several factors, such as age, race, skin condition, and collection system. Although it may seem to be more difficult to obtain an adequate sweat sample in very young infants, studies have shown no statistically significant difference in the proportion of insufficient samples in patients younger than 6 weeks when compared with patients older than 6 weeks.[37] Collection systems vary with regard to insufficient samples, especially in young infants (e.g., there is a higher failure rate associated with collection using Macroduct coils than with collection onto gauze or filter paper).[44] If an adequate sweat sample is not obtained, the test can be repeated as soon as is practical because the rate of sweating can vary from day to day. To ensure adequate sweat production, the analyst should check that the reagents are within the expiration date and that the size of the stimulation area corresponds to the size of the collection surface.

Skin Reactions

Burns to the patient's skin after iontophoresis are extremely rare but can occur at either electrode. If the burn occurs at the site of pilocarpine stimulation, sweat should not be collected. Pilocarpine urticaria associated with sweat testing is also rare but has been reported.[61]

To minimize the potential for burns, the analyst should:

1. Keep the electrode surfaces clean. Copper electrodes should be cleaned after every use with emery cloth to remove surface oxidation.
2. Attach the electrodes firmly. Maintain a wet interface with the skin during iontophoresis. When using liquid reagents on gauze or filter paper, ensure that they are thoroughly saturated. When using gel reagents, a drop of type I distilled water can be applied to the gel surface.
3. Prevent bare metal of the electrode from touching the skin. The gauze or filter paper pads should be slightly larger than the electrodes. When using gel reagents, do not use Pilogel disks that have a crack or structural defect in them.
4. Limit iontophoretic current. At the beginning of iontophoresis, slowly raise the current, and do not exceed 4.0 mA current.

Sources of Error in Sweat Testing

Unreliable methodology, technical errors, and errors in interpretation can all lead to erroneous sweat test results. Methods that do not quantitate sweat collected or do not have an established minimum sample volume or weight are subject to false-negative results because an adequate sweat rate cannot be ensured.

Other problems with sweat testing include errors of evaporation, contamination, and errors in dilution, instrument calibration, sample identification, and result reporting. These errors occur more frequently in institutions performing relatively few tests.[103] Laboratories with a low testing volume for sweat analysis should consider discontinuing the test and referring patients to accredited CF care centers for testing and evaluation. Interpretation errors with the sweat test include lack of knowledge about the laboratory method, failure to repeat borderline and positive results, failure to repeat negative test results when inconsistent with the clinical picture, and failure to repeat testing in patients diagnosed as CF who do not follow the expected clinical course. Malnutrition, dehydration, eczema, and rash can increase sweat electrolytes, whereas edema and the administration of mineralocorticoids can decrease sweat electrolytes.[89]

Sweat Testing Quality Assurance

High-quality sweat testing includes selecting appropriate methodology, having a sufficient testing volume to ensure familiarity with the test, and limiting the testing personnel to a small number of well-trained individuals. An effective quality assurance program for sweat analysis encompasses preanalytical, analytical, and postanalytical factors.

Preanalytical Quality Assurance

Physicians should be aware of the clinical spectrum of CF and appropriately order a sweat test on patients suspected of the disorder. Because of the significant preanalytical variation associated with sweat testing, duplicate testing from two body sites is recommended.[26] Most sweat chloride concentrations agree within 5 mmol/L on bilateral testing. Each laboratory should establish a required level of agreement for bilateral results. It has been suggested that when the sweat chloride concentration is less than 60 mmol/L the duplicate tests should agree within 10 mmol/L, and when the chloride concentration exceeds 60 mmol/L the tests should agree within 15 mmol/L.[79] Stimulation and collection procedures should minimize the opportunity for evaporation and contamination of the sweat sample. The patient's skin at the collection site should be free of inflammation or rash.

Analytical Quality Control

To monitor the accuracy and precision of the analytical process, two levels of controls should be performed every day when patient samples are analyzed. One control should reflect the concentration of sweat chloride concentration in a non-CF patient and the other control should reflect the concentration of sweat chloride found in a CF patient. The controls should be performed in parallel with patient samples and the results should fall within a predetermined range before patient results can be reported. Both short- and long-term quality control should be monitored.

An important part of a quality assurance plan includes the external validation of sweat analysis accuracy through participation in proficiency testing. The CAP offers a proficiency testing program consisting of six specimens per year. Participants receive feedback concerning their performance on these specimens relative to others in their peer group.

Postanalytical Quality Assurance

The results of the sweat test must be interpreted in light of the patient's clinical presentation by a physician knowledgeable about CF. There are several conditions other than CF that are associated with elevations in sweat electrolytes (Box 27-1). These conditions usually are distinguishable from CF based on the patient's clinical presentation.

BLOOD GASES AND pH

Clinical management of respiratory and metabolic disorders often depends on rapid, accurate measurements of oxygen and carbon dioxide in blood. Vigorous measures to support life in patients with cardiopulmonary impairment depend largely on assisted ventilation using mixtures of gases that are tailored in response to laboratory blood gas and acid-base results. Determination of blood gases also plays an important part in the detection of acid-base imbalance and in monitoring therapy. Modern instruments for blood gas determinations are simple to operate and, with meticulous maintenance and quality control, are capable of rapid turnaround of very reliable laboratory data. Details of the patho-

BOX 27-1 Diseases Other than Cystic Fibrosis Associated With an Elevated Sweat Electrolyte Concentration

Anorexia nervosa
Atopic dermatitis
Autonomic dysfunction
Ectodermal dysplasia
Environmental deprivation
Familial cholestasis
Fucosidosis
Glucose-6-phosphate dehydrogenase deficiency
Glycogen storage disease: type 1
Hypogammaglobulinemia
Klinefelter's syndrome
Long-term prostaglandin E_1 infusion
Mauriac syndrome
Mucopolysaccharidosis type 1
Nephrogenic diabetes insipidus
Nephrosis
Protein calorie malnutrition
Pseudohypoaldosteronism
Psychosocial failure to thrive
Untreated adrenal insufficiency
Untreated hypothyroidism

From National Committee for Clinical Laboratory Standards: Sweat Testing: Sample Collection and Quantitative Analysis: Approved Guideline. NCCLS Document C34-A2. Villanova, PA, National Committee for Clinical Laboratory Standards, 2000, p. 30.

physiology of blood gases in relation to respiration and acid-base disorders are discussed in detail in Chapter 46.

The recommended nomenclature in this area of analysis has been finalized by the NCCLS,[77] but because alternative nomenclatures exist[51] and are in common use, some of these are also summarized in Box 27-2.

BEHAVIOR OF GASES

Determination of gas pressures in expired air or blood depends on the application of certain physical principles (Table 27-4). The partial pressure of a gas dissolved in blood is by definition equal to the partial pressure of the gas in an imaginary ideal gas phase in equilibrium with the blood. At equilibrium, the partial pressure (tension) of a gas is the same in erythrocytes and plasma, so that the partial pressure of a gas is the same in whole blood and plasma. The partial pressure of a gas in a gas mixture is defined as the substance fraction of gas (mole fraction) times the total pressure. The tension of a gas in a liquid is, in fact, a measure of the chemical activity of the gas in the liquid. In the physicochemical literature, it is called the *fugacity.*

Various spaces where gases are present include the ambient environment (room air), the bronchial tree and alveoli of the patient, and the measuring chamber of a laboratory instrument. In all these spaces, atmospheric (baro-

BOX 27-2 Conversion Factors, Prefixes, Symbols, and Descriptors Used in Discussions of Gases Measured in Blood and Expired Air[*67,77]

Conversion Factors

1 mm Hg = 0.133 kPa
1 kPa = 7.5 mm Hg
kPa: 1 kilopascal = 1000 pascal. The pascal is the SI derived unit of pressure; it equals 1 Newton/m^2 (see also Chapter 1)

General Prefixes

P: partial pressure or tension
Usage: PO_2, PCO_2, PH_2O
Alternative: pO_2
S: saturation fraction
Usage: SO_2
Alternative: sO_2
c: substance concentration
Usage: ctO_2 for concentration of total O_2
Usage: $ctCO_2$ for concentration of total CO_2
Usage: $cHCO_3^-$ for concentration of bicarbonate
d: dissolved gas, used with substance concentration (*c*)
t: total, used with substance concentration (*c*), thus $ctCO_2 = HCO_3^- + cdCO_2$
Specimen origin is indicated by lower case letters. Whole blood and plasma are distinguished by capitals.

a: arterial	B: blood
v: venous	P: plasma
c: capillary	

Usage: PO_2(aB), for partial pressure of O_2 in arterial blood

Prefixes Associated with External Respiration

V: volume of air or blood (unit, L)
$\dot{V}$: volume rate (unit, L/min)
F: substance fraction, also called mole fraction
E: expired air
I: inspired air
A: alveolar air
Usage: $\dot{V}$(A) means alveolar ventilation; and $\dot{V}$(B) cardiac output; FO_2(I) fraction of O_2 in inspired air; PO_2(A) partial pressure of O_2 in alveolar air; and PCO_2(E) partial pressure of CO_2 in expired air.

Other Descriptors

BTPS: *Body Temperature* (37 °C or 310.16 K) and ambient *Pressure*, fully *Saturated* (PH_2O = 47 mm Hg or 6.25 kPa)
STPD: *Standard Temperature* (0 °C or 273.16 K) and standard *Pressure* (760 mm Hg or 101.08 kPa) of *Dry* gas
Amb: ambient atmosphere (unit is atm, atmosphere)
B: barometric (atmospheric)
BTPS: Usage: *P*(amb), *P*(Amb)
SVP: *Saturated Vapor Pressure*, the vapor pressure of water. SVP_T means SVP at a specified temperature, e.g., $SVP_{37\,°C}$ = 47 mm Hg; PH_2O(saturated)
ATPS: *Ambient Temperature* and *Pressure*, *Saturated* with water vapor

*This list is not complete, but is presented to facilitate interpretation of terms used in the text and to illustrate various forms that may be encountered in the literature.

TABLE 27-4 Physical Principles Applied in Blood Gas Measurements

Boyle's law: The volume of an ideal gas at a constant temperature varies inversely with the pressure exerted to contain it.	$V \propto 1/P$
Charles' (Gay-Lussac's) law: The volume of an ideal gas at a constant pressure varies directly with its absolute temperature.	$V \propto T$
Avogadro's hypothesis: Equal volumes of different ideal gases at the same temperature and pressure contain the same number of molecules.	$n_i/V_i = n_j/V_j$
Dalton's law: The total pressure exerted by a mixture of ideal gases is the sum of the partial pressures of each of the gases in the mixture.	$P = \Sigma P_i$
Henry's law: The amount of a sparingly soluble gas dissolved in a liquid is proportional to the partial pressure of the gas over the liquid.	$c = \alpha \times P$

metric) pressure, P(Amb), is the prevailing pressure, and partial pressures of each of the gases present in these spaces must add up to the value of P(Amb), which will vary with altitude and barometric pressure. Scientific convention reduces measurements of gas volumes made at P(Amb) to standard temperature (0 °C or 273.16 K) and pressure (760 mm Hg or 101.325 kPa) for dry gas (STPD) to make experimental data transferable. However, in blood gas work, the standard is that measurements of partial pressure are always made at body temperature (usually 37 °C), at P(Amb), and in the presence of saturated water vapor (PH_2O = 47 mm Hg). Use of this BTPS convention (see Box 27-2) has the following practical effects:

1. It relates laboratory data for blood gases strictly to the geographical location of the patient, so that reference intervals become altitude dependent.
2. It assumes a standard body temperature of 37 °C and that the measuring device also holds the sample of blood at exactly 37 °C. This assumption requires special concern for thermal stability of the instrument. Just as important, it implies that in circumstances such as *imposed* hypothermia, when a patient's temperature is not 37 °C, blood gas values determined at 37 °C might need to be corrected to the actual body temperature to obtain an estimate of blood gas partial pressures in the patient. Temperature corrections are addressed later in this section.
3. It recognizes that the partial pressures of measured gases in the blood coexist with a constant and standard saturated vapor pressure (SVP), which is identical for both the calibration conditions of the instrument and measurement conditions of the blood sample.

Boyle's and Charles' laws and Avogadro's hypothesis are combined in what is called the *general gas equation:*

$$P = (nRT)/V$$

where

P = pressure in units of millimeters of mercury (mm Hg)
n = Hg or kilopascals (kPa)
V = volume in liters in which an ideal gas is contained
T = temperature in degrees kelvin (0 °C = 273.16 K)
n = number of moles of gas, and
R = gas constant

The SI unit of P is the pascal (Pa). However, millimeters of mercury (also called *torr*) has continued to remain popular (see Box 27-2 for conversion factors). Use of SI units does have a practical advantage in that 1 atm almost equals 100 kPa (1 atm = 101.325 kPa). Partial pressures expressed in kilopascals are therefore very close estimates of percentages of the gases in the mixture at 1 atm. Pressure, P (or p), may mean either total pressure, as in the expression P(Amb) for the mixture of gases in ambient air, or partial pressure in blood, as in PO_2(aB). Numerical value and units of R differ depending on the units used for P, so that:

$$R = 62.36\text{ mm Hg} \times \text{L} \times {}^\circ\text{K}^{-1} \times \text{mol}^{-1}$$

or

$$R = 8.31\text{ kPa} \times \text{L} \times {}^\circ\text{K}^{-1} \times \text{mol}^{-1}$$

After rearranging terms and evaluating n as 1 mol and P as 760 mm Hg, the volume of 1 mol of a pure ideal gas at 0 °C (no water vapor) is 22.4 L. The general gas equation is the justification for accepting partial pressures of gases in blood as estimators of their concentrations. However, PO_2 is related only to the concentration of dissolved O_2 (cdO_2) in the blood and PCO_2 to the concentration of dissolved CO_2 ($cdCO_2$) in the blood (see Henry's law, Table 27-4.) In fact, the total concentration of O_2 in blood ctO_2 is the sum of concentrations of dissolved O_2 and of O_2 bound to hemoglobin, with dO_2 being a small component of tO_2 (see Hemoglobin Saturation section later in this chapter). The total concentration of CO_2 ($ctCO_2$) is defined operationally as the sum of concentrations of dissolved CO_2, carbonic acid, HCO_3^-, undissociated bicarbonate, and carbonate ion.

Dalton's law (see Table 27-4) may be written for room air as

$$P(\text{Amb}) = PO_2 + PCO_2 + PN_2 + PH_2O + PX$$

where PX is that of any other gas in the air sample.

However, for gases in solution, Dalton's law does not apply. That is, the sum of partial pressures of all the dissolved gases may be lower than, equal to, or higher than the measured pressure of the solution. For instance, if the sum of gas tensions is significantly higher than the pressure of the solution, bubbles may form, as they can in the blood of divers surfacing from the deep (giving rise to a condition known as "the bends") or in a cold blood sample being warmed for analysis. Dalton's law of partial pressures remains important, however, for calibration and control of the measuring devices.

Consider a calibrator gas certified to contain 15% O_2 (L/L or mol/mol) and 5% CO_2, the remainder being N_2. The mole fractions (or *F*) of the gases in the dry mixture are 0.15, 0.05, and 0.80, respectively. This mixture, after saturation with water vapor at 37 °C (to mimic a patient's blood or alveolar air), is introduced into a blood gas instrument's measuring chamber (held at 37 °C to mimic a patient's body temperature) for the purpose of calibrating the instrument for subsequent measurements of gases in patients' samples. If the local barometric pressure, *P*(Amb), on this occasion is 747 mm Hg, then the humidified calibrator gas is present in the chamber at ambient, barometric pressure, such that

$$P(\text{Amb}) = 747\text{ mm Hg} = PO_2 + PCO_2 + PN_2 + PH_2O$$

To set the instrument to the PO_2 and PCO_2 of the calibrator gas, we must first account for PH_2O at 37 °C, which is equal to SVP of water, 47 mm Hg. Therefore

$$P(\text{Amb}) - PH_2O = PO_2 + PCO_2 + PN_2$$
$$= 747 - 47 = 700\text{ mm Hg}$$

If *P*(Amb) corrected for PH_2O represents the sum of partial pressures for the dry gases whose mole fractions we know, we can calculate the exact PO_2 and PCO_2 values for the calibrator gas, under the circumstances of measurement, and then enter these calibrator values into the instrument:

$$PO_2 = 700 \times 0.15 = 105\text{ mm Hg}$$
$$PCO_2 = 700 \times 0.05 = 35\text{ mm Hg}$$

The law of partial pressure is also applied in defining gas mixtures used to determine $PO_2(0.5)$ or P_{50} and other derived quantities and to control instrumentation with tonometered samples.

Henry's law predicts the amount of dissolved gas in a liquid in contact with a gaseous phase (see Table 27-4). The concentration (mol/L) of free dissolved gas (dG) in blood (B) is calculated:

$$c\text{dG(B)} = \alpha\text{G(B)} \times P\text{G(B)}$$

where αG(B) is the coefficient of solubility for the gas in blood at 37 °C.

The coefficient for O_2 in blood, αO_2, is 0.00140 (mol/L)/mm Hg (the corresponding coefficient for the volume-volume relationship is 31 μL/L/mm Hg). Therefore when arterial PO_2 is normal (100 mm Hg) the concentration of dissolved O_2 in arterial blood, cdO_2, is 0.140 mmol/L, which is a very small proportion of the ctO_2 content in blood (~9 mmol/L), the bulk of which is O_2 bound by hemoglobin. Increasing the O_2 fraction of inspired air to 100% or increasing the pressure of inspired air, as in a hyperbaric chamber, forces more O_2 into a solution. In therapy with pure O_2, when PO_2 may rise to 640 mm Hg, the cdO_2 could be as high as 0.9 mmol/L. In hyperbaric treatment, an arterial PO_2 of 2500 mm Hg (~3.2 atm) is equivalent to cdO_2 of 3.5 mmol/L. Prediction of concentrations of cdO_2 in these therapies is useful because tissue oxygenation by dissolved O_2 becomes increasingly important when hemoglobin-mediated O_2 delivery is impaired.

The $cdCO_2$ can be calculated in the same way: αCO_2 at 37 °C in plasma = 0.0306 mmol/L/mm Hg. Thus at a PCO_2 of 40 mm Hg, the $cdCO_2 = 40 \times 0.0306 = 1.224$ mmol/L. In the determination of blood gases, PCO_2 is determined along with blood pH. As will be subsequently explained, these two parameters in conjunction with the Henderson-Hasselbalch equation permit the calculation of HCO_3^-, as follows:

$$\log c\text{HCO}_3^- = \text{pH} - pK' + \log[PCO_2 \times \alpha CO_2(\text{P})]$$

The antilog is then taken to derive $cHCO_3^-$.

Application of the Henderson-Hasselbalch Equation in Blood Gas Measurements

Carbon dioxide and water react to form carbonic acid, which in turn dissociates to hydrogen ions and HCO_3^-.

$$CO_2 + H_2O \overset{K_{\text{hydration}}}{\rightleftharpoons} H_2CO_3 \overset{K_{\text{dissociation}}}{\rightleftharpoons} H^{\oplus} + HCO_3^{\ominus}$$

Thus the total concentration of CO_2 ($ctCO_2$), the concentration of bicarbonate ($cHCO_3^-$), the concentration of dissolved CO_2 ($cdCO_2$), and H^+ ion concentration (cH^+) are interrelated. The constant *K* for the hydration reaction is 2.29×10^{-3} (p*K* = 2.64 at 37 °C), whereas the constant *K* for the dissociation of carbonic acid is 2.04×10^{-4} (p*K* = 3.69).

In the classical formulation, Henderson (1908), using concentrations for bicarbonate, CO_2, and H^+ and assuming the concentration of water to be constant, combined these two reactions and incorporated the constant *K′* with a value of 4.68×10^{-7}, and thus a p*K′* of 6.33 at 37 °C:

$$K' = cH^+ \times cHCO_3^- / cdCO_2$$

The concentration of dissolved CO_2 *includes* the small amount of undissociated (dissolved) carbonic acid. It can be expressed as $cdCO_2 = \alpha \times PCO_2$, where α is the solubility coefficient for CO_2. $cHCO_3^-$ then represents $ctCO_2$ minus $cdCO_2$, which includes carbonic acid. The "bicarbonate" concentration by this definition includes undissociated sodium bicarbonate, carbonate ($NaCO_3$) and carbamate (carbamino-CO_2; $RCNHCOO^-$), which are present in exceedingly small amounts in plasma.

If the Henderson equation is rearranged and $cdCO_2$ is replaced by $\alpha \times PCO_2$, the following equation results:

$$cH^+ = K' \times \alpha \times PCO_2 / cHCO_3^-$$

In 1916 Hasselbalch showed that a logarithmic transformation of the equation was a more useful form, and used the symbols pH (= $-\log cH^+$) and pK' (= $-\log K'$). pH is defined as the negative log of the *activity* of H^+ (aH^+), which is the entity actually measured with pH meters. The resulting Henderson-Hasselbalch equation becomes

$$pH = pK' + \log\left[cHCO_3^- / (\alpha \times PCO_2)\right]$$

or

$$pH = pK' + \log\{[ctCO_2 - (\alpha \times PCO_2)]/(\alpha \times PCO_2)\}$$

K' is the apparent, overall (combined) dissociation constant for carbonic acid. It is *apparent* because concentrations are used rather than activities and *overall* because both the $cdCO_2$ and the concentration of carbonic acid are used. K' depends not only on the temperature but also on the ionic strength of the solution.

For blood at 37 °C, the normal mean value is pK'(P) = 6.103, with a normal biological standard deviation (SD) of about ±0.0015, mainly caused by variations in ionic strength. The solubility coefficient for CO_2 gas, α, also varies with the composition of the solution. For pure water at 37 °C, the solubility coefficient $\alpha = 0.0329\,\text{mmol} \times L^{-1} \times \text{mm Hg}^{-1}$, and for normal plasma at 37 °C it is $0.0306\,\text{mmol} \times L^{-1} \times \text{mm Hg}^{-1}$, with a biological SD of about $\pm 0.0003\,\text{mmol} \times L^{-1} \times \text{mm Hg}^{-1}$.

Inserting pK' and α for normal plasma at 37 °C, the Henderson-Hasselbalch equation takes the following form:

$$pH = 6.103 + \log\frac{cHCO_3^-}{0.0306 \times PCO_2}$$

or

$$pH = 6.103 + \log\frac{ctCO_2 - 0.0306 \times PCO_2}{0.0306 \times PCO_2}$$

where PCO_2 is measured in millimeters of mercury and $cHCO_3^-$ and $ctCO_2$ are measured in millimoles per liter. Taking the antilogarithm, combining the constants, and expressing $[H^+]$ in nmol/L, the equation becomes

$$cH^+ = 24.1 \times \frac{PCO_2}{cHCO_3^-}$$

If normal values are substituted in the equation,

$$cH^+ = 24.1 \times \frac{40}{25.4}\,\text{nmol/L} = 38.0\,\text{nmol/L}$$

Clearly, by measuring any two of the four parameters, PCO_2 or $cdCO_2$, pH, $ctCO_2$, or $cHCO_3^-$, and using the Henderson-Hasselbalch equation with the above appropriate values for pK' and α, the other two parameters may be calculated. Although used as constants, these values must be recognized as means and susceptible to biological variation. Changes in ionic strength of ±20% cause changes in pK' between 6.08 and 6.12. Variations in pK' of plasma also occur with temperature (pK will decrease 0.0026 per 1 °C increase and decrease slightly with increasing pH). For most clinical purposes, these variations of pK' can be ignored. However, in pathological cases with markedly deviant ionic strength, the change in pK' may be significant. The value of α is affected by the presence of increased salts or proteins in solution (value decreases) or lipids (value increases). For instance, in lipemic plasma, the value of α may be 0.033 or even higher. Thus parameters calculated on the assumption that pK' and α are invariant may have significant error under certain pathological circumstances, and several authors suggest caution in using values calculated from blood gas analyzers in extremely ill patients and in children.[75,87] For instance, one study showed that in 17 of 51 adult intensive care unit patients, the calculated and measured tCO_2 values differed by >10%,[75] whereas another showed differences >20% in 27 of 107 pediatric intensive care unit patients.[87] Nevertheless, with both pH and PCO_2 measured electrochemically, $cHCO_3^-$, $cdCO_2$, and $ctCO_2$ are routinely calculated by algorithms in the microprocessors of most blood gas instruments. One advantage of such a calculated value is that it essentially reflects the *activity* of HCO_3^- (i.e., bicarbonate concentration is reported as if measured with an ISE) in the *water* phase of plasma, and thus it is not affected by the electrolyte exclusion effects, as other nondirect measurements of HCO_3^- may be.

OXYGEN IN BLOOD

The total O_2 content (ctO_2) of a blood sample is the sum of the concentrations of hemoglobin-bound O_2 and of dissolved O_2. At a blood ctO_2 of 9 mmol/L, the cdO_2 is only approximately 0.14 mmol/L, and the rest of the O_2 is associated with hemoglobin as oxyhemoglobin (O_2Hb). The O_2Hb is defined as erythrocyte hemoglobin with O_2 reversibly bound to Fe^{2+} of its heme group. Each mole of hemoglobin-Fe^{2+} binds 1 mol of O_2. In erythrocytes, hemoglobin exists as a tetramer (64,456 g/mol), but when expressing Hb concentration in moles per liter, it is reported as the concentration of monomer (16,114 g/mol). Thus 1 L of blood with a normal hemoglobin concentration (cHb) of 9.3 mmol/L (~15 g/dL or 150 g/L) carries 9.3 mmol of O_2 at STPD if all hemoglobin is in the form of O_2Hb.

Thus 1 g of hemoglobin is capable of binding 1.39 mL (0.062 mmol) of O_2 at STPD. This value is referred to as the specific O_2 binding capacity of hemoglobin A (Hb A, the normal adult gene product). Hb A reversibly binds O_2 at its heme moiety and also binds biological effectors at other allosteric sites on the molecule. Methemoglobin (MetHb), carboxyhemoglobin (COHb), sulfhemoglobin (SulfHb), and cyanmethemoglobin are forms of hemoglobin that are not capable of reversible binding of O_2 caused by chemical alterations of the heme moiety (see Chapter 31). These chemically altered hemoglobins are collectively termed *dyshemoglobins.* Another group of abnormal hemoglobins have genetically determined changes in their amino acid sequence that can alter the allosteric binding properties of the molecule and thus affect O_2 affinity. These hemoglobins are collectively referred to as hemoglobin variants or hemoglobinopathies. More than 500 hemoglobin variants have been described,[7,17] with sickle cell hemoglobin (Hb S) as just one example.

Uptake of O_2 by the blood in the lungs is governed primarily by the PO_2 of alveolar air and by the ability of O_2 to diffuse freely across the alveolar membrane into the blood. At the PO_2 normally present in alveolar air (~102 mm Hg) and with a normal membrane and normal hemoglobin A, more than 95% of hemoglobin will bind O_2. At a $PO_2 > 110$ mm Hg, more than 98% of normal hemoglobin A binds O_2. When all hemoglobin is saturated with O_2, further increase in the PO_2 of alveolar air simply increases the concentration of dO_2 in the arterial blood.

Delivery of O_2 by the blood to the tissue is governed by the large gradient between PO_2 of the arterial blood and that of the tissue cells, and by the dissociation of O_2Hb in the erythrocytes at the lower PO_2 of the blood–tissue cell interface.

Three properties of the arterial blood are essential to ensure adequate O_2 delivery to the tissue:

1. Arterial PO_2 must be sufficiently high (~90 mm Hg) to create a diffusion gradient from the arterial blood to the tissue cells. Low arterial PO_2 (hypoxemia) results in tissue hypoxia (O_2 starvation).
2. The O_2-binding capacity of the blood must be normal (i.e., the concentration of hemoglobin capable of binding and releasing O_2 must be normal). Decreased Hb concentration may cause so-called anemic hypoxia.
3. The hemoglobin must be able to bind O_2 in the lungs yet release it at the tissue. In other words, the affinity of hemoglobin for O_2 must be normal. Too great an affinity of hemoglobin for O_2 may cause "affinity-based" tissue hypoxia, in which O_2 is not released at the capillary-tissue interface (see later in this chapter).

The PO_2 at the venous end of the capillaries should stay around 38 mm Hg, and thus the normal arteriovenous difference in PO_2 is 50 to 60 mm Hg. This corresponds to a normal delivery of 2.3 mmol of O_2 to the tissue per liter of blood.

Hemoglobin Oxygen Saturation

Before discussing the factors that affect Hb affinity for O_2, it is important to define the concept of hemoglobin oxygen saturation (SO_2):

$$SO_2 = \frac{\text{Oxygen content}}{\text{Oxygen capacity}}$$

This is the fraction (percentage) of the functional hemoglobin that is saturated with oxygen and is essentially an indirect means of estimating the PO_2. However, at least three different approaches exist for determining oxygen "saturation," and although each is distinct, they are often used interchangeably to determine "oxygen saturation." These three terms, hemoglobin oxygen saturation (SO_2), fractional oxyhemoglobin (FO_2Hb), and an estimated oxygen saturation (O_2Sat), have distinct definitions set by the NCCLS.[77] The ambiguous use of these three terms is due to the fact that in healthy subjects with normal amounts of normal hemoglobin, the values for all three entities are very similar. However, the assumptions made for normal, healthy subjects can lead to erroneous conclusions in seriously ill patients and those with dyshemoglobins or hemoglobin variants when these values are used interchangeably.

Spectrophotometric methods are used to determine O_2Hb and HHb,[72] and SO_2 is calculated according to

$$SO_2 = \frac{cO_2Hb}{cO_2Hb + cHHb}$$

where cO_2Hb is the concentration of oxyhemoglobin, $cHHb$ the concentration of deoxyhemoglobin, and the sum of oxyhemoglobin and deoxyhemoglobin represents all hemoglobin capable of reversibly binding O_2. SO_2 is usually expressed as a percent in the United States, but may also be expressed as a decimal fraction of 1.00.

SO_2 is most often determined by simple pulse oximetry, a spectrophotometric approach that can determine oxyhemoglobin and reduced hemoglobin (HHB) but not COHb, MetHb, or SulfHb. These devices measure absorbance at 660 and 940 nm for which O_2Hb and HHb have unique absorbance patterns. These are usually bedside monitors used for monitoring HbO_2 saturation and serve this purpose extremely well. However, use of SO_2 in the initial evaluation of a patient with dyshemoglobins or other abnormal hemoglobins can be very misleading. For instance, in a comatose patient with 15% COHb, the SO_2 by simple pulse oximetry might read 0.95, whereas the fraction of oxyhemoglobin would in reality only be 0.80. Thus it seems reasonable to assess for the presence of dyshemoglobins before using SO_2 for clinical purposes. The reference interval for SO_2 from healthy adults is 0.94 to 0.98 (94% to 98%).[101]

Another expression of oxygen "saturation" is the fractional oxyhemoglobin (FO_2Hb), which is calculated as:

$$FO_2Hb = \frac{cO_2Hb}{ctHb}$$

where the concentration of total hemoglobin $ctHb$ equals the sum of O_2Hb, HHb, COHb, MetHb, and SulfHb. This value requires determination of all hemoglobin species and can be performed on a co-oximeter or on some modern blood gas analyzers, such as those from Instrumentation Laboratories or Radiometer. These instruments prepare a hemolysate from whole blood by sonication and by spectrophotometer determine the total amount of hemoglobin and the percent of each of the aforementioned species. This is accomplished by using monochromatic light at 6 to 128 fixed wavelengths between 535 and 670 nm and measuring absorbance at each of the wavelengths. Newer co-oximeters from Bayer Diagnostics and AVL use a diode array and the Radiometer ABL 700 series uses 128 wavelengths. Because each species of hemoglobin has its own absorbance pattern, a microcomputer can calculate the percent of each one. The reference interval for FO_2Hb is 0.90 to 0.95 (90% to 95%).

The microprocessors of blood gas instruments sometimes estimate the oxygen saturation (SO_2) from measured pH, PO_2, and hemoglobin with the use of empirical equations.[99] If used at all, this value should be clearly referred to as an estimated SO_2, but it is frequently reported as and referred to as "O_2Sat." Calculated values such as "O_2Sat" should be interpreted with reservation because the algorithmic approach assumes normal O_2 affinity of the hemoglobin, normal 2,3-diphosphoglycerol (2,3-DPG) concentrations, and the absence of dyshemoglobins. Such calculated estimates have been found to vary as much as 6% saturation from measured values.[90] Because of this, the NCCLS has discouraged the use of estimated values.[77]

Decreases in arterial FO_2Hb indicate either a low arterial PO_2 or an impaired ability of hemoglobin to bind O_2. The amount of O_2 that the blood can carry is determined by three major factors: the PO_2, which reflects how much O_2 is dissolved in the blood; the amount of normal (effective) hemoglobin available in erythrocytes; and the affinity of the available hemoglobin for O_2. Decreases in PO_2 indicate a reduced ability of O_2 to diffuse from alveolar air into the blood. This can be due either to hypoventilation or to increased venoarterial shunting that is secondary to cardiac or pulmonary insufficiency. In either case, the result is a right-to-left shunting of blood that has not reached equilibrium with the alveolar air. This results in a decreased PO_2 and an increased PCO_2. Decreases in the concentration of total hemoglobin can result from a decreased number of erythrocytes that contain a normal concentration of hemoglobin (normochromic anemia) or a decreased mean cell concentration of hemoglobin in the erythrocytes (hypochromic anemia). Decreased FO_2Hb hemoglobin can also occur as a result of poisonings that convert part of the hemoglobin into the species COHb, MetHb, SulfHb, or cyanmethemoglobin, which cannot properly bind or exchange O_2. Clinically, it is important to distinguish between arterial hypoxemia (decreased arterial PO_2 and decreased SO_2 or FO_2Hb because of decreased availability of O_2) and cyanosis (decreased FO_2Hb because of abnormally high concentrations of reduced hemoglobin or chemically altered hemoglobin incapable of carrying O_2). Note that in the cyanosis setting, measurement of SO_2 or an estimated SO_2 ("O_2Sat") could be normal if the cyanosis is due to the presence of metHb or COHb.

The oxygen concentration of blood (ctO_2) is the sum of O_2 bound to hemoglobin and cdO_2. Originally, ctO_2 was determined by blood collected anaerobically and treated with ferricyanide reagent to liberate O_2 from hemoglobin under negative pressure to release all free O_2 from solution. The oxygen binding capacity was the amount of O_2 in the same sample determined in the same manner after the blood had been equilibrated with a gas mixture sufficiently rich in O_2 to saturate the blood with O_2. Blood gas analyzers determine ctO_2 by the following calculation[77]:

$$ctO_2(\text{mL/dL}) = FO_2Hb \times bO_2 \times ctHb(\text{g/dL}) + (\alpha O_2) \times (PO_2)$$

where bO_2 equals 1.39 mL/g and αO_2, the solubility coefficient of O_2 at 37 °C and STPD, equals 0.0031 (mL/dL)/mm Hg = 0.00140 (mmol/L)/mm Hg. Note that this calculation is based on FO_2Hb and $ctHb$. If SO_2 is used, it is necessary to use the effective hemoglobin concentration (i.e., to subtract the concentration of any dyshemoglobins present from the concentration of $ctHb$). Thus on initial patient presentation, determination of any dyshemoglobins may be necessary to obtain an accurate value for ctO_2 for its use in subsequent calculations.

Hemoglobin-Oxygen Dissociation

The degree of association or dissociation of O_2 with hemoglobin is determined by PO_2 and the affinity of hemoglobin for O_2. When the SO_2 of blood is determined over a range of PO_2 and plotted against PO_2, a sigmoidal curve called the O_2 dissociation curve is obtained. The *shape* of the curve arises from the increasing efficiency with which HHb molecules bind more O_2 once some O_2 has been bound ("cooperativity"; see also Chapter 31). The *location* of the curve relative to the PO_2 required to achieve a particular concentration of SO_2 in the blood is a function of the affinity of the hemoglobin for O_2.

The affinity of hemoglobin for O_2 depends on five factors: temperature, pH, PCO_2, concentration of 2,3-DPG, and the presence of minor hemoglobins, such as COHb and metHb. Dissociation of O_2 in relation to 2,3-DPG concentration and abnormal hemoglobin proteins, such as fetal hemoglobin (Hb F), thalassemias, and other hemoglobinopathies, is discussed in Chapter 31. Note that Figure 46-7 illustrates the effect of different concentrations of 2,3-DPG on the SO_2-PO_2 relationship. This chapter describes the effects of temperature, pH, and PCO_2 on dissociation behavior.

The graph in Figure 27-3 illustrates the effect of plasma pH on the O_2 dissociation curve (the Bohr effect). Similar graphs can be made for variations of PCO_2, 2,3-DPG, and temperature. The shifting locations of the curves are described in the third column of the chart in Figure 27-3, with increasing affinity for O_2 shifting the curve to the left. These sigmoidal curves, however, are difficult to use when quantitative estimates of the amount of shift are desired, when calculating the PO_2 at which 50% of Hb is binding O_2 (P_{50}). The Hill logit-log transform (illustrated as the Hill plot, Figure 27-3, *B*) converts the curvilinear dissociation function into a linear function. The slope of the linear function, called the *Hill slope*, is essentially constant at 2.7 for an SO_2 between 40% and 80%.

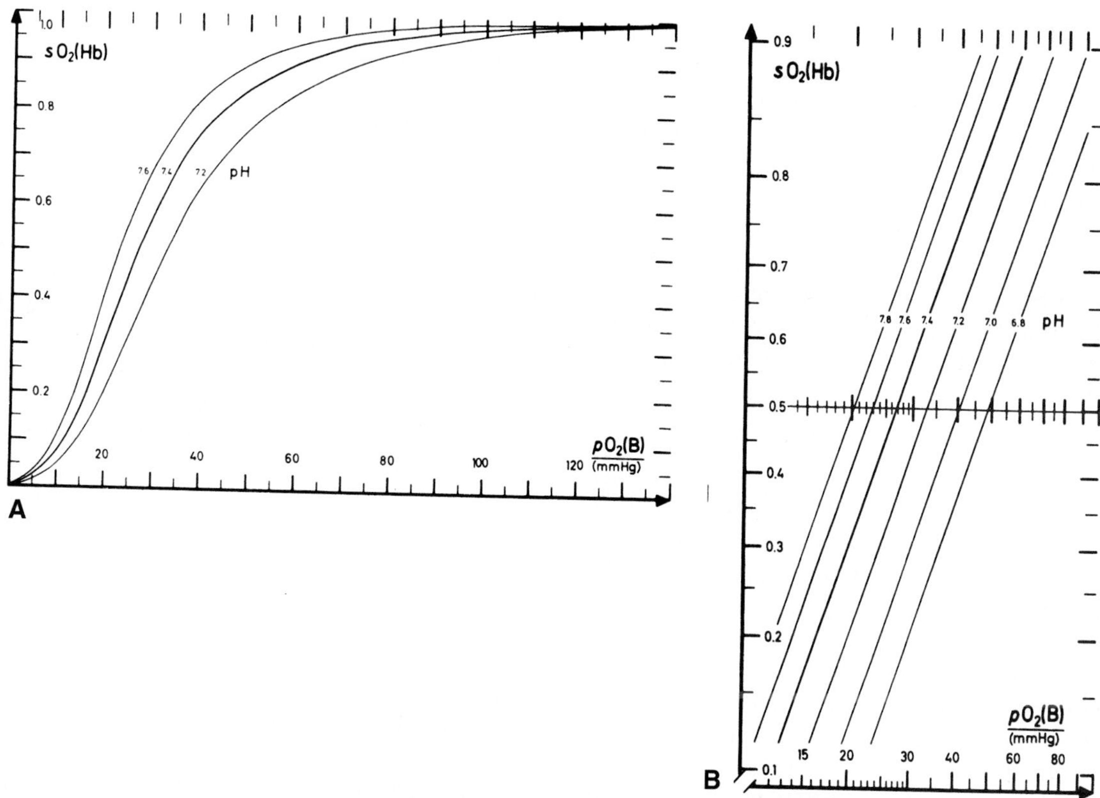

Deviation from Standard Conditions	Shift in Dissociation Curve	Affinity of Hemoglobin for O_2	Coefficient of Change*
pH(P) > 7.4	←	↑	$\frac{\Delta \log PO_2}{\Delta pH(P)} = -0.46$
pH(P) < 7.4	→	↓	
Temperature			
>37 °C	→	↓	$\frac{\Delta \log PO_2}{\Delta T} = +0.024\ K^{-1}$
<37 °C	←	↑	
PCO_2 > 40 mm Hg	→	↓	$\frac{\Delta \log PO_2}{\Delta \log PCO_2} = +0.02$
PCO_2 < 40 mm Hg	←	↑	
*c*DPG(E)			
>normal	→	↓	$\frac{\Delta \log PO_2}{\Delta(cDPG(E)/c^*)} = +0.04$
<normal	←	↑	

Figure 27-3 A, Oxygen dissociation curves for human blood with different plasma pH, but constant PCO_2 of 40 mm Hg, a 2,3-diphosphoglycerol concentration in erythrocytes of 5.0 mmol/L, and temperature at 37 °C. **B,** A Hill plot. Conditions are the same as in **A.** *DPG,* 2,3-diphosphoglycerol.

*The coefficients given in this chart are the basis for the correction of measured PO_2; their application to P_{50} correction is discussed in the text contained on the Evolve site that accompanies this book. The effect of pH(P) to shift the dissociation curve is called the *Bohr effect*; the coefficient above for $\Delta \log PO_2/\Delta pH(P)$ applies to conditions when the PCO_2 is 40 mm Hg and changes in pH(P) are due to changes in concentrations of noncarbonic acids and bases. If, however, the changes in pH(P) are being caused by changes in PCO_2, then the absolute value of the coefficient is greater, i.e., $\Delta \log PO_2/\Delta pH(P) = -0.49$. The coefficients for the Bohr effect are specified for PO_2 of whole blood but use the pH of plasma, pH(P). The coefficient for DPG effect is based on the DPG concentration in the erythrocytes *c*DPG(E).

$c^* = 1$ mmol/L.

The linear transforms of the dissociation curves have allowed linear coefficients of change (fourth column of the chart in the legend to Figure 27-3) to be determined for each of the factors that shift dissociation curves, and hence the lines on the Hill plot. These coefficients find application, singly or in combination, for correcting measured PO_2 or calculated P_{50} for the effects of different temperature, PCO_2, pH, and 2,3-DPG concentrations.

Determination of P_{50}

P_{50} is defined as the PO_2 for a given blood sample at which the hemoglobin of the blood is half saturated with O_2. The measured value of P_{50} differs from the standard value of P_{50} by some amount determined by the extent that pH differs from 7.40, PCO_2 differs from 40 mm Hg, temperature differs from 37 °C, and 2,3-DPG differs from 5.0 mmol/L. The value of P_{50} therefore becomes a measure of change of the hemoglobin affinity because of the factors that affect it. A procedure for determining P_{50} is available on the Evolve site that accompanies this book.[7,56,91,95,101] The procedure uses the principle that:

$$\log P_{50} = \log PO_2 - \text{logit } SO_2/2.7$$

where logit $SO_2 = \log[SO_2/(1 - SO_2)]$ and 2.7 is the Hill slope.

The P_{50} reference intervals for adults, measured at 37 °C and corrected to pH(P) of 7.4, are 25 to 29 mm Hg. For newborn infants, the interval is 18 to 24 mm Hg because of the presence of fetal Hb (Hb F).

Clinical Significance

Increased values for P_{50} indicate displacement of the O_2 dissociation curve to the right (i.e., a decreased affinity of the hemoglobin for O_2). The chief causes are hyperthermia, acidemia, hypercapnia, high concentrations of 2,3-DPG, or presence of a hemoglobin variant with decreased O_2 affinity. The physiological effects of decreased affinity of hemoglobin are small. In general, the affinity is still sufficient to allow the hemoglobin to bind adequate amounts of O_2 in the lungs. Low affinity facilitates dissociation of O_2Hb at the peripheral tissue cell. Indeed, in anemia, low affinity (as a result of increases in 2,3-DPG) is a desirable compensatory mechanism.

Low values for P_{50} signify displacement of the O_2 dissociation curve to the left (i.e., increased affinity of hemoglobin). The main causes are hypothermia, acute alkalemia, hypocapnia, low concentration of 2,3-DPG, increased COHb and MetHb, or a hemoglobin variant. Decreases of 2,3-DPG are commonly observed in acid states that have persisted for more than a few hours. The initial increase in P_{50} caused by the acidemia is gradually compensated for by a decrease in 2,3-DPG so that P_{50} then falls to lower than normal values. The physiological consequence of increased affinity of hemoglobin for O_2 is less efficient dissociation of O_2Hb at the peripheral tissue and lower tissue PO_2.

TONOMETRY

Tonometry is the process of exposing a liquid to a gas phase in such a way that each gas in the gaseous phase partitions to an equilibrium between the liquid and gas. This equilibration, in effect, imparts the PCO_2 and PO_2 of the equilibrating gas to the blood to which it is exposed within the tonometer. Equilibration by tonometry uses gases of known fractional composition, humidified at 37 °C to give a saturated water vapor pressure of 47 mm Hg. The PCO_2 or PO_2 of such gases is calculated according to Dalton's law (see section on behavior of gases). Tonometry is used to treat blood samples for various special studies that are requested only rarely in most hospital settings and for preparing quality control material in whole blood. Direct determination of P_{50} and of standard bicarbonate are two applications of tonometry.

Tonometry may be achieved by simple homemade assemblies or by commercially available equipment. Some commercially available tonometers use a thin-film technique. It consists of a glass or plastic cup fitted on a shaft and enclosed in a humidified chamber whose temperature is maintained at 37 °C. A few milliliters of blood is placed in the cup, and gas flow is initiated to continuously flush the inside surface of the cup with the humidified gas. A controller unit causes the cup to rotate rapidly and periodically in short bursts, so that the blood in the cup is thrown in a thin layer over the inside walls. Another form of tonometry is the bubble technique. It uses a syringe that is specially constructed to allow gas to be introduced and humidified through the plunger. During tonometry, the syringe is laid in a thermostatically controlled aluminum heat block. Additional detail on tonometry and its applications can be found in a previous edition of this textbook. Reference conditions for tonometry have been recommended by a committee of the International Federation of Clinical Chemistry and Laboratory Medicine (IFCC).[49]

DETERMINATION OF PCO_2, PO_2, AND PH

The instruments used for determination of PCO_2, PO_2, and pH are highly automated. Proper specimen collection and handling are critical for accurate determinations.

Specimens

Whole blood is the most likely specimen for a clinical laboratory to receive for gas analysis and may be obtained from any site accessible to vascular catheterization or entry. These sites commonly are the vessels of the extremities, but special studies may require access to the chambers of the heart and great vessels of the chest. Analysts should recognize that some specimens are difficult to obtain and should be handled with utmost care. Sometimes the volume of the specimen collected for analysis, particularly from premature neonates, has to be as small as possible without sacrificing specimen quality and analytical accuracy.

Differences in measured blood gas values between arterial and venous are most pronounced for PO_2. In fact, PO_2 is the only clinical reason for the more difficult arterial collections. PO_2 is generally 60 to 70 mm Hg lower in venous blood after O_2 is released in the capillaries, whereas PCO_2 is 2 to 8 mm Hg higher in venous blood. pH is generally only 0.02 to 0.05 pH units lower in a venous sample.

Quality assurance of blood analysis for gases and pH is dependent on control of preanalytical error (i.e., on proper collection and handling of the specimen) and on control of the analytical instrument and testing process. Because laboratory personnel do not always control collection of arterial or venous specimens, they must work closely and cooperatively with physicians, nurses, respiratory therapists, and other personnel who obtain these samples. Guidelines for controlling preanalytical errors have been published by the NCCLS.[77]

Arterial puncture carries a slight medical risk and under no circumstances should it be undertaken by anyone who has not been properly trained to perform it. Arterial puncture is always done with a syringe and needle. No tourniquet is used, and no pull or very gentle pull is applied to the plunger of the syringe as the arterial blood pressure pushes blood into the syringe. An NCCLS-approved standard, H-11A3, describes appropriate procedures.

Venous blood for measuring blood gases and pH is best collected with a needle and syringe, although some laboratories also accept specimens drawn to a complete fill of an evacuated tube containing a dry heparin salt. In the collection of venous blood from an arm vein, the specimen should be obtained after release of a tourniquet, and the patient should not be allowed to flex the fingers or clench the fist. Prolonged application of a tourniquet and/or muscular activity will decrease venous PO_2 and pH. Placement of indwelling catheters with heparin locks for short- and long-term intravenous therapies is common and the catheter can serve as a port for the specimen collection if it is thoroughly flushed with blood (usually 5× the catheter volume) before the specimen is drawn. Failure to flush the lock properly has unpredictable effects on measured quantities and is frequently indicated by bizarre, nonphysiological results.

Arterial or venous specimens are best collected anaerobically with lyophilized heparin anticoagulant in sterile syringes with capacities of 1 to 5 mL. Although in theory glass syringes are preferred to prevent the exchange of gases through the syringe wall, most blood gas syringes today are plastic and the exchange of gas that occurs within 1 hour is trivial. Lyophilized heparin is preferable to liquid heparin because the liquid heparin, which has atmospheric PO_2 and PCO_2 values, dilutes the sample, with the effect being greatest when the syringe is not completely filled. If liquid heparin is used, the size of the syringe, the concentration and volume of liquid heparin, and the volume of blood drawn into the syringe are important. Adequate anticoagulation (~0.05 mg heparin/mL blood) can be achieved by drawing enough liquid heparin solution into the syringe in such a way as to wet the interior of the barrel over the maximum inner surface area of the syringe and ejecting air and excess heparin in such a way as to leave the dead space of the syringe filled with heparin. The syringe dead space is roughly 0.1 mL, and thus when a sterile heparin solution of 500 U/mL (5 mg/mL) is used, the dead space will hold 0.5 mg of heparin. In a 1-mL syringe, or if only 1 mL of blood is drawn into a 3- or 5-mL syringe, the blood will be diluted with up to 10% heparin solution. An increasing ratio of heparin to blood (Table 27-5) can have an increasingly marked effect on measured PCO_2 and the parameters calculated from it.[35] In one study, dilution with 10% heparin having an atmospheric

TABLE 27-5 Changes in pH, PCO_2, Base Excess, PO_2, and Actual Bicarbonate With Different Volumes of Heparin Solution in Venous Samples

	Percentage Volume of Heparin Solution in Blood			
	2	4	10	20
pH	7.37	7.37	7.37	7.36
PCO_2 (mm Hg)	51.0	48.8*	44.2*	39.0†
PO_2 (mm Hg)	32.2	35.2	36.8	38.2
Actual HCO_3^- (mmol/L)	29	28‡	25	22†

From Hutchison AS, Ralston SH, Dryburgh FJ, et al. Too much heparin: Possible source of error in blood gas analysis. Br Med J 1983;287:1131-2. Significance of difference from percentage volume of 2: *$p < 0.01$; $^{\dagger}p < 0.001$; $^{\ddagger}p < 0.05$.

PCO_2 of 0.25 mm Hg led to a 10- to 20-mm Hg decrease in blood PCO_2.[45] Before analysis, mixing of the sample by simple but vigorous rolling of the syringe between the palms is usually adequate to establish the desired homogeneity whether liquid or lyophilized heparin is used.

Anaerobic technique for collection means no or minimal exposure of blood to atmospheric air. The PCO_2 of dry air is about 0.25 mm Hg, which is much less than that of blood (~40 mm Hg). Thus the CO_2 content and PCO_2 of blood exposed to air will decrease, and blood pH, which is a function of PCO_2, will rise. The PO_2 of atmospheric air (~155 mm Hg) is approximately 60 mm Hg higher than that of arterial blood and approximately 120 mm Hg higher than that of venous blood. Therefore blood from patients breathing room air that is exposed to atmospheric air gains O_2. In contrast, blood with PO_2 exceeding 150 mm Hg, as will occur in patients undergoing O_2 therapy, loses O_2 on exposure to air. Even with care in sample handling, blood can be exposed to air simply from the air in the needle and the syringe hub dead space. Error will be minimal if the resulting bubble is ejected immediately upon removing the needle from the puncture site. The potential effect of small bubbles on blood gas results was clearly demonstrated in one study in which a 100-μL bubble of room air was added to 10, 2-mL blood samples with PO_2 values between 25 and 40 mm Hg. In these samples, PO_2 increased an average of 4 mm Hg in only 2 minutes, whereas PCO_2 decreased 4 mm Hg.[74] Numerous small air bubbles have similar effects. Thus when a full syringe is disconnected from a needle or cannula, it should be held tip up, a drop of blood ejected from it, and a tightly fitting cap placed on the tip of the hub.

Arterialized capillary blood is sometimes an acceptable alternative to arterial blood when blood losses need to be minimized, when an arterial cannula is not available, or to prevent repeated arterial puncture. Freely flowing cutaneous blood originates in the arterioles and corresponds closely to arterial blood in composition. However, arterialized capillary blood is not acceptable when systolic blood pressure is less than 95 mm Hg, in cases of vasoconstriction, from patients on O_2 therapy, from newborns during the first few hours after birth, or in newborns with respiratory distress syndrome. These situations pose a particular risk of admixture with blood from the venules, resulting in erroneously low PO_2 values. Capillary puncture should be preceded by warming the selected skin puncture site for 10 minutes to achieve vasodilation and adequate blood flow through local capillaries. For collection from the finger of a child or adult or from an infant's heel, warming may be accomplished by immersing the arm or leg in water warmed to 45 °C. The first blood drop to appear should be wiped away, and subsequent free-forming drops taken up in a capillary collection tube containing lyophilized heparin. Only free-flowing blood provides a satisfactory sample, and taking up the drops as soon as they form minimizes aerobic exposure. Appropriate capillary tubes hold 70 to 300 μL of blood, and the larger-diameter tubes require mixing. A flea (a slender wire approximately 5 mm in length) is immediately inserted after filling, and a magnet is used to move the flea back and forth.

Transport and analysis of specimens should be prompt. Physicians who use blood gas and pH measurements in acute care management usually require very rapid turnaround times between specimen acquisition and reporting of results. Ideally, specimens should never be stored before analysis. However, delayed analysis of up to 1 hour will have a minimal effect on reported values from most samples. The pH of freshly drawn blood decreases on standing at a rate of 0.04 to 0.08 pH unit/hr at 37 °C, 0.02 to 0.03/hr at 22 °C, and <0.01/hr at 4 °C. The decrease in pH is accompanied by a corresponding decrease in glucose and an equivalent increase in lactate. PCO_2 increases by ~5 mm Hg/hr at 37 °C, 1 mm Hg/hr at 22 °C, and only ~0.5 mm Hg/hr at 2 °C to 4 °C. The primary cause of these changes is glycolysis by leukocytes, platelets, and reticulocytes. In freshly drawn blood with a normal PO_2 that is maintained anaerobically, cell respiration causes PO_2 to decrease at a rate of ~2 mm Hg/hr at room temperature but 5 to 10 mm Hg/hr at 37 °C. Adverse effects of glycolysis and respiration on pH, $ctCO_2$, PO_2, and PCO_2 of blood can best be prevented by analysis within 30 minutes after collection. If analysis must be delayed or if circumstances create a risk of delay, the syringe or tube containing the blood should be immersed in a mixture of ice and water until analysis is possible. Under these conditions, changes are negligible because glycolysis is inhibited. However, if plastic syringes are stored in ice water there is a risk of significant increases in PO_2, when the actual blood PO_2 is low, because of diffusion of the gas through the plastic. With state-of-the-art blood gas instrumentation, introduction of a chilled sample carries little risk of low-temperature effect on measurements because the thermal equilibration of the sample to 37 °C is rapid and complete.

The aforementioned small changes in values that can be expected with delays in analysis are true *only* when the white blood cell count (WBC) is normal or only slightly elevated. Glycolysis and the resulting effects on pH, PO_2, and PCO_2 increase dramatically with markedly elevated WBC, such as occurs in leukemia. Experiments have shown that PO_2 decreases 20 mm Hg in just 2 minutes and 40 mm Hg in only 5 minutes with WBC values greater than 100,000/μL.[20,46] Indeed, with these types of WBC values, it is virtually impossible to overcome this effect. Even after immersing the sample in ice, thermal equilibrium takes at least 3 to 5 minutes, allowing significant PO_2 loss before the contents reach 2 °C. The only alternative to obtain accurate blood gas values on such patients is immediate on-site analysis by use of a point-of-care device or by taking the blood gas analyzer to the patient.

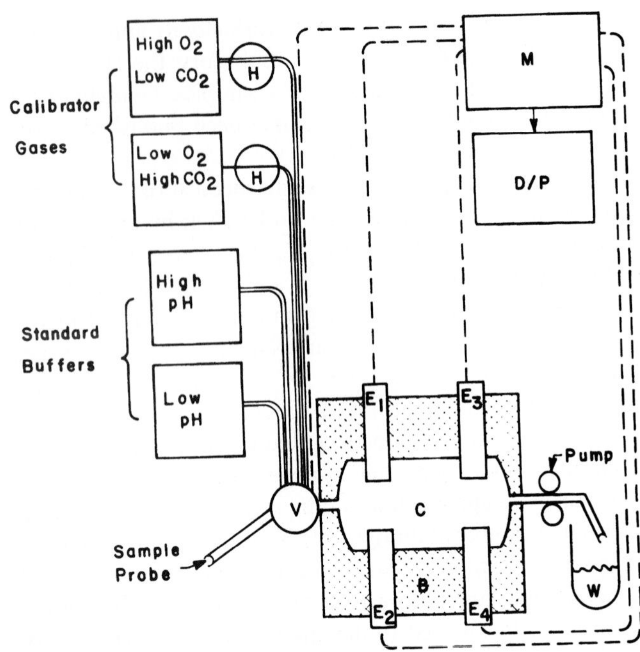

Figure 27-4 Diagram of blood gas instrumentation. *H*, Humidification device; *V*, valve; *C*, chamber; *B*, constant temperature bath at 37 °C; *W*, waste; *M*, microprocessor; *D/P*, display/printer. E (electrodes) where E_1 is PO_2, E_2 PCO_2, E_3 pH, and E_4 reference for pH.

Instrumentation

Reference methods for blood gas and electrolyte determinations have been described in detail by the IFCC.[67] A schematic diagram characteristic of a typical instrument is shown in Figure 27-4. Electrochemical principles and structural features of electrodes are discussed in Chapter 4. Prominent manufacturers of blood gas equipment include Roche Scientific Corp., Bayer Diagnostics, Instrumentation Laboratory, Nova Biomedical, and Radiometer America, Inc. Readers are referred to these manufacturers for details and operational features of specific instruments.

Recent developments in instrumentation have included "stat. profile" equipment for point-of-care or bedside testing.[36,112] Almost all manufacturers now produce small, portable, stand-alone, easy-to-operate instruments designed for "satellite lab" operations, and some hand-held devices that use disposable electrodes, such as the I-STAT instrument, are also available.[36] Such instruments often combine measurement systems for blood gases and pH with ISEs for electrolytes, glucose, urea nitrogen, and hematocrit or hemoglobin. Although design and construction may differ significantly from those used in laboratory instrumentation, the principles of analysis, especially for blood pH and gases, are not novel. Readers are referred to the manufacturers' literature and to Chapter 12 for a discussion of POCT.

The operation of a traditional blood gas instrument begins with the operator presenting a blood specimen at the sample probe. A keyboard-entered command to sample a specimen initiates uptake of the sample through the probe by a peristaltic pump that loads the chamber with 60 to 150 µL of the fluid sample. The pump is under microprocessor control to pause after admission of the sample to let the sample reside in the chamber long enough to allow thermal equilibration and for the measurements to be completed. On completion of measurement, the pump pushes the sample to waste, while output is being made available on a display, a printed tape, and often to a laboratory information system through an interface.

The instrument (see Figure 27-4) is designed so that a manually or microprocessor actuated valve (V) admits calibrator gases, standard buffers, or a sample to a small chamber (C) maintained by a fluid or metal bath (B) to a constant temperature of 37 °C ± 0.1 °C. Measuring and reference electrodes (E) protrude into this chamber. In the pH calibration phase of the instrument, high pH standard buffer and low pH standard buffer are alternately admitted into the chamber and electronic responses of the upper and lower limits of a linear pH curve are established. In the gas calibration phase, gas mixtures with high and low fractional concentrations of O_2 and CO_2 are alternately admitted into the chamber and electronic responses of the upper and lower limits of linear PO_2 and PCO_2 curves are set. In the measurement phase, an anaerobically collected blood sample is admitted.

Most instruments are designed to be self-calibrating. Under the command of the microprocessor, calibrator gases and buffers are cycled at short intervals through the chamber, and electronic responses are continually monitored and reset to the constants initially entered for high and low PCO_2 and PO_2 and high and low pH of the calibrator materials. In the United States, the regulations written for the Clinical Laboratory Improvement Amendments of 1988 (CLIA '88) mandate one point calibration every 30 minutes or within 30 minutes of every patient's sample and two point calibrations every 8 hours.

Electrodes

The tip of the pH measuring electrode is made of H^+-sensitive glass (see Chapter 4), and aside from specialized construction and miniaturization for application in the blood gas chamber, most pH measuring and reference electrodes differ little from those of free-standing pH meters.

Construction of PCO_2 and PO_2 electrodes is shown in Figures 4-4 and 4-8. The gas electrodes are fitted at the tip with gas-permeable membranes held in place with O-rings. Inside these membranes are electrolyte solutions in contact with the measuring and reference elements of the electrode. The membrane of the PCO_2 electrode usually consists of Teflon or silicone rubber approximately 25 µm thick. The electrolyte solution is a thin film containing sodium bicarbonate at 0.005 mol/L and sodium chloride (NaCl) at 0.1 mol/L saturated with AgCl. A spacer of nylon net or cellophane lies between the solution and the H^+-sensitive glass of the measuring element proper. As CO_2 diffuses from the sample into the electrolyte solution, the slight rise in $[H^+]$ from its hydration reaction is measured as ΔpH by an especially sensitive potentiometer and is transformed to $\Delta \log PCO_2$ electronically.

The membrane of a PO_2 electrode in a standard blood gas analyzer is usually ~20-µm thick polypropylene. The electrolyte solution is a thin film of phosphate buffer saturated with AgCl but also containing KCl, and is in contact with the polarized platinum cathode and the Ag/AgCl anode. As O_2 diffuses into the electrolyte, it reacts with the cathode to cause current to flow; the generated current is measured. The sensitivity ($\Delta I/\Delta PO_2$, change in current per millimeter of mercury) of a PO_2 electrode with a polypropylene membrane is around 20 pA/mm Hg. Most point-of-care analyzers use disposable electrodes, eliminating the necessity to change membranes.

Optical Approaches to Blood Gas Measurement

Optical approaches to measuring pH and blood gas parameters have recently been used in some newer point-of-care devices. These devices use single-use, dry chemistry cartridges to determine pH, PO_2, PCO_2, and in some cases electrolytes. The OPTI Critical Care Analyzer device from Osmetech, Inc. uses a series of fluorescent sensor molecules that are specific for the different gases, electrolytes, or glucose. The NPT7 from Radiometer is another point-of-care device that uses optical technologies for pH and blood gas measurement.[12] PCO_2 is determined by infrared absorbance at three wavelengths, 4228, 4268 and 4308 nm, with 4268 nm being the peak absorbance for CO_2 in plasma. The PO_2 sensor in this device uses a phosphorescent dye dissolved in a polyvinyl chloride (PVC) membrane. The dye is a Pd complex of a porphyrin molecule, and the instrument detects quenching of the phosphorescence by O_2 (see Figure 27-5). Finally the NPT7 measures pH with a pH-sensitive dye and performs co-oximetry with a 128 wavelength spectrophotometer.[12] It is likely that these types of single-use, dry chemistry approaches will become more popular in POCT. The challenges inherent to this or other types of POCT are discussed in Chapter 12.

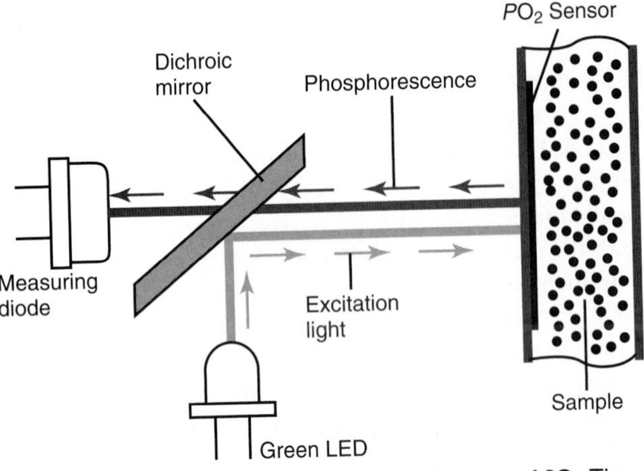

Figure 27-5 The optical system for measurement of PO_2. The optical system for PO_2 is based on the ability of O_2 to reduce the intensity and lifetime of phosphorescence from a phosphorescent dye that is in contact with the sample. The optical system comprises a green (519-nm peak) light-emitting diode (LED, that emits light, which is reflected by a dichroic mirror onto the PO_2 sensor. Because of the phosphorescence, red light (672-nm peak) is emitted back through the dichroic mirror and onto a photodetector. *(From Boalth N, Wandrup J, Larsson L, et al. Blood gases and oximetry: calibration-free new dry chemistry and optical technology for near-patient testing. Clin Chim Acta 2001;307:225-33.)*

Significant Figures of Results

Contemporary instruments commonly display pH readings to three decimal places and PCO_2 and PO_2 readings to one decimal place. The pH should be reported to two decimal places, and PCO_2 and PO_2 as integers (when the unit is mm Hg).

Calibration

Because electrodes are not stable over long periods of time, frequent calibration of pH, PCO_2, and PO_2 is required.

The pH measurement system is calibrated against primary standard buffers admitted either manually or automatically into the sample chamber. The buffers are phosphate solutions that should meet National Institutes of Standards and Technology (NIST) specifications. Calibration buffers meeting NIST specifications are available from the manufacturer of an instrument, usually in containers of appropriate size and shape for mounting as a reservoir on the instrument. The pH values of the low and high calibrator buffers are set by the manufacturer but always lie close to 6.8 and 7.4 at 37 °C. The tolerance of the specified values should be less than or equal to an SD of ±0.003 to achieve SDs of ±0.005 to ±0.01 in measuring blood pH. Unopened containers should be stored at room temperature. When visual observation or an instrument display warns of low concentrations in the reservoir, recommended practice is to replace the reservoir with a newly opened container rather than to replenish fluid in the current one. Pooling several almost empty containers is not recommended.

PCO_2 and PO_2

Calibration of the gas measurement systems is made against gases of known O_2 and CO_2 composition, admitted into the sample chamber. Compressed gases, with a certificate of analysis provided by the manufacturer, are most used as primary standards. Pure O_2, CO_2, and N_2 may be obtained in individual tanks and mixed as desired with a precision gas mixer in the blood gas laboratory, but this is seldom done today. The "low gas" mixture for calibration usually has a fractional composition of 5% CO_2, 0% O_2, and 95% N_2. The "high gas" mixture has a fractional composition of 10% CO_2, 20% O_2, and 70% N_2. These compositions correspond roughly to a calibration range of 38 to 76 mm Hg for PCO_2 and 0 to 152 mm Hg for PO_2.

The mode of calibration is determined by the design of the instrument. Most instruments contain a barometer or a transducer responsive to *P*(Amb) so that barometric pressure is always known to the microprocessor. With such instruments, only a keyboard entry of the fractional composition of O_2 and CO_2 in low and high calibrator gas mixtures needs to be made. Today, most analyzers autocalibrate without the necessity for user input. The microprocessor will calculate the values for PO_2 and PCO_2 (according to Dalton's law) for gases saturated with water vapor at 37 °C.

Liquid-Gas Difference of a PO_2 Electrode

When calibration gases are used to standardize a system, a particular property of the PO_2 electrode needs to be considered. This property is called the *liquid-gas* or *blood-gas difference*.

PO_2 and PCO_2 electrodes are alike in that gas diffusing from a liquid or gaseous sample passes through a gas-permeable membrane into an enclosed electrolyte solution that is in contact with measuring and reference elements. In both electrodes, the rate of diffusion of a gas through the membranes is slower from a liquid phase than from a gaseous phase. However, PCO_2 and PO_2 electrodes use different principles of measurement. Because CO_2 is not consumed by the PCO_2 electrode, the rate of its diffusion through the membrane is not limiting, and equilibrium is achieved between the PCO_2 of the sample and the inner bicarbonate solution. Thus the PCO_2 electrode senses PCO_2 to the same extent whether the sample is liquid and diffusion is slow or the sample is gaseous with faster diffusion.

By contrast, O_2 passing the membrane of a PO_2 electrode enters an irreversible reaction at a polarized cathode so that current generated by the reaction is proportional to the amount of O_2 reduced. The amount of O_2 available for consumption depends on the rate of diffusion of O_2 through the membrane. A steady state is achieved when the rate of diffusion equals the rate of reduction. Thus the electrode responds to a greater degree to O_2 diffusing from a gaseous phase than from a liquid phase.

The liquid-gas difference for a PO_2 electrode becomes significant when an electrode is calibrated with gas but used to measure PO_2 in blood. The difference is usually expressed as a ratio of PO_2 (gas sample) to PO_2 (liquid sample). For most electrodes, the ratio is commonly 1.02 to 1.06. For routine clinical work, a ratio of 1.04 is frequently assumed rather than determined. For the highest accuracy of blood PO_2 analysis, the ratio for a particular electrode can be determined with tonometered blood versus the same gaseous mixture and applied as a correction factor to measured PO_2.

Quality Assurance

The elements of good quality assurance of blood gas and pH measurements include proper maintenance of the instrument, use of control materials, verifying electrode linearity, checking barometer accuracy, and accurately measuring temperature.

Maintenance of Instrumentation

Sophistication of contemporary equipment and availability of high-quality calibrator materials have made reliable and accurate determination of blood pH and gases primarily a matter of meticulous maintenance and control of the equipment and proper collection and handling of specimens. Software programs of the instrument's microprocessor often provide display warnings and diagnostic routines that alert the operator and assist in the trouble-shooting process. Nevertheless, regular maintenance and close adherence to the manufacturer's recommended procedures are essential for satisfactory operation. The frequency with which maintenance should be scheduled is in direct proportion to the volume of analyses performed in the laboratory. The manufacturer's suggested schedule should be considered a minimum guideline, with experience relied on to indicate maintenance frequency.

Cleanliness of the sample chamber and path is especially important. Automatic flushing to cleanse the sample chamber and path after each blood sample measurement is a feature of most instruments without disposable electrodes. When it is not, then manual modes of flushing recommended by the manufacturer should be faithfully practiced. Despite proper flushing, however, complete or partial clogging of the chamber or path or both may occur. Frequency of clogging is often related to the number of heparinized capillary blood samples that are analyzed. Fibrin threads and small clots may be present in the specimen or may form while the sample resides in the warm chamber. If allowed to remain, they can affect subsequent measurements or calibrations by interfering with the contact of blood, buffers, or gases with electrode membranes. Visibility of the path through the heat sink is helpful for detecting clogs, dirt, and bubbles. Bubbles that fail to rinse out can be a particular problem if they settle on an electrode.

Prompt and reliable service by the manufacturer or an in-house biomedical engineer is essential for a laboratory performing many analyses per day. Also important is ready availability of goods from the manufacturer or from laboratory supply houses, such as calibrator materials (pH buffers and gases of certified quality), replacement membranes, and small parts for the maintenance of electrodes.

Proficiency testing mandated by federal law in the United States (CLIA '88) has assumed new importance for quality control of blood gas analysis. These rules became effective in January, 1991, and set criteria for satisfactory interlaboratory performance as follows: pH, target value ±0.04; PO_2, target value ±3 SD; and PCO_2, target value ±8% or ±5 mm Hg, whichever is greater. The risks of failure in a testing event are greatest for PCO_2, according to a computer model.[34] The significance of proficiency testing and the penalties for failure place a new incentive on faithful performance of internal control measures and effective response to failures of quality control. At the same time, pressures to control costs have raised the question of how often and how many concentrations of control materials are necessary to monitor intralaboratory performance effectively. The facile answer is as often and as many concentrations as it takes to maintain confidence in the measurement systems. The regulatory answer per CLIA '88 is one concentration of control every 8 hours, with the entire range of control concentrations covered in every 24-hour period. The CAP requires at least two concentrations of controls every 8 hours. In many laboratories, however, the practical answer is to run on every instrument in use, at least once per shift, three concentrations of control for pH, PO_2, and PCO_2, and always on completion of maintenance and troubleshooting procedures.

Newer analyzers, particularly the smaller satellite lab and point-of-care instruments, frequently have an "auto quality control (QC)" feature or use "electronic QCs."[109] Auto QC consists of on board QC material that is automatically analyzed by the instrument at designated intervals that fulfill regulatory requirements. Electronic QC is most common in devices with disposable electrode cartridges and consists of cartridges that verify the electronic specification of the instruments. To be acceptable to most regulatory agencies these electronic QC systems must provide a quantitative result rather than just a qualitative "ok" or "not ok."[109] Although both of these features are very user friendly, ensure proper instrument performance, and are approved by regulatory agencies, there is debate as to how well they can ensure the quality of the entire analytical performance. Such approaches do not assess operator performance or sample handling conditions that can affect blood gas results. The NCCLS has recently published a guideline for electronic QC and other alternative QC approaches for devices that use disposable electrodes.[76] For further discussion of these issues see Chapter 12 on POCT.

Control Materials

Traditionally, QC materials can be commercial blood-based fluids or aqueous fluids. Alternatively, independent standard buffers can be used for pH control and tonometered whole blood for PCO_2 and PO_2 control.

Blood-Based and Fluorocarbon-Based Control Materials. Commercial blood-based control material usually consists of tanned human erythrocytes suspended in buffered medium and sealed in vials with a gas mixture of known O_2 and CO_2 content. Nonblood fluorocarbon materials with O_2-carrying properties similar to those of blood are also available. These products usually are made at three concentrations of pH, PCO_2, and PO_2. Unopened, these types of control material have the advantages of a long shelf life in the refrigerator; 20 to 28 days for the tanned erythrocytes and even longer for the others. The buffered medium allows for control of pH along with that of PO_2 and PCO_2. Within-day and day-to-day consistency in the lifetime of a given lot have been reported to be excellent; within-day coefficients of variation over the range of concentrations were 1% to 2% for pH, PCO_2, and PO_2.

Aqueous Fluid Control Materials. These materials consist of a buffered medium sealed in vials with gas mixtures; the fluid is equilibrated with the gas by vigorous shaking by hand for a prescribed length of time immediately before the vial is opened, and a sample is admitted to the instrument. Coefficients of variation of 0.1% for pH, 2.5% for PCO_2, and 3.2% for PO_2 are common for these types of materials. The disadvantages of aqueous controls stem from their dissimilarity to blood. Lower viscosity and surface tension confer different washout characteristics and impair their ability to reflect clogging. Greater electrical conductivity reduces their effectiveness to detect inadequate grounding, and lower thermal coefficients make them slower to detect failures of temperature control. These disadvantages are most apparent with respect to PO_2, where a fluorocarbon-based matrix is superior. Nevertheless, aqueous commercial controls are far and away the most commonly used. In some laboratories, tonometered controls are used as adjuncts to commercial controls, but this is becoming rare because of the reliability and ease of use of modern blood gas analyzers.

Tonometered Whole Blood. Quality control of PO_2 and PCO_2 by tonometered blood is considered the method of choice because the control material most nearly approximates patients' samples in its interaction with gas electrodes. Tonometered blood is acknowledged to have greater sensitivity for detecting deterioration of the gas-permeable membranes of electrodes than do aqueous fluid controls. The substantial disadvantages are the time required for tonometry, particularly if two or three concentrations of control are desired; difficulties in frequently obtaining fresh, normal blood samples; the necessity for repeated calculation (and risk of miscalculation) of PCO_2 and PO_2 of the equilibrating gases; the necessity to keep special gas mixtures; and its inapplicability to control pH measurement. To prepare tonometered (gas-equilibrated) samples for use as controls, NCCLS Document C46-A recommends a fresh, single-source blood specimen.[77] Because of the difficulties in obtaining and measuring tonometric samples, the NCCLS recommends for laboratories where tonometry is not directly available that there be an arrangement with nearby laboratories or the manufacturer to make tonometric samples available when necessary.[77]

Quality Control Data. Data obtained from assays of blood gas and pH control materials may be handled in the same way as data from other clinical chemistry determinations (i.e., mean, SD, and coefficient of variation, and control and confidence limits for construction of Levey-Jennings plots). As stability of commercial aqueous control materials is generally several months, vendors often provide data reduction programs that standardize and simplify documentation. However, the resulting reports are temporally delayed and are most useful for meeting accreditation requirements as opposed to real-time corrective or preventive action. They are however useful to compare long-term performances with other laboratories. Equally important features of quality assurance to an active blood gas service are the "sixth sense" of practiced operators for detecting subtle manifestations of deterioration of instrument performance and the suspicion of trouble expressed by clinicians.

Barometer

A barometer, whether built into the instrument or free standing, should periodically be checked for accuracy. Because the classic mercury-filled barometer has become a rarity in clinical laboratories, the most reliable reference is local *P*(Amb) as recorded by the nearest official meteorological station, obtained by a phone call or via the Internet, and corrected for any altitude difference.

Temperature Control

Because an exact temperature of 37 °C is essential for the accurate measurement of blood gases and pH, state-of-the-art instrumentation is furnished with thermal sensors embedded in the heat sink around the measuring chamber and communicating to the microprocessor. Audible or visible alarms signal deviation of temperature outside of preset tolerances (usually 37 °C ± 0.1 °C). Also of value is to use temperature-sensitive buffers, such as HEPES or TES, in pH quality assurance procedures.

Sources of Analytical Error

General causes of analytical error are calibration of the instrument with incorrect set points for pH buffers or calibrator gases, degraded calibration materials, failure of temperature control of the measurement chamber, or a dirty sample chamber or path. Incorrect calibration may arise from wrong entries made for buffer or gas values into the microprocessor, from incorrect manual calculations of PCO_2 and PO_2 values by Dalton's law for calibrator gases, or from using gases that are dry because the humidification device is not working properly.

A source of error for the PO_2 electrode is using it in a range above 500 mm Hg when it has not been calibrated for use in this range. Measurements of PO_2 are particularly sensitive to temperature error. To keep systematic error to 1%

to 2%, the temperature control at 37 °C must be within ±0.1 °C. The PO_2 electrode liquid gas difference can introduce a 2% to 6% error. This error will be less when a liquid-gas correction factor is incorporated into the algorithm that generates results. Gases other than O_2 present in a blood sample may affect performance of the PO_2 electrode. The anesthetic gases halothane and nitrous oxide have a direct effect because both can be reduced at the polarized cathode in competition with O_2. Under most circumstances, however, these effects are small and can be ignored.

Reference Intervals[101]

Reference intervals for arterial blood PO_2, SO_2, PCO_2, and pH are extensively described in Chapter 56. Arterial blood PO_2, low at birth, rises to an adult concentration of 83 to 108 mm Hg. An empirical relationship of age to PO_2 is given by the following equation:

$$PO_2, \text{mm Hg} \simeq (-0.27 \times \text{age}\,[\text{y}]) + 104$$

The cause of the fall in PO_2 with age is a gradual increase in pulmonary venoarterial shunting. Values for PO_2 and PCO_2 will decrease with increasing altitude but compensatory mechanisms keep pH values the same. Saturation fraction, SO_2(aB), may be as low as 0.40 at birth but thereafter is 0.95 to 0.98. The FO_2 is 0.90 to 0.95 in healthy adults. The P_{50} corrected to pH 7.40 is 18 to 24 mm Hg for newborns and 24 to 29 mm Hg for adults.

Arterial blood PCO_2 ranges at sea level are somewhat lower for infants than for adults. The range for adults is 35 to 45 mm Hg. Values decrease with altitude above sea level at a rate of 3 mm Hg/km (5 mm Hg/mile). A physiological change occurs with change in posture; PCO_2 is 2 to 4 mm Hg higher for a sitting or standing person than for one in the supine position. During pregnancy, PCO_2 falls gradually to a mean of about 28 mm Hg just before term.

Arterial blood pH, in the first few hours of life, may vary over a range of 7.09 to 7.50, but thereafter is 7.35 to 7.45. The pH of arterial plasma, separated anaerobically at 37 °C, is 0.01 to 0.03 units greater than that of a corresponding whole blood sample, but the difference is not physiological. It arises instead from the effect of erythrocytes on the junction potential of the pH electrodes.

Temperature Correction of Measured pH, PCO_2, and PO_2

In the Henderson-Hasselbalch equation, pK' and α are used as constants for a temperature of 37 °C. The temperature-controlled sample chamber of an instrument is specified to be 37 °C ± 0.1 °C, and it is at that temperature that all measurements of pH and partial pressure of gases are made. The body temperature of a febrile patient may be elevated to 40 °C to 41 °C, or a patient may be made hypothermic for cardiopulmonary bypass surgery and have a temperature as low as 23 °C. Most blood gas instruments, on keyboard entry of a patient's actual temperature, can calculate and present temperature-corrected pH and PCO_2 and calculated values derived from the temperature-corrected primary data. Algorithms used by some manufacturers in their instruments have been listed,[6] and these are very similar or identical to the algorithms shown in Table 27-6 and specified by the NCCLS.[77]

TABLE 27-6 Temperature Correction Formulas Recommended by the NCCLS[77]

pH	$\text{pH} = \text{pH}_m + [-0.0147 + 0.0065(7.4 - \text{pH}_m)](t - 37)$
PCO_2	$PCO_2 = PCO_{2,m}10^{0.019(t-37)}$
PO_2	$PO_2 = PO_{2,m}10^{\left[\frac{(5.49 \times 10^{-11} PO_2^{3.88}) + 0.071}{(9.72 \times 10^{-9} PO_2^{3.88}) + 2.30}\right](t-37)}$

Correction of pH and PCO_2 to the actual temperature of the patient is usually omitted in states of hyperthermia. The magnitude of correction for 40 °C (104 °F) would be +0.045 for pH, and +13% for PCO_2. Therefore correction of PCO_2 can be important if the value is to be used in pulmonary gas exchange studies such as shunt calculations, but unnecessary for the clinical management of assisted ventilation. However, significant disagreement exists with respect to hypothermic states. There are two basic strategies used by anesthetists for managing hypothermia patients. In the pH-stat. method, the measured pH is corrected to the actual body temperature of the patient and then maintained as close to 7.4 as possible by introducing 3% to 5% CO_2 in the inhaled ventilator gas. Alternatively, in the α-stat. strategy, uncorrected values are used to keep the pH and PCO_2 close to the 37 °C reference value.[97] In most situations, the α-stat. method is used, primarily since it is technically easier to perform and may be slightly safer.[97] However, in children undergoing deep hypothermia and circulatory arrest, the pH-stat. strategy has been shown to be more effective at protecting the brain, and is the recommended strategy.[52]

The equation shown in Table 27-6 illustrates the complexity of the calculation to correct PO_2 to the patient's body temperature. Complexity is unavoidable because at PO_2 less than 100 mm Hg ($SO_2 \leq 0.95$), the hemoglobin-O_2 dissociation curve is shifted to the left by the decrease in temperature and by the concomitant rise in pH (see Figure 27-3). For temperature corrections of PO_2 between 100 and 400 mm Hg, accurate formulas become even more complicated.[2] The most accurate calculation of the temperature variation of PO_2 is made by iterative calculations when the only necessary parameters are the temperature coefficients of the P_{50} and the solubility coefficient of O_2 (αO_2). Several analyzers perform such calculations.

As an example of the impact of body temperature on PO_2 values, the following is given as an example. If at 37 °C and an SO_2 of 95% a patient's PO_2 is 75 mm Hg, the PO_2 would be 28 mm Hg at 22 °C. Despite the dramatic and seemingly clinically significant difference, the total oxygen content of the blood obviously does not change with temperature. Furthermore, Severinghaus has shown that SO_2 changes by less than 2% between 0 °C and 42 °C[94] depending on the initial SO_2. Thus it has been recommended that PO_2 be reported at 37 °C and not temperature corrected except when the values are to be used in pulmonary gas exchange studies.[6] Others prefer to refer all values, along with temperature-specific reference intervals, to the patient temperature.

Taken together, prudent policy for the laboratory might be to generate and report temperature-corrected results for pH and PCO_2 only on the specific request of the physician. Furthermore, as per NCCLS recommendation, temperature-corrected results should never be reported without the original results measured at 37 °C.[77]

CONTINUOUS AND NONINVASIVE MONITORING OF BLOOD GASES

Obtaining arterial, venous, or capillary blood is an invasive procedure, and test results reflect conditions pertaining only to a single point in time. Repetitive sampling in intensive or acute care management carries risks, including infection and vascular complications. In premature infants particularly, repeated sampling imposes an undesirable blood loss. Decisive action during intensive cardiopulmonary care or cardiac surgery often demands either continuous monitoring or discrete real-time data for blood gases.

Extensive discussion of noninvasive and continuous modes of monitoring is beyond the purview of this text. However, laboratorians must be aware of them, because blood samples and standard analytical equipment remain the reference for monitoring the effectiveness of such devices, and because responsibility for quality assessment and review for them is often assigned to the clinical laboratory. Indeed, some regulatory agencies, such as the CAP, have developed guidelines for laboratory oversight of "alternative test systems" that include transcutaneous and in vivo monitoring devices. Such guidelines state that "in some cases traditional approaches to management, quality control, etc. may not be directly applicable but that systems must be in place to ensure that accurate results are generated."[21]

Pulse oximeters that continuously monitor SO_2Hb are common and generally reliable.[70] Older pulse oximeters were susceptible to error depending on placement and motion but newer technology has made these devices very reliable.[13,33] Transcutaneous monitoring of PCO_2 and PO_2 is a noninvasive continuous monitoring approach that has been around for more than 30 years and has had particular value and general success in neonatal and pediatric care.[11,54,71] These devices consist of gel-encased self-adhesive electrodes that heat the skin to 43 °C to 44 °C to arterialize the capillaries and facilitate diffusion of O_2 through the skin.[98] Although the electrodes differ considerably in appearance from those used on blood gas instrumentation, they operate on exactly the same electrochemical principle.

Transcutaneous monitoring of PO_2 can vary widely depending on whether the site of application reflects arterial, capillary, or venous blood flow. However, because there is little difference between arterial and venous PCO_2, transcutaneous monitoring of PCO_2 is less problematic and pulse oximeters can often serve as a surrogate for PO_2. Transcutaneous monitoring works best in areas of thin skin thus its popularity in neonates, and in settings of normovolemia. Decreased tissue perfusion and hypovolemia can make these devices unreliable. Nevertheless, their correlations with arterial blood gases are reasonable (r values ranging from 0.7 to 0.8) and they have been recommended for trending and monitoring. However, it is recommended that baseline arterial values be obtained before commencing noninvasive monitoring. Transcutaneous monitoring can also be used to monitor local tissue perfusion after certain surgical procedures and trauma.[86,98]

Transcutaneous PCO_2 values can be up to 80% higher than corresponding capillary or arterial blood values[54] of which 40% to 50% of the difference can be explained by the difference in the temperatures of measurement (44 °C versus 37 °C). Guidelines for transcutaneous measurement of PO_2 and PCO_2 have been published by a committee of the IFCC.[50]

In addition to monitoring PO_2 and PCO_2, new inline devices that also monitor pH, electrolytes, and hematocrit have recently been introduced to the market.[10] The VIA LVM Monitor (Metracor Technologies) is one of these and consists of a single-use inline cartridge consisting of six conventional electrodes. The cartridge is attached to an arterial line and upon operator command withdraws ~1.5 mL of blood into the cartridge where analysis takes place. The analytical time is about 60 seconds after which the blood is returned via the arterial line. Cartridges undergo a two-point calibration before being placed in service and a single-point calibration is used to flush the sensors after each analysis. Analysis can be repeated every five minutes and it is claimed that cartridges can be used for up to 72 hours. In a multicenter study results from 1414 paired sample measurements showed good agreement and correlation for results from an inline monitor compared with traditional laboratory methods.[10] A similar continuous inline analyzer that uses fiber optic technology is the Paratrend 7 from Agilent Technologies. The future of such devices will likely depend on cost versus benefits to patient care and outcomes.

REFERENCES

1. Abel JE. The physical background to freezing-point osmometry and its medical-biological applications. Amer J Med Electronics 1963;2:32-41.
2. Adams AP, Hahn CEW. Principles and practice of blood gas analysis. London: Franklin Scientific Projects, 1979.
3. Adams PC, Woodhouse KW, Adela M, et al. Exaggerated hypokalemia in acute myeloid leukemia. Br Med J 1962;282:1034-5.

4. Albrink MJ, Hald PM, Man, EB, et al. Displacement of serum water by lipids of hyperlipemic serum: A new method for the rapid determination of serum water. J Clin Invest 1955;34:1483-8.
5. Apple FS, Koch DD, Graves S, Ladenson JH. Relationship between direct-potentiometric and flame-photometric measurement of sodium in blood. Clin Chem 1982;28:1931-5.
6. Ashwood ER, Kost G, Kenny M. Temperature correction of blood gas and pH measurements. Clin Chem 1983;29:1877-85.
7. Bain B. Hemoglobinopathy diagnosis. Oxford: Blackwell Science, Inc. 2001.
8. Berry MN, Mazzachi RD, Pejakovic M, Peake MJ. Enzymatic determination of potassium in serum. Clin Chem 1989;35:817-20.
9. Berry MN, Mazzachi, RD, Pejakovic M, Peake MJ. Enzymatic determination of sodium in serum. Clin Chem 1988;34:2295-8.
10. Billman GF, Hughes AB, Dudall GG, et al. Clinical performance of an in-line, ex-vivo point-of-care monitor: A multicenter study. Clin Chem 2002;48:2030-43.
11. Binder N, Atherton H, Thorkelsson T, Hoath SB. Measurement of transcutaneous carbon dioxide in low birthweight infants during the first two weeks of life. Am J Perinatol 1994;11:237-41.
12. Boalth NB, Wandrup J, Larsson L, et al. Blood gases and oximetry: calibration-free new dry chemistry and optical technology for near-patient testing. Clin Chim Acta 2001;307:225-33.
13. Bohnhorst B, Peter CS, Poets CF. Pulse oximeters' reliability in detecting hypoxemia and bradycardia: Comparison between a conventional and two new generation oximeters. Crit Care Med 2000;28: 1565-8.
14. Brand PLP, Gerritsen J, van Aalderen WM. A baby with eczema and an abnormal sweat test. Lancet 1996;348:932.
15. Bruns DE, Ladenson JH, Scott MG. Hyponatremia. N Engl J Med 2000;343:886-7 (letter).
16. Brydon WG, Roberts LB. The effect of hemolysis on the determination of plasma constituents. Clin Chim Acta 1972;41:435-8.
17. Bunn HF, Forget BG, eds. Hemoglobin: molecular, genetic and clinical aspects. Philadelphia: WB Saunders, 1986.
18. Burtis CA, Ashwood ER, eds. Tietz textbook of clinical chemistry, 3rd ed. Philadelphia: WB Saunders, 1999.
19. Caprilli R, Sopranzi N, Colaneri O, et al. Salt-losing diarrhea in idiopathic proctocolitis. Scand J Gastroenterol 1978;13:331-5.
20. Chillar RK, Belman MJ, Farbstein M. Pseudohypoxemia due to leukemia and thrombocytosis [Letter]. N Engl J Med 1980;302:584.
21. College of American Pathologists Checklist for Point of Care Testing POC.09800, November, 2002.
22. Comprehensive Chemistry Survey Set C-A. 2003 CAP Surveys. Chicago, IL: College of American Pathologists, 2003.
23. Costello P, Kubasik NP, Brody HE, et al. Multilayer film analysis: Evaluation of ion-selective electrode slides. Clin Chem 1983;29:129-32.
24. Cotlove E. Determination of chloride in biological materials. *In:* Methods of biochemical analysis. Vol. 12. D Glick, ed. New York: Interscience Publishers, 1964:277-391.
25. Creer MH, Ladenson J. Analytical errors due to lipidemia. Lab Med 1983;14:351-5.
26. Cystic Fibrosis Foundation Center Committee: Sweat Testing Guidelines. Bethesda, MD: Cystic Fibrosis Foundation (http://www.cff.org), 2005.
27. Cystic Fibrosis Foundation Center: Directors Update #1. Bethesda, MD, Cystic Fibrosis Foundation (http://www.cff.org), 1993
28. Cystic Fibrosis Foundation: Patient Registry 2000. Annual Report. Bethesda, MD, Cystic Fibrosis Foundation, 2001.
29. Daoud EWR, McClellan AC, Scott MG. Positive interferences with the Ektachem total CO_2 assay from therapy with topical cerous nitrate. Clin Chem 1990;36:1521-2.
30. Denning CR, Huang NN, Cuasay LR, et al. Cooperative study comparing three methods of performing sweat tests to diagnose cystic fibrosis. Pediatrics 1980;66:752-7.
31. Don BR, Sebastian A, Cheitlin M, et al. Pseudohyperkalemia caused by fist clenching during phlebotomy. N Engl J Med 1990;322:1290-2.
32. Duncan A, Young DS. Measurements of serum colloid pressure are of limited usefulness. Clin Chem 1982;28:141-5.
33. Durbin CG, Rostow SK. More reliable oximetry reduces the frequency of arterial blood gas analysis and hastens weaning after cardiac surgery. A prospective, randomized trial of the clinical impact of a new technology. Crit Care Med 2002;30: 1735-40.
34. Ehrmeyer SS, Laessig RH. A computer model to translate federal proficiency testing performance standards for pH/blood gases into intralaboratory precision and accuracy requirements. *In:* Methodology and clinical applications of blood gases, pH, electrolytes and sensor technology. Vol. 12. International Federation of Clinical Chemistry. RF Moran, AL VanKessel, eds. Utrecht, The Netherlands: MVI Publishing, 1990:3-18.
35. Eichhorn JH. Inaccuracy in blood gas/pH measurements caused by the blood sample. J Med Technol 1985;2:1-6.

36. Erickson KA, Wilding P. Evaluation of a novel point of care system, the I-STAT portable clinical analyzer. Clin Chem 1993;39:283-7.
37. Farrell PM, Koscik RE. Sweat chloride concentrations in infants homozygous or heterozygous for F508 cystic fibrosis. Pediatrics 1996;97:524-8.
38. Frier BM, Steer CR, Baird JD, et al. Misleading plasma electrolytes in children with severe hyperlipidaemia. Arch Dis Child 1980;55:771-5.
39. Gibson LE, diSant'Agnese PA. Studies of salt excretion in sweat. J Pediatr 1963;62:855-67.
40. Gleeson M, Henry RL. Sweat sodium or chloride. Clin Chem 1991;37:112.
41. Goodman JT, Vincent J, Rosen I. Serum potassium changes in blood clots. Am J Clin Pathol 1954;24:111-3.
42. Graber M, Subramani K, Corish D, Schwab A. Thrombocytosis elevates serum potassium. Am J Kidney Dis 1988;12:116-20.
43. Hall NP, Cornelius MJ, Keys AJ. The enzymatic determination of bicarbonate and CO_2 in reagents and buffer solutions. Anal Biochem 1983;132:152-7.
44. Hammond KB, Turcios NL, Gibson LE. Clinical evaluation of the macroduct sweat collection system and conductivity analyzer in the diagnosis of cystic fibrosis. J Pediatr 1994;124:255-60.
45. Hansen JE, Simmons DH. A systematic error in the determination of blood PCO_2. Amer Rev Resp Dis 1977;115:1061.
46. Hess CE, Nichols AB, Hunt WB, Suratt PM. Pseudohypoxemia secondary to leukemia and thrombocytosis. N Engl J Med 1979;301:361-3.
47. Hubl W, Wejbora R, Shafti-Keramet I, et al. Enzymatic determination of sodium, potassium and chloride in abnormal (hemolyzed, icteric, lipemic, paraproteinemic, or uremic) serum samples compared with indirect determination with ion-selective electrodes. Clin Chem 1994;40:1528-31.
48. Ingram RH, Jr, Seki M. Pseudohyperkalemia with thrombocytosis. N Engl J Med 1962;267:895-900.
49. International Federation of Clinical Chemistry, Committee on pH, Blood Gases and Electrolytes: An Approved IFCC Recommendation. IFCC method (1988) for tonometry of blood: Reference materials for PCO_2 and PO_2. Clin Chim Acta 1989;185: S17-24.
50. International Federation of Clinical Chemistry, Committee on pH, Blood Gases and Electrolytes: Guidelines for transcutaneous PO_2 and PCO_2 measurement. Ann Biol Clin 1990;48:39-43.
51. Joint Committee on Pulmonary Nomenclature, American College of Chest Physicians and American Thoracic Society: Pulmonary terms and symbols: A report of the AACP-ATS. Chest 1967;67:583-93.
52. Jonas R, Bellinger D, Rappaport L, et al. Relation of pH strategy and developmental outcome after hypothermic circulatory arrest. J Thorac Cardiovasc Surg 1993;106:362-8.
53. Kimura S, Asari S, Hayashi S, et al. New enzymatic method with tryptophanase for determining potassium in serum. Clin Chem 1992;38:44-7.
54. Kost GJ, Chow, JL, Kenny MA. Transcutaneous carbon dioxide for short-term monitoring of neonates. Clin Chem 1983;29:1534-6.
55. Kumar A, Chapoteau E, Czech BP, et al. Chromogenic ionophore-based methods for spectrophotometric assay of sodium and potassium in serum and plasma. Clin Chem 1988;34:1709-12.
56. Kwant G, Oeseburg B, Zijlstra WG. Reliability of the determination of whole-blood oxygen affinity by means of blood-gas analyzers and multiwavelength oximeters. Clin Chem 1989;35:773-7.
57. Ladenson JH, Apple FS, Aguanno JJ, et al. Sodium measurements in multiple myeloma: Two techniques compared. Clin Chem 1982;28:2383-6.
58. Ladenson JH. Non-analytical sources of variation in clinical chemistry results. *In:* Gradwohl's clinical laboratory methods and diagnosis. AC Sonnenwirth, L Jarett, eds. St. Louis: CV Mosby, 1980:149-92.
59. Law WT, Ertingshausen G. A novel reagent and method for determination of chloride in serum with a centrifugal analyzer. Clin Chem 1980;26: 1874-7.
60. LeGrys VA. Sweat testing for the diagnosis of cystic fibrosis: Practical considerations. J Pediatr 1996;129:892-7.
61. LeGrys VA, Retsch-Bogart G. Urticaria associated with the pilocarpine iontophoresis sweat test. Pediatr Pulmol 1977;24:296-7.
62. LeGrys VA. Assessment of sweat testing practices for the diagnosis of cystic fibrosis. Arch Pathol Lab Med 2001;125:1420-4.
63. LeGrys VA. Common errors in sweat testing reporting for cystic fibrosis. Lab Med 2002;33:21-3.
64. LeGrys VA. Data from University of North Carolina Cystic Fibrosis Center sweat testing results [unpublished], 1997.
65. Lewandrowski K, Kratz A. Case records of the Massachusetts General Hospital: Normal reference laboratory values. N Engl J Med 1999;339:1063-72.
66. Maas AH, Kofstad J, Siggaard-Andersen O, et al., eds. Ionized calcium, sodium, and potassium by ion-selective electrodes. Vol. 5. Proceedings of the first meeting of the European working group on ion-selective electrodes. IFCC Workshop, Oslo, 1983. Copenhagen: Private Press, 1984.
67. Maas AH. IFCC reference methods for measurement of pH, gases and electrolytes in blood: Reference materials. Eur J Clin Chem Clin Biochem 1991;29:253-61.
68. Maas AH, Siggaard-Andersen O, Weisberg HF, et al. Ion-selective electrodes for sodium and potassium: A

new problem of what is measured and what should be reported. Clin Chem 1985;31:482-5.
69. Mercier DE, Feld RD, Witte DL. Comparison of dew-point and freezing point osmometry. Amer J Med Technol 1978;44:1066-9.
70. Miyasaka K. Pulse oximetry in the management of children in the PICU. Anesthesia and Analgesia 2002;94:544-56.
71. Monaco F, McQuitty JC. Transcutaneous measurement of carbon dioxide partial pressure in sick neonates. Crit Care Med 1981;9:756-8.
72. Moran RF. The laboratory assessment of oxygenation. J Intern Fed Clin Chem 1993;5:147.
73. Morissette MP. Colloid osmotic pressure: Its measurement and clinical value. Can Med Assoc J 1977;116:897-900.
74. Mueller RG, Lang GE. Blood gas analysis: effects of air bubbles in syringe and delay in estimation. Br Med J Clin Res 1982;285:1659.
75. Natelson S, Nobel D. Effect of the variation of pK of the Henderson-Hasselbalch equation on values obtained for total CO_2 calculated from PCO_2 and pH values. Clin Chem 1977;23:767-9.
76. National Committee for Clinical Laboratory Standards. Quality Management for unit-use testing: proposed guideline EP18-P. Wayne, PA: National Committee for Clinical Laboratory Standards, 1999.
77. National Committee for Clinical Laboratory Standards: Blood gas and pH analysis and related measurements: Approved guideline C46-A. Wayne PA: National Committee for Clinical Laboratory Standards, 2001.
78. National Committee for Clinical Laboratory Standards: Standardization of Sodium and Potassium Ion-Selective Electrode Systems to the Flame Photometric Reference Method: Approved Standard C29-AZ. Wayne, PA: National Committee for Clinical Laboratory Standards, 1995.
79. National Committee for Clinical Laboratory Standards: Sweat Testing: Sample Collection and Quantitative Analysis: Approved Guideline. NCCLS Document C34-A2. Wayne, PA: National Committee for Clinical Laboratory Standards, 2000.
80. Nijsten MWN, deSmet BJ, Dofferhoff ASM. Pseudohyperkalemia and platelet counts. N Engl J Med 1991;325:1107.
81. Nosanchuk JS, Stull R, Keefner R. The effect of substitution of plasma for serum on chemistry stat turnaround time. Lab Med 1991;22:465-9.
82. Occupational Exposure to Bloodborne Pathogens: Occupational Safety and Health Administration (OSHA) Final Rule. Fed. Reg. 1991;56:64004-182.
83. Oesch U, Ammann D, Simon W. Ion-selective membrane electrodes for clinical use. Clin Chem 1985;32:1448-59.
84. Oliver TK, Young GA, Bates GD, et al. Factitial hyperkalemia due to icing before analysis. Pediatr 1966;38:900-2.
85. Quiles R, Fernandez-Romero JM, Fernandez E, et al. Automated enzymatic determination of sodium in serum. Clin Chem 1993;39:500-3.
86. Ribhallia SV. Developments in transcutaneous blood gas monitoring: A review. J Med Eng Technol 1991;15:143.
87. Rosan RC, Enlander D, Ellis J. Unpredictable error in calculated bicarbonate during pediatric intensive care: The elusion of fixed pK. Clin Chem 1983;29:69.
88. Rosenstein BJ. Interpreting sweat tests in the diagnosis of cystic fibrosis. J Respir Dis 1990;11:519-28.
89. Rosenstein BJ, Cutting GR. The diagnosis of cystic fibrosis: A consensus statement. J Pediatr 1998;132:589-95.
90. Salyer JW, Chatburn RL, Dolcini DM. Measured vs calculated oxygen saturation in a population of pediatric intensive care patients. Respir Care 1989;34: 342-8.
91. Samaja M, Mosca A, Luzzana M, et al. Equations and nomograms for the relationship of human blood *p*50 to 2,3-diphosphoglycerate, CO_2, and H^+. Clin Chem 1981;27:1856-61.
92. Schales O, Schales SS. A simple and accurate method for the determination of chloride in biological fluids. J Biol Chem 1941;140:879-84.
93. Schulz IJ. Micropuncture studies of the sweat formation in cystic fibrosis patients. J Clin Invest 1969;48:1470-7.
94. Severinghaus JW. Simple accurate equations for human blood O_2 dissociation computations. J Appl Physiol 1979;46:599-602.
95. Siggaard-Andersen M, Siggaard-Anderson O. Oxygen status algorithm, version 3, with some applications. Acta Anaesthesiol Scand. Suppl 1995;107:13-20.
96. Southgate JH, Collins JS, Short SM. Comparison of colorimetric potassium method with flame photometry and ion-selective electrodes. Ann Clin Biochem 1991;28:412-3.
97. Tallman R. Acid-base regulation, alpha-stat, and the Emperor's new clothes. J Cardiothorac Vasc Anesth 1997;11:282-8.
98. Tatevossian RG, Wo CCJ, Velmahos GC, et al. Transcutaneous oxygen and CO2 as early warning of tissue hypoxia and hemodynamic shock in critically ill emergency patients. Crit Care Med 2000;28: 2248-53.
99. Thomas LJ. Algorithms for selected blood acid-base and blood gas calculations. J Appl Physiol 1972;33:154-8.
100. Tietz NW, ed. Textbook of clinical chemistry. 1st ed. Philadelphia: WB Saunders, 1986.
101. Tietz NW, ed. Clinical guide to laboratory tests. 3rd ed. Philadelphia: WB Saunders, 1995.

102. Tietz NW, ed. Fundamentals of clinical chemistry. 2nd ed. Philadelphia, WB Saunders, 1976.
103. Tocci PM, McKey RM. Laboratory confirmation of cystic fibrosis. Clin Chem 1976;22:1841-4.
104. Wang T, Diamandis EP, Lane A, et al. Variability in selectivity of Hitachi ion-selective electrodes. Clin Biochem 1994;27:37-44.
105. Warhol RM, Eichenholz A, Mulhausen RO. Osmolality. Arch Intern Med 1965;116:743-9.
106. Watson MA, Scott MG. Clinical utility of biochemical analysis of cerebrospinal fluid. Clin Chem 1995;41:343-60.
107. Waugh WH. Utility of expressing serum sodium per unit of water in assessing hyponatremia. Metabolism 1969;18:706-12.
108. Webster HL. Laboratory diagnosis of cystic fibrosis. CRC Crit Rev Clin Lab Sci 1983;18:313-38.
109. Westgard JO. Electronic quality control, the total testing process and the total quality control system. Clin Chim Acta 2001;307:45-8.
110. Wolf AV. Aqueous solutions and body fluids. New York: Hoeber Medical Division, Harper & Row, 1966.
111. www.wescor.com/biomedical/html/sweat-chek.html (accessed January 24, 2003).
112. Zaloga GP, Hill TR, Strickland RA, et al. Bedside blood gas and electrolyte monitoring in critically ill patients. Crit Care Med 1989;17:920-5.

CHAPTER 28

Hormones*

Michael Kleerekoper, M.D., F.A.C.E., F.A.C.B.

A hormone is a chemical substance produced in the body by an organ, cells of an organ, or scattered cells, having a specific regulatory effect on the activity of an organ or organs.[15] They are produced at one site in the body and exert their action(s) at distant sites through what is called the *endocrine* system. It is increasingly recognized that many hormones exert actions locally through what is termed the *paracrine* system. Finally, some hormones exert their action on the cells of origin, regulating their own synthesis and secretion via an *autocrine* system. The classic endocrine hormones include insulin, thyroxine, and cortisol. Neurotransmitters and neurohormones are examples of the paracrine system, and certain growth factors that stimulate synthesis and secretion of true hormones from the same cell are examples of an autocrine system.

Table 28-1 lists hormones that are commonly measured in clinical practice plus a few others to illustrate concepts. Biochemical, clinical, and analytical information for specific hormones and cytokines may be found in Chapters 22, 25, and 48 to 54.

CLASSIFICATION

Hormones are classified as (1) polypeptides or proteins, (2) steroids, or (3) derivatives of amino acids.

Polypeptide or Protein Hormones

Adrenocorticotropic hormone (ACTH), insulin, and parathyroid hormone (PTH) are examples of polypeptide or protein hormones. They are generally water soluble and circulate freely in plasma as the whole molecule or as active or inactive fragments. The half-life of these hormones in plasma is quite short (10 to 30 minutes or less), and wide fluctuations in their concentration may be seen in several physiological and pathological circumstances. These hormones initiate their response by binding to cell membrane receptors (on or in the membrane) and exciting a "second messenger" system, which continues the specific actions of these hormones.

Steroid Hormones

Steroid hormones (e.g., cortisol and estrogen) are hydrophobic and insoluble in water. These hormones circulate in plasma, reversibly bound to transport proteins (e.g., cortisol-binding globulin and sex-hormone binding globulin) with only a small fraction free or unbound available to exert physiological action.[5,8,17] The half-life of steroid hormones is 30 to 90 minutes. Free steroid hormones, being hydrophobic, enter the cell by passive diffusion and bind with intracellular receptors either in the cytoplasm or the nucleus.[3]

Amino Acid–Related Hormones

Thyroxine and catecholamine are examples of hormones that are derived from amino acids; they are water soluble and circulate in plasma either bound to proteins (thyroxine) or free (catecholamines). Thyroxine binds avidly to three binding proteins and has a half-life of about 7 to 10 days, and the free and unbound catecholamines such as epinephrine have a very short half-life of a minute or less. As do the water-soluble peptide and protein hormones, these hormones interact with membrane-associated receptors and use a second messenger system.

RELEASE AND ACTION OF HORMONES

The physiological functions of hormones have been broadly categorized into those that (1) affect growth and development, (2) exert homeostatic control of metabolic pathways, and (3) regulate the production, use, and storage of energy. The descriptions below illustrate examples of these functions and mechanisms of control of hormone secretion.

*The author gratefully acknowledges the original contribution by Dr. Ronald J. Whitley on which portions of this chapter are based.

TABLE 28-1 Selected Hormones and Frequently Measured Hormone Precursors and Cytokines

Endocrine Organ and Hormone	Chemical Nature of Hormone	Major Sites of Action	Principal Actions
Hypothalamus			
Thyrotropin-releasing hormone (TRH)	Peptide (3 aa, Glu-His-Pro)[a]	Anterior pituitary	Release of TSH and prolactin (PRL)
Gonadotropin-releasing hormone (Gn-RH) or luteinizing hormone-releasing hormone (LH-RH)	Peptide (10 aa)	Anterior pituitary	Release of LH and FSH
Corticotropin-releasing hormone (CRH)	Peptide (41 aa)	Anterior pituitary	Release of ACTH and β-lipotropic hormone (LPH)
Growth hormone-releasing hormone (GH-RH)	Peptides (40, 44 aa)	Anterior pituitary	Release of growth hormone (GH)
Somatostatin[b] (SS) or growth hormone-inhibiting hormone (GH-IH)	Peptides (14 and 28 aa)	Anterior pituitary	Suppression of secretion of many hormones (e.g., GH, TSH, gastrin, vasoactive intestinal polypeptide [VIP], gastric inhibitory polypeptide [GIP], secretin, motilin, glucagon, and insulin)
Prolactin-releasing peptide	Peptide (20 aa)	Anterior pituitary	Release of PRL
Prolactin releasing/inhibiting factor	Dopamine	Anterior pituitary	Suppression of synthesis and secretion of PRL
Anterior Pituitary Lobe			
Thyrotropin or thyroid-stimulating hormone (TSH)	Glycoprotein heterodimer[c] (α, 92 aa; β, 112 aa)	Thyroid gland	Stimulation of thyroid hormone formation and secretion
Follicle-stimulating hormone (FSH)	Glycoprotein, heterodimer[c] (α, 92 aa; β, 117 aa)	Ovary	Growth of follicles with LH, secretion of estrogens, and ovulation
		Testis	Development of seminiferous tubules; spermatogenesis
Luteinizing hormone (LH)	Glycoprotein, heterodimer[c] (α, 92 aa; β, 121 aa)	Ovary	Ovulation; formation of corpora lutea; secretion of progesterone
		Testis	Stimulation of interstitial tissue; secretion of androgens
PRL	Peptide (199 aa)	Mammary gland	Proliferation of mammary gland; initiation of milk secretion; antagonist of insulin action
Growth hormone (GH) or somatotropin	Peptide (191 aa)	Liver	Production of IGF-I (promoting growth)
		Liver and peripheral tissues	Antiinsulin and anabolic effects
Corticotropin or adrenocorticotropin (ACTH)	Peptide (39 aa)	Adrenal cortex	Stimulation of adrenocortical steroid formation and secretion
β-Endorphin (β-END)[bh]	Peptide (31 aa)	Brain	Endogenous opiate; raising of pain threshold and influence on extrapyramidal motor activity

TABLE 28-1 Selected Hormones and Frequently Measured Hormone Precursors and Cytokines—*Continued*

Endocrine Organ and Hormone	Chemical Nature of Hormone	Major Sites of Action	Principal Actions
Anterior Pituitary Lobe—Cont'd			
α-Melanocyte-stimulating hormone (α-MSH)	Peptide (13 aa)	Skin	Dispersion of pigment granules, darkening of skin
Leu-enkephalin (LEK)[b,h] and met-enkephalin (MEK)[b,h]	Peptide (5 aa)	Brain	Same as β-endorphin
Posterior Pituitary Lobe			
Vasopressin or ADH	Peptide (9 aa)	Arterioles Renal tubules	Elevation of blood pressure; water reabsorption
Oxytocin	Peptide (9 aa)	Smooth muscles (uterus, mammary gland)	Contraction; action in parturition and in sperm transport; ejection of milk
Pineal Gland			
Serotonin or 5-hydroxytryptamine (5-HT)	Indoleamine	Cardiovascular, respiratory, and gastrointestinal systems; brain	Neurotransmitter; stimulation or inhibition of various smooth muscles and nerves
Melatonin	Indoleamine	Hypothalamus	Suppression of gonadotropin and GH secretion; induction of sleep
Thyroid Gland			
Thyroxine (T_4) and triiodothyronine (T_3)	Iodoamino acids	General body tissue	Stimulation of oxygen consumption and metabolic rate of tissue
Calcitonin or thyrocalcitonin	Peptide (32 aa)	Skeleton	Uncertain in humans
Parathyroid Gland			
Parathyroid hormone (PTH) or parathyrin	Peptide (84 aa)	Kidney	Increased calcium reabsorption, inhibited phosphate reabsorption; increased production of 1,25-dihydroxycholecalciferol
		Skeleton	Increased bone resorption
Adrenal Cortex			
Aldosterone	Steroid	Kidney	Salt and water balance
Androstenedione[d]	Steroid	Hormone precursor	Converted to estrogens and testosterone
Cortisol	Steroid	Many	Metabolism of carbohydrates, proteins, and fats; antiinflammatory effects; others
Dehydroepiandrosterone (DHEA) and dehydroepi-androstenedione sulfate (DHEAS)	Steroids	Hormone precursors	Converted to estrogens and testosterone
17-Hydroxyprogesterone	Steroid	Hormone precursor	Converted to cortisol

Continued.

TABLE 28-1 Selected Hormones and Frequently Measured Hormone Precursors and Cytokines—*Continued*

Endocrine Organ and Hormone	Chemical Nature of Hormone	Major Sites of Action	Principal Actions
Adrenal Medulla			
Norepinephrine and epinephrine	Aromatic amines	Sympathetic receptors	Stimulation of sympathetic nervous system
Epinephrine		Liver and muscle, adipose tissue	Glycogenolysis Lipolysis
Ovary			
Activin A	Peptides[e] 2 β_A subunits	Pituitary, ovarian follicle	Stimulates release of FSH; enhances FSH action; inhibits androgen production by theca cells
Activin B	Peptides[e] 2 β_B subunits beta	See activin A above	See activin A above
DHEA and DHEAS	Steroids	Hormone precursors	Converted to androstenedione
Estrogens	Phenolic steroids	Female accessory sex organs Bone	Development of secondary sex characteristics Control of skeletal maturation et al
Follistatin	Peptides (288 aa, 315 aa)	Pituitary, ovarian follicles	Inhibits FSH synthesis and secretion by binding activin
Inhibin A	Peptide (α subunit and β_A subunit)	Hypothalamus, ovarian follicle	Inhibits FSH secretion; stimulates theca cell androgen production
Inhibin B	Peptide (α subunit and β_B subunit)	See inhibin A above	See inhibin A above
Progesterone	Steroid	Female accessory reproductive structure	Preparation of the uterus for ovum implantation, maintenance of pregnancy
Relaxin	Peptide[f]	Uterus	Inhibition of myometrial contraction
Testis			
Inhibin B	See above	Anterior pituitary, hypothalamus	Control of LH and FSH secretion
Testosterone	Steroid	Male accessory sex organs	Development of secondary sex characteristics, maturation, and normal function
Placenta			
Estrogens	See above	See above	See above
Progesterone	See above	See above	See above
Relaxin	See above	See above	See above
Chorionic gonadotropin (CG) or choriogonadotropin	Glycoprotein, heterodimer[c] (α, 92 aa; β, 145 aa)	Same as LH	Same as LH; prolongation of corpus luteal function
Placental growth hormone (GH-V)	Peptides (22 & 26 kD)	Same as GH	Same as GH
Chorionic somatomammotropin (CS) or placental lactogen (PL)	Peptide (191 aa)	Same as PRL	Same as PRL

TABLE 28-1 Selected Hormones and Frequently Measured Hormone Precursors and Cytokines—*Continued*

Endocrine Organ and Hormone	Chemical Nature of Hormone	Major Sites of Action	Principal Actions
Pancreas			
Amylin	Peptide (37 aa)	Pancreas	Inhibits glucagon and insulin secretion
Glucagon	Peptide (29 aa)	Liver	Glycogenolysis
Insulin	Peptide[g]	Liver, fat, muscle	Regulation of carbohydrate metabolism; lipogenesis
Pancreatic polypeptide (PP)	Peptide (36 aa)	Gastrointestinal tract	Increased gut motility and gastric emptying; inhibition of gallbladder contraction
Somatostatin (SS)	Peptide (14 aa)	Pancreas	Inhibition of secretion of insulin, glucagon
Gastrointestinal Tract			
Gastrin[h]	Peptide (17 aa)	Stomach	Secretion of gastric acid, gastric mucosal growth
Ghrelin[h] (GHRP)	Peptide (28 aa)	Anterior pituitary	Secretion of GH
Secretin	Peptide (27 aa)	Pancreas	Secretion of pancreatic bicarbonate and digestive enzymes
Cholecystokinin-pancreozymin (CCK-PZ)[h]	Peptide (33 aa)	Gallbladder and pancreas	Stimulation of gallbladder contraction and secretion of pancreatic enzymes
Motilin	Peptide (22 aa)	Gastrointestinal tract	Stimulation of gastrointestinal motility
VIP[h]	Peptide (28 aa)	Gastrointestinal tract	Neurotransmitter; relaxation of smooth muscles of gut and of circulation; increased release of hormones and secretion of water and electrolytes from pancreas and gut
GIP	Peptide (42 aa)	Gastrointestinal tract	Inhibition of gastric secretion and motility; increase of insulin secretion
Bombesin[h]	Peptide (14 aa)	Gastrointestinal tract	Stimulation of release of various hormones and pancreatic enzymes, smooth muscle contractions and hypothermia, changes in cardiovascular and renal function
Neurotensin[h]	Peptide (13 aa)	Gastrointestinal tract and hypothalamus	Uncertain
Substance P (SP)[h]	Peptide (11 aa)	Gastrointestinal tract and brain	Sensory neurotransmitter, analgesic; increase in contraction of gastrointestinal smooth muscle; potent vasoactive hormone; promotion of salivation, increased release of histamine

Continued.

TABLE 28-1 Selected Hormones and Frequently Measured Hormone Precursors and Cytokines—*Continued*

Endocrine Organ and Hormone	Chemical Nature of Hormone	Major Sites of Action	Principal Actions
Kidney			
1,25-$(OH)_2$ cholecalciferol	Sterol	Intestine Bone	Facilitation of calcium and phosphorus absorption; increase in bone resorption in conjunction with PTH
		Kidney	Increase in reabsorption of filtered calcium
Erythropoietin	Peptide (165 aa)	Bone marrow	Stimulation of red cell formation
Renin-angiotensin-aldosterone system	Peptides (renin, 297 aa; Ang I, 10 aa; Ang II, 8 aa, produced from Ang I by angiotensin converting enzyme)	Renin (from kidney) catalyzes hydrolysis of angiotensinogen (from liver, 485 aa) to ang I in the intravascular space	Ang II increases blood pressure and stimulates secretion of aldosterone (see adrenal)
Liver			
IGF-I, formerly called somatomedin	Peptide (70 aa)	Most cells	Stimulation of cellular and linear growth
IGF-II	Peptide (67 aa)	Most cells	Insulin-like activity
Thymus			
Thymosin and thymopoietin	Peptides (28 and 49 aa)	Lymphocytes	Maturation of T lymphocytes
Heart			
Atrial natriuretic peptide (ANP, Atriopeptin)	Peptide with an intrachain disulfide bond (28 aa)	Vascular, renal, and adrenal tissues	Regulation of blood volume and blood pressure
B-type natriuretic peptide (BNP)	Peptide with an intrachain disulfide bond (32 aa)	Vascular, renal, and adrenal tissues	Regulation of blood volume and blood pressure
Adipose Tissue			
Adiponectin	Peptide oligomers of 30 kD subunits	Muscle Liver	Increases fatty acid oxidation Suppresses glucose formation
Leptin	Peptide (167 aa)	Hypothalamus	Inhibition of appetite, stimulation of metabolism
Resistin	Peptide (94 aa)	Liver	Insulin resistance
Multiple Cell Types			
Estrogens	See above	See above	See above
Galanin	Peptide (30 aa)	Brain, pancreas, gastrointestinal (GI) tract	Regulates food intake, memory, and cognition; inhibits endocrine and exocrine secretions of pancreas; delays gastric emptying; prolongs colonic transport times

TABLE 28-1 Selected Hormones and Frequently Measured Hormone Precursors and Cytokines—*Continued*

Endocrine Organ and Hormone	Chemical Nature of Hormone	Major Sites of Action	Principal Actions
Multiple Cell Types—Cont'd			
Parathyroid hormone-related peptide (PTH-RP)	Peptides (139, 141, 173 aa)	Kidney, bone	Physiological function conjectural; PTH-like actions; tumor marker
Growth factors (e.g., epidermal growth factor, fibroblast growth factor, transforming growth factor family, platelet-derived growth factor, nerve growth factors)	Peptides	Many	Stimulation of cellular growth
Monocytes/Lymphocytes/Macrophages			
Cytokines (e.g., interleukins 1-18, tumor necrosis factor, interferons)	Peptides	Many	Stimulation or inhibition of cellular growth; other

[a]*aa,* Amino acid residues.
[b]Also produced by gastrointestinal tract and pancreas.
[c]Glycoprotein hormones composed of two dissimilar peptides. The α-chains are similar in structure or identical; the β-chains differ among hormones and confer specificity.
[d]Androstenedione is also produced in the ovary and testis.
[e]Each activin and inhibin is found in multiple forms.
[f]Two chains linked by two disulfide bonds: α, 24 aa; β, 29 aa.
[g]Two chains linked by two disulfide bonds: α, 21 aa; β, 30 aa.
[h]Also produced in the brain.

Growth and Development

Normal growth and development of the whole human organism is dependent on the complex integrative function of many hormones including gonadal steroids (estrogen and androgen), growth hormone, cortisol, and thyroxine. Several pituitary hormones are responsible specifically for the growth and development of endocrine glands themselves and thus are responsible for control of synthesis and secretion of other hormones. Those other hormones can provide negative feedback on secretion of the pituitary hormones. Other regulators of the secretion of the pituitary hormones include circadian rhythms and a hypothalamic pulse generator that controls the pulsatile secretion of gonadotropins. Examples of hormones of the anterior pituitary gland include the following:

- Gonadotropins (luteinizing hormone [LH] and follicle-stimulating hormone [FSH]) that regulate the development, growth, and function of the ovary and testis (see Chapter 53). The ovarian and testicular hormones in turn regulate pubertal growth; the development and maintenance of secondary sex characteristics; the growth, development, and maintenance of the skeleton and muscles; and distribution of body fat.
- ACTH that regulates the growth of the adrenal glands and the synthesis and secretion of adrenal gland hormones (see Chapters 50 and 51).
- Thyroid-stimulating hormone (TSH) that regulates the growth of the thyroid gland and the iodination of amino acids to produce the thyroid hormones triiodothyronine and thyroxine (see Chapter 52).[1]

Homeostatic Control of Metabolic Pathways

The metabolic pathways under hormonal control are diverse and complex. The following important examples illustrate the feedback control of hormone secretion, which is critical for homeostasis:

- Regulation of blood glucose: In response to a glucose load, there is prompt release of insulin from the pancreas, which regulates the dispersal of glucose into cells (fat, muscle, liver, and brain) for the metabolism necessary to produce energy from glucose (see Chapter 25). As circulating glucose concentrations thus return to preload levels, insulin secretion slows. A number of counter-regulatory hormones come into play to further regulate this process to ensure that blood glucose levels do not become too low. These include glucagon, cortisol, epinephrine, and growth hormone.
- Regulation of serum calcium (see Chapter 49): The calcium-sensing receptor (CaSR) on the parathyroid gland recognizes the ambient concentration of ionized calcium, which in turn regulates synthesis and secretion of PTH. When ionized calcium concentrations fall

(so imperceptibly that most analytical methods could not detect the change), PTH synthesis and secretion are stimulated. This additional PTH will attempt to restore serum ionized calcium by enhancing renal tubular reabsorption of calcium and also calcium efflux from the skeleton. PTH also catalyzes the synthesis of the renal hormone calcitriol (1,25-dihydroxycholecalciferol), which acts on the gut to increase intestinal absorption of calcium. These very rapid responses of PTH and calcitriol quickly restore ionized calcium concentration to a level where the CaSR is no longer activated and both PTH and calcitriol synthesis and secretion return to basal levels.

- Water and electrolyte metabolism is regulated by aldosterone from the adrenal gland, renin from the kidney, and vasopressin (antidiuretic hormone [ADH]) from the posterior pituitary gland (see Chapters 45 and 46).

Regulation of the Production, Use, and Storage of Energy

Under normal conditions, regulation of energy production, use, and storage is under tight hormonal control. Under conditions of changing demands that require more energy (e.g., exercise, starvation, infection or trauma, and emotional stress), many hormones are up regulated to control not only circulating levels of nutrients but also the metabolism of these nutrients into necessary energy. This very complex activity, which may involve hormones from different organs as already alluded to in the preceding section, is also under neurological control, with a number of neuroendocrine hormones participating actively in this integrative metabolic process, which affects most organs in the body and modulates, for example, heart rate, sweating, fertility, and reproduction.

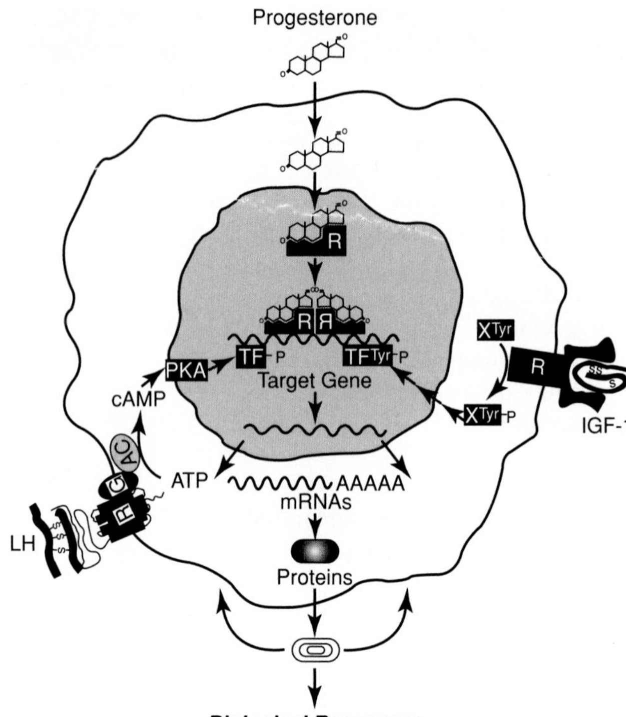

Figure 28-1 Hormonal signaling by cell-surface and intracellular receptors. The receptors for the water-soluble polypeptide hormones, LH, and insulin-like growth factor (IGF)-I, are integral membrane proteins located at the cell surface. They bind the hormone using extracellular sequences and transduce a signal by the generation of second messengers, cAMP for the LH receptor, and tyrosine-phosphorylated substrates for the IGF-I receptor. Although effects on gene expression are indicated, direct effects on cellular proteins (e.g., ion channels), are also observed. In contrast, the receptor for the lipophilic steroid hormone progesterone resides in the cell nucleus. It binds the hormone, and becomes activated and capable of directly modulating target gene transcription. *Tf,* Transcription factor; *R,* receptor molecule. *(From Conn PM, Melmed S. Textbook of endocrinology. Towanta NJ: Humana Press; 1997.)*

ROLE OF HORMONE RECEPTORS

The "unique" or specific action of a hormone on its target tissue is a function of the interaction between the hormone and its receptor. As discussed above, there are several types of hormone-receptor interaction.[3,5,8,17] The hormone-receptor complex provides the very high specificity of the action of the hormone, allowing the target tissue to accumulate the hormone from among all the molecules to which it is exposed. This is essential since hormones generally circulate in picomolar or nanomolar concentrations (10^{-9} to 10^{-12} mol/L).

Hormone receptors may be on the cell surface or intracellular within the cytoplasm or nucleus.

Cell-Surface Receptors

Peptide hormones bind to cell-surface receptors and the conformational change resulting from this binding activates an effector system, which is in turn responsible for the downstream actions of the hormone (Figure 28-1).[11,12] For most peptide hormones, the intracellular effector that is activated by the hormone-receptor interaction is a specific G-protein (guanyl-nucleotide-binding protein)[4,10,13,18] and the receptors are called G-protein–coupled receptors (GPCR, Figure 28-2). GCPRs are heptahelical molecules with seven membrane-spanning domains. The amino terminus is extracellular and the carboxy terminus is intracellular. The major structural classes of GPCRs have been identified, each containing receptors for specific subsets of hormones (Figure 28-3). Group I is the largest group containing receptors for many peptide hormones and catecholamines. Group II contains receptors for the family of gastrointestinal hormones (secretin, glucagons, and vasoactive intestinal polypeptide). Group III contains the CaSR and the glutamate receptor. Stimulation of a G-protein initiates the intracellular processes of signal transduction that characterize the specific action of the hormone. G-proteins are composed of α, β, and γ subunits and are classified according to the α subunit, of

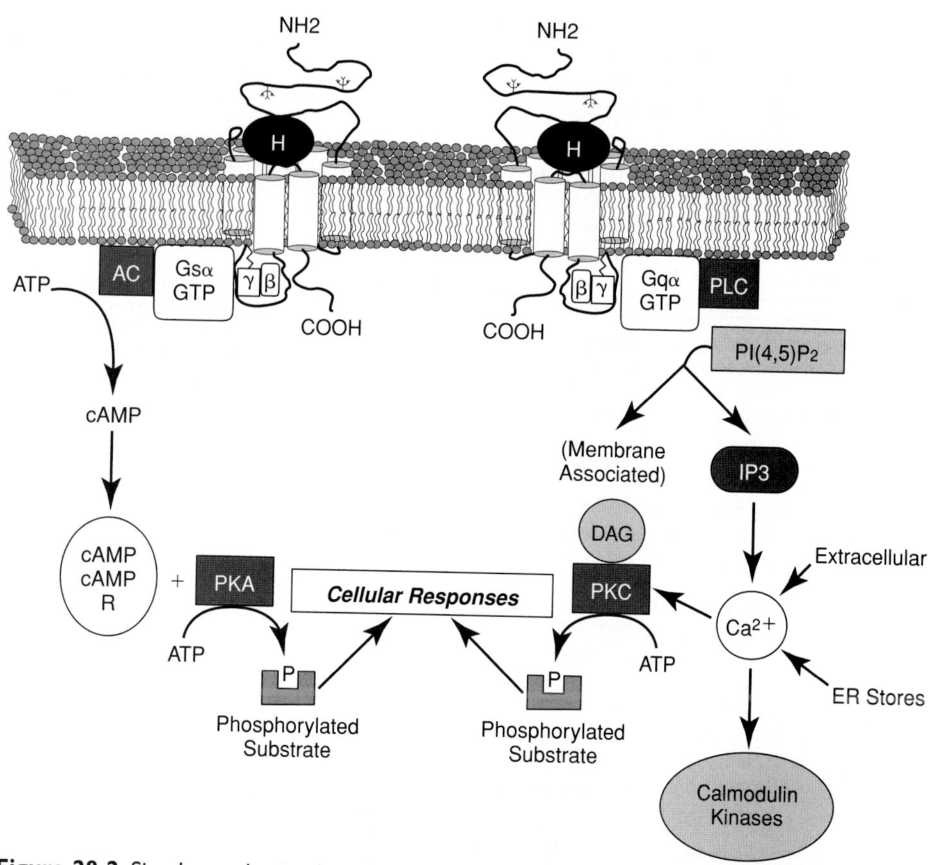

Figure 28-2 Signal transduction by cell-surface receptors that are coupled to G-proteins. Two seven-transmembrane domains, coupled to different G-proteins (G_S, and G_q) are shown. Activation of G_S leads to stimulation of the effector enzyme adenylate cyclase and the production of a cAMP second messenger, causing the activation of protein kinase A (PKA) and the initiation of potential phosphorylation cascades. Activation of G_q leads to stimulation of the effector enzyme phospholipase C-β and the production of IP3 and diacylglycerol (DAG) second messengers, one effect of which is to activate protein kinase C (PKC) and initiate a potential phosphorylation cascade. *(From Conn PM, Melmed S, eds. Textbook of endocrinology. Towanta NJ: Humana Press; 1997.)*

which 20 have been identified to date (Figure 28-3). G-proteins may stimulate adenylate cyclase (G_s type of G-proteins) or inhibit adenylate cyclase (G_i type). The many classes of GPRCs and G-proteins briefly described in this section provide some beginning insight into the mechanisms responsible for the specificity of hormone action. Some non-peptide hormones also use cell-surface receptors.

Intracellular Receptors

Lipid-soluble hormones are transported in plasma bound to carrier proteins with only a small fraction of the hormone being in the free or unbound state. The free hormone enters the cell via passive diffusion and binds to intracellular receptors in the cytoplasm or, more often, the nucleus (Figure 28-1). These receptors are characterized by a hormone-binding domain, a deoxyribonucleic acid (DNA)–binding domain, and an amino-terminal variable domain. Just as the interaction of protein or polypeptide hormones with cell-surface receptors changes the conformation of the receptor protein, the binding of a lipid-soluble hormone with its specific hormone-binding domain on the intracellular receptor changes the molecular conformation of the intracellular receptor. This conformational change, or activation of the receptor, enables the hormone-receptor complex to bind to specific regulatory DNA sequences of a target gene, permitting control of specific gene expression (Figure 28-2).[7]

POSTRECEPTOR ACTIONS OF HORMONES

Cellsurface and intracellular receptors have different post-receptor actions.

Cell-Surface Receptors

Once GPCRs are occupied by a hormone, the G-protein subunits begin a cascade of activation of specific enzymes that generate molecules that serve as second messengers to effect the hormone response. The best known of these are adenylyl cyclase, which generates cyclic adenosine monophosphate (cAMP), and phospholipase C, which generates both

G Protein-Coupled Receptor Superfamily

Family A:	*Receptors Related to Rhodopsin and the β-Adrenergic Receptor*
Group I:	Olfactory, Adenosine, Melanocortin Rs
Group II:	Adrenergic, Muscarinic, Serotonin, DA Rs
Group III:	Neuropeptide Rs and Vertebrate Opsins
Group IV:	Bradykinin R and Invertebrate Opsins
Group V:	Peptide and GP Hormone, Chemokine Rs
Group VI:	Melatonin and Orphan Rs

Family B:	*Receptors Related to the Calcitonin and Parathyroid Hormone Receptors*
Group I:	Calcitonin, Calcitonin-like, CRF Rs
Group II:	PTH and PTHrP Rs
Group III:	Glucagon, Secretin, VIP, GHRH Rs

Family C:	*Receptors Related to the Metabotropic Glutamate Receptors*
Group I:	Metabotropic Glutamate Rs
Group II:	Extracellular Calcium Ion Sensor Rs

Family D:	*Receptors Related to the STE2 Pheromone Receptor*
Group I:	Alpha Factor Pheromone Rs

Family E:	*Receptors Related to the STE3 Pheromone Receptor*
Group I:	A Factor Pheromone Rs

Family F:	*Receptors Related to the cAMP Receptor*
Group I:	Dictyostelium cAR1-4 Rs

A

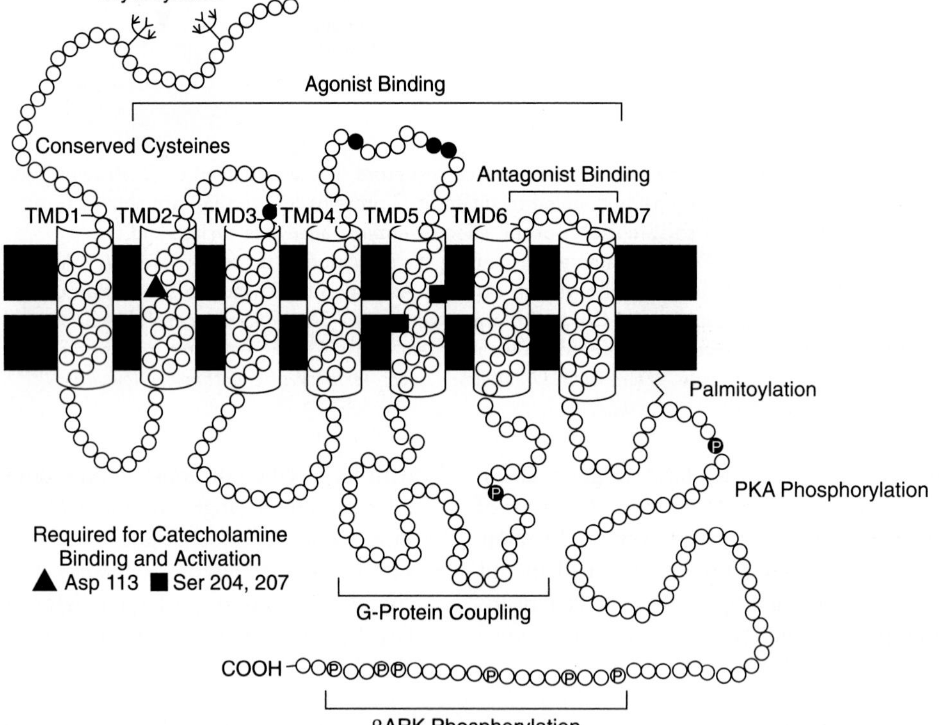

B

Figure 28-3 Classification and basic architecture of cell-surface receptors that couple to G-proteins. Panel A lists the major families and groups of GPCRs. The mammalian receptors are confined to families A, B, and C. Family A is the largest and includes the diverse odorant receptors and prototypic: GPCRs, such as rhodopsin and the β-adrenergic receptor. Panel B shows a schematic structure of one of the most extensively characterized GPCRs, the β-adrenergic receptor. Major structural features are indicated and are expanded on in the text. *(From Conn PM, Melmed S. eds. Textbook of endocrinology. Towanta NJ: Humana Press; 1997.)*

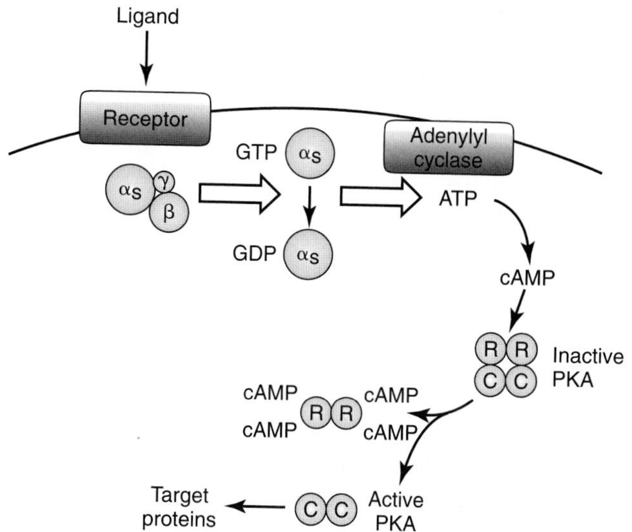

Figure 28-4 Signaling by G_S. *(From Conn PM, Melmed S, eds. Textbook of endocrinology. Towanta NJ: Humana Press; 1997.)*

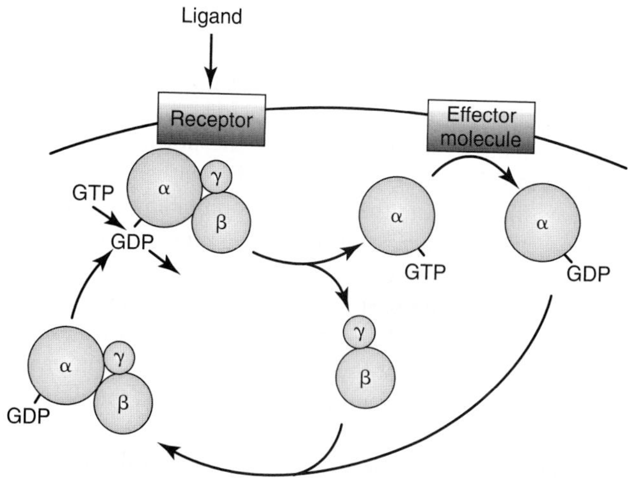

Figure 28-5 The G-protein cycle. *(From Conn PM, Melmed S, eds. Textbook of endocrinology. Towanta NJ: Humana Press; 1997.)*

inositol 1,4,5 trisphosphate (IP_3) and diacylglycerol. The production of second messengers, and the subsequent magnitude of the effect of the hormone, is a function of the amount of hormone bound to the GPRC. The binding of a small number of hormone molecules on the cell surface leads to the production of many molecules of the second messenger, thus amplifying the signal sent by the hormone (which can be thought of as the first messenger).

cAMP-dependent protein kinases are a family of enzymes that, in the presence of cAMP, phosphorylate a number of intracellular enzymes and other proteins to activate or inactivate the function of these enzymes and proteins thereby regulating their function. As a further means of regulating hormone action, these cAMP-dependent kinases consist of two catalytic and two regulatory subunits (Figure 28-4). The regulatory subunits exist as a dimer that can bind two molecules of cAMP, and the binding of cAMP releases the catalytic subunits, which are then activated as phosphorylating enzymes. When cAMP is removed from the regulatory subunit, this dimer is not able to associate two catalytic subunits and amplify the signal of the hormone.

Phospholipase C acts on inositol phospholipids within the cell membrane to produce IP_3, which opens up ion channels to facilitate entry of calcium into the cytoplasm where it acts as a messenger, and diacylglycerol, which modulates protorn kinase C activity.

The insulin receptor represents a somewhat different class of cell-surface receptors that contain intrinsic hormone-activated tyrosine kinase activity and do not otherwise involve a second messenger.[16] The insulin receptor is the prototype of this type of receptor and consists of two α and two β subunits joined by disulfide bridges. The extracellular, hormone-binding domains are the α subunits, and the β subunits are intracellular. They contain an ATP binding site and a catalytic kinase domain through which tyrosine kinase is activated immediately upon insulin binding to the receptor.

Since hormones largely serve a regulatory function, there are of necessity many self-limiting steps in the above processes. Without these self-limiting processes, hormone action would continue unabated. For cAMP, cessation of hormone action involves the inactivation of G-protein stimulation of adenylate cyclase by guanosine triphosphate (GTP)ase (Figure 28-5). In the absence of hormone interaction with the GPCR (basal or unstimulated state) G_s is bound to guanosine diphosphate (GDP). Once the hormone is bound to the receptor, GDP is released from G_s and replaced by GTP and the G_s-GTP complex activates adenylate cyclase. The G_s-GTP complex is inactivated by GTPase, restoring the G_s-GDP state, which cannot stimulate formation of cAMP until further hormone binding to the GPCR takes place. Within a few minutes (or less) of the hormone-GPCR interaction and the initiation of hormone action, the receptor is phosphorylated by protein kinase A and protein kinase C. This phosphorylation of the hormone receptor permits internalization of the complex from the cell surface into the cytoplasm where dephosphorylation occurs, permitting degradation of the hormone and recycling of the GPCR to its original transmembrane location, awaiting coupling with more hormone.

Intracellular Receptors

As noted, lipid-soluble hormones bind to the hormone-binding domain of cytosolic or nuclear receptors.[11,12] This results in a conformational change that enables the hormone-receptor complex to bind to specific regulatory DNA sequences in the 5′ end of the target gene.[7] The binding specificity of the (hormone-bound) receptor for specific regions of the DNA of the target gene is determined by zinc finger structures in the receptor's DNA-binding domain. It is the binding of the hormone-receptor complex to DNA regulatory elements that either enhances or represses gene transcription. The messenger ribonucleic acid (RNA) that is either enhanced or diminished by the hormone-receptor binding to the target gene regulates the synthesis of specific proteins that mediate the hormone's physiological actions. The system is further regulated by the presence or absence of co-activators or co-repressors of gene expression. In addition, many actions of hormones that bind to intracellular receptors are rapid and do not depend on synthesis of protein, suggesting that these hormone-receptor complexes exert actions by mechanisms different from binding to DNA.

From these descriptions, one can begin to deduce both the complexity and specificity of hormone action both in terms of an "on and/or off" concept and in terms of an "effect-size" concept.

CLINICAL DISORDERS OF HORMONES

Although several chapters of this textbook detail a variety of endocrine disorders, a brief introduction is appropriate here. In general, endocrine diseases result from either a deficiency or an excess of a single hormone or several hormones, or from resistance to the action of hormones. Hormone deficiency can be congenital or acquired and hormone excess can be from endogenous overproduction (from within the body) or exogenous overmedication. Hormone resistance can occur at several levels, but can most simply be characterized as receptor mediated, postreceptor mediated, or at the level of the target tissue. The clinical manifestations will depend on the hormone system affected and the type of abnormality.

Diabetes mellitus (DM) is an example of an endocrine disorder; it is the most common endocrine disorder in the United States (see Chapter 25). It is classified as either type 1 or type 2. DM type 1 results from a failure of the pancreas to secrete insulin even though the pancreas is otherwise normal. Type 2 is the most common form of DM and results from end-organ resistance to the action of insulin that, in this case, is secreted from the pancreas in abundant amounts and circulates at high concentrations. Secondary DM occurs when a nonendocrine disease, such as pancreatitis, destroys the pancreas including the insulin secreting cells. The biochemical hallmark of DM is hyperglycemia.

In contrast to diabetes, there are uncommon, insulin-producing tumors of the pancreas (insulinomas) in which the production of insulin is not regulated by the blood glucose concentration and the biochemical hallmark of the tumors is hypoglycemia. Thus hyperglycemia can be present when there is either insulin deficiency or insulin excess, and insulin excess can accompany both hyperglycemia and hypoglycemia. This simple illustration underscores the homeostatic and/or regulating nature of the endocrine system.

MEASUREMENTS OF HORMONES AND RELATED ANALYTES

Hormones are measured by a variety of analytical techniques including bioassay, receptor assay, immunoassay, and instrumental techniques, such as mass spectrometry interfaced with either liquid or gas chromatography. A general overview of these techniques is given here. Analytical details for individual hormones using such techniques are found in the discussion of the individual hormones in their respective chapters.

BIOASSAY TECHNIQUES

Bioassays are based on observations of physiological responses specific for the hormone being measured. In vivo bioassays usually involve the injection of test materials (such as blood or urine from a patient) into suitably prepared animals; target gland responses, such as growth or steroidogenesis, are then measured. In vitro bioassays involve the incubation of tissue, membranes, dispersed cells, or permanent cell lines in a defined culture medium, with subsequent measurement of an appropriate hormone response. Most in vitro bioassays measure responses proximal or distal to a second messenger, such as stimulation of cAMP formation. Bioassays tend to be imprecise and are rarely necessary in clinical medicine.

RECEPTOR-BASED ASSAYS

Receptor assays depend on the in vitro interaction of a hormone with its biological receptor. In this type of assay, unlabeled hormone displaces trace amounts of radioactively labeled hormone from receptor sites. A second approach is to measure a response, such as production of cAMP, when a test sample is added to a preparation that includes the receptor and necessary cofactors. In general, receptor assays are simpler to perform and have greater sensitivity than bioassays. Receptor assays also have an advantage over immunoassays in that they reflect the biological function of a hormone, namely the capacity to combine with specific receptor sites. By contrast, immunoassays may measure active hormone and inactive prohormone, hormone polymer, and metabolites when all share a common antigenic determinant or set of determinants. In general, receptor assays are not as sensitive as immunoassays, and enzymes in the biological specimen may degrade the receptor or destroy the labeled tracer. The added complexity and lability of receptor preparations also contribute to the limited application of these assays in the routine clinical laboratory.

IMMUNOASSAY TECHNIQUES

Immunoassays employing antibodies are widely used to quantify hormones (see Chapter 9). Currently, labeled-antibody (immunometric) assays with nonisotopic labels are the method of choice for measuring most hormones, especially peptides and proteins. Immunometric assays use saturating concentrations of two or more antibodies (often monoclonal) that are prepared against different epitopes of the protein molecule. One of the two antibodies is usually attached to a solid phase separation system and extracts the hormone from the serum specimen. The second antibody is linked to a signal molecule, which is then measured. The resultant signal is used to quantify the bound hormone.

Instrumental Techniques

Mass spectrometers (see Chapter 7) coupled with gas and liquid chromatographs (see Chapter 6) are powerful qualitative and quantitative analytical tools that are widely used to measure hormones.[2,6,9,14] Technical advancements in mass spectrometry have resulted in the development of matrix-assisted laser desorption/ionization (MALDI) and electrospray ionization techniques that allow sequencing of peptides and mass determination of picomole quantities of analytes.

Compared with older methods, tandem mass spectrometry offers greater analytical sensitivity, accuracy, and speed, and may allow simultaneous determination of multiple hormones related to a clinical condition.[14]

REFERENCES

1. Brent GA. The molecular basis of thyroid hormone action. N Engl J Med 1994;331:847-53.
2. Chace DH. Mass spectrometry in the clinical laboratory. Chem Rev 2001;101:445-77.
3. Edwards DP. The role of co-activators and co-repressors in the biology and mechanism of action of steroid hormone receptors. J Mammary Gland Biol Neoplasia 2000;5:307-24.
4. Farfel Z, Bourne HR, Iiri T. The expanding spectrum of G protein disease. N Engl J Med 1999;340:1012-20.
5. Funder JW. Mineralocorticoids, glucocorticoids, receptors and response elements. Science 1993;259: 1132-3.
6. Giese RW. Measurement of endogenous estrogens: analytical challenges and recent advances. J Chromatogr A 2003;1000:401-12.
7. Glass CK. Differential recognition of target genes by nuclear receptor monomers, dimers, and heterodimers. Endocr Rev 1994;15:391-407.
8. Klinge CM. Estrogen receptor interaction with estrogen response elements. Nucleic Acids Res 2001;29:2905-19.
9. Lagerstedt SA, O'Kane DJ. Measurement of plasma free metanephrine and normetanephrine by liquid chromatography-tandem mass spectrometry for diagnosis of pheochromocytoma. Clin Chem 2004;50: 603-11.
10. Lefkowitz RJ. G proteins in medicine. N Engl J Med 1995;332:186-7.
11. Mangelsdorf DJ, Thummel C, Beato M, Herrlich P, Schutz G, Umesono K et al. The nuclear receptor superfamily: the second decade. Cell 1995;83:835-9.
12. McKenna NJ, Lanz RB, O'Malley BW. Nuclear receptor coregulators: cellular and molecular biology. Endocr Rev 1999;20:321-44.
13. Neer EJ. Heterotrimeric G proteins: Organizers of transmembrane signals. Cell 1995;80:249-57.
14. Nelson RE, Grebe SK, O'Kane DJ, Singh RJ. Liquid chromatography-tandem mass spectrometry assay for simultaneous measurement of estradiol and estrone in human plasma. Clin Chem 2004;50:373-84.
15. Newman WA. Dorland's Illustrated Medical Dictionary, 30th Ed. Philadelphia: WB Saunders, 2003.
16. Olefsky JM. The insulin receptor: A multifunctional protein. Diabetes 1990;39:1009-16.
17. Pike AC, Brzozowski AM, Hubbard RE. A structural biologist's view of the oestrogen receptor. J Steroid Biochem Mol Biol 2000;74:261-8.
18. Vaughan M. Signaling by heterotrimeric G proteins minireview series. J Biol Chem 1998;273:667-13.

CHAPTER 29

Catecholamines and Serotonin

Thomas G. Rosano, Ph.D., Graeme Eisenhofer, Ph.D., and Ronald J. Whitley, Ph.D.

Catecholamines and serotonin are biogenic amines that serve as transmitters of neuronal or hormonal signals in a wide range of physiological processes. Epinephrine, norepinephrine, and dopamine are naturally occurring catecholamines that play important roles as neurotransmitters in the central nervous system or as peripheral neurotransmitters and hormonal signals in the sympathoadrenal medullary system. Epinephrine is critical, along with norepinephrine and dopamine, in maintaining the body's homeostasis and in responding to acute and chronic stress, through an orchestration of cardiovascular, metabolic, glandular, and visceral organ activities. Serotonin also serves as a neurotransmitter in the central nervous system and a modulator of vascular and gastrointestinal functions in the periphery. Abnormal production of catecholamines or serotonin may occur in a number of neuroendocrine tumors where clinical signs and symptoms reflect the pharmacological properties of the secreted amines. Clinical measurement of the biogenic amines or their metabolites aids in tumor detection and monitoring, and analytical advances have produced sensitive and specific laboratory methods that are available for clinical practice. In this chapter, we provide an overview of important aspects of biochemistry, pathophysiology, and analytical methodology for clinical assessment of catecholamines, serotonin, and their metabolites.

CHEMICAL STRUCTURE

Chemical structures of catecholamines produced naturally in humans are shown in Figure 29-1. *Epinephrine* (adrenaline), *norepinephrine* (noradrenaline), and *dopamine* are phenylethylamines with hydroxylation on positions three and four of the benzene ring and with an ethylamine moiety on position one. Hydroxyl and methyl substitution on the ethylamine side chain distinguishes the individual catecholamines both in structure and function. The catecholamines demonstrate varying degrees of alkaline instability in biological fluids and their dihydroxybenzene or catechol structure is sensitive to oxidative formation of quinones in the presence of air and light. A number of pharmaceutical and designer drugs with the basic phenylethylamine structure, but lacking dihydroxylation, also have effects on the sympathetic nervous system and are called sympathomimetic agents.

Serotonin with its indoleamine structure, as also shown in Figure 29-1, is distinct from the catecholamines but is also an important naturally occurring biogenic amine. Serotonin is produced widely in animal and plant kingdoms and is structurally related to melatonin, the principal indoleamine produced by the pineal gland. A number of natural or synthetic congeners of serotonin have biological effects ranging from cerebral vasoconstrictors (e.g., sumatriptan) to hallucinogens (e.g., *N,N*-dimethyltryptamine).

Although structurally distinct, the catecholamines and serotonin have related biometabolism, as described in the next section, and each serves as an important monoamine neurotransmitter or neurohormone in health and disease.

BIOSYNTHESIS, RELEASE, AND METABOLISM

The catecholamines and serotonin share similar pathways of biosynthesis and metabolism, including in some steps, the same enzymes. Catecholamines and serotonin are sequestered and stored in vesicular granules from where they are released into the extracellular environment by calcium-dependent exocytosis. Termination of the physiological effects of both the catecholamines and serotonin is dependent on active uptake processes, facilitated by specific

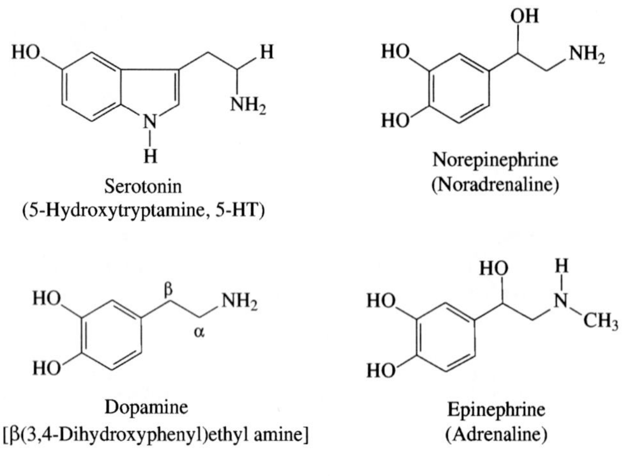

HO H NH₂ N H

Serotonin
(5-Hydroxytryptamine, 5-HT)

OH HO NH₂ HO

Norepinephrine
(Noradrenaline)

HO β NH₂ α HO

Dopamine
[β(3,4-Dihydroxyphenyl)ethyl amine]

HO H HO N CH₃ HO

Epinephrine
(Adrenaline)

Figure 29-1 Chemical structure of the catecholamines and serotonin.

plasma membrane transport proteins. Irreversible inactivation occurs after cellular uptake by metabolism, mainly by deamination and *O*-methylation for catecholamines, and by deamination for serotonin.

BIOSYNTHESIS

Catecholamines are synthesized from the amino acid tyrosine, and serotonin from tryptophan as shown in Figure 29-2. The rate-limiting step in catecholamine biosynthesis involves conversion of tyrosine to 3,4-dihydroxyphenylalanine (L-dopa) by the enzyme, tyrosine hydroxylase.[186] A related enzyme, tryptophan hydroxylase, catalyzes conversion of tryptophan to 5-hydroxytryptophan in the first step of serotonin synthesis.

Tissue sources of catecholamines are principally dependent on the presence of tyrosine hydroxylase, which is largely confined to dopaminergic and noradrenergic neurons of the central nervous system, and to sympathetic nerves and chromaffin cells of the adrenal medulla and paraganglia in the periphery. Similarly, sources of serotonin are largely dependent on the presence of tryptophan hydroxylase in central nervous system serotonergic neurons, the pineal gland, and some peripheral endocrine tissue, particularly enterochromaffin cells of the digestive tract. Platelets also contain large amounts of serotonin, but this is derived from serotonin synthesized in enterochromaffin cells of the gastrointestinal tract.[235]

Both tyrosine and tryptophan hydroxylases belong to a small family of monooxygenases, that also includes phenylalanine hydroxylase; all three enzymes require tetrahydrobiopterin as a substrate to drive the hydroxylation reaction.[74] Deficiencies in the enzymes responsible for formation and recycling of tetrahydrobiopterin result in variant forms of phenylketonuria and hyperphenylalaninemia characterized by low levels of monoamine neurotransmitters and severe neurological abnormalities.[132]

Conversion of L-dopa to dopamine and of 5-hydroxytryptophan to serotonin are both catalyzed by

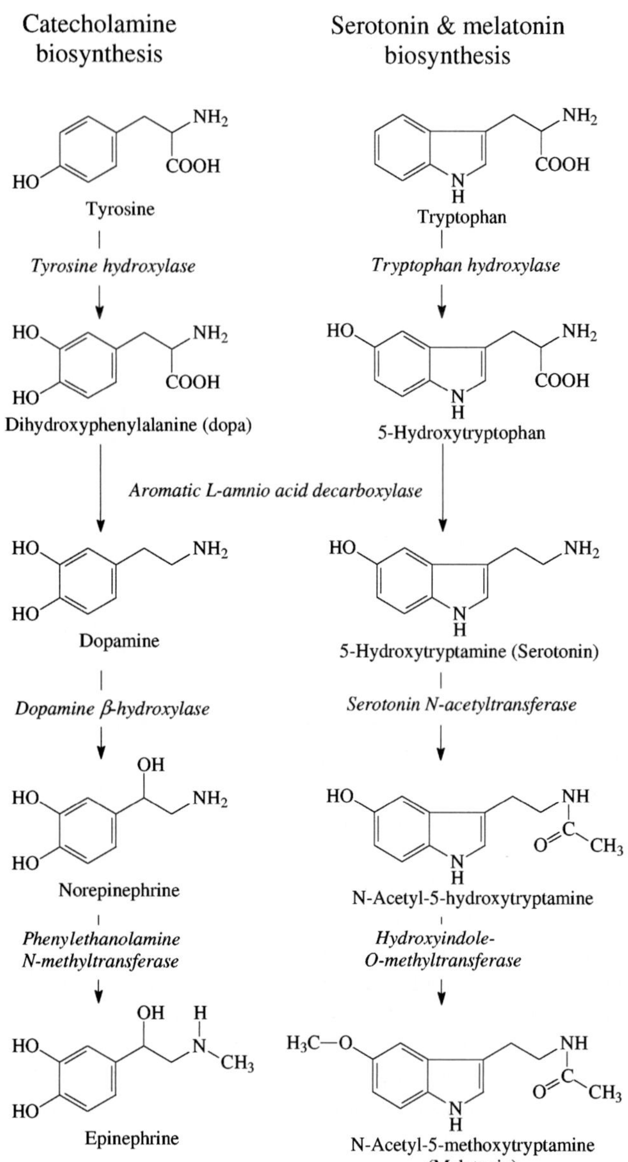

Figure 29-2 Biosynthesis of catecholamines and serotonin, and metabolism of serotonin to melatonin.

aromatic-L-amino acid decarboxylase (Figure 29-2), an enzyme with a wide tissue distribution and broad substrate specificity for aromatic amino acids. The enzyme requires pyridoxal-5-phosphate as a cofactor. The dopamine and serotonin formed in the cytoplasm by aromatic-L-amino acid decarboxylase are then transported into vesicular storage granules where the amines are available for exocytotic release as the principal neurotransmitters of central nervous system dopaminergic and serotonergic neurons.

The dopamine formed in noradrenergic neurons and chromaffin cells is further converted to norepinephrine by dopamine β-hydroxylase, a copper-containing enzyme that requires molecular oxygen and ascorbic acid for activity. The enzyme has a unique presence in vesicular storage granules, either bound to the vesicular membrane or present in the soluble matrix core. The noradrenergic neurochemical phenotype of central noradrenergic neurons and peripheral sympathetic nerves depends on both translocation of dopamine into storage granules and the presence of dopamine β-hydroxylase.

The additional presence of phenylethanolamine *N*-methyltransferase in adrenal medullary chromaffin cells leads to further conversion of norepinephrine to epinephrine (Figure 29-2). Since phenylethanolamine *N*-methyltransferase is a cytosolic enzyme, this step depends on leakage of norepinephrine from vesicular storage granules into the cell cytoplasm and the transfer of a methyl group from *S*-adenosylmethionine to norepinephrine. Epinephrine is then translocated into chromaffin granules where the amine is stored, awaiting release.

Melatonin is synthesized from serotonin in the pineal gland by two highly specific enzymes, the first step catalyzed by serotonin-*N*-acetyltransferase and the second by hydroxyindole-*O*-methyltransferase. Synthesis of melatonin in the pineal gland is regulated by the 24-hour light-dark cycle, resulting in pronounced diurnal fluctuations in production, with higher melatonin levels at night associated with induction of sleep.

Conversion of tyrosine to L-dopa by tyrosine hydroxylase and of tryptophan to 5-hydroxytryptophan by tryptophan hydroxylase represents pivotal points for regulating synthesis and maintaining stores of catecholamines and serotonin in response to changes in monoamine turnover associated with variations in exocytotic release. Rapid activation of tyrosine hydroxylase is achieved by phosphorylation of serine residues at the regulatory domain, under the control of multiple Ca^{2+} and cyclic adenosine monophosphate (cAMP)–dependent pathways influenced by changes in nerve activity and actions of peptides and other coactivators.[185,265] Feedback inhibition by catecholamines provides a further mechanism for short-term regulation of enzyme activity. Long-term regulation involves induction of synthesis of the enzyme at the transcriptional level. Similar though less well understood mechanisms are involved in the regulation of tryptophan hydroxylase.[165] Synthesis of serotonin is also controlled by the availability of tryptophan precursor derived exclusively from the diet.[260] Tyrosine, in contrast, has dietary sources and is also formed by hydroxylation of phenylalanine.

Administration of catecholamine metabolic precursors and drugs that block catecholamine biosynthetic pathways has several therapeutic uses. Alpha-methyl-L-tyrosine or metyrosine (Demser) is an analog of tyrosine that inhibits tyrosine hydroxylase, thereby decreasing catecholamine stores. The drug is used to control high blood pressure in patients with pheochromocytoma, particularly those with extensive metastatic disease, or preoperatively in patients with large or highly active tumors. Alpha-methyl-L-dopa (Aldomet) is an analog of L-dopa and a prodrug that is converted to alpha-methyl-dopamine and alpha-methyl-norepinephrine. The antihypertensive actions of the agent appear to result from central nervous system–mediated inhibition of sympathetic outflow. L-dopa is used to treat Parkinson's disease and is usually co-administered with an inhibitor of peripheral L-aromatic amino acid decarboxylase, such as carbidopa or benserazide.

Storage and Release

Storage of catecholamines and serotonin in vesicular granules is facilitated by two vesicular monoamine transporters, both of which are expressed in endocrine cells and one only in neurons.[103] Both transporters have a wide specificity for different monoamine substrates.

The driving force for vesicular monoamine transport is provided by an adenosine triphosphate (ATP)–dependent vesicular membrane proton pump, which maintains an H^+ electrochemical gradient between cytoplasm and granule matrix.[224] Disruption of this gradient in situations of energy depletion and lowered intracellular pH, such as occurs with ischemia, anoxias or cyanide poisoning, result, in a rapid and massive loss of monoamines from storage vesicles into the neuronal cytoplasm.

Contrary to usual depictions, vesicular stores of catecholamines and serotonin do not exist in a static state until exocytotic release. Rather, vesicular stores of monoamines exist in a highly dynamic equilibrium with the surrounding cytoplasm, with passive outward leakage of monoamines into the cytoplasm counterbalanced by inward active transport under the control of vesicular monoamine transporters (Figure 29-3). The magnitude and highly dynamic nature of this process can be appreciated by consideration of the effects of the drug reserpine, which blocks the ability of vesicular monoamine transporters to move monoamines from the cytoplasm into vesicles. Leakage of monoamines from vesicles is then no longer counterbalanced by vesicular translocation and stores of monoamines are rapidly depleted.

Monoamines share the acid environment of the storage granule matrix with ATP, peptides, and proteins, the most well known of which are the chromogranins.[195] The chromogranins are ubiquitous components of secretory vesicles and their widespread presence among endocrine tissue has led to their measurement in plasma as useful albeit relatively nonspecific markers of neuroendocrine tumors, including pheochromocytomas and carcinoid tumors.[194]

Catecholamines are stored in several types of vesicular granules that differ in size and type of protein and peptide components. In rat and bovine adrenal medulla there are two populations of chromaffin cells with morphologically distinct vesicles that preferentially store either norepinephrine or epinephrine and that release the two catecholamines differentially in response to different stimuli.[249] In sympathetic nerves there are large and small dense core vesicles, the latter believed to be formed by retrieval of membranes of large dense core vesicles after exocytosis.[50]

The process of exocytosis occurs at specialized locations on nerve endings or sympathetic varicosities dictated by the

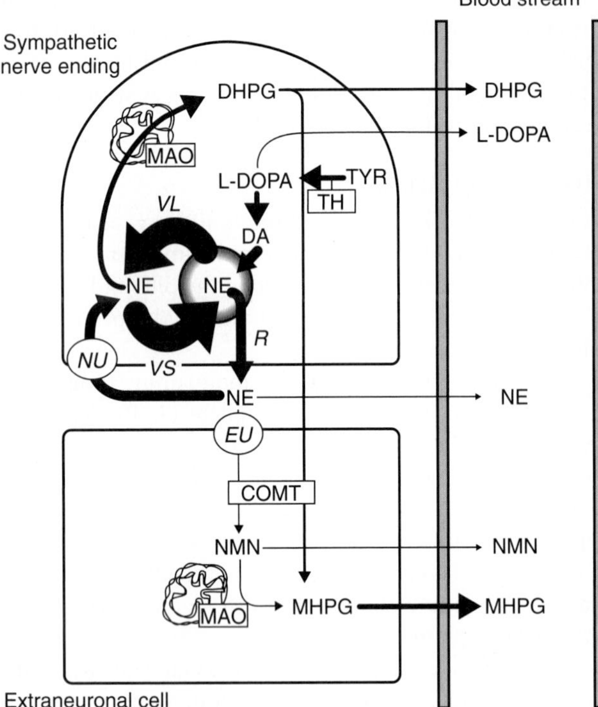

Figure 29-3 Schematic diagram illustrating the dynamics of synthesis, exocytotic release (R), neuronal reuptake (NU), extraneuronal uptake (EU), vesicular leakage (VL), vesicular sequestration (VS), and metabolism of norepinephrine (NE) in sympathetic nerve endings in relation to extraneuronal tissue and the bloodstream. Relative magnitudes of the various processes are reflected by the relative sizes of arrows. *TH,* Tyrosine hydroxylase; *MAO,* monoamine oxidase; *COMT,* catechol-*O*-methyltransferase; *TYR,* tyrosine; *L-dopa,* 3,4-dihydroxyphenylalanine; *DA,* dopamine; *DHPG,* 3,4-dihydroxyphenylglycol; *NMN,* normetanephrine; *MHPG,* 3-methoxy-4-hydroxyphenylglycol.

cell-surface expression of specialized docking proteins that interact with other proteins on the surface of secretory vesicles.[121] The process is stimulated by an influx of Ca^{2+}, which in neurons is primarily controlled by nerve impulse–mediated membrane depolarization, and in adrenal medullary cells by acetylcholine release from innervating splanchnic nerves. The wide range of voltage-, receptor-, G-protein–, and second messenger–operated Ca^{2+} channels provides numerous points for regulation of Ca^{2+}-triggered exocytosis. Consequently a variety of peptides, neurotransmitters, and humoral factors provide additional mechanisms for stimulation of exocytosis or may act to modulate nerve impulse–stimulated release of monoamines. Dopamine, norepinephrine, and serotonin also modulate their own release through occupation of autoreceptors. Regulation of monoamine release and synthesis is closely coordinated, thereby ensuring that there is appropriate replenishment of the amines lost because of exocytosis.[187]

Neuronal release of catecholamines and serotonin may also occur by calcium-independent nonexocytotic processes involving increased loss of monoamines from storage vesicles into the cytoplasm and reversal of the normal inward carrier-mediated transport to outward transport of monoamines into the extracellular environment. Examples of this process include the release of catecholamines induced by tyramine and amphetamine. Excessive release of catecholamines that accompanies hypoxic ischemia in part occurs by a similar mechanism.

Uptake and Metabolism

Since the enzymes responsible for metabolism of catecholamines have intracellular locations, the primary mechanism limiting the lifespan of catecholamines in the extracellular space is uptake by active transport, not metabolism by enzymes (Figure 29-3). Uptake is facilitated by transporters that belong to two large families of proteins with mainly neuronal or extraneuronal locations.[54] Neuronal uptake of monoamines involves the dopamine transporter at dopaminergic neurons, the norepinephrine transporter at noradrenergic neurons, and the serotonin transporter at serotonergic neurons. These same transporters are also present at some nonneuronal locations, including adrenal chromaffin cells, endothelial cells of the lungs, specialized cells of the gastrointestinal tract, and on some blood cells, such as platelets. However, most uptake of monoamines at nonneuronal locations is facilitated by a second set of proteins belonging to the organic cation transporter family. These latter transporters are expressed exclusively at extraneuronal locations and act on a broader range of substrates than the plasma membrane monoamine transporters expressed at neuronal locations.

The neuronal monoamine transporters provide the principal mechanism for rapid termination of the signal in neuronal transmission, whereas the transporters at extraneuronal locations are more important for limiting the spread of the signal and for clearance of catecholamines from the bloodstream. For the norepinephrine released by sympathetic nerves, about 90% is removed back into nerves by neuronal uptake, 5% is removed by extraneuronal uptake, and 5% escapes these processes to enter the bloodstream. In contrast, for the epinephrine released directly into the bloodstream from the adrenals, about 90% is removed by extraneuronal monoamine transport processes that are particularly important in the liver. The presence of these highly active transport processes means that monoamines are rapidly cleared from the bloodstream with a circulatory half-life of less than 2 minutes.

In addition to terminating the actions of released monoamines, the plasma membrane monoamine transporters present at neuronal locations function in sequence with vesicular monoamine transporters to recycle catecholamines for rerelease (Figure 29-3). Thus most of the norepinephrine released and recaptured by sympathetic nerves is sequestered back into storage vesicles, thereby substantially reducing the requirements for synthesis of new transmitter.

Plasma membrane monoamine transporters also function as part of metabolizing systems, requiring the additional

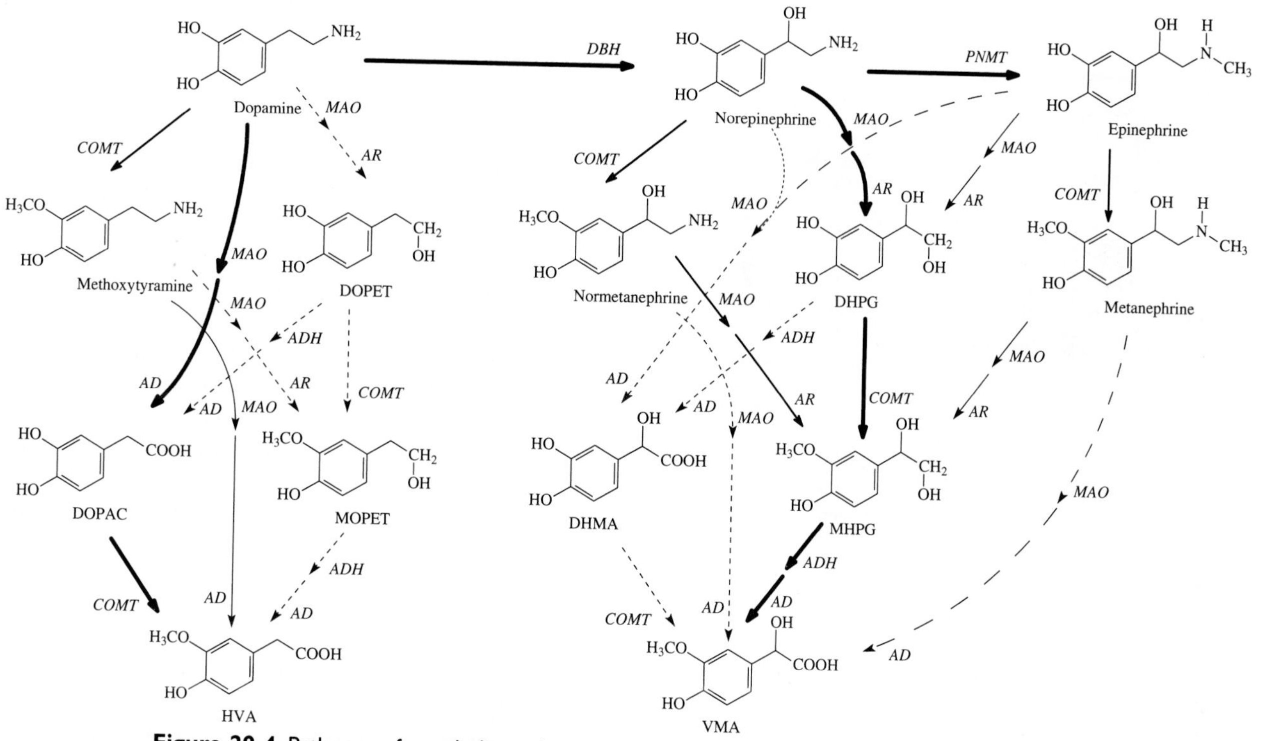

Figure 29-4 Pathways of metabolism of catecholamines. Enzymes responsible for each pathway are shown at the head of arrows. Solid arrows indicate the major pathways whereas dotted arrows indicate pathways of negligible importance. Pathways of sulfate conjugation—which are particularly important for metabolism of dopamine, normetanephrine, metanephrine, 3-methoxytyramine, and 3-methoxy-4-hydroxyphenylglycol—are not shown. *DBH*, Dopamine β-hydroxylase; *PNMT*, phenylethanolamine-*N*-methyltransferase; *MAO*, monoamine oxidase; *COMT*, catechol-*O*-methyltransferase; *AR*, aldose or aldehyde reductase; *AD*, aldehyde dehydrogenase; *ADH*, alcohol dehydrogenase; *DOPET*, 3,4-dihydroxyphenylethanol; *DOPAC*, 3,4-dihydroxyphenylacetic acid; *MOPET*, 3-methoxy-4-hydroxyphenylethanol; *HVA*, homovanillic acid; *DHPG*, 3,4-dihydroxyphenylglycol; *DHMA*, 3,4-dihydroxymandelic acid; *MHPG*, 3-methoxy-4-hydroxyphenylglycol; *VMA*, vanillylmandelic acid.

actions of enzymes for irreversible inactivation of the released amines. For both neuronal and extraneuronal metabolizing systems, inactivation of catecholamines and serotonin occurs in a series arrangement with uptake followed by metabolism.

Metabolism of catecholamines occurs by a multiplicity of pathways catalyzed by an array of enzymes resulting in a wide variety of metabolites (Figure 29-4).[60] Deamination of catecholamines by monoamine oxidase (MAO) yields reactive aldehyde intermediate metabolites that are further metabolized to either deaminated acids by aldehyde dehydrogenase, or to deaminated glycols by aldehyde or aldose reductase. The aldehyde intermediate formed from dopamine is a good substrate for aldehyde dehydrogenase, but not aldehyde or aldose reductase. In contrast, the aldehyde intermediate formed from the β-hydroxylated catecholamines norepinephrine and epinephrine is a good substrate for aldehyde or aldose reductase, but is a poor substrate for aldehyde dehydrogenase. Therefore norepinephrine and epinephrine are both preferentially deaminated to 3,4-dihydroxyphenylglycol (DHPG), the alcohol metabolite. Deamination to the deaminated acid metabolite, 3,4-dihydroxymandelic acid (DHMA), is not a favored pathway.

Catechol-*O*-methyltransferase (COMT) is responsible for the second major pathway of catecholamine metabolism, catalyzing *O*-methylation of dopamine to methoxytyramine, norepinephrine to normetanephrine, and epinephrine to metanephrine. COMT is not present in monoamine-producing neurons, which contain exclusively MAO, but is present along with MAO in most extraneuronal tissue. The membrane-bound isoform of COMT, which has high affinity for catecholamines, is especially abundant in adrenal chromaffin cells. As a result of the preceding and other differences in the expression of metabolizing enzymes, catecholamines produced at neuronal and adrenal medullary locations follow different neuronal and extraneuronal pathways of metabolism (Figure 29-5).

Neuronal pathways are quantitatively far more important than extraneuronal pathways for metabolism of the catecholamines synthesized at neuronal locations, such as the norepinephrine produced in sympathetic nerves. The

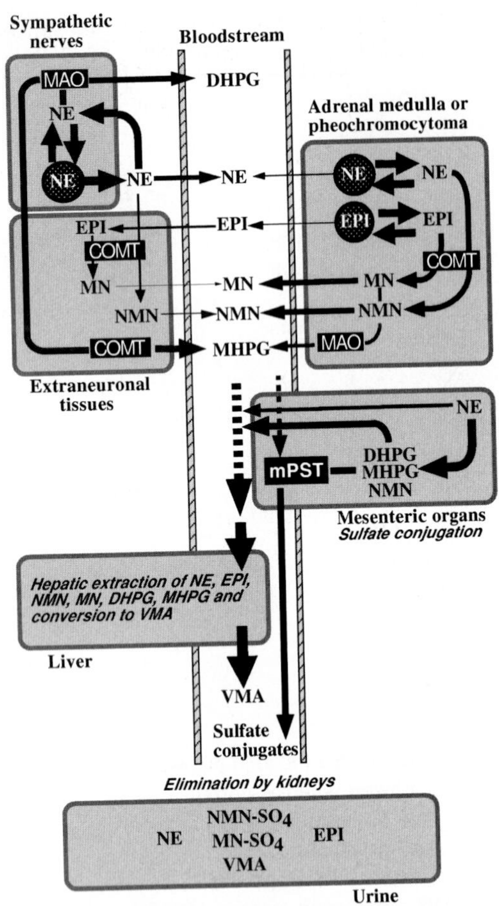

Figure 29-5 Schematic diagram illustrating the regional pathways of norepinephrine and epinephrine metabolism. Most norepinephrine is released and metabolized within sympathetic nerves, including up to one half produced in sympathetic nerves of mesenteric organs. Sulfate conjugation of catecholamines and catecholamine metabolites, particularly 3-methoxy-4-hydroxyphenylglycol (MHPG), occurs mainly in mesenteric organs, whereas production of vanillylmandelic acid (VMA) occurs mainly in the liver. *MAO*, Monoamine oxidase; *COMT*, catechol-*O*-methyltransferase; *SULT1A3*, sulfotransferase type 1A3; *NE*, norepinephrine; *EPI*, epinephrine; *NMN*, normetanephrine; *MN*, metanephrine; *DHPG*, 3,4-dihydroxy-phenylglycol; *MHPG*, 3-methoxy-4-hydroxyphenylglycol; *VMA*, vanillylmandelic acid; *NMN-SO$_4$*, normetanephrine sulfate; *MN-SO$_4$*, metanephrine sulfate; *MHPG-SO$_4$*, 3-methoxy-4-hydroxyphenylglycol sulfate.

reasons for this are twofold. First, much more norepinephrine released by sympathetic nerves is removed by neuronal uptake than by extraneuronal uptake. Second, under resting conditions, much more of the norepinephrine metabolized intraneuronally is derived from transmitter leaking from storage vesicles than from transmitter recaptured after exocytotic release. Thus most of the norepinephrine produced in the body is metabolized initially to DHPG, mainly from transmitter deaminated intraneuronally after leakage from storage vesicles or after release and reuptake. Most circulating DHPG is derived from sympathetic nerves, with relatively small contributions from the brain (<5%) and adrenals (<7%).

DHPG is further *O*-methylated by COMT in nonneuronal tissue to 3-methoxy-4-hydroxyphenylglycol (MHPG), a metabolite also produced to a limited extent by deamination of normetanephrine and metanephrine (Figure 29-5). Compared with DHPG, the latter *O*-methylated metabolites are produced in small amounts, and only at extraneuronal locations, with the single largest source representing adrenal chromaffin cells, accounting for more than 90% of circulating metanephrine and 24% to 40% of circulating normetanephrine.[64] Within the adrenals, normetanephrine and metanephrine are produced similarly to DHPG in sympathetic nerves, from norepinephrine and epinephrine leaking from storage granules into the chromaffin cell cytoplasm.

The MHPG produced from DHPG and metanephrines is either sulfate conjugated or metabolized to vanillylmandelic acid (VMA) by the sequential actions of hepatic alcohol dehydrogenase and aldehyde dehydrogenase. At least 90% of the VMA formed in the body is produced in the liver, mainly from hepatic uptake and metabolism of circulating DHPG and MHPG.[22]

In contrast to production of VMA, production of homovanillic acid (HVA) from dopamine depends mainly on *O*-methylation of the deaminated metabolite of dopamine, 3,4-dihydroxyphenylacetic acid (DOPAC), and to a lesser extent on deamination of methoxytyramine, the *O*-methylated metabolite of dopamine (Figure 29-4). As a result, HVA is formed in multiple tissues, with about 30% of circulating and urinary HVA arising from mesenteric organs and up to 20% from the brain.

With the exception of VMA, all the catecholamines and their metabolites are metabolized to sulfate conjugates by a specific sulfotransferase isoenzyme (SULT1A3). In humans, a single amino acid substitution confers the enzyme with particularly high affinity for dopamine and the *O*-methylated metabolites of catecholamines, including normetanephrine, metanephrine, and methoxytyramine.[48] The SULT1A3 isoenzyme is found in high concentrations in gastrointestinal tissues, which therefore represent a major source of sulfate conjugates.

In humans, VMA and the sulfates and glucuronide conjugates of MHPG represent the main end products of norepinephrine and epinephrine metabolism (Table 29-1). HVA and conjugates of HVA are the main metabolic end products of dopamine metabolism. These end products and the other conjugates are eliminated mainly by urinary excretion. As a result, their circulatory clearance is slow and plasma concentrations high relative to those of the precursor amines.

Serotonin is not a substrate for COMT and follows simpler pathways of metabolism than those for catecholamines (Figure 29-6). Deamination of serotonin to the aldehyde intermediate is preferentially followed by oxidation to 5-hydroxyindoleacetic acid (5-HIAA) catalyzed by

TABLE 29-1 Average Urinary Excretion of Catecholamines and Metabolites*

	Amount Excreted, µmol/day (µg/day)	Percent of Total from Norepinephrine and Epinephrine
Epinephrine (free)	0.03 (5)	0.1
Norepinephrine (free)	0.18 (30)	0.5
Epinephrine and norepinephrine (conjugated)	0.59 (100)	1.7
Metanephrine (free and conjugated)	0.33 (65)	1.0
Normetanephrine (free and conjugated)	0.55 (100)	1.6
Dihydroxyphenylglycol (free and conjugated)	1.26 (215)	3.7
3-Methoxy-4-hydroxyphenylglycol (free and conjugated)	10.9 (2000)	32.0
Vanillylmandelic acid (free)	20.2 (4000)	59.3
Dopamine (free)	1.50 (225)	
Dopamine (conjugated)	2.80 (700)	
Methoxytyramine (free and conjugated)	0.80 (130)	
Dihydroxyphenylacetic acid (free and conjugated)	7.5 (1300)	
Homovanillic acid	37.9 (6900)	

*Average values in human subjects. Modified from data in references 144, 151, and 233.

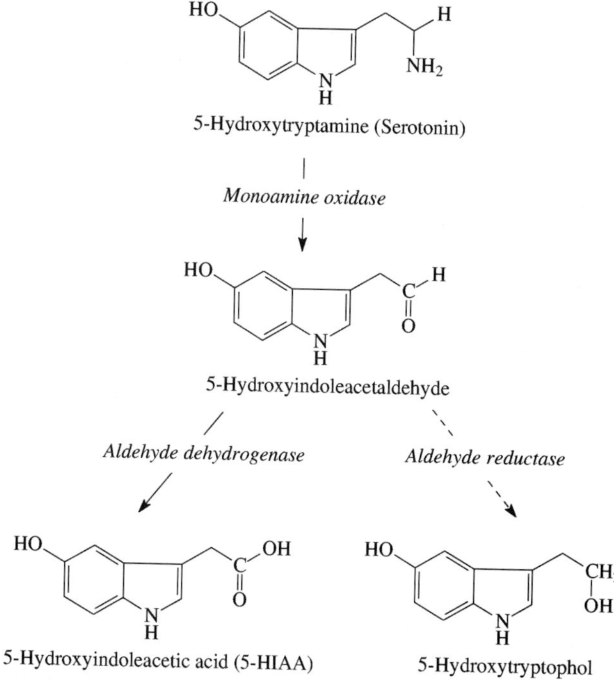

Figure 29-6 Metabolism of serotonin to 5-hydroxyindoleacetic acid (5-HIAA) and 5-hydroxytryptophol.

aldehyde dehydrogenase. Reduction to 5-hydroxytryptophol (5-HTOL) normally represents a relatively minor pathway, so that the major urinary excretion product of serotonin metabolism is 5-HIAA. Metabolism through these pathways is altered by consumption of ethyl alcohol, which through changes in the redox state leads to increased formation of 5-HTOL. Increases in ratios of 5-HTOL to 5HIAA in urine therefore provide a useful marker of alcohol abuse.

PHYSIOLOGY OF CATECHOLAMINE AND SEROTONIN SYSTEMS

The physiological and behavioral actions of catecholamines and serotonin provide a foundation for understanding disorders of monoamine excess or deficiency. Major sites of catecholamine and serotonin synthesis and action are listed in Table 29-2 for both central and peripheral nervous systems. The table provides an anatomic framework showing the location of adrenergic, dopaminergic, and serotonergic systems and the varying modes of signal transmission by the monoamines.

Catecholamines and serotonin regulate physiological events at the cellular level by interaction with families of cell-surface receptors. Adrenergic receptors, classified as α_1 (subtypes $\alpha_{1a,b,d}$), α_2 (subtypes $\alpha_{2a,b,c}$), β_1, β_2, and β_3 subcategories, initiate cellular events in response to epinephrine and norepinephrine.[35] Compared with norepinephrine, epinephrine demonstrates greater or equal affinity for α_1 and α_2 receptors, and equivalent potency with β_1 receptors. For β_2 receptor activation, epinephrine is tenfold to fiftyfold more potent than norepinephrine, and norepinephrine is tenfold more active toward β_3 receptors.[106] Dopamine has known pharmacological reactivity with α_1 and α_2 adrenergic receptors but transmits central and peripheral nerve signals primarily by selective interaction with a family of dopaminergic receptors designated as D_1, D_2, D_3, D_4, and D_5 subtypes.[82] An even larger family of serotonergic receptors subtypes ($5\text{-HT}_{1A,B,D,E,F}$, $5\text{-HT}_{2A\text{-}C}$, 5-HT_3, 5-HT_4, $5\text{-HT}_{5A\text{-}B}$, 5-HT_6, 5-HT_7) has been identified by histological and molecular

TABLE 29-2 Location of Monoamine Production and Action in the Body

	Site of Monoamine Production	Mode of Transmission	Tissue Location of Monoamine Action
Epinephrine	Adrenal medulla (chromaffin cells)	Hormonal	Cardiac muscle, smooth muscle, and widespread effects on cellular metabolism
Norepinephrine	Peripheral sympathetic ganglia and varicosities of autonomic nervous system	Neuroeffector cell junction	Effector tissue including cardiac muscle, smooth muscle, vascular endothelium, and exocrine glands
	Adrenal medulla (chromaffin cells)	Hormonal	Primarily cardiac and smooth muscle
	Brainstem (locus caeruleus and reticular formation)	Neuronal synapse	Widespread central nervous system (CNS) neuronal connections
Dopamine	Midbrain (substantia nigra)	Neuronal synapse	Neuronal connections in cerebral striatum
	Midbrain (ventral tegmentum)	Neuronal synapse	Cerebral mesolimbic and mesocortical neuronal connections
	Diencephalon (hypothalamus)	Neuronal synapse	Pituitary gland
	Retina	Neuronal synapse	Neuronal connections within the retina
	Olfactory bulb	Neuronal synapse	Neuronal connections within the olfactory bulb
	Gastrointestinal tract	Autocrine/paracrine	Regulation of bicarbonate secretion, gut motility, sodium handling, exocrine secretions
	Kidney (synthesized from circulating L-dopa)	Autocrine/paracrine	Regulation of natriuresis
Serotonin	Brainstem (raphe nucleus)	Neuronal synapse	Widespread CNS neuronal connections
	GI (enterochromaffin cells)	Hormonal (paracrine)	Gastrointestinal smooth muscle
	GI (enterochromaffin cells)	Platelet uptake/release	Platelets, vascular smooth muscle

techniques.[113] Receptors, including α_2-adrenergic, 5-HT_{1A}, 5-HT_{1B}, and 5-HT_{1D}, may serve as autoreceptors by turning off the release of their respective neurotransmitters via a negative feedback mechanism. The major physiological effects of catecholamines and serotonin, as outlined in the next section, are explained in part by these diverse receptor interactions that occur in function-specific locations throughout the vasculature and organ systems of the body.

Central Nervous System

Norepinephrine, dopamine, and serotonin represent only about 1% to 2% of the total neurotransmitters in the brain but serve an important role in autonomic (involuntary), somatic (voluntary), and information processing functions.[250] As neurotransmitters, they are produced primarily in regions of the brainstem (medulla oblongata, pons, and midbrain) by neurons with axons that project to defined, and sometimes widespread, areas of the brain or spinal cord. Although our understanding of central adrenergic, dopaminergic, and serotoninergic systems is incomplete, their role in central nervous system function and dysfunction is increasingly evident with important diagnostic and therapeutic implications.

Most norepinephrine synthesis in the brain takes place in the locus caeruleus of the pons and in the reticular formation of the medulla oblongata. About half of the norepinephrine is produced in the locus caeruleus by only a small nucleus of neurons that may respond in unison to sensory input signals.[188] The norepinephrine-producing neurons in the lower brainstem send diffuse axonal projections throughout the brain as high as the cerebral cortex. They also send descending fibers to the spinal cord where they synapse with preganglionic sympathetic neurons that communicate with the peripheral sympathetic nervous system. The norepinephrine-producing neurons of the brainstem process incoming sensory signals. They participate in regulating the activity of the sympathetic nervous system and the overall state of attention and vigilance. A predominant function of norepinephrine systems in the brain is response to stress. Stress-induced stimuli activate the brainstem production of norepinephrine with synaptic release and neuroactivation throughout many areas of the brain and spinal cord.

Dopamine is also an important neurotransmitter in the central nervous system. Dopamine accounts for more than half of the catecholamine production of the brain but its distribution and function are markedly different from norepinephrine. Dopamine neurotransmission is involved in processing sensory signals and in regulating hormonal release. Dopaminergic neurons in the retina and olfactory bulb have ultrashort projections that transmit signals within these neuronal centers for vision and smell. Neurons in the arcuate nucleus of the hypothalamus have projecting fibers that release dopamine in the portal vessels, exerting a key neuroendocrine inhibition on prolactin and thyroid-stimulating hormone release and as effects on other hormones of the pituitary gland.[201]

Dopamine is also produced by neurons in the substantia nigra and ventral tegmentum. The ventral tegmental area modulates diverse forebrain functions such as cognitive activity through axonal projection to the prefrontal cortex and reward seeking behavior via axonal fibers sent to limbic structures of the brain.[225] Consequently, disturbances in dopamine production and release from these areas of the brain are involved in a number of important neurological and psychiatric disorders, with dopamine receptors serving as key pharmacological targets for antipsychotic drug development.[227] In addition, dopaminergic neurons in the substantia nigra project into the corpus striatum to form an important nigrostriatal system, which regulates the initiation and maintenance of motor function. Control by this system over extrapyramidal (involuntary) movement is evidenced by the loss of motor control when nigrostriatal neurons degenerate in Parkinson's disease.[111]

Serotonin, like norepinephrine, is produced by small clusters of neurons in the brainstem regions but serves a diverse range of behavioral and physiological functions.[237] Neurons in the raphe nuclei of the pons and upper brainstem are a primary source of brain serotonin and project axonal fibers throughout the brain and spinal cord. Physiological and behavioral processes that may be influenced by this extensive serotonergic system include memory, learning, feeding behavior, sleep patterns, thermoregulation, pain modulation, cardiovascular function, and hypothalamic regulation of pituitary hormones. Each of the 14 known subtypes of serotonin receptors has distinct patterns of distribution in the brain and accounts for the diverse cognitive, behavioral, and physiological responses.[6] Raphe projections to the subcortical regions of the cerebral hemisphere (amygdala and hippocampus) activate receptors that influence mood and anxiety. The success in pharmacological manipulation of serotonin levels and selective receptor responses in the brain clearly indicates the importance of the central serotonergic system.[126] Buspirone, for example, reduces anxiety behavior by activation of serotonin autoreceptors in the subcortical areas of the brain, thus reducing serotonin release. Hypoactivity of the serotonergic system, on the other hand, plays an important role in depression. Selective serotonin reuptake inhibitors such as fluoxetine, paroxetine, and sertraline are effective agents in the treatment of this form of central serotonergic deficiency.[199]

Serotonin is also involved in hormonal regulation. Serotonin-releasing nerve fibers that originate in raphe nuclei and terminate in the hypothalamus exert a circadian influence on pituitary-adrenal function by stimulating hypothalamic corticotropin-releasing hormone and signaling other hormonal events mediated by enhanced prolactin and growth hormone release.[201] Serotonin also influences overall blood flow to the brain as evidenced by serotonin's vasoconstrictive effects on carotid vasculature and the beneficial pharmacological effect of a serotonergic agonist, sumatriptan, in the treatment of migraine.

Serotonin and catecholamine functions in the central nervous system are both diverse and complex, and direct assessment of central neurotransmitters by clinical laboratory methods is currently limited. The effects, however, of central serotonergic, dopaminergic, and serotonergic systems on metabolic and hormonal function are routinely measured in the clinical laboratory, and many of the therapeutic and illicit drugs that modulate central monoamine neurotransmission are monitored by laboratory techniques in a wide range of clinical settings.

Sympathetic Nervous System

In the peripheral nervous system, norepinephrine is an important neurotransmitter in the sympathetic branch of the autonomic system. Sympathetic nerve transmission operates below the level of consciousness in controlling physiological function of many organs and tissues of the body. The sympathetic system plays a particularly important role in regulating cardiovascular function in response to postural, exertional, thermal, and mental stress. With sympathetic activation, the heart rate is increased, peripheral arterioles are constricted, skeletal arterioles are dilated, and the blood pressure is elevated. In addition, sympathetic nerve stimulation dilates pupils; inhibits smooth muscles of the intestines, bronchi, and bladder; and closes the sphincters. Sympathetic signals work in balance with the parasympathetic portion of the autonomic nervous system to maintain a stable internal environment.

The hypothalamus, which integrates autonomic and neuroendocrine systems, has a controlling influence over sympathetic outflow from brainstem centers and the spinal cord. Afferent or incoming sensory signals originate from pressure, stretch, chemical, pain, and temperature receptors located in visceral organs and vessels. Afferent nerve impulses enter the central nervous system either to form the efferent component of local reflex arcs within the spinal cord or to ascend to higher centers such as the hypothalamus, where afferent signals are integrated with other neural pathways. Efferent or outgoing responses are transmitted by preganglionic sympathetic neurons that exit the spinal cord between the first thoracic and second lumbar segments. The exiting fibers converge on sympathetic ganglia chains along the spinal column or in visceral ganglia and activate multiple postganglionic neurons by releasing the neurotransmitter acetylcholine. The terminal branches of the postganglionic fibers that project from these ganglia into target organs have varicosities that form a rich ground plexus for synaptic contact with a large number of effector cells in glands and muscle fibers.

Most sympathetic postganglionic nerves liberate norepinephrine as their neurotransmitter. In limited locations, sympathetic nerve endings release acetylcholine, such as some sweat glands that undergo a noradrenergic to cholinergic switch during development.[223] In addition, dopamine is an important neurotransmitter in renal, coronary, mesenteric, and cerebrovascular beds.[85] Preganglionic sympathetic fibers also innervate the adrenal medulla, stimulating release of epinephrine from chromaffin cells as a circulating hormone.

The relative contribution of individual organs to overall sympathetic activity has been inferred from data on the release of norepinephrine into plasma.[3,64,67] Plasma norepinephrine is derived primarily from postganglionic sympathetic neurons with little contribution from the central nervous system or hormonal release from the adrenal medulla. In the resting state, the overall rate of norepinephrine spillover to the systemic circulation is in the order of 200 to 600 ng/min. Because of intervening neuronal and extraneuronal removal processes, this spillover represents less than 10% of the total norepinephrine released by sympathetic nerves. Turnover of norepinephrine, representing a loss mainly caused by metabolism, is driven primarily in the resting state by leakage of norepinephrine from vesicles into the neuronal axoplasm. Major contributors to basal sympathetic outflow, based on spillover measurements, include the gastrointestinal (GI) tract (~37%), kidney (~25%), and skeletal muscle (~11%). The heart, liver, lungs, and skin each contribute less than 10%. Alterations in norepinephrine spillover occur in response to physiological and pathological states. Exercise, overeating, low salt intake, upright position, mental stress, and aging increase sympathetic outflow. Increased spillover is also found in disorders such as cardiac failure, hypertension, and depression. Reduction in baseline norepinephrine overflow from the heart has also been shown in autonomic insufficiency and syncope, consistent with sympathetic denervation or depressed sympathetic activity in these disorders.

The physiological response to sympathetic activity in individual organs is dependent not only upon the rate of neurotransmitter release from postganglionic nerve varicosities but also the type of adrenergic receptors and their location in tissue. Vascular and organ-specific responses are classified in Table 29-3 by subcategory of interaction with adrenergic receptors. In peripheral target organs, α_1 and β_1 adrenergic receptors appear strategically located in the immediate vicinity of nerve terminals for rapid postsynaptic smooth muscle, secretion, and endocrine activation via sympathetic signals from the brain. Postsynaptic β_2 adrenergic receptors in the heart also allow rapid sympathetic neuroactivation. Extrajunctional α_2 and β_2 receptors that are remote from sympathetic nerve terminals in vascular smooth muscle or platelets may be preferentially influenced by circulating catecholamines, such as epinephrine produced by the adrenal gland.[106]

An earlier concept of the sympathetic nervous system functioning primarily as an all-or-none responder to fight or flight has been challenged by studies indicating more specific organ responses to sympathetic activation.[122,182] Thermal and pain sensors, for example, result in a sympathetic response

TABLE 29-3 Direct Effects of Adrenergic Activation on Some Organ Systems Based on Receptor Subtype

Receptor Subtype (Relative Potency)	Tissue Location (Response)	
α_1-adrenergic (NE ≤ E)	Heart (increased force) Veins (constriction) Adrenergic sweat glands (secretion) Urinary bladder sphincter (contraction) Spleen capsule (contraction)	Arterioles (constriction) Pupils (dilation) GI sphincters (contraction) Uterus in pregnancy (contraction) Penis (ejaculation)
α_2-adrenergic (NE ≤ E)	Arterioles (constriction) GI motility and tone (decreased) Pancreatic islet cell secretion (inhibit)	Adipocytes (inhibit lipolysis) Intestinal secretions (inhibit) Platelet aggregation (stimulate)
β_1-adrenergic (NE = E)	Heart (increased rate and force) Adipocytes (stimulate lipolysis)	Kidney (renin release)
β_2-adrenergic (NE << E)	Heart (increased rate and force) Gallbladder and ducts (relaxation) Adipocytes (stimulate lipolysis)	Arterioles (dilation) GI motility and tone (decreased) Bronchial muscle (dilation)
β_3-adrenergic (NE > E)	Adipocytes (stimulate lipolysis)	

Modified from references 106 and 147. The distribution of the six α_1 ($\alpha_{1a,b,d}$) and α_2 ($\alpha_{2a,b,c}$) subtypes is not completely understood and therefore not included in the table. For receptor locations in the central nervous system, refer to vonBohlen und Bohlen O, Dermietzel R. Neurotransmitters and neuromodulators. Handbook of receptors and biological effects. Darmstadt FRG, 2002.[250]

that differs markedly from the physiological response to the baroreceptor signals produced by changes in blood pressure. An increase in environmental temperature reduces sympathetic tone in peripheral vascular beds, thereby resulting in vasodilation and increased heat losses by radiation from the surface of the body. Pain receptor stimulation from surgical incision in anesthetized humans causes a proportionate increase in cutaneous vasoconstriction.[228] In a postural change from supine to upright, however, baroreceptors signal both cardiac and vascular responses via the sympathetic nerves. In the heart, sympathetic release of norepinephrine increases the rate and force of cardiac muscle contractions, ultimately increasing cardiac output. In skin and mucosa, sympathetic activation causes vasoconstriction with a resultant increase in blood pressure and redistribution of blood to visceral organs. Therefore although global sympathetic activation clearly operates in extreme conditions of stress, the differential control of sympathetic output is continually adapting cardiovascular and other organ functions in support of behavioral and environmental changes.

Adrenal Medullary System

Although often considered a part of the sympathetic nervous system, the adrenal medulla produces and secretes a different catecholamine, epinephrine, with different functions from the norepinephrine secreted by sympathetic nerves.[56] The adrenal medulla and sympathetic nerves are also regulated separately, often in divergent directions in response to different forms of stress.

The human adrenal glands overlie the superior poles of the kidneys. Each gland consists of an outer part, the lipid-rich cortex, and a thin inner central medulla containing chromaffin cells. The adrenal medulla is up to 2 mm thick and takes about one tenth of the entire weight of the gland. Blood is supplied to the adrenal medulla by direct arterial supply and from vessels draining from the cortex to the medulla. The latter supply provides an important source of adrenocortical steroids for regulation of adrenal medullary function. The neural input to the adrenal medulla includes direct innervation by cholinergic fibers that pass through the sympathetic paravertebral chain from preganglionic sympathetic cell bodies of the spinal cord.

A characteristic feature of adrenal medullary chromaffin cells is the presence of numerous catecholamine storage granules ranging in size from 100 to 300 nm in diameter. These granules turn brown when exposed to potassium bichromate solutions, ammoniacal silver nitrate, or osmium tetroxide because of the oxidation and polymerization of epinephrine and norepinephrine. This process is known as the "chromaffin reaction," hence the terms chromaffin cells and chromaffin granules. At least two kinds of adrenal medullary chromaffin cells have been identified in most animal species based on differences in chromaffin granules. Norepinephrine-producing chromaffin cells possess dense-core granules eccentrically located in the vesicle, and cells storing epinephrine have less electron-dense homogenous granules.

The human adrenal medulla produces mainly epinephrine, which as a hormone, is secreted directly into the bloodstream to act on cells distant from sites of release. As outlined previously, epinephrine and norepinephrine have overlapping but also different potencies of effect on α- and β-adrenergic receptors. The proximity of sites of norepinephrine and epinephrine release to adrenoceptors also determines differences in adrenoceptor-mediated responses to the two catecholamines. Because of these factors, epinephrine exerts its effects on different populations of adrenoceptors than norepinephrine. As a circulating hormone, epinephrine acts potently on β_2-adrenergic receptors of the skeletal muscle vasculature, causing vasodilation. In contrast, norepinephrine released locally within the vasculature causes α_1-adrenoceptor–mediated vasoconstriction. Increases in circulating epinephrine during stress may contribute to skeletal muscle vasodilatory responses, but appear to play little role in other cardiovascular changes, including increases in heart rate. Thus despite the potent hemodynamic actions of epinephrine, the adrenal medulla appears to play a minimal role in cardiovascular regulation compared with sympathetic nerves.

Epinephrine released from the adrenal glands is more important as a metabolic than as a hemodynamic regulatory hormone.[45] In particular, epinephrine stimulates lipolysis, ketogenesis, thermogenesis, and glycolysis and raises plasma glucose levels by stimulating glycogenolysis and gluconeogenesis. Epinephrine also has potent effects on pulmonary function, causing β_2-adrenoceptor–mediated dilation of airways. Circulating norepinephrine, in minor part derived from the adrenal medulla and functioning as a hormone, may have additional metabolic actions, but appears to have little importance for cardiovascular regulation compared with the higher concentrations of the amine at sympathoneuroeffector sites.

Despite the apparent importance of the adrenal medulla in homeostasis, particularly regulation of metabolism, the medulla in contrast to the adrenal cortex is not vital for survival. Studies in adrenalectomized subjects clearly show that both hemodynamic and glucose-counter-regulatory responses to insulin-hypoglycemia, exercise, and other manipulations remain intact despite absence of epinephrine responses.[46,105] This contrasts with the severe disturbances of blood pressure regulation accompanying loss of sympathetic nerves.

Compared with the sympathetic nervous system, the adrenal medulla makes a relatively minor contribution to the overall production and turnover of catecholamines (Table 29-4).

However, because phenylethanolamine-*N*-methyltransferase (PNMT) is expressed mainly in adrenal chromaffin cells, more than 90% of circulating epinephrine is derived from the adrenal medulla. This contrasts with

TABLE 29-4 Contribution of the Adrenals to Circulating Catecholamines and Metabolites

	Adrenals (pmol per min)	Total Body (pmol per min)	Adrenal Contribution (%)
Catecholamines			
Epinephrine	979	1075	91%
Norepinephrine	274	3953	7%
Dopamine	6	>290	<2%
Metabolites			
Metanephrine	449	494	91%
Normetanephrine	91	392	23%
DHPG	665	13,964	5%
DOPAC	300	>4120	<7%

circulating norepinephrine, more than 90% of which is derived from sympathetic nerves.

Apart from catecholamines, adrenal medullary chromaffin cells produce, store, and secrete a wide array of neuropeptides and proteins. Peptides include enkephalins, β-endorphin, neuropeptide Y, substance P, vasoactive intestinal peptide, neurotensin, galanin, atrial natriuretic peptide, pituitary adenylate cyclase-activating peptide, adrenomedullin, and corticotrophin. These peptides are secreted together with the catecholamines and may be involved in a local autocrine or paracrine regulation of adrenal medullary and cortical function. The major soluble proteins within chromaffin vesicles belong to the family of granins, which consist of several secretory acidic glycoproteins, the major representative being chromogranin A.

Peripheral Dopaminergic System

Dopamine is usually thought of as a neurotransmitter in the brain or as an intermediate in the production of norepinephrine and epinephrine in the periphery. It has been presumed that these sources account for the large amounts of dopamine and dopamine metabolites excreted in urine. The contribution of the brain to circulating levels and urinary excretion of dopamine metabolites is, however, now known to be relatively minor. Also, in sympathetic nerves and the adrenal medulla most dopamine is converted to norepinephrine. Therefore other sources and functions of dopamine in the periphery must be considered. Emerging evidence suggests the presence of a third peripheral catecholamine system, in which dopamine functions not as a neurotransmitter or circulating hormone, but as an autocrine or paracrine substance.[91]

In the kidneys, dopamine is now an established autocrine and/or paracrine effector substance contributing to the regulation of sodium excretion.[33] Unlike neuronal catecholamine systems, production of dopamine in the kidneys is largely independent of local synthesis of L-dopa by tyrosine hydroxylase. Thus renal denervation does not affect urinary dopamine excretion. Instead, production of dopamine in the kidneys depends mainly on proximal tubular cell uptake of L-dopa from the circulation. The L-dopa is then converted to dopamine by aromatic amino acid decarboxylase, the activity of which is up regulated by a high-salt diet and down regulated by a low-salt diet.

The presence of a renal dopamine paracrine-autocrine system explains the considerable amounts of free dopamine excreted in the urine.[258] Most derives from renal uptake and decarboxylation of circulating L-dopa and reflects the plasma levels of this amino acid and the function of the renal dopamine paracrine-autocrine system.

Although the kidneys represent the major source of urinary free dopamine, this source does not account for the larger amounts of excreted dopamine metabolites, such as HVA and dopamine sulfate. Findings of large arterial-to-portal venous increases in plasma concentrations of dopamine and its metabolites have indicated that substantial amounts of dopamine are produced and metabolized in the GI tract and other mesenteric organs.[55]

The substantial production and metabolism of dopamine in the human GI tract appear to reflect functions of dopamine as an enteric neuromodulator or paracrine and/or autocrine substance. Dopamine and dopamine receptor agonists stimulate bicarbonate secretion and protect against ulcer formation, whereas dopamine antagonists augment secretion of gastric acid and promote ulcer development.[76] Dopamine also appears to influence GI motility, sodium transport, and gastric and intestinal submucosal blood flow. In the pancreas, dopamine may modulate secretion of digestive enzymes and bicarbonate.

Morphological studies have demonstrated the presence of cells in the GI tract that contain dopamine and express components of dopamine signaling pathways, including catecholamine biosynthetic enzymes and specific dopamine receptors and transporters.[173] In the stomach, tyrosine hydroxylase is expressed in epithelial cells, including acid-secreting parietal cells. In the small intestine, cells of the lamina propria, including immune cells, also express tyrosine hydroxylase. The enzyme is additionally found in pancreatic exocrine cells.

The high rates of dopamine production by mesenteric organs cannot be accounted for by local extraction and decarboxylation of circulating L-dopa. Thus unlike the kidneys, where dopamine is produced mainly from circulating L-dopa, in the GI tract, production of dopamine requires the presence of tyrosine hydroxylase or other sources of L-dopa.

Consumption of food increases plasma concentrations of L-dopa, dopamine, and dopamine metabolites, particularly dopamine sulfate, indicating that dietary constituents may also represent an important source of peripheral dopamine.[94] Such a source does not, however, account for the substantial amounts of dopamine produced in peripheral tissue outside of the digestive tract, or of that produced in digestive tissue of fasting individuals. In particular, plasma concentrations of both L-dopa and dopamine sulfate remain high even after a 3-day fast. It is now clear that dopamine sulfate is mainly produced in the GI tract from both dietary and locally synthesized dopamine. This is consistent with findings that the GI tract contains high concentrations of the SULT1A3. Production of sulfate conjugates in the digestive tract appears to provide an enzymatic "gut-blood barrier," for detoxifying dietary biogenic amines and delimiting physiological effects of locally produced dopamine.

Enteric Nervous System

The enteric nervous system (ENS) is defined as an independent and integrated system of neurons and supporting cells located in the GI tract, gallbladder, and pancreas. It is the largest division of the autonomic nervous system and contains about the same number of neurons as the spinal cord. The ENS is composed of two networks or plexuses of intrinsic neurons, the myenteric plexus and the submucous plexus. Both are imbedded in the wall of the gut and extend from the esophagus to the anus. These networks contain more than 100 million sensory neurons, interneurons, and motor neurons. The myenteric plexus lies between the longitudinal and circular layers of intestinal smooth muscle and controls propulsive movements (peristalsis). The submucous plexus innervates glandular epithelium, intestinal endocrine cells, and submucosal blood vessels. This network senses the environment within the lumen, regulates local blood flow, and controls epithelial cell secretion.

The ENS is connected to the central nervous system by extrinsic parasympathetic and sympathetic motor neurons, and by extrinsic spinal and vagal sensory neurons. Through these bidirectional connections, the ENS can be monitored and modified.[5,96] Despite the presence of these extrinsic nerve connections, the ENS can also function autonomously in some intestinal regions. Neural transmission within the ENS is controlled by a large variety of neurotransmitters and neuromodulatory peptides, such as serotonin, norepinephrine, acetylcholine, ATP, and nitric oxide.[168] Most of these substances are also found in the brain. In addition to its function as a neurotransmitter within the ENS, serotonin also acts as a local paracrine molecule, participating in mucosal sensory transduction. More than 95% of the body's serotonin is located within the GI tract, with most being synthesized and stored in enterochromaffin cells in the gut mucosa. Serotonin is released from these cells in response to mechanical or chemical stimuli such as the passage of food, which in turn stimulates both intrinsic (via 5-HT_{1P} and 5-HT_4 receptors) and extrinsic (via 5-HT_3) vagal sensory nerve fibers.[80] Intrinsic sensory neurons activated by serotonin stimulate the peristaltic reflex and secretion, whereas extrinsic sensory neurons initiate bowel sensations such as nausea, vomiting, abdominal pain, and bloating. The paracrine actions of serotonin are terminated by uptake into epithelial cells by the same serotonin transporter used in serotonergic neurons.

Serotonin modulates numerous physiological and behavioral systems in the human body and is involved in a wide variety of clinical disorders. In the ENS, for example, serotonin plays pivotal roles in the pathogenesis of the carcinoid syndrome and the irritable bowel syndrome.[112] Differences in serotonin receptor subtypes provide a strong rationale for using pharmaceutical agents that selectively act on serotonin receptors in the treatment of these clinical disorders.[1]

CLINICAL APPLICATIONS

Catecholamines and serotonin have an important role in health and disease. For example, excess catecholamines are associated with stress, a fall in blood pressure or blood volume, thyroid hormone deficiency, congestive heart failure, and arrhythmias, and low levels of catecholamines are seen in idiopathic postural hypotension. Increased concentrations of circulating serotonin have been implicated in several pathological conditions, including chronic tension headache, hypertension, schizophrenia, Duchenne's muscular dystrophy, and preeclampsia. Although investigational measurement of catecholamines, serotonin, and their metabolites has been used in a range of pathophysiological processes, clinical laboratory measurement of the amines and their metabolites is primarily used in the diagnosis of neuroendocrine tumors. Catecholamine-secreting neurochromaffin tumors include pheochromocytomas, paragangliomas, and neuroblastomas; carcinoids are serotonin-secreting tumors. Measurement of catecholamines is also useful in the diagnosis of a number of autonomic and genetic disorders that will also be covered in this section.

Pheochromocytoma

Pheochromocytomas are catecholamine-producing tumors that arise from chromaffin cells of the adrenal medulla. Excluding neuroblastomas, about 10% of catecholamine-producing tumors arise from extraadrenal sympathochromaffin tissue, usually in the abdomen, and are known as paragangliomas. Most other paragangliomas arise from parasympathetic tissue in the chest and neck and do not produce appreciable amounts of catecholamines.[169]

Pheochromocytomas and catecholamine-producing paragangliomas are treacherous tumors that will almost invariably cause devastating cardiovascular complications and death if not recognized and properly treated. Thus once such a tumor is suspected, it is imperative that appropriate biochemical tests are employed for accurate diagnosis.

The presence of a pheochromocytoma is usually suspected because of signs and symptoms that reflect the biological effects of catecholamines released by the tumor. Hypertension is the most common sign and can be sustained or paroxysmal. Symptoms include headache, palpitations, diaphoresis, pallor, dyspnea, nausea, attacks of anxiety, and generalized weakness. Although headache, palpitations, and sweating are nonspecific symptoms, their presence with hypertension should arouse immediate suspicion of the tumor. Signs and symptoms that occur in paroxysms reflect episodic catecholamine secretion. Paroxysmal attacks usually last less than an hour with intervals between attacks varying widely and as infrequent as once every few months. Pronounced but transient symptoms usually accompany such attacks, whereas symptoms are usually less pronounced when hypertension is sustained. For more detail on the clinical presentation and other aspects of pheochromocytoma, the reader is referred to the text of Manger and Gifford.[161] Pheochromocytomas are rare, occurring in less than 0.2% of patients with hypertension. However, because of the high prevalence of hypertension and the wide spectrum of symptoms produced by pheochromocytomas, many of which occur in other clinical conditions, pheochromocytomas must be considered in many patients with and without hypertension. Patients with a high risk for pheochromocytoma, in whom testing may be carried out independently of the presence of signs and symptoms, include those with a family or previous history of the tumor, or the finding of an adrenal incidentaloma.

Most pheochromocytomas are sporadic, but a significant proportion, perhaps as many as 25%, occur in several familial tumor syndromes.[190] Pheochromocytomas in multiple endocrine neoplasia type 2 (MEN 2a or 2b) result from mutations of the ret protooncogene. In MEN 2a, there is often coexistence of medullary thyroid cancer or C-cell hyperplasia and parathyroid adenoma or hyperplasia. In MEN 2b, hyperparathyroidism is rare, but patients often present with mucosal neuromas, thickened corneal nerves, and alimentary tract ganglioneuromatosis. In von Hippel-Lindau syndrome (VHL), family-specific mutations of the VHL tumor suppressor gene determine the varied clinical presentation of tumors, including retinal angiomas, central nervous system hemangioblastomas, pheochromocytomas, and tumors in the kidneys, pancreas, and testis. Familial paragangliomas (some catecholamine producing) occur secondary to mutations of genes for several succinate dehydrogenase enzymes. In addition to paragangliomas, these familial conditions also include a predisposition to adrenal pheochromocytomas. Neurofibromatosis type 1 is the most common familial condition coexisting with pheochromocytoma, which occurs in about 1% of patients with the condition. Periodic testing for pheochromocytomas in patients with the first 3 of the above 4 familial syndromes is now recommended as part of a routine screening and surveillance plan.

Although mostly benign, about 10% to 15% of pheochromocytomas are malignant. There is a higher risk of malignant pheochromocytomas in patients with large or extraadrenal primary tumors.[125] Diagnosis of a malignant pheochromocytoma is not possible based on histopathological features, but instead requires evidence of metastatic lesions (e.g., in liver, lungs, lymphatic nodes, and bones). Metastases can occur more than 20 years after removal of an apparently benign solitary tumor. Therefore all patients with a previous history of the tumor are at risk for recurrent or malignant disease and should undergo periodic screening for the tumor.

Adrenal masses are present in 6% or more of the older population. Most are benign adenomas, but up to 10% represent pheochromocytomas. With escalation in the use of computed tomography and magnetic resonance imaging, there has been an increasing frequency in incidental findings of adrenal masses during imaging procedures for unrelated conditions. These adrenal incidentalomas represent another situation in which biochemical testing for pheochromocytomas is now recommended, irrespective of the presence of the usual signs and symptoms of the tumor.[97]

Biochemical evidence of excessive catecholamine production is crucial for diagnosis of pheochromocytoma, and has traditionally relied on measurements of urinary catecholamines, metanephrines, and VMA.[218] Most patients with hypertension and symptoms caused by active pheochromocytomas have large increases in these analytes, making the tumor relatively easy to diagnose. Problems occur in those patients in whom hypertension is paroxysmal and where there may be negligible catecholamine secretion between episodes. False-negative test results are, however, more commonly encountered in patients with "silent pheochromocytomas" in whom testing is carried out, not because of signs or symptoms, but because of an adrenal incidentaloma or as part of a routine surveillance plan for recurrent or hereditary pheochromocytomas. In one study involving 35 patients with hereditary pheochromocytomas, rates of false-negative results for plasma and urinary catecholamines, urinary total metanephrines, and urinary VMA ranged from 29% to 53%; six patients (17%) had normal results for all four tests.[63]

Another problem common to biochemical tests used for diagnosis of a pheochromocytoma is that a positive result does not necessarily establish a tumor. False-positive results must always be expected when the upper reference limit for a test is set at anything less than the 100% confidence intervals of a reference population.

The above limitations in sensitivity and specificity of biochemical tests are compounded by the large numbers of patients commonly tested for pheochromocytomas, very few of whom have the tumor. The low pretest prevalence of pheochromocytomas means that false-positive biochemical results usually far outnumber true-positive results, making it difficult to unequivocally confirm the tumor in the vast majority of patients with positive results.

With issues of sensitivity and specificity in mind and consideration of the potential dangers and rarity of a pheochromocytoma, the most important consideration in choice of biochemical tests is their reliability for detecting and excluding the tumor. In a pheochromocytoma, a missed diagnosis caused by false-negative results can have catastrophic consequences for the patient. In contrast, false-positive results can be refuted by further tests. Therefore suitably sensitive biochemical tests remain the first choice in the initial workup of a patient suspected of harboring a pheochromocytoma.

Findings that none of the traditionally used biochemical tests could reliably detect all cases of pheochromocytomas led to recommendations that biochemical testing should include a combination of measurements of catecholamines and catecholamine metabolites. VMA is excreted in urine in large amounts, which makes measurement of this metabolite a simple, easy to implement, and time-honored test for diagnosis of pheochromocytomas. Numerous studies have now made it clear, however, that measurements of urinary VMA provide a relatively insensitive diagnostic test with limited value for initial testing for pheochromocytomas. Therefore the usual recommendation has been that biochemical testing should include measurements of urinary or plasma catecholamines and urinary metanephrines.

With the development of liquid chromatographic methods sensitive enough to measure the low levels of free metanephrines in plasma there has been increased emphasis on these measurements for diagnosis of pheochromocytomas.[155,213] Studies from three independent groups have now shown that measurements of plasma free metanephrines provide a superior method for diagnosis of pheochromocytomas than other commonly used tests of catecholamine excess.[157,211,221] In the largest of these studies,[157] involving biochemical testing in more than 1000 patients, including 214 with pheochromocytomas, measurements of plasma free metanephrines and urinary fractionated metanephrines provided the highest diagnostic sensitivities, but the plasma test provided higher diagnostic specificity than the urine test. Receiver-operating characteristic curves showed that a single test of plasma free metanephrines provided higher diagnostic efficacy than all other tests, even when carried out in combination. Based on these findings it was proposed that a single test of plasma free metanephrines is sufficient for initial testing, and prevents the increased chance of false-positive results associated with multiple tests. Measurements of plasma free metanephrines have also been recommended for all patients with adrenal incidentaloma.[97]

The basis for the high diagnostic efficacy of plasma free metanephrines is explained by several factors: (1) plasma free metanephrines are produced by metabolism of catecholamines within pheochromocytomas, a process that occurs continuously and independently of variations in catecholamine release by tumors[61]; (2) normally only small amounts of metanephrines are produced in the body, and these are relatively unresponsive to sympathoadrenal activation compared with the parent amines[57]; and (3) VMA and the metanephrines commonly measured in urine are different metabolites from the free metanephrines measured in plasma, and are produced in different parts of the body by metabolic processes not directly related to the tumor itself.[60]

Urinary metanephrines are usually measured after a deconjugation step and largely reflect levels of sulfate-conjugated metanephrines produced outside of tumor tissue. The sulfate conjugates of normetanephrine and metanephrine are present in plasma at twentyfold to thirtyfold higher concentrations than the free metanephrines, and are the main form eliminated in urine. Plasma and urinary concentrations of deconjugated metanephrines are therefore easier to measure than the free metanephrines. Provided that liquid chromatographic steps for fractionated measurement of normetanephrine and metanephrine are used, measurement of the deconjugated metabolites provide diagnostic sensitivity that approaches that of measurement of plasma free metanephrines. The main drawback appears to be lower diagnostic specificity. This is particularly problematic in patients with renal insufficiency, in whom plasma concentrations of the deconjugated metanephrines are strongly elevated.[181] In contrast, since the circulatory clearance of free metanephrines by extraneuronal uptake is a rapid process largely independent of renal function, false-positive test results for the free metabolites are less of a problem.

The high diagnostic sensitivity of measurements of plasma free or urinary fractionated normetanephrine and metanephrine makes these tests the most suitable choice for the initial work up of a patient with a suspected pheochromocytoma. Negative results by these tests virtually exclude a pheochromocytoma, whereas negative results by other tests do not. Exceptions include small or microscopic (<1 cm) tumors encountered during routine screening or tumors that do not synthesize norepinephrine and epinephrine.

Increases in plasma free or urinary fractionated metanephrines, such as normetanephrine and metanephrine, are usually high enough to conclusively establish the presence of most cases of pheochromocytomas. However, where increases are of smaller magnitude, false-positive results remain difficult to distinguish from true-positive results and additional biochemical testing is necessary. Ideally, such testing should conclusively establish the presence of a pheochromocytoma before imaging studies are undertaken and the patient is committed to surgery.

Before further biochemical testing is initiated, consideration should be given to eliminating possible causes of false-positive results. These may occur because of inappropriate sampling conditions (e.g., blood sampling in nonfasting states or without a preceding 20 minute period of supine rest) or because of medications. The latter may involve direct analytical interference, such as co-chromatography of acetaminophen in high-performance liquid chromatography (HPLC) measurements of plasma normetanephrine. Usually, however, such sources of interference can be detected by careful inspection of chromatograms. More common causes of false-positive results are drugs that activate the sympathoadrenal system or influence the disposition of catecholamines. Tricyclic antidepressants and phenoxybenzamine (Dibenzyline) are particularly problematic, in one study accounting for 41% of all false-positive elevations of plasma normetanephrine and 44% to 45% of false-positive elevations of urinary and plasma norepinephrine.[59] Tricyclic antidepressants presumably increase levels of norepinephrine and normetanephrine by blocking reuptake of norepinephrine, thereby increasing the amounts available for *O*-methylation and that escape into the circulation. Phenoxybenzamine is a nonselective alpha-adrenergic blocking agent commonly used to treat patients with a pheochromocytoma. Presumably the drug elevates norepinephrine and normetanephrine by attenuating alpha$_2$-adrenoceptor–mediated feedback inhibition of norepinephrine release, possibly combined with reflexive sympathetic activation.

After the potential confounding influence of medications or other causes of false-positive results have been eliminated, some consideration should be given to the choice of additional biochemical tests and patterns of results necessary for more firmly establishing or refuting the diagnosis of a pheochromocytoma. When initial testing yields elevations in plasma normetanephrine, metanephrine, or both amines, this may be corroborated by a similar pattern of results after additional measurements of urinary normetanephrine and metanephrine. Conversely, when initial testing yields positive results for urinary fractionated metanephrines, additional measurements of plasma free metanephrines are useful.

Patterns of increases in plasma free metanephrines and catecholamines can also be useful for confirming pheochromocytomas in patients in whom initial tests of free metanephrines are positive but insufficiently elevated for a firm diagnosis.[59] More specifically, patients with a pheochromocytoma usually have larger relative increases in metanephrines than of the parent catecholamines, whereas patients with false-positive results caused by sympathoadrenal activation usually have larger increases in catecholamines than metanephrines.

The clinical presentation of the patient is also important to consider when interpreting patterns of biochemical results. Patients with tumors that produce large amounts of epinephrine (and also metanephrine) may present with hyperglycemia, dyspnea, and pulmonary edema, signs and symptoms reflecting the potent actions of epinephrine on glucose metabolism and pulmonary physiology. Such patients are also more likely to present with alternating hypotension and hypertension and to have symptoms that occur paroxysmally compared with patients with tumors that produce only norepinephrine (and hence also only normetanephrine). Pheochromocytomas associated with VHL disease produce exclusively norepinephrine and normetanephrine, whereas those occurring in patients with MEN 2 produce epinephrine and are best detected by increases in plasma free metanephrine, with or without accompanying increases in normetanephrine.[65]

Increases in plasma or urinary concentrations of L-dopa, dopamine, and methoxytyramine are not sensitive or specific markers of pheochromocytomas. However, when such increases accompany large increases in norepinephrine and normetanephrine, the pattern suggests metastatic disease. Pheochromocytomas that produce exclusively dopamine are extremely rare, but can be found in patients with paragangliomas, particularly where these have metastasized.

When biochemical testing continues to yield equivocal results, the clonidine suppression test may be useful for further confirming or excluding pheochromocytomas. As originally introduced by Bravo et al,[21] this test was designed to distinguish patients with increases in plasma catecholamines caused by pheochromocytomas from those with increases caused by sympathetic activation. By activating alpha$_2$-adrenoceptors in the brain and on sympathetic nerve endings, clonidine suppresses norepinephrine release by sympathetic nerves. Decreases in elevated plasma norepinephrine after clonidine therefore suggest sympathetic activation, whereas lack of decrease suggests a pheochromocytoma.

A problem with the clonidine suppression test is that patients with normal or mildly increased plasma levels of norepinephrine may have clonidine-induced decreases in plasma norepinephrine, despite the presence of a pheochromocytoma.[230,241] This is particularly troublesome since such patients represent those in whom it is most difficult to conclusively diagnose a pheochromocytoma. Additional measurements of plasma normetanephrine before and after clonidine have therefore been proposed to offer a useful method to overcome this limitation.[59] In a study involving 48 patients with and 49 patients without pheochromocytomas, lack of decrease and elevated plasma levels of norepinephrine or normetanephrine after clonidine confirmed pheochromocytomas with high specificity (98% to 100%). However, of 48 patients with pheochromocytomas, 16 had normal levels or decreases of norepinephrine after clonidine. In contrast, plasma normetanephrine remained elevated after clonidine in all but 2 patients, indicating higher sensitivity (96% versus 67%) and more reliable diagnosis using normetanephrine than norepinephrine responses to clonidine. Box 29-1 outlines the clonidine suppression test protocol with these added testing recommendations.

BOX 29-1 Protocol for Clonidine Suppression Test

Principle: Clonidine activates α_2-adrenergic receptors in the brain and sympathetic nerve endings to suppress norepinephrine release by sympathetic nerves without effect on catecholamine release from pheochromocytomas.

Indication: The test is used to discriminate patients with pheochromocytomas from patients with false-positive test results for catecholamines or metabolites in either plasma or urine.

Procedure: The test is best performed in the morning after an overnight fast. The patient remains recumbent throughout the entire procedure. A forearm venous cannula is placed for baseline and 3-hour blood sampling during the procedure. After at least 20 minutes of supine rest, a baseline blood sample is drawn in a heparinized tube. Clonidine, 4.3 µg/kg of body weight, is then given orally, and a repeat blood sample is drawn 3 hours later. The samples are analyzed for plasma catecholamines, with plasma normetanephrine measurement also recommended.

Interpretation: For optimum clinical specificity, a positive result highly suggestive of a pheochromocytoma includes an elevation of norepinephrine and normetanephrine at 3 hours and a failure to suppress norepinephrine more than 50% and normetanephrine more than 40 % below the baseline plasma level.

Modified from Bravo EL, Tarazi RC, Fouad FM, Vidt DG, Gifford RW, Jr. Clonidine-suppression test: a useful aid in the diagnosis of pheochromocytoma. N Engl J Med 1981;305:623-6, with additional recommendations for normetanephrine testing and interpretation from Eisenhofer G, Goldstein DS, Walther MM, Friberg P, Lenders JW, Keiser HR, Pacak K. Biochemical diagnosis of pheochromocytoma: How to distinguish true- from false-positive test results. J Clin Endocrinol Metab 2003;6:2656-66.

NEUROBLASTOMA

A neuroblastoma is a malignant neoplasm characterized in most cases by overproduction of catecholamines and their metabolites. It is a tumor of postganglionic sympathetic neurons and, like a pheochromocytoma, is of neural crest origin. Unlike pheochromocytomas, neuroblastomas rarely occur in adults[100] and are almost exclusively a pediatric cancer. Neuroblastomas account for approximately 7% of cancer in childhood and are the most common malignancy diagnosed in the first year of life.[98,99] The incidence of neuroblastomas is approximately 10 cases per million children, resulting worldwide in about 10,000 new cases per year.[166] Although familial cases have been reported,[148] the vast majority of neuroblastomas appear to develop sporadically.

The anatomic location of the primary tumor in neuroblastomas parallels the sympathetic nervous system, as predicted from its neuronal origin. The majority of tumors are intraabdominal, arising in the adrenal gland or the upper abdomen, and less frequent locations include the chest, neck, or pelvis regions. Approximately 60% of neuroblastomas are extra adrenal, compared with only about 10% of pheochromocytomas. Metastases in disseminated neuroblastomas may involve bone marrow, bone, lymph nodes, liver, and less frequently the skin, testis, and intracranial structures.

The biological behavior of a neuroblastoma ranges from regression and maturation to an aggressive course with an unfavorable outcome. Neuroblastomas are most notable for a subset of cases with complete regression or maturation to ganglioneuroma, a benign neoplasm. The high rate of neuroblastoma detection in infant screening programs compared with clinically diagnosed cases has also been explained by spontaneous tumor maturation.[110] The majority of clinically diagnosed tumors, however, are aggressive and have an unfavorable outcome.

The clinical stage of the disease (localized versus disseminated) is an important prognostic factor. Patients with early more localized stages of disease, or infants less than age 1 with a localized primary tumor and dissemination limited to skin, liver, and/or bone marrow, are considered to have a better prognosis than other stages.[23] Age at diagnosis is also important in predicting the course of the disease, with infants diagnosed with neuroblastomas in the first year of life having better survival rates.[42] Other factors, including expression of the N-*myc* (also known as *MYCN*) proto-oncogene and unfavorable histological classification, have been associated with an aggressive course of the disease. Unfortunately the overall incidence of metastatic neuroblastoma at the time of diagnosis is approximately 60%, and the need for earlier detection of children with the progressive disseminating tumors remains a diagnostic challenge.

Hypertension and other signs of sympathetic overactivity are uncommon in a neuroblastoma, in contrast with the sustained or paroxysmal hypertension associated with a pheochromocytoma. Patients commonly present with a tumor mass and clinical signs from compression effects on neighboring structures or hematological abnormalities from bone marrow involvement. The low incidence of hypertension and other signs of sympathetic overactivity may be attributed to the characteristic pattern of tumor storage and release of catecholamine and their metabolites. Catecholamine storage capacity in neuroblastoma cells is limited, as evidenced by electron microscopic findings of few secretory granules in comparison with pheochromocytoma cells.[118] Inefficient storage, coupled with excess production of catecholamines, may lead to an increase in the intracellular metabolism of the catecholamines and the release of mainly inactive metabolites. Hypertension, although rare, does occur in some patients with neuroblastomas, and an abundance of secretory granules has been noted in neuroblastoma tissue from some tumors.[176,254]

Laboratory evidence of a functional catecholamine-producing tumor is important in the clinical evaluation when a neuroblastoma is suspected. The catecholamine and metabolite secretion patterns, however, may differ markedly among patients with the tumor. Neuroblastoma cells have the capacity to synthesize dopamine and norepinephrine, depending upon their degree of metabolic maturity, but like postganglionic sympathetic neurons, lack phenylethanolamine *N*-methyltransferase and do not produce epinephrine. Because of variability in catecholamine production and metabolism in neuroblastomas there is no single reliable marker of catecholamine overproduction, and a combination of catecholamine and/or metabolites is often measured in the diagnostic evaluation.

VMA and HVA are the most widely used determinations in both the clinical setting and in screening programs for diagnosis of a neuroblastoma. Elevated urinary excretion of HVA and VMA is the result of excess tumor production of dopamine and norepinephrine, respectively. A small diurnal variation in HVA and VMA excretion and a positive correlation between random and 24-hour urine test results allow the convenient use of random urine specimens, with results expressed as the ratio of catecholamine metabolites to creatinine excretion. Clinical sensitivity in the range of 90% has been reported for urinary HVA and VMA testing by some centers.[152,245] Others have, however, reported a lower rate of neuroblastoma detection. In a large neuroblastoma screening program, in which the population with negative screening results was tracked for occurrence of neuroblastomas, an elevation in VMA, HVA, or both acid metabolites detected only 73% of the tumors.[222] Patients with early stage disease have the highest rate of false-negative test results,[207] and screening programs have been generally unsuccessful in reducing the rate of metastatic neuroblastoma in the population.[110]

Additional markers of catecholamine overproduction have been employed to improve the biochemical detection of neuroblastomas. Free dopamine may be abnormal in urine from neuroblastoma patients with VMA and HVA excretion.[29,196,214] Combined testing for VMA, HVA, and dopamine may therefore improve tumor detection, and in 1993 an international consensus report on neuroblastoma diagnosis added dopamine to the list of acceptable measurements to document the adrenergic nature of the tumor.[23] Plasma measurements of dopamine and L-dopa, the amino acid precursor of dopamine, may also have clinical value and allow the alternate use of plasma.[66,93,102] Measurement of methylated metabolites, especially normetanephrine, has also been explored.[29] When urinary normetanephrine, metanephrine, methoxytyramine, dopamine, norepinephrine, VMA, and HVA were measured, clinical sensitivity for detection of neuroblastomas was 97% to 100% when results of normetanephrine testing were coupled either with VMA in the infants or with HVA in children greater than age 1.[180] Even with an extended panel of catecholamines and metabolite measurements, a low incidence of nonsecreting tumors continues to be identified and should be considered in the interpretation of a negative test result.

The pattern of catecholamine metabolism is associated with important biological and genetic prognostic factors in neuroblastomas. Lower excretion rates of VMA, HVA, dopamine, and norepinephrine are found more often in infants with early stages of the disease, which may explain the lower clinical sensitivity of VMA and HVA testing reported in patients with an early stage neuroblastoma. Elevated levels of catecholamines and their metabolites in urine, on the other hand, are related to aggressive behavior.[264] The prognostic value of VMA and HVA levels, however, has been studied; when disease stage and age at diagnosis are taken into account, the level of VMA and HVA did not have any additional prognostic significance.[42]

The relative excretion of catecholamines and their metabolites may also point to an unfavorable outcome in neuroblastomas. Immature metabolic patterns have been observed in neuroblastoma tumor tissue, based on excretion of dopamine or HVA relative to norepinephrine or VMA. A high ratio of HVA/VMA, dopamine/VMA, or dopamine/norepinephrine indicates a relative deficiency in beta hydroxylation with a reduction in tumor cell conversion of dopamine to norepinephrine. The immature metabolic pattern has been associated with aggressive tumor behavior and other unfavorable prognostic factors,[119,152,264] but the clinical application of metabolic patterns has not been established.

Finally, clinical specificity in detecting neuroblastomas with catecholamine and metabolite measurements may be influenced by the choice of laboratory methods, dietary interference, and other catecholamine-overproduction conditions. Significant advances in the analytical specificity of laboratory methods have reduced much of the exogenous interference, and histopathology remains the ultimate diagnostic criterion for distinguishing neuroblastomas from pheochromocytomas or other catecholamine-producing neurogenic tumors, such as ganglioneuromas and ganglioneuroblastomas.

Dysautonomias and Genetic Disorders

Dysautonomias are conditions in which altered function of the autonomic nervous system adversely affects health.[92] Such conditions range from more common transient episodes in otherwise healthy people (e.g., neurocardiogenic syncope), to progressive neurodegenerative diseases (e.g., multiple system atrophy), and to even more rare genetic disorders, such as dopamine β-hydroxylase deficiency (Table 29-5).

Dysautonomias also range from mechanistically straightforward disorders in which altered autonomic function plays a primary pathophysiological role (e.g., pure autonomic failure), to conditions in which altered autonomic function worsens an independent pathophysiological state (e.g., cardiac failure), and to more mysterious disorders in which the involvement of the autonomic nervous system is less clear (e.g., chronic fatigue syndrome). Abnormalities of blood pressure control represent the common presenting clinical features of the dysautonomias. In those involving

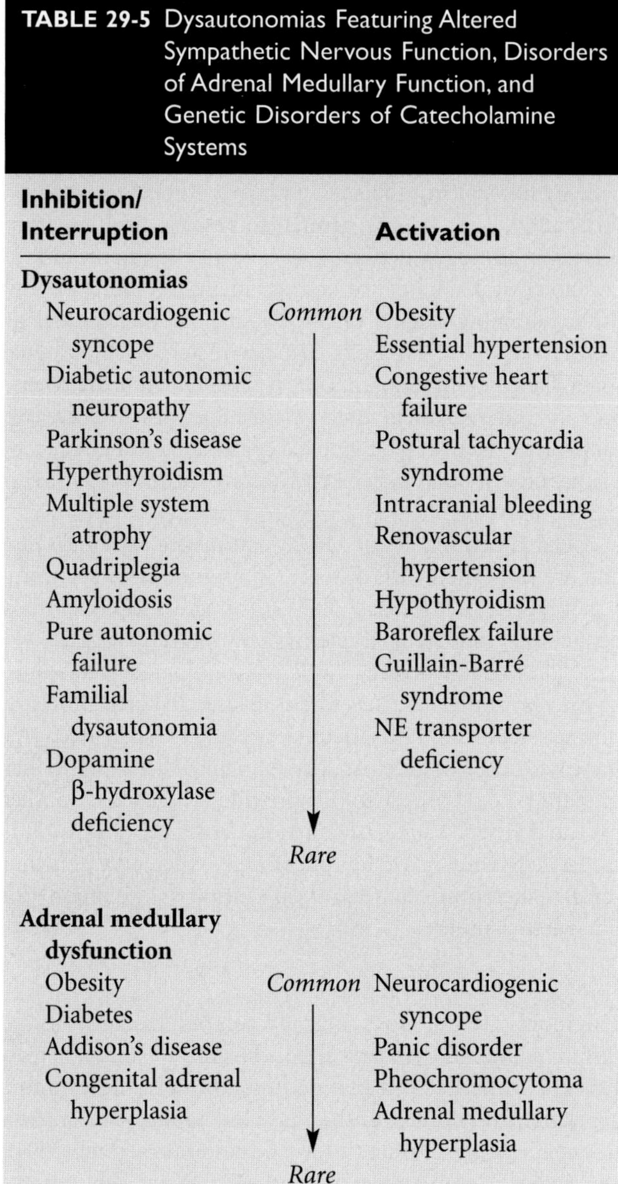

TABLE 29-5 Dysautonomias Featuring Altered Sympathetic Nervous Function, Disorders of Adrenal Medullary Function, and Genetic Disorders of Catecholamine Systems

Inhibition/ Interruption		Activation
Dysautonomias		
Neurocardiogenic syncope	*Common*	Obesity
Diabetic autonomic neuropathy	↓	Essential hypertension
Parkinson's disease		Congestive heart failure
Hyperthyroidism		Postural tachycardia syndrome
Multiple system atrophy		Intracranial bleeding
Quadriplegia		Renovascular hypertension
Amyloidosis		Hypothyroidism
Pure autonomic failure		Baroreflex failure
Familial dysautonomia		Guillain-Barré syndrome
Dopamine β-hydroxylase deficiency		NE transporter deficiency
	Rare	
Adrenal medullary dysfunction		
Obesity	*Common*	Neurocardiogenic syncope
Diabetes	↓	Panic disorder
Addison's disease		Pheochromocytoma
Congenital adrenal hyperplasia		Adrenal medullary hyperplasia
	Rare	

Genetic disorders (not included above): tyrosine hydroxylase deficiency; dopa-responsive dystonia; dihydropteridine reductase deficiency; aromatic L-amino acid decarboxylase deficiency; Menkes' disease; monoamine oxidase deficiency.

inhibition or interruption of sympathetic outflow, the presenting clinical feature is usually hypotension, particularly orthostatic hypotension. In those involving sympathetic activation, there is often hypertension—and in some, excessive increases in heart rate upon standing.

In most dysautonomias, altered or deranged sympathetic nervous function is evident from measurements of plasma or urinary levels of norepinephrine or norepinephrine metabolites. The most well-known dysautonomias, in which measurements of norepinephrine provide useful and even crucial information for diagnosis, involve the autonomic failure syndromes, particularly pure autonomic failure and multiple system atrophy.[167] The most important debilitating clinical manifestation in both conditions is orthostatic hypotension. In their most severe forms, patients are unable to remain in the upright posture for even a few minutes. The basis of the disorder involves failure of neurogenic vasoconstrictor responses secondary to defective sympathoneural release of norepinephrine. In pure autonomic failure, the lesion is postganglionic, involving degeneration of sympathetic nerves and lack of norepinephrine release, whereas in multiple system atrophy, the lesion is preganglionic and sympathetic nerves are present but do not release norepinephrine appropriately. The two syndromes can therefore be diagnosed based on measurements of catecholamines. In both there are usually absent or significantly attenuated increases in plasma concentrations of norepinephrine in response to assumption of upright posture. In pure autonomic failure, levels of norepinephrine and its metabolites are usually severely decreased, reflecting loss of sympathetic nerves. In contrast, in multiple system atrophy resting levels of catecholamines and catecholamine metabolites may be normal or even increased.

In addition to altered sympathetic function in dysautonomias, there are also clinical conditions involving dysfunction of the adrenal medulla (Table 29-5). According to a view promulgated by Canon,[35] the sympathetic and adrenal medullary systems function as a single emergency system. It has now, however, become increasingly clear that sympathetic and adrenal medullary systems are regulated separately and often in divergent directions.[56] This is illustrated by the relatively common clinical conditions of obesity and neurocardiogenic syncope. Sympathetic nervous activation in obesity is implicated to contribute to obesity-related hypertension, whereas decreased epinephrine release may participate in the changes in fatty acid metabolism and energy metabolism that accompany and contribute to weight gain. In neurocardiogenic syncope, β-adrenoceptor–mediated vasodilation—resulting from increased circulating epinephrine—combined with reduced α-adrenoceptor–mediated vasoconstriction, caused by withdrawal of sympathetic tone, are both implicated in contributing to orthostatic hypotension.

With the exception of pure autonomic failure and pheochromocytomas, abnormalities in plasma or urinary levels of catecholamines in most of the above disorders, particularly those that are more common, are usually subtle and not easily interpreted. Plasma or urinary levels of catecholamines and catecholamine metabolites in such conditions have mainly been measured for purposes of research, to better characterize and understand the particular disorder. Resulting improved understanding of such disorders, combined with advances in measurement techniques and improved ability to interpret different patterns of neurochemical results, will likely lead to increasing use of measurements of catecholamines and catecholamine metabolites for routine diagnostic and prognostic purposes. This is becoming particularly apparent for the conditions that have a hereditary basis or are due to de novo mutations of specific genes, in which advances in molecular genetics are enabling precise identification of the genetic abnormality.[90]

Familial dysautonomia, dopamine β-hydroxylase deficiency, norepinephrine transporter deficiency, and congenital adrenal hyperplasia include dysautonomias or conditions associated with adrenal medullary dysfunction in which the specific genetic abnormalities have been identified. There are also other disorders involving mutations of genes coding for proteins involved in catecholamine synthesis and metabolism in which the clinical manifestations do not clearly involve the sympathoadrenal systems or may be so globally severe that abnormalities of autonomic or adrenal medullary function are obscured (Table 29-5).

Deficiencies of tyrosine hydroxylase or of enzymes involved in production of tetrahydrobiopterin cofactor (e.g., dopa-responsive dystonia) usually result in presentation of severe neurological abnormalities in early childhood. Depending on the exact mutation, deficiencies of tyrosine hydroxylase can involve moderate to severe loss of enzyme activity, most accurately diagnosed by low cerebrospinal fluid levels of catecholamine metabolites, such as MHPG and HVA, but normal levels of 5-HIAA.[19,20] In the autosomal dominant form of dopa-responsive dystonia (Segawa disease), failure to synthesize tetrahydrobiopterin cofactor leads to a similar clinical and neurochemical phenotype as in the rarer tyrosine hydroxylase deficiency syndrome.[226] In contrast to classical forms of tetrahydrobiopterin deficiency, characterized by phenylketonuria (e.g., dihydropteridine reductase deficiencies), deficiencies of guanosine triphosphate (GTP) cyclohydrolase responsible for dopa-responsive dystonia are not accompanied by hyperphenylalaninemia and require diagnosis by measurements of pterins and pterin metabolism, in addition to measurements of catecholamine metabolites.[14]

Patients with aromatic L-amino acid decarboxylase deficiency present with clinical and biochemical manifestations that overlap those of the tyrosine hydroxylase deficiency states described previously. However, this deficiency state is characterized by additional decreases in CSF and urinary levels of 5-HIAA.[114] Also, levels of L-dopa in urine, plasma, and cerebrospinal fluid are increased, and not decreased as in the other deficiency states. Levels of 5-hydroxytryptophan are similarly increased.

The major clinical feature of patients with deficiency of dopamine β-hydroxylase is orthostatic hypotension caused by reduced synthesis and release of norepinephrine by sympathetic nerves.[9] The deficiency is characterized neurochemically by decreased levels of norepinephrine and norepinephrine metabolites and increased levels of dopamine and dopamine metabolites. Diagnosis is best achieved from an increased ratio of plasma dopamine to norepinephrine. Copper deficiency in Menkes' disease is due to defects in the gene coding for a copper-transporting adenosine triphosphatase.[129] Because dopamine β-hydroxylase is a copper-dependent enzyme, the deficiency is associated with decreased activity of the enzyme and reduced production of norepinephrine from dopamine. Prompt diagnosis at childbirth is essential for copper-replacement therapy, and is best achieved from measurements of ratios of plasma concentrations of DOPAC or L-dopa to DHPG.

Congenital adrenal hyperplasia is a relatively common genetic disorder that occurs secondary to deficiencies of certain enzymes, usually 21-hydroxylase, responsible for synthesis of cortisol.[172] The disorder is characterized clinically by adrenal insufficiency with or without salt wasting, virilization, and in girls genital ambiguity resulting from increased androgen levels. As a result of the importance of adrenocortical steroids for adrenal medullary function and for maintaining activity of phenylethanolamine *N*-methyltransferase, the disorder is also characterized by adrenal medullary hypofunction and decreased epinephrine release and intraadrenal metabolism to metanephrine. Decreased plasma levels of metanephrine provide a biomarker of disease severity that may be useful for prognosis and directing therapy.[38]

Isolated deficiencies of MAO A and B are extremely rare and are associated with distinct clinical and neurochemical phenotypes.[154] Deficiency of MAO A is associated with a behavioral disorder characterized by increased aggressiveness. Plasma and urinary levels of deaminated metabolites of catecholamines are severely decreased, whereas levels of normetanephrine and metanephrine are increased. An increased ratio of plasma normetanephrine to DHPG has therefore been proposed to provide a sensitive marker for the deficiency state. In contrast, deficiency of MAO B is associated with a mild phenotype, the only biochemical alteration is increased urinary excretion of phenylethylamine.

Carcinoid

Carcinoids are the most common tumors arising from the diffuse neuroendocrine system of the GI tract and pancreas. Derived primarily from enterochromaffin cells, these tumors are widely distributed in the body but found with greatest frequency in the GI tract (74%) and respiratory tract (25%). Carcinoids are often classified as APUDomas (*a*mine *p*recursor *u*ptake and *d*ecarboxylation) because of the ability of enterochromaffin cells to take up and decarboxylate amino acid precursors of biogenic amines. In this regard, carcinoid tumors share certain pathological and biological similarities with pheochromocytomas.

The usual carcinoid tumor is solid and yellow-tan in appearance. Tumor cells exhibit a monotonous morphology, with pink granular cytoplasm and round nuclei with infrequent mitoses. Most carcinoids can be recognized by their reactions to silver stains and to neuroendocrine cell markers, such as chromogranin and neuron-specific enolase. Ultrastructurally, carcinoids possess numerous membrane-bound, electron-dense neurosecretory granules. These granules contain peptide hormones and bioactive amines, which can occasionally be identified by immunocytochemical techniques.

Carcinoid tumors are traditionally classified according to their presumed origin from the embryonic foregut (bronchus, lung, stomach, duodenum, and pancreas), midgut (ileum, jejunum, appendix, and proximal colon), or hindgut (rectum and distal colon).[146] The most common sites for these tumors are the bronchus and/or lung (33%), ileum and/or jejunum (20%), rectum (10%), and appendix (8%).[177] A new classification system has also been proposed that takes into account variations in histopathological characteristics.[31] The overall incidence of clinically significant carcinoids in the United States has been estimated to be 1 to 2 cases per 100,000 persons. Carcinoid tumors may develop in all age groups, but they appear most frequently in adults, with a mean age of 63 for tumors of the small intestine and respiratory tract.[124] Clinically, most patients are asymptomatic until metastases are present. Bowel obstruction and abdominal pain are the most frequent presenting symptoms.

Carcinoid tumors show aggressive malignant behavior depending on the origin, depth of penetration, and size of the primary tumor.[123] Most rectal carcinomas are found incidentally at endoscopy. They are often less than 1 cm and have a low rate of metastasis, even though they may show extensive local spread. Carcinoids of the appendix are seen in about 1 in every 300 appendectomies. Almost all are less than 1 cm, and distant metastasis is rare. By contrast, 90% of intestinal carcinoids that penetrate halfway through the muscle wall will have spread to lymph nodes and distant sites at the time of diagnosis. More than 70% of intestinal carcinoids 1 to 2 cm in diameter metastasize to the liver. Fortunately, most carcinoid tumors grow slowly, and patients may live for many years. The 5-year survival rate of patients with carcinoids of the appendix is about 99%. Patients with carcinoids in the small intestine have a 5-year survival rate of about 50%.

As with normal gut endocrine cells, carcinoids synthesize, store, and release a variety of hormones and biogenic amines. One of the best characterized of these substances is serotonin. Carcinoid tumors also produce and secrete other biologically active substances, including histamine, kallikrein, bradykinins, tachykinins, prostaglandins, dopamine, and norepinephrine. Production of these substances varies in relation to the tissue origin of the tumor.[192] For example, midgut carcinoids release large quantities of serotonin into the circulation, whereas tumors derived from the foregut secrete primarily 5-hydroxytryptophan (5-HTP) (a serotonin precursor) and histamine rather than serotonin.[135] Primary hindgut carcinoids usually show no secretory activity. In some instances, carcinoid tumors may coexist with other endocrine tumors that produce gastrin, insulin, adrenocorticotropic hormone (ACTH), and catecholamines. Gastric foregut carcinoids may be associated with MEN 1.[32]

Secretion of vasoactive substances into the systemic circulation plays an important role in the development of the carcinoid syndrome. The full-blown syndrome associated with the humoral manifestations of these tumors is striking but uncommon, usually occurring only after metastasis to the liver and release of these substances directly into the systemic circulation. The classic clinical presentation of the carcinoid syndrome includes pronounced flushing (especially on the face and neck), diarrhea, bronchoconstriction, and eventual right-sided valvular heart failure. Overproduction of serotonin is found in 90% to 100% of patients with the carcinoid syndrome and is thought to be responsible for the diarrhea by its known effects on gut motility and fluid secretion. Serotonin receptor antagonists relieve the diarrhea in most cases. The pathophysiology of carcinoid flushing is not yet known, but tachykinins, bradykinins, and histamine may be mediators. Somatostatin analogues reduce circulating levels of these vasodilators. The causative agents of bronchoconstriction are also unknown, but tachykinins and bradykinins are likely mediators.

The clinical chemical evaluation of the carcinoid syndrome relies on measurements of serotonin and its metabolites in body fluids and tissue.[133] In patients with the typical carcinoid syndrome, 5-HTP is converted to serotonin and stored in tumor secretory granules and in platelets. A small amount of serotonin remains in plasma, but most is converted to 5-HIAA, which is excreted in urine. These patients have increased blood and platelet serotonin levels and increased urinary 5-HIAA. However, some foregut carcinoid tumors lack the aromatic L-amino acid decarboxylase and secrete 5-HTP rather than serotonin into the bloodstream.[193] Patients with these tumors have normal serotonin concentrations in blood and in platelets, but urinary levels are increased because 5-HTP is converted to serotonin in the kidney; urinary 5-HIAA levels may be slightly elevated.

Patients with serotonin-producing carcinoid tumors usually have striking increases in urinary 5-HIAA excretion (at least tenfold), but occasionally elevations are smaller. False-positive elevations can occur if the patient ingests serotonin-rich foods or medications, such as bananas, pineapples, chocolate, walnuts, pecans, kiwi fruit, plums, avocados, and cough medicines containing guaifenesin.[72,138] Conversely, alcohol, aspirin, and other drugs can suppress 5-HIAA levels. Patients should avoid these agents during 24-hour urine collections. Incomplete or excess 24-hour urine collections may be more accurately assessed in terms of a creatinine ratio. Fasting plasma 5-HIAA has been proposed as a convenient replacement for urine collections.[52]

The upper limit of the normal reference interval for urinary 5-HIAA excretion is variably defined and may be as low as 6 mg/day (30 µmol/day) if dietary and medicinal intake are controlled, or as high as 15 mg/day (80 µmol/day) to reduce false-positive results.[191] At an intermediate value of 10.7 mg/day (56 µmol/day), urinary 5-HIAA has a reported 77% sensitivity and 97% specificity for carcinoid disease.[34] To exclude the presence of a carcinoid tumor, lower cutoff values may be preferred (higher sensitivity); to confirm the presence of a carcinoid tumor, higher cutoff values (higher specificity) would be indicated.

Most physicians rely on the measurement of 5-HIAA to diagnose carcinoid syndrome. But when a patient strongly suspected for carcinoid syndrome shows normal or borderline increases in urinary 5-HIAA, documentation of elevated serotonin levels in platelets, plasma, whole blood, or urine may help establish the diagnosis.[134] Platelet serotonin has been reported to be more sensitive than urinary 5-HIAA for detecting carcinoids that produce small or moderate amounts of serotonin, such as foregut and hindgut carcinoids and midgut carcinoids with a low tumor volume.[171] Also, platelet serotonin levels are not affected by the patient's diet. Platelets can be saturated at high serotonin secretion rates, however, and 5-HIAA is often preferred for monitoring high serotonin production.

Attempts are being made to identify more sensitive and specific markers for carcinoids. For example, measurement of chromogranin A in serum is reported to be more sensitive than urinary 5-HIAA in detecting carcinoid tumors and may reflect tumor size, but specificity is lower.[193] Plasma levels of neuron-specific enolase, neuropeptide K, and substance P have also been suggested as diagnostic and prognostic markers in carcinoid tumors.

ANALYTICAL METHODOLOGY

Numerous methods have been proposed for the determination of catecholamines, serotonin, and their metabolites in biological fluids. In clinical practice, laboratory determinations are performed primarily for diagnosis and follow-up of patients with catecholamine- or serotonin-secreting tumors. Most laboratories measure urinary free catecholamines, metanephrine, normetanephrine, and VMA in the evaluation of pheochromocytomas, and plasma catecholamine measurements are used in some medical centers and plasma metanephrines have been applied more recently. For detection of neuroblastomas, urinary HVA and VMA are most commonly ordered in clinical practice, but other catecholamine metabolites and dopamine are also measured. Diagnostic evaluation of patients with carcinoid tumor routinely involves the measurement of 5-HIAA, and the measurement of serotonin in platelets and urine has been advocated. In this section, we focus on current clinical laboratory methods with attention to sample preparation, current analytical techniques, and reference intervals. Protocols for selected methods used in current practice are available on this book's accompanying Evolve site, found at http://evolve.elsevier.com/Tietz/textbook.[216] Earlier fluorometric, spectrophotometric, and radioenzymatic methods are briefly addressed, with more extensive coverage in an earlier work by Rosano and co-workers.[218]

Catecholamines and Metabolites

HPLC, coupled with electrochemical or fluorometric detection, now provides the most widely used assay method for measurements of urinary or plasma catecholamines in the routine clinical laboratory.[58,183,218] Once equipment is purchased and trained staff are in place, the technique can provide reliable, reproducible, and relatively rapid measurements of large numbers of samples at minimum cost per sample. Problems with interference from drugs or dietary constituents are relatively easy to identify by careful inspection of chromatograms. Consistent sources of interference are usually remedied by simple changes to chromatographic conditions. A large number of different HPLC methodologies have been described, each requiring a preanalytical extraction step to concentrate (plasma) and cleanup (plasma and urine) the sample.

In contrast to the catecholamines, measurements of urinary metanephrines and VMA are still based in some routine laboratories on the early spectrophotometric assays developed by Pisano, Crout, and others in the late 1950s and early 1960s.[204,205] Despite subsequent development of a variety of preanalytical cleanup and extraction procedures, these assays remain susceptible to analytical interference. They are also restricted to measurements in urine. Another limitation for spectrophotometric or fluorometric assays of urinary metanephrines is that these methods do not allow separate (fractionated) measurements of normetanephrine and metanephrine.

Tests of urinary total metanephrines, as measured by spectrophotometric assays, are best abandoned in favor of measurement methods that incorporate a chromatographic step to fractionate normetanephrine and metanephrine and allow their separate measurement. Since significant numbers of pheochromocytomas produce mainly or solely only one of the two metabolites, separate measurements help to ensure that small or mild increases in one metabolite are not diluted by the normal levels of the other. Additionally the chromatographic step provides an additional level of selectivity, thereby minimizing analytical interference. Although HPLC with electrochemical detection provides the most widely available measurement method for urinary fractionated metanephrines, newer methods involving mass spectrometry are likely to offer further improvement. These methods, including gas chromatography–mass spectrometry and liquid chromatography–tandem mass spectrometry,[36,44,242] should provide higher analytical specificity than HPLC methods, which with continuing improvements in instrumentation and cost should become more widely applicable for diagnostic purposes.

Collection and Storage of Samples

The conditions under which plasma or urine samples are collected can be crucial to the reliability and interpretation of test results. Many clinicians prefer 24-hour collections of urine over blood sampling since the former avoids many of the rigid sampling conditions associated with blood collections and is more convenient for clinical staff to implement. However, 24-hour collections of urine are not always easily, conveniently, or reliably collected by patients, particularly pediatric patients. Also, influences of diet and sympathoadrenal activation associated with physical activity or changes in posture are not as easily controlled for as they are for blood collections.

Because of the possible errors resulting from incomplete 24-hour urine collections or uncontrolled influences of physical activity, some investigators advocate spot or overnight urine collections.[104,131,202] Correction for differences in duration of collection is achieved by normalizing catecholamine or catecholamine metabolite excretion against urinary creatinine excretion. Additional considerations for urine collected under these conditions include dietary protein, muscle mass, level of physical activity, and time of day, all of which impact creatinine excretion and may further confound interpretation of results.[27,47,189,252]

Studies on the stability of catecholamines in urine and plasma have yielded mixed results with variable recommendations on appropriate preservatives and methods of collection.* Elaborate techniques for sample preservation as recommended in earlier years now appear to be largely unnecessary. Variable findings may be explained by autooxidation, particularly at alkaline pH, or deconjugation, particularly at low pH—two processes with opposing effects on levels of free amines. The general recommendation is that catecholamines in urine samples are best preserved with hydrochloric acid (HCl) to maintain urine acid. Aliquots are best stored frozen over protracted periods of time at −80 °C to further minimize autooxidation and deconjugation. Similarly, blood samples are best collected into tubes containing heparin or ethylenediaminetetraacetic acid (EDTA) as an anticoagulant and stored on ice before centrifugation at 4 °C, with separation of plasma for further storage at −80 °C.

Interferences from and Influences of Diet and Drugs

Dietary constituents or drugs can either cause direct analytical interference in assays or influence the physiological processes that determine plasma and urinary levels of catecholamines and catecholamine metabolites. In the former circumstances, the interference can be highly variable depending on the particular measurement method. In the latter circumstances, interference is usually of a more general nature and independent of the measurement method (Table 29-6).

Development of new drugs, variations in assay techniques, and continuing improvements in analytical procedures often make it difficult to identify which directly interfering medications should be avoided for a given analytical test. More readily identifiable and generalized sources of interference that are independent of the particular assay method tend to be associated with drugs that have primary actions on catecholamine systems. Because of the importance of these systems as therapeutic targets, such drugs represent a relatively common source of false-positive results.

Tricyclic antidepressants in particular are a major source of false-positive results for measurements of norepinephrine and normetanephrine in plasma or urine.[59] Presumably this is due to the primary inhibitory actions of these agents on monoamine reuptake. The result is an increased escape of norepinephrine from sympathetic nerve terminals into the bloodstream.[68,248]

Other medications that can cause significant interference but that are less commonly encountered during testing for pheochromocytomas include L-dopa, Sinemet, alpha-methyldopa (Aldomet), and MAO inhibitors. L-dopa that is used alone or as carbidopa (Sinemet) for the treatment of Parkinson's disease is an alumina-extractable catechol and the direct precursor of dopamine. The drug can therefore interfere directly with catecholamine assays and is also converted by catecholamine synthesizing and metabolizing enzymes to catecholamine products and metabolites with additional interfering actions.[40,210] Similarly the antihypertensive agent alpha-methyldopa is metabolized by catecholamine biosynthetic and metabolizing enzymes to alpha-methyldopamine, alpha-methylnorepinephrine, and other products, which in some but not all assays can result in significant interference.[49,184] Because active cellular uptake and not metabolism is the main determinant of catecholamine clearance, inhibitors of MAO have little effect on plasma or urinary catecholamines.[54] However, by blocking the main pathway for catabolism of the *O*-methylated catecholamine metabolites, MAO inhibitors can cause substantial increases in plasma levels and urinary excretion of normetanephrine and metanephrine.[62,251]

Reference Intervals

Interpretation of a biochemical test result as normal or abnormal depends on availability of valid reference intervals (see Chapter 16). For tests of a single analyte, such as VMA, it can be expected that at least 2.5% of patients without pheochromocytomas will have values for the analyte above the upper reference limit and 2.5% below the lower reference limit. Up to a 5% incidence of false-positive results might be expected for tests of pairs of analytes, such as norepinephrine and epinephrine in tests of urinary or plasma catecholamines or normetanephrine and metanephrine in tests of plasma free or urinary fractionated metanephrines. False-positive rates usually, however, tend to be higher than expected; this is likely due to reduced control over sampling conditions and sources of interference or differences in clinical characteristics of reference and patient populations.

Use of appropriately matched reference populations can be important for effective diagnosis of monoamine-producing tumors among different populations of patients tested for such tumors. Urinary and plasma levels of catecholamines and metanephrines show different ranges in hypertensives or hospitalized patients compared with normotensive healthy volunteers,[142,183,219] children compared with adults,[183,214,256] and males compared with females.[57,79] Also, levels of catecholamines and metanephrines in 24-hour urine specimens and plasma are not normally distributed.[156,219] Normalization of distributions, usually achiev-

*References 16, 18, 175, 203, 220, 255.

able by logarithmic transformation, is therefore useful for establishment of valid reference intervals.

Patients with hypertension tend to have higher plasma and 24-hour urinary levels of catecholamines and metanephrines than normotensives.[57,89,142,153] Use of reference intervals established in hypertensive rather than normotensive populations therefore minimizes the likelihood of false-positive results in patients tested for pheochromocytomas because of signs and symptoms. However, these same reference intervals are not necessarily appropriate for patients with pheochromocytomas who are normotensive and asymptomatic and tested for the tumor because of a hereditary predisposition or a finding of an adrenal incidentaloma. In some of these patients, the tumor may be too small to produce large enough amounts of catecholamines or catecholamine metabolites for a positive test result using reference intervals established in hypertensive or hospital patient populations. For these patient populations, use of reference intervals established in normotensive healthy volunteers may be more appropriate.

Reference intervals for plasma and urinary catecholamines and catecholamine metabolites also differ according to sex and age. Females have lower plasma concentrations of epinephrine and metanephrine than males.[57] Similarly, 24-hour urinary outputs of catecholamines and metanephrines are lower in women than men[79,128]; for epinephrine this difference remains significant when values are normalized for creatinine excretion.[79] Plasma levels of norepinephrine and normetanephrine increase with advancing age in adults, whereas plasma levels of epinephrine and metanephrine are little affected.[57] Age-related increases in 24-hour urinary outputs of norepinephrine and normetanephrine have also been reported,[128,153] but not consistently by all studies.[79] In general, the influences of age

TABLE 29-6 Drug-Induced Increases in Catecholamines and Metanephrines

	CATECHOLAMINES		METANEPHRINES	
	NE	EPI	NMN	MN
Tricyclic antidepressants				
Amitriptyline (Elavil), imipramine (Tofranil), nortriptyline (Aventyl)	+++	–	+++	–
α-Blockers (nonselective)				
Phenoxybenzamine (Dibenzyline)	+++	–	+++	–
α-Blockers (α_1-selective)				
Doxazosin (Cardura), terazosin (Hytrin), prazosin (Minipress)	+	–	–	–
β-Blockers				
Atenolol (Tenormin), metoprolol (Lopressor), propranolol (Inderal), labetalol* (Normodyne)	+	+	+	+
Calcium channel antagonists				
Nifedipine (Procardia), amlodipine (Norvasc), diltiazem (Cardizem), verapamil (Calan)	+	+	–	–
Vasodilators				
Hydralazine (Apresoline), isosorbide (Isordil, Dilatrate), minoxidil (Loniten)	+	–	unknown	
Monoamine oxidase inhibitors				
Phenelzine (Nardil), tranylcypromine (Parnate), selegiline (Eldepryl)	–	–	+++	+++
Sympathomimetics				
Ephedrine, pseudoephedrine (Sudafed), amphetamines, albuterol (Proventil)	++	++	++	++
Stimulants				
Caffeine (coffee,* tea), nicotine (Tobacco), theophylline	++	++	unknown	
Miscellaneous				
Levodopa, carbidopa (Sinemet)*	++	–	unknown	
Cocaine	++	++	unknown	

+++, substantial increase; ++, moderate increase; +, mild increase if any; –, little or no increase.
*Indicates a drug that can also cause direct analytical interference with some methods. Adapted in part from references 59 and 263.

and sex on adult reference intervals are minor and perhaps only relevant to consider for patients with borderline normal or abnormal biochemical test results.

Of greater importance than the age- and sex-related differences in adults are the much larger differences in plasma concentrations and urinary outputs of catecholamines and their metabolites in children compared with adults. Because of the dynamic changes that occur throughout childhood, and also because of the difficulty of obtaining complete urine collections, a standard practice for biochemical testing in children is to normalize excretion of catecholamines and metanephrines to that of creatinine. When this is done, ratios of urinary catecholamines or metanephrines to creatinine show a decrease with age through childhood.[30,163,214] It is therefore imperative that age-appropriate reference intervals be used for biochemical testing in children.

Another patient population in which the usual reference intervals are often invalid and in which diagnosis of a catecholamine-producing tumor can prove particularly difficult involves patients with renal failure.[18,238] In end-stage renal failure, urine collections may be impossible, and even in less severely affected patients results of 24-hour urine testing are difficult to interpret.[179] Impaired renal function results in dramatic increases in plasma concentrations of VMA and sulfate-conjugated metanephrines, rendering these tests invalid.[164,181] In contrast, since the circulatory clearance of plasma catecholamines and free metanephrines is largely independent of renal function, measurements of these analytes in plasma represent the most appropriate tests for diagnosis of pheochromocytomas in renal failure.[84] Nevertheless, plasma levels of catecholamines and free metanephrines tend to be elevated more in patients with renal failure than in normal and hypertensive populations. Also, dietary and medication-associated interferences with chromatographic analysis tend to be much more pronounced in patients with renal failure, making it difficult to obtain reliable results.

Plasma Catecholamines

Highly sensitive, specific, and reliable assay methods are required for measuring the normally very low concentrations of epinephrine, norepinephrine, and dopamine in plasma. Both unconjugated (free) and sulfoconjugated catecholamines circulate in human plasma and are increased in plasma from patients with pheochromocytomas.[209] Clinical measurement of the active free form is preferred because of the potential influence of diet on the conjugated fraction.

The earliest chemical assays were fluorometric methods, but radioenzymatic, radioimmunoassay (RIA), enzyme immunoassay (EIA), HPLC, and gas-liquid chromatography (GLC) methods with flame ionization, electron capture, or mass spectrometric detection have also been reported. Currently, HPLC assays are commonly employed for the determination of epinephrine and norepinephrine in plasma.[17,108,143] However, HPLC methods do require preliminary extraction and concentration of plasma to measure the very low levels of catecholamines found in normal subjects. The most common pretreatment involves alumina extraction, with or without a cation-exchange step; boric acid gels provide an alternate approach for selective adsorption of catecholamines. Organic solvents, acid deproteinization, ultrafiltration, and other solid phase extraction procedures can also be used to pretreat samples.[107,212] Many HPLC procedures analyze the plasma extract using reversed-phase chromatography with ion-pairing reagents; others use cation-exchange HPLC columns to separate the extracted amines. Electrochemical detection using amperometric or coulometric measurement is commonly used to quantify the catecholamines; detection limits are similar to those of radioenzymatic methods. HPLC separation can also be coupled to fluorescence detection, but precolumn or postcolumn derivatization techniques are required to enhance sensitivity and specificity. Automated procedures have been described that are sensitive, precise, and suitable for routine clinical applications; manual pretreatment may or may not be required.[53,130,262]

A method for measuring plasma free catecholamines based on HPLC with amperometric detection is available on this book's accompanying Evolve site and representative adult reference intervals[243] for plasma catecholamines are shown in Table 29-7.

Plasma Metanephrines

The metanephrines, normetanephrine and metanephrine, and the *O*-methylated metabolite of dopamine, methoxytyramine, are present in plasma in free and sulfate or glucuronide conjugated forms. Plasma concentrations of the conjugates are twentyfold to thirtyfold higher than those of the free metabolites. Rather than reflecting differences in rates of formation, the higher plasma levels of conjugated

TABLE 29-7 Plasma Catecholamine Reference Intervals for Adults

Position	Norepinephrine pg/mL (pmol/L)	Epinephrine pg/mL (pmol/L)	Dopamine pg/mL (pmol/L)
Supine (30 min)	110-410 (650-2423)	<50 (<273)	<87 (<475)
Sitting (15 min)	120-680 (709-4019)	<60 (<328)	<87 (<475)
Standing (30 min)	125-700 (739-4137)	<90 (<491)	<87 (<475)

metabolites reflect their relatively slow circulatory clearance by renal extraction and elimination in the urine.[88] This contrasts with the free metabolites, which are cleared rapidly from the bloodstream by active extraneuronal uptake mechanisms throughout tissue of the body.

The free *O*-methylated amine metabolites are present in plasma at picomolar concentrations that have made their accurate measurement technically difficult. Measurements of plasma metanephrines therefore represent relatively recent developments. The first method enabling accurate measurement of plasma free normetanephrine involved a radioenzymatic assay in which normetanephrine was converted to ^{3}H-labeled metanephrine using preparations of the enzyme phenylethanolamine-*N*-methyltransferase, incubated with ^{3}H-methyl-labeled *S*-adenosylmethionine.[141] This method, however, did not allow measurements of metanephrine or methoxytyramine, and therefore had limited clinical utility.

The first HPLC methods for measuring plasma metanephrines in the early 1990s featured an acid-hydrolysis step similar to that used for routine measurements of urinary metanephrines.[181] These measurements of plasma deconjugated (free plus conjugated) metanephrines indicated promise for diagnosis of pheochromocytomas. Very high levels of the deconjugated metabolites were also found in patients with renal failure.

An HPLC method for the more difficult measurement of plasma free metanephrines was first described in 1993.[155] This method, like those involving measurements of plasma or urinary deconjugated metanephrines, requires a preanalytical cation-exchange extraction and purification step. The low plasma concentrations of free metanephrines present several technical challenges. In particular, low levels of interfering substances, such as acetaminophen, tend to be more troublesome to measurements of plasma concentrations of the free metabolites than to the higher deconjugated metabolites. Consequently, there is a necessity for a more rigorous preanalytical extraction and purification procedure than required for the deconjugated metabolites. The requirement for high analytical sensitivity also requires a specialized electrochemical detection system and relatively pulse-free solvent delivery system. Optimal separation of the *O*-methylated amines from potentially interfering substances is best achieved using relatively long chromatographic run times of up to 40 minutes, a limiting factor for sample throughput.

Despite the above difficulties and limitations, the original HPLC method for measurement of plasma free metanephrines has been reproduced and improved upon in numerous clinical laboratories. Improvements include a method that is free from interference from the commonly used pain medication acetaminophen.[213] Such developments have been driven by increasing recognition of the high diagnostic sensitivity of measurements of plasma free metanephrines for detection of pheochromocytomas. There remains a continuing necessity for further improvements in assay technology that will increase robustness of the method and more widely advance portability of the method to the routine clinical chemistry laboratory. This need is being met by commercial development of HPLC kit methods and technical advances in measurement methods. Liquid chromatography coupled with tandem mass spectrometry represents one such advance offering considerable promise for analytically specific, high-throughput measurements suitable for the routine clinical chemistry laboratory.[216] Improvements in detection sensitivity have already extended application of this method from measurements of urinary deconjugated metanephrines[242] to the much lower levels of free metanephrines in plasma. Representative reference intervals for plasma concentrations of free and deconjugated (free plus conjugated) metanephrines in normotensive and hypertensive adults and in normotensive children are shown in Table 29-8.

TABLE 29-8 Reference Intervals for Plasma Free and Deconjugated Metanephrines in Normotensive and Hypertensive Adults and in Normotensive Children

	FREE METANEPHRINES		DECONJUGATED METANEPHRINES	
	Normetanephrine	**Metanephrine**	**Normetanephrine**	**Metanephrine**
Hypertensive adults				
pg/mL	24-145	12-72	755-5623	327-2042
nmol/L	0.13-0.79	0.06-0.37	4.1-30.7	1.7-10.4
Normotensive adults				
pg/mL	18-101	12-67	624-3041	328-1837
nmol/L	0.10-0.55	0.06-0.34	3.4-16.6	1.7-9.3
Normotensive children				
pg/mL	22-83	10-95	851-2398	380-1995
nmol/L	0.12-0.45	0.05-0.48	4.7-13.1	1.9-10.1

Plasma L-dopa, DOPAC, and DHPG

HPLC measurements of plasma catechols are usually limited to dopamine, norepinephrine, and epinephrine. However, with an alumina adsorption extraction procedure it is also possible to simultaneously measure several other catechols by HPLC[58] or microchip electrophoresis.[240] These catechols include DHPG, the deaminated metabolite of norepinephrine and epinephrine; DOPAC, the deaminated metabolite of dopamine; and 3,4-dihydroxyphenylalanine (L-dopa), the immediate precursor of dopamine. All are present in plasma at concentrations many fold higher than the catecholamines, making their detection relatively simple once appropriate chromatographic separation is achieved.

Each of the above catechols can provide unique and useful clinical information about the function of peripheral catecholamine systems.[87] DHPG in plasma is almost exclusively derived from deamination of norepinephrine in sympathetic nerves. These measurements therefore provide information about the activity of MAO. Decreases in plasma DHPG combined with reciprocal increases in normetanephrine, as assessed by plasma DHPG/normetanephrine ratios, provide a particularly useful method for identifying patients with deficiencies of MAO. DHPG is derived in part from deamination of the norepinephrine recaptured by sympathetic nerves and in part from leakage of the transmitter from storage vesicles into the sympathetic axoplasm. Provided appropriate procedures are employed to distinguish the two sources, measurements of DHPG can therefore be used to evaluate norepinephrine transporter function and assess the state of sympathoneural transmitter stores.

Since DHPG is derived almost exclusively from sympathetic nerves, it has also been proposed that these measurements might be useful for distinguishing patients with high plasma norepinephrine concentrations caused by sympathetic activation from those with high norepinephrine concentrations caused by a pheochromocytoma.[24] Unfortunately, because some pheochromocytomas produce significant quantities of DHPG,[233] use of plasma norepinephrine/DHPG ratios has turned out to have limited value for diagnosis of pheochromocytomas.

Approximately 8% of the L-dopa synthesized in sympathetic nerves is not converted to dopamine, but instead escapes into the bloodstream. Plasma concentrations of L-dopa therefore provide information about the activity of tyrosine hydroxylase, the rate-limiting enzyme in catecholamine synthesis.[95] Changes in plasma L-dopa also occur in a variety of disorders that feature derangements in catecholamine synthesis. Patients with neuroblastomas can have extremely high plasma L-dopa levels.[66,93] Elevated plasma L-dopa concentrations occasionally also occur in patients with pheochromocytomas, particularly patients with malignant disease.[93] Small amounts of circulating L-dopa also appear to be derived from melanocytes, where the amino acid is produced during phase I melanogenesis. Thus highly elevated plasma L-dopa levels can occur in patients with melanoma, particularly where this is associated with development of metastases.[69,158] Increases in plasma L-dopa also occur in patients with deficiencies of aromatic L-amino acid decarboxylase, and decreases occur in inherited disorders featuring impaired tyrosine hydroxylase activity.

Although simultaneous measurements of plasma L-dopa, DHPG, and the catecholamines offer considerable clinical utility, adoption of the method in the routine clinical chemistry laboratory is limited by several technical problems. First, separation of all the catechols and of DHPG from the solvent front requires relatively low mobile phase concentrations of organic modifiers. This consequently leads to long chromatographic run times that limit high throughput of more of the commonly requested catecholamines. Second, interference from uric acid presents a problem to measurement of DHPG by most amperometric detectors. This problem can be overcome using a coulometric electrode system for irreversible oxidation of uric acid with detection of catechols at a reducing instead of the more commonly used oxidizing potential. Third, recoveries of DHPG, L-dopa, and DOPAC from alumina tend to be lower than for the catecholamines, presenting some problem to their accurate measurement. This latter problem can be resolved by use of minimum quantities of alumina, close attention to types and strengths of acids used in the elution of catechols from the alumina, and additional correction for differences in recoveries from the internal standard.[109]

Alternatives to simultaneous measurements of the various plasma catechols include methods for individual measurements more suitable for specific applications. Examples include HPLC measurements of L-dopa and 3-*O*-methyldopa in Parkinson's disease or malignant melanoma.[8,13,158]

Representative reference intervals for plasma concentrations of L-dopa, DOPAC, and DHPG in normotensive adults are shown in Table 29-9.

Urinary Free Catecholamines

Urinary catecholamines represent a quantitatively small but diagnostically important component of the catecholamine excretion products. Catecholamines are excreted in the urine as free amines and as glucuronide and sulfate conjugates. As with plasma measurements, total urinary catecholamines (conjugated and unconjugated forms) may be measured by

TABLE 29-9 Reference Intervals for Plasma Concentrations of L-Dopa, DOPAC, and DHPG in Normotensive Adults

L-Dopa	DOPAC	DHPG
1042-2366 pg/mL (5.3-12.0 nmol/L)	674-2636 pg/mL (4.0-15.7 nmol/L)	797-1208 pg/mL (4.7-7.1 nmol/L)

TABLE 29-10 Urinary Catecholamine Reference Intervals

	Age (yr)	Epinephrine	Norepinephrine	Dopamine
Daily Excretion µg/d (nmol/d)	0-1	0-2.5 (0-14)	0-10 (0-59)	0-85 (0-555)
	1-2	0-3.5 (0-19)	1-17 (6-100)	10-140 (65-914)
	2-4	0-6.0 (0-33)	4-29 (24-171)	40-260 (261-1697)
	4-7	0.2-10 (1-55)	8-45 (47-266)	65-400 (424-2612)
	7-10	0.2-10 (1-55)	13-65 (77-384)	65-400 (424-2612)
	10-15	0.5-20 (3-109)	15-80 (89-473)	65-400 (424-2612)
	>15	0.5-20 (3-109)	15-80 (89-473)	65-400 (424-2612)
Excretion Relative to Creatinine µg/g Creatinine	0-1	up to 0.38	up to 0.31	up to 1.29
	1-4	up to 0.08	up to 0.29	up to 1.22
	4-10	up to 0.09	up to 0.11	up to 0.72
	10-18	up to 0.06	up to 0.11	up to 0.45
	>18	up to 0.04	up to 0.11	up to 0.35

hydrolyzing the sample before assay, but free amines are routinely measured because they are least affected by dietary catechols.[178]

Earlier fluorometric methods for analysis of urinary free catecholamines have been replaced by HPLC methods that allow selective quantitation of epinephrine, norepinephrine, and dopamine. Preliminary extraction of urine is still required and numerous preanalytical cleanup techniques are available. An alumina extraction procedure is typically coupled with ion-exchange or adsorption chromatography. Alumina pretreatment usually involves a batch extraction technique in which catechols are first adsorbed at pH 8.6 and then eluted with boric acid, which forms a complex with *cis*-diol groups. Purification on boric acid affinity gels provides an alternative procedure for selective adsorption of catecholamines.

Electrochemical detection with ion-pairing adaptations of reversed-phase chromatography is the most common methodology, and ion pairing with alkyl sulfonates or sulfates is generally used to enhance retention of cationic amine moieties on lipophilic stationary phases.[58,183,218] Potential analytical interference, depending upon chromatographic conditions, has been reported with α-methyldopa,[183] acetaminophen,[257] labetalol,[71] and captopril.[43] By varying the sample preparation procedures, metanephrines and VMA[77,200] may be co-analyzed along with the catecholamines. Alternate use of ion-exchange chromatography coupled with electrochemical detection offers separatory and sensitivity advantages, especially in detecting small tumors that preferentially secrete epinephrine.[11,170,259] More recently, tandem mass spectrometry methodology has been developed with high throughput capability and the added specificity resulting from tandem mass spectral detection.[149]

Representative reference intervals for unconjugated catecholamines, based on 24-hour outputs[183] and creatinine excretion,[214] in normotensive children and adults are shown in Table 29-10. Diagnostic testing based on overnight rather than on 24-hour urine collection has been suggested as a sensitive diagnostic index of autonomous catecholamine secretion by a pheochromocytoma.[124] However, reference intervals must be established for these studies because excretion of catecholamines varies during the sleep-wake cycle.[218]

Urinary Fractionated Metanephrines

Normetanephrine and metanephrine are metabolic products of norepinephrine and epinephrine, respectively, and are formed by the action of catechol-*O*-methyltransferase without deamination. As a result of active neuronal reuptake and deamination of norepinephrine, normetanephrine normally represents <5% of the total norepinephrine excretion products in urine. Metanephrine, however, even with its lower urinary concentration relative to normetanephrine, represents a major excretion product of epinephrine.[144] The metanephrines are excreted in both conjugated and unconjugated forms.[26] Unlike the catecholamines, total metanephrine excretion is not significantly influenced by diet.[178] As a result, the total metanephrines are routinely measured after acid hydrolysis or sulfatase pretreatment.

Selective quantitation of metanephrine and normetanephrine by HPLC techniques[7,197,229] is preferred and should be used in place of earlier spectrophotometric methods. Isolation of metanephrines from the urine is usually accomplished with ion-exchange chromatography. Weak cation-exchange resins are primarily used, although some procedures use a combination of strong and weak cation exchange to enhance recovery. Differential solvent extraction methods (e.g., using ethyl acetate and cyclohexane) can also be applied to remove potential interference. Although native fluorescence and ultraviolet absorption can

TABLE 29-11 Urinary Metanephrine and Normetanephrine Reference Intervals

	METANEPHRINE		NORMETANEPHRINE	
Age	**µg/day**	**µg/g Creatinine**	**µg/day**	**µg/g Creatinine**
0-3 mo	5.9-37	202-708	47-156	1535-3355
4-6 mo	6.1-42	156-572	31-111	737-2194
7-9 mo	12.0-41	150-526	42-109	592-1046
10-12 mo	8.5-101	148-65	123-103	271-1117
1-2 yr	6.7-52	40-526	32-118	350-1275
2-6 yr	11-99	74-504	50-111	104-609
6-10 yr	54-138	121-319	47-176	103-452
10-16 yr	39-242	46-307	53-290	96-411
Adult	74-297		105-354	

be used to detect the metanephrine concentrations, most HPLC procedures are based on electrochemical detection. Column conditions and stationary phases vary; typical applications include reversed-phase chromatography with ion-pairing reagents and silica-based cation-exchange chromatography. Drug interference, which may falsely increase the HPLC-based estimation of normetanephrine, has been reported for viloxazine[10] and acetaminophen.[257] Labetalol and buspirone (BuSpar) may also interfere with metanephrine analysis,[71] and treatment with α-methyldopa results in additional chromatographic peaks.[41,59,120] A fractionated metanephrine method, performed by HPLC coupled with tandem mass spectrometry, offers the advantages of short chromatographic run time, high sample throughput, and elimination of drug interference.[242]

Table 29-11 shows representative reference intervals for metanephrine and normetanephrine in children and adults.[243] One-hour excretion of metanephrines has also been used in the detection of pheochromocytomas but diurnal variation in metanephrine excretion[232,239] must be considered when short collection intervals are used.

Urinary Vanillylmandelic Acid

Vanillylmandelic Acid (VMA) is a major catecholamine metabolite formed by the actions of catechol-O-methyltransferase and MAO. It is excreted by the kidney and represents an average of 40% to 50% of the urinary excretion production of norepinephrine and epinephrine. Norepinephrine is the major source of VMA, with metabolism through MHPG as the major pathway.[25,144] VMA is not significantly conjugated and therefore is measured without a hydrolysis step. VMA was first isolated and identified in the urine of a patient with a pheochromocytoma,[13] and its analysis is commonly performed to detect the presence of pheochromocytomas and neuroblastomas.

Earlier spectrophotometric methods for determination of VMA are relatively nonspecific and have been replaced by gas chromatography or more commonly by HPLC methods. Gas chromatographic methods with flame ionization or mass spectrometric detection that have been applied to the determination of VMA are highly specific and can simultaneously determine VMA and HVA.[22,70,244] HPLC is, however, the most frequently used chromatographic method, featuring isocratic reversed-phase separation with electrochemical, spectrophotometric, fluorometric, or postcolumn detection.[73,78,215] Anion-exchange chromatography has been used effectively to isolate VMA from urine before HPLC analysis.[12] HPLC applications are relatively free of interference and may provide simultaneous measurement of VMA and other metabolites.[37,199,234] A liquid chromatography–tandem mass spectrometry method for determination of VMA has been developed and introduced into clinical laboratory practice.[159]

Representative reference intervals for VMA excretion in normotensive children and adults,[206] based on both 24-hour urine and creatinine output, are listed in Table 29-12.

Urinary Homovanillic Acid

Homovanillic acid (HVA) is the principal urinary metabolite of L-dopa and dopamine. It has particular relevance to the diagnosis and management of neuroblastomas. HVA can be assayed using several spectrophotometric and chromatographic methods. Most of the earlier photometric procedures were based on the nonspecific reaction of nitrosonaphthol with biogenic amines. However, many compounds interfere with these assays, and earlier spectrophotometric methods have been replaced by chromatographic methods, such as gas chromatography,[22] gas chromatography–mass spectrometry,[70] and HPLC. HPLC methods are the most popular and most applications employ reversed-phase column chromatography and detection of the HVA peak by ultraviolet, fluorescence spectrometry,[4,83] or amperometry[12,15,28,234] techniques. HPLC methods with electrochemical detection are sensitive, show little interference from endogenous or exogenous organic acids, and may provide simultaneous measurement of VMA and other metabolites.

TABLE 29-12 Urinary VMA Reference Intervals

Age (yr)	mg/d	µmol/d	mg/g creatinine	mmol/mol creatinine
3-6	1.0-2.6	5-13	4.0-10.8	2.3-6.2
6-10	2.0-3.2	10-16	4.0-7.5	2.3-4.3
10-16	2.3-5.2	12-26	3.0-8.8	1.7-5.0
16-83	1.4-6.5	7-33		

TABLE 29-13 Urinary HVA Reference Intervals

Age (y)	mg/d	µmol/d	mg/g creatinine	mmol/mol creatinine
3-6	1.4-4.3	8-24	5.4-15.5	3.4-9.6
6-10	2.1-4.7	12-26	4.4-11.5	2.7-7.1
10-16	2.4-8.7	13-48	3.3-10.3	2.0-6.4
16-83	1.4-8.8	8-48		

Representative reference intervals for HVA,[243] based on 24-hour urine and creatinine excretion in normotensive children and adults, are listed in Table 29-13.

SEROTONIN AND METABOLITES

Serotonin

A variety of analytical methods have been used for the determination of serotonin in body fluids and tissue.[133] The oldest assays involved the extraction of serotonin from interfering compounds and quantitation by spectrofluorometric procedures using the native fluorescence of serotonin ($\lambda ex = 300$ nm, $\lambda em = 340$ nm at neutral pH). Derivatization with Ninhydrin or *o*-phthalaldehyde increased the sensitivity and selectivity of these fluorometric methods. More specific and precise methods have subsequently been introduced, including radioenzymatic assay, RIA, EIA, gas chromatography, and HPLC. Reagent and/or test kits based on some of these techniques are available commercially.

HPLC with either fluorometric[2,34,150] or electrochemical[139,140] detection is the most frequently used chromatographic method. HPLC techniques have been developed for measuring serotonin separately or adapted for simultaneous measurement of metabolically related indoles, such as 5-HTP and 5-HIAA. Preliminary extraction and deproteinization are required before analysis, and several choices are available. Organic solvent extraction was one of the first methods used to isolate serotonin, but solvent partition has been largely replaced by procedures that employ cation-exchange resins. Other solid phase extraction procedures have also been employed, such as reversed-phase chromatography using disposable cartridges of ODS-silica. A number of methods simply deproteinize with perchloric acid or trichloroacetic acid before injecting the sample directly onto the HPLC column.

Most HPLC assays employ octadecylsilyl (C18) reversed-phase columns, although strong cation-exchange columns have also been used. The chromatography is usually performed with an isocratic mobile phase at an acid pH that contains an organic modifier and perhaps an ion-pair reagent.[160] Serotonin is protonated in the pH range of 3 to 6, and addition of an anionic ion-pair reagent creates an uncharged conjugate, which enhances the affinity of serotonin for the hydrophobic stationary phase. For measurements of very small amounts of serotonin or for specialized projects, HPLC with amperometric or coulometric detection is often favored over fluorometric detection. Serotonin is readily oxidized electrochemically, and the current that flows is proportional to concentration. For serotonin, the oxidation potential is below 0.6 V, which reduces the risk of electrochemical interference by other compounds. If other tryptophan metabolites are analyzed simultaneously, however, higher oxidation potentials are required. The lower limit of detection, defined as the lowest injected amount that produces a signal-to-noise ratio of 3, is typically 20 nmol/L for whole blood serotonin and 1 nmol/L for platelet-free plasma serotonin.[208] Interassay reproducibility, expressed as a coefficient of variation, is about 6% at a serotonin level of 1140 nmol/L.

To enhance analytical sensitivity, some HPLC procedures incorporate precolumn derivatization with fluorescent[127] and chemiluminescent[117] reagents, thereby achieving detection limits in the femtomole range. Completely automated analyses of serotonin have been described, and some systems incorporate direct injection and online solid phase extraction.[136] For laboratories that may not have the equipment, staff, or experience to measure serotonin by HPLC, alternative technologies based on RIA and EIA are available as commercial test kits. These procedures are highly sensitive and

TABLE 29-14 Serotonin Reference Intervals

Biological Sample	Mass Units	Conversion Factor	Molar Units	Reference
Whole blood	50-200 ng/mL	×5.68	280-1140 nmol/L	243
	88-1230 ng/10^9 platelets	×0.00568	0.5-7.0 nmol/10^9 platelets	34
Serum	30-200 ng/mL	×5.68	170-1140 nmol/L	116
Urine	60-167 μg/day	×5.68	340-950 nmol/24 hr	137
	38-101 μg/g creatinine	×0.653	25-66 μmol/mol creatinine	134
CSF	1.0-2.1 ng/mL	×5.68	5.7-12.0 nmol/L	133
Platelet-rich plasma	670 ± 150 ng/10^9 platelets	×0.00568	3.81 ± 0.87 nmol/10^9 platelets	138
Isolated platelets	620 ± 233 ng/10^9 platelets	×0.00568	3.52 ± 1.32 nmol/10^9 platelets	208
Platelet-poor plasma	0.93 ± 0.67 ng/mL	×5.68	5.3 ± 3.8 nmol/L	198

can measure low concentrations of serotonin in different specimens.[140]

Serotonin can be measured in whole blood, serum, platelet-rich plasma, platelet-poor plasma (i.e., platelet-free plasma), isolated platelet pellets, urine, and CSF. Most blood serotonin is stored in the platelets and is easily released during sample preparation. For whole blood serotonin, venous blood (10 mL) is drawn into a tube containing potassium EDTA as an anticoagulant, gently mixed, placed on ice, and transferred to a storage tube. An aliquot of blood is then removed for a platelet count; alternatively, a simultaneous EDTA blood sample can be collected. Antioxidants such as ascorbic acid or metabisulfite are conveniently added to the storage tube when a fluorometric detection system is used. Blood serotonin samples are stored frozen at −20 °C, preferably within 2 hours after collection.

Platelet-rich plasma samples are prepared from whole blood by centrifuging at 120*g* for 30 minutes at 4 °C[171] or at 200*g* for 15 minutes at room temperature.[208] To prevent lowering the serotonin concentration, platelet-rich plasma is prepared within 1 hour after the blood is collected and placed on ice. An aliquot of platelet-rich plasma is removed for a platelet count. Platelet-poor plasma and platelet pellets are prepared from measured aliquots of the platelet-rich sample plasma by centrifuging at 4500*g* for 10 minutes at 4 °C[198] (or at 1000*g* for 30 minutes at room temperature).[208] To reduce the probability of platelet rupture, samples should never be frozen before the cell-free plasma is obtained. Plasma and pellets are stored frozen at −20 °C and analyzed within 1 to 2 weeks after collection.

Serum samples are conveniently collected in serum separation tubes (SST) tubes. Blood clotting releases serotonin from platelets; samples should be centrifuged within 1 hour after collection and stored frozen at −20 °C. Twenty-four-hour urine samples are collected in 2-L brown polypropylene bottles containing 250 mg each of sodium metabisulfite and EDTA as preservatives. Samples are acidified to pH 4 with acetic acid before freezing.

Whole blood measurement of serotonin is popular because time-consuming isolation of platelets is not required. In general, serotonin levels in whole blood, collected with EDTA anticoagulant, better represent peripheral blood concentrations than serum serotonin, although the latter are often recommended for pediatric patients. Whole blood serotonin concentrations, expressed in nmol/L, are higher while standing than supine because of an increase in platelets.[208] For meaningful comparisons, whole blood serotonin determinations should be corrected for platelet count. Several types of anticoagulants have been studied for their ability to prevent release of serotonin from platelets; potassium EDTA gave better results than citrate in platelet-free plasma.[174] Unlike 5-HIAA, serotonin measurements are not significantly influenced by short-term ingestion of serotonin-rich foods.[138] Platelet serotonin is age dependent; elderly subjects have higher values than newborns but lower values than children and adults.[75] Representative reference intervals are shown in Table 29-14 for biological fluids.

5-Hydroxyindoleacetic Acid (5-HIAA)

Qualitative and quantitative analyses of 5-HIAA in urine were first described in 1955. Historically, two photometric methods for qualitative screening were used. The nitroso-naphthol-nitrous acid procedure[86,246] was more specific and widely used than the dimethylaminobenzaldehyde (Ehrlich's aldehyde) procedure. These qualitative screening tests, however, are no longer recommended since they are insensitive and susceptible to interference.

Like serotonin, 5-HIAA is strongly fluorescent, and a number of fluorometric procedures have been developed for quantitative analysis. Fluorescence can then be measured directly or after derivatization with *o*-phthalaldehyde.

Rapid developments in analytical techniques have led to the introduction of more selective and sensitive methods for quantitating 5-HIAA in urine and plasma, including gas chromatography, immunoassay, HPLC, and liquid chromatography–tandem mass spectrometry (LC-MS–MS). At present, HPLC is the most widespread method for measuring 5-HIAA in the clinical laboratory and has largely replaced the photometric and fluorometric methods.

TABLE 29-15 Adult Reference Intervals for Plasma and Urinary 5-HIAA

Biological Sample	Mass Units	Conversion Factor	Molar Units	Reference
Urine	1-7 mg/d	×5.23	6-37 μmol/day	217
	0-6.6 mg/g creatinine	×0.592	0-3.9 μmol/mmol creatinine	231
Plasma	5.2-13.4 ng/L	×5.23	27-70 nmol/L	52

Numerous HPLC methods have been described for measuring 5-HIAA, either separately or in combination with other clinically interesting substances.[51] Most procedures employ reversed-phase, paired-ion separations under optimized isocratic conditions. Alkyl-bonded silica, such as octadecysilyl (C18), is often used as the hydrophobic stationary phase, and an organic-aqueous buffer mixture at an acid pH is frequently used as the polar mobile phase.

Electrochemical detection using amperometric or coulometric measurement is preferred for specific measurement of small quantities of 5-HIAA; a modification of the method developed by Chou and Jaynes[39] is is available on this book's accompanying Evolve site. Like serotonin, the oxidation potential for 5-HIAA is below 0.6 V and must be optimized for each application. Very few interfering compounds are electrochemically active at such low voltage potentials. But if detection of 5-HIAA with other indoles and catecholamines is desired, then hydrodynamic voltammograms for each analyte should be studied to select the minimum potential that achieves maximum specificity.[247] Some HPLC systems use fluorometric detection, with or without derivatization, for a less demanding measurement of 5-HIAA.[231] A method combining fluorometric and electrochemical detection has also been described.[236]

Preliminary extraction of 5-HIAA may be used as an initial purification step before HPLC analysis. Organic solvents, anion-exchange resins, and other solid phase extraction procedures have all been used.[253] For many systems, direct injection of urine onto the analytical column is a common practice,[15,101] and samples are often merely diluted with a buffer to protect the HPLC system from contamination. Methods that analyze 5-HIAA without prior sample cleanup rely on the selectivity of the HPLC separation combined with fluorescence or electrochemical detection to provide the requisite specificity.

For measurement of 5-HIAA in plasma, HPLC methods with electrochemical[261] or fluorescence detection[34] have been described. The latter uses diethyl ether for preliminary extraction of heparinized plasma. The internal standard and 5-HIAA are then separated by gradient elution on a C18 column and detected with a spectrofluorometer (excitation wavelength, 280 nm; emission wavelength, 345 nm). This method is linear to 190 ng/L, and the interassay precision, expressed as a coefficient of variation, is less than 6% at a 5-HIAA concentration of 30 ng/L.

Alternative technologies based on immunoassay and tandem mass spectrometry are available for quantitating 5-HIAA. A ready-to-use competitive EIA kit has been developed for measuring chemically derivatized 5-HIAA.[115] In this procedure, dichloromethane is used to convert 5-HIAA to its methyl ester during sample preparation. This methylated derivative competes with biotin-labeled 5-HIAA for a limited number of binding sites of an antibody immobilized on microtiter plates. After incubation, the wells are washed to remove unbound biotin-labeled HIAA and then incubated with antibiotin alkaline phosphatase before a p-nitrophenyl phosphate substrate is added. The amount of biotinylated HIAA bound to the antibody is inversely proportional to the 5-HIAA concentration. This EIA method shows excellent correlation with HPLC, and interassay reproducibility coefficient of variation (CV) is about 7% at a 5-HIAA level of 7.5 mg/L.

LC-MS–MS methods for the determination of 5-HIAA in urine have been developed.[145,162] one of which uses an automated solid phase extraction, isocratic LC elution, and quantification against a stable isotope-labeled internal standard.[145] With these procedures, sample preparation is automated, chromatographic interferences are eliminated, and analytical time is reduced (2 minutes per sample).

Sample collection and storage protocols are an important consideration in testing plasma or urine by the instrumental techniques discussed above. For determination of 5-HIAA in plasma, a blood specimen is collected with heparin as an anticoagulant after an overnight fast. The separated plasma is stored frozen at −20 °C until analysis, since plasma stored at 4 °C for 7 days showed an 8% average increase in 5-HIAA concentration.[34] For urinary measurement of 5-HIAA, a 24-hour specimen is recommended, since 5-HIAA concentrations in random urine are extremely variable. Shorter (or longer) collection times may be acceptable provided results are expressed per milligram of creatinine. Because 5-HIAA is light sensitive, urine should be collected in a 2-L brown polypropylene container. As 5-HIAA is unstable at alkaline pHs,[4] a stabilizing preservative is recommended to prevent urine from becoming alkaline (e.g., 0.5 g boric acid; 10 mL HCl, 6 mol/L; 25 mL glacial acetic acid). Most importantly, the specimen should be refrigerated during collection. On receipt in the laboratory, the urine specimen is thoroughly mixed and the total volume measured and recorded. If the specimen is not collected with an acid preservative, then the pH of the urine may now be adjusted to between 2 and 3 by addition of HCl, 6 mol/L. Acidified urine can be stored at 4 °C for 2 to 4 weeks and for longer periods of time at −20 °C.

Dietary instruction for the patient may reduce potential exogenous interferences. For example, dietary sources of 5-hydroxyindoles (e.g., walnuts, bananas, avocados, eggplants, pineapples, plums, and tomatoes) should be restricted 3 to 4 days before and during urine collection. If possible, patients should abstain from all known medications that may cause an apparent increase (glycerol guaiacolate, mephenesin, phenacetin, and acetaminophen) or decrease in 5-HIAA levels (methenamine, phenothiazine tranquilizers, homogentisic acid, acetic acid, and levodopa). Whereas serotonin-containing foods clearly alter urinary 5-HIAA results, fasting plasma 5-HIAA results are not affected by foods high in hydroxyindole content. Representative reference intervals used in the interpretation of plasma and urinary 5-HIAA are shown in Table 29-15.

REFERENCES

1. Aghajaranian G, Sanders-Bush E. Serotonin. In: Nemeroff C, ed. Neuropsychopharmacology The Fifth Generation of Progress, Vol. Philadelphia: Lippincott Williams & Wilkins, 2002:15-34.
2. Anderson GM, Feibel FC, Cohen DJ. Determination of serotonin in whole blood, platelet-rich plasma, platelet-poor plasma and plasma ultrafiltrate. Life Sci 1987;40:1063-70.
3. Aneman A, Eisenhofer G, Olbe L, Dalenback J, Nitescu P, Fandriks L, Friberg P. Sympathetic discharge to mesenteric organs and the liver. Evidence for substantial mesenteric organ norepinephrine spillover. J Clin Invest 1996;97:1640-6.
4. Anton AH, Berk AI. Evaluation and improvement of homovanillic acid methodology, and a critique of liquid chromatography with electrochemical detection. Clin Chem 1987;33:600-3.
5. Aziz Q, Thompson DG. Brain-gut axis in health and disease. Gastroenterology 1998;114:559-78.
6. Barnes NM, Sharp T. A review of central 5-HT receptors and their function. Neuropharmacology 1999;38:1083-152.
7. Bertani-Dziedzic LM, Krstulovic AM, Dziedzic SW, Gitlow SE, Cerqueira S. Analysis of urinary metanephrines by reversed-phase high-performance liquid chromatography and electrochemical detection. Clin Chim Acta 1981;110:1-8.
8. Betto P, Ricciarello G, Giambenedetti M, Lucarelli C, Ruggeri S, Stocchi F. Improved high-performance liquid chromatographic analysis with double detection system for L-dopa, its metabolites and carbidopa in plasma of parkinsonian patients under L-dopa therapy. J Chromatogr 1988;459: 341-9.
9. Biaggioni I, Goldstein DS, Atkinson T, Robertson D. Dopamine-beta-hydroxylase deficiency in humans. Neurology 1990;40:370-3.
10. Bieva CJ, Ladmirant IH, Scheirs I, Dardenne JP. Administered viloxazine interferes in liquid-chromatographic assay of normetanephrines. Clin Chem 1987;33:1677-8.
11. Binder SR, Biaggi ME. Analysis of urinary catecholamines by high-performance liquid chromatography in the presence of labetalol metabolites. J Chromatogr 1987;385:241-7.
12. Binder SR, Sivorinovsky G. Measurement of urinary vanilmandelic acid and homovanillic acid by high-performance liquid chromatography with electrochemical detection following extraction by ion-exchange and ion-moderated partition. J Chromatogr 1984;336:173-88.
13. Blandini F, Martignoni E, Pacchetti C, Desideri S, Rivellini D, Nappi G. Simultaneous determination of L-dopa and 3-O-methyldopa in human platelets and plasma using high-performance liquid chromatography with electrochemical detection. J Chromatogr B Biomed Sci Appl 1997;700:278-82.
14. Bonafe L, Thony B, Leimbacher W, Kierat L, Blau N. Diagnosis of dopa-responsive dystonia and other tetrahydrobiopterin disorders by the study of biopterin metabolism in fibroblasts. Clin Chem 2001;47:477-85.
15. Bonfigli AR, Coppa G, Testa R, Testa I, De Sio G. Determination of vanillylmandelic, 5-hydroxyindoleacetic and homovanillic acid in urine by isocratic liquid chromatography. Eur J Clin Chem Clin Biochem 1997;35:57-61.
16. Boomsma F, Alberts G, van Eijk L, Man in 't Veld AJ, Schalekamp MA. Optimal collection and storage conditions for catecholamine measurements in human plasma and urine. Clin Chem 1993;39:2503-8.
17. Bouloux PM, Perrett D. Interference of labetalol metabolites in the determination of plasma catecholamines by HPLC with electrochemical detection. Clin Chim Acta 1985;150:111-7.
18. Box JC, Braithwaite MD, Duncan T, Lucas G. Pheochromocytoma, chronic renal insufficiency, and hemodialysis: a combination leading to a diagnostic and therapeutic dilemma. Am Surg 1997;63:314-6.
19. Brautigam C, Steenbergen-Spanjers GC, Hoffmann GF, Dionisi-Vici C, van den Heuvel LP, Smeitink JA, Wevers RA. Biochemical and molecular genetic characteristics of the severe form of tyrosine hydroxylase deficiency. Clin Chem 1999;45:2073-8.
20. Brautigam C, Wevers RA, Jansen RJ, Smeitink JA, de Rijk-van Andel JF, Gabreels FJ, Hoffmann GF. Biochemical hallmarks of tyrosine hydroxylase deficiency. Clin Chem 1998;44:1897-904.
21. Bravo EL, Tarazi RC, Fouad FM, Vidt DG, Gifford RW, Jr. Clonidine-suppression test: a useful aid in the diagnosis of pheochromocytoma. N Engl J Med 1981;305:623-6.
22. Brewster MA, Berry DH, Moriarty M. Urinary 3-methoxy-4-hydroxyphenylacetic (homovanillic) and

3-methoxy-4-hydroxymandelic (vanillylmandelic) acids: gas-liquid chromatographic methods and experience with 13 cases of neuroblastoma. Clin Chem 1977;23:2247-9.

23. Brodeur GM, Pritchard J, Berthold F, Carlsen NL, Castel V, Castelberry RP, et al. Revisions of the international criteria for neuroblastoma diagnosis, staging, and response to treatment. J Clin Oncol 1993;11:1466-77.
24. Brown MJ. Simultaneous assay of noradrenaline and its deaminated metabolite, dihydroxyphenylglycol, in plasma: a simplified approach to the exclusion of phaeochromocytoma in patients with borderline elevation of plasma noradrenaline concentration. Eur J Clin Invest 1984;14:67-72.
25. Brown RT, Polinsky RJ, Kopin IJ. Interconversion of O-methylated norepinephrine metabolites in humans. J Lab Clin Med 1987;110:119-24.
26. Buu NT, Angers M, Chevalier D, Kuchel O. A new method for the simultaneous analysis of free and sulfoconjugated normetanephrine, metanephrine, and 3-methoxytyramine in human urine by HPLC with electrochemical detection. J Lab Clin Med 1984;104:425-32.
27. Calles-Escandon J, Cunningham JJ, Snyder P, Jacob R, Huszar G, Loke J, Felig P. Influence of exercise on urea, creatinine, and 3-methylhistidine excretion in normal human subjects. Am J Physiol 1984;246: E334-8.
28. Candito M, Nagatsu T, Chambon P, Chatel M. High-performance liquid chromatographic measurement of cerebrospinal fluid tetrahydrobiopterin, neopterin, homovanillic acid and 5-hydroxindoleacetic acid in neurological diseases. J Chromatogr B Biomed Appl 1994;657:61-6.
29. Candito M, Thyss A, Albertini M, Deville A, Politano S, Mariani R, Chambon P. Methylated catecholamine metabolites for diagnosis of neuroblastoma. Med Pediatr Oncol 1992;20:215-20.
30. Canfell PC, Binder SR, Khayam-Bashi H. Pediatric reference intervals for normetanephrine/ metanephrine. Clin Chem 1986;32:222-3.
31. Capella C, Heitz PU, Hofler H, Solcia E, Kloppel G. Revised classification of neuroendocrine tumours of the lung, pancreas and gut. Virchows Arch 1995;425:547-60.
32. Caplin ME, Buscombe JR, Hilson AJ, Jones AL, Watkinson AF, Burroughs AK. Carcinoid tumour. Lancet 1998;352:799-805.
33. Carey RM. Theodore Cooper Lecture: Renal dopamine system: paracrine regulator of sodium homeostasis and blood pressure. Hypertension 2001;38:297-302.
34. Carling RS, Degg TJ, Allen KR, Bax ND, Barth JH. Evaluation of whole blood serotonin and plasma and urine 5-hydroxyindole acetic acid in diagnosis of carcinoid disease. Ann Clin Biochem 2002;39: 577-82.
35. Caron MG, Lefkowitz RJ. Catecholamine receptors: structure, function, and regulation. Recent Prog Horm Res 1993;48:277-90.
36. Chan E, Ho P. High-performance liquid chromatography/atmospheric pressure chemical ionization mass spectrometric method for the analysis of catecholamines and metanephrines in human urine. Rapid Commun Mass Spectrom 2001;14:1959-64.
37. Chan YP, Siu TS. Simultaneous quantitation of catecholamines and O-methylated metabolites in urine by isocratic ion-pairing high-performance liquid chromatography with amperometric detection. J Chromatogr 1988;459:251-60.
38. Charmandari E, Eisenhofer G, Mehlinger SL, Carlson A, Wesley R, Keil MF, et al. Adrenomedullary function may predict phenotype and genotype in classic 21-hydroxylase deficiency. J Clin Endocrinol Metab 2002;87:3031-7.
39. Chou PP, Jaynes PK. Determination of urinary 5-hydroxyindole-3-acetic acid using solid-phase extraction and reversed-phase high-performance liquid chromatography with electrochemical detection. J Chromatogr 1985;341:167-71.
40. Collinson PO, Kind PR, Slavin B, Weg MW, Sandler M. False diagnosis of phaeochromocytoma in patients on Sinemet. Lancet 1984;1:1478-9.
41. Cook FJ, Chandler DW, Snyder DK. Effect of buspirone on urinary catecholamine assays. N Engl J Med 1995;332:401.
42. Cotterill SJ, Pearson AD, Pritchard J, Foot AB, Roald B, Kohler JA, Imeson J. Clinical prognostic factors in 1277 patients with neuroblastoma: results of The European Neuroblastoma Study Group 'Survey' 1982-1992. Eur J Cancer 2000;36:901-8.
43. Crawford GA, Gyory AZ, Gallery ED, Kelly D. HPLC of urinary catecholamines in the presence of labetalol, captopril, and alpha-methyldopa. Clin Chem 1990;36:1849.
44. Crockett DK, Frank EL, Roberts WL. Rapid analysis of metanephrine and normetanephrine in urine by gas chromatography-mass spectrometry. Clin Chem 2002;48:332-7.
45. Cryer PE. Adrenaline: a physiological metabolic regulatory hormone in humans? Int J Obes Relat Metab Disord 1993;17 Suppl 3:S43-6; discussion S68.
46. Cryer PE, Tse TF, Clutter WE, Shah SD. Roles of glucagon and epinephrine in hypoglycemic and non-hypoglycemic glucose counterregulation in humans. Am J Physiol 1984;247:E198-205.
47. Curtis G, Fogel M. Creatinine excretion: diurnal variation and variability of whole and part-day measures. A methodologic issue in psychoendocrine research. Psychosom Med 1970;32:337-50.

48. Dajani R, Cleasby A, Neu M, Wonacott AJ, Jhoti H, Hood AM, et al. X-ray crystal structure of human dopamine sulfotransferase, SULT1A3. Molecular modeling and quantitative structure-activity relationship analysis demonstrate a molecular basis for sulfotransferase substrate specificity. J Biol Chem 1999;274:37862-8.
49. Davidson DF. Urinary catecholamine assay by HPLC: in vitro interference by some drugs. Ann Clin Biochem 1988;25 (Pt 5):583-4.
50. De Potter WP, Partoens P, Strecker S. Noradrenaline storing vesicles in sympathetic neurons and their role in neurotransmitter release: an historical overview of controversial issues. Neurochem Res 1997;22:911-9.
51. Deacon AC. The measurement of 5-hydroxyindoleacetic acid in urine. Ann Clin Biochem 1994;31 (Pt 3):215-32.
52. Degg TJ, Allen KR, Barth JH. Measurement of plasma 5-hydroxyindoleacetic acid in carcinoid disease: an alternative to 24-h urine collections? Ann Clin Biochem 2000;37 (Pt 5):724-6.
53. Dutton J, Hodgkinson AJ, Hutchinson G, Roberts NB. Evaluation of a new method for the analysis of free catecholamines in plasma using automated sample trace enrichment with dialysis and HPLC. Clin Chem 1999;45:394-9.
54. Eisenhofer G. The role of neuronal and extraneuronal plasma membrane transporters in the inactivation of peripheral catecholamines. Pharmacol Ther 2001;91:35-62.
55. Eisenhofer G, Aneman A, Friberg P, Hooper D, Fandriks L, Lonroth H, et al. Substantial production of dopamine in the human gastrointestinal tract. J Clin Endocrinol Metab 1997;82:3864-71.
56. Eisenhofer G, Ehrhart-Bornstein M, Bornstein SR. The adrenal medulla: physiology and pathophysiology. In: Govoni S, ed. Handbook of the autonomic nervous system in health and disease, Vol. New York: Marcel Dekker, Inc, 2003:185-224.
57. Eisenhofer G, Friberg P, Pacak K, Goldstein DS, Murphy DL, Tsigos C, et al. Plasma metadrenalines: do they provide useful information about sympatho-adrenal function and catecholamine metabolism? Clin Sci (Lond) 1995;88:533-42.
58. Eisenhofer G, Goldstein DS, Stull R, Keiser HR, Sunderland T, Murphy DL, Kopin IJ. Simultaneous liquid-chromatographic determination of 3,4-dihydroxyphenylglycol, catecholamines, and 3,4-dihydroxyphenylalanine in plasma, and their responses to inhibition of monoamine oxidase. Clin Chem 1986;32:2030-3.
59. Eisenhofer G, Goldstein DS, Walther MM, Friberg P, Lenders JW, Keiser HR, Pacak K. Biochemical diagnosis of pheochromocytoma: How to distinguish true- from false-positive test results. J Clin Endocrinol Metab 2003;88:2656-66.
60. Eisenhofer G, Huynh TT, Hiroi M, Pacak K. Understanding catecholamine metabolism as a guide to the biochemical diagnosis of pheochromocytoma. Rev Endocr Metab Disord 2001;2:297-311.
61. Eisenhofer G, Keiser H, Friberg P, Mezey E, Huynh TT, Hiremagalur B, et al. Plasma metanephrines are markers of pheochromocytoma produced by catechol-O-methyltransferase within tumors. J Clin Endocrinol Metab 1998;83:2175-85.
62. Eisenhofer G, Lenders JW, Harvey-White J, Ernst M, Zametkin A, Murphy DL, Kopin IJ. Differential inhibition of neuronal and extraneuronal monoamine oxidase. Neuropsychopharmacology 1996;15:296-301.
63. Eisenhofer G, Lenders JW, Linehan WM, Walther MM, Goldstein DS, Keiser HR. Plasma normetanephrine and metanephrine for detecting pheochromocytoma in von Hippel-Lindau disease and multiple endocrine neoplasia type 2. N Engl J Med 1999;340:1872-9.
64. Eisenhofer G, Rundquist B, Aneman A, Friberg P, Dakak N, Kopin IJ, et al. Regional release and removal of catecholamines and extraneuronal metabolism to metanephrines. J Clin Endocrinol Metab 1995;80:3009-17.
65. Eisenhofer G, Walther MM, Huynh TT, Li ST, Bornstein SR, Vortmeyer A, et al. Pheochromocytomas in von Hippel-Lindau syndrome and multiple endocrine neoplasia type 2 display distinct biochemical and clinical phenotypes. J Clin Endocrinol Metab 2001;86:1999-2008.
66. Eldrup E, Clausen N, Scherling B, Schmiegelow K. Evaluation of plasma 3,4-dihydroxyphenylacetic acid (DOPAC) and plasma 3,4-dihydroxyphenylalanine (DOPA) as tumor markers in children with neuroblastoma. Scand J Clin Lab Invest 2001;61:479-90.
67. Esler M, Jennings G, Lambert G, Meredith I, Horne M, Eisenhofer G. Overflow of catecholamine neurotransmitters to the circulation: source, fate, and functions. Physiol Rev 1990;70:963-85.
68. Esler MD, Wallin G, Dorward PK, Eisenhofer G, Westerman R, Meredith I, et al. Effects of desipramine on sympathetic nerve firing and norepinephrine spillover to plasma in humans. Am J Physiol 1991;260:R817-23.
69. Faraj BA, Camp VM, Murray DR, Kutner M, Hearn J, Nixon D. Plasma L-dopa in the diagnosis of malignant melanoma. Clin Chem 1986;32:159-61.
70. Fauler G, Leis HJ, Huber E, Schellauf C, Kerbl R, Urban C, Gleispach H. Determination of homovanillic acid and vanillylmandelic acid in neuroblastoma screening by stable isotope dilution GC-MS. J Mass Spectrom 1997;32:507-14.
71. Feldman JM. Falsely elevated urinary excretion of catecholamines and metanephrines in patients receiving labetalol therapy. J Clin Pharmacol 1987;27: 288-92.

72. Feldman JM, Lee EM. Serotonin content of foods: effect on urinary excretion of 5-hydroxyindoleacetic acid. Am J Clin Nutr 1985;42:639-43.
73. Felice LJ, Kissinger PT. Modification of the Pisano method for vanilmandelic acid using high pressure liquid chromatography. Clin Chim Acta 1977;76:317-20.
74. Fitzpatrick PF. Tetrahydropterin-dependent amino acid hydroxylases. Annu Rev Biochem 1999;68:355-81.
75. Flachaire E, Beney C, Berthier A, Salandre J, Quincy C, Renaud B. Determination of reference values for serotonin concentration in platelets of healthy newborns, children, adults, and elderly subjects by HPLC with electrochemical detection. Clin Chem 1990;36:2117-20.
76. Flemstrom G, Safsten B. Role of dopamine and other stimuli of mucosal bicarbonate secretion in duodenal protection. Dig Dis Sci 1994;39:1839-42.
77. Foti A, Kimura S, DeQuattro V, Lee D. Liquid-chromatographic measurement of catecholamines and metabolites in plasma and urine. Clin Chem 1987;33:2209-13.
78. Fujita K, Maruta K, Ito S, Nagatsu T. Urinary 4-hydroxy-3-methoxymandelic (vanillylmandelic) acid, 4-hydroxy-3-methoxyphenylacetic (homovanillic) acid, and 5-hydroxy-3-indoleacetic acid determined by liquid chromatography with electrochemical detection. Clin Chem 1983;29:876-8.
79. Gerlo EA, Schoors DF, Dupont AG. Age- and sex-related differences for the urinary excretion of norepinephrine, epinephrine, and dopamine in adults. Clin Chem 1991;37:875-8.
80. Gershon MD. Review article: roles played by 5-hydroxytryptamine in the physiology of the bowel. Aliment Pharmacol Ther 1999;13 Suppl 2:15-30.
81. Giles HG, Meggiorini S. Stability of catecholamines in urine. Clin Chem 1983;29:595.
82. Gingrich JA, Caron MG. Recent advances in the molecular biology of dopamine receptors. Annu Rev Neurosci 1993;16:299-321.
83. Gironi A, Seghieri G, Niccolai M, Mammini P. Simultaneous liquid-chromatographic determination of urinary vanillylmandelic acid, homovanillic acid, and 5-hydroxyindoleacetic acid. Clin Chem 1988;34:2504-6.
84. Godfrey JA, Rickman OB, Williams AW, Thompson GB, Young WF, Jr. Pheochromocytoma in a patient with end-stage renal disease. Mayo Clin Proc 2001;76:953-7.
85. Goldberg LI. Dopamine receptors and hypertension. Physiologic and pharmacologic implications. Am J Med 1984;77:37-44.
86. Goldenberg H. Specific photometric determination of 5-hydroxyindoleacetic acid in urine. Clin Chem 1973;19:38-44.
87. Goldstein DS, Eisenhofer GF, Kopin IJ. Sources and significance of plasma levels of catechols and their metabolites in humans. J Pharmacol Exp Ther 2003;305:800-11.
88. Goldstein DS, Holmes C, Sharabi Y, Brentzel S, Eisenhofer G. Plasma levels of catechols and metanephrines in neurogenic orthostatic hypotension. Neurology 2003;60:1327-32.
89. Goldstein DS, Lake CR. Plasma norepinephrine and epinephrine levels in essential hypertension. Fed Proc 1984;43:57-61.
90. Goldstein DS, Lenders JW, Kaler SG, Eisenhofer G. Catecholamine phenotyping: clues to the diagnosis, treatment, and pathophysiology of neurogenetic disorders. J Neurochem 1996;67:1781-90.
91. Goldstein DS, Mezey E, Yamamoto T, Aneman A, Friberg P, Eisenhofer G. Is there a third peripheral catecholaminergic system? Endogenous dopamine as an autocrine/paracrine substance derived from plasma DOPA and inactivated by conjugation. Hypertens Res 1995;18 Suppl 1:S93-9.
92. Goldstein DS, Robertson D, Esler M, Straus SE, Eisenhofer G. Dysautonomias: clinical disorders of the autonomic nervous system. Ann Intern Med 2002;137:753-63.
93. Goldstein DS, Stull R, Eisenhofer G, Sisson JC, Weder A, Averbuch SD, Keiser HR. Plasma 3,4-dihydroxyphenylalanine (dopa) and catecholamines in neuroblastoma or pheochromocytoma. Ann Intern Med 1986;105:887-8.
94. Goldstein DS, Swoboda KJ, Miles JM, Coppack SW, Aneman A, Holmes C, et al. Sources and physiological significance of plasma dopamine sulfate. J Clin Endocrinol Metab 1999;84:2523-31.
95. Goldstein DS, Udelsman R, Eisenhofer G, Stull R, Keiser HR, Kopin IJ. Neuronal source of plasma dihydroxyphenylalanine. J Clin Endocrinol Metab 1987;64:856-61.
96. Goyal RK, Hirano I. The enteric nervous system. N Engl J Med 1996;334:1106-15.
97. Grumbach MM, Biller BM, Braunstein GD, Campbell KK, Carney JA, Godley PA, et al. Management of the clinically inapparent adrenal mass ("incidentaloma"). Ann Intern Med 2003;138:424-9.
98. Gurney JG, Davis S, Severson RK, Fang JY, Ross JA, Robison LL. Trends in cancer incidence among children in the U.S. Cancer 1996;78:532-41.
99. Gurney JG, Ross JA, Wall DA, Bleyer WA, Severson RK, Robison LL. Infant cancer in the U.S.: histology-specific incidence and trends, 1973 to 1992. J Pediatr Hematol Oncol 1997;19:428-32.
100. Hasegawa T, Hirose T, Ayala AG, Ito S, Tomaru U, Matsuno Y, et al. Adult neuroblastoma of the retroperitoneum and abdomen: clinicopathologic distinction from primitive neuroectodermal tumor. Am J Surg Pathol 2001;25:918-24.

101. Helander A, Beck O, Wennberg M, Wikstrom T, Jacobsson G. Determination of urinary 5-hydroxyindole-3-acetic acid by high-performance liquid chromatography with electrochemical detection and direct sample injection. Anal Biochem 1991;196:170-3.
102. Helson L, Johnson GA, Smith R. DOPA metabolism in neuroblastoma. Med Pediatr Oncol 1980;8:317-22.
103. Henry JP, Sagne C, Bedet C, Gasnier B. The vesicular monoamine transporter: from chromaffin granule to brain. Neurochem Int 1998;32:227-46.
104. Heron E, Chatellier G, Billaud E, Foos E, Plouin PF. The urinary metanephrine-to-creatinine ratio for the diagnosis of pheochromocytoma. Ann Intern Med 1996;125:300-3.
105. Hoelzer DR, Dalsky GP, Schwartz NS, Clutter WE, Shah SD, Holloszy JO, Cryer PE. Epinephrine is not critical to prevention of hypoglycemia during exercise in humans. Am J Physiol 1986;251:E104-10.
106. Hoffman B, Taylor P. Neurotransmission. The autonomic nervous system. In: Linmbird L, ed. The Pharmacologic Basis of Therapeutics, Vol. New York: McGraw-Hill, 2001:115-53.
107. Hollenbach E, Schulz C, Lehnert H. Rapid and sensitive determination of catecholamines and the metabolite 3-methoxy-4-hydroxyphen-ethyleneglycol using HPLC following novel extraction procedures. Life Sci 1998;63:737-50.
108. Holly JM, Makin HL. The estimation of catecholamines in human plasma. Anal Biochem 1983;128:257-74.
109. Holmes C, Eisenhofer G, Goldstein DS. Improved assay for plasma dihydroxyphenylacetic acid and other catechols using high-performance liquid chromatography with electrochemical detection. J Chromatogr B Biomed Appl 1994;653:131-8.
110. Honjo S, Doran HE, Stiller CA, Ajiki W, Tsukuma H, Oshima A, Coleman MP. Neuroblastoma trends in Osaka, Japan, and Great Britain 1970-1994, in relation to screening. Int J Cancer 2003;103:538-43.
111. Hornykiewicz O. Parkinson's disease and the adaptive capacity of the nigrostriatal dopamine system: possible neurochemical mechanisms. Adv Neurol 1993;60:140-7.
112. Horwitz BJ, Fisher RS. The irritable bowel syndrome. N Engl J Med 2001;344:1846-50.
113. Hoyer D, Martin G. 5-HT receptor classification and nomenclature: towards a harmonization with the human genome. Neuropharmacology 1997;36:419-28.
114. Hyland K, Clayton PT. Aromatic L-amino acid decarboxylase deficiency: diagnostic methodology. Clin Chem 1992;38:2405-10.
115. IBL G. 5-HIAA ELISA. Instructions for Use. Hamburg, Germany 2001.
116. IBL G. Serotonin in Plasma/Serum/Whole Blood. Vol.: Instruction Manual, 1997: Munich, Germany.
117. Ishida J, Takada M, Hitoshi N, Iizuka R, Yamaguchi M. 4-Dimethylaminobenzylamine as a sensitive chemiluminescence derivatization reagent for 5-hydroxyindoles and its application to their quantification in human platelet-poor plasma. J Chromatogr B Biomed Sci Appl 2000;738:199-206.
118. Itoh T, Omori K. Biosynthesis and storage of catecholamines in pheochromocytoma and neuroblastoma cells. J Lab Clin Med 1973;81:889-96.
119. Izbicki T, Bozek J, Perek D, Wozniak W. Urinary dopamine/noradrenaline and dopamine/vanillylmandelic acid ratios as a reflection of different biology of adrenergic clones in children's neuroblastic tumors. J Pediatr Surg 1991;26:1230-4.
120. Jackman GP. A simple method for the assay of urinary metanephrines using high performance liquid chromatography with fluorescence detection. Clin Chim Acta 1982;120:137-42.
121. Jahn R, Sudhof TC. Synaptic vesicles and exocytosis. Annu Rev Neurosci 1994;17:219-46.
122. Janig W, Habler HJ. Specificity in the organization of the autonomic nervous system: a basis for precise neural regulation of homeostatic and protective body functions. Prog Brain Res 2000;122:351-67.
123. Jensen R. Endocrine tumors of the gastrointestinal tract and pancreas. In: Jameson J, ed. Harrison's Principles of Internal Medicine, Vol. 15th ed. New York: McGraw-Hill, 2001:593-603.
124. Jensen R, Doherty G. Carcinoid tumors and the carcinoid syndrome. In: Rosenberg S, ed. Cancer: Principles and Practice of Oncology, Vol. 6. 6th ed. Philadelphia: Lippincott Williams & Wilkins, 2001:1813-33.
125. John H, Ziegler WH, Hauri D, Jaeger P. Pheochromocytomas: can malignant potential be predicted? Urology 1999;53:679-83.
126. Jones BJ, Blackburn TP. The medical benefit of 5-HT research. Pharmacol Biochem Behav 2002;71:555-68.
127. Kai M, Iida H, Nohta H, Lee MK, Ohta K. Fluorescence derivatizing procedure for 5-hydroxytryptamine and 5-hydroxyindoleacetic acid using 1,2-diphenylethylenediamine reagent and their sensitive liquid chromatographic determination. J Chromatogr B Biomed Sci Appl 1998;720:25-31.
128. Kairisto V, Koskinen P, Mattila K, Puikkonen J, Virtanen A, Kantola I, Irjala K. Reference intervals for 24-h urinary normetanephrine, metanephrine, and 3-methoxy-4-hydroxymandelic acid in hypertensive patients. Clin Chem 1992;38:416-20.
129. Kaler SG, Holmes CS, Goldstein DS. Dopamine beta-hydroxylase deficiency associated with mutations in a copper transporter gene. Adv Pharmacol 1998;42:66-8.
130. Kamahori M, Taki M, Watanabe Y, Miura J. Analysis of plasma catecholamines by high-performance liquid chromatography with fluorescence detection:

simple sample preparation for pre-column fluorescence derivatization. J Chromatogr 1991;567:351-8.
131. Kaplan NM, Kramer NJ, Holland OB, Sheps SG, Gomez-Sanchez C. Single-voided urine metanephrine assays in screening for pheochromocytoma. Arch Intern Med 1977;137:190-3.
132. Kaufman S. Genetic disorders involving recycling and formation of tetrahydrobiopterin. Adv Pharmacol 1998;42:41-3.
133. Kema IP, de Vries EG, Muskiet FA. Clinical chemistry of serotonin and metabolites. J Chromatogr B Biomed Sci Appl 2000;747:33-48.
134. Kema IP, de Vries EG, Schellings AM, Postmus PE, Muskiet FA. Improved diagnosis of carcinoid tumors by measurement of platelet serotonin. Clin Chem 1992;38:534-40.
135. Kema IP, de Vries EG, Slooff MJ, Biesma B, Muskiet FA. Serotonin, catecholamines, histamine, and their metabolites in urine, platelets, and tumor tissue of patients with carcinoid tumors. Clin Chem 1994;40:86-95.
136. Kema IP, Meijer WG, Meiborg G, Ooms B, Willemse PH, de Vries EG. Profiling of tryptophan-related plasma indoles in patients with carcinoid tumors by automated, on-line, solid-phase extraction and HPLC with fluorescence detection. Clin Chem 2001;47:1811-20.
137. Kema IP, Schellings AM, Hoppenbrouwers CJ, Rutgers HM, de Vries EG, Muskiet FA. High performance liquid chromatographic profiling of tryptophan and related indoles in body fluids and tissues of carcinoid patients. Clin Chim Acta 1993;221:143-58.
138. Kema IP, Schellings AM, Meiborg G, Hoppenbrouwers CJ, Muskiet FA. Influence of a serotonin- and dopamine-rich diet on platelet serotonin content and urinary excretion of biogenic amines and their metabolites. Clin Chem 1992;38:1730-6.
139. Kissinger PT, Bruntlett CS, Shoup RE. Neurochemical applications of liquid chromatography with electrochemical detection. Life Sci 1981;28:455-65.
140. Kluge H BM, Reuter R, Werner S, Zahlten W, Prudlo J. Serotonin in platelets: comparative analyses using new enzyme immunoassay and HPLC test kits and the traditional fluorimetric procedure. J Lab Med 1999;23:360-4.
141. Kobayashi K, DeQuattro V, Kolloch R, Miano L. A radioenzymatic assay for plasma normetanephrine in man and patients with pheochromocytoma. Life Sci 1980;26:567-73.
142. Kobayashi K, Kolloch R, Dequattro V, Miano L. Increased plasma and urinary normetanephrine in young patients with primary hypertension. Clin Sci (Lond) 1979;57 Suppl 5:173s-6s.
143. Koch DD, Polzin GL. Effect of sample preparation and liquid chromatography column choice on selectivity and precision of plasma catecholamine determination. J Chromatogr 1987;386:19-24.
144. Kopin IJ. Catecholamine metabolism: basic aspects and clinical significance. Pharmacol Rev 1985;37:333-64.
145. Kroll CA, Magera MJ, Helgeson JK, Matern D, Rinaldo P. Liquid chromatographic-tandem mass spectrometric method for the determination of 5-hydroxyindole-3-acetic acid in urine. Clin Chem 2002;48:2049-51.
146. Kulke MH, Mayer RJ. Carcinoid tumors. N Engl J Med 1999;340:858-68.
147. Kurz T, Yamada KA, DaTorre SD, Corr PB. Alpha 1-adrenergic system and arrhythmias in ischaemic heart disease. Eur Heart J 1991;12 Suppl F:88-98.
148. Kushner BH, Gilbert F, Helson L. Familial neuroblastoma. Case reports, literature review, and etiologic considerations. Cancer 1986;57:1887-93.
149. Kushnir MM, Urry FM, Frank EL, Roberts WL, Shushan B. Analysis of catecholamines in urine by positive-ion electrospray tandem mass spectrometry. Clin Chem 2002;48:323-31.
150. Kwarts E, Kwarts J, Rutgers H. A simple paired-ion liquid chromatography assay for serotonin in cerebrospinal fluid, platelet-rich plasma, serum and urine. Ann Clin Biochem 1984;21 (Pt 5):425-9.
151. Landsberg L, Young J. Catecholamines and the adrenal gland. In: Foster DW, ed. Williams textbook of endocrinology. 8th ed. WB Saunders, 1992:636.
152. Laug WE, Siegel SE, Shaw KN, Landing B, Baptista J, Gutenstein M. Initial urinary catecholamine metabolite concentrations and prognosis in neuroblastoma. Pediatrics 1978;62:77-83.
153. Lehmann M, Keul J. Urinary excretion of free noradrenaline and adrenaline related to age, sex and hypertension in 265 individuals. Eur J Appl Physiol Occup Physiol 1986;55:14-8.
154. Lenders JW, Eisenhofer G, Abeling NG, Berger W, Murphy DL, Konings CH, et al. Specific genetic deficiencies of the A and B isoenzymes of monoamine oxidase are characterized by distinct neurochemical and clinical phenotypes. J Clin Invest 1996;97:1010-9.
155. Lenders JW, Eisenhofer G, Armando I, Keiser HR, Goldstein DS, Kopin IJ. Determination of metanephrines in plasma by liquid chromatography with electrochemical detection. Clin Chem 1993;39:97-103.
156. Lenders JW, Keiser HR, Goldstein DS, Willemsen JJ, Friberg P, Jacobs MC, et al. Plasma metanephrines in the diagnosis of pheochromocytoma. Ann Intern Med 1995;123:101-9.
157. Lenders JW, Pacak K, Walther MM, Linehan WM, Mannelli M, Friberg P, et al. Biochemical diagnosis of pheochromocytoma: which test is best? JAMA 2002;287:1427-34.

158. Letellier S, Garnier JP, Spy J, Bousquet B. Determination of the L-DOPA/L-tyrosine ratio in human plasma by high-performance liquid chromatography. Usefulness as a marker in metastatic malignant melanoma. J Chromatogr B Biomed Sci Appl 1997;696:9-17.
159. Magera MJ, Thompson AL, Matern D, Rinaldo P. Liquid chromatography-tandem mass spectrometry method for the determination vanillylmandelic acid in urine. Clin Chem 2003;49:825-6.
160. Mailman RB, Kilts CD. Analytical considerations for quantitative determination of serotonin and its metabolically related products in biological matrices. Clin Chem 1985;31:1849-54.
161. Manger WM, Gifford RW. Clinical and Experimental Pheochromocytoma. 2nd ed. Cambridge, Mass: Blackwell Science, 1996.
162. Manini P, Andreoli R, Cavazzini S, Bergamaschi E, Mutti A, Niessen WM. Liquid chromatography-electrospray tandem mass spectrometry of acidic monoamine metabolites. J Chromatogr B Biomed Sci Appl 2000;744:423-31.
163. Marchese N, Canini S, Fabi L, Famularo L. Paediatric reference values for urinary catecholamine metabolites evaluated by high performance liquid chromatography and electrochemical detection. Eur J Clin Chem Clin Biochem 1997;35:533-7.
164. Marini M, Fathi M, Vallotton M. [Determination of serum metanephrines in the diagnosis of pheochromocytoma]. Ann Endocrinol (Paris) 1994;54:337-42.
165. Martinez A, Knappskog PM, Haavik J. A structural approach into human tryptophan hydroxylase and its implications for the regulation of serotonin biosynthesis. Curr Med Chem 2001;8:1077-91.
166. Massimo L. Neuroblastoma: a challenge for pediatric oncology of the third millennium. Ann N Y Acad Sci 2002;963:59-62.
167. Mathias CJ, Polinsky RJ. Separating the primary autonomic failure syndromes, multiple system atrophy, and pure autonomic failure from Parkinson's disease. Adv Neurol 1999;80:353-61.
168. Mayer EA, Chang L, Lembo T. Brain-gut interactions: implications for newer therapy. Eur J Surg Suppl 1998:50-5.
169. McNicol AM. Differential diagnosis of pheochromocytomas and paragangliomas. Endocr Path 2001;12:407-15.
170. Mefford IN. Lauroyl sarcosine: a weak cation-exchange reagent for on-column modification of reversed-phase material. J Chromatogr 1987;393:441-6.
171. Meijer WG, Kema IP, Volmer M, Willemse PH, de Vries EG. Discriminating capacity of indole markers in the diagnosis of carcinoid tumors. Clin Chem 2000;46:1588-96.
172. Merke DP, Chrousos GP, Eisenhofer G, Weise M, Keil MF, Rogol AD, et al. Adrenomedullary dysplasia and hypofunction in patients with classic 21-hydroxylase deficiency. N Engl J Med 2000;343:1362-8.
173. Mezey E, Eisenhofer G, Hansson S, Harta G, Hoffman BJ, Gallatz K, et al. Non-neuronal dopamine in the gastrointestinal system. Clin Exp Pharmacol Physiol Suppl 1999;26:S14-22.
174. Middelkoop CM, Dekker GA, Kraayenbrink AA, Popp-Snijders C. Platelet-poor plasma serotonin in normal and preeclamptic pregnancy. Clin Chem 1993;39:1675-8.
175. Miki K, Sudo A. Effect of urine pH, storage time, and temperature on stability of catecholamines, cortisol, and creatinine. Clin Chem 1998;44:1759-62.
176. Misugi K, Misugi N, Newton WA, Jr. Fine structural study of neuroblastoma, ganglioneuroblastoma, and pheochromocytoma. Arch Pathol 1968;86:160-70.
177. Modlin IM, Sandor A. An analysis of 8305 cases of carcinoid tumors. Cancer 1997;79:813-29.
178. Moleman P. Effect of diet on urinary excretion of unconjugated catecholamines and some of their metabolites in healthy control subjects and depressed patients. Clin Chim Acta 1990;189:19-24.
179. Molvalilar S, Kocak N. Excretion of vanillylmandelic acid in renal insufficiency. Lancet 1972;2:1263.
180. Monsaingeon M, Perel Y, Simonnet G, Corcuff JB. Comparative values of catecholamines and metabolites for the diagnosis of neuroblastoma. Eur J Pediatr 2003;162:397-402.
181. Mornex R, Peyrin L, Pagliari R, Cottet-Emard JM. Measurement of plasma methoxyamines for the diagnosis of pheochromocytoma. Horm Res 1991;36:220-6.
182. Morrison SF. Differential control of sympathetic outflow. Am J Physiol Regul Integr Comp Physiol 2001;281:R683-98.
183. Moyer TP, Jiang NS, Tyce GM, Sheps SG. Analysis for urinary catecholamines by liquid chromatography with amperometric detection: methodology and clinical interpretation of results. Clin Chem 1979;25:256-63.
184. Munion GL, Seaton JF, Harrison TS. HPLC for urinary catecholamines and metanephrines with alpha-methyldopa. J Surg Res 1983;35:507-14.
185. Nagatsu T. Tyrosine hydroxylase: human isoforms, structure and regulation in physiology and pathology. Essays Biochem 1995;30:15-35.
186. Nagatsu T, Levitt M, Udenfriend S. Tyrosine hydroxylase, the initial step in norepinephrine biosynthesis. J Biol Chem 1964;239:2910-17.
187. Nagatsu T, Stjarne L. Catecholamine synthesis and release. Overview. Adv Pharmacol 1998;42:1-14.
188. Nestler EJ, Alreja M, Aghajanian GK. Molecular control of locus coeruleus neurotransmission. Biol Psychiatry 1999;46:1131-9.

189. Neubert A, Remer T. The impact of dietary protein intake on urinary creatinine excretion in a healthy pediatric population. J Pediatr 1998;133:655-9.
190. Neumann HP, Bausch B, McWhinney SR, Bender BU, Gimm O, Franke G, et al. Germ-line mutations in nonsyndromic pheochromocytoma. N Engl J Med 2002;346:1459-66.
191. Nuttall KL, Pingree SS. The incidence of elevations in urine 5-hydroxyindoleacetic acid. Ann Clin Lab Sci 1998;28:167-74.
192. Oberg K. Neuroendocrine gastrointestinal tumours. Ann Oncol 1996;7:453-63.
193. Öberg K. Carcinoid tumors, carcinoid syndrome, and related disorders. In: Polonsky K, ed. Williams Textbook of Endocrinology, Vol. 10th ed. Philadelphia: Saunders, 2003:1857-76.
194. Oberg K, Stridsberg M. Chromogranins as diagnostic and prognostic markers in neuroendocrine tumours. Adv Exp Med Biol 2000;482:329-37.
195. O'Connor DT, Wu H, Gill BM, Rozansky DJ, Tang K, Mahata SK, et al. Hormone storage vesicle proteins. Transcriptional basis of the widespread neuroendocrine expression of chromogranin A, and evidence of its diverse biological actions, intracellular and extracellular. Ann N Y Acad Sci 1994;733:36-45.
196. O'Meara A, Tormey W, FitzGerald RJ, Fitzgibbon M, Kenny D. Interpretation of random urinary catecholamines and their metabolites in neuroblastoma. Acta Paediatr 1994;83:88-92.
197. Orsulak PJ, Kizuka P, Grab E, Schildkraut JJ. Determination of urinary normetanephrine and metanephrine by radial-compression liquid chromatography and electrochemical detection. Clin Chem 1983;29:305-9.
198. Ortiz J, Artigas F, Gelpi E. Serotonergic status in human blood. Life Sci 1988;43:983-90.
199. Ortiz J, Artigas F. Effects of monoamine uptake inhibitors on extracellular and platelet 5-hydroxytryptamine in rat blood: different effects of clomipramine and fluoxetine. Br J Pharmacol 1992;105:941-6.
200. Parker NC, Levtzow CB, Wright PW, Woodard LL, Chapman JF. Uniform chromatographic conditions for quantifying urinary catecholamines, metanephrines, vanillylmandelic acid, 5-hydroxyindoleacetic acid, by liquid chromatography, with electrochemical detection. Clin Chem 1986;32:1473-6.
201. Patel YC. Neurotransmitters and hypothalamic control of anterior pituitary function. In: Jameson JL, ed. Endocrinology, Vol 1. Philadelphia: WB Saunders Company, 2001:183-200.
202. Peaston RT, Lennard TW, Lai LC. Overnight excretion of urinary catecholamines and metabolites in the detection of pheochromocytoma. J Clin Endocrinol Metab 1996;81:1378-84.
203. Pettersson J, Hussi E, Janne J. Stability of human plasma catecholamines. Scand J Clin Lab Invest 1980;40:297-303.
204. Pisano J. A simple analysis of normetanephrine and metanephrine in urine. Clin Chim Acta 1960;5:406-14.
205. Pisano J, Crout R, Abraham D. Determination of 3-methoxy-4-hydroxymandelic acid in urine. Clin Chim Acta 1962;7:285-9.
206. Premel-Cabic A, Turcant A, Allain P. Normal reference intervals for free catecholamines and their acid metabolites in 24-h urines from children, as determined by liquid chromatography with amperometric detection. Clin Chem 1986;32:1585-7.
207. Pritchard J, Barnes J, Germond S, Hartman O, deKraker J, Lewis I, et al. Stage and urine catecholamine metabolite excretion in neuroblastoma. Lancet 1989;1:514-5.
208. Pussard E, Guigueno N, Adam O, Giudicelli JF. Validation of HPLC-amperometric detection to measure serotonin in plasma, platelets, whole blood, and urine. Clin Chem 1996;42:1086-91.
209. Puyo AM, Levin GM, Armando I, Barontini MB. Free and conjugated plasma catecholamines in pheochromocytoma patients with and without sustained hypertension. Acta Endocrinol (Copenh) 1986;113:111-7.
210. Quinn N, Carruthers M. False positive diagnosis of phaeochromocytoma in a patient with Parkinson's disease receiving levodopa. J Neurol Neurosurg Psychiatry 1988;51:728-9.
211. Raber W, Raffesberg W, Bischof M, Scheuba C, Niederle B, Gasic S, et al. Diagnostic efficacy of unconjugated plasma metanephrines for the detection of pheochromocytoma. Arch Intern Med 2000;160:2957-63.
212. Raggi MA, Sabbioni C, Casamenti G, Gerra G, Calonghi N, Masotti L. Determination of catecholamines in human plasma by high-performance liquid chromatography with electrochemical detection. J Chromatogr B Biomed Sci Appl 1999;730:201-11.
213. Roden M, Raffesberg W, Raber W, Bernroider E, Niederle B, Waldhausl W, Gasic S. Quantification of unconjugated metanephrines in human plasma without interference by acetaminophen. Clin Chem 2001;47:1061-7.
214. Rosano TG. Liquid-chromatographic evaluation of age-related changes in the urinary excretion of free catecholamines in pediatric patients. Clin Chem 1984;30:301-3.
215. Rosano TG, Brown HH. Liquid-chromatographic assay for urinary 3-methoxy-4-hydroxymandelic acid, with use of a periodate oxidative monitor. Clin Chem 1979;25:550-4.
216. Rosano TG, Eisenhofer G, Whitley R. Selected methods for the determination of catecholamines,

serotonin and their metabolites. In: Burtis CA, Ashwood ER, Bruns DE, ed. Web site for Tietz textbook of clinical chemistry and molecular diagnostics, 4th ed. Philadelphia: Saunders, 2005, http://evolve.elsevier.com/Tietz/textbook/.

217. Rosano TG, Meola JM, Swift TA. Liquid-chromatographic determination of urinary 5-hydroxy-3-indoleacetic acid, with fluorescence detection. Clin Chem 1982;28:207-8.
218. Rosano TG, Swift TA, Hayes LW. Advances in catecholamine and metabolite measurements for diagnosis of pheochromocytoma. Clin Chem 1991;37:1854-67.
219. Ross GA, Newbould EC, Thomas J, Bouloux PM, Besser GM, Perrett D, Grossman A. Plasma and 24 h-urinary catecholamine concentrations in normal and patient populations. Ann Clin Biochem 1993;30 (Pt 1):38-44.
220. Rumley AG. The in vitro stability of catecholamines in whole blood. Ann Clin Biochem 1988;25 (Pt 5):585-6.
221. Sawka AM, Jaeschke R, Singh RJ, Young WF, Jr. A comparison of biochemical tests for pheochromocytoma: measurement of fractionated plasma metanephrines compared with the combination of 24-hour urinary metanephrines and catecholamines. J Clin Endocrinol Metab 2003;88:553-8.
222. Schilling FH, Spix C, Berthold F, Erttmann R, Fehse N, Hero B, et al. Neuroblastoma screening at one year of age. N Engl J Med 2002;346:1047-53.
223. Schotzinger RJ, Landis SC. Cholinergic phenotype developed by noradrenergic sympathetic neurons after innervation of a novel cholinergic target in vivo. Nature 1988;335:637-9.
224. Schuldiner S, Shirvan A, Linial M. Vesicular neurotransmitter transporters: from bacteria to humans. Physiol Rev 1995;75:369-92.
225. Schultz W, Tremblay L, Hollerman JR. Reward prediction in primate basal ganglia and frontal cortex. Neuropharmacology 1998;37:421-9.
226. Segawa M. Hereditary progressive dystonia with marked diurnal fluctuation. Brain Dev 2000;22 Suppl 1:S65-80.
227. Sesack SR, Carr DB. Selective prefrontal cortex inputs to dopamine cells: implications for schizophrenia. Physiol Behav 2002;77:513-7.
228. Shimoda O, Ikuta Y, Nishi M, Uneda C. Magnitude of skin vasomotor reflex represents the intensity of nociception under general anesthesia. J Auton Nerv Syst 1998;71:183-9.
229. Shoup RE, Kissinger PT. Determination of urinary normetanephrine, metanephrine, and 3-methoxytyramine by liquid chromatography, with amperometric detection. Clin Chem 1977;23:1268-74.
230. Sjoberg RJ, Simcic KJ, Kidd GS. The clonidine suppression test for pheochromocytoma. A review of its utility and pitfalls. Arch Intern Med 1992;152: 1193-7.
231. Skrinska V, Hahn S. High-performance liquid chromatography of 5-hydroxyindole-3-acetic acid in urine with direct sample injection. J Chromatogr 1984;311:380-4.
232. Smith E. Metanephrine and normetanephrine in human urine: method and results. J Lab Clin Med 1962;60:212-23.
233. Smythe GA, Edwards G, Graham P, Lazarus L. Biochemical diagnosis of pheochromocytoma by simultaneous measurement of urinary excretion of epinephrine and norepinephrine. Clin Chem 1992;38:486-92.
234. Soldin SJ, Hill JG. Simultaneous liquid-chromatographic analysis for 4-hydroxy-3-methoxymandelic acid and 4-hydroxy-3-methoxyphenylacetic acid in urine. Clin Chem 1980;26:291-4.
235. Stoltz JF. Uptake and storage of serotonin by platelets. In: VanHoutte PM, ed. Serotonin and the cardiovascular system. New York: Raven Press, 1985: 37-42.
236. Stroomer AE, Overmars H, Abeling NG, van Gennip AH. Simultaneous determination of acidic 3,4-dihydroxyphenylalanine metabolites and 5-hydroxyindole-3-acetic acid in urine by high-performance liquid chromatography. Clin Chem 1990;36:1834-7.
237. Struder HK, Weicker H. Physiology and pathophysiology of the serotonergic system and its implications on mental and physical performance. Part I. Int J Sports Med 2001;22:467-81.
238. Stumvoll M, Radjaipour M, Seif F. Diagnostic considerations in pheochromocytoma and chronic hemodialysis: case report and review of the literature. Am J Nephrol 1995;15:147-51.
239. Taniguchi K, Kakimoto Y, Armstrong M. Quantitative determination of metanephrine and normetanephrine in urine. J Lab Clin Med 1964;64:469-84.
240. Tanyanyiwa J, Abad-Villar EM, Hauser PC. Contactless conductivity detection of selected organic ions in on-chip electrophoresis. Electrophoresis 2004;25: 903-8.
241. Taylor HC, Mayes D, Anton AH. Clonidine suppression test for pheochromocytoma: examples of misleading results. J Clin Endocrinol Metab 1986;63:238-42.
242. Taylor RL, Singh RJ. Validation of liquid chromatography-tandem mass spectrometry method for analysis of urinary conjugated metanephrine and normetanephrine for screening of pheochromocytoma. Clin Chem 2002;48:533-9.
243. Tietz NW. Clinical Guide to Laboratory Tests. 3rd ed. Philadelphia: WB Saunders, 1995.
244. Tuchman M, Crippin PJ, Krivit W. Capillary gas-chromatographic determination of urinary

homovanillic acid and vanillylmandelic acid. Clin Chem 1983;29:828-31.

245. Tuchman M, Ramnaraine ML, Woods WG, Krivit W. Three years of experience with random urinary homovanillic and vanillylmandelic acid levels in the diagnosis of neuroblastoma. Pediatrics 1987;79: 203-5.
246. Udenfriend S, Titus E, Weissbach H. The identification of 5-hydroxy-3-indoleacetic acid in normal urine and a method for its assay. J Biol Chem 1955;216:499-505.
247. Vaarmann A, Kask A, Maeorg U. Novel and sensitive high-performance liquid chromatographic method based on electrochemical coulometric array detection for simultaneous determination of catecholamines, kynurenine and indole derivatives of tryptophan. J Chromatogr B Analyt Technol Biomed Life Sci 2002;769:145-53.
248. Veith RC, Lewis N, Linares OA, Barnes RF, Raskind MA, Villacres EC, et al. Sympathetic nervous system activity in major depression. Basal and desipramine-induced alterations in plasma norepinephrine kinetics. Arch Gen Psychiatry 1994;51:411-22.
249. Vollmer RR. Selective neural regulation of epinephrine and norepinephrine cells in the adrenal medulla—cardiovascular implications. Clin Exp Hypertens 1996;18:731-51.
250. vonBohlen und Halbach O, Dermietzel R. Neurotransmitters and neuromodulators. Handbook of receptors and biological effects. Darmstadt FRG, 2002.
251. Waldmeier PC, Antonin KH, Feldtrauer JJ, Grunenwald C, Paul E, Lauber J, Bieck P. Urinary excretion of O-methylated catecholamines, tyramine and phenyl-ethylamine by volunteers treated with tranylcypromine and CGP 11305 A. Eur J Clin Pharmacol 1983;25:361-8.
252. Wang ZM, Gallagher D, Nelson ME, Matthews DE, Heymsfield SB. Total-body skeletal muscle mass: evaluation of 24-h urinary creatinine excretion by computerized axial tomography. Am J Clin Nutr 1996;63:863-9.
253. Warburton R, Keevil B. Urinary 5-hydroxyindoleacetic acid by high-performance liquid chromatography with electrochemical detection. Ann Clin Biochem 1997;34 (Pt 4):424-6.
254. Weinblatt ME, Heisel MA, Siegel SE. Hypertension in children with neurogenic tumors. Pediatrics 1983;71:947-51.
255. Weir TB, Smith CC, Round JM, Betteridge DJ. Stability of catecholamines in whole blood, plasma, and platelets. Clin Chem 1986;32:882-3.
256. Weise M, Merke DP, Pacak K, Walther MM, Eisenhofer G. Utility of plasma free metanephrines for detecting childhood pheochromocytoma. J Clin Endocrinol Metab 2002;87:1955-60.
257. Wilson SP, Kamin DL, Feldman JM. Acetaminophen administration interferes with urinary metanephrine (and catecholamine) determinations. Clin Chem 1985;31:1093-4.
258. Wolfovitz E, Grossman E, Folio CJ, Keiser HR, Kopin IJ, Goldstein DS. Derivation of urinary dopamine from plasma dihydroxyphenylalanine in humans. Clin Sci (Lond) 1993;84:549-57.
259. Wu AH, Gornet TG. Preparation of urine samples for liquid-chromatographic determination of catecholamines: bonded-phase phenylboronic acid, cation-exchange resin, and alumina adsorbents compared. Clin Chem 1985;31:298-302.
260. Wurtman RJ, Hefti F, Melamed E. Precursor control of neurotransmitter synthesis. Pharmacol Rev 1980;32:315-35.
261. Yeung PK, Buckley SJ, Pedder SC, Dingemanse J. Determination of 3,4-dihydroxyphenylacetic acid and 5-hydroxyindoleacetic acid in human plasma by a simple and rapid high-performance liquid chromatography assay. J Pharm Sci 1996;85:451-3.
262. Yoshimura M, Komori T, Nakanishi T, Takahashi H. Estimation of sulphoconjugated catecholamine concentrations in plasma by high-performance liquid chromatography. Ann Clin Biochem 1993;30 (Pt 2):135-41.
263. Young WF, Jr. Pheochromocytoma: issues in diagnosis & treatment. Compr Ther 1997;23:319-26.
264. Zambrano E, Reyes-Mugica M. Hormonal activity may predict aggressive behavior in neuroblastoma. Pediatr Dev Pathol 2002;5:190-9.
265. Zigmond RE, Schwarzschild MA, Rittenhouse AR. Acute regulation of tyrosine hydroxylase by nerve activity and by neurotransmitters via phosphorylation. Annu Rev Neurosci 1989;12:415-61.

CHAPTER 30

Vitamins and Trace Elements*

Alan Shenkin, Ph.D., Malcolm Baines, F.R.S.C., F.R.C.Path., Gordon S. Fell, Ph.D., F.R.C.Path., and T.D.G. Lyon, B.Sc., Ph.D.

Adequate supplies of vitamins and trace elements are extremely critical in maintaining the health and development of humans. These nutrients occupy the attention of those concerned with the physical well being of a public made increasingly aware of the need for the quality and the quantity of their dietary intake. The general principle regarding assessment of nutritional status is to determine the extent to which the metabolic demand for nutrients has been or is currently being met by the supply. In clinical practice, this requires balancing supply and demand.

Accurate assessment of supply and intake is a complex procedure. In practice, a crude estimate of intake can be obtained from a careful clinical history taken by an experienced practitioner or from a food frequency questionnaire that summarizes the content of the individual's diet over several days, depending on how frequently particular typical foods are consumed.[54] A more accurate quantitative assessment usually requires a minimum of three days recording of a complete dietary diary, which is subsequently analyzed using a computer program with reference tables of the nutritional contents of most foods.[414] Unfortunately, estimates of the portion size, amounts consumed, and actual nutritional composition of the food consumed may be inaccurate. In addition, the disease process also affects the amount actually consumed and absorbed, further reducing the accuracy of the estimate of nutritional intake.

Currently, the requirements for most nutrients to maintain health are now fairly well characterized and available in reports from the Institute of Medicine (IOM) of the National Academies (http://www.iom.edu).[170-174] However, the effects of disease may increase demands. For example, hypermetabolism, as a result of trauma or infection, increases the need for protein and energy[145,349] and for the vitamin and trace element cofactors necessary for their metabolism.[526] Increased losses from the gut, kidney, skin, or dialysis also may increase the overall demand for these nutrients.

An estimate of supply also is obtained from a careful dietary history, especially if performed by a dietician, together with knowledge of any artificial nutritional supplements or therapy that may have been provided enterally or intravenously. Table 30-1 summarizes the Recommended Dietary Allowance (RDA) made in the United States and the Population Reference Intakes (from the European community) for vitamins and trace elements. These levels are expected to be present in the normal diet of healthy adults. Table 30-1 also summarizes the range of amounts present in 2000 kcal of most tube feeds used in nutritional support. It is clear that the amounts used enterally are greater than the oral amounts recommended in health to meet the increased needs resulting from the preexisting deficiencies and increased ongoing requirements as a result of disease. The amounts recommended for supply during intravenous nutrition are also summarized in Table 30-1. For the trace elements, these amounts are generally less than the oral and/or enteral requirements to allow for the reduced absorption enterally. For the vitamins, these levels are usually greater than the oral and/or enteral requirements to allow for the effects of disease.

In an attempt to improve accuracy of assessment of nutritional status, clinicians often turn to the laboratory to

*The authors gratefully acknowledge the original contributions of Donald B. McCormick, Harry L. Green, George G. Klee, and David B. Milne, on which portions of this chapter are based.

TABLE 30-1 Oral and Intravenous Micronutrient Intakes for Adults

	RDA (USA)	PRI (Europe)	Amount in 2000 Kcal Tube Feed[521]	IV Intake[9,10,243,519]
Vitamins				
A μg	900	700	1000-2160	1000
D μg	5-15	0-10	8.5-14.6	5
E mg	15	0.4/g PUFA	20-64	10
K μg	120	100-200	150	
Thiamine mg	1.2	1.1	1.4-3.4	6
Riboflavin mg	1.3	1.6	2-6	3.6
Pyridoxine mg	1.3	1.5	2-13.8	6
Niacin mg	16	18	18-45	40
Folate μg	400	200	340-880	600
B_{12} μg	2	1.4	3-15	5
Pantothenic acid μg	5*	3-12†	7-20	15
Biotin μg	30*	15-100	100-660	60
Ascorbic acid mg	90	45	100-300	200
Trace Elements				
Zinc mg	11	9.5	13-36	3.2-6.5
Copper mg	0.9	1.1	2-3.4	0.3-1.3
Selenium μg	55	55	30-130	40-100
Chromium μg	25	30-200	10-20	
Molybdenum μg	45*	74-240	19	
Manganese mg	2-3*	1-10†	2.4-8	0.05-0.2

Reference intakes for infants and children are age and weight dependent and are summarized in various sources.[170,172,174,207,530]
RDA, Recommended dietary allowance (U.S.)[170,172,174]; *PRI*, population reference intake (Europe);[463] *PUFA*, polyunsaturated fatty acids.
*Adequate intake.
†Acceptable range.

provide a result that may reflect the net balance of supply and demand.[198,524,526] Clinical laboratorians need to be aware of where such tests are useful and how to place the results of laboratory tests into the context of the clinical situation of the patient.* It is important to be aware of the limitations of laboratory tests, especially in acutely ill patients.

NUTRITIONAL ASSESSMENT AND MONITORING

In this brief overview, the nutrients used in nutritional assessment and in monitoring will be briefly discussed.†

*A discussion of the Laboratory's role in nutritional assessement plus a number of case studies are available on this book's accompanying Evolve site, found at http://evolve.elsevier.com/Tietz/textbook/.

†A number of anthropometric and biochemical techniques and methods are used to assess nutritional status. They are discussed in an earlier edition of this textbook. (Veldee MS. Nutritional assessment, therapy, and monitoring. In: Burtis CA, Ashwood ER, eds. Tietz textbook of clinical chemistry, 3rd edition. Philadelphia: WB Saunders, 1999:1380-88.)

Protein-Energy Status

In clinical practice, only a few laboratory tests are of value in the assessment of protein-energy status.[524,527] It is particularly important to recognize that serum protein concentrations are not helpful in sick patients with any form of inflammatory process (see Chapter 20). Although serum albumin is often measured and reported as an indicator of protein-energy status, factors such as increased transcapillary escape[164] and reduced hepatic synthesis make it of little value as a nutritional marker. Serum albumin is, however, a valuable prognostic marker and is frequently used as part of prognostic indices.[88] Short half-life proteins, such as transthyretin (prealbumin) also may be of some limited value in patients with no inflammatory response.[164,265]

Assessment of nitrogen balance may be used to provide information on recent protein-energy status. This requires careful 24-hour urine collection and estimation of total nitrogen content[213,313] or urea nitrogen (from which total nitrogen can usually be approximately estimated).[191] With a reasonable calculation of protein (nitrogen) intake, intake minus urine output (together with some unmeasured losses) gives an estimate of nitrogen balance. In practice, however, such measurements are now rarely required except when (1) patients appear to have excessive losses, (2) they are failing to respond to what appears to be adequate nutritional support therapy, or (3) a novel therapy is being evaluated for its effectiveness in limiting catabolism or stimulating anabolism.

Vitamin and Trace Element Status

The measurement of vitamin and trace element levels is frequently helpful in nutritional assessment. The relative value of such tests is increased by the fact that clinical assessment of their status is often poor.

Although requirements for vitamins and trace elements are known in health (Table 30-1), the effects of illness on these requirements are poorly understood and quantified. However, it is now apparent that as an individual develops progressively more severe depletion in vitamin or trace element status, the person passes through a series of stages with biochemical or physiological consequences. The metabolic or physiological penalty of such suboptimal nutritional status is usually not clear, but the assumption remains that the suboptimal metabolism is likely to have detrimental effects (e.g., subclinical deficiency of folic acid is associated with an increase in serum homocysteine concentration, which is an independent risk factor for coronary artery disease—see Chapter 26).[607] Similarly, subclinical deficiency of chromium may be associated with impaired glucose tolerance in certain types of diabetes.[13]

The time course for the development of a subclinical deficiency state varies for each individual vitamin and trace element and depends on the nature and amount of body stores. Moreover, the extent of depletion necessary before there are significant biochemical, physiological, or histological changes is poorly characterized. The consequences of an inadequate intake are more clearly delineated in Figure 30-1. There is progression from optimal tissue status through a period of initial depletion until a period of subclinical deficiency is reached with a variety of biochemical and nonspecific physiological effects. In some cases there may also be certain nonspecific histological changes that may put the individual at risk of tissue damage or neoplastic change. It is only when there is a persistent mismatch of intake and demand that eventually a full-blown clinical deficiency state develops.

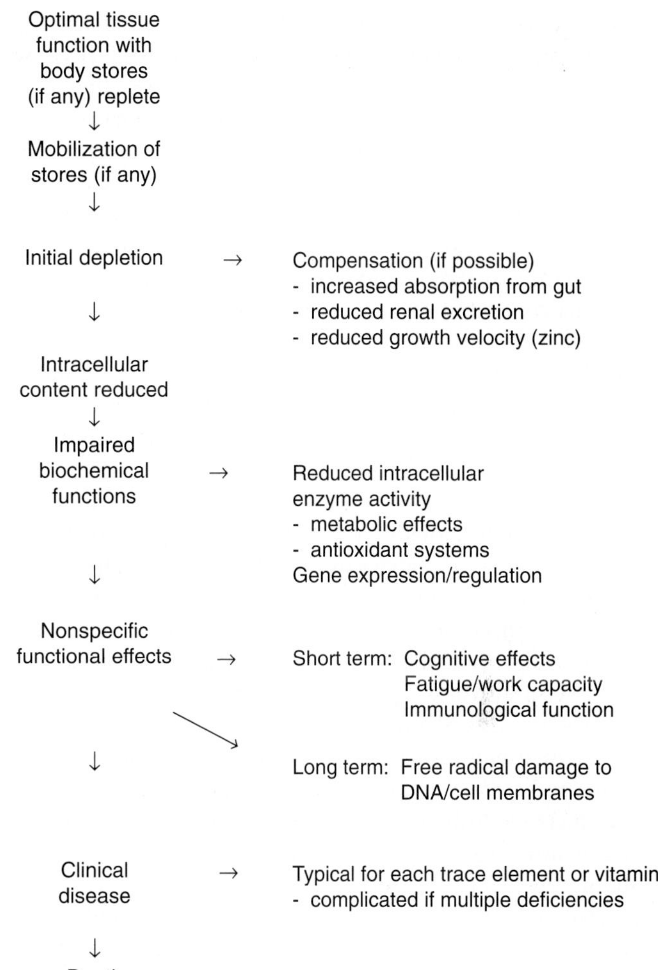

Figure 30-1 Consequences of inadequate mineral or trace element intake. *(From Shenkin A, Allwood MC. Trace elements and vitamins in adult intravenous nutrition. In: Rombeau JL, Rolandelli RH, eds. Clinical nutrition: Parenteral nutrition. Philadelphia: WB Saunders Co, 2001:60-79.)*

Enzymes or Metabolites

Determination of the effective functioning of particular enzymes or metabolic pathways potentially may be useful in demonstrating adequacy of provision. Enzymes in plasma that may be helpful in this regard are glutathione peroxidase as an index of selenium status, and red cell enzymes, such as transketolase (thiamine), glutathione reductase (riboflavin) or transaminase (pyridoxine), or glutathione peroxidase (selenium) are all widely used. Methyltetrahydrofolate reductase is involved in metabolism of homocysteine, hence assessment of plasma homocysteine is a useful measure of folate status through the indirect assessment of the action of this enzyme system.

Markers of Antioxidant Status

As it is practically impossible to measure all the biologically active antioxidants in human samples, the concept of a "global" assessment of antioxidant capacity has proved attractive.[223,224] A number of methods have therefore been developed to assess this capacity and for use in clinical research. Most of the methods use one of two main approaches to the measurement, either the quenching or delayed production of a stable, measurable radical species, or the reductant properties of the antioxidants against a radical cation or a metal ion.[499] These are usually standardized with the water-soluble vitamin E analogue Trolox. An example of the former is the total radical-trapping antioxidant parameter (TRAP) assay, which uses the stable radical species 2,2′-azinobis(3-ethylbenzthiazolinesulfonate) ($ABTS^+$) and an example of the latter is the ferric reducing ability of plasma (FRAP) assay.[43] Because these methods use different reaction principles, the same antioxidant can have different contributions to each assay, and it is for this reason that the use of more than one method is recommended for any study.[451] Vitamins that can contribute to plasma antioxidant capacity are ascorbate (up to 24% of the measured capacity), α-tocopherol (up to 10% of measured capacity), and β-carotene, though at typical plasma concentrations of around 0.5 μmol/L, the contribution of β-carotene—as with most fat-soluble vitamins—to a total antioxidant capacity of around 1000 μmol/L is minimal.

A disadvantage of many methods of total antioxidant capacity measurement is the variable contribution of common plasma constituents, particularly albumin and urate, to the measured concentration.[197] Changes in circulating concentrations of these molecules caused by acute phase changes or changes in renal function can alter measured values without reflecting changes in antioxidant vitamin concentration. This problem can be largely overcome by the use of the "antioxidant gap," a derived value that subtracts the Trolox equivalence of albumin and urate from the measured total antioxidant capacity.[389]

In an attempt to assess the functional adequacy of vitamins and trace elements involved in antioxidant pathways, products of oxidative metabolism can be measured. Those frequently used are malondialdehyde or F_2 isoprostanes, both of which give an indication of oxidation of polyunsaturated fatty acids within cells.[223] Increasing the provision of individual antioxidants or cocktails of vitamins and trace elements can lead to a reduction in production of these metabolites that can be measured in serum or urine. Such tests have not yet reached widespread application primarily because the interpretation of results is difficult. Also, knowledge of the appropriate amount of oxidative activity that is linked to particular outcomes has not yet been identified. This is especially important since there have been few clinical studies demonstrating benefit from provision of increased amounts of antioxidants.[42,167]

Analytical Factors

A number of analytical factors must be considered when assessing the status of each nutrient. They include reference intervals, concentrations of markers in plasma and tissue, and their measurement in urine.

Reference Intervals

As for all laboratory tests, interpretation of tests of nutritional status requires access to relevant reference intervals and an understanding of the factors that may alter them. Ethnic origin and geographic variation might affect the typical diet and its chemical composition, and the fiber or phytate content may alter the bioavailability of minerals. In early infancy, the liver matures, leading to an increase in serum copper, whereas dietary changes in milk and weaning are associated with changes in plasma selenium. Seasonal variations may alter the reference intervals of vitamins, especially vitamin D. Time of sampling is also important, since zinc and iron concentrations tend to be higher in fasting than fed individuals and are therefore usually lower in the afternoon.

Plasma Concentrations

Concentrations of vitamins and trace elements are measured most often in plasma or serum; this provides a reliable index of status for only a few of them (e.g., vitamin B_{12} or vitamin D). For others (e.g., folate or selenium), their concentrations only may reflect the adequacy of recent intake. An excessive provision of elements such as manganese and chromium may also be detected by high serum concentrations.[154,520]

For some vitamins or trace elements, serum measurement is limited in value, especially in seriously ill patients. This is partly a result of the lack of correlation between the amount of nutrient in the plasma compartment with the amount within the intracellular compartment in most body tissue. For example, there may be substantial stores of particular vitamins or trace elements in individual tissue (e.g., vitamin A in the liver), but mobilization into the plasma is affected by the availability of the appropriate binding proteins or by metabolism. Also, there are differences in the content of individual vitamins or trace elements between tissues, and the serum concentration will not reflect these differences. Furthermore, and particularly important, is the fact that the concentration in plasma can alter rapidly when an acute phase response (APR) to trauma or infection leads to redistribution of metals between body compartments[523]; there is increased synthesis of metallothionein, leading to the uptake of zinc into the liver, and increased synthesis of ferritin causing uptake of iron.[119,475] The result is a fall in plasma concentration of both zinc and iron. These changes in plasma concentration clearly do not reflect changes in whole body status.

There are also changes in the binding proteins in plasma as a result of the disease process. Since serum albumin falls in association with any acute illness, this inevitably leads to a fall in plasma zinc concentration. Similarly a reduction in retinol-binding-protein concentration as part of the APR or protein malnutrition also leads to a fall in serum retinol levels, whatever the amount of retinol stores within the liver.

Some patients may be relatively stable, with little APR to injury, infection, or other inflammatory disease. If this is the case, it may be possible to interpret the plasma concentrations of elements such as zinc, copper, and iron, or vitamins such as vitamin C or B_6 that would all be affected by an APR.[347] Of particular relevance is the trend in concentration of a trace element or vitamin in relation to the magnitude of the APR changes. Repeated measurements of a rapid response acute phase protein, such as C-reactive protein (CRP), together with trace elements, may therefore be helpful as part of the nutritional assessment.

Tissue Concentrations

Tissue concentrations of vitamins or trace elements are rarely measured in nutritional assessments because of the lack of availability of suitable tissue; however, where such tissue is available, measurement may be helpful (e.g., copper analysis on liver biopsy of patients with suspected Wilson's disease).

More commonly, certain types of cells from blood samples may be obtained and can provide useful information. For example, red cell folate is commonly used as a marker of folate status, and leukocyte vitamin C is a better marker of vitamin C status than plasma concentration.[495] Because of the difficulty of preparation of pure populations of cells, cellular measurements are usually only used within a research environment.

Urine Measurements

For most vitamins and trace elements, their measurement in urine is rarely helpful since most are not under homeostatic control, and excretion may be a direct reflection of intake rather than active retention in the face of whole body deficiency. High levels of excretion of certain water-soluble vitamins or trace elements may indicate ingestion of large amounts of supplements.

VITAMINS

Vitamins are organic compounds required in trace amounts (in microgram to milligram quantities per day) in the diet for health, growth, and reproduction. It is commonly understood that vitamins are natural materials that can be isolated from organisms (such as plants that can synthesize most of these compounds) or that can be chemically synthesized. Additionally, there are synthetic analogues and derivatives of vitamins designed to serve as inhibitors (e.g., amethopterin as an antifolate) and others that substitute in part for the natural vitamin (e.g., 8-ethylriboflavin for riboflavin). Only small amounts of vitamins are required for the functional, often catalytic (co-enzymatic) roles they serve, in contrast to the relatively large amounts of such macronutrients as protein, lipid, and carbohydrate, which constitute the bulk of the ingesta that serve primarily as sources for energy and reconstitution of body mass.

Historically, vitamin groups such as A, B, and D bear an Arabic subscript number following the letter either to designate structural and functional similarity (e.g., A_1 [retinol] and A_2 [3-dehydroretinol]) or to indicate the approximate order in which they are identified as the members of the so-called B-complex (e.g., B_1 [thiamine] and B_2 [riboflavin]). Common chemical names, which are receiving greater use, give a better indication of the types of compounds involved. These often reflect the presence of some specific atom (*thia*mine), prime functional group (pyridox*amine*), or even a larger portion of the molecular structure (phyllo*quinone*). Parts of some names reflect functional properties (chole*calciferol*).

Another classification pertains to the relative solubility of vitamins. Those of the "fat-soluble" group (A, D, E, and K) are more soluble in organic solvents, whereas the B-complex group vitamins and vitamin C are "water soluble." This general separation based on solubility is useful not just for purposes of noting gross physical properties but also as a reminder that the fat-soluble vitamins are absorbed, transported, and stored for longer periods of time and in a manner generally similar to that for fats. Most water-soluble vitamins share the fate of other solutes more compatible with an aqueous, physiological medium; this includes a lesser tendency to be retained for long periods of time in the body and a greater loss by way of urinary excretion. Additionally a general functional difference also exists, since the water-soluble vitamins function as coenzymes for several important enzymatic reactions in both mammals and microorganisms. By contrast, the fat-soluble vitamins generally do not function as coenzymes and are rarely used by microorganisms.

Table 30-2 provides a list of 13 known vitamins and vitameric groups essential to humans.

VITAMIN A

Vitamin A serves many important functions in the body, with its role in vision being of particular significance.

Chemistry

Vitamin A is the nutritional term for the group of compounds with a 20-carbon structure containing a methyl-substituted cyclohexenyl ring (β-ionone ring) and an isoprenoid side chain (Figure 30-2), with either a hydroxyl group (retinol), an aldehyde group (retinal), a carboxylic acid group (retinoic acid), or an ester group (retinyl ester) at the terminal C15.

Retinol, the principal vitamin A vitamer, can be oxidized reversibly to retinal—which shares all the biological activity of retinol—or further oxidized to retinoic acid, which shows some of its biological activity. The principal storage forms of vitamin A are retinyl esters, particularly palmitate. The term retinoids refers to retinol, its metabolites, and synthetic analogues with similar structure. Included in the vitamin A family are some dietary carotenoids (C40 polyisoprenoid compounds) that are classified as provitamin A because they are cleaved biologically to yield retinol. Although around 1000 compounds with carotenoid structure have been identified,[366] only around 50 possess provitamin A activity, with the principal dietary compounds being β-carotene, α-carotene, and β-cryptoxanthin. Vitamin A compounds are yellowish oils or low-melting-point solids (depending on isomeric purity) that are practically insoluble in water but soluble in organic solvents and mineral oil. Vitamin A is sensitive to oxygen and ultraviolet light, which induces a greenish fluorescence with an absorbance peak at 325 nm. The structure for the most common and effective provitamin A, *β-carotene,* is also given in Figure 30-2. This compound is an orange-to-purple, water-insoluble solid that is oxidized in

TABLE 30-2 Vitamins Required by the Human

Common Name	Trivial Chemical Name	General Roles	Symptoms of Deficiency or Disease	Direct and Indirect Assays
Fat Soluble				
Vitamin A	Retinol, retinal, retinoic acid	Vision, growth, reproduction	Nyctalopia, xerophthalmia, keratomalacia	Photometric, HPLC, fluorimetric, RIA
Vitamin D_2, D_3	Ergocalciferol Cholecalciferol	Modulation of Ca^{2+} metabolism, calcification of bone and teeth	Rickets (young), osteomalacia (adult)	CPB, HPLC, RIA
Vitamin E	Tocopherols, tocotrienols	Antioxidant for unsaturated lipids, neurological and reproductive functions	Lipid peroxidation, including red blood cell fragility, hemolytic anemia (premature, newborn)	Photometric, HPLC, erythrocyte hemolysis
Vitamin K_1, K_2	Phylloquinones Menaquinones	Blood clotting, osteocalcins	Increased clotting time, hemorrhagic disease (infant)	HPLC, prothrombin time, RIA (abnormal prothrombin, PIVKA Test)
Water Soluble				
Vitamin B_1	Thiamine	Carbohydrate metabolism, nervous function	Beriberi, Wernicke-Korsakoff syndrome	Fluorimetric, transketolase, HPLC
Vitamin B_2	Riboflavin	Oxidation-reduction reactions	Angular stomatitis, dermatitis, photophobia	Fluorimetric, HPLC, glutathione reductase
Vitamin B_6	Pyridoxine, pyridoxal, pyridoxamine	Amino acid, phospholipid, and glycogen metabolism	Epileptiform convulsions, dermatitis, hypochromic anemia	HPLC, aspartate transaminase, urine pyridoxic acid
Niacin niacinamide	Nicotinic acid, nicotinamide	Oxidation-reduction reactions	Pellagra	Fluorometric, HPLC, nicotinamide coenzymes
Folic acid	Pteroylglutamic acid	Nucleic acid and amino acid biosynthesis	Megaloblastic anemia, neural tube defects	CPB, microbiological, homocysteine
Vitamin B_{12}	Cyanocobalamin	Amino acid and branched-chain keto acid metabolism	Pernicious and megaloblastic anemia, neuropathy	CPB, microbiological, RIA, methylmalonate
Biotin	—	Carboxylation reactions	Dermatitis	Microbiological, CPB, carboxylases, avidin binding
Pantothenic acid	—	General metabolism, acetyl and acyl transfer	Burning feet syndrome	Microbiological, RIA, CPB/HPLC
Vitamin C	Ascorbic acid	Connective tissue formation, antioxidant	Scurvy	Photometric, HPLC, enzymatic

HPLC, High-performance liquid chromatography; *RIA*, radioimmunoassay; *CPB*, competitive protein binding; *PIVKA Test*, proteins induced by or involved in vitamin K antagonism or absence.

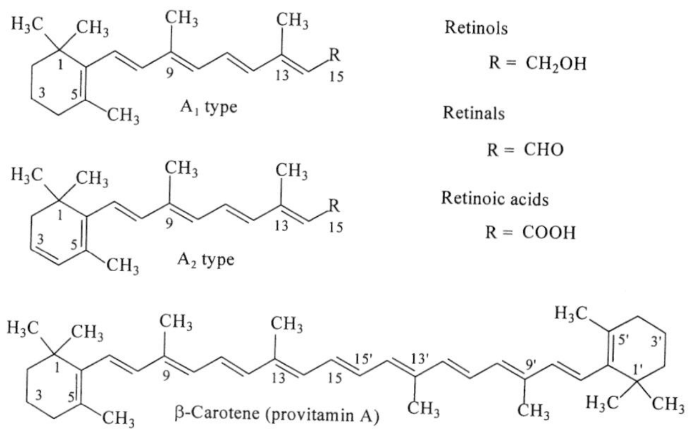

Figure 30-2 Vitaminic forms of A_1, A_2, and β-carotene.

air to inactive products. The other carotenes, cryptoxanthin and β-apocarotenals, are asymmetrical with only one β-ionone ring and yield less vitamin A activity.

Dietary Sources

Preformed vitamin A is obtained from animal-derived foods such as liver, other organ meats, and fish oils. Other sources are full cream milk, butter, and fortified margarines. The provitamin A carotenoids are obtained from yellow to orange pigment fruits and vegetables, and green leafy vegetables. Good sources are pumpkin, carrots, tomatoes, apricots, grapefruit, lettuce, and most green vegetables.[359] The U.S. National Health and Nutrition Examination Survey (NHANES-II) indicated that approximately 25% of the vitamin A requirement was provided by carotenoids and about 75% by preformed retinol.[59]

Absorption, Transport, Metabolism, and Excretion

Preformed vitamin A, most often in the form of retinyl ester, or carotenoids are subject to emulsification and mixed micelle formation by the action of bile salts before being transported into the intestinal cell. Here the retinyl esters are moved across the mucosal membrane and hydrolyzed to retinol within the cell to then be reesterified by cellular retinol-binding protein II and packaged into chylomicra, which then enter the mesenteric lymphatic system and pass into the systemic circulation.[409] A small amount of the ingested retinoid is also converted into retinoic acid in the intestinal cell. The efficiency of absorption of preformed vitamin A is high at between 70% and 90%.[533]

Carotenoids, also in micellular form, are absorbed into the duodenal mucosal cells by passive diffusion. The efficiency of absorption of carotenoids is much lower than for vitamin A, between 9% and 22%,[423] and is subject to a large number of variables, including carotenoid type, the amount in the meal, matrix properties, nutrient status, and genetic factors.[560] Once inside the mucosal cell, β-carotene is principally converted to retinal by the enzyme β-carotene-15, 15′-dioxygenase, the retinal being converted by retinal reductase to retinol and esterified, though it can also be cleaved eccentrically to β-apocarotenals, which can be further degraded to retinal or retinoic acid. The newly synthesized retinyl esters, from both preformed vitamin A and carotenoids, along with exogenous lipids and nonhydrolyzed carotenoids then pass with chylomicrons via the lymphatic system to the liver, where uptake by parenchymal cells again involves hydrolysis. In the liver, retinol is bound with retinol-binding protein (RBP, MW ~ 21,000 Da) and transthyretin (thyroxine-binding prealbumin) (MW ~ 55,000 Da) in a 1:1:1 complex of sufficient size to prevent loss by glomerular filtration and returned to the circulation, or it is stored as esters in the stellate cells. Delivery of retinol to the tissue is controlled by the availability of the vitamin A–protein complex in the circulation, though this control mechanism can be bypassed by large doses of retinol.

Retinoic acid from the intestinal mucosa is transported bound to serum albumin via the portal vein. Retinoic acid cannot be significantly reduced to retinal but is rapidly metabolized in tissue, such as liver, to yield more polar catabolites (e.g., 5,6-epoxyretinoic acid) and conjugates, such as retinoyl β-glucuronide, that are excreted. A small amount of retinoic acid undergoes enterohepatic circulation after intestinal hydrolysis of the glucuronide is excreted in the bile.

Functions

The participation of retinal in vision is considered the most important physiological function of vitamin A. All-*trans*-retinol is the predominant circulating form of vitamin A. Cells of the retina isomerize this to the 11-*cis* alcohol that is reversibly dehydrogenated to 11-*cis* retinal. This sterically hindered geometrical isomer of the aldehyde combines as a lysyl-linked Schiff base with suitable proteins (e.g., opsin) to generate photosensitive pigments such as rhodopsin. Illumination of such pigments causes photoisomerization and the release of all-*trans*-retinal and the protein, a process that couples the large conformational change to ion flux and optic nerve transmission. The all-*trans*-retinal is isomerized to the 11-*cis* isomer, which again combines with the liberated protein to reconstitute the photo pigment in a visual cycle shown in Figure 30-3. The pyridine nucleotide-dependent dehydrogenase (reductase) can also reduce the all-*trans*-retinal to all-*trans*-retinol.

Other functions of vitamin A include its role in reproduction, growth and embryonic development, and immune function, many of them mediated through the binding of retinoic acid to specific nuclear receptors that regulate genomic expression. In normal growth, and in the maintenance of the integrity of epithelial cells, retinoic acid acts through the activation of retinoic acid receptors (RAR) and retinoid X receptors (RXR) in the nucleus to regulate various genes that encode for structural proteins, enzymes, extracellular matrix proteins, and RBPs and receptors.[361] In vertebrate embryonic development, vitamin A requirement (mediated via RARs and RXRs) begins at the time of formation of the primitive heart circulation and specification

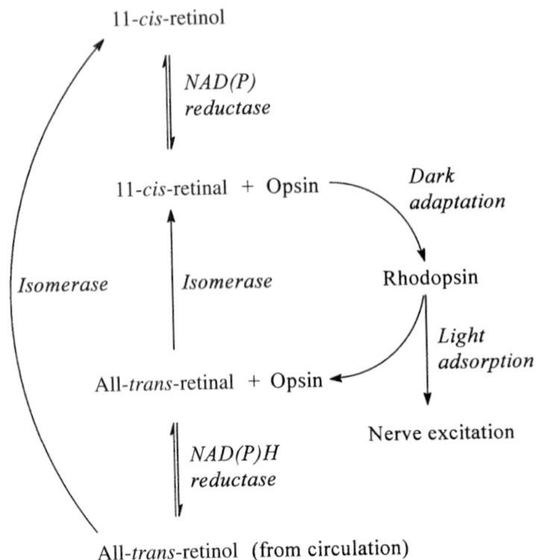

Figure 30-3 Participation of A vitamers in the visual cycle.

of the hindbrain,[639] and is later required for normal development of the limbs, heart, eyes, and ears.[134] Vitamin A deficiency impairs innate immunity by impeding normal regeneration of mucosal barriers damaged by infection, and by diminishing the function of neutrophils, macrophages, and natural killer cells. It is also required for adaptive immunity and plays a role in the development of both T-helper cells and B cells.[546] Retinol, its metabolites and synthetic retinoids, have protective effects against the development of certain types of cancer by blocking tumor promotion, by inhibiting proliferation, by inducing apoptosis, by inducing differentiation, or by a combination of these actions.[420] Finally, synthetic retinoids have been used successfully, both topically and systemically, to treat severe acne and other skin disorders of abnormal keratinization.

Some caution is required, however, regarding the use of vitamin A or β-carotene supplements since they appear to be of no benefit in reducing the incidence of gastrointestinal cancer and indeed may increase the incidence of lung cancer and mortality in certain other cancers.[55a,432a,566a]

Requirements and Reference Nutrient Intakes

Historical studies in adult humans have suggested that intakes of retinol of 500 to 600 μg/day are required to maintain adequate blood concentrations and to prevent all deficiency symptoms. The relative contribution of β-carotene and other provitamin A carotenoids to achieving this goal has undergone much revision as our knowledge has developed. In the older system of international units (IU), now largely redundant, a ratio for equivalence of activity of 1:2:4 for retinal:β-carotene:other provitamin A carotenoids was used, but this was superseded in 1967 by the retinol equivalent (RE), devised by a Food and Agriculture/World Health Organization (WHO) Expert Committee and proposing an equivalence ratio of 1:6:12. However, a 1999 study using stable isotopes of β-carotene[268] and a subsequent 2003 study[593] led the Food and Nutrition Board of the U.S. Institute of Medicine to recommend the retinol activity equivalent (RAE) as the basis of calculation of retinol intake. In this system, a ratio equivalence of 1:12:24 is recommended (i.e., 12μg β-carotene or 24μg mixed carotenoids has the same biological activity as 1μg retinol). Using this system, current RDAs for vitamin A are 900 μg RAE for men 19 years and older; 700 μg RAE for women 19 years and older, with up to 770 μg RAE/day in pregnancy and up to 1300 μg RAE/day in lactation; 300 to 900 μg RAE for children 1 to 18 years, dependent upon age and sex; and for infants an adequate intake (AI) of 400 μg RAE at 0 to 6 months and 500 μg RAE from 7 to 12 months.[174]

Intravenous Supply

The recommended provision of vitamin A to adults during intravenous nutrition (IVN), whether this is partial or total parenteral nutrition (TPN), is 1000 μg retinol. This is usually provided as retinol palmitate and is supplied either with other fat-soluble vitamins in a mixture dissolved in a fat emulsion for intravenous feeding or is designed to be compatible with a mixture of all vitamins suitable for addition to other water-soluble nutrients.[519]

Deficiency

Vitamin A deficiency primarily affects infants and children, and its prevalence is subject to WHO surveillance.[627] Risk factors include poverty, low birth weight, poor sanitation, malnutrition, infection, and parasitism. Because hepatic accumulation of vitamin A occurs during the last trimester of pregnancy, preterm infants are relatively vitamin A deficient at birth. Providing a daily oral intake of vitamin A that meets the RDA of 400 μg RAE is therefore important. Infants with birth weights of less than 1500 g (those under 30 weeks gestation) have virtually no hepatic vitamin A stores and are at risk of vitamin A deficiency. Shenai and co-workers[518] and others[68,206] have observed that (1) bronchopulmonary dysplasia (BPD), a debilitating, chronic lung disease that mimics some histological features of vitamin A deficiency, is common; (2) intramuscular injections of 630 μg RAE every 2 days can reduce the incidence of BPD; (3) vitamin A (retinol) delivered in TPN solutions may be adsorbed into the inner walls of the plastic administration sets; however, this loss can be minimized by the use ethylene vinyl acetate rather than polyvinyl chloride; (4) blood levels of vitamin A decline during TPN, often reaching concentrations of 10 to 15 μg/dL (normal, 20 to 65 μg/dL) unless adequate supplements are given.

Fat malabsorption, particularly caused by celiac disease or chronic pancreatitis, and protein-energy malnutrition predispose to vitamin A deficiency. Liver disease diminishes RBP synthesis, and ethanol abuse leads both to hepatic injury and to a competition with retinol for alcohol dehydrogenase, which is necessary for the oxidation of retinol to retinal and retinoic acid.[328] Vitamin A deficiency may lead to anemia, though the precise mechanism is not known.[513]

The clinical features of vitamin A deficiency are degenerative changes in eyes and skin, and poor dark adaptation or *night blindness* (nyctalopia) followed by degenerative changes in the retina. *Xerophthalmia,* in which the conjunctiva becomes dry with small gray plaques with foamy surfaces (Bitot's spots), develops. These lesions are reversible with vitamin A administration. More serious effects of deficiency are known as *keratomalacia* and cause ulceration and necrosis of the cornea that lead to perforation, prolapse, endophthalmitis, and blindness. Usually, there are associated skin changes, which include dryness, roughness, papular eruptions, and follicular hyperkeratosis. The general change is atrophy of certain specialized epithelia, followed by metaplastic hyperkeratinization.

Toxicity

Although vitamin A metabolism is tightly regulated, toxic effects of hypervitaminosis A can occur as a result of ingestion of excess vitamin or as a side effect of inappropriate therapy.[620] Hypervitaminosis A occurs after the liver storage of retinol and its esters exceeds 3000 μg/g tissue, after ingestion of greater than 30,000 μg/day for months or years, or if plasma vitamin A levels exceed 140 μg/dL (4.9 μmol/L). The elderly are more susceptible to vitamin A toxicity at lower doses, as exposure to retinyl esters is longer because of delayed postprandial clearance of lipoproteins.[483] Symptoms of acute toxicity from a single massive dose present as abdominal pain, nausea, vomiting, severe headaches, dizziness, sluggishness, and irritability, followed within a few days by desquamation of the skin and recovery. Chronic toxicity from moderately high doses taken for protracted periods is characterized by bone and joint pain, hair loss, dryness and fissures of the lips, anorexia, benign intracranial hypertension, weight loss, and hepatomegaly. The administration of doses up to threefold the RDA for several years resulted in classic histological changes of hepatotoxicity in 41 patients.[195] Infants given excess vitamin A over months to years can develop intracranial features, typically bulging fontanelle, and skeletal abnormalities at doses of 5500 to 6750 μg/day.[439]

Epidemiological and experimental evidence has supported the view that high vitamin A intake in humans, acting via 13-*cis*-retinoic acid, is teratogenic.[318] The critical period of susceptibility is the first trimester of pregnancy, and the primary abnormalities derive from the cranial neural crest (CNC) cells. A 1995 study of almost 23,000 pregnant women found that those who ingested more than 4500 μg/day of preformed vitamin A were at greater risk of delivering infants with malformations of CNC cell origin than women consuming less than 1500 μg/day.[478] A further intriguing association, supported in part by epidemiological studies, is that between excessive vitamin A intake and reduction in bone mineral density (BMD). Two studies of 175 Scandinavian women showed that a consistent loss in BMD at 4 sites was associated with increased preformed vitamin A intake.[376,386] Intake levels of vitamin A exceeding 1500 μg/day were associated with these changes, although 2 U.S. studies showed no increased bone mineral loss at preformed vitamin A intakes of up to 2000 μg/day.[183,257]

The findings of these and other studies have led the Food and Nutrition Board of the U.S. Institute of Medicine to recommend a tolerable upper intake level of 3000 μg/day of preformed vitamin A for men of 19 years and older, with lower levels for women of child-bearing age, infants, children, and adolescents. Carotenemia results from a chronic excessive intake of carotene-rich foods, principally carrots. This condition, in which yellowing of skin is observed, is benign, because the excess carotene is deposited rather than converted to vitamin A.

Laboratory Assessment of Status

Although measurement of the plasma concentration of vitamin A is the most convenient and widely used assessment of vitamin A status, it is not an ideal indicator because it does not decline until liver stores become critically depleted, which is thought to be at a concentration of approximately 20 μg/g liver. Early chemical methods, which may remain in use if high-performance liquid chromatography (HPLC) is not available, include the Carr-Price photometric method, which uses antimony trichloride in chloroform as the reagent, and the later Neeld-Pearson method, which uses trifluoroacetic acid to produce a blue pigment with the conjugated double bonds of vitamin A (and the carotenoids). Both methods use volatile or corrosive reagents, are nonspecific for vitamin A, are time consuming and difficult to automate, and require large sample volumes. To improve specificity and sensitivity, later methods used solvent extraction and other separation techniques, with fluorometric or spectrophotometric measurement.[585] HPLC has brought enhanced (1) specificity, (2) lowered limit of detection (less than 0.07 μmol/L), (3) accuracy (using primary standards, reference materials, and quality assurance schemes), and (4) reproducibility (between batch coefficients of variation of 10% or better).[572] Both normal-phase and reverse-phase techniques have been used.[109,373]

In the normal-phase HPLC, compounds to be separated are adsorbed to microparticulate silica gel and eluted in the order of least polar to most polar. Acceptable separation and quantitative yields of neutral and charged retinoids are obtained. Reverse-phase HPLC is preferable for acid-sensitive compounds such as 5,6-epoxyretinoic acid. Photometric, electrochemical, and mass spectrophotometric detectors have been used.

As retinol circulates in plasma as a 1:1:1 complex with RBP and transthyretin, both of these hepatically produced proteins have been measured as an indicator of vitamin A status. RBP has been measured by radial immunodiffusion or nephelometry (see Chapter 20), but its circulating concentration may be limited by inadequate dietary protein, energy, or zinc, all of which are necessary for RBP synthesis. Another confounding factor in the assessment of vitamin A status is the effect of the APR. Both RBP and transthyretin are negative acute phase proteins and thus inflammatory changes will result in transient falls in both proteins and in plasma retinol. To distinguish inflammatory from nutritional causes of reduced plasma retinol concentrations, it may be necessary to measure high-sentivity CRP.[510]

Because circulating retinol concentrations do not always correlate with total body stores of vitamin A, indirect tests have been employed to assess these stores. The relative-dose-response test, described first by Loerch et al,[341] requires 2 blood samples to be collected, one before and one 5 hours after a physiological dose of vitamin A. In vitamin A–depleted subjects there is a rapid, large, and sustained rise in serum retinol concentration, which contrasts with a lower, more shallow rise in vitamin A–sufficient subjects. A modified-relative-dose-response test (using 3,4 didehydroretinyl [DR] acetate rather than retinyl acetate and measuring the DR/retinol ratio after 5 hours) has been used by other workers to assess the vitamin A status of preschool Indonesian children[561] of lactating and nonlactating Indonesian women[562] and also in a population of well-nourished American children.[563] Quantitative assessment of total body stores may be made by using deuterated-retinol-dilution techniques, but these require long periods (about 3 weeks) for equilibration. In 2003 Ribaya-Mercado and colleagues developed a predictive mathematical formula that does not require serum isotope equilibration, allowing blood sampling to be made 3 days after isotope dosing.[466]

Reference Intervals

Guidance reference intervals for serum vitamin A are 20 to 40 μg/dL (0.70 to 1.40 μmol/L) for 1- to 6-year-old children; 26 to 49 μg/dL (0.91 to 1.71 μmol/L) for 7- to 12-year-old children; 26 to 72 μg/dL (0.91 to 2.51 μmol/L) for 13- to 19-year-old adolescents; and 30 to 80 μg/dL (1.05 to 2.80 μmol/L) for adults.[339,574] Values above 30 μg/dL (1.05 μmol/L) are associated with appreciable reserves in the liver and correlate well with vitamin A intake. Within the reference interval, values for men are generally about 20% higher than those for women.

By HPLC, the reference interval for serum β-carotene is 10 to 85 μg/dL (0.19 to 1.58 μmol/L).[574] Elevated levels are found in hypothyroid patients in whom conversion to vitamin A is decreased and in patients with hyperlipemia associated with diabetes mellitus.

VITAMIN D

Vitamin D plays an essential role as a hormone in the control of calcium and phosphorus metabolism. It is discussed in detail in Chapter 49.

VITAMIN E

Vitamin E in an antioxidant that acts as a scavenger for molecular oxygen and free radicals. It also has a role in cellular respiration.

Chemistry

Vitamin E is the nutritional term for the group of naturally occurring tocopherols and tocotrienols that have biological activity similar to RRR-α-tocopherol (formerly d-α-tocopherol).[385] Both groups have a common 6-chromanol nucleus substituted with methyl groups at positions 2 and 8 and with a phytyl tail of isoprenoid units at position 2. The isoprenoid chain is saturated in the tocopherols, but unsaturated at positions 3′, 7′, and 11′ for tocotrienols (Figure 30-4). The Greek letter prefixes α, β, γ, and δ indicate the presence or absence of methyl groups at positions 5 and 7. The tocopherols have three asymmetric carbon atoms in the isoprenoid chain, giving eight optical isomers. The naturally occurring tocopherols occur as the RRR forms, whereas the synthetic compounds are of the racemic SR forms. Synthetic vitamin E contains about 12.5% of RRR-α-tocopherol together with seven other tocopherol isomers that are less biologically active. Tocopherol and tocotrienols are viscous oils at room temperature, soluble in fat solvents, and insoluble in aqueous solutions although there exists a water-soluble analogue (Trolox-6-hydroxy-2, 5, 7, 8-tetramethylchroman-2-carboxylic acid). Also, tocopherol and tocotrienols are stable to acid and heat in the absence of oxygen, but labile to oxygen in alkaline solutions and to ultraviolet light.

Dietary Sources

The principal sources of dietary vitamin E are oils and fats, particularly wheat germ oil and sunflower oil, grains, and nuts.[33] Meats, fruits, and vegetables contribute little vitamin E. Gamma-tocopherol is the major form of vitamin E in many plant seeds in the U.S. diet, but is present at only one quarter to one tenth of the concentration of α-tocopherol in human plasma.[282,286]

Absorption, Transport, Metabolism, and Excretion

In the presence of bile, vitamin E is absorbed from the small intestine.[107] Most forms of vitamin E are absorbed nonselectively and are secreted in chylomicron particles along with triacylglycerol and cholesterol. Some of this chylomicron-

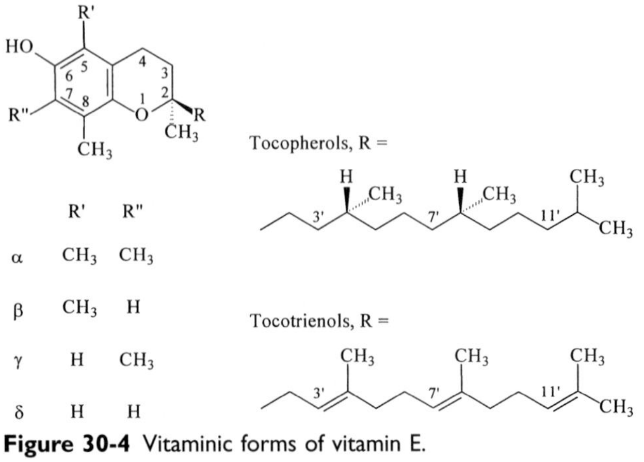

	R'	R"
α	CH_3	CH_3
β	CH_3	H
γ	H	CH_3
δ	H	H

Figure 30-4 Vitaminic forms of vitamin E.

bound vitamin E is transported and delivered to the peripheral tissue (mainly adipose tissue) with the aid of lipoprotein lipase. The liver takes up the chylomicron remnants where the α-tocopherol is incorporated into very low-density lipoprotein (VLDL)s by α-tocopherol transfer protein (α-TTP), enabling further distribution of α-tocopherol throughout the body. Plasma vitamin E is further delivered to the tissue by low-density lipoprotein (LDL) and high-density lipoprotein (HDL).[286] The specificity of α-TTP for α-tocopherol is probably responsible for its preferential storage in most tissue. Vitamin E is excreted via the bile, in the urine as tocopheronic acid and its β-glucuronide conjugate, as carboxyethyl hydroxychromans (CEHC), and by unknown routes.[507] Degradation of vitamin E has been reviewed by Brigelius-Flohe and colleagues.[75]

Functions

Historically, vitamin E has been recognized as necessary for neurological and reproductive functions, for protecting the red cell from hemolysis, and for prevention of retinopathy in premature infants.[75] Inhibition of free-radical chain reactions of lipid peroxidation is the most thoroughly defined role of vitamin E.[285] This occurs mainly within the polyunsaturated fatty acids of membrane phospholipids. Tocopherols and tocotrienols inhibit lipid peroxidation largely because they scavenge lipid peroxyl radicals faster than the radical can react with adjacent fatty acid side chains or membrane proteins. The resultant tocopheryl or tocotrienyl radicals may then react with further peroxyl radicals to produce tocopherones (nonradicals), or be regenerated by transferring an electron to ascorbate to form the ascorbyl radical. Thus vitamins E and C act synergistically to reduce lipid peroxidation (Figure 30-5).[102] Many epidemiological surveys have shown an association between reduced vitamin E intake (and other dietary factors) and increase in chronic disease incidence, particularly cardiovascular disease and cancer,[196,310,468,543] though intervention studies have produced mixed results. The Cambridge Heart Antioxidant Study[545] showed a significant 47% reduction in nonfatal myocardial infarction (MI) in the vitamin E treatment (400 or 800 IU per day) arm of a placebo-controlled study involving subjects with existing heart disease, whereas the Gruppo Italiano Studio Sopravvivenza Infarcto (GISSI) trial,[215] also involving secondary prevention, produced only a small but insignificant reduction in risk of death, nonfatal MI, or stroke in those given 300 mg per day of synthetic vitamin E versus the

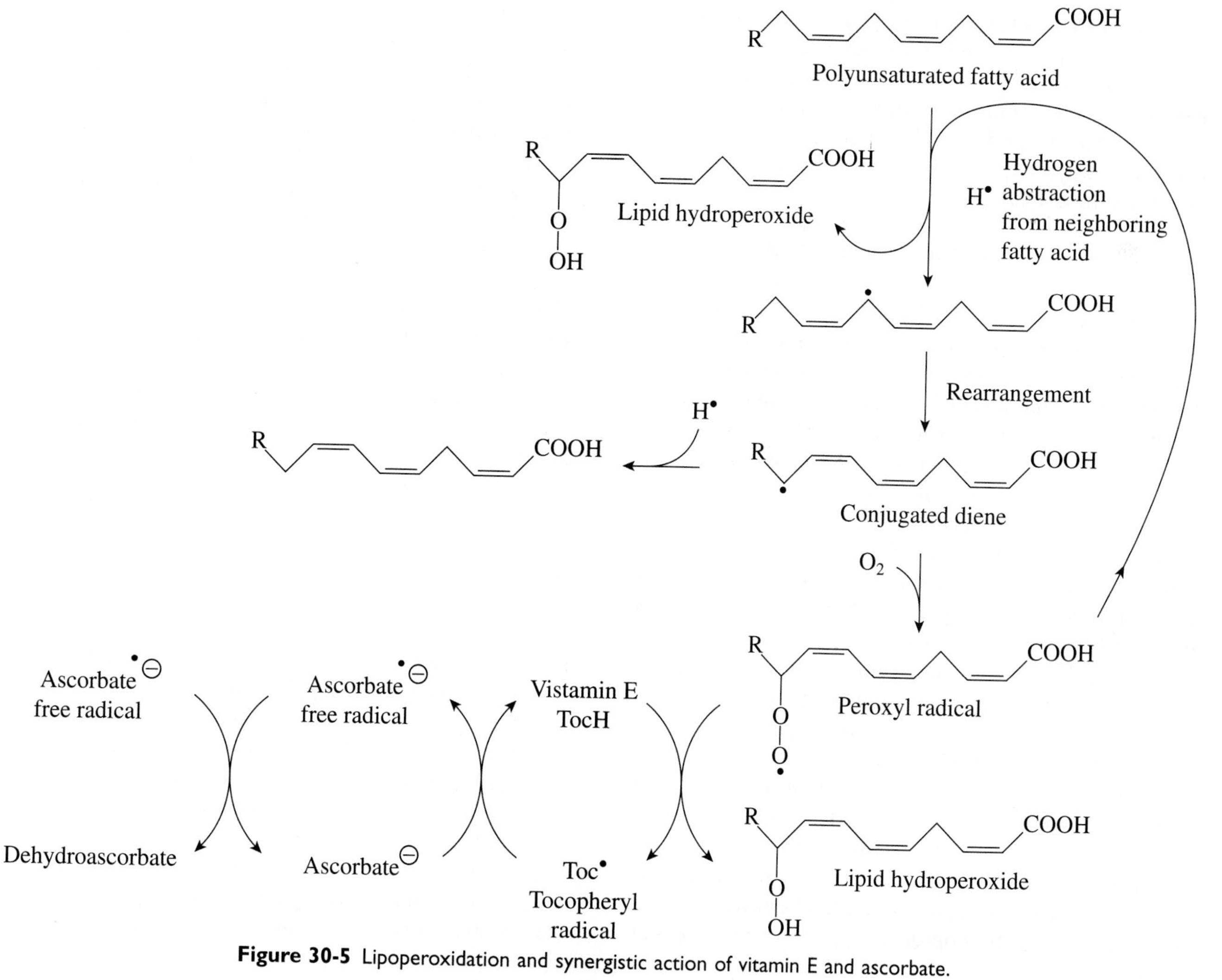

Figure 30-5 Lipoperoxidation and synergistic action of vitamin E and ascorbate.

control group. In 2002 the UK Heart Protection Study of 20,536 subjects with existing coronary disease, other occlusive disease, or diabetes showed that supplementation with vitamin E (600 mg), vitamin C (250 mg), and β-carotene (20 mg) during a period of 5 years produced no significant reduction in any type of vascular disease, cancer, or other major outcome, when compared with placebo.[240] A meta-analysis of clinical trials suggests that the response to vitamin E may be dose dependent—trials using 400 mg or less showed very slight or no benefit, whereas those using more than 400 mg per day showed a significant increase in all cause mortality.[387a] Any influence of vitamin E on disease progression may therefore be in primary prevention rather than secondary intervention, but there is also growing concern about possible harmful effects of high dose supplements.

Beyond its antioxidant properties, α-tocopherol inhibits protein kinase C and 5-lipoxygenase and activates protein phosphatase 2A and diacylglycerol kinase at the posttranslational level. Some genes (coding for CD36, α-TTP, α-tropomyosin, and collagenase) are affected by α-tocopherol at the transcriptional level. α-Tocopherol also induces inhibition of cell proliferation, platelet aggregation, and monocyte adhesion, which are thought to be due to direct interaction of α-tocopherol with cell components.[75,467] Properties independent of α-tocopherol have been ascribed to γ-tocopherol. These include the inhibition of cyclooxygenase activity, thus conferring antiinflammatory properties, and the natriuretic property of its main metabolite, γ-CEHC (2,7,8-trimethyl-2-(β-carboxyethyl)-6-hydroxychroman), not shared by α-CEHC.[286]

Requirements and Reference Nutrient Intakes

The requirement for vitamin E is related to the polyunsaturated fatty acid content of cellular structures and therefore depends on the nature and quantity of dietary fat that affect such composition. Hence the minimum adult requirement for vitamin E is not certain but is probably not more than 3 to 4 mg (4.5 to 6 IU) for RRR-α-tocopherol per day for those who ingest a diet containing the minimum of essential fatty acids (3% of calories).[172] Because vitamin E activity is derived from a series of tocopherols and tocotrienols in usual mixed diets, calculations based on their abundance and activity relative to the biologically most active RRR-α-tocopherol are used. The milligrams of β-tocopherol are multiplied by 0.5, those of γ-tocopherol by 0.1, and those of α-tocotrienol by 0.3. Their sum plus milligrams of α-tocopherol accounts for the milligrams of α-tocopherol equivalents. It has been estimated that a range of 7 to 13 mg of α-tocopherol equivalents (10 to 20 IU) can be expected in balanced diets supplying 1800 to 3000 kcal. This intake will maintain plasma concentrations of total tocopherols within the reference interval of 0.5 to 1.2 mg/dL, which also ensures an adequate concentration in all tissue.[53] Some investigators claim that the ratio of circulating α-tocopherol to total lipids (or triglycerides or β-lipoproteins) is a more accurate indicator of tissue vitamin E status than circulating α-tocopherol alone.

RDA for vitamin E was increased in the year 2000 by 50% from 10 to 15 mg/day for adults by the U.S. Food and Nutrition Board.[172] Most European reference intakes are related to the polyunsaturated fatty acid intake.[117] The changes in the United States were accompanied by some debate, critics arguing that this amount could not be met by the usual North American diet.[256,576] For infants up to 6 months, an AI of 4 mg/day was proposed, for infants 7 to 12 months an AI of 5 mg/day and the RDA for children 1 to 18 years was set at 6 to 15 mg/day, dependent upon age.[172] Another departure in the newer recommendations was that the daily requirement be met by RRR-α-tocopherol alone as the other forms of vitamin E are not converted to α-tocopherol and are poorly recognized by the α-tocopherol transfer protein in the liver.

Intravenous Supply

The recommended amount of vitamin E to be supplied intravenously to adults is 10 mg as α-tocopherol.[243] This is rather lower than the oral provision, but takes into account the fact that it is completely delivered into the blood stream.

Deficiency

Premature and low birth weight infants are particularly susceptible to development of vitamin E deficiency, because placental transfer is poor and infants have such limited adipose tissue where much of the vitamin is normally stored.[53] Signs of deficiency include irritability, edema, and hemolytic anemia. The anemia reflects the shortened life span of erythrocytes with fragile membranes; it does not respond to iron therapy, which may aggravate the condition. Although symptoms of vitamin E deficiency are rare in children and adults, deficiency can occur in some conditions. Fat malabsorption states, such as cystic fibrosis and chronic cholestasis in children, can cause neuropathy[537] and hemolytic anemia[621] as can the genetic disorder abetalipoproteinemia (within which vitamin E is transported).[404] Mutations of the gene coding for α-TTP lead to very low plasma α-tocopherol concentrations and cause neurological symptoms, including cerebellar ataxia.[506] Plasma concentrations may only be normalized by administering large amounts (up to 2 g/day) of vitamin E.

Toxicity

Excess vitamin E intake is usually only achieved by dietary supplementation. Such supplementation is contraindicated in subjects with coagulation defects caused by vitamin K deficiency or those receiving anticoagulant drugs. The U.S. Food and Nutrition Board has recommended a tolerable upper limit of 1000 mg/day of vitamin E for adults of 19 years and older, based on the absence of hemorrhagic toxicity in animal models,[172] though this has been challenged on the grounds that in those regularly taking aspirin this intake may be associated with an increased risk of bleeding.[256] A

1992 comprehensive review of tolerance and safety of vitamin E suggested that intakes of up to 3000 mg/day were safe; reversible side effects of gastrointestinal symptoms, increased creatinuria, and impairment of blood coagulation are seen at intakes of 1000 to 3000 mg/day.[298] However, as noted above, long term use of intakes of more than 400 mg per day may cause increased mortality.

Laboratory Assessment of Status

Assessment of vitamin E status has been achieved by functional methods, such as protection of erythrocyte hemolysis on addition of peroxide[151] or the inhibition of lipid peroxidation products (malondialdehyde, thiobarbituric acid-reactive substances, ethane, or pentane)[591] or by direct measurement of vitamin E concentration in tissue (erythrocytes, lymphocytes, or platelets) or serum. Early direct methods used photometric or fluorometric measurement often based on the Emmerie-Engel procedure in which tocopherol is oxidized to tocopheryl quinone by $FeCl_3$ and the resultant Fe^{2+} coupled with α,α'-dipyridyl to form a red color. Later, chromatographic methods were used, including thin layer and gas liquid, which had the ability to separate the tocopherols and tocotrienols, but these were labor intensive and time consuming. HPLC is presently the method of choice for quantitation of tocopherols in serum as it has the advantage of accuracy (by the use of primary standards) and reproducibility (between-batch coefficients of variation of 7% or better) and the ability to quantitate multiple analytes, including vitamin A and some carotenoids, in a single analytical run.[573,634] Both α- and γ-tocopherols are the principal vitamers seen, though others may be detected with minor modifications to the analytical conditions.

Reference Intervals

Guidance reference intervals for serum or plasma (heparin) vitamin E are 0.1 to 0.5 mg/dL (2.3 to 11.6 μmol/L) for premature neonates[20]; 0.3 to 0.9 mg/dL (7 to 21 μmol/L) for children (1 to 12 years)[339]; 0.6 to 1.0 mg/dL (14 to 23 μmol/L) for adolescents (13 to 19 years); and 0.5 to 1.8 mg/dL (12 to 42 μmol/L) for adults.[595]

VITAMIN K

Vitamin K promotes clotting of the blood and is required for the conversion of several clotting factors and prothrombin, and is of growing interest in bone metabolism.

Chemistry

Compounds in the vitamin K series are 2-methyl-1,4-napthoquinones, which are substituted with side chains at carbon 3. *Phylloquinone* (K_1 type) synthesized in plants and the *menaquinones* (K_2 type) of bacterial origin are the two principal natural classes of vitamin K (Figure 30-6). The principal vitamin K_1 (phylloquinone) bears a saturated, phytol, 20-carbon side chain derived from 4 isoprenoid units; this is the main K vitamin produced by plants and is the major dietary form for humans.[517] K_2 shows greater variation, but an all-*trans*-farnesylgeranylgeranyl, 35-carbon chain of 7 isoprenoid units is typical; these are produced in humans by the large bowel bacterial mass, though their contribution to vitamin K status remains a matter of dispute. Several synthetic analogues and derivatives have been used in human nutrition; most relate to or derive from *menadione* (K_3), which lacks a side-chain substituent at position 3, but which can be converted to menaquinone (MK) (e.g., MK-4, where 4 is the number of isoprenoid side chains) by addition of the side chain in the liver. The K vitamins are insoluble in water but dissolve in organic fat solvents. They are destroyed by alkaline solutions and reducing agents and are also sensitive to ultraviolet light.

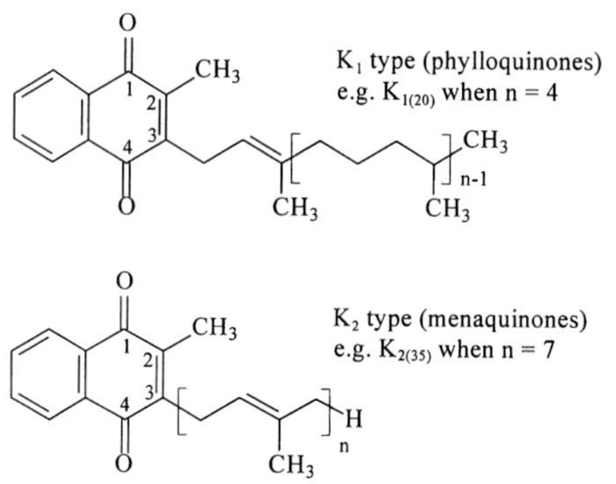

K_1 type (phylloquinones) e.g. $K_{1(20)}$ when n = 4

K_2 type (menaquinones) e.g. $K_{2(35)}$ when n = 7

Figure 30-6 Vitaminic forms of vitamin K.

Dietary Sources

The main dietary sources of the phylloquinones are green vegetables, margarines, and plant oils, whereas some menaquinones are obtained from cheese, other milk products, and eggs.[509]

Absorption, Transport, Metabolism, and Excretion

The absorption of natural vitamin K from the small intestine into the lymphatic system is facilitated by bile, as is true for other fat-soluble materials.[66,160] Efficiency of absorption varies from 15% to 65% as reflected by recovery in lymph within 24 hours. Vitamins K_1 and K_2 are bound to chylomicrons for transport from mucosal cells to the liver. Menadione (K_3) is more rapidly and completely absorbed from the gut before entering the portal blood. In liver, intracellular distribution is mostly in the microsomal fraction, where phenylation of menadione to form K_2 occurs. Release of vitamin K to the blood stream allows association with circulating β-lipoproteins for transport to other tissue. Significant levels of vitamin K have been noted in the spleen and skeletal muscle.

Within metabolically active and vitamin K–using tissue, especially liver, a microsomal vitamin K cycle exists (Figure 30-7).[237] The vitamin (quinone) is normally reduced by a thiol-sensitive flavoprotein system to the hydroquinone, which then can couple to the oxygen- and carbon dioxide–using γ-carboxylation of glutamyl residues in specific pro-

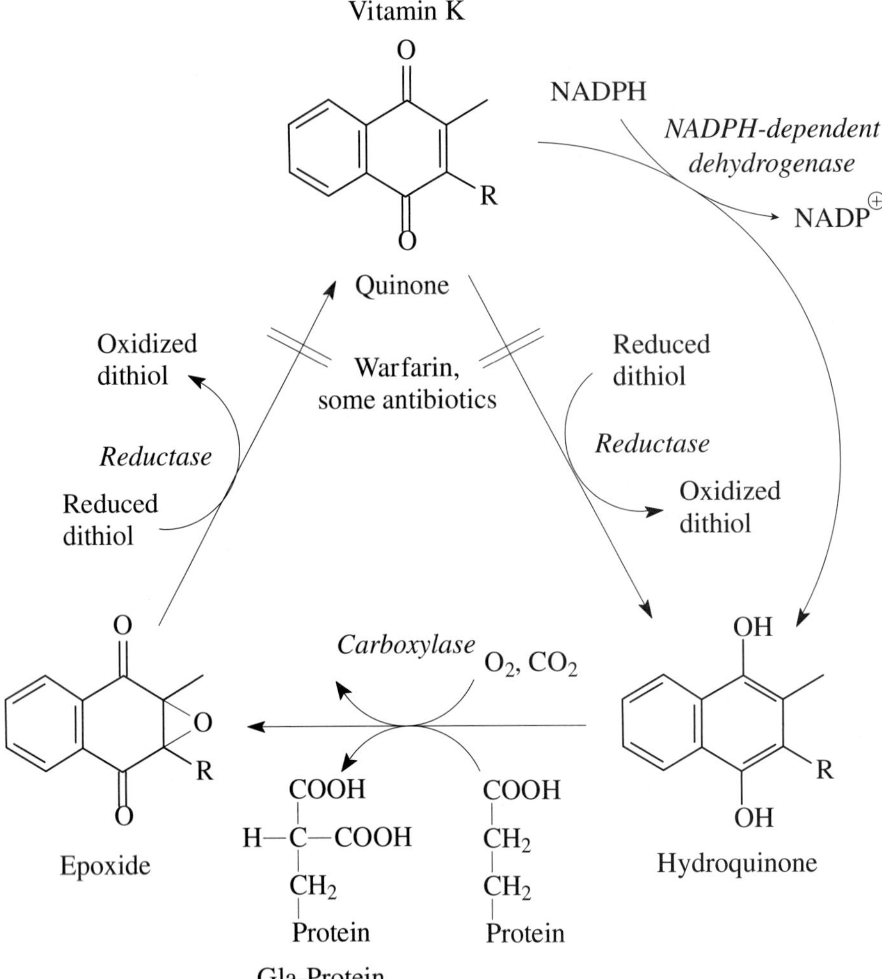

Figure 30-7 Metabolic cycling of vitamin K, the effect of warfarin, and the formation of Gla proteins.

teins (e.g., prothrombin).[160] The 2,3-epoxide of vitamin K that is subsequently formed is reduced to the starting vitamin K quinones, a process that can be antagonized by such vitamin K antagonists as warfarin.

Only traces of urinary metabolites of vitamins K_1 and K_2 appear in urine a considerable portion of vitamin K_3 (menadione) is conjugated at the hydroquinone level to form β-glucuronide and sulfate esters, which are excreted.

Functions

The essential and most thoroughly defined role of vitamin K is as a cofactor to vitamin K–dependent carboxylase, an enzyme necessary for the posttranslational conversion of specific glutamyl residues in target proteins to γ-carboxyglutamyl (Gla) residues. This γ-carboxylation increases the affinity of these proteins for calcium.[48] The antihemorrhagic function of vitamin K depends upon the formation of the Gla proteins prothrombin (factor II), proconvertin (factor VII), plasma thromboplastin component (factor IX), and Stuart factor (factor X), which together with two other hemostatic vitamin K–dependent proteins, proteins C and S and Ca^{2+}, initiate a process to form thrombin that then catalyzes the conversion of fibrinogen to a fibrin clot.[413]

Proteins that contain γ-carboxyglutamyl are also abundant in bone tissue, with osteocalcin accounting for up to 80% of the total γ-carboxyglutamyl content of mature bone. Many epidemiological studies, such as the 1999 Nurses' Health Study[161] and a 2000 study,[62] have shown an association between low vitamin K intakes and hip fracture risk, but not bone mineral density (BMD) measurements. Intervention studies have shown that vitamin K can increase BMD in osteoporotic subjects and reduce fracture rates,[531] though these studies have used menaquinone-4 in pharmacological rather than physiological doses. The improvement in bone markers was accompanied by a significant fall in the concentration of undercarboxylated osteocalcin in the treated groups. There is also evidence that vitamins K and D may act synergistically in maintaining bone density.[273]

A further major Gla protein, matrix Gla protein (MGP)—containing 5 residues of γ-carboxyglutamic acid—is found in vascular smooth muscle, bone, and many soft tissues (heart, kidney, and lungs). It is thought that MGP accumulates at sites of calcification, including calcified aortic valves and bone, and is a potent inhibitor of calcification. In experimental studies with mice lacking the gene coding for MGP, calcification of the arteries was observed that led to hemorrhagic death of the animals as a result of blood vessel rupture.[352] Results from studies such as these have led to suggestions that vitamin K could play a role in vascular disease, though as yet clinical evidence is sparse.

Requirements and Reference Nutrient Intakes

Although the human gut bacteria synthesize large amounts of menaquinones, and such compounds are found in the liver in concentrations up to 10 times those of phylloquinones, the absorption of these compounds has been difficult to demonstrate and dietary restriction of vitamin K does lead to evidence of inadequacy, as demonstrated by undercarboxylation of vitamin K–dependent proteins.[160] Thus dietary reference intakes for vitamin K have recently been revised by the Food and Nutrition Board of the U.S. Institute of Medicine. Current recommendations are 120 μg/day for men over 18 years; 90 μg/day for women older than 18 years, including those pregnant or lactating; 30 to 75 μg/day for children 1 to 18 years, dependent upon age; 2.0 μg/day for infants up to 6 months; and 2.5 μg/day for infants between 7 and 12 months, the latter requirements being met by mature breast milk.[174] The dietary intake of phylloquinone in North American and most European populations studied has been estimated at around 150 μg/day for subjects over 55 years and around 80 μg/day for younger subjects, though intakes in the Netherlands have been reported to be 2 to 3 times higher than these estimates.[509]

Intravenous Supply

In the United States, whether vitamin K should be included in preparations of vitamins for use in TPN is controversial. Although this has been standard in Europe for many years,[522] the long-standing recommendation from the American Medical Association was not to include vitamin K, since this would complicate the provision of adequate warfarin therapy in those patients who require anticoagulation.[9] However, 2003 requirements of the Food and Drug Administration (FDA) have specified that vitamin K should be included in vitamin supplements for both infants and adults, making the judgment that the physiological and practical benefits of regular provision outweigh any problems in readjusting warfarin dosage.[243] The adult recommended intravenous (IV) dose is 150 μg/day, which is provided as phytonadione.

Deficiency

Although vitamin K deficiency in the adult is uncommon, the risk is increased for fat malabsorption states (bile duct obstruction, cystic fibrosis, and chronic pancreatitis) and liver disease.[314] Risk is also increased by the use of drugs that interfere with vitamin K metabolism, such as the coumarin anticoagulants (e.g., warfarin) and antibiotics containing the *N*-methylthiotetrazole side chain (e.g., cephalosporin).[516] Other at-risk groups are hospitalized patients with poor nutrient intakes or those receiving TPN, when fat-soluble vitamin supplements may not fully meet requirements. Conversely, ingestion of supraphysiological doses of vitamins A and E has also been reported to induce vitamin K deficiency, probably by competitive mechanisms.[432] Defective blood coagulation and demonstration of abnormal noncarboxylated prothrombin are at present the only well-established signs of vitamin K deficiency.

Hemorrhagic disease of the newborn can develop readily because of (1) poor placental transfer of vitamin K, (2) hepatic immaturity leading to inadequate synthesis of coagulation proteins, and (3) the low vitamin K content of early breast milk. Prothrombin levels during this period are only about 25% of the adult levels. Severe diarrhea and antibiotics used to suppress diarrhea readily exacerbate the situation, so prothrombin levels can drop below 5% of the adult level and bleeding can occur. This condition is routinely prevented by the prophylactic administration of 0.5 to 1.0 mg of phylloquinone intramuscularly, or 2.0 mg given orally immediately after birth.

Toxicity

The use of high doses of naturally occurring vitamin K (K_1 and K_2) appears to have no untoward effect; however, menadione (K_3) treatment can lead to the formation of erythrocyte cytoplasmic inclusions known as Heinz bodies and hemolytic anemia.[406] With severe hemolysis, increased bilirubin formation and undeveloped capacity for its conjugation may produce kernicterus in the newborn.

As no adverse effects associated with vitamin K consumption from food or supplements have been reported in humans or animals, the U.S. Institute of Medicine has reported that a quantitative risk assessment cannot be performed, and thus a UL cannot be derived for vitamin K.[174]

Laboratory Assessment of Status

Because of its relatively low plasma concentration (approximately 50 times lower than vitamin D and at least 10^3 times lower than vitamins A or E), vitamin K has long presented an analytical challenge. For this reason, vitamin K status has traditionally been assessed by functional methods, primarily by its effect on clotting time. The "prothrombin time" (PT) is assessed by adding to recalcified plasma a portion of tissue thromboplastin and measuring the clotting time against a normal control sample. In vitamin K deficiency, the PT may rise above 30 seconds (normal: 10 to 14 seconds), and at least 2 seconds beyond the control time. Attempts at cross-laboratory standardization have led to the introduction of the Internationalized Normal Ratio (INR), where the PT is expressed as a fraction of the control time. A more sensitive (1000-fold) assessment of vitamin K status with respect to prothrombin can be made by the immunoassay of des-γ-carboxy prothrombin, or undercarboxylated prothrombin, PIVKA-II (protein induced by vitamin K absence or antagonism).[58] Concentrations of PIVKA-II of greater than

2 ng/mL have been considered to indicate vitamin K deficiency.[314] A newer measurement of deficient γ-carboxylation, plasma undercarboxylated osteocalcin, was developed in 1995[539] and has been shown to correlate individually with PIVKA-II and plasma phylloquinone concentrations and has a better correlation with plasma phylloquinone than PIVKA-II.[540] In this 1995 study of biochemical indices of vitamin K nutritional status in a healthy adult population, and a later one looking at changes in response to dietary phylloquinone,[538] the urinary γ-carboxyglutamic acid/creatinine ratio was measured by derivatization, HPLC separation, and fluorometric detection[229] and also shown to be sensitive to changes in dietary phylloquinone intake. This marker may have advantages in epidemiological surveys as a less invasive sample.

The direct measurement of plasma phylloquinone is probably the best indicator of vitamin K status and has been shown to correlate well with intake.[538] HPLC methods have been reviewed,[515] and typically require 0.5 to 2.0 mL of serum or plasma. Protein precipitation and lipid extraction (often into hexane), followed by solvent evaporation; preparative HPLC (to isolate vitamin K from other lipids); reevaporation of the vitamin K–rich fraction; dilution in the mobile phase; and further HPLC, with either electrochemical or fluorometric detection[281] often after postcolumn reduction, are required. Typical between-batch imprecision values are coefficient of variation (CV)s of 11% to 18% with limits of detection of lower than 50 pmol/L. An external quality assessment scheme (EQAS) is available in the UK.

Reference Interval

A guidance reference interval for plasma vitamin K is 0.13 to 1.19 ng/mL (0.29 to 2.64 nmol/L).[574]

VITAMIN B_1—THIAMINE

Thiamine, also known as vitamin B_1, forms the coenzyme thiamine pyrophosphate (TPP). It is required for the essential decarboxylation reactions catalyzed by the pyruvate and 2-oxoglutarate complexes.

Chemistry

The structure of *thiamine* (vitamin B_1) (3-[4-amino-2-methyl-pyrimidyl-5-methyl]-4-methyl-5-[β-hydroxy-ethyl]thiazole) is that of a pyrimidine ring, bearing an amino group, linked by a methylene bridge to a thiazole ring (Figure 30-8). The thiazole has a primary alcohol side chain at C5, which can be phosphorylated in vivo to produce thiamine phosphate esters, the most common of which is thiamine pyrophosphate (TPP) (also known as thiamine diphosphate, cocarboxylase). Monophosphate and triphosphate esters also occur. The basic vitamin is isolated or synthesized and handled as a solid thiazolium salt (e.g., thiamine chloride hydrochloride). Thiamine is somewhat heat labile, particularly in alkaline solutions, where base attack occurs at C2 of the thiazolium ring.

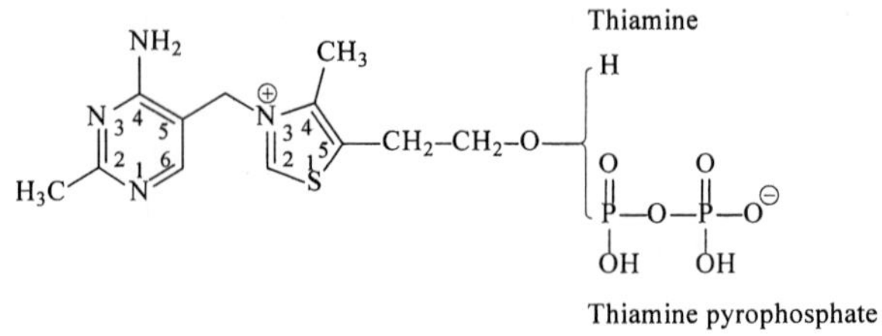

Figure 30-8 Thiamine and the pyrophosphate coenzyme.

Dietary Sources

Small amounts of thiamine and its phosphates are present in most plant and animal tissue, but more abundant sources are unrefined cereal grains, liver, heart, kidney, and lean cuts of pork. The enrichment of flour and derived food products, particularly breakfast cereals, has considerably increased the availability of this vitamin.

Absorption, Transport, Metabolism, and Excretion

Thiamine absorption occurs primarily in the proximal small intestine[317] by both a saturable (thiamine transporter) process at low concentration (1 μmol/L, or lower) and by simple passive diffusion beyond that, though percentage absorption diminishes with increased dose. The absorbed thiamine undergoes intracellular phosphorylation, mainly to the pyrophosphate, but at the serosal side 90% of the transferred thiamine is in the free form.[469] Thiamine uptake is enhanced by thiamine deficiency and reduced by thyroid hormone, diabetes, and ethanol ingestion. The gene for the specific thiamine transporter has been identified, and the transporter cloned.[166] Thiamine is carried by the portal blood to the liver. The free vitamin occurs in the plasma, but the coenzyme, TPP, is the primary cellular component. Approximately 30 mg is stored in the body with 80% as the pyrophosphate, 10% as triphosphate, and the rest as thiamine and its monophosphate. About half of the body stores are found in skeletal muscles, with much of the remainder in heart, liver, kidneys, and nervous tissues (including the brain, which contains most of the triphosphate).

The three tissue enzymes known to participate in formation of the phosphate esters are (1) thiaminokinase (a pyrophosphokinase), which catalyzes formation of TPP and adenosine monophosphate (AMP) from thiamine and adenosine triphosphate (ATP); (2) TPP-ATP phosphoryltransferase (cytosolic 5′-adenylic kinase),[297] which forms the triphosphate and adenosine diphosphate from TPP and ATP; and (3) thiamine triphosphatase, which hydrolyzes TPP to the monophosphate. Although thiaminokinase is widespread, the phosphoryl transferase and membrane-associated triphosphatase are mainly in nervous tissue.

Using radio-labeled thiamine probes, a study of thiamine metabolism at normal loads produced an estimated half-life of thiamine of 9.5 to 18.5 days, and showed a large number of breakdown products in the urine.[17] Several of these urinary catabolites are shown in Figure 30-9.

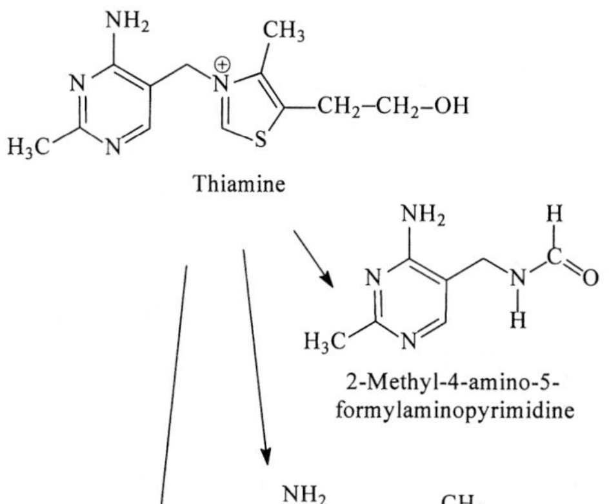

Figure 30-9 Principal urinary catabolites of thiamine.

Functions

Thiamine is required by the body as the pyrophosphate (TPP) in two general types of reaction, the oxidative decarboxylation of α-keto acids catalyzed by dehydrogenase complexes and the formation of α-ketols (ketoses) as catalyzed by transketolase, and as the triphosphate (TTP) within the nervous system. TPP functions as the Mg^{2+}-coordinated coenzyme for so-called "active aldehyde" transfers in multienzyme dehydrogenase complexes that affect decarboxylative conversion of α-keto (2-oxo) acids to acyl-coenzyme A (acyl-CoA) derivatives, such as pyruvate dehydrogenase and α-ketoglutarate dehydrogenase. These are often localized in the mitochondria, where efficient use in the Krebs tricarboxylic acid (citric acid) cycle follows.

Three types of subunit proteins constitute such dehydrogenase complexes: (1) a TPP-dependent decarboxylase, which converts the α-keto acid to an α-hydroxyalkyl-TPP complex; (2) a transacylase core, which contains lipoyl residues that are acylated by the α-hydroxyalkyl-TPP; and (3) a flavin adenine dinucleotide (FAD)–dependent dihydrolipoyl dehydrogenase, which reoxidizes the reduced lipoyl residues produced after transfer of their acyl functions to reduced CoA. In addition to energy and an ultimate ATP supply derived from reactions in the Krebs cycle, the initial pyruvate dehydrogenase–catalyzed step provides acetyl-CoA as a biosynthetic precursor to other essential compounds, such as lipids and acetylcholine of the parasympathetic nervous system.

Transketolase is a TPP-dependent enzyme found in the cytosol of many tissues, especially liver and blood cells, in which principal carbohydrate pathways exist. In the pentose phosphate pathway, which additionally supplies reduced nicotinamide-adenine dinucleotide phosphate (NADPH) necessary for biosynthetic reactions, this enzyme catalyzes the reversible transfer of a glycoaldehyde moiety from the first two carbons of a donor ketose phosphate to the aldehyde carbon of an aldose phosphate.

Although thiamine as its pyrophosphate contributes to nervous system composition and function in such essential reactions as energy production and biosynthesis of lipids and acetylcholine, a further specific, noncofactor role for thiamine has been proposed in excitable cells. Here, TTP is thought to be involved in the regulation of ion channels, specifically chloride channels of large unitary conductance, the so called maxi-Cl channels.[50] TTP may also act as a phosphate donor for the phosphorylation of proteins, suggesting a potential role in cell signaling.[356] A subacute necrotizing encephalomyelopathy is seen in patients with Leigh syndrome, resulting from the presence of an inhibitor of TPP-ATP phosphoryl transferase,[559] and consequent reduction in TTP concentration.

Requirements and Reference Nutrient Intakes

Because thiamine is necessary mainly for the metabolism of carbohydrates, fats, and alcohol, there is a direct correlation of need with the amount of metabolizable food intake. There is a greater requirement under situations in which metabolism is increased (e.g., in the normal conditions of increased muscular activity, pregnancy, and lactation, or in the abnormal cases of protracted fever, posttrauma, and hyperthyroidism.)[559] Clinical signs of deficiency in adults can be prevented with intakes of thiamine above 0.15 to 0.2 mg/1000 kcal, but 0.35 to 0.4 mg/1000 kcal may be closer to a level necessary to maintain urinary excretion and TPP-dependent erythrocyte transketolase activity within normal reference intervals.[170] With further considerations of average caloric intakes and activities in different age groups, the most recent recommendations of RDA, expressed as mg/day, are 1.2 mg/day for males 19 years and older and 1.1 mg/day for females 19 years and older.[170] The requirement for pregnant women increases early in pregnancy and then remains constant; an additional allowance of 0.3 mg/day is recommended. The lactating woman secretes 0.1 to 0.2 mg of thiamine per day in milk, so an additional 0.3-mg/day allowance is suggested. Based on the thiamine content of human milk and with an increment considered to provide a margin of safety, 0.2 mg/day is the allowance for infants up to 6 months, and 0.3 mg/day for infants 7 to 12 months. Increases above this are suggested for growing children.

Intravenous Supply

Traditionally the intravenous recommendation was for 3 mg/day for adults, usually provided as thiamine hydrochloride, but also as thiamine mononitrate or tetrahydrate. In the 2000 FDA recommendations, this has been increased to 6 mg/day,[243] recognizing the likelihood of increased demands for thiamine caused by the hypercatabolism in such patients, and the very serious potential complications of deficiency.[599]

Deficiency

The causes of thiamine deficiency[66] include inadequate intake caused by diets largely dependent on milled, nonenriched grains, such as rice and wheat, or by the ingestion of raw fish containing microbial thiaminases,[148] which hydrolytically destroy the vitamin in the gastrointestinal tract. Tea may contain antithiamine factors that have been detected in certain other plant extracts. Chronic alcoholism often leads to thiamine deficiency caused by reduced intake, impaired absorption, impaired use, and reduced storage[570] and may lead clinically to the Wernicke-Korsakoff syndrome. Other at-risk groups include those receiving parenteral nutrition without adequate thiamine supplementation,[408,476] elderly patients taking diuretics,[551] and patients undergoing long-term renal dialysis.[259]

Beriberi is the disease resulting from thiamine deficiency. Clinical signs of thiamine deficiency primarily involve the nervous and cardiovascular systems.[558,559] In the adult, symptoms most frequently observed are mental confusion, anorexia, muscular weakness, ataxia, peripheral paralysis, ophthalmoplegia, edema (wet beriberi), muscle wasting (dry beriberi), tachycardia, and an enlarged heart. In infants, symptoms appear suddenly and severely, often involving cardiac failure and cyanosis. Commonly the distinction between wet (cardiovascular) and dry (neuritic) manifestations of beriberi relates to duration and severity of the deficiency, the degree of physical exertion, and caloric intake.[622] The wet or edematous condition results from severe physical exertion and high carbohydrate intake, whereas the dry or polyneuritic form stems from relative inactivity with caloric restriction during the chronic deficiency. The three major physiological derangements that typically involve the cardiovascular system are peripheral vasodilatation leading to a high-output state, biventricular myocardial failure, and retention of sodium and water, leading to edema. Nervous system involvement includes peripheral neuropathy, Wernicke's encephalopathy, and the amnesic psychosis of Korsakoff's syndrome. More rarely, but especially in seriously ill patients in hospitals, an acute form of cardiac failure has been described (Shoshin beri-beri), which may be fatal, but is successfully and rapidly reversed with high-dose intravenous thiamine.[599]

There are several thiamine-responsive disorders caused by genetic mutation. In thiamine-responsive megaloblastic anemia (TRMA), the gene has been mapped and cloned and designated "SLC19A2" as a member of the solute carrier gene super family. Mutations of this gene, the product of which is a membrane protein that transports thiamine with submicromolar affinity, have been found in all TRMA kindreds studied.[416,459] Thiamine-responsive pyruvate dehydrogenase complex deficiency, presenting with lactic acidosis, can be caused by a point mutation within the thiamine pyrophosphate-binding region,[407] and a thiamine-responsive branched-chain keto acid dehydrogenase complex deficiency, presenting as a form of maple syrup urine disease, is caused by mutations in the E1 alpha subunit of the enzyme complex.[628] Therapeutic doses of 5 to 20 mg of thiamine daily have proved beneficial in these cases.

Toxicity

As there are no reports of adverse effects from consumption of excess thiamine from food and supplements (supplements of 50 mg/day are widely available without prescription), and the data are inadequate for a quantitative risk assessment, no UL has been defined for thiamine.[170] However, as stimulators of transketolase enzyme synthesis such as thiamine support a high rate of nucleic acid ribose synthesis necessary for tumor cell survival, chemotherapy resistance, and proliferation, some concern has been expressed that thiamine supplementation of common food products may contribute to increased cancer rates in the Western world.[64] There is, however, little evidence to support this assumption. Rarely, individuals given high-dose intravenous thiamine in treatment of beriberi have developed anaphylaxis, the frequency being about 1 : 100,000.

Laboratory Assessment of Status

As a thiamine deficiency develops, there is a rather rapid loss of the vitamin from all tissue except the brain. The decrease of TPP in the erythrocyte roughly parallels the decrease of this coenzyme in other tissue. During this time, thiamine levels in urine fall to near zero; the urinary metabolites remain high for some time before decreasing.

Historically, assessment of thiamine status was by animal bioassay (the correction of bradycardia in thiamine-deficient rats) and later by microbiological assays using the fungus *Phycomyces blakesleeanus*, yeast fermentation, or bacteria of the *Staphylococcus, Streptococcus,* or *Lactobacillus* species. Some bacterial microbiological assays are still in use in the food industry. Early chemical methods were often based upon the production of a fluorophore, thiochrome, when thiamine is oxidized with ferricyanide in alkaline solution, a property that is used in some modern chromatographic methods.

Because the basic biological function of thiamine is to act as the pyrophosphate cofactor in a number of enzyme systems, two differing approaches to assessment of status became available. The analyte, either free or phosphorylated, can be measured directly in a suitable body fluid or tissue or its properties as an enzymatic cofactor can be exploited in a functional assay. Both approaches have their advantages and disadvantages, and a consensus as to which is the more useful has not been achieved; the two are probably complementary, each supplying some, but not all, of the information necessary to assess thiamine adequacy (Table 30-3).

The most commonly used enzyme for the functional assay is transketolase. Transketolase catalyzes two reactions in the pentose phosphate pathway (Figure 30-10). As an enzyme within the erythrocyte, transketolase is independent of nonspecific changes in the extracellular plasma. As vitamin B_1 deficiency becomes more severe, (1) thiamine becomes limiting in the body cells, (2) the amount of the coenzyme is depleted, and (3) the transketolase activity subsequently diminishes. The "TPP effect" measures the extent of depletion of the transketolase enzyme for coenzyme by assaying enzyme activity before and after TPP supplementation. The percent increase in activity is defined as the TPP effect or activation coefficient. Several methods are available to measure transketolase activity. In the Brin procedure,[77] activities of holo forms and apo forms of transketolase in erythrocyte hemolysates are measured before and after addition of TPP, by photometric determinations of the amount of ribose-5′-phosphate used or hexose-6-phosphate formed. This method is reliable but time consuming. In an alternative method, the rate of formation of glyceraldehyde-3-P is measured indirectly by a coupled reaction in a system containing excess triosephosphate isomerase (TIM), glycerolphosphate dehydrogenase (GD), and NADH.[536] Glyceraldehyde-3-P is converted by TIM to dihydroxyacetone-P, which in the presence of GD and NADH is reduced to glycerol-1-P. The rate of NADH oxidation, measured at 340 nm, is proportional to the transketolase activity. Kinetic methods such as these have been automated with consequent improvements in throughput and precision.[401]

TABLE 30-3 Relative Merits of Direct (Erythrocyte Thiamine Pyrophosphate) or Functional (Erythrocyte Transketolase) Measurements in Assessing Thiamine Status

Erythrocyte Thiamine Pyrophosphate	Erythrocyte Transketolase Activation
Advantages • Pure standard available • Precise and robust methodology • More stable when frozen • Depletes at rate similar to other organs • Methodology (HPLC) allows measurement of other forms of thiamine • Can detect tissue accumulation	**Advantages** • May correlate better with clinical conditions in repleted patients • Large database established
Disadvantages May normalize very early with parenteral treatment	**Disadvantages** • Depletion of apoenzyme may be nonnutritional (e.g., liver disease, diabetes) • Variants may have abnormal binding • May be influenced by cofactor deficiencies (e.g., magnesium) • Difficult to standardize, less robust • Derived activation coefficient reduces precision

The transketolase activation test is in reality two tests: one a measurement of basal activity and the other the degree to which the basal activity can be increased by exogenous thiamine pyrophosphate, and each may be influenced by different factors. There is evidence that chronic deficiency states of thiamine may down regulate synthesis of the apoenzyme.[473] In comparison studies against erythrocyte TPP concentrations, better correlations were obtained with basal activity rather than the activation coefficient.[24]

Other potential disadvantages of the transketolase test are reductions in apoenzyme synthesis in diseases other than thiamine deficiency (diabetes,[181] liver disease[156]), reduced apoenzyme to coenzyme binding with apotransketolase variants,[289] lack of stability relative to TPP on processing and storage,[453] lack of a standard or EQAS, and variations in published upper limits for the activation coefficient from 15.5% to 40%. The main advantages of the transketolase test are that it is widely used, has a relatively large database and body of experience, and is claimed to correlate better with clinical conditions in alcoholic patients being repleted with thiamine.[258]

Direct measurement of circulating thiamine concentration may be made in plasma, erythrocytes, or whole blood. The plasma (or serum) concentration is thought to reflect recent intake and is mainly unphosphorylated thiamine at low concentration (around 10 to 20 nmol/L). Because the erythrocyte contains approximately 80% of the total thiamine content of whole blood,[503] mainly as the pyrophosphate,[304] and erythrocyte thiamine stores deplete at a similar rate to other major organs,[76] HPLC measurement of TPP in erythrocytes is a good indicator of body stores. Typical HPLC methods include a protein precipitation step, precolumn or postcolumn formation of the fluorophore; thiochrome, usually with alkaline ferricyanide; and isocratic separation.[23,555] The method is easily standardized with pure thiamine pyrophosphate, has good precision (interbatch CVs of 5% to 8%), acceptable limits of detection (around 10 nmol/L), and the analyte is stable at −70 °C for at least 7 months and at room temperature for 48 hours.[24] Whole blood samples may be analyzed in a manner similar to washed erythrocytes and have the advantage of simpler sample handling, but are subject to variable plasma dilution. However, a good correlation has been obtained between erythrocyte and whole blood TPP concentrations, particularly when whole blood TPP included a correction for hemoglobin (Hb). At the time of writing, no EQAS are available for thiamine analysis.

Determination of the urinary excretion of thiamine in a 4-hour specimen, especially with comparison of excretion before and after a test load, is helpful in differentiating among extremes of thiamine status. However, as with most assessments based on amount of water-soluble vitamins in urine, excretion can be influenced considerably by dietary intake, absorption, and other factors. Measurements of certain urinary metabolites, notably thiamine acetic acid, have also been suggested as reflecting thiamine status.[412]

Reference Intervals

Reference intervals for thiamine and its esters depend upon whether (1) erythrocytes, whole blood, or plasma are used as a sample; (2) cellular concentrations are expressed per liter of packed red cells or grams of Hb; and (3) mass or SI units are used. Some guidance intervals are, for erythrocyte transketolase activity 0.75 to 1.30 U/g Hb (48.4 to 83.9 kU/mol Hb) and for percent TPP effect (activation), 0 to 15% is normal, 16% to 25% marginally deficient and >25% severely deficient with clinical signs. For direct TPP concentration measurements, typical intervals are 173 to 293 nmol/L erythrocytes and 90 to 140 nmol/L whole blood,[168] or 280 to 590 ng/g Hb in erythrocytes and 275 to 675 ng/g Hb in whole blood.[555]

VITAMIN B_2—RIBOFLAVIN

Riboflavin, also known as vitamin B_2, is an essential component of FAD and flavin mononucleotide (FMN)—coenzymes that are involved in many redox reactions.

Chemistry

Vitamin B_2 refers to riboflavin and its related metabolites, which act as cofactors to several reduction-oxidation enzymes. The parent compound—riboflavin, 7,8-dimethyl-10-[1′-D-ribityl]isoalloxazine)—is a yellow fluorescent compound whose major physiological role is to act as a precursor for FMN (riboflavin-5′-phosphate) and FAD. FMN is formed from riboflavin by flavokinase-catalyzed phosphorylation, and FAD is formed from FMN and ATP by the action of FAD synthetase, also called pyrophosphorylase (Figure 30-11).[470] FAD is further converted by covalent bonding to form various tissue flavoproteins.[384] Flavins are stable during exposure to heat but are decomposed by light, which causes photodegradation of the D-ribitol side chain at position 10 of the isoalloxazine ring system to ultimately yield lumiflavin (7,8,10-trimethylisoalloxazine) under alkaline conditions and lumichrome (7,8-dimethylalloxazine) at all pH values, especially in neutral-to-acidic solutions. Flavins are chemically and biologically reduced to nearly colorless compounds that rapidly reoxidize on exposure to air (oxygen).

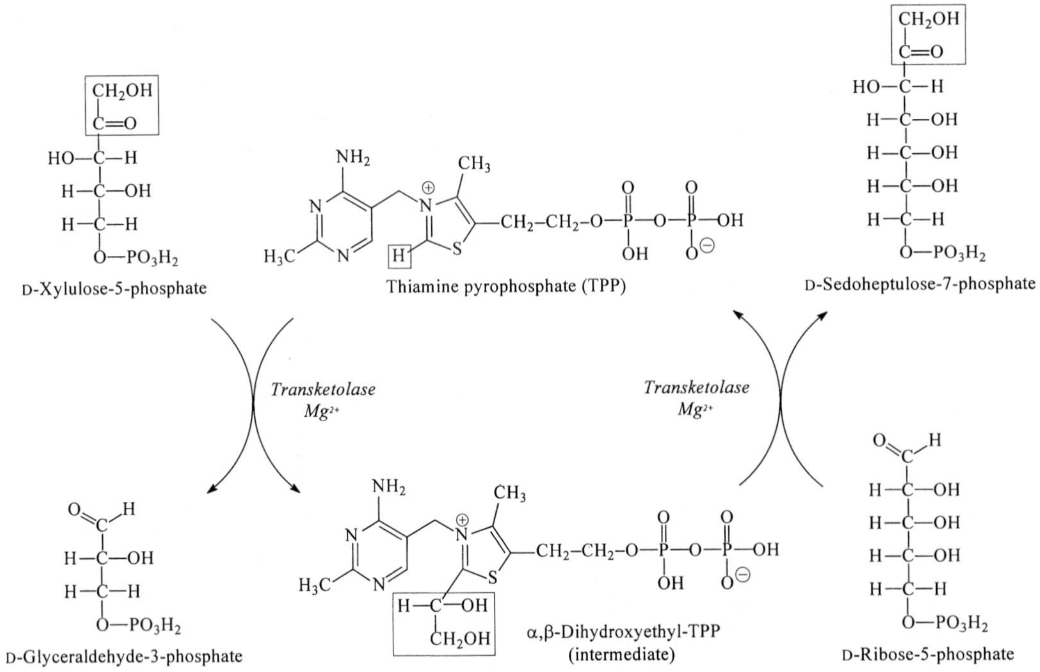

Figure 30-10 The transketolase reaction.

Dietary Sources

Rich sources of the coenzyme forms of the vitamin are liver, kidney, and heart. Many vegetables are also good sources, but cereals are rather low in flavin content. However, current practices of fortification and enrichment of cereal products have made these significant contributors to the daily requirement. Milk, from cows[480] and humans,[479] is a good source of the vitamin, but considerable loss can occur from exposure to light during pasteurization and bottling or as a result of irradiation to increase the vitamin D content.

Absorption, Transport, Metabolism, and Excretion

Most dietary riboflavin is taken in as a complex of food protein with the coenzymes FMN and FAD. These coenzymes are released from noncovalent attachment to proteins as a consequence of gastric acidification. Nonspecific action of pyrophosphatase and phosphatase on the coenzyme occurs in the upper gut.[370] The vitamin is primarily absorbed in the proximal small intestine by a saturable transport system that is rapid and proportional to intake before leveling off at doses near 27 mg riboflavin per day.[636] Bile salts appear to facilitate the uptake, and a modest amount of the vitamin circulates via the enterohepatic system.[470] Active transport at lower levels of intake was thought to be sodium ion–dependent and involve phosphorylation, though later work has suggested that uptake is independent of sodium ions.[488] The transport of flavins in human blood involves loose binding to albumin and tight binding to a number of globulins, with the major binding being to several classes of immunoglobulins (IgA, IgG, and IgM).[266,377] Pregnancy increases the concentration of carrier protein for riboflavin,[411] which results in a higher rate of riboflavin uptake at the maternal surface of the placenta.[123] The uptake of riboflavin into the cells of organs, such as liver, is facilitated, possibly requiring a specific carrier, at physiological concentrations, but can be by diffusion at higher concentrations.[67] Metabolic interconversions of flavins at the cellular level are outlined in Figure 30-12. Conversion of riboflavin to coenzymes occurs within the cellular cytoplasm of most tissue but particularly in the small intestine, liver, heart, and kidney. The obligatory first step is the ATP-dependent phosphorylation of the vitamin catalyzed by flavokinase. The FMN product can be complexed with specific apoenzymes to form several functional flavoproteins, but the larger quantity is further converted to FAD in a second ATP-dependent reaction catalyzed by FAD synthetase (pyrophosphorylase). Biosynthesis of flavocoenzymes, particularly at the flavokinase step, is probably tightly regulated. Thyroxine and triiodothyronine stimulate FMN and FAD synthesis in mammalian systems.[324] FAD is the predominant flavocoenzyme present in tissue where it is mainly complexed with numerous flavoprotein dehydrogenases and oxidases. Some FAD (less than 10%) can also become covalently linked to any of 5 specific amino acid residues of a few important apoenzymes.[142] Examples include the 8α-N(3)-histidyl FAD within succinate dehydrogenase and 8α-S-cysteinyl FAD within monoamine oxidase, both of mitochondrial localization. Turnover of covalently attached flavocoenzymes requires intracellular proteolysis, and further degradation of the coenzymes involves nonspecific pyrophosphatase cleavage of FAD to FMN and AMP, and further action by nonspecific phosphates on FMN and AMP. Because there is little storage of riboflavin as such, the urinary excretion reflects dietary intake. Milk contains reasonable quantities of the vitamin and lesser amounts of coenzyme, principally FMN. Smaller amounts of side-chain degradation products, such as lumichrome, 10-formylmethylflavin, and 10-(2′-hydroxyethyl)flavin, and ring-altered compounds are also excreted and may largely result from the action of intestinal

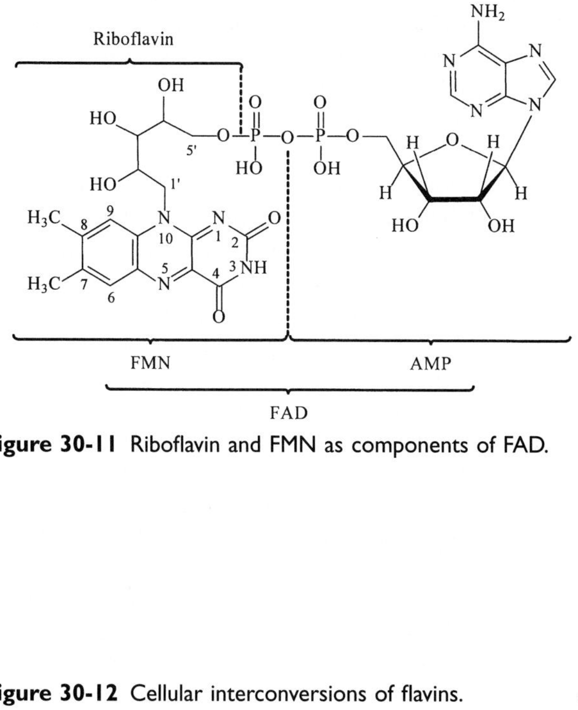

Figure 30-11 Riboflavin and FMN as components of FAD.

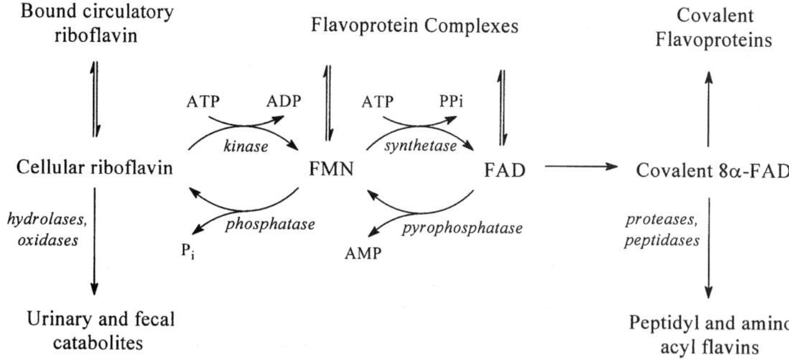

Figure 30-12 Cellular interconversions of flavins.

microorganisms.[104] Traces of 8α-flavin peptides and catabolites are found in urine and feces.

Functions

Riboflavin, as its coenzyme derivatives, is involved in a large variety of chemical reactions. These derivatives are capable of both one- and two-electron transfer processes, and play a pivotal role in coupling the two-electron oxidation of most organic substrates to the one-electron transfer of the respiratory chain,[364] thus being involved in energy production. They also function as electrophiles and nucleophiles, with covalent intermediates of flavin and substrate frequently being involved in catalysis. Flavoproteins catalyze dehydrogenation reactions, hydroxylations, oxidative decarboxylations, deoxygenations, and reductions of oxygen to hydrogen peroxide.[470] The chemical versatility of the flavoproteins is clearly controlled by specific interactions with the proteins with which they are bound.[364] Other major functions of riboflavin include drug metabolism in conjunction with the cytochrome P-450 enzymes and lipid metabolism.

Flavins also have both prooxidative and antioxidative functions. They are thought to contribute to oxidative stress through the ability to produce superoxide[364] and to catalyze the production of hydrogen peroxide. As an antioxidant, FAD is a coenzyme to glutathione reductase in the regeneration of reduced glutathione from oxidized glutathione, necessary for the removal of lipid peroxides. Riboflavin deficiency is associated with increased lipid peroxidation.[141] Flavins have also been linked with apoptosis[364] and have homocysteine-lowering properties, FAD being a cofactor to methylenetetrahydrofolate reductase in the remethylation of homocysteine.[394] Newer therapeutic uses of riboflavin are in the prophylaxis of migraine attacks[500] and in the treatment of lactic acidosis caused either by the use of nucleoside reverse transcriptase inhibitors in patients with the acquired immunodeficiency syndrome[179] or by genetic defects in the mitochondrial respiratory chain, such as in Leigh disease.[431]

Requirements and Reference Nutrient Intakes

Assessment of riboflavin status has been made on the basis of the relationship of dietary intake to overt signs of hyporiboflavinosis, urinary excretion of the vitamin, erythrocyte riboflavin content, and erythrocyte glutathione reductase activity.[170] Calculations have been based on protein allowances, energy intakes, and metabolic body size, but these do not differ significantly because they are interdependent. At least 0.5 mg of riboflavin per 1000 kcal is required by the adult, and 0.6 mg/1000 kcal constitutes the allowance suggested for all ages. Based on considerations such as these, the current RDA has been set at 1.3 mg/day for men of 19 to 70 years of age and older, and 1.1 mg/day for women in the same age group. Children 1 to 3 years old have an RDA of 0.5 mg/day, increasing to 0.6 mg/day up to age 8. From 8 to 18 years, RDAs progressively approach adult levels. Because pregnant women tend to excrete less riboflavin as pregnancy progresses and additionally exhibit FAD stimulation of erythrocyte glutathione reductase activity, recommended allowances call for an additional 0.3 mg/day during pregnancy. During lactation, between 18 and 80 μg of riboflavin are secreted daily into every 100 mL of human milk. Assuming that an infant will ingest an average of 750 mL of milk per day during its first 6 months and 600 mL/day for the next 6 months, this secretion rate translates into an ingestion of between 100 and 600 μg of riboflavin per day. Further assuming that 70% of maternally ingested riboflavin is used for milk production, these data suggest that the present RDA for lactating women should be increased by an additional 400 to 500 μg/day. Accordingly the RDA for lactating women has been set at 1.6 mg/day.[170]

Intravenous Supply

The recommended intravenous supply of riboflavin in adults is 3.6 mg/day.[9] Riboflavin in TPN mixtures may be subject to degradation under exposure to ultraviolet light, so bags containing riboflavin should either contain fat emulsion or be covered to provide protection from light.[519]

Deficiency

Although riboflavin has a wide distribution in foodstuffs, many people live for long periods on low intakes, and consequently, minor signs of deficiency are common in many parts of the world. In addition to poor intake, functional deficiency can be induced by diseases such as hypothyroidism and adrenal insufficiency that inhibit the conversion of riboflavin to its coenzyme derivatives and by drugs such as chlorpromazine, imipramine, and amitriptyline that have a similar tricyclic structure to riboflavin—the anticancer drug doxorubicin and the antimalarial quinacrine.[140,437] Excess ethanol ingestion interferes with both the digestion and absorption of riboflavin.[441]

Because flavin coenzymes are widely distributed in intermediary metabolism, the consequences of deficiency may be widespread. Because riboflavin coenzymes are involved in the metabolism of folic acid, pyridoxine, vitamin K, and niacin,[471] deficiency will affect enzyme systems other than those requiring flavin coenzymes. With increasing riboflavin deficiency, tissue concentrations of FMN and FAD fall, as does flavokinase activity, thus further decreasing FMN concentrations. FMN concentrations are decreased proportionally more than FAD concentrations. Decreases in the activities of enzymes requiring FMN generally follow the fall in tissue concentrations, whereas the FAD-dependent enzymes are more variably affected.[83]

The deficiency syndrome is characterized by sore throat, hyperemia, edema of the pharyngeal and oral mucous membranes, cheilosis, angular stomatitis, glossitis (magenta tongue), seborrheic dermatitis, and normochromic, normocytic anemia associated with pure red blood cell aplasia of the bone marrow. However, some of these symptoms, such as glossitis and dermatitis, when encountered in the field may have resulted from other complicating deficiencies.

Toxicity

Probably as a result of its limited solubility and limited gastric absorption, no adverse effects have been associated with ingestion of riboflavin appreciably above RDA levels. One study reported no short-term side effects in 49 patients treated with 400 mg/day of riboflavin with meals for at least 3 months.[500] Because of a lack of data for risk assessment, no tolerable upper intake level has been proposed for riboflavin.[170]

Laboratory Assessment of Status

Riboflavin status is assessed by (1) determination of urine riboflavin excretion, (2) a functional assay using the activation coefficient of stimulation of the enzyme glutathione reductase by FAD, or (3) direct measurement of riboflavin or its metabolites in plasma or erythrocytes. The advantages and disadvantages of functional or direct methods have been discussed in the section on thiamine.

Urinary riboflavin can be measured using fluorometric and microbiological procedures, but for specificity, HPLC combined with fluorometric detection is the method of choice.[104] Under conditions of adequate intake, the amount excreted per day is more than 120 μg or 80 μg/g creatinine. The rate of excretion expressed as μg/g creatinine is greater for children than for adults. Conditions causing negative nitrogen balance and the administration of antibiotics and certain psychotropic drugs (phenothiazine derivatives) increase urinary riboflavin as a consequence of tissue depletion and displacement. A load return test may augment the reliability, but is more cumbersome.

A commonly used method for assessing riboflavin status uses the determination of FAD-dependent glutathione reductase activity in freshly lysed erythrocytes.[495] This enzyme-based assay has been chosen for the majority of surveys of riboflavin status. Most methods measure the rate of change of absorbance at 340 nm caused by the oxidation of NADPH and have been automated to give rapid throughputs and CVs of less than 2% within run, though some have used fluorescence detection with increased sensitivity.[90] Potential problems are that in long-standing riboflavin deficiency the apoenzyme activity may be reduced, possibly leading to a misleading activation coefficient calculation, and that in patients with glucose-6-phosphate deficiency, a misleadingly low activation coefficient may be measured, possibly caused by enhanced binding of FAD to the apoenzyme.[450]

Direct measurement of riboflavin, FMN, and FAD in plasma or erythrocytes may be made by HPLC, usually with fluorescence detection after protein precipitation[90] or by capillary zone electrophoresis with laser-induced fluorescence detection (CZE-LIF).[438] In a study of riboflavin status and FMN and FAD concentrations in plasma and erythrocytes from elderly subjects at baseline and after low-dose riboflavin supplementation, using both activation coefficient measurements and CE-LIF, it was concluded that concentrations of all B_2 vitamers except plasma FAD are potential indicators of vitamin B_2 status, and that plasma riboflavin and erythrocyte FMN may be useful in the assessment of vitamin B_2 status in population studies.[262]

Reference Intervals

The reference interval for erythrocyte riboflavin using a fluorometric method[311] is 10 to 50 μg/dL (266 to 1330 nmol/L).[574] The reference interval for serum or plasma levels of riboflavin is 4 to 24 μg/dL (106 to 638 nmol/L).[186,574] Guidance reference intervals for the activation coefficient of erythrocyte glutathione reductase by FAD are 1.20 (adequacy), 1.21 to 1.40 (marginal deficiency), and 1.41 and above (deficiency).[32]

VITAMIN B_6—PYRIDOXINE, PYRIDOXAMINE, AND PYRIDOXAL

Pyridoxine (pyridoxol), pyridoxamine, and *pyridoxal* are the three natural forms of vitamin B_6. They are converted to pyridoxal phosphate, which is required for the synthesis, catabolism, and interconversion of amino acids.

Chemistry

The vitamin B_6 group comprises three natural forms: *pyridoxine* (pyridoxol) *(PN), pyridoxamine (PM),* and *pyridoxal (PL),* which are 4-substituted 2-methyl-3-hydroxyl-5-hydroxymethyl pyridines (Figure 30-13). During metabolic conversions, each vitamer becomes phosphorylated at the 5-hydroxymethyl substituent. Although both pyridoxamine-5′-phosphate (PMP) and pyridoxal-5′-phosphate (PLP, P-5′-P) interconvert as coenzyme forms during aminotransferase (transaminase)-catalyzed reactions, PLP is the coenzyme form that participates in the large number of B_6-dependent enzyme reactions.

Dietary Sources

Vitamin B_6 is widely distributed in animal and plant tissues where the phosphorylated forms, and particularly PLP, predominate. Meats, poultry, and fish are good sources, as are yeast, certain seeds, bran, and bananas; somewhat more limited sources are milk, eggs, and green leafy vegetables.[295] In the United States and some other countries, fortified ready-to-eat cereals are the main dietary source of vitamin B_6. The common commercial form of the vitamin is pyridoxine hydrochloride, which is a water-soluble, white, crystalline solid. Solutions of the B_6 vitamers are decomposed by light, especially in the ultraviolet region at neutral to alkaline pH. The reactive aldehyde function of PLP leads to significant loss during thermal processing of foods.[210]

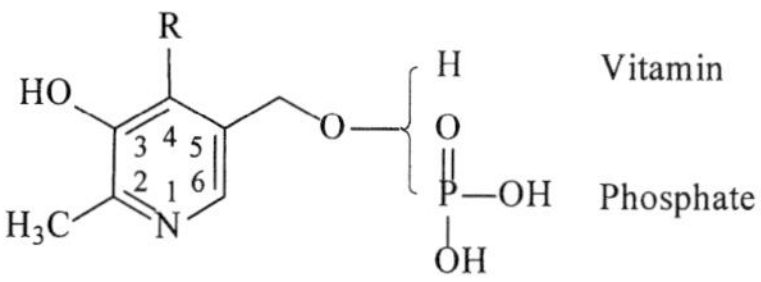

Figure 30-13 Free and phosphorylated forms of vitamin B_6. R = CH_2OH for pyridoxine, CH_2NH_2 for pyridoxamine, and CHO for pyridoxal.

Absorption, Transport, Metabolism, and Excretion

Food sources of animal origin contain mainly PLP with some PMP, whereas plant sources also contain pyridoxine-5′-glucoside, which is absorbed in a different manner. The phosphorylated sources are hydrolyzed by the intraluminal action of intestinal alkaline phosphatase, but pyridoxine-5′-glucoside is less effectively hydrolyzed by nonspecific glycosidase within cells, and some pyridoxine-5′-glucoside can be absorbed intact and hydrolyzed in various tissues.[251] The nonphosphorylated vitamers are readily absorbed by the mucosal cells by a process of passive diffusion, which does not appear to be limited by load.[227] Here, as in other cells requiring vitamin B_6, the unphosphorylated vitamers may be "metabolically trapped" as the phosphorylated forms by cytoplasmic pyridoxal kinase responsible for catalyzing the ATP-dependent phosphorylation of all three vitamin forms. Transport to the liver via the portal vein is by the unphosphorylated form.

Figure 30-14 shows the intracellular metabolism of vitamin B_6. Most cells contain a cytosolic FMN-dependent, pyridoxine (pyridoxamine)-5′-phosphate oxidase responsible for catalyzing the oxygen-dependent conversion of pyridoxine phosphate and pyridoxamine phosphate to PLP (and hydrogen peroxide).[578] PLP can enter directly into subcellular organelles, such as hepatocyte mitochondria,[351] and can bind for catalytic function with numerous specific apoenzymes throughout the cell. The erythrocyte, in addition, traps PLP as a conjugate Schiff base with hemoglobin.[375] Vitamin B_6 in muscle accounts for 80% of body stores, mostly as PLP bound to glycogen phosphorylase.[56] Total body stores of vitamin B_6 are thought to be about 1 mmole.

Release of free vitamin, mainly pyridoxal, occurs when physiological nonsaturating levels of vitamin are absorbed. Here the phosphates are hydrolyzed by nonspecific alkaline phosphatase located on the plasma membrane of cells. Some PLP is also released into the circulation by the liver.[578] Because the reactive aldehyde is capable of forming Schiff bases with amino groups, PLP in plasma is more tightly complexed to proteins—mostly albumin—than is pyridoxal, which forms an intramolecular hemiacetal between the 4-formyl and 5-hydroxymethyl functions. Although PLP is the principal tissue form of vitamin B_6 and pyridoxal constitutes much of the circulating vitamin, the main catabolite excreted in urine is 4-pyridoxic acid (4-PA), which is formed by the action of the FAD-dependent general liver aldehyde oxidase and especially by NAD-specific aldehyde dehydrogenase, which is found in most tissue.

Functions

As coenzyme PLP, vitamin B_6 functions in more than 100 reactions that embrace the metabolism of macronutrients, such as proteins, carbohydrates, and lipids.[326,369] Especially diverse are PLP-dependent enzymes that are involved in amino acid metabolism. By virtue of the ability of PLP to condense its 4-formyl substituent with the α-amino group of an amino acid to form an azomethine (Schiff base) linkage, a conjugated double-bond system, extending from the α-carbon of the amino acid to the pyridinium nitrogen in PLP, results in reduced electron density about the α-carbon. This configuration potentially weakens each of the bonds from the amino acid α-carbon to the adjoined hydrogen, carboxyl, and side-chain functions. A given apoenzyme then locks in a particular configuration of the coenzyme-substrate compound, such that maximal overlap of the bond to be broken will occur with the resonant, coplanar, electron-withdrawing system of the coenzyme complex. Aminotransferases affect rupture of the α-hydrogen bond with the ultimate formation of an α-keto acid and pyridoxamine-5′-phosphate; this reversible reaction provides an interface between amino acid metabolism and that of ketogenic and glucogenic reactions (see Chapter 21).

Other examples of PLP-requiring enzymes are the amino acid decarboxylases that lead to formation of amines, including several that are functional in nervous tissue (e.g., epinephrine, norepinephrine, serotonin, and γ-aminobutyrate); cysteine desulfhydrase and serine hydroxymethyltransferase, which use PLP to effect the loss or transfer of amino acid side chains; phosphorylase, which catalyzes phosphorolysis of the α-1,4-linkages of glycogen; and cystathione beta-synthase in the transsulfuration pathway of homocysteine. Additionally the biosynthesis of heme depends on the early

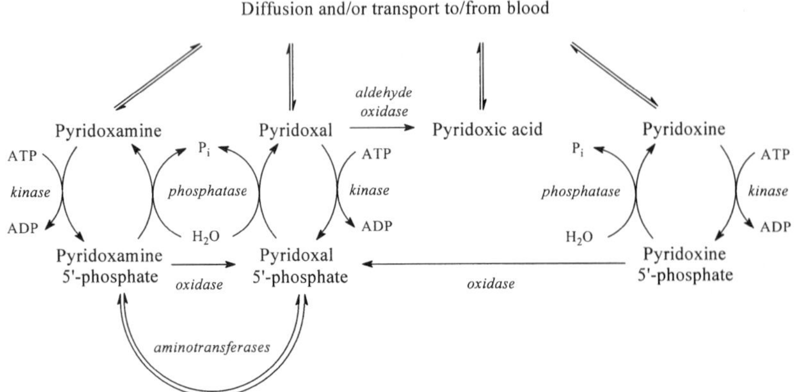

Figure 30-14 Metabolism of vitamin B_6.

formation of 5-aminolevulinate from PLP-dependent condensation of glycine and succinyl-CoA, followed by decarboxylation, and an important role in lipid metabolism is the PLP-dependent condensation of L-serine with palmitoyl-CoA to form 3-dehydrosphinganine, a precursor of sphingomyelins. Therapeutically, vitamin B_6 has been used in the treatment of some intractable seizures in neonates and infants,[204] in other vitamin B_6–responsive inborn errors of metabolism,[41] and in the carpal tunnel syndrome.[254]

Requirements and Reference Nutrient Intakes

Requirements for vitamin B_6 are complicated by (1) differences in protein intake, (2) the probable provision of a fraction of the necessary quantity through bacterial synthesis in the intestinal tract, (3) the use of alcohol and oral contraceptives, and (4) the infrequent cases in which extra requirements are apparent.[169,327] Estimates of requirements with some margin of safety have been based on the production and cure of clinical signs of deficiency but more often on biochemical parameters. The latter include the determination of the urinary excretion of vitamin B_6 and 4-PA or xanthurenic acid after a tryptophan load test, the plasma levels of PLP, and red blood cell transaminase activity.[170] A ratio of 0.016 mg of vitamin B_6/g of protein intake has been suggested for normal adults and may be extrapolated to children and adolescents. Recommendations (1998) have proposed RDAs of 0.5 mg/day for children 1 to 3 years, 0.6 mg/day for children 4 to 8 years, 1.0 mg/day for children 9 to 13 years, 1.3 mg/day for boys 14 to 18 years, 1.3 mg/day for men to age 50 years, and 1.7 mg/day for men over 50 years. Girls 14 to 18 years have an RDA of 1.2 mg/day; women 19 to 50 years, 1.3 mg/day; and women over 50 years, 1.5 mg/day.[170] An addition of 0.6 mg B_6 per day is suggested for pregnant women to match the increased protein allowance during gestation. During lactation, an additional 0.5 mg/day is recommended to accommodate for extra protein intake and provide a level of 0.10 to 0.25 mg/L of the vitamin in milk, which is adequate for the breast-fed infant.

Intravenous Supply

The recommended intravenous supply of vitamin B_6 has been increased from 4 mg/day to 6 mg/day for adults to ensure adequate amounts in patients who are sometimes receiving quite large amino acid intakes.[243] This is usually provided as pyridoxine hydrochloride.

Deficiency

A deficiency of vitamin B_6 alone is uncommon, and it is more usual to expect the problem to occur in association with deficits in other vitamins of the B-complex. As with other water-soluble vitamins that function as coenzymes, the relative affinity of the coenzyme for a given apoenzyme and the extent to which a particular holoenzyme-catalyzed reaction is essential are reflected in the progressive symptomatology of deficiency of the vitamin. Investigations of the consequences of vitamin B_6 deficiency in the human use diets deficient in the vitamin and/or diets containing an antagonist, usually 4′-deoxypyridoxine.[112] There are, however, instances in which drug interactions have led to hypovitaminosis of B_6.[371] The antituberculosis drug isoniazid (isonicotinic acid hydrazide) forms hydrazones with pyridoxal and PLP. As with other "carbonyl reagents," such compounds not only cause loss by displacement and urinary excretion, but the Schiff bases formed with pyridoxal inhibit pyridoxal kinase,[372] and the PLP Schiff bases may additionally inhibit some PLP-dependent enzymes.[578] Penicillamine (β-dimethyl cysteine), used in treatment of patients with Wilson's disease in an attempt to decrease the damaging levels of copper found in liver, inactivates PLP by forming a thiazolidine derivative.[280] Other drugs that can cause vitamin B_6 deficiency include the antiparkinsonian drugs benserazide and carbidopa, which react by forming hydrazones,[40] and theophylline.[200]

There are several vitamin B_6–responsive inborn errors of metabolism[41] that include (1) cases of infantile convulsions in which the apoenzyme for glutamate decarboxylase has a poor affinity for the coenzyme; (2) a type of chronic anemia in which the number but not morphological abnormality of erythrocytes is improved by pyridoxine supplementation; (3) xanthurenic aciduria in which affinity of the mutant kynureninase for PLP is decreased; (4) primary cystathioninuria caused by similarly defective cystathionase; and (5) homocystinuria in which there is less of the normal cystathionine synthetase.[403] In these cases increased levels (200 to 1000 mg/day) of administered vitamin B_6 are required for life.[477] Low vitamin B_6 status (together with low vitamin B_{12} and folate status) in humans has been linked to hyperhomocysteinemia and as an independent risk factor for cardiovascular disease.[121,316]

Biochemical markers of vitamin B_6 deficiency occur early and become more marked as the deficiency progresses.[327,495,578] Plasma levels of PLP and urinary output of B_6 and 4-PA decrease within 1 week of removal of vitamin from the diet. Because liver kynureninase activity is decreased, there is increased xanthurenic acid in urine. Aminotransferase activity in serum and red blood cells also decreases. Clinically, electroencephalographic abnormalities appear within 3 weeks and epileptiform convulsions are a common finding in young vitamin B_6–deficient subjects. In addition, skin changes occur, including dermatitis with cheilosis and glossitis. Hematological manifestations may include a decrease in the number of circulating lymphocytes and possibly a normocytic, microcytic, or sideroblastic anemia.

Toxicity

Although no adverse effects have been observed with high intakes of vitamin B_6 from food sources, high oral supplemental doses can have neurotoxic and photosensitive effects. The first reported cases in humans were a series of 7 patients who had taken between 2 and 6 g of pyridoxine per day for up to 40 months. Four of these patients were unable to walk and all showed severe sensory neuropathy of the extremities, though the majority of the symptoms were reversed on stopping the pyridoxine.[497] None of the subsequent studies showed any evidence of sensory nerve damage at intakes below 200 mg/day. Based on the end point of development of sensory neuropathy, 1998 recommendations have set a tolerable upper intake level of 100 mg/day for adults.[170]

Laboratory Assessment of Status

As with the other B vitamins that act as coenzymes, biochemical assessment of vitamin B_6 can be made by direct chemical analysis of the vitamer or its metabolites, or by functional means. Measurements that have been used are PLP in plasma or red cells, its metabolite 4-PA in urine or plasma, the activity and activation coefficient of the red cell aminotransferases (aspartate and alanine), and the tryptophan load metabolite excretion test.[32] As no single marker adequately reflects status, a combination of these markers offers the best approach.

Direct assessment was originally made by microbiological techniques using specific strains of *Saccharomyces carlsbergensis* for all 3 natural vitamers, *Enterococcus faucium* for pyridoxal and pyridoxamine, and *Lactobacillus casei* for pyridoxal. Levels of 20 μg of vitamin B_6 per gram creatinine in urine are considered indicative of marginal or inadequate dietary intake of the vitamin. Plasma PLP and plasma or urine 4-PA are most commonly measured by HPLC, PLP with fluorescence detection following precolumn fluorophore formation either as a semicarbazone,[582] or a pyridoxic acid phosphate,[387] and 4-PA with its natural fluorescence. During deficiency, the level of 4-PA will drop well below the normal level of at least 0.8 mg/day in urine. Using ion-pair reversed-phase chromatography,[63] plasma vitamin B_6 vitamers (PLP, PL, PN, PMP, PM, and 4-PA) were measured in 90 patients undergoing coronary angiography before and after treatment with pyridoxine, 40 mg daily for up to 84 days. PLP, 4-PA, and to a lesser degree PL were found to be the predominant B_6 metabolites in pretreatment plasma. After treatment, PN was also detectable, and PN and PL showed the largest increases in concentration. Increases in plasma concentrations of PLP, PL, and 4-PA occurred within 3 days of supplementation and were steady for the remainder of the study period. Other direct measurements have used recombinant enzyme technology. A homogenous, nonradioactive recombinant enzymatic method for PLP has been described that uses 5 μL of plasma, has a detection limit of 5 nmol/L, and may be applicable to adaptation to an automated analyzer.[228]

Functional assessment of vitamin B_6 status may be made by measuring the activity of red cell aspartate (or alanine) aminotransferase, and its activation coefficient on incubation with PLP, though as the apoenzyme is highly unsaturated with PLP, the results obtained have more variability than corresponding methods for vitamins B_1 and B_2 and are thus considered less useful. Activation coefficients of less than about 1.5 for aspartate aminotransferase and 1.2 for alanine aminotransferase are considered normal but may depend somewhat on the assay method used. Measurement of urinary tryptophan metabolites, particularly xanthurenic acid, following an oral load (2 to 5 g) of L-tryptophan, is one of the most common indices used in studies of vitamin B_6 nutriture, because changes can be recognized early and measurements are relatively easy. Amounts of xanthurenate well above the normal (about 25 mg/day) are seen in vitamin B_6 deficiency. Levels of other metabolites, such as kynurenic acid and 3-hydroxykynurenine, are also increased.

Reference Intervals

A guidance reference interval for plasma PLP is 5 to 30 ng/mL (20 to 121 nmol/L).[464] Plasma levels less than 5 ng/mL (20 nmol/L) are judged deficient. Guidance values for other vitamin B_6 metabolites have been published elsewhere.[495]

VITAMIN B_{12}—CYANOCOBALAMIN

Vitamin B_{12}, also known as cyanocobalamin, is a water-soluble hematopoietic vitamin that is required for the maturation of erythrocytes.

Chemistry

Vitamin B_{12} is one of the most structurally complex small molecules produced by nature, whose biosynthetic pathway has been extensively studied and elucidated.[613] The generic term vitamin B_{12} refers to a group of physiologically active substances chemically classified as cobalamins or corrinoids. They are composed of tetrapyrrole rings surrounding central cobalt atoms and nucleotide side chains attached to the cobalt. The cobalamin tetrapyrrole ring, exclusive of cobalt and other side chains, is called a corrin. All compounds containing this corrin nucleus are corrinoids. The cobalt-corrin complex is termed cobamide. In cobalamins, 5,6-dimethylbenzimidazole riboside is bound to the cobalt atom by one of its imidazole nitrogens and its 2′-ribose carbon is linked with an ester of aminoisopropanol and propionic acid to the corrin ring (Figure 30-15).

Cobalamins differ in the nature of additional side groups bound to cobalt. Examples are methyl (methylcobalamin), 5′-deoxyadenosine (deoxyadenosyl [short form, adenosyl] cobalamin, or coenzyme B_{12}), hydroxyl (hydroxocobalamin), H_2O (aquocobalamin, or vitamin B_{12b}), and cyanide (cyanocobalamin). Cyanocobalamin is a stable compound that forms dark red, needlelike crystals; it is the reference compound for measuring serum cobalamin concentration. Less stable serum cobalamins may be converted to this compound for quantitation. The predominant physiological form of cobalamin in serum is methylcobalamin, whereas that in cytosols is adenosylcobalamin. It is recommended that the term vitamin B_{12} be used as the generic descriptor for all corrinoids exhibiting qualitatively the biological activity of cyanocobalamin.[126] Cyanocobalamin has a molecular weight of 1355 Da and a solubility of 12 g/L in water at 20 °C. It is also soluble in lower alcohols and aliphatic acids, but is insoluble in acetone, ether, and chloroform. It is grad-

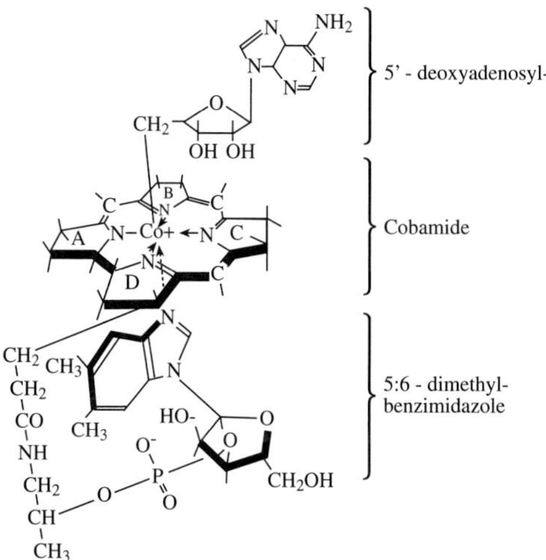

Figure 30-15 The structure of 5′-deoxyadenosyl cobalamin. *(Modified from Chanarin I: The megaloblastic anemias, 2nd edition, Oxford: Blackwell Scientific, 1979.)*

ually destroyed on exposure to light.[126] Aqueous solutions of cyanocobalamin exhibit a distinctive absorption spectrum with maxima at 278, 361, and 550 nm, with absorptivity coefficients of 115, 207, and 63 at these maxima, respectively. The spectrum is independent of pH but changes when cyanocobalamin binds to intrinsic factor (IF). Because of its stability in aqueous solutions and its distinct absorption spectrum, accurate concentrations of cyanocobalamin can be prepared and used as calibrators for the measurement of serum cobalamin levels.

Dietary Sources

All vitamin B_{12} is ultimately the product of microbial synthesis, and because plants do not use the vitamin, the main dietary sources are meat and meat products, dairy products, fish and shellfish, and fortified ready-to-eat cereals.[170]

Absorption, Transport, Metabolism, and Excretion

The uptake of vitamin B_{12} from the intestine into the circulation is a complex mechanism, involving five separate vitamin B_{12}–binding molecules, receptors, and transporters.[484] The vitamin B_{12} released from food in the stomach is bound to haptocorrin (R protein, a salivary protein), and travels with it into the intestine where the haptocorrin is digested by pancreatic enzymes. The liberated vitamin B_{12} then binds to IF, a glycoprotein with a molecular weight of approximately 50 kDa, which is produced by the gastric mucosa. When the vitamin B_{12}–IF complex reaches the distal ileum, it is bound by receptors on the surface of mucosal epithelial cells and then enters the cells. Within the mucosal epithelial cells, the vitamin B_{12}–IF complex is dissociated with the vitamin B_{12}, then binding with transcobalamin II (TcII). The B_{12}-TcII complex is then transported across the cell membrane bound to a TcII-receptor and then released into the plasma of the mucosal capillaries and subsequently to the blood in the portal vein.[222] Almost all of the vitamin B_{12} is taken up by hepatocytes as the blood in the portal vein passes through the liver. It is stored in the liver and released to plasma to meet physiological demands. If the quantity of vitamin B_{12} exceeds the capacity of hepatocyte receptors, most of the excess is excreted by the kidneys. Normally, approximately 1 mg of vitamin B_{12} is stored in the liver, a quantity equivalent to the daily metabolic requirement for 2000 days. Thus when the dietary supply of vitamin B_{12} is interrupted or mechanisms of absorption are impaired, vitamin B_{12} deficiency does not become evident for 5 years or more.

IF is a glycoprotein with a molecular weight of approximately 50 kDa, secreted by the parietal cells of the stomach. Many other substances can bind vitamin B_{12}, but no other known substance has the property of transporting it across the intestinal wall. One molecule of IF binds one molecule of vitamin B_{12}. The gastric secretion of IF is stimulated by food, histamine, and gastrin; it is inhibited by vagal blockade. The ileal receptor for the IF–vitamin B_{12} complex has an association constant of approximately 5×10^9 mol/L between pH 6.4 and 8.4. The binding does not appear to be specific for the configuration of the vitamin B_{12} molecule, because complexes of IF with various analogues of vitamin B_{12} bind equally well to the ileal receptors.

The most important vitamin B_{12} transport protein in plasma is TcII, a β-globulin. It is synthesized mainly in the liver but also in other tissue. TcII is a polypeptide with a molecular weight of approximately 43 kDa; it has a single vitamin B_{12} binding site per molecule.[511] TcII is less specific for vitamin B_{12} than is IF; it also binds cobalamins that are physiologically inactive. TcII transports vitamin B_{12} to receptors on cell membranes throughout the body. Binding is very rapid: if TcII–vitamin B_{12} is injected intravenously, it is almost completely cleared in one passage through tissue, mostly by the liver.[222] The TcII–vitamin B_{12} complex enters the cell by pinocytosis. Lysosomal proteolysis degrades TcII and releases the vitamin B_{12}. Unbound vitamin B_{12} can also enter the tissue cells, but the process is much less efficient.[222]

Two types of vitamin B_{12} binders are found in human gastric juice, one with slow (S) and one with rapid (R) mobility in zone electrophoresis. The slow component is IF, and the rapid component is R protein. Immunologically identical R proteins are found in plasma, amniotic fluid, milk, saliva, ascitic fluid, and granulocytes. However, this granulocyte-derived protein can be differentiated from the other R proteins electrophoretically. It is called *transcobalamin III,* whereas the R protein from other sources is designated *transcobalamin I.* Collectively, these two binders are called *cobalophilins.* They are glycoproteins with molecular weights between 60 and 150 kDa. Heterogeneity of R proteins may be due to variations in the carbohydrate moieties (sialic acid residues) rather than in the apoproteins. They have one binding site per molecule and bind vitamin B_{12} analogues to some extent. In gastric juice at pH 2, the cobalophilins have much greater affinity than IF and bind almost all vitamin B_{12}. It has been postulated that cobalophilins aid in host defense against bacteria by depriving them of access to vitamin B_{12}. However, the physiological function of these proteins is unknown.

Vitamin B_{12} is continually secreted in the bile, but most of this is reabsorbed and available for metabolic functions. If circulating vitamin B_{12} concentrations exceed the binding capacity of the blood, the excess will be excreted in the urine, but in most circumstances the highest losses of vitamin B_{12} occur through the feces.

Functions

Vitamin B_{12} is required in coenzyme form for more than 12 different enzyme systems.[36] In humans it is required in (1) adenosylcobalamin, coenzyme to L-methylmalonyl-CoA mutase in the conversion of L-methylmalonyl CoA to succinyl-CoA; and (2) methylcobalamin, coenzyme to methionine synthase in the conversion of homocysteine to methionine. In the former reaction (Figure 30-16), the mutase is a mitochondrial matrix enzyme that binds 2 mol of adenosyl-cobalamin (Cbl) per dimer[350] and participates in a complex reaction using radical chemistry.[27] The conversion of L-methylmalonyl-CoA to succinyl-CoA links propionyl-CoA, which is formed from amino acids, such as valine, isoleucine, and methionine, and odd-chain fatty acids with the tricarboxylic acid (TCA) cycle. Congenital defects of the mutase synthesis or inability to synthesize adenosyl-Cbl result in life-threatening methylmalonic aciduria and metabolic ketoacidosis. In the latter reaction (Figure 30-16), methylcobalamin serves as an intermediate in the transfer of a methyl group from 5-methyltetrahydrofolate to homocysteine for the formation of methionine. Methionine is required for the protein synthesis and as the methyl donor, *S*-adenosylmethionine. Congenital defects in methionine synthase or the synthesis of methyl-Cbl result in severe hyperhomocysteinemia.[158]

Requirements and Reference Nutrient Intakes

The total body stores of vitamin B_{12} are estimated to be between 2 and 5 mg in the adult man,[4] of which about 1 mg is in the liver and a smaller amount in the kidney. There is thought to be a daily obligatory loss of vitamin B_{12} of about 0.1% of body pool, irrespective of size,[246] suggesting that a daily requirement to maintain stores would be 2 to 5 µg. The daily diet of Western countries contains between 5 and 30 µg of vitamin B_{12}, with average ingestion being 7 to 8 µg/day by adult men and 4 to 5 µg/day by adult women. Additional small amounts may be available from vitamin B_{12} synthesis by intestinal microorganisms. Of the amount ingested, between 1 and 5 µg is absorbed.

The RDA for vitamin B_{12} is based on the amount necessary for the maintenance of hematological status and normal serum vitamin B_{12} concentrations, and assumes 50% absorbance of ingested vitamin B_{12}. The RDA for adults (19 to 50 years) has been set at 2.4 µg/day, with an increase to 2.6 µg/day in pregnancy and to 2.8 µg/day in lactation. RDAs for children are 0.9 µg/day at 1 to 3 years, 1.2 µg/day at 4 to 8 years, 1.8 µg/day at 9 to 13 years, and 2.4 µg/day at 14 to 18 years. Because 10% to 30% of older persons may be unable to absorb naturally occurring vitamin B_{12}, it is recommended that those older than 50 years meet their RDA mainly by consuming foods fortified with vitamin B_{12} or with a vitamin B_{12}–containing supplement.[170]

Intravenous Supply

The recommended intravenous intake for adults is 5 µg/day as cyanocobalamin, an amount in excess of the oral recommendation that will more than meet requirements.[9]

Deficiency

Deficiency of vitamin B_{12} in humans is associated with megaloblastic anemia and neuropathy. The most common cause of vitamin B_{12} deficiency is *pernicious anemia,* an autoimmune disease in which chronic atrophic gastritis results from antibodies to gastric parietal cells and IF, directed against gastric parietal cell H^+/K^+-ATPase.[575] A 1996 population study showed that 1.9% of persons over 60 years old have undiagnosed pernicious anemia, though the diagnosis is made most commonly in young to middle-aged black women (mean age 53 years) and in middle-aged to elderly whites.[94] Pernicious anemia may also occur in children because of either failure of IF secretion or secretion of biologically inactive IF. Other groups at risk of vitamin B_{12} deficiency include those (1) older than 65 years of age; (2) with malabsorption; (3) who are vegetarians; (4) with autoimmune disorders; (5) taking prescribed medication known to interfere with vitamin absorption or metabolism, including nitrous oxide, phenytoin, dihydrofolate reductase inhibitors, metformin, and proton pump inhibitors; and (6) infants with suspected metabolic disorders.

1. Adenosylcobalamin-dependent, L-methylmalonyl–CoA mutase reaction

$$\text{L-methylmalonyl-CoA} \rightleftharpoons \text{Succinyl-CoA}$$

2. Methylcobalamin-dependent, methionine synthase reaction

$$CH_3\text{-Cob(III)alamin} + \text{homocysteine} \rightarrow \text{Cob(I)alamin} + \text{methionine}$$

$$\text{Cob(I)alamin} + \text{5-methyltetrahydrofolate} \rightarrow CH_3\text{-Cob(III)alamin} + \text{tetrahydrofolate}$$

Figure 30-16 Participation of cobalamin coenzymes in human metabolism.

Intestinal malabsorption of vitamin B_{12} may be caused by gastrectomy or ileal resection, with an inverse relationship between the length of ileum resected and the absorption of vitamin B_{12}. Other causes of malabsorption are tropical sprue, inflammatory disease of the small intestine, intestinal stasis with overgrowth of colonic bacteria, which consume the vitamin B_{12} ingested by the host, and HIV infection. Another cause of vitamin B_{12} malabsorption is failure to extract cobalamin from food. Some patients fail to absorb cobalamin bound to food, whereas absorption of nonfood-bound cobalamin in the Schilling test is unimpaired. This is particularly a problem in patients with compromised gastric status[92] or early in the course of development of pernicious anemia.

Vegetarians have a lower intake of vitamin B_{12} than omnivores, and though clinical signs of deficiency are uncommon, biochemical markers of status indicate functional vitamin B_{12} deficiency. In a study of 66 lactovegetarians or lacto-ovo vegetarians, 29 vegans, and 79 omnivores, the incidence of low holotranscobalamin II was 77%, 92%, and 11%, respectively, in the 3 groups; of elevated methylmalonic acid, 68%, 83%, and 5%; and of elevated total homocysteine, 38%, 67%, and 16%. Consequently, these results indicate that the health aspects of prolonged hyperhomocysteinemia may have to be addressed.[245]

A large number of disorders are associated with cobalamin deficiency in infancy or childhood. Of these, the most commonly encountered is the Imerslund-Graesbeck syndrome, a condition that is characterized by inability to absorb vitamin B_{12}, with or without IF, and proteinuria. It appears to be due to an inability of intestinal mucosa to absorb the vitamin B_{12}–IF complex. The second most common of these is congenital deficiency of gastric secretion of IF. Very rarely, congenital deficiency of vitamin B_{12} in a breast-fed infant is due to deficiency of vitamin B_{12} in maternal breast milk as a result of unrecognized pernicious anemia in the mother. This is rare because most women with undiagnosed and untreated pernicious anemia are infertile. Additionally, there are some rare methylmalonic acidemias (acidurias) caused by inborn errors in homocysteine and methionine metabolism that are responsible for disorders in vitamin B_{12} status.[157]

The hematological effects of vitamin B_{12} deficiency are indistinguishable from those of folate deficiency. The classical morphological changes in the blood, in approximate order of appearance are: hypersegmentation of neutrophils, macrocytosis, anemia, leukopenia, and thrombocytopenia, with megaloblastic changes in bone marrow accompanying the peripheral blood changes. The cause of the hematological abnormalities is thought to be the imbalance of decreased deoxyribonucleic acid (DNA) synthesis and adequate ribonucleic acid (RNA) synthesis caused by the secondary block in folate metabolism caused by the vitamin B_{12} deficiency.[7] Many immature cells die in the bone marrow, possibly by apoptosis, leading to a release of bilirubin and lactate dehydrogenase (LD) into the blood. This is termed ineffective erythropoiesis. All of the bone marrow lesions can be reversed by vitamin B_{12} treatment.

In addition to hematological changes, vitamin B_{12} deficiency can lead to a demyelinating disorder of the central nervous system in man. Serious and often irreversible neurological disorders can occur, such as burning pain or loss of sensation in the extremities, weakness, spasticity and paralysis, confusion, disorientation, and dementia. This condition has been given the name *subacute combined degeneration of the spinal cord.* Neurological symptoms may occur without any discernible hematological changes in the blood, and indeed an intriguing inverse relationship between the hematological and the neurological has been observed.[239] The incidence of neurological complications is between 75% and 90% of all individuals with clinically observable vitamin B_{12} deficiency, and may in about 25% of cases be the only clinical manifestation of deficiency. The mechanism of the disorder is uncertain though there is some indirect evidence that suggests that disorders of both enzyme systems requiring vitamin B_{12} coenzymes are necessary before neurological symptoms occur.[158] The response of neurological symptoms to vitamin B_{12} replacement is often dependent upon the duration of the symptoms. Vitamin B_{12} deficiency may also be associated with other mainly gastrointestinal complications, such as glossitis of the tongue, appetite and weight loss, flatulence and constipation, mental changes, and infertility.[7]

Toxicity

No adverse effects have been associated with excess vitamin B_{12} intake from food or supplements in healthy people. Daily oral doses of up to 2 mg of cyanocobalamin can be used for treatment of deficiency in those who can tolerate oral supplementation.[320] There are insufficient data in the literature to propose a tolerable upper intake level for vitamin B_{12}.[170]

Laboratory Assessment of Status

Both direct and indirect (functional) methods are available for assessing vitamin B_{12} status. The indirect tests include assays for urinary and serum concentrations of methylmalonic acid, plasma homocysteine, the deoxyuridine suppression test, and the vitamin B_{12} absorption test. Cytochemical staining of red blood cell (RBC) precursors and the test for IF blocking antibodies are also ancillary methods for assessing vitamin B_{12} status.

Microbiological, competitive protein binding (CPB), and immunometric assays have been used for the quantitation of serum vitamin B_{12}. The microbiological assays have largely been replaced by the other, more convenient and precise methods though they remain reference methods for the determination of biologically active vitamin B_{12}. The most widely used procedures use either *Euglena gracilis, Lactobacillus leishmannii,* or a mutant of *Escherichia coli,* though each of these organisms is susceptible to growth inhibition by antibiotics or other drugs, such as methotrexate, that may be in a patient's serum. Furthermore, these assays require at least 24 hours to establish adequate growth of the microorganism. However, the use of microtiter enzyme-linked immunosorbent assay (ELISA) plate technology has increased the utility of some microbiological assays.[301]

Commercial kits are available for the CPB assays of vitamin B_{12}. The vitamin B_{12} binder used is often nonhuman IF, usually obtained from hog stomach. If the IF is not highly purified, it may contain R proteins, which bind not only vitamin B_{12} but also related metabolically inactive compounds, giving higher values. IF must therefore be either highly purified or have cobinamide (a vitamin B_{12} analogue) added to the IF to saturate all binding sites on the R proteins. Cobinamide is not bound by IF.

In a widely used CPB assay, vitamin B_{12} (cobalamin) competes with ^{57}Co-labeled cobalamin for a limited number of binding sites on IF. Some assays require a preliminary step in which the specimen is boiled in a buffered solution containing dithiothreitol, KCN, and ^{57}Co-labeled tracers to release vitamin B_{12} from endogenous binding proteins. Alternatively, other procedures irreversibly denature endogenous binding proteins by increasing the pH from 12 to 13 and then readjusting the pH to 9.3 before the binding reagent is added. Subsequent separation of bound and free folate and vitamin B_{12} is achieved by contact with dextran-coated charcoal, which absorbs the free (unbound) molecules, leaving protein-bound vitamin B_{12} in the solution.

Most immunometric methods use solid phase separation by immobilizing the IF binder on beads or magnetic particles. The free vitamin B_{12} then remains in the supernatant, and the bound analytes become part of the solid phase suspension. For simultaneous folate/vitamin B_{12} measurement, a gamma-scintillation counter that discriminates between the energy levels of ^{57}Co (for vitamin B_{12}) and ^{125}I (for folate) must be used.

Multiple automated and semiautomated systems are available for measuring vitamin B_{12} and folate, using, for example, chemiluminescence as a signal. The assays are standardized with a 7.5-minute incubation, magnetic particle separation, and acridium ester signal. The precision of automated systems allows specimens to be analyzed in singlet while maintaining CVs less than those found for the mean of duplicates of radioimmunoassays.

Indirect tests assess the functional adequacy of vitamin B_{12}. Serum methylmalonic acid concentration is increased when a lack of adenyl-Cbl causes a block in the conversion of methylmalonyl-CoA to succinyl-CoA. It is a sensitive test of status, being often the first analyte to be raised in subclinical vitamin B_{12} deficiency.[496] It has a further advantage in that it is unaffected by folate deficiency. Early methods for methylmalonic acid lacked sensitivity and specificity, a situation that has been resolved by the adoption of gas chromatographic–mass spectrometric methods,[542] though these require specialized handling. Plasma total homocysteine concentration is a sensitive indicator of vitamin B_{12} status, because methyl-Cbl is required for the remethylation of homocysteine to methionine, but is not specific, being elevated in deficiency of folate and vitamin B_6 and vitamin B_{12}. Plasma concentrations of total homocysteine can be reliably measured by HPLC with fluorescent or electrochemical detection, and enzymatic and capillary gas chromatography–mass spectroscopy methods.[495] Plasma samples for homocysteine analysis must be obtained soon after venipuncture to reduce preanalytical increases that occur on standing, though these can be minimized by the use of a fluoride–ethylenediaminetetraacetic acid (EDTA) tube. The increased screening of plasma total homocysteine concentrations as an independent risk factor for cardiovascular disease (see Chapter 26) may lead to the recognition of further cases of subclinical vitamin B_{12} deficiency.

The measurement of holotranscobalamin II is potentially useful as a specific marker of biologically available vitamin B_{12}, because only cobalamin bound to TcII is specifically available for uptake by all cells. Other methods have been described for the measurement of holotranscobalamin in serum, one using an immobilized monoclonal antibody to human transcobalamin, followed by measurement of released cobalamin by CPB.[584] This method is currently available as a commercial kit. The other method uses magnetic beads coated with cobalamin to precipitate apotranscobalamin followed by measurement of the holotranscobalamin in the supernatant by ELISA.[417] Though these methods are claimed to be precise and simple to perform, there remains doubt over the interpretation of the measured concentrations,[93] and over their sensitivity and specificity in the diagnosis of vitamin B_{12} deficiency.[342]

The deoxyuridine suppression test measures the effect of prior addition of deoxyuridine on the uptake of radiolabeled thymidine into the DNA of cultured bone marrow cells, peripheral blood lymphocytes, or whole blood. Normal samples that contain vitamin B_{12} can convert deoxyuridine to thymidine and therefore do not take up as much thymidine. Samples from patients who are deficient in vitamin B_{12} show less suppression than in normal patients. Because it is relatively time consuming, the deoxyuridine suppression test is not widely available for use as a diagnostic test.[556]

The Schilling test is primarily a test of vitamin B_{12} absorption and not of status, but it permits differentiation of causes of vitamin B_{12} deficiency (pernicious anemia or intestinal malabsorption). The proportion absorbed from orally administered ^{57}Co- or ^{58}Co-labeled vitamin B_{12} is measured by determining the radioactivity in feces, urine, or serum or by externally scanning the liver. The usual procedure is to measure radioactivity in a 24-hour urine sample, which is collected after oral administration of 0.5 μg of radioactive Co-labeled vitamin B_{12} after an overnight fast. In normal individuals, 8% or more of the dose administered is excreted in the urine, whereas in people with pernicious anemia, less than 7% (often 0% to 3%) is excreted. A confirmatory test for lack of IF requires ingestion of vitamin B_{12} and IF.[74]

Reference Intervals

Depending on the laboratory and the procedure used, reference intervals can vary widely. The WHO, in their report in 1968, defined a serum vitamin B_{12} concentration of less than 150 ng/L (110 pmol/L) as deficient, and one of 201 ng/L (147 pmol/L) or higher[619] as acceptable. A dietary and nutritional survey of British adults in 1990 published a reference interval of 206 to 678 ng/L (151 to 497 pmol/L).[209] The changes in serum vitamin B_{12} concentration as a function of age in healthy adults have been the subject of contradictory reports. Data from a study population in the United States (Framingham Study) showed an increased prevalence (40.5% of 222 subjects) of low serum vitamin B_{12} concentration (<258 pmol/L) in elderly subjects than in a control group of younger subjects (17.9% incidence).[335] Vitamin B_{12} concentrations within the reference interval may not necessarily reflect adequate vitamin B_{12} status, because serum concentrations may be maintained at the expense of tissue stores. Conversely, low serum vitamin B_{12} concentrations may not be indicative of vitamin B_{12} deficiency. Most of the vitamin B_{12} in serum is bound to TcI, which is released by granulocytes and has no functional role in transport of vitamin B_{12} to cells. Low serum vitamin B_{12} concentration may be due to a reduction in TcI as a consequence of low total granulocyte mass. This has been observed in benign neutropenia, multiple myeloma, and leukemic reticuloendotheliosis and may be expected in other conditions in which the bone marrow is hypoplastic, aplastic, or replaced by malignant cells.

Serum methylmalonic acid concentrations below 376 nmol/L have been considered acceptable in an elderly U.S. population,[335] as have concentrations below 320 nmol/L in a group of older Dutch subjects.[589]

VITAMIN C—ASCORBIC ACID

Vitamin C (L-ascorbic acid) serves as a reducing agent in several important hydroxylation reactions in the body.

Chemistry

As shown in Figure 30-17, the term vitamin C refers to all molecules that exhibit antiscorbutic properties in humans and includes both ascorbic acid and its oxidized form, dehydroascorbic acid (DHA). The vitamin C redox system comprises these molecules and the free radical intermediate, monodehydroascorbic acid,[288] the product of one-electron oxidation of ascorbic acid. L-ascorbic acid is the enol form of 2-oxo-L-gulofuranolactone, the enolic hydroxyl on ring carbon 3 having a pK_a of 4.2 and conferring its acidic nature. The vitamin is a white, crystalline solid that is readily soluble in water. Acidic solutions (below pH 3) show absorption maximum at 245 nm, whereas solutions of the ionized material (above pH 5) have an absorption peak at 265 nm. Ascorbic acid is a relatively strong reductant with an E_0' (pH 7) of +0.58 volt. The dehydro form is more labile than the reduced form to hydrolytic ring opening to yield 2,3-diketo-L-gulonic acid, which is not antiscorbutic.

L-Ascorbic acid Dehydroascorbic acid

Figure 30-17 L-ascorbic and dehydroascorbic acids. *(Modified from Row PB: Inherited disorders of folate metabolism. In Stanbury JB, Wyngaarden DS (eds): The metabolic bases of inherited disease, 5th edition, New York: McGraw-Hill, 1983.)*

Dietary Sources

Plants and most animals possess the ability to synthesize the vitamin from D-glucose via the lactones of D-glucuronic and L-gulonic acids; however, some mammals, including the human, lack L-gulonolactone oxidase, the enzyme that catalyzes the formation of 2-keto-L-gulonolactone, which spontaneously tautomerizes to L-ascorbic acid. Excellent sources of the vitamin are citrus fruits, berries, melons, tomatoes, green peppers, broccoli, brussels sprouts, and leafy green vegetables.[548] Losses during processing, especially with heat and aerobic conditions, can be considerable.

Absorption, Transport, Metabolism, and Excretion

Gastrointestinal absorption of ascorbic acid occurs by a combination of sodium-dependent active transport at low concentrations and by simple diffusion at high concentrations.[482] Between 70% and 90% of a usual dietary intake of ascorbic acid (up to 180 mg/day) is absorbed, falling to 50% or less at loads greater than 1 g/day.[292] The absorbed ascorbic acid moves rapidly from the intestinal cell into blood by a process of facilitated diffusion.[358] Ascorbate uptake by cells is mediated by specific transporters, ascorbate by the sodium-dependent transporters SVCT 1 and SVCT 2 and DHA via the facilitated-diffusion glucose transporters GLUT 1, 3, and 4.[332] Vitamin C is found in most tissues, but glandular tissues, such as the pituitary, adrenal cortex, corpus luteum, and thymus, have the highest amounts and the retina has 20 to 30 times the plasma concentration. DHA, once transported intracellularly, is reduced to ascorbate, and in plasma vitamin C exists predominantly as the ascorbate ion. Many cells, particularly the hepatic cells, neutrophils, mononuclear phagocytes, osteoblasts, and erythrocytes, are capable of DHA uptake and recycling to ascorbate, which maintains a human body pool of up to 2 g.[292] The biological half-life of vitamin C in an individual ranges from 8 to 40 days, with an average of about 16 days. Vitamin C is conserved during periods of low intake, absorption becoming maximum with minimum urinary excretion. Excretion of unchanged ascorbate occurs increasingly with increased dosage, with almost all of an injected dose more than 500 mg being excreted over 24 hours.[331] DHA that is not recycled may be irreversibly delactonized to 2,3-diketogulonic acid and further degraded to oxalic acid for urine excretion. Other catabolic products of 2,3-diketogulonic acid are L-lyxonic acid, L-xylose, and L-threonic acid.

Functions

Ascorbic acid acts as a cofactor for a number of mixed function oxidases in processes in which it promotes enzyme activity by maintaining metal ions in their reduced form (particularly iron and copper). Its most clearly established and critical functional role is as a cofactor for protocollagen hydroxylase, the enzyme responsible for hydroxylation of prolyl and lysyl residues within nascent peptides in connective tissue proteins.[288] Among these are collagen and related proteins, which comprise intercellular material of cartilage, dentin, and bone. Ascorbate is also involved in (1) carnitine biosynthesis serving as a cofactor to 6-*N*-trimethyl-L-lysine hydrolase; (2) γ-butyrobetaine hydrolase, which converts γ-butyrobetaine to carnitine; (3) the degradation of tyrosine via 4-OH phenylpyruvate dioxygenase; (4) the synthesis of adrenal hormones via dopamine β-hydroxylase; (5) the biosynthesis of corticosteroids and aldosterone; (6) the hydroxylation of cholesterol in the formation of bile acids; and (7) folate metabolism and leukocyte functions. Nonheme iron absorption, as Fe^{2+}, is also enhanced by simultaneous ingestion of the vitamin.[261]

Ascorbic acid is one of the most effective water-soluble antioxidants in biological fluids[182] and can scavenge physiologically important reactive oxygen species and reactive nitrogen species. Both ascorbate and the ascorbyl radical have low reduction potentials[82] and react with most other biologically relevant radicals. The ascorbyl radical is relatively stable because of resonance stabilization of the unpaired electron. Ascorbate can regenerate other small molecule antioxidants, including α-tocopherol, reduced glutathione, urate, and β-carotene from their respective radical species, and may therefore prevent oxidative damage to biological macromolecules, including DNA, lipids, and proteins. There has been concern that in certain situations of vitamin supplementation ascorbic acid acts as a prooxidant.[444] However, this has been disputed by other workers.[95] It has also been recognized that dehydroascorbate has important intracellular properties that are different from, but sometimes complementary to, those of ascorbate.[130,623]

Requirements and Reference Nutrient Intakes

The amount of vitamin C sufficient to alleviate and cure the clinical signs of scurvy is only 10 mg/day, which is probably near the minimum requirement in man. This amount, however, is not adequate to maintain near saturation of tissue in the adult human male, who has a body pool of 1.5 to 2 g and shows clinical symptoms of deficiency when this total pool falls below about 300 mg.[25,252] Acknowledgment of functions of vitamin C beyond the antiscorbutic, particularly the antioxidant function, has led to the development of the concept of the optimal nutrition state, and the intake required to achieve this. Current recommendations of the U.S. Institute of Medicine about estimated average requirements and RDAs has reflected this approach.[425] The RDA for adult males, older than 19 years and beyond 70 years, has been set at 90 mg/day, and the corresponding RDA for women at 75 mg/day. To provide for fetal needs, an additional 10 mg/day is recommended for the pregnant woman to offset the decrease in plasma vitamin C level during pregnancy. A lactating woman should receive an additional 45 to 50 mg/day, because an average of 18 to 22 mg may be secreted in 600 to 700 mL of milk. Children 1 to 3 years have an RDA of 15 mg/day; those 4 to 8 years, an RDA of 25 mg/day; boys aged 9 to 13, an RDA of 45 mg/day; and those 14 to 18 years, an RDA of 75 mg/day. Corresponding values for girls are 45 and 65 mg/day, respectively. No RDA is given for infants up to 1 year old; instead AI levels of 40 mg/day up to 6 months and 50 mg from 7 to 12 months are recommended. Some special groups, such as smokers, should take an additional 35 mg/day.[353]

Intravenous Supply

The recommended IV intake for adult patients receiving TPN was 100 mg for many years,[9] but this has now been increased to 200 mg/day.[243] This reflects the expected increased requirements for wound healing and for antioxidant activity.

Deficiency

Protracted deficiency of vitamin C leads to the classic disease of scurvy, which still occurs in developed countries. Those most at risk of the disease include (1) elderly men, particularly those who live alone; (2) those with alcohol dependence and smokers; (3) those taking unbalanced diets; (4) some mentally ill patients; (5) renal failure patients undergoing peritoneal dialysis or hemodialysis; and (6) some patients with cancer.[149] The lack of vitamin C causes an inability to form adequate intercellular substance in connective tissue and is reflected in swollen, tender, and often bleeding or bruised loci at joints and in other areas where structurally weakened tissue cannot withstand stress. Infantile scurvy, also known as Barlow's disease, exhibits a bayonet-rib syndrome. The gums are livid and swollen, cutaneous bleeding often begins on the lower thighs as perifollicular hemorrhages, and large spontaneous bruises (ecchymoses) may arise almost anywhere on the body. Ocular hemorrhages, drying of salivary and lacrimal glands, parotid swelling, femoral neuropathy, edema of the lower extremities, and psychological disturbances have also been described. Some scorbutic patients may develop anemia, display radiological changes characteristic of osteoporosis, or die suddenly from heart failure. Diseases of vitamin C deficiency that might reflect its role as an antioxidant include an increased risk of coronary heart disease, as demonstrated in a cohort of Finnish men,[425] and an increased risk of death by stroke in a cohort of elderly British people.[193]

Toxicity

Vitamin C is generally well tolerated by healthy subjects, and ingestion of supplements of 2 to 4 g/day—as taken by some for the prevention or amelioration of the common cold—is usually without hazard, though gastrointestinal irritation has been experienced.[253] Other potential but rare adverse effects include increased oxalate excretion and kidney stone formation, increased uric acid excretion, excess iron absorption, lowered vitamin B_{12} levels, systemic conditioning and "rebound" scurvy, and prooxidant effects in the presence of free Fe^{3+} or Cu^{2+} ions.[172] Ingestion of amounts of vitamin C above 200 mg/day shows little increase in plasma steady-state concentrations and suggests that overload of vitamin C is unlikely. Consideration of such data has led the Food and Nutrition Board of the U.S. Institute of Medicine to propose a tolerable upper intake level for vitamin C to be 2 g/day for adults older than 19 years.[135]

Laboratory Assessment of Status

There are at present no useful functional tests of vitamin C adequacy, thus laboratory assessment of status is made by direct measurement of plasma, urine, or tissue concentrations of ascorbic acid, total vitamin C, or (rarely) metabolite. Because ascorbic acid is readily oxidized by dissolved oxygen at a neutral pH, plasma samples should be treated with a metal-chelating and protein-precipitating acid, such as metaphosphoric acid, soon after a phlebotomy. Samples so treated may be stored at −80 °C for several years.[32] Plasma ascorbate concentration is considered to be a reliable indicator of ascorbate intake[276] and has been measured photometrically by oxidation with 2,4-dinitrophenylhydrazine to form the red *bis*-hydrazone or with 2,4-dichlorophenol-indophenol, which is reduced to a colorless form.[548] A more specific approach is to use the enzyme ascorbate oxidase to convert ascorbate to dehydroascorbate, which is then coupled with o-phenylene diamine to form a product that is measured fluorometrically[606] or at 340 nm on an automated analyzer.[325] HPLC methods have the potential advantage of specificity, but are generally more time consuming. Detection may be by precolumn derivatization to the fluorescent quinoxaline, or by electrochemical or coulometric means. Care must be taken during the analysis to prevent oxidation of the ascorbate before detection, because a sulfhydryl donor, such as dithiothreitol or homocysteine, should be added to the sample and mobile phase.[32] With suitable sample preparation, both ascorbic acid and total vitamin C, and by difference, DHA may be measured together by HPLC[360] or gas chromatography–mass spectrometry.[131] Leukocyte ascorbic acid is considered to be a better indicator of body stores than plasma ascorbate, but has not been widely adopted because of the large sample volume requirement, the difficulty of automating the analysis, the influence of fluctuating leukocyte numbers, and the relative difficulty of the analysis. Urinary excretion and RBC concentrations have not been found to be specific and useful indices of vitamin C status; however, urinary levels of ascorbic acid, especially following a load test, can be helpful in the clinical diagnosis of scurvy.

Reference Intervals

With adequate intake of vitamin C, plasma concentrations of total vitamin (ascorbic acid plus dehydroascorbic acid) are between 0.4 and 1.5 mg/dL (23 to 85 μmol/L). The lower limit value may be seen in some cases with subclinical vitamin C deficiency and in older individuals. A value lower than 0.2 mg/dL (11 μmol/L) is considered deficient. The guidance reference interval for vitamin C levels in leukocytes is 20 to 53 μg/10^8 leukocytes (1.14 to 3.01 fmol/leukocyte). A value in leukocytes of less than 10 μg/10^8 leukocytes (0.57 fmol/leukocyte) is considered deficient.[548]

BIOTIN

Biotin (also known as vitamin H) is the prosthetic group for a number of carboxylation reactions (e.g., pyruvate, acetyl-CoA, propionyl Co-A, and decarboxylases).

Chemistry

Biotin is *cis*-tetrahydro-2-oxothieno[3,4-*d*]-imidazoline-4-valeric acid (Figure 30-18). The vitamin in most organisms occurs mainly bound to protein. The ε-amino group of the lysyl side chain of protein is linked via an amide function, involving the carboxyl group of the valeryl side chain of biotin. In addition, some biotin is linked noncovalently as a complex with avidin, a protein in egg white.

Dietary Sources

Good sources of biotin include liver, kidney, pancreas, eggs, yeast, and milk. Cereal grains, fruits, most vegetables, and meat are poor sources.[114] The ureido ring and the ionizable carboxyl group of biotin allow modest solubility of the white crystalline solid in aqueous solution, especially at an alkaline pH. Oxidizing agents convert the thioether to sulfoxides and sulfones, which do not have biotin activity.

Absorption, Transport, Metabolism, and Excretion

Biotin in the diet is largely protein bound, and digestion of these proteins by gastrointestinal enzymes produces biotinyl peptides, which may be further hydrolyzed by intestinal biotinidase to release biotin. Avidin, a protein found in raw egg whites, binds biotin tightly and prevents its absorption. The peptide biocytin (ε-N-biotinyl lysine) is resistant to hydrolysis by proteolytic enzymes in the intestinal tract but together with biotin is readily absorbed.[637] A biotin carrier, the sodium-dependent multivitamin transporter (SMVT)

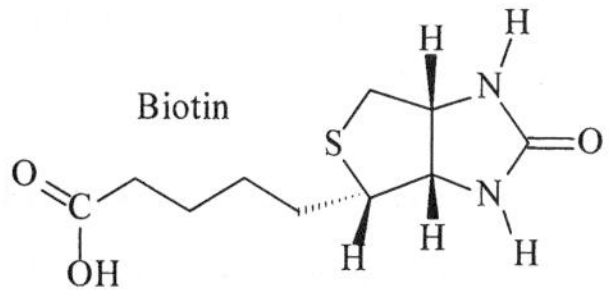

Figure 30-18 Biotin.

for which pantothenic acid and lipoate compete,[449] is located in the intestinal brush border membrane and transports biotin against a sodium ion concentration gradient. The enzyme biocytinase (biotin amidohydrolase) in plasma and erythrocytes catalyzes the hydrolysis of biocytin to yield free biotin. Biotin is cleared from the circulating blood more rapidly in deficient than in normal mammals; it is taken up by such tissues as liver, muscle, and kidney and is localized in cytosolic and mitochondrial carboxylases. Covalent attachment of biotin to apoenzymes involves ATP-dependent conversion of the vitamin to biotinyl-5′-adenylate followed by condensation of the biotinyl moiety with ε-amino groups of specific lysyl residues in apoenzymes preformed from subunits. The enzymes responsible for catalyzing the formation of the ε-N-biotinyl-L-lysyl (biocytinyl) moiety of proteins are holoenzyme synthetases.

About half of the absorbed biotin is excreted as the metabolites bisnorbiotin, occurring from β-oxidation of the valeric acid side chain, and biotin sulfoxide, occurring from the oxidation of the sulfur in the heterocyclic ring.[635] The circulating plasma and urinary excretion patterns show a ratio of 3:2:1 for biotin, bisnorbiotin, and biotin sulfoxide. Minor metabolites are bisnorbiotin methyl ketone and biotin sulfone. Careful balance studies in humans, where perhaps only 1 mg is the total body content, showed that urinary excretion of biotin often exceeded dietary intake, and that in all cases, fecal excretion was as much as three to six times greater than dietary intake because of microfloral biosynthesis.

Functions

The principal biochemical function of biotin in man is as a cofactor for carboxylation reactions. Five carboxylases are currently found in human tissue[487]; one of these, an acetyl-CoA carboxylase, is inactive and may act as a storage vehicle for biotin.[532] The others are carboxylases for acetyl-CoA, propionyl-CoA, β-methylcrotonyl-CoA, and pyruvate. These enzymes operate via a common mechanism, which involves phosphorylation of bicarbonate by ATP to form carbonyl phosphate, followed by transfer of the carboxyl group to the sterically less hindered nitrogen of the biotin moiety. The resulting N(1)-carboxybiotinyl enzyme can then exchange the carboxylate function with a reactive center in a substrate. With cytosolic acetyl-CoA carboxylase, the product is malonyl-CoA, used for fatty acid biosynthesis. In mitochondria, pyruvate carboxylase catalyzes formation of oxaloacetate, which together with acetyl-CoA forms citrate. The other carboxylases are involved in the metabolism of odd-numbered fatty acids and branched-chain fatty acids.[635] Research showing altered gene expression during biotin deficiency and new enzymatic activities of the enzyme biotinidase is confirming earlier suggestions of a role for biotin in the regulation of gene expression.[374]

Requirements and Reference Nutrient Intakes

At present there are insufficient scientific data to make recommendations of RDAs for biotin. Intestinal microflora make a significant contribution to the body pool of available biotin, making determination of the dietary requirement difficult. Mean urinary excretion, reflective of dietary intake, ranges from 6 to 50 μg/day for adults who ingest 28 to 100 μg/day. Consideration of urinary excretion of both biotin and the metabolite 3-hydroxyisovalerate[397] has led to recommendations on AI, rather than requirements.[170] The suggested AI for adults 19 years and older is 30 μg/day; for adolescents 14 to 18 years, 25 μg/day; for children 9 to 13 years, 20 μg/day; for children 4 to 8 years, 12 μg/day; for children 1 to 3 years, 8 μg/day; and for infants less than 1 year, 0.7 μg/kg of body weight. An additional 5 μg/day is recommended for the lactating mother. Those receiving hemodialysis or peritoneal dialysis, or with a biotinidase deficiency, would require more.

Intravenous Supply

The recommended supply of biotin to adults during TPN is 60 μg/day.[9]

Deficiency

Biotin deficiency is uncommon but may be seen (1) with prolonged consumption of raw egg whites, (2) in TPN without biotin supplementation, and (3) in patients with a genetic deficiency of biotinidase. The first two situations may be complicated by effects on gut flora that produce biotin.[487] Symptoms include anorexia, nausea, vomiting, glossitis, pallor, depression, and a dry scaly dermatitis.[91] Based on urinary excretion patterns of 3-hydroxyisovaleric acid, (Figure 30-19) concern has been expressed about marginal biotin deficiency in pregnancy, because this has been shown to be teratogenic in several mammalian species.[396] Significantly lowered urinary excretion or circulating blood levels have also been found in alcoholics, patients with achlorhydria, and among the elderly and some athletes.[61] Finally, there are rather rare genetic enzyme defects, such as in holoenzyme synthetase (reflected in inadequate conversion of apocarboxylases to holocarboxylases) and propionyl-CoA carboxylase (reflected in a distinguishing acidemia).[635]

Toxicity

No adverse effects of biotin in doses of up to 300 times a normal dietary intake have been reported, as in patients with biotinidase deficiency.[624] Tolerable upper intake levels for biotin have not been set, because there are insufficient data.[170]

Laboratory Assessment of Status

Traditionally, biotin has been measured in biological samples by microbiological assay, where whole blood is first digested with papain or acid hydrolysis to release free biotin, samples of which are then added to a biotin-deficient medium inoculated with a test organism, such as *Lactobacillus plantarum*.[502] Other methods for unbound biotin include avidin-binding assays, where a competitive protein-binding radioassay is set up with ^{3}H-labeled biotin, or a nonradioactive enzyme-linked sorbent assay using streptavidin as the

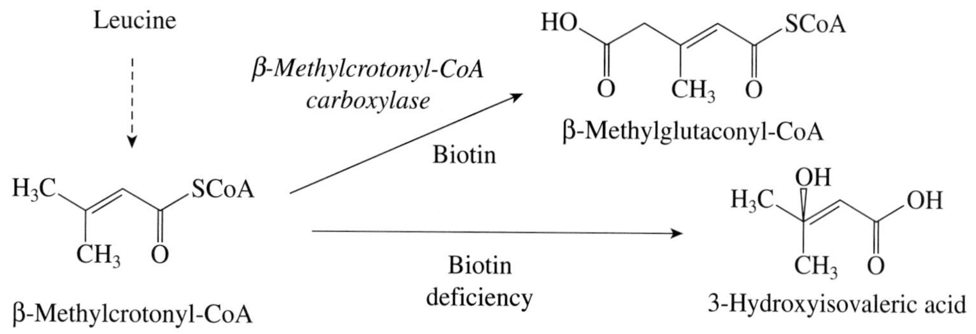

Leucine

β-Methylcrotonyl-CoA carboxylase

Biotin

β-Methylglutaconyl-CoA

β-Methylcrotonyl-CoA

Biotin deficiency

3-Hydroxyisovaleric acid

Figure 30-19 Formation of 3-hydroxyisovaleric acid under conditions of biotin deficiency.

binding agent.[502,614] Generally, biotin content of red cells is similar to that of plasma for a given method, but there is often poor agreement between methods, which may relate to the specificity of the methods employed.[495] Urinary excretion of biotin and 3-hydroxyisovaleric acid appears to be a better indicator of biotin status than blood concentrations. This was shown in a study of experimental biotin deficiency, when both urinary biotin and metabolites, measured by HPLC separation followed by an avidin-binding assay, and urinary 3-hydroxyisovaleric acid, measured by gas chromatography–mass spectrometry, showed significant changes whereas serum biotin concentration did not.[397] Functional markers of biotin status are being increasingly investigated. Lymphocyte propionyl-CoA carboxylase, measured by an optimized assay that is based on the incorporation of labeled $H^{14}CO_3^-$, has been shown to be an early and sensitive indicator of biotin deficiency in a rat model,[395] in patients on prolonged TPN without biotin,[598] and in children with protein-energy malnutrition.[597]

Reference Intervals

Typical reference interval values for whole blood biotin by a microbiological method are 0.5 to 2.20 nmol/L, mean 1.31 nmol/L. Deficiency is considered likely below 0.5 nmol/L.[502] Reference values for other metabolites and fluids have been published elsewhere.[495]

FOLIC ACID

Folic acid serves as a carrier of one-carbon groups in many metabolic reactions. It is required for the biosynthesis of compounds such as choline, serine, glycine, purines, and deoxythymidine monophosphate (dTMP).

Chemistry

Folate and *folic acid* are generic terms for a family of compounds that function as coenzymes in the processing of one-carbon units and that are derived from pteroic acid (*Pte*), to which one or more molecules of glutamic acid are attached. Pteroic acid is composed of a pteridine ring joined to a *p*-aminobenzoic acid residue (Figure 30-20). In basic solution, this substance has absorption maxima at 256, 282, and 365 nm and is fluorescent. When pteroic acid is conjugated with one molecule of L-glutamic acid, pteroylglutamic acid (PteGlu) is formed, and this can be reduced to dihydrofolic acid (H_2PteGlu or DHF/FH_2,) with hydrogens in positions 7 and 8, or to tetrahydrofolate (H_4PteGlu or THF/FH_4) with hydrogens in positions 5, 6, 7, and 8. Only the reduced forms are biologically active. Other folate derivatives have multiple glutamic acid residues ($H_4PteGlu_n$), when *n*, the number of glutamate residues, may be 1 to 7. Biochemically, these polyglutamates are similar to monoglutamates, but the former function as the natural coenzymes. Multiple forms of folic acid occur with substitutions of functional groups, such as methyl, formyl, methylene, hydroxymethyl, and others at nitrogen atoms in the pteroic acid residue, usually N^5 or bridging N^5 and N^{10}. Although various forms of folic acid are normally present in human serum and other body fluids, the principal form is 5-methyltetrahydrofolate. This is slowly oxidized in alkaline solution, but this is reversed by adding ascorbic acid. It is relatively stable in acid solutions but unstable when exposed to light.

Dietary Sources

The principal food sources of folate are liver, spinach, and other dark green leafy vegetables, legumes, such as kidney and lima beans, and orange juice, although in countries where cereal fortification with folate is established, this is often the major source of dietary folate.[21,549] Since the U.S. FDA program of fortification of all enriched grain products with folic acid (140 μg per 100 g) began in 1996, study populations have shown a doubling of mean plasma folate concentrations and significant falls in total homocysteine concentration, though data are not available as yet to show if the incidence of neural tube defects (NTDs), the primary purpose of the fortification, has been reduced.[279]

Absorption, Transport, Metabolism, and Excretion

Folate is absorbed from dietary sources, such as those listed above, mainly as reduced methyl- and formyl-tetrahydropteroylpolyglutamates. The bioavailability of folate from food sources is variable and dependent upon factors such as incomplete release from plant cellular structure, entrapment in food matrix during digestion, inhibition of deglutamation by other dietary constituents, and possibly the degree of polyglutamation.[211,491] The bioavailability of supplemental folic acid is greater than that of food folate, and may be as high as 100% for folic acid supplements taken on an empty stomach compared with about 50% for food folates.[170] Polyglutamate forms of folate present in food are first converted to monoglutamates, by pteroylpolyglutamate hydrolase, in the intestinal mucosa. Absorption of the monoglutamyl folates at low concentration occurs by a saturable transport process with an acidic pH optimum (pH around 5), with an additional apparently nonsaturable absorption mechanism when intestinal folate concentrations exceed 5 to 10 µmol/L.[363] After cellular uptake, most of the folate is reduced and methylated and enters the circulation as 5-methyltetrahydrofolate (5-MTHF), circulating loosely bound to albumin or to a lesser degree to a high-affinity folate-binding protein. Uptake by certain cells (kidney, placenta, and choroid plexus) occurs by membrane-associated folate-binding proteins that act as folate receptors, and the reduced folate carrier, a member of the SLC19 family, facilitates uptake by most tissue.[365] Once within the cell, 5-MTHF is demethylated and converted to the polyglutamyl form by folylpolyglutamate synthase, which helps to retain folate within the cell, because it is unable to cross cell membranes. For release into the circulation, the polyglutamates are reconverted to monoglutamates by polyglutamate hydrolase.

Folic acid and vitamin B_{12} metabolism are linked by the reaction that transfers a methyl group from 5-MTHF to cobalamin. In cases of cobalamin deficiency, folate is "trapped" as 5-MTHF and is "metabolically dead." It cannot be recycled as tetrahydrofolate (THF) back into the folate pool to serve as the main one-carbon unit acceptor for many biochemical reactions. Eventually, cellular depletion of MTHF ensues, causing a reduction in thymidylic acid synthesis, which in turn results in megaloblastic anemia and neuropathies. This concept is supported by the fact that THF corrects the megaloblastic anemia in patients with congenital methylmalonic aciduria and homocystinuria, whereas it is not corrected with methyltetrahydrofolate. However, some investigators have suggested that vitamin B_{12} is required for the conversion of folic acid to the formyl form and that formyltetrahydrofolates are the natural substrates for forming folate polyglutamates.

Protein-free plasma folate is filtered at the glomerulus and most is reabsorbed by the proximal renal tubules. Consequently, intact urinary folate is only a small percentage of intake. Folate is predominantly excreted by catabolism following cleavage of the C9-N10 bond to produce *p*-aminobenzoylpolyglutamates, which are then hydrolyzed to monoglutamates and *N*-acetylated before excretion. Biliary excretion of folate has been estimated at about 100 µg/day, but much of this is reabsorbed in an enterohepatic circulation. Fecal losses have been studied by radiolabeling and have been found to be similar in type and quantity to urinary losses.[315]

Functions

Folate coenzymes, together with coenzymes derived from vitamins B_{12}, B_6, and B_2, are essential for one-carbon metabolism. Biochemically, a carbon unit from serine or glycine is

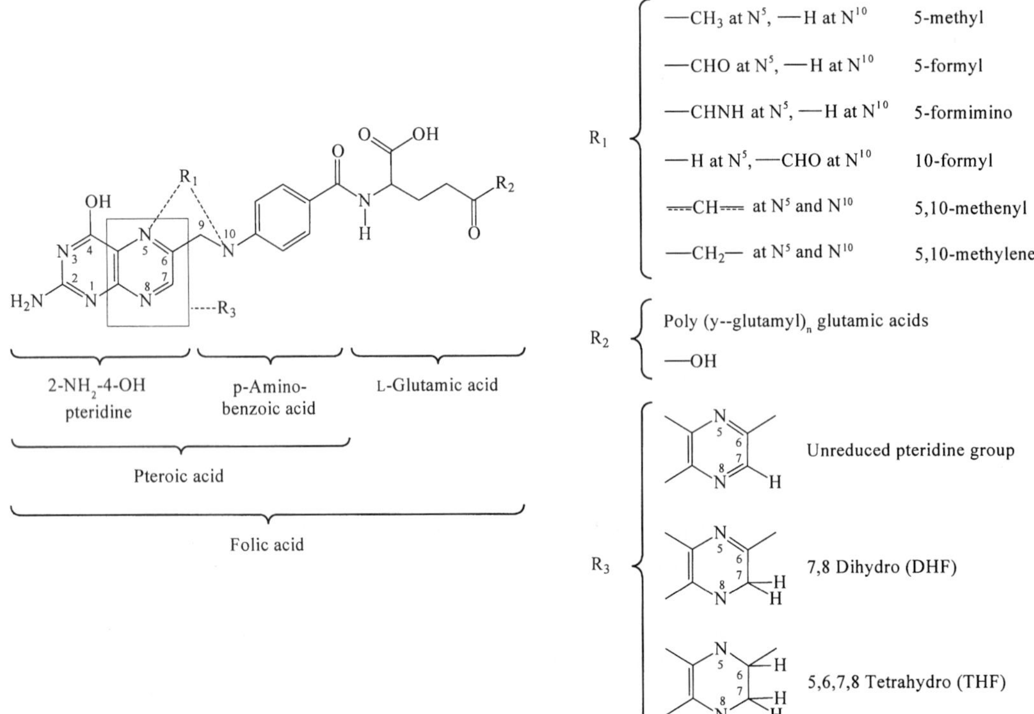

Figure 30-20 Structure and relationships of folic acid and its derivatives.

transferred to THF to form methylene-THF, which is then (1) used in the synthesis of thymidine (and incorporation into DNA), (2) oxidized to formyl-THF for use in the synthesis of purines (precursors of RNA and DNA), or (3) reduced to methyl-THF, which is necessary for the methylation of homocysteine to methionine. Much of this methionine is converted to S-adenosylmethionine, a universal donor of methyl groups to DNA, RNA, hormones, neurotransmitters, membrane lipids, and proteins.[512] Some of these reactions are illustrated in Figure 30-21. Different folates are involved in these reactions, depending on the chemical state of the single carbon fragments transferred:

Reaction	Group Transferred	Folic Acid Derivative
Serum/glycine metabolism	Methylene ($-CH_2-$)	N^5, N^{10}-Methylene THF/FH_4
Histidine catabolism	Formimino ($-CHNH$)	N^5-Formimino THF/FH_4
Thymidylate synthesis	Methylene ($-CH_2-$)	N^5, N^{10}-Methylene THF/FH_4
Methionine synthesis	Methyl ($-CH_3$)	N^5-Methyl THF/FH_4
Purine synthesis	Methenyl ($=CH-$)	N^5, N^{10}-Methenyl THF/FH_4
	Formyl ($-CHO$)	N^{10}-Formyl THF/FH_4

1. Serine-Glycine Metabolism

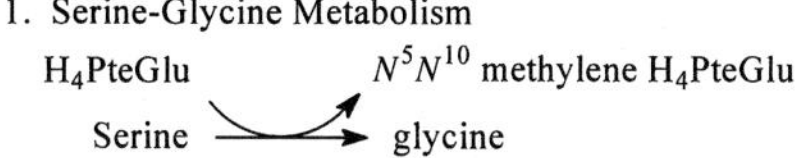

2. Histidine Catabolism

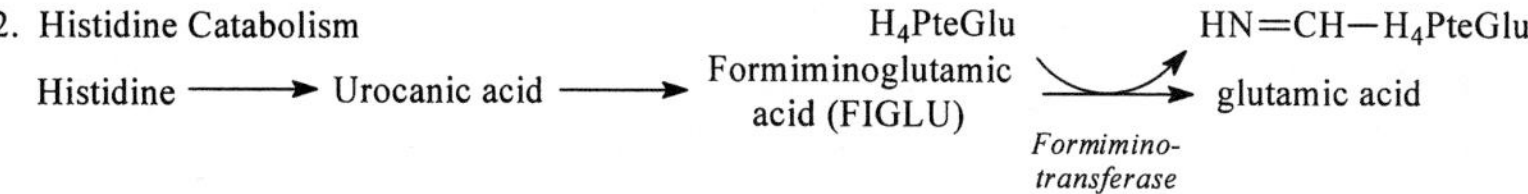

3. Thymidylate Synthesis

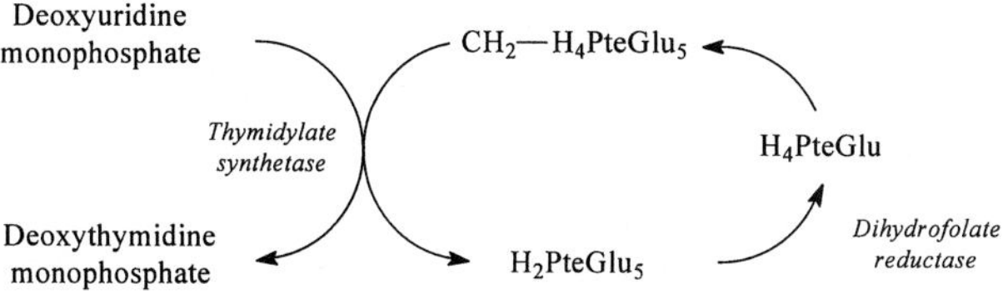

Figure 30-21 The 5 major metabolic functions of folate in human cells.

4. Methionine Synthesis

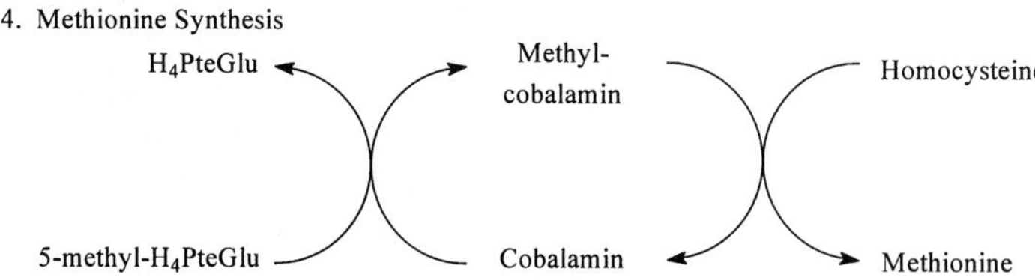

5. Purine Synthesis

a. Introduction of carbon 8 of purine nucleus

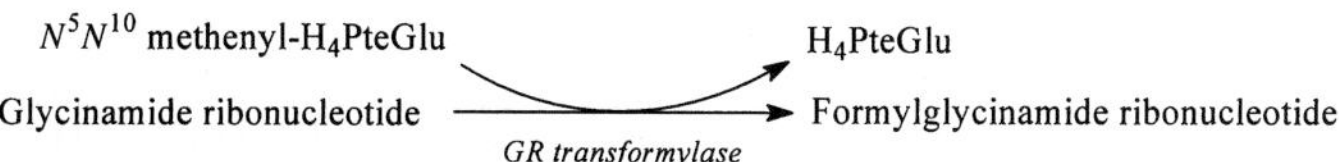

b. Closure of purine nucleus by addition of carbon 2

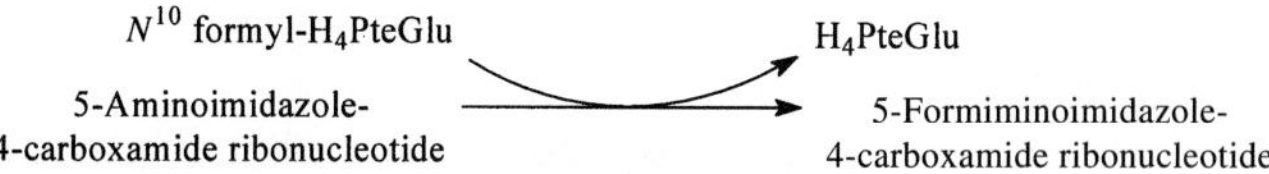

The interconversion of these forms of folic acid takes place through various electron transfer reactions facilitated by specific enzyme systems and coenzymes, such as the reduced forms of flavin-adenine dinucleotide ($FADH_2$) and NADPH. The conversion between the N^5-, N^{10}-methylene form and N^{10}-formyl forms is readily reversible, but the reduction of methylene to methyl and reduction of free THF to formyltetrahydrofolate is essentially irreversible. Conversion of N^5-methyltetrahydrofolate back to free THF may require cobalamin.

The role of folic acid in the metabolism of homocysteine has received increased interest recently.[631] Elevations of plasma homocysteine concentrations have been shown to be independent risk factors for coronary artery disease[460,583] and probably cerebrovascular disease (see Chapter 26).[399] The involvement of folate in its coenzyme forms with homocysteine and methionine metabolism is summarized in Figure 30-22. Folate is the principal micronutrient determinant of homocysteine status,[323] and supplementation with folate has been used as a treatment modality to reduce circulating homocysteine concentrations. Primary (fasting) homocystinemia can be treated with 0.5 to 5.0 mg/day of folic acid,[592] with an expectation of an approximate 25% fall in baseline concentration.[205]

Requirements and Reference Nutrient Intakes

Based on folate concentrations in liver biopsy samples, and assuming that the liver contains about half of all body stores, total body stores of folate are estimated to be between 12 and 28 mg.[618] Kinetic studies that show both fast-turnover and very-slow-turnover folate pools indicate that about 0.5% to 1% of body stores are catabolized or excreted daily,[212] suggesting a minimum daily requirement of between 60 and 280 μg to replace losses. In calculating nutritional requirement, the concept of dietary folate equivalents (DFE) has been used to adjust for the nearly 50% lower bioavailability of food folate compared with supplemental folic acid, such that 1 μg DFE = 0.6 μg of folic acid from fortified food = 1 μg of food folate = 0.5 μg folic acid supplement taken on an empty stomach.[170] Before the fortification program of cereal grains with folic acid conducted between 1988 and 1994, the median intake of folate from food in the United States was approximately 250 μg/day; this figure is expected to increase by about 100 μg/day after fortification. Recommendations

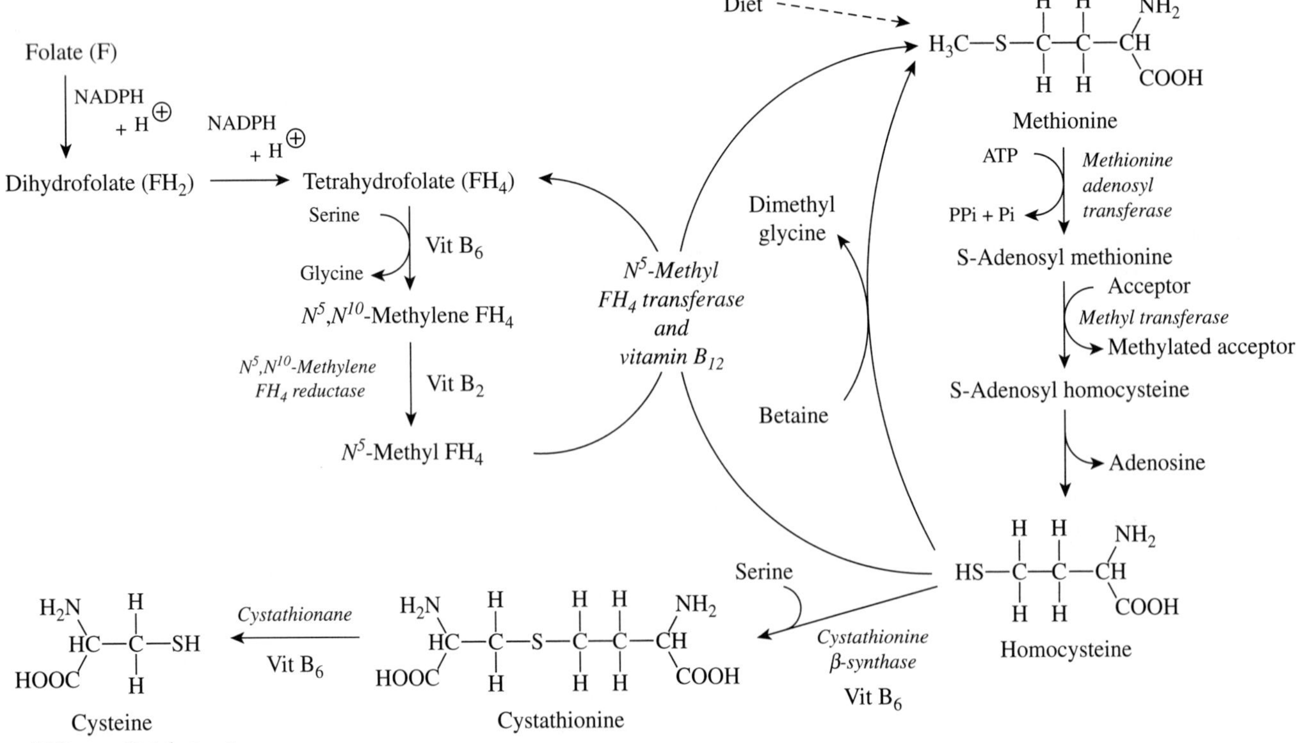

Figure 30-22 Metabolism of homocysteine and methionine.

on dietary reference intakes by the U.S. Institute of Medicine made in 1998 have shifted the emphasis away from prevention of deficiency and toward the concept of optimal health.[170] There is also an increased awareness of the contribution of micronutrient intake to genomic stability.[155] Current RDAs of the U.S. Institute of Medicine are 400 µg/day DFE for adults 19 years and older, and also for adolescents between 14 and 18 years; 300 µg/day DFE for children 9 to 13 years; 200 µg/day DFE for children 4 to 8 years; and 150 µg/day DFE for children 1 to 3 years. An adequate intake for infants of 0 to 6 months is set at 65 µg/day DFE and at 80 µg/day DFE for infants 7 to 11 months. Based on maintenance of erythrocyte folate concentrations during pregnancy, the RDA for pregnant women of all ages is set at 600 µg/day DFE, and at 500 µg/day DFE for lactating women of all ages.[22,170]

Intravenous Supply

The previous adult recommendation for intravenous supply of folic acid of 400 µg/day has been increased to 600 µg/day, as part of the requirements set by the FDA.[243]

Deficiency

Deficiency of folate may result from (1) the absence of intestinal microorganisms (gut sterilization), (2) poor intestinal absorption (e.g., after surgical resection or in celiac disease or sprue), (3) insufficient dietary intake (including chronic alcoholism), (4) excessive demands (as in pregnancy, liver disease, and malignancies), (5) administration of antifolate drugs (e.g., methotrexate), and (6) anticonvulsant therapy (that can increase folate requirements, especially during pregnancy).[334] Inadequate folate intake leads first to decreased serum folate concentration, then a decrease in erythrocyte folate concentration, an increase in plasma homocysteine, and then megaloblastic changes in the bone marrow and other tissue.[170] Megaloblastic anemia (characterized by large, abnormally nucleated erythrocytes in the bone marrow) is the major clinical manifestation of folate deficiency, although sensory loss and neuropsychiatric changes may also occur. Deficiency of folate and iron may coexist in malnourished people, in which case the macrocytosis of RBCs, otherwise typical of folic acid deficiency, is not observed.

Pregnancy brings increased demand upon folate stores because of increased DNA synthesis and one-carbon transfer reactions and low serum folate concentrations in pregnancy are associated with adverse outcomes, including preterm delivery, infant low birth weight, and fetal growth retardation.[501] Additionally, many observational studies have confirmed a reduction in risk of NTDs with periconceptual folic acid supplementation.[65] In a large controlled intervention trial conducted in two regions of China and involving approximately 250,000 women, a daily supplement of 400 µg of folic acid taken at least 80% of the time was associated with an 85% risk reduction of NTDs in an area of high baseline frequency and a 40% reduction in an area of low baseline frequency.[49] Current suggestions are that women planning pregnancy should take at least 400 µg/day, although an intake of 5 mg of folic acid daily is recommended, especially for those with a previous history of NTD.[608] Although the etiology of NTDs is probably multifactorial, involving more than one aspect of folate use,[29] one factor that contributes to this and other folate-requiring conditions is genetic polymorphism.

The most extensively studied polymorphic alleles are those of 5,10-methylenetetrahydofolate reductase (MTHFR), the enzyme responsible for the irreversible reduction of 5,10-MTHF to 5-methyltetrahydrofolate (5-MTHF), the methyl donor of homocysteine to methionine. A single point C to T mutation at base pair 677 (C677T), causing a substitution of valine for alanine, leads to a thermolabile protein with reduced enzymatic activity. The homozygous T/T enzyme has an incidence of around 12% in Asian and Caucasian populations, and a loss of enzyme activity of about 50%, and the heterozygous C/T variant can have an incidence of up to 50% in some populations, with a lesser degree of enzyme inactivity.[69,294]

This variant, and a second with an A to C substitution at base pair 1298 (A1298C), with its effects on folate metabolism and intracellular folate availability, may increase the risk of chromosomal aberrations, and its link with leukemia has been reviewed.[472] A further enzyme involved in folate metabolism, methionine synthase, has also been shown to have at least two relatively prevalent polymorphisms, though these are thought to be benign.[105] The absorption of folate from polyglutamyl folate food sources is thought to be reduced by a variant of glutamate carboxypeptidase II because of a H475Y substitution.[132]

Lower than normal serum folate concentrations have been reported in patients with psychiatric disorders. In two studies, about one third of psychiatric patients had low RBC folate levels, with most of the low values being in depressed patients. Another study reported an inverse correlation between serum folate levels and the duration of depressive illness. Limited evidence suggests that folate may have a role as a supplement to other treatments for depression.[566]

Toxicity

No adverse effects have been reported from the consumption of folate-fortified foods, thus any signs of toxicity are associated with supplemental folate. Most of the limited evidence suggests that excessive folate supplementation, typically in doses up to 10 mg/day, though some have gone to 500 mg/day, can precipitate or exacerbate neuropathy in vitamin B_{12}–deficient subjects, and it is this endpoint that has been used to set a tolerable upper intake level of 1 mg/day from fortified food or supplements for adults.[170] One recognized complication of folate supplementation is to "mask" vitamin B_{12} deficiency, because the associated anemia responds to folate alone. This may delay treatment of the deficiency, allowing neurological abnormalities to progress.

Laboratory Assessment of Status

Folate status may be reliably assessed by direct measurement of serum and erythrocyte or whole blood concentrations, and its metabolic function as coenzyme assessed by metabolite concentrations, such as plasma homocysteine (see Chapters 20 and 26). Serum folate concentrations are considered indicative of recent intake and not of tissue stores, but serial measurements have been used to confirm adequate intake. Whole blood or erythrocyte folate concentrations are more indicative of tissue stores and have been shown to have a moderate correlation with liver folate concentrations taken through a biopsy.[170] Because folate is taken up only by the developing erythrocyte in the bone marrow and not by the mature cell, erythrocyte concentrations reflect folate status over the 120-day lifespan of the cell. Urine folate excretion is not considered to be a sensitive indicator of folate status.[495]

CPB assays have now largely replaced microbiological procedures for the measurement of serum, whole blood, or erythrocyte folate, though the use of microtiter 96-well plates has enabled microbiological assay using *Lactobacillus casei* to be partly automated.[427] The binder used in the CPB folate assay is a protein that occurs naturally in milk, called β-lactoglobulin or milk folate binder, commonly used together with a radioactive ^{125}I-folate label, though nonisotopic fluorescence and bioluminescence labels are becoming more popular. One commercial assay uses selective protein binding coupled to ion capture, followed by fluorescence assay. However, because problems of standardization and intermethod agreement persist with CPB assays, more specific analytical techniques have been developed, including HPLC with electrochemical or mass-spectrometric detection.[32]

Several analytes are known to be indicative of folate metabolism. Plasma total homocysteine increases when there is a deficiency of 5-MTHF, such that the methylation of homocysteine to methionine is compromised. However, though plasma homocysteine is considered to be a sensitive functional indicator, it is not specific because its concentration can be influenced by deficiency of other vitamins (B_6 and B_{12}) involved in the metabolism of homocysteine. Similarly the methylation of DNA is dependent upon adequate 5-MTHF. A sensitive new method for the rapid detection of abnormal methylation patterns in global DNA patterns has been reported and may have promise as a functional marker,[445] as may the measurement of the degree of uracil incorporation into DNA, 5,10-methylene THF being required for the conversion of deoxyuridine monophosphate (dUMP) to dTMP by thymidylate synthetase.[60]

Reference Intervals

Because of methodological differences, reference values for folate are method dependent. The data collected from the NHANES of 1988 to 1994 in the United States, in which almost 3000 blood samples were analyzed, produced reference intervals of 2.6 to 12.2 µg/L (6.0 to 28.0 nmol/L) for serum folate and 103 to 411 µg/L (237 to 945 nmol/L) for erythrocyte folate. Biochemical deficiency has been defined as a concentration of <1.4 µg/L (<3.2 nmol/L) for serum folate and <110 µg/L (<253 nmol/L) for erythrocyte folate.[+]

Niacin and Niacinamide

Niacin and niacinamide (nicotinamide and nicotinic acid amide) are converted to the ubiquitous redox coenzymes nicotinamide-adenine dinucleotide $(NAD)^+$ and nicotinamide-adenine dinucleotide phosphate $(NADP)^+$.

Chemistry

The term niacin refers to nicotinic acid (pyridine-3-carboxylic acid), its amide nicotinamide, and derivatives that show the same biological activity as nicotinamide. A distinction between the two primary vitamin forms has to be considered, however, when considering some aspects of their metabolism and especially their different pharmacological actions at high doses. Structures of both vitamers and the two coenzyme forms containing the nicotinamide moiety are given in Figure 30-23.

Dietary Sources

Nicotinamide-adenine dinucleotide (NAD; diphosphopyridine nucleotide) and nicotinamide-adenine dinucleotide phosphate (NADP; also termed triphosphopyridine nucleotide) represent most of the niacin activity found in good sources that include yeast, lean meats, liver, and poultry.[101] Milk, canned salmon, and several leafy green vegetables contribute lesser amounts but are still sufficient to prevent deficiency. Additionally, some plant foodstuffs, especially cereals such as corn and wheat, contain niacin bound to various peptides and sugars in forms nutritionally not readily available (niacinogens or niacytin).[274] Because tryptophan is a precursor of niacin, protein provides a considerable portion of niacin equivalent. As much as two thirds of niacin required by adults can be derived from tryptophan metabolism via nicotinic acid ribonucleotide

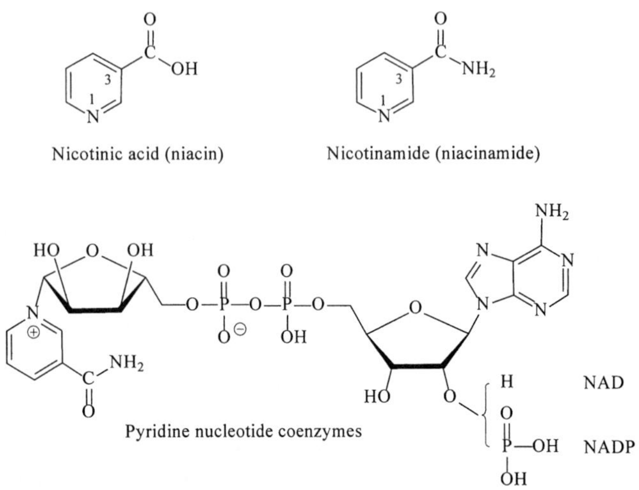

Nicotinic acid (niacin)

Nicotinamide (niacinamide)

Pyridine nucleotide coenzymes

NAD

NADP

Figure 30-23 Niacin, niacinamide, and coenzyme.

to NAD and NADP. It has been found that 60 mg of tryptophan can provide the equivalent of 1 mg of niacin in the adult. In countries where fortification of processed cereals is practiced, this may provide up to 20% of niacin intake.[274]

Free forms of the vitamin are white, stable solids that are quite soluble in water. The oxidized coenzymes are labile to alkali, whereas the reduced (dihydro) coenzymes are labile to acid. Reduction of the oxidized coenzymes commonly occurs by addition of a hydride ion to the *para* (4) position of the nicotinamide ring, with simultaneous formation of a solvated proton. NADH and NADPH (but not NAD and NADP) absorb light in the near ultraviolet region (339 nm). This forms the basis for many biochemical assays.

Absorption, Transport, Metabolism, and Excretion

Dietary NAD and NADP are hydrolyzed by enzymes, such as NAD glycohydrolase, in the intestinal mucosa to release nicotinamide, which together with any nicotinic acid is rapidly absorbed in both the stomach and intestine by an Na^+-dependent facilitated diffusion at low concentrations and passive diffusion at higher concentrations.[35] Nicotinamide is the main circulating form in the plasma, either postabsorption or by release from hydrolyzed liver NAD, and this can be taken up by most tissue requiring NAD by simple diffusion, though there is evidence of a facilitated transport in the erythrocyte.[319]

Once inside blood, kidney, brain, and liver cells both nicotinic acid and nicotinamide are converted to the coenzyme forms. The first step involves the cytosolic phosphoribosyltransferase-catalyzed reaction of nicotinate or nicotinamide with 5-phosphoribosyl-1-pyrophosphate to form pyrophosphate and nicotinic acid ribonucleotide or nicotinamide ribonucleotide, respectively.[367] An additional source of nicotinic acid ribonucleotide is from the action of quinolate phosphoribosyltransferase on quinolinate formed from tryptophan. The efficiency of this pathway is under nutritional and hormonal regulation, with deficiency of vitamin B_6 (riboflavin) and iron slowing the conversion—and protein, tryptophan, energy, and niacin restriction increasing the efficiency.[274] Nicotinic acid ribonucleotide from whatever source is converted to deamido-NAD by an adenylyltransferase catalyzed attachment of the AMP moiety from ATP, and the deamido compound subsequently reacts with glutamine and a cytosolic ATP–dependent synthetase step to yield NAD, glutamate, and phosphate. Nicotinamide mononucleotide is directly converted by the adenylyltransferase to NAD. NADP is formed by a kinase-catalyzed phosphorylation of NAD. In the tissue, most of the vitamin is present as nicotinamide in NAD and NADP, although the liver may contain a significant fraction of the free vitamin. There is little storage of niacin as such.

Excess niacin is excreted mainly as the N-methylnicotinamide (NMN), after methylation in the liver, and the two oxidation products of NMN, N-methyl-2-pyridone-5-carboxamide, and N-methyl-4-pyridone-carboxamide.[402]

Functions

Niacin is essential as the coenzymes NAD and NADP in which nicotinamide acts as an electron acceptor or hydrogen donor in a large number of redox reactions. Many of the enzymes function as dehydrogenases and catalyze such diverse reactions as the conversion of alcohols (often sugars and polyols) to aldehydes or ketones, hemiacetals to lactones, aldehydes to acids, and certain amino acids to keto acids.[367] The common mechanism of operation involves the stereospecific abstraction of a hydride ion from substrate, with *para* addition to one or the other side of carbon 4 in the pyridine ring of the nucleotide coenzyme. The second hydrogen of the substrate group oxidized is concomitantly removed as a proton and ultimately exchanges as a hydronium ion. Most dehydrogenases using NAD or NADP function reversibly. Glutamate dehydrogenase, for example, favors the oxidative direction, whereas others, such as glutathione reductase, preferentially catalyze reduction. In addition to redox reactions, NAD is also a substrate for three classes of enzymes that cleave the β-N-glycosylic bond of NAD to free nicotinamide and catalyze the transfer of adenosine diphosphate (ADP)-ribose.[321] One such enzyme, poly(ADP-ribose) polymerase-1 (PARP-1), is involved in base excision repair and is thought to be important for genomic stability.[219] Nicotinic acid, when used as a pharmaceutical agent, has important antiatherogenic properties. It effectively lowers triglycerides, raises HDL cholesterol, and shifts LDL particles to a less atherogenic phenotype.[270]

Requirements and Reference Nutrient Intakes

Requirements for niacin are expressed as niacin equivalents (NE), which take account of the contribution of tryptophan derived from protein. Earlier estimates of niacin requirements were based on energy expenditure, reflecting the biological function of the niacin coenzymes in the oxidation of fuel molecules. However, current recommendations merely reflect the fact that different age groups and sexes have, on average, different energy expenditure and that no directly relevant studies have linked energy intake or expenditure with niacin requirement.[170] The median intake of preformed niacin from food in the United States is 28 mg for men and 18 mg for women. A study of two Canadian populations showed corresponding values of 41 mg and 28 mg per day. Additionally the average U.S. diet supplies between 0.7 and 1.1 g of tryptophan per day.[410] Based on niacin metabolite excretion data, current RDA for males 19 years to more than 70 years are 16 mg/day of NE, and for women of the same age, 14 mg/day. An increase of 4 NE per day during pregnancy is recommended and an increase of 3 NE daily for lactation will offset the preformed niacin lost in milk. Human milk contains approximately 0.17 mg of niacin and 22 mg of tryptophan/dL or 70 kcal, and these amounts are adequate to meet niacin needs of the infant. Adequate intakes of 2 mg/day of preformed niacin and 4 mg/day NE have been extrapolated from adult requirements for infants of 0 to 6 months and 7 to 12 months, respectively. RDAs are set at

6 mg/day for children 1 to 3 years, 8 mg/day for children 4 to 8 years, 12 mg/day for boys and girls 9 to 13 years, 14 mg/day for girls 14 to 18 years, and 16 mg/day for boys 14 to 18 years.[170]

Intravenous Supply

The recommended supply to adult patients receiving TPN is 40 mg/day in the form of nicotinamide.[9] This increase above the oral recommendations will ensure an adequate intake to match increased energy expenditure.

Deficiency

Pellagra is the classic deficiency disease of the human that has been most often found among those who subsist chiefly on corn (maize), which is low in both niacin and tryptophan.[474] Although its pathogenesis has been attributed to a deficiency of these two factors, other associated complicating factors are a lack of pyridoxal-5-phosphate, FAD, and iron, which are functional in the conversion of tryptophan to niacin and the presence of mycotoxins elaborated by mold infestations, mainly by *Fusarium*.[622] Pellagra is also an occasional secondary manifestation of *carcinoid syndrome,* in which up to 60% of tryptophan is catabolized to 5-OH tryptophan and serotonin; *Hartnup disease,* an autosomal recessive disorder in which several amino acids, including tryptophan, are poorly absorbed; and in treatment with the antituberculous drug isoniazid, which competes with pyridoxal-5-phosphate.

The typical presentation of pellagra is that of a chronic wasting disease associated with dermatitis, dementia, and diarrhea. The characteristic erythematous dermatitis is bilateral and symmetrical and occurs on skin areas exposed to sunlight. Mental changes include fatigue, insomnia, and apathy, which precede an encephalopathy characterized by confusion, disorientation, hallucination, loss of memory, and eventually frank organic psychoses. The diarrhea, when it occurs, reflects a widespread inflammation of the intestinal mucous surfaces, including a bright red tongue; other gastrointestinal manifestations include achlorhydria, glossitis, stomatitis, and vaginitis.

Toxicity

Although no toxic effects have been associated with niacin intake from naturally occurring foods, the use of supplements and pharmacological doses of niacin has produced adverse effects in some subjects. In disorders of reduced tryptophan availability, such as Hartnup syndrome and carcinoid syndrome, daily niacin doses of 40 to 200 mg may be required, and in the treatment of dyslipidemias nicotinic acid in doses up to 6 g daily may be used. Such doses are commonly associated with vascular dilation or "flushing," a burning, tingling sensation of the face (that may be reddened), arms, and chest, and is thought to be mediated by prostaglandins. This may be modulated by gradual increments of the drug and by taking with meals. Other side effects of high-dose niacin treatment are pruritus, nausea, vomiting, and diarrhea, though these symptoms often abate with continued therapy. Additional effects are abnormal glucose tolerance, hyperuricemia, peptic ulcer, hepatomegaly, jaundice, and increased serum aminotransferases. In a study of 814 patients on a combination extended-release niacin preparation (maximum dose, 2 g), flushing caused intolerance in 10% of those studied, hepatotoxicity was seen in 0.5%, and myopathy was not reported.[398] The symptoms of flushing have been taken as an end point sign in the formulation of a tolerable upper intake level for niacin. This has been set at 35 mg/day for adults of 19 years and older, with lower levels for children and adolescents.[170]

Laboratory Assessment of Status

At present, no blood markers are commonly used as indicators of niacin status. Most assessments of niacin nutriture have been based on measurement of the 2 urinary metabolites, N′-methylnicotinamide and N′-methyl-2-pyridone-5-carboxamide. Normally, adults excrete 20% to 30% of their niacin in the form of methylnicotinamide and 40% to 60% as the pyridone. An excretion ratio of pyridone to methylnicotinamide of 1.3 to 4.0 is thus normal, but latent niacin deficiency is indicated by a value below 1.0. As depletion occurs, the pyridone is absent for weeks before clinical signs are noted, and the methylnicotinamide excretion falls to a minimum at about the time that clinical signs are evident.[495] HPLC methods are currently the methods of choice,[492,529] though some capillary electrophoresis methods have been developed.[272] However, the measurement of 2-pyridone and N′-methylnicotinamide concentrations in plasma may provide a more reliable metabolite ratio than urine measurements. A newer approach that may prove valuable is the ratio of NAD/NADP in erythrocytes and plasma tryptophan. A ratio of NAD/NADP below 1.0 would be indicative of a risk of developing niacin deficiency.[188]

Reference Intervals

A guidance reference interval for the excretion rate of N^1-methylnicotinamide is 2.4 to 6.4 mg/day (17.5 to 46.7 μmol/day) or 1.6 to 4.3 mg/g creatinine (11.7 to 31.4 μmol/g creatinine).[277,495]

Pantothenic Acid

Pantothenic acid is a component of coenzyme A (CoA) and is required for the metabolism of fat, protein, and carbohydrate via the citric acid cycle.

Chemistry

Pantothenic acid is of ubiquitous occurrence in nature, where it is synthesized by most microorganisms and plants from pantoic acid (D-2,4-dihydroxy-3,3-dimethylbutyric acid) derived from L-valine, and β-alanine derived from L-aspartate. Addition of cysteamine at the C-terminal end and phosphorylation at C4 of pantoic acid forms 4′-phosphopantetheine, which serves as a covalently attached prosthetic group of acyl carrier proteins, and, when attached

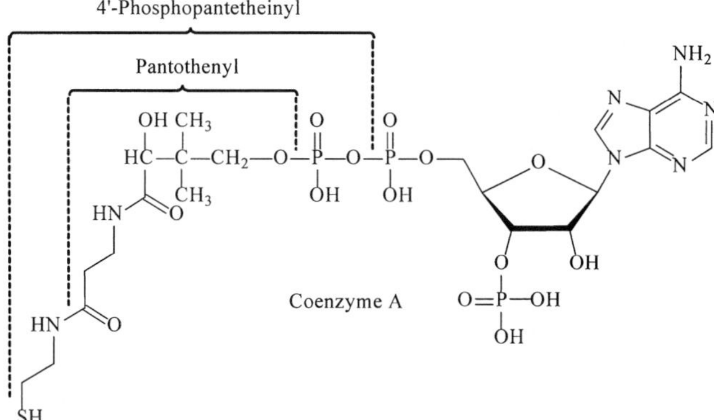

Figure 30-24 Pantothenate and 4′-phosphopantetheine as components of CoA.

to ribose 3′-phosphate and adenine, CoA as shown in Figure 30-24. Pantothenic acid is a hygroscopic, viscous oil, which is easily destroyed by heat, especially at extremes of pH. The most common commercial synthetic form is the calcium salt.

Dietary Sources

Pantothenic acid is widely distributed in foods, mostly within CoA-containing compounds, and is particularly abundant in animal sources, legumes, and whole grain cereals. Excellent food sources (100 to 200 μg/g dry weight) include egg yolk, kidney, liver, and yeast. Fair sources (35 to 100 μg/g) include broccoli, lean beef, skimmed milk, sweet potatoes, and molasses. More than one half of the pantothenate in wheat may be lost during manufacture of flour, and up to one third is lost during cooking of meat.[170,443]

Absorption, Transport, Metabolism, and Excretion

Pantothenic acid is taken in as dietary CoA compounds and 4′-phosphopantetheine and hydrolyzed by pyrophosphatase and phosphatase in the intestinal lumen to dephospho-CoA, phosphopantetheine, and pantetheine. This is further hydrolyzed to pantethenic acid. The vitamin is primarily absorbed as pantothenic acid by a saturable process at low concentrations and by simple diffusion at higher ones. The saturable process is facilitated by a sodium-dependent multivitamin transporter, for which biotin and lipoate compete.[449] After absorption, pantothenic acid enters the circulation and is taken up by cells in a manner similar to its intestinal adsorption. The synthesis of CoA from pantothenate is regulated by pantothenate kinase, which itself is subject to negative feedback from the products CoA and acyl-CoA.[553] The steps involved were outlined above. Pantothenic acid is excreted in the urine after hydrolysis of CoA compounds by enzymes that cleave phosphate and the cysteamine moieties. Only a small fraction of pantothenate is secreted into milk and even less into colostrum.

Functions

Pantothenic acid has two major metabolic roles, the first as part of CoA and the other as the prosthetic group of the acyl-carrier protein (ACP). In the former role, CoA is primarily involved in acetyl and acyl transfer reactions in catabolic processes of carbohydrate, lipid, and protein chemistry. Examples of these are the acetylation of sugars, phospholipid, isoprenoid, and steroid biosynthesis and protein acetylation.[388] Acetyl-CoA that derives from the metabolism of carbohydrates, fats, and amino acids can acetylate compounds, such as choline and hexosamines to produce essential biochemicals; it can also condense with other metabolites, such as oxaloacetate, to supply citrate and cholesterol. As the 4′-phosphopantetheine moiety of ACP, the phosphodiester-linked prosthetic group uses the sulfhydryl terminus to exchange with malonyl-CoA to form an ACP-S malonyl thioester, which can chain elongate during fatty acid biosynthesis.[368] In a 1998 study, pantothenic acid was found to protect rats against some deleterious effects of gamma radiation.[534] In a 2001 study, it was found to have antioxidant properties, thereby protecting lymphocytes against ultraviolet light–induced apoptosis.[535] Pantothenic acid used pharmaceutically may have benefits of lowering cholesterol, enhancing athletic performance, and relieving the symptoms of rheumatoid arthritis.[388]

Requirements and Reference Nutrient Intakes

A number of studies have estimated the dietary intake of pantothenic acid in humans to be 4 to 7 mg/day, which seems sufficient for normal health.[299,564] Urinary excretion of pantothenic acid on a typical American diet averages 2.6 mg/day,[564] but may range from 2 to 7 mg/day in adults consuming 5 to 7 mg/day and is strongly dependent on intake; another 1 to 2 mg/day is lost in feces. The primary criterion used to estimate an AI for pantothenic acid is whether its intake is adequate to replace urinary excretion. It has been set at 5 mg/day for adolescents 14 years to 18 years and for adults.[170] Children 1 year to 13 years have AIs extrapolated from adult values, and infants have AIs reflecting intake from human milk, which contains approximately 2 mg/L. An additional 1 mg/day is suggested in pregnancy and an additional 2 mg/day is suggested for lactating mothers.

Intravenous Supply

The recommended intravenous supply for adults is 15 mg/day of dexpanthenol.[9]

Deficiency

The widespread availability of pantothenic acid in food is commensurate with its many roles and makes an uncomplicated dietary deficiency of pantothenate unlikely in humans. Symptoms have been produced in a few volunteers who have received ω-methylpantothenic acid as an antagonist[251] and in people fed semisynthetic diets virtually free of pantothenate.[187] Subjects became irascible and developed postural hypotension and rapid heart rate on exertion, epigastric distress with anorexia and constipation, numbness and tingling of the hands and feet, hyperactive deep tendon reflexes, and weakness of finger extensor muscles. The eosinopenic response to adrenocorticotropic hormone was impaired. More severe deficiency in animals leads to adrenocortical failure. Historically, pantothenic acid deficiency has been associated with the syndrome of "burning feet," experienced by prisoners in the second World War in Asia, and relieved only by pantothenic acid supplementation, and not by other B-group vitamins.[201]

Toxicity

There are no reports of adverse effects, with the exception of occasional mild diarrhea, with oral pantothenic acid in doses as high as 20 g/day.[457,553] In the absence of evidence of toxicity, a tolerable upper intake level cannot be derived for pantothenic acid.

Laboratory Assessment of Status

There are no convenient or reliable functional tests of pantothenic acid status, thus assessment is made by direct measurement of whole blood or urine pantothenic acid concentrations. Urine measurements are perhaps the easiest to conduct and interpret, and concentrations are closely related to dietary intake.[495] Whole blood measurements are preferred to plasma, which contains only free pantothenic acid and is insensitive to changes in pantothenic acid intake. Concentrations of pantothenic acid in all of the above fluids can be measured by microbiological assay, most commonly using *Lactobacillus plantarum*. Whole blood must first be treated with an enzyme preparation to release pantothenic acid from CoA.[26] Other techniques that have been used to measure pantothenic acid in human samples include radioimmunoassay[629] and gas chromatography.[508] Other techniques that have been developed include gas chromatography–mass spectrometry[28] and a stable isotope dilution assay.[486] CoA and ACP can be measured by enzymatic methods.[109]

Reference Intervals

Urinary excretion of pantothenic acid of less than 1 mg/day is considered abnormally low. Suspicion of inadequate intake is further supported if whole blood levels are less than 100 μg/L. A guidance reference interval for pantothenic acid in whole blood or serum is 344 to 583 μg/L (1.57 to 2.66 μmol/L),[143] and for urinary excretion is 1 to 15 mg/day (5 to 68 μmol/day).[629]

TRACE ELEMENTS

The term "trace element" was originally used to describe the residual amount of inorganic analyte quantitatively determined in a sample. Increased analytical sensitivity now allows the accurate determination of most inorganic micronutrients present at very low concentrations in body fluids and tissue. Those present at (μg/dL) in body fluids and in tissue (mg/kg) are however still widely referred to as "trace elements" and those found at ng/dL or μg/kg as the "ultratrace elements." The corresponding dietary requirements are quoted in mg/day or μg/day, respectively.

The biological effects of deficiency disease define the essential trace elements. For example, an element is considered essential when the signs and symptoms induced by a deficient diet are uniquely reversed by an adequate supply of the particular trace element under investigation.[378,428]

For iron, iodine, cobalt (as cobalamins), selenium, copper, and zinc there are clinical examples of reversible deficiency disease. For these elements there is enough known about their biochemical functions to explain their importance in human nutrition. For others, such as manganese, chromium, molybdenum, and vanadium, their importance remains to be fully accepted in clinical practice. Still other elements such as bromine, fluorine, cadmium, lead, strontium, lithium, and tin have been claimed by at least one investigator to be essential for one or more animal species as demonstrated by dietary deprivation studies.

Classification

This wide range of biologically active elements has led to a suggestion for classification beyond "essentiality" into the additional categories pharmacologically beneficial and nutritionally beneficial or possibly essential.[419]

Pharmacologically Beneficial

Trace elements in this category would include fluoride used for protection against dental caries and lithium salts used in the treatment of manic depression. The dosages required for a beneficial pharmacological effect greatly exceed the amounts of these elements normally found in food.

Nutritionally Beneficial or Possibly Essential

For some trace elements, continued suboptimal dietary intake—in the presence of physiological, nutritional, or other metabolic stress—may eventually have a detrimental effect. Then additional dietary supplementation may have a "health restorative" effect. Such effects are most clearly demonstrated in experimental animals. Examples include the effects of boron in the presence of vitamin D depletion,[260] or the need for increased vanadium when there is either an experimentally induced deficient or excess supply of dietary iodine.[588]

Dose-Effect Relationships

At low intakes of the recognized essential trace elements, deficiency disease may be seen, and then with increasing dietary supply a plateau region of optimal supply is reached. Still higher intakes will result in adverse toxic effects. The concentration window separating beneficial dietary intake from toxic intake varies depending upon the element in question, and on the nature of the chemical species present in the diet. This is similar to the dose-effect relationship described for the organic micronutrients (Figure 30-25). Therefore the RDA is set at amounts that are sufficient to prevent deficiency. A tolerable upper intake value that will

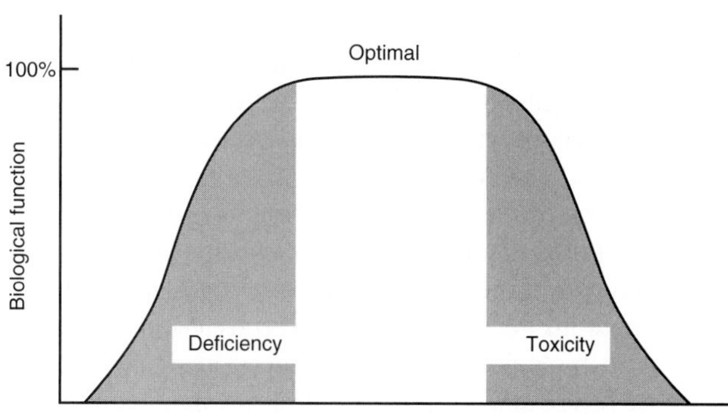

Figure 30-25 Model of the relationship between tissue concentration and intake of an essential nutrient and dependent biological function.

prevent toxicity is also proposed for the inorganic micronutrients of known importance to human health.[174]

Reversal of clinical signs and symptoms by supplementation with a single trace element or with micronutrient mixtures has been used as indirect evidence of a preexisting deficiency. Growth velocities in children, regain of lean body mass, rate of wound healing, resistance to infection, and alterations in cognitive function can be assessed. However, many confounding factors, in particular the presence of disease or of other nutritional deficits, can affect the interpretation of changes in these indices.

Reductions of metalloenzyme activity induced by the deficiency may be partially or wholly restored by effective treatment. Reversal of hematological and immune function laboratory abnormalities can also be used, as can hormonal changes induced by the deficiency.

Chemistry

Trace elements interact with available ligands, mainly the electron donors nitrogen, sulfur, and oxygen to form a wide variety of chemical complexes or species. Some metals such as Fe, Cu, Mo, and Cr are stable in more than one valence state and participate in biologically important oxidation-reduction reactions.[180] The transition metals with an incompletely filled *3d*-orbital (Fe, Cu, and Co) coordinate with a large number of groups to form stable complexes. Zinc lies at the end of the first transition series in the periodic table. Zn^{2+}, with a complete *3d* electron shell, is a particularly stable ion with unique biological functions. Reviews of the biological chemistry of the essential elements are available.[180,428]

Biochemistry/Homeostasis

Most aspects of intermediary metabolism require essential trace elements in the form of metalloenzymes that have a range of catalytic properties. Specific metalloproteins are required for the transport and safe storage of very reactive metal ions, such as Fe^{3+} or Cu^{2+}. Examples are metallothionein (Cu, Zn), transferrin, ferritin and hemosiderin (Fe), and ceruloplasmin (Cu).

Homeostatic controls are required to regulate the supply of essential trace elements to tissue cells in the face of varying dietary intakes. These involve regulation of intestinal absorption, specific transport systems in peripheral blood, uptake and storage mechanisms in tissue, and control of excretion. The principal excretory route for some important trace metals (Zn, Cu) is in feces both by regulation of initial absorption and by resecretion into the intestinal tract in bile and other intestinal fluids. For the halides (iodide and fluoride) excess intake is primarily excreted in urine. For others (Se, B, Mo, and Cr) urinary output is also important. Losses of trace elements by other routes, through hair and/or nails, skin cell desquamation, and in sweat, are generally minor, although studies have been published measuring such losses.[275] Similarly menstrual iron loss or seminal fluid zinc loss could be important in specialized studies.

Combinations of poor dietary supply, intestinal malabsorption because of the antagonistic effects of other trace elements, or blockage of uptake by substances like phytate—together with increased excretory losses as a result of disease, injury, and infection—can result in overt, symptomatic trace element deficiency disease.[47] Liver disease, inflammatory bowel disease, and renal disease will affect trace element absorption and excretion to a variable extent and may cause an acquired deficiency disease.

Catabolic responses to injury, infection, and malignant disease can result in increased essential trace element losses in feces and in urine, and burn injury causes extensive losses in exudates through the damaged skin.[45]

If postsurgical patients, especially those with short bowel syndrome, require prolonged periods of nasogastric tube feeding or intravenous feeding and are treated with nutrient regimens lacking sufficient inorganic micronutrients, they will develop symptomatic deficiency disease. Clinical cases of trace element deficiency have been described for copper, zinc, selenium, and chromium.[525]

Inborn Errors

Although genetic defects in the metabolism of trace elements are rare, they are nonetheless important because of the information they have provided as to homeostatic control mechanisms. This in turn has led to development of effective therapeutic strategies. The most commonly investigated disorders are those affecting iron (hemochromatosis), copper (Wilson's disease and Menkes' syndrome), zinc (acrodermatitis enteropathica), and molybdenum (molybdenum cofactor disease).

Interactions

The physiological interaction between different essential trace elements and also with the other essential major minerals can have significant effects on health. Such interactions are mostly considered as affecting the intestinal bioavailability of nutrients from various diets. The complex interactions that were investigated systematically in animal studies have been important in trying to understand the mechanisms of absorption by the intestinal mucosal cells, an area that is still poorly defined. Both synergistic and antagonistic effects on bioavailability have been given a theoretical basis by the observation that ions with similar electronic configurations in their outer orbit are likely to interact competitively. For example, there is strong interaction between zinc and copper and also between molybdenum and tungsten.[249]

The ability of zinc ions to block copper absorption, possibly by formation of intestinal metallothionein that strongly binds copper, has led to its use in pharmacological doses in the management of Wilson's disease.[73] Similarly molybdate ion can form insoluble copper-molybdate complexes in the intestine that limit copper absorption. The detrimental effects of organic phosphate (phytic acid) in limiting zinc absorption are aggravated by excess dietary calcium, probably by formation of a highly insoluble Ca-Zn-phytate complex. The subject of these and other interactions has been reviewed.[428]

Synergistic interactions occur in other tissues and can have important biological and clinical consequences. For example, the interaction between selenium and iodine has been investigated.[528] It is known that deiodinases are selenoproteins and that they remove iodine from T_4 to produce the biologically active T_3. Also the selenoprotein glutathione peroxidase is active in the thyroid in the destruction of excess hydrogen peroxide and is therefore important in thyroid hormone production. In certain areas of the world, combined selenium and iodine deficiency can occur and affect treatment; provision of selenium may be necessary to correct hypothyroidism, but also may precipitate its onset.[19,528]

Selenium deficiency in experimental animal studies is exacerbated by vitamin E depletion. The antioxidant properties of tocopherol and glutathione peroxidase are similar and can to some extent overlap, although this is highly species dependent.[550]

Zinc and vitamin A are also interrelated, and it appears that zinc depletion limits the bioavailability of vitamin A. Controlled studies found that combined zinc and vitamin A supplementation is more clinically effective than vitamin A alone or zinc alone in controlling diarrhea and minimizing respiratory infections.[455]

Experimentally, it is usual to conduct animal and human studies using depletion of one essential element at a time. It is likely that in vivo the circumstances causing depletion of one essential element will be accompanied by varying degrees of depletion of other micronutrients, and that the possibility of interactions and synergistic effects should be considered when designing therapies.

Laboratory Assessment of Trace Element Status

As understanding of underlying biochemical intracellular mechanisms increases for a particular trace element, the determination of the active species becomes of increased importance.[390,567] For iodine, assay of the thyroid hormones and of their control and feedback systems has largely replaced direct determination of the element. Cobalamin (vitamin B_{12}) is measured in body fluids by immunoassay rather than by a nonspecific cobalt determination. This process is gradually extending to other trace elements, because metalloenzymes and protein species are proposed as indices of Fe, Zn, Cu, and Se status.

For several of the "ultratrace" elements (Cr, Mo, and V), insufficient information is currently available as to the critical molecular species underlying their biological actions. Direct methods for determining total trace element concentrations in biological samples are therefore required. This can pose severe analytical difficulties, and may require specialist laboratory facilities, with appropriate techniques employed to reduce sample contamination.[390]

Dietary intakes of trace elements can be assessed for individual patients or population groups by direct dietary analysis and by taking dietary histories. The estimated intakes can then be compared with the current dietary reference values.

Direct measurement of total dietary intake over several days together with measurement of all outputs in urine, feces, or by other routes can be used to estimate positive or negative balances. Because of the intrinsic difficulty of ensuring complete collection of all materials with minimal contamination, metabolic balance studies can have systematic errors.[380]

The net intake can be also be estimated by using exogenous and endogenous labeling of representative diet with radio or stable isotopes of the trace element under investigation. These research methods can give valuable insights as to the bioavailability of nutrients and the efficiency of uptake by the intestinal tract from particular diets.[436]

Analytical Considerations

Analytical factors that have to be considered in the measurement of trace elements include (1) specimen requirements, (2) preanalytical factors, (3) collection equipment, and (4) analytical methodology.

Specimen Requirements

Direct determination of trace elements is made in many types of specimens including whole blood, blood plasma or serum, leukocytes, urine, saliva, cerebrospinal fluid (CSF), breast milk, and sweat. Tissue samples may be obtained by needle biopsy (liver, bone,) or following an autopsy. Hair and nail samples offer a noninvasive means of sampling tissue and are used to assess toxic metal exposure. Measurements of hair and nails for essential elements may be of value on a group basis during studies of severely depleted populations but are of limited value in the investigation of individual hospital patients. Problems of external contamination from environmental pollution, cosmetics, shampoos, and other sources are difficult to control.[220]

The most commonly submitted samples for direct trace element analysis are of whole blood, blood plasma, or serum. Plasma protein levels of the relevant carrier proteins transferrin (Fe), albumin (Zn), ceruloplasmin (Cu), and selenoprotein P (Se) can give useful additional information.

The concentration of essential trace elements in nucleated cells can be determined in various types of leukocytes and in platelets; this is a direct measure of intracellular trace element levels. However, separation of different types of white cells and platelets in whole blood is subject to serious problems of contamination before trace element analysis.[392]

Problems from prolonged storage of samples can arise and short-term storage at 4 °C to 10 °C with a rapid turnaround analytical time is good practice. Repeated freezing and thawing of blood plasma and other types of material can lead to precipitation of proteins and nonhomogeneous samples.

Preanalytical Factors

There are numerous variables that can affect trace element determinations before the analysis of the sample is undertaken and these require careful control. Guidelines giving details of sample collection procedures, and procedures for limitation of contamination in a range of sample types, are available for essential and toxic trace elements.[338,390] Age, sex, ethnic origin, time of sampling in relation to food intake, time of day and year, history of medication, tobacco usage, and other factors should be recorded when establishing reference intervals from healthy control populations.

For hospital patients with infections, and after accidental injury or postsurgery, the systemic inflammatory response will affect the concentration of essential elements in circulating blood independently of nutritional status. For example, the APR causes increased permeability of capillaries and transfer of certain plasma carrier proteins and their trace metals into interstitial space. Hepatic synthesis of some plasma proteins, the so-called acute phase proteins, is also induced, so that these proteins increase in concentration in plasma, together with any metals that they carry (e.g., ceruloplasmin and copper). Moreover, there are marked changes in the kinetics of elements, with altered rates of transfer to and from the tissue. Knowledge of the effect of disease on metal kinetics and distribution is therefore essential.[523]

Collection Equipment

The choice of container for samples is important, since contamination from rubber, cork, and colored plastics can be a problem. For blood plasma, collection plastic tubes with lithium heparin as an anticoagulant are suitable for most analyses. For blood serum, plain glass containers can be used. For the ultratrace metals (Mn, Cr), special arrangements have to be made to collect blood via plastic cannulae or silanized steel needles, and then the sample is placed into acid-washed containers. "Trace metal" vacutainers are available commercially. It is good practice to run dilute acid blanks through all the containers and collection systems to ensure that all batches remain as free from contamination as possible.

For random urine samples and for tissue biopsy samples, a plain plastic container is preferable with no added preservative. For 24-hour urine collections, polyethylene bottles should be used with glacial acetic acid as the preservative. It is important that the urine collections should not be made into disposable fiber or stainless steel containers.

For further details and advice, specialist laboratories should be consulted (e.g., in the United States, the United States Department of Agriculture (USDA), Beltsville Agricultural Research Center (BARC), Washington D.C.,[424] or the U.S. Department of Agriculture, Agriculture Research Service Human Nutrition Research Center, Grand Forks, N.D.[393] UK and European readers may wish to consult the Supra Area Assay Service[494] or the Scottish Trace Element and Vitamin Laboratory).[577] These sites have links to other specialist laboratories.

Analytical Methodology

An analytical method used for the determination of trace and ultratrace elements in biological specimens must be (1) sensitive, (2) specific, (3) precise, (4) accurate, and (5) relatively fast. The detection limits of such methods are very important because concentrations of trace or ultratrace elements in some samples are in the nanogram per gram to microgram per gram range. In practice, the concentration of a trace or ultratrace element should be about at least 10 times the detection limit of the method, thus ensuring sufficient accuracy and precision.

Analytical techniques used for clinical trace metal analysis include photometry, atomic absorption spectrophotometry (AAS), inductively coupled plasma optical emission (ICP-OES), and inductively coupled plasma mass spectrometry (ICP-MS). Other techniques, such as neutron activation analysis (NAA) and x-ray fluorescence (XRF), and electrochemical methods, such as anodic stripping voltammetry (ASV), are used less commonly. For example. NAA requires a nuclear irradiation facility and is not readily available and ASV requires completely mineralized solutions for analysis, which is a time-consuming process.

Photometry

The principals of photometric measurements are discussed in Chapter 3. When applied to the analysis of trace elements, photometric methods are based on the use of a color-forming reagent; however, they are not specific for a particular metal. Interferences also occur in hemolyzed, lipemic, and icteric samples. In practice, the technique lacks sufficient sensitivity for all but the more abundant trace elements, such as iron, zinc, and copper. Many photometric methods for zinc and copper have been described[1,71,255,357] and kits for them are available commercially.

Atomic Absorption Spectrophotometry

AAS is a widely used method for the determination of Zn and Cu in serum and has largely replaced less specific photometric methods. (The principles of AAS are detailed in Chapter 3 and elsewhere,[55,127] and Delves has written a useful review on the application of AAS to clinical pathology.)[128]

Unfortunately the technique lacks the sensitivity to measure Cu in urine and the more sensitive but technically more demanding electrothermal atomization atomic absorption spectrometry (ETA-AAS) is required. In this technique, sample volumes as small as 10 µl are sequentially volatilized and atomized in a graphite tube. This technique is useful in situations in which the sample volume is limiting (e.g., premature babies) or for elements in which increased analytical sensitivity is required, such as selenium or manganese. Significant analytical errors can result from nonspecific optical absorption in the graphite tube and are caused by matrix components being volatilized along with the analyte atoms. Optical background correction systems using a deuterium lamp or employing the Zeeman effect are now standard components in ETA-AAS instrumentation (see Chapter 3). Flame and electrothermal AS are therefore widely used, but these are single element techniques and as such the methods for different elements have to be run sequentially, which can be wasteful in terms of time and sample.

Inductively Coupled Plasma-Optical Emission Spectrometry (ICP-OES)

ICP-OES is replacing AAS in some laboratories. Major changes to ICP-OES instrumentation that have led to this trend in replacement include (1) use of conventionally or radially viewed plasmas, which can now be viewed axially thereby greatly improving sensitivity; (2) replacement of monochromators with echelle spectrometers; (3) replacement of photomultiplier detectors with charge-coupled detectors (CCD), which have the ability to capture the whole echellogram and thereby deliver truly simultaneous analysis over the entire spectrum; and (4) use of vacuum or argon purged optics, allowing measurement down to and including the primary aluminum line at 167 nm.

With up-to-date ICP-OES, the elements Ca, Mg, Zn, Cu, Fe, and Al can be determined in a single analysis.[103,454] Apart from its multielement capabilities and increased sensitivity, ICP-OES also offers a wide dynamic range (e.g., three orders of magnitude for most elements) that allows simultaneous analyses to be obtained on a single diluted aliquot of sample. The high temperature of the plasma, 7500 °C, renders the technique largely free of chemical interferences, but matrix effects, background, and spectral interferences are greater than those in AAS. This is especially true of the axially viewed plasma in which emission from metal oxides may be observed. However, it is expected that sophisticated algorithms built into the software of modern instruments will overcome most problems. Axially and radially viewed ICP has been compared with respect to signal/background ratio, matrix effects, and sodium and calcium interferences.[70,139]

Inductively Coupled Plasma-Mass Spectrometry (ICP-MS)

This technique is more sensitive than either ETA-AAS or ICP-OES and is now the method of choice for ultratrace elements. The spectra are simpler than those of ICP-OES, but isobaric and polyatomic interferences do occur. Polyatomic interferences are more likely at masses <80. As ICP-MS can also be used to measure stable isotopes, it is used for conducting stable isotope tracer experiments and isotope dilution analysis. The principles of mass spectrometry are discussed in Chapter 7 and several textbooks are available on ICP-MS.[248,565] Clinical applications of ICP-MS have been described and reviewed.[452]

Quality Assurance Considerations

Because methods for trace element analyses are not standardized and are disposed to matrix effects and contamination problems, quality assurance measures must be incorporated into trace element analysis schemes. An effective quality assurance scheme for trace or ultratrace element analyses requires incorporation of the following into each batch of analysis: (1) reagent blanks, (2) replicate analyses to assess precision, (3) calibrators of the trace elements of interest in the expected concentration range of the specimens analyzed, and (4) a control or reference solution with known or certified concentrations of the trace elements to be determined to assess accuracy and batch-to-batch precision. The reference material should be of the same matrix type and contain approximately the same amounts of analyte as the specimens. Many different control or reference materials that contain certified amounts of trace elements are available. For quality control of trace element determinations in tissue specimens, reference materials of different biological matrices that have certified values for most macro and trace elements are available from the National Institute of Standards and Technology, Office of Standard Reference Materials in Washington, D.C. and from the Institute for Reference Materials and Measurements (IRMM) in Geel, Belgium (see Chapter 1).

A specimen pool that has been characterized by more than one laboratory can be conveniently and reliably used for quality control. Aliquots of such a pool should be stored frozen in tightly capped polypropylene tubes, with a minimum of headspace. No changes in zinc or copper concentrations were seen in serum samples frozen for up to 50 days.[163] Frozen pool samples can also be used to assess day-to-day precision of methods. Thawed specimens should be well mixed before sampling because analytical errors are caused by metal concentration gradients in unmixed thawed specimens. Recovery studies of elements from samples containing known quantities of added analyte are useful at intervals, for assessing accuracy and linearity, but such studies do not have to be performed daily. It is also recommended that trace elements participate in one or more EQAS. Organizations providing such schemes are listed in Box 30-1 and compilations of reference intervals have been published.[178,601]

Individual Trace Elements

Trace elements include chromium, cobalt, copper, fluoride, iron, manganese, molybdenum, selenium, and zinc.

Chromium

Chromium (Cr), which occurs naturally in various crustal materials, is a transitional element with many industrial

BOX 30-1 Organizations Providing Proficiency Testing and Quality Assurance Programs for Trace Element Testing Laboratories

The College of American Pathologists
325 Waukegan Road
Northfield IL 60093-2750
USA
Contact: Survey Coordinator
www.cap.org
Phone: (800) 323-4040

Laboratoire de toxicologie humaine
Institute National de Sante Publique du Quebec
945, ave Wolfe, Sainte-Foy Quebec G1V 5B3
Canada
ctq@inspq.qc.ca
www.inspq.qc.ca
Phone: (418) 650-5115
Fax: (418) 654-2148

Societe Francaise de Biologie Clinique (SFBC)
Laboratoire de Biochemie C
CHRU Grenoble- B.P. 217
38043 Grenoble Cedex 9
France
INRS-Service TMPC-B.P.27
54501 Vandoevre-les-Nancy
francois.baruthio@inrs.fr
Phone: (33) 83 50 20 00
Fax: (33) 83 50 20 19

SKZL (Foundation for Quality Assessment in Clinical Laboratories), Section Multi Component Analysis
Beatrix Park 1
NL-7101 BN Winterswijk
Netherlands
Phone +31 543 544774
Fax: +31 543 524265

Trace Elements Proficiency Testing Program
New York State Department of Health
Wadsworth Centre, PO Box 509
Albany, NY 12201-0509
USA
lead@wadsworth.org
www.wadsworth.org/testing/lead/index.htm
Phone: (518) 474-5475
Fax: (518) 473-7586

Guildford Trace Elements External Quality Assessment Scheme (TEQUAS)
Robens Institute, University of Surrey
Guildford GU2 5XH
UK
A.Taylor@surrey.ac.uk
Phone: +44 1483 502742
Fax: +44 1483 503517

METOS scheme, Department of Clinical Biochemistry, National Institute of Health
Viale Regina Elena, 299-00161 Roma
Italy
m.patria@iss.it
Phone: +39 6 49902559/31
Fax: +39 6 4461961/8380

Institut und Poliklinik fur Arbeits-, Sozial-und Umweltmedizin
Schillerstr. 25, D-91054
Erlingen
Germany
Tobias.weiss@rzmail.uni-erlangen.de
www.g-equas.de
Phone: 09131-85 22 37 4
Fax: 09131-85 61 26

uses and is discharged into the environment as industrial waste.

Chemistry

Chromium (atomic number 24, atomic weight 51.99) is a transition metal that occurs in biology with valence 3^+ or 6^+, each having markedly different properties. Trivalent Cr^{3+} is a d^3 cation, which usually forms octahedral complexes with slow ligand exchange. The element has no redox or acid-base properties.[180] It is considered an essential trace element that enhances the action of insulin.[382] Hexavalent Cr^{6+} is a strong oxidant and can cause tissue damage,[587] although the toxic Cr^{6+} ion is normally rapidly reduced to Cr^{3+} during contact with foodstuffs and gastric contents.

The molecular composition of a biologically active form of Cr^{3+} found in brewer's yeast, known as glucose tolerance factor (GTF), is not established. The structure of the Cr^{3+} bioactive molecule is thought to be the octahedral chromium complex, with two molecules of nicotinic acid having four coordination sites linked to glutamic acid, glycine, and cysteine, but attempts to isolate and purify the substance have not been successful. It is not clear whether GTF in brewer's yeast is better used than inorganic chromium in relation to insulin activation.[430]

Dietary Sources

Estimates of the amount of chromium in foodstuffs vary, partly because of analytical difficulties, but also because of contamination during contact with stainless steel during food processing, storage, and cooking. Processed meats, whole grain products, green beans, broccoli, and some spices are relatively good sources, but fruit and dairy products are not. Foodstuffs with high amounts of sucrose or fructose are intrinsically low in chromium and furthermore these sugars may promote urine loss. The estimated dietary intake for adults in the United States varies from 20 to 30 μg/day. Supplements containing chromium are taken by about 8% of adults in the United States and the NHANES III survey estimated that this added 23 μg Cr per day.[174]

Absorption, Transport, Metabolism, and Excretion

Intestinal absorption of Cr^{3+} is low, ranging from 0.4% to 2.5%, so fecal output is mainly unabsorbed dietary chromium. Absorption is increased marginally by ascorbic acid, amino acids, oxalate, and other dietary factors. After absorption, chromium binds to plasma transferrin with an affinity similar to that of iron.[231] It then concentrates in human liver, spleen, other soft tissue, and bone.[333] Urine chromium output is around 0.2 to 0.3 μg/day, the amount excreted being to some extent dependent upon intake. Paradoxically, urine output appears to be relatively increased at low dietary levels. Thus 2% is lost in urine at an intake of 10 μg/day, but only 0.5% at an intake of 40 μg/day.[14] Both running and resistive exercise increases urine chromium excretion.[15,481]

Functions

Severely chromium-deficient rats have impaired growth, reduced lifespan, corneal lesions, and alterations in carbohydrate, lipid, and protein metabolism. Supplementation with inorganic chromium restored glucose tolerance in these animals. Repetition of laboratory studies on experimental animals by other groups gave inconsistent results. Claims of benefits from chromium supplementation in diabetic patients, the elderly, and malnourished children were published but also not confirmed by others. It was later realized that analytical methods for chromium determination used in some of the earlier studies were orders of magnitude too high because of contamination of samples before analysis. Also, ineffective background optical correction was used in the graphite furnace AAS systems then available.[217,596] However, many of the important biological observations made in those early investigations have since been confirmed using more accurate analytical techniques.[381]

The biochemical mechanism that allows chromium to potentiate the actions of insulin receptors on cell membranes has been intensively investigated.[603] It is now suggested that a low molecular weight intracellular octapeptide (LMWCr), also known as chromodulin, binds Cr^{3+} and enhances the response of insulin receptors. Chromodulin binds four Cr^{3+} ions and then locates on cell membranes near to the site of insulin receptors. The structure of chromodulin has been examined by a variety of advanced spectroscopic techniques and the complex shown to possess a unique type of multinuclear assembly, with the chromium centers having an octahedral coordination with oxygen-based ligands.[278]

Chromodulin, first described in the 1980s, has been isolated from liver, kidney, and other tissues in several species of experimental animals. Its proposed mode of action is (1) the inactive insulin receptors on cell membranes are converted to an active form by binding circulating insulin; (2) this binding stimulates the movement into cells of chromium bound to plasma transferrin; (3) chromium then binds to apoLMWCr, converting it to an active form that then binds to the insulin receptors and potentiates kinase activity; (4) as plasma glucose and insulin fall to normoglycemic levels, the LMWCr factor is released from the cell to terminate its effects. It is thought that the released chromodulin is the naturally occurring form of chromium in urine.[111]

Requirements and Reference Nutrient Intakes

Because there has not been sufficient evidence to set an estimated average requirement (EAR), an AI based on estimated intakes has been set at 35 μg Cr per day for men and 25 μg Cr per day for women. No tolerable upper limit was set for dietary Cr^{3+} intake.[174]

Intravenous Supply

It is now advised that patients on short-term TPN (<1 to 3 months) receive 10 to 20 μg Cr per day. Those on long-term TPN who are clinically and biochemically stable may be receiving enough chromium via contamination of their nutrients.[11]

Commercial multielement intravenous additives will usually contain about 10 to 30 μg Cr. When high concentrations of glucose (20% to 50%) are given intravenously as the main energy source, increased losses of chromium in urine may occur. Urinary losses could be monitored (although this is rarely done) and input increased especially if signs of unexplained glucose intolerance are seen. However, there also have been reports that excessive amounts of chromium may have been given to children and adults during TPN, with possible detrimental effects on renal function.[221,329]

Deficiency

Clinical signs of human chromium deficiency were first clearly described in patients receiving parenteral nutrition for a prolonged period using a nutritional regimen that did not supply sufficient chromium.[11] Only a few case histories been have published.[81,184,284] All had similar presentations, with previously stable patients developing insulin-resistant glucose intolerance, weight loss, and in some cases neurological deficits. Addition of substantial amounts of Cr^{3+} to the intravenous regimen (150 to 200 μg/day) reversed glucose intolerance and reduced insulin requirements with eventual improvement in the neurological disorders.

It was later noted that a patient on TPN who developed glucose intolerance and neuropathy also had been receiving metronidazole. Baseline serum chromium concentrations were seemingly increased. Yet treatment with 250 μg chromium chloride intravenously for 2 weeks resulted in rapid clinical remission, and normal nerve conduction was restored within 3 weeks.[600]

These cases, although rare, influenced the U.S. Food and Nutrition Board to designate chromium as an essential trace element.[174] It is not clear why there have been so few cases of clinical chromium deficiency in comparison with zinc, copper, and selenium, but this might relate to chromium contamination of infusion fluids, especially in the amino acid mixture.[520]

Clinical Significance

Chromium is thought to play a role in impaired glucose tolerance, diabetes, and cardiovascular disease.

Impaired Glucose Tolerance and Diabetes. More than 15% of adults aged 40 to 74 are thought to have impaired glucose tolerance and it has been suggested that poor chromium nutritional status may be a factor.[174] However, the variability of dietary chromium intake and the lack of an easily usable laboratory or clinical marker to identify those patients with poor chromium status create difficulties. A metaanalysis investigated 15 randomized controlled trials that reported adequate data on the effect of chromium on glucose, insulin, and glycated Hb A_{1c}. Of the 618 participants, 193 had type 2 diabetes and 425 of the subjects were either in good health or had only impaired glucose tolerance.[8] The authors concluded that there was no effect from chromium on glucose or insulin in nondiabetic participants and that the data for persons with diabetes are inconclusive. Consequently, large scale trials are required.

A controlled trial of higher doses (250 µg and 1000 µg of chromium) as chromium picolinate was conducted in China on 180 type 2 diabetic subjects. This trial did find improvements in glucose handling and reduction in glycosylated hemoglobin.[13] Benefit was also found in previous studies on populations of malnourished children in Jordan, Nigeria, and Turkey. It is possible that other interacting dietary depletions may aggravate chromium deficiency in these populations.[382]

It has now been suggested that short-term dosage of <1000 µg Cr per day may be a useful additional treatment for type 2 diabetes. Monitoring of kidney function and clinical assessment of any dermatological changes are advised.[485] Anderson maintains that chromium supplementation has been shown to improve glucose handling in all the main types of diabetes.[12] The dosages used suggest a pharmacological role for chromium and potential toxicity has to be considered and therapeutic benefit.[283] Chromium therapy in the control and prevention of diabetes is therefore of considerable interest and the subject of much controversy.[293]

Glucose Intolerance in the Elderly. Glucose intolerance is age related and chromium supplementation trials in the elderly have been conducted with variable results.[430] The inability to determine which of the elderly trial subjects was initially chromium depleted makes it difficult to interpret the findings. If the observations can be confirmed and there is an age-related decrease in the chromium concentration in hair, sweat, and blood serum, then there is a necessity for further studies in the elderly.[125]

Cardiovascular Disease. Chromium depletion has long been thought to be associated with an increased cardiovascular risk.[379,504] A double-blind 12-week study of 23 healthy adult men showed that 200 µg chromium (as chromium chloride) increased HDL cholesterol and decreased insulin levels.[465] Other reports of favorable lipid responses to chromium supplementation have also been published.[2,244] Abnormal lipid profiles are found in patients with type 2 diabetes and may be associated with an increased risk of cardiovascular disease. However, additional larger-scale studies are necessary to confirm the effects of chromium on risk factors for cardiovascular disease.[430]

Toxicity

Hexavalent chromium (6^+) is a recognized carcinogen, and industrial exposure to fumes and dusts containing this metal is associated with increased incidence of lung cancer, dermatitis, and skin ulcers. Environmental health risks arise from soil contamination by Cr^{6+} waste disposal sites left by the leather tanning and dyestuff industries.[587] Cr^{6+} is more efficiently absorbed than Cr^{3+} and its toxicity and carcinogenic effects involve reduction to $Cr^{5+}$and Cr^{3+} by cysteine, with the formation of intracellular DNA adducts.[638] Cr^{3+}species are relatively nontoxic partly because of their poor intestinal absorption and rapid excretion in urine.

However, chromium picolinate is a widely used dietary supplement and this compound has been reported to cause renal and hepatic damage when used at high doses.[100] Patients with preexisting renal or liver disease may be at particular risk from adverse effects. Vincent[604] has found that chromium picolinate has a different intracellular pathway from other forms of Cr^{3+}. There may be benefits from chromium picolinate in relation to diabetes control,[13] but the claims that this supplement can promote body fat loss and muscle mass gain have not been substantiated.[604]

Laboratory Assessment of Status

A beneficial response of glucose-intolerant patients to chromium supplementation is presently the only means of confirming chromium deficiency. No practicable method of assessing intracellular chromium depletion is yet available and there is no consistently reliable animal model for chromium deficiency. Furthermore, it has been known from early animal experiments that circulating chromium is not in equilibrium with physiologically important reserves.[381] It has been shown in late pregnancy that serum chromium concentration does not correlate with glucose intolerance, insulin resistance, or serum lipids.[216]

A possibly useful test has been proposed that uses radioactive $^{51}Cr^{6+}$ to label red cells. The ion is then reduced to Cr^{3+} and the amount bound to cell membranes is dependent upon the initial amount of Cr^{3+} present, which in turn is a reflection of the adequacy of chromium nutritional status. The test was applied to 25 type 2 diabetes patients and 35 controls. No difference was found, and it was concluded that chromium nutrition has only a minor role in this condition.[615]

Direct determination of chromium in diet, in oral and intravenous nutritional support regimens, and in blood plasma or serum can only be carried out if great care is taken to prevent contamination before and during analysis.[430] Sample collection procedures have to avoid any contact with stainless steel, so all-plastic phlebotomy systems or siliconized steel needles should be used, and samples should be stored in acid washed containers. Acid digestion of diet samples in sealed pressure vessels using microwave heating may be necessary to reduce background effects and also to prevent losses of volatile chromium compounds. Specialist trace element laboratories employing ICP-MS and stable chromium isotopes[602] now offer improved analytical sensitivity and allow tracer methods for metabolic studies.[436]

The detection of increased amounts of chromium in urine is a confirmation of recent occupational or environmental exposure to excess chromium. It also may be useful to monitor urine chromium in trials that use pharmacological dosages of chromium, both to confirm compliance and to detect potential toxicity. This is possible using available graphite furnace AAS instrumentation.[217,225]

Reference Values

Very low values are now considered as normal for serum (0.1 to 0.2 µg/L, 2 to 3 nmol/L) and for urine <0.2 µg Cr per L (<3 nmol/L). Thus the detection of deficiency by direct analysis is difficult.[430,596]

Cobalt

Cobalt (Co) is essential for humans only as an integral part of vitamin B_{12} (cobalamin). No other function for cobalt in the human body is known. Details of vitamin B_{12} biochemistry and function are discussed above. Microflora of the human intestine cannot use cobalt to synthesize physiologically active cobalamin. The human vitamin B_{12} requirement must be supplied by the diet. Free (nonvitamin B_{12}) cobalt does not interact with the body vitamin B_{12} pool.

Copper

Copper (Cu) is an important trace element and is associated with a number of metalloproteins. It is present in biological systems in both the 1^+ and 2^+ valence states.

Chemistry

Copper (atomic number 29, atomic weight 63.54) has Cu^{1+} and Cu^{2+} oxidation states in biological systems; the facile exchange between these ions gives the element important redox properties. Because of their high electron affinities, these ions are the most strongly bound to organic molecules of all the essential trace metals. Copper in biological material is complexed with proteins, peptides, and other organic ligands. An elaborate series of binding and transport proteins inside cells protects the genome from copper-generated free radical attack.[336] This keeps the concentration of free copper in the cytoplasm very low (around 10^{-15} mol/L.) Copper bioinorganic chemistry evolved concurrently with that of molecular oxygen. Numerous blue-colored copper-containing proteins, most of which are oxidases, are located outside the cytoplasm on the surface of cell membranes or in vesicles. However, the copper metalloenzyme superoxide dismutase (SOD) protects against random free radical damage both in the cytoplasm and in blood plasma. Paradoxically, it was the ability of copper ions to generate free radicals that led to the evolutionary development of the extracellular matrix by polymerization and cross-linking of low molecular weight substrates. This allowed the formation of collagen, chitin, and other structural proteins essential for the development of multicellular life forms.[180]

Dietary Sources

The copper content of food is variable and can be affected by applications to crops of copper-containing fertilizers and fungicidal sprays. Also the use of copper-containing cooking vessels contributes to total intake. The metal is most plentiful in organ meats, such as liver and kidney, with relatively high amounts also being found in shellfish, nuts, whole grain cereals, bran, and all cocoa-containing products. Lower amounts of copper are found in white meats and in dairy products, especially cow's milk. The median intake of copper in the United States is around 1.0 to 1.6 mg/day.[174]

Absorption, Transport, Metabolism, and Excretion

Copper absorption mainly occurs in the small intestine, although gastric uptake has been shown to occur to a smaller extent. Some copper may also be incorporated by inhalation and skin absorption. The extent of intestinal copper absorption varies with dietary copper content and is around 50% at low copper intakes (<1 mg Cu per day) but only 20% at higher intakes (>5 mg Cu per day).[580] Copper intestinal uptake is pH dependent and relatively efficient. Absorption is reduced by other dietary components, such as zinc (via metallothionein), molybdate, and iron, and increased by amino acids and by dietary sodium.[230]

Absorbed copper is transported to the liver in portal blood bound to albumin, where it is incorporated by the hepatocytes into cuproenzymes and other proteins and then exported in peripheral blood to tissue and organs. Although two thirds of the 80 to 100 mg total body copper content is located in the skeleton and muscle, the liver is the key organ in copper homeostasis.[580] More than 90% of the copper exported from the liver into peripheral blood is in the form of the glycoprotein ceruloplasmin, which has a blue color when separated from other plasma proteins. Its structure can be studied by electron paramagnetic resonance spectroscopy and other spectroscopic techniques.[355] It is a positive acute phase reactant and increases during infection and after tissue injury. Ceruloplasmin also increases in pregnancy and during use of oral contraceptives, leading to a rise in serum copper concentration. A smaller amount of copper in plasma (<10%) is bound to albumin by specific peptide sequences and this copper is in equilibrium with plasma amino acids. This fraction may be important for cellular uptake.

An overview of copper metabolism is illustrated in Figure 30-26.[230]

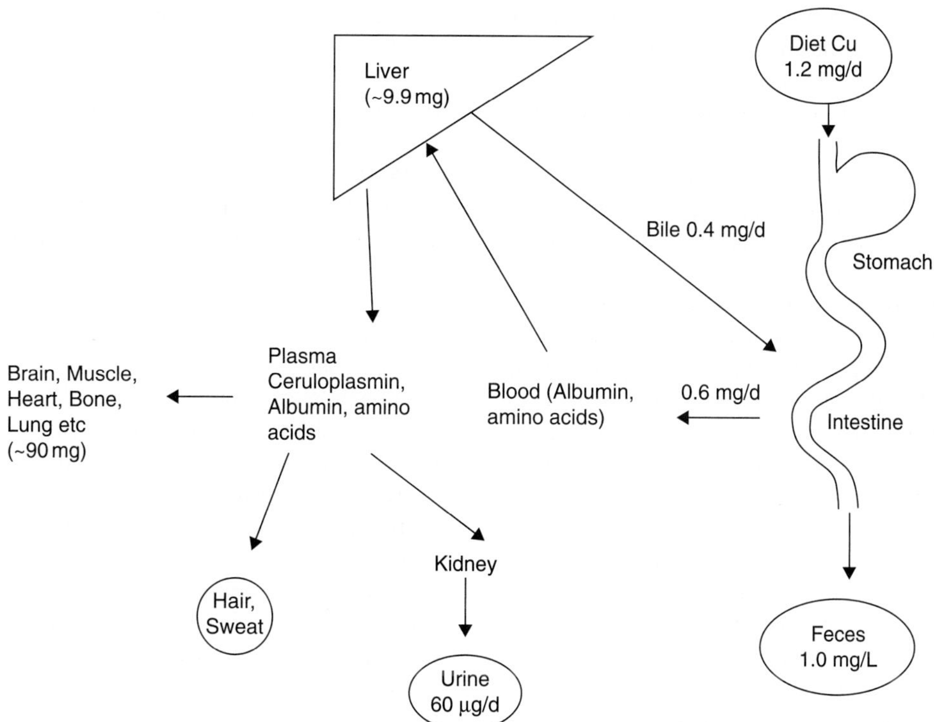

Figure 30-26 Metabolism of copper. *(Modified from Harris ED. Copper. In: O'Dell BL, Sunde RA, eds. Handbook of nutritionally essential mineral elements. New York: Marcel Dekker, 1997:231-73.)*

Between 0.5 and 2.0 mg of copper per day is excreted via bile into feces. Patients with cholestatic jaundice or other forms of liver dysfunction are therefore at risk of copper accumulation caused by failure of excretion. Copper losses in urine and sweat are <3% of dietary intake. Urine copper output is normally less than 60 μg/day.

Functions

Copper is a catalytic component of numerous enzymes and is also a structural component of other important proteins in humans, animals, plants, and microorganisms.[180,230,337] Some of those considered of potential importance in human biochemistry are briefly described below.

Energy Production. Cytochrome c oxidase is a multi-subunit complex containing copper and iron. Located on the external face of mitochondrial membranes, the enzyme catalyzes a four-electron reduction of molecular oxygen, establishing a high-energy proton gradient across the inner mitochondrial membrane, which is necessary for ATP production. Cytochrome c and cytochrome c oxidase are essential for oxidative phosphorylation that is the basis of intracellular energy production.

Connective Tissue Formation. Protein-lysine 6-oxidase (lysyl oxidase) is a cuproenzyme that is essential for stabilization of extracellular matrixes, specifically the enzymatic cross-linking of collagen and elastin. Complex mechanisms involve the deamination of lysine and hydrolysine residues at specific extracellular sites. The enzyme is highly associated with connective tissue and located in the aorta, dermal connective tissue, fibroblasts, and the cytoskeleton of many other cells.

Iron Metabolism. Copper-containing enzymes—namely ferroxidase I (ceruloplasmin) and ferroxidase II, and the recently described hephaestin in the enterocyte—oxidize ferrous iron to ferric iron. This allows incorporation of Fe^{3+} into transferrin and eventually into hemoglobin. Ferroxidase II is a yellow protein, the importance of which in iron metabolism is not as well characterized as that of ceruloplasmin.

Central Nervous System. Dopamine monooxygenase (DMO) is an enzyme that requires copper as a cofactor and uses ascorbate as an electron donor. This enzyme catalyzes the conversion of dopamine to norepinephrine, the important neurotransmitter. There are soluble and membrane-bound forms of the enzyme, the latter being found in the chromaffin granules of the adrenal cortex. Monoamine oxidase, one of the numerous amine oxidases, is a copper-containing enzyme that catalyzes the degradation of serotonin in the brain and is also involved in the metabolism of the catecholamines.

The formation of the phospholipids necessary for myelin sheath formation is affected by cytochrome c oxidase depletion. It is now known that the prion protein (PrP) binds Cu II and may be involved in copper regulation within the brain.[86]

Melanin Synthesis. Tyrosinase is a copper-containing enzyme that is present in melanocytes and catalyzes the synthesis of melanin. Starting with L-dopa as a substrate, tyrosinase catalyzes multiple oxidative steps to produce the melanin biopigments pheomelanin and eumelanin.

Antioxidant Functions. Both intracellular and extracellular SODs are copper- and zinc-containing enzymes, able to convert superoxide radicals to hydrogen peroxide, which can be subsequently removed by catalase and other antioxidant defenses. The plasma protein ceruloplasmin also binds copper ions and thus prevents oxidative damage from free copper ions, which can generate hydroxyl radicals.

Regulation of Gene Expression and Intracellular Copper Handling. Copper-dependent proteins act as transcription factors for specific genes, such as those regulating SOD and catalase. Metallothionein synthesis is controlled by copper-responsive transcription factors, and this protein is important in regulating the intracellular distribution of copper.[581] Additional specialized proteins act as "copper chaperones" to deliver copper to intracellular sites and prevent oxidative damage by free copper ions.[162]

Inborn Errors of Copper Metabolism. Menkes' syndrome is caused by a defective gene that regulates the metabolism of copper in the body. Wilson's disease is inherited as an autosomal recessive trait having a defect in the metabolism of copper, with accumulation of copper in the liver, brain, kidney, cornea, and other tissues. Investigation of these rare genetic defects has been of great value in uncovering details of the control of copper transport. Copper-transporting P-type ATPases, known as ATP7A and ATP7B, are essential factors in maintaining copper balance.[120,617] Impaired intestinal transport of copper caused by a mutation in the ATP7A gene leads to the severe copper deficiency disease seen in Menkes' syndrome. Defects in the ATP7B gene affect both incorporation of copper into ceruloplasmin and copper excretion via bile. This results in a toxic accumulation of copper and is the basis of Wilson's disease.

Another genetic defect results in failure of hepatic synthesis of ceruloplasmin (aceruloplasminemia), which is a neurodegenerative disease. Retinal damage, secondary iron overload, and insulin-dependent diabetes present in the fourth to fifth decade of life.[232,242]

Requirements and Reference Nutrient Intakes

The recommended dietary intake for adults is 0.9 mg/day. This is close to the lower limit of 1.0 mg/day found in dietary surveys and has led to suggestions that marginal copper depletion could be found in the U.S. population.[309] The tolerable upper limit is 10 mg/day.[174]

Intravenous Supply

The usual adult supply of copper intravenously varies from 0.3 to 1.3 mg/day (5 to 20 µmol/day), the higher amounts being required in those patients with preexisting depletion or biliary losses and lower amounts in those with cholestasis.

Deficiency

Malnourished Infants. When malnourished infants with a history of chronic diarrhea were rehabilitated using a formula based upon cow's milk, they developed an iron-resistant anemia, neutropenia, and other hematological disorders and bone lesions.[118] Copper supplementation of milk feeds reversed these abnormalities and addition of 2.5 mg Cu per day is now advised.[118]

Premature Infants. Most of the accumulation of copper in the fetal liver occurs in the last 3 months of pregnancy, and premature infants fed formula lacking sufficient copper are at risk of deficiency disease since they lack adequate liver copper stores. Hematological abnormalities and easily fractured brittle bones have been described.[345] The radiographic changes in infants with copper deficiency include osteopenia and metaphyseal spurs.[214] As noted above, formulas based on cow's milk require copper supplementation. Monitoring of plasma copper is advisable and results should be related to postnatal age; at 4 weeks mean values are 42 µg/dL (6.6 µmol/L), rising to 55 µg/dL (8.7 µmol/L) by 14 weeks.[87]

Nutritional Support. Adults and children fed intravenously without addition of sufficient copper to the nutrient regimen develop symptomatic copper deficiency. The hematological changes of hypochromic anemia and neutropenia are reversed by copper supplementation.[189,190] Similar effects have been reported during prolonged enteral feeding via jejunostomy.[89] Children may also develop the typical bone changes mentioned above.

Menkes' Syndrome. The history and aspects of the diagnosis and therapy of this condition have been reviewed.[291] It is a rare condition (1/100,000 live births), the mutation is X-linked, and typically occurs in male infants at 2 to 3 months. They present with loss of previously normal development, hypotonia, seizures, and failure to thrive. Physical changes in the hair (pili torti), in facial appearance, and neurological abnormalities suggest the diagnosis. Low levels of copper in plasma, liver, and brain occur because of impaired intestinal copper absorption. Local first line tests would be finding plasma copper of <10 µmol/L, ceruloplasmin <220 mg/L, and demonstration of pili torti by microscopic examination of hair. Further tests can demonstrate failure of isotopic copper egress from cultured fibroblasts and show plasma catecholamine abnormalities. Placental copper measurement and direct mutation analysis are additional investigative procedures. Deficiency of the copper enzyme DMO in CSF is thought to be an important finding that allows early diagnosis. The effectiveness of therapy with parenteral copper histidine is debatable, although success has been claimed in less severely affected cases, especially if treatment is started early.[108]

Malabsorption Syndromes. Patients at risk include those with celiac disease, tropical sprue, cystic fibrosis, and short bowel syndrome. Excessive intake of oral zinc supplements can cause anemia and hematological abnormalities in the absence of occult blood loss.[218,263] The copper deficiency is caused by zinc induction of metallothionein in the intestinal mucosa, which then sequesters dietary copper, blocking its absorption.

Cardiovascular Disease. Animal studies show that severe copper deficiency causes cardiac damage, but the abnormality differs from that seen in human cardiovascular disease. The myocardium is hypertrophied and may rupture in animal models. Coronary artery pressure is decreased, but in human ischemic disease it is increased.[124] The role of copper in human cardiovascular disease is controversial, although much supporting evidence for a positive link with low dietary copper intake has been published.[309]

Epidemiological surveys have also shown that increased plasma copper values are a positive cardiovascular risk factor. A U.S. study of 4400 adult men and women found that those with plasma copper values in the two highest quartiles had the greatest risk of dying from cardiovascular disease.[176] An increase in plasma ceruloplasmin and hence plasma copper may be a nonspecific response to the inflammation of arteries found in arteriosclerosis. It is known that the ceruloplasmin hepatic messenger RNA (mRNA) increases during inflammation and that this is induced by interleukin 6. Insulin is now also known to be involved in the transcriptional regulation of ceruloplasmin synthesis.[199,514]

Toxicity

As mentioned above, Wilson's disease is a genetic disorder of copper metabolism that causes an increase in copper to toxic levels.[152,203] The problems of diagnosis and appropriate laboratory investigations have been reviewed.[159,192]

The incidence of Wilson's disease is estimated to be 1/30,000 live births with a carrier frequency of 1/90 in the general population. The presentation is highly variable, so adolescents or young adults with otherwise unexplained liver disease or neurological symptoms should be screened, especially where there is a family history of suspected Wilson's disease. Initial local investigations would include plasma copper and ceruloplasmin, which will usually be low (less than 50 µg/dL, 8 µmol Cu per L, and less than 200 mg/L ceruloplasmin). Although the total plasma copper is decreased, the nonceruloplasmin bound fraction is increased, allowing deposition of copper in the brain, eyes, and kidneys.

Slit lamp eye examination may detect copper deposits in the eye (Kayser-Fleischer rings) and there may be abnormalities in liver function tests with an increased urine copper output (>500 µg Cu per L). Liver biopsy for copper analysis is useful in suspected cases and results above 250 µg/g Cu dry weight are usually found (normal 8 to 40 µg Cu per g dry weight). Failure of copper incorporation into plasma ceruloplasmin can also be demonstrated using an oral dose of stable ^{65}Cu isotope.[354] This may be helpful in excluding Wilson's disease when other tests are equivocal. Gene tracking and mutation detection are now possible, but since several hundred mutations exist this may not be informative.

Diagnosis can be difficult in the Wilson's disease cases presenting with acute liver failure.[490,544] Prompt diagnosis is important since urgent liver transplantation may be required.[498] In these cases, a greatly increased plasma copper will be found but without an appropriately increased ceruloplasmin. The unbound plasma copper fraction can increase to more than 80% of the total plasma copper (normal 5% to 10%). The excess copper is released from the necrotic liver and causes intravascular hemolysis and renal failure.[429]

The chronic form of Wilson's disease is treated by oral chelating agents, such as penicillamine and trientine, that remove excess copper from tissue and increase urine copper excretion.[609] Oral administration of zinc salts or ammonium molybdate, which block copper intestinal absorption, has also been successful.[73]

Toxicity can also arise directly from copper contamination of diet and water supplies. Acute poisoning has been recorded following accidental or intentional ingestion of copper sulfate. Guidelines for the maximum copper content of drinking water have been suggested and they vary from about 1 to 3 mg Cu per L. Children may be genetically sensitive to copper in drinking water and develop chronic liver disease,[405] as is found in Indian children exposed to a copper-contaminated diet.[557] Environmental aspects of copper toxicity and the impact upon human health have been reviewed.[147,169]

Laboratory Assessment of Status

Several well-controlled dietary deprivation studies have demonstrated the utility of the clinical laboratory in providing measures of copper status. For example, plasma copper and ceruloplasmin assays are convenient and widely used to confirm severe copper deficiency. However, they are not sensitive indicators in marginal copper depletion.

Since about 90% of plasma copper is bound to ceruloplasmin, factors that increase the hepatic synthesis of ceruloplasmin, such as an APR or the oral contraceptive pill, will increase plasma copper independently of dietary copper intake.[199] In premature infants with liver immaturity and low ceruloplasmin synthesis, plasma copper values below 30 µg/L (<5 µmol Cu per L) suggest the necessity for increased copper input.

Dietary depletion studies using low copper diets have demonstrated a decrease in plasma copper and then a return upon dietary supplementation; however, plasma copper values remained largely within the reference interval.[580] It is suggested that the ratio of immunologically to enzymatically measured ceruloplasmin may be a useful index of marginal copper depletion. This ratio, which is the specific activity of ceruloplasmin, will be low in marginal copper depletion. Apoceruloplasmin increases in blood serum during copper depletion and this will contribute to the total ceruloplasmin assay. The enzymatic activity decreases even in marginal copper depletion. The specific activity of ceruloplasmin is therefore sensitive to copper status and is not affected by age, sex, or hormonal influences.[390] In a study of copper depletion, a low copper diet (0.57 mg/day) was fed to 12 post menopausal women for 35 days followed by supplementation for 35 days (2 mg/day).[391] Responsive markers were red cell SOD, platelet cytochrome oxidase, red cell glutathione peroxidase, and clotting factor VIII. Although of potential value for detecting marginal copper depletion, these measurements are not in widespread use because of sample instability and lack of standardized methods.[390]

Urine copper decreases during dietary deprivation, but the change from an already low basal value is small, and difficulties in reliable collection and with sample contamination make this of limited use.

Clinically, copper status should therefore be investigated initially by measurement of serum copper and assessment of the APR and interpreted in the light of clinical and drug information.

Reference Intervals

For adults plasma copper is usually in the interval 70 to 140 μg/dL (10 to 22 μmol/L). Values in women of childbearing age and especially in pregnancy are higher. For adults a plasma copper below 50 μg/dL (8 μmo/L) and for infants below 30 μg/dL (5 μmol/L) indicates probable copper depletion. Urine copper output is normally less than 60 μg/24 hr (<1.0 μmol/24 hr) and values above 200 μg/24 hr (3 μmo/L) are found in Wilson's disease. A copper concentration in a liver biopsy sample of >250 μg Cu per g dry weight (normally 8 to 40 μg/g dry weight) is indicative of Wilson's disease, in the absence of other causes of cholestatic disease.

Manganese

Manganese (Mn) is present in biological systems bound to protein in either the 2^+ or 3^+ valence state. It is associated mainly with the formation of connective and bony tissue, with growth and reproductive functions, and with carbohydrate and lipid metabolism.

Chemistry

Manganese (atomic number 25, atomic weight 54.94) is a first transition series metal ($3d^5s^2$) and is next to iron in the periodic table. Of the 11 oxidation states available chemically to manganese, only Mn^{2+} and Mn^{3+} are found in biological systems, mostly bound to protein. The Mn^{2+} ion with an unpaired electron is paramagnetic and can be detected in tissue by magnetic resonance imaging. The bioinorganic chemistry of manganese is complex and detailed accounts have been published.[180,322]

Dietary Sources

Manganese-rich sources include whole grain foods, nuts, leafy vegetables, soy products, and teas. Average intake in the United States is about 2 mg/day, with median values for adult men being 2.2 mg/day, range 0.3 to 8.3 mg/day; and for women median 1.8 mg/day, range 0.3 to 5.9 mg/day (NHANES III). Vegetarian diets containing high amounts of whole grains and nuts can supply more than 10 mg/day.[174]

Absorption, Transport, Metabolism, and Excretion

Dietary manganese is absorbed from the small intestine by mechanisms that may have a pathway common to that of iron. Manganese absorption increases at low dietary intakes and decreases at higher intakes, with tracer studies suggesting absorption efficiencies of 2% to 15%. Diets high in iron, calcium, magnesium, phosphates, fiber, phytic acid, oxalate, and tannins from tea can reduce the absorption of manganese.

Once absorbed, manganese is transported in portal blood to the liver bound to albumin and then exported to other tissue bound to transferrin and possibly to α_2 macroglobulin. Excretion of manganese is primarily via bile into feces, with urine output being very low and not sensitive to dietary intake.[322]

Functions

Manganese is a constituent of many important metalloenzymes and also acts as a nonspecific enzyme activator. Mn^{2+} ions can be replaced by Mg^{2+}, Co^{2+}, and other cations during the activation of some enzymes.[322] Some important manganese-dependent enzymes are discussed below.

Superoxide Dismutase (SOD). Manganese-dependent SOD is a mitochondrial enzyme and is an important factor in limiting oxygen toxicity; it is one of the most studied enzymes in human biochemistry. The enzyme catalyzes the breakdown of the superoxide radical O_2^- to H_2O_2, which is then removed by catalase and glutathione peroxidase. The half-life of this enzyme in blood serum is longer than that of the cytoplasmic Cu, Zn SOD.

Pyruvate Carboxylase. This enzyme has manganese firmly in its structure and acts together with phosphoenol pyruvate (PEP) carboxykinase, an enzyme that is activated by manganese ions. These enzymes are required to catalyze the formation of PEP from pyruvate, a key reaction in the hepatic synthesis of glucose.

Arginase. Arginase is the terminal enzyme in the urea cycle, hydrolyzing L-arginine to urea and ornithine, completing the deamination of amino acids. Arginase is most concentrated in the liver, but is also found in other tissues. The structure of the enzyme isolated from rat liver shows it to have a unique binuclear manganese cluster.[296] The activity of arginase affects the production of nitric oxide by limiting the availability of L-arginine required for the synthesis of nitric oxide synthetase. This relationship has been investigated in a number of diverse diseases, including asthma and schizophrenia.[383,630]

Glycosyl Transferases. These enzymes are responsible for the sequential addition of carbohydrate molecules to proteins to form proteoglycans, and ultimately connective tissue and cartilage. They are therefore important for the structural integrity of bone and skin, and for normal wound healing.

Requirements and Reference Nutrient Intakes

Because of lack of information on manganese dietary requirements, the Food and Nutrition Board has set an AI level for adults at 2.3 mg/day for males and 1.8 mg/day for females. A tolerable upper intake limit of 11 mg/day was set for adults based on no observed effect for

Western diets. For infants the UL could not be set because of lack of data. There is concern about the potential toxicity of manganese for infants whose immature hepatic development reduces the biliary excretion of excess manganese. Therefore, the only dietary source of manganese in the age group 0 to 12 months should be from normal diet or from a formula.[174]

Deficiency

Overt manganese deficiency has not been documented in humans eating natural diets. However, in numerous animal studies, signs of experimentally induced manganese deficiency include impaired growth and reproductive function, skeletal abnormalities, impaired glucose tolerance, and impaired cholesterol synthesis.[322] A child on long-term TPN lacking in manganese developed signs of bone demineralization and impaired growth that were reversed by supplementation.[422] A volunteer male was deprived of vitamin K and inadvertently of manganese when fed a diet with only 0.34 mg Mn per day for 6.5 months. Effects included a low plasma cholesterol, dermatitis, color changes in hair, and reduced blood-clotting function not responsive to vitamin K. Supplementation with manganese gradually reversed these symptoms.[137] Seven young men fed experimental diets low in manganese developed skin lesions and low plasma cholesterol.[185]

Prolidase deficiency in infants is a rare genetic disorder that causes (1) skin ulceration, (2) mental retardation, (3) increased urinary excretion of iminodipeptides, (4) recurrent infections, and (5) splenomegaly; it is known to be associated with abnormalities of manganese biochemistry. Red cells have an increased amount of manganese although serum manganese is normal. Red cell arginase activity is less than half of normal, suggesting a defect in the supply of manganese for enzyme activation.[343,346]

Various unrelated medical conditions have been observed to be associated with lowered serum or whole blood manganese. These include osteoporosis, diabetes mellitus, and epilepsy.[247] The clinical relevance of such observations is uncertain.

Toxicity

The occupational health hazard from prolonged exposure to manganese-containing dust or fumes is well recognized (see Chapter 35). Neurological symptoms resembling Parkinson's disease develop slowly over a period of months or years. The health risks from long-term, low-level manganese exposure have been reviewed.[208]

Of concern is the possibility that patients with severe liver disease may have neurological and behavioral signs of manganese neurotoxicity because of failure to excrete manganese in bile. Manganese deposition in the globus pallidus during liver failure results in T_1-weighted magnetic resonance signal hypersensitivity. By causing deficits in neurotransmitter production, manganese ions may be partially responsible for the symptoms of postsystemic hepatic encephalopathy.[238] Deposition of manganese in the brain has been demonstrated in children with biliary atresia[264] and in adult cirrhotic patients.[541]

Patients receiving manganese intravenously during TPN have also shown evidence of manganese retention and deposition in the midbrain and brainstem, especially those with cholestasis. Typical symptoms are of a parkinsonian-like tremor and abnormalities of gait.[144] Children have also been observed to accumulate manganese in the globus pallidus and brainstem, although with nonspecific symptoms.[433] A study on adults compared the effects of increasing doses of manganese of 0, 1, 2, and 20 µmol/day in patients receiving home parenteral nutrition.[554] A high correlation was found between blood manganese, magnetic resonance imaging (MRI) intensity, and T_1 values in the globus pallidus. A dose of 1 µmol/day (55 µg/day) caused no abnormalities in MRI measurements and blood manganese remained within the reference interval.

In a study of 30 patients receiving long-term home IV nutrition, whole blood manganese was increased (>3.8 µg/L, 210 nmo/L) in 26 patients and plasma manganese in 23 (>4 µg/L, 23 nmol/L) patients. None of the patients had signs of neurological disease. In a control group of patients with cholestatic disease, but not receiving IVN, whole blood manganese was within the reference interval.[611] This suggests that cholestasis alone will not lead to increased blood manganese, and the main reason for high blood concentrations in patients on IV nutrition is excess provision, with this being made worse if cholestasis also exists. Infants (0 to 12 months) requiring IVN are at particular risk because of immature hepatic function. In a group of 57 children receiving IVN,[154] 11 had both cholestasis and increased blood manganese and one had a movement disorder. Four of these 11 patients died and whole blood manganese was very high (11 to 33.5 µg/L, 615 to 1840 nmol/L) in the 7 survivors. Manganese supplements were reduced or withdrawn, and after 4 months blood manganese had declined to 11.6 µg/L (643 nmol/L). During the same period, serum bilirubin also declined significantly. The long-term outcome of manganese deposition has been investigated in two children on long-term TPN who initially had MRI scan abnormalities and raised whole blood manganese.[290] After reduction of manganese input, they were followed for a 3-year period with improvement in MRI scan abnormalities and a fall in whole blood manganese. No neurological signs were found, and the children developed normally. It is now recommended that only 1 µg Mn per kg (18 nmol/kg) be administered during TPN in infants and no more than 1 to 2 µmol/day (55 to 110 µg/day) in adults.

All patients requiring prolonged IVN, especially those who have cholestasis, should be monitored for evidence of manganese retention.

Laboratory Assessment of Status

There is a necessity to balance the need for adequate manganese nutrition against the potential risk from toxicity.[208] This necessitates monitoring of manganese status in at-risk patients. Whole blood manganese levels are not responsive to dietary depletion, but measurement of serum manganese, lymphocyte Mn SOD activity, and blood arginase are potentially useful when assessing possible nutritional depletion, although these are rarely performed in clinical practice. Whole blood manganese and serum manganese in combination with brain MRI scans and neurological assessment are used to detect excessive exposure. Manganese in whole blood and plasma or serum is determined by standard graphite furnace AAS methods.[390,435]

Plastic cannulae should be used for phlebotomy, and hemolysis should be prevented during sample separation. Whole blood has about 10 times as much manganese as plasma or serum and is not as affected by contamination from steel needles during sample collection. This makes measurement of whole blood manganese the most widely used method in clinical laboratory practice for monitoring manganese status.

Reference Intervals

The reference interval for serum manganese is 0.5 to 1.3 μg/L (9 to 24 nmol/L). The reference interval for whole blood manganese is 5 to 15 μg/L (90 to 270 nmol/L). Increases in serum manganese to >5.4 μg/L (>30 nmol/L) or blood manganese to >20 μg/L (>360 nmol/L) are indices of manganese retention.

Molybdenum

The essential need for molybdenum (Mo) by animals and humans is based on its incorporation into metalloenzymes.

Chemistry

Molybdenum (atomic number 42, atomic weight 95.94) is a metal in the second transition series. The element can have a number of oxidation states but the most stable in biological systems is Mo^{6+} as found in molybdate (MoO_4^{2-}). Molybdenum has the highest atomic number of the essential trace metals. There is a close parallel between molybdenum, tungsten, and vanadium chemistry. Molybdenum enzymes are ecologically vital, facilitating important carbon, nitrogen, and sulfur cycles.[180]

Dietary Sources

Legumes, such as peas, lentils, and beans, are good sources along with grains and nuts, whereas meats, fruits, and many vegetables are relatively poor sources.[174] The average dietary intake is 76 to 109 μg Mo per day for U.S. adults.

Absorption, Transport, Metabolism, and Excretion

Molybdenum is efficiently absorbed over a wide range of dietary intakes mainly as molybdate, although competitive inhibition of absorption by sulfate reduces intestinal uptake. Concentrations in whole blood are about 1.0 μg/L (10 nmol/L) and some 80% to 90% or more of molybdenum in whole blood is bound to red cell proteins. Transport of the smaller amount in blood plasma may involve α_2-macroglobulin.[174] Urine output directly reflects the dietary intake of molybdenum, stable isotope studies at high and low levels of intake indicating renal homeostatic regulation.[579,616]

Functions

Several important mammalian enzymes, such as sulfite oxidase, xanthine dehydrogenase, and aldehyde oxidase, require molybdenum as a cofactor. This organic component is a molybdopterin complex.[307] Sulfite oxidase is probably the most important enzyme in relation to human health. This enzyme catalyzes the last step in the degradation of sulfur amino acids, oxidizing sulfite to sulfate and transferring electrons to cytochrome c. Xanthine dehydrogenase and aldehyde oxidase hydroxylate a number of heterocyclic substances, such as purines, pteridines, and others.[287]

Requirements and Reference Nutrient Intakes

The RDA for Mo has been set at 45 μg Mo per day for adults, which is below the estimated average dietary intake.[174]

Deficiency

Molybdenum deficiency has not been observed in healthy people consuming a normal diet. A single case report[3] described a patient receiving prolonged parenteral nutrition during treatment for severe Crohn's disease who developed an intolerance to intravenous amino acids, especially L-methionine. Clinical signs included tachycardia, visual defects, neurological irritability, and eventually coma. The symptoms improved on discontinuing amino acid infusion. Biochemical abnormalities included high plasma methionine and low plasma uric acid levels. There was an increased urinary sulfite, thiosulfate, and other abnormalities of urinary sulfur output, with a low excretion of uric acid and xanthine metabolites, suggesting defects in sulfite oxidase and xanthine oxidase. Treatment with ammonium molybdate (300 μg/day) improved the clinical and biochemical abnormalities.

The lack of further reports of this nature suggests that for most patients there is sufficient molybdenum present as a contaminant in the TPN fluids. Nonetheless, it is now common to include a small amount of molybdenum (19 μg/day, 0.2 μmol/day) in trace element additive mixtures.

There are also very rare recessive inherited diseases that result from defects in the biosynthesis of molybdenum cofactor; in most cases they result in early childhood death. First symptoms are failure to thrive and seizures; in later stages lens dislocations are noted together with cerebral atrophy. Disease-causing mutations have been located, and the possibility of gene therapy is being investigated.[461,462]

Biochemical diagnosis can be made by detection of excess sulfite in urine using the Merckoquant sulfite dipstick test (Merck KGaA, Darmstadt, Germany). Samples should not be evaluated until at least 10 days after birth and should be tested within 10 minutes of collection. Another type of molybdenum cofactor deficiency can be confirmed by finding a low plasma uric acid. Specialized centers can offer biochemical prenatal diagnosis on chorionic villi samples.[307]

Toxicity

Molybdenum compounds have low toxicity in humans. There are some reports of increased blood uric acid in occupational exposures and also in Armenian populations that have an abnormally high dietary intake (10 to 15 mg Mo per day). A single report of acute toxicity from self-administration of 300 to 800 μg Mo per day was not confirmed by later studies on healthy men given as much as 1500 μg Mo per day for 24 days.[247]

Excess molybdenum intake induces copper deficiency in ruminants by blockading copper absorption through formation of an insoluble thiomolybdate-copper complex. This has suggested the use of ammonium molybdate in the management of Wilson's disease.[73] There is also speculation that the blockade of copper absorption using molybdate may influence new blood vessel formation (angiogenesis) during tumor growth.[72]

Laboratory Assessment of Status

Whole blood and serum or plasma molybdenum concentrations are too low to be used for the detection of deficiency. However, urinary output is responsive to increases or decreases of input. Measuring urate or sulfite in the urine is the most available means of confirming molybdenum cofactor disorders or possible molybdenum deficiency by detecting changes in sulfur and purine metabolism. Until recently only neutron activation analysis (NAA) had sufficient sensitivity to measure molybdenum in biological samples.[602] With the availability of ICP-MS, studies using stable molybdenum isotopes are now possible, and this has been used to investigate absorption and excretion of molybdenum during depletion and repletion studies.[579]

Reference Intervals

There is about 0.5 μg Mo per L (5 nmol/L) in plasma or serum and about 1 μg Mo per L (10 nmol/L) in whole blood.[602] Urine molybdenum values determined by ICP-MS vary from 40 to 60 μg/L, the amount determined being influenced by recent dietary intake.[271]

Selenium

Selenium (Se) is an essential element for humans, being a constituent of the enzyme glutathione peroxidase and believed to be closely associated with vitamin E in its functions.

Chemistry

Selenium (atomic number 34, atomic weight 78.96) is a nonmetal and has several chemical forms and valences. Selenium is in group VI of the periodic table, and therefore it has a bioinorganic chemistry that is related to sulfur.[180,550] The most important biologically active compounds contain selenocysteine, where selenium is substituted for sulfur in cysteine. Now considered to be the twenty-first amino acid, selenocysteine is incorporated into proteins by the specific codon UGA, which was previously thought to be solely a stop codon.[236] Selenomethionine is synthesized by plants but not in animals or humans. Since it is biologically identical to methionine sharing the same metabolic pathways, selenomethionine is nonspecifically incorporated into the general protein pool and is present in major proteins, such as albumin and hemoglobin. Selenium in selenomethionine makes up about half of the total dietary intake and is made available for selenocysteine synthesis when the methionine pathways catabolize selenomethionine. Ingested selenium compounds selenate, selenite, selenocysteine, and selenomethionine are metabolized largely via selenide that may be associated with a chaperone protein before being converted to selenophosphate, which is an important precursor in the synthesis of selenocysteine proteins (Figure 30-27).[550]

Dietary Sources

Selenium enters the food chain mainly as selenomethionine from plants that take the element up from the soil but do not appear to use it. The soil content of selenium is highly variable and can be low in volcanic soils when soluble salts are leached out by ground water. Soils in parts of China and New Zealand are particularly low in selenium. Acid soils, where insoluble selenium complexes can be formed with iron and aluminum, occur in some parts of Europe, resulting in low available soil selenium. The geographical source of plant and animal foodstuffs determines the level of dietary intake. In the United States and Canada, wheat and other cereal products are a good source of selenium; average intakes in North America range from 80 to 220 μg Se per day, whereas in the UK dietary intake is about 30 to 60 μg/day.[30] Intakes in China are as low as 11 μg/day and in New Zealand 28 μg/day.[84]

Absorption, Transport, Metabolism, and Excretion

Intestinal absorption of the various dietary forms of selenium is efficient but is not regulated. The inorganic salts selenite and selenate used as dietary supplements and in food fortification are almost completely absorbed, but much of the selenate ion is rapidly excreted in urine.[179a] Selenium from inorganic salts is more rapidly incorporated into glutathione peroxidase and other selenoproteins than selenium from organic sources containing selenomethionine. However, selenium-enriched yeast containing the organic forms is considered less toxic and is widely used as a dietary supplement.[172]

Whole body selenium is about 15 mg, as estimated by direct tissue analysis and radioisotope techniques, with the tissue concentration of selenium being highest in the kidney and the liver followed by the other organs. Radioisotope-labeled selenium accumulates initially in the liver, kidneys, and lungs. Selenium present in some selenocysteine proteins appears to be a functional reserve. When dietary selenium is limited, synthesis of glutathione peroxidase (GSHP)x-1 is

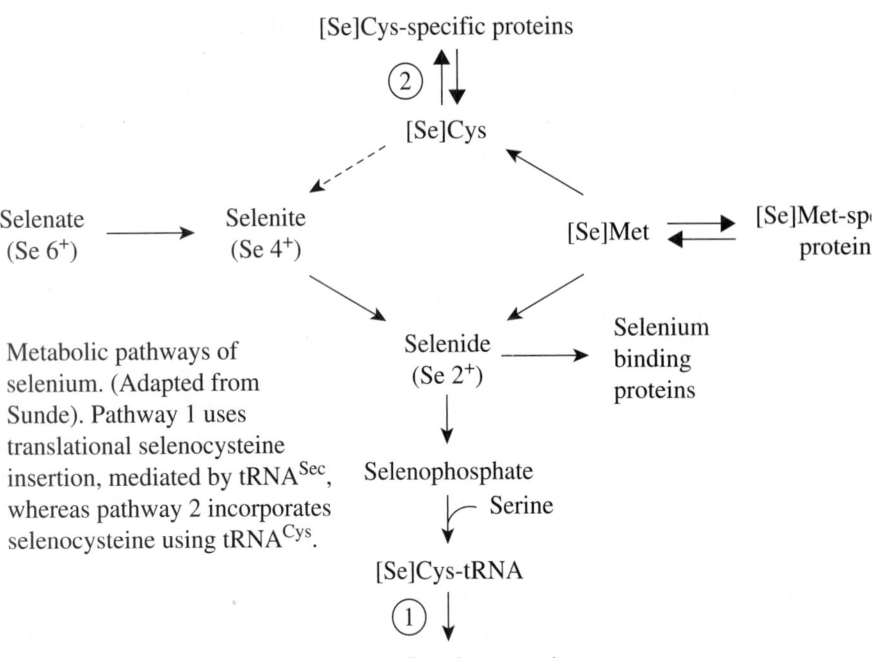

Figure 30-27 Metabolic pathways of selenium.

down regulated, making selenium available for synthesis of other proteins.[172]

The concentrations of selenium in whole blood and in plasma and/or serum are related to dietary intake. About 50% to 60% of the total plasma selenium is present as the protein selenoprotein P, a highly basic protein having multiple histidine residues and about 10 atoms of selenium per molecule.[550] Around 30% of plasma selenium is present as glutathione peroxidase (GSHPx-3) and the remainder is incorporated into albumin as selenomethionine.[234]

Urinary output of selenium is the major route of excretion and reflects recent dietary intake. The amounts excreted vary widely ranging from less than 20 µg Se per L to above 1000 µg Se per L, depending upon the geographical origins of the food.[6]

Functions

Thirty or more biologically active selenocysteine-containing proteins are now identified. More than 15 have been purified and their biological function investigated.[79,550] Some of the most important ones are listed below.

Glutathione Peroxidase (GSHPx). This enzyme has four isoforms, GSHPx-1 in red cells, GSHPx-2 in gastrointestinal mucosa, blood plasma GSHPx-3, and the cell membrane located GSHPx-4. These enzymes use the reducing power of glutathione to remove an oxygen atom from hydrogen peroxide and lipid hydroperoxides. They may also be involved in regulation and formation of arachidonic metabolites derived from hydroperoxides.[18]

Iodothyronine Deiodinase. Type I, II, and III isoforms of this enzyme are responsible for conversion of the precursor hormone T_4 to the active hormone T_3.[79] Type I, thyroxine-5-deiodinase, is located in the liver, kidney, and muscle and is responsible for more than 90% of plasma T_3 production. Pituitary, brain, and brown adipose tissue contain the Type II and III deiodinases.[550]

Thioredoxin Reductases. Three isoforms catalyze the NADPH-dependent reduction of thioredoxin and are important in maintaining the intracellular redox state.

Selenophosphate Synthetase. This enzyme is required for the intracellular synthesis of selenoproteins via a monoselenium phosphate intermediate.

Selenoprotein P. This protein is the major selenium-containing protein in blood plasma, may be a transport protein for the element, and has an antioxidant function.[85]

Selenoprotein W. This is a selenoprotein found in skeletal muscle that is reduced in concentration in white muscle disease in animals.[550] Deficiencies in the production of these selenoproteins, especially the glutathione peroxidases, are likely to be related to signs and symptoms of selenium deficiency disease.

Requirements and Reference Nutrient Intakes

It is now proposed,[172] after review of Chinese and New Zealand supplementation studies, that the RDA for selenium is set at 55 µg/day for adults. On this basis, dietary surveys in North America do not indicate that selenium deficiency is likely in the general population. However, in many countries in Europe, intakes are now close to or below 55 µg/day, and selenium dietary provision may now be suboptimal.[458]

Intravenous Supply

There is uncertainty about the most appropriate intake, but given the above figures for dietary requirement, intravenous requirement is unlikely to be less than 40 μg/day (0.5 μmol/day), and in many adult patients, especially the more seriously ill, it may be 100 μg/day (1.3 μmol/day) or more.

Deficiency

The role of selenium in human medicine has been reviewed.[84,458] Animal studies in the 1950s demonstrated the nutritionally beneficial effects of selenium by showing that there was a selenium-responsive liver necrosis in vitamin E–deficient rats. There are important selenium-dependent diseases in farm animals, such as white muscle disease in sheep and cattle, and myopathy of cardiac and skeletal muscle in lambs and calves. In these animals, some cause of oxidative stress, such as increased physical activity or vitamin E deficiency—together with dietary selenium deficiency—is required to elicit the disease.

Severe Deficiency. Symptomatic selenium deficiency has been well characterized in Keshan disease and nutritional depletion in hospital patients.

Keshan Disease. Conclusive evidence for a role for selenium in human nutrition came with publication of the results of large-scale trials in China that show the protective effect of selenium supplementation on children and young adults suffering from an endemic cardiomyopathy. This was observed in areas of the country (Keshan region) with low soil selenium levels.[550]

Kashin-Beck Disease. A type of severe arthritis is described in parts of China and neighboring areas of Russia where soil selenium is particularly low. However, trials of selenium supplementation were not conclusive and other unidentified factors may be present.

Nutritional Depletion in Hospital Patients. Selenium was one of the last essential trace elements to be accepted as nutritionally important, with more attention being given to its potential toxicity. There was initially inadequate selenium provision in specialized diets used to treat inborn errors[590] and during long-term parenteral nutrition,[594] leading to cases of deficiency. Symptomatic cases continue to be reported, although the need for selenium supplementation during nutritional support is well established. Symptoms of severe deficiency include muscle weakness.[302] Cases involving cardiomyopathy, which is usually fatal and resembles Keshan disease,[340,633] and macrocytosis and pseudoalbinism in children[605] have been described.

Marginal Deficiencies. Marginal selenium deficiencies are thought to be involved in thyroid function, immune function, reproductive disorders, mood disorders, inflammatory conditions, cardiovascular disease, viral virulence, and cancer chemoprevention.

Thyroid Function. Selenium and other trace elements are necessary for normal thyroid function since the important deiodinase enzymes are selenoproteins.[19] Three children with biochemical and clinical signs of hypothyroidism were successfully treated by oral selenium therapy.[442] Although the deiodinases are not thought to be significantly affected in marginal selenium depletion, it has been observed that endemic goiter in Sri Lanka, which is resistant to iodine supplementation, occurs in areas with low soil selenium.[177] Similarly, endemic thyroid disease in Zaire may be related to the combination of iodine and selenium depletion. Care must be taken since the stimulation of thyroid hormone metabolism may induce hypothyroidism.

The low T_3 syndrome observed after major trauma may also be related to changes in selenium status affecting the activity of iodothyronine deiodinase, with selenium supplements reversing most of the biochemical abnormalities found in thyroid function tests.[46]

Immune Function. Deficiency of selenium is accompanied by loss of immunocompetence and this is related to the reduction of selenoproteins in the liver, spleen, and lymph nodes. Both cell-mediated immunity and B-cell function are impaired.

Considerable selenium losses in wound exudates following severe burns have been recorded, and supplementation of a mixture of selenium, zinc, and copper leads to a reduction in respiratory infections.[47] Supplementation, even in apparently selenium-adequate individuals, has some immune function stimulatory effects, including improvement in natural killer cell activity and increases in IL-2 receptor expression.[458] It has been speculated that the increased infection rates in acquired immunodeficiency syndrome (AIDS) patients may be related to selenium depletion and this may even influence the progression from human immunodeficiency virus (HIV) positivity to the AIDS syndrome.[34]

Reproductive Disorders. Adequate selenium supply is necessary for successful reproduction in a variety of farm animals. Various studies have looked at the situation in humans. Male fertility could be affected by selenium depletion insofar as it is necessary for testosterone synthesis and to maintain sperm viability.[458]

Mood Disorders. The brain is reported to receive a priority supply of selenium during dietary depletion and/or repletion studies in animals and the turnover of neurotransmitters is altered. This has led to extensive studies of the role of selenium and other antioxidants in senility of the elderly, in epilepsy in children, and in Alzheimer's disease. Marginal selenium depletion has been associated with anxiety, confusion, and hostility, and improvements have been claimed following supplementation.[458]

Inflammatory Conditions. Many conditions associated with inflammation and increased oxidative stress could be influenced by selenium status.[16] Positive effects from supplementation studies in arthritis and in pancreatitis have been reported. Low serum selenium values are found in asthma, and some limited clinical trial studies show benefits from supplementation.[458] In a small trial in patients in intensive care with systemic inflammatory response syndrome (SIRS), high-dose selenium supplements over 9 days were associated with reduced incidence of renal failure and reduced mortality in the most severely ill.[16]

Cardiovascular Disease. The protective role of selenium against cardiovascular disease has been extensively investigated, but with no conclusive findings.[165,458] The low soil selenium concentration in Finland resulted in locally grown food having low selenium content. This together with concerns about the high incidence of coronary disease in parts of the country led to selenium fortification of agricultural fertilizers.[312] Although an impressive decline in coronary disease mortality was found between 1972 and 1992, the benefits were linked primarily to other major diet and lifestyle changes.[440]

Viral Virulence. It is now considered possible that an unusually virulent strain of the Coxsackie virus is part of the cause of cardiomyopathy in selenium-depleted regions of China. This is consistent with the marked seasonal variations in the incidence of the disease.

It is known that nutritional depletion will impair the immune responses and increase the lethalness of viruses and other infectious agents. A series of experimental studies on mice have shown that a nonlethal form of Coxsackie B (CVB 3/O) converted to a virulent strain when inoculated into selenium-deficient mice.[39] Inoculation of selenium-adequate mice with the mutated virus then caused myocarditis. Sequencing the DNA from the altered virus showed that there were 6 nucleotide changes that corresponded to nucleotide sequences in the genome of a virulent strain of the virus. Further evidence came from experiments with GSPHx knockout mice. More than half of these mice infected with the nonlethal CVB/3O virus developed myocarditis but none of the wild type controls were affected. The virus recovered from these affected mice showed genome changes similar to those found in virulent strains of the virus. It is thought that the selenium-deficient host altered the viral pathogen, probably involving oxidative stress in the tissue of the depleted animals. Further animal studies[38] have demonstrated that a mild strain of influenza virus exhibits increased virulence when given to selenium-deficient mice. New viruses continue to appear through the evolution of existing viruses and these may be lethal strains. RNA viruses are known to mutate easily and lack proof-reading systems and repair mechanisms.[37,330,415]

There is speculation that a similar process can occur in regions of the world, such as parts of Africa, where the human population has depletions of selenium and other micronutrients and is intermittently exposed to viral diseases. There is as yet no direct evidence that similar processes do occur in human populations. However, an epidemic of optic and peripheral neuropathy in Cuba that affected more than 50,000 individuals was shown to be associated with deficiencies of several micronutrients, including selenium. Supplementation of the population with a multicomponent micronutrient mixture coincided with the subsidence of the disease.[37]

Cancer Chemoprevention. Although not primarily a nutritional issue, there is interest in the role of selenium supplementation in the prevention of certain types of cancer. Experimental work on animals shows that chemical carcinogenesis is modified by selenium. Also, epidemiological surveys have found a link between cancer incidence and soil selenium content, suggesting a higher incidence of certain cancers in individuals with a low selenium intake.[116] Large-scale trials in China, conducted on more than 130,000 individuals, compared one township (20,847 people) having a high risk for viral hepatitis B and liver cancer with four control townships in the same area. The high-risk population received selenium-enriched table salt and in an 8-year follow-up the average incidence of liver cancer was reduced by 35%. There was no reduction in incidence in the control populations. Studies on 226 people with chronic hepatitis B found that a controlled trial of selenium-enriched yeast reduced the development of liver cancer during a 2-year follow-up period.[632]

It now seems likely that selenium supplementation above the minimum dietary requirement has a role in cancer prevention, particularly in relation to prostatic cancer.[110] The mechanism is not established, but in selenium-adequate subjects the excess selenium may produce a low molecular weight methylated selenium compound that has chemopreventive properties.[115,116] A large selenium and vitamin E cancer prevention study, known as the Selenium and Vitamin E Cancer Prevention Trial (SELECT) study, will carry out controlled trials on more than 32,000 men to establish if there is a beneficial effect.[308]

Toxicity

Areas of China and the United States have high amounts of selenium in soil, and locally produced food contains excess selenium. Clinical signs of selenosis are garlic odor in the breath, hair loss, and nail damage.[172] The tolerable upper limit has been set at 400 μg/day for adults and less for children. There have been reported cases of toxicity from self-administered dosages. Because of a manufacturing error, 13 individuals taking supplements containing 27.3 mg (27,300 μg) per tablet showed clinically significant selenium toxicity.[247]

Laboratory Assessment of Status

Early animal studies and human population surveys used whole blood as the main indicator of selenium status. Whole blood selenium can be determined after acid digestion using a fluorometric method.[235] The more convenient carbon furnace atomic absorption spectroscopy (CFAAS) assay for plasma and/or serum selenium is now the most widely used procedure.[194] The main components of plasma selenium are extracellular glutathione peroxidase (GSHPx-3) and selenoprotein P.

Red cell GSPHx-1 and plasma GSPHx-3 are assayed by enzymatic methods using a variety of peroxide substrates,[550] with tertiary-butyl peroxide being a commonly used substrate since it is not as affected by catalase as is hydrogen peroxide.[51] The values obtained are dependent on the substrate used and the reaction conditions. During selenium supplementation studies, the plateau reached in plasma GSPHx-3 activity has been used to assess minimum dietary requirements.[172]

The effects of different forms of inorganic and organic selenium supplementation upon GSPHx activity in blood lymphocytes, granulocytes, platelets, and erythrocytes have been described in a trial on 45 human volunteers.[80] Some changes were acute and transient, whereas cytosolic GSHPx activity (GSHPx-1) increased gradually in both treatment groups over 28 days.

In patients receiving TPN at home, the time course for development of deficiency and repletion of enzyme activity has been studied.[113] After 1 year on TPN without selenium supplements, all patients had low plasma selenium and red cell GSHPx, and cellular metabolism of exogenous hydrogen peroxide was also impaired. With replacement of selenium as selenious acid, there was a rapid increase in GSHPx-3 within the first 24 hours, reaching normal levels within 1 to 2 weeks. Platelet GSHPx also returned to normal in 1 to 2 weeks, whereas polymorph GSHPx was more variable but normalized in about 3 weeks. Red cell GSHPx took 3 to 4 months to recover, consistent with the need for formation of these cells in the presence of selenium.

The major selenium-containing plasma protein selenoprotein P can be determined by immunological methods.[5] The production of monoclonal antibodies to selenoprotein P has been described[489] and used to study the structure and function of the protein and to quantify it. It is also possible to separate selenoprotein P from other plasma proteins by heparin affinity chromatography followed by CFAAS selenium analysis.[234] Selenoprotein P concentration in plasma responds rapidly to supplementation and has been used in nutritional studies of Chinese populations to confirm the adequacy of intake.[250]

Plasma selenoprotein P, plasma GSPHx-3, and total plasma selenium concentration are all lowered by the APR to injury or infection.[418] This effect should be considered when interpreting plasma selenium values in postoperative patients or those with infection or inflammatory disease.

Hair and nail selenium analysis can be useful as a measure of long-term dietary selenium intake. Selenium being a sulfur analogue, it is incorporated into the sulfur-rich keratin of hair and nails. One study showed a correlation between toenail selenium, blood selenium, and dietary intake.[344] In a study of a 10-year old child receiving TPN who developed selenium-responsive muscle weakness, hair analysis was used to help assess selenium dosage.[568] An analytical method using microwave-assisted acid digestion of hair and nails, followed by CFAAS selenium analysis, has been described.[233] In a small study using this procedure, values for hair and nail selenium in healthy UK people were found to be 0.32 to 0.76 μg/g (n = 25) and 0.17 to 0.66 μg/g (n = 27), respectively. However, for population studies, use of selenium-containing hair preparations will affect the hair selenium results and this would have to be carefully assessed and controlled.

Urine selenium output is mainly a reflection of the recent dietary input and has not been extensively employed in population surveys.

In summary, there are many possible markers for selenium status. In practice, measurement of plasma selenium or GSHPx provides a good estimate of status and in particular the adequacy of recent intake, provided they are interpreted in the knowledge of changes in the APR. For a better index of long-term intake, platelet, red cell, or neutrophil GSHPx, or hair or nail selenium can also be measured.

Reference Intervals

The reference interval for selenium in whole blood, plasma or serum, hair, and nails should be established locally, since these indices are affected by dietary selenium intake. Plasma selenium adult values lie in the interval 63 to 160 μg/L (0.8 to 2.0 μmol/L). Values of less than 40 μg Se per L (0.5 μmol/L) indicate probable selenium depletion.

Values in children are lower and in the UK are[569] 16 μg/L to 71 μg/L (0.2 to 0.9 μmo/L) for <2-year-olds; 40 μg/L to 103 μg/L (0.5 to 1.3 μmol/L) for 2- to 4-year-olds; and 55 μg/L to 134 μg/L (0.7 to 1.7 μmol/L) for 4- to 16-year-olds. Cut-off values of less than 8 μg/L (0.1 μmol/L) in neonates are strongly suggestive of selenium depletion. Increased plasma values are found in suspected selenium toxicity and results above 5 μmol/ (400 μg/L) are an indication of excess intake.

Red cell glutathione peroxidase activity (GSHPx-1) in adults varies from 13 to 25 U/g Hb, whereas values in children are slightly lower.[569] Local age-related reference intervals are again required.

Zinc

The discovery of a variety of zinc (Zn) related clinical disorders has directly demonstrated the importance of zinc in human nutrition. It is second to iron as the most abundant trace element in the body.

Chemistry

Zine (atomic number 30, atomic weight 65.39) lies at the end of the first transition series. Zn^{2+} with a filled 3*d* electron shell is a particularly stable ion. The bioinorganic chemical features of zinc, which underlie the very diverse biological functions of this trace metal, include its relatively high abundance compared with other trace elements. Zinc has fast ligand exchange kinetics and flexible coordination geometry, and is a good electron acceptor (strong Lewis acid), with no redox reactions. There is a hypothesis that zinc ions, present in the cytoplasm at 10^{-11} mol/L and in equilibrium with numerous zinc metalloenzymes and transcription factors, can act as a "master hormone," particularly in relation to cell division and growth.[180] There are no naturally colored zinc complexes and this may have delayed the recognition of the biological importance of zinc until the development of suitable atomic spectroscopic methods that could be applied to biological samples and used as probes to identify and study metalloproteins.[96]

Dietary Sources

Zinc is widely distributed in food mainly bound to proteins. The bioavailability of dietary zinc is dependent upon the digestion of these proteins to release zinc and allow it to bind to peptides, amino acids, phosphate, and other ligands within the intestinal tract. The most available dietary sources of zinc are red meat and fish, whereas white meats and flesh from young animals provide less zinc. Wheat germ and whole bran are good sources but their zinc content is reduced by milling and food processing. The median intake for men in the United States is about 14 mg/day and for women 9 mg/day.[174]

Absorption, Transport, Metabolism, and Excretion

Regulation of the net intestinal uptake of zinc is by control of absorption efficiency in the face of variable dietary zinc input and ranges from 20% to 50% of the dietary content. At an intake of 12.2 mg Zn per day, the fractional absorption was 26%, but at the very low intake of 0.23 mg Zn per day this increased to 100%. These and other measurements were made on 12 male volunteers using stable ^{67}Zn tracer to assess zinc homeostasis and plasma zinc kinetics.[306] Estimates of zinc absorption have also been compared using four different stable isotope techniques.[348] It was concluded that a double isotopic tracer ratio method is accurate and is recommended as a practicable procedure. Using this method, the fraction of dietary zinc absorbed was equivalent to 30% ± 10%. Fine control of net absorption is by secretion of endogenous zinc into the intestinal lumen from pancreatic fluid and other intestinal fluids.[305] Such losses range from less than 1 mg/day on a low zinc diet to more than 5 mg/day on a zinc-rich diet. The ability to conserve dietary zinc by limiting intestinal loss can allow a positive metabolic balance even at low dietary zinc intakes. Interaction with other dietary constituents such as phytate, calcium, and iron reduce, the net absorption of zinc significantly so that diets high in phytate and calcium reduce the growth rate of young rats.

In human diets, leavening of bread and exposure of cereals to wet heat lower the phytate content, increasing zinc availability. Other factors, such as dietary fiber and a constituent of beans, can also lower zinc intestinal absorption but to a lesser extent.[106] Iron at supplemental dosages (up to 65 mg/day) may decrease zinc absorption so that pregnant and lactating women taking iron may require zinc supplementation.[426]

Absorbed zinc is transported to the liver by the portal circulation where active incorporation into metalloenzymes and plasma proteins such as albumin and α_2-macroglobulin occurs. Blood plasma contains less than 1% of the total body content of zinc and lies within a narrow concentration interval 80 to 120 µg/dL (12 to 18 µmol/L). About 80% of plasma zinc is associated with albumin and most of the rest tightly bound in the high molecular protein α_2-macroglobulin.[175] The zinc on albumin is in equilibrium with plasma amino acids (mostly histidine and cysteine) and this small (<1%) ultrafilterable fraction may be important in cellular uptake mechanisms (Figure 30-28).[106]

Total adult body content of zinc is about 2 to 2.5 g and the metal is present in the cells of all metabolically active tissue and organs. About 55% of the total is found in muscle and approximately 30% in bone.[106] The prostate, semen, and the retina have particularly high local concentrations of zinc. Almost all zinc in a red cell is in the form of carbonic anhydrase so that red cell zinc concentration is about 10 times higher than plasma. Hemolysates normally have about 50 µg Zn per g Hb, and total leukocyte zinc is normally about 100 ± 25 µg/10^{10} cells.

Fecal excretion includes both unabsorbed dietary zinc and zinc resecreted into the gut. The total amount normally equals the total dietary intake and is of the order of 10 to 15 mg/day in healthy populations. In contrast, urine output of zinc is normally only about 0.5 mg/day, but this can increase markedly during catabolic illness. The release of intracellular contents from skeletal muscle has been established as the source of the excess urinary zinc in the postoperative period, using zinc radiotracer labeling. Two patients took an oral dose of 5 µCi radioactive ^{65}Zn about a month before elective surgery for total hip replacement, allowing incorporation of the tracer into skeletal muscle. Urine output of radioactive zinc, total zinc, and total nitrogen was measured before operation and daily for 3 weeks after surgery. There was a large increase in the excretion of all of these, the peaks occurring at 10 days. There was a good correlation between radioactive zinc and total zinc in the urine of both patients, suggesting skeletal muscle as the source.[153] Urine zinc also increases more than threefold during short-term total starvation, as a result of release from skeletal muscle and excretion of ketone bodies.[146]

Functions

More than 300 zinc metalloenzymes occur in all six categories of enzyme systems. Important examples in human tissue include carbonic anhydrase, alkaline phosphatase, RNA and DNA polymerases, thymidine kinase carboxypeptidases, and alcohol dehydrogenase. The key roles of zinc in protein and nucleic acid synthesis explain the failure of growth and impaired wound healing observed in individuals with zinc deficiency. In some enzymes, such as Cu and Zn SOD, structural stability is ensured by zinc protein binding and the catalytic activity of the enzyme by the active copper site. Classifications of zinc enzymes, their structure and mode of action have been detailed in various texts.[106,180] Proteins can form domains able to bind tetrahedral zinc atoms by coordination with histidine and cysteine to form folded structures that have become known as "zinc fingers."[44] These biologically active molecules have important roles in gene expression by acting as DNA-binding transcription factors and play a key role in developmental biology and also

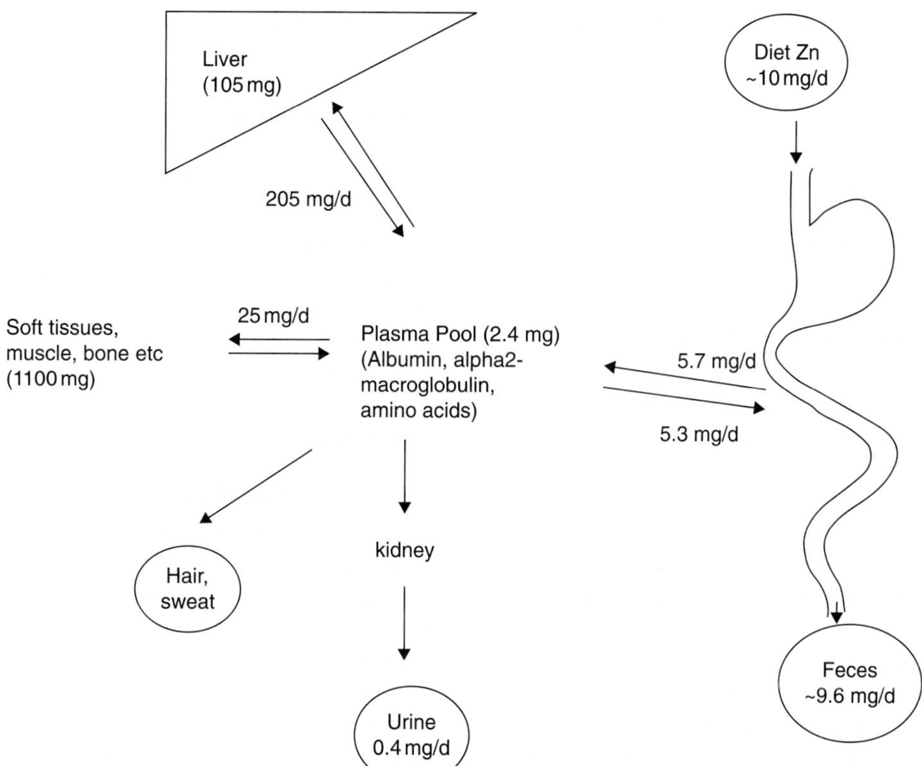

Figure 30-28 Summary of zinc metabolism.

in the regulation of steroid, thyroid, and other hormone synthesis.[150,586] Zinc binding to the metal response factor MTF1 activates metallothionein (Mt) expression. This multifunctional, low molecular weight protein (9000 to 10,000 Da) has a high content of cysteine and reversibly binds zinc. Mt is important in intracellular zinc trafficking and helps to maintain intracellular zinc concentrations. Hepatic synthesis of Mt is induced by interleukin-1, interleukin-6, and glucocorticoids in response to infection, trauma, and other stressors.[106,505]

Requirements and Reference Nutrient Intakes

In the United States, the Dietary Reference Intake (DRI) for zinc is 11 mg/day for men and 8 mg/day for women. Infants and young children need smaller amounts. Increased amounts are required during pregnancy and lactation. Strict vegetarians may need as much as 50% more zinc per day because of the increased phytic acid and fiber in their diet.[174]

Intravenous Supply

Stable adult patients require 2.5 to 4.0 mg/day (40 to 60 µmol/day), but in those who are depleted or who have increased gastrointestinal losses, the requirement is about 6 mg/day (100 µmol/day).

Clinical Deficiency

As might be expected from the multiple biochemical functions of zinc, the clinical presentation of deficiency disease is varied, nonspecific, and related to the degree and duration of the depletion.[226,305,446] Signs and symptoms include depressed growth with stunting; increased incidence of infection, possibly related to alterations in immune function; diarrhea; altered cognition; defects in carbohydrate use; reproductive teratogenesis; skin lesions; alopecia; eyesight defects; and other adverse clinical outcomes.

Effects on Growth. It has been claimed that dietary zinc deficiency is prevalent in countries worldwide where a cereal-based diet high in phytate and fiber but low in animal protein is common.[448] This could affect as many as 2 billion people and may be a major public health issue comparable with the recognized deficiencies of iron and iodine. In children, reduced growth and other developmental abnormalities are reversible by zinc supplementation. A meta-analysis of some 37 intervention trials shows that zinc supplementation has a significant effect upon linear growth and weight regain.[78] Studies have also shown that lean tissue retention and protein synthesis are increased if zinc is added to therapeutic regimens used in famine relief, especially when soya-based formulations with a high phytate content were being used as a protein source.[202]

It is known that the zinc in human breast milk is efficiently absorbed because of the presence of factors such as picolinate and citrate. However, the total quantity of zinc in breast milk is related to maternal nutritional status, and there is a physiological decline in the zinc content of "mature milk" after about 6 months lactation. Although cases of symptomatic zinc deficiency have been reported in breast-fed infants,[241,267] the need for zinc supplementation for women in low-income countries during pregnancy is controversial. Reduction of neonatal morbidity and incidence of infections is reported in some studies, but the large-scale introduction of the zinc supplementation of pregnant women necessitates more controlled trials.[434]

Acrodermatitis Enteropathica. Acrodermatitis enteropathica (AE) is characterized by periorificial and acral dermatitis, alopecia, and diarrhea. Patients with this disorder have abnormally low blood zinc levels (<30 µg/dL); symptoms are reversed by oral zinc supplementation, with this being diagnostic.[31] This formerly fatal condition is an autosomal recessive inborn error affecting zinc absorption from the intestinal mucosa, but the location of the gene defect has not yet been identified.

Parenteral Nutrition. When clinical techniques were developed for TPN in the 1960s and 1970s, the early sources of amino acids were based on whole protein hydrolysates that had zinc and other trace elements present as contaminants. When these were replaced with mixtures of synthetic amino acids in the 1980s, this necessitated the addition of trace element additives. Some patients requiring intravenous feeding after surgery are likely to be significantly zinc depleted because of poor oral intake before and after surgery. They may also have increased zinc losses from the intestinal tract via diarrhea and in urine from catabolism of muscle during periods of negative nitrogen balance. Diarrhea, mental depression, dermatitis, delayed wound healing, and alopecia are seen during the anabolic period of weight regain when there is insufficient zinc in the nutritional regimen to support tissue repair.[300] Provision of adequate zinc intravenously to achieve a positive zinc balance is associated with improvement in nitrogen balance.[625] Routine provision of 100 µmol/day (6.5 mg) in the IVN regimen is normally adequate in stable patients,[527] but increased amounts of zinc and other micronutrients are required in the most severely injured patients.[526]

Infectious Disease. Zinc depletion impairs immunity[446] and has a direct effect on the gastrointestinal tract,[547] which increases the severity of enteric infections. A placebo-controlled trial of zinc supplementation (10 to 20 mg/day) of 1240 children ages 6 to 30 months was conducted in North India. There was a substantial reduction in the incidence of both severe and prolonged diarrhea in the treated group.[52] A review of controlled trials of zinc supplementation of children in low-income countries found significant clinical benefits.[57] Six out of nine trials in cases of persistent diarrhea claimed improvement; in five trials in respiratory disease, there was a lower rate of infection. Some caution is required with the doses of zinc employed. In a study of severely malnourished children, those treated with doses of 3 to 6 mg Zn per kg had a significantly increased mortality compared with those given 1.0 to 1.5 mg Zn per kg.[136] Interaction with vitamin A is important, since in populations at risk of zinc and vitamin A deficiency, provision of zinc alone increased the incidence of respiratory infection, but when vitamin A was also added, respiratory infections were decreased.[455]

Other Conditions. Other groups of individuals are considered to be at risk either from a marginal dietary deficiency or from an acquired deficiency secondary to disease. These groups would include female adolescents during pregnancy and lactation. Also affected may be patients with malabsorption syndrome, inflammatory bowel disease, alcoholic liver disease, and anorexia nervosa.[305] A significant proportion of cases of sickle cell anemia have clinical signs and symptoms and some laboratory abnormalities of zinc deficiency. These patients respond well to zinc supplementation.[447]

Subclinical Effects of Deficiency

When zinc deficiency is not severe enough to cause clinical signs and symptoms, it may still have a subclinical effect on immune function, the synthesis and action of hormones, and neurological function.

Immune Function. Patients with zinc deficiency in the Middle East were known to die before the age of 25 because of various infections and parasitic disease. In zinc deficiency, there is a reduction in the activity of serum thymulin, the thymus-specific hormone that is involved in T-cell function, and an imbalance develops between Th1 and Th2 helper cells. The lytic activity of natural killer cells also decreases. Moreover, zinc is also necessary for intracellular binding of tyrosine kinase to the T-cell receptors CD-4 and CD-8, which are required for T-lymphocyte activation. These complex changes result in an impairment of cell-mediated immunity and may be the basis for increased infection rates seen in marginal zinc depletion.[446]

There have been suggestions that zinc supplements may be beneficial in reducing the severity or duration of the common cold. Studies have been inconsistent, putative benefits small, and given the doses of zinc used, a high incidence of side effects was encountered.[362]

Hormones. Zinc is thought to have a role in the synthesis and actions of many hormones, via zinc transcription factors. Zinc depletion is associated with low circulating concentrations of testosterone, free T_4, insulin-like growth factor (IGF)-1, and thymulin.[446] Both plasma IGF-1 and growth velocity increase in zinc-supplemented children.[421]

Neurological Effects. Severe zinc deficiency is known to affect mental well-being, with varying degrees of confusion and depression being consistent with zinc enzymes having important activity in brain development and function. The history of zinc in relation to the brain and possible relevance to human disease has been reviewed.[122,493]

Toxicity

Clinical effects of ingestion of a zinc-contaminated diet are abdominal pain, diarrhea, nausea, and vomiting (see Chapter 35). Single doses of 225 to 450 mg of Zn can induce vomiting, with milder forms of gastrointestinal upset being reported at 50 to 150 mg Zn/day, (dosages that were initially used in therapy). More than 60 mg Zn per day can result in copper depletion by causing intestinal blockade of intestinal absorption. The U.S. Nutrition Board has set the tolerable upper level of intake for adults at 40 mg/day.[174]

Laboratory Assessment of Status

Although plasma zinc determination is insensitive to dietary zinc intake and subject to a variety of influences, it remains the most widely used laboratory test to confirm severe deficiency and to monitor adequacy of zinc provision, especially if interpreted together with changes in serum albumin and the APR. No feasible laboratory procedures are established for clearly identifying populations with marginal zinc depletion. The clinical and biochemical responses to zinc supplementation are therefore used to postulate a marginally zinc-depleted state.

Plasma Zinc. Plasma samples are preferred to serum for zinc analysis because of possible zinc contamination from erythrocytes, platelets. and leukocytes during clotting and centrifugation. Plasma zinc levels are most commonly measured by FAAS, although photometric methods are available.

A study using stable zinc isotope tracers during experimental induction of acute zinc depletion (0.23 mg Zn per day) found that the plasma zinc level took 5 weeks to decline to 65% of the baseline values, and that the observed fall was caused by a reduction in zinc release from the most slowly turning over zinc pool.[306] Care has to be taken in controlling numerous preanalytical factors that will lower plasma zinc independently of dietary intake. These include collection of sample in relation to meals, time of day, and use of steroid-based medications, such as the contraceptive pill. Any cause of hypoalbuminemia will also lower plasma zinc. Plasma albumin is a negative acute phase reactant and is redistributed into interstitial spaces from the plasma pool during infection, after trauma, and in chronic disease. The induction of hepatic Mt synthesis during the APR, and subsequent sequestering of zinc, further lowers the plasma level.[523] It is therefore essential to consider plasma zinc results along with plasma albumin and plasma CRP or another marker of the APR.

Blood Cell Zinc. Some investigators have suggested that the zinc content of white cells and platelets better reflects tissue zinc.[571,610] The zinc content of neutrophils, lymphocytes, and platelets has been shown to decline more rapidly than plasma zinc in experimental studies of zinc depletion in humans.[446] However, the relatively large volume of blood required and problems with contamination make large-scale application to patients in the hospital or to population surveys difficult, especially in studies involving children.

Zinc in Hair. Low hair zinc has been associated with poor growth in children, and has been used as a criterion for initiating supplementation studies.[174] However, variables such as hair growth rate and external contamination from hair dyes and cosmetics can cause inconsistent results. Results from individual patients are difficult to interpret.

Zinc-Dependent Enzymes. Despite the large number of zinc metalloenzymes that have been identified, no single enzyme assay has yet found acceptance as an indicator of zinc status. This may be due to avid retention of zinc by these enzymes, even in the face of dietary zinc depletion, and to difficulties with reproducible measurements of activity. However, bone-specific alkaline phosphatase, extracellular SOD, lymphocytes, and plasma 5-nucleotidase appear to be responsive to zinc intake.[626]

Metallothionein. The determination of Mt in red cells and MT mRNA in circulating monocytes is considered of probable value since Mt falls in zinc deficiency. However, the clinical use of these measurements is not yet confirmed by large-scale investigations of depleted populations.[626]

Urine Zinc. There is a slight fall in the urinary excretion of zinc during dietary deficiency. Difficulties of sample contamination during collection make this of limited practical value. Increases in urine zinc are, however, an important source of loss in the severely injured catabolic patient, although measurement is rarely required except in research studies.

Reference Intervals

Serum zinc concentrations are generally 5% to 15% higher than plasma because of osmotic fluid shifts from the blood cells when various anticoagulants are used. Plasma zinc concentrations exhibit both circadian and postprandial fluctuations. Concentrations decrease after food and are higher in the morning than in the evening.

A reference interval, for clinical guidance, is 80 to 120 µg/dL (12 to 18 µmol/L).

Fasting morning values of plasma zinc below 70 µg/dL (10.7 µmol/L) on more than one occasion require further investigation. Results below 30 µg/dL (5 µmol/L) suggest likely deficiency. Urine zinc excretion lies in the range from 0.2 to 1.3 mg/24 hr (3 to 21 µmol/24 hr).

OTHER POSSIBLY ESSENTIAL ELEMENTS

More than 15 additional trace elements are considered by some investigators to have a potentially important role in human medicine. A review by Nielsen considers these in detail and discusses emerging concepts of "essentiality."[419] For some such as lead, cadmium, arsenic, aluminum, and nickel, the clinical laboratory will primarily consider them as toxic elements (see Chapter 35). Others, such as lithium and fluoride, are classified as pharmacologically beneficial and monitoring of dosage may be required. Some elements can be considered "nutritionally beneficial" and are reported to produce "restorative health effects" at lower dosages. Evidence comes mainly from animal studies when dietary depletion of the element is combined with other metabolic, hormonal, or physiological "stressors."

For a few elements (boron, silicon, and vanadium), the circumstantial evidence is considered to be strong, although no agreed biochemical mechanism is established. For this reason the DRI report,[174] which considered in detail the nutritional aspects of arsenic, boron, nickel, silicon, and vanadium, was unable to establish dietary recommendations. For boron, silicon, and vanadium, it was noted that measurable responses in humans have been observed during variations in the dietary intake of these elements. There is promotion of these and other elements by the supplement industry and the clinical chemist may be asked for advice and possibly for monitoring of dosage in cases of suspected toxicity. AAS, ICP-OES, and ICP-MS methods can be applied to the determination of most of these elements in biological samples.[390]

The contamination of TPN solutions by small amounts of metals, such as Al, Pb, Cd and Ni, could also be a problem, as could the lack of others, such as Si, B, and V, when very long-term nutritional support is required.

Fluoride

Fluoride (Fl) is the most widely used of the "pharmacologically beneficial trace elements" in the area of public health. Dental caries has been described as the last major epidemic of preventable bacterial disease and dental decay leads to tooth loss, nutritional problems, and systemic infections.[97]

Dietary Sources

Many studies over the last 50 years have established that addition of fluoride to drinking water reduces the incidence of tooth decay, and more than 60% of the U.S. population now uses fluoridated water. Clinical studies from 1950 to 1980 in 20 different countries found that adding fluoride to community water supplies, within the interval 0.7 mg to 1.2 mg/L, reduced the incidence of caries by 40% to 50% in primary (infant) teeth and by 50% to 60% in permanent teeth.[129] The subject is controversial and there is opposition to "mass medication" with fluoride. Reviews of the benefits and the risks associated with the use of fluoride are available.[97-99,247,400]

Fluoride supplementation of salt, sugar, and milk has also been used in areas where fluoride is not added to water supplies.

Function

The fluoride ion can exchange for hydroxyl in the crystal structure of apatite, a main component of skeletal bone and teeth. This stabilizes the regenerating tooth surface. Fluoride is available from saliva and may also be released from dental plaque at low pH.[98] Initially, benefit was considered solely to be for the erupting teeth of children, but topical effects on adult teeth are now also thought to reduce decay. There is some initial evidence from small studies that pharmacological doses of fluoride may reduce the incidence of bone fracture in patients with osteoporosis. However, a metaanalysis of fluoride therapy from 11 controlled studies on 1429 subjects found that although this increased lumbar bone density, the incidence of vertebral fractures was not significantly decreased.[247]

Absorption, Transport, Metabolism, and Excretion[99]

Fluoride ions are absorbed from both the stomach and the small intestine. The soluble salts are efficiently absorbed, and the peak increase of fluoride in blood plasma is within 1 hour of ingestion. Ions are rapidly cleared from plasma into tissue in exchange with anions, such as hydroxyl, citrate, and carbonate. At least 95% of the 2.6 g of total body fluoride is located in bones and teeth. Almost 90% of excess fluoride is excreted in urine.

Toxicity

Dental fluorosis is the mottling of enamel in the erupting teeth of children and it is now estimated to affect around 20% of the population. This can be a disfiguring condition and occurs in a higher proportion of children than initially expected.[612] This is possibly due to the ingestion of fluoride-containing toothpaste by children. It is suggested that "pediatric" toothpastes with lower fluoride content be made available in areas where there is existing fluoridation of the water supply.[98]

Occupational exposure to inhaled fluoride dusts in cryolite workers during aluminum refining has resulted in severe bone abnormalities, but safety equipment now limits such exposure. No cases of skeletal fluorosis are attributed to use of controlled fluoridation of water supplies.[99] However, skeletal fluorosis may occur in areas of the world where naturally occurring drinking water has high levels of fluoride, such as China and the Indian subcontinent. It is thought that exposure to fluoride intakes of 10 to 25 mg/day for 10 years or more may result in skeletal fluorosis, but other nutritional factors may make these populations more susceptible.[247]

A number of diverse adverse effects have been attributed to water fluoridation. Investigators have found no convincing evidence of increased rates of cancer, heart disease, kidney disease, liver disease, presenile dementia, birth defects, or Down syndrome.[247]

Laboratory Assessment of Status

Laboratory analysis of drinking water may be required to assess possible fluoride excess in natural well waters and may also be necessary during incidents of failure of the equipment used to treat drinking water. The determination of fluoride in urine can be used to assess exposure to different sources of fluoride.[303] For drinking water and urine, direct determination using a fluoride-specific electrode is employed. For food, feces, and tissue, prior separation of fluoride from the sample matrix is required using a Conway diffusion procedure.[99] The combination of the fluoride-electrode with flow injection has allowed a rapid and sensitive method to be used for serum and urine fluoride analysis.[269]

Reference Intervals

Concentrations of fluoride in body fluids and tissue will vary widely depending upon the fluoride content of drinking water and input from diet, toothpaste, and mouth rinses. For urine, a guideline interval is 0.2 mg to 3.2 mg/L (10.5 to 168 µmol/L).

Boron

Boron (B) may be the next element to be recognized as essential in human nutrition. The evidence is largely circumstantial because there is no clear biological function for boron in humans.

Function

Responses to dietary deprivation of boron have been described with alterations in calcium metabolism, brain function, and energy production.[419] The responses from a low dietary boron intake (0.25 mg/2000 kcal) for 63 days and the effects of supplementation with 3.0 mg/day included increases in 25-hydroxycholecalciferol, decreases in calcitonin, decreased serum glucose, and increased serum triglycerides among other biochemical changes.[419] Some of the effects were more evident when dietary copper was marginal and magnesium inadequate. There is a necessity for further research to clarify the role of boron in human and animal physiology and to establish a dietary requirement.[133]

Dietary Sources

It is thought that the acceptable safe range of boron intake is from 1 to 13 mg/day, and there is evidence that some people are consuming less than 1 mg/day. Plant foods, especially fruits, leafy vegetables, nuts, and legumes, are good sources, whereas meat, fish, and dairy products are not.[419]

Absorption, Transport, Metabolism, and Excretion

More than 90% of dietary boron is absorbed as boric acid, $B(OH)_3$, and transported in blood in this neutral form, which may be readily excreted in urine.

Laboratory Assessment of Status

Problems with contamination and losses of volatile boron compounds during sample preparation have limited the reliable documentation of boron concentrations in human tissue and body fluids.[138] A complex technique involving a porous graphite column—inductively coupled plasma-atomic emission spectrophotometry (ICP-AES)—and an ICP time of flight mass spectrometer (TOF-MS) has been developed for investigations of boron neutron capture in cancer therapy.[552] Adaptation of this method to nutritional studies of boron should be possible.

REFERENCES

1. Abe A, Yamashita S, Noma A. Sensitive, direct colorimetric assay for copper in serum. Clin Chem 1989;35:552-4.
2. Abraham AS, Brooks BA, Eylath U. The effects of chromium supplementation on serum glucose and lipids in patients with and without non-insulin-dependent diabetes. Metabolism 1992;41:768-71.
3. Abumrad NN, Schneider AJ, Steel D, Rogers LS. Amino acid intolerance during prolonged total parenteral nutrition reversed by molybdate therapy. Am J Clin Nutr 1981;34:2551-9.
4. Adams JF, Tankel HI, MacEwan F. Estimation of the total body vitamin B12 in the live subject. Clin Sci 1970;39:107-13.
5. Akesson B, Bellew T, Burk RF. Purification of selenoprotein P from human plasma. Biochim Biophys Acta 1994;1204:243-9.
6. Alaejos MS, Romero CD. Urinary selenium concentrations. Clin Chem 1993;39:2040-52.
7. Allen RH. Megaloblastic anemias. In: Goldman L, Bennett JC, eds. Cecil Textbook of Medicine. Philadelphia: WB Saunders Co, 2000:859-67.
8. Althuis MD, Jordan NE, Ludington EA, Wittes JT. Glucose and insulin responses to dietary chromium supplements: a meta-analysis. Am J Clin Nutr 2002;76:148-55.
9. American Medical Association DoFaN. Multivitamin preparations for parenteral use: A statement by the Nutrition Advisory Group. J Parenter Enteral Nutr 1979;3:258-62.
10. American Medical Association DoFaN. Working conference on parenteral trace elements. Bull N Y Acad Med 1984;60:1115-212.
11. Anderson RA. Chromium and parenteral nutrition. Nutrition 1995;11:83-6.
12. Anderson RA. Chromium in the prevention and control of diabetes. Diabetes Metab 2000;26:22-7.
13. Anderson RA, Cheng N, Bryden NA, Polansky MM, Cheng N, Chi J, Feng J. Elevated intakes of supplemental chromium improve glucose and insulin variables in individuals with type 2 diabetes. Diabetes 1997;46:1786-91.
14. Anderson RA, Kozlovsky AS. Chromium intake, absorption and excretion of subjects consuming self-selected diets. Am J Clin Nutr 1985;41:1177-83.
15. Anderson RA, Polansky MM, Bryden NA, Roginski EE, Patterson KY, Reamer DC. Effect of exercise (running) on serum glucose, insulin, glucagon, and chromium excretion. Diabetes 1982;31:212-6.
16. Angstwurm MW, Schottdorf J, Schopohl J, Gaertner R. Selenium replacement in patients with severe systemic inflammatory response syndrome improves clinical outcome. Crit Care Med 1999;27:1807-13.
17. Ariaey-Nejad MR, Balaghi M, Baker EM, Sauberlich HE. Thiamin metabolism in man. Am J Clin Nutr 1970;23:764-78.
18. Arthur JR. The glutathione peroxidases. Cell Mol Life Sci 2000;57:1825-35.
19. Arthur JR, Beckett GJ. Thyroid function. Br Med Bull 1999;55:658-68.
20. Baeckert PA, Greene HL, Fritz I, Oelberg DG, Adcock EW. Vitamin concentrations in very low birth weight

infants given vitamins intravenously in a lipid emulsion: measurement of vitamins A, D, and E and riboflavin. J Pediatr 1988;113:1057-65.
21. Bailey LB, Moyers S, Gregory JF III. Folate. In: Bowman BA, Russell RA, eds. Present Knowledge in Nutrition. Washington: ILSI Press, 2001:214-29.
22. Bailey LB. New standard for dietary folate intake in pregnant women. Am J Clin Nutr 2000;71:1304S-7S.
23. Baines M. Improved high performance liquid chromatographic determination of thiamin diphosphate in erythrocytes. Clin Chim Acta 1985;153:43-8.
24. Baines M, Davies G. The evaluation of erythrocyte thiamin diphosphate as an indicator of thiamin status in man, and its comparison with erythrocyte transketolase activity measurements. Ann Clin Biochem 1988;25 (Pt 6):698-705.
25. Baker EM, Hodges RE, Hood J, Sauberlich HE, March SC, Canham JE. Metabolism of 14C- and 3H-labeled L-ascorbic acid in human scurvy. Am J Clin Nutr 1971;24:444-54.
26. Ball GFM. Pantothenic acid. Water-soluble vitamin assays in human nutrition. New York: Chapman and Hall, 1994.
27. Banerjee R, Vlasie M. Controlling the reactivity of radical intermediates by coenzyme B(12)-dependent methylmalonyl-CoA mutase. Biochem Soc Trans 2002;30:621-4.
28. Banno K. Measurement of pantothenic acid and hopantenic acid by gas chromatography-mass spectroscopy. Methods Enzymol 1997;279:213-9.
29. Barber RC, Lammer EJ, Shaw GM, Greer KA, Finnell RH. The role of folate transport and metabolism in neural tube defect risk. Mol Genet Metab 1999;66: 1-9.
30. Barclay MN, MacPherson A, Dixon J. Selenium content of a range of UK foods. J Food of Composition and Analysis 1995;8:307-8.
31. Barnes PM, Moynahan EJ. Zinc deficiency in acrodermatitis enteropathica: multiple dietary intolerance treated with synthetic diet. Proc R Soc Med 1973;66:327-9.
32. Bates CJ. Vitamin analysis. Ann Clin Biochem 1997;34 (Pt 6):599-626.
33. Bauernfeind JC. The tocopherol content of food and influencing factors. CRC Crit Rev Food Sci Nutr 1977;8:337-82.
34. Baum MK, Miguez-Burbano MJ, Campa A, Shor-Posner G. Selenium and interleukins in persons infected with human immunodeficiency virus type 1. J Infect Dis 2000;182 Suppl 1:S69-S73.
35. Bechgaard H, Jespersen S. GI absorption of niacin in humans. J Pharm Sci 1977;66:871-2.
36. Beck WS. Cobalamin (vitamin B12). In: Rucker RB, Suttie JW, McCormick DB, Machlin LJ, eds. Handbook of vitamins. New York: Marcel Dekker, Inc, 2001:463-512.
37. Beck MA. Nutritionally induced oxidative stress: effect on viral disease. Am J Clin Nutr 2000;71: 1676S-81S.
38. Beck MA, Levander OA, Handy J. Selenium deficiency and viral infection. J Nutr 2003;133: 1463S-7S.
39. Beck MA, Shi Q, Morris VC, Levander OA. Rapid genomic evolution of a non-virulent coxsackievirus B3 in selenium-deficient mice results in selection of identical virulent isolates. Nat Med 1995;1:433-6.
40. Bender DA. Effects of benserazide, carbidopa and isoniazid administration on tryptophan-nicotinamide nucleotide metabolism in the rat. Biochem Pharmacol 1980;29:2099-104.
41. Bender DA. Non-nutritional uses of vitamin B6. Br J Nutr 1999;81:7-20.
42. Bender DA. Daily doses of multivitamin tablets. BMJ 2002;325:173-4.
43. Benzie IF, Strain JJ. The ferric reducing ability of plasma (FRAP) as a measure of "antioxidant power": the FRAP assay. Anal Biochem 1996;239:70-6.
44. Berg JM, Shi Y. The galvanization of biology: a growing appreciation for the roles of zinc. Science 1996;271:1081-5.
45. Berger MM, Cavadini C, Chiolero R, Dirren H. Copper, selenium, and zinc status and balances after major trauma. J Trauma 1996;40:103-9.
46. Berger MM, Reymond MJ, Shenkin A, Rey F, Wardle C, Cayeux C et al. Influence of selenium supplements on the post-traumatic alterations of the thyroid axis: a placebo-controlled trial. Intensive Care Med 2001;27:91-100.
47. Berger MM, Spertini F, Shenkin A, Wardle C, Wiesner L, Schindler C, Chiolero RL. Trace element supplementation modulates pulmonary infection rates after major burns: a double-blind, placebo-controlled trial. Am J Clin Nutr 1998;68:365-71.
48. Berkner KL. The vitamin K-dependent carboxylase. J Nutr 2000;130:1877-80.
49. Berry RJ, Li Z, Erickson JD, Li S, Moore CA, Wang H et al. Prevention of neural-tube defects with folic acid in China. China-U.S. Collaborative Project for Neural Tube Defect Prevention [corrected; erratum to be published]. N Engl J Med 1999;341:1485-90.
50. Bettendorff L. A non-cofactor role of thiamine derivatives in excitable cells? Arch Physiol Biochem 1996;104:745-51.
51. Beutler E, Blume KG, Kaplan JC, Lohr GW, Ramot B, Valentine WN. International Committee for Standardization in Hematology: recommended methods for red-cell enzyme analysis. Br J Hematol 1977;35:331-40.
52. Bhandari N, Bahl R, Taneja S, Strand T, Molbak K, Ulvik RJ et al. Substantial reduction in severe diarrheal morbidity by daily zinc supplementation in young north Indian children. Pediatrics 2002;109:e86.

53. Bieri JG, Evarts RP. Tocopherols and polyunsaturated fatty acids in human tissues. Am J Clin Nutr 1975;28:717-20.
54. Bingham SA, Welch AA, McTaggart A, Mulligan AA, Runswick SA, Luben R et al. Nutritional methods in the European Prospective Investigation of Cancer in Norfolk. Public Health Nutr 2001;4:847-58.
55. Bings NH, Bogaerts A, Broekaert JA. Atomic spectroscopy. Anal Chem 2002;74:2691-711.
55a. Bjelakovic G, Nikolova D, Simonetti R, Gluud C. Antioxidant supplements for prevention of gastrointestinal cancers-systematic review and meta-analysis. Lancet 2004;364:1219-28.
56. Black AL, Guirard BM, Snell EE. The behavior of muscle phosphorylase as a reservoir for vitamin B6 in the rat. J Nutr 1978;108:670-7.
57. Black RE. Zinc deficiency, infectious disease and mortality in the developing world. J Nutr 2003;133:1485S-9S.
58. Blanchard RA, Furie BC, Kruger SF, Waneck G, Jorgensen MJ, Furie B. Immunoassays of human prothrombin species which correlate with functional coagulant activities. J Lab Clin Med 1983;101:242-55.
59. Block G, Dresser CM, Hartman AM, Carroll DM. Nutrient sources in the American Diet: quantitative data from the NHANES-II Survey. I Vitamins and minerals. Am J Epidemiol 1985;122:13-26.
60. Blount BC, Mack MM, Wehr CM, MacGregor JT, Hiatt RA, Wang G et al. Folate deficiency causes uracil misincorporation into human DNA and chromosome breakage: implications for cancer and neuronal damage. Proc Natl Acad Sci U S A 1997;94:3290-5.
61. Bonjour JP. Biotin in man's nutrition and therapy—a review. Int J Vitam Nutr Res 1977;47:107-18.
62. Booth SL, Tucker KL, Chen H, Hannan MT, Gagnon DR, Cupples LA et al. Dietary vitamin K intakes are associated with hip fracture but not with bone mineral density in elderly men and women. Am J Clin Nutr 2000;71:1201-8.
63. Bor MV, Refsum H, Bisp MR, Bleie O, Schneede J, Nordrehaug JE et al. Plasma vitamin B6 vitamers before and after oral vitamin B6 treatment: a randomized placebo-controlled study. Clin Chem 2003;49:155-61.
64. Boros LG. Population thiamine status and varying cancer rates between western, Asian and African countries. Anticancer Res 2000;20:2245-8.
65. Botto LD, Moore CA, Khoury MJ, Erickson JD. Neural-tube defects. N Engl J Med 1999;341:1509-19.
66. Bowman BA, Russell RM. Present knowledge in nutrition, 8th ed. Washington DC: International Life Sciences Institute, 2001.
67. Bowman BB, McCormick DB, Rosenberg IH. Epithelial transport of water-soluble vitamins. Annu Rev Nutr 1989;9:187-99.
68. Brandt RB, Mueller DG, Schroeder JR, Guyer KE, Kirkpatrick BV, Hutcher NE, Ehrlich FE. Serum vitamin A in premature and term neonates. J Pediatr 1978;92:101-4.
69. Brattstrom L, Wilcken DE, Ohrvik J, Brudin L. Common methylenetetrahydrofolate reductase gene mutation leads to hyperhomocysteinemia but not to vascular disease: the result of a meta-analysis. Circulation 1998;98:2520-6.
70. Brenner IB, Zander A, Cole M, Wiseman A. Comparison of axially and radially viewed inductively coupled plasmas for multi-element analysis: effect of sodium and calcium. J Anal Atom Spectrom 1997;12:897-906.
71. Brenner AJ, Harris ED. A quantitative test for copper using bicinchoninic acid. Anal Biochem 1995;226: 80-4.
72. Brewer GJ. Copper control as an antiangiogenic anticancer therapy: lessons from treating Wilson's disease. Exp Biol Med (Maywood) 2001;226:665-73.
73. Brewer GJ, Hedera P, Kluin KJ, Carlson M, Askari F, Dick RB et al. Treatment of Wilson disease with ammonium tetrathiomolybdate: III. Initial therapy in a total of 55 neurologically affected patients and follow-up with zinc therapy. Arch Neurol 2003;60:379-85.
74. Brigden ML. Schilling test still useful in pernicious anemia? Postgrad Med 1999;106:37-8.
75. Brigelius-Flohe R, Kelly FJ, Salonen JT, Neuzil J, Zingg JM, Azzi A. The European perspective on vitamin E: current knowledge and future research. Am J Clin Nutr 2002;76:703-16.
76. Brin M. Erythrocyte as a biopsy tissue for functional evaluation of thiamine adequacy. JAMA 1964;187: 762-6.
77. Brin M, Tai M, Ostashever AS, Kalinsky H. The effect of thiamine deficiency on the activity of erythrocyte hemolysate transketolase. J Nutr 1960;71:273-81.
78. Brown KH, Peerson JM, Rivera J, Allen LH. Effect of supplemental zinc on the growth and serum zinc concentrations of prepubertal children: a meta-analysis of randomized controlled trials. Am J Clin Nutr 2002;75:1062-71.
79. Brown KM, Arthur JR. Selenium, selenoproteins and human health: a review. Public Health Nutr 2001;4:593-9.
80. Brown KM, Pickard K, Nicol F, Beckett GJ, Duthie GG, Arthur JR. Effects of organic and inorganic selenium supplementation on selenoenzyme activity in blood lymphoctyes, granulocytes, platelets and erythrocytes. Clin Sci (Lond) 2000;98:593-9.
81. Brown RO, Forloines-Lynn S, Cross RE, Heizer WD. Chromium deficiency after long-term total parenteral nutrition. Dig Dis Sci 1986;31:661-4.
82. Buettner GR. The pecking order of free radicals and antioxidants: lipid peroxidation, alpha-tocopherol,

and ascorbate. Arch Biochem Biophys 1993;300: 535-43.

83. Burch HB, Combs AM, Lowry OH, Padilla AM. Effects of riboflavin deficiency and realimentation on flavin enzymes of tissues. J Biol Chem 1956;223: 29-45.
84. Burk RF. Selenium: recent clinical advances. Curr Opin Gastroenterol 2001;17:162-6.
85. Burk RF, Hill KE, Motley AK. Selenoprotein metabolism and function: evidence for more than one function for selenoprotein P. J Nutr 2003;133: 1517S-20S.
86. Burns CS, Aronoff-Spencer E, Legname G, Prusiner SB, Antholine WE, Gerfen GJ et al. Copper coordination in the full-length, recombinant prion protein. Biochemistry 2003;42:6794-803.
87. Burns J, Forsyth JS, Paterson CR. Factors associated with variation in plasma copper levels in preterm infants of very low birth weight. Eur J Pediatr 1993;152:240-3.
88. Buzby GP, Mullen JL, Matthews DC, Hobbs CL, Rosato EF. Prognostic nutritional index in gastrointestinal surgery. Am J Surg 1980;139:160-7.
89. Camblor M, De La Cuerda, Breton I, et al. Copper deficiency with pancytopenia due to enteral nutrition through jejunostomy. Clinical Nutrition 1997;16: 129-31.
90. Capo-chichi CD, Gueant JL, Feillet F, Namour F, Vidailhet M. Analysis of riboflavin and riboflavin cofactor levels in plasma by high-performance liquid chromatography. J Chromatogr B Biomed Sci Appl 2000;739:219-24.
91. Carlson GL, Williams N, Barber D, et al. Biotin deficiency complicating long-term total parenteral nutrition in an adult patient. Clinical Nutrition 1995;14:186-90.
92. Carmel R. Subtle and atypical cobalamin deficiency states. Am J Hematol 1990;34:108-14.
93. Carmel R. Measuring and interpreting holo-transcobalamin (holo-transcobalamin II). Clin Chem 2002;48:407-9.
94. Carmel R. Prevalence of undiagnosed pernicious anemia in the elderly. Arch Intern Med 1996;156:1097-100.
95. Carr A, Frei B. Does vitamin C act as a pro-oxidant under physiological conditions? FASEB J 1999;13:1007-24.
96. Centre for Biochemical and Biophysical Science and Medicine. www.hms.harvard.edu/bbsm/vallee.htm. 2005.
97. Centres for Disease Control. Achievements in public health 1900-1999: Fluoridation of drinking water to prevent dental caries. MMWR 1999;48:933-40.
98. Centres for Disease Control. Recommendations for using Fluoride to Prevent and Control Dental Caries in the United States. MMWR 2001;50:1-42.
99. Cerklewski FL. Fluoride. In: O'Dell BL, Sunde RA, eds. Handbook of nutritionally essential mineral elements. New York: Marcel Dekker, 1997:583-602.
100. Cerulli J, Grabe DW, Gauthier I, Malone M, McGoldrick MD. Chromium picolinate toxicity. Ann Pharmacother 1998;32:428-31.
101. Cervantes-Laureen D, McElvaney NG, Moss J. Niacin. In: Shils ME, Olson JA, Shike M, Ross AC, eds. Modern Nutrition in Health and Disease. Baltimore: Williams and Wilkins, 1999:401-11.
102. Chan AC. Partners in defense, vitamin E and vitamin C. Can J Physiol Pharmacol 1993;71:725-31.
103. Chappuis P, Poupon J, Rousselet F. A sequential and simple determination of zinc, copper and aluminium in blood samples by inductively coupled plasma atomic emission spectrometry. Clin Chim Acta 1992;206:155-65.
104. Chastain JL, McCormick DB. Flavin catabolites: identification and quantitation in human urine. Am J Clin Nutr 1987;46:830-4.
105. Chen LH, Liu ML, Hwang HY, Chen LS, Korenberg J, Shane B. Human methionine synthase. cDNA cloning, gene localization, and expression. J Biol Chem 1997;272:3628-34.
106. Chesters JK. Zinc. In: O'Dell BL, Sunde RA, eds. Handbook of Nutritionally Essential Mineral Elements. New York, Basel, Hong Kong: Marcel Dekker, 1997:185-230.
107. Chow CK. Vitamin E. In: Machlin LJ, ed. Handbook of vitamins. New York: Marcel Dekker, 1991: 165-98.
108. Christodoulou J, Danks DM, Sarkar B, Baerlocher KE, Casey R, Horn N et al. Early treatment of Menkes disease with parenteral copper-histidine: long-term follow-up of four treated patients. Am J Med Genet 1998;76:154-64.
109. Chytil F, McCormick DB. Vitamins and coenzyme. Methods in enzymology. Orlando: Academic Press Inc, 1986:Part Hpp.
110. Clark LC, Combs GF, Jr., Turnbull BW, Slate EH, Chalker DK, Chow J et al. Effects of selenium supplementation for cancer prevention in patients with carcinoma of the skin. A randomized controlled trial. Nutritional Prevention of Cancer Study Group. JAMA 1996;276:1957-63.
111. Clodfelder BJ, Emamaullee J, Hepburn DD, Chakov NE, Nettles HS, Vincent JB. The trail of chromium(III) in vivo from the blood to the urine: the roles of transferrin and chromodulin. J Biol Inorg Chem 2001;6:608-17.
112. Coburn SP. The chemistry and metabolism of the vitamin B6 antagonist, 4-deoxypyridine. Boca Raton, FL: CRC Press, 1981.
113. Cohen HJ, Brown MR, Hamilton D, Lyons-Patterson J, Avissar N, Liegey P. Glutathione peroxidase and selenium deficiency in patients receiving home par-

enteral nutrition: time course for development of deficiency and repletion of enzyme activity in plasma and blood cells. Am J Clin Nutr 1989;49: 132-9.
114. Combs GF. Biotin. The Vitamins. Fundamental Aspects in Nutrition and Health. San Diego: Academic Press, 1992:350-65.
115. Combs GF, Jr., Clark LC, Turnbull BW. An analysis of cancer prevention by selenium. Biofactors 2001;14:153-9.
116. Combs GF, Jr., Gray WP. Chemopreventive agents: selenium. Pharmacol Ther 1998;79:179-92.
117. Commission of the European Communities. Report of the scientific committee for food (31st series). 1992.
118. Cordano A. Clinical manifestations of nutritional copper deficiency in infants and children. Am J Clin Nutr 1998;67:1012S-6S.
119. Cousins RJ, Leinart AS. Tissue-specific regulation of zinc metabolism and metallothionein genes by interleukin 1. FASEB J 1988;2:2884-90.
120. Cox DW, Moore SD. Copper transporting P-type ATPases and human disease. J Bioenerg Biomembr 2002;34:333-8.
121. Cravo ML, Gloria LM, Selhub J, Nadeau MR, Camilo ME, Resende MP et al. Hyperhomocysteinemia in chronic alcoholism: correlation with folate, vitamin B-12, and vitamin B-6 status. Am J Clin Nutr 1996;63:220-4.
122. Cuajungco MP, Lees GJ. Zinc metabolism in the brain: relevance to human neurodegenerative disorders. Neurobiol Dis 1997;4:137-69.
123. Dancis J, Lehanka J, Levitz M. Placental transport of riboflavin: differential rates of uptake at the maternal and fetal surfaces of the perfused human placenta. Am J Obstet Gynecol 1988;158:204-10.
124. Danks DM. Copper deficiency in humans. Annu Rev Nutr 1988;8:235-57.
125. Davies S, McLaren HJ, Hunnisett A, Howard M. Age-related decreases in chromium levels in 51,665 hair, sweat, and serum samples from 40,872 patients–implications for the prevention of cardiovascular disease and type II diabetes mellitus. Metabolism 1997;46:469-73.
126. Davis RE. Clinical chemistry of vitamin B12. Adv Clin Chem 1985;24:163-216.
127. Dean JR, Ando DJ, Metcalf E. Atomic absorption & plasma spectroscopy. New York: John Wiley & Sons, 1997.
128. Delves HT. Atomic absorption spectroscopy in clinical analysis. Ann Clin Biochem 1987;24: 529-51.
129. DePaola DP. Nutrition in relation to dental medicine. In: Shils ME, Olson JA, Shihe M, Ross AC, eds. Modern Nutrition in Health and Disease. Baltimore, MD: Williams and Wilkins, 1999:1099-124.
130. Deutsch JC. Dehydroascorbic acid. J Chromatogr A 2000;881:299-307.
131. Deutsch JC, Kolhouse JF. Ascorbate and dehydroascorbate measurements in aqueous solutions and plasma determined by gas chromatography-mass spectrometry. Anal Chem 1993;65:321-6.
132. Devlin AM, Ling EH, Peerson JM, Fernando S, Clarke R, Smith AD, Halsted CH. Glutamate carboxypeptidase II: a polymorphism associated with lower levels of serum folate and hyperhomocysteinemia. Hum Mol Genet 2000;9:2837-44.
133. Devrian TA. The physiological effects of dietary boron. Crit Rev Food Sci Nutr 2003;43:219-31.
134. Dickman ED, Smith SM. Selective regulation of cardiomyocyte gene expression and cardiac morphogenesis by retinoic acid. Dev Dyn 1996;206:39-48.
135. Dietary Reference Intakes for Vitamin C, Vitamin E, Selenium and Carotenoids. Washington DC: National Academy Press, 2000.
136. Doherty CP, Sarkar MA, Shakur MS, Ling SC, Elton RA, Cutting WA. Zinc and rehabilitation from severe protein-energy malnutrition: higher-dose regimens are associated with increased mortality. Am J Clin Nutr 1998;68:742-8.
137. Doisy EA Jr. Micronutrient controls on biosynthesis of clotting proteins and cholesterol. In: Hemphill DD, ed. Trace substances in environmental health. Columbia, MO: University of Missouri, 1973:193-9.
138. Downing RG, Strong PL, Hovanec BM, Northington J. Considerations in the determination of boron at low concentrations. Biol Trace Elem Res 1998;66: 3-21.
139. Dubuisson C, Poussel E, Mermet J-M. Comparison of axially and radially viewed inductively coupled plasma emission spectrometry in terms of signal-to-background ratio effects. J Anal Atom Spectrom 1997;12:281-6.
140. Dutta P. Disturbances in glutathione metabolism and resistance to malaria: current understanding and new concepts. J Soc Pharm Chem 1993;2:11-48.
141. Dutta P, Seirafi J, Halpin D, Pinto J, Rivlin R. Acute ethanol exposure alters hepatic glutathione metabolism in riboflavin deficiency. Alcohol 1995;12:43-7.
142. Edmondson DE, Newton-Vinson P. The covalent FAD of monoamine oxidase: structural and functional role and mechanism of the flavinylation reaction. Antioxid Redox Signal 2001;3:789-806.
143. Eissenstat BR, Wyse BW, Hansen RG. Pantothenic acid status of adolescents. Am J Clin Nutr 1986;44:931-7.
144. Ejima A, Imamura T, Nakamura S, Saito H, Matsumoto K, Momono S. Manganese intoxication during total parenteral nutrition. Lancet 1992;339:426.

145. Elia M. Metabolic response to starvation, injury and sepsis. In: Payne-James J, Grimble G, Silk D, eds. Artificial nutrition support in clinical practice. London: GMM, 2001:1-24.
146. Elia M, Crozier C, Neale G. Mineral metabolism during short-term starvation in man. Clin Chim Acta 1984;139:37-45.
147. Environmental Health Criteria 200. Copper. 1998. WHO Geneva.
148. Evans WC. Thiaminases and their efffect on animals. In: Munson PL, Glover J, Diczfalusy U, et al, eds. Vitamins and Hormones. New York: Academic Press, Inc, 1975:467-504.
149. Fain O, Mathieu E, Thomas M. Scurvy in patients with cancer. BMJ 1998;316:1661-2.
150. Falchuk KH. The molecular basis for the role of zinc in developmental biology. Mol Cell Biochem 1998;188:41-8.
151. Farrell PM, Bieri JG, Fratantoni JF, Wood RE, di Sant'Agnese PA. The occurrence and effects of human vitamin E deficiency. A study in patients with cystic fibrosis. J Clin Invest 1977;60:233-41.
152. Fatemi N, Sarkar B. Molecular mechanism of copper transport in Wilson disease. Environ Health Perspect 2002;110 Suppl 5:695-8.
153. Fell GS, Fleck A, Cuthbertson DP, Queen K, Morrison C, Bessent RG, Husain SL. Urinary zinc levels as an indication of muscle catabolism. Lancet 1973;1:280-2.
154. Fell JM, Reynolds AP, Meadows N, Khan K, Long SG, Quaghebeur G et al. Manganese toxicity in children receiving long-term parenteral nutrition. Lancet 1996;347:1218-21.
155. Fenech M. Micronutrients and genomic stability: a new paradigm for recommended dietary allowances (RDAs). Food Chem Toxicol 2002;40:1113-7.
156. Fennelly J, Frank O, Baker H, Leevy CM. Red blood cell-transketolase activity in malnourished alcoholics with cirrhosis. Am J Clin Nutr 1967;20:946-9.
157. Fenton WA, Rosenberg LE. Disorders of proprionate and methylmalonate metabolism. In: Scriver CS, Beaudet AL, Sly WS, Valle DR, eds. The metabolic and molecular basis of inherited disease. New York: McGraw-Hill, 1995:1423-49.
158. Fenton WA, Rosenberg LE. Inherited disorders of cobalamin transort and metabolism. In: Scriver CR, Beaudet AL, Sly WS, Valle DR, eds. The metabolic and molecular bases of inherited disease. New York: McGraw-Hill, 1995:3129-49.
159. Ferenci P, Caca K, Loudianos G, Mieli-Vergani G, Tanner S, Sternlieb I et al. Diagnosis and phenotypic classification of Wilson disease. Liver 2003;23:139-42.
160. Ferland G. Vitamin K. In: Bowman BA, Russell RA, eds. Present knowledge in nutrition. Washington: ILSI Press, 2001:164-72.
161. Feskanich D, Weber P, Willett WC, Rockett H, Booth SL, Colditz GA. Vitamin K intake and hip fractures in women: a prospective study. Am J Clin Nutr 1999;69:74-9.
162. Field LS, Luk E, Culotta VC. Copper chaperones: personal escorts for metal ions. J Bioenerg Biomembr 2002;34:373-9.
163. Fisher GL, Davies LG, and Rosenblatt LS. The effects of container composition, storage duration, and temperature on serum mineral levels. La Fleur. National Bureau of Standards, TS, p 58. Symposium on Accuracy in Trace Analysis, Proceedings of the 6th IMR Symposium, 422. 1975. National Bureau of Standards, Special Publication.
164. Fleck A, Raines G, Hawker F, Trotter J, Wallace PI, Ledingham IM, Calman KC. Increased vascular permeability: a major cause of hypoalbuminaemia in disease and injury. Lancet 1985;1:781-4.
165. Fleming CR, Lie JT, McCall JT, O'Brien JF, Baillie EE, Thistle JL. Selenium deficiency and fatal cardiomyopathy in a patient on home parenteral nutrition. Gastroenterology 1982;83:689-93.
166. Fleming JC, Tartaglini E, Steinkamp MP, Schorderet DF, Cohen N, Neufeld EJ. The gene mutated in thiamine-responsive anemia with diabetes and deafness (TRMA) encodes a functional thiamine transporter. Nat Genet 1999;22:305-8.
167. Fletcher RH, Fairfield KM. Vitamins for chronic disease prevention in adults: clinical applications. JAMA 2002;287:3127-9.
168. Floridi A, Pupita M, Palmerini CA, Fini C, Alberti FA. Thiamine pyrophosphate determination in whole blood and erythrocytes by high performance liquid chromatography. Int J Vitam Nutr Res 1984;54:165-71.
169. Food and Agriculture Organisation, World Health Organisation. Joint FAO/WHO Expert Consultation on Human Vitamin and Mineral Requirements. 1998. Bangkok, Thailand: 2000 Rome.
170. Food and Nutrition Board IOM. Dietary Reference Intakes for Thiamin, Roboflavin, Niacin, Vitamin B6, Folate, Vitamin B12, Pantothenic Acid, Biotin, and Choline. Washington, DC: National Academy Press, 1998.
171. Food and Nutrition Board IOM. Dietary Reference Intakes for Calcium, Phosphorus, Magnesium, Vitamin D and Fluoride. Washington, DC: National Academy Press, 1999.
172. Food and Nutrition Board IOM. Dietary Reference Intakes for Vitamin C, Vitamin E, Selenium, and Carotenoids. Washington, DC: National Academy Press, 2000.
173. Food and Nutrition Board IOM. Dietary Reference Intakes for Energy, Carbohydrate, Fiber, Fat, Fatty Acids, Cholesterol, Protein, and Amino Acids. Washington, DC: National Academy Press, 2002.

174. Food and Nutrition Board IOM. Dietary Reference Intakes for Vitamin A, Vitamin K, Arsenic, Boron, Chromium, Copper, Iodine, Iron, Manganese, Molybdenum, Nickel, Silicon, Vanadium, and Zinc. Washington, DC: National Academy Press, 2002.
175. Foote JW, Delves HT. Albumin bound and alpha 2-macroglobulin bound zinc concentrations in the sera of healthy adults. J Clin Pathol 1984;37:1050-4.
176. Ford ES. Serum copper concentration and coronary heart disease among US adults. Am J Epidemiol 2000;151:1182-8.
177. Fordyce FM, Johnson CC, Navaratna UR, Appleton JD, Dissanayake CB. Selenium and iodine in soil, rice and drinking water in relation to endemic goitre in Sri Lanka. Sci Total Environ 2000;263:127-41.
178. Forrer R, Gautschi K, Lutz H. Simultaneous measurement of the trace elements Al, As, B, Be, Cd, Co, Cu, Fe, Li, Mn, Mo, Ni, Rb, Se, Sr, and Zn in human serum and their reference ranges by ICP-MS. Biol Trace Elem Res 2001;80:77-93.
179. Fouty B, Frerman F, Reves R. Riboflavin to treat nucleoside analogue-induced lactic acidosis. Lancet 1998;352:291-2.
179a. Francesconi K A, Pannier F. Selenium Metabolites in Urine: A Critical Overview of Past Work and Current Status. Clin Chem 2004;50:2240-53.
180. Frausto Da Silva JJR, Williams RJP. The biological chemistry of the elements. *The inorganic chemistry of life*, 2nd ed. Oxford: Oxford University Press, 2001.
181. Fredrich W. Thiamine. Vitamins. Berlin: de Gruyter, 1988:341-94.
182. Frei B, Stocker R, England L, Ames BN. Ascorbate: the most effective antioxidant in human blood plasma. Adv Exp Med Biol 1990;264:155-63.
183. Freudenheim JL, Johnson NE, Smith EL. Relationships between usual nutrient intake and bone-mineral content of women 35-65 years of age: longitudinal and cross-sectional analysis. Am J Clin Nutr 1986;44:863-76.
184. Freund H, Atamian S, Fischer JE. Chromium deficiency during total parenteral nutrition. JAMA 1979;241:496-8.
185. Friedman BJ, Freeland-Graves JH, Bales CW, Behmardi F, Shorey-Kutschke RL, Willis RA et al. Manganese balance and clinical observations in young men fed a manganese-deficient diet. J Nutr 1987;117:133-43.
186. Fritz I, Said H, Harris C, et al. A new sensitive assay for plasma riboflavin using high performance liquid chromatography. J Am Coll Nutr 1987;6:454.
187. Fry PC, Fox HM, Tao HG. Metabolic response to a pantothenic acid deficient diet in humans. J Nutr Sci Vitaminol (Tokyo) 1976;22:339-46.
188. Fu CS, Swendseid ME, Jacob RA, McKee RW. Biochemical markers for assessment of niacin status in young men: levels of erythrocyte niacin coenzymes and plasma tryptophan. J Nutr 1989;119:1949-55.
189. Fuhrman MP, Herrmann V, Masidonski P, Eby C. Pancytopenia after removal of copper from total parenteral nutrition. J Parenter Enteral Nutr 2000;24:361-6.
190. Fujita M, Itakura T, Takagi Y, Okada A. Copper deficiency during total parenteral nutrition: clinical analysis of three cases. J Parenter Enteral Nutr 1989;13:421-5.
191. Fuller NJ, Elia M. Inadequacy of urinary urea for estimating nitrogen balance. Ann Clin Biochem 1990;27: 510-1.
192. Gaffney D, Fell GS, O'Reilly DS. ACP Best Practice No 163. Wilson's disease: acute and presymptomatic laboratory diagnosis and monitoring. J Clin Pathol 2000;53:807-12.
193. Gale CR, Martyn CN, Winter PD, Cooper C. Vitamin C and risk of death from stroke and coronary heart disease in cohort of elderly people. BMJ 1995;310:1563-6.
194. Gardiner PH, Littlejohn D, Halls DJ, Fell GS. Direct determination of selenium in human blood serum and plasma by electrothermal atomic absorption spectrometry. J Trace Elem Med Biol 1995;9: 74-81.
195. Geubel AP, De Galocsy C, Alves N, Rahier J, Dive C. Liver damage caused by therapeutic vitamin A administration: estimate of dose-related toxicity in 41 cases. Gastroenterology 1991;100:1701-9.
196. Gey KF. Prospects for the prevention of free radical disease, regarding cancer and cardiovascular disease. Br Med Bull 1993;49:679-99.
197. Ghiselli A, Serafini M, Natella F, Scaccini C. Total antioxidant capacity as a tool to assess redox status: critical view and experimental data. Free Radic Biol Med 2000;29:1106-14.
198. Gidden F, Shenkin A. Laboratory support of the clinical nutrition service. Clin Chem Lab Med 2000;38:693-714.
199. Gitlin JD. Transcriptional regulation of ceruloplasmin gene expression during inflammation. J Biol Chem 1988;263:6281-7.
200. Glenn GM, Krober MS, Kelly P, McCarty J, Weir M. Pyridoxine as therapy in theophylline-induced seizures. Vet Hum Toxicol 1995;37:342-5.
201. Glusman M. The syndrome of "burning feet" (nutritional myalgia) as a manifestation of nutritional deficiency. Am J Med 1947;3:211-23.
202. Golden BE, Golden MH. Effect of zinc on lean tissue synthesis during recovery from malnutrition. Eur J Clin Nutr 1992;46:697-706.
203. Gollan JL, Gollan TJ. Wilson disease in 1998: genetic, diagnostic and therapeutic aspects. J Hepatol 1998;28 Suppl 1:28-36.

204. Gospe SM. Pyridoxine-dependent seizures: findings from recent studies pose new questions. Pediatr Neurol 2002;26:181-5.
205. Graham IM, O'Callaghan P. Vitamins, homocysteine and cardiovascular risk. Cardiovasc Drugs Ther 2002;16:383-9.
206. Greene HL, Philips BL, Franck L, et al. Persistently low blood retinol levels during and after enteral feeding of very low birth weight infants. Examination of losses into intravenous administration sets and a method of prevention by addition to a lipid emulsion. Pediatrics 1987;79:892-200.
207. Greene HL, Hambidge KM, Schanler R, Tsang RC. Guidelines for the use of vitamins, trace elements, calcium, magnesium, and phosphorus in infants and children receiving total parenteral nutrition: report of the Subcommittee on Pediatric Parenteral Nutrient Requirements from the Committee on Clinical Practice Issues of the American Society for Clinical Nutrition. Am J Clin Nutr 1988;48:1324-42.
208. Greger JL. Nutrition versus toxicology of manganese in humans: evaluation of potential biomarkers. Neurotoxicology 1999;20:205-12.
209. Gregory J, Foster K, Tyler H, and Wiseman M. The Dietary and Nutritional Survey of British Adults. Office of Population Censuses and Surveys.Social Survey Division. 1990. London, HMSO.
210. Gregory JF, Kirk JR. Vitamin B6 in foods: assessment of stability and bioavailability. 72. 1978. Washington DC: National Academy of Sciences. Human Vitamin B6 Requirements.
211. Gregory JF III. Case Study: Folate bioavailability. J Nutr 2001;131:1376S-82S.
212. Gregory JF, III, Williamson J, Liao JF, Bailey LB, Toth JP. Kinetic model of folate metabolism in nonpregnant women consuming [2H2]folic acid: isotopic labeling of urinary folate and the catabolite para-acetamidobenzoylglutamate indicates slow, intake-dependent, turnover of folate pools. J Nutr 1998;128:1896-906.
213. Grimble GK. Nitrogen analysis in the clinical laboratory. Laboratory Practice 1990;39:71-5.
214. Grunebaum M, Horodniceanu C, Steinherz R. The radiographic manifestations of bone changes in copper deficiency. Pediatr Radiol 1980;9:101-4.
215. Gruppo Italiano per lo Studio della Sopravvivenza nell'Infarto miocardico. Dietary supplementation with n-3 polyunsaturated fatty acids and vitamin E after myocardial infarction: results of the GISSI-Prevenzione trial. Lancet 1999;354:447-55.
216. Gunton JE, Hams G, Hitchman R, McElduff A. Serum chromium does not predict glucose tolerance in late pregnancy. Am J Clin Nutr 2001;73:99-104.
217. Guthrie BE, Wolf WR, Veillon C. Background correction and related problems in the determination of chromium in urine by graphite furnace atomic absorption spectrometry. Anal Chem 1978;50: 1900-2.
218. Gyorffy EJ, Chan H. Copper deficiency and microcytic anemia resulting from prolonged ingestion of over-the-counter zinc. Am J Gastroenterol 1992;87:1054-5.
219. Hageman GJ, Stierum RH. Niacin, poly(ADP-ribose) polymerase-1 and genomic stability. Mutat Res 2001;475:45-56.
220. Hair Analysis Panel Discussion. Exploring the State of the Science. www.atsdr.cdc.gov/HAC/hair_analysis, 2005.
221. Hak EB, Storm MC, Helms RA. Chromium and zinc contamination of parenteral nutrient solution components commonly used in infants and children. Am J Health Syst Pharm 1998;55:150-4.
222. Hall CA. The transport of vitamin B12 from food to use within the cells. J Lab Clin Med 1979;94:811-6.
223. Halliwell B, Gutteridge JMC. Free radicals in biology and medicine, 3rd ed. Oxford: Oxford University Press, 1999.
224. Halliwell B. Antioxidants and human disease: a general introduction. Nutr Rev 1997;55:S44-S49.
225. Halls DJ, Fell GS. Faster determination of chromium in urine by atomic absorption spectrometry. J Anal At Spectrom 1988;3:105-9.
226. Hambidge M. Human zinc deficiency. J Nutr 2000;130:1344S-9S.
227. Hamm MW, Mehansho H, Henderson LM. Transport and metabolism of pyridoxamine and pyridoxamine phosphate in the small intestine of the rat. J Nutr 1979;109:1552-9.
228. Han Q, Xu M, Tang L, Tan X, Tan X, Tan Y, Hoffman RM. Homogeneous, nonradioactive, enzymatic assay for plasma pyridoxal 5-phosphate. Clin Chem 2002;48:1560-4.
229. Haroon Y. Rapid assay for gamma-carboxyglutamic acid in urine and bone by precolumn derivatization and reversed-phase liquid chromatography. Anal Biochem 1984;140:343-8.
230. Harris ED. Copper. In: O'Dell BL, Sunde RA, eds. Handbook of nutritionally essential mineral elements. New York, Basel, Hong Kong: Marcel Dekker, 1997:231-73.
231. Harris DC. Different metal-binding properties of the two sites of human transferrin. Biochemistry 1977;16:560-4.
232. Harris ZL. Aceruloplasminemia. J Neurol Sci 2003;207:108-9.
233. Harrison I, Littlejohn D, Fell GS. Determination of selenium in human hair and nail by electrothermal atomic absorption spectrometry. J of Analytical Atomic Spectroscopy 1995;10:215-9.
234. Harrison I, Littlejohn D, Fell GS. Distribution of selenium in human blood plasma and serum. Analyst 1996;121:189-94.

235. Harrison I, Littlejohn D, Fell GS. Improved molecular fluorescence method for the determination of selenium in biological samples. Analyst 1996;121:1641-6.
236. Hatfield DL, Gladyshev VN. How selenium has altered our understanding of the genetic code. Mol Cell Biol 2002;22:3565-76.
237. Hauschka PV, Lian JB, Gallop PM. Vitamin K and mineralisation. Trends Biochem Sci 1978;3:75.
238. Hazell AS, Butterworth RF. Hepatic encephalopathy: An update of pathophysiologic mechanisms. Proc Soc Exp Biol Med 1999;222:99-112.
239. Healton EB, Savage DG, Brust JC, Garrett TJ, Lindenbaum J. Neurologic aspects of cobalamin deficiency. Medicine (Baltimore) 1991;70:229-45.
240. Heart Protection Study Collaborative Group. MRC/BHF Heart Protection Study of antioxidant vitamin supplementation in 20,536 high-risk individuals: a randomised placebo-controlled trial. Lancet 2002;360:23-33.
241. Heinen F, Matern D, Pringsheim W, Leititis JU, Brandis M. Zinc deficiency in an exclusively breast-fed preterm infant. Eur J Pediatr 1995;154:71-5.
242. Hellman NE, Gitlin JD. Ceruloplasmin metabolism and function. Annu Rev Nutr 2002;22:439-58.
243. Helphingstine CJ, Bistrian BR. New Food and Drug Administration requirements for inclusion of vitamin K in adult parenteral multivitamins. J Parenter Enteral Nutr 2003;27:220-4.
244. Hermann J, Arquitt A, Stoecker BJ. Effect of chromium supplementation on plasma lipids, apolipoproteins and glucose in elderly subjects. Nutr Res 1994;14:671-4.
245. Herrmann W, Schorr H, Obeid R, Geisel J. Vitamin B-12 status, particularly holotranscobalamin II and methylmalonic acid concentrations, and hyperhomocysteinemia in vegetarians. Am J Clin Nutr 2003;78:131-6.
246. Heyssel RM, Bozian RC, Darby WJ, Bell MC. Vitamin B12 turnover in man. The assimilation of vitamin B12 from natural foodstuff by man and estimates of minimal daily dietary requirements. Am J Clin Nutr 1966;18:176-84.
247. Higdon J. An evidence-based approach to vitamins and minerals. New York; Stuttgart: Thieme, 2003.
248. Hill S. Inductively coupled plasma spectrometry and its applications. Boca Raton: CRC Press, 1999.
249. Hill CH, Matrone G. Chemical parameters in the study of in vivo and in vitro interactions of transition elements. Fed Proc 1970;29:1474-81.
250. Hill KE, Xia Y, Akesson B, Boeglin ME, Burk RF. Selenoprotein P concentration in plasma is an index of selenium status in selenium-deficient and selenium-supplemented Chinese subjects. J Nutr 1996;126:138-45.
251. Hodges RE, Bean WB, Ohlson MA, Bleiler R. Human pantothenic acid deficiency produced by omega-methyl pantothenic acid. J Clin Invest 1959;38: 1421-5.
252. Hodges RE, Hood J, Canham JE, Sauberlich HE, Baker EM. Clinical manifestations of ascorbic acid deficiency in man. Am J Clin Nutr 1971;24:432-43.
253. Hoffer A. Ascorbic acid and toxicity. N Engl J Med 1971;285:635-6.
254. Holm G, Moody LE. Carpal tunnel syndrome: current theory, treatment, and the use of B6. J Am Acad Nurse Pract 2003;15:18-22.
255. Homsher R, Zak B. Spectrophotometric investigation of sensitive complexing agents for the determination of zinc in serum. Clin Chem 1985;31:1310-3.
256. Horwitt MK. Critique of the requirement for vitamin E. Am J Clin Nutr 2001;73:1003-5.
257. Houtkooper LB, Ritenbaugh C, Aickin M, Lohman TG, Going SB, Weber JL et al. Nutrients, body composition and exercise are related to change in bone mineral density in premenopausal women. J Nutr 1995;125:1229-37.
258. Howard JM. Assessment of vitamin B(1) status. Clin Chem 2000;46:1867-8.
259. Hung SC, Hung SH, Tarng DC, Yang WC, Chen TW, Huang TP. Thiamine deficiency and unexplained encephalopathy in hemodialysis and peritoneal dialysis patients. Am J Kidney Dis 2001;38:941-7.
260. Hunt CD. The biochemical effects of physiologic amounts of dietary boron in animal nutrition models. Environ Health Perspect 1994;102 Suppl 7:35-43.
261. Hunt JR, Mullen LM, Lykken GI, Gallagher SK, Nielsen FH. Ascorbic acid: effect on ongoing iron absorption and status in iron-depleted young women. Am J Clin Nutr 1990;51:649-55.
262. Hustad S, McKinley MC, McNulty H, Schneede J, Strain JJ, Scott JM, Ueland PM. Riboflavin, flavin mononucleotide, and flavin adenine dinucleotide in human plasma and erythrocytes at baseline and after low-dose riboflavin supplementation. Clin Chem 2002;48:1571-7.
263. Igic PG, Lee E, Harper W, Roach KW. Toxic effects associated with consumption of zinc. Mayo Clin Proc 2002;77:713-6.
264. Ikeda S, Sera Y, Yoshida M, Ohshiro H, Uchino S, Oka Y et al. Manganese deposits in patients with biliary atresia after hepatic porto-enterostomy. J Pediatr Surg 2000;35:450-3.
265. Ingenbleek Y, Young VR. Significance of transthyretin in protein metabolism. Clin Chem Lab Med 2002;40:1281-91.
266. Innis WS, McCormick DB, Merrill AH, Jr. Variations in riboflavin binding by human plasma: identification of immunoglobulins as the major proteins responsible. Biochem Med 1985;34:151-65.
267. Inoue K, Kito M, Kato S, Osawa M, Okuda H, Yabuta K, Maeda T. A case of acquired zinc deficiency in a

mature breast-fed infant. J Perinat Med 1998;26: 495-7.
268. International Vitamin A Consultative Group. Bioavailability of dietary carotenoids: current concepts. Washington DC: ILSI Press, 1999.
269. Itai K, Tsunoda H. Highly sensitive and rapid method for determination of fluoride ion concentrations in serum and urine using flow injection analysis with a fluoride ion-selective electrode. Clin Chim Acta 2001;308:163-71.
270. Ito MK. Niacin-based therapy for dyslipidemia: past evidence and future advances. Am J Manag Care 2002;8:S315-S322.
271. Iversen BS, Menne C, White MA, Kristiansen J, Christensen JM, Sabbioni E. Inductively coupled plasma mass spectrometric determination of molybdenum in urine from a Danish population. Analyst 1998;123:81-5.
272. Iwaki M, Murakami E, Kakehi K. Chromatographic and capillary electrophoretic methods for the analysis of nicotinic acid and its metabolites. J Chromatogr B Biomed Sci Appl 2000;747:229-40.
273. Iwamoto J, Takeda T, Ichimura S. Effect of combined administration of vitamin D3 and vitamin K2 on bone mineral density of the lumbar spine in postmenopausal women with osteoporosis. J Orthop Sci 2000;5:546-51.
274. Jacob RA. Niacin. In: Bowman BA, Russell RM, eds. Present knowledge in nutrition. Washington, DC: ILSI Press, 2001:199-206.
275. Jacob RA, Sandstead HH, Munoz JM, Klevay LM, Milne DB. Whole body surface loss of trace metals in normal males. Am J Clin Nutr 1981;34:1379-83.
276. Jacob RA, Skala JH, Omaye ST. Biochemical indices of human vitamin C status. Am J Clin Nutr 1987;46:818-26.
277. Jacob RA, Swendseid ME, McKee RW, Fu CS, Clemens RA. Biochemical markers for assessment of niacin status in young men: urinary and blood levels of niacin metabolites. J Nutr 1989;119:591-8.
278. Jacquamet L, Sun Y, Hatfield J, Gu W, Cramer SP, Crowder MW et al. Characterization of chromodulin by X-ray absorption and electron paramagnetic resonance spectroscopies and magnetic susceptibility measurements. J Am Chem Soc 2003;125:774-80.
279. Jacques PF, Selhub J, Bostom AG, Wilson PW, Rosenberg IH. The effect of folic acid fortification on plasma folate and total homocysteine concentrations. N Engl J Med 1999;340:1449-54.
280. Jaffe IA. The antivitamin B 6 effect of penicillamine: clinical and immunological implications. Adv Biochem Psychopharmacol 1972;4:217-26.
281. Jakob E, Elmadfa I. Rapid HPLC assay for the assessment of vitamin K1, A, E and beta-carotene status in children (7-19 years). Int J Vitam Nutr Res 1995;65: 31-5.
282. Janiszowska W, Pennock JF. The biochemistry of vitamin E in plants. Vitam Horm 1976;34:77-105.
283. Jeejeebhoy KN. The role of chromium in nutrition and therapeutics and as a potential toxin. Nutr Rev 1999;57:329-35.
284. Jeejeebhoy KN, Chu RC, Marliss EB, Greenberg GR, Bruce-Robertson A. Chromium deficiency, glucose intolerance, and neuropathy reversed by chromium supplementation, in a patient receiving long-term total parenteral nutrition. Am J Clin Nutr 1977;30:531-8.
285. Jialal I, Grundy SM. Effect of combined supplementation with alpha-tocopherol, ascorbate, and beta carotene on low-density lipoprotein oxidation. Circulation 1993;88:2780-6.
286. Jiang Q, Christen S, Shigenaga MK, Ames BN. gamma-tocopherol, the major form of vitamin E in the US diet, deserves more attention. Am J Clin Nutr 2001;74:714-22.
287. Johnson JL. Molybdenum. In: O'Dell BL, Sunde RA, eds. Handbook of nutritionally essential mineral elements. New York, Basel, Hong Kong: Marcel Dekker, 1997:413-38.
288. Johnston CS. Vitamin C. In: Bowman BA, Russell RM, eds. Present knowledge in nutrition. Washington DC: ILSI Press, 2001.
289. Kaczmarek MJ, Nixon PF. Variants of transketolase from human erythrocytes. Clin Chim Acta 1983;130:349-56.
290. Kafritsa Y, Fell J, Long S, Bynevelt M, Taylor W, Milla P. Long-term outcome of brain manganese deposition in patients on home parenteral nutrition. Arch Dis Child 1998;79:263-5.
291. Kaler SG. Metabolic and molecular bases of Menkes disease and occipital horn syndrome. Pediatr Dev Pathol 1998;1:85-98.
292. Kallner A, Hartmann D, Hornig D. Steady-state turnover and body pool of ascorbic acid in man. Am J Clin Nutr 1979;32:530-9.
293. Kalman DS. Chromium picolinate and type 2 diabetes. Am J Clin Nutr 2003;78:192-3.
294. Kang SS, Zhou J, Wong PW, Kowalisyn J, Strokosch G. Intermediate homocysteinemia: a thermolabile variant of methylenetetrahydrofolate reductase. Am J Hum Genet 1988;43:414-21.
295. Kant AK, Block G. Dietary vitamin B-6 intake and food sources in the US population: NHANES II, 1976-1980. Am J Clin Nutr 1990;52:707-16.
296. Kanyo ZF, Scolnick LR, Ash DE, Christianson DW. Structure of a unique binuclear manganese cluster in arginase. Nature 1996;383:554-7.
297. Kaplowitz T. Thiamin triphosphate synthesis in animals. In: Kobayashi T, ed. Proceedings of the 1st International Congress on Vitamins and Biofactors in Life Sciences. Tokyo: Centre for Academic Publications Japan, 1992:383-6.

298. Kappus H, Diplock AT. Tolerance and safety of vitamin E: a toxicological position report. Free Radic Biol Med 1992;13:55-74.
299. Kathman JV, Kies C. Pantothentic acid status of free living adolescents and young adults. Nutr Res 1984;4:245-50.
300. Kay RG, Tasman-Jones C, Pybus J, Whiting R, Black H. A syndrome of acute zinc deficiency during total parenteral alimentation in man. Ann Surg 1976;183:331-40.
301. Kelleher BP, Broin SD. Microbiological assay for vitamin B12 performed in 96-well microtitre plates. J Clin Pathol 1991;44:592-5.
302. Kelly DA, Coe AW, Shenkin A, Lake BD, Walker-Smith JA. Symptomatic selenium deficiency in a child on home parenteral nutrition. J Pediatr Gastroenterol Nutr 1988;7:783-6.
303. Ketley CE, Cochran JA, Lennon MA, O'Mullane DM, Worthington HV. Urinary fluoride excretion of young children exposed to different fluoride regimes. Community Dent Health 2002;19:12-7.
304. Kimura M, Itokawa Y. Determination of thiamine and its phosphate esters in human and rat blood by high-performance liquid chromatography with post-column derivatization. J Chromatogr 1985;332:181-8.
305. King JC, Keen CL. Zinc. In: Shils ME, Olson JA, Shihe M, Ross AC, eds. Modern nutrition in health and disease. Baltimore: Williams and Wilkins, 1999: 223-39.
306. King JC, Shames DM, Lowe NM, Woodhouse LR, Sutherland B, Abrams SA et al. Effect of acute zinc depletion on zinc homeostasis and plasma zinc kinetics in men. Am J Clin Nutr 2001;74:116-24.
307. Kisker C, Schindelin H, Rees DC. Molybdenum-cofactor-containing enzymes: structure and mechanism. Annu Rev Biochem 1997;66:233-67.
308. Klein EA, Lippman SM, Thompson IM, Goodman PJ, Albanes D, Taylor PR, Coltman C. The selenium and vitamin e cancer prevention trial. World J Urol 2003;21:21-7.
309. Klevay LM. Trace element and mineral nutrition in ischemic hart disease. In: Bogden JD, Klevay LM, eds. Clinical nutrition of the essential trace elements and minerals. Totowa, New Jersey: Humana Press, 2000:251-71.
310. Knekt P, Reunanen A, Jarvinen R, Seppanen R, Heliovaara M, Aromaa A. Antioxidant vitamin intake and coronary mortality in a longitudinal population study. Am J Epidemiol 1994;139:1180-9.
311. Knoblock E, Hodr R, Janda J, et al. Spectrofluorimetric micromethod for determining riboflavin in the blood of newborn babies and their mothers. Int J Vitam Nutr Res 1979;49:144-51.
312. Koivistoinen P, Huttunen JK. Selenium in food and nutrition in Finland. An overview on research and action. Ann Clin Res 1986;18:13-7.
313. Konstantinides FN. Nitrogen balance studies in clinical nutrition. Nutr Clin Pract 1992;7:231-8.
314. Krasinski SD, Russell RM, Furie BC, Kruger SF, Jacques PF, Furie B. The prevalence of vitamin K deficiency in chronic gastrointestinal disorders. Am J Clin Nutr 1985;41:639-43.
315. Krumdieck CL, Fukushima K, Fukushima T, Shiota T, Butterworth CE, Jr. A long-term study of the excretion of folate and pterins in a human subject after ingestion of 14C folic acid, with observations on the effect of diphenylhydantoin administration. Am J Clin Nutr 1978;31:88-93.
316. Kuller LH, Evans RW. Homocysteine, vitamins, and cardiovascular disease. Circulation 1998;98:196-9.
317. Laforenza U, Patrini C, Alvisi C, Faelli A, Licandro A, Rindi G. Thiamine uptake in human intestinal biopsy specimens, including observations from a patient with acute thiamine deficiency. Am J Clin Nutr 1997;66:320-6.
318. Lammer EJ, Chen DT, Hoar RM, Agnish ND, Benke PJ, Braun JT et al. Retinoic acid embryopathy. N Engl J Med 1985;313:837-41.
319. Lan SJ, Henderson LM. Uptake of nicotinic acid and nicotinamide by rat erythrocytes. J Biol Chem 1968;243:3388-94.
320. Lane LA, Rojas-Fernandez C. Treatment of vitamin b(12)-deficiency anemia: oral versus parenteral therapy. Ann Pharmacother 2002;36:1268-72.
321. Lautier D, Lagueux J, Thibodeau J, Menard L, Poirier GG. Molecular and biochemical features of poly (ADP-ribose) metabolism. Mol Cell Biochem 1993;122:171-93.
322. Leach RM, Harris ED. Manganese. In: O'Dell BL, Sunde RA, eds. Handbook of nutritionally essential mineral elements. New York, Basel, Hong Kong: Marcel Dekker, 1997.
323. Lee BJ, Lin PT, Liaw YP, Chang SJ, Cheng CH, Huang YC. Homocysteine and risk of coronary artery disease: Folate is the important determinant of plasma homocysteine concentration. Nutrition 2003;19:577-83.
324. Lee SS, McCormick DB. Thyroid hormone regulation of flavocoenzyme biosynthesis. Arch Biochem Biophys 1985;237:197-201.
325. Lee W, Roberts SM, Labbe RF. Ascorbic acid determination with an automated enzymatic procedure. Clin Chem 1997;43:154-7.
326. Leklem JE. Vitamin B6. In: Ziegler EE, Filer LJ, eds. Present knowledge in nutrition. Washington DC: ILSI Press, 1996:174-83.
327. Leklem JE. Vitamin B6. In: Shils ME, Olson JA, Shihe M, Ross AC, eds. Modern nutrition in health and disease. Baltimore, MD: Williams and Williams, 1999:413-21.
328. Leo MA, Lieber CS. Alcohol, vitamin A, and beta-carotene: adverse interactions, including hepatotoxic-

ity and carcinogenicity. Am J Clin Nutr 1999;69:1071-85.
329. Leung FY, Galbraith LV. Elevated serum chromium in patients on total parenteral nutrition and the ionic species of contaminant chromium. Biol Trace Elem Res 1995;50:221-8.
330. Levander OA. Involvement of Selenium in the Regulation of Viral Virulence. ML Moxon Honorary Lectures, SpecialCircular.ohioline.ag.ohio-state.edu/sc167/sc_08, 167-199. 2003.
331. Levine M, Conry-Cantilena C, Wang Y, Welch RW, Washko PW, Dhariwal KR et al. Vitamin C pharmacokinetics in healthy volunteers: evidence for a recommended dietary allowance. Proc Natl Acad Sci USA 1996;93:3704-9.
332. Liang WJ, Johnson D, Jarvis SM. Vitamin C transport systems of mammalian cells. Mol Membr Biol 2001;18:87-95.
333. Lim TH, Sargent T, III, Kusubov N. Kinetics of trace element chromium(III) in the human body. Am J Physiol 1983;244:R445-R454.
334. Lindenbaum J, Allen RH. Clinical spectrum and diagnosis of folate deficiency. In: Bailey LB, ed. Folate in health and disease. New York: Marcel Dekker, 1995:43-74.
335. Lindenbaum J, Rosenberg IH, Wilson PW, Stabler SP, Allen RH. Prevalence of cobalamin deficiency in the Framingham elderly population. Am J Clin Nutr 1994;60:2-11.
336. Linder MC. Copper and genomic stability in mammals. Mutat Res 2001;475:141-52.
337. Linder MC, Hazegh-Azam M. Copper biochemistry and molecular biology. Am J Clin Nutr 1996;63:797S-811S.
338. Lockitch G, Fasset JD, Gerson B, et al. Control of preanalytical variation in trace element determinations. Approved Guideline NCCLS 1997;17:1-30.
339. Lockitch G, Halstead AC, Wadsworth L, Quigley G, Reston L, Jacobson B. Age- and sex-specific pediatric reference intervals and correlations for zinc, copper, selenium, iron, vitamins A and E, and related proteins. Clin Chem 1988;34:1625-8.
340. Lockitch G, Taylor GP, Wong LT, Davidson AG, Dison PJ, Riddell D, Massing B. Cardiomyopathy associated with nonendemic selenium deficiency in a Caucasian adolescent. Am J Clin Nutr 1990;52:572-7.
341. Loerch JD, Underwood BA, Lewis KC. Response of plasma levels of vitamin A to a dose of vitamin A as an indicator of hepatic vitamin A reserves in rats. J Nutr 1979;109:778-86.
342. Loikas S, Lopponen M, Suominen P, Moller J, Irjala K, Isoaho R et al. RIA for serum holo-transcobalamin: method evaluation in the clinical laboratory and reference interval. Clin Chem 2003;49:455-62.
343. Lombeck I, Wendel U, Versieck J, van Ballenberghe L, Bremer HJ, Duran R, Wadman S. Increased manganese content and reduced arginase activity in erythrocytes of a patient with prolidase deficiency (iminodipeptiduria). Eur J Pediatr 1986;144:571-3.
344. Longnecker MP, Stampfer MJ, Morris JS, Spate V, Baskett C, Mason M, Willett WC. A 1-y trial of the effect of high-selenium bread on selenium concentrations in blood and toenails. Am J Clin Nutr 1993;57:408-13.
345. Lonnerdal B. Copper nutrition during infancy and childhood. Am J Clin Nutr 1998;67:1046S-53S.
346. Lopes I, Marques L, Neves E, Silva A, Taveira M, Pena R et al. Prolidase deficiency with hyperimmunoglobulin E: a case report. Pediatr Allergy Immunol 2002;13:140-2.
347. Louw JA, Werbeck A, Louw ME, Kotze TJ, Cooper R, Labadarios D. Blood vitamin concentrations during the acute-phase response. Crit Care Med 1992;20:934-41.
348. Lowe NM, Woodhouse LR, Matel JS, King JC. Comparison of estimates of zinc absorption in humans by using 4 stable isotopic tracer methods and compartmental analysis. Am J Clin Nutr 2000;71:523-9.
349. Lowry SF. Modulating the metabolic response to injury and infection. Proc Nutr Soc 1992;51:267-77.
350. Ludwig ML, Matthews RG. Structure-based perspectives on B12-dependent enzymes. Annu Rev Biochem 1997;66:269-313.
351. Lui A, Lumeng L, Li TK. Metabolism of vitamin B6 in rat liver mitochondria. J Biol Chem 1981;256:6041-6.
352. Luo G, Ducy P, McKee MD, Pinero GJ, Loyer E, Behringer RR, Karsenty G. Spontaneous calcification of arteries and cartilage in mice lacking matrix GLA protein. Nature 1997;386:78-81.
353. Lykkesfeldt J, Christen S, Wallock LM, Chang HH, Jacob RA, Ames BN. Ascorbate is depleted by smoking and repleted by moderate supplementation: a study in male smokers and nonsmokers with matched dietary antioxidant intakes. Am J Clin Nutr 2000;71:530-6.
354. Lyon TD, Fell GS, Gaffney D, McGaw BA, Russell RI, Park RH et al. Use of a stable copper isotope (65Cu) in the differential diagnosis of Wilson's disease. Clin Sci (Lond) 1995;88:727-32.
355. Machonkin TE, Zhang HH, Hedman B, Hodgson KO, Solomon EI. Spectroscopic and magnetic studies of human ceruloplasmin: identification of a redox-inactive reduced Type 1 copper site. Biochemistry 1998;37:9570-8.
356. Makarchikov AF, Wins P, Janssen E, Wieringa B, Grisar T, Bettendorff L. Adenylate kinase 1 knockout mice have normal thiamine triphosphate levels. Biochim Biophys Acta 2002;1592:117-21.

357. Makino T. A simple and sensitive colorimetric assay of zinc in serum using cationic porphyrin. Clin Chim Acta 1999;282:65-76.
358. Malo C, Wilson JX. Glucose modulates vitamin C transport in adult human small intestinal brush border membrane vesicles. J Nutr 2000;130:63-9.
359. Mangels AR, Holden JM, Beecher GR et al. Carotenoid content of fruits and vegetables. An evaluation of analytical data. J Am Diet Assoc 1993;93:284-9.
360. Margolis SA, Paule RC, Ziegler RG. Ascorbic and dehydroascorbic acids measured in plasma preserved with dithiothreitol or metaphosphoric acid. Clin Chem 1990;36:1750-5.
361. Marrill J, Idres N, Capron CC, et al. Retinoic acid metabolism and mechanism of action: a review. Curr Drug Metab 2003;93:284-9.
362. Marshall I. Zinc for the common cold (Cochrane Methodology Review). The Cochrane Library 2003;4.
363. Mason JB. Intestinal transport of monoglutamyl folates in mamalian systems. In: Picciano MF, Stokstad ELR. Gregory JF, eds. Folic acid metabolism in health and disease. New York: Wiley-Liss, 1990: 47-64.
364. Massey V. The chemical and biological versatility of riboflavin. Biochem Soc Trans 2000;28:283-96.
365. Matherly LH, Goldman DI. Membrane transport of folates. Vitam Horm 2003;66:403-56.
366. Mayne ST. Beta-carotene, carotenoids, and disease prevention in humans. FASEB J 1996;10:690-701.
367. McCormick DB. Biochemistry of coenzymes. In: Meyers RA, ed. Encyclopedia of molecular biology and molecular medicine. New York, VC: 1996: 396-406.
368. McCormick DB. Biochemistry of coenzymes—pantothenic acid. In: Meyers RA, ed. Encyclopedia of molecular biology and molecular medicine. New York, VC: 1996.
369. McCormick DB. Biochemistry of coenzymes—pyridoxine B6. In: Meyers RA, ed. Encyclopedia of molecular biology and molecular medicine. New York, VC: 1996:396-406.
370. McCormick DB. Riboflavin. In: Shils ME, Olson JA, Shihe M, Ross AC, eds. Modern nutrition in health and disease. Baltimore, MD: Williams and Wilkins, 1999:391-9.
371. McCormick DB. Vitamin B6. In: Bowman BA, Russell RA, eds. Present knowledge in nutrition. Washington DC: ILSI Press, 2001:207-13.
372. McCormick DB, Snell BA. Pyridoxal phosphokinases: II. Effect of inhibitors. J Biol Chem 1961;236:2085-8.
373. McCormick DB, Wright LD. Vitamins and coenzyme. Methods in enzymology. New York: Academic Press Inc, 1980:part Fpp.
374. McMahon RJ. Biotin in metabolism and molecular biology. Annu Rev Nutr 2002;22:221-39.
375. Mehansho H, Henderson LM. Transport and accumulation of pyridoxine and pyridoxal by erythrocytes. J Biol Chem 1980;255:11901-7.
376. Melhus H, Michaelsson K, Kindmark A, Bergstrom R, Holmberg L, Mallmin H et al. Excessive dietary intake of vitamin A is associated with reduced bone mineral density and increased risk for hip fracture. Ann Intern Med 1998;129:770-8.
377. Merrill AH, Froehlich JA, McCormick DB. Isolation and identification of alternative riboflavin-binding proteins from human plasma. Biochem Med 1981;25:198-206.
378. Mertz W. Trace elements in human and animal nutrition, 5th ed. New York: Academic Press, 1987.
379. Mertz W. Trace minerals and atherosclerosis. Fed Proc 1982;41:2807-12.
380. Mertz W. Use and misuse of balance studies. J Nutr 1987;117:1811-3.
381. Mertz W. Chromium research from a distance: from 1959 to 1980. J Am Coll Nutr 1998;17:544-7.
382. Mertz W. Interaction of chromium with insulin: a progress report. Nutr Rev 1998;56:174-7.
383. Meurs H, Maarsingh H, Zaagsma J. Arginase and asthma: novel insights into nitric oxide homeostasis and airway hyperresponsiveness. Trends Pharmacol Sci 2003;24:450-5.
384. Mewies M, McIntire WS, Scrutton NS. Convalent attachment of flavin adenine dinucleotide (FAD) and flavin mononucleotide (FMN) to enzymes: the current state of affairs. Protein Sci 1998;7:7-20.
385. Meydani M. Vitamin E. Lancet 1995;345:170-5.
386. Michaelsson K, Holmberg L, Mallmin H, Sorensen S, Wolk A, Bergstrom R, Ljunghall S. Diet and hip fracture risk: a case-control study. Study Group of the Multiple Risk Survey on Swedish Women for Eating Assessment. Int J Epidemiol 1995;24:771-82.
387. Millart H, Lamiable D. Determination of pyridoxal 5′-phosphate in human serum by reversed phase high performance liquid chromatography combined with spectrofluorimetric detection of 4-pyridoxic acid 5′-phosphate as a derivative. Analyst 1989;114:1225-8.
387a. Miller ER, Pastor-Barriuso R, Dalal D, Riemersma RA, Appel LJ, Guallar E. Meta-analysis: High-dosage Vitamin E supplementation may increase all cause mortality. Ann Int Med 2005;142: in press.
388. Miller JW, Rogers LM, Rucker RB. Pantothenic acid. In: Bowman BA, Russell RA, eds. Present knowledge in nutrition. Washington DC: ILSI Press, 2001:253-60.
389. Miller NJ, Johnston JD, Collis CS, Rice-Evans C. Serum total antioxidant activity after myocardial infarction. Ann Clin Biochem 1997;34 (Pt 1):85-90.
390. Milne DB. Laboratory assessment of trace elements and mineral status. In: Bogden JD, Klevay LM, eds. Laboratory assessment of trace elements and minerals. Totowa, New Jersey: Humana Press, 2000:69-90.

391. Milne DB, Nielsen FH. Effects of a diet low in copper on copper-status indicators in postmenopausal women. Am J Clin Nutr 1996;63:358-64.
392. Milne DB, Ralston NV, Wallwork JC. Zinc content of cellular components of blood: methods for cell separation and analysis evaluated. Clin Chem 1985;31: 65-9.
393. Mineral Analysis Laboratory Grand Forks Human Nutrition Center. www.gfhnrc.ars.usda.gov. 2005.
394. Moat SJ, Ashfield-Watt PA, Powers HJ, Newcombe RG, McDowell IF. Effect of riboflavin status on the homocysteine-lowering effect of folate in relation to the MTHFR (C677T) genotype. Clin Chem 2003;49:295-302.
395. Mock DM, Mock NI. Lymphocyte propionyl-CoA carboxylase is an early and sensitive indicator of biotin deficiency in rats, but urinary excretion of 3-hydroxypropionic acid is not. J Nutr 2002;132: 1945-50.
396. Mock DM, Quirk JG, Mock NI. Marginal biotin deficiency during normal pregnancy. Am J Clin Nutr 2002;75:295-9.
397. Mock NI, Malik MI, Stumbo PJ, Bishop WP, Mock DM. Increased urinary excretion of 3-hydroxyisovaleric acid and decreased urinary excretion of biotin are sensitive early indicators of decreased biotin status in experimental biotin deficiency. Am J Clin Nutr 1997;65:951-8.
398. Moon YS, Kashyap ML. Niacin extended-release/Lovastatin: combination therapy for lipid disorders. Expert Opin Pharmacother 2002;3:1763-71.
399. Morris MS. Folate, homocysteine, and neurological function. Nutr Clin Care 2002;5:124-32.
400. Mouatt B. Health and fitness series–2. Dental decay and the case for fluoride. J Fam Health Care 2003;13:34-6.
401. Mount JN, Heduan E, Herd C, Jupp R, Kearney E, Marsh A. Adaptation of coenzyme stimulation assays for the nutritional assessment of vitamins B1, B2 and B6 using the Cobas Bio centrifugal analyser. Ann Clin Biochem 1987;24 (Pt 1):41-6.
402. Mrochek JE, Jolley RL, Young DS, Turner WJ. Metabolic response of humans to ingestion of nicotinic acid and nicotinamide. Clin Chem 1976;22:1821-7.
403. Mudd SH. Pyridoxine-responsive genetic disease. Fed Proc 1971;30:970-6.
404. Muller DP, Lloyd JK. Effect of large oral doses of vitamin E on the neurological sequelae of patients with abetalipoproteinemia. Ann N Y Acad Sci 1982;393:133-44.
405. Muller T, Muller W, Feichtinger H. Idiopathic copper toxicosis. Am J Clin Nutr 1998;67:1082S-6S.
406. Munday R, Smith BL, Munday CM. Effects of butylated hydroxyanisole and dicoumarol on the toxicity of menadione to rats. Chem Biol Interact 1998;108:155-70.
407. Naito E, Ito M, Yokota I, Saijo T, Matsuda J, Ogawa Y et al. Thiamine-responsive pyruvate dehydrogenase deficiency in two patients caused by a point mutation (F205L and L216F) within the thiamine pyrophosphate binding region. Biochim Biophys Acta 2002;1588:79-84.
408. Nakasaki H, Ohta M, Soeda J, Makuuchi H, Tsuda M, Tajima T et al. Clinical and biochemical aspects of thiamine treatment for metabolic acidosis during total parenteral nutrition. Nutrition 1997;13:110-7.
409. Napoli JL. A gene knockout corroborates the integral function of cellular retinol-binding protein in retinoid metabolism. Nutr Rev 2000;58:230-6.
410. National Research Council CoDA. Recommended dietary allowances, 10th ed. Washington, DC: National Academy of Sciences, 1989.
411. Natraj U, George S, Kadam P. Isolation and partial characterisation of human riboflavin carrier protein and the estimation of its levels during human pregnancy. J Reprod Immunol 1988;13:1-16.
412. Neal RA. Vitamin deficiencies: Thiamin. Hansen RG and Munro HN. 129. 1970. Nashville, GSMHA and National Institute of Health. Proc. Workshop on Problems of Assessment and Alleviation of Malnutrition in the US.
413. Nelsestuen GL, Shah AM, Harvey SB. Vitamin K-dependent proteins. Vitam Horm 2000;58:355-89.
414. Nelson M. Methods and validity of dietary assessment. In: Garrow JS, James WPT, Ralph A, eds. Human nutrition and dietetics. Edinburgh: Churchill Livingstone, 2000:311-31.
415. Nelson HK, Shi Q, Van Dael P, Schiffrin EJ, Blum S, Barclay D et al. Host nutritional selenium status as a driving force for influenza virus mutations. FASEB J 2001;15:1846-8.
416. Neufeld EJ, Fleming JC, Tartaglini E, Steinkamp MP. Thiamine-responsive megaloblastic anemia syndrome: a disorder of high-affinity thiamine transport. Blood Cells Mol Dis 2001;27:135-8.
417. Nexo E, Christensen AL, Hvas AM, Petersen TE, Fedosov SN. Quantification of holo-transcobalamin, a marker of vitamin B12 deficiency. Clin Chem 2002;48:561-2.
418. Nichol C, Herdman J, Sattar N, O'Dwyer PJ, St JO, Littlejohn D, Fell G. Changes in the concentrations of plasma selenium and selenoproteins after minor elective surgery: further evidence for a negative acute phase response? Clin Chem 1998;44:1764-6.
419. Nielsen FH. Possibly essential trace elements. In: Bogden JD, Klevay LM, eds. Clinical nutrition of the essential trace elements and minerals. Totowa, New Jersey: Humana Press, 2000:11-36.
420. Niles RM. Recent advances in the use of vitamin A (retinoids) in the prevention and treatment of cancer. Nutrition 2000;16:1084-9.

421. Ninh NX, Thissen JP, Collette L, Gerard G, Khoi HH, Ketelslegers JM. Zinc supplementation increases growth and circulating insulin-like growth factor I (IGF-I) in growth-retarded Vietnamese children. Am J Clin Nutr 1996;63:514-9.
422. Norose N, Terai M, Norose K. Manganese deficiency in a child with very short bowel syndrome receiving long-term parenteral nutrition. J Trace Elem Exp Med 1992;5:100-1.
423. Novotny JA, Dueker SR, Zech LA. Compartmental analysis of the dynamics of B-carotene metabolism in an adult volunteer. J Lipid Res 1995;36:1825-38.
424. Nutrient Requirements and Functions Laboratory Beltsville Agriculture Research Centre. www.barc.usda.gov/bhnrc/nrfl/nrflres.html. 2005.
425. Nyyssonen K, Parviainen MT, Salonen R, Tuomilehto J, Salonen JT. Vitamin C deficiency and risk of myocardial infarction: prospective population study of men from eastern Finland. BMJ 1997;314:634-8.
426. O'Brien KO, Zavaleta N, Caulfield LE, Wen J, Abrams SA. Prenatal iron supplements impair zinc absorption in pregnant Peruvian women. J Nutr 2000;130: 2251-5.
427. O'Broin S, Kelleher B. Microbiological assay on microtitre plates of folate in serum and red cells. J Clin Pathol 1992;45:344-7.
428. O'Dell BL, Sunde RA. Handbook of nutritionally essential mineral elements. New York: Marcel Dekker, 1997.
429. O'Donnell JG, Watson ID, Fell GS, Allison ME, Russell RI, Mills PR. Wilson's disease presenting as acute fulminant hepatic failure. Scott Med J 1990;35:118-9.
430. Offenbacker GE, Xavier Pi-Sunyer Stoecker BJ. Chromium. In: O'Dell BL, Sunde RA, eds. Handbook of nutritionally essential mineral elements. New York, Basel, Hong Kong: Marcel Dekker, 1997: 389-412.
431. Ogle RF, Christodoulou J, Fagan E, Blok RB, Kirby DM, Seller KL et al. Mitochondrial myopathy with tRNA(Leu(UUR)) mutation and complex I deficiency responsive to riboflavin. J Pediatr 1997;130:138-45.
432. Olson RE. The function and metabolism of vitamin K. Annu Rev Nutr 1984;4:281-337.
432a. Omenn GS, Goodman GE, Thornquist MD, Balmes J, Cullen MR, et al. Effects of a combination of beta-carotene and vitamin A on the lung cancer incidence, total mortality, and cardiovascular mortality in smokers and asbestos-exposed workers. N Engl J Med 1996;334:1150-55
433. Ono J, Harada K, Kodaka R, Sakurai K, Tajiri H, Takagi Y et al. Manganese deposition in the brain during long-term total parenteral nutrition. J Parenter Enteral Nutr 1995;19:310-2.
434. Osendarp SJ, West CE, Black RE. The need for maternal zinc supplementation in developing countries: an unresolved issue. J Nutr 2003;133: 817S-27S.
435. Ottaway JM, Halls DJ. Determination of Manganese in Biological Materials. Pure and Appl Chem 1986;1307-16.
436. Patterson KY, Veillon C. Stable isotopes of minerals as metabolic tracers in human nutrition research. Exp Biol Med (Maywood) 2001;226:271-82.
437. Pelliccione N, Pinto J, Huang YP, Rivlin RS. Accelerated development of riboflavin deficiency by treatment with chlorpromazine. Biochem Pharmacol 1983;32:2949-53.
438. Perez-Ruiz T, Martinez-Lozano C, Sanz A, Bravo E. Determination of riboflavin, flavin mononucletide and flavin adenine dinucleotide in biological tissues by capillary zone electrophoresis and laser-induced fluorescence detection. Electrophoresis 2001;22: 1170-4.
439. Persson B, Tunell R, Ekengren K. Chronic vitamin A intoxication during the first half year of life. Acta Paediatr Scand 1965;54:49-60.
440. Pietinen P, Vartiainen E, Seppanen R, Aro A, Puska P. Changes in diet in Finland from 1972 to 1992: impact on coronary heart disease risk. Prev Med 1996;25:243-50.
441. Pinto J, Huang YP, Rivlin RS. Mechanisms underlying the differential effects of ethanol on the bioavailability of riboflavin and flavin adenine dinucleotide. J Clin Invest 1987;79:1343-8.
442. Pizzulli A, Ranjbar A. Selenium deficiency and hypothyroidism: a new etiology in the differential diagnosis of hypothyroidism in children. Biol Trace Elem Res 2000;77:199-208.
443. Plesofsky-Vig N. Pantothentic acid. In: Shils ME, Olson JA, Shihe M, Ross AC, eds. Modern nutrition in health and disease. Baltimore, MD: Williams and Wilkins, 1999:423-32.
444. Podmore ID, Griffiths HR, Herbert KE, Mistry N, Mistry P, Lunec J. Vitamin C exhibits pro-oxidant properties. Nature 1998;392:559.
445. Pogribny I, Yi P, James SJ. A sensitive new method for rapid detection of abnormal methylation patterns in global DNA and within CpG islands. Biochem Biophys Res Commun 1999;262:624-8.
446. Prasad AS. Effects of zinc deficiency on immune functions. Journal of Trace Elements in Experimental Medicine 2000;13:1-20.
447. Prasad AS. Zinc deficiency in patients with sickle cell disease. Am J Clin Nutr 2002;75:181-2.
448. Prasad AS. Zinc deficiency. BMJ 2003;326:409-10.
449. Prasad PD, Ganapathy V. Structure and function of mammalian sodium-dependent multivitamin transporter. Curr Opin Clin Nutr Metab Care 2000;3:263-6.
450. Prentice AM, Bates CJ, Prentice A, Welch SG, Williams K, McGregor IA. The influence of G-6-PD

activity on the response of erythrocyte glutathione reductase to riboflavin deficiency. Int J Vitam Nutr Res 1981;51:211-5.
451. Prior RL, Cao G. In vivo total antioxidant capacity: comparison of different analytical methods. Free Radic Biol Med 1999;27:1173-81.
452. Pruszkowski E, Neubauer K, Thomas R. An overview of clinical applications by inductively coupled plasma mass spectometry. Atomic Spectroscopy 1998;19:115.
453. Puxty JA, Haskew AE, Ratcliffe JG, McMurray J. Changes in erythrocyte transketolase activity and the thiamine pyrophosphate effect during storage of blood. Ann Clin Biochem 1985;22 (Pt 4):423-7.
454. Rahil-Khazen R, Henriksen H, Bolann BJ, Ulvik RJ. Validation of inductively coupled plasma atomic emission spectrometry technique (ICP-AES) for multi-element analysis of trace elements in human serum. Scand J Clin Lab Invest 2000;60:677-86.
455. Rahman MM, Wahed MA, Fuchs GJ, Baqui AH, Alvarez JO. Synergistic effect of zinc and vitamin A on the biochemical indexes of vitamin A nutrition in children. Am J Clin Nutr 2002;75:92-8.
456. Raiten DJ, Fisher KD. Assessment of folate methodology used in the Third National Health and Nutrition Examination Survey (NHANES III, 1988-1994). J Nutr 1995;125:1371S-98S.
457. Ralli EP, Dumm ME. Relation of pantothenic acid to adrenal cortical function. Vitam Horm 1953;11: 133-58.
458. Rayman MP. The importance of selenium to human health. Lancet 2000;356:233-41.
459. Raz T, Labay V, Baron D, Szargel R, Anbinder Y, Barrett T et al. The spectrum of mutations, including four novel ones, in the thiamine-responsive megaloblastic anemia gene SLC19A2 of eight families. Hum Mutat 2000;16:37-42.
460. Refsum H, Ueland PM, Nygard O, Vollset SE. Homocysteine and cardiovascular disease. Annu Rev Med 1998;49:31-62.
461. Reiss J. Genetics of molybdenum cofactor deficiency. Hum Genet 2000;106:157-63.
462. Reiss J, Johnson JL. Mutations in the molybdenum cofactor biosynthetic genes MOCS1, MOCS2, and GEPH. Hum Mutat 2003;21:569-76.
463. Reports of the Scientific Committee for Food, Commission of the European Communities. 31st Series. 1992.
464. Reynolds RD. Nationwide assay of vitamin B6 in human plasma by different methods. Fed Proc 1983;42:665.
465. Riales R, Albrink MJ. Effect of chromium chloride supplementation on glucose tolerance and serum lipids including high-density lipoprotein of adult men. Am J Clin Nutr 1981;34:2670-8.
466. Ribaya-Mercado JD, Solon FS, Dallal GE, Solomons NW, Fermin LS, Mazariegos M et al. Quantitative assessment of total body stores of vitamin A in adults with the use of a 3-d deuterated-retinol-dilution procedure. Am J Clin Nutr 2003;77: 694-9.
467. Ricciarelli R, Zingg JM, Azzi A. The 80th anniversary of vitamin E: beyond its antioxidant properties. Biol Chem 2002;383:457-65.
468. Rimm EB, Stampfer MJ, Ascherio A, Giovannucci E, Colditz GA, Willett WC. Vitamin E consumption and the risk of coronary heart disease in men. N Engl J Med 1993;328:1450-6.
469. Rindi G, Laforenza U. Thiamine intestinal transport and related issues: recent aspects. Proc Soc Exp Biol Med 2000;224:246-55.
470. Rivlin RS. Riboflavin. In: Bowman BA, Russell RM, eds. Present knowledge in nutrition. Washington DC: ILSI Press, 2001:191-8.
471. Rivlin RS, Pinto JT. Riboflavin (vitamin B2). In: Rucker R, Suttie JW, McCormick DB, Machlin LJ, eds. Handbook of vitamins. New York: Marcel Dekker, 2001.
472. Robien K, Ulrich CM. 5,10-Methylenetetrahydrofolate reductase polymorphisms and leukemia risk: a HuGE minireview. Am J Epidemiol 2003;157: 571-82.
473. Rodriguez MR. [Importance of water-soluble vitamins as regulatory factors of genetic expression]. Rev Invest Clin 2002;54:77-83.
474. Roe DA. A plague of corn. Ithaca, New York: Cornell University Press, 1973.
475. Rogers JT, Bridges KR, Durmowicz GP, Glass J, Auron PE, Munro HN. Translational control during the acute phase response. Ferritin synthesis in response to interleukin-1. J Biol Chem 1990;265:14572-8.
476. Romanski SA, McMahon MM. Metabolic acidosis and thiamine deficiency. Mayo Clin Proc 1999;74:259-63.
477. Rosenberg LE. Vitamin-responsive inherited diseases affecting the nervous system. Res Publ Assoc Res Nerv Ment Dis 1974;53:263-72.
478. Rothman KJ, Moore LL, Singer MR, Nguyen US, Mannino S, Milunsky A. Teratogenicity of high vitamin A intake. N Engl J Med 1995;333:1369-73.
479. Roughead ZK, McCormick DB. Flavin composition of human milk. Am J Clin Nutr 1990;52:854-7.
480. Roughead ZK, McCormick DB. Qualitative and quantitative assessment of flavins in cow's milk. J Nutr 1990;120:382-8.
481. Rubin MA, Miller JP, Ryan AS, Treuth MS, Patterson KY, Pratley RE et al. Acute and chronic resistive exercise increase urinary chromium excretion in men as measured with an enriched chromium stable isotope. J Nutr 1998;128:73-8.

482. Rumsey SC, Levine M. Absorption, transport and disposition of ascorbic acid in humans. J Nutr Biochem 1998;9:116-30.
483. Russell RM. The vitamin A spectrum: from deficiency to toxicity. Am J Clin Nutr 2000;71:878-84.
484. Russell-Jones GJ, Alpers DH. Vitamin B12 transporters. Pharm Biotechnol 1999;12:493-520.
485. Ryan GJ, Wanko NS, Redman AR, Cook CB. Chromium as adjunctive treatment for type 2 diabetes. Ann Pharmacother 2003;37:876-85.
486. Rychlik M. Quantification of free and bound pantothenic acid in foods and blood plasma by a stable isotope dilution assay. J Agric Food Chem 2000;48:1175-81.
487. Said HM. Biotin: the forgotten vitamin. Am J Clin Nutr 2002;75:179-80.
488. Said HM, Ma TY. Mechanism of riboflavin uptake by Caco-2 human intestinal epithelial cells. Am J Physiol 1994;266:G15-G21.
489. Saito Y, Watanabe Y, Saito E, et al. Production and application of monoclonal antibodies to himan selenoprotein P. Journal of Health Science 2001;47:346-52.
490. Sallie R, Katsiyiannakis L, Baldwin D, Davies S, O'Grady J, Mowat A et al. Failure of simple biochemical indexes to reliably differentiate fulminant Wilson's disease from other causes of fulminant liver failure. Hepatology 1992;16:1206-11.
491. Sanderson P, McNulty H, Mastroiacovo P, McDowell IF, Melse-Boonstra A, Finglas PM, Gregory JF, III. Folate bioavailability: UK Food Standards Agency workshop report. Br J Nutr 2003;90:473-9.
492. Sandhu JS, Fraser DR. Measurement of niacin metabolites in urine by high pressure liquid chromatography. A simple, sensitive assay of niacin nutritional status. Int J Vitam Nutr Res 1981;51:139-44.
493. Sandstead HH, Frederickson CJ, Penland JG. History of zinc as related to brain function. J Nutr 2000;130:496S-502S.
494. SAS Trace Element Laboratories. www.sas-centre.org. 2005.
495. Sauberlich HE. Laboratory tests for the assessment of nutritional status, 2nd ed. Boca Raton, FL: CRC Press, 1999.
496. Savage DG, Lindenbaum J, Stabler SP, Allen RH. Sensitivity of serum methylmalonic acid and total homocysteine determinations for diagnosing cobalamin and folate deficiencies. Am J Med 1994;96:239-46.
497. Schaumburg H, Kaplan J, Windebank A, Vick N, Rasmus S, Pleasure D, et al. Sensory neuropathy from pyridoxine abuse. A new megavitamin syndrome. N Engl J Med 1983;309:445-8.
498. Schilsky ML, Scheinberg IH, Sternlieb I. Liver transplantation for Wilson's disease: indications and outcome. Hepatology 1994;19:583-7.
499. Schlesier K, Harwat M, Bohm V, Bitsch R. Assessment of antioxidant activity by using different in vitro methods. Free Radic Res 2002;36:177-87.
500. Schoenen J, Lenaerts M, Bastings E. High-dose riboflavin as a prophylactic treatment of migraine: results of an open pilot study. Cephalalgia 1994;14:328-9.
501. Scholl TO, Johnson WG. Folic acid: influence on the outcome of pregnancy. Am J Clin Nutr 2000;71:1295S-303S.
502. Schrijver J, van Breederode N, van ben Berg H, Bitsch R. Biotin in whole blood by microbiological assay: biotin in plasma or urine by RIA. In: Fidanza F, ed. Nutritional status assessment: A manual for population studies. London: Chapman & Hall, 1991:296-303.
503. Schrijver J, Speek AJ, Klosse JA, van Rijn HJ, Schreurs WH. A reliable semiautomated method for the determination of total thiamine in whole blood by the thiochrome method with high-performance liquid chromatography. Ann Clin Biochem 1982;19:52-6.
504. Schroeder HA, Nason AP, Tipton IH. Chromium deficiency as a factor in atherosclerosis. J Chronic Dis 1970;23:123-42.
505. Schroeder JJ, Cousins RJ. Interleukin 6 regulates metallothionein gene expression and zinc metabolism in hepatocyte monolayer cultures. Proc Natl Acad Sci U S A 1990;87:3137-41.
506. Schuelke M, Mayatepek E, Inter M, Becker M, Pfeiffer E, Speer A et al. Treatment of ataxia in isolated vitamin E deficiency caused by alpha-tocopherol transfer protein deficiency. J Pediatr 1999;134:240-4.
507. Schultz M, Leist M, Petrzika M, Gassmann B, Brigelius-Flohe R. Novel urinary metabolite of alpha-tocopherol, 2,5,7,8-tetramethyl-2(2′-carboxyethyl)-6-hydroxychroman, as an indicator of an adequate vitamin E supply? Am J Clin Nutr 1995;62:1527S-34S.
508. Schulze zur WE, Hesse C, Hotzel. [The gas chromatographic determination pantothenic acid in urine (author's transl)]. Z Klin Chem Klin Biochem 1974;12:498-503.
509. Schurgersl LJ, Geleijnse JM, Grobee DE, et al. Nutritional intake of vitamin K1 (phylloquinone) and K2 (memoquinone) in the Netherlands. J Nutr Environ Med 1999;9:115-22.
510. Schweigert FJ. Inflammation-induced changes in the nutritional biomarkers serum retinol and carotenoids. Curr Opin Clin Nutr Metab Care 2001;4:477-81.
511. Seetharam B, Li N. Transcobalamin II and its cell surface receptor. Vitam Horm 2000;59:337-66.
512. Selhub J. Folate, vitamin B12 and vitamin B6 and one carbon metabolism. J Nutr Health Aging 2002;6:39-42.

513. Semba RD, Bloem MW. The anemia of vitamin A deficiency: epidemiology and pathogenesis. Eur J Clin Nutr 2002;56:271-81.
514. Seshadri V, Fox PL, Mukhopadhyay CK. Dual role of insulin in transcriptional regulation of the acute phase reactant ceruloplasmin. J Biol Chem 2002;277:27903-11.
515. Shearer MJ. Measurement of phylloquione (vitamin K1) in serum and plasma by HPLC. In: Fidanza F, ed. Nutritional status assessment—A manual for population studies. London: Chapman and Hall, 1991: 214-20.
516. Shearer MJ. Vitamin K metabolism and nutriture. Blood Rev 1992;6:92-104.
517. Shearer MJ. The roles of vitamins D and K in bone health and osteoporosis prevention. Proc Nutr Soc 1997;56:915-37.
518. Shenai JP, Kennedy KA, Chytil F, Stahlman MT. Clinical trial of vitamin A supplementation in infants susceptible to bronchopulmonary dysplasia. J Pediatr 1987;111:269-77.
519. Shenkin A, Allwood MC. Trace elements and vitamins in adult intravenous nutrition. In: Rombeau JL, Rolandelli RH, eds. Clinical nutrition: Parenteral nutrition. Philadelphia: WB Saunders Co, 2001: 60-79.
520. Shenkin A, Fell GS, Halls DJ, et al. Essential trace element provision to patients receiving home intravenous nutrition in the United Kingdom. Clinical Nutrition 1986;5:91-7.
521. Shenkin A. Adult micronutrient requirements. In: Payne-James J, Grimble G, Silk D, eds. Artificial nutrition support in clinical practice. London: GMM, 2001:193-212.
522. Shenkin A. Vitamin and essential trace element recommendations during intravenous nutrition: theory and practice. Proc Nutr Soc 1986;45:383-90.
523. Shenkin A. Trace elements and inflammatory response: implications for nutritional support. Nutrition 1995;11:100-5.
524. Shenkin A. Impact of disease on markers of macronutrient status. Proc Nutr Soc 1997;56:433-41.
525. Shenkin A. Micronutrients in adult nutritional support: requirements and benefits. Curr Opin Clin Nutr Metab Care 1998;1:15-9.
526. Shenkin A. Micronutrients in the severely-injured patient. Proc Nutr Soc 2000;59:451-6.
527. Shenkin A, Cederblad G, Elia M, Isaksson B. International Federation of Clinical Chemistry. Laboratory assessment of protein-energy status. Clin Chim Acta 1996;253:S5-59.
528. Sher L. Role of thyroid hormones in the effects of selenium on mood, behavior, and cognitive function. Med Hypotheses 2001;57:480-3.
529. Shibata K, Onodera M, Kawada T, Iwai K. Simultaneous micro-determination of serotonin and 5-hydroxyindole-3-acetic acid with 5-hydroxy-N omega-methyltryptamine, as an internal standard, in biological materials by high-performance liquid chromatography with electrochemical detection. J Chromatogr 1988;430:381-7.
530. Shils ME, Brown RO. Parenteral nutrition. In: Shils ME, Olson JA SM, Ross AC, eds. Modern nutrition in health and disease. Baltimore: Williams & Wilkins, 1999:1657-88.
531. Shiraki M, Shiraki Y, Aoki C, Miura M. Vitamin K2 (menatetrenone) effectively prevents fractures and sustains lumbar bone mineral density in osteoporosis. J Bone Miner Res 2000;15:515-21.
532. Shriver BJ, Roman-Shriver C, Allred JB. Depletion and repletion of biotinyl enzymes in liver of biotin-deficient rats: evidence of a biotin storage system. J Nutr 1993;123:1140-9.
533. Sivakumar B, Reddy V. Absorption of labelled vitamin A in children during infection. Br J Nutr 1972;27:299-304.
534. Slyshenkov VS, Omelyanchik SN, Moiseenok AG, Trebukhina RV, Wojtczak L. Pantothenol protects rats against some deleterious effects of gamma radiation. Free Radic Biol Med 1998;24:894-9.
535. Slyshenkov VS, Piwocka K, Sikora E, Wojtczak L. Pantothenic acid protects jurkat cells against ultraviolet light-induced apoptosis. Free Radic Biol Med 2001;30:1303-10.
536. Smeets EH, Muller H, de Wael J. A NADH-dependent transketolase assay in erythrocyte hemolysates. Clin Chim Acta 1971;33:379-86.
537. Sokol RJ, Butler-Simon N, Heubi JE, Iannaccone ST, McClung HJ, Accurso F et al. Vitamin E deficiency neuropathy in children with fat malabsorption. Studies in cystic fibrosis and chronic cholestasis. Ann N Y Acad Sci 1989;570:156-69.
538. Sokoll LJ, Booth SL, O'Brien ME, Davidson KW, Tsaioun KI, Sadowski JA. Changes in serum osteocalcin, plasma phylloquinone, and urinary gamma-carboxyglutamic acid in response to altered intakes of dietary phylloquinone in human subjects. Am J Clin Nutr 1997;65:779-84.
539. Sokoll LJ, O'Brien ME, Camilo ME, Sadowski JA. Undercarboxylated osteocalcin and development of a method to determine vitamin K status. Clin Chem 1995;41:1121-8.
540. Sokoll LJ, Sadowski JA. Comparison of biochemical indexes for assessing vitamin K nutritional status in a healthy adult population. Am J Clin Nutr 1996;63:566-73.
541. Spahr L, Butterworth RF, Fontaine S, Bui L, Therrien G, Milette PC et al. Increased blood manganese in cirrhotic patients: relationship to pallidal magnetic resonance signal hyperintensity and neurological symptoms. Hepatology 1996;24: 1116-20.

542. Stabler SP, Marcell PD, Podell ER, Allen RH, Lindenbaum J. Assay of methylmalonic acid in the serum of patients with cobalamin deficiency using capillary gas chromatography-mass spectrometry. J Clin Invest 1986;77:1606-12.
543. Stampfer MJ, Hennekens CH, Manson JE, Colditz GA, Rosner B, Willett WC. Vitamin E consumption and the risk of coronary disease in women. N Engl J Med 1993;328:1444-9.
544. Steindl P, Ferenci P, Dienes HP, Grimm G, Pabinger I, Madl C et al. Wilson's disease in patients presenting with liver disease: a diagnostic challenge. Gastroenterology 1997;113:212-8.
545. Stephens NG, Parsons A, Schofield PM, Kelly F, Cheeseman K, Mitchinson MJ. Randomised controlled trial of vitamin E in patients with coronary disease: Cambridge Heart Antioxidant Study (CHAOS). Lancet 1996;347:781-6.
546. Stephensen CB. Vitamin A, infection, and immune function. Annu Rev Nutr 2001;21:167-92.
547. Sturniolo GC, Mestriner C, D'Inca RD. Trace element and mineral nutrition in gastrointestinal disease. In: Bogden JD, Klevay LM, eds. Clinical nutrition of the essential trace elements and minerals. Totowa, New Jersey: Humana Press, 2000:289-307.
548. Suaberlich HE. Vitamin C. In: ed. Laboratory tests for the assessment of nutritional status. Boca Raton, FL: CRC Press, 1999.
549. Subar AF, Block G, James LD. Folate intake and food sources in the US population. Am J Clin Nutr 1989;50:508-16.
550. Sunde RA. Selenium. In: O'Dell BL, Sunde RA, eds. Handbook of nutritionally essential mineral elements. New York, Basel, Hong Kong: Marcel Dekker, 1997:493-557.
551. Suter PM, Vetter W. Diuretics and vitamin B1: are diuretics a risk factor for thiamin malnutrition? Nutr Rev 2000;58:319-23.
552. Svantesson E, Capala J, Markides KE, Pettersson J. Determination of boron-containing compounds in urine and blood plasma from boron neutron capture therapy patients. The importance of using coupled techniques. Anal Chem 2002;74:5358-63.
553. Tahiliani AG, Beinlich CJ. Pantothenic acid in health and disease. Vitam Horm 1991;46:165-228.
554. Takagi Y, Okada A, Sando K, Wasa M, Yoshida H, Hirabuki N. Evaluation of indexes of in vivo manganese status and the optimal intravenous dose for adult patients undergoing home parenteral nutrition. Am J Clin Nutr 2002;75:112-8.
555. Talwar D, Davidson H, Cooney J, St JO'Reilly D. Vitamin B(1) status assessed by direct measurement of thiamin pyrophosphate in erythrocytes or whole blood by HPLC: comparison with erythrocyte transketolase activation assay. Clin Chem 2000;46:704-10.
556. Tamura T, Soong SJ, Sauberlich HE, Hatch KD, Cole P, Butterworth CE, Jr. Evaluation of the deoxyuridine suppression test by using whole blood samples from folic acid-supplemented subjects. Am J Clin Nutr 1990;51:80-6.
557. Tanner MS. Role of copper in Indian childhood cirrhosis. Am J Clin Nutr 1998;67:1074S-81S.
558. Tanphaichitr V. Thiamine. In: Shils ME, Olson JA, Shihe M, Ross AC, eds. Modern nutrition in health and disease. Baltimore, MD: Williams and Wilkins, 1999:381-90.
559. Tanphaichitr V. Thiamine. In: Machlin LJ, ed. Handbook of Vitamins. New York: Marcel Dekker, 2001:275-316.
560. Tanumihardjo SA. Factors influencing the conversion of carotenoids to retinol: bioavailability to bioconversion to bioefficacy. Int J Vitam Nutr Res 2002;72:40-5.
561. Tanumihardjo SA, Koellner PG, Olson JA. The modified relative-dose-response assay as an indicator of vitamin A status in a population of well-nourished American children. Am J Clin Nutr 1990;52:1064-7.
562. Tanumihardjo SA, Muherdiyantiningsih, Permaesih D, Dahro AM, Muhilal, Karyadi D, Olson JA. Assessment of the vitamin A status in lactating and nonlactating, nonpregnant Indonesian women by use of the modified-relative-dose-response (MRDR) test. Am J Clin Nutr 1994;60:142-7.
563. Tanumihardjo SA, Muhilal, Yuniar Y, Permaesih D, Sulaiman Z, Karyadi D, Olson JA. Vitamin A status in preschool-age Indonesian children as assessed by the modified relative-dose-response assay. Am J Clin Nutr 1990;52:1068-72.
564. Tarr JB, Tamura T, Stokstad EL. Availability of vitamin B6 and pantothenate in an average American diet in man. Am J Clin Nutr 1981;34:1328-37.
565. Taylor HE. Inductively coupled emission and mass spectrometry: Practices and techniques. San Diego: Academic Press, 2000.
566. Taylor MJ, Carney S, Geddes J, Goodwin G. Folate for depressive disorders. Cochrane Database Syst Rev 2003;CD003390.
566a. Taylor PR, Greenwald P. Nutritional interventions in cancer preventions. J Clin Oncol 2005,10;23:333-45.
567. Templeton DM. The importance of trace element speciation in biomedical science. Anal Bioanal Chem 2003;375:1062-6.
568. Terada A, Nakada M, Nakada K, Yamate N, Tanaka Y, Yoshida M, Yoshida K. Selenium administration to a ten-year-old patient receiving long-term total parenteral nutrition (TPN)–changes in selenium concentration in the blood and hair. J Trace Elem Med Biol 1996;10:1-5.
569. Thomas AG, Miller V, Shenkin A, Fell GS, Taylor F. Selenium and glutathione peroxidase status in paediatric health and gastrointestinal disease. J Pediatr Gastroenterol Nutr 1994;19:213-9.

570. Thompson AD. Mechanisms of vitamin deficiency in chronic alcohol misuse and the development of the Wernicke-Korsakoff syndrome. Alcohol Alcohol 2000;35 Suppl 1:2-7.
571. Thompson RP. Assessment of zinc status. Proc Nutr Soc 1991;50:19-28.
572. Thurnham DI, Smith E, Flora PS. Concurrent liquid-chromatographic assay of retinol, alpha-tocopherol, beta-carotene, alpha-carotene, lycopene, and beta-cryptoxanthin in plasma, with tocopherol acetate as internal standard. Clin Chem 1988;34:377-81.
573. Thurnham DI, Smith E, Flora PS. Concurrent liquid-chromatographic assay of retinol, alpha-tocopherol, beta-carotene, alpha-carotene, lycopene, and beta-cryptoxanthin in plasma, with tocopherol acetate as internal standard. Clin Chem 1988;34:377-81.
574. Tietz NW. Clinical guide to laboratory tests, 3rd ed. Philadelphia: WB Saunders Co, 1995.
575. Toh BH, van Driel IR, Gleeson PA. Pernicious anemia. N Engl J Med 1997;337:1441-8.
576. Traber MG. Vitamin E: too much or not enough? Am J Clin Nutr 2001;73:997-8.
577. Trace Element and Micronutrient Unit NHS Scotland. www.trace-element.org.uk. 2005.
578. Tryfiates GP. Vitamin B6 metabolism and role in growth. Westport, CT: Food and Nutrition Press, Inc, 1980.
579. Turnlund JR, Keyes WR, Peiffer GL. Molybdenum absorption, excretion, and retention studied with stable isotopes in young men at five intakes of dietary molybdenum. Am J Clin Nutr 1995;62:790-6.
580. Turnlund JR, Keyes WR, Peiffer GL, Scott KC. Copper absorption, excretion, and retention by young men consuming low dietary copper determined by using the stable isotope 65Cu. Am J Clin Nutr 1998;67:1219-25.
581. Uauy R, Olivares M, Gonzalez M. Essentiality of copper in humans. Am J Clin Nutr 1998;67:952S-9S.
582. Ubbink JB, Serfontein WJ, de Villiers LS. Stability of pyridoxal-5-phosphate semicarbazone: applications in plasma vitamin B6 analysis and population surveys of vitamin B6 nutritional status. J Chromatogr 1985;342:277-84.
583. Ueland PM, Refsum H, Beresford SA, Vollset SE. The controversy over homocysteine and cardiovascular risk. Am J Clin Nutr 2000;72:324-32.
584. Ulleland M, Eilertsen I, Quadros EV, Rothenberg SP, Fedosov SN, Sundrehagen E, Orning L. Direct assay for cobalamin bound to transcobalamin (holo-transcobalamin) in serum. Clin Chem 2002;48:526-32.
585. Underwood BA. Methods for assessment of vitamin A status. J Nutr 1990;120 Suppl 11:1459-63.
586. Urnov FD. A feel for the template: zinc finger protein transcription factors and chromatin. Biochem Cell Biol 2002;80:321-33.
587. US Department of Health and Human Services. Case studies in environmental medicine. Chromium Toxicity. Course SS3048 Agency for Toxic Substances and Disease Registry, Publication No ASTDR-HE-CS-2001-0005, 2000.
588. Uthus EO, Nielsen FH. Effect of vanadium, iodine and their interaction on growth, blood variables, liver trace elements and thyroid status indices in rats. Magnes Trace Elem 1990;9:219-26.
589. van Asselt DZ, de Groot LC, van Staveren WA, Blom HJ, Wevers RA, Biemond I, Hoefnagels WH. Role of cobalamin intake and atrophic gastritis in mild cobalamin deficiency in older Dutch subjects. Am J Clin Nutr 1998;68:328-34.
590. van Bakel MM, Printzen G, Wermuth B, Wiesmann UN. Antioxidant and thyroid hormone status in selenium-deficient phenylketonuric and hyperphenylalaninemic patients. Am J Clin Nutr 2000;72:976-81.
591. Van Gossum A, Shariff R, Lemoyne M, Kurian R, Jeejeebhoy K. Increased lipid peroxidation after lipid infusion as measured by breath pentane output. Am J Clin Nutr 1988;48:1394-9.
592. van Guldener C, Stehouwer CD. Homocysteine-lowering treatment: an overview. Expert Opin Pharmacother 2001;2:1449-60.
593. van Lieshout M, West CE, van Breemen RB. Isotopic tracer techniques for studying the bioavailability and bioefficacy of dietary carotenoids, particularly beta-carotene, in humans: a review. Am J Clin Nutr 2003;77:12-28.
594. van Rij AM, McKenzie JM, Thomson CD, Robinson MF. Selenium supplementation in total parenteral nutrition. J Parenter Enteral Nutr 1981;5:120-4.
595. Vatassery GT, Krezowski AM, Eckfeldt JH. Vitamin E concentrations in human blood plasma and platelets. Am J Clin Nutr 1983;37:1020-4.
596. Veillon C. Analytical chemistry of chromium. Sci Total Environ 1989;86:65-8.
597. Velazquez A, Teran M, Baez A, Gutierrez J, Rodriguez R. Biotin supplementation affects lymphocyte carboxylases and plasma biotin in severe protein-energy malnutrition. Am J Clin Nutr 1995;61:385-91.
598. Velazquez A, Zamudio S, Baez A, Murguia-Corral R, Rangel-Peniche B, Carrasco A. Indicators of biotin status: a study of patients on prolonged total parenteral nutrition. Eur J Clin Nutr 1990;44:11-6.
599. Velez RJ, Myers B, Guber MS. Severe acute metabolic acidosis (acute beriberi): an avoidable complication of total parenteral nutrition. J Parenter Enteral Nutr 1985;9:216-9.
600. Verhage AH, Cheong WK, Jeejeebhoy KN. Neurologic symptoms due to possible chromium deficiency in long-term parenteral nutrition that closely mimic metronidazole-induced syndromes. J Parenter Enteral Nutr 1996;20:123-7.

601. Verieck J, Cornelis R. Trace element in human plasma or serum. CRC Press, 1989.
602. Verseick J, Cornelis R. Normal levels of trace elements in human blood plasma or serum. Analytical Chimica Acta 1980;116:217-54.
603. Vincent JB. The biochemistry of chromium. J Nutr 2000;130:715-8.
604. Vincent JB. The potential value and toxicity of chromium picolinate as a nutritional supplement, weight loss agent and muscle development agent. Sports Med 2003;33:213-30.
605. Vinton NE, Dahlstrom KA, Strobel CT, Ament ME. Macrocytosis and pseudoalbinism: manifestations of selenium deficiency. J Pediatr 1987;111:711-7.
606. Vuilleumier JP, Keck E. Flourimetric assay of vitamin C in biological materials, using a centrifugal analyser with fluorescence attachment. J Micronutr Anal 1989;5:25-34.
607. Wald DS, Law M, Morris JK. Homocysteine and cardiovascular disease: evidence on causality from a meta-analysis. BMJ 2002;325:1202.
608. Wald NJ, Law MR, Morris JK, Wald DS. Quantifying the effect of folic acid. Lancet 2001;358:2069-73.
609. Walshe JM. Treatment of Wilson's disease: the historical background. QJM 1996;89:553-5.
610. Wang H, Prasad AS, Dumouchelle F. Zinc in platelets, lympohocytes and granulocytes by flameless atomic absorption spectrophotometry. J Micronutrient Anal 1989;5:181-90.
611. Wardle CA, Forbes A, Roberts NB, Jawhari AV, Shenkin A. Hypermanganesemia in long-term intravenous nutrition and chronic liver disease. J Parenter Enteral Nutr 1999;23:350-5.
612. Warren JJ, Levy SM. Current and future role of fluoride in nutrition. Dent Clin North Am 2003;47: 225-43.
613. Warren MJ, Raux E, Schubert HL, Escalante-Semerena JC. The biosynthesis of adenosylcobalamin (vitamin B12). Nat Prod Rep 2002;19:390-412.
614. Wellenberg GJ, Banks JN. Enzyme linked sorbent assay to quantify d-biotin in blood. J Sci Fd Agric 1993;63:1-5.
615. Wells IC, Claassen JP, Anderson RJ. A test for adequacy of chromium nutrition in humans–relation to type 2 diabetes mellitus. Biochem Biophys Res Commun 2003;303:825-7.
616. Werner E, Roth P, Heinrichs U, Giussani A, Cantone MC, Zilker TH et al. Internal biokinetic behaviour of molybdenum in humans studied with stable isotopes as tracers. Isotopes Environ Health Stud 2000;36: 123-32.
617. Wessling-Resnick M. Understanding copper uptake at the molecular level. Nutr Rev 2002;60:177-9.
618. Whitehead VM. Polygammaglutamyl metabolites of folic acid in human liver. Lancet 1973;1:743-5.
619. WHO Scientific Group. Nutritional Anemias. World Health Organisation Technical Report Series No 405. 1968. Geneva, World Health Organisation.
620. Wiegand VW, Hartmann S, Hummler H. Safety of vitamin A: recent results. Int J Vitam Nutr Res 1998;68:411-6.
621. Wilfond BS, Farrell PM, Laxova A, Mischler E. Severe hemolytic anemia associated with vitamin E deficiency in infants with cystic fibrosis. Implications for neonatal screening. Clin Pediatr (Phila) 1994;33:2-7.
622. Wilson JD. Disorders of vitamins: Deficiency, excess, and errors of metabolism. In: Petersdorf RG, Adams RD, Braunwald E, et al, eds. Harrison's principles of internal medicine. New York: McGraw-Hill Book Company, 1991.
623. Wilson JX. The physiological role of dehydroascorbic acid. FEBS Lett 2002;527:5-9.
624. Wolf B, Heard GS. Biotinidase deficiency. In: Barness L, Oski F, eds. Advances in pediatrics. Chicago: Medical Book Publishers, 1991:1-21.
625. Wolman SL, Anderson GH, Marliss EB, Jeejeebhoy KN. Zinc in total parenteral nutrition: requirements and metabolic effects. Gastroenterology 1979;76: 458-67.
626. Wood RJ. Assessment of marginal zinc status in humans. J Nutr 2000;130:1350S-4S.
627. World Health Organisation. The global prevalence of vitamin A deficiency. 1995. Geneva. Micronutrient Series document WHO/NUT/95.3.
628. Wynn RM, Davie JR, Chuang JL, Cote CD, Chuang DT. Impaired assembly of E1 decarboxylase of the branched-chain alpha-ketoacid dehydrogenase complex in type IA maple syrup urine disease. J Biol Chem 1998;273:13110-8.
629. Wyse BW, Wittwer C, Hansen RG. Radioimmunoassay for pantothenic acid in blood and other tissues. Clin Chem 1979;25:108-10.
630. Yanik M, Vural H, Kocyigit A, Tutkun H, Zoroglu SS, Herken H et al. Is the arginine-nitric oxide pathway involved in the pathogenesis of schizophrenia? Neuropsychobiology 2003;47:61-5.
631. Young IS, Woodside JV. Folate and homocysteine. Curr Opin Clin Nutr Metab Care 2000;3:427-32.
632. Yu SY, Zhu YJ, Li WG. Protective role of selenium against hepatitis B virus and primary liver cancer in Qidong. Biol Trace Elem Res 1997;56:117-24.
633. Yusuf SW, Rehman Q, Casscells W. Cardiomyopathy in association with selenium deficiency: A case report. J Parenter Enteral Nutr 2002;26:63-6.
634. Zaman Z, Fielden P, Frost PG. Simultaneous determination of vitamins A and E and carotenoids in plasma by reversed-phase HPLC in elderly and younger subjects. Clin Chem 1993;39:2229-34.
635. Zempleni J. Biotin—Present Knowledge in Nutrition. In: Bowman BA, Russell RA, eds. Present knowledge in nutrition. Washington: ILSI Press, 2001.

636. Zempleni J, Galloway JR, McCormick DB. Pharmacokinetics of orally and intravenously administered riboflavin in healthy humans. Am J Clin Nutr 1996;63:54-66.
637. Zempleni J, Mock DM. Bioavailability of biotin given orally to humans in pharmacologic doses. Am J Clin Nutr 1999;69:504-8.
638. Zhitkovich A, Quievryn G, Messer J, Motylevich Z. Reductive activation with cysteine represents a chromium(III)-dependent pathway in the induction of genotoxicity by carcinogenic chromium(VI). Environ Health Perspect 2002;110 Suppl 5:729-31.
639. Zile MH. Function of vitamin A in vertebrate embryonic development. J Nutr 2001;131:705-8.

CHAPTER 31

Hemoglobin, Iron, and Bilirubin*

Trefor Higgins, M.Sc., Ernest Beutler, M.D., and Basil T. Doumas, Ph.D.

Hemoglobin (Hb), iron, and bilirubin are analytes that collectively may be viewed in terms of a manufacturing process in which the raw material (iron) is incorporated with other raw materials in a multistage complex process leading to a finished product (Hb). This finished product has a limited lifespan after which degradation into the waste product (bilirubin) occurs. Within this process many exquisite biochemical control, conservation, and synthesis mechanisms are found. This process may be disrupted by a deficiency in the supply of raw material, lack of control or synthesis mechanisms, excessive loss of finished product, or excessive conversion to or deficiency in the elimination of waste products. These disruptions are manifest in the clinical disorders of iron deficiency anemias, liver disease, and various genetic diseases—including Crigler-Najjar and Gilbert syndromes, hemoglobinopathies, and thalassemias.

Reliable analytical methods for the measurement of these analytes were among the first to be developed for routine use in the clinical laboratory. Laboratory analysis has contributed significantly to our understanding of the physiological role of these analytes and continues to be crucial in the diagnosis of diseases associated with disruptions in supply, synthesis, and elimination of these parameters.

HEMOGLOBIN

Hb is a hemoprotein whose primary function is to transport oxygen from the lungs to the body tissue. It was first isolated in 1849 and was the first oligomeric protein to be characterized by ultracentrifugation and to have its (1) molecular mass accurately determined; (2) physiological function described; and (3) following the 25-year study of Max Perutz and colleagues in Cambridge, its structure defined by x-ray crystallography.[138] In 1949 Linus Pauling and H. Itano[135] showed that the Hb from patients with sickle cell disease differed from normal Hb by having two to four more net positive charges. From 1956 to 1959 Vernon Ingram published a series of four papers that identified the reasons for the charge difference by locating the single amino acid difference between Hb from normal individuals and those with sickle cell disease and so described the first hemoglobinopathy.[85-88]

Thalassemias and hemoglobinopathies are clinical disorders related to Hb pathophysiology. Regarding the former, inadequate production of α- or β-globin chains results in α- or β-thalassemia, respectively. Modifications in the amino acid sequence of either the α- or β-chains results in hemoglobinopathies.

BIOCHEMISTRY

Hemoglobin is a globular protein with a diameter of 6.4 nm and a molecular weight of approximately 64,500 Da. As shown in Figure 31-1, Hb consists of four globin subunits arranged to resemble a thick-walled shell with a small central cavity. Each globin chain is looped about itself to form a pocket or cleft in which the heme group nestles. Normally, this heme pocket is formed entirely by nonpolar (hydrophobic) amino acids. The heme moiety is suspended within this pocket by an attachment of its iron atom to the imidazole group of the proximal histidine (position 92 of the β-chain [β92] or position 87 of the α-chain [α87]). The imidazole group of the distal histidine (β63 or α58) is also in contigu-

*The authors gratefully acknowledge the original contributions of Virgil F. Fairbanks and George G. Klee (hemoglobin and iron) and Keith G. Tolman and Robert Rej (bilirubin) upon which portions of this chapter are based.

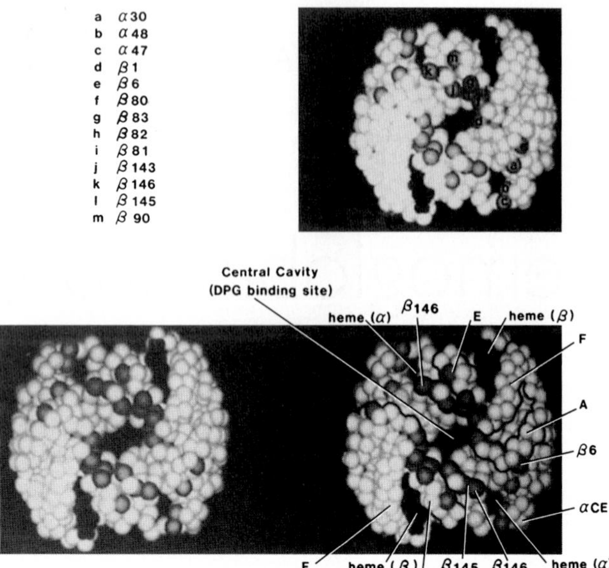

Figure 31-1 Model of the Hb tetramer with the β-chain subunits facing the reader. Amino acids are represented as spherules. Those that are shaded affect Hb mobility in citrate agar gel. Spherules labeled *d, j, k,* and *l* in the upper panel constitute the 2,3-diphosphoglycerate binding site and are important in regulation of the oxygen affinity of Hb. The lower panel is a stereo pair for three-dimensional viewing. To obtain the three-dimensional effect, hold the illustration at arm's length. The β-globin chains appear to be between the reader and the more distant α-chains. On the right, some of the segments of the β-globin chain have been outlined, and segments and critical components have been marked. β146 is the COO^- end of the β-chain; β6 is the site of amino acid substitutions responsible for Hbs S and C. *(From Winter WP, Yodh J. Interaction of human hemoglobin and its variants with agar. Science 1983;221:175-8. Copyright 1983 by the American Association for the Advancement of Science.)*

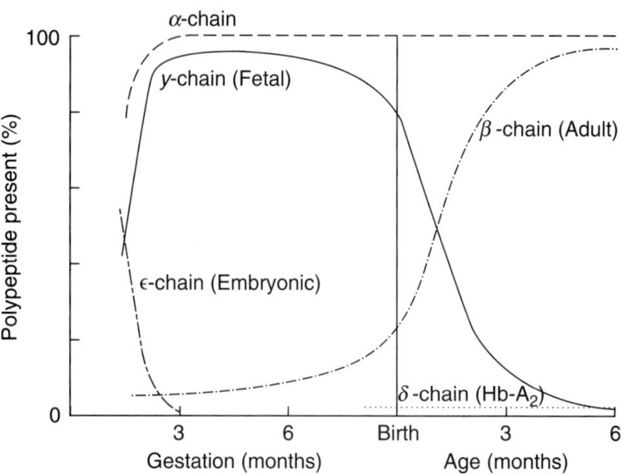

Figure 31-2 Changes in relative proportions of globin chains at various stages of embryonic, fetal, and postnatal life. *(Reprinted from Huehns ER, Dance N, Beaven GH, Hecht F, Motulsky AG. Human embryonic hemoglobins. Cold Spring Harbor Symp Quant Biol 1965;29:327-331.)*

ity with the iron of heme, but it appears to swing in and out of this position to permit the passage of O_2 into and out of the Hb molecule. The four iron atoms are in the divalent state, whether Hb is oxygenated or deoxygenated.

Globin Structure of Normal and Fetal Hemoglobin

In normal human adults, Hb A is composed of two normal α- and two normal β-polypeptide chains and is represented symbolically as $\alpha_2\beta_2$; it represents at least 96% of the total Hb contained in a sample of whole blood. Hb A_2 is typically about 2.5% to 3.0% of total Hb; it contains two α- and two δ-chains and is designated as $\alpha_2\delta_2$. *Fetal Hb (Hb F)* predominates during fetal life but rapidly diminishes during the first year of postnatal life. In normal adults, less than 1% of Hb is Hb F. It consists of two α- and two γ-chains ($\alpha_2\gamma_2$).

In early embryonic life, the yolk sac produces the globin chains zeta (ζ) and epsilon (ε). These globin chains combine to form the major embryonic hemoglobins Hb Gower 1($\zeta_2\varepsilon_2$) and 2($\alpha_2\varepsilon_2$) and Hb Portland 1($\zeta_2\gamma_2$) and 2($\zeta_2\beta_2$). Production of the ζ-chain ceases at a gestational age of approximately 4 months (Figure 31-2). Production of α- and γ-chains start at about 6 weeks gestation, with Hb F (fetal hemoglobin, $\alpha_2\gamma_2$) increasing in concentration to become the major Hb found in the fetus. Glycine or alanine may be found at position 136 of the γ-chain in the fetus, giving rise to two distinct γ-chains designated $^{G}\gamma$ and $^{A}\gamma$, respectively. Formation of Hb A ($\alpha_2\beta_2$) commences at about 28 weeks gestation and at birth can form up to 15% of the total Hb, with the remainder of the Hb consisting mainly of Hb F with a very small amount of Hb A_2. The production of the γ-chain declines after birth, and normal adult Hb F values are usually obtained by 1 year of age but may be elevated until 2 years of age.

Protein Structure

As with all proteins, the function of Hb is dictated by its primary, secondary, tertiary, and quaternary structure.

Primary Structure. The α- and non–α-globin chains of Hb are 141 and 146 amino acid residues in length, respectively. There is some sequence homology, with 64 individual amino acid residues in identical positions in both α- and β-chains. The β-chain differs from the δ- and γ-chains by 39 and 10 residues, respectively. The amino terminal of the β-globin chain is the site of attachment of glucose (Hb A_{1c}), urea, and salicylate.[30] The carboxy terminal amino acid of the β-chain is tyrosine and can function as a part of salt bridges. Although there are no disulfide bonds, there are six –SH groups (from cysteine at positions α104, β93, and 112). The γ-chain has a glycine amino terminal and the alkali resistance of Hb F is attributed to the presence of threonine and tryptophan at positions 112 and 130 of the γ-chain, respectively. The γ-chain is unique in that it is the only globin chain to be susceptible to acetylation and acetylated Hb F is a prominent feature in cord and neonatal blood and may form as much as 25% of the total Hb.

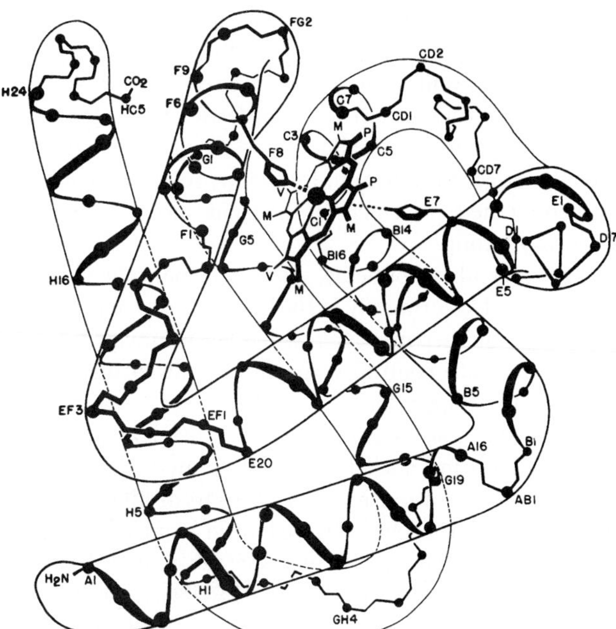

Figure 31-3 Structure of the Hb subunit. Chains of amino acids in spiral or helical segments are linked by short, nonhelical segments. The helical segments are designated A through H. In this illustration, amino acids are designated in accordance with the helical or nonhelical segment in which they occur. *(From Dickerson RE. X-ray analysis and protein structure. In: Neurath H, Ed. The Proteins: composition, structure and function. 2nd ed. Vol. 2. New York: Academic Press, 1964:603-778.)*

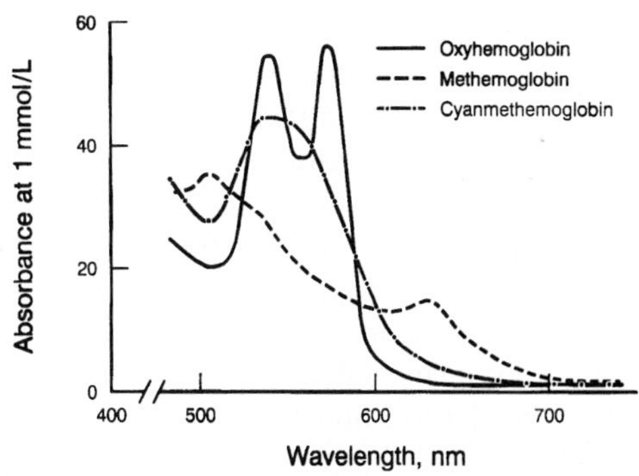

Figure 31-4 Spectrophotometric absorption curves for oxyhemoglobin, methemoglobin, and cyanmethemoglobin (authors' data). Oxyhemoglobin and cyanmethemoglobin are used in measuring the Hb concentration. The peak at 630 nm, which is distinctive for methemoglobin, is abolished by addition of cyanide, and the resultant decrease in absorbance is directly proportional to the methemoglobin concentration. All heme proteins exhibit their maximum absorbance in the Soret band region of 400 to 440 nm. Because the absorbance of Hb in the Soret region is approximately 10 times the absorbance at 540 nm, the Soret peaks have been omitted from this diagram. The absorbance curve for methemoglobin is greatly influenced by small changes in pH. The curve given here was obtained at a pH of 6.6.

Secondary Structure. Approximately 75% to 80% of the polypeptide chains of the α- and non–α-chains are arranged in helices, with the remainder forming non-helical turns. The β-chain of Hb A is arranged into eight helices identified as A through H (Figure 31-3). In contrast, the α-chain is missing an equivalent of the D helix and so has only seven helices. Nomenclature within the helices identifies the helix and position within the helix of the amino acid residue (e.g., F3 is the third amino residue in the F helix). Amino acid residues in the peptide chains that join adjacent helices are described by the identification of the two adjacent helices and position of the residues within the joining peptide. For example, EF3 would be the third residue in the peptide joining the E and F helices.

Tertiary Structure. The tertiary structure of Hb refers to the arrangement of the helices into a three-dimensional, pretzel-like structure. The heme group, located in a crevice between the E and F helices, is attached to histidine residues in each globin chain. This attachment is essential to maintaining the secondary and tertiary structure of the globin chains.

Quaternary Structure. The quaternary structure of Hb results from the attachment of the four globin chains to each other. Strong $\alpha_1\beta_1$ and $\alpha_2\beta_2$ dimeric bonds hold the molecule in a stable form. The tetrameric $\alpha_1\beta_2$ and $\alpha_2\beta_1$ bonds make significant contributions to the stability of the structure. The shifting, rotation, and sliding in the quaternary structure result in a number of physiological effects, including the sigmoid oxygen dissociation curve and the Bohr effect.

Modified Hemoglobins

In addition to the Hbs discussed above, carboxyhemoglobin, methemoglobin, and sulfhemoglobin are other Hbs whose structure has been environmentally or chemically modified.

Each of the modified Hbs has a characteristic spectral pattern as shown in Figure 31-4. These spectral characteristics form the basis of analysis in the many co-oximeters and blood gas analyzers that provide, in a single analysis, the simultaneous quantitative measurement of carboxyhemoglobin, methemoglobin, and sulfhemoglobin. The spectral scans are performed using multidiode arrays covering a wide range of wavelengths followed by patented calculations that discriminate between the normal and modified Hbs.

Carboxyhemoglobin

Carboxyhemoglobin is formed by the preferential attachment of carbon monoxide over oxygen to Hb. Carboxyhemoglobin concentrations (usually expressed as a carboxyhemoglobin saturation) have been known to reach 20% in individuals who are exposed to significant workplace concentrations of carbon monoxide. For example, police directing traffic at busy intersections and workers in radiator and welding shops have high carboxyhemoglobin concentrations at the end of the working day. The ability to perform heavy manual work or complex tasks is impaired at carboxyhemoglobin concentrations of 10% or less.[31] Faulty home furnaces and automobile exhaust systems can produce large amounts of carbon monoxide, sometimes with tragic results. Carboxyhemoglobin saturation levels in the range of 15% to 25% may be associated with dizziness, headaches, and nausea, and greater than 50% saturation is considered life threatening.[162] Following removal of the exposed individual from the carbon monoxide source, there is a slow decline in carboxyhemoglobin concentration in keeping with the half-life of 4 to 5 hours at sea level.[163]

Methemoglobin

The iron of heme is normally in the reduced ferrous state (Fe^{2+}). Under alkaline conditions, the iron is oxidized to the ferric state (Fe^{3+}) by toxic agents, such as nitrates (found in some well waters), aniline dyes, chlorates, drugs—such as quinones, phenacetin, sulfonamides—or local anesthetics, such as procaine, benzocaine, and lidocaine. This oxidation converts the heme to hematin[183] and the Hb to methemoglobin. Patients with methemoglobin are cyanotic, since methemoglobin is unable to reversibly bind oxygen. Methemoglobin is normally reduced to Hb in the cell by the reduced form of nicotinamide-adenine dinucleotide (NADH)-cytochrome reductase system.

Hereditary methemoglobinemia is a rare condition first described in Europeans but later found in individuals of many racial backgrounds. Familial methemoglobinemia in an autosomal recessive mode of transmission is due to a deficiency in the enzyme NADH-cytochrome b5 reductase. Hb variants that stabilize the ferric iron state are associated with an autosomal dominant familial methemoglobinemia. Methemoglobinemia is treated by the administration of ascorbic acid or methylene blue.

Sulfhemoglobin

Sulfhemoglobin is produced by the reaction of sulfur-containing compounds with heme to form an irreversible chemical alteration and oxidation of Hb by the introduction of sulfur in one or more of the porphyrin rings. The most common cause of sulfhemoglobinemia is exposure to drugs[27]—such as phenacetin and sulfonamides with H_2S, the foul smelling component of sour gas—as a secondary cause. Sulfhemoglobin cannot transport oxygen, and cyanosis is noted at low concentrations.

Biosynthesis

The biosynthesis of Hb requires the biosynthesis of both heme and the globin polypeptide chains.

Heme Biosynthesis

Heme, ferrous protoporphyrin IX, consists of four pyrrole rings surrounding an iron atom with four of the six electron pairs of iron attached to the nitrogen atoms in the pyrrole rings (see Chapter 32). One of the remaining electron pairs attaches to a histidine residue in a globin chain, and the other pair is available for binding and transporting an oxygen molecule. The latter electron pair is protected from oxidation by the surrounding nonpolar amino acid residues of the globin chain. Hemin results from the relatively easy oxidation of the iron of heme from the ferrous to the ferric state.[183] To remain electrically neutral, a halide molecule, usually chloride, becomes attached to hemin. In alkaline solution hematin is formed by the replacement of the halide atom of hemin by a hydroxyl group.

The biosynthesis of heme, shown schematically in Figure 31-5, takes place primarily in the bone marrow and the liver and is an eight-step process[141] with each step involving a different genetically controlled enzyme. Details of this process are given in Chapter 32.

Heme synthesis is controlled by a regulatory negative feedback loop in which heme inhibits the activity of ferrochelatase and acquisition of iron from the transport protein transferrin. The decrease in iron acquisition leads to a decrease in iron uptake into the cell with subsequent decrease in δ-aminolevulinic acid and heme production. Iron deficiency and increased erythropoietin synthesis lead to the combination of the iron regulatory proteins with the iron-responsive elements in the transferrin receptor protein messenger ribonucleic acid (mRNA). This combination in turn leads to protection of the mRNA from degradation with subsequent increased uptake of iron into erythroid cells because of the increased expression of transferrin receptors on the cell membrane.

Globin Synthesis

The genes that control the α-like and ζ-globin chains are located in a cluster on chromosome 16 at position 16p13.3, which is near to the chromosome 16 telomere (Figure 31-6). The α-like gene extends over 28 kb and contains, reading from the upstream (5′) end to the downstream (3′) end of the DNA segment, an embryonic α-like ζ-globin gene, a hypervariable region (HVR), a pseudo–ζ-gene, a pair of pseudo–α-genes, a pair of functional α-globin genes, an unexpressed α-like θ gene, and finally another hypervariable region. Alpha-thalassemia arises from the deletion of one or more α-globin genes. Deletion of all four genes and subsequent production of Hb Bart's is incompatible with life.

The β-, γ-, and δ-globin genes are clustered closely together on chromosome 11 (Figure 31-6). Reading from the 5′ end, the gene sequence is an ε-gene followed by a two γ-genes (designated Gγ and Aγ, respectively), a pseudo–ψβ-gene, a δ-gene, and another β-gene. Therefore two genes determine the γ-chain, with one gene each determining the δ- and β-chains. There is substantial variability between individuals and groups in the α- and β-genes, with the most frequent being multiples of the ζ-, ψζ-, and α-genes.

In common with all genes, the globin genes consist of exons (coding sequences) and introns (intervening noncoding sequences), with codons (triplets of nucleotides) coding for specific amino acids. The globin genes have three exons and two introns with a promoter region (specific for the globin chain) at the 5′ end of each gene. The transcription

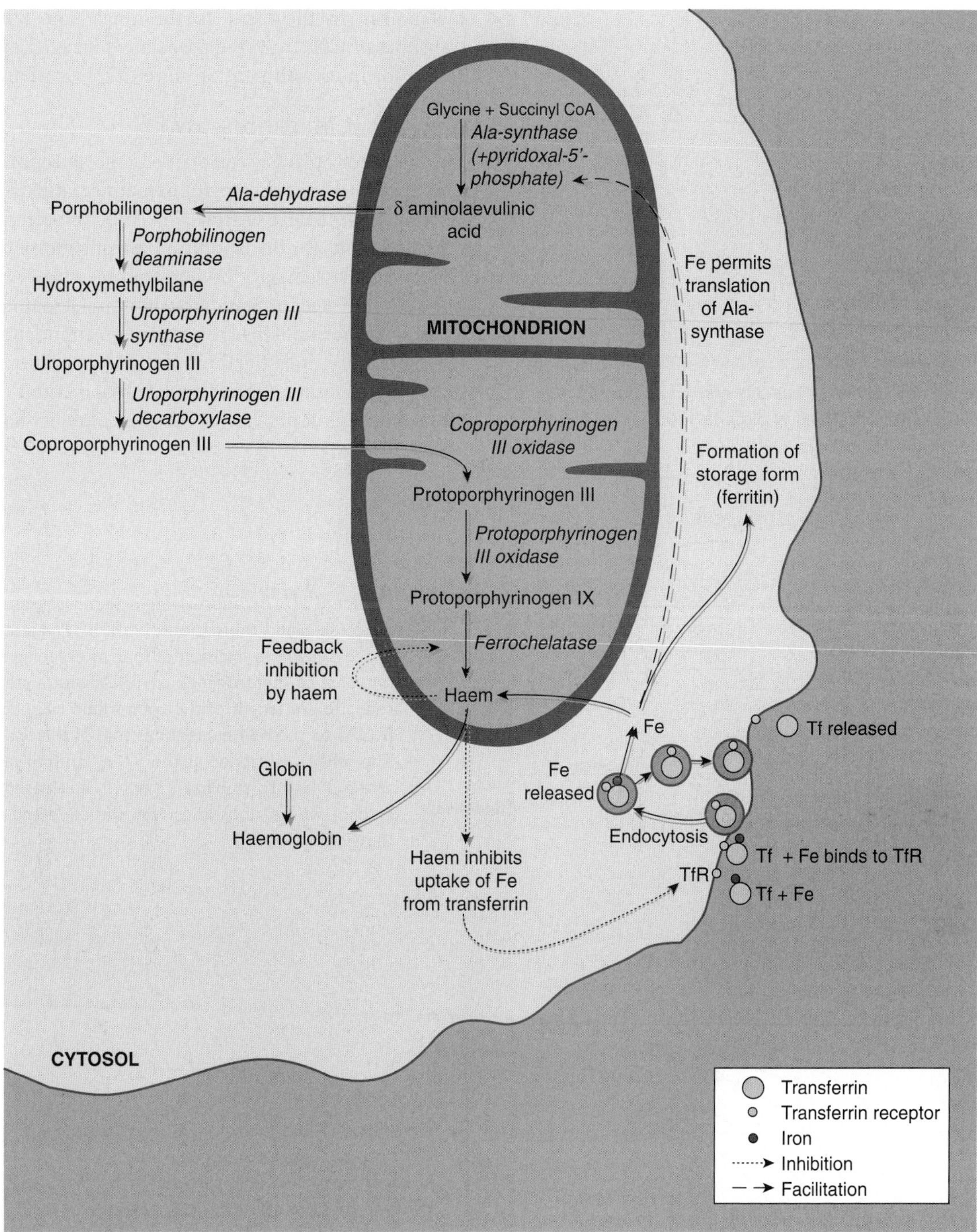

Figure 31-5 Heme synthesis. *(From Bain BJ: Haemoglobinopathy diagnosis. London: Blackwell, 2001.)*

and translation processes are the same as in any other synthesis of amino acid chains (Figure 31-7).

Physiological Role

The iron of heme is in the ferrous state and is able to combine reversibly with oxygen to act as the major oxygen-carrying moiety. The term cooperativity is used to describe the interaction of globin chains in such a way that oxygenation of one heme group enhances the probability of oxygenation of the other heme group. The Bohr effect refers to the reduction of oxygen affinity with a decrease in pH from the physiological range (7.35 to 7.45) to 6.0 and is another result of this cooperativity. As the pH of the tissue decreases as a result of the presence of the end products of anaerobic metabolism, CO_2 and carbonic acid, the delivery of oxygen to the exercising tissue is enhanced. The influence of pH on the oxygen dissociation of oxygen is shown in Figure 31-8. Carbon dioxide reversibly combines with the amino terminal groups of Hb to form carbamated Hb, facilitating the removal of about 10% of the CO_2 formed as a result of

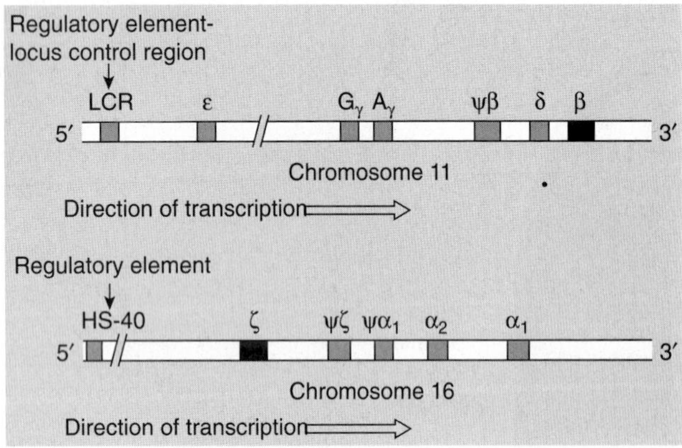

Figure 31-6 α- and β-gene globin clusters. *(From Bain BJ: Haemoglobinopathy diagnosis. London: Blackwell, 2001.)*

metabolism in the tissue to the lungs. The removal and transport of CO_2 from the tissue are enhanced by the preference for the attachment of more CO_2 by carbamated Hb.

ANALYTICAL METHODOLOGY

The laboratory plays a crucial role in the detection and characterization of the hemoglobinopathies and thalassemias discussed in the next sections.[4] There have been several recommendations for the laboratory investigation of abnormal Hbs and thalassemias.[29,73,89] For example, the 1978 International Committee for Standardization in Hematology expert panel on abnormal Hbs has prepared recommendations for the laboratory investigation of these conditions.[91] In its initial investigation, (1) a complete blood count (CBC), (2) electrophoresis at pH 9.2, (3) tests for solubility and sickling,

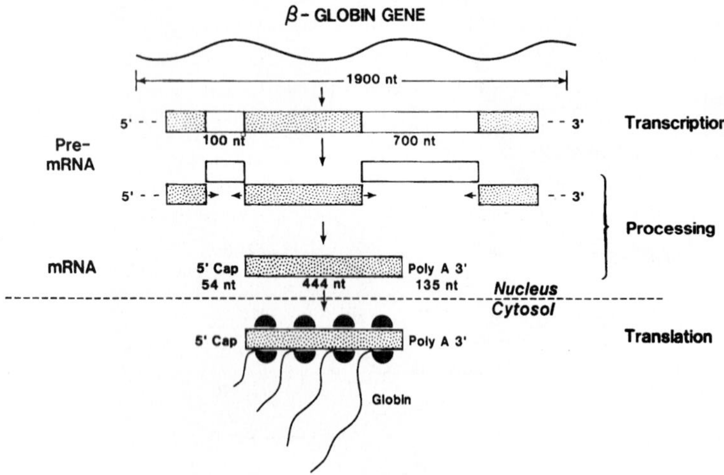

Figure 31-7 An abbreviated scheme of transcription, processing, and translation of mRNA. This complicated process involves excision of long intervening segments (introns) of "heterogeneous" RNA, with a stepwise reduction in length of the transcribed ribonucleic acid (RNA) to the 444 nucleotides (nt) of the final mRNA. The mRNA is capped at the 5′ end and polyadenylated at the 3′ end to stabilize it, then it is released into cytosol, where ribosomes read the code and assemble the globin chains.

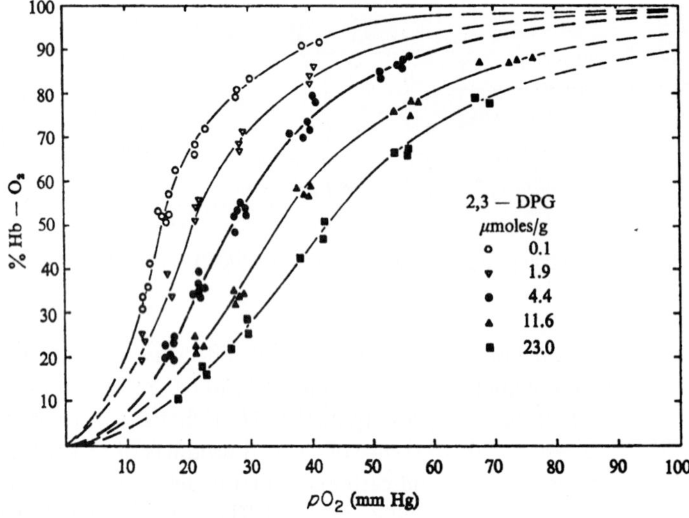

Figure 31-8 Normal oxygen dissociation curve of Hb. Changes in 2,3-diphosphoglycerate (2,3-DPG) concentration in the erythrocyte greatly influence the position of the curve. As the concentration of 2,3-DPG increases, the curve shifts to the right. *(From Duhm J. The effect of 2,3-DPG and other organic phosphates on the Donnan equilibrium and the oxygen affinity of human blood. In. Roth M, Astrup P. Eds. Oxygen affinity of hemoglobin and red cell acid base status [Alfred Benzon Symposium, IV], Copenhagen, Denmark: Alfred Benzon Foundation, 1972.)*

and (4) the quantification of Hb A_2 and Hb F were recommended. If an abnormal Hb was found as a result of these initial tests, further tests including electrophoresis at pH 6.2, globin chain separation, and isoelectric focusing were recommended by the panel. If the presence of an unstable Hb or Hb with altered oxygen affinity was suspected, then heat and isopropanol stability tests were recommended. Although new techniques have replaced some of these tests, the approach of using multiple assays in the initial investigation of hemoglobinopathies and thalassemias has shown merit and is used in many laboratories involved in the investigation of these disorders. In addition to the above tests, the iron status of the patient should be known either by measurement of ferritin or by iron/total iron binding capacity/saturation index. Information on the ethnicity and/or nationality of the patient, when allowed under patient confidentiality rules, may provide useful information since thalassemias (e.g., β-thalassemia in individuals of Mediterranean origin) and certain hemoglobinopathies (e.g., Hb S trait and homozygous S in African-Americans) are associated with certain ethnic and/or national groups.

Red blood cells (RBCs) and their indices, Hb, and related compounds are measured by several different types of analytical techniques and methods.

Preferred Specimen

The preferred blood sample is one collected with either K or Na salts of ethylenediaminetetraacetic acid (EDTA) as the anticoagulant. To minimize the formation of degradation products, which are especially noticeable as small bands eluting with similar retention time as Hb A_{1c} and Hb F on high-performance liquid chromatography (HPLC) analysis, testing should be performed within 5 days of collection and samples should be stored at 4 °C.

Analytical Techniques

Analytical techniques used to measure RBCs and their indices, Hb, and related compounds include determining a CBC, electrophoresis, immunoassay, molecular techniques, and sensitive separation techniques, such as HPLC, capillary electrophoresis, mass spectrometry, and deoxyribonucleic acid (DNA) analysis.

Complete Blood Count

The complete blood count (CBC) (1) counts RBCs, white blood cells, and platelets; (2) measures Hb; (3) estimates the red cells' volume, and (4) sorts the white blood cells into subtypes. Knowledge of red cell indices and the appearance of the peripheral blood film are vital to the diagnosis of both α- and β-thalassemias. Hemoglobinopathies have a lesser impact on the red cell indices but may present abnormal red cell morphology on the peripheral blood film. In thalassemias, the Hb concentration and the mean corpuscular volume (MCV), an index of cell size, are decreased, sometimes markedly, whereas in hemoglobinopathies both are often normal. One study recommends that an MCV of less than 72 fL (reference interval ~80 to 100 fL)[99] is maximally sensitive and specific for the presumptive diagnosis of thalassemia. However, the use of an MCH (mean corpuscular hemoglobin) value less than 27 pg (reference interval ~26 to 35 pg)[119] has been recommended as the decision point to further investigate for iron deficiency anemia and thalassemia. The rationale for the selection of MCH over MCV as the decision point for further investigation is the potential increase of up to 5 fL in MCV in samples more than 24 hours old.

The RBC is either in the upper half of or above the reference interval in thalassemias but within the reference interval in most hemoglobinopathies without a coinherited thalassemia. In contrast the RBC is low in iron deficiency anemias and anemia of chronic disease and is proportionally related to the decrease in Hb concentration. The red cell distribution width (RDW), a measure of the variation in the size of the RBC (anisocytosis), tends to be above the reference interval in iron deficiency anemias and other microcytic anemias. The RDW in thalassemias is usually within the reference interval, reflecting the uniformity of the red cell size. However, in Hb H disease and δβ-thalassemia the RDW is moderately increased.

In thalassemias the RBCs in the peripheral blood smear are hypochromic and microcytic. The characteristic sickle or crescent-shaped RBCs are seen (Figure 31-9) in the peripheral blood smear of patients who are homozygous for Hb S (sickle cell disease) and target cells are seen in blood smears from patients who are homozygous for Hb E (Figure 31-9) and Hb C. In addition, lip cells and crystalline inclusions (Hb C cells) may be found in peripheral blood smears from individuals who are homozygous for Hb C. These findings are less uniformly present than the typical morphological features of sickle cell disease.

There are several formulas, using parameters from the CBC, to calculate a thalassemic index used to differentiate iron deficiency from thalassemia.[99] Although none have proved to be totally satisfactory in all clinical situations and may not add significant information over the use of the MCV alone in selecting cases for further investigation, many laboratories use these calculations as an adjunct to the CBC parameters. One such formula[72] is

$$\text{Discriminant Factor (DF)} = (\text{MCV} \times \text{MCV}) \times \frac{\text{RDW}}{\text{Hb}} \times 100$$

A DF of <65 is associated with thalassemia minor and a value >75 is associated with iron deficiency anemia. Values between 65 and 75 are classified as equivocal and may indicate a combined iron deficiency anemia with an underlying thalassemia.

The CBC parameters are very often the first indication that the patient might have either a thalassemia or a hemoglobinopathy however, these data are not sufficient to make even a presumptive diagnosis. In addition; the iron status of the patient, as measured with either ferritin or iron/iron

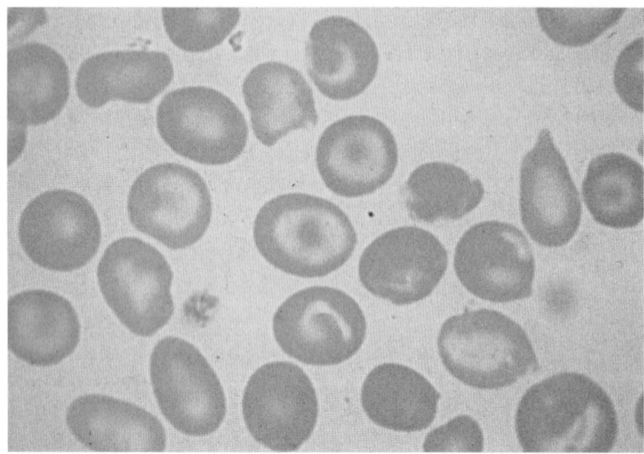

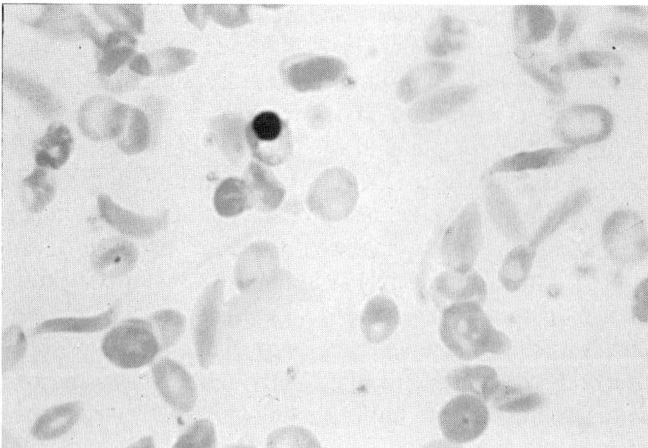

Figure 31-9 Peripheral blood smear from patients with homozygous Hb E (a) and homozygous Hb S (b).

binding/saturation index tests (see the next section), can help in differentiating iron deficiency anemia from anemia of chronic disease and thalassemia. However, ferritin is elevated in acute phase reactions, and iron deficiency can mask an underlying thalassemia.

An algorithm[126] based on the MCV, MCH, Hb A_2, and Hb F quantifications has been advocated to better discriminate between β-thalassemia minor, iron deficiency, δβ-thalassemia, and hereditary persistence of fetal hemoglobin (HPFH).[131]

Electrophoresis

Electrophoresis (see Chapter 5) under alkaline conditions (pH 9.2) is the most common initial screening method for the detection and preliminary identification of hemoglobinopathies. Several media, including paper and cellulose acetate, have been used although agarose[119] is now the medium of choice and the one usually supplied commercially. A pH 9.2 barbital buffer is the most common buffer system. Visualization of the separated Hb bands is achieved by using a protein-binding stain, such as Amido Black or Ponceau S. Hemoglobin bands stain blue with Amido Black and reddish pink with Ponceau S. Following clearing of excess stain, the Hb bands on the agarose media are clearly seen against the clear background. Figure 31-10 shows an alkaline electrophoresis gel stained with Amido Black. Quantification by densitometry of the Hb A_2 and F bands on alkaline electrophoresis, although commonly performed by laboratories, is not recommended by the College of American Pathologists in the hemoglobinopathy survey critiques[98] because of high analytical imprecision resulting from limitations of densitometry in measuring low levels of staining.

The Hbs migrate according to electrical charge, with Hb H moving the fastest (closest to the anode). The order of migration (fastest to slowest) is Hb H, Hb N, Hb I, Hb J, Hb A, Hb F, Hb S, and Hb C. Hemoglobins D and G co-migrate with Hb S, and Hbs E, O, and A_2 co-migrate with Hb C. Hemoglobin Constant Spring migrates slightly toward the cathode.

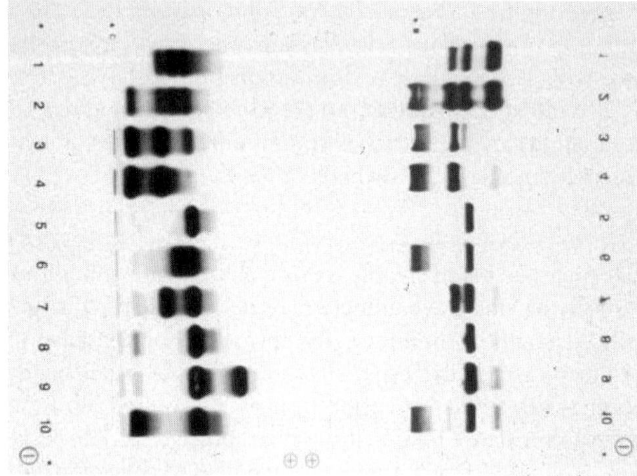

Figure 31-10 Alkaline and acid electrophoresis of various hemoglobinopathies. Lane 1, Hb S, Hb FA control; Lane 2, HB S, Hb F, HbCA control; Lane 3, transfused SC disease; Lane 4, SC disease; Lane 5, Hb A (normal); Lane 6, Hb Presbyterian; Lane 7, Hb S; Lane 8, raised Hb A_2 (β-thalassemia trait); Lane 9, Hb J Baltimore; Lane 10, Hb C.

Electrophoresis at pH 6.4 using a citrate buffer is performed when an abnormal band is noted on alkaline Hb electrophoresis. Agarose is the preferred medium, with Acid Violet the preferred stain. Figure 31-10 shows the same Hb variants performed on agarose electrophoresis at pH 6.4 and stained with Acid Violet. The order of migration (cathode to anode, fastest to slowest) is Hb F, Hb A, Hb S, and Hb C. Hemoglobins D, G, I, J, O, A_2, and E co-migrate with Hb A.

Based on positions of the bands in acid and alkaline electrophoresis, a presumptive identification of the Hb variant may be made. For example, bands are found on alkaline electrophoresis in both A and C positions. On acid electrophoresis if bands are found in the A and C positions, then a presumptive identification of Hb C trait may be made, as this pattern is characteristic. However, if a band is found only in the A position on acid electrophoresis, then a presumptive identification of Hb E may be made. If bands are found in the C position on alkaline electrophoresis and between the S and A positions on acid electrophoresis, then a presumptive identification of Hb O may be made. Further testing is required to determine if the Hb O is Hb O Arab, O Indonesia, or O Padova. Fairbanks[56] described a numbering system for the most common Hb bands on alkaline electrophoresis (Hb H = 1, Hb A = 5, Hb S = 9, Hb C = 13) that allowed the position of a band to be described more exactly than the commonly used descriptive term "between S and A positions." Unfortunately, this system has not found universal acceptance. Laboratories should keep a bank of electrophoretic data obtained to help in future identification of unusual Hb variants

Specific types of electrophoresis that are used for Hb analysis include isoelectric focusing, electrophoresis, and capillary electrophoresis.

Isoelectric Focusing Electrophoresis. Isoelectric focusing electrophoresis (IEF)[34,170] has higher resolving power than conventional electrophoresis, but is more expensive, time consuming, and technique dependent to perform (see Chapter 5). Commercial IEF gels are made of cellulose acetate or polyacrylamide with the pH gradient produced by the inclusion of amphoteric materials of different pH values in bands in the gel. Locations of the Hb bands are identified using stains similar to those used in conventional electrophoresis. The bands or zones produced by IEF (Figure 31-11) are better defined than conventional electrophoresis, and reliable quantification of the separated Hbs at high concentrations using densitometry may be made. Quantification of Hb A_2 and Hb F at low concentrations, however, is imprecise and not recommended. The Hb elution pattern in IEF is similar to that of alkaline Hb electrophoresis except that Hb D and Hb G are resolved from each other and from Hb S. Historically, IEF has been used extensively to identify and characterize Hb variants; however, it is less used now because of the previously mentioned limitations.

Capillary Isoelectric Focusing Electrophoresis. Capillary isoelectric focusing electrophoresis* combines the detection sensitivity of capillary electrophoresis (see Chapter 5) with the resolution qualities and existing extensive data on Hb variant separation by immunoelectrophoresis (IEP) and the automated sampling and digital data acquisition techniques developed for chromatography. With it, the hemolysate is introduced into the capillary chamber using low pressure injection and then focused at high voltage (typically ~30 kV and 0.5 to 1.5 μA) during which it is essential to maintain adequate cooling. The separated Hbs are then eluted, using low-pressure and simultaneous voltage, past either a single wavelength spectrophotometric detector set to read at 415 nm or a dual wavelength detector set at 415 and 450 nm. In routine use, the Hbs are typically separated within 15 minutes, but the elution time may be extended if the presence of abnormal Hb is suspected. Hb variants[77] are identified by comparison of the isoelectric point (pI) values and migration times of the unknown, using Hb A as the reference peak, with known controls and published data. Quantification is based on the integration of the measured absorbance of the bands, and accurate results have been obtained for Hb A_2 and Hb F concentrations.

*References 45, 70, 77, 78, 113, 158a, 165, 167a.

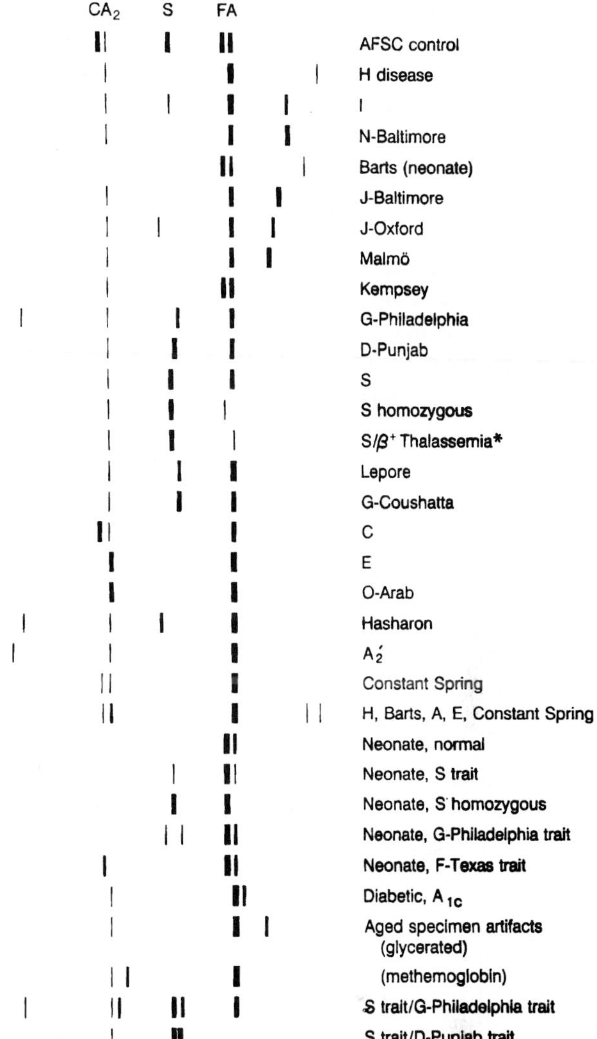

Figure 31-11 A diagram of isoelectric focusing patterns for a variety of Hb variants. The conditions shown represent heterozygotes (traits) unless otherwise indicated. The width of the bars approximates the relative density of the bands observed. The acid anodic (pH 6) side is to the right, and the alkaline cathodic (pH 8) side is to the left. The same pattern is observed in homozygous patients with Hb S disease who have received Hb A by transfusion.

High-Performance Liquid Chromatography

HPLC using a column packed with cation-exchange resin[68,130-133,145,170] provides, in a single analytical protocol, the quantification of Hbs F and A_2 (see Chapter 6 for a detailed discussion of HPLC). With it, the initial identification of an Hb variant on the basis of the elution time may be made. It has also been used to detect α-thalassemia phenotypes.

After injection and subsequent adsorption onto the particles of cation-exchange resin, molecules of Hb are eluted using gradient elution. Detection of the eluted Hbs is achieved by monitoring the effluent solvent stream using a dual wavelength photometer (usually set to measure at wavelengths of 415 and 690 nm). The technique is precise for the quantification of both Hb F and Hb A_2, and presumptive identification of the common Hb variant may be made. These features have made HPLC the method of choice for hemoglobinopathy and thalassemia screening for many laboratories including those performing neonatal hemoglobinopathy screening. Figure 31-12 shows the separation on a commercial system of several Hb variants.

Several commercial methods are available but lack the resolution achieved by noncommercial methods. A noncommercial HPLC method has been described with the retention time and relative concentration of 40 common Hb variants listed.[130] This system requires a longer time of analysis, provides superior resolution, and overcomes the problem of co-elution of several Hb variants that occurs with commercial systems. For example, with one commercial system, Hbs E, Osu-Christianborg, G-Coushatta, Lepore, and G-Copenhagen co-elute with Hb A_2, making Hb A_2

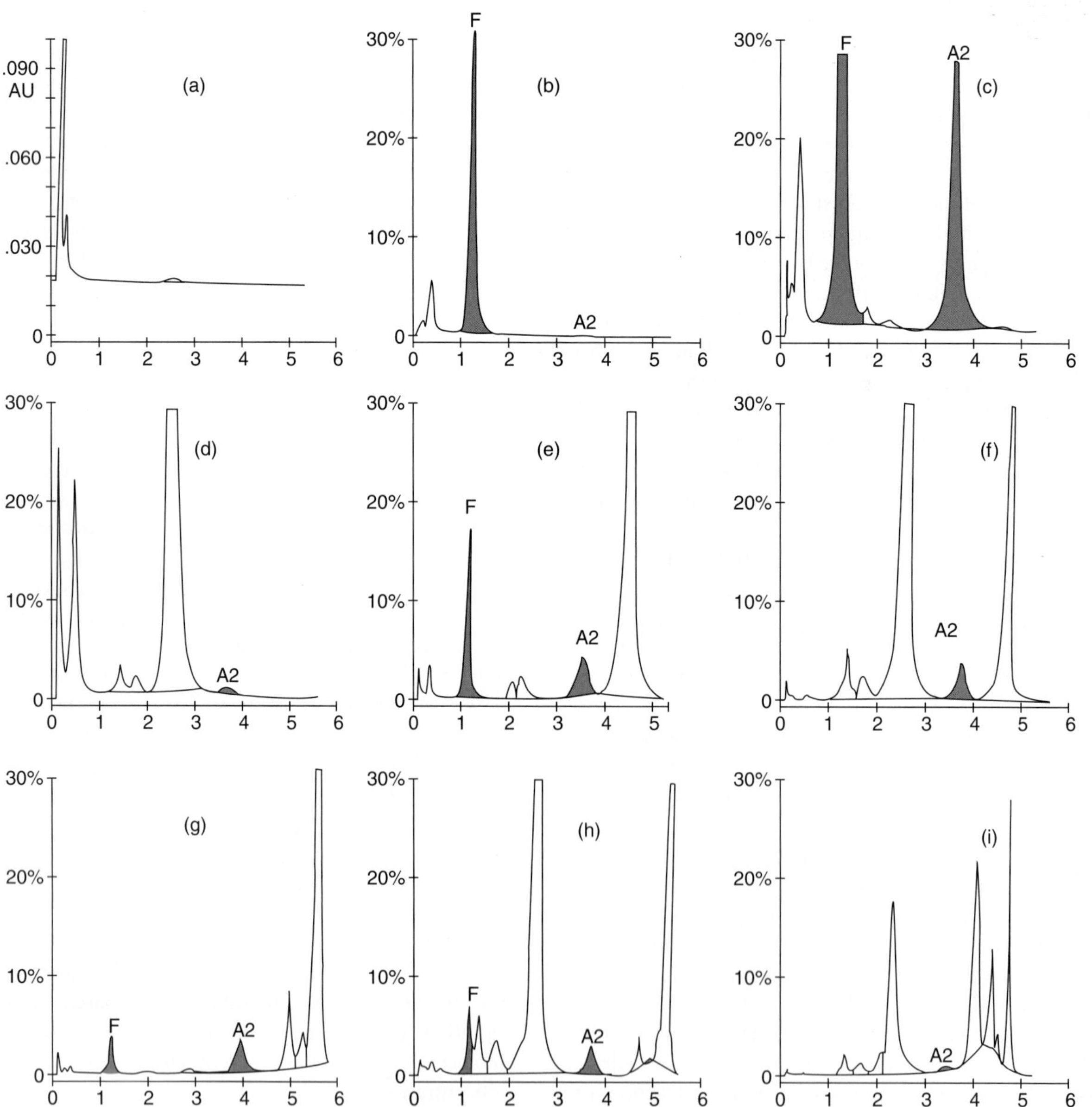

Figure 31-12 HPLC chromatograms obtained on the Bio-Rad Variant β-Thal short program for *a,* Hb Bart's; *b,* $β^0$-thalassemia major; *c,* B^+-thalassemia homozygous E; *d,* Hb H; *e,* homozygous S; *f,* S trait; *g,* homozygous C; *h,* C trait; *i,* Hb S-Hb G Philadelphia. *(From Clarke GM, Trefor N, Higgins TN. Laboratory Investigation of Hemoglobinopathies and Thalassemias: Review and Update. Clin Chem 2000;46: 1284-90.)*

quantification and definitive identification of the Hb variants impossible.[44]

Other chromatographic problems, such as a rising baseline, have resulted in Hb A_2 concentration being falsely low in Hb D patients.[47,155] However, this may be corrected mathematically to produce a more accurate result. Patients with Hb S have falsely increased Hb A_2 concentrations caused by the co-elution of glycated Hb S with Hb A_2.[166] Diagnosis of co-inheritance of β-thalassemia with Hb S, a combination that is not unusual, may be compromised by this false increase in Hb A_2. However, knowledge of the concentration of Hb A_2 is not essential in making the diagnosis of β^0- or β^+-thalassemia in these patients. In a case of β^0 thalassemia (β-thalassemia major) no δ-globin chain is produced, and the electrophoretic pattern and HPLC closely resemble those of a homozygous Hb S patient (large Hb F and Hb S peaks with no Hb A peak). In β^+-thalassemia (β-thalassemia intermedia), the concentration of Hb S is greater than that of Hb A, a situation that is only seen otherwise in recently transfused patients who have sickle cell disease. Co-inheritance of β-thalassemia minor and Hb S may be diagnosed in these patients by setting the upper limit of the reference interval at 5.0%.[82] Capillary zone electrophoresis and microcolumn methods have been described that eliminate the interference of glycated Hb S with Hb A_2 quantification.

The use of relative elution time rather than absolute elution time in initial identification of an unknown Hb variant is useful and recommended.[145] The reference Hb ideally is one that is found in low concentrations in most individuals. In this regard Hb A_2 is probably the most useful as a reference point despite the number of co-eluting Hb variants.

The elution time of the Hb may change slightly with increasing Hb variant concentration. For example, Hb F concentrations obtained by HPLC are often lower than those from the alkaline denaturation and/or spectrophotometric methods that are often quoted in standard hematology texts and used for the diagnosis of juvenile myelomonocytic leukemia (JMML) and monosomy 7 syndrome. However, caution should be used in interchanging Hb F concentrations obtained by HPLC with other methods.

It should be noted that hemoglobinopathies may interfere with glycated hemoglobin (GHb) analysis, as results may be falsely increased or decreased, depending on the particular method and the hemoglobinopathy.[30,154] Hemoglobin variants that cannot be separated from Hb A or Hb A_{1c} will produce spuriously increased or decreased results by ion-exchange HPLC.

Electrospray Mass Spectroscopy

Electrospray mass spectrometry (see Chapter 7) is becoming the method of choice for the complete characterization of newly discovered Hb variants.[19-21,143] With it, the mass of the variant, whether the variant is an α- or β-chain variant, the possible location and identity of the amino acid residue substitution, and the quantity of variant present may be derived.

To analyze a sample with this technique, the globin chains are first separated by conventional methods and then isolated by semipreparative HPLC. The isolated fractions are further concentrated using a variety of techniques including membrane filtration. The fraction containing the mutant globin chain is digested using specific endopeptidases that selectively cut at certain amino acid residues of the globin chain. The resultant digested peptide fragments are further separated by preparative HPLC and the mutant peptide sequenced using Edman degradation. Another portion of the digested globin chains is entered into the electrospray mass spectrometer, and the resultant mass spectrum provides information on the mass of the mutant globin chain, which can be then used to provisionally identify the substituted amino acid. For Hb Rambam,[20] the mass spectrum of the β-globin chains shows the mass of the normal β-chain to be 15,867 Da and the mass of the mutant β-chain to be 15,925 Da. The increase in mass of 58 in the mutant β-globin chain may be attributed to a change in amino acid residue from glycine (MW 75 Da) to aspartic acid (MW 133 Da).

DNA Analysis

DNA analysis is used in the investigation of thalassemias and hemoglobinopathies to identify, in populations with a known high incidence of disease, those specific individuals at risk and who may benefit from genetic counseling. For example, DNA analysis has been used to:

1. Diagnose α^0- and α^+-thalassemia[8,26,177]
2. Investigate potentially life-threatening disorders of Hb synthesis in the fetus and is performed at less than 10 weeks gestation on chorionic villus[126] samples
3. Characterize the β-thalassemia genotype*
4. Screen at-risk populations for clinically significant Hb variants[69,159]
5. Distinguish between conditions that have similar, laboratory, and clinical presentation but are due to different genetic conditions[123]

The Southern blot analysis of genomic DNA using α- and ζ-primers is widely used in the investigation of α-thalassemias, especially in the identification of individuals with α^0-thalassemia. Polymerase chain reaction (PCR), using allele-specific primers, is used by reference laboratories in the identification of common β-thalassemia mutations and some hemoglobinopathies. Gene sequencing information may supplement these techniques in some cases.

Specific Tests

Tests that are used to measure Hbs and related analytes include those for Hb H, Hb S, unstable Hbs, and globin chains.

Determining Hemoglobin H

Hb H is an insoluble tetramer consisting of four β-globin chains and arises in α-thalassemia in which there is a

*References 69, 79, 83, 105, 157, 176.

decreased production of α-globin chains caused by nonexpression of three of the four α-globin genes and a subsequent excess of β-globin chains. If these tetramers are oxidized, precipitation occurs, which may be viewed microscopically. In the laboratory, this oxidation is achieved by staining unfixed cells with new methylene blue or brilliant cresyl blue at 37 °C. The inclusion of positive and negative controls with each batch of Hb H preparations is essential because there is substantial batch-to-batch variability in the dye.[74] There is controversy on the necessity to perform this test on freshly collected blood and whether the test should be performed on all suspected α-thalassemia cases.

In Hb H disease, 30% to 100% of the red cells contain inclusions, which have been described as looking like "golf balls" (Figure 31-13). In α-thalassemia minor (one functional α-gene) as few as 1 cell with inclusions per 1000 to 10,000 red cells may be seen, and the diagnosis of α-thalassemia minor cannot be definitively made in the absence of Hb H inclusions. The presence of Hb H inclusions may serve as confirmation of a presumptive diagnosis of α^0-thalassemia (α-thalassemia major) or Hb H disease.

Precipitate patterns resembling Hb H inclusions may arise from staining of reticulin and Howell-Jolly bodies and other protein and nucleic acid entities. Hb H inclusions may also be very rare and difficult to detect when there is increased reticulocytosis.

Hb H detection by this method is laborious to perform and is quite subjective. However, for the detection of the two α-gene *cis* deletion (–/αα) of α^0-thalassemia, the test is reported to have a clinical sensitivity of 0.47 and a specificity of 0.99.[100]

Sickling Tests

Sickling tests are useful in confirming the presence of Hb S in a sample following initial electrophoresis at alkaline pH. When fully oxygenated Hb S is fully soluble but when deoxygenated, polymerization occurs, forming insoluble tactoids, which deform the red cells in a characteristic rigid sickle shape. In the laboratory, deoxygenation and lysis of the RBCs is achieved by the use of a solution of sodium metabisulfite in a phosphate buffer. The addition of the sodium metabisulfite reagent to an Hb S–containing blood sample causes turbidity. This turbidity is visualized by holding a lined card or a card with writing on it behind the reaction test tube (Figure 31-14). In positive samples lines or letters cannot be seen whereas in negative samples lines or letters are clearly visible. Both a positive and negative control should be performed with each test. The hematocrit of the blood sample to be tested should be measured and if less than 15% the amount of blood used in the test should be doubled because a low Hb concentration is a demonstrated cause of falsely negative sickling screens. Lipemic samples and samples with a monoclonal protein (M-protein) may give a false-positive result. Hb C Harlem and Hb Memphis ($\alpha 23(B4)^{Glu \rightarrow Gln}$) also give a positive result in this procedure and therefore it is essential to identify the Hb present in all positive tests by other techniques. The test is quite subjective and the combination of two identification techniques, such as HPLC and alkaline electrophoresis, may eliminate the necessity to perform this test on a routine basis.

Tests for Unstable Hemoglobins

These tests use either heat or isopropanol to precipitate the unstable Hb and must be performed on fresh blood. There are more than 100 unstable Hbs resulting mainly from the interchange of nonpolar amino acid residues for polar amino acid residues in positions in either the α- or β-globin chain associated with the heme cleft. Hb Hasharon ($\alpha 47(CD)^{Asp \rightarrow His}$), an Hb variant found in Ashkenazi Jews,

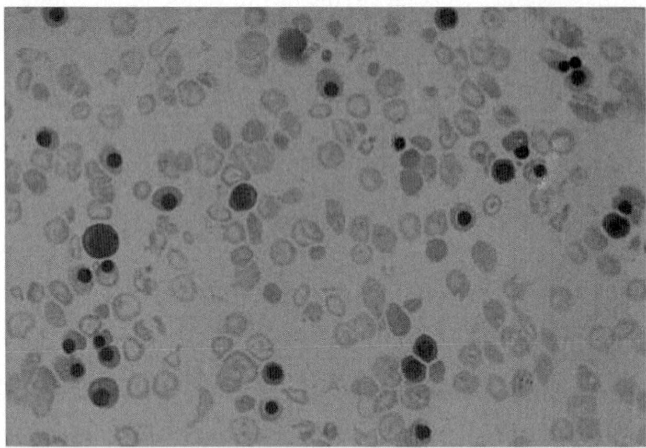

Figure 31-13 Peripheral blood smear of an individual with β^0-thalassemia. *(Courtesy Dr. G. Clarke, Dynacare Kasper Medical Laboratories.)*

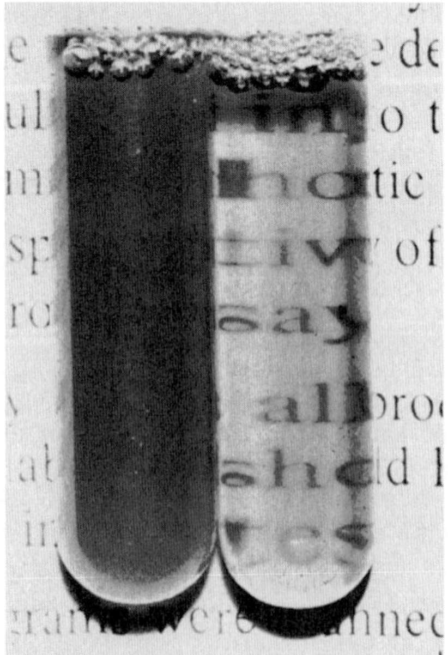

Figure 31-14 Solubility test for Hb S. Deoxyhemoglobin S *(left tube)* is insoluble in 2.3 mol/L phosphate buffer. By contrast, normal hemolysate *(right tube)* is sufficiently transparent that print can easily be read through it.

results from the substitution of the nonpolar amino acid residue histidine for the polar aspartic acid residue at position 47 of the α-chain. In conventional nomenclature, Hb Hasharon should be written as $\alpha 47(CE5)^{Asp \rightarrow His}$; however, to maintain uniformity with the β-, γ-, and δ-globin chains the term CD is used to designate the corresponding inter-helical segment of the α-chain, which does not have a D segment.

Nonpolar isopropanol weakens the internal bonds within Hb, decreasing the stability of the Hb molecule. Normal hemoglobin (Hb A) precipitates within 40 minutes at 37 °C in the presence of a 17% solution of isopropanol in a pH 7.4 TRIS buffer. Unstable Hbs usually precipitate within 5 minutes under these conditions. Both a positive and negative control should be included with each analysis, although a positive control may not always be readily available. An umbilical cord blood or neonatal sample, not fresh, may be an acceptable alternative as a positive control. At the time of reading, the negative control should be clear, and the positive control should have some flocculation.

Normal Hb is stable when heated to 50 °C. However, unstable Hbs precipitate to varying extents when similarly treated. A hemolysate of the sample in a pH 7.4 TRIS-phosphate buffer is divided into two aliquots. One is stored at 4 °C, the other is heated at 50 °C for 2 hours. Both samples are then centrifuged and Hb quantification is performed on each supernatant. The quantification of the unstable Hb is calculated using the following formula:

$$\% \text{ Unstable hemogobin} = \frac{\text{Hb}(4\,°\text{C}) - \text{Hb}(50\,°\text{C})}{\text{Hb}(4\,°\text{C})} \times 100$$

Frequently, both heat and isopropanol stability tests are performed when a suspected unstable Hb variant is investigated. Unstable Hb variants may not appear on HPLC or electrophoresis, especially if the variant is unstable enough to precipitate before analysis by these techniques.

Globin Chain Analysis

In this analysis, the globin chains and heme in a red cell lysate are first dissociated using urea and dithiothreitol. The dissociated globin chains are then separated electrophoretically at both an alkaline and acid pH (Figure 31-15). HPLC may also be used for separation. Globin chains are identified by comparison of retention times and/or electrophoretic mobility with known reference materials or published data. Globin chain analysis is an adjunct to methods described earlier and in many laboratories has been discontinued and replaced with either HPLC or capillary isoelectric focusing.

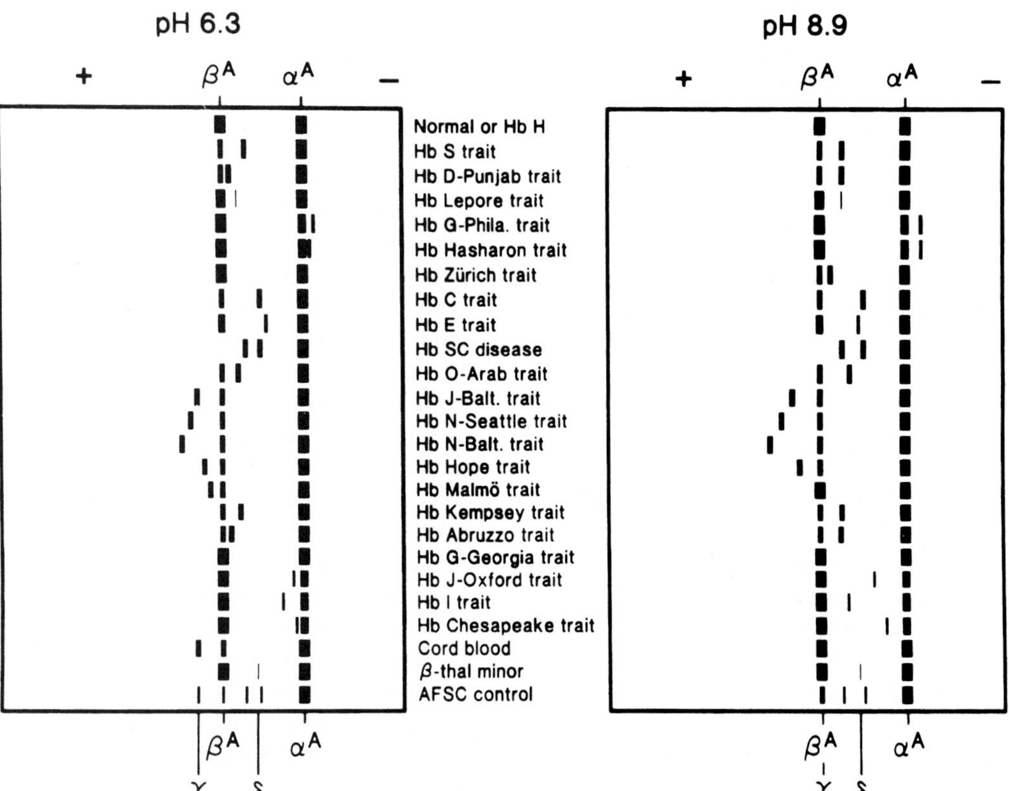

Figure 31-15 Comparison of electrophoretic mobilities of globin chains derived from Hb variants in urea buffers, 8 mol/L. The *left panel* shows separation at pH 6.3, and the *right panel* shows separation at pH 8.9. Results are shown for all common and some uncommon Hb variants. Because most of the variants are in specimens from people who are heterozygotes, the normal β^A- and α^A-globin chains are also present and serve as position markers.

Clinical Significance

The thalassemias and hemoglobinopathies are clinical disorders related to Hb pathophysiology. Although they may have similar clinical manifestations,[44] such as anemia of varying severity, they form two distinct disease groups of genetic origin. For example, the thalassemias originate from insufficient globin chain production instigated by a variety of causes, including gene deletion, nonsense mutations, or from mutations that affect the transcription or stability of mRNA products. The name thalassemia is derived from the Greek word for sea, *thalassa,* because all the early cases of β-thalassemia were described in children of Mediterranean origin.

Hemoglobinopathies, the most common single gene disorder in the world, are structural Hb variants arising from mutations in the globin genes, which result in substitutions or disruptions in the normal amino acid residue sequence in one or more of the globin chains of Hb.

Thalassemias

Thalassemias are identified by the globin chain in which there is a production deficiency. For example, α- and β-thalassemias result from a deficiency in α- and β-globin chain production, respectively. They are further classified depending on the extent of globin chain production and the resultant severity of the anemia.

α-Thalassemias

The α-thalassemias arise from deficiencies in the production of the α-globin chains and are caused by deletions or (less frequently) point mutations in one or more of the four α-globin genes. By convention, the term α^0-thalassemia is used when the two deleted α-globin chain genes are in the same gene cluster. This is sometimes described as a *cis* deletion and is written as (–/αα). The term α^+-thalassemia is used when the two deleted α-globin chain genes are on opposite gene clusters. It is sometimes described as a *trans* deletion and is written (–α/–α). A single α-gene deletion (αα/–α) is called α-thalassemia trait or α-thalassemia minor. Point mutations are much less frequent, currently numbering less than 40. The conventional nomenclature for these point mutations α-thalassemias is $\alpha^T\alpha$ or $\alpha\alpha^T$. The α-thalassemias range in clinical presentation from conditions that are incompatible with life to slight anemia or clinically and hematologically single-gene silent deletions. The severity of the anemia reflects the number of deleted genes. The α-thalassemias occur worldwide and are particularly prevalent in South East Asia, Southern China, Mediterranean countries (particularly Greece and the Greek Cypriot part of Cyprus), India, the Middle East, and the islands of the South Pacific.

Individual types of α-thalassemias are discussed below.

Hb Bart's. Hb Bart's results from deletion of all four α-globin genes with the subsequent inability to produce any α-globin chains that leads to failure of synthesis of Hbs A, F, or A_2. In the fetus there is an excess of γ-globin chains that join together to form unstable tetramers known as Hb Bart's (γ^4). Mothers carrying a fetus with Hb Bart's usually present clinically between 20 and 26 weeks gestation with pregnancy-induced hypertension and polyhydramnios. Ultrasound of the fetus shows hydrops. Severe anemia (Hb usually <80 g/L) is noted on a fetal blood sample obtained by cordocentesis. It is important to rule out other causes for the hydropic fetus by performing TORCH (*to*xoplasmosis, *r*ubella, *c*ytomegalovirus, and *h*erpes simplex) testing.

HPLC analysis of a cordocentesis blood sample shows one or two very sharp and narrow peaks at the injection point on the chromatogram (Figure 31-12, *a*). The major band is Hb Bart's with a smaller band attributed to Hb Portland. There is a complete absence of Hb F. Alkaline electrophoresis shows a band migrating at or close to the solvent front (Hb Bart's) with another band in the Hb A position (Hb Portland).

Hb Bart's hydrops fetalis is almost invariably fatal,[43] with some fetuses dying in utero and others surviving a few hours after birth. Treatment using intrauterine transfusion has had very limited success, with potential complications in the children of growth retardation and severe brain damage, which may possibly be related to long-standing intrauterine anemia.

Laboratory investigation of the parents of fetuses with Hb Bart's shows a normal HPLC pattern with normal Hb F and A_2 quantification. Parental analysis typically shows a decreased level of Hb, decreased MCH, and MCV with the blood smear showing hypochromic, microcytic red cells. The Hb H test may be positive in one or both parents. A two α-gene *cis*-deletion (–/αα) or three gene deletion (–/–α) is seen in genetic testing of both parents. This requirement restricts the incidence of Hb Bart's to a much smaller population than would be expected based on the worldwide distribution of two α-gene deletions, as the presence of *trans* deletions in both parents would not give rise to a four gene deletion in the offspring. Hb Bart's is relatively common in South East Asia, particularly in Thailand, the Philippines, and Hong Kong where there is a high prevalence of the $-^{SEA}$ deletion.

Hb H Disease. This disorder is usually caused by a three α-globin gene deletion (–/–α) and is characterized by a chronic anemia of variable severity. Individuals with the nondeletional Hb H disease ($\alpha^T\alpha$/–) are usually more severely affected and are more likely to require transfusion therapy than those with the deletional Hb H disease. There is a significant underproduction of α-globin chains and subsequent joining of free β-globin chains to form the insoluble β-globin chain tetramer Hb H. HPLC analysis of a hemolysate from an individual with Hb H disease shows two bands with low retention times forming a doublet together with a normal Hb A band. Hb F and Hb A_2 concentrations are within the reference interval (Figure 31-12, *d*). Electrophoresis at alkaline pH shows a fast moving band together with a band in the Hb A position that possibly has reduced staining when compared with other samples run concurrently. The CBC shows a moderately reduced level of Hb, and

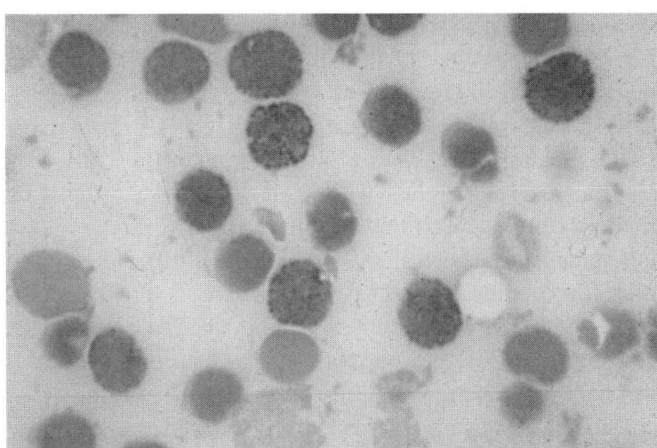

Figure 31-16 Hb H preparation showing punctate inclusions on a patient with Hb H disease.

markedly reduced MCV and MCH with slightly raised RBC count. Iron studies are normal although the ferritin may be raised. The Hb H preparation is positive, with many cells with typical punctate inclusions (Figure 31-16).

Iron therapy is not indicated, and transfusion therapy is usually unnecessary except in acute illness, in pregnancy, and with exposure to oxidant drugs, which destabilizes Hb H, causing precipitation of the somewhat insoluble protein. Genetic counseling is recommended to prospective parents who have Hb H disease.

α-Thalassemia Major. α-Thalassemia major is the result of a two α-chain gene deletion. These deletions may be on the same gene (–/αα, α^0-thalassemia) described as a *cis* deletion or on different genes (–α/–α, α^+-thalassemia) described as a *trans* deletion. The CBC of affected individuals shows a mildly reduced level of Hb with low MCV and MCH. HPLC analysis shows no abnormal Hb peaks and the Hb F and Hb A_2 concentrations are within the reference interval. Hb H preparation may show a rare cell with punctate inclusions. Iron studies are normal. In the routine clinical laboratory, the diagnosis of α-thalassemia major is based on exclusion criteria rather than definitive tests. The presence of thalassemic indices in a patient with normal Hb A_2 and Hb F quantifications is very often the only basis for many diagnoses of α-thalassemia major, particularly in the setting of a positive family history. A photometric enzyme-linked immunosorbent assay (ELISA) for the identification of adult carriers of the ($-^{SEA}$) α^0-thalassemia deletion has been described.[100] This method is based on the measurement of minuscule amounts of embryonic ζ-cells present in these adult carriers. Not all α-thalassemia deletions have continued ζ-chain production and so a negative test is not diagnostic of α-thalassemia major. This test could be useful in screening individuals at risk for giving birth to a fetus with Hb Bart's hydrops fetalis.

α-Thalassemia Trait. α-Thalassemia trait describes a single α-globin chain gene deletion (–α/αα). A single α-globin gene deletion is frequently clinically and hematologically silent. A CBC of an individual with this trait shows a normal or marginally decreased Hb level, MCV, and MCH. Iron studies are normal, and no abnormal Hb peaks are seen on HPLC analysis.

β-Thalassemias

The β-thalassemias result from a reduction in the synthesis of the β-globin chain[127] and are commonly found in the Mediterranean region, Africa, the Middle East, South East Asia—especially the Southern provinces of China including Hong Kong, the Indian subcontinent, the Malay peninsula, Burma, and Indonesia.[179] Frequency of gene distribution is estimated at 3% to 10% in some populations. The high frequency of β-thalassemia in the tropics is thought to reflect an advantage of heterozygotes against *Plasmodium falciparum* malaria. More than 200 β-thalassemia mutations have been described; however, in each ethnic group a relatively small number of mutations account for the majority of cases (the ratio most often quoted is 20 or fewer mutations account for 80% or more of the cases). Clinical manifestations of β-thalassemia range from mild anemia to severe life-threatening disease requiring lifelong transfusions.

β^0-Thalassemia (β-Thalassemia Major). Sometimes called Cooley's anemia after the physician[181] who in 1925 first described the condition in the children of Italian and Greek immigrants in New York by noting that these children failed to grow, had frequent infections, appeared pale and malnourished, had splenomegaly, and had facial bone changes.

β-Thalassemia major results from mutations that interfere with translation or are involved in the initiation, elongation, or termination of globin chain synthesis. Mutations that interfere with translation account for almost 50% of all the β-thalassemia mutations. Included in this are frame shift or nonsense mutations that produce premature termination codons that result in incomplete translation of the β-globin gene and nonproduction of the β-globin chain resulting in β^0-thalassemia.

Clinical presentation is usually at less than 1 year of age with features that include small size for age, abdominal girth expansion, and failure to thrive. Physical examination of the subject may reveal frontal bossing[146] (a rounded eminence on the forehead) caused by thickening of the cranial bones, pallor, and prominence of the cheek bones, which, in older children, obscures the base of the nose and exposes the teeth. These features are a result of marrow expansion (up to a thirtyfold increase) caused by ineffective erythropoiesis with production of highly unstable α-globin tetramers leading to increased plasma volume and the formation of extramedullary erythropoietic tissue, especially in the thorax and paraspinal region. The spleen, liver, and heart may be enlarged also because of extramedullary hematopoiesis.

Typical CBC results include severe anemia with the Hb concentration between 30 and 65 g/L, MCV 48 to 72 fL, and the mean corpuscular hemoglobin concentration (MCHC) 230 to 320 g/L. On the peripheral blood smear, a characteristic markedly abnormal RBC morphology is noted, which includes a large number of microcytes, numerous target cells, which may have a bridge joining the central and peripheral pigment zones, polychromasia and occasional spherocytes, schistocytes, and nucleated red cells. Anisocytosis is noted, the diameter of the RBC ranges from 3 to 15 μm with little pigment, and there is shape distortion. Prominent basophilic stippling is noted. RBC osmotic fragility is frequently observed. A typical peripheral blood on a patient with β^0 thalassemia is shown in Figure 31-16.

The white blood cell (WBC) and platelet counts are usually normal. Ferritin is usually within the upper half of the reference interval, and the total bilirubin is mildly elevated with a borderline elevation in the conjugated fraction. Urinalysis frequently shows increased urobilinogen or urobilin concentration and is often colored dark brown to black because of the presence of dipyroles and mesobilifuscin. The latter features reflect ineffective hematopoiesis with intramedullary red cell destruction. HPLC analysis (Figure 31-12, *b*) shows a major Hb F peak with an absence of an Hb A peak and variable Hb A_2 (range 1% to 5.9%, mean 1.7%) peak. Electrophoresis at alkaline and acid pH shows a dominant band in the F position on both gels.[7]

Family studies on both parents and siblings should be performed and the classical β-thalassemia minor pattern described later in the chapter should be found in the parents. The siblings may be either normal or have β-thalassemia minor. A family case history is seen in Figure 31-17.

Transfusion together with iron chelation is the only therapy, and splenectomy is frequently performed. Following splenectomy inclusion, bodies consisting of denatured α-chains can be observed in the blood smear following staining with methyl violet. Puberty is often delayed, incomplete, or completely absent. In boys there may be active spermatogenesis, and Leydig cell function is normal. In the older chronically transfused patient, iron overload is a common feature. Diabetes mellitus and hypoparathyroidism are frequent sequelae. Numerous cardiopulmonary conditions, including pericarditis and myocardial hemosiderosis, are the leading causes of death in transfused patients, and are frequently associated with β^0-thalassemia.

β^+-Thalassemia (β-Thalassemia Intermedia). With this disorder, there is a significant reduction in the production of β-globin chain with subsequent reduction in the quantity of Hb A present, which is attributed to a wide variety of geno-

TEST/REF	INDEX PAT 7 MO F	MOTHER 33 YRS	FATHER 40 YRS	SIBLING 3 YR F
HB	↓ 72 G/L	↓ 114	↓ 132	122
REF	105-135	120-160	135-175	115-135
RBC	↓ 3.23 (10^{12}/L)	5.19	↑ 6.61	4.42
REF	3.70-5.30	4.10-5.20	4.50-6.00	3.90-5.30
MCV	↓ 69 fL	↓ 68	↓ 63	80
REF	70-86	80-100	80-100	75-87
MCH	↓ 22 pg	↓ 22	↓ 20	28
REF	26-35	26-35	26-35	26-35
HBA	↓ 0.00	0.94	↑ 0.93	0.96
REF	0.94-0.98	0.94-0.98	0.94-0.98	0.94-0.98
HBA2	0.030	↑ 0.054	↑ 0.058	0.030
REF	<0.03	<0.03	<0.03	<0.03
HBF	0.97	<0.01	<0.01	<0.01
REF	<0.10	<0.01	<0.01	<0.01

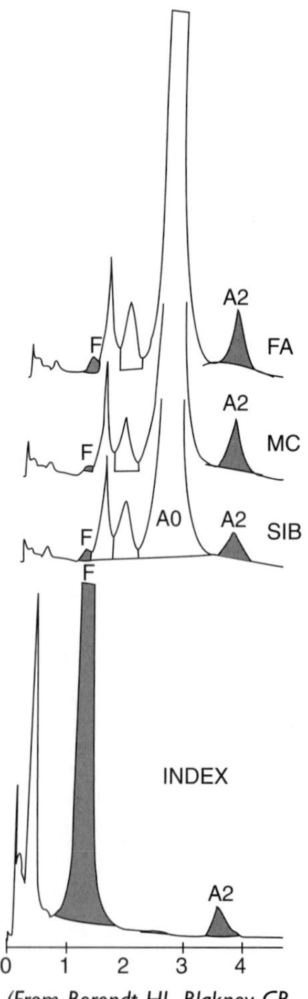

Figure 31-17 HPLC chromatograms and CBC results from a family study of a child with B^0-thalassemia. *(From Berendt HL, Blakney GB, Clarke GM, Higgins TN. A case of β-thalassemia major detected using HPLC in a child of Chinese ancestry Clin Biochem 2000;33:311-13.)*

types. There are many different causes for β^+-thalassemia, with variations in one or two β-globin genes. The clinical severity in individuals with variations in two β-globin chains is much less than when there is a variation in only one gene, a condition sometimes called dominant β-thalassemia. There is a reduction in the severity of the clinical features with the coinheritance of α-thalassemia. β^+-thalassemia is found in Mediterranean countries, especially in the Eastern Mediterranean.

Clinical presentation varies from symptoms similar to β^0-thalassemia to those associated with β-thalassemia trait. Transfusions are usually not necessary, and hydroxyurea therapy is frequently used to increase the production of Hb F and to mitigate disease symptoms.

HPLC analysis shows a large Hb F peak with a reduced Hb A peak. Hb A_2 is above the reference interval at concentrations greater than those associated with β-thalassemia minor. Bands in the A and F positions are seen on electrophoresis at both alkaline and acid pH. The Hb is significantly reduced (60 to 100 g/L). The peripheral blood smear shows the same features as β^0-thalassemia, including anisocytosis, hypochromia, target cells, basophilic stippling, and nucleated RBCs.

β-Thalassemia Minor (β-Thalassemia Trait). Patients with β-thalassemia minor are very often asymptomatic except at times of hematopoietic stress, such as infections or pregnancy, when they may require, in extreme situations, blood transfusions because of the development of anemia. The CBC on patients with β-thalassemia trait shows low normal or decreased Hb level and hematocrit, decreased MCV (<72 fL) and MCH (<27 pg), and normal RDW. The discriminant factor is <60 pg. However, for patients with liver disease and β-thalassemia, the MCV and MCH may be in the low end of the reference interval.

The peripheral blood smear shows microcytic RBCs with occasional hypochromia, poikilocytosis, and target cells.

The diagnosis of β-thalassemia minor, with appropriate indices in the CBC, is dependent on the finding of a raised Hb A_2 concentration (>3.5%). Iron deplete individuals should become iron replete before a definitive diagnosis of β-thalassemia is made as the Hb A_2 may be falsely low.[109] HPLC is the preferred method for this quantification since densitometric scanning of the Hb A_2 band on an alkaline electrophoresis gel is not recommended because of poor precision and accuracy. In 30% to 40% of all cases of β-thalassemia minor, the Hb F will also be raised (>1.0%). The lifespan of the RBC may be reduced, and diabetics may show a lower Hb A_{1c} compared with normal individuals with equivalent glycemic control. The β-thalassemia mutation may be identified either by Southern blot using mutation specific probes or by gap-PCR.

δβ-Thalassemia. Deletion of both δ- and β-genes results in δβ-thalassemia. Both heterozygous and homozygous conditions have been described. It is found in a variety of ethnic groups but is most prevalent in countries of the Eastern Mediterranean, especially Greece and Italy, and is the result of one of eight mutations that have been described to date. CBC analysis shows a reduced level of Hb (80 to 135 g/L) with low normal or marginally reduced MCV and MCH. HPLC analysis shows an Hb A peak with a reduced Hb A_2 concentration and raised Hb F concentration.

The exception to the preceding description is the Sardinian type of δβ-thalassemia in which there are thalassemic indices on the CBC (low MCV and MCH, normal RDW) with a normal Hb A_2 concentration and an Hb F concentration between 15% and 20%. Hb Lepore is sometimes classified as a δβ-thalassemia because of a reduction in the production of both δ- and β-globin chains or as an Hb variant because of the presence of an abnormal globin chain.

Hereditary Persistence of Fetal Hemoglobin (HPFH). The term hereditary persistence of Hb F is used to describe a group of genetic conditions in which the concentration of Hb F is increased above the upper limit of the reference interval because of the reduction of β-globin synthesis and a compensatory increase in δ-globin synthesis. Two major classes, heterocellular and deletional, of HPFH have been described. Several deletional variants of HPFH have been described, including Greek, Indian, Italian, Corfu, and black.

In black HPFH the Hb F is raised to between 10% and 36% of the total Hb with normal Hb A_2 concentrations. The Hb, MCV, and MCH are within the reference intervals. It is clinically innocuous and asymptomatic. Similarly, there are no clinical abnormalities associated with Greek HPFH although the concentration of Hb F is in the range of 15% to 25%.

Nondeletional HPFH, sometimes named heterocellular HPFH, describes a group of presentations in which the increase of Hb F is distributed heterogeneously among the red cells in otherwise normal individuals. The Hb F concentration varies between 1% and 13% of the total Hb heterozygotes and 19% to 21% in homozygotes. There are no clinical or hematological abnormalities.

Hemoglobinopathies

Although more than 900 hemoglobinopathies have been described, only 9 have some clinical significance. Recent immigration from regions with a high frequency of hemoglobinopathies (South East Asia or Africa) to regions (Western Europe, Central and South America, and Canada) that had low frequencies has increased the incidence of hemoglobinopathies in these areas. The incidental and fortuitous finding of a hemoglobinopathy in the HPLC analysis for the quantification of Hb A_{1c} has increased both the number and incidence of Hb variants.* Several Hb variants (e.g., Hb Rambam, Niigata, and Camden) interfere with HPLC methods for quantifying Hb A_{1c}.

---

*References 36, 41, 81, 156, 175, 178.

Nomenclature

Hb variants are named using letters (Hbs S, D, E, etc.), the family name of the index case (Hb Lepore), the place of discovery of the variant or place of origin of the propositus (Hb Edmonton) or the name of the river (Hb Saale)[21] flowing through the city in which the propositus lived. In some cases both a letter and name are used as in Hb J-Baltimore, indicating the Hb is classified as having electrophoretic mobility similar to other J Hbs but differs from them in amino acid sequence and was originally discovered in Baltimore. The term AS trait (sometimes abbreviated to S trait) is used to describe a heterozygous state in which one of the β-globin chains is S and the other is A. In instances in which no normal β-globin chain is present (e.g., Hb SD) the β-globin chain present in the higher concentration is usually, although not always, placed first. A systematic nomenclature system is now used alongside the variant name to describe the affected chain and location on the chain and the amino acid substitution. For example, Hb Spanish Town ($\alpha 27(B8)^{Glu \rightarrow Val}$), a Hb variant named after a district in Kingston, Jamaica and found in Jamaicans of African descent, results from a substitution of valine for glutamic acid in position 27 of the α-globin chain, which is located in position 8 of the B helix of the α-chain.

Classification of Hemoglobin Variants

Hb variants are classified according to the type of mutation. Single point mutations in α-globin chain give rise to a substitution of one amino acid residue. As an example Hb San Diego ($\beta 109(G11)^{Val \rightarrow Met}$) has a methionine residue instead of the normal valine at position 109 of the β-chain. Hemoglobin C Harlem ($\beta 6(A3)^{Glu \rightarrow Val}$;$\beta 73(E17)^{Asp \rightarrow Asn}$) is an example of an Hb variant in which two amino acid residues are substituted, namely valine replacing glutamic acid at position 6 and asparagine replacing aspartic acid at position 73 of the β-chain. Hemoglobin C Harlem is electrophoretically similar to Hb C but behaves like Hb S in every other aspect including clinical manifestation. *Deletion* Hb variants arise from the deletion of one to five amino acid residues in the globin chain. Hb Vicksburg ($\beta 75(E19)^{Leu \rightarrow 0}$) is an example in this category of Hb having a deletion of leucine in position 75 of the β-chain. *Insertion* Hbs arise from an insertion of one to three amino acid residues into the globin chain. Hemoglobin Grady is an example in this category having an insertion of a three amino acid residue sequence (glutamine-phenylalanine-threonine) between positions 118 and 119 of the α-chain. *Deletion-insertion* Hbs arise from the deletion of a portion of the normal amino acid residue sequence and the insertion of another sequence with resultant lengthening or shortening of the globin chain. An example of this type of Hb variant is Hb Montreal in which the three normal amino acid residues between positions 72 and 76 of the β-globin chain are replaced with a four amino acid residue sequence. *Elongation* Hbs result from a single base pair mutation or frameshift at the 3′ end of exon 3 or the 5′ end of exon 1 of the α_2- or the β-globin chain. The elongation hemoglobin, Hb Constant Spring (named after an ethnic Chinese family from the Constant Spring district of Jamaica), has an additional 31 amino acid residues joined at position 142 (the carboxy terminal) of the α-chain. *Fusion* Hbs result from the fusion of either an α- or β-globin chain with a portion of another globin chain. Hemoglobin Lepore-Hollandia results from the fusion of the first 22 amino acid residues of the δ-chain, with the amino acid sequence from position 50 onward of normal β-globin. For the latter four categories, the systematic name is long and cumbersome, prompting the universal use of the variant name rather than the systematic nomenclature.

Types of Hemoglobin Variants

In α-chain variants, the variant usually forms less than 25% of the total Hb since the mutation typically occurs only in one of the four genes that code for the α-globin chain. For β-chain variants in the heterozygous state, the variant forms greater than 25% but less than 50% of the total Hb. Based on the mutation of only one of the β-globin chain genes, the β-chain variant should form 50% of the total Hb. However, the formation of Hb A is favored in almost all cases over the variant Hb. This information can be used to categorize an unknown Hb variant as either an α- or β-globin chain variant.

Hb VarDatabase is a relational database of Hb variants and thalassemia mutations and may be accessed at the web site http://globin.cse.psu.edu/hbvar/menu.html.

Hemoglobin S ($b6(A3)^{Glu/EVal}$). Hb S, either in the heterozygous or homozygous state, is the most widespread of the Hb variants and arises from a substitution of valine for glutamic acid at position 6 in the A helix of the β-globin chain. Hb S is found in high frequency in West and North Africa, the Middle East (especially Saudi Arabia), and the Indian subcontinent. Approximately 8% of African-Americans are heterozygous for Hb S, and homozygous Hb S is found in 1 in 500 newborns in this group. Four haplotypes originating from different geographic locations have been described. The widespread distribution of the single point gene mutation responsible for the synthesis of Hb S in areas where *P. falciparum* malaria is endemic is due to the protection of Hb S heterozygotes from the worst manifestations of the malaria.

Homozygous Hemoglobin S (HbSS). In homozygous Hb S, a valine for glutamic acid substitution occurs on both β-globin chains because of the inheritance of mutated β-globin chain genes from both parents. The condition is described as "sickle cell anemia or sickle cell disease" because of the sickle shaped RBCs that occur when there is a "sickle cell crisis" and is sometimes written as $\beta^S\beta^S$.[154a]

HPLC analysis (Figure 31-12, *e*) of a hemolysate of an individual homozygous for Hb S shows no Hb A peak with a small Hb A_2 peak. The apparent Hb A_2 concentration may be falsely increased because of the presence of glycated Hb S. Hemoglobin S forms 85% to 90% of the total Hb. The Hb F concentration is variable, with females having higher concentrations than men and is somewhat, although not exclusively, haplotype dependent. The highest Hb F concentrations (10% to 25%) are found in individuals from the Middle East and the Indian subcontinent with the Arab-Indian haplotype. Low Hb F concentrations (5% to 6%) are found in the West African Cameroon (sometimes called Senegal) haplotype. The remaining haplotypes, the Benin and Bantu, have Hb F concentrations in the range of 6% to 7%. Increased concentrations of Hb F mitigate to some extent the clinical manifestations of sickle cell anemia. Electrophoresis (Figure 31-10) at both alkaline and acid pH shows a single large band in the Hb S position with small bands at the Hb A_2 and Hb F positions. The sickle cell screen test is positive.

CBC analysis of an individual homozygous for Hb S indicates a moderate to a major decreased Hb level (60 to 100 g/L) with a normal to increased MCV and MCH. In individuals with a concurrent thalassemia, the Hb is further decreased and both the MCV and MCH are lowered. In the neonate the peripheral blood smear shows the occasional sickle and target cells and Howell-Jolly bodies. As a patient's age increases, these features of hyposplenism become increasingly evident. In the adult the percentage of sickle cells observed can be as much as 30% to 40%. In the setting of a sickle cell crisis, fewer sickle cells may be present than when the individuals are clinically well. Howell-Jolly bodies, target cells, Pappenheimer bodies, boat-shaped cells, and nucleated RBCs are noted. The platelet count and neutrophil counts are elevated. Sometimes blister cells in which the Hb appears to be present in only one half of the cell is observed.

Heterozygous Hemoglobin S (HbS Trait). HPLC analysis (Figure 31-12, *f*) of a hemolysate of a blood sample from an individual who is heterozygous for Hb S shows peaks in the Hb A and S positions, with 40% of the total Hb found in the Hb S peak. Hb S concentrations <30% are suggestive of a co-inheritance of α-thalassemia. Hb F concentration is variable. Electrophoresis (Figure 31-10) at both alkaline and acid pH shows bands in the A and S positions

CBC analysis from an individual who is heterozygous for Hb S shows a slightly decreased level of Hb, and typically sickle cells are not seen on the peripheral blood film. Patients are often asymptomatic, and the first time an individual is diagnosed as heterozygous for Hb S (sickle cell trait) is often when an Hb A_{1c} analysis is requested on the individual or when a family study is initiated for genetic counseling. In the United States there are neonatal screening programs designed specifically to detect both heterozygous and homozygous Hb S in newborns. Although individuals with sickle cell trait are clinically asymptomatic, genetic counseling should be considered because co-inheritance of two β-globin gene abnormalities may contribute to a sickle cell disorder. Both α- and β-thalassemia can be co-inherited with heterozygous Hb S.

Hemoglobin SC (Hb SC Disease). SC disease arises when both β-globin chains are substituted at position 6 with either valine (Hb S) or lysine (Hb C). On HPLC analysis peaks are noted in the S and C positions, with the S peak forming the majority of the Hb present.

Electrophoresis (Figure 31-10) at both alkaline and acid pH shows bands in the S and C positions, and the sickling test is positive.

Hemoglobin SD. Hb S may be coinherited with Hb D (SD disease). Individuals with this disease have similar but milder clinical presentation when compared with that of sickle cell disease (Hb SS). HPLC analysis shows two peaks, one in the Hb S position forming approximately 38% to 42% of the total Hb and the other in the Hb D position forming 43% to 45% of the total Hb. The Hb F concentration is usually within the reference interval although concentrations as high as 14% have been observed in some individuals with SD disease. Alkaline electrophoresis shows a band in the S position. Acid electrophoresis shows bands in the S and A positions. The sickling test is positive. CBC analysis shows a greatly decreased level of Hb with normal to slightly elevated MCV. Target, boat-shaped, nucleated, red, and sickle cells—together with anisocytosis and poikilocytosis—are noted on the peripheral blood smear.

Hemoglobin S/O Arab. Co-inheritance of Hb S and Hb O Arab presents a similar or somewhat milder clinical presentation to sickle cell disease and is found in the Middle East and North Africa.

One or more abnormal α-globin chains can combine with Hb S. In African-Americans and West Africans the combination of Hb G Philadelphia ($\alpha 68(E17)^{Asn \rightarrow Lys}$) with Hb S is prevalent. HPLC analysis (Figure 31-12, *i*) on blood samples from these individuals shows at least two major peaks and two smaller peaks. The two major peaks are due to the combination of the normal α-chain with the normal β-chain and the abnormal α-chain with the normal β-chain. The two smaller peaks are due to the combination of the normal α-chain with the abnormal β-chain and the abnormal α-chain with the abnormal β-chain. Electrophoresis at alkaline pH shows major bands in the A and S positions with a minor band in the C position. At acid pH, bands are seen in the A and S positions. CBC analysis gives a slightly decreased Hb level with normal MCV and MCH. α- or β-thalassemia can be co-inherited with Hb G Philadelphia and Hb S. In these cases, CBC analysis results in markedly decreased MCV and MCH with reduced Hb concentration.

Hemoglobin C ($b6(A3)^{Glu \rightarrow Lys}$). Hb C arises from a substitution of lysine for glutamic acid at position 6 of the β-globin chain. Hb C may be found in the homozygous (Hb C disease, $\beta^C\beta^C$) or heterozygous (Hb C trait) states. Hb C is commonly found in West Africa and the Caribbean. It is the second most commonly studied, after Hb S, of all Hb variants. HPLC analysis (Figure 31-12, *g*) on samples from individuals with homozygous Hb C shows a large peak in the C position, with Hb C forming 90% to 95% of the total Hb. Hb F concentrations are variable. Glycated Hb C is found as a small peak eluting before the Hb C peak. The ratio of the elution times of glycated Hb C to Hb C is the same as that of Hb A_{1c} and Hb A. Electrophoresis at alkaline and acid pH shows a single band in the C position.

Mild to moderate anemia is the most common clinical presentation. CBC analysis shows normal or slightly decreased Hb levels with a normochromic and normocytic red cell morphology. An increase in polychromasia may be present, and the reticulocytes may contribute to an increase in the MCV. The peripheral blood smear shows numerous target cells with occasional nucleated RBCs and characteristic irregular contracted red cells (sometimes called pyknocytes). Hb C crystals may be seen, and bilirubin concentrations may be slightly elevated. Red cell survival and osmotic fragility are decreased.

Heterozygous Hemoglobin C (Hb C Trait). HPLC analysis (Figure 31-12, *h*) and electrophoresis at both alkaline and acid pH (Figure 31-10) on blood samples from individuals who are heterozygous for Hb C show bands in the A and C positions with Hb C forming 30% to 40% of the total Hb. CBC analysis may show target cells and is generally normochromic with the MCV near the lower limit of the reference interval.

Heterozygous Hb C individuals are usually asymptomatic. Genetic counseling may be useful where prospective parents have abnormalities in the β-globin gene.

Hb C may be co-inherited with both α- and β-thalassemia, and the concentration of Hb C is related to the number of functioning α-genes. With only two functioning α-genes, the Hb C concentration can fall to 32% of the total Hb. Co-inheritance of Hb C with either β^0- or β^+-thalassemia results in moderately severe anemia with splenomegaly. The Hb F concentration is increased.

Hemoglobin D Punjab (b121(GH4)$^{Glu \rightarrow Gln}$). Hb D Punjab is an Hb variant in which glutamic acid at position 121 of the β-globin chain is replaced with glutamine. The names Hb D Los Angeles or Hb D Punjab are used to describe this variant, with the former name used more in North America and the latter in the United Kingdom. Hb D Punjab is found in the Punjab region of the Indian subcontinent especially in Sikhs of the Lycus Valley. Large scale immigration from this area to the United Kingdom, the United States and Canada has widened the distribution of Hb D Punjab. Hb D Punjab is also found in Caucasians whose foreparents lived in the Indian subcontinent in the time of the British Raj. Hemoglobin D Punjab is found in the heterozygous (Hb D Punjab trait) and homozygous (Hb D Punjab disease, $\beta^D\beta^D$) states.

HPLC analysis of blood from an individual with homozygous Hb D Punjab shows normal or marginally raised Hb F and Hb A_2 peaks with a large peak in the Hb D position forming >90% of the total Hb. Electrophoresis at alkaline pH shows a band in the S position, which migrates to the A position in acid electrophoresis. CBC analysis shows a mild decrease in Hb levels, MCV, and MCH with target cells observed in the blood smear. Patients present clinically with mild anemia.

HPLC analysis on individuals with Hb D Punjab trait shows two peaks, one at the A position and the other at the D position, with Hb D forming 30% to 40% of the total Hb. The Hb F and Hb A_2 concentrations are within or slightly above the reference intervals. Electrophoresis at alkaline pH shows two bands, one in the A position and the other in the S position. On electrophoresis at acid pH, a single band in the A position is noted. HPLC is the preferred method for identification of Hb D, because a similar electrophoretic pattern, on both alkaline and acid pH, is seen with Hb G. CBC analysis is unremarkable except for the presence of target cells on the blood smear.

Individuals with Hb D Punjab trait are clinically asymptomatic.

Co-inheritance of Hb D Punjab (both heterozygous and homozygous states) with β-thalassemia is common. CBC analysis on these patients shows decreased levels of Hb with markedly decreased MCV and MCH. Target and irregular contracted cells together with hypochromia and anisocytosis are seen on the blood smear. The quantification of Hb A_2 in individuals with coinheritance of Hb D Punjab and β-thalassemia presents a challenge to the laboratory since HPLC analysis underestimates the Hb A_2 concentration because of an unstable rising baseline in these individuals. Although not normally recommended, quantification of Hb A_2 by densitometry on alkaline electrophoresis may be the only method available to many laboratories. CBC analysis shows a greatly decreased level of Hb with low MCV and MCH. The blood smear shows target and contracted cells with hypochromia and anisocytosis.

Individuals with coinheritance of Hb D Punjab and β-thalassemia present with a notable compensated anemia.

Hemoglobin D Iran (b22(B4)$^{Glu \rightarrow Gln}$). Hb D Iran is a β-globin chain variant in which glutamine replaces glutamic acid at position 22 of the β-globin chain.

On HPLC analysis peaks are seen in the A and A_2 positions with the quantification for HbA_2 far above that normally expected. Alkaline electrophoresis shows two bands, one in the A position and the other in the S position. On acid electrophoresis a single band in the A position is noted.

Individuals with Hb D Iran are asymptomatic.

Hemoglobin E (b26(B8)$^{Glu \rightarrow Lys}$). Hb E is a β-chain variant with lysine replacing glutamic acid at position 26 of the β-globin chain. More individuals have the Hb variant Hb E than any other variant. Hb E is found in both the homozygous and heterozygous states and combined with β-thalassemia. It is widespread in the Far East including Southern China, Cambodia, Thailand, and Laos. Hb E is increasingly found in the United States and Canada caused by immigration from this area.

HPLC analysis of blood from individuals with homozygous Hb E (Hb E disease, $\beta^E\beta^E$) shows a single peak (>90% of the total Hb) co-eluting with Hb A_2. Hemoglobin F is within or marginally above the reference interval. On alkaline electrophoresis a single band is noted in the C position, which migrates to the A position in acid electrophoresis.

CBC analysis shows normal to marginally decreased Hb levels with low MCV and MCH. Target cells are noted in the peripheral blood smear. Iron studies are normal.

Homozygous Hb E individuals are usually asymptomatic although slight anemia may be present.

HPLC analysis of blood from individuals with heterozygous Hb E shows two peaks, one in the A position and the other in the A_2 position. Hb E forms approximately 30% of the total Hb. CBC analysis shows normal Hb levels and occasionally low MCV. Target cells are noted in the peripheral blood smear. Iron studies are normal.

Heterozygous Hb E individuals are usually asymptomatic although slight anemia may be present.

The co-inheritance of Hb E and thalassemia produces an anemia of variable severity. The HPLC on a patient with co-inheritance of β-thalassemia and homozygous E is shown in Figure 31-12, *c*. Co-inheritance of homozygous Hb E and β-thalassemia leads to a severe anemia with greatly reduced Hb levels, MCV, and MCH with increased Hb F concentration. Numerous target cells are noted on the peripheral blood smear together with microcytosis, anisocytosis, hypochromia, and a few nucleated red cells. Iron studies are normal. In the most severe cases, the clinical presentation is similar to that of β^0-thalassemia, and transfusion may be the only therapy. Co-inheritance of heterozygous Hb E with α-thalassemia produces a less severe anemia with low Hb and MCV and MCH. Target cells are noted on the peripheral blood smear together with microcytosis and hypochromia. Patients who are pregnant may need to be monitored closely although transfusion is not usually required.

The quantification of Hb A_2, which is important in the diagnosis of possible coinheritance of β-thalassemia with Hb E, provides a challenge to the laboratory since Hb E and Hb A_2 co-elute. Molecular studies are the only satisfactory method to establish coinheritance of Hb E and β-thalassemia, although the severity of the disease, family studies, and an increased Hb F may lead to a suspicion of coinheritance.

Hemoglobin O Arab (b121(GH4)$^{Glu \rightarrow Lys}$). Hb O Arab is a β-chain variant with lysine replacing glutamic acid at position 121 of the β-globin chain. Hb O Arab is found in a wide variety of ethnic groups in North Africa and Eastern Europe and is not confined, nor is it even common, among Arab populations. Hb O Arab has been found in both the heterozygous and homozygous states.

HPLC analysis of blood from an individual with homozygous Hb O Arab shows a single band between the S and C positions, with Hb O Arab forming >90% of the total Hb. Electrophoresis at alkaline pH shows a band close to the C position. On electrophoresis at acid pH, a band between the A and S positions (but closer to A) is seen. CBC analysis shows a normal or marginally low Hb level, MCV, and MCH. The peripheral blood smear shows slight microcytosis.

There are no unusual hematological features on individuals with heterozygous Hb O Arab. HPLC analysis on blood from these individuals shows two peaks, one in the A position and the other eluting close to the C position and forming 30% to 40% of the total Hb. Electrophoresis at alkaline electrophoresis shows bands in the A and close to the C position. On acid electrophoresis, two bands are noted: one in the A position and the other in a position between the A and S positions.

Hybrid Hemoglobins. Hybrid Hbs, or crossover Hbs, describe a group of Hb variants in which one of the globin chains is a hybrid of amino acid sequences of two other globin chains. The term crossover Hb is sometimes used because there is a point in the amino acid sequence in which there is a crossover from the amino acid sequence of one globin chain to another globin chain. Individuals with these hybrid Hb variants present with the clinical features and laboratory findings, particularly in their CBC, that are similar to thalassemia. The production of the hybrid globin chain is reduced. Hb Lepore is the prototypical hybrid Hb.

Hemoglobin Lepore. Hb Lepore is classified as a δβ-hybrid Hb variant on the basis that the non–α-chain is a hybrid of δ- and β-globin chains. It is unique in that it is the only hemoglobinopathy named after the family name of the index case. Delta-beta hybrid Hbs arise because there are deletions of part of the 3′ portion of the δ-globin gene and in the 5′ portion of the β-globin chain with a resultant formation of a δβ-fusion gene. Three distinct variations of Hb Lepore have been described. In Hb Lepore-Hollandia (δβ-hybrid [δ through 22; β from 50]), a variant found in Canada and Papua New Guinea, there is fusion of the first 22 amino acid residues of the δ-globin chain with the amino acids from position 50 onwards of the β-globin chain. In Hb Lepore-Baltimore (δβ-hybrid [δ through 50: β from 86]), found mainly in individuals of Spanish ancestry, the first 50 amino acid residues of the δ-globin chain are fused with the amino acid residues from position 86 of the β-globin chain. In Hb Lepore-Boston-Washington (δβ-hybrid [δ through 87; β from 116]), the most common Hb Lepore, the first 87 amino acid residues of the δ-globin chain are fused with the amino acid residues from position 116 onwards of the β-globin chain. Hb Lepore-Boston-Washington, sometimes called Hb Lepore-Boston, is found mainly in individuals of Italian descent although it has been found in individuals from Eastern Europe.

HPLC analysis of blood from individuals with Hb Lepore shows a greatly raised Hb A_2 level with a marginally reduced Hb A concentration. The Hb A_2 concentration is usually greater than 10% of the total Hb and is falsely increased because of the co-elution of Hb A_2 and Hb Lepore. Electrophoresis at alkaline pH shows a band in the S position for Hb Lepore-Boston-Washington and in a position between the A and S positions for the other Hb Lepore variants. At acid pH there is a single band in the A position for all Hb Lepore variants.

CBC analysis shows a greatly reduced level of Hb, MCV, and MCH for homozygotes for Hb Lepore. The hematological findings are very similar to β-thalassemia major or intermedia. CBC analysis on heterozygotes shows a slightly reduced MCV and MCH. The hematology findings are very similar to β-thalassemia trait. Iron studies are normal in both heterozygotes and homozygotes. The similarity of the hematology in Hb Lepore and β-thalassemia makes the careful review of the HPLC and electrophoretic analysis essential to distinguish the two. The two key pieces of evidence to distinguish between the two are the finding of a greatly raised Hb A_2 on HPLC analysis and a small band in the S position on electrophoresis at alkaline pH.

Elongation Hemoglobins. Elongation Hbs, of which there are 13, include seven α-chain and six β-chain variants, result from the lengthening of either the C or N terminus of either globin chain. The most important, from a clinical perspective, are the five C terminal α-chain variants in which the terminal codon TAA is changed and there is an addition of an amino acid sequence. The prototypical elongation Hb is Hb Constant Spring. In this variant the C terminal TAA codon is changed to CAA in the α_2-gene and there is an addition of a 31 amino acid sequence at the C terminal end to give an α-globin chain length of 173 amino acid residues rather than the normal 142 residue length. This increase in the length results in instability of the Hb variant, and synthesis of this elongated globin chain is reduced. Hemoglobin Constant Spring is found in South East Asia especially in Vietnam, Cambodia, and Laos and is found in both the heterozygous and homozygous states.

Patients with Hb Constant Spring present with slightly reduced Hb, MCV, and MCH with hypochromia and microcytosis in the peripheral blood smear. Iron studies are often normal.

The instability of Hb Constant Spring presents a challenge to the laboratory diagnosis of this variant. The blood used for analytical procedures should be as fresh as possible, and samples greater than 24 hours old should not be used. HPLC analysis of blood from individuals with Hb Constant Spring shows a small peak in the C position, which forms approximately 4% to 6% of the total Hb in the homozygote and 1% to 3% in the heterozygote. On electrophoresis at alkaline pH, a small band migrating cathodally to the application point may be seen. This electrophoretic mobility is unique in that it is the only Hb variant that moves toward the cathode rather than the anode.

Hemoglobin Constant Spring is commonly found in combination with α^0-thalassemia especially the $-^{SEA}$ mutation. The clinical presentation of this combination results in a severe form of Hb H disease.

IRON

Normally, very small quantities of iron are present in most cells of the body, in plasma, and in other extracellular fluids, and the body rigorously conserves its iron supply, so that less than 0.1% of the body iron content is lost daily, mostly in desquamated cells.

BIOCHEMISTRY

Distribution

Body iron is distributed into a number of different compartments that include Hb, storage iron, tissue iron, myoglobin, and a labile pool. The average amount of iron in these compartments is summarized in Table 31-1.

Hemoglobin

One mL of erythrocytes contains 1 mg of iron. In a 70-kg male the red cell mass is about 2 L, therefore it contains about 2 g of Hb iron.[10]

Storage Iron

Iron is stored in the body in the form of ferritin and hemosiderin.

Ferritin. Ferritin consists of a protein shell surrounding an iron core,[23,76] and hemosiderin is formed when ferritin is broken down in secondary lysosomes.[6,180] Hemosiderin therefore appears to represent the end point of the intracellular storage iron pathway. Ferritin consists of an apoferritin shell and an interior ferric oxyhydroxide $(FeOOH)_x$ crystalline core. The apoferritin shell is composed of 24 subunits, which are either L (light) or H (heavy) ferritin chains. The proportion of light chains to heavy chains differs from tissue to tissue (Figure 31-18). The shell is 12 to 13 nm in diameter, and its interior cavity is 7 to 8 nm in diameter. Only ferrous iron is taken up by ferritin, and it is oxidized by a catalytic site on the H chain. The H chains contain small intrasubunit channels, which may be used by iron entering the cavity. The exact composition of the FeOOH core crystal is somewhat different in different species and contains different amounts of phosphates. In humans it is a ferrihydrite ($5\ Fe_2O_3 \cdot 9\ H_2O$). Release of iron from ferritin is probably nonenzymatic and may involve reduction by reduced flavin mononucleotide or other reducing substances. The resultant Fe^{2+} leaves the crystal and diffuses out through a pore of the ferritin shell.

TABLE 31-1 Average Iron Content of Compartments in an Average 70-kg Male (Based on Estimates)

Compartment	Iron Content (mg)	Total Body Iron (%)
Hb iron	2000	67
Storage iron (ferritin, hemosiderin)	1000	27
Myoglobin iron	130	3.5
Labile pool	80	2.2
Other tissue iron	8	0.2
Transport iron	3	0.08

From Fairbanks VF, Beutler E. Iron metabolism. In: Beutler E, Lichtman MA, Coller BS, Kipps TJ, Seligsohn U, eds. Williams hematology. New York: McGraw-Hill, 2001:295-304.

Ferritin is found in nearly all cells of the body. In hepatocytes of the liver and in the macrophages of the marrow and other organs, ferritin provides a reserve of iron readily available for formation of Hb and other heme proteins, in a form in which the iron is shielded from body fluids, so that it is unable to produce oxidative damage, as would be the case if it were in ionic form. In men the total body content of stored iron, mostly as ferritin, is approximately 800 mg; in healthy women, it ranges up to 200 mg. Minute quantities of ferritin are also present in serum in concentrations proportional to total body stored iron. This ferritin differs from tissue ferritin in that it is glycosylated, contains mostly L chains, and is poor in iron, representing mostly apoferritin. Liver injury and a large number of pathological processes result in release of relatively large amounts of ferritin into plasma.

Hemosiderin. *Hemosiderin* is aggregated, partially deproteinized ferritin. In contrast to ferritin, hemosiderin is insoluble in aqueous solutions, a difference that has traditionally been used to distinguish these two iron storage compounds. Iron is only slowly released from hemosiderin, possibly because it occurs in relatively large aggregates and therefore has a much smaller surface/volume ratio. Like ferritin, hemosiderin normally is found predominantly in cells of the liver, spleen, and bone marrow.

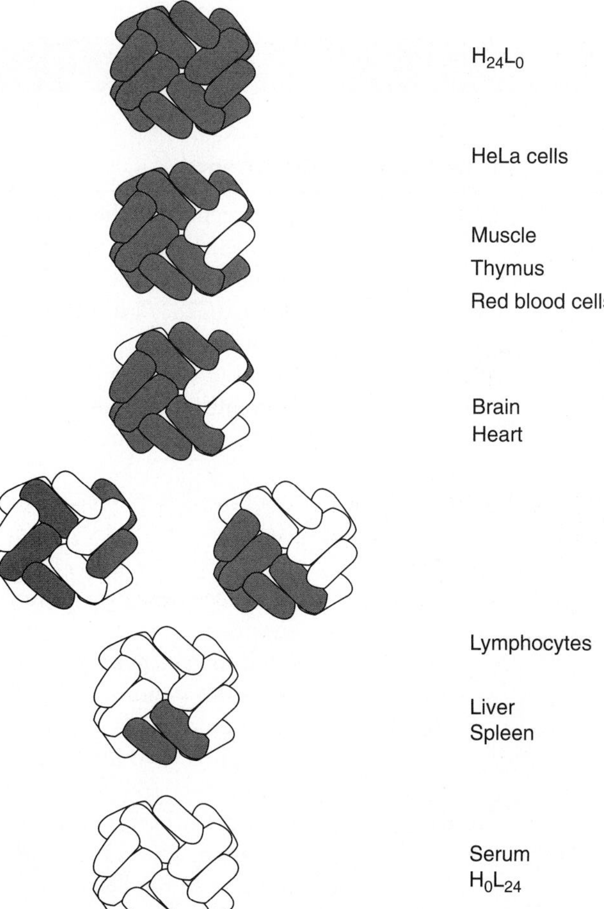

Figure 31-18 Schematic representation of the subunit structure of ferritins from various tissues. *(From Harrison PM, Arosio P. The ferritins: molecular properties, iron storage function and cellular regulation. Biochim Biophys Acta 1996;1275:161-203.)*

Tissue Iron

Numerous cellular enzymes and coenzymes require iron, either as an integral part of the molecule or as a cofactor. Notable are the *peroxidases* and *cytochromes,* all of which, like Hb, are heme proteins. Other enzymes, such as *aconitase* and *ferredoxin,* have iron that is coordinated with sulfur in a so-called iron-sulfur cluster. Nearly half of the enzymes of the *Krebs cycle* contain iron. These enzymes and coenzymes, which appear in all nucleated cells of the body, are referred to collectively as the *tissue iron compartment.* The tissue iron compartment normally amounts to approximately 8 mg. Although a small compartment, it is metabolically critical. Some iron enzyme activities diminish early in the course of iron deficiency.[58]

Myoglobin

Myoglobin very closely resembles a single Hb subunit. Because myoglobin does not form tetramers, it lacks the allosteric properties of Hb.

Labile Pool

Approximately 80 mg of iron is found in the labile pool. This compartment has no clear anatomical location; rather it is a concept derived from kinetic measurements with radiolabeled iron.[94]

Transport

Iron is transported from one organ to another by a plasma iron transport protein, *apotransferrin.* This β_1-globulin with a molecular weight of 75,000 Da has two iron binding sites per molecule. Each of these sites may bind one Fe^{3+} ion together with one ion of HCO_3^-. The apotransferrin-Fe^{3+} complex is called *transferrin.* Normally, there is a total of approximately 2.5 mg of iron in plasma. Particularly under abnormal conditions, such as in patients with thalassemia, a small amount of iron that is not bound to apotransferrin is found in the plasma.[28,80] When transferrin binds to the *transferrin receptor* of cells the transferrin-receptor complex is internalized into a vacuole that becomes acidified, releasing the iron from transferrin. The apotransferrin is then transported back to the cell surface, ready to transport another transferrin molecule to the interior of the cell. This series of reactions has been designated *the transferrin cycle.* The transferrin receptor forms a complex with the HFE protein, producing minor kinetic changes in transferrin binding.[106,134] The significance of this association in the regulation of iron homeostasis is not fully understood.

Regulation of Iron Homeostasis

The amount of iron loss from the body depends only minimally upon the iron burden; regulation of body iron content is therefore achieved almost entirely by modulating the amount of iron absorbed from the upper intestinal tract.

Normal Iron Balance

The average American diet provides 10 to 15 mg of iron daily, mostly in the form of the heme proteins, Hb, and myoglobin, in meat. In the past, a significant component of iron in the diet consisted of inorganic iron leached from iron utensils. Normally, approximately 1 mg of iron is absorbed each day. Absorption occurs principally in the duodenum. Heme is absorbed directly as such. To be absorbed, inorganic iron must be in the ferrous state (Fe^{2+}).

Proteins That Affect Iron Homeostasis

In spite of extensive research efforts, the mechanism by which the body normally regulates its iron content remains a mystery. However, a considerable number of proteins that appear to play a role in iron homeostasis have been discovered; mutations of these proteins in humans and/or their targeted disruption or overproduction in mice can be shown to result either in iron overload or in iron deficiency. Table 31-2 summarizes the effects of some of these proteins on iron homeostasis. The exact role of each of these proteins is not fully understood, but a widely adopted schema of the participation of some of them in iron transport across the intestinal mucosal cell is illustrated in Figure 31-19.

ANALYTICAL METHODOLOGY

A number of methods are used to measure iron and related analytes. These include methods for serum iron, iron binding capacity, transferrin saturation, and serum ferritin.

Methods for Serum Iron, Iron Binding Capacity, and Transferrin Saturation[62,90,144]

Principle

With serum iron assays, iron is (1) released from transferrin by decreasing the pH of the serum, (2) reduced from Fe^{3+} to Fe^{2+}, and (3) complexed with a chromogen such as bathophenanthroline or ferrozine. Such iron-chromogen complexes have an extremely high absorbance at the appropriate wavelength, which is proportional to iron concentration.

TABLE 31-2 Proteins That Affect Iron Homeostasis and Man and Mouse

Protein	Effect of Deficiency	REFERENCES: Human Data	REFERENCES: Murine Data	Comments
HFE	Increased Fe	59	9,107,188	Most patients with hereditary hemochromatosis are homozygous for the 845 A > G (C282Y) mutation of this gene
β_2-Microglobulin	Increased Fe		49,153	Believed to function by preventing transport of *HFE* to membrane
Transferrin	Increased Fe	2,15	169	
Transferrin receptor-1	Lethal increased CNS Fe	Unknown	107	
Transferrin receptor-2	Increased Fe	33	65	
Ferroportin (SLC11A3)	Increased Fe	66,125,150		Dominant inheritance of iron overload
Hephaestin	Fe deficiency	Unknown	173	Sex-linked gene deletion is cause of *sla* mouse
Nramp1 (SLC11A1)	Alters iron distribution in macrophages	Unknown	186	Deficiency increases susceptibility to infection in mice
Nramp2 (DMT-1)	Fe deficiency	Unknown	63,64	The naturally occurring mutations found in the *mk* mouse and the Belgrade rat are the same
Ceruloplasmin	Fe increased	123	75	Brain accumulation and neurological disease
Hepcidin	Fe increased	151	122,140	

Optical characteristics of bathophenanthroline, of ferrozine, and of alternative chromogens are shown in Table 31-3. The assay may be performed manually or in an automated fashion by any of several commercially available methods.

The serum unsaturated iron binding capacity and total iron binding capacity (TIBC) are determined by addition of sufficient Fe^{3+} to saturate iron binding sites on transferrin. The excess Fe^{3+} is removed (e.g., by adsorption with light magnesium carbonate [$MgCO_3$] powder), and the assay for iron content is then repeated. From this second measurement, the TIBC is obtained. Transferrin saturation is calculated as follows:

$$\text{Transferrin saturation (\%)} = \frac{100 \times \text{serum iron}}{\text{TIBC}}$$

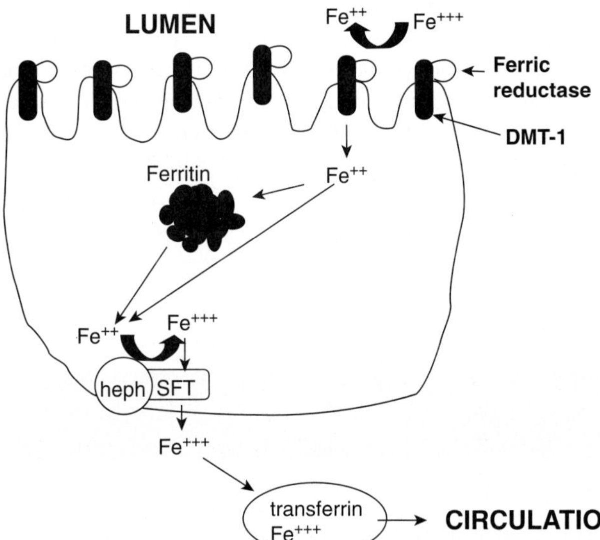

Figure 31-19 Schematic representation of some of the steps that may occur when iron is transported from the intestinal lumen to the blood. *Heph,* Hephaestin; *SFT,* stimulator of iron transport; *DMT-1,* divalent metal transporter-1.

Reference Intervals

Normal reference values differ by as much as 35% between commercial methods. Therefore a generic reference interval can no longer be stated. Many of the commercially available methods appear to underestimate the true value of serum iron concentration by 25% or more, and some appear to be unreliable at concentrations of serum iron less than 30 μg/dL (5 μmol/L). Methods that include deproteinization, either by precipitation or by dialysis, consistently appear to provide results that are substantially higher than those results obtained by methods that do not include a step of deproteinization. From a practical standpoint, if an automated commercial method is used, it is advised that a laboratory independently define its own reference intervals.

Clinical Relevance

The serum iron concentration refers to the Fe^{3+} bound to serum transferrin and does not include the iron contained in serum as free Hb. The serum iron concentration is decreased in many but not all patients with iron deficiency anemia and in chronic inflammatory disorders such as acute infection, immunization, and myocardial infarction (Table 31-4). Serum iron concentration diminishes especially in patients who are beginning to respond to specific hematinic therapy for anemias of other causes such as treatment of pernicious anemia with cyanocobalamin. Acute or recent hemorrhage, including that caused by blood donation, results in low serum iron concentration. Serum iron con-

TABLE 31-3 Characteristics of Some Chromogens Used in Iron Assays

Chromogen			
Common Name	**Chemical Name**	**Absorbance Maximum of Fe^{2+} Complex (nm)**	**Molar Absorbance of Fe^{2+} Complex**
Bathophenanthroline disulfonate, sodium	4,7-bis(4-phenyl sulfonic acid)-1,10-phenanthroline, sodium salt	534	22.14×10^3
Tripyridyl triazine	2,4,6-tripyridyl-*s*-triazine	593	22.6×10^3
Ferrozine	3-(2-pyridyl)-5,6-bis(4-phenyl sulfonic acid) 1,2,4 triazine, sodium salt	562	28.0×10^3
Terosite	2,6-bis(4-phenyl-2,2-pyridyl)-4-phenyl pyridine	583	30.2×10^3

Modified from Carter P. Spectrophotometric determination of serum iron at the submicrogram level with a new reagent (ferrozine). Anal Biochem 1971;40:450-8.

centration decreases during menstruation. Use of hormonal contraceptives raises serum iron concentration, but on cessation of contraceptive hormone intake, serum iron concentration decreases as much as 30% concurrently with uterine bleeding.

Greater than normal concentrations of serum iron occur in iron loading disorders such as hemochromatosis, in patients with aplastic anemia, in acute iron poisoning in children, and after oral ingestion of iron medication or parenteral iron administration or acute hepatitis. For example, one 0.3-g tablet of ferrous sulfate ingested by an adult may raise the serum iron concentration by 300 to 500 µg/dL (50 to 90 µmol/L).

Because normally only about one third of the iron binding sites of transferrin are occupied by Fe^{3+}, serum transferrin has considerable reserve iron binding capacity. This is called the serum unsaturated iron binding capacity. The TIBC is a measurement of the maximum concentration of iron that transferrin can bind. The serum TIBC varies in disorders of iron metabolism. It is often increased in iron deficiency and decreased in chronic inflammatory disorders or malignancies, and it is often decreased also in hemochromatosis.

Comments and Precautions

1. Except when atomic absorption spectroscopy is used, hemolysis has very little effect on the serum iron assay results because Hb iron is not released from heme by acid treatment. However, when serum specimens show marked hemolysis, a small amount of iron may be liberated from Hb. Such sera should be rejected.
2. Many factors influence serum iron concentration and TIBC. Changes that may be observed in various physiological or pathological conditions are listed in Table 31-4. Day-to-day variation is quite notable in healthy people. A distinct diurnal variation results in serum iron concentrations being lower in the afternoon than morning and quite low in the evening (as low as 10 to 20 µg/dL [2 to 4 µmol/L] in healthy people). Because of the numerous causes of low serum iron concentration, results must be interpreted with caution. Furthermore, many people with mild iron deficiency have normal values for serum iron concentration and TIBC.
3. Because of the great quantities of iron in the environment, scrupulous care is necessary to ensure that glassware, water, and reagents do not become contaminated with iron.

TABLE 31-4 Conditions Known to Affect Serum Iron Concentration, Total Iron Binding Capacity, and Transferrin Saturation

Condition	Effect
Diurnal variation	Normal values in morning; low values in midafternoon; very low values near midnight
Menstrual cycle	Premenstrually, elevated values (SI increased by 10%-30%); at menstruation, low values (SI decreased by 10%-30%)
Pregnancy	May elevate SI owing to increased progesterone; may lower SI owing to iron deficiency
Ingestion of iron (including iron-fortified vitamins)	High values; may raise SI by +54 µmol/L (+300 µg/dL) and Tsat to 100%
Oral contraceptives (progesterone-like)	High values; may raise SI to >36 µmol/L (>200 µg/dL) and Tsat to 75%; also elevates TIBC
Iron contamination of syringe, vacutainer tube, or other glassware (phenomenon may be rare, sporadic, very difficult to prove)	High values; e.g., SI >30 µmol/L (>170 µg/dL); Tsat of 75%-100%
Iron dextran injection	Very high values; SI may be >180 µmol/L (>1000 µg/dL), Tsat 100%, probably from circulating iron dextran; effect may persist for several weeks
Hepatitis	Very high values; SI may be >180 µmol/L (>1000 µg/dL) owing to hyperferritinemia from hepatocyte injury
Acute inflammation (respiratory infection), abscess, immunization, myocardial infarction	Low or normal SI; normal or low Tsat
Chronic inflammation or malignancy	Low or normal SI; normal or low Tsat
Iron deficiency	Low or normal SI; low or normal Tsat; increased TIBC
Iron overload (hemochromatosis)	High SI; high Tsat; normal or low TIBC

From Fairbanks VF. Laboratory testing for iron status. Hosp Pract 1991;26:19.
SI, Serum iron concentration; *TIBC,* total iron binding capacity; *Tsat,* transferrin saturation.

4. Serum transferrin concentration may be estimated from the TIBC by the following relationship:

$$\text{Serum transferrin (g/L)} = 0.007 \times \text{TIBC } (\mu g/dL)$$

The relationship is not entirely linear because a small portion of iron in serum is bound to other proteins. Therefore the calculated TIBC values are slightly higher than the amount of transferrin-bound iron. These small differences, however, are of no practical consequence. Immunoassays are available for assay of serum transferrin concentration. Results of the immunological measurement of transferrin concentration correlate with those of the TIBC assay. A slight advantage for the immunoassay of transferrin is that the required volume per specimen is much smaller.

Methods for Serum Ferritin

Principle

Serum ferritin assay may be performed by any of several methods, including immunoradiometric assay, ELISA, and immunochemiluminescent and immunofluorometric methods. Reagents for this assay are available in kit form and in automated immunoassay instruments from several manufacturers. The manufacturers' instructions should be followed.

Reference Intervals

Reference intervals for serum ferritin levels are summarized in Table 31-5. However, considerable variation in reference values has been observed with different methods for serum ferritin assay. Consequently, reference intervals must be determined for each laboratory.

Clinical Relevance

Ferritin is present in the blood in very low concentration. Although it is an acute phase protein, under normal conditions it roughly reflects the body iron content. The circulating protein is iron poor and largely consists of iron-poor, glycosylated L chains; it is largely apoferritin. The plasma ferritin concentration declines very early in the development of iron deficiency, long before changes are observed in blood Hb concentration, RBC size, or serum iron concentration. Thus measurement of serum ferritin concentration can serve as a very sensitive indicator of iron deficiency that is uncomplicated by other concurrent disease. Alternatively a large number of chronic diseases result in increased serum ferritin concentration.[142] These diseases include chronic infections; chronic inflammatory disorders, such as rheumatoid arthritis or renal disease; heart disease; and numerous malignancies, especially lymphomas, leukemias, breast cancer, and neuroblastoma. In patients who have any of these chronic disorders together with iron deficiency, serum ferritin concentration is often normal. An increase in plasma ferritin concentration occurs in viral hepatitis or after toxic liver injury as a result of release of ferritin from damaged liver cells. Plasma ferritin concentration is also increased in patients with iron storage disease and is used to gauge the effectiveness of phlebotomy therapy. However, as a screening test for detection of early iron overload, measurement of serum ferritin concentration appears to be less sensitive than measurement of serum iron concentration, TIBC, and percent transferrin saturation.

Comments and Precautions

1. Replicate same-day assays on the same specimen should have a coefficient of variation (CV) of ± 4% for ferritin concentrations of 100 to 300 μg/L and ±10% for ferritin concentrations of 10 to 20 μg/L.
2. Because precision decreases at very high serum ferritin concentration, all specimens with results exceeding 80 μg/L should be diluted with diluting sera to the 200- to 400-μg/L range and repeated. Any specimen with greater than a 7% difference between duplicate assay results should be reassayed.
3. A high-dose hook effect that is similar to a prozone phenomenon formerly complicated interpretation of serum ferritin assays; specimens with actual ferritin concentration exceeding 1000 μg/L could exhibit count rates that would be obtained at normal serum ferritin concentration. Fortunately, currently available reagents no longer result in the hook effect when serum ferritin concentration is high.

TABLE 31-5 Reference Intervals for Serum Ferritin

	ng/mL	μg/L
Newborn	25-200	25-200
1 mo	200-600	200-600
2-5 mo	50-200	50-200
6 mo-15 yr	7-140	7-140
Adult man	20-250	20-250
Adult woman	20-200	20-200
Iron overload[182]		
Adult male	>400	>400
Adult female	>200	>200

From Tietz NW, (ed). Clinical guide to laboratory tests, 3rd ed. Philadelphia: WB Saunders Co, 1995.

Method for Red Cell Volume and Hemoglobin Content

MCV and MCHC are the red cell indices used to characterize the blood of patients with anemia (see Chapter 11). Laser light scattering is used to measure the hemoglobin content and concentration of individual red cells.[120] This is an early indicator of iron deficiency. Its usefulness is limited in patients with MCV values of >100 fL, but in others it compares favorably with other measurements of iron status.[42,54,114,164]

Method for Serum Transferrin Receptor

The cell membranes of the developing RBC precursors in bone marrow are very rich in transferrin receptors, to which the iron-transferrin complex binds before it is internalized and the iron is released from transferrin in the cytosol. The number of transferrin receptors increases in the presence of iron deficiency and decreases in iron excess. These variations in the quantity of transferrin receptors in erythropoietic tissue are also reflected in changes in serum transferrin receptor, but to a large extent the serum transferrin receptor levels reflect the amount of erythropoietic activity, regardless of the iron status of the patient.

CLINICAL SIGNIFICANCE

Iron deficiency and iron overload are the major disorders of iron metabolism. There are, in addition, many diseases in which abnormal distribution of iron may play primary or secondary roles. Included are such disorders as hyperferritinemia with cataracts,[148] aceruloplasminemia, GRACILE syndrome,[58,60,148] neuroferritinopathy,[46] atransferrinemia, and possibly neurodegenerative disease such as Parkinsonism, Hallervorden-Spatz syndrome, and Alzheimer's disease.[160] These latter disorders will not be discussed further here.

Iron Deficiency

Iron deficiency is one of the most prevalent disorders of humans.[39] It is particularly a disease of children, of young women, and of older people, but it occurs in people of all ages and all social strata. In children it is frequently caused by dietary deficiency, because milk has a low iron content. In adults it is almost always the result of chronic blood loss or childbearing.[58]

Many different measurements have been advocated for the diagnosis of iron deficiency. Originally, emphasis was placed upon the red cell indices; hypochromic anemia was generally considered a synonym for iron deficiency in the first half of the twentieth century. Subsequently the staining of the marrow for iron measurement of the serum iron and the iron binding capacity, serum ferritin, and erythrocyte protoporphyrin became practical, and were used and studied extensively for their ability to diagnose iron deficiency. Circulating transferrin receptor and reticulocyte Hb levels also have been found to have diagnostic value. Of all of these tests, the marrow iron is probably the most reliable but the least practical for any but patients with complex diagnostic problems. However, even it can be misleading (1) when the sample size or observer skill is insufficient,[5] (2) in patients who have been treated with iron by the parenteral route, (3) where stainable iron may be present in the face of deficiency,[128] and (4) in patients with myeloproliferative disease.[40,161]

Although most methods very readily identify severe, uncomplicated iron deficiency, the large number of tests that have been advocated for the diagnosis of iron deficiency is a reflection of the fact that none by itself is sufficient to detect mild iron deficiency or iron deficiency in a clinically complex setting. Receiver operator characteristic curves (ROC) confirm that no one method is superior, and that different studies differ in the conclusions that they draw regarding advantages of one method over another.[61,114,167,172]

Iron Overload

Hemosiderosis, hemochromatosis, and some anemias are conditions associated with iron overload and iron storage diseases.

Hemosiderosis

Hemosiderosis is a term used to imply iron overload without associated tissue injury. It occurs locally in sites of bleeding or inflammation, and may be widespread in persons who have been given large amounts of iron, either as iron medication or as blood transfusions.

Hemochromatosis

Hemochromatosis is a condition in which the body accumulates excess amounts of iron; it is one of the most common genetic diseases in humans. The symptoms of hemochromatosis include the "classic triad" of bronzing of the skin, cirrhosis, and diabetes. Other manifestations include cardiomyopathies and arrhythmias, endocrine deficiencies, and possibly arthropathies.

Secondary hemochromatosis is the consequence of the increased administration and absorption of iron. The administration of iron includes that given with the transfusions that are required in certain anemic patients and the ill-advised and unfortunate administration of iron to anemic patients who are not actually iron deficient. The most common causes of secondary hemochromatosis are thalassemia major and acquired myelodysplastic states, but there are many other circumstances in which secondary iron overload occurs, including pyruvate kinase deficiency and congenital dyserythropoietic anemias.

Hereditary hemochromatosis is the most common hereditary form of hemochromatosis. It results from hereditary abnormalities of proteins that regulate iron hemostasis. In recent years, the genetic lesions responsible for many forms of the disease have been discovered. It is an adult onset disorder, formerly called *primary hemochromatosis* or *idiopathic hemochromatosis,* which is linked to the HLA loci on chromosome 6.

Other forms of hemochromatosis include a severe, early onset form, designated *juvenile hemochromatosis,* and an iron storage disease in which storage takes place largely in macrophages, *African iron overload* and *ferroportin deficiency.* An effort has been made recently to classify hereditary forms of hemochromatosis as types 1 through 5, but this does not serve to clarify our understanding of the disorders and inaccurately groups iron storage disease with different etiologies into the same "type." This classification will therefore not be employed here.

Hereditary Hemochromatosis. Hereditary hemochromatosis is the classical disorder of iron overload.[32] It is due to an inborn error of iron absorption; the precise mechanism remains unknown. Approximately 80% of whites of Northern European origin are homozygotes for a common mutation of the *HFE* gene. This mutation (845 G > A; C282Y) is a common polymorphism in Northern Europe.

Some 10% to 15% of Northern Europeans are heterozygous for this mutation and therefore about 5/1000 are homozygotes. Although it has been shown to associate with the transferrin receptor, the mechanisms by which it causes increased iron absorption are not understood. The biochemical penetrance of the homozygous state for the major (C282Y) mutation is fairly high; more than 50% of such individuals have elevated transferrin saturations and/or ferritin levels[12,13] and about 10% have elevated serum glutamic oxaloacetic transaminases levels. Although some investigators have maintained that many or most homozygotes are seriously affected[32,129] numerous recent studies show that the clinical penetrance of the homozygous state is very low, probably of the order of 1%,[3,13,92,139] and there is no significant effect on lifespan.[174] Rarely, hereditary hemochromatosis results from mutations in the transferrin receptor-2 gene.[149] This type of hemochromatosis is indistinguishable from classical hereditary hemochromatosis caused by a mutation in the *HFE* gene.

Juvenile Hemochromatosis. Juvenile hemochromatosis is a rare disorder that resembles hereditary hemochromatosis clinically, but that has a much earlier average age of onset and a greater tendency to develop endocrine and cardiac manifestations than does hereditary hemochromatosis. It too is inherited, although the mutation is not in the *HFE* gene, but rather in an as-yet-unidentified gene on chromosome 1q[152] or in hepcidin.[151]

A dominantly inherited form of iron storage disease results from mutations in ferroportin (SLC11A3).[37,50,124,125] Here iron storage occurs primarily in macrophages, not in liver parenchyma. Iron accumulation appears to be more common in Africans than Europeans, and although diet may play a major role, it is thought that there is also a genetic predisposition that may account for the increased iron burden.[71]

Anemias With Iron Storage

The most common cause of iron overload is thalassemia, particularly in the parts of the world where it is prevalent (see earlier section). Indeed, the cardiac complications of iron overload are among the most common causes of death in β-thalassemia major. *Sideroblastic anemias* are a group of iron-loading disorders, many of which are of unknown cause. In a hereditary type of this disorder, there is deficiency of erythroid specific 5-aminolevulinic acid synthetase in RBC precursors because of mutations involving the X-linked gene that encodes this enzyme.[38] Iron storage is common in patients with congenital dyserythropoietic anemia[11,158] and may be found in patients with red cell enzyme deficiencies, particularly pyruvate kinase deficiency.[48]

BILIRUBIN

Bilirubin is the orange-yellow pigment derived from senescent red blood cells. It is extracted and biotransformed mainly in the liver, and excreted in bile and urine. The chemistry, biochemistry, and analytical methodology for bilirubin and related compounds are reviewed in this section.

Chemistry

Bilirubin was discovered by Virchow in 1849 in blood extravasates; he called the yellow pigment "hematoidin." The term "bilirubin" was coined by Stadeler in 1864, and in 1874 Tarchanoff demonstrated the direct association of bile pigments to Hb. In 1942 Fisher and Plieninger synthesized bilirubin IXα and proposed the structure shown in the upper portion of Figure 31-20. This linear tetrapyrrolic structure of the bilirubin molecule was accepted for more than 30 years. However, an important and puzzling chemical property of the bilirubin molecule is its insolubility in water and its solubility in a variety of nonpolar solvents. The solubility of bilirubin in nonpolar, lipid solvents is not predicted from this linear tetrapyrrole structure, because the two propionic acid side chains would be expected to make the bilirubin molecule highly polar and therefore water soluble.

The overall chemical structure of bilirubin was established by x-ray crystallography.[24] According to this work, bilirubin assumes a ridge-tiled configuration stabilized by six intramolecular hydrogen bonds. Two additional important structural features have also been noted: (1) a so-called Z-Z *(trans)* conformation for the double bonds between carbons 4 and 5 and 15 and 16, and (2) an involuted hydrogen-bonded structure in which the propionic acid–carboxylic acid groups are hydrogen bonded to the nitrogen atoms of the pyrrole rings (Figure 31-20, bottom). These bonds sta-

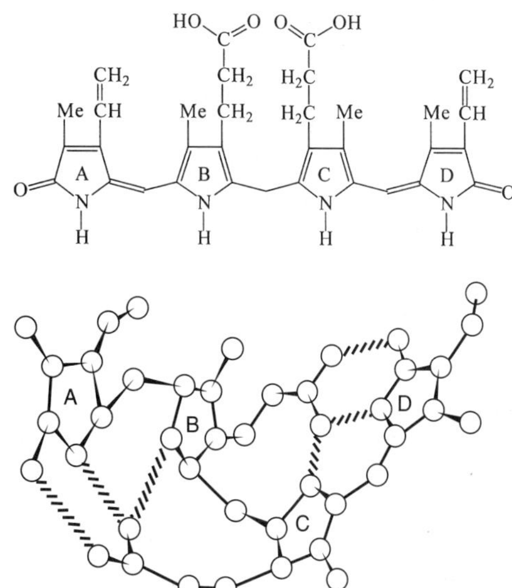

Figure 31-20 Bilirubin IXα structure. *Top,* The unfolded or linear tetrapyrrole structure showing the Z bonds. *Bottom,* The folded conformation showing extensive internal hydrogen bonding. *(Reprinted by permission of Elsevier Science Publishing Co., Inc., from Schmid, R. Bilirubin metabolism: State of the art. Gastroenterology 1978;74:1307-12, with permission from the American Gastroenterological Association.)*

bilize the Z-Z configuration of bilirubin and prevent its interaction with polar groups in aqueous media. When exposed to light, the Z-Z configuration is converted to the E-E *(cis)* conformation and to other combinations, namely 4E-15Z and 4Z-15E. The E-E conformation and other E-containing isomers do not permit the degree of internal hydrogen bonding that occurs in the Z-Z conformation and are therefore more water soluble than in the Z-Z conformation. Thus light-exposed forms of bilirubin are more water soluble and readily excreted in the bile. This is the rationale for irradiating jaundiced newborns with 450 nm light.[117]

The bilirubin molecule in the crystalline state takes, as mentioned above, the form of a ridge tile rather than a linear tetrapyrrole, with the ridge being along the line C8-C10-C12. In this configuration, rings A and B lie in one plane and rings C and D in another, with a 98° angle between the two rings. The preferred conformation of bilirubin in aqueous solution at pH 7.4 is not known, but the occurrence of a hydrogen-bonded structure in aqueous solution would explain some of the unique chemical properties of bilirubin IXα. For example, the addition of hydrogen bond–breaking chemicals—such as caffeine, methanol, ethanol, urea, or surface active agents—is required for unconjugated bilirubin to react with diazo reagent. These reagents likely act by breaking internal hydrogen bonds of the bilirubin molecule, allowing it to react with diazotized sulfanilic acid or other diazo compounds. In contrast, bilirubin IXα monoglucuronide and diglucuronide are quite soluble in water and react readily with diazo reagents. The bulky glucuronic acid moiety precludes conjugated bilirubin from undergoing internal hydrogen bond formation. Bilirubin glucuronides, being water soluble, are readily excreted in the bile and urine, whereas unconjugated bilirubin is not.

Bilirubin deriving from natural sources consists almost entirely (99%) of the IXα. Bilirubins IXβ and IXδ, arising from the cleavage of the β- and δ-methene bridges, consist of less than 0.5% of bilirubin isolated from bile. However, bilirubin reference materials available from commercial sources, and from the National Institute of Standards and Technology (Standard Reference Material 916a) contain variable amounts of IIIα and XIIIα isomers.[115] The two isomers are formed by cleavage of bilirubin IXα at the central methylene bridge; subsequent recombination of the two different dipyrrole units gives a mixture of the three isomers. This isomerization of bilirubin occurs in aqueous solution at acidic or neutral pH, but not when bilirubin is bound to albumin.[116]

BIOCHEMISTRY

Bilirubin IXα is produced from the catabolism of protoporphyrin IX by a microsomal heme oxygenase. The tetrapyrrolic product of the ring opening at the α-methene bridge is the green pigment biliverdin, which is subsequently reduced to bilirubin by the reduced form of nicotinamide adenine dinucleotide phosphate (NADPH)–dependent, cytosolic enzyme biliverdin reductase (Figure 31-21). For each mole of heme catabolized by this pathway, one mole each of carbon monoxide, bilirubin, and ferric iron is produced. Daily bilirubin production from all sources in man averages from 250 to 300 mg. Approximately 85% of the total bilirubin produced is derived from the heme moiety of Hb released from senescent erythrocytes that are destroyed in the reticuloendothelial cells of the liver, spleen, and bone marrow. The remaining 15% is produced from RBC precursors destroyed in the bone marrow (so-called ineffective erythropoiesis) and from the catabolism of other heme-containing proteins, such as myoglobin, cytochromes, and peroxidases.

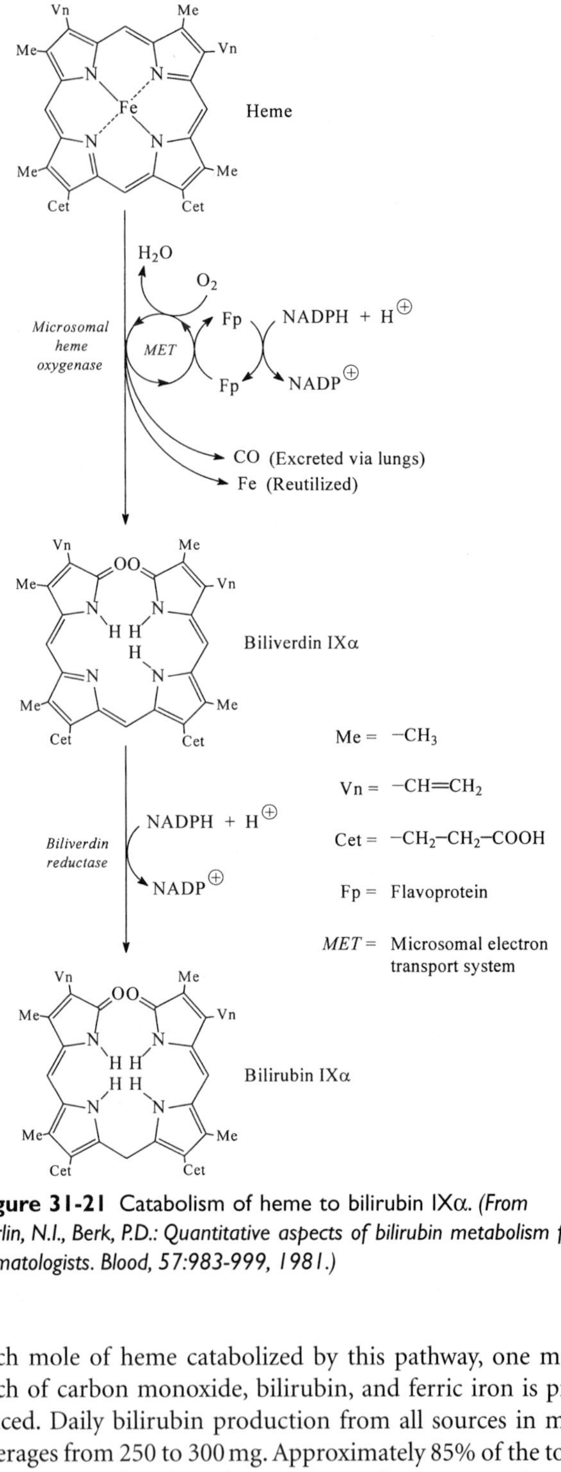

Figure 31-21 Catabolism of heme to bilirubin IXα. *(From Berlin, N.I., Berk, P.D.: Quantitative aspects of bilirubin metabolism for hematologists. Blood, 57:983-999, 1981.)*

In blood, bilirubin is bound to albumin ($K_d \sim 10^{-8}$ mol/L) and transported to the liver. Bilirubin then dissociates from

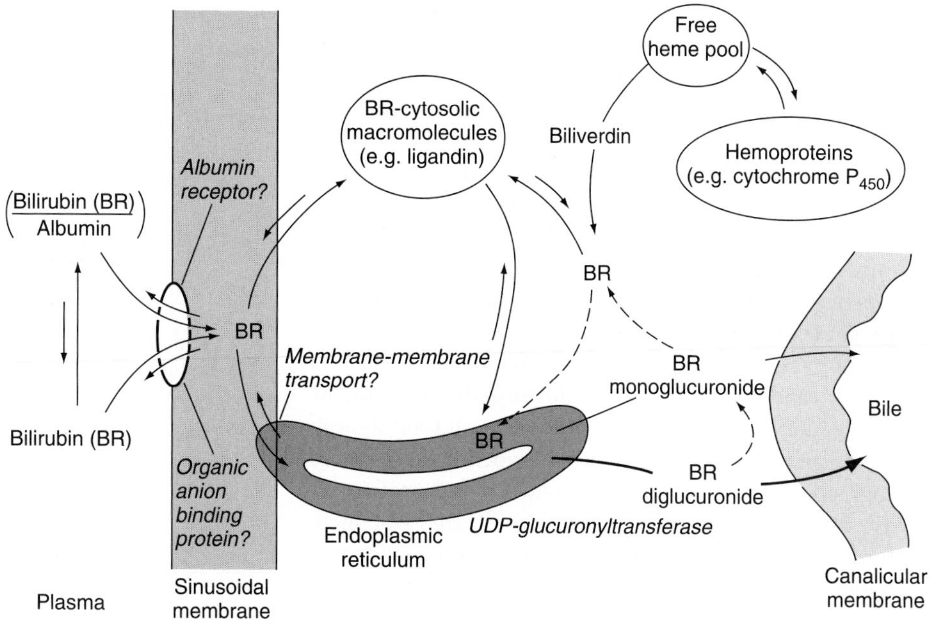

Figure 31-22 Bilirubin uptake, metabolism, and transport in the hepatocyte. *(From Gollan JL, Schmid R. In Popper H, Schaffner F, Eds. Progress in liver diseases, Vol. 7, Chapter 15. Philadelphia: WB Saunders Company, 1982.)*

albumin by an unknown process at the sinusoidal membrane of the hepatocyte. It is then transported across the membrane (Figure 31-22). Once inside the liver cells, bilirubin is reversibly bound to soluble proteins known as ligandins or protein Y. Ligandins are cytosolic proteins of the glutathione-S-transferase gene family and constitute ~5% of the total protein of human liver cytosol. Ligandin also binds a variety of other compounds, such as steroids, bromsulfthalein (BSP), indocyanine green, and some carcinogens. Ligandin likely plays an important role in the processing of these compounds; it may increase the net efficiency of uptake by retarding the reflux of these substances back to plasma.

Inside the hepatocytes, bilirubin is rapidly conjugated with glucuronic acid to produce bilirubin monoglucuronide and diglucuronide, which are then excreted into bile (see Figure 33-22). The microsomal enzyme bilirubin uridine diphosphate (UDP)–glucuronyltransferase (EC 2.4.1.17) catalyzes the formation of bilirubin monoglucuronide. It is not certain whether the conversion of the monoglucuronide to the diglucuronide is catalyzed by the same enzyme or by another enzyme located in or near the canaliculus. The excretion of conjugated bilirubin into bile against a marked concentration gradient is thought to be an energy-dependent, active-transport process.

In adults, virtually all bilirubin excreted in bile is in the form of glycosidic conjugates; glucuronides account for ~95% of them and glucosides and xylosides constitute the remainder. Of the glucuronides, diglucuronide is the major fraction (~90%) and monoglucuronide the minor fraction (~10%).

Bilirubin glucuronides are not substantially reabsorbed in the intestine. Rather, they are hydrolyzed by the catalytic action of β-glucuronidase from the liver, intestinal epithelial cells, and bacteria. This unconjugated bilirubin is then reduced by anaerobic intestinal microbial flora to form a group of three colorless tetrapyrroles collectively called *urobilinogens.* In each of these three bilirubin reduction products, all bridge carbons are in the saturated (methylene) form. The urobilinogens differ from one another in the degree of hydrogenation of the vinyl side chains and in the two end pyrrole rings; urobilinogens contain 6, 8, or 12 more hydrogen atoms than does bilirubin and are named *stercobilinogen, mesobilinogen,* and *urobilinogen,* respectively. Up to 20% of the urobilinogen produced daily is reabsorbed from the intestine and enters the enterohepatic circulation. Most of the reabsorbed urobilinogen is taken up by the liver and is reexcreted in the bile; a small fraction (2% to 5%) enters the general circulation and appears in urine. In the lower intestinal tract, the three urobilinogens spontaneously oxidize at the middle methylene bridge to produce the corresponding bile pigments stercobilin, mesobilin, and urobilin, which are orange-brown and the major pigments of stool. Approximately 50% of the conjugated bilirubin excreted in bile is metabolized to products other than the urobilinogens. The detailed structure of these metabolites has not been characterized.

Analytical Methodology

Several analytical techniques are used to measure bilirubin and metabolites in serum, urine, and feces.*

Serum Bilirubin

The reaction of bilirubin with diazotized sulfanilic acid, known as the diazo reaction, discovered by Ehrlich in 1883

*Methodologal details for methods discussed in this section are included in this book's accompanying Evolve site, found at http:/evolve.elsevier.com/Tietz/textbook/.

and applied to the measurement of bilirubin in serum and bile by van den Bergh and Muller in 1916, is the basis of the most widely used methods for measuring bilirubin. The observation that in sera from jaundiced infants the reaction was slow and required an accelerator to proceed and it was fast in bile and in adult sera without addition of ethanol led to the terms "direct" and "indirect" bilirubin. The chemical nature of direct and indirect bilirubins was elucidated by Billing, Cole, and Lathe in the mid-1950s.[18] They isolated by an open column reversed phase chromatography on siliconized kieselguhr (cellite or diatomaceous earth) three bilirubin fractions, unconjugated bilirubin (indirect reacting fraction), and bilirubin monoglucuronide and diglucuronide (direct reacting fractions). Kuenzle and colleagues[97] were the first to successfully use an open-column chromatography technique that did not involve a deproteinization step. Four bilirubin fractions were obtained: unconjugated bilirubin (α-bilirubin), monoconjugated bilirubin (β-bilirubin), diconjugated bilirubin (γ-bilirubin), and a fraction bound strongly to protein (δ-bilirubin). The last fraction was clearly distinct from the albumin-bilirubin complex that exists in serum.

Diazo Methods

The most widely used chemical methods for bilirubin measurement are those based on the diazo reaction.[108a] In this reaction, diazotized sulfanilic acid (the diazo reagent) reacts with bilirubin to produce two azodipyrroles (azopigments) (Figure 31-23), which are reddish purple at neutral pH and blue at low or high pH values. Van den Bergh and Muller[171] applied this reaction to the quantitation of bilirubin in serum. They described the fraction of bilirubin that reacted with the diazo reagent in the absence of alcohol as the direct bilirubin fraction and used the term indirect bilirubin for the difference between total bilirubin (found after the addition of alcohol to the reaction mixture) and the direct bilirubin fraction. Numerous variations of the van den Bergh method have been developed. All use one of a variety of "accelerators," which like alcohol, facilitate the reaction of unconjugated (indirect) bilirubin with the diazo reagent; the most commonly used accelerators are caffeine,[93] dyphylline,[118] and a number of surface active agents. The diazo method of Malloy and Evelyn,[112] which uses methanol as an accelerator, has substantial matrix effects, negative interference by Hb, turbidity due to protein precipitation by methanol, and a relatively long reaction time.[52] This method, which has been virtually abandoned, is mentioned here for historical reasons only.

The diazo method described by Jendrassik and Grof in 1938[93] and later modified by Doumas and colleagues[137] gives results for serum total bilirubin that are reproducible and reliable. In this procedure, an aqueous solution of caffeine and sodium benzoate serves as the accelerator. Studies on the mechanism by which the caffeine-benzoate solution facilitates the reaction of unconjugated bilirubin with the diazo reagent have provided strong, albeit indirect, evidence that

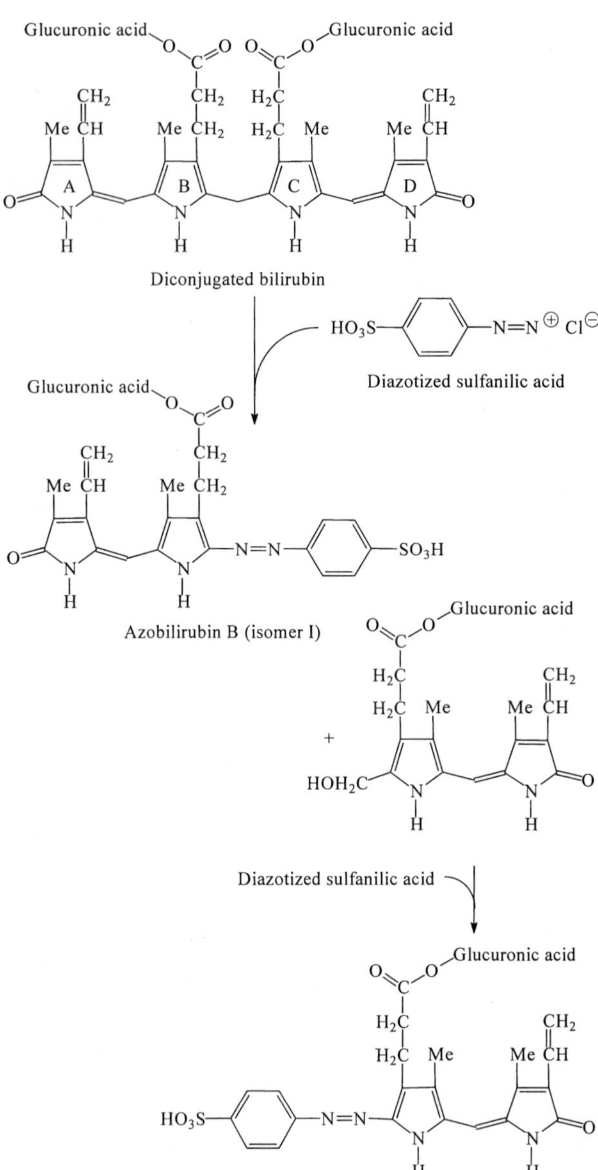

Figure 31-23 The reaction of bilirubin glucuronide with diazotized sulfanilic acid to produce isomers I and II of azobilirubin B. Unconjugated bilirubin reacts in the same way to produce isomers I and II of azobilirubin A.

caffeine, and perhaps benzoate, displaces unconjugated bilirubin from its association sites on albumin. This occurs by (1) formation of hydrogen bonds between bilirubin and caffeine,[67,101] thus making bilirubin water soluble, or (2) complex formation and disruption of the bilirubin internal hydrogen bonds. By use of samples prepared by addition of unconjugated bilirubin and authentic human diconjugated bilirubin to low-bilirubin pooled sera—and a nuclear magnetic resonance technique—Lo and Wu[108] have shown that the modified Jendrassik-Grof total bilirubin assay detects unconjugated and diconjugated bilirubin quantitatively (as unconjugated bilirubin equivalents). This method has acceptable transferability among laboratories and is currently the method of choice.

Other methods for determining bilirubin include direct spectrophotometric measurement of total bilirubin in serum using analysis of a two-component system (i.e., measuring absorbance at two wavelengths and solving a system of two simultaneous equations). This approach is applicable to sera from healthy neonates because only unconjugated bilirubin is present in such sera. Correction for oxyhemoglobin is necessary, because it is invariably present in sera from neonates (For further details see Analytical Methods in this book's accompanying Evolve site, found at http:/evolve.elsevier.com/Tietz/textbook/.

High-Performance Liquid Chromatography

HPLC methods have also been developed that allow for relatively rapid separation and quantification of the four bilirubin fractions. HPLC has been helpful in detecting and separating the various bilirubin photoisomers produced during phototherapy in newborns and thus in elucidating the mechanism by which phototherapy lowers the concentration of bilirubin in the newborn blood.[117] There are several versions of HPLC for analysis of bilirubin fractions. In the method of Blanckaert,[22] bilirubin conjugates, but not unconjugated bilirubin, are converted to the corresponding bilirubin methyl esters by base-catalyzed transesterification in methanol followed by extraction with chloroform. With this procedure, the α-, β-, and γ-bilirubin fractions are recoverable, but the δ-fraction (delta-bilirubin) remains in the denatured protein pellet that is produced by the chloroform extraction. In the HPLC method of Lauff and coworkers,[103] all four bilirubin fractions remain in solution after a step that involves salting out globulins with sodium sulfate. Both methods require the use of dim incandescent or yellow light to minimize photodegradation of the various bilirubin species. A simple and fast HPLC method has been published by Adachi et al[1]; the method uses a Micronex RP-30 column, which does not require salting out of globulins or chemical transformation of the bilirubin conjugates. This method separates serum bilirubin into five fractions; the fifth fraction eluted between the monoglucuronide and the unconjugated bilirubin is the Z,E or the E,Z photoisomer. The elution sequence is the same as in the procedure of Lauff.[103]

Additional studies indicated that the δ-bilirubin fraction consists of one or more bilirubin species that are covalently bound to albumin.[104] Existence of covalent linkage is supported by the fact that the associated bilirubin species are not released from the albumin fraction by treatment with strong acid or base or a variety of strong denaturing agents, by hydrolysis with proteolytic enzymes, or by boiling in methanol. The δ-bilirubin reacts directly with diazotized sulfanilic acid. The discovery of δ-bilirubin has solved the mystery of the persisting high bilirubin concentrations, mostly direct reacting, in patients with intrahepatic or obstructing jaundice long after hepatitis has subsided or obstruction has been relieved. It is the slowest fraction to clear from serum because it follows the catabolism of albumin, which has a half-life of approximately 19 days.

From HPLC analyses of a large number of sera from patients with various liver disorders, Wu and colleagues[185] found the following proportions of the four bilirubin fractions in cholestatic sera: 27% (8% to 55%) unconjugated bilirubin, 24% (8% to 37%) monoconjugated bilirubin, 13% (7% to 21%) diconjugated bilirubin, and 37% (1% to 77%) δ-bilirubin.

HPLC has been very helpful in elucidating the nature of the bilirubin species occurring naturally in blood or formed during phototherapy. Clinically, it offers little, if any, aid to the physician in the differential diagnosis of jaundice, because knowing the percentage of each of the bilirubin fractions in blood is of no diagnostic value. It cannot be considered as a reference method for measuring total bilirubin in blood, because its accuracy and precision are inadequate. The method is calibrated with unconjugated bilirubin with the untested assumption that the other three bilirubin fractions have molar absorptivities identical to that of the calibrator,[102] when in fact this is not known. Furthermore, errors in the measurement of the four species may be cumulative and may result in a large total error, and the method is insensitive at total bilirubin concentrations below 1 mg/dL (17 μmol/L) and too laborious for routine clinical analysis. Some of the δ-bilirubin may be lost during pretreatment of samples.

A capillary electrophoresis method for measuring the different types of bilirubin has been developed by Wu and his associates.[184]

Enzymatic Methods

Enzymatic methods for total and direct bilirubin and for bilirubin conjugates with glucuronic acid are based on the oxidation of bilirubin with bilirubin oxidase to biliverdin with molecular oxygen.[121] Near pH 8 and in the presence of sodium cholate and sodium dodecylsulfate, all four bilirubin fractions are oxidized to biliverdin, which is further oxidized to purple and finally colorless products. The decrease in absorbance, at 425 or 460 nm, is proportional to the concentration of total bilirubin. Results by the bilirubin oxidase method were in good agreement with those obtained by the Jendrassik-Grof procedure.[136] Direct bilirubin is measured at pH 3.7 to 4.5; at this pH range, the enzyme oxidizes bilirubin conjugates and δ-bilirubin, but not unconjugated bilirubin.[51,96] At pH 10 the enzyme oxidizes selectively the two glucuronides.[53,96] δ-bilirubin is not oxidized at all, and only 5% of the unconjugated bilirubin is measured as conjugates.[53]

Transcutaneous Measurement of Bilirubin

This noninvasive approach for measuring bilirubin was introduced by Yamanouchi et al.[187] The first bilirubinometer (icterometer) was a reflectance photometer, which used two filters to correct for the color of Hb and required measurements at eight body sites. Efforts to improve the accuracy of such measurements have been successful and led to the development of devices of acceptable performance. Recent reports indicate that at least one of these devices (Bili*Check* ($SpectR_x$ Inc., Norcross, Ga.) provides results that are within ±2 mg/dL of those obtained by a diazo procedure.[16,147] Another study found that the Bili*Check* underestimated serum bilirubin when its concentration was >10 mg/dL (170 µmol/L).[55]

Although transcutaneous bilirubin measurements may not substitute for laboratory quantitative determinations, they provide instantaneous information, reduce the necessity for serum bilirubin determinations, spare infants the trauma of heel sticks, and save money.[111] Furthermore, they are useful in determining whether in a jaundiced infant it is necessary to draw blood to guide treatment, such as phototherapy or exchange transfusion. Another application is predicting those babies that require follow-up according to the "hour-specific" serum bilirubin nomogram by Bhutani et al.[17]

Urine Bilirubin

Because only conjugated bilirubin is excreted in urine, its presence indicates conjugated hyperbilirubinemia. The most commonly used method for detecting bilirubin in urine involves the use of a dipstick impregnated with a diazo reagent. Dipstick methods can detect bilirubin concentrations as low as 0.5 mg/dL.

A fresh urine specimen is required because bilirubin is unstable when exposed to light and room temperature, and it may be oxidized to biliverdin (which is diazo negative) at the normally acidic pH of the urine. If the test is delayed, the sample must be protected from light and stored at 2 °C to 8 °C for no longer than 24 hours. The reagent strip (Chemstrip, Roche Diagnostics; Multistix, Bayer Corp.) is immersed into the urine specimen for no longer than 1 second and is read 60 seconds later. During this time bilirubin reacts with a diazo reagent, yielding a pink to red-violet color, the intensity of which is proportional to the bilirubin concentration. The reaction mechanism for urinary conjugated bilirubin is the same as that described in Figure 31-23 except that 2,6-dichlorobenzene-diazonium-tetrafluoroborate is substituted for diazotized sulfanilic acid in the Chemstrip, and 2,4-dichloroaniline diazonium salt in the Multistix. Another commonly used test, more sensitive than the Multistix, is the Ictotest reagent tablet (Bayer Corporation); in this semiquantitative procedure the diazo reagent is *p*-nitrobenzenediazonium-*p*-toluenesulfonate.

The Chemstrip and Multistix strips for bilirubin in urine are highly specific tests and have a low incidence of false-positive results. However, medications that color the urine red or that give a red color in an acid medium, such as phenazopyridine, can produce a false-positive reading. Large quantities of ascorbic acid or of nitrite also worsen the detection limit of the test. In practice, bilirubin is rarely measured in urine.

Urobilinogen in Urine and Feces

An increase in urobilinogen in the urine occurs whenever hepatocellular function is decreased or there is an excess of urobilinogen in the gastrointestinal (GI) tract that exceeds the liver's capacity to reexcrete it. Examples of such conditions are viral hepatitis, cirrhosis, and hemolysis. In contrast, when biliary excretion of bilirubin (e.g., cholestasis) is impaired, urinary excretion of urobilinogen decreases owing to the limited delivery of bilirubin to the gut. The clay-colored or chalky white stool of patients with cholestatic jaundice results from decreased bilirubin reaching the GI tract and the subsequent low quantities of metabolites produced. These disturbances of urobilinogen excretion are the basis for the historical use of urobilinogen analysis in urine and feces as an index of liver disease. However, urobilinogen measurement is of little help in the modern evaluation of liver disease, because it does not add to the diagnostic information obtained from the commonly performed tests described in the section on diagnostic strategy. A brief description of the measurement of urobilinogen in urine and feces can be found in the 3rd edition of this textbook on page 1137.

CLINICAL SIGNIFICANCE

Defects in bilirubin metabolism resulting in jaundice can occur at each step of the metabolic pathway (see Figure 31-22). The disorders are usually classified as (1) inherited disorders of bilirubin metabolism and (2) jaundice of the newborn. All of these disorders are characterized by predominant elevations in either conjugated or unconjugated bilirubin in the absence of other abnormal liver tests. It is only in these disorders that bilirubin fractionation is clinically useful.

Patients are occasionally seen with isolated elevations in bilirubin concentration. In most cases this is due to inherited disorders of bilirubin metabolism, familial hyperbilirubinemia, or hemolysis. It is not difficult to distinguish hemolysis severe enough to cause hyperbilirubinemia, because the patient with hemolysis will have many other disease manifestations. An algorithm for differentiating the familial causes of hyperbilirubinemia is presented in Figure 31-24. Isolated hyperbilirubinemia was discussed in a previous section on disorders of bilirubin metabolism.

Inherited Disorders of Bilirubin Metabolism

Inherited disorders of bilirubin metabolism include Gilbert's, Crigler-Najjar (Type I), Crigler-Najjar (Type II), Lucey-Driscoll, Dubin-Johnson, and Rotor's syndromes.

Gilbert Syndrome

Gilbert syndrome is a benign condition manifested by mild unconjugated hyperbilirubinemia. This abnormality, affecting 3% to 5% of the population, is clinically important, because it is often misdiagnosed as chronic hepatitis. The serum concentration of bilirubin fluctuates between 1.5 and 3 mg/dL (26 and 51 µmol/L) and tends to increase with

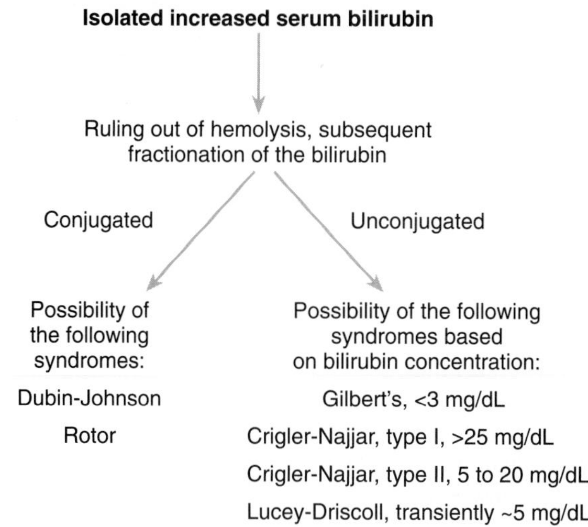

Figure 31-24 Algorithm for differentiating the familial causes of hyperbilirubinemia.

fasting. Hepatic glucuronyltransferase activity is low as a consequence of a mutation in the bilirubin-UDP-glucuronosyltransferase (*UGT1A1*) gene. In the vast majority of patients, this mutation is a repeat in the promoter, so that there are seven rather than the "normal" six ATs.[25] Occasionally, subjects with only five and as many as eight repeats are encountered; the transcription of the gene is inversely proportional to the number of repeats,[14] so that bilirubin levels tend to be higher in those patients with the largest number of repeats in the promoter. In Asia, Gilbert syndrome has sometimes been found to be caused by a single point mutation in exon 1 of the *UGT1A1* gene.[95] Gilbert syndrome is easily distinguished from chronic hepatitis by the absence of anemia and bilirubin in urine, and by normal liver function tests. The condition is probably inherited as an autosomal recessive trait. Despite the fact that total biliary bilirubin is reduced, there is an increase in the ratio of bilirubin monoglucuronide to diglucuronide, suggesting that there is also a defect in the conversion of bilirubin monoglucuronide to diglucuronide.

Patients with Gilbert syndrome may be predisposed to acetaminophen toxicity since acetaminophen is primarily metabolized by glucuronidation. The diagnosis is usually made by chance on routine medical examination or when jaundice occurs following an intercurrent infection or fasting. Special diagnostic tests are occasionally necessary and include demonstrating a rise in bilirubin on fasting and a fall in bilirubin upon taking phenobarbital. No treatment is needed, but patients must be reassured that they do not have liver disease.

Crigler-Najjar Syndrome (Type I)

Crigler-Najjar syndrome type I is a rare disorder caused by complete absence of UDP-glucuronyltransferase and manifested by very high levels of unconjugated bilirubin (25 to 50 mg/dL). It is inherited as an autosomal recessive trait. Most patients die of severe brain damage caused by kernicterus (encephalopathy related to increased bilirubin that leads to permanent brain damage) within the first year of life. Phlebotomy and plasmapheresis can reduce the serum bilirubin, but encephalopathy usually develops. Early liver transplantation is the only effective therapy.

Crigler-Najjar Syndrome (Type II)

This is a rare autosomal dominant disorder characterized by a partial deficiency of UDP-glucuronyltransferase. Unconjugated bilirubin is usually 5 to 20 mg/dL (85 to 340 μmol/L). Unlike the Crigler-Najjar syndrome type I, type II responds dramatically to phenobarbital and a normal life can be expected.

Lucey-Driscoll Syndrome

Lucey-Driscoll syndrome is a familial form of unconjugated hyperbilirubinemia caused by a circulating inhibitor of bilirubin conjugation. The hyperbilirubinemia is mild and lasts for the first 2 to 3 weeks of life.

Dubin-Johnson Syndrome

Dubin-Johnson syndrome is a benign, autosomal recessive condition characterized by jaundice with predominantly elevated conjugated bilirubin and a minor elevation of unconjugated bilirubin. Excretion of various conjugated organic anions and bilirubin, but not bile salts, into bile is impaired, reflecting the underlying defect in canalicular excretion. Intravenous cholangiography does not show the gallbladder, but a ^{99m}Tc-hepatobiliary iminodiacetic acid (HIDA) scan does. There is a derangement in the excretion of urinary coproporphyrin; the normal ratio of coproporphyrin I to III is reversed. The liver has a characteristic greenish black appearance and liver biopsy reveals a dark brown pigment in hepatocytes and Kupffer's cells that looks like lipofuscin but is probably melanin. Serum alanine aminotransferase and alkaline phosphatase are usually normal, and pruritus is absent. The condition is benign, although patients may develop jaundice during pregnancy or while taking oral contraceptives.

Rotor Syndrome

Rotor syndrome is another form of conjugated hyperbilirubinemia similar to Dubin-Johnson syndrome but without pigment in the liver. The gallbladder is seen on intravenous cholecystography. Total urinary coproporphyrins are elevated, with about two thirds being coproporphyrin I. The prognosis is excellent.

Jaundice in the Neonate

Disorders that cause jaundice in the neonate are classified as either unconjugated or conjugated hyperbilirubinemia (see Box 31-1).[121a]

Unconjugated Hyperbilirubinemia

Unconjugated hyperbilirubinemia poses a risk for development of kernicterus (acute bilirubin encephalopathy), espe-

Box 31-1 Physiological Classification of Jaundice

Unconjugated Hyperbilirubinemia

Increased Production of Unconjugated Bilirubin from Heme

- Hemolysis
  - Hereditary
  - Acquired
- Ineffective erythropoiesis
- Rapid turnover of increased RBC mass (in the neonate)

Decreased Delivery of Unconjugated Bilirubin (in Plasma) to Hepatocyte

- Right-sided congestive heart failure
- Portacaval shunt

Decreased Uptake of Unconjugated Bilirubin Across Hepatocyte Membrane

- Competitive inhibition
  - Drugs
  - Others
- Gilbert's syndrome
- Sepsis, fasting

Decreased Storage of Unconjugated Bilirubin in Cytosol (Decreased Y and Z Proteins)

- Competitive inhibition
- Fever

Decreased Biotransformation (Conjugation)

- Neonatal jaundice (physiological)
- Inhibition (drugs)
- Hereditary (Crigler-Najjar)
  - Type I (complete enzyme deficiency)
  - Type II (partial deficiency)
- Hepatocellular dysfunction
- Gilbert's syndrome

Conjugated Hyperbilirubinemia (Cholestasis)

Decreased Secretion of Conjugated Bilirubin into Canaliculi

- Hepatocellular disease
  - Hepatitis
  - Cholestasis (intrahepatic)
- Dubin-Johnson and Rotor's syndromes
- Drugs (estradiol)

Decreased Drainage

- Extrahepatic obstruction
  - Stones
  - Carcinoma
  - Stricture
  - Atresia
- Sclerosing cholangitis
- Intrahepatic obstruction
  - Drugs
  - Granulomas
  - Primary biliary cirrhosis
  - Bile duct paucity
  - Tumors

cially in low-birth-weight infants. Kernicterus refers to a neurological syndrome that results in brain damage owing to deposition of bilirubin in the basal ganglia and brainstem nuclei. In term infants the early symptoms of kernicterus are poor feeding, lethargy, and vomiting; later opisthotonos (backward arching of the trunk), seizures, and death may follow. Seventy percent of affected infants die within the first week and the remaining have severe brain damage. This syndrome can be prevented by phototherapy and exchange transfusion in infants with elevated unconjugated bilirubin concentrations.

Causes of unconjugated hyperbilirubinemia in the neonate are physiological jaundice of the newborn, hemolytic disease, and breast milk hyperbilirubinemia.

Physiological Jaundice of the Newborn. Babies frequently become jaundiced within a few days of birth, a condition known as physiological jaundice of the newborn. Bilirubin levels reach a peak within 3 to 5 days of birth and remain elevated for less than 2 weeks. Bilirubin is usually less than 5 mg/dL, with 90% unconjugated. Factors contributing to physiological jaundice are (1) an increased bilirubin load in the newborn because the RBCs have a shortened lifespan, (2) the appearance of "shunt" bilirubin, which is bilirubin derived from ineffective erythropoiesis or non-RBC sources, (3) decreased conjugation of bilirubin owing to a relative lack of glucuronyl transferase (conjugating enzyme) in the first few days following birth, (4) increased absorption of bilirubin in the intestine owing to beta-glucuronidase in meconium, which hydrolyzes bilirubin conjugates to unconjugated bilirubin that can be passively reabsorbed, and (5) exposure of breast-feeding infants to pregnanediol, nonesterified fatty acids, and other inhibitors of bilirubin conjugation present in the breast milk.

Bilirubin concentrations of 13 mg/dL (222 μmol/L) or greater occurred in 6% of 2297 infants who weighed more than 2500 g.[110] Physiological jaundice is generally not harmful, but bilirubin levels above 10 mg/dL (170 μmol/L) coupled with prematurity, low serum albumin, acidosis, and substances that compete for the binding sites of albumin (e.g., ceftriaxone, sulfisoxazole, and aspirin) may increase the risk for kernicterus. Physiological jaundice of the newborn is treated with phototherapy; the infant is exposed to light of approximately 450 nm that disrupts the intramolecular hydrogen bonds in the bilirubin molecule and yields a number of photoisomers that are more water-soluble than the Z,Z-isomer and thus excreted in the bile.[117] Exchange transfusions are rarely necessary.

Hemolytic Disease. Hemolytic disease in the newborn results from maternal-fetal incompatibility of Rhesus blood factors in which the maternal Rh-negative blood becomes sensitized by either a previous pregnancy with an Rh-positive fetus or an Rh-positive blood transfusion. The infant becomes jaundiced with unconjugated bilirubin in the first or second day of life and is susceptible to kernicterus. The diagnosis is confirmed by a Coombs' test in the infant, an Rh-positive blood in the infant and Rh-negative blood in the mother. Other rare inherited hemolytic anemias, such as glucose-6-phosphate dehydrogenase (G6PD) deficiency, may also lead to unconjugated hyperbilirubinemia.

Breast Milk Hyperbilirubinemia. This type of hyperbilirubinemia affects about 30% of breast-fed newborns. It is due to α-glucuronidase in breast milk, which hydrolyzes conjugated bilirubin in the intestine. The unconjugated bilirubin, being more lipophilic, is passively absorbed. The condition lasts for a few weeks and is treated by discontinuing breast feeding.

Conjugated Hyperbilirubinemias

These syndromes are characterized by hyperbilirubinemia in which the conjugated bilirubin exceeds 1.5 mg/dL (24 μmol/L). The most important are idiopathic neonatal hepatitis and biliary atresia. Diagnosing the cholestatic syndromes may be difficult. The family history may be helpful in diagnosing α_1-antitrypsin deficiency, cystic fibrosis, galactosemia, hereditary fructose intolerance, and tyrosinosis. Serum tyrosine and α_1-antitrypsin levels should be obtained. Urinary nonglucose-reducing substances are obtained if galactosemia is suspected; the diagnosis is confirmed by the absence of the enzyme UDP galactose-1-phosphate uridyl transferase in cells and tissues, such as RBCs and liver. Serological tests may be necessary for hepatitis A, B, and C, and for adenovirus, coxsackievirus, cytomegalovirus, herpes simplex, rubella, and *Toxoplasma.* Liver biopsy may be performed, but the liver tends to look similar, with giant cells and extramedullary erythropoiesis dominating in both hepatitis and cholestatic syndromes. The typical features of periportal red hyaline globules seen with periodic acid-Schiff (PAS) stain that are characteristic for α_1-antitrypsin deficiency are usually not seen early in the course of the disorder. An HIDA isotope scan is essential for determining the patency of the biliary tree. Percutaneous or endoscopic cholangiography may be done in patients with equivocal HIDA scan results.

Conjugated hyperbilirubinemia is seen fairly often in the newborn as a complication of parenteral nutrition.

Idiopathic Neonatal Hepatitis

About 75% of cases of hepatitis in the neonate are idiopathic giant cell hepatitis, a disorder of unknown etiology characterized by cholestatic jaundice. There is a familial trend that may reflect an autosomal recessive inheritance. Jaundice appears within the first 2 weeks. The child initially appears well and gains weight. The liver and spleen then become enlarged and stools become pale. Serum aminotransferases are usually >400 U/L; the prothrombin time is prolonged. Liver biopsy reveals characteristic giant cells with hepatocyte acinar formation. Cholestasis is prominent. It is important to rule out extrahepatic biliary obstruction, such as occurs in biliary atresia, with an HIDA scan.

The treatment is supportive, with adequate nutrition and correction of hypoprothrombinemia. The prognosis is favorable, with 90% of infants surviving without sequelae.

Biliary Atresia

Biliary atresia is a heterogeneous group of acquired disorders that involve either the extrahepatic or intrahepatic bile ducts. Possible etiologies include cytomegalovirus, reovirus III, Epstein-Barr virus, rubella virus, α_1-antitrypsin deficiency, Down syndrome, and trisomy 17 or 18.

Extrahepatic biliary atresia may involve all or part of the extrahepatic biliary tree. The gallbladder is usually absent. Involvement of the hepatic or common duct leads to the characteristic syndrome of severe cholestatic jaundice. It occurs in 1 in 10,000 births, with females more commonly affected than males. Jaundice and pruritus usually appear in the first week. Stools are pale and the urine is tea colored. Jaundice is deep, but the aminotransferases are only mildly elevated. If jaundice persists beyond 14 days of age, a direct or conjugated bilirubin measurement must be performed to exclude biliary atresia. If it is elevated, the urine should be tested for bile and the stool color inspected; if the color is not green or yellow, biliary atresia is likely. Early identification of this condition is essential if these infants are to benefit from the operation of portoenterostomy, which should be performed no later than 60 days after birth.[84] If portoenterostomy is not successful, liver transplantation is the treatment of choice. Children rarely live beyond 3 years unless the lesion is surgically correctable.

Intrahepatic biliary atresia is characterized by a paucity of intrahepatic bile ducts. Jaundice usually appears within the first few days of life. Serum bilirubin is elevated and serum cholesterol may be very high and lead to the formation of xanthomas. The hepatic histology is nonspecific, showing bile duct paucity, giant cells, inflammation, and fibrosis. Survival into adolescence is common, although growth is usually retarded.

A syndromatic variant, *Alagille syndrome,* has similar features but is an autosomal dominant condition with a characteristic triangular face, skeletal abnormalities, retinal pigmentation, and pulmonary stenosis.

Treatment of intrahepatic biliary atresia is symptomatic, with intramuscular replacement of vitamins A, D, and E. Medium chain triglycerides that do not need bile acids for absorption provide calories in patients with partial atresia. Cholestyramine may relieve pruritus. Ursodeoxycholic acid reduces serum enzyme activities and relieves pruritus in some patients.

REFERENCES

1. Adachi Y, Inufusa H, Yamashita M, Kambe A, Yamazaki K, Sawada Y, et al. Clinical application of

bilirubin fractionation by simplified liquid chromatography. Clin Chem 1988;34:385-8.

2. Asada-Senju M, Maeda T, Sakata T, Hayashi A, Suzuki T. Molecular analysis of the transferrin gene in a patient with hereditary hypotransferrinemia. J Hum Genet 2002;47:355-9.
3. Åsberg A, Hveem K, Kruger O, Bjerve KS. Persons with screening-detected haemochromatosis: as healthy as the general population? Scand J Gastroenterol 2002;37:719-24.
4. Bains B. Laboratory techniques for the identification of abnormalities of globin chain synthesis. In: Bain BJ, ed. Haemoglobinopathy diagnosis. London: Blackwell Science, 2001:20-48.
5. Barron BA, Hoyer JD, Tefferi A. A bone marrow report of absent stainable iron is not diagnostic of iron deficiency. Ann Hematol 2001;80:166-9.
6. Bell SH, Weir MP, Dickson DP, Gibson JF, Sharp GA, Peters TJ. Mossbauer spectroscopic studies of human haemosiderin and ferritin. Biochim Biophys Acta 1984;787:227-36.
7. Berendt HL, Blakney GB, Clarke G, Higgins TN. A case of β thalassemia major detected using HPLC in a child of Chinese ancestry. Clin Biochem 2000;33: 311-3.
8. Berfstrome Jones AC, Doon A. Evaluation of a single-tube multiplex polymerase chain reaction screen for detection of common alpha thalassemia genotypes in a clinical laboratory. Am J Clin Path 2002;118:18-24.
9. Beutler E. Commentary. Targeted disruption of the HFE gene. Proc Natl Acad Sci USA 1998;95:2033-4.
10. Beutler E. Production and destruction of erythrocytes. In: Beutler E, Lichtman MA, Coller BS, Kipps TJ, Seligsohn U, eds. Williams hematology. New York: McGraw-Hill, 2001:355-68.
11. Beutler E. The congenital dyserythropoietic anemias. In: Beutler E, Lichtman MA, Coller BS, Kipps TJ, Seligsohn U, eds. Williams hematology. New York: McGraw-Hill, 2001:413-7.
12. Beutler E, Felitti V, Gelbart T, Ho N. The effect of HFE genotypes in patients attending a health appraisal clinic. Ann Intern Med 2000;133:329-37.
13. Beutler E, Felitti VJ, Koziol JA, Ho NJ, Gelbart T. Penetrance of the 845G→A (C282Y) HFE hereditary haemochromatosis mutation in the USA. Lancet 2002;359:211-18.
14. Beutler E, Gelbart T, Demina A. Racial variability in the UDP-glucuronosyltransferase 1 (*UGT1A1*) promoter: A balanced polymorphism for regulation of bilirubin metabolism? Proc Natl Acad Sci USA 1998;95:8170-4.
15. Beutler E, Gelbart T, Lee P, Trevino R, Fernandez MA, Fairbanks VF. Molecular characterization of a case of atransferrinemia. Blood 2000;96:4071-4.
16. Bhutani VK, Gourley GR, Adler S, Kreamer B, Dalin C, Johnson LH. Noninvasive measurement of total serum bilirubin in a multiracial predischarge newborn population to assess the risk of severe hyperbilirubinemia. Pediatrics 2000;106:E17.
17. Bhutani VK, Johnson L, Sivieri EM. Predictive ability of a predischarge hour-specific serum bilirubin for subsequent significant hyperbilirubinemia in healthy term and near-term newborns. Pediatrics 1999;103: 6-14.
18. Billing BH, Cole PG, Lathe GH. The excretion of bilirubin as a glucuronide giving the direct van den Bergh reaction. Biochemical J 1957;65:774-83.
19. Bissé E, Schauber C, Zorn N, Epting T, Eigel A, Van Dorselaer A, et al. Hemoglobin Görwihl ($\alpha_L\beta_2$5 (A_2) Pro→Ala), an electrophoretically silent variant with impaired glycation. Clin Chem 2003;49:137-43.
20. Bissé E, Zorn N, Eigel A, Lizama M, Huaman-Guillen P, März W. Hemoglobin Rambam (β 69 (E 13) Gly→Asp, a pitfall in the assessment of diabetic control-characterization by electrospray mass spectrometry and HPLC. Clin Chem 1998;44: 2172-7.
21. Bisse E, Zorn N, Heinrichs I, Eigel A, Van Dorsselaert A, Weiland H, et al. Characterization of a new electrophoretically silent hemoglobin variant. J Biol Chem 2000;275:21380-4.
22. Blanckaert N. Analysis of bilirubin and bilirubin mono- and di-conjugates. Determination of their relative amounts in biological samples. Biochem J 1980;185:115-28.
23. Blouquit Y, Delanoe GJ, Lacombe C, Arous N, Cayre Y, Peduzzi J, et al. Structural study of hemoglobin Hazebrouck, beta 38(C4)Thr→Pro. A new abnormal hemoglobin with instability and low oxygen affinity. FEBS Lett 1984;172:155-8.
24. Bonnett R, Davis E, Hursthouse MB. The structure of bilirubin. Nature 1976;262:327-8.
25. Bosma PJ, Chowdhury JR, Bakker C, Gantla S, de Boer A, Oostra BA, et al. The genetic basis of the reduced expression of bilirubin UDP-glucuronosyltransferase 1 in Gilbert's syndrome. N Engl J Med 1995;333:1171-5.
26. Bowie LJ, Reddy PL, Nagabhushan M, Sevigny P. Detection of α thalassemia by multiplex polymerase chain reaction. Clin Chem 1994;40:2260-6.
27. Brandebury RO, Smith HL. Sulfhemoglobinemia: a study of 63 clinical cases. Am Heart J 1951;42:582.
28. Breuer W, Ermers MJJ, Pootrakul P, Abramov A, Hershko C, Cabantchik ZI. Desferrioxamine-chelatable iron, a component of serum non-transferrin-bound iron, used for assessing chelation therapy. Blood 2001;97:792-8.
29. British Committee for Standards in Haematology. Guidelines for hemoglobinopathy screening. Clin Lab Haematol 1988;10:87-94.
30. Bry L, Chen PC, Sacks DB. Effects of hemoglobin variants and chemically modified derivatives on

assays for glycohemoglobin. Clin Chem 2001;47: 153-63.

31. Buchwald H. A rapid and sensitive method for estimating carbon monoxide in blood and its application in problem areas. J Am Ind Hygine Assoc 1969;30:564-9.
32. Bulaj ZJ, Ajioka RS, Phillips JD, LaSalle BA, Jorde LB, Griffen LM, et al. Disease-related conditions in relatives of patients with hemochromatosis. N Engl J Med 2000;343:1529-35.
33. Camaschella C, Roetto A, Cali A, De Gobbi M, Garozzo G, Carella M, et al. The gene TFR2 is mutated in a new type of haemochromatosis mapping to 7q22. Nature Genet 2000;25:14-15.
34. Campbell M, Henthorn JS, Davies SC. Evaluations of cation-exchange HPLC compared with isoelectric focusing for neonatal hemoglobinopathy screening. Clin Chem 1999;45:969-75.
35. Carter P. Spectrophotometric determination of serum iron at the submicrogram level with a new reagent (ferrozine). Anal Biochem 1971;40:450-8.
36. Caruso D, Du Riva L, Giavarini F, Galli G, Brambilla S, Luraschi P, et al. A hemoglobin variant found during glycohemoglobin measurement, identified as Hb Toulon (α77 (EF6) Pro→Hia) by random mass spectroscopy. Hemoglobin 2002;26:197-9.
37. Cazzola M, Cremonesi L, Papaioannou M, Soriani N, Kioumi A, Charalambidou A, et al. Genetic hyperferritinaemia and reticuloendothelial iron overload associated with a three base pair deletion in the coding region of the ferroportin gene (SLC11A3). Br J Haematol 2002;119:539-46.
38. Cazzola M, May A, Bergamaschi G, Cerani P, Ferrillo S, Bishop DF. Absent phenotypic expression of X-linked sideroblastic anemia in one of two brothers with a novel ALAS2 mutation. Blood 2002;100:4236-8.
39. Centers for Disease Control and Prevention. Iron deficiency–United States, 1999-2000. MMWR Morb Mortal Wkly Rep 2002;51:897-9.
40. Cervantes F, Rozman C, Brugues R, Llanas I. Iron stores in chronic granulocytic leukemia at presentation. Scand J Haematol 1984;32:469-74.
41. Chen D, Crimmins DL, Hsu FF, Lindberg FF, Scott M. Hemoglobin Raleigh as the cause of falsely increased hemoglobin A_{1c} in an automated ion-exchange HPLC method. Clin Chem 1998;44: 1296-301.
42. Chuang CL, Liu RS, Wei YH, Huang TP, Tarng DC. Early prediction of response to intravenous iron supplementation by reticulocyte haemoglobin content and high-fluorescence reticulocyte count in haemodialysis patients. Nephrol Dial Transplant 2003;18:370-7.
43. Chur DH, Waye JS. Hydrops fetalis caused by alpha thalassemia: an emerging health care problem. Blood 1998;91:2213-22.
44. Clarke GM, Higgins TN. Laboratory investigation of hemoglobinopathies and thalassemias: Review and update. Clin Chem 2000;46:1284-90.
45. Cotton F, Lin C, Fontaine B, Gulbu B, Jansens J, Ventongen F. Evaluation of a capillary electrophoresis method for routine determination of hemoglobins A_2 and F. Clin Chem 1999;46:237-43.
46. Crompton DE, Chinnery PF, Fey C, Curtis AR, Morris CM, Kierstan J, et al. Neuroferritinopathy: a window on the role of iron in neurodegeneration. Blood Cells Mol Dis 2002;29:522-31.
47. Dash S. HbA_2 in subjects with HbD. Clin Chem 1998;44:2381-2.
48. De Braekeleer M, St-Pierre C, Vigneault A, Simard H, De Medicis E. Hemochromatosis and pyruvate kinase deficiency. Report of a case and review of the literature. Blut 1991;62:188-9.
49. de Sousa M, Reimao R, Lacerda R, Hugo P, Kaufmann SH, Porto G. Iron overload in beta 2-microglobulin-deficient mice. Immunol Lett 1994;39:105-11.
50. Devalia V, Carter K, Walker AP, Perkins SJ, Worwood M, May A, Dooley JS. Autosomal dominant reticuloendothelial iron overload associated with a 3-base pair deletion in the ferroportin 1 gene (SLC11A3). Blood 2002;100:695-7.
51. Doumas BT, Perry B, Jendrzejczak B, Davis L. Measurement of direct bilirubin by use of bilirubin oxidase. Clin Chem 1887;33:1349-53.
52. Doumas BT, Perry BW, Sasse EA, Straumfjord JV. Standardization in bilirubin assays: Evaluation of selected methods and stability of bilirubin solutions. Clin Chem 1973;19:984-93.
53. Doumas BT, Yein F, Perry B, Jendrzejczak B, Kessner A. Determination of the sum of bilirubin sugar conjugates in plasma by bilirubin oxidase. Clin Chem 1999;45:1255-60.
54. Enders HM. Evaluating iron status in hemodialysis patients. Nephrol Nurs J 2002;29:366-70.
55. Engle WD, Jackson GL, Sendelbach D, Manning D, Frawley WH. Assessment of a transcutaneous device in the evaluation of neonatal hyperbilirubinemia in a primarily Hispanic population. Pediatrics 2002;110:61-7.
56. Fairbanks V. Tables of hemoglobin variants. In: Fairbanks VF, ed. Hemoglobinopathies and Thalassemias. New York: BC Decker, 1980:247-260.
57. Fairbanks VF, Beutler E. Iron metabolism. In: Beutler E, Lichtman MA, Coller BS, Kipps TJ, Seligsohn U, eds. Williams Hematology. New York: McGraw-Hill, 2001:295-304.
58. Fairbanks VF, Brandhagen DJ. Disorders of iron storage and transport. In: Beutler E, Lichtman MA, Coller BS, Kipps TJ, Seligsohn U, eds. Williams Hematology. New York: McGraw-Hill, 2001: 489-502.

59. Feder JN, Gnirke A, Thomas W, Tsuchihashi Z, Ruddy DA, Basava A, et al. A novel MHC class I-like gene is mutated in patients with hereditary haemochromatosis. Nature Genet 1996;13:399-408.
60. Fellman V. The GRACILE syndrome, a neonatal lethal metabolic disorder with iron overload. Blood Cells Mol Dis 2002;29:444-50.
61. Fernandez-Rodriguez AM, Guindeo-Casasus MC, Molero-Labarta T, Dominguez-Cabrera C, Hortal C, Perez-Borges P, et al. Diagnosis of iron deficiency in chronic renal failure. Am J Kidney Dis 1999;34: 508-13.
62. Fielding J. Iron. In: Cook JD, ed. Methods in Hematology. New York: Churchill Livingstone, 1980:15-43.
63. Fleming MD, Romano MA, Su MA, Garrick LM, Garrick MD, Andrews NC. Nramp2 is mutated in the anemic Belgrade (b) rat: evidence of a role for nramp2 in endosomal iron transport. Proc Natl Acad Sci USA 1998;95:1148-53.
64. Fleming MD, Trenor CC3, Su MA, Foernzler D, Beier DR, Dietrich WF, Andrews NC. Microcytic anaemia mice have a mutation in Nramp2, a candidate iron transporter gene. Nature Genet 1997;16:383-6.
65. Fleming RE, Ahmann JR, Migas MC, Waheed A, Koeffler HP, Kawabata H, et al. Targeted mutagenesis of the murine transferrin receptor-2 gene produces hemochromatosis. Proc Natl Acad Sci USA 2002;99:10653-8.
66. Fleming RE, Sly WS. Ferroportin mutation in autosomal dominant hemochromatosis: loss of function, gain in understanding. J Clin Invest 2001;108:521-2.
67. Franzini C, Cattozzo G. Low affinity complex between bilirubin and caffeine. Clin Chem 1987;33:597-9.
68. Fucharoen S, Winichagoon P, Wisedpanichkiy B S-N, Sriphanich R, Oncoung W, Wuangsapaya W, et al. Prenatal and post natal diagnosis of thalassemias and hemoglobinopathies by HPLC. Clin Chem 1998;44:740-8.
69. Gemignani F, Perra C, Landi S, Canzian F, Kury A, Tõnisson N, et al. Reliable detection of β thalassemia and G6PD mutations by a DNA microarray. Clin Chem 2002;48:2051-4.
70. Gerritsma, Sinnige D, Drieze C, Sittrop B, Houtsma P, Hulshort-Jansen N, Huisman W. Qualitative and quantitative analysis of hemoglobin variants using capillary zone electrophoresis. Ann Clin Biochem 2000;37:380-9.
71. Gordeuk V, Mukiibi J, Hasstedt SJ, Samowitz W, Edwards CQ, West G, et al. Iron overload in Africa. Interaction between a gene and dietary iron content. N Engl J Med 1992;326:95-100.
72. Green R, King R. A new red cell discriminant incorporating volume dispersion for differentiating iron deficiency anemia from thalassemia minor. Blood Cells 1989;15:481-495.
73. Guidelines for the investigation of the α and β thalassemia traits. The thalassemia working party of the BCSH General Hematology Task Force. J Clin Pathol 1994;47:289-95.
74. Hall RB, Haga JA, Guerra CG, Castleberry SM, Hichman JR. Optimizing the detection of hemoglobin H disease. Lab Med 1995;26:736-41.
75. Harris ZL, Durley AP, Man TK, Gitlin JD. Targeted gene disruption reveals an essential role for ceruloplasmin in cellular iron efflux. Proc Natl Acad Sci USA 1999;96:10812-7.
76. Harrison PM, Arosio P. The ferritins: molecular properties, iron storage function and cellular regulation. Biochim Biophys Acta 1996;1275:161-203.
77. Hempe JM, Craver RD. Separation of hemoglobin variants with similar change by capillary isoelectric focussing: value of isoelectric point for identification of common and uncommon hemoglobin variants. Electrophoresis 2000;21:738-43.
78. Hempe JM, Craver RD. Quantification of hemoglobin variants by capillary isoelectric focussing. Clin Chem 1994;40:2288-95.
79. Herrmann MM, Dobrowolski SF, Wittwer CT. Rapid β globin genotyping by multiplexing proble melting temperature and color. Clin Chem 2000;46:425-8.
80. Hershko C, Peto TEA. Non-transferrin plasma iron. Br J Haematol 1987;66:149-51.
81. Honda SAA, Bhagavan NV, Sugiyama CE, Gallatry CR, Dublis R, Flegal I, Rios CN, Scottonini AG. Hemoglobinopathies detected by CBC analysis and HPLC hemoglobin A_{1C} analysis. Lab Med 1994;25:1976-81.
82. Howanitz JH, Howanitz PJ, Chauhan YP. Influences of CBC results and HPLC hemoglobin S measurements on criteria for diagnosis of beta thalassemia. Clin Chem 2003;496(s):A18.
83. Huisman THJ. Combination of β chain abnormal hemoglobins with each other or with β thalassemia determinants with known mutations: influence of phenotype. Clin Chem 1997;43:1850-6.
84. Hussein M, Howard ER, Mieli-Vergani G, Mowat AP. Jaundice at 14 days of age: exclude biliary atresia. Arch Dis Child 1991;66:1177-9.
85. Ingram VM. A specific chemical difference between globins of normal and sickle-cell anemia hemoglobins. Nature 1956;178:792-4.
86. Ingram VM. Gene mutations in human hemoglobin: the chemical difference between normal and sickle cell hemoglobin. Nature 1957;180:326-8.
87. Ingram VM. The chemical difference between normal and sickle cell hemoglobin. Biochem Biophys Acta 1959;36:402-11.
88. Ingram VM. The comparison of normal human and sickle-cell hemoglobin by "Finger Printing". Biochem Biophys Acta 1958;28:539-45.

89. International Committee for standardization in haematology. ISCH Expert panel for neonatal screening of haemologlobinopathies. Clin Lab Haematol 1988;10:335-45.
90. International Committee for Standardization in Haematology. The measurement of total and unsaturated iron binding capacity in serum. Br J Haematol 1978;38:281-94.
91. International committee for standardization in hematology. Recommendations of a system for a system for identifying abnormal hemoglobins. Blood 1978;50:1065-7.
92. Jackson HA, Carter K, Darke C, Guttridge MG, Ravine D, Hutton RD, et al. HFE mutations, iron deficiency and overload in 10 500 blood donors. Br J Haematol 2001;114:474-84.
93. Jendrassik L, Grof P. Vereinfachte photometrische Methoden zur Bestimmung des Blutbilirubins. Biochem Z 1938;297:81-9.
94. Kakhlon O, Cabantchik ZI. The labile iron pool: characterization, measurement, and participation in cellular processes. Free Radic Biol Med 2002;33:1037-46.
95. Koiwai O, Nishizawa M, Hasada K, Aono S, Adachi Y, Mamiya N, et al. Gilbert's syndrome is caused by a heterozygous missense mutation in the gene for bilirubin UDP-glucuronosyltransferase. Hum Mol Genet 1995;4:1183-6.
96. Kosaka A, Yamamoto C, Morishita Y, Nakane K. Enzymatic determination of bilirubin fractions in serum. Clin Biochem 1987:20:451-8.
97. Kuenzle CC, Maier C, Rutner JR. The nature of four bilirubin fractions from serum and of three bilirubin fractions from bile. J Lab Clin Med 1966;67:294-306.
98. Lafferty J. College of American Pathologists hemoglobinopathy survey HG-B. Chicago, IL: College of American Pathologists, 1999.
99. Lafferty JD, Crowther MA, Ali MA, Levine ML. The evaluation of various mathematical RBC indices and their efficacy in discriminating between thalassemic and non-thalassemic microcytosis. Am J Clin Path 1996;106:201-5.
100. Lafferty JD, Crowther MD, Waye JS, Chui DHK. A reliable screening test to identify adult carriers of the ($-^{SEA}$) alpha°-thalassemia deletion A J Clin Path 2000;114:927-31.
101. Landis JB, Pardue HL. Kinetics of the reaction of unconjugated and conjugated bilirubins with p-diazobenzenesulfonic acid, Clin Chem 1978;24: 1690-9.
102. Lauff JJ, Kasper ME, Ambrose RT. Quantitative liquid chromatographic estimation of bilirubin species in pathological serum. Clin Chem 1983;29:800-5.
103. Lauff JJ, Kasper ME, Ambrose RT. Separation of bilirubin species in serum and bile by high performance reverse-phase liquid chromatography. J Chromatogr 1981;226:391-402.
104. Lauff JJ, Kasper ME, Wu TW, Ambrose RT. Isolation and preliminary characterization of a fraction of bilirubin in serum that is firmly bound to protein. Clin Chem 1982;28:629-37.
105. Le Denmat C, Duchassaing D. Rapid diagnosis of β thalassemia mutations in Mediterraneans by PCR and restriction analysis of natural or created sites. Clin Biochem 1997;30:433-7.
106. Lebrón JA, Bennett MJ, Vaughn DE, Chirino AJ, Snow PM, Mintier GA, et al. Crystal structure of the hemochromatosis protein HFE and characterization of its interaction with transferrin receptor. Cell 1998;93:111-23.
107. Levy JE, Montross LK, Andrews NC. Genes that modify the hemochromatosis phenotype in mice. J Clin Invest 2000;105:1209-16.
108. Lo DH, Wu TW. Assessment of the fundamental accuracy of the Jendrassik and Grof total and direct bilirubin assays. Clin Chem 1983;29:31-6.
108a. Lo SF, Doumas BT, Ashwood ER. Performance of bilirubin determinations in US laboratories—revisited. Clin Chem 2004;50:190-4. Epub 2003 Nov 18.
109. Madan N, Sikka MK, Sharma R, Rusia U. Phenotypic expression of hemoglobin A_2 beta thalassemia trait with iron deficiency. Ann Hematol 1998;77:93-6.
110. Maisels MJ, Gilford K. Normal bilirubin levels in the newborn and the effect of breast feeding. Pediatrics 1986;78:837-45.
111. Maisels MJ, Kring E. Transcutaneous bilirubinometry decreases the need for serum bilirubin measurements and saves money. Pediatrics 1997;99:599-601.
112. Malloy HT, Evelyn KA. The determination of bilirubin with the photoelectric colorimeter. J Biol Chem 1937;119:481-90.
113. Mario N, Baudin B, Aussel C, Giboudeau J. Capillary isoelectric focussing and high-performance cation-exchange chromatography compared for qualitative and quantitative analysis of hemoglobin variants. Clin Chem 1997;43:2137-42.
114. Mast AE, Blinder MA, Lu Q, Flax S, Dietzen DJ. Clinical utility of the reticulocyte hemoglobin content in the diagnosis of iron deficiency. Blood 2002;99: 1489-91.
115. McDonagh AF, Assisi F. Commercial bilirubin: a trinity of isomers. FEBS Lett., 1971;18:315-17.
116. McDonagh AF, Assisi. The ready isomerization of bilirubin IX-a in aqueous solution. Biochem J 1972;129:797-800.
117. McDonagh AF, Palma LA, Lightner DA. Blue light and bilirubin excretion. Science 1980;208:145-51.
118. Michaelsson M. Bilirubin determination in serum and urine. Scnd J Clin Lab Invest 1961;13(Suppl. 56).
119. Milner PF, Gooden HM. Rapid Citrate-agar electrophoresis in routine screening for hemoglobinopathies using a simple hemolysate. Am J Clin Path 1975;64:58-64.

120. Mohandas N, Kim YR, Tycko DH, Orlik J, Wyatt J, Groner W. Accurate and independent measurement of volume and hemoglobin concentration of individual red cells by laser light scattering. Blood 1986;68:506-13.
121. Murao S, Tanaka N. Isolation and identification of a microorganism producing bilirubin oxidase. Agric Biol Chem 1982:46:2031-4.
121a. Newman TB, Liljestrand P, Escobar GJ. Combining clinical risk factors with serum bilirubin levels to predict hyperbilirubinemia in newborns. Arch Pediatr Adolesc Med 2005;159:113-9.
122. Nicolas G, Bennoun M, Devaux I, Beaumont C, Grandchamp B, Kahn A, Vaulont S. Lack of hepcidin gene expression and severe tissue iron overload in upstream stimulatory factor 2 (USF2) knockout mice. Proc Natl Acad Sci USA 2001;98:8780-5.
123. Nittis T, Gitlin JD. The copper-iron connection: Hereditary aceruloplasminemia. Semin Hematol 2002;39.
124. Njajou OT, de Jong G, Berghuis B, Vaessen N, Snijders PJ, Goossens JP, et al. Dominant Hemochromatosis Due to N144H Mutation of SLC11A3: Clinical and Biological Characteristics. Blood Cells Mol Dis 2002;29:439-43.
125. Njajou OT, Vaessen N, Joosse M, Berghuis B, van Dongen JW, Breuning MH, et al. A mutation in SLC11A3 is associated with autosomal dominant hemochromatosis. Nature Genet 2001;28:213-14.
126. Old JM. Screening and genetic diagnosis of haemoglobin disorders Blood Reviews 2003;17:43-53.
127. Olivieri N. The β thalassemias. N Engl J Med 1999; 341:99-109.
128. Olsson S, Lundvall O, Weinfeld A. Availability of iron stores built up by iron dextrin as studied with desferrioxamine and phlebotomy. Acta Med Scand 1972;191:49-56.
129. Olynyk JK, Cullen DJ, Aquilia S, Rossi E, Summerville L, Powell LW. A population-based study of the clinical expression of the hemochromatosis gene. N Engl J Med 1999;341:718-24.
130. Ou C-N, Rognerud CL. Diagnosis of hemoglobinopathies electrophoresis vs HPLC. Clin Chem Acta 2001;313:187-94.
131. Ou C-N, Rognerud CL. Liquid chromatography in diagnosis of rare hemoglobin variant (Hb Chicago) and its combination with HbS: Hb Chicago/S trait and Hb Chicago/sickle cell disease. Clin Chem 1996;42:774-6.
132. Ou C-N, Rognerud CL. Rapid analysis of hemoglobin variants by cation-exchange HPLC. Clin Chem 1993;39:820-4.
133. Papadea C, Cate JC. Identification of quantification of hemoglobins A, F, S and C by automated chromatography. Clin Chem 1996;42:57-63.
134. Parkkila S, Waheed A, Britton RS, Bacon BR, Zhou XY, Tomatsu S, et al. Association of the transferrin receptor in human placenta with HFE, the protein defective in hereditary hemochromatosis. Proc Natl Acad Sci USA 1997;94:13198-202.
135. Pauling L, Itano HA, Singer SJ, Wells IC. Sickle Cell anemia, a molecular disease. Science 1949;110:543-8.
136. Perry B, Doumas BT, Buffone G, Glick M, Ou CN, Ryder K. Measurement of total bilirubin by use of bilirubin oxidase. Clin Chem 1986:32:329-32.
137. Perry BW, Doumas BT, Bayse DD, Butler T, Cohen A, Fellows N, et al. A candidate reference method for determination of bilirubin in serum. Test for transferability. Clin Chem 1983;29:297-301.
138. Peurtz MF, Muirhead H, Cox J, Goaman LCG. Three dimensional Fourier synthesis of horse oxyhemoglobin at 2.8A resolution: the atomic model. Nature 1968;219:133-9.
139. Phatak PD, Ryan DH, Cappuccio J, Oakes D, Braggins C, Provenzano K, et al. Prevalence and penetrance of HFE mutations in 4865 unselected primary care patients. Blood Cells Mol Dis 2002;29:41-7.
140. Pigeon C, Ilyin G, Courselaud B, Leroyer P, Turlin B, Brissot P, Loreal O. A new mouse liver-specific gene, encoding a protein homologous to human antimicrobial peptide hepcidin, is overexpressed during iron overload. J Biol Chem 2001;276:7811-9.
141. Ponka P. Tissue-specific regulation of iron metabolism and heme synthesis: distant contact mechanisms in erythroid cells. Blood 1997;89:1-25.
142. Reeves WB, Haurani FI. Clinical applicability and usefulness of ferritin measurements. Ann Clin Lab Sci 1980;10:529-35.
143. Reynolds TM, Harvey TC, Green BN, Smith A, Hartland AJ. Hemoglobin Wayne in a British family: identification by electrospray ionization/mass spectrometry. Clin Chem 2002;48:2261-3.
144. Rice EW, Fenner HE. Study of the ICSH proposed reference method for serum iron assay: Obtaining optically clear filtrates and substitution of ferrozine. Clin Chim Acta 1974;53:391-3.
145. Rioux, Godart C, Huntrel D, Mathis M, Bimet C, Bardakjian J, et al: Cation-exchange HPLC evaluated for presumptive identification of hemoglobin variants. Clin Chem 1997;43:34-9.
146. Rioya L, Grot R, Garabedian M, Cournot-Witmer G. Bone disease in children with homozygous beta thalassemia. Bone Miner 1990;8:69-86.
147. Robertson A, Kazmierczak S, Vos P. Improved transcutaneous bilirubinometry: Comparison of SpectRx Bili Check and Minolta Jaundice Meter JM-102 for estimating total serum bilirubin in a normal newborn population. J Perinatology 2002;22:12-14.
148. Roetto A, Bosio S, Gramaglia E, Barilaro MR, Zecchina G, Camaschella C. Pathogenesis of hyperferritinemia cataract syndrome. Blood Cells Mol Dis 2002;29:532-5.

149. Roetto A, Daraio F, Alberti F, Porporato P, Cali A, De Gobbi M, et al. Hemochromatosis Due to Mutations in Transferrin Receptor 2. Blood Cells Mol Dis 2002;29:465-70.
150. Roetto A, Merryweather-Clarke AT, Daraio F, Livesey K, Pointon JJ, Barbabietola G, et al. A valine deletion of ferroportin 1: A common mutation in hemochromatosis type 4? Blood 2002;100:733-4.
151. Roetto A, Papanikolaou G, Politou M, Alberti F, Girelli D, Christakis J, et al. Mutant antimicrobial peptide hepcidin is associated with severe juvenile hemochromatosis. Nature Genet 2003;33:21-2.
152. Roetto A, Totaro A, Cazzola M, Cicilano M, Bosio S, D'Ascola G, et al. Juvenile hemochromatosis locus maps to chromosome 1q. Am J Hum Genet 1999;64:1388-93.
153. Rothenberg BE, Voland JR. β2 Knockout mice develop parenchymal iron overload: A putative role for class I genes of the major histocompatibility complex in iron metabolism. Proc Natl Acad Sci USA 1996;93:1529-34.
154 Sacks DS. Hemoglobin variants and hemoglobin A_{1c} analysis: Problem solved? Clin Chem 2003;49: 1245-47.
154a. Sarnaik SA. Sickle cell diseases: current therapeutic options and potential pitfalls in preventive therapy for transcranial Doppler abnormalities. Pediatr Radiol 2005; [Epub ahead of print].
155. Schendl WJ, Lipp RW, Trinker M, Hopmeirer P. Hemoglobin D (β 121 (C-H4) Glu→Gln) causing falsely low and high HbA_2 values in HPLC. Clin Chem 1998;44:1999-2000.
156. Schnedl HJ, Reisinger EC, Pieber TR, Lipp RW, Schreiber F, Hopmeier P, et al. Hemoglobin Sherwood Forest detected by high performance liquid chromatography for hemoglobin A_{1C}. Am J Clin Path 1995;104:444-6.
157. Shaji RV, Edison ES, Poonkuzhali B, Srivastava A, Chandy M. Rapid detection of β-globin gene mutations and polymorphisms by temporal temperature gradient gel electrophoresis. Clin Chem 2003;49:777-81.
158. Shalev H, Kapleushnik Y, Haeskelzon L, Degani O, Kransnov T, Sphilberg O, et al. Clinical and laboratory manifestations of congenital dyserythropoietic anemia type I in young adults. Eur J Haematol 2002;68:170-4.
158a. Shihabi ZK, Hinsdale ME. Simplified hemoglobin chain detection by capillary electrophoresis. Electrophoresis 2005;26:581-5 [Epub ahead of print].
159. Simsek M, Darr S, Ojeli H, Bayami R. Improved diagnosis of sickle cell mutation by a robust amplification refractory polymerase chain reaction. Clin Biochem 1999;32:677-80.
160. Sipe JC, Lee P, Beutler E. Brain iron metabolism and neurodegenerative disorders. Dev Neurosci 2002;24:188-96.
161. Sokal JE, Sheerin KA. Decreased stainable marrow iron in chronic granulocytic leukemia. Am J Med 1986;81:395-9.
162. Stewart RD. The effect of carbon monoxide on humans. Ann Rev Pharm 1975;15:405-22.
163. Stewart RD, Baretta LR, Platte, Stewart EB, Kalbfleisch JH, Van Yserloo B, et al. Carboxyhemoglobin levels in American blood donors. J Am Med Assoc 1974;229:1187-95.
164. Stoffman N, Brugnara C, Woods ER. Use of reticulocyte hemoglobin content (CHR) measurement in screening for iron deficiency. J Adolesc Health 2003;32:132.
165. Sugano M, Hidaka H, Yamauchi K, Nakabayashi T, Higuchic Y, Fujita K, et al. Analysis of hemoglobin and globin chain variants by a commonly used capillary isoelectric focussing method. Electrophoresis 2000;21:3016-9.
166. Suh DD, Krauss JS, Bures K. Influenic of hemoglobin S adducts on HbA_2 quantification by HPLC. Clin Chem 1996;42:1113-14.
167. Tessitore N, Solero GP, Lippi G, Bassi A, Faccini GB, Bedogna V, et al. The role of iron status markers in predicting response to intravenous iron in haemodialysis patients on maintenance erythropoietin. Nephrol Dial Transplant 2001;16:1416-23.
167a. Tian H, Emrich CA, Scherer JR, Mathies RA, Andersen PS, Larsen LA, et al. High-throughput single-strand conformation polymorphism analysis on a microfabricated capillary array electrophoresis device. Electrophoresis 2005; [Epub ahead of print].
168. Tietz NW (ed). Clinical guide to laboratory tests, 3rd ed. Philadelphia: WB Saunders Co, 1995.
169. Tenor CC, Campagna DR, Sellers VM, Andrews NC, Fleming MD. The molecular defect in hypotransferrinemic mice. Blood 2000;96:1113-18.
170. Turpeinen U, Siplia I, Antila P, Kayalainen U, Kuronen B, Kalteklnen N, et al. Two α chain variants, Hb Broussais and Hb Cemenelum, characterized by cation HPLC, iso-electric focussing and peptide sequencing. Clin Chem 1995;41:532-6.
171. van den Bergh AAH, Muller P. Uber eine direkte und eine indirekte Diazo-reaktion auf Bilirubin. Biochem Z 1916;77:90-103.
172. van Tellingen A, Kuenen JC, de Kieviet W, van Tinteren H, Kooi ML, Vasmel WL. Iron deficiency anaemia in hospitalised patients: value of various laboratory parameters. Differentiation between IDA and ACD. Neth J Med 2001;59:270-9.
173. Vulpe CD, Kuo YM, Murphy TL, Cowley L, Askwith C, Libina N, et al. Hephaestin, a ceruloplasmin homologue implicated in intestinal iron transport, is defective in the sla mouse. Nature Genet 1999;21:195-9.
174. Waalen J, Felitti VJ, Gelbart T, Ho NJ, Beutler E. Penetrance of hemochromatosis. Blood Cells Mol Dis 2002;29:418-32.

175. Wallace C, Arfay AA, Salkie ML, Crockford PM. Spurious levels of glycated hemoglobin due to the presence of unsuspected hemoglobin variants Can J Diab Care 1994;18:16-20.
176. Wang W, Kham SKY, Yeo G-H, Quah T-C, Chong SS. Multiplex minisequencing screen for common Southeast Asian and Indian β thalassemia mutations. Clin Chem 2003;49:209-213.
177. Wang W, Ma ESK, Chan AYY, Chui DHK, Chong SS. Multiple minisequencing screen for seven Southeast Asian non-deletional α-thalassemia mutations. Clin Chem 2003;49:800-3.
178. Watanabe T, Kato K, Yamada D, Midorikawa S, Sato W, Shiga M, et al. A nondiabetic case of hemoglobin variant (Hb Nigata) with inappropriately high and low HbA_{1c} titers detected by different methods. Clin Chem 1998;44:1502-4.
179. Weatherall DJ, Clegg JB. Thalassemia; a global public health problem. Nat Med 1996;2:847-9.
180. Weir MP, Gibson JF, Peters TJ. Biochemical studies on the isolation and characterization of human spleen haemosiderin. Biochem J 1984;223: 31-8.
181. Whipple GH, Bradford WL. Mediterranean disease thalassemia (erythroblastic anemia of Cooley): associated pigment abnormalities simulating hemochromatosis. J Pediatr 1936;9:279-311.
182. Witte DL, Crosby WH, Edwards CQ, Fairbanks VF, Mitros FA. Hereditary hemochromatosis. Clin Chim Acta 1996;245:139-200.
183. Wright RO, Lewander WJ, Woolf AD. Methemoglobinemia: etiology, pharmacology, and clinical management. Ann Emerg Med 1999;34:646-56.
184. Wu N, Sweedler JV, Lin M. Enhanced separation and deletion of serum bilirubin species by capillary electrophoresis using a mixed anionic surfactant-protein buffer system with laser-induced fluorescence detection. J Chromatogr B Biomed Appl 1994;654:185-91.
185. Wu TW, Dappen GM, Powers DM, Lo DH, Rand RN, Spayd RW. The Kodak Ektachem clinical chemistry slide for measurement of bilirubin in newborns: Principles and performance. Clin Chem 1982;28:2366-72.
186. Wyllie S, Seu P, Goss JA. The natural resistance-associated macrophage protein 1 Slc11a1 (formerly Nramp1) and iron metabolism in macrophages. Microbes Infect 2002;4:351-9.
187. Yamanouchi I, Yamauchi Y, Igarashi I. Transcutaneous bilirubinometry: Preliminary studies of noninvasive bilirubin meter in the Okayama National Hospital. Pediatrics 1980;65:195-202.
188. Zhou XY, Tomatsu S, Fleming RE, Parkkila S, Waheed A, Jiang J, et al. HFE gene knockout produces mouse model of hereditary hemochromatosis. Proc Natl Acad Sci USA 1998;95:2492-7.

CHAPTER 32

Porphyrins and Disorders of Porphyrin Metabolism*

Allan C. Deacon, B.Sc., Ph.D., Dip.C.B., F.R.C.Path., Sharon D. Whatley, Ph.D., and George H. Elder, M.D.

The porphyrias are a group of diseases in which there is deficiency in one of the enzymes of heme biosynthesis leading to the overproduction of intermediates of the pathway.[76a] These intermediates are excreted in excessive amounts in urine, feces, or both. The clinical consequences depend on the nature of the heme precursors that accumulate. In the acute porphyrias, excess porphyrin precursors (5-aminolevulinic acid [ALA] and porphobilinogen) are associated with potentially fatal acute neurovisceral attacks, which are often provoked by a range of commonly prescribed drugs, hormonal factors, alcohol, starvation, stress, or infection. In the nonacute porphyrias, and in those acute porphyrias in which the skin may be affected, accumulation of porphyrins results in photosensitization and skin lesions. Diagnosis depends on laboratory investigation to demonstrate the pattern of heme precursor accumulation specific for each type of porphyria and requires examination of appropriate specimens for the key metabolites using adequately sensitive and specific methods.

Technical advances in the field of molecular genetics make it possible to investigate many porphyrias at the molecular level. Although not essential for diagnosis of symptomatic cases, these techniques are becoming increasingly valuable for the investigation of families with porphyria.

PORPHYRIN CHEMISTRY

Before discussing the porphyrin synthesis and disorders of porphyrin metabolism, porphyrin structure, nomenclature, and chemical characteristics are reviewed.

STRUCTURE AND NOMENCLATURE

The basic porphyrin structure consists of four monopyrrole rings connected by methene bridges to form a tetrapyrrole ring (Figure 32-1).[15] Many porphyrin compounds are known but only a limited number are of clinical interest. The porphyrin compounds of relevance to the porphyrias (Table 32-1) differ in the substituents occupying the peripheral positions 1 through 8. Variation in the distribution of the same substituents around the peripheral positions of the tetrapyrrole ring gives rise to porphyrin isomers, which are usually depicted by Roman numerals (i.e., I, II, III etc.). The reduced form of a porphyrin is known as a porphyrinogen (see Figure 32-1) and differs by the absence of six hydrogens (four from the methylene bridges and two from ring nitrogens). Porphyrinogens are unstable in vitro and are spontaneously oxidized to the corresponding porphyrins. Under the lower oxygen tension of the cell, porphyrinogens are stable and form intermediates of the heme biosynthetic pathway; aromatization to protoporphyrin at the penultimate step requires an enzyme.

CHELATION OF METALS

The arrangement of four nitrogen atoms in the center of the porphyrin ring enables porphyrins to chelate various metal ions. Protoporphyrin that contains iron is known as heme; ferroheme refers specifically to the Fe^{2+} complex and ferriheme to Fe^{3+}. Ferriheme associated with a chloride counter ion is known as hemin, or hematin when the counter ion is hydroxide.

SPECTRAL PROPERTIES

Porphyrins were named from the Greek root for "purple" (porphyra) and owe their color to the conjugated double-bond structure of the tetrapyrrole ring. The porphyrinogens

*The authors gratefully acknowledge the original contributions of Drs. Robert F. Labbe and Kern L. Nuttall, on which portions of this chapter are based.

have no conjugated double bonds and are therefore colorless. Porphyrins show a particularly strong absorbance near 400 nm, often called the Soret band. When exposed to light in the 400-nm region, porphyrins display a characteristic orange-red fluorescence in the range of 550 to 650 nm. Absorbance and fluorescence are altered by substituents around the porphyrin ring and by metal binding. Zinc chelation shifts the fluorescence peak of protoporphyrin to shorter wavelengths and reduces the fluorescence intensity. The strong binding of iron alters the character of protoporphyrin to the extent that heme lacks significant fluorescence.

SOLUBILITY

Porphyrins are only marginally soluble in water. The differing solubilities of individual porphyrins are of importance not only in the design of analytical methods for their extraction and/or fractionation but in determining the route of excretion from the body. At pH 7, the carboxyl groups are ionized, and the molecule has a net negative charge. Below pH 2 the pyrrole nitrogens and the carboxyl groups become protonated so that the molecule has a net positive charge. At physiological pH, the solubility of a given porphyrin is determined by the number of substituent carboxyl groups. Uroporphyrin has eight carboxylate groups and is the most soluble porphyrin in aqueous media. Protoporphyrin has only two carboxylate groups and is essentially insoluble in water, but dissolves readily in lipid environments and binds readily to the hydrophobic regions of proteins, such as albumin. Coproporphyrin, with four carboxylate groups, has intermediate solubility.

Traditional extraction methods for porphyrins have two steps: first, extraction into an acidified organic solvent, followed by a second or back extraction into aqueous acid. The initial extraction takes advantage of the fact that at pH 3 to 5 (near to their isoelectric point) porphyrins are less soluble in aqueous media and move into the organic phase. Coproporphyrin and protoporphyrin are readily extracted into diethyl ether, but the more highly carboxylated porphyrins (uroporphyrin and heptacarboxylate porphyrin) require the use of a more hydrophilic solvent, such as cyclohexanone or butanol. The back extraction induces porphyrin compounds to move back into the aqueous solution by decreasing the pH to less than 2. This pH shift causes the protonation of the pyrrolenine nitrogens and carboxylate groups, thereby reversing the solubility characteristics of porphyrins. Compounds such as heme and chlorophyll in which the pyrrole nitrogens are tightly bound to iron and magnesium, respectively, remain uncharged at low pH and trapped in the organic layer.

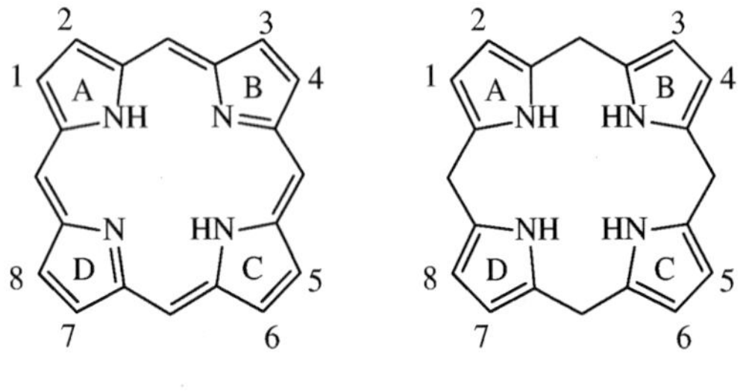

Porphyrin Porphyrinogen

Figure 32-1 Porphyrin and porphyrinogen structures; numbers 1 to 8 represent various substituents, the nature and order of which determine the type of porphyrin or porphyrinogen (Table 32-1). Numbering system and ring designations are based on the Fischer system. A revised system formulated by the International Union of Pure and Applied Chemistry-International Union of Biochemistry (IUPAC-IUB) Joint Commission on Biochemical Nomenclature is appropriate for more complex needs.[104]

TABLE 32-1 Substituents Around the Macrocycle in Porphyrins of Clinical Importance

Position	1	2	3	4	5	6	7	8
Uroporphyrin-I	C_m	C_{et}	C_m	C_{et}	C_m	C_{et}	C_m	C_{et}
Uroporphyrin-III	C_m	C_{et}	C_m	C_{et}	C_m	C_{et}	C_{et}	C_m
Heptacarboxylate porphyrin-III	C_m	C_{et}	C_m	C_{et}	C_m	C_{et}	C_{et}	Me
Hexacarboxylate porphyrin-III	Me	C_{et}	C_m	C_{et}	C_m	C_{et}	C_{et}	Me
Pentacarboxylate porphyrin-III	Me	C_{et}	Me	C_{et}	C_m	C_{et}	C_{et}	Me
Coproporphyrin-III	Me	C_{et}	Me	C_{et}	Me	C_{et}	C_{et}	Me
Coproporphyrin-I	Me	C_{et}	Me	C_{et}	Me	C_{et}	Me	C_{et}
Isocoproporphyrin	Me	Et	Me	C_{et}	C_m	C_{et}	C_{et}	Me
Dehydroisocoproporphyrin	Me	Vn	Me	C_{et}	C_m	C_{et}	C_{et}	Me
Deethylisocoproporphyrin	Me	H	Me	C_{et}	C_m	C_{et}	C_{et}	Me
Protoporphyrin	Me	Vn	Me	Vn	Me	C_{et}	C_{et}	Me
Pemptoporphyrin	Me	H	Me	Vn	Me	C_{et}	C_{et}	Me
Deuteroporphyrin	Me	H	Me	H	Me	C_{et}	C_{et}	Me
Mesoporphyrin	Me	Et	Me	Et	Me	C_{et}	C_{et}	Me

C_m, carboxymethyl (—CH_3COOH); C_{et}, carboxyethyl (—CH_2CH_2COOH); *Me*, methyl (—CH_3); *Et*, ethyl (—CH_2CH_3); *Vn*, vinyl (—$CH_2 = CH_2$).

HEME BIOSYNTHESIS

The complex tetrapyrrole ring structure of heme is built up in a stepwise fashion from the very simple precursors succinyl-CoA and glycine (Figure 32-2).[24] The pathway is present in all nucleated cells. From measurements of total bilirubin production,[4] it has been estimated that daily synthesis of heme in humans is 5 to 8 mmol/kg body weight. Of this, 70% to 80% occurs in the bone marrow and is used for hemoglobin synthesis. Approximately 15% is synthesized in the liver and is used to produce cytochrome P-450, mitochondrial cytochromes, and other hemoproteins. The pathway is compartmentalized, with some steps occurring in the mitochondrion and others in the cytoplasm. Little is known about the transport of intermediates across the mitochondrial membrane, and no transport defect has yet been reported in the porphyrias.

ENZYMES OF HEME BIOSYNTHESIS

The genes for all the enzymes of human heme biosynthesis have been characterized (Table 32-2), and the structures of 5-aminolevulinic acid dehydratase (ALAD), hydroxymethylbilane synthase (HMBS), uroporphyrinogen-III synthase (UROS), uroporphyrinogen decarboxylase (UROD), and ferrochelatase (FECH) have been determined by x-ray crystallography.[47,94,97,153,158]

5-Aminolevulinate Synthase (EC 2.3.1.37), ALAS

ALAS is the initial enzyme of the pathway and catalyzes the formation of ALA from succinyl-CoA and glycine. The enzyme is mitochondrial and requires pyridoxal phosphate as a cofactor, which forms a Schiff base with the amino group of glycine at the enzyme surface. The carbanion of the Schiff base displaces Co enzyme A from succinyl-CoA with the formation of α-amino-β-ketoadipic acid, which is then decarboxylated to ALA. The activity of ALAS is rate limiting as long as the catalytic capacities of other enzymes in the pathway are normal.

5-Aminolevulinic Acid Dehydratase (EC 4.2.1.24), ALAD

ALAD (also known as porphobilinogen synthase) is a cytoplasmic enzyme that catalyzes the formation of the monopyrrole porphobilinogen (PBG) from two molecules of ALA with elimination of two molecules of water. The enzyme requires zinc ions as a cofactor and reduced sulfhydryl groups at the active site and is therefore susceptible to inhibition by lead.

Hydroxymethylbilane Synthase (EC 2.5.1.61), HMBS

HMBS (also known as porphobilinogen [PBG] deaminase) is a cytoplasmic enzyme that catalyzes the formation of one molecule of the linear tetrapyrrole 1-hydroxymethylbilane (HMB; also known as preuroporphyrinogen) from four molecules of PBG with the release of four molecules of ammonia.[149] The former enzyme committee designation for HMBS was EC 4.3.1.8, but in 2003 the enzyme was redesignated as EC 2.5.1.61. The enzyme has two molecules of its own substrate: PBG, attached covalently to the apoenzyme as a prosthetic group.[138] The enzyme is susceptible to allosteric inhibition by intermediates further down the heme biosynthetic pathway, notably coproporphyrinogen-III and protoporphyrinogen-IX.[101]

Uroporphyrinogen-III Synthase (EC 4.2.1.75), UROS

UROS is a cytoplasmic enzyme that rearranges and cyclizes HMB to form uroporphyrinogen-III.[149] Each pyrrole ring of HMB contains a methylcarboxylate and an ethylcarboxylate substituent, which are in the same orientation. By the rotation of none, one, or two alternate or two adjacent pyrrole rings it is possible to arrive at four different isomers. Apart

TABLE 32-2 Human Enzymes and Genes of Heme Biosynthesis

Enzyme	Monomer Mol Wt (kDa)*†	Chromosomal Location of Gene	Gene Size (kb)	# Exons	Expression
ALAS1	70.6	3p21.1	17	12	Ubiquitous
ALAS2	64.6	Xp11.21	22	11	Erythroid cells
ALAD	36.3	9q34	13	13	Ubiquitous and erythroid-specific mRNAs
HMBS	37.0	11q24.1-24.2	10	15	Ubiquitous and erythroid-specific isoforms
UROS	29.5	10q25.2-26.3	34	10	Ubiquitous and erythroid-specific mRNAs
UROD	40.8	1p34	3	10	Ubiquitous
CPO	40.3	3q12	14	7	Ubiquitous
PPOX	50.8	1q21-23	5	13	Ubiquitous
FECH	47.8	18q21.3	45	11	Ubiquitous

*ALAD is a homooctamer, HMBS and UROS are monomers, all other enzymes are homodimers.
†Molecular weights for ALAS1, ALAS2, CPO, and FECH include presequences that are cleaved during mitochondrial import.

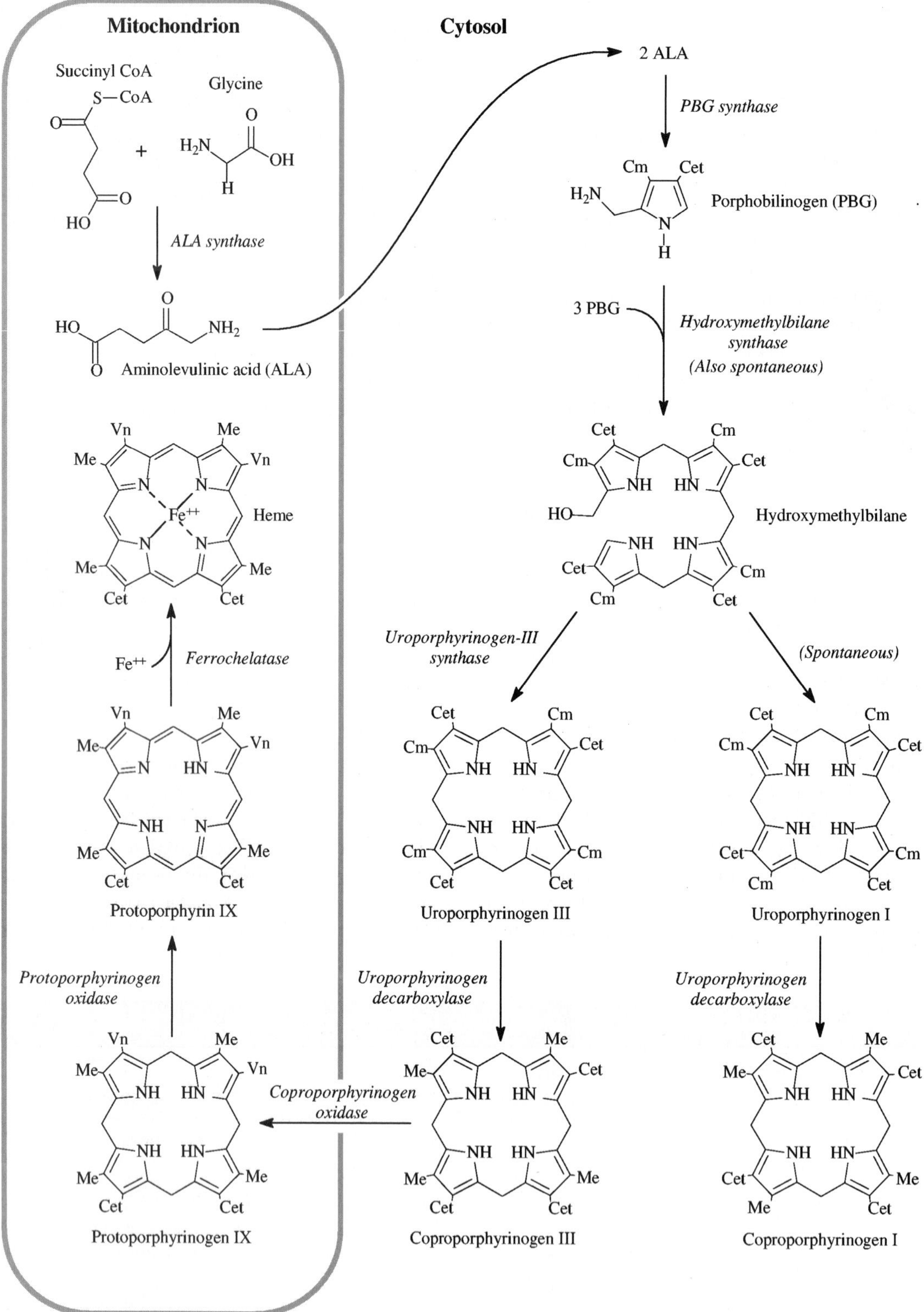

Figure 32-2 Biosynthetic pathway of porphyrins and heme. C_{et}, —CH_2CH_2COOH; C_m, —CH_2COOH; Me, —CH_3; Vn, —$CH=CH_2$.

from closing the ring structure, the enzyme rotates the D-ring via a spirane intermediate,[3] producing the type-III isomer—this is vital since only this isomer contributes to heme biosynthesis. HMB is unstable and in those porphyrias in which excess HMB accumulates, cyclization occurs nonenzymatically with the formation of the type-I isomer. Normally, only minimum amounts of uroporphyrinogen-I are formed.

Uroporphyrinogen Decarboxylase (EC 4.1.1.37), UROD

This is the last cytoplasmic enzyme in the pathway and catalyzes the decarboxylation of all four carboxymethyl groups to form the tetracarboxylic coproporphyrin. The enzyme will use both the I and III isomers of uroporphyrinogen as substrate. Decarboxylation commences on ring D and proceeds stepwise through rings A, B and C with formation of heptacarboxylate, hexacarboxylate, and pentacarboxylate intermediates at a single active site.[74] A UROD deficiency causes accumulation of these intermediates in addition to its substrate, uroporphyrinogen. At high substrate concentrations, decarboxylation occurs by a random mechanism.[95]

Coproporphyrinogen Oxidase (EC 1.3.3.3), CPO

CPO is situated in the intermembrane space of mitochondria and catalyzes the sequential oxidative decarboxylation of the 2- and 4-carboxyethyl groups to vinyl groups to produce the more lipophilic protoporphyrinogen-IX, with formation of a tricarboxylic intermediate, harderoporphyrinogen.[88] Oxygen is required as the oxidant. The enzyme requires sulfhydryl groups for activity, making it a target for inhibition by metals.[155] The enzyme is specific for the type-III isomer, so that metabolism of the I-series of porphyrins does not occur beyond coproporphyrinogen-I. The product of the enzyme differs from the substrate in that the replacement of two of the carboxyethyl groups by vinyl groups has introduced a third substituent into the molecule. Therefore the number of possible isomeric forms increases, and conventionally the numbering system changes so that the III isomer becomes the IX isomer. Because of increasing complexity, this Roman numeral designation is no longer recommended above IV.[104] In UROD-deficient states, one of the ethylcarboxylate groups of the accumulated pentacarboxylate porphyrinogen is decarboxylated by an unknown mechanism to form the isocoproporphyrin series of porphyrins.

Protoporphyrinogen Oxidase (EC 1.3.3.4), PPOX

PPOX is a flavoprotein located in the inner mitochondrial membrane and catalyzes the removal of six hydrogens (four from methylene bridges and two from ring nitrogens) to form protoporphyrin-IX. This involves a three-step, six-electron flavin adenine dinucleotide (FAD)–dependent oxidation that consumes molecular oxygen.[24] Nonenzymatic oxidation also occurs in vitro. However, under the oxygen tension in the cell, PPOX is essential for the oxidation to occur. The protoporphyrin produced is the only porphyrin that functions in the heme pathway. Other porphyrins are produced by nonenzymatic oxidation and represent porphyrinogens that have irreversibly escaped from the pathway.

Ferrochelatase (EC 4.99.1.1), FECH

FECH (also known as heme synthase) is an iron-sulfur protein[158] located in the inner mitochondrial membrane. This enzyme inserts ferrous iron into protoporphyrin to form heme. During this process, two hydrogens are displaced from the ring nitrogens. Other metals in the divalent state will also act as substrate,[85] yielding the corresponding chelate (e.g., incorporation of Zn^{2+} into protoporphyrin to yield zinc protoporphyrin). In iron-deficient states Zn^{2+} successfully competes with Fe^{2+} in developing red cells so that the concentration of zinc protoporphyrin in erythrocytes increases. Furthermore, other dicarboxylic porphyrins will also serve as substrates (e.g., mesoporphyrin).

EXCRETION OF HEME PRECURSORS

Normally, only minute amounts of heme precursors accumulate. The route of excretion largely depends on solubility. The porphyrin precursors ALA and PBG are water soluble and are excreted almost exclusively in urine. Uroporphyrinogen, with eight carboxylate groups, is readily water soluble and is also excreted via the kidney. The last intermediate of the pathway, protoporphyrin (and also protoporphyrinogen), which has only two carboxylate groups, is insoluble in water and is excreted in the feces via the biliary tract. The other porphyrins are of intermediate solubility and appear in both urine and feces. Coproporphyrinogen-I is taken up and excreted by the liver in preference to the III isomer so that coproporphyrinogen-I predominates in feces and coproporphyrinogen-III in urine. All porphyrinogens in the urine or feces are slowly oxidized to the corresponding porphyrins. Reference intervals for porphyrins and their precursors in urine, feces, and blood are given in Table 32-3.

Once in the gut, porphyrins are susceptible to modification by gut flora. The two vinyl groups of protoporphyrin are reduced to ethyl groups, hydrated to hydroxyethyl groups, or removed, giving rise to a variety of secondary porphyrins. Gut flora can also metabolize heme (whether of dietary heme, as components from cells sloughed off from the lining of the gut, or resulting from gastrointestinal bleeding) to produce a variety of dicarboxylic porphyrins.[6] Furthermore, some bacteria are capable of de novo synthesis of porphyrins.

REGULATION OF HEME BIOSYNTHESIS

Heme supply in all tissue is controlled by the activity of mitochondrial ALAS, the first enzyme of the pathway. There are two isoforms of ALAS. The ubiquitous isoform, ALAS1, is encoded by a gene on chromosome 3p21 and expressed in all tissue. Since it has a half-life of only about an hour, changes in its rate of synthesis produce short-term alterations in enzyme concentration and cellular ALAS activity. Synthesis of ALAS1 is under negative feedback control by

TABLE 32-3 Adult Reference Intervals

Specimen	Analyte	Reference interval
Urine	Porphobilinogen	<10 μmol/L[45]
		<1.5 μmol/mmol creatinine[8]
	Total porphyrin	20-320 nmol/L[29]
		<35 nmol/mmol creatinine[8]
	Uroporphyrin	0.8-3.1 μmol/mmol creatinine[6]
	Heptacarboxylate porphyrin	<0.9 μmol/mmol creatinine[6]
	Coproporphyrin-I	1.2-5.7 μmol/mmol creatinine[6]
	Coproporphyrin-III	4.8-23.8 μmol/mmol creatinine[6]
	%Coproporphyrin-III*	68-86[6]
Feces	Total porphyrin	10-200 nmol/g dry wt[92]
	Coproporphyrin-I	1.1-5.5 nmol/g feces[6]
	Coproporphyrin-III	0.2-2.5 nmol/g feces[6]
	%Coproporphyrin-III*	16-35[6]
	Total dicarboxylate porphyrin	0.5-12.8 nmol/g feces[6]
Erythrocytes	Total porphyrin	0.4-1.7 μmol/L erythrocytes[45]

**%Coproporphyrin-III*, (coproporphyrin-III/coproporphyrin [I + III]) × 100%

Urinary porphyrin: creatinine ratios are higher in children weighing less than 30 kg or less than 9 years old.[10]

heme.[99] In the liver, but not most other tissue, ALAS1 is induced by a wide range of drugs and chemicals that induce microsomal cytochrome P-450 dependent oxidases (CYPs). This effect is probably mediated mainly by direct transcriptional activation by drug-responsive nuclear receptors[51] rather than being secondary to depletion of an intracellular regulatory heme pool as a consequence of use of heme for CYP assembly. Induction of ALAS1 is prevented by heme, which acts by destabilizing messenger ribonucleic acid (mRNA) for ALAS1, by blocking mitochondrial import of pre-ALAS1, and possibly by inhibiting transcription.[99]

The erythroid isoform, ALAS2, is encoded by a gene on chromosome Xq21-22 and is expressed only in erythroid cells. Its activity is regulated by two distinct mechanisms.[119] Transcription is enhanced during erythroid differentiation by the action of erythroid-specific transcription factors, and mRNA concentrations are regulated by iron. Iron deficiency in erythroid cells promotes specific binding of iron regulatory proteins to an iron-responsive element in the 5′ untranslated region (UTR) of ALAS2 mRNA with consequent inhibition of translation.

ABNORMALITIES OF PORPHYRIN METABOLISM

Abnormalities of porphyrin metabolism are caused by inherited defects in the genes of the biosynthetic pathway enzymes, diseases called the porphyrias, or by conditions (e.g., lead toxicity) that affect the enzymatic activity in subjects with normal heme synthesis genes.

The Porphyrias

The porphyrias are a group of metabolic disorders that result from partial deficiencies of the enzymes of heme biosynthesis[1] (Table 32-4). All are inherited in monogenic patterns, apart from some forms of porphyria cutanea tarda (PCT) and rare types of erythropoietic porphyria. Each type of porphyria is defined by the association of characteristic clinical features with a specific pattern of accumulation of heme precursors that reflects increased formation of substrates for the enzyme that is deficient in that type of porphyria (Table 32-5).

The porphyrias are characterized clinically by two main features: skin lesions on sun-exposed areas and acute neurovisceral attacks, typically comprising abdominal pain, peripheral neuropathy, and mental disturbance. The skin lesions are caused by porphyrin-catalyzed photodamage of which singlet oxygen is the main mediator.[118] Acute attacks are associated with increased formation of ALA from induced activity of hepatic ALAS1 and partial hepatic heme deficiency, often in response to induction of hepatic cytochrome P450s (CYPs) by drugs and other factors. The relationship of these biochemical changes to the neuronal dysfunction that underlines all the clinical features of the acute attack is uncertain.[105] ALA may act as a neurotoxin; heme deficiency in the liver may interfere with the synthesis of neurotransmitters, the action of heme-dependent enzymes in the nervous system may be impaired, or one or more of these effects may act together.

In Table 32-4 the porphyrias are divided into the acute porphyrias, in which acute neurovisceral attacks occur, and the nonacute porphyrias. Other classifications include division into hepatic (acute intermittent porphyria [AIP], hereditary coproporphyria [HCP], variegate porphyria [VP], and PCT) and erythropoietic (congenital erythropoietic porphyria [CEP], erythropoietic protoporphyria [EPP]) porphyrias according to the main site of overproduction of

TABLE 32-4 The Main Types of Human Porphyria

Disorder	Defective Enzyme	Prevalence*	Neurovisceral Crises	Skin Lesions	Inheritance
Acute Porphyrias					
ALA dehydratase deficiency porphyria (ADP)	ALAD	–	+	–	AR
AIP	HMBS	1-2:100,000	+	–	AD
HCP	CPO	1-2:10^6	+	+[†‡]	AD
VP	PPOX	1:250,000	+	+[†‡]	AD
Nonacute Porphyrias					
CEP	UROS	1:10^6	–	0.001[‡]	AR
PCT	UROD	1:25,000	–	+[‡]	Complex
EPP	FECH	1:130,000	–	+[§]	AR (20% AD) Complex (mainly AD)

*Estimated prevalence of clinically overt disease in the United Kingdom.
[†]Skin lesions and neurovisceral crises may occur alone or together.
[‡]Fragile skin, bullae.
[§]Acute photosensitivity without fragile skin, bullae.
AR, Autosomal recessive; *AD*, autosomal dominant.

TABLE 32-5 The Porphyrias: Patterns of Overproduction of Heme Precursors During Clinically Overt Phase of Disease

Porphyria	Urine PBG/ALA	Urine Porphyrins	Fecal Porphyrins	Erythrocyte Porphyrins	Plasma Fluorescence Emission Peak
ADP	ALA	Copro III	Not increased	Zn-proto	—
AIP	PBG > ALA	Mainly uroporphyrin from PBG	Normal, or slight increase in Copro, Proto[a]	Not increased	615-620 nm[b]
CEP	Not increased	Uro I, Copro I	Copro I	Zn-proto, Proto, Copro I, Uro I	615-620 nm
PCT	Not increased	Uro, Hepta[c]	Isocopro, Hepta[c]	Not increased	615-620 nm
HCP	PBG > ALA[d]	Copro III, uroporphyrin from PBG	Copro III	Not increased	615-620 nm[b]
VP	PBG > ALA[d]	Copro III, uroporphyrin from PBG	Proto IX > Copro III, X-porphyrin	Not increased	624-628 nm
EPP	Not increased	Not increased	+/–Proto[e]	Proto	626-634 nm[f]

[a]Total porphyrin may be increased because of presence of excess uroporphyrin.[127]
[b]Not always increased during acute attack.
[c]Other methylcarboxylate substituted porphyrins are increased to a smaller extent; uroporphyrin is a mixture of type I and III isomers; heptacarboxylate porphyrin is mainly type III.
[d]PBG and ALA may be normal when only skin lesions are present.
[e]Not increased in about 40% of patients.
[f]Protoporphyrin bound to globin (if there is hemolysis in the sample) has a peak at 626-628 nm.

heme precursors, or into cutaneous and acute porphyrias, but both of these classifications make some porphyrias difficult to place.

Acute Porphyrias

The acute porphyrias include ALA dehydratase deficiency porphyria (ADP), AIP, VP, and HCP. These disorders are autosomal dominant except for ADP, which is autosomal recessive.

Biochemistry and Molecular Genetics

The inherited defect in each of the autosomal dominant acute porphyrias (AIP, VP, and HCP, Table 32-4) is a mutation leading to complete or near complete inactivation of one of the pairs of allelic genes that encode the enzyme whose partial deficiency causes the disorder. Enzyme activities are therefore half of normal in all tissue in which they are expressed, reflecting the activity of the normal gene *trans* to the mutant allele. Heme supply is maintained at normal or near normal levels by up regulation of ALAS, with a consequent increase in the substrate concentration for the defective enzyme. These compensatory changes vary between tissues, being most prominent in the liver and undetectable in most other organs, and between individuals. Thus in all autosomal dominant acute porphyrias, some individuals show no evidence of overproduction of heme precursors, and others have biochemically manifest disease with or without clinical symptoms.

Low clinical penetrance is a prominent feature of all the autosomal dominant acute porphyrias. Family studies indicate that about 80% of affected individuals are asymptomatic throughout life. Surveys of blood donors suggest that the AIP gene may be present in as many as 1 in 1500 of the population.[111] For all three disorders, the gene frequency is sufficiently high for rare "homozygous" variants of AIP, HCP, or VP to occur in individuals who are homozygotes or compound heterozygotes for disease-specific mutations[41,89] and for the same person to have two separate types of porphyria.

All the autosomal dominant acute porphyrias show extensive allelic heterogeneity.[38,44,63,89,103] More than 200 disease-specific mutations have been identified in AIP and more than 120 in VP (Human Gene Mutation Database: www.hgmd.org). About 3% of families with AIP have HMBS mutations that impair expression of the ubiquitous isoform and therefore do not decrease activity in erythroid cells. All other mutations in the autosomal dominant acute porphyrias affect all tissue. Most are restricted to one or a few families, but founder mutations are present in some populations and explain the high frequency of VP in South Africans of Dutch descent and of AIP in Sweden.[42,89]

About 25% of patients with overt acute porphyria have no family history of the disease. Such sporadic presentation is a reflection of the high prevalence of mutations in the population; acute porphyria caused by de novo mutation is uncommon.

Unlike the other acute porphyrias, ADP is an autosomal recessive disorder. Patients are compound heterozygotes or homozygotes for a range of mutations in the ALAD gene. The prevalence of heterozygous carriers may be as high as 2% in some populations.[96]

Clinical Features

The life-threatening, acute neurovisceral attacks that occur in AIP, VP, and HCP are clinically identical.[42,64,89] Acute attacks are more common in women, usually occurring first between the ages of 15 and 40, and are very rare before puberty. Their main clinical features are summarized in Table 32-6. The clinical features of ADP, which has been reported in only six families, are similar but may start in childhood.[132]

Acute attacks almost always start with abdominal pain that rapidly becomes very severe but is not accompanied by other signs of an acute surgical condition. Pain may also be present in the back and thighs and may occasionally be most severe in these regions. Signs of autonomic neuropathy, such as vomiting, constipation, tachycardia, and hypertension, are frequent. When convulsions occur, they are often caused by hyponatremia. Pain may dissipate within a few days, but in severe cases a predominant motor neuropathy develops that may progress to flaccid quadriparesis. Persistent pain and vomiting may lead to weight loss and malnutrition. The acute phase may be accompanied by mental confusion with abrupt changes in mood, hallucinations, and other psychotic features. However, these mental disturbances disappear with remission. Persistent psychiatric illness is not a feature of the acute porphyrias, though mild anxiety or depression may be present in some patients.[106] Abdominal pain usually resolves within 2 weeks, but recovery from neuropathy may take many months and is not always complete. Most patients have one or a few attacks followed by complete recovery and prolonged remission. About 5% have repeated acute attacks, which in women may be premenstrual.

TABLE 32-6 Clinical Features of an Acute Neurovisceral Attack of Porphyria

Symptom/Sign	Percent of Acute Attacks
Abdominal pain	97
Nonabdominal pain	25
Vomiting	85
Constipation	46
Psychological symptoms	8
Convulsions	5
Muscle weakness	8
Sensory loss	2
Hypertension (diastolic > 85 mm Hg)	64
Tachycardia (> 80/min)	65
Hyponatremia (< 135 nmol/L)	37

Data from Elder GH, Hift RJ. Treatment of acute porphyria. Hosp Med 2001;62:422-8.

Precipitating factors can be identified in about two thirds of patients who present with acute attacks. The most important are drugs, alcohol—especially binge drinking—the menstrual cycle, pregnancy, calorie restriction, infection, and stress. Drugs known to provoke acute attacks include barbiturates, sulfonamides, progestogens, and most anticonvulsants, but many others have been implicated in the precipitation of acute attacks.[1,72,89] Many of these precipitating factors induce hepatic CYPs.

Skin lesions similar to those of PCT and other bullous porphyrias are present in about 80% of patients with clinically manifest VP (Table 32-4). About 60% of patients with this condition present with skin lesions alone.[152] The skin is less commonly affected in HCP; skin lesions without an acute attack are uncommon and usually provoked by intercurrent cholestasis.[102]

Long-term complications of acute porphyria include chronic renal failure, hypertension, and hepatocellular carcinoma.[1,89]

Treatment

As soon as an attack of acute porphyria is suspected as the cause of illness, drugs and other potential provoking agents should be withdrawn and supportive treatment started using drugs that are known to be safe.[43] Opiates are usually required to control pain. Addition of chlorpromazine or promazine may help to reduce the requirement for analgesics. Patients are prone to severe hyponatremia, and careful administration of any intravenous fluids, with avoidance of hypotonic solutions, is essential. If hyponatremia develops, it should be corrected slowly because patients with acute porphyria are particularly susceptible to cerebral edema and osmotic demyelination. Adequate caloric intake must be maintained, preferably by giving carbohydrate-rich supplements orally or if necessary via a nasogastric tube. When vomiting prevents enteral administration, 100 g of dextrose per day given intravenously as a 5% solution in normal saline should suffice.

Unless the attack is mild and clearly resolving, specific treatment with intravenous heme should be started as soon as the diagnosis has been established.[43,89,109] This treatment increases the concentration of heme in the liver, thus decreasing the activity of ALAS1 and the formation of ALA and PBG. The effect of treatment may be monitored by measuring these metabolites, but this is not essential because clinical improvement is the required end point. Heme administration will not reverse an established neuropathy. If heme preparations are not available, hepatic ALA synthase activity can be decreased by carbohydrate loading,[13] but this treatment is less effective than intravenous heme and more difficult to administer.

Repeated attacks are difficult to control. Cyclical premenstrual attacks in women may be prevented by suppression of ovulation with gonadorelin analogues,[1,43] but most patients require repeated courses of intravenous heme. In one patient with AIP, orthotopic liver transplantation led to immediate and prolonged remission with restoration of PBG excretion to normal.[141]

Management of Families

Diagnosis of autosomal dominant acute porphyria should be followed by investigation of the patient's family to identify affected, often asymptomatic, relatives so that they can be advised to avoid factors known to provoke potentially fatal acute attacks. Presymptomatic diagnosis also has the benefit that specific treatment can be started promptly if an attack does develop without delay while a diagnosis is sought. Though attacks are very rare before puberty, children should be tested at as young an age as is practicable to ensure that their status is known by the time they reach puberty and to enable the very low risk for affected children to be further reduced. Counseling to reduce the risk of an acute attack should include comprehensive information about the disease, including specific advice to guide selection of safe drugs, and provision of jewelry or some other means to identify the individual as having an acute porphyria.

Nonacute Porphyrias

The nonacute porphyrias include PCT, CEP, and EPP.

Porphyria Cutanea Tarda

PCT is by far the most common porphyria.[38,41] The annual incidence of new cases in the United Kingdom is between 2 and 5 per million of the population.[41] The disease occurs at all ages in both sexes with onset usually during the fifth and sixth decades.

Clinical Features

Lesions on sun-exposed skin, particularly the backs of the hands, forearm, and face, are present in all patients. These lesions are identical to those seen in the other bullous porphyrias (Table 32-4). Increased mechanical fragility of the skin, with trivial trauma leading to erosions, is present in virtually all patients. Subepidermal bullae, hypertrichosis of the face, and patchy pigmentation are also common. Erosions and bullae heal slowly to leave atrophic scars, milia, and depigmented areas. Patchy or diffuse sclerodermatous changes are less common and, unlike the other skin lesions, may affect areas of the trunk that are not exposed to sun.

The skin lesions are often the first sign of underlying liver cell damage. Clinically, overt liver disease is uncommon, but minor alterations in biochemical tests of liver function are present in more than 50% of patients. Needle biopsy of the liver reveals hepatic siderosis in most patients, usually accompanied by minor histopathological abnormalities: mild fatty infiltration, focal necrosis of hepatocytes, and inflammation of portal tracts. Cirrhosis is unusual, being present in less than 15% of patients, but carries a high risk of hepatocellular carcinoma.

The combination of skin lesions with liver damage is strongly associated with alcohol abuse, estrogens, infection with hepatotropic viruses, particularly hepatitis C (HCV), and mutations in the hemochromatosis (HFE) gene.[14,38] Hepatic iron overload and at least one of the other associated factors are present in almost all patients. Between 8% and 79% of patients have antibodies to HCV, the prevalence being highest in the United States and southern Europe and lowest in Western Europe. About 20% of patients of Northern European descent are homozygous for the C282Y mutation in the HFE gene, but in spite of having the genotype of genetic hemochromatosis, very few show clinical evidence of iron overload. However, increased serum ferritin concentrations and other biochemical indicators of iron overload are common in PCT irrespective of the HFE genotype, suggesting that the origin of hepatic iron overload is multifactorial. PCT may also occur in association with other disorders, notably chronic renal failure, systemic lupus erythematosus, and hematological malignancies. In addition, rare cases of a PCT-like syndrome resulting from production of porphyrins by primary hepatic tumors have been described.[112]

Pathogenesis and Molecular Genetics

PCT results from a decrease in activity of UROD in the liver, which leads to overproduction of uroporphyrin and other carboxymethyl-substituted porphyrinogens. These autooxidize to porphyrins, which accumulate in the liver and skin where they act as photosensitizers and are excreted in urine and bile. Two main types of PCT can be identified by measurement of UROD activity in liver and extrahepatic tissue, and analysis of the UROD gene. About 80% of patients have the sporadic (type-I) form of PCT in which the enzyme defect is restricted to the liver, and the UROD gene appears to be normal. Typically, there is no family history of PCT, but rare cases are clustered in families (type-III PCT). The rest have familial (type-II) PCT. In this form, mutation of one UROD gene leads to half of normal UROD activity in all tissue, which is inherited in an autosomal dominant manner.[113] As with the other autosomal dominant porphyrias, clinical penetration of familial PCT is low and there is considerable allelic heterogeneity, with each of the more than 50 mutations described being present in only one or a few families. A rare variant of familial PCT, hepatoerythropoietic porphyria (HEP), in which UROD mutations, some of which have also been found in familial PCT, are present on both alleles, has been described.[38,41] PCT may also be caused by exposure to certain polyhalogenated aromatic hydrocarbons, such as hexachlorobenzene[23] and 2,3,7,8-tetrachlorodibenzo-p-dioxin.[38]

In families with familial PCT, half-normal enzyme activity is not by itself sufficient to cause clinically overt disease. Further inactivation of UROD in the liver seems to be required, and the process responsible for this inactivation appears also to be responsible for inactivation of hepatic UROD in sporadic PCT and in toxic PCT caused by chemicals.[38,44] The inactivation process decreases catalytic activity without impairing immunoreactivity, is iron dependent, and is reversible. Current evidence from experimental models of PCT suggests that UROD is inactivated by an inhibitor that is produced by iron-dependent oxidation of a substrate of the UROD reaction, possibly mediated by hepatic CYPs, particularly CYP1A2. The putative inhibitor has not yet been identified.

Treatment

In addition to protection of the skin from sunlight, there are two specific treatments for PCT: depletion of hepatic iron stores by repeated phlebotomy or other means, and low-dose oral chloroquine.[131] In patients with chronic renal failure and PCT, hepatic iron stores can be decreased by erythropoietin with or without phlebotomy.

Congenital Erythropoietic Porphyria

CEP is the least common but most severe of the cutaneous porphyrias.[53,147] The prevalence is less than one per million in the United Kingdom. This disorder is also known as Günther disease.

Clinical Features

The clinical features range in severity from hydrops fetalis with death in utero—through the onset in infancy of severe skin lesions with transfusion-dependent hemolytic anemia—to mild skin lesions, resembling PCT, that do not start until adult life. Late-onset cases may also develop in association with hematological malignancy, particularly myelodysplasia.[80]

Most patients present in early infancy. Blisters on skin exposed to the sun or other sources of ultraviolet A (UVA) radiation, and reddish-brown staining of diapers by urinary porphyrins, are common early signs. The skin lesions resemble those of PCT but are more severe and persistent throughout life. With age, progressive scarring, particularly if erosions become infected, and atrophic changes lead to photomutilation with erosions of the terminal phalanges; destruction of ears, nose, and eyelids; and alopecia. Accumulation of porphyrin in bone is visible as erythrodontia—brownish-red teeth that fluoresce in UVA light. The skin changes are usually accompanied by hemolytic anemia and splenomegaly. Hemolysis may be fully compensated or mild but, in some patients, anemia is severe enough to require repeated transfusion.

Molecular Pathology

CEP is an autosomal recessive disease. Patients are homoallelic or heteroallelic for mutations in the UROS gene that decrease UROS activity (Table 32-2). Decreased UROS activity leads to massive overproduction of uroporphyrinogen-I and other isomer-I series of porphyrins, mainly in the bone marrow. Porphyrins accumulate in erythrocytes, and their precursors are released into the plasma as these cells die.

Most patients are heteroallelic unless their parents are consanguineous. More than 30 separate mutations have been identified; C73R is at a mutation "hot spot" in the gene and has been found on 34% of alleles investigated to date. Genotype and/or phenotype comparisons show some correlation.[33] Patients who are homozygous for C73R have particularly severe disease; in compound heterozygotes, the effect of C73R is modified by the nature of the mutation on the other allele. Other mutations are associated with mild disease.

Treatment

Protection against sunlight and prevention of skin infections are essential. Sunscreen ointments may occasionally provide some benefit, but physical avoidance of UVA radiation is usually necessary. Hypertransfusion and activated charcoal to decrease the enterohepatic circulation of porphyrin, hydroxyurea, intravenous heme, and antioxidant preparations have also been used to suppress erythropoiesis and porphyrin formation or to ameliorate the effects of porphyrin accumulation but none has been shown to have a reliable, long-term effect.[33,53,147] Hemolytic anemia may require repeated transfusion and infusion of deferoxamine to prevent iron overload.

At present the only curative treatment is allogeneic bone marrow transplantation. Gene therapy by introduction of a normal UROS gene into the patient's hematopoietic stem cells remains under development.[147]

Erythropoietic Protoporphyria

EPP is characterized by life-long acute photosensitivity caused by accumulation of protoporphyrin-IX in the skin.[22,146] The absence of fragile skin, subepidermal bullae, and hypertrichosis distinguishes it clinically from all other cutaneous porphyrias.

Clinical Features

Patients present with acute photosensitivity, normally between the ages of 1 and 6, and both sexes are equally affected. Once a child within an EPP family reaches the age of 14, the risk of developing acute photosensitivity becomes very low. Onset during adult life is very rare; most cases have been associated with myelodysplasia.[2]

Exposure to sun is followed, usually within 5 to 30 minutes, by an intensely painful, burning, prickling, itching sensation in the skin, most frequently on the face and backs of the hands. Symptoms persist for several hours or occasionally days and are not relieved by shielding the skin from light. Patients characteristically seek relief by plunging their hands into water or covering their skin with wet towels. Young children may become very distressed by the pain. The skin may appear normal throughout although there is often erythema, which may be followed by edematous swelling with crusting. These changes usually subside within a few hours so that by the time the child reaches the physician there is nothing to be seen, and the episode may be dismissed as severe sunburn. Subsequent exposure to sunlight provokes a similar reaction. Recurrent episodes lead to chronic skin changes that are often minor and hard to detect. Typical lesions are shallow linear scars over the bridge of the nose and elsewhere on the face, and the skin may become thickened and waxy, especially over the knuckles. Symptoms tend to be more severe during spring and summer and may improve during pregnancy.

The most severe complication of EPP is progressive hepatic failure that is caused by accumulation of protoporphyrin in the liver.[22,146] About 20% of patients have abnormal biochemical tests of liver function, particularly increased aspartate aminotransferase, but only 2% to 5% of patients develop liver failure. EPP may also increase the risk of cholelithiasis, the formation of gallstones being promoted by high concentrations of protoporphyrin in the bile.

Clinically significant anemia is unusual. About 25% of patients have a mild, hypochromic, microcytic anemia, which may be accompanied by sideroblastic changes in erythroid precursor cells.

Molecular Pathology and Genetics

The primary biochemical abnormality in EPP is decreased *FECH* activity. Although this decrease is present in all tissue, the excess protoporphyrin is formed mainly in erythroid cells. Accumulation of protoporphyrin in the liver is the result of failure of the liver to excrete the increased load it receives from release of protoporphyrin from erythrocytes and their immediate precursors.

The mode of inheritance of EPP is complex but has recently been clarified by enzymatic and molecular studies of families.[63] Molecular analysis has identified more than 60 disabling mutations of the *FECH* gene that are inherited in EPP families in an autosomal dominant pattern. Within these families, *FECH* activities in patients with overt disease are lower than the half-normal activities in their asymptomatic relatives with the same mutation. Thus a decrease in *FECH* activity to less than 50% of normal appears to be essential for development of sufficient overproduction of protoporphyrin to produce symptoms. In most families, this further decrease is produced by inheritance of a low expression *FECH* allele *trans* to the severe mutation.[63] The low expression allele is a polymorphic *FECH* variant present in about 10% of the Western European population. Substitution of a T nucleotide by a C nucleotide at a polymorphic site in intron 3 (IVS3-48C/T) enhances use of an alternative splice site, leading to increased formation of an unstable, untranslated mRNA and reduction of *FECH* expression by about 25%. This pattern of inheritance has been described as autosomal dominant with modulation by expression of the wild type of FECH allele.[63] Uncommon autosomal recessive cases of EPP have also been reported.[22]

At present, genetic analysis does not enable patients at risk from liver disease to be identified with certainty. Patients with null mutations or autosomal recessive disease may be at greater risk than those with missense mutations *trans* to a low expression allele.[107]

Treatment

Acute photosensitivity can be controlled by avoidance of sunlight, suitable clothing, and reflectant sunscreens, if these are cosmetically acceptable. Some patients are helped by production of a photoprotectant tan by measures such as narrowband ultraviolet B (UVB) phototherapy or dihydroxyacetone ointment. Oral β-carotene, which acts as a singlet oxygen quencher, is effective in some patients. Doses should be sufficient to maintain a plasma concentration of 6 to 8 μg/L.[146]

At present there is no reliable method for predicting liver failure in EPP. All patients should have at least annual biochemical tests of liver function. Persistent abnormalities should be investigated by liver biopsy and further treatment considered if even mild hepatocellular necrosis and fibrosis are present. Once liver failure develops, liver transplantation becomes the only treatment but protoporphyrin may reaccumulate in the transplanted liver.[70]

Abnormalities of Porphyrin Metabolism Not Caused by Porphyria

Abnormalities of porphyrin metabolism, excretion, or both may occur in the absence of porphyria caused by a number of other diseases that need to be considered when interpreting data from patients in whom porphyria is suspected.[9,45,69]

Lead Toxicity

Lead exposure increases urinary ALA and coproporphyrin-III excretion and causes accumulation of Zn-protoporphyrin in erythrocytes. The definitive test for lead toxicity is measurement of blood lead, but occasionally lead exposure is responsible for porphyria-like symptoms and may be an unexpected finding when investigating patients for suspected porphyria.[79]

Increased ALA excretion is secondary to inhibition of ALAD caused by lead displacing zinc at its catalytic center. Two isoenzymes (ALAD1 and ALAD2) are produced from the ALAD gene by alternative splicing activated by two non-translated codominant alleles 1 and 2.[78] The ALAD2 isoenzyme is more electronegatively charged than ALAD1 so that its affinity for lead is higher.[151] As a consequence, individuals with the ALAD2 genotype are more susceptible to lead toxicity.[140] Furthermore, individuals who are heterozygous for ALAD deficiency appear to be at increased risk from lead exposure.[37]

Lead also leads to the increased excretion of coproporphyrin-III in urine. CPO requires sulfhydryl groups for activity and so is potentially a target for inhibition by lead. The increased levels of red cell zinc-protoporphyrin (ZPP) associated with lead exposure are probably not caused by inhibition of *FECH* because inhibition of this enzyme requires higher lead concentrations than those usually encountered following lead exposure. The current view is that lead exposure creates an intracellular iron deficiency (perhaps by affecting iron transport into the cell or inhibition of iron reductase) so that zinc replaces iron as a substrate for *FECH*.[84] Once formed, erythrocyte ZPP remains elevated for the life of the red cell. Since the half-life of an erythrocyte is longer than that of blood lead, monitoring of lead workers requires both whole-blood lead and ZPP testing. ZPP measurement also has the advantage that there is no interference from lead contamination via the skin when the blood sample is collected, especially if a finger-prick sample is used.

Other Toxic Exposures

Secondary coproporphyrinuria has also been described because of the toxic effects of alcohol,[139] arsenic,[54] and other heavy metals.[156]

Hereditary Tyrosinemia Type-I

Succinylacetone, which accumulates in this disease, has a structural resemblance to ALA and is therefore a competitive inhibitor of ALAD.[134] Consequently, its substrate ALA accumulates and excess amounts are excreted in urine. Patients with hereditary tyrosinemia suffer neurological crises very similar to attacks of acute porphyria.[120] They can be treated with heme infusions.[121]

Renal Disorders

Impaired glomerular function reduces the clearance of those water-soluble porphyrins normally excreted in the urine. Furthermore, these porphyrins are poorly cleared by dialysis and, as a consequence, plasma porphyrins are raised in end-stage renal failure.[48]

Hepatobiliary Disorders

In obstructive jaundice, cholestatic jaundice, hepatitis, and cirrhosis there is an increased excretion of predominantly coproporphyrin-I, because liver disease causes a diversion of the secretion of coproporphyrin-I from the biliary to the renal route.[36,124]

In the Dubin-Johnson syndrome there is increased urinary excretion of coproporphyrin-I and a reduced excretion of coproporphyrin-III.[50,82] In Rotor's syndrome, urinary excretion of coproporphyrin-I is increased with normal coproporphyrin-III excretion,[50,154] and in Gilbert's disease there is increased urinary excretion of both isomers.

Hematological Disorders

In iron deficiency anemia, zinc acts as an alternative substrate for FECH, leading to increased ZPP. Increased red cell protoporphyrin (mostly ZPP) may also occur in sideroblastic, megaloblastic, and hemolytic anemias.[100]

Diet, Bacteria, and Gastrointestinal Bleeding

The dicarboxylic porphyrin fraction of feces contains protoporphyrin and other dicarboxylic porphyrins derived from it by bacterial reduction or removal of vinyl side groups. Additional protoporphyrin and other dicarboxylic porphyrins may be formed by the action of gut flora on heme-containing proteins derived from the diet or gastrointestinal hemorrhage.[6,126] Even minor gastrointestinal hemorrhage, particularly if occurring high in the gut, which may not give rise to a positive occult blood test, can markedly increase the concentration of dicarboxylic porphyrins in feces.[142] Confusion with EPP may occur when associated iron deficiency increases erythrocyte total porphyrin and when skin lesions from some other cause are present, or with VP when coexisting liver disease causes coproporphyrinuria. Porphyria can be excluded when no porphyrin fluorescence is detectable on fluorescence emission spectroscopy of plasma. Porphyrins may also come directly from the diet and there is one report of consumption of brewer's yeast producing a fecal porphyrin profile indistinguishable from VP.[91]

PSEUDOPORPHYRIA

The term "pseudoporphyria" was originally applied to patients with PCT-like skin lesions in whom no abnormality of accumulation or excretion of porphyrins could be demonstrated.[65,67] Many drugs are potent photosensitizers and may produce porphyria-like lesions.[65] Plasma porphyrin concentrations are often raised in dialysis patients without porphyria because of impaired excretion of these molecules and inefficient clearance by dialysis.[48] Even in the absence of biochemical evidence of porphyria, dermatological problems commonly affect dialysis patients and often share common features of PCT (melanosis, actinic elastosis, fragility, and bullae).[59,137] The levels of plasma porphyrin seen in dialysis patients are often much higher than normal but rarely approach those found in patients with active skin lesions caused by PCT.[60] Nevertheless, the term "dialysis porphyria" has been coined for these patients even though it is unlikely that raised porphyrins are responsible for the skin lesions. Genuine PCT may occur in dialysis patients, and some of the cases of dialysis porphyria in the literature have not been adequately investigated to exclude PCT. These patients are often anuric, and without the benefit of urinary analysis, careful evaluation of plasma and fecal porphyrins[60] is necessary to distinguish pseudoporphyria from PCT and acute porphyrias in which skin lesions may occur.

LABORATORY DIAGNOSIS OF PORPHYRIA

A number of clinical situations exist that benefit from laboratory testing for heme precursors. These include patients with symptoms of acute porphyria, typical cutaneous lesions, and relatives of patients known to have porphyria.

PATIENTS WITH SYMPTOMS OF PORPHYRIA

The clinical features of the porphyrias are insufficiently specific to enable their diagnosis without laboratory investigation. In patients with current symptoms caused by porphyria, it is always possible to demonstrate excessive production of heme precursors. Diagnosis depends on demonstrating specific patterns of overproduction of heme precursors (Table 32-5) and is usually straightforward provided appropriate specimens are examined for the relevant intermediates using adequately sensitive techniques.[11,29,45,144] Acute attacks of porphyria are always associated with excess excretion of PBG, ALA, or both. Patients having cutaneous symptoms caused by porphyria always have an excessive production of porphyrins. DNA and enzyme studies give no information about disease activity, are rarely necessary to confirm the diagnosis in clinically overt porphyria, and are mainly of use for family studies.

Patients With Acute Neurovisceral Symptoms

Three strategies exist when testing patients with acute neurovisceral symptoms that depend on the clinical setting: (1) investigating the acute attack, (2) diagnosing the cause, and (3) investigating possible acute porphyria when the patient is in remission.

Investigation During a Suspected Acute Attack

The one essential investigation in patients with suspected acute porphyria is an adequately sensitive test for excess urinary PBG.[8,29] Failure to correctly diagnose an attack of acute porphyria not only delays appropriate life-saving treatment but may result in the patient being subjected to the risk of unnecessary surgery or administration of porphyrinogenic drugs, which may further aggravate the attack with potentially fatal consequences. On the other hand, a false diagnosis of porphyria may be just as serious by delaying vital surgery or other treatment and may also lead to analgesic (including opiate) misuse and dependency.

Measurement of urinary total porphyrin by itself is unhelpful and may be misleading. Concentrations are usually increased when PBG is present in excess, owing to in vitro polymerization of PBG to uroporphyrin. But increases in hepatobiliary disease, alcohol abuse, and other disorders are common.[69,100] During an attack, PBG excretion is grossly elevated, and the increase is usually in excess of 10 times the upper reference limit. Normal PBG, at a time when symptoms are present, excludes all acute porphyrias, except the very rare ADP, as their cause. In AIP, PBG usually remains elevated for weeks or even months after an attack. However, in VP or HCP, PBG may rapidly return to normal (sometimes within days) once the attack starts to resolve. Therefore if a suspected attack is entering remission or if clinical suspicion of acute porphyria persists, analysis of fecal and plasma porphyrins, with measurement of ALA if these are normal, is advisable even if PBG excretion is normal. Increased urinary PBG requires careful evaluation, since although the patient clearly has an acute porphyria, the disease may not be the cause of current symptoms. Some patients with AIP have very high rates of PBG excretion in the absence of symptoms, and there is poor correlation between urinary PBG and symptoms, with no "threshold" above which symptoms appear. PBG excretion increases during an acute attack, but detection of this change requires information about the patient's baseline excretion. Even though a high urinary PBG excretion increases the likelihood that porphyria is responsible for symptoms, the final diagnosis must always be made on clinical grounds.

If increased urinary PBG was found by a qualitative and/or semiquantitative screening test, then this finding must be confirmed by a specific, quantitative method to eliminate the possibility of a false-positive test result.[98] This is best done on the original urine specimen (ideally stored frozen) since by the time a repeat is obtained, PBG may have returned to normal.

Testing for ALA is often performed along with PBG. Both are typically elevated in the acute porphyrias, although ALA is increased to a lesser extent. Inclusion of ALA allows lead poisoning and ADP to be detected, but the risk of missing these conditions is very low if total urinary porphyrin is measured in addition to PBG. Furthermore, measurement of ALA is more susceptible to interference.[81]

Differentiation Between the Acute Porphyrias

The management of the attack is the same regardless of the type of porphyria, so further investigation is not a matter of urgency. Differentiation between the acute porphyrias is essential for the selection of appropriate tests to use for family studies; the absence of skin lesions does not exclude VP or HCP (Table 32-4). If total fecal porphyrin is normal, then VP and HCP are excluded and the patient must have AIP. Assay of red cell HMBS activity is not essential and may mislead. If total fecal porphyrin is raised, porphyrins should be fractionated by a high-performance liquid chromatography (HPLC) technique capable of resolving coproporphyrin isomers.[90] In HCP, coproporphyrin-III is grossly elevated and protoporphyrin-IX minimally raised or normal. In VP, protoporphyrin-IX (and other dicarboxylate porphyrins) are raised, and there is a smaller increase in coproporphyrin (with the type-III isomer predominating) (Table 32-5). It is important to remember that protoporphyrin-IX and other dicarboxylate porphyrins may arise by the action of gut flora on heme[6] (whether the heme is of dietary origin or the result of gastrointestinal bleeding) and directly from the diet. There has been a report of excess consumption of brewer's yeast resulting in a fecal porphyrin profile indistinguishable from VP.[91] Therefore if the fecal porphyrin pattern resembles VP, plasma should be examined by fluorescence emission spectroscopy for the characteristic fluorescence maximum at 624 to 628 nm (Table 32-5).[117] If the fecal porphyrins (supplemented by plasma fluorescence emission spectroscopy) do not confirm VP or HCP (i.e., the raised fecal porphyrins are of dietary origin) then again the patient must have AIP. Assay of leukocyte coproporphyrinogen oxidase or protoporphyrinogen oxidase (the enzymes deficient in HCP and VP, respectively) is technically difficult, unnecessary, and may mislead. Analysis of urinary porphyrins is unhelpful in differentiating between the acute porphyrias.

Investigation During Clinical Remission

Sometimes the laboratory is asked to make a retrospective diagnosis of porphyria after the patient has fully recovered from an attack or as the cause of a chronic neuropsychiatric disorder some time after the onset of the illness. The first step is to quantify urinary PBG: screening tests are too insensitive for this purpose. Fecal porphyrin is measured (to exclude HCP) and plasma fluorescence emission spectroscopy performed (to exclude VP). If all of these tests are negative, it is very unlikely that symptoms are and/or were due to porphyria. However, it is difficult to exclude porphyria after long periods (i.e., several years) of clinical remission. Depending upon the degree of clinical suggestion, enzyme and DNA studies may be pursued but are often unrewarding.

Patients With Cutaneous Symptoms

The skin lesions of the cutaneous porphyrias are always accompanied by overproduction of porphyrins. The route of investigation should be dictated by the clinical presentation (Table 32-4).

Patients Complaining of Acute Photosensitivity

For suspected EPP, the essential investigation is measurement of whole blood (or erythrocyte) porphyrin using a sensitive fluorometric method. Screening tests using solvent extraction of blood or fluorescence microscopy of erythrocytes[123] are unreliable and should not be used.[27] If the erythrocyte and/or whole blood porphyrin concentration is within normal limits, EPP is excluded. If the concentration is increased, it is important to determine whether the increase is caused by free protoporphyrin, as in EPP, or ZPP, as in iron deficiency and lead toxicity. This requires extraction with a neutral solvent, such as ethanol[55] or acetone,[68] to prevent the demetalation caused by strong acids, followed by fluorescence spectroscopy or HPLC to distinguish free protoporphyrin from ZPP (fluorescence emission maxima 630 nm and 587 nm, respectively). Measurement of fecal protoporphyrin has no place in the diagnosis of EPP. Even if raised, erythrocyte porphyrin analysis is essential to exclude an increase caused by the action of gut flora on heme from the diet or from gastrointestinal bleeding.

Patients With Bullae/Fragility/Scarring

There are four main porphyrias in which clinically indistinguishable skin lesions occur (Table 32-4). The porphyrins that accumulate vary in solubility, and therefore testing both urine and feces is useful. Total urinary and fecal porphyrin should be measured by a spectrophotometric[8,27] or fluorometric[8] method, with adequate sensitivity and plasma porphyrins determined by fluorescence emission spectroscopy.[25,58] In practice, fecal analysis is often unnecessary because the two most common bullous porphyrias, PCT and VP, can be identified by analysis of urine and plasma (Table 32-5). If these tests are normal, then porphyria is excluded as the cause of any active skin lesions. Any increase in total urinary or fecal porphyrin should be further investigated by determination of individual porphyrins using a technique capable of resolving all porphyrins of clinical interest—including isomers.[90] Older separation methods based on solvent fractionation are unreliable.[30] The pattern observed in each of these porphyrias is unique (Table 32-5).

In PCT, excretion and plasma porphyrin concentrations return to normal during remission, with the proportions of individual porphyrins in urine and feces remaining abnormal for longer than total porphyrin concentrations. Thus in a patient whose skin lesions have healed, and whose total urinary and fecal porphyrin concentrations are normal, determination of individual porphyrins may reveal the diagnosis. The plasma fluorescence scan in VP and fecal coproporphyrin-III excretion in HCP remain abnormal for many years after clinical remission.

Relatives of Patients With Porphyria

Depending on the type of porphyria, screening relatives may be indicated.

Presymptomatic Diagnosis of Autosomal Dominant Acute Porphyrias

Screening family members to identify asymptomatic individuals who have inherited AIP, VP, or HCP, and are therefore at risk for acute attacks, is an essential part of management of families with these disorders. Screening may be carried out by metabolite measurement, enzyme assay, DNA analysis, or a combination of these approaches. The most sensitive metabolite assays for the presymptomatic diagnosis of each disorder are listed in Table 32-7.[7,71,77,93] These tests are almost always normal before puberty and therefore are not suitable for the investigation of children. In addition, urinary PBG excretion in AIP and the plasma fluorescence scan in VP may often be normal in asymptomatic adults shown by DNA analysis to be affected (Table 32-7). Measurement of the activity of the defective enzyme is more sensitive, but both sensitivity and specificity are limited by the overlap between activities in disease and in the normal population.[42,77,89] Erythrocyte HMBS assay is widely used for the presymptomatic diagnosis of AIP.[77]

Mutation detection by DNA analysis is specific and much more sensitive than biochemical methods.[42,52,77,89,120] It is therefore fast replacing other methods, particularly since it has the additional advantage of enabling asymptomatic disease to be excluded with certainty. However, it depends on prior identification of a disease-specific mutation in the family under investigation. In the 5% or so of families in which a mutation cannot be identified, gene tracking using intragenic single nucleotide polymorphisms (SNPs) may be helpful but requires at least two unequivocally affected family members.[35]

Other Porphyrias

Family investigation has a more limited role in the clinical management of other porphyrias. In PCT, the autosomal dominant familial form can be identified by erythrocyte UROD assay[108] or mutational analysis,[21,41] but there is as yet no evidence that family studies are necessary unless requested by anxious relatives.[40] However, patients of Northern European origin should be tested for the C282Y mutation in the hemochromatosis (*HFE*) gene and the families of homozygotes investigated for hemochromatosis. In EPP, testing the unaffected parent for the presence of the IVS3-48C low expression *FECH* allele is helpful for assessing the risk that a future child will have clinically overt disease.[63] Asymptomatic individuals from EPP families may wish to know whether they have inherited a severe *FECH* mutation, and thus have the potential to transmit the disease. FECH assay and/or mutation identification is required for this purpose[63,103]; erythrocyte protoporphyrin concentrations are rarely unequivocally abnormal in such individuals.

In the autosomal recessive porphyrias, CEP and ADP, screening families for asymptomatic carriers is not normally helpful, because the low carrier frequency in the general population makes the risk of transmission to the next generation very low. For severe homozygous or compound heterozygous porphyrias, such as CEP, ADP, HEP, and homozygous AIP, prenatal diagnosis may be indicated and has been reported for CEP[56] and HEP.[57]

ANALYTICAL METHODS

The analytical methods used in conjunction with porphyrias are described here briefly. Full descriptions are available on this book's accompanying Evolve site, found at http://evolve.elsevier.com/Tietz/textbook/.

Methods for Metabolites

The metabolite methods include those for ALA, PBG, and urinary, fecal, plasma, and blood porphyrins.

TABLE 32-7 Presymptomatic Diagnosis of Autosomal Dominant Acute Porphyrias: Metabolite Measurements in Asymptomatic Individuals With Porphyria Proven by Mutational Analysis

Porphyria	Metabolite	No. Individuals	Sensitivity	Specificity
AIP	Urine PBG*	84†	43%	100%
HCP	Fecal copro isomer I/III ratio†	11‡	64%	100%
VP	Plasma porphyrin fluorescence	109†	62%	100%

*Greater than 10.2 μmol/L.
†Aged 15 years or more.
‡Aged 7 years or more.

Specimen Collection and Stability

All samples must be protected from light; urinary porphyrin concentrations can decrease by up to 50% if kept in the light for 24 hours. Urinary porphyrins and PBG are best analyzed in fresh, random (10 to 20 mL) samples collected without preservative. Very dilute urine (creatinine less than 4 mmol/L) is unsuitable for analysis.

Although, with the exception of CEP, urine is often of normal color in the nonacute porphyrias, during the acute attack urine may be a reddish color because of the nonenzymatic condensation of PBG to uroporphyrins and other pigments.

Twenty-four-hour collections offer little advantage, delay diagnosis, and increase the risk of losses during the collection period. PBG and porphyrins are stable in urine in the dark at 4 °C for up to 48 hours and for at least a month at −20 °C. Specimens for ALA estimation should be promptly refrigerated. Urine specimens can be stored at 4 °C in the dark for at least 2 weeks without significant loss of ALA,[125] and frozen specimens are stable for weeks.[12] Whereas PBG is more stable around pH 8 to 9, ALA is more stable around pH 3 to 4, although more acidic environments notably reduce ALA stability.

About 5 to 10 g wet weight of feces is adequate for porphyrin measurements. Diagnostically, important changes in concentration are unlikely to occur with 36 hours at room temperature and samples are stable for many months at −20 °C.

Blood, anticoagulated with ethylenediaminetetraacetic acid (EDTA), shows no loss of protoporphyrin for up to 8 days at room temperature and for at least 8 weeks at 4 °C in the dark.

Available Methods for Porphyrin Precursors

PBG and ALA are water soluble and concentrate in the urine, and are therefore measured almost exclusively in the urine in the clinical laboratory. PBG is in general the more important of the precursors, whereas ALA is used more as a supplemental test.

Porphobilinogen

Most methods for PBG are based on the reaction of Ehrlich's reagent (dimethylaminobenzaldehyde in acidic solution) with the α-methene carbon of the pyrrole ring to form a colored product variously described as "rose red" or "magenta," which has a characteristic absorption spectrum with a peak at 553 nm and a shoulder at 540 nm. Porphyrins do not contain any α-methene hydrogens and so do not react. Some other substances in urine either react with the reagent to give red products, notably urobilinogen, inhibit the reaction, or are pigmented themselves and so mask the red chromogen.[25,160] All need to be removed. This is best achieved by ion-exchange chromatography (first described by Mauzerall and Granick[98]) but methods for accurate quantification of PBG based on this procedure are time consuming. More sensitive methods based on HPLC[76] and tandem-mass spectrophotometry (MS)[49] are available.

Qualitative screening tests in which urine is reacted directly with Ehrlich's reagent and assessed visually for the formation of the red chromogen (e.g., the Watson-Schwartz[150] and Hoesch[87] tests) are convenient but have been criticized for poor detection limits and interferences, even when solvent extraction has been used to separate the PBG-Ehrlich compound from the urobilinogen-Ehrlich complex.[16,17,27,135]

The Mauzerall-Granick method has been modified in attempts to produce an alternative that is acceptable for screening purposes. Buttery et al[18,19] avoided the use of columns by employing batchwise treatment with resin, and visually compared the final color with that of a surrogate calibrator. Blake et al[8] eliminated the centrifugation steps by using resin-filled syringes with detachable filters and compared the final color with a range of artificial calibrators. These modifications reduced the time taken to perform the test to 10 minutes and produced a semiquantitative result. A commercial kit based on Blake's method is available (Trace PBG Kit; Alpha Laboratories, Eastleigh, Hampshire, UK) and appears to be more analytically sensitive and specific for initial screening than qualitative, solvent extraction procedures.[32] A 2002 innovation uses resin-filled nylon sacs.[61]

If a qualitative screening test is used, it is essential to include appropriate controls and confirm all positive test results using a specific quantitative method.[29]

5-Aminolevulinic Acid

ALA can be measured directly[62] but is converted more usually into an Ehrlich's-reacting pyrrole by condensation with a reagent such as acetylacetone after separation from PBG by two-stage anion exchange chromatography. A method for the measurement of PBG and ALA, based on that of Mauzerall and Granick, is available commercially (Bio-Rad Laboratories, Hercules, Calif.). An alternative photometric method has been proposed[20] for more rapid testing.

Compared with PBG procedures, interferences are much more common with ALA. For example, the acetylacetone derivatization step can form a compound with penicillin that reacts with Ehrlich's reagent.[81]

Method for the Determination of Porphobilinogen in Urine

The PBG procedure described on the Evolve site that accompanies this book uses commercially available ion-exchange columns, but some laboratories might prefer to prepare an ion-exchange resin themselves.[18,19,135] PBG in the resin eluate reacts with Ehrlich's reagent to form a colored product that is scanned in a spectrometer.

Reference intervals are given in Table 32-3. Scanning the spectrum of the product is essential if interferences are to be identified. Imipenem, for example, often gives a peak at 580 nm with Ehrlich's reagent.[148] The coefficient of variation at the cutoff of 9 μmol/L is approximately ± 10%, but becomes considerably less precise at lower concentrations. For this reason, very dilute urines (creatinine <1.5 μmol/L) are unsuitable.

Urinary PBG that is raised at least 2 to 3 times the upper reference limit is diagnostic of an acute porphyria. However, porphyria is not necessarily the cause of symptoms (see discussion in the section on investigation of acute porphyria). Further investigation is necessary to identify the type of porphyria. Normal PBG excretion in the presence of symptoms provides very strong evidence against those symptoms being caused by acute porphyria.

Analysis of Porphyrins in Urine and Feces

Methods for porphyrin fractionation are complex and time consuming and not available in every laboratory. For this reason, simple qualitative screening tests are often used to exclude the majority of specimens that do not require further investigation from the few that justify fractionation of the individual porphyrins. Screening tests in which extracts of urine or feces are examined visually for typical red-pink fluorescence of porphyrins lack sensitivity and should not be used.[27] Methods based on spectrophotometric scanning of acidified urine or fecal extracts for the presence of the Soret band are recommended and yield semiquantitative information.[29] Quantitative fluorometric methods are also available.[8]

All methods for the fractionation of porphyrins are based on the different solubilities of individual porphyrins caused by their different β-substituents and to a lesser extent on the substituent order around the macrocycle. Thus methods include differential extraction with solvents, paper and thin layer chromatography, and HPLC.[45,129] Solvent extraction methods should not be used, because they yield only limited and sometimes misleading information.[30] Reversed-phase HPLC is the current method of choice and separates all porphyrins of clinical interest, including isomers and metal chelates, without the need for prior methylation.[5,75,124] Spectrophotometric or fluorometric detection can be used; the latter has superior sensitivity and specificity is preferred.

Semiquantitative Method for Total Porphyrin in Urine

This simple method for total urine porphyrins uses scanning spectrometry and is described fully on the Evolve site that accompanies this book A typical spectrum is shown in Figure 32-3.

Reference values are given in Table 32-3. The method is reproducible but only semiquantitative. The detection limit depends on the amount of background absorbance but concentrations of approximately 50 nmol/L should be detected in urine of normal color. Ideally, concentrations should be expressed as a ratio to creatinine concentration to correct for urine concentration.

Very occasionally, urine contains substances that produce a very high background absorbance, making identification of any peak in the 400-nm region difficult. Such samples require analysis by alternative methods, such as HPLC.

Increased concentrations require further investigation to identify individual porphyrins; porphyria should not be diagnosed on the basis of increased total porphyrin alone.

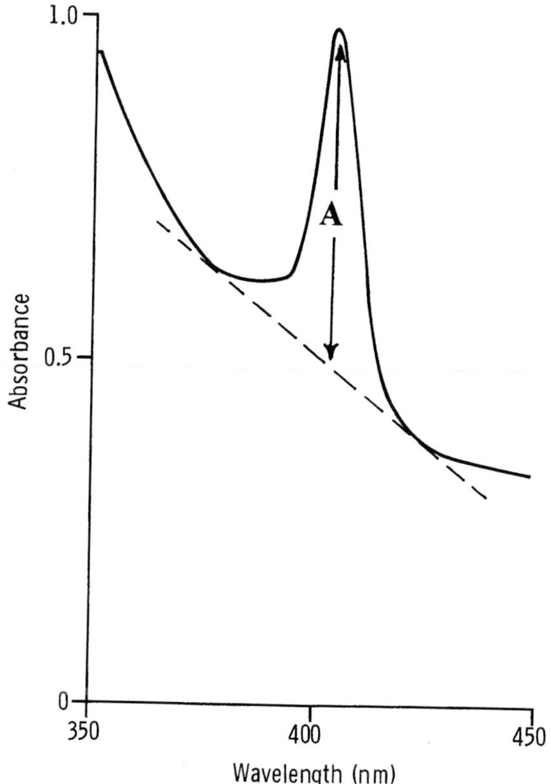

Figure 32-3 Absorption spectrum of acidified urine showing the procedure for the measurement of corrected absorbance *(A)* of the porphyrin peak.

Semiquantitative Method for Total Porphyrin in Feces

This simple method for total fecal porphyrins uses scanning spectrometry after extraction[26,92] and is described fully on the Evolve site that accompanies this book.

Reference values are given in Table 32-3. The expression of concentration on a dry weight basis corrects for the moisture content of feces. Total fecal porphyrin determined by this method, unlike most tests based on solvent extraction, includes uroporphyrin.[127]

Very occasionally, feces contain substances that produce a very high background absorbance, making identification of any peak in the 400-nm region difficult. Such samples require analysis by alternative methods, such as HPLC.

Increased total fecal porphyrin concentration requires further investigation by fractionation, identification, and quantification of individual porphyrins using a technique, such as HPLC, that resolves coproporphyrin I and III isomers. Porphyria should never be diagnosed on the basis of raised total fecal porphyrin alone.

HPLC Fractionation of Porphyrins in Urine and Feces

This complex method for urine and fecal porphyrins uses sample preparation, HPLC separation, and fluorometric detection.[122] It is described in detail on the Evolve site that accompanies this book. The samples are assayed with and without addition of calibrator to assist with fluorometric peak identification.

Figure 32-4 shows typical profiles from patients with various types of porphyria.

In addition to the biosynthetic porphyrins, several isocoproporphyrins may be found in feces of patients with PCT,[39] some of which may not be completely resolved.

For diagnostic purposes, quantification of individual porphyrins is rarely necessary, particularly if the concentrations are clearly elevated. Table 32-5 shows expected findings in the various types of porphyria, and reference values for individual porphyrin fractions are given in Table 32-3. There is considerable variation in the reference values quoted in the literature,[145] probably a consequence of the difficulties in calibration.

The extraction method for fecal porphyrins results in some interference with the chromatography caused by a proportion of the diethyl ether dissolving in the aqueous phase. As a result an extra peak elutes just before the uroporphyrin position. This peak contains any uroporphyrin in the sample, up to 50% of the heptacarboxylate porphyrins and smaller amounts of hexacarboxylate and pentacarboxylate porphyrins.

Methods for Blood Porphyrins

The methods described below require a spectrofluorometer fitted with a red-sensitive photomultiplier. If such equipment is not available locally, samples should be referred to a specialized laboratory because erythrocyte and plasma measurements are required rarely for the urgent assessment of acutely ill patients.

Determination of Erythrocyte Total Porphyrin

This method for erythrocyte total porphyrin uses double extraction and fluorometry.[8,114,115] It is described in detail on the Evolve site that accompanies this book.

Reference intervals are given in Table 32-3. Total erythrocyte porphyrin concentrations are increased in EPP, CEP, the rare homozygous variants of the autosomal dominant porphyrias, iron deficiency, hemolytic anemia, some other forms of anemia, and lead poisoning. A normal total porphyrin concentration excludes the diagnosis of EPP. Distinction between EPP and other causes of increased erythrocyte total porphyrin concentration requires differentiation between protoporphyrin and its zinc chelate because the acidic condition of this assay dissociates the zinc chelate and provides only a measure of total porphyrin.

Qualitative Determination of Zinc-Protoporphyrin and Protoporphyrin

This qualitative method for ZPP and protoporphyrin uses extraction and fluorometry.[55] It is described in detail on the Evolve site that accompanies this book.

Emission peaks for ZPP and free protoporphyrin are 587 nm and 630 nm, respectively. If the main peak is at 587 nm, EPP is excluded, whereas a pronounced predominance of the peak at 630 nm confirms the diagnosis of EPP (see Figure 32-5). With experience, this test can be used to screen for EPP without the necessity for quantitative analysis. It is possible to quantify both ZPP and protoporphyrin by measuring the peak heights at 587 nm and 630 nm above a constructed baseline if calibrator solutions of both protoporphyrins are prepared, providing allowance is made for a contribution of fluorescence from ZPP at the maximum for free protoporphyrin.[28] A limitation of this method is that the efficiency of the extraction of ZPP is only about 50%.[28]

Analysis of Plasma Porphyrins

Plasma porphyrins may be determined by fluorescence emission spectroscopy of saline-diluted plasma[25,58,117] or deproteinized extracts,[93] or by HPLC.[73] The first of these methods has the advantages of simplicity and including porphyrins that are bound covalently to plasma proteins and is detailed below.

Fluorescence Emission Spectroscopy of Plasma Porphyrins

This method detects the fluorescent emission of plasma porphyrins when excited at 405 nm.[58,117] It is described in detail on the Evolve site that accompanies this book.

Figure 32-6 shows typical fluorescence emission maximum wavelengths for the cutaneous porphyrias. The plasma in VP contains porphyrin covalently bound to protein with a fluorescence emission maximum at 624 to 628 nm.[117] In other porphyrias, porphyrin is noncovalently bound to albumin and hemopexin.[83] A normal fluorescence emission scan in plasma from a patient with clinically active skin lesions excludes all cutaneous porphyrias as their cause.[31,58] The scan may become normal in PCT and HCP as skin lesions heal, and the diagnosis may be missed unless individual porphyrins are also measured in urine and feces from such patients. In addition, the scan may be abnormal during an acute attack of AIP or HCP in the absence of skin lesions and is always abnormal in clinically manifest VP, whether skin lesions are present or not (Table 32-5).

The plasma porphyrin concentration may be increased in conditions in which porphyrin excretion is impaired, such as renal failure and cholestasis. Although plasma porphyrin concentrations are usually higher in chronic renal failure with PCT than in renal failure alone,[116] unequivocal diagnosis of PCT in this situation is best achieved by fecal porphyrin analysis[60] or fractionation of plasma porphyrins by HPLC.[73]

Enzyme Measurements

Assay of the individual enzymes of the heme biosynthetic pathway is rarely required for the investigation of patients with symptoms of porphyria. However, measurement of enzyme activities is useful for family studies when the individual mutation cannot be identified or when DNA analysis is not available, and for the identification of subtypes such

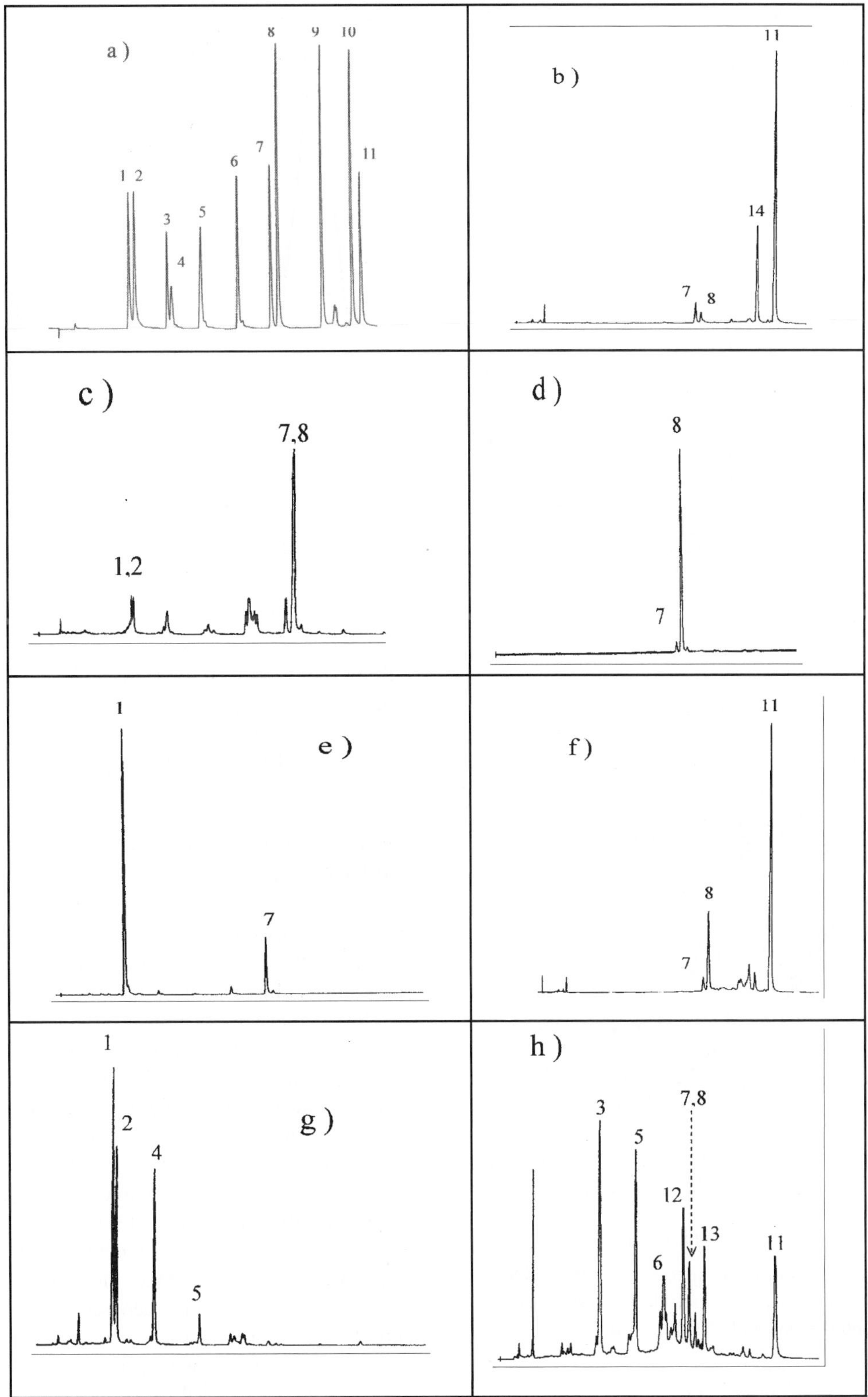

Figure 32-4 Representative HPLC chromatograms for *(a)* working standard; *b,* normal feces; *c,* normal urine; *d,* feces—hereditary coproporphyria; *e,* urine—congenital erythropoietic porphyria; *f,* feces—variegata porphyria; *g,* urine—porphyria cutanea tarda; and *h,* feces—porphyria cutanea tarda chromatographic conditions as described in the appendix on the Evolve site that accompanies this book. Peaks are: *1,* uroporphyrin-I; *2,* uroporphyrin-III; *3,* heptacarboxylate porphyrin-I; *4,* heptacarboxylate porphyrin-III; *5,* hexacarboxylate porphyrin; *6,* pentacarboxylate porphyrin; *7,* coproporphyrin-I; *8,* coproporphyrin-III; *9,* deuteroporphyrin-IX; *10,* mesoporphyrin-IX; *11,* protoporphyrin-IX; *12,* hydroxyisocoproporphyrin; *13,* isocoproporphyrin; *14,* pemptoporphyrin-IX.

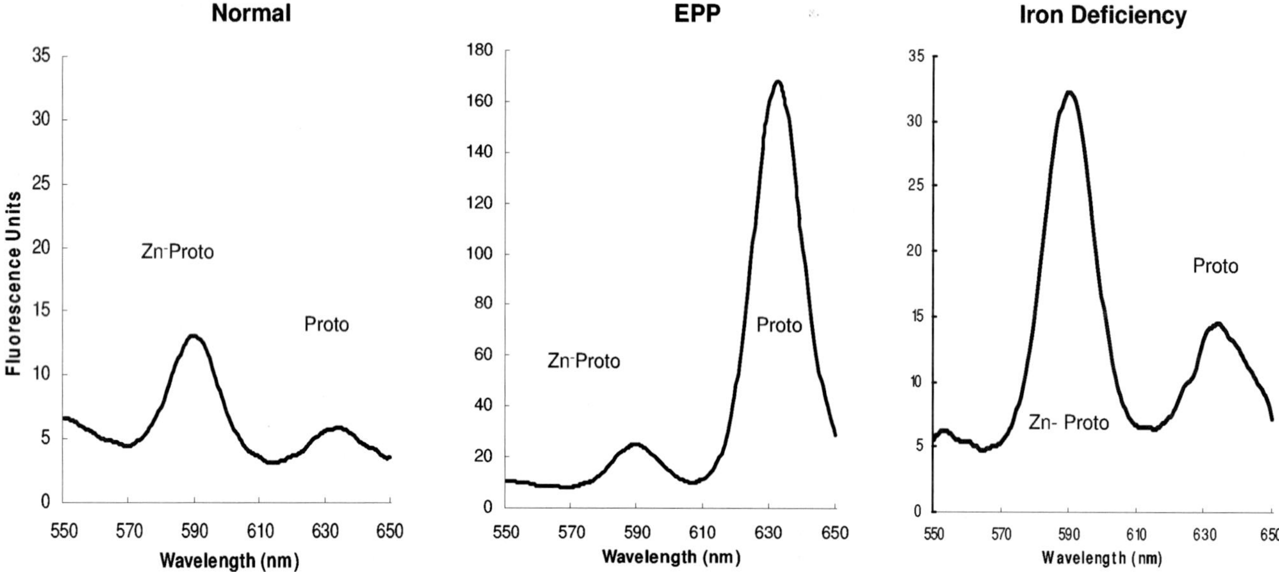

Figure 32-5 Fluorescence emission spectra (excitation at 405 nm) of ethanolic extracts of erythrocytes from a normal individual and patients with EPP or iron deficiency. Note that different scales are used.

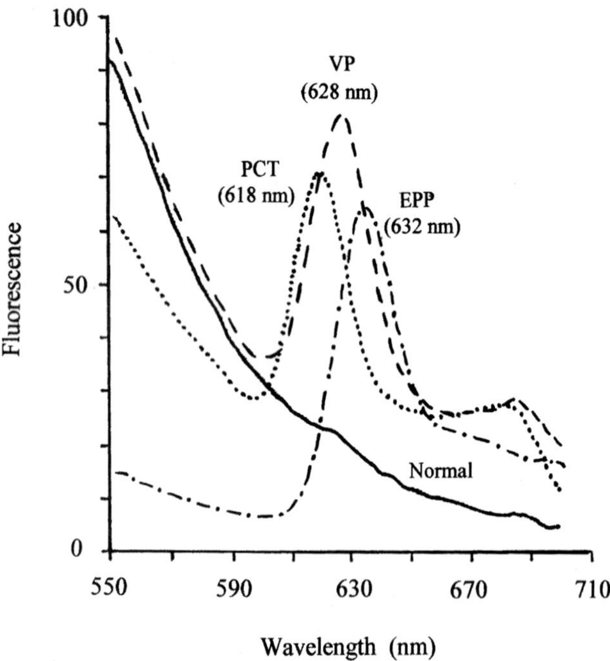

Figure 32-6 Fluorescence emission spectra (excitation 405 nm) of dilutions in phosphate buffered saline (PBS) of plasma from a normal individual and patients with various porphyrias.

as nonerythroid AIP and "homozygous" forms of autosomal dominant porphyrias. Erythrocytes are a convenient source of cytoplasmic enzymes (ALAD, HMBS, UROS, and UROD)[33,46,56,133] but assay of the mitochondrial enzymes (CPO, PPOX, and FECH)[34,66,128] requires nucleated cells, such as leukocytes or cultured fibroblasts.[25] Assays for enzymes that use porphyrin*ogens* as substrates are particularly difficult because the substrate is unstable, has to be prepared in situ and, particularly with protoporphyrinogen, undergoes nonenzymatic oxidation during the assay. However, erythrocyte HMBS measurement is relatively straightforward and will be described in detail.

Assay of Erythrocyte Hydroxymethylbilane Synthase Activity

This enzymatic assay determines the amount of porphyrinogens formed from an excess of added PBG over the course of 30 minutes. It is described in detail on the Evolve site that accompanies this book.

The reference interval for this method[157] (mean ± 2 standard deviation [SD]) is 20 to 42 nmol uroporphyrin per milliliter of erythrocytes per minute at 37 °C.

HMBS activity is usually below the reference interval in AIP, except in the uncommon nonerythroid form; but there is overlap between activities in AIP and normal individuals.[120] After exclusion of families with nonerythroid AIP, HMBS activity has been reported to have a sensitivity of 84% and a specificity of 77% for detection of AIP in patients without symptoms.[52] In France the prevalence of abnormally low HMBS activities in the general population is about 1 in 800.[111]

For family studies, where the incidence of AIP is quite high, the predictive values of positive and negative test results are reasonable, and HMBS assay is helpful, although not foolproof, in assigning AIP status. In the general population, where the incidence of disease-specific mutations in the *HMBS* gene is in the order of 1 in 15,000, the predictive values are too low for the test to be of any value.

HMBS activity falls markedly as red cells age, so that any shift in their age distribution will be reflected in measured activity. Increased erythropoiesis may raise activity sufficiently to mask an inherited deficiency. Measurement of erythrocyte HMBS activity is therefore not reliable for the presymptomatic detection of AIP in subjects who are hematologically abnormal, have received a recent blood transfusion, or are less than 1 year old. Activity may also be increased in liver disease and in chronic alcohol abuse.

DNA Analysis

Screening families for porphyria by DNA analysis is a two-stage process. First, the mutation that causes porphyria in the family under investigation needs to be identified by analysis of DNA from a family member in whom the diagnosis of a specific type of porphyria has been established unequivocally. Second, that patient's relatives are then screened for the mutation. The first part of this process is the more complex. Because most mutations are restricted to one or a few families, identification of a mutation in a new family almost always requires analysis of the entire gene or at least all exons with their flanking intronic sequences and the promoter region. Initial testing for a single mutation is worthwhile only in those countries where founder mutations predominate, for example, VP in South Africa and AIP in Sweden.

Mutation Detection

Two main approaches are used to analyze a gene for the presence of a mutation (see also Chapter 37). The gene may either be screened to find the region that contains the mutation, and then only that region sequenced to identify the mutation, or all regions of the gene likely to contain the mutation may be sequenced directly. Prior screening considerably decreases the amount of sequencing that is required, but this is becoming a less important consideration as DNA sequencing becomes cheaper and more straightforward with development of ever better automated fluorescence sequencers.

Denaturing gradient gel electrophoresis (DGGE), single-strand conformational polymorphism (SSCP) analysis, heteroduplex analysis, and denaturing HPLC have all been used to screen the *HMBS* and other porphyria genes for mutations.* DGGE is currently the most widely used technique and is very sensitive† but requires gradient gels and polymerase chain reaction (PCR) primers with guanine cytosine (GC) extensions. Denaturing HPLC, though still requiring amplification of the gene in small fragments (about 500 bp), is rapid, simple, and robust. It has been shown to have high sensitivity for detection of mutations in many genes[159] and has the potential to replace DGGE as the method of choice.

Once the mutation that causes porphyria in a family has been identified, relatives are then screened for its presence either by using one of the screening methods listed above, by direct sequencing of the region containing the mutation, or by some other mutation-specific method (see Chapter 37).

A method for identifying mutations in the human *HMBS* gene by direct sequencing is described later in this chapter. The method can be adapted for other porphyria genes by using the appropriate amplification and sequencing primers. Primer sequences have been published for the *PPOX*,[151] *CPO*[102], *UROD*[103], *FECH*[107], and *UROS*[33] genes.

*References 21, 86, 102, 103, 110, 111, 120, 130, 136, 143, 151, 152.

†References 21, 110, 120, 130, 143, 151.

Mutation Analysis of the Human *HMBS* Gene by Direct Sequencing

PCR is used to amplify some of the exons of the *HMBS* gene, which are then sequenced using the Sanger method. If no mutations are found, the remaining exons and the 5′ intron are evaluated. If a mutation is found in an exon, it is re-sequenced in the reverse direction.

In a prospective study of 198 unrelated patients with proven AIP, this method detected a mutation in 97% of patients. Almost all mutations were detected by sequencing in one direction only; only rarely was sequencing in the opposite direction required to reveal an abnormality. Because amplified genomic DNA is sequenced directly, without subcloning, the risk of PCR artifacts is very low and is essentially eliminated by sequencing a new PCR product in the opposite direction to confirm each mutation. Complete gene deletions and large partial deletions that prevent the binding of primers are not detected by this method, because only the normal allele will be amplified for sequencing. Such deletions or mutations that lie outside the regions that are sequenced may explain the failure to find an abnormality in all patients.

In most countries, about one third of the mutations that are identified will not have been reported previously in AIP and may represent rare polymorphisms rather than disease-specific mutations. Criteria that suggest that such novel mutations cause disease include production of a frameshift or stop codon, the absence of any other sequence abnormality in the gene, segregation with disease, and nonconservative change of an amino acid residue that is conserved between species and/or known to have a functional role in catalysis. Mutations of consensus bases in splice sites are also likely to be disease specific, but ideally all putative splicing defects should be confirmed by analysis of mRNA. Proof that a missense mutation causes disease may require expression and characterization of the mutant enzyme in a prokaryotic or eukaryotic vector.

Identification of a Functional Polymorphism in *FECH* Gene

The method is described in detail on the Evolve site that accompanies this book. It tests for the presence of the IVS3-48C FECH allele. This allele causes decreased expression of FECH because substitution of the T nucleotide at IVS3-48 by a C nucleotide leads to enhanced use of an alternative splice site with increased formation of an unstable mRNA for FECH.[63]

The IVS3-48C allele is carried by about 12% of the Western European population. If it is not present in the partner of a patient with overt EPP, and they have not previously had a child with overt EPP, the risk that the couple will have a child with overt EPP is less than 1 in 50, whereas if it is present, the risk is about 1 in 4. Investigation for the presence of the IVS3-48C allele in the parents of a child with overt EPP is usually not helpful because in such families the risk of overt EPP in subsequent children is 1 in 4, irrespective of whether the unaffected partner carries the low expression allele. Testing a newborn child for the low expression allele may also be useful for predicting the child's risk of later developing symptoms.

RERERENCES

1. Anderson KE, Sassa S, Bishop DF, Desnick RJ. Disorders of heme biosynthesis: X-linked sideroblastic anemia and the porphyrias. In: Scriver CR, Beaudet AL, Sly WS and Valle D, eds. The metabolic and molecular basis of inherited disease, 8th ed. New York: McGraw-Hill, 2000:2961-3062.
2. Aplin C, Whatley SD, Thompson P, Hoy T, Fisher P, Singer C, et al. Late-onset erythropoietic porphyria caused by a chromosome 18q deletion in erythroid cells. J Invest Dermatol 2001;117:1647-9.
3. Battersby AR, Fookes CJ, Matcham GW, McDonald E. Biosynthesis of the pigments of life: formation of the macrocycle. Nature 1980;285:17-21.
4. Berk PD, Rodkey FL, Blaschke TF, Collison HA, Waggoner JG. Comparison of plasma bilirubin turnover and carbon monoxide production in man. J Lab Clin Med 1974;83:29-36.
5. Beukeveld GJJ, Nagel AW, de Ruyter-Buitenhuis AW, Kwarts EW, Wolthers BG. Determination of porphyrins in blood, urine and faeces by means of HPLC and its application to establishing porphyrias. Biochim Clin 1987;11:203-13.
6. Beukeveld GJ, Wolthers BG, van Saene JJ, de Haan TH, de Ruyter-Buitenhuis LW, van Saene RH. Patterns of porphyrin excretion in feces as determined by liquid chromatography; reference values and the effect of flora suppression. Clin Chem 1987;33:2164-70.
7. Blake D, McManus J, Cronin V, Ratnaike S. Fecal coproporphyrin isomers in hereditary coproporphyria. Clin Chem 1992;38:96-100.
8. Blake D, Poulos V, Rossi R. Diagnosis of porphyria—recommended methods for peripheral laboratories. Clinical Biochemical Reviews 1992;13(suppl 1):S1-24.
9. Bleiberg J, Wallew M, Brodkin K et al. Industrially acquired porphyria. Arch Dermatol 1964;89:793-7.
10. Bloom KE, Zaider MF, Morledge LJ, Poh-Fitzpatrick MB. Urinary porphyrin excretion in normal children and adults. Am J Kidney Dis 1991;18:483-9.
11. Bossenmailer I, Cardinal R. Stability of δ-aminolaevulinic acid and porphobilinogen in urine under varying conditions. Clin Chem 1968;14:610-4.
12. Bossenmailer I, Cardinal R. Stability of δ-aminolaevulinic acid and porphobilinogen in urine under varying conditions. Clin Chem 1968;14:610-4.
13. Brodie MJ, Moore MR, Thompson GG, Goldberg A. The treatment of acute intermittent porphyria with laevulose. Clin Sci Mol Med 1977;53:365-71.
14. Bulaj ZJ, Phillips JD, Ajioka RS, Frankilin MR, Griffen LM, Guinee DJ, et al. Hemochromatosis genes and other factors contributing to the pathogenesis of porphyria cutanea tarda. Blood 2000;95:1565-71.
15. Burnham BF. The chemistry of porphyrins. Semin Haematol 1968;5:296-322.
16. Buttery JE, Carrera AM, Pannall PR. Reliability of the porphobilinogen screening assay. Pathology 1990;22:197-8.
17. Buttery JE, Carrera AM, Panall PR. Analytical sensitivity and specificity of two screening methods for urinary porphobilinogen. Ann Clin Biochem 1990;27:165-6.
18. Buttery JE, Chamberlain BR, Beng CG. A sensitive method for screening for urinary porphobilinogen. Clin Chem 1989;35:2311-2.
19. Buttery JE, Stuart S. Measurement of porphobilinogen in urine by a simple resin method with use of a surrogate standard. Clin Chem 1991;37:2133-6.
20. Buttery JE, Stuart S, Panall PR. An improved direct method for the measurement of urinary δ-aminolaevulinic acid. Clin Biochem 1995;28:477-80.
21. Christiansen L, Ged C, Hombrados I, Brons-Poulsen J, Fontanellas A, de Verneuil H, et al. Screening for mutations in the uroporphyrinogen decarboxylase gene using denaturing gradient gel electrophoresis. Identification and characterization of six novel mutations associated with familial PCT. Hum Mutat 1999;14:222-32.
22. Cox TM. Protoporphyria. In: Kadish KM, Smith KM, Guilard R, eds. The porphyrin handbook, vol. 14, Medical aspects of porphyrias, Amsterdam: Academic Press, 2003:121-150.
23. Cripps DJ, Peters HA, Gocmen A, Dogrmici I. Porphyria turcica due to hexachlorobenzene—A 20 to 30 year follow-up study on 204 patients. Brit J Dermatol 1984;111:413-22.
24. Dailey HA. Enzymes of heme biosynthesis. J Biol Inorg Chem 1997;2:411-7.
25. De Rooij FWM, Edixhoven A, Wilson JHP. Porphyria: a diagnostic approach. In: Kadish KM, Smith KM, Guilard R, eds. The porphyrin handbook, vol. 14, Medical aspects of porphyrias, Amsterdam: Academic Press, 2003:211-46.
26. Deacon AC. Fecal porphyrin screening [Letter]. Clin Chem 1990;36:1383.
27. Deacon AC. Performance of screening tests for porphyria. Ann Clin Biochem 1998;25:392-7.
28. Deacon AC, Asadipour A, Peters TJ. Spectrofluorometric determination of erythrocyte protoporphyrins

[Abstract]. In: Association of Clinical Biochemists. Proceedings of the National Meeting—Focus '98, 1998:33.
29. Deacon AC, Elder GH. ACP Best Practice No 165. Front line tests for the investigation of suspected porphyria. J Clin Pathol 2001;54:500-7.
30. Deacon AC, Ledden JA. Limitations of solvent fractionation techniques for urinary and faecal porphyrins. Ann Clin Biochem 1998;35:314-6.
31. Deacon AC, Marsden TJ. Which front-line test for cutaneous porphyria? [Abstract]. In: Association of Clinical Biochemists: Proceedings of the National Meeting—Focus 2001, London 2001:35.
32. Deacon AC, Peters TJ. Identification of acute porphyria: evaluation of a commercial screening test for porphobilinogen. Ann Clin Biochem 1998;35: 726-32.
33. Desnick RJ, Aplin KH. Congenital erythropoietic porphyria: advances in pathogenesis and treatment. Br J Haematol 2002;117:779-95.
34. Deybach JC, Da Silva V, Nordman Y. The inherited enzymatic defect in porphyria variegate. Hum Genet 1981;58:425-8.
35. Deybach JC, Puy H. Acute intermittent porphyria: from clinical to molecular aspects. In: Kadish KM, Smith KM, Guilard R, eds. The porphyrin handbook, vol. 14, Medical aspects of porphyrias. Amsterdam: Academic Press, 2003:23-42.
36. Doss M, Tiepermann von R, Jendrychowsky A et al. Diagnostic significance of urinary coproporphyrin isomer analysis. In: Doss M, Nawroccki P., eds. Supplement to the proceedings of the I. International porphyrin meeting on porphyrins in human diseases. University of Marburg, 1975;1:257-63.
37. Dyer J, Garrick DP, Inglis A, Pye IF. Plumboporphyria (ALAD deficiency) in a lead worker: A scenario for potential diagnostic confusion. Brit J Industr Med 1993; 50:1119-21.
38. Elder GH. Porphyria cutanea tarda and related disorders. In: Kadish KM, Smith KM, Guilard R, eds. The porphyrin handbook, vol. 14, Medical aspects of porphyrias. Amsterdam: Academic Press, 2003:67-92.
39. Elder GH. Differentiation of porphyria cutanea tarda symptomatica from other types of porphyria by measurement of isocoproporphyrin in faeces. J Clin Pathol 1975;28:601-7.
40. Elder GH. Hepatic porphyrias in children. J Inherited Metabolic Dis 1997;20:237-46.
41. Elder GH. Porphyria cutanea tarda. Seminars in liver disease 1998;18:67-76.
42. Elder GH, Hift RJ, Meissner PN. The acute porphyrias. Lancet 1997;349:1613-7.
43. Elder GH, Hift RJ. Treatment of acute porphyria. Hosp Med 2001;62:422-8.
44. Elder GH, Roberts AG. Uroporphyrinogen decarboxylase. J Bioenerg Biomembr 1994;27:207-14.
45. Elder GH, Smith SG, Smyth SJ. Laboratory investigation of the porphyrias. Ann Clin Biochem 1990;27:395-412.
46. Elder GH, Wyvill PC. Measurement of uroporphyrinogen decarboxylase using porphyrinogens prepared by chemical reduction. Enzyme 1982;28:186-95.
47. Erskine PT, Senior A, Awan SJ, Lambert R, Lewis G, Tickle IJ, et al. X-ray structure of 5-aminolaevulinate dehydratase, a hybrid aldolase. Nature Struct Biol 1997;4:1025-31.
48. Fontanellas A, Coronel F, Santos JL, Herrero JA, Moran MJ, Guerra P, et al. Heme biosynthesis in uremic patients on CAPD or hemodialysis. Kidney Int 1994;45:220-3.
49. Ford RE, Magera MJ, Kloke KM, Chezick PA, Fauq A, McConnell JP. Quantitative measurement of porphobilinogen in urine by stable-isotope dilution liquid chromatography-tandem mass spectrometry. Clin Chem 2001;47:1627-32.
50. Frank M, Doss M, Carvalho DG. Diagnostic and pathogenetic implication of urinary coproporphyrin excretion in the Dubin-Johnson syndrome. Hepatogastroenterology 1990;37:147-51.
51. Fraser DJ, Podvinec M, Kaufmann MR, Meyer UA. Drugs mediate the transcriptional activation of 5-aminolaevulinic acid synthase (ALAS1) gene via the chicken xenobiotic-sensing nuclear receptor (CXR). J Biol Chem 2002;277:34717-26.
52. Fraunberg M von und zu, Timonen K, Mustajoki P, Kauppinen R. Clinical and biochemical characteristics and genotype-phenotype correlation in Finnish variegate porphyria patients. Eur J Hum Genet 2002;10:649-57.
53. Fritsch C, Bolsen K, Ruzicka T, Goerz G. Congenital erythropoietic porphyria. J Am Acad Dermatol 1997;36:594-610.
54. Garcia-Vargas GG. Urinary porphyrins and heme biosynthetic enzyme activities measured by HPLC in arsenic toxicity. Biomed Chormatogr 1996;10: 278-84.
55. Garden JS, Mitchell DG, Jackson KW. Improved ethanol extraction procedure for determining zinc protoporphyrin in whole blood. Clin Chem 1977;23:264-9.
56. Ged C, Morea-Gady I, Taire L et al. Prenatal diagnosis in congenital erythropoietic porphyria by metabolic measurement and DNA mutation analysis. Prenatal Diagnosis 1996;16:83-6.
57. Ged C, Ozalla D, Herrero C, Lecha M, Mendez M, de Verneuil H, et al. Description of a new mutation in hepatoerythropoietic porphyria and prenatal exclusion of a homozygous fetus. Arch Dermatol 2002;138:957-60.
58. Gibbs NK, Traynor N, Ferguson J. Biochemical diagnosis of the cutaneaous porphyrias: five years experi-

ence of plasma spectrofluorimetry. Brit J Dermatol 1995; 135(suppl 45):18.

59. Gibson GE, McGinnity E, McGrath PM, Carmody M, Walshe J, Donohoe J, et al. Cutaneous abnormalities and metabolic disturbance of porphyrins in patients on maintenance dialysis. Clin Exp Dermatol 1997;22:124-7.
60. Glynne P, Deacon AC, Goldsmith D, Pusey C, Clutterbuck E. Bullous dermatoses in end-stage renal failure: porphyria or pseudoporphyria? Am J Kidney Dis 1999;34:155-60.
61. Gorchein A. Testing for porphobilinogen in urine. Clin Chem 2002;48:564-6.
62. Gorchein A. Determination of delta-aminolaevulinic acid in biological fluids by gas-liquid chromatography with electron-capture detection. Biochem J 1984; 219:883-9.
63. Gouya L, Puy H, Robreau AM, Lamoril J, Da Silva V, Grandchamp B, et al. The penetrance of autosomal dominant erythropoietic protoporphyria is modulated by expression of wild type FECH. Nat Genet 2002;30:23-7.
64. Grandchamp B. Acute intermittent porphyria. Semin Liver Dis 1998;18:17-24.
65. Green JJ, Manders SM. Pseudoporphyria. J Am Acad Dermatol 2001;44:100-8.
66. Guo R, Lim CK, Peters TJ. Accurate and specific HPLC assay of coproporphyrinogen oxidase activity in human peripheral lymphocytes. Clin Chim Acta 1988;177:245-52.
67. Harber C, Bickers DR. Porphyria and pseudoporphyria. J Invest Dermatol 1984; 82:207-9.
68. Hart D, Piomelli S. Simultaneous quantitation of zinc protoporphyrin and free protoporphyrin in erythrocytes by acetone extraction. Clin Chem 1981;27: 220-2.
69. Hindmarsh JT, Oliveras L, Greenway DC. Biochemical differentiation of the porphyrias. Clin Biochem 1999;32:609-19.
70. Hift R, Meissner P. Miscellaneous abnormalities in porphyrin production and disposal. In: Kadish KM, Smith KM, Guilard R, eds. The porphyrin handbook, vol. 14, Medical aspects of porphyrias. Amsterdam: Academic Press, 2003:151-68.
71. Hift RJ, Davidson BP, van der Hooft C, Meissner DM, Meissner PN. Plasma fluorescence scanning and fecal porphyrin analysis for the diagnosis of variegate porphyria: precise determination of sensitivity and specificity with detection of protoporphyrinogen oxidase mutations as a reference standard. Clin Chem 2004; 50:915-23.
72. Hift RJ, Meissner P, Moore MR. Porphyria: a toxicogenetic disease. In: Kadish KM, Smith KM, Guilard R, eds. The porphyrin handbook, vol. 14, Medical aspects of porphyrias. Amsterdam: Academic Press, 2003:303-38.
73. Hindmarsh JT, Oliveras L, Greenway DC. Plasma porphyrins in the porphyrias. Clin Chem 1999;45:1070-6.
74. Jackson AH, Sancovich HA, Ferramola AM, Evans N, Games DE, Matlin SA, et al. Macrocyclic intermediates in the biosynthesis of porphyrins. Phil Trans Roy Soc 1976;273:191-206.
75. Jacob K, Doss M. Excretion pattern of faecal coproporphyrin isomers I-IV in human porphyrias. Eur J Clin Chem Clin Biochem 1995;33:893-901.
76. Jamani A, Pudek M, Schreiber WE. Liquid-chromatographic assay of urinary porphobilinogen. Clin Chem 1989;35:471-5.

76a. Kauppinen R. Porphyrias. Lancet 2005;365:241-52.

77. Kauppinen R, Fraunberg M. Molecular and biochemical studies of acute intermittent porphyria in 196 patients and their families. Clin Chem 2002;48:1891-1900.
78. Kaya AH, Plewinska M, Wong DM, Desnick RJ, Wetmur JG. Human delta-aminolaevulinate dehydratase (ALAD) gene: structure and alternative splicing of the erythroid and housekeeping mRNAs. Genomics 1994;19:242-8.
79. Kean RW, Deacon AC, Delves HT, Moreton JA, Frost PG. Indian herbal remedies for diabetes as a cause of lead poisoning. Postgrad Med J 1994;70:113-4.
80. Kontos A, Ozog D, Bichakjian C, Lim HW. Congenital erythropoietic porphyria associated with myelodysplasia presenting in a 72-year old man: report of a case and review of the literature. Br J Dermatol 2003;148:160-4.
81. Kornfield JM, Ullman WW. Penicillin interference with the determination of δ-aminolaevulinic acid. Clin Chim Acta 1973;46:187-90.
82. Koskelo P, Mustajoki P. Altered coproporphyrin-isomer excretion in patients with the Dubin-Johnson syndrome. Int J Biochem 1980;12:975-8.
83. Koskelo P, Muller-Eberhard U. Interaction of porphyrins with proteins. Seminars in Hematology 1977;14:221-6.
84. Labbe RF. Lead poisoning mechanisms. Clin Chem 1990;36:1870-1.
85. Labbe RF, Rettmer RL. Zinc protoporphyrin: A product of iron-deficient erythropoiesis. Semin Haematol 1989;26:40-6.
86. Lam CW, Poon PM, Tong SF, Lo AW, Lai CK, Choi KL, et al. Novel mutation and polymorphisms of the HMBS gene detected by denaturing HPLC. Clin Chem 2001;47:343-6.
87. Lamon J, With T, Redeker A. The Hoesch test: bedside screening for urinary PBG inpatients with suspected porphyria. Clin Chem. 1974;20:1438-40.
88. Lamoril J, Puy H, Gouga, Rosipal R, Da Silva V, Grandchamp B, et al. Neonatal hemolytic anemia due to inherited harderoporphyria: clinical characteristics and molecular basis. Blood 1998;91:1453-7.

89. Lamoril J, Puy H, Whatley SD, Martin C, Woolf JR, Da Silva V, et al. Characterization of mutations in the CPO gene in British patients demonstrates absence of genotype-phenotype correlation and identifies relationship between hereditary coproporphyria and harderoporphyria. Am J Hum Genet 2001; 68:1130-8.
90. Lim CK, Peters TJ. Urine and faecal porphyrin profiles by reversed-phase high-performance liquid chromatography in the porphyrias. Clin Chim Acta 1984;139:55-63.
91. Lim CK, Rideout JM, Peters TJ. Pseudoporphyria associated with consumption of brewer's yeast. Brit Med J 1984;288:1640-2.
92. Lockwood WH, Poulos V, Rossi E, Curnow DH. Rapid procedure for fecal porphyrin assay. Clin Chem 1985;31:163-7.
93. Long C, Smyth SLS, Woolf J, Murphy GM, Finlay AY, Newcombe RG, et al. Detection of latent variegate porphyria by fluorescence emission spectroscopy of plasma. Brit J Dermatol 1993;129:9-13.
94. Louie GV, Brownlie PD, Lambert R, Cooper JB, Blundell TL, Wood SP, et al. Structure of porphobilinogen deaminase reveals a flexible multidomain polymerase with a single catalytic site. Nature 1992;359:33-9.
95. Luo J, Lim CK. Order of uroporphyrinogen-III decarboxylations on incubation of porphobilinogen and uroporphyrinogen-III with erythrocyte uroporphyrinogen decarboxylase. Biochem J 1993;289, 519-523.
96. Maruno M, Furuyama K, Akagi R, Horie Y, Meguro K, Garbaczewski L, et al. Highly heterogeneous nature of delta-aminolevulinate dehydratase (ALAD) deficiencies in ALAD porphyria. Blood 2001;97: 2972-8.
97. Matthews MA, Schubert HL, Whitby FG, Alexander KJ, Schadick K, Bergonia HA, et al. Crystal structure of human uroporphyrinogen III synthase. EMBO J 2001;21:5832-9.
98. Mauzerall D, Granick S. The occurrence and determination of δ-aminolaevulinic acid and porphobilinogen in urine. J Biol Chem 1956;219:435-46.
99. May BK, Dogra SC, Sadlon TJ, Bhasker CR, Cox TC, Bottomley SS. Molecular regulation of heme biosynthesis in higher vertebrates. Prog Nucleic Acid Res Mol Biol 1995;51:1-51.
100. McColl KEL, Godberg A. Abnormal porphyrin metabolism in diseases other than porphyria. Clinics in Haematology 1980;9:427-45.
101. Meissner P, Adams P, Kirsch R. Allosteric inhibition of human lymphoblast and purified PBG-deaminase by protoporphyrinogen and coproporphyrinogen. J Clin Invest 1991;91:1436-44.
102. Meissner P, Hift R, Corrigall A. Variegate porphyria. In: Kadish KM, Smith KM, Guilard R, eds. The porphyrin handbook, vol. 14, Medical aspects of porphyrias. Amsterdam: Academic Press, 2003:93-120.
103. Mendez M, Sorkin L, Rossetti MV, Astrin KH, del C Batlle AM, Parera VE, et al. Familial porphyria cutanea tarda: characterization of seven novel uroporphyrinogen decarboxylase mutations and frequency of common hemochromatosis alleles. Am J Hum Genet 1998;63:1363-75.
104. Merritt JE, Loening KL. Nomenclature of tetrapyrroles. Eur J Biochem 1982;108:1-30.
105. Meyer UA, Schuurmans MM, Lindberg RLP Acute porphyrias: pathogenesis of neurological manifestations. Semin Liver Dis 1998;18:43-52.
106. Millward LM, Kelly P, Deacon AC et al. Self-rated psychosocial consequences and quality of life in the acute porphyrias. J Inherited Metabolic Diseases 2001;24:733-47.
107. Minder EI, Gouya L, Schneider-Yin X, Deybach JC. A genotype-phenotype correlation between null allele mutations in the ferrochelatase gene and liver complication in patients with erythropoietic protoporphyria. Cell Mol Biol 2002;48:91-6.
108. Mukerji SK, Pimstone NR. Uroporphyrinogen decarboxylases from human erythrocytes: purification, complete separation and partial characterization of the two isoenzymes. Int J Biochem 1992;24:105-19.
109. Mustajoki P, Nordmann Y. Early administration of heme arginate for acute porphyric attacks. Arch Intern Med 1993;153:2004-8.
110. Nissen H, Petersen NE, Mustajoki S, Hansen TS, Mustajoki P, Kauppinen R, et al. Diagnostic strategy, genetic diagnosis and identification of a new mutation in acute intermittent porphyria by denaturing gradient gel electrophoresis. Hum Mutat 1997;9: 122-30.
111. Nordmann Y, Puy H, Da Silva V, Simonin S, Robreau AM, Bonaiti C, et al. Acute intermittent porphyria: prevalence of mutations in the porphobilinogen deaminase gene in blood donors in France. J Intern Med 1997;242:213-7.
112. O'Reilly K, Snape J, Moore MR. Porphyria cutanea tarda resulting from primary hepatocellular carcinoma. Clin Exp Dermatol 1988;13:44-8.
113. Phillips JD, Parker TL, Schubert HL, Whitby FG, Hill CP, Kushner JP. Functional consequences of naturally occurring mutations in human uroporphyrinogen decarboxylase. Blood 2001;98:3179-85.
114. Piomelli S. A micromethod for free erythrocyte porphyrins: The FPP test. J Lab Med 1973;81:932-40.
115. Piomelli S. Free erythrocyte porphyrin in the detection of undue absorption of lead and of iron deficiency. Clin Chem 1977;23:264-9.
116. Poh-Fitzpatrick MB, Sosin AE, Bemis J. Porphyrin levels in plasma and erythrocytes of chronic hemodialysis patients. J Am Acad Dermatol 1982;7:100-4.
117. Poh-Fitzpatrick MB. A plasma fluorescence marker for variegate porphyria. Arch Dermatol 1980;116:543-7.

118. Poh-Fitzpatrick MB. Clinical features of the porphyrias. Clinics in Dermatology 1998;16:251-64.
119. Ponka P. Tissue-specific regulation of iron metabolism and heme synthesis: distinct control mechanisms in erythroid cells. Blood 1997;89:1-25.
120. Puy H, Deybach JC, Lamoril J, Robreau AM, Da Silva V, Gouya L, et al. Molecular epidemiology and diagnosis of PBG deaminase gene defects in acute intermittent porphyria. Am J Hum Genet 1997;60:1373-83.
121. Rank JM, Pascual-Leone A, Payne W, Glock M, Freese D, Sharp H, et al. Hematin therapy for the neurologic crisis of tyrosinemia. J Pediatr 1991;118:136-9.
122. Rimington C. Spectral absorption coefficients of some porphyrins in the Soret-band region. Biochem J 1960;75:620-3.
123. Rimington C, Cripps DJ. Biochemical and fluorescence-microscopy screening tests for erythropoietic protoporphyria. Lancet 1 1965;1:624-6.
124. Rocchi E, Gibertini P, Santunione V, Balli F, Ventura E. Faecal and urinary coproporphyrin isomers in biliary atresia and neonatal hepatitis. Ric Clin Lab 1980;10:509-10.
125. Roels H, Lauwerys R, Buchet JP, Berlin A, Smeets J. Comparison of four methods for determination of δ-aminolaevulinic acid in urine, and evaluation of critical factors. Clin Chem 1974;20:753-60.
126. Rose IS, Young GP, St John DJ, Deacon MC, Blake D, Henderson RW. Effect of ingestion of hemoproteins on fecal excretion of hemes and porphyrins. Clin Chem 1989;35:2290-6.
127. Rossi E. Increased fecal porphyrins in acute intermittent porphyria. Clin Chem 1999;45:281-3.
128. Rossi E, Costin KA, Garcia-Webb P. Ferrochelatase activity in human lymphocytes as quantified by a new high-performance liquid-chromatography method. Clin Chem 1988;34:2481-5.
129. Rossi E, Curnow DH. Porphyrins. In: Lim CK ed. HPLC of small molecules. Oxford: IRL Press, 1986:261-303.
130. Rufenacht UB, Gouya L, Schneider-Yin X, Puy H, Schafer BW, Aquaron R, et al. Systematic analysis of molecular defects in the ferrochelatase gene from patients with erythropoietic protoporphyria. Am J Hum Genet 1998;62:1341-52.
131. Sarkany, RE. The management of porphyria cutanea tarda. Clin Exp Dermatol 2001;26:225-32.
132. Sassa S. ALAD porphyria. Seminars in Liver Disease 1998;18:95-101
133. Sassa S. δ-aminolaevulinic acid dehydratase assay. Enzyme 1982;28:133-45.
134. Sassa S, Kappas A. Hereditary tyrosinemia and the heme biosynthetic pathway: profound inhibition of delta-aminolevulinic acid dehydratase activity by succinylacetone. J Clin Invest 1983;71:625-34.
135. Schreiber WE, Jamani A, Pudek MR. Screening tests for porphobilinogen are insensitive. Am J Clin Pathol 1989;92:644-9.
136. Schreiber WE, Rozon C, Fong F, Jamani A. Detection of polymorphisms and mutations in the porphobilinogen deaminase gene by nonisotopic SSCP. Chem 1994;40:1982-3.
137. Seubert S, Seubert A, Rumpf KW, Kiffe H. A porphyria cutanea trada-like distribution pattern of porphyrins in plasma, hemodialysate, hemofiltrate, and urine of patients on chronic hemodialysis. J Invest Dermatol 1985;85:107-9.
138. Shoolingin-Jordan PM, Warren MJ, Awan SJ. Dipyrromethane cofactor assembly of porphobilinogen deaminase: formation of apoenzyme and preparation of holoenzyme. Methods Enzymol 1997;281:327-36.
139. Sieg T, Doss MO, Kandels H, Schneider J. Effect of alcohol on δ-aminolaevulinic acid dehydratase and porphyrin metabolism in man. Clin Chim Acta 1991;202:211-8.
140. Sithisarankul P, Schwartz BS, Lee BK, Kelsey KT, Strickland PT. Aminolevulinate dehydratase genotype mediates plasma levels of the neurotoxin, 5-aminolaevulinic acid, in lead exposed workers. Am J Ind Med 1997;32:15-20.
141. Soonawalla ZF, Orug T, Badminton MN, Elder GH, Rhodes JM, Bramhall SR, et al. Liver transplantation as a cure for acute intermittent porphyria. Lancet 2004;363:705-6.
142. St John DJ, Young GP, McHutchison JG, Deacon MC, Alexeyeff MA. Comparison of the specificity and sensitivity of Hemoccult and HemoQuant in screening for colorectal neoplasia. Ann Intern Med 1992;117:376-82.
143. Tchernitchko D, Lamoril J, Puy H, Robreau AM, Bogard C, Rosipal R, et al. Evaluation of mutation screening by heteroduplex analysis in acute intermittent porphyria. Clin Chim Acta 1999; 279:133-43.
144. Thunell S, Harper P, Brock A, Peterson NE. Porphyrins, porphyrin metabolism and porphyrias. II. Diagnosis and monitoring in the acute porphyrias. Scan J Clin Lab Invest 2000;60:541-59.
145. Tietz NW., Ed: Clinical Guide to Laboratory Tests. 3rd ed. Philadelphia, WB Saunders Co., 1995.
146. Todd DJ. Erythropoietic protoporphyria. British J Dermatol 1994;131:751-66.
147. Verneuil H de, Ged C, Moreau-Gaudry F. Congenital erythropoietic porphyria. In: Kadish KM, Smith KM, Guilard R, eds. The porphyrin handbook, vol. 14, Medical aspects of porphyrias. Amsterdam: Academic Press, 2003:43-66.
148. Verstraeten L, Ledoux MC, Moos B, Callebaut B, Cornu G, Hassoun A. Interference of Tienam in the colorimetric determination of 5-aminolevulinic acid

and porphobilinogen in serum and urine. Clin Chem 1992;38:2557-8.
149. Warren MJ, Scott AI. Tetrapyrrole assembly and modification into the ligands of biologically functional cofactors. Trends Biochem Sci 1990;15:486-91.
150. Watson CJ, Schwartz S. A simple test for urinary porphobilinogen. Proc Soc Exp Biol 1941;47:393-4.
151. Wetmur JG, Kaya AH, Plewinska M, Desnick RJ. Molecular characterization of the human aminolaevulinate dehydratase 2 (ALAD2) allele: implications for molecular screening of individuals for genetic susceptibility to lead poisoning. Am J Hum Gen 1991;49:757-63.
152. Whatley SD, Puy H, Morgan RR, Robreau A-M, Roberts AG, Nordmann Y, et al. Variegate porphyria in western Europe: Identification of PPOX gene mutations in 104 families, extent of allelic heterogeneity, and absence of correlation between phenotype and type of mutation. Am J Hum Genet 1999;65:984-94.
153. Whitby FG, Phillips JD, Kushner JP, Hill CP. Crystal structure of human uroporphyrinogen decarboxylase. EMBO Journal 1998;17:2463-71.
154. Wolkoff AW, Wolpert E, Pascasio FN, Atrias JM. Rotor syndrome, a distinct inheritable pathophysiologic entity. Am J Med 1976;60:173-9.
155. Woods JS, Miller HD. Quantitative measurement of porphyrins in biological tissues and evaluation of tissue porphyrins during toxicant exposures. Fundam Appl Toxicol 1993;21:291-7.
156. Woods JS, Martin MD, Naleway CA, Echeverria D. Urinary porphyrin profiles as a biomarker of mercury exposure: Studies on dentists with occupational exposure to mercury vapour. J Toxicol Environ Health 1993;40:235-46.
157. Wright DJ, Lim CK. Simultaneous determination of hydroxymethylbilane synthase and uroporphyrinogen-III synthase in erythrocytes by HPLC. Biochem J 1983;213:85-8.
158. Wu CK, Dailey HA, Rose JP, Burden A, Sellers VM, Wang BC. The 2.0 A structure of human ferrochelatase, the terminal enzyme of heme biosynthesis. Nat Struct Biol 2000;8:156-160.
159. Xiao M, Oefner PJ. Denaturing high performance chromatography: a review. Hum Mutat 2001;17:439-74.
160. Young D. Effect of drugs on clinical laboratory tests. 5th Ed. Vol 1, Listing by test. Washington: AACC press, 2000:642-3.

USEFUL WEBSITES

American Porphyria Foundation: http://www.porphyriafoundation.com (2005).

Canadian Porphyria Foundation: http://www.cpf-inc.ca (2005).

European Porphyria Initiative: http://www.porphyriaeurope.com (2005).

French Porphyria Center: http://www.porphyries.com.fr (2005).

CHAPTER 33

Therapeutic Drugs and Their Management

Thomas P. Moyer, Ph.D., and Leslie M. Shaw, Ph.D.

Therapeutic drug management (TDM) is a multidisciplined clinical activity initiated by the physician ordering laboratory quantification of drug concentration in a biological fluid to assess therapeutic compliance, efficacy, or to elucidate—the cause of drug-induced toxicity. The medical professionals involved in TDM include the ordering physician, clinical laboratorian, clinical pharmacologist, and nurses involved in medication delivery.

The limitations of empirical drug dosing such as standard or fixed dose regimens have long been recognized by physicians, who have responded with all of their clinical skills and knowledge of basic pharmacology to individualize each patient's drug dosage. TDM offers the physician a scientific rather than empiric approach to selecting a drug regimen to optimize therapy. The practice of TDM facilitates improved response to therapy by providing the prescribing physician with objective information about drug disposition; TDM describes a patient's pharmacokinetic status at the moment of specimen collection.

Pharmacokinetics is the science that describes the relationship between drug dose and the time course of drug absorption, distribution, and elimination that results in a specific drug concentration in biological systems.[93,119,150] Clinical pharmacokinetics involves the application of mathematical relationships to predict whether a drug concentration quantified at a specific time reflects normal or abnormal distribution and metabolism in a unique patient. Abnormal evaluation derived by this exercise may be the result of significant factors such as genetics, drug-drug interaction, organ failure, or patient noncompliance. Clinical pharmacokinetics can also be applied to predict appropriate change in dose or dosing interval to allow for safe and effective treatment and to attain optimal response to the drug as quickly as possible. It is important therefore for the clinician and laboratorian to understand not only how to quantify drugs in biological specimens but how these results are used to achieve effective drug therapy. As mentioned earlier, TDM is a multidisciplinary approach that relies on the cooperative efforts of the physician, nurse, pharmacologist, pharmacist, and clinical laboratorian.

To be effective, TDM requires the acquisition of a valid specimen followed by timely determination of the drug concentration in the specimen and interpretation of results in the context of dose, time of last dose, and other drugs present. Results should be reported or collated with the dosing schedule so that they may be interpreted in a pharmacokinetic context.

Knowledge of the impact of genetics on drug disposition developed rapidly in the late 1990s and continues to develop in the early 2000s. This knowledge field as it relates to drug disposition has become known as pharmacogenomics. TDM and pharmacogenomics are highly interactive disciplines used in conjunction to elucidate the overall pharmacokinetic status of an individual patient. While the basic concepts of pharmacogenomics are outlined elsewhere in this text (Chapter 43), the specific aspects of the discipline that relate to the interpretation of TDM results are included in this chapter. Reviews by O'Kane[101] and Weinshilboum,[147] and the Internet website offered by Flockhart[37] are good sources for additional information.

This chapter focuses on the laboratory's role in the discipline of TDM. Excellent descriptions of the roles of the physician and consulting pharmacologist are presented in Melmon and Morrelli's *Basic Principles in Therapeutics,*[81] Goodman and Gilman's *The Pharmacological Basis of Therapeutics,*[51] and Mandell and colleagues' *Principles and Practice of Infectious Diseases.*[78] The *Physicians' Desk Reference* (PDR), published annually by Medical Economics

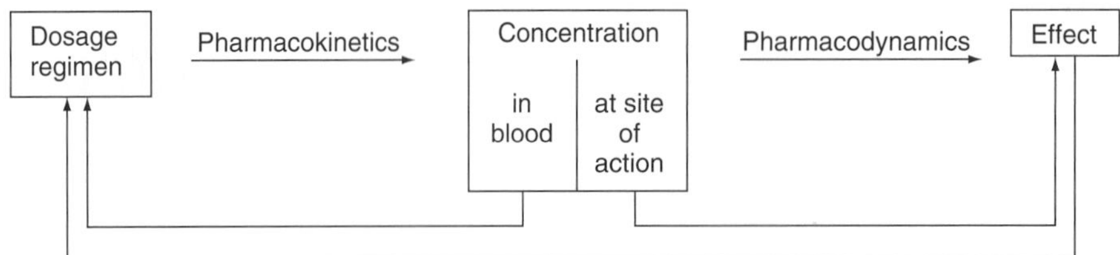

Figure 33-1 Conceptual relationship between pharmacodynamics and pharmacokinetics.

of Montvale, New Jersey, is also an excellent source of dosing guidance and pharmacokinetic information.

DEFINITIONS

Pharmacology comprises that body of knowledge surrounding chemical agents and their effects on living processes. This is a broad field, and it has traditionally been confined to those drugs that are useful in the prevention, diagnosis, and treatment of disease. *Pharmacotherapeutics* is that part of pharmacology concerned primarily with the application or administration of drugs to patients for the purpose of prevention and treatment of disease. For this aspect of medical practice to be effective, the pharmacodynamic and pharmacokinetic properties of drugs should be understood.

Pharmacodynamics encompasses the processes of interaction of pharmacologically active substances with target sites, and the biochemical and physiological consequences leading to therapeutic or adverse effects.[29] For many drugs, the ultimate effect or mechanism of action at the molecular level is understood poorly, if at all. However, effects at the cellular or organ system level or in the whole body are relatively well understood and can usually be related to dose of the drug.

Pharmacokinetics describes the processes of the uptake of drugs by the body, the biotransformations they undergo, the distribution of the drugs and their metabolites in tissue, and the elimination of the drugs and their metabolites from the body. Clinical pharmacokinetics is the discipline that applies the principles of pharmacokinetics to safe and effective therapeutic management of an individual patient. It is this aspect of pharmacology that most strongly influences the interpretation of TDM results and that is dealt with in more detail in this chapter.

Note that the term "pharmacology" relates to the broad knowledge of the systemic effects of a drug; "pharmacodynamics" refers to the interaction of a drug at its site of action; and "pharmacokinetics" is a mathematical description of drug disposition. These terms are quite different and should not be used interchangeably.

Figure 33-1 illustrates the conceptual relationship between pharmacodynamics and pharmacokinetics. The former relates drug concentration at the site of action to the observed magnitude of the effect. Pharmacokinetics, on the other hand, relates dose, dosing interval, and route of administration (regimen) to drug concentration in the blood. For more complete discussions of these basic concepts, the reader is encouraged to review standard textbooks of pharmacology.[51,81,87,88,119]

Toxicology is the subdiscipline of pharmacology concerned with adverse effects of chemicals on living systems. Toxic effects and mechanisms of action may be different from therapeutic effects and mechanisms for the same drug. Similarly, at the high dose of drugs at which toxic effects may be produced, rate processes are frequently altered compared with those at therapeutic doses. For these reasons, the terms *toxicodynamics* and *toxicokinetics* are now applied to these special situations.

BASIC CONCEPTS

The pharmacological effect of a drug is elicited by direct interaction of the drug with a receptor controlling a specific function or by a drug-mediated alteration of the physiological process regulating the function; this is known as the mechanism of action. In a given tissue, the site at which a drug acts to initiate events leading to a specific biological effect is called the *site of action* of the drug. For most drugs, the intensity and duration of the observed pharmacological effect are proportional to the concentration of the drug at the receptor, predicted by pharmacokinetics.

Mechanism of Action

The *mechanism of action* of a drug is the biochemical or physical process occurring at the site of action to produce the pharmacological effect. Drug action is usually mediated through a receptor. Cellular enzymes and structural or transport proteins are important examples of drug receptors. Nonprotein macromolecules may also bind drugs, resulting in altered cellular functions controlled by membrane permeability or DNA transcription. Some drugs are chemically similar to important natural endogenous substances and may compete for binding sites. In addition, some drugs may block formation, release, uptake, or transport of essential substances. Others may produce an effect by interacting with relatively small molecules to form complexes that actively bind to receptors. These and other examples of receptor binding are more completely discussed in pharmacology texts.*

*References 51, 81, 87, 88, 93, 119.

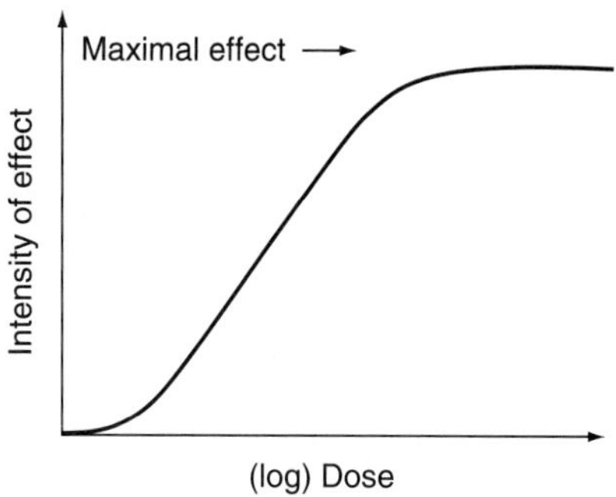

Figure 33-2 The log dose-effect relationship. The plateau (maximum effect) is likely due to saturation at the receptor.

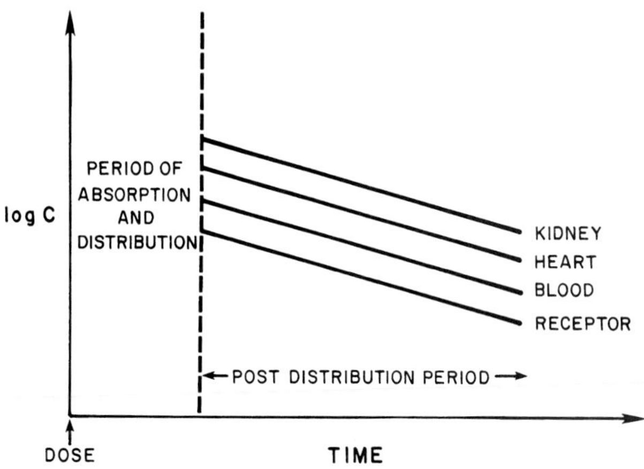

Figure 33-3 Property of kinetic homogeneity. Blood concentration of drug correlates with, but may not be equal to, the concentration in tissue and at the receptor site.

Although the exact molecular interactions that describe the mechanism of action remain obscure for many drugs, theoretical models have been developed to explain them. One concept postulates that a drug binds to intracellular macromolecular receptors through ionic and hydrogen bonds and van der Waals forces. This theoretical model further postulates that if the drug-receptor complex is sufficiently stable and able to modify the target system, an observable pharmacological response will occur. As Figure 33-2 illustrates, the response is dose dependent until a maximum effect is reached. The plateau may be due to saturation at the receptor or overload of a transport process.

The utility of monitoring drug concentration is based on the premise that pharmacological response correlates with the concentration of the drug at the site of action (receptor). Measurement of the concentration at the receptor site in a patient is technically impractical, if not impossible. However, studies have shown that for many drugs a strong correlation exists between the serum drug concentration and the observed pharmacological effect. In addition, years of relating blood concentrations to drug effects have demonstrated the clinical utility of drug concentration information. One must nevertheless always keep in mind that a serum drug concentration does not necessarily equal the concentration at the receptor; it merely reflects it. However, for pharmacokinetic studies it is assumed that changes in drug concentration in blood (or serum) versus time are proportional to changes in local concentrations at the receptor site or in body tissue. This assumption is sometimes called the *property of kinetic homogeneity* and is applicable to all pharmacokinetic models in postabsorptive and postdistributive phases of the time course. Figure 33-3 illustrates that property for a hypothetical compound. Parallel concentrations (log C) are expected in blood at the receptor and in tissue as time passes. Figure 33-3 is hypothetical; the absolute concentration of a drug in various tissues is highly variable from drug to drug.

The property of kinetic homogeneity is an important assumption in TDM because it is the basis on which all therapeutic and toxic concentration reference values are established. Measurable concentration ranges collectively define a

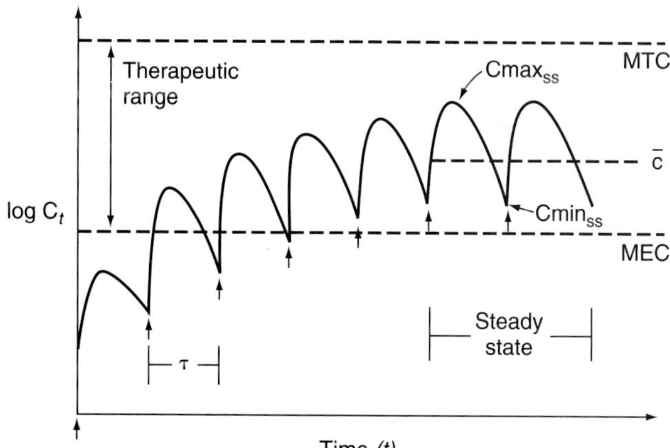

Figure 33-4 The peak, median, and trough drug concentrations increase with multiple identical doses administered once each half-life until they reach steady state. For most drugs, it takes five to seven half-lives to reach steady state. At steady state, optimal peak and trough concentrations are less than the MTC and greater than the MEC. The range of values between MEC and MTC is referred to as the "therapeutic range." C_{maxss} and C_{minss}, maximum and minimum steady-state concentrations; $\bar{C}$, average steady-state concentration; τ, dosing interval; *D*, dose; *MTC*, minimum toxic concentration; *MEC*, minimum effective concentration. *(Modified from Gilman AG, Goodman L, Gilman A, Eds. The pharmacological basis of therapeutics, 6th ed. New York: Macmillan, 1980. Reproduced with permission of The McGraw-Hill Companies.)*

therapeutic range (Figure 33-4) that represents the relationship between *minimum effective concentration* (MEC) and *minimum toxic concentration* (MTC). In the optimal dosing cycle, the *trough blood concentration* (the lowest concentration achieved just before the next dose) should not fall below the MEC, and the *peak blood concentration* (the highest concentration achieved within the dosing cycle) should not rise higher than the MTC. This is usually achieved by adminis-

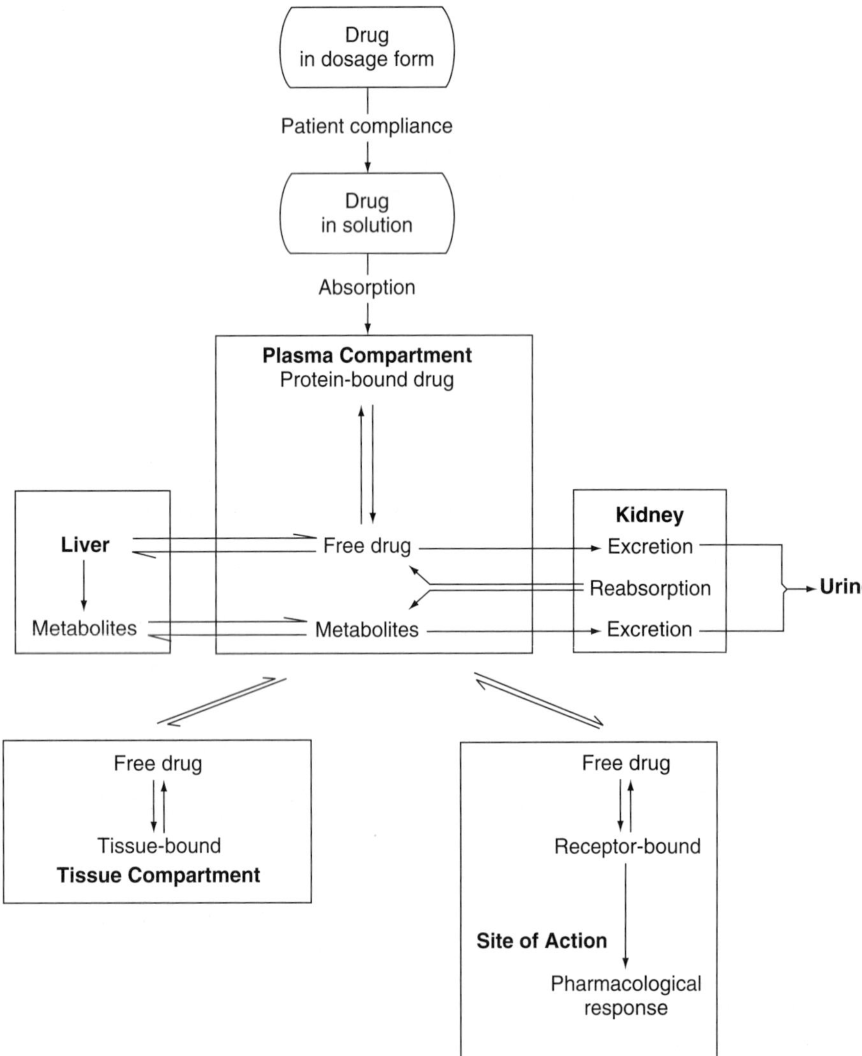

Figure 33-5 Factors affecting plasma drug concentration. *Absorption:* Drug must be formulated to ensure bioavailability for absorption from the gastrointestinal tract or other administration site. *Metabolism:* Drug is converted to a more soluble compound (metabolite), which may be pharmacologically active or inactive. Metabolism may occur in tissue other than the liver. *Excretion:* The more water-soluble drugs and their metabolites are usually excreted in urine. Excretion may also occur via bile, feces, saliva, and expired air. *Tissue storage:* The drug may be stored in tissue that exhibits no pharmacological response to it; side effects may occur from drug interaction with a specific physiological system. *Site of action:* Free drug binds to the receptor and produces pharmacological response. The number and type of receptors to which the drug is bound determine the intensity and duration of the observed response. *(Modified from Pippenger CE. TDM: Principles of drug utilization. Syva Monitor. San Jose: Syva Co. November, 1978:1,3-5.)*

tering the drug once every half-life, denoted by τ in Figure 33-4. Multiple dosing regimens should achieve *steady-state* serum drug concentrations consistently greater than the MEC and less than the MTC within the therapeutic range. Steady state is the point at which the body concentration of the drug is in equilibrium with the rate of dose administered and the rate of elimination. Blood concentrations greater than the MTC put patients at risk for toxicity; concentrations less than the MEC put them at risk for the disorder that the drug is supposed to treat. MTC and MEC are useful guidelines in therapy; this concept is incorporated into tables presented later in this chapter summarizing specific drug data. Doses must be planned to achieve therapeutic concentrations, and these must be monitored to guide adjustment of dose if necessary. The smaller the difference between MEC and MTC, the smaller the therapeutic index and the more likely TDM will be necessary. The key concept to remember is that the MEC and MTC define the therapeutic range for most drugs.

Pharmacokinetics

As defined previously, pharmacokinetics is the study of the rate processes of absorption, distribution, biotransformation, and excretion of drugs, poisons, and chemicals of both exogenous and endogenous origin. Figure 33-5 depicts in detail the many factors affecting drug concentration and pharmacological response.

In pharmacokinetics, mathematical approaches are used to predict or describe certain events, usually for calculating a dosing regimen or predicting the serum drug concentration after a given drug dose. The mathematical tools most often used in clinical pharmacokinetics are compartmental models and model-independent relationships.

Compartmental Models

Compartmental models have been the foundation of pharmacokinetic data analysis. The compartmental approach is presented here to facilitate definition of important pharmacokinetic parameters. Compartmental models are determin-

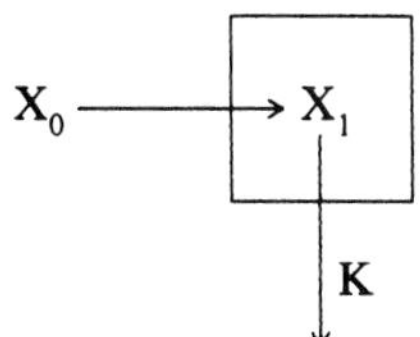

Figure 33-6 A one-compartment pharmacokinetic model.

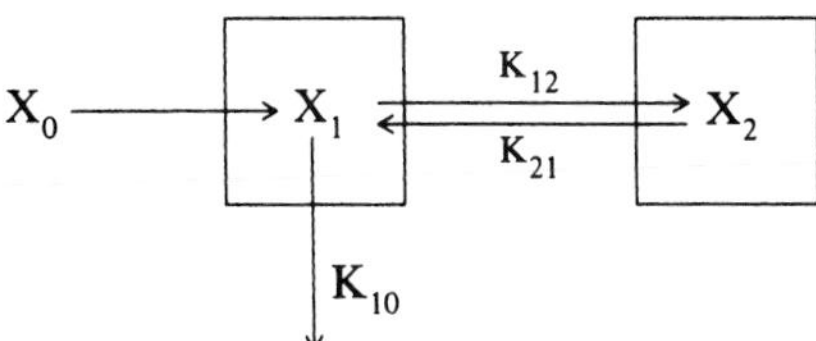

Figure 33-7 A two-compartment pharmacokinetic model.

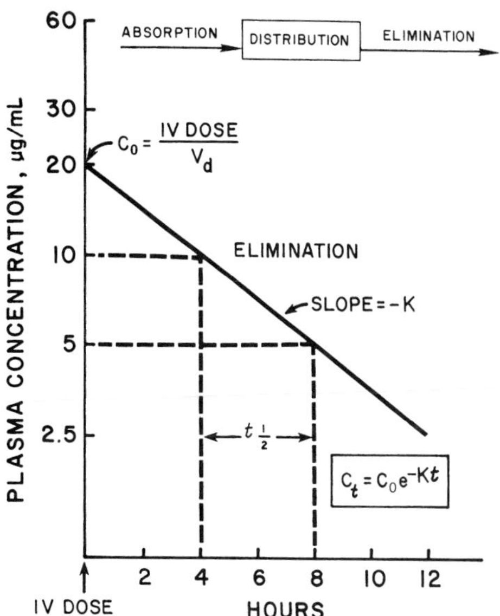

Figure 33-8 Drug concentration in plasma after intravenous administration of a single dose. The data show mono-exponential decline, which describes a one-compartment model.

istic in nature; drug concentration and time determine or define the model. The number and values of compartments assigned to the model have no true physiological meaning or anatomical reality. The intravascular fluid compartment (blood) usually is the anatomical reference compartment. The advantage of intravascular fluid as the reference compartment is the ease with which it may be sampled to provide a definitive profile of blood concentration of drug versus time. The actual number of compartments can be quite extensive. However, for the sake of simplicity, one-, two-, and three-compartment models are used most often.

In a one-compartment model, the body is considered as a single compartment (Figure 33-6). It is assumed that after introduction of a drug, the substance is rapidly and uniformly distributed throughout the body. Such a model is frequently applied to water-soluble antibiotics, such as gentamicin. In contrast, the two-compartment model (Figure 33-7) accounts for an initial decline of drug concentration in the reference compartment because of distribution from the plasma into vascularized tissue (the second compartment). The three-compartment model mimics a system like the two-compartment model with a third reservoir, such as adipose tissue or cellular nuclei, in which the drug resides over the long term. In Figures 33-6 and 33-7, X_0 represents the drug dose given and therefore the amount of drug in the system at zero time; X_1 the amount of drug in the central or reference compartment; and X_2 the amount of drug in the peripheral compartment in the case of the two-compartment model. The *k*s are first-order rate constants; k and k_{10} are elimination rate constants, because they describe the rates at which the drug leaves the reference compartment and is lost from the system. k_{12} and k_{21} are transfer rate constants describing, for the two-compartment model only, rates at which the drug is exchanged between compartments within the system. Figure 33-8 illustrates graphically the relationship between log of concentration and time for the one-compartment model. The curve in Figure 33-8 is described by the following equation:

$$C_t = C_0 e^{-kt} \tag{1}$$

where C_0 is the initial plasma concentration of the drug; C_t is the blood concentration of the drug as a function of time; and k is the first-order elimination rate constant. C_0 is estimated by extrapolating the line shown in Figure 33-8 to zero time. From knowledge of C_0 and k, one can theoretically predict C at any time (C_t), or one can determine k, and C_0, and C_t either graphically or mathematically. As shown later, most drugs are administered in repetitive doses rather than in a single bolus.

Figure 33-9 illustrates the more complex kinetics demonstrated by the two-compartment model. The curve is described by the following equation:

$$C_t = Ae^{-\alpha t} + Be^{-\beta t} \tag{2}$$

where the rate constant alpha (α) is the slope of the curve during the phase in which the drug is being distributed, referred to as the *distribution phase.* Beta (β) is the slope of the curve during the phase in which the drug is being eliminated by metabolism and excretion (assuming that distribution is complete) and is derived by extrapolating the *elimination phase* of the curve in Figure 33-9 to time = 0, which would have existed if distribution had been immediate and complete. A is an estimate, using the method of residuals, of the theoretical plasma concentration at time = 0 made immediately after intravenous injection of a bolus of drug. B is derived by extrapolation of the terminal slope line to time = 0. The method of residuals merely corrects the

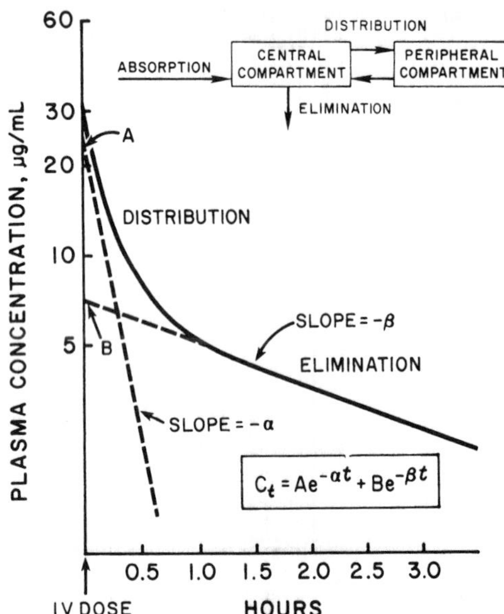

Figure 33-9 Decline of plasma concentration versus time after intravenous administration of a drug best characterized by a two-compartment model.

measured plasma level for the amount of drug distributed into tissue (as estimated on the extrapolated slope).

For simplicity, the intravenous bolus one-compartment model is used for illustrative purposes. After introduction of an intravenous bolus dose (D_0) into the single compartment, the drug is assumed to distribute instantaneously through all fluids and tissues of the body. The property of kinetic homogeneity is also assumed.

In TDM, it is preferable to work with concentrations of a drug in this homogeneous compartment, so D_1 (amount of drug in the compartment) is divided by a volume term. This volume term is called apparent *volume of distribution,* or V_d. It is not a real volume in the physiological sense, but instead is a proportionality constant to translate the absolute amount of drug present in the compartment into its concentration relative to a volume.

The V_d can be determined easily for the one-compartment model. When $t = 0$ (the time the drug bolus is introduced), D_0, the amount of drug given and corrected for bioavailability (f), is equal to the amount of drug in the compartment; the blood concentration (C_0) is

$$C_0 = \frac{D_0 \times f}{V_d} \quad (3)$$

Reorganization of this relationship provides the mathematical description of volume of distribution

$$V_d = \frac{D_0 \times f}{C_0} \quad (4)$$

The units of V_d are usually liters (L) or liters per kilogram of body weight (L/kg). Although V_d is a mathematical term and not a real physiological parameter, it is useful for contrasting degrees to which different types of drugs distribute. For instance, the polar hydrophilic drug gentamicin has a $V_d = 0.2$ L/kg, whereas the nonpolar lipophilic drug digoxin has a $V_d = 10$ L/kg. Gentamicin is concentrated in the blood, whereas digoxin is predominantly distributed into tissue.

Using the same assumptions, the first-order elimination rate constant can be determined. Referring to Figure 33-8, note that the relation between C_t and time is a natural logarithmic function where

$$\ln C_t = \ln C_0 - kt \quad (5)$$

Given a zero time blood drug concentration (C_0), a nonzero time concentration (C_t), and a defined time (t), then k can be readily determined either algebraically, graphically, or with appropriate software. For example, in a graphical plot of ln C_t versus t, the slope of the linear relationship is $-k$. The elimination rate constant k represents the fraction of drug removed per unit of time and has units of reciprocal time (min^{-1}, h^{-1}, day^{-1}). The overall elimination rate constant (k) includes the renal constant (k_{CR}), the biliary constant (k_{CB}), the metabolic constant (k_{CM}), and others such that $k = k_{CR} + k_{CB} + k_{CM}$.

The elimination rate constant (k) can be related to another parameter, half-life (τ), by the following equation:

$$\tau_{1/2} = \frac{0.693}{k} \quad (6)$$

Half-life (τ) is usually defined as the time required for the amount of drug in blood to decline to one half of a measured value. Figure 33-8 demonstrates how the half-life can be rapidly determined from a semilog plot of drug concentration versus time. Two or more successive concentrations collected at times t_1 and t_2 are required for the estimate of k used in the calculation of half-life

$$k = \frac{\ln C_{t_1} - \ln C_{t_2}}{t_2 - t_1} \quad (7)$$

If the measured half-life differs markedly from reported values for the drug in question, a component of elimination is likely to be the cause (i.e., decreased k_{CR} in renal impairment or decreased k_{CB} or k_{CM} in liver dysfunction).

Total body clearance (Cl_T) is defined as the theoretical total volume of blood, serum, or plasma completely cleared of drug per unit of time. It is usually expressed in units of mL/min, L/hr, mL/min/kg, or L/hr/kg. Like the elimination rate constant, Cl_T is the sum total of all the clearances contributed by each elimination route (i.e., $Cl_T = Cl_{CR} + Cl_{CB} + Cl_{CM} + \ldots$). Clearance is a most important parameter, because it provides a better representation than does k of the body's ability to eliminate a drug. In addition, Cl_T has more physiological meaning and is readily used to relate the dosing rate to steady-state concentration.

Clearance is mathematically related to V_d and k as

$$Cl_T = V_d k \quad (8)$$

Actual calculation of clearance is made using the pharmacokinetic approach of deriving the *a*rea *u*nder the *c*urve (AUC) from the time versus concentration curves shown in Figures 33-8 and 33-9. Clearance is described by

$$Cl_T = \frac{D_0 \times f}{\text{AUC}} \tag{9}$$

where AUC is the *a*rea *u*nder the *c*urve described by the plasma concentration versus the time histogram and integrated over time from zero to infinity.

In TDM, we are rarely concerned with a drug administered as a single, one-time intravenous bolus. Drugs administered repetitively pose the usual therapeutic situations. Figure 33-3 shows that a drug repetitively administered at a fixed dosing interval will accumulate in the body until a steady-state condition exists. Note that the normal dosing cycle is once each half-life (τ). *Steady state* is defined as that point in the dosing scheme when the amount entering the circulation (governed by the dosing rate) equals the amount eliminated (governed by the elimination rate).

Assuming first-order elimination, five to seven half-lives of a drug are required to reach 97% to 99% of a steady-state value. At steady state, assuming τ is constant, the profiles of concentration versus time should be superimposable from dose to dose.

Steady-state drug concentration (C_{ss}) at any time during a dosing interval is described by equation (10)

$$C_{ss} = \frac{(D_0 \times f)e^{-kt}}{V_d(1 - e^{-kt})} \tag{10}$$

In TDM, the maximum ($C_{max\text{-}ss}$) and minimum ($C_{min\text{-}ss}$) steady-state concentrations are often of primary interest (see Figure 33-3). Hence, the following equations are more useful:

$$C_{max\ SS} = \frac{D_0 \times f}{V_d(1 - e^{-kt})} \tag{11}$$

$$C_{min\ SS} = \frac{(D_0 \times f)e^{-kt}}{V_d(1 - e^{-kt})} \tag{12}$$

Again, recall that equations (10) through (12) apply only to dosing by repeated intravenous bolus. They are useful only when D_0, f, V_d, k, τ, and t (dosing intervals) are known.

Model-Independent Relationships

Model-independent relationships are frequently used in evaluation of clinical pharmacokinetics, because there are fewer relationships to remember, fewer restrictive assumptions, a more general insight into elimination mechanisms, and easier computations. However, model-independent relationships are not without their disadvantages; conceptualization of compartments or physiological spaces may be lost, specific information that may be clinically relevant or pertinent to mechanisms of distribution or elimination can be lost, and the difficulty can be increased in constructing profiles of concentration versus time.

The most frequently used model-independent approach applies the concept of median blood concentration, C (see Figure 33-3) and is described by

$$C = \frac{D_0 \times f}{Cl_T \times \tau} \tag{13}$$

This equation may be used for any drug. The equation is most useful when the half-life of a drug is much greater than t, the dosing interval.

Drug Disposition

Many factors have a profound influence on the pharmacokinetics of drugs and consequently on a patient's pharmacological response (Box 33-1). For example, the consideration of the patient's history, with particular emphasis on their pathophysiological state and adjunct drug therapy, is essential at the initiation of drug therapy and TDM. Other important factors include how a drug is absorbed, distributed, metabolized, cleared by the liver, biotransformed, and excreted.

Absorption

Most drugs administered continually to patients over a long period of time are administered extravascularly. Although intramuscular and subcutaneous routes are used, the oral route accounts for administration of most of the extravascular doses. The absorption process depends on the drug dissociating from its dosing form, dissolving in gastrointestinal fluids, and then diffusing across biological membrane barriers into the bloodstream. The rate and extent of drug absorption may vary considerably depending on the nature of the drug itself (e.g., solubility, pK_a), on the matrix in which it is present, and on the physiological environment (e.g., pH, gastrointestinal motility, vascularity).

The fraction of a drug that is absorbed into the systemic circulation is referred to as its *bioavailability.* The bioavailability (f) of a given drug is usually calculated by comparing, in the same subjects, the area under the plasma concentration-time curve (AUC) of an equivalent dose of the intravenous form and oral form

$$f = \frac{\text{AUC}_{\text{oral}}}{\text{AUC}_{\text{iv}}} \tag{14}$$

The bioavailability of a particular drug, if the drug is to be useful, must be great enough so that the active component will pass in sufficient amount and in a desirable time from the gut into the systemic circulation. Bioavailability is typically greater than 70% for drugs to be orally useful. An exception would be a case in which the lumen of the gastrointestinal tract is the site of drug action (e.g., antibiotics used to sterilize the gut). Low bioavailability would then be considered advantageous.

Some drugs that are rapidly and completely absorbed nevertheless have low bioavailability to the systemic circula-

BOX 33-1 Factors That Influence Drug Disposition in Humans

Demographic Factors
- Age category (premature infant, neonate, infant, prepubescent and postpubescent child, adult, elderly adult)
- Weight
- Gender
- Race
- Genetic constitution

Disease-Related Factors
- Liver disease (cirrhosis, hepatitis, cholestasis)
- Kidney disease
- Thyroid disorders (hypothyroidism or hyperthyroidism)
- Cardiovascular disease (arrhythmias, congestive heart failure)
- Gastrointestinal disease or disorder (sprue or other malabsorption syndromes, peptic ulcer, colitis)
- Cancer
- Surgery
- Burns
- Nutritional status (cachectic or anorexic states)

Extracorporeal Factors
- Hemodialysis
- Peritoneal dialysis
- Cardiopulmonary bypass
- Hypothermia or hyperthermia

Chemical and Environmental Factors Influencing:

Absorption of Drug
- Food or co-administered drug affecting extent and rate of absorption

Distribution of Drug
- Co-administered drug affecting binding to plasma proteins or tissue receptors

Metabolism of Drug
- Food intake (carbohydrates, proteins, lipids) competing for metabolizing systems
- Co-administration of drug that induces metabolizing enzymes (e.g., phenobarbital)
- Co-administration of drug that inhibits metabolizing enzymes (e.g., cimetidine)

Excretion of Drug
- Co-administration of drug that competes for renal tubular secretory paths (e.g., probenecid or penicillin)
- Changes in urinary flow rate
- Co-administration of compounds that enhance tubular reabsorption (e.g., sodium bicarbonate or phenobarbital)

tion. This is true of drugs with a high *hepatic extraction rate.* After oral administration, drugs that are absorbed in the lumen of the small intestine are carried by the portal vein directly to the liver. A drug with a high hepatic extraction rate may be extensively metabolized by the liver before it reaches the systemic circulation. This phenomenon is called the *first-pass effect.*

In addition to the extent of absorption, the rate of absorption is important. The absorption of a drug is generally considered a first-order process, and the absorption rate constant of a drug is usually much greater than its elimination rate constant. By manipulating their formulations (e.g., theophylline, quinidine) to produce "slow-" or sustained-release products, the apparent rate of absorption of many drugs can be controlled. For example, formulations that provide sustained release permit drugs taken orally to be taken at less frequent intervals. Conditions that may influence the extent or rate of drug absorption include abnormal gastrointestinal motility; diseases of the stomach, and the small and large intestine; gastrointestinal infections; radiation; food; and interaction with other substances in the gastrointestinal tract. One should be particularly aware of co-administered drugs that directly affect gut absorption, such as antacids, kaolin, sucralfate, cholestyramine, and antiulcer medications, and co-administration of morphine, which slows gut motility.

Distribution

After a drug enters the vascular compartment, it interacts with various blood constituents and is carried by various transport processes to different body organs and tissues. The overall process is referred to as *distribution.* The factors determining the distribution pattern of a drug are: (1) binding of the drug to circulating blood components, (2) binding to fixed receptors, (3) passage of the drug through membrane barriers, and (4) the ability to dissolve in structural or storage lipids. Molecular weight, pK_a, lipid solubility, and other physical and chemical properties of the drug also are important determinants of distribution.

Once a drug enters the systemic circulation, it distributes and comes to equilibrium with many of the blood components. One of these clinically significant groups is plasma proteins. An equilibrium exists between a *free* and protein-*bound* drug. It is generally believed that only the free fraction of the drug is available for distribution and elimination. In addition, only the free drug is available to cross cellular membranes or to interact with the drug receptor to elicit a biological response. Therefore changes in the protein-binding characteristics of a drug can have a profound influence on the distribution and elimination of a drug and on the manner in which steady-state concentrations are interpreted. Each drug has its own characteristic protein-binding pattern that depends on its physical and chemical properties. As a general rule, however, acidic drugs are bound primarily to albumin, and basic drugs primarily to globulins, particularly α_1-acid glycoprotein (AAG). Some drugs bind to both albumin and globulins.

Depending on its affinity for plasma proteins, a drug may be either tightly or loosely bound. A weakly bound drug can be displaced from its protein sites by a drug with a greater affinity for the plasma protein-binding sites. For example, phenytoin and valproic acid, drugs that are frequently co-administered for epilepsy, compete with each other as they bind to albumin. Because valproic acid is present at higher concentration, its mass causes a significant shift of phenytoin from bound to free form. Protein binding of a drug also depends on the physical characteristics of the plasma proteins and on the presence or absence of fatty acids or other drugs in the blood. Fatty acids can displace a drug from its protein-binding sites; tightly bound drugs are not displaced, but a weakly bound drug can be displaced quite rapidly by free fatty acids present in increased concentrations. It is important to recognize that even though the total drug concentration may remain unchanged, displacement of a drug from its plasma protein-binding sites elevates free drug concentrations and can result in clinical toxicity.

Anything that alters the concentration of free drug in the plasma ultimately alters the amount of drug available to enter tissue and interact with specific receptor systems. Disease states can alter free drug concentrations. For example, the composition of plasma is altered by an increase in nonprotein nitrogen compounds in uremia, by acid-base and electrolyte imbalances, and often by a decrease in albumin; free drug concentrations are frequently elevated. Patients may experience adverse effects that are a direct consequence of the increased free drug concentrations. If one monitors total plasma drug concentration in these patients, little change might be noted because the total concentration remains unchanged, or may even decrease, while the free fraction may increase significantly. Marked alterations of free drug concentration are not detected because the total drug concentration may not be dramatically different from that observed in healthy patients. For example, phenytoin is 90% bound and 10% free in healthy subjects. In uremic patients, 20% to 30% of the total plasma concentration of phenytoin may be free. If one considers a healthy patient who has a total plasma phenytoin concentration of 15 µg/mL, the free phenytoin concentration is likely to be 1.5 µg/mL. If a uremic patient has a total concentration of 15 µg/mL, the free drug concentration may be 4.5 µg/mL. A free phenytoin concentration of 4.5 µg/mL is sufficient to precipitate severe phenytoin side effects, including lethargy and increased seizure frequency. Therefore, in uremic patients, it is advisable to quantify free phenytoin concentrations and adjust the drug dose to maintain free phenytoin concentration at approximately 2.0 µg/mL.

Alteration of protein concentration in response to acute stress can alter free drug concentration. For example, after myocardial infarction, there is a rapid rise in AAG concentration. Lidocaine is used to control arrhythmias because of the infarction, but lidocaine is a basic drug that is highly bound to AAG. Doses of lidocaine adequate to control arrhythmia immediately after infarction are likely to become ineffective 48 to 72 hours later because the higher concentration of AAG that occurs after infarction diminishes the amount of free drug available to tissue. The arrhythmia reappears and because the total lidocaine plasma concentration necessary to control the arrhythmia seems to be in the toxic range, the lidocaine dose is decreased when in reality it should be increased to maintain the optimal free concentration.

Some drugs exhibit saturation of the available plasma protein-binding sites at optimal total drug concentrations. For example, disopyramide binding is concentration dependent and varies widely from patient to patient. Consequently, its total concentration and the observed clinical responses vary markedly from patient to patient. Valproic acid is also a drug that shows saturation at concentrations greater than 100 µg/mL. Thus, an increase of total plasma valproic acid concentration from 100 to 125 µg/mL represents a significant increase in the free valproic concentration.

Any change in normal physiological status can alter free drug concentrations and thus change the distribution of drugs between plasma and tissue. Geriatric patients often exhibit hypoalbuminemia with a notable decrease in protein-binding sites for drugs. In the elderly, the classical signs of drug intoxication are not usually apparent; instead, the clinical symptoms of drug intoxication are manifested as impaired cognitive function—particularly confusion. Elderly patients may be considered senile when in reality an increased free drug concentration is affecting their cognitive ability. Reduction of drug dose to decrease the free drug concentrations may result in dramatic improvements in these patients' personalities.

Estimation of the free drug concentration will continue to be of interest to TDM. Ultrafiltration techniques are useful in satisfying this need. However, it should be remembered that laboratory measurements now only *estimate* the free drug concentration in circulating blood. Artifacts introduced in drawing, processing, and storing blood can modify dissociation equilibria for some drugs. Despite these drawbacks, free drug estimations by ultrafiltration are superior to estimations of free drug concentration based on measurements in saliva. Few drugs show a strong correlation between salivary concentration and free drug concentration in plasma. In addition, collection of saliva from acutely ill patients is difficult.

Metabolism

The rate of the enzymatic process to metabolize a drug can be estimated using the Michaelis-Menten equation

$$\frac{dC}{dt} = \frac{V_{max} \times C}{K_m \times C} \quad (15)$$

where V_{max} is the maximum velocity of the reaction; K_m, the Michaelis-Menten constant is the drug concentration at which the rate of metabolism is one half of the maximum; and C is the blood drug concentration.

Drugs are usually administered to achieve concentrations in the blood considerably below the K_m of a particular drug. Therefore if K_m is much greater than C, equation (15) can be simplified to

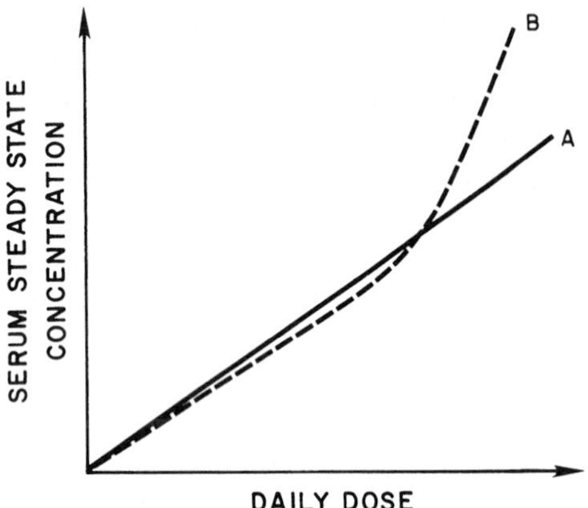

Figure 33-10 Dose-response curves. *Line A* illustrates the linear relationship between serum drug concentration and total daily dose of a drug that displays first-order kinetics typical of most drugs. *Line B* illustrates the dose-response relationship for a drug that displays capacity-limited kinetics because of a saturable enzyme or transport mechanism; in this situation, serum concentration becomes independent of total daily dose, and the relationship of drug concentration to dose becomes nonlinear. *(Modified from Pippenger CE. Practical pharmacokinetic applications. Syva Monitor, San Jose:Syva Co, January, 1979:1-4.)*

$$\frac{dC}{dt} = \frac{V_{max} \times C}{K_m} \quad (16)$$

and V_{max}/K_m can be written as the constant, k, such that

$$\frac{dC}{dt} = kC \quad (17)$$

where k is a simple first-order rate constant for the metabolic elimination. In other words, the rate of metabolism is proportional to the concentration of a drug. *First-order kinetics* are characteristic of the metabolism of most drugs.

In the event that the rate of metabolism approaches V_{max}, the rate becomes independent of concentration and thus descriptive of a *zero-order* process. Several drugs, notably phenytoin, salicylate, ethanol, and theophylline, cannot be characterized by simple first-order kinetics. Instead, the rate of metabolism of these compounds is said to be *capacity-limited* or *nonlinear,* meaning clearance or the apparent half-life changes with changes in concentration. Figure 33-10 (curve *B*) shows how a dose-response curve may be linear (first order) until the capacity of some pathway is reached; it then becomes nonlinear. Equations (10) and (13) have shown the relationship between plasma concentration, total body clearance, half-life, and dose. Therefore, important clinical considerations arise when a patient is treated with a drug that displays nonlinear kinetics. First, changes in dosing result in disproportionate changes in steady-state drug concentrations so that titration to appropriate serum levels must be approached conservatively. Secondly, because both clearance and apparent half-life of the drug change with increasing drug concentration, the length of time required to reach a new steady-state concentration is prolonged.

All of the equations previously described for predicting dose or concentration assume linear kinetic systems; they are therefore not adaptable to treatment with drugs that display nonlinear kinetics. Using a linearized Michaelis-Menten equation, methods for predicting phenytoin dose and concentration have been developed and applied to individual drug dosing regimens.

Hepatic Clearance

For those drugs dependent solely on hepatic elimination, total body clearance (Cl_T) equals hepatic clearance (Cl_H). When the liver is considered from a purely physiological perspective, the hepatic clearance is determined by the hepatic blood flow (Q) and the hepatic extraction fraction (E).

$$Cl_H = Q \times E \quad (18)$$

The hepatic extraction fraction of a drug reflects the affinity of a particular drug for hepatic microsomal enzymes; E can be found experimentally or calculated by the following equation:

$$E = \frac{C_a - C_e}{C_a} \quad (19)$$

where C_a is the concentration of the drug in blood entering the liver, and C_e is the concentration of the drug in the hepatic venous effluent. For drugs that possess a high extraction fraction, hepatic clearance approaches hepatic blood flow (Q). The total body clearance of highly extracted drugs primarily depends on hepatic blood flow for their elimination. These drugs usually have low bioavailability because of the first-pass effect described earlier. Lidocaine is an example of such a drug. The clearance of low-extracted drugs is less dependent on blood flow and more dependent on the quantity and quality of the hepatic microsomal enzymes. Total body clearance of these drugs is affected by hepatic function, enzyme inducers and inhibitors, and changes in free drug concentration. A review on this subject is available.[119]

Biotransformation

The liver is the principal organ responsible for xenobiotic metabolism. One of its major roles is to convert lipophilic nonpolar molecules to more polar water-soluble forms. The drug molecule (a xenobiotic) can be modified by phase I reactions, which alter chemical structure by oxidation, reduction, or hydrolysis; or by phase II reactions, which conjugate the drug (glucuronidation or sulfation) to create more water-soluble forms. Typically, both phase I and phase II reactions occur. Most drug metabolism takes place in the microsomal fraction of the hepatocytes, where many environmental chemicals and endogenous biochemicals (xenobiotics) are also processed by the same mechanisms.

Enzymes of the hepatic microsomal system can be induced or inhibited. Enzyme induction and inhibition have greatest significance for drugs with low to moderate hepatic extraction fractions.

Microsomal enzyme induction leads to an increase in the activity of enzymes present, most commonly through increases in the mass quantity of the oxidizing enzymes. The many isoenzymes of cytochrome P_{450} are affected variably by different enzyme-inducing drugs. For example, phenobarbital and theophylline and polycyclic hydrocarbons induce enzyme activity differently. Two classical and clinically relevant enzyme inducers can be contrasted.

Phenobarbital Induction

Phenobarbital represents the type of enzyme inducer with broad induction effects. After a latency period, production of cytochrome P_{450}, cytochrome P_{450} reductase, and related enzymes is increased. In addition, liver weight, hepatic blood flow, bile flow, and production of hepatic proteins also all increase. This induction apparently increases the P_{450} isoenzyme mass for which debrisoquin is a substrate, because the hepatic clearance of debrisoquin is increased after phenobarbital administration. This enzyme is referred to as cytochrome P_{450}-2D6 (Cyp 2D6). Phenobarbital induction has little effect on theophylline clearance, suggesting a different isoenzyme for theophylline metabolism.

Theophylline and Polycyclic Hydrocarbons Induction

Theophylline and polycyclic hydrocarbons in tobacco smoke (3-methylcholanthrene) represent a second type of enzyme inducer with broad induction effects. They induce CyP 1A in which no change in P_{450} reductase occurs and a different terminal oxidase appears. After this type of induction, the clearance of theophylline but not that of antipyrine is increased. These substances have served as prototypes for the classification of enzyme inducers. Obviously, when patients are on a drug with a narrow therapeutic index, their dosing regimen would need to be adjusted should a known enzyme-inducing drug be added to or deleted from their therapy.

Because the drug-metabolizing enzymes of the liver and gastrointestinal tract are nonspecific and interact with a wide variety of endogenous and exogenous substances, it is not surprising that the presence of one drug inhibits the metabolism of a second drug that is co-administered. Several general mechanisms have been proposed to describe these events. They include substrate competition, competitive or noncompetitive inhibition, product inhibition, and repression (where the amount of enzyme is reduced by either decreased synthesis or increased degradation). Most drug-drug interactions probably fall into the categories of substrate competition or competitive or noncompetitive inhibition. Examples of xenobiotics that have been shown to significantly inhibit drug metabolism include antiretrovirals, cimetidine, erythromycin, fluconazole, grapefruit juice, and verapamil. As with enzyme inducers, the addition or deletion of an inhibitory drug in a patient's drug therapy requires appropriate TDM and dose adjustment of the affected drug. TDM allows one to monitor these processes and adjust dosing accordingly.

The role of TDM becomes particularly apparent for drugs that undergo hepatic or gastrointestinal metabolism. Wide variability in the rate of metabolism of any given drug exists not only in different patients in the general population but also in the same patient at different times and in different circumstances. This variability is due to factors such as age, weight, gender, genetics, exposure to environmental substances, diet, co-administered drugs, and disease. Furthermore, there is no acceptable, endogenous, biochemical marker by which hepatic or gastrointestinal function, and consequently hepatic or gastrointestinal capability for drug clearance, can be routinely assessed before drug therapy is initiated.

The biotransformation of drugs may produce metabolites that are pharmacologically active. In such instances, the metabolite should also be measured because it is contributing to the effect of the drug on the patient. Primidone and procainamide are examples of such drugs. If the metabolite is inactive, it need not be measured, but steps should be taken to ensure that it does not interfere in the analytical process.

Excretion

Excretion of drugs or chemicals from the body can occur through biliary, intestinal, pulmonary, or renal routes. Although each of these represents a possible mechanism of drug elimination, renal excretion is a major pathway for the elimination of most water-soluble drugs or metabolites and is important in TDM. Alterations in renal function may have a profound effect on the clearance and apparent half-life of the parent compound or its active metabolite(s); decreased renal function causes elevated serum drug concentrations and increases the pharmacological response.

Kidney function, in contrast to liver function, is readily and reliably evaluated by estimation of creatinine clearance (see Chapter 24). Creatinine is a metabolic product of muscle metabolism and is produced at a constant rate by the body. It is primarily eliminated from the body by the kidneys through the glomerular filtration mechanism. Renal clearance of creatinine at 120 mL/min approximates the glomerular filtration rate of 90 to 130 mL/min. Therefore measurement of creatinine clearance on a routine basis provides an effective tool to evaluate kidney function. A strong correlation has been shown to exist between creatinine clearance and the total body clearance or elimination rate constant of those drugs primarily dependent on the kidneys for their elimination. Examples of drugs whose therapeutic use is adjusted to account for changes in creatinine clearance include amikacin, digoxin, gentamicin, tobramycin, and vancomycin.

Clinical Utility

TDM is most valuable when the drug in question is used chronically and has a narrow therapeutic index. A number of advantages can be realized by a TDM program.

1. Noncompliance can be recognized. Many patients, especially those with chronic disease, require prolonged drug therapy. The problem of compliance is particularly evident with patients who are characteristically free of pain or in unusual discomfort as with epilepsy, asthma, hypertension, mild heart disease, and transplantation. Patients may develop a sense that their disease has been cured and they no longer need the drug. The end results of noncompliance are exacerbation of the existing disorder and treatment failure. Greenstein reported in 1998 the results of a large, multicenter study that estimated 23% noncompliance with chronic therapy for a life-threatening disorder.[46] Shemesh has reported that the best means to document noncompliance is the assessment of blood concentration.[127] Drug concentration values provide positive feedback to physicians regarding patient compliance, allowing for identification of the noncomplying patient.
2. Patients undergoing changes in drug disposition characteristics can be recognized. Occasionally, the disposition pattern of drugs in particular individuals may change from the average patient population parameters. Aberrant disposition may be attributable to an effect of a drug or disease state not previously recognized. The clinical condition and individual metabolism of patients may not only differ from one to another but may change in the same patient during treatment. Both the pharmacokinetic disposition and the pharmacodynamic response to a given drug dose in individual patients may vary widely as a direct consequence of genetic influences. Studies of these genetic factors (pharmacogenetics) have clearly demonstrated that all aspects of pharmacokinetics and pharmacodynamics are under genetic control. One of the frequent examples of such a change can be seen when adolescents progress through puberty—most drug disposition parameters change, requiring frequent dose and dosing interval adjustment, guided by TDM.
3. Therapeutic drug regimens can be adjusted during periods of continuous physiological change. Normal alterations in physiological state, as in pregnancy or aging, or continuous pathophysiological or hemodynamic changes as consequences of disease, surgical treatment of disease, and the healing process complicate assessment of drug dose needs.
4. Baseline concentrations associated with an optimal therapeutic regimen can be identified. After a patient has undergone an extensive workup to define an appropriate therapeutic regimen, a physician can establish a baseline drug concentration at which the patient responds well. Should the patient's response change significantly in the future, the physician can rapidly document whether the patient has been compliant or whether a new disease state may be altering the pharmacodynamics or pharmacokinetics of a drug.
5. The most appropriate drug-dosing regimens can be initiated and maintained for a particular patient.

ANALYTICAL CONSIDERATIONS

The evolution of TDM has been facilitated by the development of rapid, sensitive, and specific analytical techniques. These technical advances have driven the growth of the fields of pharmacology, biopharmaceutics, and pharmacokinetics.

Analytical Techniques

Analytical techniques that are used to measure therapeutic drugs includes immunoassay and instrumental techniques, such as chromatographic and electrophoretic procedures, and the so-called "hyphenated techniques," where chromatographs are coupled with a mass spectrometer.*

Immunoassay

Radioimmunoassay (RIA) techniques permit quantification of drug concentration in microliter volumes of serum at nanograms per milliliter concentrations. However, the complexity of this technique, long turnaround time, problems, with waste disposal, and lack of RIA for a wide variety of drugs have prevented its widespread adoption for routine drug assays. Few RIAs now are used for TDM.

Proliferation of TDM to all laboratories and physicians was achieved with the development of the nonisotopic immunoassay (see Chapter 9). Numerous systems have evolved to provide this technology in both the clinical laboratory and physician's office. The major advantages of these systems are their microcapability, specificity, rapidity, ease of performance, and adaptation to automated analyzers (see Chapter 11).

Instrumental Methods

Gas-liquid chromatography (GLC) permits separation of parent drug from metabolite(s) and differentiation from co-administered drugs and endogenous compounds. It has the ability to separate and quantify several drugs within a given class of drugs.[122] Disadvantages of GLC include the need for (1) a relatively large volume of sample to achieve biologically important sensitivity and (2) chemical derivatization to ensure that the analytes have the prerequisite volatility. Advances in the development of mass spectrometer detectors (GC/MS) and application of capillary columns have increased the sensitivity of the instruments to such an extent that drug analysis can now be routinely performed on microliter (μL) volumes of sample.

High-performance liquid chromatography (HPLC) techniques offer versatility with minimal sample preparation. Its specificity and sensitivity, relatively small sample requirements, and the ease of operation make HPLC a practical alternative to GLC. HPLC has also been adapted to the simultaneous quantification of a large variety of drugs and

*Several analytical methods and case studies for therapeutic drugs are found on this book's accompanying Evolve site, found at http://evolve.elsevier.com/Tietz/textbook/.

their metabolites (see Chapter 6 and a review by Sadeg and colleagues[120] for a discussion of chromatographic techniques). Capillary electrophoresis, a relatively new technique (see Chapter 5), has been used to measure a variety of drugs,[104,137] including caffeine,[118] various cardiac drugs,[99] felbamate,[128] and gabapentin.[41]

The combination of HPLC with tandem mass spectrometers (LC/MS/MS) has revolutionized the analytical approach to TDM. This technology allows for direct analysis of biological specimens with minimal sample preparation, high sensitivity, specificity, precision, and high throughput.

Issues of Concern

Analytical issues of continuing concern for a TDM service include the following:

1. Assay methods used for TDM should be accurate and reproducible. All clinical laboratories with a TDM service should be actively involved in an internal quality control and external proficiency testing program. In addition, sample volume and assay turnaround time should be considered in selecting the most appropriate analytical method.
2. Each laboratory should inform the medical staff about therapeutic and toxic concentration ranges, analytical method (when appropriate), action values, required sample volume, and collection tube specifications.
3. Guidelines should be available for ideal sample schedules for each individual drug monitored. Steady-state trough concentrations usually are most desirable; however, other sample schedules may be appropriate, depending on the properties of the drug or the individual needs of the patient.
4. The time and date of collection of the drug sample and of the last dose should be noted. To assess steady-state conditions, the length of time a patient has been on a particular regimen should be known. In vitro conditions affecting stability of the drug in a sample (e.g., penicillin or heparin and aminoglycoside antibiotics) or the assay specificity (e.g., presence of hemolysis) should be considered for sample handling procedures.
5. Because laboratory reports become part of a patient's chart, it is useful to devise a reporting format that incorporates all of the data necessary for interpretation (drug formulation, frequency and amount, plasma concentration, time of dose, time of draw, and other drugs coadministered).

SPECIFIC DRUG GROUPS

Drugs that are routinely monitored are conveniently classified by the kind of therapy they support (e.g., antibiotics, control of epilepsy, management of respiratory or cardiac function, suppression of immune response). An analytical method for one drug in a grouping is often applicable to other drugs in the same grouping. The following discussion is organized in accordance with classifications commonly recognized. Note that some drugs, such as salicylate and nitroprusside (assessed by the quantification of thiocyanate), are discussed in Chapter 34.

Antiepileptic Drugs

Many antiepileptic drugs are used to treat seizures (Table 33-1). Most are analyzed collectively by either GLC or HPLC[68] or individually analyzed by immunoassay. The advantage of HPLC or GLC is that simultaneous analyses can be accomplished. Immunoassay procedures are less labor intensive and are usually quicker than HPLC or GLC for a single analyte; however, analysis of multiple antiepileptics or metabolites requires additional assays. For example, GLC[38] and HPLC[43] methods allow for the simultaneous measure of several common anticonvulsants. Immunoassay, however, is the mainstay of monitoring these drugs in most clinical laboratories.

Carbamazepine

Carbamazepine, proprietary name *Tegretol,* is used in the treatment of generalized tonic-clonic, partial, and partial-complex seizures. It is also used for the treatment of pain associated with trigeminal neuralgia. Like phenytoin, carbamazepine modulates the synaptic sodium channel, which prolongs inactivation, reducing the ability of the neuron to respond at high frequency.[51] The physiological effect of this action is reduction in central synaptic transmission, aiding in control of abnormal neuronal excitability. Carbamazepine also has an antidiuretic effect, reducing concentrations of antidiuretic hormone.

After oral administration, carbamazepine is slowly but erratically absorbed with wide individual variability. Over 80% of the drug is protein bound.. The elimination half-life early in therapy is approximately 24 hours. With chronic therapy, the enzyme cytochrome P_{450} 3A4 (CyP 3A4) and its associated drug transporter P-glycoprotein (Pg)—responsible for metabolism—are induced, and the elimination half-life is reduced to 15 to 20 hours. Because hepatic metabolism is the principal means by which plasma concentration is reduced, any reduction in liver function results in drug accumulation.

The therapeutic concentration range for optimal pharmacological effect of carbamazepine is 4 to 12 µg/mL. Toxicity associated with excessive carbamazepine ingestion occurs at plasma concentrations in excess of 15 µg/mL and is characterized by symptoms of blurred vision, paresthesia, nystagmus, ataxia, drowsiness, and diplopia. Side effects unrelated to plasma concentration include development of an urticarial rash, which usually disappears on discontinuation of the drug, and hematological depression (leukopenia, thrombocytopenia, and aplastic anemia).

The active metabolite of carbamazepine is carbamazepine-10,11-epoxide formed by action of CyP 3A4. This metabolite has been found to accumulate in children to concentrations equivalent to carbamazepine. It may contribute to symptoms of intoxication in children who have a thera-

TABLE 33-1 Pharmacokinetic Parameters of Antiepileptic Drugs

Drug	Minimum Effective Concentration (MEC) (μg/mL)	Minimum Toxic Concentration (MTC) (μg/mL)	Average Half-Life (hr)	Average Volume of Distribution (L/kg)	Average Oral Bioavailability (%)	Average Protein Binding (%)	Important Metabolizing Enzymes
Carbamazepine	4	12	15-20	1.4	70	75	CyP 3A4, Pg
Carbamazepine-10,11-epoxide	0.4	4	7	NA	NA	50	CyP 2C19
Clonazepam	0.015	0.06	25	3.2	98	85	
Ethosuximide	40	100	30-60	0.7	NA	0	UGT
Felbamate	40	120	14-21	0.8	90	25	CyP 2D6
Gabapentin	2	12	5-9	0.8	60	0	CyP 2D6
Lamotrigine	1	8	20-30	1.2	98	60	CyP 2C19, UGT
Levetiracetam	3	63	7		100		CyP 2C19
Mephobarbital	1	5	30	NA	NA	50	CyP 2C19
Methsuximide	0.01	0.04	3	NA	NA	NA	
Oxcarbazepine metabolite (MHC)	6-10		8-10	0.8			UGT
Normethsuximide	10	40	30				
Phenobarbital	15 (children) 20 (adults)	35 (children) 40 (adults)	70 (children) 90 (adults)	1.0	90	40-60	CyP 2C9, 2C19 UGT
Phenytoin	10 (free: 1.0)	20 (free: 2.0)	~20	0.6	90	90	CyP 2C9, 2C19 UGT
Primidone	5	12	15	0.7	92	20	CyP 2C9, 2C19
Tiagabine	0.005	0.52	7-9			96	CyP 2C19
Topiramate	2	12	18-23				CyP 2C19
Valproic acid	50 (free: 5)	100 (free: 10)	12-16 (adults) 8 (children)	0.2	100	93	CyP 2C19
Zonisamide	10	30	50-70	1.4	50	50	CyP 2C19

NA, Not applicable.

peutic plasma concentration of the parent drug. Because carbamazepine is metabolized by CyP 3A4, drugs that induce this enzyme (erythromycin, oxcarbazepine, phenytoin, and St. John's Wort) increase the rate of clearance of carbamazepine.

Co-administration of erythromycin, phenytoin, or valproic acid increases the rate of metabolism of carbamazepine, reducing the blood concentration. Itraconazole and grapefruit juice interfere with CyP 3A4, increasing carbamazepine levels.

Because of carbamazepine's relatively long half-life, the specimen yielding the most useful information is the one representing the trough concentration, although in the case of suspected mild intoxication, the peak value of the plasma concentration correlates more closely with toxicity. The peak specimen should be collected 4 to 8 hours after the oral dose.

Ethosuximide

Ethosuximide, proprietary name *Zarontin,* is used for the treatment of absence seizures characterized by brief loss of consciousness. Ethosuximide reduces the flow of calcium through T-type calcium channels in the synapse of thalamic neurons; because thalamic neurons are the main source of 3-Hz spike-wave rhythms in absence seizures, reduction of calcium flow slows the rate of these seizure-inducing pulses.

Ethosuximide is readily absorbed from the gastrointestinal tract. In children its half-life is approximately 33 hours, although this may be prolonged in adults. The drug is cleared mainly by metabolism as the hydroxyethyl metabolite and the glucuronide ester (metabolized by UDP-glucuronosyltransferase–UGT, or sulfate ester metabolized by sulfotransferase—ST) of the hydroxyethyl metabolite; the exact cytochrome enzyme isomer has not been identified. The trough specimen yields the most useful information regarding therapeutic efficacy. The optimal therapeutic concentration of ethosuximide is 40 to 100 μg/mL. Toxicity related to an excessive blood concentration of ethosuximide is rare. Symptoms of gastrointestinal distress, lethargy, dizziness, and euphoria may be encountered early in therapy, but patients usually become tolerant to these symptoms.

Levetiracetam

Levetiracetam *(Keppra)* is approved for adjunctive therapy and treatment of partial onset seizures in adults with epilepsy. Levetiracetam is 100% bioavailable. Once absorbed, it is <10% bound to protein and has a volume of distribution of 1.0 L/kg. Following an oral dose, it reaches maximum concentration in 1 hour. The clearance half-life is 7 ± 1 hour and clearance is 0.96 mL/min/kg predominantly by renal elimination of the parent drug. Twenty-four percent of the parent drug undergoes hepatic metabolism by CyP 2C19 to an inactive carboxylic acid metabolite. Levetiracetam is cleared predominantly by renal function. A 40% reduction in levetiracetam clearance is expected is expected if the creatinine clearance is <30 mL/min. Prepubescent children clear levetiracetam 40% faster than adults. There are no pharmacokinetic interactions between levetiracetam and other antiepileptic drugs.

In adults, maximum blood concentration correlates with dose. The minimal effective serum concentration for seizure control is 3 µg/mL. Peak therapeutic serum concentrations of 10 to 63 µg/mL occur 1 hour after dose. Trough therapeutic concentrations occurring just before the next dose range from 3 to 34 µg/mL.[8]

Toxicity effects known to be associated with levetiracetam use include decreased RBC count and hematocrit, decreased neutrophil count, somnolence, asthenia, and dizziness. These toxicities may be associated with blood concentrations in the therapeutic range. Co-administration of cimetidine will interfere with the test, producing artifactually increased measurements of levetiracetam. The laboratory can identify the presence of cimetidine, and laboratory reports will reflect cimetidine interference if it is detected.

Oxcarbazepine

Oxcarbazepine (OCBZ—*Trileptal*) has been approved for therapy of partial seizures with and without secondarily generalized seizures in adults and as adjunctive therapy for partial onset seizures in children ages 4 to 16. OCBZ is a prodrug that is almost immediately and completely metabolized to 10-hydroxy-10,11-dihydrocarbamazepine known as monohydroxycarbamazepine (MHC), the metabolite responsible for OCBZ's therapeutic effect. Reductase enzymes not subject to induction catalyze the conversion of OCBZ to MHC. MHC is cleared as the glucuronide conjugate formed by action of UGT. MHC selectively induces CyP 3A4 enzymes responsible for the metabolism of estrogens, immunosuppressants, and the dihydropyridine calcium-channel blockers. Carbamazepine activates UGT, enhancing the rate of clearance of MHC.

The metabolism of OCBZ is extensive; about 96% of the dose is excreted in the urine as metabolites, less than 1% as unchanged drug, and about 27% as free MHC. The majority of the dose is recovered as the glucuronide ester of either OCBZ or MHC, approximately 9% and 49%, respectively. The apparent volume of distribution of MHC is 0.8 L/kg. Approximately 40% of MHC is bound to serum proteins, predominantly to albumin. The elimination half-life is 1.0 to 2.5 hours for OCBZ and 8 to 10 hours for MHC. MHC shows a linear and dose-proportional increase (based on OCBZ dose) in the range of 300 to 2700 mg/day. Since MHC is cleared predominantly by the kidney, the daily dosage of OCBZ given to patients with creatinine clearance <30 mL/min should be half that given to patients with normal renal function.[45]

Steady-state MHC concentrations in a trough specimen collected just before the next dose correlate with the OCBZ dose. Trough monitoring is recommended for assessment of compliance or to verify dose adequacy. Optimal response to OCBZ occurs when trough MHC concentration is in the range of 6 to 10 µg/mL.[45] Peak plasma concentration of MHC occurs 4 to 6 hours after dose. Because carbamazepine activates UGT, patients taking carbamazepine concomitantly with OCBZ have significantly lower MHC concentrations than patients not receiving carbamazepine. Toxicity effects associated with OCBZ includes hyponatremia, dizziness, somnolence, diplopia, fatigue, nausea, vomiting, ataxia, abnormal vision, abdominal pain, tremor, dyspepsia, and abnormal gait. These toxicities may be observed when blood concentrations are in the therapeutic range. Serum sodium concentration below 125 mmol/L and decreased T4 have been seen in patients treated with MHC.

Phenobarbital

Phenobarbital is used in the treatment of all seizures except absence seizures, and is known by a wide variety of proprietary names and found in combination with many other drugs. It is used for treatment of generalized tonic-clonic, partial, focal motor, temporal lobe, and febrile seizures. It is also known to reduce synaptic transmission, resulting in decreased excitability of the entire nerve cell, inducing sedation. Phenobarbital potentiates synaptic inhibition through action on the γ-aminobutyric acid-A ($GABA_A$) receptor by increasing the duration of chloride flow into the synapse.[52] The end result is an increase in seizure threshold and inhibition of the spread of discharges from the epileptic foci.

Absorption of oral phenobarbital is slow but complete. The time at which peak plasma concentrations are reached is widely variable and ranges from 4 to 10 hours after the dose. Phenobarbital is 40% to 60% bound to plasma proteins. CyP 2C19 is the primary hepatic enzyme involved in metabolism, producing an elimination half-life of 70 to 100 hours; metabolism is age dependent (children average 70 hours, geriatric patients 100 hours). Because hepatic metabolism is the primary organ of elimination, reduced liver function results in prolonged half-life.

The optimally effective therapeutic concentration of phenobarbital is between 15 and 40 µg/mL.[35] The predominant side effect observed in adults at blood concentrations greater than 40 µg/mL is sedation, although tolerance to this effect develops with chronic therapy.

Phenobarbital is metabolized by CyP 2C19 to *p*-hydroxyphenobarbital, which is largely excreted as the glucuronide (by UGT). When renal and hepatic function are decreased, patients experience decreased clearance of the drug. Alcohol, carbamazepine, other barbiturates, and rifampin induce oxidative enzymes (CyP 2C19 and 2C9); this induction results in increased metabolism of phenytoin, reduced serum concentration of phenobarbital, and a reduced pharmacological effect. Drugs such as chloramphenicol, cimetidine, disulfiram, isoniazid, omeprazole, and topiramate compete with phenobarbital metabolism. Elimination of phenobarbital may be decreased in the presence of valproic acid and salicylate if reduction in urinary pH occurs. During chronic administration of either valproate or salicylate, the concentration of phenobarbital may increase 10% to 20%, and a dose adjustment may be necessary to avoid intoxication. Phenobarbital induces mixed-function oxidative enzymes (CyP 2B6), resulting in increased metabolism of other xenobiotics after approximately 1 to 2 weeks of therapy.

Because of the long elimination half-life of phenobarbital, the blood concentration does not change rapidly. Therefore a serum specimen collected late in the dose interval (trough) is representative of the overall effect. Results from specimens collected 2 to 4 hours after the dose can be misleading, because they may be construed to be the peak concentration when in actuality they precede the peak. Table 33-1 summarizes pharmacokinetic data of the anticonvulsant drugs.

Phenytoin

Phenytoin (diphenylhydantoin), most commonly available as *Dilantin* but also available in generic form, is used in the treatment of primary or secondary generalized tonic-clonic seizures, partial or complex-partial seizures, and status epilepticus. The drug is not effective for absence seizures. Phenytoin acts by modulating the synaptic sodium channel by prolonging inactivation, which reduces the ability of the neuron to respond at high frequency.[51] The physiological effect of this action is reduction in central synaptic transmission, aiding in control of abnormal neuronal excitability.

Phenytoin is not readily soluble in aqueous solutions. When administered by intramuscular injection, most of the dose precipitates at the site of injection and is then slowly absorbed. A prodrug called fosphenytoin *(Cerebyx)* allows intramuscular injection of phenytoin and has increased aqueous solubility for intramuscular injection.[112] After injection, it is rapidly converted to phenytoin. Absorption of oral phenytoin is slow and sometimes incomplete. Variations in the drug preparation have been blamed for low bioavailability. Once absorbed, the drug is tightly bound to protein (90% to 95%). As with all drugs, the pharmacological effect of phenytoin is directly related to the amount present in the free (unbound) state. Only free phenytoin is available to cross biological membranes and interact at biologically important binding sites. The degree of protein binding can be reduced by the presence of other drugs, anemia, and hypoalbuminemia, which occurs regularly in the elderly. In these conditions, an increased effect is observed at the same total drug concentration as in plasma from normal patients.

The optimal therapeutic concentration for seizure control without side effects is 10 to 20 μg/mL. In a large population study, Buchthal and colleagues found a 50% response rate in patients with plasma concentrations greater than 10 μg/mL and an 86% suppression of seizure activity at concentrations exceeding 15 μg/mL.[12] These concentrations also serve as reasonable guidelines when the drug is used as a cardiac antiarrhythmic agent. Free phenytoin concentrations of 1 to 2 μg/mL are optimal. Total phenytoin concentrations in excess of 20 μg/mL do not usually enhance seizure control and are often associated with nystagmus and ataxia. Total phenytoin plasma concentrations in excess of 35 μg/mL have been shown to actually precipitate seizure activity. A side effect of phenytoin not related to plasma concentration is development of gingival hyperplasia.

Phenytoin is metabolized by hepatic microsomal hydroxylating enzymes by CyP 2C19 and 2C9. The principal metabolite is 5-(*p*-hydroxyphenyl)-5-phenylhydantoin, which is excreted principally as a glucuronide ester (by UGT). Other minor metabolites are of minimal clinical importance. Hepatic metabolism of phenytoin may become saturated within the therapeutic range. Once metabolism is saturated, small dose increments result in large changes in blood concentration (see Figure 33-10); this phenomenon partially explains the wide variation in dose among patients that is required to accomplish a therapeutic effect.[66] Because of this saturation phenomenon, first-order kinetics do not apply to phenytoin at blood concentrations in excess of 5 μg/mL.

The time to collect the specimen is determined by the reason for monitoring. If a patient displays any symptoms of intoxication, then the peak blood concentration is of interest. This specimen is collected 4 to 5 hours after the dose, although the peak level may be delayed up to 8 hours if the drug is given in conjunction with food or drugs that increase stomach acidity. If the principal question at hand is adequate therapy, then the trough concentration is more useful; that specimen is collected just before the next dose is given.

A number of drug interactions result in alteration of the disposition of phenytoin. Alcohol, carbamazepine, other barbiturates, and rifampin induce oxidative enzymes (CyP 2C19 and 2C9); this induction results in increased metabolism of phenytoin, reduced serum concentration of both total and free phenytoin, and reduced pharmacological effect. Drugs such as chloramphenicol, cimetidine, disulfiram, isoniazid, omeprazole, and topiramate compete with phenytoin metabolism, resulting in an increase of both total and free phenytoin concentrations and enhancement of the pharmacological effect. Salicylate, valproic acid, phenylbutazone, sulfisoxazole, and sulfonylureas compete with phenytoin for serum protein-binding sites. The end result is diminished total serum concentration of phenytoin while the free phenytoin concentration and pharmacological effect remain approximately the same. The interest in monitoring the free phenytoin concentration is in response to these altered protein-binding states.

Primidone

Primidone, proprietary name *Mysoline,* is effective in the treatment of tonic-clonic and partial seizures. The mechanism of action of this drug is similar to that described for phenobarbital, and the therapeutic effect is due partially to the accumulation of its major metabolite, phenobarbital, created by the action of CyP 2C19. A second metabolite of primidone, phenylethylmalonamide, created by the action of CyP 2C9 also has some antiepileptic activity.

Primidone is rapidly and completely absorbed after oral administration. Once absorbed, it is not highly protein bound and it has a half-life of approximately 10 hours. Disposition of the drug is known to be affected by the drugs that alter CyP 2C19 and 2C9 metabolism and by diseases that alter phenobarbital disposition.

The optimal therapeutic concentration of primidone has been established as 5 to 12 µg/mL. Because phenobarbital is an active metabolite of primidone, concurrent analysis of phenobarbital is required for complete result interpretation. The previously defined therapeutic range for phenobarbital applies to adequate primidone therapy. The phenobarbital concentrations rise gradually over a period of 1 to 2 weeks after therapy is initiated. Toxicity due to accumulation of primidone occurs at serum concentrations in excess of 15 µg/mL and is usually associated with symptoms of sedation, nausea, vomiting, diplopia, dizziness, ataxia, and a phenobarbital concentration greater than 40 µg/mL. Specimen collection is dictated by the same rules that apply to phenobarbital; the trough concentration is most useful.

Co-administration of acetazolamide with primidone results in decreased gastrointestinal absorption of primidone and subsequent diminished plasma concentrations. Primidone administered in association with phenytoin produces a modest elevation of the phenobarbital/primidone ratio because phenytoin competes with the hepatic hydroxylating enzymes associated with phenobarbital's metabolism. Co-administration of valproic acid, for the same reasons outlined for phenobarbital, causes a modest increase in both primidone and phenobarbital serum concentrations.

Topiramate

Topiramate *(Topamax)* is a broad spectrum, antiepileptic drug. It has sodium channel blocking activity and it potentiates the activity of gamma-aminobutyric acid (GABA), and inhibits the potentiation of the glutamate receptor. Because of this range of activities, topiramate blocks seizure spread rather than raising seizure potential.

Topiramate is routinely administered orally, absorbed rapidly, and metabolized minimally, but its disposition is affected by CyP 2C19. Serum concentrations of other anticonvulsant drugs are not significantly affected by the concurrent administration of topiramate, with the exception in individual patients on phenytoin who exhibit increased phenytoin plasma concentrations after addition of topiramate. Co-administration of phenytoin or carbamazepine decreases topiramate serum concentrations. Changes in cotherapy with phenytoin or carbamazepine (e.g., addition or withdrawal) for patients stabilized on topiramate therapy may require topiramate dose adjustment. As with other renally eliminated anticonvulsant drugs, patients with impaired renal function exhibit decreased renal clearance.

Peak serum blood concentration of topiramate is achieved 2 to 3 hours after dosing. Peak concentrations in the range of 9.0 to 12 µg/mL indicate that the dose is appropriate to achieve optimal antiepileptic activity. The minimum blood concentration, achieved just before the next dose, should be >2.0 µg/mL to ensure adequate antiepileptic protection. Concentrations <2.0 µg/mL indicate that the dose is either suboptimal or administered too infrequently.[103] Topiramate may be quantified by immunoassay or GLC-FID.

Valproic Acid

Valproic acid, brand name *Depakene* or *Depakote*, is used for treatment of absence seizures. It has also been shown to be useful against tonic-clonic and partial seizures when used in conjunction with other antiepileptic agents, such as phenobarbital or phenytoin. The drug inhibits the enzyme GABA transaminase, resulting in an increase in the concentration of GABA in the brain. GABA is a potent inhibitor of presynaptic and postsynaptic discharges in the central nervous system. Valproic acid also modulates the synaptic sodium channel by prolonging inactivation, which reduces the ability of the neuron to respond at high frequency. This action gives it some activity against tonic-clonic seizures.[51]

Valproic acid is rapidly and almost completely absorbed after oral administration. Peak concentrations occur 1 to 4 hours after an oral dose. The principal metabolite, 2-*n*-propyl-3-ketopentanoic acid, is created by action of CyP 2C19 and has anticonvulsant activity comparable to that of valproic acid, although this metabolite does not accumulate in plasma; the exact cytochrome enzyme isomer involved in metabolism has not been identified. The single-dose half-life is 16 hours in healthy adults, but this decreases to 12 hours on chronic therapy and may be as short as 8 hours in children. In neonates and in hepatic disease, when metabolism is reduced, the half-life becomes prolonged. Valproic acid is highly protein bound (93%). In circumstances when competition for protein binding increases, such as in uremia, cirrhosis, or concurrent drug therapy, the percent of free valproic acid increases.

The minimum effective therapeutic concentration of valproic acid is 50 µg/mL. Concentrations in excess of 100 µg/mL have been associated with hepatic toxicity and acute toxic encephalopathy. Glycine has been observed to accumulate in patients on valproic acid therapy.

Clearance of valproic acid is rapid, presenting a dosing dilemma. The dose must be adequate to provide a plasma concentration >40 µg/mL while avoiding concentrations in excess of 100 µg/mL. The ideal specimen for monitoring blood concentration is the one drawn just before the next dose, usually early in the morning to confirm that an adequate dose has been prescribed before bedtime. Dosing is particularly problematic in young children who might sleep for more than one complete half-life of the drug.

Valproic acid modulates the action of various other common antiepileptic drugs. It inhibits the nonrenal clearance of phenobarbital, resulting in elevated phenobarbital levels. It competes with phenytoin for protein-binding sites. The free phenytoin concentration remains approximately the same, but the total phenytoin in the plasma decreases. Because the free phenytoin concentration remains unchanged, the pharmacological effect is retained. Other common antiepileptic drugs that induce hepatic oxidative enzymes result in increased valproic acid clearance; this increased clearance rate requires a higher dose to maintain effective therapeutic levels.

γ-Aminobutyric Acid Analogs/Agonists

Studies of benzodiazepines that occurred in the 1970s led to knowledge of the GABA receptor, a membrane-bound protein complex on the surface of dedicated neural and glial cells that operate as inhibitory neurotransmitters. Activation of these cells serves to restrain neuronal excitation. Absence of or decreased GABA control of neurotransmission is one cause of seizure activity. These studies led to the development of drugs that act to increase the activity of GABA receptors, either by increasing GABA concentration or by directly interacting with the GABA receptor. Felbamate, gabapentin, lamotrigine, tiagabine, and zonisamide are examples of such drugs.

Felbamate

Felbamate, proprietary name *Felbatol,* was approved for primary or adjunctive therapy of partial seizures. Its use is limited to those patients who fail other drug treatments, because felbamate carries with it a substantial risk of aplastic anemia and liver failure that is not related to the blood level. Biweekly monitoring of complete blood count, serum aminotransferases, and bilirubin is recommended to detect early onset of these side effects. Felbamate is particularly effective in control of Lennox-Gastaut syndrome.

Felbamate is completely absorbed from the gastrointestinal tract. The drug is 30% bound to plasma proteins, and optimal blood concentrations for felbamate range from 40 to 120 μg/mL.[26] It is eliminated by hepatic metabolism (CyP 2D6), with its half-life ranging from 14 to 21 hours.[26] Felbamate saturates metabolism when the concentration exceeds 120 μg/mL; at that concentration, metabolism converts from first order to zero order. HPLC is commonly used for felbamate analysis.[116,128]

Gabapentin

Gabapentin, proprietary name *Neurontin,* is a chemical analog of GABA that promotes the release of GABA. It does not interact directly with the GABA receptor, nor does it inhibit glutamic acid decarboxylase, the enzyme that usually controls cellular concentration of GABA. Gabapentin has been proven effective for treatment of drug-resistant partial seizures.[113]

Absorption of oral gabapentin is complete. Gabapentin is 10% bound to plasma proteins, and its elimination half-life is 5 to 9 hours. The optimally effective therapeutic concentration of gabapentin is between 2 and 12 μg/mL.[10,26] Side effects observed in adults at blood concentrations greater than 12 μg/mL are somnolence, ataxia, dizziness, and fatigue. The drug does not undergo hepatic metabolism, and it does not activate any metabolic enzymes, so co-administration of gabapentin with other drugs does not affect their concentrations. Co-administration with antacids is known to reduce absorption of gabapentin by approximately 20%. HPLC is used to quantify gabapentin.[53]

Lamotrigine

Lamotrigine, proprietary name *Lamictal,* is not a GABA analog, but binds to the GABA receptor; it is therefore considered a GABA agonist. Lamotrigine acts like phenytoin and carbamazepine, blocking repetitive nerve firings induced by depolarization of spinal cord neurons. The FDA approved lamotrigine for adjunctive therapy of partial seizures.

Lamotrigine is satisfactorily tolerated and completely absorbed from the gastrointestinal tract after oral administration. It is 60% bound to plasma proteins. Optimal response occurs when the trough blood level is between 1 and 2 μg/mL, and the peak level ranges from 5 to 8 μg/mL.[18,26] Half-life ranges from 20 to 30 hours. Elimination occurs through metabolism by UGT; the metabolite is the glucuronide ester. Co-administration with CyP 2C19–inducing drugs such as phenobarbital, phenytoin, or carbamazepine results in reduced lamotrigine concentration—dosage increases of approximately 30% are required to maintain optimal blood concentration.

Lamotrigine is a potent inhibitor of dihydrofolate reductase. Folate concentrations are decreased when this drug is administered. If folate replacement is not implemented, rash and anemia may be experienced when lamotrigine is at its therapeutic concentration. Lamotrigine has also been associated with development of severe rash (Stevens-Johnson syndrome) in approximately 1% of patients receiving lamotrigine. These side effects are not drug concentration related.

Dizziness, ataxia, diplopia, blurred vision, nausea, and vomiting are signs of toxicity that occur when the blood level exceeds 10 μg/mL. A chromatographic method for analysis of lamotrigine has been reported.[42]

Tiagabine

Tiagabine, proprietary name *Gabitril,* is indicated as adjunctive therapy in adults and children for treatment of partial seizures. It is frequently administered to patients receiving at least one concomitant antiepileptic drug. Tiagabine is a selective blocker of GABA uptake into presynaptic neurons. Tiagabine binds to recognition sites associated with the GABA uptake carrier. By this action, tiagabine blocks GABA uptake into presynaptic neurons, permitting more GABA to be available for receptor binding on the surface of postsynaptic cells.

Tiagabine has an elimination half-life of 7 to 9 hours. In patients receiving CyP 3A4 inducing anti-epileptic drugs (AEDs), the elimination half-life decreases to 4 to 7 hours. Phenytoin, phenobarbital, and carbamazepine are CyP 3A4 inducers. Valproic acid and gabapentin are not. Tiagabine is not considered to be a CyP 3A4 inducer.[130]

Tiagabine reaches peak serum concentration approximately 45 minutes following an oral dose in the fasting state. Pediatric patients reach peak concentration at approximately 2.4 hours.[49] Tiagabine is well absorbed, with food slowing the absorption rate but not altering the extent of absorption (high fat diet prolongs peak serum concentrations to about 2.5 hours). Tiagabine is >95% absorbed, with oral bioavailability of about 90%. Tiagabine pharmacokinetics are linear over the typical dose range of 2 to 24 mg. Tiagabine is 96% bound to human plasma proteins, mainly to serum albumin and alpha-1-acid glycoprotein. Co-administration with valproic acid reduces protein binding to 94%, increasing the free fraction of tiagabine by 40%.[8]

Trough tiagabine serum concentrations vary from 5 to 35 ng/mL in most patients receiving therapeutic doses and are proportional to dose. A single 4 mg dose administered to a child produced a peak serum concentration in the range of 52 to 108 ng/mL. At steady state, an adult receiving 40 mg per day is expected to have peak serum concentration in the range of 110 to 260 ng/mL, and an adult receiving 80 mg per day is expected to have peak serum concentration in the range of 220 to 520 ng/mL. Serum concentrations >800 ng/mL indicate excessive dosing associated with adverse effects such as asthenia, ataxia, difficulty concentrating, and depression.

Zonisamide

Zonisamide, proprietary name *Zonegran,* is a sodium and calcium channel blocker. It also binds to the GABA receptor, but does not produce a chloride influx. Approved for adjunct treatment of partial seizures that do not respond to a single drug, zonisamide is satisfactorily tolerated but not completely absorbed from the gastrointestinal tract after oral administration; bioavailability averages 50%. It is 50% bound to plasma proteins. Optimal response occurs when the peak level ranged from 10 to 30 μg/mL.[72] Half-life ranges from 50 to 70 hours. Elimination occurs through metabolism by Cyp 2C19. Co-administration with CyP 2C19–inducing drugs such as phenobarbital, phenytoin, or carbamazepine results in reduced zonisamide concentration.[40] Chromatographic methods for analysis of zonisamide have been reported.[61,94]

Miscellaneous, Infrequently Used Antiepileptic Drugs

Benzodiazepines, mephobarbital, and succinimides have antiepileptic activity. However, they are infrequently prescribed for this purpose.

Benzodiazepines

Benzodiazepines interact at the $GABA_A$ receptor to increase the duration of chloride flow into the synapse.[51] The end result is an increase in seizure threshold and inhibition of the spread of discharges from the epileptic foci.

Diazepam, proprietary name *Valium,* is frequently used in emergency situations to gain control in status epilepticus. Unfortunately, tolerance to diazepam at the GABA receptor develops rapidly, and diazepam becomes ineffective within 2 to 3 days. Diazepam is therefore not used for long-term control of seizure disorders.

Clonazepam, proprietary name *Clonopin,* is a benzodiazepine with chemical structure closely related to diazepam. The mechanism of action is the same as described for diazepam, but tolerance does not develop as rapidly as with diazepam. Clonazepam is currently approved for use in absence seizures, infantile spasms, akinetic seizures, and Lennox-Gastaut syndrome. Plasma concentrations associated with maximal effectiveness of the drug range from 15 to 60 ng/mL. At concentrations higher than 80 ng/mL, no additional seizure protection is observed, and toxicity (drowsiness and ataxia) ensues. The most suitable methods adaptable to routine analysis are based on GLC with electron capture detection,[30] although HPLC methods also are effective.[1]

Mephobarbital

The antiepileptic activity of mephobarbital, proprietary name *Mebaral,* is due to its principal metabolite, phenobarbital. Metabolism is through hepatic CyP 2C19, induced by phenobarbital. Thus long-term therapy results in multiphasic elimination profiles of the drug. Early in therapy, high concentrations (>5 μg/mL) of mephobarbital and low concentrations (<10 μg/mL) of phenobarbital may be observed. After enzymatic induction, the pattern shifts to one in which phenobarbital predominates (20 to 40 μg/mL) and mephobarbital is a minor constituent (1 to 3 μg/mL) at equilibrium. Effective therapeutic monitoring can be accomplished only after a steady state has been achieved by administering a constant dose for at least 21 days. Mephobarbital concentration is usually determined by chromatography as described for phenobarbital methods. It should be noted that mephobarbital in most immunoassays cross-reacts to some degree with phenobarbital.

Succinimides

Three succinimides have proved useful in the control of absence seizures: ethosuximide (proprietary name *Zarontin*), methsuximide (proprietary name *Celontin*), and phensuximide (proprietary name *Milontin*). Ethosuximide is widely used and is reviewed elsewhere in this chapter. Methsuximide and phensuximide are less commonly used and monitored.

Both methsuximide and phensuximide are active in control of absence seizures and seizures of temporal lobe

TABLE 33-2 Pharmacokinetic Parameters of Cardioactive Drugs

Drug	Minimum Effective Concentration (MEC) (μg/mL*)	Minimum Toxic Concentration (MTC) (μg/mL*)	Average Half-Life (hr)	Average Oral Volume of Distribution (L/kg)	Average Bioavailability (%)	Important Protein Binding (%)	Metabolizing Enzymes
Amiodarone	1.0	2.0	45 days†	60	45	99	CyP 3A4, Pg
Digoxin	0.5 ng/mL*	0.8 ng/mL*	40	5	70	25	CyP 3A4, Pg
Disopyramide	2.0	5.0	8	0.6	83	45-70*	CyP 2D6
Flecainide	0.2	1.0	14	5	70	45	CyP 2D6
Lidocaine	1.5	6.0	1.8	1.1	35	70	CyP 2D6 CyP 3A4, Pg
Mexiletine	0.7	2.0	10	5	90	60	CyP 2D6
Procainamide	4.0	12.0	6	1.9	83	20	NAT1
N-Acetylprocainamide	12.0	18.0	8				
Propafenone	0.2	1.0	6	2.0	40	90	CyP 2D6
Propranolol	0.020	0.10	4	4.0	25	90	CyP 1A2, 2D6
Quinidine	2.0	5.0	6	2.7	80	85	CyP 3A4, Pg
Tocainide	6.0	15.0	12	3	90	10	CyP 2D6

*Except where noted in text.
†See text.

origin, but phensuximide has been found to be less effective because of its short half-life. Methsuximide is effective because it is metabolized to an active metabolite that is stable and has a long half-life. Steady-state serum concentrations of methsuximide and normethsuximide on a standard adult dose of 900 mg/d range from 0.01 to 0.040 μg/mL and 10 to 40 μg/mL, respectively.

Cardioactive Drugs

Pharmacokinetic parameters of digoxin and other cardioactive drugs are summarized in Table 33-2. Digoxin, disopyramide, lidocaine, procainamide, and quinidine are usually quantified by immunoassay. HPLC methods to quantify the other cardioactive drugs are reviewed in a previous edition of this chapter.[91]

Amiodarone

Amiodarone, proprietary name *Cordarone,* is used to control supraventricular and ventricular tachyarrhythmias. The drug is of interest as a substitute for other class I antiarrhythmics, such as procainamide or quinidine, because it has a very long elimination half-life (45 days). The effective serum concentration of the drug, measured 24 hours after a single daily dose, ranges from 1.0 to 2.0 μg/mL.[117] The drug is indicated for control of ventricular tachycardia and fibrillation resistant to other forms of therapy. Amiodarone is extensively metabolized by the CyP 3A4 system; its metabolism is significantly affected by co-administration with carbamazepine, erythromycin, phenytoin, rifampin, and St. John's Wort. In addition, the presence of amiodarone will prolong metabolism of several drugs including cyclosporine, digoxin, protease inhibitors, sirolimus (Siro), tacrolimus (Tac), and verapamil.

Amiodarone is a structural analog of thyroxine, and much of its toxicity is related to interactions that occur at thyroid hormone receptors. Pulmonary fibrosis is a frequent adverse effect that is related to dose, and drug level doses <200 mg/day and maintenance of peak levels <2 μg/mL can help avoid this life-threatening side effect.

Digoxin

Digoxin, proprietary name *Lanoxin,* is one of a group of cardiac glycosides obtained from digitalis plants (e.g., *Digitalis lanata*). It restores the force of cardiac contraction in congestive heart failure and is also used in the management of supraventricular tachycardias. The drug binds to the extracytoplasmic side of the α-subunit of membrane-bound Na^+-K^+-ATPase, inhibiting both cellular Na^+ efflux, and K^+ influx in myocardial cells. This reduces the sodium/potassium gradient in the Purkinje's fibers of the atrial, junctional, and ventricular myocardium, resulting in a decreased transmembrane potential. Inhibition of Na^+-K^+-ATPase is postulated to enhance movement of calcium ions in the cell, increasing calcium ion availability and improving cardiac contractility.

At low concentrations, digoxin causes the atrium to be less electrically excitable. Moderate concentrations of digoxin are required to reduce the rate of depolarization in the spontaneously depolarizing conductive fibers (Purkinje's fibers), and toxic concentrations of digoxin are necessary to diminish depolarization of the ventricular myocardium. Disagreement over the clinical value of digoxin measurements and the failure of the digoxin concentration to correlate with clinical toxicity are usually related to aberrations in serum and tissue concentrations of sodium, potassium, magnesium, and calcium. Increased sensitivity to digoxin is noted in states of hypokalemia, hypomagnesemia, and hypercalcemia, which make establishment of the true therapeutic concentration of digoxin difficult because all parameters are interactive.

Absorption of digoxin is variable and dependent on the drug formulation. The *U.S. Pharmacopeia* requires more than 65% of digoxin in tablet form to dissolve in 60 minutes. In plasma, digoxin is 25% protein bound. Digoxin is concentrated in tissue. In a steady state, the concentration of digoxin in cardiac tissue is 15 to 30 times that of plasma. Accumulation of digoxin in tissue lags behind the plasma concentration. For example, although the peak plasma concentration is reached 2 to 3 hours after the oral dose, the peak tissue concentration occurs 6 to 10 hours after an oral dose. Although pharmacological effects and toxicity correlate with tissue concentration rather than plasma concentration, the effective and safe therapeutic plasma concentration of digoxin ranges from 0.8 to 2.0 ng/mL.[102] (However, this range has recently been questioned, with a suggestion that maintenance of digoxin in the range of 0.5 to 0.8 ng/mL is most efficacious.)[114] Clinically, the effective range for digoxin is not determined at the peak plasma concentration but rather at the time of peak tissue concentration. Thus to ensure a correlation between plasma concentration and tissue concentration, the appropriate time to collect the specimen is 8 hours or more after the dose. Results from specimens collected earlier than 8 hours after the dose are misleading, because they do not correlate with tissue concentrations.

Digoxin *toxicity* is characterized by nonspecific symptoms of nausea, vomiting, anorexia, and predominance of green/yellow visual distortion. Cardiac symptoms of intoxication include multiform premature ventricular contractions (PVCs), ventricular bigeminy, ventricular tachycardia, and ventricular fibrillation. Combinations of decreased conduction and increased automaticity may result in paroxysmal atrial tachycardia with atrioventricular node block and nonparoxysmal junction tachycardia. These symptoms are frequently observed when the blood concentration exceeds 2 ng/mL in adults. Children tolerate higher concentrations and do not usually exhibit toxicity until the digoxin concentration exceeds 4 ng/mL. The relationship between the blood level of digoxin and clinical and toxic response is presented in Figure 33-11.[74]

Elimination of digoxin follows first-order kinetics; 50% to 70% is excreted unchanged or in the form of digoxigenin monosaccharides or disaccharides in the urine. A small amount is metabolized to dihydrodigoxin and also excreted by the kidneys. The remainder is found in the stool as digoxigenin and its saccharides. As a result, digoxin toxicity develops more frequently and lasts longer in patients with renal impairment. Dose requirements are decreased in patients with renal disease. In 1979, Bresnahan and Vlietstra presented a simple method for calculating dosage based on creatinine clearance and uses the concepts outlined in equation (13).[11] Digoxin is metabolized by CyP 3A4 and is transported out of cells via the P-glycoprotein transporter (Pg); co-administration of cyclosporine, protease inhibitors, quinidine, Siro, Tac, or verapamil prolongs the rate of clearance of digoxin, requiring dose adjustment.

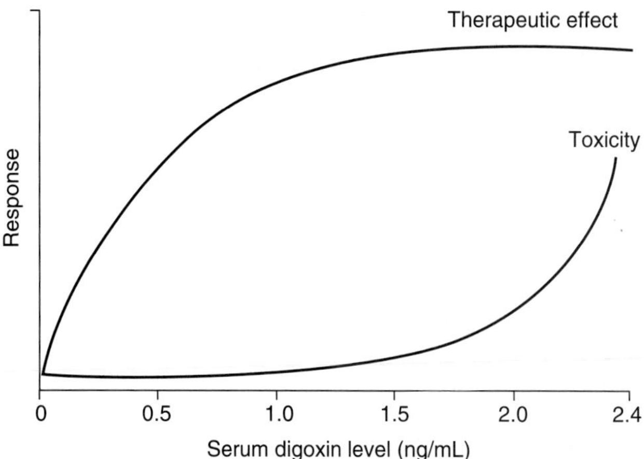

Figure 33-11 Relationship between digoxin concentration and response, showing that the therapeutic effect occurs at low concentration, whereas the onset of toxicity occurs exponentially as the concentration increases.

Decreased gastrointestinal absorption of digoxin occurs with sprue and small intestinal resections, high-fiber diets, hyperthyroidism, and situations of increased gastrointestinal motility. A more dangerous situation develops secondary to the interaction of quinidine and digoxin,[70] resulting in an increase in the digoxin concentration.

Nonisotopic immunoassays (see Chapter 9) are the standard for measuring and monitoring digoxin levels. Accurate results have been obtained with small sample sizes (e.g., 10 to 50 μL serum) and short incubation times (e.g., 8 to 30 minutes). In the typical immunoassay, patient samples, controls, and calibrators containing digoxin are placed in assay tubes with a constant amount of immobilized digoxin antibody. During an incubation period, the digoxin from the specimen binds to the antibodies. In most assays, the remaining unbound digoxin antibodies left after the preliminary incubation are washed and then reacted with a labeled digoxin analog followed by a short, fixed-time incubation. The amount of label bound to the immobilized antibody decreases in proportion to the increasing amounts of unlabeled digoxin from the original specimen. Levels of digoxin in the samples are then determined by relating the amount of bound label in each tube to a calibration curve constructed from appropriate calibrators. For more detailed instructions on these techniques, the protocol for the specific procedure used should be consulted.

Note: Digitoxin is infrequently prescribed; however, serum levels should be evaluated in patients suspected of having digitalis intoxication with nondetectable digoxin levels. Digoxin immunoassay procedures cross-react only minimally with digitoxin, requiring that a digitoxin-selective antibody be substituted in the assay.

Disopyramide

Disopyramide, proprietary name *Norpace,* is used for maintenance of sinus rhythm in patients with atrial flutter and atrial fibrillation and for prevention of ventricular tachycardia and fibrillation. The mechanism of action of disopyramide is similar to that of quinidine, and the drug can be used as replacement therapy for quinidine when quinidine side effects are intolerable.

Disopyramide is nearly completely absorbed, and a small fraction undergoes first-pass hepatic metabolism. In the blood, disopyramide binds to plasma proteins. Binding is highly variable among individuals and also depends on the concentration of disopyramide; the higher the concentration, the greater the free fraction. Thus toxicity develops rapidly as the drug concentration increases. The elimination half-life is 4 to 8 hours. Elimination is by renal clearance and hepatic metabolism. Metabolism has a minor role in elimination, but with renal insufficiency, clearance is prolonged, causing accumulation of disopyramide.

Optimal antiarrhythmic effect is accomplished at plasma concentrations of 2.0 to 5.0 µg/mL. The relationship between clinical response and optimal therapeutic concentration is confused by a decrease in protein binding, which occurs as plasma concentration of disopyramide rises.[24] Disopyramide binds variably to serum proteins; binding ranges from 45% to 70% at 2 µg/mL total serum concentration and 30% to 45% at 5 µg/mL.

Disopyramide is metabolized to nordisopyramide (monodealkylated) by the action of CyP 2D6; nordisopyramide has antiarrhythmic activity approximately 25% that of disopyramide. Under normal circumstances, nordisopyramide accumulates to concentrations ranging from 0.2 to 1.0 µg/mL, and the compound does not accumulate out of proportion to disopyramide in situations of reduced hepatic or renal function. Therefore little additional therapeutic information is gained by monitoring nordisopyramide.

The predominant side effects of disopyramide are anticholinergic and include dry mouth, urinary hesitancy, and constipation. These symptoms occur at plasma concentrations exceeding 4.5 µg/mL. Cardiac toxicity is usually associated with blood concentrations greater than 10 µg/mL and is characterized by atrioventricular node blockage, bradycardia, and asystole. Because of the wide degree of variability of protein binding, interindividual differences in the blood concentration at which these symptoms develop are great. Disopyramide is analyzed by HPLC or immunoassay.

Flecainide

Flecainide, proprietary name *Tambocor,* is a sodium channel blocker with cardiac activity like disopyramide. The drug has significant toxicity in patients with myocardial infarction and has therefore fallen out of favor. For those patients who fail to respond to other sodium channel blockers, it might be a drug of last resort.

Flecainide is completely absorbed. It has an elimination half-life of 10 to 17 hours. Elimination occurs by hepatic metabolism (CyP 2D6) and renal clearance. Drugs affecting the CyP 2D6 will interfere with flecainide metabolism. Optimal response occurs when serum levels are in the range of 200 to 1000 ng/mL.[34] HPLC methods for measuring flecanide have been developed.[91]

Lidocaine

Lidocaine, proprietary name *Xylocaine,* is the drug of choice for the initial therapy of PVCs and the prevention of ventricular arrhythmias. Lidocaine is contraindicated when bradycardias and severe atrioventricular node block appear after myocardial infarction. Lidocaine shortens the action potential refractory period in these fibers and does so at concentrations less than those required to exert pharmacological effects at other sites, such as the ventricular myocardium.

Because lidocaine undergoes nearly complete first-pass hepatic metabolism by CyP 3A4 and 2D6 when administered orally, it is administered only as an intravenous or intramuscular injection. Once in the blood, it is 50% bound to protein, mainly to AAG and albumin. Clearance of lidocaine is very rapid. The distribution half-life is ~0.5 hour, and the elimination half-life is 1 to 1.5 hours. Reduced hepatic function impairs clearance and causes prolonged elimination and accumulation of the drug. This is due both to reduced blood flow to the liver (seen in heart failure) and to decreased metabolism of lidocaine. The end effect is lidocaine intoxication if the dose is not adjusted to account for this decreased metabolic rate.

The relationship between optimal blood concentration of lidocaine and its clinical effect is best interpreted in light of the greatest likelihood of therapeutic success, therapeutic failure, or toxicity for selective concentration increments. Blood concentrations less than 1.5 µg/mL are rarely effective. Concentrations ranging from 1.5 to 6.0 µg/mL are usually effective and are rarely associated with any form of central nervous system or cardiovascular toxicity. Concentrations ranging from 4 to 6 µg/mL may be needed for suppressing arrhythmias but may be associated with mild central nervous system depression and slight QRS widening on the electrocardiogram. Concentrations ranging from 6 to 8 µg/mL are acceptable only if alternative therapy is not possible, because these levels have been associated with significant central nervous system depression and atrioventricular node blockage. Concentrations exceeding 8 µg/mL are commonly associated with seizure activity, significant hypotension, and life-threatening decreased cardiac output.

Lidocaine has two metabolites formed by action of Cyp 2D6 and 3A4 that are detected in plasma, monoethylglycinexylidide (MEGX) and glycinexylidide (GX). MEGX and lidocaine have nearly identical toxic equivalency, and the sum total of lidocaine and MEGX concentration averaged 18.7 µg/mL (ranging from 17.9 to 28.0 µg/mL) in patients experiencing lidocaine-induced convulsions. Substitution of MEGX for lidocaine resulted in the same mean concentration for the equivalent convulsive activity.

Because lidocaine is most commonly administered as a constant infusion after a loading dose, the time to collect the specimen is determined by the reason for monitoring. If the blood concentration is intended to document an adequate concentration early in therapy, the specimen should be collected 30 minutes after the loading dose, or 5 to 7 hours after therapy is initiated if no loading dose is given (five half-lives after start of therapy). If a patient shows diminished mental status, QRS widening, or other toxic symptoms, the specimen should be collected as close to the episode as possible and analysis performed immediately, because these symptoms present a potentially life-threatening situation (onset of severe lidocaine intoxication).

The total plasma concentration of lidocaine is a result of clearance of the drug and is modulated by hepatic function. There is little impact on clearance in renal disease. In situations of decreased organ perfusion, clearance is reduced and increased blood concentrations of lidocaine should be expected; reduced dosing is appropriate in these circumstances. The principal binding protein of lidocaine, AAG, has been demonstrated to accumulate after myocardial infarction. The result of accumulation of this protein is reduction of free lidocaine, which reduces the pharmacological effect of the drug. Lidocaine is usually analyzed by immunoassay, and MEGX and GX by HPLC.

Mexiletine

Mexiletine, proprietary name *Mexitil,* is used for control of ventricular dysrhythmias. It undergoes hepatic metabolism by CyP 2D6. The therapeutic concentration varies from 0.7 to 2.0 μg/mL. The drug exhibits a high degree of oral bioavailability, is approximately 60% protein bound, and is predominantly cleared by the kidneys. Mexiletine has a large volume of distribution (5 L/kg), indicating that it is highly tissue bound. Myocardial infarction and uremia reduce renal clearance, resulting in an increase in half-life. Mexiletine toxicity occurs at concentrations greater than 2 μg/mL and is characterized by tremor, dizziness, ataxia, dysarthria, diplopia, nystagmus, confusion, and hypotension.

Procainamide

Procainamide, proprietary name *Pronestyl,* is used for therapy of PVCs, ventricular tachycardia, atrial fibrillation, and paroxysmal atrial tachycardia. Its mechanism of action is similar to that of quinidine in that it increases the threshold membrane potential by blocking potassium outflow, reducing excitability and contraction velocity in Purkinje's fibers and ventricular muscle.

Absorption of procainamide is rapid and complete. Peak plasma concentrations after oral administration are reached within 0.75 to 1.5 hours if the drug is given in capsule form or within 1 to 3 hours if given in tablet form. Once absorbed, procainamide is about 20% bound to plasma proteins. Excretion of procainamide depends on hepatic metabolism by *N*-acetyltransferase (NAT1) and renal clearance; therefore alteration in either organ function leads to accumulation of procainamide and its metabolites. The half-life is 3 to 4 hours in healthy adults.

The concentration at which procainamide blocks PVCs and inhibits ventricular tachycardia ranges from 4 to 12 μg/mL, although patients are able tolerate concentrations higher than this for short periods of time. Studies by Meyerburg[82] suggest that patients experiencing chronic PVCs can tolerate blood concentrations as high as 16 μg/mL to reduce PVCs to a reasonable number. Minimum plasma concentrations of 8 μg/mL were required for protection against sustained ventricular tachycardia.

The issue of the ideal therapeutic concentration for procainamide is complicated by one of its metabolites, *N*-acetylprocainamide (NAPA), having antiarrhythmic activity similar to procainamide. This compound has been shown to accumulate in patients with impaired renal function and fast acetylators.[32] The optimal therapeutic concentration of NAPA is not well defined. The drug is used in Europe, where the maximum tolerable concentration of NAPA in the absence of procainamide is 30 μg/mL. Co-analysis of NAPA is necessary to provide a complete assessment of therapy or define metabolic status. Fast acetylators have concentrations of NAPA equal to or exceeding those of procainamide in a specimen collected 3 hours after administration, whereas slow acetylators have procainamide present at greater than twice the NAPA concentration in a specimen collected during the same time interval. Because the effects of procainamide and NAPA are cumulative, peak plasma concentrations of procainamide should be limited to 8 to 12 μg/mL, and peak concentrations of procainamide plus NAPA should not exceed 30 μg/mL. Interpretation of results requires knowledge of a patient's cardiac status. Given concentrations may be intolerable in some patients, whereas others may require higher levels for control of PVCs.

Symptoms of intoxication include (1) bradycardia, (2) prolongation of the QRS interval, (3) atrioventricular block, and (4) induced arrhythmias. These symptoms occur at blood concentrations of procainamide and NAPA exceeding 30 μg/mL. Hypotension sometimes encountered in procainamide therapy is not related to excessive plasma concentration. The development of systemic lupus erythematosus associated with procainamide therapy is not related to plasma concentration but is associated with the acetylator status of the patient; slow acetylators predominate in the group in whom the syndrome develops.

Propafenone

Propafenone, proprietary name *Rythmol,* is an antiarrhythmic drug that has α-adrenergic receptor blocking properties and minor calcium antagonistic activity. It undergoes extensive first-pass metabolism by CyP 2D6 with a half-life of approximately 6 hours. Its clinical efficacy is maintained through formation of metabolites (primarily 5-hydroxy-propafenone) that are more pharmacologically active than the parent drug and have longer plasma half-lives (11 to 24 hours). It is occasionally useful to measure the serum concentration of propafenone to document patients' compliance. Normal response to the drug occurs when the serum concentration is in the range of 0.2 to 1.0 μg/mL.[51] Toxicity related to propafenone occurs when the blood concentration exceeds 2 μg/mL and is expressed as gastrointestinal upset, central nervous system irritability, and skin reactions.

Propranolol

Propranolol is used in the treatment of arrhythmias of atrial and ventricular origin, angina pectoris, myocardial infarction, and hypertension. It is a nonselective β-blocker with action on cardiac receptors (β_1) and on vascular and bronchial smooth muscle receptors (β_2). Propranolol's principal effect is to reduce the heart rate, thus relieving angina, and to slow conduction at the atrioventricular node, reducing the ventricular rate in patients with atrial fibrillation. It is included here as representative of other β-blockers, such as acebutalol, prindolol, esmolol, flestolol, metoprolol, nadolol, and sotalol, which are like propranolol.

Although propranolol is well absorbed, it undergoes such a high degree of first-pass hepatic metabolism that its final bioavailability is low (20% to 40%), widely variable between individuals, and dose dependent (the higher the dose, the greater the bioavailability). In the plasma, propranolol is highly protein bound (95%) to albumin and AAG. Elimination half-life is 3 to 4 hours. Elimination is predominantly by CyP 1A2 and 2D6 metabolism; therefore, reduced hepatic function or reduced blood flow to the liver causes accumulation of propranolol.

There is a close relationship between slowing of the heart rate and blood concentration.[107] In specimens collected 2 hours after dosing for 2 days with 40 mg of drug four times daily, complete β-adrenergic blockade (equated with suppression of the adrenergic component of exercise-induced tachycardia) correlated with a blood concentration of 100 ng/mL. Blood concentrations in specimens collected 8 hours after the dose, associated with approximately 60% β-adrenergic blockage, ranged from 10 to 40 ng/mL. The same study also documented a close correlation between the blood concentration and the degree of heart rate slowing, suggesting that observation of the heart rate serves as an adequate means to monitor the therapeutic efficacy, precluding blood measurements in most patients. There is virtually no relationship between plasma concentration of propranolol and the hypotensive effect of the drug.

Propranolol and other β-blockers have been analyzed by HPLC using the native fluorescence of the molecule for detection.

Quinidine

Quinidine, available as either quinidine sulfate or quinidine gluconate, is used in the treatment of atrial premature contraction, paroxysmal supraventricular tachycardia, supraventricular tachyarrhythmia, PVCs, and ventricular tachycardia and in prophylactic treatment after myocardial infarction. It is also used with care in the treatment of atrial fibrillation and atrial flutter, although this treatment is commonly accompanied by the administration of either digoxin or a β-blocker (propranolol) to provide atrioventricular node blockade. These pharmacological responses appear to be based on a mechanism of action involving blockade of cholinergic neurotransmission, which results in depression or abolition of ectopic impulse generation, an increase in the duration of action potential of sinoatrial node cells, and most important, prolongation of the effective refractory period of atrial, ventricular, and Purkinje's fibers.

Absorption of quinidine is complete and rapid. Peak serum concentrations are reached in 1.5 to 2 hours after oral intake, unless the slow-release preparation (quinidine gluconate) is used. Peak plasma concentrations are attained 4 to 5 hours after quinidine gluconate administration, and the trough concentration occurs 1 to 2 hours after the next administration. Once absorbed, quinidine is 80% protein bound. Metabolism of quinidine is by CyP 3A4. Clearance of quinidine depends on adequate hepatic and renal function. Reduction of either of these two functions results in accumulation of the drug. Renal clearance is a function of urine pH. If the urine is alkaline or if a patient has renal tubular acidosis, clearance is reduced.

A strong correlation has been shown to exist between blood concentration of quinidine and optimal pharmacological response.[88] The optimal therapeutic concentration for quinidine is 2 to 5 μg/mL. Quinidine toxicity is usually observed at concentrations exceeding 8 μg/mL and is characterized by symptoms of cinchonism, tinnitus, lightheadedness, giddiness, and cardiovascular toxicity, including PVCs and atrioventricular node block. The predominant toxic effect is gastrointestinal distress, including nausea, vomiting, anorexia, and abdominal discomfort. Hypersensitivity reactions associated with quinidine are not related to blood concentration.

Clearance of quinidine depends on CyP 3A4. Induction of this system by drugs such as carbamazepine, phenytoin, and St. John's Wort leads to enhanced clearance of quinidine. Diminished organ perfusion, CyP 3A4 inhibition by grapefruit juice or erythromycin, or co-administration with protease inhibitors results in decreased clearance. Quinidine itself has been reported to dilate peripheral blood vessels, resulting in mild to moderate hypotension and reduced clearance over the short term. Quinidine affects the rate of clearance of digoxin. Quinidine is analyzed by either HPLC or immunoassay. Fluorescence techniques should be considered obsolete.

Tocainide

Tocainide, proprietary name *Tonocard,* has electrophysiological properties similar to lidocaine. It is useful in the management of ventricular arrhythmias typified by a prolonged QT interval. Tocainide has the advantage over lidocaine in that it can be taken orally, and it has a relatively long half-life (13 to 16 hours). Optimal response to tocainide

TABLE 33-3 Pharmacokinetic Parameters of Bronchodilator Drugs

Drug	Minimum Effective Concentration (MEC) (μg/mL)	Minimum Toxic Concentration (MTC) (μg/mL)	Average Half-Life (hr)	Average Volume of Distribution (L/kg)	Average Oral Bioavailability (%)	Average Protein Binding (%)	Important Metabolizing Enzymes
Caffeine	8	14	5 30 (neonates)	0.6	100	35	CyP 1A2
Theophylline	8	20	7-10 (adults) 3-5 (children)	0.5	95	55	CyP 1A2

occurs when the blood concentration is in the range of 6 to 15 μg/mL.[77] At therapeutic concentrations, tocainide is 10% protein bound, does not undergo significant first-pass metabolism, but is metabolized by CyP 2D6. It has a volume of distribution of 3 L/kg, but undergoes significant hepatic metabolism and renal clearance. Toxicity associated with tocainide occurs at concentrations in excess of 15 μg/mL and is characterized by gastrointestinal disturbance, central nervous system irritability culminating in convulsions, and cardiopulmonary depression. HPLC is the method most commonly used for tocainide quantification.

Congestive heart failure and uremia reduce renal clearance and the volume of distribution and increase the clearance half-life. Tocainide is not highly protein bound, so it does not exhibit the protein-binding phenomenon described for lidocaine after myocardial infarction. Clinically, the dose should be reduced proportionally to glomerular filtration to maintain therapeutic levels.

Verapamil

Verapamil, proprietary name *Calan,* is a calcium channel blocker that is effective in the treatment of various cardiovascular disorders, including angina (classical and variant), arrhythmias (paroxysmal supraventricular tachycardia), atrial flutter, atrial fibrillation, hypertrophic cardiomyopathy (idiopathic hypertrophic subaortic stenosis), hypertension, congestive heart failure, and Raynaud's phenomenon, along with the preservation of ischemic myocardium and the treatment of migraine headaches.

There is a good correlation between cardiac responsiveness and blood concentration.[50] The effective blood concentration of verapamil ranges from 50 to 250 ng/mL. CyP 3A4 and 1A2 metabolize verapamil; it is a potent inhibitor of CyP 3A4. Sinus bradycardia and heart block occurring at blood concentrations exceeding 250 ng/mL characterized toxic symptoms. All subjects studied showed atrioventricular block at concentrations exceeding 450 ng/mL. HPLC is the method used for quantification of this drug.

Other Cardioactive Drugs

Diuretics and angiotensin-converting enzyme inhibitors are being used to treat cardiac problems.[51] In general, pharmacological effects of these new diuretics and angiotensin-converting enzyme inhibitors are monitored by physiological function rather than by measuring blood levels.

BRONCHODILATORS

Drugs used as bronchodilators include the β-adrenergic agonists, caffeine, and theophylline. Pharmacokinetic details of some bronchodilators are summarized in Table 33-3.

β-Adrenergic Agonists

β-Adrenergic agonists, such as albuterol, bitolterol, isoproterenol, metaproterenol, pirbuterol, and terbutaline in the inhaled form, have become the treatment of choice for a short-acting approach to relief of asthma. These drugs are very effective at providing rapid bronchodilation without significant cardiac or systemic effects. Because they are administered in the vapor form, have short time of action, and produce little toxicity, measurement of blood levels offers little clinical benefit; patient response provides a convenient form of monitoring therapy.

Caffeine

A minor metabolite of theophylline in adults, caffeine has been shown to accumulate to significant concentrations in neonates. Caffeine itself is an effective inhibitor of apnea, which may explain the lower therapeutic concentration required for control of neonatal apnea. Therapy with caffeine alone has also been demonstrated as effective in the treatment of neonatal apnea; it is gaining popularity because of caffeine's long half-life in neonates (>30 hours). Caffeine is metabolized by CyP 1A2; this enzyme is not active in neonates. The optimal therapeutic concentration of caffeine in this situation ranges from 8 to 14 μg/mL. Caffeine is measured by HPLC or immunoassay.

Theophylline

Theophylline, available under many proprietary names, relaxes bronchial smooth muscles to relieve or prevent asthma. The therapeutic effect of theophylline is likely due to antagonism of adenosine receptors in smooth muscle, whereas the toxic effects are due to inhibition of cyclic nucleotide phosphodiesterase. With increased use of β-adrenergic agonists, and because of the considerable toxicity associated with it, theophylline is now considered

TABLE 33-4 Pharmacokinetic Parameters of Commonly Monitored Antibiotic Drugs

Drug	Minimum Effective Concentration (MEC)* (μg/mL)	Minimum Toxic Concentration (MTC) (μg/mL)	Average Half-Life (hr)	Average Volume of Distribution (L/kg)	Average Oral Bioavailability (%)	Average Protein Binding (%)
Amikacin	25	35	2.5	0.3		5
Ciprofloxacin	<0.2	4	4	2	100	40
Chloramphenicol	10	25	3	0.9	75-90	53
Gentamicin	<5	8	2.5	0.3		5
Kanamycin	25	35	2.1	0.25		0
Sulfonamides, all	75	125	6-10	0.2	100	70-90
Tobramycin	<5	8	2	0.3		<10
Vancomycin	20	40	6	0.5		<10

*Organism sensitivity studies (minimum inhibitory concentration; see text) define the minimum effective concentration.

an alternative therapy used only in treatment of persistent asthma when albuterol or its analogs are not effective.[132]

Theophylline is readily absorbed after oral, rectal, or parenteral administration. If the drug is taken orally without food, the blood concentration peaks within 2 hours. If it is administered with food or as the slow-release formula, peak concentrations occur 3 to 5 hours after the dose. Once absorbed, it is 50% protein bound. Theophylline is metabolized by CyP 1A2, which is highly active in children and in adults who smoke. In these people, the half-life ranges from 3 to 4 hours. Nonsmoking adults in good health have an elimination half-life averaging 9 hours. The half-life in neonates and in adults with congestive heart failure can be prolonged to 20 to 30 hours, depending on the degree of liver immaturity or loss of liver function. Co-administration of cimetidine, ciprofloxacin, and ticlopidine will reduce the clearance of theophylline.

The relationship between serum concentration and prevention of symptoms of chronic asthma has been documented.[52] There is a proportional relationship between forced expiratory volume and theophylline concentration, with the optimum therapeutic effect occurring at concentrations ranging from 8 to 20 μg/mL. Suppression of exercise-induced bronchospasm in asthmatic patients occurs at concentrations exceeding 10 μg/mL and is optimal at 15 μg/mL. Neonatal apnea treated with theophylline responds to slightly lower concentrations, ranging from 5 to 10 μg/mL. Relaxation of bronchial smooth muscle is directly proportional to blood concentration and continues at concentrations greater than 20 μg/mL. When the blood level exceeds 20 μg/mL, the secondary side effects become significant.

Theophylline clearance is a function of a metabolic process that is dose dependent. At serum concentrations greater than 20 μg/mL, small dose increases lead to disproportionately large increases in serum concentration and intoxication. Symptoms of theophylline toxicity include nausea, vomiting, headache, diarrhea, irritability, and insomnia. Transient central nervous system stimulation occurring at initial administration is not directly related to blood concentration. This effect diminishes with chronic use. Serious toxicity characterized by cardiac arrhythmias and seizures is usually associated with serum concentrations in excess of 30 μg/mL. Once seizure activity begins, the final prognosis is very poor. Morbidity is reported in nearly all patients, and mortality can be as high as 50%.[157]

Immunoassay is the standard method for the determination of theophylline. Theophylline, caffeine, and dyphylline have been simultaneously quantified by HPLC.

ANTIBIOTICS

Antibiotics that require TDM include aminoglycosides, chloramphenicol, sulfonamides, vancomycin, trimethoprim, β-lactams, and tetracyclines. Pharmacokinetic details of these antibiotics are summarized in Table 33-4. Aminoglycosides and vancomycin are quantified by immunoassay. Other antibiotics have been measured by HPLC.

Aminoglycosides

Aminoglycosides are polycationic agents that kill aerobic gram-negative bacteria. They act by binding to the 30S ribosomal subunit of bacterial mRNA, thereby inhibiting protein synthesis. They are inactive under anaerobic conditions because an oxygen-dependent active transport mechanism is involved in the transfer of aminoglycosides across the bacterial cell wall. The aminoglycoside class of drugs includes amikacin, gentamicin, kanamycin, neomycin, netilmicin, sisomicin, streptomycin, and tobramycin.

The aminoglycosides are a very polar group of compounds and are thus poorly absorbed from the intestinal tract. They are routinely administered intravenously or intramuscularly to achieve a high degree of bioavailability.

TABLE 33-5 Minimal Inhibitory Concentrations of Antibiotics*

Antibiotic	Susceptible (μg/mL)	Intermediate (μg/mL)	Resistant (μg/mL)
Amikacin	<16	32	>64
Chloramphenicol	<8	16	>32
Gentamicin	<4	<8	>12
Kanamycin	<16	32	>64
Tobramycin	<4	8	>16
Vancomycin	<4	8-16	>32

Data from Methods for Dilution Antimicrobial Susceptibility Tests for Bacteria That Grow Aerobically. 4th ed. M7-A4. Approved Standard. Wayne, PA: National Committee for Clinical Laboratory Standards, 1997.
*Values are for organisms other than *Haemophilus* spp, *Neisseria gonorrhoeae,* and *Streptococcus* spp.

TABLE 33-6 Normal Effective Concentrations of Antibiotics (μg/mL)

Drug	Peak (μg/mL)	Peak Pulse Dosing (μg/mL)	Trough (μg/mL)	Toxic (μg/mL)*
Amikacin	25-35	40-60	4-8	>35
Chloramphenicol	10-25	NA	10	>25
Gentamicin	5-8	20-24	1-2	>10
Kanamycin	25-35	NA	4-8	>35
Sulfonamides	75-125	NA	>75	>300
Tobramycin	5-8	20-24	1-2	>10
Trimethoprim	5-8	NA		>50
Vancomycin	20-40	NA	5-10	>80

NA, Not applicable.
*Note: Does not apply to pulse dosing.

When administered directly into the blood, they rapidly distribute to the extracellular fluid but do not cross cell membranes or bind to plasma proteins; this behavior is consistent with their unusually low volume of distribution. Most tissues and nonrenal or hepatic secretions contain very small concentrations of aminoglycosides, the exceptions being the renal cortex, where the drug is concentrated, and bile because of active hepatic secretion. The drugs are mainly excreted by glomerular filtration. Elimination half-lives are short, ranging from 2 to 3 hours. Because clearance is highly dependent on renal function, any impairment of glomerular filtration causes accumulation of these drugs.

Therapy with antimicrobial agents differs from the approach used for most other drugs discussed in this chapter. With them, the goal is to achieve a concentration in plasma such that the bacteria are killed but the host remains undamaged. Because the organisms treated are variable and can become resistant to certain drugs, treatment with specific aminoglycoside agents should always be directed by susceptibility testing. Effective minimal inhibitory concentrations of these drugs are listed in Table 33-5.

A limit to the blood concentration of aminoglycosides has been recommended, although considerable variability is reported regarding the relationship of blood concentration to later onset of toxicity.[78] Renal tubular necrosis and degeneration of the auditory nerve are the side effects most frequently experienced after exposure to high concentrations of aminoglycosides. Both peak and trough specimens are required to monitor toxicity. Table 33-6 identifies target maximum peak and trough serum concentrations; in this mode of monitoring, the intent of therapy should be to dose the patient in such a manner that the peak concentration does not exceed these limits. In a large surgical patient survey in which dosing was carried out under controlled conditions, limited nephrotoxicity was experienced when the peak serum concentration of gentamicin was maintained below 8 μg/mL.[155]

Dose corrections must be made in patients with compromised renal function because these patients have prolonged half-life and slower elimination. Guidelines have been prepared (Table 33-7) that allow application of creatinine clearance to estimate adequate initial dose.[121] This

TABLE 33-7 Useful Guidelines for Gentamicin Dose Calculated from Lean Body Weight and Creatinine Clearance

1. Select loading dose in mg/kg (lean weight) to provide peak serum level desired. Approximate peak levels from commonly used loading doses are indicated below.

Loading Dose	Expected Peak Serum Concentration Based on 30-min IV Infusion, (μg/mL)
2.0 mg/kg	6-8
1.75 mg/kg*	5-7
1.5 mg/kg	4-6
1.25 mg/kg	3-5
1.0 mg/kg	2-4

2. Select maintenance dose (as percentage of chosen loading dose) to continue peak serum levels indicated above according to patient's creatinine clearance (*Ccr*) and desired dosing interval.

	Percentage of Loading Dose Required for Dosage Interval Selected†		
Ccr	8 hr	12 hr	24 hr
90	90	—	—
80	88	—	—
70	84	—	—
60	79	91	—
50	74	87	—
40	66	80	—
30	57	72	92
25	51	66	88
20	45	59	83
15	37	50	75
10	29	40	64
7	24	33	55
5	20	28	48
2	1	20	35
0	9	13	25

From Hull JH, Sarubbi FA. Gentamicin serum concentrations: Pharmacokinetic predictions. Ann Intern Med 1976; 85:188.
*Recommended for most moderate to severe systemic infections.
†Shaded areas indicate suggested dosage intervals.

should then be followed up by quantification of the blood concentration and dose adjustment following the method outlined by Gilbert.[44]

Toxicity associated with aminoglycosides manifests as delayed-onset vestibular and cochlear sensory cell destruction and acute renal tubular necrosis. The degree and severity of cell damage are variable among the various drugs, but they all cause cell damage if the concentrations exceed the limits listed in Table 33-4. Unfortunately, the guidelines identified in Table 33-6 do not guarantee the avoidance of toxicity; a small number of patients experience toxic effects regardless of the concentration. Fortunately, most patients reverse the toxic effects without direct intervention if the toxicity is associated with reasonable blood concentrations (see Table 33-7). Irreparable loss of vestibular, cochlear, or renal function usually correlates with administration of one of the aminoglycosides at elevated blood concentrations for periods longer than 2 weeks.

Aminoglycosides display peak concentration–dependent killing of microorganisms. Clinically, the therapeutic goal is to achieve peak concentrations 10 times the minimum inhibitory concentration (MIC) of the organism. Once per day dosing of two or more times the usual 48-hour dose (known as pulse dosing) may minimize the development of adaptive resistance, and nephrotoxicity may be decreased or delayed. Target peak concentrations are typically more than twice the target concentrations for the usual 48-hour dosing regimen (see Table 33-6). Reports of reactions similar to endotoxemia (chills, rigors, fever, hypotension, tachycardia, and respiratory distress) have been associated with once daily therapy. Most studies with pulse dosing of aminoglycosides have been performed in patients with low failure rates in urinary tract infections or abdominal and/or pelvic infections. These patient groups may be good candidates for pulse dosing. Patients who are critically ill or who are suspected to have considerably higher than normal volumes of distribution may not achieve desired peak concentrations. Quantification of the drug concentration at 2 hours after the end of a 1 hour infusion and an 8 to 12 hour concentration after the first dose can be used to calculate individual patient pharmacokinetic parameters (e.g., extrapolated peak and trough, half-life, etc.) and the dose optimized. See Case Study No. 3 on this book's accompanying Evolve site, found at http://evolve.elsevier.com/Tietz/textbook/ for an example of how to perform these calculations.

Heparin has been implicated as a deactivator of gentamicin by formation of an inactive complex. This complex, although biologically inactive, retains some structural resemblance to the initial aminoglycoside and cross-reacts with antibodies to the specific aminoglycoside. Heparin concentrations encountered in therapeutic antithrombotic therapy are less than 3 units/mL, making an in vivo complication unlikely. However, specimen collection tubes containing heparin (1000 units/mL) may lead to complex formation, a phenomenon that could interfere with some immunoassay procedures. In practice, aminoglycoside antibiotics are measured by immunoassay.

Chloramphenicol

Chloramphenicol, proprietary name *Chloromycetin* and others, is used as a bactericidal agent. It acts by binding to the 50S ribosomal subunit of bacteria mRNA, and inhibits protein synthesis in prokaryotic organisms. Use of this drug depends on its relative toxicity against the microorganism versus the host. The drug is used against gram-negative bacteria such as *Haemophilus influenzae, Neisseria meningitidis, Neisseria gonorrhoeae, Salmonella typhi,* all *Brucella* species, *Bordetella pertussis, Vibrio cholerae,* and *Shigella.* These organisms all are susceptible to a serum concentration of 6 μg/mL. Organisms that are susceptible to a concentration of 12 μg/mL are *Escherichia coli, Klebsiella pneumoniae, Pseudomonas pseudomallei, Chlamydia,* and *Mycoplasma.*

Chloramphenicol is rapidly absorbed in the gastrointestinal tract. Peak serum concentrations occur 1 to 2 hours after the oral dose. In plasma, chloramphenicol is approximately 50% protein bound and is cleared with a half-life of 2 to 3 hours. Peak serum concentrations after administration of chloramphenicol palmitate or succinate occur 4 to 6 hours after the dose. Chloramphenicol distributes to all tissues, and it concentrates in the cerebrospinal fluid. The drug is actively metabolized by the liver by NAT1 and UGT. Thus chloramphenicol accumulates in cases of hepatic disease. Renal disease does not dramatically reduce clearance.

Toxicity associated with chloramphenicol therapy includes blood dyscrasias and cardiovascular collapse; both show a modest relationship to blood concentration. Other blood concentration–related toxicities include anemia, characterized by maturation arrest in the marrow; cytoplasmic vacuolation of early erythroid and myeloid cells; reticulocytopenia; and increases in both serum iron and serum iron–binding capacity. These symptoms all are associated with serum concentrations in excess of 25 μg/mL. Development of aplastic anemia is not related to dose or blood concentration. Cardiovascular collapse, which occurs primarily in newborns, has been related to a total serum chloramphenicol concentration in excess of 50 μg/mL. An oral dose of 50 mg/kg/d results in an optimal peak serum concentration of 10 to 25 μg/mL in a healthy adult.

Procedures for the determination of chloramphenicol concentrations in blood serum include HPLC and immunoassay. Methods for chloramphenicol determination must be able to differentiate between the prodrug forms, chloramphenicol palmitate or succinate, and their active metabolite, chloramphenicol. (An HPLC method for measuring chloramphenicol is included on this book's accompanying Evolve site, found at http://evolve.elsevier.com/Tietz/textbook/.)

Fluoroquinolones

Fluoroquinolones, characterized by ciprofloxacin, gatifloxacin, levofloxacin, and moxifloxacin (Figure 33-12), have antibiotic activity against gram-positive (*Streptococcus pneumoniae* and *pyogenes, Staphylococcus aureus,* and *Enterococcus faecalis*); gram-negative (*Escherichia coli, Haemophilus influenzae, Moraxella catarrhalis, Klebsiella pneumoniae,* and *Pseudomonas aeruginosa*); and atypical pathogens (*Chlamydia pneumoniae, Mycoplasma pneumoniae,* and *Legionella pneumophila*). They are administered orally at doses varying from 200 to 800 mg twice per day. Maximum serum concentrations are attained 1 to 2 hours after oral dosing. Peak serum concentrations after a standard dose average 1 to 4 μg/mL. Trough concentrations at 12 hours after dose are >0.2 μg/mL.

Fluoroquinolones distribute into most tissues with an apparent volume of distribution of 1.5 to 2 L/kg. They have serum half-lives of ~4 hours and renal clearance of ~6 mL/min/kg; clearance is reduced in renal failure. They are ~40% protein bound and metabolized by hepatic conjugation (UGT); they undergo little phase I metabolism. Symptoms of toxicity include restlessness, diarrhea, and gastrointestinal upset. Skin rash may be a sign of sensitivity to fluoroquinolones.

Because fluoroquinolones have a wide therapeutic index and dose-dependent toxicity, routine drug monitoring is not indicated. Monitoring fluoroquinolone concentration is indicated in renal failure, which will cause fluoroquinolones to accumulate. Optimal response occurs when serum concentration exceeds 1.5 μg/mL. Activity is maintained as long as the trough concentration is >0.2 μg/mL. Co-administration with antacids, ferrous sulfate, food, or sucralfate reduces absorption by 30% to 60%. Co-administration with morphine reduces absorption by >50%.

Sulfonamides

Sulfonamides act by competitively antagonizing bacterial use of *p*-aminobenzoic acid, which is important in the synthesis of folic acid. Therefore, organisms dependent on self-

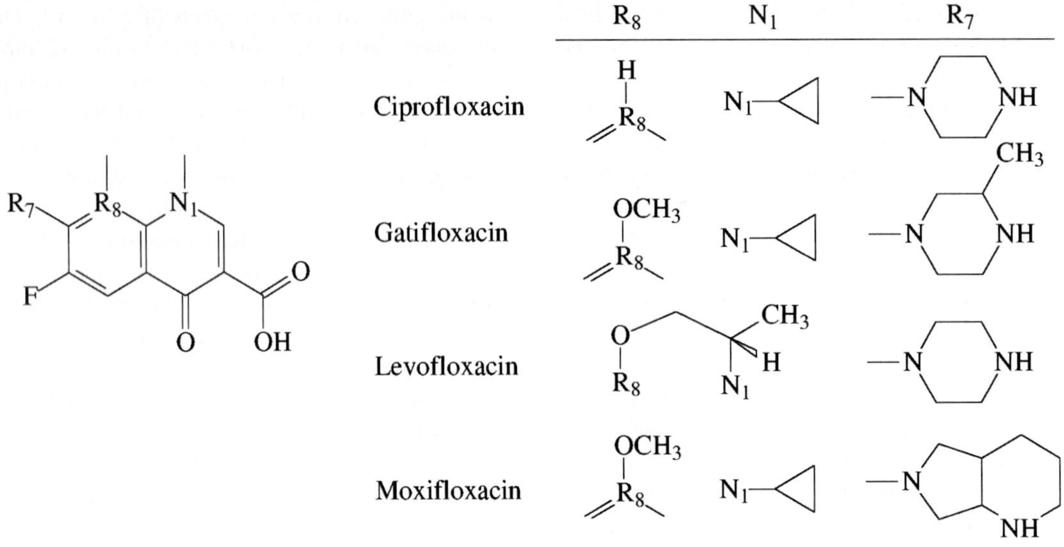

Figure 33-12 Chemical structures of fluoroquinolones.

synthesized folic acid for growth are susceptible to sulfonamides. Sulfonamides are used against common urinary tract pathogens such as *E. coli, Klebsiella, Enterobacter, Proteus mirabilis,* and indole-positive *Proteus* species. They are not used for infections caused by *Pseudomonas aeruginosa.* The sulfonamides are active against *H. influenzae, Streptococcus pneumoniae, Shigella flexneri,* and *Shigella sonnei* isolated from the middle ear or bronchial secretions.

The sulfonamides are nearly completely absorbed from the gastrointestinal tract. Once absorbed they are bound to protein (60% to 90%), mainly to albumin, and are distributed to all tissue. Metabolism is by *N*-acetylation, with the products having no antimicrobial activity.

Blood dyscrasias associated with sulfonamide use are not related to dose or blood concentration of the drug. The predominant toxicity associated with sulfonamide use is the formation and deposition of crystalline aggregates in the kidney, ureter, and bladder. The safe and effective peak concentration of these drugs in serum (75 to 125 μg/mL) is well separated from the serum concentration at which crystallization in the urinary tract occurs. Serum concentrations in excess of 300 μg/mL maintained for prolonged periods of time have been associated with such crystal formation. The method of choice for quantification of sulfonamides is HPLC.[43]

Vancomycin

Vancomycin is a glycopeptide that has bactericidal action against gram-positive bacteria and some gram-negative cocci. Vancomycin is used because of its activity against methicillin-resistant staphylococci and corynebacteria. It has thus become popular for treatment of endocarditis and sepsis caused by these organisms.

Although the drug is poorly absorbed when given orally, a 1-g dose given intravenously every 12 hours accomplishes a peak blood concentration of 20 to 40 μg/mL and a trough concentration of 5 to 10 μg/mL. It has an average elimination half-life of 5 to 6 hours. Blood concentration–related toxicity involves the auditory nerve. Concentrations less than 30 μg/mL are rarely associated with this development. Toxicities not related to dose or blood concentration are rare and include fever, phlebitis, and pain at the infusion site. In patients with impaired renal function, the serum concentration may increase to toxic levels because of reduced clearance. Immunoassay is the standard technique for monitoring concentration.

Miscellaneous Antibiotic Drugs

Trimethoprim is administered as a combination drug with sulfamethoxazole. The drug is excreted in proportion to sulfamethoxazole; it is not toxic and therefore is not commonly monitored. Sulfa determination may be used to establish compliance.

Adverse reactions to β-*lactams* (penicillins and cephalosporins) are not related to dose or blood concentrations. They are commonly administered in doses 10 to 100 times greater than necessary to inhibit organism growth, and appropriate dosing may be guided by susceptibility testing. Patient compliance and evaluation of patients with renal impairment are the most likely reasons to monitor the blood concentration.

Tetracyclines are broad-spectrum antibiotics. They are not highly toxic, and therefore, like the β-lactams, the need to monitor their serum concentrations is limited to monitoring patient compliance and adjusting dose in patients with impaired renal function.

Table 33-8 lists pharmacokinetic data for other antibiotics.[78]

TABLE 33-8 Pharmacokinetic Data for Other Antibiotics

	Serum Concentration for Selected Doses		Serum Half-Life (hr) (for Creatinine Clearance [mL/min])	
Drug	**Dose (g)**	**Peak Serum (μg/mL)**	**Creatinine Clearance >80**	**Creatinine Clearance <10**
Penicillins				
Amoxicillin	0.5 po	5.5-11.0	0.7-1.4	7.4-21
Ampicillin	0.5 po	3-6	0.7-1.4	7.4-21
	2.0 IV	47		
Azlocillin	2 IV	165	1	5
Carbenicillin	3 IV	278	0.8-1	9.4-23.4
Cloxacillin	0.5 po	7-15	0.4-0.8	0.8-2.3
Dicloxacillin	0.5 po	10-18	0.6-0.8	1-2.2
Methicillin	1 IV	59.8	0.4-0.5	4-6
Mezlocillin	1 IV	64-143	0.7-1.3	1.6-14
	2 IV	161-364		
Nafcillin	0.5 IV	40	0.5-1.5	1.8-2.8
Oxacillin	0.5 po	2.6-3.9	0.3-0.8	0.5-2
Penicillin G	2 mU q2h IV	20	0.4-0.9	6-20
Penicillin V	0.25 po	2.3-2.7	0.5	7-10
Piperacillin	4 IV	389-484	0.6-1.3	2.1-6
Temocillin	1 IV	160	4.5-5	18-27
Ticarcillin	2 IV	200-218	0.9-1.3	13.5-16.2
Cephalosporins				
First Generation				
Cefadroxil	1 po	24-35	1.1-2	20-25
Cefazolin	1 IV	188	1.2-2.2	18-36
Cephalexin	0.5 po	15-18	0.5-1.2	5-30
Cephalothin	1 IM	15-21	0.5-0.9	3-8
	1 IV	30		
Cephapirin	1 IV	67	0.6-0.9	2.4
Cephradine	0.5 po	15-18	0.7-2	8-15
Second Generation				
Cefaclor	0.5 po	13-15	0.5-1	2.8
Cefamandole	2 IV	214	0.5-2.1	12-18
Cefotetan	2 IV	237	2.8-4	12-30
Cefoxitin	1 IM	22-24	0.7-1	13-22
	2 IV	221		
Cefprozil	0.5 po	8.2-10.4	0.9-1	5.9
Cefuroxime	0.75 IV	51.1	1-2	20
Third Generation				
Cefixime	0.4 po tablets	3.7	2.4-4	11.5
Cefoperazone	2 IV	253	1.6-2	2-2.5
Cefotaxime	1 IV	102.4	0.9-1	
Cefpodoxime	0.2 po	2.3	1.9-3	9.8
Ceftazidime	1 IV	69	1.4-2	12-35
Ceftizoxime	2 IV	132	1.4-1.8	25-35
Ceftriaxone	2 IV	223-276	5.4-10.9	12.2-18.2
Moxalactam	1 IV	60-100	2	20
	2 IV	150-200		

Continued.

TABLE 33-8 Pharmacokinetic Data for Other Antibiotics—*Continued*

	Serum Concentration for Selected Doses		Serum Half-Life (hr) (for Creatinine Clearance [mL/min])	
Drug	**Dose (g)**	**Peak Serum (µg/mL)**	**Creatinine Clearance >80**	**Creatinine Clearance <10**
β-Lactams				
Aztreonam	2 IV	204-255	1.3-2.2	6-9
Carumonam	2	300	1.3-1.7	11.3
Imipenem	0.5 IV	21-58	0.8-1	3-5
Loracarbef	0.4 po capsules	14	1	32
Tetracyclines				
Doxycycline	0.1 IV	2.5	14-24	18-30
Tetracycline	0.5 po	3-4.3	6-12	57-120
Azalides and Macrolides				
Azithromycin	0.5 po	0.09-0.44	79	
Clarithromycin	0.5 po	2-3	5-7	
Clindamycin	0.6 IV	10	2-3	2-3.5
Erythromycin	0.25 po	0.1-2	1.5-2	6
Metronidazole	7.5 mg/kg	26	6-14	8-15
Fusidic Acid				
Fusidic acid	0.5 po	14-38		
Quinolones and Urinary Tract Agents				
Ciprofloxacin	0.75 po	2.5-4.3	3-5	5-10
Nalidixic acid	1 po	20-40	1.1-2.5	>1
Norfloxacin	0.4 po	1.3-1.9	2.3-4	6-7
Antimycobacterial Agents				
Ethambutol	25 mg/kg po	2-5	3	>7
Isoniazid	7 mg/kg po	4.5	0.5-4	2-10
Pyrazinamide	0.5 po	9-12	10-16	
Rifampin	0.6 IV	17.5	2-5	2-5
Streptomycin	1 IM	25-50	2-3	up to 110
Antifungal Agents				
Amphotericin B	0.03 IV	1	>24	>24
Itraconazole	0.2 po	2.3/3.5	21-60	
Ketoconazole	0.2 po	4.2	8	8
Miconazole	0.522 IV	6	0.4-2.4	
Antiviral Agents				
Acyclovir	0.8 po	1.6	2.1-3.5	19.5
	5 mg/kg IV	7.7		
Ganciclovir	5 mg/kg IV	6.6-8.3	2.5-3.6	10
Vidarabine	10 mg/kg IV	3-6	1.5-3.3	

Data from Mandell GL, Bennett JE, Dolin R, Eds. Principles and practice of infectious disease, 4th ed. New York: Churchill Livingstone, 1995.
IV, Intravenous; *IM,* intramuscular; *po,* oral; *NA,* data not available.

TABLE 33-9 Pharmacokinetic Parameters of Antiretroviral Drugs

Drug	Minimum Effective Concentration (MEC) (μg/mL)	Minimum Toxic Concentration (MTC) (μg/mL)	Average Half-Life (hr)	Average Oral Bioavailability (%)	Average Protein Binding (%)	Important Metabolizing Enzymes
Delavirdine	3-8	14-16	5-7	70	99	
Didanosine (ddI)	0.1-0.3	1.2-2.4	1.5	40	<5	
Efavirenz	0.5	2.9	40-55		99	CyP 2B6, 3A4, Pg
Indinavir	0.1	8-10	1.8	60		CyP 3A4, Pg
Lamivudine (3TC)	1-2	5-8	5-7	80	<5	
Nelfinavir	1-3	3-4	3-5	90	98	CyP 2C19, 3A4, Pg
Nevirapine	3-8	10-15	30	93	60	
Ritonavir	1-6	8-14	3-5	70	98	CyP 3A4, Pg
Saquinavir	0.05-0.2	0.5-2.5	12	15	98	CyP 3A4, Pg
Zalcitabine (ddC)	<0.005	0.025	2	80	<5	
Zidovudine (AZT)	<0.02	1.2-1.8	1	65	25	

Antiretrovirals

Successful treatment of human immunodeficiency virus (HIV-1) infection has been achieved through successful implementation of highly active antiretroviral therapy, frequently referred to as HAART. This involves simultaneous administration of both nucleoside and nonnucleoside reverse transcriptase inhibitors and one or more protease inhibitors. The common nucleoside reverse transcriptase inhibitors are the thymidine analogs didanosine (ddI), lamivudine (3TC), and zalcitabine (ddC); and the non-thymidine analogs abacavir (Ziazen), stavudine (d4T), and zidovudine (AZT). The nonnucleoside reverse transcriptase inhibitors include delavirdine, efavirenz, and nevirapine. The protease inhibitors include indinavir, nelfinavir, ritonavir, and saquinavir. Response to therapy is monitored by quantification of HIV-RNA copies (viral load) and CD-4+ T-lymphocyte count. Successful therapy is indicated when viral load is reduced to <50 copies/mL and CD-4+ count >500 per mL.

Because treatment success is highly dependent upon adherence to therapy and development of viral resistance is potentiated by noncompliance, patients must be continuously reminded to adhere to their dosing schedules at all times. Drug monitoring is used as a tool to assess patient compliance. Aggressive counseling would be indicated if the blood concentration of the prescribed drugs becomes nondetectable. Pharmacokinetic parameters of antiretrovirals are outlined in Table 33-9. A method to quantify antiretrovirals, with recommended reference intervals, has been published.[92] Tandem MS is becoming the method of choice for monitoring HAART because it is less prone to interference by the common multidrug combinations.[145]

Antipsychotic Drugs

Drugs used in psychiatric care that are commonly monitored include antidepressants, some neuroleptics, and lithium. Pharmacological parameters of these antipsychotic drugs are shown in Table 33-10.

Antidepressants

Antidepressants are used to treat endogenous depression characterized by depressed mood, feelings of guilt, appetite suppression, insomnia, weight change, diminished ability to concentrate, loss of interest or pleasure in usual activities, and decreased sexual drive. In more severe cases, depersonalized behavior, paranoid behavior, obsessive-compulsive behavior, and suicidal tendencies are obvious. The antidepressants include (1) amino ketones (bupropion [*Wellbutrin*]), cyclohexanols (venlafaxine [*Effexor*]), (2) dibenzoxazepines (amoxapine [*Asendin*]), (3) diphenylamines (fluoxetine [*Prozac*]), (4) naphthalenamines (sertraline [*Zoloft*]), (5) tetracyclics (maprotiline [*Ludiomil*]), (6) triazoles (paroxetine [*Paxil*], and trazodone [*Desyrel*]), and (7) tricyclics (amitriptyline [*Elavil*], clomipramine [*Anafranil*], desipramine [*Norpramine*], doxepin [*Sinequan*], imipramine [*Tofranil*], nortriptyline [*Pamelor*], protriptyline [*Vivactil*], and trimipramine [*Surmontil*]).

Endogenous depression implies that there is no apparent organic or societal cause of these behavior changes. Treatment of depression with the tricyclic or tetracyclic depressants results in pharmacological activity through inhibition of the reuptake of catecholamines in the central nervous system. The end result is a positive effect on mood. The optimal therapeutic concentrations and important pharma-

TABLE 33-10 Pharmacokinetic Parameters of Antipsychotic Drugs

Drug	Minimum Effective Concentration (MEC) (ng/mL)	Minimum Toxic Concentration (MTC) (ng/mL)	Average Half-Life (hr)	Average Volume of Distribution (L/kg)	Average Oral Bioavailability (%)	Average Protein Binding (%)	Important Metabolizing Enzymes
Amitriptyline	80	250	21	15	50	95	CyP 2C19, 2D6, 3A4, Pg
Amoxapine	200	600	8			90	
Bupropion	25	100	12	7		84	CyP 2B6, 2D6, 3A4, Pg
Clozapine	100	600	8			97	CyP 1A2, 3A4
Doxepin	150	250	17	20	27	90	CyP 2C19, 2D6, 3A4, Pg
Fluoxetine	90	300	55	35	60	95	CyP 2C19, 2D6, 3A4, Pg
Haloperidol	1	10	18	18	60	65	CyP 1A2, 2D6
Imipramine	150	250	12	18	40	90	CyP 2C19, 2D6, 3A4, Pg
Lithium	0.6 mmol/L	1.2 mmol/L	22	0.8	100	0	
Maprotiline	200	600	40				
Nefazodone	25	2500	3	NA	95	99	CyP 2C19
Nortriptyline	50	150	30	18	50	92	CyP 2C19, 3A4, Pg
Olanzapine	10	1000	30	15	90	93	CyP 1A2, UGT
Paroxetine	30	70	21	13	90	95	CyP 2D6
Protriptyline	70	260	80	22	75	92	CyP 2C19, 2D6, 3A4, Pg
Quetiapine	Not Known	Not Known	10	10	10	83	Cyp 2D6, 3A4, Pg
Sertraline	NA	300	26	76		98	CyP 2C19, 2D6
Trazodone	800	1600	7	1	75	93	CyP 2C19, 2D6, 3A4, Pg
Trimipramine	100	300	NA	NA	NA	90	CyP 2C19, 2D6, 3A4, Pg
Venlafaxine	70	250	5	6.5	92	27	CyP 2D6, Pg

**NA*, Not applicable.

cokinetic parameters of antidepressants are listed in Table 33-10.

Tricyclic Antidepressants

Tricyclic antidepressants are nearly completely absorbed from the gastrointestinal tract but undergo first-pass hepatic metabolism, so their ultimate bioavailability is variable. Because these drugs slow gastrointestinal activity and gastric emptying, their absorption may be delayed. Once absorbed, they are highly protein and tissue bound, resulting in large apparent volumes of distribution. Peak plasma concentrations are reached from 2 to 12 hours after the oral dose. Metabolism is by CyP 2C19, 2D6, and 3A4 *N*-demethylation and aromatic ring hydroxylation, followed by conjugation (UGT). If the drug administered is the tertiary tricyclic amine (amitriptyline, doxepin, and imipramine), metabolism causes accumulation of the respective secondary amine (nortriptyline, nordoxepin, and desipramine). These substances have generally equal pharmacological activity and accumulate to concentrations approximately (but variably) equal to the parent drug. The hydroxylated metabolites have little pharmacological activity. Taking factors such as variable bioavailability, high volume of distribution, variable metabolic activity, and generation of pharmacologically active metabolites into consideration, it is not surprising that patient response to these drugs is widely variable. Determining the serum concentration gives the physician the assurance that a patient has been properly dosed.

Drugs such as cimetidine, chloramphenicol, haloperidol, methylphenidate, and phenothiazines generally inhibit hepatic oxidative enzymes. Inhibition of end-product metabolism of the tertiary tricyclic antidepressants results in a greater accumulation of the secondary amine metabolite (amitriptyline is metabolized to nortriptyline, doxepin to nordoxepin, imipramine to desipramine), because conversion to the aromatic ring hydroxylated metabolites is blocked. Co-administration of perphenazine with a tricyclic antidepressant causes accumulation of the secondary amine to concentrations two to four times normal, with onset of toxicity occurring at the expected blood concentrations.

Tricyclic antidepressants show a good correlation between therapeutic response and serum concentration. A linear relationship between clinical improvement and serum concentration is noted for most of these drugs, the exception being nortriptyline, which has a specific therapeutic window. A serum concentration of nortriptyline below or above the concentration range of 50 to 150 ng/mL correlates with worsening of moods. The other antidepressants do not display this effect; the upper limit of the optimum blood concentration for these other antidepressants is limited by the onset of toxicity. Toxicity is expressed as dry mouth and perspiration, signs that may also occur with depression. Thus it is difficult to differentiate between mild toxicity caused by the drug and the disease that is being treated. More serious toxicity is expressed as atrioventricular node block, characterized by a widening of the electrocardiographic QRS interval. Onset occurs at serum concentrations ranging from 800 to 1200 ng/mL, and the severity of intoxication is related to the serum concentration. The relationship between serum concentration and cardiac toxicity diminishes with time after intoxication as the drug is absorbed into tissues. Despite this toxicity, the tricyclic antidepressants remain very important drugs in the treatment of depression.

Numerous methods have been published for analysis of tricyclic antidepressants. These drugs present various problems to the clinical laboratory: (1) the therapeutic serum concentration is 10 to 100 times lower than that of other commonly monitored drugs, and thus to be clinically useful, the method must be able to measure serum concentrations <50 ng/mL; (2) these drugs have metabolites that must also be measured; and (3) these drugs are structurally similar to common sleep inducers, antihistamines, and many over-the-counter medications used for appetite suppression, which are potential interferences. Of the many hundreds of methods published, only a few have satisfactorily overcome these obstacles.

Analysis by gas chromatography-mass spectrometry (GC/MS) using selected ion monitoring is the reference method.[9] Methods for trazodone[141] and amoxapine[21] are also available. HPLC has been successfully used for analysis of tricyclic antidepressants, although separation and selectivity are problems with this technique.[80]

Selective Serotonin Reuptake Inhibitors

Selective serotonin reuptake inhibitors (SSRIs) are frequently prescribed medications. Their therapeutic actions are diverse, ranging from efficacy in depression to obsessive-compulsive disorder, panic disorder, bulimia, and other conditions.[131] They include bupropion, fluoxetine, nefazodone, paroxetine, and miscellaneous other drugs.

Bupropion. Bupropion is a weak blocker of serotonin, norepinephrine, and dopamine. Bupropion is rapidly absorbed, reaching peak level within 2 hours of oral administration. It is thought to undergo considerable first-pass metabolism, although studies have not been done to confirm this because the drug is not available in intravenous form. It is estimated that bioavailability ranges from 5% to 20%. Bupropion is metabolized by CyP 3A4, 2B6, and 2D6. Major metabolites include the hydroxylated morphinol-metabolite and the *threo*-amino alcohol metabolite. The half-life of bupropion ranges from 8 to 24 hours. On a typical daily dose (100 to 250 mg), bupropion serum levels correlate with dose and are in the range of 25 to 100 ng/mL. Methods to measure serum concentration have been developed.[134]

Fluoxetine. Fluoxetine (and other nontricyclic antidepressants) acts by inhibiting serotonin uptake in the central nervous system. The drug has fewer antagonistic effects on muscarinic, histaminic, and α-adrenergic receptors than the tricyclic antidepressants, allowing it to be used with fewer side effects. Fluoxetine is metabolized by CyP 3A4, 2D6, and 2C19. Fluoxetine has a very long half-life (48 hours), and its active metabolite, norfluoxetine, is eliminated with a half-life of 180 hours. Optimal response to fluoxetine occurs when the plasma concentration is in the range of 90 to 300 ng/mL.[110] Norfluoxetine is usually present at approximately the same concentration as fluoxetine. The drug undergoes significant hepatic metabolism, and blood levels are affected by liver disease. Compromised renal function has little effect on the excretion rate of fluoxetine.

Nefazodone. Nefazodone is an antidepressant that inhibits neuronal uptake of serotonin and norepinephrine. Nefazodone is a 5-HT_2 antagonist that is rapidly absorbed and has low bioavailability (20%) because it undergoes first-pass metabolism. In March of 2004, the U.S. FDA issued a Public Health Advisory that called attention to reports of both suicidal ideation and suicide attempts in children taking antidepressant drugs such as nefazodone for the treatment of major depressive disorder (MDD). Because of several cases of liver toxicity, nefazodone (Serzone) was taken off the market in June of 2004. An HPLC method with electrochemical detection has been published for the analysis of nefazodone.[39]

Paroxetine. Paroxetine is a selective serotonin reuptake inhibitor with demonstrated clinical utility as an antidepressant. Paroxetine is completely absorbed after oral ingestion and reaches peak steady-state levels of 30 to 70 ng/mL in approximately 5 hours. It undergoes hepatic metabolism by Cyp 2D6, has a half-life of 21 hours, and metabolites are inactive. Steady-state concentrations of paroxetine on a typical dose of 20 mg/day are achieved in 10 days. Clinical response appears to be related to serum concentration[110] and a chromatographic method is available.[48]

Other SSRIs. The antidepressants amoxapine, fluoxetine, sertraline, trazodone, and venlafaxine do not have the same degree of cardiac toxicity that plagues the tricyclic and tetracyclic antidepressants. Treatment with doses slightly greater than normal does not predispose the patient to major toxicity. Therefore monitoring levels of these drugs is not required to avoid toxic side effects. However, if the patient is not responding to the drug as expected, monitoring the level may be useful in demonstrating noncompliance. A variety of methods are available for measuring these antidepressants in body fluids.[80]

Lithium

Lithium, whose proprietary names include *Eskalith, Lithane, Lithonate,* and others, is administered as lithium carbonate and used for treatment of the manic phase of affective disorders, mania, and manic-depressive illness. It is postulated to act by enhancing reuptake of catecholamines, thereby reducing their concentration in the neuronal junction. This produces a sedating effect on the central nervous system. Lithium also modulates the distribution of sodium, calcium, and magnesium in nerve cells, which reduces the rate of glucose metabolism that effects nerve function. The actual mechanism of action of lithium in affecting mania remains theoretical.

Absorption of lithium from the gastrointestinal tract is complete, with peak plasma concentration reached 2 to 4 hours after an oral dose. This cation does not bind to protein. Lithium elimination is biphasic; during the first phase, 30% to 40% of the dose of lithium is cleared, with an apparent half-life of 24 hours. During the second phase, the remainder of lithium incorporated into the cellular ion pool is cleared, exhibiting a half-life of 48 to 72 hours. Clearance is predominantly a function of the kidneys, where active reabsorption occurs. Reduced renal function causes prolonged clearance times.

The optimal therapeutic response to lithium has not been related to a specific serum concentration. However, toxicity is related to serum concentration and consequently serum lithium concentrations are monitored to ensure patient compliance and to avoid intoxication. It has been recommended that a standardized 12-hour postdose serum lithium concentration be used to assess adequate therapy.[91] The interval of 1.0 to 1.2 mmol/L was identified as the optimal trough therapeutic concentration. Concentrations of 1.2 to 1.5 mmol/L signified a warning range, and a concentration in excess of 1.5 mmol/L *in a specimen drawn 12 hours after the dose* indicates a significant risk of intoxication. Early symptoms of intoxication include apathy, sluggishness, drowsiness, lethargy, speech difficulties, irregular tremors, myoclonic twitchings, muscle weakness, and ataxia. These symptoms, although not life threatening, are uncomfortable for patients and indicate that the onset of life-threatening seizures is imminent.

Lithium excretion parallels that of sodium. It readily passes the glomerular membrane and is reabsorbed in the proximal convoluted tubules. In situations in which patients are vulnerable to dehydration (fever, watery stools, vomiting, loss of appetite, and hot weather), the potential for lithium intoxication is increased. In dehydration, the proximal tubular response to reabsorption of sodium (and lithium) is reduction of clearance. Increased reabsorption of lithium leads to increased blood concentration of lithium. Severe intoxication, characterized by muscle rigidity, hyperactive deep tendon reflexes, and epileptic seizures, is usually associated with lithium concentrations in excess of 2.5 mmol/L.

The concentration of lithium in serum, plasma, urine, or other body fluids has been determined by flame emission photometry, atomic absorption spectrometry, or electrochemically using an ion-selective electrode. Serum analysis, the most useful specimen for lithium monitoring, is most commonly quantified by automated spectrophotometric assay.

Other Antipsychotic Drugs

Psychotic patients are most often treated with clozapine, haloperidol, lithium, olanzapine, or one of the phenothiazines, or a combination of these drugs. Because response to these drugs is unpredictable and patients are difficult to control, monitoring serum concentration may aid in adjusting therapy. Numerous methods to measure the serum concentration of the various neuroleptic agents have been reported.[23]

Quantitative procedures for haloperidol and phenothiazines suffer from a major drawback: they are too specific. The major problem encountered with monitoring these drugs is the number of active metabolites of each. Numerous metabolites have been reported for the common phenothiazines, most of which have some pharmacological activity.[19] Thus therapeutic monitoring of these drugs requires co-analysis of numerous metabolites, an option that is analytically problematic, and reference materials for most of the metabolites are not available.

Clozapine

Clozapine, proprietary name *Clozaril,* is an effective antipsychotic drug that inhibits dopamine binding at the D-1 and D-2 receptors, and more actively binds at limbic binding sites than at striatal sites. Clozapine undergoes hepatic metabolism by CyP 3A4 and 1A2 to yield numerous, inactive metabolites; the serum half-life of clozapine is 4 to 12 hours. On a typical daily dose (100 mg bid), clozapine is 97% bound to plasma proteins. Patients respond to the drug when trough serum concentrations of clozapine are in the range of 100 to 600 ng/mL, and methods of analysis have been described.[69]

Clozapine is likely to produce agranulocytosis in approximately 1% of patients who receive the drug. This toxicity is an exposure-related event that occurs regardless of blood level. For this reason, use of clozapine is limited to schizophrenic patients who do not respond to conventional treatment. Biweekly monitoring of white cell count is required in all patients prescribed this drug.

Olanzapine

Olanzapine, a thienobenzodiazepine with proprietary name *Zyprexa,* is a serotonin and dopamine antagonist with antimuscarinic activity. It also blocks histamine receptors. It is completely absorbed to reach peak concentrations in the range of 1000 ng/mL in 6 hours. Olanzapine has a half-life averaging 35 hours. It is 93% protein bound. Olanzapine is cleared by CyP 1A2 metabolism to inactive desalkyl amine and by UGT to *N*-glucuronide metabolites. An HPLC method with electrochemical detection for measuring olanzapine has been published.[16]

Quetiapine

Quetiapine, a dibenzothiazepine with proprietary name *Seroquel,* is an antipsychotic drug similar to clozapine; it inhibits dopamine binding at the D-1 and D-2 receptors. It is completely absorbed to reach peak concentrations in the range of 1000 ng/mL in 6 hours. Quetiapine has a half-life averaging 5 hours. It is 80% protein bound. Quetiapine is cleared by CyP 2C9 and 2C19 metabolism to inactive desalkyl amine metabolites. Quetiapine is likely to produce liver function abnormalities in a small number of patients who receive the drug; evaluation of liver function should be performed regularly on patients prescribed quetiapine.

ANTIMETABOLITES

Methotrexate and thiopurines are antimetabolites and representative of several drugs that interrupt cell cycling that

TABLE 33-11 Key Pharmacokinetic Parameters of Methotrexate

Drug	Minimum Toxic Concentration at 24 hrs After Dose (μmol/L)	Minimum Toxic Concentration at 48 hrs After Dose (μmol/L)	Minimum Toxic Concentration at 72 hrs After Dose (μmol/L)	Average Half-Life at 100 μmol/L (hr)	Average Half-Life at 10 μmol/L (hr)	Average Half-Life at 1 μmol/L (hr)
Methotrexate	>10	>1	>0.1	1.8	8.4	>10

are used to treat neoplastic diseases; their use may require TDM.

Methotrexate

Methotrexate has proved useful in the (1) management of acute lymphoblastic leukemia in children; (2) management of choriocarcinoma and related trophoblastic tumors in women[36]; (3) management of carcinomas of the breast, tongue, pharynx, and testes; (4) maintenance of remission in leukemia; and (5) treatment of severe, debilitating psoriasis. High-dose methotrexate administration followed by leucovorin rescue is effective in treatment of carcinoma of the lung and osteogenic sarcoma. Intrathecal administration is effective in treating meningeal leukemia or lymphoma. Table 33-11 lists pharmacokinetic parameters for methotrexate.

Methotrexate inhibits DNA synthesis by decreasing availability of pyrimidine nucleotides. Methotrexate competitively inhibits the enzyme dihydrofolate reductase, thus decreasing the concentrations of the tetrahydrofolate essential to the methylation of the pyrimidine nucleotides and consequently the rate of pyrimidine nucleotide synthesis. Leucovorin, a folate analog, is used to rescue host cells from methotrexate inhibition; as a synthetic substrate for dihydrofolate reductase, leucovorin administration allows resumption of tetrahydrofolate-dependent synthesis of pyrimidines and reinitiation of DNA synthesis. Methotrexate is a nonspecific cytotoxin, and prolongation of blood levels appropriate to killing tumor cells may lead to severe, unwanted cytotoxic effects such as myelosuppression, gastrointestinal mucositis, and hepatic cirrhosis.

Serum concentrations of methotrexate are commonly monitored during high-dose therapy (>50 mg/m^2) to identify the time at which active intervention by leucovorin rescue should be initiated. Criteria for blood concentrations indicative of a potential for toxicity after single-bolus, high-dose therapy are as follows:[115]

1. Methotrexate concentration greater than 10 μmol/L 24 hours after dose.
2. Methotrexate concentration greater than 1 μmol/L 48 hours after dose.
3. Methotrexate concentration greater than 0.1 μmol/L 72 hours after dose.

Characteristically, blood concentrations are monitored at 24, 48, and 72 hours after the single dose, and leucovorin is administered when methotrexate levels are inappropriately high for a postdose phase. The route of elimination for methotrexate is primarily renal excretion. During the period of high blood levels, particular attention must be paid to maintaining output of a large volume of alkaline urine. The pK_a of methotrexate is 5.5; thus small decreases in urine pH result in significant reduction in its solubility. Keeping urinary pH alkaline diminishes the risks of intratubular precipitation of the drug and obstructive nephropathy during the treatment period. Monitoring blood levels therefore provides the basis for decisions for timing of initiation and continuance of leucovorin treatment and for managing urinary pH.

Methotrexate has been measured in biological specimens using a wide variety of techniques. RIA and the folate reductase inhibition techniques have been used, but nonisotopic immunoassays are now the method of choice.[3] Liquid chromatographic procedures have also been developed to allow for co-analysis of the drug and its metabolites.[7]

Thiopurines

The thiopurine drug mercaptopurine, and its prodrug azathioprine, are used as to treat neoplasias such as leukemia. Thiopurines are metabolized by thiopurine *S*-methyltransferase (TPMT) to form *S*-methylthiopurines, which are further metabolized to *S*-methylthiopurine nucleosides, the very short-lived active agent. Approximately 1% of Caucasians are homozygous for an allele variant of TPMT that expressed no activity. Patients expressing minimal TPMT activity shunt thiopurine to an alternate metabolic pathway, resulting in accumulation of thiopurine nucleosides, which cause cytotoxicity. Patients at risk for thiopurine intoxication can be identified by monitoring TPMT phenotypic enzymatic activity,[146] genotype,[147] or thiopurine nucleotide concentration.[106] Table 33-11 lists pharmacokinetic parameters for thiopurines.

Other Antimetabolites

For various reasons, purine and pyrimidine drugs have not been routinely monitored outside of clinical trials. Cytosine arabinoside; 5-fluorouracil; 5-fluorodeoxyuridine and its monophosphate, 5-azacytidine; and 2,2 difluorodeoxycytidine, which are all antimetabolites like methotrexate, have been extensively studied. Analytical methods have also been developed, but little relationship between circulating blood level and therapeutic efficacy has been found to justify routine monitoring. Alkylating agents such as cyclophosphamide are metabolically converted to active compounds with lifespans of only seconds before they interact with tissue and are destroyed. Measurement of active metabolite would be extremely useful but is obviously impractical. Actinomycin and doxorubicin have toxic effects (bone marrow suppression and dermatitis) that are both immediate and long acting and that appear to relate not to a circulating blood concentration but to dose mass and length of exposure. Definition of specific dosing regimens for these drugs is currently of more concern than is control of circulating concentration. Cisplatin, easily measurable by platinum analysis, causes renal toxicity that may be related to both blood levels and length of exposure, although monitoring is not common.

Immunosuppressants

Immunosuppressants are drugs capable of suppressing immune responses. They are used to treat autoimmune disease, allergy, multiple myeloma, and chronic nephritis, and in organ transplantation. For example, immunosuppressants that are used to provide maintenance immunosuppression in solid organ and bone marrow transplant patients include cyclosporine, everolimus (Ever), mycophenolic acid (MPA), Siro, and Tac (Figure 33-13).

History of Immunosuppressant Therapy

Patterns of use of immunosuppressive drugs in transplant patients have changed through the decades.[139] From 1954 to 1962, referred to as the "Experimental Era," there were few transplants performed; the incidence of acute rejection during the first year following transplant surgery was 80% and the 1-year graft survival was 40%, and the search was on to find acceptable immunosuppression techniques. The successful use of azathioprine combined with corticosteroid from 1962 to 1983, the "Azathioprine Era," made widespread kidney transplantation possible. The rates and severity of acute rejection (65% acute rejection) were high, as was the graft loss rate (60% with 1-year survival). The "Cyclosporine Era" (1983 to 1995) provided for significant improvement of outcomes (45% acute rejection, 85% with 1-year survival), and routine transplantation of organs other than kidneys was instituted with a relatively fixed drug regimen. The recognition, in early clinical trials, that cyclosporine has a narrow therapeutic index and highly variable pharmacokinetics in renal transplant patients led to the development of immunoassay[14] and HPLC methods for quantification.[89] It was during this era that therapeutic drug monitoring of cyclosporine became a standard of practice, and set the stage for the evolution of this practice for the other major maintenance immunosuppressants. Introduction of Tac in 1994 and mycophenolate mofetil in 1995 opened the most recent era. The introduction of Siro in 1999 and Ever in 2004 provided a major addition to this era.

Drug regimens used in the current era for maintenance immunosuppression vary widely according to the transplanted organ, especially the choice and dosing strategy for calcineurin inhibitors (cyclosporine or Tac).[22,55,56,58,86] In 2002 the United Network for Organ Sharing (UNOS) reported that the following combinations of maintenance immunosuppressants were used in newly transplanted patients: (1) Tac + MPA + corticosteroids; (2) cyclosporine + Siro + corticosteroids; (3) cyclosporine + MPA + corticosteroids; and (4) Tac + Siro + corticosteroids. (It is anticipated that Ever can be substituted for Siro.) All of these drugs have narrow therapeutic indices and their pharmacokinetics are highly variable in transplant patients, particularly in the early posttransplant period. They require close supervision with TDM guiding dosage adjustments to minimize the risks of opportunistic infections, lymphoproliferative disease, and serious drug-specific toxicities from excessive immunosuppression and rejection from too little immunosuppression.

Corticosteroids are dosed according to empiric guidelines whereas cyclosporine, Tac, MPA, Siro, and Ever are dosed to achieve and maintain target concentrations in blood (cyclosporine, Tac, Siro, Ever) or plasma (MPA). In today's practice—which often includes reduction of the calcineurin inhibitor, dosing, and target concentrations or elimination of corticosteroid within the first posttransplant year—the demand for tighter and better control of immunosuppressant concentrations is heightened requiring more involvement of laboratorians to help in the demanding process to provide optimal immunosuppression.

Cyclosporine

Cyclosporine, proprietary names *Sandimmune* (cyclosporine) and *Neoral*, is a cyclic peptide composed of 11 amino acids, some of novel structure, isolated from the fungus *Trichoderma polysporum* (Figure 33-13). The compound has been shown effective in suppressing acute rejection in recipients of allograft organ transplants. Cyclosporine is approved for use in renal, cardiac, hepatic, pancreatic, and bone marrow transplants.

The activation and proliferation of T lymphocytes are considered to be the basic cellular immune responses leading ultimately to rejection of transplanted tissue in the absence of effective immunosuppression. An important effect of T cell activation is production of the Ca^{2+}/calmodulin-activated form of the serine/threonine phosphatase calcineurin. The latter is responsible for the activation and nuclear translocation of a number of transcription factors, such as nuclear factor of activated T (NFAT) cells.

Cyclosporine provides maintenance immunosuppression by inhibition of the activation of T lymphocytes via a multifaceted mechanism.[105] The drug, a fat soluble 11 amino acid cyclic polypeptide, crosses the lymphocyte membrane freely where it forms a pharmacologically active complex with the intracellular immunophilin receptor cyclophilin. This complex, but not cyclosporine by itself, inhibits the Ca^{2+}/calmodulin-activated form of serine/threonine phosphatase calcineurin, thereby inhibiting the activation of NFAT cells. The latter action is considered to be the key step

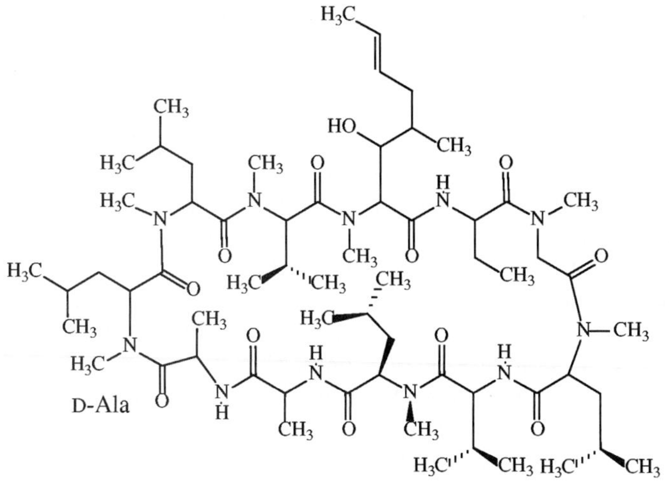

Cyclosporin A
$C_{62}H_{109}N_{11}O_{12}$ M.W. = 1204

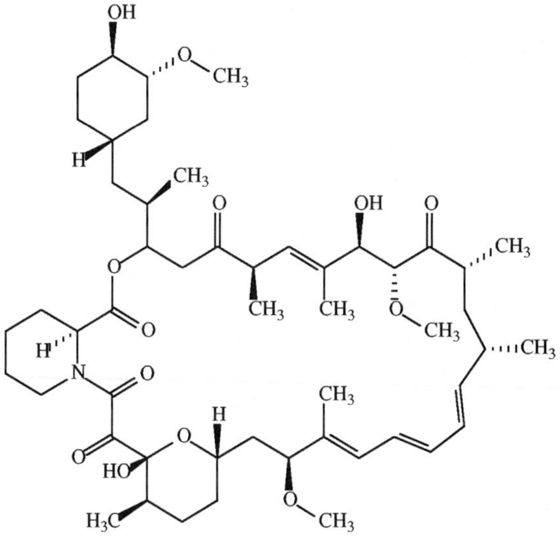

Sirolimus
$C_{51}H_{79}NO_{13}$ M.W. = 914.2

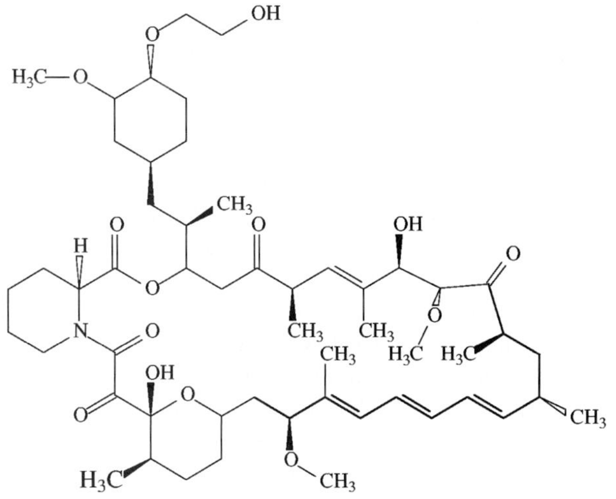

Everolimus
$C_{53}H_{83}NO_{14}$ M.W. = 958.3

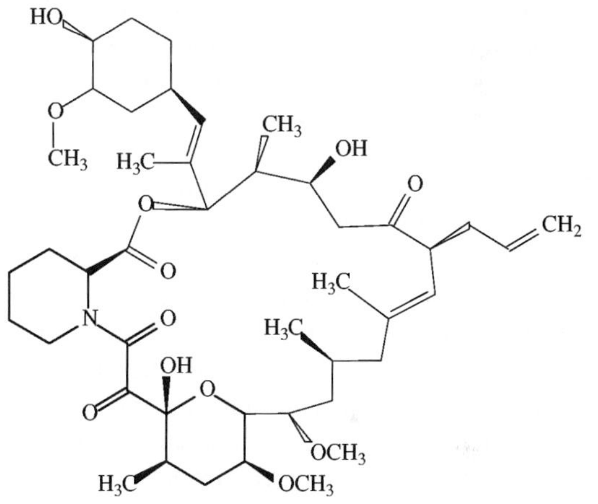

Tacrolimus
$C_{44}H_{69}NO_{12}$ M.W. = 804.0

Figure 33-13 Chemical structures of cyclosporine, sirolimus, tacrolimus, and everolimus.

that leads to several important effects of cyclosporine on the activated T lymphocytes. Although cyclosporine inhibits the peptidylprolyl isomerase activity of cyclophilin, this action has not been shown to affect T cell activation.[109]

Inhibition of activation of NFAT mediated by cyclosporine leads to the downregulation of transcription of cytokine genes for cytokines such as IL-2, IL-3, IL-4, and IL-12; inflammatory mediators such as TNFα; and growth factors such as granulocyte and/or macrophage colony stimulating factor (see Chapter 22). Inhibition of calcineurin by the cyclosporine/cyclophilin complex produces other important intracellular effects that contribute to the overall immunosuppressive effect. The intracellular mechanism(s) by which cyclosporine produces side effects—such as the acute nephrotoxic effects including reduced renal blood flow, afferent arteriolar vasoconstriction, decreased glomerular filtration rate, and increased renal vascular resistance—remains unknown. It is likely that inhibition by cyclosporine/cyclophilin of calcineurin-mediated processes in kidney tissue is responsible for these effects.

Absorption of cyclosporine in the form of Sandimmune is highly variable, ranging from 5% to 40%. Whole-blood concentration correlates with the degree of immunosuppression and toxicity, but there is a poor relationship between dose and blood concentration. A microemulsion form of cyclosporine, Neoral, has more reproducible absorption—averaging 40%—and exhibits better correlation between dose, blood level, and clinical response.[60] In addition to

Neoral and Sandimmune, there are three generic forms of cyclosporine approved for use by the U.S. Food and Drug Administration (FDA). Although considered therapeutically equivalent to Neoral, the excipients differ from that of Neoral or Sandimmune. The chemical structure of these is equivalent to that of cyclosporine; however, close therapeutic drug monitoring is recommended when switching from one formulation to another in view of the very limited availability of peer-reviewed, published data on the generics.[108]

Immunosuppression requires trough whole-blood concentrations of at least 100 ng/mL. A consensus report notes that trough whole-blood concentrations exceeding 600 ng/mL were associated with hepatic, renal, neurological, and infective complications.[64] Strategies for reducing the toxicity of cyclosporine and other immunosuppressive drugs have been published that suggest that therapeutic trough blood concentrations of cyclosporine for renal transplants are 100 to 300 ng/mL, whereas 200 to 350 ng/mL is used as the target concentration for cardiac, hepatic, and pancreatic transplants.[126] Simultaneous immunosuppression with low-dose prednisone and either MPA or Siro allows the patient to enjoy a good response to cyclosporine at lower concentration; some renal transplant patients obtain a satisfactory response with trough cyclosporine levels of 70 ng/mL.[73]

The limitations of trough concentration monitoring of cyclosporine were recognized by Kahan, who showed that the dose interval AUC of the drug provided a more precise estimate of drug exposure and better predictive performance for estimation of risks for acute rejection or toxicity.[62] However, the impracticality of measurement of a full AUC using a series of samples collected over the 12-hour dose interval prevented this more accurate and precise determination of cyclosporine exposure from ever becoming a widely used monitoring test. A new approach is based on the association of most of the variability in cyclosporine pharmacokinetics during the first few hours following oral administration. This approach measures either the area under the blood cyclosporine concentration-time curve in the first 4 hours postdose[6] or measures the blood cyclosporine concentration at 2 hours postdose, known as C2 monitoring.[20] The latter approach promises to provide for more precise targeting of cyclosporine exposure.[86]

Cyclosporine is slowly absorbed, and peak concentrations are reached in 4 to 6 hours. Cyclosporine is 90% protein bound and concentrated in erythrocytes.[149] The degree of concentration in erythrocytes is temperature dependent in vitro; for this reason, measurement of plasma concentration is not recommended.[54] The optimal specimen for analysis is whole blood. The elimination profile of cyclosporine is biphasic. An early elimination phase with an apparent half-life that typically ranges from 3 to 7 hours is followed by a slower elimination phase with an apparent half-life ranging from 18 to 25 hours. The volume of distribution is 17 L/kg. Cyclosporine undergoes extensive metabolism by CyP 3A4. Many of the 31 known metabolites of cyclosporine are inactive.[151] One of the major metabolites, hydroxylated at the number 1 amino acid, retains approximately 10% of the immunosuppressive activity of the parent compound.

Many drugs alter the disposition of cyclosporine. Drugs that inhibit cytochrome P450 3A enzyme activity and block P-glycoprotein (Pg) have been found to decrease cyclosporine metabolism and reduce the barrier to absorption from the gastrointestinal tract, thereby causing increased blood concentration. The latter was recognized in 1999 as very important, together with CyP 3A, as a natural barrier to absorption of xenobiotics.[4,47] Examples include the calcium channel blockers verapamil, diltiazem, and nicardipine; azole antifungal drugs fluconazole, itraconazole, voriconazole, and ketoconazole; and antibiotics, such as erythromycin. All prolong metabolism of cyclosporine and reduce the barrier to absorption sufficiently to increase the risk of nephrotoxicity.[84] Co-administration of phenytoin, phenobarbital, carbamazepine, and rifampin results in induction of CyP 3A enzymes and Pg, which, respectively, increase the rate at which cyclosporine is metabolized in the gastrointestinal tract and liver, and the countertransport of the drug, thereby reducing significantly the bioavailability of the parent drug.[64] Intravenous administration of sulfadimidine and trimethoprim decreases cyclosporine concentrations.

The first procedure available for analysis of cyclosporine was an RIA developed by Sandoz Pharmaceuticals, the producer of cyclosporine. This immunoassay exhibits approximately 30% cross-reactivity with inactive metabolites, and the test is now considered obsolete. Nonisotopic immunoassays have been developed for whole-blood analysis.[27,79,86] HPLC methods have been developed and are used now by many laboratories.[89] A practical HPLC tandem mass spectrometry method is included on this book's accompanying Evolve site, found at http://evolve.elsevier.com/Tietz/textbook/.

Everolimus

Ever, proprietary name *Certican* and also known as *SDZ RAD*, is a rapamycin analog with potent immunosuppressive activity when used in conjunction with CyA. Structurally, Ever is a semisynthetic lipophilic macrocyclic lactone macrolide (Figure 33-13). Like Siro (see below), Ever forms a complex with intracellular immunophilin FK-BP12 that modulates the immune response by combining with the specific cell-cycle regulatory protein mTOR and inhibiting its activation. This inhibition results in suppression of cytokine-driven T lymphocyte proliferation, inhibiting the progression from the G_1 to the S phase of the cell cycle. Ever is metabolized through oxidation by CyP 3A in the gastrointestinal tract and liver. At least 20 metabolites have been identified.[97]

Cyclosporine inhibits the metabolism of Ever, requiring Ever dose reduction when co-administered with CyA; simultaneous administration of CyA and Ever is expected to be the usual approach to immunosuppression. Ever does not affect CyA metabolism. The primary side effect of concern with Ever therapy is hyperlipidemia.[31]

Ever is administered orally as an oral microsuspension. Ever is rapidly absorbed from the gastrointestinal tract, with the average time to reach maximal concentration in whole blood of about 3 hours.[98] Low bioavailability is predicted by extensive intestinal and hepatic metabolism by CYP3A and countertransport by the multidrug efflux pump Pg in the gastrointestinal tract. This absorption barrier varies considerably from patient to patient and within-patient and is the site of clinically important drug-drug and drug-food interactions. The apparent elimination half-life of Ever is 24 hours. Proportionality between dose and blood concentration increases with a greater dose,[31] and higher dosing appears to increase bioavailability. Steady-state trough blood concentration on a 3 mg/day dose in an adult is likely to be in the range of 3 to 20 ng/mL.[31,97] A detailed description of an HPLC/MS/MS method to quantify Ever blood concentration is included on this book's accompanying Evolve site, found at http://evolve.elsevier.com/Tietz/textbook/.

Mycophenolate Mofetil

Mycophenolate mofetil (MMF), proprietary name *CellCept,* is the 2-morpholinoethyl ester prodrug form of the active immunosuppressant MPA (Figure 33-14). The latter is a fermentation product of several *Penicillium* species that has antifungal, antibacterial, antitumor, and immunosuppressive activity in animal models.[111] Following the demonstration of its immunosuppressive efficacy in human renal transplant patients and in combination with cyclosporine and corticosteroids, formal clinical trials were conducted. In 1995 MMF was approved by the U.S. FDA for this use.

MPA is a reversible and uncompetitive inhibitor of inosine monophosphate dehydrogenase (IMPDH). A very important characteristic of proliferating lymphocytes is the greatly increased rate of de novo purine biosynthesis. The sustained and markedly increased rate of guanine nucleotide production catalyzed by IMPDH is the rate limiting step in de novo purine biosynthesis that cannot be provided by the salvage pathway in proliferating lymphocytes.[33] Thus the proliferative response of activated T cells is dependent on a continuous and increased supply of intracellular guanine nucleotide pool. T cell proliferation is arrested by the suppression of guanine nucleotide production when IMPDH is inhibited by MPA. The mechanism of action whereby MPA produces its immunosuppressive effect in proliferating T lymphocytes is thus clearly distinct from that of the calcineurin inhibitors: cyclosporine or Tac, and Siro.

MMF is rapidly hydrolyzed by widely distributed esterases in blood and tissues to produce MPA. The rate limiting step in the clearance of MPA is its conversion to the phenolic glucuronide metabolite MPAG (Figure 33-14) via

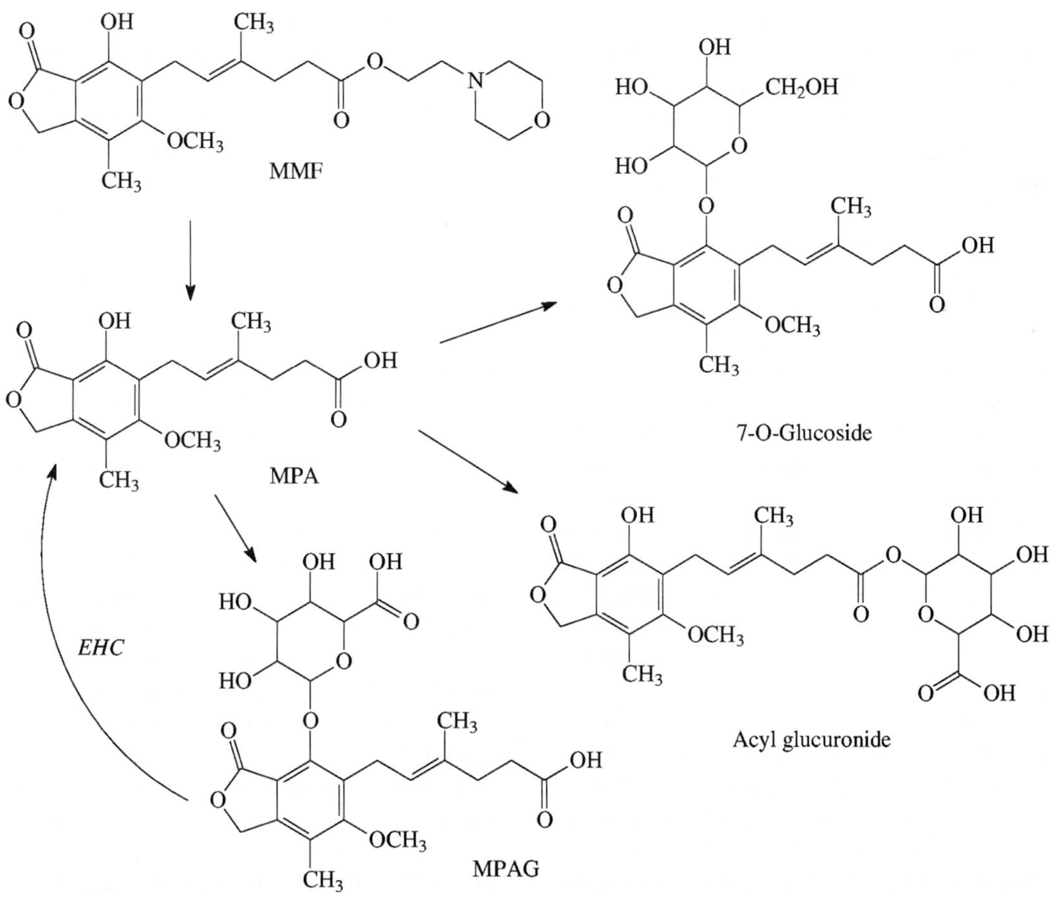

MMF

MPA

7-O-Glucoside

Acyl glucuronide

MPAG

EHC

Figure 33-14 Chemical structures and metabolic pathways of mycophenolate mofetil (MMF), mycophenolic acid (MPA), and mycophenolate glucuronide (MPAG).

the catalytic action of UGT in the liver, gastrointestinal tract, and possibly other tissues, such as kidney. MPAG is the primary metabolite of MPA and is pharmacologically inactive.[67] The acyl glucuronide and 7-O-glucoside are metabolites that are produced in much smaller quantities than either MPA or MPAG.[129] The glucoside metabolite has no pharmacological activity, but the acyl glucuronide is under evaluation for its potential toxic effects.[148] MPAG is cleared by the kidney and accumulates to as much as several hundred–fold higher plasma concentration as the steady-state trough concentration of MPA in uremic patients.[123-125]

MPA usually reaches maximal concentrations within an hour of the time of oral administration of MMF.[13] Distribution of the drug is rapid and essentially complete in most patients within 2 to 3 hours of administration.[13] In whole blood, >99.9% of the drug is in the plasma compartment.[100] MPA's clearance is affected by (1) glucuronidation, (2) enterohepatic circulation (EHC), and (3) the quantity of its free fraction. EHC is considered to be a significant contributor to the dose interval kinetics of MPA, especially the post-distribution phase of the concentration-time curve. The contribution of EHC to the MPA AUC is about 37%, ranging from 10% to 61%, based on the effect of concomitant administration of cholestyramine.[13] The appearance of a secondary MPA concentration peak anywhere from 4 to 12 hours following the morning dose of MMF is believed to result from EHC.

MPA is avidly and extensively bound to human serum albumin. In stable transplant patients, the MPA free fraction ranges from 1% to 3%.[100] When one or more of the following conditions are present, the MPA free fraction will increase significantly:

1. Early poor kidney function in renal transplant patients
2. Chronic renal failure
3. Low serum albumin concentration
4. Hyperbilirubinemia
5. Liver transplant patients in the early posttransplant period

Increased free fraction will cause an increased clearance of MPA, resulting in lower total MPA concentrations that return to baseline values when the condition that caused the change in free fraction becomes normal.[124] In chronic renal failure, however, the total MPA concentration is often within the guidelines for effective immunosuppression, but the free concentrations can be substantially elevated—placing the patient at increased risk for overimmunosuppression.[54,65,83] It is hypothesized that chronic uremia causes reduction in the intrinsic clearance that results in zero order kinetics for MPA clearance.

The primary sites and effects of drug-drug interactions involving other medications and MPA are likely to be decreased absorption in the gastrointestinal tract, inhibition of enterohepatic cycling, and inhibition of transport of the primary phenolic glucuronide metabolite. Meal consumption just before oral intake of MMF delays absorption, causing a reduction in the maximal concentration by about 25%. Administration of antacids containing magnesium and aluminum hydroxides has been reported to reduce peak concentration of MPA by 33% and AUC by 17%. The two interactions with the greatest reported effects are cholestyramine and ferrous sulfate.[13,85] Cholestyramine produces a 40% reduction in the MPA AUC when co-administered with MMF. The common iron supplement ferrous sulfate lowers the MPA AUC by about 90%. Long-term effects of this drug interaction are under investigation. It has been suggested that corticosteroids cause enhanced clearance of MPA via induction of UGT activity.[15] This is based on the observed 33% increase in the dose-corrected MPA trough concentration in a cohort of stable renal transplant patients at 12 months, following corticosteroid withdrawal, compared with the value at 6 months during maintenance therapy with corticosteroids.[15] Further investigation will be required to establish whether or not there is a direct cause-effect relationship in transplant patients. Corticosteroids have been shown to induce UGT activity in animal models. Inhibition of transport of MPAG from liver into bile is the presumed mechanism for the significant lowering of MPA concentration and raising of MPAG concentration by concomitant cyclosporine.[140] This drug-drug interaction results in MPA AUC values, adjusted for MMF dose, that are approximately 45% higher in patients on concomitant Tac versus those on concomitant cyclosporine.

HPLC methods with UV detection for MPA quantification are in common use in clinical pharmacokinetic studies and in clinical laboratories.[5,138] An immunoassay has been developed and is in routine use in centers outside the United States.[144] Validated HPLC assays with mass spectrometric detection have been developed and are particularly useful for the accurate measurement of free MPA concentration.[125] A new method that uses IMPDH, the natural target receptor of MPA, is in development.[28] Inhibition of IMPDH activity by MPA in an aliquot of patient serum or plasma is the basis for this method.

Sirolimus

Siro, proprietary name *Rapamune,* and formerly known as Rapamycin, is a macrocyclic antibiotic with immunosuppressive activity.[57] It is a fermentation product of the actinomycete *Streptomyces hygroscopicus,* which was isolated from soil samples collected on Rapa Nui (Easter Island) following a search for novel antifungal agents. Structurally, Siro is a lipophilic macrocyclic lactone composed of a 31-membered macrolide ring (Figure 33-13). It was shown to possess antifungal, antitumor, and immunosuppressive activity in animal model studies.[96] Subsequently, following discovery of its efficacy for the prophylaxis of acute rejection in renal transplant patients, formal clinical trials were undertaken; in 1999 Siro was approved for this indication by the U.S. FDA.

The complex of Siro and the intracellular immunophilin FK-BP12 modulates the immune response by combining with the specific cell-cycle regulatory protein mTOR and inhibiting its activation. This inhibition results in suppression of cytokine driven T lymphocyte proliferation, inhibiting the progression from the G_1 to the S phase of the cell cycle.[75] Metabolism of Siro by the human body is driven by oxidative metabolism by CyP 3A in the gastrointestinal tract and liver. There are at least 7 metabolites characterized as 41-O- and 7-O-demethyl, several hydroxy, hydroxy-demethylated, and didemethylated Siro.

Siro is administered orally as an oral solution in a vehicle containing a combination of phosphatidylcholine, propylene glycol, monoglycerides, ethanol, soy fatty acids, ascorbyl palmitate, and polysorbate 80 with a Siro concentration of 1 mg/mL. A 1 mg tablet formulation was recently approved, but this formulation is not bioequivalent to the oral solution. However, the two are clinically equivalent at a 2-mg dose based on comparable rates of efficacy failure graft loss or death. Siro is rapidly absorbed from the gastrointestinal tract, with the average time to reach maximal concentration in whole blood of about 2 hours.[156] The average bioavailability of Siro is 15%.[153] The low bioavailability is attributable to extensive intestinal and hepatic metabolism by CYP3A and to countertransport by the multidrug efflux pump Pg in the gastrointestinal tract.[95] This absorption barrier varies considerably from patient to patient and within-patient and is the site of clinically important drug-drug and drug-food interactions.

Siro distributes primarily into blood cells (95%), with only 3% and 1% distributing into plasma, lymphocytes, and granulocytes, respectively.[152] The extensive and avid binding of Siro to the ubiquitously distributed intracellular FK-binding proteins accounts for the high blood to plasma Siro concentration ratio. Approximately 2.5% of the Siro within the plasma fraction is unbound.[95]

The relationship between Siro whole blood trough concentrations has been investigated in renal transplant patients who received concomitant full dose cyclosporine and corticosteroid therapy. According to this study, the minimum effective Siro concentration—below which there is a significant increase in risk for acute rejection—is 4 to 5 ng/L.[63] The threshold concentration of 13 to 15 ng/L was identified, above which the risks for the concentration-related side effects of thrombocytopenia (<100,000 platelets/mm^3), leukopenia (<4000 leukocytes/mm), and hypertriglyceridemia (>300 mg/dL serum triglycerides) are increased.[63]

HPLC methods with MS, MS/MS, and UV detection have been validated and are in use in laboratories worldwide.[59,136] An immunophilin binding assay was developed for Siro measurement[25] and an investigational microparticle enzyme immunoassay was used in two phase III clinical trials.[95] Currently, there is no available automated immunoassay, although assays of this type are in development.

Tacrolimus

Tac, proprietary name *Prograf* and formerly known as *FK506*, is a macrolide lactone isolated from *Streptomyces tsukubaensis* in 1984 and is a potent immunosuppressant, which consists of a 23-membered carbon ring and a hemiketal-masked α,β-diketoamide function (Figure 33-13). Tac is approved for prophylaxis of organ rejection in patients receiving allogeneic liver transplants and for use as an immunosuppressant in kidney transplantation. This potent immunosuppressant has been used effectively in other solid organ transplant patients for prevention of graft-versus-host-disease in allogeneic stem cell transplant recipients and in pancreatic islet transplantation.

As with cyclosporine and Siro, Tac exerts its immunosuppressive effect following the formation of a complex with immunophilins. The complex of Tac and FK-BP12 in lymphocytes suppresses the synthesis of cytokines and inflammatory mediators by the same mechanisms (see Cyclosporine section for details and references).

Cytochrome P450 3A is primarily responsible for Tac metabolism and nine metabolites have been isolated from human blood and rat bile, or produced in vitro by human or animal liver microsomes. Tac metabolites in the blood of liver and kidney transplant patients totaled 42% to 45% of the Tac concentration. All of the metabolites, except for 31-O-desmethyl Tac, a minor Tac metabolite, have little immunosuppressive activity. The latter has in vitro immunosuppressive activity comparable with that of the parent drug. The total immunosuppressive activity of the metabolites is therefore negligible in transplant patients. However, in liver transplant patients with hyperbilirubinemia, there can be significant high bias in the immunoassay results because of metabolite accumulation that results from impaired bile clearance.[76]

Tac is most often administered by the oral route in capsules as a solid dispersed in hydroxypropylmethylcellulose. A solution for injection is available. The absorption from the small intestine is generally low, averaging 25%—but highly variable from patient to patient, ranging from 4% to 93%—and changes with time following transplant surgery.[142] Low Tac bioavailability, such as cyclosporine and Siro, is due to the presence of CyP 3A4/5 and the multidrug efflux pump Pg in the small intestinal enterocytes. The combination of this drug metabolizing enzyme and the drug efflux pump are thought to form a natural barrier to the absorption of xenobiotics in the gastrointestinal tract. The extensive interpatient range of bioavailability is likely due to the wide range of CYP3A4/5 catalytic activity and the amount of Pg per unit of weight of small intestine. Since many other drugs are substrates for these two systems, the gastrointestinal tract is an important site for many drug-drug interactions involving Tac.[17]

The distribution in blood is characterized by an extensive uptake by cells. The whole blood–to-plasma ratio varies from 15 to 35. The high affinity of Tac for FK-binding proteins and their rich presence in blood cells account for this distribution. Approximately 99% of Tac in plasma is bound to proteins, primarily α_1-acid glycoprotein, lipoproteins, albumin, and globulins.[154] The major route of elimination is

TABLE 33-12 Pharmacokinetic Parameters of Immunosuppressant Drugs

Drug	Minimum Effective Concentration (MEC) (ng/mL)	Minimum Toxic Concentration (MTC)* (ng/mL)	Average Half-Life (hr)	Average Volume of Distribution (L/kg)	Average Oral Bioavailability (%)	Average Protein Binding (%)	Important Metabolizing Enzymes
Cyclosporin A†	100	350†	8.4	3-5	30	90	CyP 3A4, Pg
Everolimus	3	20†	24	NA	NA	NA	CyP 3A4, Pg
Mycophenolic acid	2 µg/mL	12 µg/mL	18	4	94	97	UGT
Sirolimus	6	20†	13	2.6	NA	NA	CyP 3A4, Pg
Tacrolimus	6	20†	21	0.85	15	85	CyP 3A4, Pg

NA, Not applicable.
*Trough concentration.
†Refers to data for Neoral.

fecal excretion of metabolites. Elimination half-life of Tac is variable. Average half-life values of 12 hours and 19 hours have been reported in liver and renal transplant patients. Tac pharmacokinetic parameters are summarized in Table 33-12.

As for cyclosporine and Siro, many drugs interact with Tac by either inducing the production of CyP 3A4/5 and Pg or by competitively blocking the Tac binding site on these. A comprehensive review on this subject has been published.[17]

The relationship between Tac dose, trough blood concentration, and clinical outcomes—including acute rejection, nephrotoxicity, and toxicity requiring dose reduction—was investigated in a prospective multicenter study in liver transplant patients.[90] A significant inverse correlation between Tac trough blood concentration and the risk of acute rejection during the first week following liver transplantation was shown using logistic regression analysis. Nephrotoxicity and other side effects were also significantly correlated with increasing Tac trough blood concentrations during this time period. Receiver operator characteristic curve analyses showed that Tac trough blood concentrations could differentiate between toxicity and nonevents.[143]

A number of specific and sensitive HPLC/MS methods have been developed.[2,17,71,133,135] An immunoassay for Tac measurement is also available.

CLINICAL APPLICATIONS

Three case studies that apply the clinical principles and the pharmacology data described in this chapter are presented on this book's accompanying Evolve site, found at http://evolve.elsevier.com/Tietz/textbook/. They present typical problems the clinician and clinical laboratorian are faced with in daily practice.

REFERENCES

1. Akerman KK, Jolkkonen J, Parviainen M, Penttila I. Analysis of low-dose benzodiazepines by HPLC with automated solid-phase extraction. Clin Chem 1996; 42:1412-6.
2. Alak AM. Measurement of tacrolimus (FK506) and its metabolites: A review of assay development and application in therapeutic drug monitoring and pharmacokinetic studies. Ther Drug Monit 1997;19:338-51.
3. Albertioni F, Rask C, Eksborg S, Poulsen JH, Pettersson B, Beck O, et al. Evaluation of clinical assays for measuring high-dose methotrexate in plasma. Clin Chem 1996;42:39-44.
4. Ambudkar SV, Dey S, Hrycyna CA, Ramachandra M. Biochemical, cellular, and pharmacological aspects of the multidrug transporter. Ann Rev Pharmacol Toxicol 1999;39:361-98.
5. Baldelli S, Murgia S, Merlini S, Zenoni S, Perico N, Remuzzi G, et al. High-performance liquid chromatography with ultraviolet detection for therapeutic drug monitoring of everolimus. J Chromatogr B Analyt Technol Biomed Life Sci 2005;816:99-105.
6. Belitsky P, Dunn S, Johnston A, Levy G. Impact of absorption profiling on efficacy and safety of cyclosporin therapy in transplant recipients. Clin Pharmacokinet 2000;39:117-25.
7. Belz S, Frickel C, Wolfrom C, Nau H, Henze G. High-performance liquid chromatographic determination of methotrexate, 7-hydroxymethotrexate, 5-methyltetrahydrofolic acid and folinic acid in serum and cerebrospinal fluid. J Chromatogr B Biomed Appl 1994;661:109-18.
8. Benedetti MS. Enzyme induction and inhibition by new anti-epileptic drugs: A review of human studies. Fund Clin Pharma 2000;14:301-19.
9. Biggs JT, Holland WH, Chang S, Hipps PP, Sherman WR. Electron beam ionization mass fragmentographic analysis of tricyclic antidepressants in human plasma. J Pharm Sci 1976;65:261-8.
10. Blum RA, Comstock TJ, Sica DA, Schultz RW, Keller E, Reetze P, et al. Pharmacokinetics of gabapentin in subjects with various degrees of renal function. Clin Pharmacol Ther 1994;56:154-9.

11. Bresnahan JF, Vliestra RE. Digitalis glycosides. Mayo Clin Proc 1979;54:675-84.
12. Buchthal F, Svensmark O, Schiller PJ. Clinical and electroencephalographic correlations with serum levels of diphenylhydantoin. Arch Neurol 1960; 2:624-30.
13. Bullingham RE, Nicholls AJ, Kamm BR. Clinical pharmacokinetics of mycophenolate mofetil. Clin Pharmacokinet 1998;34:429-55.
14. Calne RY, White DJ, Thiru S, Evans DB, McMaster P, Dunn DC, et al. Cyclosporin A in patients receiving renal allografts from cadaver donors. Lancet 1978; 2:1323-7.
15. Cattaneo D, Perico N, Gaspari F, Gotti E, Remuzzi G. Glucocorticoids interfere with mycophenolate mofetil bioavailability in kidney transplantation. Kidney Int 2002;62:1060-7.
16. Chiu JA, Franklin RB. Analysis and pharmacokinetics of olanzapine (LY170053) and two metabolites in rat plasma using reversed-phase HPLC with electrochemical detection. J Pharm Biomed Anal 1996; 14:609-15.
17. Christians U, Jacobsen W, Benet LZ, Lampen A. Mechanisms of clinically relevant drug interactions > associated with tacrolimus. Clin Pharmacokinet 2002; 41:813-51.
18. Cohen AF, Land GS, Breimer DD, Yuen WC, Winton C, Peck AW. Lamotrigine, a new anticonvulsant: Pharmacokinetics in normal humans. Clin Pharmacol Ther 1987;42:535-41.
19. Cohen BM, Herschel M, Aoba A. Neuroleptic, antimuscarinic, and anticholinergic activity of chlorpromazine, thioridazine and their metabolites. Psychiatry Res 1979;1:199-208.
20. Cole E, Midtvedt K, Johnston A, Pattison J, O'Grady C. Recommendations for the implementation of Neoral C(2) monitoring in clinical practice. Transplantation 2002;73:S19-22.
21. Cooper TB, Kelly RG. GLC analyses of loxapine, amoxapine, and their metabolites in serum and urine. J Pharm Sci 1979;68:216-9.
22. Cristillo AD, Bierer BE. Identification of novel targets of immunosuppressive agents by cDNA-based microarray analysis. J Biol Chem 2002;277:4465-76.
23. Dahl SG. Plasma level monitoring of antipsychotic drugs: Clinical utility [Review] Clin Pharmacokinet 1986;11:36-61.
24. David BM, Madsen BW, Ilett KF. Plasma binding of disopyramide. Br J Clin Pharmacol 1980;9:614-8.
25. Davis DL, Soldin SJ. Identification of ubiquitin as an immunophilin. Biochem Biophys Res Commun 2000; 277:325-9.
26. Devinsky O, Vasquez B, Luciano D. New antiepileptic drugs for children: Felbamate, gabapentin, lamotrigine, and vigabatrine. J Child Neurol 1994;9(Suppl): S33-45.
27. Dias VC, Legatt DF, Yatscoff RW. The EMIT Cyclosporine Assay: development of application protocols for the Boehringer Mannheim Hitachi 911 and 917 analyzers. Clin Biochem 1997;30:155-62.
28. Dorn AR, Mountain LD, Phillips M, et al. Roche Diagnostics automated clinical analyzer enzyme/receptor assay for mycophenolic acid measurement in transplant patient samples [Abstract]. Ther Drug Monit 2003;25:510.
29. Duffus JH. Glossary for chemists of terms used in toxicology. Pure Appl Chem 1993;65:2003-122.
30. Edelbroeck PM, De Wolff FA. Improved micromethod for determination of underivatized clonazepam in serum by gas chromatography. Clin Chem 1978;24:1774-7.
31. Eisen HJ, Tuzcu EM, Dorent R, Kobashigawa J, Mancini D, Valantine-von Kaeppler HA, et al. Everolimus for the prevention of allograft rejection and vasculopathy in cardiac transplant recipients. N Engl J Med 2003;349:847-58.
32. El-Yazigni A, Chaley K., Martin CR. A simplified and rapid test for acetylator phenotyping by use of the peak height ratio of two urinary caffeine metabolites. Clin Chem 1989;35:848-51.
33. Eugui EM, Allison A. Immunosuppressive activity of mycophenolate mofetil. Ann NY Acad Sci 1993; 685:309-29.
34. Evers J, Eichelbaum M, Kroemer HK. Unpredictability of flecainide plasma concentrations in patients with renal failure: Relationship to side effects and sudden death. Ther Drug Monit 1994;16:349-51.
35. Feely J, Wilkinson GR, McAllister CB, Wood AJJ. Increased toxicity and reduced clearance of lidocaine by cimetidine. Ann Intern Med 1982;96:592-4.
36. Ferrari S, Sassoli V, Orlandi M, Strazzari S, Puggioli C, Battistini A, et al. Serum methotrexate (MTX) concentrations and prognosis in patients with osteosarcoma of the extremities treated with a multidrug neoadjuvant regimen. J Chemother 1993;5:135-41.
37. Flockhart D. 2005, at http://medicine.iupui.edu/flockhart/table.htm.
38. Foerster EH, Dempsey J, Garriott JC. A gas chromatographic procedure for acid and neutral drugs in blood. J Anal Toxicol 1979;3:87-91.
39. Franklin M. Determination of nefazodone and its metabolites in plasma by high-performance liquid chromatography with coulometric detection. J Pharm Biomed Anal 1993;11:1109-13.
40. Fukuoka N, Tsukamoto T, Uno J, Kimura M, Morita S. Influence of coadministered antiepileptic drugs on serum zonisamide concentrations in epileptic patients: quantitative analysis based on suitable transforming factor. Biol Pharm Bull 2003;26:1734-8.
41. Garcia LL, Shihabi ZK, Oles K. Determination of gabapentin in serum by capillary electrophoresis. J Chromatogr B Biomed Appl 1995;669:157-62.

42. George S, Wood AJ, Braithwaite, RA. Routine therapeutic monitoring of lamotrigine in epileptic patients using a simple and rapid high performance liquid chromatographic technique. Ann Clin Biochem 1995; 32:584-8.
43. Gerson B, Anhalt JP. High-pressure liquid chromatography and therapeutic drug monitoring. Chicago: American Society of Clinical Pathologists, 1980:172.
44. Gilbert DN Aminoglycosides. In: Mandell GL, Bennett JE, Dolin R, eds. Principles and practice of infectious diseases, 4th ed. New York: Churchill Livingstone, 1995:279-306.
45. Gonzalez-Esquivel DF, Ortega-Gavilan M, Alcantara-Lopez G, Jung-Cook H. Plasma level monitoring of oxcarbazepine in epileptic patients. Arch Med Res 2000;31:202-5.
46. Greenstein S, Siegal B. Compliance and noncompliance in patients with a functioning renal transplant A multicenter study. Transplantation 1998;66:1718-26.
47. Guengerich FP. Cytochrome P-450 3A4: Regulation and role in drug metabolism. Ann Rev Pharmacol Toxicol 1999;39:1-17.
48. Gupta RN. Column liquid chromatographic determination of paroxetine in human serum using solid-phase extraction. J Chromatogr B Biomed Appl 1994; 661:362-5.
49. Gustavson LE, Boellner SW, Granneman GR, Qian JX, Guenther HJ, el-Shourbagy T, et al. A single-dose study to define tiagabine pharmacokinetics in pediatric patients with complex partial seizures. Neurology 1997;48:1032-7.
50. Harder S, Thurmann P, Siewert M, et al. Concentration/effect relationship and enantio-selective analysis of verapamil in hypertensive patients. J Cardiovasc Pharmacol 1992;19:665-9.
51. Hardman JG, Limbird LE, Molinoff PB, Ruddon RW, Gilman AG, Eds. Goodman & Gilman's the pharmacological basis of therapeutics, 10th ed. New York: McGraw-Hill, 2001.
52. Hendeles L, Weinberger M. Theophylline: Therapeutic use and serum concentration monitoring. In: Taylor WJ, Finn AL, Eds. Individualizing drug therapy. New York: Gross, Townsend, and Frank, 1981:32-65.
53. Hengy H, Ernst-Ulrich K. Determination of gabapentin in plasma and urine by high performance liquid chromatography and pre-column labeling for ultraviolet detection. J Chromatog 1985;341:473-8.
54. Holt DW. Monitoring mycophenolic acid. Ann Clin Biochem 2002;39:173-83.
55. Holt DW. Therapeutic drug monitoring of immunosuppressive drugs in kidney transplantation. Curr Opin Nephrol Hypertens 2002;11:657-63.
56. Holt DW, Armstrong VW, Griesmacher A, Morris RG, Napoli KL, Shaw LM. International Federation of Clinical Chemistry/International Association of Therapeutic Drug Monitoring and Clinical Toxicology working group on immunosuppressive drug monitoring. Ther Drug Monit 2002;24:59-67.
57. Holt DW, Denny K, Lee TD, Johnston A. Therapeutic monitoring of sirolimus: its contribution to optimal prescription. Transplant Proc 2003;35:157S-161S.
58. Holt DW, Johnston A. Monitoring Immunosuppressive Drugs: Has It a Future? Ther Drug Monit 2004; 26:244-7.
59. Holt DW, Lee T, Jones K, Johnston A. Validation of an assay for routine monitoring of sirolimus using HPLC with mass spectrometric detection. Clin Chem 2000;46:1179-83.
60. Hoppu K, Jalanko H, Laine J, Holmberg C. Comparison of conventional oral cyclosporine and cyclosporine microemulsion formulations in children with a liver transplant. Transplantation 1996;62:66-71.
61. Johannessen SI, Battino D, Berry DJ, Bialer M, Kramer G, Tomson T, Patsalos PN. Therapeutic drug monitoring of the newer antiepileptic drugs. Ther Drug Monit 2003;25:347-63.
62. Kahan BD, Welsh M, Rutzky LP. Challenges in cyclosporine therapy: the role of therapeutic monitoring by area under the curve monitoring. Ther Drug Monit 1995;17:621-4.
63. Kahan BD, Napoli KL, Kelly PA, Podbielski J, Hussein I, Urbauer DL, et al. Therapeutic drug monitoring of sirolimus: Correlations with efficacy and toxicity. Clin Transplant 2000;14:97-109.
64. Kahan BD, Shaw LM, Holt D, Grevel J, Johnston A. Consensus document: Hawk's Cay meeting on therapeutic monitoring of cyclosporine Clin Chem 1990; 36:1510-6.
65. Kaplan B, Meier-Kriesche HU, Friedman G, Mulgaonkar S, Gruber S, Korecka M, et al. The effect of renal insufficiency on mycophenolic acid protein binding. J Clin Pharmacol 1999;39:715-20.
66. Koch-Weser J. Serum drug concentrations and therapeutic guides. N Engl J Med 1972;287:227-31.
67. Korecka M, Nikolic D, van Breemen RB, Shaw LM. Inhibition of inosine monophosphate dehydrogenase by mycophenolic acid glucuronide is attributable to the presence of trace quantities of mycophenolic acid. Clin Chem 1999;45:1047-50.
68. Kouno Y, Ishikura C, Homma M, Oka K. Simple and accurate high-performance liquid chromatographic method for the measurement of three antiepileptics in therapeutic drug monitoring. J Chromatogr 1993; 622:47-52.
69. Kronig MH, Munne RA, Szymanski S, Safferman AZ, Pollack S, Cooper T, et al. Plasma clozapine levels and clinical response for treatment-refractory schizophrenic patients. Am J Psychiatry 1995;152:179-83.
70. Leahey EB Jr, Reiffel JA, Drusin RE, Heissenbuttel RH, Lovejoy WP, Bigger JT Jr. Interaction between quinidine and digoxin. JAMA 1978;240:533-4.

71. Lensmeyer G, Poquette MA. Therapeutic monitoring of tacrolimus concentrations in blood: semi-automated extraction and liquid chromatography-electrospray ionization mass spectrometry. Ther Drug Monit 2001;20:239-49.
72. Leppik I, Shellenberger K. Zonisamide pharmacokinetics: direct relationship between oral dose and blood levels. Epilepsia 1999;40:286.
73. Leung LY, Lim H-K, Hicks D, et al. Metabolite characterization in rat and human liver microsomal incubations and trough whole blood of renal transplant patients treated with sirolimus, cyclosporine, and prednisone [Abstract]. ISSX Proc 1996;10:366.
74. Lewis RP. Digitalis. In: Leier CV ed. Cardiotonic drugs: A clinical survey. New York: Marcel Dekker Inc, 1987:85-150.
75. Macdonald A, Scarola J, Burke JT, Zimmerman JJ. Clinical pharmacokinetics and therapeutic drug monitoring of sirolimus. Clin Therapeutics 2000;22(Suppl B):B101-21.
76. MacFarlane GD, Scheller DG, Ersfeld DL, Shaw LM, Venkatarmanan R, Sarkozi L, et al. Analytical validation of the PRO-Trac II ELISA for the determination of tacrolimus (FK-506) in whole blood. Clin Chem 1999;45:1449-58.
77. Maloney JD, Nissen RG, McColgan JM. Open clinical studies at a referral center: chronic maintenance tocainide therapy in patients with recurrent sustained ventricular tachycardia refractory to conventional antiarrhythmic agents. Am Heart J 1980;100:1023-30.
78. Mandell GL, Bennett JE, Dolin R, Eds. Principles and practice of infectious diseases, 5th ed New York: Churchill Livingstone, 2000.
79. McBride JH, Kim SS, Rodgerson DO, Reyes AF, Ota MK. Measurement of cyclosporine by liquid chromatography and three immunoassays in blood from liver, cardiac, and renal transplant recipients. Clin Chem 1992;38:2300-6.
80. McIntyre IM, King CV, Skafidis S, Drummer OH. Dual ultraviolet wavelength high-performance liquid chromatographic method for the forensic or clinical analysis of seventeen antidepressants and some selected metabolites. J Chromatogr 1993;621:215-23.
81. Melmon MF, Morelli HF, Hoffman BB, Nierenberg DW, Eds. Melmon & Morelli's clinical pharmacology: Basic principles in therapeutics, 4th ed New York: McGraw-Hill, 2000.
82. Myerburg RJ, Kessler KM, Kiem I, Pefkaros KC, Conde CA, Cooper D, et al. Relationship between plasma levels of procainamide suppression of premature ventricular complexes and prevention of recurrent ventricular tachycardia. Circulation 1981; 64:280-90.
83. Meier-Kriesche HU, Shaw LM, Korecka M, Kaplan B. Pharmacokinetics of mycophenolic acid in renal insufficiency. Ther Drug Monit 2000;22:27-30.
84. Morgenstern GR, Powles R, Robinson B, McElwain TJ. Cyclosporin interaction with ketoconazole and melphalan. Lancet 1982;2:1342.
85. Morii M, Ueno K, Ogawa A, Kato R, Yoshimura H, Wada K, et al. Impairment of mycophenolate mofetil absorption by iron ion. Clin Pharm Ther 2000;68: 613-6.
86. Morris RG, Holt DW, Armstrong VW, Griesmacher A, Napoli KL, Shaw LM. Analytic aspects of cyclosporine monitoring, on behalf of the IFCC/IATDMCT Joint Working Group. Ther Drug Monit 2004;26:227-30.
87. Moyer TP, Boeckx RC. Applied therapeutic drug monitoring, Vol. 1. Washington DC: AACC Press, 1982.
88. Moyer TP, Boeckx RC. Applied therapeutic drug monitoring, Vol 2. Review and Case Studies. Moyer TP, Boeckx RC, Eds. Washington DC: AACC Press, 1984.
89. Moyer TP, Johnson P, Faynor SM, Sterioff S. A review of drug monitoring problems and presentation of a simple, accurate liquid chromatographic procedure that solves these problems. Clin Biochem 1986; 19:83-9.
90. Moyer TP, Post GR, Sterioff S, Anderson CF. Cyclosporine nephrotoxicity is minimized by adjusting dosage on the basis of drug concentration in blood. Mayo Clin Proc 1988;63:241-7.
91. Moyer TP, Therapeutic drug monitoring In: Burtis CA, Ashwood ER, eds. Tietz textbook of clinical chemistry, 3rd Ed. WB Saunders Co: Philadelphia, PA, 1999:862-905.
92. Moyer TP, Temesgen Z, Enger R, Estes L, Charlson J, Oliver L, Wright A. Drug monitoring of antiretroviral therapy for HIV-1 infection: method validation and results of a pilot study. Clin Chem 1999;45:1465-76.
93. Mungall DR. Applied clinical pharmacokinetics. New York: Raven Press, 1983.
94. Nakamura M, Hirade K, Sugiyama T, Katagiri Y. High-performance liquid chromatographic assay of zonisamide in human plasma using a non-porous silica column. J Chromatogr B Biomed Sci Appl 2001; 755:337-41.
95. Napoli KL, Taylor PJ. From beach to bedside: History of the development of sirolimus. Ther Drug Monit 2001;23:559-86.
96. Napoli KL, Wang M, Stepkowski SM, Kahan, BD. Distribution of sirolimus in rat tissue. Clin Biochem 1997;30:135-42.
97. Nashan B. Review of the proliferation inhibitor everolimus. Expert Opin Investig Drug 2002; 11:1842-50.
98. Neumayer HH, Paradis K, Korn A, Jean C, Fritsche L, Budde K, Winkler M, et al. Entry-into-human study with the novel immunosuppressant SDZ RAD in stable renal transplant recipients. J Clin Pharmacol 1999;48:694-703.

99. Nguyen NT, Siegler RW. Capillary electrophoresis of cardiovascular drugs. J Chromatogr A 1996;735: 123-50.
100. Nowak I, Shaw LM. Mycophenolic acid binding to human serum albumin: Characterization and relation to pharmacodynamics. Clin Chem 1995;41:1011-17.
101. O'Kane DJ, Weinshilboum RM, Moyer TP. Pharmacogenomics and reducing the frequency of adverse drug events. Pharmacogenomics 2003;4:1-4.
102. Packer M, Gheorghiade M, Young JB, Costantini PJ, Adams KF, Cody RJ, et al. Withdrawal of digoxin from patients with chronic heart failure treated with angiotensin-converting enzyme inhibitors. N Engl J Med 1993;329:1-7.
103. Perucca E. Pharmacokinetic profile of topiramate in comparison with other new anti-epileptic drugs. Epilepsia 1996;37(Suppl 2):S8-13.
104. Pesek JJ, Matyska MT. Separation of tetracyclines by high-performance capillary electrophoresis and capillary electrochromatography. J Chromatogr A 1996; 736:313-20.
105. Pette M, Pette DF, Muraro PA, Martin R, McFarland HF. In vitro modulation of human, autoreactive MBP-specific CD4+ T-cell clones by cyclosporin. A J Neuroimmunol 1997;76:91-9.
106. Pike NG, Franklin CL, Mays DC, Lipsky JL, Lowry PW, Sandborn WJ. Improved methods for determining the concentration of 6-thioguanine nucleotides and 6-methylmercaptopurine nucleotides in blood. J Chromatogr 2001;757:1-9.
107. Pine M, Favrot L, Smith S, McDonald K, Chidsey CA. Correlation of plasma propranolol concentration with therapeutic response in patients with angina pectoris. Circulation 1975;52:886-9.
108. Pollard S, Nashan B, Johnston A, Hoyer P, Belitsky P, Keown P, et al. A pharmacokinetic and clinical review of the potential clinical impact of using different formulations of cyclosporin A. Clin Ther 2003;5:1654-69.
109. Rao A, Luo C, Hogan PG. Transcription factors of the NFAT family: regulation and function. Annu Rev Immunol 1997;15:707-47.
110. Preskorn SH. Pharmacokinetics of antidepressants: Why and how they are relevant. J Clin Psychiatry 1993;54(Suppl J):14-34.
111. Quinn CM, Bugeja VC, Gallagher JA, Whittaker PA. The effect of mycophenolic acid on the cell cycle of Candida albicans. Mycopathologia 1990;111:165-8.
112. Ramsay RE, Wilder BJ, Uthman BM, Garnett WR, Pellock JM, Barkley GL, et al. Intramuscular fosphenytoin (Cerebyx) in patients requiring a loading dose of phenytoin. Epilepsy Res 1997;28:181-7.
113. Ramsay RE. Clinical efficacy and safety of gabapentin. Neurology 1994;44:S23-32.
114. Rathore SF, Curtis JP, Wang Y, et al. Association of serum digoxin concentration and outcomes in patients with heart Failure. JAMA 2003;289:871-8.
115. Relling MV, Fairclough D, Ayers D, Crom WR, Rodman JH, Pui CH, et al. Patient characteristics associated with high-risk methotrexate concentrations and toxicity. J Clin Oncol 1994;12:1667-72.
116. Remmel RE, Miller SA, Graves NM. Simultaneous assay for felbamate plus carbamazepine, phenytoin, and their metabolites by liquid chromatography. Ther Drug Monit 1990;12:90-6.
117. Riva E, Gerna M, Neyroz P, Urso R, Bartosek I, Guaitani A. Pharmacokinetics of amiodarone in man. J Cardiovasc Pharmacol 1982;4:264-9.
118. Rodopoulos N, Norman A. Determination of caffeine and its metabolites in urine by high-performance liquid chromatography and capillary electrophoresis. Scand. J Clin Lab Invest 1994;54:305-15.
119. Rowland M, Tozer TN. Clinical pharmacokinetics: Concepts and application. Philadelphia: Lea & Febiger, 1995.
120. Sadeg N, Francois G, Petit B, Dutertre-Catella H, Dumontet M. Automated liquid-chromatographic analyzer used for toxicology screening in a general hospital: 12 months' experience. Clin Chem 1997; 43:498-504.
121. Sarubbi FA, Hull JH. Amikacin serum concentrations Prediction of levels and dosage guidelines. Ann Intern Med 1978;89:612-18; and Gentamicin serum concentrations: Pharmacokinetic predictions. Ann Intern Med 1976;85:183-9.
122. Sharpe PC, Morrow J, Trimble ER. An audit of therapeutic drug monitoring anticonvulsants. Ulster Med J 1995;64:151-6.
123. Shaw LM, Holt DW, Oellerich M, Meiser B, van Gelder T. Current issues in therapeutic drug monitoring of mycophenolic acid: Report of a roundtable discussion. Ther Drug Monit 2001;23:305-15.
124. Shaw LM, Kaplan B, Brayman KL. Introduction and overview. Clin Ther 2000;22(Suppl B):B1-13.
125. Shaw LM, Korecka M, van Breeman R, Nowak I, Brayman KL. Analysis, pharmacokinetics and therapeutic drug monitoring of mycophenolic acid. Clin Biochem 1998;31:323-8.
126. Shaw LM, Kaplan B, Kaufman D. Toxic effects of immunosuppressive drugs: Mechanisms and strategies for controlling them. Clin Chem 1996;42:1316-21.
127. Shemesh E, Shneider BL, Savitzky JK, et al. Medication adherence in pediatric and adolescent liver transplant recipients. Pediatrics 2004;113:825-32.
128. Shihabi ZK, Oles KS. Felbamate measured in serum by two methods: HPLC and capillary electrophoresis. Clin Chem 1994;40:1904-8.
129. Shipkova M, Armstrong VW, Wieland E, Niedmann PD, Schutz E, Brenner-Weiss G, et al. Identification of glucoside and carboxyl-linked glucuronide conjugates of mycophenolic acid in plasma of transplant recipients treated with mycophenolate mofetil. Br J Pharmacol 1999;126:1075-82.

130. So EL, Wolff D, Graves NM, Leppik IE, Cascino GD, Pixton GC, et al. Pharmacokinetics of tiagabine as add-on therapy in patients taking enzyme-inducing antiepilepsy drugs. Epilepsy Res 1995;22:221-6.
131. Stahl SM. Mechanism of action of serotonin selective reuptake inhibitors. Serotonin receptors and pathways mediate therapeutic effects and side effects. J Affect Disord 1998;51:215-35.
132. Stoloff SW. The changing role of theophylline in pediatric asthma. Am Fam Physician 1994;49:839-44.
133. Streit F, Armstrong VW, Oellerich M. Rapid liquid chromatography-tandem mass spectrometry routine method for simultaneous determination of sirolimus, everolimus, tacrolimus, and cyclosporin A in whole blood. Clin Chem 2002;48:955-8.
134. Sweet RA, Pollock BG, Kirshner M, Wright B, Altieri LP, DeVane CL. Pharmacokinetics of single- and multiple-dose bupropion in elderly patients with depression. J Clin Pharmacol 1995;35:876-84.
135. Taylor PJ, Salm P, Lynch SV, Pillans PI. Simultaneous quantification of tacrolimus and sirolimus in human blood by high performance liquid chromatography-tandem mass spectrometry. Ther Drug Monit 2000; 21:608-12.
136. Taylor PJ, Johnson AG. Quantitative analysis of sirolimus (rapamycin) and its metabolites in blood by high performance liquid chromatography-electrospray tandem mass spectrometry. J Chromatography 1998;718:251-7.
137. Thormann W, Zhang CX, Schmutz A. Capillary electrophoresis for drug analysis in body fluids. Ther Drug Monit 1996;18:506-20.
138. Tsina I, Chu F, Hama K, Kaloostian M, Tam YL, Tarnowski T, Wong B. Manual and automated (robotic) high-performance liquid chromatography methods for the determination of mycophenolic acid and its glucuronide in human plasma. J Chromatogr B Biomed App 1996;675:119-29.
139. UNOS Market Share Report. Immunosuppression practice and trends. 2005, Chapter 4, www.unos.org.
140. van Gelder T, Hilbrands LB, Vanrenterghem Y, Weimar W, de Fijter JW, Squifflet JP, et al. A randomized double-blind, multicenter plasma concentration controlled study of the safety and efficacy of oral mycophenolate mofetil for the prevention of acute rejection after kidney transplantation. Transplantation 1999;68:261-6.
141. Vatassery GT, Holden LA, Hazel DK, Dysken MW. Determination of trazodone and its metabolite, 1-m-chlorophenyl-piperazine, in human plasma and red blood cell samples by HPLC. Clin Biochem 1997; 30:149-54.
142. Venkataramanan R, Swaminathan A, Prasad T, Jain A, Zuckerman S, Warty V, et al. Clinical pharmacokinetics of tacrolimus. Clin Pharmacokinet 1995;29: 404-30.
143. Venkataramanan R, Shaw LM. Clinical utility of monitoring tacrolimus blood concentrations in liver transplant patients. J Clin Pharmacol 2001;41: 542-51.
144. Vogl M, Weigel G, Seebacher G, Griesmacher A, Laufer G, Muller MM. Evaluation of the EMIT mycophenolic acid assay from Dade Behring. Ther Drug Monit 1999;21:638-43.
145. Volosov A, Alexander C, Ting L, Soldin SJ. Simple rapid method for quantification of antiretrovirals by liquid chromatography—tandem mass-spectrometry. Clin Biochem 2002;35:99-103
146. Weinshiboum RM, Sladek SL. Mercaptopurine pharmacogenetics: Monogenetic inheritance of erythrocyte thiopurine methyltransferase activity. Am J Hum Genet 1980;32:651-2.
147. Weinshiboum RM. Inheritance and drug response. N Engl J Med 2003;48:529-37.
148. Wieland E, Shipkova M, Schellhaas U, Schutz E, Niedmann PD, Armstrong VW, et al. Induction of cytokine release by the acyl glucuronide of mycophenolic acid: A link to side effects? Clin Biochem 2000; 33:107-13.
149. Winkler M, Ringe B, Baumann J, Loss M, Wonigeit K, Pichlmayr R. Plasma vs whole blood for therapeutic drug monitoring of patients receiving FK 506 for immunosuppression. Clin Chem 1994;40:2247-53.
150. Winter ME. Basic Clinical Pharmacokinetics. 3rd ed. Koda-Kimble, MA, Young LY, Eds., San Francisco, Applied Therapeutics, Inc., 1994.
151. Yatscoff RW, Rosano TG, Bowers LD. The clinical significance of cyclosporine metabolites. Clin Biochem 1991;24:23-35.
152. Yatscoff R, LeGatt D, Keenan R, Chackowsky P. Blood distribution of rapamycin. Transplantation 1993; 56:1202-6.
153. Yatscoff RW, Boeckx R, Holt DW, Kahan BD, LeGatt DF, Sehgal S, et al. Consensus guidelines for therapeutic drug monitoring of rapamycin: report of the consensus panel. Ther Drug Monit 1995;17:676-80.
154. Zahir H, Nand RA, Brown KF, Tattam BN, McLachlan AJ. Validation of methods to study the distribution and protein binding of tacrolimus in human blood. J Pharmacol Toxicol Methods 2001;46:27-35.
155. Zaske DE, Cipolle RJ, Strate RG. Gentamicin dosage requirements: Wide interpatient variations in 242 surgery patients with normal renal function. Surgery 1980;87:164-9.
156. Zimmerman JJ, Kahan BD. Pharmacokinetics of sirolimus in stable renal transplant patients after multiple oral dose administration. J Clin Pharmacol 1997;37:405-15.
157. Zwillich CW, Sutton FD, Neff TA, Cohn WM, Matthay RA, Weinberger MM. Theophylline-induced seizures in adults: Correlation with serum concentrations. Ann Intern Med 1975;82:784-7.

CHAPTER 34

Clinical Toxicology*

William H. Porter, Ph.D.

Toxicology is a broad, multidisciplinary science whose goal is to determine the effects of chemical agents on living systems. *Clinical toxicology* is a division of toxicology and is defined as the analysis of drugs, metals, and other chemical agents in body fluids and tissue for the purpose of patient care. Such analyses are often necessary for the diagnosis and management of acute drug overdose and acute exposure to chemicals of unknown origin from the patient's environment.

This chapter focuses primarily on the analytes a laboratorian encounters in clinical toxicology and on analytical techniques used to measure them. Because a comprehensive discussion of all the aspects of toxicology is beyond the scope of this chapter, the clinical significance and toxicity of only a select number of common drugs, drugs of abuse, and other chemicals are discussed. For additional information, readers are referred to several excellent texts on toxicology, including *Clinical Management of Poisoning and Drug Overdose,*[185] *Ellenhorn's Medical Toxicology: Diagnosis and Treatment of Human Poisoning,*[136] *Casarett and Doull's Toxicology: The Basic Science of Poisons,*[247] *Clinical Toxicology of Commercial Products,*[177] *Goodman and Gilman's The Pharmacologic Basis of Therapeutics,*[189] and *Goldfrank's Toxicologic Emergencies,* and to Chapters 30 and 35 where some of the more toxic metals are discussed.[75]

BASIC INFORMATION

In practice, it is not possible nor necessary to test for all of the hundreds or thousands of clinical toxins that may be encountered. In reality up to 24 drugs or agents account for 80% or more of intoxication treated in most emergency departments.[328,471] Moreover, some drugs are encountered very infrequently in some locations but with relatively high frequency in others. For example, phencyclidine (PCP) use is almost nonexistent in some areas but is responsible for a relatively high number of intoxications in a few large metropolitan cities. Thus the scope of clinical toxicology testing provided by the laboratory will depend on the pattern of local drug use and on the available resources of the institution and should be developed in consultation with the appropriate clinical staff.[270]

The value of drug and/or substance testing (screening) is well established (1) in the workplace, (2) for some athletic competitions, (3) to monitor drug use during pregnancy, (4) to evaluate drug exposure and/or withdrawal in newborns, (5) to monitor patients in pain management and drug abuse treatment programs, and (6) to aid in the prompt diagnosis of toxicity for a select number of drugs or agents for which a specific antidote or treatment modality is required (Table 34-1). In many other instances of drug toxicity, the value of drug screening, especially on an emergency basis, is more controversial.[65,139,239,314,388] It is argued that often drug toxicity is recognizable based on history and clinical signs and symptoms (see section on Toxic Syndromes), that treatment is general and supportive (Box 34-1) and therefore not influenced by results of drug screens, and that drug screen results often are not available soon enough to add valuable information. However, the clinical history is not always available or reliable, not all patients present with symptomatology clearly recognizable as drug or substance intoxication, and symptomatology may be complicated and confusing in instances of multiple drug overdose.[198,239,256,365] Moreover, it is clearly important to rule in or rule out drug toxicity as a possible etiology for patients with altered mental status or coma of unknown origin or for patients with seizures. For instance, a negative drug screen is helpful in the differential evaluation of a comatose patient eventually diagnosed with meningitis. For other patients, the results of drug testing may confirm the diagnosis or be valuable for follow-up counsel-

*The author gratefully acknowledges original contributions by Dr. Tom P. Moyer, upon which portions of the chapter are based.

TABLE 34-1 Antidote or Specific Treatment for Intoxication

Toxin	Antidote/Treatment
Acetaminophen	*N*-Acetylcysteine (Mucomyst)
Aluminum	Deferoxamine
Anticholinergic agents	Physostigmine
Arsenic	Dimercaprol, 2,3-dimercaptosuccinic acid, D-penicillamine
Barbiturates	Charcoal hemoperfusion, multiple-dose oral activated charcoal, alkaline diuresis (phenobarbital only)
Benzodiazepines	Flumazenil
Beta-blockers	Glucagon
Calcium channel blockers	Calcium
Carbamazepine	Multiple-dose oral activated charcoal; charcoal hemoperfusion
Carbon monoxide	Oxygen (normobaric or hyperbaric)
Cyanide	Amyl nitrite, sodium nitrite, sodium thiosulfate
Digoxin	Digibind (Fab fragments)
Ethylene glycol, methanol	Ethanol, hemodialysis, fomepizole (4-methylpyrazol)
Iron	Deferoxamine
Isoniazid	Pyridoxine
Isopropanol	Hemodialysis
Lead	Calcium disodium edetate, dimercaprol, 2,3-dimercaptosuccinic acid
Lithium	Hemodialysis
Mercury	Dimercaprol, 2,3-dimercaptosuccinic acid, D-penicillamine
Nitrites, nitrates	Methylene blue
Opioids	Naloxone
Organophosphate or carbamate insecticide	Atropine, pralidoxime (controversial for carbamates)
Salicylates	Bicarbonate, hemodialysis, alkaline diuresis
Theophylline	Multiple-dose oral activated charcoal, charcoal hemoperfusion
Tricyclic antidepressants	Bicarbonate

Data from references 9, 43, 137, 155, 268, 404.

BOX 34-1 General Supportive Measures in Treatment of Drug Overdose

1. Maintain airway, adequate ventilation, and oxygenation; provide tracheal intubation if required.
2. Maintain adequate cardiovascular function—intravenous crystalloid solutions and vasopressors (e.g., dopamine, norepinephrine) if required.
3. If comatose, administer glucose, thiamine, naloxone, and oxygen.
4. For seizures, administer diazepam, phenytoin.
5. Decontaminate gastrointestinal system—perform gastric lavage; induce vomiting if appropriate (syrup of ipecac); administer activated charcoal; administer cathartic (sodium sulfate, magnesium sulfate, or sorbitol); perform whole-bowel irrigation (isotonic polyethylene glycol electrolyte solution).

Data from references 43, 141, 155, 268, 404.

ing or treatment; in the latter instances, drug screens may not be required emergently.

Approaches to drug testing range from the provision of just a few specific tests (e.g., acetaminophen, salicylate, ethanol, digoxin, and iron) to additional targeted groups of drugs (e.g., stimulant panel and coma panel) or to a more comprehensive general drug screen that might include 100 or so drugs and/or substances. For all of these situations, it is important that the laboratory communicate with the physician concerning the scope (and limitation) of the service and the proper timing and selection of specimens; when possible, the laboratory should assist with interpretation of results. At a minimum, the laboratory request slip should clearly state the drugs that it has the capability of detecting. Otherwise, the report of a "negative" result for a drug screen could be misleading.

Clinical Considerations

To operate effectively, the laboratory requires a prerequisite amount of clinical information to guide ordering of the correct tests and to ensure that interpretation of results is complete and accurate. For example, the physician should provide the following information with the laboratory request:

1. The time and date of the suspected exposure and any indications from the patient or patient's family that might aid in identification of the toxin. The laboratory personnel must also have knowledge of the time that the specimens were collected.

2. Assessment of the physical state of the patient at the time of presentation, which should include the following:
   a. Vascular status (including measurement of blood pressure and pulse rate)
   b. Respiratory status (hypoventilation or hyperventilation)
   c. Temperature (presence of hypothermia or hyperthermia)
   d. Neurological status (determination of whether the patient is alert, comatose, or hyperactive or has neuropathy, cholinergic activity, or Babinski's sign)
   e. Cardiac status (determination of heart rate, electrocardiogram pattern, and QRS interval)
   f. Gastrointestinal (GI) status (presence of severe GI distress, vomiting, or diarrhea)

As described in the section Toxic Syndromes and discussed later in this chapter, each of these symptoms suggests a certain group of toxins. Such information is useful to guide test selection and interpretation of results. Realistically, physicians do not always have time or are not willing to provide such information. This clinical information is not necessary for test selection if the laboratory provides solely a broad-spectrum drug screen or provides symptom-related drug screens (coma panel and stimulant panel) selectable by the physician. However, such information still aids test interpretation. Because toxidrome assessment may be flawed by clinical inexperience, multidrug overdose, or delayed onset of action, an expert toxicology committee of the National Academy of Clinical Biochemistry discourages establishment of toxidrome-based drug screen panels.[491]

Analytical Considerations

Because of the wide range of drugs of interest, no single analytical technique is adequate for broad-spectrum drug detection. Therefore several analytical approaches in combination are generally required. These may include simple, inexpensive, and rapid spot tests; immunoassays (see Chapter 9); and chromatographic and/or mass spectrometric techniques (see Chapters 6 and 7), including thin-layer chromatography (TLC), high-performance liquid chromatography (HPLC), gas chromatography (GC), gas chromatography-mass spectrometry (GC-MS or GC-MS-MS), and liquid chromatography-mass spectrometry (LC-MS or LC-MS-MS).[442] Moreover, because of the innumerable drugs, metabolites, and endogenous substances that may be encountered, positive identification based on the results of a single analytical technique is generally not sufficiently definitive. Sound laboratory practice dictates the use of a second or confirmatory procedure that preferably is based on different analytical principles. Currently, GC-MS is the most widely used definitive confirmatory procedure. Confirmatory testing is mandatory for forensic drug testing (e.g., workplace drug testing).

Speed of analysis, or turnaround time (TOT), is a critical issue in clinical toxicology. A drug analysis that requires several hours to complete or that is not available at all hours of the day is of little value in a clinical emergency. On the other hand, a rapid test that provides false information could result in erroneous diagnostic and therapeutic decisions. Quantitative determinations in serum are important for acetaminophen, salicylate, ethanol, methanol, isopropanol, ethylene glycol, carbamazepine, phenytoin, valproic acid, phenobarbital, iron, transferrin (or unsaturated iron binding capacity), lithium, theophylline, and digoxin, and in whole blood for carboxyhemoglobin and methemoglobin. Results for these determinations should be available within 1 hour of specimen receipt.[491] For many other drugs, their serum concentration and the severity of toxicity do not correlate sufficiently to warrant obtaining quantitative information. In these cases, qualitative identification in urine is generally sufficient.

The proper selection of analytical methods and the interpretation of results requires a knowledge of the pharmacology and pharmacokinetics of the toxins of interest. For example, the potential hepatotoxicity of acetaminophen is related to the concentration of unmetabolized drug. Therefore, appropriate analytical methods for acetaminophen should measure only parent drug and not inactive metabolites. Moreover, quantitation of serum acetaminophen or salicylate before completion of the absorptive phase may be misleading in instances of overdose. Morphine is excreted in urine largely as morphine-3-glucuronide. The most sensitive detection of morphine necessitates a prior hydrolysis (acid or enzymatic) or methods that will directly measure the conjugate (e.g., immunoassay). Detection of the unique heroin metabolite, 6-monoacetylmorphine, distinguishes heroin use from ingestion of poppy seeds as the cause of a positive urine test for morphine.

Toxic Syndromes

Toxic syndromes ("toxidromes") are clinical syndromes that are essential for the successful recognition of poisoning patterns. A toxidrome is the constellation of clinical signs and symptoms that suggests a specific class of poisoning. The most important toxidromes are (1) anticholinergic, (2) cholinergic, (3) opioid and opioid withdrawal, (4) sedative-hypnotic and sedative-hypnotic withdrawal, and (5) sympathomimetic. Symptoms for these toxidromes are listed in Table 34-2.

Autonomic Nervous System

Many drugs commonly ingested in overdose cause dysfunction (agonistic or antagonistic) of the autonomic nervous system, the clinical consequences of which provide important clues to the clinician for diagnosis and treatment and also help guide the laboratory in the selection of appropriate tests.[135,256,276,328,404]

Biologically, the autonomic nervous system controls many physiological functions, including respiration, circulation, metabolism, digestion, secretions, and body temperature.[200] The *sympathetic* and *parasympathetic systems* are the two major divisions of the autonomic nervous system. In general, they are antagonistic (one stimulates while the other

TABLE 34-2 Symptoms of the Important Toxidromes

Toxidrome	Symptom
Anticholinergic	Agitation
	Blurred vision
	Choreoathetosis
	Decreased bowel sounds
	Dry skin
	Fever
	Flushing
	Hallucinations
	Ileus
	Lethargy/coma
	Mydriasis
	Myoclonus
	Psychosis
	Seizures
	Tachycardia
	Urinary retention
Cholinergic	Bradycardia
	Bronchorrhea
	Defecation
	Emesis
	Gastrointestinal distress (diarrhea)
	Lacrimation
	Salivation
	Urination
Opioid	Bradycardia
	Decreased bowel sounds
	Hypotension
	Hypothermia
	Lethargy/coma
	Miosis
	Shallow respirations
	Slow respiratory rate
Opioid withdrawal	Anxiety
	Diaphoresis
	Diarrhea with increased bowel sounds
	Fever
	Hypertension
	Irritability
	Lacrimation
	Muscle ache and spasm
	Mydriasis
	Nausea, vomiting
	Piloerection
	Restlessness
	Rhinorrhea
	Tachycardia
	Tachypnea
	Tremor
	Yawning
Sedative-hypnotic	Ataxia
	Blurred vision
	Confusion
	Delirium
	Diplopia
	Dysesthesias
	Hallucinations
	Hypotension
	Lethargy/coma
	Nystagmus
	Paresthesias
	Respiratory depression
	Sedation
	Slurred speech
Sedative-hypnotic, ethanol withdrawal	Agitation
	Anxiety
	Confusion
	Diaphoresis
	Dysphoria
	Fever
	Hallucinations
	Hypertension
	Insomnia
	Irritability
	Muscle spasm
	Nausea and vomiting
	Restlessness
	Seizures
	Tachycardia
	Tremor
Sympathomimetic	Agitation
	Diaphoresis
	Excessive motor activity
	Excessive speech
	Hallucinations
	Hypertension
	Hyperthermia
	Insomnia
	Restlessness
	Tachycardia
	Tremor

inhibits), and most organs are enervated by both, although not with equal tone. Norepinephrine is the neurotransmitter for postganglionic sympathetic fibers (adrenergic) that enervate skin, eyes, heart, lungs, GI tract, exocrine glands, and some neuronal tracts in the central nervous system (CNS). Physiological responses to activation of the adrenergic system are complex and depend on the type of receptor (α_1, α_2, β_1, β_2) activated, some of which are excitatory and others that have opposing inhibitory responses. These membrane-spanning adrenergic receptors are coupled to cytoplasmic surface GTP-binding regulatory proteins (G-proteins). Receptor activation results in GTP-mediated G-protein activation. The activated G-protein reacts with cell effectors, which may be enzymes such as adenyl cyclase or phospholipase C, or with multimeric transmembrane ion channels selective for Ca^{2+} or K^+. The resultant alterations (increase or decrease) in intracellular cAMP, Ca^{2+}, or K^+ ions leads to membrane hyperpolarization (inhibitory), depolarization (excitatory), or—for example—smooth muscle contraction. Other sympathetic neurotransmitters are dopamine, present in the extrapyramidal tracts in the CNS, and epinephrine, present in the adrenal medulla. Stimulation of the sympathetic nervous system produces CNS excitation (agitation, anxiety, tremors, delusions, and paranoia), headache, seizures, hypertension, mydriasis (dilated pupils), hyperpyrexia, and diaphoresis. In severe cases, hypotension, cardiac arrhythmias, and coma may occur. Examples of drugs that cause a *sympathomimetic* response include amphetamine, methhamphetamine, 3,4-methylenedioxymethamphetamine (MDMA), cocaine, PCP, lysergic acid diethylamide (LSD), ephedrine, pseudoephedrine, phenylpropanolamine, and caffeine. Some laboratories provide a stimulant drug screen panel designed to detect several of these drugs.

Acetylcholine is the neurotransmitter active in parasympathetic neurons (CNS and postganglionic peripheral), in autonomic ganglia (both sympathetic and parasympathetic), and in peripheral somatic nerves that enervate skeletal muscle (neuromuscular junction). Cholinergic responses may be subdivided into *muscarinic* (activated by muscarine) and *nicotinic* (activated by nicotine), depending on acetylcholine receptor type. Muscarinic receptors are G-protein coupled and are present in all autonomic ganglia, in postganglionic parasympathetic synapses, and in cortical and subcortical neurons. Muscarinic receptors are blocked by atropine. Nicotinic receptors are pentameric membrane-spanning ligand-gated Na^+ and Ca^{+2} ion channels and are prominent in all autonomic ganglia and at the neuromuscular end plate; they are blocked by tubocurarine but not atropine. Substances that activate muscarinic and/or nicotinic receptors are referred to as parasympathomimetic, cholinergic, or cholinomimetic. Activation of muscarinic receptors results in miosis, salivation, lacrimation, nausea and vomiting, bradycardia, increased GI motility, micturition, increased bronchial secretions and bronchoconstriction, hypotension, and diaphoresis. Two mnemonics have been developed to help recall muscarinic symptoms: DUMB BELS (**d**iarrhea, **u**rination, **m**iosis, **b**radycardia, and **b**ronchorrhea-**b**ronchoconstriction, **e**mesis, **l**acrimation, **s**weating-**s**alivation)[135] and SLUDGE (**s**alivation, **l**acrimation, **u**rination, **d**efecation, **GI** distress, **e**mesis-eye findings, miosis).[92]

Agents that cause these symptoms include organophosphate and carbamate insecticides (cholinesterase inhibitors),[379] pilocarpine, physostigmine, and certain species of mushrooms that contain muscarine.

Activation of nicotinic receptors initially stimulates postjunctional response but at high dose produces inhibition. Symptoms of activation of nicotinic cholinergic receptors at the neuromuscular junction include muscular twitching, weakness, and paralysis; stimulation of nicotinic receptors at sympathetic ganglia causes hypertension, tachycardia, and mydriasis. Agents that result in symptoms of both muscarinic and nicotinic cholinergic stimulation include organophosphate, carbamate, and nicotine-containing insecticides.

Anticholinergic Induced

Anticholinergic agents produce a syndrome somewhat similar to that associated with stimulation of sympathetic neurons (inhibition of cholinergic response leads to unopposed sympathomimetic activity). These symptoms include agitation, delirium, coma, tachycardia, hypertension, elevated temperature, and mydriasis. Important additional anticholinergic symptoms that distinguish this syndrome from the sympathomimetic syndrome are urinary retention; decreased bowel sounds; dry, flushed skin; and dry mouth. A mnemonic phrase will help the reader remember these symptoms: "red as a beet, dry as a bone, mad as a hatter, hot as stone, bowel and bladder lose their tone, and the heart runs alone."[422] Substances that cause the anticholinergic syndrome include antihistamines, atropine, cyclic antidepressant drugs, phenothiazines, anti-Parkinson's drugs, skeletal muscle relaxants, scopolamine, and several plants that contain so-called belladonna alkaloids (atropine or scopolamine), such as jimsonweed.

Opioid Induced

Another important toxic syndrome is that caused by *opioids.* This toxidrome includes coma, respiratory depression, bradycardia, hypotension, hypothermia, miosis, pulmonary edema, decreased bowel sounds, and decreased reflexes. Common causes of this syndrome, in which CNS depression is a cardinal sign, include morphine, codeine, oxycodone, hydrocodone, hydromorphone, propoxyphene, pentazocine, methadone, and meperidine. The toxidrome caused by *sedative-hypnotic drugs* and *ethanol* is similar to that for the opioids, except that sedative-hypnotic drugs generally produce miosis initially but then in later stages of coma cause mydriasis. Ethanol intoxication typically causes mydriasis. Included in this category of drugs are the benzodiazepines, barbiturates, γ-hydroxybutyrate (GHB), meprobamate, ethchlorvynol, glutethimide, methaqualone, and ethanol. Some laboratories provide a drug screen panel, variously known as a coma panel, narcotic panel, or sedative-hypnotic panel, designed to detect many drugs that produce these symptoms.

Abstinence Syndromes

Chronic use of certain drugs results in tolerance to some of their pharmacological effects and thus to accelerated doses to achieve desired responses. Abrupt discontinuance of drugs in individuals who have developed tolerance may lead to an abstinence or *withdrawal syndrome*, which tends to be opposite to the original effects produced by the drugs. For example, symptoms of sedative-hypnotic and alcohol withdrawal include dilated pupils, sweating, tachycardia, increased blood pressure, nausea, vomiting, muscle spasm, insomnia, anxiety, irritability, increased temperature, tremor, hallucinations, and seizures. With the exception of seizures and hallucinations, opioid withdrawal shares other features of alcohol or sedative-hypnotic withdrawal. Additional features characteristic of opioid withdrawal include yawning, lacrimation, rhinorrhea, piloerection, diarrhea, and muscle ache. Withdrawal from chronic cocaine use causes dysphoria, somnolence, fatigue, depression, and bradycardia.[333] Elicitation of a withdrawal response is evidence of physical drug dependence. Barbiturate or ethanol withdrawal may be so severe as to be life-threatening. Laboratory confirmation of the nature of the withdrawal syndrome may help initiate proper treatment.

Other toxic syndromes will be discussed in subsequent sections of the chapter.

SCREENING PROCEDURES FOR DETECTION OF DRUGS

Screening procedures are designed for the relatively rapid and generally qualitative detection of drugs or other toxic substances. In general, screening tests have adequate sensitivity but may not be highly specific. Thus a negative result yielded by a screening procedure rules out the presence of clinically significant concentrations of a particular analyte with reasonable certainty. Because of possible interferences, a positive result should be considered "presumptive positive" and should be confirmed by an alternate procedure of greater specificity. Screening procedures may be designed to detect a particular drug or drug class. Tests for such purposes include simple visual color tests (spot tests), determination of serum osmol gap, and immunoassays. Screening procedures capable of detecting a broad range of drugs and metabolites generally involve the use of some type of a separation technique, such as planar chromatography (TLC), GC, or HPLC.

Spot Tests

Spot tests are rapid, easily performed, noninstrumental qualitative procedures that provide presumptive evidence for the presence of tested drugs. Any positive response must be followed by testing with a more specific method. They are valuable to rule out the presence of drugs or to suggest (but not prove) the presence of a drug of a particular group. Spot tests are now less frequently employed, some largely replaced by rapid immunoassays that may be performed at the point-of-care or in the central laboratory.) Methods for the spot test detection of acetaminophen,[49,359,424] salicylate,[424,452] phenothiazines,[160] and ethchlorvynol[193] are found in the Chapter 34 Appendix that is located on this book's accompanying Evolve site, found at http://evolve.elsevier.com/Tietz/textbook/. A more extensive list of spot tests can be found in a previous edition of this textbook.[53]

Determination of Volatiles by Serum Osmol Gap

The principal osmotically active constituents of serum are Na^+, Cl^-, HCO_3^-, glucose, and urea. Several empirical formulas based on the measurement of these substances have been used to calculate the serum osmolality. One commonly used formula is[174,350]:

$$\text{mOsm/kg} = \left[1.86\,\text{Na}^+\,(\text{mmol/L}) + \frac{\text{glucose (mg/dL)}}{18}\right] + \frac{\text{urea N (mg/dL)}}{2.8} + 0.93$$

The difference between the actual osmolality, measured by freezing-point depression, and the calculated osmolality is referred to as *delta-osmolality,* or the *osmol gap.* Normally, the osmol gap is <10 mOsm/kg. Alcohols, acetone, and ethylene glycol, when present at significant concentrations, increase actual serum osmolality and would thus result in an increased osmol gap (>10 mOsm/kg). Volatile substances are not detected when osmolality is measured with a vapor pressure osmometer. Therefore for the purpose of determining the osmol gap, only osmolality measurements based on freezing-point depression are acceptable. The determination of the osmol gap is a rapid means to detect exogenous, nonionized osmolutes present at milligram-per-deciliter concentrations.

Each 100 mg/dL of ethanol in serum results in a delta-osmolality of 21.7 mOsm/kg.[349] By considering this predictable effect of ethanol on the serum osmolality, it is possible to determine what portion of an increased osmol gap is due to ethanol. A significant residual osmol gap (>10 mOsm/kg) would suggest the possible presence of isopropanol, methanol, acetone, or ethylene glycol. A nomogram that relates serum ethanol concentration and osmol gap is available to assist with this interpretation.[349] Alternatively, the contribution of ethanol to the measured osmolality can be calculated (ethanol, mg/dL ÷ 4.6) and included in the preceding formula for delta osmolality calculation; these calculations may be programmed on a calculator or minicomputer.[348] This information, in conjunction with the presence or absence of metabolic acidosis or serum acetone, can be helpful to the clinician if specific measurements of alco-

TABLE 34-3 Laboratory Findings Characteristic of Ingestion of Alcohols

Alcohol	Osmol Gap	Metabolic Acidosis With Anion Gap	Serum Acetone	Urine Oxalate
Ethanol	+	−	−	−
Methanol	+	+	−	−
Isopropanol	+	−	+	−
Ethylene glycol	+	+	−	+

hols other than ethanol and of ethylene glycol are not available on an emergency basis (Table 34-3). It must be realized that substances administered to patients such as mannitol (osmotic diuretic) and propylene glycol (solvent for diazepam and phenytoin) may increase serum osmolality. Moreover, this screening method is insensitive to low yet clinically significant concentrations of ethylene glycol (<50 mg/dL) and methanol (<30 mg/dL).[349] After ingestion of methanol, some patients may have increased osmol gaps not entirely accounted for by the presence of methanol.[266,306]

Immunoassay

Different types of immunoassay are useful methods to screen specimens for drugs (see Chapters 9 and 33). They include enzyme-multiplied immunoassay technique (EMIT), fluorescence polarization immunoassay (FPIA), cloned enzyme donor immunoassay (CEDIA), kinetic microparticle immunoassay (Abuscreen Online), and radioimmunoassay (RIA). In some cases, these assays are relatively specific for a single drug (e.g., PCP or propoxyphene), but in others, several drugs of a similar class are detected (e.g., opiates, barbiturates, β-phenylethylamines ["amphetamines"]). The detection limit for various members of a class of drugs (e.g., opiates) or the degree of cross-reactivity for similar drugs (e.g., sympathomimetic amines) varies, and each manufacturer of immunoassay reagents should be consulted for specific information. These assays are easy to perform, the results are "semi-quantitative" (higher or lower than a predetermined calibrator cut-off concentration) rather than subjective (e.g., TLC), and they generally have low detection limits (0.02 to 1.0 μg/mL). Several nonisotopic immunoassays (e.g., EMIT, CEDIA, Online, and FPIA) have been automated (see Chapter 11). A number of portable, noninstrumental immunoassay-based drug detection devices are available for nonlaboratory, point-of-care (POC) use (see section On-Site Drug Testing). Test principles for these devices include solid phase enzyme immunoassay, microparticle capture immunochromatography, latex agglutination-inhibition, or gold microparticle capture immunoassay.

For comprehensive clinical (emergency) drug screening, immunoassays complement chromatographic procedures (TLC and GC), because they detect the drugs that would require hydrolysis before chromatography (e.g., morphine-3-glucuronide and oxazepam glucuronide), that may require a separate extraction (e.g., benzoylecgonine), or that have high TLC detection limits (e.g., PCP).

For drug abuse detection, immunoassays are the methods of choice for initial screening (see later section on Drugs of Abuse).

Planar Chromatography

Planar chromatography, commonly known as thin-layer chromatography (TLC), is a versatile procedure that requires no instrumentation and thus is operationally relatively simple and inexpensive (see Chapter 6). However, its application to drug screening requires considerable experience and skill to recognize drug and metabolite patterns and the various detection color hues. With this technique, a large number of drugs may be detected; it may be applied to the analysis of serum, gastric contents, or urine. Urine, however, is the specimen of choice, because most drugs and drug metabolites are present in urine in relatively high concentrations. Although the detection limit varies for each drug and with the conditions of extraction and detection, it is generally on the order of 0.5 to 4.0 μg/mL. Procedures for drug screening using conventional TLC plates have been described.[39,49,67,72,159] Most TLC plates used for drug detection are coated with silica gel. Although these plates may be prepared in the analyst's laboratory, most find it advantageous to purchase commercial precoated plates. After extraction and specimen spotting, the TLC plates are developed with appropriate solvents to achieve chromatographic resolution. The drugs and metabolites are then visualized as spots by their fluorescence or ultraviolet absorbance and by their color development with a combination of reagent sprays or dip solutions. Identification is made by co-chromatographing reference compounds with the unknowns followed by comparison of their relative migration distances (known as R_f values) and detection characteristics with those of the unknowns.

Although some laboratories use a single TLC plate for drug screening, it is advantageous to use as many as three separate plates per urine specimen.[67,72] Different developing solvents may then be used to separate drugs more effectively in the acidic-neutral and the basic drug classes. In addition, the sequential application of multiple spray reagents to a single TLC plate results in diffusion of spots and increases the complexity of interpretation. Some commonly used drug detection reagents and their preparation are:

Ninhydrin. Reacts with drugs that contain primary or secondary amines, such as amphetamine and other sympathomimetic amines. Dissolve 100 mg ninhydrin in 100 mL of acetone. Prepare fresh reagent for each test.

Mercuric sulfate. Forms white precipitate with barbiturates, glutethimide, and phenytoin. Suspend 5 g of mercuric oxide in 100 mL of water. Add, while mixing, 20 mL of concentrated sulfuric acid. Cool and dilute to 250 mL with water. This reagent is stable indefinitely at room temperatures in a closed container.

Diphenylcarbazone. Reacts with barbiturates, glutethimide, and phenytoin to form blue or purple spots. Dissolve 10 mg of diphenylcarbazone in 50:50 chloroform: acetone. Reagent will remain stable for 1 month at room temperature when stored in a brown bottle.

Iodoplatinate. Forms various colors with tertiary amine compounds. Dissolve 1.0 g platinic chloride in about 50 mL of water. Dissolve 10 g of potassium iodide in about 200 mL of water. Add the potassium iodide solution to the platinic chloride solution and dilute to 500 mL with water. Store in a dark bottle. Solution will remain stable for 6 months.

Dragendorff's reagent. Methaqualone forms an orange color; most drugs form a brown color. Dissolve 2.2 g of bismuth subnitrate in 25 mL of glacial acetic acid and add 100 mL of water. Dissolve 50 g of potassium iodide in 125 mL of water. Combine 10 mL of each of these solutions with 20 mL of glacial acetic acid and 100 mL of water. Store in dark bottle. Reagent will remain stable for 6 months.

Absorption of ultraviolet light (254 nm). For determination of benzodiazepines, barbiturates, and methaqualone.

Fluorescence of long ultraviolet light (366 nm). For determination of benzodiazepines, quinine, and quinidine.

The TLC plates most commonly used in clinical toxicology laboratories are designed for convenient and rapid specimen application, solvent migration, and detection. The example presented here is the commercially available Toxi-Lab system manufactured by Varian (Lake Forest, Calif.). The plates are made of glass microfibers impregnated with silicic acid. Specimen application is facilitated by the rapid evaporation of the solvent in the extract in the presence of a glass fiber disk. During evaporation, the specimen is absorbed onto the disk, which is then placed in a prepunched hole on the TLC strip. Thus time-consuming specimen spotting is avoided. Moreover, disks containing reference drugs are already in place on the TLC strips.

Extraction tubes prefilled with buffer salts and solvents are provided. It is necessary only to add ~5 mL of urine and extract by mixing. Acid and neutral drugs are extracted at pH 4.5 and basic-neutral drugs at pH 9.0. Each extract is concentrated onto a specimen application disk.

The chromatographic strip for acidic-neutral drugs contains application disks that have 11 reference drugs already preabsorbed into them (Figure 34-1, *A* and Color Plate 1). After placing the disk containing the absorbed unknown specimen in the precut hole, the strip is developed in chloroform : ethyl acetate (60 : 40) that contains a trace of ammonium hydroxide. The strips are dried and then dipped into three color development solutions: diphenylcarbazone, silver nitrate, and mercuric sulfate. Barbiturates, phenytoin, glutethimide, and ethinamate appear as blue spots. When observed under long ultraviolet light (366 nm), the barbiturates absorb light (form a dark spot), whereas diazepam fluoresces. Identification is made by direct comparison of the properties of the unknown spots with those of the reference drugs.

The chromatographic strips for basic drugs contain a reference disk that has a total of 26 preabsorbed reference drugs (see Figure 34-1, *B* and Color Plate 1). The disk containing extracted and absorbed drugs from the unknown is placed on the chromatographic strip, which is then developed with methanol : water : ethyl acetate solution (2 : 1 : 58) containing a trace of ammonium hydroxide. After drying, the strip is saturated with formaldehyde vapor and then dipped into sulfuric acid. Many basic drugs form a variety of colors. Upon dipping the plate in water, the color for some drugs disappears, some drugs change color, and some drugs form a color for the first time. The plate is then viewed under long ultraviolet light (366 nm), and fluorescent spots are noted. Finally the plate is dipped into a modified Dragendorff's reagent, which produces a brown color for most drugs. The R_f values and color development or fluorescence at each of the four stages are compared for the reference drugs and the unknown(s). Important information on expected metabolite patterns for many drugs is provided by the manufacturer. The entire procedure may be completed in approximately 30 to 40 minutes.

Gas Chromatography

Also known as gas liquid chromatography, GC is relatively rapid, is capable of resolving a broad spectrum of drugs, and is widely used for qualitative and quantitative drug analysis.[150] Capillary columns, because of their high efficiency, have become the most commonly used analytical columns for drug detection by GC (see Chapter 6). In many instances, nonderivatized drugs have good GC properties when capillary columns are used; in some instances, derivatization to a less polar or more volatile compound is necessary. Common detectors for drug detection by GC are flame ionization and alkali flame ionization (nitrogen phosphorus) detectors and mass spectrometers, which provide the greatest accuracy of identification. An automated method for general drug screening by GC-MS spectrometry has been published.[367] A screening method based on GC with flame ionization detection is included in the Chapter 33 Appendix that is found on the book's accompanying Evolve site (http://evolve.elsevier.com/Tietz/textbook/).

TOXI-LAB® B WORKSHEET

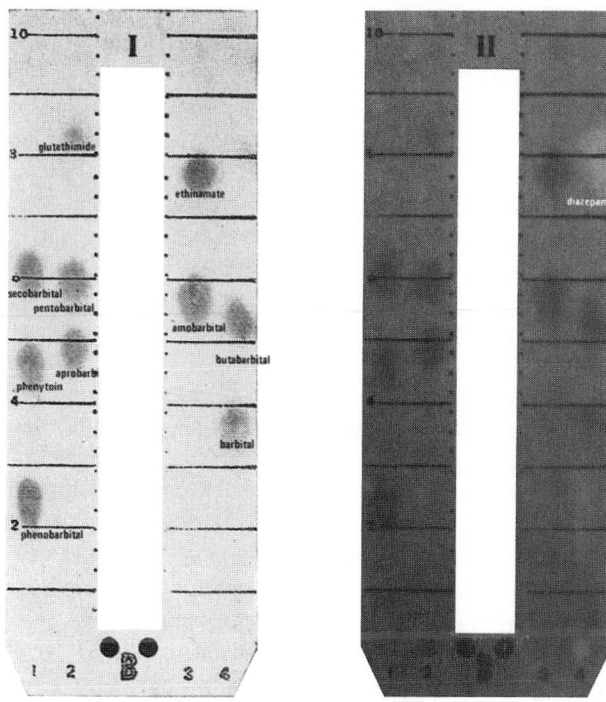

TOXI-LAB® A WORKSHEET

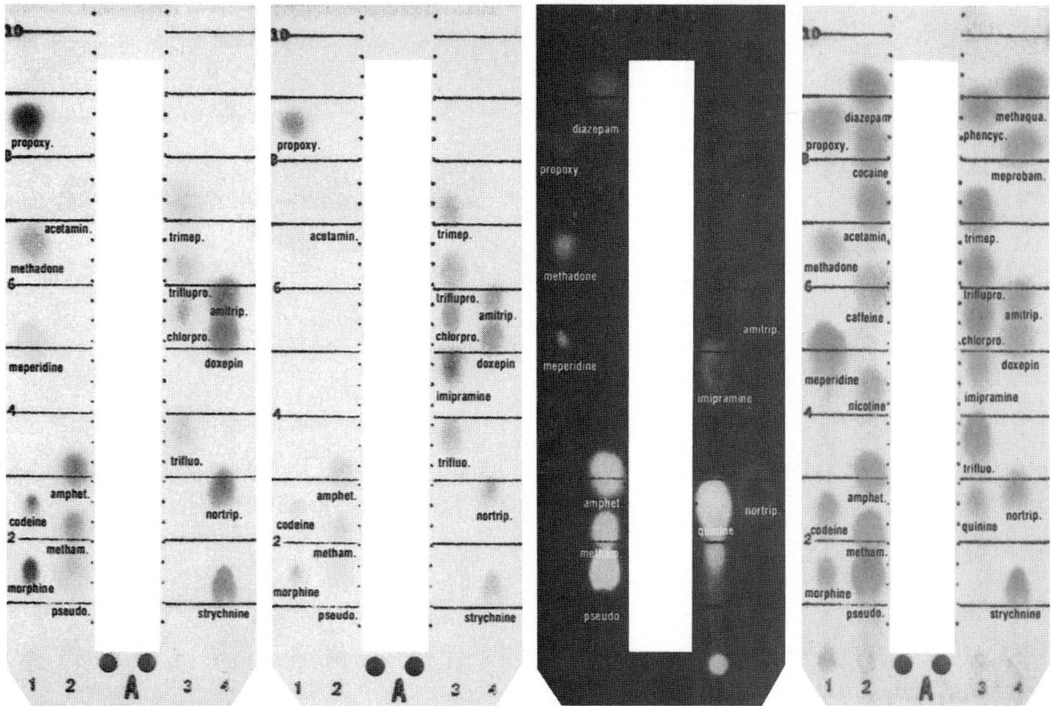

Some variation in the color and position of the drug spots is normal.

Figure 34-1 Examples of TLC plates used in drug screening: basic drugs (B Worksheet) and acidic, neutral drugs (A Worksheet). (See Color Plate 1.) *(Reproduced with permission of Toxi-Lab, Inc., Irvine, Calif.)*

HIGH-PERFORMANCE LIQUID CHROMATOGRAPHY

The resolving power of HPLC (see Chapter 6) for separating widely divergent chemical constituents has been applied to the complex challenge of comprehensive drug screening in biological fluids. Advantages of HPLC over GC include the ability to analyze polar compounds without derivatization (e.g., morphine and benzoylecgonine) and thermally labile drugs (e.g., chlordiazepoxide). In 1991 a chromatographic retention time database for drugs became available.[59] Moreover the advent of detectors that can provide a spectral scan of compounds as they elute from the column has greatly increased the discriminatory power of this technique. Screening procedures for 225 to 370 drugs have been reported that use gradient elution with reverse-phase columns and spectral scanning with diode-array detectors.[59,290,455] An isocratic, HPLC system with diode-array spectral scanning has been reported for the detection and quantitation of about 30 basic drugs and/or metabolites in serum.[377]

A commercial, completely automated HPLC system designed for drug screening is available (REMEDi; Bio-Rad Laboratories, Hercules, Calif.) and has been evaluated in a general hospital setting.[389] This system uses four columns in series and column switching techniques to extract, separate, and perform a spectral scan on eluted drugs. Identification of about 300 drugs and metabolites is based on computer matching of retention time and spectra with comparable data stored in the drug library. Quantitation of identified drugs may also be performed. This device has also been adapted to a tandem mass spectrometry for the identification of a broad spectrum of drugs in urine.[153]

Liquid chromatography-single quadruple mass spectrometry (LC-MS) has also been applied to drug screening in serum.[442,460]

PHARMACOLOGY AND ANALYSIS OF SPECIFIC DRUGS AND TOXIC AGENTS

The toxic, pharmacological, biochemical, and analytical characteristics of several individual drugs and toxins are discussed in this section.

AGENTS THAT CAUSE CELLULAR HYPOXIA

Carbon monoxide and methemoglobin-forming agents interfere with oxygen transport, resulting in cellular hypoxia. Cyanide interferes with oxygen use and therefore causes an apparent cellular hypoxia.

Carbon Monoxide

Carbon monoxide (CO) is a colorless, odorless, tasteless gas that is a product of incomplete combustion of carbonaceous material. Common exogenous sources of carbon monoxide include cigarette smoke, gasoline engines, and improperly ventilated home heating units. Small amounts of carbon monoxide are produced endogenously in the metabolic conversion of heme to biliverdin.[264] This endogenous production of carbon monoxide is accelerated in hemolytic anemias.[287]

Toxic Effects

When inhaled, carbon monoxide combines tightly with the heme Fe^{2+} of hemoglobin to form carboxyhemoglobin. The binding affinity of hemoglobin for carbon monoxide is about 250 times greater than that for oxygen. Therefore high concentrations of carboxyhemoglobin limit the oxygen content of blood. Moreover, the binding of carbon monoxide to a hemoglobin subunit increases the oxygen affinity for the remaining subunits in the hemoglobin tetramer. Thus at a given tissue PO_2 value, less oxygen dissociates from hemoglobin when carbon monoxide is also bound, shifting the hemoglobin-oxygen dissociation curve to the left. Consequently, carbon monoxide not only decreases the oxygen content of blood, but also decreases oxygen availability to tissue, thereby producing a greater degree of tissue hypoxia than would an equivalent reduction in oxyhemoglobin due to hypoxia alone.[216,446] Carbon monoxide may also bind to other heme proteins, such as myoglobin and mitochondrial cytochrome oxidase a_3; this may limit oxygen use when tissue PO_2 is very low.[171,216]

The toxic effects of carbon monoxide are a result of hypoxia. Organs with high oxygen demand, such as the heart and brain, are most sensitive to hypoxia and thus account for the major clinical sequelae of carbon monoxide poisoning. A general correlation between blood carboxyhemoglobin concentration and clinical symptoms is given in Table 34-4. It must be emphasized that the carboxyhemoglobin concen-

TABLE 34-4 Carboxyhemoglobin Effects

Carboxyhemoglobin (%)	Response
10	Shortness of breath on vigorous muscular exertion
20	Shortness of breath on moderate exertion, slight headache
30	Decided headache, irritation, ready fatigue, and disturbance of judgment
40-50	Headache, confusion, collapse, and fainting on exertion
60-70	Unconsciousness, respiratory failure, and death if exposure is continued
80	Rapidly fatal
Over 80	Immediately fatal

From Deichmann WB, Gerarde HW. Symptomatology and therapy of toxicological emergencies. New York: Academic Press Inc, 1964.

tration, although helpful in diagnosis, does not always correlate with the clinical findings or prognosis.[324,392] Factors other than carboxyhemoglobin concentration that contribute to the toxicity include length of exposure, metabolic activity, and underlying disease, especially cardiac or cerebrovascular disease. Moreover, low carboxyhemoglobin concentrations relative to the severity of poisoning may be observed if the patient was removed from the carbon monoxide–contaminated environment several hours before blood sampling.

One of the more insidious effects of carbon monoxide poisoning is the delayed development of neuropsychiatric sequelae, which may include personality changes, motor disturbances, and memory impairment. These manifestations do not correlate either with the length of exposure or the maximum blood carboxyhemoglobin concentration but are more likely if patients experienced a deep coma.[25]

Treatment for carbon monoxide poisoning involves removal of the individual from the contaminated area and the administration of oxygen. The half-life of carboxyhemoglobin is 5 to 6 hours when the patient breathes room air; it is reduced to about 1.5 hours when he or she breathes 100% oxygen. In severe cases, hyperbaric oxygen treatment at 2 to 3 atmospheres is recommended, if available. In the latter instance, the carboxyhemoglobin half-life is reduced to about 25 minutes.[446] Hyperbaric oxygen therapy may reduce the incidence of neurological manifestations after exposure.[300] Hyperbaric oxygen therapy has been recommended when the carboxyhemoglobin concentration exceeds 25%.[178] It has been suggested that decisions should not be made to institute hyperbaric oxygenation based solely on the carboxyhemoglobin concentration owing to the inconsistent correlation between such a measurement and clinical severity.[300,324] However, this therapy is recommended for any patient with loss of consciousness, significant neurological symptoms, cardiovascular complications, or severe acidosis regardless of the carboxyhemoglobin concentration.[212]

Analytical Methodology

Carbon monoxide may be released from hemoglobin and then measured by GC, or it may be determined indirectly as carboxyhemoglobin by spectrophotometry. Gas chromatographic methods are accurate and precise even for very low concentrations of carbon monoxide. The spectrophotometric methods are rapid, convenient, accurate, and precise, except at very low concentrations of carboxyhemoglobin (<2% to 3%).

Gas chromatographic methods measure the carbon monoxide content of blood. When blood is treated with potassium ferricyanide, carboxyhemoglobin is converted to methemoglobin, and the carbon monoxide is released into the gas phase. Measurement of the released carbon monoxide may be performed by GC using a molecular sieve column and a thermal conductivity detector.[124] A lower detection limit is achieved by incorporating a reducing catalyst (e.g., nickel) between the GC column and the detector to convert carbon monoxide to methane. The methane may then be detected with a flame ionization detector.[182] A very low detection limit may also be achieved by the use of a heated mercuric oxide reaction chamber between the GC column and an ultraviolet light detector. As carbon monoxide elutes from the column, it reacts with mercuric oxide to form mercury gas, which has a high molar absorptivity at 254 nm.[463] In practice, the carbon monoxide binding capacity is also determined after an aliquot of the blood specimen is treated with carbon monoxide to saturate the hemoglobin. The results are then expressed as percent of carboxyhemoglobin:

$$\% \text{ HbCO} = \frac{\text{CO content}}{\text{CO capacity}} \times 100$$

GC methods are accurate and precise and are considered to be reference procedures. Normal values for carboxyhemoglobin in rural nonsmokers are about 0.5%; for urban nonsmokers, 1% to 2%; and for smokers, 5% to 6%.[27] Values may be increased by about 3% in hemolytic anemias.[287]

Spectrophotometric methods rely on the characteristic spectral absorption properties of carboxyhemoglobin.[501] Of several such methods, the most popular are based on automated, multiwavelength measurements of several hemoglobin species. Commercially available instruments (Instrumentation Laboratories' Co-Oximeter [Lexington, Mass.], Radiometer's OSM 3 Hemoximeter [Copenhagen, Denmark], Bayer Diagnostics Co-Oximeter [Tarrytown, N.Y.], and Roche Diagnostic's AVL Co-Oxylite [Indianapolis]) perform absorption measurements on blood specimens at 4 to 7 wavelengths and then compute the concentration of deoxyhemoglobin, oxyhemoglobin, carboxyhemoglobin, and methemoglobin based on a series of matrix coefficients. A more advanced optical system is based on a 128-wavelength spectrometer (ABL 700; Radiometer, Copenhagen, Denmark).

The spectrophotometric methods generally compare favorably with gas chromatographic procedures at carboxyhemoglobin concentrations greater than 2% to 3%, but their precision is poor below these levels.[463] Therefore, they are sufficiently accurate and precise for measurement of carbon monoxide after exogenous exposure but are too insensitive to detect the increased endogenous production of carbon monoxide that occurs in hemolytic anemias.

Fetal hemoglobin has slightly different spectral properties than adult hemoglobin. Consequently, falsely high carboxyhemoglobin values of 4% to 7% may occur when blood from neonates is measured by some spectrophotometric methods.[464] Moreover, erroneous results may occur with lipemic specimens and in the presence of methylene blue (see section on Methemoglobin-Forming Agents). These interferences are eliminated or greatly minimized by Radiometer's ABL 700.

The automated, multicomponent spectrophotometric methods for the determination of carboxyhemoglobin and other hemoglobin species are the most rapid and convenient. A spectrophotometric procedure for carboxyhemoglobin[444] applicable to manual spectrophotometers is included in the the Chapter 34 Appendix that is found on the book's accompanying Evolve site (http://evolve.elsevier.com/Tietz/textbook/). This procedure provides results that are in agreement with those of a gas chromatographic[334] and of an automated, multiwavelength spectrophotometric method.[202]

Cyanide

Hydrocyanic acid, often referred to as *prussic acid* or as *cyanide* when in the ionized state (CN^-), is a colorless, odorless gas released when anything containing ionically bound or complexed CN^- is exposed to acid. Burning of urea foam produces formaldehyde and hydrocyanic acid; fires in homes with urea foam insulation represent a significant source of exposure.

Toxic Effects

When inhaled, hydrocyanic acid is rapidly absorbed across alveolar capillaries into blood where it binds to hemoglobin. The hydrocyanic acid bound in the erythrocyte is in equilibrium with free hydrocyanic acid in the serum at a ratio of 10:1. Cyanide in serum readily crosses all biological membranes and avidly binds to heme iron (Fe^{3+}) in the cytochrome a-a_3 complex within mitochondria.[398,462] When bound to cytochrome a-a_3, CN^- is a competitive inhibitor and causes uncoupling of oxidative phosphorylation. Patients exposed to toxic levels of cyanide exhibit rapid onset of symptoms typical of cellular hypoxia—flushing, headache, tachypnea, dizziness, and respiratory depression—which progress rapidly to coma, seizure, complete heart block, and death if the dose is sufficiently large. Symptoms are usually dose related and correlate strongly with CN^- concentration.[9] Treatment requires rapid identification of CN^- as the intoxicant followed by administration of sodium nitrite to cause formation of methemoglobin, which avidly binds and clears CN^-, and thiosulfate (a sulfur donor) to enhance clearance via metabolism.

Cyanide is metabolized by the ubiquitous enzyme rhodanase to thiocyanate (SCN^-), drawing on the body's sulfur-donor pool for substrate to convert CN^- to SCN^-. Thiocyanate is relatively inert and is cleared by the kidney. The conversion of CN^- to SCN^- occurs slowly relative to the pharmacological action of CN^-, so measurement of SCN^- is of use in monitoring clearance but not very useful in assessing acute CN^- exposure. In an acute exposure, the patient experiences symptoms of toxicity with high blood CN^- levels, but the serum SCN^- level remains low until 12 to 24 hours later.[9,312]

Administration of nitroprusside to control acute hypertension contributes to the total body pool of CN^- and complicates the interpretation of the blood CN^- concentration. Nitroprusside ($Fe[CN]_5NO$) avidly binds to hemoglobin in erythrocytes; at equilibrium, the amount of CN^- that is bound in the erythrocyte owing to nitroprusside as compared with that of the serum is 200:1, approximately 20 times that found in the erythrocyte if the exposure were due to ionic CN^-. These patients do not exhibit CN^- toxicity unless they are unable to clear the drug. Measurement of SCN^- is the recommended procedure to monitor nitroprusside therapy, because measurement of blood CN^- will be confounded by all the nitroprusside in the erythrocyte.

The normal CN^- concentration is less than 0.2 μg/mL of whole blood because of the presence of CN^- in foods such as dark green vegetables and nuts that contain cyanogenic glycosides (e.g., amygdalin), and the use of tobacco products that contain CN^-. Normal SCN^- concentration in serum is less than 4 μg/mL, but smokers may have serum SCN^- levels as high as 10 μg/mL. Patients with acute exposure are likely to have high blood CN^- levels and low serum SCN^- concentrations. The patient likely becomes comatose when blood CN^- level is greater than 2 μg/mL, and levels greater than 5 μg/mL are lethal. Patients receiving nitroprusside therapy, however, may have blood CN^- concentrations as high as 50 to 100 μg/mL without symptoms of toxicity.[12]

Analytical Methodology

Following microdiffusion, whole blood CN^- is measured by photometric analysis[10,112] or by ion-selective electrode analysis.

A spectrophotometric procedure for measuring cyanide is included in the Chapter 34 Appendix that is found on this book's accompanying Evolve site (http://evolve.elsevier.com/Tietz/textbook/).[10] In this method, a sealed, two-well microdiffusion cell is used to separate hydrocyanic acid from blood by mixing a sample of whole blood with strong acid in a sealed chamber and allowing the hydrocyanic acid gas generated to be absorbed into a strong base located in another part of the sealed chamber. One well of the cell contains the blood specimen and strong acid (unmixed until the cell is sealed), and the other well contains a strong base to absorb the hydrocyanic acid gas. After the hydrocyanic acid is collected in the aqueous base medium, pyridine, barbituric acid, and chloramine-T are added to generate a red complex, with the intensity of the color proportional to the concentration of CN^-. A good-quality spectrophotometer is required to measure the absorbance. Quick and easy methods for serum SCN^- analysis have been described.[461]

Methemoglobin-Forming Agents

The heme iron in hemoglobin is normally in the ferrous state (Fe^{2+}). When oxidized to the ferric state (Fe^{3+}), methemoglobin is formed, and this form of hemoglobin cannot bind oxygen. The principal physiological system to maintain hemoglobin iron in the reduced state is NADH-methemoglobin reductase (diaphorase I) (Figure 34-2). The NADH for this enzyme is supplied by normal glycolysis (Embden-Meyerhof pathway). A minor pathway for methemoglobin reduction involves NADPH-methemoglobin reductase (diaphorase II), and the NADP for this enzyme reaction is derived from the hexose-monophosphate shunt. Congenital

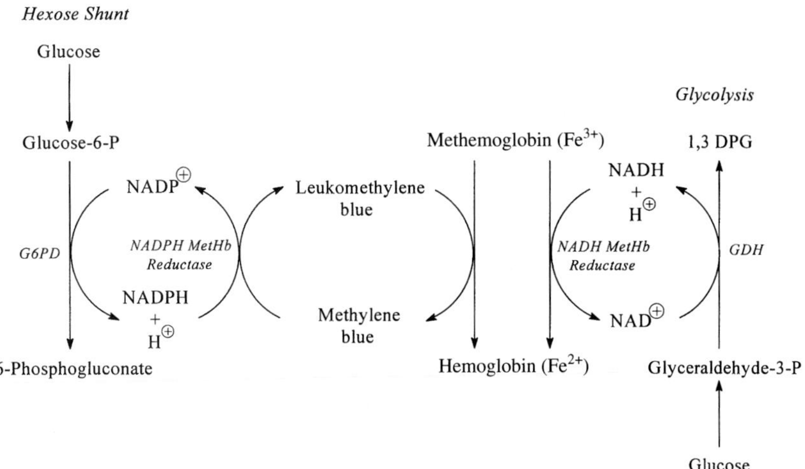

Figure 34-2 Enzymatic pathways for methemoglobin reduction.

TABLE 34-5 Acquired Causes of Methemoglobinemia

Drugs	Chemical Agents
Amyl nitrite	Aniline
Benzocaine	Aniline dyes
Chloroquine	Butyl nitrite
Dapsone	Chlorobenzene
Lidocaine	Naphthalene
Nitroglycerin	Nitrates
Phenacetin	Nitrites
Phenazopyridine	Nitrophenol
Primaquine	Nitrous oxide
Sulfonamides	

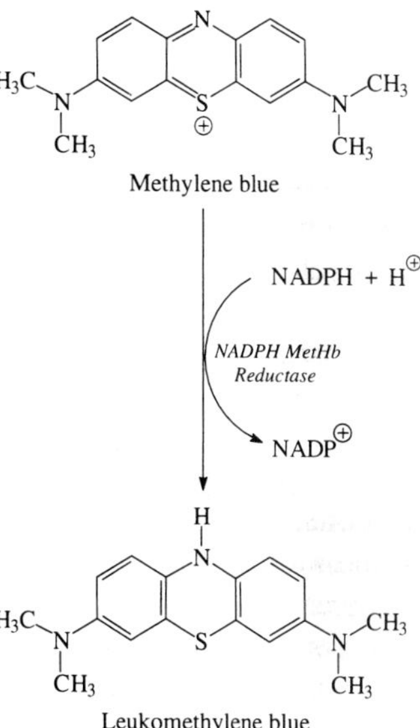

Figure 34-3 Participation of methylene blue as an electron acceptor in the NADPH-dependent methemoglobin reductase reaction.

methemoglobinemia may result from a deficiency of NADH–methemoglobin reductase or more rarely from hemoglobin variants (hemoglobin M) in which heme iron is both more susceptible to oxidation and more resistant to reduction by the methemoglobin reductase system.

Toxic Effects

An acquired (toxic) methemoglobinemia may be caused by a number of drugs and chemicals (Table 34-5).

The normal concentration of methemoglobin is <1.5% of total hemoglobin. In otherwise healthy individuals, methemoglobin levels up to 20% cause only cyanosis. Concentrations between 20% and 50% may cause dyspnea, exercise intolerance, fatigue, weakness, and syncope. More severe symptoms of dysrhythmias, seizures, metabolic acidosis, and coma are associated with methemoglobin concentrations of 50% to 70%, and levels >70% may be lethal.[376] All of these symptoms are a consequence of hypoxia associated with the diminished O_2 content of the blood and with a decreased O_2 dissociation from hemoglobin species in which some, but not all, subunits contain heme iron in the ferric state (i.e., shift of dissociation curve to the left). The PO_2 is normal in these patients and therefore so is the calculated hemoglobin oxygen saturation. Thus, a normal PO_2 in a cyanotic patient is a significant indication for the possible presence of methemoglobinemia. The direct measurement of methemoglobin is important in these cases and may be performed by the manual spectrophotometric method of Evelyn and Malloy or by automated multiwavelength measurements with a co-oximeter (see section on Carbon Monoxide).

Specific therapy for toxic methemoglobinemia involves the administration of methylene blue, which acts as an electron transfer agent in the NADPH–methemoglobin reductase reaction and thereby increases the activity of this system several fold (Figure 34-3).[376] Methylene blue and sulfhemoglobin cause spectral interference in the measurement of methemoglobin with some co-oximeters[240,499] but not with the Evelyn-Malloy method.[240]

Analytical Methodology

Methemoglobin is measured manually[240] or by automated multiwavelength measurements with a co-oximeter. As methemoglobin is not stable at room temperature, specimens should be kept on ice or refrigerated but not frozen.[240] The stability of methemoglobin at 4 °C has not been well studied. Some sources indicate significant decreases in methemoglobin concentrations after 4 to 8 hours,[269] whereas others report little or no change after 24 hours.[240] Freezing results in an increase in methemoglobin concentration.[240]

ALCOHOLS

Several alcohols are toxic and medically important. They include ethanol, methanol, and isopropanol.

Alcohols of Toxicological Interest

Ethanol is a widely used and often abused chemical substance. Consequently the measurement of ethanol is one of the more frequently performed tests in the toxicology laboratory. Although less frequently encountered, it is important to include methanol, isopropanol, and acetone (a metabolite of isopropanol) in a test battery for alcohols for proper evaluation of the acutely intoxicated patient.

Ethanol

The principal pharmacological action of ethanol is CNS depression. The CNS effects vary, depending on the blood ethanol concentration, from euphoria and decreased inhibitions (≤50 mg/dL) to increased disorientation and incoordination (100 to 300 mg/dL) and then to coma and death (>400 mg/dL) (Table 34-6). A blood alcohol concentration of 100 mg/dL was previously established as the statutory limit for operation of a motor vehicle in most states in the United States. A new federal mandate requires that this limit be lowered to 80 mg/dL by 2004. Not all individuals experience the same degree of CNS dysfunction at similar blood alcohol levels. Moreover, the CNS actions of ethanol are more pronounced when the blood ethanol concentration is increasing (absorptive phase) than when it is declining (elimination phase), partly because of the phenomenon of acute tolerance.[176] In addition, heavy alcohol use leads to a more chronic form of tolerance. When consumed with other CNS depressant drugs, ethanol exerts a potentiation or synergistic depressant effect. This can occur at relatively low alcohol concentrations, and a number of deaths have resulted from combined ethanol and drug ingestion.[168]

The pharmacological mechanisms for the CNS depressant actions of ethanol are complex and incompletely understood, but probably involve both enhancement of major inhibitory neurons and impairment of excitatory neurons. The principal CNS inhibitory neuronal system is mediated by the neurotransmitter γ-aminobutyric acid (GABA). When GABA binds to its postsynaptic receptor subtype $GABA_A$, this oligomeric ion-gated complex "opens" to allow inward flux of Cl^-, leading to membrane hyperpolarization and subsequent decreased electrical response. This GABA-mediated inhibitory response is enhanced by ethanol and other CNS depressant drugs, such as barbiturates, benzodiazepines, and most general anesthetic agents. A major CNS excitatory response is mediated by the neurotransmitter glutamate. Ethanol inhibits the excitatory response mediated by a Ca^{2+} ion-gated glutamate receptor subtype termed the *N*-methyl-D-aspartate (NMDA) receptor. Additionally, central adrenergic stimulation may be indirectly inhibited by ethanol via its enhancement of the activity of phenylethanolamine-*N*-methyltransferase (PNMT), the enzyme responsible for the extraneuronal conversion of norepinephrine to epinephrine. Epinephrine in turn activates presynaptic α_2-receptors, which inhibit the release of norepinephrine. The aforementioned chronic tolerance to ethanol is considered to be mediated by ethanol-induced increased responsiveness and upregulation in the synthesis of NMDA receptors, by a concomitant downregulation and desensitization of $GABA_A$ receptors, and by downregulation of the presynatic α_2-adrenergic receptors. Largely because of these adaptive changes, abrupt withdrawal from chronic, heavy ethanol use leads to a physical abstinence syndrome, which has prominent features of CNS excitation. Included among these withdrawal symptoms are anxiety, irritability, insomnia, muscle tremor and cramps, seizures, hallucinations, and increased temperature, blood pressure, and heart rate.

Ethanol is metabolized principally by liver alcohol dehydrogenase to acetaldehyde, which is subsequently oxidized to acetic acid by aldehyde dehydrogenase. The rate of elimination of ethanol from blood generally approximates a zero-order process. Although this rate varies among individuals, it averages about 15 mg/dL/h (ranging from 11 to 22 mg/dL/h) for males and 18 mg/dL/h (ranging from 11 to 22 mg/dL/h) for females.[125] At both low (<20 mg/dL)[465] and high (>300 mg/dL) ethanol concentrations, the elimination becomes more nearly first-order and is accelerated at high concentrations (e.g., ~22 mg/dL/h at ~300 mg/dL).[58] The elimination rate is also influenced by drinking practice (e.g., alcoholics have average elimination rates of about 30 mg/dL/h).[480]

Ethanol is a teratogen, and alcohol consumption during pregnancy can result in the baby being born with fetal alcohol spectrum disorders (FASD). FASD is an umbrella term describing the range of effects that can occur in an individual whose mother drank alcohol during pregnancy (http://www.nofas.org). These effects may include physical, mental, behavioral, and/or learning disabilities with possible lifelong implications. The term FASD is not intended for use as a clinical diagnosis. Other alcohol-related conditions include alcohol-related neurodevelopmental disorder (ARND) and alcohol-related birth defects (ARBD). As many as 12,000 infants are born each year with FAS, and three times as many have ARND or ARBD. FAS, ARND, and ARBD affect more newborns every year than Down syndrome, cystic fibrosis, spina bifida, and sudden infant death syndrome combined (http://www.nofas.org). FAS, ARND,

TABLE 34-6 Stages of Acute Alcoholic Influence/Intoxication

Blood Alcohol Concentration (g/100 mL)	Stage of Alcoholic Influence	Clinical Signs/Symptoms
0.01-0.05	Subclinical	Influence/effects not apparent or obvious Behavior nearly normal by ordinary observation Impairment detectable by special tests
0.03-0.12	Euphoria	Mild euphoria, sociability, talkativeness Increased self-confidence; decreased inhibitions Diminution of attention, judgment, and control Some sensory-motor impairment Slowed information processing Loss of efficiency in finer performance tests
0.09-0.25	Excitement	Emotional instability; loss of critical judgment Impairment of perception, memory, and comprehension Decreased sensory response; increased reaction time Reduced visual acuity, peripheral vision, and glare recovery Sensory-motor incoordination; impaired balance Drowsiness
0.18-0.30	Confusion	Disorientation, mental confusion; dizziness Exaggerated emotional states (fear, rage, grief, etc.) Disturbances of vision (diplopia, etc.) and of perception of color, form, motion, dimensions Increased pain threshold Increased muscular incoordination; staggering gait; slurred speech Apathy, lethargy
0.25-0.40	Stupor	General inertia; approaching loss of motor functions Markedly decreased response to stimuli Marked muscular incoordination; inability to stand or walk Vomiting; incontinence of urine and feces Impaired consciousness; sleep or stupor
0.35-0.50	Coma	Complete unconsciousness; coma; anesthesia Depressed or abolished reflexes Subnormal temperature Impairment of circulation and respiration Possible death
0.45+	Death	Death from respiratory arrest

Reprinted with permission of KM Dubowski, 1997.

and ARBD are 100% preventable when a woman completely abstains from alcohol during her pregnancy.

Methanol

Methanol is used as a solvent in a number of commercial products, as a constituent of antifreeze and window cleaning fluids, and as a component of canned fuel. It may be consumed by alcoholics intentionally as an ethanol substitute or accidentally when present as a contaminant in illegal whiskey. Accidental ingestions have occurred in children.

The CNS effects of methanol are substantially less severe than those of ethanol. Methanol is oxidized by liver alcohol dehydrogenase (at about one tenth the rate of ethanol) to formaldehyde. Formaldehyde in turn is rapidly oxidized by aldehyde dehydrogenase to formic acid, which may cause serious acidosis and optic neuropathy, resulting in blindness or death.[296,298] Serum formate concentrations correlate better with the degree of acidosis and the severity of CNS and ocular toxicity than do serum methanol concentrations.[410] Therefore some investigators recommend the measurement of serum formate to assess the severity of toxicity and to guide appropriate therapy in cases of methanol ingestion. Treatment for methanol intoxication may include the administration of ethanol or preferably fomepizole to inhibit the metabolism of methanol, sodium bicarbonate therapy to help alleviate the metabolic acidosis, folate administration to enhance folate-mediated metabolism of formate, and the use of hemodialysis to enhance clearance of methanol and formate.[22]

Headspace gas chromatographic analysis is the method of choice for the measurement of methanol. An adaptation of this technique may be used to measure formate, the toxic metabolite of methanol, after esterification to methyl formate. These methods are included in the Chapter 34 Appendix that is found on the book's accompanying Evolve site (http://evolve.elsevier.com/Tietz/textbook/). An enzymatic assay based on formate dehydrogenase has also been reported.[54]

Isopropanol

Isopropanol is readily available to the general population as a 70% aqueous solution for use as rubbing alcohol. It has about twice the CNS depressant action as ethanol, but it is not as toxic as methanol.

Isopropanol has a short half-life ($t_{1/2}$) of 1 to 6 hours, as it is rapidly metabolized by alcohol dehydrogenase to acetone, which is eliminated much more slowly ($t_{1/2}$, 17 to 27 hours), primarily in alveolar air and urine.[115,228,313,326] Therefore concentrations of acetone in serum often exceed those of isopropanol during the elimination phase following isopropanol ingestion (Figure 34-4). Acetone has CNS depressant activity similar to that of ethanol, and because of its longer half-life, it prolongs the apparent CNS effects of isopropanol.

Severe isopropanol intoxication, like that of ethanol, can result in coma or death. Appropriate therapy in such cases includes hemodialysis. The therapeutic administration of ethanol is not indicated for isopropanol intoxication.

Isopropanol and its metabolite, acetone, may be determined by headspace gas chromatography or by NMR spectroscopy.[313] A headspace gas chromatographic method is included in the Chapter 34 Appendix that is found on the book's accompanying Evolve site (http://evolve.elsevier.com/Tietz/textbook/).

Analysis of Alcohols*

Similar techniques are used to measure alcohol in blood, serum, saliva, or urine and for postmortem specimens (e.g. vitreous fluid and skeletal muscle). Determination of ethanol in expired air requires specialized breath alcohol analyzers (see section on Breath Alcohol).

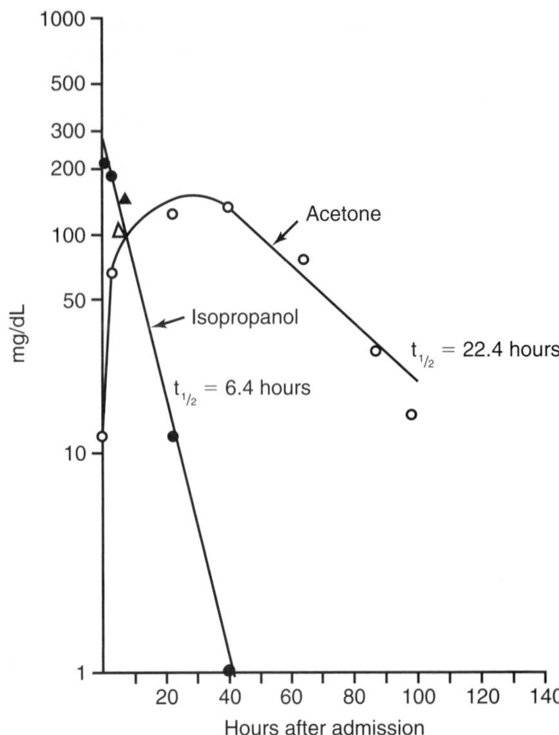

Figure 34-4 Isopropanol and acetone concentrations in serum after an acute overdose of isopropanol. Closed and open circles indicate serum isopropanol and acetone concentrations, respectively. Isopropanol and acetone concentrations in spinal fluid are indicated by closed and open triangles, respectively. *(From Natowicz M, Donahue J, Gorman L, Kane M, McKissick J, Shaw L. Pharmacokinetic analysis of a case report of isopropanol intoxication. Clin Chem 1985; 31:326-8.)*

Blood Alcohol

Suitable blood-related specimens for the determination of alcohols are serum, plasma, or whole blood. The venipuncture site should be cleansed with an alcohol-free disinfectant, such as aqueous benzalkonium chloride (Zephiran).

Alcohol distributes into the aqueous compartments of blood, and because the water content of serum (~98%) is greater than that of whole blood (~86%), results indicating higher alcohol levels are obtained with serum. Experimentally the serum:whole blood ethanol ratio is 1.14 (1.09 to 1.18) and varies slightly with hematocrit.[479] Several states have enacted laws that define intoxication while driving a motor vehicle under the influence of alcohol based on whole blood ethanol concentrations. Some states do not specify the specimen type. Therefore laboratories that perform alcohol determinations should make clear the choice of specimen.

Because of the volatile nature of alcohols, specimens must be kept capped to avoid evaporative loss to the atmosphere. Blood may be stored, when properly sealed, for 14 days at room temperature or at 4 °C, with or without preservative.[481] For longer storage or for nonsterile postmortem specimens,

*In this section, the term "alcohol" is defined as ethanol unless otherwise indicated.

sodium fluoride should be used as a preservative to prevent a decrease or occasionally an increase (via fermentation) in ethanol concentration.

To measure ethanol in blood, enzymatic analysis is the method of choice for many laboratories. In this method, ethanol is measured by oxidation to acetaldehyde with NAD^+, a reaction catalyzed by alcohol dehydrogenase (ADH). With this reaction, formation of NADH, measured at 340 nm, is proportional to the amount of ethanol in the specimen. The reaction is driven almost completely to the right by use of excess NAD^+ and ADH and agents such as semicarbazide or tris (hydroxymethyl) aminomethane to trap acetaldehyde as it is formed.[165]

Under most assay conditions, ADH is reasonably specific for ethanol. Interference, relative to ethanol, is generally about 7% for isopropanol, 3% for methanol, and 4% for ethylene glycol.[165] Reagent kits for use with manual spectrophotometers or automated analyzers are available from several manufacturers. Some manufacturers (Dade-Behring [*aca*], Abbott [TDx], Dade-Behring [EMIT]) claim interference from isopropanol, methanol, acetone, and ethylene glycol to be less than 1%.

Serum (or plasma) is the most common specimen for ethanol analysis by ADH methods; the method also performs well with urine or saliva. In some methods, whole blood may be used directly,[77] but in others, a precipitation step may be required before analysis to avoid interference from hemoglobin.[166] These methods generally compare closely with gas chromatographic methods.[77,176]

Ethanol assays using ADH, especially those that are fully automated, are convenient for clinical laboratories that do not have gas chromatographic instrumentation. The specificity for ethanol must be clearly communicated to physicians treating acutely intoxicated patients. Otherwise, very low or negative ethanol values might be misinterpreted as "alcohol" in a patient who ingested methanol or isopropanol. Ethanol measurements may be used in conjunction with the osmol gap to screen for possible presence of significant quantities of methanol, isopropanol, or ethylene glycol (see Determination of Volatiles by Serum Osmol Gap). A head space gas chromatographic method for alcohols (acetone) is included in the Chapter 34 Appendix that is found on the book's Evolve site (http://evolve.elsevier.com/Tietz/textbook/).

Breath Alcohol

Statutory laws for driving under the influence of alcohol were originally based on the concentration of ethanol in venous whole blood. Because the collection of blood is invasive and requires intervention by medical personnel, the determination of alcohol in expired air has long been the mainstay of evidential alcohol measurements.[188,229,299] There is also growing clinical interest in the determination of breath alcohol at the point-of-care. The fundamental principle for use of breath analysis is that alcohol in capillary alveolar blood rapidly equilibrates with alveolar air in a ratio of approximately 2100:1 (blood:breath). Therefore breath alcohol expressed as g/210 L is approximately equivalent to g/dL of alcohol in whole blood. This blood-breath ratio may actually be closer to 2300:1 but in any case is variable. Nevertheless, in the United States evidential breath alcohol measurements are based on the ratio of 2100:1. The lower blood-breath ratio will predict a slightly lower than actual blood alcohol concentration and its use therefore is not prejudicial. To alleviate the confusion and uncertainty surrounding the conversion from breath to blood alcohol concentration, the traffic laws in the United States have been amended to read "alcohol concentration shall mean either grams of alcohol per 100 milliliters of blood or grams per 210 liters of breath."[299] Before breath analysis, a waiting period of 15 minutes is required to allow for clearance of any residual alcohol that may have been present in the mouth (e.g., very recent drinking, the use of alcohol-containing mouthwash, or vomiting alcohol-rich gastric fluid).

During the period of active alcohol absorption (30 to 120 minutes before peak venous blood alcohol concentration), the alcohol concentration in arterial blood may be higher than that in peripheral venous blood.[75] Consequently, breath alcohol concentration may also be higher than that in venous blood during this absorption phase, because end-expiratory air equilibrates with pulmonary arterial blood. The potential consequences of performing breath alcohol analysis during the absorption phase have been the subject of considerable debate.[227,230]

In the interest of public safety, the U.S. Department of Transportation (DOT) has mandated breath alcohol testing in addition to screening for drugs of abuse in urine (see section on Drugs of Abuse) for commercial transportation employees.[450,451] If the breath alcohol concentration is between 0.02 and 0.04 g/210 L for duplicate measurements (within 30 minutes), an employee is not allowed to resume safety-sensitive duties for 8 hours (24 hours for motor vehicle drivers). If the concentration is 0.04 g/210 L or greater, the employee is suspended from duty until evaluation by substance abuse professionals has been obtained and appropriate follow-up testing has been initiated.

Several commercial evidential breath alcohol measurement devices are available. The principle of measurement is either infrared absorption spectrometry (most common), dichromate-sulfuric acid oxidation-reduction (photometric), GC (flame ionization or thermal conductivity detection), electrochemical oxidation (fuel cell), or metal-oxide semiconductor sensors.[188,229] A list has been published of DOT-approved breath alcohol devices.[123,451] Some of these devices are approved for screening only. In this case, the second or "confirmatory" breath alcohol determination must be performed with an approved evidential breath alcohol analyzer. Breath alcohol devices may also be used for the medical evaluation of patients at the point of care (e.g., emergency department). A Fourier transform infrared point-of-care breath analyzer capable of measurement of ethanol, methanol, and isopropanol performed well in the evaluation and management of patients with methanol poisoning.[260]

Saliva Alcohol

Because saliva (increasingly referred to as oral fluid) may be easily and noninvasively collected, there is growing interest in its use for ethanol measurements and for the detection of drugs of abuse (see Drugs of Abuse). Ethanol distributes between blood and saliva by passive diffusion largely according to the water content of these fluids (85% w/v for whole blood; 99% for saliva).[233] Experimentally the ethanol concentration in saliva is about 9% higher than in whole blood,[233] a value slightly lower than predicted based on their respective water content; the ethanol concentration in serum and saliva would be predicted to be about the same based on their similar water content. The concentration time profiles for ethanol in blood, breath, and saliva are all similar.[232,233]

A small test device, Q.E.D. Saliva Alcohol Test (OraSure Technologies, Bethlehem, Pa.), has been developed to measure ethanol in saliva. Saliva is absorbed onto a swab, which is then inserted into the test cartridge. Ethanol measurement is based on an ADH reaction coupled with a diaphorase-mediated color indicator reaction, which provides for visual end-point detection on a thermometer-like scale after a 2-minute incubation.

This device was evaluated and determined to provide results in agreement with those for breath or venous blood ethanol.[232] The Q.E.D. is suited for on-site use in the emergency department, in the workplace, and potentially at the roadside. It is approved by the DOT for alcohol screening.[449] Although designed for measurement of alcohol in saliva, the Q.E.D. provides accurate measurements for serum ethanol as well.[117]

The ON-SITE alcohol test card device (Roche Diagnostic Systems, Branchburg, N.J.), for the qualitative measurement of ethanol in saliva or urine is also based on an ADH-diaphorase coupled detection scheme. This test card is designed to produce a positive response for ethanol concentrations greater than 0.02 g/dL. This device is also approved by the DOT for screening.[449]

A third DOT-approved device (Alco-Screen 02, Chematics, Inc., North Webster, Ind.) consists of a plastic test strip suitable for insertion under the subject's tongue or into collected saliva. After saturation of the reaction pad with saliva and a 2-minute incubation period, an ADH-diaphorase coupled indicator color bar becomes visible if the ethanol concentration is 0.02 g/dL or greater.

The flow of saliva is largely under the control of the parasympathetic nervous system. Collection of saliva may therefore be difficult from individuals who experience anticholinergic symptomatology (e.g., dry mouth associated with tricyclic antidepressant overdose). In addition, salivary flow may be impaired in some alcoholics.[129]

Urine Alcohol

Urine has been used as an alternate, less invasive specimen for the determination of alcohol, compared with blood. During the postabsorptive phase following alcohol ingestion, the concentration of alcohol in urine is roughly 1.3 times of that in blood.[75] Calculations of blood alcohol concentration from that determined in urine based on this average urine-blood alcohol ratio are admissible in some jurisdictions. However, the use of urine alcohol measurements for this purpose is discouraged by some authors, because the ratio of 1.3 is highly variable, and the urine alcohol concentration represents an average of the blood alcohol concentration during the time period in which urine collected in the bladder. A better correlation of urine with blood alcohol concentration is obtained by first emptying the bladder and then collecting urine after 20 to 30 minutes.

There is renewed interest in urine alcohol testing in conjunction with testing urine for drugs of abuse (see Drugs of Abuse). For this purpose, the detection of alcohol in urine represents ingestion of alcohol within the previous ~8 hours. Urine is not an approved specimen for alcohol measurement by the DOT.

Postmortem Alcohol

Alcohol is measured in postmortem blood and vitreous humor. Muscle has been proposed as a useful alternative specimen to postmortem blood.[167]

ANALGESICS (NONPRESCRIPTION)

Analgesics are substances that relieve pain without causing loss of consciousness. When used in excess, analgesics such as acetaminophen and salicylate can result in a toxic response.

Acetaminophen

Acetaminophen has analgesic and antipyretic actions. In common with the group of drugs referred to as nonsteroidal antiinflammatory drugs (NSAIDs: e.g., aspirin, ibuprofen, and indomethacin), acetaminophen's pharmacological actions are related to its competitive inhibition of cyclooxygenase enzymes, resulting in decreased production of prostaglandins, which are important mediators of inflammation, pain (low-to-moderate), and fever.[382] Contrary to other NSAIDs, acetaminophen has very weak antiinflammatory activity, a consequence of its weak inhibition of peripheral tissue cyclooxygenase compared with that in the brain. In normal dose, acetaminophen is safe and effective, but it may cause severe hepatic toxicity or death when consumed in overdose quantities. Less frequently, nephrotoxicity may also occur. The initial clinical findings in acetaminophen toxicity are relatively mild and nonspecific (nausea, vomiting, and abdominal discomfort) and thus are not predictive of impending hepatic necrosis, which typically begins 24 to 36

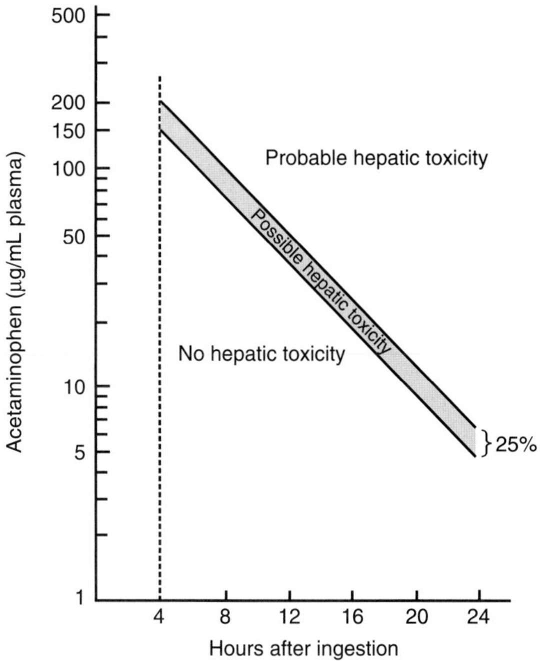

Figure 34-5 Rumack-Matthew nomogram. *(From Rumack BH, Matthew H. Acetaminophen poisoning and toxicity. Pediatrics 1975;55:871-6. Reproduced by permission of Pediatrics.)*

hours after a toxic ingestion and becomes most severe by 72 to 96 hours.[360] Although uncommon with severe overdose, coma and metabolic acidosis may occur before development of hepatic necrosis.[154] Antidotal therapy with *N*-acetylcysteine (NAC; Mucomyst) (see below) is most effective when administered well before hepatic injury occurs as signified by elevations of AST and ALT. Thus the measurement of serum acetaminophen concentration becomes paramount for proper assessment of the severity of overdose and for making appropriate decisions for antidotal therapy. A useful nomogram is available that relates serum acetaminophen concentration and time following acute ingestion to the probability of hepatic necrosis (Figure 34-5).[386]

There are several qualifications concerning the use of this nomogram. First, blood samples should not be obtained earlier than 4 hours after ingestion to ensure that absorption is complete. Second, the nomogram applies only to acute and not chronic ingestions. Toxicity from chronic ingestion of acetaminophen or other drugs is cumulative and typically occurs at lower blood concentrations than in acute overdose. Third, the nomogram is not useful if the time of ingestion is unknown (within ± 2 hours) or is considered unreliable. In this case, two or more samples taken at 2- to 3-hour intervals may be used to estimate the acetaminophen elimination half-life. Hepatotoxicity is more probable when the acetaminophen half-life is greater than 4 hours, and hepatic coma is likely when the half-life is greater than 12 hours. Some,[373] but not all,[413] investigators believe the half-life to be a better predictor of hepatotoxicity than interpretation based on a single serum concentration. Fourth, serial determination of serum levels (e.g., every 2 hours) is warranted if extended-release medication has been ingested (Tylenol Extended Relief), because the time to reach peak serum concentration may be delayed beyond 4 hours.[180,438] Serial serum levels are also required when there has been co-ingestion of drugs that may delay gastric emptying (e.g., propoxyphene, present in combination with acetaminophen in Darvocet-N).[445] In this case, if the history is reliably known, clinical presentation (e.g., opioid toxidrome) and drug screen results should alert the physician to the need for serial monitoring. Fifth, alcoholic patients, fasting or malnourished patients, and patients on chronic therapy with microsomal enzyme-inducing drugs (anticonvulsants) may have increased susceptibility to acetaminophen hepatotoxicity,[63,90,400,411,475] presumably as a result of induction of cytochrome P_{450} (see below) and, in the case of alcoholics or fasting patients, depletion of glutathione (see below). In these cases, it has been proposed that the decision line in the nomogram be lowered by 50% to 70%.[411,415] Others do not advocate any change in the therapeutic decision line for such patients with acute ingestion. These risk factors may be more important in chronic acetaminophen poisoning. Although therapeutic guidelines for chronic acetaminophen poisoning have not been established, one recommended approach is to administer NAC if AST is elevated in symptomatic patients or if AST is >2-fold upper reference limit and acetaminophen >10 µg/mL for asymptomatic patients.[51]

Acetaminophen is normally metabolized in the liver to glucuronide (50% to 60%) and sulfate (~30%) conjugates.[161] A smaller amount (~10%) is metabolized by a cytochrome P_{450} mixed-function oxidase pathway that is thought to involve formation of a highly reactive intermediate (*N*-acetylbenzoquinoneimine)[311] (Figure 34-6). This intermediate normally undergoes electrophilic conjugation with glutathione and then subsequent transformation to cysteine and mercapturic acid conjugates of acetaminophen. With acetaminophen overdose, the sulfation pathway becomes saturated, and consequently a greater portion is metabolized by the P_{450} mixed-function oxidase pathway. When the tissue stores of glutathione become depleted, arylation of cellular molecules by the benzoquinoneimine intermediate leads to hepatic necrosis.[311]

Specific therapy for acetaminophen overdose is the administration of NAC, which probably acts as a glutathione substitute.[70] NAC may also provide substrate to replenish hepatic glutathione[108] or to enhance sulfate conjugation[279] or both. The time of administration of NAC is critical. Maximum efficacy is observed when NAC is administered within 8 hours, but efficacy then declines sharply between 18 and 24 hours after ingestion.[412] The antidote may have some beneficial effects even after liver injury has occurred, presumably by its ability to improve tissue oxygen delivery and use.[191] An initial loading dose (140 mg/kg) of NAC should be followed by 17 maintenance doses (70 mg/kg) given every 4 hours. A shorter treatment with only five maintenance doses was proposed in 2003.[496] If the serum acetaminophen results

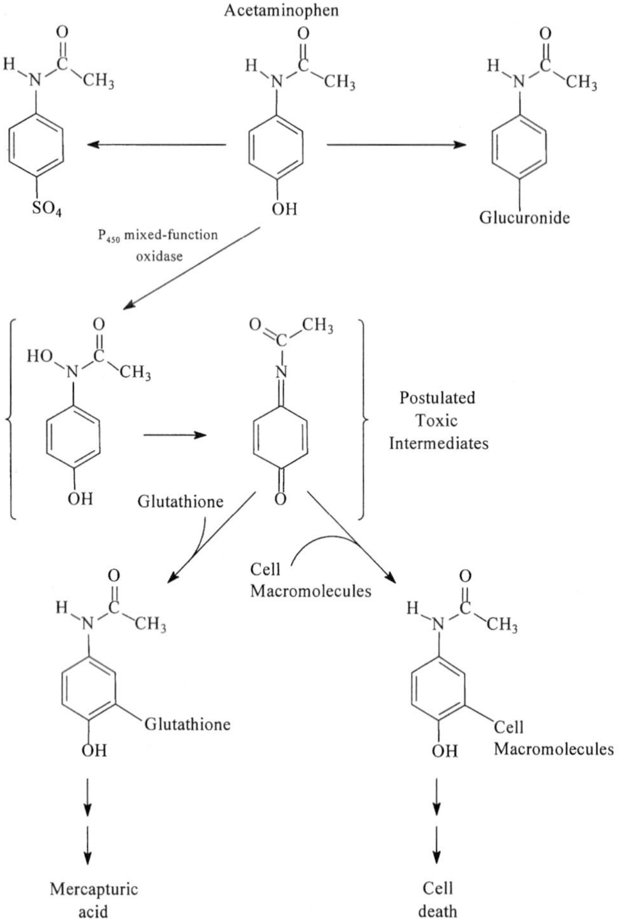

Figure 34-6 Pathways of acetaminophen metabolism. *(From Mitchell JR, Thorgeirsson SS, Potter WZ, Jollow DJ, Keiser H. Acetaminophen-induced hepatic injury: Protective role of glutathione in man and rationale for therapy. Clin Pharmacol Ther 1974; 16:676.)*

are not available locally within 8 hours of suspected ingestion, treatment with NAC should begin. This treatment may be discontinued if belated assay results indicate that it is not warranted.

Many photometric methods are available for the determination of acetaminophen.[66,478] In general, these methods are relatively easy to perform but may be subject to a number of interferences.[66] Some methods measure the nontoxic metabolites and the potentially toxic parent acetaminophen and thus may produce especially misleading results. Therefore only methods specific for parent acetaminophen should be used.[371] Immunoassays for acetaminophen, such as EMIT (Dade-Behring, Palo Alto, Calif.), FPIA (Abbott Laboratories, North Chicago, Ill.), and particle-enhanced turbimetric inhibition immunoassay (Beckman Coulter, Brea, Calif.) are widely used because they are rapid, easily performed, and accurate. A different approach uses arylacylamide amidohydrolase for hydrolysis of acetaminophen (but not conjugates) to *p*-aminophenol and acetate. Subsequent color formation depends on reaction of the generated *p*-aminophenol with 8-hydroxyquinoline[320] or *o*-cresol.[375] Adaptations of this enzyme assay are used on the VITROS (Johnson & Johnson Clinical Diagnostics, Rochester, N.Y.) and other automated chemistry analyzers.[68] Arylacylamide amidohydrolase methods are susceptible to interference by NAC,[301] bilirubin,[50] and IgM monoclonal immunoglobulins.[210] Most chromatographic methods are highly accurate and therefore may be considered reference procedures; however, they are more difficult to perform, especially on an emergency basis. A reference HPLC procedure[368] is included in the Chapter 34 Appendix that is found on this book's accompanying Evolve site (http://evolve.elsevier.com/Tietz/textbook/). A qualitative, one-step lateral flow immunoassay (cutoff 25 µg/mL) suitable for point-of-care application is available (SureStep, Applied Biotech, San Diego).

Salicylate

Acetylsalicylic acid (aspirin) has analgesic, antipyretic, and antiinflammatory properties. These therapeutic benefits derive from its ability to inhibit biosynthesis of prostaglandins by acetylation of active site serine and subsequent irreversible inhibition of cyclooxygenase enzymes (COX-1; COX-2 isoenzymes).[382] Salicylate, the metabolite of aspirin, also reduces prostaglandin synthesis by uncertain mechanisms. Because of these therapeutic benefits and the general lack of serious side effects at normal doses, aspirin is widely available and frequently consumed. Therapeutic serum salicylate concentrations are generally lower than 60 mg/L for analgesic-antipyretic effects, and 150 to 300 mg/L for antiinflammatory actions.[382]

Aspirin also interferes with platelet aggregation and thus prolongs bleeding time. The platelet inhibitory effect is a consequence of aspirin's ability to acetylate and irreversibly inhibit platelet cyclooxygenase, thereby reducing the formation of thromboxane A_2, a potent mediator of platelet aggregation. Platelets have little or no capacity for protein synthesis ; therefore, the duration of this enzyme inhibition is for the normal life span of the platelets (8 to 11 days).[385] Because of this platelet inhibitory activity, low-dose aspirin has been recommended as prophylactic therapy for some individuals at risk for thromboembolic disease.[352,428] There is an epidemiological association between aspirin ingestion and Reye's syndrome in children and adolescents with viral infections (e.g., varicella and influenza).[211] Aspirin use is therefore contraindicated in these patients.

The absorption of normal doses of regular aspirin from the GI tract is generally rapid, with peak serum concentration achieved within 2 hours.[382] This peak value may be delayed for 12 hours or longer for enteric-coated or slow-release formulations.[253] Moreover, toxic doses of aspirin may form concretions or bezoars and produce pylorospasm, thereby delaying absorption. Serum salicylate in such instances may not reach maximum concentration for 6 hours or longer,[122] an important consideration when the assessment of the severity of toxicity is based on such measurements.

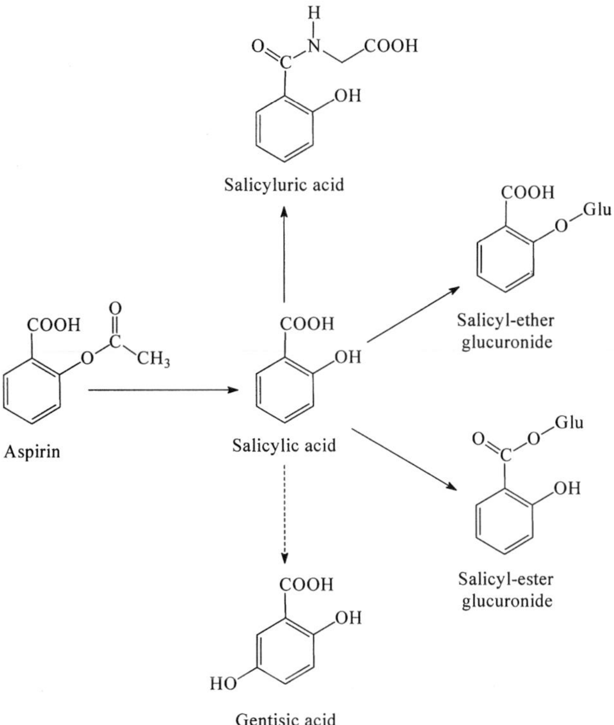

Figure 34-7 Metabolism of aspirin. (Glu, glucuronide.)

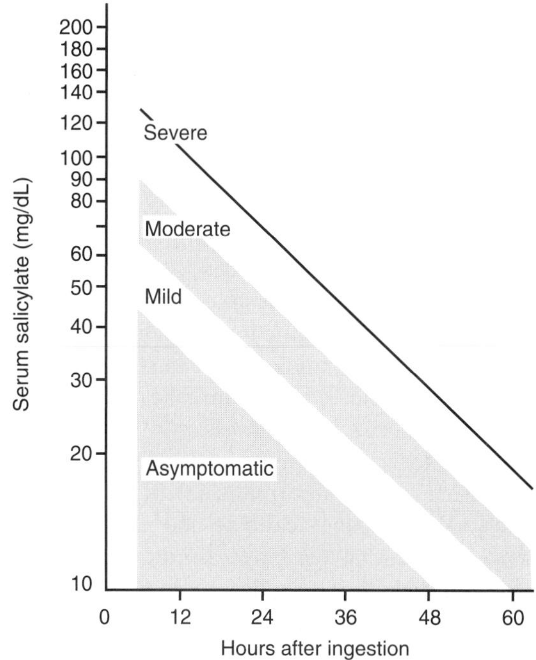

Figure 34-8 Nomogram for estimating the severity of acute salicylate intoxication. *(From Done AK. Salicylate intoxication: Significance of measurements of salicylate in blood in cases of acute ingestion. Pediatrics 1960; 26:800. Reproduced by permission of Pediatrics.)*

Once absorbed, aspirin has a very short half-life ($t_{1/2}$ = 15 min) because of its rapid hydrolysis to salicylate. Salicylate is eliminated mainly by conjugation with glycine to form salicyluric acid and to a lesser extent with glucuronic acid to form phenol and acyl glucuronides (Figure 34-7). A very small amount is hydroxylated to gentisic acid. These metabolic pathways may become saturated even at high therapeutic doses. Consequently, serum salicylate concentration may increase disproportionately with dosage. At high therapeutic or toxic doses, the salicylate elimination half-life is prolonged (15 to 30 hours versus 2 to 3 hours at low dose), and a much larger portion of the dose is excreted in urine as salicylate.[382]

Salicylates directly stimulate the central respiratory center and thereby cause hyperventilation and respiratory alkalosis. Moreover, salicylates cause uncoupling of oxidative phosphorylation. As a result, heat production (hyperthermia), oxygen consumption, and metabolic rate may be increased. In addition, salicylates enhance anaerobic glycolysis but inhibit Krebs cycle and transaminase enzymes, all of which lead to accumulation of organic acids and thus to metabolic acidosis.[459]

The primary acid-base disturbance observed with salicylate overdosage depends on age and severity of intoxication. Respiratory alkalosis predominates in children over age 4 and in adults, except in very severe cases that may progress through a mixed respiratory alkalosis–metabolic acidosis to metabolic acidosis. In 97 adult patients who had plasma salicylate concentrations greater than 700 mg/L, 19% were found to have respiratory alkalosis, 61% had combined respiratory alkalosis and metabolic acidosis, and 15% had metabolic acidosis. Mortality was associated with acidemia.[85] In children under age 4, the initial period of respiratory alkalosis is very brief and therefore may not be observed; in such cases, metabolic acidosis predominates.[459] CNS depression is more pronounced when acidemia is severe, a consequence of increased brain uptake of nonionized salicylic acid. Respiratory acidosis, a result of severe CNS depression or pulmonary edema, may sometimes occur and is indicative of a poor prognosis.

The symptoms of salicylate intoxication include tinnitus, diaphoresis, hyperthermia, hyperventilation, nausea, vomiting, and acid-base disturbances. CNS effects include lethargy, disorientation, and in severe cases, coma and seizures. Tinnitus may occur at salicylate concentrations greater than 200 mg/L, but more serious toxic manifestations are generally not evident unless the salicylate concentration exceeds 300 mg/L.[382]

Measurement of serum salicylate concentration is important for assessment of the severity of intoxication. A nomogram that relates serum salicylate concentration and time after ingestion with the severity of intoxication was developed by Done[122] (Figure 34-8), primarily for use with pediatric patients. The nomogram applies only to acute ingestion of salicylate and should not be used to estimate severity of chronic toxicity. The nomogram is less useful for adult patients,[127] who tend to have less severe acidemia (mixed respiratory alkalosis–metabolic acidosis) than young children (acidosis). Moreover, interpretation of the nomogram is complicated in instances of mixed drug ingestion. For these reasons, use of this nomogram is discouraged by some toxicologists.

Aspirin absorption may be delayed when overdose quantities are consumed, especially of enteric-coated or slow-release preparations. This must be considered when interpreting serum salicylate values, especially for specimens obtained earlier than 6 hours after ingestion. Repeat testing within 2 to 3 hours is recommended to ensure that absorption is complete; subsequent testing provides an indication of effectiveness of therapeutic intervention. Because of the aforementioned complications, proper assessment of salicylate intoxication requires sound clinical evaluation in combination with serum salicylate levels.

Treatment for salicylate intoxication is directed toward (1) decreasing further absorption, (2) increasing elimination, and (3) correcting acid-base and electrolyte disturbances. Activated charcoal binds aspirin and prevents its absorption. Elimination of salicylate may be enhanced by alkaline diuresis and in severe cases by hemodialysis.[459] Sodium bicarbonate may be given to alleviate metabolic acidosis. Indications for hemodialysis include serum salicylate >1000 mg/L, severe CNS depression, intractable metabolic acidosis, hepatic failure with coagulopathy, and renal failure.[156]

A urine drug screen may be helpful to recognize the presence of drugs from combination medications with aspirin (e.g., antihistamines, sympathomimetic amines, and propoxyphene) or that otherwise are co-ingested.

Classic methods for the measurement of salicylate in serum are based on the method of Trinder.[452] These procedures rely on the reaction between salicylate and Fe^{3+} to form a colored complex that is measured at 540 nm. To lessen endogenous background interference, either a protein precipitation step or a serum blank is necessary. Nevertheless, blank readings equivalent to about 20 to 25 mg/L are generally observed. Moreover, interference by salicylate metabolites, endogenous compounds, and some drugs, especially structurally related drugs such as diflunisal (difluorophenyl salicylate),[393] may occur. Azide, present as a preservative in some commercial control sera, also causes interference. Despite these limitations, photometric methods continue to be successfully used to assess salicylate overdose. In a comparative study with 115 patient specimens, Trinder method results agreed very closely with those of a reference HPLC procedure.[220] However, significant interference with the Trinder method was observed for one patient who consumed an overdose of dichloralphenazone. Thus for best interpretation of test results, as much information as possible should be obtained regarding drug ingestion history.

Other methods for salicylate quantitation include fluorescent polarization immunoassay[238] and a salicylate hydroxylase–mediated photometric procedure[321] (Figure 34-9). These procedures are subject to some of the same interferences as is the Trinder method, but the salicylate hydroxylase method is considered more specific.[321] This enzyme method has been adapted to automated analyzers, such as the Synchron (Beckman Coulter). Gas and liquid chromatographic methods are the most specific methods for salicylate,[81,378] but their general availability, especially for emergency use, is limited and probably not necessary.[393,434]

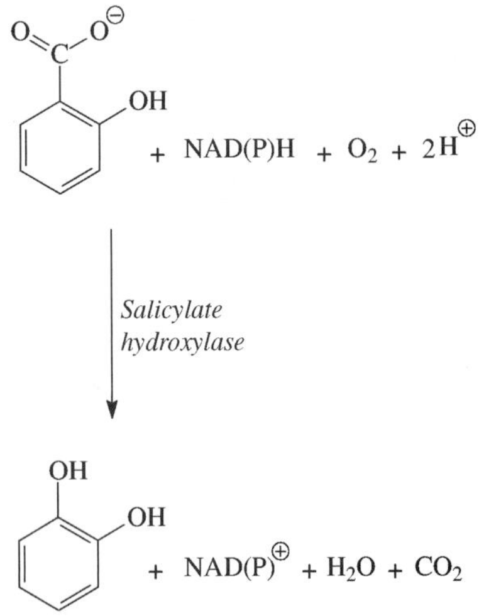

Figure 34-9 Salicylate hydroxylase–mediated oxidative decarboxylation of salicylate.

Because of its ease of performance and wide acceptance, the photometric method of Trinder[132] for measuring salicylates is included in the Chapter 34 Appendix that is found on this book's accompanying Evolve site (http://evolve.elsevier.com/Tietz/textbook/). In addition, an HPLC method[81] suitable for pharmacokinetic studies or for therapeutic monitoring of salicylate is also included. A qualitative spot test based on the Trinder reaction is also on the Evolve site (http://evolve.elsevier.com/Tietz/textbook/). A qualitative, one-step lateral flow immunoassay (cutoff 100 mg/L) suitable for point-of-care application is commercially available (Applied Biotech, San Diego).

Drugs Related to the Anticholinergic Toxidrome

While the tricyclic antidepressants, the phenothiazines, and the antihistamines have divergent therapeutic applications, in overdose they often share similar anticholinergic and antihistaminic toxidromes as principal components of their overall toxic effects. These overlapping toxicities are likely related to their common methyl or dimethyl aminoethyl ($—CH_2CH_2N[CH_3]_2$; $—CH_2CH_2NHCH_3$) moieties, which are structurally related to similar groups in acetylcholine ($—CH_2CH_2N[CH_3]_3$) and histamine ($—CH_2CH_2NH_2$).

Tricyclic Antidepressants

Tricyclic antidepressants represent a class of drugs widely prescribed for the treatment of endogenous depression and neuralgic pain, migraine headache, enuresis, and attention deficit disorder (see Chapter 33). Tricyclic antidepressants include imipramine, amitriptyline, and their N-

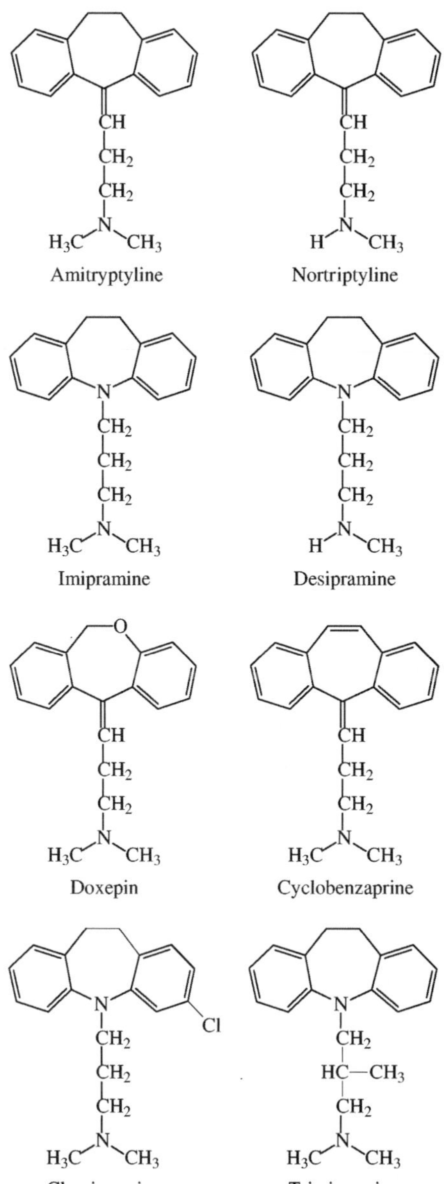

Figure 34-10 Structure of some tricyclic antidepressants and the muscle relaxant cyclobenzaprine.

demethylated derivatives, desipramine and nortriptyline; clomipramine; doxepin; and trimipramine (Figure 34-10). Other cyclic antidepressant drugs include amoxapine and maprotiline.

Tricyclic antidepressants block neuronal uptake of norepinephrine and variably serotonin (those with tertiary amine side chains), and the degree of inhibition seems to correlate with antidepressant activity. However, the block in amine uptake occurs shortly after drug administration, whereas the antidepressant effects generally require several weeks to develop.[20,250,337] Thus the mechanism of action is incompletely understood and may involve changes in presynaptic and postsynaptic neurogenic amine receptor response. In addition to their mood-elevating actions, tricyclic antidepressants also have sedative effects that may be related to antihistamine activity in the CNS. Tertiary amines (amitriptyline, doxepin, and imipramine) produce greater sedation than the secondary amines. Cyclic antidepressants also exert central and peripheral anticholinergic effects and peripheral α_1-adrenergic blockade.

Because of their continued use, narrow therapeutic range, and the nature of the illness for which they are typically prescribed, tricyclic antidepressants may cause severe or fatal toxicity.[138,278,357,419] For example, in March of 2004 the U.S. FDA issued a Public Health Advisory because of both suicidal ideation and suicide attempts in children taking antidepressant drugs for the treatment of major depressive disorder.

The antimuscarinic actions of tricyclic antidepressants are responsible for side effects frequently experienced even at therapeutic doses and are therefore commonly present in overdose. These effects include tachycardia, hyperpyrexia, dilated pupils, dry skin and mouth, flushing, decreased GI motility, and urinary retention.

The CNS manifestations of tricyclic antidepressant overdose may vary from mild agitation or drowsiness to delirium, coma, respiratory depression, or seizures. These manifestations are thought to result in part from central anticholinergic and antihistaminic actions of these drugs.

Cardiovascular toxicity is the most serious manifestation of tricyclic antidepressant overdose and accounts for the majority of fatalities. Tricyclic antidepressants inhibit Na^+ entry via sodium channels in the myocardium, which results in decreased conductivity, decreased contractility, and arrhythmia (quinidine-like effect). In addition, their anticholinergic and sympathomimetic (inhibition of norepinephrine uptake) effects contribute to dysrhythmias. In mild overdose, these effects result in tachycardia and slight increase in blood pressure. With more severe overdose, serious arrhythmias and conduction delays may develop, of which the most distinct feature is prolongation of the QRS interval in the electrocardiogram. In addition, cardiac output decreases, which coupled with peripheral vasodilation (α_1-adrenergic blockade) leads to life-threatening hypotension. Death often results from arrhythmias or hypotension. The cardiotoxic manifestations may occur within a few hours of overdose, or they may be delayed for 24 hours or longer. It is important to recognize that a patient's symptomatology (perhaps initially only mild anticholinergic effects) is due to tricyclic antidepressants so that a proper period of monitoring for delayed and possibly catastrophic cardiotoxicity can be followed. Thus laboratory identification of these drugs, especially in the absence of a reliable history, provides crucial information.

In addition to general supportive measures (gastric lavage, activated charcoal, and IV fluids), therapy for tricyclic antidepressant overdose includes administration of $NaHCO_3$ for dysrhythmias (alkalinization causes tricyclic antidepressants to dissociate from the membrane sodium channels and Na^+ provides a favorable gradient for Na^+ channel activated membrane depolarization). Physostigmine, a reversible cholinesterase inhibitor, can effectively reverse the central and peripheral anticholinergic manifestations of tricyclic antidepressant toxicity. However, its use is generally contraindicated in tricyclic antidepressant overdose because of the risk of enhancing cardiac conduction delays, which may result in asystole. Hemodialysis or hemoperfusion is not beneficial because the tricyclic antidepressant drugs have a large volume of distribution and are extensively bound to plasma proteins.

Newer, safer drugs that are selective inhibitors of serotonin reuptake [e.g., fluoxetine (Prozac), sertraline (Zoloft), and paroxetine (Paxil)] have no or minimal antimuscarinic, antihistaminic, or adverse cardiovascular effects. They are now the drugs of choice for treatment of depressive disorders.

Tricyclic antidepressants may be measured quantitatively in serum by chromatographic methods (most commonly HPLC) or by immunoassay (EMIT; FPIA; see Chapter 33). These immunoassays may also be used for qualitative or semiquantitative detection of tricyclic antidepressants, which are useful for screening. Immunoassays are rapid and relatively easy to perform but may be subject to interference by other drugs, such as chlorpromazine,[347] thioridazine,[387] cyproheptadine,[476] cyclobenzaprine,[347] and diphenhydramine.[425] Tricyclic antidepressants are adequately detected in urine, using TLC (e.g., Toxi-Lab) and by colloidal gold immunoassay (Triage, BioSite Diagnostics, San Diego). In cases of overdose, qualitative identification (serum or urine) is sufficient, because the severity of intoxication is more reliably indicated by an increase in the QRS interval (>100 ms) than by the serum concentration.[57]

Cyclobenzaprine, a tricyclic amine structurally very similar to amitriptyline (see Figure 34-10), is used as a centrally acting skeletal muscle relaxant. Like amitriptyline, cyclobenzaprine causes sedation, produces central and peripheral muscarinic blockade, and potentiates adrenergic actions. In overdose, cyclobenzaprine may cause a typical anticholinergic toxidrome and cardiac arrhythmias, hypotension, and coma. However, cyclobenzaprine overdose is not as frequent nor as lethal as amitriptyline overdose.

The analytical distinction between amitriptyline and cyclobenzaprine is often difficult. Cyclobenzaprine cross-reacts with immunoassays for tricyclic antidepressants (EMIT, TDx, and Triage) and generally co-elutes or co-migrates with amitriptyline in HPLC and TLC. However, cyclobenzaprine and amitriptyline have different ultraviolet spectra; therefore, they may be distinguished by HPLC using a diode array detector by either multiwavelength scanning (e.g., Remidi)[119,366] or dual-wavelength discrimination.[119] Although these two drugs co-migrate using the Toxi-Lab system, they may be distinguished by differences in fluorescence at stage III (amitriptyline fluoresces pink whereas cyclobenzaprine fluoresces orange).[40] Finally, amitriptyline and cyclobenzaprine are well resolved using capillary column GC (Figure 34-11) and may be distinguished by careful examination of their respective mass spectra (ratio of 202/215 amu ions differ) (Figure 34-12).[486]

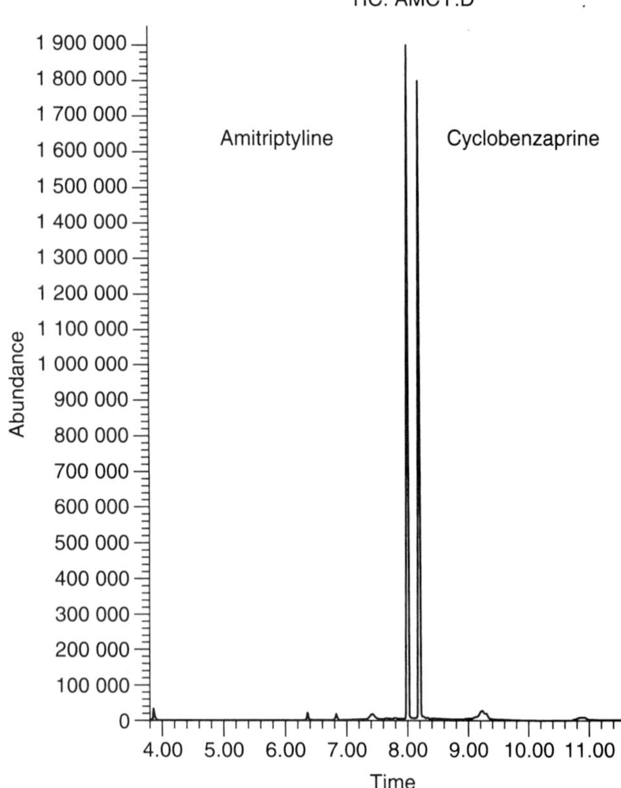

Figure 34-11 Total-ion chromatogram for amitriptyline and cyclobenzaprine. Time = minute.

Phenothiazines

Phenothiazines are tricyclic compounds that have chemical and pharmacological properties in common with the tricyclic antidepressant drugs (Figure 34-13; see also previous section on Tricyclic Antidepressants). They are primarily used for their neuroleptic (behavior modifying) properties in the treatment of severe psychiatric illness (psychoses and mania). In addition, phenothiazines are administered to control nausea and vomiting, for sedation, and for potentiation of analgesia and general anesthesia.[21]

The phenothiazines inhibit dopaminergic receptors in the CNS, a property thought to account for their neuroleptic effect.[21] In addition, phenothiazines inhibit muscarinic, α-adrenergic, histaminic, and serotonergic receptors, which accounts for many of their toxic or undesirable side effects.

The principal manifestations of phenothiazine toxicity involve the CNS and cardiovascular system.[21,37,286] Signs of CNS toxicity include sedation, coma, respiratory depression (uncommon), seizures, hypothermia or hyperthermia, and extrapyramidal movement disorders (acute dystonia, parkinsonism, akathisia, tardive dyskinesia, and neuroleptic malignant syndrome); the extrapyramidal symptoms result from an imbalance between inhibitory dopamine and

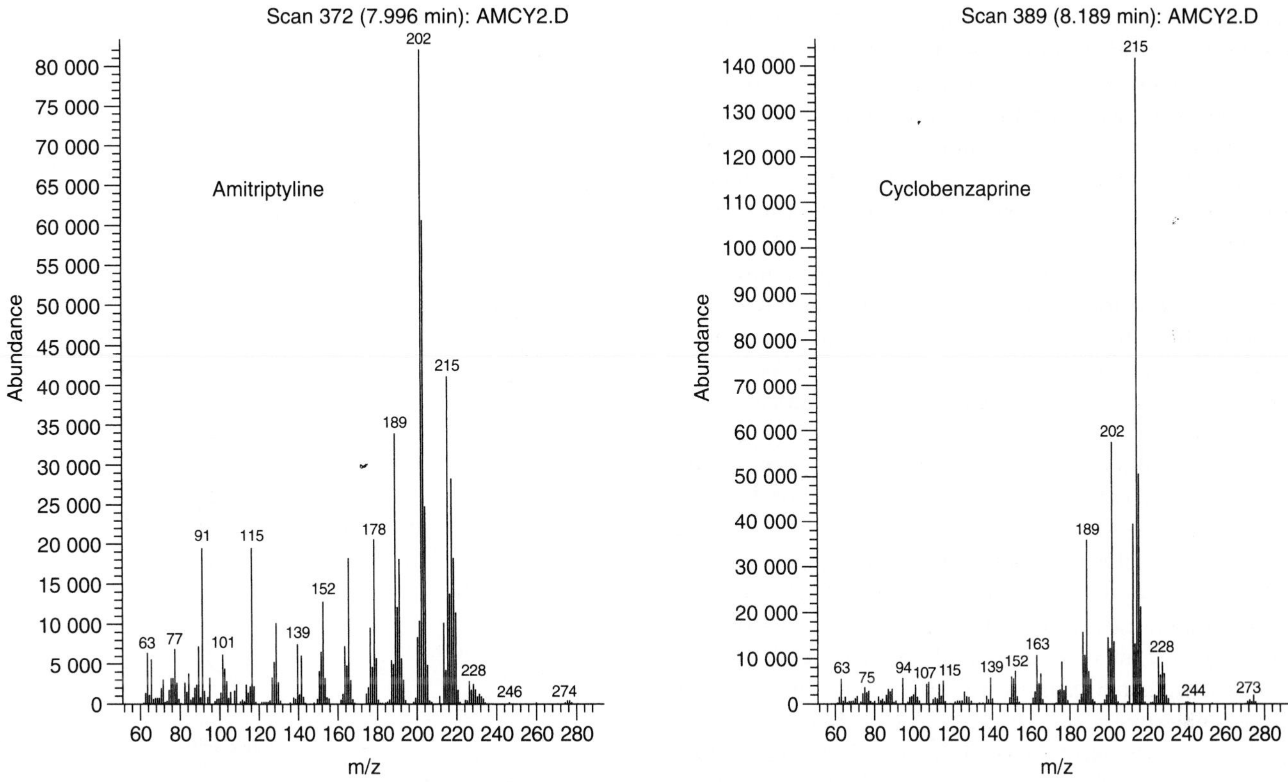

Figure 34-12 Mass spectra for amitriptyline and cyclobenzaprine. The spectra were scanned from 60 to 500 amu to avoid the large, dominant 58 amu ion present in each.

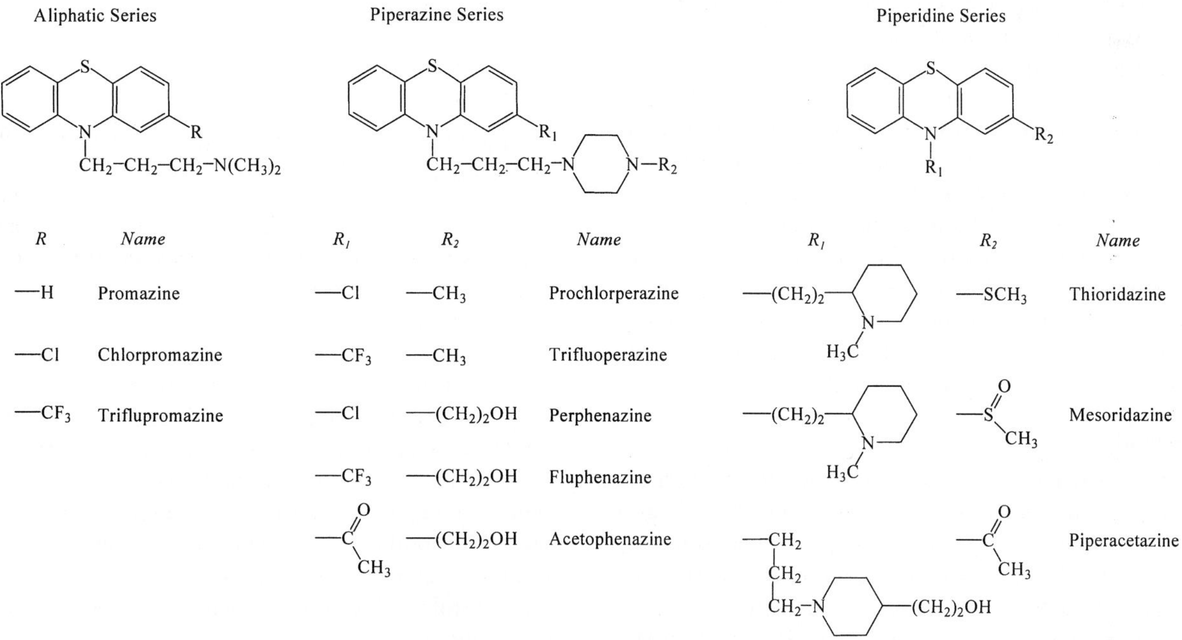

Figure 34-13 Chemical structure of representative phenothiazines.

excitatory acetylcholine responses within the extrapyramidal motor system. The cardiovascular effects include orthostatic or frank hypotension and arrhythmias, a consequence of the quinidine-like depressant action on the myocardium and α-adrenergic blockade. Additional peripheral antimuscarinic manifestations include decreased bowel sounds, urinary retention, skin flushing, blurred vision, and dry mouth.

The cardiovascular, CNS, and anticholinergic symptoms of phenothiazine toxicity are similar to, but generally much less severe than, those for the tricyclic antidepressants. Phenothiazines are relatively safe, and few deaths have occurred when toxic doses have been ingested alone. Much more severe toxicity occurs when phenothiazines are co-ingested with tricyclic antidepressant drugs or other CNS depressant drugs, such as ethanol, opioids, barbiturates, or benzodiazepines.

Therapy for phenothiazines is generally supportive and similar to that for tricyclic antidepressant overdose. Physostigmine can reverse the central and peripheral anticholinergic manifestations of phenothiazines; however, because these manifestations are rarely life-threatening and because physostigmine may cause severe bradycardia or asystole it is not recommended for treatment of phenothiazine overdose. Because of the large volume of distribution and extensive protein binding, hemodialysis or hemoperfusion is not beneficial for phenothiazine overdose.

The phenothiazines are extensively metabolized by the liver to a number of metabolites, some of which are pharmacologically active. Less than 1% of a dose is excreted unchanged in the urine. The correlation between dose, serum concentration, and pharmacological effect is poor; therapeutic drug monitoring[470] or serum quantitation in instances of overdose is not warranted.[37,286] Qualitative detection of phenothiazines or their metabolites in urine is sufficient to document ingestion for symptomatic patients. Suitable methods of detection include TLC (e.g., Toxi-Lab) and the spot test using the Forrest reagent (potassium dichromate, sulfuric acid, perchloric acid, and nitric acid).[53] The ability to also detect other co-ingested drugs, such as opioids, tricyclic antidepressants, barbiturates, and benzodiazepines, is important to alert the physician to the enhanced potential for severe toxicity from their combined ingestion.

Antihistamines

Histamine released from mast cells plays an important physiological role in immediate hypersensitivity and allergic responses. In addition, histamine functions as a neurotransmitter in the CNS and it is a potent stimulus for gastric acid secretion. These actions depend on the interaction of histamine with two types of receptors, H_1 and H_2.[69] H_1 and H_2 receptors are coupled via G proteins to phospholipase C and adenylyl cyclase, respectively. The principal H_2 receptor response is stimulation of gastric acid secretion, whereas other actions of histamine (e.g., smooth muscle contraction, vasodilation, increased capillary permeability, pain, and itching) are primarily mediated by H_1 receptors.

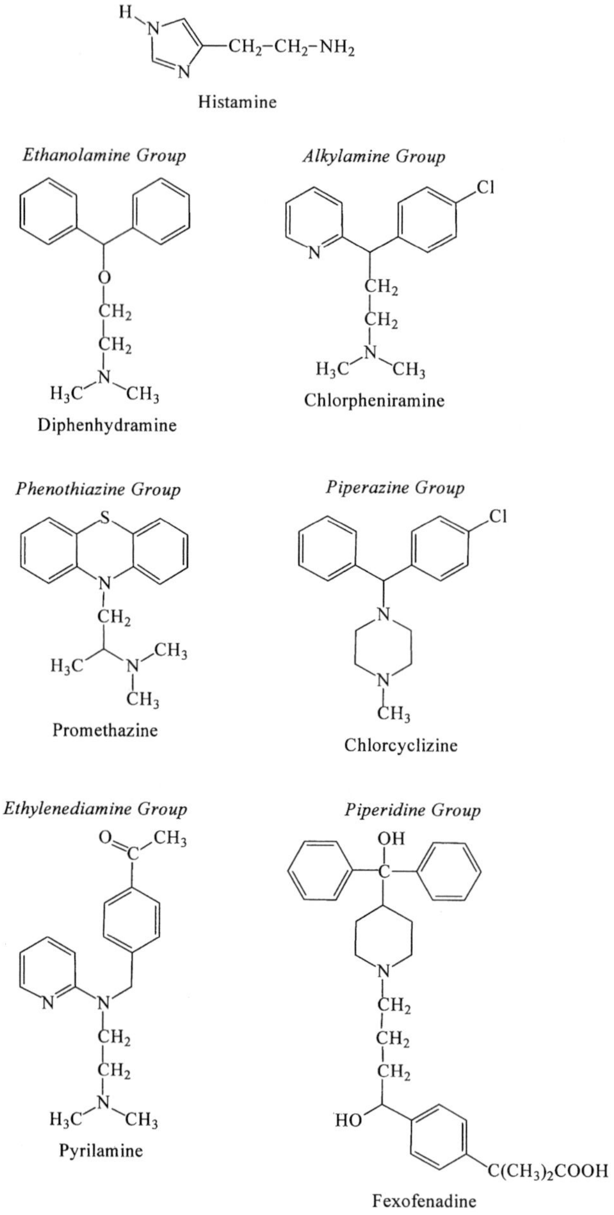

Figure 34-14 Chemical structure of histamine and representative H_1 antagonists.

The antihistamine drugs are classified as H_1 or H_2 antagonists, based on their principal receptor site binding.[69] The H_1 antagonists contain a substituted ethylene amine (—$CH_2CH_2NR_2$—), in common with both histamine (Figure 34-14) and acetylcholine (Figure 34-15); therefore they exhibit both antihistaminic and anticholinergic pharmacological actions. The second-generation H_1 antagonists, such as fexofenadine (Allegra), have very little anticholinergic activity.

The therapeutic actions of H_1 antagonists include smooth muscle relaxation, decreased bronchial secretions, decreased allergic response, and sedation. They are therefore used to treat immediate hypersensitivity reactions, as cold remedies, to suppress motion sickness, and for sedation (the second-generation H_1 antagonists [e.g., fexofenadine] do not pene-

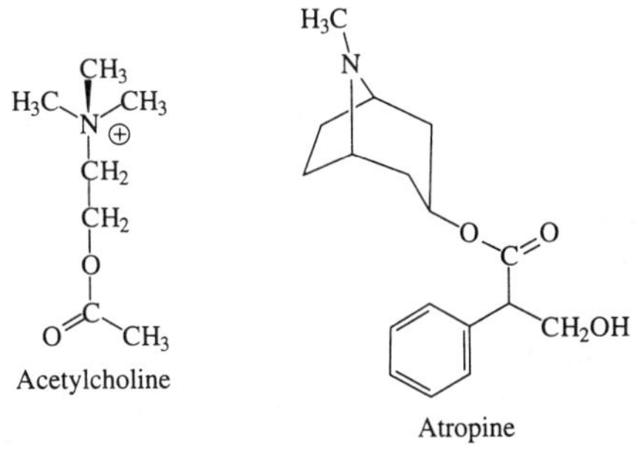

Figure 34-15 Structure for the neurotransmitter acetylcholine and its antagonist, atropine.

trate the blood-brain barrier well and therefore do not cause sedation). The H_2 antagonists are widely used to treat peptic ulcer disease. The most prominent H_2 antagonists are cimetidine (Tagamet), ranitidine (Zantac), famotidine (Pepcid), and nizatidine (Axid).

The principal manifestations of overdose due to H_1 antagonists are CNS depression or stimulation and anticholinergic symptoms.[69,246,473] Symptoms of CNS depression include sedation, drowsiness, ataxia, and coma. CNS stimulation, more common in children, results in excitement, hallucinations, toxic psychosis, delirium, and convulsions. The antimuscarinic toxidrome includes dry mouth, flushed dry skin, urinary retention, sinus tachycardia, dilated pupils, blurred vision, and fever. Death may occur because of respiratory depression or cardiovascular collapse.

Treatment for H_1 antagonist overdose is general and supportive (e.g., gastric lavage and activated charcoal).[246,473] Hemodialysis or hemoperfusion is not efficacious because these drugs have a large volume of distribution and are highly protein bound. Physostigmine may be used cautiously if central and peripheral anticholinergic symptoms are prominent, and there is no evidence of cardiac conduction delays (electrocardiogram; no evidence [history or drug screen] of exposure to drugs that can cause conduction delays [e.g., cocaine, tricyclic antidepressants, phenothiazines, and procainamide]).

Antihistamines are present in prescription and nonprescription forms, alone or in combination with analgesics, such as aspirin and acetaminophen. In instances of overdose, a urine drug screen that detects salicylate, acetaminophen, and the antihistamines is helpful, especially when the source of intoxication is unknown. The detection of either analgesic in the urine of a symptomatic patient should lead to their quantitation in serum to assess their potential toxicity (see sections on Salicylate and Acetaminophen). Quantitation of antihistamines in serum is not useful, because there is a poor correlation between dose, drug level, and degree of toxicity.[473]

Overall the antihistamines are relatively safe. However, their CNS depressant actions are enhanced by co-ingestion of ethanol, sedative-hypnotic drugs, and opioids; their anticholinergic actions are potentiated by co-ingestion of tricyclic antidepressants and phenothiazines. Therefore the detection of any of these drugs in combination on a urine drug screen should alert the physician to a potentially more serious intoxication.

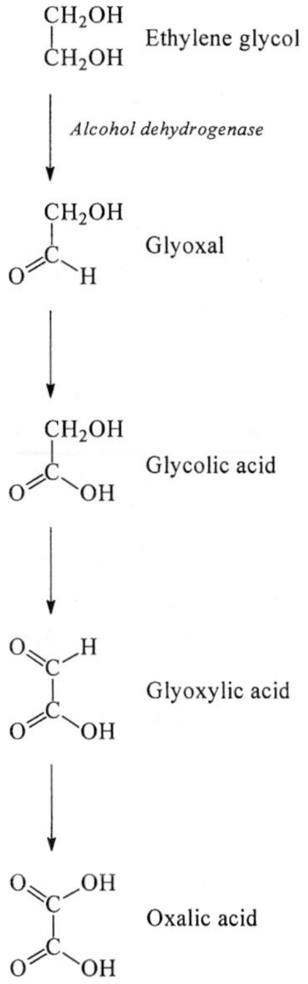

Figure 34-16 Metabolism of ethylene glycol.

Ethylene Glycol

Ethylene glycol, present in antifreeze products, may be ingested accidentally or for the purpose of inebriation or suicide. Ethylene glycol itself is relatively nontoxic, and its initial CNS effects resemble those of ethanol. However, metabolism of ethylene glycol by ADH results in the formation of a number of acid metabolites, including oxalic acid and glycolic acid (Figure 34-16).

These acid metabolites are responsible for much of the toxicity of ethylene glycol,[199,219] the clinical manifestations of which include neurological abnormalities (CNS depression; in severe cases, coma and convulsions), severe metabolic acidosis, acute renal failure, and cardiopulmonary failure.[280] The serum concentration of glycolic acid correlates more closely with clinical symptoms and mortality than does the concentration of ethylene glycol.[199,369] Because of the rapid elimination of ethylene glycol ($t_{1/2}$ ~3 hours), its serum concentration may be low or undetectable at a time when that for glycolic acid remains elevated.[164,199,369] Thus the determination of both ethylene glycol and glycolic acid provides useful clinical and confirmatory analytical information in cases of ethylene glycol ingestion. Other laboratory findings commonly observed with ethylene glycol poisoning include increased serum osmol and anion gaps, decreased serum calcium, and the presence of calcium oxalate crystals in the urine. The decreased serum calcium results from calcium oxalate deposition in tissue or from a possible interference in normal parathyroid hormone response[409] or both.

Early recognition of ethylene glycol intoxication and thus of the need for timely therapeutic intervention is important because of the compound's short half-life (about 3 hours). Blood concentration of ethylene glycol may decline rapidly during the first 24 hours following ingestion.[361] Therefore relatively low serum concentrations (0.05 to 2 g/L) may be observed in serious intoxication if several hours have elapsed between the time of ingestion and that of blood sampling. In such cases, the measurement of glycolic acid is especially important. Serum concentrations associated with deaths from ethylene glycol ingestion have ranged from 0.06 to 4.3 g/L,[29,369] highlighting the lack of correlation between ethylene glycol concentration and severity of toxicity. It is thus impossible to define a serum ethylene glycol concentration associated with a high probability of death. Contrarily, a mortality rate of 33% occurred when serum glycolic acid was >10 mmol/L in a study of 41 patients; 94% of survivors with glycolic acid >10 mmol/L developed acute renal failure.[369]

Appropriate therapy for ethylene glycol intoxication includes administration of fomepizole (4-methylpyrazole) or ethanol to competitively inhibit the ADH-mediated metabolism of ethylene glycol, aggressive therapy with sodium bicarbonate to help alleviate the acidosis, and hemodialysis or forced diuresis to enhance the removal of ethylene glycol and acid metabolites.[23,64,205] A serum ethanol concentration of ~100 mg/dL is sufficient to saturate ADH and thus prolongs the elimination half-life of ethylene glycol from ~3 hours (metabolism and renal excretion) to about 17 hours (renal excretion).[361] Administration of ethanol or preferably fomepizole is generally recommended when the serum ethylene glycol concentration is greater than 0.2 g/L.[23] Hemodialysis effectively removes ethylene glycol and glycolic acid and is recommended when the serum ethylene glycol concentration is greater than 0.5 g/L, with severe metabolic acidosis (pH <7.25 to 7.30), or with renal failure, regardless of the serum ethylene glycol concentration.[23] Serum glycolic acid ≥10 mmol/L predicts with high probability acute renal failure and the need for hemodialysis, whereas those patients with levels <10 mmol/L likely only require adequate antimetabolite therapy.[64,369] In the absence of glycolic acid measurements, an anion gap >20 mmol/L or pH <7.3 predicts acute renal failure in known ethylene glycol ingestions somewhat less reliably.[369] Patients with initial serum ethylene glycol concentration of 6.5 g/L,[361] 5.6 g/L,[429] 8.1 g/L,[369] and 18.9 g/L[225] survived because of early therapy with ethanol infusion and hemodialysis.

Ethylene glycol intoxication is relatively rare, but when it does occur, it is important for the laboratory to provide rapid (<2 hours) analytical support. A GC-MS method is included in the Chapter 34 Appendix that is found on this book's accompanying Evolve site (http://evolve.elsevier.com/Tietz/textbook/); it allows for the simultaneous determination of ethylene glycol and glycolic acid.[370] It is relatively simple and rapid, and it is free from interference by propylene glycol (a diluent for parenteral drugs, such as diazepam and phenytoin) or 2,3-butanediol (may be present in serum from some alcoholics); these glycols may interfere with the determination of ethylene glycol in some chromatographic procedures.[231] A comparable procedure using flame ionization detection has also been described.[494] Ethylene glycol may be rapidly measured with the use of glycerol dehydrogenase,[52,289] but these enzyme methods are subject to interference by glycerol,[52,291] propylene glycol,[3,291] 2,3-butanediol,[291,308,330] β-hydroxybutyrate,[52] and high concentrations of lactate and lactate dehydrogenase.[133] A serum osmol gap >10 mmol/L may be a nonspecific indicator of the presence of ethylene glycol (see section on Screening Methods).[23,369]

Toxic Metals/Iron

Several toxic metals, including arsenic, iron, lead, and mercury, are discussed in Chapters 30 and 35. Their measurement in urine, blood, and hair (in some cases) is valuable to help diagnose acute or chronic metal poisoning. Specific therapy for these toxins is listed in Table 34-1. Because the assessment of acute iron overdose requires emergency laboratory support, it is discussed in this chapter.

When severe acute iron intoxication occurs in children, significant morbidity or death may result.[358a] The limited physiological regulation of iron absorption from the GI tract may become overwhelmed with acute ingestion of large doses of iron. In such instances, the likelihood of iron toxicity is enhanced because no specific mechanisms exist for iron elimination. The initial toxic effects on the GI tract are a result of a direct corrosive action of iron on the mucosa, which may cause mucosal edema, infarction, ulceration, or hemorrhage. As a result, clinical symptoms of nausea, vomiting, abdominal pain, diarrhea, hematemesis, and melena may be evident. The systemic actions of excess iron affect the cardiovascular system, general metabolic functions, the liver, and the CNS. The cardiovascular effects of iron toxicity include decreased cardiac output, venous pooling of blood, and capillary leakage, all of which may lead to hypotension, shock, cyanosis, lethargy, tachycardia, and lactic acidosis. Within the liver, excess iron may cause swelling or necrosis of hepatocytes, resulting in abnormal liver function tests and a coagulopathy. Moreover, iron may accumulate within hepatic mitochondria and promote oxygen–free radical formation, lipid peroxidation of mitochondrial membranes, and interference with the electron transport system. Consequently, dysfunction of the Krebs cycle and oxidative phosphorylation lead to metabolic acidosis and secondarily cause hyperglycemia. The effects on the CNS range from lethargy and obtundation to frank coma. These effects may be secondary to cardiovascular, hepatic, and metabolic toxicity and to a direct CNS action of iron.

Specific treatment for iron toxicity involves administration of deferoxamine to chelate unbound iron.[358a] The deferoxamine–Fe complex is then excreted in the urine, often resulting in a characteristic vin rose color. The decision to administer deferoxamine is based on the history, clinical symptoms, and measurement of serum iron. In general, only mild toxicity is evident when the serum iron is below 300 μg/dL, and deferoxamine administration is normally not necessary. When the serum iron reaches 500 μg/dL, serious systemic toxicity is likely and may be fatal at concentrations of 1000 μg/dL or greater. Serum iron should be measured on admission and again 4 to 6 h after ingestion when absorption should be complete and the maximum serum level obtained. Serial measurement of serum iron is warranted if sustained–release medication has been ingested or if large bezoars are evident by abdominal x-ray.

Iron toxicity is presumably not likely unless the total serum iron concentration exceeds the total iron–binding capacity (TIBC; see Chapter 31). Thus, measurement of TIBC would be important in cases of iron poisoning but is discouraged because of methodological limitations.[382a,440a] In the determination of TIBC, excess iron is added to serum to bind all available iron-binding sites. Excess unbound iron is then removed by an absorbent material (e.g., $MgCO_3$) prior to measurement of bound iron. In the presence of excess endogenous iron, this absorbent material may be inadequate to remove all unbound iron, resulting in a falsely elevated TIBC. However, this limitation does not apply to the homogenous measurement of the unbound iron-binding capacity (UIBC), at least up to a total iron of 500 μg/dL,[382a] or to the immunochemical determination of transferrin, both of which may be performed on automated general chemistry analyzers. The TIBC (μg/dL) is equal to UIBC (μg/dL) + Fe (μg/dL) or to transferrin (mg/dL) × 1.43. Outcome-based validation of these derived TIBC measures in acute iron toxicity remains to be performed. Nevertheless, an expert toxicology committee of the National Academy of Clinical Biochemistry recommends their determination for the evaluation of iron toxicity.[491] Other general laboratory parameters that are considered helpful in the assessment of iron toxicity include WBC > 15,000 × 10^9/L and a serum glucose >150 mg/dL.

Deferoxamine interferes with photometric measurements of iron and UIBC,[382a] an important consideration if serum iron and UIBC measurements are used to monitor therapy with deferoxamine. Deferoxamine has a short $t_{1/2}$ (~1 h); therefore, a delay of at least 4 h after deferoxamine administration would be appropriate before measurements of serum iron and UIBC are repeated.

Organophosphate and Carbamate Insecticides

Acetylcholine is an essential neurotransmitter that affects parasympathetic synapses (autonomic and CNS), sympathetic preganglionic synapses, and the neuromuscular junction (see also prior section on Toxic Syndromes). Hydrolysis of acetylcholine by acetylcholinesterase, which is present in nerve tissue, normally limits the duration of action of this neurotransmitter and allows for normal synaptic function. Organophosphate (e.g., Malathion, Parathion, Diazinon, Dursban) and carbamate (e.g., Sevin and Furadan) insecticides (Figure 34-17) exert their toxicity by inhibiting the action of acetylcholinesterase and thereby causing a pronounced cholinergic response.[24,78,92,140,437] Enzyme inhibition is the consequence of phosphorylation (organophosphates) or carbamylation (carbamates) of the cholinesterase-active site serine hydroxyl group. The resulting alkylphosphorylserine bond undergoes spontaneous hydrolysis with subsequent enzyme reactivation at very slow to essentially nonexistent rates, depending on the size of the alkyl groups. Moreover, some phosphorylated enzyme complexes, especially those with a secondary alkyl group, lose an alkyl group at variable rates (generally 24 to 48 hours) to form a phosphoryl oxyanion serine bond that is completely resistant to even pharmacologically mediated hydrolysis (Figure 34-18). This dealkylation reaction, termed enzyme "aging," is probably mediated by enzyme active-site histidine and glutamate side chains.[401] In contrast to the phosphoryl-serine bond, the carbamyl-serine bond undergoes spontaneous hydrolysis with regeneration of enzyme activity (24 to 48 hours). For this reason and because of poor CNS penetration, carbamate insecticide neurotoxicity is less severe and of shorter duration than that for the organophosphates.

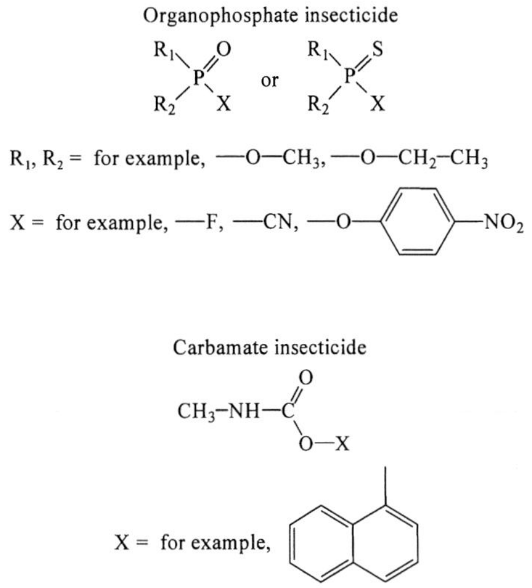

Organophosphate insecticide

$R_1R_2P(=O)X$ or $R_1R_2P(=S)X$

R_1, R_2 = for example, —O—CH_3, —O—CH_2—CH_3

X = for example, —F, —CN, —O—C_6H_4—NO_2

Carbamate insecticide

CH_3—NH—C(=O)—O—X

X = for example, (naphthyl)

Figure 34-17 General chemical structures for organophosphate and carbamate insecticides.

Excess synaptic acetylcholine stimulates muscarinic receptors (peripheral and CNS) and stimulates but then depresses or paralyzes nicotinic receptors.[437] Activation of peripheral muscarinic receptors causes signs and symptoms described by the mnemonics SLUDGE or DUMB BELS, defined earlier.

The CNS neurotoxic effects include restlessness, agitation, lethargy, confusion, slurred speech, seizures, coma, cardiorespiratory depression, or death.

Stimulation or paralysis of nicotinic receptors at the neuromuscular junction causes muscle fasciculations, cramping, weakness, and respiratory muscle paralysis; stimulation of

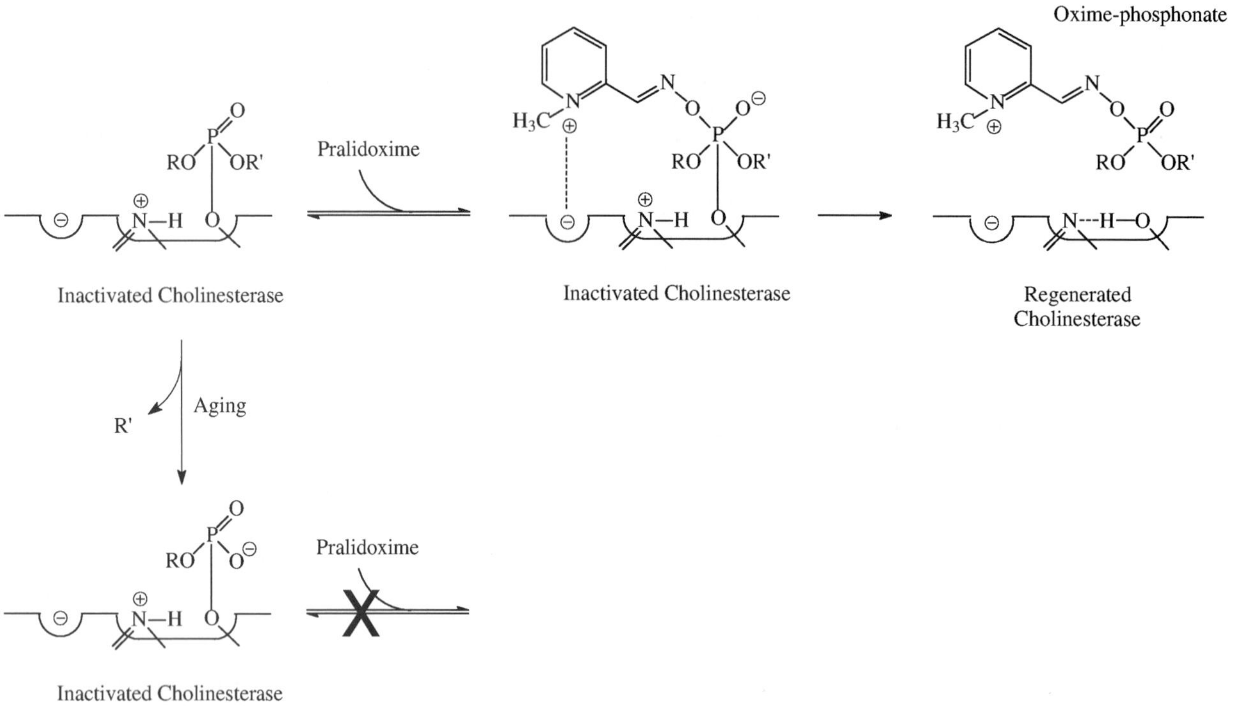

Figure 34-18 Reactivation of phosphorylated acetylcholinesterase by pralidoxime; formation of "aged" phosphorylated enzyme, which does not reactivate. The active site catalytic triad of serine, histidine, and glutamate is depicted by —OH, =NH—, and a negative charge, respectively.

nicotinic receptors at sympathetic ganglia results in hypertension, tachycardia, pallor, and mydriasis.

The actual signs and symptoms observed depend on the balance of muscarinic and nicotinic receptor activation. While miosis (muscarinic action) is most common, it may not always be present, and indeed mydriasis (nicotinic action) may occur. Likewise tachycardia (nicotinic effect) may be present rather than bradycardia (muscarinic action). Death most commonly results from respiratory failure, a consequence of nicotinic receptor–mediated muscle paralysis, combined with muscarinic-facilitated bronchorrhea, bronchoconstriction, and CNS depression.

Specific therapy for organophosphate and carbamate insecticide poisoning includes the administration of atropine (see Figure 34-15) to block the muscarinic (but not nicotinic) actions of acetylcholine. In addition, pralidoxime is given to reactivate cholinesterase. Pralidoxime binds to the cholinesterase catalytic site and via nucleophilic attack by its oxime group, dephosphorylates or decarbamylates the serine group (Figure 34-18). Pralidoxime is ineffective in reactivating the "aged" form of the phosphorylated enzyme. The administration of pralidoxime may not be necessary in cases of carbamate insecticide poisoning because carbamylated cholinesterase spontaneously reactivates within a few hours. In fact, pralidoxime is considered contraindicated in these cases by some authors, because cholinesterase inhibition by carbaryl (Sevin), but not other carbamates, may be enhanced by pralidoxime. Others administer pralidoxime in either case, because the particular insecticide ingested may not be known.[78,92] A more potent bisquaternary oxime, obidoxime, is available outside the United States.

Three neurological sequelae of organophosphate poisoning may occur after the initial cholinergic crisis has responded to atropine and oxime therapy. In what is referred to as intermediate syndrome,[403] paralysis of proximal limb muscles, neck flexors, cranial nerves, and respiratory muscles may occur 24 to 96 hours following cholinergic resolution. Respiratory muscle paralysis may be severe enough to result in death. This phenomenon, caused by excessive nicotinic receptor stimulation, may result from redistribution of lipophilic organophosphates from adipose tissue and/or from inadequate oxime therapy. In another syndrome, organophosphate-induced delayed neuropathy (OPIDN),[1] weakness of extremities, ataxia, and eventually paralysis may occur 1 to 3 weeks following severe intoxication. Respiratory muscles are not affected. It is believed that this peripheral neuropathy is the consequence of phosphorylation and inhibition of an axonal-membrane enzyme that is designated neuropathy target esterase. Alternatively, phosphorylation and activation of a Ca^{2+}/calmodulin kinase may in turn enhance proteolysis of neuronal cytoskeletal proteins and cause structural changes in neurofilaments, resulting in impaired axonal transport.[1] Finally, extrapyramidal symptoms similar to Parkinson's disease have very rarely occurred several days after cholinergic crisis resolution. A favorable response was observed with an antiparkinsonian agent.[14]

Acetylcholinesterase similar to that in nerve tissue is also present in erythrocytes, and its measurement is useful for the diagnosis of organophosphate or carbamate insecticide poisoning (see Chapter 21). A different cholinesterase, butyrylcholinesterase (pseudocholinesterase), is present in serum and is also inhibited by these insecticides. The activity of butyrylcholinesterase declines and returns to normal more rapidly than that for the red cell enzyme.

Butyrylcholinesterase is synthesized in the liver, and its serum activity is influenced by liver disease and other acute or chronic illness. Thus red cell cholinesterase activity theoretically should correlate more closely with the degree of neurotoxicity. In acute poisoning, symptoms generally begin when cholinesterase activity is inhibited by about 50% of the lower limits of normal and this degree of inhibition is of diagnostic value. However, the degree of cholinesterase inhibition generally does not correlate well with the clinical severity of poisoning. Interpretation of test results is made more difficult because of considerable individual variability of normal levels.

Measurement of serum butyrylcholinesterase activity is easier to perform than that for red cell cholinesterase and thus is more likely to be performed in hospital clinical laboratories (see Chapter 21). These measurements are useful for the diagnosis of acute ingestions or for monitoring chronic exposure. They may be less useful in instances of carbamate insecticide poisoning because of spontaneous enzyme activity regeneration. Therapy for acute ingestion is guided by history and clinical presentation, not by cholinesterase activity. However, monitoring serum butyrylcholinesterase activity may have prognostic value in organophosphate poisoning.[15] The most definitive means of determining organophosphate or carbamate insecticide exposure is by measurement of their urinary metabolites, generally by GC-MS[379] or GC-MS-MS.[62] Such determination is not necessary nor generally available for emergency management of acutely poisoned patients.

Drugs of Abuse

Drug use and abuse are widespread in society, and public awareness has been heightened as to their impact on public safety and on lost productivity in industry. To resolve these issues, governmental, industrial, educational, and sports agencies are increasingly requiring drug testing of prospective and existing employees, students, and participants in professional and amateur athletics. Moreover, drug abuse during pregnancy is of concern, both medically and socially. Testing for drugs of abuse may also be a medical requirement for (1) organ transplantation candidates, (2) pain management clinics, (3) drug abuse treatment programs, and (4) psychiatric programs.[358] Drug testing for these purposes represents a significant activity for toxicology laboratories.

Testing for drugs of abuse usually involves testing a single urine specimen for a number of drugs. It should be noted, however, that a single urine drug test detects only fairly recent drug use; it cannot differentiate casual use from chronic drug abuse. The latter requires sequential drug testing and clinical evaluation. Moreover, urine drug testing cannot determine degree of impairment, the dose of drug taken, or the exact time of use. Many of these issues were described in detail at the 1987 Arnold O. Beckman Conference[126] and in a report by the Committee on Substance Abuse Testing.[258] Because of these and other limitations of testing for drugs in urine, there is growing interest in the use of alternate biological specimens for drug testing (see section on Alternate Specimens).

Drug testing results for nonmedical purposes may be the sole evidence for punitive action or denial of individual rights. Therefore this testing should be considered a forensic toxicology activity, requiring the highest standards of analytical methodology, specimen security, and documentation. Moreover, laboratories engaged in this testing should be appropriately certified by the Substance Abuse and Mental Health Service Administration (SAMHSA)* of the U.S. Department of Health and Human Services or the Forensic Urine Drug Testing program sponsored jointly by the American Association for Clinical Chemistry and the College of American Pathologists.

Several techniques are used during the collection of a urine specimen or subsequently in the laboratory to guard against attempts by a donor to alter the specimen in a manner that may prevent drug detection. These tactics may include the exchange of urine from a drug-free individual, or dilution of the specimen to below cutoff limits with tap or toilet water, by excessive consumption of water, or by use of a diuretic. Also, readily available adulterants, such as detergent, bleach, salt, alkali, ammonia, or acid, may be added to the specimen in an attempt to interfere with immunoassay screening procedures. Other more sophisticated adulterants specifically marketed to avoid drug detection include glutaraldehyde (Urine Aid; Clear Choice), nitrite (Klear; Whizzies), chromate (Urine Luck; Sweet Pee's Spoiler), and a combination of peroxide and peroxidase (Stealth). These adulterants also interfere with immunoassays to variable degrees and the oxidizing agents (nitrite, chromate, and peroxide/peroxidase) may result in destruction of morphine, codeine, and the principal metabolite resulting from marijuana use, thus interfering with their GC-MS confirmation as well as immunoassays.[†]

Direct observation of urine collection is the most stringent means to guard against specimen exchange or adulteration. However, an individual's right to privacy and dignity must be weighed against the need for the highest degree of certainty of specimen integrity. Alternative measures to prevent specimen adulteration include a (1) limitation on clothing or other personal belongings allowed in the specimen collection area, (2) addition of coloring agent to toilet water, and (3) inactivation of the hot water tap. In addition, a number of validity checks for specimen integrity may be made at the collection site and at the testing site. Validity testing criteria have been established by the DHHS for the

*Formerly the National Institute on Drug Abuse (NIDA).

[†]References 98, 99, 353, 354, 453, 454, 488.

TABLE 34-7 Specimen Validity Check Reagents

	pH	Creatinine	Specific Gravity	Nitrite	Glutaraldehyde	Chromate	Bleach	Oxidants	Peroxidase/ Oxidants
Test Strips									
Adulta Check 6	✓	✓		✓	✓	✓		✓	
Adulta Check 10	✓*	✓	✓	✓	✓	✓	✓	✓	✓
Intect 7	✓	✓	✓	✓	✓	✓	✓		
Mask Ultra Screen	✓	✓	✓	✓			✓		
Liquid[†]									
SVT	✓	✓	✓	✓	✓	✓	✓	✓	✓
Detect Test	✓	✓	✓	✓		✓			

*pH 5-9; pH 2-12.
[†]Separate reagent for each analyte.

drug testing program mandated for U.S. federal employees.[432] According to these criteria, the specimen must be examined for unusual color, odor, foaming, or precipitate and its temperature should be 90 °F to 100 °F (32 °C to 38 °C) when determined within 4 minutes of collection. A specimen is reported as dilute when the specific gravity is >1.0010 but <1.0030 and the creatinine >2 mg/dL but ≤20 mg/dL. Although specimen recollection is not mandated, the employer may require direct observation of the next regular urine collection. A substituted specimen is defined by a specific gravity ≤1.0010 or ≥1.0200 and creatinine <2 mg/dL, whereas an adultered urine is one with pH <3 or ≥11, nitrite >500 µg/mL (much lower concentrations occur with some urinary tract infections), or if a specific adulterant is detected and confirmed. A specimen is invalid if the pH is ≥ 3 < 4.5 or ≥ 9 < 11, if the creatinine and specific gravity are inconsistent, if nitrite is ≥ 200 < 500 µg/mL, or if the presence of other adulterants is suspected. In such cases, the urine specimen is rejected and generally not tested for drugs. The finding of a substituted or an adulterated specimen is deemed equivalent to a refusal to test and would result in the removal of the individual from safety-sensitive duties. Commercial reagents for validity testing are available in both test strip and liquid form (Table 34-7).

The urine should be collected in tamper-proof specimen cups, and a chain of custody maintained to identify all individuals involved in specimen collection, transfer, and testing. Specimens that test positive should be stored frozen for a minimum of 1 year. Detailed information on the collection and processing of specimens for drug testing has been described in the federal rules for employee drug testing[432,433] and in the federal regulations promulgated by the Department of Transportation[4] and the Nuclear Regulatory Commission.[206]

Workplace drug testing generally is restricted to alcohol (see section on alcohols) and a few drugs that have a high abuse potential, some of which are illicit. Depending on the nature of the testing program, this may involve testing for a select number of the following drugs or drug classes:

Amphetamine/methamphetamine
Barbiturates
Benzodiazepines
Cannabinoids
Cocaine
LSD
Methylenedioxyamphetamine (MDA)
Methylenedioxymethamphetamine (MDMA)
Methylenedioxyethylamphetamine (MDEA)
Methadone
Opiates
PCP
Propoxyphene

Drugs given in italics are included in a panel for testing employees of the U.S. government.[432] This panel is also used in many other testing programs and because of their widespread use is known as the "NIDA five."

Testing programs for participants engaged in athletic competition are typically much more extensive and include assays for a larger group of drugs, including stimulants, β-blockers, diuretics, and anabolic steroids. A listing of the banned drugs included in the Olympic testing programs can be found on the Canadian Center for Ethics in Sports web page (http://www.cces.ca).

Initial screening tests for the previously listed drugs are typically immunoassays (e.g., EMIT, FPIA, CEDIA, microparticle immunoassay, and RIA; see Chapter 9). These assays are calibrated at established cutoff concentrations. Specimens yielding responses greater than the cutoff (threshold) value are considered positive, whereas values below the cutoff are considered negative. Cutoff values are not synonymous with assay detection limits. Instead the

TABLE 34-8 U.S. Government Drug Detection Cutoff Concentrations

	Immunoassay (ng/mL)		GC-MS (ng/mL)	
Drug or Drug Class	**HHS/DOT**	**DOD**	**HHS/DOT**	**DOD**
Amphetamines	1000	500		
Amphetamine			500	500
Methamphetamine			500*	500*,†
MDA				500
MDMA				500
MDEA				500
Barbiturates		200		
Amobarbital				200
Butalbital				200
Pentobarbital				200
Secobarbital				200
Cannabinoids	50	50		
THC-COOH			15	15
Cocaine metabolites	300	150		
Benzoylecgonine			150	100
LSD		0.5		0.2
Opiates	2000	2000		
Morphine			2000	4000
Codeine			2000	2000
6-Acetylmorphine			10	10
PCP	25	25	25	25

Data from Fed Reg 1988;53:11963; Fed Reg 1994;59:29908-81; Fed Reg 1997;62:51118-20; Irving J. Drug testing in the military: Technical and legal problems. Clin Chem 1988;34:637-40; Liu RH. Evaluation of common immunoassay kits for effective workplace drug testing. In Liu RH, Goldberger BA, Eds. Handbook of workplace drug testing. Washington DC: AACC Press, 1995:70; Newberry RJ. Drug urinalysis testing levels. Department of Defense Memorandum, 1997.

GC-MS, Gas chromatography-mass spectrometry; *HHS,* Department of Health and Human Services; *DOT,* Department of Transportation; *DOD,* Department of Defense; *MDA,* methylenedioxyamphetamine; *MDMA,* methylenedioxymethamphetamine; *MDEA,* methylenedioxyethylamphetamine; *PCP,* phencyclidine; *LSD,* lysergic acid diethylamide; *THC-COOH,* 11-nor-Δ^9-tetrahydrocannabinol-9-carboxylic acid.

*Also requires presence of amphetamine (≥200 ng/mL).

†Requires chiral analysis; S(+)-methamphetamine >20% of total.

cutoff is established higher than the detection limit (to ensure reliable measurement) but low enough to detect drug use within a reasonable time frame.

Immunoassays may not be specific for the tested drug. Similar drugs may result in a positive test; for example, pseudoephedrine, present in cold medications, may produce a positive response in immunoassays designed to detect amphetamine and methamphetamine. Therefore it is imperative that positive screening tests be confirmed by an alternate, more definitive test. The most widely accepted method for drug confirmation is GC-MS. For further discussion of this technique, the reader is referred to Chapter 7. Liquid chromatography-tandem mass spectrometry is also used for rapid detection of drugs of abuse.[60,331,472]

For confirmation, quantitative drug measurements are performed using selective ion monitoring with GC-MS. Cutoff values for confirmation are established at or generally below cutoff values for the initial screening tests (Table 34-8; also see Table 34-9 for newly proposed cutoff values). The result may be reported as positive or negative relative to the cutoff value. However, the actual concentration may be helpful when interpreting morphine and codeine results (discussed later in this chapter) and when monitoring individuals enrolled in drug treatment programs. In the latter case, subjects who test positive but who have decreasing values on sequential testing may be judged abstinent, whereas those whose values suddenly increase are likely noncompliant. For this purpose, it is essential to normalize the drug concentration to urine creatinine level (nanograms of drug per milligram of creatinine). This will help compensate for fluctuations in absolute drug concentration related to physiological variation in urine dilution or concentration.[47,294]

In the following sections, the pharmacological and analytical aspects of commonly measured drugs will be discussed. Several different extraction and derivatization procedures have been used for confirmation of these drugs by GC-MS. Several of these methods are briefly described below and in more detail on this book's accompanying Evolve site (http://evolve.elsevier.com/Tietz/textbook/).

TABLE 34-9 SAMHSA Draft Guidelines for Drug Assay Cutoff Values

	Urine ng/mL	Oral Fluid ng/mL	Sweat ng/patch	Hair pg/mg
Initial Test				
THC metabolite[a]	50	4[b]	4	1
Cocaine metabolite	150	20	25	500
Opiates[c]	2000	40	25	200
PCP	25	10	20	300
Amphetamines[d]	500	50	25	500
MDMA	500	50	25	500
Confirmatory Test				
THC parent		2	1	
THC metabolite	15			0.05
Cocaine				500[e]
Benzoylecgonine(BE) 100	8[e,f]	25[e,f]	50[e]	
Morphine	2000	40	25	200
Codeine	2000	40	25	200
6-AM	10[g]	4	25	200[g,h]
PCP	25	10	20	300
Amphetamine	250	50	25	300
Methamphetamine	250[i]	50[j]	25[j]	300[k]
MDMA	250	50	25	300
MDA	250	50	25	300
MDEA	250	50	25	300

Substance Abuse and Mental Health Administration draft guidelines for federal workplace testing program. http://workplace.samhsa.gov/ResourceCenter/DT/FA/GuidelinesDraft4.htm (Accessed March 2005).

[a] Δ^9-THC-COOH.

[b] Parent and metabolite.

[c] Initial test for 6-AM allowed at cutoffs of 10 ng/mL (urine), 4 ng/mL (oral fluid), 25 ng/patch (sweat), and 200 pg/mg (hair).

[d] S(+)-methamphetamine calibrator.

[e] Cocaine ≥ cutoff and BE/cocaine ≥0.05 or cocaethylene ≥50 pg/mg or norcocaine ≥50 pg/mg.

[f] Cocaine or BE.

[g] May be reported alone if initial and confirmatory tests are above cutoffs.

[h] Must contain morphine ≥200 ng/mg.

[i] Must contain amphetamine ≥100 ng/mL.

[j] Must contain amphetamine ≥ limit of detection (LOD).

[k] Must contain amphetamine ≥50 ng/mg.

Amphetamine, Methamphetamine, and Related Sympathomimetic Amines

Amphetamine and methamphetamine (Figure 34-19) are CNS stimulant drugs that have limited legitimate pharmacological use.[201] They are used to treat narcolepsy, obesity, and attention-deficit hyperactivity disorders. However, they produce an initial euphoria and have a high abuse potential. Other sympathomimetic amines that also have high potential for abuse include the "designer" amphetamines, ephedrine, pseudoephedrine, phenylpropanolamine, and methylphenidate (Ritalin).

Pharmacological Response

Amphetamine and Methamphetamine. These drugs are sympathomimetic amines that have a stimulating effect on both the central and peripheral nervous systems. They (1) increase blood pressure, heart rate, body temperature, and motor activity, (2) relax bronchial muscle, and (3) depress the appetite. Abuse of these drugs may lead to strong psychic dependence, marked tolerance, and mild physical dependence associated with tachycardia, increased blood pressure, restlessness, irritability, insomnia, personality changes, and the severe form of chronic intoxication psychosis similar to schizophrenia. These unpleasant responses reinforce the repetitive use of the drugs to maintain the "high." In extreme cases, addicts may have "speed runs," in which large intravenous (IV) doses are used for several days during which they do not sleep or eat. This is followed, when exhaustion intervenes, by prolonged sleep for 1 or more days after which they awaken hungry but depressed, leading to repetition of the cycle.[2] Tolerance and psychological dependence develop with repeated use of amphetamines.[201] Long-

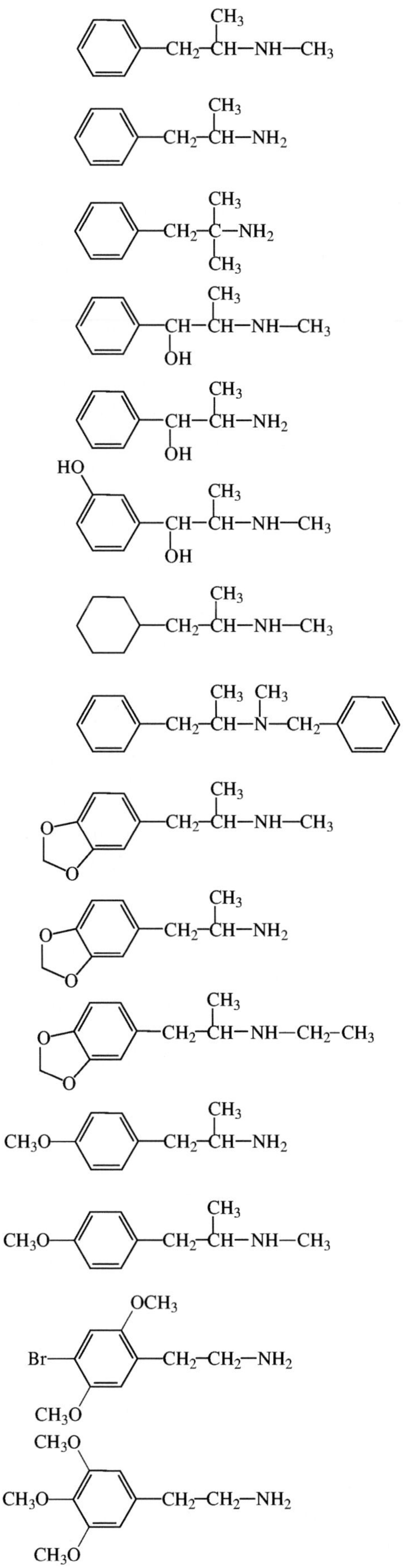

Methamphetamine

Amphetamine

Phentermine

Ephedrine/Pseudoephedrine*

Phenylpropanolamine

Phenylephrine

Propylhexedrine

Benzphetamine

Methylenedioxy-methamphetamine (MDMA)

Methylenedioxyamphetamine (MDA)

Methylenedioxyethylamphetamine (MDEA)

Paramethoxyamphetamine (PMA)

Paramethoxymethamphetamine (PMMA)

4-Bromo-2,5-dimethoxyphenyl-ethylamine (2 C-B)

Mescaline

Figure 34-19 Chemical structure of sympathomimetic amines. *Ephedrine and pseudoephedrine are diastereoisomers.

term effects may include depression and impaired memory and motor skills, probably caused by a decrease in dopamine transporters and by damage to dopaminergic and serotonergic neurons (see below).

The CNS stimulatory effects of amphetamine and methamphetamine result from their ability to enhance presynaptic release of the neurotransmitter catecholamines norepinephrine and dopamine at low to moderate dose and of serotonin at high dose and to a lesser degree to inhibit their neuronal reuptake.[201] Consequently the neurotransmitter content in the synaptic cleft is increased, resulting in enhanced postsynaptic activation. The CNS effects of norepinephrine are less well understood compared with its peripheral manifestation, but it is believed to contribute to increased mental alertness, lack of fatigue, and an anorectic effect. Dopamine regulates feeling of pleasure, emotion, motivation, and movement. It is thought to be responsible for the euphoria associated with amphetamine use. Excessive dopaminergic activity may produce acute choreoathetosis (random involuntary muscle movements) and paranoid psychosis. Serotonin modulates mood, emotion, sleep, cognition, appetite, pain sensation, temperature regulation, motor activity, sensory perception, sexual behavior, and pituitary release of antidiuretic hormone (ADH). Excessive serotonergic stimulation may lead to what is referred to as the serotonin syndrome. Symptoms of the serotonin syndrome include shivering, myoclonus (muscle spasm), muscle rigidity, tremor, hyperthermia, tachycardia, diaphoresis, hypertension progressing to hypotension, agitation, seizures, and coma. If untreated, lactic acidosis, rhabdomyolysis, myoglobinuria, acute renal failure, hepatic failure, and adult respiratory syndrome may ensue. Excessive activation of serotonergic neurons is a prominent feature of most hallucinogenic drugs (e.g., MDMA, LSD, PCP). Peripheral adrenergic activation may result in increased blood pressure, cardiac arrhythmias, diaphoresis, and mydriasis.

The optical isomers of amphetamine and methamphetamine exhibit stereoselective pharmacological properties. The CNS activity of S(+)-amphetamine is three to four times greater than of R(−)-amphetamine, but the latter drug has more potent cardiovascular effects than the former.[201] Moreover, amphetamine is metabolized primarily by oxidative deamination, a process that is stereoselective for S(+)-amphetamine.[73] Consequently, the elimination half-life for R(−)-amphetamine may be as much as 40% longer than that for S(+)-amphetamine.[468] In addition to hepatic metabolism, amphetamine is eliminated as unchanged drug in urine; the extent of such elimination is dependent on urine pH. Normally, about 30% of a dose is excreted unchanged, but this may vary from as much as 70% in acid urine to as low as 1% in alkaline urine.[26] The elimination half-life (renal excretion and hepatic metabolism) also varies with urine pH from 7 to 14 hours at acid pH to 18 to 34 hours at alkaline pH.[157] These effects of urine pH on the elimination of unchanged amphetamines are a consequence of tubular reabsorption of nonionized but not ionized amphetamine (pK_a 9.9).

The CNS effects of S(+)-methamphetamine are about 10 times greater than those of R(−)-methamphetamine, but the latter drug has greater vasoconstrictive properties than the former.[152,201] Because of the minimal CNS activity and thus low abuse potential, R(−)-methamphetamine is included in some nonprescription nasal inhalants (e.g., Vick's) for its vasoconstrictive properties.

A significant portion of a methamphetamine dose is eliminated unchanged in urine in a pH-dependent manner similar to that for amphetamine. In addition, methamphetamine is metabolized in liver primarily by hydroxylation and, to a lesser extent, by *N*-demethylation to amphetamine. Following methamphetamine ingestion, amphetamine is present in urine at a concentration that is roughly 10% of that for methamphetamine. The overall metabolism, including formation of amphetamine, is to some degree enantioselective for S(+)-methamphetamine.[46,73] Thus when racemic methamphetamine is ingested, urine specimens contain relatively more R(−)-methamphetamine than S(+)-methamphetamine, but a greater amount of S(+)-amphetamine than R(−)-amphetamine (Figure 34-20).[96,203]

Recreational use of methamphetamine and amphetamine congeners (so-called "designer" amphetamines) has had a resurgence in popularity, especially among young people who participate in all night dance parties called "raves" and in nightclubs.[11,447] At these events, loud, high-tempo "techno" music is played with a variety of strobe-type or other light effects and pyrotechnic displays. Various drugs, referred to as "club drugs," are commonly used at these events to enhance energy for prolonged partying and/or dancing (e.g., all night), to distort or enhance the visual and auditory sensations, and to promote social and physical interactions. The moniker "club drug" does not imply that recreational use is restricted to this social environment.

Designer Amphetamines. MDMA (3,4-methylenedioxymethamphetamine) is the most popular of the amphetamine-like "club drugs" and is known as ecstasy (Figure 34-19). Other "designer" amphetamines include 3,4-methylenedioxyethylamphetamine (MDEA; "Eve"), 3,4-methylenedioxyamphetamine (MDA), which is also a

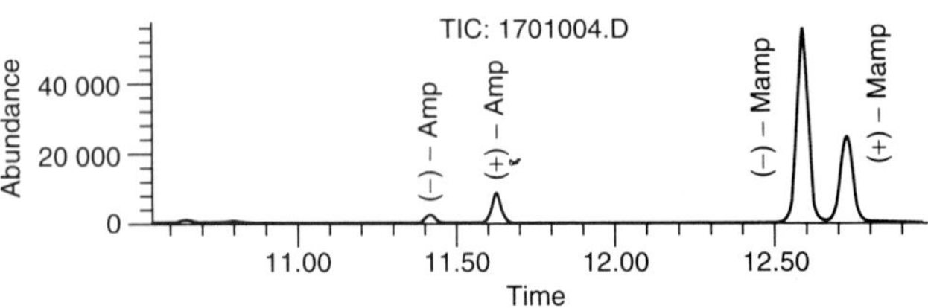

Figure 34-20 Chromatographic separation of amphetamine and methamphetamine stereoisomers after their reaction with R(−)-α-methoxy-α-trifluoromethyl-phenylacetyl chloride to form corresponding diastereoisomers. (−)-Amp and (+)-Amp, R(−)-, and S(+)-amphetamine, respectively. (−)-Mamp and (+)-Mamp, R(−)-, and S(+)-methamphetamine, respectively. This urine specimen is from an individual believed to have ingested racemic methamphetamine.

metabolite of MDMA; and 4-bromo-2,5-dimethoxyphenylethylamine (Nexus; 2 C-B).[172] Paramethoxyamphetamine (PMA) is an especially toxic designer amphetamine, which has resulted in several deaths from its unsuspected ingestion as an ecstasy substitute.[251]

MDMA has structural features in common with methamphetamine and the protypical hallucinogenic agent, mescaline (Figure 34-19), which is derived from the peyote cactus. MDMA produces a greater presynaptic release of serotonin than norepinephrine or dopamine. Consequently, it has considerably less CNS stimulant activity but greater hallucinogenic properties compared with methamphetamine. MDMA produces euphoria, enhanced pleasure and sociability, and heightened sensual arousal. Adverse effects include confusion, ataxia, restlessness, poor concentration, and psychoses. At higher doses, central and peripheral adrenergic responses similar to those described for amphetamine/methamphetamine ensue. Long-term consequences of its abuse include changes in mood, sleep disturbance, anxiety, and impairment in cognition and memory. These neuropsychiatric manifestations are a likely consequence of permanent damage to serotonergic neurons. Because of their popularity, abuse potential, and serious short- and long-term toxicity, SAMHSA has proposed to include MDA, MDMA, and MDEA in the mandatory federal workplace drug testing program.[432]

MDMA is a chiral compound in which the S(+)-enantiomer possesses the greater pharmacological activity. MDMA undergoes stereoselective demethylation to MDA, with the rate of conversion of S(+)-MDMA to S(+)-MDA exceeding that for R(−)-MDMA to R(−)-MDA. Consequently, the concentrations in urine of R(−)-MDMA and S(+)-MDA are greater than those for S(+)-MDMA and R(−)-MDA subsequent to ingestion of racemic MDMA.[148,197]

In overdose, the toxic manifestations of amphetamine, methamphetamine, and MDMA have features of adrenergic excess and the serotonin syndrome. These symptoms include dizziness, tremor, irritability, hypertension progressing to hypotension, diaphoresis, mydriasis, cardiac arrhythmias, muscle rigidity, and if severe, hyperthermia, seizures, coma, and cerebral hemorrhage.[82,201] Agitation, muscle rigidity, hyperthermia, and diaphoresis, in combination, may lead to life-threatening dehydration and rhabdomyolysis with subsequent lactic acidosis, acute renal failure, and disseminated intravascular coagulopathy (DIC). Death most commonly results from hyperthermia, dysrhythmias, and cerebral hemorrhage. Dance club participants who ingest methamphetamine or MDMA are at increased risk of severe dehydration, rhabdomyolysis, and renal failure as a result of the intense physical exertion, hyperthermia, and excessive sweating. To guard against these toxic manifestations, these individuals ingest copious amounts of water, which combined with sodium loss in sweat and stimulation of ADH release by serotonin, especially in the case of MDMA, may result in profound hyponatremia with the potential to cause cerebral edema and seizures.

Treatment for sympathomimetic amine overdose involves general supportive measures. Acid diuresis will enhance the elimination of the amphetamines, but its use is controversial[91,185] and is certainly not without the risk of renal failure from precipitation of myoglobin (enhanced at acid pH) in renal tubules (myoglobinuria is the result of rhabdomyolysis).

Ephedrine and Pseudoephedrine. These amines are diastereoisomeric adrenergic agonists. Ephedrine causes more prominent bronchodilation (β-adrenergic action) than pseudoephedrine and is present in some nonprescription medications for the treatment of asthma. Many dietary supplements contain ephedra, the herbal form of ephedrine. These products are widely marketed for weight loss and are also used by some athletes who believe they enhance performance. Ephedra, containing pills have been sold as a safe "herbal ecstasy." Adverse effects of ephedrine and ephedra include elevated blood pressure, palpitations, agitation, psychiatric disturbances, myocardial infarction, seizures, cerebral hemorrhage, and death.[405] Adverse reactions are more likely with high dose, when co-ingested with caffeine or other stimulant drugs, or with preexisting cardiovascular disease or seizure disorders. A ban on ephedra sales has been instituted in the United States; it is also banned for athletic competition by the National Football League, the National Collegiate Athletic Association, and the International Olympic Committee.

Pseudoephedrine is used for its vasoconstrictive properties (α-adrenergic action) as a nasal decongestant in a wide variety of cold remedies. Both 1R,1S(−)-ephedrine and 1S,1S(+)-pseudoephedrine have been popular starting products for the synthesis of S(+)-methamphetamine.[282] Because of this, the quantity per purchase of products containing these drugs is now restricted.

Phenylpropanolamine (PPA). Until recently, PPA was widely available in a number of nonprescription cold medications and diet control products. Adverse effects are similar to those described for ephedrine. In response to an FDA warning of increased risk of hemorrhagic stroke, especially in women, PPA has been withdrawn from the market by most manufacturers. Before this withdrawal, PPA was another popular starting product for synthesis of S(+)-methamphetamine.[282] PPA is also a metabolite of ephedrine and pseudoephedrine.

Methylphenidate (Ritalin). Ritalin is a sympathomimetic agent with psychostimulant properties similar to S(+)-amphetamine. It is widely used to treat attention deficit hyperactivity disorder (ADHD) in children and adults. There has been increasing diversion and abuse of methylphenidate among children and adults for its stimulant and purported aphrodisiac properties. In overdose, the clinical effects of methylphenidate are similar to those of amphetamine. Relatively few cases of serious overdose have been reported.

Methylphenidate is rapidly metabolized to ritalinic acid (Figure 34-21), which accounts for 60% to 89% of a dose

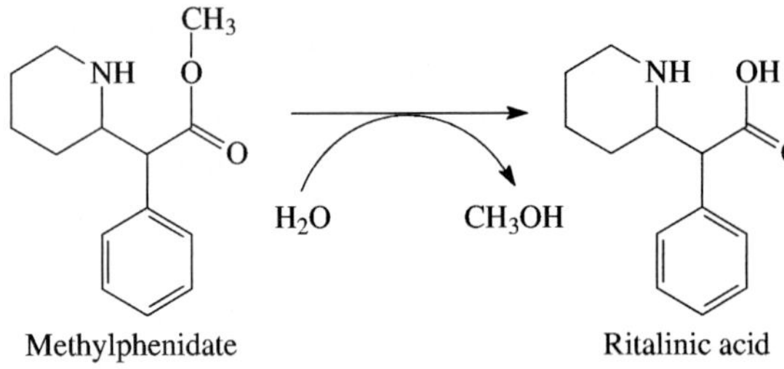

Methylphenidate → Ritalinic acid (H_2O, CH_3OH)

Figure 34-21 Metabolism of methylphenidate.

excreted in 24 hours. Less than 1% of the dose is excreted as the parent drug.[34]

The detection of methylphenidate compliance or abuse by urine drug assay is problematic, a phenomenon that may foster its abuse among individuals who are subjected to urine drug testing. Detection of the parent drug is made difficult by its generally low concentration, and ritalinic acid, present in much higher concentration, is difficult to extract and analyze by gas chromatographic techniques. It does not form a stable N,O-di-trimethylsilyl derivative, a probable consequence of the general instability of N-trimethylsilyl derivatives and the spatial proximity of the —NH and —COOH groups (Figure 34-21). Ritalinic acid may be analyzed directly by LC-tandem mass spectrometry,[134] or by GC-MS after sequential reactions with MSTFA and MBTFA to form the N-trifluoroacetyl,O-trimethylsilyl ester[134] or after methylation to re-form methylphenidate. Ritalinic acid may be isolated from urine using a dehydration procedure then methylated with dimethylformamide dimethyl acetal and the resulting methylphenidate analyzed by GC-MS.

Analytical Methodology[406]

The initial screening test for amphetamine and methamphetamine is typically immunoassay. For confirmation of a presumptive positive test, a quantitative drug measurement is performed using GC-MS.

Immunoassay. Immunoassays for amphetamine and methamphetamine have variable cross-reactivities with other sympathomimetic amines, such as ephedrine, pseudoephedrine, phenylpropanolamine, phentermine, methylenedioxyamphetamine (MDA), methylenedioxyethylamphetamine (MDEA), and methylenedioxymethamphetamine (MDMA) (see Figure 34-19). Many immunoassays are less reactive with MDA, MDMA, and MDEA compared with amphetamine and methamphetamine. A multiplex CEDIA assay has been introduced that employs a combination of separate monoclonal antibodies to amphetamine, methamphetamine, and MDMA.[285] At the proposed new SAMHSA screening cutoff of 500 ng/mL (Table 34-9), this assay has good sensitivity and specificity for these drugs compared with GC-MS. A single assay for MDMA based on enzyme multiplied immunoassay technology (DRI reagent) is also available along with on-site, single use test devices (see section on On-Site Drug Testing). False-positive results, due to the phenothiazine drugs chlorpromazine and promethazine, have been reported using the EMIT assay[421]; chloroquine produced false-positive response with CEDIA amphetamine reagent.[284] For forensic application, confirmation of immunoassay positive test results by GC-MS is mandatory. Liquid chromatography-tandem mass spectrometry is applicable for sensitive and specific direct detection of MDMA and MDA in urine.[331]

Chiral discrimination of methamphetamine isomers may be necessary to distinguish use of nonprescription nasal inhalants (R[−]-methamphetamine) from illicit use of S(+)-methamphetamine. Some immunoassays have high specificity for S(+)-methamphetamine. However, definitive enantio-discrimination requires the use of a chiral derivatization reagent to form diastereomers of R- and S-methamphetamine, which may be resolved using conventional GC-MS (see Figure 34-20).[94,152,209] The Department of Defense requires chiral resolution of methamphetamine isomers. For the test to be considered positive for illicit methamphetamine use, S(+)-methamphetamine must be >20% of the total methamphetamine content (Table 34-8).

Several prescription drugs are metabolized to methamphetamine (and subsequently to amphetamine) or to amphetamine.[95] For instance, selegiline (Eldepryl), used to treat Parkinson's disease, is metabolized to R(−)-methamphetamine and R(−)-amphetamine. The (+)-isomer of benzphetamine (Didrex®), administered as an anorectic agent, is also metabolized to methamphetamine and amphetamine, presumably the S(+)-isomers. Chiral discrimination would rule out illicit use of methamphetamine in the case of selegiline but not benzphetamine. However, benzphetamine is a schedule III drug, so its use without a prescription is illicit. Other prescription drugs, not legally available in the United States, that are metabolized to methamphetamine (and amphetamine) include dimethylamphetamine, famprofazone, fencamine, and furfenorex; those metabolized to amphetamine include amphetaminil, clobenzorex, ethylamphetamine, fenethylline, fenproporex, mefenorex, mesocarb, and prenylamine.

Gas Chromatography-Mass Spectrometry. A positive screening result for amphetamine or methamphetamine (or MDA, MDEA, and MDMA) obtained by immunoassay is confirmed by GC-MS analysis of the urine specimen. A GC-MS method for amphetamine and methamphetamine that can be adapted to include MDA, MDMA, and MDEA is included in the Chapter 34 Appendix that is found on this book's accompanying Evolve site (http://evolve.elsevier.com/Tietz/textbook/). With this method, it should be noted that specimens containing ephedrine or pseudoephedrine occasionally have been reported to test positive for methamphetamine when 4-carbethoxyhexafluorobutyryl chloride (4-CB) is used as a derivatizing reagent.[443]

To guard against a false-positive report of methamphetamine owing to the presence of ephedrine or pseudoephedrine, SAMHSA regulations require identification of methamphetamine (cutoff, 500 ng/mL) and of its metabolite, amphetamine (cutoff, 200 ng/mL). Amphetamine-4-CB is not formed from α-hydroxyamines. However, the requirement for amphetamine ≥200 ng/mL may not be satisfied in some cases of known methamphetamine ingestion, especially during the initial 12 hours postdose period, leading to false-negative results.[457,490] To increase detection rate for amphetamine and methamphetamine, SAMHSA has proposed[432] a reduction of the screening and confirmation cutoff from 1000 ng/mL and 500 ng/mL to 500 ng/mL and 250 ng/mL, respectively. Methamphetamine would require the presence of at least 100 ng/mL amphetamine metabolite for a positive result. In a 2002 study,[345] these lower cutoff values increased the detection rate for methamphetamine by 48% compared with current cutoff values. Moreover, the highest detection rate for methamphetamine was achieved by use of the 250 ng/mL cutoff with elimination of the amphetamine requirement. In the described procedure, periodate oxidation before derivatization destroys α-hydroxyamines and therefore eliminates possible false report of methamphetamine owing to their presence.[147]

Barbiturates

The barbiturates have a low therapeutic index and a relatively high abuse potential. Because of their rapid onset and short duration of action, the short- to intermediate-acting barbiturates are used as sedative-hypnotics (amobarbital, butabarbital, butalbital, pentobarbital, and secobarbital) and are those most commonly abused. The longer acting barbiturates (mephobarbital and phenobarbital), used primarily for their anticonvulsant properties, are rarely abused.

Pharmacological Response

Barbiturates suppress CNS neuronal activity and thus have sedative and hypnotic properties.[186] This CNS suppression is a result of barbiturate-enhanced activation of the inhibitory GABA-ergic neuronal system mediated by the neurotransmitter γ-aminobutyric acid (GABA).[86] Postsynatic $GABA_A$ receptors are multisubunit transmembrane Cl^- conductance channels, which when activated by GABA open to allow flow of Cl^- into the neuron, with subsequent hyperpolarization and inhibition of electrical transmission. At low dose, some barbiturates bind to the $GABA_A$ receptors and enhance their response to GABA. At a higher dose, barbiturate binding results in prolonged opening of the Cl^- channel, without the necessity for GABA binding. In addition, barbiturates suppress excitatory glutamate-responsive AMPA (alpha-amino-3-OH-4-isoxozole propionic acid) ion-gated receptor subtypes.

Because of their low therapeutic index and high potential for abuse, the barbiturates have largely been replaced by the safer benzodiazepines for sedative and hypnotic purposes. Nevertheless, they continue to be available for this purpose or in combination with other analgesic, antihypertensive, antiasthmatic, antispasmodic, or antidiuretic drugs. The combination of barbiturates, such as butalbital with analgesic preparations, is ironic. Not only do barbiturates lack analgesic properties, but at low doses they antagonize the effects of analgesics. Phenobarbital is effective as an anticonvulsant drug (see Chapter 33), and short- and ultrashort-acting barbiturates (Table 34-10) are used for IV anesthesia. Anesthetic doses of barbiturates, such as pentobarbital, are also used to reduce intracranial pressure from cerebral edema associated with head trauma, surgery, or cerebral ischemia.[295] For the induction of this therapeutic coma, sufficient pentobarbital is administered IV to achieve a serum pentobarbital concentration between about 20 and 50 μg/mL. Therefore appropriate analytical methods are necessary to monitor serum pentobarbital concentrations in these circumstances. Moreover, barbiturates continue to be subject to abuse and are a source of intentional or, less commonly, accidental drug intoxication. Measurement of the common barbiturates in serum or urine can aid in the diagnosis and management of barbiturate intoxication.

The general formula for barbiturates is given in Table 34-10. Any change in the constituents at position five that confers an increase in lipid solubility typically results in increased onset of action, decreased duration of action, and increased potency. Moreover an increase in hydrophobic properties also leads to more rapid and extensive hepatic metabolic clearance and thus to decreased urinary elimination of an unchanged drug.

The classification of barbiturates as "ultrashort-acting," "short-acting," "intermediate-acting," and "long-acting" refers to the duration of effect and not to the elimination half-life. The duration of action is determined by the rate of distribution into brain and subsequent redistribution to other tissues.[86]

The major manifestations of barbiturate intoxication are CNS, cardiovascular, and respiratory depression. Severe intoxication results in coma, hypothermia, hypotension, and cardiorespiratory arrest.

Appropriate treatment for barbiturate intoxication includes general cardiopulmonary support and measures to prevent further drug absorption and to enhance elimination. Urine alkalinization may enhance the elimination of long-acting barbiturates (e.g., phenobarbital and barbital) but has little effect on intermediate-, short-, or ultrashort-acting barbiturates.

Once filtered by the glomerulus, a nonionized drug may be appreciably reabsorbed by the tubules. The goal of alkalinization is to maintain the urine pH between 7.5 and 8.5. In this pH range, a large fraction of an acidic drug will be ionized, and its elimination in urine will thus be enhanced.

For urine alkalinization to be effective, the drug should have low plasma protein binding, be appreciably eliminated in urine as an unchanged drug, and have a pK_a below 7.4. From an examination of Table 34-10, only phenobarbital (and other long-acting barbiturates [e.g., barbital]) fulfills these criteria. The primary route of elimination of ultra-short-, short-, and intermediate-acting barbiturates is by hepatic metabolism. Thus with the exception of aprobarbital, only small amounts are eliminated in urine as an unchanged drug. Moreover, at pH 8.0, only about 50% of a

TABLE 34-10 Characteristics of Barbiturates

(General structure: barbituric acid ring with N1–H, C2=O, N3–H, C4=O, C6=O, and substituents R1 and R2 at C5)

Barbiturate	Duration of Action (hr)	Half-life (hr)	Therapeutic Concentration (μg/mL)	Toxic Concentration (μg/mL)	% Protein Bound	% Excreted Unchanged in Urine	pK_a	R_1	R_2
Ultrashort-Acting									
Thiopental*	0.5	6-7	1-5 (hypnotic) 7-130 (anesthesia)	>10	75-90	0.3	7.6	$—CH_2CH_3$	$—CH(CH_3)CH_2CH_2CH_3$
Short-Acting									
Butalbital	3-4	34-42	–	–	26	3	7.9	$—CH_2CH{=}CH_2$	$—CH_2CH(CH_3)CH_3$
Pentobarbital	3-4	15-30	1-5	>10	65	1	7.9	$—CH_2CH_3$	$—CH(CH_3)CH_2CH_2CH_3$
Secobarbital	3-4	19-34	1-2	>5	46-70	5	7.9	$—CH_2CH{=}CH_2$	$—CH(CH_3)CH_2CH_2CH_3$
Intermediate-Acting									
Amobarbital	6-8	8-42	1-5	>10	59	1-3	7.9	$—CH_2CH_3$	$—CH_2CH_2CH(CH_3)CH_3$
Aprobarbital	6-8	14-34	–	–	55-70	13-24	8.1	$—CH_2CH{=}CH_2$	$—CH(CH_3)CH_3$
Butabarbital	6-8	34-42	–	–	26	5-9	7.9	$—CH_2CH_3$	$—CH(CH_3)CH_2CH_3$
Long-Acting									
Phenobarbital	10-12	40-140	15-40	>65	45-50	25-33	7.2	$—CH_2CH_3$	$—C_6H_5$

Data from Baselt RC. Disposition of toxic drugs and chemicals in man. 7th ed. Foster City, CA: Biomedical Publications, 2004; Tietz NW, Ed. Clinical guide to laboratory tests. Philadelphia: WB Saunders Co, 1995; and Physician's desk reference. 56th ed. Montvale, NJ: Medical Economics, 2002.
*Oxygen at position 2 is replaced by sulfur.

short- or intermediate-acting barbiturate (pK_a 7.9 to 8.1) is ionized, whereas phenobarbital (pK_a 7.2) is about 85% ionized. Hemodialysis is effective in increasing the elimination of all barbiturates. However, it is more effective for long-acting barbiturates than for shorter-acting barbiturates because of differences in their lipid solubility and protein binding. Whereas urine alkalinization may increase the elimination of phenobarbital somewhat, it is considerably less effective than the process referred to as GI dialysis, which is mediated by the repeated oral administration of activated charcoal (multiple-dose activated charcoal, MDAC).[9,131]

The rationale for MDAC therapy is that drug secreted into the GI tract (along with a previously unabsorbed drug) is bound by charcoal and thus cannot be reabsorbed. Drugs that are amenable to this process are ones that have a small volume of distribution, low protein binding, and a prolonged elimination $t_{1/2}$ following overdose. Currently, MDAC is recommended only for the treatment of serious phenobarbital, theophylline, carbamazepine, quinine, and dapsone overdose.[9]

The barbiturates undergo extensive hepatic metabolism in which the C5 substituents are transformed to alcohols, phenols, ketones, or carboxylic acids; these metabolites may be excreted in urine in part as glucuronide conjugates. For some barbiturates (amobarbital and phenobarbital), *N*-glucosylation is an additional important metabolic trans-

TABLE 34-11 Urinary Excretion of Barbiturates and Metabolites

	PERCENT SINGLE DOSE EXCRETED IN URINE			
Barbiturate	**Parent**	**Hydroxy Derivatives**	***N*-Glucosyl Derivatives**	**Carboxylic Acids**
Amobarbital	1-3	30-50	29	5
Aprobarbital	8-18			
Butabarbital	5-9	2-3		24-34
Butalbital*	3	60		
Pentobarbital	1	88		
Phenobarbital	25-33	18-19	24-30	
Secobarbital	5	50		

From Baselt, R.C.: Disposition of Toxic Drugs and Chemicals in Man. 7th ed. Foster City, Calif., Biomedical Publications, 2004.
*In dogs; excretion in humans unknown.

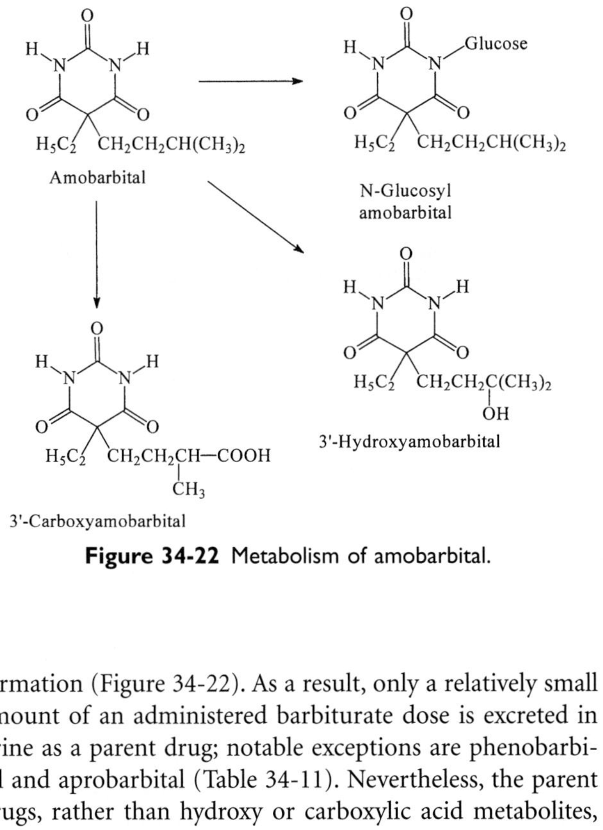

Amobarbital

N-Glucosyl amobarbital

3'-Hydroxyamobarbital

3'-Carboxyamobarbital

Figure 34-22 Metabolism of amobarbital.

formation (Figure 34-22). As a result, only a relatively small amount of an administered barbiturate dose is excreted in urine as a parent drug; notable exceptions are phenobarbital and aprobarbital (Table 34-11). Nevertheless, the parent drugs, rather than hydroxy or carboxylic acid metabolites, are targeted for detection in urine screening and confirmation procedures. This analytical approach is generally successful for barbiturates, because these drugs are ingested in sufficiently high doses to allow detection of unmetabolized drug in urine.

Analytical Methodology

Methods are available for detecting barbiturate overdose and abuse. To detect overdose, semiquantitative immunoassays suitable for detection of barbiturates in serum are available and useful for this purpose. Capillary GC is also useful for this purpose, and a capillary GC procedure is described in the Chapter 34 Appendix that is found on this book's accompanying Evolve site (http://evolve.elsevier.com/Tietz/textbook/). Barbiturate overdoses are also detected in urine by TLC (e.g., Toxi-Lab) or by immunoassay. To detect barbiturate abuse by analyzing urine specimens, immunoassay and GC-MS are the methods of choice for screening and confirmation, respectively.

Immunoassay. Commercial immunoassays for barbiturates include EMIT, FPIA, Triage, DPC RIA, Abuscreen Online, Abuscreen RIA, and CEDIA. All use secobarbital as the calibrator at a cutoff concentration of either 200 or 300 ng/mL. The degree of cross-reactivity of other barbiturates varies with each assay.[281] Little information is known concerning cross-reactivity with barbiturate metabolites, except for *p*-hydroxyphenobarbital, which is detected by several of the immunoassays.[281] The detection period in urine following ingestion of barbiturates varies somewhat with different assays and depends on the pharmacological properties of the drugs. The short- to intermediate-acting barbiturates may generally be detected for 1 to 4 days following use; long-acting barbiturates, such as phenobarbital, may be detected for several weeks after chronic use.[181]

Capillary Gas Chromatography. To detect barbiturate overdose, a serum sample can be analyzed for several barbiturates using the capillary GC technique described in the Chapter 34 Appendix that is found on this book's accompanying Evolve site (http://evolve.elsevier.com/Tietz/textbook/). In this method, aprobarbital is first added to an aliquot of the sample as an internal standard. Barbiturates in the aliquot are then extracted twice with diethyl ether, and the ether is dehydrated with solid sodium sulfate and then evaporated to dryness. The residue is dissolved in 50 μL of ethyl acetate, and an aliquot is injected into the gas chromatograph.

Gas Chromatography-Mass Spectrometry. In practice, a positive screening result for barbiturates obtained by immunoassay is confirmed by GC-MS analysis of the urine specimen. A GC-MS method for barbiturates is included in the Chapter 34 Appendix that is found on this book's accompanying Evolve site (http://evolve.elsevier.com/Tietz/textbook/).

In this method, a urine specimen that tests positive for barbiturates by immunoassay is extracted (liquid-liquid). The extract is then dried and treated with *N,N*-dimethylformamide dimethyl acetal to form methyl derivatives of the barbiturates. Following addition of a buffer, the methylated barbiturates are extracted with hexane and analyzed by GC-MS. Pentobarbital-D_5 and phenobarbital-D_5 are used as internal standards for quantitation.

Benzodiazepines

Benzodiazepines are any of a group of compounds having a common molecular structure and acting similarly as depressants of the CNS.

Pharmacological Response

Benzodiazepines have anxiolytic, sedative-hypnotic, muscle relaxant, and anticonvulsant properties. They are among the most commonly prescribed drugs in the western hemisphere because of their efficacy, safety, low addiction potential, minimal side effects, and high public demand for sedative and anxiolytic agents; they have largely replaced barbiturates for sedative-hypnotic use.[86,149,288] Thirteen benzodiazepines are currently approved for use in the United States (Table 34-12). Qualitatively, they all have similar pharmacological effects. Specific clinical applications are largely determined by differences in onset and duration of action and by quantitative differences in their clinical effects. One member of this class, alprazolam, has been used for the treatment of depression. Another benzodiazepine, flunitrazepam (Figure 34-23), is approved for use in many countries but not the United States. However, it has illegally entered the United States (especially Texas and Florida) and has been illicitly sold to the drug-abusing community. In addition, because of its potent sedative-hypnotic action, especially in combination with alcohol, and its ability to induce short-term amnesia, it has gained notoriety as a "date rape" pill.

Benzodiazepines are typically administered orally, and the rate of absorption is the principal determinant of the rate of onset and the intensity of action. Highly lipophilic benzodiazepines (diazepam and flurazepam) are rapidly absorbed (time to peak serum concentration <1.2 hours), and less lipophilic compounds (oxazepam and temazepam) are more

TABLE 34-12 Benzodiazepine Characteristics

Compound (Trade Name)	Therapeutic Uses	$t_{1/2}$ (hr)	Main Urinary Metabolite
Alprazolam (Xanax)	Anxiety; depression	8-14	α-hydroxy glucuronide
Chlordiazepoxide (Librium, others)	Anxiety; alcohol withdrawal; preanesthetic medication	6-27; active metabolites	Oxazepam glucuronide
Clorazepate (Tranxene, others)	Anxiety; seizure disorders	2 (prodrug)* active metabolite	Oxazepam glucuronide
Diazepam (Valium, others)	Anxiety; status epilepticus, muscle relaxation; preanesthetic medication	30-56	Oxazepam glucuronide
Lorazepam (Ativan)	Anxiety; preanesthetic medication	8-25	Lorazepam glucuronide
Oxazepam (Serax)	Anxiety	5-15	Oxazepam glucuronide
Estazolam (Prosom)	Insomnia	10-24	4-hydroxy glucuronide
Flurazepam† (Dalmane)	Insomnia	2-3; active metabolite, 50-100	N^1-hydroxy ethyl glucuronide
Quazepam (Doral)	Insomnia	6-10	2-oxo-3-hydroxy glucuronide
Temazepam (Restoril)	Insomnia	5-17	Temazepam glucuronide
Triazolam (Halcion)	Insomnia	2-3	α-hydroxy glucuronide
Clonazepam (Klonopin)	Seizure disorders	20-60	7-amino-3-hydroxy conjugates
Midazolam (Versed)	Preanesthetic and intraoperative medication	1-4	α-hydroxy glucuronide

Data from Baselt RC. Disposition of toxic drugs and chemicals in man. 7th ed. Foster City CA: Biomedical Publications, 2004; Charney DS, Michic SJ, Harris RA. Hypnotics and sedatives. In Hardman JG, Limbird LE, Gilman AG, eds. Goodman and Gilman's The pharmacological basis of therapeutics, 10th ed. New York: McGraw-Hill, 2001:399-427.

*Converted to nordiazepam by gastric HCl.

†Active metabolite, *N*-desalkylflurazepam.

slowly absorbed (time to peak serum concentration 2 to 3 hours).[86,149]

Following GI absorption or IV administration, benzodiazepines are rapidly distributed to the CNS. Subsequently, benzodiazepines are more slowly redistributed from the CNS to more poorly perfused tissue, such as adipose tissue and muscle. The rate of this redistribution is an important determinant of the duration of action of benzodiazepines and, like that for GI absorption, is largely determined by drug lipophilicity, with the more lipophilic drugs, such as midazolam and triazolam, having the shortest duration of action. Additional factors that influence the duration of benzodiazepine action are hepatic metabolism and acute tolerance, resulting in decreased response to benzodiazepines with continued drug exposure.

Benzodiazepines undergo hepatic oxidation and conjugation, often forming metabolites with pharmacological activity (Figures 34-23 through 34-27). Several benzodiazepines are metabolized to oxazepam, which is then excreted as the inactive glucuronide. Others are inactivated by glucuronidation as the only (lorazepam) or most important (temazepam) metabolic transformation. In some cases, metabolic transformations occur before the drug reaches significant concentrations in the systemic circulation. For example, clorazepate is decarboxylated to nordiazepam by stomach acid, and flurazepam and prazepam are converted to active metabolites by hepatic first-pass metabolism.[86,149]

Benzodiazepines with the shortest elimination half-life ($t_{1/2}$) generally have the shortest duration of action. In some cases, an active metabolite may have a $t_{1/2}$ longer than the parent drug and thus contributes to a longer duration of action. For instance, flurazepam has a $t_{1/2}$ of 2 to 3 hours, but its active metabolite, desalkylflurazepam, has a $t_{1/2}$ of 50 to 100 hours. These pharmacokinetic properties in part determine the primary clinical applications for some benzodiazepines. For instance midazolam ($t_{1/2}$ = 1 to 4 hours) is used for preanesthetic sedation or for sedation for endoscopic procedures because of its rapid onset and short duration of action.

Benzodiazepines useful to treat anxiety generally have an intermediate to long elimination $t_{1/2}$ (alprazolam and diazepam), and those primarily used as anticonvulsants (clonazepam) have a long $t_{1/2}$. Elimination $t_{1/2}$ is clearly not the sole determinant of duration of action of benzodiazepines. In some cases, the rate of drug redistribution from the CNS may be an even more important factor. For instance, midazolam ($t_{1/2}$ = 1 to 4 hours) and diazepam ($t_{1/2}$ = 30 to 56 hours) were demonstrated to have equivalent recovery times for single-dose, short-term sedation.[13] For this application, the distribution kinetics for diazepam are more significant than elimination $t_{1/2}$.

Benzodiazepines act on the CNS by potentiating the action of the major endogenous CNS inhibitory neurotransmitter, γ-aminobutyric acid (GABA).[86,149] Benzodiazepines bind to $GABA_A$-receptor sites and thereby enhance GABA-mediated chloride transmembrane conductance, which results in hyperpolarization and diminished neural electrical discharge. The remarkable safety of benzodiazepines compared with barbiturates is probably related to their activation of the endogenous GABA effect. Conversely, high doses of barbiturates increase neural chloride conductance independent of GABA.

Some degree of tolerance and physical dependence may develop after prolonged use of benzodiazepines.[408] A withdrawal syndrome similar to that for barbiturates and alcohol may be observed, but it is generally less severe, less frequent,

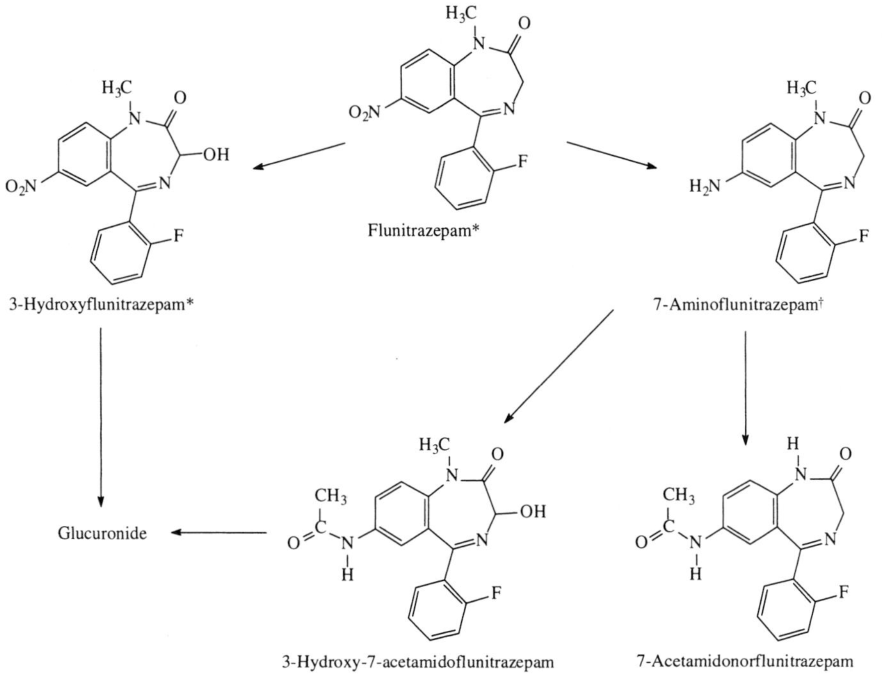

3-Hydroxyflunitrazepam*

Flunitrazepam*

7-Aminoflunitrazepam†

Glucuronide

3-Hydroxy-7-acetamidoflunitrazepam

7-Acetamidonorflunitrazepam

Figure 34-23 Metabolic transformation of flunitrazepam.
*Not approved for use in the United States.
†Principal metabolite in urine.

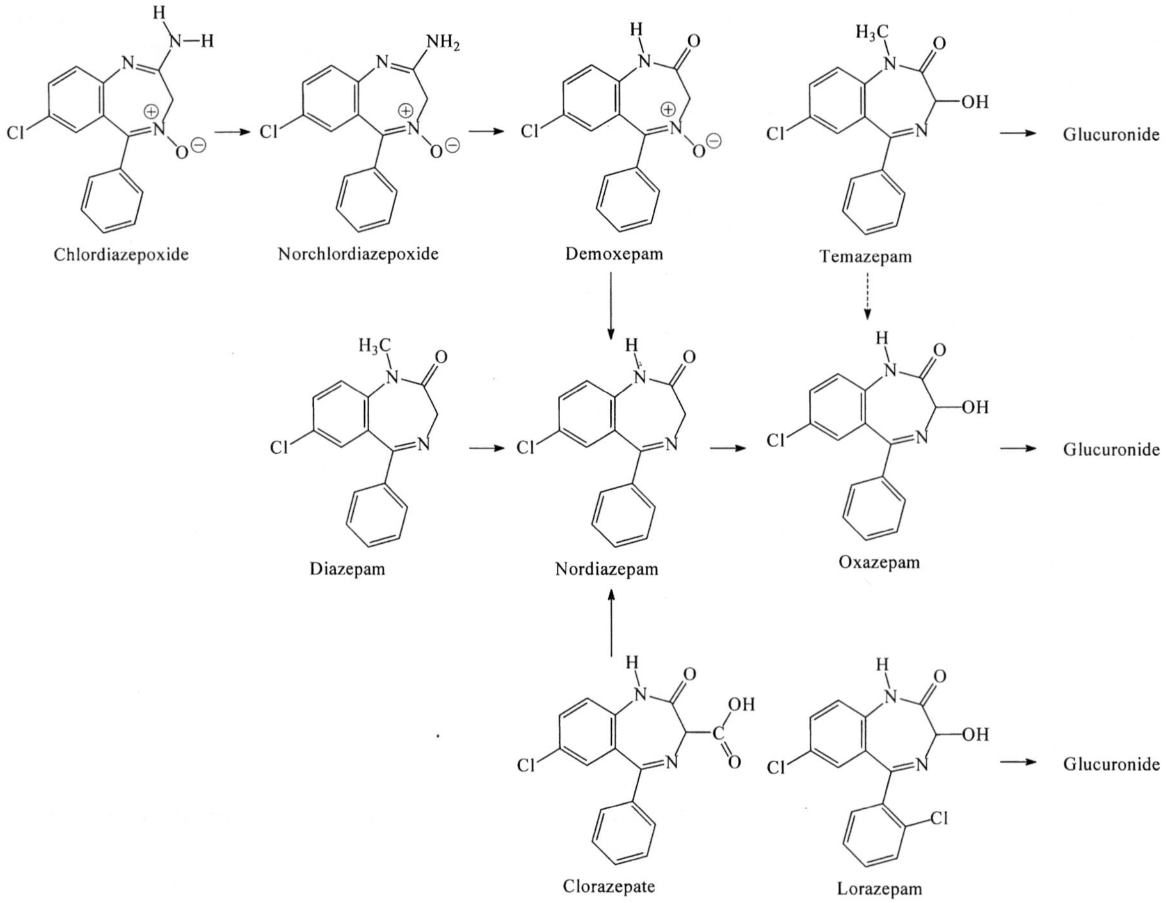

Chlordiazepoxide → Norchlordiazepoxide → Demoxepam

Temazepam → Glucuronide

Diazepam → Nordiazepam → Oxazepam → Glucuronide

Clorazepate

Lorazepam → Glucuronide

Figure 34-24 Metabolic transformation of chlordiazepoxide, diazepam, and related 1,4-benzodiazepines.

Flurazepam → N-1-Hydroxyethylflurazepam → N-1-Desalkylflurazepam → N-1-Desalkyl-3-hydroxyflurazepam → Glucuronide

Glucuronide

Quazepam → 2-Oxoquazepam → 3-Hydroxy-2-oxoquazepam → Glucuronide

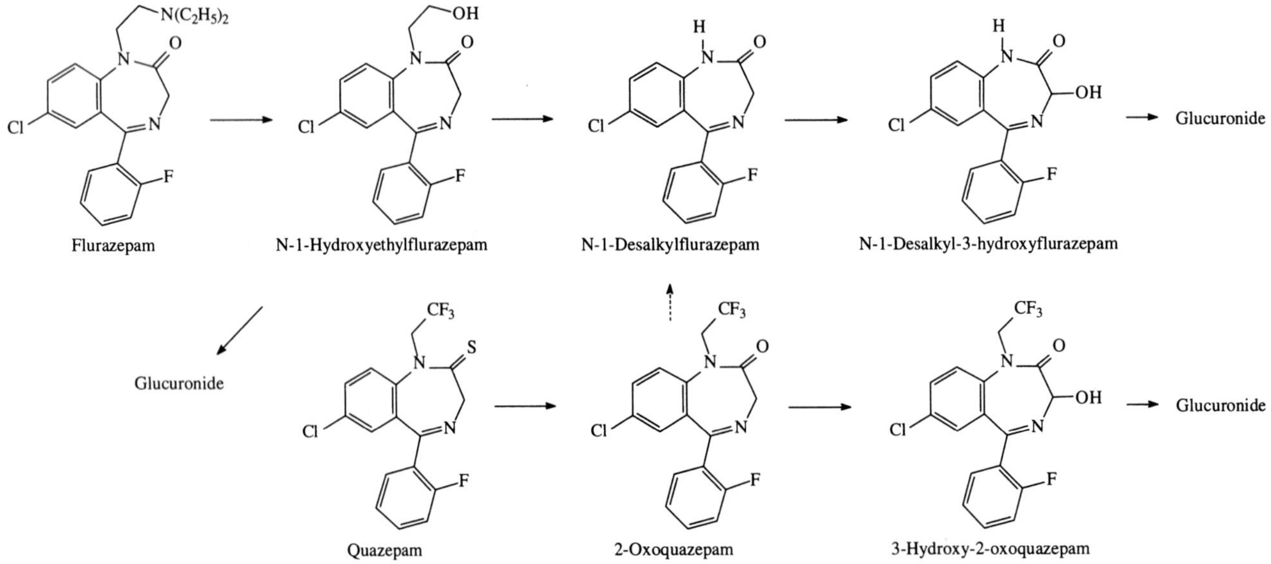

Figure 34-25 Metabolic transformation of flurazepam and related 1,4-benzodiazepines.

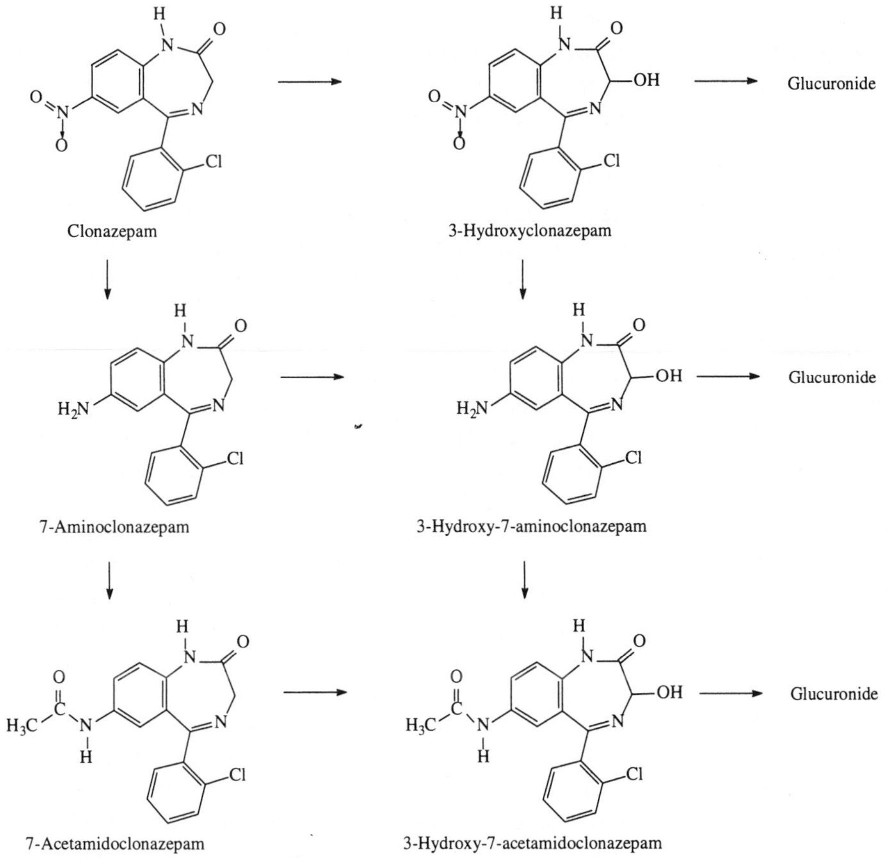

Clonazepam → 3-Hydroxyclonazepam → Glucuronide

7-Aminoclonazepam → 3-Hydroxy-7-aminoclonazepam → Glucuronide

7-Acetamidoclonazepam → 3-Hydroxy-7-acetamidoclonazepam → Glucuronide

Figure 34-26 Metabolic transformation of clonazepam.

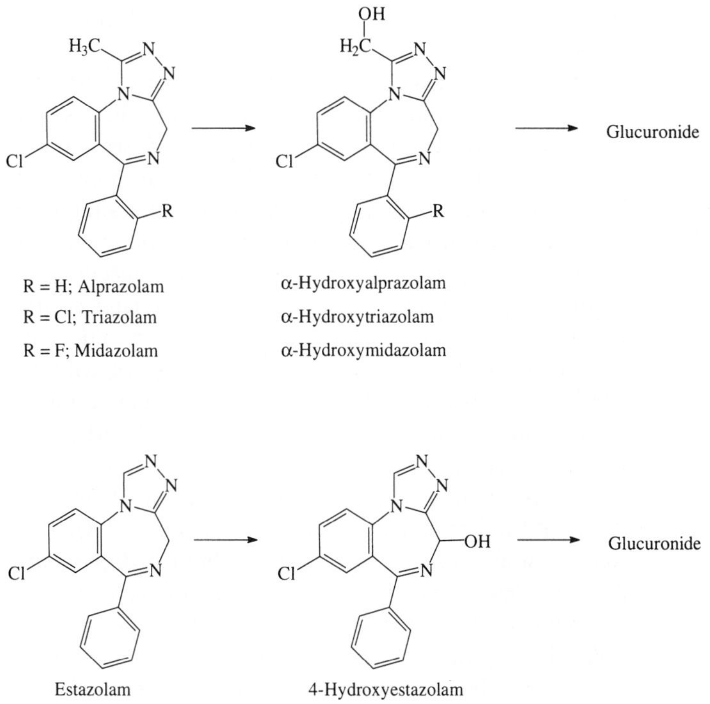

R = H; Alprazolam → α-Hydroxyalprazolam → Glucuronide

R = Cl; Triazolam → α-Hydroxytriazolam

R = F; Midazolam → α-Hydroxymidazolam

Estazolam → 4-Hydroxyestazolam → Glucuronide

Figure 34-27 Metabolic transformation of some triazolobenzodiazepines.

and not as prolonged.[149] These symptoms may include anxiety, apprehension, tremors, muscle weakness, anorexia, nausea, vomiting, dizziness, hyperthermia, and convulsions. The frequency and severity of withdrawal symptoms are greater for the most rapidly eliminated benzodiazepines, with longer duration of therapy (>4 months), with higher doses, and with abrupt discontinuation of the drug.[149,288] Withdrawal symptoms may be especially severe for alprazolam. Tolerance to some effects of benzodiazepines may occur. Tolerance is believed to result from an adaptation of the GABA-receptors to continued benzodiazepine exposure, whereby their response is diminished. This leads to the need for higher doses to achieve the desired effect.

Despite their widespread use, abuse of benzodiazepines is relatively low and is more likely to occur in individuals who abuse other drugs or alcohol. However, as a result of their widespread use, benzodiazepine intoxication is not uncommon. Benzodiazepine CNS toxicity is generally mild to moderate and may be manifest as drowsiness, slurred speech, ataxia, and occasionally coma. More serious toxic effects causing respiratory depression or cardiovascular compromise are infrequent. Indeed, few well-documented deaths have been attributed to benzodiazepine intoxication alone.

Treatment for benzodiazepine intoxication is supportive; respiratory assistance is generally only necessary when benzodiazepines are co-ingested with other CNS depressants, such as alcohol. Because of extensive protein binding (85% to 95%) and a large volume of distribution (1 to 3 L/kg), hemodialysis or hemoperfusion is not effective. Flumazenil (Figure 34-28), a benzodiazepine antagonist, quickly improves the clinical condition in cases of benzodiazepine overdose but is probably not necessary for most cases.[204] In instances of coma secondary to multiple drug overdose, removal of the benzodiazepine contribution by flumazenil may avoid the need for intubation and ventilatory assistance. Moreover a trial dose of flumazenil may aid in the diagnosis of benzodiazepine overdose and possibly avoid other procedures, such as a computed tomography scan. Caution is needed when administering flumazenil in cases of mixed tricyclic antidepressant–benzodiazepine overdose, because adverse effects have been reported, including precipitation of seizures and cardiac arrhythmias. Therefore it may be prudent to perform a screening test for tricyclic antidepressants before administration of flumazenil. Flumazenil is not detected by immunoassays for benzodiazepines.[316]

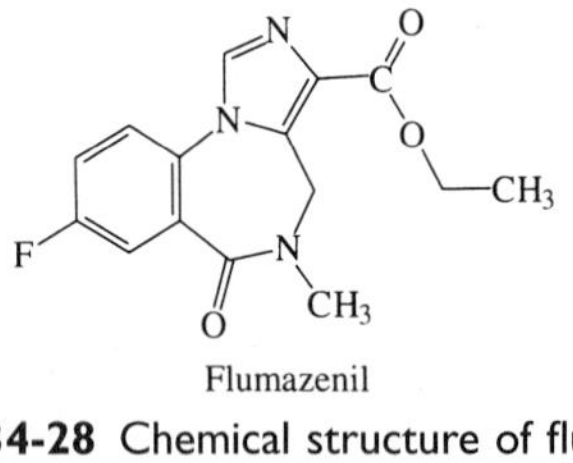

Flumazenil

Figure 34-28 Chemical structure of flumazenil.

Analytical Methodology

Benzodiazepines may be identified and quantified in serum, generally by HPLC, but such quantitative information is not warranted in cases of benzodiazepine overdose because serum levels are not predictive of severity of intoxication.[149] However, a urine or serum immunoassay screening test for benzodiazepines is valuable to aid in the evaluation of patients with an unknown cause of CNS depression.

To detect abuse, the initial screening test for benzodiazepines is typically immunoassay. For confirmation of a presumptive positive test, a quantitative drug measurement is performed using GC-MS.

Immunoassay. Several commercial immunoassay systems are available for the detection of a wide variety of benzodiazepines and metabolites (e.g., EMIT, Roche Abuscreen Online, FPIA, CEDIA, BioSite Triage, and DPC RIA). These immunoassays differ somewhat in their ability to detect the various benzodiazepines, their metabolites, and glucuronide conjugates. The response with the EMIT, FPIA, Online, and CEDIA assays for several benzodiazepines is enhanced by prior hydrolysis of urine with β-glucuronidase[407]; hydrolysis is most important to ensure detection of oxazepam, temazepam, nordiazepam, and lorazepam.* The CEDIA and Online methods have been adapted for automated online hydrolysis.[45,307,384] The Triage test device uses monoclonal antibodies selected for their reactivity with the benzodiazepine glucuronide conjugates; glucuronidase hydrolysis would actually decrease the test's detection limit with this device.[249] The detection time in urine following benzodiazepine use is extremely variable and depends on a number of factors, including the immunoassay system, inclusion of glucuronidase hydrolysis, the benzodiazepine ingested, the dose, and the duration of drug use. Long-acting benzodiazepines (diazepam, chlordiazepoxide, and clorazepate) are given in relatively large doses and may be detected for several days to weeks or even months following chronic use. Short-acting benzodiazepines (alprazolam and triazolam) are used in lower doses and might only be detected for a few days. The analytical specificity of benzodiazepine immunoassays is good; few false-positive results have been reported. Oxaprozin (a nonsteroidal anti-inflammatory drug) causes a positive response with the EMIT, FPIA, Triage, and CEDIA benzodiazepine assays.[329] False-negative results are common, especially when the immunoassay is performed without prior glucuronide hydrolysis. In one large study conducted in 2002,[61] the sensitivity and specificity for EMIT, compared with GC-MS, were 67% and 100%, respectively, without hydrolysis and 87% and 96%, respectively, with enzyme pretreatment.

The detection of flunitrazepam (Rohypnol) is especially challenging because of the low therapeutic and illicit doses, and the low degree of cross-reactivity of most immunoassays with the principal urinary metabolite, 7-

*References 44, 45, 61, 303, 305, 307, 384, 418.

aminoflunitrazepam.[390,423,467,469] As for other benzodiazepines, prior glucuronidase hydrolysis may improve immunoassay detection.[390] ELISA methods with high selectivity for 7-aminoflunitrazepam and improved sensitivity have been developed.[467,469] In the absence of a sufficiently sensitive immunoassay, direct analysis of 7-aminoflunitrazepam by GC-MS is indicated in suspected cases of flunitrazepam ingestion (e.g., suspected "date rape").

Gas Chromatography-Mass Spectrometry. A positive screening result for benzodiazepines obtained by immunoassay is confirmed by GC-MS analysis of the urine specimen. A GC-MS method for benzodiazepines is included in the Chapter 34 Appendix that is found on the book's accompanying Evolve site (http://evolve.elsevier.com/Tietz/textbook/).

Cannabinoids

Cannabinoids are a group of C_{21} compounds found in the plant species *Cannabis sativa.* The principal psychoactive cannabinoid is Δ^9-tetrahydrocannabinol (THC) (Figure 34-29). THC is typically consumed by smoking marijuana, which is a mixture of crushed leaves, flowers, and sometimes stems from the cannabis plant. Hashish, the dried, resinous secretions of the plant, may also be smoked. Hashish generally has a higher content of THC than does marijuana.

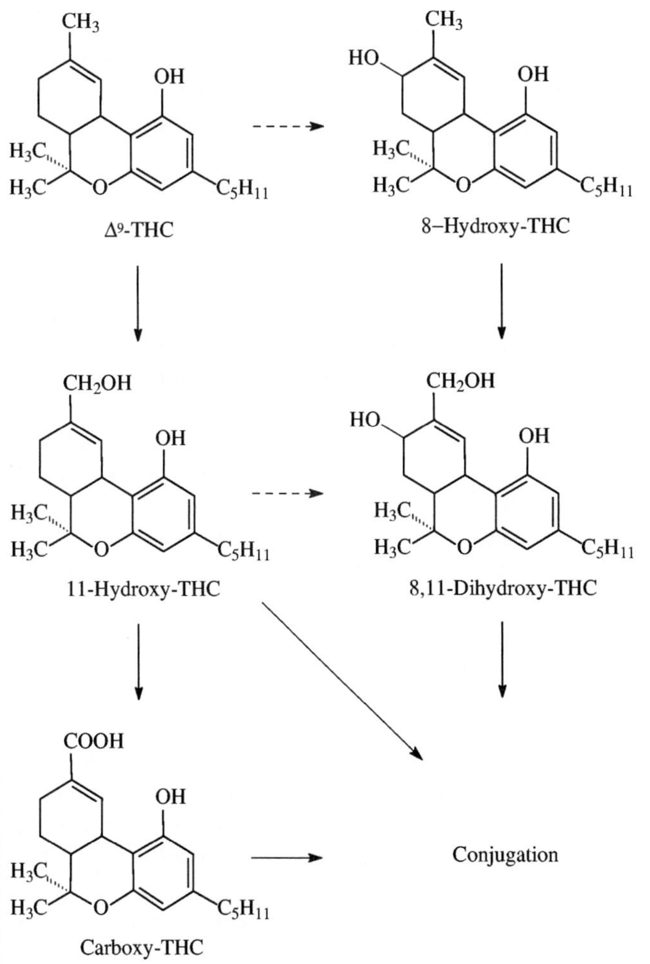

Δ9-THC

8–Hydroxy-THC

11-Hydroxy-THC

8,11-Dihydroxy-THC

Carboxy-THC

Conjugation

Figure 34-29 Principal metabolic route for THC in humans.

Pharmacological Response

The major psychoactive effects of THC are euphoria and a sense of relaxation and well-being. These effects occur within minutes of smoking marijuana, reach a peak in about 15 to 30 minutes, and may persist for 2 to 4 hours.[121,235] Associated with this "high" are a loss of short-term memory and impairment of intellectual performance (recall, reading comprehension, ability to concentrate, and mathematical problem solving). Moreover, psychomotor skills may be sufficiently impaired to adversely affect automobile or airplane operating performance.[235] Some controversy exists concerning the degree of impairment of performance much beyond 4 hours after marijuana use. Even greater uncertainty surrounds the long-term negative health effects of chronic marijuana use. Tolerance and a mild degree of physical dependence may develop after chronic marijuana and hashish use.

Endogenous cannabinoid receptors have been identified in brain and on B lymphocytes and macrophages.[16] They are transmembrane G-protein coupled receptors with signal transduction pathways, which involve modulation of adenyl cyclase, inhibition of voltage-dependent Ca^{2+} channels, and activation of K^+ channels. Subsequent to recognition of these receptors, two endogenous cannabimimetic eicosanoids, arachidonylethanolamide (anandamide) and 2-arachidonyl-glycerol, have been identified.[16,297] These receptors are postulated to be involved in modulation of mood, memory, cognition, movement, pain recognition, thermoregulation, appetite, and immune response.

After inhalation of marijuana smoke, THC is rapidly absorbed through the lungs and reaches peak blood concentration within minutes; thereafter, blood concentration rapidly declines to about 10% of peak levels within 1 to 2 hours. This rapid decline in THC concentration is a result of its facile distribution to tissue such as brain, fat, and muscle. The rapid tissue distribution phase, a consequence of the lipophilic nature of THC, is followed by a slow redistribution of THC back into the blood stream and subsequent hepatic elimination. The terminal elimination half-life of THC is about 1 day in casual marijuana users and 3 to 5 days in chronic users.[224,235] The peak psychoactive effects of THC generally lag behind the peak blood concentration by about 20 to 30 minutes.[121] Undoubtedly the concentration of THC in venous blood poorly reflects the THC concentration in the brain.

Although marijuana is the most frequently used illicit drug, it does have some limited legitimate medicinal use. Dronabinol (Marinol) contains synthetic THC and is used to treat anorexia and nausea in AIDS patients, nausea and vomiting associated with chemotherapy, and asthma and glaucoma.[343]

Nine U.S. states have legalized the use of marijuana for medical purposes. However, marijuana trafficking remains

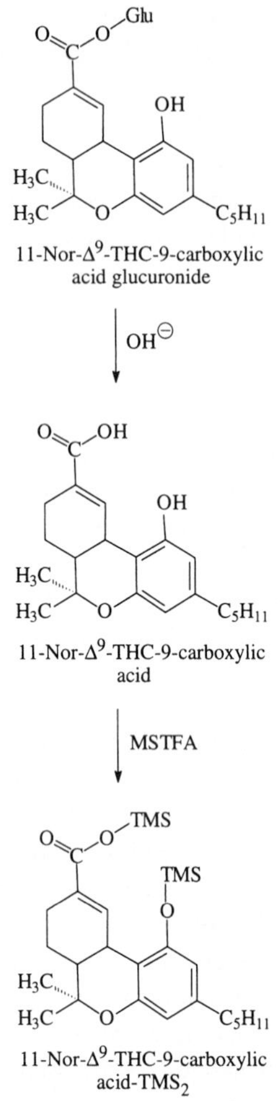

11-Nor-Δ^9-THC-9-carboxylic acid glucuronide

$OH^{\ominus}$

11-Nor-Δ^9-THC-9-carboxylic acid

MSTFA

11-Nor-Δ^9-THC-9-carboxylic acid-TMS_2

Figure 34-30 Chemical structure of derivatives of THC metabolites. *Glu,* Glucuronide.

a crime under federal law. Measurement in urine of the carboxylic acid metabolite of Δ^9-tetrahydrocannabivarin (C3 homologue of THC), present in cannabis but not in dronabinol, has been proposed as a means to distinguish ingestion of marijuana from that of Marinol.[144]

Analytical Considerations

The initial screening test for THC is typically immunoassay. For confirmation of a presumptive positive test, a quantitative drug measurement is performed using GC-MS.

Immunoassay. THC is extensively metabolized to a large number of compounds, most of which are inactive. The principal urinary metabolite is 11-nor-Δ^9-tetrahydrocannabinol-9-carboxylic acid (THC-COOH) and its glucuronide conjugate (see Figure 34-30). Immunoassays designed to screen urine samples for marijuana use measure this and other THC metabolites. These assays are calibrated with THC-COOH, but because of cross-reactivity with many other THC metabolites, quantitative results based on them are 1.5 to 8 times greater than the actual concentration of THC-COOH as determined by GC-MS.[226] Therefore immunoassay results are interpreted as THC-COOH equivalents.

Because of the slow release of THC from tissue storage sites, urine may test positive for THC metabolites (>20 ng/mL THC-COOH equivalents) for 2 to 5 days after last marijuana use by infrequent smokers; some individuals may test positive for as long as 10 days. Chronic smokers may test positive for 3 to 4 weeks after abstinence.[38,399] Some heavy smokers may remain positive for up to 46 days and may require as long as 77 days to test negative for 10 consecutive days.[142] Therefore, a positive urine test for THC-COOH can only be interpreted to indicate past marijuana use (immediate to several weeks) and is unrelated to impairment.

Due to fluctuations in fluid excretion, the concentration of THC metabolites in urine may suddenly increase rather than decline or may vary between positive and negative values when sequentially measured during the terminal elimination phase after abstinence. In this case, an increase in metabolite concentration could falsely imply reuse of marijuana. Therefore, to better monitor abstinence, the concentration of THC-COOH should be expressed per milligram of creatinine.[38,47,261,262] Increases of 0.5[207] and 1.5[293] in the THC-COOH to creatinine ratio between two specimens collected at least 24 hours apart have been proposed as criteria to indicate reuse. The specimen-ratio criterion of 0.5 has the higher sensitivity and would be better applied for monitoring in drug treatment programs. However, the 1.5 ratio criterion has very high specificity (low false-positive) and would be more appropriate if punitive action is anticipated.[163,207]

Legitimate concern has been raised about the possibility of "passive inhalation" of sufficient sidestream marijuana smoke from nearby users to result in a positive urine cannabinoid test. It has been demonstrated that such can occur but under rather unrealistic conditions.[102] Under more normal circumstances, passive inhalation did not result in a urine THC-COOH concentration in excess of 12 ng/mL.[102,323] Nevertheless, as a precaution against passive inhalations resulting in a positive test, some laboratories screen for urine cannabinoids at a cutoff concentration of 100 ng/mL THC-COOH equivalents. However, at this cutoff value, test sensitivity in one study was only 47% when compared with that for GC-MS (cutoff value, 15 ng/mL THC-COOH). Test sensitivity increased to 93% at a cutoff value of 20 ng/mL THC-COOH equivalents.[414] The U.S. federally mandated screening cutoff was reduced from 100 ng/mL to 50 ng/mL THC-COOH equivalents.[292] One study demonstrated that such a reduction in screening cutoff resulted in a 23% to 54% increase in test sensitivity, depending on immunoassay, with only a slight decrease (1.0% to 2.6%) in test specificity.[208] A 1997 study suggests that consideration should be given to lowering the values listed for Δ^9-THC-COOH in Table 34-8.[482]

Seeds and oil from the hemp plant (also a variety of *Cannabis sativa* L) contain Δ^9-tetrahydrocannabinol. Consumption as nutritional supplements of hemp-seed oil with relatively high THC content may result in a positive urine test for THC-COOH,[267,431] thus prompting a "hemp defense" as explanation for the test result. Since 1998, the hemp industry has made an effort to reduce the THC content of these products by including a wash step before seed processing. Repeated daily ingestion of hemp oil with current lower THC content is not likely to result in a positive urine test for THC-COOH at SAMHSA cutoffs,[271] but it is possible.[183] In 2001, the DEA included any product that contains THC under the Schedule I controlled substance classification,[214] thus negating the "hemp defense."

Gas Chromatography-Mass Spectrometry. A positive screening result for THC obtained by immunoassay is confirmed by GC-MS analysis of the urine specimen. A GC-MS method for THC is included in the Chapter 34 Appendix that is found on this book's accompanying Evolve site (http://evolve.elsevier.com/Tietz/textbook/).

Cocaine

Cocaine is an alkaloid present in the leaves of the coca plant that grows in South America. The drug has a long history of human consumption, beginning with its use by ancient South American civilizations, followed by its initial incorporation in a popular cola drink (discontinued in the early 1900s), and continuing to its current popularity as a recreational drug.[179,222]

Pharmacological Response

Cocaine is a potent CNS stimulant that elicits a state of increased alertness and euphoria[179,222] with its actions similar to those of amphetamine but of shorter duration. These CNS effects are thought to be largely associated with the ability of cocaine to block dopamine reuptake at nerve synapses and thereby prolong the action of dopamine in the CNS. It is this response that leads to recreational abuse of cocaine. Cocaine also blocks the reuptake of norepinephrine at presynaptic nerve terminals; this produces a sympathomimetic response (including an increase in blood pressure, heart rate, and body temperature). Cocaine is effective as a local anesthetic and vasoconstrictor of mucous membranes and is therefore used clinically for nasal surgery, rhinoplasty, and emergency nasotracheal intubation.

For recreational use, cocaine (hydrochloride salt) is often administered by nasal insufflation ("snorting") or less frequently, intravenously. Cocaine is more volatile when converted from the salt to the freebase; therefore freebase cocaine may be inhaled by smoking. This latter route of administration results in a rapid onset of action. It has gained increased popularity owing to the ready availability of the freebase cocaine form known as "crack." Consequently the number of emergency room admissions related to cocaine toxicity has increased.[109,179]

The CNS and cardiovascular effects of cocaine exhibit acute tolerance, with its effects more pronounced when the concentration of cocaine in blood is increasing than when it is at a similar but decreasing concentration.[8,222] Thus a clockwise hysteresis is observed when the blood concentration of cocaine is plotted against its CNS or cardiovascular effects over time. This phenomenon mitigates against attempts to correlate isolated blood concentration values with psychomotor effects. Because rate of change is probably more significant than absolute concentration, the psychomotor stimulant effects of cocaine are dependent both on dose and on route of administration, with IV administration and smoking resulting in the most rapid rate of increase in concentration.

Acute cocaine toxicity produces a sympathomimetic response that may result in mydriasis, diaphoresis, hyperactive bowel sounds, tachycardia, hypertension, hyperthermia, hyperactivity, agitation, seizures, or coma. Sudden death due to cardiotoxicity may occur following cocaine use. Death may also occur following the sequential development of hyperthermia, agitated delirium, and respiratory arrest. Excited delirium and extreme physical activity may lead to rhabdomyolysis, acute renal failure, and disseminated intravascular coagulopathy.

Cocaine is rapidly hydrolyzed by separate liver esterases to the inactive metabolites ecgonine methyl ester and benzoylecgonine (Figure 34-31). Ecgonine methyl ester may also be formed by the action of serum butyrylcholinesterase, and cocaine may be converted to benzoylecgonine by spontaneous hydrolysis. The formation of benzoylecgonine has often been attributed entirely to spontaneous hydrolysis, but it has clearly been shown to be mediated mainly by a liver carboxyesterase.[116] This latter enzyme, in the presence of ethanol, catalyzes transesterification of cocaine (benzoylecgonine methyl ester) to cocaethylene (benzoylecgonine ethyl ester). Cocaethylene possesses the same CNS stimulatory activity as cocaine in experimental animals.[196] Ethanol and cocaine are commonly co-abused, and it is speculated that formation of cocaethylene may cause enhanced CNS stimulation and therefore lead to reinforcement of the co-abuse. Cocaethylene may also result in enhanced cardiotoxicity; it is more lethal than cocaine in experimental animals.[195] Cocaethylene is not infrequently present in urine or serum of hospital patients who test positive for benzoylecgonine.[18,492] When "crack" cocaine is smoked, a pyrolysis product, anhydroecgonine methyl ester, is formed and may be detected in urine.[217,346]

The elimination half-life for cocaine ranges from 0.5 to 1.5 hours, for ecgonine methyl ester from 3 to 4 hours, and for benzoylecgonine from 4 to 7 hours.[5-7] The principal urinary metabolites are benzoylecgonine and ecgonine methyl ester. Only small amounts of cocaine are excreted in urine. The elimination half-life for cocaethylene is 2.5 to 6 hours,[19,218,221] considerably longer than that for cocaine. This longer elimination half-life may contribute to cocaethylene's toxicity.

Analytical Methodology

The initial screening test for cocaine (benzoylecgonine) is typically immunoassay. For confirmation of a presumptive

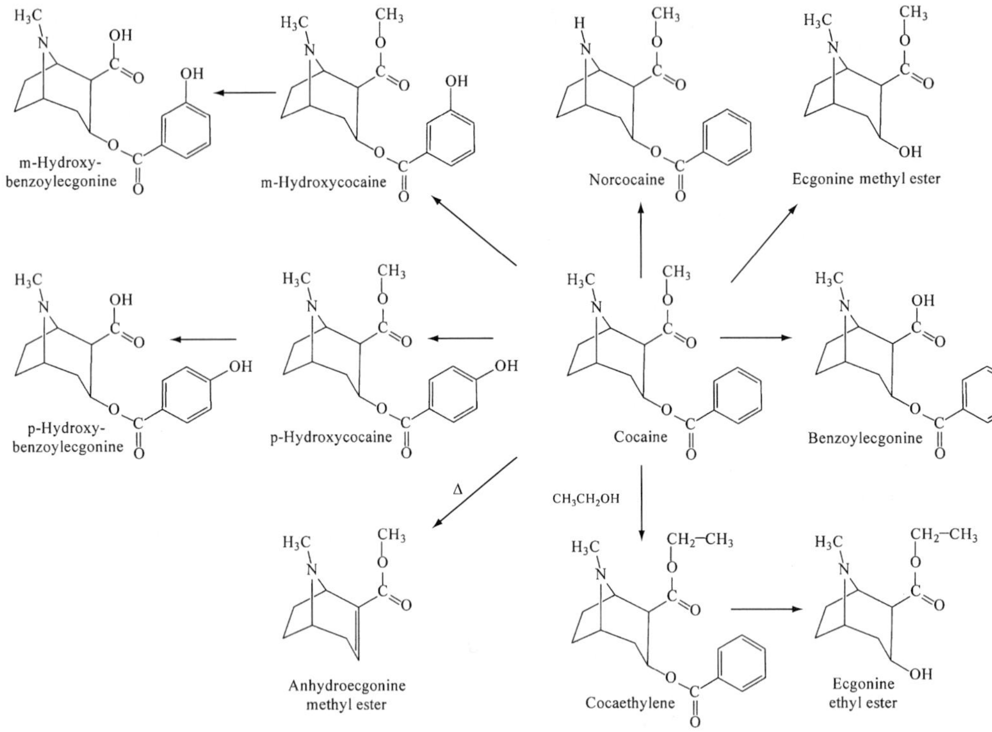

Figure 34-31 Metabolism and pyrolysis of cocaine.

positive, a quantitative drug measurement is performed using GC-MS.

Immunoassay. Screening immunoassays (e.g., Dade-Behring [EMIT], Abbott [FPIA]) are designed for the detection of benzoylecgonine. These assays have a 300-ng/mL cutoff and detect benzoylecgonine excretion for 1 to 3 days following cocaine use. However, for chronic heavy cocaine users, the detection time may extend to 10 to 22 days following the last dose,[474] apparently because of tissue storage of cocaine. Ordinarily cocaine may be detected in urine by chromatographic methods for only about 8 to 12 hours after use, but in heavy chronic users, this detection period may be 4 to 5 days.[104] These facts should be considered when interpreting the results of a urine drug test for individuals in drug treatment programs. A positive urine drug test for benzoylecgonine beyond 3 days after the last dose does not necessarily indicate continued use. For such purposes, it is better to monitor quantitatively the urinary excretion of benzoylecgonine, normalized to creatinine, over time.[47,440] Drug abstinence would be indicated by decreasing urinary excretion of cocaine metabolites. However, creatinine normalization may not always reliably indicate reuse.[374]

In meconium, *m*- and *p*-hydroxybenzoylecgonine (normally minor metabolites in adult urine) significantly contribute to the benzoylecgonine immunoreactivity.[346,427]

The consumption of Peruvian coca tea, which is not legally imported into the United States, may result in a positive urine test for benzoylecgonine.[187]

Gas Chromatography-Mass Spectrometry. A positive screening result for benzoylecgonine obtained by immunoassay is confirmed by GC-MS analysis of the urine specimen. A GC-MS method for benzoylecgonine is included in the Chapter 34 Appendix that is found on this book's accompanying Evolve site (http://evolve.elsevier.com/Tietz/textbook/). This method uses normalized ion ratios as this compensates for any changes in the mass spectrometer ion source at the time of analysis[55] and either a single or multiple calibrators.[151,394]

Gamma-Hydroxybutyrate (GHB)

Gamma-hydroxybutyrate (γ-hydroxybutyrate/GHB) is a naturally occurring metabolite of γ-aminobutyric acid (GABA) and like GABA, it may possess CNS neuroinhibitory activity via specific GHB receptors.

Pharmacological Response

GHB was investigated as an anesthetic agent but was discontinued because of its lack of analgesia and because of adverse side effects including seizures. It is used outside the United States to treat alcohol and opioid withdrawal and was recently approved in the United States under the name Xyrem for the treatment of narcolepsy.

When ingested, GHB stimulates dopamine release, leading to pleasurable effects such as euphoria, muscle relaxation, and heightened sexual desire.[48,113] It also has CNS depressant effects resulting in sedation and hypnosis. Because GHB was reported to enhance growth hormone release, it has been used as a steroid alternative by body builders and athletes. Athletes also have used GHB as a sleep aid because they believe it promotes rapid recovery from vigorous repetitive competition. These properties and the availability of GHB in dietary supplements led to growing recreational abuse of the drug. GHB has become popular as a euphorigenic club drug, most often used in combination with alcohol and also with MDMA or cocaine to "mellow" their adverse stimulant properties. Its rapid onset and hypnotic and short-term amnestic properties have resulted in the use of GHB for drug-facilitated sexual assault (date rape drug).

The FDA removed GHB from consumer products in 1990 in response to its increasing abuse and danger. This action led to its replacement by γ-butyrolactone (GBL), a GHB precursor (Figure 34-32) that is also used as a chemical cleaning agent and solvent. GBL is more rapidly absorbed and has greater bioavailability compared with GHB.[420] GBL is also readily converted ex vivo to GHB by its treatment with an alkaline solution. Health supplement products containing GBL (e.g., RenewTrient, Revivarant, Reinforce) have also now been removed from the market only to be replaced by another GHB precursor, 1,4-butanediol (Figure 34-32),[500] also present in household cleaning agents and industrial solvents. GHB itself has a number of colorful street names including liquid ecstasy, easy lay, zonked, and Georgia home boy. Diet supplements that contain 1,4-butanediol include SomatoPro and Revitalize Plus.

Toxic manifestations of GHB or its precursors include nausea and vomiting, bradycardia, hypotension, coma, seizures, and severe but not prolonged respiratory depression.[113,274,309] Periods of agitation may be interspersed between apnea and unresponsiveness. It is uncertain whether this agitation is a direct GHB effect or a consequence of co-ingested stimulant drugs. Deaths have been reported but are almost always associated with co-ingestion of alcohol or other drugs.

GHB is rapidly absorbed from the GI tract and its onset of action is extremely rapid. Loss of consciousness may occur within 15 to 30 minutes. The duration of response is also short, typically 1 to 3 hours for normal dose and 2 to 4 hours with excessive dose. Overdose leading to coma and respiratory depression requiring assisted ventilation generally resolves in <6 hours. Frequent use of GHB in high dose may produce tolerance and dependence despite its short duration of action. A withdrawal syndrome consisting of tremor, agitation, paranoia, delirium, hallucinations, confusion, tachycardia, and hypertension may follow cessation from chronic heavy use.[130]

The CNS depressant effects of GHB may result from its interaction with endogenous GHB receptors and with $GABA_B$ receptors.[48] The latter are G-protein coupled receptors distinct from the $GABA_A$ receptors for depressant drugs, such as benzodiazepines and barbiturates. Of note, patients with GHB overdose do not respond to the opioid antagonist naloxone or to the benzodiazepine antagonist flumazenil. Fomepizole, an inhibitor of alcohol dehydrogenase, is likely beneficial for patients who ingest 1,4-butanediol.[420]

Analytical Methodology

Immunoassays for GHB are not currently available. Thus chromatographic techniques (usually GC-MS) are required for analysis. GHB is rapidly eliminated ($t_{1/2}$ ~ 30 minutes) and therefore the detection period is <6 to 8 hours in plasma and <10 to 12 hours in urine. In drug-facilitated sexual assault cases, low GHB concentrations may be observed in urine (1.0 to 610 mg/dL).[302] Because GHB is produced endogenously, it is important to establish an appropriate analytical cutoff above which only exogenous GHB is mea-

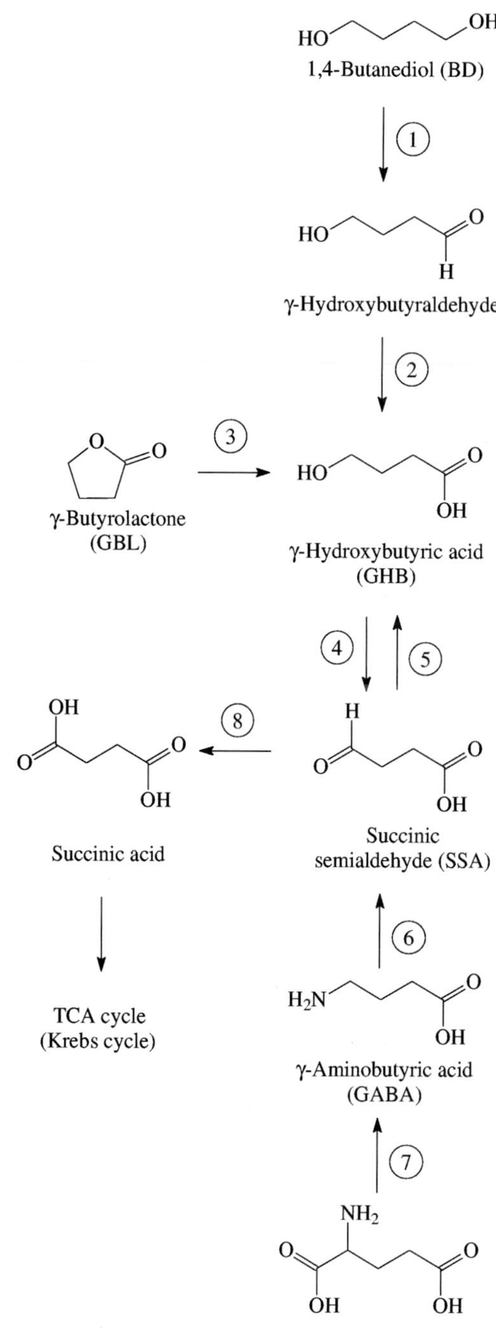

Figure 34-32 Metabolism of γ-hydroxybutyrate and its precursors. *1,* alcohol dehydrogenase; *2,* aldehyde dehydrogenase; *3,* lactonase; *4,* GHB dehydrogenase; *5,* SSA reductase; *6,* GABA transaminase; *7,* glutamate decarboxylase; *8,* SSA dehydrogenase.

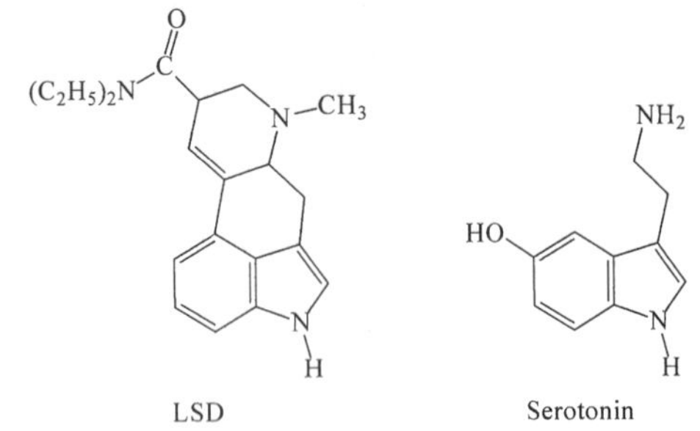

Figure 34-33 Chemical structure of LSD and serotonin.

sured. In urine, endogenous levels are well below 1.0 mg/dL and this is the recommended analytical cutoff.[265,495]

A GC-MS method for measuring GBH is included in the Chapter 34 Appendix that is found on this book's accompanying Evolve site (http://evolve.elsevier.com/Tietz/textbook/). In this method, a urine specimen is treated with acidified acetonitrile and then dehydrated by evaporation. GHB is converted to its bis-trimethylsilyl derivative and analyzed using GHB-D_6 as internal standard.

Lysergic Acid Diethylamide (LSD)

LSD shares structural features with serotonin (5-hydroxytryptamine; Figure 34-33), a major CNS neurotransmitter and neuromodulator.[456,487] LSD is synthesized from D-lysergic acid, a naturally occurring ergot alkaloid found in the fungus *Claviceps purpurea,* which grows on wheat and other grains. During synthesis, some LSD epimerizes to iso-LSD, which is inactive (Figure 34-33).

Pharmacological Response

LSD is an extremely potent psychedelic indolealkylamine.[32] The drug LSD binds to serotonin receptors in the CNS and acts as a serotonin agonist. The principal psychological effects of LSD are perceptual distortions of colors, sound, distance, and shape; depersonalization and loss of body image; and rapidly changing emotions from ecstasy to depression or paranoia. These hallucinogenic actions of LSD are stereoselective, elicited only by the D-isomer.[487] There has been a resurgence in the use of LSD, previously popular as a drug of abuse during the 1960s. The Department of Defense includes LSD among the drugs for which urine testing is required (see Table 34-8).

The physiological effects of LSD are related to its sympathomimetic actions and include mydriasis (most frequent and consistent), tachycardia, increased body temperature, diaphoresis, and hypertension; at higher doses, parasympathomimetic actions may be observed (e.g., salivation, lacrimation, nausea, and vomiting [muscarinic actions]). Neuromuscular effects may include paresthesia, muscle twitches, and incoordination (nicotinic actions).[456,487]

The most common adverse effects of LSD are panic attacks. In addition, unpredictable recurrence of hallucinations (flashbacks) may occur weeks or months after last drug use and LSD may elicit psychotic reactions (thought disorders, hallucinations, depression, and depersonalization). LSD is used illicitly because of its hallucinogenic effects. There is no evidence that repeated LSD use results in dependence or withdrawal symptoms.[456,487]

Popular dosage forms include powder, gelatin capsule, tablet, or LSD-impregnated sugar cubes, filter paper, or postage stamps. The drug is rapidly absorbed from the GI tract; the effects begin within 40 to 60 minutes, peak at about 2 to 4 hours, and subside by 6 to 8 hours. The elimination $t_{1/2}$ is about 3 hours. The metabolism of LSD in humans is incompletely understood, but 2-oxo-3-hydroxy-LSD is present in urine at concentrations 10- to 43-fold greater than LSD (Figure 34-34).[363,364,380] *N*-demethyl-LSD is also present in urine specimens, but at concentrations approximately equivalent to those of LSD. The other metabolites described in Figure 34-34 are among those identified in animals, but as yet not conclusively identified in man. Iso-LSD is not a metabolite but is formed by nonenzymatic epimerization of LSD during synthesis or during storage of urine at alkaline pH and elevated temperature.[391]

The clinical effects of LSD ingestion are usually benign and require no medical intervention. However, panic attacks may be severe and require treatment with diazepam; LSD-induced psychosis may be treated with haloperidol. Rare cases of massive overdose have resulted in life-threatening hyperthermia, rhabdomyolysis, acute renal failure, hepatic failure, DIC, respiratory arrest, and coma. Few if any well-documented deaths directly related to LSD ingestion have been reported.

Analytical Considerations

Because of the very high potency of LSD and therefore low typical dose (~50 µg) and its rapid and extensive metabolism (Figure 34-34), only about 1% to 2% of the drug is excreted unchanged in urine.[380] Thus detection of LSD presents an especially difficult analytical challenge. Even with sensitive assays, the detection window for LSD is generally only 12 to 24 hours.[380]

Immunoassays targeted to detect LSD at the usual cutoff concentration of 500 pg/mL include DPC RIA, Roche Abuscreen RIA, CEDIA, EMIT, KIMS, and ELISA. Confirmation is typically performed by GC-MS[162,355] at the U.S. Department of Defense established cutoff concentration of 200 pg/mL. Not unexpectedly, immunoassays are less specific for LSD compared with GC-MS. Although the metabolites 2-oxo-3-hydroxy-LSD and *N*-demethyl LSD generally cross react only when present at about 100 to 200 times that for LSD,[477] other as yet identified metabolites may potentially account for some instances of nonconfirmed positive immunoassay response.[97,489] However, true false-positive results due to various therapeutic drugs occur, especially with the EMIT assay.[97,381,477] The detection window may be extended, perhaps twofold to threefold, by including 2-oxo-3-hydroxy-LSD in the confirmatory test using sensitive techniques such as GC-MS-MS,[380] LC-MS-MS,[248,364] or

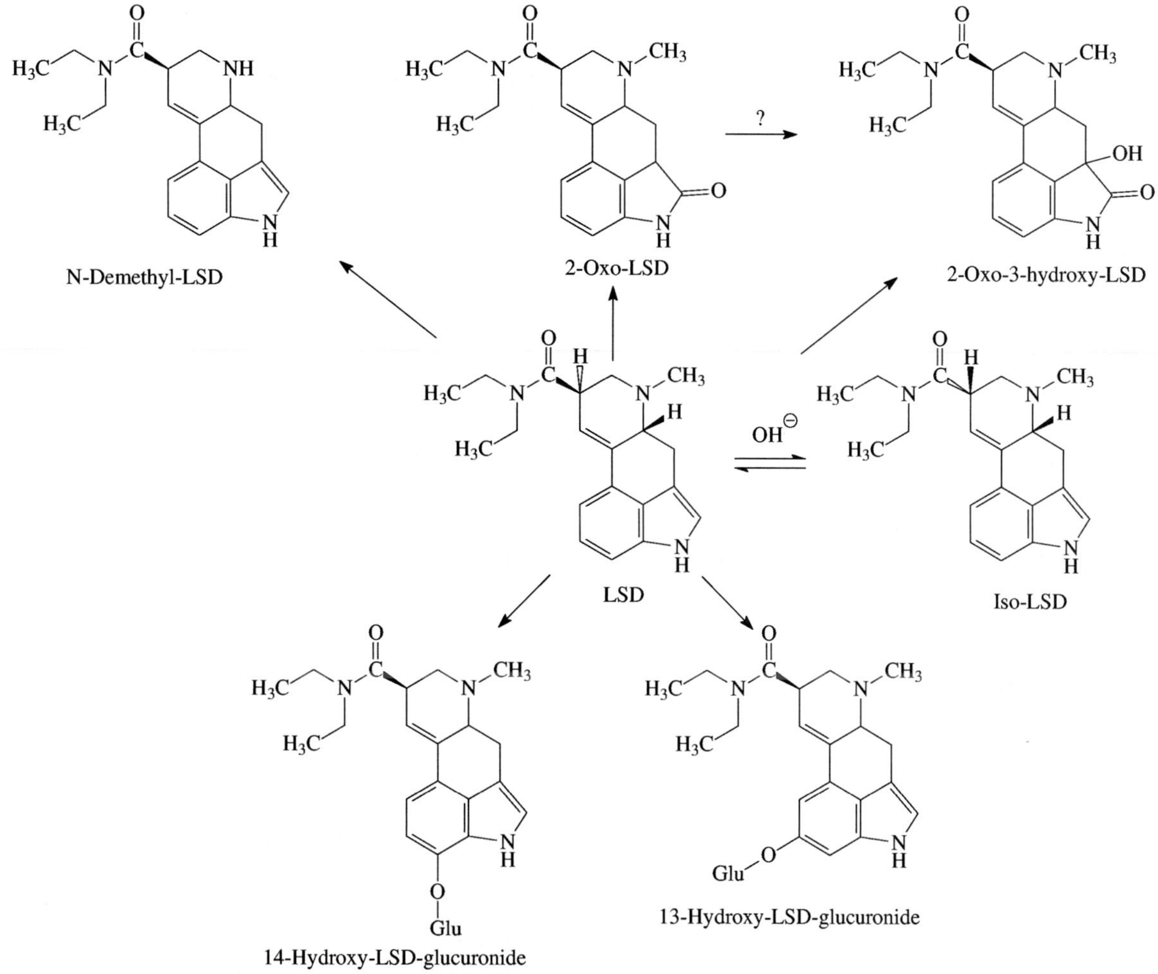

Figure 34-34 Metabolism of LSD.

LC-MS.[363] Likewise, detection of iso-LSD in addition to LSD may also extend the detection interval.[93] Urine specimens should be protected from sunlight, bright fluorescent light, or elevated temperature at alkaline pH in order to avoid degradation of LSD[275] and 2-oxo-3-hydroxy-LSD or epimerization of LSD to iso-LSD.[275,391]

Opioids/Opiates

Opioid is a general term applied to all substances with morphine-like properties. The term opiate is used to describe naturally occurring or semisynthetic analgesic alkaloids derived from opium, the dried milky juice from the unripe seeds of the poppy plant. Morphine is the principal and prototypical analgesic alkaloid of opium. Opium also contains smaller amounts of codeine. Some important semisynthetic derivatives of morphine include heroin, oxycodone, hydrocodone, oxymorphone, hydromorphone, and levorphanol. Codeine may also be synthesized by 3-methylation of morphine. Synthetic agents with morphine-like properties include propoxyphene, methadone, meperidine, and fentanyl (Figure 34-35).[184]

Pharmacological Response

Opiates are used clinically because of their analgesic properties. Opiates also cause sedation, euphoria, respiratory depression, orthostatic hypotension, diminished intestinal motility, nausea, and vomiting. The major manifestations of morphine overdose are coma, miosis (pinpoint pupils), and respiratory depression. Pulmonary edema often is a complication of morphine overdose, and death may result from cardiopulmonary arrest. Treatment for morphine overdose includes administration of the opiate antagonist naloxone (Narcan), which dramatically reverses the effects of morphine.[184]

Endogenous opioid receptors have been identified, cloned, and sequenced. They are members of the trimeric G-protein-binding superfamily, which are coupled to signal transduction via adenyl cyclase, and to Ca^{2+} and K^+ ion-channel transport.[184] Three major receptor subtypes are known (mu, kappa, and delta). Mu (μ) receptor activation results in sedation, euphoria (via dopamine release), analgesia, respiratory depression, and GI dysmoility. Kappa (κ) receptors mediate spinal analgesia, miosis (via acetylcholine

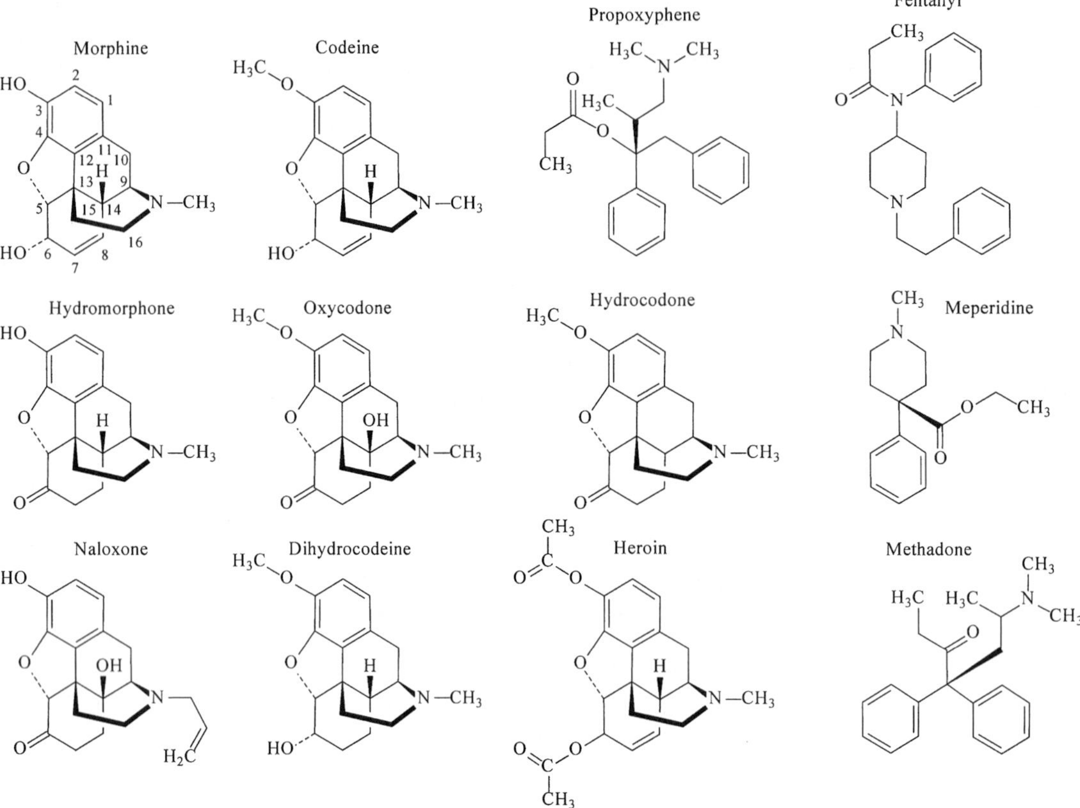

Figure 34-35 Chemical structures of representative opioids and of the opioid antagonist naloxone.

release), diuresis (inhibition of ADH release), and a dysphoric response. Delta (δ) receptors are responsible for brain and spinal analgesia. Some opioids (e.g., codeine and hydrocodone) are effective antitussive agents, but the central receptors responsible for this action have not been clearly identified. Most opioid agonist are rather nonselective in binding to the receptor subtypes. Naloxone (Narcan) and naltrexone (Trexan) are opioid receptor antagonists. Endogenous ligands for these receptors are peptides referred to as endorphins. They are believed to mollify pain and produce euphoria. The "runner's high" subsequent to intense physical activity is considered to be endorphin mediated.

Because of their analgesic and euphorigenic properties, opiates have a high abuse potential. Chronic use of morphine leads to tolerance and to both physical and psychological dependence. Withdrawal from morphine addiction may be treated by the administration of methadone, a long-lasting, orally active opiate. Over time, the goal is to replace opiate use with methadone, and then gradually wean addicts from the methadone. Other therapeutic agents for treating morphine addiction include naltrexone, a long-acting opiate antagonist; levo-α-acetylmethadol (LAAM), a long-acting (~4 days) agonist; and clonidine, a central α_2-adrenergic agonist antihypertensive agent with CNS actions similar to opiates.[327] Buprenorphine, a partial μ receptor agonist and weak κ receptor antagonist, has recently been approved for treatment of opioid addiction.[424a]

Heroin (diacetylmorphine) is the form of morphine most favored by opiate abusers because of its rapid onset of action. It is generally administered by IV or subcutaneous injection or, less frequently, by smoking or nasal insufflation.[417] Heroin itself is not active, but it is rapidly converted ($t_{1/2} <$ 6 min) to 6-acetylmorphine, which in turn is hydrolyzed ($t_{1/2} <$ 40 min) to morphine (Figure 34-36).[30,215] Both 6-acetylmorphine and morphine are pharmacologically active. Morphine (average elimination $t_{1/2} \approx$ 2 hours; range, 1 to 8 hours) is inactivated mainly by glucuronide conjugation at the 3-hydroxyl (phenolic)group.[173] The average elimination half-life for morphine-3-glucuronide is 3 to 4 hours following IV,[173] 8 hours following intramuscular,[310] and 9 to 10 hours after oral morphine administration.[173] In addition to morphine-3-glucuronide, smaller amounts of morphine-6-glucuronide are also formed. However, unlike morphine-3-glucuronide, which is inactive, morphine-6-glucuronide has even more potent analgesic activity than morphine.[338,339] Moreover, the elimination $t_{1/2}$ for both glucuronides is similar but longer than for morphine[173]; therefore morphine-6-glucuronide accumulates in serum to greater concentrations than morphine. Thus morphine-6-glucuronide contributes to the analgesic and toxic effects of morphine, especially for patients with renal failure. Of the total morphine in urine, about 90% is morphine-3-glucuronide (50% to 75% of the morphine dose), and about 10% is free morphine.[35,372]

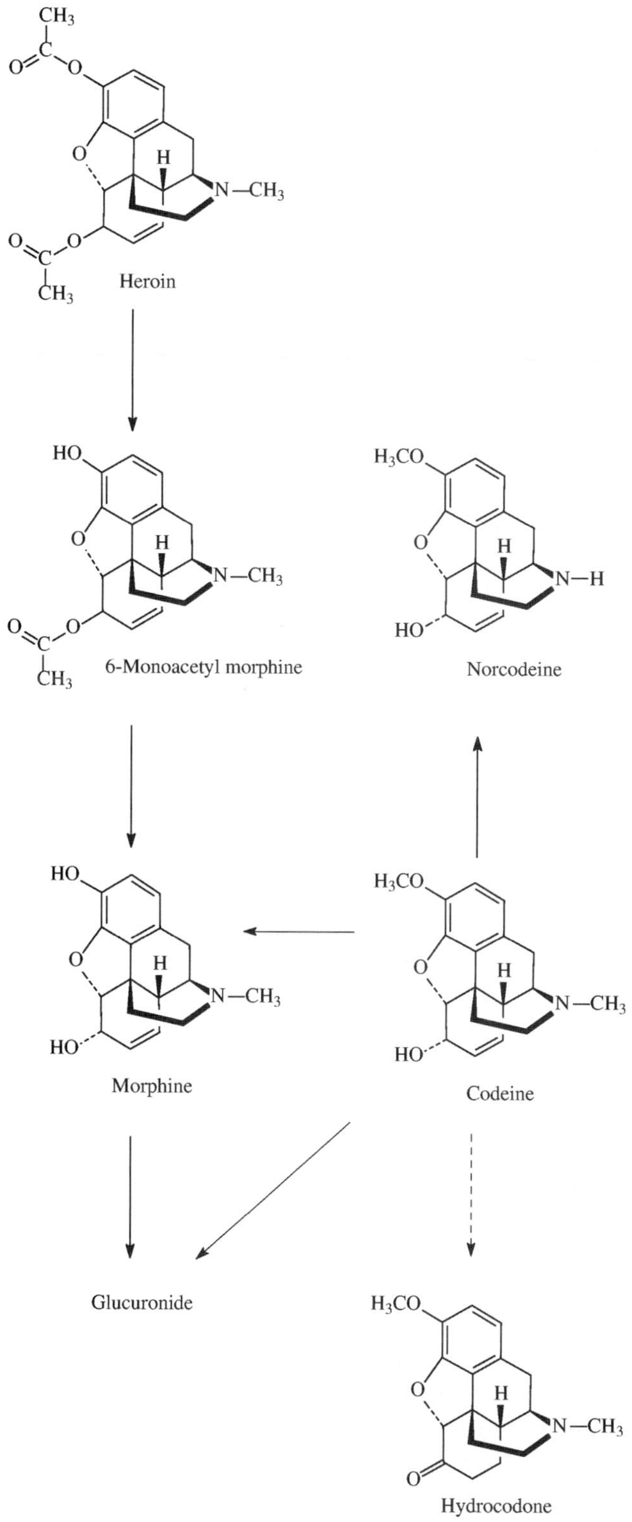

Figure 34-36 Metabolism of heroin and codeine.

Codeine has only about one tenth the analgesic potency of morphine; this is a consequence of the blocked phenolic hydroxyl group, which prohibits binding to opioid μ-receptors. A small amount of codeine (10%) is converted to morphine (see Figure 34-36), which accounts for the analgesic properties of codeine.[184] This 0-demethylation is mediated by the cytochrome P_{450} isoform, CYP 2D6, which exhibits genetic polymorphism. Slow metabolizers produce very small amounts of morphine and thus experience no analgesia, whereas fast metabolizers experience a greater than expected analgesic effect.[497] A similar amount of norcodeine is formed by *N*-demethylation.[28] Hydrocodone is a minor metabolite.[344] Thus both codeine and morphine may be detected in urine following codeine ingestion. In addition, hydrocodone may also be detected in low concentration (~100 ng/mL) when urine codeine concentration is high (>5000 ng/mL).[344] Codeine is frequently combined with nonopiate analgesic agents (e.g., aspirin and acetaminophen); it is also an effective antitussive agent in some cough medicines.

Acetylcodeine is a common contaminant of heroin; thus both codeine and morphine may frequently be detected in urine following heroin use. Since morphine is a codeine metabolite, legitimate codeine use has been purported as explanation for a urine drug test positive for morphine and codeine when in fact heroin was used. In the case of heroin, the concentration of morphine exceeds that of codeine, whereas the reverse is true within the first 24 hours following codeine use. However, a reversal in the codeine:morphine ratio may occur in the late elimination period (>24 hours) subsequent to codeine administration.[106,372] This is a consequence of the longer terminal elimination phase for morphine compared with that for codeine. Dutt and coworkers have proposed a ratio of codeine:morphine >0.5 to be indicative of codeine use when the urine morphine concentration is >200 ng/mL; for morphine concentrations <200 ng/mL, any level of codeine would suggest its use.[128] These guidelines may not always be reliable in the late elimination phase.[83] With this cutoff, some subjects may test positive for morphine (>300 ng/mL) but negative for codeine (<300 ng/mL), even though codeine had been ingested.[106] Thus it is not always possible to distinguish between legitimate codeine use (e.g., from a cough preparation) and heroin or morphine abuse based on the codeine:morphine ratio in urine. A high degree of certainty for the ingestion of codeine only is provided by urine codeine >5000 ng/mL, with a codeine to morphine ratio <0.5.[83,263] Likewise the detection of the 6-acetylmorphine metabolite of heroin or of the 6-acetylcodeine heroin contaminant provides evidence for heroin use. However, the detection period for these acetyl derivatives is relatively short (~8 to 12 hours).[105,426] Contrary to measurements in urine, the plasma concentrations of morphine and codeine may more clearly distinguish between heroin and codeine use. Following a single dose of codeine, the plasma codeine concentration exceeded that for morphine (codeine:morphine >1.0) during the entire 23 hours postdose detection period.[254] With heroin use, the expected ratio is <1.0.[80]

The consumption of foods that contain poppy seeds (e.g., cakes, muffins, rolls, and bagels) may result in significant urinary excretion of morphine and codeine.[194,430] Obviously, this may cause false incrimination of illicit opiate use as determined by drug testing programs. ElSohly and coworkers[143] proposed guidelines to eliminate poppy seed ingestion as the source of a positive urine opiate test. According to these guidelines, any of the following findings would eliminate poppy seed ingestion as the principal opiate source: morphine level >5000 ng/mL; codeine level >300 ng/mL; morphine:codeine ratio less than 2; morphine level >1000 ng/mL with no codeine. However, these guidelines may not always be reliable, because the consumption of poppy seed streusel was reported to result in urine samples with concentrations of morphine >5000 ng/mL and of codeine >300 ng/mL.[402] The morphine:codeine ratio, however, was always greater than 2. A lower morphine:codeine ratio would indicate codeine use and thus eliminate poppy seed ingestion as the opiate source. Detection of the heroin metabolite 6-acetylmorphine (see Figure 34-36) would also eliminate poppy seed ingestion.[105,322] However, 6-acetylmorphine is rapidly eliminated, so its detection in urine is limited to earlier than 24 hours (perhaps <8 hours) after heroin use.[105] Therefore the absence of 6-acetylmorphine does not rule out heroin or, of course, morphine use. To avoid some of the issues concerning poppy seed ingestion and the legitimate use of opiate medications, the Department of Defense established confirmatory cutoff concentrations of 4000 ng/mL morphine and 2000 ng/mL codeine, and also requires testing for 6-monoacetylmorphine (see Table 34-8). The Department of Health and Human Services likewise increased the screening and confirmatory cutoff concentrations from 300 ng/mL to 2000 ng/mL for morphine and codeine and also requires testing for 6-acetylmorphine (cutoff, 10 ng/mL).[84] Nevertheless, in the absence of 6-acetylmorphine, even these morphine cutoffs may not always eliminate poppy seed consumption. A 2003 study reported that the consumption of poppy seeds with unusually high morphine content resulted in a peak urine morphine concentration of 10,000 ng/mL.[441] For clinical purposes, the 300 ng/mL (or lower) cutoff is appropriate. From the foregoing discussion, it is obvious that caution is required when interpreting the results of a positive urine test for morphine and codeine.

Hydromorphone and oxymorphone are semisynthetic opiates that have about 8 to 10 times the potency of morphine. Hydromorphone has greater oral bioavailability than morphine; oxymorphone has limited IV use for postsurgical analgesia. Hydrocodone, oxycodone, and dihydrocodeine are 3 to 10 times more potent than codeine, and, like codeine, they have relatively good oral bioavailability. Hydrocodone is metabolized to hydromorphone and dihydrocodeine (Figure 34-37). This conversion is mediated by CYP 2D6, which exhibits genetic polymorphism. Rapid metabolizers form a greater amount of the more potent hydromorphone compared with slow metabolizers. The metabolite transformations for dihydrocodeine and oxycodone are presented in Figures 34-38 and 34-39, respectively. The elimination $t_{1/2}$ for all of these opiates is slightly longer than that for morphine, ranging from about 2.5 to 5 hours.[28,184]

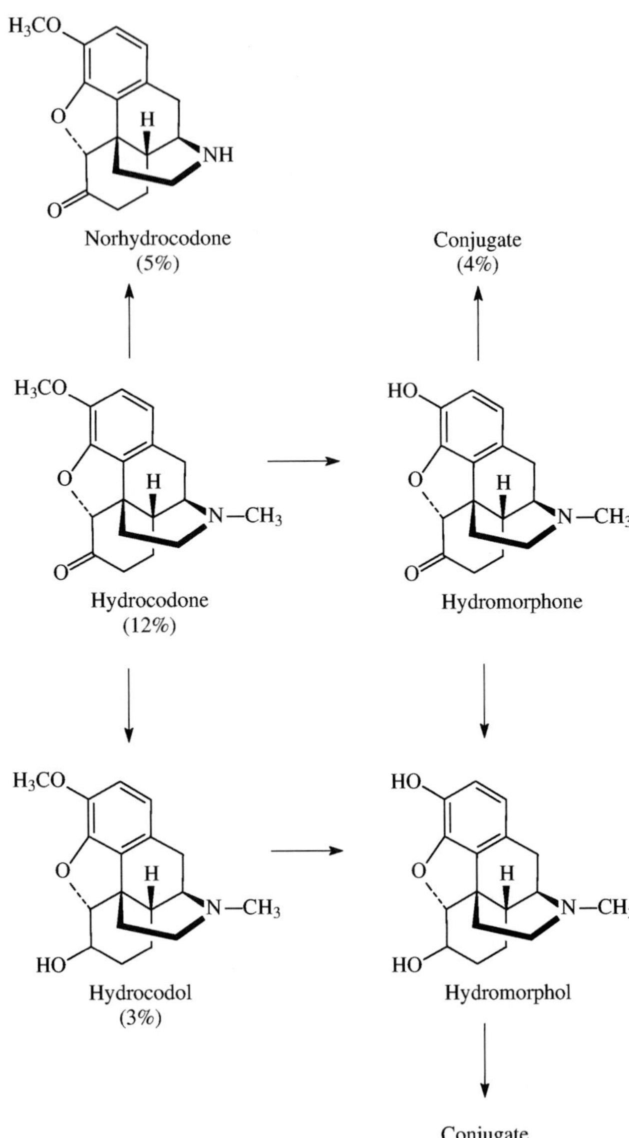

Figure 34-37 Hydrocodone and hydromorphone metabolic transformations. The figures in parenthesis are percent of a dose of hydrocodone excreted in urine. Rapid metabolizers excrete more hydromorphone conjugates (5.9%) compared with slow metabolizers (1.0%). Hydrocodol and hydromorphol exist as 6-α and β-stereiosomers. 6-α-hydrocodol is dihydrocodeine; 6-α-hydromorphol is dihydromorphine. For hydromorphone administration, 6% of the dose is excreted as the free parent drug and 30% as conjugates. Only trace amounts of hydromorphol conjugates are formed.

As for codeine, oxycodone is frequently formulated in combination with aspirin (Percodan) or acetaminophen (Percocet and Tylox). Therefore the detection of either salicylate or acetaminophen along with codeine or oxycodone in the urine of patients who display an opiate toxidrome should lead to the measurement of salicylate or acetaminophen in serum to assess their toxicity (see Salicylate and Acetaminophen sections). Alternatively, empiric quantitive serum acetaminophen and salicylate determinations are

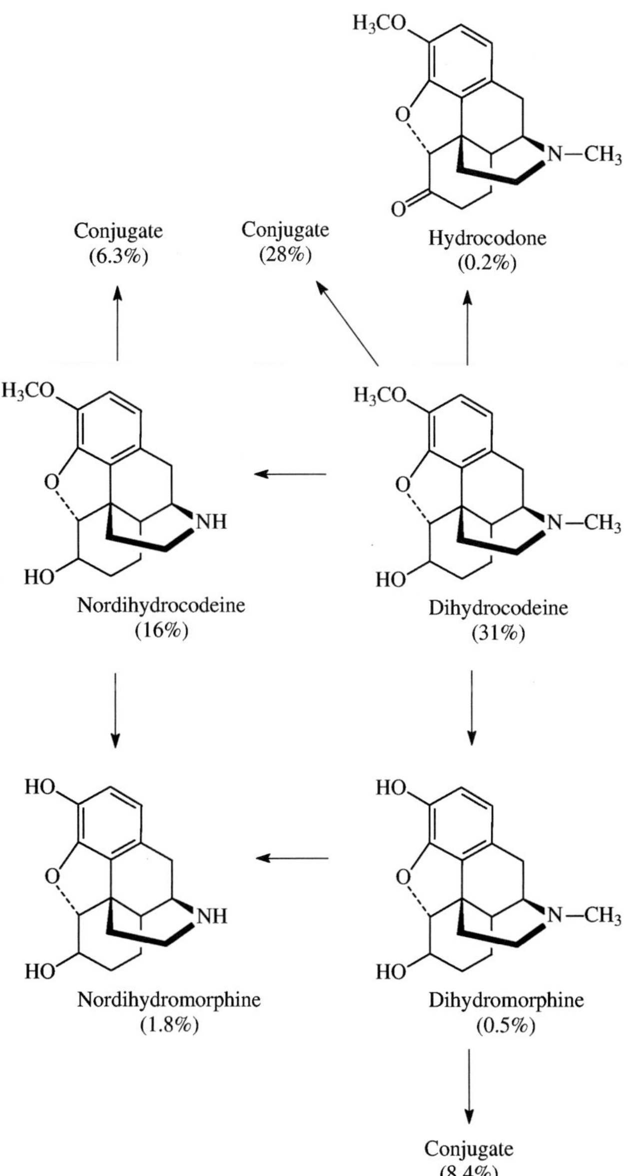

Figure 34-38 Metabolism of dihydrocodeine. Values in parentheses are percent of dose excreted in urine.

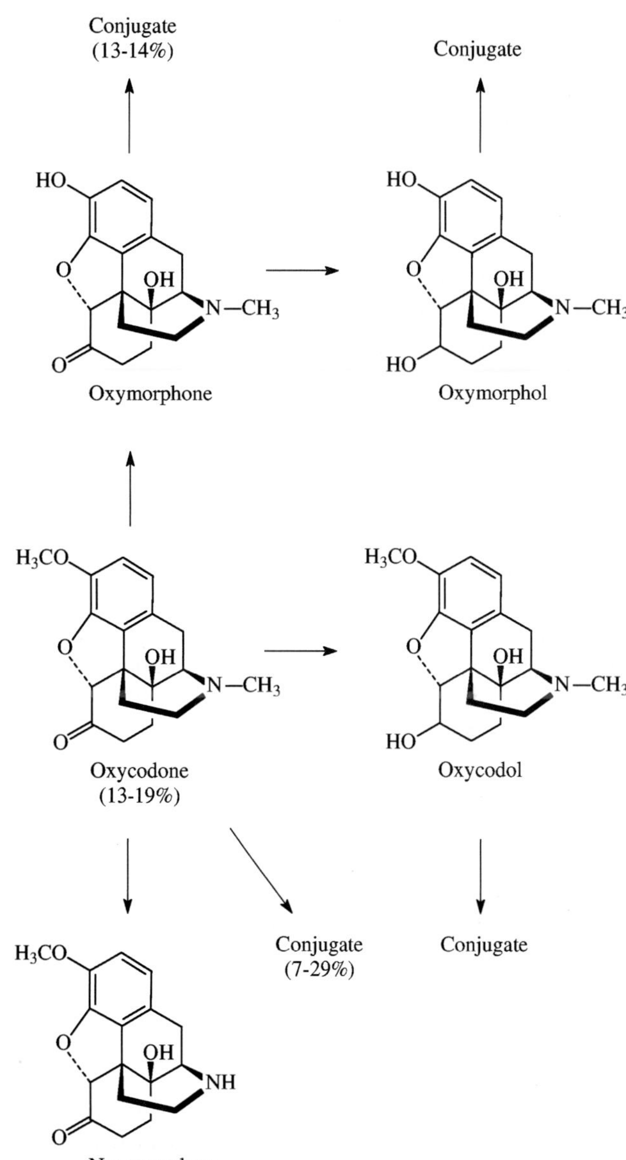

Figure 34-39 Metabolism of oxycodone and oxymorphone. Values in parentheses are percent of oxycodone dose excreted in urine. For oxymorphone dose, 1.9% is excreted as the parent drug, 44% as conjugates, and 3% as oxymorphol.

appropriate for patients with the opioid toxidrome. Non-combination oxycodone is also available in immediate and extended release dosage form. The later (OxyContin) is a very effective oral analgesic for patients with chronic pain (e.g., cancer patients). Illicit diversion of OxyContin has led to especially severe drug abuse, addiction, and several deaths in certain regions of the United States. The pills may be chewed or crushed to release for immediate availability the entire dose, which is intended for extended release over a 12-hour period. In some cases, the crushed pill may be snorted or solubilized for IV injection.

In pain management programs, urine drug testing is often employed to monitor compliance, diversion, or substitution for the prescribed drugs. Based on the results of such tests, an individual may be dismissed from the program. It is important for drug-testing laboratories to communicate relevant aspects of the metabolic interconversion of opiates to physicians responsible for these programs. Otherwise the detection of hydromorphone and dihydrocodeine in addition to prescribed hydrocodone (Figure 34-37) may be falsely interpreted as substitution. Likewise a urine specimen that contains prescribed codeine plus its morphine metabolite or very low concentrations (~100 ng/mL) of the minor hydrocodone metabolite (detected when codeine is >5000 ng/mL) should not be interpreted as heroin and/or morphine or hydrocodone use. Alternatively a urine specimen that tests negative for prescribed codeine but positive for hydromorphone or hydrocodone would clearly indicate substitution.

Monitoring compliance for oxycodone in pain management programs is problematic because of the low cross-reactivity of oxycodone in most opiate immunoassays (e.g., >5000 ng/mL oxycodone for positive result with EMIT assay using a 300 ng/mL morphine cutoff). In this instance, a false-negative opiate immunoassay test may lead to an accusation of oxycodone diversion. The direct determination of oxycodone by GC-MS is more appropriate to monitor compliance for this drug. Alternatively a new, single use, lateral-flow immunoassay test device (see also section on On-Site Drug Test) is available for the initial detection of oxycodone at 100 ng/mL cutoff (Rapid One OXY; American Bio Medica Corp, New York).

Analytical Methodology

The initial screening test for opiates is most often immunoassay. For confirmation of a presumptive positive test, a quantitative drug measurement is performed using GC-MS.[383]

Immunoassay. Immunoassays are rapid, convenient procedures for screening urine specimens for opiates. For clinical application, a cutoff of 300 ng/mL morphine (or morphine equivalents) is commonly used to distinguish negative from positive urine specimens whereas a cutoff of 2000 ng/mL is mandated by SAMHSA for workplace drug screening. The commercial immunoassays for opiates are designed primarily for the detection of morphine and codeine. The degree of cross-reactivity with morphine-3-glucuronide and with other opiates varies among the immunoassays. In general, cross-reactivity with oxycodone and oxymorphone is very low.[281,416] False-positive responses for some immunoassays have resulted from dextromethorphan, diphenhydramine, ephedrine/pseudoephedrine, doxylamine, chlorpheniramine, brompheniramine,[418] quinolone antibiotics,[17,304] and rifampin.[114,458]

The detection period following morphine or codeine use varies somewhat with the dose, the cutoff concentration for the immunoassay, and the degree of cross-reactivity with the glucuronide conjugates. In general, urine specimens test positive for 1 to 3 days following morphine (or heroin) or codeine use when assayed at a cutoff of 300 ng/mL. At a cutoff of 2000 ng/mL, the detection period following single-dose heroin decreased from 24 to 48 hours (300 ng/mL cutoff) to 12 to 24 hours but test specificity increased.[458] The applicability of the higher cutoff has been challenged by the finding of 6-monoacetylmorphine in a high percentage of specimens with morphine <2000 ng/mL in cases of heroin-associated death.[317]

Gas Chromatography-Mass Spectrometry. A positive screening result for opiates obtained by immunoassay is confirmed by GC-MS analysis of the urine specimen.[383] A GC-MS method is included in the Chapter 34 Appendix that is found on this book's accompanying Evolve site (http://evolve.elsevier.com/Tietz/textbook/).

Dextromethorphan

Dextromethorphan is structurally related to the opioids, but it does not bind to opioid receptors at normal dose and is thus devoid of analgesic activity.[327] The (−) isomer of dextromethorphan, levorphan (not available in the United States), is a potent opioid analgesic, and an example of the stereoselective nature of opioid receptor binding.

Dextromethorphan does have antitussive activity comparable with that of codeine. It is present in a number of cough medications, often in combination with antihistamines, nasal decongestants, aspirin, and acetaminophen. At very high dose, dextromethorphan may cause lethargy or somnolence, agitation, ataxia, nystagmus, diaphoresis, and hypertension.[332,484,498] The abuse of dextromethorphan, especially by adolescents and teenagers who refer to it as "DMX," has become widespread in some locations. Abusers describe feelings of euphoria; dissociative effects, such as a sense of floating; and hallucinations. Discontinuation of the drug is frequently followed by dysphoria and depression. Most preparations contain dextromethorphan as the bromide salt. Excessive ingestion of dextromethorphan may result in bromide poisoning and in a negative serum anion gap consequent to the disproportional response to bromide with common methods for chloride analysis.

Dextromethorphan is metabolized to dextrophan (Figure 34-40) by the cytochrome P_{450} isozyme 2D6 (CYP 2D6), which exhibits genetic polymorphism. Dextrophan also lacks analgesic activity, but it does retain antitussive action. Dextrophan may be responsible for the more pleasant psychotropic effects of high dose dextromethorphan, whereas the parent drug may cause dysphoria, sedation, and ataxia.[498] Thus poor metabolizers (deficient in CYP 2D6 activity) may be less prone and extensive metabolizers more prone to continue the abuse of dextromethorphan.

Dextrophan and to a lesser degree dextromethorphan bind to the PCP and ketamine binding site on the *N*-methyl-D-aspartate (NMDA) receptor, which probably accounts for their similar dissociative psychotropic actions[327] (see Phencyclidine and Ketamine).

Dextrophan is the enantiomer of levorphanol, a potent opioid agonist available in the United States (Levo-Dromoran). Unless chiral analytical techniques are used, these enantiomers cannot be resolved. Drug testing laboratories that use conventional chromatographic techniques should not report a finding of levorphanol only, but should instead report dextrophan/levorphanol with a comment on their isomeric relationship and on the origin of dextrophan. This is especially important for pain management drug screening in which a false report of levorphanol may result in dismissal from the program. This report duality is advisable even when parent dextromethorphan is also detected. Savvy abusers of levorphanol conceivably may co-ingest dextromethorphan to conceal use of levorphanol. If such is suspected, chiral resolution of dextrophan and levorphanol would then be necessary.

Dextromethorphan cross-reacts with most immunoassays for opioids.[418]

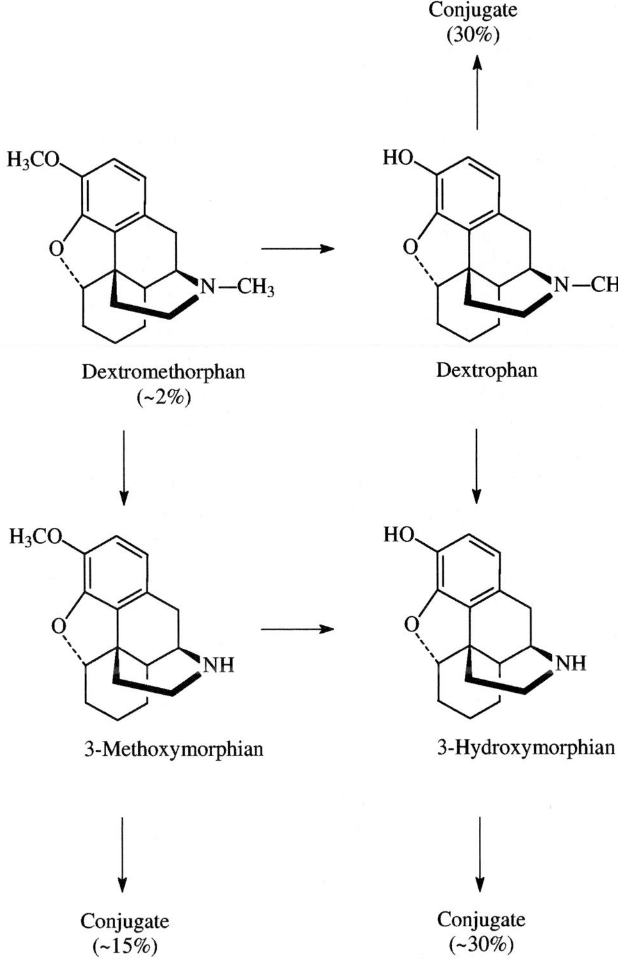

Figure 34-40 Metabolism of dextromethorphan. Values in parenthesis are percent of dose excreted in urine.

Methadone

Methadone is an opioid with similar structure to propoxyphene (see Figure 34-35).

Pharmacological Response

The major pharmacological actions of methadone, mediated by μ- and δ-receptor interactions, are similar to those of other opioids and include analgesia, sedation, respiratory depression, miosis, antitussive effects, and constipation. Methadone is administered as a racemic mixture (R,S-[±]-methadone), but the analgesic activity is due almost entirely to the R(−)-isomer. When administered intramuscularly, methadone and morphine have equivalent analgesic potency. In contrast to morphine, methadone retains about 50% of its intramuscular analgesic potency when taken orally.[184]

Methadone is rapidly absorbed from the GI tract with an onset of action within 30 to 60 minutes. The elimination $t_{1/2}$ is long (15 to 55 hours) compared with morphine ($t_{1/2}$ = 1 to 8 hours). Because of the longer elimination $t_{1/2}$, methadone accumulates in blood and tissue following repeated doses, and this presumably contributes to its relatively long duration of action (6 to 8 hours).[184,268]

Methadone is used clinically (1) for relief of pain, (2) to treat opioid abstinence syndrome, and (3) to treat heroin addicts in an attempt to wean them from illicit IV drug use.[439]

Tolerance to the effects of methadone develops with repeated doses, but more slowly than is true for morphine. Likewise, withdrawal develops more slowly and is generally less intense but more prolonged than morphine withdrawal. Withdrawal symptoms include weakness, anxiety, insomnia, abdominal discomfort, sweating, and hot and cold flashes.[184]

In overdose, methadone causes CNS and respiratory depression, miosis, bradycardia, hypotension, circulatory collapse, hypothermia, coma, seizures, and pulmonary edema (although less frequently than morphine). Treatment for methadone overdose includes supportive measures to maintain adequate respiration and blood pressure, and the administration of the opioid antagonist naloxone to reverse the effects of methadone.[268,485] If repeated administration of naloxone is required, patients should be monitored for 48 to 72 hours following overdose. Dialysis is not an effective treatment modality, because methadone has a large volume of distribution (V_d = 4 to 5 L/kg) and is highly protein bound (87%).[184]

Methadone is metabolized in the liver primarily to 2-ethylidene-1,5-dimethyl-3,3-diphenylpyrrolidine (EDDP) and 2-ethyl-5-methyl-3,3-diphenylpyrroline (EMDP) (Figure 34-41). The principal urinary excretion products are methadone (5% to 50% of dose) and EDDP (3% to 25% of dose); relatively more methadone (pK_a 8.62) than EDDP is excreted when urine is acidic.[33] Monitoring compliance in methadone maintenance programs with urine drug testing may be confounded by the declining dose over time and the pH-dependent urinary excretion of methadone. For such purpose, measurement of EDDP was more effective than methadone in a large study.[170] Moreover, a methadone-positive, EDDP-negative specimen would indicate specimen spiking by a noncompliant patient.

Analytical Methodology

The initial screening test for methadone is typically immunoassay. For confirmation of a presumptive positive test, a quantitative drug measurement is performed using GC-MS.

Immunoassay. Screening immunoassays for methadone include DPC (RIA), EMIT, CEDIA, TDx, and Roche Abuscreen. A typical assay cutoff concentration is 300 ng/mL. No cross-reactivity with EDDP or EDMP has been reported; however, (−)-α-acetylmethadol (LAAM),[89] a long-acting methadone analog, and verapamil metabolites[277] may cross-react in some assays. Methadone may generally be detected in urine for up to 72 hours following ingestion. Immunoassays specific for EDDP are available (CEDIA; DRI).

Gas Chromatography-Mass Spectrometry. A positive screening result for methadone obtained by immunoassay is confirmed by GC-MS analysis of the urine specimen. A GC-MS method for methadone is included in the Chapter 34 Appendix that is found on this book's accompanying Evolve site (http://evolve.elsevier.com/Tietz/textbook/).

Propoxyphene

Propoxyphene is an opioid structurally similar to methadone (see Figure 34-35).

Pharmacological Response

Propoxyphene is a widely prescribed narcotic analgesic with a potency approximately one-half that of codeine when each is orally administered. Typical oral doses of propoxyphene have about the same analgesic effect as 600 mg aspirin.[184] Only the (+)-isomer (Darvon, others) binds to μ receptors to produce analgesia; the (−)-isomer (Novrad; appropriately the mirror image spelling of Darvon) is devoid of analgesic activity but is effective as an antitussive agent. Propoxyphene is prescribed most often as a combination with acetaminophen or aspirin.[184]

Propoxyphene is rapidly absorbed and undergoes extensive hepatic first-pass metabolism to norpropoxyphene (Figure 34-42). The elimination $t_{1/2}$ for propoxyphene is about 15 hours (8 to 24), and that for norpropoxyphene is 27 hours (24 to 34). Norpropoxyphene may contribute to the analgesic and cardiotoxic effects of propoxyphene.[36]

Propoxyphene overdose may result in nausea, vomiting, and drowsiness or in more severe cases, CNS depression, convulsion, respiratory depression, and cardiovascular collapse. Cardiac arrhythmia atypical for opioid overdose is a consequence of blockade of myocardial Na^+ channels, primarily by norpropoxyphene (similar to tricyclic antidepressant cardiotoxicity). Death, usually a result of respiratory depression and cardiac arrhythmia, is more common when propoxyphene is ingested with another CNS depressant, such as alcohol.[184,327]

Propoxyphene and norpropoxyphene may be quantified in serum by GC or HPLC, but because of the poor correlation between serum concentration and degree of impairment or prognosis, such quantitative information is generally not helpful in cases of propoxyphene overdose. However, their qualitative identification in urine may be useful to help confirm or establish the cause of a patient's symptomatology. Because propoxyphene is frequently taken in combination with acetaminophen or aspirin, quantitation

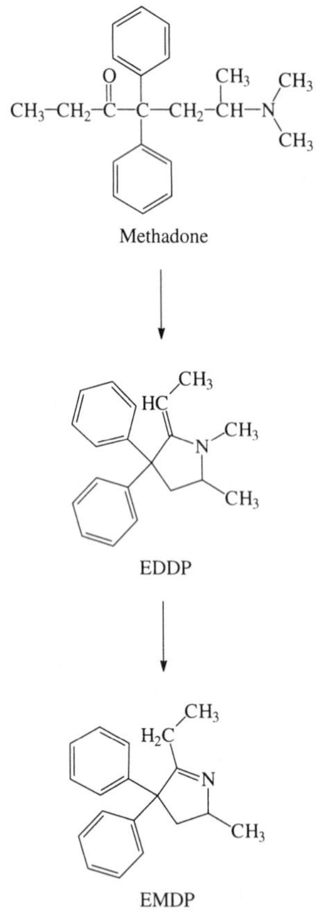

Methadone

EDDP

EMDP

Figure 34-41 Metabolism of methadone.

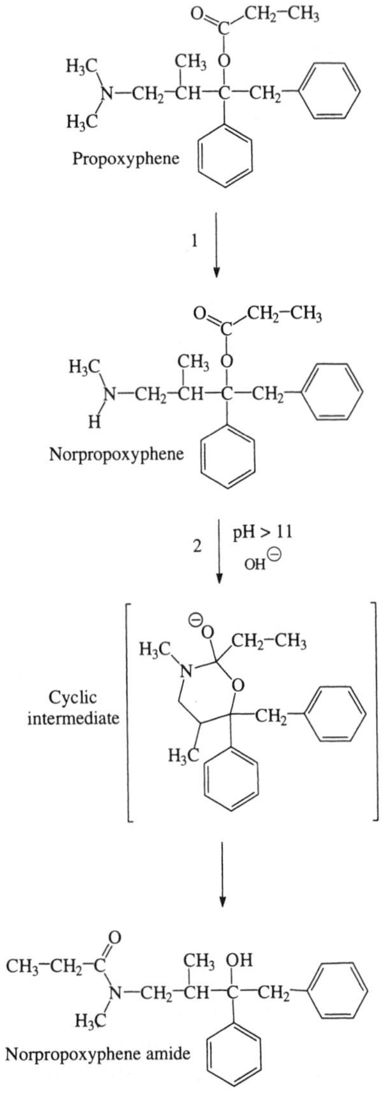

Propoxyphene

1

Norpropoxyphene

2 pH > 11 OH⊖

Cyclic intermediate

Norpropoxyphene amide

Figure 34-42 *1*, *N*-Demethylation of propoxyphene; 2, Base-catalyzed conversion of norpropoxyphene to norpropoxyphene amide.

of acetaminophen and salicylate in serum is advisable to assess their possible toxicity.

Naloxone is effective in reversing the CNS and respiratory depressant actions of propoxyphene but has little effect on the cardiotoxicity. The latter may be treated with $NaHCO_3$ to reverse the Na^+-channel inhibition (a similar therapeutic rationale applies to the treatment of tricyclic antidepressant cardiotoxicity). Because propoxyphene has a large volume of distribution (10 to 18 L/kg) and is highly protein bound (70% to 80%), hemodialysis is of little value in instances of serious overdose. Forced diuresis likewise is of little value because only about 1% is eliminated in urine as unchanged propoxyphene.

Analytical Methodology

The initial screening test for propoxyphene is typically immunoassay. For confirmation of a presumptive positive test, a quantitative drug measurement is performed using GC-MS.

Immunoassay. Immunoassays for propoxyphene (EMIT, CEDIA, FPIA) are designed for the detection of the parent drug; cross-reactivity with norpropoxyphene, present in much greater concentration than the parent drug, is weak, especially for EMIT. In general, propoxyphene may be detected for about 2 days following use. Diphenhydramine may produce a false-positive response with EMIT.[395]

Gas Chromatography-Mass Spectrometry. A positive screening result for propoxyphene obtained by immunoassay is confirmed by GC-MS analysis of the urine specimen for norpropoxyphene. Because norpropoxyphene is present in urine at considerably greater concentrations than propoxyphene, and because the latter has poor gas chromatographic characteristics, confirmation analysis by GC-MS is directed at the determination of norpropoxyphene after its conversion to norpropoxyphene amide. A GC-MS method for norpropoxyphene is included in the Chapter 34 Appendix that is found on this book's accompanying Evolve site (http://evolve.elsevier.com/Tietz/textbook/).

Phencyclidine and Ketamine

Phencyclidine (PCP) is a potent veterinary analgesic and anesthetic; it is sometimes used illicitly by humans in cases of drug abuse, leading to serious psychological disturbances. Ketamine is a rapid-acting general anesthetic and anesthesia adjunct, administered intramuscularly and intravenously.

Pharmacological Response

PCP and ketamine share common structural features (Figures 34-43 and 34-44) and possess similar pharmacological actions. They are classified as dissociative anesthetics because they cause functional dissociation of pain perception, consciousness, movement, and memory.[335] Thus an anesthetic dose produces profound analgesia, but the indi-

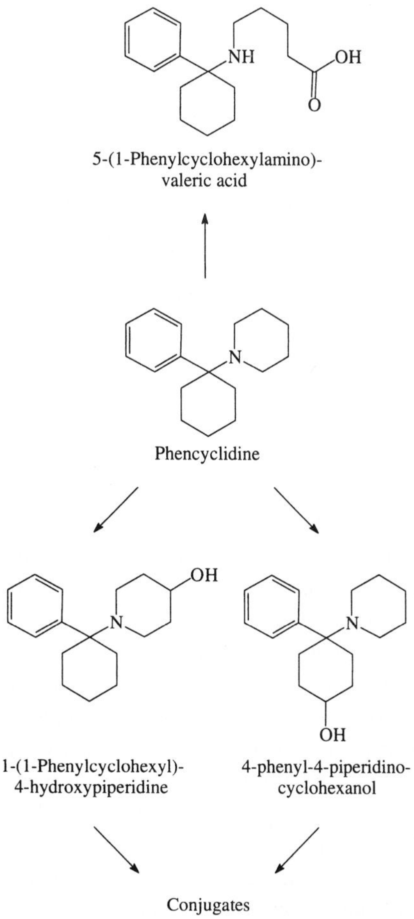

5-(1-Phenylcyclohexylamino)-valeric acid

Phencyclidine

1-(1-Phenylcyclohexyl)-4-hydroxypiperidine

4-phenyl-4-piperidino-cyclohexanol

Conjugates

Figure 34-43 Metabolism of PCP.

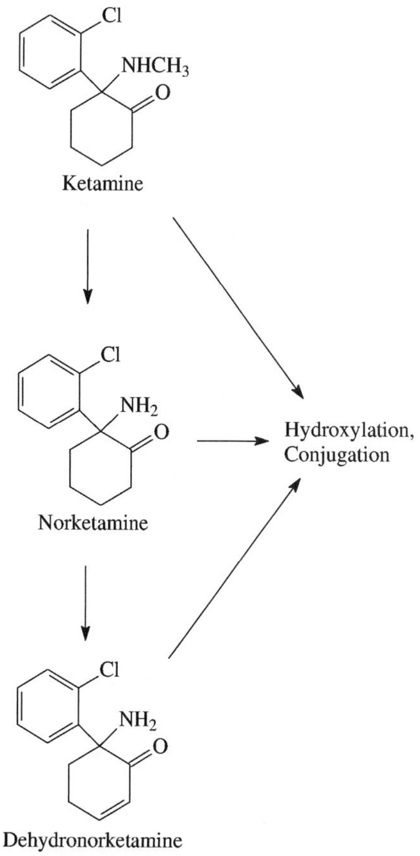

Ketamine

Norketamine

Dehydronorketamine

Hydroxylation, Conjugation

Figure 34-44 Metabolism of ketamine.

viduals are in an amnestic and cataleptic state with eyes open, are able to move limbs involuntarily, and have minimal respiratory or cardiovascular depression. Because some individuals experience acute psychosis and dysphoria during emergence from PCP-induced anesthesia, it was quickly withdrawn from clinical use. Ketamine has about one tenth the potency of PCP, a shorter duration of action, and less prominent emergence reactions, especially in children. Its use in humans is largely limited to pediatrics, but it is widely applied in veterinary medicine.

Most anesthetic agents activate CNS inhibitory $GABA_A$ receptors, glycine-gated Cl^- channel receptors, or nicotinic receptors (acetylcholine-gated Na^+ channels). PCP and ketamine are unique as they act by inhibiting the excitatory glutaminergic system by binding to an *N*-methyl-D-aspartate (NMDA) receptor site to produce noncompetitive allosteric inhibition of glutamate binding.[335] Additional actions include euphoria, elevated blood pressure, tachycardia, and bronchodilation, consequences of inhibition of dopamine and norepinephrine synaptic reuptake. At a higher dose, GABA-ergic and central nicotinic actions may produce sedation, lethargy, coma, and respiratory depression. Additionally, central and peripheral muscarinic and nicotinic response may cause miosis or mydriasis, diaphoresis, increased salivation, bronchorrhea, blurred vision, and urinary retention.

The acronym PCP is derived from the chemical name for PCP, 1-(1-**p**henyl**c**yclohexyl)-**p**iperidine or more colorfully from its designation during the 1960s as the "**p**eace **p**ill". PCP is used recreationally for its mind-altering or "out of body" experience. Adverse effects are complex and unpredictable. In addition to those previously cited, these include dysphoria, ataxia, nystagmus, agitation, anxiety, paranoia, amnesia, seizures, muscle rigidity, hostility, delirium, delusions of grandeur, and hallucinations. A sense of superhuman strength coupled with the lack of pain perception may lead to excessive physical exertion and accidental or intentional self-induced trauma, which in some cases may lead to rhabdomyolysis and myoglobinuric renal failure. Thus PCP-related deaths most often are secondary to these adverse behavioral drug effects. Recreational use of PCP has declined since the 1980s but continues to be a problem in some large metropolitan cities.

With repeated use of PCP, psychological dependence may develop, but tolerance or withdrawal syndrome is not profound.

The drug is rapidly absorbed from the GI tract. This form of ingestion is difficult to regulate and results therefore in the highest probability of overdose or "bad trips." Thus, smoking (PCP sprinkled on tobacco, parsley leaves, or marijuana) is now the most popular mode of ingestion, because users may self-titrate the most dangerous effects of PCP.[487] Once absorbed, PCP is extensively metabolized by the liver (~90% of a dose); only 10% to 15% is excreted unchanged in the urine. The principal metabolites excreted in urine are the glucuronide conjugates of hydroxylated metabolites (~25% to 30%), 5-(1-phenylcyclohexyl-amino) valeric acid (~15%), and unidentified polar metabolites (~40%)[107] (Figure 34-43).[107]

PCP is a lipophilic weak base (pK_a ~8.5). It is secreted into and "trapped" in ionized form in the acidic gastric fluid where concentrations may be 20 to 50 times greater than in serum; subsequently, PCP is reabsorbed in the alkaline duodenum.[487] This gastroenterohepatic recirculation probably contributes to the typical waxing and waning of clinical effects of PCP and, along with its large V_d of 5 to 7 L/kg, partly explains PCP's long elimination $t_{1/2}$ (20 to 50 hours), long duration of action (24 to 48 hours), and prolonged urinary excretion after the last dose (1 to 2 weeks; longer with chronic use).[487]

Treatment of PCP toxicity is supportive. Severe agitation or seizures may respond to diazepam; severe psychoses may require a neuroleptic drug, such as haloperidol.[487] For the most serious cases, continuous nasogastric suction to help remove PCP may be beneficial; urine acidification to hasten elimination has been advocated by some but is controversial.[335]

Ketamine (known on the street as vitamin K, Special K, Super K, cat valium) has become popular as a "club drug" for its PCP- and LSD-like mood altering hallucinogenic effects (referred to as "K-land"), but at higher dose it may cause an "out of body" or "near-death" experience referred to as the "K-hole." Its anesthetic and amnestic properties reportedly have resulted in its use as a date-rape drug.[11] Ketamine is metabolized to norketamine, which has about one third the activity of ketamine, and to dehydronorketamine, which may also be active (Figure 34-44).[31,113]

Analytical Methodology

The initial screening test for PCP is typically immunoassay. For confirmation of a presumptive positive test, a quantitative drug measurement is performed using GC-MS.[158] Immunoassays for ketamine are not available. Ketamine, norketamine, and dehydronorketamine may be determined by GC-MS or LC-MS.[318]

Immunoassay. Quantification of PCP in serum is not helpful in the diagnosis or management of PCP toxicity, because there is low correlation between drug concentration and drug effects.[335] However, qualitative identification of PCP in urine is useful to help diagnose PCP toxicity. For this purpose, PCP-specific immunoassays are rapid and generally are more sensitive than thin-layer chromatography. Whether or not PCP is included in a general urine drug screen depends on applicable regulations and on the prevalence of PCP use in the local community. In some locations, the prevalence of PCP use may be too low to warrant routine screening for PCP. Immunoassays for PCP (e.g., EMIT, FPIA, CEDIA, Roche Abuscreen) are generally reliable; false positives have been reported because of high concentrations of dextromethorphan,[56] diphenhydramine,[272] and thioridazine.[283,466] Confirmation of immunoassay-positive specimens using an alternate technique (e.g., GC-MS) is therefore necessary.

Gas Chromatography-Mass Spectrometry. PCP is required to be included in U.S. government–regulated drug abuse screening programs (see Table 34-8); nongovernmental screening programs may elect to include PCP in drug abuse screens, depending on the local probability of PCP use. Initial screening by immunoassay, if positive, is followed by confirmation using GC-MS. A GC-MS method for PCP is included in the Chapter 34 Appendix that is found on this book's accompanying Evolve site (http://evolve.elsevier.com/Tietz/textbook/).

Detection of Drugs of Abuse Using Other Types of Specimens

Urine is currently the most common specimen for detection of drugs of abuse. However, the window of detectability in urine is generally limited to a few days following drug use. In addition, the collection of urine may require some invasion of privacy and loss of dignity, and urine specimens are subject to adulteration or manipulation to evade detection. For these reasons, alternate biological specimens that may avoid some of these limitations have been investigated.[76]

Meconium

Alcohol and drug use during pregnancy is a significant social and medical issue. One study estimated that approximately 11% of women have used illicit drugs during pregnancy[88]; another reported that 15% of the pregnant women studied had used alcohol or illicit drugs.[87] Infants born to mothers who used illicit drugs have an increased rate of perinatal morbidity, mortality, and neurobehavioral problems. Prevention of drug use during pregnancy and proper treatment of drug-exposed infants depend on recognition (detection) of drug use or exposure. Because maternal self-reporting is not reliable, it has been suggested that urine drug testing be performed for high-risk populations as part of standard prenatal care.[100] However, urine testing of the mother or newborn is able to detect only recent drug use (within a few days before birth), and urine collection from newborns may be problematic. For these reasons, Ostrea and co-workers pioneered drug testing using meconium, the fecal material present in the newborn's stool during the first 2 to 3 days, and presented evidence for an improved drug detection rate compared with urine.[342]

Meconium begins to form during the second trimester and continues to accumulate until birth. Drugs are believed to be deposited in meconium via fetal bile excretion and from swallowed amniotic fluid, which contains drug and drug metabolites eliminated in the fetal urine. Testing meconium may therefore provide historical evidence of maternal drug use anytime during the last two trimesters. The greater utility of meconium drug testing compared with urine has been confirmed by others.[74,273,325] Other investigators have suggested that detection limit of the assay is more important than specimen type and that urine test results comparable to meconium will be achieved by lowering the typical screening cutoff for urine testing.[79,120,192,259]

Whereas meconium is more easily collected from newborns than urine, it is considerably more difficult to analyze. Meconium is a heterogeneous, gelatinous material from which drugs must be extracted before analysis by immunoassay and confirmation by GC-MS.[146] It should be noted that drug extraction from meconium using inorganic acids, methanol, or any other alcohol is protected by U.S. patents.[340,341]

Studies on meconium have raised new issues concerning fetal versus maternal drug metabolism. For instance, while *m*-hydroxybenzoylecgonine and *p*-hydroxybenzoylecgonine are present in lesser amounts in adult urine than benzoylecgonine, they are major contributors to the benzoylecgonine immunoreactivity in meconium.[346,427] It is unclear whether these findings represent a difference in fetal cocaine metabolism or are the result of placental transfer of these metabolites. Likewise, concordance between immunoassay screening for marijuana metabolites and GC-MS confirmation for THC-COOH (see Cannabinoids) is considerably less for meconium than for urine, because meconium contains greater amounts of 11-hydroxy-Δ^9-THC and 8β,11-dihydroxy-Δ^9-THC metabolites.[145,146]

As for adult urine, cocaethylene may be detected in meconium, and its presence indicates maternal use of ethanol and cocaine (see section on Cocaine). Significant alcohol use during pregnancy may be indicated by measurement of fatty acid ethyl esters in meconium.[315]

Meconium drug testing is growing but is far less standardized than urine drug testing. Assay cutoff limits and units (ng/g meconium or ng/mL of extract) may vary, and suitable reference or control materials are not yet available. Cutoff limits proposed by SAMHSA are presented in Table 34-9.

Hair

Since the 1970s, hair has been analyzed for trace metals for purposes of assessing nutritional status. However, (1) lack of standardized procedures (collection, preparation, and analysis), (2) lack of reference limits, and (3) problems due to environmental contamination have limited the success of hair analysis for this purpose. However, the analysis of lead, arsenic, and mercury in hair is an established and accepted method of assessing prior toxic exposure to these metals (see Chapter 35).

The analysis of drugs in human hair was described by Baumgartner et al in 1979.[41] Since then, there has been increasing interest in the analysis of hair for the purpose of detecting drug use.[42,190,213,241,243] Hair is advantageous as a biological specimen, because it is easily obtained without loss of privacy or dignity (unless pubic hair is obtained), and it is not easily altered or manipulated to avoid drug detection. Moreover, once deposited in hair, drugs are very stable; therefore prior drug use may be detected for several months. Because hair grows at a relatively constant rate (0.3 to 0.4 mm/d), the potential exists for segmental hair analysis to provide a "chronicle" of prior drug use.

The mechanisms by which drugs are deposited in hair are not well understood but may include transfer from blood to the growing hair shaft, transfer from sweat and sebum (some sweat glands empty into hair follicles), and environmental contamination.[236] Factors that may affect the deposition of drugs in hair also are not well established but may include the rate of hair growth, anatomical location of hair, type of hair, hair color (melanin content), effects of various hair treatments, and environmental contamination, especially for drugs that are smoked (marijuana, cocaine, heroin, and PCP).

Drugs, when deposited in hair, are generally present in relatively low concentrations (pg/mg-ng/mg); thus sensitive analytical techniques are required for detection. Moreover, parent drug is generally present in greater amount than metabolites. Parent drug–specific RIA procedures have most commonly been used for drug detection in hair. Some immunoassays designed primarily for urine drug testing and therefore that may have greatest reactivity with metabolites are of limited use for hair analysis. Confirmation of immunoassay results, generally by GC-MS, GC-MS-MS, or LC-MS-MS, remains a requisite for any forensic application of hair drug testing. These techniques may also be suitable for initial qualitative drug abuse screening[351] and for direct sequential hair analysis without prior immunoassay.[255]

For drug detection, hair offers potential advantages compared with urine, but much additional research will be necessary before hair analysis becomes applied generally. A better understanding of the disposition kinetics of drugs in hair is needed; methods of washing, extraction or digestion, and analysis will all have to be more standardized; cutoff limits will have to be agreed upon; and suitable quality control and proficiency test materials will have to be developed. Toward these goals, SAMHSA has proposed draft drug cutoff values for hair analysis (Table 34-9).

Sweat

Drugs may be excreted in sweat and, as for hair, the parent drug is generally present in a greater amount than metabolites.[213,242] Moreover, sweat excretion may be an important mechanism by which drugs enter hair.[101]

Sweat patch collection devices that resemble an adhesive bandage may be worn for several days to several weeks, during which drug, if present, accumulates in the absorbent pad in the patch while water vapor escapes through the semipermeable covering.[245] Thus sweat drug testing offers the possibility to monitor drug use over extended periods of time without the need for frequent collection of urine.[71] Sweat drug testing would be particularly advantageous for monitoring drug use in correctional institutions or in drug rehabilitation programs.[244] Cutoff values currently proposed by SAMHSA are listed in Table 34-9.

Saliva (Oral Fluid)

The measurement of drugs in saliva is of interest both for purposes of therapeutic drug monitoring and for the detection of illicit drug use.[213,397] Compared with urine, saliva is easy to obtain, with less invasion of privacy and ease of adulteration. Saliva is an ultrafiltrate of plasma; therefore drug concentration in it reflects the free or active fraction and may more closely reflect drug effect than is possible with urine measurements. The transfer of drug from blood to saliva is influenced by drug protein binding, pK_a, lipid solubility, and blood pH (saliva is more acidic than blood). In general, drugs are present in saliva in lower concentration and may be detected for a shorter time period compared with urine.[396,397] Detection of drugs in saliva therefore indicates recent drug use. Moreover, saliva drug concentration may correlate with degree of impairment, except when buccal contamination may have occurred because of oral ingestion, smoking, or snorting of the drug. The SAMHSA draft cutoff values for drugs in saliva are presented in Table 34-9; they have been validated by a large study.[103] (See also Alcohols for a discussion of ethanol measurements in saliva.)

ON-SITE DRUG TESTING

On-site drug test devices for urine and saliva are designed for easy, rugged, and portable use by nontechnical personnel.[336] Although they are relatively simple to use, proper training of nonlaboratory users is important for optimal performance.[169,234,252]

Many on-site devices are commercially available for urine drug testing and at least six for saliva drug testing. They are noninstrumental immunoassay test devices that are designed for use at the site of collection with results available within 3 to ~10 minutes and are variously configured to detect only one drug or as many as 10 drugs simultaneously. The spectrum of drugs tested includes tricyclic antidepressants, barbiturates, benzodiazepines, methadone, MDMA (MDA and MDEA), oxycodone, and the traditional SAMHSA or NIDA 5. As previously cited, such devices are also available for measurement of acetaminophen and salicylate in serum or whole blood. Evaluations for some of these test devices for urine* and saliva[319,362] have been published. A comprehensive review of on-site drug testing is also available.[356] (Also see earlier section on Alcohols for discussion of on-site alcohol testing).

The assay principles of these on-site test devices are briefly summarized with some selected product listings.

SEQUENTIAL COMPETITIVE BINDING MICROPARTICLE CAPTURE IMMUNOASSAY

The Triage (BioSite Diagnostics, San Diego) is an example of a on-site test device that uses a sequential, two-step, competitive binding microparticle capture immunoassay. In this device, drug–colloidal gold microparticles compete with the drug in urine for drug-specific first antibody. The mixture is then transferred onto a membrane that contains an immo-

*References 110, 111, 118, 237, 252, 356, 435, 436, 448, 483, 493.

bilized, drug-specific second antibody. If a drug is present at concentrations above the threshold, the insufficient first antibody is available to combine with all drug–gold particle conjugates. These drug conjugates then bind to an immobilized second antibody to form a colored band, which appears after washing the membrane to remove unbound drug conjugate. If drug is absent or present below threshold concentration, the first antibody combines with all drug–gold particles, which then prevents their subsequent binding to the second antibody. In this case, no colored band is formed. Ligand-conjugated control microparticles and antiligand antibodies are included and the membrane configured to provide both positive internal control (adequate transfer of reagents) and negative internal control (inadequate incubation time).

Homogenous Microparticle Capture Immunochromatography

The underlying principle of one-step, solid-phase immunochromatography (also known as lateral flow immunoassay) is the inhibition of antigen-antibody capture on a porous membrane by a drug present in the specimen. Different applications of this measurement concept have been commercialized.

One approach used by a number of on-site drug testing devices may be characterized as homogenous microparticle capture immunochromatography. In this technique, a drug conjugate is immobilized on the porous membrane and drug-specific antibody, coated on colored microparticles, is present in the specimen application portion of the membrane. When specimen is applied, it moves along the membrane by capillary action; in the process, the antibody-coated microparticles are mobilized.

If drug is present above threshold concentration, the limited antibody binding sites on the colored microparticles are all saturated; these particles cannot react with immobilized drug conjugate and therefore no colored band appears at the test line (positive test). If drug is absent or present below threshold concentration, the microparticles are captured by the immobilized drug conjugate to form a colored band at the test line (negative test). For internal quality control, microparticles not bound at the test line progress to a control line where they are captured by the immobilized antibody (e.g., antimouse or anti BSA if the microparticles are also coated with BSA).

A number of devices are based on this test format including First Check (Worldwide Medical Corp, Irvine, Calif.), microLine (Drug Screening Systems Inc., Blackwood, N.J.), Ontrak TesTcup (Roche Diagnostics, Cherry Hill, N.J.), Verdict (Editek, Inc., Burlington, N.C.), Visualine II (Sun Biomedical Laboratories, Cherry Hill, N.J.), and StarTox (Starplex Scientific, Ontario, Canada).

A variation of the microparticle capture approach is designed to allow visualization of the colored microparticles not captured by the immobilized drug. The intensity of the color, compared with a reference chart, determines test status. This approach is used in the Frontline device (Roche Diagnostics).

Some on-site drug test devices use dye-conjugated, drug-specific antibodies in place of microparticles. Otherwise, test principles are the same as those for the microparticle capture immunoassay. Test devices in this format include AccuSign (Princeton Biomeditech Corp., Princeton, N.J.) and Syva Rapid Test (Dade Behring, Newark, Del.).

Yet another variation reverses the capture configuration. In this case, drug-specific antibody is immobilized on the membrane and the dye-conjugated drug is contained in the application zone. Test principles otherwise remain the same. Examples with this format include Status DS and Status Stik (LifeSign, Somerset, N.J.).

Solid Phase Competitive Sequential Enzyme Immunoassay

A solid phase competitive enzyme immunoassay is used by a number of on-site drug testing devices, including the EZ-Screen (Editek, Inc., Burlington, N.C.), I.D. Block (International Diagnostic Systems Corp., St. Joseph, Mich.), and Target (V-Tech, Inc., Pomona, Calif.). In these devices, drug in urine competes with a drug-enzyme conjugate for a limited number of drug-specific, membrane-immobilized antibody binding sites. After reaction, the membrane is washed to remove unbound drug-enzyme conjugate, and enzyme substrate is added. Because of the competitive nature of the assay, color formation is inversely proportional to urine drug concentration (i.e., higher drug concentrations result in less binding of drug-enzyme conjugate and therefore less color formation).

Latex-Agglutination-Inhibition Immunoassay

The Abuscreen Ontrak (Roche Diagnostic Systems, Branchburg, N.J.) is an example of an on-site device that uses a latex-agglutination-inhibition immunoassay. In this type of assay, drug in urine and drug-latex particle conjugates compete for a limited number of drug-specific antibody binding sites. If drug is absent or below threshold concentration, drug-latex particle conjugates react with antibody and are agglutinated. When the drug is present above threshold, insufficient antibody binding sites are available for reaction with drug-latex conjugates, and their agglutination is thus inhibited.

REFERENCES

1. Abou-Donia MB, Lapadula DM. Mechanisms of organophosphorus ester-induced delayed neurotoxicity: type I and type II. Ann Rev Pharmacol Toxicol 1990;30:405-40.
2. Albertson TE, Van Hoozen BF, Allen RP. Amphetamines. In: Haddad LM, Shannon MW, Winchester JF, eds. Clinical management of poisoning and drug overdose, 3rd ed. Philadelphia: WB Saunders Co, 1998:560-8.

3. Allen K, Hamlin C. Interference in a rapid enzymatic method for ethylene glycol. Ann Clin Lab Sci 1993; 23:321. (abstract).
4. Allen MJ Procedures for transportation workplace drug testing programs. Fed Reg 1989;54:49854-84. (http://www.dot.gov/ost/dapc/NEW_DOCS/part40_complete_20041109_A.doc).
5. Ambre J, Fischman M, Ruo T-I. Urinary excretion of ecgonine methyl ester, a major metabolite of cocaine in humans. J Anal Toxicol 1984;8:23-5.
6. Ambre J, Ruo TI, Nelson J, Belknap S. Urinary excretion of cocaine, benzoylecgonine, and ecgonine methyl ester in humans. J Anal Toxicol 1988;12:301-6.
7. Ambre J. The urinary excretion of cocaine and metabolites in humans: A kinetic analysis of published data. J Anal Toxicol 1985;9:241-5.
8. Ambre JJ, Belknap SM, Nelson J, Ruo TI, Shin SG, Atkinson AJ Jr. Acute tolerance to cocaine in humans. Clin Pharmacol Ther 1988;44:1-8.
9. American Academy of Clinical Toxicology and European Association of Poisons Centers and Clinical Toxicologists position statement: Multiple-dose oral activated charcoal. J Toxicol Clin Toxicol 1999; 37:731-51.
10. Ames MA, Moyer TP, Kovach JS, Moertel CG, Rubin J. Pharmacology of amygdalin (laetrile) in cancer patients. Cancer Chemother Pharmacol 198;6:51-7.
11. An Overview of Club Drugs, Drug Intelligence Brief, DEA, Feb 2000.
12. Apple FS, Lowe MC, Googins MK, Kloss J. Serum thiocyanate concentrations in patients with normal or impaired renal function receiving nitroprusside. Clin Chem 1996;42:1878-9 (Letter).
13. Ariano RE, Kassum DA, Aronson KJ. Comparison of sedative recovery time after midazolam versus diazepam administration. Crit Care Med 1994; 22:1492-6.
14. Arima H, Sabue K, So M, Morishima T, Ando H, Katsuya H. Transient and reversible parkinsonism after acute organophosphate poisoning. J Toxicol Clin Toxicol 2003;41:67-70.
15. Aygun D, Doganay Z, Altintop L, Guven H, Onar M, Deniz T, et al. Serum acetylcholinesterase and prognosis of acute organophosphate poisoning. J Toxicol Clin Toxicol 2002;40:903-10.
16. Axelrod J, Felder CC. Cannabinoid receptors and their endogenous agonist, amandamide. Neurochem Res 1998;23:575-81.
17. Baden LR, Horowitz G, Jacoby H Eliopoulos GM. Quinolones and false-positive urine screening for opiates by immunoassay technology. JAMA 2001; 286:3115-9.
18. Bailey DN. Cocaethylene (ethylcocaine) detection during toxicological screening of a university medical center patient population. J Anal Toxicol 1995; 19:247-50.
19. Bailey DN. Serial plasma concentrations of cocaethylene, cocaine and ethanol in trauma victims. J Anal Toxicol 1993;17:79-83.
20. Baldessarini RJ. Drugs and the treatment of psychiatric disorders. Depression and anxiety disorders. In: Hardman JG, Limbird LE, Gilman AG, eds. Goodman and Gilman's the pharmacological basis of therapeutics. 10th ed. New York: McGraw-Hill, 2001:447-83.
21. Baldessarini RJ Tarazi FI. Drugs and the treatment of psychiatric disorders. Psychosis and mania.In: Hardman JG, Limbird LE, Gilman AG, eds. Goodman and Gilman's the pharmacological basis of therapeutics. 10th ed. New York: McGraw-Hill, 2001:485-520.
22. Barceloux DG, Bond GR, Krenzelok EP, Cooper H, Vale JA. American Academy of Clinical Toxicology practice guidelines on the treatment of methanol poisoning. J Toxicol Clin Toxicol 2002;40:415-46.
23. Barceloux DG, Krenzelok EP, Olson K, Watson W. American Academy of Clinical Toxicology practice guidelines on the treatment of ethylene glycol poisoning. J Toxicol Clin Toxicol 1999;37:537-60.
24. Bardin PG, van Eeden SF, Moolman JA, Foden AP, Joubert JR. Organophosphate and carbamate poisoning. Arch Int Med 1994;154:1433-41.
25. Bartlett R. Carbon monoxide poisoning. In: Haddad LM, Shannon MW, Winchester JF, eds. Clinical management of poisoning and drug overdose, 3rd ed. Philadelphia: WB Saunders Co, 1998:885-98.
26. Baselt RC. Amphetamine. In: Disposition of toxic drugs and chemicals in man. 7th ed. Foster City, CA: Biomedical Publications, 2004:66-9.
27. Baselt RC. Carbon monoxide. In: Disposition of toxic drugs and chemicals in man, 7th ed. Foster City, CA: Biomedical Publications, 2004:175-8.
28. Baselt RC. In: Disposition of toxic drugs and chemicals in man, 7th ed. Foster City, CA: Biomedical Publications, 2004:344, 546, 550, 829.
29. Baselt RC. Ethylene glycol. In: Disposition of toxic drugs and chemicals in man, 7th ed. Foster City, CA: Biomedical Publications, 2004:425-8.
30. Baselt RC. Heroin In: Disposition of toxic drugs and chemicals in man, 7th ed. Foster City, CA: Biomedical Publications, 2004:532-6.
31. Baselt RC. Ketamine In: Disposition of toxic drugs and chemicals in man, 7th ed. Foster City, CA: Biomedical Publications, 2004:586-8.
32. Baselt RC. Lysergic acid diethylamide. In: Disposition of toxic drugs and chemicals in man, 7th ed. Foster City, CA: Biomedical Publications, 2004:629-31.
33. Baselt RC. Methadone. In: Disposition of toxic drugs and chemicals in man, 7th ed. Foster City, CA: Biomedical Publications, 2004:678-82.
34. Baselt RC. Methylphenidate. In: Disposition of toxic drugs and chemicals in man, 7th ed. Foster City, CA: Biomedical Publications, 2004:728-30.

35. Baselt RC. Morphine. In: Disposition of toxic drugs and chemicals in man, 7th ed. Foster City, CA: Biomedical Publications, 2004:759-63.
36. Baselt RC. Propoxyphene. In: Disposition of toxic drugs and chemicals in man, 7th ed. Foster City, CA: Biomedical Publications, 2004:953-6.
37. Bass, RR, Vargas, J. The antipsychotic drugs. In: Haddad LM, Shannon MW, Winchester JF, eds. Clinical management of poisoning and drug overdose, 3rd ed. Philadelphia: WB Saunders Co, 1998: 780-93.
38. Bastiani RJ. Urinary cannabinoid excretion patterns. In: Agurell S, Dewey WL, Willette RE eds. The cannabinoids: Chemical, pharmacologic, and therapeutic aspects. San Diego, Academic Press, Inc, 1984:263-80.
39. Bastos ML, Kananen GE, Monforte JR, Sunshine I. TLC of basic organic drugs. In: Sunshine I ed. Methodology for analytical toxicology. Boca Raton, FL, CRC Press, Inc, 1975:434-42.
40. Bateh RP. Distinguishing cyclobenzaprine and amitriptyline. J Anal Toxicol 1987;11:235 (Letter).
41. Baumgartner AM, Jones PF, Baumgartner WA, Black CT.Radioimmunoassay of hair for determining opiate-abuse histories. J Nucl Med 1979;20:748-52.
42. Baumgartner WA, Hill VA. Hair analysis for drugs of abuse: Decontamination issues. In: Sunshine I ed. Recent developments in therapeutic drug monitoring and clinical toxicology. New York: Marcel Dekker Inc, 1992:577-97.
43. Bayer MJ, McKay C. Advances in poison management. Clin Chem 1996;42:1361-6.
44. Beck O, Lafolie P, Hjemdahl P, Borg S, Odelius G, Wirbing P. Detection of benzodiazepine intake in therapeutic doses by immunoanalysis of urine: Two techniques evaluated and modified for improved performance. Clin Chem 1992;38:271-5.
45. Beck O, Lin Z, Brodin K, Borg S, Hjemdahl P. The Online screening technique for urinary benzodiazepines: Comparison with EMIT, FPIA and GC-MS. J Anal Toxicol 1997;21:554-7.
46. Beckett AH, Rowland M. Urinary excretion kinetics of methylamphetamine in man. J Pharm Pharmacol 1965;17(suppl):1095-145.
47. Bell R, Taylor EH, Ackerman B, Pappas AA. Interpretation of urine quantitative 11-nor-Δ^9-tetrahydrocannabinol-9-carboxylic acid to determine abstinence from marijuana smoking. Clin Toxicol 1989;27: 109-15.
48. Bernasconi R, Mathivet P, Bischoff S, Marescaux C. Gamma-hydroxybutyric acid: an endogenous neuromodulator with abuse potential? Trends Pharmacol Sci 1999;20:135-41.
49. Berry DJ, Grove J. Emergency toxicological screening for drugs commonly taken in overdose. J Chromatogr 1973;80:205-19.
50. Bertholf RL, Johannsen LM, Bazooband A, Mansouri V. False-positive acetaminophen results in a hyperbilirubinemic patient. Clin Chem 2003;49:695-8.
51. Bizovi KE, Smilkstein MJ. Acetaminophen. In: Goldfrank LR, Flomenbaum NE, Lewin NA, Howland MA, Hoffman RS, Nelson LS, eds. Goldfrank's toxicologic emergencies, 7th ed. New York: McGraw-Hill, 2002:480-501.
52. Blandford DE, Desjardins RP. A rapid method for measurement of ethylene glycol. Clin Biochem 1994; 27:25-30.
53. Blanke RV, Decker WJ. Analysis of toxic substances. In: Textbook of Clinical Chemistry. NW Tietz, Ed Philadelphia: WB Saunders Co, 1986: 1670-744.
54. Blomme B, Lheureux P, Gerlo E, Maes V. Cobas Mira S endpoint enzymatic assay for plasma formate. J Anal Toxicol 2001;25:77-9.
55. Bodor G, Roggeman R, Turk J. Variations in abundance of the molecular ion of the derivatized cocaine metabolite benzoylecgonine. Clin Chem 1990; 36:742-7.
56. Boeckx RL. False positive EMIT DAU PCP assay as a result of an overdose of dextromethorphan. Clin Chem 1987;33:974-5 (abstract).
57. Boehnert MT, Lovejoy FH. Value of the QRS duration versus the serum drug level in predicting seizures and ventricular arrhythmias after an acute overdose of tricyclic antidepressants. N Eng J Med 1985; 313:474-9.
58. Bogusz M, Poch J, Stasko W. Comparative studies on the rate of ethanol elimination in acute poisoning and in controlled conditions. J Forensic Sci 1977; 22:446-51.
59. Bogusz M, Wu M. Standard HPLC/DAD system, based on retention indices and spectral library, applicable for systematic toxicological screening. J Anal Toxicol 1991;15:188-97.
60. Bogusz MJ, Maier R-D, Krüger K-D, Kohls U. Determination of common drugs of abuse in body fluids using one isolation procedure and liquid chromatography-atmospheric-pressure chemical-ionization mass spectrometry. J Anal Toxicol 1998;22:549-58.
61. Borrey D, Meyer E, Duchateau L, Lambert W, Van Peteghem C, De Leenheer A.. Enzymatic hydrolysis improves the sensitivity of Emit screening for urinary benzodiazepines. Clin Chem 2002;48: 2047-9.
62. Bravo R, Driskell WJ, Whitehead, Jr RD, Needham LL, Barr DB. Quantitation of dialkyl phosphate metabolites of organophosphate pesticides in human urine using GC-MS-MS with isotopic internal standards. J Anal Toxicol 2002;26:245-52.
63. Bray GP, Harrison PM, O'Grady JG, Tredger JM, Williams R. Long term anticonvulsant therapy worsens outcome in paracetamol induced fulminant hepatic failure. Hum Exp Toxicol 1992;11:265-72.

64. Brent J, McMartin K, Phillips S, Burkhart KK, Donovan JW, Wells M,, et al. Fomepizole for the treatment of ethylene glycol poisoning. N Eng J Med 1999;340:832-8.
65. Brett AS. Implications of discordance between clinical impression and toxicology analysis in drug overdose. Arch Intern Med 1988;148:437-41.
66. Bridges RR, Kinniburgh DW, Keehn BJ, Jennison TA. An evaluation of common methods for acetaminophen quantitation for small hospitals. Clin Toxicol 1983;20:1-17.
67. Broussard LA, Fendley TW, Pellegrino L. Screening procedures: 1. Multiple drugs by thin-layer chromatography. In: Frings CS, Faulkner WR eds. Selected methods of emergency toxicology, Vol 11. Washington DC, AACC Press. 1986:13-21.
68. Brown J, Murphy D, MacEachem M. Development of an enzymatic acetaminophen reagent and application on Hitachi and Cobas analyzers. Clin Chem 1996; 42:S150 (abstract).
69. Brown NJ, Roberts LJ II. Histamine, bradykinin and their antagonists In: Hardman JG, Limbird LE, Gilman AG, eds. Goodman and Gilman's the pharmacological basis of therapeutics, 10th ed. New York: McGraw-Hill, 2001:645-67.
70. Buckpitt AR, Rollins DE, Mitchell JR. Varying effects of sulfhydryl nucleophiles on acetaminophen oxidation and sulfhydryl adduct formation. Biochem Pharmacol 1979;28:2941-6.
71. Burns M, Baselt RC. Monitoring drug use with a sweat patch: and experiment with cocaine. J Anal Toxicol 1995;19:41-8.
72. Butler TJ. Thin-layer chromatography. In: Thoma JJ, Bondo PB, Sunshine I eds. Guidelines for analytical toxicology programs, Vol I. Boca Raton, FL, CRC Press, Inc, 1977:217-49.
73. Caldwell J. The metabolism of amphetamines in mammals. Drug Metab Rev 1976;5:219-80.
74. Callahan CM, Grant TM, Phipps P, Clark G, Novack AH, Streissguth AP, et al. Measurement of gestational cocaine exposure: sensitivity of infants' hair, meconium, and urine. J Pediatr 1992;120:763-8.
75. Caplan YH. Blood, urine, and other fluid and tissue specimens for alcohol analyses. In: Garriott JC ed. Medicological aspects of alcohol. Tucson, AZ: Lawyers & Judges Publishing Co, 1996:137-50.
76. CaplanYH, Goldberger BA. Alternative specimen for workplace drug testing. J Anal Toxicol 2001; 25:396-9.
77. Caplan YH, Levine B. Evaluation of the Abbott TDx-radiative energy attenuation (REA) ethanol assay in a study of 1105 forensic whole blood specimens. J Forensic Sci 1987;32:55-61.
78. Carlton FB, Simpson, WM Jr, Haddad LM. The Organophosphates and Other Insecticides. In: Haddad LM, Shannon MW, Winchester JF, eds. Clinical management of poisoning and drug overdose, 3rd ed. Philadelphia: WB Saunders Co, 1999: 836-45.
79. Casanova OQ, Lombardero N, Behnke M, Eyler FD, Conlon M, Bertholf RL. Detection of cocaine exposure in the neonate. Arch Pathol Lab Med 1994; 118:988-93.
80. Ceder G, Jones AW. Concentration ratios of morphine to codeine in blood of impaired drivers as evidence of heroin use and not medication with codeine. Clin Chem 2001;47:1980-4.
81. Cham BE, Johns D, Bochner F, Imhoff DM, Rowland M. Simultaneous liquid-chromatographic quantitation of salicylic acid, salicyluric acid, and gentisic acid in plasma. Clin Chem 1979;25:1420-5.
82. Chan P, Chen JH, Lee MH, Deng JF. Fatal and nonfatal methamphetamine intoxication in the intensive care unit. Clin Toxicol 1994;32:147-55.
83. Chang B-L, Huang M-K. Urinary excretion of codeine and morphine following the administration of codeine containing cold syrup. J Anal Toxicol 2000; 24:133-9.
84. Changes to the testing cutoff levels for opiates for Federal workplace drug testing programs. Fed Regi 1995;60(221):57587-9; Fed Reg 1997;62(189): 51118-20.
85. Chapman BJ, Proudfoot AT. Adult salicylate poisoning: Deaths and outcome in patients with high plasma salicylate concentrations. QJ Med 1989; 72:699-707.
86. Charney DS, Mihic SJ, Harris RA. Hypnotics and sedatives. In: Hardman JG, Limbird LE, Gilman AG, eds. Goodman and Gilman's the pharmacological basis of therapeutics, 10th ed. New York: McGraw-Hill, 2001:399-427.
87. Chasnoff IJ, Landress HJ, Barrett ME. The prevalence of illicit-drug or alcohol use during pregnancy and discrepancies in mandatory reporting in Pinellas County, Florida. N Engl J Med 1990;322:1202-6.
88. Chasnoff IJ. Drug use and women: Establishing a Standard of Care. Ann N Y Acad Sci 1989;562:208-10.
89. Cheever ML, Armendariz GA, Moody DE. Detection of methadone, LAAM, and their metabolites by methadone immunoassay. J Anal Toxicol 1999; 23:500-5.
90. Cheung L, Potts RG, Meyer KC. Acetaminophen treatment nomogram. N Engl J Med 1994;330:1907-8 (Letter).
91. Chiang WK, Goldfrank LR. Amphetamines. In: Goldfrank LR, Flomenbaum NE, Lewin NA, Howland MA, Hoffman RS, Nelson LS, eds. Goldfrank's toxicologic emergencies, 7th ed. New York: McGraw-Hill, 2002:1020-33.
92. Clark RF. Insecticides: Organic phosphorus compounds and carbamates. In: Goldfrank LR, Flomenbaum NE, Lewin NA, Howland MA, Hoffman RS, Nelson LS, eds. Goldfrank's toxicologic

emergencies, 7th ed. New York: McGraw-Hill 2002:1346-60.

93. Clarkson ED, Lesser D, Paul BD. Effective GC-MS procedure for detecting iso-LSD in urine after base-catalyzed conversion to LSD. Clin Chem 1998; 44:287-92.
94. Cody JT. Determination of methamphetamine enantiomer ratios in urine by gas chromatography-mass spectrometry. J Chromatogr 1992;580:77-95.
95. Cody JT. Important issues in testing for amphetamine. In: Liu RH, Goldberger BA eds. Handbook of workplace drug testing. Washington, DC: AACC Press, 1995:239-88.
96. Cody JT, Schwarzhoff R. Interpretation of methamphetamine and amphetamine enantiomer data. J Anal Toxicol 1993;17:321-6.
97. Cody JT, Valtier S. Immunoassay analysis of lysergic acid diethylamide. J Anal Toxicol 1997;21:459-64.
98. Cody JT, Valtier S Effects of Stealth™ adulterant on immunoassay testing for drugs of abuse. J Anal Toxicol 2001;25:466-70.
99. Cody JT, Valtier S, Kuhlman J Analysis of morphine and codeine in samples adulterated with Stealth.™ J Anal Toxicol 2001;25:572-5.
100. Colmorgen GHC, Johnson C, Zazzarino MA, Durinzi K. Routine urine drug screening at the first prenatal visit. Am J Obstet Gynecol 1992;166:588-90.
101. Cone EJ, Hillsgrove MJ, Jenkins AJ, Keenan RM, Darwin WD. Sweat testing for heroin, cocaine and metabolites. J Anal Toxicol 1994;18:298-305.
102. Cone EJ, Johnson RE, Darwin WD, Yousefnejad D, Mell LD, Paul BD, et al. Passive inhalation of marijuana smoke: Urinalysis and room air level of delta-9-tetrahydrocannabinol. J Anal Toxicol 1987; 11:89-96.
103. Cone EJ, Presley L, Lehrer M, Seiter W, Smith M, Kardos KW, et al. Oral fluid testing for drugs of abuse: positive prevalence rates by Intercept™ immunoassay screening and GC-MS-MS confirmation and suggested cutoff concentrations. J Anal Toxicol 2002;26:541-6.
104. Cone EJ, Weddington WW Jr. Prolonged occurrence of cocaine in human saliva and urine after chronic use. J Anal Toxicol 1989;13:65-8.
105. Cone EJ, Welch P, Mitchell JM, Paul BD. Forensic drug testing for opiates: I. Detection of 6-acetylmorphine in urine as an indicator of recent heroin exposure: Drug and assay considerations and detection times. J Anal Toxicol 1990;15:1-7.
106. Cone EJ, Welch P, Paul BD, Mitchell JM. Forensic drug testing for opiates: III. Urinary excretion rates of morphine and codeine following codeine administration. J Anal Toxicol 1991;15:161-6.
107. Cook CE, Perez-Reyes M, Jeffcoat AR, Brine DR. Phencyclidine disposition in humans after small doses of radiolabeled drug. Fed Proc 1983;42:2566.
108. Corcoran GB, Racz WJ, Smith CV, Mitchell JR. Effects of N-acetylcysteine on the disposition and metabolism of acetaminophen in mice. J Pharmacol Exp Ther 1985;232:857-63.
109. Cregler LL, Mark H. Medical complications of cocaine abuse. N Engl J Med 1986;315:1495-1500.
110. Crouch DJ, Frank JF, Farrell LJ, Karsch HM, Klaunig JE. A multiple-site laboratory evaluation of three on-site urinalysis drug-testing devices. J Anal Toxicol 1998;22:493-502.
111. Crouch DJ, Hersch RK, Cook RF, Frank JF, Walsh JM. A field evaluation of five on-site drug-testing devices. J Anal Toxicol 2002;26:493-9.
112. Cruz-Landeria A, López-Rivadulla M, Concheiro-Carro L, Fernández-Gómez P, Tabernero-Duque MJ. A new spectrophotometric method for the toxicological diagnosis of cyanide poisoning. J Anal Toxicol 2000;24:266-70.
113. Curry SC, Mills KC, Graeme KA. Neurotransmitters. In: Goldfrank LR, Flomenbaum NE, Lewin NA, Howland MA, Hoffman RS, Nelson LS, eds. Goldfrank's toxicologic emergencies, 7th ed. New York: McGraw-Hill, 2002:154-5.
114. Daher R, Haidar JH, Al-Amin H. Rifampin interference with opiate immunoassay. Clin Chem 2002; 48:203-4 (Letter).
115. Daniel DR, McAnalley BH, Garriott JC. Isopropyl alcohol metabolism after acute intoxication in humans. J Anal Toxicol 1981;5:110-2.
116. Dean RA, Christian CD, Sample RH, Bosron WF. Human liver cocaine esterases: Ethanol-medicated formation of ethylcocaine. FASEB J 1991;5:2735-9.
117. DeKeijzer MH, Korf H, Kusters R. Salivary reagent stick measure serum ethanol concentrations. Clin Chem 1996;42:985-6 (Letter).
118. de la Torre R, Domingo-Salvany A, Badia R, Gonzalez G, McFarlane D, San L, et al. Clinical evaluation of the Triage® analytical device for drugs-of-abuse testing. Clin Chem 1996;42:1433-8.
119. Demorest DM. Distinguishing cyclobenzaprine from amitriptyline and imipramine by liquid chromatography with UV multi-wavelength or full-spectrum detection. Blood levels of cyclobenzaprine in emergency screens. J Anal Toxicol 1987;11:133 (Letter).
120. Dohnal J, Bowie L, Lewis D. Assay sensitivity more important than specimen type when screening neonates for cocaine exposure. Clin Chem 1995; 41:S128 (abstract).
121. Domino LE, Domino SE, Domino EF. Relation of plasma delta-9-THC concentrations to subjective "high" in marijuana users: A review and reanalysis. In: Agurell S, Dewey WL, Willette RE eds. The cannabinoids: Chemical, pharmacologic, and therapeutic aspects. San Diego, Academic Press Inc, 1984:245-61.

122. Done AK. Salicylate intoxication: Significance of measurements of salicylate in blood in cases of acute ingestion. Pediatrics 1960;26:800-7.
123. Dubowski KM, Caplan YH. Alcohol testing in the workplace. In: Garriott JC ed. Medicolegal aspects of alcohol. Tucson, AZ: Lawyers & Judges Publishing Co, 1996:439-75.
124. Dubowski KM, Luke JL. Measurement of carboxyhemoglobin and carbon monoxide in blood. Ann Clin Lab Sci 1973;3:53-65.
125. Dubowski KM. Human pharmacokinetics of alcohol. Alcohol Tech Rep 1976;5:55-63.
126. Dubowski KM. Proceedings of the 1987 Arnold O Beckman Conference. Clin Chem 1987;33:5B-112B.
127. Dugandzic RM, Tierney MG, Dickinson GE, Dolan MC, McKnight DR. Evaluation of the validity of the Done nomogram in the management of acute salicylate intoxication. Ann Emerg Med 1989;18:1186-90.
128. Dutt MC, Lo DS-T, Ng DLK, Woo S-O. Gas chromatographic study of the urinary codeine-to-morphine ratios in controlled codeine consumption and in mass screening for opiate drugs. JChromatogr 1983;267:117-24.
129. Dutta SK, Orestes M, Vengulekur S, Kwo P. Ethanol and human saliva: effect of chronic alcoholism on flow rate, composition, and epidermal growth factor. Am J Gastroenterol 1992;87:350-4.
130. Dyer JE, Roth B, Hyma BA. Gamma-hydroxybutyrate withdrawal syndrome. Ann Emerg Med 2001;37: 147-53.
131. Ebid A-H-I, Abdel-Rahman HM. Pharmacokinetics of phenobarbital during certain enhanced elimination modalities to evaluate their clinical efficacy in management of drug overdose. Ther Drug Monit 2001; 23:209-16.
132. Eckfeldt JH, Nelson KM. Salicylate determined with a microcentrifugal analyzer, and compared with DuPont aca, Trinder, and liquid-chromatographic methods. Clin Chem 1983;29:839-41.
133. Eder AF, Dowdy YG, Gardiner JA, Wolf BA, Shaw LM. Serum lactate and lactate dehydrogenase in high concentrations interfere in enzymatic assay of ethylene glycol. Clin Chem 1996;42:1489-91.
134. Eichhorst J,Etter M,Lepage J, Lehotay DC. Urinary screening for methylphenidate(Ritalin) abuse: a comparison of liquid chromatography-tandem mass spectrometry, gas chromatography-mass spectrometry, and immunoassay methods. Clin Bichem 2004; 37:175-83.
135. Ellenhorn MJ, Schonwald S, Ordog G, Wasserberger J. The Clinical Approach. In: Ellenhorn MJ ed. Medical toxicology: Diagnosis and treatment of human poisoning. 2nd ed. Baltimore, Lippincott Williams & Wilkins,1997:3-46.
136. Ellenhorn MJ, Schonwald S, Ordog G, Wasserberger J. Medical toxicology: Diagnosis and treatment of human poisoning. 2nd ed. Baltimore, Lippincott Williams & Wilkins, 1997.
137. Ellenhorn MJ, Schonwald S, Ordog G, Wasserberger J. Antidotes. In: Ellenhorn MJ ed. Medical toxicology, Diagnosis and treatment of human poisoning. 2nd ed. Baltimore, Lippincott Williams & Wilkins, 1997: 89-105.
138. Ellenhorn MJ, Schonwald S, Ordog G, Wasserberger J. Cyclic antidepressants. In: Ellenhorn MJ ed. Medical toxicology, Diagnosis and treatment of human poisoning. 2nd ed. Baltimore, Lippincott Williams & Wilkins, 1997:624-50.
139. Ellenhorn MJ. Medical toxicology: A primer for the medicolegal age. Clin Toxicol 1978;13:439-62.
140. Ellenhorn MJ, Schonwald S, Ordog G, Wasserberger J. Pesticides. In: Ellenhorn MJ ed. Medical toxicology, Diagnosis and treatment of human poisoning. 2nd ed. Baltimore, Lippincott Williams & Wilkins, 1997:1614-63.
141. Ellenhorn MJ, Schonwald S, Ordog G, Wasserberger J. Supportive Care. In: Ellenhorn MJ ed. Medical toxicology, Diagnosis and treatment of human poisoning. 2nd ed. Baltimore, Lippincott Williams & Wilkins, 1997:106-27.
142. Ellis GM Jr, Mann MA, Judson BA, Schramm NT, Tashchian A. Excretion patterns of cannabinoid metabolites after last use in a group of chronic users. Clin Pharmacol Ther 1985;38:572-8.
143. ElSohly HN, ElSohly MA, Stanford DF. Poppy seed ingestion and opiate urinalysis: A closer look. J Anal Toxicol 1990;14:308-10.
144. ElSohly MA, DeWit H, Wachtel SR, Feng S, Murphy TP. Δ^9-tetrahydrocannabivarin as a marker for the ingestion of marijuana versus Marinol ®: results of a clinical study. J Anal Toxicol 2001;25:565-71.
145. ElSohly MA, Feng S. Δ^9-THC metabolites in meconium: identification of 11-OH–Δ^9 - THC, 8β, 11-diOH– Δ^9 –THC, and 11–nor–Δ^9–THC–9–COOH as major metabolites of Δ^9 THC. J Anal Toxicol 1998; 22:329-35.
146. ElSohly MA, Stanford DF, Murphy TP, Lester BM, Wright LL, Smeriglio VL, et al. Immunoassay and GC-MS procedures for the analysis of drugs of abuse in meconium. J Anal Toxicol 1999;23:436-45.
147. ElSohly MA, Stanford DF, Sherman D, Shah H, Bernot D, Turner CE. A procedure for eliminating interferences from ephedrine and related compounds in the GC/MS analysis of amphetamine and methamphetamine. J Anal Toxicol 1992;16:109-11.
148. Fallon JK, Kicman AT, Henry JA, Milligan PJ, Cowan DA, Hutt AJ Stereospecific analysis and enantiomeric disposition of 3,4-methylenedioxymethamphetamine (ecstasy) in humans. Clin Chem 1999;45:1058-69.
149. Farrell SE, Roberts JR. Benzodiazepines. In: Haddad LM, Shannon MW, Winchester JF, eds. Clinical man-

agement of poisoning and drug overdose, 3rd ed. Philadelphia: WB Saunders Co, 1998:609-27.

150. Fenton J, Schaffer M, Chen NW, Bermes EW Jr. A comparison of enzyme immunoassay and gas chromatography/mass spectrometry in forensic toxicology. J Forensic Sci 1980;25:314-9.
151. Finkle BS, Black D, Blanke RV, Butler TJ, Jones GR, Sample RH. Analysis for commonly abused drugs in urine at selected threshold ("cutoff") concentrations. Clin Chem 1991;37:586-7.
152. Fitzgerald RL, Ramos JM Jr, Bogema SC, Poklis A. Resolution of methamphetamine stereoisomers in urine drug testing: Urinary excretion of R(−)-methamphetamine following use of nasal inhalers. J Anal Toxicol 1988;12:255-9.
153. Fitzgerald RL, Rivera JD, Herold DA. Broad spectrum drug identification directly from urine, using liquid chromatography-tandem mass spectrometry. Clin Chem 1999;45:1224-34.
154. Flanagan RJ, Mant TGK. Coma and metabolic acidosis in severe acute paracetamol poisoning. Human Toxicol 1986;5:179-82.
155. Flomenbaum NE, Goldfrank LR, Weisman RS, Lewin NA, Howland MA, Hoffman RS, et al. General management of the poisoned or overdosed patient. In: Goldfrank LR, Flomenbaum NE, Lewin NA, Howland MA, Hoffman RS, Nelson LS, eds., Goldfranks toxicology emergencies, 7th ed. New York: McGraw-Hill, 2002:25-41.
156. Flomenbaum NE. Salicylates In: Goldfrank LR, Flomenbaum NE, Lewin NA, Howland MA, Hoffman RS, Nelson LS, eds. Goldfrank's toxicologic emergencies, 7th ed. New York: McGraw-Hill, 2002:507-18.
157. Foltz RL, Fentiman AF, Foltz RB. GC/MS Assays for Abused Drugs in Body Fluids. National Institute on Drug Abuse. Research Monograph 32. Publication (ADM) 80-1014. Washington, DC, US Department of Health and Human Services. 1980:150-64.
158. Foltz RL, Fentiman AF, Foltz RB. GC/MS Assays for Abused Drugs in Body Fluids. National Institute on Drug Abuse. Research Monograph 32. Publication (ADM)80-1014. Washington, DC, US Department of Health and Human Services. 1980:25-38.
159. Forney R. Modified Davidow TLC drug screening procedure. In: Sunshine I ed. Methodology for analytical toxicology. Boca Raton, CRC Press Inc. 1975:443-7.
160. Forrest IS, Forrest FM. Urine color test for the detection of phenothiazines. Clin Chem 1960;6:11-5.
161. Forrest JAH, Clements JA, Prescott LF. Clinical pharmacokinetics of paracetamol. Clin Pharmacokinet 1982;7:93-107.
162. Francom Francom P, Andrenyak D, Lim HK, Bridges RR, Foltz RL, Jones RT. Determination of LSD in urine by capillary column gas chromatography and electron impact mass spectrometry. J Anal Toxicol 1988;12:1-8.
163. Fraser AD, Worth D. Urinary excretion profiles of 11-nor-9-carboxy-Δ^9-tetrahydrocannabinol: A Δ^9-THCCOOH to creatinine ratio study. J Anal Toxicol 1999;23:531-4.
164. Fraser AP, MacNeil W. Colorimetric and gas chromatographic procedures for glycolic acid in serum: the major toxic metabolite of ethylene glycol. Clin Toxicol 1993;31:397-405.
165. Gadsden RH, Taylor EH, Steindel SJ. Ethanol in biological fluids by enzymic analysis. In: Frings CS, Faulkner WR eds. Selected methods of emergency toxicology, Vol 11. Washington DC, AACC Press. 1986:63-5.
166. Gadsden RH. Study of forensic and clinical source hemoglobin interference with the DuPont aca ethanol method. Ann Clin Lab Sci 1986;16:399-406.
167. Garriott JC. Skeletal muscle as an alternative specimen for alcohol and drug analysis. J Forensic Sci 1991;36:60-9.
168. Garriott JC. Pharmacology and toxicology of ethyl alcohol. In: Garriott JC ed. Medicolegal aspects of alcohol. Tucson, AZ: Lawyers & Judges Publishing Co Inc, 1996:35-63.
169. George S, Braithwaite RA. Use of on-site testing for drugs of abuse. Clin Chem 2002;48:1639-1646.
170. George S, Parmar S, Meadway C, Braithwaite RA. Application and validation of a urinary methadone metabolite (EDDP) immunoassay to monitor methadone compliance. Ann Clin Biochem 2000; 37:350-354.
171. Ginsberg, MD. Carbon monoxide intoxication: Clinical features, neuropathy and mechanisms of injury. Clin Toxicol, 23:281-288, 1985.
172. Giroud C, Augsburger M, Rivier L, Mangin P, Sadeghipour F, Varesio E, et al. 2C-B: a new psychoactive phenylethylamine recently discovered in ecstasy tablets sold on the Swiss black market. J Anal Toxicol 1998;22:345-54.
173. Glare PA, Walsh TD. Clinical pharmacokinetics of morphine. Ther Drug Monit 1991;13:1-23.
174. Glasser DS. Utility of the serum osmol gap in the diagnosis of methanol or ethylene glycol ingestion. Ann Emerg Med 1996;27:343-6.
175. Goldfrank LR, Flomenbaum NE, Lewin NA, Howland MA, Hoffman RS, Nelson LS, eds. Goldfrank's toxicologic emergencies, 7th ed. New York: McGraw-Hill, 2002.
176. Goldstein DB. Pharmacology of alcohol. New York, Oxford University Press, 1983:80.
177. Gosselin RE, Smith RP, Hodge HC, Braddock JE, eds: Clinical toxicology of commercial products, 5th ed. Baltimore, Williams & Wilkins, 1984.
178. Gozal D, Ziser A, Shupak A, Melamed Y. Accidental carbon monoxide poisoning. Clin Pediatr 1985; 24:132-5.

179. Grabowski J, ed: Cocaine: Pharmacology, effects, and treatment of abuse. National Institute on Drug Abuse;. Research Monograph 50, Publication (ADM)84-1326, US Department of Health and Human Services, Washington, DC. 1984.
180. Graudins A, Aaron CK, Linden CH. Overdose of extended-release acetaminophen. N Engl J Med 1995; 333:196 (Letter).
181. Green KB, Isenschmid DS. Medical review officer interpretation of urine drug test results. In: Liu RH, Goldberger BA, eds. Handbook of workplace drug testing. Washington, DC: AACC Press, 1995:321-53.
182. Guillot JG, Weber JP, Savole JY. Quantitative determination of carbon monoxide in blood by headspace gas chromatography. J Anal Toxicol 1981;5:264-6.
183. Gustafson RA, Levine B, Stout PR, Klette KL, George MP, Moolchan ET, Huestis MA. Urinary cannabinoid detection times after controlled oral administration of Δ^9-tetrahydrocannabinol to humans. Clin Chem 2003;49:1114-24.
184. Gutstein HB, Akil H. Opioid analgesics In: Hardman JG, Limbird LE, Gilman AG, eds. Goodman and Gilman's the pharmacological basis of therapeutics, 10th ed. New York: McGraw-Hill, 2001:569-619.
185. Haddad LM, Shannon MW, Winchester JF, eds. Clinical management of poisoning and drug overdose, 3rd ed. Philadelphia: WB Saunders Co, 1998.
186. Haddad LM, Winchester JF. Barbiturates. In: Haddad LM, Shannon MW, Winchester JF, eds: Clinical management of poisoning and drug overdose, 3rd ed. Philadelphia: WB Saunders Co, 1998:521-7.
187. Hammett-Stabler CA, Winecker RE, Garside D, Ropero-Miller JD Consumption of imported Peruvian tea leads to positive urine results for cocaine and its metabolites. Clin Chem 2003;49:A121.
188. Harding P. Methods for breath analysis. In: Garriott JC, ed. Medicolegal aspects of alcohol. Tucson, AZ: Lawyers & Judges Publishing Co., 1996:181-217.
189. Hardman JG, Limbird LE, Gilman AG, eds. Goodman and Gilman's the pharmacologic basis of therapeutics, 10th ed. New York: McGraw-Hill, 2001.
190. Harkey MR, Henderson GL. Hair analysis for drugs of abuse. In: Baselt RC, ed. Advances in analytical toxicology Vol 11. Chicago, Year Book Medical Publishers, Inc, 1989:298-329.
191. Harrison PM, Wendon JA, Gimson AE, Alexander GJ, Williams R. Improvement by acetylcysteine of hemodynamics and oxygen transport in fulminant hepatic failure. N Engl J Med 1991;324:1852-7.
192. Hattab EM, Goldberger BA, Johannsen LM, Kindland PW, Ticino F, Chronister CW, Bertholf RL Modification of screening immunoassays to detect sub-threshold concentrations of cocaine, cannabinoids, and opiates in urine: use for detecting maternal and neonatal drug exposures. Ann Clin Lab Sci 2000; 30:85-91.
193. Haux P. Ethchlorvynol (placidyl) estimation in urine and serum. Clin Chim Acta 1972;43:139-41.
194. Hayes, LW, Krasselt, WG, Mueggler, PA. Concentrations of morphine and codeine in serum and urine after ingestion of poppy seeds. Clin Chem, 36:806-8, 1987.
195. Hearn WL, Rose S, Wagner J, Ciarleglio A, Mash DC. Cocaethylene is more potent than cocaine in mediating lethality. Pharmacol Biochem Behav 1991;39: 531-3.
196. Hearn WL, Flynn DD, Hime GW, Rose S, Cofino JC, Mantero-Atienza E, et al. Cocaethylene: a unique cocaine metabolite displays high affinity for the dopamine transporter. J Neurochem 1991;56: 698-701.
197. Hensley D, Cody JT. Simultaneous determination of amphetamine, methamphetamine, methylenedioxyamphetamine (MDA), methylenedioxymethamphetamine (MDMA), and methylenedioxyethylamphetamine (MDEA) enantiomers by GC-MS. J Anal Toxicol 1999;23:518-523.
198. Hepler BR, Sutheimer CA, Sunshine I. The role of the toxicology laboratory in emergency medicine II: Study of an integrated approach. Clin Toxicol 1984/85;22:503-28.
199. Hewlett TP, McMartin KE, Lauro AJ, Ragan FA. Ethylene glycol poisoning: The value of glycolic acid determinations for diagnosis and treatment. Clin Toxicol 1986;24:389-402.
200. Hoffman BB, Taylor P. Neurotransmission: The autonomic and somatic motor nervous systems. In: Hardman JG, Limbird LE, Gilman AG, eds. Goodman and Gilman's the pharmacological basis of therapeutics, 10th ed. New York: McGraw-Hill, 2001:115-53.
201. Hoffman BB. Catecholamines, sympathomimetic drugs and adrenergic receptor antagonists. In: Hardman JG, Limbird LE, Gilman AG, eds. Goodman and Gilman's the pharmacological basis of therapeutics 10th ed. New York: McGraw-Hill, 2001:215-68.
202. Holmes EW, Covault HP, Sabapathy T. Carboxyhemoglobin by spectrophotometry. In: Frings CS, Faulkner WR, eds. Selected methods of emergency toxicology, Vol 11. Washington DC, AACC Press. 1986:53-6.
203. Hornbeck CL, Czarny RJ. Retrospective analysis of some L-methamphetamine/L-amphetamine urine data. J Anal Toxicol 1993;17:23-5.
204. Howland MA. Flumazenil In: Goldfrank LR, Flomenbaum NE, Lewin NA, Howland MA, Hoffman RS, Nelson LS, eds. Goldfrank's toxicologic emergencies, 7th ed. New York: McGraw-Hill, 2002:946-51.
205. Howland MA. Fomepizole. In: Goldfrank LR, Flomenbaum NE, Lewin NA, Howland MA, Hoffman RS, Nelson LS, eds. Goldfrank's toxicologic emergencies, 7th ed. New York: McGraw-Hill, 2002: 999-1003.

206. Hoyle JC. Fitness-for-duty programs. Fed Reg 1988; 54:24468-508. (http://www.nrc.gov/reactors/operating/ops-experience/fitness-for-duty-programs/history.html)
207. Huestis MA, Cone EJ Differentiating new marijuana use from residual drug excretion in occasional marijuana users. J Anal Toxicol 1998;22:445-54.
208. Huestis MA, Mitchell JM, Cone EJ. Lowering the federally mandated cannabinoid immunoassay cutoff increases true-positive results. Clin Chem 1994; 40:729-33.
209. Hughes RO, Bronner WE, Smith ML. Detection of amphetamine and methamphetamine in urine by gas chromatography/mass spectrometry following derivatization with (−)–menthyl chloroformate. J Anal Toxicol 1991;15:256-9.
210. Hullin DA An IgM paraprotein causing a falsely low result in an enzymatic assay for acetaminophen. Clin Chem 1999;45:155-6. (Letter).
211. Hurwitz ES, Barrett MJ, Bregman D, Gunn WJ, Schonberger LB, Fairweather WR, et al. Public Health Service study on Reye's syndrome and medications: Report of the pilot phase. N Engl J Med 1985; 313:849-57.
212. Hyperbaric Oxygen Therapy Committee, Hyperbaric Oxygen Therapy. Committee Report, Hampson, NB (ed), Undersea and Hyperbaric Medical Society, Kensington, MD, 1999.
213. Inoue T, Seta S, Goldberger BA. Analysis of drugs in unconventional samples. In: Liu RH, Goldberger BA eds. Handbook of Workplace Drug Testing. Washington, DC: AACC Press, 1995:131-58.
214. Interpretation of listing of "tetrahydrocannabinol" in Schedule I (Interpretive Rule). Fed Regt 2001;66:195; 51530-44.
215. Inturrisi CE, Max MB, Foley KM, Schultz M, Shin SU, Houde RW. The pharmacokinetics of heroin in patients with chronic pain. N Engl J Med 1984; 310:1213-7.
216. Jackson DL, Menges H. Accidental carbon monoxide poisoning. JAMA 1980;243:722-74.
217. Jacob P III, Lewis ER, Elias-Baker BA, Jones RT. A pyrolysis product, anhydroecgonine methyl ester (methylecgonidine), is in the urine of cocaine smokers. J Anal Toxicol 1990;14:353-7.
218. Jacob P, Mendelson JE, Jones RT, Benowitz NL. Formation and elimination kinetics of cocaethylene in humans. Clin Pharmacol Ther 1993;53:174.
219. Jacobsen D, Overbo S, Ostborg J, Sejersted OM. Glycolate causes the acidosis in ethylene glycol poisoning and is effectively removed by hemodialysis. Acta Med Scand 1984;216:409-16.
220. Jarvie DR, Heyworth R, Simpson D. Plasma salicylate analysis: A comparison of colorimetric, HPLC and enzymatic techniques. Ann Clin Biochem 1987; 24:364-73.
221. Jatlow P. Cocaethylene: pharmacologic activity and clinical significance. Ther Drug Monit 1993;15:533-6.
222. Jatlow PI. Drug of abuse profile: Cocaine. Clin Chem 1987;33:66B-71B.
223. Joern WA. Surface absorption of the urinary marijuana carboxy metabolite: The problem and a partial solution. J Anal Toxicol 1992;16:401 (Letter).
224. Johansson E, Agurell S, Hollister LE, Halldin MM. Prolonged apparent half-life of Δ^1-tetrahydrocannabinol in plasma of chronic marijuana users. J Pharm Pharmacol 1988;40:374-5.
225. Johnson B, Meggs WJ, Bentzel CJ. Emergency department hemodialysis in a case of severe ethylene glycol poisoning. Ann Emerg Med 1999;33:108-10.
226. Jones AB, ElSohly HN, Aragat ES, ElSohly MA. Analysis of the major metabolite of Δ^9-tetrahydrocannabinol in urine: IV. A comparison of five methods. J Anal Toxicol 1984;8:249-51.
227. Jones AW (Reply by Simpson G). Concerning accuracy and precision of breath-alcohol measurements. Clin Chem 1987;33:1701-6.
228. Jones AW. Elimination half-life of acetone in humans: case reports and review of the literature. J Anal Toxicol 2000;24:8-9.
229. Jones, AW. Measurement of alcohol in blood and breath for legal purposes. In: Crow KE, Batt RD, eds. Human metabolism of alcohol. Vol I. Pharmacokinetics, medicolegal aspects, and general interests. Boca Raton, FL: CRC Press, 1989:71-99.
230. Jones AW (Reply by Simpson G). Reliability of breath-alcohol measurements during the absorption phase. Clin Chem 1987;128-2130 (Letter).
231. Jones AW, Nilsson L, Gladh SA, Karlsson K, Beck-Friis J. 2,3-Butanediol in plasma from an alcoholic mistakenly identified as ethylene glycol by gas-chromatographic analysis. Clin Chem 1991;1453-5.
232. Jones AW. Measuring ethanol in saliva with the QED enzymatic test device: Comparison of results with blood and breath alcohol concentrations. J Anal Toxicol 1995;19:169-74.
233. Jones AW. Pharmacokinetics of ethanol in saliva: comparison with blood and breath alcohol profiles, subjective feelings of intoxication, and diminished performance. Clin Chem 1993;39:1837-44.
234. Jones B, Bachner P. Q-Probe-Bedside glucose monitoring data analysis and critique. Northfield, IL, College of American Pathologists, 1991:5-15.
235. Jones RT. Drug of abuse profile: Cannabis. Clin Chem 1987;33:72B-81B.
236. Joseph RE Jr, Höld KM, Wilkins DG, Rollins DE, Cone EJ Drug testing with alternative matrices II. Mechanisms of cocaine and codeine deposition in hair. J Anal Toxicol 1999;23:396-408.
237. Kadehjian LJ Performance of five non-instrumented urine drug-testing devices with challenging near-cutoff specimens. J Anal Toxicol 2001;25:670-9.

238. Karnes HT, Beightol LA. Evaluation of fluorescence polarization immunoassay for quantitation of serum salicylates. Ther Drug Monit 1985;7:351-4.
239. Kellermann AL, Fihn SD, LoGerto JP, Copass MK. Impact of drug screening in suspected overdose. Ann Emerg Med 1987;16:1206-16.
240. Kelner M, Bailey DN. Mismeasurement of methemoglobin ("methemoglobin revisited"). Clin Chem 1985;31:168-9 (Letter).
241. Kidwell DA, Blank DL. Hair analysis: Techniques and potential problems. In: Sunshine I ed. Recent developments in therapeutic drug monitoring and clinical toxicology. New York: Marcel Dekker Inc., 1992: 555-63.
242. Kidwell DA, Holland JC, Athanaselis S. Testing for drugs of abuse in saliva and sweat. J Chromatogr B 1998;713:111-35.
243. Kintz P ed. Drug Testing in Hair. Boca Raton, FL: CRC Press Inc, 1996.
244. Kintz P, Brenneisen R, Bundeli P, Mangin. Sweat testing for heroin and metabolites in a heroin maintenance program. Clin Chem 1997;43:736-9.
245. Kintz P, Tracqui A, Jamey C, Mangin P. Detection of codeine and phenobarbital in sweat collected with a sweat patch. J Anal Toxicol 1996;20:197-201.
246. Kirk MA. Anticholinergics and Antihistamines. In: Haddad LM, Shannon MW, Winchester JF, eds. Clinical management of poisoning and drug overdose, 3rd ed. Philadelphia: WB Saunders Co, 1998:641-9.
247. Klaassen CD, Amdur MO, Doull J, eds. Casarett and Doull's Toxicology: The Basic Science of Poisons. 5th ed. New York: McGraw-Hill, 1996.
248. Klette KL, Horn CK, Stout RP, Anderson CJ LC-MS analysis of human urine specimens for 2-oxo-3-hydroxy LSD: method validation for potential interferants and stability study of 2-oxo-3-hydroxy LSD under various storage conditions. J Anal Toxicol 2002;26:193-200.
249. Koch TR, Raglin RL, Kirk S, Bruni JF. Improved screening for benzodiazepine metabolites in urine using the Triage™ panel for drugs of abuse. J Anal Toxicol 1994;18:168-72.
250. Koch-Weser J. Tricyclic antidepressants. N Engl J Med 1978;16:1106-9.
251. Kraner JC, MCCoy DJ, Evans MA, Evans LE, Sweeney BJ Fatalities caused by the MDMA-related drug paramethoxyamphetamine. J Anal Toxicol 2001;25: 645-8.
252. Kranzler HR, Stone J, McLaughlin L. Evaluation of a point-of-care testing product for drugs of abuse;testing site is a key variable. Drug and Alcohol Dependence 1995;40:55-62.
253. Krenzelok EP, Kerr F, Proudfoot AT. Salicylate toxicity. In: Haddad LM, Shannon MW, Winchester JF, eds.: Clinical management of poisoning and drug overdose, 3rd ed. Philadelphia: WB Saunders Co, 1998: 675-87.
254. Kronstand R, Jones AW. Concentration ratios of codeine-to-morphine in plasma after a single oral dose (100 mg) of codeine phosphate. J Anal Toxicol 2001;25:486-7.
255. Kronstrand R, Nyström I, Josefsson M, Hodgins S. Segmental ion spray LC-MS-MS analysis of benzodiazepines in hair of psychiatric patients. J Anal Toxicol 2002;26:479-84.
256. Kulig K. Initial management of ingestions of toxic substances. N Engl J Med 1992;326:1677-81.
257. Kushmir M, Jones C, Struempler R, Urry FM. Eliminating interferences of related compounds in opiates GC/MS analysis. Clin Chem 1996;42:S218.
258. Kwong, TC, Chamberlain RT, Frederick DL, Kapur B, Sunshine I. Critical issues in urinalysis of abused substances: Report of the substance-abuse testing committee. Clin Chem 1988;34:605-32.
259. Kwong TC, Ryan RM. Detection of intrauterine illicit drug exposure by newborn drug testing. Clin Chem 1997;43:235-42.
260. Laakso O, Haapala M, Jaakkola P, Laaksonen R, Luomanmaki K, Nieminen J, et al FT-1R breath test in the diagnosis and control of treatment of methanol intoxications. J Anal Toxicol 2001;25: 26-30.
261. Lafolie P, Beck O, Blennow G, Boreus L, Borg S, Elwin CE, et al. Importance of creatinine analysis of urine when screening for abused drugs. Clin Chem 1991; 37:1927-31.
262. Lafolie P, Beck O, Hjemdahl P, Borg S. Using relation between urinary cannabinoid and creatinine excretions to improve monitoring of abuser adherence to abstinence. Clin Chem 1994;40:170-1 (Letter).
263. Lafolie P, Beck O, Lin Z, Albertoni F, Boréus L. Urine and plasma pharmacokinetics of codeine in healthy volunteers: implications for drugs-of-abuse testing. J Anal Toxicol 1996;20:541-6.
264. Landaw, I A, Winchell, H I. Endogenous production of carbon-14 labeled carbon monoxide: An in vivo technique for the study of heme catabolism. J Nucl Med 1966;7:696-707.
265. Le Beau MA, Christenson RH, Levine B, Darwin WD, Huestis MA. Intra- and interindividual variations in urinary concentrations of endogenous gamma-hydroxybutyrate. J Anal Toxicol 2002;26:340-6.
266. LeGatt DF, Audette RJ, Blakney G, Vaughan D. Excess serum osmolality after ingestion of methanol: The exception, not the rule. Clin Chem 1991;37:1802-4.
267. Lehmann T, Sager F, Brenneisen R. Excretion of cannabinoids in urine after ingestion of Cannabis seed oil. J Anal Toxicol 1997;21:373-5.
268. Leikin JB, Paloucek FP. Methadone. In: Leikin JB ed. Leikin & Paloucek's poisoning & toxicology handbook 3rd Hudson, OH: Lexi-Comp, Inc, 2002:806-8.

269. Leikin JB, Paloucek FP. Methemoglobin. In: Leikin JB ed. Leikin & Paloucek's Poisoning & Toxicology Handbook, 3rd ed Hudson, OH: Lexi-Comp, Inc, 2002:814.
270. Leikin JB. Management of drug overdose. Medical Update for Psychiatrists. 1996:41-60.
271. Leson G, Pless P, Grotenhermen F, Kalant H, ElSohly MA. Evaluating the impact of hemp food consumption on workplace drug tests. J Anal Toxicol 2001; 25:691-8.
272. Levine BS, Smith ML. Effects of diphenhydramine on immunoassay of phencyclidine in urine. Clin Chem 1990;36:1258 (Letter).
273. Lewis DE, Moore CM, Leikin JB, Kolle, A. Meconium analysis for cocaine: a validation study and comparison with paired urine analysis. J Anal Toxicol 1995; 19:148-50.
274. Li J, Stokes SA, Woeckener A. A tale of novel intoxication: seven cases of γ-hydroxybutyric acid overdose. Ann Emerg Med 1998;31:723-8.
275. Li Z, McNally AJ, Wang H, Salmone SJ Stability study of LSD under various storage conditions. J Anal Toxicol 1998;22:520-5.
276. Liang HK. Clinical evaluation of the poisoned patient and toxic syndromes. Clin Chem 1996;42: 1350-1355.
277. Lichtenwalner MR, Mencken T, Tully R, Petosa M. False-positive immunochemical screen for methadone attributable to metabolites of verapamil. Clin Chem 1998;44:1039-41.
278. Liebelt EL, Francis PD. Cyclic Antidepressants. In: Goldfrank LR, Flomenbaum NE, Lewin NA, Howland MA, Hoffman RS, Nelson LS, eds. Goldfrank's toxicologic emergencies, 7th ed. New York: McGraw-Hill, 2002:847-64.
279. Lin JH, Levy G. Sulfate depletion after acetaminophen administration and replenishment by infusion of sodium sulfate or N-acetylcysteine in rats. Biochem Pharmacol 1981;30:2723-5.
280. Linnanvuo-Laitinen M, Huttunen K. Ethylene glycol intoxication. Clin Toxicol 1986;24:167-74.
281. Liu RH. Evaluation of common immunoassay kits for effective workplace drug testing. In: Handbook of Workplace Drug Testing. RH Liu, BA Goldberger, Eds Washington, DC: AACC Press, 1995:67-129.
282. Logan BK. Amphetamines: an update on forensic issues. J Anal Toxicol 2001;25:400-4.
283. Long C, Crifasi J, Maginn D. Interference of thioridazine (Mellaril) in identification of phencyclidine. Clin Chem 1996;42:1885-6 (Letter).
284. Lora-Tamayo C, Tena T, Rodriquez A, Moreno D. High concentration of chloroquine in urine gives positive result with amphetamine CEDIA reagent. J Anal Toxicol 2002;26:58 (Letter).
285. Loor R, Lingenfelter C, Wason PP, Tang K, Davoudzadeh. Multiplex assay of amphetamine, methamphetamine, and ecstasy drug using CEDIA technology. J Anal Toxicol 2002;26:267-73.
286. LoVecchio F, Lewin LA. Antipsychotics. In: Goldfrank LR, Flomenbaum NE, Lewin NA, Howland MA, Hoffman RS, Nelson LS, eds. Goldfrank's toxicologic emergencies, 7th ed. New York: McGraw-Hill, 2002: 875-84.
287. Lundh B, Cavallin-Stahl E, Mercke C. Heme catabolism, carbon monoxide production and red cell survival in anaemia. Acta Med Scand 1975;197:161-71.
288. Mackler SA, Schweizer E. Benzodiazepines as anxiolytic agents: the risks of long-term treatment. Hospital Practice 1992; September 30, 109-16.
289. Mahly M, Lardet G, Vallon JJ. Automated Cobas Mira kinetic enzymatic assay for ethylene glycol applied to emergency situations. J Anal Toxicol 1994;18:269-71.
290. Maier RD, Bogusz M. Identification power of a standardized HPLC-DAD system for systematic toxicological analysis. J Anal Toxicol 1995;19:79-83.
291. Malandain H, Cano Y. Interference of glycerol, propylene glycol, and other diols in enzymatic assay of ethylene glycol. Clin Chem 1995;41:S120 (abstract).
292. Mandatory guidelines for federal workplace drug testing programs. Fed Reg 1994;59:29908-81.
293. Manno JE, Ferslew KE, Manno BR. Urine excretion patterns of cannabinoids and the clinical application of the EMIT-dau cannabinoid urine assay for substance abuse treatment. In: Agurell S, Dewey WL, Willette RE eds. The cannabinoids: Chemical, pharmacologic, and therapeutic aspects. San Diego: Academic Press Inc, 1984:281-90.
294. Manno JE. Interpretation of urinalysis results. In: Hawks RL, Chiang CN eds. Urine Testing for Drugs of Abuse. National Institute on Drug Abuse, Research Monograph 73, publication (ADM)87-1481, Washington, DC: US Department of Health and Human Services, 1986:54-61.
295. Marshall LP, Smith RW, Shapiro DM. The outcome with aggressive treatment in severe head injuries: Part II. Acute and chronic barbiturate administration in management of head injury. J Neurosurg 1979;50: 26-30.
296. Martin-Amat G, McMartin KE, Hayreh MS, Tephly TR. Methanol poisoning: Ocular toxicity produced by formate. Toxicol Appl Pharmacol 1978;45:201-5.
297. Martin BR, Mechoulam R, Razdan RK. Discovery and characterization of endogenous cannabinoids. Life Sci 1999;65:573-95.
298. Martin KE, Ambre JJ, Tephly TR. Methanol poisoning in human subjects. Role for formic acid accumulation in the metabolic acidosis. Am J Med 1980;68:414-8.
299. Mason MF, Dubowski KM. Breath as a specimen for analysis for ethanol and other low molecular weight alcohols. In: Garriott JC ed. Medicolegal aspects of alcohol. Tucson, AZ: Lawyers & Judges Publishing Co. 1996:171-80.

300. Mathieu D, Nolf M, Durocher A, Saulnier F, Frimat P, Furon D, et al. Acute carbon monoxide poisoning: Risk of late sequelae and treatment by hyperbaric oxygen. Clin Toxicol 1985;23:315-24.
301. Mayer M, Salpeter L. More on interference of N-acetylcysteine in measurement of acetaminophen. Clin Chem 1998;44:892-3 (Letter).
302. McCusker RR, Paget-Wilkes H, Chronister CW, Goldberger BA, ElSohly MA. Analysis of gamma-hydroxybutyrate (GHB) in urine by gas chromatography-mass spectrometry. J Anal Toxicol 1999;23: 301-5.
303. Meatherall R. Benzodiazepine screening using EMIT II® and TDx®: urine hydrolysis pretreatment required. J Anal Toxicol 1994;18:385-90.
304. Meatheral R, Dai J False-positive EMIT II opiates from ofloxacin. Ther Drug Monit 1997;19:98-9.
305. Meatherall R, Fraser AD. Comparison of four immunoassays for the detection of lorazepam in urine. Ther Drug Monit 1998;20:673-5.
306. Meatherall R, Krahn J. Excess serum osmolality after ingestion of methanol. Clin Chem 1990;36:2004-7.
307. Meatherall RC, Fraser AD. CEDIA dau benzodiazepine screening assay: a reformulation. J Anal Toxicol 1998;22:270-3.
308. Mégarbane B, Fompeydie D, Garnier R, Baud FJ. Treatment of a 1,4-butanediol poisoning with fomepizole. J Toxicol Clin Toxicol 2002;40:77-80.
309. Miró O, Nogué S, Espinosa G, To-Figueras J, Sánchez M. Trends in illicit drug emergencies: the emerging role of gamma-hydroxybutyrate. J Toxicol Clin Toxicol 2002;40:129-35.
310. Mitchell JM, Paul BD, Welch P, Cone EJ. Forensic drug testing for opiates. II. Metabolism and excretion rate of morphine in humans after morphine administration. J Anal Toxicol 1991;15:49-53.
311. Mitchell JR, Thorgeirsson SS, Potter WZ, Jollow DJ, Keiser H. Acetaminophen-induced hepatic injury: Protective role of glutathione in man and rationale for therapy. Clin Pharmacol Ther 1974;16:676-84.
312. Moertel CG, Ames MM, Kovach JS, Moyer TP, Rubin JR, Tinker JH. A pharmacologic and toxicological study of amygdalin. JAMA 1981;245:591-4.
313. Monaghan MS, Olsen KM, Ackerman BH, Fuller GL, Porter WH, Pappas AA. Measurement of serum isopropanol and the acetone metabolite by proton nuclear magnetic resonance: application to pharmacokinetic evaluation in a simulated overdose model. J Toxicol Clin Toxicol 1995;33:141-9.
314. Montague RE, Grace RF, Lewis JH, Shenfield GM. Urine drug screens in overdose patients do not contribute to immediate clinical management. Ther Drug Monit 2001;23:47-50.
315. Moore C, Jones J, Lewis D, Buchi K. Prevalence of fatty acid ethyl esters in meconium specimens. Clin Chem 2003;49:133-6.
316. Moore JD. Pharmacology, use, and monitoring of flumazenil, a benzodiazepine antagonist. AACC TDM/TOX 1993;14:57-62.
317. Moore KA, Addison J, Levine B, Smialek JE. Applicability of opiate cutoffs to opiate intoxication cases. J Anal Toxicol 2001;25:657-8 (Letter).
318. Moore KA, Sklerov J, Levine B, Jacobs, AJ. Urine concentrations of ketamine and norketamine following illegal consumption. J Anal Toxicol 2001;25: 583-8.
319. Moore L, Wicks J, Spiehler V, Holgate R. Gas chromatography-mass spectrometry confirmation of Cozart RapiScan saliva methadone and opiates tests. J Anal Toxicol 2001;25:520-4.
320. Morris HC, Overton PD, Ramsay JR, Campbell RS, Hammond PM, Atkinson T, et al. Development and validation of an automated enzyme assay for paracetamol (acetaminophen). Clin Chem Acta 1990;187:95-104.
321. Morris HC, Overton PD, Ramsay JR, Campbell RS, Hammond PM, Atkinson T, et al. Development and validation of an automated, enzyme-mediated colorimetric assay of salicylate in serum. Clin Chem 1990;36:131-5.
322. Mule SJ, Casella GA. Rendering the "poppy-seed defense" defenseless: Identification of 6-monoacetylmorphine in urine by gas chromatography/mass spectroscopy. Clin Chem 1988;34:1427-30.
323. Mule SJ, Lomax P, Gross SJ. Active and realistic passive marijuana exposure tested by three immunoassays and GC/MS in urine. J Anal Toxicol 1988;12:113-16.
324. Myers RAM, Britten JS. Are arterial blood gases of value in treatment decisions for carbon monoxide poisoning? Crit Care Med 1989;17:139-42.
325. Nair P, Rothblum BA, Hebel R. Neonatal outcome in infants with evidence of fetal exposure to opiates, cocaine and cannabinoids. Clin Pediatr 1994;33:280-5.
326. Natowicz M, Donahue J, Gorman L, Kane M, McKissick J, Shaw L. Pharmacokinetic analysis of a case of isopropanol intoxication. Clin Chem 1985;31:326-8.
327. Nelson LS. Opioids. In: Goldfrank LR, Flomenbaum NE, Lewin NA, Howland MA, Hoffman RS, Nelson LS, eds. Goldfrank's toxicologic emergencies, 7th ed. New York: McGraw-Hill, 2002:901-23.
328. Nice A, Leikin JB, Maturen A, Madsen-Konczyk LJ, Zell M, Hryhorczuk DO. Toxidrome recognition to improve efficiency of emergency urine drug screens. Ann Emerg Med 1988;17:676-80.
329. Nishikawa T, Kamijo Y, Ohtani H, Fraser AD. Oxaprozin interference with urinary benzodiazepine immunoassays and noninterference with receptor assay. J Anal Toxicol 1999;23:125-6.
330. Nisson L, Jones AW. 2,3-Butanedial: a potential interfering substance in the assay of ethylene glycol

by an enzymatic method. Clin Chem Acta 1992;208: 225-9.

331. Nordgren HK, Beck O. Direct screening of urine for MDMA and MDA by liquid chromatography-tandem mass spectrometry. J Anal Toxicol 2003;27:15-19.
332. Nordt SP. "DXM": A new drug of abuse? Ann Emerg Med 1998;31:794-5 (Letter).
333. O'Brien C. Drug addiction and drug abuse. In: Hardman JG, Limbird LE, Gilman AG, eds. Goodman and Gilman's the pharmacological basis of therapeutics, 10th ed. New York: McGraw-Hill, 2001:621-42.
334. Ocak A, Valentour JC, Blanke RV. The effects of storage conditions on the stability of carbon monoxide in postmortem blood. J Anal Toxicol 1985;9: 202-6.
335. Olmedo R. Phencyclidine and ketamine. In: Goldfrank LR, Flomenbaum NE, Lewin NA, Howland MA, Hoffman RS, Nelson LS, eds. Goldfrank's toxicologic emergencies, 7th ed. New York: McGraw-Hill, 2002:1034-45.
336. On-site drug testing. Jenkins AJ, Goldberger BA (eds). Humana Press, Totowa, NJ, 2002.
337. Orsulak PJ. Mission impossible. Understanding clinical pharmacology and use of antidepressant drugs. In-service Training and Continuing Education, American Association for Clinical Chemistry 1988;10:7-17.
338. Osborne R, Joel S, Trew D, Slevin M. Morphine and metabolite behavior after different routes of morphine administration: demonstration of the importance of the active metabolite morphine-6-glucuronide. Clin Pharmacol Ther 1990;47: 12-19.
339. Osborne R, Thompson P, Joel S, Trew D, Patel N, Slevin M. The analgesic activity of morphine-6-glucuronide. Br J Clin Pharmacol 1992;34:130-8.
340. Ostrea EM. Method for detecting maternally transferred drug metabolites in newborn infants. US Patent 5,015,589, May 14, 1991.
341. Ostrea EM. Method of detecting maternally transferred drug metabolites in newborn infants. US Patent 5,185,267. February 9, 1993.
342. Ostrea EM Jr, Brady MJ, Parks PM, Asensio DC, Naluz A. Drug screening of meconium in infants of drug-dependent mothers: An alternative to urine testing. J Pediatr 1989;115:474-7.
343. Otten EJ. Marijuana In: Goldfrank LR, Flomenbaum NE, Lewin NA, Howland MA, Hoffman RS, Nelson LS, eds. Goldfrank's toxicologic emergencies, 7th ed. New York: McGraw-Hill, 2002:1054-8.
344. Oyler JM, Cone EJ, Joseph, Jr RE, Huestis MA. Identification of hydrocodone in human urine following controlled codeine administration. J Anal Toxicol 2000;24:530-5.
345. Oyler JM, Cone EJ, Joseph, Jr RE, Moolchain ET, Huestis MA. Duration of detectable methamphetamine and amphetamine excretion in urine after controlled oral administration of methamphetamine to humans. Clin Chem 2002;48:1703-14.
346. Oyler J, Darwin WD, Preston KL, Suess P, Cone EJ. Cocaine disposition in meconium from newborns of cocaine-abusing mothers and urine of adult drug users. J Anal Toxicol 1996;20:453-62.
347. Pankey S, Collins C, Jaklitsch A, Izutsu A, Hu M, Pirio M, et al. Quantitative homogeneous enzyme immunoassays for amitriptyline, nortriptyline, imipramine, and desipramine. Clin Chem 1986;32:768-72.
348. Pappas AA, Gadsden RH Jr, Gadsden RH Sr, Groves WE. Computerized calculation of osmolality and its automatic comparison with observed serum ethanol concentration. Am J Clin Pathol 1982;77:449-51.
349. Pappas AA, Gadsden RH, Porter WH, Mullins RE. Osmolality of serum for evaluating the acutely intoxicated patient. In: Frings CS, Faulkner WR eds. Selected methods of emergency toxicology, Vol 11. Washington DC: AACC Press. 1986:85-8.
350. Pappas AA, Gasden RH, Taylor EH. Serum osmolality in acute intoxication. A prospective study. Am J Clin Path 1985;84:74-9.
351. Paterson S, McLachlan-Troup N, Cordero R, Dohnal M, Carman S. Qualitative screening for drugs of abuse in hair using GC-MS. J Anal Toxicol 2001;25:203-8.
352. Patrono C. Aspirin as an antiplatelet drug. N Engl J Med 1994;330:1287-94.
353. Paul BD, Jacobs A. Effects of oxidizing adulterants on detection of 11-nor-Δ^9-THC-9-carboxylic acid in urine. J Anal Toxicol 2002;26:460-3.
354. Paul BD, Martin KK, Maguilo J, Jr, Smith ML. Effects of pyridinium chlorochromate adulterant (Urine Luck) on testing for drugs of abuse and a method for quantitative detection of chromium(VI) in urine. J Anal Toxicol 2000;24:233-37.
355. Paul BD, Mitchell JM, Burbage R, Moy M, Sroka R. Gas chromatographic-electron-impact mass fragmentometric determination of lysergic acid diethylamide in urine. J Chromatogr 1990;529:103-12.
356. Peace MR, Poklis JL, Tarnai LD, Poklis A. An evaluation of the OnTrak Testcup®-er on-site urine drug testing device for drugs commonly encountered from emergency departments. J Anal Toxicol 2002;26: 500-3.
357. Pentel PR, Keyler DE, Haddad LM. Tricyclic antidepressants and selective serotonin reuptake inhibitors. In: Haddad LM, Shannon MW, Winchester JF, eds.: Clinical management of poisoning and drug overdose, 3rd ed. Philadelphia: WB Saunders Co, 1998:437-51.
358. Perrone J, De Roos F, Jayaraman S, Hollander JE. Drug screening versus history in detection of substance use in ED psychiatric patients. Am J Emerg Med 2001;19:49-51.

358a. Perrone J. Iron. In: Goldfrank LR, Flomenbaum NE, Lewin NA, Howland MA, Hoffman RS, Nelson LS, eds. Goldfrank's toxicologic emergencies, 7th ed. New York: McGraw-Hill, 2002:548-57.
359. Perrone J, Hollander JE, Shaw L, De Roos F. Predictive properties of a qualitative urine acetaminophen screen in patients with self-poisoning. J Toxicol Clin Toxicol 1999;37:769-72.
360. Perry H, Shannon MW. Acetaminophen. In: Haddad LM, Shannon MW, Winchester JF, eds. Clinical management of poisoning and drug overdose, 3rd ed. Philadelphia: WB Saunders Co, 1998:664-74.
361. Peterson CD, Collins AJ, Himes JM, Bullock ML, Keane WF. Ethylene glycol poisoning: Pharmacokinetics during therapy with ethanol and hemodialysis. N Engl J Med 1981;304:21-3.
362. Pichini S, Navarro M, Farre M, Ortuno J, Roset PN, Pacifici R, et al. On-site testing of 3,4-methylenedioxymethamphetamine (Ecstasy) in saliva with Drugswipe and Drugread: a controlled study in recreational users. Clin Chem 2002;48:174-6.
363. Poch GK, Klette KL, Anderson C. The quantitation of 2-oxo-3-hydroxy lysergic acid diethylamide (O-H-LSD) in human urine specimens, a metabolite of LSD: comparative analysis using liquid chromatography-selected ion monitoring mass spectrometry and liquid chromatography-ion trap mass spectrometry. J Anal Toxicol 2000;24:170-9.
364. Poch GK, Klette KL, Hallare DA, Manglicmot MG, Czarmy RJ, McWhorter LK, et al. The detection of metabolites of LSD in human urine specimens: 2-oxo-3-hydroxy LSD, a prevalent metabolite of LSD. J Chromatogr 1999;724:23-33.
365. Pohjola-Sintonen S, Kivisto KT, Vuori E, Lapatto-Reiniluoto O, Tiula E, Neuvonen PJ. Identification of drugs ingested in acute poisoning: correlation of patient history with drug analyses. Ther Drug Monit 2000;22:749-52.
366. Poklis A, Edinboro LE. REMEDi drug profiling system readily distinguishes between cyclobenzaprine and amitriptyline in emergency toxicology urine specimens. Clin Chem 1992;38:2349-50 (Letter).
367. Polettini A, Groppi A, Vignali C, Montagna M. Fully-automated systematic toxicologic analysis of drugs, poisons, and metabolites in whole blood, urine and plasma by gas chromatography-full scan mass spectrometry. J Chromatogr 1998;713:265-79.
368. Porter WH, Dorie LD, Rutter PW, et al. Acetaminophen by liquid chromatography. In: Frings CS, Faulkner WR eds. Selected methods of emergency toxicology, Vol 11. Washington DC: AACC Press. 1986:33-6.
369. Porter WH, Rutter PW, Bush BA, Pappas AA, Dunnington JE. Ethylene glycol toxicity: the role of serum glycolic acid in hemodialysis. J Toxicol Clin Toxicol 2001;39:607-15.
370. Porter WH, Rutter PW, Yao HH. Simultaneous determination of ethylene glycol and glycolic acid in serum by gas chromatography-mass spectrometry. J Anal Toxicol 1999;23:591-7.
371. Porter WH, Stewart MJ, Chambers AM, Watson ID. In acetaminophen assay, only unconjugated drug should be measured. Clin Chem 1984;30:1884-5.
372. Posey BL, Kimble SN. High-performance liquid chromatographic study of codeine, norcodeine, and morphine as indicators of codeine ingestion. J Anal Toxicol 1984;8:68-74.
373. Prescott LF, Roscoe P, Wright N, Brown SS. Plasma-paracetamol half-life and hepatic necrosis in patients with paracetamol overdose. Lancet 1971;1:519-22.
374. Preston KL, Epstein DH, Cone EJ, Wtsadik AT, Huestis MA, Moolchan ET. Urinary elimination of cocaine metabolites in chronic users during cessation. J Anal Toxicol 2002;26:393-400.
375. Price CP, Hammond PM, Scawen MD. Evaluation of an enzymatic procedure for the measurement of acetaminophen. Clin Chem 1983;29:358-61.
376. Price D. Methemoglobinemia. In: Goldfrank LR, Flomenbaum NE, Lewin NA, Howland MA, Hoffman RS, Nelson LS, eds. Goldfrank's toxicologic emergencies, 7th ed. New York: McGraw-Hill, 2002: 1438-49.
377. Puopolo PR, Volpicelli SA, Johnson DM, Flood JG. Emergency toxicology testing (detection, confirmation, and quantification) of basic drugs in serum by liquid chromatography with photodiode array detection. Clin Chem 1991;37:2124-30.
378. Rance MJ, Jordan BJ, Nichols JD. A simultaneous determination of acetylsalicylic acid, salicylic acid and salicylamide in plasma by gas-liquid chromatography. J Pharm Pharmacol 1975;27:425-9.
379. Remaley AT, Hicks DG, Kane MD, Shaw LM. Laboratory assessment of poisoning with a carbamate insecticide. Clin Chem 1988;34:1933-6.
380. Reuschel SA, Percey SE, Liu S, Eades DM, Foltz RL. Quantitative determination of LSD and a major metabolite, 2-oxo-3-hydroxy-LSD, in human urine by solid-phase extraction and gas chromatography-tandem mass spectrometry. J Anal Toxicol 1999;23:306-12.
381. Ritter D, Cortese CM, Edwards LC, Baker JL, Chung HD, Long C. Interference with testing for lysergic acid diethylamide. Clin Chem 1997;43:635-7.
382. Roberts LJ, II, Morrow JD. Analgesic-antipyretic and antiinflammatory agents and drugs employed in the treatment of gout. In: Hardman JG, Limbird LE, Gilman AG, eds. Goodman and Gilman's the pharmacological basis of therapeutics, 10th ed. New York: McGraw-Hill, 2001:687-731.
382a. Roberts WL, Smith PT, Martin WJ, Rainey PM. Performance characteristics of three serum iron and

total iron-binding capacity methods in acute iron overdose. Am J Clin Pathol 1999;112:657-64.

383. Ropero-Miller JD, Lambing MK, Winecker RE. Simultaneous quantitation of opioids in blood by GC-EI-MS analysis following deproteination, detautomerization of keto analytes, solid-phase extraction, and trimethylsilyl derivatization. J Anal Toxicol 2002;26:524-8.
384. Ropero-Miller JD, Garside D, Goldberger BA. Automated on-line hydrolysis of benzodiazepines improves sensitivity of urine screening by a homogeneous enzyme immunoassay. Clin Chem 1997;43:1659-60.
385. Roth GJ, Majerus PW. The mechanism of the effect of aspirin on human platelets: I. Acetylation of a particulate fraction protein. J Clin Invest 1975;56:624-32.
386. Rumack BH, Matthew H. Acetaminophen poisoning and toxicity. Pediatrics 1975;55:871-6.
387. Ryder KW, Glick MR. The effect of thioradizine on the Automatic Clinical Analyzer serum tricyclic antidepressant screen. J Clin Pathol 1986;86:248-9.
388. Rygnestad T, Aarstad K, Gustafsson K, Jenssen U. The clinical value of drug analyses in deliberate self-poisoning. Hum Exper Toxicol 1990;9:221-30.
389. Sadeg N, Francois G, Petit B, Dutertre-Catella H, Dumontet M. Automated liquid-chromatographic analyzer used for toxicology screening in a general hospital: 12 month's experience. Clin Chem 1997;43:498-504.
390. Salamone SJ, Honasoge S, Brenner C, McNally AJ, Passarelli J, Goc-Szkutnicka, et al. Flunitrazepam excretion patterns using the Abuscreen OnTrak and OnLine immunoassays: Comparison with GC-MS. J Anal Toxicol 1997;21:341-5.
391. Salomone SJ, Li Z, McNally AJ, Vitone S, Wu RS. Epimerization studies of LSD using ^{1}H nuclear magnetic resonance (NMR) spectroscopy. J Anal Toxicol 1997;21:492-7.
392. Sanchez R, Fosarelli P, Felt B, Greene M, Lacovara J, Hackett F. Carbon monoxide poisoning due to automobile exposure: Disparity between carboxyhemoglobin levels and symptoms of victims. Pediatrics 1988;82:663-6.
393. Sarma L, Wong SHY, DellaFera S. Diflunisal significantly interferes with salicylate measurements by FPIA-TDx and UV-VIS aca Methods. Clin Chem 1985;31:1922-3.
394. Schep RA. Precision and accuracy in the quantitation of carboxytetrahydrocannabinol by isotope dilution gas chromatography/mass spectrometry. J Anal Toxicol 1990;14:296-300.
395. Schneider S, Wenning R. Interference of diphenhydramine with the EMIT II immunoassay for porpoxyphene. J Anal Toxicol 1999;23:637-8 (Letter).
396. Schramm W, Craig PA, Smith RH, Berger GE. Cocaine and benzoylecgonine in saliva, serum, and urine. Clin Chem 1993;36:481-7.
397. Schramm W, Smith RH, Craig PA, Kidwell DA. Drugs of abuse in saliva. A review. J Anal Toxicol 1992;16:1-9.
398. Schulz V. Clinical pharmacokinetics of nitroprusside, cyanide, thiosulphate and thiocyanate. Clin Pharmacokinet 1984;9:239-51.
399. Schwartz RH, Hawks RL. Laboratory detection of marijuana use. JAMA 1985;254:788-92.
400. Seeff LB, Cuccherini BA, Zimmerman HJ, Adler E, Benjamin SB. Acetaminophen hepatotoxicity in alcoholics: A therapeutic misadventure. Ann Intern Med 1986;104:399-404.
401. Segall Y, Waysbort D, Barak D, Ariel N, Doctor BP, Grunwald J, et al. Direct observation and elucidation of the structure of aged and nonaged phosphorylated cholinesterases by ^{31}P NMR spectroscopy. Biochemistry 1993;32:13441-50.
402. Selavka CM. Poppy seed ingestion as a contributing factor to opiate-positive urinalysis results: The Pacific perspective. J Forensic Sci 1991;36:685-96.
403. Senanayake N, Karalliedde L. Neurotoxic effects of organorphosphorus insecticides. N Engl J Med 1987;316:761-3.
404. Shannon MW, Haddad LM. The emergency management of poisoning. In: Haddad LM, Shannon MW, Winchester JF, eds.: Clinical management of poisoning and drug overdose, 3rd ed. Philadelphia: WB Saunders Co, 1998:2-31.
405. Shekelle PG, Hardy ML, Morton SC, Maglione M, Mojica WA, Suttorp MJ, et al. Efficacy and safety of ephedra and ephedrine for weight loss and athletic performance. A meta-analysis. JAMA 2003;289:1537-45.
406. Shippe RL, Kippenberger DJ. Retrospective study of urinalysis for dl-amphetamine and dl-methamphetamine analysis under current Department of Defense Guidelines. J Anal Toxicol 2000;24:450-2.
407. Simonsson P, Liden A, Lindberg S. Effect of β-glucuronidase on urinary benzodiazepine concentrations determined by fluorescence polarization immunoassay. Clin Chem 1995;41:920-3.
408. Simpson RJ, Power KG, Wallace LA, Butcher MH, Swanson V, Simpson EC. Controlled comparison of the characteristics of long-term benzodiazepine users in general practice. Br J Gen Pract 1990;40:22-6.
409. Simpson E. Some aspects of calcium metabolism in a fatal case of ethylene glycol poisoning. Ann Clin Biochem 1985;22:90-3.
410. Sjersted OM, Jacobsen D, Ovrebo S, Jansen H. Formate concentrations in plasma from patients poisoned with methanol. Acta Med Scand 1983;213:105-10.

411. Smilkstein MJ, Douglas DR, Daya MRl. Acetaminophen poisoning and liver function. N Engl J Med 1994;331:1310-11 (Letter).
412. Smilkstein MJ, Knapp GL, Kulig KW, Rumack BH. Efficacy of oral N-acetylcysteine in the treatment of acetaminophen overdose: Analysis of the national multicenter study (1976-1985). N Engl J Med 1988;319:1557-62.
413. Smilkstein MJ, Rumack BH. Elimination half-life ($T_{1/2}$) as a predictor of acetaminophen-induced hepatotoxicity. Vet Human Toxicol 1994;36:377 (abstract).
414. Smith DE, Gutgesell ME, Schwartz RH, Thorne MM, Bogema S. Federal guidelines for marijuana screening should have lower cutoff levels: A comparison of results from immunoassays and gas chromatography-mass spectrometry. Arch Pathol Lab Med 1989;113:1299-300.
415. Smith JAE, Hine ID, Beck P, Routledge PA. Paracetamol toxicity: is enzyme induction important? Human Toxicol 1986;5:383-5.
416. Smith ML, Hughes RO, Levine B, Dickerson S, Darwin WD, Cone EJ. Forensic drug testing for opiates. VI. Urine testing for hydromorphone, hydrocodone, oxymorphone, and oxycodone with commercial opiate immunoassays and gas chromatography-mass spectrometry. Clin Chem 1995;41:18-26.
417. Smith ML, Shimomura ET, Summers J, Paul BD, Jenkins AJ, Darwin WD, et al. Urinary excretion profiles for total morphine, free morphine, and 6-acetylmorphine following smoked and intravenous heroin. J Anal Toxicol 2001;25:504-14.
418. Smith ML, Shimomura ET, Summers J, Paul BD, Nichols D, Shippee R, et al. Detections time and analytical performance of commercial urine opiate immunoassays following heroin administration. J Anal Toxicol 2000;24:522-9.
419. Smith RK, O'Mara K. Tricyclic antidepressant overdose. J Family Pract 1982;15:247-53.
420. Smith SW, Topliff AR, Danigellis Ml. CDC MMWR: Adverse events associated with ingestion of gamma-butyrolactone-Minnesota, New Mexico, and Texas, 1998-1999. JAMA 1999;281:979-80.
421. Smith-Kielland A, Olsen KM, Christophersen AS. False-positive results with EMIT® II amphetamine/methamphetamine assay in users of common psychotropic drugs. Clin Chem 1995;41:952-3.
422. Snook CP. Overdose and poisoning: Physiological responses. In: Professional practice in toxicology: A review. Washington, DC: AACC Press, 1993.
423. Snyder H, Schwenzer KS, Pearlman R, McNally AJ, Tsilimidos M, Salamone SJ, et al. Serum and urine concentrations of flunitrazepam and metabolites, after a single oral dose, by immunoassay and GC-MS. J Anal Toxicol 2001;25:699-704.
424. Song W, Gao BL, Dou C. One step immunoassay for the detection of acetaminophen and salicylate in serum, plasma and whole blood. Clin Chem 2001;47A 189 (Abstract).
424a. Sporer KA. Buprenorphine: a primer for emergency physicians. Ann Emerg Med 2004;43:580-4.
425. Sorisky A, Watson DC. Positive diphenhydramine interference in the EMIT-ST® assay for tricyclic antidepressants in serum. Clin Chem 1986;32:715 (Letter).
426. Staub C, Marset M, Mino A, Mangin P. Detection of acetylcodeine in urine as an indicator of illicit heroin use: method validation and results of a pilot study. Clin Chem 2001;47:301-7.
427. Steele BW, Bandstra ES, Wu NC, Hime GW, Hearn WL. m-Hydroxybenzoyl-ecgonine: An important contributor to the immunoreactivity in assays for benzoylecogonine in meconium. J Anal Toxicol 1993;17:348-52.
428. Steering Committee of the Physicians' Health Study Research Group: Final report on the aspirin component of the ongoing Physicians' Health Study. N Engl J Med 321:129-35, 1989.
429. Stokes JB, Aueron F. Prevention of organ damage in massive ethylene glycol ingestion. JAMA 1980;243:2065-6.
430. Struempler RE. Excretion of codeine and morphine following ingestion of poppy seeds. J Anal Toxicol 1987;11:97-9.
431. Struempler RE, Nelson G, Urry FM. A positive cannabinoids workplace drug test following ingestion of commercially available hemp seed oil. J Anal Toxicol 1997;21:283-5.
432. Substance Abuse and Mental Health Administration. Mandatory guidelines and proposed revisions to mandatory guidelines for federal workplace testing programs. Fed Reg 2004;19644-732. (http://workplace.samhsa.gov)
433. Sullivan M. Mandatory guidelines for federal workplace drug testing programs. Fed Reg 1988; 53:11970-89.
434. Sutherland DE, Lott JA, Marenberg S. Salicylate by spectrophotometry. In: Frings CS, Faulkner WR eds. Selected methods of emergency toxicology, Vol 11. Washington DC: AACC Press. 1986:89-92.
435. Swartz JG, Hurd IL, Carnahan JJ: Determination of tricyclic antidepressants for ED analysis. Am J Emerg Med 1994;12:513-6.
436. Taylor EH, Oertli EH, Wolfgang JW, Mueller E. Accuracy of five on-site immunoassay drugs-of-abuse testing devices. J Anal Toxicol 1999;23:119-24.
437. Taylor P. Anticholinesterase agents. In: Hardman JG, Limbird LE, Gilman AG, eds. Goodman and Gilman's the pharmacological basis of therapeutics, 10th ed. New York: McGraw-Hill, 2001:175-91.
438. Temple AR, Mrazik TJ. More on extended-release acetaminophen. N Engl J Med 1995;333:1508 (Letter).

439. Tennant F, Shannon J. Cocaine abuse in methadone maintenance patients is associated with low serum methadone concentrations. J Addict Dis 1995;14: 67-74.
440. Tennant F, Shannon J. Quantitative urine testing: A new tool for diagnosing and treating cocaine use. Postgrad Med 1989;86:107-14.
440a. Tenebein M, Yatscoff RW. The total iron-binding capacity in iron poisoning. Is it useful? Am J Dis Child 1991;145:437-9.
441. Thevis M, Opfermann G, Schänzer W. Urinary concentrations of morphine and codeine after consumption of poppy seeds. J Anal Toxicol 2003; 27:53-6.
442. Thevis M, Opfermann G, Schanzer W. Liquid Chromatography/electrospray ionization tandem mass spectrometric screening and confirmation methods for beta 2-agonists in human or equine urine. J Mass Spectrom 2003;38:1197-206.
443. Thurman EM, Pedersen MJ, Stout RL, Martin T. Distinguishing sympathomimetic amines from amphetamine and methamphetamine in urine by gas chromatography/mass spectrometry. J Anal Toxicol 1992;16:19-27.
444. Tietz NW, Fiereck EA. The spectrophotometric measurement of carboxyhemoglobin. Ann Clin Lab Sci 1973;3:36-42.
445. Tighe TV, Walter FG. Delayed toxic acetaminophen level after initial four hour nontoxic level. Clin Toxicol 1994;32:431-4.
446. Tomaszewski C. Carbon monoxide. In: Goldfrank LR, Flomenbaum NE, Lewin NA, Howland MA, Hoffman RS, Nelson LS, eds. Goldfrank's toxicologic emergencies, 7th ed. New York: McGraw-Hill, 2002:1478-91.
447. Tong T, Boyer EW. Club drugs, smart drugs, raves, and circuit parties: an overview of the club scene. Ped Emerg Care 2002;18:216-18.
448. Towt J, Tsai SC, Hernandez MR, Klimov AD, Kravec CV, Rouse SL, et al. Ontrak Testcup. A novel, on-site, multi-analyte screen for the detection of abused drugs. J Anal Toxicol 1995;19:504-10.
449. Transportation Department, National Highway Traffic Safety Administration. Highway Safety Programs;Conforming products list of screening devices to measure alcohol in bodily fluids. Fed Reg 2001;66:22639-40.
450. Transportation Department, National Highway Traffic Safety. Procedures for transportation workplace drug and alcohol testing programs. Fed Reg 2000;65:79462;Fed Reg 2001;65:41944;http://www.dot.gov/ost/dapc/main/Part40_complete_20040318.doc.
451. Transportation Department, National Highway Traffic Safety Administration. Highway safety programs;Model specifications for devices to measure breath alcohol. Fed Reg 2002;67:62091-4.
452. Trinder P. Rapid determination of salicylate in biological fluids. Biochem J 1954;57:301-3.
453. Tsai S-CJ, ElSohly MA, Dubrovsky T, Twarowska B, Towt J, Salamone SJ. Determination of five abused drugs in nitrite-adulterated urine by immunoassays and gas chromatography mass spectrometry. J Anal Toxicol 1998;22:474-80.
454. Tsai JSC, ElSohly MA, Tsai S-F, Murphy TP, Twarowska B, Salamone SJ. Investigation of nitrite adulteration on the immunoassay and GC-MS analysis of cannabinoids in urine specimens. J Anal Toxicol 2000;24:708-14.
455. Turcant A, Premel-Cabic A, Cailleux A, Allain P. Toxicological screening of drugs by microbore high-performance liquid chromatography with photodiode-array detection and ultraviolet spectral library searches. Clin Chem 1991;37:1210-15.
456. Tucker JR, Ferm RP. Lysergic acid diethylamide and other hallucinogens. In: Goldfrank LR, Flomenbaum NE, Lewin NA, Howland MA, Hoffman RS, Nelson LS, eds. Goldfrank's toxicologic emergencies, 7th ed. New York: McGraw-Hill, 2002:1046-53.
457. Valentine JL, Kearns GL, Sparks C, Letzig LG, Valentine CR, Shappell SA, et al. GC-MS determination of amphetamine and methamphetamine in human urine for 12 hours following oral administration of dextromethamphetamine: lack of evidence supporting the established forensic guidelines for methamphetamine confirmation. J Anal Toxicol 1995;19:581-90.
458. van As H, Stolk LML. Rifampicin cross-reacts with opiate immunoassay. J Anal Toxicol 1999;23:71 (Letter).
459. Veltri JC, Thompson MIB. Salicylates. In: Skoutakis VA ed. Clinical toxicology of drugs: Principles and practice. Philadelphia: Lea & Febiger, 1982:227-43.
460. Venisse N, Marquet P, Duchoslav E, Dupuy JL, Lachâtre G. A general unknown screening procedure for drugs and toxic compounds in serum using liquid chromatography-electrospray-single quadrupole mass spectrometry. J Anal Toxicol 2003;27:7-14.
461. Vesey CJ, Kirk CJC. Two automated methods for measuring plasma thiocyanate compared. Clin Chem 1985;31:270-4.
462. Vesey CJ, Wilson J. Red cell cyanide. J Pharm Pharmacol 1978;30:20-6.
463. Vreman HJ, Mahoney JJ, Van Kessel AL, Stevenson DK. Carboxyhemoglobin as measured by gas chromatography and with the IL 282 and 482 CO-Oximeter. Clin Chem 1988;34:2562-66.
464. Vreman HJ, Ronquillo RB, Ariagno RL, Schwartz HC, Stevenson DK. Interference of fetal hemoglobin with the spectrophotometric measurement of carboxyhemoglobin. Clin Chem 1988;34:975-7.
465. Wagner JG, Wilkinson PK, Sedman AJ. Elimination of alcohol from human blood. J Pharmacol 1976; 65:152-4.

466. Walberg CB, Gupta RC. Quantitation of phencyclidine in urine by enzyme immunoassay. J Anal Toxicol 1982;6:97.
467. Walshe K, Barrett AM, Kavanagh PV, McNamara SM, Moran C, Shattock AG. A sensitive immunoassay for flunitrazepam and metabolites. J Anal Toxicol 2000; 24:296-9.
468. Wan SH, Matin SB, Azarnoff DL. Kinetics, salivary excretion of amphetamine isomers, and effect of urinary pH. Clin Pharmacol Ther 1978;23:585-90.
469. Wang PH, Liu C, Tsay WI, Li JH, Liu RH, Wu TG, et al. Improved screen and confirmation test of 7-aminoflunitrazepam in urine specimens for monitoring flunitrazepam (Rohypnol) exposure. J Anal Toxicol 2002;26:411-18.
470. Waraska J, Nagle JD. A critical assessment of antipsychotic drug monitoring. Clinics Lab Med 1987; 7:435-52.
471. Warner A. Cost-effective toxicology testing. In-Service Training and Continuing Education, American Association for Clinical Chemistry 1996;17(2): February.
472. Weinmann W, Svoboda M. Fast screening for drugs of abuse by solid-phase extraction combined with flow-injection ion spray-tandem mass spectrometry. J Anal Toxicol 1998;22:319-28.
473. Weisman RS. Antihistamines and decongestants. In: Goldfrank LR, Flomenbaum NE, Lewin NA, Howland MA, Hoffman RS, Nelson LS, eds. Goldfrank's toxicologic emergencies, 7th ed. New York: McGraw-Hill, 2002:535-43.
474. Weiss RG, Gawin FH. Protracted elimination of cocaine metabolites in long-term high dose cocaine abusers. Am J Med 1988;85:879-80.
475. Whitcomb DC, Block GD. Association of acetaminophen hepatotoxicity with fasting and ethanol use. JAMA 1994;272:1845-50.
476. Wians FH Jr, Norton JT. False-positive serum tricyclic antidepressant screen with cyproheptadine. Clin Chem 1993;39:1355-6 (Letter).
477. Wiegand RF, Klette KL, Stout PR, Gehlhausen JM. Comparison of EMIT II ®, CEDIA®, and DPC ® RIA assays for the detection of lysergic acid diethylamide in forensic urine samples. J Anal Toxicol 2002; 26:519-23.
478. Wiener K. A review of methods for plasma paracetamol estimation. Ann Clin Biochem 1978;15:187-96.
479. Winek CL, Carfagna M. Comparison of plasma, serum, and whole blood ethanol concentrations. J Anal Toxicol 1987;11:267-8.
480. Winek CL, Murphy KL. The rate and kinetic order of ethanol elimination. Forensic Sci Int 1984;25: 159-66.
481. Winek CL, Paul LJ. Effect of short-term storage conditions on alcohol concentrations in blood from living human subjects. Clin Chem 1983;29:1959-60.
482. Wingert W. Lowering cutoffs for initial and confirmation testing for cocaine and marijuana: Large-scale study of effects on the rates of drug-positive results. Clin Chem 1997;43:100-3.
483. Wennig R, Moeller MR, Haguenoer JM, Marocchi A, Zoppi F, Smith BL, et al. Development and evaluation of immunochromatographic rapid tests for screening of cannabinoids, cocaine, and opiates in urine. J Anal Toxicol 1998;22:148-55.
484. Wolfe TR, Caravati EM. Massive dextromethorphan ingestion and abuse. Am J Emerg Med 1995;13: 174-6.
485. Wolff K. Characterization of methadone overdose: clinical considerations and the scientific evidence. Ther Drug Monit 2002;24:457-70.
486. Wong ECC, Koenig J, Turk J. Potential interference of cyclobenzaprine and norcyclobenzaprine with HPLC measurement of amitriptyline and nortriptyline: Resolution by GC-MS analysis. J Anal Toxicol 1995;19:218-24.
487. Wright RO, Woolf AD. Phencyclidine. In: Haddad LM, Shannon MW, Winchester JF, eds.: Clinical management of poisoning and drug overdose, 3rd ed. Philadelphia: WB Saunders Co, 1998:552-9.
488. Wu AHB, Bristol B, Sexton K, Cassella-McLane GC, Holtman V, Hill DW. Adulteration of urine by "Urine Luck." Clin Chem 1999;45:1051-7.
489. Wu AHB, Feng Y-J, Pajor A, Gornet TG, Wong SS, Forte E, Brown J. Detection and interpretation of lysergic acid diethylamide results by immunoassay screening of urine in various testing groups. J Anal Toxicol 1997;21:181-4.
490. Wu AHB, Johnson KG, Wong SS. Impact of revised NIDA guidelines for methamphetamine testing in urine. Clin Chem 1992;38:2352-3.
491. Wu AHB, McKay C, Broussard LA, Hoffman RS, Kwong TC, Moyer TP, et al. National Academy of Clinical Biochemistry laboratory medicine practice guidelines: recommendations for the use of laboratory tests to support poisoned patients who present to the Emergency Department. Clin Chem 2003;49:357-9.
492. Wu AHB, Onigbinde TA, Johnson KG, Wimbash GH. Alcohol-specific cocaine metabolites in serum and urine of hospitalized patients. J Anal Toxicol 1992;16:132-6.
493. Yang JM, Lewandrowski KB. Urine drugs of abuse testing at the point-of-care: clinical interpretation and programmatic considerations with specific reference to the Syva Rapid Test (SRT). Clin Chim Acta 2001;307:27-32.
494. Yao HH, Porter WH. Simultaneous determination of ethylene glycol and its major toxic metabolite, glycolic acid, in serum by gas chromatography. Clin Chem 1996;42:292-7.

495. Yeatman DT, Reid K. A study of urinary endogenous gamma-hydroxybutyrate (GHB) levels. J Anal Toxicol 2003;27:40-2.
496. Yip L, Dart RC. A 20-hour treatment for acute acetaminophen overdose. N Engl J Med 2003;384:2471-2 (Letter).
497. Yue QY, Hasselström J, Svensson JO, Säwe J Pharmacokinetics of codeine and its metabolite in Caucasian healthy volunteers: comparison between extensive and poor hydroxylators of debrisoquine. Br J Clin Pharmacol 1991;31:635-42.
498. Zawertailo LA, Kaplan HL, Busto UE, Tyndale RF, Sellers EM. Psychotropic effects of dextromethorphan are altered by CYP2D6 polymorphism: a pilot study. J Clin Psychopharmacol 1998;18:332-7.
499. Zoppi F, Brenna S, Fumagall C, Marocchi A. Discrimination among dyshemoglobins: analytical approach to a toxicological query. Clin Chem 1996;42:1300-02 (Letter).
500. Zvosec DL, Smith SW, McCutcheon JR, Spillane J, Hall BJ, Peacock EA. Adverse events, including death, associated with the use of 1, 4-butanediol. N Engl J Med 2001;344:87-94.
501. Zwart A, van Kampen EJ, Zizlstra WG. Results of routine determination of clinically significant hemoglobin derivatives by multicomponent analysis. Clin Chem 1986;32:972-8.

ADDITIONAL READING

Badia R, de la Torre R, Corcione S, Segura J. Analytical approaches of European Union laboratories to drugs of abuse analysis. Clin Chem 1998;44:790-99.

Biologic markers in urinary toxicology. National Washington DC: Academy Press, 1995.

Brandenberger H, Maes RA, eds. Analytical toxicology for clinical, forensic, and pharmaceutical chemists. New York: Walter De Gruyter, 1997.

Descotes J. Human toxicology. New York: Elsevier Science, 1996.

De Vries J, Hollinger MA, Niesink RJ. Textbook of toxicology: Principles and applications. Boca Raton, FL: CRC Press, 1996.

Drummer OH. Postmortem toxicology of drugs of abuse. Forensic Sci Int 2004;142:101-13.

Duffus JH. Glossary for chemists of terms used in toxicology: IUPAC recommendations 1993. Pure Appl Chem 1993;65:2003-133.

Ellenhorn MJ, Schonwald S, Ordog G, Wasserberger J. Ellenhorn's medical toxicology, diagnosis and treatment of human poisoning, 2nd ed. Baltimore: Williams & Wilkins, 1997.

Flanagan RJ. Guidelines for the interpretation of analytical toxicology results and unit of measurement conversion factors. Ann Clin Biochem 1998;35:261-8.

Haddad LM, Shannon MW, Winchester JF, eds. Clinical management of poisoning and drug overdose 3rd ed. Philadelphia: WB Saunders Co, 1998.

Haschek WM, Rousseaux CG. Fundamentals of toxicologic pathology. San Diego: Academic Press, 1996.

Lewis RA. Dictionary of toxicology. Boca Raton, FL: Lewis Publishers, 1996.

Lu FC. Basic toxicology: Fundamentals, target organs, and risk assessment 3rd ed. Bristol, PA: Taylor & Francis, 1996.

Massaro EJ. Handbook of human toxicology. Boca Raton, FL: CRC Press, 1997.

Raharjo TJ, Verpoorte R. Methods for the analysis of cannabinoids in biological materials: a review. Phytochem Anal 2004;15:79-94.

Rea WJ. Chemical sensitivity: Tools for diagnosis & methods of treatment Vol 4, Boca Raton, FL: Lewis Publishers, 1996.

Ryan RP, Terry CE. Toxicology desk reference: The toxic exposure & medical monitoring index Vol 1-3, Bristol, PA: Taylor & Francis, 1996.

Streissguth A. Fetal alcohol syndrome: A guide for families and communities. Baltimore: Paul Brookes Publishing, 1997.

Trout GJ, Kazlauskas R. Sports drug testing—an analyst's perspective. Chem Soc Rev 2004;33:1-13. Epub 2003 Dec 08.

Verstraete AG. Detection times of drugs of abuse in blood, urine, and oral fluid. Ther Drug Monit 2004;26: 200-5.

Viccellio P. Handbook of emergency toxicology 2nd ed. Philadelphia: Lippincott-Raven Publishers, 1997.

Williams P. Principles of toxicology. New York: Van Nostrand Reinhold, 1997.

CHAPTER 35

Toxic Metals

Thomas P. Moyer, Ph.D., Mary F. Burritt, Ph.D., and John Butz, B.A.

Metals have been recognized as toxins for centuries. Arsenic poisoning was a favored way to dethrone royalty in the Renaissance era. Mercury poisoning was common in eighteenth century Europe associated with generation of felt from beaver pelts to make the popular top hat. The hat makers displayed behavioral changes typical of those resulting from mercury exposure, leading to common use of the phrase "mad as a hatter." In the 1950s a tragic case of mercury poisoning occurred in the Minamata Bay of Japan where large quantities of industrial mercury were dumped into the bay. Over 3000 victims have been recognized as having "Minamata disease," a syndrome that is characterized by symptoms of methylmercury poisoning.[59] In 1971 mercury contamination of seed grain caused 6000 deaths in Iraq.

BASIC CONCEPTS

Important questions to consider for metal toxicity are: (1) Is the metal of concern toxic? (2) What is the prevalence associated with the metal of concern? (3) What are the signs and symptoms of exposure to that metal? (4) Is the degree of exposure known? (5) Do adequate analytical techniques exist to measure the metal? (6) Are appropriate tissues available to quantify the metal?

Section I of this chapter addresses these questions. Section II focuses on the unique characteristics of the more common metals known to be associated with toxicity. Readers are referred to Casarett's and Doull's *Toxicology*[96] for detail on rare metal toxicities.

Prevalence of Metal-Based Toxicity

As the twenty-first century begins, one would expect that metal toxicities would be well known and avoidable. However, humans encounter elemental toxins frequently, with chronic, low-concentration exposure occurring more frequently in individuals than in large population groups. Concern continues regarding low-concentration exposure to lead and the effect such exposure has on mental development in the young. Arsenic is common in our environment, and individuals are occasionally exposed because of a lack of knowledge of the household products they are using. Many insecticides contain arsenic as an active ingredient; careless use of these products can lead to significant exposure. Arsenic is frequently identified as the cause of peripheral neuropathy among patients who have been unsuspectingly exposed. Ground water contaminated with arsenic in the Bengal basin of Bangladesh exceeding WHO safety limits because of leaching from bedrock presents a serious health risk to the large population living in that region.* Cadmium is used to manufacture brightly colored paint pigments; painters who fail to use adequate respiratory protection while spray painting with these products can experience significant exposure. Cadmium is also a significant toxin in tobacco products.[81] Mercury has been shown to leach from dental amalgams.[137] Initially, this finding caused considerable concern; however, later studies have failed to find a causal relationship.[6,78,172] Studies have indicated that apoptotic pathways are initiated by metals such as arsenic, cadmium, chromium, nickel, and beryllium and possibly lead, antimony, and cobalt.[135]

Although rare, manufacturing errors can cause production of products that contain toxic metals. In the early 1960s, a Canadian beer brewery accidentally contaminated a large lot of its product with cobalt. The product was sold to and consumed by the public, resulting in an outbreak of renal disease and cardiomyopathy. In this type of situation, the U.S. Public Health Service is often called in to identify the cause of an outbreak of unusual symptoms. The clinical laboratory should be prepared to support these types of investigations.

*References 1, 15, 86, 89, 93, 154, 166, 173.

One study of a large outpatient general medicine population ($N = 329{,}000$) places perspective on the issue of the role of toxic metals in disease.[118] From among a group of human subjects representing a broad spectrum of all disease types, with some concentration of tertiary care patients, 1986 patients (0.6% of the total population) were identified as having some physical finding or exposure concern indicating reason for further examination for metals. Of these, 152 cases (0.05% of the original population) were singled out by laboratory testing as cases of high suspicion that metals were involved. Of these, 32 cases (0.01% of the population, or 1 in 9700) ultimately were proven to have metal toxicities. Eighteen of these cases were arsenic related, two were cadmium related, seven were lead related, and five were mercury related.

The incidence of metal poisoning in this population attributable to arsenic, cadmium, lead, or mercury poisoning appears to be of the same scale as the more common inborn errors of metabolism, such as neonatal hypothyroidism and phenylketonuria, and is the same order of magnitude as the incidence of adult-onset hemochromatosis, a disease for which mandatory screening has been suggested. Screening for these diseases is indicated because they are treatable, and treatment significantly reduces long-term morbidity. The same can be said for metal toxicities. When identified early, disease caused by metal exposure is readily treatable with good outcome. Conversely, if exposure is not identified and reduced, serious and sometimes irreparable damage to the nervous, renal, and cardiovascular systems can occur.

TABLE 35-1 Conditions in Which Metal Toxicity Can Be a Causative Factor

Metal	Condition
Aluminum	In dialysis encephalopathy or dementia
Arsenic	When the patient reports bilateral pain radiating from feet to leg
Cadmium	Renal disease in aerosol painters
Copper-zinc deficiency	Induced loss of wound healing
Lead	In children under age 2 living in older homes
Manganese	Onset of parkinsonism under age 50
Mercury	Acute changes in behavior, impaired speech, visual field constriction, hearing loss, and somatosensory
Selenium (deficiency)	In patients undergoing total parenteral nutrition
Thallium	Acute hair loss
Zinc (deficiency)	Burn patients exhibiting erythema

Diagnosing Toxicity

Confirming the diagnosis of metal toxicity is difficult because signs and symptoms are similar to a number of other diseases. Diagnosis of metal toxicity requires demonstration of all of the following three factors: (1) a source of metal exposure must be evident, (2) the patient must demonstrate signs and symptoms typical of the metal, and (3) abnormal metal concentration in the appropriate tissue must be evident.

If one of these features is absent, one cannot make a conclusive diagnosis of metal toxicity. The laboratory plays a key role in this process, and appropriate specimen collection coupled with accurate analysis can make a major difference in correct diagnosis.

In clinical practice, analysis of toxic elements should always be considered in the clinical workup of the patient with (1) renal disease of unexplained origin, (2) bilateral peripheral neuropathy, (3) acute changes in mental function, (4) acute inflammation of the nasal or laryngeal epithelium, or (5) a history of exposure. Certain elements should be considered as the active, causative, or deficient agent in specific circumstances (Table 35-1).

Classification of Metals

Some metals are essential for life (see Chapter 30), but if an individual's exposure exceeds a certain threshold, toxicity may develop. Nonessential metals can be toxic even at low concentrations. Review of the periodic table provides some insight into the determination of a metal's potential toxicity (Figure 35-1).

Elements in groups IA and IIA in rows three through five of the periodic table generally fit the role of essential elements. The gastrointestinal tract and dermis are very effective at regulating the body burden of these compounds—it is very difficult to cause toxicity by one of these elements unless the element is injected directly into the vascular system. Elements in groups IB through VIIB and VIII in row four of the periodic table are generally essential for life but required at low concentrations; many are protein cofactors required for activity. The gastrointestinal tract and dermis regulate intake to some degree, but overload will induce passive diffusion that can lead to excessive concentrations and toxicity. Elements in row five and below are classified as nonessential (or if essential, are required at picomolar concentrations or less). As one moves from right to left across the periodic table, the elements become more prevalent and therefore have greater potential to induce toxicity. Elements in groups IB and IIB in rows six and seven and group IIIA through VIA in rows four to six are of particular interest as toxins, because they have electron configuration that allows them to bond covalently with sulfur. Later in this chapter, this characteristic is identified as a significant factor in the

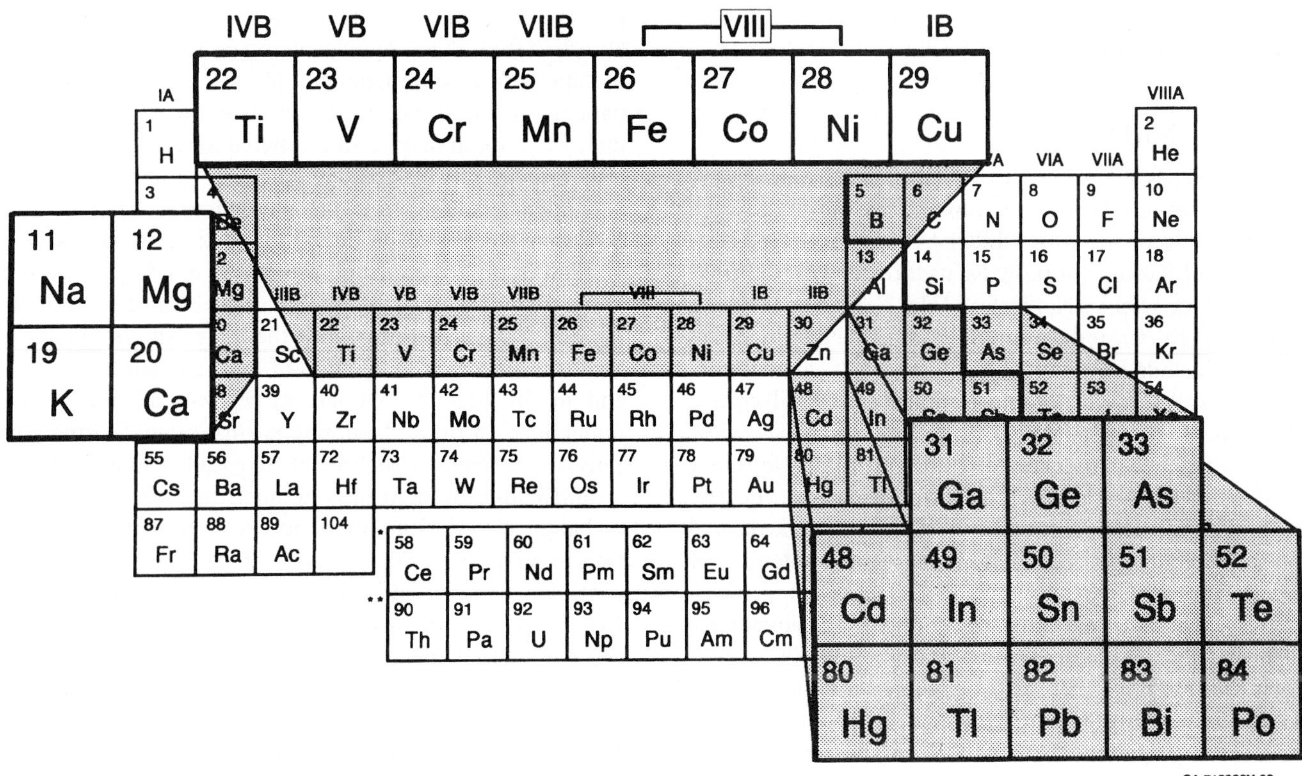

Figure 35-1 Periodic table, with emphasis on toxic elements.

mechanism of action of the group of metals often referred to as "heavy metals."* These include arsenic, cadmium, lead, mercury, and thallium, all toxins of considerable concern. Elements in VIIA (halides) are essential for life but toxic when present in excess. Group VIIIA, the inert elements, are toxic in the gas phase because they can cause anoxia; their inert characteristic is the cause of their toxicity.

Occupational Monitoring

Employees are frequently monitored when working in an environment where exposure to toxic metals is a possibility.† The most common form of monitoring involves quantification of airborne concentrations of metals in the production process. Threshold limit values for airborne concentrations and time-interval exposure concentrations are defined by the U.S. National Institute for Occupational Safety and Health (NIOSH) to ensure worker safety. Workers may also be monitored by quantification of biological samples. The most common sample used is a random urine sample, and results are expressed in concentration units for the metal of interest per gram of creatinine to normalize for excretion volume variances. Only cadmium has defined urine excretion concentrations set by a U.S. federal agency to ensure worker safety.[127] Additional technical and regulatory information about toxic metals is available at the Occupational Safety and Health Administration (OSHA) web site (http://www.osha.gov/SLTC/metalsheavy/index.html).

The World Health Organization (WHO) and OSHA have defined blood concentrations for lead that are designed to warn employers when workers are overexposed.[143] Safety limits for other metals have been set by professional organizations, such as the American Conference of Governmental Hygienists.[53]

Analytical Methods

Atomic absorption spectrometry with flame (AA-F) or electrothermal atomization furnace (AA-ETA), inductively coupled plasma-emission spectroscopy (ICP-ES), inductively coupled plasma-mass spectrometry (ICP-MS), and high-performance liquid chromatography-mass spectrometry (LC-MS) are state-of-the-art analytical techniques used to measure metals in biological fluids. They are specific and sensitive and provide the clinical laboratory with the capability to measure a broad array of metals at clinically significant concentrations. For example, ICP-MS is used to measure several metals simultaneously.[26,113,124] Photometric assays are also available but require large volumes of sample and have limited analytical performance. Spot tests are also

*The International Union of Pure and Applied Chemistry (IUPAC) considers the term "heavy metal" to be both meaningless and misleading, and recommends that it no longer be used. (Duffus, JH. "Heavy metals" a meaningless term? IUPAC Technical Report. Pure Appl Chem 2002;74:793-807.)

†References 22, 25, 41, 75, 90, 149, 182.

available but should be considered obsolete because they are error prone, often yielding false-positive results.[133]

SPECIFIC METALS

Certain metals are known to be toxic when humans are exposed to elevated concentrations and five metals are listed in the top 20 of the 2003 CERCLA* Priority List of Hazardous Substances (http://www.atsdr.cdc.gov/cxcx3.html). They include arsenic (No. 1), lead (No. 2), mercury (No. 3), cadmium (No. 7), and chromium (No. 17). Other metals of concern include aluminum, beryllium, cobalt, copper, iron, manganese, nickel, platinum, selenium, silicon, silver, and thallium. The Agency for Toxic Substances and Disease Registry (ATSDR) produces "toxicological profiles" for many of these metals on their website (http://www.atsdr.cdc.gov/toxpro2.html). These hazardous substances are ranked based on their frequency of occurrence, toxicity, and potential for human exposure.

Several of these metals are also considered essential trace elements and are discussed also in Chapter 30. Risk assessments for essentiality versus toxicity for chromium, copper, iodine, iron, manganese, molybdenum, selenium, and zinc have been performed by several U.S. governmental and private organizations.[72]

Methods for aluminum, arsenic, lead, mercury, and selenium are included in the Appendix to Chapter 35 located on this book's accompanying Evolve site, found at http://evolve.elsevier.com/Tietz/textbook/.

ALUMINUM

Aluminum (Al) is an extremely light, whitish, lustrous, metallic element, obtainable from bauxite or clay. Aluminum compounds are used chiefly for their antacid and astringent properties. In 1972 Alfrey and colleagues first described an encephalopathy that was observed in patients undergoing prolonged hemodialysis for renal failure.[2] The disease was characterized by abnormal speech, myoclonic jerks, and convulsions. Patients with these signs also showed a predominance of osteomalacic fractures.[178] Since then, it has become well understood that exposure of patients in renal failure to Al-laden dialysis water, Al-containing oral phosphate binders, and Al-laden albumin administered during dialysis is the primary cause of these signs of Al toxicity. Aluminum is also a developmental toxicant if administered parenterally.[54]

Under normal physiological conditions, the usual daily dietary intake of 5 to 10 mg of Al is completely excreted. This excretion is accomplished by avid filtration of Al from the blood by the glomerulus of the kidney. Patients in renal failure lose this ability and are candidates for Al toxicity. The dialysis process is not highly effective at eliminating Al and can be a significant source of exposure.[3] Furthermore, it is a common practice to administer Al-based gels orally to patients in renal failure to reduce the amount of phosphate absorbed from their diet to avoid excessive phosphate accumulation. A small fraction of this Al may be absorbed; patients in renal failure accumulate this Al. Following dialysis, albumin may be administered to replace that which is removed during dialysis. Some albumin products have high Al content resulting from the pharmaceutical purification process of passing the product through Al silicate filters.

Aluminum accumulates in blood if not filtered by the kidney; it avidly binds to proteins, such as transferrin, and is rapidly distributed throughout the body. Aluminum overload leads to the accumulation of Al at two sites: in bone[27] and in the brain.[58] In bone, Al replaces calcium at the mineralization front, disrupting normal osteoid formation. This can be readily visualized histologically using Goldner's stain. Deposition of Al in bone interrupts normal calcium exchange; the calcium in bone becomes unavailable for resorption into blood, a process under the physiological control of parathyroid hormone (PTH) and 1,25 dihydroxy vitamin D. Aluminum binding to calcium binding sites in the parathyroid gland causes an abnormal physiological response by the parathyroid gland, which results in the biochemical profile that is virtually diagnostic of Al overload disease—abnormally low PTH for the degree of renal failure present combined with high serum Al.[110]

The normal physiological action of PTH on bone is blunted in patients with renal failure, because their renal cells are not synthesizing the 1,25 dihydroxy vitamin D required for normal PTH action. It is typical for patients in renal failure to have high serum PTH values; this represents secondary hyperparathyroidism, the normal physiological response to vitamin D deficit. Deposition of Al at the bone mineralization front and binding to parathyroid calcium receptors interferes with this physiologic process. The usual parathyroid response to these conditions decreases secretion of PTH. The result is lower-than-expected serum PTH concentration for the degree of renal disease present.

McCarthy has defined a biochemical profile that is characteristic of Al overload disease.[110] In human subjects with normal renal function, serum Al concentration is normally lower than 6 μg/L. Patients in renal failure invariably have serum Al concentrations well above this amount. Clinical guidelines published in 2003[57] suggest that patients with no signs or symptoms of osteomalacia or encephalopathy are likely to have serum Al concentrations <20 μg/L and PTH whole molecule concentrations >16 pmol/L, typical for secondary hyperparathyroidism associated with renal failure. Patients with signs and symptoms of osteomalacia or encephalopathy typically have serum Al concentrations >60 μg/L and PTH concentrations lower than <16 pmol/L; these laboratory parameters indicate Al-related bone disease. Patients with serum Al concentrations >20 μg/L but <60 μg/L were identified as candidates for likely onset of Al-related bone disease; these patients required aggressive efforts to reduce their daily Al exposure. A graphic presentation of these concepts is presented in Figure 35-2. Efforts to reduce

*CERCLA: Comprehensive Environmental Response, Compensation, and Liability Act (or Superfund).

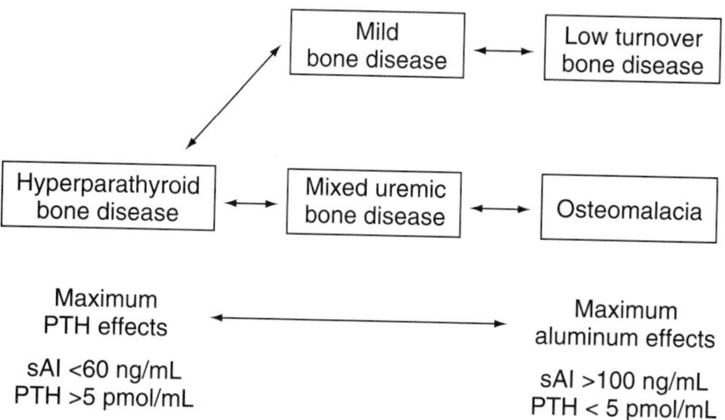

Figure 35-2 Aluminum's effect on bone physiology.

Al intake include switching from Al-containing phosphate binders to calcium-containing phosphate binders, ensuring that dialysis water contains less than 10 µg/L of Al, and ensuring that the albumin used during postdialysis therapy is Al-free.

Aluminum toxicity has also been linked with oral exposure as a result of Al-containing pharmaceutical products such as Al-based phosphate binders or antacid intake.[138] As over-the-counter antacids are an important source for human Al exposure from a quantitative point of view, patient information leaflets in Europe contain warnings of possible Al toxicity.[138]

Interest in the role of Al in Alzheimer's disease (AD) was raised when Perl observed that Al accumulates in the neurofibrillary tangle of patients with AD.[129] He concluded that the focal accumulation of Al had an association with neurofibrillary degeneration in the hippocampal neurons that might play a role in the development of AD. Although a cause-and-effect relationship between accumulation of Al in brain and AD has yet to be conclusively demonstrated,[142] studies have clearly shown an increased concentration of Al in the brain.[30,85,151] It is possible that accumulation of Al in the neurofibrillary tangle of AD patients is a secondary finding associated with the disease but not directly related to the cause. Glycosylation of beta amyloid likely plays a role in AD and may provide for structural alteration of protein that increases Al binding.[61,85] A 2002 review discusses the role of Al as a risk factor for developing Alzheimer's disease.[162]

Aluminum-related bone disease can be diagnosed and treated with deferoxamine, an avid chelator of both iron and Al. The deferoxamine infusion test is useful for the ultimate diagnosis of Al overload disease, and the drug has demonstrated utility for treating acute Al overload.[50,57,114]

Collection of specimens for serum Al analysis can be a complicating factor. Most of the common evacuated blood collection devices used in phlebotomy today have rubber stoppers that are made of Al silicate. Puncture of the rubber stopper for blood collection is sufficient to contaminate the sample with Al to produce an abnormal concentration of Al. Typically, blood collected in standard evacuated blood tubes will be contaminated by 20 to 60 µg/L of Al; this can be readily demonstrated by collecting blood from a normal volunteer into a standard evacuated phlebotomy tube. Special evacuated blood collection tubes are required for Al testing.[116] These tubes are readily available from commercial suppliers and should always be used. Failure to pay attention to this issue can result in the generation of abnormal results because of sample contamination, which can lead to misinterpretation and misdiagnosis.

Analysis of Al can be routinely performed by inductively coupled plasma (ICP) mass spectrometry (ICP-MS). Alternatively, atomic absorption spectrometry with electrothermal atomization may be employed, but considerable attention must be paid to matrix interferences.

Antimony

Antimony (Sb) compounds have been known since ancient Egyptian times and were used as cosmetics by the women of that era. In the sixteenth century, Sb preparations were thought to be wonder drugs and in the nineteenth century were prescribed for a number of conditions. Antimony compounds are used today as the standard treatment against parasitic diseases, such as leishmaniasis, schistosomiasis, and bilharziasis.[32]

Pure metallic Sb is not used in industry because it is very brittle; however, alloys of Sb are used in a number of fields of technology. For example, addition of Sb to lead, tin, and copper increases the hardness of these metals when used as electrodes, bullets, type metal for printing, and ball bearings. Other uses include fire-resistant chemicals, pigments, and dyes.

Antimony is not an essential metal. Workplace exposure to Sb dust over a period of years leads to pneumoconiosis. The size of the dust particles of Sb trioxide significantly increases the occurrence of pneumoconiosis, with the smaller particles being more dangerous. The workers at greatest danger are those in underground facilities and metal production. Smoking may also contribute to the respiratory problems.[10] Symptoms of acute exposure include a metallic taste, headache, nausea, and dizziness; after a short interval, vomiting, diarrhea, and intestinal spasms occur. The severity of the symptoms depends on both the dose and route of administration. In chronic intoxication, adverse health effects include cardiac arrhythmias, upper respiratory and ocular irritation, spontaneous abortions, premature births, and dermatitis.[51] Lymphocytosis, eosinophilia, and a reduction in leukocyte and platelet counts are also seen and indicate damage to the liver and spleen. The inability of the blood to clot is seen when a lethal dose of Sb is received. Breathing is shallow and irregular, and death is almost always due to respiratory paralysis.[9] There is evidence supporting an increased risk for the development of lung cancer in Sb smelter workers, but the effect may be multifactorial due, for example, to the presence of arsenic in the work environment.[10,44] It is important to remember that when intoxication occurs with metallic Sb, the effect is due not just to the

Sb, but also the lead, arsenic, and other metals that may accompany it.[9]

ARSENIC

Arsenic (As) is perhaps the best known of the metal toxins, having gained notoriety from its extensive use by Renaissance nobility as an antisyphilitic agent and an antidote against acute arsenic poisoning, as chronic administration of low doses protects against acute poisoning by massive doses.[130] This agent was memorably used in the well-known tale "Arsenic and Old Lace"[92] as a means of terminating undesirable acquaintances. Even today, As is still a dangerous toxicant as evidenced by the Bangladesh incidence where several hundred persons had been poisoned by drinking ground water contaminated with As leaching from bedrock.* In fact, as mentioned earlier, arsenic is listed as the No. 1 toxicant on the U.S. CERCLA Priority List of Hazardous Substances (http://www.atsdr.cdc.gov/cxcx3.html). It is also still found in some insecticides.

Arsenic exists in a number of toxic and nontoxic forms.[165] The toxic forms are the inorganic species As^{3+}, also denoted as As(III), the more toxic As^{5+}, also known as As(V), and their partially detoxified metabolites, monomethylarsine (MMA) and dimethylarsine (DMA). Detoxification occurs in the liver as As^{5+} is reduced to As^{3+} and then methylated to MMA and DMA.[186] As a result of these detoxification steps, As^{3+} and As^{5+} are found in the urine shortly after ingestion, whereas MMA and DMA are the species that predominate more than 24 hours after ingestion. Urinary As^{3+} and As^{5+} concentrations peak at approximately 10 hours and return to normal 20 to 30 hours after ingestion. Urinary MMA and DMA concentrations normally peak at about 40 to 60 hours and return to baseline 6 to 20 days after ingestion.[117] The half-life of inorganic As in blood is 4 to 6 hours with a half-life of the methylated metabolites of 20 to 30 hours. Serum concentrations of As are elevated for only a short time after administration, after which As rapidly disappears into the large body phosphate pool. Abnormal serum As concentrations are detected for only a few hours (<4 hours) after ingestion. The structures of these and related As species are shown in Figure 35-3.

Nontoxic forms of As are present in many foods. Arsenobetaine and arsenocholine are the two most common forms of organic As that are found in food.[99] The foods that most commonly contain significant concentrations of organic As are shellfish and other predators in the seafood chain (e.g., cod and haddock). Consequently the rate of As excretion in normal people is 0 to 120 µg per 24-hour specimen. Following ingestion, arsenobetaine and arsenocholine undergo rapid renal clearance to become concentrated in the urine. Organic As is completely excreted within 1 to 2 days after ingestion, and there are no residual toxic metabolites. The apparent half-life of organic As is 4 to 6 hours. Consumption of seafood before collection of a urine sample for As testing is likely to result in an elevation of the concentration of As reported to be found in the urine; this can be clinically misleading.

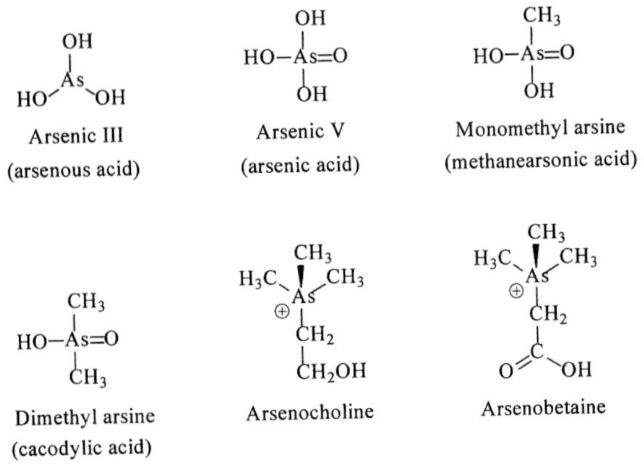

*References 1, 15, 86, 89, 93, 154, 166, 173.

Arsenic III (arsenous acid) — Arsenic V (arsenic acid) — Monomethyl arsine (methanearsonic acid)

Dimethyl arsine (cacodylic acid) — Arsenocholine — Arsenobetaine

Figure 35-3 Structures of arsenic species.

The toxicity of As is due to three different mechanisms, two of which are related to energy transfer. Arsenic avidly binds to dihydrolipoic acid, a necessary cofactor for pyruvate dehydrogenase. Absence of the cofactor inhibits the conversion of pyruvate to acetyl coenzyme A, the first step in gluconeogenesis. Arsenic also competes with phosphate for reaction with ADP, resulting in formation of the lower energy ADPAs rather than ATP. Arsenic also binds with any hydrated sulfhydryl group on protein, distorting the three-dimensional configuration of the protein and thus causing it to lose activity. Arsenic is also a known carcinogen, but the mechanism of this effect is not definitively known.[37] British antilewisite (BAL) is an effective antidote for treating As intoxication; the active agent in BAL is dimercaprol, a sulfhydryl-reducing agent. This suggests that the primary mechanism of action of As's toxicity is related to sulfhydryl binding. Arsenic also interferes with the activity of several enzymes of the heme biosynthetic pathway.[68] There is also evidence of an increased risk of bladder, skin, and lung cancers following consumption of water with high As contamination[18,145] and lung cancer from smoking. In addition, a causal association has been established between exposure to environmental tobacco smoke and lung cancer, with a relative risk in the order of 1.2.[18,120]

To distinguish among toxic inorganic species and nontoxic organic species of As of seafood origin, high-performance liquid chromatographic (HPLC) techniques that separate the various species of As in biological fluids and tissues have been developed.[158] A relatively simple method of separation using liquid-liquid extraction has also been reported.[7] A typical finding in a urine specimen with total 24-hour excretion of As of 350 µg/24 hours is that greater than 95% is present as the organic, nontoxic seafood species and that less than 5% is present as the inorganic, toxic species. Such a finding indicates that the elevated total As concentration was likely due to ingestion of seafood.

Hair analysis is frequently used to document time of As exposure.[83] Arsenic circulating in the blood will bind to protein by formation of a covalent complex with sulfhydryl groups of the amino acid cysteine. Because As has a high affinity for keratin, which has high cysteine content, the As concentration in hair or nails is higher than in other tissue. Several weeks after exposure, transverse white striae, called "Mees' lines," may appear in the fingernails; this is caused by denaturation of keratin by metals such as As, cadmium, lead, and mercury. Because hair grows at a rate of approximately 0.5 cm/mo, hair collected from the nape of the neck can be used to document recent exposure. Axillary or pubic hair is used to document long-term (6 months to 1 year) exposure. Hair As >1 µg/g dry weight indicates excessive exposure. In one study, the highest hair As observed was 210 µg/g dry weight in a case of chronic exposure that was the cause of death.[83]

Serum is the least useful specimen for identifying As exposure. Serum concentrations of As are elevated for only a short time after administration, after which As is bound to protein[187] and rapidly disappears into the large body phosphate pool, as the body treats As like phosphate, incorporating it wherever phosphate would be incorporated. Absorbed As is rapidly circulated and distributed into tissue storage sites. Abnormal serum As concentrations are detected for only a few hours (<4 hours) after ingestion. This test is useful only to document an acute exposure when the As is likely to be >100 ng/mL for a short period of time. Normally, serum As is <35 ng/mL.

Arsenic also has been accurately analyzed by ICP/MS.[26,124] The specimen is prepared in dilute acid containing gallium as an internal standard and aspirated directly into the argon plasma. Mass response from the argon plasma is monitored for As (75 m/z), gallium (70 m/z), and $^{16}O^{35}Cl$ (51 m/z) to allow for correction for $^{40}Ar^{35}Cl$ (75 m/z) interference. The operator must be aware of the potential for interference from argon chloride. A correction is made by accounting for chloride by measuring 51 m/z and subtracting that residual from 75 m/z.[124] Urine is the sample of choice for As analysis because As is excreted predominantly by the kidney where it becomes concentrated. An ICP-MS method for quantifying As in urine is included in the appendix for this chapter, which is found on the book's accompanying Evolve site (http://evolve.elsevier.com/Tietz/textbook/). Atomic absorption methods are also available.[7]

Beryllium

Beryllium (Be) is an alkaline earth metal found in the earth's crust at an approximate concentration of 3 to 5 mg/kg; it is poisonous and not necessary for human health. Beryllium alloys are lightweight, stiff, and highly electrically conductive. Beryllium as pure metal, Be alloys, and ceramics are used in a wide range of applications, including dental appliances, golf clubs, nonsparking tools, wheelchairs, satellite and spacecraft manufacture, circuit board production, and nuclear power, and in weapons as a neutron modulator.

The general population is exposed to Be through food and drinking water although the concentrations are low and of no clinical consequence. The major route by which Be enters the body is via the respiratory tract, and industrial exposure usually occurs from inhalation and ingestion of Be dust. Inhaled Be compounds are cleared very slowly from the lungs. Soluble compounds are absorbed to a much greater degree than those such as Be oxide, which are much less soluble. Beryllium salts are strongly acidic when dissolved in water and this is thought to be a major toxic effect on human tissue. Absorbed Be accumulate in the skeleton. Renal clearance is very slow. Beryllium can inhibit a variety of enzyme systems including alkaline phosphatase, acid phosphatase, phosphoglycerate mutase, hexokinase, and lactate dehydrogenase.[144]

Acute exposure is rare, usually caused by an industrial accident or explosion, and typically results in chemical pneumonitis. Chronic Be exposure in the workplace has led to occupational health concerns because of its potential to cause a progressive and potentially fatal respiratory condition called chronic Be disease (CBD) characterized by the formation of granulomas resulting from an immune reaction to Be particles in the lung.[49] Studies have suggested that the size of the Be particles affects not only the site of deposition but also the amount deposited. This in turn may influence the clearance rate and thus the time of contact between the immune cells and Be.[97] Several years ago, researchers noted that blood and lung cells from CBD patients proliferated when exposed to Be in culture. This assay has been refined and is offered as the Be lymphocyte proliferation test (BeLPT). Unfortunately, because of the nature of the test and the variability from lab to lab, the BeLPT can produce false-negative and problematic results.[49,108] Efforts have begun by several groups to standardize the assay. Despite these issues, the BeLPT in bronchoalveolar cells is part of the current "gold standard" diagnosis for CBD.[144] The clinical course of chronic Be disease is variable and the prognosis is unpredictable. Studies suggest, but do not conclusively link, Be exposure and lung cancer in humans.[73]

Cadmium

Cadmium (Cd) is a byproduct of zinc and lead smelting. It is used in industry in electroplating, in the production of nickel-based rechargeable batteries, as a common pigment in organic-based paints, and in tobacco products. Breathing the fumes of Cd vapors leads to nasal epithelial deterioration and pulmonary congestion resembling chronic emphysema.[81] A common source of chronic exposure is spray painting of organic-based paints without the use of a protective breathing apparatus. Auto repair mechanics represent a work group that has significant opportunity for exposure to Cd.

The toxicity of Cd resembles the other metals (arsenic, mercury, and lead) in that it attacks the kidney; renal dysfunction with proteinuria of slow onset (over a period of years) is the typical presentation.[63,150] Chronic exposure to Cd causes accumulated renal damage.[150] Breathing the fumes of Cd vapors leads to nasal epithelial deterioration and pulmonary congestion resembling chronic emphysema. Cadmium toxicity is expressed via formation of protein-Cd adducts that change the conformational structure of the protein, causing it to denature. This protein denaturation occurs at the site of highest concentration—in the alveoli if exposure is due to dust inhalation and in the proximal tubule of the kidney, because this is a major route of excretion.

In 1992 the NIOSH mandated that employees exposed to Cd in the workplace be monitored using the quantification of urine Cd and creatinine, expressing the results of μg of Cd per gram of creatinine.[127] This is based on the finding that renal damage caused by Cd exposure can be detected by increased Cd excretion relative to creatinine. Cadmium excretion >3 μg Cd/g of creatinine indicates significant exposure to Cd. Results >15 μg Cd/g of creatinine are considered indicative of severe exposure. Urine Cd is a more specific measure of Cd exposure than are other markers of renal function, such as β_2-microglobulin, retinol-binding protein, or *N*-acetyl glucosaminidase.[174]

Normal blood Cd concentration is less than 5 ng/mL, with most concentrations being in the interval of 0.5 to 2 ng/mL. Moderately increased blood Cd (3 to 7 ng/mL) may be associated with tobacco use.[80] Acute toxicity is observed when the blood concentration exceeds 50 ng/mL. Usual daily excretion of Cd is less than 3 μg/day. Collection of urine samples using a rubber catheter can result in elevated results, because rubber contains trace amounts of Cd that are extracted as urine passes through it. Brightly colored plastic urine collection containers should be avoided because the pigment in the plastic may be Cd-based. Cadmium concentrations also increase with age and may be involved with senescence.[16] Cadmium is usually quantified by atomic absorption spectrometry, but it can also be accurately quantified by ICP-MS.[124]

CHROMIUM

Occupational exposure to chromium (Cr) represents a significant health hazard.[5,126] Chromium is used extensively in the manufacture of stainless steel, in chrome plating, in the tanning of leather, as a dye for printing and textile manufacture, as a cleaning solution, and as an anticorrosive in cooling systems. The toxic form of Cr is Cr^{6+} (Cr[VI]), which is quite rare; a strong oxidizing environment is required to convert the common form Cr^{3+} (Cr[III]) to Cr^{6+}, as might be found when Cr^{3+} is exposed to high temperatures in the presence of oxygen or during high-voltage electroplating. Inhalation of the vapors of Cr^{6+} causes erosion of the epithelium of the nasal passages and produces squamous-cell carcinomas of the lung.[40,126] Cr^{6+} is very lipid soluble and readily crosses cell membranes, whereas Cr^{3+} is rather insoluble and does not readily cross membranes. Clinically, monitoring biological specimens for Cr^{6+} is neither practical nor clinically useful to detect Cr toxicity, as the instant it enters a cell, it is reduced to nontoxic Cr^{3+}.[169] Instead, monitoring the air at the manufacturing site for Cr^{6+} is the usual way to test for Cr^{6+} exposure. Quantification of total Cr in urine can be used to assess exposure to total Cr but does not indicate that the specific exposure was to Cr^{6+}. Atomic absorption spectrometry is commonly used to measure Cr concentrations in body fluids.[152]

Chromium has also been known as the "glucose tolerance factor." Chromium is required for insulin activity.[115] Work from the 1970s suggested Cr deficiency as a cause of diabetes, but this theory has been refuted as an artifact of specimen collection anomalies.[24] A 1994 study demonstrated that Cr concentrations in normoglycemic subjects are essentially the same as those in hypoglycemic subjects.[95] Existing technology cannot measure Cr deficiency, because the lower limit of the reference interval of Cr in blood challenges the detection limit (0.2 ng/mL) of atomic absorption techniques.

COBALT

Cobalt (Co) is rare but widely distributed in the environment. Cobalt is an essential element, although Co deficiency has not been reported in humans. Cobalt is the essential cofactor in vitamin B_{12}. Quantification of active vitamin B_{12} (see Chapter 30) is the usual way to assess nutritional status; quantification of serum, blood, or urine Co concentration is not the typical means of assessing vitamin B_{12} status.

Cobalt is found in metal alloys that (1) are very hard, (2) have high melting points, and (3) are resistant to oxidation.[47,102] Occupational exposure occurs during production and machining of these metal alloys and can lead to interstitial lung disease.[121] Cardiomyopathy and renal failure are symptomatic of acute Co exposure; this was exemplified by an incidence of mass population exposure to Co when beer contaminated with the metal was consumed.[163] Quantification of urinary Co is an effective means of identifying individuals with excessive exposure.

Cobalt is not highly toxic, but large enough doses will produce pulmonary edema, allergy, nausea, vomiting, hemorrhage, and renal failure. Chronic symptoms include pulmonary syndrome, skin irritation, allergy, gastrointestinal irritations, nausea, cardiomyopathy, hematological disorders, and thyroid abnormalities.[100] The inhalation of dust during machining of Co alloyed metals can lead to interstitial lung disease.[121] Improperly handled, ^{60}Co can cause radiation poisoning from exposure to gamma radiation. Cobalt exposure alone may not lead to toxicity and must be considered within the context of exposure to multiple metals.[102]

Cobalt is quantified in biological tissues by atomic absorption spectrometry[157] and by ICP-MS.[26]

COPPER

The homeostasis and analysis of copper (Cu) are discussed in Chapter 30. Copper ingestion has been found to lead to serious toxicity,[66,79] and it may be encountered as a pesticide. Also, Cu is one of the active agents in marine antifouling paints and as a wood preservative is used with green "treated" wood containing high concentrations of Cu and As. Ingestion of either of these sources produces severe gastrointestinal upset with severe irritation of the epithelial layer of the gastrointestinal tract, hemolytic anemia, centrilobular hepatitis with jaundice, and renal damage. Excess Cu ingestion interferes with absorption of zinc[148] and can lead to zinc deficiency, which is frequently characterized by slow healing. The classical presentation of Cu toxicosis is represented by the genetic disease of Cu accumulation known as Wilson's disease.[105] This disease is typified by hepatocellular damage (increased transferases) and/or changes in mood and behavior because of accumulation of Cu in central neurons. The genetic basis for this disease has been identified.[78A]

IRON

The homeostasis and analysis of iron (Fe) are reviewed in Chapters 30. Iron supplements are used frequently to maintain an adequate body burden of Fe. Occasionally, ingestion exceeds the needed daily requirement, resulting in Fe toxicity.[23,43] Acute ingestion of more than 0.5 g of Fe can produce severe irritation of the epithelial lining of the gastrointestinal tract and result in hemosiderosis, which may develop into hepatic cirrhosis. The presence of excessive amounts of Fe in serum *and* urine defines this diagnosis. Although yet to be proven, chronic iron overload is thought to be linked to cancer[87] and atherosclerosis.[184]

LEAD

Lead (Pb) is a metal commonly found in the environment. It can be an acute and chronic toxin.[103] Lead is present at high concentration (up to 35% w/w) in many paints manufactured before 1970. The Pb content of paints intended for household use was limited to <0.5% in 1972, but Pb is still found in paint products intended for nondomestic use and in artists' pigments. Ceramic products for use in homes, such as dishes or bowls, available from noncommercial suppliers (such as local artists) can contain significant amounts of Pb, which can be leached from the ceramic by weak acids, such as vinegar and fruit juices. Leaded crystal contains up to 10% Pb, which can be leached during long-term storage of acidic fluids, such as fruit juice. Lead is also found in dirt from areas adjacent to homes painted with Pb-based paints and on highways where it has accumulated from the use of leaded gasoline in automobiles. Use of leaded gasoline has diminished significantly since the introduction of unleaded gasoline, which has been required in personal automobiles in the United States since 1978. Lead is also found in soil near abandoned industrial sites where Pb may have been used. Water transported through Pb or Pb-soldered pipe contains some Pb, with higher concentrations found in water that is weakly acidic. Some foods (e.g., moonshine distilled in Pb pipes) and some traditional home medicines also contain Pb.[34] Exposure to Pb from any of these sources by ingestion, inhalation, or dermal contact can cause significant toxicity.

A typical diet in the United States contributes approximately 300 μg of Pb per day, of which 1% to 10% is absorbed; children may absorb as much as 50% of the dietary intake. The fraction of Pb absorbed is enhanced by nutritional deficiency. The majority of the daily intake is excreted in the stool after direct passage through the gastrointestinal tract. Although a significant fraction of the absorbed Pb is rapidly incorporated into bone and erythrocytes, Pb is ultimately distributed among all tissues. Lipid-dense tissues, such as the central nervous system, are particularly sensitive to organic forms of Pb. All Pb absorbed is ultimately excreted in bile or urine. Soft-tissue turnover of Pb occurs within approximately 120 days.[17]

Lead expresses its toxicity by several mechanisms that are described graphically in Figure 35-4. It avidly inhibits amino levulinic acid dehydratase (ALAD), one of the enzymes that catalyze synthesis of heme from porphyrin. Inhibition of ALAD causes accumulation of protoporphyrin in erythrocytes (see Chapter 32), which is a significant marker for Pb exposure. Anemia caused by the lack of heme is frequently observed in Pb toxicity. Lead also is an electrophile that avidly forms covalent bonds with the sulfhydryl group of cysteine in proteins. Thus proteins in all tissue exposed to Pb will have Pb bound to them. Keratin in hair contains a high fraction of cysteine relative to other amino acids and avidly binds Pb; hair analysis for Pb is a good marker for exposure. Some proteins become labile as Pb binds with them because Pb causes the tertiary structure of the protein to change; cells of the nervous system are particularly susceptible to this effect. Some Pb-bound proteins change their tertiary configuration sufficiently so that they become antigenic; renal tubular cells are particularly susceptible to this effect because they are exposed to relatively high Pb concentrations during clearance.

The development of Pb toxicity follows a progressive pattern. Figure 35-5 describes this progression through a series of symptoms.[146] The finding that Pb contributes significantly to decreased intellectual capability in the very

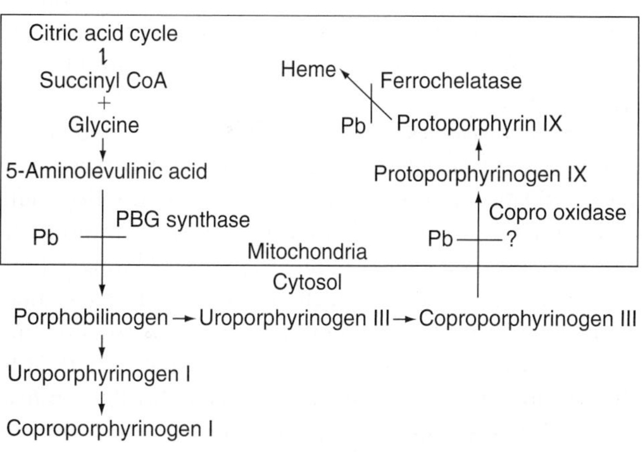

Figure 35-4 Erythropoietic effects of lead.

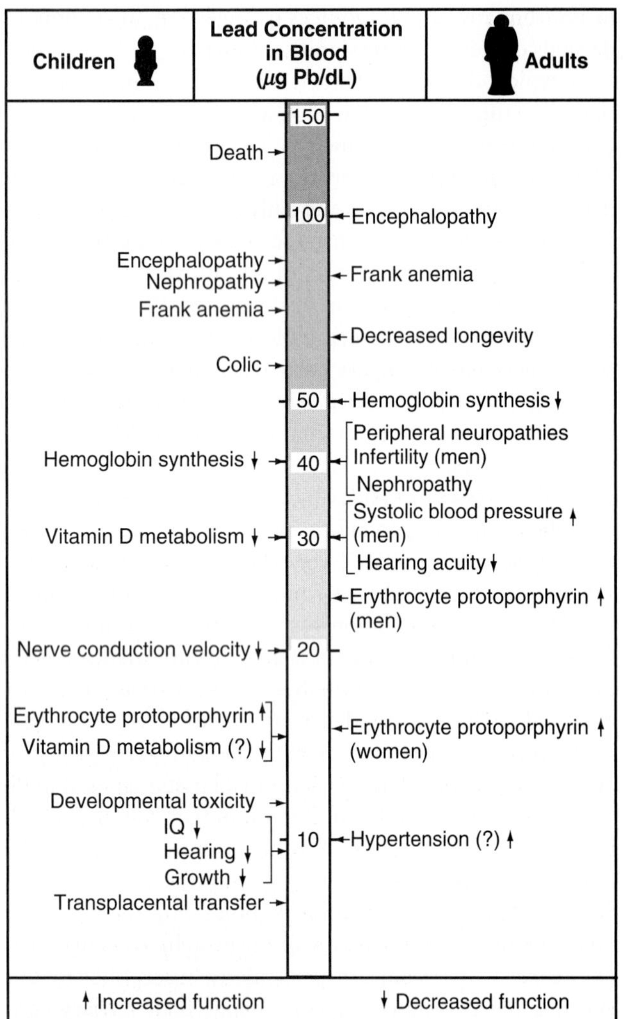

Figure 35-5 Effects of inorganic lead on children and adults (lowest observable adverse effect concentrations). *(From Royce SE, Needleman HL, Eds. Case studies in environmental medicine: Lead toxicity. Washington DC: US Public Health Service, ATSDR, 1990.)*

young is of particular concern.[132] Young children are particularly prone to the effects of Pb because they have greater opportunity for exposure.[8] Children tend to spend a lot of time on the floor. In older homes that have been previously treated with Pb-based paints, Pb-laden paint chips and dust accumulate on the floor, which children are likely to ingest.

The definitive test for Pb toxicity is measurement of blood Pb.[143] Over the past 3 decades, studies have shown an inverse relationship between blood Pb concentrations and children's IQ at increasingly lower Pb concentrations. In response, the CDC has continued to lower the upper limit of normal for children, which is now stated at less than 10 μg/dL. It is also important to note that the median blood Pb concentration is children fell from 15 μg/dL in 1978 to 2 μg/dL in 1999 because of measures such as the removal of Pb from gasoline.[140] Consequently, renewed interest in determining safe blood Pb concentrations resulted in additional studies.[139] These studies assessed the intellectual impairment in children with Pb concentration below 10 μg/dL. Preliminary data have indicated that there is an inverse relationship between Pb concentrations and children's IQ even at blood Pb concentrations below 10 μg/dL.[31] If additional studies show similar findings, it may be appropriate to review the current reference interval for blood Pb concentrations in children.

The WHO has defined whole blood Pb concentrations greater than 30 μg/dL in adults as indicative of significant exposure. Lead concentrations greater than 60 μg/dL require chelation therapy. Similar to the situation seen in children, adult blood Pb concentrations have dropped to a mean value of 1.4 μg/dL for ages 20 to 49 and a mean value of 1.9 μg/dL for ages 50 to 69.[125] Given the decreasing blood Pb concentrations in adults, it may be important to revisit the recommendations regarding Pb exposure. Studies have shown a number of adverse health effects in adults exposed to Pb at concentrations below existing regulatory exposure limits. These include hypertension, adverse reproductive outcomes, and subtle central nervous system problems.[21,153,168] In 2000 the CDC recommended that, as a preventive health measure, blood Pb concentrations in exposed workers be reduced to <25 μg/dL by the year 2010.[171]

Erythrocyte protoporphyrin concentrations are not a sensitive indicator of low-concentration Pb exposure[101] but are definitive markers for Pb overdose; an erythrocyte protoporphyrin concentration greater than 60 μg/dL is a significant indicator of Pb exposure (see Chapter 32). Serum ALAD concentrations are also a useful indicator for medium to high concentrations of Pb exposure; however, they do not correlate with low concentrations of Pb exposure.[35] Serum Pb analysis is of very limited utility, because Pb concentrations are abnormal only for a short period of time after exposure.[35] Normally the hair Pb content is lower than 5 ug/g; hair Pb concentration greater than 25 μg/g indicates severe Pb exposure. Quantification of urine excretion rates either before[11] or after chelation therapy[180] has been used as an indicator of Pb exposure. However, blood Pb levels have the strongest correlation with toxicity.

Avoidance of continued exposure to Pb is paramount when blood Pb concentrations exceed acceptable limits. Severe Pb toxicity may require chelation therapy using BAL, administered intravenously. Oral dimercaprol has become a standard therapy and is being used in the outpatient setting for all except those with the most severe Pb poisoning.[74] Although chelation therapy is effective in reducing blood Pb concentrations, a 2003 study indicated that chelation therapy given to preschool children with Pb concentrations in the range of 20 to 44 μg/dL showed no beneficial effect on tests of cognition or behavior.[140] Likewise, there are no placebo-controlled, randomized studies that demonstrate a positive impact on therapeutic outcome from chelation therapy in adults, only improvement in symptoms and decreased mortality.[98] Therefore, prevention may be the only real solution.

Analysis of Pb is routinely performed by either ICP-MS[26,124] or electrothermal atomic absorption spectrometry. EDTA anticoagulated blood is the specimen of choice for Pb analysis, because Pb is concentrated in the erythrocytes. Sodium heparin may also be used; however, samples that are not analyzed within 48 hours are frequently clotted and must be rejected. Care must be taken when obtaining capillary blood. Surface contamination, insufficient collection volume, and inadequate mixing with EDTA result in frequent sample rejection. Urinalysis can also be performed; urine quantification correlates with exposure.

If ICP-MS is used to measure Pb levels,[26,124] care must be taken to sum the masses of 206, 207, and 208 m/z to account for the natural isotopic variation of Pb in the environment. Failure to sum masses can skew results above or below the actual concentration, as the isotopic abundance of a particular mass in the calibrator might not match the sample. However, this isotopic variation can be exploited to determine the source of Pb exposure. By determining the relative abundances of Pb in blood and also of potential sources of exposure (e.g., paint chips and soil), a matching pattern can be identified. The exposure source with the same ratio of major Pb isotopes as the blood should then be avoided or removed from the patient's environment.

An ICP-MS method for quantifying Pb in whole blood is included in the appendix for this chapter that is found on the book's accompanying Evolve site (http://evolve.elsevier.com/Tietz/textbook/).

MANGANESE

Manganese (Mn) is ubiquitous in the environment. Specifically, manganese is (1) a binding agent in red brick, (2) present in most steel alloys as an anticorrosive, (3) used extensively in laboratories as a cleaning agent for glassware, and (4) a common pigment in paints and glazes. Humans exhibit toxicity to Mn when exposed to large quantities of dust containing the metal, which can occur in mining, ore crushing, the machining of Mn alloys, and the construction and destruction of brick. After chronic exposure, Mn accumulates in the substantia nigra of the brain, causing a Parkinson-like neurodegenerative disorder known as manganism.[28,52,112] Manganese toxicity has also been observed in children receiving long-term parenteral nutrition.[62]

Blood or urine Mn concentrations are good indicators of exposure.[104] Adult reference values for blood Mn are 0.4 to 1.1 ng/mL (7.0 to 20.0 nmol/L) for serum or plasma and 7.7 to 12.1 ng/mL (140 to 220 nmol/L) for whole blood. Typical daily excretion of Mn in urine is from 0.2 to 0.5 µg/day. However, approximately 5% of normal people excrete up to 2 µg of the metal per day, probably because of greater than average exposure.

Most of the Mn in daily diets is not absorbed. Because Mn-containing dust is common, contamination of urine with the metal can easily occur. Trace contamination of acid preservatives used for stabilizing the urine has also been observed. Manganese is quantified by electrothermal atomization atomic absorption spectrometry[122] or by ICP-MS.[26]

MERCURY

Annually, the atmosphere and surface of the earth are exposed to approximately 36,000 tons of mercury (Hg), a product of the natural outgassing of rock (30,000 tons/yr), from industry used in electrolysis, in electrical switches, and as a fungicide (6000 tons/yr); and incorporated into dental amalgams (90 tons/yr).[161]

There is considerable opportunity for Hg exposure in our environment. Mercury is used as a conductor in many electrical switches; most home thermostats contain elemental Hg in a glass bulb to serve as a temperature switch. Mercury is used extensively in the pulp and paper industry as a whitener; the effluents from paper plants are a known source of Hg. Mercury is commonly used in industry as a catalyst in the synthesis of plastics and is frequently found in antifouling and latex paints because it is a potent fungicide. Mercury is approximately 50% of the mass of dental amalgams.[137] The single largest source of Hg in the environment is natural outgassing from granite rock; this source accounts for approximately 80% of all Hg accumulation in the environment.

Mercury is essentially nontoxic in its elemental form (Hg^0). In the absence of any chemical or biological system that chemically alters Hg^0, it can be consumed orally without any significant side effects. However, once Hg^0 is chemically modified to the ionized, inorganic species, Hg^{2+}, it becomes toxic. Further bioconversion to an alkyl Hg, such as methyl Hg (CH_3Hg^+), yields a very toxic species of Hg that is highly selective for lipid-rich tissue, such as the neuron.[42] The relative order of toxicity is as follows:

$$Hg^0(\text{Nontoxic}) < Hg^{2+} \ll CH_3Hg^+(\text{Very toxic})$$

Mercury can be chemically converted from the elemental state to the ionized state; in industry, this is frequently accomplished by exposing Hg^0 to a strong oxidant, such as chlorine. Elemental Hg can also be bioconverted to both Hg^{2+} and alkyl Hg by microorganisms that exist both in the normal human gut and in the bottom sediment of lakes and rivers. When Hg^0 enters bottom sediment, it is absorbed by bacteria, fungi, and related microorganisms; these organisms metabolically convert it to Hg^{2+}, CH_3Hg^+, $(CH_3)_2Hg$, and similar species. Consequently the methyl mercurials are accumulated in the aquatic food chain and reach their highest levels in predatory fish.[33,39]

As a consequence of methylmercury accumulating in the aquatic food chain, most human exposure to mercury happens through the eating of contaminated fish, shellfish, and sea mammals.[33,167] In adults, cases of methylmercury poisoning are characterized by the focal degeneration of neurons in regions of the brain such as the cerebral cortex and cerebellum. Depending on the degree of in utero exposure, methylmercury may result in effects ranging from fetal death to subtle neurodevelopmental delays. Consequently, because pregnant women, women of childbearing age, and young children are particularly at risk, the U.S. Food and Drug Administration recommends that they avoid eating shark, swordfish, mackerel, and tilefish.[60] However, no definitive consensus has been reached to date on the safety level of maternal exposure during pregnancy.

Mercury toxicity is expressed in three ways. First, Hg^{2+} avidly reacts with sulfhydryl groups of protein, causing a change in the tertiary structure of the protein with subsequent loss of the biological activity associated with that protein; because Hg^{2+} becomes concentrated in the kidney during the regular clearance processes, this is the target organ that experiences the greatest toxicity. Secondly, with the tertiary change noted previously, some proteins become immunogenic, eliciting a proliferation of B-lymphocytes that generate immunoglobulins to bind the new antigen (collagen tissue are particularly sensitive to this). Thirdly, alkyl Hg species, such as methylmercury, are particularly lipophilic and avidly bind to proteins in lipid-rich tissue, such as neurons; myelin is particularly susceptible to disruption by this mechanism.[38,185] Mercury has also been found to alter porphyrin excretion patterns.[181]

Experience with Hg poisoning has been gained from investigation of the 1951 to 1963 industrial dumping of Hg-laden waste sludge into Minamata Bay, Japan. Fish in Minamata Bay became heavily laden with Hg through the food chain. The local human population whose diet was dependent on fish from the bay exhibited symptoms of methylmerecury poisoning, which include ataxia, impaired speech, visual field constriction, hearing loss, and somatosensory change, characterized histologically by cerebral cortex necrosis.[170] Collectively, these symptoms have become known as Minamata disease.[59]

In the late 1980s, the public became concerned about exposure to Hg from dental amalgams.[76,137] However, later studies have failed to confirm a causal relationship.[6,78,172] Basic to the initial concerns was the fact that restorative dentistry used a Hg-silver amalgam for approximately 90 years as a filling material. In 1989 Hahn showed that there is a small (2 to 20 μg/day) release of Hg^0 from amalgam when it is mechanically manipulated, such as by chewing.[76] The normal bacterial flora present in the mouth convert a fraction of Hg^{2+} to CH_3Hg^+; the latter has been shown to be incorporated into body tissue. In addition, the habit of gum chewing can cause release of Hg from dental amalgams at concentrations greatly above normal. Hanson noted in 1991 the release of up to 100 μg/day of Hg in several human subjects who had the typical placement of dental amalgams (weighing approximately 800 mg each) after chewing gum for 8 hours.[77]

Concerns have also been raised about the possible relationship between Hg exposure from vaccines and autistic disorders. In the United States, the prevalence of autism has risen from 1 in approximately 2500 in the mid 1980s to 1 in approximately 300 children in the mid1990s.[70] Several investigators believe that this rise is because of the Hg that is present in vaccines as the preservative thimerosal (sodium ethyl mercury thiosulfate).[12-14,46,70,71] However, this causality has been questioned by numerous other studies who have not been able to confirm this relationship.* In 2001 the Committee on Immunization Safety Review of the Board on Health Promotion and Disease Prevention of the Institute of Medicine (IOM) initiated a study to review the connection between Hg-containing vaccines and neurodevelopmental disorders, including autism. The committee has issued several reports and in their eighth and final one in 2004, they reported that the hypothesis was biologically plausible, but that there was insufficient evidence to accept or reject a causal connection and recommended a comprehensive research program.[88] The findings of this report have been challenged,[14] and it has even been recommended that thimerosal be removed from all vaccines in the United States.[71] Some Scandinavian countries have already removed it from their vaccines.[94,160]

Dietary sources can also contribute to Hg body burden, as many foods contain Hg. For example, commercially distributed fish considered safe for consumption contain less than 0.3 μg/g, but some game fish contain more than 2 μg/g and if consumed on a regular basis, contribute to significant body Hg loads.

Analysis of blood, urine, and hair for Hg levels is used to determine exposure. The quantity of Hg found in blood and urine correlates with degree of toxicity, and hair analysis is used historically to document the time of peak exposure. However, it should be noted that hair analysis for metals in general is difficult because of contamination. Normal whole blood Hg concentration is usually lower than 10 μg/L. Figure 35-6 shows a distribution of blood concentrations seen in a large population composed of unaffected, healthy individuals.[124] Individuals who have mild occupational exposure (e.g., dentists) may routinely have whole blood Hg concentrations of up to 15 μg/L.[56] Significant exposure is indicated when the whole blood Hg concentration is greater than 50 μg/L (if exposure is to methylmercury) or greater than 200 μg/L (if exposure is to Hg^{2+}). The WHO safety standard for daily exposure of Hg is 45 μg per day, with a daily urine excretion exceeding 50 μg/day indicating significant exposure. Normally, hair contains less than 1 μg/g of Hg; greater amounts indicate increased exposure. Treatment with BAL or penicillamine will mobilize Hg, allowing for its excretion in the urine. Therapy is usually monitored by following urinary excretion of Hg; therapy may be terminated after the daily urine excretion rate falls below 50 μg/L.

An ICP-MS method for quantifying Hg in biological specimens is included in the appendix for this chapter that is found on this book's accompanying Evolve site http://evolve.elsevier.com/Tietz/textbook/).

*References 20, 71, 82, 94, 107, 119, 160, 176.

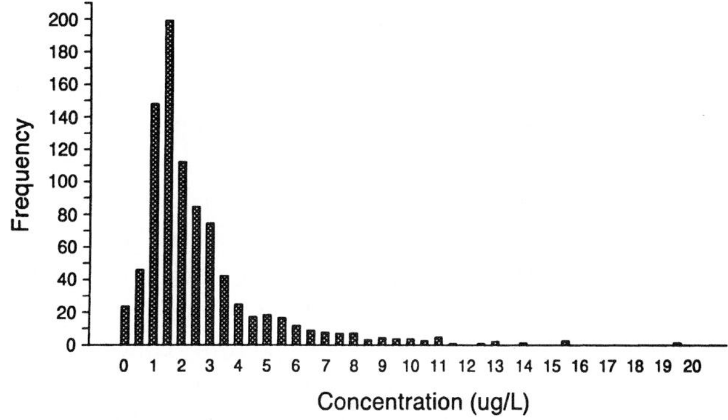

Figure 35-6 Distribution of blood mercury in a healthy population.

NICKEL

Nickel (Ni) is frequently used in the production of metal alloys (which are popular for their anticorrosive and hardness properties), in Ni-based rechargeable batteries, and as a catalyst in the hydrogenation of oils. Elemental Ni is nontoxic except that it will induce inflammation at point of contact.[134] It is likely that Ni is essential for life at very low concentrations. Nickel carbonyl ($Ni[CO]_4$), used in petroleum refining, is one of the most toxic chemicals known to humans.[155] Nickel carbonyl is absorbed after inhalation, readily crosses all biological membranes, and noncompetitively inhibits ATPase and RNA polymerase.* Patients exposed to Ni carbonyl exhibit rapid onset of pulmonary congestion and inability to oxygenate hemoglobin, followed by development of lesions of the lung, liver, kidney, adrenal glands, and spleen.[91,106] Other compounds of Ni have been found to be toxic in the rat.[133]

Patients undergoing dialysis are exposed to Ni and accumulate Ni in blood and other organs. There appear to be no adverse health effects from this exposure.[123] Nickel is quantified by electrothermal atomic absorption spectrometry.[123]

PLATINUM

A variety of platinum (Pt)-containing antineoplastic agents are used in chemotherapy, typified by cisplatin (*cis*-dichlorodiammineplatinum dihydrate).[29,55] All of these compounds have some nephrotoxicity that is related to the concentration of Pt circulating in the blood.[48] Although it is not common to measure Pt concentrations in all patients receiving cisplatin therapy, quantification of Pt concentrations in patients with reduced renal function can help identify whether the Pt is the cause of the compromised renal function. Peak serum concentrations greater than 1 μg/mL but less than 1.5 μg/mL correlate with little nephrotoxicity and good therapeutic response.[67] Either AA-ETA or ICP-MS can be used to measure Pt.[4]

SELENIUM

Selenium (Se) is an essential element and may play a role in mitigating biological damage caused by arsenic and cadmium exposure.[128] It is a cofactor required to maintain glutathione peroxidase activity, an enzyme that catalyzes the degradation of organic hydroperoxides. The absence of Se correlates with a loss of glutathione peroxidase activity and is associated with damage to cell membranes because of the accumulation of free radicals. In humans, cardiac muscle is the tissue most susceptible to Se deficiency; with cell membrane damage, normal cells are replaced with fibroblasts.[64] This condition is known as *cardiomyopathy* and is characterized by an enlarged heart consisting of predominantly nonfunctioning fibrotic tissue.

The normal daily dietary intake of Se is 0.01 to 0.04 ppm, which is similar to the typical content of the metal in soil (0.05 ppm) and sea water (0.09 ppm). Excessive exposure occurs when daily intake exceeds 0.4 ppm.[183] Selenium accumulates in biological tissue such that the normal concentration in human blood serum is 95 to 160 ng/mL (0.15 ppm). In the state of Se deficiency associated with loss of glutathione peroxidase activity, the serum concentration is less than 40 ng/mL.[136]

Selenium deficiency among people who consume food from only a particular region can be related to low soil content of the metal in that region; the soil of the Keshan region of China is noted for this characteristic. Children living in the Keshan region who receive no Se supplement develop cardiomyopathy. Deficiency is also related to use of total parenteral nutrition, which is therapy administered to patients who have no functional bowel (e.g., those who have undergone surgical removal of the small and large intestines because of cancer) or who have acute inflammatory bowel disease, such as Crohn's disease (see Chapter 48). Selenium supplementation to raise serum concentration above 90 ng/mL is the usual practice in these patients, and serum monitoring on a semiannual basis is performed to ensure adequacy of supplementation.

Selenium toxicity has been observed in animals when daily intake exceeds 0.44 ppm.[183] Teratogenic effects are frequently noted in the offspring of animals living in regions where Se soil content is high, such as in south central South Dakota and the northern coastal regions of California.[159] Selenium toxicity in humans is not known to be a significant problem except in acute overdose cases, and Se is not classified as a human teratogen. Selenium is found in many over-the-counter vitamin preparations because its antioxidant activity is thought to be anticarcinogenic.[175] There is no substantiating evidence that Se inhibits cancer development.[159]

Selenium may be quantified by ICP-MS,[26] or alternatively by atomic absorption spectrometry, after the specimen is

*Of historical note, an epidemic occurred in 1976 in Philadelphia that became known as "legionnaires' disease." Before the cause was identified as microbiological, serious consideration was given to the possibility that the cause was nickel carbonyl, because the presentation of the patients resembled that expected for those exposed to this toxic metal complex.

mixed with matrix modifier. An ICP-MS procedure for measuring selenium in serum is presented in the appendix for Chapter 35 found on this book's accompanying Evolve site at http://evolve.elsevier.com/Tietz/textbook/.

Silicon

Silicon (Si) is the most abundant element in our environment; it constitutes 26% of the earth's crust. From the toxicological viewpoint, several forms of Si are of interest, including amorphous oxides of Si (e.g., asbestos) and methylated polymers of Si (e.g., silicone).

Inhalation of asbestos-containing dust leads to deposition of asbestos fibers in the pulmonary alveoli.[120] These fibers are needle-shaped spicules approximately 150 µm in length and up to 15 µm in diameter. When these fibers are inhaled, they deposit in the alveoli where they are surrounded by macrophages and become coated with protein and mucopolysaccharide to form "asbestos bodies." The diagnosis of asbestosis is made by interpretation of a chest x-ray by a qualified radiologist, demonstration of asbestos in sputum, and documentation of asbestos bodies in a lung biopsy by electron microscopy.[69,141] Direct analysis of lung tissue for Si is not useful, because all lung tissue is infiltrated with Si, most of which is not asbestos. Thus direct analysis for Si cannot distinguish asbestosis from normal background Si.

Concern about the use of silicone in implants and about its possible toxicity have come to public attention based on reports of a high prevalence of connective tissue disease associated with breast augmentation.[19,45] Silicone appears to induce a response from polymorphonuclear cells and macrophages that bind small particles of silicone and transport them to lymph nodes, where they can accumulate.[156] Other studies do not support a rheumatological role for silicone.[65,147,179] Quantification of blood[131] or tissue concentrations[111] correlates with the presence of implants but not with symptoms of joint disease.

Silver

The clinical interest in silver (Ag) analysis is limited to two applications: (1) monitoring burn patients treated with Ag sulfadiazine and (2) monitoring patients treated with Ag-containing nasal decongestants. In both cases, Ag deposits in many organs, including the subepithelium of skin and mucous membranes, producing a syndrome called *argyria* (graying of the skin). Argyria is associated with growth retardation, hemopoiesis, cardiac enlargement, degeneration of the liver, and destruction of renal tubules. The normal concentration of serum Ag is less than 2 ng/mL. Typical Ag concentrations observed in serum of unaffected patients during treatment range up to 300 ng/mL, and their urine output can be as high as 550 µg/day.[177]

Thallium

Thallium (Tl) is a byproduct of lead smelting. Interest in Tl derives primarily from its use as a rodenticide; accidental exposure represents the most likely source of exposure. Additionally, environmental concerns are growing because thallium is a waste product of coal combustion and the manufacturing of cement.[84] Thallium is rapidly absorbed via ingestion, inhalation, and skin contact. It is considered to be as toxic as lead and mercury and has similar sites of action.[84,109,164] The mechanism of Tl toxicity is (1) competition with potassium at cell receptors to affect ion pumps, (2) inhibition of DNA synthesis, (3) binding to sulfhydryl groups on proteins in neural axons, and (4) concentration in renal tubular cells to cause necrosis. Patients exposed to high doses of Tl (>1 g) demonstrate alopecia (hair loss), peripheral neuropathy and seizures, and renal failure.[69] Normal serum concentrations are less than 10 ng/mL, and normal daily urine excretion is less than 10 µg/day. Exposed patients can have serum concentrations as high as 50 µg/mL, with urine output in excess of 500 µg/day. The long-term prognosis from such an exposure is poor.[36]

REFERENCES

1. Alam MG, Snow ET, Tanaka A. Arsenic and heavy metal contamination of vegetables grown in Samta village, Bangladesh. Sci Total Environ 2003;308 83-96.
2. Alfrey AC, Mitchell JM, Burks J, et al. Syndrome of dyspraxia and multifocal seizures associated with chronic hemodialysis. Trans Am Soc Artif Intern Organs 1972;18:257-61.
3. Alfrey AC. Aluminum toxicity in patients with chronic renal failure. Ther Drug Monit 1993;15: 593-7.
4. Allain P, Berre S, Mauras Y, Le Bouil A. Evaluation of inductively coupled mass spectrometry for the determination of platinum in plasma. Biol Mass Spectrom 1992;21:141-3.
5. Alpoim MC, Geraldes CF, Oliveira CR, Lima MC. Molecular mechanisms of chromium toxicity: Oxidation of hemoglobin. Biochem Soc Trans 1995;23:241S.
6. Bates MN, Fawcett J, Garrett N, Cutress T, Kjellstrom T. Health effects of dental amalgam exposure: a retrospective cohort study. Int J Epidemiol 2004;33:894-902. May 20 [Epub ahead of print].
7. Bavazzano P, Perico A, Rosendahl K, Apostoli P. Determination of urinary arsenic by solvent extraction and electrothermal atomic absorption spectroscopy. J Anal At Spectrom 1996;11:521-4.
8. Bellinger DC. Lead. Pediatrics 2004;113 (4 Suppl):1016-22.
9. Bencze K. Antimony. In: Seiler HG, Sigel A, Sigel H, eds. Handbook on metals in clinical and analytical chemistry. New York: Marcel Dekker Inc, 1994:227-36.
10. Berg JE. Antimony. Nordic Expert Group, Skyberg, K. Arbete Och Halsa 1998;11:37.
11. Berger OG, Gregg DJ, Succop PA. Using unstimulated urinary lead excretion to assess the need for chelation

in the treatment of lead poisoning. J Pediatr 1990;116:46-51.
12. Bernard S, Enayati A, Redwood L, Roger H, Binstock T. Autism: a novel form of mercury poisoning. Med Hypotheses 2001;56:462-71.
13. Bernard S, Enayati A, Roger H, Binstock T, Redwood L. The role of mercury in the pathogenesis of autism. Mol Psychiatry 2002;7 Suppl 2:S42-3.
14. Blaxill MF, Redwood L, Bernard S. Thimerosal and autism? A plausible hypothesis that should not be dismissed. Med Hypotheses 2004;62:788-94.
15. Bhattacharyya R, Chatterjee D, Nath B, Jana J, Jacks G, Vahter M. High arsenic groundwater: mobilization, metabolism and mitigation–an overview in the Bengal Delta Plain. Mol Cell Biochem 2003;253: 347-55.
16. Bin QH, Garfinkel D. The cadmium toxicity hypothesis of aging: A possible explanation for the zinc deficiency hypothesis of aging. Med Hypotheses 1994;42:380-4.
17. Binder S, Falk H, eds. Strategic plan for the elimination of childhood lead poisoning: Report to the Risk Management Subcommittee, Committee to Coordinate Environmental Health and Related Programs. Atlanta GA: Centers for Disease Control, 1991.
18. Boffetta P, Nyberg F. Contribution of environmental factors to cancer risk. Br Med Bull 2003;68:71-94.
19. Bondurant S, Ernster V, Herdman R, Editors. Safety of silicone breast implants. Committee on the Safety of Silicone Breast Implants, Washington DC: Institute of Medicine, 1999.
20. Borchers AT, Keen CL, Shoenfeld Y, Silva J Jr, Gershwin ME. Vaccines, viruses, and voodoo. J Investig Allergol Clin Immunol 2002;12:155-68.
21. Borja-Aburto VH, Hertz-Picciotto I, Rojas Lopez M. Blood lead levels measured prospectively and the risk of spontaneous abortion. Am J Epidemiol 1999;50:590-7.
22. Borska L, Fiala Z, Smejkalova J, Tejral J. Health risk of occupational exposure in welding processes I. Genotoxic risk. Acta Medica (Hradec Kralove) 2003;46: 25-9.
23. Britton RS, Ramm GA, Olynyk J, Singh R, O'Neill R, Bacon BR. Pathophysiology of iron toxicity. Adv Exp Med Biol 1994;356:239-53.
24. Brune D, Aitio A, Nordberg G, Vesteberg O, Gerhardsson L. Normal concentrations of chromium in serum and urine—a TRACY project. Scand J Work Environ Health 1993;19 Suppl 1:39-44.
25. Buchancova J, Knizkova M, Hyllova D, Vrlik M, Mesko D, Klimentova G, et al. Content of the selected trace elements (Al, As, Cd, Cu, Fe, Hg, Mn, Ni, Pb, Zn) in blood, urine and hair of blood donors without occupational exposure to these metals. Cent Eur J Publ Health 1994;2:82-7.
26. Burritt MF, Butz JA. (Modified from Forrer R, Guatschi K, Lutz H. Simultaneous measurement of trace element Al, As, B, Be, Cd, Co, Cu, Fe, Li, Mn, Mo, Ni, Rb, Se, Sr, and Zn in human serum and their reference ranges by ICP-MS. Biological Trace Element Research 2001;80:77-93.
27. Bushinsky DA, Sprague SM, Hallegot P, Girod C, Chabala JM, Levi-Setti R. Effects of aluminum on bone surface ion composition. J Bone Mineral Res 1995;10:1988-97.
28. Butterworth RF, Spahr L, Fontaine S, Layrargues GP. Manganese toxicity, dopaminergic dysfunction and hepatic encephalopathy. Metab Brain Dis 1995;10:259-67.
29. Calvert H, Judson I, van der Vijgh WJ. Platinum complexes in cancer medicine: Pharmacokinetics and pharmacodynamics in relation to toxicity and therapeutic activity. Cancer Surv 1993;17:189-217.
30. Campbell A. The potential role of aluminum in Alzheimer's disease. Nephrol Dial Transplant 2002;17 Suppl 2:17-20.
31. Canfield RL, Henderson CR, Cory-Slechta DA, et al: Intellectual impairment in children with blood lead concentrations below 10 µg per deciliter. NEJM 2003;348:1517-26.
32. Carrio J, de Colmenares M, Riera C, Gallego M, Arboix M, Portus M. Leishmania infantum: stage specific activity of pentavalent antimony related with the assay conditions. Exp Parasitol 2000;95: 209-14.
33. Castoldi AF, Coccini T, Manzo L. Neurotoxic and molecular effects of methylmercury in humans. Rev Environ Health 2003;18:19-31.
34. Chadzynski L. Manual for the identification and abatement of environmental lead hazards. Washington DC: Division of Maternal and Child Health. US Public Health Service, June 1986.
35. Chalevelakis G, Bouronikou H, Yalouris AG, Economopoulos T, Athanaselis S, Raptis S. Delta-Aminolaevulinic acid dehydratase as an index of lead toxicity: Time for a reappraisal? Eur J Clin Invest 1995;25:53-8.
36. Chandler HA, Archbold GP, Gibson JM, O'Callaghan P, Marks JN, Pethybridge RJ. Excretion of a toxic dose of thallium. Clin Chem 1990;36:1506-9.
37. Chiou HY, Hsueh YM, Liaw KF, Horng SF, Chiang MH, Pu YS, et al. Incidence of internal cancers and ingested inorganic arsenic: a seven-year follow-up study in Taiwan. Cancer Research 1995;55:1296-1300.
38. Clarkson TW, Magos L, Myers GJ. The toxicology of mercury—current exposures and clinical manifestations. N Engl J Med 2003;359:1731-7.
39. Clarkson TW, Strain JJ. Nutritional factors may modify the toxic action of methyl mercury in fish-eating populations. J Nutr 2003;133(5 Suppl 1): 1539S-43S.

40. Cohen MD, Kargacin B, Klein CB, Costa M. Mechanisms of chromium carcinogenicity and toxicity. Crit Rev Toxicol 1993;23:255-81.
41. Cornelis R. Recommendations of the International Union of Pure and Applied Chemistry concerning analytical quality criteria in the biological monitoring of toxic metals. Scand J Work Environ Health 1993;19 Suppl 1:14-8.
42. Costa LG, Aschner M, Vitalone A, Syversen T, Soldin OP. Developmental neuropathology of environmental agents. Annu Rev Pharmacol Toxicol 2004;44:87-110.
43. Crichton RR, Ward RJ. Iron species in iron homeostasis and toxicity. Analyst 1995;120:693-7.
44. Criteria Group for Occupational Standards: Scientific basis for Swedish occupational standards XXI. Consensus for antimony compounds. Arbete Och Halsa 2000;22:1-14.
45. Cuellar ML, Gluck O, Molina JF, Gutierrez S, Garcia C, Espinoza R. Silicone breast implant-associated musculoskeletal manifestations. Clin Rheumat 1995;14:667-72.
46. Davidson PW, Myers GJ, Weiss B. Mercury exposure and child development outcomes. Pediatrics 2004;113(4 Suppl):1023-9.
47. De Boeck M, Kirsch-Volders M, Lison D. Cobalt and antimony: genotoxicity and carcinogenicity. Mutat Res 2003;533:135-52.
48. Deegan PM, Nolan C, Ryan MP, Basinger MA, Jones MM, Hande KR. The role of the renin-angiotensin system in cisplatin nephrotoxicity. Renal Failure 1995;17:665-74.
49. Deubner DC, Goodman MG, Iannuzzi J. Variability, predictive value, and uses of the beryllium blood lymphocyte proliferation test (BLPT): preliminary analysis of the ongoing workforce survey. Appl Occup Environ Hyg 2001;16:521-6.
50. D'Haese PC, Couttenye MM, Goodman WG, Lemoniatou E, Digenis P, Sotornik I, et al. Use of the low-dose deferoxamine test to diagnose and differentiate between patients with aluminum-related bone disease, increased risk for aluminum toxicity, or aluminum overload. Nephr Dialy Transplant 1995;10:1874-84.
51. Dickerson OB. Antimony, arsenic and their compounds. In: Zenx C, Dickerson OB, Horvath EP, eds. Occupational medicine, 3rd Ed. St Louis: Mosby-Year Book Inc, 1994:466-73.
52. Dobson AW, Erikson KM, Aschner M. Manganese neurotoxicity. Ann N Y Acad Sci 2004;1012:115-28.
53. Documentation of the threshold limit values and biological exposure indices, 6th ed. Cincinnati, OH, American Conference of Governmental Industrial Hygienists, 1991.
54. Domingo JL. Reproductive and developmental toxicity of aluminum: A review. Neurotoxicol Teratol 1995;17:515-21.
55. Dubey S, Schiller JH. Chemotherapy for advanced non-small cell lung cancer. Hematol Oncol Clin North Am 2004;18:101-14.
56. Echeverria D, Heyer NJ, Martin MD. Behavioral effects of low-level exposure to elemental Hg among dentists. Neurotoxicol Teratol 1995;17:161-8.
57. Eknoyan G, Levin A, Levin NW. Clinical practice guidelines for bone metabolism and disease in chronic kidney disease. Am J Kid Dis 2003;42: S7-S201.
58. Erasmus RT, Savory J, Wills MR, Herman MM. Aluminum neurotoxicity in experimental animals. Ther Drug Monit 1993;15:588-92.
59. Eto K. Minamata disease. Neuropathology 2000;20 Suppl:S14-19.
60. Evans EC. The FDA recommendations on fish intake during pregnancy. J Obstet Gynecol Neonatal Nurs 2002;31:715-20.
61. Exley C, Schley L, Murray S, Hackney CM, Birchall JD. Aluminum, beta-amyloid and non-enzymatic glycosylation. FEBS Letters 1995;364:182-84.
62. Fell JM, Reynolds AP, Meadows N, Khan K, Long SG, Quaghebeur G, et al. Manganese toxicity in children receiving long-term parenteral nutrition. Lancet 1996;347:1218-21.
63. Fels LM, Bundschuh I, Gwinner W, et al. Early urinary markers of target nephron segments as studied in cadmium toxicity. Kidney Int Suppl 1994;47:S81-8.
64. Fleming CR, McCall JT, O'Brien JF, Forsman RW, Ilstrup DM, Petz J. Selenium status in patients receiving home parenteral nutrition. J Parenteral Enteral Nutr 1984;8:258-62.
65. Gabriel SE, O'Fallon WM, Kurland LT, Beard CM, Woods JE, Melton LJ 3rd. Risk of connective-tissue diseases and other disorders after breast implantation. N Engl J Med 1994;330:1697-702.
66. Gaetke LM, Chow CK. Copper toxicity, oxidative stress, and antioxidant nutrients. Toxicology 2003;189:147-63.
67. Gamelin E, Allain P, Maillart P, Turcant A, Delva R, Lortholary A, et al. Long-term pharmacokinetic behavior of platinum after cisplatin administration. Cancer Chemother Pharmacol 1995;37:97-102.
68. Garcia-Vargas GG, Hernandez-Zavala A. Urinary porphyrins and heme biosynthetic enzyme activities measured by HPLC in arsenic toxicity. Biomed Chromatogr 1996;10:278-84.
69. Gardner DE, Crapo JD, Massaro EJ, eds. Toxicology of the lung. New York: Raven Press, 1988.
70. Geier DA, Geier MR. An assessment of the impact of thimerosal on childhood neurodevelopmental disorders. Pediatr Rehabil 2003;6:97-102.
71. Geier DA, Geier MR. A comparative evaluation of the effects of MMR immunization and mercury doses from thimerosal-containing childhood vaccines on

the population prevalence of autism. Med Sci Monit 2004;10:PI33-9. Epub 2004 Mar 01.
72. Goldhaber SB. Trace element risk assessment: essentiality vs. toxicity. Regul Toxicol Pharmacol 2003;38:232-42.
73. Gordon T, Bowser D. Beryllium: Genotoxicity and carcinogenicity. Mutat Res 2003;533:99-105.
74. Graziano JH, Lolacono NJ, Meyer P. Dose response study of oral 2,3-dimercaptosuccinic acid in children with elevated blood lead concentrations. J Pediatr 1988;113:751-7.
75. Grimsrud TK, Berge SR, Martinsen JI, Andersen A. Lung cancer incidence among Norwegian nickel-refinery workers 1953-2000. J Environ Monit 2003;5:190-7.
76. Hahn LJ, Kloiber R, Vimy MJ, Takahashi Y, Lorscheider FL. Dental "silver" tooth fillings: A source of mercury exposure revealed by whole-body image scan and tissue analysis. FASEB J 1989;3:2641-6.
77. Hanson M, Pleva J. The dental amalgam. A review. Experientia 1991;47:9-22.
78. Hansen G, Victor R, Engeldinger E, Schweitzer C. Evaluation of the mercury exposure of dental amalgam patients by the Mercury Triple Test. Occup Environ Med 2004;61:535-40.
78A. Harris ZL, Gitlin JD. Genetic and molecular basis for copper toxicity. Am J Clin Nutr 1996;63:836S-41S.
79. Hasan N, Emery D, Baithun SI, Dodd, S. Chronic copper intoxication due to ingestion of coins: A report of an unusual case. Hum Exper Toxicol 1995;14:500-2.
80. Herber RFM. Cadmium In: Seiler HG, Sigel A, Sigel H, eds. Handbook on metals in clinical and analytical chemistry. New York: Marcel Dekker Inc, 1994:292.
81. Hertz-Picciotto I, Hu SW. Contribution of cadmium in cigarettes to lung cancer: an evaluation of risk assessment methodologies. Arch Environ Health 1994;49:297-302.
82. Hessel L. Mercury in vaccines. Bull Acad Natl Med. 2003;187:1501-10.
83. Hindmarsh JT, McCurdy RF. Clinical and environmental aspects of arsenic toxicity. Crit Rev Clin Lab 1986;23:315-47.
84. Hoffman RS. Thallium toxicity and the role of Prussian blue in therapy. Toxicol Rev 2003;22:29-40.
85. Hollosi M, Shenm ZM, Perczel A, Fasman GD. Stable intrachain and interchain complexes of neurofilament peptides: A putative link between Al^{3+} and Alzheimer disease. Proc Nat Acad Sci 1994;91:4902-6.
86. Hoque BA, Hoque MM, Ahmed T, Islam S, Azad AK, Ali N, et al. Demand-based water options for arsenic mitigation: an experience from rural Bangladesh. Public Health 2004;118:70-7
87. Huang X. Iron overload and its association with cancer risk in humans: evidence for iron as a carcinogenic metal. Mutat Res 2003;533:153-71.
88. Institute of Medicine Report. Immunization safety review: Vaccines and autism. Immunization Safety Review Committee, Board on Health Promotion and Disease Prevention. Washington DC: The National Academy Press, 2004. (http://books.nap.edu/catalog/10997.html).
89. Islam R, Salminen R, Lahermo P.W. Arsenic and other toxic elemental contamination of groundwater, surface water and soil in Bangladesh and its possible effects on human health. Env Geochem Health 2000;22:33-53.
90. Jarup L. Hazards of heavy metal contamination. Br Med Bull 2003;68:167-82.
91. Kasprzak KS, Sunderman FW Jr, Salnikow K. Nickel carcinogenesis. Mutat Res 2003;533:67-97.
92. Kesserling J. Arsenic and Old Lace: A comedy. New York, Random House, Inc, 1941.
93. Khan MM, Sakauchi F, Sonoda T, Washio M, Mori M. Magnitude of arsenic toxicity in tube-well drinking water in Bangladesh and its adverse effects on human health including cancer: evidence from a review of the literature. Asian Pac J Cancer Prev. 2003;4:7-14.
94. Kimmel SR. Vaccine adverse events: separating myth from reality. Am Fam Physician 2002;66:2113-20.
95. Kitapci F, Dilmen U, Akyol O, Toppare M, Kaya IS, Senses DA, et al. Plasma chromium levels in hypoglycemic preterm, full-term and in intrauterine-growth-retarded babies. Biol Neonate 1994;66: 267-71.
96. Klaasen CD. Principles of Toxicology. In Klassen CD, ed. Casarett's & Doull's toxicology: The basic science of poisons, 6th Ed. New York: McGraw-Hill, 2001: 11-34.
97. Kolanz ME, Madl AK, Kelsh MA, Kent MS, Kalmes RM, Paustenbach DJ. A comparison and critique of historical and current exposure assessment method for beryllium: Implications for evaluating risk of chronic beryllium disease. Appl Occup Environ Hyg 2001;6:593-614.
98. Kosnett MJ. Lead. In: Ford MD, Delaney KA , Ling LJ, Erickson T, eds, Clinical toxicology. New York: WB Saunders 2001:723-36.
99. Lawrence JF, Michalik P, Tam G, Conacher HBS. Identification of arsenobetaine and arsenocholine in Canadian fish and shellfish by high-performance liquid chromatography with atomic absorption detection and confirmation by fast atom bombardment mass spectrometry. J Agri Food Chem 1981;34: 315-19.
100. Léopold T, Lejeune R. Cobalt. In: Seiler HG, Sigel A, Sigel H, eds. Handbook on metals in clinical and analytical chemistry. New York: Marcel Dekker Inc, 1994:333-8.
101. Leung FY, Bradley C, Pellar TG. Reference intervals for blood lead and evaluation of zinc protoporphyrin

as a screening test for lead toxicity. Clin Biochem 1993;26:491-6.

102. Lison D, Lauwerys R. Cobalt bioavailability from hard metal particles: Further evidence that cobalt alone is not responsible for the toxicity of hard metal particles. Arch Toxicol 1994;68:528-31.
103. Lockitch G. Perspectives on lead toxicity. Clin Biochem 1993;26:371-81.
104. Lucchini R, Selis L, Folli D, Apostoli P, Mutti A, Vanoni O, et al. Neurobehavioral effects of manganese in workers from a ferroalloy plant after temporary cessation of exposure. Scand J Work Environ Health 1995;21:143-9.
105. Ludwig J, Moyer TP, Rakela J. The liver biopsy diagnosis of Wilson's disease. Methods in pathology. Am J Clin Pathol 1994;102:443-6.
106. Lumb GD, Sunderman FW Sr. The problem of latency in the development of tumors following exposure to nickel compounds. Sci Total Environ 1994;148:85-90.
107. Madsen KM, Lauritsen MB, Pedersen CB, Thorsen P, Plesner AM, Andersen PH, et al. Thimerosal and the occurrence of autism: Negative ecological evidence from Danish population-based data. Pediatrics 2003;112:604-6.
108. Maier LA. Beryllium health effects in the era of the beryllium lymphocyte proliferation test. Appl Occup Environ Hyg 2001;16:514-20.
109. Malbrain ML, Lambrecht GL, Zandijk E, Demedts PA, Neels HM, Lambert W, et al. Treatment of severe thallium intoxication. J Toxicol Clin Toxicol 1997;35:97-100.
110. McCarthy JT, Milliner DS, Kurtz SB, Johnson WJ, Moyer TP. Interpretation of serum aluminum values in dialysis patients. Am J Clin Pathol 1986;86:629-36.
111. McConnell JP, Moyer TP, Nixon DE, Schnur PL, Salomao DR, Crotty TB, et al. Determination of silicon in breast and capsular tissue from patients with breast implants performed by inductively coupled plasma emission spectroscopy: Comparison with tissue histology. Am J Clin Pathol 1997;107:236-46.
112. Mergler D, Huel G, Bowler R, Iregren A, Belanger S, Baldwin M, et al. Nervous system dysfunction among workers with long-term exposure to manganese. Environ Res 1994;64:151-80.
113. Michalke B. Element speciation definitions, analytical methodology, and some examples. Ecotoxicol Environ Saf 2003;56:122-39.
114. Milliner DS, Nebeker HG, Ott SM, Andress DL, Sherrard DJ, Alfrey AC, et al. Use of the deferoxamine infusion test in the diagnosis of aluminum-related osteodystrophy. Ann Intern Med 1984;101:775-80.
115. Morris BW, Griffiths H, Kemp GJ. Effect of glucose loading on concentrations of chromium in plasma and urine of healthy adults. Clin Chem 1988;34:1114-16.
116. Moyer TP, Mussman GV, Nixon DE. Blood-collection device for trace and ultra-trace metal specimens evaluated. Clin Chem 1991;37:709-14.
117. Moyer TP. Testing for arsenic. Mayo Clin Proc 1993;68:1210-11.
118. Moyer TP. Incidence of heavy metal toxicity in a clinical population (abstract). 4th International Conference on Therapeutic Drug Monitoring and Toxicology, Vienna, Austria, 1994.
119. Nelson KB, Bauman ML. Thimerosal and autism? Pediatrics 2003;111:674-9.
120. Neuberger JS, Field RW. Occupation and lung cancer in nonsmokers. Rev Environ Health 2003;18: 251-67.
121. Nemery B, Lewis CP, Demedts M. Cobalt and possible oxidant-mediated toxicity. Sci Total Environ 1994;150:57-64.
122. Neve J, Leclerq N. Factors affecting determination of manganese in serum by atomic absorption spectrometry. Clin Chem 1991;37:723-8.
123. Nixon DE, Moyer TP, Squillace DP, McCarthy JT. Determination of serum nickel by graphite furnace atomic absorption spectrometry with Zeeman-effect background correction: Values in a normal population and a population undergoing dialysis. Analyst 1989;114:1671-4.
124. Nixon DE, Moyer TP. Routine clinical determination of lead, arsenic, cadmium, mercury, and thallium in urine and whole blood by inductively coupled plasma mass spectrometry. Spectrochim Acta 1996;51B: 13-25.
125. NHANES. National Health and Nutrition Examination Survey, Hyattsville Maryland: US Department of Health and Human Services, Centers for Disease Control and Prevention, National Center for Health Statistics, 1999.
126. O'Brien TJ, Ceryak S, Patierno SR. Complexities of chromium carcinogenesis: Role of cellular response, repair and recovery mechanisms. Mutat Res 2003;533:3-36.
127. Occupational exposure to cadmium. Fed Regist 1992;57:42:102-42, & 462.
128. Patrick L. Toxic metals and antioxidants: Part II. The role of antioxidants in arsenic and cadmium toxicity. Altern Med Rev 2003;8:106-28.
129. Perl DP. Alzheimer's disease: X-ray spectrometric evidence of aluminum accumulation in neurofibrillary tangle-bearing neurons. Science 1980;208:297-9.
130. Peters GR, McCurdy RF, Hindmarsh JT. Environmental aspects of arsenic toxicity. Crit Rev Clin Lab Sci 1996;33:457-93.
131. Peters W, Smith D, Lugowski S, McHugh A, Keresteci A, Baines C. Do patients with silicone-gel breast implants have elevated levels of blood silicon compared with control patients? Ann Plast Surg 1995;34:343-7.
132. Pocock SJ, Smith M, Baghurst P. Environmental lead and children's intelligence: A systematic review of the epidemiological evidence. Br Med J 1994;309: 1189-97.

133. Porter WH, Moyers TP. Clinical Toxicology. In: Burtis CA, Ashwood ER, eds. Tietz textbook of clinical chemistry, 2nd ed. Philadelphia: WB Saunders, 1994:1155-235.
134. Probst P, Kuntzlin D, Fleischer B. TH2-type infiltrating T cells in nickel-induced contact dermatitis. Cellul Immunol 1995;165:134-40.
135. Pulido MD, Parrish AR. Metal-induced apoptosis: Mechanisms. Mutat Res 2003;533:227-41.
136. Rannem T, Ladefoged K, Hylander E, Christiansen J, Laursen H, Kristensen JH, et al. The effect of selenium supplementation on skeletal and cardiac muscle in selenium-depleted patients. J Parenteral Enteral Nutr 1995;19:351-55.
137. Reinhardt JW. Risk assessment of mercury exposure from dental amalgams. J Public Health Dent 1988;48:172-7.
138. Reinke CM, Breitkreutz J, Leuenberger H. Aluminium in over-the-counter drugs: Risks outweigh benefits? Drug Saf 2003;26:1011-25.
139. Rifai N, Cohen G, Wolf M, Cohen L, Faser C, Savory J, et al. Incidence of lead poisoning in young children from inner-city, suburban, and rural communities. Ther Drug Monit 1993;15:71-4.
140. Rogan WJ, Ware JH. Exposure to lead in children—How low is low enough? N Engl J Med 2003;348: 1515-16.
141. Roggli VL, Pratt PC, Brody AR. Asbestos content of lung tissue in asbestos associated diseases: A study of 110 cases. Br J Ind Med 1986;43:18-28.
142. Rondeau V. A review of epidemiologic studies on aluminum and silica in relation to Alzheimer's disease and associated disorders. Rev Environ Health 2002;17:107-21.
143. Roper WL, Houk VN, Falk H, Binder S. Preventing lead poisoning in young children: A statement by the Centers for Disease Control. Atlanta, GA: Centers for Disease Control. US Department of Health and Human Services publication PB92-155076/HDM, 1991.
144. Rossman MD. Beryllium. In: Seiler HG, Sigel A, Sigel H, eds. Handbook on metals in clinical and analytical chemistry. New York: Marcel Dekker Inc, 1994:259-67.
145. Rossman TG. Mechanism of arsenic carcinogenesis: An integrated approach. Mutat Res 2003;533:37-65.
146. Royce SE, Needleman HL, eds. Case studies in environmental medicine: Lead toxicity. Washington DC: US Public Health Service, ATSDR, 1990.
147. Sanchez-Guerrero J, Colditz GA, Karlson EW, Hunter DJ, Speizer FE, Liang MH. Silicone breast implants and the risk of connective-tissue diseases and symptoms. N Engl J Med 1995;332:1666-70.
148. Sandstead HH. Requirements and toxicity of essential trace elements, illustrated by zinc and copper. Am J Clin Nutr 1995;61:621S-24S.
149. Satarug S, Baker JR, Urbenjapol S, Haswell-Elkins M, Reilly PE, Williams DJ, et al. A global perspective on cadmium pollution and toxicity in non-occupationally exposed population. Toxicol Lett 2003;137:65-83.
150. Satoh M, Koyama H, Kaji T, Kito H, Tohyama C. Perspectives on cadmium toxicity research. Tohoku J Exp Med 2002;196:23-32
151. Savory J, Huang Y, Herman MM, Wills MR. Quantitative image analysis of temporal changes in tau and neurofilament proteins during the course of acute experimental neurofibrillary degeneration: Non-phosphorylated epitopes precede phosphorylation. Brain Res 1996;707:272-81.
152. Schermeier AJ, O'Connor LH, Pearson KH. Semi-automated determination of chromium in whole blood and serum by Zeeman electrothermal atomic absorption spectrophotometry. Clin Chem Acta 1985;152:123-34.
153. Schwartz J. Lead, blood pressure and cardiovascular disease in men. Archives Environ Health 1995;50: 31-7.
154. Serre ML, Kolovos A, Christakos G, Modis K. An application of the holistochastic human exposure methodology to naturally occurring arsenic in Bangladesh drinking water. Risk Anal 2003;23:515-28.
155. Shi Z. Nickel carbonyl: Toxicity and human health. Sci Total Environ 1994;148:293-8.
156. Shons AR, Schubert W. Silicone breast implants and immune disease: An overview. Ann Plast Surg 1992;28:491-501.
157. Slavin W. Graphite furnace AAS for biological materials. The Science of the Total Environment 1998;71:17-35.
158. Spall WD, Lynn JG, Andersen JL, Valdez JG, Gurley LR. High-performance liquid chromatographic separation of biologically important arsenic species utilizing on-line inductively coupled argon plasma atomic absorption spectrometric detection. Anal Chem 1986;58:1340-3.
159. Spallholz JE. On the nature of selenium toxicity and carcinostatic activity. Free Radical Biol Med 1994;17:45-64.
160. Stehr-Green P, Tull P, Stellfeld M, Mortenson PB, Simpson D. Autism and thimerosal-containing vaccines: Lack of consistent evidence for an association. Am J Prev Med 2003;25:101-6.
161. Stopford W. Industrial exposure to mercury. In: Nriagu JO, ed. The biogeochemistry of mercury in the environment. Amsterdam: Elsevier-North Holland, 1979:367-97.
162. Suay Llopis L, Ballester Diez F. Review of studies on exposure to aluminum and Alzheimer's disease. Rev Esp Salud Publica 2002;76:645-58.
163. Sullivan J, Parker M, Carson SB. Tissue Co content in beer drinker's myocardiopathy. J Lab Clin Med 1968;71:893-8.
164. Tabandeh H, Crowston JG, Thompson GM. Ophthalmologic features of thallium poisoning. Am J Ophthalmol 1994;117:243-5.

165. Tabocova S, Hunter ES III, Gladen BC. Developmental toxicity of inorganic arsenic in whole embryo: Culture oxidation state, dose, time, and gestational age dependence. Toxicol Appl Pharmacol 1996;138:298-307.
166. Tareq SM, Safiullah S, Anawar HM, Rahman MM, Ishizuka T. Arsenic pollution in groundwater: A self-organizing complex geochemical process in the deltaic sedimentary environment, Bangladesh. Sci Total Environ 2003;313:213-26.
167. Tollefson L, Cordle F. Methylmercury in fish: A review of residue levels, fish consumption and regulatory action in the United States. Environ Health Perspect 1986;68:203-8.
168. Torres-Sanchez LE, Berkowitz G, Lopez-Carrillo L. Interuterine lead exposure and preterm birth. Environ Res 1999;81:297-301.
169. Tsalev DL, Zaprianov ZK, Eds. Atomic absorption spectrometry in occupational and environmental health practice. Boca Raton: CRC Press, 1984.
170. Tubaki T, Irukayam K. Minamata disease. Amsterdam: Elsevier, 1976.
171. US Department of Health and Human Services. Healthy people 2010: Understanding and improving health, 2nd ed Washington, DC: US Government Printing Office, 2000.
172. Vamnes JS, Lygre GB, Gronningsaeter AG, Gjerdet NR. Four years of clinical experience with an adverse reaction unit for dental biomaterials. Community Dent Oral Epidemiol 2004;32:150-7.
173. van Geen A, Ahmed KM, Seddique AA, Shamsudduha M. Community wells to mitigate the arsenic crisis in Bangladesh. Bull World Health Organ 2003;81:632-8.
174. van Sittert NJ, Ribbens PH, Huisman B, Lugtenburg D. A nine year follow up study of renal effects in worker exposed to cadmium in a zinc ore refinery. Br J Indust Med 1996;50:603-12.
175. Vernie LN. Selenium in carcinogenesis. Biochem Biophys Acta 1984;738:203-17.
176. Verstraeten T, Davis RL, DeStefano F, Lieu TA, Rhodes PH, Black SB, et al. Vaccine Safety Datalink Team. Safety of thimerosal-containing vaccines: A two-phased study of computerized health maintenance organization databases. Pediatrics 2003;112:1039-48.
177. Wan AT, Conyers RAJ, Coombs CJ, Masterton JP. Determination of silver in blood, urine, and tissues of volunteers and burn patients. Clin Chem 1991;37:1683-7.
178. Ward MK, Pierides AM, Fawcett P. Dialysis encephalopathy syndrome. Proc EDTA 1976;13: 348-54.
179. Weinzweig J, Schnur PL, McConnell JP, Harris JB, Petty PM, Moyer TP, et al. Silicon analysis of breast and capsular tissue from patients with saline or silicone gel breast implants: II. Correlation with connective-tissue disease. Plast Reconstr Surg 1998;101:1836-41.
180. Weinberger HL, Post EM, Schneider T, Helu B, Friedman J. An analysis of 248 initial mobilization tests performed on an ambulatory basis. Am J Dis Child 1987;141:1266-70.
181. Woods JS. Altered porphyrin metabolism as a biomarker of mercury exposure and toxicity. Can J Physiol Pharmacol 1996;74:210-15.
182. Yaghi B, Abdul-Wahab SA. Assessment of lead, zinc, copper, nickel and chromium in total suspended particulate matter from the workplace in Al-Rusayl Industrial Estate, Oman. J Environ Monit 2003;5: 950-2.
183. Yang G, Zhou R. Further observations on the human maximum safe dietary selenium intake in a seleniferous area of China. J Trace Elem Electroly in Health Dis 1994;8:159-65.
184. Zacharski LR, Gerhard GS. Atherosclerosis: A manifestation of chronic iron toxicity? Vasc Med 2003; 8:153-5.
185. Zalups RK, Lash LH. Advances in understanding the renal transport and toxicity of mercury. J Toxicol Environ Health 1994;42:1-44.
186. Zakharyan RA, Sampayo-Reyes A, Healy SM, Tsaprailis G, Board PG, Liebler DC, et al. Human monomethylarsonic acid reductase is a member of the glutathione-S-transferase superfamily. Chem Res Toxicol 2001;14:1051-7.
187. Zhang X, Cornelis R, De Kimpe J, Mees L, Lameire N. Study of arsenic-protein binding in serum of patients on continuous ambulatory peritoneal dialysis. Clin Chem 1998;44:141-7.

ADDITIONAL READING

Carre V, Aubriet F, Scheepers PT, Krier G, Muller JF. Potential of laser ablation and laser desorption mass spectrometry to characterize organic and inorganic environmental pollutants on dust particles. Rapid Commun Mass Spectrom 2005;19:871-80 [Epub ahead of print].

Clarkson TW, Magos L, Myers GJ. The toxicology of mercury–current exposures and clinical manifestations. N Engl J Med 2003;349:1731-7.

Eisler R. Health risks of gold miners: A synoptic review. Environ Geochem Health 2003;25:325-45.

Eisler R. Arsenic hazards to humans, plants, and animals from gold mining. Rev Environ Contam Toxicol 2004;180:133-65.

Marcotrigiano GO, Storelli MM. Heavy metal, polychlorinated biphenyl and organochlorine pesticide residues in marine organisms: Risk evaluation for consumers. Vet Res Commun 2003;27 Suppl 1:183-95.

Walker JD, Enache M, Dearden JC. Quantitative cationic-activity relationships for predicting toxicity of metals. Environ Toxicol Chem 2003;22:1916-35.

SECTION V

Molecular Diagnostics and Genetics

CHAPTER 36

Principles of Molecular Biology and Approaches to Nucleic Acid Isolation

*Y.M. Dennis Lo, M.A., D.M., D.Phil., F.R.C.P., F.R.C.Path., and Rossa W.K. Chiu, M.B.B.S., Ph.D., F.R.C.P.A.**

Molecular diagnostics represents one of the most rapidly developing areas in clinical chemistry. Advances in the field have been made possible by our improved understanding of molecular biology and genetics and of their relationships with human diseases, and the development of powerful technologies for the analysis of nucleic acids. The chapters in this section attempt to provide an overview of the important advances in molecular diagnostics. The fundamental concepts in molecular biology are reviewed in this chapter. Molecular diagnostic techniques and operational requirements are discussed in Chapters 37 and 38, respectively. The subsequent chapters focus on key areas of molecular diagnostics, specifically hematological malignancies (Chapter 39), inherited diseases (Chapter 40), identity assessment (Chapter 41), infectious diseases (Chapter 42), and pharmacogenetics (Chapter 43).

LANDMARK DEVELOPMENTS IN GENETICS AND MOLECULAR DIAGNOSTICS

Amazing developments in biotechnology have taken place in the late twentieth century.[38] For example, we have witnessed the decoding of the human genome, cloning of organisms, and progress in stem cell research and gene therapy. Many of these advances would not have been possible without the many earlier landmark discoveries that unveiled the mysteries of genetics and paved the way for modern molecular diagnostics.[2,31] Genetics began modestly when Mendel experimented with garden peas. His findings, published in 1866 and suggesting the concepts of alleles and genes as discrete units of heredity, essentially captured the most fundamental concepts in inheritance. In 1910 Morgan revealed that the units of heredity are contained within chromosomes, but it was Avery in 1944 who confirmed through studies on bacteria that it was DNA that carried the genetic information. Franklin and Wilkins studied DNA by x-ray crystallography, which subsequently led to the unraveling of the double-helical structure of DNA by Watson and Crick in 1953. In the 1960s Smith demonstrated that DNA can be cleaved by restriction enzymes, which Arber had discovered earlier and which facilitated the subsequent development of recombinant DNA technologies. Nathans furthered the work on restriction enzymes and was the first to construct a genetic map. In 1975 the Southern blot was invented, which allowed the detection of specific DNA sequences. Soon after, in 1977, DNA-sequencing methodologies were developed, and the first complete DNA sequence of an organism, a bacteriophage, was published. Prenatal genetic diagnosis of sickle cell disease was first shown to be feasible by Kan and Chang in 1981. Mullis and co-workers developed the polymerase chain reaction (PCR) in 1985. DNA microarrays, which allow the simultaneous interrogation of gene transcripts, became a reality in 1996. Remarkably, the draft human genome sequence was released in 2001 and completed in 2003.

*The authors gratefully acknowledge the original contributions of Drs. Elizabeth R. Unger and Margaret A. Piper, upon which portions of this chapter are based.

This is a brief account of a fraction of the many great discoveries that shaped modern genetics and molecular diagnostics. We shall now start the discussion of the principles of molecular biology beginning with the Watson and Crick model of DNA and, for the readers who persist in the journey, the chapter shall end with discussion of the greatest biotechnological achievement of mankind of our time, the Human Genome Project.

NUCLEIC ACID CHEMISTRY, BIOCHEMISTRY, AND BIOLOGY

Nucleic acids form the repository for hereditary information and provide the means of translating that information into the cellular machinery of life. Detailing the structure and function of nucleic acids has been a central theme of molecular biology; a review of nucleic acid chemistry and biochemistry is fundamental to further discussions on nucleic acid diagnostic tests.

MOLECULAR COMPOSITIONS AND STRUCTURES OF DNA AND RNA

The physicochemical properties and function of nucleic acids are largely governed by the compositions and structures of DNA and RNA. A single molecule of DNA is a polymer consisting of a backbone of invariant composition and of side groups arranged in a variable sequence. The polymer is synthesized from monomers (nucleotides) composed of the sugar deoxyribose, a phosphate residue, and a purine or pyrimidine base. The purines are *adenine* (A) and *guanine* (G), and the pyrimidines are *cytosine* (C) and *thymine* (T) (Figure 36-1). The four nucleotide building blocks of DNA are abbreviated dATP (deoxyadenine-triphosphate), dGTP (deoxyguanine-triphosphate), dCTP (deoxycytosine-triphosphate), and dTTP (deoxythymine-triphosphate), respectively. Nucleotides are joined by phosphodiester bonds that link the 5′-phosphate group of one to the 3′-hydroxyl group of the next (Figure 36-2). There are no 3′-3′ or 5′-5′ linkages; thus the sugar and phosphate moieties compose the nonspecific portions of the molecule. The sequence of the bases varies from molecule to molecule and uniquely identifies each DNA polymer, which as discussed later, determines the identity and function of the protein or RNA products that the DNA encodes.

Although the purines and pyrimidines are of different compositions and sizes, when in the proper orientation, adenine forms hydrogen bonds with thymine and guanine forms hydrogen bonds with cytosine to form planar structures of similar dimensions (Figure 36-1). This and the fact that the base portion of each nucleotide is hydrophobic contributes to the energetically favorable secondary structure of DNA as it is found in its native form: a right-handed, double-stranded helix. The planar *base pairs* stack in the inside of the helix, 10 bases per turn, whereas the hydrophilic sugar-phosphate backbone forms noncovalent bonds with surrounding water molecules. For the two DNA polymers to form the proper hydrogen bonds between the bases, two requirements must be fulfilled: the polymers must run in opposite directions *(antiparallel)* as defined by the free hydroxyl groups at each end (3′-5′ vs. 5′-3′), and the sequences of each molecule must be such that A:T and G:C hydrogen bonds are always formed *(base pairing).* Two DNA strands that meet this requirement are called *complementary.*

Owing to base pairing and the double-helical conformation, double-stranded DNA (dsDNA) is an exceptionally stable molecule. Retention of the base pairs in the inner portion of the helix prevents disruption by water molecules. The helical conformation places each monomer in an identical orientation within the molecule and forms the same secondary bonds as every other monomer. This secondary bonding contributes to the overall stability. Because the base

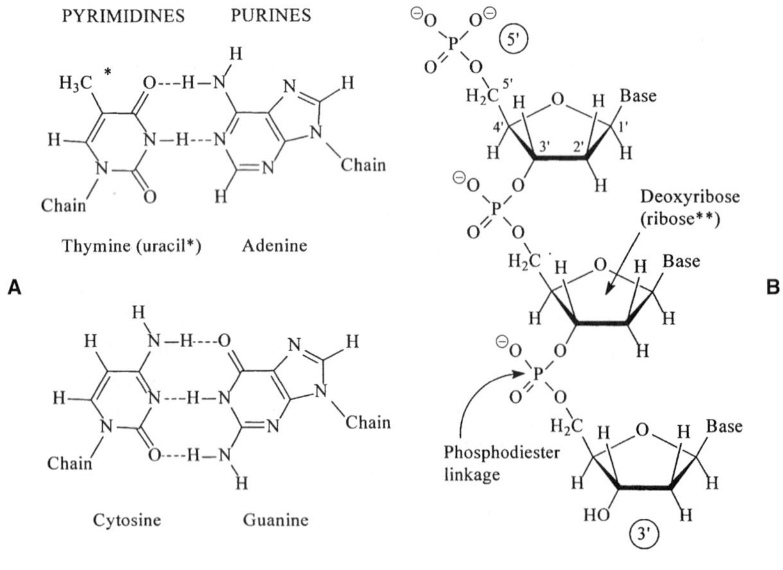

Figure 36-1 Purine and pyrimidine bases and the formation of complementary base pairs. *Dashed lines* indicate the formation of hydrogen bonds. (In RNA, thymine is replaced by uracil, which differs from thymine only in its lack of the methyl group.) *(Modified from Piper, M.A., Unger, E.R.: Nucleic Acid Probes: A Primer for Pathologists. Chicago, ASCP Press, 1989.)*

pairs are of similar size, the helix retains a constant angle of rotation and avoids distortion. All of these features dictate that all dsDNA molecules, regardless of base sequence, retain the same shape and size within a pH range of approximately 4 to 9. Outside these limits, the base pair bonds are disrupted and the helix unwinds.[90]

RNA is chemically very similar to DNA but differs in important ways. The sugar unit is ribose with an added hydroxyl group at the 2′ position, and the methylated pyrimidine *uracil* (U) replaces thymine. RNA exists in various functional forms but typically as a single-stranded polymer that is much shorter than DNA and that has an irregular three-dimensional structure. Research from recent years has revealed that RNA conformations are not random structures and the folding mechanism of RNA molecules is complex.[19,99] The secondary structure adopted by an RNA molecule is to a large extent related to its nucleotide sequence. The secondary structure for particular RNA sequences can be as regular as the secondary structure of a protein. It is now known that RNA molecules can further interact to form complex tertiary structures, which are intimately related to novel functions of RNA, such as the catalytic activity of ribozymes.[19,99]

CHROMOSOME STRUCTURE

DNA molecules are extremely long and in the eukaryotic cell are maintained in orderly and compact three-dimensional structures. Each diploid human cell contains two full complements of the human genome, each copy consisting of approximately 3.2 billion nucleotides. This vast amount of genetic material is organized into 23 homologous chromosome pairs, with each pair contributed by a homolog of maternal origin and the other of paternal origin. Each chromosome is a highly-ordered structure of a single dsDNA molecule, compacted many times with the aid of structural DNA-binding proteins. The chromosomal arrangement of human DNA not only allows the packaging of the vast human genome into the limited physical dimensions of the cell nucleus, but also governs one of the Mendelian laws of inheritance on independent assortment whereby genes located on different chromosomes recombine at random from one generation to the next. In addition, as will be discussed later, the structural organization of the human genome is intimately related to the control of DNA transcription, replication, recombination, and repair.[2,37,46]

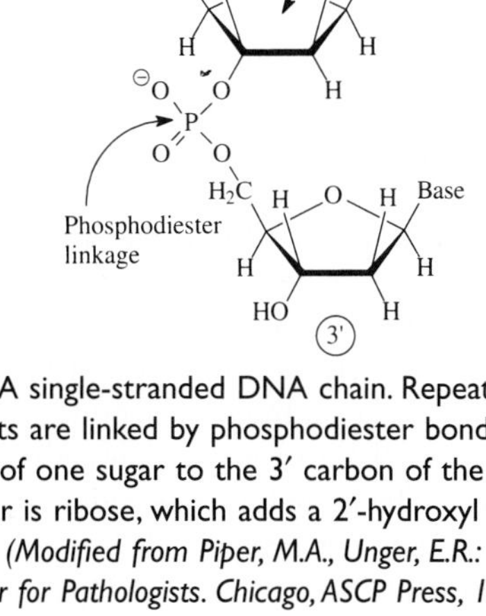

Nuclear DNA in conjunction with its associated structural proteins, including histone and nonhistone proteins, is known as *chromatin*. Chromatin is arranged and organized in a hierarchical fashion where the degree of condensation increases with higher levels of structural organization. The *nucleosome* represents the most basic level of chromatin organization and is present as repeated units along the full length of each chromosome. Each nucleosome unit consists of a nucleosome core particle and 20 to 80 base pairs of linker DNA, which spans between adjacent nucleosomes.[70] A nucleosome core particle involves 146 base pairs of dsDNA tightly wound around an octamer of histone proteins, two each of four histone proteins, namely H2A, H2B, H3, and H4.[71] The linker DNA segments are associated with the linker histone H1. Nucleosomes are further packed in successive levels of complexity wherein the most compact stage,[37] chromatin, appears as discrete mitotic chromosomes as seen in the metaphase of a cell cycle. Integrity of the nucleosomal structure is crucial to the maintenance of the higher-order arrangements of chromatin.[70]

Chromatin condensation is a dynamic process that changes in a coordinated fashion in association with the cell cycle. In general, chromatin is much less condensed during interphase, at which time DNA is replicated. However, the extent of chromatin condensation during interphase varies among regions of the genome. Genomic regions that are rich in genes are in general less compactly organized and are termed *euchromatin*. Regions that are gene-poor or span over transcriptionally silent genes are more densely packed and are called *heterochromatin*. Our understanding of the biological role of heterochromatin and the mechanisms that govern its formation and assembly has improved in recent years. Heterochromatin is important for the maintenance of specialized chromatin structures, X-chromosome inactivation in females, maintenance of genome stability by stabilizing repetitive DNA sequences, and regulation of gene expression.[33] Eukaryote chromosomes contain two specialized regions of heterochromatin, namely the centromeres and telomeres. The former plays an important role in directing the movement of chromosomes between daughter cells during cell division, while the latter contains repetitive nucleotide sequences that are located on and protect the ends of chromosomes. Besides the large centromeric or

Figure 36-2 A single-stranded DNA chain. Repeating nucleotide units are linked by phosphodiester bonds that join the 5′ carbon of one sugar to the 3′ carbon of the next. (In RNA, the sugar is ribose, which adds a 2′-hydroxyl to deoxyribose.) *(Modified from Piper, M.A., Unger, E.R.: Nucleic Acid Probes: A Primer for Pathologists. Chicago, ASCP Press, 1989.)*

telomeric blocks of heterochromatin, smaller domains of heterochromatin are scattered throughout the genome and are associated with the control of gene expression. The assembly of heterochromatin starts at the most basic level of chromatin organization, the nucleosomes, and involves DNA methylation, histone modifications, noncoding RNAs, and sequence-specific DNA binding proteins.[33] The functional implications of the structural organization of chromatin will be discussed further below.

Replication, Transcription, and Translation

Each time a cell divides, the entire DNA content of that cell must be faithfully duplicated, so that the total complement of hereditary information (the *genome* of the organism) is retained in each daughter cell. This process is called *replication*. Owing to the laws of base pairing (i.e., adenine pairs only with thymine, and guanine only with cytosine), the sequence of a single strand of DNA dictates the sequence of its complementary strand. Replication proceeds in a *semi-conservative* fashion, with the two parent strands of a dsDNA molecule each serving as the template for the synthesis of a daughter strand. The duplicated dsDNA molecules produced in this manner are each composed of one parent strand and one daughter strand. For replication to occur, the original double-stranded helix must be separated, which is an energetically unfavorable event. This is accomplished with a combination of DNA-specific proteins and enzymes, and synthesis of both daughter strands proceeds as the parent strands separate. Replication is initiated at multiple sites during this process, but each origin of replication is used only once during a single cell cycle.

Daughter strands are synthesized by *DNA polymerase III*, an enzyme that reads the parent template and attaches nucleotides to the growing daughter strand according to the base-pairing rules of dsDNA. DNA polymerase III begins synthesis at the replication fork, the point of strand separation, with a short RNA primer that base-pairs to the parent template. Later, this primer is excised and replaced with DNA by the DNA repair enzyme, *DNA polymerase I*. Because DNA polymerase III synthesizes DNA only in the 5′-3′ direction, one daughter strand is synthesized continuously, whereas the other must be synthesized discontinuously. The fragments on the discontinuous strand are then joined by the *DNA ligase* enzyme. Many other proteins are involved in unwinding and stabilizing the parent strands for synthesis, in protecting single-stranded regions, in recognizing initiation sites, and in synthesizing the RNA primer. In addition to synthetic capabilities, the DNA polymerases possess an exonuclease or "proofreading" function: When an incorrect nucleotide is added to the growing polymer, a conformational change brings the chain in contact with the exonuclease portion of the enzyme, which excises the incorrect nucleotide. This helps maintain the integrity of the original DNA sequence.

The information in DNA is arranged in units specifying production of proteins and RNA molecules required for cellular function. These units, called *genes*, include coding regions specifying the amino acid sequence of a protein and the regulatory regions controlling the rate and timing of that protein's production. The production of proteins is mediated by RNA molecules that carry the information for specific proteins from the DNA in the nucleus to the cytoplasm, where the proteins are synthesized. These are *messenger RNAs* (mRNAs). The process of transferring the sequence information from the coding regions of DNA to the RNA message is called *transcription*.

Like replication, transcription requires separation of the duplex DNA strands and uses a polymerase to copy the template DNA strand. For transcription, the polymerase is *RNA polymerase II*, which binds to sequences in the regulatory region of the gene called the *promoter*. Promoters occur approximately 100 bases "upstream" (i.e., at the 5′ end) from the initiation site of transcription where the first ribonucleotide unit is paired with the template (uracil pairs with adenine). Promoters are usually rich in thymine and adenine in repeating patterns and have been referred to as a *TATA box*. Initiation of transcription requires many protein cofactors to bind to RNA polymerase to form the active initiation complex. Other regions of DNA known as *enhancers* may interact with the initiation complex to stimulate or repress transcription. Regulation of transcription is the primary mechanism cells use to control gene expression.[88]

Transcription continues until chain termination occurs in response to specific sequences. The RNA transcript quickly detaches from the template DNA because restoration of the DNA-DNA duplex is energetically more favorable than retaining the DNA-RNA hybrid or a segment of ssDNA. The end product is a complementary sequence of ribonucleotides that contains the information necessary for protein synthesis. However, additional modifications are required before mRNA can be exported to the cytoplasm where protein synthesis takes place.[2] The 5′ end is modified by the addition of 7-methyl guanosine residues to form a structure called a *cap*. The 3′ end is modified by the addition of multiple adenine bases, called the *poly A tail*. Both caps and tails are necessary for translation of mRNA into protein, and the poly-A tail may also stabilize the mRNA molecule. Noncoding regions termed *introns* are excised from the mRNA by a molecular complex termed a *spliceosome*. These complexes are composed of multiple small nuclear ribonucleoprotein particles (snRNPs). Spliceosomes mediate the cleavage and ligation of RNA at specific recognition sequences. After the introns are removed, the mRNA contains *exons*, or coding sequences, and is transported into the cytoplasm.

Translation is the process whereby the mRNA sequence directs the amino acid sequence during protein synthesis. Twenty-one amino acids are involved in protein synthesis and each is specified by a three-nucleotide sequence known as a *codon*. Because there are 64 possible codons, most amino acids are specified by more than one codon. In addition, two codons do not code for amino acids but always signal termination of protein synthesis (stop codons), and one codon,

TABLE 36-1 The Genetic Code (Translation of mRNA to Amino Acids During Protein Synthesis)

Nucleotide Position in the Codon					
1st	**2nd**	**3rd**			
		U	C	A	G
U	U	Phenylalanine	Phenylalanine	Leucine	Leucine
	C	Serine	Serine	Serine	Serine
	A	Tyrosine	Tyrosine	Stop	Stop
	G	Cysteine	Cysteine	Selenocysteine*	Tryptophan
C	U	Leucine	Leucine	Leucine	Leucine
	C	Proline	Proline	Proline	Proline
	A	Histidine	Histidine	Glutamine	Glutamine
	G	Arginine	Arginine	Arginine	Arginine
A	U	Isoleucine	Isoleucine	Isoleucine	Methionine
	C	Threonine	Threonine	Threonine	Threonine
	A	Asparagine	Asparagine	Lysine	Lysine
	G	Serine	Serine	Arginine	Arginine
G	U	Valine	Valine	Valine	Valine
	C	Alanine	Alanine	Alanine	Alanine
	A	Aspartic acid	Aspartic acid	Glutamic acid	Glutamic acid
	G	Glycine	Glycine	Glycine	Glycine

*The codon UGA can code for either selenocysteine or stop.

UGA, codes for either a stop or for selenocysteine, depending on the adjacent sequences or RNA-binding proteins.[36] The genetic code is shown in Table 36-1. Translation takes place on *ribosomes,* which are ribonucleoprotein complexes that function as protein synthesis factories. A ribosome binds to the initiation site on mRNA to form an initiation complex. During synthesis, codons are "read" by *transfer RNA* (tRNA), short RNA molecules that have a sequence complementary to an amino acid codon *(anticodon),* and are bound to the amino acid molecule specified by the codon. As synthesis proceeds, the appropriate tRNA anticodon base-pairs with the next mRNA codon. An enzyme on the ribosome then catalyzes the formation of a peptide bond between the amino acid bound to the tRNA and the growing protein chain. The previous tRNA is released and the next tRNA is added. The ribosome moves along the mRNA until a stop codon is reached and synthesis is complete. The ribosome and the protein product are then dissociated from the mRNA. More than one ribosome can move along an mRNA molecule at a time, forming a *polyribosome.*

Genetics and Epigenetics

Genetic and epigenetic phenomena are intimately related. In general, genetic events are related to the sequence information of DNA, and thus include the consequences of the transmission of a particular DNA sequence (e.g., the inheritance of DNA mutations or polymorphisms) or the acquisition of DNA sequence variations (e.g., the accumulation of somatic mutations in aging or cancer development). These genetic issues are discussed in some of the subsequent chapters. On the other hand, there have been inconsistent views regarding the definition of epigenetics.[34] In most circumstances, epigenetics encompasses processes that alter gene function or its interpretation by mechanisms other than those that rely on DNA sequence change.[39] Practically, epigenetics has evolved to include the study of DNA methylation, genomic imprinting, histone modification, chromatin remodeling, and others.[75] Most of these processes add another dimension to gene expression control.

DNA methylation refers to the addition of a methyl group to the fifth carbon position of cytosine residues in CpG dinucleotides. Approximately 80% of all CpG dinucleotides in the human genome are methylated and these mainly include isolated CpG dinucleotides and clusters, termed CpG islands, in nonpromoter DNA repeat elements.[75] These patterns of methylation are faithfully reproduced during DNA replication by maintenance DNA methyltransferases (DNMT1), so that the methylation pattern is inherited by daughter cells at cell division. In addition, DNA methylation is implicated in growth and development of organisms. After embryo fertilization, the genome becomes demethylated (except imprinted loci, see discussion later in this chapter) to pave the way for the establishment of developmentally related patterns of DNA methylation by de novo DNA methyltransferases (DNMT3a and DNMT3b). Genomic imprinting and gene dosage compensation of X-linked genes in females are also mediated by DNA methylation. Genomic imprinting is an epigenetic phenomenon whereby the genetic function of particular alleles is determined by whether it is paternally or maternally inherited. The human insulin-like growth factor-2 H19 *(IGF2-H19)* locus on chromosome 15 is an example of an imprinted locus whereby the disomic inheritance of either the paternal or maternal allele results in significantly different clinical outcomes, namely Prader-Willi and Angelman syndromes, respectively (see Chapter 40, Inherited Diseases). Differential methylation of the imprinted locus from the time of germ cell development allows the recognition of the parental origin of the imprinted alleles by the cellular processes.

Besides growth and development, DNA methylation is a well-recognized epigenetic phenomenon that mediates gene silencing.[43] With the exception of CpG islands within DNA repeat elements, other CpG islands, particularly those found in promoter regions of active genes, are unmethylated in the homeostatic state. If, on the contrary, the promoter CpG islands become hypermethylated, the genes would become transcriptionally silenced. Aberrant hypermethylation of gene promoters, particularly those of tumor suppressor genes and genes involved in DNA repair, is a well-known phenomenon in tumor development.[42] The methylation of gene promoters has been shown to hinder the association of methylation-sensitive transcription factors, thus preventing gene activation. In addition, hypermethylated sites attract the binding of methyl-CpG binding proteins, such as methyl-CpG binding protein 2 (MECP2) and methyl-CpG binding domain proteins (MBD1 and MBD2), which further block the association of a number of transcription factors.[42] More importantly, it is now appreciated that these methyl-CpG binding proteins have the ability to recruit histone deacetylases, a phenomenon that leads to deacetylation of histones and that ultimately represses transcription.

As discussed, histones are an integral part of nucleosomes, the basic repeating structural unit of chromatin. The amino termini of histone proteins can be modified post-translationally by processes that include acetylation, methylation, phosphorylation, and ubiquination.[46] Acetylation of the lysines on the amino termini of histones H3 and H4 by histone acetyltransferases decreases histone-DNA interaction and improves the accessibility of DNA to transcriptional activation. On the contrary, histone deacetylation by histone deacetylases promotes the formation of compact nucleosomes, leading to repression of transcription. Histone deacetylation is in fact a key component to the assembly of heterochromatin, the transcriptionally inactive chromatin.[33] Methylation of the ninth amino acid residue, lysine, on histone H3 generates a binding site for heterochromatin protein (HP1) and thus is another key event in heterochromatin formation.[103] Phosphorylation of the tenth amino acid, serine, on histone H3 is important for chromosome condensation and mitosis.

Besides the histone modifications, nucleosomes can be remodeled by ATP-dependent processes, including octamer sliding, DNA looping, and histone substitution.[46] Octamer sliding allows the relocation of histone octamers to adjacent DNA segments. DNA looping refers to the mechanism whereby the DNA segment originally wrapped around the nucleosome could be unlooped. Histone substitution allows the replacement of octamer subunits with variant histones. Consequently, nucleosomes are dynamic structures that can be remodeled according to the transcriptional demands of the cell. Furthermore, energy-dependent processes also exist that facilitate the remodeling of higher-order chromatin structures with implications on genetic events, such as DNA transcription, replication, repair, and recombination.[75] In summary, gene function is moderated by an interrelated web of epigenetic mechanisms. The interdependency between the control of gene function or expression and the structural organization of chromatin can be appreciated from the dual structural and functional effects of CpG methylation, histone modification, heterochromatin formation, and nucleosomal and chromatin remodeling.

NUCLEAR AND MITOCHONDRIAL GENOMES

Up to this point we have focused our attention on the nuclear genome only. Yet, in fact, it is not the only genome in the cell, the mitochondrial genome being the other important genetic component of eukaryotic cells. The human mitochondrial genome is a circular piece of DNA 16.5 kb in length.[107] Mitochondrial DNA is transmitted between generations by maternal inheritance, with the mitochondria coming from the oocytes and not (usually) from sperm. Multiple copies of mitochondrial DNA are present within each mitochondrion and each cell contains a variable number of mitochondria depending on the energy requirements of the particular cell type. Thus certain cell types may contain up to several thousand copies of mitochondrial DNA.[87,93] This greater abundance, compared with that of nuclear DNA, makes mitochondrial DNA attractive for tests for which sample DNA is limited (e.g., crime scenes, pathogen detection, and paleontology). Mitochondrial DNA is double-stranded for most of its length except at the replication and transcription control region (the D-loop). Unlike the nuclear genome, the mitochondrial genome is not packaged into nucleosomal units. Instead, it has a unique structural organization, which researchers have just begun to unravel.[1,4] It encodes for 13 polypeptides, all involved in the oxidative phosphorylation pathway; two ribosomal RNAs (rRNAs); and all of the 22 tRNAs required for mitochondrial protein synthesis. Several other proteins are also required for normal mitochondrial function and are encoded by nuclear genes.

The mutation rate of mitochondrial DNA is 10 to 20 times higher than that of nuclear DNA. This high rate has been viewed as a result of the poor fidelity of mitochondrial DNA polymerase.[41,55] Germ-line mutations in the mitochondrial genome generally lead to neurodegenerative and/or myopathic diseases, such as MELAS (myopathy, encephalopathy, lactic acidosis, and strokelike episodes) and Leber's hereditary optic neuropathy.[55] Somatic mutations, on the other hand, are associated with aging and cancer development.[108] Consequent to the accumulation of sequence variations, more than one population of mitochondrial DNA sequences may be present in a cell. This state is termed *heteroplasmy* as opposed to homoplasmy in which the cell contains a homogeneous population of mitochondrial genomes. When performing genetic analysis for mitochondrial DNA, a note of caution is warranted on the potential problems related to the presence of nuclear pseudogenes, which are DNA segments in the nuclear genome with significant homology to the mitochondrial genome.[110] The close resemblance of the nuclear and mitochondrial DNA segments may result in the false-positive detection of mitochondrial DNA sequences[109] and thus the specificity of PCR systems for mitochondrial DNA detection needs to be carefully evaluated.[82] Disorders associated with mitochondrial DNA and tests for the disorders are discussed in Chapter 40.

Circulating Nucleic Acids

Apart from studies in the field of virology, most molecular analyses have been performed on DNA and RNA that have been extracted from cells. In the 1940s, however, intriguing data appeared that pointed toward the existence of cell-free DNA and RNA in the plasma of human subjects.[73] However, apart from a handful of reports,[52-54] the field of circulating nucleic acids remained largely dormant until the 1990s. Since that time, interest in cell-free DNA has grown rapidly, largely because of its potential to provide new tools in molecular diagnostics.

Cancer DNA in Plasma

In 1994 two groups simultaneously reported the presence of tumor-associated oncogene mutations in DNA in the plasma and serum of cancer patients.[96,105] These reports were rapidly followed by the detection of other cancer-associated molecular changes in DNA found in plasma and serum, including microsatellite alterations,[10,76] oncogene amplifications,[11] epigenetic changes,[24,111,112] mitochondrial mutations,[80] and viral nucleic acids.[64,74] The detection and quantification of circulating tumor-derived DNA in plasma and serum have been shown to allow the detection,[64] monitoring,[58,66,100] and prognostication of a variety of cancers.[6,44,63]

The mechanism through which DNA is released into the plasma and serum has generally been thought to be because of cell death,[40] probably through a combination of apoptosis and necrosis. Consistent with this view, circulating DNA in cancer patients has been shown to consist mainly of short DNA fragments.[7,32] The functional implication of circulating tumor DNA remains unclear, although provocative hypotheses have been proposed regarding the possibility that such DNA may mediate “genometastasis.”[29,30]

Fetal DNA in Maternal Plasma

The presence of tumor-derived DNA in the plasma of cancer patients has inspired researchers to look for other types of circulating nucleic acids. In particular, the similarity between the placenta and a malignant neoplasm[97] has led to the discovery of cell-free fetal DNA in the plasma and serum of pregnant women.[65] Fetal DNA has been shown to be present in the plasma of almost all pregnant women, from the early first trimester onward,[21] and to be present in increasing concentrations as gestation progresses.[67] Following delivery, fetal DNA is cleared rapidly from maternal plasma, with an apparent half-life on the order of 16 minutes.[69]

The discovery of cell-free fetal DNA in maternal plasma and serum has opened up new possibilities for noninvasive prenatal diagnosis. Fetal DNA is readily detectable in maternal plasma, but most of the DNA in maternal plasma is still of maternal origin.[67] Thus most workers in the field have attempted to detect unique genetic markers that the fetus has inherited from the father (e.g., Y chromosomal markers for a male fetus). This technology has now been used for the noninvasive prenatal diagnosis of a number of conditions, including sex-linked disorders,[21] RhD status,[59] congenital adrenal hyperplasia,[12] achondroplasia,[89] and β-thalassemia.[13] Fetal RhD status determination in RhD-negative women has been adopted as a routine service by several laboratories.[26] In addition to the qualitative mutation analyses of fetal DNA in maternal plasma, quantitative aberrations have also been reported in a number of pregnancy-associated disorders, including preeclampsia,[61,115] preterm labor,[56] trisomy 21,[51,60] hyperemesis gravidarum,[92] and invasive placentation.[91] These data have generally been produced by the measurement of fetal-derived Y chromosomal DNA sequences in the plasma or serum of women carrying male fetuses. Thus if a gender- and polymorphism-independent fetal-specific marker could be developed in the future, fetal DNA measurement might be used as an additional analyte for prenatal screening.

Other Applications of Circulating DNA

Apart from oncology and fetomaternal medicine, plasma DNA also has other applications in molecular diagnostics. In a situation analogous to the presence of a fetus in a preg-nant woman, DNA derived from a transplanted organ has also been detected in the plasma of the transplant recipient.[68,72] It has been hypothesized that a measurement of graft-derived DNA concentration might provide a noninvasive method for monitoring graft rejection, analogous to the situation of urine DNA measurement following kidney transplantation.[113,114] In addition, the association between plasma DNA and cell death[27,28] has also prompted investigators to measure circulating DNA concentration in various conditions associated with tissue injury, including pulmonary embolism,[104] trauma,[48,62,85] myocardial infarction,[8] and stroke.[86]

Plasma RNA

The detection of cell-free DNA in plasma has prompted investigators to see if cell-free RNA may also be present in the plasma. This was first achieved through the detection of tumor-derived RNA, including tumor-associated viral RNA[57] and a tissue-specific mRNA transcript,[47] in the plasma and serum of cancer patients. Since then a number of RNA targets, including telomerase components[9,23] and multiple epithelial mRNA transcripts,[94] have been detected in the plasma and serum of patients suffering from a variety of cancers.

One apparent paradox in the detection of RNA in plasma is the well-known lability of RNA. Indeed, if purified RNA is added to plasma, the RNA molecules are largely degraded within a matter of seconds.[101] However, when endogenous plasma RNA is studied, the RNA molecules have been shown to be remarkably stable, with concentrations remaining unchanged for extended periods at room temperature.[101] The stability of endogenous plasma RNA has recently been shown to be related to the fact that such RNA molecules appear to be associated with particulate matter.[78] One possible nature of such particulate matter is apoptotic bodies.[35]

Fetal RNA has been found in the plasma of pregnant women.[83] Recently, the placenta has been shown to be a major organ responsible for the release of fetal RNA into maternal plasma.[79] Thus placental mRNA transcripts, such as human placental lactogen,[79] the beta-subunit of human chorionic gonadotropin,[79] and corticotrophin releasing hormone,[77] have been detected in maternal plasma. Through the use of expression microarray analysis, literally hundreds of new fetal RNA markers potentially suitable for maternal plasma detection could be developed.[102] The quantitative analysis of placental mRNA in maternal plasma has the potential to be used in the monitoring of pregnancy-associated disorders such as preeclampsia.[25,77]

Apart from cancer and pregnancy, circulating RNA has also been detected in patients with acute trauma.[84] It is expected that further clinical applications will be forthcoming during the next few years.

NUCLEIC ACID ISOLATION

Many of the key advances in understanding of DNA and RNA have been achieved by study of purified nucleic acids. In the molecular diagnostic laboratory, some tests can be performed directly on samples of biological fluids, but techniques for isolation of nucleic acids often are critical.

DNA Isolation

Extraction of DNA and/or RNA is a key preliminary step to subsequent molecular analysis. Quite a number of protocols have been developed over the years. In selecting the most appropriate protocol for one's laboratory, some of the issues worth considering include the specimen type and volume required, yield, purity, size of the isolated nucleic acids, ease of operation, throughput, cost, and whether the protocol involves the use of hazardous reagents or is amenable to automation. With the advent of PCR, molecular analyses could be performed on a variety of specimens, including whole blood, plasma, serum, tissue biopsies, cultured cells, buccal swabs, cerebrospinal fluids, amniotic fluids, paraffin-embedded tissue, and so on. Although there are a variety of commercial protocols available for DNA extraction, most protocols can be classified into a few categories that involve either liquid- or solid-phase extraction. In general, solid-phase extraction methods are more commonly used because of the relative ease of operation, the ability to process large batches of specimens, high reproducibility, and adaptability to automation. However, solution-based methods are still favored when large quantities of DNA or large sample volumes are involved.

Because the phosphate esters of the nucleic acid backbone are strong acids and exist as anions at neutral pH, DNA is soluble in water up to about 1% of weight of solute per volume of solution and can be precipitated by the addition of alcohol. Alcohol precipitation has therefore been used in many nucleic acid extraction protocols. In general, most DNA extraction protocols involve an initial step of cell lysis whereby both the cellular and nuclear membrane envelopes are disrupted. Cellular proteins are then removed by salt precipitation or degraded enzymatically. An additional step of RNase digestion is optional. The genomic DNA that remains in solution is then precipitated by the addition of alcohol. The DNA precipitate is isolated and rehydrated. The resultant DNA extract can be stored until subsequent analysis. For the solution-based protocols, cellular and protein debris is usually separated from the soluble DNA fraction by solvent extraction through the use of solvents with different solubility constants. The well-known phenol-chloroform protocols are based on this principle. After the DNA is precipitated by alcohol, the DNA pellet is isolated by manual removal of the excess alcohol solution. Careful attention to this step is required to prevent the inadvertent removal of the DNA pellet, which can be quite fine or loose in some instances. Before rehydration of the DNA pellet, it is air-dried to remove the remaining drops of alcohol. Because of the number of manual steps involved, the sample throughput of these solution-based methods is limited.

On the other hand, solid-phase extraction methods are more robust. These methods involve the use of either silica membranes or magnetic particles. Both methods take advantage of the reversible binding of DNA with the respective solid phases. Silica can bind nucleic acids in a reversible manner dependent on the ionic strength of the environment.[95] Silica-based methods usually involve the impregnation of silica onto a filter, which is housed in a plastic column. After cell lysis and protein digestion, DNA is precipitated by the addition of alcohol. The solution is then allowed to pass through the silica-impregnated filter, which binds and purifies the DNA from other debris present in the alcohol solution. Either centrifugation or vacuum manifolds can be used for the filtration step. The bound DNA is usually washed and subsequently eluted using nuclease-free water or low ionic strength buffers. Similarly, methods based on the use of magnetic particles allow the isolation and purification of alcohol-precipitated DNA from other debris by placing the solution under a magnetic field whereby DNA molecules precoated with magnetic beads are retained. The magnetic beads are subsequently removed from the purified DNA before the final elution step. Both the silica-based and magnetic particle–based methods are applicable to various scales of operation. Isolated columns can be used for the extraction of a small number of specimens. The 96-well plate formats are available from some commercial providers, and allow the processing of specimens at medium throughput. Moreover, the protocols can be further adapted for use on automated platforms for large-scale processing.[22,50]

RNA Isolation

RNA analysis and therefore RNA extraction are required for studies on gene expression. RNA molecules are generally less stable than DNA because unlike DNA, RNA is not protected by a stable double-helical conformation and in addition, RNA is subject to alkaline hydrolysis via its 2′-hydroxyl group of the ribose moiety. Although both DNA and RNA can be degraded enzymatically by DNA- and RNA-specific nucleases (DNase and RNase, respectively), RNases are nearly ubiquitous, making it much more difficult to work with native RNA molecules in the laboratory. Thus certain issues warrant special attention when one works with RNA, including its extraction.[20] Because of the inherent instability of RNA, clinical specimens intended for RNA analysis should either be processed promptly in the fresh state; preserved by the immediate addition of preservation agents, such as RNA*later*™ (Ambion®, Austin, TX); or snap-frozen by liquid nitrogen. The number of freeze-thaw cycles should be minimized and this is equally applicable to solutions of extracted RNA. Utmost care is needed to prevent RNase contamination and this includes the use of RNase-free reagents, RNase-free plastic ware, and the cleaning or decontamination of the working surfaces and equipment with RNase-free detergents or chemicals. Water treated with diethylpyrocarbonate (DEPC) for the inactivation of RNase should be used. As the DNA sequence of eukaryotic genes differs from their mRNA counterparts only by the presence of introns, there exists a possibility in which both DNA and RNA segments are co-amplified in specimens contaminated with DNA. Therefore care must be taken to avoid DNA contamination. Alternatively, DNA digestion by DNase I treatment is commonly incorporated as an additional step during the process of RNA purification.

The underlying principles for RNA extraction are essentially identical to those of DNA isolation and purification. Both solution-based and solid-phase extraction protocols are available. Similarly, RNA molecules are first released by lysis of cells; isolated and purified from the protein and lipid debris, either by phenol-chloroform extraction or reversible binding to silica; and precipitated by use of alcohol. However, the composition of lysis buffers typically includes phenol (e.g., Trizol, Invitrogen, Carlsbad, Calif.), sodium dodecyl sulfate, or guanidinium salts, as these buffers not only lyse cells directly, but also inhibit RNase effectively.[14] The successful isolation of high quality RNA is thus dependent to some extent on the degree of cellular exposure to these denaturants. Therefore tissue specimens need to be ground to a fine powder form before lysis. To prevent RNA degradation during grinding, the procedure should be performed on either snap-frozen tissue or specimens preserved with RNA stabilizing agents.[20] The above procedures are relevant to the isolation of total RNA, which comprises mRNAs, rRNAs, small nuclear RNAs, and tRNAs. However, protocols have been developed for the isolation of mRNA, which are based on the capture of the polyadenylated tails on the 3′ ends of mRNA by hybridization to cellulose-bound oligo(dT) molecules.[20]

Assessment of Nucleic Acid Yield and Quality

Nucleic acid molecules absorb ultraviolet light maximally at 260 nm owing almost entirely to the constituent bases. Thus DNA or RNA yield can be quantified by spectrophotometric measurement of the absorbance at 260 nm. Alternatively, isolated nucleic acids can be subjected to agarose gel electrophoresis and their yield quantified by densitometric measurements.

Both spectrophotometric and densitometric methods can be used for the assessment of the quality of the extraction of DNA and RNA. Purity can be evaluated by assessing the ratio of the absorbances at 260 nm and 280 nm (A_{260}/A_{280}), the latter reflecting the presence of the aromatic amino acids in contaminating protein. Values greater than 1.8 indicate minimal contamination with protein. The sizes of the isolated genomic DNA can be estimated by gel electrophoresis. Total RNA integrity can be assessed by estimating the size distribution of the extracted RNA and the appearances of the 18S and 28S rRNA peaks. With RNase degradation, the RNA size distribution will be shifted toward the smaller fragments and the rRNA peaks would become less discernible. Similarly, high quality mRNA preparations isolated by oligo(dT)-cellulose should display broad size ranges.

In assessing the yield and quality of DNA/RNA extracts, electrophoretic methods provide better precision and more information regarding quality, for instance the size distribution of the isolated DNA/RNA. Yet, these methods generally require significantly higher amounts of the extracted sample when compared with spectrophotometric assessment. However, automated analyzers that use prefabricated chips with microfluidic channels and are designed for the electrophoresis of microvolumes of DNA and RNA have become available.[81] These instruments allow the sensitive and precise quantification and qualitative assessment of nucleic acids.

Techniques for analysis of nucleic acids are described in the next chapter.

THE HUMAN GENOME PROJECT

The Human Genome Project is the biggest biological project ever undertaken by mankind. Apart from its ambitious goal of deciphering the 3 billion base pairs that make up the human genetic code, it also represents a model for the planning, organization, and execution of large-scale biological projects.[16,17] The first serious discussion of the feasibility of such a project can be traced back to the mid 1980s. In 1988 a special committee of the U.S. National Research Council of the U.S. National Academy of Sciences formulated a 15-

year human genome project, costing some $200 million a year. A genetic map with 1 cM resolution was accomplished in September 1994. A physical map involving 52,000 sequence-tagged sites (STSs) was completed in October 1998. The final journey to the completion of this project was marked by a highly publicized race between a publicly funded group of investigators and a private effort. The public effort, undertaken by the International Human Genome Sequencing Consortium, consisted of investigators from 20 centers located in six countries: the United States, the United Kingdom, Japan, China, France, and Germany. The completion of a draft sequence was announced June 26, 2000, and it was published in two landmark papers, one from the public team and one from the private team, in February 2001.[49,106] The final sequence was accomplished in April 2003, with 99.99% sequencing accuracy, with no gaps.

The human genome consists of 3.2 Gb of DNA. Among these sequences, some 2.95 Gb consists of weakly staining, potentially gene-rich euchromatic regions. Only some 1.1% to 1.4% is sequence that encodes proteins. Over half of the DNA consists of various types of repeated sequences. The number of genes in the human genome has been estimated to be between 26,000 and 31,000. These estimates provide an interesting comparison with the 6000 genes estimated for a yeast cell, 13,000 for a fruit fly, 18,000 for a worm, and 26,000 for a plant.[3] With the basic sequence decoded, the project that awaits biologists would be the even more difficult task of elucidating the biological functions of these stretches of DNA.

An understanding of our genetic heritage has the potential of providing a quantum leap in our understanding of the biology of life. It would also greatly enhance our ability to elucidate the molecular basis of diseases. For example, through the data generated from the Human Genome Project, new disease-associated genes are being discovered almost every week, as compared with the early multiyear efforts that resulted in the identification of the genes responsible for each single-gene disorder, such as cystic fibrosis.[45] Developments in the genome project have also given us enhanced ability to develop tests for the molecular diagnosis of numerous diseases. In the longer term, these developments also provide new targets for the pharmaceutical industry.

Apart from its scientific merits, it is important to realize the enormous nonscientific implications of the Human Genome Project. It was visionary for the early proponents of the Human Genome Project to set aside part of the budget of the project to study the social, legal, and ethical implications of this project.[15] The most commonly expressed fear by the public is that genetic information may be used in ways that could harm people, such as barring them from getting insurance, employment, or other social opportunities. Important steps have been taken by legislators to safeguard against genetic discrimination, such as the passing of the Genetic Information Nondiscrimination Act by the U.S. Senate in 2003.[18]

The Human Genome Project can be regarded as a foundation on which future large-scale biological projects can be built.[17] One important extension of our knowledge of the human genome is a detailed understanding of the heritable variation in the human genome. One class of such variations is the single nucleotide polymorphisms (SNPs). A public project, the International HapMap Project, has been launched to study the patterns of linkage disequilibrium and haplotypes across the human genome and to characterize SNPs.[98] Another large-scale project is the Encyclopedia of DNA Elements (ENCODE) Project (http://www.genome.gov/ENCODE/), which aims to identify all of the functional elements in the human genome. A feasibility study involving 1% of the human genome has been done. Our understanding of life is likely to be expanded in a synergistic manner by related efforts, such as the Human Epigenome Project,[5] which aims to elucidate all of the methylation sites in the 30,000 human genes in approximately 200 samples, and the rapidly growing field of proteomics. The twenty-first century will likely be the century when a key biological revolution will take place.

REFERENCES

1. Alam TI, Kanki T, Muta T, Ukaji K, Abe Y, Nakayama H, et al. Human mitochondrial DNA is packaged with TFAM. Nucleic Acids Res 2003;21:1640-5.
2. Alberts B, Johnson A, Lewis J, Raff M, Roberts K, Walter P. Molecular biology of the cell. 4th ed. New York: Garland Science, 2002.
3. Baltimore D. Our genome unveiled. Nature 2001;409:814-16.
4. Bogenhagen DF, Wang Y, Shen EL, Kobayashi R. Protein components of mitochondrial DNA nucleoids in higher eukaryotes. Mol Cell Proteomics 2003;2:1205-16.
5. Bradbury J. Human Epigenome Project-Up and Running. PLoS Biol 2003;1:E82.
6. Chan ATC, Lo YMD, Zee B, Chan LYS, Ma BB, Leung SF, et al. Plasma Epstein-Barr virus DNA and residual disease after radiotherapy for undifferentiated nasopharyngeal carcinoma. J Natl Cancer Inst 2002;94:1614-19.
7. Chan KCA, Zhang J, Chan ATC, Lei KI, Leung SF, Chan LYS, et al. Molecular characterization of circulating EBV DNA in the plasma of nasopharyngeal carcinoma and lymphoma patients. Cancer Res 2003;63:2028-32.
8. Chang CP, Chia RH, Wu TL, Tsao KC, Sun CF, Wu JT. Elevated cell-free serum DNA detected in patients with myocardial infarction. Clin Chim Acta 2003;327:95-101.
9. Chen XQ, Bonnefoi H, Pelte MF, Lyautey J, Lederrey C, Movarekhi S, et al. Telomerase RNA as a detection marker in the serum of breast cancer patients. Clin Cancer Res 2000;6:3823-6.
10. Chen XQ, Stroun M, Magnenat JL, Nicod LP, Kurt AM, Lyautey J, et al. Microsatellite alterations in

plasma DNA of small cell lung cancer patients. Nature Med 1996;2:1033-5.
11. Chiang PW, Beer DG, Wei WL, Orringer MB, Kurnit DM. Detection of erbB-2 amplifications in tumors and sera from esophageal carcinoma patients. Clin Cancer Res 1999;5:1381-6.
12. Chiu RWK, Lau TK, Cheung PT, Gong ZQ, Leung TN, Lo YMD. Noninvasive prenatal exclusion of congenital adrenal hyperplasia by maternal plasma analysis: a feasibility study. Clin Chem 2002;48:778-80.
13. Chiu RWK, Lau TK, Leung TN, Chow KCK, Chui DKH, Lo YMD. Prenatal exclusion of beta-thalassaemia major by examination of maternal plasma. Lancet 2002;360:998-1000.
14. Chomczynski P, Sacchi N. Single-step method of RNA isolation by acid guanidinium thiocyanate-phenol-chloroform extraction. Anal Biochem 1987;162:156-9.
15. Clayton EW. Ethical, legal, and social implications of genomic medicine. N Engl J Med 2003;349:562-9.
16. Collins FS, Green ED, Guttmacher AE, Guyer MS. A vision for the future of genomics research. Nature 2003;422:835-47.
17. Collins FS, Morgan M, Patrinos A. The human genome project: lessons from large-scale biology. Science 2003;300:286-90.
18. Collins FS, Watson JD. Genetic discrimination: time to act. Science 2003;302:745.
19. Conn GL, Draper DE. RNA structure. Curr Opin Struct Biol 1998;8:278-85.
20. Connolly MA, Clausen PA, Lazar JG. RNA purification. In: Dveksler GS, ed. PCR Primer: A laboratory manual. 2nd ed. New York: Cold Spring Harbor Laboratory Press, 2003:117-33.
21. Costa JM, Benachi A, Gautier E. New strategy for prenatal diagnosis of X-linked disorders. N Engl J Med 2002;346:1502.
22. Costa JM, Ernault P. Automated assay for fetal DNA analysis in maternal serum. Clin Chem 2002;48:679-80.
23. Dasi F, Lledo S, Garcia-Granero E, Ripoll R, Marugan M, Tormo M, et al. Real-time quantification in plasma of human telomerase reverse transcriptase (hTERT) mRNA: a simple blood test to monitor disease in cancer patients. Lab Invest 2001;81:767-9.
24. Esteller M, Sanchez-Cespedes M, Roesll R, Sidransky D, Baylin SB, Herman JG. Detection of aberrant promoter hypermethylation of tumor suppressor genes in serum DNA from non-small cell lung cancer patients. Cancer Res 1999;59:67-70.
25. Ferguson-Smith MA. Placental mRNA in maternal plasma: prospects for fetal screening. Proc Natl Acad Sci U S A 2003;100:4360-2.
26. Finning KM, Martin PG, Soothill PW, Avent ND. Prediction of fetal D status from maternal plasma: introduction of a new noninvasive fetal RHD genotyping service. Transfusion 2002;42:1079-85.
27. Fournie GJ, Courtin JP, Laval F, Chale JJ, Pourrat JP, Pujazon MC, et al. Plasma DNA as a marker of cancerous cell death. Investigations in patients suffering from lung cancer and in nude mice bearing human tumours. Cancer Lett 1995;91:221-7.
28. Fournie GJ, Martres F, Pourrat JP, Alary C, Rumeau M. Plasma DNA as cell death marker in elderly patients. Gerontology 1993;39:215-21.
29. Garcia-Olmo D, Garcia-Olmo DC. Functionality of circulating DNA: the hypothesis of genometastasis. Ann N Y Acad Sci 2001;945:265-75.
30. Garcia-Olmo D, Garcia-Olmo DC, Ontanon J, Martinez E, Vallejo M. Tumor DNA circulating in the plasma might play a role in metastasis. The hypothesis of the genometastatis. Histol Histopathol 1999;14:1159-64.
31. Garwin L, Lincoln T. A century of *Nature*: twenty-one discoveries that changed science and the world. Chicago: The University of Chicago Press, 2003.
32. Giacona MB, Ruben GC, Iczkowski KA, Roos TB, Porter DM, Sorenson GD. Cell-free DNA in human blood plasma: length measurements in patients with pancreatic cancer and healthy controls. Pancreas 1998;17:89-97.
33. Grewal SI, Moazed D. Heterochromatin and epigenetic control of gene expression. Science 2003;301:798-802.
34. Griesmer J. What is "epi" about epigenetics? Ann N Y Acad Sci 2002;981:97-110.
35. Hasselmann DO, Rappl G, Tilgen W, Reinhold U. Extracellular tyrosinase mRNA within apoptotic bodies is protected from degradation in human serum. Clin Chem 2001;47:1488-9.
36. Hatfield DL, Gladyshev VN. How selenium has altered our understanding of the genetic code. Mol Cell Biol 2002;22:3565-76.
37. Horn PJ, Peterson CL. Molecular biology. Chromatin higher order folding—wrapping up transcription. Science 2002;297:1824-7.
38. Isaacson W. The biotech century. Time 1999 Jan 11:42-3.
39. Jablonka E, Lamb MJ. The changing concept of epigenetics. Ann N Y Acad Sci 2002;981:82-96.
40. Jahr S, Hentze H, Englisch S, Hardt D, Fackelmayer FO, Hesch RD, et al. DNA fragments in the blood plasma of cancer patients: quantitations and evidence for their origin from apoptotic and necrotic cells. Cancer Res 2001;61:1659-65.
41. Johnson AA, Johnson KA. Fidelity of nucleotide incorporation by human mitochondrial DNA polymerase. J Biol Chem 2001;276:38090-6.
42. Jones PA, Baylin SB. The fundamental role of epigenetic events in cancer. Nat Rev Genet 2002;3:415-28.
43. Jones PA, Takai D. The role of DNA methylation in mammalian epigenetics. Science 2001;293:1068-70.

44. Kawakami K, Brabender J, Lord RV, Groshen S, Greenwald BD, Krasna MJ, et al. Hypermethylated APC DNA in plasma and prognosis of patients with esophageal adenocarcinoma. J Natl Cancer Inst 2000;92:1805-11.
45. Kerem B, Rommens JM, Buchanan JA, Markiewicz D, Cox TK, Chakravarti A, et al. Identification of the cystic fibrosis gene: genetic analysis. Science 1989;245:1073-80.
46. Khorasanizadeh S. The nucleosome: from genomic organization to genomic regulation. Cell 2004;116:259-72.
47. Kopreski M, Benko FA, Kwak LW, Gocke CD. Detection of tumor messenger RNA in the serum of patients with malignant melanoma. Clin Cancer Res 1999;5:1961-5.
48. Lam NYL, Rainer TH, Chan LYS, Joynt GM, Lo YMD. Time course of early and late changes in plasma DNA in trauma patients. Clin Chem 2003;49:1286-91.
49. Lander ES, Linton LM, Birren B, Nusbaum C, Zody MC, Baldwin J, et al. Initial sequencing and analysis of the human genome. Nature 2001;409:860-921.
50. Leb V, Stocher M, Valentine-Thon E, Holzl G, Kessler H, Stekel H, et al. Fully automated, internally controlled quantification of hepatitis B Virus DNA by real-time PCR by use of the MagNA Pure LC and LightCycler instruments. J Clin Microbiol 2004;42:585-90.
51. Lee T, LeShane ES, Messerlian GM, Canick JA, Farina A, Heber WW, et al. Down syndrome and cell-free fetal DNA in archived maternal serum. Am J Obstet Gynecol 2002;187:1217-21.
52. Leon SA, Ehrlich GE, Shapiro B, Labbate VA. Free DNA in the serum of rheumatoid arthritis patients. J Rheumatol 1977;4:139-43.
53. Leon SA, Shapiro B, Servi P, Parsons RG. A comparison of DNA and DNA-binding protein levels in malignant disease. Eur J Cancer 1981;17:533-8.
54. Leon SA, Shapiro B, Sklaroff DM, Yaros MJ. Free DNA in the serum of cancer patients and the effect of therapy. Cancer Res 1977;37:646-50.
55. Leonard JV, Schapira AH. Mitochondrial respiratory chain disorders I: mitochondrial DNA defects. Lancet 2000;355:299-304.
56. Leung TN, Zhang J, Lau TK, Hjelm NM, Lo YMD. Maternal plasma fetal DNA as a marker for preterm labour. Lancet 1998;352:1904-5.
57. Lo KW, Lo YMD, Leung SF, Tsang YS, Chan LYS, Johnson PJ, et al. Analysis of cell-free Epstein-Barr virus associated RNA in the plasma of patients with nasopharyngeal carcinoma. Clin Chem 1999;45: 1292-4.
58. Lo YMD, Chan LYS, Chan ATC, Leung SF, Lo KW, Zhang J, et al. Quantitative and temporal correlation between circulating cell-free Epstein-Barr virus DNA and tumor recurrence in nasopharyngeal carcinoma. Cancer Res 1999;59:5452-5.
59. Lo YMD, Hjelm NM, Fidler C, Sargent IL, Murphy MF, Chamberlain PF, et al. Prenatal diagnosis of fetal RhD status by molecular analysis of maternal plasma. N Engl J Med 1998;339:1734-8.
60. Lo YMD, Lau TK, Zhang J, Leung TN, Chang AM, Hjelm NM, et al. Increased fetal DNA concentrations in the plasma of pregnant women carrying fetuses with trisomy 21. Clin Chem 1999;45:1747-51.
61. Lo YMD, Leung TN, Tein MS, Sargent IL, Zhang J, Lau TK, et al. Quantitative abnormalities of fetal DNA in maternal serum in preeclampsia. Clin Chem 1999;45:184-8.
62. Lo YMD, Rainer TH, Chang LYS, Hjelm NM, Cocks RA. Plasma DNA as a prognostic marker in trauma patients. Clin Chem 2000;46:319-23.
63. Lo YMD, Chan ATC, Chan LYS, Leung SF, Lam CW, Huang DP, et al. Molecular prognostication of nasopharyngeal carcinoma by quantitative analysis of circulating Epstein-Barr virus DNA. Cancer Res 2000;60:6878-81.
64. Lo YMD, Chan LYS, Lo KW, Leung SF, Zhang J, Chan ATC, et al. Quantitative analysis of cell-free Epstein-Barr virus DNA in plasma of patients with nasopharyngeal carcinoma. Cancer Res 1999;59:1188-91.
65. Lo YMD, Corbetta N, Chamberlain PF, Rai V, Sargent IL, Redman CW, et al. Presence of fetal DNA in maternal plasma and serum. Lancet 1997;350:485-7.
66. Lo YMD, Leung SF, Chan LYS, Chan ATC, Lo KW, Johnson PJ, et al. Kinetics of plasma Epstein-Barr virus DNA during radiation therapy for nasopharyngeal carcinoma. Cancer Res 2000;60:2351-5.
67. Lo YMD, Tein MS, Lau TK, Haines CJ, Leung TN, Poon PM, et al. Quantitative analysis of fetal DNA in maternal plasma and serum: implications for noninvasive prenatal diagnosis. Am J Hum Genet 1998;62:768-75.
68. Lo YMD, Tein MSC, Pang CCP, Yeung CK, Tong KL, Hjelm NM. Presence of donor-specific DNA in plasma of kidney and liver-transplant recipients. Lancet 1998;351:1329-30.
69. Lo YMD, Zhang J, Leung TN, Lau TK, Chang AM, Hjelm NM. Rapid clearance of fetal DNA from maternal plasma. Am J Hum Genet 1999;64:218-24.
70. Luger K. Structure and dynamic behavior of nucleosomes. Curr Opin Genet Dev 2003;13:127-35.
71. Luger K, Mader AW, Richmond RK, Sargent DF, Richmond TJ. Crystal structure of the nucleosome core particle at 2.8 A resolution. Nature 1997;389: 251-60.
72. Lui YYN, Woo KS, Wang AYM, Yeung CK, Li PKT, Chau E, et al. Origin of plasma cell-free DNA after solid organ transplantation. Clin Chem 2003;49: 495-6.

73. Mandel P, Métais P. Les acides nucléiques du plasma sanguin chez l'homme. C. R. Acad. Sci. Paris 1948;142:241-3.
74. Mutirangura A, Pornthanakasem W, Theamboonlers A, Sriuranpong V, Lersanguansinchi P, Yenrudi S, et al. Epstein-Barr viral DNA in serum of patients with nasopharyngeal carcinoma. Clin Cancer Res 1998;4:665-9.
75. Nakao M. Epigenetics: interaction of DNA methylation and chromatin. Gene 2001;278:25-31.
76. Nawroz H, Koch W, Anker P, Stroun M, Sidransky D. Microsatellite alterations in serum DNA of head and neck cancer patients. Nature Med 1996;2:1035-7.
77. Ng EKO, Leung TN, Tsui NBY, Lau TK, Panesar NS, Chiu RWK, et al. The concentration of circulating corticotropin-releasing hormone mRNA in maternal plasma is increased in preeclampsia. Clin Chem 2003;49:727-31.
78. Ng EKO, Tsui NBY, Lam NYL, Chiu RWK, Yu SC, Wong SC, et al. Presence of filterable and nonfilterable mRNA in the plasma of cancer patients and healthy individuals. Clin Chem 2002;48:1212-17.
79. Ng EKO, Tsui NBY, Lau TK, Leung TN, Chiu RWK, Panesar NS, et al. mRNA of placental origin is readily detectable in maternal plasma. Proc Natl Acad Sci USA 2003;100:4748-53.
80. Nomoto S, Yamashita K, Koshikawa K, Nakao A, Sidransky D. Mitochondrial D-loop mutations as clonal markers in multicentric hepatocellular carcinoma and plasma. Clin Cancer Res 2002;8: 481-7.
81. Panaro NJ, Yuen PK, Sakazume T, Fortina P, Kricka LJ, Wilding P. Evaluation of DNA fragment sizing and quantification by the Agilent 2100 bioanalyzer. Clin Chem 2000;46:1851-3.
82. Parfait B, Rustin P, Munnich A, Rotig A. Co-amplification of nuclear pseudogenes and assessment of heteroplasmy of mitochondrial DNA mutations. Biochem Biophys Res Commun 1998;247:57-9.
83. Poon LLM, Leung TN, Lau TK, Lo YMD. Presence of fetal RNA in maternal plasma. Clin Chem 2000;46:1832-4.
84. Rainer TH, Lam NYL, Tsui NBY, Ng EKO, Chiu RWK, Joynt GM, et al. Effects of filtration on glyceraldehyde-3-phosphate dehydrogenase mRNA in the plasma of trauma patients and healthy individuals. Clin Chem 2004;50:206-8.
85. Rainer TH, Lo YMD, Chan LYS, Lam NYL, Lit LCW, Cocks RA. Derivation of a prediction rule for posttraumatic organ failure using plasma DNA and other variables. Ann N Y Acad Sci 2001;945: 211-20.
86. Rainer TH, Wong LK, Lam W, Yuen E, Lam NYL, Metreweli C, et al. Prognostic use of circulating plasma nucleic acid concentrations in patients with acute stroke. Clin Chem 2003;49:562-9.
87. Robin ED, Wong R. Mitochondrial DNA molecules and virtual number of mitochondria per cell in mammalian cells. J Cell Physiol 1988;136:507-13.
88. Rosenthal N. Regulation of gene expression. N Engl J Med 1994;331:931-3.
89. Saito H, Sekizawa A, Morimoto T, Suzuki M, Yanaihara T. Prenatal DNA diagnosis of a single-gene disorder from maternal plasma. Lancet 2000;356:1170.
90. Sambrook J, Russell DW. Molecular cloning: a laboratory manual. 3rd ed. New York: Cold Spring Harbor Laboratory Press, 2001.
91. Sekizawa A, Jimbo M, Saito H, Iwasaki M, Sugito Y, Yukimoto Y, et al. Increased cell-free fetal DNA in plasma of two women with invasive placenta. Clin Chem 2002;48:353-4.
92. Sekizawa A, Sugito Y, Iwasaki M, Watanabe A, Jimbo M, Hoshi S, et al. Cell-free fetal DNA is increased in plasma of women with hyperemesis gravidarum. Clin Chem 2001;47:2164-5.
93. Shuster RC, Rubenstein AJ, Wallace DC. Mitochondrial DNA in anucleate human blood cells. Biochem Biophys Res Commun 1988;155:1360-5.
94. Silva JM, Dominguez G, Silva J, Garcia JM, Sanchez A, Rodriguez O, et al. Detection of epithelial messenger RNA in the plasma of breast cancer patients is associated with poor prognosis tumor characteristics. Clin Cancer Res 2001;7:2821-5.
95. Smith C, Otto P, Bitner R, Shiels G. DNA purification. In: Dveksler GS, ed. PCR primer: A laboratory manual. 2nd ed. New York: Cold Spring Harbor Laboratory Press, 2003:87-115.
96. Sorenson GD, Pribish DM, Valone FH, Memoli VA, Bzik DJ, Yao SL. Soluble normal and mutated DNA sequences from single-copy genes in human blood. Cancer Epidemiol Biomarkers Prev 1994;3: 67-71.
97. Strickland S, Richards WG. Invasion of the trophoblasts. Cell 1992;71:355-7.
98. The International HapMap Consortium. The International HapMap Project. Nature 2003;426: 789-96.
99. Thirumalai D. Native secondary structure formation in RNA may be a slave to tertiary folding. Proc Natl Acad Sci U S A 1998;95:11506-8.
100. To EWH, Chan KCA, Leung SF, Chan LYS, To KF, Chan ATC, et al. Rapid clearance of plasma Epstein-Barr virus DNA following surgical treatment of nasopharyngeal carcinoma. Clin Cancer Res 2003;9:3254-9.
101. Tsui NBY, Ng EKO, Lo YMD. Stability of endogenous and added RNA in blood specimens, serum, and plasma. Clin Chem 2002;48:1647-53.
102. Tsui NBY, Chim SSC, Chiu RWK, Lau TK, Ng EKO, Leung TN, et al. Systematic microarray-based identification of placental mRNA in maternal plasma:

towards non-invasive prenatal gene expression profiling. J Med Genet 2004;41:461-7.
103. Urnov FD. Methylation and the genome: the power of a small amendment. J Nutr 2002;132:2450S-2456S.
104. Vargo JS, Becker DM, Philbrick JT, Schoonover FW, Davis JS. Plasma DNA. A simple, rapid test for aiding the diagnosis of pulmonary embolism. Chest 1990;97:63-8.
105. Vasioukhin V, Anker P, Maurice P, Lyautey J, Lederrey C, Stroun M. Point mutations of the N-Ras gene in the blood plasma DNA of patients with myelodysplastic syndrome or acute myelogenous leukaemia. Br J Haematol 1994;86:774-9.
106. Venter JC, Adams MD, Myers EW, Li PW, Mural RJ, Sutton GG, et al. The sequence of the human genome. Science 2001;291:1304-51.
107. Wallace DC. Mitochondrial disease in man and mouse. Science 1999;283:1482-8.
108. Wallace DC. A mitochondrial paradigm for degenerative diseases and ageing. Novartis Found Symp 2001;235:247-63; discussion 263-6.
109. Wallace DC, Stugard C, Murdock D, Schurr T, Brown MD. Ancient mtDNA sequences in the human nuclear genome: a potential source of errors in identifying pathogenic mutations. Proc Natl Acad Sci U S A 1997;94:14900-5.
110. Woischnik M, Moraes CT. Pattern of organization of human mitochondrial pseudogenes in the nuclear genome. Genome Res 2002;12:885-93.
111. Wong IH, Lo YMD, Zhang J, Liew CT, Ng MH, Wong N, et al. Detection of aberrant p16 methylation in the plasma and serum of liver cancer patients. Caner Res 1999;59:71-3.
112. Wong IH, Zhang J, Lai PB, Lau WY, Lo YMD. Quantitative analysis of tumor-derived methylated p16INK4a sequences in plasma, serum, and blood cells of hepatocellular carcinoma patients. Clin Cancer Res 2003;9:1047-52.
113. Zhang J, Tong KL, Li PK, Chan AY, Yeung CK, Pang CC, et al. Presence of donor-and recipient-derived DNA in cell-free urine samples of renal transplantation recipients: urinary DNA chimerism. Clin Chem 1999;45:1741-6.
114. Zhong XY, Hahn D, Troeger C, Klemm A, Stein G, Thomson P, et al. Cell-free DNA in urine: a marker for kidney graft rejection, but not for prenatal diagnosis? Ann N Y Acad Sci 2001;945:250-7.
115. Zhong XY, Laivuori H, Livingston JC, Ylikorkala O, Sibai BM, Holzgreve W, et al. Elevation of both maternal and fetal extracellular circulating deoxyribonucleic acid concentrations in the plasma of pregnant women with preeclampsia. Am J Obstet Gynecol 2001;184:414-19.

CHAPTER 37

Nucleic Acid Techniques*

Carl T. Wittwer, M.D., Ph.D., and Noriko Kusukawa, Ph.D.

The tools of molecular diagnostics allow analysis of medically important sequence variations despite an always-present background of complex genomic structure. We begin this chapter by considering the organization of human, bacterial, and viral genomes, and the spectrum of variations in nucleic acids that are of medical concern. We will then describe the enzymes that allow us to process nucleic acids into forms that are amenable to analytical interrogation. We then discuss amplification techniques that are often necessary to allow observation of the alterations of interest or to quantify a specific nucleic acid sequence in a sample. Then the tools used to detect or visualize nucleic acids are discussed. Finally specific methodologies are described that allow identification, quantification, and/or segregation of individual nucleic acid species.

Developers of molecular diagnostic techniques are extremely competitive. Converts to one technique, instrument, or probe design often adopt a religious fervor and commitment. In this chapter, we have avoided cute trade names that, in our opinion, do not belong in the scientific literature. To misquote the Bard's fool, ". . . if you think our presentation less familiar, please accept that our intent was not to offend, perhaps inspection of the references will mend."

GENOMES AND NUCLEIC ACID ALTERATIONS

Before discussing nucleic acid alterations that are of medical interest, we review and expand on the description of the structure of genomes presented in Chapter 36. We emphasize concepts that are important when developing and using the techniques of molecular diagnostics.

Human Genome

As mentioned in the previous chapter, each human cell contains two copies of a 3.2-billion-member sequence code of nucleic acids on 46 chromosomes. Box 37-1 lists statistics for the human genome and the types of variation found in the genetic sequence that are important in clinical diagnostics.

Three quarters of human DNA is *intergenic* or between genes. More than 60% of this intergenic sequence consists of "parasitic" DNA regions of transposable elements 100 to 11,000 bases in length. Between 2 million and 3 million of these elements are present in each copy of the genome. They contribute to genetic recombination and chromosome structure, and provide an evolutionary record of mutation and selection.

Intergenic DNA also carries most of the simple sequence repeats (SSRs) present in the genome. These repeats are known as *microsatellites* or *short-tandem repeats* (STRs) when the repeat unit is 1 to 13 bases, and *minisatellites* or *variable number of tandem repeats* (VNTRs) when the repeat unit is 14 to 500 bases. SSRs are critical markers in genetic linkage studies, and in forensic or medical identity testing. They are formed by slippage during replication and are highly polymorphic between individuals. The most common SSRs are dinucleotide repeats such as ACACAC and ATAT. On average, approximately one SSR occurs every 2000 bases.

One quarter of the human genome consists of genes. There are about 30,000 genes in the human genome. The average gene covers 27,000 bases, but only about 1300 of these bases code for amino acid sequence. These coding regions, or exons, are interspersed throughout the gene. On average, there are about nine exons per gene. The noncoding areas between exons are known as *introns.* Within a gene, 95% of the sequence is covered by introns, while only 5%

*Parts of this chapter are based on the original contributions by Elizabeth R. Unger, Ph.D., M.D., and Margaret A. Piper, Ph.D., M.P.H.: Nucleic Acid Biochemistry and Diagnostic Applications (2nd and 3rd editions). These contributions are thankfully acknowledged.

BOX 37-1 The Human Genome and Its Sequence Variation

The Human Genome: 3.2 billion base pairs, 23 chromosome pairs (47-245 million base pairs per chromosome)

Genes (25%)		*Intergenic Sequences (75%)*	
24%	Intron sequences	45%	Parasitic (transposon-derived repeats)
1.1-1.4%	Exon sequences	5%	Segmental duplications
		3%	Simple sequence repeats (SSRs, STRs)
		22%	Other

Number of genes: ~30,000
Average gene:
- 27,000 base pairs
- 9 exons
- 1340 bases of coding sequence
- 446 amino acids

Sequence Alterations: 99.9% identity (1 difference every 1250 bases between randomly selected haploid genomes)

Single Nucleotide Polymorphisms (SNPs): identified every 100-300 bases

97% Noncoding
3% Within exons

Disease-Causing Mutations

70% SNPs
- 49% Missense (amino acid substitution)
- 11% Nonsense (termination)
- 9% Splicing
- <1% Regulatory

23% Small insertions/deletions
7% Gross lesions (large insertions/deletions, repeats, rearrangements, complex)

Epigenetic Alterations

Variable initiation
Alternative splicing
Methylation (regulation)
Histone phosphorylation, methylation, acetylation

Data compiled from the Human Gene Mutation Database[93] and Lander et al.[51]

consists of coding sequence within exons. Coding sequences comprise only 1.1% to 1.4% of the total genome.

Sequence Variation Within the Human Genome

If you compare the genome from any two individuals, you will find on average one difference every 1250 bases (i.e., approximately 99.9% of the sequence is identical between randomly chosen copies of the genome). The most common sequence variations are single base changes, also known as *single nucleotide polymorphisms* or SNPs. Millions of SNPs have been described, and many new SNPs continue to be reported. Some SNPs are common in the population with allele frequencies of 0.1 to 0.5 (i.e., present in 10 to 50 of every 100 copies studied), though others are very rare. Although an SNP has been identified every 100 to 300 bases, many of these are not found frequently in the population. The vast majority of SNPs (97%) occur in noncoding regions; only 3% of SNPs are associated with exons.

Sequence Variations That Cause Human Disease

Many of the sequence variations in the genome do not affect human health. For example, SNPs and SSRs found in the intergenic sequence are rarely associated with disease. Similarly, most of the SNPs in introns, except for splicing and regulatory mutations, are not known to affect gene function. In addition, some of the SNPs within exons are silent alterations that do not code for a change in amino acid sequence because of the redundancy in the genetic code. Still other SNPs in exons code for amino acid changes that do not affect protein function. Even such silent SNPs may nonetheless be of considerable medical interest as genetic markers. (See also Chapter 40, Inherited Diseases.)

Single Nucleotide Polymorphisms

Of the sequence alterations that are known to cause disease (and we will use the word *mutations* specifically for these types of alterations), about 70% are SNPs, followed in frequency by small insertions/deletions and gross lesions (see Box 37-1). Most of these SNPs are *missense* mutations and cause an amino acid substitution, while significantly fewer are *nonsense* mutations that change an amino acid code to a termination code resulting in premature polypeptide chain termination. Approximately 9% of disease-causing mutations are SNPs that alter the splicing sites located just outside of an exon, resulting in altered concatenation of coding sequences. Finally, less than 1% of known disease-causing mutations are SNPs that affect the regulatory efficiency of transcription by altering promoter/enhancer regions in introns or the stability of the RNA transcript.

Insertion, Deletions, Rearrangements, and Short-Tandem Repeats

The small insertion/deletion mutations account for about 23% of the nucleic acid sequence alterations that cause disease. An insertion refers to the presence of extra bases while deletion implies the absence of certain bases in comparison to a reference sequence. Insertion and deletion mutations often result in a shift of the codon reading frame, resulting in altered amino acid sequence downstream of the mutation—commonly followed by chain termination from a nonsense codon. *Indels* are deletions followed by insertions (e.g., replacement of AGGTC by TG).

The remaining mutations are mostly larger lesions and comprise only 7% of human mutations. These include whole gene duplications and deletions, SSR expansions (e.g., trinucleotide repeat expansions), gene rearrangements (e.g., B- and T-cell gene rearrangements), and complex polymorphic loci related to health and disease (e.g., HLA).

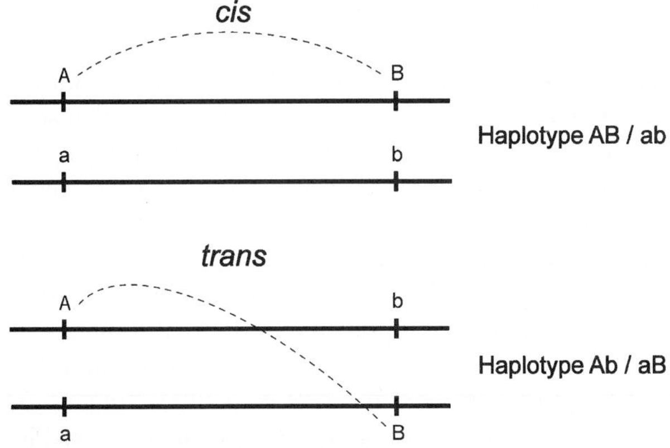

Figure 37-1 Schematic diagram of haplotypes. Two polymorphic sites reside on each of the two chromosomes of a chromosome pair. At a polymorphic site, one of two or more DNA sequences may be present. In the schematic, one site on each chromosome may have either the sequence (allele) designated as "A" or the sequence variation (allele) called "a." The other site may have either the sequence (allele) designated as "B" or the sequence variation called "b." The possible *haplotypes* are: AB/ab in which allele A and allele B are on the same chromosome (in which case A and B are said to be in *cis*), or Ab/aB in which allele A and B are on different chromosomes (and are referred to as being in *trans*).

Examples of mutations in human genes are discussed in more detail in Chapter 40, Inherited Diseases.

Haplotypes

Often, sequence variants are inherited together in a contiguous block, or *haplotype.* A schematic representation of haplotypes (and *alleles*) and an explanation are given in Figure 37-1 and its legend.

Disease associations may depend not on any particular mutation but on the overall effect of several linked alleles that define the haplotype. For example, enzyme function depends on the haplotype that defines the amino acid sequence in the protein. When the haplotype linkage of alleles is strong (e.g., in the example in Figure 37-1, when allele A is always found with allele B on the same chromosome) genotype determination at a single locus may identify the haplotype (and disease association) with high confidence. By contrast, methods for determining the *cis/trans* phase of alleles at distant loci are necessary when the haplotype linkage is weak and also when the disease association and/or haplotype linkage is first being established. Haplotypes may be defined by the phases of many polymorphic loci.

Alterations in Mitochondrial DNA

Most human genetic material is present in two copies, with the exception of the unpaired sex chromosome in males and mitochondrial DNA. The presence of only a single copy of genes on the X and Y chromosome in males leads to well-known sex-linked disorders. In contrast, the 16,500 bp mitochondrial genome is present in over 1000 copies per cell, constituting about 0.3% of human DNA. Allele fractions may vary over a wide range when all mitochondria in a cell are considered. That is, mutations in mitochondrial DNA are *heteroplasmic,* meaning the ratio of wild-type to mutant alleles within a cell can vary almost continuously, sometimes resulting in a wide range of symptoms even when only one mutation is involved. See Chapter 40 for discussion of disease associated with mutations in mitochondrial DNA.

Numerical Gene Alterations and Cellular DNA content

Sometimes genes or even chromosomes are present in more than two copies. If extra copies of genes lose their function, they are known as pseudogenes. It is important to distinguish pseudogenes from functional genes since sequence variations in pseudogenes are seldom of clinical importance. Some very important genes are present in many copies so that overall protein expression is not affected if a chance mutation occurs in one copy. Most genes, however, are present in two copies and the normal gene dosage is two. When these genes, such as *HER-2-neu,* are present in more than two functional copies, the genes are said to be *amplified.* As a result, more mRNA transcripts and protein are usually made, resulting in cellular abnormalities and possible progression to cancer. Many cancers and some genetic disorders are correlated with abnormal (increased or decreased) chromosome numbers or *aneuploidy.* The specific chromosomal alterations can be determined by cytogenetics, or the overall DNA content can be determined by flow cytometry.

Human Epigenetic Alterations

In addition to the sequence alterations considered above, epigenetic alterations, including alternative splicing and methylation, affect gene expression. (See the heading "Genetics and Epigenetics" in the preceding chapter for descriptions and discussion.) Even though the number of genes may be limited to 30,000, variable transcription initiation and exon splicing is estimated to produce about 90,000 mRNA transcripts and protein products.

Methylation of cytosine to form 5-methylcytosine occurs frequently; about 70% of CpG dinucleotides in the human genome are methylated. Although not inherited, interest in this "5th base" has increased recently as correlations with cancer have been reported.[50] CpG islands are about 1000 bases in length and are often found near the 5′-end of genes. These regions consist of clusters of CG dinucleotides that are usually not methylated in normal cells. However, CpG methylation correlates with condensed chromatin structure and promoter inactivation; an important example occurs in tumor-suppressor genes.

As described in the preceding chapter (Chapter 36), DNA is associated with proteins in nucleosomes.[42] Gene expression can be altered by histone phosphorylation, acetylation, and methylation. Our understanding of epigenetic alterations and their relation to disease is rapidly developing.

Bacterial Genomes and Sequence Alterations

Bacterial genomes are considerably less complex than human or other eukaryotic genomes. Common bacteria have only one chromosome, usually a circular DNA double helix of 4 million to 5 million base pairs, about 1000 times less than the amount of DNA in a human cell. About 90% of the DNA in bacteria codes for protein. There are no introns, but there are multiple small intergenic regions, dispersed throughout the genome, that carry repetitive sequences. The common bacterium *Escherichia coli* contains about 4300 genes.

In addition to the large circular chromosome that carries essential genes, bacteria also carry accessory genes in smaller circles of double-stranded DNA known as plasmids. Plasmids range in size from 1000 to over 1 million base pairs. Plasmids are important in molecular diagnostics as they often encode pathogenic factors and antibiotic resistance.

The bacterial repertoire of DNA can be altered by: (1) gain or loss of plasmids; (2) single-base changes, small insertions, and deletions as in eukaryotic genomes; and (3) larger segmental rearrangements, including inversions, deletions, and duplications. Some genes, such as those for ribosomal RNA, are present in many copies and can be used to identify different species of bacteria. In addition, the intergenic repetitive sequences can serve as multiple targets for oligonucleotide probes, enabling the generation of unique DNA profiles or fingerprints for individual bacterial strains.

Viral Genomes and Sequence Alterations

Viral genomes are considerably less complex than bacterial genomes. Common viruses that infect humans vary in size from about 5000 to 250,000 bases, or 20 to 1000 times less than the amount of nucleic acid in *E. coli.* Because viruses use the host's cellular machinery, they do not need as many genes. Small viruses may encode only several genes, but the larger viruses can encode hundreds. The viral genome consists of either DNA or RNA, and the nucleic acid may be single-stranded or double-stranded, linear, or circular with one or multiple fragments and/or copies per viral particle. As in bacteria, there are no introns. In fact in some viruses, the exons overlap with different reading frames coding different products from the same nucleic acid sequence. Noncoding regions are usually present at the terminal ends of linear genomes. Repeat segments are often found as terminal or internal repeats and may be inverted.

Sequence alterations in viruses are common. Areas of high sequence variation may be interspersed between conserved domains. Higher frequencies of variation can be correlated with lower polymerase fidelity and may allow escape from antibody recognition and from antiviral drugs. Common mutations in viruses include point mutations, insertions, and deletions. Sequence diversity within a viral species may be so great that consensus sequences for molecular typing are difficult to find.

NUCLEIC ACID ENZYMES

Nucleic acid enzymes are critical tools for the techniques used in molecular diagnostics. Common enzymes that act on nucleic acids include those that synthesize longer polymers and those that degrade nucleic acid into shorter fragments. These enzymes are critical for DNA replication and RNA transcription and must be present in all cells that replicate. In addition to general-function enzymes, a variety of unique enzymes, found in bacteria and viruses, act on specific nucleic acid sequences. Many of these enzymes have been purified and synthesized in vitro, sometimes "engineered" with alterations that improve their performance or stability (e.g., at high temperatures needed to dissociate double-stranded DNA in laboratory tests). Our ability to manipulate nucleic acids in vitro with these enzymes has made modern molecular biology possible. They are also used extensively in nucleic acid diagnostics, including sample preparation, probe labeling, signal generation, and amplification of targets and probes.

Nucleases are enzymes that hydrolyze one or more phosphodiester bonds in nucleic acid polymers. Nucleases may require a free hydroxyl end (exonucleases), with specificity for the 3′ or 5′ end, or may act only on internal bonds (endonucleases). For example, some probe techniques are based on 5′-exonuclease activity that cleaves nucleic acids between two fluorescent labels. Nucleases can be DNA- or RNA-specific and may act on only double- or single-stranded polymers. For example, DNAse I digests double-stranded DNA (dsDNA) and S1 nuclease acts only on single-stranded DNA (ssDNA). DNase I can be used to specifically degrade DNA in nucleic acid mixtures when only RNA is of interest. RNAses are very stable enzymes that are common laboratory contaminants.

Restriction endonucleases are found in bacteria; these enzymes prevent replication of foreign DNA.[90] Their action is sequence-specific, requiring recognition sequences of usually 4 to 10 nucleotides on a double-stranded DNA molecule. At each location where this sequence is found, the enzyme cuts both strands in a reproducible manner, resulting in either staggered or blunt-end cuts. For example, *Eco*RI is a restriction enzyme from *E. coli* that recognizes the 6-base sequence GAATTC and cuts between the G and the A on both strands, producing a staggered cut:

5′ . . . G/AATTC . . . 3′
3′ . . . CTTAA/G . . . 5′

Note that "blunt end" cuts would be produced if the enzyme hydrolyzed the bond between A and T.

Restriction enzymes are used for digesting large strands of DNA into smaller fragments and for preparing DNA from different sources to be joined together in cloning procedures. *Nicking enzymes* are restriction enzymes that cut only one strand of double-stranded nucleic acid.

Ligases catalyze the formation of phosphodiester linkages between two nucleic acid chains.[44] DNA ligases are not sequence-specific and require the presence of a complementary template. In contrast, RNA ligases used in mRNA processing do not require a template but are sensitive to sequence.

Polymerases catalyze the synthesis of complementary nucleic acid polymers using a parent strand as a template.[43] In vitro, these enzymes can extend an oligonucleotide primer that is annealed to a template strand. Extension requires that the 3′OH of the extending end is free, and that nucleotide triphosphates (NTPs) are present. Extension stops if you run out of template or NTPs, or if no 3′OH groups are available at the extending end. Thermostable polymerases, such as *Thermus aquaticus (Taq)* DNA polymerase, are essential reagents for the automation of many nucleic acid amplification procedures.

Reverse transcriptase is found in retroviruses and catalyzes the synthesis of DNA from either an RNA or a DNA template.[5] Retroviruses have RNA genomes, and reverse transcriptase activity thus is required as part of their replication. In vitro, reverse transcriptase is used to make complementary DNA *(cDNA)* copies of RNA in samples and may be used for cloning, probe preparation, and nucleic acid assays.

AMPLIFICATION TECHNIQUES

Achieving adequate detection limits is a central concern for clinical applications of nucleic acid analysis. Techniques that increase the amount of either the target, the detection signal, or the probe are referred to as "amplification methods." Examples of amplification methods are listed in Table 37-1. In target amplification, the nucleic acid region around the area of interest is copied many times by in vitro methods. Areas outside the target are not amplified. In signal amplification, the amount of target stays the same, but the signal is increased by one of several methods, including sequential hybridization of branching nucleic acid structures and

TABLE 37-1 Amplification Techniques

Techniques	Amplification Type	Enzymes Needed	Thermal Cycling
Polymerase chain reaction (PCR)[85]	Target	DNA polymerase (thermostable)	Yes
Ligase chain reaction (LCR)[105]	Target	DNA ligase (thermostable)	Yes
Transcription-based amplification system (TAS)[47]	Target	Reverse transcriptase RNA polymerase	Yes
Transcription-mediated amplification (TMA)[40]; self-sustained sequence replication (3SR)[30]; nucleic acid sequence-based amplification (NASBA)[18]	Target	Reverse transcriptase RNA polymerase RNase H	No
Strand displacement amplification (SDA)[101]	Target	*Hinc*II DNA polymerase I (exonuclease deficient)	No
Loop-mediated amplification (LAMP)[71]	Target	DNA polymerase	No
Linked linear amplification (LLA)[81]	Target	DNA polymerase (thermostable)	Yes
Whole genome amplification (WGA) or multiple displacement amplification (MDA)[21]	Target	ϕ29 DNA polymerase	No
Antisense RNA amplification (aRNA)[77]	Target	T4 DNA polymerase Klenow S1 nuclease T7 polymerase	No
Branched DNA (bDNA)[17]	Signal	Alkaline phosphatase	No
Serial invasive signal amplification[32]	Signal	Cleavase	No
Q-beta replicase (QBR)[60]	Probe	Q-beta replicase	No
Rolling circle amplification (RCA)[6,59]; ramification amplification (RAM)[114]	Probe	T4 gene 32 protein ϕ29 DNA polymerase DNA ligase (RAM)	No
Isothermal oligo amplification[100]	Probe	*Bst*NBI nicking enzyme DNA polymerase (exonuclease deficient)	No

continuous enzyme action on substrate that may be recycled. Finally, in probe amplification the probe (or a product of the probe) is amplified only in the presence of the target. Amplification techniques can often achieve over a million-fold amplification in less than an hour.

Polymerase Chain Reaction (PCR) —Target Amplification

When the amount of target nucleic acid is increased by synthetic in vitro methods, target amplification is said to occur. The polymerase chain reaction (PCR)[85] is the best known and most widely applied of the target amplification methods. Because of the commercial availability of thermostable DNA polymerases, kits, and instrumentation, this method has been widely adopted in research and is also routinely used in the clinical laboratory.

Details of the PCR Process

PCR requires a thermostable DNA polymerase, nucleotides of each base (collectively referred to as *dNTPs*), the target sequence, and a pair of oligonucleotides (referred to as *primers*) complementary to opposite strands flanking the sequence to be detected. In the first step, target duplexes are denatured into single strands by heat (Figure 37-2). When the mixture is cooled, primers provided in great excess (usually over a million times the concentration of the initial target) specifically anneal to complementary sequences on the target. Once the primers are annealed, the action of the polymerase synthesizes two additional DNA strands containing the primers as the 5′ ends. The primers are placed close enough together so that the polymerase extends each strand far enough to include the priming site of the other primer. Usually, the optimal temperature for polymerization is at an intermediate temperature between the denaturation and annealing temperatures. The second cycle also begins with denaturation, but now there are twice as many strands (the original genomic DNA and the extension products from the first cycle) available for primer annealing and subsequent polymerization or extension. The temperature cycling is continued among (typically) three temperatures: a high temperature sufficient to denature the target sequence, a low temperature that allows annealing of the primers to the target, and a third temperature optimal for polymerase extension. The instrument that takes samples through the multiple steps of changing temperature is known as a *thermocycler.*

Repetitive thermocycling results in the exponential accumulation of the short product (consisting of primers and all intervening sequences). If the efficiency of each cycle is optimal, the number of target sequences doubles each cycle (efficiency = 2.0). PCR efficiency depends on the primers and the temperature-cycling conditions, along with the

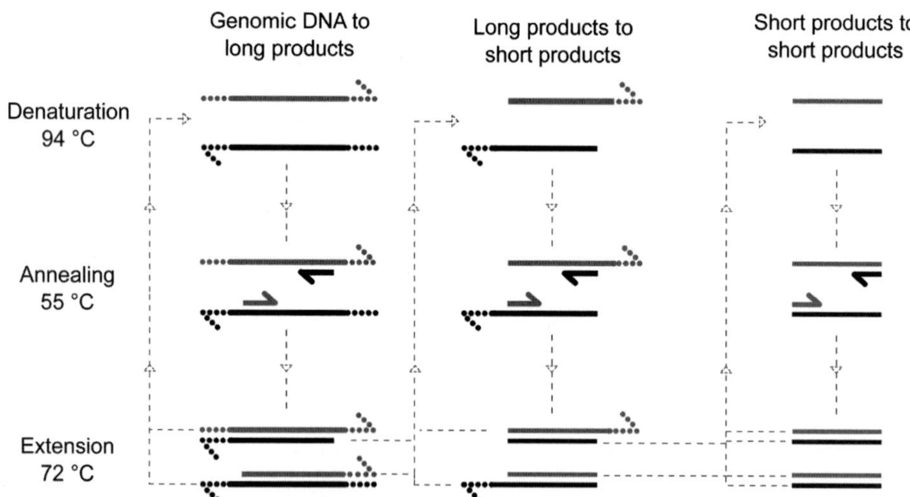

Figure 37-2 Schematic diagram of the polymerase chain reaction (PCR). Repetitive cycles of denaturation, annealing, and extension are paced by temperature cycling of the reaction. Two primers (indicated as short segments) anneal to opposite template strands (long gray and black lines) to define the region to be amplified. Extension occurs from the 3′-ends (indicated with half arrow heads). In each cycle, genomic DNA is denatured and annealed to primers that extend in opposite directions across the same region, producing long products of undefined length. Long products generated by extension of one of the primers anneal to the other primer during the next cycle, producing short products of defined length. Any short products present also produce more short products. After n cycles, up to 2^n new copies of the amplified region are present [n long products and ($2^n - n$) short products] plus 1 (original) genomic copy. A similar approach can be used to amplify RNA targets by initial reverse transcription of the RNA template to produce the DNA template.

presence or absence of polymerase inhibitors. Amplified products accumulate exponentially in the beginning cycles of PCR. At some point, however, the efficiency of amplification falls and, eventually the amount of product plateaus (Figure 37-3) either from exhaustion of components or from competition between primer and product annealing (i.e., the single strands of product are at such high concentrations that they anneal to each other rather than to the primers). The S-curve shape is similar to the logistic model for population growth. In a typical PCR reaction using 0.5 μM of each primer, the maximum DNA concentration achievable is about 10^{11} copies/μL.

With the addition of an initial reverse-transcriptase step to form cDNA from RNA in the sample, RNA targets can also be successfully amplified into DNA copies. The reverse transcription and DNA amplification steps are usually catalyzed by two different polymerases, but some thermostable enzymes (such as the *Tth* polymerase) have both DNA polymerase and reverse transcription activities, so that both steps can be performed in the same tube with the same enzyme.

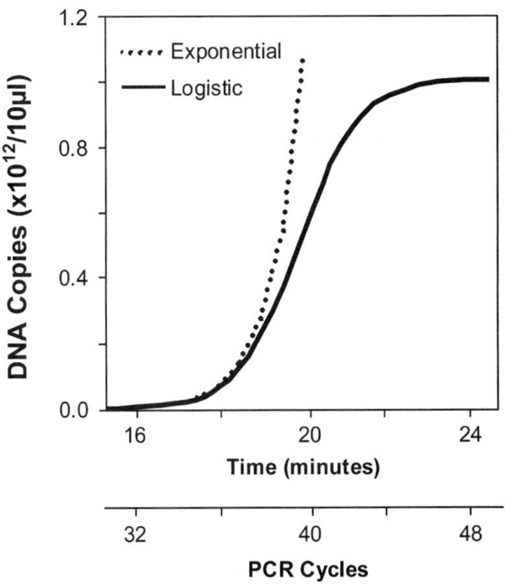

Figure 37-3 Exponential and logistic curves for DNA amplified by PCR. A doubling time of 30 seconds is assumed for PCR. That is, given the equation $N_t = N_0e^{rt}$, in which N_t is the amount of DNA at time t and N_0 is the initial amount of the DNA, r is 1.386 min^{-1} for PCR. A carrying capacity of 10^{11} copies of PCR product per μL was used assuming that the reaction is primer limited at one third the primer concentration (initially at 0.5 μM, or 1×10^{11} primer molecule pairs per μL). Starting with only one target copy, it takes only 23 minutes (46 cycles) to amplify the target to saturation. *(Modified with permission of the publisher from Wittwer CT, Kusukawa N. Real-time PCR. In Persing DH, Tenover FC, Versalovic J, Tang YW, Unger ER, Relman DA, White TJ (eds.), Molecular Microbiology: Diagnostic Principles and Practice, Washington, DC: ASM Press, 2004:71-84. © 2004 ASM Press.)*

After amplification, the products can be detected by various methods. Simple gel electrophoresis with ethidium bromide staining may suffice. When greater accuracy is required, one of the primers can be fluorescently labeled so that after PCR the fragments are accurately sized on a *DNA sequencing* device. Alternatively, some form of hybridization assay can be used to verify or analyze the amplified product. Automated methods are always attractive and closed-tube methods are particularly advantageous in the clinical laboratory. Adding a fluorescent dye or probe before amplification allows thermocyclers equipped with optical detection to analyze the reaction as it progresses (real-time PCR) or after the reaction is complete (endpoint measurement) without need to process the sample for a separate analysis step.

PCR Kinetics and Rapid Cycling

It is natural to think about PCR in terms of three events—denaturation of double-stranded target, annealing of target and primers, and extension of the DNA strand from the primer—occurring at three temperatures, each requiring a certain amount of time. Indeed, it is common to perform PCR by holding the reaction mixture at three different temperatures (for instance, denaturation at 94 °C, annealing at 55 °C, and extension at 72 °C). Standard thermocycling instruments that use conical tubes focus on accurate temperature control of the heating block at equilibrium, not on the dynamic control of the sample temperature. As a result, sample temperatures are not well defined during transitions, and long cycle times have become standard to ensure that the sample reaches target temperatures. Reproducibility between instruments and manufacturers is poor and PCR often takes 2 to 4 hours to complete a typical 30-cycle amplification.

The kinetics of PCR suggest that *rapid transitions* between temperatures and *continuous* changing of temperature (i.e., with minimal or no pauses in the rate of change of temperature to create temperature plateaus) provide a better paradigm of PCR amplification (Figure 37-4). Denaturation, annealing, and extension are very rapid reactions as shown by experiments in capillaries.[107] The use of temperature "spikes" at denaturation and annealing, instead of extended temperature plateaus, allows for rapid cycling with the appropriate instrumentation. The actual time required for PCR depends on the size of the product, but when it is less than 500 bp, a 30-cycle amplification is easily completed in 15 minutes. Furthermore, rapid amplification improves specificity. Consider PCR amplification of a 536 bp fragment of β-globin amplified at different cycling speeds (Figure 37-5). With conventional slow cycling, many nonspecific products are generated (cycling profile A). These products disappear as the cycling time is decreased (profiles B, C, and D). In fact, amplification yield and product specificity are optimal when denaturation and annealing times are minimal.

Initial denaturation of genomic DNA may be required before PCR cycling, depending on how the DNA sample was prepared. Either boiling the sample or an initial

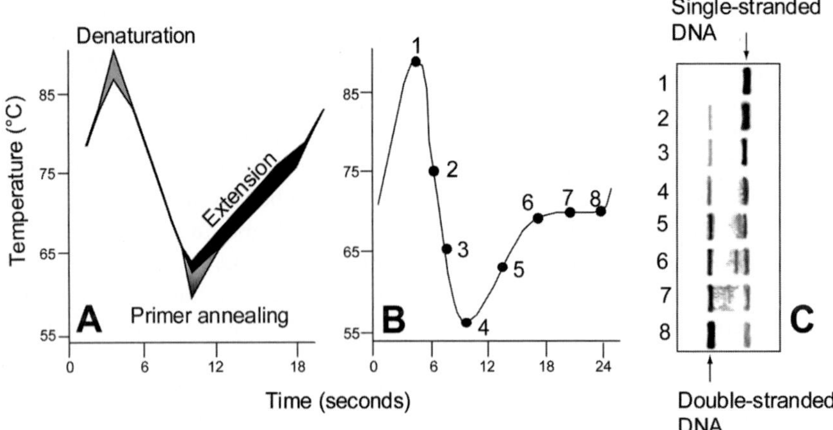

Figure 37-4 A visual demonstration of PCR kinetics. The three phases of PCR (denaturation, annealing, and extension) occur as the temperature is continuously changing (panel A). Toward the end of PCR temperature cycling, the reaction contains single- and double-stranded PCR products. When different points of the cycle are sampled (by snap-cooling the mixture in ice water, panel B) and analyzed, the transition from denatured single-stranded DNA to double-stranded DNA is revealed as a continuum (panel C). Progression of the extension reaction can be followed by additional bands appearing between the single- and double-stranded DNA (time points 5 to 7). *(Modified with permission from Wittwer CT, Herrmann MG: Rapid thermal cycling and PCR kinetics. In: PCR Applications. M Innis, D Gelfand, J Sninsky, eds., San Diego: Academic Press, 1999:211-229. © 1999 Academic Press.)*

denaturation step of 5 to 10 seconds before PCR cycling may be necessary. During PCR, however, there is no need to hold the denaturation temperature at all. Even for long PCR products, denaturation is complete in less than 1 second after the denaturation temperature is reached. Anything greater than a denaturation time of "0" only serves to degrade the polymerase. If longer denaturation times are required, either the sample is not reaching temperature or heat-activated polymerases are being used.

Product specificity is optimal when annealing times are less than 1 second. Longer annealing times may be required if the primer concentrations are low. The required extension time for each cycle depends on the length of the PCR product. Extension is not instantaneous, although it is much faster than common practice would suggest. Extension rates of *Taq* polymerase under optimal conditions are 50 to 100 bases per second. Use of a 5 to 10 minute final extension is not rational. Products can be as small as 40 bp to about 40 kb. To amplify products longer than 5 kb, mixtures of polymerases that include some 3′-exonuclease activity to edit mismatched nucleotides are usually used.

Instead of separate annealing and extension temperatures, both processes can be carried out at the same temperature, resulting in two-temperature, instead of three-temperature, cycling. Although this simplifies the demand on instrumentation and programming, it limits the choice of primers and requires a longer extension time at suboptimal temperatures.

PCR Optimization and Primer Design

In addition to the temperature-cycling conditions, the specificity of PCR depends on the choice of primers and the Mg^{++} concentration. The choice of primers often dictates the quality and success of the amplification reaction. To select primers, the sequence of the target must be known. Some guidelines for primer selection are intuitive and helpful:

1. Avoid primers that anneal to themselves or to other primers. Particularly avoid complementarity at the 3′-end of primers, and especially do not use a primer that has reciprocal 3′-end complementation.
2. Choose primers that are specific to your target. Avoid simple sequence repeats and common repeated sequences, such as *Alu* repeats. If your target has close relatives, design your primers so that they will anneal only to your intended target. Targets that you want to avoid include pseudogenes (for genomic DNA) and related bacterial or viral strains (for microorganisms).
3. Avoid primers that have sequence complementary to internal sequences of the intended product, especially at the 3′-ends of the primers.
4. Use primers between 18 and 25 bases that are matched in melting temperature (Tm) to each other. A primer greater than 17 bases long has a good chance of being unique in the human genome.
5. Unless you have a reason to amplify longer targets, choose a product length less than 500 bases. Shorter products amplify with higher efficiency.

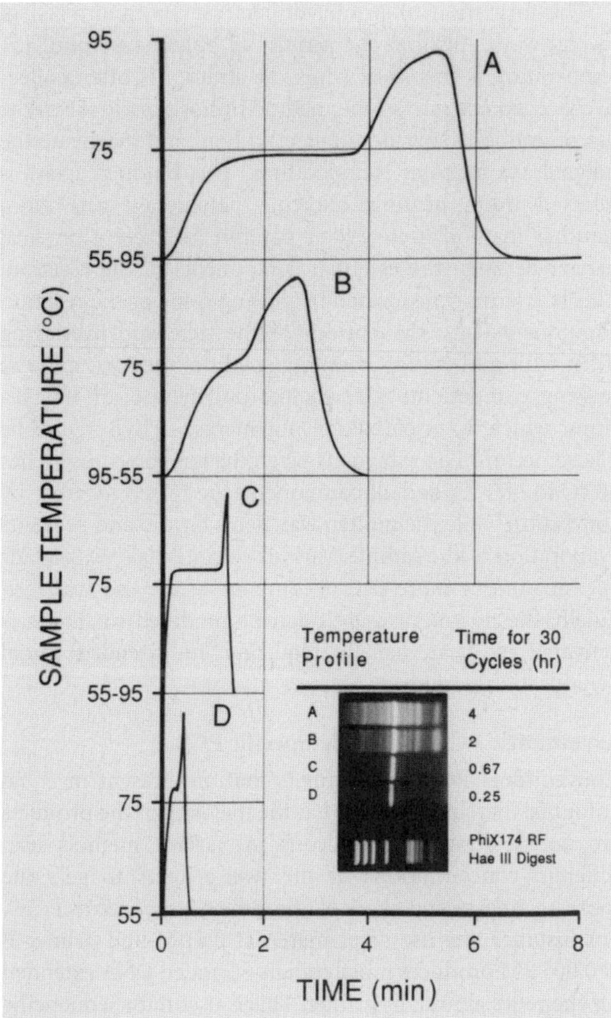

Figure 37-5 Rapid PCR improves product specificity. Samples were cycled 30 times through profiles A, B, C, and D. Increased specificity of amplification of a 534 bp β-globin fragment is seen with faster cycles (C and D). *(Reprinted by permission of the publisher from Wittwer CT, Garling DJ: Rapid cycle DNA amplification: time and temperature optimization. BioTechniques 1991, 10:76-83. © 1991 Eaton Publishing.)*

6. As a final test, do a search for sequences similar to your primers that are present in the background DNA likely to be present in your assay (http://www.ncbi.nlm.nihgov/BLAST/). Many primer selection programs are available, both commercially and freely obtained over the Internet. However, none of the selection rules used have been empirically tested.

With the human genome sequenced, it should be possible to vastly improve primer selection. Given two primers, an entire genome search for mispriming sites could rule out primer pairs with the potential to produce undesired PCR products. For exponential PCR, priming sites must be oriented appropriately within a close distance. The desired target can be favored by choosing a small product size and rapid cycling.

Detection Limits of PCR

When PCR is performed under optimal conditions, a single copy of the target can be detected. At the end of a 30-cycle amplification, a single target molecule in a tube will multiply up to a billion copies. In reality, however, we need to take into account the statistical probability of getting that single copy into the reaction tube as determined by the Poisson distribution. If a dilute solution of template is distributed among test tubes such that, on average, one target copy will be present per tube, 37% of the tubes will have no target, 37% will have one target, and the remainder will have more than one. If there is an average of two copies per tube, approximately 14% of the tubes will have no template and will provide a false-negative result. About five copies on average are necessary for 99% of the tubes to include at least one copy. This limitation of low copy analysis holds true for any amplification technique.

3′-end of PCR Products

Taq DNA polymerase and other polymerases have a terminal transferase activity that results in the nontemplated addition of a single nucleotide to the 3′-ends of PCR products. In the presence of all four dNTPs, dATP is preferentially added. This means that some percentage of the double-stranded products generated by PCR will not have blunt ends but a protruding A at the 3′-end. Although this does not influence most detection protocols, it can complicate some systems with high detection sensitivity and size resolution. On the other hand, this feature is useful for high-efficiency cloning and ligation of PCR products.[117]

Contamination Control for PCR (False-Positive Results)

Because PCR can detect a single molecule of target sequence, a small amount of contamination in a sample can easily produce a false-positive result. The greatest potential for contamination comes from the product of the amplification reaction, referred to as the *amplicon* (used interchangeably with *PCR product*). After amplification, each reaction mixture may contain as many as 10^{12} copies of the amplicon. Thus minute aerosol droplets contain more than enough target for robust amplification. Amplicon can contaminate reagents, pipettes, and glassware. It is easy to turn a laboratory into a Dr. Seuss fiasco.[89] Experience has dictated the use of laboratory procedures that minimize contamination by amplicons.[49] These include the use of physically separated areas for preamplification and postamplification steps, positive-displacement pipettes to minimize aerosol contamination, and the use of prealiquoted reagents. The most effective way of all is to not let the product out of the tube. Methods that perform amplification, detection, and characterization in a closed tube eliminate the risk of product contamination. Even with these precautions, a negative control or blank (all reactants minus target DNA) is one of the most important controls for PCR.

In combination with the precautions listed above, chemical modifications can be made to the amplicon so it becomes an unsuitable template for further amplification. One of the commonly practiced chemical modifications is to substitute deoxyuridine 5′ triphosphate (dUTP) for deoxythymidine 5′ triphosphate (dTTP) in amplification reactions, which results in incorporation of U in place of T in the amplified product. A bacterial enzyme, uracil-*N*-glycosylase (UNG), degrades DNA that contains U. Because U is not normally found in DNA, only amplicons will be susceptible to degradation by UNG treatment. During a brief incubation step before amplification, uracil-containing DNA strands that are carried over from previous amplifications are enzymatically degraded and cannot serve as substrates for further amplification. UNG is then inactivated during the first denaturation cycle, so newly formed amplicon can accumulate normally during the reaction. However, UNG may regain activity, even after multiple cycles of amplification, if the temperature of the reaction mixture drops below 55 °C. Residual UNG activity may also affect the detection limit (and the sensitivity of quantitative PCR assays) if amplified products are held at room temperature before detection.

Inhibition Control for PCR (False-Negative Results)

PCR is a resilient process and does not require highly purified nucleic acid. In practice, however, clinical samples may contain unpredictable amounts of impurities that can inhibit polymerase activity. To ensure reliable amplification, some form of nucleic acid purification is often used. The idiosyncratic nature of PCR inhibitors within clinical specimens requires demonstration that the sample (or preparation of nucleic acid purified from it) will allow amplification. A control nucleic acid sequence, usually different from the target, can be added to the sample (or extract from the sample). Failure to amplify this control indicates that further purification of the sample is required to remove inhibitors of the reaction.

Hot Start Techniques

PCR sensitivity and specificity can be compromised by the formation of unintended low molecular weight artifacts. This process is initiated before PCR when the primers, template, and polymerase are all together at temperatures below the annealing temperature of PCR. Even at low temperatures, if a primer momentarily anneals to another primer or to an undesired target region, *Taq* DNA polymerase may extend the complex. If the extension product, in turn, is primed and extended, then unintended, double-stranded products can be formed (e.g., primer dimers) that serve as amplification templates throughout the reaction. Primer-dimers can be distinguished from the intended target by their molecular weight or melting temperature, but they also influence the efficiency of the intended amplification and decrease the sensitivity of the assay.

The formation of primer-dimers can be minimized in several ways. All limit the activity of polymerase until the temperature is increased (thus the strategy is often collectively called *hot start*). One method of hot start involves the use of antibody (or an aptamer) to bind and inactivate the polymerase at room temperature. The binding agent is released upon heating, allowing polymerase activation. Another method uses wax or paraffin to create a physical barrier between the essential components in the reaction. This barrier may be created by putting some of the reaction components into the bottom of the tube and overlaying them with molten wax. Cooling solidifies the wax, and the missing components (usually the polymerase, or magnesium, which is essential for polymerase activity) can be placed on top. The wax melts when the temperature reaches 60 °C to ~80 °C, and all components are mixed together by convection while the molten wax floats on top and prevents evaporation of the sample. Various commercially wax beads encasing one or more critical components are also available. Finally the polymerase itself can be modified so that it is activated by heat, usually requiring an extended initial denaturation period.

Asymmetric PCR and Allele-Specific PCR

Conventional PCR uses primers that are present in equal amounts, thereby ensuring that the majority of the products are double-stranded amplicons. A variant method uses different concentrations of the two primers to generate more of one strand than of the other *(asymmetric PCR)*. For instance, the use of primer A at 0.5 μM and primer B at 0.005 μM produces mostly single-stranded DNA extended off the more abundant primer. This is useful for sequencing purposes or making single-stranded probes. Yield of the product, however, may be low. With less extreme ratios (e.g., primer A at 0.5 μM and primer B at 0.2 μM), the yield is mostly preserved, with one strand produced in enough excess to make it more available for probe hybridization.

Another variant method called *allele-specific PCR* enables preferential amplification of one genetic allele over another. The 3′-end of one primer is placed at the polymorphic site and is extended only if it is completely complementary to the target. This strategy is used for distinguishing a gene from its pseudogenes and for genotyping of SNPs. Allele-specific PCR is also the most common method used for determining haplotypes.[63]

Other Forms of Target Amplification

A large number of other methods of target amplification have been described. Short descriptions of some of these methods follow, with citations of sources of further information.

Ligase Chain Reaction

The ligase chain reaction (LCR)[105] uses four oligonucleotides and a DNA ligase. Two of the oligonucleotides anneal directly adjacent to each other on the target. When they are joined (ligated), they form a target for the remaining two oligonucleotides (and vice versa). As in PCR, temperature cycling is used and the target is ideally doubled each cycle. The ligase chain reaction requires that the exact sequence of the region to be amplified is known.

Transcription-Based Amplification Methods

Transcription-based amplification methods are modeled after the replication of retroviruses. These methods are known by various names including nucleic acid sequence–based amplification (NASBA),[18] transcription-mediated amplification (TMA),[29,40] and self-sustained sequence replication (3SR) assays.[30] Isothermal target amplification, using the collective activities of reverse transcriptase, RNase H, and RNA polymerase, is common to these methods. As illustrated in Figure 37-6, the method may be applied to single-stranded RNA or double-stranded DNA targets. A reverse transcriptase is used to synthesize a cDNA strand from the template RNA with a primer that has an RNA polymerase promoter sequence as a 5′-tail. The RNA strand of the RNA/DNA duplex is then digested with RNAse H, followed by synthesis of double-stranded DNA with an opposing primer. The promoter sequence on the double-stranded DNA then promotes transcription of multiple copies of single-stranded RNA by the RNA polymerase, completing the cycle. As in PCR, all reagents can be included in one mixture and amplification is exponential with completion in less than an hour. Unlike PCR, these methods do not require temperature cycling (except for an initial heat denaturation if a DNA template is used). The method is particularly advantageous when the target is RNA (e.g., HIV and HCV in blood bank nucleic acid testing).

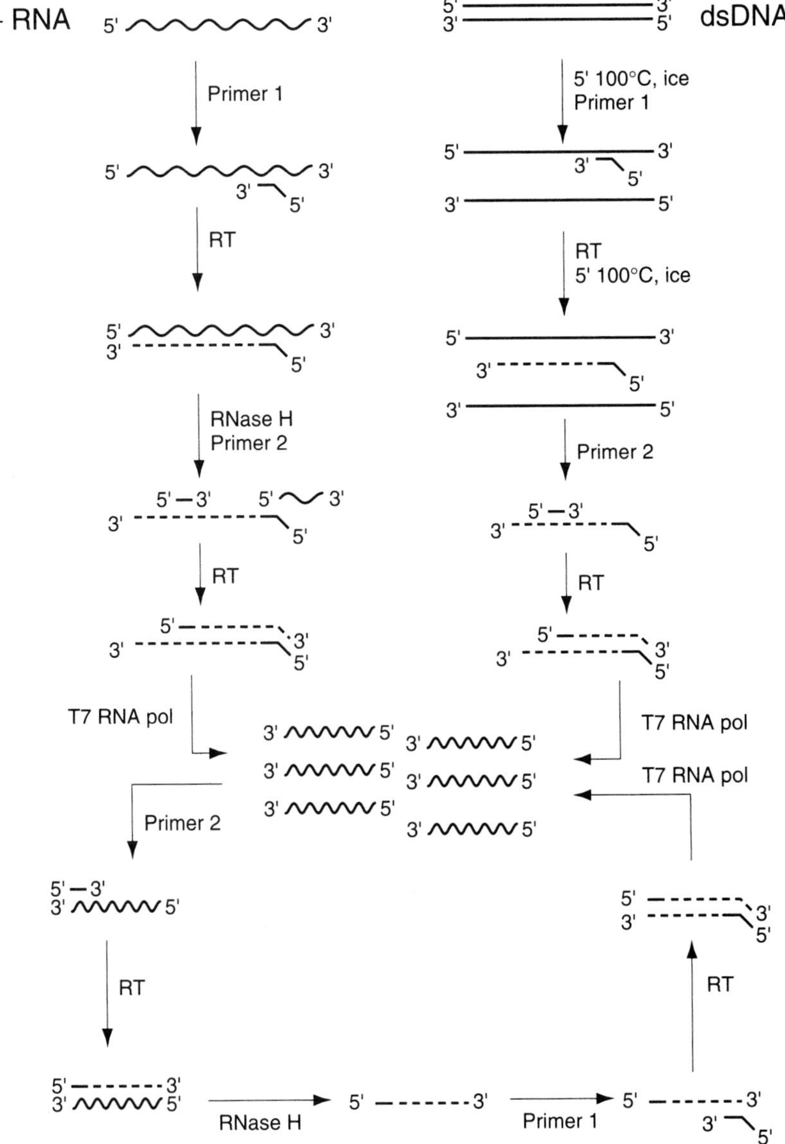

Figure 37-6 Schematic diagram of the nucleic acid sequence–based amplification (NASBA) method applied to single-stranded RNA and double-stranded (ds)DNA. The method is based on an extension of primer 1 (containing a T7 promoter) by reverse transcriptase (RT), degradation of the RNA strand by RNase H (or heat denaturation for double-stranded DNA), synthesis of the second strand of DNA by reverse transcriptase, and RNA synthesis by T7 RNA polymerase (pol). With RNA synthesis, the system enters the cyclic phase. *Solid lines,* DNA; *dashed lines,* newly synthesized DNA; *wavy lines,* RNA. *(Reprinted by permission of the publisher from vanGemen B, Kievits T, Nara P, et al.: Qualitative and quantitative detection of HIV-1 RNA by nucleic acid sequence-based amplification. AIDS, 7(Suppl 2):S107-S110, 1993. © 1993 Rapid Science Publishers.)*

Strand Displacement Amplification

Another isothermal amplification technique is strand displacement amplification (SDA).[101] After heat denaturation of DNA in the presence of four primers, dCTP, dGTP dUTP, and a modified deoxynucleotide (dATPαS), two enzymes are added, an exonuclease-deficient polymerase and a restriction enzyme. The two flanking primers that enter into exponential amplification have a restriction site added to their 5′ end and get nicked by the restriction enzyme, allowing displacement of strands that can in turn be primed, extended, and nicked. Deoxy-ATPαS is used so that the restriction sites include a hemiphosphorothioate linkage to allow single-strand nicking, instead of cutting through double strands.

Loop-Mediated Amplification

The target amplification methods presented so far produce a defined length of RNA or DNA according to the placement of the primers. In loop-mediated isothermal amplification (LAMP), multiple populations of repeated DNA structures in the shape of a stem and loop (stem-loops) are produced, and concatenated structures of variable length and branching are generated.[71] After DNA denaturation, the process is isothermal, requiring four primers and a polymerase. Two of the primers each recognize two distinct sequences on the target DNA, resulting in loops forming at the end of extension products. Repeated strand displacement DNA synthesis results in the final mixture of products.

Linked Linear Amplification

If two PCR primers include elements that cannot be replicated, an exponential expansion is reduced to arithmetic accumulation. However, if multiple nested sets of internal primers (also nonreplicable) are included, product accumulation (at least in theory) can approach that of PCR. This process is known as linked linear amplification. It requires a polymerase, several sets of nested primer pairs, and thermal cycling similar to PCR.[81]

Whole Genome and Whole Transcriptome Amplification

Instead of specific amplification of one target to improve sensitivity, methods that amplify all genomic DNA or mRNAs are useful when the target is in short supply. For example, *multiple-displacement amplification* uses exonuclease-resistant random hexamers and a highly processive polymerase to amplify DNA nonspecifically.[21] Initial DNA denaturation is not necessary and the reaction proceeds isothermally. Similarly, messenger RNA can be generically amplified with a poly(T) primer modified with an RNA polymerase promoter.[77] After reverse transcription, second-strand DNA synthesis, and transcription, antisense RNA is produced. Both whole genome and antisense RNA amplification are also useful as nucleic acid purification methods before amplification or detection.

OTHER APPROACHES TO AMPLIFICATION

It is not always necessary to amplify the target DNA sequence or a cDNA sequence complementary to an RNA target. Instead of target amplification, both signal amplification and probe amplification can be used.

Signal Amplification: Branched-Chain DNA

Instead of increasing the concentration of target, signal amplification techniques use nucleic acids to magnify the detection signal. The branched-chain DNA (bDNA) method is one of these techniques in common use. The bDNA approach hybridizes the target nucleic acid to multiple capture probes affixed to a microtiter well.[99] This is followed by hybridization to a series of "extender," "preamplifier," and amplifier probes. The final, highly branched amplifier probe includes multiple copies of signal-generating enzymes that act on a chemiluminescent substrate to produce light. The use of nucleotide analogs isoC and isoG may be used to increase specificity of the signaling cascade.

Serial Invasive Amplification

When two probes overlap on one target, an "invasive" cleavage reaction can be catalyzed by certain structure-specific nucleases. The cleaved fragment, in turn, can cause invasive cleavage of a secondary probe in the shape of a hairpin. The hairpin probe can be designed as a fluorogenic indicator by using a reporter/quencher pair of dyes that are separated by cleavage. This serial sequence of events (primary invasion and cleavage, followed by secondary invasion and cleavage of an indicator probe) is known as the serial invasive signal amplification reaction.[32] After DNA denaturation, cooling, and the addition of enzyme are completed, the reaction is run at a temperature at which both the primary and secondary reactions recycle.

Probe Amplification—Q-beta Replicase

Q-beta replicase is a method in which the concentration of probe increases if the target is present. Similar to target amplification, a large amount of nucleic acid product makes detection much easier. An RNA probe is replicated exponentially in the presence of the RNA-directed RNA polymerase, Q-beta replicase.[60] The probe is a recombinant RNA hybrid that includes sequence complementary to the target embedded in a naturally occurring template for the enzyme.

Rolling Circle Amplification

If a primer is annealed to a closed circle of DNA in the presence of a processive, displacing polymerase, the complement of the circle will be synthesized over and over again with displacement of the tandem repeats.[59] If two primers are used in opposite orientation, progressively more complex branches will be formed in an exponential reaction. Rolling circle amplification is triggered by formation of the circle by ligation of the two ends of a linear probe on template DNA. Ligation may happen directly, after polymerization through a gap, or after annealing of an additional, allele-specific oligonucleotide.

Isothermal Oligo Amplification

Short oligonucleotides, 8 to 16 bases in length, can be linearly produced at a constant temperature in the presence of a polymerase and a nicking enzyme.[100] The replication can be exponential if the amplification template is in excess and contains two complementary copies of the signal oligonucleotide. The signal oligonucleotide, or trigger, is originally produced by hybridization of a "trigger template" to the target, generating the oligonucleotide trigger by extension and nicking.

Endpoint Quantification in Amplification Assays

Amplification assays can produce both qualitative answers (yes/no, more or less abundant than reference materials) and quantitative answers (the original concentration of target sequence in the sample). In order to use the amplification process for quantitative assessments, many variables need to be carefully controlled. Variations in extraction efficiency, presence of enzyme inhibitors, lot-to-lot variation in enzyme and reagent performance, and day-to-day variation in reaction and detection conditions need to be addressed in methods that attempt to yield a quantitative result.

Quantitative analysis at the end point of amplification is usually carried out by use of calibrators with known amounts of target or a target-mimic. Quantification of sample nucleic acid may be determined by comparison with an *internal standard* of known amount that is added at the time of sample processing to control for efficiency of nucleic acid purification. These internal standards can be DNA fragments, plasmids, or RNA packaged into synthetic phage or virus particles to mimic the assay of real viruses (so called *armored RNA*[102]). One such strategy uses a *competitor* template, which is amplified by the target primers but generates an amplicon with sequence or size different from that of the expected amplicon. This competitor template is added in varying amounts to replicates of the sample before amplification. When the target and competitor are present at equal concentrations, the amounts of the two different products will also be the same. The competitor is present in the same tube as the sample, so any variation in enzyme activity affects both products identically. This method is not frequently used in clinical applications because of the requirement for multiple assays on each patient sample.

Real-time PCR is a simpler and more powerful approach to quantification than endpoint assays. The reaction is monitored each cycle, and the profiles of the curves are used to calculate initial target concentrations. Real-time PCR is described in further detail in later sections of this chapter.

DETECTION TECHNIQUES

Molecular diagnostics creates requirements for detection techniques used in two rather different tasks:

- Generic measurement or visualization of nucleic acid
- Discrimination and measurement of specific nucleic acid sequences

The latter task usually involves the use of reporter molecules and labeled probes.

Generic Measurement and Visualization of Nucleic Acids

To measure or visualize nucleic acids generically, two approaches are used: ultraviolet absorbance and dye staining.

UV Absorbance

Nucleic acid molecules absorb ultraviolet light maximally at 260 nm owing almost entirely to the constituent bases. This property can be used to measure the nucleic acid content of a solution. DNA double helices have lower molar absorptivity than would be measured from the equivalent number of nucleotide monomers, and when DNA is denatured into single strands (ssDNA) (e.g., by extremes of heat or pH) absorptivity increases.[72] If a double-stranded DNA preparation is pure, a 50 mg/L solution has an absorbance of 1.0 at 260 nm. Single-stranded nucleic acids (DNA or RNA) have a greater absorbance, so only about 30 mg/L gives an absorbance of 1.0. More precise estimates for oligonucleotides are based on dinucleotide contributions reviewed later in this chapter. It is common to assess the purity of a nucleic acid preparation by its ratio of absorbances at 260 nm and 280 nm *(260:280 ratio)*. In contrast to nucleic acids, proteins absorb maximally at 280 nm. A pure preparation of nucleic acid should have a 260:280 ratio of 1.7 to 2.0. Lower values suggest significant protein contamination.

Fluorescent Staining of Nucleic Acids

Although absorbance measurements are simple and precise, they are not sensitive. Fluorescent stains that bind to nucleic acid are 1000 to 10,000 times more sensitive than absorbance measurements. The best known example of a nucleic acid dye is ethidium bromide, a positively charged, intercalating dye for double-stranded DNA and to a lesser extent, single-stranded DNA and RNA. Cyanine dyes, such as SYBR Green I, are also popular stains for nucleic acids, as they do not fluoresce unless they are bound to nucleic acids, thus providing very low background. With the appropriate optics, single molecules of DNA can be visualized with cyanine-based nucleic acid stains.[75] Nucleic acid dyes can detect DNA and RNA in gels, or in solution (such as in real-time PCR).

Reporter Molecules and Labeled Probes

Ultraviolet absorbance and fluorescent dyes in themselves do not discriminate between different nucleic acid sequences (i.e., they are not sequence-specific). Specificity in nucleic acid assays almost always comes from the hybridization of two complementary nucleic acid strands. Many reporter molecules can be covalently attached or incorporated into nucleic acid probes. The use of these probes can reveal the physical presence or location of sequences complementary to the nucleic acid portion of the probe.

Radioactivity

The first probes used in nucleic acid detection were radioactively labeled. Radioactive labels are still favored in some research settings because of the sensitivity obtained with probes of high specific activity. The most frequently used isotopic labels are ^{32}P and ^{33}P, which are incorporated into the probe by enzymatic reactions. *Nick translation* is a classical method of labeling double-stranded DNA fragments. Nicks are introduced randomly into each strand of DNA by DNase I, and the resulting 3′-OH groups form priming sites for DNA polymerase. Labeled nucleotides are incorporated as the polymerase extends the strand by digesting and removing the unlabeled strand. Another method of labeling double-stranded DNA is *random priming,* in which the nucleic acid is denatured and allowed to anneal with short hexamer oligonucleotides of random sequence. The 3′ end of an annealed hexamer forms the initiation site for the DNA polymerase, which incorporates labeled nucleotides using single-stranded regions of the DNA as the template. Labeled nucleic acid can also be synthesized by PCR, or if a labeled RNA is desired, it can be prepared by use of a double-stranded DNA fragment containing a promoter sequence for RNA polymerase and incorporating radiolabeled ribonucleotides by transcription.

Additional enzymatic reactions are useful for labeling oligonucleotides. T4 polynucleotide kinase may be used to label the 5′ end of an oligonucleotide with ^{32}P or ^{33}P. Alternatively, terminal deoxynucleotidyl transferase (TdT) can be used to add labeled nucleotides onto the 3′ end in a *tailing* reaction. No template is required, and the number and type of nucleotides can be controlled by the reaction conditions. This results in a somewhat longer probe than the original oligonucleotide, with additional labeled bases at the 3′ end. The sensitivity that is achieved with radioactive nucleic acid probes is largely determined by the extent of incorporation of the radiolabel. Radioactively labeled probes have a short half-life limited by isotopic decay and radiolysis of the nucleic acid. This inherent instability, along with concerns of radioisotope safety and disposal, restricts the use of radioactive probes in the clinical laboratory. (See Chapter 1 for further descriptions and discussion of radioactivity.)

Indirect Probe Detection

The first practical example of nonisotopic probe labeling used a biotin-labeled analog of dUTP.[52] Despite the altered steric configuration, this nucleotide is incorporated by both DNA polymerase and terminal transferase. Other functional groups, such as digoxigenin, may also be used as affinity labels through chemical linkage to a dUTP and incorporation into polynucleotides. Alternatively, oligonucleotide probes can be labeled during synthesis with biotin or amino linkers for subsequent attachment to indicator molecules. Labels at either the 5′ or 3′ end of the molecule are usually preferred because central modifications may interfere with hybridization.

Biotin and other affinity labels do not generate detectable signals on their own. However, they can initiate signal amplification mediated by high-affinity binding with antibodies, or in the case of biotin, with avidin or streptavidin. These binding molecules can be linked to enzymes—such as horseradish peroxidase or alkaline phosphatase—connecting a single target to a single enzyme. Enzyme activity is monitored according to the enzyme substrate used (chemiluminescent, colorimetric, or fluorescent).

Affinity labels can be used to capture and localize targets to an area of a solid support. For example, biotinylated probes can be affixed to a streptavidin-coated surface. After incubation with the target nucleic acid, a second probe is added, which is either directly labeled with fluorescence or conjugated through an affinity label to an enzyme. Any background or nonspecific localization of reagents results in amplification of an undesired signal along with the desired signal, and these methods usually require multiple separation and washing steps to decrease the background.

Nucleic acids can also be linked to organic indicator molecules that emit light when exposed to certain chemicals (chemiluminescence). For example, when acridinium esters are exposed to hydrogen peroxide at high pH, light is emitted.[69] Bioluminescence occurs when biomolecules produce light through catalysis of certain substrates. Alkaline phosphatase and peroxidase are examples of enzymes that can act on luminescent substrates to emit light. Luciferase is another example of a bioluminescent molecule. Luciferase has been used as an indicator of ATP generation in pyrosequencing (see the Alternatives to Electrophoresis section later in this chapter). Electrochemiluminescence is initiated at an electrode surface in the presence of certain chelates of ruthenium (II). Once activated by charge transfer, chemiluminescence occurs.[10] For further discussion of these detection techniques, see Chapter 3 on Optical Techniques.

Fluorescent Labels

Advances in oligonucleotide synthesis and fluorescence detection systems have made fluorescently labeled probes the preferred reporter for nucleic acid analysis. Many fluorescent labels are now available, allowing color multiplexing for applications such as DNA sequencing, fragment length analysis, DNA arrays, and real-time PCR (all reviewed later in this chapter). Techniques such as fluorescence polarization, fluorescence resonance energy transfer (FRET), and fluorescence quenching can provide additional detection specificity. Fluorescence polarization can be used to distinguish free from bound label, if the molecular rotation of the probe changes upon binding.[48] Molecular rotation primarily depends upon the size of the molecule, so binding of a small probe onto a large target results in a polarization increase that can be measured. FRET techniques depend on the distance between two spectrally distinct fluorescent labels. The two labels are either brought closer together through hybridization, or end up farther apart, often through hydrolytic cleavage of a dual-labeled probe.[109] Finally, fluorescence quenching or augmentation can occur with hybridization of a fluorescent oligonucleotide to its target. The effect depends on the specific fluorescent dye and the inherent quenching from G residues in the target and/or probe.[19,67] Alternatively, quenching moieties can be purposely incorporated into the probe.[54,97] For further discussion, see Chapter 3, Optical Techniques.

Electrochemical Reporters

Electrochemical detection of nucleic acids is an area of continued research. A hybridization event can be detected by a redox indicator molecule that recognizes the DNA duplex, or by other hybridization-induced changes in electrochemical parameters, such as conductivity or capacitance. (See Chapter 4 for further discussion of electrochemistry and sensors.) One design attaches an oligonucleotide to an electrode surface. If the complementary target is present, it binds to this oligonucleotide and to an electroactive reporter oligonucleotide labeled with ferrocenyl derivatives that can be detected by voltammetry.[98] Another design also uses a tethered oligonucleotide, a target, and a reporter probe, although the reporter probe is attached to a metal nanoparticle that changes the conductivity between electrodes.[74] Although labeled probes are usually used, detection with unlabeled probes has also been demonstrated. An unlabeled oligonucleotide anchored to a field-effect sensor can be used to detect hybridization to the target by an increase in the local charge.[25] Although the techniques are very interesting, it is difficult to make electronic methods sensitive and specific enough so that nucleic acid amplification is not required.

DISCRIMINATION TECHNIQUES

Three general categories of nucleic acid discrimination techniques will be reviewed:

- Electrophoretic separation: Provides physical separation of individual nucleic acid species based on molecular weight and shape.
- Alternatives to electrophoresis: Determines the size or sequence of nucleic acid without use of electrophoresis. Examples are high-performance liquid chromatography (HPLC) and mass spectrometry.
- Hybridization assays: Provides visualization of specific nucleic acids out of a background, usually by use of probes.

Some techniques use both electrophoresis and hybridization.

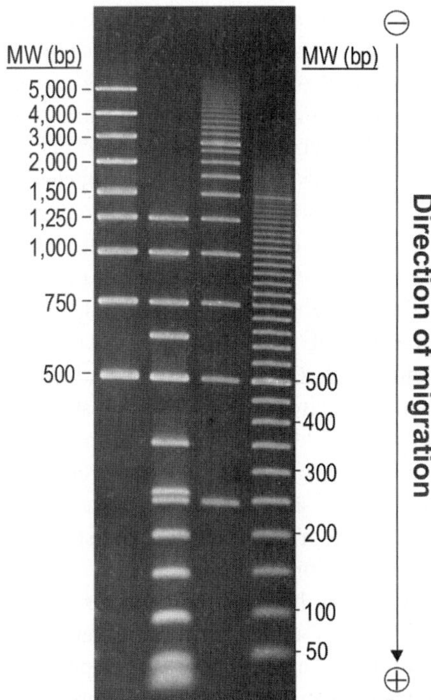

Figure 37-7 A photograph of multiple DNA fragments after agarose gel electrophoresis (1% w/v, SeaKem LE agarose gel) showing the separation of double-stranded DNA molecules by size. *(Photograph courtesy of Cambrex Bio Science Rockland, Inc., Rockland, Maine.)*

ELECTROPHORESIS

Electrophoresis is the most commonly used method for DNA and RNA analysis. Both DNA and RNA are negatively charged and will migrate toward the anode (the positively charged electrode) when an electrical field is present within an appropriately buffered solution. Separation of different nucleic acids occurs when mixtures are allowed to travel through a neutral sieving polymer under the electrical field. Separation is primarily based on molecular weight, with smaller molecules traveling faster through the polymer than larger ones (Figure 37-7). When very large molecules (≥50 kb) have to be separated, pulsed electrical fields are employed to help move these molecules through the polymer matrix.[61] Separation also occurs based on the physical conformation, or shape, of the molecule. For instance, single-stranded molecules may fold into secondary structures, and double-stranded molecules may form heteroduplexes, nicked or superhelical circular structures. Separation based on shape can provide useful information, but it can also confuse size-based analysis. For instance, because RNA generally has a high degree of secondary structure, electrophoresis of RNA is usually performed under denaturing conditions to abolish these structures. Electrophoresis of DNA is performed under nondenaturing or denaturing conditions depending on the application. The result of an electrophoretic separation provides the basis of interpretation of many clinical assays.

Agarose and *polyacrylamide* are the two types of polymers commonly used in electrophoresis. Several chemical variants of the polymers are commercially available and are tailored for different separation ranges and applications. The choice of polymer and polymer concentration (usually expressed as % w/v) is dictated by (1) the size of nucleic acid to be separated, (2) the resolution that is required, and (3) how you will visualize and analyze the result. Using various concentrations, an agarose gel can separate nucleic acid fragments as small as 20 bp to over 10 Mb (10,000 kb), including chromosomes of yeast, fungi, and parasites. But it is generally suited for low-resolution separation (2% to 5% differences in size). Agarose polymers are cast in trays (often commercially supplied as precast gels) and submerged in buffer. The gels are permeable to fluorescent nucleic acid–binding dyes, and results of electrophoresis are recorded by a photographic image of the stained gel under ultraviolet illumination.

Polyacrylamide polymers are suited for high-resolution separation (down to about 0.1% size differences) of short molecules (up to about 2 kb), and are the primary polymer for single-stranded nucleic acid separation, such as *DNA sequencing*. Polyacrylamide is used either as a linear polymer solution, which is filled in capillaries *(capillary electrophoresis)*, or as cross-linked gels, which are cast between two plastic or glass plates *(slab gel electrophoresis)*. Polyacrylamide gels are permeable to fluorescent stains, and also suitable for silver staining of nucleic acids. In addition, the optical clarity of polyacrylamide polymers makes them ideal for visualizing emission signals from fluorescently labeled fragments using laser-induced fluorescence detection.

Table 37-2 lists common electrophoresis-based techniques described further in this section.

Restriction Fragment Length Polymorphism

DNA extracted from a cell is extremely long, and is usually cut into shorter fragments before electrophoresis to aid the analysis. Restriction endonucleases cut double-stranded DNA into fragments of reproducible size; the same enzyme produces the same fragments in different specimens if the specimens contain the same DNA sequence. If an alteration in the DNA abolishes or creates a cleavage site recognized by the enzyme (or changes the spacing between two cleavage sites), then electrophoresis of digested fragments will reveal those changes (or polymorphisms) in fragment length: hence the name *restriction fragment length polymorphism* (RFLP).

PCR/RFLP

Many sequence alterations are on fragments that can be amplified by PCR, making RFLP analysis very simple. After PCR, the products are digested with one or more restriction enzymes and analyzed by electrophoresis. For example, if a sample has a mutation that disrupts an enzyme recognition site, this can be distinguished from a sample that does not have the mutation. Such an assay will produce one uncut PCR fragment when the mutation is present, and two shorter fragments when the mutation is absent (Figure 37-8). If the mutation is present as a heterozygote (one normal and one mutant copy of DNA), then one long and two shorter fragments will be observed. Usually it is possible to design the assay so that the fragments can be easily resolved by agarose electrophoresis and visualized by staining the gel with a fluorescent DNA-binding dye, such as ethidium bromide. One variant of this method uses reverse-transcribed mRNA, which lacks the introns that would be present in the DNA. In this way, multiple exons can be analyzed in one PCR reaction.

PCR Product Length Analysis

Some DNA alterations involve sequence insertions, deletions, rearrangements, and changes in the number of repeat sequences (such as STRs and VNTRs). If these alterations reside within a fragment that can be amplified reliably by PCR, then variation in the length of the amplified fragment will indicate these structural alterations. Enzyme digestion is

TABLE 37-2 Commonly Used Electrophoresis-Based Techniques

Techniques Using Electrophoresis	Detection/ Scanning of Polymorphisms
PCR/Restriction fragment length polymorphism (RFLP)	Detection
PCR (RT-PCR) fragment analysis	Detection
Southern blotting	Detection
Northern blotting	Detection
Heteroduplex migration assay (CSGE)	Scanning
Single-strand conformation polymorphism analysis (SSCP, SSCA)	Scanning
Denaturing gradient gel electrophoresis (DGGE)	Scanning
Temperature-gradient electrophoresis (TGGE and TGCE)	Scanning
DNA sequencing	Detection
Single-nucleotide extension assay (SNE)	Detection
Oligo-ligation assay (OLA)	Detection

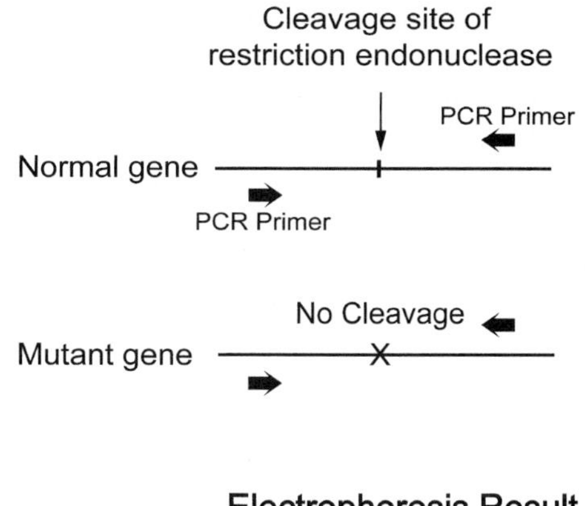

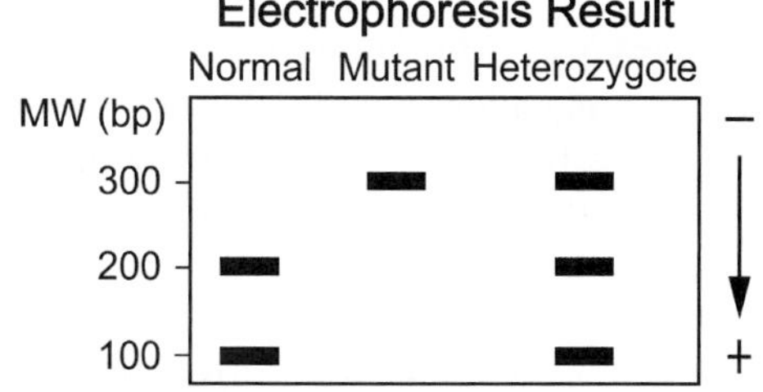

Figure 37-8 An example of PCR-RFLP. A DNA fragment amplified by PCR carries a site (a unique sequence of generally four or more bases) that is recognized and cleaved by a restriction endonuclease. If the mutation is present, this site is altered and is no longer recognized by the enzyme. Electrophoresis reveals that the fragment from a normal specimen was indeed cut by the enzyme, generating two fragments shorter than the original length, while the fragment from a homozygous mutant was not cut and the original length of the amplicon is preserved. In a heterozygous mutant, both the original fragment and the shorter fragments are visible.

not necessary in many of these assays. The length differences may be large and easily picked up with agarose gel electrophoresis or small enough to require a denaturing polyacrylamide matrix. Fluorescent labels may be incorporated into the product during the PCR to simplify detection of the fragment lengths. These techniques are most widely used in diagnosis of fragile X syndrome (See Chapter 40, Inherited Diseases) and in identity assessment (Chapter 41).

Direct analysis of PCR products by electrophoresis (without enzyme digestion) can also allow the final interpretation of an assay in which the presence of an amplification product is directly diagnostic (e.g., for the presence of a bacterium, virus, or fungus, in a specimen). The specificity of the amplification reaction is verified by the known size of the fragment. Internal negative and positive controls are employed to control for potential contamination and to establish detection sensitivity.

Direct PCR product analysis by electrophoresis is also frequently used in the clinical laboratory to query the quality of intermediary steps prior to the assay. (For example, was the nucleic acid isolated successfully? How well was it purified? Did the amplification work? How specific was the PCR? And so on).

Southern Blotting

When a DNA alteration spans a large region that is not easily amplified by PCR, Southern blotting (or Southern blot analysis) can be used to detect the alteration (Figure 37-9). The original sample DNA (rather than an amplified fragment) is digested by a restriction endonuclease, separated by agarose electrophoresis, and transferred to a solid support followed by selective visualization of fragments by hybridization of labeled probes. A nylon or nitrocellulose membrane

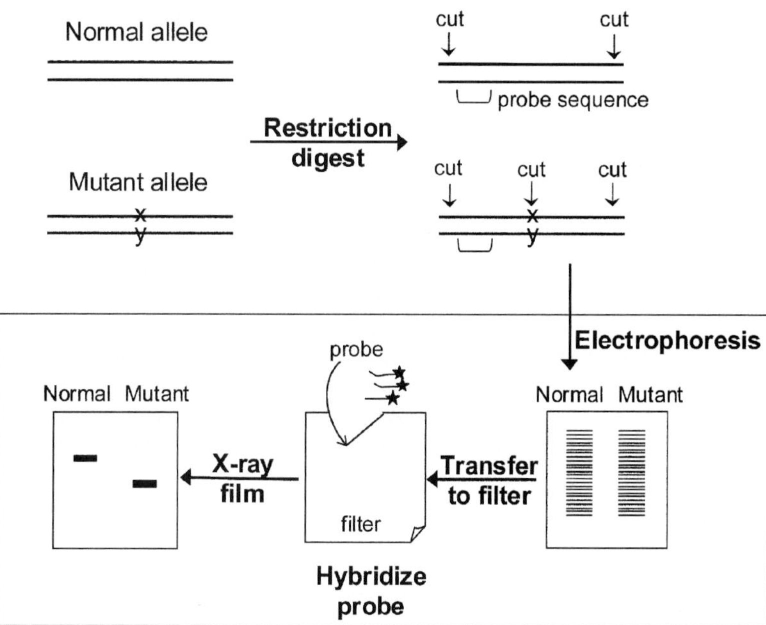

Figure 37-9 Schematic of Southern blotting. Genomic DNA is isolated from a normal specimen and from a mutant specimen carrying the polymorphic allele (x,y). The mutant allele generates a new site that is recognized by the enzyme. The normal specimen does not have this site. After restriction enzyme digestion of genomic DNA, both samples are separated by agarose electrophoresis. At this point, no discrete bands are visible over the background of many fragments that are generated by the enzyme. DNA is transferred to a filter and hybridized with a short DNA probe that is radioactively labeled. This probe hybridizes to the genomic sequence on one side of the polymorphic site. After exposing the filter to x-ray film, a smaller, digested band is seen in the specimen with the mutant allele compared with the larger fragment seen in the normal specimen.

(or filter) is usually used as the support. Details of the transfer process differ, but most methods use acid treatment to fragment the DNA (thus making it smaller and easier to elute from the gel), followed by base denaturation (single strands bind to membranes much more efficiently) and neutralization. Original methods of transfer relied on capillary action, with the filter placed in contact with the gel and absorbent paper stacked on top to blot the transfer buffer and DNA onto the filter. Typically, this process was allowed to proceed overnight. Vacuum or pressure systems can be used to speed the transfer. After transfer, DNA is permanently immobilized on the filter by baking or ultraviolet cross-linking. The filter is then incubated with a single-stranded probe that forms a stable complex with its complementary target affixed on the filter. If the original DNA was of good quality and if restriction enzyme treatment was complete, the fragments of interest can be visualized on film (autoradiographic or chemiluminescent) or directly on the filter (colorimetric) (see Figure 37-9). Ten to 50 µg of genomic DNA is usually sufficient for detection. The procedure was named after its inventor, E. M. Southern.[92] Southern blot analysis reveals polymorphisms in the DNA sequence based on the RFLP profile made visible by probes. It can also detect large structural alterations, such as deletions, duplications, insertions, and rearrangements. Southern blotting is labor-intensive and takes much longer than PCR.

Northern Blotting

Northern blotting was not named for its inventor, but as a companion technique that uses RNA rather than DNA as the test nucleic acid. RNA is transferred from the gel after electrophoresis onto a solid support followed by hybridization with a specific labeled probe. Because RNA molecules have defined lengths and are much shorter than genomic DNA, it is not necessary to cleave RNA before electrophoresis. However, because of the secondary structure of RNA, it is necessary to perform electrophoresis under denaturing conditions, usually formaldehyde/formamide buffers in agarose gels. RNA extracted from cells consists primarily of ribosomal and transfer RNA. Messenger RNA comprises only 1% to 2% of total cellular RNA. After electrophoresis and staining, undegraded RNA reveals two clearly visible bands of ribosomal RNA. Electrophoresis of about 10 µg of RNA is usually sufficient to see the mRNA of interest after hybridization with a probe. Northern blotting provides information about the size of mRNA transcripts. While only semiquantitative, the relative concentration of a particular transcript can be estimated by reference to a constitutively expressed control transcript, such as actin.

Heteroduplex Migration Analysis

Heteroduplex migration analysis (also called conformation-sensitive gel electrophoresis, CSGE) reveals the presence of mutations by the altered electrophoretic mobility of a double-stranded DNA fragment that contains one or more mismatched bases (a heteroduplex) versus one that is perfectly matched (a homoduplex). Originally described as a PCR artifact,[66] heteroduplex migration analysis has become a popular mutation-scanning technique, primarily because of its technical simplicity. Double-stranded DNA generated by PCR is denatured, then allowed to reanneal, and electrophoresed under slightly denaturing conditions (e.g., 15% urea, 40 °C) on polyacrylamide gels (often with special gel preparations that are available for this application). Detection is performed by silver staining of the gel, or by fluorescence detection if one of the PCR primers is labeled. Heteroduplexes usually tend to migrate more slowly than homoduplexes during electrophoresis (Figure 37-10). While mutant alleles are often present as heterozygotes in a clinical specimen, homozygous mutations require mixing with wild-type DNA for the mutations to be detected.

The ability of this technique to detect polymorphisms is relatively good, and the presence of a single nucleotide polymorphism in a fragment as large as 600 bp can be detected.

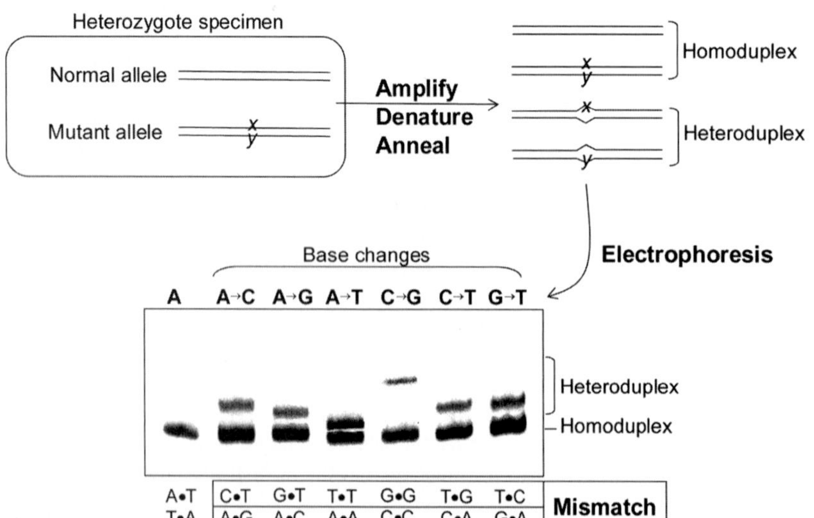

Figure 37-10 A schematic of heteroduplex migration analysis. When amplified DNA from a heterozygous specimen is denatured and cooled, the fragments reanneal in four combinations. Electrophoresis on a specialized polyacrylamide gel reveals the presence of heteroduplexes by extra band(s) appearing above the homoduplex band.

The principal factor influencing the sensitivity of this technique to base changes is the combination of the mismatched bases. Greater mobility differences (relative to the homoduplex) occur in the order of G:G/C:C > A:C/T:G = A:G/T:C > A:A/T:T.[34] This and other mutation-scanning methods are useful when a wide variety of sequence alterations might be present. Particularly when most of the samples tested are wild-type ("normal"), it is more economical to scan for the presence of mutations before performing specific genotyping or DNA sequence analysis.

Single-Strand Conformation Polymorphism Analysis

Single-strand conformation polymorphism analysis (SSCP, or SSCA) is another electrophoresis technique used to scan for unknown variants in nucleic acid sequence. Similar to heteroduplex analysis, it first requires PCR amplification. The amplicon is then diluted, denatured with heat and formamide, and the resulting single-stranded DNA is separated by nondenaturing polyacrylamide electrophoresis (usually run at 4 °C). During electrophoresis, the single-stranded molecules fold into three-dimensional structures according to their primary sequence. Electrophoretic mobility then becomes a function of size and shape of the folded single-stranded molecules. If the sequence of a reference sample differs from that of the fragment being tested, even by only a single nucleotide, it is possible that at least one of the strands, if not both, will adopt different conformations and exhibit a unique banding pattern (Figure 37-11). Since its introduction in 1989,[73] SSCP has emerged as one of the most popular mutation-detection strategies. Results can be visualized by silver staining of the gel or by fluorescent detection using labeled primers during PCR. Unlike heteroduplex migration analysis, there is no need to mix reference materials to detect the presence of a homozygous mutant specimen. Reports on the sensitivity of the SSCP technique have been variable, and detection rates seem influenced by the G + C content of the fragment and the assay conditions.[35] Different conditions may be required to detect all mutations, making multiple runs sometimes necessary for one target sequence. Furthermore the results of SSCP are difficult to interpret when one sequence gives rise to multiple single-stranded conformations, some of which may be difficult to see, depending on the amplification and electrophoresis conditions. It is also difficult to establish reliable protocols for fragments greater than ~200 bp.

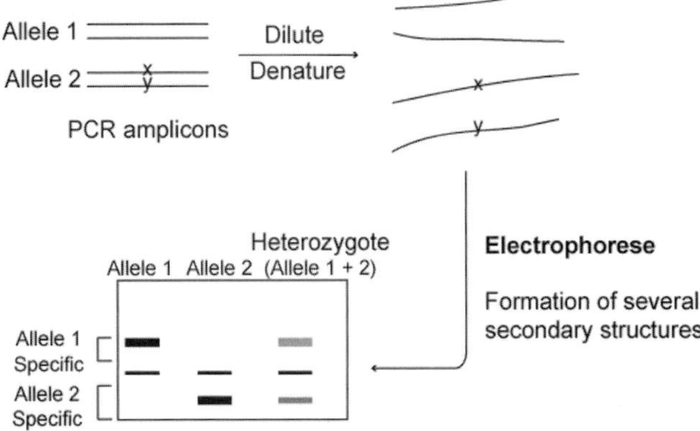

Figure 37-11 A schematic of single-strand conformation polymorphism analysis (SSCP). PCR amplicons carrying the polymorphic site (shown as x and y) are diluted and then denatured to form single-stranded fragments. When the fragments are electrophoresed, they assume secondary structures. When conditions are right, polymorphisms are detected by differential band patterns compared with a known sample.

Denaturing Gradient Gel Electrophoresis

Denaturing gradient gel electrophoresis (DGGE) is yet another technique to scan for unknown variants in nucleic acid sequence. Separation of a PCR product is performed at a constant temperature with a gel that includes a concentration gradient of denaturants, such as urea, along the direction of electrophoresis. If the sequence of the PCR product is known, the detection rate of mutations can reach 100%. However, creating identical gels is challenging, making routine implementation difficult. Depending on the melting characteristics of the product, it may be necessary to attach an artificial GC-rich sequence *(GC clamp)* to one end of the fragment to provide optimum separation.[15]

Temperature-Gradient Electrophoresis

Temperature gradient electrophoresis is an analog of DGGE. Instead of using denaturants, a spatial or temporal temperature gradient is used to provide the denaturing effect. Initial designs placed an electrophoresis gel over an insulated metal plate with a linear temperature gradient established perpendicular or parallel to the direction of electrophoresis (temperature gradient gel electrophoresis, or TGGE).[82] Separation occurs according to size, shape, and thermal stability of the nucleic acids. If the temperature gradient is established perpendicular to the direction of electrophoresis, intramolecular conformational changes show up as continuous transition curves, while strand-separation leads to discontinuous transitions. Heteroduplexes are detected by a shift of the transition curves to lower temperatures.

Temperature gradients can also be applied during capillary electrophoresis.[55] A portion of the capillary array is placed inside a heating chamber whose temperature is computer controlled to generate a gradual heat ramp (typically a 10 °C ramp at 0.5 °C to ~0.7 °C/min). Similar to the heteroduplex migration assay, PCR products are first denatured, reannealed, and then injected into the capillary. The electrophoresis polymer solution contains an intercalating dye and nucleic acids are detected by fluorescence. The presence of a heteroduplex is detected by a change in the peak profile, which under certain conditions may show all four possible duplexes as peaks[26] (Figure 37-12). The sensitivity of this technique for detecting the presence of heteroduplexes is very good, and many samples can be run at once. However, as with heteroduplex migration analysis, a homozygous mutant sample is difficult to discriminate from a homozygous normal sample without mixing the two together to form heteroduplexes.

DNA Sequencing

DNA sequencing,[24] once strictly a research technique, is now routinely performed in the clinical laboratory. The actual nucleic acid sequence of a DNA fragment can be determined and compared with a reference sequence with an error rate of 0.1% (one misidentified base in 1000). Often the sequence is analyzed on both strands (sense and antisense), which will provide even greater accuracy. Any deviation from the reference sequence is identified using computer programs matching the sequences. Base changes resulting in an altered amino acid code, stop codons, deletions, or insertions can be identified. The most common sequencing strategy uses PCR in the first step to amplify the region of interest, followed by a variation of the chain-termination reaction developed by F. Sanger in the late 1970s.[86] This reaction (also referred to as the Sanger reaction) generates fragments that are terminated at various lengths by the incorporation of one of the four dideoxynucleotide base analogs (Figure 37-13) during extension from the sequencing primer (Figure 37-14). Dideoxynucleotides lack the 3′ hydroxyl group (OH) and the 2′OH on the pentose ring, and because DNA chain growth requires the addition of deoxynucleotides to the 3′OH group, incorporation of this base analog terminates chain growth. The most common method for generating these terminated fragments is *cycle sequencing,* repeating the steps of annealing, chain extension and termination, and denaturation by temperature cycling, similar to PCR. The fragments generated are tagged with a fluorescent dye (by use of either labeled primers or labeled terminator dideoxynucleotides), then separated by denaturing polyacrylamide gel or capillary electrophoresis, and detected by fluorescence detection as the fragments travel past the detector (Figure 37-15). When fluorescently labeled primers are used, four tubes are needed for separate termination reactions. If only one color is used, then each termination reaction mixture is electrophoresed in a separate lane or capillary. If four colors are used, then the termination reactions can be combined before electrophoresis and only one capillary is necessary. Alternatively, the use of four terminators of different colors makes it possible to streamline the process down to one tube for the termination reactions and one capillary. About 600 bases can be resolved in a 2½-hour run on a capillary electrophoresis instrument. DNA sequencing is most commonly used in infectious disease testing, such as genotyping of HIV for drug resistance and of HCV to establish prognosis and appropriate therapy. Whole-gene sequencing for the detection of disease-causing mutations is still an expensive proposition, whether it is for population screening (in which the majority of samples will not have a mutation) or even for patients affected with the disease. Therefore, in genetic testing, DNA sequencing is often performed only after an initial *mutation scanning assay* has determined the exons that need to be sequenced or otherwise genotyped.

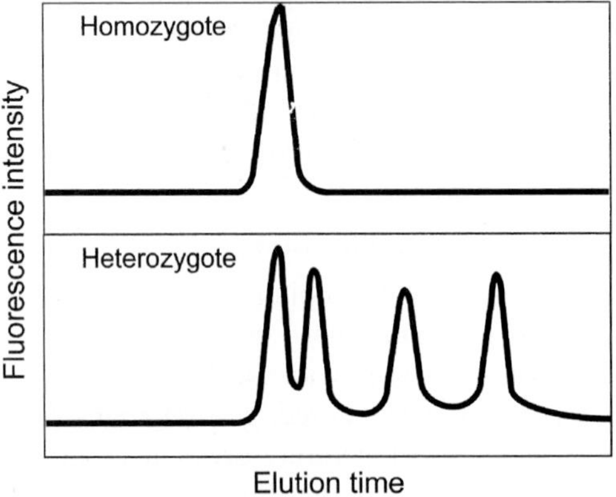

Figure 37-12 An example of temperature-gradient capillary electrophoresis (TGCE). The PCR fragments are denatured and annealed before the electrophoresis (see diagram in Figure 37-10). Only one peak is visible for the PCR fragment of a normal homozygous specimen, whereas all four possible duplexes are visible and separated from each other in a heterozygous mutant specimen. The shape of the elution profile (rather than the elution time) is used to compare unknowns with control samples.

Single Nucleotide Extension Assay

Also known as *single-base primer extension* or *minisequencing,* single nucleotide extension (SNE) assays involve the

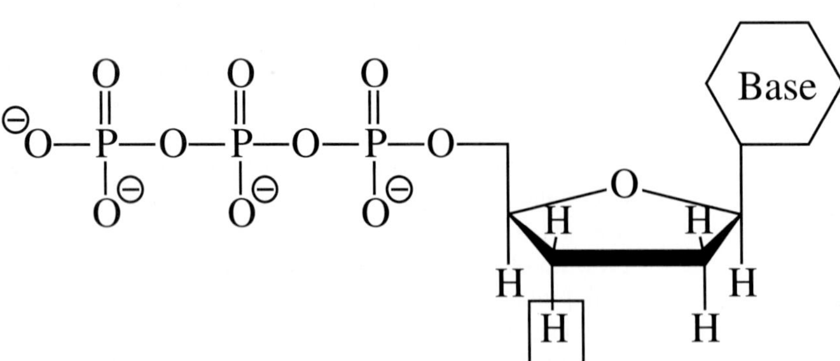

Figure 37-13 A dideoxynucleotide. Notice the absence of the 3′-OH that is usually present in standard deoxynucleotides.

annealing of an oligonucleotide primer to a single-stranded PCR amplicon at a location that is immediately adjacent to, but does not include, the site of the SNP, followed by enzymatic extension of the primer in the presence of polymerase and dideoxynucleotide terminators without dNTPs. Each of the four terminators is labeled with a unique label so that it is possible to detect which base was incorporated. SNE assays can be multiplexed on automated DNA sequencing instruments by varying the lengths of the primers so that each SNP is resolved by size in one electrophoresis run. There are also many nonelectrophoresis methods to read out the results of an SNE assay, including colorimetric detection on microtiter plates, product-capture detection systems on DNA microarrays, bead hybridization assays detected by flow cytometry, solution-based fluorescence polarization detection systems, and mass spectrometry. SNE assays are useful when the gene of interest contains a relatively large number of disease-causing SNPs. SNE assays do not work well if there are polymorphisms in the primer-binding site. Nor will they detect polymorphisms at a position other than immediately adjacent to the 3′ end of the primer.

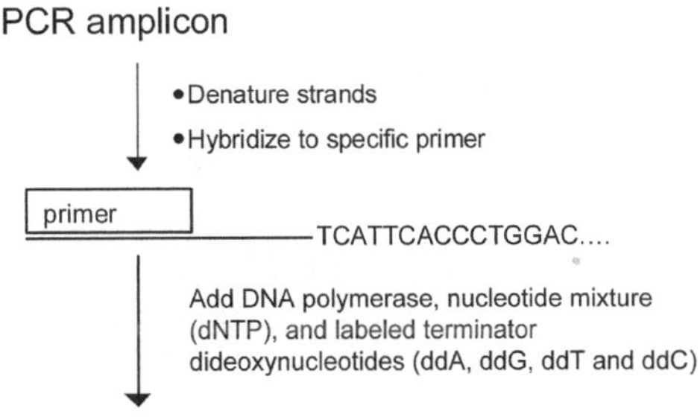

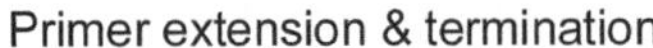

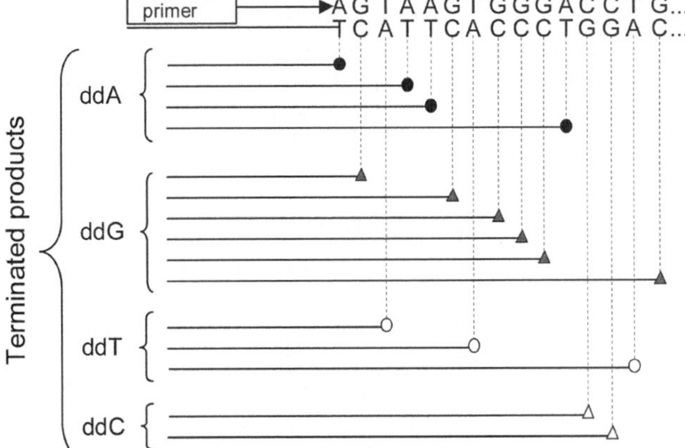

Figure 37-14 The chain-termination reaction (Sanger). A PCR amplicon is denatured and then hybridized to a specific oligonucleotide primer. As the DNA polymerase extends the primer by incorporating bases (dNTPs) complementary to the template, it occasionally incorporates a terminator base analog (ddA, ddG, ddT, or ddC) that stops further extension. The result is a mixture of extended products with varying lengths. Each terminator base may be labeled with one of four different fluorescent tags (shown as different symbols in the diagram). Alternatively, the primer can carry four different fluorescent tags in individual chain-termination reactions (containing only one ddNTP) performed in separate tubes. The original procedure incorporated a radioactive dNTP during extension, allowing monochromatic detection of the truncated fragments that were electrophoresed in four separate lanes, each for one of the terminator bases (see Figure 37-15).

Oligo Ligation Assay

Another assay format frequently used in the clinical laboratory for SNP detection is the oligo ligation assay (OLA). Two oligonucleotide probes are hybridized to adjacent sequences of amplified target DNA, with the known SNP site positioned at the end of one probe (Figure 37-16). DNA ligase covalently joins the two probes only if both probes are perfectly hybridized to the target including the polymorphic base. A probe matching the normal base and another probe matching the mutant base are usually prepared. These two can be discriminated by differential electrophoretic mobility by varying the number of modifying tail units attached. These tails were initially noncomplementary poly A or poly C tails but now consist of pentaethylene oxide (PEO) units. The probe hybridizing to both alleles (the *common probe*) provides the reporter molecule, usually a fluorescent label. Multiplexing of SNP detection is achieved by attaching different fluorescent labels to the common probes and also varying the numbers of tail units on the allele-specific probes. Following ligation, probes for multiple SNP sites are separated by denaturing polyacrylamide electrophoresis in the presence of labeled size standards.

ALTERNATIVES TO ELECTROPHORESIS

Newer technologies that replace assays traditionally performed by electrophoresis are emerging, some of which are attractive alternatives for the clinical laboratory as they achieve analysis of nucleic acids with less hands-on time and with far greater throughput because of automation. These include pyrosequencing, mass spectrometry, and HPLC.

Pyrosequencing

Pyrosequencing[84] is a method to determine the nucleic acid sequence of short segments without the use of electrophoresis. A sequencing primer is hybridized to a single-stranded template that is usually generated by PCR. Four enzymes, a DNA polymerase, ATP sulfurylase, luciferase and apyrase, and two substrates—adenosine 5′ phosphosulfate and luciferin—are included in the reaction mixture (Figure 37-17). One of the four dNTPs is added to the reaction (dATPαS is substituted for dATP because it is incorporated by the polymerase but is not a luciferase substrate). If the base is complementary to the template strand, DNA polymerase catalyzes its incorporation. Each incorporation event is accompanied by release of a pyrophosphate (PPi) so that the quantity of PPi produced is equimolar to the

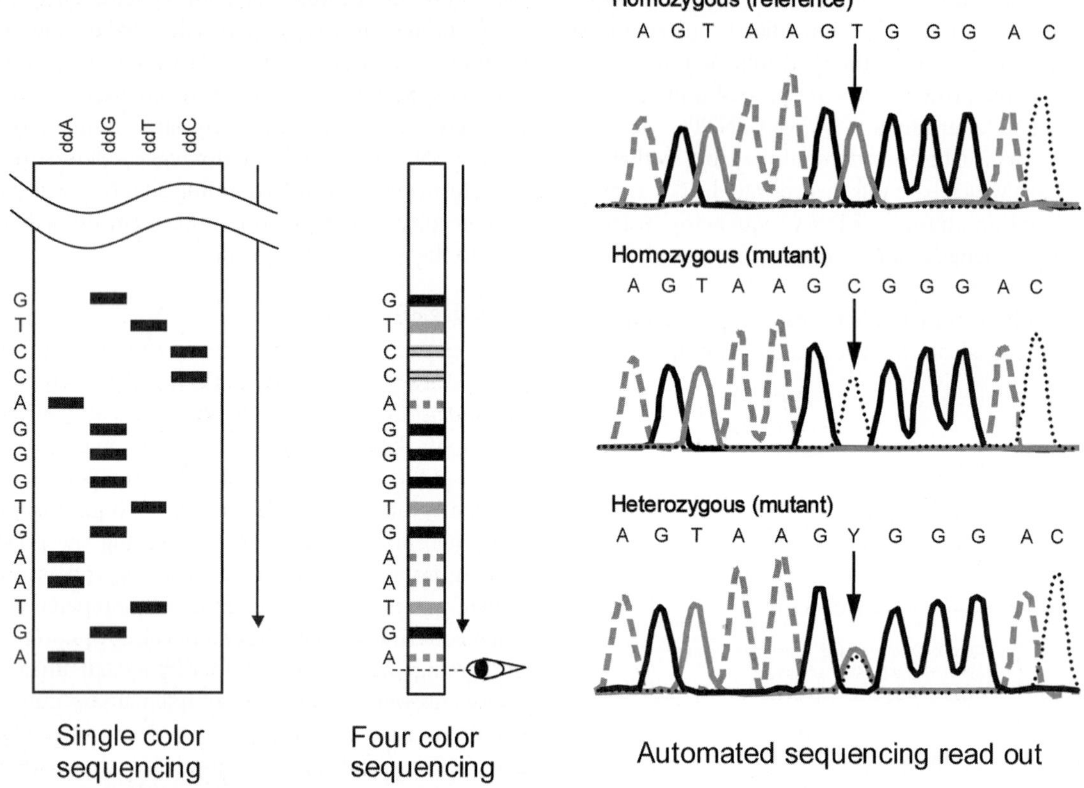

Figure 37-15 Schematic of DNA sequencing. Extension products generated by the chain-termination (Sanger) reaction are separated using four lanes (if only one label is used), or using one lane (if different color dyes are used for each of the terminator reactions). The four-color strategy is amenable to automated end-point fluorescence detection (shown by the eye icon) for both slab gel and capillary electrophoresis. The direction of fragment migration is from top to bottom. Sequence read is from bottom to top in the gels, and from left to right for the automated sequence. Examples of a reference sample (homozygous T at the polymorphic site), a mutant sample (homozygous C), and a heterozygous mutant sample (T and C) are shown.

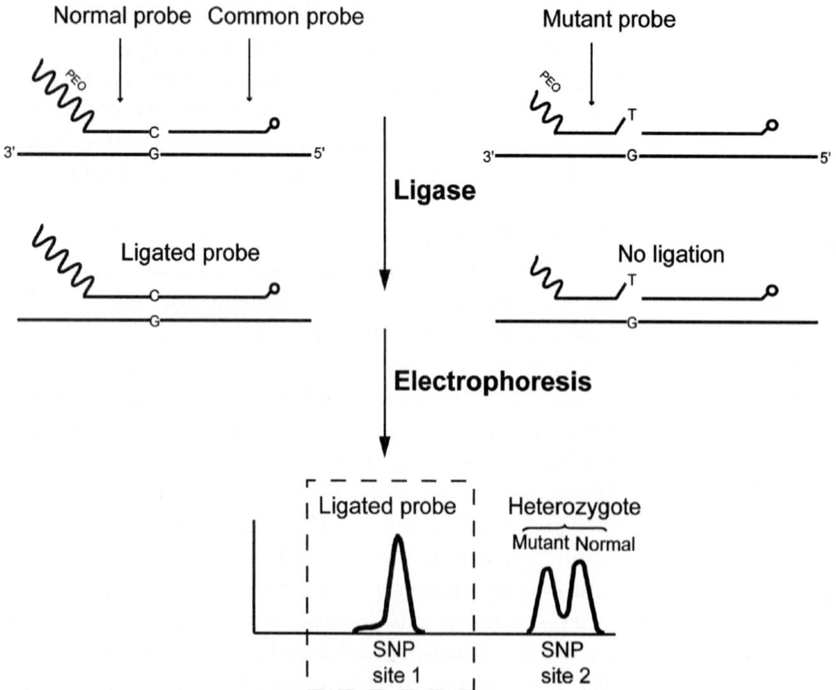

Figure 37-16 Oligo ligation assay. A probe specific to the normal allele (C) is shown hybridized onto a normal DNA sample (G). This probe also is attached to a mobility modifying tail (PEO). Hybridized next to the normal-allele probe is the common probe that is labeled with a fluorescent tag. In the presence of ligase, the two probes are covalently joined to generate a longer probe. The mutant-allele specific probe (T) with a shorter PEO tail also hybridizes to the normal DNA sample but is not ligated to the common probe because of the mismatched base at its 3′ end. Electrophoresis and end-point, laser-induced detection reveals the ligated normal-allele probe, which can be differentiated from the significantly shorter common probe alone (not shown on the graph) or from a ligated mutant-allele probe because of the different lengths of PEO tails. Multiple SNP sites can be analyzed in one electrophoresis assay by varying the tail lengths (e.g., SNP site 2 in graph), or by use of multicolor fluorescence tags.

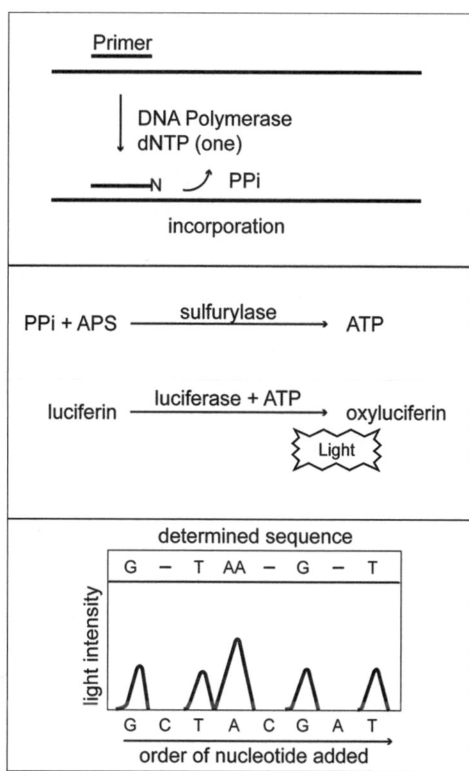

Figure 37-17 Schematic of pyrosequencing. Individual dTNPs are added one by one to the single-stranded template, a primer, and a polymerase. Pyrophosphate is generated if the dNTP is complementary to the next base on the template *(top)*. Any pyrophosphate produced reacts with adenosine-5′-phosphosulfate (APS) to produce ATP, which in turn generates light in the presence of luciferase *(middle)*. The sequence can be determined from the order of dTNP addition and the intensity of light produced.

amount of incorporated nucleotide. The release of PPi is monitored by conversion of PPi and adenosine 5′ phosphosulfate into ATP by the ATP sulfurylase, and ATP in turn drives conversion of luciferin into oxyluciferin, which generates visible light. The light produced is proportional to the number of nucleotides incorporated. Apyrase, which is a nucleotide-degrading enzyme, continuously degrades ATP and unincorporated dNTP. This switches off the light in preparation for the next dNTP addition. As the process is repeated by adding one dNTP at a time, the complementary DNA strand is built and the nucleotide sequence is determined (see Figure 37-17). Because the technique can be automated, it is useful when the sequences of a large number of short segments need to be determined.

Mass Spectrometry

Matrix-assisted laser-desorption ionization time-of-flight (MALDI-TOF) mass spectrometry can be used to detect sequence polymorphisms.[14,79] With mass spectroscopy, no label is necessary because the alleles differ in mass. After isolation of genomic DNA, a specific DNA fragment including the polymorphic site is amplified by PCR. Heat-labile alkaline phosphatase is added to the reaction to dephosphorylate any residual nucleotides, preventing future incorporation and interference with the primer extension assay. Samples are then heated to inactivate the alkaline phosphatase. An extension primer is hybridized directly or closely adjacent to the polymorphic site. Appropriate unlabeled deoxynucleotides and/or dideoxynucleotides are incorporated through the polymorphic site and terminated with the incorporation of a dideoxynucleotide generating allele-specific diagnostic product of different mass. Salt is removed from the sample, and ~10 nL of it is spotted onto an array coated with 3-hydroxypicolinic acid. This is placed into the MALDI-TOF, which measures the mass of the extension products. Once the mass is determined, the genotype is determined (Figure 37-18). Despite its complexity, automated systems processing 384 to 1536 samples at once are available.

High-Performance Liquid Chromatography

HPLC is commonly used for separating and purifying oligonucleotides. Separation is usually based on ion-pair, reversed-phase chromatography and is particularly useful for purifying fluorescently labeled probes guided by absorbance and fluorescent elution profiles.

A more recent variant of this technology is denaturing HPLC (dHPLC). Denaturing HPLC is run at a single elevated temperature to partially denature double-stranded DNA. Similar to heteroduplex migration analysis, dHPLC analyzes a mixture of PCR amplicons that are denatured and reannealed, revealing the presence of heteroduplexes as additional peaks that are shifted in retention compared with the homoduplex sample.[113] To separate double-stranded DNA, alkylated nonporous poly (styrene-divinylbenzene) resins are used, with a hydroorganic eluent containing an amphiphilic ion (e.g., triethylammonium ion) and a small hydrophilic counter-ion (e.g., acetate). Retention of double-stranded DNA is governed by electrostatic interactions between the positive triethylammonium ions adsorbed to the resin and the negative phosphodiester groups of DNA. An increase in the concentration of organic solvent (e.g., acetonitrile) in the mobile phase results in desorption of the amphiphilic ions and the double-stranded DNA. UV is often used for detection; thus PCR amplicons do not have to be labeled. The system can also be connected to a multicolor laser–induced fluorescence scanner or a mass spectrometer. The limitations of dHPLC include the need to establish specific temperatures for distinct types of mismatches and that samples must be run sequentially, one at a time.

Hybridization Assays—Principles

The second major category of nucleic acid discrimination techniques is *hybridization*. All hybridization assays are based on the ability of single-stranded nucleic acids to form specific double-stranded hybrids. The process requires (1)

Chain-termination Reaction
With ddATP & dCTP, dGTP, dTTP

5' primer
3' TGT • • → A TGT • •

5' primer
3' CGT • • → GCA CGT • •

Mass Spectrometry

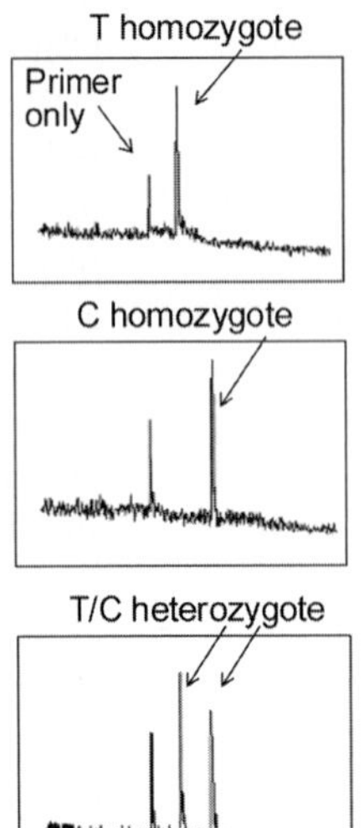

Figure 37-18 Sequence polymorphism analysis by mass spectrometry. The *underlined* base is the polymorphic site in the template (T or C). Single-stranded template is primed and extended in the presence of three dNTPs and one ddNTP, producing fragments of different mass depending on the sequence. The boxed "A" in this example indicates the incorporated terminator adenine base. The mass of terminated products is precisely measured by MALDI-TOF mass spectrometric data (relative intensity versus m/z).

that probe and target nucleic acids are mixed under conditions that allow for specific complementary base pairing and (2) that there is a method to detect any resulting double-stranded nucleic acids. A *probe* indicates a nucleic acid whose identity is known, and the *target* or *sample* is a nucleic acid whose identity or abundance is revealed by hybridization. In some of the methods discussed here, hybridization occurs between a target in solution and a probe that is tethered to a solid surface. In *homogeneous* or *real-time* techniques, both the probes and the targets are in solution, and hybridization and detection occur without washing steps. Some of the homogeneous methods also monitor the dissociation of hybridized duplexes under controlled heating, revealing the identities of the hybridized duplexes by *melting curve* signatures.

As with any assay, both positive and negative controls are necessary for validation of hybridization assays. A positive control is one known to contain sequences complementary to the probe. They are used to establish that sample preparation is adequate to release target for the assay and to ensure that the probe will hybridize to the target under the assay conditions. The positive control may also be used to monitor the detection limit of the assay if it is chosen near the lower limit of detection. A negative control (i.e., one known not to contain sequences complementary to the probe) is used to monitor specificity of the probe-target interactions, and to detect the presence of positive contamination if any is present. Negative controls also allow monitoring of the background signal generated.

Hybridization Thermodynamics

The thermodynamically favored structure of DNA under physiological conditions is an ordered double-stranded helix formed of two separate DNA molecules held together by noncovalent interactions. The duplex structure is most stable when all opposing bases are complementary, allowing for maximal hydrogen bonding and base stacking. The noncovalent binding between two DNA strands is both specific (i.e., sequence-dependent) and reversible. Denaturing agents (such as high temperature [>90 °C], formamide, or extremes of pH) favor dissociation of the double-stranded molecule into two separate random coils (see Figure 37-19). On removal of the denaturant, single strands attempt to rejoin to re-form duplexes, strongly favoring interactions that maximize complementary base pairing. Because tempera-

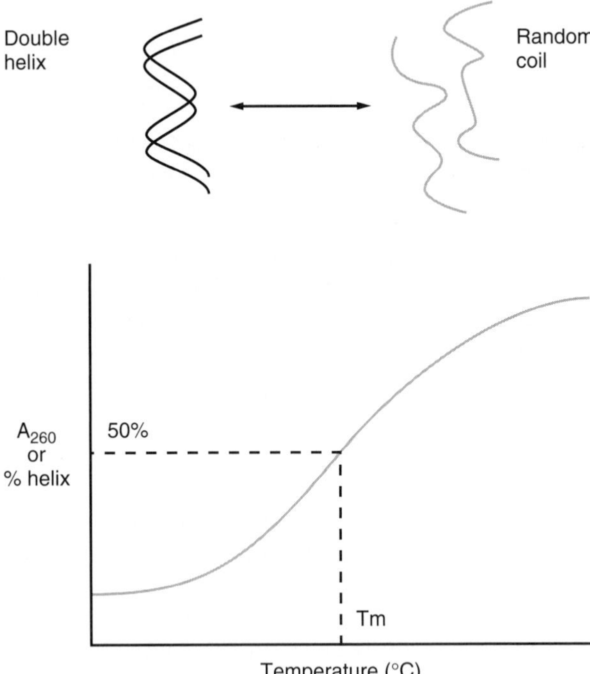

Figure 37-19 Melting curve of double-helical nucleic acid. *(Modified with permission from Piper MA, Unger ER: Nucleic Acid Probes: A Primer for Pathologists. Chicago, ASCP Press, 1989.)*

ture is the denaturant most easily manipulated, double- to single-strand transformation is referred to as *melting*, and the temperature at which one half of the DNA is melted is referred to as the *melting temperature*, or *Tm*, of the duplex. Duplexes with mismatched base pairs are less stable than those with a perfect sequence match and thus melt at a lower temperature. The reverse process, in which two complementary strands recombine to form a stable duplex molecule, is referred to as *annealing* or *hybridization*. Hybridization can occur between DNA strands, RNA strands, and strands of nucleic acid analogs (such as peptide nucleic acids, also known as PNA[70]), in all combinations.

Stringency and Mismatches

The conditions of the hybridization reaction define the degree of base pair mismatch that will be tolerated in a duplex structure. The tolerance (or lack thereof) for mistakes in base pairing is referred to as the *stringency* of the hybridization reaction. Conditions of high stringency (low salt concentration, high formamide level, and high temperature) require exact base pairing. As the stringency of the hybridization assay is lowered (by increasing salt concentrations, lowering formamide level, and lowering temperature), increasing numbers of base pair mismatches are tolerated in a duplex structure. The stringency of the hybridization reaction is determined by the environment during the hybridization reaction and the subsequent washing steps designed to remove nonspecifically interacting nucleic acid.

Conventional hybridizations were performed in the presence of empirically determined ingredients selected to modulate the stringency of the reaction and to favor interaction of nucleic acid molecules through specific base pair hydrogen bonds rather than charge interactions. The components varied widely but included buffers, salts, denaturants such as formamide, high-molecular-weight polymers, carrier DNA or RNA, and various "magic" ingredients designed to reduce background (such as detergents, bovine serum albumin, skim milk, and ficoll). Such a complex mixture was conveniently referred to as a hybridization *cocktail*. The ionic strength was often determined by the concentration of a "saline sodium citrate" (SSC) buffer with a standard 1 × concentration of 0.15 mol/L NaCl and 0.015 mol/L sodium citrate (pH 7.0). In contemporary real-time PCR and melting analysis, the hybridization solution is the buffer in which PCR occurs, and there are no separate washing steps.

Hybridization Kinetics

The kinetics of solution-phase hybridizations are second order, being proportional to the concentrations of both hybridizing strands.[103] The rate-limiting step is nucleation, where a small number of base pairs are formed in the correct orientation, followed by a rapid "zippering" of complementary sequences. In the case of a probe present in great excess to the target, hybridization proceeds as a pseudofirst order reaction, depending only on the concentration of the target. However, the time required to hybridize the probe to a given fraction of the target remains proportional to the probe concentration. For example, during PCR the concentration of primers is much greater than that of the target, and the reaction rate during each annealing step depends on the concentration of available single-stranded product, but the time required to anneal primers to a certain fraction of the target is proportional to the primer concentration.

The availability of nucleic acids for hybridization can also be an issue. In PCR, primer annealing competes with the formation of double-stranded product. As the concentration of product increases during PCR, some double-stranded product is formed before primer annealing can occur (see Figure 37-4). Similarly, when double-stranded probes are used at high concentrations, probe self-annealing interferes with probe-target hybridization. Available hybridization sites can also be limited by intramolecular secondary structure of the probe or target (e.g., as seen in SSCP).

In addition to probe concentration and availability, the length of the probe and the complexity of the nucleic acids affect hybridization rates. Rates are directly proportional to the square root of the probe length and inversely proportional to complexity, defined as the total number of base pairs present in nonrepeating sequences. Mismatches up to about 10% have little effect on hybridization rates.

The rate of the hybridization reaction is influenced by many factors in the reaction environment, most notably temperature and ionic strength. Above the Tm, no stable hybrids are present, although transient complexes may form. As the temperature is lowered below the Tm, hybridization rates increase until a broad maximum occurs about 20 °C to 25 °C below the Tm. Hybridization rates also increase with the ionic strength. Divalent cations like Mg^{++} have a much stronger effect than monovalent cations like Na^+ or K^+.

When the nucleic acid target or probe is immobilized on a solid support, the kinetics of hybridization are even more complex. Many of the preceding observations still hold true, but the rate and extent of solid-phase hybridization are lower than with solution-phase hybridization. Depending on the concentrations of the reactants, solid-phase hybridization can be either nucleation-limited or diffusion-limited. Optimal efficiency of solid-phase hybridization is achieved under conditions that facilitate diffusion of the probe to the support and that favor hybridization over strand-reassociation if double-stranded probes are used. This usually means a small volume of hybridization solution and relatively low probe concentrations. In practice, solid-phase hybridization assays are empirically designed. Time of hybridization and probe concentration are the two variables most frequently adjusted in the assay. Conditions that tend to maximize the extent of hybridization and minimize the background or nonspecific attachment of the probe are selected.

Probes

In a hybridization assay, the probe is analogous in its role and importance to the antibody in an immunoassay. As mentioned earlier, a probe is the nucleic acid whose identity is known and is used to reveal the identity or abundance of a target or sample. Like antibodies in immunoassays, probes can be unlabeled or labeled with one of a variety of reporter molecules, depending on the technique used to detect hybridization. Probes may be cloned (recombinant), generated by PCR, or synthesized (oligonucleotides). They may be DNA, RNA, PNA, and single-stranded or double-stranded. Selection, purification, and labeling of probes are crucial to success of hybridization assays.

Cloned Probes

Cloned probes consist of a known segment of DNA inserted into a plasmid vector that is propagated by growth in a bacterium. Many different plasmid vectors are now available; pBR322 was one of the first in common use.[11] The probe may consist of the entire plasmid DNA (insert plus vector sequences), or the insert may be purified from the vector sequences. The latter method is obviously more cumbersome but may result in reduced background. The resulting probe is a double-stranded DNA probe and it must be denatured before use.

Some vectors contain RNA promoter regions adjacent to the inserted DNA sequence. These regions permit generation of RNA transcripts from the DNA insert. Because only one strand is copied during the RNA synthesis, single-stranded RNA probes are generated. Controlling the orientation of the insert in relation to the promoter region allows the production of transcripts in the "sense" direction (i.e., same as mRNA) or "antisense" direction (i.e., complementary to mRNA).

PCR-Generated Probes

PCR-generated probes are simple to prepare.[39] During amplification, the PCR product typically is labeled with nucleotides that are radioactive, are fluorescent, or have attached affinity labels. If desired, single-stranded probes can be obtained by using a biotin-labeled primer, followed by solid-phase separation with streptavidin.

Oligonucleotide Probes

Oligonucleotide probes are even easier to obtain than PCR-generated probes. These probes are usually 15 to 45 bases of single-stranded nucleic acid that are chemically synthesized to a specified base sequence. Most commonly, they are DNA, but RNA and PNA oligonucleotides can also be used. Automated, efficient, and accurate methods of synthesis continue to lower the cost of production. Sequence information is now routinely available in public databases (e.g., the NIH genetic sequence database, GenBank[8]) and a similarity check for probe sequence can be performed using public algorithms (e.g., BLAST). Probe sequences must be carefully chosen to minimize cross-hybridization with pseudogenes (eukaryotes) or related species (bacteria and viruses). The melting temperature of the probe should allow both favorable hybrid stability and discrimination between related sequences under the stringency of the assay. Oligonucleotide probes are often prepared with covalent attachment of a reporter molecule (such as fluorescent dyes) or affinity labels that allow them to be attached to solid supports. Probes used in homogeneous (real-time) PCR are usually oligonucleotides with a fluorescent label.

Estimating Tm of Oligonucleotide Probes

Significant recent progress in nearest neighbor stability calculations now allows probe Tm estimation to within 2 °C. A unified thermodynamic database has been compiled,[87] and new parameters for all possible single mismatches[1-4,76] and dangling ends have been estimated.[12] Many software programs and Web sites are available for in silico Tm estimation.

Purity of Labeled Oligonucleotide Probes

The purity of labeled oligonucleotide probes is an important factor for success in hybridization assays and critical in homogeneous PCR assays. Commercial oligonucleotides with a fluorescent label are of variable purity. End users are well advised to assess the concentration and purity of all fluorescently labeled probes before use. A good method is to first calculate the predicted absorbance coefficient (usually referred to in tables by the older term "extinction coefficient") of the oligonucleotide at 260 nm ($e_{260(\text{oligo})}$) using nearest-neighbor absorbance values. These values have been tabulated[13] and are also used by many software programs to calculate the related value, nmol per absorbance unit at 260 nm, or nmol/$A_{260(\text{oligo})}$, which can be converted into the extinction coefficient by the formula $e_{260(\text{oligo})} = 10^6/(\text{nmol}/A_{260(\text{oligo})})$. Next the concentration of the fluorescent label (C_{fluor}) can be calculated from the extinction coefficients provided in the literature or by the supplier

$$C_{\text{fluor}} = A_{\lambda\text{max of fluor}}/e_{\lambda\text{max of fluor}}$$

The concentration of the fluorescently labeled oligonucleotide is calculated as

$$C_{\text{oligo}} = [A_{260} - (A_{\lambda\text{max of fluor}} \times e_{260(\text{fluor})}/e_{\lambda\text{max of fluor}})]/e_{260(\text{oligo})}$$

This equation takes into account the A_{260} contribution from the fluorophore. Similar equations for more than one label can be derived. The concentrations of fluorophore and oligonucleotide should be nearly equal (i.e., the ratio of fluorophore to oligonucleotide should be near 1). Acceptable ratios are between 0.8 and 1.2. Ratios less than 0.8 suggest incomplete labeling or destruction of the attached dye. Ratios greater than 1.2 suggest the presence of free dye. A ratio near 1 is a necessary but not a sufficient criterion of a pure probe. Co-elution of the A_{260} peak and the fluorescence peak on reversed-phase HPLC is additional evidence of purity.

Hybridization Assays—Examples

Hybridization reactions can be divided into two broad categories: *solid-phase,* in which either probe or target is tethered

TABLE 37-3 Hybridization Assays

Solid-Phase Hybridization	• Dot-blot and line-probe assays • Arrays (microarrays and medium-density arrays) • In situ hybridization • Southern and Northern blotting (reviewed earlier)
Solution-Phase Hybridization	• Real-time (or homogeneous) PCR • PCR melting analysis • Other classical techniques

to a solid support while the other is in solution, and *solution-phase* hybridizations, in which both are in solution (Table 37-3). Somewhat surprisingly, nucleic acids bound on a solid matrix can still bind complementary nucleic acids. Solid-phase assays are useful because multiple samples can be processed together, facilitating control, washing, and separation procedures. Hybridization on a solid support is, however, less efficient than solution-hybridization and the kinetics are slower and more difficult to predict. Both solid-phase and liquid-phase assays are used routinely in the clinical laboratory. Solid-phase assays include dot blots, line probes, arrays, in situ hybridization, and Southern and Northern blotting.

Several classical hybridization methods used probe-target hybridization in solution, followed by either the removal of the unbound labeled probe (by exclusion chromatography or electrophoresis) or capture of the probe-target hybrid (by hydroxyapatite, magnetic particles, or other affinity capture methods). The signal from the labeled probe-target complex was then measured. For example, *hybrid capture* methods use a bound antibody that is specific for RNA-DNA hybrid molecules that are formed during solution-phase hybridization of a DNA sample and an unlabeled RNA probe. The assay can be adapted to a microtiter plate format for automation of washing and detection.

Recently, solution hybridization has been combined with amplification, detection, and quantification and analysis all in the same tube. These homogeneous, closed-tube, real-time assays do not require any additions, washing, or separation steps.

Dot-Blot and Line-Probe Assays

Conventional hybridization assays on membranes are known as dot blots or line probes, depending on the geometry of the individual spots. The nucleic acids are applied with suction, using a commercially available manifold that results in a shape that is either round (dot) or elongated (line or slot). After immobilization, the membrane is incubated with complementary nucleic acid at a constant temperature, followed by one or more washes to discriminate matched from mismatched nucleic acid. The method allows multiple probe-target hybridizations to be carried out simultaneously under identical conditions.

Two general formats are used for these assays: either multiple samples are affixed to the solid support and interrogated by a small number of probes ("sample-down"), or multiple probes are attached to the support and a small number of samples is used ("probe-down") (Figure 37-20). In the sample-down format, purified nucleic acid or amplified fragments from multiple samples are immobilized on the support.

In the probe-down format, unlabeled probes bound to the filter are allowed to interact directly with a specimen that carries the label (a technique also known as "reverse dot blot"). Alternatively, instead of having to label the sample, a set of secondary probes can be used for signal generation. Signal probes remain attached to the filter only through sample-mediated hybridization; the sample nucleic acid forms a sandwich between the immobilized probe and the signal-generating probe. Similar assays have been developed substituting microtiter plate wells for filters. This requires chemical modification of the plastic wells to bind short DNA probes at one end, allowing the bound probes to hybridize to sample, but this approach is more amenable to automation of washing and detection.

Results of a dot-blot or line-probe assay are usually qualitative: if hybridization has occurred, a signal is generated at the specified spot and a simple yes/no interpretation is given. As the number of probes or samples increases, it becomes challenging to find a hybridization condition that provides high stringency for all probe-target combinations.

Arrays

Extending further the concept of increasing the level of parallelism in hybridization assays, microarrays (also called DNA arrays or DNA chips) were introduced in the mid1990s.[88] Compared with dot-blot and line-probe assays, spot sizes in microarrays are decreased (typically to less than 200 microns in diameter) such that one array can contain thousands of spots. This dimensional change requires specialized detection equipment, software, and informatics to analyze the data. Microarrays are fabricated on solid surfaces (generally on glass, but sometimes on other supports, such as gel pads or coated gold surfaces) either by in situ synthesis of oligonucleotides or by physical spotting of probes with the aid of robotic arraying equipment or electronic addressing. (Hybridization arrays and fabrication of "chips" have been described in Chapter 10 and will not be further described here.) Because of its massively parallel capability, microarrays have attracted tremendous interest among researchers who wish to monitor the whole genome (or at least a significant portion of the genome) for (1) identification of sequence polymorphisms and mutations and (2) quantification of gene expression. The development of expressed-sequence-tag (EST) clone libraries has greatly contributed to the advancement of gene expression microarrays. ESTs are short sequences that are expressed in certain

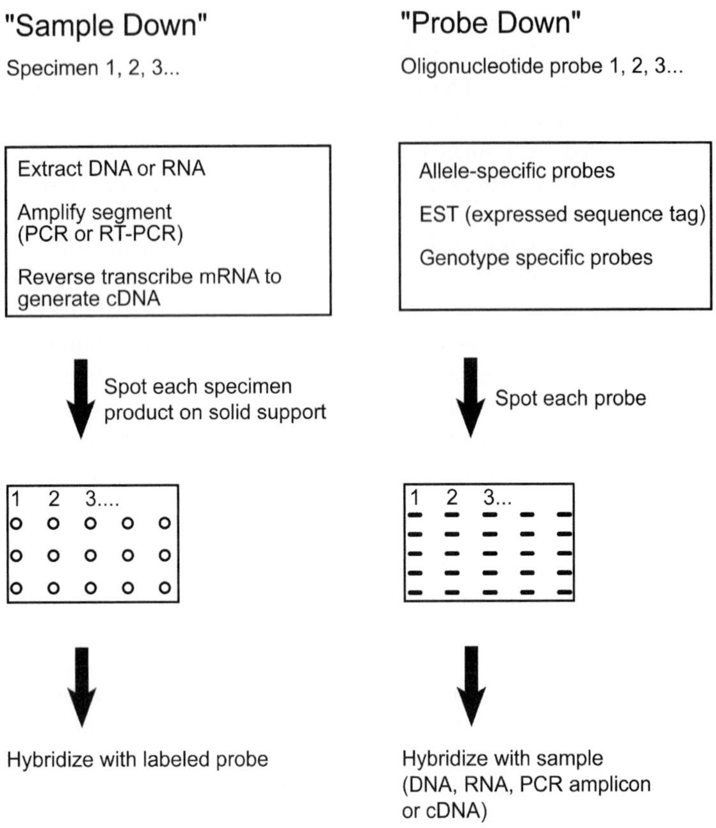

"Sample Down"

Specimen 1, 2, 3...

Extract DNA or RNA

Amplify segment (PCR or RT-PCR)

Reverse transcribe mRNA to generate cDNA

Spot each specimen product on solid support

1 2 3....

Hybridize with labeled probe

"Probe Down"

Oligonucleotide probe 1, 2, 3...

Allele-specific probes

EST (expressed sequence tag)

Genotype specific probes

Spot each probe

1 2 3...

Hybridize with sample (DNA, RNA, PCR amplicon or cDNA)

Figure 37-20 Two modes of dot-blot and line-probe assays. In the "sample-down" mode, DNA, cDNA, RNA, or amplified products are attached to the solid support and hybridized to labeled probes in solution. Alternatively, different probes are spotted onto the support ("probe-down") and the sample is in solution.

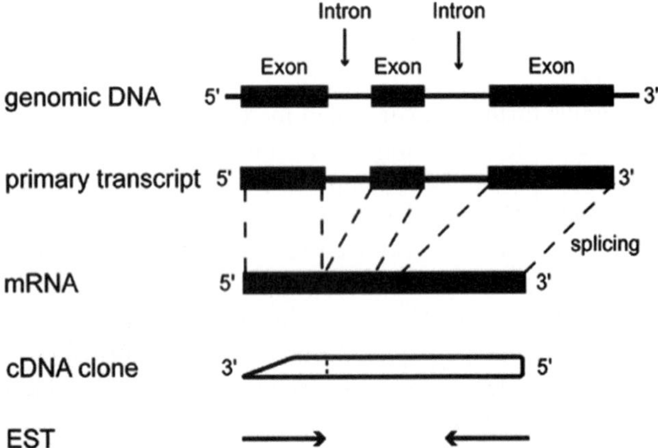

Figure 37-21 Expressed sequence tags (ESTs) can be used as probes to identify expressed genes by hybridizing to mRNA or cDNA.

cells, tissues, or organs at different developmental stages (Figure 37-21). An example of a two-color comparative EST microarray used in gene expression studies is shown in Figure 37-22. Studying gene expression in tumors can lead to the discovery of new diagnostic or prognostic markers and novel therapeutic targets. For example, characteristic patterns of gene expression can classify breast tumors into clinically relevant subgroups.[91] Expression microarrays have also identified specific signaling pathways in follicular lymphoma transformation, suggesting therapeutic targets.[23] The promise of microarrays is accompanied by challenges, including the need for strict requirements for controls and good experimental design.

Following the advent of high-density microarrays, arrays of lower density were introduced that still process more hybridization reactions than classical dot-blot or line-probe formats. Sometimes called *medium-density arrays,* these tools are emerging in the clinical laboratory for genetic disease, oncology, and pharmacogenetic testing of specimens for multiple mutations. Many companies are involved in the supply of microarray and medium-density array systems, and the industry is moving swiftly.[33,38] The arrays do not need to be attached to a two-dimensional surface as long as their "address" can be decoded. For example, microspheres can be coded by fluorescence intensity in two different channels, while fluorescence in a third channel monitors hybridization. All channels can be read simultaneously using a flow cytometer.[41] Some characteristics of arrays are listed in Table 37-4. A literature survey of array technology and applications has been published.[45]

In Situ Hybridization

In situ hybridization is a specialized type of solid-support assay in which morphologically intact tissue, cells, or chromosomes affixed to a glass microscope slide provide the

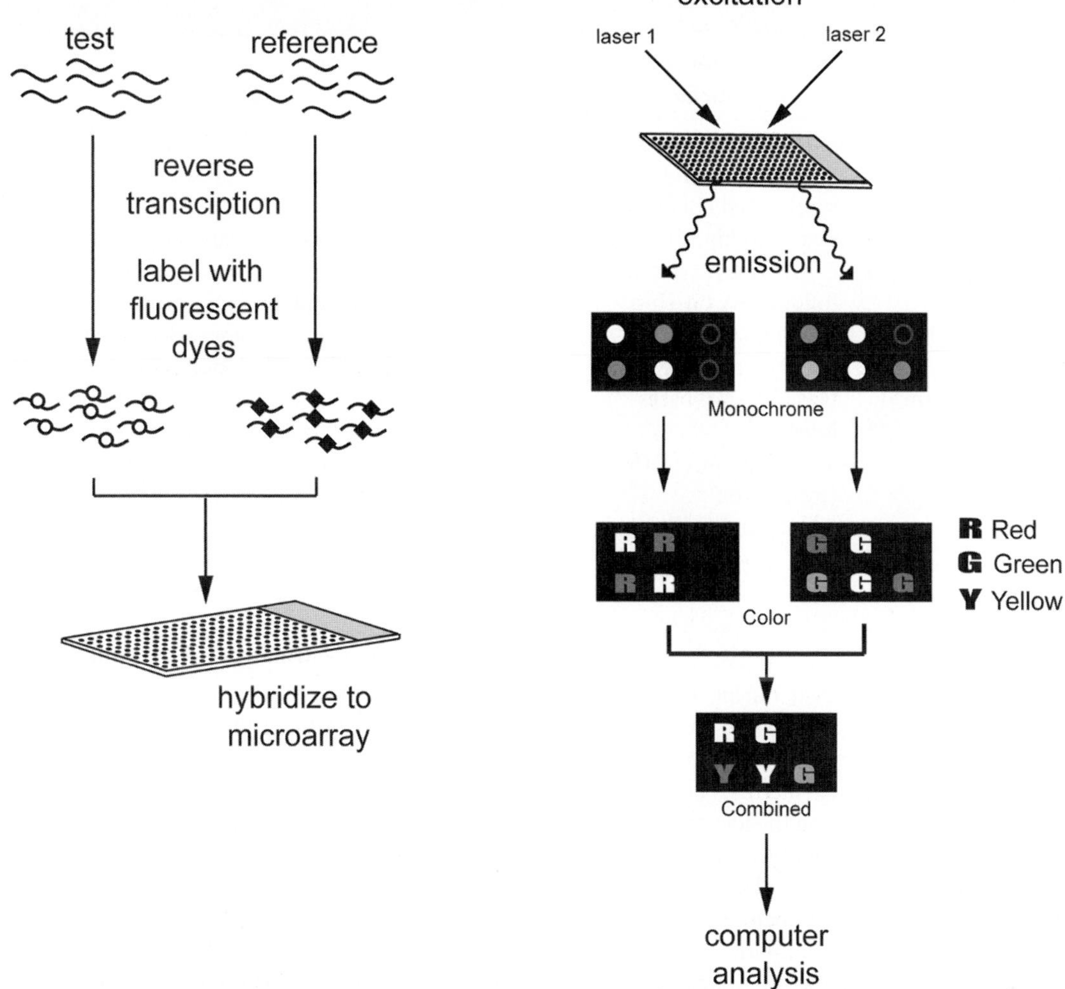

Figure 37-22 A two-color microarray experiment. An array of DNA clones representing expressed-sequence tags (ESTs) is affixed to a glass slide. Messenger RNAs in the test and reference specimen are converted into differentially labeled cDNA by reverse transcription and incorporation of two different fluorescent dyes. The two samples are hybridized together onto the array. The array is washed, and the image is captured twice, each time with a laser of a wavelength that excites one of the dyes but not the other. The monochromatic images are then converted to two colors (green for the test sample [G], and red for the reference [R]), and the images are combined. If the abundance of cDNA is the same in each of the two samples, then the composite spot will be shown as yellow [Y]. If one is in greater abundance, then that color will be preserved. Upregulation and downregulation of gene expression are then analyzed by software.

matrix for hybridization. The process is analogous to immunohistochemistry except that nucleic acids instead of antibodies are used as probes. The strength of the method lies in linking morphological evaluation with detection of specific nucleic acid sequences. When fluorescent probes are applied to metaphase chromosome spreads or interphase nuclei the technique is referred to as fluorescent in-situ hybridization or *FISH*. Detecting numerical aberrations or translocations of chromosomes can be achieved rapidly. FISH can also be combined with immunohistochemistry so that information on both the amount of protein expression and the gene dosage can be obtained on the same slide. In tissue, in situ hybridization is appropriate when localization of a target is important. However, experience in histopathology is necessary for accurate interpretation. In situ hybridization can provide information on the level of mRNA expression, but not on the size or structure of the mRNA. As might be expected, hybridization within a tissue matrix is more variable than in solution or on well-characterized chemical surfaces.

TABLE 37-4 Microarrays and Medium-Density Arrays

Type of Array Surface	What Is Tethered on the Array Surface	Hybridization	Detection
Glass (microscope slides, silicon wafers) Chemically coated transducers (gold electrodes, gold-coated piezoelectric crystals) Microelectrodes coated with gel pad Microsphere beads (4 μm diameter, stained with fluorescent dye)	Oligonucleotide probes (20 to ~80-mers) are synthesized either in situ (on-chip) or by conventional synthesis followed by on-chip immobilization Expressed-sequence tags (200-500 bases long) Sample DNA or cDNA (by electronic addressing)	Typically the array is exposed to labeled sample DNA or labeled sample cDNA (and less frequently to labeled probes), hybridized, and the identity/abundance of complementary sequences is determined	Fluorescence detection: confocal or laser scanning devices, CCD cameras, near-infrared imaging, surface plasmon resonance imaging, flow cytometry (for microspheres) Other: electronic detection, mass spectrometry

Real-Time PCR

In real-time PCR, data are collected during nucleic acid amplification rather than at a single endpoint. The technique uses fluorescent reporter molecules and instrumentation that records fluorescence during thermal cycling. The data obtained provide information on the identity, quantity, and sequence of the nucleic acid sample. Fluorescent dyes or probes capable of signaling the relative quantity of DNA are added to the PCR mixture before amplification. The same reaction tube is used for amplification and fluorescence monitoring, and there are no sample transfers, reagent additions, or gel separation steps, thereby eliminating the risk of product contamination in subsequent reactions. Because the process is simple and fast, real-time PCR is replacing many conventional techniques in the clinical laboratory.

Real-time PCR was first described using ethidium bromide to monitor the accumulation of a double-stranded PCR product with the fluorescence signal recorded once each cycle.[36,37] If target DNA is present, the fluorescence increases. How early during PCR one begins to see a signal depends on the initial amount of target DNA, and this provides a systematic method of quantification. Further, when fluorescence is continuously monitored as the temperature is raised, a melting curve can be generated. Often the first derivative of this melting curve is plotted to visually aid a person in determining the position of the melting temperature. Melting analysis can be used to verify the identity of the amplified product and to detect sequence variants down to a single base (Figure 37-23). Real-time PCR and melting analysis can be considered as "dynamic" hybridization assays in which the formation or dissociation of the probe-target duplex (or product duplex) is monitored in real time.

Dyes and Probe Formats for Real-Time PCR

Many different fluorescent reporter systems are used in real-time PCR, and some of the more common ones are shown in Figure 37-24. Many methods use probes with sequences complementary to the target. Others rely on the specificity afforded by PCR primers, and some have the additional option of melting analysis to verify the melting temperature of the probe or product.

Double-Stranded DNA Binding Dyes

Although ethidium bromide was the first dye used in real-time PCR, SYBR Green I is more commonly used today. Introduced to real-time PCR in 1997,[109] SYBR Green I has fluorescent properties similar to those of fluorescein, allowing the use of commonly available real-time optics. Both ethidium bromide and SYBR Green I exhibit an increase in fluorescence when bound to double-stranded DNA (see Figure 37-24, row one), but the performance of SYBR Green I in real-time PCR surpasses ethidium bromide because of the very low background fluorescence of the free dye, and because it can better distinguish double strands from single strands of nucleic acids.[110] SYBR Green I is commonly used for real-time quantification when the specificity of a probe is not needed and the cost of probes can be avoided.

Fluorescently Labeled Primers

Labeled primers can also be used to monitor PCR. In one system, a primer with a 5′-hairpin is labeled with a fluorophore and a quencher so that fluorescence is quenched in the hairpin conformation. When the primer straightens out during PCR, fluorescence increases[68] (see Figure 27-24, row six). If the sequence of the primer is carefully considered, the quencher moiety is not necessary.[67] Nonhairpin primers

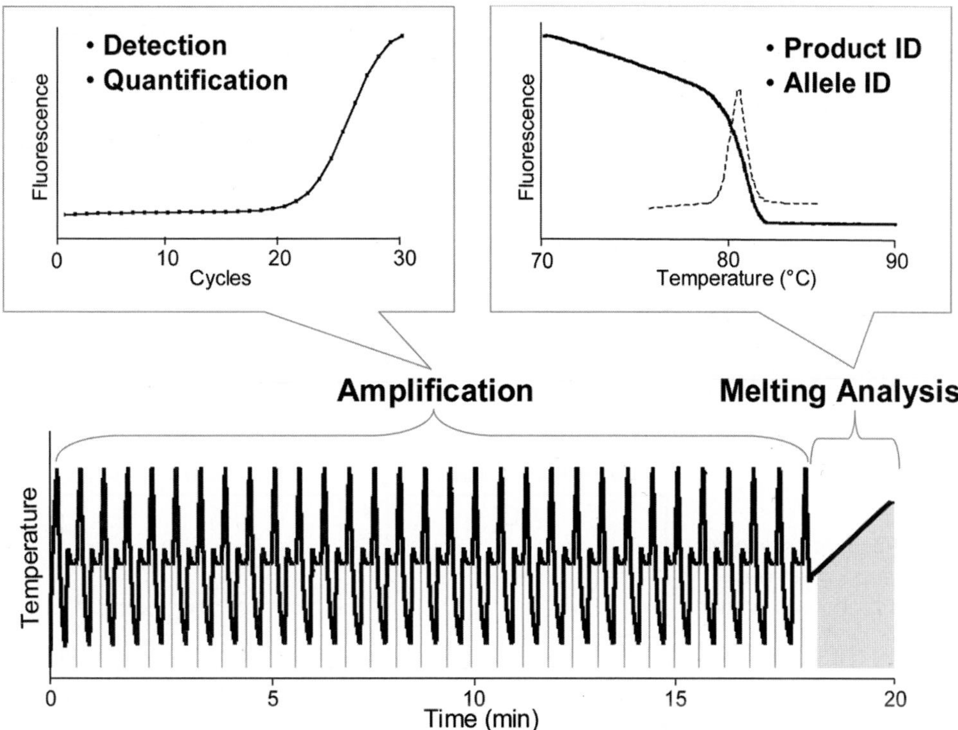

Figure 37-23 Real-time monitoring during amplification and melting analysis. The bottom panel shows a typical rapid-cycle temperature profile that is followed by a temperature ramp for melting analysis. When a signal is monitored during amplification once each cycle *(dotted lines)*, it provides information on the presence or absence of specific target sequences and allows quantification of the target. When a signal is monitored continuously through the melting phase *(shaded area)*, it can provide information that verifies target identification or establishes genotype. *(Modifed with permission of the publisher from Wittwer CT, Kusukawa N. Real-time PCR. In Persing DH, Tenover FC, Versalovic J, Tang YW, Unger ER, Relman DA, White TJ (eds.), Molecular Microbiology: Diagnostic Principles and Practice, Washington, DC: ASM Press, 2004:71-84.)*

with a single label can also be used for detection and genotyping because of changes in fluorescence that occur with hybridization.[31]

One advantage of fluorescently labeled primers over dsDNA dyes is that multiplexing is possible. However, with both dsDNA dyes and labeled primers, reaction specificity depends on the specificity of the primers. Any double-stranded product that is formed will be detected, including primer-dimers. Therefore, hot start techniques, temperature discrimination by collecting real-time data at a high temperature, and melting curve analysis to confirm the desired product are useful.

Probe-Specific Detection

The use of fluorescent probes in PCR provides an additional level of specificity to the process. Fluorescent probes that hybridize to PCR products during amplification change fluorescence by two possible mechanisms: (1) a covalent bond between two dyes is broken by hydrolysis or made through ligation, or (2) the fluorescence change follows reversible hybridization of the probe to the target. Following this distinction, when an irreversible covalent bond is involved, the probes are called *hydrolysis probes.* When probes reversibly change fluorescence on duplex formation, they are called *hybridization probes.* One major difference between the two probe types is that melting analysis is possible with hybridization probes, but not with hydrolysis probes.

Hybridization Probes. These probes change fluorescence upon hybridization, usually by fluorescence resonance energy transfer.[53,109] Two interacting fluorophores may be placed on adjacent probes (see Figure 37-24, row two), or one may be placed on a primer and the other on a probe (see Figure 37-24, row three). Only one probe with one fluorophore may be necessary if the fluorescence is quenched by deoxyguanosine residues.[19] Another single-labeled probe design uses thiazole orange attached to a peptide nucleic acid.[94] In each of these designs, the fluorescence change of hybridization probes is reversible with melting.

Hydrolysis Probes. A fluorophore-labeled probe can be synthesized with a quencher located in a position that allows

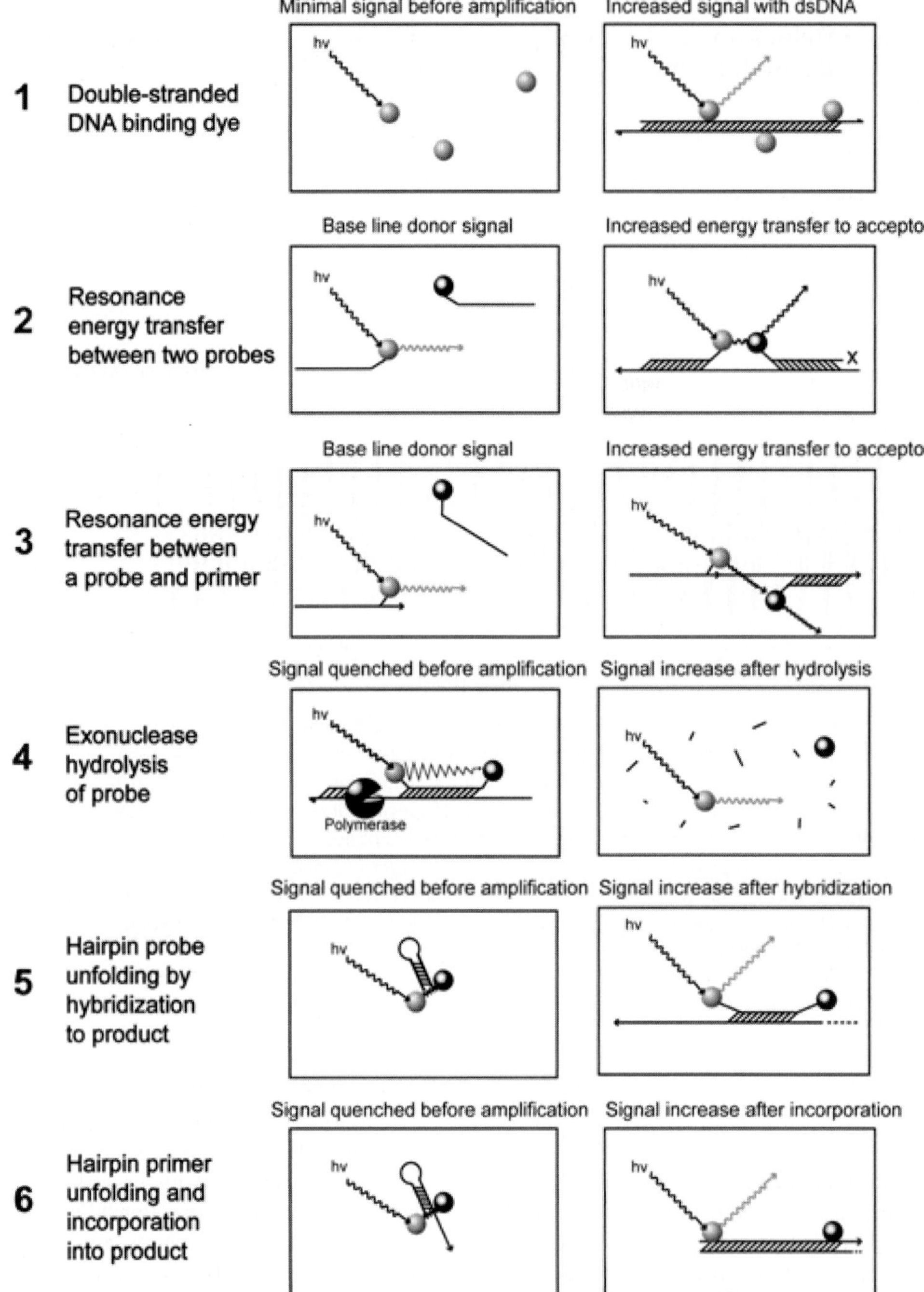

Figure 37-24 Common probes and dyes for real-time PCR. *(1)* Double-stranded DNA dyes show a significant increase in fluorescence when bound to DNA (*hv* = excitation light). *(2)* Adjacent hybridization probes. Fluorescence resonance energy transfer (FRET) is illustrated between a donor and acceptor fluorophore. The "x" indicates phosphorylation of the 3′ terminus of the probe to prevent polymerase extension. *(3)* FRET between a labeled primer and a single hybridization probe. *(4)* Hydrolysis probes are cleaved between the reporter and quencher, resulting in increased fluorescence. *(5)* Hairpin probes are quenched in the native conformation, but increase in fluorescence when hybridized. *(6)* Hairpin primers retain their native, quenched conformation until they are incorporated into a double-stranded product. *(Modified with permission of the publisher from Pritham GH, Wittwer CT: Continuous fluorescent monitoring of PCR. J Clin Lig Assay 1998, 21:404-412. © 1998 Clinical Ligand Assay Society, Inc.)*

it to quench the fluorescence from the fluorophore. If the probe is hydrolyzed during PCR between the fluorophore and the quencher, fluorescence will increase. The most common implementation uses the 5′-exonuclease activity of the DNA polymerase to hydrolyze the probe and dissociate the labels (see Figure 37-24, row four). This method has been simplified by putting the fluorophores on opposite ends of the probe.[58] Hybrid-stabilizing agents, such as a minor-groove binder, can be added to the probe to make the system more robust.[46] Dual-labeled probes can also be cleaved using a DNAzyme (a DNA molecule that acts as a catalyst) generated during PCR.[96] Finally, irreversible ligation can also be used for homogeneous genotyping with a fluorescent readout.[16] Hydrolysis probes generate fluorescence through changes in covalent bonds. The change in fluorescence signal is irreversible, and melting analysis of the hydrolyzed probe is not useful.

Mixed Mechanism Probes. Several probe systems appear to function by both hydrolysis and hybridization mechanisms. These include hairpin probes, self-probing amplicon primers, and displacement probes. A hairpin probe functions similarly to a hairpin primer in that it is designed to increase in fluorescence when the distance between the quencher and the reporter increases upon target hybridization (see Figure 37-24, row five). Similarly, primers that result in self-probing amplicons have a hairpin that separates quencher from reporter when hybridized.[104] Competitive displacement probes separate quencher and reporter by competitive hybridization.[56] However, in all three cases, polymerases with exonuclease activity are usually used and the labeled probes are potential substrates for exonuclease cleavage. Indeed, the fluorescence versus cycle number plots often resemble irreversible hydrolysis rather than reversible hybridization (Figure 37-25). Conversely, many exonuclease probes, especially probes labeled on each end, show significant hybridization signals.[58]

Detection and Quantification in Real-Time PCR

When fluorescence is monitored once each cycle in the presence of SYBR Green I, the data closely follow the expected logistic shape discussed earlier (see Figures 37-3 and 37-25 top left). However, with hydrolysis probes, fluorescence is cumulative and continues to increase even after the amount of product reaches a plateau (see Figure 37-25, top middle). In contrast, reactions monitored with hybridization probes may show a decrease in fluorescence at high cycle number[112] (see Figure 37-25, top right). Despite differences in curve shape, all real-time systems follow the amount of product being produced during PCR, and this information is used for detection and quantification.

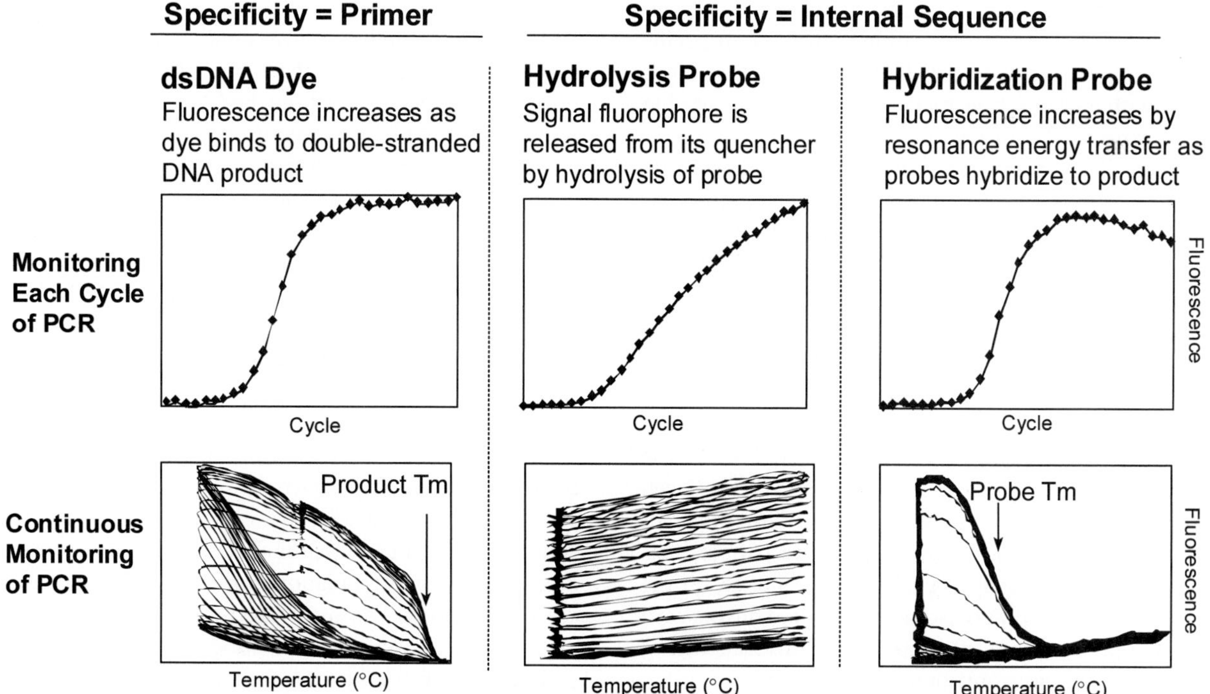

Figure 37-25 Monitoring in real time. The top row shows data collected once each PCR cycle, and the bottom row shows data collected continuously (5 times per second) during all PCR cycles. Three different reporter systems are shown. *(Modified with permission of the publisher from Wittwer CT, Kusukawa N. Real-time PCR. In Persing DH, Tenover FC, Versalovic J, Tang YW, Unger ER, Relman DA, White TJ (eds.), Molecular Microbiology: Diagnostic Principles and Practice, Washington, DC: ASM Press, 2004:71-84.)*

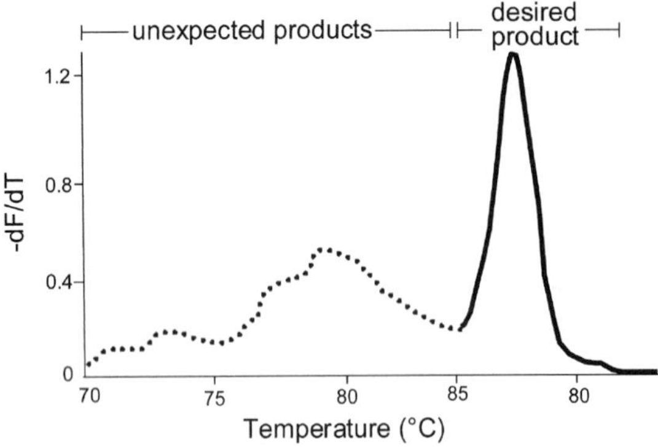

Figure 37-26 First-derivative melting curve showing the target (at high Tm, *solid line*) and nonspecific PCR products (at lower Tm, *dotted line*). *(Modified by permission of the publisher from Morrison TB, Weiss JJ, and Wittwer CT: Quantification of low-copy transcripts by continuous SYBR Green I monitoring during amplification. Biotechniques, 1998, 24:954-63. © 1998 Eaton Publishing.)*

Detection

A fluorescent signal that increases during PCR and follows one of the expected curve shapes suggests that the specific target is present and was amplified. In contrast, a signal that stays at background even after 40 to ~50 PCR cycles suggests that the target is absent and that no amplification occurred. Algorithms that analyze the entire curve are more robust than simple threshold methods.[110] Adequate positive controls (to rule out inhibitory factors) and adequate negative controls (to rule out product contamination and nonspecific signal generation) are necessary. If the fluorescent signal is reversible with hybridization, melting analysis can be used to verify the expected Tm of the probe or product.

When specificity of the assay depends upon the specificity of the primers ("primer-specific detection," as is the case when DNA dyes or labeled primers are used), the possibility of unexpectedly amplifying other targets or primer-dimers is a concern. One way to eliminate or decrease the detection of unexpected targets is to acquire fluorescence during each cycle at a temperature just below the melting transition of the expected target. To illustrate the concept, Figure 37-26 shows a first-derivative melting curve of products at the end of a PCR that generated unexpected products along with the desired product. The signal was generated with SYBR Green I, a dye that detects all double-stranded DNA. The plot reveals both lower Tm species that are unexpected products and a single Gaussian-shaped peak that is centered on the target's predicted Tm. If fluorescence is acquired during each cycle at (in this case) 85 °C, the unexpected products will be denatured and will not contribute to the signal.

Multiplexing of detection is possible with probes that are labeled with different-color dyes or with probes that have different melting temperatures. For example, probe multiplexing can be used to detect the presence of more than one infectious organism, or to discriminate an internal control template from the target.

TABLE 37-5 Correlation Between PCR Efficiency and Amplification Curve Spacing

PCR Efficiency	Cycles/Log [DNA]*
2.0	3.32
1.9	3.59
1.8	3.92
1.7	4.34
1.6	4.90
1.5	5.68

From Wittwer CT, Kusukawa N. Real-time PCR. In Persing DH, Tenover FC, Versalovic J, Tang YW, Unger ER, Relman DA, White TJ (eds.), Molecular Microbiology: Diagnostic Principles and Practice, Washington, DC: ASM Press, 2004:71-84. © 2004 ASM Press.
*The number of cycles that separates each decade difference in initial template concentration (Cycles/log [DNA]) is 1/log (efficiency). The calibration curve slope is the negative of this value (−1/log (efficiency)), assuming the log [initial template] is plotted on the *x*-axis as the independent variable, and cycle number is plotted on the *y*-axis as the dependent variable.

Quantification

Real-time PCR offers a convenient and systematic approach to quantification by monitoring the amount of product each cycle. Perhaps the most popular clinical use of real-time PCR is in the assessment of viral load, particularly for HIV and HCV. The clinical need for quantification is well established and real-time methods give rapid and precise answers. However, other amplification systems, particularly transcription-based and branched DNA methods, are also popular in this highly competitive field. Additional quantitative applications of real time PCR include quantification of mRNAs (after reverse transcription) in gene-expression studies and assessment of gene dosage in genetics and oncology.

One of the advantages of real-time PCR is its large dynamic range. Figure 37-27, *A* shows an extended range of external calibrators in a typical real-time PCR. As the initial template concentration increases, the curves shift to earlier cycles. The extent of the shift depends on the PCR efficiency (Table 37-5). The cycle at which fluorescence rises above background correlates inversely with the log of the initial template concentration (Figure 37-27, *B*). This "cycle" is actually a *virtual* cycle that includes a fractional component determined by interpolation, which can be calculated by several methods. The most precise of these methods is to take the *second derivative* of the curve and determine the cycle number from the maximum point (Figure 37-28). The second derivative of the amplification curve is estimated numerically with Savitzky-Golay polynomials.[78] The second derivative is derived from the shape of the curves and there is no need to adjust baselines or worry about normalizing the fluorescence values. Other methods include *threshold analysis* where a fluorescence level is selected that intersects

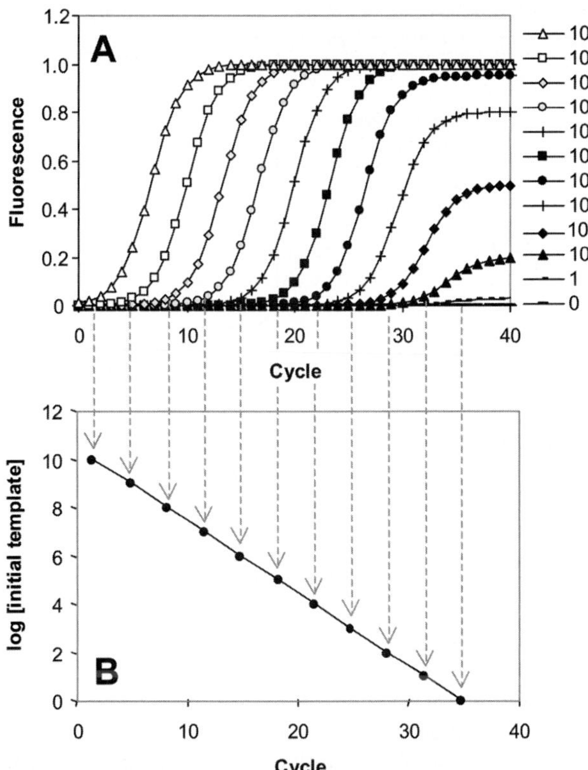

Figure 37-27 Quantification by real-time PCR. Shown are typical real-time curves for amplification reactions of varying initial target concentrations (panel A), and the log of the initial concentration plotted against the cycle number at which the signal rises above background (panel B) as calculated by the second derivative maximum (see Figure 37-28). *(Modified with permission of the publisher from Wittwer CT, Kusukawa N. Real-time PCR. In Persing DH, Tenover FC, Versalovic J, Tang YW, Unger ER, Relman DA, White TJ (eds.), Molecular Microbiology: Diagnostic Principles and Practice, Washington, DC: ASM Press, 2004:71-84.)*

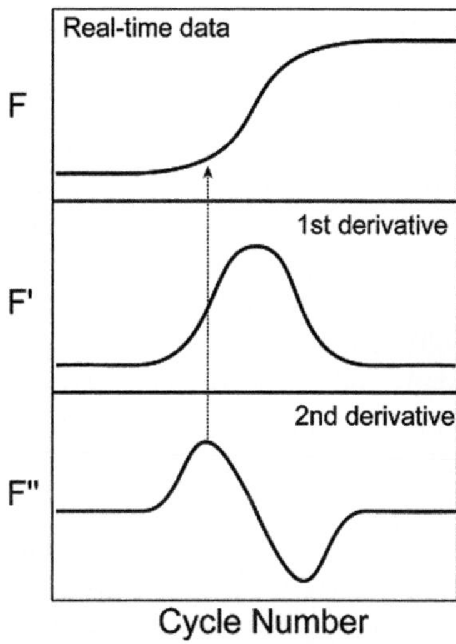

Figure 37-28 Finding the cycle number at which fluorescence rises above background. Real-time fluorescence data (F) from the amplification reaction are shown with the first (F′) and second (F″) derivatives. The maximum of the second derivative corresponds to a defined point on the real-time data where the curve starts to rise. *(Modified with permission of the publisher from Wittwer CT, Kusukawa N. Real-time PCR. In Persing DH, Tenover FC, Versalovic J, Tang YW, Unger ER, Relman DA, White TJ (eds.), Molecular Microbiology: Diagnostic Principles and Practice, Washington, DC: ASM Press, 2004:71-84.)*

with the amplification curves. The fractional cycle number of each curve is found by interpolation and is known as the *cycle threshold* or C_t. However, when the sample fluorescence does not reach the threshold (as may happen with low copy samples), quantification is not possible. The fractional cycle number can also be determined by *fitting points to an exponential.* The number of points in the log-linear portion of each amplification curve is found by inspection on a log-linear plot. The intersection of a line through these points and a set fluorescence level is known as the *crossing point,* or C_p. In both the C_t and C_p methods, it is necessary to adjust the fluorescence baseline before comparing different samples. In some cases, subtraction of a no-template control may eliminate irrelevant signals. Usually an early cycle interval is chosen (e.g., cycles 5 to 10) to represent the baseline. In *arithmetic adjustment,* all baselines are adjusted to zero by subtracting a curve-specific constant. In *proportional adjustment,* the baseline is first adjusted to 1.0 by dividing by a curve-specific constant, followed by subtraction of 1.0 from all points to bring the baseline to zero. Amplification curves can also be *normalized* to between 0.0 and 1.0 with the equation $F_{normalized} = (F_{measured} - F_{min})/(F_{max} - F_{min})$.

Accuracy and Precision

The accuracy of real-time PCR quantification depends not only on the method chosen to analyze the curves, but also on the quality of calibrators used. Purified PCR products quantified by spectrophotometry are easily obtained. When serially diluted, these calibrators can accurately quantify the amount of target in human genomic DNA.[78] Alternatively, purified plasmids or genomic DNA can be used as calibrators. Limiting dilution analysis to determine the amount of "amplifiable" DNA is seldom necessary.[64] The precision of quantitative real-time PCR depends on the copy number. When the initial target concentration is low, imprecision is high. Part of the variance comes from stochastic limitations as defined by the Poisson distribution as described earlier. In addition, the PCR efficiency may be more variable at low copy numbers.

Melting Analysis

Not only can amplification, detection, and quantification be performed by homogeneous hybridization, but detailed genotyping information can also be obtained. Genotyping is best performed in the same tube by monitoring the melting of hybridized duplexes during controlled heating, producing a melting curve signature for the duplex. Such a signature monitors duplex binding over of a range of temperatures in contrast to the single-temperature analysis of conventional hybridization techniques, such as dot blots or microarrays. The advantages of complete melting curves also apply when considering only homogeneous techniques. For example, methods that rely on hydrolysis for signal generation and/or those that acquire data only at one temperature generally result in more genotyping errors.[95] Amplification and melting analysis is a powerful combination of techniques that only requires temperature control and sampling of fluorescence. Many other genotyping techniques require complex separation and/or detection equipment after PCR. Real-time PCR with melting curve analysis allows detection, quantification, and genotyping in less than 30 minutes (see Figure 37-23) without ancillary processing or additional equipment. A book series has been published on methods and applications of rapid-cycle, real-time PCR.[22,62,80,108]

When fluorescence is monitored continuously within each cycle of PCR, the hybridization characteristics of PCR products and probes can be observed. In the plots of fluorescence versus temperature (see Figure 37-25, bottom panels), fluorescence is monitored five times a second during rapid-cycle PCR.[109] With SYBR Green I, the melting characteristics of the amplified DNA can identify the product.[83] No hybridization information is revealed with hydrolysis probes, whereas the melting of hybridization probes is readily apparent. Probe melting occurs at a characteristic temperature that can be exploited to confirm target identity and to analyze sequence alterations under the probe. For routine testing in the clinical laboratory, a single melting curve is usually performed at the end of PCR instead of monitoring hybridization throughout the entire PCR process (see Figure 37-23).

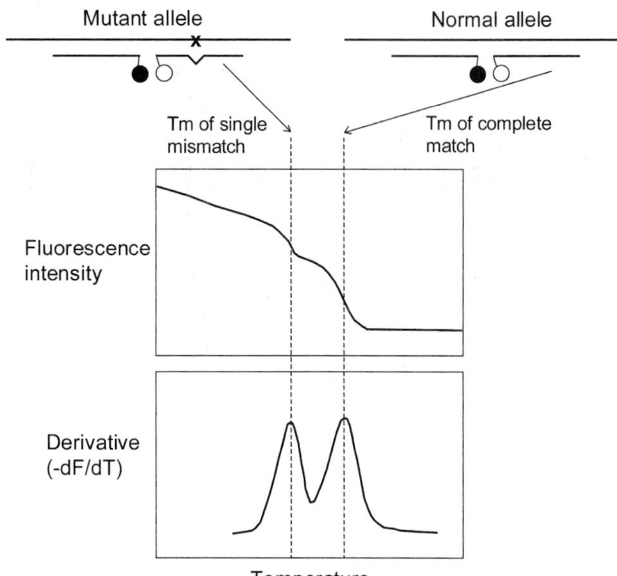

Figure 37-29 Melting curve SNP genotyping. A heterozygous specimen with an SNP under the probe is amplified and melted. Two temperature transitions are visible, one from the mutant allele that is mismatched with the probe and melts at a lower temperature, and one from the normal allele that is completely matched with the probe and melts at a higher temperature. The derivative plot shows the melting temperatures of both the mutant-probe and the normal-probe duplexes as peaks. *(Modified with permission of the publisher from Bernard PS, Pritham GH, Wittwer CT: Color multiplexing hybridization probes using the apolipoprotein E locus as a model system for genotyping. Anal Biochem 1999, 273:221-228. © 1999 Academic Press.)*

Melting Protocols

Immediately after the last PCR cycle, the samples are momentarily denatured (90 °C to 94 °C) cooled to about 10 °C below the Tm range of interest, and finally heated at a ramp rate of 0.1 °C to 0.3 °C while continuously monitoring fluorescence. When hybridization probes are used, the cooling protocol should maximize formation of probe-target duplexes while minimizing formation of the duplex PCR product. Minor primer asymmetry (1:2 to 1:4) and use of 5′-exonuclease–deficient polymerases may be helpful. Rapid cooling (at rates of ~20 °C/sec) to 10 °C above the Tm interest range, followed by slow cooling at 0.1 °C to 1.0 °C/s to 10 °C below the interest range, favors probe-target duplex formation of all alleles.

SNP Detection by Melting Curve Analysis

A hybridization probe-pair placed over a heterozygous polymorphism is shown in Figure 37-29. The reporter probe is complementary to the normal allele. As the temperature is increased, the mismatched mutant hybrid melts first, giving the first transition, followed by the matched normal hybrid. The melting temperatures of both hybrids are easily seen in the derivative plot generated by numerical Savitzky-Golay polynomial estimation.[78] A well-optimized probe design will provide a Tm difference of 8 °C to ~10 °C for a single base mismatch under the probe. The calculation for the baseline in the derivative plot assumes that there are two stable states of fluorescence, one on each side of the transitional region, that depend linearly on temperature (as does fluorescence from a pure fluorophore in solution). After baseline subtraction, each transition can be quantified by fitting multiple Gaussian curves by nonlinear least squares regression.

SNP genotyping by melting curve analysis can be achieved with a variety of probe and dye methods. The top row of Figure 37-30 shows the design of traditional hybridization probe pairs[9] and the results of homozygous wild-type, mutant, and heterozygous samples that are well discriminated from each other. Virtually the same result can be achieved by use of a single hybridization probe in which the fluorescent signal is quenched on the free probe, but dequenched as it forms a hybrid with the target (second row)[7]. The third row shows a design in which no probe is used, and the signal is provided by either a labeled primer that is incorporated into the amplicon[31] or a DNA binding dye[57]; the melting profile of the PCR product is used for genotyping. Finally, the last row shows a design with

require PCR. Allele-specific PCR can be linked to hydrolysis of a dual-labeled probe by formation of a double flap gap.[65] Finally, ligation can be used to join two ends of a long, single "padlock" probe if and only if both ends perfectly anneal to adjacent sites on the target. The resulting circle can be amplified by rolling circle amplification.

CONCLUSION

Molecular diagnostics remains a trendy, developing field in laboratory medicine. Current progress in nucleic acid techniques is extraordinary, driven by the promise of great return. Can drug therapy be tailored to each individual by appropriate molecular tests? Can diagnostic biochips parallel the microelectronics revolution, continuing to provide more information at less expense? Will complete genome sequencing for individual predisposition testing become a reality? Although we are still years away from the Star Trek tricorder, the time for immediate personalized diagnostics will come. To boldly explore these new frontiers, current and future analysis techniques will provide the starship. Indeed the rate-limiting factor is usually in establishing the biological correlations, not the sophistication of the techniques to analyze nucleic acid. Nevertheless, simple, powerful, and cost-effective techniques will get us there sooner.

Techniques for molecular analysis often require multiple steps, including sample preparation, amplification, and analysis. As a result, successful automation is critical for their routine adoption in the clinical laboratory. However, to corruptly paraphrase Henry David Thoreau in Civil Disobedience—"I heartily adhere to the motto: The best automation is not needing to automate." The simplest techniques are often the best. As for immunoassays, methods that require separation and washing steps are being replaced with nonseparation methods that are rapid and homogeneous. These and other simple methods hold great promise for the clinical laboratory.

REFERENCES

1. Allawi HT, SantaLucia J Jr. Nearest neighbor thermodynamic parameters for internal G.A mismatches in DNA. Biochemistry 1998;37:2170-9.
2. Allawi HT, SantaLucia J Jr. Nearest-neighbor thermodynamics of internal A.C mismatches in DNA: sequence dependence and pH effects. Biochemistry 1998;37:9435-44.
3. Allawi HT, SantaLucia J Jr. Thermodynamics and NMR of internal G.T mismatches in DNA. Biochemistry 1997;36:10581-94.
4. Allawi HT, SantaLucia J Jr. Thermodynamics of internal C.T mismatches in DNA. Nucleic Acids Res 1998;26:2694-701.
5. Baltimore D. Viral RNA-dependent DNA polymerase. 1970. Biotechnology 1992;24:3-5.
6. Baner J, Nilsson M, Mendel-Hartvig M, Landegren U. Signal amplification of padlock probes by rolling circle replication. Nucleic Acids Res 1998;26:5073-8.
7. Bennett CD, Campbell MN, Cook CJ, Eyre DJ, Nay LM, Nielsen DR, et al. The Lighttyper™: high-throughput genotyping using fluorescent melting curve analysis. Biotechniques 2003;34:1288-92, 94-5.
8. Benson DA, Karsch-Mizrachi I, Lipman DJ, Ostell J, Rapp BA, Wheeler DL. GenBank. Nucleic Acids Res 2002;30:17-20.
9. Bernard PS, Ajioka RS, Kushner JP, Wittwer CT. Homogeneous multiplex genotyping of hemochromatosis mutations with fluorescent hybridization probes. Am J Pathol 1998;153:1055-61.
10. Blackburn GF, Shah HP, Kenten JH, Leland J, Kamin RA, Link J, et al. Electrochemiluminescence detection for development of immunoassays and DNA probe assays for clinical diagnostics. Clin Chem 1991;37:1534-9.
11. Bolivar F, Rodriguez RL, Greene PJ, Betlach MC, Heyneker HL, Boyer HW. Construction and characterization of new cloning vehicles. II. A multipurpose cloning system. Gene 1977;2:95-113.
12. Bommarito S, Peyret N, SantaLucia J Jr. Thermodynamic parameters for DNA sequences with dangling ends. Nucleic Acids Res 2000;28:1929-34.
13. Borer P. Handbook of biochemistry and molecular biology. In: Fasman GD, ed. Boca Raton, Fla: CRC Press, 1975:589.
14. Braun A, Little DP, Koster H. Detecting CFTR gene mutations by using primer oligo base extension and mass spectrometry. Clin Chem 1997;43:1151-8.
15. Cariello NF, Scott JK, Kat AG, Thilly WG, Keohavong P. Resolution of a missense mutant in human genomic DNA by denaturing gradient gel electrophoresis and direct sequencing using in vitro DNA amplification: HPRT Munich. Am J Hum Genet 1988;42:726-34.
16. Chen X, Livak KJ, Kwok PY. A homogeneous, ligase-mediated DNA diagnostic test. Genome Res 1998;8:549-56.
17. Collins ML, Irvine B, Tyner D, Fine E, Zayati C, Chang C, et al. A branched DNA signal amplification assay for quantification of nucleic acid targets below 100 molecules/ml. Nucleic Acids Res 1997;25:2979-84.
18. Compton J. Nucleic acid sequence-based amplification. Nature 1991;350:91-2.
19. Crockett AO, Wittwer CT. Fluorescein-labeled oligonucleotides for real-time PCR: using the inherent quenching of deoxyguanosine nucleotides. Anal Biochem 2001;290:89-97.
20. de Kok JB, Wiegerinck ET, Giesendorf BA, Swinkels DW. Rapid genotyping of single nucleotide polymorphisms using novel minor groove binding DNA oligonucleotides (MGB probes). Hum Mutat 2002;19:554-9.

21. Dean FB, Hosono S, Fang L, Wu X, Faruqi AF, Bray-Ward P, et al. Comprehensive human genome amplification using multiple displacement amplification. Proc Natl Acad Sci U S A 2002;99:5261-6.
22. Dietmaier W, Wittwer C, Sivasubramanian N. Rapid cycle real-time PCR: methods and applications: genetics and oncology. Berlin: Springer,2002:205 pp.
23. Elenitoba-Johnson KS, Jenson SD, Abbott RT, Palais RA, Bohling SD, Lin Z, et al. Involvement of multiple signaling pathways in follicular lymphoma transformation: p38-mitogen-activated protein kinase as a target for therapy. Proc Natl Acad Sci U S A 2003;100:7259-64.
24. Franca LT, Carrilho E, Kist TB. A review of DNA sequencing techniques. Q Rev Biophys 2002;35: 169-200.
25. Fritz J, Cooper EB, Gaudet S, Sorger PK, Manalis SR. Electronic detection of DNA by its intrinsic molecular charge. Proc Natl Acad Sci U S A 2002;99:14142-6.
26. Gao Q, Yeung ES. High-throughput detection of unknown mutations by using multiplexed capillary electrophoresis with poly(vinylpyrrolidone) solution. Anal Chem 2000;72:2499-506.
27. Germer S, Higuchi R. Single-tube genotyping without oligonucleotide probes. Genome Res 1999;9:72-8.
28. Germer S, Holland MJ, Higuchi R. High-throughput SNP allele-frequency determination in pooled DNA samples by kinetic PCR. Genome Res 2000;10:258-66.
29. Giachetti C, Linnen JM, Kolk DP, Dockter J, Gillotte-Taylor K, Park M, et al. Highly sensitive multiplex assay for detection of human immunodeficiency virus type 1 and hepatitis C virus RNA. J Clin Microbiol 2002;40:2408-19.
30. Guatelli JC, Whitfield KM, Kwoh DY, Barringer KJ, Richman DD, Gingeras TR. Isothermal, in vitro amplification of nucleic acids by a multienzyme reaction modeled after retroviral replication. Proc Natl Acad Sci U S A 1990;87:1874-8.
31. Gundry CN, Vandersteen JG, Reed GH, Pryor RJ, Chen J, Wittwer CT. Amplicon melting analysis with labeled primers: a closed-tube method for differentiating homozygotes and heterozygotes. Clin Chem 2003;49:396-406.
32. Hall JG, Eis PS, Law SM, Reynaldo LP, Prudent JR, Marshall DJ, et al. Sensitive detection of DNA polymorphisms by the serial invasive signal amplification reaction. Proc Natl Acad Sci U S A 2000;97:8272-7.
33. Heller MJ. DNA microarray technology: devices, systems, and applications. Annu Rev Biomed Eng 2002;4:129-53.
34. Highsmith WE Jr, Jin Q, Nataraj AJ, O'Connor JM, Burland VD, Baubonis WR, et al. Use of a DNA toolbox for the characterization of mutation scanning methods. I: construction of the toolbox and evaluation of heteroduplex analysis. Electrophoresis 1999;20:1186-94.
35. Highsmith WE Jr, Nataraj AJ, Jin Q, O'Connor JM, El-Nabi SH, Kusukawa N, Garner MM. Use of DNA toolbox for the characterization of mutation scanning methods. II: evaluation of single-strand conformation polymorphism analysis. Electrophoresis 1999;20:1195-203.
36. Higuchi R, Dollinger G, Walsh PS, Griffith R. Simultaneous amplification and detection of specific DNA sequences. Biotechnology (N Y) 1992;10:413-17.
37. Higuchi R, Fockler C, Dollinger G, Watson R. Kinetic PCR analysis: real-time monitoring of DNA amplification reactions. Biotechnology (N Y) 1993;11: 1026-30.
38. Holloway AJ, van Laar RK, Tothill RW, Bowtell DD. Options available—from start to finish—for obtaining data from DNA microarrays II. Nat Genet 2002;32 Suppl:481-9.
39. Hopfenbeck JA, Holden JA, Wittwer CT, Kjeldsberg CR. Digoxigenin-labeled probes amplified from genomic DNA detect T-cell gene rearrangements. Am J Clin Pathol 1992;97:638-44.
40. Jonas V, Alden MJ, Curry JI, Kamisango K, Knott CA, Lankford R, et al. Detection and identification of *Mycobacterium tuberculosis* directly from sputum sediments by amplification of rRNA. J Clin Microbiol 1993;31:2410-16.
41. Kellar KL, Iannone MA. Multiplexed microsphere-based flow cytometric assays. Exp Hematol 2002;30:1227-37.
42. Khorasanizadeh S. The nucleosome: from genomic organization to genomic regulation. Cell 2004;116:259-72.
43. Kornberg A, Baker TA. DNA replication, 2nd Edition, New York: WH, Freeman and Company, 1992: 101-273.
44. Kornberg A, Baker TA. DNA replication, 2nd Edition, New York: WH Freeman and Company, 1992:307-322.
45. Kricka LJ, Fortina P. Microarray technology and applications: an all-language literature survey including books and patents. Clin Chem 2001;47: 1479-82.
46. Kutyavin IV, Afonina IA, Mills A, Gorn VV, Lukhtanov EA, Belousov ES, et al. 3′-minor groove binder-DNA probes increase sequence specificity at PCR extension temperatures. Nucleic Acids Res 2000;28:655-61.
47. Kwoh DY, Davis GR, Whitfield KM, Chappelle HL, DiMichele LJ, Gingeras TR. Transcription-based amplification system and detection of amplified human immunodeficiency virus type 1 with a bead-based sandwich hybridization format. Proc Natl Acad Sci U S A 1989;86:1173-7.
48. Kwok PY. SNP genotyping with fluorescence polarization detection. Hum Mutat 2002;19:315-23.
49. Kwok S, Higuchi R. Avoiding false positives with PCR. Nature 1989;339:237-8.

50. Laird PW. The power and the promise of DNA methylation markers. Nat Rev Cancer 2003;3:253-66.
51. Lander ES, Linton LM, Birren B, Nusbaum C, Zody MC, Baldwin J, et al. Initial sequencing and analysis of the human genome. Nature 2001;409:860-921.
52. Langer PR, Waldrop AA, Ward DC. Enzymatic synthesis of biotin-labeled polynucleotides: novel nucleic acid affinity probes. Proc Natl Acad Sci U S A 1981;78:6633-7.
53. Lay MJ, Wittwer CT. Real-time fluorescence genotyping of factor V Leiden during rapid-cycle PCR. Clin Chem 1997;43:2262-7.
54. Lee LG, Connell CR, Bloch W. Allelic discrimination by nick-translation PCR with fluorogenic probes. Nucleic Acids Res 1993;21:3761-6.
55. Li Q, Liu Z, Monroe H, Culiat CT. Integrated platform for detection of DNA sequence variants using capillary array electrophoresis. Electrophoresis 2002;23:1499-511.
56. Li Q, Luan G, Guo Q, Liang J. A new class of homogeneous nucleic acid probes based on specific displacement hybridization. Nucleic Acids Res 2002;30:E5.
57. Liew MA, Pryor R, Palais R, Meadows C, Erali M, Lyon E, Wittwer CT. Genotyping of single nucleotide polymorphisms by high-resolution melting of small amplicons. Clin Chem 2004:50:1156-64.
58. Livak KJ, Flood SJ, Marmaro J, Giusti W, Deetz K. Oligonucleotides with fluorescent dyes at opposite ends provide a quenched probe system useful for detecting PCR product and nucleic acid hybridization. PCR Methods Appl 1995;4:357-62.
59. Lizardi PM, Huang X, Zhu Z, Bray-Ward P, Thomas DC, Ward DC. Mutation detection and single-molecule counting using isothermal rolling-circle amplification. Nat Genet 1998;19:225-32.
60. Lomeli H, Tyagi S, Pritchard CG, Lizardi PM, Kramer FR. Quantitative assays based on the use of replicatable hybridization probes. Clin Chem 1989;35: 1826-31.
61. Maule J. Pulsed-field gel electrophoresis. Mol Biotechnol 1998;9:107-26.
62. Meuer SC, Wittwer C, Nakagawara K. Rapid cycle real-time PCR: methods and applications. Berlin: Springer,2001:408 pp.
63. Michalatos-Beloin S, Tishkoff SA, Bentley KL, Kidd KK, Ruano G. Molecular haplotyping of genetic markers 10 kb apart by allele-specific long-range PCR. Nucleic Acids Res 1996;24:4841-3.
64. Morrison TB, Weis JJ, Wittwer CT. Quantification of low-copy transcripts by continuous SYBR Green I monitoring during amplification. Biotechniques 1998;24:954-8, 60, 62.
65. Moser MJ, Marshall DJ, Grenier JK, Kieffer CD, Killeen AA, Ptacin JL, et al. Exploiting the enzymatic recognition of an unnatural base pair to develop a universal genetic analysis system. Clin Chem 2003;49:407-14.
66. Nagamine CM, Chan K, Lau YF. A PCR artifact: generation of heteroduplexes [Letter]. Am J Hum Genet 1989;45:337-9.
67. Nazarenko I, Pires R, Lowe B, Obaidy M, Rashtchian A. Effect of primary and secondary structure of oligodeoxyribonucleotides on the fluorescent properties of conjugated dyes. Nucleic Acids Res 2002;30:2089-195.
68. Nazarenko IA, Bhatnagar SK, Hohman RJ. A closed tube format for amplification and detection of DNA based on energy transfer. Nucleic Acids Res 1997;25:2516-21.
69. Nelson NC, Cheikh AB, Matsuda E, Becker MM. Simultaneous detection of multiple nucleic acid targets in a homogeneous format. Biochemistry 1996;35:8429-38.
70. Nielsen PE. PNA technology. Methods Mol Biol 2002;208:3-26.
71. Notomi T, Okayama H, Masubuchi H, Yonekawa T, Watanabe K, Amino N, Hase T. Loop-mediated isothermal amplification of DNA. Nucleic Acids Res 2000;28:E63.
72. Nucleic acids in chemistry and biology. New York: IRL Press at Oxford University Press, 1990:446 pp.
73. Orita M, Iwahana H, Kanazawa H, Hayashi K, Sekiya T. Detection of polymorphisms of human DNA by gel electrophoresis as single-strand conformation polymorphisms. Proc Natl Acad Sci U S A 1989;86:2766-70.
74. Park SJ, Taton TA, Mirkin CA. Array-based electrical detection of DNA with nanoparticle probes. Science 2002;295:1503-6.
75. Perkins TT, Quake SR, Smith DE, Chu S. Relaxation of a single DNA molecule observed by optical microscopy. Science 1994;264:822-6.
76. Peyret N, Seneviratne PA, Allawi HT, SantaLucia J Jr. Nearest-neighbor thermodynamics and NMR of DNA sequences with internal A.A, C.C, G.G, and T.T mismatches. Biochemistry 1999;38:3468-77.
77. Phillips J, Eberwine JH. Antisense rna amplification: a linear amplification method for analyzing the mrna population from single living cells. Methods 1996;10:283-8.
78. Press WH, Teukolsky SA, Vetterling WT, Flannery BP. Salvitsky-Golay smoothing filters. In: Numerical recipes in C: the art of scientific computing. New York: Cambridge University Press, Cambridge England, 1992:650-5.
79. Pusch W, Wurmbach JH, Thiele H, Kostrzewa M. MALDI-TOF mass spectrometry-based SNP genotyping. Pharmacogenomics 2002;3:537-48.
80. Reischl U, Wittwer C, Cockerill F. Rapid cycle real-time PCR—methods and applications: microbiology and food analysis. Berlin: Springer, 2002:258 pp.

81. Reyes AA, Ugozzoli LA, Lowery JD, Breneman JW III, Hixson CS, Press RD, Wallace RB. Linked linear amplification: a new method for the amplification of DNA. Clin Chem 2001;47:31-40.
82. Riesner D, Steger G, Zimmat R, Owens RA, Wagenhofer M, Hillen W, et al. Temperature-gradient gel electrophoresis of nucleic acids: analysis of conformational transitions, sequence variations, and protein-nucleic acid interactions. Electrophoresis 1989;10:377-89.
83. Ririe KM, Rasmussen RP, Wittwer CT. Product differentiation by analysis of DNA melting curves during the polymerase chain reaction. Anal Biochem 1997;245:154-60.
84. Ronaghi M, Uhlen M, Nyren P. A sequencing method based on real-time pyrophosphate. Science 1998;281:363, 5.
85. Saiki RK, Gelfand DH, Stoffel S, Scharf SJ, Higuchi R, Horn GT, et al. Primer-directed enzymatic amplification of DNA with a thermostable DNA polymerase. Science 1988;239:487-91.
86. Sanger F, Nicklen S, Coulson AR. DNA sequencing with chain-terminating inhibitors. Proc Natl Acad Sci U S A 1977;74:5463-7.
87. SantaLucia J Jr. A unified view of polymer, dumbbell, and oligonucleotide DNA nearest-neighbor thermodynamics. Proc Natl Acad Sci U S A 1998;95:1460-5.
88. Schena M, Shalon D, Davis RW, Brown PO. Quantitative monitoring of gene expression patterns with a complementary DNA microarray. Science 1995;270:467-70.
89. Seuss. The cat in the hat comes back! In: Beginner Books. New York, 1958
90. Smith HO. Nucleotide sequence specificity of restriction endonucleases. Science 1979;205:455-62.
91. Sorlie T, Tibshirani R, Parker J, Hastie T, Marron JS, Nobel A, et al. Repeated observation of breast tumor subtypes in independent gene expression data sets. Proc Natl Acad Sci U S A 2003;100:8418-23.
92. Southern EM. Detection of specific sequences among DNA fragments separated by gel electrophoresis. J Mol Biol 1975;98:503-17.
93. Stenson PD, Ball EV, Mort M, Phillips AD, Shiel JA, Thomas NS, et al. Human gene mutation database (HGMD): 2003 update. Hum Mutat 2003;21:577-81.
94. Svanvik N, Stahlberg A, Sehlstedt U, Sjoback R, Kubista M. Detection of PCR products in real time using light-up probes. Anal Biochem 2000;287: 179-82.
95. Teupser D, Rupprecht W, Lohse P, Thiery J. Fluorescence-based detection of the CETP TaqIB polymorphism: false positives with the TaqMan-based exonuclease assay attributable to a previously unknown gene variant. Clin Chem 2001;47:852-7.
96. Todd AV, Fuery CJ, Impey HL, Applegate TL, Haughton MA. DzyNA-PCR: use of DNAzymes to detect and quantify nucleic acid sequences in a real-time fluorescent format. Clin Chem 2000;46: 625-30.
97. Tyagi S, Bratu DP, Kramer FR. Multicolor molecular beacons for allele discrimination. Nat Biotechnol 1998;16:49-53.
98. Umek RM, Lin SW, Vielmetter J, Terbrueggen RH, Irvine B, Yu CJ, et al. Electronic detection of nucleic acids: a versatile platform for molecular diagnostics. J Mol Diagn 2001;3:74-84.
99. Urdea MS, Horn T, Fultz TJ, Anderson M, Running JA, Hamren S, et al. Branched DNA amplification multimers for the sensitive, direct detection of human hepatitis viruses. Nucleic Acids Symp Ser 1991:197-200.
100. Van Ness J, Van Ness LK, Galas DJ. Isothermal reactions for the amplification of oligonucleotides. Proc Natl Acad Sci U S A 2003;100:4504-9.
101. Walker GT, Linn CP, Nadeau JG. DNA detection by strand displacement amplification and fluorescence polarization with signal enhancement using a DNA binding protein. Nucleic Acids Res 1996;24: 348-53.
102. WalkerPeach CR, Winkler M, DuBois DB, Pasloske BL. Ribonuclease-resistant RNA controls (Armored RNA) for reverse transcription-PCR, branched DNA, and genotyping assays for hepatitis C virus. Clin Chem 1999;45:2079-85.
103. Wetmur JG. DNA probes: applications of the principles of nucleic acid hybridization. Crit Rev Biochem Mol Biol 1991;26:227-59.
104. Whitcombe D, Theaker J, Guy SP, Brown T, Little S. Detection of PCR products using self-probing amplicons and fluorescence. Nat Biotechnol 1999;17: 804-7.
105. Wiedmann M, Wilson WJ, Czajka J, Luo J, Barany F, Batt CA. Ligase chain reaction (LCR)—overview and applications. PCR Methods Appl 1994;3:S51-64.
106. Willmore C, Holden JA, Zhou L, Tripp S, Wittwer CT, Layfield LJ. Detection of c-kit activating mutations in gastrointestinal stromal tumors by high-resolution amplicon melting analysis. Am J Clin Path 2004;122:206-16.
107. Wittwer CT, Garling DJ. Rapid cycle DNA amplification: time and temperature optimization. Biotechniques 1991;10:76-83.
108. Wittwer CT, Hahn M, Kaul K. Rapid cycle real-time PCR—methods and applications: quantification. Berlin: Springer, 2004:223 pp.
109. Wittwer CT, Herrmann MG, Moss AA, Rasmussen RP. Continuous fluorescence monitoring of rapid cycle DNA amplification. Biotechniques 1997;22:130-1, 4-8.
110. Wittwer CT, Kusukawa N. Real-time PCR. In: Persing DH, Tenover FC, Relman DA, White TJ, Tang YW, Versalovic J, Unger ER, eds. Diagnostic molecular

microbiology: principles and applications. Washington: ASM Press, 2004:71-84.

111. Wittwer CT, Reed GH, Gundry CN, Vandersteen JG, Pryor RJ. High-resolution genotyping by amplicon melting analysis using LCGreen. Clin Chem 2003;49:853-60.
112. Wittwer CT, Ririe KM, Andrew RV, David DA, Gundry RA, Balis UJ. The Lightcycler™: a microvolume multisample fluorimeter with rapid temperature control. Biotechniques 1997;22:176-81.
113. Xiao W, Oefner PJ. Denaturing high-performance liquid chromatography: a review. Hum Mutat 2001;17:439-74.
114. Zhang DY, Zhang W, Li X, Konomi Y. Detection of rare DNA targets by isothermal ramification amplification. Gene 2001;274:209-16.
115. Zhou L, Myers A, Vandersteen JG, Wang L, Wittwer CT. Closed-tube genotyping with unlabeled oligonucleotide probes and a saturating DNA dye. Clin Chem 2004;50:1328-35.
116. Zhou L, Vandersteen J, Wang L, Fuller T, Taylor M, Palais B, Wittwer CT. High-resolution DNA melting curve analysis to establish HLA genotypic identity. Tissue Antigens 2004;64:156-64.
117. Zhou MY, Gomez-Sanchez CE. Universal TA cloning. Curr Issues Mol Biol 2000;2:1-7.

CHAPTER 38

Design and Operation of the Molecular Diagnostics Laboratory

Anthony A. Killeen, M.D., Ph.D.

INTRODUCTION

The design and operation of a molecular diagnostics laboratory have much in common with other areas of the clinical laboratories. The purpose of this chapter is to highlight specific issues that are unique to a molecular diagnostics laboratory, both in design and operation.

Centralization or Decentralization?

Molecular techniques are of importance in clinical diagnostics in most disciplines of laboratory medicine and pathology and their applications will continue to grow in essentially all areas of testing. These considerations raise a fundamental question in the design of a laboratory system: should each discipline that uses molecular techniques have its own molecular laboratory space or is a centralized molecular laboratory a more suitable model to deliver molecular testing services? The answer will depend to a large degree on local factors, but has significant implications for the overall costs and efficiencies of providing molecular testing services. The major argument in favor of centralization is the efficiencies achieved through sharing of equipment, reagents, personnel, and space. On the other hand, the adoption of molecular techniques in areas as diverse as microbiology and inherited diseases requires a broad range of specialist skills and knowledge that may be difficult to develop in a centralized laboratory. In addition, certain molecular tests may be integral to the activities of another laboratory, thereby precluding their performance in a central molecular testing facility. For example, many hospital laboratories use a dual system in which a central laboratory performs tests in areas such as molecular genetics and molecular oncology, whereas molecular techniques for advanced microbial identification and characterization are performed in the existing microbiology laboratory.

Choosing a Test Menu

Factors that influence the decision to offer a test include the local demand, the resources available to perform the test, the skills and interests of the personnel, particularly the laboratory director, the likelihood of the test being financially viable, and whether the test is, in whole or part, patented or has other intellectual property restrictions.

Local demand for testing will most likely come from clinicians who are looking for tests to help with patient diagnosis and management. Such demands should be carefully evaluated to ensure that clinician expectations can be reasonably met in a cost-effective manner. Higher volume tests tend to improve the overall financial stability of a laboratory because the fixed costs become a smaller proportion of the individual test cost. Conversely, it seldom makes financial sense to offer low-volume tests unless reimbursements are sufficiently high to cover the costs. However, volumes may increase if the laboratory can become a regional or national referral center for a test. If a clinician has expertise in a clinical area that stimulates test ordering, it is possible that offering a laboratory test may enhance the ability of the clinical service to attract increased recognition, more patients, research support, and other external funding. Thus what seems at first to be a low-volume test may with time become an important item in the laboratory's and institution's repertoire. A further consideration in selecting the test menu is the ability to deliver acceptable turnaround times. Expectations for turnaround time, and therefore the frequency with which tests must be performed, vary with the analyte. For example, tests for infectious agents usually require a shorter turnaround time than do tests for chronic, inherited diseases. Expectations of a short turnaround time tend to increase the analytical cost per sample, while at the same time indicate the need to offer a test in house rather than send samples to an external laboratory.

SPACE AND DESIGN CONSIDERATIONS

The major consideration in the physical layout of a molecular diagnostics laboratory, other than adequate space, is a design that prevents or helps control contamination. The use of polymerase chain reaction (PCR) and other target amplification methodologies can introduce an important source of laboratory error, namely, contamination of the laboratory with amplicons from previous reactions. These can be introduced in the laboratory environment when a tube containing amplicons is opened and a small amount of the solution becomes an aerosol. Without careful laboratory technique, amplicons can be spread to new samples and reagents by airborne droplets, gloves, skin, pens, paper, and pieces of equipment, such as pipettes. Because each amplicon can be replicated in a subsequent amplification reaction, an amplicon that contaminates a new patient sample or a reagent solution can lead to an erroneous result, usually a false-positive determination. Contamination of the laboratory by amplicons is a serious problem that often requires extensive decontamination and every precaution should be taken to prevent this problem.

Historically the design of the laboratory has been an important factor in controlling contamination, and the most common design feature that is unique to the molecular diagnostics laboratory has been use of separate rooms for set up and analysis of target amplification reactions. Some laboratory designs also incorporate a positive pressure air control system to prevent airflow from the analysis room to the sample set up or reagent preparation rooms. The air from the analysis room may be vented directly to the exterior of the laboratory building. Such design features can be implemented more easily when planning new construction than when attempting to adapt space in an older building for use as a molecular diagnostics laboratory. If multiple rooms are unavailable, consideration should be given to using laminar flow hoods that contain an ultraviolet light. UV-induced cross-linking of DNA can minimize the effects of amplicon contamination during sample set up.

Other methods to avoid contamination involve meticulous laboratory practice by personnel. The flow of operations from sample receipt to amplified product analysis involves a sequential series of steps that tend from "clean" to "contaminated." It therefore follows that there should be no movement of reagents or equipment in the reverse direction to this flow. For example, pipettes that are used in the post-PCR area should never be introduced into a pre-PCR area. Laboratory coats that are worn in the post-PCR area should be removed before entering a pre-PCR area. Gloves should be discarded after use in the post-PCR area. Laboratory benches should be regularly cleaned using amplicon decontaminating agents, such as solutions of bleach.

Modifications to the procedures used can also reduce contamination. Reagent strategies, such as the use of uracil in PCR reactions combined with preincubation of samples with uracil *N*-glycosylase (UNG), can minimize the risk of contamination.[11] Commercially available systems have been developed that use a closed analytical system (i.e., reaction tubes that are analyzed without being opened). Finally, there are alternative laboratory methods to PCR that do not involve target amplification. These include several methods generally known as "signal amplification" techniques.[8] Depending on the laboratory space (particularly if only limited space is available) and the desired test menu, use of such techniques may be preferable to target amplification methods.

OPERATIONAL CONSIDERATIONS

As mentioned previously, only operational details that are specific for a molecular diagnostics laboratory are discussed here. Many of these involve regulatory issues that are relevant to practice within the United States and may vary between jurisdictions. They are provided here for general guidance.

Documents, Records, Sample Retention

Compared to past laboratory testing, newer molecular testing sometimes has unique information needs and sample storage requirements. Requisitions, consent, records, and sample retention are reviewed in this section.

Requisitions

As with all requests for testing, the requisition form should indicate patient identifying information, the ordering physician's name and contact information, the sample type, the time of collection, and the test to be performed. For genetic testing, it is common that the requisition form will solicit information on relevant family history that is often provided as a hand-drawn pedigree diagram. Such information can be essential for test interpretation and should be available to the testing laboratory.

Consent for Genetic Testing and Privacy of Medical Records

Much more attention is given in the medical literature to the need for informed consent for genetic testing than to most areas of laboratory testing. The principal reason for this is that by testing for inherited disorders, information may be obtained that has diagnostic or risk implications for other family members. In addition, genetic testing may indicate a high probability of development of symptomatic disease later in life in patients who appear well at the time of testing. Patients and families may be stigmatized by a diagnosis of genetic disease and may suffer discrimination in employment and in insurability. Although the number of documented cases of such discrimination is few, the fear of adverse consequences of genetic testing is quite common. For these reasons, obtaining informed consent for genetic testing is a common practice and is required by law in many states.[6]

Record Keeping

Under current U.S. federal guidelines, the following records must be retained for at least 2 years for all laboratory testing: specimen requisitions, patient test results and reports, instrument printouts, accession records, quality control records, instrument maintenance records, proficiency testing records, and quality improvement records. Laws concerning records for paternity and forensic testing vary by state; it is the responsibility of the director to assure all applicable regulations are met.

Retention of Extracted Nucleic Acids

Under current federal law, there is no minimum length of time for which an extracted sample of DNA or RNA must be stored after analysis is complete, although regulations do exist for retention of the primary sample. Because extracted samples tend to be of small volume (measured in microliters), many laboratories retain samples indefinitely. However, some states, acting out of concerns for genetic privacy, have proposed or enacted legislation that requires destruction of samples for genetic testing after analysis is complete. These laws vary widely and often specify exceptions (e.g., for samples used in forensic work). Laboratory directors are responsible for following the requirements of their own jurisdictions.

PERSONNEL

The qualifications of personnel are determined by regulatory agencies and by the availability of suitable staff. In the United States, the qualifications for director, technical supervisor, and medical technologists are provided in the Clinical Laboratory Improvement Amendments.[1]

Directorship

The laboratory director should be qualified to direct a high-complexity laboratory. Under current U.S. regulations, federal law requires no formal experience in molecular diagnostics. However, because of the need to issue an interpretation of many molecular diagnostic test results, the director should ideally have training that includes experience in at least one major area of molecular laboratory activity, such as molecular genetics, oncology, infectious diseases, or identity testing. The expertise of the director may need to be complemented by additional personnel with appropriate training, including associate directors with expertise in areas of relevance to the test menu (e.g., hematopathology, genetics, and microbiology).

Technical Personnel

The most suitable educational background for a medical technologist in a molecular diagnostics laboratory is completion of a medical technology training program, including training or experience in molecular diagnostics. However, few medical technology programs produce graduates with specific skills in molecular diagnostics, and thus there is often a need for extensive on-the-job training of newly hired personnel.

Individuals with skills in molecular biology but without formal training in medical technology may be an alternative source of personnel in some geographical areas, but their employment may be contingent on local legal standards for employment within a clinical laboratory (e.g., state licensure requirements). Such individuals often have a strong theoretical background and possibly extensive laboratory experience (often in a research setting), but it is important to recognize that there are specific skills acquired in a formal medical technology program and that the clinical laboratory is a different environment than a research laboratory. This is particularly true in the areas of quality control and abiding by standard procedures.

RESULT REPORTING

Specific guidelines for reporting molecular pathology test results in the United States can be found in the "Molecular Pathology Checklist" from the College of American Pathologists (CAP).[2] In general, information that should be included in reports of genetic testing include details of the methods used including all probes and restriction enzymes, the locus and mutations tested, the findings, and an interpretive report. When mutation testing is incomplete because not all possible disease-causing mutations are examined, the report should indicate the false-negative rate. For example, the recommended panel for cystic fibrosis carrier screening in the U.S. population includes a basic set of only 25 of the >1000 known mutations. This abbreviated panel can detect 80% to 85% of mutations in Caucasians. The false-negative rate for mutation identification is therefore 15% to 20%. In the case of an individual with a negative test result, the report should include a Bayesian estimate of the posterior risk of carrying a mutation.[5]

Where genetic testing is based on linked genetic markers, the report should indicate the false-negative and false-positive rates arising from recombination between the test locus and the disease locus. This can be inferred from the known genetic distance between the loci.

In the case of some genetic diseases, the genotype-phenotype relationship varies with the mutation and the pattern of inheritance (e.g., dominant versus recessive) and the report should include an appropriate discussion of the findings relevant to the observed mutations. For example, some mutations in *CYP21* (the steroid 21-hydroxylase gene)–such as the common gene deletion mutation–are associated with severe, classic congenital adrenal hyperplasia (an autosomal recessive disorder) whereas other mutations, such as V281L, in the same gene are associated with the late-onset form of the disease, which is characterized by milder symptoms of androgen excess in females.[7] In the case of Huntington disease (an autosomal dominant disorder), expansions of the pathogenic trinucleotide repeat in the range of 35 to 39 repeats are associated with a later age of onset than are mutations of ≥40 repeats.[9] Information on mutation-specific phenotypes, penetrance, and pattern of inheritance should be described. It is also common practice to include in reports of genetic testing a statement that genetic counseling may be appropriate for the patient and family.

Laboratories that perform genetic studies occasionally encounter families in which the laboratory findings are inconsistent with the reported paternity. These situations should be discussed with the clinician or genetic counselor to determine whether specimens were correctly labeled and the family relationships accurately reported on the requisition form. If there is a possibility of a sample mix-up, new samples should be obtained. In cases of demonstrated nonpaternity, it may not be possible to determine the risk of a genetic disease to an offspring and the report should indicate this. The issue of nonpaternity or undisclosed adoption is clearly one that has to be approached with great discretion by the genetic counselor or other professional who is responsible for communication of the test result to the patient or family.

It is not uncommon for patients, fearing discrimination, to request that genetic testing be performed without informing their health insurance companies and without having the results entered into the medical record. In such situations, the genetics results are often stored in a shadow chart maintained by the patient's physician in a private office or similar location. This practice is problematic for various reasons. First, a complete medical record may be needed in an emergency, and the absence of essential medical information may delay appropriate medical therapy. Storing portions of the record in separate locations undermines the integrity and usefulness of the medical record. In addition, as a practical matter, the reason for a clinic visit and some mention of the test result usually appears elsewhere in the medical record (e.g., in correspondence between physicians), and therefore the degree to which a test result can be truly sequestered from the formal medical record is probably limited. Also, from a legal perspective, the medical record includes all information relevant to a patient's care, even if that information is stored in an alternative location. The entire medical record should be available to authorized personnel.

The immediate resolution to these issues is to ensure that the complete medical record is secured and that hospital employees and others access only information that is needed for patient care. All employees should be made aware of policies related to confidentiality of patient records and the importance of adhering to principles of patient privacy. In the United States, this is not just an ethical requirement, but also a legal one under the Health Insurance Portability and Accountability Act of 1996 (HIPAA).[3] Respect of patient privacy should make the use of shadow records unnecessary. More global solutions to fears of genetic discrimination require introduction of legislation that forbids such discrimination, particularly in employment and insurability.[10]

Use of Analyte-Specific Reagents

In the United States, laboratory methods that involve the use of analyte-specific reagents (which include many molecular test methods) necessitate a disclaimer on test reports. The language should include the statement that "this test was developed and its performance characteristics determined by (laboratory name). It has not been cleared or approved by the U.S. Food and Drug Administration."[4] This statement is not required for tests that have been cleared by the FDA for use in clinical diagnostics. The language of the statement may be misinterpreted by some insurance payers as meaning that the test was performed for research purposes. To avoid this misperception, many laboratories include an additional statement to the effect that the test was not performed as a research test or that approval is not required by the FDA. Specific wording addressing this is recommended by the CAP molecular pathology inspection checklist.[2]

Correlation With Other Laboratory Results

For testing in areas such as molecular oncology, inherited disorders, and posttransplantation bone marrow engraftment, it is common that other testing is performed on the sample. This may include morphology studies, flow cytometry, or cytogenetic evaluation. Where possible, the results of molecular diagnostic tests should be compared with those from other tests to ensure that results are consistent, or that inconsistent results are fully investigated before a final report is issued. Such practice should be an integral component of the laboratory's quality assurance program.

Quality Assurance and Quality Improvement

Assuring the quality of reagents and test results is reviewed in this section.

Testing of New Reagents

Because of the relatively high reliance on in-house developed assays in molecular diagnostics laboratories, it is still quite common for laboratories to produce their own reagents. Careful preparation of all reagents is essential; however, certain reagents such as PCR primers and Southern blot probes are particularly critical. Commonly, these are produced by the laboratory or by commercial suppliers that may vary in the degree of process control of the reagent manufacturing. Before any reagent is placed into service, it is necessary to verify that it performs to specification. The most straightforward way to do this is by comparing the results obtained with the new reagent lot with those from a previous lot. This comparison should contain known positive and negative controls or as many of the possible genotypes as are available. Additional validation steps can be taken: in the case of Southern blot probes that are cloned in plasmids, it may be possible to verify the identity of the probe by examining the restriction digestion pattern of the plasmid or by sequencing the cloned insert. In the case of PCR primers, the sequence of the PCR product can be determined to confirm that the expected gene sequence is being amplified. The laboratory should retain documentation on the locus, sequence, origin, restriction map, presence of polymorphisms, presence of cross-hybridizing bands, and other relevant information for each probe or primer set that it uses. Such information can be invaluable in resolving unusual or unexpected results.

Quality Control

As a matter of routine quality assessment, control specimens that test the entire preanalytic, analytic, and postanalytic process should be used. For example, in the area of microbiology or oncology testing, positive and negative control samples should be analyzed with any patient samples and taken through the extraction, amplification, and detection portions of the analysis to assure that established limits of detection and/or quantification are being met. Any amplification reaction should include a blank control that contains all reagents but not an amplifiable template as a means to identify amplicon contamination.

Laboratories that perform genetic testing for mutations should have control materials containing known mutations or wild type of alleles that are analyzed on a regular basis to confirm that the analytical method is producing accurate results; at least one sample should be included in every patient run. For certain genetic tests, where there are a limited number of known mutations, it may be possible to include both mutation and wild type of controls with each analytical run. However, many genes of interest include a large number of mutations, so that it is not always practical to run a control for each mutation with every analytical run. In such a situation, a reasonable compromise must be achieved that ensures that the analytical method can detect all mutations. This might be accomplished, for example, by testing all control samples when new lots of critical reagents are first placed in service, and thereafter by rotating a different set of mutation controls with each run. Control materials containing known mutations can be obtained from several sources. These include cell and DNA repositories, such as the one maintained by Coriel Laboratories, and synthesized control materials, such as oligonucleotides. Analytical methods that produce quantitative results e.g., for HIV-1 viral load measurement, should include appropriate calibrators and controls. Sources of calibrators and controls include commercial manufacturers and in-house developed materials.

Proficiency Testing

Although proficiency testing (PT) is discussed in Chapter 19, some additional comments regarding PT in the molecular diagnostics laboratory are necessary. The major PT program in the United States is provided by the CAP. U.S. laboratories that hold a certificate under the Clinical Laboratory Improvement Act must be enrolled in an acceptable PT program if one is available. Because of the limited number of tests that are covered in organized PT programs, it is often necessary for laboratories to perform some other means of PT. These must be performed at least semiannually. If no formal PT program exists, acceptable alternatives include participation in ungraded PT challenges, sample exchange with other laboratories performing the test, split sample analysis with another in-house method or by another technologist using the same method, testing of assayed materials, regional pools, and clinical validation by chart review or other means. Wherever possible, the PT program should cover the entire testing process. In the case of molecular diagnostics, this should include nucleic acid extraction, sample analysis, and interpretation of the results, including (if appropriate) Bayesian calculation of risk. The results of all PT challenges must be documented and reviewed by the laboratory director or designee.

SUMMARY

The design and operation of a molecular diagnostics laboratory have several unique aspects that differ from other clinical laboratories. The choice of a central facility versus discipline-specific molecular diagnostics laboratories will have a large impact on overall cost and efficiencies. In choosing a test menu, careful attention should be paid to costs, reimbursement, expected volumes, turnaround times, and the expertise required of personnel. The use of target amplification methods requires careful attention to laboratory design and workflow.

Operational details that are specific to a molecular diagnostics laboratory include regulatory issues related to genetic information that may vary between jurisdictions, personnel qualifications, and availability, and the ability to report genetic results that are based on Bayesian calculations. Use of appropriate quality control materials and participation in a proficiency testing program that challenges all phases of the analytical process are essential for successful operation of a molecular diagnostics laboratory.

REFERENCES

1. Clinical Laboratory Improvement Amendments. http://www.cms.hhs.gov/clia/ (accessed July 20, 2004).
2. College of American Pathologists. Checklist for Molecular Pathology Inspections. http://www.cap.org/apps/docs/laboratory_accreditation/checklists/molecular_pathology_december2003.pdf (accessed July 20, 2004).
3. Department of Health and Human Services, Centers for Medicare & Medicaid Services, The Health Insurance Portability and Accountability Act of 1996 (HIPAA) http://www.cms.hhs.gov/hipaa (accessed August 19, 2004).

4. Department of Health and Human Services, Food and Drug Administration. Medical devices; classification/reclassification; restricted devices; analyte specific reagents. Final rule. Fed Register. 1997(Nov 21); 62243-45 [21CFR809, 21CFR864] http://www.fda.gov/cdrh/oivd/index.html (accessed August 19, 2004).
5. Grody WW, Cutting GR, Klinger KW, Richards CS, Watson MS, Desnick RJ. Laboratory standards and guidelines for population-based cystic fibrosis carrier screening. Genet Med 2001;3:149-54.
6. Johnson A, Genetic Privacy. Genetics Brief, National Conference of State Legislatures, Denver, CO, 2002 http://www.ncsl.org/programs/health/genetics/Geneticprivacy.pdf (accessed July 20, 2004).
7. Keegan CE, Killeen AA. An overview of molecular diagnosis of steroid 21-hydroxylase deficiency. J Mol Diagn 2001;32:49-54.
8. Killeen AA. Principles of Molecular Pathology. Totowa, NJ: Humana Press, 2004.
9. Kremer B, Goldberg P, Andrew SE, Theilmann J, Telenius H, Zeisler J, et al. A worldwide study of the Huntington's disease mutation. The sensitivity and specificity of measuring CAG repeats. N Engl J Med 1994;330:1401-6.
10. Silvers A, Stein MA. Human rights and genetic discrimination: protecting genomics' promise for public health. J Law Med Ethics 2003;31:377-89.
11. Udaykumar, Epstein JS, Hewlett IK. A novel method employing UNG to avoid carry-over contamination in RNA-PCR. Nucleic Acids Res 1993;21:3917-8.

CHAPTER 39

Molecular Genetics and Diagnosis of Hematopoietic Neoplasms

Kojo S.J. Elenitoba-Johnson, M.D.

The hematopoietic neoplasms are a diverse group of malignancies that traditionally have been diagnosed by use of a variety of ancillary techniques. Important advances over the last few decades have elucidated the biological bases for the development of these diseases. The hematopoietic malignancies include the lymphomas, leukemias, and plasma cell dyscrasias. These diseases represent neoplastic proliferations of the hematopoietic system and are characterized by monoclonality, clonal progression, clonal dominance, and suppression of normal clones.

The *leukemias* are malignant neoplasms that are primarily bone marrow– and peripheral blood–based. Thus the diagnostic material in these cases is typically obtained from the bone marrow or the peripheral blood. The leukemias are classified according to a putative lineage commitment or stage of differentiation (e.g., myeloid, myelomonocytic, lymphoblastic, lymphoid, etc.) and clinicopathological characteristics, such as disease onset and aggressiveness of clinical course (acute versus chronic). Simply stated, the tumor cells in acute leukemias consist mainly of immature or blast cells with limited differentiation. By comparison, a significant proportion of the neoplastic cells in the chronic leukemias are mature and differentiated.

The *lymphomas* are neoplasms of B-, T- or natural killer cells, and characteristically present as tumorous enlargements of peripheral lymphoid or extranodal tissues. As with the leukemias, the lymphomas are subclassified into distinct clinicopathological entities based on lineage, cell of origin and/or putative normal counterpart, and degree of differentiation. Despite their designation as primarily tissue-based neoplasms, malignant lymphomas may involve the bone marrow or peripheral blood. Conversely, leukemic proliferations may occur in tissue as extramedullary tumorlike nodules or masses (extramedullary myeloid tumors) or in the peripheral blood.

This chapter reviews the diagnostic techniques that are routinely used in molecular diagnostic laboratories for the detection and quantification of the distinctive molecular genetic abnormalities that are characteristic of several hematopoietic neoplasms. Identification of the fundamental aberrations involved in the genesis of lymphomas and leukemias has permitted the development of tumor-specific therapeutic interventions and molecular tests, which serve as important adjuncts in the specific diagnosis, choice of therapy, monitoring, and overall management of patients affected with hematological malignancies. This chapter is by no means an exhaustive listing of these tests, but an attempt has been made to illustrate the utility of the more common techniques with a prototypical example in each case. Where relevant, some detail is provided into the physiology or pathogenesis of specific neoplasms that provides insights into the molecular basis for the particular assay design. The most commonly performed molecular tests for the evaluation of hematopoietic neoplasms are tests for rearrangement of antigen-receptor genes and analyses for recurrent chromosomal translocations. In many cases the genetic markers are exploited as unique markers for specific categories of hematological neoplasia, and hence receive the most attention in this chapter.

ANTIGEN-RECEPTOR GENE REARRANGEMENTS FOR DETERMINATION OF CLONALITY

The histological features that distinguish benign reactive lymphocytic proliferations from malignant populations can be subtle and somewhat subjective. The introduction of molecular biological techniques into diagnostic pathology has refined lymphoma diagnostics and classification. B- and T-lymphocytes exhibit the unique property of rearrangement of the immunoglobulin (Ig) and T-cell receptor (TCR) genes, respectively. The immunoglobulin and T-cell receptor genes encode the amino acid sequences of the polypeptides that constitute the corresponding antigen receptor. The antigen-receptor molecules mediate antigen recognition and are responsible for the specificity of the normal immune response. B-lymphocytes are the mediators of humoral response and produce immunoglobulins, while the T-lymphocytes are the mediators of the cellular response. Because each reactive lymphocyte carries a unique antigen-receptor gene sequence, identification of clonal populations arising from a parent malignant lymphocyte becomes feasible since the malignant population is characteristically monoclonal. Tests for monoclonality were originally developed using the Southern blotting hybridization (SBH) methodology, which remains the gold standard for specificity for detection of clonality throughout a broad range of lymphoid malignancies (Table 39-1). More recently, SBH has been complemented by polymerase chain reaction (PCR)–based strategies.

MOLECULAR GENETIC BASIS FOR IMMUNOGLOBULIN-GENE REARRANGEMENTS

Humoral immunity is achieved by the cognitive and effector functions provided by B-lymphocytes. Immunoglobulins (Ig) are produced exclusively by B-lymphocytes, and constitute the hallmark of the humoral response. Ig molecules are heterodimeric polypeptides consisting of two identical 50 to 70 kD heavy chains associated with two identical light chains (κ or λ) of approximately 23 kD. The Ig chains are linked by noncovalent forces and interchain disulfide bridges, and together form a bilaterally symmetrical structure. The heavy and light chain proteins encoded by their corresponding genes consist of a tandem series of homologous segments, comprising approximately 110 amino acid residues. These segments undergo folding into 12 kD domains with single intrachain disulfide bridges. Heavy chains contain one variable (V) and three constant (C) domains, while light chains contain one N-terminal V and one C domain. In both heavy and light chains, the V domain consists of four relatively invariable framework regions of 15 to 30 amino acids separated by three 9- to 12-amino acid–long hypervariable or complementarity determining regions (CDR). In both heavy and light chains, the CDR3 region is the farthest away from the N-terminus and exhibits the greatest sequence variability among the three CDRs. The C-terminal region of secreted Ig molecules binds to complement components and Fc receptors. The genes encoding the Ig proteins are the target for DNA-based studies for clonality assessment.

The organization of Ig genes in the germline is fundamentally similar in all species studied. Genes encoding the two light chains, κ and λ, and the locus containing the various heavy chain genes are located on different chromosomes. To generate the large number of antibody molecules necessary, B-cells have evolved a unique strategy that involves recombination of germline-encoded immunoglobulin gene segments and a somatic hypermutation mechanism that further diversifies the reactivities of the rearranged antigen-receptor molecules.[114] The three immunoglobulin gene loci—for IgH, Igκ, and Igλ—are located at chromosomes 14q32, 2p12, and 22q11, respectively. In the germline configuration, all antigen-receptor genes consist of discontinuous DNA segments, which are referred to as variable (V), diversity (D), joining (J), and constant (C) regions. While both the Ig heavy and light chain genes contain V, J, and C regions, only the IgH genes contain D regions (Figure 39-1). The IgH gene contains approximately 51 V_H segments, 27 D_H segments, 9 J_H segments, and 11 C_H genes. The IgH V_H segment genes can be categorized into seven families based on the relatedness of the DNA sequences.

The ability of the immunoglobulin genes to undergo recombination in a manner analogous to shuffling of cards affords the capacity to achieve an enormous primary Ig repertoire of 10^9 sequences (Figure 39-2). The region coding

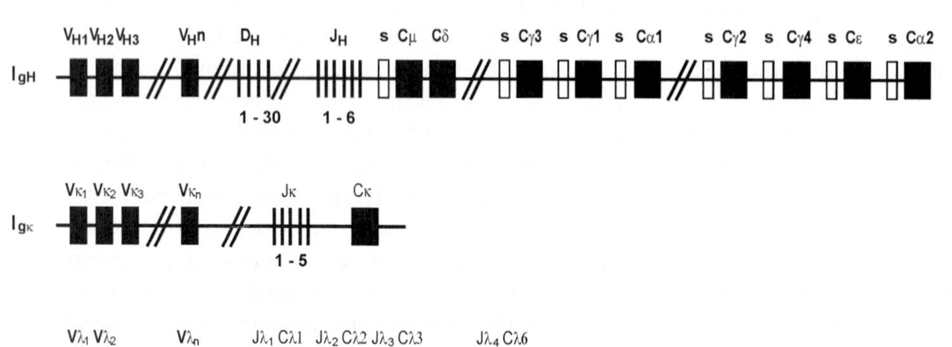

Figure 39-1 Schematic representation of the germline configurations of the antigen-receptor gene loci. Immunoglobulin heavy chain (IgH), immunoglobulin kappa (Igκ), and lambda (Igλ) light chains. Each gene comprises several variable (V), joining (J), and constant (C) segments. Note that the IgH gene contains diversity (D) gene segments. Switch regions are indicated by S.

Table 39-1 Detection Frequency of Antigen-Receptor Gene Rearrangements by Southern Blot Analysis

	Cases With Antigen-Receptor Gene Rearrangement (%)					
	Immunoglobulin Genes			T-Cell Receptor Genes		
	IgH	Igκ	Igλ	TCRβ	TCRγ	TCRδ
B-cell Neoplasms						
Precursor B-cell acute lymphoblastic leukemia/lymphoma	100	40-50	20-25	20-30	50-60	70-80
Chronic lymphocytic leukemia/ small lymphocytic lymphoma	10	100	30	<10	<10	<10
Prolymphocytic leukemia	100	100	30	Rare	Rare	NA
Hairy cell leukemia/variant	100	100	30-50	Rare	NA	NA
Lymphoplasmacytic lymphoma/ immunocytoma	100	100	30	Rare	NA	NA
Marginal zone B-cell lymphoma						
Low-grade, B-cell lymphoma of mucosa-associated lymphoid tissue	100	100	30	<10	Rare	NA
Splenic marginal zone lymphoma	100	100	30	0	NA	NA
Mantle-cell lymphoma	100	100	50	Rare	NA	NA
Follicular lymphoma	100	100	30	<10	<10	<10
Diffuse large B-cell lymphoma	100	100	30	<10	<10	NA
Burkitt lymphoma	100	100	30-40	Rare	Rare	NA
Plasma-cell myeloma	90	90	30	10	10	NA
T-cell Neoplasms						
Precursor T-cell acute lymphoblastic leukemia/lymphoma	20	Rare	Rare	90-95	90-95	>95
Chronic lymphocytic leukemia/ prolymphocytic leukemia	<10	0	0	100	100	>90
Large granular lymphocytic leukemia						
T cell	Rare	0	0	>90	>90	>90
Natural-killer cell	0	0	0	0	0	0
Peripheral T-cell lymphoma, unspecified	<10	Rare	0	>90	>90	>90
Peripheral T-cell lymphoma, specific variants						
Adult T-cell leukemia/lymphoma	<10	0	0	100	>90	>90
Nasal-T/NK lymphoma	0	0	0	<10	0	Rare
Angioimmunoblastic T-cell lymphoma	20	10-20	10-20	90	90	90
Intestinal T-cell lymphoma	0	0	0	100	NA	NA
Anaplastic large cell lymphoma	10	Rare	0	60-70	60-70	90
Hepatosplenic T-cell lymphoma	0	0	0	70-80	70-80	80-90
Subcutaneous panniculitis-like T-cell lymphoma	0	0	0	>90	>90	50
Mycosis fungoides/Sézary syndrome	0	0	0	70-80	70-80	>90

for human Ig C contains 11 C region segments, which define 9 functional immunoglobulin classes and subclasses (IgM, IgD, IgG1, IgG2, IgG3, IgG4, IgA1, IgA2, and IgE). The C region genes are initially uninvolved in the rearrangement process but are subsequently juxtaposed to the VDJ complex during RNA splicing. Incorporation of the C regions into the rearranged VDJ recombination permits *class switching* (i.e., the specific V(D)J rearrangement can be expressed as an IgG, IgA, or other Ig classes). Following the formation of a productive IgH rearrangement, the light chain loci undergo a similar recombination process involving the joining of V to J segments, since there are no D segments present in the light chain loci.[26]

The Igκ light chain gene is located on chromosome 2p11-13, and contains approximately 76 Vκ genes, 5 Jκ segments, and 1 Cκ gene. There is a κ-deleting sequence (element) present 3′ to the Cκ region. In Igλ-expressing B-cells in which the Igκ genes are not productively rearranged, the κ-deleting element undergoes rearrangement such that the Cκ locus is deleted. The Igλ light chain is situated on chromosome 22q11, and consists of 70-71 Vλ genes with 7-11 Jλ and 7-11 Cλ genes arranged in tandem. The Cλ locus is polymorphic and may be present in one to nine copies per allele in different individuals. The hierarchy of the rearrangement events is such that both alleles of the heavy chain rearrange before the light chain genes; the kappa (κ) light chain locus usually is productively rearranged before the lambda light chain genes. Thus the immunoglobulin lambda (λ) light chain gene is not favored for clonality analysis because it frequently rearranges after the kappa light chain gene. In addition, because the majority of clonal rearrangements of the immunoglobulin heavy chain gene can be detected in up to 95% of clonal processes, it has become customary to perform only Southern blot analysis for the IgH locus in many laboratories.

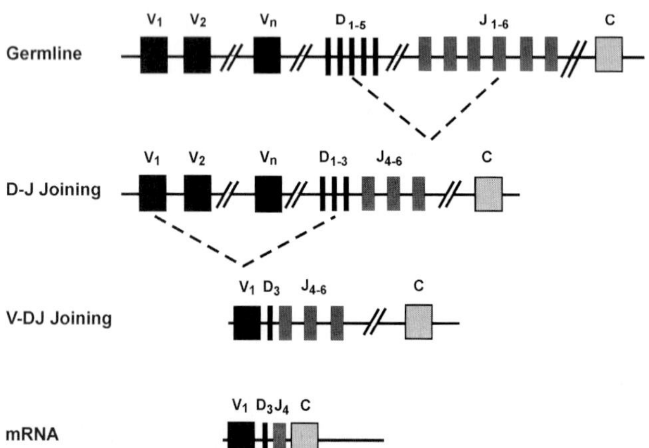

Figure 39-2 Schematic representation of antigen-receptor gene rearrangement mechanism using the IgH chain locus as a model. There is an initial DJ joining in a partial/incomplete recombination, followed by a VDJ joining to complete the rearrangement. The C regions are included at the mRNA level via RNA splicing to form a V(D)JC transcript.

Molecular Genetic Basis for T-Cell Receptor Gene Rearrangements

A process similar to that described for the Ig genes occurs in the TCR genes, with the notable exception of the absence of a somatic hypermutation mechanism in TCR gene rearrangements. The developmental hierarchy of TCR genes is such that the TCR-δ gene is the first to rearrange, followed by the TCRγ, TCRβ, and then the TCRα genes.[24] The TCR-δ gene is located on chromosome 14q11, and contains up to six Vδ segments, only two or three Dδ segments, and three Jδ segments. It is located within the TCR-α gene, immediately 3′ to the last TCR-Vα gene and 5′ to the TCR-Jα segments. This location is important since productive rearrangements of the TCRδ gene lead to expression of the γ/δ TCR. In the event that the TCRδ rearrangement is non-productive, Vα to Jα rearrangements obligatorily require that the TCRδ be deleted.

As previously indicated, the TCRδ gene (Figure 39-3) is located on band 14q11, flanks the TCRα gene on either side, and contains several Vα segments. An extensive J region comprises up to 50 Jα genes and 1 Cα locus. By virtue of the architectural disposition of the TCRα and δ loci, rearrangement of a Vα segment to a Jα segment typically leads to deletion of the intervening TCRδ loci. T-cells undergoing such rearrangements may then go on to express the TCR-α/β protein. The TCRβ gene is located on band 7q34 and contains 75 to 100 Vβ segments, flanked at the 3′ end by two Dβ, Jβ, and Cβ regions. For each region, there is one Dβ segment, with six or seven Jβ segments, and one Cβ segment. Rearrangements may occur within or between segments (e.g., Vβ1 to Jβ1 or Vβ2 to Jβ1). There is extensive sequence homology between the Cβ1 and Cβ2 segments. This phenomenon is exploited in the use of a consensus Cβ probe when Southern blotting of the TCR genes is used for clonality assessment. The TCRγ gene is located on band 7q15, and contains about 12-15 Vγ segments and 2 Jγ genes.[22] The

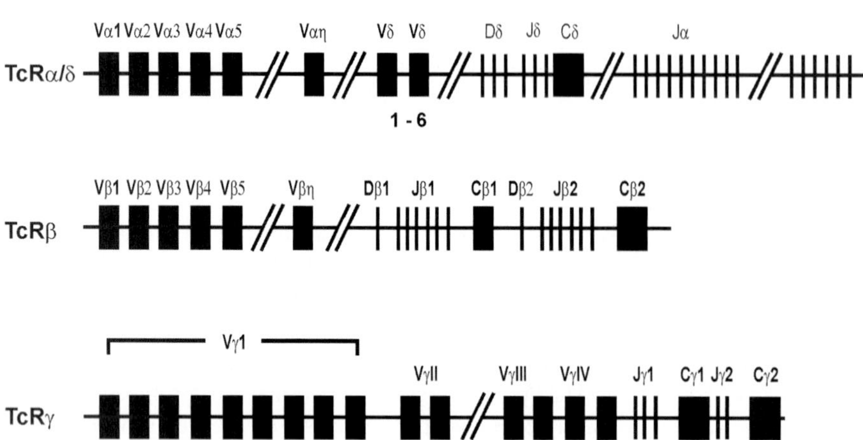

Figure 39-3 T-cell receptor (TCR) genes consist of α/δ-, β-, and γ-chain genes. The architectural configurations are similar to that of the Ig loci. Note that only the TCRβ- and δ- genes contain diversity (D) regions.

simple structure of the architecture of this gene favors its use as a target for TCR receptor PCR, whereas consensus primers are designed to encompass the relatively few Vγ and the Jγ genes.

Southern Blot Hybridization Analysis for Antigen-Receptor (Ig or TCR) Gene Rearrangements

In this procedure, high-quality total cellular DNA extracted from a fresh or flash-frozen specimen is subjected to digestion by bacterial restriction endonucleases, which produce DNA fragments encompassing the Ig or TCR gene region segments to be interrogated (Figures 39-4 and 39-5). The enzyme-digested ("restricted") DNA from each enzyme is subjected to gel electrophoresis and transferred by blotting and immobilized on a membrane. A labeled-probe complementary to the Ig J region segment is hybridized to the membrane. Clonal rearrangements are recognized by the identification of one or two novel rearranged bands that are distinct from the germline pattern obtained with a benign sample or placental DNA. One or two novel rearranged (nongermline) bands may be identifiable depending on whether there is a clonal monoallelic or biallelic rearrangement (Figure 39-6).

Materials suitable for Southern blot analysis include fresh tissue or aspiration biopsy material, as long as sufficient cellular material can be obtained from the specimen of interest. Ethanol-fixed tissue can also be used. However,

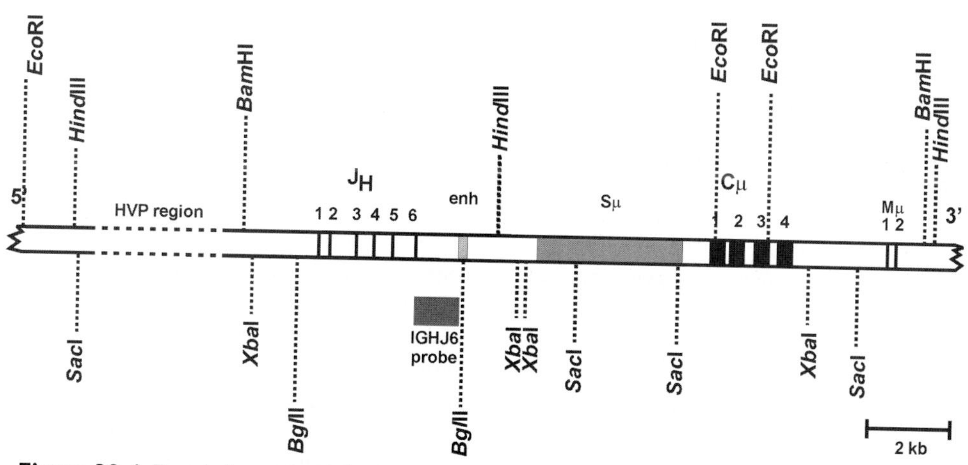

Figure 39-4 Restriction map of the IgH chain locus. The sites of the enzyme restriction sites determine the sizes of the fragments that are visualized using the IgHJ6 probe as illustrated (e.g., BamHI, XbaI, and BglII enzymes yield 16 kb, 6.2 kb, and 3.8 kb fragments, respectively). Restriction patterns different from the germline patterns are indicative of a novel rearrangement event.

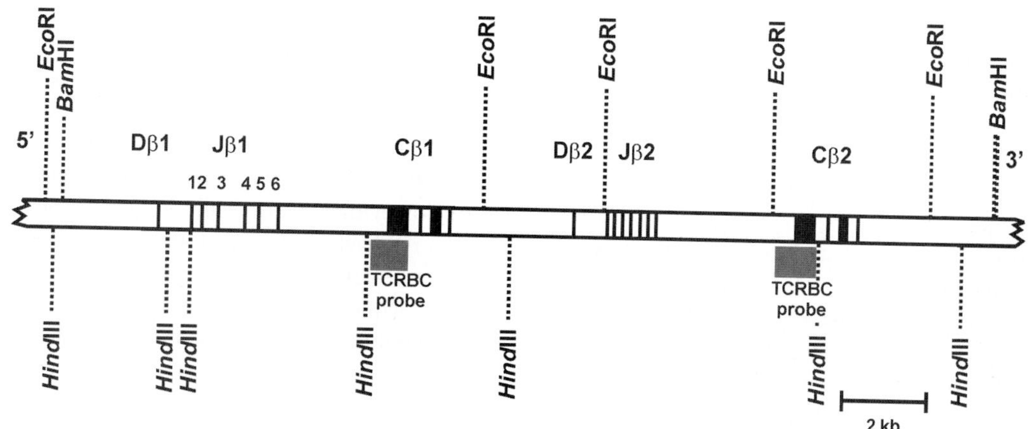

Figure 39-5 Restriction map of the TCRβ chain locus. The probe is complementary to the TCRβ constant region. There is extensive sequence homology between the Cβ1 and Cβ2 segments. Thus the Cβ probe hybridizes to both the Cβ1 and Cβ2 segments, thereby resulting in two germline band signals for all enzymes depicted except BamHI. The EcoRI site located between the Cβ1 and Jβ2 segments is notoriously resistant to digestion and may yield a partial digest with a band of 8.0 kb in size.

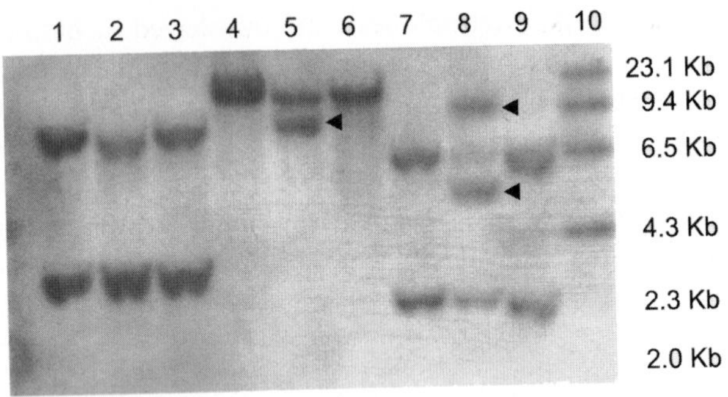

Figure 39-6 Southern blot hybridization analysis for clonal rearrangements of the TCRβ chain locus. DNA samples extracted from two different patients with a suspected diagnosis of T-cell lymphoma are assessed. Lanes 1 to 3 represent the EcoRI digests. Lanes 4 to 6 show the BamHI digests, and lanes 7 to 9 demonstrate the HindIII digests from both samples run side by side. Lane 10 shows the DNA size marker. Lanes 1, 4, and 7 show the restriction patterns in the germline control (placenta) using the EcoRI, BamHI, and HindIII enzymes, respectively. DNA from patient 1 (Lanes 2, 5, and 8) shows a germline pattern using EcoRI, but novel rearrangements (arrowheads) using BamHI and HindIII. Patient 2 (lanes 3, 6, and 9) shows a germline pattern in all three enzyme digests. Accordingly, sample 1 is scored as showing evidence for a monoclonal T-cell population, and sample 2 is scored as showing evidence of a polyclonal T-cell population.

formalin-fixed tissue yields DNA of insufficient quality to permit reliable Southern blotting because of cross-linking of proteins to DNA. A Southern blot hybridization assay using three enzymes requires approximately 1.5×10^7 cells (approximately 15 μg of intact total cellular DNA). Hypothetically, all of the antigen-receptor genes could be used as potential targets for the assessment of clonality, but only the immunoglobulin heavy and light chain and the TCR beta chain loci have gained widespread use. The T-cell TCRα locus is impractical, because it contains several J segments that are distributed widely, and thus would pose practical challenges in the optimization of assays for multiple probes. Evaluation of the TCRγ and δ loci is also not favored because they have only a limited number of V segments such that even reactive T-cell populations may yield confusing nongermline bands.

The diagnostic hallmark of a clonal population is the presence of a nongermline novel rearranged band (see Figure 39-6); but nongermline bands do not always indicate monoclonality. Single nucleotide polymorphisms (SNPs) may create or abolish restriction enzyme recognition sites thus yielding novel restriction banding patterns. In this scenario, digestion with a different restriction endonuclease would yield a germline configuration. The potential of SNPs to confound the interpretation of Southern blot studies justifies testing with up to three or more enzymes for the unequivocal assignment of monoclonality. Incomplete digestion by a restriction enzyme can also result in a nongermline band that does not indicate monoclonality. This is typically evident in the control sample (placental DNA) and invalidates the significance of any such band in the test sample.

Clonal rearrangements of either the Ig or TCR genes have also been used to ascertain the lineage of hematological neoplasms that do not express B- or T-cell specific markers. Intuitively, clonal rearrangements of the Ig genes would indicate B-cell processes, and clonal rearrangements of the TCR genes would indicate T-cell processes. However, some malignant lymphomas (notably lymphoblastic) and leukemias (especially acute leukemias) may demonstrate both Ig and TCR rearrangements. Further, up to 20% of acute myeloid leukemias (AMLs) may demonstrate rearrangements of either the Ig or TCR genes.[19,51,60] Hence, lineage is best assigned using a combination of immunophenotypic and molecular studies.

Polymerase Chain Reaction Analysis of Antigen-Receptor Gene Rearrangements

Although analysis by SBH for detection of antigen-receptor gene rearrangements is recognized as the "gold standard" for the assessment of clonality, PCR-based assays have become the mainstay for the detection of rearrangements of the Ig and TCR genes in many molecular diagnostic laboratories. SBH is not only labor-intensive and time-consuming, but it requires a substantial quantity of "intact" DNA (with full-length or nearly full-length copies of the gene or genes of interest), making it less amenable to use for specimens with suboptimal DNA quality (as is the case with fixed paraffin-embedded tissue samples). PCR is well suited for such specimens, which constitute the majority of samples analyzed in the clinical laboratory.

The application of PCR for the identification of clonality entails the use of consensus V-region and J-region primers and in vitro amplification of DNA across the V(D)J junction followed by evaluation of the PCR products by gel electrophoresis or other methods for analysis of the uniformity of PCR-generated fragments. In the germline configuration, these V- and J-region segments are located several kilobases apart and would not be amplifiable. However, the V(D)J recombination brings the VDJ segments into close proximity and thereby permits amplification of products that are less than 80 to 350 bases depending on the primers used. The V-region primers are typically designed to be complementary to the relatively conserved framework regions (I, II, or III), and the J-region primer is typically complementary to consensus sequences present across all six J regions in the immunoglobulin heavy chain gene. Similar strategies exist for the light chain genes as well, but the rate of detection of clonal rearrangements is lower and hence the IgH-PCR is favored. Use of framework III consensus primers provides the highest rate of detection, but can be complemented with increased diagnostic sensitivity afforded by the inclusion of framework II and/or framework I primer-mediated IgH-PCR for clonality. Among the T-cell assays, the TCRγ-PCR is the most informative. In these assays, monoclonal populations yield one or two dominant bands (Figure 39-7). Poly-

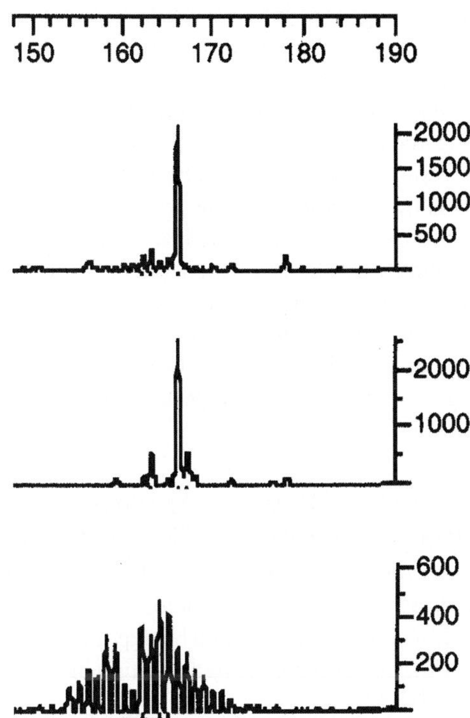

Figure 39-7 Polymerase chain reaction (PCR) analysis for clonal rearrangements of the antigen-receptor gene loci. PCR analysis of the TCR γ-chain locus is shown. The upper and middle panels show duplicate assays with monoclonal capillary electrophoretic peaks of identical size (~166 bp) in both replicates. The bottom panel shows a polyclonal pattern.

clonal cells, each of which carries a unique rearrangement with slightly different band sizes, demonstrate a ladder or smear pattern on gel electrophoresis.[67,109] Following completion of PCR, the PCR products are analyzed by gel electrophoresis.[34,113] The PCR products are most commonly visualized by ultraviolet transillumination of ethidium bromide–stained gels. Agarose and polyacrylamide gels are most commonly used for resolution of PCR products. Agarose gels have the advantages of being relatively inexpensive and easy to make, but they provide inferior resolution of PCR products, such that products of similar size can be difficult to distinguish. Polyacrylamide gels offer significantly better product resolution and can be configured to reliably discriminate bands differing in size by as little as three bases. This is often highly useful in the assessment of PCR products for antigen-receptor gene rearrangement assays. Even further resolution may be achieved by supplementation of size fractionation with additional parameters. Denaturing gradient gel electrophoresis and temperature-gradient gel electrophoresis achieve finer resolution of PCR products by exploiting the sequence-specific and melting characteristics of double-stranded DNA.[47] The incorporation of denaturants, such as formamide or urea in gradient gels, or modulation of the temperature can further increase resolution based on the melting temperature (Tm) of the DNA sequence rather than on size. Radioisotopic detection is an alternative to ethidium bromide detection. The PCR primers could be labeled with radioisotopes, the PCR products analyzed by electrophoresis, and the PCR products visualized by autoradiography. Ultraviolet transillumination of ethidium bromide–stained gels is more popular than radioisotope-based methods, because it is easier to perform and poses fewer hazards with regard to handling and disposal of radioactive wastes. A successful PCR exhibits PCR products in the expected size range, appropriate results in the positive and negative controls, and absence of bands in the template-free (H_2O) control.

PCR-based clonality assays are less sensitive in detecting all of the possible clonal rearrangements than is SBH analysis, which approaches 100% if sufficient restriction enzymes and a variety of probes are used. Depending on the assay and the lymphoid neoplasm tested, PCR-based clonality studies may show false-negative rates of 10% to 40% when compared with SBH. A reason frequently cited to explain the high false-negative rate for PCR is that, in contrast to SBH, PCR does not detect partial DJ rearrangements, wherein the V- and J-region genes are not approximated to one another and are too distant for conventional PCR to generate an amplification product. Secondly, the consensus primers in PCR tests are incapable of hybridizing to all of the different V regions, any one of which could be potentially present in any one neoplasm. Of particular importance to the Ig genes, somatic mutations occurring within the Ig V-region genes also result in decreased ability for the consensus V-region primers to anneal optimally to the V-region genes in the template DNA. Thus lymphoid neoplasias such as follicular lymphoma with a high somatic hypermutation rate yield lower positive rates by PCR-based Ig clonality tests.[103,104] Most of these difficulties can be overcome by use of multiple primer sets. In the event of a negative PCR result, SBH analysis may be performed if sufficient high-quality genomic DNA is available. The main drawback for PCR is the marked propensity for contamination. Thus various strategies for contamination control, such as maintaining separate DNA extraction and amplification rooms, use of laminar flow hoods, and incorporation of uracil DNA glycosylase into PCR, generally should be employed to prevent contamination problems.

The ability to detect a rare, aberrant DNA species in a background of normal DNA (often referred to as "sensitivity" of the PCR-based tests) is dependent on the particular application. For antigen-receptor gene rearrangement studies, PCR can detect a monoclonal population in a background of 10^2 to 10^3 polyclonal cells of the same phenotype (B- or T-cells). By comparison, PCR can detect one cell harboring a chromosomal translocation within a background of 10^5 to 10^6 cells negative for the translocation.[76]

LYMPHOMA-SPECIFIC RECURRENT CHROMOSOMAL TRANSLOCATIONS

The immunoglobulin gene rearrangement process, which is integral to the normal development of B-cells and the elaboration of an appropriate immune response, is susceptible to abnormal translocation of foreign genes. Translocation of these genes is associated with their deregulation, which is integral to the development of lymphoid neoplasia. A translocation typically involves the transfer of a piece of one chromosome to a different chromosome. Nonrandom chromosomal translocations are frequently observed in hematological neoplasia and in many cases are characteristic of a specific type of leukemia or lymphoma.

The translocations typically result in one of two genetic consequences.

1. The translocation may juxtapose an oncogene and an antigen-receptor gene, leading to dysregulated expression of the oncogene and increased concentration of the oncoprotein. This is the mechanism most frequently seen in malignant lymphomas, and is exemplified by the t(14;18)(q32;q21) that is characteristic of follicular lymphoma. The translocation juxtaposes the *bcl-2* gene (18q21) and the IgH gene (14q32), leading to overexpression of the *bcl-2* gene and increased *bcl-2* mRNA and protein.[116]
2. Alternatively the chromosomal translocation leads to the in-frame juxtaposition of two different genes, with resultant creation of a novel chimeric gene. This mechanism is most commonly observed in the leukemias and less commonly in malignant lymphomas. In the t(2;5)(2p23;q35) seen in anaplastic large cell lymphoma, an abnormal fusion gene (*NPM-ALK*) is formed and is central to pathogenesis.[80] Similarly, a t(11;18)(q21;q21) is seen in a subset of extranodal, marginal-zone B-cell lymphomas of mucosa-associated lymphoid tissue. This translocation forms an abnormal *API-MLT1* chimeric fusion that is implicated in the molecular pathogenesis of the malignant lymphoma.[27]

Reverse-transcription-PCR is well suited for the diagnostic detection of such chimeric fusions, because the fusion product is often within the size range that can be amplified by conventional PCR. Secondly, many of the translocation breakpoints are widely dispersed and not clustered. If DNA were to be considered as the template for such PCR, it would best be performed as a long-distance (LD) PCR protocol. LD PCR protocols, however, are unsuitable for many types of clinical samples, such as paraffin-embedded material, that characteristically do not contain high-quality, intact genomic DNA.

A list of the common chromosomal translocations, the participating genes, and the associated lymphomas is provided in Table 39-2.

Southern Blot Hybridization Analysis for the Detection of Chromosomal Translocations

SBH analysis is an excellent method for the detection of chromosomal translocations. A sequence-specific probe to the gene of interest is used for SBH analysis as described for the antigen-receptor genes. Detection of a pattern in which bands of different sizes than are seen in the germline configuration of the gene of interest would suggest the presence of a translocation. It should be noted that this method does not identify the translocation partner of the gene of interest. As with the antigen-receptor gene rearrangement, studies by SBH single nucleotide polymorphisms at enzyme restriction sites may result in nongermline patterns that may be misinterpreted as translocations. In this scenario, use of a different restriction enzyme will correctly show the gene locus to be of germline size. The labor-intensive nature of SBH and the requirement for high-quality DNA have diminished its popularity for routine detection of chromosomal translocations in the clinical laboratory. PCR continues to gain increasing use for the routine detection of recurrent chromosomal translocations.

Polymerase Chain Reaction Analysis for Detection of Chromosomal Translocations

The polymerase chain reaction is a methodology that is very well suited for the analysis of chromosomal translocations, particularly when the translocation breakpoints are clustered and the sequences flanking the translocation breakpoints are well characterized.

t(14;18)(q32;21)—*BCL-2*/JH Aberration

The t(14;18)(q32;21) that is characteristic of follicular lymphoma exemplifies the utility of PCR in the detection of a chromosomal translocation that is characteristic of a specific form of non-Hodgkin lymphoma. The t(14;18) is a balanced reciprocal translocation involving the *BCL-2* gene (18q21) and the IgH locus (14q32). The *BCL-2* gene consists of three exons and two introns.[106] There are up to four different regions on 18q21 where the breakpoints are frequently located. The 18q21 breakpoints in the majority of translocations are clustered in the *major breakpoint cluster* region (MBR). The MBR is a 150 bp sequence located within the 3′-untranslated region of exon 3 of the *BCL-2* gene and harbors approximately 60% of the breakpoints found in follicular lymphoma.[115,124] Another 20% of follicular lymphomas harbor t(14;18) aberrations in which the breakpoint is located at the *minor cluster* region, which is located 30 kb further 3′ to the *BCL-2* gene. An additional cluster of breakpoints located at the *variant cluster region* located 5′ upstream to the *BCL-2* gene harbors approximately 5% of the breakpoints found in follicular lymphoma (Figure 39-8).[95] More an *intermediate cluster region* (ICR) has been described with additional 18q21 breakpoints associated with follicular lymphoma.[1] Although initial studies comparing conventional cytogenetics, Southern blot, and PCR-based methods for detection of the t(14;18) (not including the ICR) have shown that 86% of the cases were identified by Southern blotting and 75% by PCR,[57] the inclusion of PCR assays targeting the ICR improves the detection rate for the t(14;18) by PCR.[1] Figure 39-9 (Color Plate 2) shows fluorescence in situ hybridization (FISH) analysis demonstrating the t(14;18) in a sample that tested negative by

Table 39-2 Common Recurrent Chromosomal Aberrations in Human Malignant Lymphoma

Cytogenetic Abnormality	Genes or Loci (@) Involved	Disease	Clinical Features	Frequency of Abberation (%)
t(14;18)(q32;q21)	*BCL2/IGH@*	FL	Indolent	~90
t(2;18)(p12;q21)	*IGK@/BCL2*	FL	Indolent	<5
t(3;14)(q27;q32)	*BCL6/IGH@*	FL	Indolent	~10
t(11;14)(q13;q32)	*BCL1/IGH@*	MCL	Aggressive	>90
Trisomy 3	Unknown	MZBCL-MALT	Indolent	Variable
t(11;18)(p21;q21)	*API2*/MLT	MZBCL	Indolent	50
t(1;14)(p22;q32)	*BCL10/IGH@*	MZBCL	Indolent	*
t(9;14)(p13;q32)	*PAX-5/IGH@*	LPL	Indolent-Aggressive	*
t(8;14)(q24;q32)	*MYC/IGH@*	Burkitt lymphoma	Highly Aggressive	75
t(2;8)(p12;q24)	*MYC/IGK@*	Burkitt lymphoma	Highly Aggressive	15
t(8;22)(q24;q11)	*MYC/IGL@*	Burkitt lymphoma	Highly Aggressive	10
t(3;14)(q27;q32)	*BCL6/IGH@*	DLBCL	Aggressive	~30
t(14;18)(q32;q21)	*BCL2/IGH@*	DLBCL	Aggressive	30
Amplification 9p	*REL*	PMLBCL	Aggressive	*
Del 13q14	Unknown	B-CLL	Indolent	25-50
Trisomy 12	Unknown	B-CLL	Indolent	30
t(11;14)(q13;q32)	*BCL1/IGH@*	B-PLL	Aggressive	*
t(2;5)(p23;q35)	*NPM/ALK*	ALCL,T/NK	Aggressive	~40
Inv 14(q11;q32) or complex translocations involving both chromosomes 14	Unknown	T-PLL	Aggressive	75
Isochromosome 7q	Unknown	Hepatosplenic γ/δ	Aggressive	*
Trisomy 8	Unknown	Hepatosplenic γ/δ	Aggressive	*

Note that IGK and IGL are symbols for genes Igκ and Igλ, respectively.
FL, Follicular lymphoma; *MCL*, Mantle-cell lymphoma; *MZBCL*, marginal-zone B-cell lymphoma; *MALT*, mucosa-associated lymphoid tissue; *LPL*, lymphoplasmacytic lymphoma; *DLBCL*, diffuse large B-cell lymphoma; *PMLBCL*, primary mediastinal large B-cell lymphoma; *B-CLL*, B-chronic lymphocytic leukemia; *PLL*, prolymphocytic leukemia; *ALL*, acute lymphoblastic leukemia; *ALCL*, anaplastic large-cell lymphoma; *NK*, natural killer.
*An insufficient number of patients were studied to permit accurate assessment of percentage of tumors with the cytogenetic aberration indicated.

PCR. An important caveat to note is that the t(14;18) has been detected in benign tonsils, in reactive lymph nodes,[5,71] and in the peripheral blood of normal blood donors.

t(11;14)(q13;32)—*BCL-1*/JH Aberration

The t(11;14)(q13;32) abnormality is characteristic of mantle cell lymphoma,[70,123] but rare in other types of malignant lymphoma. This translocation juxtaposes the *BCL-1* locus on 11q13 with the immunoglobulin heavy chain gene enhancer locus at 14q32.[117] Structurally, there are multiple breakpoints on chromosome 11. The most frequently involved location on 11q13 is the major translocation cluster (MTC) region, which is located 110 kb 5′ to the *BCL-1* locus.[117] Other breakpoints occurring within minor translocation cluster regions have also been described 3′ to the major translocation cluster but 5′ to the *BCL-1* locus (Figure 39-10).[94] The *BCL-1* gene consists of five exons covering a genomic distance of approximately 15 kb.[81] The gene encodes cyclin D1, which regulates cellular transition from G1 to S phase. Despite the diversity of the breakpoints flanking the *BCL-1* gene, the t(11;14) does not lead to disruption of the coding region of the *BCL-1* gene. Consequently, the expression of cyclin D1 is qualitatively normal, but quantitatively increased. One of the practical consequences of the multiple breakpoints in mantle cell lymphoma is that approximately 70% of cases of mantle cell lymphoma can be demonstrated to harbor the t(11;14) by Southern blotting analysis using multiple probes for detection of the various breakpoints.[126] By comparison, most published PCR protocols only detect approximately 40% of t(11;14) anomalies in mantle cell lymphoma (Figure 39-10), and the majority of these are clustered in the MTC.[126] This is in notable contrast to DNA fiber FISH, which reportedly may detect up to 95% of t(11;14) aberrations, making FISH the most sensitive method for detection of this abnormality.[118]

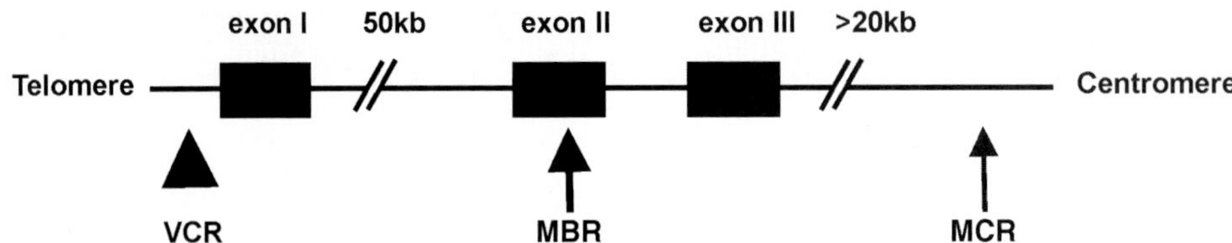

Figure 39-8 Schematic representation of the organization of the *BCL-2* gene and most frequent breakpoints on chromosome 18q21 involved in the t(14;18). The *BCL-2* exons are represented as rectangles. MBR represents the major breakpoint cluster region where approximately 50% to 60% of the breakpoints occur. MCR represents the minor breakpoint cluster region where 20% to 25% of the breakpoints may be found. VCR represents the variant cluster region where 5% to 20% of the breakpoints may be found.

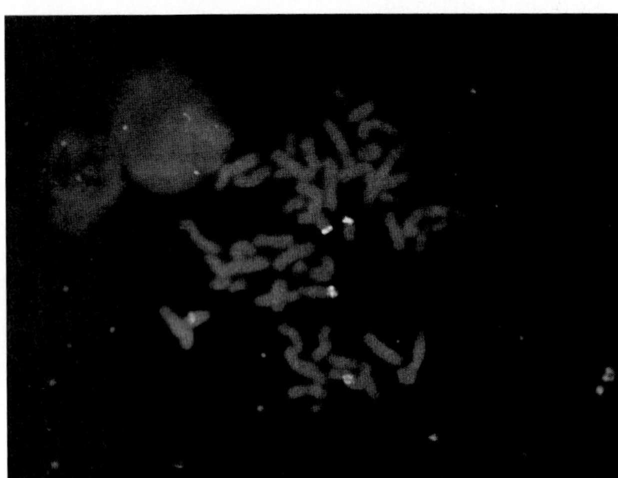

Figure 39-9 Fluorescence in situ hybridization for the t(14;18) anomaly on metaphase spreads of a case of follicular lymphoma. The immunoglobulin heavy chain sequences on 14q32 *(red)* when juxtaposed to the *bcl-2* sequences on 18q21 *(green)* yield a yellow fusion signal indicative of the presence of the t(14;18). (See Color Plate 2.)

MOLECULAR GENETICS OF LEUKEMIAS

As indicated previously, human leukemias are characterized by recurrent genetic abnormalities that can be used as genetic markers of the specific leukemia. The genetic abnormalities are most often recurrent chromosomal translocations, which result in chimeric fusions leading either to a differentiation block or enhancement of proliferation. The chronic leukemias of myeloid derived cells are characterized by constitutive activation of tyrosine kinases whose primary effect is to confer an excessive proliferative signal and an increased survival advantage. An example of this is the t(9;22), which results in the *BCR-ABL* chimeric fusion that is characteristic of chronic myelogenous leukemia (CML). Inhibition of the activated tyrosine kinase is a bona fide therapeutic option as has been demonstrated with imatinib mesylate (Gleevec) in CML. By comparison, the chromosomal translocations in the acute myeloid leukemias typically result in loss-of-function aberrations within transcription factors that lead to maturational arrest or differentiation blocks at early stages of hematopoietic development. The preponderance of evidence suggests that the genetic aberrations leading to maturational arrest in the acute myeloid leukemias are by themselves insufficient to cause leukemia. However, the concomitant occurrence of cooperating mutations in the *RAS* and the tyrosine kinase genes *FLT3* and *C-KIT* permits progression to a frank leukemia. In either case, the presence of the genetic aberrations provides a target for disease detection, monitoring, and potential gene-specific therapy. A comprehensive list of translocations and the fusions in acute leukemias is in Table 39-3 with French-American-British classification designations. The most frequently employed technique for the detection of the chimeric transcripts in the molecular laboratory is RT-PCR. In addition, the prevalence of specific genetic mutations often requires that screening for such mutations be performed in the diagnostic laboratory. While it is recognized that the definitive method for the detection of the point mutations is sequencing, a variety of techniques may be used for screening for the presence of point mutations (e.g., single-strand conformation polymorphism analysis,[86,111] denaturation gradient gel electrophoresis,[12] or fluorescence real-time PCR-based melting curve analysis).[35]

ACUTE MYELOID LEUKEMIAS

The translocations that occur in the acute myeloid leukemias (AML) target transcription factors or transcriptional coactivators. The transcription factors are involved in the differentiation of the hematopoietic cells, and disruption of their normal function by the translocation leads to developmental arrest and maturational block at immature stages of differentiation. The targeted transcription factors include the retinoic acid receptor alpha (RARα) in acute promyelocytic leukemia and several members of the core binding factor (CBF) complex. CBF is a transcription factor that consists of heterodimers, including a DNA-binding component known as *AML1* (*RUNX1/CBFA2/PEBP2A*), and a subunit CBFβ that activates the transcription of *AML1*. CBF is targeted in the t(8;21)[39] aberration, which results in the AML/*ETO* fusion that is characteristic of AML with differentiation (AML FAB-M2). CBF is similarly targeted in the inv(16), which leads to the CBFβ/SMMHC found in a subset of AML patients.[72] The multilineage importance of CBF is manifest in a subset of precursor B-cell acute lymphoblastic leukemias, where it is targeted in the t(12;21) that leads to

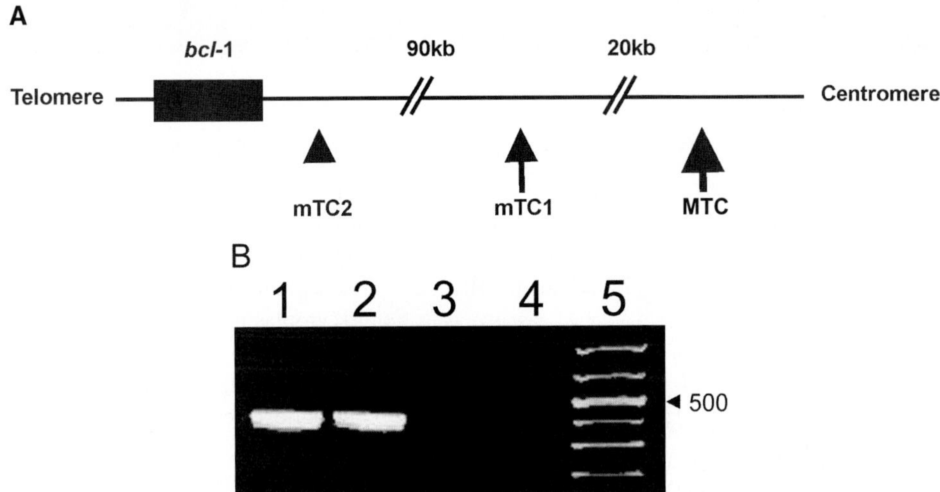

Figure 39-10 A, Schematic representation of the organization of the of the *bcl-1* gene on chromosome 11q13 and the breakpoint regions associated with the t(11;14). The *bcl-1* gene is represented as a white rectangle. The relative locations of the major translocation cluster (MTC) where up to 40% of the breakpoints are clustered and the minor translocation cluster regions (mTC1 and mTC2) are indicated. The size of the amplified PCR product may vary depending on the location of the breakpoints. **B,** PCR analysis and agarose gel electrophoresis for the detection of t(11;14). The primers were directed against the MTC of *bcl-1*. Lane 1 represents a positive control with a band at ~450 bp. Lane 2 is the patient sample with a positive band also at ~450 bp. Lane 3 contains a negative control (reactive tonsil). Lane 4 represents a no-template (H_2O) control. Lane 5 shows the size marker.

the *TEL/AML1* fusion.[45] All of the chimeric proteins that result from the chimeric fusions are dominant negative inhibitors of CBF-mediated transcription.[43,54] The transcriptional repression of the CBF target genes caused by the CBF-chimeric proteins partly involves the recruitment of the histone deacetylase complex.

By comparison, acute promyelocytic leukemia is characterized by translocations involving the *RARA* gene (Table 39-3). These translocations result in a block of myeloid differentiation at the promyelocytic stage. It has been shown that the maturational arrest is due in part to the recruitment of the nuclear co-repressor/histone deacetylase complex. The ability of all-*trans* retinoic acid (ATRA) to bind to *PML*/RARα, resulting in the release of the nuclear co-repressor complex, partly explains the ability of ATRA to relieve the maturational block in promyelocytes that is central to the development of acute promyelocytic leukemia.

t(8;21)(q22;q22)—*AML1-ETO*

The t(8;21)(q22;q22) is found in approximately 7% of de novo AML, and is more common in young individuals. The translocation is found in 20% to 40% of AMLs of the FAB-M2 subtype.[4] It has also been reported infrequently in M1 and M4 subtypes, and in rare cases of therapy associated AML. The translocation leads to the fusion of the *AML1* gene (acute myeloid leukemia 1 gene), also known as *CBFA2* (core binding factor subunit A2), or *PEBP2a* (polyoma enhancer binding protein 2 subunit a) to the *ETO* gene (8;21), also known as *MTG8* (myeloid translocation gene on chromosome 8) and *RUNX1T1*.

The t(8;21) portends a good prognosis in cases of de novo AML, with a favorable response to treatment with cytosine arabinoside.[82] The *AML1-ETO* chimeric fusion is detectable by RT-PCR in the vast majority of t(8;21)-positive AMLs, thus making RT-PCR a good choice for detection of the t(8;21) in clinical samples. The *AML1-ETO* fusions join exon 5 of *AML1* to exon 2 of *ETO* (Figure 39-11), and the fusion transcript can also be detected in complex translocations in a significant proportion of cases that are t(8;21) negative by conventional cytogenetics.[4,78] Specifically, RT-PCR has been reported to detect *AML1-ETO* fusions in 8% to 12% of AML.[4,66,78] Interestingly the *AML1-ETO* fusion transcript may be detected using sensitive end-point PCR assays several years after chemotherapy or a bone marrow transplant (BMT), thus limiting its predictive value for relapse in affected patients.[59] Quantitative studies using recently developed real-time PCR protocols (Figure 39-12 [Color Plate 3]) may provide a better indication of an increase in transcript copies and hence disease recurrence.

t(15;17)(q22;q21)—*PML-RARα*

The t(15;17) is the characteristic molecular abnormality in acute promyelocytic leukemia (APL), which is classified as AML FAB-M3. This abnormality is present in virtually all cases of APL, which constitutes 5% to 10% of all AMLs. The t(15;17) results in juxtaposition of the putative transcription factor *PML* on 15q22[13,74] to the retinoic acid receptor-α gene on 17q21.[89] The breakpoints on chromosome 17 are confined to a 15 kb fragment within intron 2 of the *RARα* locus. The breakpoints on chromosome 15 are more varied, with

Table 39-3 Common Recurrent Chromosomal Aberrations in Human Leukemia

Chromosomal Abnormalities	Genes or Loci (@) Involved	Disease	Clinical Features	Frequency of Genetic Alteration (%)
t(9;22)(q34;q11)	*BCR/ABL (p210)*	CML	Good prognosis	95
t(12;21) cryptic	*TEL/AML1*	Precursor B-cell ALL	Good prognosis	20-25
t(9;22)(q34;q11)	*BCR/ABL (p190)*	Precursor B-cell ALL	Poor prognosis	5-20
t(1;19)(q23;p13)	*E2A/PBX*	Precursor B-cell ALL	Pre-B phenotype (cytoplasmic μ), poor response to anti-metabolites	3-6
t(4;11)(q21;q23)	*MLL/AF4*	Precursor B-cell ALL	Mixed lineage, infants, poor prognosis leukocytosis	3
t(11;19)(q23;p13)	*MLL/ENL*	Precursor B-cell ALL	Leukocytosis	<1
t(8;14)(q24;q32)	*MYC/IGH@*	B-ALL	FAB L3, mature B-cell phenotype extramedullary disease	85
t(2;8)(p12;q24)	*MYC/IGK@*	B-ALL	FAB L3, mature B-cell phenotype extramedullary disease	10
t(8;22)(q24;q11)	*MYC/IGL@*	B-ALL	FAB L3, mature B-cell phenotype extramedullary disease	5
None	*TAL1* deletion	Precursor T-cell ALL	Extramedullary disease, CD2+, CD10–	25
t(1;14)(p32;q11)	*TRD@/TAL1*	Precursor T-cell ALL	Extramedullary disease, CD2+, CD10–	3
t(1;7)(p32;q35)	*TRB@/TAL1*	Precursor T-cell ALL	Extramedullary disease, CD2+, CD10–	<1
t(8;14)(q24;q11)	*TRA@/MYC*	Precursor T-cell ALL	Extramedullary disease	2
t(11;14)(p15;q11)	*TRD@/RBTN1*	Precursor T-cell ALL	Extramedullary disease	<1
t(11;14)(p13;q11)	*TRD@/RBTN2*	Precursor T-cell ALL	Extramedullary disease	7
t(10;14)(q24;q11)	*TRD@/HOX11*	Precursor T-cell ALL	Extramedullary disease	4
t(1;7)(p34;q34)	*TRB@/LCK*	Precursor T-cell ALL	Extramedullary disease	1
t(8;13)(p11;q11-12)	*FGFRI/ZNF198*	Precursor T-cell ALL	Eosinophilia	<1
t(8;21)(q22;q22)	*AML1/ETO*	AML	AML-FAB M2	10-15 (30% of AML M2)
inv(16)(p13;q22)	*CBFβ/MYH11*	AML	FAB M4EO	10
t(6;9)(p23;q34)	*DEK/CAN*	AML	Basophilia	2
t(9;11)(p22;q23)	*MLL/AF9*	AML	FAB M4-M5, infants	5
t(8;16)(p11;p13)	*MOZ/CBP*	AML	FAB M4, M5	<1
t(7;11)(p15;p15)	*NUP98/HOXA9*	AML	FAB M2, M4	1
t(3;5)(q25;q34)	*NPM/MLF 1*	AML	Myelodysplastic syndrome	1
t(15;17)(q22;q21)	*PML/RARA*	AML	FAB M3, coagulopathy, good retinoic acid response	7 (75% of AML M3)
t(11;17)(q23;q21)	*PLZF/RARA*	AML	FAB M3, coagulopathy, poor retinoic acid response	<1
t(5;17)(q32;q21)	*NPM/RARA*	AML	FAB M3, coagulopathy, poor retinoic acid response	<1

CML, Chronic myelogenous leukemia; *ALL,* acute lymphoblastic leukemia; *AML,* acute myelogenous leukemia; *p210 and p190,* chimcric proteins (see text); *FAB* (with L3, M3, M4EO, etc), French-American-British classifications; *TRB@, TRD@,* T-cell receptor β and δ loci.
*Estimated frequency per clinical disease category.

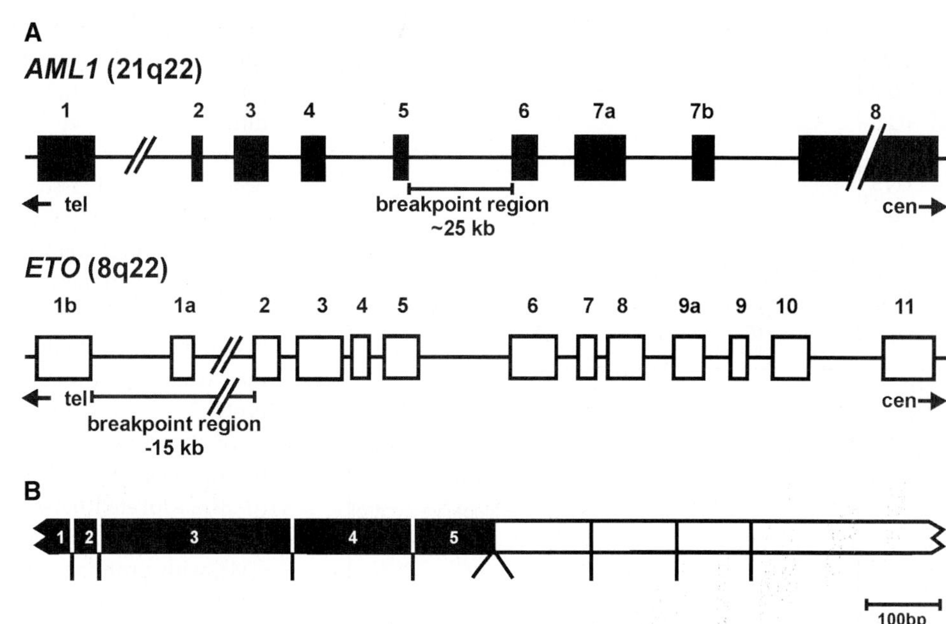

Figure 39-11 Schematic representation of the organization of the *AML1* (21q22) and the *ETO* genes (8q22) involved in the t(8;21) anomaly that is characteristic of FAB AML-M2. The centromeric (c) and telomeric (tel) directions are indicated. In panel A, the exons of the *AML1* gene are depicted in black rectangles; the exons of the *ETO* gene are depicted in white rectangles. In panel B, the configuration of the *AML1/ETO* chimeric fusion is shown. The numbers below the fusion transcript indicate the position of the first nucleotide in the exon involved, or the last nucleotide of the exon immediately 5′ to the fusion.

involvement of three or more breakpoint cluster distinct regions (bcr) (Figure 39-13, *A*). These include intron 6 (*bcr* 1), which is involved in approximately 55% of cases; exon 6 (*bcr* 2), which is involved in 5% of cases; and intron 3 (*bcr* 3), which is involved in 40% of cases. Similar to the scenario seen in the t(9;22) leading to the *BCR-ABL* fusion, the different breakpoints on *PML*, the alternatively spliced transcripts, and usage of two different polyadenylation sites further give rise to a greater variety of *PML-RARα* fusion transcripts of different sizes (Figure 39-13, *B*).[10] Recognition of these varied transcripts is important in the design of diagnostic RT-PCR assays that are capable of detecting the majority of t(15;17) fusions (Figure 39-13, *B*). In this regard, most assays have been directed at the *PML-RARα* fusion, since the reciprocal (*RARα-PML*) fusion is not detectable in some cases of APL. The *PML-RARα* chimeric protein contributes to leukemogenesis by blocking the differentiation of myeloid cells at the level of promyelocytes. Persistent detection of *PML-RARα* transcripts in a treated patient is an ominous indication of a tendency relapse. The recent availability of quantitative real-time protocols provides an opportunity for sensitive and specific monitoring of consecutive samples at appropriate intervals for the identification of patients with high relapse potential.

Chronic Leukemias of Myeloid/Monocytic Lineage

The chronic myeloid leukemias are characterized by translocations that lead to constitutive activation of tyrosine kinases. As mentioned earlier, the most common of these is the t(9;22)(q34;q11), resulting in the *BCR/ABL* fusion that is characteristic of CML. Up to seven different chromosomal translocations are associated with the chronic leukemias of myeloid/monocytic lineage, but all are characterized by the formation of a chimeric fusion with a carboxyterminal tyrosine kinase domain and an oligomerization motif in the amino terminus of the fusion protein. The oligomerization motif is important for the constitutive activation of the tyrosine kinase, which transforms the hematopoietic cells and confers them with ligand-independent growth potential.

t(9;22)(q34;q11)—*BCR-ABL* Aberration

The t(9;22), also known as the Philadelphia chromosome, is the diagnostic hallmark of CML and is found in virtually 100% of cases. The translocation is also found in up to 20% to 50% of acute lymphoblastic leukemias (ALLs) in adults, in 2% to 10% of childhood ALLs, in rare cases of malignant lymphoma, and in myeloma.[11,62-64,75] The t(9;22) results in the juxtaposition of 3′ sequences on the *c-ABL* tyrosine kinase proto-oncogene (9q34), to the 5′ sequences of the breakpoint cluster region *BCR* gene (22q11). The t(9;22) results in the formation of two hybrid genes: *BCR-ABL* on the derivative chromosome 22, and *ABL-BCR* on the derivative chromosome 9.[25] The *BCR-ABL* fusion encodes a chimeric protein with constitutively activated tyrosine kinase activity. While the breakpoints on chromosome 9 are relatively constant and 5′ to exon 2 of *c-ABL*, the breakpoints on chromosome 22 are quite variable and within the *BCR* gene (Figure 39-14).[53,62] Depending on the location of the breakpoint, the fusion protein resulting from the *BCR-ABL* fusion could vary in size from 190 to 230 kDa. Up to 95% of CMLs, 30% to 50% of adult t(9;22) positive ALLs, and 20% to 30% of childhood t(9;22)-positive ALLs harbor breakpoints in the m-*BCR* region of the *BCR* gene.[48,87,91,101] The *BCR* breakpoints in virtually all of the CML cases occur in the 9.0 kb region between exons 13 and 15 (also known as b2 and b4, respectively). Fusion is

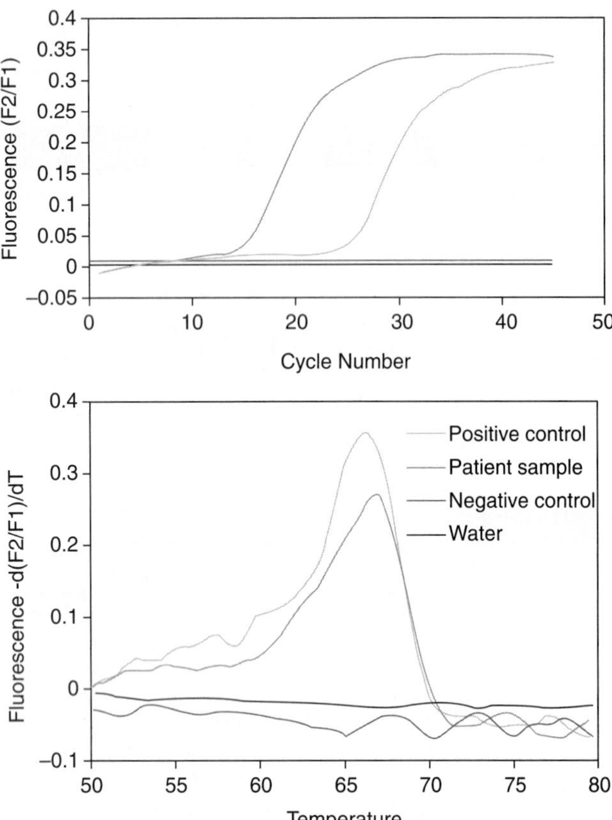

Figure 39-12 Real-time PCR detection of *AML1/ETO* fusion transcript. Real-time PCR detection was performed using a sequence-specific hybridization probe format with oligonucleotide probes labeled with fluorescein as the donor fluorophore and LCRed640 as the acceptor. Postamplification melting analysis was performed to provide confirmation of amplicon identity through the probe melting temperature. Panel A shows the fluorescence (F) versus cycle number (C) on the LightCycler™ (Roche Diagnostics). The characteristic three-phase profiles of amplification curves are recognizable (i.e., initial lag, exponential or log/linear, and the final plateau phase). The red curve represents the positive amplification signal for the t(8;21) in the Kasumi cell line positive control. The blue curve represents the patient sample also showing the presence of the *AML1/ETO* fusion. The green line represents a negative control (placental cDNA), and the black line is the no-template (H_2O) control. Panel B shows the derivative melting curves with positive melting peaks at ~65°C in both the Kasumi cell line positive control and the patient sample. Both the negative and water controls show flat lines indicating the absence of the t(8;21) *AML1/ETO* product. (See Color Plate 3.)

to a breakpoint located in the large intron between exons 1b and 2 of the *ABL* gene[20] (Figure 39-14). The resulting *BCR-ABL* transcript measures 8.5 kb and contains either *BCR* exon b2 or b3 and *ABL* exon 2 (exon a2). This transcript encodes the 210 kDa *BCR-ABL* chimeric protein ($p210^{BCR/ABL}$). The most common fusions found in CML are b3-a2 fusions, accounting for 55% of the *BCR-ABL* junctions, and b2-a2 (40%).[107] Less frequently (5%), both the b3-a2 and b2-a2 fusions may occur as a result of alternative splicing.[107] Thus far, there appear to be no significant prognostic differences between p210-positive CMLs with different transcripts.[107]

In rare cases of CML, the breakpoint in the *BCR* gene occurs at the ALL-associated m-*BCR,* which leads to the generation of the $p190^{BCR/ABL}$ fusion protein.[105] p190-positive CML patients characteristically exhibit relative and absolute monocytosis in peripheral blood reminiscent of chronic myelomonocytic leukemia.[77] Another distinct but rare fusion that has been described in t(9;22)-positive CML is one that results in the formation of a large 230 kDa fusion protein as a consequence of a fusion between exon 19 (c3) of *BCR* and exon 2 (a2) of *ABL*. The *BCR* breakpoints for this fusion are located in the micro breakpoint cluster region (μ-*BCR*) located between exons 19 and 20 (see Figure 39-14). The p230 fusion is characteristic of a peculiar form of CML with prominent neutrophilic proliferation. The clinical course of p230-positive CML is reportedly indolent in the majority of cases.[88]

Another distinct breakpoint cluster region in the *BCR* gene has been uniquely associated with t(9;22)-positive ALLs.[53] Up to 60% of t(9;22)-positive ALL carry translocations in which the breakpoints are located in a distinct region known as the "minor breakpoint cluster region" (m-*BCR*). m-*BCR* is located between the two alternative exons and exon 2 (see Figure 39-14). The *ABL* breakpoints are located in the large intron between exon 1b and exon 2 of the *ABL* gene (see Figure 39-14). The resulting e1-a2 fusion encodes a 190 kD *BCR-ABL* chimeric protein[21] that is expressed mostly in *ALLs,* and rather infrequently as the exclusive *BCR-ABL* transcript in CML.[96,105] On the other hand, the remaining 40% of t(9;22)-positive ALLs may express the p210 *BCR-ABL* fusion, thus indicating its relative lack of specificity. A significant number of CML cases also express low levels of e1-a2 transcripts in addition to p210 via an alternative splicing mechanism.[23,56,96,119]

Conventional cytogenetics, FISH, and RT-PCR have been reliably used for the laboratory detection of the t(9;22). RT-PCR detection is possible in up to 95% of cases, and may detect up to 10% of cases missed by conventional cytogenetics,[23] and is an important modality for minimal residual disease detection. Recently, quantitative real-time PCR-based approaches have improved the ability to detect and quantify *BCR-ABL* transcripts in CML patients[32,61] (Figure 39-15 [Color Plate 4]). The recent availability the tyrosine kinase inhibitor imatinib mesylate for CML is an important development in the treatment of CML[31,32] and further underscores the importance of methods for sensitive and specific identification and quantification of the *BCR-ABL* fusions in patients with a clinical suspicion of a CML.

t(9;22) in Acute Lymphoblastic Leukemia

The t(9;22) has emerged as a sine qua non for the diagnosis of CML, and the recent development of novel tyrosine kinase inhibitor therapy portends a favorable prognosis. By con-

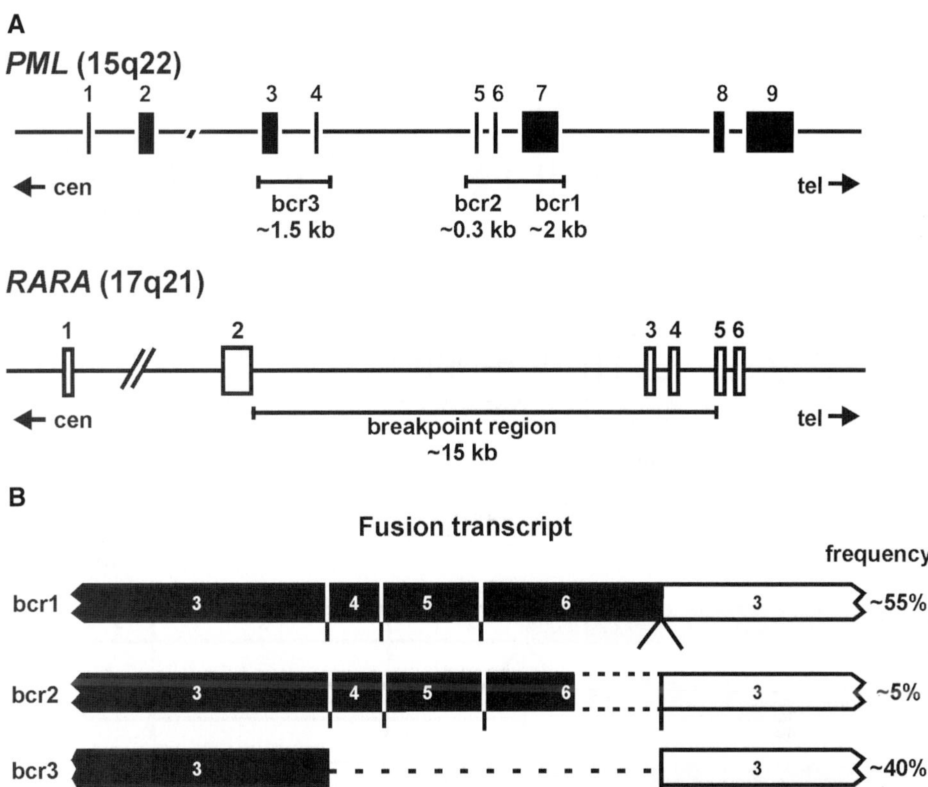

Figure 39-13 Schematic representation of the organization of the *PML* (15q22) and *RARα* (17q11) genes involved in the t(15;17) anomaly, which is characteristic of FAB AML-M3. The centromeric (c) and telomeric (tel) directions are indicated. In panel A, the exons of the *PML* gene are depicted in black rectangles, and the exons of the *RARα* gene are depicted in white rectangles. In panel B, the configuration of the *PML-RARα* chimeric fusions are shown.

trast, the presence of the t(9;22) is an independent poor prognostic factor in ALLs.[41,102,125]

Use of Reverse-Transcription Polymerase Chain Reaction in Chromosomal Translocations

Reverse-transcription polymerase chain reaction (RT-PCR) is particularly indicated in the detection of chromosomal translocations wherein the breakpoints are widely dispersed with large intervening introns between the juxtaposed fragments that limit the practicality of conventional PCR. As RT-PCR begins with synthesis of complementary (cDNA) from mRNA (with use of oligo-dT priming, random hexamers, or gene-specific primers), the template for the PCR is not the genomic DNA, but the complementary DNA derived from the reverse-transcribed RNA. RT-PCR for identification of a characteristic chromosomal translocation will be addressed later using the example of the t(9;22), which is present in virtually 100% of cases of chronic myeloid leukemias and in a smaller subset of acute lymphoblastic leukemias.

Real-Time Polymerase Chain Reaction Methods

The PCR assays traditionally used in the study of hematological malignancies have entailed a two-step procedure comprising an initial amplification reaction, followed by analysis of the PCR products in a separate process. PCR product analysis has generally entailed size fractionation by gel electrophoresis and product visualization by ultraviolet (UV) illumination of ethidium bromide–stained gels or by chemiluminescent or radioisotopic detection. The recent advent of real-time PCR techniques now permits PCR amplification with simultaneous monitoring of product accumulation.[55] Real-time PCR methodologies employ variations of fundamental fluorescence chemistries to monitor product accumulation. Higuchi et al introduced the incorporation of a double-stranded DNA (dsDNA) binding dye (ethidium bromide) into amplification reactions, with fluorescence monitoring at each cycle for quantitative analysis.[55] Such real-time PCR assays using dsDNA-binding dyes, such as ethidium bromide and SYBR Green I, are relatively inexpensive and easy to use, but suffer the drawback that they do not offer specificity beyond that inherent in the PCR. In poorly optimized reactions, the nonspecific dsDNA binding dye- or intercalator-based assays can yield false-positive results. It is thus important to carefully optimize primer design to discourage primer-dimer and nonspecific product formation.[16]

For studies of hematological malignancies, the sequence-specific fluorescence probe–based systems provide the advantage of an important further test for identification of the sequence of interest by virtue of hybridization of fluorescently labeled internal probes to the amplified target sequence.[127] The most commonly used sequence-specific chemistries include the exonuclease (TaqMan), the linear hybridization probe, and the hairpin-based (Molecular Beacon) systems. (See Chapter 37 for further information on nucleic acid techniques.)

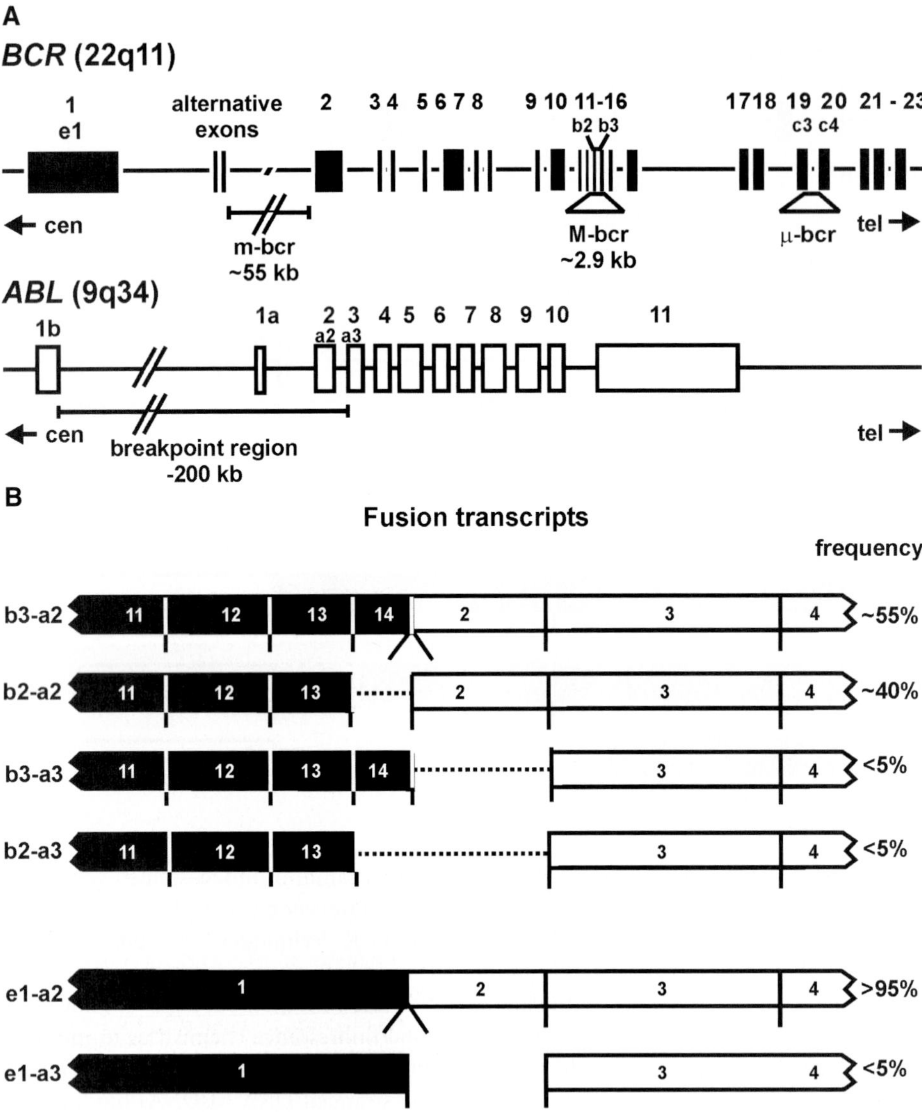

Figure 39-14 Schematic representation of the *BCR* (22q11) and *ABL* (9q34) genes involved in the t(9;22), which is characteristic of all CMLs and a subset of *ALLs*. The centromeric (cen) and telomeric (tel) directions are indicated. The relative positions of the major breakpoint cluster (M-*BCR*), the minor breakpoint cluster (m-*BCR*), and the micro breakpoint cluster regions (µ-*BCR*) are shown. The previously used alternative nomenclature for the *BCR* and *ABL* exons is included where relevant. In panel A, the exons of the *BCR* genes are depicted in black rectangles, and those of the *ABL* genes are depicted in white rectangles. In panel B, the configuration and varieties of the *BCR-ABL* chimeric fusions seen in CML are shown. In the lower part of panel B, the configuration and varieties of the *BCR-ABL* fusions seen in *ALL* are shown. The e1-a2 transcript is most commonly detected in t(9;22)-positive *ALL*, while the b3-a2 and b2-a2 fusions are the most commonly detected in CML.

Quantification

Real-time PCR is particularly advantageous for the quantitative analysis of nucleic acid sequences. Previously, quantitative PCR was based on end-point or competitive assays that measured band intensities in ethidium bromide–stained gels, or hybridization-based approaches using radioisotopic labeling and densitometry.[120] Fluorescence-based, real-time PCR assays characteristically demonstrate three phases: an initial background phase, an exponential or logarithmic phase, and a plateau phase. The exponential phase starts after the background phase and occurs when product accumulation rises significantly above background levels, and ends at the beginning of the plateau phase. The plateau phase occurs as a result of a combination of factors, including the accumulation of reaction products, ineffective polymerase activity, and competition of the accumulated PCR product for the oligonucleotide primers. The onset of the log-linear phase is inversely related to the abundance of the target of interest at the beginning of the PCR. By using calibrators with known quantities of a specific target, a calibration curve can be plotted with a crossing threshold (y-axis) against log concentration (x-axis) for the target of interest. The crossing threshold for a control and specific gene targets in unknown samples can be derived from their PCRs and read off the calibration curve to yield a copy number for the target transcript. By contrast, traditional methods require multiple amplification reactions in several tubes, which is labor-intensive and could lead to inaccurate results.

ONCOGENE AND TUMOR SUPPRESSOR GENE MUTATIONS IN HEMATOPOIETIC MALIGNANCIES

The concomitant occurrence of additional genetic aberrations and chromosomal translocations is common in hematological malignancies. The *RAS* oncogene is one of the most frequently mutated genes in cancer,[14] and is mutated in up

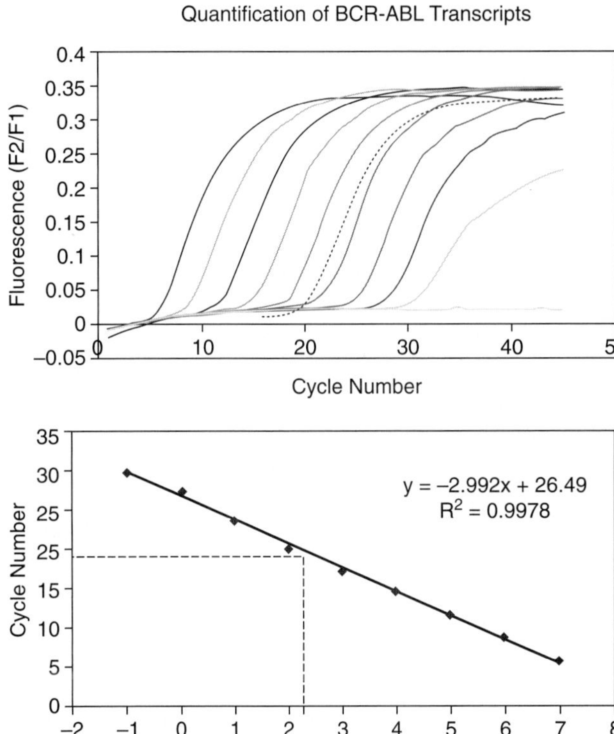

Figure 39-15 Real-time quantitative PCR of *BCR-ABL* transcripts. Serial log dilutions of the plasmids containing the *BCR-ABL* transcripts. Real-time PCR provides a remarkable dynamic range of quantification (10^9 to 10^0 template copies) in this example. The upper panel shows the amplification curves obtained using the *BCR-ABL* containing plasmids and an unknown patient sample depicted as a dotted line. Note the regular ~3.3-cycle interval between log dilutions. The lower panel shows a standard curve (linear regression of cycle number versus log template concentration). As indicated by the dotted line in the lower panel, the cycle threshold (onset of the log-linear phase of the amplification curve) can be used to quantitate the copy number of the target in the tested sample. (See Color Plate 4.)

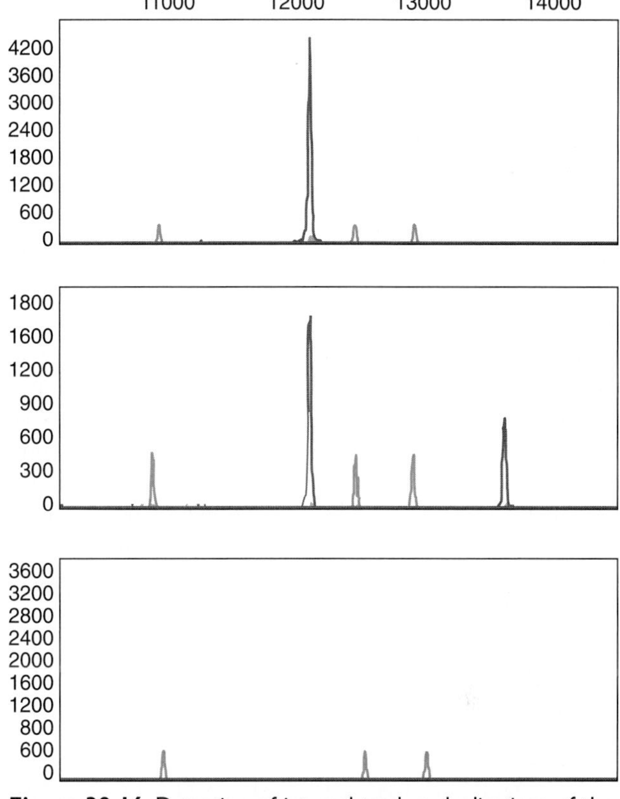

Figure 39-16 Detection of internal tandem duplications of the *FLT3* gene by PCR and capillary gel electrophoresis of PCR products. Capillary electropherograms show clear resolution of PCR products. The x-axis represents the sizes of PCR products and the y-axis shows the fluorescence intensity, which correlates with the abundance of the PCR product. The upper panel shows a wild type of pattern (blue peak). The middle panel shows an additional peak of greater size than the wild-type peak (blue peak on the left). The blue peak on the right represents a *FLT3* internal tandem duplication. The lower panel shows the size markers (red peaks) also present in the upper and middle panels. (See Color Plate 5.)

to 25% to 44% of hematopoietic malignancies and myelodysplastic syndromes (MDS).[7] The presence of *RAS* mutations has been reported to portend a worse prognosis in patients with AML and MDS.[84,85] The mutations are clustered in "hot spots" occurring at codons 12, 13, or 61, rendering them fairly easy to detect using different strategies for mutation detection, such as single strand conformation polymorphism analysis (SSCP) and denaturing gradient gel electrophoresis (DGGE).

Mutations of another tyrosine kinase, *FLT3*, have been described in acute myeloid leukemias.[83,128] The majority of these mutations are internal tandem duplications (ITDs) within the juxtamembrane domain (JMD) of the gene, and are present in up to 24% of AML cases. ITDs have been identified in all FAB subtypes of AML, most frequently in acute promyelocytic leukemia (AML FAB-M3). Figure 39-16 (Color Plate 5) shows an example of an *FLT3* ITD detected by PCR and capillary electrophoresis in a case of acute myeloid leukemia, which also demonstrated the presence of the *PML-RARA* fusion transcript. The presence of the ITD was inferred by the larger PCR product size (Figure 39-16 [Color Plate 5]) and was subsequently confirmed by sequencing. Additional mutations distinct from the ITDs occurring in the JMD have been described in a subset of AMLs. The most common of these is a base substitution occurring at the codon for aspartic acid residue 835 in the activation loop of *FLT3*. D835 mutations have been identified in 7% of AML, 3% of MDS, and 3% of ALLs.[128] If *FLT3* ITDs and activation mutations are combined, *FLT3* may be the most frequently mutated gene in acute myeloid leukemia. Mutations in the activation loop of another receptor tyrosine kinase *C-KIT* have been reported in mast cell proliferations,[73] and in a small proportion of AMLs.[17]

The *P53* gene is a tumor suppressor gene that encodes a nuclear phosphoprotein/transcription factor, which regulates diverse cellular processes, including DNA repair, cell-cycle arrest, and apoptosis. p53 inactivation is associated with genomic instability, and deregulated cell cycle entry and progression. The p53 gene is the most commonly mutated tumor suppressor gene in cancer. p53 mutations are commonly present in a variety of hematological disorders, including blast crisis in CML, AML, MDS,[68,122] and adult T-cell leukemia/lymphoma.[97] p53 mutations are also implicated in the histological transformation of follicular lymphoma into diffuse large B-cell lymphoma[98] and have been described in a small subset of cases of Hodgkin lymphoma.[37] p53 mutations correlate with resistance to chemotherapy and portend a worse prognosis.[122] The p53 mutations are localized mainly to mutational "hot spots" in exons 5 to 8 and may be single base substitutions, deletions, or insertions. Dominant negative inactivation of critical p53 protein function can be achieved by a mutation on one allele, since the wild type protein can dimerize with mutated proteins, resulting in functional impairment of p53 protein activity.[44] DGGE,[49] constant denaturant gel electrophoresis,[12] and SSCP[37] have been used with great success for the detection of p53 mutations and can serve as effective screening tools in the molecular laboratory.

MINIMAL RESIDUAL DISEASE DETECTION AND MONITORING

The occurrence of characteristic genetic aberrations and the uniqueness of antigen-receptor gene rearrangements in lymphoid neoplasia provide an attractive opportunity for the exploitation of the high sensitivity and specificity of molecular techniques for the detection of minimal residual disease and therapeutic monitoring. The sensitivity and specificity of molecular techniques in being capable of detecting one aberrant cell in a background of 10^{3-6} are superior to those provided solely by clinical or microscopic examination.

PCR-based studies have enjoyed their greatest utility for the detection of clonal antigen-receptor rearrangements and recurrent chromosomal translocations. In antigen-receptor gene rearrangements, clonal identity may be established either by designing sequence-specific primers for the unique antigen-receptor rearrangement, or by sequencing the PCR product from the subsequent sample.

The ideal scenario for the analysis of antigen-receptor rearrangements for monitoring of minimal residual disease (MRD) requires identification of the sequence of the specific clonal antigen-receptor gene rearrangement in the tumor of interest, followed by clonality analysis and sequencing of the initial and subsequent samples. The antigen-receptor gene rearrangement sequences of the initial and subsequent biopsies are compared for sequence homology. Alternatively, tumor-specific antigen-receptor primers may be designed for amplification of the subsequent sample, with successful amplification being considered evidence of clonal identity.

MRD testing using antigen-receptor PCR-based monitoring is especially significant in the pediatric population in patients with acute lymphoblastic leukemia/lymphoma.[79] The detection of clonal rearrangements of the antigen-receptor genes at the end of induction therapy has been shown to be predictive of a high relapse potential.[40,121] In addition, the demonstration of persistent positivity in successive analyses is a good indicator of future clinical relapse, while persistent negativity is indicative of a durable remission.[110]

The detection of chromosomal aberrations by PCR-based methods continues to evolve as a tool for MRD detection. Indeed the clinical significance of the qualitative detection of chromosomal translocations has been the subject of intense study with varying implications depending on the natural biology of the hematological disorder (if present), the specific clinical context, the translocation detected, or the methodology employed. For instance, t(14;18) has been detected in the peripheral blood and reactive lymphoid tissues of healthy individuals, leading to uncertainty about the significance of the qualitative detection of the t(14;18).[30,71] Similarly, highly sensitive PCR assays have detected the t(9;22) in the peripheral blood of otherwise healthy elderly individuals.[9,15]

The implications of qualitative detection of translocations vary with the translocation detected. For instance, there is a very high risk of relapse associated with the detection of residual *PML-RARα* transcripts after therapy.[28,29] By contrast, the t(8;21) *AML1-ETO* fusion may be detected in patients who have sustained and durable clinical remissions following treatment. The *AML1-ETO* fusion may be also detected in patients who have undergone chemotherapy or bone marrow transplantation.[59,65] On the other hand, the detection of the t(9;22) *BCR-ABL* fusion transcript is most prognostically significant for relapse if conversion to positivity occurs within 6 to 12 months of treatment. The predictive value of the presence of the chimeric transcripts can be affected by therapy-associated factors, such as graft-versus-host disease and type of transplant.[92] Nevertheless, persistent molecular negativity for the *BCR-ABL* transcript is indicative of good response to therapy and favors a durable remission.

The recent availability of quantitative real-time PCR-based assays for the quantitative detection of specific genetic alterations holds great promise in the quantification of tumor burden, response to therapy, and relapse potential. Appropriately done, the tests should be performed at a series of regular and successive time-points during the management of the disease. This approach is more apt to identify increasing, decreasing, or stabilizing trends in the abundance of the translocation product in tested samples. Figure 39-15 (Color Plate 4) show a quantitative RT-PCR study for the *BCR-ABL* transcript that incorporates several calibrators for the determination of the number of copies of the fusion transcript present in the sample. An alternative approach involves the determination of the ratio of the expression levels of the fusion transcript being tested against that of a stably expressed house-keeping gene, and monitoring the changes that ensue over time.

DETECTION OF VIRAL GENOMES

Viruses involved in the pathogenesis of abnormal proliferations of hematopoietic cells include the human T-cell leukemia virus type I found in adult T-cell leukemia/lymphoma and Kaposi-sarcoma herpesvirus/human herpesvirus-8 (KSHV/HHV8) seen in Kaposi sarcoma, primary effusion lymphoma, and multicentric Castleman's disease.[18] All of these viruses can be detected using the standard molecular biology techniques described in this chapter. PCR is commonly used because of its speed and ease of performance. Primer design should take into consideration the propensity for shared sequences within related viruses. Optimal specificity can be obtained by designing primers to unique portions of the genome of the virus of interest. Because of its well-established role in the pathogenesis of a variety of lymphoproliferative disorders, Epstein-Barr virus (EBV) and its detection are discussed below as an example of a virus that may be detected by in situ hybridization.

EPSTEIN-BARR VIRUS

EBV was identified in 1964 by Epstein, Achong, and Barr in cultured cells obtained from a malignant lymphoma described by Dennis Burkitt.[38] EBV was subsequently identified by Werner Henle and colleagues as the cause of infectious mononucleosis.[52] EBV is a lymphotropic virus that has been associated with several malignant neoplasms including endemic Burkitt lymphoma, nasopharyngeal carcinoma, nasal T/NK-type lymphoma, and some subtypes of Hodgkin lymphoma. EBV is also implicated in the pathogenesis of the majority of posttransplant lymphoproliferative disorders.[58]

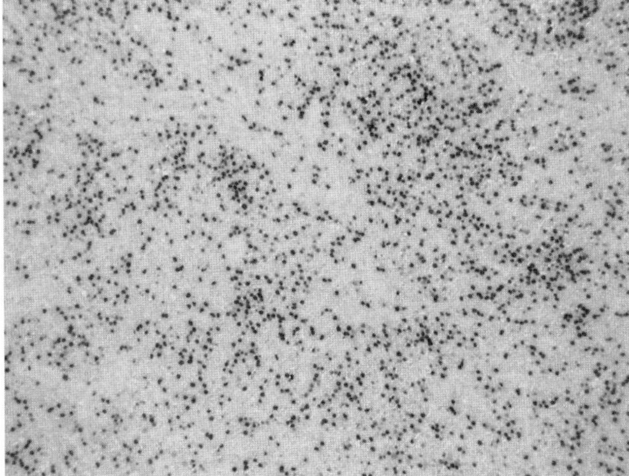

Figure 39-17 In situ hybridization (ISH) for the Epstein-Barr virus (EBV). ISH hybridization for EBV shows numerous positive signals (dark-blue spots) for EBV using the EBER-1 probe. The tissue sample was obtained from a solid-organ transplant patient who developed widespread nodal and extranodal masses. The positive reaction for EBV in this assay supports a diagnosis of posttransplant lymphoproliferative disease. (See Color Plate 6.)

Figure 39-17 (Color Plate 6) shows an example of positive EBV in situ hybridization in a case of posttransplant lymphoproliferative disease.

EBV is an enveloped icosahedral virus containing a double-stranded DNA genome of 172 kb with more than 100 open reading frames, potentially encoding an equivalent number of proteins.[6] The precise size of each virion varies from particle to particle because of the presence of tandemly repeated sequences, each 500 bp long, present in the virus termini. Viral tropism is mediated via attachment of the gp350/220 viral envelope protein to the complement receptor type 2 C3d (CR2) or CD21.[42,112] The virus exhibits tropism for B-cells, some T-cells, dendritic cells, and epithelial cells. After infection, typically via the oropharyngeal mucosa, EBV undergoes lytic replication in vivo. In the lytic replication, the linear genome is duplicated, assembled into viral capsid, and eliminated from the cell by budding or lysis. By contrast, B-cells are efficiently immortalized by EBV in vitro. In immortalized cells, the viral genome is circularized by fusion of the termini (episomal), and the viral infection is latent with lack of production of viral particles. In the latent phase, viral replication occurs coordinately with host cell division. During latent infection, 11 genes are actively transcribed, including 6 nuclear antigens (EBNA-1, -2, -3A, -3B, -3C, -LP), 3 membrane proteins (latent membrane proteins LMP-1, -2A and -2B), and 2 EBV-encoded small non-polyadenylated RNAs (EBER-1/-2).[3] The EBERs are present at very high copy numbers in the nuclei of latently infected cells.[69] The abundance of this transcript makes it attractive for detection of latent EBV infection in cells and tissue specimens by in situ hybridization (see Figure 39-17 [Color Plate 6]). Three latency patterns of expression have been described that relate to the expression of latency gene products. In latency pattern I, exemplified by Burkitt lymphoma cells, EBNA-1 is the only antigen that is expressed. In latency pattern II (exemplified by Hodgkin lymphoma), EBNA-1 and LMP-1 are expressed, and in latency pattern III (exemplified by posttransplant lymphoproliferative disease), all nuclear and latent membrane antigens are expressed. Based on the premise that one virion infects one host cell, and each virion has a unique number of terminal repeats with each episome being exactly replicated in all of its progeny, the clonality status of different cell populations has been assessed using probes complementary to the EBV termini by SBH analysis.[50] Genomic probes that are complementary to sequences adjacent to the EBV termini (called terminal repeat region probes) are used. In this assay, a specimen yielding a single size of episomal EBV DNA is considered monoclonal. This is based on the premise that all of the cells arose from a parent cell containing the same EBV DNA episome that was replicated in the progeny. By contrast, a sample yielding various sized episomes, with a ladder pattern in which fragments differ by 500 bp, is indicative of a polyclonal population wherein each progenitor cell harbored a different EBV DNA episome.[90] An obvious advantage of using EBV terminal repeat probes for assessment of clonality is that it can also be used for assessment of clonality in EBV-positive nonhematopoietic neoplasms (e.g., nasopharyngeal carcinoma) in which antigen-receptor gene rearrangements are not informative.[90] EBV in situ hybridization using probes targeting the EBER-1 transcript has contributed significantly to the identification of EBV in several hematopoietic and nonhematopoietic disorders.

IN SITU HYBRIDIZATION

The ability to visualize the cellular localization of different gene products is an important aspect of molecular biology and pathology. In situ hybridization (ISH) permits identification of the exact cellular location of target DNA or RNA in cytological preparations or microscopic sections. ISH uses a nucleic acid (DNA or RNA) probe that is complementary to the gene sequence of interest. The probe may be labeled by nonisotopic or radioisotopic methods. ISH hybridization of fixed paraffin-embedded tissue sections entails initial dissolution of paraffin in xylene and serial rehydration in aqueous solutions of ethanol with decreasing ethanol contents ("graded ethanols"). For DNA targets, the tissue section is subjected to denaturation, followed by application of the probe for hybridization. Several washing steps with modulation of stringency (temperature, ionic/salt concentration) are necessary to ensure specificity of the hybridization. Development of signals indicative of specific hybridization depends on the system used. Colorimetric detection using the avidin-biotin system and peroxidase chemistry with a substrate (e.g., diaminobenzidine) yielding a visible precipitate is currently favored for light microscopic applications.

ISH is versatile and can be used for the detection of viral targets and for a number of other diagnostic tests including in the assessment of B-cell clonality by light chain restriction. Recent developments that have led to widespread utility of ISH include the development of nonfluorescent chromophore in situ hybridization protocols that permit the ISH analysis of a variety of targets using the light microscope.[8]

POTENTIAL OF MICROARRAYS IN MOLECULAR DIAGNOSTICS OF HEMATOLOGICAL MALIGNANCIES

The recent advent of high-density oligonucleotides or cDNA array formats that permit the simultaneous evaluation of the expression status of thousands of genes in a single hybridization experiment promises to revolutionize the molecular diagnosis of hematological malignancies. Microarrays are prepared by immobilization of nucleic acid sequences onto glass slides.[99,100] In the cDNA hybridization format, the expression level of a transcript in one sample is compared with that in another sample in a competitive hybridization. The mRNA from the samples of interest is extracted and reverse transcribed to produce cDNA. cDNA from each sample is labeled with a different fluorophore—such as Cy5, which emits in the red spectrum, and Cy3, which emits in the green spectrum. The labeled samples are mixed and hybridized to the array. The hybridization signals are captured by a laser confocal microscope scanner. The ratio of Cy5/Cy3 fluorescence for each gene (i.e., red versus green) is computed and yields data that reflect the relative levels of expression of the interrogated gene in the test and the reference samples.

The technique provides an impressive dynamic range for quantification of several genes in a single experiment, and permits the determination of profiles that reflect the molecular signature of a specific tumor category. Integration of the vast amounts of information obtained from microarray experiments requires the use of sophisticated bioinformatics tools and algorithms to obtain biologically meaningful information.[33,46,93] Microarrays have been used in class distinction,[46] class discovery,[2] and class prognostication of outcomes in processes with distinct expression profiles.[2,108] More recently, microarray analysis has been employed in the elucidation of molecular and cellular signaling pathways that are involved in the pathogenesis of hematopoietic malignancies.[36] The potential of this technology to reveal novel markers for accurate disease diagnosis and prognosis, and markers of chemoresistance or predictors of rapid response to therapy makes it attractive for molecular diagnostics of these conditions. It is envisaged that smaller, highly predictive gene sets will be assembled in disease-related diagnostic "chips" for the assessment of specific categories of hematological malignancies and other diseases.

CONCLUSIONS

Hematopoietic neoplasms are associated with distinctive molecular aberrations that are amenable to diagnostic detection. In addition, the identification of the molecular abnormality in many cases also carries important prognostic information and disease-specific implications for treatment. The choice of methodology depends on the nature of the aberration being evaluated, the nature of the available samples, and the sensitivity afforded by the available methodologies. Technical issues aside, the potential contribution of a test must be evaluated for each patient individually. Most importantly, molecular tests should be used as adjunctive tools in the evaluation of the patient, and should never be used in isolation without consideration of clinical findings. The management of a patient should incorporate the entire complement of available clinical and diagnostic information, including flow cytometry and morphological findings on peripheral blood, biopsies, and bone marrow aspirates. Ideally, all this information could be analyzed and synthesized to produce a final diagnostic report that incorporates these findings.

REFERENCES

1. Albinger-Hegyi A, Hochreutener B, Abdou MT, Hegyi I, Dours-Zimmerman MT, Kurrer MO, et al. High

frequency of t(14;18)-translocation breakpoints outside of major breakpoint and minor cluster regions in follicular lymphomas: improved polymerase chain reaction protocols for their detection. Am J Pathol 2002;160:823-32.
2. Alizadeh AA, Eisen MB, Davis RE, Ma C, Lossos IS, Rosenwald A, et al. Distinct types of diffuse large B-cell lymphoma identified by gene expression profiling. Nature 2000;403:503-11.
3. Anagnostopoulos I, Hummel M. Epstein-Barr virus in tumours. Histopathology 1996;29:297-315.
4. Andrieu V, Radford-Weiss I, Troussard X, Chane C, Valensi F, Guesnu M, et al. Molecular detection of t(8;21)/AML1-ETO in AML M1/M2: correlation with cytogenetics, morphology and immunophenotype. Br J Haematol 1996;92:855-65.
5. Aster JC, Kobayashi Y, Shiota M, Mori S, Sklar J. Detection of the t(14;18) at similar frequencies in hyperplastic lymphoid tissues from American and Japanese patients. Am J Pathol 1992;141:291-9.
6. Baer R, Bankier AT, Biggin MD, Deininger PL, Farrell PJ, Gibson TJ, et al. DNA sequence and expression of the B95-8 Epstein-Barr virus genome. Nature 1984;310:207-11.
7. Beaupre DM, Kurzrock R. RAS and leukemia: from basic mechanisms to gene-directed therapy. J Clin Oncol 1999;17:1071-9.
8. Beck RC, Tubbs RR, Hussein M, Pettay J, Hsi ED. Automated Colorimetric In Situ Hybridization (CISH) Detection of Immunoglobulin (Ig) Light Chain mRNA Expression in Plasma Cell (PC) Dyscrasias and Non-Hodgkin Lymphoma. Diagn Mol Pathol 2003;12:14-20.
9. Biernaux C, Loos M, Sels A, Huez G, Stryckmans P. Detection of major bcr-abl gene expression at a very low level in blood cells of some healthy individuals. Blood 1995;86:3118-22.
10. Biondi A, Rambaldi A, Pandolfi PP, Rossi V, Giudici G, Alcalay M, et al. Molecular monitoring of the myl/retinoic acid receptor-alpha fusion gene in acute promyelocytic leukemia by polymerase chain reaction. Blood 1992;80:492-7.
11. Bloomfield CD, Goldman AI, Alimena G, Berger R, Borgstrom GH, Brandt L, et al. Chromosomal abnormalities identifying high-risk and low-risk patients with acute lymphoblastic leukemia. Blood 1986;67:415-20.
12. Borresen AL, Hovig E, Smith-Sorensen B, Malkin D, Lystad S, Andersen TI, et al. Constant denaturant gel electrophoresis as a rapid screening technique for p53 mutations. Proc Natl Acad Sci U S A 1991;88:8405-9.
13. Borrow J, Goddard AD, Sheer D, Solomon E. Molecular analysis of acute promyelocytic leukemia breakpoint cluster region on chromosome 17. Science 1990;249:1577-80.
14. Bos JL. ras oncogenes in human cancer: a review. Cancer Res 1989;49:4682-9.
15. Bose S, Deininger M, Gora-Tybor J, Goldman JM, Melo JV. The presence of typical and atypical BCR-ABL fusion genes in leukocytes of normal individuals: biologic significance and implications for the assessment of minimal residual disease. Blood 1998;92:3362-7.
16. Brownie J, Shawcross S, Theaker J, Whitcombe D, Ferrie R, Newton C, Little S. The elimination of primer-dimer accumulation in PCR. Nucleic Acids Res 1997;25:3235-41.
17. Care RS, Valk PJ, Goodeve AC, Abu-Duhier FM, Geertsma-Kleinekoort WM, Wilson GA, et al. Incidence and prognosis of c-KIT and FLT3 mutations in core binding factor (CBF) acute myeloid leukaemias. Br J Haematol 2003;121:775-7.
18. Cesarman E, Knowles DM. Kaposi's sarcoma-associated herpesvirus: a lymphotropic human herpesvirus associated with Kaposi's sarcoma, primary effusion lymphoma, and multicentric Castleman's disease. Semin Diagn Pathol 1997;14:54-66.
19. Cheng GY, Minden MD, Toyonaga B, Mak TW, McCulloch EA. T cell receptor and immunoglobulin gene rearrangements in acute myeloblastic leukemia. J Exp Med 1986;163:414-24.
20. Chissoe SL, Bodenteich A, Wang YF, Wang YP, Burian D, Clifton SW, et al. Sequence and analysis of the human ABL gene, the BCR gene, and regions involved in the Philadelphia chromosomal translocation. Genomics 1995;27:67-82.
21. Clark SS, McLaughlin J, Crist WM, Champlin R, Witte ON. Unique forms of the abl tyrosine kinase distinguish Ph1-positive CML from Ph1-positive ALL. Science 1987;235:85-8.
22. Cossman J, Uppenkamp M, Sundeen J, Coupland R, Raffeld M. Molecular genetics and the diagnosis of lymphoma. Arch Pathol Lab Med 1988;112:117-27.
23. Costello R, Lafage M, Toiron Y, Brunel V, Sainty D, Arnoulet C, et al. Philadelphia chromosome-negative chronic myeloid leukaemia: a report of 14 new cases. Br J Haematol 1995;90:346-52.
24. Davey MP, Bongiovanni KF, Kaulfersch W, Quertermous T, Seidman JG, Herschfield MS, et al. Immunoglobulin and T-cell receptor gene rearrangement and expression in human lymphoid leukemia cells at different stages of maturation. Proc Natl Acad Sci U S A 1986;83:8759-63.
25. de Klein A, van Kessel AG, Grosveld G, Bartram CR, Hagenmeijer A, Bootsma D, et al. A cellular oncogene is translocated to the Philadelphia chromosome in chronic myelocytic leukaemia. Nature 1982;300:765-7.
26. de Villartay JP, Hockett RD, Coran D, Korsmeyer SJ, Cohen DI. Deletion of the human T-cell receptor delta-gene by a site-specific recombination. Nature 1988;335:170-4.

27. Dierlamm J, Baens M, Wlodarska I, Stefanova-Ouzounova M, Hernandez JM, Hossfeld DK, et al. The apoptosis inhibitor gene API2 and a novel 18q gene, MLT, are recurrently rearranged in the t(11;18)(q21;q21)associated with mucosa-associated lymphoid tissue lymphomas. Blood 1999;93:3601-9.
28. Diverio D, Pandolfi PP, Rossi V, Biondi A, Pelicci PG, Lo Coco F. Monitoring of treatment outcome in acute promyelocytic leukemia by RT-PCR. Leukemia 1994;8 Suppl 2:S63-5.
29. Diverio D, Rossi V, Avvisati G, De Santis S, Pistilli A, Pane F, et al. Early detection of relapse by prospective reverse transcriptase-polymerase chain reaction analysis of the PML/RARalpha fusion gene in patients with acute promyelocytic leukemia enrolled in the GIMEMA-AIEOP multicenter "AIDA" trial. GIMEMA-AIEOP Multicenter "AIDA" Trial. Blood 1998;92:784-9.
30. Dolken G, Illerhaus G, Hirt C, Mertelsmann R. BCL-2/JH rearrangements in circulating B cells of healthy blood donors and patients with nonmalignant diseases. J Clin Oncol 1996;14:1333-44.
31. Druker BJ, Talpaz M, Resta DJ, Peng B, Buchdunger E, Ford JM, et al. Efficacy and safety of a specific inhibitor of the BCR-ABL tyrosine kinase in chronic myeloid leukemia. N Engl J Med 2001;344:1031-7.
32. Druker BJ, Tamura S, Buchdunger E, Ohno S, Segal GM, Fanning S, et al. Effects of a selective inhibitor of the Abl tyrosine kinase on the growth of Bcr-Abl positive cells. Nat Med 1996;2:561-6.
33. Eisen MB, Spellman PT, Brown PO, Botstein D. Cluster analysis and display of genome-wide expression patterns. Proc Natl Acad Sci U S A 1998;95:14863-8.
34. Eisenstein BI. The polymerase chain reaction. A new method of using molecular genetics for medical diagnosis. N Engl J Med 1990;322:178-83.
35. Elenitoba-Johnson KS, Bohling SD, Wittwer CT, King TC. Multiplex PCR by multicolor fluorimetry and fluorescence melting curve analysis. Nat Med 2001;7:249-53.
36. Elenitoba-Johnson KS, Jenson SD, Abbott RT, Palais RA, Bohling SD, Lin Z, et al. Involvement of multiple signaling pathways in follicular lymphoma transformation: p38-mitogen-activated protein kinase as a target for therapy. Proc Natl Acad Sci U S A 2003;100:7259-64.
37. Elenitoba-Johnson KS, Medeiros LJ, Khorsand J, King TC. P53 expression in Reed-Sternberg cells does not correlate with gene mutations in Hodgkin's disease. Am J Clin Pathol 1996;106:728-38.
38. Epstein MA, Achong BG, Barr YM. Virus particles in cultured lymphoblasts from Burkitt's lymphoma. Lancet 1964;1:702-3.
39. Erickson P, Gao J, Chang KS, Look T, Whisenant E, Raimondi S, et al. Identification of breakpoints in t(8;21) acute myelogenous leukemia and isolation of a fusion transcript, AML1/ETO, with similarity to Drosophila segmentation gene, runt. Blood 1992;80:1825-31.
40. Evans PA, Short MA, Owen RG, Jack AS, Forsyth PD, Shiach CR, et al. Residual disease detection using fluorescent polymerase chain reaction at 20 weeks of therapy predicts clinical outcome in childhood acute lymphoblastic leukemia. J Clin Oncol 1998;16: 3616-27.
41. Faderl S, Kantarjian HM, Talpaz M, Estrov Z. Clinical significance of cytogenetic abnormalities in adult acute lymphoblastic leukemia. Blood 1998;91: 3995-4019.
42. Fingeroth JD, Weiss JJ, Tedder TF, Strominger JL, Biro PA, Fearon DT. Epstein-Barr virus receptor of human B lymphocytes in the C3d receptor CR2. Proc Natl Acad Sci U S A 1984;81:4510-4.
43. Frank R, Zhang J, Uchida H, Meyers S, Heibert SW, Nimer SD. The AML1/ETO fusion protein blocks transactivation of the GM-CSF promoter by AML1B. Oncogene 1995;11:2667-74.
44. Galmarini CM, Falette N, Tabone E, Levrat C, Britten R, Voorzanger-Rousselot N, et al. Inactivation of wild-type p53 by a dominant negative mutant renders MCF-7 cells resistant to tubulin-binding agent cytotoxicity. Br J Cancer 2001;85:902-8.
45. Golub TR, Barker GF, Bohlander SK, Heibert SW, Ward DC, Bray-Ward P, et al. Fusion of the TEL gene on 12p13 to the AML1 gene on 21q22 in acute lymphoblastic leukemia. Proc Natl Acad Sci U S A 1995;92:4917-21.
46. Golub TR, Slonim DK, Tamayo P, Huard C, Gaasenbeek M, Mesirov JP, et al. Molecular classification of cancer: class discovery and class prediction by gene expression monitoring. Science 1999;286:531-7.
47. Greiner TC, Raffeld M, Lutz C, Dick F, Jaffe ES. Analysis of T cell receptor-gamma gene rearrangements by denaturing gradient gel electrophoresis of GC-clamped polymerase chain reaction products. Correlation with tumor-specific sequences. Am J Pathol 1995;146:46-55.
48. Groffen J, Stephenson JR, Heisterkamp N, de Klein A, Bartram CR, Grosveld G. Philadelphia chromosomal breakpoints are clustered within a limited region, bcr, on chromosome 22. Cell 1984;36:93-9.
49. Guldberg P, Nedergaard T, Nielsen HJ, Olsen AC, Ahrenkiel V, Zeuthen J. Single-step DGGE-based mutation scanning of the p53 gene: application to genetic diagnosis of colorectal cancer. Hum Mutat 1997;9:348-55.
50. Gulley ML, Raphael M, Lutz CT, Ross DW, Raab-Traub N. Epstein-Barr virus integration in human lymphomas and lymphoid cell lines. Cancer 1992;70:185-91.

51. Ha K, Minden M, Hozumi N, Gelfand EW. Immunoglobulin gene rearrangement in acute myelogenous leukemia. Cancer Res 1984;44:4658-60.
52. Henle G, Henle W, Diehl V. Relation of Burkitt's tumor-associated herpes-type virus to infectious mononucleosis. Proc Natl Acad Sci U S A 1968;59: 94-101.
53. Hermans A, Heisterkamp N, von Linden M, van Baal S, Meijer D, van der Plas D, et al. Unique fusion of bcr and c-abl genes in Philadelphia chromosome positive acute lymphoblastic leukemia. Cell 1987;51:33-40.
54. Heibert SW, Sun W, Davis JN, Golub T, Shurtleff S, Bujis A, et al. The t(12;21) translocation converts AML-1B from an activator to a repressor of transcription. Mol Cell Biol 1996;16:1349-55.
55. Higuchi R, Fockler C, Dollinger G, Watson R. Kinetic PCR analysis: real-time monitoring of DNA amplification reactions. Biotechnology (N Y) 1993;11: 1026-30.
56. Hochhaus A, Lin F, Reiter A, Skladny H, Mason PJ, van Rhee F, et al. Quantification of residual disease in chronic myelogenous leukemia patients on interferon-alpha therapy by competitive polymerase chain reaction. Blood 1996;87:1549-55.
57. Horsman DE, Gascoyne RD, Coupland RW, Coldman AJ, Adomat SA. Comparison of cytogenetic analysis, southern analysis, and polymerase chain reaction for the detection of t(14;18) in follicular lymphoma. Am J Clin Pathol 1995;103:472-8.
58. Hsieh WS, Lemas MV, Ambinder RF. The biology of Epstein-Barr virus in post-transplant lymphoproliferative disease. Transpl Infect Dis 1999;1:204-12.
59. Jurlander J, Caligiuri MA, Ruutu T, Baer MR, Strout MP, Oberkircher AR, at al. Persistence of the AML1/ETO fusion transcript in patients treated with allogeneic bone marrow transplantation for t(8;21) leukemia. Blood 1996;88:2183-91.
60. Kitchingman GR, Rovigatti U, Mauer AM, Melvin S, Murphy SB, Stass S. Rearrangement of immunoglobulin heavy chain genes in T cell acute lymphoblastic leukemia. Blood 1985;65:725-9.
61. Kreuzer KA, Lass U, Bohn A, Landt O, Schmidt CA. LightCycler technology for the quantitation of bcr/abl fusion transcripts. Cancer Res 1999;59:3171-4.
62. Kurzrock R, Gutterman JU, Talpaz M. The molecular genetics of Philadelphia chromosome-positive leukemias. N Engl J Med 1988;319:990-8.
63. Kurzrock R, Kloetzer WS, Talpaz M, Blick M, Walters R, Arlinghaus RB, Gutterman JU. Identification of molecular variants of p210bcr-abl in chronic myelogenous leukemia. Blood 1987;70:233-6.
64. Kurzrock R, Shtalrid M, Gutterman JU, Koller CA, Walters R, Trujillo JM, Talpaz M. Molecular analysis of chromosome 22 breakpoints in adult Philadelphia-positive acute lymphoblastic leukemia. Br Haematol 1987;67:55-9.
65. Kusec R, Laczika K, Knobl P, Friedl J, Greinix H, Kahls P, et al. AML1/ETO fusion mRNA can be detected in remission blood samples of all patients with t(8;21) acute myeloid leukemia after chemotherapy or autologous bone marrow transplantation. Leukemia 1994;8:735-9.
66. Langabeer SE, Walker H, Rogers JR, Burnett AK, Wheatley K, Swirsky D, et al. Incidence of AML1/ETO fusion transcripts in patients entered into the MRC AML trials. MRC Adult Leukaemia Working Party. Br J Haematol 1997;99:925-8.
67. Lehman CM, Sarago C, Nasim S, Comerford J, Karcher DS, Garrett CT. Comparison of PCR with southern hybridization for the routine detection of immunoglobulin heavy chain gene rearrangements. Am J Clin Pathol 1995;103:171-6.
68. Lepelley P, Preudhomme C, Vanrumbeke M, Quesnel B, Cosson A, Fenauz P. Detection of p53 mutations in hematological malignancies: comparison between immunocytochemistry and DNA analysis. Leukemia 1994;8:1342-9.
69. Lerner MR, Andrews NC, Miller G, Steitz JA. Two small RNAs encoded by Epstein-Barr virus and complexed with protein are precipitated by antibodies from patients with systemic lupus erythematosus. Proc Natl Acad Sci U S A 1981;78:805-9.
70. Leroux D, Le Marc'Hadour F, Gressin R, Jacob MC, Keddari E, Monteil M, et al. Non-Hodgkin's lymphomas with t(11;14)(q13;q32): a subset of mantle zone/intermediate lymphocytic lymphoma? Br J Haematol 1991;77:346-53.
71. Limpens J, de Jong D, van Krieken JH, Price CG, Young BD, van Ommen GJ, Kluin PM. Bcl-2/JH rearrangements in benign lymphoid tissues with follicular hyperplasia. Oncogene 1991;6:2271-6.
72. Liu P, Tarle SA, Hajra A, Claxton DF, Marlton P, Freedman M, et al. Fusion between transcription factor CBF beta/PEBP2 beta and a myosin heavy chain in acute myeloid leukemia. Science 1993;261:1041-4.
73. Longley BJ, Jr., Metcalfe DD, Tharp M, Wang X, Tyrell L, Lu SZ, et al. Activating and dominant inactivating c-KIT catalytic domain mutations in distinct clinical forms of human mastocytosis. Proc Natl Acad Sci U S A 1999;96:1609-14.
74. Longo L, Pandolfi PP, Biondi A, Rambaldi A, Mencarelli A, Lo Coco F, et al. Rearrangements and aberrant expression of the retinoic acid receptor alpha gene in acute promyelocytic leukemias. J Exp Med 1990;172:1571-5.
75. Maurer J, Janssen JW, Thiel E, van Denderen J, Ludwig WD, Aydemir U, et al. Detection of chimeric BCR-ABL genes in acute lymphoblastic leukemia by the polymerase chain reaction. Lancet 1991;337:1055-8.
76. Medeiros LJ, Carr J. Overview of the role of molecular methods in the diagnosis of malignant lymphomas. Arch Pathol Lab Med 1999;123:1189-207.

77. Melo JV, Myint H, Galton DA, Goldman JM. P190BCR-ABL chronic myeloid leukaemia: the missing link with chronic myelomonocytic leukaemia? Leukemia 1994;8:208-11.
78. Mitterbauer M, Kusec R, Schwarzinger I, Haas OA, Lechner K, Jaeger U. Comparison of karyotype analysis and RT-PCR for AML1/ETO in 204 unselected patients with AML. Ann Hematol 1998;76: 139-43.
79. Moppett J, Burke GA, Steward CG, Oakhill A, Goulden NJ. The clinical relevance of detection of minimal residual disease in childhood acute lymphoblastic leukaemia. J Clin Pathol 2003;56:249-53.
80. Morris SW, Kirstein MN, Valentine MB, Dittmer KG, Shapiro DN, Saltman DL, Look AT. Fusion of a kinase gene, ALK, to a nucleolar protein gene, NPM, in non-Hodgkin's lymphoma. Science 1994;263: 1281-4.
81. Motokura T, Arnold A. PRAD1/cyclin D1 proto-oncogene: genomic organization, 5′ DNA sequence, and sequence of a tumor-specific rearrangement breakpoint. Genes Chromosomes Cancer 1993;7: 89-95.
82. Mrozek K, Heinonen K, de la Chapelle A, Bloomfield CD. Clinical significance of cytogenetics in acute myeloid leukemia. Semin Oncol 1997;24:17-31.
83. Nakao M, Yokota S, Iwai T, Kaneko H, Horiike S, Kashima K, et al. Internal tandem duplication of the flt3 gene found in acute myeloid leukemia. Leukemia 1996;10:1911-18.
84. Neubauer A, Dodge RK, George SL, Davey FR, Silver RT, Schiffer CA, et al. Prognostic importance of mutations in the ras proto-oncogenes in de novo acute myeloid leukemia. Blood 1994;83:1603-11.
85. Neubauer A, Greenberg P, Negrin R, Ginzton N, Liu E. Mutations in the ras proto-oncogenes in patients with myelodysplastic syndromes. Leukemia 1994;8:638-41.
86. Orita M, Iwahana H, Kanazawa H, Hayashi K, Sekiya T. Detection of polymorphisms of human DNA by gel electrophoresis as single-strand conformation polymorphisms. Proc Natl Acad Sci U S A 1989;86:2766-70.
87. Paietta E, Racevskis J, Neuberg D, Rowe JM, Goldstone AH, Wiernik PH. Expression of CD25 (interleukin-2 receptor alpha chain) in adult acute lymphoblastic leukemia predicts for the presence of BCR/ABL fusion transcripts: results of a preliminary laboratory analysis of ECOG/MRC Intergroup Study E2993. Eastern Cooperative Oncology Group/Medical Research Council. Leukemia 1997;11:1887-90.
88. Pane F, Frigeri F, Sindona M, Luciano L, Ferrara F, Cimino R, et al. Neutrophilic-chronic myeloid leukemia: a distinct disease with a specific molecular marker (BCR/ABL with C3/A2 junction). Blood 1996;88:2410-14.
89. Petkovich M, Brand NJ, Krust A, Chambon P. A human retinoic receptor which belongs to the family of nuclear receptors. Nature 1987;330:444-50.
90. Raab-Traub N, Flynn K. The structure of the termini of the Epstein-Barr virus as a marker of clonal cellular proliferation. Cell 1986;47:883-9.
91. Radich J, Gehly G, Lee A, Avery R, Bryant E, Edmands S, et al. Detection of bcr-abl transcripts in Philadelphia chromosome-positive acute lymphoblastic leukemia after marrow transplantation. Blood 1997;89:2602-9.
92. Radich JP, Gehly G, Gooley T, Bryant E, Clift RA, Collins S, et al. Polymerase chain reaction detection of the BCR-ABL fusion transcript after allogeneic marrow transplantation for chronic myeloid leukemia: results and implications in 346 patients. Blood 1995;85:2632-8.
93. Ramaswamy S, Tamayo P, Rifkin R, Mukherjee S, Yeang CH, Angelo M, et al. Multiclass cancer diagnosis using tumor gene expression signatures. Proc Natl Acad Sci U S A 2001;98:15149-54.
94. Rimokh R, Berger F, Delsol G, Charrin C, Bertheas MF, French M, et al. Rearrangement and overexpression of the BCL-1/PRAD-1 gene in intermediate lymphocytic lymphomas and in t(11q13)-bearing leukemias. Blood 1993;81:3063-7.
95. Rimokh R, Gadoux M, Bertheas MF, Berger F, Garoscio M, Deleage G, et al. FVT-1, a novel human transcription unit affected by variant translocation t(2;18)(p11;q21) of follicular lymphoma. Blood 1993;81:136-42.
96. Saglio, Pane F, Gottardi E, Frigeri F, Buonaiuto MR, Guerrasio A, et al. Consistent amounts of acute leukemia-associated P190BCR/ABL transcripts are expressed by chronic myelogenous leukemia patients at diagnosis. Blood 1996;87:1075-80.
97. Sakashita A, Hattori T, Miller CW, Suzushima H, Asou N, Takatsuki K, Koeffler HP. Mutations of the p53 gene in adult T-cell leukemia. Blood 1992;79:477-80.
98. Sander CA, Yano T, Clark HM, Harris C, Longo DL, Jaffe ES, Raffeld M. p53 mutation is associated with progression in follicular lymphomas. Blood 1993;82:1994-2004.
99. Schena M, Shalon D, Davis RW, Brown PO. Quantitative monitoring of gene expression patterns with a complementary DNA microarray. Science 1995;270:467-70.
100. Schena M, Shalon D, Heller R, Chai A, Brown PO, Davis RW. Parallel human genome analysis: microarray-based expression monitoring of 1000 genes. Proc Natl Acad Sci U S A 1996;93:1064-19.
101. Schlieben S, Borkhardt A, Reinisch I, Ritterbach J, Janssen JW, Ratei R, et al. Incidence and clinical outcome of children with BCR/ABL-positive acute lymphoblastic leukemia (ALL). A prospective RT-

PCR study based on 673 patients enrolled in the German pediatric multicenter therapy trials ALL-BFM-90 and CoALL-05-92. Leukemia 1996;10: 957-63.

102. Secker-Walker LM, Craig JM, Hawkins JM, Hoffbrand AV. Philadelphia positive acute lymphoblastic leukemia in adults: age distribution, BCR breakpoint and prognostic significance. Leukemia 1991;5:196-9.
103. Segal GH, Jorgensen T, Masih AS, Braylan RC. Optimal primer selection for clonality assessment by polymerase chain reaction analysis: I. Low grade B-cell lymphoproliferative disorders of nonfollicular center cell type. Hum Pathol 1994;25:1269-75.
104. Segal GH, Jorgensen T, Scott M, Braylan RC. Optimal primer selection for clonality assessment by polymerase chain reaction analysis: II. Follicular lymphomas. Hum Pathol 1994;25:1276-82.
105. Selleri L, von Lindern M, Hermans A, Meijer D, Torelli G, Grosveld G. Chronic myeloid leukemia may be associated with several bcr-abl transcripts including the acute lymphoid leukemia-type 7 kb transcript. Blood 1990;75:1146-53.
106. Seto M, Jaeger U, Hockett, RD, Graninger W, Bennett S, Goldman P, Korsmeyer SJ. Alternative promoters and exons, somatic mutation and deregulation of the Bcl-2-Ig fusion gene in lymphoma. Embo J 1988;7:123-31.
107. Shepherd P, Suffolk R, Halsey J, Allan N. Analysis of molecular breakpoint and m-RNA transcripts in a prospective randomized trial of interferon in chronic myeloid leukaemia: no correlation with clinical features, cytogenetic response, duration of chronic phase, or survival. Br J Haematol 1995;89:546-54.
108. Shipp MA, Ross KN, Tamayo P, Weng AP, Kutok JL, Aguiar RC, et al. Diffuse large B-cell lymphoma outcome prediction by gene-expression profiling and supervised machine learning. Nat Med 2002;8: 68-74.
109. Sioutos N, Bagg A, Michaud GY, Irving SG, Hartmann DP, Siragy H, et al. Polymerase chain reaction versus Southern blot hybridization. Detection of immunoglobulin heavy-chain gene rearrangements. Diagn Mol Pathol 1995;4:8-13.
110. Steenbergen EJ, Verhagen OJ, van Leeuwen EF, van den Berg H, Behrendt H, Slater RM, et al. Prolonged persistence of PCR-detectable minimal residual disease after diagnosis or first relapse predicts poor outcome in childhood B-precursor acute lymphoblastic leukemia. Leukemia 1995;9:1726-34.
111. Suzuki Y, Orita M, Shiraishi M, Hayashi K, Sekiya T. Detection of ras gene mutations in human lung cancers by single-strand conformation polymorphism analysis of polymerase chain reaction products. Oncogene 1990;5:1037-43.
112. Tanner J, Weis J, Fearon D, Whang Y, Kieff E. Epstein-Barr virus gp350/220 binding to the B lymphocyte C3d receptor mediates adsorption, capping, and endocytosis. Cell 1987;50:203-13.
113. Templeton NS. The polymerase chain reaction. History, methods, and applications. Diagn Mol Pathol 1992;1:58-72.
114. Tonegawa S. Somatic generation of antibody diversity. Nature 1983;302:575-81.
115. Tsujimoto Y, Crossman J, Jaffe E, Croce CM. Involvement of the bcl-2 gene in human follicular lymphoma. Science 1985;228:1440-3.
116. Tsujimoto Y, Gorham J, Crossman J, Jaffe E, Croce CM. The t(14;18) chromosome translocations involved in B-cell neoplasms result from mistakes in VDJ joining. Science 1985;229:1390-3.
117. Tsujimoto Y, Yunis J, Onorato-Showe L, Erikson J, Nowell PC, Croce CM. Molecular cloning of the chromosomal breakpoint of B-cell lymphomas and leukemias with the t(11;14) chromosome translocation. Science 1984;224:1403-6.
118. Vaandrager JW, Schuuring E, Zwikstra E, de Boer CJ, Kleiverda KK, van Krieken JH, et al. Direct visualization of dispersed 11q13 chromosomal translocations in mantle cell lymphoma by multicolor DNA fiber fluorescence in situ hybridization. Blood 1996;88:1177-82.
119. van Rhee F, Marks DI, Lin F, Szydlo RM, Hochhaus A, Treleaven J, et al. Quantification of residual disease in Philadelphia-positive acute lymphoblastic leukemia: comparison of blood and bone marrow. Leukemia 1995;9:329-35.
120. Wang AM, Doyle MV, Mark DF. Quantitation of mRNA by the polymerase chain reaction. Proc Natl Acad Sci U S A 1989;86:9717-21.
121. Wasserman R, Galili N, Ito Y, Silber JH, Reichard BA, Shane S, et al. Residual disease at the end of induction therapy as a predictor of relapse during therapy in childhood B-lineage acute lymphoblastic leukemia. J Clin Oncol 1992;10:1879-88.
122. Wattel E, Preudhomme C, Hecquet B, Vanrumbeke M, Quesnel B, Dervite I, et al. p53 mutations are associated with resistance to chemotherapy and short survival in hematologic malignancies. Blood 1994;84:3148-57.
123. Weisenburger DD, Sanger WG, Armitage JO, Purtilo DT. Intermediate lymphocytic lymphoma: immunophenotypic and cytogenetic findings. Blood 1987;69:1617-21.
124. Weiss LM, Warnke RA, Sklar J, Cleary ML. Molecular analysis of the t(14;18) chromosomal translocation in malignant lymphomas. N Engl J Med 1987;317: 1185-9.
125. Westbrook CA, Hooberman AL, Spino C, Dodge RK, Larson RA, Davey F, et al. Clinical significance on the BCR-ABL fusion gene in adult acute lymphoblastic leukemia: a Cancer and Leukemia Group B Study (8762). Blood 1992;80:2983-90.

126. Williams ME, Swerdlow SH, Rosenberg CL, Arnold A. Chromosome 11 translocation breakpoints at the PRAD1/cyclin D1 gene locus in centrocytic lymphoma. Leukemia 1993;7:241-5.
127. Wittwer CT, Hermann MG, Moss AA, Rasmussen RP. Continuous fluorescence monitoring of rapid cycle DNA amplification. Biotechniques 1997;22:130-1, 4-8.
128. Yamamoto Y, Kiyoi H, Nakano Y, Suzuki R, Kodera Y, Miyawaki S, et al. Activating mutation of D835 within the activation loop of FLT3 in human hematologic malignancies. Blood 2001;97:2434-9.

CHAPTER 40

Inherited Diseases

Cindy L. Vnencak-Jones, Ph.D.

Since the first description of the use of the polymerase chain reaction (PCR) for the diagnosis of sickle cell anemia in 1985, numerous applications of PCR have been described.[38,503] The invention of PCR coupled with advances in computer technology and the chemistry of fluorescent molecules have revolutionized the field of human genetics and enabled the accelerated completion of the Human Genome Project. In more recent years, the Internet has enhanced the growth of this discipline and aided in a phenomenal number of discoveries by enabling rapid exchange of information and unrestricted communication among investigators around the world.

This chapter will review deoxyribonucleic acid (DNA) testing for some of the more common inherited autosomal recessive, autosomal dominant, and X-linked genetic diseases, and discuss testing of several mitochondrial, imprinting, and complex diseases. Since molecular testing for inherited diseases has impacted virtually every discipline of clinical medicine, the reader should refer to other chapters within this textbook for discipline-specific diseases, including inherited disorders of erythrocyte enzymes (see Chapter 21) and inborn errors of carbohydrate metabolism (see Chapter 25). In this rapidly evolving area of diagnostic testing, although testing for the same disease occurs in many clinical laboratories, multiple methodologies can be used to achieve the same sensitivity and specificity. Similar to other areas of laboratory medicine, the methodology chosen by the DNA laboratory is determined by the expected volume for the test, the availability of personnel to perform the assay, the current instrumentation within the laboratory, and the accessibility of funds for capital equipment.

In conjunction with the scientific discoveries that have been made in the area of human genetics, equally explosive has been the public awareness of DNA and genetic diseases through the media and the Internet. During the next 20 years, we as scientists and as a society will debate various issues. Which genetic tests will be used for routine carrier or diagnostic screening? Who has a right to know the results of genetic testing? The insurance company? The employer? Will knowledge of this information cause discrimination or stigmatization? Once we begin to unravel the interaction between genetic and environmental factors, can insurance or healthcare coverage be denied to the person who engages in a lifestyle likely to cause disease based on their genetic predisposition? How will the healthcare system absorb the cost of these expensive assays? Can the healthcare community be trained to understand complex principles of genetics and provide comprehensive counseling? Can a person's genetic makeup predisposing them to aberrant behavior provide a defense in a court of law? To what extent will manipulation of genetic material be tolerated in our society? Will most couples undergo in vitro fertilization and preimplantation genetic screening to choose the embryo with the most desirable genes? Will cloning be allowed? Will embryonic stem cell research be routine? Although it is difficult to predict what the future will bring, one thing is clear: the future will be both scientifically and intellectually stimulating, yet no doubt controversial.

DISEASES WITH MENDELIAN INHERITANCE

Autosomal Recessive Diseases

An individual with an autosomal recessive disease has inherited two abnormal alleles at a given locus by receiving one mutant allele from each carrier parent, and the disease-causing gene is on one of the autosomes (1 to 22) and not a sex chromosomes (X or Y). Typically the carrier parent with one abnormal allele has no clinical features of the disease yet possesses a 50% risk of donating the mutant allele to his or her offspring. Matings in which both partners are carriers of an abnormal allele have a 25% chance of having a child with both normal alleles, a 50% chance of having a child that has received only one abnormal allele, and a 25% chance of having an affected child. The affected patient may be homozygous for a specific mutation by receiving the same mutation from each parent or may be a compound heterozygote having received a different mutation within the gene from each parent. Regardless of the mechanism, the end result is the same; the patient has no normal allele. However, the specific mutations present in the patient can affect the clinical severity of the disease. In pedigrees illustrating autosomal recessive disorders, both males and females are equally affected, and for rare diseases, consanguinity is likely to be observed.

Cystic Fibrosis

Cystic fibrosis (CF) is one of the most common autosomal recessive diseases in people of Northern European ancestry with an estimated incidence in the United States of about 1 in 3200 and a carrier frequency of about 1 in 29.[236] The frequency of the disease within other ethnic populations is much lower with an estimated incidence of 1 in 9200 in U.S. Hispanics, 1 in 10,900 in Native Americans, 1 in 15,000 in African Americans, and 1 in 31,000 in Asian Americans.[236] CF is a multisystem disorder affecting the pulmonary, gastrointestinal, and reproductive organs. However, the phenotypic expression of the disease is heterogeneous, ranging from meconium ileus and severe respiratory disease in infants to mild pulmonary symptoms and no evidence of gastrointestinal problems even in adulthood. Morbidity and mortality of the disease are most related to mucus accumulation; recurrent infections with unusual pathogens, such as *Pseudomonas aeruginosa;* and excessive inflammation in the lung. Although in the past, CF resulted in death in early childhood for most patients, the U.S. Cystic Fibrosis Foundation reported in September 2000 that the median survival age among 22,301 patients ranging from 1 month to 74 years was 32.2 years, with about 40% of patients living past the age of 18.[125] This represents a significant increase from just 1 decade earlier (1990) when data from 17,857 patients showed the median age at 12.5 years, with about 33% of patients representing adults.[180] The increased survival age is largely caused by organ transplantation, improved nutrition, and new drug therapies and is likely to continue to increase with the potential of successful gene therapy to the lung during the next decade.[148]

The severity and frequency of the disease led to an intensive search for the gene. The gene was mapped to 7q31 (long arm of chromosome 7, banding region 31) in 1985 and was subsequently cloned in 1989.* The CF gene is extremely large, containing 27 exons and producing a transcript of approximately 6.5 kb. It codes for the CF transmembrane conductance regulator protein (CFTR) of 1480 amino acids. CFTR consists of two repeated motifs, each containing six hydrophobic transmembrane domains and one hydrophilic intracellular nucleotide-binding fold connected by a highly charged regulatory domain site.[481] The molecule is located within the lipid bilayer, predominantly at the apical membrane of secretory epithelial cells where it serves as a cyclic adenosine monophosphate (cAMP)–activated chloride ion channel to regulate chloride ion conductance.[15,44] In addition to chloride conductance, the molecule is involved in transport of sodium, potassium, and ATP from the intracellular compartment to the extracellular surface.[515,552] A routine sweat chloride concentration determination is considered necessary for the diagnosis of CF (>60 mmol/L in childhood; >40 mmol/L older than 15 years), although some patients with *CFTR* mutations may have borderline or even normal results.[112,147,200,257,544] These atypical patients may have only congenital bilateral absence of the vas deferens (CBAVD), pancreatitis, pulmonary disease, or nasal polyps. Thus although the diagnosis of CF can easily be made in patients with characteristic clinical features and abnormal sweat chloride concentrations, in patients with atypical presentation, mutations in the *CFTR* gene cannot be excluded without complete sequence analysis of the gene. The wide clinical diversity among CF patients in part is because of varying effects on the CFTR protein caused by more than 1000 mutations identified in the *CFTR* gene thus far.[126] However, it is also possible that the "nonclassic" CF phenotype is caused by factors other than mutations in the *CFTR* gene.[222]

Since CF is an autosomal recessive disorder, the CF patient must have two mutant *CFTR* alleles to develop the disease. Some mutations are "private" and unique to a family, and others may be common among CF patients. Patients will be homozygous with two copies of the same mutation or will represent a compound heterozygote with one copy of one mutation and one copy of a second mutation. Although the type and location of the mutation vary in their effect on *CFTR* and ultimately affect the phenotype of the patient, environmental factors and less characterized modifier genes also appear to be important in modulating the CF disease phenotype.* The *CFTR* genotype and clinical phenotype are most closely related for pancreatic involvement and least closely related for pulmonary manifestations of the disease.[152,652] Idiopathic juvenile patients with chronic pancreatitis have almost five times the expected carrier frequency of *CFTR* mutations, perhaps suggesting that *CFTR* carriers are predisposed to pancreatitis in the presence of other undefined pathogenetic factors, or perhaps these represent atypical patients with CF whose second gene mutation was not identified.[579] Further, although CBAVD is considered the primary congenital form of CF, most patients with CBAVD do not have two *CFTR* mutations[112]; only 19 of 102 patients had two detectable *CFTR* mutations, and 54 patients had only one detectable *CFTR* mutation.[112] Interestingly, 34 of these 54 (63%) had a rare DNA variant in intron 8 (called 5T, a sequence of five thymidines) in their second allele that is present in <5% of the general population. When present, the 5T variant affects the efficiency of exon 9 splicing and without exon 9, the chloride channel is

*References 300, 306, 409, 481, 490, 581.

*References 4, 90, 149, 213, 314, 497, 505, 509, 653.

not functional. In 29 CBAVD patients, no *CFTR* mutations were identified, but 7 (24%) had the 5T variant. Thus in CBAVD, the 5T variant allele is present and in *trans* (on the opposite allele) with a second *CFTR* mutation or is associated with the more common 7T allele when it is in *cis* (on the same allele) with *CFTR* mutation R117H (i.e., with R, arginine, in place of H, histidine, at amino acid 117). Interestingly, if the 5T allele is in *cis* with mutation R117H, it is associated with a classic CF phenotype rather than CBAVD.[301]

The types of mutations in *CFTR* can illustrate the association of the genotype with the phenotype. Mutations can be divided into five classes. Patients with class 1 mutations have defects in protein production, and class 2 mutations are associated with defective processing of CFTR. In both cases, CFTR trafficking to the cell membrane does not occur, and both class 1 and class 2 mutations are typically associated with a severe phenotype. Class 3 and 4 mutations have CFTR expression at the cell membrane, but channel activity is reduced. Class 3 mutations can be associated with a more severe phenotype and result from defective regulation, and class 4 mutations can be mild and result from defective conduction. Class 5 mutations are associated with abnormal splicing of the *CFTR* messenger ribonucleic acid (mRNA) and may be associated with a severe phenotype (621 + 1G>T) or a mild phenotype (2789 + 5G>A). The most common mutation, deltaF508, seen in about 70% of CF chromosomes in Caucasians of Northern European descent, affects processing of CFTR and prevents its trafficking to the apical membrane.[111] Prevalent mutations G542X and W1282X cause premature translation termination and thus truncation of the protein.[237] The frequently observed mutation G551D results in CFTR that reaches the apical membrane but that improperly regulates the chloride channel.[623]

DNA testing for the identification of *CFTR* mutations is performed for a variety of reasons (Box 40-1). DNA testing is performed to confirm the diagnosis of disease in patients with equivocal sweat chloride results or in instances when insufficient material is collected. Alternatively, in the known CF patient, mutation analysis can be requested to help predict the prognosis since some genotype-phenotype correlations exist. At the same time, identifying the mutations segregating in a family enables preimplantation diagnosis or prenatal testing for subsequent pregnancies and carrier or diagnostic testing for other at-risk family members. Similarly, state-sponsored newborn screening programs have detected infants with CF and at the same time have identified at-risk family members and enabled genetic testing.[626] In addition, newborn screening allows for early diagnosis and intervention of patients, which has been associated with reduced severity of lung disease and increased survival.[218,619] Some families referred for prenatal CF testing have no family history of CF. Rather, in these families, hyperechogenic bowel was diagnosed in the fetus on routine ultrasonography. In one study of 209 fetuses, 7 were subsequently given the diagnosis of CF, which is about 84 times the estimated risk of CF in the general population.[394]

BOX 40-1 Referrals for *CFTR* Mutation Analysis

Confirm diagnosis
Determine prognosis
Family member testing
Newborn screening
Preconception couples
Expectant couples
Prenatal testing—at-risk fetus
Prenatal testing—echogenic bowel
Preimplantation diagnosis
Infertile male with CBAVD
Semen and oocyte donors

The most challenging and controversial DNA testing for CF is carrier screening for preconception and expectant couples. Carrier screening in these circumstances was recommended in October 2001 by the American College of Obstetricians and Gynecologists (ACOG) in conjunction with the American College of Medical Genetics (ACMG).[12] With the heterogeneity of *CFTR* mutations, testing for more than 1000 mutations in this population would be a daunting task. For this reason, a core panel of 25 mutations was proposed as a minimum standard for CF carrier screening. The mutations initially proposed included those with an estimated prevalence of at least 0.1% of CF mutant alleles; this yields a CF carrier detection rate of about 88% for non-Hispanic Caucasians.[12,220] Slight variations in the reported frequencies of these mutations in nonHispanic Caucasian alleles have recently been described, but the overall detection rate remains at about 88%[438] (Table 40-1). The intent of the screening panel was to identify individuals at risk for classical CF, not CBAVD, and thus it is recommended that the 5T and/or 7T or 9T status be evaluated only in the presence of mutation R117H.

The standard of care recommended by the ACOG is to offer CF testing to preconception or expectant couples, a very large group of people. The social and technical issues surrounding this testing are complex. Various methods are commercially available to reduce the number of laboratories performing “home brew” assays, and standards and guidelines for *CFTR* mutation testing have been proposed[477] (Figure 40-1 and Color Plate 7). Further standardization for reporting of these complex results has been recommended, although adherence to these standards is not ideal.[17,220]

Social issues associated with population screening for this genetic disease are in part rather specific to this program (such as the enormous number of mutations in this huge gene), but many others are illustrative of issues that surround genetic testing in general. The issues surrounding this program include: (1) the inability to detect CF carriers with *CFTR* mutations other than the 25 included in the screening

TABLE 40-1 ACMG/ACOG Mutation Panel for Preconception and Prenatal CF Carrier Screening With Frequency of Each Mutation in Non-Hispanic CF Caucasian Alleles*

Mutation	Frequency (%)
ΔF508	72.42
G542X	2.28
G551D	2.25
621 + 1G>T	*1.57
W1282X	1.50
N1303K	1.27
R553X	0.88
ΔI507	0.87
R117H	0.70
3849 + 10kbC>T	0.58
2789+5G>A	0.48
1717 – 1G>A	0.48
R347P	0.45
711 + 1G>T	0.43
R560T	0.38
3659delC	0.34
A455E	0.34
G85E	0.29
R1162X	0.23
2184delA	0.17
1898 + 1G>A	0.16
R334W	0.14
I148T	0.09
3120 + 1G>A	0.08
1078delT	0.02
TOTAL	88.40

*Frequencies represent the "average" frequency of the mutation as determined from the comparison of two data sets by Palomaki et al.[438]

panel, (2) the need for appropriate genetic counseling of patients before their consenting to the analysis, (3) the need for proper understanding of the possibility of a false-negative result, (4) stigmatization of being a "carrier" of a genetic disease, (5) threats to confidentiality of results, (6) effects on health insurability, and (7) possible increase in the number of abortions following the identification of previously unknown affected fetuses. In addition to these social and/or ethical issues, opposition to this screening panel has also arisen over the set of mutations included in the panel because those currently selected underrepresent the mutations found in minorities.[165,201,249,253-254] It is likely that mutations in the *CFTR* screening panel will change as carrier screening evolves and the program is critically evaluated.[548-549]

Hereditary Hemochromatosis

Hereditary hemochromatosis (HH) is an autosomal recessive disorder of iron regulation that can result in excess iron deposition in otherwise healthy tissue. Affected individuals can absorb approximately 3 to 4 mg of iron per day compared with the normal rate of 1 to 2 mg per day. Symptoms associated with this disease occur during mid to late adulthood, but the diagnosis of HH is often delayed, because the early symptoms of weakness, lethargy, joint pain, and abdominal pain are nonspecific. Complications of the disease include hepatic cirrhosis, diabetes mellitus, hypopituitarism, hypogonadism, arthritis, and cardiomyopathy.[29,458,641] The incidence of the disease is estimated to be about 1 in 200 to 400, making HH one of the most common genetic disorders known. However, the phenotypic expression of the disease is dependent on other genetic and environmental factors. The disease is more common in men than women presumably because of the protective effect of iron loss during menstruation and pregnancy. In addition, although regular blood donation is protective against HH, increased alcohol consumption, dietary iron, or vitamin C, an enhancer of iron uptake, increases the likelihood of symptoms in the presence of an affected genotype.[459] Laboratory testing for hemochromatosis most often includes determination of transferrin saturation [(serum iron/total iron binding capacity) × 100] and serum ferritin with a saturation >55% to 60% considered abnormal for men, >45% to 50% abnormal for women, serum ferritin >400 µg/L (400 ng/mL) abnormal for men, and >200 µg/L (200 ng/mL) abnormal for women. These tests may be ordered singly or in combination. Subsequently a liver biopsy often follows to determine the amount of stainable iron and the degree of injury.[635] Management of the disease includes therapeutic phlebotomy and dietary avoidance of medicinal iron, mineral supplements, excess vitamin C, and uncooked seafoods.[39]

In 1976 Simon et al reported an association of human leukocyte antigen (HLA)-A3 and HLA-B14 antigens with idiopathic hemochromatosis, which suggested that the HH gene was located near the major histocompatibility complex (MHC) on chromosome 6p (short arm of chromosome 6).[409,532] Classic genetic studies confirmed linkage of the HH gene to the HLA locus, and in 1996 Feder et al cloned the HH gene, *HFE*.[172,288,321] Although *HFE* remains the primary gene associated with hemochromatosis, other genes have been mapped or cloned that are associated with dominantly inherited hemochromatosis (*SLC11A3, ferroportin1, and H-ferritin*) and with juvenile and rare autosomal recessive (*TFR2*) forms of hemochromatosis. Additional genes associated with iron metabolism likely exist.*

The *HFE* gene protein, HFE, encodes a β_2-microglobulin-asociated protein with structural resemblance to MHC class I proteins. The *HFE* gene contains seven exons spanning about 12 kb, and the 4.1 kb mRNA is widely expressed with some suggestion of higher expression in the liver and intestine, major sites of iron metabolism in the body, and to

*References 97, 298, 424, 489, 496, 617.

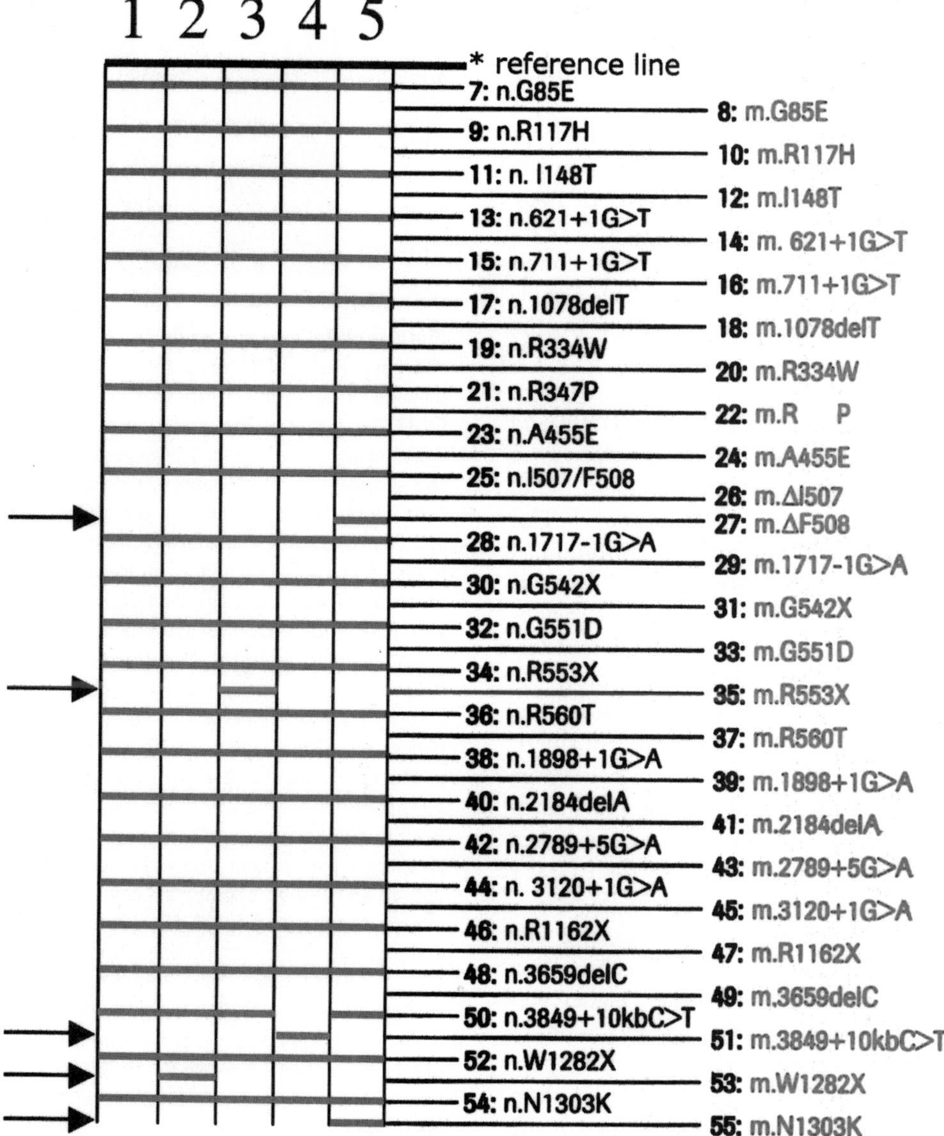

Figure 40-1 CF mutation-detection assay CF Gold 1.0 developed by Roche Diagnostics Corp. Thirty to 45 ng of patient DNA is amplified in a multiplex amplification reaction. Amplicons are denatured and hybridized to membrane-bound oligonucleotide probes specific for 25 normal (n) and corresponding mutant (m) alleles. Lane 1 represents the pattern obtained from patient DNA in which none of the 25 common mutations is present; bands detected correspond only to normal alleles. Lane 2 represents the pattern obtained from patient DNA in which mutation W1282X is present in one allele, since bands corresponding to both nW1282X and mW1282X are present. In lane 3, mutation R553X is present in one allele since bands corresponding to mR553X and nR553X are present. Lanes 2 and 3 could represent CF carriers or could represent DNA from patients with CF for whom only one of their two mutations is identified. In the latter case, the second disease-causing mutation must be a mutation other than one of the 25 represented in this panel. Conversely, lane 4 represents patient DNA in which two copies of mutation 3849 + 10kbC>T are detected. Note that no band corresponding to n3849 + 10kbC>T is present. Lane 5 represents DNA from a CF patient who is a compound heterozygote with mutation delta F508 present on one allele and mutation N1303K present on the second mutant allele. Detection of 5, 7, or 9 T polymorphism in intron 8 has not been determined in these patients but can be performed by this assay. The strip contains oligonucleotide probes for the determination of this polymorphism in patient DNA above the reference line. However, before testing, this part of the strip is removed and is only performed as a reflex test if mutation R117H is detected. (See Color Plate 7.)

a lesser degree in the brain.[172] Normal HFE binds to the transferrin receptor and reduces its affinity for iron-loaded transferrin.[173,326,504] Interestingly, although HFE is widely expressed in the gastrointestinal tract, the most abundant immunohistochemical staining for the protein is in the crypt enterocytes, where it has a distinct intracellular localization suggesting that its function is to sense the level of body iron stores and regulate, rather than directly participate in, iron absorption.[439,614] *HFE* knockout mice exhibit profound abnormalities in iron homeostasis and likewise have significantly decreased iron uptake from the plasma by the duodenum.[578,651]

A founder effect, suggested by linkage disequilibrium between HLA haplotypes and the *HFE* gene, was confirmed in two studies by the identification of homozygosity for a common mutation, G-to-A base pair substitution, in 148 of 178 (83%) and 121 of 147 (82.3%) HH patients.[61,172] This mutation results in a cysteine-to-tyrosine substitution at amino acid 282 (C282Y) in HFE and disrupts disulfide bridges required for normal interaction with β_2-microglobulin on the cell surface and allows for high-affinity transferrin binding to the uncomplexed transferrin receptor.[172-174] The allele frequency of this mutation is 0.05 in Caucasians, 0.01 in Hispanics, and as low as 0.0067 in African Americans.[454] Although carriers of this mutation have been reported to have a twofold increased risk for acute myocardial infarction compared with noncarriers, they do not have higher transferrin saturation or ferritin than C282Y noncarriers.[384,584]

A second base substitution of C-to-G in exon 2 and resulting in a histidine (H) to aspartic acid (D) substitution at codon 63 (H63D) has been identified in a higher percentage of C282Y-negative HH patients than would be expected based on the frequency of this mutation in the population.[172] This mutation is observed in 89% of HH chromosomes that do not have mutation C282Y compared with a frequency of 15% to 17% in Caucasian control *HFE* genes.[172,454] HFE, with this alteration, is expressed at the cell surface, but its interaction with the transferrin receptor is altered, resulting in more iron deposition within the cell.[173,615] The frequency of mutation H63D is lower in African Americans (0.026) and Hispanics (0.10).[454] Mutation H63D is associated with an increased risk of developing a mild form of hemochromatosis, but appears to have little effect for causing disease when inherited by itself (wild type and/or H63D), which represents 2.5% of HH chromosomes, or when two copies of the mutation are inherited (H63D/H63D), which is seen in 1.4% of HH patients.[351] Although many compound heterozygotes (C282Y/H63D) in the general population are asymptomatic, H63D may contribute to disease when inherited with mutation C282Y since 4.5% of HH patients have this genotype, although interestingly, these patients display variability in liver histological findings and iron indices.[59,287,296,351,512]

More recently a third common mutation in the *HFE* gene has been reported that is associated with a mild form of hemochromatosis.[25,264,397] This A-to-T mutation results in a serine-to-cysteine substitution at codon 65 (S65C) in exon 2 and is in close proximity in the gene to the previously described H63D mutation. In one study, mutation S65C was detected in 2.49% of normal controls yet was identified in 10 of 128 (7.8%) of HH chromosomes that coded for neither C282Y nor H63D.[397] Thus although C282Y is the primary mutation in *HFE* associated with HH, compound heterozygotes C282Y-H63D and C282Y-S65C have an increased risk of developing HH, thus suggesting their role in the development of HH.

DNA analysis of the *HFE* gene is done using a variety of methodologies and in most laboratories includes testing for mutations C282Y and H63D (Figure 40-2). Once *HFE* mutation analysis has confirmed the cause of HH in the patient, transferrin saturation (TS), serum ferritin, and DNA testing of at-risk family members can identify those who may benefit from earlier treatment and dietary restrictions.[88]

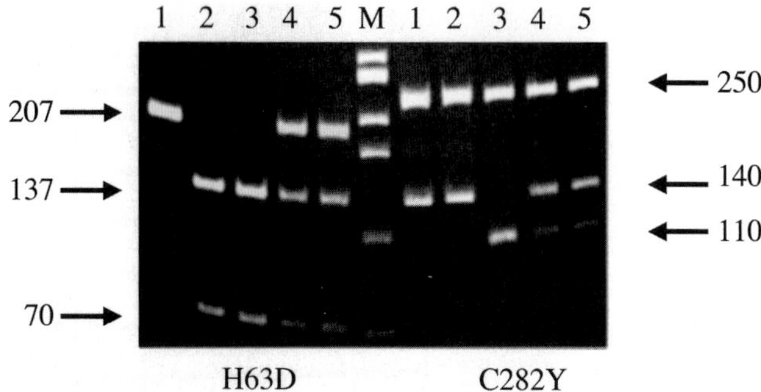

Figure 40-2 Detection of mutations H63D and C282Y in the *HFE* gene. Patient DNA is amplified by PCR using oligonucleotide primer pairs that flank either mutation H63D or C282Y, respectively. For detection of mutation H63D, 207 bp PCR products are digested with restriction endonuclease *BclI* and subjected to electrophoresis on a 5% polyacrylamide gel *(left)*. Mutation H63D results from a C-to-G base substitution and destroys a *BclI* site thereby preventing digestion of 207 bp fragments into 137 bp and 70 bp fragments. Detection of mutation C282Y uses digestion of 390-bp amplified products with restriction endonuclease *RsaI* and electrophoresis on a 5% polyacrylamide gel *(right)*. Mutation C282Y results from a G-to-A base substitution and creates an *RsaI* site within the amplicons cleaving 140-bp fragments to 110-bp and 30-bp fragments. In patient one *(lanes 1)*, the H63D-specific 207-bp amplification products are not digested with *BclI* to yield wild-type bands of 137 bp and 70 bp, thereby indicating that the restriction site has been lost in both alleles. Conversely the C282Y-specific amplicons from patient one yield exclusively wild-type bands of 250-bp and 140-bp fragments. Genotype for patient one is interpreted as mutation H63D, wild-type C282Y on both alleles. Genotype for patient two *(lanes 2)* is wild-type H63D, wild-type C282Y on both alleles. Genotype for patient three *(lanes 3)* is wild-type H63D, m C282Y on both alleles. Patient four *(lanes 4)* is a compound heterozygote with mH63D, wild-type C282Y on one allele and wild-type H63D, mC282Y on the second allele. *Lanes 5* represents control DNA heterozygous for mutations H63D and C282Y.

HH is illustrative of common problems in screening for genetic disorders. Since HH is a common disorder with clinical symptoms that can be prevented with easy and inexpensive early intervention, population-based screening for HH has been considered.[92,116] If DNA-based testing were to be used in an attempt to identify HH patients, stigmatization and discrimination in *HFE*-positive patients could result. Moreover, because of incomplete penetrance, many people with mutations will neither have nor ever develop iron overload.[5,60,433] Phenotypic measurements of transferrin saturation or serum ferritin could be more appropriate than genotypic studies for population-based screening for HH, but these results can also be misleading since iron overload can occur from a host of other conditions unrelated to hemochromatosis and mutations in *HFE*.[635] For these reasons and others, national population-based screening programs have not been implemented. However, a comprehensive, multicenter, 5-year, multiethnic study involving 100,000 adults is in progress to evaluate the prevalence, genetic, and environmental factors associated with HH and the personal and societal impact of screening and diagnosis. The information obtained from this Hemochromatosis and Iron Overload Screening (HEIRS) study will assist in determining policy regarding the feasibility, logistics, and associated benefits of population screening.[368]

Carbamyl Phosphate Synthetase I Deficiency

Carbamyl phosphate synthetase I (CPSI) deficiency is an autosomal recessive inborn error of metabolism with an estimated incidence of about 1 in 62,000 in the United States to as low as 1 in 800,000 in Japan.[85,405] The frequency of the disease may actually be higher in regions of the world with a higher percentage of consanguineous matings, and reported frequencies do not account for the undiagnosed neonates that die in the first few days of life. The affected newborn appears clinically normal but within the first 24 to 72 hours develops vomiting and lethargy, and as blood ammonia levels continue to rise, coma and death are imminent unless treatment is initiated immediately. Although a delay in diagnosis and treatment is associated with a worse prognosis, the disease is rare, the symptoms are rather nonspecific, and diagnosis is often delayed. The condition can be first interpreted as sepsis. Once the diagnosis is made, sodium benzoate and sodium phenylacetate can be started,[554,582] and hemodialysis may be required to further reduce ammonia levels and prevent irreversible brain damage and death arising from cerebral edema.[163,554] Prospective treatment in at-risk patients to prevent hyperammonemia improves neurological outcome.[355,654] Laboratory findings include increased plasma ammonia; low plasma urea; decreased or absent plasma citrulline and arginine; normal urine orotic acid; and normal urine organic acids.[543] The diagnosis is confirmed by a liver biopsy for measurement of CPSI activity. In most patients, CPSI enzyme activity less than 20% of controls is consistent with CPSI deficiency, and activity less than 5% results in neonatal presentation. However, a few patients have been reported with partial CPSI activity that was associated with late or adult presentation.[95,269,342,508,636] The chronic phase of the disease is treated with a nitrogen-restricted diet, citrulline, and chronic sodium phenylbutyrate to reduce the blood ammonia.[57] Management of this urea cycle disorder is complex and is most effective with immediate intervention and a multidisciplinary effort.[554] Liver transplantation can be an effective form of treatment.[629]

The *CPSI* gene is mapped to 2q35, spans >120 kb, comprises 38 exons, and consists of a 123-nucleotide 5′-untranslated region, an open reading frame of 4500 nucleotides, and 1123 nucleotides in the 3′-untranslated region.[409,555-556] Exons range in size from 56 to 260 bp in length, and introns range from 415 to 21,160 bp.[556] The *CPSI* gene encodes a 165 kD proenzyme that is transported into the mitochondria, where it is cleaved into the functional 160 kD form.[239] CPSI is present in the mitochondrial matrix of hepatocytes and epithelial cells of the intestinal mucosa.[502] CPSI catalyzes the first step of the urea cycle by converting ammonia and bicarbonate to carbamyl phosphate.[500] Through a series of enzymatic reactions, the toxic ammonia molecule is converted to the nontoxic water-soluble urea containing two amino groups, which is excreted as urine. In the absence of CPSI or any of the other urea cycle enzymes, a hyperammonemic crisis ensues, and associated neurological tissue destruction and/or death occurs.

In contrast to DNA testing for hereditary hemochromatosis, which is a widespread disorder with only three common mutations, or CF, a frequent disease with more than 1000 mutations, CPSI deficiency represents a rare disorder with no common mutations. Rather, heterogeneous mutations throughout the gene have been described including missense, deletion, insertion, and splicing mutations.[24,177,272,472,553] Heterogeneous mutations for a rare disease make clinical testing for CPSI deficiency challenging. With a relatively low volume of specimens received annually, a clinical laboratory cannot batch specimens to improve the efficiency of testing, because turnaround times would not be acceptable. Thus it is not feasible for a clinical laboratory to sequence the very large *CPSI* gene in every family to identify the private mutations segregating in that family. For these reasons, DNA testing in a clinical laboratory for CPSI deficiency most often involves indirect testing or linkage studies using highly polymorphic microsatellite repeat markers (Figure 40-3 and Color Plate 8). Further DNA testing is not used to make or confirm the diagnosis, but rather to determine the haplotype of the microsatellite markers flanking the abnormal *CPSI* genes segregating with the disease in each family. Once this has been determined, haplotype analysis can be performed on a subsequent at-risk fetus to determine its status with regard to CPSI deficiency.

To initiate these studies, once the diagnosis of CPSI deficiency has been confirmed by enzymatic studies on the affected child, or is strongly suspected from abnormal laboratory results, DNA specimens are collected from the parents

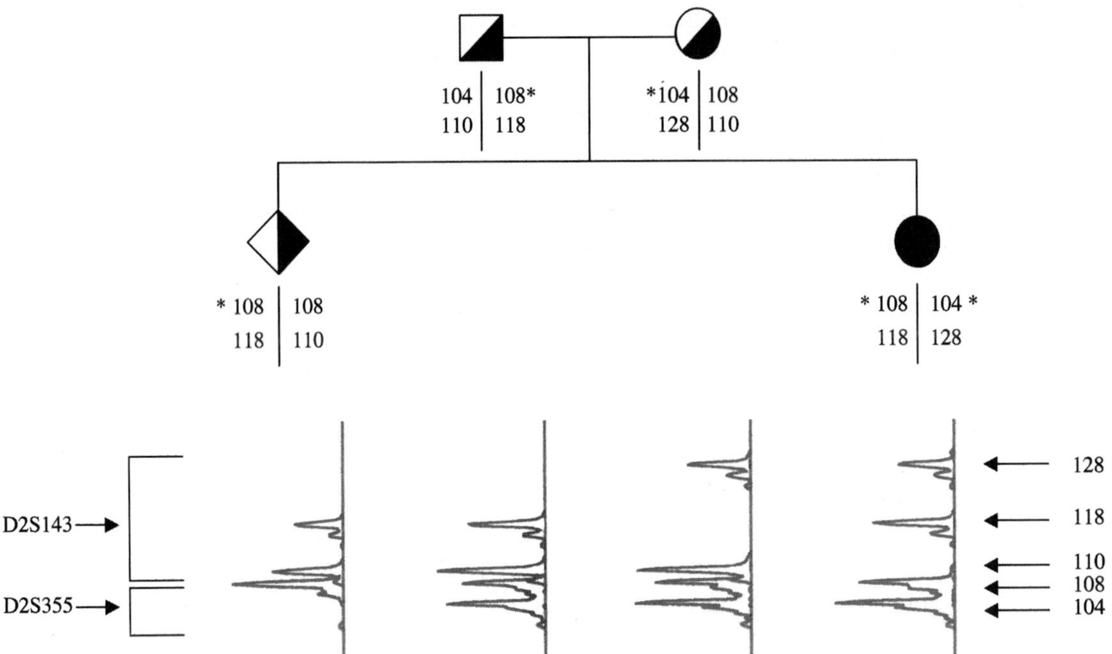

Figure 40-3 Electropherograms illustrating prenatal DNA-linkage studies on a family with CPSI deficiency D2S355 and D2S143 represent dinucleotide markers 4 centimorgans 5′ (D2S355) and 3 centimorgans 3′ (D2S143) to the *CPSI* gene, respectively. DNA samples from the affected child, parents, and fetus are amplified by PCR using oligonucleotide primer pairs specific for each marker, with one primer of each pair labeled with a fluorescent dye. Amplicons are subjected to electrophoresis on a 5% denaturing polyacrylamide gel on an ABI 377 DNA sequencer and analyzed using GeneScan software 3.1b3. The maternal haplotype donated to the affected child is 104,128, indicating that the mother's 108,110 allele is not linked to an abnormal *CPSI* gene. The paternal allele donated to the affected child is 108,118, indicating that the father's 104,110 allele is in repulsion with CPSI deficiency. The maternal allele donated to the fetus is 108,110. This allele is not linked to an abnormal *CPSI* gene. The paternal allele donated to the fetus is 108,118. This allele is linked to an abnormal *CPSI* gene. These results indicate that the fetus is a carrier of CPSI deficiency but is not affected. (See Color Plate 8.)

and the affected child. If the affected child died before collection of a peripheral blood sample, paraffin-embedded autopsy material can be submitted for analysis. Within days, *CPSI*-linked DNA markers for the family are analyzed, markers for which the family is informative are identified, and the accuracy of future prenatal linkage studies is determined. When the family ultimately requests future prenatal testing, either chorionic villus tissue or cultured chorionic villus tissue or amniocytes from the fetus are submitted for analysis. Within a few days, the fetal DNA is tested with the DNA markers for which the family is informative, and a diagnosis regarding the CPSI deficiency of the fetus is known. In most instances, the accuracy of the results approaches 99%.

Although considered highly accurate and rapidly applicable to all families regardless of the CPSI mutation, linkage studies can be problematic.

- First, linkage studies cannot determine the diagnosis of the affected child, but rather rely upon additional laboratory testing and clinical findings to identify this disease in the patient. An *accurate diagnosis* of CPSI deficiency is essential before initiating DNA studies. For example, if the diagnosis in the affected child is incorrect and a disease-causing mutation is present in a gene other than *CPSI*, then linkage studies using DNA markers flanking the *CPSI* gene to predict the status of an at-risk fetus are totally irrelevant and will lead to erroneous conclusions. In such cases, a second child inheriting the same *CPSI* haplotypes from each parent may be misinterpreted as affected; the pregnancy may be terminated when, tragically, the fetus was normal. Alternatively, if the second child inherits different *CPSI* haplotypes from each parent, the fetus may be misinterpreted as being normal when in fact the fetus may have inherited the same unknown disease-causing mutation(s) as the previously affected child with an inaccurate diagnosis of CPSI deficiency.
- A second requirement for linkage studies is that the family structure must be accurately reported. Since the microsatellite repeat markers used in the analysis are highly polymorphic, cases of *alternative paternity* are likely to be detected. Nonetheless, if the father of the affected child shared similar haplotypes with the father of the fetus,

misinterpretation of the results would occur. This scenario could result in the termination of a normal pregnancy.

- Third, because of the chance of *genetic recombination* between the *CPSI* gene and the linked, flanking polymorphic markers, the possibility of recombination exists and with that the possibility of an incorrect diagnosis for the fetus. This could result in the birth of a second affected child despite the fact that the haplotypes of the two affected children differ, or a normal pregnancy may be terminated if, through genetic recombination, the fetus shares the same haplotype but is unaffected.
- Last, although highly polymorphic, the possibility exists that one or both parents are *not informative* (i.e., heterozygous) for one or more of the DNA markers thereby preventing prenatal studies on future at-risk pregnancies or compromising the accuracy of future prenatal results.

Although less commonly performed now, prenatal testing for CPSI deficiency can be performed by measuring CPSI activity in tissue from a fetal liver biopsy specimen.[399,519,644]

Autosomal Dominant Diseases

In autosomal dominant conditions, a single abnormal allele is sufficient to cause disease despite the presence of a normal allele. An individual with an autosomal dominant disease may have inherited an abnormal allele from an affected parent, or alternatively the mutant allele may have risen de novo as a new mutation during gametogenesis in an unaffected parent. The disease-causing gene is on one of the autosomes (1 to 22) and not on a sex chromosome (X or Y). An affected individual possesses a 50% risk of donating the mutant allele to an offspring. Different mutations within the gene have varying effects on the protein so that affected patients can have variability in clinical expression of the disease. In some instances, known mutant gene carriers have no clinical symptoms of the disease, a phenomenon referred to as reduced penetrance, yet possess a 50% chance of having an affected child. Differences in phenotypic expression of the disease are most likely explained by the effect of other genes (modifier genes) and/or environmental influences. In pedigrees illustrating autosomal dominant inheritance, both males and females are affected, and male-to-male transmission is observed.

Achondroplasia

Achondroplasia is the most common form of human genetic dwarfism and is inherited as an autosomal dominant trait with complete penetrance. It is characterized by short-limbed dwarfism (rhizomelic form), macrocephaly, frontal and biparietal bossing, bowing of the lower extremities, and normal intelligence. Infants with this disease can die within the first year of life from central apnea caused by compression at the craniocervical junction; homozygous disease is most often lethal.[211,415,444] Children undergoing surgical decompression of the craniocervical junction have decreased mortality and demonstrate improvement in neurological function. The mean standard deviation (SD) adult height is 131 (5.6) cm for men and 124 (5.9) cm for women. The life expectancy is about 10 years less than that for the general population.[246] During the first 5 years of life, affected children are at risk of death from compression of the brainstem and/or the upper cervical spinal cord. Deaths in adults between 25 and 54 years of age are most often attributed to cardiovascular problems. Achondroplasia has an incidence of about 0.5 to 1.5 per 10,000 births and has been reported in individuals from different races and ethnic groups.[434]

More than 90% of patients are born to parents of normal height. These patients represent sporadic cases arising from new mutations, a phenomenon associated with advanced paternal age.[415,630] However, in one unusual report, two siblings with achondroplasia born to unaffected parents were a result of germline mosaicism from the mother since, although she had no clinical features of achondroplasia, a mutant allele was detected in DNA extracted from her peripheral blood.[252] In a second remarkable case, two affected siblings sharing a 4p haplotype derived from their unaffected father were born to normal-sized parents, suggesting that either two de novo, independent, sporadic events had occurred, or paternal gonadal mosaicism was present.[540] This "paternal effect" has been thought to occur because of lifelong spermatogonial stem cell divisions and thus an increase in production of mutant sperm as the male grows older.[124] However, recent data generated from examining sperm DNA from donors of different ages did not illustrate an exponential increase in mutation with age, indicating that sperm mutation frequency cannot explain an effect of paternal age in achondroplasia.[573]

The gene for achondroplasia was mapped to the telomeric region of chromosome 4p (4p16.3) in 1994 using linkage studies on multigenerational families.[186,409,604] Subsequently the fibroblast growth factor receptor 3 gene (*FGFR3*), mapped to this region and previously considered as a candidate gene for Huntington's disease (HD), was evaluated as a candidate gene for achondroplasia and reported to have mutations in patients with achondroplasia.[527,570] The *FGFR3* protein product, FGFR3, contains three extracellular immunoglobulin-like domains, a single transmembrane domain, and an intracellular tyrosine kinase domain.[294] FGFR3 is a tyrosine kinase receptor, which when bound to 1 of 23 fibroblast growth factors (FGFs) coupled with heparin sulfate–bearing proteoglycans on the cell surface, induces dimerization of receptor monomers, activates tyrosine kinase activity, and promotes phosphorylation of key tyrosine residues in the cytoplasmic domain, which in turn induces multiple signaling pathways.[271,564] Precisely which FGFs serve as ligands for FGFR3 is not known, and FGFR3 may use different FGFs at different stages of development and at different locations of the growth plate. The target genes for FGFR3 are not well characterized, but FGFR3 is thought to negatively regulate chondrocyte proliferation and differentiation.[117,139]

The primary mutation in achondroplasia results in a defect in internalization and degradation of the mutant receptor. Thus it is retained on the cell surface and has uncontrolled and prolonged activation in chondrocytes.[388] Hence, chondrocyte maturation and terminal differentiation are inhibited. Following the discovery of the association between achondroplasia and *FGFR3* mutations, other similar gain-of-function mutations at other sites within this gene have been identified as the cause of less common forms of dwarfism, including thanatophoric dysplasia types I and II and hypochondroplasia.[49-50,463,494,566]

In the original report identifying the *FGFR3* gene as the cause of achondroplasia, 15 of 16 patients had a G-to-A transition mutation at nucleotide 1138 (G1138A), and the only patient that did not have this mutation instead had a G-to-C transversion mutation at the same position (G1138C).[527] Both mutations result in a glycine-to-arginine substitution in the transmembrane domain of FGFR3 at codon 380. The frequency of the G-to-A transition mutation at codon 380 in achondroplasia patients is well documented.[48,493] This base pair may be prone to mutation, because a cytosine residue in a CpG dinucleotide is known to be a hot spot for transition mutations.[36,64,151] If the cytosine residue is methylated (i.e., as 5-methylcytosine), it can spontaneously deaminate to thymine to introduce the change from a G:C base pair to an A:T base pair in subsequent replications of DNA. Since >98% of *FGFR3* mutations causing achondroplasia are G1138A, and about 1% are G1138C, DNA testing includes direct mutation analysis for both mutations. Testing can be performed postnatally to confirm the diagnosis of achondroplasia. In addition, prenatal DNA testing may be requested by unaffected couples with an affected child representing a sporadic case, although the risk for germline mosaicism is considered low, and their risk of a second affected child is minimal. Pregnancies involving mating between two affected individuals are not uncommon. Prenatal DNA testing can be requested by these couples who have a 25% chance of having a child homozygous for this condition. This presents difficult choices for the couple. In one study, attitudes of affected individuals and relatives toward abortion based on prenatal diagnosis indicated that if the fetus was determined to be homozygous for this condition, 40% would consider termination compared with 41% that would not; 19% were unsure of what they would do.[210] In this same study, if the fetus was heterozygous for a mutation causing achondroplasia, 5% would consider termination and 86% would not; 8% were unsure what they would do. Lastly, if the fetus was determined to be normal and not to have received a mutation causing this disease, 90% responded that they would not consider termination of the pregnancy but 3% would; 6% were unsure of what their decision might be.

Charcot-Marie-Tooth Disease

Charcot-Marie-Tooth (CMT) disease, sometimes referred to as hereditary motor and sensory neuropathies (HMSN), refers to a genetically heterogeneous group of hereditary neuropathies characterized by chronic motor and sensory polyneuropathy and demonstrating all patterns of mendelian inheritance.[54,69]

The most common form of CMT, type 1A, is one of the most common autosomal dominant disorders in man, with an estimated incidence of 1 in 2500. This disease is characterized by progressive distal muscle atrophy and weakness, depressed or absent deep tendon reflexes, high-arched feet, decreased nerve conduction velocity (generally <35 to 40 m/s), and nerve demyelination as visualized on biopsy specimens. The age of onset is within the first decade of life in 50% of patients and before the age of 20 in 70% of patients.[65] However, despite a common genetic abnormality, phenotypic manifestations of the disease are variable even within the same family, suggesting the influence of environmental factors or modifier genes at other loci.[65,330] Lastly, as in achondroplasia, the phenotype of patients who are homozygous for two abnormal CMT genes, having inherited an abnormal CMT gene from each of their parents, is more severe despite having nerve conduction velocities similar to heterozygotes or those with one abnormal allele.[551]

In studies of extended families with CMT, the gene was mapped to the short arm of chromosome 17 and specifically localized to 17p11.2-p12 (short arm of chromosome 17 between banding regions 11.2 and 12).[376,409,466,594-595] Further, some DNA markers in this region detected a duplication in the DNA of affected individuals within families and in unrelated CMT patients.[232,347] The peripheral myelin protein gene, *PMP22*, was identified as a candidate gene for CMT type 1A in 1992.[442] *PMP22* is contained within a 1.5 Mb monomer unit that is flanked by several low-copy repeat sequences.[450] A duplication of the gene is associated with disease and results from unequal meiotic crossing over caused by misalignment of homologous sequences. Breakpoints within the repeated sequences are variable between patients, but 76% occur within a 1.7 kb "hot spot" for recombination where the DNA sequences are 98% homologous.[475] The reciprocal deletion of this crossover resulting in the loss of an allele and only one copy of the *PMP22* gene is associated with a different condition, hereditary neuropathy with liability to pressure palsies (HNPP).[108] Although the vast majority of patients with CMT type 1A have *PMP22* gene duplications, point mutations have also been reported to cause disease.[484,589] Interestingly, one such mutation is the same mutation identified in the spontaneously occurring neurological mouse mutants, *Trembler-J.*

A duplication of *PMP22* results in an extra copy of the gene (altered *gene dosage*) and overexpression of the PMP22 protein, which is considered the causative event for disease. Interestingly, patients with trisomy 17p (three copies of the short arm of chromosome 17), who would have an altered *PMP22* copy number, also have clinical features consistent with CMT.[109,348] PMP22 is a 160–amino acid transmembrane glycoprotein that contains four transmembrane hydrophobic regions and two extracellular domains with the amino and C termini exposed to the cytosol. It is predominantly localized in the compact portion of myelin.[127] PMP22 is predominantly expressed in myelinating Schwann cells of the peripheral nervous system where it is important in myelination and myelin stability and acts as a negative modulator of Schwann cell growth.[403,538,657] From studies on transgenic mice, it has been proposed that when overexpressed, PMP22 accumulates in a late-Golgi and/or plasma-membrane compartment and uncouples myelin assembly from the underlying program of Schwann cell differentiation.[422]

The *PMP22* gene duplication associated with CMT type 1A can be detected by use of Southern blot analysis, fluorescence in situ hybridization (FISH) on interphase cells, or PCR.[27,30,383,518,550] Detection of the CMT 1A duplication or HNPP deletion can be made by observing unique PCR products not seen in normal controls, which represent junction fragments formed from the recombination event between *PMP22* flanking repeated sequences.[550] Alternatively the detection of three (CMT 1A) or conversely one (HNPP) allele, rather than the expected two seen in normal control DNA following amplification of multiple microsatellite repeat markers in this region, offers another rapid and accurate use of PCR.[30,323,518] These methods are useful for clinical testing, but as a result of gene patents and exclusive license agreements for clinical DNA testing for CMT 1A, testing is available only at one laboratory in the United States.[196,332]

In families in which the duplication has been identified, testing of asymptomatic adult relatives is possible, and testing of a minor is discouraged. Prenatal testing for this nonlethal, clinically variable, adult-onset disorder would be possible but requires in-depth genetic counseling to review the ethical and psychological aspects of such studies.[55] In the suspected patient with no family history and in which no gene duplication has been identified, the risk of transmission of the disorder to their offspring is less clear. The patient could have a de novo point mutation in *PMP22* not detected or have an affected father but be unaware that the diagnosis is caused by alternative paternity; the patient could have CMT caused by an autosomal recessive or an X-linked gene or have a disorder arising from an environmental effect.

Huntington's Disease

HD is an autosomal dominant, late-onset neurodegenerative disorder with an incidence of about 1 in 10,000 in most populations of European origin. The disease is progressive and characterized by frequent involuntary, rapid movements (chorea) and dementia with a median survival time of 15 to 18 years after the onset of symptoms.[243] The mean age of onset is in the decade between 35 and 44 years, but approximately 25% of patients first display symptoms after the age of 50, and about 10% of patients have juvenile HD with the age of onset before 20 years.[243,402] In the first few years of the disease, symptoms include mood disturbances, cognitive deficits, clumsiness, and impairment of voluntary movement.[243] The next stage of the disease is associated with

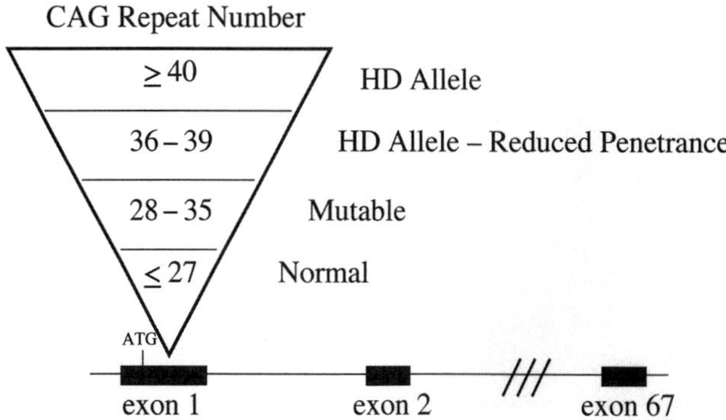

Figure 40-4 Schematic representation of the polyglutamine-encoding CAG repeat in exon 1 of the HD gene and associated alleles. A CAG-repeat number ≤27 is considered normal. CAG-repeat numbers of 28 to 35 are "mutable" and although they are not associated with an abnormal phenotype, these alleles are prone to meiotic expansion to an HD allele. CAG repeats of 36 to 39 are considered HD alleles but with reduced penetrance, indicating that both unaffected and affected patients have been reported with alleles of this size. CAG repeats ≥40 are associated with HD with complete penetrance.

slurred speech (dysarthria), hyperreflexia, chorea, gait abnormalities, and behavioral disturbances including intermittent explosiveness, apathy, aggression, alcohol abuse, sexual dysfunction and deviations, and increased appetite.[183] As the disease advances, bradykinesia, rigidity, dementia, dystonia, and dysphagia are present. In the late stages of HD, weight loss, sleep disturbances, and incontinence occur.

In 1983 Gusella et al reported linkage between DNA marker D4S10 on the short arm of chromosome 4 and HD based on studies from a large kindred in Venezuela.[226] Subsequently, more DNA markers were identified, and the region of the genome containing the HD gene was narrowed to 4p16.3 (short arm of chromosome 4 band 16.3).* Through an international collaborative effort and 10 years after its initial localization, the HD gene, *IT15,* was cloned.[274] The molecular basis of HD was determined to be expansion of a glutamine-encoding CAG trinucleotide repeat and was subsequently confirmed in a worldwide study by the identification of expanded CAG repeat alleles in HD patients from 565 families representing 43 national or ethnic groups.[309] In this initial international study, the median CAG-repeat length was reported to be 44 in affected patients and 18 in controls. Normal CAG repeats range from 10 to 27, repeats of 28 to 35 are considered "mutable," repeats of 36 to 39 are associated with reduced penetrance of the disease, and repeats of 40 or greater are associated with HD[11] (Figure 40-4). No environmental or genetic factors associated with the penetrance of the HD are known.[499]

New mutations for HD (the presence of an affected individual in the absence of a family history) occur from expan-

*References 42, 119, 202, 352, 409, 622.

sion of CAG-mutable alleles and occur almost exclusively through expansion during paternal transmission.[208] Although mutable alleles are present in about 1% of the population, it appears that flanking DNA sequences may influence the instability of these alleles by enhancing the formation of hairpin loop structures.[114,209] In addition, single sperm analysis studies have demonstrated 11% instability (9% expansions and 2.5% contractions) in CAG repeats of 30 compared with 0.6% instability (contractions only) seen in average sized alleles of 15 to 18 repeats.[329] These studies indicated that there is an increase in instability as the repeat number increases. This concept is further supported by the observations that CAG repeats of 36 showed 53% instability, and CAG repeats from 38 to 51 had instability ranging from 92% to 99%. As in fragile X syndrome, instability of the CAG repeat is also likely to occur through replication slippage caused by formation of hairpin loop structures.[209]

The number of CAG repeats is inversely correlated with the age at onset of the disease. Patients with onset as early as 2 years of life have a repeat number approaching 100 or greater and late-onset-disease patients have repeat numbers of 36 to 39.*

The onset of symptoms occurs at progressively younger ages in successive generations of affected families, a pattern called anticipation. Anticipation is explained by meiotic expansion of the unstable CAG repeat during transmission by the affected parent, resulting in an even higher CAG-repeat number in the offspring and an earlier age of onset. In addition, although 69% of affected father-child pairs show expansion, only 32% of affected mother-child pairs demonstrate expansion. Further, <2% of maternal expansions result in a change of >5 repeats, whereas up to 21% of paternal transmissions increase by >7 repeats.[308] An increase in the CAG-repeat number is also associated with more rapid progression of disease and greater neuropathological severity in the striatum.[189,449] Interestingly, however, homozygotes with two expanded CAG-repeat alleles do not have more severe disease than heterozygotes.[309,401,625]

The HD gene protein, huntingtin (htt), consists of 3144 amino acids, is ubiquitously expressed in all tissue, and predominantly resides in the cytoplasm with lesser amounts in the nucleus.[133,227,267,575,602] In neurons, htt is associated with synaptic vesicles and microtubules and is abundant in dendrites and nerve terminals. Huntingtin interacts with multiple proteins functioning in intracellular trafficking and cytoskeletal organization, thereby suggesting its role in these activities.† Expansion of the CAG repeats results in elongation of the *N*-terminal glutamine tract and triggers the preferential loss of striatal neurons.[335]

The precise mechanism of disease progression has not been elucidated. However, expanded alleles are effectively transcribed and translated, but as a result of the increase in glutamine residues, the protein is misfolded.[510] Thus abnormal folding may result in aberrant protein-protein interaction of mutant htt with any of its protein partners and could contribute to the pathogenesis of HD. In addition, truncated fragments of mutant htt, containing the amino terminus with expanded polyglutamine repeats, accumulate to form large aggregates in the nucleus (nuclear inclusions) and in other subcellular compartments.[141,325,346] The aggregates are thought to be toxic to the cell and may also sequester proteins essential for cell viability (e.g., transcription factors) or may trigger degradation of specific factors through the ubiquitin-proteasome-dependent pathway.*

DNA testing for HD is performed by use of PCR so that the exact CAG-repeat number can be determined.[274] Soon after the initial report, it was discovered that the accuracy of determining the CAG-repeat number by PCR was compromised by the inclusion of a polymorphic CGG repeat immediately downstream from the CAG repeat. Since the CGG repeat was contained within the amplified sequence, the length of the amplicon could be altered and overestimated.[20,498] Upon this discovery, a new primer pair was identified that flanked the CAG repeat, yet excluded the problematic polymorphic CGG repeat and provided accurate assessment of the CAG-repeat number.[621] However, in contrast to earlier years when PCR involved the use of ^{32}P labeled primers for this and similar assays, currently the most common methodology for this assay involves the use of PCR with fluorescently labeled primers[609] (Figure 40-5 and Color Plate 9). In addition, guidelines for diagnostic testing by clinical labs with reference to standardization and interpretation have been proposed.[11]

Besides the technical and interpretive difficulties associated with HD testing, many ethical issues exist as well, primarily as they relate to presymptomatic testing (Box 40-2). The first policy statement on ethical issues relating to genetic testing for HD was adopted in 1989 at a joint meeting with representatives from the International Huntington Association and the World Federation of Neurology.[279] At this time, the gene had not yet been cloned, and predictive testing was performed using linkage studies; the asymptomatic patient was quoted the likelihood of inheriting the mutant allele. These tests were less than perfect and provided, at best, results in only 60% to 75% of families. Moreover, the possibility of recombination allowed erroneous predictions to occur.[244,400] In other families, living affected members were not available, or markers were not informative. Once the gene was cloned and direct mutation analysis was possible, risk assessments were reversed in a small percentage of patients.[9]

Following the cloning of the gene and the availability of direct mutation analysis, guidelines for predictive testing were reevaluated and proposed by the International Huntington Association and the World Federation of Neurology Research Group on Huntington's Chorea.[280] Direct predic-

*References 19, 81, 153, 274, 309, 537.

†References 34, 161, 336-338, 375, 533, 612, 620.

*References 291, 365, 428, 461, 471, 529, 642.

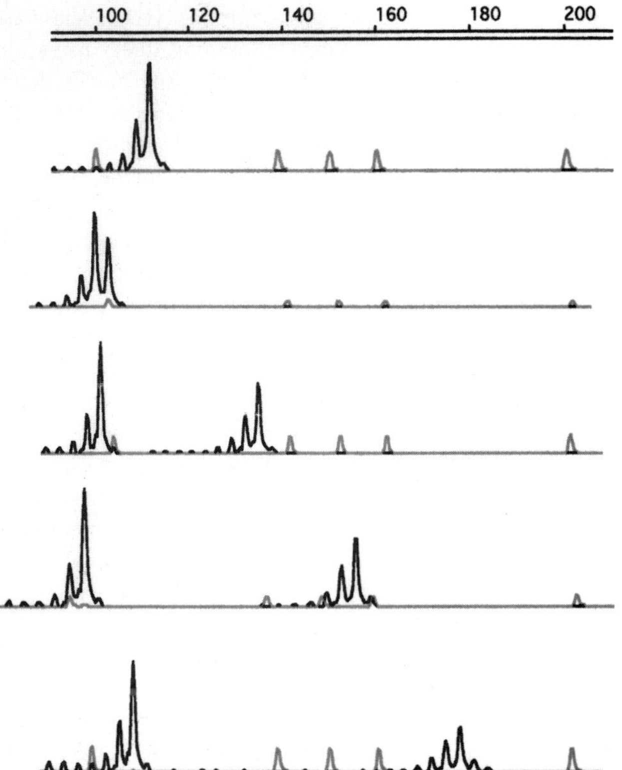

Figure 40-5 Electropherograms representing various patterns observed in patients referred for HD testing. The polyglutamine-encoding CAG repeat in exon 1 is amplified by PCR using flanking oligonucleotide primers, one of which is labeled with a fluorescent dye. Amplicons are subjected to electrophoresis on a 5% denaturing polyacrylamide gel on an ABI 377 DNA sequencer and analyzed using GeneScan software 3.1 b3. Amplicons 100 bp in length contain 18 CAG repeats and flanking DNA. Patient one *(row 1, top)* has amplicons 112 bp in length and has 22 CAG repeats on both HD alleles. Patient two *(row 2)* has 97 bp and 100 bp amplicons, corresponding to CAG repeats of 17 and 18. The diagnosis of HD can be ruled out in these two patients. Patient three *(row 3)* has 97 bp and 133 bp amplicons corresponding to CAG repeats of 17 and 29. The results would not support a diagnosis of HD. However, a CAG repeat of 29 is mutable and can undergo meiotic expansion to an HD allele. Patient four *(row 4)* has CAG repeats of 19 and 38 as depicted by amplicons 103 bp and 160 bp in length. In the symptomatic patient, these results would support the diagnosis of HD. However, in the presymptomatic patient, the phenotype of this HD allele with reduced penetrance cannot be predicted with certainty. Patient five *(row 5)* has CAG repeats of 21 and 44 since amplicons 109 bp and 178 bp in length were detected. These results would confirm the diagnosis of HD. Genetic counseling regarding the implications of the DNA findings in patients three, four, and five is indicated. (See Color Plate 9.)

tive testing was preferred over linkage studies and was readily accepted by the HD community.[28] The approach used for HD has become the model for predictive testing for late-onset diseases, and similar formats have been applied to other late-onset inherited diseases, including autosomal dominant cerebellar ataxias, and less common, dominantly inherited, fatal familial insomnia.[207,588] If an HD-causing expanded CAG-repeat allele is identified in the asymptomatic patient (≥40 years), the median age of onset in HD patients with the patient's corresponding CAG-repeat number can be quoted to the patient.[81] Predictive testing should be performed only on adults and only with informed consent. Informed consent implies that the patient has been thoroughly counseled and clearly understands both the advantages and disadvantages of knowing the results. Advantages of having this test include but are not limited to the removal of uncertainty regarding whether they have or have not inherited the mutant allele and the feeling of relief for those who have not inherited a mutant HD allele. This information can help patients appropriately plan their personal and career paths. Disadvantages of knowing this information include but are not limited to: (1) the feeling of "survivor's guilt" in those who learn that they have not inherited a mutant allele and other family members have; (2) fear from learning that they have inherited a mutant HD allele and will develop this incurable disease; (3) risk of discrimination in employment or health insurance coverage if the results are disclosed; (4) worry that they possess a 50% chance of passing this gene on to their offspring; and (5) uncertainty of developing disease if they have inherited a mutant HD allele containing 36 to 39 CAG repeats.

Importantly the guidelines indicate that the patient should be accompanied by a trusted friend or loved one throughout the counseling and testing procedure. This person can provide stability to the patient by being able to intimately speak to the patient about the situation and discuss the information shared at the counseling sessions. Most importantly, as a part of this process, the partner will be present when the results of the testing are revealed and

BOX 40-2 Ethical Issues Associated With Presymptomatic DNA Testing for HD

Patients must be 18 years of age.
The decision to proceed with testing must be voluntary and informed.
Genetic counseling regarding benefits/pitfalls of testing is required.
A support partner is needed for the patient for counseling and the testing process.
Diagnosis of HD in family should be confirmed by DNA testing before presymptomatic testing.
Psychiatric assessment of patient is necessary before testing.
Follow-up genetic counseling is recommended after delivery of results.
Discrimination by insurance carriers or employers may occur following completion of testing.
Prenatal testing of fetus is controversial; preimplantation diagnosis is available.

can provide comfort and support as needed both then and in the following days, weeks, or months. Ultimately, however, it is the patient's decision to proceed with this testing and to accept both the benefits and pitfalls of knowing this information. The patient's decision to proceed must be his or hers, without coercion from family members, clinicians, friends, or employers.

Since catastrophic events, such as suicides or attempted suicides, can follow predictive testing, a psychiatric assessment is often part of the testing protocol for the safety of the patient.[10] Before performing the mutation studies, it is important that the patient be considered mentally stable since the HD test results can precipitate depression. The results of the psychiatric evaluation can influence the time of the DNA test, postponing it until such time when the patient is considered mentally able to deal with the possibly devastating news.

If possible before testing, the diagnosis of HD should be confirmed in an affected member of the family to be certain that the disease in the family is indeed HD. Excluding HD cannot rule out a different dominantly inherited neurodegenerative disease in the family for which the patient likely retains a risk of development. Since HD is a delayed-onset disease, as the asymptomatic at-risk patient ages, the risk of testing positive with an expanded CAG repeat decreases.[240] Thus should the patient elect not to have predictive testing, the genetic counselor can provide information regarding the probability that an HD mutation exists, which based on the individual's age, may provide some comfort to the patient.

Prenatal testing for HD is another complicated issue associated with this disease and may not be provided in all laboratories that perform routine HD testing. If a molecular genetics laboratory chooses not to provide prenatal testing (e.g., because of the possibility of termination of a pregnancy for a late-onset disorder or because it constitutes presymptomatic testing of the child should the parents choose not to terminate), it is the responsibility of the laboratory to identify an alternative source of testing to which the patient can be referred. Before the cloning of the HD gene, prenatal testing was performed using linkage studies, and the likelihood that the child would develop HD was "excluded" if the child had inherited an HD haplotype from an unaffected grandparent.[379,586] The concept of exclusion testing was difficult to understand, however, and not all families were heterozygous for the DNA markers thereby making the test inconclusive. In some instances, the status of the parent at risk for developing the disease was also revealed. Moreover, testing could in theory lead to abortion of 50% of fetuses who had not inherited HD but rather had inherited the normal HD allele from the affected grandparent. To eliminate some of the controversy of prenatal testing for HD, preimplantation genetic testing (PGT) can be performed. In PGT in vitro fertilization is used to produce embryos that then have a biopsy performed for analysis of their HD genes. Once PCR has been used to determine the HD CAG-repeat numbers, only embryos with normal HD alleles are implanted. This methodology, combining direct mutation analysis and PGT, eliminates the necessity for prenatal testing to determine the HD status of the fetus since the HD alleles of the fetus are known to be normal, and the need for termination of a pregnancy is eradicated. Further, this can also be performed without disclosing the HD status of the asymptomatic, yet at-risk parent. However, this approach of nondisclosure PGT can pose ethical problems to the testing personnel.[78] In some testing centers, PGT may be performed by direct mutation analysis in families for which the at-risk parent is knowledgeable regarding his or her carrier status, and embryos with only normal HD alleles are implanted. Alternatively, in families in which the parent is unaware of his or her HD status, PGT can be performed using exclusion testing whereby only embryos who have not inherited an affected grandparent allele are implanted, and the size of the HD CAG-repeat number is not determined.[78,520-521]

X-Linked Diseases

In X-linked diseases, the mutant allele resides on the X chromosome. In X-linked recessive diseases, females are carriers of the disease with one normal and one mutant allele but typically are not affected. Males receiving the mutant allele from their mothers and having only one X chromosome have no normal allele and thus are affected. All daughters of affected males are carriers of a mutant allele. Carrier females have a 25% chance of transmitting their normal allele to a son, a 25% chance of having an affected son, a 25% chance of having a daughter who carries the mutant allele, and a 25% chance of having a daughter who receives her normal allele. In the absence of a family history, an affected male can have a mutant allele that rose de novo as a new mutation during the formation of the egg. Roughly one third of all cases of X-linked disorders represent new mutations indicating that the mother is not a carrier of a mutant allele and not at risk for subsequent affected children. In pedigrees associated with X-linked recessive conditions, typically only males are observed, and male-to-male transmission of the disease is not seen. In less frequent X-linked dominant diseases, one copy of the mutant allele is sufficient to cause disease despite the presence of a normal allele. Further, in males with only a mutant allele, these diseases are often lethal.

Hemophilia A

Hemophilia A is an X-linked recessive bleeding disorder caused by a deficiency of coagulation factor VIII (FVIII) and affects approximately 1 in 10,000 males worldwide. The disease is characterized by prolonged bleeding after injuries or surgery, renewed bleeding after the initial bleeding has ceased, and in severe cases, spontaneous bleeding into the joints. The severity of the disease is determined by the amount of FVIII coagulant activity present in the plasma; mild, moderate, and severe disease have corresponding FVIII activity levels of 5% to 30%, 1% to 5%, and <1% of control, respectively. In the patient with severe or moderate hemophilia A disease, the activated partial thromboplastin time (aPTT) will be prolonged while all other routine coagulation test results are normal. In patients with mild hemophilia A disease, however, aPTT is often normal. The age of diagnosis is typically earlier in cases with severe disease and a family history.[106] Although most patients with severe disease are diagnosed in the first year of life, patients with mild disease may not be diagnosed until several years later. Although hemophilia A is an X-linked disease and typically presents in males, females with the disease have been reported. Carrier females can present with severe disease caused by skewed X-chromosome inactivation in which the X chromosome with the mutant *FVIII* gene is not inactivated, or alternatively the female may have a mutant *FVIII* gene on each of her X chromosomes.[391,517,590,633]

The *FVIII* gene is positioned on Xq28 (long arm of the X chromosome band 28) and was cloned in 1984.[205,409] The gene spans more than 186,000 base pairs and includes 26 exons.[21] A plethora of nucleotide substitutions, gene deletions, insertions, and rearrangements throughout the *FVIII* gene have been reported in patients with hemophilia. The variability accounts for much of the clinical heterogeneity that is observed with this disease.[393,583] Interestingly, although routine screening of the coding, splice junctions, promoter region, and polyadenylation site of the gene could detect the mutation in the majority of patients with mild to moderate disease, the disease-causing mutation in about half of the patients with severe disease remained elusive for several years.[258]

In 1993 a common inversion mutation was identified in approximately 45% of patients with severe disease.[319,414] The inversion mutation arose from genetic recombination between a small intronless gene within intron 22, gene A, and one of two additional copies of the gene A located approximately 500 kb upstream from the *FVIII* gene. The mechanism for the inversion involves flipping of the tip of the X chromosome allowing pairing between homologous sequences and genetic recombination between one of the upstream copies of gene A and the copy of gene A within intron 22. Consequently the *FVIII* gene is divided into two parts, with exons 1 to 22 widely separated and in an opposite orientation and thus inverted from exons 23 to 26. The majority (>75%) of inversion mutations involve the distal copy of gene A upstream from the *FVIII* gene as compared with the adjacent proximal copy of gene A.[319] Rossiter et al showed that this genetic recombination between homologous intragenic and extragenic copies of gene A occurred as a new mutation predominantly during male meiosis with a male-to-female ratio of 302 : 1.[492] Since during male meiosis Xq is unpaired with a homologue, it is able to flip on itself for an intrachromosomal recombination event. The role of this mutation as a primary cause of severe hemophilia A disease was subsequently confirmed by the analysis of DNA from patients with hemophilia from around the world.[22] Additionally, this mutation has been identified in the Chapel Hill dog colony with hemophilia A disease and presumably arose from the same mechanism of genetic recombination between homologous sequences.[344] Although the causative mutation in the majority of patients can be identified through a combination of various screening techniques, in 1% to 2% of patients the causative *FVIII* gene mutation is not identified.[305] These may represent patients with mutations in upstream regulatory sequences or at other gene loci whose proteins interact with the FVIII molecule.

FVIII is synthesized as a single polypeptide chain of 2351 amino acid residues and an approximate weight of 280 kD.[599] The encoded FVIII protein is predominantly produced in the liver, circulates in the plasma, and is stabilized through noncovalent binding to the complex multimeric glycoprotein von Willebrand's factor (vWF). In the intrinsic coagulation pathway, proteolytic activation of FVIII by small amounts of thrombin frees it from vWf, where it then participates as a cofactor with activated factor IX to catalyze the conversion of factor X to factor Xa.[168] Factor Xa hydrolyzes and activates prothrombin to thrombin. As the concentration of thrombin increases, FVIIIa is ultimately cleaved by thrombin and inactivated. This dual action of thrombin on FVIII regulates the formation of the FVIIIa, IXa, and X complex and thus regulates the clotting cascade. A deficiency of coagulation FVIII then leads to uncontrolled bleeding. The treatment for bleeding episodes is intravenous infusions of FVIII concentrate as quickly as possible to prevent pain, disability, and chronic joint disease. Children with severe hemophilia can be given prophylactic infusions of FVIII concentrate to maintain their clotting activity above 1% and decrease the number of spontaneous bleeding episodes.[349] As a result, clotting factor consumption has increased dramatically over the years and is quite costly but has significantly decreased hemophilic arthropathy.[178] However, management of 15% to 33% of severe and moderately affected patients is complicated by antibody formation to exogenous FVIII caused by repeated infusions. The antibodies can rapidly neutralize infused FVIII. Interestingly the antibodies produced by many patients have hydrolytic activity toward FVIII.[318] Management of the disease was further complicated in hemophilia patients who had contracted human immunodeficiency virus (HIV) and/or hepatitis C virus (HCV) from contaminated plasma-derived FVIII concentrates in the early 1980s. Fortunately, with mandatory and improved screening for these and other viruses, these products are considerably safer, but fears are not completely alleviated.[26] For these reasons, there is great interest in gene therapy for the treatment of hemophilia; several clinical trials have been completed, and others are underway.[387,628] Thus far low levels of FVIII expression have been observed in all trials and have been associated with clinical improvement.

In the mid1980s, after the discovery of the *FVIII* gene and before our current technology of rapid DNA sequencing, DNA testing for hemophilia A primarily involved the use of linkage studies and restriction fragment length polymorphisms to determine the carrier status of at-risk females in the family and to perform prenatal testing.[23,634] Although accurate, these studies could be complicated by (1) the large number of family members required for participation in the analysis, (2) a limited number of alleles for each marker (limiting the chance that key members of the family would be informative [i.e., heterozygous] for a given marker), and (3) genetic recombination between the informative marker and the *FVIII* gene mutation, which could affect the accuracy of the results. Moreover, in the absence of a family history, the carrier status of the mother of a sporadic case was uncertain (though as many as two thirds of these mothers might be carriers). PCR and the analysis of polymorphic microsatellite repeats within the *FVIII* gene increased the number of families in which linkage studies could be performed and significantly improved turnaround times.[320]

The most significant improvement in DNA testing was the identification of the inversion mutation in families with severe disease and the ability to offer direct mutation analysis as opposed to linkage studies.[290,610] As a result, the carrier status of the mother of a sporadic case with a detectable inversion mutation could now be determined with certainty, and her risk for another affected son could be precisely predicted to be 25% (Figure 40-6). In addition, prenatal and carrier testing results would be completely informative and accurate and would not be subjected to inaccuracy caused by the possibility of genetic recombination. Subsequently a PCR assay for the detection of the inversion mutation was developed. It eliminated the necessity for labor-intensive and expensive Southern blot analysis and significantly improved turnaround times.[340-341] For clinical samples, if the patient has a negative test result for a common inversion mutation, DNA sequence analysis of the *FVIII* gene is typically performed, and the turnaround time is about 4 to 8 weeks. Once the mutation segregating in the family has been identified, direct mutation testing for prenatal studies or the carrier status for other at-risk females in the family is available with a usual turnaround time of 2 weeks.[196]

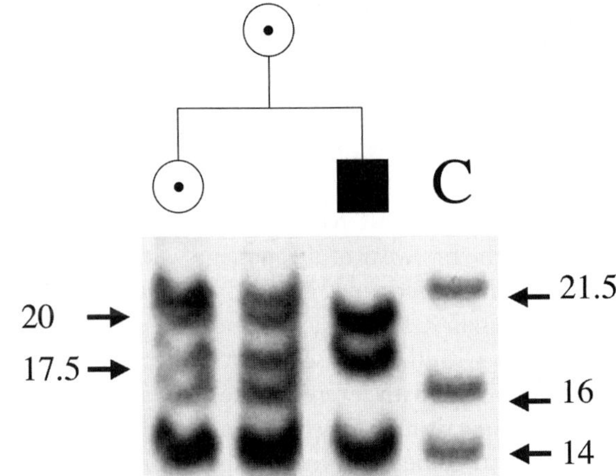

Figure 40-6 Southern blot analysis for the detection of a common inversion mutation present in the DNA of about 50% of patients with severe hemophilia A disease. Patient DNA is digested with restriction endonuclease *BclI*, blotted to a nylon membrane, and hybridized with a ^{32}P-labeled probe corresponding to sequences in intron 22 of the factor VIII gene. Autoradiography was at −70 °C for 24 hours. Normal control DNA (*lane C*) yields bands 21.5 kb, 16 kb, and 14 kb in length. The pattern observed for the affected male (*shaded box*) in this family yields an altered banding pattern with bands of 20 kb, 17.5 kb, and 14 kb. Bands of these sizes confirm the presence of an inversion mutation resulting from homologous recombination between a copy of gene A within intron 22 of the factor VIII gene and the distal copy of gene A 5′ to the factor VIII gene. DNA analysis of the patient's mother and sister indicates that they are carriers of the inversion mutation with bands at 21.5 kb, 16 kb, and 14 kb generated from their wild-type allele and bands at 20 kb, 17.5 kb, and 14 kb generated from their mutant allele. Identification of the inversion mutation in this family will facilitate accurate carrier screening in other at-risk females in this family.

Duchenne's Muscular Dystrophy

Duchenne's muscular dystrophy (DMD) is an X-linked recessive disorder characterized by progressive skeletal muscle wasting. The incidence of DMD is about 1 in 3500 male births, making it the most common severe neuromuscular disease in man. The onset of DMD is typically before 3 years of age with gait difficulty, progressive myopathic weakness with pseudohypertrophy of calves, and grossly elevated serum creatine kinase (CK) as a result of degenerating fibers. Electromyography and muscle biopsy are used to confirm the diagnosis. In Wales, newborn screening of plasma creatine kinase has been used to identify affected males before the onset of clinical signs and to prevent delay in the diagnosis.[440] In this scenario, after informed parental consent, if the diagnosis is made at this time, immediate pediatric and genetic services can be offered to the families.

Most DMD patients are wheelchair bound between 10 and 15 years of age. Continual degeneration and regeneration of muscle eventually lead to the replacement of muscle tissue by adipose and connective tissue, causing progressive disease; death usually occurs before the age of 30 from respiratory or cardiac failure. Carrier females can be asymptomatic or have varying degrees of clinical symptoms depending on the degree of inactivation of the X chromosome harboring the mutant DMD gene in the various tissues where the DMD protein is expressed.[266] Females with severe disease most often result from a carrier female with skewed lyonization or an X-autosome translocation involving the *DMD* gene.*

Cytogenetic abnormalities in DMD patients and DNA linkage studies localized the DMD locus to Xp21 (the short arm of the X chromosome band 21).† Mixing DNA enhanced for X-linked genes from a 49,XXXXY cell line with DNA

*References 77, 217, 478, 606, 645, 647.

†References 31, 131, 184, 217, 409, 606, 647.

from a patient with DMD and a cytogenetic deletion in Xp21, Kunkel et al cleverly used subtraction hybridization to clone the DNA corresponding to the patient's deletion.[316] The deleted region was cloned because during the hybridization, the X-linked sequences from the cell line had no complementary sequences with which to anneal in the patient's DNA and thus were available for cloning. Subsequently, this cloned DNA was found to detect deletions in DMD patients.[315,385] A complete 14 kb cDNA transcript was eventually cloned from fetal skeletal muscle and was used to detect deletion mutations in 53 of 104 patients.[307]

The *DMD* gene is the largest gene in the human genome known to date, spans 2.2 megabases (Mb), contains 79 exons, and has multiple promoter regions.[138,261] The protein product, dystrophin with 3685 amino acids, has a molecular weight of 427 kD and represents approximately 0.002% of total striated muscle protein. Dystrophin is a cytoskeletal protein associated with a protein complex, dystrophin-associated protein complex (DAPC), which in skeletal muscle plays a structural role connecting the actin cytoskeleton to the extracellular matrix, stabilizing the sarcolemma during repeated cycles of contraction and relaxation, and transmitting force generated in the muscle sarcomeres to the extracellular matrix.[154,571] Without dystrophin, an integral component of DAPC, sarcolemmal integrity is compromised. As a result, there is an influx of extracellular calcium triggering calcium-activated proteases and fiber necrosis.[547] Other roles for DAPC have also been proposed, indicating that several mechanisms may be involved in the DMD phenotype.[229,467,470,506] Gene expression studies of diseased and normal muscle have revealed the overexpression of genes involved in muscle structure and regeneration processes.[242,425] Further characterization of the genetic profiles between normal and diseased muscle may help elucidate the molecular mechanisms underlying the dystrophic changes and muscle hypertrophy seen in DMD patients. Although not yet reality, technological advances in many areas of science and medicine suggest that gene therapy for DMD lies in the not so distant future.[104,485]

Because of the tremendous size (2.2 Mb), complexity (8 promoters), and diversity of mutations within the *DMD* gene, DNA testing for DMD presents a challenge for clinical laboratories.[331] Although DNA testing is often not required for diagnosis, because findings on immunohistochemical studies on a biopsy of muscle tissue are considered as diagnostic, identification of the mutation causing the disease in a family is required for carrier detection of at-risk females and for prenatal testing. Intragenic deletions, most often encompassing multiple exons, represent about 60% to 65% of all mutations, affect the translational reading frame of the protein, and lead to a truncated and nonfunctional protein. Duplications of gene sequences are observed in about 5% of patients. Both deletions and duplications can be rapidly detected by use of a combination of multiplex PCR reactions. Electrophoretic gels of the amplified DNA will show the loss of a band or bands or an increased intensity of one or more bands.[46,105] Duplications in affected males and carrier females and deletions in carrier females can be more difficult to observe but can be detected using an endogenous internal standard.[273,464] Detection of the remaining 30% of mutations is tedious, labor intensive, and often beyond the scope of most clinical laboratories. Many of these mutations are within noncoding parts of the gene and are private (i.e., unique to a single patient).[465] Such *DMD* gene mutations have been detected by use of one of a variety of reported techniques, including denaturing gradient gel electrophoresis, protein truncation test, heteroduplex analysis, single-strand confirmation polymorphism, and DNA sequencing.[146,181,192,373,465]

Becker muscular dystrophy (BMD), a milder and less common form of muscular dystrophy with an estimated incidence of 1 in 18,500 births, is an allelic variation of DMD caused by different mutations within the *DMD* gene.[45,94,118,262,643] About 55% of BMD patients have deletions within the dystrophin locus, with those having deletions around the distal rod domain of dystrophin (exons 45 to 60) showing a more classic BMD phenotype and in some cases even remaining free of symptoms until their 50s. However, BMD patients with deletions involving the amino-terminal domain of dystrophin (exons 1 to 9) have a more severe phenotype with an earlier age of onset and a more rapid progression of disease. Patients with X-linked dilated cardiomyopathy (DCM) have also been shown to have mutations at the dystrophin locus.[175,378,396,435] The pattern of mutations in dystrophin causing DCM is less well characterized, with alterations reported in various regions including the promoter region, exon:intron junction splice sites, and various exons throughout the gene.

For DMD or BMD families in which no deletion or duplication is detected, carrier and prenatal testing can be offered by clinical laboratories using DNA linkage studies. However, since the intragenic recombination frequency for this gene is estimated to be about 12%, these studies require the use of both multiple intragenic and 5′ and 3′ flanking markers for an accurate carrier or prenatal result.[3] Particularly difficult are sporadic cases of DMD or BMD in which no other family member with DMD or BMD is known and no mutation in the affected individual is detected. Generally, one third of sporadic cases are thought to represent a new mutation in the mother's gamete from which that individual was derived. Thus neither the mother nor female siblings would be carriers, and the risk to the mother for a second affected son would be considered minimal.

In 1987 Bakker et al first described the phenomenon of germline mosaicism in which no *DMD* gene mutation is present in lymphocyte DNA, but *DMD* gene mutations are present in the germline tissue.[32] Presumably these mutations occur during mitosis in germline proliferation and explain the report of multiple affected children of women whose lymphocyte DNA contains no *DMD* mutations.

In mutation-negative families, carrier assessment involves measurement of serum CK activity and linkage studies.[276]

Carrier assignment, however, is not perfected. Linkage studies are complex, require participation of multiple family members, and are confounded by inaccuracy caused by meiotic recombination or germline mosaicism. Serum CK is, by definition, above the reference interval (defined as the 95th percentile of a healthy reference group of age-matched women) in ~1 of 20 noncarrier women. Moreover, serum CK decreases in DMD carrier women as they age. Thus for DMD and/or BMD families, identification of the mutation in the family best enables rapid and accurate direct mutation analysis for carrier and prenatal testing in that family.

Fragile X Syndrome

Fragile X syndrome is one of the most commonly inherited forms of mental retardation, with an estimated incidence of 1 in 3500 males and 1 in 9000 females.[123] The name of the condition reflects the cytogenetic abnormality of a breakpoint or fragile site in the X chromosome. The clinical syndrome was first described by Martin and Bell in 1943 in a family with sex-linked mental retardation in both males and females who had no dysmorphic features.[360] The disease was later redefined by Lubs, who noted the presence of a marker X chromosome in the leukocytes of some mentally retarded males following incubation of cells in cell culture media depleted of folate and thymidine; the marker segregated with mental retardation in the family.[345] The chromosomal locus for this fragile site would later be localized to Xq27.3 (the long arm of the X chromosome band 27.3).[241,409] Common clinical features associated with fragile X syndrome are mental retardation, delayed motor and speech development, macroorchidism, long face, prominent forehead and jaw, large ears, flat feet, and abnormal behavioral characteristics that include hyperactivity, hand flapping, temper tantrums, persevering speech patterns, poor eye contact, and occasionally autism.[136] These features are often less frequent and milder in affected females than in affected males because of random X inactivation of their abnormal fragile X gene and expression of their normal gene in half of their tissue.

As a sex-linked disease, fragile X syndrome has a complicated inheritance pattern. Affected females are heterozygous for the mutation, and unaffected males can transmit the mutation through the family. For this reason, Sherman et al proposed that fragile X syndrome was an X-linked dominant disorder with reduced penetrance (79% for males and 35% for females), but the penetrance of the disease appeared to increase in subsequent generations within a family.[524,526] The mechanism of this "Sherman paradox" was resolved when the gene causing fragile X syndrome, *FMR1* (Fragile X Mental Retardation) was cloned in 1991.[47,310,430,607,646] *FMR1* was the first gene discovered to cause disease through an expansion of an unstable trinucleotide repeat sequence. The unstable CGG repeat is located in the 5′-untranslated region of the *FMR1* gene in exon 1. The gene spans 38 kb, contains 17 exons, and encodes a 4.4 kb transcript.[156] Alleles contain blocks of CGG repeats usually 7 to 13 repeats in length, which can be interspersed with single AGG repeats.[317,539] Allelic diversity results from the variable number and lengths of these CGG-repeat blocks. There are no distinct boundaries separating the repeat number categories, however. Normal alleles have 5 to 45 repeats; gray zone alleles have 46 to 54; premutation alleles have 55 to 200; and full mutation expansion alleles contain >200 repeats[354] (Figure 40-7). Individuals with a normal number of CGG repeats do not have fragile X syndrome nor are they at risk of having an affected child. Individuals with 46 to 54 repeats represent alleles in the upper range of normal or a smaller than average premutation allele. These individuals do not have fragile X syndrome, yet may have a slightly increased risk of repeat instability and expansion to a full mutation in their offspring in some families. Premutation alleles are unstable and can expand to a larger allele in the premutation range when

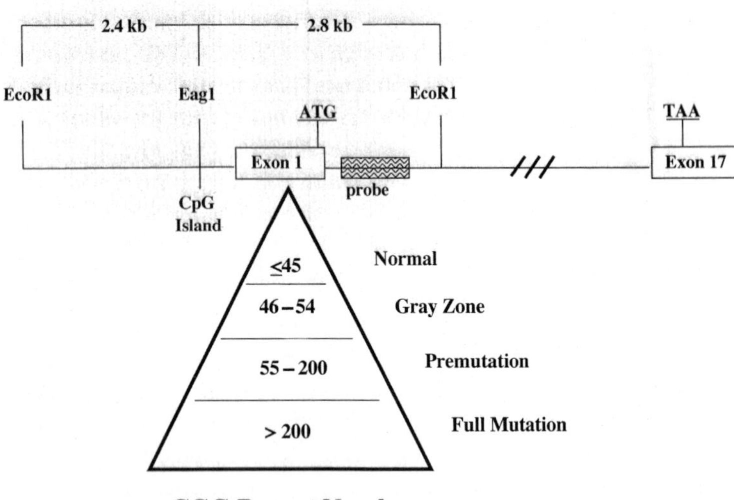

Figure 40-7 Schematic representation of the CGG repeat in exon 1 of *FMR1* and associated alleles. A CGG-repeat number less than or equal to 45 is normal. A CGG-repeat number of 46 to 54 is in the gray zone and has been reported to expand to a full mutation in some families. A CGG-repeat number of 55 to 200 is considered a premutation allele and is prone to expansion to a full mutation during female meiosis. A CGG-repeat number in excess of 200 is considered a full mutation and is diagnostic of fragile X syndrome.

TOXI-LAB® B WORKSHEET

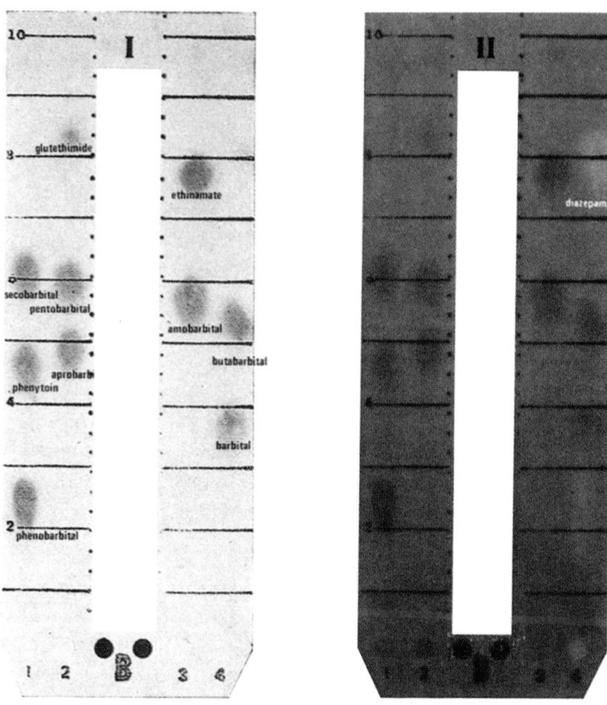

TOXI-LAB® A WORKSHEET

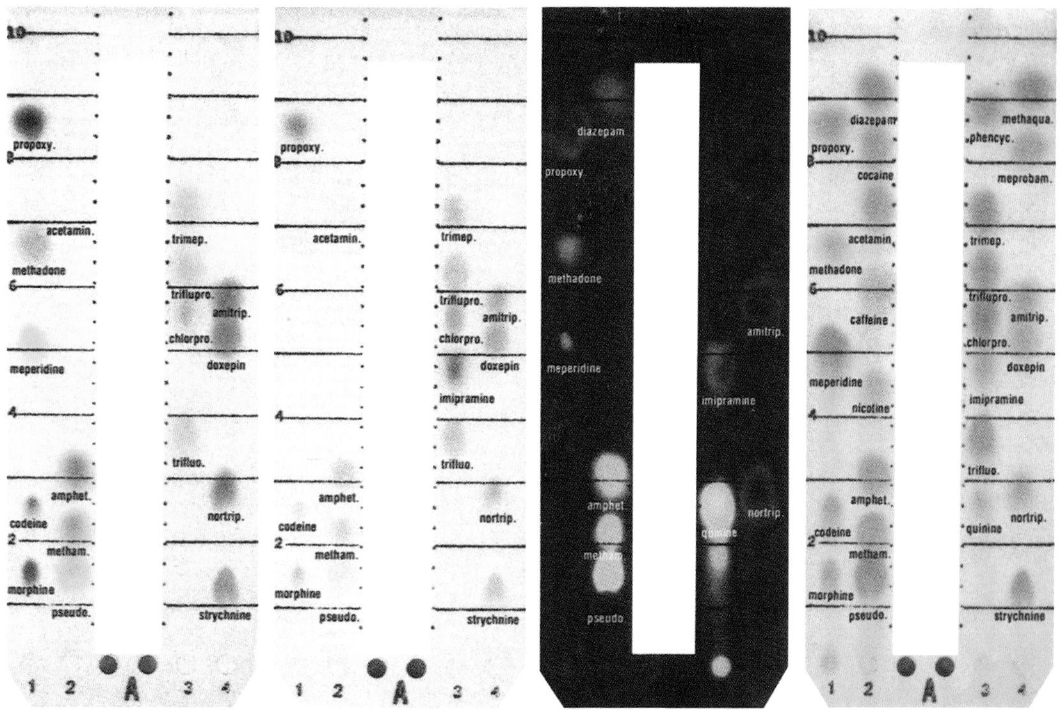

Some variation in the color and position of the drug spots is normal.

Color Plate I Examples of TLC plates used in drug screening: basic drugs (B Worksheet) and acidic, neutral drugs (A Worksheet). (See Figure 34-1.) *(Reproduced with permission of Toxi-Lab, Inc., Irvine, Calif.)*

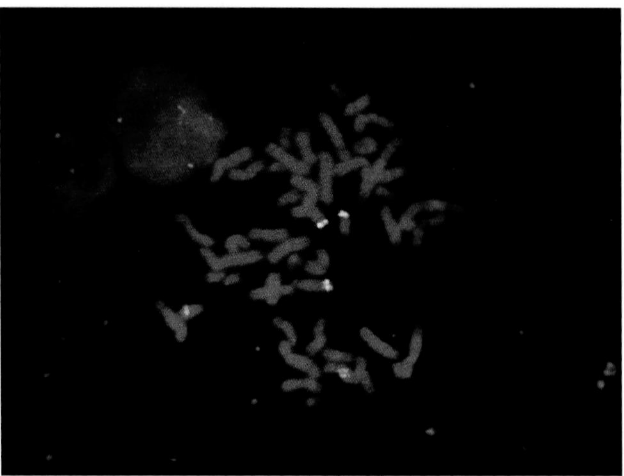

Color Plate 2 Fluorescence in situ hybridization for the t(14;18) anomaly on metaphase spreads of a case of follicular lymphoma. The immunoglobulin heavy chain sequences on 14q32 *(red)* when juxtaposed to the *bcl-2* sequences on 18q21 *(green)* yield a yellow fusion signal indicative of the presence of the t(14;18). (See Figure 39-9.)

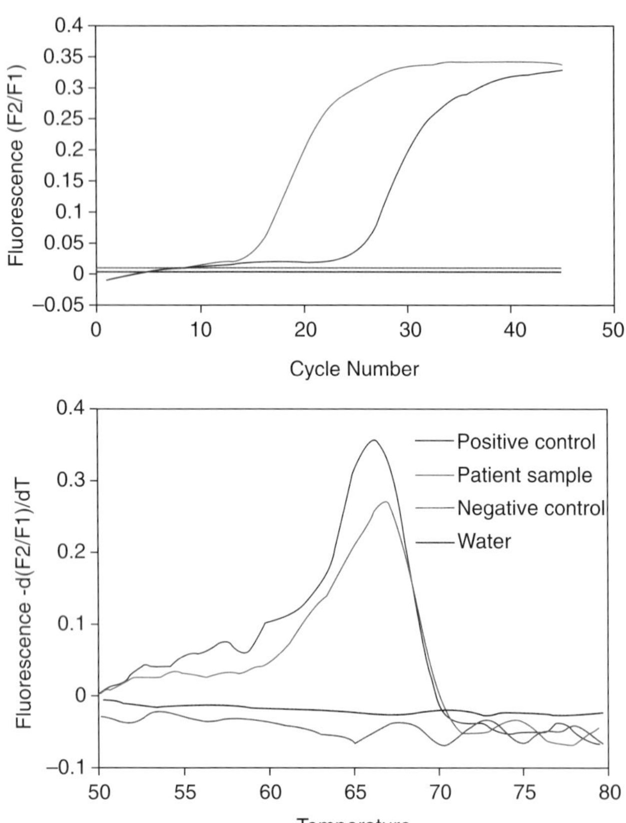

Color Plate 3 Real-time PCR detection of *AML1/ETO* fusion transcript. Real-time PCR detection was performed using a sequence-specific hybridization probe format with oligonucleotide probes labeled with fluorescein as the donor fluorophore and LCRed640 as the acceptor. Postamplification melting analysis was performed to provide confirmation of amplicon identity through the probe melting temperature. Panel A shows the fluorescence (F) versus cycle number (C) the LightCycler™ (Roche Diagnostics). The characteristic three-phase profiles of amplification curves are recognizable (i.e., initial lag, exponential or log/linear, and the final plateau phase). The red curve represents the positive amplification signal for the t(8;21) in the Kasumi cell line positive control. The blue curve represents the patient sample also showing the presence of the *AML1/ETO* fusion. The green line represents a negative control (placental cDNA), and the black line is the no-template (H_2O) control. Panel B shows the derivative melting curves with positive melting peaks at ~65°C in both the Kasumi cell line positive control and the patient sample. Both the negative and water controls show flat lines indicating the absence of the t(8;21) *AML1/ETO* product. (See Figure 39-12.)

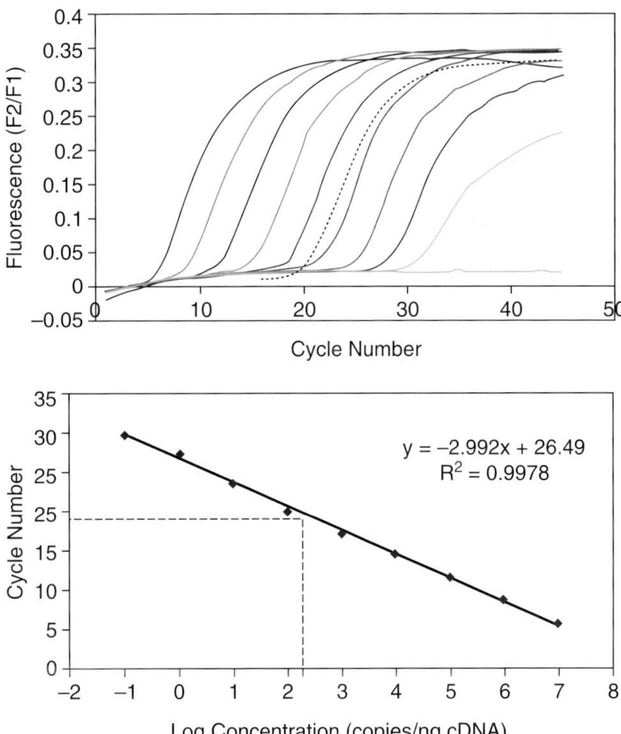

Color Plate 4 Real-time quantitative PCR of *BCR-ABL* transcripts. Serial log dilutions of the plasmids containing the *BCR-ABL* transcripts. Real-time PCR provides a remarkable dynamic range of quantification (10^9 to 10^0 template copies) in this example. The upper panel shows the amplification curves obtained using the *BCR-ABL* containing plasmids and an unknown patient sample depicted as a dotted line. Note the regular ~3.3-cycle interval between log dilutions. The lower panel shows a standard curve (linear regression of cycle number versus log template concentration). As indicated by the dotted line in the lower panel, the cycle threshold (onset of the log-linear phase of the amplification curve) can be used to quantitate the copy number of the target in the tested sample. (See Figure 39-15.)

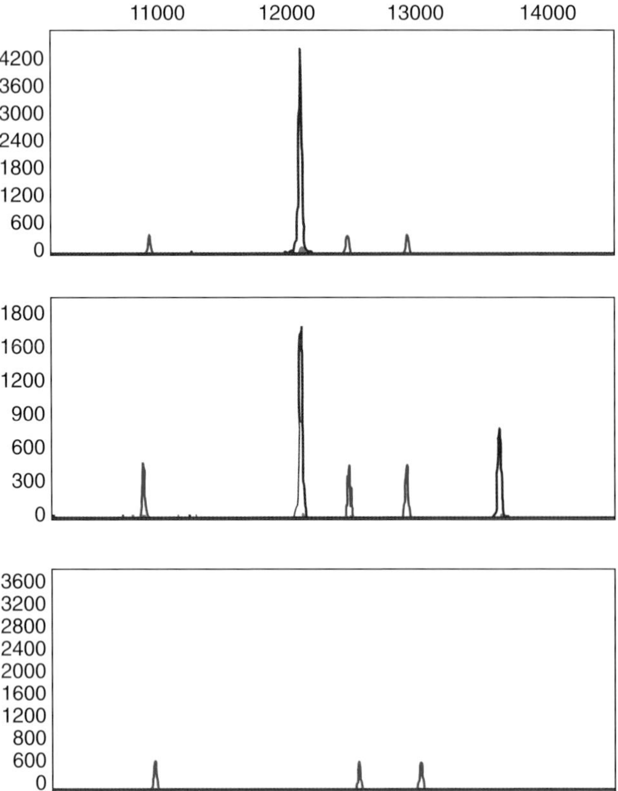

Color Plate 5 Detection of internal tandem duplications of the *FLT3* gene by PCR and capillary gel electrophoresis of PCR products. Capillary electropherograms show clear resolution of PCR products. The x-axis represents the sizes of PCR products and the y-axis shows the fluorescence intensity, which correlates with the abundance of the PCR product. The upper panel shows a wild type of pattern *(blue peak)*. The middle panel shows an additional peak of greater size than the wild-type peak *(blue peak on the left)*. The blue peak on the right represents a *FLT3* internal tandem duplication. The lower panel shows the size markers *(red peaks)* also present in the upper and middle panels. (See Figure 39-16.)

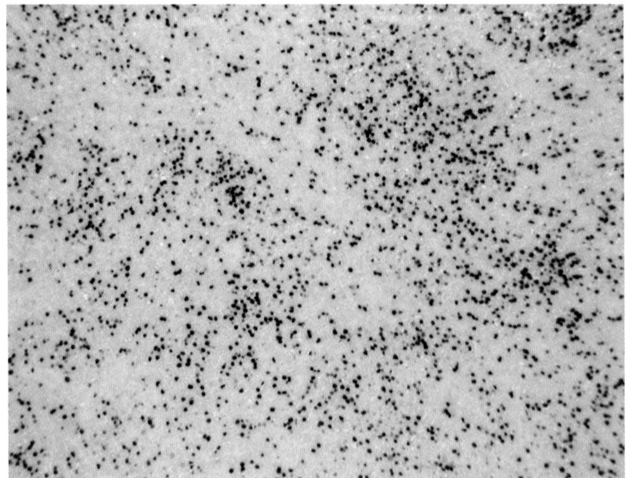

Color Plate 6 In situ hybridization (ISH) for the Epstein-Barr virus (EBV). ISH hybridization for EBV shows numerous positive signals *(dark-blue spots)* for EBV using the EBER-1 probe. The tissue sample was obtained from a solid-organ transplant patient who developed widespread nodal and extranodal masses. The positive reaction for EBV in this assay supports a diagnosis of posttransplant lymphoproliferative disease. (See Figure 39-17.)

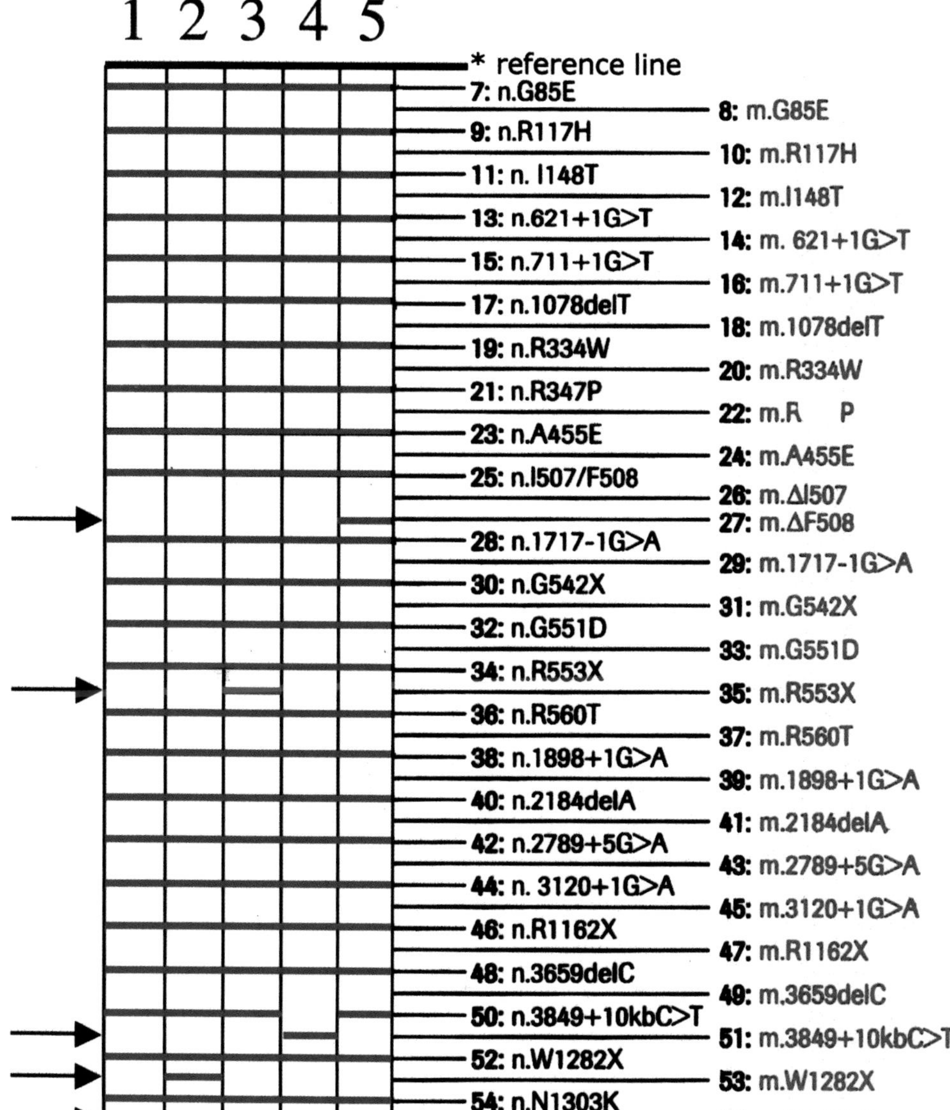

Color Plate 7 CF mutation-detection assay CF Gold 1.0 developed by Roche Diagnostics Corp. Thirty to 45 ng of patient DNA is amplified in a multiplex amplification reaction. Amplicons are denatured and hybridized to membrane-bound oligonucleotide probes specific for 25 normal (n) and corresponding mutant (m) alleles. Lane 1 represents the pattern obtained from patient DNA in which none of the 25 common mutations is present; bands detected correspond only to normal alleles. Lane 2 represents the pattern obtained from patient DNA in which mutation W1282X is present in one allele, since bands corresponding to both nW1282X and mW1282X are present. In lane 3, mutation R553X is present in one allele since bands corresponding to mR553X and nR553X are present. Lanes 2 and 3 could represent CF carriers or could represent DNA from patients with CF for whom only one of their two mutations is identified. In the latter case, the second disease-causing mutation must be a mutation other than one of the 25 represented in this panel. Conversely, lane 4 represents patient DNA in which two copies of mutation 3849 + 10kbC>T are detected. Note that no band corresponding to n3849 + 10kbC>T is present. Lane 5 represents DNA from a CF patient who is a compound heterozygote with mutation delta F508 present on one allele and mutation N1303K present on the second mutant allele. Detection of 5, 7, or 9 T polymorphism in intron 8 has not been determined in these patients but can be performed by this assay. The strip contains oligonucleotide probes for the determination of this polymorphism in patient DNA above the reference line. However, before testing, this part of the strip is removed and is only performed as a reflex test if mutation R117H is detected. (See Figure 40-1.)

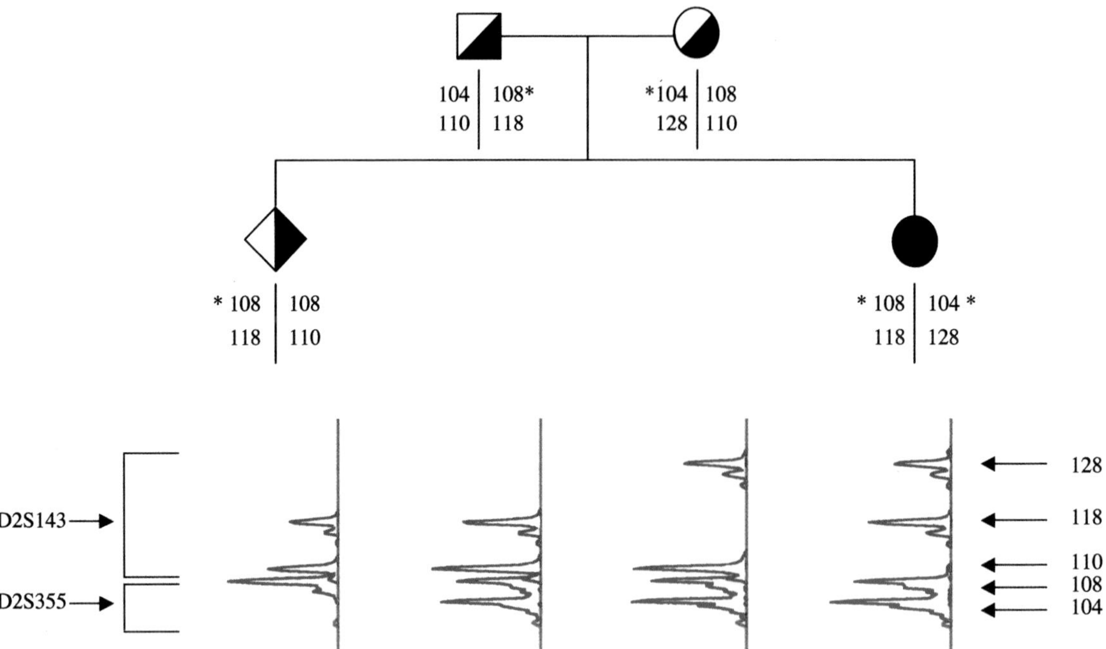

Color Plate 8 Electropherograms illustrating prenatal DNA-linkage studies on a family with CPSI deficiency D2S355 and D2S143 represent dinucleotide markers 4 centimorgans 5′ (D2S355) and 3 centimorgans 3′ (D2S143) to the *CPSI* gene, respectively. DNA samples from the affected child, parents, and fetus are amplified by PCR using oligonucleotide primer pairs specific for each marker, with one primer of each pair labeled with a fluorescent dye. Amplicons are subjected to electrophoresis on a 5% denaturing polyacrylamide gel on an ABI 377 DNA sequencer and analyzed using GeneScan software 3.1b3. The maternal haplotype donated to the affected child is 104,128, indicating that her 108,110 allele is not linked to an abnormal *CPSI* gene. The paternal allele donated to the affected child is 108,118, indicating that his 104,110 allele is in repulsion with CPSID. The maternal allele donated to the fetus is 108,110. This allele is not linked to an abnormal *CPSI* gene. The paternal allele donated to the fetus is 108,118. This allele is linked to an abnormal *CPSI* gene. These results indicate that the fetus is a carrier of CPSID but is not affected. (See Figure 40-3.)

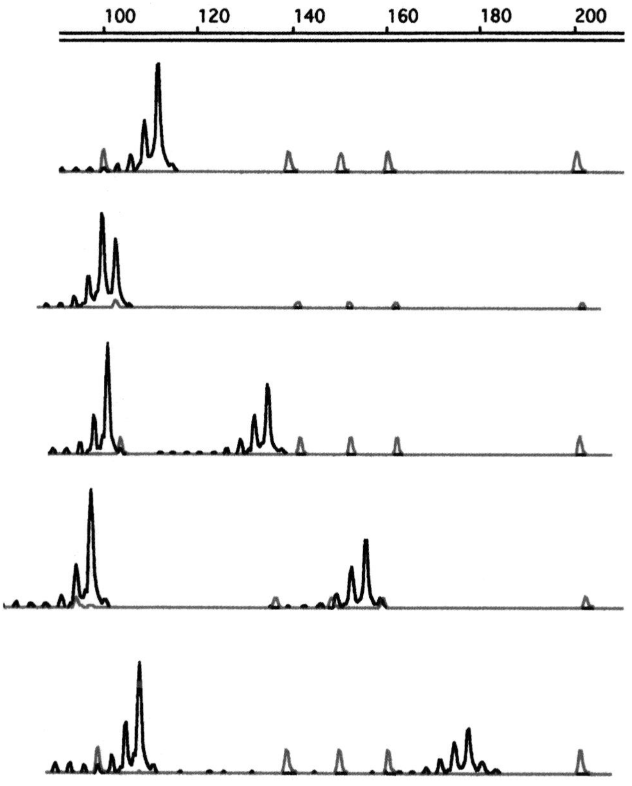

Color Plate 9 Electropherograms representing various patterns observed in patients referred for HD testing. The polyglutamine-encoding CAG repeat in exon 1 is amplified by PCR using flanking oligonucleotide primers, one of which is labeled with a fluorescent dye. Amplicons are subjected to electrophoresis on a 5% denaturing polyacrylamide gel on an ABI 377 DNA sequencer and analyzed using GeneScan software 3.1 b3. Amplicons 100 bp in length contain 18 CAG repeats and flanking DNA. Patient one *(row 1)* has amplicons 112 bp in length and has 22 CAG repeats on both HD alleles. Patient two *(row 2)* has 97 bp and 100 bp amplicons, corresponding to CAG repeats of 17 and 18. The diagnosis of HD can be ruled out in these two patients. Patient three *(row 3)* has 97 bp and 133 bp amplicons corresponding to CAG repeats of 17 and 29. The results would not support a diagnosis of HD. However, a CAG repeat of 29 is mutable and can undergo meiotic expansion to an HD allele. Patient four *(row 4)* has CAG repeats of 19 and 38 as depicted by amplicons 103 bp and 160 bp in length. In the symptomatic patient, these results would support the diagnosis of HD. However, in the presymptomatic patient, the phenotype of this HD allele with reduced penetrance cannot be predicted with certainty. Patient five *(row 5)* has CAG repeats of 21 and 44 since amplicons 109 bp and 178 bp in length were detected. These results would confirm the diagnosis of HD. Genetic counseling regarding the implications of the DNA findings in patients three, four, and five is indicated. (See Figure 40-5.)

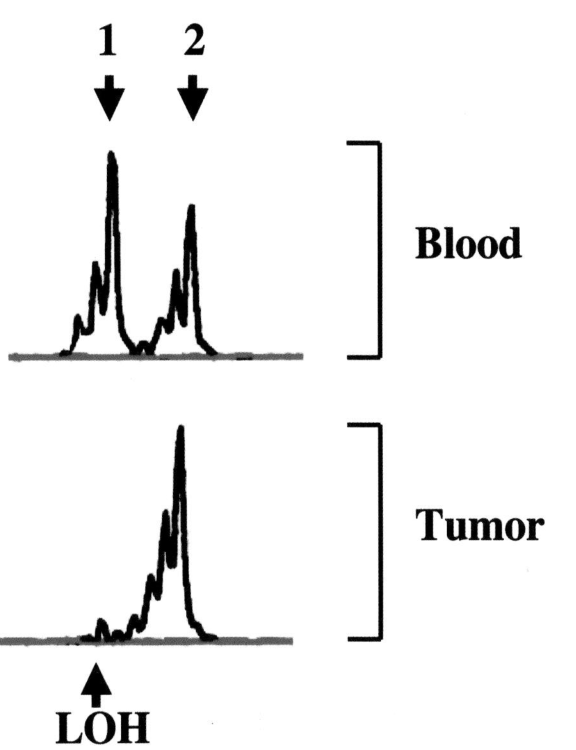

Color Plate 10 Electropherograms illustrating LOH in tumor DNA. Patient DNA is extracted from the peripheral blood and tumor tissue and amplified by PCR using an oligonucleotide primer pair specific for a polymorphic, microsatellite repeat locus contained within the chromosomal region thought to be deleted during tumorigenesis. One of the primers within the pair is labeled with a fluorescent dye. Amplicons are subjected to electrophoresis on a 5% denaturing polyacrylamide gel in an ABI DNA sequencer and analyzed using GeneScan software 3.1 b3. Constitutive DNA from the patient's blood illustrates heterozygosity for this marker with amplicons represented by alleles 1 and 2. In DNA from the tumor, a single peak representing a typical homozygous pattern is observed. Thus there is LOH in tumor DNA. This loss signifies the loss of the second allele and also indicates the loss of this region on the chromosome. (See Figure 40-11.)

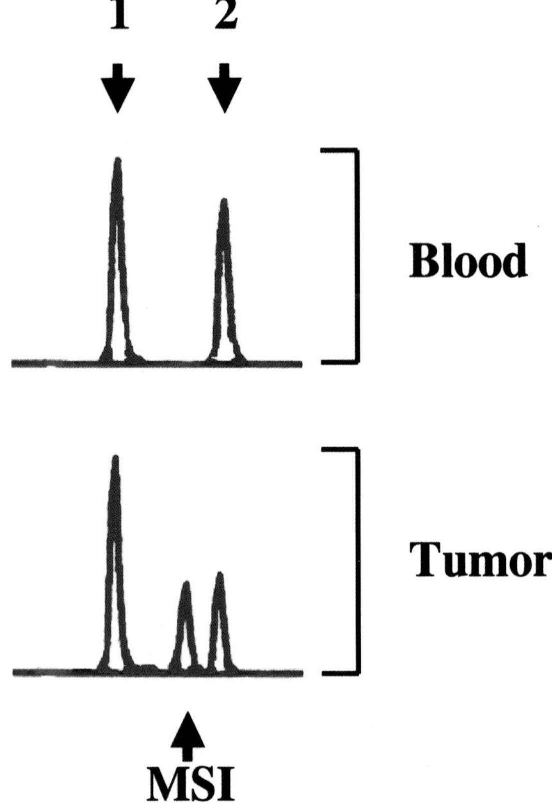

Color Plate 11 Electropherograms illustrating MSI in tumor DNA. Patient DNA is extracted from the peripheral blood and tumor tissue and amplified by PCR using an oligonucleotide primer pair specific for a microsatellite repeat locus. One of the primers within the pair is labeled with a fluorescent dye. Amplicons are subjected to electrophoresis on a 5% denaturing polyacrylamide gel in an ABI DNA sequencer and analyzed by GeneScan software 3.1 b3. Constitutive DNA from the patient's blood illustrates heterozygosity for this marker with amplicons represented by alleles 1 and 2. In DNA from the tumor, in addition to constitutive alleles 1 and 2, amplicons representing DNA fragments of a different size are present; these indicate a change in repeat number for one of the alleles. Because of dysfunctional MMR enzymes, mistakes occurring during the replication of microsatellite repeat sequences resulting in expansions or contractions of the repeat number remain unrepaired. In this case, a contraction in the repeat number of allele 2 has occurred. (See Figure 40-12.)

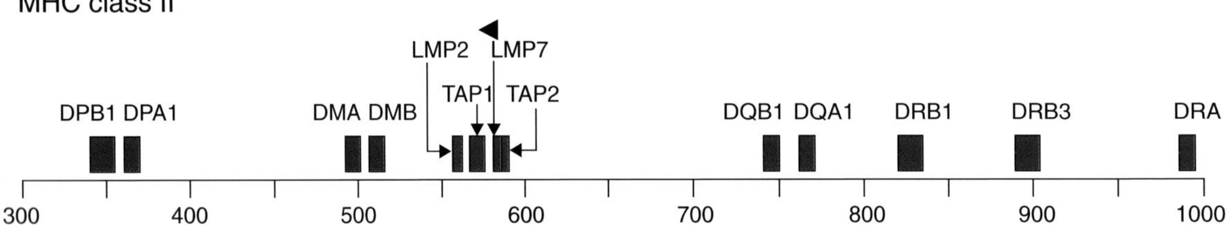

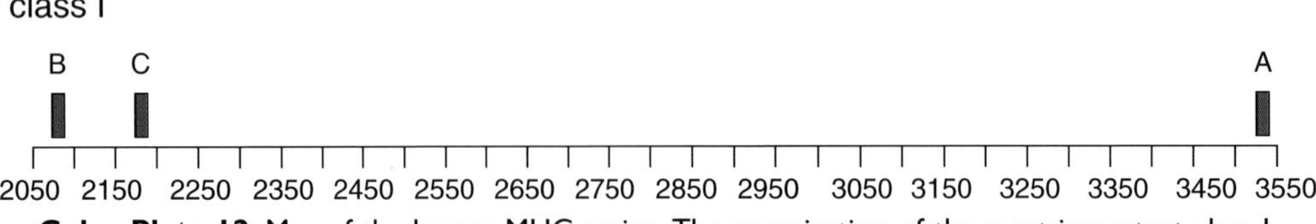

Color Plate 12 Map of the human MHC region. The organization of the most important class I and class II genes of the MHC is shown, with approximate genetic distances given in thousands of base pairs (kb). Genes are ordered from telomere to centromere. Not shown are MHC class III genes, which map between class I and class II genes. (See Figure 41-2.)

transmitted or can expand to a full mutation allele and an offspring with fragile X syndrome.[426] Although rare, premutation alleles have been reported to undergo rather drastic contractions (82 to 33, 95 to 35, 145 to 43, 130 to 10, and 70 to 54).[84,426] The recent establishment of transgenic mice with CGG-repeat instability similar to that seen in humans should facilitate a better understanding of this phenomenon.[40,72] Premutation carrier females have a higher prevalence of premature ovarian failure (POF) as compared with females with normal CGG-repeat numbers in the general population.[120,441,513] Interestingly, full mutation carrier females and their noncarrier sisters appear to have no increased risk for POF.[523] Moderate CGG expansion seen in premutation carrier females may affect neurocognitive functioning related particularly to attention-related tasks.[51,545] Further, despite overexpression of *FMR1* in premutation carriers, the FMR1 protein, FMRP, appears to be significantly diminished, suggesting reduced translation efficiency.[299] Thus diminished FMRP levels in premutation carriers are negatively correlated with the repeat number, and overexpression of *FMR1* has a positive correlation with the repeat number. The risk of CGG expansion from a premutation to a full mutation allele is dependent on several factors including the number of pure uninterrupted CGG repeats, the number and position of interspersed AGG repeats, haplotype background, and less, well-characterized heritable factors.[93,155-157,251,427,525] In a large collaborative study among 13 laboratories in eight countries and involving >1500 premutation carrier females, the smallest premutation alleles shown to expand contained 59 repeats with no AGG interruptions.[426] Most data from humans suggest that expansion occurs before zygote formation, but the possibility of CGG expansion occurring very early in embryogenesis cannot be excluded.[356,392] Expansions of premutations to full mutations are largely confined to transmissions from females to offspring and are thought to occur from slippage during DNA replication of the lagging strand as a result of hairpin formation within the expanded CGG-repeat sequence.[190] Transmission of premutation repeat alleles in males remained stable in 16% of transmissions, decreased in size in 22% of transmissions, and expanded to a larger premutation allele in 62% of transmissions.[427] Premutation carrier fathers of premutation carrier females, or normal transmitting males, were previously thought to have a fairly normal phenotype with no clinical features of fragile X syndrome, although these males may have large ears and deficits in nonverbal tasks, which now too may be explained by reduced levels of FMRP.[299,343] Further, older premutation carrier males may exhibit a neurodegenerative syndrome characterized by progressive intention tremor, parkinsonism, and generalized brain atrophy.[230,285] Although FMRP is decreased, increased concentrations of *FMR1* transcript may represent a gain-of-function effect and possibly play a role in this premutation tremor and/or ataxia syndrome.[285] Recently, mice with premutation CGG repeats in the *FMR1* gene have been shown to have intranuclear inclusions in distinct regions of the brain, suggesting the role of the *FMR1* gene in this process and providing a possible explanation of clinical features observed in symptomatic premutation carriers.[631] Although expansion of a premutation to a full mutation is associated with maternal transmission, the sex of the fetus has no apparent effect on this process.[426]

The fragile X phenotype occurs following expansion of the CGG repeat, hypermethylation, and histone deacetylation of the adjacent CpG island in the promoter region of the *FMR1* gene, transcriptional silencing of the gene, and ultimately no production of FMRP.[47,115,456,560] *FMR1* mRNA is highly expressed in the testis and in the fetal and adult brain.[2,259] FMRP is an RNA-binding protein with two RNA-binding motifs and is associated with translating polyribosomes as a part of a large ribonucleoprotein complex.[35,176,534] Thus in cells from fragile X patients, hundreds of mRNAs exhibit abnormal translational profiles.[83] Recent studies on the *Drosophila* homologue of FMRP have indicated that FMRP mediates translation repression through RNA interference.[99,102,282,364] Males with full expansion alleles but incomplete methylation—"mosaic males"—may have severe mental retardation or a milder phenotype.[366,495] Although in vitro reactivation of the *FMR1* gene has been reported by inducing DNA demethylation and the reassociation of acetylated histones, reactivation of *FMR1* may not be enough to restore FMRP concentrations because transcripts with large repeats are not translated efficiently.[113,299]

Although CGG expansion is the mechanism of disease in greater than 99% of all cases, a point mutation within the gene (I304N) and deletions have also been reported to cause disease in males presenting with a clinical phenotype of fragile X syndrome.[132,194,235,565] DNA testing for fragile X syndrome using Southern blot analysis of peripheral blood enables detection of all possible genotypes (though not of all causes of fragile X as detected by cytogenetics [Figure 40-8]). PCR analysis with capillary electrophoresis is used to complement the testing by providing the precise CGG-repeat number. (It may also be used as the first test, but when it fails to resolve two alleles in a female or to identify an allele in a male the sample must be tested by Southern blot analysis because an expanded allele may be present that is too large to be amplified.) Chorionic villus samples or amniotic fluid can be tested, but the methylation pattern expected in adult tissue may be absent.

As expected, as the CGG-repeat length increases, the risk of expansion from a premutation to a full mutation in premutation carrier females increases. This information is most useful for determining the risk of an affected offspring during genetic counseling of a premutation carrier female. Although a woman with premutation CGG repeat of 55 to 59 is given about a 5% risk of expansion to a full mutation, a woman with a repeat length of 70 to 79 is given a 31% risk of expansion, and a woman with a CGG-repeat length >100 is given close to a 100% chance of expansion.[426] The American College of Human Genetics has published guidelines for testing in the laboratory.[354]

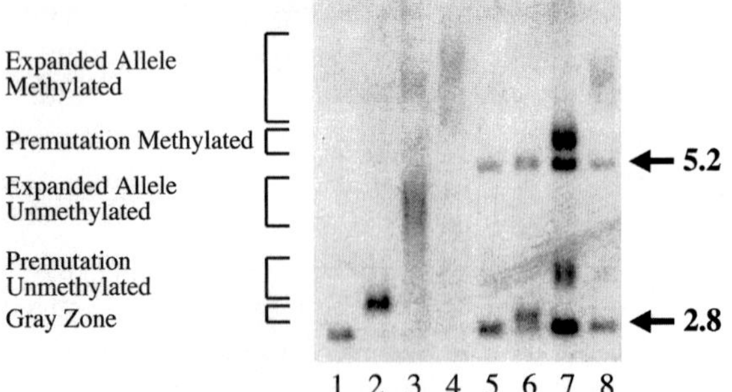

Figure 40-8 Southern blot analysis for the diagnosis of fragile X syndrome. Patient DNA is simultaneously digested with restriction endonucleases *EcoR*I and *Eag*I, blotted to a nylon membrane, and hybridized with a ^{32}P-labeled probe adjacent to exon 1 of *FMR1* (see Figure 40–7). *Eag*I is a methylation-sensitive restriction endonuclease that will not cleave the recognition sequence if the cytosine in the sequence is methylated. Normal male control DNA with a CGG-repeat number of 22 on his single X chromosome *(lane 1)* generates a band about 2.8 kb in length corresponding to *Eag*I-*EcoR*I fragments (see Figure 40–7). Normal female control DNA with a CGG-repeat number of 20 on one X chromosome and a CGG-repeat number of 25 on her second X chromosome *(lane 5)* generates two bands, one at about 2.8 kb and a second at 5.2 kb. *EcoR*I-*EcoR*I fragments approximately 5.2 kb in length represent methylated DNA sequences characteristic of the lyonized chromosome in each cell that is not digested with restriction endonuclease *Eag*I. DNA in lane 2 contains a *FMR1* CGG-repeat number of 90 and is characteristic of a normal transmitting male. The banding pattern observed in lane 3 is representative of a mosaic male with a single X chromosome with a full mutation (>200 repeats). However, the full mutation in some cells is unmethylated; in other cells, the full mutation is fully methylated, hence the term mosaic. In those cells in which the full mutation is unmethylated, digestion by both *Eag*I and *EcoR*I occurs, and in those cells in which the full mutation is fully methylated, digestion of the DNA by *Eag*I is inhibited. The banding pattern observed in lane 4 is diagnostic of a male with fragile X syndrome illustrating the typical expanded allele fully methylated in all cells. Lane 6 is characteristic of a female with a normal allele and a CGG-repeat number of 29 and a larger gray zone allele with a CGG-repeat number of 54. Lane 7 is the banding pattern observed from a premutation carrier female with one normal allele having a CGG-repeat number of 23 (band at about 2.8 kb) and a second premutation allele with CGG repeats of 120 to about 200 (band at about 3.1 kb). In premutation carrier females, in cells in which the X chromosome with the premutation allele is lyonized, the normal 5.2 kb *EcoR*I-*EcoR*I band is larger because of the increased CGG-repeat number and is about 5.5 kb in length. Lane 8 is diagnostic of a female with fragile X syndrome with one full expansion mutation allele that is completely methylated and transcriptionally silenced on one X chromosome but with a second normal allele with a CGG-repeat number of 33.

DISEASES WITH NONMENDELIAN INHERITANCE

Mitochondrial DNA Diseases

Mitochondria are organelles present in the cytoplasm of all eukaryotic cells of animals, higher plants, and some microorganisms. Mitochondria generate energy for the cellular processes by producing adenosine triphosphate (ATP) through oxidative phosphorylation (OXPHOS); they are important in maintaining calcium homeostasis and play a role in apoptosis.[191,453,468,535] The matrix of the mitochondrion is surrounded by a cardiolipin-rich inner membrane, and both are enclosed by a second outer membrane. Within the matrix are copies of the mitochondrial genome, mitochondrial deoxyribonucleic acid (mtDNA). Each mitochondria contains between about 2 and 10 copies of mtDNA, so with hundreds of mitochondria per cell, an estimated 10^3 to 10^4 copies of mtDNA exist within each cell, with brain, skeletal, and cardiac muscle having particularly high concentrations. The mtDNA is a double-stranded, circular molecule containing 16,569 base pairs that encodes 37 genes including: two ribosomal RNAs (rRNA), 22 transfer RNAs (tRNA), and 13 subunits required for the OXPHOS system, with seven belonging to complex I, one to complex III, three to complex IV, and two to complex V.[16,144] The majority of the subunits involved in the OXPHOS system are nuclear encoded as are several nuclear gene products that regulate mitochondrial gene expression.[225,611] Interestingly the mitochondrial genetic code is slightly different from the universal code. For example, in mtDNA, TGA codes for tryptophan rather than a termination codon, and all mitochondrial-encoded polypeptides contain codons requiring only the mitochondrial-encoded 22 tRNA molecules for translation rather than the 31 predicted by Crick's wobble hypothesis.[37] The high copy number of mtDNA per cell coupled with a small genome and unique sequence variations between individuals makes mtDNA sequence analysis an ideal tool for forensic studies.[372,587]

Mitochondria-related diseases can result from mutations in nuclear DNA or, as first reported in 1988, can result from mutations in the mitochondrial genome.* However, mitochondrial genetics are different from mendelian genetics in several aspects. First, all mtDNA is maternally inherited. With mature oocytes having the highest mtDNA copy number per cell at 10^5 and sperm having the lowest mtDNA copy number per cell at 10^2 after fertilization, sperm mtDNA is selectively degraded so that only maternal mtDNA remains. Thus if a mother is carrying an mtDNA mutation, it will be transmitted to all of her children, but only her daughters can transmit the disease to their offspring. Although this is considered the rule, paternal mtDNA inheritance has been reported and may result from incomplete degradation of sperm mtDNA in early embryogenesis.[514] If an mtDNA mutation arises, it will exist among

*References 223, 265, 511, 558, 616, 649.

a population of normal mtDNA. This coexistence of normal and mutant mtDNA copies within the same cell is referred to as *heteroplasmy* and is the second unique feature of mitochondrial genetics. Thirdly, during cell division, the proportion of normal and mutant mtDNA can shift as mitochondria and their accompanying genomes are partitioned into daughter cells. Thus in development and differentiation, the proportion of normal and mutant mtDNA can vary among cells and tissue within the body. Lastly the percentage of mutant mtDNA required within a cell, tissue, or organ system to result in a deleterious phenotype is referred to as the *threshold effect.* The threshold for disease varies between people, energetic requirements for tissue, and the mtDNA mutation. As is evident, genetic counseling for families with mtDNA disorders is complicated by the inability to accurately predict phenotype caused by the phenomena of heteroplasmy and threshold effect.[572]

Two types of mtDNA mutations exist, those that affect mitochondrial protein synthesis (tRNA and rRNA genes) and those within the protein-encoding genes themselves.[144,212] Direct sequencing of mtDNA is considered the gold standard for mutation detection, but this methodology may be unable to detect a low percentage of mutant mtDNA in a heteroplasmic state. Recently a simple and effective method referred to as temporal temperature-gradient gel electrophoresis coupled with PCR and DNA sequencing has been described that can detect heteroplasmic mutations as low as 4%.[637] Although mtDNA mutations are now associated with a significant number of inherited diseases, acquired mtDNA deletions are associated with the aging process, and mitochondrial dysfunction is associated with neurodegenerative diseases.[53,121,436,562] The most likely cause of somatic mtDNA mutations is via damage by oxygen free radicals produced as by-products of aerobic metabolism.[14,479]

Leber Hereditary Optic Neuropathy

Leber hereditary optic neuropathy (LHON) is the most common mitochondrial disease and the first linked to maternal inheritance through a mutation in the mtDNA.[616] LHON is characterized by bilateral subacute loss of central vision caused by focal degeneration of the retinal ganglion cell layer and of the optic nerve.[357] After initial symptoms, both eyes are usually affected within 6 months. Approximately 50% to 60% of males and only 8% to 32% of females who possess the mtDNA mutation will actually develop this optic neuropathy.[417] Nuclear-encoded factors that affect mtDNA expression, mtDNA products, or mitochondrial metabolism may modify the phenotypic expression of LHON.[418] Genetic counseling in LHON is complicated in that the amount of mutant mtDNA transmitted by heteroplasmic females cannot be predicted, and testing cannot predict which individuals will develop visual symptoms.[275]

LHON is a disorder caused by OXPHOS deficiency. Although more than 27 mutations have been associated with this disease, mtDNA mutations G3460A, G11778A, and T14484C represent 95% of those identified.[353] Mutation G11778A was the first described, is the most common, and accounts for at least 50% of cases. In most affected individuals, LHON mutations appear to be homoplasmic, with only mutant mtDNA detected, but in 15% of cases, the mutations are heteroplasmic, with a mixture of both normal and mutant mtDNA detected.[536,608] Each of the common mutations affects a subunit of the nicotinamide adenine dinucleotide : ubiquinone oxidoreductase in complex I of the OXPHOS pathway. The mechanism by which these mutations cause the LHON phenotype is not well understood.[418]

Clinical DNA testing for these mutations is widely available and typically involves PCR amplification coupled with restriction endonuclease analysis and gel electrophoresis.[18,398] If the patient's mtDNA is negative for the three common mutations, testing for other mtDNA mutations associated with LHON should be considered.[167,398] DNA sequencing of all of the mtDNA-encoded complex I genes or of the entire mitochondrial genome may be required but should be employed only when clinical suspicion for LHON is high.[18,418]

Leigh Syndrome

Leigh syndrome (LS), or subacute necrotizing encephalomyelopathy, is a progressive neurodegenerative disorder that eventually leads to death. In contrast to LHON, patients present within the first few years of life with hypotonia, failure to thrive, psychomotor regression, ocular movement abnormalities, ataxia, and brainstem and basal ganglia dysfunction caused by severe dysfunction of mitochondrial energy metabolism. The clinical phenotype for LS is variable in patients with the same pathogenic mtDNA mutation and largely results from differences in the percentage of mutant mtDNA among organs and tissues within an individual[98,580] (Figure 40-9).

LS exhibits genetic heterogeneity, with disease-causing mutations identified in both nuclear and mtDNA, making both mendelian and maternal patterns of inheritance possible for this syndrome.[143] Mutations in mtDNA genes *ATPase6* (complex V), ND5 (complex I), and $tRNA^{Lys}$, or nuclear-encoded genes affecting pyruvate dehydrogenase or respiratory chain enzyme complexes I, II, and IV have been reported.* The most common biochemical abnormality associated with LS is deficiency of cytochrome c oxidase caused by defects in the assembly of complex IV. The protein products from the *SURF-1* and *COX 10* genes play an important role in the assembly of complex IV, and mutations in these genes follow an autosomal recessive mode of inheritance.

Clinical testing for mitochondrially inherited LS uses direct sequencing of mtDNA-encoded genes. Because of the genetic heterogeneity of nonmitochondrially inherited LS and the need for mutation screening for a number of genes,

*References 7, 76, 363, 451, 561, 568, 574, 577, 591-592.

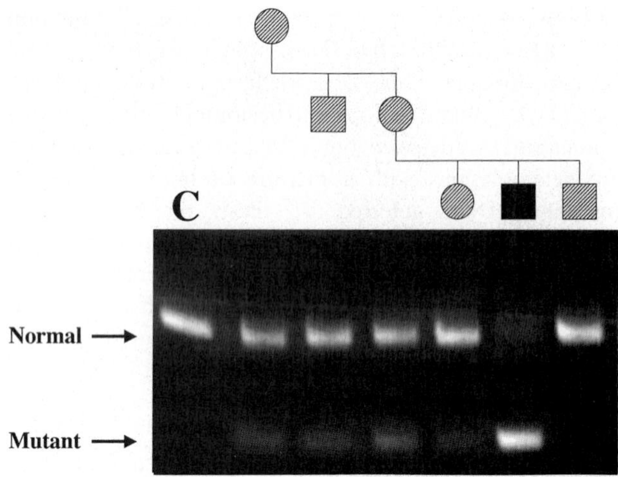

Figure 40-9 Detection of varying degrees of heteroplasmy for mtDNA mutation A8344G in a family with Leigh syndrome.[441] Mitochondrial DNA was extracted from a peripheral blood specimen from an affected male with Leigh syndrome and from family members. Mitochondrial DNA was amplified using an oligonucleotide primer pair that flanks mitochondrial mutation A8344G. The A-to-G base substitution creates a *Nae* I recognition site (GCCGGC), which is not present in normal control mtDNA (C). Amplicons from each member of the family and the control were digested with *Nae* I and subjected to gel electrophoresis. The virtual absence of undigested amplicons in the affected male indicates the presence of almost 100% mutant mtDNA in the cells from this specimen and coincides with the severe phenotype of Leigh syndrome in this patient.[441] In contrast, his sister, mother, and grandmother with 30%, 40%, and 20% mutant mtDNA suffer only from migraine headaches. His uncle, with 30% mutant mtDNA present, suffers with attention-deficit-hyperactivity disorder and learning disabilities. Heteroplasmy, or variation in the percentage of normal and mutant mitochondria, largely explains the observed phenotypic differences in this family. *(Figure courtesy of Thomas W. Prior, Ph.D., Depts of Pathology and Neurology, Ohio State University, Columbus, Ohio.)*

clinical testing for LS is limited and not currently available in the United States.[196]

IMPRINTING

Imprinting refers to the differential marking or "imprinting" of specific paternally and maternally inherited alleles during gametogenesis, resulting in differential expression of those genes. Such imprints on the DNA during gametogenesis must be maintained through DNA replication in the somatic cells of the offspring, must be reversible from generation to generation, and must influence transcription. DNA methylation is the primary mechanism for genomic imprinting. The number of imprinted genes in the human genome is estimated to be less than 200, and most are clustered around imprinting control centers. Alterations in normal imprinting patterns can result in disease.

Prader-Willi and Angelman Syndromes

Prader-Willi syndrome (PWS) is characterized by hypotonia, obesity, short stature, small hands and feet, motor and mental retardation, and hypogonadism. The syndrome is also associated with specific behavioral and psychopathological characteristics, which present challenging management issues.[140,412] The disorder is relatively frequent, with an incidence of 1 in 10,000 to 15,000. Angelman syndrome (AS) is characterized by severe mental retardation, inappropriate bouts of laughter, absence of speech, gait ataxia, frequently microcephaly, and seizures. The incidence of AS is estimated at about 1 in 12,000 to 20,000. As apparent from their characteristic physical findings, PWS and AS are clinically distinct syndromes; yet each results from one of several possible genetic changes involving chromosomal region 15q11-q13 (long arm of chromosome 15 within banding regions 11 and 13).[409,419] Within this 4-megabase (Mb) region, 2 Mb are imprinted, with gene expression dependent on parental origin. PWS results from the loss of paternally expressed genes in this region, and AS results primarily from the loss of a maternally expressed gene in this region.

The primary candidate gene for PWS is the paternally expressed *SNURF-SNRPN* locus.[206,419,437] There is extensive DNA methylation at the CpG island upstream from this locus on the maternal allele resulting in transcriptional silencing of this locus. The *SNURF-SNRPN* is a complex locus that contains a *cis*-acting regulatory region referred to as the imprinting center (IC), which controls resetting of parental imprints in the 15q11-13 region during gametogenesis and two polypeptides, SmN and SNURF, and a small nucleolar RNA (snoRNA), *HBII-13*.* SmN is involved in mRNA splicing in the brain, and SNURF (*SNRPN* Upstream Reading Frame) is found in the nucleus, contains 71 amino acids, may bind RNA, and has a C-terminal motif similar to ubiquitin. HBII-13 is encoded from within intron 12 of SNURF and modifies RNA, perhaps mRNA and rRNA and snRNA. In addition, multiple imprinted and paternal-only expressed genes have also been identified in this region including *NDN,* which encodes necdin, a protein important for neuronal differentiation and a suppressor for cell proliferation; *IPW,* which encodes a 2.2 kb RNA but is not translated into a polypeptide; *MKRN3,* which encodes makorin ring zinc-finger protein 3; and *MAGEL2,* which encodes melanoma antigen-like gene 2.[295,328,406,624] These expressed genes may have additive roles in the phenotype of PWS.[420] The loss of normally expressed paternal genes in 15q11-q13 resulting in PWS can occur by several mechanisms. Most commonly, PWS (65% to 70%) results from a de novo deletion encompassing this area following unequal homologous recombination involving repeated homologous sequences in this region. The subsequent zygote would be monosomic for these genes by possessing only the maternal copy. Alternatively, 25% to 30% of PWS is caused by uniparental disomy.

*References 62, 103, 214, 431, 501, 559.

In this scenario, although two copies of the genes located in 15q11-q13 exist, both are maternal in origin, arising in most cases from meiosis I nondisjunction and subsequent loss of the third, paternal-derived chromosome 15 through mitotic loss postzygotically. This mechanism of chromosome loss rescues the zygote from trisomy 15, a condition that is incompatible with life.[486] Although in this situation the fetus is genetically complete with two chromosome 15s (disomy), both chromosomes are, however, from the same parent (uniparental) with a loss of paternal-expressed loci in the critical imprinted region 15q11-q13. In about 5% of cases, PWS can result from microdeletions encompassing the paternal IC. Or in some cases, there is no detectable DNA mutation, but rather there is an abnormal imprint.[86-87] A microdeletion containing the IC prevents this *cis*-acting control center from resetting the imprint in the germline. These mutations, if present on the maternal chromosome of phenotypically normal fathers, will be transmitted to offspring as the paternal chromosome and result in a child with PWS. Lastly, less than 1% of PWS cases are caused by chromosomal rearrangements disrupting the genes in the 15q11-q13 region.[557]

The primary maternally expressed gene in the PWS and/or AS critical region is *UBE3A,* although a second gene, *ATP10C,* has been shown to display predominantly maternal expression in brain and lymphocytes.[304,374] The *UBE3A* gene is almost exclusively expressed in the brain, contains 16 exons, and encodes an E3 ubiquitin ligase involved in the ubiquitination pathway for degradation of a diverse range of protein substrates.[260] The lack of ubiquitination could result in the inability to degrade or functionally alter targeted proteins. Similar to PWS, 70% of AS patients have a deletion of the critical 15q11-q13 region. However, unlike PWS in which a deletion on the paternal allele causes PWS, in AS a deletion encompassing this region on the maternal chromosome 15 yields the clinically distinct AS phenotype. Recently an inversion mutation was identified in the mother of four of six AS patients with a deletion in this region.[203] It is likely that the presence of these inverted DNA sequences in these women predisposed this region to deletions in their offspring by interfering with normal homologous synapses, or pairing of homologous chromosomes, during meiosis. AS patients with a deletion have a more severe phenotype possibly because of haploinsufficiency of nonimprinted *UBE3A* adjacent and co-deleted genes. In 7% of AS patients, phenotypic expression of the syndrome occurs as a result of uniparental disomy because of the inheritance of two copies of a paternal chromosome 15 in contrast to the normal inheritance of one paternal and one maternal allele. As a consequence, with both paternal *UBE3A* genes silenced, there is no functional UBE3A protein. In 3% of AS patients, an imprinting defect has been described.[86,270] A cytogenetic rearrangement has been detected in about 1% of AS cases, and in 11% of cases, a mutation in the *UBE3A* gene itself has been reported.[164] Although these mutations can arise de novo, they can be silently transmitted through several generations. For example, if a *UBE3A* mutation rose de novo on a paternal allele transmitted to a son, the son could transmit the mutation to a son or daughter to result in a normal phenotype. However, although this son could again transmit the silenced *UBE3A* mutation to his offspring, his sister could donate her mutated *UBE3A* paternally derived allele to her offspring, and the child would have AS. Lastly, in about 11% of AS patients, the etiology of the disease has not been established.

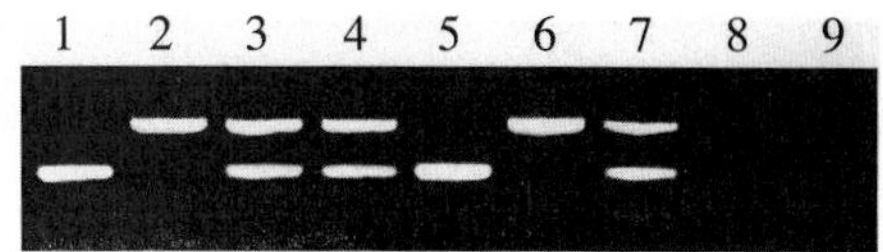

Figure 40-10 Methylation-specific PCR assay for the diagnosis of PWS and AS. Extracted DNA is treated with sodium bisulfate before amplification using multiplex PCR and oligonucleotide primers specific for modified DNA.[482] Normal individuals show amplicons representing their methylated maternal allele and amplicons from their unmethylated paternal allele. PWS patients show only the maternal allele and AS patients show only the paternal allele. Results observed following PCR amplification and gel electrophoresis of patients referred for PWS and AS testing. Patient DNA with patterns diagnostic of AS *(lanes 1 and 5),* PWS *(lanes 2 and 6),* and patients referred for AS or PWS but who have normal methylation patterns *(lanes 3 and 4)* are shown. Normal control DNA patterns and a negative control reaction in which no template DNA was added are indicated in lanes 7 and 8, respectively. No amplification products are observed in unmodified normal control DNA *(lane 9),* illustrating the specificity of the PCR primers specifically for sodium bisulfate modified DNA. *(Figure courtesy of Jack Tarleton, Ph.D., Director of Genetics Laboratory, Fullerton Genetics Center, Mission Hospitals, Asheville, N.C.)*

Diagnostic testing for individuals suspected of having AS or PWS can involve a variety of methodologies.[13] Further, determining the genetic mechanism for the cause of the disease is important for determining recurrence risks for the family.[89] Under most circumstances, initiating testing with methylation-specific PCR (mPCR) is one scenario that can be used and may be the most cost-effective approach[386] (Figure 40-10). In methylation-specific PCR, genomic DNA is treated with sodium bisulfite before PCR to convert unmethylated cytosine residues to uracil without altering the methylated cytosine residues (those silenced in the 15q11-13 region). The subsequent PCR reactions use oligonucleotide primers specific to DNA strands that contain either uracil (unmethylated) or cytosine (methylated).[312,603] Methylation-specific PCR provides a rapid and reliable diagnostic test to rule out PWS or AS. If the result is negative, >99% of PWS and about 80% of AS patients can be ruled out. PWS patients with a chromosomal rearrangement disrupting the genes in this area will not be identified by this test. Similarly, AS patients with a *UBE3A* mutation, a chromosome rearrangement disrupting the genes in the region, or AS resulting from an unknown etiology will not be diagnosed with this

TABLE 40-2 Molecular Mechanisms and Tests for Prader-Willi and Angelman Syndromes*

Molecular Mechanism	Angelman Syndrome (Frequency)	Prader-Willi Syndrome (Frequency)	Methylation-Specific PCR Result	Possible Detection Methods
Deletion (~4 Mb) of chromosome 15q11-13	70% (maternal)	65%-70% (paternal)	Abnormal	High-resolution cytogenetics or FISH
Uniparental disomy	7% (paternal)	25%-30% (maternal)	Abnormal	PCR for microsatellite analysis
Imprinting center defect	3%	~5%	Abnormal	IC sequencing
UBE3A mutation (specific to AS)	11%	N/A	Normal	UBE3A sequencing
Chromosomal rearrangement in chromosome 15q11-13 region	<1% (maternal)	<1% (paternal)	Normal	High-resolution cytogenetics or FISH
No detectable abnormality	~11%	Very few cases	Normal	N/A

*Modified from a table prepared by Allison Presley, MD, University of Virginia.

methodology. However, if the result is positive, FISH studies can be performed to detect a deletion within 15q11-13, and/or uniparental disomy DNA testing should be done to determine the genetic mechanism of disease for appropriate genetic counseling of the family. The mechanisms and tests for PWS and AS are summarized and contrasted in Table 40-2.

Complex Diseases

A complex or multifactorial inheritance pattern indicates interaction of one or more genes with one or more environmental factors. Multifactorial diseases can be more prevalent in some families with several affected family members, but the disease does not follow typical mendelian inheritance patterns. Disease may present in multiple family members because of the sharing of similar disease-predisposing alleles and often the sharing of similar daily habits, routines, and diet. The degree of genetic and environmental contribution to a disease process varies among complex diseases, and identification of the causative genetic and environmental factors is challenging. Further, it is difficult to assess the relative importance of genetic and environmental influences in the development of a disease, though twin studies are often used. Among twins who were raised together, a greater concordance of disease among monozygotic (MZ) twins—who share all of their genes—than in dizygotic (DZ) twins, who share 50% of their genes, provides strong evidence of a genetic component to the disease. Conversely, disease concordance <100% in MZ twins is strong evidence that nongenetic factors play a role in the disease. Examples of largely adult-onset complex diseases include type 1 diabetes, multiple sclerosis, Parkinson disease, hypertension, alcoholism, and thrombophilia.

Thrombophilia

Deep vein thrombosis (DVT) occurs in about 1 per 1000 individuals, and complications from DVT, including pulmonary embolism, account for about 50,000 deaths per year.[531] Venous thrombosis is caused by a disruption of normal hemostasis caused by the interaction of one or more genes and environmental factors and/or acquired conditions, including use of oral contraceptives, trauma, obesity, immobility, pregnancy, age, or surgery.[250] Although the protein products of many genes are involved in the anticoagulation and coagulation pathway and are involved in the regulation of hemostasis, mutations in the factor V and prothrombin genes are associated with DVT, represent the most frequent genetic cause of thrombophilia, and are common in the population.[58,457] Further, patients with both mutations have an increased risk of a recurrent DVT and may require different management than patients with only one of the two mutations.[134] Consistent with that of a complex disease, despite the presence of these mutations and some environmental and/or acquired factors, it is impossible to predict a patient's clinical course even within members of the same family. Thus venous thrombosis illustrates our lack of understanding in the interaction of known and uncharacterized risk factors in predisposition to a complex disease.

Activated protein C in conjunction with its cofactor, protein S, plays a key role in the anticoagulant system by inactivating membrane-bound factors Va and VIIIa. The inability to inactivate procoagulant factors Va or VIIIa could disturb hemostasis, heighten the coagulation pathway, increase the generation of thrombin, and promote clot formation. In 1993 Dahlback reported familial thrombophilia caused by resistance to activated protein C (APC).[129] In 1994

Bertina et al observed linkage of the factor V gene and the APC resistance phenotype and reported a G-to-A base substitution at nucleotide 1691 in exon 10 of the factor V gene.[58] This nucleotide change results in an arginine-to-glutamine substitution at codon 506 (R506Q) in the factor V protein. Cleavage at the arginine residue at codon 506 by APC is the initial step of inactivation of the activated factor V protein, causing it to display a decreased affinity for factor Xa.[128,297,358] As a result, there is reduced efficiency in catalyzing the activation of prothrombin to alpha-thrombin.[358] However, substitution with a glutamine residue at this site prolongs inactivation of this molecule by APC by approximately tenfold, thereby shifting the balance of hemostasis to favor coagulation and increasing thrombin production.[248] Interestingly, this mutation is quite common in the Caucasian population of Northern European descent, with a frequency of 3% to 5%, but is essentially absent in Asian, African, or Australian populations.[58,268,474,480] This phenomenon is thought to result from the fact that the G-to-A mutation occurred as a single event approximately 21,000 to 34,000 years ago after the evolutionary divergence of non-Africans from Africans and of Caucasians from Mongoloids.[655] Heterozygous carriers have a 7.9-fold increased relative risk of thrombosis compared with a ninety-onefold increased risk for homozygotes.[491] The risk for thrombosis is increased in the presence of other genetic or environmental and/or acquired factors.[70,162,197,362,596] The mean age of onset of symptoms associated with thrombosis is 44 years for heterozygotes and 31 years in homozygotes.[491] Further, although transmitted as a dominant trait—with carriers of this mutation possessing a lifelong risk—and because thrombophilia is a complex disease resulting from the interaction of both genetic and environmental and/or acquired factors, many heterozygote carriers can remain asymptomatic.[216,491]

In 1996 Poort et al described a genetic variant in the 3′-untranslated region of the prothrombin gene in 18% of patients with a documented family history of venous thrombosis.[457] In a population-based case control study, this common allele (G-to-A base substitution at nucleotide 20210) increased the risk of venous thrombosis 2.8-fold and was associated with increased plasma prothrombin (>1.15 kU/L). The risk of venous thrombosis is increased sixteenfold in G20210A carriers using oral contraceptives, and the risk of cerebral vein thrombosis increases 149-fold in G20210A carriers using oral contraceptives.[361-362] In the Caucasian population, this base substitution is present in 6.2% of patients with venous thrombosis compared with 2.3% of controls. This allele is thought to be largely confined to the Caucasian population, because it was not detected in 170 Japanese, nor 80 Asians, although it was reported in 1 of 256 African-American infants and 2 African-American patients with venous thrombosis.[142,185,283] Similar to the origin of factor V mutation G1691A, it is thought that the G20210A base substitution occurred as a single event after the divergence of Africans from non-Africans and of Caucasoid from Mongoloid subpopulations.[656] Prothrombin, also referred to as factor II, is the precursor of thrombin and plays a primary role in fibrin production and clot formation. The G-to-A substitution increases the processing of the 3′-end of the pre-mRNA and thus functions as a gain-of-function mutation, culminating in increased mRNA accumulation and increased synthesis of protein.[195] This aberration of RNA metabolism results in increased synthesis of prothrombin and can enhance clot formation. Note that the substitution does not change the amino acid sequence of prothrombin.

Inherited together, G1691A (factor V) and G20210A (factor II, prothrombin) convey at least a twentyfold increased risk for a venous thromboembolic event (VTE). They are commonly seen together in thrombophilia patients thus supporting the additive genetic effect associated with complex diseases.[41,101,134,160,576]

DNA testing for G1691A and G20210A in clinical laboratories is performed by any one of several methodologies with those most commonly reported being invasive cleavage of oligonucleotide probes (Invader assay), PCR coupled with restriction-endonuclease digestion and gel electrophoresis, and real-time PCR.[58,238,327,457,627] Many other techniques have been described.[33,67,150,256,443] Any testing platform is acceptable for clinical use as long as the procedure has been properly validated in the laboratory and follows appropriate quality assurance guidelines.[221] Standards for reporting of molecular diagnostic tests have been published as well, but many laboratories reporting factor V mutation results do not follow these guidelines.[17,410]

DNA-based testing for factor V may be requested on a patient following the factor V Leiden-specific functional assay (Coatest APC resistance, Chromogenix AB, Sweden) to confirm the diagnosis and to distinguish between heterozygotes and homozygotes. Similarly, DNA testing can be ordered in place of the functional assay especially for patients with lupus anticoagulant and a markedly prolonged baseline aPTT (which may interfere with the assay), or in family members of G1691A-positive patients.[648] Since there may be multiple causes of a thrombotic event, factor V and prothrombin testing is especially recommended in patients in whom a high clinical suspicion exists, such as patients with: (1) venous thrombosis or pulmonary embolism and age under 50; (2) venous thrombosis at an unusual site (hepatic, mesenteric, portal, or cerebral veins); (3) recurrent VTE; (4) VTE and a strong family history of thrombotic disease; (5) VTE in pregnant women or women taking oral contraceptives; or (6) relatives who had VTE at age less than 50 years.[221,367,462]

Benefits from DNA testing include the identification of individuals at risk for recurrent events, especially in situations that predispose to thrombosis, such as oral contraceptive use, management of pregnancy complications, or hormone replacement therapy.[135,462] In addition, DNA testing enables the identification of at-risk family members. Screening is not recommended for populations or newborns nor is prenatal screening recommended. Although factor V

R506Q represents the genetic factor in thrombophilia in greater than 50% of families with thrombosis, inherited defects in protein C, protein S, and antithrombin are detectable in approximately 10% to 15% of families with venous thrombosis. These latter, less common deficiencies can be diagnosed through laboratory assays and do not typically involve DNA testing because of the heterogeneity of mutations in these genes.[43,73,476] Mutations at two other factor V arginine-cleavage sites have been reported, but these mutations are very rare and are not part of routine DNA testing in patients.[107,632]

Inherited Breast Cancer

Mutations in the two major breast cancer genes, *BRCA1* and *BRCA2*, predispose patients to breast and ovarian cancer and to prostate and colon cancer (*BRCA1*) or pancreatic cancer (*BRCA2*). The incidence of mutations in these genes within the population is estimated to be between 1 in 500 and 1 in 1000.[563] However, the combined frequency of three common mutations in the Ashkenazi Jewish population is as high as almost 3%.[483] Breast carcinoma is second only to lung carcinoma as a cause of cancer-related death among women in the Western hemisphere, but familial breast cancer accounts for only 5% to 10% of all cases. *BRCA1* and *BRCA2* mutations are present in only about 20% of familial cases and are often associated with a younger age of onset. Recent studies suggest that the progression rate of breast neoplasia is accelerated in women who carry *BRCA1* or *BRCA2* mutations compared with other patients who have breast carcinoma with or without a family history.[6] In families in which breast cancer is segregating, but no *BRCA1* or *BRCA2* mutation has been detected, additional genes that predispose to breast cancer are likely but have yet to be identified.[600] The inability to identify breast cancer susceptibility genes in these families may reflect: (1) genetic heterogeneity in the family with mutations in several genes, (2) low penetrance of these mutations, making it difficult to distinguish family members without mutation from asymptomatic carriers in the studies, (3) an autosomal recessive mode of inheritance, or (4) breast cancer acting as a complex disease that results from the interaction of both several genes and environmental factors, thereby making it difficult to tease out the genetic component of the disease. Recently developed gene-expression assays of tumor tissue may be instrumental for classification of these families into subsets, aiding studies aimed at determining the molecular origin of these cancers.[247] Mutations in tumor-suppressor genes *TP53* or *ATM* are also associated with "familial" cancer, including breast cancer in mutation-positive females.[284,334]

Mutations in *BRCA1* and *BRCA2* are inherited in an autosomal dominant fashion, with offspring of known carriers or of affected patients possessing a 50% chance of inheriting the predisposing cancer gene mutation. Inheritance of the mutation does not convey a certainty of developing cancer nor indicate the type of cancer or the age of onset.[333] The average cumulative risk of breast cancer for mutations in either BRCA1 or BRCA2 is about 27% to age 50 and 64% to age 70.[516] Both environmental and genetic factors play a role in the development of breast or other cancers in mutation-positive patients as does the type of DNA mutation in *BRCA1* or *BRCA2*.[193,407-408,516]

Using DNA linkage studies, Hall et al mapped the gene for early onset familial breast cancer to 17q21 (long arm of chromosome 17 banding region 21).[231,409] In 1994 *BRCA1* was cloned and later confirmed by several other investigators as the susceptibility gene in breast and ovarian cancer kindreds.[100,188,377] The *BRCA1* gene spans 80 kb, is composed of 24 exons, 22 encode the 7.8-kb mRNA that is translated into a protein of 1863 amino acids. The large exon 11 (3427 bp) accounts for 61% of the coding portion of the gene. In families in whom linkage to *BRCA1* was excluded, a second susceptibility locus at 13q12-13 (long arm of chromosome 13 within banding region 12 and 13), *BRCA2*, was proposed and subsequently cloned.[409,567,638-639] The *BRCA2* gene, unrelated in sequence to *BRCA1*, spans 70 kb, contains 26 exons, encodes an 11.5-kb mRNA, and is translated into a protein of 3418 amino acids. *BRCA1* and *BRCA2* are considered tumor-suppressor genes requiring inactivation of both alleles for progression to neoplasm. In a patient with familial breast cancer, a mutant allele is inherited, and the second allele—the patient's wild-type allele—is inactivated through somatic mutation. BRCA1 and BRCA2 proteins are multifunctional, interacting with numerous other proteins in complex and separate systems involved in response to DNA damage, regulation of transcription, remodeling of chromatin, and regulation of cell growth.[130,585,605]

Mutations in *BRCA1* and *BRCA2* are heterogeneous and located throughout each gene, with more than 1600 identified to date.[79,196] Interestingly the range of mutations varies greatly among different populations, with founder mutations observed in many ethnic groups.[339,413,563] In Ashkenazi Jewish breast and ovarian cancer families, mutations 185delAG and 5382insC are the ones primarily observed in *BRCA1*, and in families in whom these mutations are not present, the identification of other *BRCA1* mutations is rare.[455] In addition, *BRCA2* mutation 6174delT has been observed in 6 of 80 (8%) Ashkenazi Jewish women diagnosed with breast cancer before age 42 as compared with 0 of 93 non-Jewish women diagnosed with breast cancer at the same age.[416] *BRCA1* mutation 943ins10 is an ancient founder mutation of West African origin, and mutation 2804delAA, estimated to have occurred about 32 generations ago, is seen in Dutch and Belgian families.[369,432,445] The *BRCA2* mutation 999del5 is common in the Icelandic population, whereas the founder *BRCA2* mutations S2835X and 5802del4 are common in Japanese breast cancer families.[278,293] In contrast, *BRCA1* and *BRCA2* mutations are less commonly associated with familial breast cancer in Taiwanese and Chinese populations.[110,650]

Testing for disease-associated mutations is made difficult by the heterogeneity of disease-causing mutations and the complexity of the *BRCA1* and *BRCA2* genes. Moreover, the clinical significance of some observed variants may be unknown and in some cases may be benign.[137] Interestingly the majority of *BRCA1* and *BRCA2* disease-associated mutations result in premature truncation of the protein and thus a loss of function. For this reason, the protein truncation test (PTT) is often employed as a screening method for mutation detection. In this methodology, multiple PCR primer pairs are designed to span the gene with each primer pair, including one primer that includes an RNA polymerase promoter and a translation initiation sequence. The resulting amplicons are incubated in an in vitro translation system, and the synthesized proteins are subjected to sodium dodecyl sulfate (SDS)–polyacrylamide gel electrophoresis for detection of truncated proteins.[263]

In addition to PTT, various other screening techniques have been described to provide maximum sensitivity in mutation detection, yet high throughput of specimens. Other common screening assays include microarrays, denaturing high-performance liquid chromatography (DHPLC), single-strand conformation polymorphism (SSCP), denaturing gradient gel electrophoresis (DGGE), heteroduplex analysis (HA), and fluorescence assisted mismatch analysis (FAMA).[228,522] More recently, other unique methods have been described as well, including allele-specific gene expression analysis (AGE), multiplex ligation-dependent probe amplification (MLPA), and restriction endonuclease fingerprinting, single-strand conformation polymorphism coupled with capillary electrophoresis.[311,389-390]

Although screening assays can detect DNA perturbations, DNA sequence (DS) analysis is required for precise identification of the base or bases involved. In many instances, a combination of screening methods is used, thereby reducing the region of the gene that requires DNA sequencing analysis. In addition, since founder mutations within various populations exist, information regarding the ethnicity of the patient may be valuable in determining the strategy for analysis, employing a method to detect those mutations most common in that population. An alternative approach is to eliminate screening of the gene and rather perform direct DS analysis of the *BRCA1* and *BRCA2* genes on each specimen. A large study concluded that DS is not the most cost-effective method available for testing.[522]

Clinical testing for *BRCA1* and *BRCA2* is primarily performed on women with breast cancer and a strong family history of breast and/or ovarian cancer or on presymptomatic women with a strong family history of breast and/or ovarian cancer for which prior identification of a *BRCA1* or *BRCA2* mutation in the family may or may not have occurred. The impact of genetic testing on these patients has been well evaluated.[75,234,371] The likelihood of identifying a *BRCA1* or *BRCA2* mutation in a patient is increased to 10% or greater if: (1) breast cancer was diagnosed in two women in the family before the age of 50; (2) breast cancer was diagnosed in women in the family before age 50, and ovarian cancer was detected in one or more women in the family; (3) breast cancer was diagnosed after the age of 50 in one woman, and ovarian cancer was detected in two or more women in the family; (4) ovarian cancer is present in two or more family members; (5) male breast cancer is present, and breast or ovarian cancer is present in the family.[488]

In presymptomatic cases, extensive genetic counseling addressing both the positive and possible negative aspects of genetic testing must be discussed with the patient before genetic testing is undertaken. Counseling often involves participation of family members, usually spouses. Based on the family history, the genetic counselor should inform the patient of the likelihood that a *BRCA1* or *BRCA2* mutation could be segregating in the family, the risk of disease(s) associated with mutations, and an overview of prevention and surveillance options available for mutation carriers.[487] Counseling may be needed for psychological issues, including the fear of cancer or medical procedures, past experiences involving loved ones with cancer, feelings of guilt about possibly transmitting a cancer-causing gene to children, and discrimination by employers or insurers if a positive test result is disclosed.[74] The continued anxiety and uncertainty with some test results should be discussed as well. For example, in some instances when DNA from an affected family member is not available for testing, the presymptomatic patient must clearly understand that a negative result could imply the inability to detect the specific *BRCA1* or *BRCA2* gene mutation segregating in the family and would not exclude the possibility of a mutation in another breast cancer–susceptibility gene that may be present in the family. Further, the possibility of identifying a DNA alteration of unclear significance and the associated uncertainty and anxiety resulting from such a finding must also be discussed. A U.S. patent has resulted in clinical testing for *BRCA1* and *BRCA2* being available exclusively at one location within the United States; both false-negative test results and variants of uncertain significance are possible.[196] The absolute control of diagnostic testing of these genes for patient care is an issue of much debate.[52]

Once an asymptomatic, mutation-positive woman has been identified, she may wish to undergo prophylactic bilateral mastectomy, oophorectomy, or specialized surveillance and prevention strategies for the early detection of both breast and ovarian cancer. The risk of breast cancer can be significantly lower in women choosing prophylactic surgery than in those opting for increased surveillance.[370]

Inherited Colon Cancer

Colorectal cancer (CRC) is the second leading cause of cancer death in the United States, with about 5% of cases associated with inherited mutations linked to colon cancer syndromes. The molecular basis of sporadic and inherited CRC involves two distinct pathways, one of chromosomal instability and one associated with microsatellite instability. The original model of chromosome instability proposed in 1990 to explain the pathogenesis of most sporadic tumors (~85%) has been further characterized to reveal a complex chain of events whereby normal colon lining (mucosa) is transformed

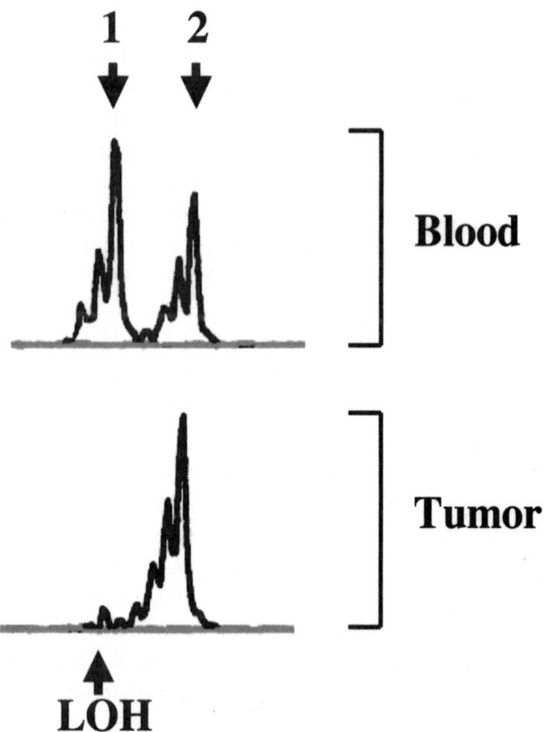

Figure 40-11 Electropherograms illustrating loss of heterozygosity (LOH) in tumor DNA. Patient DNA is extracted from the peripheral blood and tumor tissue and amplified by PCR using an oligonucleotide primer pair specific for a polymorphic, microsatellite repeat locus contained within the chromosomal region thought to be deleted during tumorigenesis. One of the primers within the pair is labeled with a fluorescent dye. Amplicons are subjected to electrophoresis on a 5% denaturing polyacrylamide gel in an ABI DNA sequencer and analyzed using GeneScan software 3.1 b3. Constitutive DNA from the patient's blood illustrates heterozygosity for this marker with amplicons represented by alleles 1 and 2. In DNA from the tumor, a single peak representing a typical homozygous pattern is observed. Thus there is LOH in tumor DNA. This loss signifies the loss of the second allele and also indicates the loss of this region on the chromosome. (See Color Plate 10.)

into adenomatous and then into malignant mucosa via the inactivation of tumor-suppressor genes and the activation of genes involved in tumor cell proliferation.[96,171]

The *chromosomal instability (CIN) pathway* begins with the loss of function of the adenomatous polyposis coli (*APC*) tumor-suppressor gene product, most often because of a somatic inactivating gene mutation on one allele followed by a chromosomal deletion encompassing the second *APC* allele and adjacent flanking DNA on chromosome 5q (Figure 40-11 and Color Plate 10). Since *APC* is involved early in the tumorigenic process, it has been referred to as the "gatekeeper."[303] The cascade of events proceeds with continued activation of the *KRAS* (Kirsten rat sarcoma virus) proto-oncogene on 12p12.1 (short arm of chromosome 12 banding region 12.1) through somatic gene mutations (most frequently occurring in codons 12, 13, or 61), which in the presence of *APC* inactivation increases growth and proliferation of the cell.[409] Subsequent inactivation of the tumor-suppressor gene *DCC* (deleted in colon cancer) and frequent loss of adjacent tumor-suppressor genes on 18q (long arm of chromosome 18) including SMAD4 and SMAD and the inactivation of tumor-suppressor gene *TP53* on 17p (short arm of chromosome 17) are identified in late adenoma and carcinoma.[409]

The *microsatellite instability (MSI) pathway* in sporadic CRC arises from mutations or altered expression of genes involved in DNA mismatch repair (MMR)[255,381,528] (Figure 40-12 and Color Plate 11). As a result of an altered and thus dysfunctional MMR system, DNA replication errors, primarily within microsatellite repeats or repetitive sequences, remain uncorrected and accumulate. Although expansion or contraction of the microsatellite-repeat number is of little significance in much of the noncoding areas of the genome, changes within coding regions of the genome and specifically within genes involved in cell growth and regulation can alter the sequences of their protein products and thus affect their function.

Inherited CRC syndromes initiate as a result of an inherited mutation in one of the genes involved in the CIN or MSI pathway. Although several CRC syndromes exist, the two most common are familial adenomatous polyposis (FAP) and hereditary nonpolyposis colorectal cancer (HNPCC).[170,286] Most interestingly, tumors in FAP kindreds and tumors displaying CIN more frequently are found in the distal part of the colon, whereas tumors in HNPCC families and tumors displaying MSI more commonly occur in the proximal part of the colon.[277]

FAP, characterized by hundreds to thousands of adenomatous polyps throughout the large bowel, is inherited in an autosomal dominant fashion. Penetrance is 80% to 100%, and the estimated incidence is 1 in 8000.[66] FAP accounts for less than 1% of CRC observed in the United States. In about 25% of cases no family history exists, indicating that these cases arise as a result of a new mutation; there is no tendency for paternal versus maternal origin of the mutated allele.[66,482] Polyps first appear during the second decade of life.[452] CRC ultimately develops approximately 10 to 15 years after the onset of polyposis, with the median age of CRC in untreated FAP patients being about 40.[66,452] Although an individual polyp is no more likely to progress to cancer than a sporadic polyp, it is the sheer number of polyps in these patients that increases the likelihood that one will progress to cancer. Further, patients with FAP are at increased risk for developing cancer of the thyroid, small intestine, stomach, and brain.[170] The gene responsible for FAP, the *APC* gene, was ultimately cloned in 1991 following linkage to chromosome 5q21 (long arm of chromosome band 21) in FAP kindreds in 1987.[68,219,302,409,423] The *APC* gene spans 8535 base pairs, contains 15 exons, and encodes a protein of 2843 amino acids with a molecular weight of about 312 kD. The APC protein is a multidomain, multifunctional protein, partici-

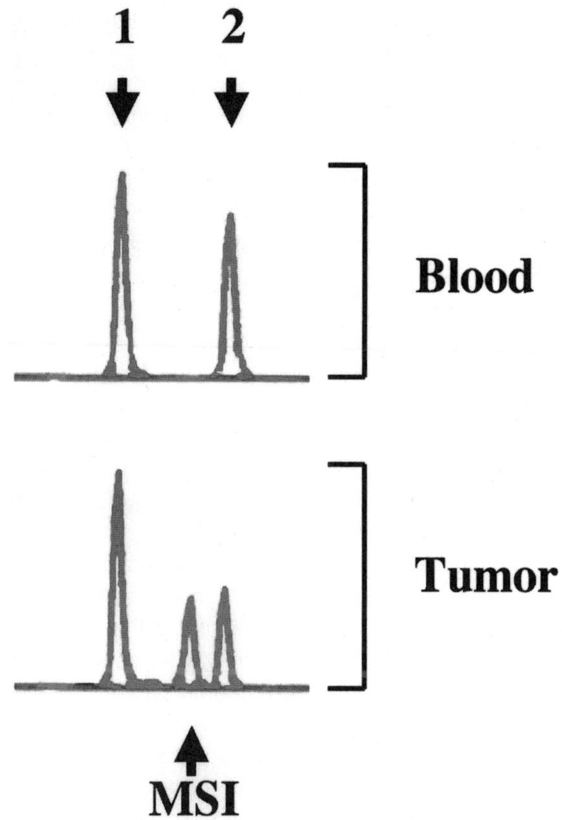

Figure 40-12 Electropherograms illustrating MSI in tumor DNA. Patient DNA is extracted from the peripheral blood and tumor tissue and amplified by PCR using an oligonucleotide primer pair specific for a microsatellite repeat locus. One of the primers within the pair is labeled with a fluorescent dye. Amplicons are subjected to electrophoresis on a 5% denaturing polyacrylamide gel in an ABI DNA sequencer and analyzed by GeneScan software 3.1 b3. Constitutive DNA from the patient's blood illustrates heterozygosity for this marker with amplicons represented by alleles 1 and 2. In DNA from the tumor, in addition to constitutive alleles 1 and 2, amplicons representing DNA fragments of a different size are present; these indicate a change in repeat number for one of the alleles. Because of dysfunctional MMR enzymes, mistakes occurring during the replication of microsatellite repeat sequences resulting in expansions or contractions of the repeat number remain unrepaired. In this case, a contraction in the repeat number of allele 2 has occurred. (See Color Plate 11.)

pating in several cellular processes, including cell adhesion and migration, signal transduction, microtubule assembly, and chromosome segregation. Best understood is the regulation of β-catenin levels through interaction with APC. β-catenin is required for binding with E-cadherin, a member of the calcium-dependent cell adhesion molecules, and is also involved in signal transduction pathways.[63,182] Mutations altering the association of β-catenin with APC minimize degradation and increase cytoplasmic levels of β-catenin; this can affect cell-cell adhesion and the transcription of genes, promoting cell proliferation (specifically *CMYC*) or inhibition of cell death.[245,395]

Studies on FAP families indicate that a wide variety of germline mutations exist; >95% result in truncated proteins, either because of a nonsense mutation (30%) or by a frameshift mutation, and most are contained within the 5′-half of the gene.[56] In germline mutations there are two hot spots at codons 1061 and 1309, with the most common mutation being an AAAAG deletion at codon 1309. These mutations leave the truncated APC protein unable to regulate β-catenin.

Genotype-phenotype correlations exist for some *APC* mutations. Patients with truncating mutations at the extreme 5′-end of the gene (codons 1 to 163) or mutations at the carboxyl-terminal end of the gene (codons 1860 to 1987) have the attenuated form of the disease, developing a smaller number of polyps (<100).* A severe phenotype is observed in patients with mutations between codons 1250 and 1464, and patients with truncating mutations between codons 1403 and 1578 are at an increased risk for extracolonic disease.[145,404] Intrafamilial and interfamilial phenotypic variability exists even in the presence of an identical mutation and may be explained by a modifier gene or genes.[122,199] The site of the inherited germline mutation appears to influence the type of somatic inactivating mutation occurring at their normal *APC* gene.[322] If the germline mutation occurs between codons 1194 and 1392, the second hit to the normal allele is likely a deletion encompassing the *APC* allele. However, if the germline mutation is outside this region, the second hit will likely result in a truncating mutation within the mutation cluster region (MCR) between codons 1286 and 1513.[322,382]

The PTT is most often used to test for mutations in a family because the majority of FAP mutations result in a truncated protein. Once a possible mutation has been detected, the region is sequenced to determine the precise identity of the mutation.[204,460] Other screening or direct detection methodologies can be used, and collectively a sensitivity of about 87% can be achieved.[359,429] If the mutation within the family can be identified, it is recommended that the family be referred for genetic counseling. DNA testing should be performed in at-risk family members as young as 10 to 12 years of age.[198] Genetic testing can significantly alter the 50% pretest risk for disease to a risk of 0% or 100%. Although DNA testing on an asymptomatic minor is typically not endorsed by the genetic community, in this scenario, early identification of the mutation in these patients will clearly impact their clinical management by initiating intense screening programs and possible prophylactic colectomy in that decade. Family members testing negative for the mutation do not have an increased risk of CRC and can avoid intensive screening programs. Further, in some FAP mutation–positive families, preimplantation genetic diagnosis has been successfully employed to prevent the birth of a child with an inherited predisposition to FAP.[473]

*References 80, 169, 187, 530, 542, 593, 618.

If the mutation in the family cannot be identified, DNA linkage studies may be useful for presymptomatic identification of at-risk family members. If the mutation in the family cannot be identified and if DNA linkage studies are not informative or available, screening is recommended with yearly sigmoidoscopy as early as age 12. Further, when repeatedly negative sigmoidoscopy results are found, the frequency of such exams can be reduced in each subsequent decade of life.

The most common inherited CRC susceptibility syndrome is HNPCC, which represents about 2% to 3% of all CRC cases. In contrast to FAP, HNPCC is characterized by a few polyps that possess an accelerated transformation potential to carcinoma in as little as 1 to 2 years. HNPCC is inherited as an autosomal dominant disorder with a penetrance of 80% to 85%. HNPCC is sometimes also referred to as Lynch syndrome for Dr. Lynch's observation of an autosomal dominant predisposition to early onset CRC of proximal involvement and cancers of other organs in two large Midwestern kindreds.[350] HNPCC patients have a lifetime risk of 70% to 80% for developing CRC, thereby suggesting a role for other factors in this disease process.[224] To assist clinicians in identifying patients in HNPCC kindreds and to help standardize the ascertainment and study of these families, the International Collaborative Group on HNPCC developed the Amsterdam criteria (AC) in 1991.[597] Basically the criteria for inclusion as an HNPCC family included at least three affected members spanning two successive generations with the diagnosis of colon cancer before the age of 50. In addition, one affected individual must be a first-degree relative of two other individuals, and because this mode of inheritance is consistent with autosomal dominant, the diagnosis of FAP must be excluded. Because some HNPCC families were excluded by these stringent criteria, and these criteria did not account for the risk to these patients for cancers of other organs as well, an expanded, more inclusive set of criteria was subsequently developed in Bethesda in 1998 and as the Amsterdam criteria II in 1999.[71,598] The expanded definition would also include a kindred with multiple family members affected with HNPCC-associated cancers of the endometrium, ovary, stomach, hepatobiliary system, small bowel, ureter, or renal pelvis with a diagnosis before age 45 and demonstrating autosomal dominant transmission between two generations. In addition, if an individual has endometrial cancer or CRC before age 45 (which is about 30 years earlier than that seen in the general population) or a colorectal adenoma diagnosed before 40 years of age, or if an individual has two HNPCC-related cancers, including synchronous and metachronous CRC or associated extracolonic cancer, the patient could meet the criteria as a possible HNPCC patient.

Mutations in six mismatch repair genes have now been linked to HNPCC. The first was mapped to 2p15-16 using large HNPCC kindreds.[447] Simultaneously, MSI was noted in a subset of sporadic CRC.[281,569] Concurrently in yeast genetics, Strand et al reported that mutations in three yeast genes involved in DNA MMR led to 100-fold to 700-fold increases in mutations in simple repetitive sequences and postulated that the human homologues of these genes may be involved in HNPCC.[546] One such gene, *hMSH2,* mapped to 2p15-16 and in fact was found to be altered in HNPCC kindreds.[179,324] Subsequently, mutations in genes *hMSH6* (2p15-16), *hMLH1* (3p21), *hPMS1* (2q31), *hPMS2* (7p22), and *hMLH3* (14q24.3) have been identified in HNPCC families, although more than 90% of HNPCC mutations are observed in *hMSH2* and *hMLH1.*[82,380,421,640]

HNPCC mutations are diverse and are located throughout these genes.[448] Almost all errors made during DNA replication are repaired through the proofreading 3′-to-5′ exonuclease activity of DNA polymerase. Uncorrected errors of mismatched bases between the two strands are repaired before cell division through the MMR proteins.[292] In addition to the repair of a mismatched base pair, the MMR system repairs "loop outs" from unmatched bases that can occur during the replication of a microsatellite or small repetitive sequences. In the case of HNPCC, a germline mutation in one of the six known MMR genes is inherited, causing one allele to be nonfunctional. In the tumor tissue of these patients, the second allele has been rendered inactive through a second mutational hit. Uncorrected somatic replication errors thus accumulate both within noncoding and insignificant locations throughout the genome and in coding regions of genes involved in cell growth and signaling and in DNA of other genes involved in DNA repair. Some targeted genes with repetitive sequences in their coding regions that have been shown to be altered in patients with MSI include transforming growth factor B type II receptor (tumor suppressor), insulin-like growth factor II receptor (tumor suppressor), *BAX* (promotes apoptosis), and *hMSH6* and *hMSH3.*[8,446,469,541]

MSI is identified in 90% of HNPCC-related CRC as opposed to only 15% to 20% of sporadic CRC.[1] MSI in sporadic CRC is attributed to inactivation of gene expression of *hMLH1* through biallelic methylation rather than as somatic mutations or loss of heterozygosity (LOH) as seen in HNPCC-related CRC.[313,601] Further, patients whose tumors demonstrate MSI have better survival and better response to chemotherapy than those whose tumors do not express MSI.[159,233] No association between tumor MSI and survival was seen, however, in young patients under the age of 30.[166]

Testing of tumor tissue for MSI (see Figure 40-12) is the initial laboratory step in investigation of HNPCC patients because MSI is a measure of MMR deficiency and indicates probable defects in MMR genes through germline and somatic changes. International guidelines for analysis of MSI in CRC recommend a panel of five markers: BAT25, BAT26, D5S346, D2S123, and D17S250.[71] MSI is characterized by the expansion or contraction of DNA sequences through the insertion or deletion of repeated sequences. If MSI is detected at two or more of the five loci, the tumor has a "high" frequency of MSI. If MSI is detected at one locus, the tumor has a "low" frequency of MSI. If MSI is not detected at any locus, the tumor is considered to be microsatellite stable.

If the family history supports the diagnosis of HNPCC and if MSI is confirmed in the tumor, DNA from the patient's blood can be referred for testing to identify the germline mutation that could be segregating in the family. Since most mutations occur in genes *MLH1* or *MSH2*, DNA sequence analysis of these genes is most often used and is considered the gold standard but is expensive. Since many mutations result in prematurely truncated proteins, PTT is sometimes used as an initial screening tool. However, optimal mutation detection in HNPCC can be achieved only by combining expert clinical selection of families with an extensive strategy to detect mutations.[613]

If a mutation is identified, at-risk adult family members could pursue presymptomatic testing if desired and if appropriate genetic counseling is supplied.[96] Similar to presymptomatic testing for other adult-onset disorders, the counseling session should include verification of the family history and discussion of the clinical course of the disease, including risks of developing the disease and issues in disease management. Discussions should be incorporated into the session, including how the patient will act upon both positive and negative results, feelings of survivor guilt or stigmatization, and the possibility of discrimination for insurance and employment. If a germline mutation is detected, a colonoscopy should be performed every 1 or 2 years or 5 years younger than the youngest age of diagnosis in the family.[411] Further, because of the high incidence of endometrial cancer associated with HNPCC, at-risk women in the family should be screened for endometrial cancer annually with endometrial aspiration biopsy and transvaginal ultrasound beginning at age 25.[91] Alternatively, if genetic testing is not pursued, relatives should begin an intensive screening program with a colonoscopy every 1 to 2 years starting between 20 and 30 years of age and then annually after age 40. If no mutation is detected in the proband, presymptomatic DNA testing for family members is not recommended. Some testing strategies may result in false-negative results caused by the inability of the assays employed to identify all mutations at these loci. However, some mutation-negative families may have germline mutations in other, yet unknown MMR genes.[289] Although detection of a mutation in a family that meets HNPCC criteria is not always possible, careful surveillance of at-risk family members in mutation-negative families is also considered critical.

REPORTING OF TEST RESULTS

As the preceding pages make clear, DNA testing for inherited diseases is complex, and it is most important to convey the results of a genetic test thoroughly. Results must be presented in a manner that can be easily and accurately understood by a professional whose expertise is not genetics because, in many instances, primary care givers will be communicating the test results to the patient. Unfortunately, however, with the increasing clinical demand for genetic testing and the increasing number of laboratories performing such tests, uniformity in communicating these complex results to referring clinicians does not exist.[17] The Molecular Pathology Laboratory Inspection Checklist of the College of American Pathologists (CAP) indicates that failure to include pertinent information within the patient report constitutes a deficiency.[507]

Based upon the CAP guidelines, a comprehensive genetic report should include the patient's name; medical record number and/or birth date; sex; ethnicity (if relevant); type of specimen and date received; specimen's laboratory identification number; laboratory test requested; name and address of laboratory performing the test; name and address of referring physician, hospital, or genetic counselor; date of report; brief interpretation of the results; and a descriptive comments section explaining the test results. Although preparation of the comments can be labor intensive, the comment section is vital to a genetic report and should include the following: (1) brief clinical history of patient (indicating the reason for referral); (2) detailed explanation of the methodology (citing literature if possible); (3) description of the patient's results; (4) sensitivity and specificity of the assay (e.g., number of mutations analyzed, percentage of mutations not detected, possibility of genetic heterogeneity, and chance of genetic recombination); (5) clinical significance of the results (e.g., recurrence risk, genotype-phenotype correlation or penetrance, with citations of literature if possible); and (6) statement that genetic counseling for the patient is recommended to discuss the implications of the results for the health and management of the patient and, when mutations are identified, to inform the patient of the potential risk of the disease to other family members.

Because many assays performed in clinical DNA laboratories have been developed by the laboratory or use commercially available "analyte specific reagents" (ASR) that are not approved by the U.S. Food and Drug Administration (FDA), reports in the United States often must include a disclaimer that states, "This test was developed and its performance characteristics determined by (laboratory name). It has not been cleared or approved by the U.S. Food and Drug Administration."[215] In addition, the CAP recommends the additional statements: "The FDA has determined that such clearance or approval is not necessary. This test is used for clinical purposes. It should not be regarded as investigational or for research. This laboratory is certified under the Clinical Laboratory Improvement Amendments of 1988 (CLIA-88) as qualified to perform high complexity clinical laboratory testing."[507] Lastly the report should be reviewed and signed by the laboratory director.

GLOSSARY

Allele—An alternative form of a gene found at a specific location on a chromosome.

Crossover—See "Recombination."

Diploid—Having a full set of (paired) chromosomes (46 chromosomes in humans, half from each parent).

DNA marker—A polymorphic locus that is easily assayed, yielding reproducible results.

DNA methylation—The addition of a methyl residue to the 5 position of the pyrimidine ring of a cytosine base to form 5-methylcytosine and most often occurring at CpG DNA sequences. DNA methylation can serve as a mode of gene regulation by preventing gene transcription.

Downstream—A DNA sequence located 3′ to another DNA sequence.

Gene deletion—A circumstance in which all or part of a gene is lost.

Gene dosage—The number of copies of a particular gene. In most cases, there are two copies of each gene, thereby producing a fixed amount of the protein product from that gene. In situations in which more or fewer copies of the gene are present, ultimately, an increase or decrease in the protein product occurs.

Gene duplication—A condition in which all or part of a gene is repeated.

Gene inversion—A rearrangement of the gene or part of the gene causing the orientation of the DNA sequences in the gene to be reversed in relation to the flanking chromosomal DNA sequences.

Haploid—Having a single set of chromosomes, as in gametes (eggs and sperm) (i.e., half the number of chromosomes in a mature somatic cell).

Linkage disequilibrium—The occurrence of two alleles from two loci inherited together on a chromosome more frequently than predicted by chance.

Linkage studies—A method using DNA markers physically adjacent to (i.e., "linked") to a disease gene. Through this "indirect" analysis, the disease gene can be tracked through a family to determine the disease status of at-risk individuals without requiring knowledge of the diseasing-causing mutation segregating in the family.

Meiosis—The two-step process of cell division that produces gametes (ova in females and sperm in males) with one half the number of chromosomes of the parent cell. Contrast with mitosis.

Mitosis—Process of cell division that produces daughter cells that are genetically identical to the parent cell with the same number of chromosomes as the parent cell. Contrast with meiosis.

Haploinsufficiency—In the presence of a loss-of-function DNA mutation, the remaining normal allele is unable to produce sufficient quantities of the specific gene's protein product, and disease results.

Homologous sequences—DNA sequences that share a similar order of DNA bases. If two sequences are 95% homologous, 95% of their bases are identical at a particular location.

Microsatellite repeat markers—Highly polymorphic DNA sequences of short repeats generally comprising <6 bases. These repeats are widely prevalent in both coding and noncoding regions of the human genome.

Nondisjunction—Failure of chromosomes to separate during cell division.

Penetrance—The percentage of individuals who carry the disease genotype and have symptoms of the disease. Complete penetrance implies that all individuals who possess the abnormal allele will develop the disease, whereas incomplete or reduced penetrance indicates that not all individuals who have the disease allele will become symptomatic. Incomplete penetrance of a disease suggests that other genetic loci and/or environmental factors can influence or modify the pathogenesis of the disease.

Primer—A short oligonucleotide designed to anneal to single-stranded DNA and from which DNA polymerase can add deoxynucleotide triphosphate (dNTPs) in a complementary fashion to the template DNA. A primer pair flanks the target DNA to be amplified in PCR and creates the specificity of the reaction.

Recombination—Crossing over between DNA sequences resulting in the exchange of information between two alleles. This process occurs in meiosis between homologous chromosomes and during mitosis between sister chromatids. Homologous recombination refers to this process when it occurs between similar sequences in corresponding regions. Crossing over between misaligned yet similar sequences is called unequal homologous recombination and results in a duplication on one allele and the reciprocal deletion on the alternate allele.

Restriction fragment length polymorphism—A polymorphism in the DNA sequence that either creates or destroys a restriction endonuclease recognition site thereby enabling detection by altering base-pair lengths of digested DNA fragments.

Skewed X-inactivation (lyonization)—A process by which inactivation of the X chromosome is not random.

REFERENCES

1. Aaltonen LA, Salovaara R, Kristo P, Canzian F, Hemminki A, Peltomaki P, et al. Incidence of hereditary nonpolyposis colorectal cancer and the feasibility of molecular screening for the disease. N Engl J Med 1998;338:1481-7.
2. Abitbol M, Menini C, Delezoide AL, Rhyner T, Vekemans M, Mallet J. Nucleus basalis magnocellularis and hippocampus are the major sites of FMR-1 expression in the human fetal brain. Nature Genet 1993;4:147-52.
3. Abbs S, Roberts RG, Mathew CG, Bentley DR, Bobrow M. Accurate assessment of intragenic recombination frequency within the Duchenne muscular dystrophy gene. Genomics 1990;7:602-6.
4. Acton JD, Wilmott RW. Phenotype of CF and the effects of possible modifier genes. Paediatr Respir Rev 2001;2:332-9.

5. Adams PC, Chakrabarti S. Genotypic/phenotypic correlations in genetic hemochromatosis: evolution of diagnostic criteria. Gastroenterology 1998;114: 319-23.
6. Adem C, Reynolds C, Soderberg CL, Slezak JM, McDonnell SK, Sebo TJ, et al. Pathologic characteristics of breast parenchyma in patients with hereditary breast carcinoma, including BRCA1 and BRCA2 mutation carriers. Cancer 2003;97:1-11.
7. Akagi M, Inui K, Tsukamoto H, Sakai N, Muramatsu T, Yamada M, et al. A point mutation of mitochondrial ATPase 6 gene in Leigh syndrome. Neuromus Dis 2002;12:53-5.
8. Akiyama Y, Iwanaga R, Saitoh K, Shiba K, Ushio K, Ikeda E, et al. Transforming growth factor B type II receptor gene mutations in adenomas from hereditary nonpolyposis colorectal cancer. Gastroenterology 1997;112:33-9.
9. Almqvist E, Adam S, Bloch M, Fuller A, Welch P, Eisenberg D, et al. Risk reversals in predictive testing for Huntington disease. Am J Hum Genet 1997;61:945-52.
10. Almqvist EW, Bloch M, Brinkman R, Craufurd D, Hayden MR, et al. A worldwide assessment of the frequency of suicide, suicide attempts, or psychiatric hospitalization after predictive testing for Huntington disease. Am J Hum Genet 1999;64:1293-1304.
11. The American College of Medical Genetics/American Society of Human Genetics Huntington Disease Genetic Testing Working Group. ACMG/ASHG Statement: Laboratory guidelines for Huntington disease genetic testing. Am J Hum Genet 1998;62: 1243-7.
12. The American College of Obstetricians and Gynecologists. Preconception and prenatal carrier screening for CF: clinical and laboratory guidelines. 2001 (http//www.acog.org).
13. The American Society of Human Genetics and American College of Medical Genetics. Test and Technology Transfer committee. ASHG/ACMG Report. Diagnostic testing for Prader-Willi and Angelman syndromes: report of the ASHG/ACMG test and technology transfer committee. Am J Hum Genet 1996;58:1085-88.
14. Ames BN, Shigenaga MK, Hagen TM. Oxidants, antioxidants, and the degenerative diseases of aging. Proc Natl Acad Sci USA 1993;90:7915-22.
15. Anderson MP, Berger HA, Rich DP, Gregory RJ, Smith AE, Welsh MJ. Nucleoside triphosphates are required to open the CFTR chloride channel. Cell 1991;67:775-84.
16. Anderson S, Bankier AT, Barrell BG, et al. Sequence and organization of the human mitochondrial genome. Nature 1981;290:457-65.
17. Andersson HC, Krousel-Wood MA, Jackson KE, Rice J, Lubin IM. Medical genetic test reporting for cystic fibrosis (deltaF508) and factor V Leiden in North American laboratories. Genet Med 2002;4:324-7.
18. Andreu AL, Marti R, Hirano M. Analysis of human mitochondrial DNA mutations. Methods Molec Biol 2003;217:185-97.
19. Andrew SE, Goldberg YP, Kremer B, Telenius H, Theilmann J, Adam S, et al. The relationship between trinucleotide (CAG) repeat length and clinical features of Huntington's disease. Nat Genet 1993;4: 398-403.
20. Andrew SE, Goldberg YP, Theilmann J, Zeisier J, Hayden MR. A CGG repeat polymorphism adjacent to the CAG repeat in the Huntington disease gene: implications for diagnostic accuracy and predictive testing. Hum Molec Genet 1994;3:65-7.
21. Antonarakis S. Molecular genetics of coagulation factor VIII gene and hemophilia A. Thromb Haemost 1995;74:322-8.
22. Antonarakis SE, Rossiter JP, Young M, Horst J, de Moerloose P, Sommer SS, et al. Factor VIII inversions in severe hemophilia A: results from an international consortium. Blood 1995;86:2206-12.
23. Antonarakis SE, Waber PG, Kittur SD, Patel AS, Kazazian HH, Mellis MA, et al. Hemophilia A: detection of molecular defects and of carriers by DNA analysis. N Engl J Med 1985;313:842-8.
24. Aoshima T, Kajita M, Sekido Y, Kikuchi S, Yasuda I, Saheki T, et al. Novel mutations (H337R and 238-362del) in the CPS1 gene cause carbamoyl phosphate synthetase I deficiency. Hum Heredity 2001;52: 99-101.
25. Asberg A, Thorstensen K, Hveem K, Bjerve KS. Hereditary hemochromatosis: the clinical significance of the S65C mutation. Genet Testing 2002;6:59-62.
26. Azzi A, De Santis R, Morfini M, Zakrzewska K, Musso R, Santagostino E, et al. TT virus contaminates first-generation recombinant factor VIII concentrates. Blood 2001;98:2571-73.
27. Baas F. Genetic diagnosis of Charcot-Marie-Tooth disease. Methods Molec Biol 2003;217:177-84.
28. Babul R, Adam S, Kremer B, Dufrasne S, Wiggins S, Huggins M, et al. Attitudes toward direct predictive testing for the Huntington disease gene. JAMA 1993;270:2321-25.
29. Bacon BR, Sadiq SA. Hereditary hemochromatosis: presentation and diagnosis in the 1990s. Am J Gastroenterol 1997;92:784-89.
30. Badano JL, Inoue K, Katsanis N, Lupski JR. New polymorphic short tandem repeats for PCR-based Charcot-Marie-Tooth disease type 1A duplication diagnosis. Clin Chem 2001;47:838-43.
31. Bakker E, Hofker MH, Goor N, Mandel JL, Wrogemann K, Davies KE, et al. Prenatal diagnosis and carrier detection of Duchenne muscular dystrophy with closely linked RFLPs. Lancet 1985;1: 655-8.

32. Bakker E, Van Broeckhoven C, Bonten EJ, van de Vooren MJ, Veenema H, Van Hul W, et al. Germline mosaicism and Duchenne muscular dystrophy mutations. Nature 1987;329:554-6.
33. Ballering LA, Bon MA, Steffens-Nakken HM, Van den Bergh FA. Chemiluminescent detection of factor V *Leiden* in a routine laboratory. Ann Clin Biochem 1996;33:259-62.
34. Bao J, Sharp AH, Wagster MV, Becher M, Schilling G, Ross CA, et al. Expansion of polyglutamine repeat in huntingtin leads to abnormal protein interactions involving calmodulin. Proc Natl Acad Sci USA 1996;93:5037-42.
35. Bardoni B, Mandel J-L. Advances in understanding of fragile X pathogenesis and FMRP function, and in identification of X linked mental retardation genes. Curr Opin Genet & Develop 2002;12:284-93.
36. Barker D, Schafer M, White R. Restriction sites containing CpG show a higher frequency of polymorphisms in human DNA. Cell 1984;36:131-8.
37. Barrell BG, Bankier AT, Drouin J. A different genetic code in human mitochondria. Nature 1979;282: 189-94.
38. Bartlett JMS, Stirling D, eds. PCR protocols, 2nd ed. Methods Mol Biol 2003;226:3-532.
39. Barton JC, McDonnell SM, Adams PC, Brissot P, Powell LW, Edwards CQ, et al. Management of hemochromatosis. Ann Intern Med 1998;129:932-9.
40. Baskaran S, Datta S, Mandal A, Gulati N, Totey SM, Anand R, et al. Instability of CGG repeats in transgenic mice. Genomics 2002;80:151-7.
41. Bavikatty NR, Killeen AA, Akel N, Normolle D, Schmaier AH. Association of the prothrombin G20210A mutation with factor V Leiden in a Midwestern American population. Am J Clin Path 2000;114:272-5.
42. Baxendale S, MacDonald ME, Mott R, Francis F, Lin C, Kirby SF, et al. A cosmid contig and high resolution restriction map of the 2 megabase region containing the Huntington's disease gene. Nat Genet 1993;4:181-6.
43. Bayston TA, Lane DA. Antithrombin: molecular basis of deficiency. Thromb Haemost 1997;78:339-43.
44. Bear CE, Li C, Kartner N, Bridges RJ, Jensen TJ, Ramjeesingh M, et al. Purification and functional reconstitution of the cystic fibrosis transmembrane conductance regulator (CFTR). Cell 1992;68:809-18.
45. Beggs AH, Hoffman EP, Snyder JR, Arahata K, Speecht L, Shapiro F, et al. Exploring the molecular basis for variability among patients with Becker muscular dystrophy: dystrophin gene and protein studies. Am J Hum Genet 1991;49:54-67.
46. Beggs AH, Koenig M, Boyce FM, Kunkel LM. Detection of 98% of DMD/BMD gene deletions by polymerase chain reaction. Hum Genet 1990;86: 45-8.
47. Bell MV, Hirst MC, Nakahori Y, MacKinnin RN, Roche A, Flint TJ, et al. Physical mapping across the fragile X: hypermethylation and clinical expression of the fragile X syndrome. Cell 1991;64:861-6.
48. Bellus GA, Hefferon TW, Ortiz de Luna RI, Hecht JT, Horton WA, Machado M, et al. Achondroplasia is defined by recurrent G380R mutations of FGFR3. Am J Hum Genet 1995;56:368-73.
49. Bellus GA, McIntosh I, Smith EA, Aylsworth AS, Kaitila I, Horton WA, et al. A recurrent mutation in the tyrosine kinase domain of fibroblast growth factor receptor 3 causes hypochondroplasia. Nat Genet 1995;10:357-9.
50. Bellus GA, Spector EB, Speiser PW, Weaver CA, Garber AT, Bryke CR, et al. Distinct missense mutations of the FGFR3 Lys650 codon modulate receptor kinase activation and the severity of the skeletal dysplasia phenotype. Am J Hum Genet 2000;67: 1411-21.
51. Bennetto L, Pennington BF, Porter D, Taylor AK, Hagerman RJ. Profile of cognitive functioning in women with the fragile X mutation. Neuropsychology 2001;15:290-299.
52. Benowitz S. European groups oppose Myriad's latest patent on *BRCA1.* J Natl Cancer Inst 2003;95:8-9.
53. Berdanier CD, Everts HB. Mitochondrial DNA in aging and degenerative disease. Mutation Res 2001;475:169-84.
54. Berger P, Young P, Suter U. Molecular cell biology of Charcot-Marie-Tooth disease. Neurogen 2002;4: 1-15.
55. Bernard R, Boyer A, Negre P, Malzac P, Latour P, Vanderberghe A, et al. Prenatal detection of the 17p11.2 duplication in Charcot-Marie-Tooth disease type 1A: necessity of a multidisciplinary approach for heterogeneous disorders. Eur J Hum Genet 2002;10:297-302.
56. Beroud C, Soussi T. APC gene: database of germline and somatic mutations in human tumors and cell lines. Nucleic Acids Res 1996;24:121-4.
57. Berry GT, Steiner RD. Long-term management of patients with urea cycle disorders. J Pediatr 2001;138:S56-61.
58. Bertina RM, Koeleman BPC, Koster T, Rosendaal FR, Dirven RJ, de Ronde H, et al. Mutation in blood coagulation factor V associated with resistance to activated protein C. Nature 1994;369:64-7.
59. Beutler E. The significance of the 187G (H63D) mutation in hemochromatosis. Am J Hum Genet 1997;61:762-4.
60. Beutler E, Felitti VJ, Koziol JA, Ho NJ, Gelbart T. Penetrance of 845G-A (C282Y) *HFE* hereditary haemochromatosis mutation in the USA. Lancet 2002;359:211-8.
61. Beutler E, Gelbart T, West C, Lee P, Adams M, Blackstone R, et al. Mutation analysis in hereditary

hemochromatosis. Blood Cells, Molec Dis 1996; 187-94.

62. Bielinska B, Blaydes SM, Buiting K, Yang T, Krajewska-Walasek M, Horsthemke B, et al. De novo deletions of SNRPN exon 1 in early human and mouse embryos result in a paternal to maternal imprint switch. Nature Genet 2000;25:74-8.
63. Bienz M. The subcellular destinations of APC proteins. Nat Rev 2002;3:328-38.
64. Bird AP. DNA methylation and the frequency of CpG in animal DNA. Nucl Acids Res 1980;8:1499-04.
65. Birouk N, Gouider R, Guern EL, Gugenheim M, Tardieu S, Maisonobe T, et al. Charcot-Marie-Tooth disease type 1A with 17p11.2 duplication: clinical and electrophysiological phenotype and factors influencing disease severity in 119 cases. Brain 1997;120: 813-23.
66. Bisgaard ML, Fenger K, Bulow S, Niebuhr E, Mohr J. Familial adenomatous polyposis (FAP): frequency, penetrance, and mutation rate. Hum Mut 1994;3: 121-5.
67. Blasczyk R, Ritter M, Thiede C, Wehling J, Hintz G, Neubauer A, et al. Simple and rapid detection of factor V Leiden by allele specific PCR amplification. Thromb Haemost 1996;75:757-9.
68. Bodmer WF, Bailey CJ, Bodmer J, Bussey HJ, Ellis A, Gorman P, et al. Localization of the gene for familial adenomatous polyposis on chromosome 5q. Nature 1987;328:614-6.
69. Boerkoel CF, Takashima H, Garcia CA, Olney RK, Johnson J, Berry K, et al. Charcot-Marie-Tooth disease and related neuropathies: mutation distribution and genotype-phenotype correlation. Ann Neurol 2002;51:190-201.
70. Bokarewa MI, Bremme K, Blomback M. Arg506-Gln mutation in factor V and risk of thrombosis during pregnancy. Br J Haematol 1996;92:473-8.
71. Boland CR, Thibodeau SN, Hamilton SR, Sidransky D, Eshleman JR, Burt RW, et al. A National Cancer Institute workshop on microsatellite instability for cancer detection and familial predisposition: development of international criteria for the determination of microsatellite instability in colorectal cancer. Cancer Res 1998;58:5248-57.
72. Bontekoe CJM, Bakker CE, Nieuwenhuizen IM, van der Linde H, Lans H, de Lange D, et al. Instability of a (CGG)98 repeat in the FMR1 promoter. Hum Molec Genet 2001;10:1693-1699.
73. Borgel D, Grandrille S, Aiach M. Protein S deficiency. Thromb Haemost 1997;78:351-6.
74. Botkin JR, Croyle RT, Smith KR, Baty BJ, Lerman C, Goldgar DE, et al. A model protocol for evaluating the behavioral and psychosocial effects of *BRCA1* testing. J Natl Cancer Insti 1996;88:872-82.
75. Botkin JR, Smith KR, Croyle RT, Baty BJ, Wylie JE, Dutson D, et al. Genetic testing for a BRCA1 mutation: prophylactic surgery and screening behavior in women 2 years post testing. Am J Med Genet 2003;118A:201-9.
76. Bougeron T, Rustin P, Birch-Machin M, Bourgeois M, Viegas-Pequignot E, Munnich A, et al. A mutation of nuclear succinate dehydrogenase gene results in mitochondrial respiratory chain deficiency. Nat Genet 1995;11:144-9.
77. Boyd Y, Buckle V, Holt S, Munro E, Hunter D, Craig I. Muscular dystrophy in girls with X; autosome translocations. J Med Genet 1986;23:484-90.
78. Braude PR, De Wert GMWR, Evers-Kiebooms E, Pettigrew RA, Geraedts JPM. Non-disclosure preimplantation genetic diagnosis for Huntington's disease: practical and ethical dilemmas. Prenatal Diag 1998;18:1422-6.
79. Breast Cancer Information Core— http://www.nhgri.nih.gov/intramuralresearch/labtransfer/bic/.
80. Brensinger JD, Laken SJ, Luce MC, Powell SM, Vance GH, Ahnen DJ, et al. Variable phenotype of familial adenomatous polyposis in pedigrees with 3′ mutation in the *APC* gene. Gut 1998;43:548-52.
81. Brinkman RR, Mezei MM, Theilmann J, Almqvist E, Hayden MR. The likelihood of being affected with Huntington disease by a particular age, for a specific CAG size. Am J Hum Genet 1997;60:1202-10.
82. Bronner CE, Baker SM, Morrison PT, Warren G, Smith LG, Lescoe MK, Kane M, et al. Mutation in the DNA mismatch repair gene homologue *hMLH1* is associated with hereditary non-polyposis colon cancer. Nature 1994;368:258-61.
83. Brown V, Jin P, Ceman S, Darnell JC, O'Donnell WT, Tenenbaum SA, et al. Microarray identification of FMRP-associated brain mRNAs and altered mRNA translational profiles in fragile X syndrome. Cell 2001;107:477-87.
84. Brown WT, Houck GE, Ding X, Zhong N, Nolin S, Glicksman A, et al. Reverse mutations in the fragile X syndrome. Am J Med Genet 1996;64:287-92.
85. Brusilow SW, Maestri NE. Urea cycle disorders: diagnosis, pathophysiology, and therapy. Adv Pediatr 1996;43:127-70.
86. Buiting K, Dittrich B, Gross S, Lich C, Farber C, Buchholz T, et al. Sporadic imprinting defects in Prader-Willi syndrome and Angelman syndrome: implications for imprint-switch models, genetic counseling and prenatal diagnosis. Am J Hum Genet 1998;63:170-80.
87. Buiting K, Saitoh S, Gross S, Dittrich B, Schwartz S, Nicholls RD, et al. Inherited microdeletions in the Angelman and Prader-Will syndromes define an imprinting centre on human chromosome 15. Nature Genet 1995;9:395-400.
88. Bulaj ZJ, Ajioka RS, Phillips JD, LaSalle BA, Jorde LB, Griffen LM, et al. Disease-related conditions in rela-

tives of patients with hemochromatosis. N Engl J Med 2000;343:1529-35.

89. Burger J, Buiting K, Dittrich B, Gross S, Lich C, Sperling K, et al. Different mechanisms and recurrence risks for imprinting defects in Angelman syndrome. Am J Hum Genet 1997;61:88-93.
90. Burke W, Aitken ML, Chen SH, Scott CR. Variable severity of pulmonary disease in adults with identical cystic fibrosis mutations. Chest 1992;102:506-9.
91. Burke W, Peterson G, Lynch P, Botkin J, Daly M, Garber J, et al. Recommendations for follow-up care of individuals with inherited predisposition to cancer. I. Hereditary nonpolyposis colon cancer. Cancer Genetics Studies Consortium. JAMA 1997;277:915-9.
92. Burke W, Thomson E, Khoury MJ, McDonnell SM, Press N, Adams PC, et al. Hereditary hemochromatosis: gene discovery and its implications for population-based screening. JAMA 1998;280:172-8.
93. Burman RW, Anoe KS, Popovich BW. Fragile X full mutations are more similar in siblings than in unrelated patients: further evidence for a familial factor in CGG repeat dynamics. Genet in Medicine 2000;2:242-8.
94. Bushby KMD, Gardner-Medwin D. The clinical, genetic and dystrophin characteristics of Becker muscular dystrophy. I. Natural history. J Neurol 1993;240:98-104.
95. Call G, Seay AR, Sherry R, Qureshi IA. Clinical features of carbamyl phosphate synthetase-I deficiency in an adult. Ann Neurol 1984;16:90-3.
96. Calvert PM, Frucht H. The genetics of colorectal cancer. Ann Intern Med 2002;137:603-12.
97. Camaschella C, Roetto A, Cali A, De Gobbi M, Garozzo G, Carella M, et al. The gene *TFR2* is mutated in a new type of hemochromatosis mapping to 7q22. Nat Genet 2000;25:14-5.
98. Carelli V, Baracca A, Barogi S, Pallotti F, Valentino ML, Montagna P, et al. Biochemical-clinical correlation in patients with different loads of the mitochondrial DNA T8993G mutation. Arch Neurol 2002;59:264-70.
99. Carthew RW. RNA interference: the fragile X syndrome connection. Current Biol 2002;12:R852-854.
100. Castilla LH, Couch FJ, Erdos MR, Hoskins KF, Calzone K, Garber JE, et al. Mutations in the BRCA1 gene in families with early-onset breast and ovarian cancer. Nature Genet 1994;8:387-91.
101. Cattaneo M, Chantarangkul V, Tailoi E, Santos JH, Tagliabue L. The G20210A mutation of the prothrombin gene in patients with previous first episodes of deep-vein thrombosis: prevalence and association with factor V G1691A, methylenetetrahydrofolate reductase C677T and plasma prothrombin levels. Thrombo Res 1999;93:1-8.
102. Caudy AA, Myers M, Hannon GJ, Hammond SM. Fragile X-related protein and VIG associate with the RNA interference machinery. Genes & Develop 2002;16:2491-6.
103. Cavaille J, Buiting K, Kiefmann M, Lalande M, Brannan CI, Horsthemke B, et al. Identification of brain-specific and imprinted small nucleolar RNA genes exhibiting an unusual genomic organization. Proc Natl Acad Sci USA 2000;97:14311-6.
104. Chamberlain JS. Gene therapy of muscular dystrophy. Hum Molec Genet 2002;11:2355-62.
105. Chamberlain JS, Gibbs RA, Ranier JE, Caskey CT. Multiplex PCR for the diagnosis of Duchenne muscular dystrophy. In: Innis MA, Gelfand DH, Sninsky JJ, White TJ, eds. PCR protocols: a guide to methods and applications. San Francisco: Academic Press, 1990:272-81.
106. Chambost H, Gaboulud V, Coatmelec B, Rafowicz A, Schneider P, Calvez T, et al. What factors influence the age at diagnosis of hemophilia? Results of the French hemophilia cohort. J Pediatr 2002;141:548-52.
107. Chan WP, Lee CK, Kwong YL, Lam CK, Liang R. A novel mutation of Arg 306 of factor V gene in Hong Kong Chinese. Blood 1998;91:1135-9.
108. Chance PF, Alderson MK, Leppig KA, Matsunami N, Smith B, Swanson PD, et al. DNA deletion associated with hereditary neuropathy with liability to pressure palsies. Cell 1993;72:143-51.
109. Chance PF, Bird TD, Matsunami N, Lensch MW, Brothman AR, Feldman GM. Trisomy 17p associated with Charcot-Marie-Tooth neuropathy type 1A phenotype: evidence for gene dosage as a mechanism in CMT1A. Neurol 1992;42:2295-99.
110. Chen ST, Chen RA, Kuo SJ, Chien YC. Mutational screening of breast cancer susceptibility gene 1 from early onset, bi-lateral, and familial breast cancer patients in Taiwan. Breast Can Res Treat 2003;77: 133-43.
111. Cheng SH, Gregory RJ, Marshall J, Paul S, Souza DW, White GA, O'Riordan CR, et al. Defective intracellular transport and processing of CFTR is the molecular basis of most cystic fibrosis. Cell 1990;63:827-34.
112. Chillon M, Casals T, Mercier B, Bassas L, Lissens W, Silber S, et al. Mutations in the cystic fibrosis gene in patients with congenital absence of the vas deferens. N Engl J Med 1995;332:1475-80.
113. Chiurazzi P, Pomponi MG, Willemsen R, Oostra BA, Neri G. In vitro reactivation of the FMR1 gene involved in fragile X syndrome. Hum Molec Genet 1998;7:109-13.
114. Chong SS, Almqvist E, Telenius H, LaTray L, Nichol K, Bourdelat-Parks B, et al. Contribution of DNA sequence and CAG size to mutation frequencies of intermediate alleles for Huntington disease: evidence from single sperm analyses. Hum Molec Genet 1997;6:301-9.
115. Coffee B, Zhang F, Warren ST, Reines D. Acetylated histones are associated with FMR1 in normal but not

fragile X-syndrome cells. Nature Genet 1999;22: 98-101.
116. Cogswell ME, Burke W, McDonnell SM, Franks AL. Screening for hemochromatosis: a public health perspective. Am J Prev Med 1999;16:134-40.
117. Colvin JS, Bohne BA, Harding GW, McEwen DG, Ornitz DM. Skeletal overgrowth and deafness in mice lacking fibroblast growth factor receptor 3. Nat Genet 1996;12:390-7.
118. Comi GP, Prelle A, Bresolin N, Moggio M, Bardoni A, Gallanti A, et al. Clinical variability in Becker muscular dystrophy. Genetic, biochemical and immunhistochemical correlates. Brain 1994;117:1-14.
119. Conneally PM, Haines JL, Tanzi RE, Wexler NS, Penchaszadeh GK, Harper PS, et al. Huntington's disease: no evidence for heterogeneity. Genomics 1989;5:304-8.
120. Conway GS, Payne NN, Webb J, Murray A, Jacobs PA. Fragile X premutation screening in women with premature ovarian failure. Hum Reprod 1998;13:1184-1187.
121. Corral-Debrinski M, Horton T, Lott MT, Shoffner JM, Beal MF, Wallace DC. Mitochondrial DNA deletions in human brain: regional variability and increase with advanced age. Nature Genet 1992;2:324-9.
122. Crabtree MD, Tomlinson IPM, Hodgson SV, Neale K, Phillips RKS, Houlston RS. Explaining variation in familial adenomatous polyposis: relationship between genotype and phenotype and evidence for modifier genes. Gut 2002;51:420-3.
123. Crawford DC, Meadows KL, Newman JL, Taft LF, Pettay DL, Gold LB, et al. Prevalence and phenotype consequence of *FRAXA* and *FRAXE* alleles in a large, ethnically diverse, special education needs population. Am J Hum Genet 1999;64:495-507.
124. Crow JF. The origins, patterns and implications of human spontaneous mutation. Nat Rev Genet 2000;1:40-7.
125. Cystic Fibrosis Foundation. Patient registry 1999. Annual data report. Bethesda, Md, September 2000.
126. Cystic Fibrosis Mutation Database. www.genet.sickkids.on.ca/cftr/.
127. D'Urso D, Muller HW. Ins and outs of peripheral myelin protein-22: mapping transmembrane topology and intracellular sorting. J Neurosci Res 1997;49:551-62.
128. Dahlback B. Inherited thrombophilia: resistance to activated protein C as a pathogenic factor of venous thromboembolism. Blood 1995;85:607-14.
129. Dahlback B, Carlsson M, Svensson PJ. Familial thrombophilia due to a previously unrecognized mechanism by poor anticoagulant response to activated protein C: prediction of a cofactor to activated protein C. Proc Natl Acad Sci USA 1993;90:1004-8.
130. Daniel DC. Highlight: BRCA1 and BRCA2 proteins in breast cancer. Microsc Res Tech 2002;59:68-83.
131. Davies KE, Pearson PL, Harper PS, Murray JM, O'Brien T, Sarfarazi M, et al. Linkage analysis of two cloned DNA sequences flanking the Duchenne muscular dystrophy locus on the short arm of the human X chromosome. Nucl Acids Res 1983;11: 2303-12.
132. De Boulle K, Verkerk AJMH, Reyniers E, Vits L, Hendrickx J, Van Roy B, et al. A point mutation in the FMR-1 gene associated with fragile X mental retardation. Nature Genet 1993;3:31-35.
133. De Rooij KE, Dorsman JC, Smoor MA, Den Dunnen JT, van Ommen GJ. Subcellular localization of the Huntington's disease gene product in cell lines by immunofluorescence and biochemical subcellular fractionation. Hum Mol Genet 1996;5:1093-99.
134. De Stefano V, Martinelli I, Mannucci PM, Paciaroni K, Chiusolo P, Casorelli I, et al. The risk of recurrent deep venous thrombosis among heterozygous carriers of both factor V Leiden and the G20210A prothrombin mutation. N Engl J Med 1999;341:801-6.
135. De Stefano V, Rossi E, Paciaroni K, Leone G. Screening for inherited thrombophilia: indications and therapeutic implications. Haematologica 2002;87: 1095-1108.
136. de Vries BBA, Halley DJJ, Oostra BA, Niermeijer MF. The fragile X syndrome. J Med Genet 1998;35: 579-589.
137. Deffenbaugh AM, Frank TS, Hoffman M, Cannon-Albright L, Neuhausen SL. Characterization of common *BRCA1* and *BRCA2* variants. Genetic Testing 2002;6:119-21.
138. Den Dunnen JJ, Grootscholten PM, Bakker E, Blonden LAJ, Ginjaar HB, Wapenaar MC, et al. Topography of the Duchenne Muscular Dystrophy (DMD) gene: FiGE and cDNA analysis of 194 cases reveals 115 deletions and 13 duplications. Am J Hum Genet 1989;45:835-47.
139. Deng C, Wynshaw-Boris A, Zhou F, Kuo A, Leder P. Fibroblast growth factor receptor 3 is a negative regulator of bone growth. Cell;1996:84:911-21.
140. Descheemaeker MJ, Vogels A, Govers V, Borghgraef M, Willekens D, Swillen A. Prader-Willi syndrome: new insights in the behavioral and psychiatric spectrum. J Intellect Disabil Res 2002;46:41-50.
141. Difiglia M, Sapp E, Chase KO, Davies SW, Bates GP, Vonsattel JP, et al. Aggregation of huntingtin in neuronal intranuclear inclusions and dystrophic neuritis in brain. Science 1997;277:1990-3.
142. Dilley A, Hooper WC, Austin H, Lally C, Wenger NK, Evatt BL. The prevalence of the prothrombin 20210 G-A variant in African Americans. Blood 1997;90:652a.
143. DiMauro S, De Vivo DC. Genetic heterogeneity in Leigh syndrome. Ann Neurol 1996;40:5-7.

144. DiMauro S, Schon EA. Mitochondrial DNA mutations in human disease. Am J Med Genet 2001;106:18-26.
145. Dobbie Z, Spycher M, Mary JL, Haner M, Guldenschuh I, Hurliman R, et al. Correlation between the development of extracolonic manifestations in FAP patients and mutations beyond codon 1403 of the APC gene. J Med Genet 1996;33:274-80.
146. Dolinsky LCB. Denaturing Gradient Gel Electrophoresis (DGGE) for mutation detection in Duchenne muscular dystrophy (DMD). Methods Molec Biol 2003;217:165-75.
147. Dreyfus DH, Bethel R, Gelfend EW. Cystic fibrosis 3849 + 10 kb C > T mutation associated with severe pulmonary disease and male fertility. Am J Respir Crit Care Med 1996;153:858-60.
148. Driskell RA, Engelhardt JF. Current status of gene therapy for inherited lung diseases. Annu Rev Physiol 2003;65:585-612.
149. Drumm ML. Modifier genes and variation in cystic fibrosis. Respir Res 2001;2:125-128.
150. Dubreuil Lastrucci RM, Dawson DA, Bowden JH, Munster M. Development of a simple multiplex polymerase chain reaction for the simultaneous detection of factor V Leiden and prothrombin 20210A mutations. Molecular Diag 1999;4:247-50.
151. Duncan B, Miller J. Mutagenic deamination of cytosine residues in DNA. Nature 1980;287:560-1.
152. Durno C, Corey M, Zielenski J, Tullis E, Tsui LC, Durie P. Genotype and phenotype correlations in patients with cystic fibrosis and pancreatitis. Gastroenterology 2002;123:1857-64.
153. Duyao M, Ambrose C, Myers R, Novelletto A, Persichetti F, Frontali M, et al. Trinucleotide repeat length instability and age of onset in Huntington's disease. Nat Genet 1993;4:387-92.
154. Ehmsen J, Poon E, Davies K. The dystrophin-associated protein complex. J Cell Sci 2002;115:2801-3.
155. Eichler EE, Hammond HA, Macpherson JN, Ward PA, Nelson DL. Population survey of the human FMR1 CGG repeat substructure suggests biased polarity for the loss of AGG interruptions. Hum Molec Genet 1995;4:2199-208.
156. Eichler EE, Holden JJA, Popovich BW, Reiss AL, Snow K, Thibodeau SN, et al. Length of uninterrupted CGG repeats determines instability in the FMR1 gene. Nat Genet 1994;8:88-94.
157. Eichler EE, Macphreson JN, Murray A, Jacobs PA, Chakravarti A, Nelson DL. Haplotype and interspersion analysis of the FMR1 CGG repeat identifies two different mutational pathways for the origin of the fragile X syndrome. Hum Molec Genet 1996;5:319-30.
158. Eichler EE, Richards S, Gibbs RJ, Nelson DL. Fine structure of the human FMR1 gene. Hum Mol Genet 1993;2:1147-53.
159. Elsaleh H, Joseph D, Grieu F, Zeps N, Spry N, Iacopetta B. Association of tumor site and sex with survival benefit from adjuvant chemotherapy in colorectal cancer. Lancet 2000;355:1745-50.
160. Emmerich J, Rosendaal FR, Cattaneo M, Margaglione M, DeStefano V, Cumming T, et al. Combined effect of Factor V Leiden and prothrombin 20210A on the risk of venous thromboembolism. Thromb Haemost 2001;86:809-16.
161. Engelender S, Sharp AH, Colomer V, Tokito MK, Lanahan A, Worley P, et al. Huntingtin-associated protein 1 (HAP1) interacts with the p150^{Glued} subunit of dynactin. Hum Molec Genet 1997;6:2205-12.
162. Faioni EM, Franchi F, Bucciarelli P, Margaglione M, De Stefano V, Castaman G, et al. Coinheritance of the HR2 haplotype in the factor V gene confers an increased risk of venous thromboembolism to carriers of factor V R506Q. Blood 1999;94:3062-6.
163. Falk MC, Knight JF, Roy LP, Wilcken B, Schell DN, O'Connell AJ, et al. Continuous venovenous haemofiltration in the acute treatment of inborn errors of metabolism. Pediatr Nephrol 1994;8:330-333.
164. Fang P, Lev-Lehman E, Tsai TF, Matsuura T, Benton CS, Sutcliffe JS, et al. The spectrum of mutations in *UBE3A* causing Angelman syndrome. Hum Molec Genet 1999;8:129-135.
165. Farrell PM, Fost N. Prenatal screening for cystic fibrosis: where are we now? J Pediatr 2002;141:758-63.
166. Farrington SM, McKinley AJ, Carothers AD, Cunningham C, Bubb VJ, Sharp L, et al. Evidence for an age-related influence of microsatellite instability on colorectal cancer survival. Int J Cancer 2002;98:844-50.
167. Fauser S, Leo-Kottler B, Besch D, Luberichs J. Confirmation of the 14568 mutation in the mitochondrial ND6 gene as causative in Leber's hereditary optic neuropathy. Opthal Genet 2002;23:191-7.
168. Fay PJ. Factor VIII structure and function. Thromb Haemost 1993;70:63-7.
169. Fearnhead NS, Britton MP, Bodmer WF. The ABC of APC. Hum Molec Genet 2001;10:721-33.
170. Fearnhead NS, Wilding JL, Bodmer WF. Genetics of colorectal cancer: hereditary aspects and overview of colorectal tumorigenesis. Brit Med Bulletin 2002;64:27-43.
171. Fearon ER, Vogelstein B. A genetic model for colorectal tumorigenesis. Cell 1990;61:759-67.
172. Feder JN, Gnirke A, Thomas W, Tsuchihashi Z, Ruddy DA, Basava A, et al. A novel MHC class I-like gene is mutated in patients with hereditary haemochromatosis. Nature Genet 1996;13:399-408.
173. Feder JN, Penny DM, Irrinki A, Lee VK, Lebron JA, Watson N, et al. The hemochromatosis gene product complexes with the transferrin receptor and lowers its

affinity for ligand binding. Proc Natl Acad Sci USA 1998;95:1472-7.

174. Feder JN, Tsuchihashi Z, Irrinki A, Lee VK, Mapa FA, Morikang E, et al. The hemochromatosis founder mutation in HLA-H disrupts B2-microglobulin interaction and cell surface expression. J Biol Chem 1997;272:14025-8.
175. Feng J, Yan J, Buzin CH, Sommer SS, Towbin JA. Comprehensive mutation scanning of the dystrophin gene in patients with nonsyndromic X-linked dilated cardiomyopathy. J Am Coll Cardiol 2002;40:1120-4.
176. Feng Y, Absher D, Eberhart DE, Brown V, Malter HE, Warren ST. FMRP associates with polyribosomes as an mRNP and the I304N mutation of severe fragile X syndrome abolishes this association. Molec Cell 1997;1:109-18.
177. Finckh U, Kohlschutter A, Schafer H, Sperhake K, Colombo JP, Gal A. Prenatal diagnosis of carbamoyl phosphate synthetase I deficiency by identification of a missense mutation in CPSI. Hum Mutat 1998;12:206-11.
178. Fischer K, Van der bom JG, Mauser-Bunschoten EP, Roosendaal G, Prejs R, et al. Changes in treatment strategies for severe haemophilia over the last 3 decades: effects on clotting factor consumption and arthropathy. Haemophilia 2001;7:446-52.
179. Fishel R, Lescoe MK, Rao MRS, Copeland NG, Jenkins NA, Garber J, et al. The human mutator gene homolog *MSH2* and its association with hereditary nonpolyposis colon cancer. Cell 1993;75:1027-38.
180. FitzSimmons SC. The changing epidemiology of cystic fibrosis. J Pediatr 1993;122:1-9.
181. Flanigan KM, von Niederhausern A, Dunn DM, Alder J, Mendall JR, Weiss RB. Rapid direct sequence analysis of the dystrophin gene. Am J Hum Genet 2003;72:931-9.
182. Foddle R. The *APC* gene in colorectal cancer. Eur J Cancer 2002;38:867-71.
183. Folstein SE. The psychopathology of Huntington's disease. Res Publ Assoc Res Nerv Ment Dis 1991;69:181-91.
184. Francke U, Ochs HD, de Martinville B, Giacalone J, Lindgren V, Disteche C, et al. Minor Xp21 chromosome deletion in a male associated with expression of Duchenne muscular dystrophy, chronic granulomatous disease, retinitis pigmentosa and McLeod syndrome. Am J Hum Genet 1985;37:250-67.
185. Franco RF, Elion J, Tavella MH, Araujo AG, Zago MA. Heterogeneous distribution of the 20210 G-A prothrombin and 677 C-T methylenetetrahydrofolate reductase mutations in different human populations: relevance for vascular disease risk. Blood 1997;90:3130a.
186. Francomano CA, Ortiz de Luna RI, Hefferon TW, Bellus GA, Turner CE, Taylor E, et al. Localization of the achondroplasia gene to the distal 2.5 Mb of human chromosome 4p. Hum Molec Genet 1994;3:787-92.
187. Friedl W, Meuschel S, Caspari R, Lamberti C, Krieger S, Sengteller M, et al. Attenuated familial adenomatous polyposis due to a mutation in the 3′ part of the *APC* gene: a clue for understanding the function of the APC protein. Hum Genet 1996;97:579-84.
188. Friedman LS, Ostermeyer EA, Szabo CI, Dowd P, Lynch ED, Rowell SE, et al. Confirmation of BRCA1 by analysis of germline mutations linked to breast and ovarian cancer in ten families. Nature Genet 1994;8:399-404.
189. Furtado S, Suchowersky O, Rewcastle B, Graham L, Klimek M, Garber A. Relationship between trinucleotide repeats and neuropathological changes in Huntington's disease. Ann Neurol 1996;39:132-6.
190. Gacy AM, McMurray CT. Influence of hairpins on template reannealing at trinucleotide repeat duplexes: a model for slipped DNA. Biochem 1998;37:9426-34.
191. Ganitkevich VY. The role of mitochondria in cytoplasmic Ca^{2+} cycling. Exper Physiol 2003;88:91-7.
192. Gardner RJ, Bobrow M, Roberts RG. The identification of point mutations in Duchenne muscular dystrophy patients by using reverse-transcription PCR and the protein truncation test. Am J Hum Genet 1995;57:311-20.
193. Gayther SA, Mangion J, Russell P, Seal S, Barfoot R, Ponder BAJ, et al. Variation of risks of breast and ovarian cancer associated with different germline mutations of the *BRCA2* gene. Nature Genet 1997;15:103-5.
194. Gedeon AK, Baker E, Robinson H, Partington MW, Gross B, Manca A, et al. Fragile X syndrome without CCG amplification has an FMR1 deletion. Nature Genet 1992;1:341-4.
195. Gehring NH, Frede U, Neu-Yilik G, Hundsdoerfer P, Vetter B, Hentze MW, et al. Increased efficiency of mRNA 3′ end formation: a new genetic mechanism contributing to hereditary thrombophilia. Nat Genet 2001;28:389-92.
196. GeneTests: Medical Genetics Information Resource (database online). A listing of research and clinical labs for disease specific referrals. www.genetests.org
197. Gerhardt A, Scharf RE, Beckmann MW, Struve S, Bender HG, Pillny M, et al. Prothrombin and factor V mutations in women with a history of thrombosis during pregnancy and the puerperium. N Engl J Med 2000;342:374-80.
198. Giardiello FM, Brensinger JD, Peterson G. American Gastroenterological Association technical review on hereditary colorectal cancer and genetic testing. Gastroenterology 2001;121:198-213.
199. Giardiello FM, Krush AJ, Peterson GM, Booker SV, Kerr M, Tong LL, et al. Phenotypic variability of familial adenomatous polyposis in 11 unrelated fami-

lies with identical *APC* gene mutation. Gastroenterology 1994;106:1542-7.
200. Gibson LE, Cooke RE. A test for the concentration of electrolytes in sweat in cystic fibrosis of the pancreas utilizing pilocarpine by iontophoresis. Pediat 1959;23: 545-9.
201. Gilbert F. Cystic fibrosis carrier screening: steps in the development of a mutation panel. Genet Testing 2001;5:223-7.
202. Gilliam TC, Tanzi RE, Haines JL, Bonner TI, Faryniarz AG, Hobbs WJ, et al. Localization of the Huntington's disease gene to a small segment of chromosome 4 flanked by D4S10 and the telomere. Cell 1987;50:565-71.
203. Gimelli G, Pujana MA, Patricelli MG, Russo S, Giardino D, Larizza L, et al. Genomic inversions of human chromosome 15q11-q13 in mothers of Angelman syndrome patients with class II (BP2/3) deletions. Hum Molec Genet 2003;12:849-58.
204. Gite S, Lim M, Carlson R, Olejnik J, Zehnbauer B, Rothschild K. A high throughput nonisotopic protein truncation test. Nat Biotech 2003;21:194-7.
205. Gitschier J, Wood WI, Goralka JM, Wion KL, Chen EY, Eaton DH, et al. Characterization of the human factor VIII gene. Nature 1984;312:326-30.
206. Glenn CC, Saitoh S, Jong MTC, Filbrandt MM, Surti U, Driscoll DJ, et al. Gene structure, DNA methylation, and imprinted expression of the human SNRPN gene. Am J Hum Genet 1996;58:335-46.
207. Goizet C, Lesca G, Durr A. Presymptomatic testing in Huntington's disease and autosomal dominant cerebellar ataxias. Neurol 2002;59:1330-6.
208. Goldberg YP, Kremer B, Andrew SE, Theilmann J, Graham RK, Squitieri F, et al. Molecular analysis of new mutations for Huntington's disease: intermediate alleles and sex of origin effects. Nat Genet 1993;5:174-9.
209. Goldberg YP, McMurray CT, Zeisler CT, Almqvist E, Sillence D, Richards F, et al. Increased instability of intermediate alleles in families with sporadic Huntington disease compared to similar sized intermediate alleles in the general population. Hum Molec Genet 1995;4:1911-8.
210. Gooding HC, Boehm K, Thompson RE, Hadley D, Francomano CA, Biesecker BB. Issues surrounding prenatal genetic testing for achondroplasia. Prenatal Diag 2002;22:933-40.
211. Gordon N. The neurological complications of achondroplasia. Brain Dev 2000;22:3-7.
212. Graff C, Bui TH, Larsson NG. Mitochondrial diseases. Best Prac & Res Clinic Obstet Gyn 2002;16:715-28.
213. Grasemann H, van's Gravesande KS, Buscher R, Knauer N, Silverman ES, Palmer LJ, et al. Endothelial nitric oxide synthase variants in cystic fibrosis lung disease. Am J Respir Crit Care Med 2003;167:390-4.
214. Gray TA, Saitoh S, Nicholls RD. An imprinted, mammalian bicistronic transcript encodes two independent proteins. Proc Natl Acad Sci USA 1999;96:5616-21.
215. Graziano C. Disclaimer now needed for analyte-specific reagents. CAP Today 1998;12:5-11.
216. Greengard JS, Eichinger S, Griffin JH, Bauer KA. Variability of thrombosis among homozygous siblings with resistance to activated protein C due to an Arg-Gln mutation in the gene for factor V. N Engl J Med 1994;331:1559-62.
217. Greenstein RM, Reardon MP, Chan TS. An X-autosome translocation in a girl with Duchenne muscular dystrophy, evidence for DMD gene localization. Pediatr Res 1977;11:475A.
218. Gregg RC, Simantel A, Farrell PM, Koscik R, Kosorok MR, Laxova A, et al. Newborn screening for cystic fibrosis in Wisconsin: comparison of biochemical and molecular methods. Pediatri 1997;99:819-24.
219. Groden J, Thliveris A, Samowitz W, Carlson M, Gelbert L, Albertsen H, et al. Identification and characterization of the familial adenomatous polyposis coli gene. Cell 1991;66:589-600.
220. Grody WW, Cutting GR, Klinger KW, Richards CS, Watson MS, Desnick RJ. Laboratory standards and guidelines for population-based cystic fibrosis carrier screening. Genet Med 2001;3:149-54.
221. Grody WW, Griffin JH, Taylor AK, Korf BR, Heit JA. American College of Medical Genetics consensus statement on factor V Leiden mutation testing. Genet Med 2001;3:139-48.
222. Groman JD, Meyer ME, Wilmott RW, Zeitlin PL, Cutting GR. Variant cystic fibrosis phenotypes in the absence of CFTR mutations. N Engl J Med 2002;347:401-7.
223. Gropman AL. Diagnosis and treatment of childhood mitochondrial diseases. Current Neurol Neuroscience Reports 2001;1:185-94.
224. Gryfe R, Kim H, Hsieh ETK, Aronson MD, Holowaty EJ, Bull SB, et al. Tumor microsatellite instability and clinical outcome in young patients with colorectal cancer. N Engl J Med 2000;342:69-77.
225. Gugneja S, Virbasius CM, Scarpulla RC. Nuclear respiratory factors 1 and 2 utilize similar glutamine containing clusters of hydrophobic residues to activate transcription. Mol Cell Biol 1996;16: 5708-16.
226. Gusella JA, Wexler NS, Conneally PM, Naylor S, Anderson MA, Tanzi RE, et al. A polymorphic DNA marker genetically linked to Huntington's disease. Nature 1983;306:234-8.
227. Gutekunst CA, Levey A, Heilman C, Waley W, Yi H, Nash N, et al. Identification and localization of huntingtin in brain and human lymphoblastoid cell lines with anti-fusion protein antibodies. Proc Natl Acad Sci USA 1995;92:8710-4.

228. Hacia JG, Brody LC, Chee MS, Fodor SPA, Collins F. Detection of heterozygous mutations in *BRCA1* using high density oligonucleotide arrays and two-colour fluorescence analysis. Nature Genet 1996;14:441-7.
229. Hack AA, Cordier L, Shoturma DI, Lam MY, Sweeney HL, McNally EM. Muscle degeneration without mechanical injury in sarcoglycan deficiency. Proc Natl Acad Sci USA 1999;96:10723-8.
230. Hagerman RJ, Leehey M, Heinrichs W, Tassone F, Wilson R, Wills J, et al. Intention tremor, parkinsonism, and generalized brain atrophy in male carriers of fragile X. Neurology 2001;57:127-30.
231. Hall JM, Lee MK, Newman B, Morrow JE, Anderson LA, Huey B, et al. Linkage of early-onset familial breast cancer to 17q21. Science 1990;250:1684-9.
232. Hallam PJ, Harding AE, Berciano J, Barker DF, Malcolm S. Duplication of part of chromosome 17 is commonly associated with hereditary motor and sensory neuropathy type 1 (Charcot-Marie-Tooth disease type 1). Ann Neurol 1992;31:570-2.
233. Halling KC, French AJ, McDonnell SK, Burgart LJ, Schaid DJ, Peterson BJ, et al. Microsatellite instability and 8p allelic imbalance in stage B2 and C colorectal cancers. J Natl Cancer Inst 1999;91:1295-303.
234. Hallowell N, Foster C, Ardern-Jones A, Eeles R, Murday V, Watson M. Genetic testing for women previously diagnosed with breast/ovarian cancer: examining the impact of *BRCA1* and *BRCA2* mutation searching. Genet Testing 2002;6:79-87.
235. Hammond LS, Macias MM, Tarleton JC, Pai GS. Fragile X syndrome and deletions in FMR1. Am J Med Genet 1997;72:430-4.
236. Hamosh A, Fitzsimmons SC, Macek M, Knowles MR, Rosenstein BJ, Cutting GR. Comparison of the clinical manifestations of cystic fibrosis in black and white patients. J Pediatr 1998;132:255-9.
237. Hamosh A, Rosenstein BJ, Cutting GR. CFTR nonsense mutations G542X and W1282X associated with severe reduction of CFTR mRNA in nasal epithelial cells. Hum Mol Genet 1992;1:542-4.
238. Happich D, Schwaab R, Hanfland P, Hoernschemeyer D. Allelic discrimination of factor V leiden using a 5′ nuclease assay. Thromb Haemost 1999;82:1294-6.
239. Haraguchi Y, Uchino T, Takiguchi M, Endo F, Mori M, Matsuda I. Cloning and sequence of a cDNA encoding human carbamyl phosphate synthetase I: molecular analysis of hyperammonemia. Gene 1991;107:335-40.
240. Harper PS, Newcombe RG. Age at onset and life table risks in genetic counseling for Huntington's disease. J Med Genet 1992;29:239-42.
241. Harrison CJ, Jack EM, Allen TD, Harris R. (1983) The fragile X: a scanning electron microscopic study. J Med Genet 1983;20:280-5.
242. Haslett JN, Sanoudou D, Kho A, Bennett RR, Greenberg SA, Kohane IS, et al. Gene expression comparison of biopsies from Duchenne muscular dystrophy (DMD) and normal skeletal muscle. Proc Natl Acad Sci USA 2002;99:15000-5.
243. Hayden MR. Huntington's chorea. London, Berlin, Heidelberg: Springer, 1981.
244. Hayden MR, Bloch M, Fahy M. Predictive testing for Huntington's disease using linked DNA markers. N Engl J Med 1988;319:583.
245. He TC, Sparks AB, Rago C, Hermeking H, Zawel L, da Costa LT, et al. Identification of c-MYC as a target of the APC pathway. Science 1998;281:1509-12.
246. Hecht JT, Francomano CA, Horton WA, Annegers JF. Mortality in achondroplasia. Am J Hum Genet 1987;41:454-64.
247. Hedenfalk I, Ringner M, Ben-Dor A, Yakhini Z, Chen Y, Chebil G, et al. Molecular classification of familial non-BRCA1/BRCA2 breast cancer. Proc Natl Acad Sci USA 2003;100:2532-7.
248. Heeb MJ, Kojima Y, Greengard JS, Griffin JH. Activated protein C resistance: molecular mechanisms based on studies using purified Gln506 — Factor V. Blood;1995:85:3405-11.
249. Heim RA, Sugarman EA, Allitto BA. Improved detection of cystic fibrosis mutations in the heterogeneous U.S. population using an expanded, pan-ethnic mutation panel. Genet in Med 2001;3:168-76.
250. Heit JA, Silverstein MD, Mohr DN, Petterson TM, O'Fallon WM, Melton LJ. Risk factors for deep vein thrombosis and pulmonary embolism: a population-based case-control study. Arch Intern Med 2000; 160:809-15.
251. Heitz D, Devus D, Imbert G, Kretz C, Mandel JL. Inheritance of the fragile X syndrome: size of the fragile X premutation is a major determinant of the transition to full mutation. J Med Genet 1992;29: 794-801.
252. Henderson S, Sillence D, Loughlin J, Bennetts B, Sykes B. Germline and somatic mosaicism in achondroplasia. J Med Genet 2000;37:956-8.
253. Henneman L, Bramsen I, Van Der Ploeg HM, Ten Kate LP. Preconception cystic fibrosis carrier couple screening: impact, understanding, and satisfaction. Genet Testing 2002;3:195-202.
254. Henneman L, Poppelaars FAM, Ten Kate LP. Evaluation of cystic fibrosis carrier screening programs according to genetic screening criteria. Genet in Med 2002;4:241-9.
255. Herman JG, Umar A, Polyak K, Graff JR, Ahuja N, Issa JPJ, et al. Incidence and functional consequences of *hMLH1* promoter hypermethylation in colorectal carcinoma. Proc Natl Acad Sci USA 1998;95: 6870-5.
256. Hessner MJ, Budish MA, Friedman KD. Genotyping of factor V G1691A (Leiden) without the use of PCR by invasive cleavage of oligonucleotide probe. Clin Chem 2000;46:1051-6.

257. Highsmith WE, Burch LH, Zhou Z, Olsen JC, Boat TE, Spock A, et al. A novel mutation in the cystic fibrosis gene in patients with pulmonary disease but normal sweat chloride concentrations. N Engl J Med 1996;331:974-80.
258. Higuchi M, Kazazian HH, Kasch L, Warren TC, McGinniss MJ, Phillips JA, et al. Molecular characterization of severe hemophilia A suggests that about half the mutations are not within the coding regions and splice junctions of the factor VIII gene. Proc Natl Aca Scu USA 1991;88:7405-9.
259. Hinds HL, Ashley CT, Sutcliffe JS, Nelson DL, Warren ST, Housman DE, et al. Tissue specific expression of FMR-1 provides evidence for a functional role in fragile X syndrome. Nature Genet 1993;3:36-42.
260. Hochstrasser M. Ubiquitin-dependent protein degradation. Annul Rev Genet 1996;30:405-39.
261. Hoffman EP, Brown RH, Kunkel LM. Dystrophin: the protein product of the Duchenne muscular dystrophy locus. Cell 1987;51:919-28.
262. Hoffman EP, Kunkel Lm. Dystrophin abnormalities in Duchenne/Becker muscular dystrophy. Neuron 1989;2:1019-29.
263. Hogervorst FBL, Cornelis RS, Bout M, van Vliet M, Oosterwijk JC, Olmer R, et al. Rapid detection of *BRCA1* mutations by the protein truncation test. Nature Genet 1995;10:208-12.
264. Holmstrom P, Marmur J, Eggertsen G, Gafvels M, Stal P. Mild iron overload in patients carrying the *HFE* S65C gene mutation: a retrospective study in patient with suspected iron overload and healthy controls. Gut 2002;51:723-30.
265. Holt IJ, Harding AE, Morgan-Hughes JA. Deletions of muscle mitochondrial DNA in patients with mitochondrial myopathies. Nature 1988;331:717-9.
266. Hoogerwaard EM, Bakker E, Ippel PF, Oosterwijk JC, Majoor-Krakauer DF, Leschot NJ, et al. Signs and symptoms of Duchenne muscular dystrophy and Becker muscular dystrophy among carriers in the Netherlands: a cohort study. Lancet 1999;353: 2116-9.
267. Hoogeveen AT, Willemsen R, Meyer R, De Rooij K, van Ommen G, Galjaard H. Characterization and localization of the Huntington disease gene product. Hum Mol Genet 1993;2:2069-73.
268. Hooper WC, Dilley A, Ribeiro MJA, Benson J, Austin H, Silva V, et al. A racial difference in the prevalence of the Arg506-Gln mutation. Thromb Res 1996;81:577-81.
269. Horiuchi M, Imamura Y, Nakamura N, Maruyama I, Saheki T. Carbamoylphosphate synthetase deficiency in an adult: deterioration due to administration of valproic acid. J Inher Metab Dis 1993;16:39-45.
270. Horsthemke B, Dittrich B, Buiting K. Imprinting mutations on human chromosome 15. Hum Mutat 1997;10:329-37.
271. Horton WA, Lunstrum GP. Fibroblast growth factor receptor 3 mutations in achondroplasia and related forms of dwarfism. Rev Endo Metab Dis 2002;3: 381-5.
272. Hoshide R, Matsuura T, Haraguchi Y, Endo F, Yoshinaga M, Matsuda I. Carbamyl phosphate synthetase I deficiency-one base substitution in an exon of the CPSI gene causes a 9-basepair deletion due to aberrant splicing. J Clin Invest 1993;91:1884-7.
273. Hu X, Ray PN, Murphy EG, Thompson MW, Worton RG. Duplicational mutation at the Duchenne muscular dystrophy locus: its frequency, distribution, origin, and phenotype: genotype correlation. Am J Hum Genet 1990;46:682-95.
274. Huntington's Disease Collaborative Research Group. A novel gene containing a trinucleotide repeat that is expanded and unstable on Huntington's disease chromosomes. Cell 1993;72:971-83.
275. Huoponen K, Puomila A, Savontaus ML, Mustonen E, Kronqvist E, Nikoskelainen E. Genetic counseling in Leber hereditary optic neuropathy (LHON). Acta Ophthalmol Scand 2002;80:38-43.
276. Hyser CL, Doherty RA, Griggs RC, Mendell JR, Polakowska R, Quirk S, et al. Carrier assessment for mothers and sisters of isolated Duchenne dystrophy cases: The importance of serum enzyme determinations. Neurol 1987;37:1476-80.
277. Iacopetta B. Are there two sides to colorectal cancer? Int J Cancer 2002;101:403-8.
278. Ikeda N, Miyoshi Y, Yoneda K, Shiba E, Sekihara Y, Moritoshi K, et al. Frequency of *BRCA1* and *BRCA2* germline mutations in Japanese breast cancer families. Int J Cancer 2001;91:83-8.
279. International Huntington Association / World Federation of Neurology. Ethical issues policy statement on Huntington's disease molecular genetics predictive test. J Med Genet 1990;27:34-8.
280. International Huntington Association (IHA) and the World Federation of Neurology (WFN) Research Group on Huntington's Chorea. Guidelines for the molecular genetics predictive test in Huntington's disease. Neurol 1994;44:1533-6.
281. Ionov Y, Peinado MA, Malkhosyan S, Shibata D, Perucho M. Ubiquitous somatic mutations in simple repeated sequences reveal a new mechanism for colonic carcinogenesis. Nature 1993;363:558-61.
282. Ishizuka A, Siomi MC, Siomi H. A Drosophila fragile X protein interacts with components of RNAi and ribosomal proteins. Genes & Develop 2002;16: 2497-508.
283. Isshiki I, Murata M, Watanabe R, Matsubara Y, Kawano K, Aoki N, et al. Frequencies of prothrombin 20210G-A mutation may be different among races-studies on Japanese populations with various forms of thrombotic disorders and healthy subjects. Blood Coagul Fibrinol 1998;9:105-6.

284. Izatt I, Greenman J, Hodgson S, Ellis D, Watts S, Scott G, et al. Identification of germline missense mutations and rare allelic variants in the ATM gene in early-onset breast cancer. Gene Chromosome Canc 1999;26:286-94.
285. Jacquemont S, Hagerman RJ, Leehey M, Grigsby J, Zhang L, Brunberg JA, et al. Fragile X premutation tremor/ataxia syndrome: molecular, clinical, and neuroimaging correlates. Am J Hum Genet 2003;72: 869-78.
286. Jass JR. Familial colorectal cancer: pathology and molecular characteristics. Lancet Oncology 2000;1:220-6.
287. Jazwinska EC, Cullen LM, Busfield F, Pyper WR, Webb SI, Powell LW, et al. Haemochromatosis and HLA-H (Letter). Nat Genet 1996;14:249-51.
288. Jazwinska EC, Lee SC, Webb SI, Halliday JW, Powell LW. Localization of the hemochromatosis gene close to D6S105. Am J Hum Genet 1993;53:347-52.
289. Jenkins Ma, Baglietto L, Dite GS, Jolley DJ, Southey MC, Whitty J, et al. After *hMSH2* and *hMLH1*-What next? Analysis of three-generational, population-based, early-onset colorectal cancer families. Int J Cancer 2002;102:166-71.
290. Jenkins PV, Collins PW, Goldman E, McCraw A, Riddell A, Lee CA, et al. Analysis of intron 22 inversions of the factor VIII gene in severe hemophilia A: implications for genetic counseling. Blood 1994;84:2197-201.
291. Jiang H, Nucifora FC, Ross CA, DeFranco DB. Cell death triggered by polyglutamine-expanded huntingtin in a neuronal cell line is associated with degradation of CREB-binding protein. Hum Molec Genet 2003;12:1-12.
292. Jiricny J, Nystrom-Lahti M. Mismatch repair defects in cancer. Curr Opin Genet Dev 2000;10:157-61.
293. Johannesdottir G, Gudmundsson J, Bergthorsson JT, Arason A, Agnarsson BA, Eiriksdottier G, et al. High prevalence of the 999del5 mutation in Icelandic breast and ovarian cancer patients. Cancer Res 1996;56:3663-5.
294. Johnson DE, Lu J, Chen H, Werner S, Williams LT. Human fibroblast growth factor receptor genes: a common structural arrangement underlies the mechanisms for generating receptor forms that differ in their third immunoglobulin domain. Molec Cell Biol 1991;11:4627-34.
295. Jong MT, Gray TA, Ji Y, Glenn CC, Saitoh S, Driscoll DJ, et al. A novel imprinted gene, encoding a RING zinc-finger protein, and overlapping antisense transcript in Prader-Willi syndrome critical region. Hum Mol Genet 1999;8:783-93.
296. Jouanolle AM, Fergelot P, Gandon G, Yaouanq J, Le Gall JY, David V. A candidate gene for hemochromatosis: frequency of the C282Y and H63D mutations. Hum Genet 1997;100:544-7.
297. Kalafatis M, Bertina RM, Rand MD, Mann KG. Characterization of the molecular defect in factor V^{R506Q}. J Biol Chem 1995;270:4053-7.
298. Kato J, Fujikawa K, Kanda M, Fukuda N, Sasaki K, Takayama T, et al. A mutation, in the iron responsive element of H ferritin mRNA, causing autosomal dominant iron overload. Am J Hum Genet 2001;69:191-7.
299. Kenneson A, Zhang F, Hagedorn CH, Warren ST. Reduced FMRP and increased FMR1 transcription is proportionally associated with CGG repeat number in intermediate-length and premutation carriers. Hum Molec Genet. 2001;10:1449-54.
300. Kerem BS, Rommens JM, Buchanan JA, Markiewicz D, Cox TK, Chakravarti A, et al. Identification of the cystic fibrosis gene: genetic analysis. Science 1989;245:1073-80.
301. Kiesewetter S, Macek M, Davis C, Curristin SM, Chu CS, Graham C, et al. A mutation in CFTR produces different phenotypes depending on chromosomal background. Nat Genet 1993;5:274-8.
302. Kinzler KW, Nilbert MC, Su LK, Vogelstein B, Bryan TM, Levy DB, et al. Identification of FAP locus genes from chromosome 5q21. Science 1991;253: 661-5.
303. Kinzler KW, Vogelstein B. Landscaping the cancer terrain. Science 1998;280:1036-7.
304. Kishino T, Lalande M, Wagstaff J. UBE3A/E6AP mutations cause Angelman syndrome. Nat Genet 1997;15:70-3.
305. Klopp N, Oldenburg J, Uen C, Schneppenheim R, Graw J. 11 hemophilia A patients without mutations in the factor VIII encoding gene. Thromb Haemost 2002;88:357-60.
306. Knowlton RG, Cohen-Haguenauer O, Van Cong N, Grezal J, Brown VA, Barker D, et al. A polymorphic DNA marker linked to cystic fibrosis is located on chromosome 7. Nature 1985;318:380-2.
307. Koenig M, Hoffman EP, Bertelson CJ, Monaco AP, Feener C, Kunkel LM. Complete cloning of the Duchenne muscular dystrophy (DMD) cDNA and preliminary genomic organization of the DMD gene in normal and affected individuals. Cell 1987;50: 509-17.
308. Kremer B, Almqvist E, Theilmann J, Spence N, Telenius H, Goldberg YP, et al. Sex-dependent mechanisms for expansions and contractions of the CAG repeat on affected Huntington disease chromosomes. Am J Hum Genet 1995;57:343-50.
309. Kremer B, Goldberg P, Andrew SE, Theilmann J, Telenius H, Ziesler J, et al. A worldwide study of the Huntington's disease mutation: The sensitivity and specificity of measuring CAG repeats. N Engl J Med 1994;330:1401-6.
310. Kremer EJ, Pritchard M, Lynch M, Yu S, Holman K, Baker E, et al. Mapping of DNA instability at the

fragile X to a trinucleotide repeat sequence p(CGG)n. Science 1991;252:1711-4.
311. Kringen P, Egedal S, Pedersen JC, Harbitz TB, Tveit KM, Berg K, et al. *BRCA1* mutation screening using restriction endonuclease fingerprinting-single-strand-confirmation polymorphism in an automated capillary electrophoresis system. Electro 2002;23: 4085-91.
312. Kubota T, Das S, Christian SL, Baylin SB, Herman JG, Ledbetter DH. Methylation-specific PCR simplifies imprinting analysis. Nature Genet 1997;16: 16-7.
313. Kuismanen SA, Holmberg MT, Salovaara R, de la Chapelle A, Peltomaki P. Genetic and epigenetic modification of *MLH1* accounts for a major share of microsatellite-unstable colorectal cancers. Am J Pathol 2000;156:1773-9.
314. Kulczycki LL, Kostuch M, Bellanti JA. A clinical perspective of cystic fibrosis and new genetic findings: relationship of CFTR mutations to genotype-phenotype manifestations. Am J Med Genet 2003;116A:262-7.
315. Kunkel LM. Analysis of deletions in DNA of patients with Becker and Duchenne muscular dystrophy. Nature 1986;322:73-7.
316. Kunkel LM, Monaco AP, Middlesworth W, Ochs H, Latt SA. Specific cloning of DNA fragments absent from the DNA of a male patient with an X-chromosome deletion. Proc Natl Acad Sci USA 1985;82:4778-82.
317. Kunst CB, Warren ST. Cryptic and polar variation of the fragile X repeat could result in predisposing normal alleles. Cell 1994;77:853-61.
318. Lacroix-Desmazes S, Mistra N, Bayry J, Villary S, Kazatchkine MD, Kaveri SV. Antibodies with hydrolytic activity towards factor VIII in patients with hemophilia A. J Immunol Methods 2002;269: 251-6.
319. Lakich D, Kazazian HH, Antonarakis SE, Gitschier J. Inversions disrupting the factor VIII gene are a common cause of severe hemophilia A. Nature Genet 1993;5:236-41.
320. Lalloz MR, McVey JH, Pattinson JK, Tuddenham EGD. Haemophilia A diagnosis by analysis of a hypervariable dinucleotide repeat within the factor VIII gene. Lancet 1991;338:207-11.
321. Lalouel JM, Le Mignon L, Simon M, Fauchet R, Bourel M, Rao DC, et al. Genetic analysis of idiopathic hemochromatosis using both qualitative (disease status) and quantitative (serum iron) information. Am J Hum Genet 1985;37:700-18.
322. Lamlum H, Iiyas M, Rowan A, Clark S, Johnson V, Bell J, et al. The type of somatic mutation at *APC* in FAP is determined by the site of the germline mutation: a new facet to Knudson's "two-hit" hypothesis. Nat Med 1999;5:1071-5.
323. Latour P, Boutrand L, Levy N, Bernard R, Boyer A, Claustrat F, et al. Polymorphic short tandem repeats for diagnosis of the Charcot-Marie-Tooth disease 1A duplication. Clin Chem 2001;47:829-37.
324. Leach FS, Nicolaides NC, Papadopoulos N, Liu B, Jen J, Parsons R, et al. Mutations of a mutS homolog in hereditary nonpolyposis colorectal cancer. Cell 1993;75:1215-25.
325. Leavitt BR, Wellington CL, Hayden MR. Recent insights into the molecular pathogenesis of Huntington disease. Semin Neurol 1999;19:385-95.
326. Lebron JA, Bennett MJ, Vaughn DE, Chirino AJ, Snow PM, Mintier GA, et al. Crystal structure of the hemochromatosis protein HFE and characterization of its interaction with transferrin receptor. Cell 1998;93:111-23.
327. Ledford M, Friedman KD, Hessner MJ, Moehlenkamp C, Williams TM, Larson RS. A multi-site study for detection of the factor V (Leiden) mutation from genomic DNA using a homogeneous invader microtiter plate fluorescence resonance energy transfer (FRET) assay. J Molec Diag 2000;2:97-104.
328. Lee S, Kozlov S, Hernandez L, Chamberlain SJ, Brannan CI, Stewart CL, et al. Expression and imprinting of MAGEL2 suggest a role in Prader-Willi syndrome and the homologous murine imprinting phenotype. Hum Mol Genet 2000;9: 1813-9.
329. Leeflang EP, Zhang L, Tavare S, Hubert R, Srinidhi J, MacDonald ME, et al. Single sperm analysis of the trinucleotide repeats in the Huntington's disease gene: quantification of the mutation frequency spectrum. Hum Molec Genet 1995;4:1519-26.
330. LeGuern E, Gouider R, Mabin D, Tardieu S, Birouk N, Parent P, et al. Patients homozygous for the 17p11.2 duplication in Charcot-Marie-Tooth disease 1A. Ann Neurol 1997;41:104-8.
331. Leiden Muscular Dystrophy pages (database online). Dystrophin (DMD) sequence variations. http://www.dmd.nl/database.html.
332. Leonard DGB. Improved method for diagnosis of Charcot-Marie-Tooth type 1A: patent pending? Clin Chem 2001;47:807-8.
333. Levy-Lahad E, Catane R, Eisenberg S, Kaufman B, Hornreich G, Lishinsky E, et al. Founder BRCA1 and BRCA2 mutations in Ashkenazi Jews in Isreal: frequency and differential penetrance in ovarian cancer and in breast-ovarian cancer families. Am J Hum Genet 1997;60:1059-67.
334. Li FP. Familial cancer syndromes and clusters. Curr Prob Cancer 1990;14:73-144.
335. Li H, Li SH, Johnston H, Shelbourne PF, Li XJ. Amino-terminal fragments of mutant huntingtin show selective accumulation in striatal neurons and synaptic toxicity. Nature Genet 2000;25: 385-9.

336. Li SH, Gutekunst CA, Hersch SM, Li XJ. Association of HAP1 isoforms with a unique cytoplasmic structure. J Neurochem 1998;71:2178-85.
337. Li XJ, Li SH, Sharp AH, Nucifora FC, Schilling G, Lanahan A, et al. A huntingtin-associated protein enriched in brain with implications for pathology. Nature 1995;378:398-02.
338. Li Y, Chin LS, Levey AI, Li L. Huntingtin-associated protein-1 interacts with Hrs and functions in endosomal trafficking. J Biol Chem 2002;277: 28212-21.
339. Liede A, Narod SA. Hereditary breast and ovarian cancer in Asia: genetic epidemiology of *BRCA1* and *BRCA2*. Hum Mut 2002;20:413-24.
340. Liu Q, Nozari G, Sommer SS. Single tube polymerase chain reaction for rapid diagnosis of the inversion hotspot of mutation in hemophilia A. Blood 1998;92:1458-9.
341. Liu Q, Sommer SS. Subcycling-PCR for multiplex long-distance amplification of regions with high and low GC content: application to the inversion hotspot in the factor VIII gene. Biotech 1998;25:1022-8.
342. Lo WD, Sloan HR, Sotos JF, Klinger RJ. Late clinical presentation of partial carbamyl phosphate synthetase I deficiency. Am J Dis Child 1993;147:267-9.
343. Loesch DZ, Hay DA, Mulley J. Transmitting males and carrier females in fragile X-revisited. Am J Med Genet 1994;51:392-9.
344. Lozier JN, Dutra A, Pak E, Zhou N, Zheng Z, Nichols TC, et al. The Chapel Hill hemophilia A dog colony exhibits a factor VIII gene inversion. Proc Natl Acad Sci USA 2002;99:12991-6.
345. Lubs H. A marker X chromosome. Am J Hum Genet 1969;21:231-44.
346. Lunkes A, Mandel Jl. A cellular model that recapitulates major pathogenic steps of Huntington's disease. Hum Molec Genet 1998;7:1355-61.
347. Lupski JR, de Oca-Luna RM, Slaugenhaupt S, Pentao L, Guzzetta V, Trask BJ, et al. DNA duplication associated with Charcot-Marie-Tooth disease type 1A. Cell 1991;66:219-32.
348. Lupski JR, Wise CA, Kuwano A, Pentao L, Parke JT, Glaze DG, et al. Gene dosage is a mechanism for Charcot-Marie-Tooth disease type 1A. Nat Genet 1992;1:29-33.
349. Lusher JM. Considerations for current and future management of haemophilia and its complications. Haemophilia 1995;1:2-10.
350. Lynch HT, Shaw MW, Magnuson CW, Larsen AL, Krush AJ. Hereditary factors in two large Midwestern kindreds. Arch Intern Med 1966;117:206-12.
351. Lyon E, Frank EL. Hereditary hemochromatosis since discovery of the HFE gene. Clinical Chem 2001;47:1147-56.
352. MacDonald ME, Anderson MA, Gilliam TC, Tranebjaerg L, Carpenter NJ, Magenis E, et al. A somatic cell hybrid panel for localizing DNA segments near the Huntington's disease gene. Genomics 1987;1:29-34.
353. Mackey DA, Oostra RJ, Rosenberg T, Nikoskelainen E, Bronte-Stewart J, Poulton J, et al. Primary pathogenic mtDNA mutations in multigeneration pedigrees with Leber hereditary optic neuropathy. Am J Hum Genet 1996;59:481-5.
354. Maddalena A, Richards CS, McGinniss MJ, Brothman A, Desnick RJ, Grier RE, et al. Technical standards and guidelines for fragile X: the first of a series of disease-specific supplements to the standards and guidelines for clinical genetics laboratories of the American College of Medical Genetics. Genet in Med 2001;3:200-5.
355. Maestri NE, Hauser ER, Bartholomew D, Brusilow SW. Prospective treatment of urea cycle disorders. J Pediatr 1991;119:923-8.
356. Malter HE, Iber JC, Willemsen R, deGraaff E, Tarleton JC, Leisti J, et al. Characterization of the full fragile X syndrome mutation in fetal gametes. Nature Genet 1997;15:165-9.
357. Man PYW, Turnbull DM, Chinnery PF. Leber hereditary optic neuropathy. J Med Genet 2002;39:162-9.
358. Mann KG, Kalafatis M. Factor V: a combination of Dr Jekyll and Mr Hyde. Blood 2003;10120-30.
359. Markey K, Axel L, Ahnen D. Basic concepts for genetic testing in common hereditary colorectal cancer syndromes. Cur Gastroenterology Reports 2002;4:404-13.
360. Martin JP, Bell J. A pedigree of mental defect showing sex-linkage. J Neurol Psych 1943;6:154-7.
361. Martinelli I, Sacchi E, Landi G, Taili E, Duca F, Mannucci PM. High risk of cerebral-vein thrombosis in carriers of a prothrombin-gene mutation and in users of oral contraceptives. N Engl J Med 1998; 338:1840-1.
362. Martinelli I, Taioli E, Bucciarelli P, Akhavan S, Mannucci PM. Interaction between the G20210A mutation of the prothrombin gene and oral contraceptive use in deep vein thrombosis. Arterioscler Thromb Vasc Biol 1999;19:700-3.
363. Mattews PM, Marchington DR, Squier M, Land J, Brown R, Brown GK. Molecular genetic characterization of an X-linked form of Leigh's syndrome. Ann Neurol 1993;33:652-5.
364. Mazroul R, Huot ME, Tremblay S, Filion C, Labelle Y, Khandjian EW. Trapping of messenger RNA by fragile X mental retardation protein into cytoplasmic granules induces translation repression. Hum Molec Genet 2002;11:3007-17.
365. McCampbell A, Taylor JP, Taye AA, Robitschek J, Li M, Walcott J, et al. CREB-binding protein sequestration by expanded polyglutamine. Hum Molec Genet 2000;9:2197-202.
366. McConie-Rosell A, Lachiewicz AM, Spiridigliozzi GA, Tarleton J, Schoenwald S, Phelan MC, et al. Evidence

that methylation of the FMR-1 locus is responsible for variable phenotypic expression of the fragile X syndrome. Am J Hum Genet 1993;53:800-9.

367. McGlennen RC, Key NS. Clinical and laboratory management of the prothrombin G20210A mutation. Arch Pathol Lab Med 2002;126:1319-25.

368. Mclaren CE, Barton JC, Adams PC, Harris EL, Acton RT, Press N, et al. Hemochromatosis and iron overload screening (HEIRS) study design for an evaluation of 100,000 primary care-based adults.

369. Mefford HC, Baumbach L, Panguluri RC, Whitfield-Broome C, Szabo C, Smith S, et al. Evidence for a *BRCA1* founder mutation in families of West African ancestry. Am J Hum Genet 1999;65: 575-8.

370. Meijers-Heijboer H, van Geel B, van Putten WLJ, Henzen-Logmans SC, Seynaeve C, Menke-Pluymers MBE, et al. Breast cancer after prophylactic bilateral mastectomy in women with a *BRCA1* or *BRCA2* mutation. N Eng J Med 2001;345:159-64.

371. Meiser B, Butow P, Friedlander M, Barratt A, Schnieden V, Watson M, et al. Psychological impact of genetic testing in women from high-risk breast cancer families. Eur J Cancer 2002;38:2025-31.

372. Melton T, Clifford S, Kayser M, Nasidze I, Batzer M, Stoneking M. Diversity and heterogeneity in mitochondrial DNA of North American populations. J Forensic Sci 2001;46:46-52.

373. Mendell JR, Buzin CH, Feng J, Yan J, Serrano C, Sangani DS, et al. Diagnosis of Duchenne dystrophy by enhanced detection of small mutations. Neurol 2001;57:645-50.

374. Mequro M, Kashiwagi A, Mitsuya K, Nakao M, Kondo I, Saitoh S, et al. A novel maternally expressed gene, ATPIOC, encodes a putative aminophospholipid translocase associated with Angelman syndrome. Nature Genet 2001;28:19-20.

375. Metzler M, Legendre-Guillemin V, Gan L, Chopra V, Kwok A, McPherson PS, et al. HIP1 functions in clathrin-mediated endocytosis through binding to clathrin and adaptor protein 2. J Biol Chem 2001;276:39271-6.

376. Middleton-Price HR, Harding AE, Monteiro C, Berciano J, Malcolm S. Linkage of hereditary motor and sensory neuropathy type I to the pericentromeric region of chromosome 17. Am J Hum Genet 1990;46:92-4.

377. Miki Y, Swensen J, Shattuck-Eidens D, Futreal PA, Harshman K, Tavtigian S, et al. A strong candidate for the breast and ovarian cancer susceptibility gene *BRCA1*. Science 1994;266:66-71.

378. Milasin J, Muntoni F, Severini GM, Bartoloni L, Vatta M, Krajinovic M, et al. A point mutation in the 5'splice site of the dystrophin gene first intron responsible for X-linked dilate cardiomyopathy. Hum Molec Genet 1996;5:73-9.

379. Millan FA, Curtis A, Mennie M, Holloway S, Boxer M, Faed MJW, et al. Prenatal exclusion testing for Huntington's disease: a problem of too much information. J Med Genet 1989;26:83-5.

380. Miyaki M, Konishi M, Tanaka K, Kikuchi-Yanoshita R, Muraoka M, Yasuno M, et al. Germline mutation of MSH6 as the cause of hereditary nonpolyposis colorectal cancer. Nat Genet 1997;17:271-2.

381. Miyakura Y, Sugano K, Konishi F, Ichikawa A, Maekawa M, Shiyoh K, et al. Extensive methylation of *hMLH1* promoter region predominates in proximal colon cancer with microsatellite instability. Gastroenterology 2001;121:1300-9.

382. Miyoshi Y, Nagase H, Ando H, Horii A, Ichii S, Nakatsuru S, et al. Somatic mutations of the APC gene in colorectal tumors: mutation cluster region in the *APC* gene. Hum Molec Genet 1992;1:229-33.

383. Mohammed MS, Shaffer LG. Fluorescence in situ hybridization (FISH) for identifying the genomic rearrangements associated with three myelinopathies. Methods Molec Biol 2003;217:219-38.

384. Moirand R, Guyader D, Mendler MH, Jouanolle AM, Le Gall JY, David V, et al. HFE based re-evaluation of heterozygous hemochromatosis. Am J Med Genet 2002;111:356-61.

385. Monaco AP, Bertelson CJ, Middlesworth W, Colletti CA, Aldridge J, Fischbeck KH, et al. Detection of deletions spanning the Duchenne muscular dystrophy locus using a tightly linked DNA segment. Nature 1985;316:842-5.

386. Monaghan KG, Wiktor A, Van Dyke DL. Diagnostic testing for Prader-Willi syndrome and Angelman syndrome: a cost comparison. Genet in Med 2002;4: 448-50.

387. Monahan PE, White GC. Hemophilia gene therapy: update. Curr Opin Hematol 2002;9:430-6.

388. Monsonego-Ornan E, Adar R, Feferman T, Segev O, Yayon A. The transmembrane mutation G380R in fibroblast growth factor receptor 3 uncouples ligand-mediated receptor activation from down-regulation. Mol Cell Biol 2000;20:516-22.

389. Montagna M, Agata S, De Nicolo A, Menin C, Sordi G, Chieco-Bianchi L, et al. Identification of *BRCA1* and *BRCA2* carriers by allele-specific gene expression (AGE) analysis. Int J Cancer 2002;98:732-6.

390. Montagna M, Dalla Palma M, Menin C, Agata S, De Nicolo A, Chieco-Bianchi L, et al. Genomic rearrangements account for more than one-third of the *BRCA1* mutations in northern Italian breast/ovarian cancer families. Hum Molec Genet 2003;12:1055-61.

391. Mori PG, Pasino M, Vadala CR, Bisogni MC, Tonini GP, Scarabicchi S. Haemophilia A in a 46, X, i(Xq) female. Br J Haematol 1979;43:143-7.

392. Moutou C, Vincent MC, BiancalanaV, Mandel JL. Transition from premutation to full mutation in

fragile X syndrome is likely to be prezygotic. Hum Molec Genet 1997;6:971-9.

393. MRC Haemostasis & Thrombosis database resource site. The haemophilia a mutation, structure, test and resource site. http://europium.csc.mrc.ac.uk
394. Muller F, Dommergues M, Simon-Bouy B, Ferec C, Oury JF, Aubry MC, et al. Cystic fibrosis screening: a fetus with hyperechogenic bowel may be the index case. J Med Genet 1998;35:657-60.
395. Munemitsu S, Albert I, Souza B, Rubenfeld B, Polakis P, et al. Regulation of intracellular B-catenin levels by the adenomatous polyposis coli (APC) tumor-suppressor protein. Proc Natl Acad Sci USA 1995;92:3046-50.
396. Muntoni F, Cau M, Ganau A, Congiu R, Arvedi G, Mateddu A, et al. Brief report: deletion of the dystrophin muscle-promoter region associated with X-linked dilated cardiomyopathy. N Eng J Med 1993;329:921-5.
397. Mura C, Raguenes O, Ferec C. HFE mutations analysis in 711 hemochromatosis probands: evidence for S65C implication in mild form of hemochromatosis. Blood 1999;93:2502-5.
398. Muralidharan K. Detection of mitochondrial DNA mutations associated with Leber Hereditary Optic Neuropathy. Methods Molec Biol 2003;217:199-205.
399. Murotsuki J, Uehara S, Okamura K, Yajima A, Oura T, Miyabayashi S. Fetal liver biopsy for prenatal diagnosis of carbamoyl phosphate synthetase deficiency. Am J Perinatology 1994;11:160-2.
400. Myers RH, Farber LA, Busella JF, Martin JB. Predictive testing for Huntington's disease using linked DNA markers. N Engl J Med 1988;319:583-4.
401. Myers RH, Leavitt J, Farrer LA, Jagadeesh J, McFarlane H, Mastromauro CA, et al. Homozygote for Huntington disease. Am J Hum Genet 1989;45: 615-8.
402. Myers RH, Sax DS, Schoenfeld M, Bird ED, Wolf PA, Vonsattrel JP, et al. Late onset of Huntington's disease. J Neurol Neurosurg Psychiatry 1985;48:530-4.
403. Naef R, Suter U. Many facets of the peripheral myelin protein PMP22 in myelination and disease. Micro Res Techniq 1998;41:359-71.
404. Nagase H, Miyoshi Y, Horii A, Aoki T, Agawa M, Utsunomiya J, et al. Correlation between the location of germ-line mutations in the *APC* gene and the number of colorectal polyps in familial adenomatous polyposis patients. Cancer Res 1992;52:4055-7.
405. Nagata N, Matsuda I, Oyanagi K. Estimated frequency of urea cycle enzymopathies in Japan. Am J Med Genet 1991;39:228-9.
406. Nakada Y, Taniura H, Uetsuki T, Inazawa J, Yoshikawa K. The human chromosomal gene for necdin, a neuronal growth suppressor, in the Prader-Willi syndrome deletion region. Gene 1998;213:65-72.
407. Narod SA, Dube MP, Klijn J, Lubinski J, Lynch HT, Ghadirian P, et al. Oral contraceptives and the risk of breast cancer in BRCA1 and BRCA2 mutation carriers. J Natl Canc Insti 2002;94:23:1773-9.
408. Nathanson KL, Shugart YY, Omaruddin R, Szabo C, Goldgar D, Rebbeck TR, et al. CGH-targeted linkage analysis reveals a possible BRCA1 modifier locus on chromosome 5q. Hum Molec Genet 2002;11: 1327-32.
409. National Center for Biotechnology Information—http://www.ncbi.nlm.nih.gov/mapview/maps.cgi?org=hum&chr=l&maps=ideogr
410. National Committee for Clinical Laboratory Standards. Molecular diagnostic methods for genetic diseases; approved guidelines. National Committee for Clinical Laboraotory Standards 2000; CCLS document MM1-A, 17.
411. National Comprehensive Cancer Network. NCCN colorectal cancer screening practice guidelines. Oncology 1999;13:152-79.
412. Nativio DG. The genetics, diagnosis and management of Prader-Willi syndrome. J Pediatr Health Care 2002;16:298-03.
413. Nauhausen S. Founder populations and their uses for breast cancer genetics. Breast Cancer Res 2000;2: 77-81.
414. Naylor J, Brinke A, Hassock S, Green PM, Giannelli F. Characteristic mRNA abnormality found in half the patients with severe haemophilia A is due to large DNA inversions. Hum Molec Genet 1993;2:1773-8.
415. Nelson FW, Hecht JT, Horton WA, Butler IJ, Goldie WD, Miner M. Neurological basis of respiratory complications in achondroplasia. Ann Neurol 1988; 24:89-93.
416. Neuhausen S, Gilewski T, Norton L, Tran T, McGuire P, Swensen J, et al. Recurrent BRCA2 6174delT mutations in Ashkenazi Jewish women affected by breast cancer. Nature Genet 1996;13:126-8.
417. Newman NJ. Leber's hereditary optic neuropathy. New genetic considerations. Arch Neurol 1993;50:540-8.
418. Newman NJ. From genotype to phenotype in Leber Hereditary Optic Neuropathy: still more questions than answers. J Neuro-Ophthalmol 2002;22:257-61.
419. Nicholls RD, Knepper JL. Genome organization, function, and imprinting in Prader-Willi and Angelman syndromes. Annu Rev Genomics Hum Genet 2001:2:153-75.
420. Nicholls RD, Saitoh S, Horsthemke B. Imprinting in Prader-Willi and Angelman syndromes. Trends in Genet 1998;14:194-200.
421. Nicolaides NC, Papadopoulos N, Liu B, Wei TF, Ruben SM, Rosen CA, et al. Mutations of two PMS homologues in hereditary nonpolyposis colon cancer. Nature 1994;371:75-80.
422. Niemann S, Sereda MW, Suter U, Griffiths IR, Nave KA. Uncoupling myelin assembly and Schwann cell differentiation by transgenic overexpression of

peripheral myelin protein 22. J Neurosci 2000;20:4120-8.

423. Nishisho I, Nakamura Y, Miyoshi Y, Miki Y, Ando H, Horii A, et al. Mutations of chromosome 5q21 genes in FAP and colorectal cancer patients. Science 1991;253:665-9.
424. Njajou OT, Vaessen N, Joosse M, Berghuis B, van Dongen JWF, Breuning MH, et al. A mutation in *SLC11A3* is associated with autosomal dominant hemochromatosis. Nat Genet 2001;28:213-4.
425. Noguchi S, Tsukahara T, Fujita M, Kurokawa R, Tachikawa M, Toda T, et al. cDNA microarray analysis of individual Duchenne muscular dystrophy patients. Hum Molec Genet 2003;12:595-600.
426. Nolin SL, Brown WT, Glicksman A, Houck GE, Gargano AD, Sullivan A, et al. Expansion of the fragile X CGG repeat in females with premutation or intermediate alleles. Am J Hum Genet 2003;72: 454-64.
427. Nolin SL, Lewis FA, Ye LL, Houck GEJ, Glicksman AE, Limprasert P, et al. Familial transmission of the FMR1 CGG repeat. Am J Hum Genet 1996;59: 1252-61.
428. Nucifora FC, Sasaki M, Peters MF, Huang H, Cooper JK, Yamada M, et al. Interference by Huntingtin and atrophin-1 with CBP-mediated transcription leading to cellular toxicity. Science 2001;291:2423-28.
429. O'Sullivan MJ, McCarthy TV, Doyle CT. Familial adenomatous polyposis: from benchside to bedside. Am J Clin Pathol 1998;109:521-6.
430. Oberle I, Rousseau F, Heitz D, Kretz C, Devys D, Hanauer A, et al. Instability of a 550-base pair DNA segment and abnormal methylation in fragile X syndrome. Science 1991;252:1097-102.
431. Ohta T, Gray TA, Rogan PK, Buiting K, Gabriel JM, Saitoh S, et al. Imprinting-mutation mechanisms in Prader-Willi syndrome. Am J Hum Genet 1999;64:397-413.
432. Olopade OI, Fackenthal JD, Dunston G, Tainsky MA, Collins F, Whitfield-Broome C. Breast cancer genetics in African Americans. Cancer 2003;97:236-45.
433. Olynyk JK, Cullen DJ, Aquilla S, Rossi E, Summerville L, Powell LW. A population based study of the clinical expression of the hemochromatosis gene. N Engl J Med 1999;341:718-24.
434. Orioli I, Castilla E, Barbosa-Neto J. The birth prevalence rates for skeletal dysplasias. J Med Genet 1986;23:328-32.
435. Oritz-Lopez R, Li H, Su J, Goytia V, Towbin J. Evidence for a dystrophin missense mutation as a cause of X-linked dilated cardiomyopathy. Circulation 1997;95:2434-2440.
436. Orth M, Schapira AHV. Mitochondrial and degenerative disorders. Am J Med Genet 2002;106:27-36.
437. Ozcelik T, Leff S, Robinson W, Donlon T, Lalande M, Sanjines E, et al. Small nuclear ribonucleoprotein polypeptide N (SNRPN), an expressed gene in the Prader-Willi syndrome critical region. Nature Genet 1992;2:265-9.
438. Palomaki GE, Haddow JE, Bradley LA, FitzSimmons SC. Updated assessment of cystic fibrosis mutation frequencies in non-Hispanic Caucasians. Genet in Med 2002;4:90-4.
439. Parkkila S, Waheed A, Britton RS, Feder JN, Tsuchihashi Z, Schatzman RC, et al. Immunohistochemistry of HLA-H, the protein defective in patients with hereditary hemochromatosis, reveals unique pattern of expression in gastrointestinal tract. Proc Natl Acad Sci USA 1997;94:2534-9.
440. Parsons EP, Clarke AJ, Bradley DM. Newborn screening for Duchenne muscular dystrophy, a psychosocial study. Arch Dis Child 2002;86:F91-5.
441. Partington MW, Moore DY, Turner GM. Confirmation of early menopause in fragile X carriers. Am J Med Genet 1996;64:370-372.
442. Patel PI, Roa BB, Welcher AA, Schoener-Scott R, Trask BJ, Pentao L, et al. The gene for the peripheral myelin protein PMP-22 is a candidate for Charcot-Marie-Tooth disease type 1A. Nature Genet 1992;1:159-65.
443. Patrushev LI, Zykiva ES, Kayushin AL, Korosteleva MD, Miroshnikov AI, Bokarew IN, et al. New DNA diagnostic system for detection of factor V *Leiden*. Thrombosis Res 1998;92:251-9.
444. Pauli RM, Horton VK, Glinski LP, Reiser CA. Prospective assessment of risks for cervicomedullary-junction compression in infants with achondroplasia. Am J Hum Genet 1995;56:732-44.
445. Peelen T, van Vliet M, Petrij-Bosch A, Mieremet R, Szabo C, von den Ouweland AMW, et al. A high proportion of novel mutations in *BRCA1* with strong founder effects among Dutch and Belgian hereditary breast and ovarian cancer families. Am J Hum Genet 1997;60:1041-9.
446. Peltomaki P. Deficient DNA mismatch repair: a common etiologic factor for colon cancer. Hum Molec Genet 2001;10:735-40.
447. Peltomaki P, Aaltonen LA, Sistonen P, Pylkkanen L, Mecklin JP, Jarvinen H, et al. Genetic mapping of a locus predisposing to human colorectal cancer. Science 1993;260;810-2.
448. Peltomaki P, Vasen HF, and the ICG-HNPCC. Mutations predisposing to hereditary nonpolyposis colorectal cancer: database and results of a collaborative study. Gastroenterology 1997;113:1146-58.
449. Penney JB, Vonsattel JP, MacDonald M, Gusella J, Myers R. CAG repeat number governs the development rate of pathology in Huntington's disease. Ann Neurol 1997;41:689-92.
450. Pentao L, Wise CA, Chinault AC, Patel PI, Lupski JR. Charcot-Marie-Tooth type 1A duplication appears to arise from recombination at repeat sequences flank-

ing the 1.5 Mb monomer unit. Nature Genet 1992;2: 292-300.

451. Pequignot MO, Dey R, Zeviani M, Tiranti V, Godinot C, Poyau A. Mutations in the *SURF1* gene associated with Leigh syndrome and cytochromecoxidase deficiency. Hum Mutation 2001;17:374-81.
452. Petersen GM, Slack J, Nakamura Y. Screening guidelines and premorbid diagnosis of familial adenomatous polyposis using linkage. Gastroenterology 1991;100:1658-64.
453. Petit PX, Zamzami N, Vayssiere JL, et al. Implication of mitochondria in apoptosis. Mol Cell Biochem 1997;174:185-8.
454. Phatak PD, Ryan DH, Cappuccio J, Oakes D, Braggins C, Provenzano K, et al. Prevalence and penetrance of HFE mutations in 4865 unselected primary care patients. Blood Cells, Molecules, Dis 2002;29:41-7.
455. Phelan CM, Kwan E, Jack E, Li S, Morgan C, Aube J, et al. A low frequency of non-founder *BRCA1* mutations in Ashkenazi Jewish breast-ovarian cancer families. Hum Mut 2002;20:352-7.
456. Pieretti M, Zhang F, Fu YH, Warren ST, Oostra BA, Caskey CT, et al. Absence of expression of the FMR1 gene in fragile X syndrome. Cell 1991;66:817-22.
457. Poort SR, Rosendaal FR, Reitsma PH, Bertina RM. A common genetic variation in the 3′-untranslated region of the prothrombin gene is associated with elevated plasma prothrombin levels and an increase in venous thrombosis. Blood 1996;88:3698-703.
458. Powell LW. Diagnosis of hemochromatosis. Semin Gastrointest Dis 2002;13:80-8.
459. Powell LW, Burt MJ, Halliday JW, Jazwinska EC. Hemochromatosis: genetics and pathogenesis. Semin Liver Dis 1996;16:55-63.
460. Powell SM. Direct analysis for familial adenomatous polyposis mutations. Mol Biotechnol 2002;20: 197-207.
461. Preisinger E, Jordan BM, Kazantsev A, Housman D. Evidence for a recruitment and sequestration mechanism in Huntington's disease. Philos Trans R Soc Lond Ser B Biol Sci 1999;354:1029-34.
462. Press RD, Bauer KA, Kujovich JL, Heit JA. Clinical utility of factor V Leiden (R506Q) testing for the diagnosis and management of thromboembolic disorders. Arch Pathol Lab Med 2002;126:1304-18.
463. Prinos P, Costa T, Sommer A, Kilpatrick MW, Tsipouras P. A common FGFR3 gene mutation in hypochondroplasia. Hum Molec Genet 1995;4:2097-2101.
464. Prior TW. Determination of gene dosage-utilization of endogenous and exogenous internal standards. Methods Molec Biol 2003;217:3-12.
465. Prior TW, Bartolo C, Pearl DK, Papp AC, Snyder PJ, Sedra MS, et al. Spectrum of small mutations in the dystrophin coding region. Am J Hum Genet 1995;57:22-33.
466. Raeymaekers P, Timmerman V, De Jonghe P, Swerts L, Gheuens J, Martin JJ, et al. Localization of the mutation in an extended family with Charcot-Marie Tooth neuropathy (HMSNI). Am J Hum Genet 1989;45:953-8.
467. Rafael JA, Townsend ER, Squire SE, Potter AC, Chamberlain JS, Davies KE. Dystrophin and utrophin influence fiber type composition and post-synaptic membrane structure. Hum Mol Genet 2000;9: 1357-67.
468. Raha S, Robinson BH. Mitochondria, oxygen free radicals, and apoptosis. Am J Med Genet 2001;106:62-70.
469. Rampino N, Yamamoto H, Ionov Y, Li Y, Sawai H, Reed JC, et al. Somatic frameshift mutations in the BAX gene in colon cancers of the microsatellite mutator phenotype. Science 1997;275:967-9.
470. Rando TA. The dystrophin-glycoprotein complex, cellular signaling, and the regulation of cell survival in the muscular dystrophies. Muscle Nerve 2001;24:1575-94.
471. Ranjan Jana N, Zemskov EA, Wang G, Nukina N. Altered proteasomal function due to the expression of polyglutamine-expanded truncated N-terminal huntingtin induces apoptosis by caspase activation through mitochondrial cytochrome c release. Hum Molec Genet 2001;10:1049-59.
472. Rapp B, Haberle J, Linnebank M, Wermuth B, Marquardt T, Harms E, et al. Genetic analysis of carbamoylphosphate synthetase I and ornithine transcarbamylase deficiency using fibroblasts. Eur J Pediatr 2001;160:283-7.
473. Rechitsky S, Verlinsky O, Chistokhina A, Sharapova T, Ozen S, Masciangelo C, et al. Preimplantation genetic diagnosis for cancer predisposition. Reprod BioMed 2002;5:148-155.
474. Rees DC, Cox M, Clegg JB. World distribution of factor V Leiden. Lancet 1995;346:1133-4.
475. Reiter LT, Murakami T, Koeuth T, Pentao L, Muzny DM, Gibbs RA, et al. A recombination hotspot responsible for 2 inherited peripheral neuropathies is located near a mariner transposon-like element. Nature Genet 1996;12:288-97.
476. Reitsma PH, Bernardi F, Doig RG, Gandrille S, Greengard JS, Ireland H, et al. Protein C deficiency: a database of mutations, 1995 update. Thrombo Haemost 1995;73:876-89.
477. Richards CS, Bradley LA, Amos J, Allitto B, Grody WW, Maddalena A, et al. Standards and guidelines for CFTR mutation testing. Genet in Med 2002;4:379-91.
478. Richards CS, Watkins SC, Hoffman EP, Schneider NR, Milsark IW, Katz KS, et al. Skewed X inactivation in a female MZ twin results in Duchenne muscular dystrophy. Am J Hum Genet 1990;46: 672-81.

479. Richter C, Park JW, Ames BN. Normal oxidative damage to mitochondrial and nuclear DNA is extensive. Proc Natl Acad Sci USA 1988;85:6465-7.
480. Ridker PM, Miletich JP, Hennekens CH, Buring JE. Ethnic distribution of factor V Leiden in 4047 men and women. JAMA 1997;277:1305-7.
481. Riordan JR, Rommens JM, Kerem BS, Alon N, Rozmahel R, Grzelczak Z, et al. Identification of the cystic fibrosis gene: cloning and characterization of complementary DNA. Science 1989;245:1066-73.
482. Ripa R, Bisgaard ML, Bulow S, Nielsen FC. De novo mutations in familial adenomatous polyposis (FAP). Eur J Hum Genet 2002;10:631-7.
483. Roa BB, Boyd AA, Volcik K, Richards CS. Ashkenazi Jewish population frequencies for common mutations in *BRCA1* and *BRCA2*. Nature Genet 1996;14:185-7.
484. Roa BB, Garcia CA, Suter U, Kulpa DA, Wise CA, Mueller J, et al. Charcot-Marie-Tooth disease type 1A: association with a spontaneous point mutation in the *PMP22* gene. N Engl J Med 1993;329:96-101.
485. Roberts ML, Dickson G. The future of Duchenne muscular dystrophy gene therapy: shrinking the *dystrophin* gene. Curr Opin Molec Therapeutics 2002;4:343-8.
486. Robinson WP, Christian SL, Kuchinka BD, Penaherrera MS, Das S, Schuffenhauer S, et al. Somatic segregation errors predominantly contribute to the gain or loss of a paternal chromosome leading to uniparental disomy for chromosome 15. Clin Genet 2000;57: 349-58.
487. Robson ME. Clinical considerations in the management of individuals at risk for hereditary breast and ovarian cancer. Cancer Control 2002;9:457-65.
488. Robson ME, Offit K. Considerations in genetic counseling for inherited breast cancer predisposition. Sem Rad Oncol 2002;12:362-70.
489. Roetto A, Totaro A, Cazzola M, Cicilano M, Bosio S, D'Ascola G, et al. Juvenile hemochromatosis locus maps to chromosome 1q. Am J Hum Genet 1999;64:1388-93.
490. Rommens JM, Iannuzzi MC, Kerem BS, Drumm ML, Melmer G, Dean M, et al. Identification of the cystic fibrosis gene: chromosome walking and jumping. Science 1989;245:1059-65.
491. Rosendaal FR, Koster T, Vandenbroucke JP, Reitsma PH. High risk of thrombosis in patients homozygous for factor V Leiden (activated protein C resistance). Blood 1995;85:1504-8.
492. Rossiter JP, Young M, Kimberland ML, Hutter P, Ketterling RP, Gitschier J, et al. Factor VIII gene inversions causing severe hemophilia A originate almost exclusively in male germ cells. Hum Molec Genet 1994;3:1035-9.
493. Rousseau F, Bonaventure J, Legeai-Mallet L, Pelet A, Rozet JM, Maroteaux P, et al. Mutations in the gene encoding fibroblast growth factor receptor-3 in achondroplasia. Nature 1994;371:252-4.
494. Rousseau F, El Ghouzzi V, Delezoide AL, Legeai-Mallet L, Le Merrer M, Munnich A, et al. Missense FGFR3 mutations create cysteine residues in thanatophoric dwarfism type I (TDI). Hum Molec Genet 1996;5:509-12.
495. Rousseau F, Heitz D, Tarleton J, MacPherson J, Malmgren H, Dahl N, et al. A multicenter study on genotype-phenotype correlations in the fragile X syndrome, using direct diagnosis with probe StB12.3: the first 2,253 cases. Am J Hum Genet 1994;55: 225-37.
496. Roy CN, Andrews NC. Recent advances in disorders of iron metabolism: mutations, mechanisms and modifiers. Hum Molec Genet 2001;10:2181-6.
497. Rubin BK. Exposure of children with cystic fibrosis to environmental tobacco smoke. N Engl J Med 1990;323:782-8.
498. Rubinsztein DC, Leggo J, Barton DE, Ferguson-Smith MA. Site of (CGG) polymorphism in the HD gene. Nature Genet 1993;5:214-5.
499. Rubinsztein DC, Leggo J, Coles R, Almqvist E, Biancalana V, Cassiman J-J, et al. Phenotypic characterization of individuals with 30-40 CAG repeats in the Huntington disease (HD) gene reveals HD cases with 36 repeats and apparently normal elderly individuals with 36-39 repeats. Am J Hum Genet 1996;59:16-22.
500. Rubio V. Structure-function studies in carbamoyl phosphate synthetases. Biochem Soc transactions 1993;21:198-202.
501. Runte M, Huttenhofer A, Gross S, Kiefmann M, Horsthemke B, Buiting K. The IC-SNURF-SNRPN transcript serves as a host for multiple small nucleolar RNA species and as an antisense RNA for UBE3A. Hum Molec Genet 2001;10:2687-2700.
502. Ryall J, Nguyen M, Bendayn M, Shore GC. Expression of nuclear genes encoding the urea cycle enzymes, carbamoyl-phosphate synthetase I and ornithine carbamyl transferase, in rat liver and intestinal mucosa. Eur J Biochem 1985;152:287-92.
503. Saiki RK, Scharf S, Faloona F, Mullis KB, Horn GT, Erlich HA, et al. Enzymatic amplification of beta-globin genomic sequences and restriction site analysis for diagnosis of sickle cell anemia. Science 1985;230:1350-4.
504. Salter-Cid L, Brunmark A, Li Y, Leturcq D, Peterson PA, Jackson MR, et al. Transferrin receptor is negatively modulated by the hemochromatosis protein HFE: Implications for cellular iron homeostasis. Proc Natl Acad Sci USA 1999;96:5434-9.
505. Salvatore F, Scudiero O, Castaldo G. Genotype-phenotype correlation in cystic fibrosis: the role of modifier genes. Am J Med Genet 2002;111:88-95.
506. Sander M, Chavoshan B, Harris SA, Iannaccone ST, Stull JT, Thomas GD, et al. Functional muscle

ischemia in neuronal nitric oxide synthase-deficient skeletal muscle of children with Duchenne muscular dystrophy. Proc Natl Acad Sci USA 2000;97:13818-23.

507. Sarewitz S, ed. Molecular Pathology Checklist, CAP Laboratory Accreditation Program. College of American Pathologists, Northfield, Ill. 2003;19-21.
508. Sassaman EA, Zartler AS, Mulick JA. Cognitive functioning in two sisters with carbamyl phosphate synthetase I deficiency. J Ped Psychol 1981;6:171-5.
509. Schechter MS, Shelton BJ, Margois PA, Fitzsimmons SC. The association of socioeconomic status with outcomes in cystic fibrosis patients in the United States. Am J Respir Crit Care Med 2001;163:1331-7.
510. Schilling G, Sharp AH, Love SJ, Wagster MV, Li SH, Stine OC, et al. Expression of the Huntington's disease (IT15) protein product in HD patients. Hum Molec Genet 1995;4:1365-71.
511. Schon EA, Bonilla E, DiMauro S. Mitochondrial DNA mutations and pathogenesis. J Bioener Biomemb 1997;29:131-49.
512. Schoniger-Hekele M, Muller C, Polli C, Wrba F, Penner E, Ferenci P. Liver pathology in compound heterozygous patients for hemochromatosis mutations. Liver 2002;22:295-301.
513. Schwartz CE, Dean J, Howard Peebles PN, Bugge M, Mikkelsen M, Tommerup N, et al. Obstetrical and gynecological complications in fragile X carriers: a multicenter study. Am J Med Genet 1994;51: 400-402.
514. Schwartz M, Vissing J. Paternal inheritance of mitochondrial DNA. N Engl J Med 2002;347:576-580.
515. Schwiebert EM, Egan ME, Hwang TH, Fulmer SB, Allen SS, Cutting WB, et al. CFTR regulates outwardly rectifying chloride channels through an autocrine mechanism involving ATP. Cell 1995;82:1063-73.
516. Scott CL, Jenkins MA, Southey M, Davis TA, Leary JA, Easton DF, et al. Average age-specific cumulative risk of breast cancer according to type and site of germline mutations in BRCA1 and BRCA2 estimated from multiple-case breast cancer families attending Australian family cancer clinics. Hum Genet 2003;112:542-51.
517. Seeler RA, Vnencak-Jones CL, Bassett LM, Gilbert JB, Michaelis RC. Severe hemophilia A in a female: a compound heterozygote with nonrandom X-inactivation. Haemophilia 1999;5:445-9.
518. Seeman P, Mazanec R, Zidar J, Hrusakova S, Ctvrteckova M, Rautenstrauss B. Charcot-Marie-Tooth disease type 1A (CMT1A) and hereditary neuropathy with liability to pressure palsies (HNPP): reliable detection of the CMT1A duplication and HNPP deletion using 8 microsatellite markers in 2 multiplex PCRs. Internatl J Molec Med 2000;6:421-6.
519. Sereni LP, Bachmann C, Pfister U, Buscaglia M, Nicolini U. Prenatal diagnosis of carbamoyl-phosphate synthetase deficiency by fetal liver biopsy. Prenatal Diag 1988;8:307-9.
520. Sermon K, De Rijcke M, Lissens W, De Vos A, Platteau P, Bonduelle M, et al. Preimplantation genetic diagnosis for Huntington's disease with exclusion testing. Eur J Hum Genet 2002;10:591-98.
521. Sermon K, Goossens V, Seneca S, Lissens W, De Vos A, Vanderborst M, et al. Preimplantation diagnosis for Huntington's disease (HD): clinical application and analysis of the HD expansion in affected embryos. Prenatal Diag 1998;18:1427-36.
522. Sevilla C, Moatti JP, Julian-Reynier C, Eisinger F, Stoppa-Lyonnet D, Bressac-de Paillerets B, Sobol H. Testing for *BRCA1* mutations: a cost-effectiveness analysis. Eur J Hum Genet 2002;10:599-606.
523. Sherman SL. Premature ovarian failure among fragile X premutation carriers: parent of origin effect? Am J Hum Genet 2000;67:11-3.
524. Sherman SL, Jacobs PA, Morton NE, Froster-Iskenius U, Howard-Peebles PN, Nielsen KB, et al. Further segregation analysis of the fragile X syndrome with special reference to transmitting males. Hum Genet 1985;69:289-99.
525. Sherman SL, Meadows KL, Ashley AE. Examination of factors that influence the expansion of the fragile X mutation in a sample of conceptuses from known carrier females. Am J Med Genet 1996;64:256-60.
526. Sherman SL, Morton NE, Jacobs PA, Turner G. The marker (X) syndrome: a cytogenetic and genetic analysis. Ann Hum Genet 1984;48:21-37.
527. Shiang R, Thompson LM, Zhu YZ, Church DM, Fielder TJ, Bocian M, et al. Mutations in the transmembrane domain of FGFR3 cause the most common genetic form of dwarfism, achondroplasia. Cell 1994;78:335-42.
528. Shibata D, Peinado MA, Ionov Y, Malkhosyan S, Perucho M. Genetic instability in repeated sequences is an early somatic event in colorectal tumorigenesis that persist after transformation. Nat Genet 1994;6:273-81.
529. Shimohata T, Nakajima T, Yamada M, Uchida C, Onodera O, Naruse S, et al. Expanded polyglutamine stretches interact with TAF (II) 130, interfering with CREB-dependent transcription. Nature Genet 2000;26:29-36.
530. Shirio L, Otterud B, Stauffer D, Lynch H, Lynch P, Watson P, et al. Alleles of the APC gene: an attenuated form of familial polyposis. Cell 1993;75:951-7.
531. Silverstein MD, Heit JA, Mohr DN, Petterson TM, O'Fallon WM, Melton LJ. Trends in the incidence of deep vein thrombosis and pulmonary embolism: a 25-year population based cohort study. Arch Intern Med 1998;158:585-93.
532. Simon M, Bourel M, Fauchet R, Genete B. Association of HLA-A3 and HLA-B14 antigens with idiopathic haemochromatosis. Gut 1976;17:332-4.

533. Singaraja RR, Hadano S, Metzler M, Givan S, Wellington CL, Warby S, et al. HIP14, a novel ankyrin domain-containing protein, links huntingtin to intracellular trafficking and endocytosis. Hum Molec Genet 2002;11:2815-28.
534. Siomi H, Siomi MC, Nussbaum RL, Dreyfuss G. The protein product of the fragile X gene, *FMR1*, has characteristics of an RNA-binding protein. Cell 1993;74:291-98.
535. Smeitink J, van den Heuvel L, DiMauro S. The genetics and pathology of oxidative phosphorylation. Nat Rev Genet 2001;2:342-52.
536. Smith KH, Johns DR, Heher KL, Miller NR. Heteroplasmy in Leber's hereditary optic neuropathy. Arch Ophthalmol 1993;111:1486-90.
537. Snell RG, MacMillan JC, Cheadle JP, Fenton I, Lazarou LP, Davies P, et al. Relationship between trinucleotide repeat expansion and phenotypic variation in Huntington's disease. Nat Gent 1993;4:393-7.
538. Snipes GJ, Suter U, Welcher AA, Shooter EM. Characterization of a novel peripheral nervous system myelin protein (PMP-22/SR13). J Biol Chem 1992;117:225-38.
539. Snow K, Doud LK, Hagerman R, Pergolizzi RG, Erster SH, Thibodeau SN. Analysis of CGG sequence at the FMR1 locus in fragile X families and in the general population. Am J Hum Genet 1993;53:1217-28.
540. Sobetzko D, Braga S, Rudeberg A, Superti-Furga A. Achondroplasia with the FGFR3 1138-g to a (G380R) mutation in two sibs sharing a 4p haplotype derived from their unaffected father. J Med Genet 2000;37:958-9.
541. Souza R, Appel R, Yin J, Wang S, Smolinski KN, Abraham JM, et al. Microsatellite instability in the insulin-like growth factor II receptor gene in gastrointestinal tumours. Nat Genet 1996;14:255-7.
542. Sovavia C, Berk T, Madlensky L, Mitri A, Cheng H, Gallinger S, et al. Genotype-phenotype correlations in attenuated adenomatous polyposis coli. Am J Hum Genet 1998;62:1290-301.
543. Steiner RD, Cederbaum SD. Laboratory evaluation of urea cycle disorders. J Pediatr 2001;138:S21-9.
544. Stern RC. The diagnosis of cystic fibrosis. N Engl J Med 1997;336:487-91.
545. Steyaert J, Legius E, Borghgraef M, Fryns JP. A distinct neurocognitive phenotype in female fragile-X premutation carriers assessed with visual attention tasks. Am J Med Genet 2003;116A:44-51.
546. Strand M, Prolla TA, Liskay RM, Petes TD. Destabilization of tracts of simple repetitive DNA in yeast by mutations affecting DNA mismatch repair. Nature 1993;365:274-6. Erratum in Nature 1994;368:569.
547. Straub V, Campbell KP. Muscular dystrophies and the dystrophin-glycoprotein complex. Curr Opin Neurol 1997;10:168-75.
548. Strom CM, Huang D, Buller A, Redman J, Crossley B, Anderson B, et al. Cystic fibrosis screening using the College panel: platform comparison and lessons learned from the first 20,000 samples. Genet Med 2002;4:289-96.
549. Strom CM, Huang D, Chen C, Buller A, Peng M, Quan F, et al. Extensive sequencing of the cystic fibrosis transmembrane regulator gene: assay validation and unexpected benefits of developing a comprehensive test. Genet Med 2003;5:9-14.
550. Stronach EA, Clark C, Bell C, Lofgren A, McKay NG, Timmerman V, et al. Novel PCR-based diagnostic tools for Charcot-Marie-Tooth type 1A and hereditary neuropathy with liability to pressure palsies. J Peripher Nerv Syst 1999;4:117-22.
551. Sturtz FG, Latour P, Mocquard Y, Cruz S, Fenoll D, LeFur JM, et al. Clinical and electrophysiological phenotype of a homozygously duplicated Charcot-Marie-Tooth (type 1A) disease. Europ Neurol 1997;38:26-30.
552. Stutts MJ, Canessa CM, Olsen JC, Hamrick M, Cohn JA, Rossier BC, et al. CFTR as a cAMP-dependent regulator of sodium channels. Science 1995;269: 847-50.
553. Summar ML. Molecular genetic research into carbamoyl-phosphate synthase I: molecular defects and linkage markers. J Inher Metab Dis (Suppl 1) 1998; 21:30-9.
554. Summar ML. Current strategies for the management of neonatal urea cycle disorders. J Pediatr 2001;138:S30-9.
555. Summar ML, Dasouki MJ, Schofield PJ, Krishnamani MRS, Vnencak-Jones C, Tuchman M, et al. Physical and linkage mapping of human carbamyl phosphate synthetase I (CPSI) and reassignment from 2p to 2q35. Cytogenet Cell Genet 1995;71:266-7.
556. Summar ML, Hall LD, Eeds AM, Hutcheson HB, Kuo AN, Willis AS, et al. Characterization of genomic structure and polymorphisms in the human carbamyl phosphate synthetase I gene. Gene 2003;311:51-7.
557. Sun Y, Nicholls RD, Butler MG, Saitoh S, Hainline BE, Palmer CG. Breakage in the SNRPN locus in a balanced 46,XY,t(15;19) Prader-Willi syndrome patient. Hum Molec Genet 1996;5:517-24.
558. Suomalainen A, Kaukonen J. Diseases caused by nuclear genes affecting mtDNA stability. Am J Med Genet 2001;106:53-61.
559. Sutcliffe JS, Nakao M, Christian S, Orstavik KH, Tommerup N, Ledbetter DH, et al. Deletions of a differentially methylated CpG island at the SNRPN gene define a putative imprinting control region. Nature Genet 1994;8:52-8.
560. Sutcliffe JS, Nelson DL, Zhang F, Pieretti M, Caskey CT, Saxe D, et al. DNA methylation represses FMR-1 transcription in fragile X syndrome. Hum Mol Genet 1992;1:397-400.

561. Sweeney MG, Hammans SR, Duchen LW, Cooper JM, Schapira AHV, Kennedy CR, et al. Mitochondrial DNA mutation underlying Leigh's syndrome: clinical, pathological, biochemical and genetic studies of a patient presenting with progressive myoclonic epilepsy. J Neurol Sci 1994;121:57-65.
562. Swerdlow RH. Mitochondrial DNA-related mitochondrial dysfunction in neurodegenerative diseases. Arch Pathol Lab Med 2002;126:271-80.
563. Szabo CI, King MC. Population genetics of *BRCA1* and *BRCA2*. Am J Hum Genet 1997;60:1013-20.
564. Szebenyi G, Fallon JF. Fibroblast growth factors as multifunctional signaling factors. Internatl Rev Cytol 1999;185:45-106.
565. Tarleton J, Kenneson A, Taylor AK, Crandall K, Fletcher R, Casey R, et al. A single base alteration in the CGG repeat region of FMR1: possible effects on gene expression and phenotype. J Med Gent 2002;39:196-200.
566. Tavormina P, Shiang R, Thompson L, Zhu Y, Wilkin D, Lachman R, et al. Thanatophoric dysplasia (types I and II) caused by distinct mutations in fibroblast growth factor receptor 3. Nat Genet 1995; 9:321-8.
567. Tavtigian SV, Simard J, Rommens J, Couch F, Shattuck-Eidens D, Neuhausen S, et al. The complete *BRCA2* gene and mutations in chromosome 13q-linked kindreds. Nature Genet 1996;12:333-7.
568. Taylor RW, Morris AAM, Hutchinson M, Turnbull DM. Leigh disease associated with a novel mitochondrial DNA ND5 mutation. Euro J Hum Genet 2002;10:141-4.
569. Thibodeau SN, Bren G, Schaid D. Microsatellite instability in cancer of the proximal colon. Science 1993;260:816-9.
570. Thompson LM, Plummer S, Schalling M, Altherr MR, Gusella JF, Housman DE, et al. A gene encoding a fibroblast growth factor receptor isolated from the Huntington Disease gene region of human chromosome 4. Genomics 1991;11:1133-42.
571. Thompson TG, Kunkel LM. Advances in muscular dystrophy: exciting new prospects for the Millennium. NeuroScience News 2000;3:4-12.
572. Thorburn DR, Hans-Henrik MD. Mitochondrial disorders: genetics, counseling, prenatal diagnosis and reproductive options. Am J Med Genet 2001;106: 102-14.
573. Tiemann-Boege I, Navidid W, Grewal R, Cohn D, Eskenaz B, Wyrobek AJ, et al. The observed human sperm mutation frequency cannot explain the achondroplasia paternal age effect. Proc Natl Acad Sci USA 2002;99:14952-57.
574. Tiranti V, Hoertnage K, Carrozzo R, Galimberti C, Munaro M, Granatiero M, et al. Mutations of SURF-1 in Leigh disease associated with cytochrome c oxidase deficiency. Am J Hum Genet 1998;63:1609-21.
575. Tolttier Y, Devys D, Imbert G, Saudou G, An I, Lutz Y, et al. Protein cellular localization of the Huntington's disease protein and discrimination of the normal and mutated form. Nat Genet 1995;10:104-10.
576. Tosetto A, Rodeghiero F, Martinelli I, De Stefano V, Missiaglia E, Chiusolo P, et al. Additional genetic risk factors for venous thromboembolism in carriers of the factor V Leiden mutation. Br J Haematol 1998;103:871-6.
577. Triepels RH, van den Heuvel L, Loeffen J. Leigh syndrome associated with a mutation in NDUFS7 (PSST) nuclear encoded subunit of complex I. Ann Neurol 1999;45:787-90.
578. Trinder D, Olynyk JK, Sly WS, Morgan EH. Iron uptake from plasma transferrin by the duodenum is impaired in the *Hfe* knockout mouse. Proc Natl Acad Sci USA 2002;99:5622-6.
579. Truninger K, Malik N, Ammann RW, Muellhaupt B, Seifert B, Muller HJ, et al. Mutations of the cystic fibrosis gene in patients with chronic pancreatitis. Am J Gastroenterol 2001;96:2657-61.
580. Tsao CY, Herman G, Boue DR, Prior TW, Lo WD, Atkin JR, et al. Leigh disease with mitochondrial DNA A8344G mutation: case report and brief review. J Child Neurol 2003;18:62-4.
581. Tsui LC, Buchwald M, Barker D, Braman JC, Knowlton R, Schumm JW, et al. Cystic fibrosis locus defined by a genetically linked polymorphic DNA marker. Science 1985;230:1954-57.
582. Tuchman M, Mauer SM, Holzknecht RA, Summar ML, Vnencak-Jones CL. Prospective versus clinical diagnosis and therapy of acute neonatal hyperammonaemia in two sisters with carbamyl phosphate synthetase deficiency. J Inher Metab Dis 1992;15: 269-77.
583. Tuddenham EGD, Schwaab R, Seehafer J, Miller DS, Gitschiver J, Higuchi M, et al. Haemophilia A: database of nucleotide substitutions, deletions, insertions and rearrangements of the factor VIII gene, 2nd ed. Nuc Acids Res 1994;22:3511-33.
584. Tuomainen TP, Kontula K, Nyyssonen K, Lakka TA, Helio T, Salonen JT. Increased risk of acute myocardial infarction in carriers of the hemochromatosis gene cyc282tyr mutation. Circulation 1999;100: 1274-9.
585. Tutt A, Ashworth A. The relationship between the roles of BRCA genes in DNA repair and cancer predisposition. Trends Molec Med 2002;8:571-6.
586. Tyler A, Quarrell OWJ, Lazarou LP, Meredith AL, Harper PS. Exclusion testing in pregnancy for Huntington's disease. J Med Genet 1990;27: 488-95.
587. Tzen CY, Wu TY, Liu HF. Sequence polymorphism in the coding region of mitochondrial genome encompassing position 8389-8865. Foren Sci Internatl 2001;120:204-9.

588. Ulm J, Vnencak-Jones CL, Bosque P. Research on familial Creutzfeldt-Jacob Disease (FCJD) resulting in presymptomatic testing: implications for the Human Genome Project. J Genet Counseling 1993; 2:9-15.
589. Valentijn LJ, Baas F, Wolterman RA, Hoogendijk JE, van den Bosch HA, Zorn I, et al. Identical point mutations of PMP-22 in Trembler-J mouse and Charcot-Marie-Tooth disease type 1A. Nature Genet 1992;2:288-91.
590. Valleix S, Vinciguerra C, Lavergne JM, Leuer M, Delpech M, Negrier C. Skewed X-chromosome inactivation in monochorionic diamniotic twin sisters results in severe and mild hemophilia A. Blood 2002;100:3034-6.
591. Valnot I, von Kleist-Retzow JC, Barrientos A. A mutation in the human heme A:farnesyltransferase gene (COX 10) causes cytochrome c oxidase deficiency. Hum Mol Genet 2000;9:1245-9.
592. van den Heuvel L, Ruitenbeek W, Smeets R, Gelman-Kohan Z, Elpeleg O, Loeffen J, et al. Demonstration of a new pathogenic mutation in human complex I deficiency: a 5 bp duplication in the nuclear gene encoding the 18kD (AQDQ) subunit. Am J Hum Genet 1998;62:262-8.
593. van der Luijt R, Meera Khan P, Vasen HFA, Breukel C, Tops CM, Scott RJ, et al. Germline mutations in the 3' part of APC exon 15 do not result in truncated proteins and are associated with attenuated adenomatous polyposis coli. Hum Genet 1996;98:727-34.
594. Vance JM, Barker D, Yamaoka LH, Stajich JM, Loprest L, Hung W-Y, et al. Localization of Charcot-Marie-Tooth 1a (CMT 1a) to chromosome 17p11.2. Genomics 9;1991:623-8.
595. Vance JM, Nicholson GA, Yamaoka LH, Stajich J, Stewart CS, Speer MC, et al. Linkage of Charcot-Marie-Tooth neuropathy type 1A to chromosome 17. Exp Neurol 1989;104:186-9.
596. Vandenbroucke JP, Koster T, Briet E, Reitsma PH, Bertina RM, Rosendaal FR. Increased risk of venous thrombosis in oral-contraceptive users who are carriers of factor V Leiden mutation. Lancet 1994;344:1453-7.
597. Vasen HF, Mecklin JP, Khan PM, Lynch HT. The International Collaborative Group on Hereditary Non-Polyposis CRC. (ICG-HNPCC). Dis Colon Rectum 1991;34:424-5.
598. Vasen HFA, Watson P, Mecklin JP, Lynch HT and The International Collaborative Group on HNPCC. New clinical criteria for Hereditary Nonpolyposis Colorectal Cancer (Lynch syndrome) proposed by the International Collaborative Group on HNPCC. Gastroenterology 1999;116:1453-6.
599. Vehar GA, Keyt B, Eaton D, Rodriguez H, O'Brien DP, Rotblat F, et al. Structure of human factor VIII. Nature 1984;312:337-42.
600. Vehmanen P, Friedman LS, Eerola H, McClure M, Ward B, Sarantaus L, et al. Low proportion of *BRCA1* and *BRCA2* mutations in Finnish breast cancer families: evidence for additional susceptibility genes. Hum Molec Genet 1997;6:2309-15.
601. Veigl ML, Kasturi L, Olechnowicz J, Ma AH, Lutterbaugh JD, Periyasamy S, et al. Biallelic inactivation of *hMLH1* by epigenetic silencing, a novel mechanism causing human MSI cancers. Proc Natl Acad Sci USA 1998;95:8698-702.
602. Velier J, Kim M, Schwarz C, Kim TW, Sapp E, Chase K, et al. Wild-type and mutant huntingtins function in vesicle trafficking in the secretory and endocytic pathways. Exp Neurol 1998;152:34-40.
603. Velinov M, Jenkins EC. PCR-based strategies for the diagnosis of Prader-Willi/Angelman syndromes. Methods in Molec Biol 2003;217:209-16.
604. Velinov M, Slaugenhaupt SA, Stoilov I, Scott CI, Gusella JF, Tsipouras P. The gene for achondroplasia maps to the telomeric region of chromosome 4p. Nat Genet 1994;6:314-7.
605. Venkitaraman AR. Cancer susceptibility and the functions of BRCA1 and BRCA2. Cell 2002;108: 171-82.
606. Verellen-Domoulin C, Freund M, de Meyer T, Laterre C, Frederic J, Thompson MW, et al. Expression of an X-linked muscular dystrophy in a female due to translocation involving Xp21 and non random X-inactivation. Hum Genet 1984;67:115-9.
607. Verkerk AJ, Pieretti M, Sutcliffe JS, Fu YH, Kuhl DP, Pizzuti A, et al. Identification of a gene (FMR-1) containing a CGG repeat coincident with a breakpoint cluster region exhibiting length variation in fragile X syndrome. Cell 1991;65:905-14.
608. Vilkki J, Savontaus ML, Nikoskelainen EK. Segregation of mitochondrial genomes in a heteroplasmic lineage with Leber hereditary optic neuroretinopathy. Am J Hum Genet 1990;47:95-100.
609. Vnencak-Jones CL. Fluorescence PCR and GeneScan analysis for the detection of CAG repeat expansions associated with Huntington's disease. Methods Molec Biol 2003;217:101-10.
610. Vnencak-Jones CL, Phillips JA, Janco RL, Cohen MP, Dupont WD, Kazazian HH, et al. Analysis of factor VIII gene inversion mutations in 166 unrelated haemophilia A families: frequency and utility in genetic counseling. Haemophilia 1996;2:18-23.
611. Vu TH, Hirano M, DiMauro S. Mitochondrial disease. Neurol Clin N Am 2002;20:809-39.
612. Waelter S, Scherzinger E, Hasenbank R, Nordhoff E, Lurz R, Goehler H, et al. The huntingtin interacting protein HIP1 is a clathrin and alpha-adaptin-binding protein involved in receptor-mediated endocytosis. Hum Molec Genet 2001;10:1807-17.
613. Wagner A, Barrows A, Wijnen JT, van der Klift H, Franken PF, Verkuijlen P, et al. Molecular analysis of

hereditary nonpolyposis colorectal cancer in the United States: High mutation detection rate among clinically selected families and characterization of an American founder genomic deletion of the *MSH2* gene. Am J Hum Genet 2003;72:1088-1100.

614. Waheed A, Parkkila S, Saarnio J, Fleming RE, Zhou XY, Tomatsu S, et al. Association of HFE protein with transferrin receptor in crypt enterocytes of human duodenum. Proc Natl Acad Sci USA 1999;96: 1579-84.
615. Waheed A, Parkkila S, Zhou XY, Tomatsu S, Tsuchihashi Z, Feder JN. Hereditary hemochromatosis: effects of C282Y and H63D mutations on association with B2-microglobulin, intracellular processing, and cell surface expression of the HFE protein in COS-cells. Proc Natl Acad Sci USA 1997;94:12384-9.
616. Wallace DC, Singh G, Lott MT, Hodge JA, Schurr TG, Lezza AMS, et al. Mitochondrial DNA mutation associated with Leber's hereditary optic neuropathy. Science 1988;242:1427-30.
617. Wallace DF, Pedersen P, Dixon JL, Stephenson P, Searle JW, Powell LW, et al. Novel mutation in *ferroportin1* is associated with autosomal dominant hemochromatosis. Blood 2002;100:692-4.
618. Walon C, Kartheuser A, Michils G, Smaers M, Lannoy N, Ngounou P, et al. Novel germline mutations in the *APC* gene and their phenotypic spectrum in familial adenomatous polyposis kindreds. Hum Genet 1997;100:601-5.
619. Wang SS, O'Leary LA, FitzSimmons SC, Khoury MJ. The impact of early cystic fibrosis diagnosis on pulmonary function in children. J Pediatr 2002;141: 804-10.
620. Wanker EE, Rovira C, Scherzinger E, Hasenbank R, Walter S, Tait D, et al. HIP-I: A huntingtin interacting protein isolated by the yeast two-hybrid system. Hum Molec Genet 1997;6:487-95.
621. Warner JP, Barron LH, Brock DJH. A new polymerase chain reaction (PCR) assay for the trinucleotide repeat that is unstable and expanded on Huntington's disease chromosomes. Molec Cellular Probes 1993;7:235-9.
622. Wasmuth JJ, Hewitt J, Smith B, Allard D, Haines JL, Skarecky D, et al. A highly polymorphic locus very tightly linked to the Huntington's disease gene. Nature 1988;332:734-6.
623. Welsh MJ, Smith AE. Molecular mechanisms of CFTR chloride channel dysfunction in cystic fibrosis. Cell 1993;73:1251-4.
624. Wevrick R, Kerns JA, Francke U. Identification of a novel paternally expressed gene in the Prader-Willi syndrome region. Hum Mol Genet 1994;3: 1877-82.
625. Wexler NS, Young AB, Tanzi RE, Travers H, Starosta-Rubinstein SS, Penney JB, et al. Homozygotes for Huntington's disease. Nature 1987;326:194-7.
626. Wheeler PG, Smith R, Dorkin H, Parad RB, Comeau AM, Bianchi DW. Genetic counseling after implementation of statewide cystic fibrosis newborn screening: two years' experience in one medical center. Genet in Med 2001;3:411-5.
627. Whitcombe D, Brownie J, Gillard HL, McKechnie D, Theaker J, Newton CR, et al. A homogeneous fluorescence assay for PCR amplicons: its application to real-time, single-tube genotyping. Clin Chem 1998;44:918-23.
628. White GC. Gene therapy in hemophilia: clinical trials update. Thromb Haemost 2001;86:172-7.
629. Whitington PF, Alonso EM, Boyle JT, Molleston JP, Rosenthal P, Emond JC, et al. Liver transplantation for the treatment of urea cycle disorders. J Inher Metab Dis 1998;21:112-8.
630. Wilkin DJ, Szabo JK, Cameron R, Henderson S, Bellus GA, Mack ML, et al. Mutations in fibroblast growth-factor receptor 3 in sporadic cases of achondroplasia occur exclusively on the paternally derived chromosome. Am J Hum Genet 1998;63:711-6.
631. Willemsen R, Hoogeveen-Westerveld M, Reis S, Holstege J, Severijnen LA, Nieuwenhuizen IM, et al. The *FMR1* CGG repeat mouse displays ubiquitin-positive intranuclear neuronal inclusions; implications for the cerebellar tremor/ataxia syndrome. Hum Molec Genet 2003;12:949-59.
632. Williamson D, Brown K, Luddington R, Baglin C, Baglin T. Factor V Cambridge: A new mutation (Arg306-Thr) associated with resistance to activated protein C. Blood 1998;91:1140-4.
633. Windsor S, Lyng A, Taylor SAM, Ewenstein BM, Neufeld EJ, Lillicrap D. Severe haemophilia A in a female resulting from two de novo factor VIII mutations. Br J Haematol 1995;90:906-9.
634. Wion KL, Tuddenham EGD, Lawn RM. A new polymorphism in the factor VIII gene for prenatal diagnosis of hemophilia A. Nucleic Acid Res 1986;14:4535-4542.
635. Witte DL, Crosby WH, Edwards CQ, Fairbanks VF, Mitros FA. Practice guideline development task force of the College of American Pathologists: hereditary hemochromatosis. Clin Chim Acta 1996;245: 139-200.
636. Wong LJ, Craigen WJ, O'Brien WE. Postpartum coma and death due to carbamoylphosphate synthetase I deficiency. Ann Intern Med 1994;120:216-7.
637. Wong LJC, Liang MH, Kwon H, Park J, Bai RK, Tan DJ. Comprehensive scanning of the entire mitochondrial genome for mutations. Clin Chem 2002;48:1901-2.
638. Wooster R, Bignell G, Lancaster J, Swift S, Seal S, Mangion J, et al. Identification of the breast cancer susceptibility gene *BRCA2*. Nature 1995;378:789-92.
639. Wooster R, Neuhausen SL, Mangion J, Quirk Y, Ford D, Collins N, et al. Localization of a breast cancer

susceptibility gene, *BRCA2*, to chromosome 13q12-13. Science 1994;265:2088-90.

640. Wu Y, Berends MJW, Sijmons RH, Mensink RGJ, Verlind E, Kooi KA, et al. A role for *MLH3* in hereditary nonpolyposis colorectal cancer. Nat Genet 2001;29:137-8.
641. Yang Q, McDonnell SM, Khoury MJ, Cono J, Parrish RG. Hemochromatosis-associated mortality in the United States from 1979-1992: An analysis of multiple-cause mortality data. Ann Intern Med 1998;129:946-53.
642. Yang W, Dunlap JR, Andrews RB, Wetzel R. Aggregated polyglutamine peptides delivered to nuclei are toxic to mammalian cells. Hum Molec Genet 2002;11:2905-17.
643. Yazaki M, Yoshida K, Nakamura A, Koyama J, Nanba T, Ohori N, et al. Clinical characteristics of aged Becker muscular dystrophy patients with onset after 30 years. Eur Neurol 1999;42:145-9.
644. Yoshino M, Nishiyori A, Koga Y, Mizushima Y, Maeshiro H, Inoue T, et al. Potential pitfall of prenatal enzymatic diagnosis of carbamoyl-phosphate synthetase I deficiency. J Inher Metab Dis 1997;20: 1-2.
645. Yoshioka M, Yorifuji T, Mituyoshi I. Skewed X inactivation in manifesting carriers of Duchenne muscular dystrophy. Clin Genet 1998;52:102-7.
646. Yu S, Pritchard M, Kremer E, Lynch M, Nancarrow J, Baker E, et al. Fragile X genotype characterized by an unstable region of DNA. Science 1991;252:1179-81.
647. Zatz M, Vianna-Morgante AM, Campos P, Diament AJ. Translocation (X;6) in a female with Duchenne muscular dystrophy, implications for the localization of the DMD locus. J Med Genet 1981;18:442-7.
648. Zehnder JL, Benson RC. Sensitivity and specificity of the APC resistance assay in detection of individuals with factor V Leiden. Am J Clin Path 1996;106: 107-11.
649. Zeviani M, Moraes CT, DiMauro S, Nakase H, Bonilla E, Schon EA, et al. Deletions of mitochondrial DNA in Kearns-Sayre syndrome. Neurology 1988;38: 1339-46.
650. Zhi X, Szabo C, Chopin S, Suter N, Wang QS, Ostrander EA, et al. *BRCA1* and *BRCA2* sequence variants in Chinese breast cancer families. Hum Mut 2002;#554 online.
651. Zhou XY, Tomatsu S, Fleming RE, Parkkila S, Waheed A, Jiang J, et al. HFE gene knockout produces mouse model of hereditary hemochromatosis. Proc Natl Acad Sci USA 1998;95:2492-7.
652. Zielenski J. Genotype and phenotype in cystic fibrosis. Respiration 2000;67:117-33.
653. Zielenski J, Corey M, Rozmahel R, Markiewicz D, Aznarez I, Casals T, et al. Detection of cystic fibrosis modifier locus for meconium ileus on human chromosome 19q13. Nat Genet 1999;22:128-9.
654. Zimmer KP, Naim HY, Koch HG, Colombo JP, Rossi R, Schmid KW, et al. Survival after early treatment for carbamyl phosphate synthetase (CPS) I deficiency associated with increase of intramitochondrial CPS I. Lancet 1995;346:1530-1.
655. Zivelin A, Griffin JH, Xiao X, Pabinger I, Samama M, Conard J, et al. A single origin for a common Caucasian risk factor for venous thrombosis. Blood 1997;89:397-402.
656. Zivelin A, Rosenberg N, Faier S, Kornbrot N, Peretz H, Mannhalter C, et al. A single genetic origin for the common prothrombotic G20210A polymorphism in the prothrombin gene. Blood 1998;92:1119-24.
657. Zoidl G, Blass-Kampmann S, D'Urso D, Schmalenbach C, Muller HW. Retroviral-mediated gene transfer of the peripheral myelin protein PMP22 in Schwann cells: modulation of cell growth. EMBO J 1995;14:1122-8.

ADDITIONAL READING

Imprinting Disorders

Clayton-Smith J, Laan L. Angelman syndrome: a review of the clinical and genetic aspects. J Med Genet 2003;40:87-95.

Goldstone AP. Prader-Willi syndrome: advances in genetics, pathophysiology and treatment. TRENDS in Endocrinology and Metabolism 2004;15:12-20.

CHAPTER 41

Identity Assessment

Thomas M. Williams, M.D.,
Victor W. Weedn, M.D., J.D.,
and Malek Kamoun, M.D., Ph.D.

Identity testing exploits variations present within the human genome to distinguish between two individuals. Identity assessment has five basic uses: (1) confirm or refute that a sample is from a specific person in forensic testing; (2) resolve questions regarding the identity of a clinical specimen; (3) select donors for a planned transplant recipient to minimize rejection and improve graft survival, via histocompatibility testing; (4) assess whether hematopoietic cells are donor- or recipient-derived following stem cell transplantation; (5) identify the parents of a child.

VARIATION IN THE HUMAN GENOME

Identity testing began with the use of serological methods to identify variations in proteins that differ among individuals. The discovery of the genetic basis for these protein differences and of genetic variability at loci not encoding proteins, coupled with technical advances, allowed the field to move to direct analysis of DNA. Genetic variation among individuals is extensive, with about 1 sequence difference for every 400 to 1000 nucleotides on autosomal chromosomes. Variants of a genetic locus in a population are referred to as alleles. A locus is said to be polymorphic when the least common allele has a frequency of ≥0.01 in a population. While several alleles may be found in a population for an autosomal locus, an individual may have at most two alleles at that locus. There are several classes of genetic variants in the genome; some are more useful than others for identity testing.

GENETIC VARIATION USEFUL IN IDENTITY TESTING

Highly repetitive sequence elements that contribute to the structure of centromeres and telomeres and hundreds of thousands of copies of transposable elements that move about the genome over time may vary among individuals. However, these repetitive sequence elements are generally not useful for identity testing. More than 1 million single nucleotide polymorphisms (SNPs) have been identified in the genome. A subset of SNPs can be identified based on the ability of a restriction endonuclease to digest double-stranded DNA at the site of the variation. These SNPs are referred to as restriction fragment length polymorphisms (RFLPs). SNPs and RFLPs have been important in genetic linkage analysis and the study of disease pathogenesis; however, they are less useful for identity testing because they usually have only two alleles.

Variable numbers of tandem repeat loci (VNTRs) or minisatellite loci consist of repeated sequences of DNA. The number of repeats varies from allele to allele. This difference can be detected as an RFLP if the locus containing the VNTR is digested with a restriction endonuclease and hybridized to a labeled DNA probe in Southern hybridization assays. VNTRs are attractive for identity testing, because the loci usually have a number of different alleles with relatively high allele frequencies. Minisatellite regions are commonly subtelomeric and have core repeats of 8- to 80-base pair lengths, resulting in DNA fragment lengths of 0.5 to >20 kilobases.

Short tandem repeat (STR) or microsatellite loci consist of DNA sequence motifs that have core repeats of two to seven base pairs.[5,13] Examples include the dinucleotide 5′ CACACACA 3′ and the tetranucleotide 5′ TTTATTTATTTA 3′. Thousands of STRs are scattered throughout the genome. Because they are flanked by unique sequences, each can be specifically amplified with the polymerase chain reaction (PCR) for analysis. In populations of individuals, multiple alleles may be present based on differences in the number of repeated motifs at the locus. STRs have many characteristics that make them ideal for identity testing: (1) They can be analyzed in fluorescent automated systems; (2) alleles can be assigned in a definitive manner following analysis; (3) STR loci are almost always transmitted in families in a Mendelian fashion; (4) the loci may have 10 or more alleles, often with

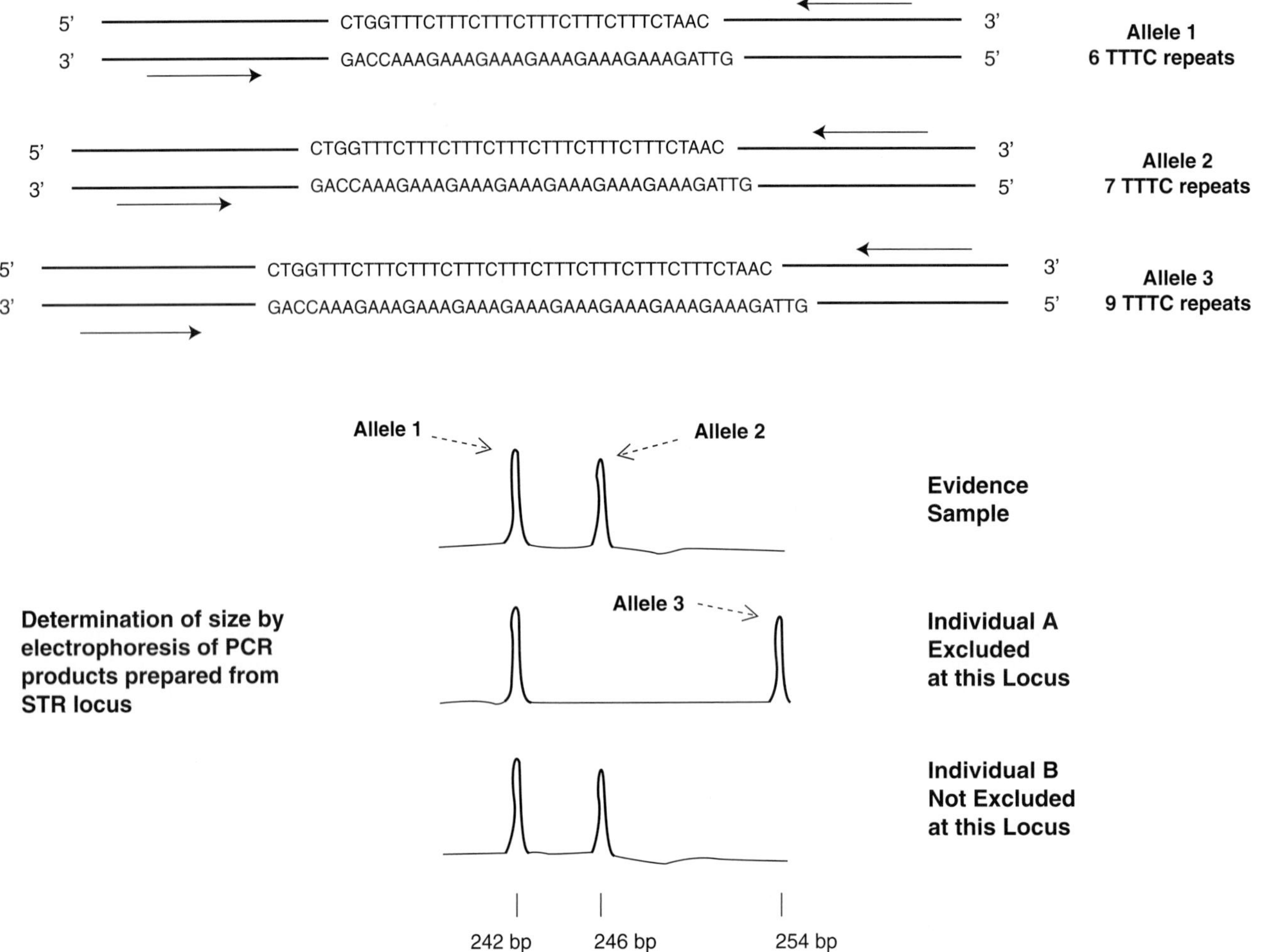

Figure 41-1 Identity testing via STR analysis. A STR locus can be specifically amplified with the PCR using primers binding to unique sequences adjacent to the repeat motif in the genome. In the example shown, the polymorphic repeat is the tetramer TTTC. Three example alleles with 6, 7, and 9 repeats at this locus are shown. The genotype for an individual or evidence sample can be determined by performing the PCR with a fluorescently labeled primer and sizing the products on a high-resolution gel with laser detection. The PCR products should differ in size from each other by multiples of 4 nt. The use of several fluorescent dyes and different-sized PCR products allows multiplexing for assessment of a number of independently segregating STR loci simultaneously.

substantial allele frequencies, making them highly informative; and (5) extensive information is available about allele frequencies in many human populations for STRs commonly used in identity testing.[6]

Commercially available STR systems employ tetrameric and pentameric repeat loci, which produce fewer artifactual bands and are characterized by roughly equal amplification of both alleles in an individual (Figure 41-1). Fragments can be labeled during the PCR amplification with fluorescently tagged primers that facilitate multiplexing.

Two special genetic regions with sufficient sequence variability for identity testing include the human leukocyte antigen (HLA) loci within the major histocompatibility complex (MHC) and the mitochondrial DNA. The HLA loci described in the Transplantation Testing section later in this chapter are interesting in that the polymorphisms are densely packed and preferentially located in the exons rather than the introns of these genes on chromosome 6. Mitochondrial genome variation is useful in forensic identity testing and is described in that section.

Exclusion of Tested Individuals

The exclusion of a tested person in identity testing is based on the presence of alleles at a locus that make it impossible for him or her to be a contributor to the tested sample. For example, if the person has the alleles j and k at the autosomal locus L, then, in the absence of mutations, it is not possible for him to be the major contributor to an evidence sample with the alleles m and n at L or to be the father of a child with the alleles m and p at L. In practice, laboratory protocols require that exclusion be based on incompatible results for at least two loci to rule out mutation events or other sources of error. In this context, "impossible" implies a situation in which samples have been collected correctly and have not been mislabeled, testing has been performed accurately, and results have been interpreted and reported appropriately.

Likelihood of Inclusion of Tested Individuals

If a tested individual has genotypes at several loci that are identical to the genotypes found in an evidence sample, then that person is not excluded as the contributor to the sample. The inclusion of a tested individual in identity testing is based on a probability calculation relying upon knowledge of the allele frequencies in human populations for the tested loci. For each locus, the likelihood that a random person of relevant ethnicity would have a genotype identical to that found in the evidence sample can be calculated. If the tested loci independently segregate during meiosis, the overall probability that a random person rather than the accused is responsible can be calculated by multiplying the likelihoods for each locus. When several loci are tested and each has many possible alleles, it becomes extremely likely that an individual whose genotypes match those found in the evidence sample is the person who contributed the DNA to the sample.

Discriminatory power is the ability of an identity testing system to distinguish an individual or group from the rest of the population. The power of discrimination of a locus or testing system should not be confused with accuracy. ABO blood group typing is accurate, but poorly discriminating, since this locus results in only a few phenotypes of generally high frequency in populations. Current identity test systems that employ a number of highly polymorphic loci may have powers of discrimination that exceed 1×10^{-10}, making it very unlikely that any unrelated individual on earth other than a nonexcluded suspect could be the source of an evidence sample. However, likelihoods of this magnitude should be viewed with knowledge that a variety of potential problems extraneous to the testing technology, involving sample collection and labeling, and test interpretation and reporting, may lead to an erroneous result.

Parentage calculations are often performed using Bayesian methods that consider the prior probability that an individual is the father of a child. It is obvious, for example, that the prior probability of a man living in Boston being the father of a co-worker's child is much greater than that of a Beijing inhabitant with no overt connection to the mother. Most crime laboratories in the United States do not report calculations using Bayesian analyses, but instead report the population phenotypic frequencies for White, Black, and Hispanic populations and sometimes a likelihood ratio that an individual is the source of a DNA specimen. When questions arise regarding assumptions that must be made during the calculation of inclusion probabilities, laboratories generally choose the conservative option that favors the accused individual.

Samples Employed for Identity Testing

Samples for identity testing can be any specimen that contains DNA. Samples obtained from an individual for paternity testing or as a reference sample to be compared with DNA prepared from evidence are usually peripheral blood or buccal mucosa. Samples useful for forensic testing, engraftment assays, and the identification of clinical samples may range from plucked hairs to bone marrow aspirates to paraffin embedded tissue. While subject to degradation over time in the presence of enzymes, acidic or basic conditions, or high temperature, DNA is a remarkably stable molecule that can be recovered and successfully analyzed from solutions, surfaces, and cells.

FORENSIC DNA TYPING

DNA testing has revolutionized criminalistics.[15,29] Only fingerprint evidence can rival the ability of DNA as trace evidence left at a scene to identify a perpetrator. As a general rule, other trace evidence merely links an article, instrument, or material to a scene. The origin of DNA-based identity testing is generally traced to a 1985 article in *Nature* by Alec Jeffreys.[14] He coined the term "DNA fingerprint" and suggested that the hybridization of DNA probes to polymorphic genetic loci could be exploited for forensic purposes. Jeffreys first applied his techniques to civil and criminal cases in England. In the United States, DNA-based identity testing was introduced via commercial laboratories and later the Federal Bureau of Investigation (FBI). Today there are approximately 200 forensic DNA typing laboratories in the United States and many other DNA laboratories around the globe.

Forensic Applications

Forensic testing differs from clinical laboratory testing in several ways: (1) The forensic question is usually one of identity rather than one of presence or absence, character, or quantity as in most clinical laboratory analysis. (2) Specimens received by forensic laboratories are much more diverse than the typical blood, fluid, and tissue samples handled by clinical laboratories. (3) Clinical samples are collected under controlled circumstances, while evidence from which DNA must be isolated may be exposed to the environment in a variety of ways. Experiments may be necessary to validate testing for a particular case. (4) Evidentiary material cannot be replenished and may be present in only trace amounts. Testing may consume the sample and thus complete or repeat testing may be impossible. (5) Forensic identity testing is scrutinized in a judicial environment requiring complete accounting for the whereabouts of evidence following its collection and strict validation of procedures. Most other laboratorians perform routine analyses of samples collected in defined ways. Forensic identity testing must contend with much more variability in samples and testing conditions.

TABLE 41-1 DNA Typing Systems and Their Characteristics

Genetic Systems	Timeframe	PCR-based	Discrimination	Comments
RFLP analysis of VNTRs	1980s-1990s	–	++++	Labor intensive
PCR dot-blots	1980s-1990s	+	+	Limited discrimination
STRs	Late 1990s to present	+	++++	Current mainstay
mtDNA	Mid1990s to present	+	++	Used in hairs, skeletons
Y-markers	Beginning use	+	++	Male DNA
Alu repeats	Not yet in use	+	++	Population marker
SNPs	Not yet in use	+	+++	Useful for samples with highly degraded DNA

Genetic Systems Used in Forensic Identification

Numerous genetic systems that are employed by forensic laboratories are summarized in Table 41-1.[3,21]

VNTR Analysis by RFLP

Jeffreys described a method to create a barcode-like DNA fingerprint based upon VNTRs. Because the probes used bind to several loci in Southern hybridization experiments and produce numerous bands per probe, they are termed "multilocus probes." In the United States, laboratories prefer single locus probe (SLP) systems that hybridize to only a single genetic locus. SLPs generally yield one or two bands on an autoradiogram per probe. SLP genetic systems are robust and generate readily interpretable bands, more precise allele frequency statistics, and less sensitivity to fragmentation of high molecular weight DNA.

RFLP testing with SLPs was the predominant method of DNA typing in most forensic laboratories throughout most of the 1990s. RFLP testing commonly employed six genetic loci: D1S7, D2S44, D4S139, D10S28, D14S13, D17S79. The resulting average discrimination for Caucasian Americans is approximately 1 in 1.2×10^{11}. However, Southern hybridization–based RFLP analysis is expensive, labor intensive, difficult to automate, and less sensitive than PCR-based methods. Furthermore, RFLP tests suffer from allele sizing imprecision, requiring that the results be binned and statistical measures of confidence employed for interpretation. Finally, RFLP is sensitive to DNA degradation—an important issue with environmentally exposed forensic specimens. RFLP tests have been largely abandoned in favor of the more efficient PCR-based assays discussed below.[4]

Short Tandem Repeats

Most identity testing performed today relies on the PCR. PCR testing is inherently sensitive, allowing routine analysis of nanogram quantities of genomic DNA and often successful testing of picogram quantities (one cell contains 5 to 10pg of DNA). The PCR underlies the characterization of STR and other loci for forensic identity testing loci described in this and later sections below.

STR testing is quick, less expensive, more forgiving with respect to technical skills needed, less sensitive to DNA degradation, and more amenable to automation in comparison with the Southern hybridization methods described above. Although less discriminating than RFLP genetic markers, STR analysis can be made as powerful as Southern RFLP analysis through the use of large numbers of informative loci.

The National Institute of Justice provided funding for the initial application of STRs in forensics. STRs were used in forensic casework during the first Persian Gulf War and were widely adopted for testing by forensic laboratories in the United Kingdom and the United States in the mid to late 1990s.

The FBI convened a panel of forensic scientists in 1998 that chose a panel of 13 STR loci for use in the National DNA Index System. These "13 core loci" have become the standard for casework and databanking for most forensic laboratories around the world (Table 41-2). They have been commercialized as kits by Promega (Madison, Wis.) and Applied Biosystems (Foster City, Calif.; a division of PerkinElmer) in a variety of formats. STRs are now routinely used in crime labs globally and typically yield discriminatory values of one in trillions to quadrillions.

Gender Markers and Y-Chromosome Markers

The amelogenin locus is useful as a gender marker. The X chromosome amelogenin gene differs from its homologue on chromosome Y by a six base pair polymorphism, allowing the distinction between individuals with 46,XY and 46,XX karyotypes. Males will display amelogenin locus heterozygosity; females will exhibit homozygosity. Reagents for assessing the amelogenin locus are incorporated in commercially available STR kits.

Y-chromosome polymorphic loci can be used as identifying loci found only in males. In this way, the male-specific DNA obtained from a vaginal swab can be typed without the usual "differential extraction" in which the DNA from

TABLE 41-2 List of Short Tandem Repeats Core Loci

	CURRENTLY AVAILABLE COMMERCIAL STR KITS			
Core Loci	**Profiler**	**Cofiler**	**Identifiler**	**Powerplex 16**
D3S1358	D3S1358	D3S1358	D3S1358	D3S1358
D5S818	D5S818		D5S818	D5S818
D7S820	D7S820	D7S820	D7S820	D7S820
D8S1170	D8S1170		D8S1170	D8S1170
D13S317	D13S317		D13S317	D13S317
D16S539		D16S539	D16S539	D16S539
D18S51	D18S51		D18S51	D18S51
D21S11	D21S11		D21S11	D21S11
CSF1PO		CSF1PO	CSF1PO	CSF1PO
FGA	FGA		FGA	FGA
THO1		THO1	THO1	THO1
TPOX		TPOX	TPOX	TPOX
vWA	vWA		vWA	vWA
			D2S1338	Penta D
			D19S433	Penta E
	Amelogenin	Amelogenin	Amelogenin	Amelogenin

The 13 STR core loci are listed against the STR systems present in the currently available commercial STR kits. Profiler, Cofiler, and Identifiler are available from Applied Biosystems, Inc. (Foster City, Calif.) and Powerplex 16 is available from Promega Corp. (Madison, Wis).

TABLE 41-3 Y-Chromosome Markers

European	European	U.S. Haplotype
Minimal Haplotype	Extended Haplotype	
DYS19	DYS19	DYS19
DYS385a/b	DYS385a/b	DYS385a/b
DYS389 I/II	DYS389 I/II	DYS389 I/II
DYS390	DYS390	DYS390
DYS391	DYS391	DYS391
DYS392	DYS392	DYS392
DYS393	DYS393	DYS393
	YCAIIa/b	
		DYS348
		DYS349

Y-chromosome markers are listed in their major haplotype groups.

spermatozoa is released after the female fraction from epithelial cells. Y-chromosome loci useful for identity testing include STRs or SNPs (described later in this chapter). Laboratories typically employ locally developed or commercially available panels of 6-20 Y-chromosome STRs for analyses (Table 41-3). Y-chromosome SNPs are in development.

Y-chromosome polymorphic loci are linked, resulting in discriminatory power significantly less than a panel of independently segregating somatic STR loci. Discriminatory values can be increased by using a large panel of Y-chromosome markers in conjunction with a large database of typed individuals.

Mitochondrial DNA

Mitochondrial genomes are circular double-stranded DNA molecules, which are 16,569 base pairs long, that are present as one or more copies within the mitochondria of a cell. Thus mitochondrial DNA (mtDNA) is present in hundreds to thousands of copies per cell. MtDNA, unlike chromosomal DNA, does not undergo meiosis and does not participate in genetic recombination events. MtDNA remains stable over generations, except for the acquisition of mutations at a rate 10 to 20 times that of nuclear DNA.

MtDNA is transmitted to children via oocytes. Although it is generally thought that mitochondrial DNA is exclusively derived from the mother, a minor contribution from the father is occasionally present, particularly in disease states. The normal state of mitochondria is generally thought to be one of "homoplasmy," in which all the mtDNA has the same sequence. However, because of mutational events, a state of "heteroplasmy" in which more than one mtDNA sequence is present in the same tissue may exist. High-level heteroplasmy is generally of the order of 30% of the mtDNA sequence before it is reported. Unrecognized low-level heteroplasmy is common. Heteroplasmy appears to be somewhat tissue-specific rather than uniform throughout the body. Thus two shed hairs may show discrepant mtDNA sequences. Due to heteroplasmy, one or two nucleotide mismatches between two individuals is not an absolute basis for exclusion of a tested individual.

In the human mitochondrial genome, only approximately 1200 bases in the region of transcription origin (15971-579), known as the "displacement loop" (D-loop) or "control region," are noncoding. This D-loop contains two hypervariable regions that contain the majority of polymorphisms useful for identity (HVI: 16024-16365, HVII: 73-340). Polymorphisms outside this region can also be employed for testing. MtDNA polymorphisms are typically identified for forensic testing via DNA sequencing of the hypervariable regions.[13] This method is expensive, labor intensive, and highly sensitive to contamination. A limited number of laboratories offer this service. More convenient hybridization technology for mtDNA testing has recently been introduced as a "linear array" by Roche Molecular Systems (Alameda, Calif.).

The mtDNA sequence obtained from a specimen is compared with the "revised Cambridge" reference sequence. Because mtDNA polymorphisms are linked, the individual polymorphism frequencies cannot be multiplied together to generate a likelihood of identity like independently segregating chromosomal locus allele frequencies. Instead the mtDNA haplotype identified in a sample is compared with those deposited in a database to derive a frequency statistic. Most mitochondrial haplotypes in the database are unique. Since the database has greater than 600 entries, it can be fairly stated that most mitochondrial haplotypes have a discriminatory value of greater than 1 in 600. However, there are 18 common haplotypes with population frequencies greater than 0.5% including a haplotype present in 7% of the population. In aggregate, these common haplotypes account for 20% of all haplotypes.

MtDNA is primarily useful in identity testing in three contexts. First, a sample may be available that contains mitochondrial but not nuclear DNA. For example, shed hairs that do not have roots generally contain only mtDNA. Second, when the DNA within a specimen, such as skeletal remains, is substantially degraded, the high copy number of mtDNA makes it more likely to yield a result than nuclear DNA. Third, mtDNA analysis may become essential when only a distant relative is available for a reference specimen. In this example, nuclear DNA requires samples from multiple close kindred, but mtDNA matching would require only a distant maternal relative.

Single Nucleotide Polymorphisms

A DNA locus whose polymorphism extends over a short region is generally preferable for identity testing, because it may remain intact and available for analysis in the face of extensive levels of DNA degradation. Loci for which a single base pair varies in a population of individuals are referred to as SNPs. These are the most common type of polymorphisms in the human genome. They are particularly amenable to automation and chip technology using hybridization, polymerase extension, or ligation reaction assays. Despite a four-base possibility, most are biallelic with a dominant and nondominant allele. A large set of SNPs must be used to obtain significant discriminatory values. SNPs are not used in forensic laboratories at this time, but are likely to be used in the near future. SNP analysis is expected to be particularly useful in identifying individuals killed in the World Trade Center collapse for whom only severely degraded DNA samples are available.

Other Systems

Other systems are also being pursued for forensic identity testing, generally for phenotypic information. The Alu family of mobile elements comprises 5% of the human genome. These elements repeatedly insert themselves into the human genome. Polymorphisms occur within these elements so that the age of the element can be inferred. The systems are inherited; the recent polymorphisms become markers of descent and older elements (without the Alu insertion site) are markers of root ancestry. Similarly, the L1 family of long interspersed elements (LINES) can be used to trace evolutionary ancestry. In combination with other genetic systems, Alu and LINE markers will provide some statistical inference about human evolution and race and ethnicity that may be helpful to investigators.

Instrumentation Used in Forensic Laboratories

Most forensic DNA testing is performed using capillary electrophoretic (CE) systems. These systems have a substantially faster run times and higher resolution than slab gels. The ABI Prism 310 Genetic Analyzer is currently the most popular instrument for forensic DNA casework, but other CE systems are also available. Instrumentation allowing "on-demand" handling of a few specimens at fast run times is convenient for most casework. High-throughput capillary instruments are used as "batch" instruments for DNA databanking operations. The ABI Prism 3100 Genetic Analyzer is available as a 4 or 16 capillary system and the ABI Prism 3700 DNA Analyzer is a 96 capillary unit. Amersham Biosciences sells the Megabace series of instruments that can be configured with 48, 96, or 384 capillaries.

Instrumentation under development for forensic testing generally focuses on a goal of miniaturization yielding ultrafast and portable assays that would be useful for field testing. Network Biosystems (Boston) is miniaturizing capillary arrays by etching microchannels into large chips, resulting in an ultrafast CE array that has run times of seconds and produces sharper bands than conventional CE instruments. Nanogen (San Diego) has produced chip technology based on "electronic stringency control" that can detect STR and SNP systems.

Quality Assurance and Accreditation in Forensic DNA Analysis

Crime labs are unregulated, except in the case of submission of DNA results to the National DNA Index System (NDIS) through the Combined DNA Index System software. The

DNA Identification Act of 1994 gave the FBI regulatory oversight of DNA profiles entered into the national database. The legislation called for a DNA Advisory Board that produced recommended standards, based largely on guidelines of the FBI's Technical Working Group on DNA Analysis Methods (TWGDAM). The Scientific Working Group on DNA Analysis Methods, which has replaced the TWGDAM, now advises the FBI Director to create standards revisions.

One aspect of the FBI/DNA Advisory Board standards is a requirement for accreditation. The National Forensic Science Technology Center and the American Society of Crime Laboratory Directors/Laboratory Accreditation Board (ASCLD/LAB) accredit crime laboratories. ASCLD/LAB requirements include minimal educational credits and experience, proficiency testing twice a year per analyst, and annual audits. All testing requires a technical and an administrative review. An additional NDIS audit is required by the FBI. Judicial scrutiny provides another layer of critical review of those cases heard in court. Defense review and challenge, however, vary greatly.

Proficiency test providers for forensic laboratories include the Collaborative Testing Service, the College of American Pathologists, Cellmark Diagnostics, and Quality Forensics.

Standard reference materials from the National Institute of Standards and Technology (NIST) are available for RFLP Profiling (SRM 2390), PCR-based Profiling DNA standard (SRM 2391b), Y-chromosome testing (SRM 2395), and mtDNA testing. Standards require annual NIST-traceable comparisons.

Statistical Interpretation

In the early days of DNA-based identity testing, significant challenges were launched regarding the interpretation of DNA typing results.[7,11,16,30] Questions included whether loci exhibit Hardy-Weinberg equilibrium and whether allele frequencies vary significantly among ethnic groups. Current forensic genetic systems have not demonstrated significant deviation from Hardy-Weinberg equilibria. The systems also show greater intragroup allelic diversity than between-group diversity. A National Research Council panel was created to address these issues.[18] The resultant report (so-called "NRC I") introduced a "ceiling principle" to ensure the conservativism of the frequency estimates, which itself generated considerable controversy. This led to NRC II, which articulated the current standards of statistical analysis.[19] Statistical formulas are routinely applied to Caucasian, Black, and Hispanic population databases. Specialized databases also exist for Native American Indian and for Pacific and African populations.

Convicted Offender Databases

All 50 states now have convicted offender databases. Initially, most databases exclusively contained sexual offenders, but the recent trend is to expand the databases to include all felons. States have begun to consider collecting DNA evidence in connection with lesser crimes, such as burglaries, to help solve these cases, to potentially interdict the progression to more serious future offenses, and to identify "hits" in the databases linked to past serious crimes. Three states (Louisiana, Texas, and Virginia) have recently adopted legislation allowing collection of DNA specimens on arrest.

DNA profiles are placed in the NDIS. If a "hit" is determined, the local crime laboratories of the involved states are put in contact to discuss details. Identifying information other than the DNA profile is not entered into the system. Uploading of DNA profiles triggers quality assurance requirements and legal constraints on the use of the DNA specimens and profiles.

The use of identity testing and linked databases in crime investigation has been aggressively pursued in the United Kingdom. U.K. forensic scientists maintain that approximately 50% of biological specimens from crime scenes result in hits in their databases, suggesting that a relatively small group of professional criminals perpetrate most crimes. They believe that DNA-based testing may be a more efficient tool for investigating crimes than traditional methods, such as canvassing neighborhoods.

Legal Issues

Early challenges to the practice and interpretation of DNA-based forensic identification have faded as the public, attorneys, and judges have become more knowledgeable about this technology. The most common challenges today involve issues regarding sample collection, preservation of the evidence, chain-of-custody documentation, and validation studies. New applications of DNA-based testing to assess ethnicity or to infer phenotypic features from evidence or to identify an assailant from very small samples, such as fingerprints,[28] are likely to cause controversy in the future.

USE OF DNA TESTING FOR THE IDENTIFICATION OF CLINICAL SPECIMENS

Identity testing can also be used to confirm the identity of a clinical or anatomic pathology laboratory patient specimen.[24,25] Occasionally, questions arise regarding the identity of specimens in the clinical laboratory. DNA prepared from a peripheral blood or buccal mucosa specimen can be compared with the pathology specimen to confirm that it is derived from the patient. The authors have encountered a variety of requests for this specialized identity service. (1) A patient lost confidence that her breast biopsy results were hers following a series of reporting errors involving the spelling of her name and her birth date. (2) A biopsy of a colonic lesion revealed adenocarcinoma. The subsequent colectomy specimen was devoid of a tumor. (3) A gastrectomy was performed after a biopsy diagnosis of adenocarcinoma. No tumor was seen in the gastrectomy specimen. (4) Multiple blocks from two breast lumpectomy procedures were processed. Because of labeling errors, it was unclear to which patient the various paraffin embedded blocks belonged. (5) A young male fractured his femur and developed osteomyelitis. Curettings from the fracture site demonstrated acute inflammation but also a fragment of tissue that appeared to be a squamous cell carcinoma.

In cases 1-4, identity testing with STRs demonstrated that all the specimens in question truly belonged to the involved patients. In case 5, testing following microdissection of the tissue fragments revealed that the squamous carcinoma "floater" was derived from another individual. The availability of identity testing in situations such as these can be a significant benefit to the involved patients and health providers.

In prenatal testing for inherited disorders, chorionic villus sampling (CVS) performed early in pregnancy is sometimes employed as a source of fetal DNA for testing. Testing for a disorder such as cystic fibrosis may reveal that the genotypes for the mother and the fetus are identical, for example that they are both heterozygous carriers of a cystic fibrosis mutation. This result is entirely consistent with the usual segregation of chromosomes during meiosis. However, there is a risk that the CVS material was not derived largely from the fetus but was decidual cells primarily from the mother. If the father is a carrier of a cystic fibrosis mutation, this may result in the failure to diagnose cystic fibrosis in a fetus. Identity testing can be employed to confirm that the tested cells have a genotype distinct from those of the mother and are a valid sample from the fetus.

TRANSPLANTATION TESTING

Obtaining well-matched tissue enhances transplanted organ and bone marrow survival. The human leukocyte antigen (HLA) alleles determine the tissue compatibility for the acceptance of transplanted allografts. HLA genes encode highly polymorphic cell surface molecules that are strong alloantigens. A kidney allograft is rejected as a result of an immune response directed against HLA alloantigens, which are expressed on the graft but are absent from the host.

GENETIC FEATURES OF HLA GENES

The HLA genes are located within a genetic complex designated as the MHC. The MHC includes about 4 Mb on the short arm of chromosome 6 (6p21.3). Many of the more than 200 genes in the MHC are involved in the regulation of the immune response.[16,20] The genes encoding the HLA class I (A, B, and C) and the class II (DR, DQ, and DP) molecules are the most polymorphic loci in the human genome (Figure 41-2 [Color Plate 12] and Table 41-4). This polymorphism made the HLA loci an attractive and powerful early resource for identity testing.

HLA genes are co-dominantly expressed and most individuals are heterozygous at the HLA class I and class II loci. Most of the sequence diversity for the HLA class I loci is located in the second and third exons and, for the class II loci, the second exon. These domains encode the peptide-binding regions of the HLA molecules. The pattern of allelic sequence diversity for both the class I and class II loci is unusual; most alleles differ from their closest neighbor by multiple substitutions, with some alleles differing in the second and third exons by as much as 15%. This pattern is suggestive of segmental exchange of nucleotide motifs between alleles of the same locus. As a result, different HLA alleles are mosaic-like combinations of a subset of all polymorphisms.[10,17]

Although a very large number of alleles (e.g., >400 for HLA-B and HLA-DRB1) can be found in the worldwide population, a much smaller number (e.g., 30 to 50 for HLA-DRB1) is present in most individual populations.

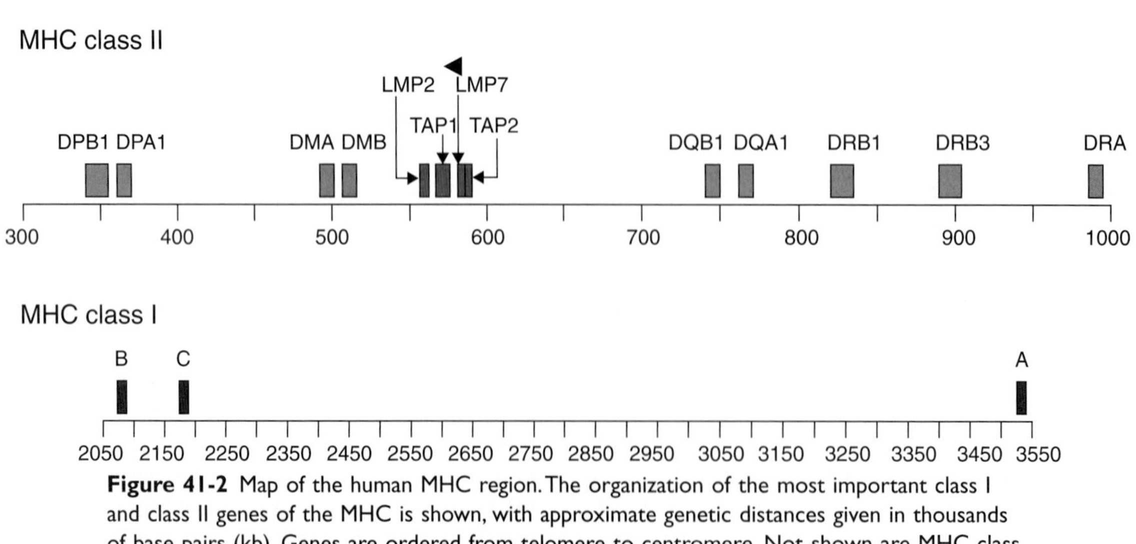

Figure 41-2 Map of the human MHC region. The organization of the most important class I and class II genes of the MHC is shown, with approximate genetic distances given in thousands of base pairs (kb). Genes are ordered from telomere to centromere. Not shown are MHC class III genes, which map between class I and class II genes. (See Color Plate 12.)

Importantly, different populations tend to have different frequency distributions of alleles and exhibit different patterns of linkage disequilibrium. This variability exists among both racial and ethnic groups.

The HLA genes exist in linkage disequilibrium, also referred to as gametic association. Gametic associations are regularly found between certain HLA alleles of A and B, C and B, B and DRB1, and DRB1 and DQB1 loci. The HLA genes are transmitted in families as haplotypes. The number of possible haplotypes is vast. However, because of linkage disequilibrium, the number of haplotypes found in a population is more limited.[8,17] Genetic recombination or crossing over in the HLA region is a relatively rare event, occurring for the most part no more than 1% per meiosis between A and B, and between B and DRB1. Recombination can also occur between A and C, and between B and C (0.6% and 0.2%, respectively).

TABLE 41-4 Names of the Most Important HLA Class I and Class II Genes and Their Encoded Polypeptide Ordered from Telomere to Centromere

Name	Encoded Polypeptide
HLA-A	Class I α-chain
HLA-C	Class I α-chain
HLA-B	Class I α-chain
HLA-DRA	DR α-chain
HLA-DRB3	DR β3-chain determining DR52 specificities
HLA-DRB1	DR β1-chain determining specificities DR1, DR2, DR3, DR4, DR5, etc.
HLA-DQA1	DQ α-chain
HLA-DQB1	DQ β-chain
TAP2	ABC (ATP binding cassette) transporter (associated with antigen presentation)
LMP7	Proteasome-related sequence (role in loading class I molecules with peptides)
TAP1	ABC (ATP binding cassette) transporter (associated with antigen presentation)
LMP2	Proteasome-related sequence (role in loading class I molecules with peptides)
HLA-DMB	DM β-chain (control peptide loading by class II molecules)
HLA-DMA	DM α-chain (control peptide loading by class II molecules)
HLA-DPA1	DP α-chain
HLA-DPB1	DP β-chain

Historical Applications of HLA Typing

HLA allele identification has been used for transplantation, forensic, parentage, and chimerism testing. The latter three are of historical interest and are discussed in this section.

Forensic DNA Testing

The first case in the United States in which DNA-based identity testing was used, *Pestinikas v. Pennsylvania* (1986), involved HLA-DQA1 oligonucleotide, dot-blot hybridization analysis for forensic identification. This commercially available DQA1 system was later modified with five additional non-HLA genetic loci, resulting in discriminatory power of approximately 1 in 2000. The relatively low discriminatory power and problems with interpreting mixtures resulted in the migration of forensic laboratories to other methods and genetic loci as described previously.

Parentage Testing

The use of the HLA loci for parentage testing has been replaced by methods described later in this chapter. The polymorphism of the loci was first inferred from antisera that distinguished among antigenic specificities. These specificities were especially numerous within the Class I loci and it was recognized that they could be exploited in identity testing. Typically, a panel of serological reagents was employed that defined HLA loci and red cell antigens. The emergence of many highly informative non-HLA polymorphic loci that could be conveniently genotyped led to a reduced utility of the HLA loci for parentage testing in the 1990s.

Chimerism

While the HLA loci can be used to study the engraftment of transplanted hematopoietic stem cells (see later in this chapter), other more convenient loci are genotyped for this purpose. These other loci are essential when the transplant donor recipient pair are HLA-identical siblings or allele-matched unrelated individuals.

Transplantation

Matching the HLA alleles of donors and recipients for renal transplantation improves long-term graft survival of kidneys from living related and unrelated donors and from deceased donors. For example, the half-life survival for a graft from an HLA-identical sibling is 23 years compared with a one haplotype–related donor with a half-life of 12.8 years.[10,26] Importantly, the effect of HLA matching remains significant even with the most recent forms of immunosuppression. The effect of HLA matching on the survival of heart and lung transplants is also statistically significant. In contrast, the effect of HLA matching for liver transplants is uncertain.

Hematopoietic cell transplantation (HCT) is employed to treat several classes of disorders. HLA compatibility between donor and recipient in HCT affects not only the ability to achieve sustained engraftment of donor HCT but also the risk of developing acute and chronic graft versus host disease (GVHD). Posttransplant risk of graft failure, GVHD, and mortality can be affected by quantitative and qualitative characteristics of donor-recipient HLA allele mismatching. In allogeneic stem cell transplantation, the donor is an individual who is genetically nonidentical and either related or unrelated to the recipient. Three different categories of donors are usually considered in the following order of preference: HLA genotypically identical siblings, HLA mismatched relatives, and unrelated donors, matched or mismatched. The goal when screening for an HLA-matched sibling donor is to identify which of any siblings have inherited the same HLA haplotypes from their parents.

HLA typing within families for transplantation sometimes leads to the discovery that the father is not the biological father of some or all of the children. There are a variety of opinions among healthcare providers about whether this possibility should be discussed with the family before testing and how or whether "false paternity" should be reported to the family.

When a matched sibling donor does not exist for a patient requiring allogeneic HCT (70% of cases), searching for extended family members or donors from an unrelated bone marrow registry would be the next option. Registries of volunteer bone marrow donors and cord blood exist in most developed countries (http://www.marrow.org). Currently, approximately 65% of patients can find an acceptable donor among the 4 million individuals registered in the U.S.-based National Marrow Donor Program (NMDP). However, patients belonging to racial groups that are not well represented in the registries have a considerably decreased probability of finding a donor (http://www.marrow.org).[3]

DNA-Based HLA Allele Identification

Most commonly used molecular diagnostic methods have been used to identify HLA alleles. Strategies based on oligonucleotide probe hybridization, DNA sequencing, and allele-specific DNA amplification have become the most common ones used currently for HLA typing. Each of these methods relies on amplification with PCR of genomic DNA of relevant regions of an HLA gene from the tested individual.[10] Samples for testing are usually peripheral blood but may be any tissue containing nucleated cells.

Typing methods involve the design of primer pairs that are able to amplify all alleles at the target HLA locus with the polymorphic sequence motifs situated between the primer sites. Laboratories usually amplify at least exons 2 and 3 of class I genes and exon 2 of class II genes. Some prepare larger amplification products that include exon 1 and/or exon 4 of class I genes. Amplification primers may be located within exons or introns. Primers positioned in introns allow complete analysis of exons and inspection of exon/intron junctions for splice site polymorphisms. Primers must be carefully chosen to attain locus-specific amplification since the HLA loci are the products of gene duplication and divergence and retain substantial homology. Further, many HLA loci have closely related pseudogenes that do not encode functional polypeptides but may result in nonspecific PCR products.[10]

The amplicons prepared are subsequently analyzed by a variety of methods. They can be hybridized to oligonucleotide probes in reverse or forward dot-blot assays. The panel of probes is chosen to cover critical polymorphic positions in the HLA gene tested. The pattern of reactivity of the panel can then be analyzed to assign allele identities.[10]

Alternatively, amplicons can be directly sequenced via dideoxynucleotide chain termination methods. This approach is increasingly attractive for allele level typing because of the large numbers of alleles known to exist at the HLA loci. The homozygous or heterozygous sequence obtained can be compared with a library of known sequences of alleles for allele assignment.[31]

A third commonly employed method, sequence-specific primer PCR (SSP-PCR) employs pairs of PCR primers chosen so that their 3′-most nucleotide or nucleotides are complementary to a polymorphic position that distinguishes an allele or an allele group from other alleles. If the individual possesses the allele(s) of interest, the PCR will lead to a product whose size and presence are typically identified by agarose gel electrophoresis or can be detected with real-time methods. A typing can be performed by choosing many pairs of primers in independent reactions to cover all allele groups.[10]

Commercial reagents and software for analysis of results are available for each of these three methods. Laboratories tailor HLA typing assays to the specific applications discussed above. Choice of methods depends upon typing volume, turnaround requirements, and the resolution needed.

Interpretation of HLA Test Results

The number of alleles at the HLA class I and class II loci, and a listing of serologically defined specificities and their allele equivalents, are available online at several Web sites (http://www.anthonynolan.com/HIG, accessed April 1, 2004 or http://www.ebi.ac.uk/imgt/hla/, accessed April 1, 2004). The alleles of each of the HLA antigens are numbered based on the original serological nomenclature. HLA alleles are now designated by a superscripted asterisk after the locus of origin and a number corresponding to the particular allele (e.g., HLA-A*0201). Parallel testing using serological and DNA genotyping of HLA alleles has led to the use of one nomenclature for the description of low-resolution typing in which the HLA assignment might include more than one possible related allele (e.g., HLA-A A*02) and a nomenclature reflecting the high-resolution allelic typing. Thus different HLA allele subtypes (e.g., for A*02) can appear indistinguishable when tested by serology or with a limited panel of nucleic acid probes so a generic or low-resolution typing is obtained. New HLA alleles are named by an international nomenclature committee. Annual HLA nomenclature reports with frequent updates are available at the Web sites listed above.

Quality Assurance and Quality Control Issues

Quality control and assurance programs for HLA testing should be similar to those for other types of PCR-based testing. The NMDP and the American Society for Histocompatibility and Immunogenetics (ASHI) maintain a cell repository of a subset of known alleles (http://www.ashi-hla.org/, accessed April 1, 2004). As in other PCR-based testing, strict measures to prevent contamination of pre-PCR areas with genomic DNA and PCR products are essential. Importantly, testing for contamination arising from products prepared in SSP-PCR can be challenging because the many PCR reactions necessary to type an individual often result in products varying in size and composition. Measures to prevent contamination in PCR-based testing have been widely described; such information is available online at the ASHI Web site.

Proficiency Testing

Several proficiency testing programs are available in the United States. These include the College of American Pathologists (CAP), ASHI, and the Southeastern Organ Procurement Foundation. Each offers comprehensive programs to assess laboratories' ability to correctly identify HLA alleles. The University of California at Los Angeles has offered an international cell exchange program for many years. Laboratories are challenged to correctly type samples that often include unusual or recently described alleles.

Accreditation and Certification of Laboratories and Professionals

Clinical histocompatibility laboratories are high complexity laboratories that must have a CLIA license in the United States. Laboratories may be inspected and accredited by CAP or ASHI. The United Network for Organ Sharing, NMDP, and CLIA have all designated ASHI with deemed status for purposes of accreditation of HLA laboratories. Laboratories are generally directed by individuals with Ph.D., M.D., or both degrees. ASHI administers a program to assess the qualifications of doctoral level individuals to direct ASHI-accredited laboratories. Directors can take a certifying examination administered by the American Board of Histocompatibility and Immunogenetics (ABHI). The ABHI also certifies laboratory staff as histocompatibility technologists and specialists. Information is available on the ASHI Web site.

CHIMERISM AND HEMATOPOIETIC CELL ENGRAFTMENT ANALYSIS

Successful HCT effectively results in chimerism with the recipient's hematopoietic cells derived from the donor. With the exception of monozygotic twins, it is virtually always possible to use polymorphic loci on chromosomes to distinguish between DNA prepared from cells derived from the recipient and cells from the donor. This is true even for siblings if enough loci are studied. Suppose the father and mother of two siblings have alleles j and k and s and t, respectively, at a locus. The likelihood that the two siblings will inherit an identical genotype such as js or jt at this locus is 1 in 4. The likelihood that the siblings will be identical for other studied loci for which the parents are similarly heterozygous is also 1 in 4. In this particular example of complete parental heterozygosity, the risk that no locus will be found at which the two siblings can be distinguished is 1 in 4^N where N is the number of independently segregating loci tested. Commercial engraftment testing reagents that include 9 to 16 independently segregating loci will virtually always reveal at least a single locus at which donor and recipient cells can be distinguished.

Methods for Performing Engraftment Analysis

Sources of DNA for engraftment testing are typically peripheral white blood cells or bone marrow aspirates. It is crucial to obtain genomic DNA samples from the recipient before the transplant to determine his or her native genotypes at the tested loci. Then posttransplant samples can be compared with "pure" specimens from the donor and from the pretransplant recipient. If a pretransplant sample from the recipient is not available, another sample such as buccal cells may be obtained. Care should be taken in interpreting results from these alternate sources, however, since donor-derived inflammatory cells may be present.

Testing can be performed on genomic DNA isolated from the entire cell population of the specimen. Alternatively, the sample can be sorted by flow cytometry or immunorosetting to assess engraftment of specific cell lineages.[12] For example, engraftment of the T-cell versus non–T-cell components can be assessed after flow cytometry sorting based on expression of the CD3 surface molecule, a T-cell marker.

DNA typing methods used in engraftment analysis are summarized in Table 41-5. These methods have evolved like those used for identity testing in general. Initial methods relied on Southern blotting to detect RFLPs or VNTRs. These labor-intensive hybridization assays have been largely replaced by PCR-based methods.

One PCR-based strategy is to amplify a series of VNTR loci with subsequent separation of the DNA fragments on polyacrylamide gels.[23] Alleles can be assigned via comparison with size standards after staining with ethidium bromide. The sensitivity of this method for detecting a small admixture of donor or recipient DNA is roughly 10%. Sensitivity can be increased to the <1% to 1% range with silver staining of the amplification products.

As described earlier in this chapter for forensic identification, fluorescent detection of PCR products derived from STR, or microsatellite loci, has been adopted by many labo-

TABLE 41-5 DNA Typing Methods Used in Engraftment Testing

Method	Description	Comment
RFLP analysis of VNTR loci	Digest genomic DNA with restriction endonuclease and detect polymorphic VNTR loci by Southern blotting	Highly informative identity testing method also used in early forensics, now discarded because of its labor-intensive nature
PCR analysis of VNTR loci	Amplify VNTR loci and size by gel electrophoresis	This assay can be quite sensitive when bands are detected by silver staining
STR analysis	Multiplex amplification of several STR loci with sizing by fluorescent detection	Becoming the standard method in the field because of the efficiency and partial automation
Cytogenetics	Interphase analysis of X and Y chromosomes with fluorescent in situ hybridization	May be useful when donor and recipient are of different genders

ratories for engraftment assays.[22] This method is attractive because of the ability to automate the assay, fewer problems associated with "stutter bands," the extensive characterization of these loci in a variety of populations, and their high degree of polymorphism. Surveys from the proficiency testing programs described below indicate that the majority of laboratories providing clinical engraftment testing currently analyze STR loci.

When the donor and recipient are of different genders, analysis of the sex chromosomes in posttransplant hematopoietic cells can be useful in engraftment testing. Cytogenetic analysis of chromosomes in interphase cells with X- and Y-specific probes may be performed with fluorescent in situ hybridization assays. The percent donor or recipient cells can be determined by assessing the ratio of cells with XX signals to those with XY signals. Alternatively PCR-based analysis of X- and Y-chromosome loci can be carried out. For example, the reappearance of Y-specific amplification products in a male whose donor was his sister may indicate relapse of a malignancy. Polymorphic loci on chromosome X can be studied similar to the autosomal STR discussed above.

Selection and Interpretation of Short Tandem Repeat Loci

Engraftment testing is accomplished by preparing genomic DNA from donor and pretransplant and posttransplant recipient specimens followed by PCR amplification of the selected STR loci. Amplification reactions are typically multiplexed using fluorescently labeled commercially available reagents as described above for forensic identity testing. Products are then separated via high resolution slab or capillary electrophoresis on an automated genetic analyzer. Comparison of DNA fragment sizes with a reference ladder allows software to assign alleles for each locus.

The analysis of a donor sample and a pretransplant recipient sample allows the laboratory to identify which STR loci are informative (nonidentical genotypes) for the pair. A posttransplant sample can then be studied. If only fluorescent peaks from the donor are observed, then the cells studied are donor in origin. Rarely, only recipient peaks will be seen, consistent with recipient origin of the cells. These assays can detect admixtures of cell populations down to approximately 3%. Therefore, results indicating that a sample is exclusively from the donor are often reported as >97% donor. If fluorescent peaks derived from both the donor and the recipient are seen, the sample must be a mixture of cells from the two individuals.

The percent recipient in a mixed sample can be calculated by summing the intensities of the informative recipient peaks and dividing by the sum of the intensities of the informative recipient and donor peaks. Many laboratories then average the percent recipient for each locus to arrive at a final result. Some laboratories run a calibration curve of artificial mixtures of donor and recipient DNA for each tested pair. Other laboratories validate the assay with calibration curves for a number of control "donor" and "recipient" mixtures, and do not run new calibration curves for each new donor-recipient pair.

Applications of Microsatellite Locus Testing to Engraftment Analysis

Several clinical questions can be answered with engraftment testing.[27] Is engraftment of donor cells proceeding well in the weeks following a stem cell transplant? In the setting of a history of successful engraftment, do subsequent studies demonstrate a resurgence of recipient-derived hematopoietic cells indicating a relapse? Has stable chimerism developed following transplantation with the production of hematopoietic cells derived from both the donor and recipient?

The correlation of engraftment testing results with the clinical history is crucial for interpretation of results. Thus appropriate communication between the engraftment testing laboratory and the transplantation team is essential.

Consultation with a hematopathologist may be helpful in interpreting results in complex cases.

A result indicating 85% donor cells and 15% recipient cells might be equally consistent with an engrafting marrow 3 weeks after transplantation or with relapse 6 months following transplantation. The date of the transplant in relation to sample collection, the conditioning regimen used before transplant, and evidence from peripheral smear or bone marrow aspirate examination may be helpful in interpreting results. Unusual history, if unknown, can cause considerable confusion. For example, some recipients may have received more than one stem cell transplant or may have had a donor who is an identical twin.

The interpretation of an engraftment result from a single sample can be difficult. Multiple samples collected at intervals after transplantation may reveal changes in the fraction of donor and recipient over time that can be correlated with the evolving clinical picture.

Proficiency Testing

Proficiency testing programs for engraftment testing are offered by the CAP and the ASHI. Challenge specimens are typically artificial mixtures of genomic DNA from two related or unrelated individuals. In both surveys, participant laboratories have demonstrated a high degree of agreement for challenge samples. The standard deviation from the mean of participant results in a 50-50 mixture of "donor" and "recipient" cells is typically ±2% to 4%. For mixtures that approach the sensitivity threshold of the assay (for example 6% recipient, 94% donor) somewhat broader standard deviations may be seen.

Quality Assurance and Quality Control

Quality control and assurance programs for engraftment testing should be similar to those for other types of identity testing. Assays may require as little as 1 ng of genomic DNA. Thus strict measures to prevent contamination of pre-PCR areas with genomic DNA and PCR products are important.

Accreditation

Accreditation of programs may be through the ASHI or the CAP. Since engraftment testing is a variant of identity testing, the standards used are often those written for paternity and other forms of identity testing. However, because engraftment testing deals with subpopulations of cells and the relative proportions of cells, organizations such as the ASHI have developed accreditation standards specifically for engraftment testing.

PARENTAGE TESTING

Questions regarding the parentage of minor and adult children arise frequently in modern society. Generally at issue is whether a particular man is the father of a child. As discussed in the chapter introduction, parentage testing allows an individual to be excluded or not excluded as the parent of a child. If not excluded, the likelihood that he is the father can be calculated. Court-ordered and privately sought parentage testing is usually performed to facilitate decisions regarding responsibility for the financial support of a child. However, there are other reasons individuals may wish to establish parentage; an example is the settlement of an estate. As discussed earlier, laboratories performing other types of identification tests for purposes unrelated to parentage (e.g., HLA typing for transplantation) should be aware of the possibility of inadvertently uncovering "false paternity."

Methods, Instrumentation, and Sample Requirements

Methods for parentage testing have evolved considerably over time similar to other human identification applications. Initial methods relied on serological techniques to identify red cell antigens, such as the ABO and the MNS groups and the highly polymorphic HLA antigens found on most cells. Since 1990 there has been a substantial migration of parentage laboratories to DNA-based methods, especially to those based on analysis of STR alleles. The significant advantages of these PCR-based assays with detection of fluorescently labeled DNA fragments on automated genetic analyzers have been discussed in the section on forensic identification. Recently SNPs have also been introduced in commercial parentage laboratories.

Selection and validation of testing methods are key issues in paternity testing. Specific requirements for paternity testing may be mandated by local laws and agreements. Thus the choice of methods and genetic systems should be based on an agreement between the client(s) and the laboratory.

Nonstandardized methods should not be used as the sole methods within a paternity testing laboratory. In addition, a nonstandard method should only be used if it can be documented that the method is used in at least one other laboratory, thus making it possible to obtain a second opinion based on repeated testing.

Like other forms of identity testing, samples for paternity testing may be any specimen containing chromosomal DNA. In practice, programs generally perform testing on peripheral blood samples or buccal smears. Buccal smears are increasingly preferred as they offer a noninvasive means of sample collection, which is especially convenient when testing minors.

Reporting of Test Results

In addition to the usual paternity test reports, laboratories are occasionally asked to provide interpretative reports when less than complete information is available. The usual report is discussed next and the interpretive reports are discussed afterwards.

Test Reports

The results should include all the information requested by the client and necessary for the interpretation of the test results and all information required by the method used. If the weight of evidence is calculated, it must be based on likelihood ratio principles, such as the paternity index.[2,9]

Exclusion of a Tested Man

Standard parentage testing involves genotyping several polymorphic loci in samples from a trio consisting of the mother, child, and presumed father. Inspection of the alleles found in the mother and the child at the genetic loci analyzed reveals alleles that must have been contributed by the child's biological father. If the accused father does not have an obligatory allele at one of the tested loci, he is excluded as the biological father. Laboratories require the absence of an obligatory allele for at least *two* loci in a tested man to exclude him as the father. The requirement of multiple loci reduces the possibility of making an error caused by a technical problem or caused by a rare mutation at one of the examined loci.

The power of an analyzed locus to exclude a tested man depends upon the number of alleles found at the locus and their allele frequencies in human populations. ABO typing can exclude a tested man but has a relatively poor probability of exclusion of about 15%. The HLA and VNTR loci have many alleles and a single locus may have greater than 90% probability of excluding a falsely accused man. The STR loci have an intermediate number of alleles. A single STR locus typically has a 30% to 60% likelihood of excluding a wrongly accused man. The ease of STR analysis makes these loci attractive for parentage testing even with their lower exclusion power. If a number of STRs that independently segregate during meiosis are studied, a cumulative probability of exclusion can be calculated based on the product of exclusion power for each tested locus. The use of 9 to 16 unlinked, and therefore independent, STRs provided in commercially available human identity reagents generally results in at least a 99% probability of exclusion of a falsely accused man.

Inclusion of a Tested Man

The alleles found at the analyzed loci may be entirely consistent with the accused man being the biological father of the child. In this case, the likelihood that he is truly the father rather than a random individual who is not excluded can be calculated. A number of assumptions underlie accurate calculations of the likeliness of paternity. Tested individuals must be properly identified, testing must be accurate, and allele frequencies in relevant populations must be well characterized.

The probability of paternity (W) and the paternity index (PI) are two closely related values that express the likelihood that the tested man is truly the father rather than another man who by chance shares alleles at a tested locus. Calculation of the PI takes into account allele frequencies at the locus in relevant populations. If multiple independent loci are analyzed, a cumulative PI based on the products of the individual loci can be calculated. Government entities typically require that the paternity index be >100 : 1 and the probability of paternity be >99% for inclusion of a man. Other evidence bearing on the probability that a man is the father before testing is performed can be integrated with test results using Bayesian analysis to calculate a posterior probability of paternity. The prior probability that an accused man is the father is typically set at 50%, but a range of likelihoods given different prior probabilities (e.g., 10% to 50%) can be calculated for comparison.

Opinions, Interpretations, and Problems

Standard parentage testing requires samples from the trio described above. However, there are many cases in which the mother, child, and putative father may not all be available for testing. If a sample cannot be obtained from the mother it may still be possible to exclude a tested man or to calculate his probability of paternity. For example, the finding of locus L genotypes 1,3 for the child and 4,5 for the tested man is inconsistent with the hypothesis that he is the father whether or not we know the mother's genotype. Similarly, when the accused man is not available, testing performed for individuals related to him may be used to calculate the likelihood that he is the biological father of the child in question.

While STRs and VNTRs are usually transmitted in a faithful Mendelian fashion, mutations can occur. A child and tested man may be encountered who share an allele at all but one of the tested loci. The possibility that the man is truly the father and that a mutation has occurred at the mismatched locus should then be entertained. If additional loci are tested with no additional genetic inconsistencies discovered, the likelihood of paternity can be calculated by considering the frequency of mutations at the mismatched locus. Alternatively, additional genotyping may reveal more exclusions, making it unlikely that the tested man is truly the father. Laboratories should apply procedures for estimating uncertainty of measurement. The measurement of uncertainty of tests should be known and should be included in the interpretation of test results.

Quality Assurance and Quality Control

The quality control and assurance measures for paternity testing are similar to those for other types of human identity testing. Positive identification of samples, prevention of DNA contamination, the use of control alleles of known size, and the validation of software employed for genetic analysis and calculation are among measures common to identity testing programs. Population distribution data for the systems used must be documented. In addition, mutation frequencies of the systems used must be documented and used appropriately.

Policy and Procedures for Resolution of Complaints

The laboratory should have a policy and procedure for the resolution of complaints received from clients or other parties. Paternity testing programs involving knowledge of sensitive family information results may be employed in legal proceedings. Samples and records including information stored electronically must be handled carefully to ensure their privacy, confidentiality, and security. Laboratory procedures for documentation of the identity of individuals contributing samples for study and the chain of custody of specimens should be very detailed.

Accreditation

Recommendations and standards for paternity testing are formulated by government agencies or professional organizations (e.g., the Standards for Parentage Testing Laboratories of the American Association of Blood Banks [AABB]). The AABB administers a laboratory inspection and accreditation program.[1] The ASHI and CAP also publish relevant standards. The CAP and AABB jointly offer a proficiency testing survey.

REFERENCES

1. American Association of Blood Banks. Standards for Parentage Testing Laboratories, 5th Edition. 2001;1-57.
2. Baur MP, Elston RC, Gurtler H, Henningsen K, Hummel K, Matsumoto H, et al. No fallacies in the formulation of the paternity index. Am J Human Genetics 1986;39:528-36.
3. Beatty PG, Mori M, Milford E. Impact of racial genetic polymorphism on the probability of finding an HLA-matched donor. Transplantation 1995;60:778-83.
4. Budowle B, Moretti T, Smith J. DNA Typing Protocols. In: Molecular Biology and Forensic Analysis, Eaton Publishing Co., Natick, MA, 2000.
5. Butler JM. Forensic DNA Typing. In: Biology and Technology behind STR Markers, Academic Press, London, 2000.
6. Butler JM, Reeder DJ. STR DNA Internet Database. http://www.cstl.nist.gov/div831/strbase (accessed April 4, 2004).
7. Chakraborty R, Kidd KK. The utility of DNA typing in forensic casework. Science 1991;254:1735-9.
8. Dawkins R, Leelayuwat C, Gaudieri S, Tay G, Hui J, Cattley S, et al. Genomics of the major histocompatibility complex: haplotypes, duplication, retroviruses and disease. Immunol Rev 1999;167:275-304.
9. Elston RC. Probability and Paternity Testing. Am J Human Genetics 1986;39:112-22.
10. Erlich HA, Opelz G, Hansen J. HLA DNA Typing and Transplantation. Immunology 2001;14:347-56.
11. Evett IW, Weir B. Interpreting DNA Evidence. In: Statistical Genetics for Forensic Scientists, Sinauer Associates, Inc., Sunderland, MA, 1998.
12. Fernandez-Aviles F, Urbano-Ispizua A, Aymerich M, Colomer D, Rovira M, Martinez C, Nadal E, Talarn C, Carreras E, Montserrat E. Serial quantification of lymphoid and myeloid mixed chimerism using multiplex PCR amplification of short tandem repeat-markers predicts graft rejection and relapse, respectively, after allogeneic transplantation of CD34+ selected cells from peripheral blood. Leukemia 2003;17:613-20.
13. Holland MM, Parsons TJ. Mitochondrial DNA sequence analysis—validation and use for forensic casework. Forensic Science Review 1999;11:21-50.
14. Jeffreys AJ, Wilson V, Thein SL. Hypervariable "minisatellite" regions in human DNA. Nature 1985;314:67-73.
15. Jeffreys AJ, Wilson V, Thein SL. Individual specific "fingerprints" of human DNA. Nature 1985;316:76-9.
16. Lander ES, Budowle B. DNA Fingerprinting dispute laid to rest. Nature 1994;371:735-8.
17. Little AM, Parham P. Polymorphism and evolution of HLA class I and II genes and molecules. Rev Immunogenet 1999;1:105-23.
18. National Research Council. DNA Technology in Forensic Science. National Academy Press, Washington, D.C., 1992.
19. National Research Council. The Evaluation of Forensic DNA Evidence. National Academy Press, Washington, D.C., 1996.
20. Rhodes DA, Trowsdale J. Genetics and molecular genetics of the MHC. Rev Immunogenet 1999;1:21-31.
21. Rudin N, Inman K. An Introduction to Forensic DNA Analysis, second edition, CRC Press, Boca Raton, FL, 2001.
22. Scharf SJ, Smith AG, Hansen JA, McFarland C, Erlich HA. Quantitative determination of bone marrow transplant engraftment using fluorescent polymerase chain reaction primers for human identity markers. Blood 1995;85:1954-63.
23. Schichman SA, Suess P, Vertino AM, Gray PS. Comparison of short tandem repeat and variable number tandem repeat genetic markers for quantitative determination of allogeneic bone marrow transplant engraftment. Bone Marrow Transplant 2002;29:243-8.
24. Shibata D. Identification of mismatched fixed specimens with a commercially available kit based on the polymerase chain reaction. Am J Clin Pathol 1993;100:666-70.
25. Tsongalis GJ, Wu AH, Silver H, Ricci A Jr. Applications of forensic identity testing in the clinical laboratory. Am J Clin Pathol 1999;112(1 Suppl 1):S93-103.
26. United Network for Organ Sharing UNOS. 2000 Annual Report, the U.S. Scientific Registry of Transplant Recipients and the Organ Procurement and Transplantation Network. Transplant data 1992-2001. Department of Health and Human Services, Health Resources and Services Administration.

27. Van Deerlin VM, Leonard DG. Bone marrow engraftment analysis after allogeneic bone marrow transplantation. Clin Lab Med 2000;20:197-225.
28. Van Oorschot RAH, Jones MK. DNA fingerprints from fingerprints. Nature 1997;387:767.
29. Weedn VW, Hicks JW. The unrealized potential of DNA testing, Research in Action, National Institute of Justice, Washington, DC, 1998.
30. Wooley J, Harmon RP. The forensic brouhaha: science or debate? Am J Human Genetics 1992;51:1164-5.
31. Wu J, Bassinger S, Griffith BB, et al. Analysis of HLA Class I Alleles via Direct Sequencing of PCR Products. ASHI Laboratory Manual, 4th Edition, 2001.

World Wide Web Sites

www.anthonynolan.com/HIG—The Anthony Nolan Trust, HLA Informatics page.

www.ashi-hla.org—American Society for Histocompatibility and Immunogenetics.

www.cstl.nist.gov/div831/strbase—National Institute of Standards and Technology, Short Tandem Repeat DNA Internet DataBase.

www.ebi.ac.uk/imgt/hla—European Bioinformatics Institute, IMGT/HLA Sequence Database.

www.marrow.org—National Marrow Donor Program.

CHAPTER 42

Molecular Methods in Diagnosis and Monitoring of Infectious Diseases

Andrea Ferreira-Gonzalez, Ph.D., and Angela M. Caliendo, M.D., Ph.D.

In the short time since their introduction, nucleic acid tests have profoundly affected the management of infectious diseases. In contrast to microbial culture methods, "molecular" methods are rapid, thus allowing early decisions about treatment to be based on data about the pathogen(s) in an individual patient. Molecular methods have provided a means to detect pathogens that could not be easily detected by traditional methods such as culture, antigen detection, or serology. By rapidly providing quantification and sequences of nucleic acids in pathogens, the methods have transformed the approaches to prediction and monitoring of response to therapy, assessing risk of disease development, and determining disease prognosis.

The first third of this chapter reviews concepts in the development and clinical implementation of molecular assays for testing in infectious disease. Readers with backgrounds in analytical techniques or molecular testing or infectious diseases may wish to use the headings in the text to identify the parts of interest to them. The later sections of the chapter describe nucleic acid testing for specific pathogens, with a new section heading for each pathogen or pair of related pathogens. These sections include discussion of the clinical utility of the testing and are focused on those pathogens for which molecular testing is considered the standard of care. Because the field is expanding rapidly, we provide links throughout the chapter to Web sites where recent developments can be monitored.

DEVELOPMENT OF MOLECULAR ASSAYS FOR INFECTIOUS DISEASES

Molecular infectious disease laboratories use methods developed by in vitro manufacturers and assays developed by individual laboratories. Complete reagent sets developed by manufacturers are provided with quality-controlled reagents that have been manufactured under Good Manufacturing Practices (GMP), and the performance of the entire molecular test has been determined for a particular clinical claim. For example, a number of reagent sets and complete systems of reagents and associated instrumentation are commercially available for the diagnosis of sexually transmitted diseases caused by *Chlamydia trachomatis* (CT) and/or *Neisseria gonorrhoeae* (GC), as are systems for monitoring disease progression in patients diagnosed with human immunodeficiency virus-1 (HIV-1) infection by quantification of HIV-1 RNA in plasma specimens. These products usually include reagents for nucleic acid isolation, amplification, and detection/quantification with a specific protocol. In the United States, they are commercialized using different labels depending upon U.S. Food and Drug Administration (FDA) status and review including FDA-approved, FDA-cleared, for research use only (RUO), or for investigational use only (IUO).

Nucleic acid–based testing for infectious diseases, as for other clinical conditions, usually involves three major steps: specimen processing, nucleic acid amplification, and product detection. Several systems automate one or two steps, and automation of all three steps in a single analyzer is expected from manufacturers in the near future. It is expected that these systems will be capable of integration with common laboratory information systems, thus creating another major advance for clinical microbiology laboratories and facilitating reporting of results in timeframes that allow more rapid institution or alteration of therapy.

Many clinical laboratories find it necessary to develop methods to detect various infectious agents for which there are no commercially available methods or systems. Laboratory-developed tests (LDT), formerly known as home-brew assays or in-house developed assays, are those assays that have been fully developed and validated by the laboratory that offers the testing. Usually, these assays use a combination of reagents that are purchased separately from various manufacturers. The analytical and clinical verification of the LDT is the responsibility of each laboratory, and this verification procedure is more complex than verification of an FDA-cleared or FDA-approved test.

Analyte-Specific Reagents

In the United States, the jurisdiction of the FDA includes reagents, equipment, and complete assays used in diagnosis or treatment of disease. The FDA introduced the term analyte-specific reagent (ASR) to refer to such reagent(s) used in LDTs that confer specificity for detecting a particular analyte.[58] ASRs include antibodies, specific receptor proteins, ligands, and oligonucleotides. Because of the importance of ASRs in infectious disease testing, we summarize key points of the regulations here.

The FDA considers LDTs medical devices subject to FDA regulatory oversight, but with very few exceptions has not executed this authority (the high complexity laboratories that develop LDTs are regulated by the Center for Medicare and Medicaid Services under the provisions of the Clinical Laboratory Improvement Act [CLIA] of 1988). With the ASR category, the FDA shifted its focus from the laboratory to the manufacturers of reagents, and proposed controls and restrictions to ensure their quality and consistency, and to clarify that a laboratory setting up these tests is responsible for the tests' performance.

Manufacturers are restricted in the distribution, use, and labeling of ASRs, and can sell them only to CLIA-certified, high-complexity laboratories. They must register and list ASRs with the FDA, follow GMP, and report adverse events that result from product failure. Most of these products are exempted from premarket review, but are subject to restricted labeling and use. The labeling of these reagents is restricted to "description of the identity and purity including source and method of acquisition of the ASR, in addition to standard information already required for general purpose reagents," with the specific disclaimer reading: "Analyte-specific reagent, analytic and performance characteristics are not established." Furthermore, manufacturers are forbidden from labeling and/or promoting ASRs, including any statements about the ASR's analytical performance, clinical performance, or diagnostic ability. Commerce of ASRs to in vitro diagnostic (IVD) manufacturers or nonclinical organizations (academic, research, and forensic settings) is exempt from the ASR rule.

The FDA has mandated that laboratories using ASRs must label their reports with the statement, "This test was developed and its performance characteristics determined by (laboratory name). It has not been cleared or approved by the U.S. Food and Drug Administration." LDTs that use primers and probes made in the laboratory are not covered by this rule. The College of American Pathologists (CAP) has suggested additional language to reflect the fact that FDA review is not required under this regulation.

When to Use a Molecular Test for an Infectious Disease

A new test should provide reliable, cost-effective, and timely results necessary for diagnosis and management. Test selection should not be based solely on cost. Performance characteristics and impact on patient care and management are critical components of the decision. New tests can improve patient care and decrease its cost as in the use of genotyping of HIV-1 to detect drug resistance.[76] This testing added a new cost, but allowed rapid and accurate determination of the potential effectiveness of expensive drugs. This improved clinical outcomes and decreased the incidence of virological failures and the total cost of treatment. The ability of molecular assays to enhance clinical care in infectious disease often arises from increased diagnostic sensitivity and specificity and shortened turnaround time.

Both clinicians and laboratorians are key players in identifying the testing needs of a medical center. The technical capabilities within the laboratory must be assessed in relation to the clinical needs. Consideration must be given to the interconnected issues of test volume, required turn-around time, and costs of performing the assay. An adequate testing volume is important to maintain proficiency of personnel and to control cost. Rapid turnaround for most tests in infectious disease implies testing of single samples rather than batches, with increased costs. As development and validation of LDTs are costly, it is best to determine if a similar assay is pending FDA review.

Patented procedures and sequence information affect decisions about testing. It is not always clear whether a technology or sequence has been patented or, if so, who owns the patent. It is thus advisable to check with the investigators who first described the sequence and to review the patent database and pending patent databases (United States Patent and Trademark Office Home Page: www.uspto.gov).

Choice of Specimen to Test and Analytical Approach

After a clinical need has been identified, a thorough literature search should be carried out to characterize the clinical utility of testing and its relation to specimen types, deoxyribonucleic acid (DNA) or ribonucleic acid (RNA) targets, and testing methodologies, whether qualitative or quantitative. For example, in distinguishing clinically significant cytomegalovirus (CMV) disease from asymptomatic CMV infection in immunocompromised individuals,[155] the detection of viral nucleic acid is not informative, and quantitative assays are necessary. Similarly the choice of RNA or DNA affects the ability to distinguish disease from nondisease status. Careful consideration should be given to the advantages and disadvantages of potential methodologies and the laboratory capabilities and the abilities necessary to ensure successful test development.

Test Development

Target sequences must be chosen to prevent cross-hybridization with other known sequences. A preliminary evaluation of published protocols or use of generic default concentrations for polymerase chain reaction (PCR) components can be a useful starting point. Modifications in assay design may be necessary depending on the specimen type. For example, if using fixed paraffin-embedded tissue as the specimen source, one might want to limit the size of the amplified product since tissue fixation can significantly affect nucleic acid quality and consequently affect the ability to amplify long nucleic acid sequences.

After initial tests, the next step is to optimize steps of the analytical process, including nucleic acid extraction, amplification, detection, and quantification. For amplification procedures, variables to be optimized may include buffer pH, nucleotide concentration, $MgCl_2$ concentration, type of polymerase, primer concentration, and annealing temperature.[74,90,191]

Preanalytical Variables

Common preanalytical variables include specimen type, specimen volume, anticoagulant, and specimen transport, storage, and handling. The type of specimen that is acceptable for testing will be largely determined by the pathogenesis of the disease and plays a key role in the performance and interpretation of the test results. Molecular assays often offer the convenience of using a small, less-invasive specimen. The diagnosis of herpes simplex virus (HSV) encephalitis is a classic example, where culture of brain biopsy has been replaced by PCR testing of a small volume of cerebrospinal fluid (CSF). Although molecular tests can detect the presence of small numbers of organisms, the probability of detection increases when a larger volume of specimen is added to the amplification reaction. This reflects in part the probability of having any organisms in the tested volume of sample. Because molecular assays do not need viable organisms for testing, more flexibility in specimen transport is possible than for culture methods.

Appropriate specimen collection and transport conditions are critical to ensure nucleic acid integrity, especially for quantitative methods, and to prevent cross-contamination of specimens. The appropriate specimen type, timing of specimen collection, and specimen handling will depend on the clinical presentation of the disease, the pathobiology of the infection, and the type of nucleic acid required for the test. The format of the molecular assay being developed may affect the amount of specimen required. Specimen transport and storage conditions are likely to vary among specimen types and between RNA and DNA tests. They will vary depending upon the need for viable or intact cells or microorganisms and must be determined by each laboratory. RNA is especially susceptible to degradation by ubiquitous enzymes. Specimens may be stable at room temperature for days or may require, for example, separation of plasma from cells within a few hours of collection and either immediate testing or storage of the plasma at −80 °C until testing is performed. Adding a known amount of purified target, microorganism, or cells to target-negative specimens can be useful in efforts to assess the preanalytical variables. Detailed written instructions for specimen collection and for handling and transport should be provided to those individuals involved in these tasks and duties.

Internal Controls

Internal controls, which are added to the clinical specimen before processing, are often used to detect the presence of inhibitors of amplification or to determine if nucleic acid degradation occurred during specimen processing. Internal controls are often synthetic segments of nucleic acid that use the same primer sequence as the target molecule, with a portion of the sequence internal to the primer binding sites that is unique to the internal control. This allows simultaneous amplification of the internal control and target, but separate detection using sequence-specific probes or physical separation of the two products by size. Internal controls and the target sequence must have the same or very similar efficiencies of amplification, and thus they must have similar length and base composition.

Failure to amplify the internal control may be due to nucleic acid degradation, inhibitors of amplification, or amplification failure. Regardless of the cause, when the internal control is not detected the assay is invalid.

A low amount of the internal control is used to avoid competition with the target in the patient specimen and to detect low levels of inhibition in the reaction. Amplification of a housekeeping gene can be used in place of an internal control when detecting or quantifying nucleic acid from a cellular specimen or tissue. However, most of the housekeeping genes are highly abundant, and thus subtle losses of nucleic acid or inhibition of amplification may not be detected. The use of RNA from a gene with a similar approximate abundance as the target sequence is preferred.

Nucleic Acid Extraction

Several commercially available manual and automated methods have been successfully applied to infectious disease testing of a wide variety of clinical specimens. These methods are rapid, usually require only a small volume of specimen, and provide more consistent results than older methods. In addition, the commercially available approaches can reduce hands-on labor requirements, and many can accommodate sample volumes ranging from 100 µL to 500 µL and even 1 mL of specimen.

Quantitative Molecular LDTs

Quantitative methods for DNA and RNA (reviewed in Chapter 37) are widely used in infectious disease testing to determine, for example, the viral load of agents such as hepatitis C virus (HCV) and HIV-1. Quantification requires a reproducible relationship between the amount of input target and the output signal from the assay. The concentration of analyte in a sample is determined by comparison of the signal from the sample with that from calibrators of known concentration. External calibrators avoid competition with the target sequence for reaction components, such as nucleotides, and can be naturally occurring—exactly matching the target of interest. The major disadvantage of external calibrators is that they are analyzed in a different reaction from the patient specimen and thus are not subject to the same reaction efficiencies or inhibition as the target sequence in the patient specimen. External calibrators are used for the quantification of HIV-1 in patient specimens using bDNA technology.[131] More recently, external calibrators have been used with good success to quantify nucleic acid present in patient specimens by real-time PCR technology.[83,103,177]

An internal calibrator can be synthesized in vitro to contain the same primer binding sequence as the target of interest, but with a different sequence internal to the primer binding sites. This allows the calibrator and the target sequence to be differentiated by using sequence-specific probes, as described above, for the internal control.

Internal calibrators compensate for inhibitors and/or loss of nucleic acid during the nucleic acid extraction procedure, but they (like internal "amplification controls") can compete with the target sequence for assay components and result in lower quantified result or no result at all. Since internal calibrators have some variation in sequence compared with the target to enable specific detection, natural analytical materials do not make good internal calibrators.

When amplifying nucleic acids from cells or tissues, amplification of a housekeeping gene may be used as an internal control and even as a calibrator. It is important to understand that these internal calibrators might be present at a much higher concentration than the target of interest and might also compete for reaction reagents, providing an inaccurate quantification of the target.

TEST VERIFICATION

Verification of a test is a complex process that can be divided in two phases: analytical and clinical verification. Analytical verification provides critical information about the performance of the test, while clinical verification establishes the clinical indications for the test. Determination of the clinical indications provides information about the appropriate settings, including disease states and populations for which the test can be used. Table 42-1 provides a list of guidelines that can be useful in developing validation programs. In addition, Table 42-2 outlines a checklist to assist in the verification process for a molecular assay.

In the United States, major differences exist between the implementation of an FDA-cleared test versus a non-FDA cleared test. As stipulated in CLIA '88,[59] laboratories implementing FDA-cleared tests need to verify the performance characteristics of the test for the indications for use. On the other hand, implementation of an LDT is a more complex process, as laboratories are required to establish the analytical verification of the test.

Analytical Verification

Laboratories must assess each LDT's detection limit (often called in regulations the "sensitivity"), specificity, accuracy, precision, and linear or reportable range. Verification of a LDT can be challenging when no standard reference material is available. Table 42-3 lists suppliers of reference materials that can be used during analytical verification and as a source of material for quality control purposes. National and international organizations are developing standard reference materials that will be useful for assay verification. The World Health Organization (WHO) recently introduced[157] a standard reference material for HCV for verification of nucleic acid tests. This lyophilized material (HCV 96/790) contains approximately 100,000 genome equivalents per milliliter and was assigned a value of 100,000 International Units (IU)/mL.[157] WHO also introduced an HIV standard, HIV 97/656. Similar to the HCV standard, it consists of a lyophilized preparation of HIV-1-genotype B virus from a plasmapheresis donation. Several laboratories have tested this material with different technologies, obtaining a mean value of 4.79 log genome equivalents/mL, which was assigned a value of 100,000 IU/mL. Finally the WHO hepatitis B virus (HBV) standard 97/746 has been assigned a value of 1 million IU/mL.[125] Reference panels calibrated to WHO standard reference material are commercially available (Table 42-3).

Some laboratories have established their own reference materials for analytical validation. Creating a reference material requires an independently established method for determining target nucleic acid concentration or, alternatively, conducting studies to compare their test with another established assay. For example, samples can be split for a comparison study with another laboratory that performs a similar molecular test. To compare results with another molecular assay, both laboratories should perform a similar assay or at a minimum test for the same target sequence. The samples for testing may be available from one of the laboratories or from an outside source, such as a collaborating laboratory, government organization (the Centers for Disease Control and Prevention [CDC], FDA, or National Institutes of Health), or a commercial supplier.

TABLE 42-1 Guidelines for Molecular Infectious Disease Testing

Organization	Guideline	Internet Address
NCCLS	MM-3-A Molecular Diagnostic Methods for Infectious Diseases	www.nccls.org
	MM-6-A Quantitative Molecular Diagnostics for Infectious Diseases	
	MM-10-P Genotyping	
FDA	Guidance for industry in the manufacture and clinical evaluation of in vitro tests to detect in vitro nucleic acid sequences of HIV-1 (draft guidance).	http://www.fda.gov/cber/gdlns/hivhcvnat.pdf
	Guidance for industry and/or FDA reviewers' staff. Pre-market approval applications for assays pertaining to hepatitis C virus (HCV) that are indicated for diagnosis or monitoring of HCV infection or associated disease (draft guidance).	http://www.fda.gov/cber/gdlns/hivhcvnat.pdf
ASM	Cumitech 31: February 1997. Verification and validation of procedures in the clinical microbiology laboratory; ASM Press.	www.asm.org
ASTM	Guide E1873-97: Standard guide for detection of nucleic acid sequences by the polymerase chain reaction technique.	www.astm.org
	Guide E2048-99: Standard guide for detection of nucleic acids of the *Mycobacterium tuberculosis* complex and other pathogenic mycobacteria by the polymerase chain reaction technique.	
AMP	Recommendations for in-house development and operation of molecular diagnostic tests.	www.ampweb.org

NCCLS, National Committee for Clinical Laboratory Standards; *FDA,* Food and Drug Administration; *AMP,* Association of Molecular Pathology; *ASM,* American Society of Microbiology; *ASTM,* American Society for Testing and Materials.

TABLE 42-2 Checklist for Verification of Molecular LDT

Name of Test	State the name of the test. Be sure that the name identifies the particular organism and/or disease/condition to be tested.
Intended use	What the test measures and for what purpose. Identify the particular microorganism and indicate the use of the test (e.g., diagnosis, prognosis, monitoring response to treatment, guiding therapy, etc.).
Indications for use	Provide clinical condition(s). Use reference standard definitions as found in OMIM.
Method category	Identify methodology used for the test.
Testing procedure	Information with regard to specimen types, specimen handling and transport procedures, nucleic acid isolation and storage, description of the test procedure, data reports, expected results, technical interpretation of results.
Test results	Representative examples of results.
Analytical verification	Analytical "sensitivity," analytical specificity, precision, and linear dynamic range.
Quality control and quality assurance	Delineate QC and QA program. Identify informal proficiency program if no HHS-approved program exists.
Assay limitations	Briefly delineate and discuss potential limitations.
Clinical data	Primary objective of the study, clinical condition evaluated, patient population, demographics, sample size estimate.
Clinical verification	Clinical sensitivity, clinical specificity, positive predictive value, negative predictive value.
Reporting of test results	Clinical interpretation.
Clinical utility	Potential clinical benefit to patient.

OMIM, Online Mendelian Inheritance in Man.

TABLE 42-3 Commercial Sources for Control and Panel Materials

Company	Available Material
Boston Biomedica Inc. (www.bbii.com)	Quantitative and qualitative controls; external run controls; quantification, verification, and performance panels for HCV, HIV, HBV, external run controls for CMV, *Chlamydia trachomatis,* and *Mycobacterium tuberculosis.*
Advanced Biotechnology Inc. (www.bioresearchonline.com/storefronts/abi.htmL)	Control DNA, virus and cell lines (HIV, HTLV, EBV, CMV, HSV, VZV, HCV, SIV, and rubella). Native and recombinant products; purified viruses, antigens, proteins, and antibodies.
Stratagene (www.stratagene.com)	Universal human reference RNA for microarray technology.
AcroMetrix (www.acrometrix.com)	External run controls, secondary reference controls, verification panels for HIV, HCV and HBV, HIV genotyping. Internet evaluation service.
National Institute for Biological Standards and Controls (www.nibsc.ac.uk)	Evaluation/statistics service, working reagents for HIV-1 RNA, HCV, HBV, HAV, parvovirus B19.
Ambion (www.ambion.com)	Armored RNA for internal controls.
American Type Culture Collection (www.attc.gov)	Bacteria, bacteriophages, cell lines and hybridomas, filamentous fungi and yeast, tissue cultures, and viruses.

Reference materials may be naturally occurring or synthetic. "Natural" reference materials are those that consist of a known analyte or known quantity of an analyte as it occurs naturally in the test matrix, purified from the test matrix, or derived by culture of the organism or cell lines. Examples used by a number of laboratories are intact virus particles, bacteria naturally containing the target in their genome, cell lines containing a specific genetic change, or intracellular RNA or DNA. "Synthetic" reference materials include single- or double-stranded DNA, or RNA manufactured in vitro, which are quantified by physical and/or biochemical methods. Such synthetic reference materials can include synthesized DNA in the form of oligonucleotides, single-stranded DNA produced by cloning recombinant phage, cloning into vectors such as plasmids, or a DNA fragment produced by a chemical or physical method from a larger DNA molecule. Synthetic RNA reference materials can be generated by in vitro transcription of DNA templates.

Assessment of analytical characteristics should use test or reference materials that are similar to the intended patient specimen and are carried through the entire process. If possible, precision studies should be performed with more than one lot or batch of reagents and/or materials. Assessment of the accuracy of molecular methods is challenging when, as often happens, the methods have lower detection limits than the established methods.[115,182,183] A well-characterized reference material can be used for accuracy studies.

The linear range of an assay is the span of analyte concentrations for which the final value output is directly proportional to the analyte concentration, with acceptable accuracy and precision. Every assay has an upper and lower limit of quantification, and the lower limit of quantification may be higher than the limit of detection for the assay. The linearity of a quantitative assay may be assessed by testing multiple replicates of at least four different concentrations of the analyte.

Analytical sensitivity (the change of signal per unit change of analyte) is determined by performing serial dilutions of an appropriate number of samples containing known amounts of the analyte. The limit of detection of virus is sometimes defined as the lowest concentration that produces a measurable signal (above background) in 95% of replicates tested. The limit of quantification is the lowest concentration of nucleic acid that can be quantified with an acceptable uncertainty; the uncertainty is often defined in terms of imprecision (coefficient of variation [CV]), which may be as high as 30% for these tests. Analytical specificity is the ability of an analytical method to detect and/or quantify what the test is intended to measure. For infectious disease testing, it is particularly important to ensure that primers and probes do not hybridize with nucleic acid from organisms present in the normal flora or those that cause a similar clinical syndrome.

The susceptibility of the assay to interfering substances must be determined. Exogenous interfering substances are introduced into the specimen, usually during specimen collection or processing. Common examples are heparin and phenol. Both inhibit amplification by polymerases. Endogenous interfering substances, such as bilirubin and lipids, can be increased by disease.

Clinical Verification

The proposed indications for use of the test should be defined before starting the clinical verification. As for any tests (see Chapter 13) the indication for use of an assay could involve the making of a diagnosis, the ruling out of a diagnosis, the provision of prognostic information, or the monitoring of disease—especially, in infectious diseases, establishing resolution of the disease. Special cases of these indications include the screening of a population (e.g., blood donors) and the confirmation of results from another assay. The first step is to formulate a clinical question (Chapter 13), which should take into account the management decision that needs to be made, the role of the method in decision-making, and the target population to which the test will be applied. Known analytical limitations (e.g., precision and linear range) should be taken into consideration when determining the clinical indication for each assay. Further details are provided in Chapters 13 and 15.

Determining the diagnostic accuracy and clinical utility (Chapters 13 and 15) of an assay can be especially difficult when the molecular assay is more sensitive than the reference standard ("gold standard") test. Viral culture, which has been considered "the gold standard" for many years, is an imperfect reference standard test. An insensitive reference standard can make the molecular assay falsely appear to have a low diagnostic specificity. This situation may require use of an expanded gold standard, including a second nonmolecular method (such as serology), a second molecular assay targeting a different region of the genome, or even clinical diagnosis to ascertain the specificity of the molecular assay. For the study of molecular testing for CT, the expanded reference standard included testing by direct fluorescent-antibody assay and/or another molecular test.

Determination of diagnostic accuracy (Chapters 13 and 15) requires attention to both the population and the type of sample, as the results for a method in a given population using a specified sample type may not apply in another population or for another sample type in the same population. Investigation of the diagnostic specificity should include samples from patients with diseases that might be confused with the indicated disease. Specimens from healthy donors are less useful unless the test is intended for screening. The clinical utility of an infectious disease test can also be affected by factors such as microbial-host interactions, microbial dynamics, variants and mutations, and replicative fitness of the microbial agent.

QUALITY CONTROL AND QUALITY ASSURANCE

Quality assurance programs (Chapter 19) address all aspects of the testing process, from test selection to interpretation and use of results. Further details for molecular testing laboratories are provided in Chapter 38. In the United States, the extent of quality assurance and quality control performed for any molecular assay depends on whether the test is FDA-cleared, is "for research use only," is being used "off-label" (for nonapproved uses), or is an LDT. In general LDTs require more extensive quality control, because the analytical performance must be established and maintained by the laboratory. As a result, LDTs require a quality control program for validating the composition, concentration, purity, and performance of critical reagents of the testing process. Tolerance limits should be established for each of these reagents and whenever possible should use a quantitative measurement to avoid subjective evaluation of the quality of the critical reagent. All new reagents should be tested in parallel or concurrently with the previous lot of reagents.

Careful selection of control material and types of controls is vital for the interpretation of test results. For molecular assays, controls may be necessary to detect inhibition of amplification, to assess adequacy of extraction of nucleic acid from the clinical specimens, or to identify degradation of nucleic acid during the extraction procedure. Negative and positive controls are necessary (and required by CLIA '88 regulations), and both must be processed in every clinical test run. The CLIA '88 final rule (published in January 2003) mandates for quantitative molecular assays a negative and two concentrations of positive control in every run. Failure to obtain the correct result for any of the controls invalidates the run. Positive controls should be at a clinically relevant concentration of the nucleic acid target sequence in a background of nucleic acid lacking the target sequence. A positive control should be present at or near the limit of detection of the assay. Positive control material that resembles a patient specimen can also be used as a nucleic acid extraction control to test the ability of the extraction procedure to successfully release the nucleic acid from the organism.

Available control materials include patient specimens that have been well characterized by a similar method, synthetic controls such as Armored RNA (Ambion Inc., Austin, Texas), or purified nucleic acid, although purified nucleic acid would not be appropriate for use as an extraction control. Armored RNA uses a bacteriophage coat around an RNA target to produce pseudoviral particles. Control material is currently available for a variety of pathogens, including HIV-1, HCV, hepatitis A virus, enterovirus, Norwalk virus, and West Nile virus. These armored RNA preparations are stable for at least 11 months and are compatible with a large number of different platforms commonly used for quantitative molecular assays. Table 42-3 lists other manufacturers of control materials.

To check for inhibitors, an internal control can be added to the sample. Alternatively, two portions of the specimen can be tested, with one of them containing an added target. For a specimen to be considered negative, the test result for the specimen amplified directly must be negative and the specimen with added nucleic acid must be positive. The amount of target nucleic acid added to the patient specimen should be close to the limit of detection of the assay, so that low levels of inhibition can be detected. The use of these controls is often discontinued if the inhibition rate is determined to be less than 1%.

Proficiency testing for molecular diagnostics laboratories remains a challenge because adequate proficiency testing programs are unavailable to cover the wide variety of molecular assays offered by a number of laboratories. The CAP offers the only proficiency program accredited for molecular infectious disease by the U.S. government. The program covers only a limited number of microorganisms and in certain instances it does not cover the number of challenges required by CLIA '88. Testing is provided for CT and GC, and HIV-1 and HCV quantitative assays, and for *Borrelia burgdorferi*, CMV, HSV, HCV genotyping, HCV RNA, HIV-1 genotyping, human papillomavirus (HPV), mec A, molecular typing-bacterial, and *Mycobacterium tuberculosis* (MTb). Proficiency testing from Acrometrix (Benencia, Calif.) for HIV-1 genotyping and HCV genotyping offers the submitting of results and retrieving of survey summaries via the Internet. The CDC also offers a Model Performance Evaluation Program for detection and quantification of HIV-1 RNA and detection of MTb.

When no external proficiency-testing program is available, laboratories can compare results on "split" samples shared with other laboratories, perform split-sample testing by an established in-laboratory method, or validate test results based on clinical diagnosis. Specific professional organizations, such as the Association for Molecular Pathology, have been instrumental in facilitating split-sample testing among laboratories through sample exchanges for their members. When exchanging samples between laboratories, it is important to identify a laboratory that uses the same procedure or one that detects the same nucleic acid sequence, and for quantitative methods to ensure similar calibration of the tests. This is important, because even viral load values from commercial assays for HIV-1 RNA can differ by as much as tenfold for any given specimen.

The procedure protocol should be written according to specific guidelines, such as those from the National Committee for Clinical Laboratory Standards (NCCLS).[126] The laboratory procedure is one of the most important aids during orientation and training of new personnel along with continuing assessment for trained personnel.

INTERPRETATION OF RESULTS

Interpretation of the results of molecular assays for infectious diseases requires an understanding of the target organism's biology and the pathogenesis of the related infectious disease(s), and the advantages and limitations of the technology used. Some of the challenges in interpreting these tests are unique to molecular tests and may be different from considerations in interpreting other microbiological tests, such as culture and serology. Such differences may relate to distinguishing viable from nonviable organisms and correlating nucleic acid detection with the presence of the disease.

Interpretation of a negative result requires the consideration of assay sensitivity and efficiencies of nucleic acid extraction and amplification. A false-negative result may be caused by inhibition of or decreased efficiency of amplification, and proper controls for this have been described above. Insufficient sample, inappropriate specimen type, inappropriate timing of sample collection, and degradation of nucleic acid during transport and handling are other sources of false-negative results.

The factors that need to be considered when interpreting a positive result include assay specificity and contamination. Here again, assay design plays a key role in result interpretation. Specificity of molecular infectious disease assays is related to the primers and probes used during amplification and detection/quantification steps. If primers allow amplification of nucleic acids from other pathogens normally present in a patient specimen, false-positive results are possible. For example, primers and probes designed for detection of *Mycoplasma pneumoniae* should not amplify or detect other microorganisms present in the normal oral flora or other common respiratory pathogens. While uncommon, problems with primer specificity have been reported; primers designed to amplify the 5′ untranslated region of the enterovirus genome have also been shown to amplify rhinovirus RNA.[153] This will not be an issue if the assay is only used for CSF, but could cause false-positive results if respiratory specimens are tested.

False-positive results can also occur as the result of carryover contamination of amplified products. This is not a problem with signal amplification methods, but can be of significant concern for target amplification methods, such as PCR, nucleic acid sequenced based amplification (NASBA), transcription-mediated amplification (TMA), and strand displacement assay (SDA). The use of real-time assays that do not require post amplification handling of the product greatly reduces the risk of carryover contamination. Cross-contamination of clinical specimens with target DNA during specimen collection, transport, and processing can occur with any method. Strict attention to good laboratory practices is needed to minimize the risk of cross-contamination.

Molecular tests for infectious diseases do not provide information regarding the viability of an organism. Nucleic acid for certain microorganisms can be found for a period of time after treatment is initiated. For example, CT DNA can be detected in the urine of patients for as long as 3 weeks after initiation of the appropriate therapy.[63] Similarly, HSV DNA can be detected in CSF of patients with encephalitis for 2 weeks or longer after initiation of acyclovir therapy.[97] Monitoring of response to therapy with qualitative assays has limited clinical utility and is best done using quantitative methods. One exception is the use of qualitative RT-PCR method to monitor response to treatment to interferon and ribavirin in HCV-positive patients. In this instance, the absence of detectable HCV RNA from plasma or serum specimen is used to define the virological response to treatment.[50,102,141]

Detection of nucleic acid of a pathogen does not ensure that the organism is the cause of the disease. The organism might be forming part of the normal flora, colonizing a specific area, or causing infection but not disease. One of the primary uses of molecular assays for CMV is for distinguishing active CMV disease from clinically insignificant CMV infection. Early studies evaluating the clinical utility of CMV DNA assays used very sensitive qualitative methods and peripheral blood mononuclear cells as the specimen of choice. As a result, CMV DNA was detected in immunocompromised patients with and without CMV disease, and even in healthy donors.[99] Several approaches have been used to overcome this shortfall and improve the clinical specificity of molecular assays for the diagnosis of active CMV disease in immunocompromised patients, including development of quantitative molecular methods, use of plasma as the specimen, and detection of CMV mRNA rather than DNA. Cutoff values have been proposed as a means to discriminate infection from clinically relevant disease.[60,111]

A common application for quantitative molecular assays is in monitoring of disease progression or response to therapy over time. To determine if changes in the quantitative values are clinically significant or due to expected fluctuations of the measurement, one must consider analytical and biological variability. For example, for the current HIV-1 viral load assays, to allow for both assay and biological variability, changes in the viral load must exceed 0.5 $\log_{10}$ (a threefold change in concentration) to represent a biologically significant change in viral replication.

REPORTING OF RESULTS

Reporting results for qualitative assays in infectious disease is simple: The nucleic acid is either present or "not detected" in the patient specimen. Further relevant information that is useful when reporting results includes the detection limit and specificity of the test and the rate of inhibition for a given specimen type, particularly for assays that do not contain an inhibition control.

Reporting of results for quantitative molecular infectious disease assays is more complex and requires understanding of intrinsic analytical variables that might affect the test results. Quantitative molecular assay results can be expressed in a variety of units, such as copies, genome equivalents, or international units of the target nucleic acid per unit of specimen. Despite all recommendations of august bodies that the unit of volume be the liter (as in SI units), the unit of volume typically used in clinical microbiology laboratories for specimens such as plasma is the milliliter. Concentrations may also be related to a number of leukocytes (e.g., 10,000) or weight of tissue. Results of viral load assays are usually reported as either copies per milliliter or $\log_{10}$ copies/mL. Reporting results as $\log_{10}$ copies/mL may help prevent overinterpretation of small changes. As with all assays, results above the dynamic range should be reported as greater than the upper limit (i.e., >100,000 copies/mL) and "negative specimens" should be reported as less than the lower limit of the assay (e.g., <400 copies/mL). The limit of detection for an assay may not be the same as the limit of quantification; in fact the limit of detection may be lower than the amount of nucleic acid that can be accurately quantified. So the analyte may be detected in a specimen, but at a concentration below the limit of quantification. These values can be reported with the comment "analyte detected, but unable to quantify." This can be confusing to clinicians; so many laboratories report these as less than the limit of quantification (i.e., <400 copies/mL).

SPECIFIC PATHOGENS

Nucleic acid testing has had a tremendous impact on the practice of infectious diseases. These tests are used in a variety of ways, including diagnosis of pathogens that do not grow using conventional methods or grow very slowly, monitoring response to therapy, assessing risk of disease development, and determining disease prognosis. This section will review nucleic acid testing as it applies to specific pathogens with a focus on those pathogens for which nucleic acid testing is considered the standard of care.

CHLAMYDIA TRACHOMATIS AND *NEISSERIA GONORRHOEAE*

CT and GC will be discussed together since several of the available nucleic acid tests for these pathogens are multiplex assays. Though both CT and GC can cause a variety of clinical infections, we will focus on genital infections.

Detection of CT is a challenging and important public health issue. CT is a major cause of genital infections, with an estimated 1 million cases occurring annually among sexually active adolescents and young adults in the United States.[67] More than half of the infections are asymptomatic.[167] Even when symptomatic, the diagnosis can be missed because the manifestations are protean. In males, CT infection may present as urethritis, epididymitis, prostatitis, or proctitis[24,124] and as cervicitis, endometritis, and urethritis in women, with 10% to 40% of infections in women progressing to pelvic inflammatory disease (PID) if untreated.[147,168] Related complications include chronic pelvic pain, ectopic pregnancies, and infertility. In the United States, CT infection is a likely cause of most secondary infertility in females. In pregnant women, there is the additional risk of transmitting the infection to the newborn during labor and delivery, leading to pneumonia or conjunctivitis in the newborn.

GC also may present in various ways, and the clinical presentations overlap those of CT. Males may have acute urethritis with discharge, epididymitis, prostatitis, and urethral strictures. In women, GC infection can produce cervicitis, which if left untreated can lead to PID, abscesses, or salpingitis.

The traditional methods for the diagnosis of CT infections include cell culture, immunofluorescent antigen detection, enzyme immunoassay, and more recently nonamplified nucleic acid detection. These traditional methods have been replaced in many laboratories with amplified nucleic acid tests because of their greater sensitivity in detecting CT from genital specimens. For GC, which was traditionally diagnosed based on culture methods that rely on selective media, nucleic acid testing does not offer a significant improvement in sensitivity compared with culture when culture is performed under ideal conditions. However, GC is a fastidious organism and is highly susceptible to extreme temperatures and desiccation, which can lead to a decreased sensitivity of culture, particularly when specimen transport is required before culturing.[88] Nucleic acid testing for GC offers a sensitive and reliable alternative to culture.

In addition to a high sensitivity and specificity, nucleic acid testing offers several advantages over conventional culture and antigen-detection methods for the diagnosis of CT and GC. Testing for both pathogens can be done on a single specimen, and for some multiplex assays, testing is performed in a single reaction. Unlike the infectious organism itself, the DNA and RNA of GC and CT are quite stable in commercial transport devices, thus accounting for some of the increased sensitivity of these assays compared with the culture. The stability of nucleic acid avoids the necessity of immediate transport to the laboratory, and specimens may be stored refrigerated or at room temperature before transport. The transport and storage requirements vary among tests, so it is important to refer to the package insert for specific details. An additional advantage of nucleic acid testing is the use of urine specimens, which for women allows testing to be done without the need for a pelvic examination. In males, urine offers a convenient and sensitive alternative to collection with a urethral swab and increases the likelihood that asymptomatic males will agree to be tested.

FDA-cleared tests for the detection of CT and GC from clinical specimens (Table 42-4) can use a variety of specimens, including cervical swabs, urethral swabs, and urine from both asymptomatic and symptomatic individuals. Not all assays are approved for all conditions, and the current assays are not FDA-cleared for oral, rectal, respiratory, or conjunctival specimens. The performance characteristics of the assays vary (details are available in the package inserts); however, some general comments can be made concerning all of the tests. The diagnostic sensitivity of the tests varies depending on the specimen type and whether the patient is asymptomatic or symptomatic. Interpretation of the results of nucleic acid testing for CT can be challenging, because many studies have shown these assays to be more sensitive than culture, which was previously used as the gold standard for clinical trials. For males, the sensitivity of testing urine specimens is nearly equivalent to testing urethral swabs.[19,36,45,86,180] A limited volume (20 mL to 50 mL) of first-passed urine is preferred, as larger volumes will lead to a decreased concentration of organism in the sample and thus reduced sensitivity. With proper specimen collection, male urethral swabs and urine specimens have a sensitivity of nearly 100% for the detection of GC or CT. For women, cervical swab specimens provide the highest sensitivity for the detection of GC and CT, with many studies showing a sensitivity of 90% to 95%.[19,45,104,144,180] Urine specimens can be used, but they generally result in a lower sensitivity than cervical swabs (75% to 85%).[36,45,100,139] An alternative to urine testing in women is the use of self-collected vaginal swabs, which have shown in some studies a sensitivity that is equal to that obtained with cervical swabs, although use of this specimen type has not been cleared by the FDA.[80]

Nucleic acid testing is not the standard of care for diagnosing CT and GC in cases of sexual abuse.[33] Some have suggested its use in cases of sexual abuse of adults if testing is done using two assays, each of which targets a different region of the genome. This is not practical for clinical laboratories, because most use only one assay and no single transport medium can be used for all of the FDA-cleared CT and GC molecular assays. For cases of sexual abuse in chil-

TABLE 42-4 Summary of FDA-Cleared Testing for *Chlamydia Trachomatis* and *Neisseria Gonorrhoeae**

Test	Assay Method	Gene Target	Comments
Amplicor® CT/NG *COBAS Amplicor® CT/NG* (Roche Diagnostics, Indianapolis)	PCR	CT: cryptic plasmid NG: M-Ngo PII†	Internal control, multiplex assays
BD ProbeTec™ ET C. trachomatis and N. gonorrhoeae amplified DNA Assay (Becton-Dickinson, Franklin Lakes, NJ)	SDA	CT: cryptic plasmid NG: Piv_{Ng} gene	Internal control
Aptima Combo® 2 Assay‡ (GenProbe, San Diego, CA)	TMA	CT: 23S rRNA NG: 16S rRNA	Multiplex assay Target capture nucleic acid extraction
HC® 2 CT ID *HC® 2 GC ID* *HC® 2 CT/GC Combo Test* (Digene Corporation, Gaithersburg, MD)	Hybrid Capture	CT: cryptic plasmid GC: genomic DNA	

C. trachomatis and *CT, Chlamydia trachomatis; N. gonorrhoeae* and *GC, Neisseria gonorrhoeae; PCR,* polymerase chain reaction; *SDA,* strand displacement assay; *TMA,* transcription-mediated amplification.

*For FDA listings of these and any newer tests, see http://www.accessdata.fda.gov/scripts/cdrh/cfdocs/cfRL/listing.cfm and use testcodes LSK and LSL for *Chlamydia* and *N. gonorrhea,* respectively.

†Cytosine DNA methyltransferase.

‡Confirmatory assays for CT and NG are also available.

dren, culture is still recommended for the detection of GC and CT. Another limitation of nucleic acid testing for the detection of CT or GC is use as a test of cure. Because DNA can persist in urine samples for up to 3 weeks after completion of therapy,[63] test of cure using nucleic acid testing is discouraged. If this must be done, then testing should be delayed for at least 3 weeks after initiating therapy.

For several of the GC assays, there is a reduced specificity because of cross-hybridization of primers with nongonococcal *Neisseria* species.[69,123] The ProbeTec test has been reported to produce false-positive results with *N. flavescens, N. lactamica, N. subflava,* and *N. cinerea,* and the Amplicor assay can produce false-positive results with *N. flavescens, N. lactamica,* and *N. sicca.* Because of cross-reactivity with these nongonococcal species of *Neisseria,* there is concern about generating false-positive results with pharyngeal specimens.[136] However, *N. cinerea, N. lactamica, N. subflava,* and *N. sicca* have also been isolated from genital mucosa, so it is also possible to generate false-positive results from genital specimens.

Other sources of false-positive results include carryover contamination of amplified product and cross-contamination during specimen collection, transport, or processing. Concerns over these issues have led to a discussion of confirmatory testing for CT and GC, since false-positive results can have psychosocial or medicolegal ramifications. False-positive results in a low-prevalence population can significantly reduce the predictive value of a positive result. For example, though the specificity of nucleic acid testing for GC or CT generally ranges from 98% to 99%, the positive predictive value may be as low as 60% to 70% in a population with a low prevalence. CDC Guidelines for STD testing[33] discuss options for confirmatory testing, including (1) testing of another specimen with a different assay that has a different target, (2) testing of the original specimen with a different assay that has a different target, (3) repeating the original test using the original specimen but with a blocking antibody or competitive probe, and (4) repeating the original test using original specimen. Confirmatory testing can be expensive and complicate work flow. Some laboratories have established gray zones or equivocal ranges for specimens with initial low-level positive results[46] and perform confirmatory testing only on such specimens. This appears to be a rational approach, since low-positive specimens are less likely to be confirmed as positive upon repeat testing—although other laboratories confirm all positive results, either using the same test or using a second assay.

False-negative results from inhibition of amplification are a consideration for both GC and CT testing and have been reported for both cervical swabs and urine specimens.[37,105,151] Inhibition rates may vary considerably depending on the amplification method and are related in part to the method used for nucleic acid extraction.[105] For tests that use a crude lysate in testing (such as the Amplicor and ProbeTec tests), inhibition rates tend to be higher than those seen with the Aptima combo test, which uses a target capture method to purify nucleic acid. For the assays that test a crude lysate, it is useful to include the internal control or amplification control to assess for inhibition of amplification. In this situation, the specimen would not be reported as negative for GC or CT unless there was amplification of the internal control. There are no clear guidelines concerning when it is appropriate to discontinue use of an internal control. However, to contain costs, some laboratories discontinue the use of the internal control if inhibition rates are less than 1%.

There is interest in performing CT and GC testing for liquid cytology specimens, because a single specimen can be used for cervical cytology (Pap smear) and for CT and GC testing.[10] The latter two tests would be performed on the liquid specimen that remained after completion of the Pap and HPV testing. However, there are several drawbacks to this approach that must be considered. The instruments used to prepare the liquid Pap smears were not designed to control for cross-contamination during processing, which may lead to false-positive results. CT and GC testing would not be performed until after the Pap smear results and HPV testing were complete, which could delay diagnosis and treatment of CT or GC infections. Moreover, there may be inadequate specimen remaining to complete CT and GC testing, thus requiring the patient to make a return visit to collect an additional sample. At this time it remains unclear how these various issues will be resolved.

Decisions regarding the choice of a specific amplification test for the detection of CT and GC should not be based solely on the cost of reagents. Other key factors to consider include test performance characteristics, such as diagnostic sensitivity and specificity, and whether the test has been cleared for urine and swab specimens in both symptomatic and asymptomatic individuals. Ideally the test should include an internal control, particularly if a crude lysate is used in the assay. Other factors to consider are degree of automation, ease of use, work flow issues, and space and equipment needs.

Human Papillomavirus

Anogenital HPV infections are common in both men and women. It is estimated that more than 24 million men and women in the United States are currently infected with HPV.[68] HPV is a sexually transmitted infection; it is most common among sexually active young women ages 15 through 25 years. In one study, cervicovaginal HPV was found in 43% of sexually active college women during a 3-year period.[78]

HPV is classified as either cutaneous or mucosal, infecting, respectively, keratinizing or nonkeratinizing epithelium. The focus of this section will be the mucosal types, which include approximately 30 types of HPV that infect the anogenital area. The types of HPV that are spread through sexual contact are classified as either low risk or high risk for progression to malignancy. There are multiple types of both low-risk and high-risk HPV. Infections with HPV can lead to a variety of outcomes, ranging from benign genital warts to penile or cervical cancer. The outcome is driven by the type of HPV. Genital warts or condyloma acuminata are caused by low-risk HPV types and have a low likelihood of progressing to malignancy.[65] Conversely, penile cancer in men and cervical cancer in women are associated with high-risk HPV infections.[12,114,186,194] Infections can, however, be transient, and progression to cancer occurs over decades.[56,176]

Until recently, the standard method for the diagnosis of cervical cancer was the detection of abnormal cells by cervical cytology (Pap smear) or biopsy. The morphological changes associated with HPV infection include atypical squamous cells of undetermined significance (ASCUS), low-grade squamous intraepithelial lesion (LSIL), and high-grade squamous intraepithelial lesion (HSIL).[150,158] The diagnosis of ASCUS using a Pap smear has an estimated prevalence of 5% to 10%, with rates as high as 20% reported in sexually active women. Not all women with ASCUS progress to cervical cancer. HPV testing now plays an important role in assessing which women with ASCUS are at the highest risk of developing cervical cancer. Current recommendations are to test all women with ASCUS for the presence of high-risk HPV. Those women testing positive for high-risk HPV DNA should be referred for colposcopy, while those patients testing negative for HPV DNA can be followed according to routine practice.[164] Another more recently recognized use of high-risk HPV testing is as a primary screening tool for all women 30 years of age and older,[96] regardless of whether they have ASCUS detected on a Pap smear. This is based on the observation that women over the age of 30 who have persistent infection with high-risk types of HPV are at the greatest risk of developing cervical cancer. Women who have a normal Pap and a negative HPV screen are at very low risk of developing cervical cancer and would require less frequent screening than those with either an abnormal Pap or a positive HPV screen. Because of the clear association of HPV with cervical cancer and the availability of high-volume HPV testing, some are questioning the role of cervical cytology as a primary screen for cervical cancer.

Proper use of HPV testing requires not only detection of the virus or viral DNA, but also classifying it as either low-risk or high-risk. Viral culture for HPV is not easily performed and not available in clinical laboratories, and cytological examination cannot distinguish between low-risk and high-risk HPV infection. This has led laboratories to rely on molecular testing for the detection and classification of HPV. Various methods are available, including detection of HPV DNA by signal amplification and PCR. Currently the only available FDA-cleared test for the detection and classification of HPV DNA is the Hybrid Capture® 2 (HC2) test (Digene Corporation, Gaithersburg, Md.). The test relies on signal amplification technology and probe hybridization. The test uses two separate pools of RNA probes: one for detecting high-risk HPV DNA and another for low-risk HPV DNA. The high-risk pool contains RNA probes specific for HPV types 16, 18, 31, 33, 35, 39, 45, 51, 52, 56, 58, 59, and 68, and the low-risk pool of RNA probes detects HPV types 6, 11, 42, 43, and 44. The test results are reported as high-risk or low-risk HPV DNA detected. There is no identification of the specific high-risk type or low-risk type. PCR-based assays for the detection and typing of HPV are used in research laboratories[43,66,95,107,181]; however, PCR-based methods are in commercial development for use in the clinical laboratory.

The HC2 test has been FDA-cleared for three indications: aiding in the diagnosis of sexually transmitted HPV infections (high-risk and low-risk test), testing of specimens from patients with ASCUS-grade cytology results to determine the need for colposcopy (high-risk test only),[44] and primary screening of women age 30 and older (high-risk test only).[96] The recommended specimen types for HPV DNA testing include cervical swabs, liquid-based cytology specimens, and cervical biopsy specimens.

One concern with the HC2 test is difficulties with reproducibility of results near the signal/cutoff ratio for a positive result. Whether these signals are due to low concentrations of HPV DNA or they represent false-positive results remains unclear. As a result of this poor repeatability, some laboratories have established an equivocal range or gray zone for the test. When a result is within the gray zone, it is reported as indeterminate or testing is repeated and reported as positive only if a positive result is found on repeat testing. A potential cause of false-positive results for high-risk HPV is that certain low-risk HPVs are detected with the high-risk probe pool. Such false-positive results are seen in specimens with high concentrations of HPV 6 or HPV 42 DNA.

Testing of liquid-based cytology specimens in the HC2 assay is viewed favorably by many clinicians, since one specimen can be collected for both the Pap smear and HPV testing. Logistical issues with this approach can be challenging to the clinical laboratory. When Pap results are used to determine which samples are tested for HPV, the laboratory may find it difficult to complete the HPV testing within 21 days of specimen collection (as required according to the package insert) if there are delays in completing or reporting the Pap smear results. There may be inadequate volume of specimen remaining after the Pap smear is complete; this is a particular problem for specimens with a low cellular content, as a greater volume of specimen is used for the Pap smear. Finally, if the HC2 testing is not performed in the cytology laboratory, the testing laboratory may experience delays in specimen receipt, again making it difficult to complete testing within 21 days of specimen collection.

Several new approaches to HPV testing are under investigation that may provide more insight into identifying those women at highest risk of progressing to cervical cancer. These include assessing if there is prognostic value in determining HPV viral load and evaluating expression of HPV E6 and E7 mRNA as a marker for viral persistence and disease progression.

Human Immunodeficiency Virus Type 1

HIV-1, the causative agent of the acquired immunodeficiency syndrome (AIDS), is an RNA virus belonging to the genus lentivirus of the family Retroviridae. The replication of the virus is complex and involves reverse transcription of the RNA genome into a double-stranded DNA molecule, with subsequent integration into the host genome. The reverse transcriptase enzyme does not have proofreading capabilities, leading to the marked genetic diversity of HIV-1. There are two distinct genetic groups: the major (M) and outlier (O) groups. Viruses in the M group are further divided into 8 subtypes or clades, designated A through H, based on the sequence diversity within the HIV-1 *gag* and *env* genes.[41] Group M virus is found worldwide, with clade B predominating in Europe and North America. Complex replication cycles and genetic diversity are two factors that influence the design and interpretation of HIV-1 molecular assays.

Viral-Load Testing

The management of persons infected with human HIV-1 has been revolutionized by both viral-load and resistance testing. With these tools, it is possible to maximize the effectiveness of antiretroviral therapy for an individual. Viral-load testing became the standard of care around 1996, followed more recently by resistance testing. The clinical utility of viral-load testing (which refers to quantifying HIV-1 RNA, usually from plasma) has been well established. Testing is used to determine when to initiate antiretroviral therapy, to monitor response to therapy, and to predict time to progression to AIDS. Higher viral loads are associated with a more rapid progression to AIDS and death.[118,119,134] Viral-load testing is used more routinely in decisions regarding when to initiate antiretroviral therapy and in monitoring response to therapy. Current treatment guidelines[192] recommend initiating therapy for individuals based on several factors, including CD4 cell count, viral loads, and symptoms. In cases in which viral loads exceed 50,000 copies/mL, therapy can be initiated regardless of CD4 cell count and the presence of symptoms.

The current standard for treating HIV-1–infected individuals is to use combinations of protease inhibitors or non-nucleoside reverse-transcriptase inhibitors with nucleoside analogs.[192] This combination therapy is often referred to as highly active antiretroviral therapy or HAART. Initial use of these effective drug combinations in individuals who have not been treated with them before ("naïve" individuals) is expected to decrease viral-load values by at least 2 $\log_{10}$ copies/mL. The goal of therapy is to achieve viral-load values below the limit of detection of currently available assays (50 copies/mL), although this is not always possible in all individuals, particularly in those with very high pretreatment viral-load values or in those who have failed in prior therapeutic regimens. Guidelines for the use of HIV-1 RNA concentrations in clinical practice have been published,[156] and are frequently updated (http://www.aidsinfo.nih.gov/, http://www.iasusa.org). In general, a plasma HIV-1 viral load should be measured before beginning therapy (baseline) and then again at 2 to 8 weeks after the initiation of therapy to determine the response to therapy. Testing is then repeated at 3- to 4-month intervals to evaluate continued effectiveness of the regimen. Any increase in viral load should be confirmed with repeat testing, as a variety of other illnesses can transiently increase viral load. When a significant increase in viral load has been documented, HIV-1 resistance testing should be considered (see below).

Molecular assays are also useful in the diagnosis of acute HIV-1 infection in neonates because maternal IgG crosses the placenta, an uninfected newborn may be seropositive into the second year of life. Both qualitative proviral DNA tests and viral-load assays are useful for the diagnosis of HIV-1 infection in newborns.[47,170,193] HIV-1 RNA testing appears to be more sensitive than proviral DNA testing for the diagnosis of acute HIV-1 infection in newborns,[47,170] though both are used in clinical practice. The diagnosis of HIV-1 infection in a newborn requires testing at two different time points, usually shortly after birth and then again at 6 weeks to several months of age.

The use of HIV-1 viral-load testing for *diagnosing* acute HIV-1 infection in adults is more controversial. The currently available viral-load assays are approved only for use in patients known to be infected with HIV-1, but they have clear utility in the diagnosis of acute infection, which is defined as the period after exposure to the virus but before seroconversion. In the "window period," the ELISA and Western blot assays are negative or indeterminate, so additional testing is necessary. Individuals with acute infection are often symptomatic with a mononucleosis type of syndrome, which may include fever, fatigue, rash, lymphadenopathy, and oral ulcers.[89] During this acute infection, the plasma concentration of viral RNA is very high, usually 10^5 to 10^7 copies/mL, and viral-load measurements are a useful diagnostic tool. Acute HIV-1 infection should be suspected in an individual presenting with appropriate symptoms and risk factors. In these individuals, testing for acute HIV-1 infection would include an enzyme-linked immunosorbent assay (ELISA) and a viral-load assay. Care must be taken to correctly interpret these test results, as individuals with acute HIV-1 infection would be expected to have a negative or indeterminate ELISA and/or Western blot, and a very high viral load (greater than 100,000 copies/mL). The concern with using viral-load testing to diagnose acute HIV infection is that false-positive results have been reported.[48] In one study the false-positive results were found when using the Versant bDNA test,[48] with false-positive results usually lower than 2000 copies/mL. Before diagnosing acute HIV infection, individuals must be educated regarding the limitations of these tests and must give informed consent to testing. To minimize the likelihood of reporting a false-positive result, repeat testing should be done on all specimens with a detectable viral load and an HIV1/2 ELISA should be obtained at the time of viral-load testing. It is critical to

TABLE 42-5 The First Quantitative HIV (Viral Load) Assays Approved by the FDA*

Test	Amplification Method	Reportable Range
Amplicor HIV Monitor v1.5 Test (Roche Diagnostics, Indianapolis, IN)	RT-PCR	Ultrasensitive: 50-100,000 copies/mL Standard: 400-750,000 copies/mL
Versant HIV-1 RNA 3.0 Assay (Bayer Diagnostics, Tarrytown, NY)	bDNA	75-500,000 copies/mL
NucliSens HIV-1 QT Assay (bioMerieux, Durham, NC)	NASBA	176-3,470,000 copies/mL

RT-PCR, Reverse transcription-polymerase chain reaction; *bDNA,* branched DNA; *NASBA,* nucleic acid sequence based amplification.
*For FDA listings of these and any newer tests, visit http://www.accessdata.fda.gov/scripts/cdrh/cfdocs/cfRL/listing.cfm and use test code MTL.

remember that patients with acute retroviral syndrome should have very high concentrations of HIV-1 RNA.

HIV-1 viral-load assays that are currently FDA-approved are listed in Table 42-5. The lower limit of quantification differs among the three assays. The reportable concentration range of each of the Amplicor assays is limited, so both an ultrasensitive and a standard version of the test are needed to cover the clinically important range of viral-load values. Viral-load assays must be able to accurately quantify the various viral subtypes. In the United States and Europe subtype B predominates, though infections with non-B subtypes are becoming more common and are certainly an important cause of HIV-1 infection globally. The Versant bDNA assay will accurately quantify HIV-1 subtypes A thru G,[85] and the Amplicor RT-PCR version 1.5 will accurately quantify subtypes A through H.[85,137,138] The earlier Amplicor assay (version 1.0) underquantified non-B subtypes[85] and has been replaced by the 1.5 assay version. The NucliSens NASBA assay underestimates concentrations of subtype G.[85,130,137] None of the currently available assays is recommended for the quantification of group O virus. Viral-load values obtained with the different assays may not always agree, so it is recommended to choose one assay when monitoring patients over time.

The available viral-load assays have an intraassay imprecision (CV) of 0.12 to 0.2 $\log_{10}$, with the Versant bDNA assay showing the best precision.[16] For the Amplicor (version 1.0) assay, the total variation was approximately 0.26 $\log_{10}$, including intraassay, interassay, and biological variation.[17] Based on this degree of variation, changes in viral load should exceed 0.5 $\log_{10}$ (threefold) to represent a biologically relevant change in viral replication. Reporting viral-load results as $\log_{10}$ copies/mL is recommended[127] and will assist in preventing clinicians from overinterpreting small changes in viral load. This is particularly important for values near the limit of quantification, where assay variability is the greatest. A variety of acute and opportunistic infections and vaccinations can transiently increase HIV-1 RNA in plasma,[53,134,169] so it is recommended not to measure viral load for monitoring of individuals who are acutely ill and those who have been recently vaccinated.

Viral-load testing is routinely performed on plasma specimens, and ethylene diamine tetraacetic acid (EDTA) is the anticoagulant of choice. Acid citrate dextrose is also an acceptable anticoagulant, but for the Amplicor and Versant assays blood anticoagulated in heparin is unacceptable. Viral-load testing can be done on specimens other than plasma, including serum, dried blood (or plasma) spots on filter paper, CSF, and genital secretions. The assays have not been validated on all of these specimen types, and testing these specimens is usually reserved for research studies. It is critical to handle clinical specimens properly to minimize the risk of RNA degradation during specimen collection and transport. Plasma should be separated within 6 hours of collection, and ideally stored at −20 °C, although plasma viral RNA is stable at 4 °C for several days. For laboratories performing testing from specimens collected at remote sites, VACUTAINER Plasma Preparation Tubes (PPTs) can be useful. The tube can be centrifuged at the collection site and shipped in the PPT tube. A gel provides a physical barrier between the plasma and cells, and tubes can be shipped without the need to transfer the plasma into a separate tube.[79]

Resistance Testing

Four general classes of antiretroviral drugs are used in clinical care: nucleoside reverse transcriptase inhibitors (NRTIs), nonnucleoside reverse transcriptase inhibitors (NNRTIs), protease inhibitors (PIs), and a new class of drug, fusion inhibitors. Viral resistance can occur with each of these classes of drug, particularly when viral replication is not maximally suppressed during therapy. The current standard of care is to use regimens that contain a combination of drugs, usually a PI or NNRTIs with several NRTIs, since resistance is less likely to occur on the complex regimens than on monotherapy.[192]

A variety of studies have evaluated the clinical utility of antiviral resistance testing in HIV-1 infected individuals. Several early prospective randomized clinical trials of genotypical resistance testing were conducted with persons who had failed therapy with multidrug regimens, including the protease inhibitors and NRTIs. In both the VIRADAPT[39,54] and GART[8] studies, the selection of the salvage regimen was determined either by the use of genotypical resistance testing (genotype arm) or by considering which antiretroviral drugs had been used in prior treatment regimens (control arm). The response rates in the genotype arms were higher than in the control arm. For example, in the VIRADAPT study, patients in the genotype arm had a greater decrease in viral load 6 months after initiating salvage therapy, and more of them (32% versus 14%) had plasma viral loads <200 copies/mL.[39,54] The Havana trial helped establish the utility of expert advice in interpreting the genotypical resistance data by comparing genotype resistance testing, expert advice, or both with the standard of care for selecting a regimen in patients failing therapy.[179] Although either genotyping or expert advice improved response compared with the control group, the best response was seen in the group receiving both genotyping and expert advice. The VIRA3001 study, a prospective randomized trial that compared standard of care to phenotypic resistance testing in patients who failed a PI-containing regimen, found a better virological outcome for patients in the phenotypic arm.[40] Although some trials of resistance testing have not shown improved clinical outcomes compared with standard of care,[72,120,122] the results of the randomized trials favor use of resistance testing.

Guidelines for the appropriate use of HIV-1 resistance testing in adults have been established by an International AIDS Society-USA panel of experts.[76] Resistance testing is recommended in patients who are failing on an initial antiretroviral regimen and in those failing after numerous regimens. In addition, resistance testing is recommended before initiating therapy for patients who have been infected within the previous 2 years. This is based on the finding that some resistance mutations can persist in plasma HIV-1 RNA for more than 12 months in untreated patients.[18] Resistance testing is also recommended in pregnant women to optimize treatment and in hopes of minimizing transmission of HIV-1 infection to the neonate. As it is possible to transmit drug-resistant virus, it is also recommended that resistance testing be done on patients presenting with acute or recent (within 12 months) HIV-1 infection, particularly if the person from whom HIV-1 was acquired ("source patient") is known and is receiving antiretroviral therapy.

Genotypic assays identify specific mutations or nucleotide changes that are associated with a decreased susceptibility to an antiviral drug. The effective use of genotypic resistance testing requires an extensive understanding of the genetics of antiretroviral resistance. There are several methods available for genotypic assays, including automated dideoxynucleoside terminator cycle sequencing, DNA hybridization using high-density microarrays, and reverse hybridization using the line probe assay. This discussion will be limited to automated sequencing methods, since this is the method used in the overwhelming majority of genotypic resistance testing performed for management of patients. The currently available assays will detect mutations in the reverse transcriptase and protease gene; modifications of existing assays will be needed to detect the resistance mutations associated with fusion inhibitors.

The initial step in genotypic assays is the isolation of HIV-1 RNA from plasma, followed by RT-PCR amplification and sequencing of the reverse transcriptase and protease genes. The analysis of the results involves sequence alignment and editing, mutation identification by comparison with a wild-type sequence, and interpretation of the clinical significance of the mutations identified. Most clinical laboratories performing genotypic resistance testing rely on commercial assays that provide reagents and software programs to assist with the interpretation of the results. Two assays have been cleared by the FDA, the Trugene HIV-1 Genotyping Kit and OpenGene DNA Sequencing System (Bayer Diagnostics Corp., Tarrytown, N.Y.) and the ViroSeq HIV-1 Genotyping System (Celera Diagnostics/Abbott Laboratories, Abbott Park, Ill.). In addition to these commercial assays, several laboratories have developed automated-cycle sequencing assays for HIV-1 resistance testing.

The interpretation of genotypic resistance testing is complex. The interpretation of resistance mutations uses "rules-based" software that takes into account cross-resistance and interactions of mutations. The commercially available systems generate a summary report that lists the various mutations that have been identified in the reverse transcriptase and protease genes, and each drug is reported as resistant, possibly resistant, no evidence of resistance, or insufficient evidence. A comprehensive discussion of the specific mutations associated with each antiretroviral drug and the interactions of mutations is beyond the scope of this chapter, but is available from a variety of sources[76,122] (http://hiv-web.lanl.gov/content/index, http://www.iasusa.org., http://hivdb.standford.edu/).

Phenotypic resistance assays measure viral replication in the presence of antiretroviral drugs. Results of phenotypic assays are typically reported as the inhibitory concentration of a drug that reduces in vitro HIV-1 replication by 50% (IC_{50}). The IC_{50} is usually reported as the fold change in IC_{50} relative to a wild-type strain. Initially, phenotypic assays required the isolation of infectious HIV-1 from a blood specimen. Newer phenotypic assays use high-throughput automated assays based on recombinant DNA technology. For these assays, HIV-1 RNA is amplified from a plasma specimen, eliminating the need for a viral isolate. This testing is not performed in clinical laboratories and the technology is available only from two commercial laboratories. For the PhenoSense assay (ViroLogic, San Francisco, Calif.), the protease and reverse transcriptase genes are amplified using RT-PCR and inserted into a modified HIV-1 vector that has a luciferase reporter-gene in place of the viral envelope gene.[140] Viral replication is measured by quantification of luciferase expression in the presence of various concentrations of antiretroviral drugs. The reproducibility of the assay is such that increases in IC_{50} of greater than 2.5-fold can be reliably detected in the assay. The other assay (Antivirogram, Virco, Mechelen, Belgium) combines patient and HIV-1 vector sequences using in vitro recombination.[75] Viral replication is measured using a reporter-gene system. Based on replicate studies performed by the company, reduced susceptibility is defined as a greater than fourfold increase in IC_{50} compared with the wild-type virus. This technical cutoff often differs from the cutoff that is associated with clinical resistance to a drug, which is referred to as the clinical cutoff. The change in IC_{50} associated with clinical failure may differ for each drug tested. For example, with the protease inhibitor lopinavir, the IC_{50} that correlates with clinical resistance may be in the range of a greater than or equal to a tenfold increase in IC_{50},[184] compared with a twofold increase for the NRTI ddI. It is likely that IC_{50} cutoffs will continue to be modified as more clinical outcomes data become available. Results of phenotypic assays include not only the change in IC_{50} value, but also an interpretation of whether there is an increase or decrease in susceptibility compared with the wild-type virus.

A "virtual phenotype" is also available commercially for assessing HIV-1 drug resistance. With a virtual phenotype, rather than performing a phenotypic assay directly, the information is inferred from the genotypic assay. The results of the genotypic assay are entered into a database containing matching genotypic and phenotypic results from thousands of clinical specimens, and the closest matching phenotypic results are averaged and reported as the virtual phenotype.

Both phenotypic and genotypic assays are used in clinical care: some clinicians prefer phenotypic testing because it is a direct measure of viral susceptibility, while others prefer genotypic testing because the development of a mutation may precede phenotypic expression of resistance.[77] Other advantages of genotypic testing include relatively rapid turnaround time (a few days), easier availability, and lower cost than phenotypic testing. Providers often use genotypic testing routinely and rely on phenotypic testing for patients who have failed multiple regimens and have very complex genotypic results. If both assays are used, it is key to remember that the results of the two assays may not agree, because the presence of a resistance mutation does not assure its expression in a phenotypic assay.

A limitation of the currently used genotypic and phenotypic assays is that they can detect only those mutants that make up at least 20% of the total viral population. Regimens chosen based on resistance testing may not always be effective because the minority populations will quickly predominate in the presence of a drug. Drug selection pressure is also needed for some resistance mutations to persist at detectable concentrations in the viral population; when the drug therapy is discontinued, the wild-type virus may quickly predominate. For this reason, it is recommended that specimens for resistance testing be obtained while the patient is on antiretroviral therapy.

The minimum viral load required for reliable resistance testing is approximately 1000 copies/mL. Because genotyping assays are especially sensitive to RNA degradation, care must be taken to properly handle the specimen after collection. Guidelines outlined for collection and transport of specimens for testing in viral-load assays should be followed for resistance testing.

Herpes Simplex Virus

HSV, a member of the herpesvirus family, is a double-stranded DNA virus. Following primary infection, the virus remains latent in sensory neurons and can be reactivated under a variety of situations, including stress, trauma, sun exposure, and various immunocompromised states. HSV types 1 and 2 produce various clinical syndromes involving the skin, eye, central nervous system (CNS), and genital tract. Although nucleic acid testing has been used to detect HSV DNA in all of these clinical manifestations, this discussion will focus on the use of HSV PCR for the diagnosis of CNS infections, since nucleic acid amplification testing is widely viewed as the standard of care for the diagnosis of these infections.

HSV causes both encephalitis and meningitis; in adults encephalitis is usually caused by infection with HSV type 1, and meningitis is most commonly caused by HSV type 2. HSV encephalitis is a severe infection with a high morbidity and mortality; treatment with acyclovir reduces the mortality from approximately 70% in untreated infections to 19% to 28%. Neurological impairment, however, is common (about 50%) in those who survive.[188,189] HSV encephalitis may reflect primary infection or reactivation of latent infection. HSV meningitis is usually a self-limited disease, which resolves during the course of several days without therapy. In some patients the disease may recur as a lymphocytic meningitis over a period of years.[178,188]

Neonatal HSV infection occurs in 1:3500 to 1:5000 deliveries in the United States.[188] It is most commonly acquired by intrapartum contact with infected maternal genital secretions and is usually caused by HSV type 2. In the newborn there are three general presentations of the disease: skin, eye, and mouth disease accounts for approximately 45% of infections, encephalitis accounts for 35%, and disseminated disease accounts for 20%. As disseminated disease is often associated with neurological disease, CNS disease occurs in about 50% of newborns with neonatal HSV infection.

HSV encephalitis cannot be distinguished clinically from encephalitis caused by other viruses such as West Nile virus, St. Louis encephalitis virus, and Eastern equine encephalitis virus. Historically the gold standard for the diagnosis of HSV encephalitis required brain biopsy with identification of HSV by cell culture or immunohistochemical staining. This approach provided high sensitivity (99%) and specificity (100%), but it required an invasive procedure, and several days elapsed before results were available. Cell culture of CSF has a sensitivity of less than 10% for the diagnosis of HSV encephalitis in adults. Tests that measure HSV antigen or antibody in CSF have sensitivities of 75% to 85%, and specificities of 60% to 90%.[188] Because of the limitations of conventional methods, there was interest in assessing the clinical utility of PCR for the detection of HSV DNA from the CSF of patients with encephalitis.

The two largest studies have compared HSV PCR on CSF specimens with a brain biopsy[6,97] in patients with suspected HSV encephalitis. The sensitivity and specificity of PCR were greater than 95%, and the sensitivity of HSV PCR did not decrease significantly until 5 to 7 days after start of therapy. PCR is positive early in the course of illness, usually within the first 24 hours of symptoms, and in some individuals HSV DNA can persist in the CSF for weeks after initiating therapy.[6,97,190]

The clinical utility of HSV PCR has also been established for the diagnosis of neonatal HSV infection. In one study,[92] HSV DNA was detected in the CSF of 76% (26 of 34) infants with CNS disease, 94% (13 of 14) with disseminated infection, and 24% (7 of 29) with skin, eye, or mouth disease. The persistence of HSV DNA in the CSF of newborns for greater than 1 week after initiating therapy is associated with a poor outcome.[106] Based on the findings, detection of HSV DNA in CSF by PCR has become the standard of care for the diagnosis of HSV encephalitis and neonatal HSV infection. In newborns with disseminated disease, HSV DNA may be detected in serum or plasma specimens, and can be a useful diagnostic tool in newborns if it is not possible to do a lumbar puncture. Though the sensitivity of HSV PCR is high, it is not 100%, so a negative PCR test may not rule out neurological disease HSV as the cause, particularly if the pretest probability is high. In this situation it is important to consider repeat testing.

As with HSV encephalitis, HSV meningitis cannot be distinguished clinically from other viral meningitides, although recurrence of viral meningitis is a strong clue that HSV may be the etiologic agent. Unlike HSV encephalitis, HSV meningitis has not been the subject of large studies evaluating the clinical utility of PCR for diagnosis. Nonetheless, as the sensitivity of cell culture of CSF specimens is only 50%, HSV PCR of CSF is commonly used in the evaluation of meningitis. It has been described as accurate in anecdotal reports.[159,178]

Currently there are no FDA-cleared assays for the detection of HSV DNA from clinical specimens, and the performance characteristics of existing assays may vary. The Light Cycler assay (Roche Diagnostics, Indianapolis, IN) is available as an analyte-specific reagent PCR assay designed for the detection of HSV DNA types 1 and 2 equally. Distinguishing between HSV types 1 and 2 may not be necessary, since the clinical management is the same for both infections. Primers used for the detection of HSV DNA commonly target the polymerase, glycoprotein B, glycoprotein D, or thymidine kinase genes. It is important that the primers not amplify DNA from other herpesviruses that are associated with neurological disease; these include cytomegalovirus, varicella zoster virus, human herpesvirus type 6, and Epstein-Barr virus.

HSV PCR assays need low detection limits (several hundred copies per milliliter of specimen) to be useful in evaluation of neurological disease. This is particularly true for the diagnosis of meningitis in which CSF concentrations of DNA tend to be lower than those seen with encephalitis. HSV neurological disease rarely occurs without an increased CSF white blood cell count or protein concentration.[162] Caution should be exercised in applying this generalization to immunocompromised individuals, as they may not mount a typical inflammatory response to HSV infection. Although HSV PCR of CSF specimens is clearly the gold standard for the diagnosis of neurological disease, results should be interpreted with caution since neither sensitivity nor specificity is 100%. Test results should always be interpreted within the context of the clinical presentation of the patient. If results do not correlate with the clinical impression, repeat testing should be performed.

ENTEROVIRUS

Enteroviruses are a diverse group of single-stranded RNA viruses belonging to the Picornavirus family. The group includes polioviruses, enteroviruses types A-D, and parechovirus (human echovirus). Numerous clinical presentations are seen with the nonpolioviruses, including acute aseptic meningitis, encephalitis, exanthems, conjunctivitis, acute respiratory disease, gastrointestinal disease, myopericarditis, and sepsislike syndrome in neonates. Diagnoses typically are based on clinical presentation and/or culture methods. Cell culture methods have several drawbacks, including the requirement to inoculate multiple cell lines, because no single cell line is optimal for all enterovirus types; the inability to grow some enterovirus types in cell culture; the limited diagnostic sensitivity of cell culture (65% to 75%); and the long turnaround time of 3 to 8 days for those enteroviruses that do grow in a cell culture.[38] The long turnaround time for the culture means that results are rarely available in a timeframe to influence clinical management. Nucleic acid testing offers several important advantages over cell culture, including improved sensitivity and turnaround time. As a result, nucleic acid testing is considered the new gold standard for the diagnosis of aseptic meningitis and neonatal sepsis syndrome caused by the enterovirus.

Two methods are used for the detection of enteroviral RNA from clinical specimens: RT-PCR and NASBA. The primers used in clinical testing most commonly target the highly conserved 5′-untranslated region of the gene (5′UTR)[152,154] and will detect polioviruses and enteroviruses. These primers will not detect echovirus types 22 and 23, which have been reclassified as parechoviruses, although these viruses can cause aseptic meningitis. In general, molecular assays have good detection limits ranging from 0.1 to 50 tissue culture infectious doses 50 (TCID50) per assay.* The assays are quite specific, but sequence similarities may allow amplification of some types of rhinoviruses.[13,185,196] As with HSV, there is no FDA-cleared assay for the detection of

*References 13, 61, 133, 145, 152, 171, 185, 196, 197.

enterovirus RNA from clinical specimens. Several ASRs are available for detection of enterovirus RNA from CSF specimens to assist laboratorians in assay development. The Enterovirus Consensus assay (Argene Biosoft, Varihles, France) uses RT-PCR technology and detects all 64 enteroviral serotypes.[13] The other available ASR assay is the NucliSens Basic Kit (bioMerieux, Boxtel, the Netherlands), which uses NASBA technology.[61,196] A clinical evaluation of the NASBA assay showed it to be more sensitive than CSF viral culture for the detection of enterovirus, and its had a specificity of 100%.[196]

The clinical utility of nucleic acid testing for the diagnosis of enteroviral infections has been documented in a variety of clinical studies,[1,2,91] with the testing showing a sensitivity equal to or greater than that of cell culture, a high specificity, and faster turnaround time than cell culture. Several studies have suggested that the introduction of molecular methods for the diagnosis of enteroviral infections in infants and pediatric patients can lead to cost savings in other parts of the hospital because of the decreased length of stay, reduction in the use of antibiotics, and reduction in imaging studies.[71,108,128,145] The cost savings may be small, however, as the typical length of stay for children with viral meningitis is short with or without use of molecular testing (personal communication, D.E. Bruns, 22 May 2004). To maximize the benefit to patient care and cost savings, testing should be available daily.

As mentioned above, many molecular assays detect rhinoviruses and most will detect polioviruses. These two factors can lead to unexpected and misleading positive results when testing respiratory or stool specimens. The diagnosis of enterovirus meningitis should be based on testing of CSF specimens, while sepsis syndrome in the neonate is best made by testing serum, plasma, or CSF samples.

Perinatal Group B Streptococcal Disease

In the 1970s Group B streptococcal (GBS) disease was the leading infectious cause of neonatal morbidity and mortality, with case rates of 2 to 3 per 1000 live births and case-fatality rates as high as 50%.[31] In 1996, consensus guidelines from the CDC, the American Academy of Pediatrics, and the American College of Obstetrics and Gynecology were issued in an effort to reduce the rate of GBS disease in newborns.[31] The guidelines called for use of intrapartum prophylactic antibiotics for GBS using either a risk-based or screening-based approach. In the risk-based approach, antibiotics were administered based on the identification of one of the following risk factors: intrapartum fever, prolonged rupture of membranes, or imminent preterm delivery. For the screening-based approach, vaginal and/or rectal cultures were collected at 35 to 37 weeks of gestation, and those women with positive cultures received intrapartum antibiotics. Since the widespread implementation of these guidelines, the number of cases of GBS disease has decreased, but GBS remains a serious cause of neonatal infection. GBS disease in the newborn is classified as either early disease, which occurs within 1 week of life and usually presents as a sepsis syndrome or pneumonia, or late disease, which is defined as that presenting at greater than 1 week of life and that presents most commonly as sepsis or meningitis.

GBS colonization of pregnant women is common, with a prevalence of 10% to 30%; colonization may be transient, chronic, or intermittent.[148] Those women who are colonized are 25 times more likely to deliver infants with early onset GBS disease.[14] The effectiveness of the 1996 guidelines for the prevention of neonatal GBS was recently reevaluated, and it was determined that the screening approach to GBS prevention was greater than 50% more effective than the risk-based approach.[160] Based on these findings, in 2002 the CDC issued updated guidelines recommending that vaginal/rectal GBS screening cultures be done on all pregnant women. The exceptions included women with a previous infant that had GBS disease or those with GBS bacteriuria during pregnancy, because these women require intrapartum antibiotics. The risk-based approach is to be used only for women with unknown GBS status at the time of labor and delivery. See the CDC guidelines[31] for a more detailed description, and refer to the CDC Web site for updates.

Methods for GBS screening cultures have been standardized and include collection of a vaginal/rectal swab and transport to the laboratory in either Aimes or Stuarts media. The specimen is then inoculated into an enrichment broth (LIM broth), incubated for 18 to 24 hours, and then subcultured onto a sheep-blood agar plate. GBS is then identified based on colony morphology, hemolysis, and latex agglutination testing. This two-step method ensures maximal sensitivity for GBD detection. GBS cultures usually require 2 to 3 days to complete. Since GBS is universally susceptible to penicillin and ampicillin, antimicrobial susceptibility testing is not routinely performed, but is needed for women with a serious allergy to penicillin.

A recent study evaluated the clinical utility of using a real-time PCR assay for the detection of GBS in pregnant women.[9] A Light Cycler assay (Roche Diagnostics, Indianapolis, IN) was compared with cultures in 112 pregnant women and was found to have a sensitivity of 97%, a specificity of 100%, and a negative and positive predictive value of 98.8% and 100%, respectively. Testing results were available within 45 minutes of the time the specimen arrived in the laboratory, which raised the possibility of offering real-time testing to women who present in labor. This could be especially useful for women who present with an unknown GBS status; based on current guidelines, these women would receive intrapartum antibiotics based on risk factors. As women without risk factors are still at risk of delivering newborns with GBS disease,[160] PCR testing would undoubtedly offer a more sensitive method for GBS detection than one based on risk factors alone. In addition, intrapartum testing would be useful in identifying women whose GBS status changes in the interval between screening culture (week 35 to 37 of gestation) and the time of delivery.

Recently a real-time PCR assay was cleared by the FDA (IDI-Strep B using the Cepheid Smart Cycler, Infection Diagnostic Inc., Quebec) for the detection of GBS from vaginal and/or rectal swabs in pregnant women. In a multicenter clinical trial, the IDI-Strep B test demonstrated a sensitivity of 94% and a specificity of 96% compared with intrapartum culture (IDI-Strep B package insert). The assay requires a few simple hands-on steps to prepare the specimen. The testing cartridge is then inserted into the Smart Cycler, and testing is complete in less than 1 hour. The test also includes an internal control to monitor for inhibition of amplification. The IDI-Strep B test offers a rapid and sensitive alternative to GBS culture. These advantages need to be balanced with the challenge of providing intrapartum test results to clinicians within 1 to 2 hours at any time of day or night, and the cost of nucleic acid testing must be compared with the cost of culture. If intrapartum testing is done, there will not be adequate time for erythromycin and clindamycin susceptibility testing, so women with severe penicillin allergies will require therapy with vancomycin. An alternative approach is to replace antepartum culture at 35 to 37 weeks of gestation with the real-time PCR assay. With the availability of an FDA-cleared test, there will be more discussion on the use of GBS PCR testing of pregnant women.

Cytomegalovirus

CMV, a member of the herpesvirus family, is a double-stranded enveloped DNA virus. CMV causes a clinically minor infection in immunocompetent individuals, but remains an important pathogen in immunocompromised individuals, including persons with AIDS, transplant recipients, and those on immune-modulating drugs. Primary infection is usually asymptomatic in immunocompetent persons, though a small percentage of individuals with CMV infection may develop a mononucleosis type of syndrome. Following the primary infection, a lifelong latent infection is established, which does not cause clinical symptoms. However, if an infected individual becomes immunocompromised, the virus can reactivate, leading to a wide variety of clinical syndromes.

The most severe CMV infections are seen in those individuals who acquire their primary infection while immunocompromised. In persons with AIDS, CMV disease rarely occurs when the CD4+ cell count is above 100 cells/mm^3; the most common clinical presentations are retinitis, esophagitis, and colitis. In transplant recipients, the occurrence and severity of CMV disease are related to the CMV serostatus of the organ donor and recipient, the type of organ transplanted, and the overall degree of immunosuppression. For example, CMV disease tends to be more severe in lung transplant recipients than in renal transplant recipients. For all types of organ recipients, the most severe disease occurs when CMV-seronegative recipients receive an organ from a CMV-seropositive donor, and the primary CMV infection occurs while the person is immunosuppressed. CMV disease can also occur in seropositive individuals whether they receive an organ from a seropositive or seronegative donor. The clinical findings associated with CMV disease in transplant recipients are diverse and include interstitial pneumonitis, esophagitis and colitis, fever, leukopenia, and less commonly retinitis and encephalitis. CMV disease also occurs in bone marrow transplant recipients.

The diagnosis of CMV disease represents a challenge because of the presence of the latent infection. Immunocompromised individuals can have an asymptomatic, clinically insignificant, low-level, persistent infection that must be distinguished from clinically important active CMV disease. The distinction can be challenging when using sensitive molecular assays that can detect small amounts of CMV DNA in clinical specimens.

Traditionally the diagnosis of CMV disease relied on the detection of CMV from clinical specimens by use of cell culture techniques in human diploid fibroblasts. Though considered the gold standard, these conventional culture methods are labor-intensive and have a long turnaround time of 1 to 3 weeks. In addition, the assays lack adequate sensitivity for detecting CMV present in blood specimens.[112,113] The rapid shell-vial culture method can provide results in 1 to 2 days and is useful for detection of CMV in tissue, respiratory, and urine specimens. However, this assay may also fail to detect CMV in blood.[112,113] Many laboratories rely on the antigenemia assay, which detects the matrix protein pp65 in polymorphonuclear cells. This semiquantitative assay is rapid, and the number of CMV antigen-positive cells correlates with the likelihood of CMV disease,[113,187] but the assay is labor-intensive, and CMV antigen is not stable in whole blood specimens for periods of greater than 24 hours.

In light of the limitations of culture and antigen detection methods, there has been great interest in using nucleic acid testing for the detection and quantification of CMV DNA from plasma and blood specimens. Qualitative and quantitative molecular assays available for this purpose are outlined in Table 42-6. The two qualitative assays that have been cleared by the FDA for detection of CMV from blood specimens are the Hybrid Capture System CMV DNA test (version 2) (Digene Corp., Gaithersburg, Md.) and the NucliSens CMV test (bioMerieux, Durham, N.C.). The Hybrid Capture assay is a signal-amplification assay that detects CMV DNA in whole blood specimens. The NucliSens assay uses NASBA technology to detect pp67 late messenger RNA in whole blood specimens. The isothermal NASBA assay detects pp67 RNA but not CMV DNA, eliminating concerns about detection of DNA in latent infection. Quantitative molecular CMV assays that are available include the Hybrid Capture assay mentioned above and the Amplicor CMV MONITOR test (Roche Diagnostics, Indianapolis), a

TABLE 42-6 CMV Tests in Clinical Use*

Test	Amplification Method	Range
Hybrid Capture System CMV DNA (version 2) (Digene Corp, Gaithersburg, Md)	Signal amplification	1400-600,000 copies/mL
Amplicor CMV Monitor Test (Roche Diagnostics, Indianapolis, IN)	PCR	400-50,000 copies/mL
NucliSens CMV Test (bioMerieux, Durham, NC)	NASBA	Qualitative
Laboratory Developed Test	PCR	Varies

RT-PCR, Reverse transcription-polymerase chain reaction; *NASBA,* nucleic acid sequence based amplification.
*For current FDA listings, see http://www.accessdata.fda.gov/scripts/cdrh/cfdocs/cfRL/listing.cfm.

DNA PCR assay (neither of which has been cleared by the FDA). CMV PCR LDTs that use standard and real-time PCR methods are also widely used in clinical laboratories. These LDTs use various specimen types, nucleic acid extraction methods, target genes, calibrators, and detection methods. As a result, viral load values obtained with the different assays may not always agree. This makes it very difficult to compare results among clinical studies that use these assays and to establish concentrations of CMV DNA that correlate with clinical disease.

The analytical performances have been evaluated for the Amplicor PCR and Hybrid Capture assays. The imprecision (expressed as standard deviations) of the assays ranges from 0.11 to 0.48 $\log_{10}$, with greater variability seen below 1000 copies/mL (3.0 $\log_{10}$ copies/mL).[25,28] In general the Amplicor assay is more reproducible than the Hybrid Capture assay.[28] Based on these data, changes in viral load (copies per milliliter) less than threefold to fivefold may not represent clinically relevant changes in viral replication.

An unsettled issue for CMV molecular assays is the appropriate specimen type for testing. Almost all assays use either plasma or whole blood, with concentrations of CMV DNA measured in whole blood higher than those measured in plasma.[146] Because pp67 RNA is intracellular, the NucliSens assay uses whole blood samples. Likewise the Hybrid Capture assay has been designed to measure CMV DNA in whole blood specimens. The Amplicor PCR assay can accommodate blood or plasma specimens. CMV DNA may be detected in whole blood or leukocytes of individuals without active CMV disease. Some studies have shown a good association between high CMV DNA concentrations in plasma and active CMV disease[27,146] and suggest that detecting CMV DNA in plasma rather than in leukocytes may provide a better correlation with clinical disease, because the detection of CMV DNA in plasma suggests active viral replication.[146] However, it is clear that CMV DNA can also be detected in the plasma in patients without active CMV disease.[26,27] In addition to specimen type, assay format may be useful in distinguishing active disease from asymptomatic infection. For example, the pp67 mRNA detected in the NucliSens assay is expressed in high concentrations in patients with active disease and is not expressed during latent infection.[121] This has been supported in studies that have shown that the NucliSens assay is positive less frequently than assays that detect CMV DNA.[64] For CMV DNA-based assays, correlation with clinical disease requires quantifying CMV DNA to establish a concentration of CMV DNA that correlates with the likelihood of disease. The concentration of DNA that predicts disease will be higher in assays that use whole blood specimens than in those that test plasma specimens.

The clinical uses of CMV molecular assays are diverse and include assisting in decisions regarding initiating preemptive therapy, diagnosis of active CMV disease, and monitoring response to therapy. *Preemptive therapy* refers to the use of a laboratory test to identify a group of individuals at higher risk for developing CMV disease. For example, all members of the group would be tested for the presence of CMV DNA in their blood or plasma, and only those testing positive would be treated. Therapy is administered before development of symptoms in an attempt to prevent the development of active disease. By contrast, with *prophylactic therapy,* all patients in the group are treated, without further stratification of risk, thus involving treatment of a greater number of patients.

Molecular assays have utility for the diagnosis of active CMV disease, because CMV DNA concentrations are higher in patients with active CMV disease than in those with asymptomatic infection.[42,60,81,149,187] A study in liver transplant recipients using the Amplicor PCR assay showed that the median peak viral load in patients with asymptomatic infection was 1850 copies/mL compared with 55,000 copies/mL for those with active disease.[81] The viral load cutoff that was most predictive of the development of active disease was between 2000 and 5000 copies/mL of plasma. A similar study in renal transplant recipients using the Hybrid Capture assay showed that the risk of developing CMV disease increased from 1.5% with a viral load of 10,000 copies/mL of blood to 73% when the viral load was 1 million copies/mL of blood.[3] It is important to note that the viral load cutoffs differed in the two studies because of the use of different assays and differences in specimen type (plasma versus whole blood).

Once active CMV disease has been diagnosed, molecular assays are useful in monitoring response to therapy. Viral-load values decrease rapidly after beginning appropriate antiviral therapy, and several studies have reported that CMV DNA is cleared from the plasma within several weeks of initiating therapy.[26,27,82] Failure of viral loads to decrease promptly should raise concerns of possible treatment failure, because persistently elevated concentrations of CMV DNA (20,000 to 70,000 copies/mL in plasma) during therapy have been seen in patients with documented resistance of CMV to the therapy.[26] Molecular assays also have clinical utility in identifying patients at risk of relapsing CMV infection. In a group of solid-organ transplant recipients,[161] those patients with a detectable viral load after completing 14 days of ganciclovir therapy for CMV infection were at increased risk of relapse. Similarly an increased risk of relapse has been shown for patients with persistent pp67 mRNA after completing a course of therapy.[135] The rate of decline in CMV DNA after initiating therapy can be used to predict risk of relapse of CMV infection. In one study, CMV DNA was cleared from the plasma in 17 days for patients without recurrent CMV disease compared with 34 days for those with evidence of recurrent disease.[82] By following viral-load concentrations weekly after initiating antiviral therapy, it may be possible to identify those at risk of recurrent disease and thus intensify therapy and possibly prevent recurrent disease.

CMV DNA concentrations are also useful in assessing the risk of developing CMV disease in persons with AIDS. In a study by Spector et al,[166] detection of CMV DNA in plasma was associated with an increased risk of developing CMV disease and an increased risk of death. In addition, each $\log_{10}$ increase in viral load (i.e., each tenfold increase in concentration) was associated with a threefold increase in the risk of developing CMV disease. The clinical importance of CMV viral load in patients was further established in patients with advanced AIDS in whom the CMV DNA load was found to be more predictive of developing CMV disease or death than HIV-1 viral load.[165] A more recent study has identified individuals with a CD4+ cell count of less than 50 cells/mm^3 and an HIV-1 viral load of greater than 10,000 copies/mL of plasma as those at greatest risk of developing end-organ CMV disease.[57] In this group of individuals, a rise in CMV DNA above the limit of detection of either the Hybrid Capture or Amplicor PCR assays was associated with the development of CMV end-organ disease. This study identifies a group of HIV-1–infected individuals that may benefit from monitoring CMV viral load and preemptive therapy for the prevention of CMV end-organ disease.

A major challenge that remains for laboratories offering these assays is the difference in results among assays. A well-characterized CMV DNA standard reference material for use in calibrating the assays could greatly assist in achieving agreement of viral-load values among different tests, thus facilitating the determination of CMV concentrations that predict or correspond to clinical events.

MYCOBACTERIUM TUBERCULOSIS

Mycobacterium tuberculosis (MTb) causes a wide range of clinical infections, including pulmonary disease, miliary tuberculosis, meningitis, pleurisy/pericarditis/peritonitis, gastrointestinal disease, genitourinary disease, and lymphadenitis. MTb infection was in steady decline in the United States until the late 1980s into the early 1990s, when the number of reported cases began to increase. This resurgence in the number of infections was related to the AIDS epidemic, homelessness, and a decreased focus on tuberculosis control programs. By the late 1990s the infection rate had declined to an all time low.[34] One group in which the infection rate continues to rise is in foreign-born persons, which is due to immigration from countries with a high prevalence of MTb infections.[34] This increase in MTb infections focused considerable attention on the development of assays for the rapid diagnosis of MTb infections, and molecular methods were at the center of this effort. The goal was to design very sensitive assays that would allow for the direct detection of MTb from clinical specimens. However, this goal has proven to be more difficult to reach than originally anticipated.

The standard methods for detection of MTb include acid-fast bacilli (AFB) smear and conventional and liquid culture methods. The AFB smear is rapid, but has a poor sensitivity of 20% to 80%.[15] Another challenge with the AFB smear is that it cannot distinguish MTb from nontuberculous mycobacteria (NTM), such as *M. avium*-complex (MAC). This distinction is important because disseminated MAC and MTb are both common infections in persons with AIDS. Culture methods for the detection of MTb are sensitive, but growth detectable by standard methods may require 6 to 8 weeks in a culture. Growth often occurs more quickly in liquid culture than with conventional methods, but can still require weeks. With these limitations of culture methods, there was great enthusiasm for nucleic acid testing as a rapid, sensitive method for detection of MTb, especially given the needs to rapidly isolate patients with active, untreated disease and to initiate prompt therapy, particularly in immunocompromised hosts.

Two nucleic acid amplification tests have been approved by the FDA for detection of MTb from clinical specimens: the Amplified *Mycobacterium tuberculosis* Direct Test (MTD test; Gen Probe, Inc., San Diego), and the Amplicor *Mycobacterium tuberculosis* Test (Roche Diagnostics, Indianapolis). The MTD test is based on transcription-mediated amplification of ribosomal RNA. The Amplicor test is based on PCR technology and the target is the 16S ribosomal RNA gene. The MTD test has broader clinical applications, because it can be used to test both AFB smear–positive and smear-negative respiratory specimens. The Amplicor test is approved only for AFB smear–positive respiratory specimens. Neither assay has been approved for nonrespiratory specimens, which limits their clinical utility for diagnosis of extrapulmonary MTb infections. This is unfortunate, because diagnosis of some of these infections is often difficult. In addition to these commercially available assays, LDTs are widely used, and a key advantage of these assays is the ability to test respiratory and nonrespiratory specimens.

Both the MTD test and the Amplicor test have a sensitivity of 95% to 98% when using AFB smear–positive respiratory specimens, and the specificity ranges from 99% to 100%. However, early studies showed that the sensitivity for AFB smear-negative specimens was ~50%.[32] Based on these data, it was clear that the test could not be used to rule out MTb infection on smear–negative respiratory specimens. This further limited the clinical utility of these tests, because it became clear that the nucleic acid testing would be used to supplement the AFB smear and culture rather than replace these testing modalities. Another limitation of the currently available nucleic acid assays is that they can be used only on specimens from patients who had not received antituberculosis therapy within the past 12 months. This limitation was included because DNA can persist in respiratory secretions (and other body fluids) for months after the mycobacteria are no longer viable.

The MTD test was subsequently reformulated and evaluated in a clinical trial comparing this test to a culture and to the probability of MTb infection as determined by a panel of experts.[87] The sensitivity and specificity of the test were 86% and 98%, respectively. The positive and negative predictive values were 91% and 97%, respectively. Based on this study, the reformulated MTD test was approved by the FDA for use on both AFB smear–positive and AFB smear–negative specimens. The CDC has established guidelines for the use of nucleic acid testing on respiratory specimens.[30,35] Patients with a positive AFB smear and a positive nucleic acid testing result should be presumed to have MTb infection, and there is no need for additional nucleic acid testing. If the sputum smear is AFB-positive, if two or three specimens are negative by nucleic acid testing, and if inhibition of amplification has been ruled out, then the patient can be presumed to have NTM infection. If the sputum specimen is AFB smear–negative and repeatedly positive by the MTD test (Note: the Amplicor test is not approved for use with smear-negative samples), then the patient can be presumed to have MTb infection. For patients with an AFB-negative smear, a negative nucleic acid test does not rule out MTb infection.

A key consideration with molecular assays is controlling for inhibition of amplification. This is particularly critical for the detection of MTb nucleic acid from respiratory specimens, because these specimen types often contain blood or glycoprotein, which can inhibit amplification. The Amplicor assay contains an internal control, and a negative result cannot be reported unless the internal control is detected. The MTD test does not contain an inhibition control, though many laboratories include such a control by adding a positive control material to a second aliquot of the clinical specimen.

An important role for molecular assays is in the diagnosis of extra-pulmonary MTb infections, such as meningitis, pleuritis, pericarditis, or peritonitis, because these infections can be very difficult to diagnose by traditional methods. The MTD and Amplicor tests have been used on CSF specimens for the diagnosis of MTb meningitis,[7,11,98] although the tests have not been approved by the FDA for this indication. In addition, PCR LDTs have been developed with the flexibility needed to test a variety of clinical specimens. As mentioned for respiratory specimens, it is critical to remember that a negative nucleic acid test result does not rule out extra-pulmonary MTb infection, and molecular assays using these complex body fluids should include an inhibition control.

Though there are considerable limitations to the currently available nucleic acid tests for the detection of MTb infection, they have a role in the clinical laboratory in that they can provide a rapid diagnosis. The goal would be to develop assays with a higher sensitivity (>99%) for AFB smear–negative specimens, because this may eliminate the need to culture specimens that are negative when tested in nucleic acid assays.

Hepatitis C Virus

HCV, an RNA virus, is a major cause of chronic liver disease. According to the National Health and Nutrition Examination Survey (NHANES) of 1988-1994, approximately 4 million Americans were infected with HCV and 2.7 million were estimated to have chronic infection. After acute infection, 80% to 85% of individuals develop a chronic infection, and 2% to 4% of these individuals develop cirrhosis and end-stage liver disease, making end-stage liver disease secondary to HCV the most common indication for liver transplantation in the United States.[129] The development of molecular testing for HCV infection has been a major advance in the clinical care of infected individuals, because the virus cannot be grown in a culture.

Detection and Quantification of HCV RNA

The applications of HCV RNA testing include assisting in the diagnosis of HCV infection, excluding HCV infection as the etiologic agent of symptoms, screening the blood supply, monitoring response to therapy, and determining the duration of therapy. Qualitative molecular assays are used to confirm the diagnosis of HCV infection, which is particularly important in distinguishing seropositive individuals who have cleared the infection from seropositive persons who have chronic infection. Individuals who have cleared the infection will not have detectable RNA, while those with persistent infection will have detectable RNA. Recent data from the CDC have shown that 95% of positive results of screening ELISA that have a signal-to-cutoff ratio (s/co) >3.8 can be confirmed as true positives.[29] For these specimens, confirmation testing is not routinely needed. For specimens with an s/co ratio of <3.8, confirmation testing should be done with either a recombinant immunoblot assay (RIBA) or by detection of HCV RNA. If HCV RNA detection is used as the confirmatory test, then RNA-negative specimens should be tested in the RIBA. This is to distinguish a false-positive ELISA result from true infection. Alternatively, repeat testing for HCV RNA should be done, because viremia may be intermittent and HCV infection should not be ruled out based on one negative HCV RNA test. Qualitative molecular assays are also used to diagnose HCV infection in infants born to HCV-infected mothers. Since maternal IgG antibody can cross the placenta, these infants can be seropositive into the second year of life. Detection of HCV RNA in the plasma or serum of the newborn shortly after birth would be diagnostic of infection. Detection of HCV RNA in plasma or serum can be a useful diagnostic test in immunocompromised individuals, such as those with end-stage HIV-1 infection, because they may not mount a normal immune response to the virus and may not be seropositive.

Qualitative HCV RNA testing is also used to define a treatment response to interferon and ribavirin combination therapy for HCV infection because these assays are very sensitive, with lower limits of detection between 5 and 50 copies/mL plasma. Response to therapy is defined as an undetectable HCV RNA after completion of therapy, while a sustained response is defined as an undetectable viral load 24 weeks after completion of therapy.[116] More recently, qualitative HCV RNA assays have been developed for screening the blood supply. HCV RNA is detectable in serum during the "window period" between infection and seroconversion (when tests for HCV antibodies are negative). As most individuals with recently acquired HCV infection are asymptomatic, testing of blood donors for HCV RNA allows identification of individuals at risk for transmitting HCV infection who would have been missed if testing were done with only serological assays. Nucleic acid testing for HCV RNA has reduced the window period by an average of 26 days.[94] By screening the blood supply with HCV antibody testing alone, it was estimated that 1 in 100,000 units contained HCV RNA, but with the addition of testing by nucleic acid amplification technology (often called NAT) for HCV, the risk is projected to be reduced to 1 in 367,000 units.[94] Data from the first 2 years of experience with nucleic acid testing of the blood supply confirmed these estimates, because 1 in 259,000 screened units was found to be HCV RNA–positive and antibody-negative.[172,173]

HCV viral-load testing can be used to predict the response to antiviral therapy. Patients with viral loads above 2 million copies/mL of plasma are less likely to respond to interferon/ribavirin therapy than those with lower viral loads.[51,116,142] Although genotype is a stronger predictor of response to therapy than viral load (see below), recent studies have shown the utility of determining the viral load after 12 weeks of therapy. Patients who fail to have a $2 \log_{10}$ drop in HCV RNA concentrations (i.e., concentrations are one one-hundredth the initial concentrations) at 12 weeks after initiating interferon and ribavirin have a 3% likelihood of responding to therapy compared with 65% for patients who do achieve a $2 \log_{10}$ drop in viral load.[62,101] By determining HCV viral load at baseline and again after 12 weeks of therapy, patients who are very unlikely to respond to therapy can be identified earlier in the course of therapy. This will allow for discontinuation of potentially toxic drugs and a reduction in the cost of therapy. On the other hand, individuals with a $2 \log_{10}$ drop in viral load will have therapy continued for either 24 or 48 weeks depending on the HCV genotype and other risk factors.

Several qualitative assays have been approved by the FDA for the detection of HCV RNA in plasma or serum specimens (Table 42-7). The Amplicor HCV test and the COBAS Amplicor HCV test (Roche Diagnostics, Indianapolis) are based on RT-PCR technology; the COBAS test allows for

TABLE 42-7 HCV RNA Tests In Clinical Use*

Test	Assay Method	Comments
Amplicor HCV Test v2.0 (Roche Diagnostics, Indianapolis)	RT-PCR	Qualitative, limit of detection 50 IU/mL
Versant HCV RNA Assay (Bayer Diagnostics, Tarrytown, NY)	TMA	Qualitative, limit of detection 5 IU/mL
In-Laboratory Developed	RT-PCR	Varies
Versant HCV RNA v3.0 Assay (Bayer Diagnostics, Tarrytown, NY)	bDNA	Quantitative, range 615-7.7 million IU/mL
Amplicor HCV Monitor Test v2.0 (Roche Diagnostics, Indianapolis)	RT-PCR	Quantitative, range 600-800,000 IU/mL
Laboratory Developed Test	RT-PCR	Quantitative, varies
Real-Time HCV Assays (ASR) (Roche Diagnostics and Abbott Diagnostics)	RT-PCR	Quantitative, range 10-50 IU/mL to 10-30 million IU/mL

For current FDA listings, see http://www.accessdata.fda.gov/scripts/cdrh/cfdocs/cfRL/listing.cfm.

RT-PCR, Reverse transcription-polymerase chain reaction; *TMA,* transcription mediated amplification; *bDNA,* branched DNA; *ASR,* analyte-specific reagent.

*Excluding molecular testing for the blood supply.

automation of the amplification and detection steps. Both versions of the Amplicor test have a lower limit of detection of 50 international units (IU)/mL. The Versant HCV RNA Qualitative Assay (Bayer Diagnostics, Tarrytown, N.Y.) uses transcription-mediated amplification (TMA) and can detect as few as 5 IU of HCV RNA/mL of HCV RNA. In addition to these tests, RT-PCR LDTs are also used in some laboratories. Two additional qualitative assays are available only for screening the blood supply: the Procleix HIV-1/HCV assay (Gen-Probe, Inc., San Diego) based on TMA technology, which is FDA-approved,[84] and the AMPLISCREEN HCV Test v2.0 (Roche Diagnostics, Indianapolis), which is an RT-PCR assay. Both assays report a lower limit of detection of less than 50 IU/mL.

Various tests are available for the quantification of HCV RNA. The Versant HCV RNA 3.0 assay (Bayer Diagnostics Corp., Tarrytown, N.Y.) is the only currently FDA-approved assay for HCV viral-load testing (Table 42-7). The assay is based on bDNA technology, and has a broad dynamic range and a lower limit of quantification of 615 IU/mL. The Amplicor HCV MONITOR test (Roche Diagnostics, Indianapolis) has a similar limit of quantification (600 IU/mL), but a much more limited linear range. Dilution of the clinical specimen is needed to measure viral loads greater than 800,000 IU/mL. Several large clinical studies evaluating the efficacy of interferon/ribavirin therapy have used an RT-PCR assay developed by the National Genetics Institute (NGI) (SuperQuant). This assay has a dynamic range of 100 to 100 million copies/mL, although dilution of the specimen is required to cover the entire dynamic range. A recent advance in HCV testing has been the availability of several real-time RT-PCR assays.[93,109] These assays have a lower limit of detection similar to those seen for the qualitative HCV assays (10 to 50 IU/mL) and a broad dynamic that allows for the accurate quantification of HCV concentrations up to 10 to 50 million IU/mL.[93] The availability of these real-time assays could allow laboratories to replace both their current qualitative and quantitative tests. At this time, real-time tests are available as ASRs from Roche Diagnostics[93] and Abbott Laboratories (Abbott Park, Ill.).

Earlier versions of the Amplicor RT-PCR and bDNA assays did not accurately quantify all genotypes of HCV,[52,73] and usually underestimated the concentrations of genotypes 2 and 3. However, the current versions of the Amplicor RT-PCR (version 2.0), Versant bDNA (version 3.0), and real-time assays accurately quantify all HCV genotypes.[52,93,110] When reporting results as copies per milliliter, the viral-load values obtained with the Versant bDNA and Amplicor RT-PCR may disagree, due in part to the use of different calibrators. The availability of an established WHO international standard has allowed standardization of HCV assays with reporting of results as IU per milliliter.[157]

The intra-assay imprecision (SDs) of the HCV Versant bDNA and Amplicor RT-PCR assays ranges from 0.05 to 0.3 $\log_{10}$; the Versant bDNA assay is more precise.[73] The biological variation of HCV viral load ranges from 0.5 $\log_{10}$ to 0.75 $\log_{10}$.[70] Based on these data, changes in HCV viral load need to exceed 1 $\log_{10}$ (i.e., a tenfold change in concentration) to represent significant changes in viral replication.

HCV Genotyping

A hallmark of HCV infection is genetic heterogeneity, resulting from the low fidelity of the RNA-dependent RNA polymerase, which frequently introduces random nucleotide errors during viral replication. These replication errors could yield 10 to 100 nucleotide changes per position per year,[49] giving rise to many genetic variants (quasispecies) of the virus in a single patient. Based on the identification of these genomic differences, HCV has been classified into six major genotypes and multiple subtypes within each genotype.[22] There are geographic differences in the distribution of HCV types. In the United States approximately two-thirds of the infections are type 1, with the remaining being predominately types 2 and 3.[55,117]

The HCV genome contains well-defined 5′- and 3′-untranslated regions (5′UTR and 3′UTR). The 5′UTR is the most conserved portion of the genome and is frequently used as the target for molecular assays, including genotyping assays.[20] The HCV genome is divided into seven areas: the core region that encodes the capsid C protein, the E1 and E2 regions that encode the envelope proteins (gp33 and gp72), and several nonstructural protein regions (NS2, NS3, NS4, and NS5). The NS5B region shows less sequence homology than the 5′UTR, and sequencing of NS5B has been successfully used for genotyping HCV.[163]

As mentioned above, the probability of response to therapy depends on genotype. In one study, ~70% of patients with genotypes 2 and 3 had a sustained response after 12 months of combination therapy compared with only 30% of patients with genotype 1,[116] and no additional benefit was obtained by treating patients with genotype 2 or 3 beyond 24 weeks. In contrast, the response rate after 24 weeks of therapy for patients with genotype 1 was 16% compared with 28% after 48 weeks of therapy. These results have been confirmed in another randomized trial[142] comparing interferon 2b plus ribavirin with a placebo in patients with chronic HCV infection. Similar results were seen in a more recent study comparing peginterferon plus ribavirin with interferon plus ribavirin. A greater percentage of patients in the peginterferon plus ribavirin arm achieved a sustained virological response compared with those patients in the interferon plus ribavirin arm (56% versus 44%), respectively.[62] In addition, patients with HCV genotypes 2 or 3 had a significantly higher rate of sustained virological response than those with genotype 1. HCV genotyping, along with pretreatment viral load, age, gender, and the presence of hepatic fibrosis, can be used to determine the duration of antiviral therapy,[143] with genotype being the strongest predictor of a sustained virological response.

Several methods have been developed for genotyping and/or subtyping HCV, but most clinical laboratories use either the reverse hybridization-based line probe assay (INNO-LiPA HCV II, manufactured in Belgium for Bayer Corp., Norwood, Mass.), or direct DNA sequencing. The INNO-LiPA assay is based on reverse hybridization of 5′UTR amplified products with genotype-specific probes.[174] This assay is convenient to use for many clinical laboratories because genotyping can be done directly from the amplicons generated in the Amplicor HCV Test (Roche Diagnostics, Indianapolis). The biotin-labeled amplified products are reverse-hybridized to the specific probes on the INNO-LiPA strips; streptavidin conjugated with alkaline phosphatase is added, followed by substrate addition. A purple/brown line develops where there is sequence homology between the biotinylated PCR products and the probe, and the genotype is determined based on the pattern of probe hybridization. The INNO-LiPA HCV II discriminates and identifies HCV genotypes 1a, 1b, 2a/c, 2b, 3a, 3b, 3c, 4, 5a, and 6a.[175] The INNO-LiPA is accurate in typing HCV, but cannot reliably subtype HCV.[4,195] There is not sufficient sequence variation in the 5′UTR to allow distinction between subtypes 2a and 2c, and reverse hybridization data of subtypes 1a and 1b may be discordant with NS5B in ~10% of cases.[175] Currently this is not a significant limitation of the assay because treatment decisions are based on viral genotype not subtype. In addition, the INNO-LiPA method is user-friendly and well suited for routine use in clinical laboratories that perform HCV genotyping.

Automated sequencing assays, both developed commercially and in-laboratory, are available to genotype HCV, and the genomic regions commonly used include 5′UTR,[20] NS5B (163), and core.[21] Sequencing methods require sequence alignment and comparison with reference sequences to determine the genotype and subtype. An HCV genotyping kit based on automated sequencing (Trugene HCV 5′NC, Bayer Diagnostics) targets the 5′NC region. Though this assay can accurately type HCV, like the INNO-LiPA assay it is unable to accurately subtype the virus.[132] When more variable regions of the virus are sequenced, such as NS5B, it is possible to determine both viral type and subtype.[163]

There have been several studies comparing the performance of the INNO-LiPA HCV II assay and automated DNA sequencing methods. One study found a 91% concordance rate between the two assays.[5] A more recent study compared the performance characteristics of the Trugene HCV assay and the INNO-LiPA.[132] Both methods were able to genotype 105 of the 106 serum specimens. There was concordance at the genotype level for 103 of 104 (99%) specimens. Sequence analysis of the NS5B region supported the INNO-LiPA result for the single genotype discrepant result. No subtype was called for 36 (34%) specimens typed by INNO-LiPA and 20 (19%) of those typed by Trugene HCV assay. Mixtures of genotypes were successfully identified with both methods, with the INNO-LiPA assay detecting populations making up at least 5% of the total population, and the Trugene HCV assays detecting populations of at least 10%. The overall performance of the two assays was similar and both assays can accurately type HCV, but neither method should be used for subtyping.[132]

A 2002 study reported on the use of real-time PCR with melting curve analysis as a method to genotype HCV.[23] Using a single pair of fluorescence resonance energy transfer (FRET) probes, it was possible to distinguish types 1a/b, 2a/c, 2b, 3a, and 4 on the basis of differences in melting temperatures. This method showed good concordance with INNO-LiPA. Of the 124 samples tested with both methods, 13 were nontypable by either of the methods; however, there was agreement for 108 of the remaining 111 samples. All three discrepant samples typed as 2a/c by melting curve analysis, while 2 of the 3 were typed as 2b by INNO-LiPA. The remaining sample typed as 1 by INNO-LiPA, which was confirmed by sequence analysis. Real-time PCR with melting curve analysis is a reliable method for typing HCV. As with other methods using the 5′UTR of the virus, it will not accurately subtype all samples.

REFERENCES

1. Abzug MJ, Loeffelholz M, Rotbart HA. Diagnosis of neonatal enterovirus infection by polymerase chain reaction. J Pediatr 1995;126:447-50.
2. Ahmed A, Brito F, Goto C, Hickey SM, Olsen KD, Trujillo M, et al. Clinical utility of the polymerase chain reaction for diagnosis of enteroviral meningitis in infancy. J Pediatr 1997;131:393-7.
3. Aitken C, Barrett-Muir W, Millar CT, Thomas J, Sheridan F, Jeffries D, et al. Use of molecular assays in diagnosis and monitoring of cytomegalovirus disease following renal transplantation. J Clin Microbiol 1999;37:2804-7.
4. Andonov A, Chaudhary R. Subtyping of hepatitis C virus isolates by a line probe assay using hybridization. J Clin Microbiol 1995;33:254-6.
5. Ansaldi F, Torre F, Bruzzone B, Picciotto A, Crovari P, Icardi G. Evaluation of a new hepatitis C virus sequencing assay as a routine method of genotyping. J Med Virol 2001;63:17-21.
6. Aurelius E, Johansson B, Skoldenberg B, Staland A, Forsgren M. Rapid diagnosis of herpes simplex encephalitis by nested polymerase chain reaction assay of cerebrospinal fluid. Lancet 1991;337:189-92.
7. Baker CA, Cartwright CP, Williams DN, Nelson SM, Peterson PK. Early detection of central nervous system tuberculosis with the gen-probe nucleic acid amplification assay: utility in an inner city hospital. Clin Infect Dis 2002;35:339-42.
8. Baxter JD, Mayers DL, Wentworth DN, Neaton JB, Hoover ML, Winters MA, et al. A randomized study of antiretroviral management based on plasma genotypic antiretroviral resistance testing in patients failing therapy. AIDS 2000;14:F83-93.

9. Bergeron MG, Ke D, Menard C, Picard FJ, Gagnon M, Bernier M, et al. Rapid detection of group B streptococci in pregnant women at delivery. N Engl J Med 2000;343:175-9.
10. Bianchi A, Moret F, Desrues JM, Champenois T, Dervaux Y, Desvouas O, et al. PreservCyt transport medium used for the ThinPrep Pap test is a suitable medium for detection of Chlamydia trachomatis by the COBAS Amplicor CT/NG test: results of a preliminary study and future implications. J CLin Microbiol 2002;40:1749-54.
11. Bonington A, Strang JI, Klapper PE, Hood SV, Rubombora W, Penny M, et al. Use of Roche AMPLICOR Mycobacterium tuberculosis PCR in early diagnosis of tuberculosis meningitis. J Clin Microbiol 1998;36:1251-4.
12. Bosch FX, Manos MM, Munoz N, Sherman M, Jansen AM, Peto J, et al. Prevalence of human papillomavirus in cervical cancer: a worldwide perspective. International biological study on cervical cancer (IBSCC) Study Group. J Natl Cancer Inst 1995;87:796-802.
13. Bourlet T, Caro V, Minjolle S, Jusselin I, Pozzetto B, Crainic R, et al. New PCR test that recognizes all human prototypes of enterovirus: application for clinical diagnosis. J Clin Microbiol 2003;41: 1750-2.
14. Boyer KM, Gotoff SP. Strategies for chemoprophylaxis of GBS early-onset infections. Antibiot Chemother 1985;35:267-80.
15. Bradley SP, Reed SL, Catanzaro A. Clinical efficacy of the amplified Mycobacterium tuberculosis direct test for the diagnosis of pulmonary tuberculosis. Am J Respir Crit Care Med 1996;153:1606-10.
16. Brambilla D, Leung S, Lew J, Todd J, Herman S, Cronin M, et al. Absolute copy number and relative change in determinations of human immunodeficiency virus type 1 RNA in plasma: effect of an external standard on kit comparisons. J Clin Microbiol 1998;36:311-4.
17. Brambilla D, Reichelderfer P, Bremer J, Shapiro DE, Hershow RC, Katzenstein DA, et al. The contribution of assay variation and biological variation to the total variability of plasma HIV-1 RNA measurements. AIDS 1999;13:2269-79.
18. Brenner BG, Routy JP, Petrella M, Moisi D, Oliveira M, Detorio M, et al. Persistence and fitness of multidrug-resistant human immunodeficiency virus type 1 acquired in primary infection. J Virol 2002;76: 1753-61.
19. Buimer M, van Doornum GJ, Ching S, Peerbooms PG, Plier PK, Ram D, et al. Detection of Chlamydia trachomatis and Neisseria gonorrhoeae by ligase chain reaction-based assays with clinical specimens from various sites: implications for diagnostic testing and screening. J Clin Microbiol 1996;34:2395-400.
20. Bukh J, Purcell R, Miller R. Sequence analysis of the 5′ noncoding region of hepatitis C virus. Proc Natl Acad Sci USA 1992;89:4942-6.
21. Bukh J, Purcell R, Miller R. Sequence analysis of the core gene of 14 hepatitis C virus genotypes. Proc Natl Acad Sci USA 1994;91:8239-43.
22. Bukh J, Purcell RH, Miller RH. At least 12 genotypes of hepatitis C virus predicted by sequence analysis of the putative E1 gene of isolates collected worldwide. Proc Natl Acad Sci USA 1993;90:8234-8.
23. Bullock GC, Bruns DE, Haverstick DM. Hepatitis C genotype determination by melting curve analysis with a single set of fluorescence resonance energy transfer probes. Clin Chem 2002;48:2147-54.
24. Burstein GR, Zenilman JM. Nongonococcal urethritis—a new paradigm. Clin Infect Dis 1999;28:S66-73.
25. Caliendo AM, Schuurman R, Yen-Lieberman B, Spector SA, Andersen J, Manjiry R, et al. Comparison of quantitative and qualitative PCR assays for cytomegalovirus DNA in plasma. J Clin Microbiol 2001;39:1334-8.
26. Caliendo AM, St George K, Kao SY, Allega J, Tan BH, LaFontaine R, et al. Comparison of quantitative cytomegalovirus (CMV) PCR in plasma and CMV antigenemia assay: clinical utility of the prototype AMPLICOR CMV MONITOR test in transplant recipients. J Clin Microbiol 2000;38:2122-7.
27. Caliendo AM, St. George K, Allega J, Bullotta AC, Gilbane L, Rinaldo CR. Distinguishing cytomegalovirus (CMV) infection and disease with CMV nucleic acid assays. J Clin Microbiol 2002;40:1581-6.
28. Caliendo AM, Yen-Lieberman B, Baptista J, Andersen J, Crumpacker C, Schuurman R, et al. Comparison of molecular tests for detection and quantification of cell-associated cytomegalovirus DNA. J Clin Microbiol 2003;41:3509-13.
29. Centers for Disease Control and Prevention. Guidelines for laboratory testing and result reporting of antibody to hepatitis C virus. MMWR 2003;52:1-15.
30. Centers for Disease Control and Prevention. Nucleic acid amplification tests for tuberculosis. MMWR 1996;45:950-2.
31. Centers for Disease Control and Prevention. Prevention of Perinatal Group B Streptococcal Disease. MMWR 2002:1-26.
32. Centers for Disease Control and Prevention. Rapid diagnostic tests for tuberculosis: what is the appropriate use? American Thoracic Society Workshop. MMWR 1997;155:1804-14.
33. Centers for Disease Control and Prevention. Sexually transmitted diseases treatment guidelines. MMWR 2002;51:1-78.
34. Centers for Disease Control and Prevention. Tuberculosis morbidity—United States, 1997. MMWR 1998;47:253-7.

35. Centers for Disease Control and Prevention. Update: Nucleic acid amplification tests for tuberculosis. MMWR 2000;49:593-4.
36. Chernesky MA, Jang D, Lee H, Burczak JD, Hu H, Sellors J, et al. Diagnosis of Chlamydia trachomatis infections in men and women by testing first-void urine by ligase chain reaction. J Clin Microbiol 1994;32:2682-5.
37. Chong S, Jang D, Song X, Mahony J, Petrich A, Barriga P, et al. Specimen processing and concentration of Chlamydia trachomatis added can influence false-negative rates in the LCx assay but not in the APTIMA Combo 2 assay when testing for inhibitors. J Clin Microbiol 2003;41:778-82.
38. Chonmaitree T, Menegus MA, Powell KR. The clinical relevance of 'CSF viral culture.' A two-year experience with aseptic meningitis in Rochester, NY. JAMA 1982;247:1843-7.
39. Clevenbergh P, Durant J, Halfon P, Giudice PD, Mondain V, Montagne N, et al. Persisting long-term benefit of genotype-guided treatment for HIV-infected patients failing HAART. The VIRADAPT study: week 48 follow-up. Antiviral Ther 2000;5: 65-70.
40. Cohen CJ, Hunt S, Sension M, Farthing C, Conant M, Jacobson S, et al. A randomized trial assessing the impact of phenotypic resistance testing on antiretroviral therapy. AIDS 2002;16:579-88.
41. Connor R, Ho D, Kuritzkes DR, Richman DD. Human immunodeficiency virus. In: Richman DD, ed. Clinical Virology, 1st ed. New York: Churchill Livingstone, 1997:707-54.
42. Cope AV, Sabin C, Burroughs A, Rolles K, Griffiths PD, Emery VC. Interrelationships among quantity of human cytomegalovirus (HCMV) DNA in blood, donor-recipient serostatus, and administration of methylprednisolone as risk factors for HCMV disease following liver transplantation. J Infect Dis 1997;176:1484-90.
43. Coutlee F, Gravitt P, Kornegay J, Hankins C, Richardson H, Lapointe N, et al. Use of PGMY primers in L1 consensus PCR improves detection of human papillomavirus DNA in genital samples. J Clin Microbiol 2002;40:902-7.
44. Cox JT, Lorincz AT, Schiffman MH, Sherman ME, Cullen A, Kurman RJ. Human papillomavirus testing by hybrid capture appears to be useful in triaging women with a cytologic diagnosis of atypical squamous cells of undetermined significance. Am J Obstet Gynecol 1995;172:946-54.
45. Crotchfelt KA, Pare B, Gaydos C, Quinn TC. Detection of Chlamydia trachomatis by the Gen-Probe AMPLIFIED Chlamydia Trachomatis Assay (AMP CT) in urine specimens from men and women and endocervical specimen from women. J Clin Microbiol 1998;36:391-4.
46. Culler EE, Caliendo AM, Nolte FS. Reproducibility of positive test results in the BDProbeTec ET system for detection of Chlamydia trachomatis and Neisseria gonorrhoeae. J Clin Microbiol 2003;41:3911-4.
47. Cunningham CK, Charbonneau TT, Song K, Patterson D, Sullivan T, Cummins T, et al. Comparison of human immunodeficiency virus 1 DNA polymerase chain reaction and qualitative and quantitative RNA polymerase chain reaction in human immunodeficiency virus 1-exposed infants. Pediatr Infect Dis J 1999;18:30-5.
48. Daar ES, Little S, Pitt J, Santangelo J, Ho P, Harawa N, et al. Diagnosis of primary HIV-1 infection. Los Angeles County Primary HIV Infection Recruitment Network. Ann Intern Med 2001;134:25-9.
49. Davis G. Hepatitis C virus genotypes and quasispecies. Am J Med 1999;107:21S-25S.
50. Davis GL. Monitoring of viral levels during therapy of hepatitis C. Hepatology 2002;36:S145-51.
51. Davis GL, Esteban-Mur R, Rustgi V, Hoefs J, Gordon SC, Trepo C, et al. Interferon alfa-2b alone or in combination with ribavirin for the treatment of relapse of chronic hepatitis C. International Hepatitis Interventional Therapy Group. N Engl J Med 1998;339: 1493-9.
52. Detmer J, Lagier R, Flynn J, Zayati C, Kolberg J, Collins M, et al. Accurate quantification of hepatitis C virus (HCV) RNA from all HCV genotypes by using branched-DNA technology. J Clin Microbiol 1996;34:901-7.
53. Donovan RM, Bush CE, Markowitz NP, Baxa DM, Saravolatz LD. Changes in virus load markers during AIDS-associated opportunistic diseases in human immunodeficiency virus-infected persons. J Infect Dis 1996;174:401-3.
54. Durant J, Clevenbergh P, Halfon P, Delgiudice P, Porsin S, Simonet P, et al. Drug-resistance genotyping in HIV-1 therapy: the VIRADAPT randomised controlled trial. Lancet 1999;353:2195-9.
55. Dusheiko G, Schmilovitz-Weiss H, Brown D, McOmish F, Yap PL, Sherlock S, et al. Hepatitis C virus genotypes: an investigation of type-specific differences in geographic origin and disease. Hepatology 1994;19:13-8.
56. Ellerbrock TV, Chiasson MA, Bush TJ, Sun XW, Sawo D, Brudney K, et al. Incidence of cervical squamous intraepithelial lesions in HIV-infected women. JAMA 2000;283:1031-7.
57. Erice A, Tierney C, Hirsch M, Caliendo AM, Weinberg A, Kendall MA, et al. Cytomegalovirus (CMV) and human immunodeficiency virus (HIV) burden, CMV end-organ disease, and survival in subjects with advanced HIV infection (AIDS Clinical Trials Group Protocol 360). Clin Infect Dis 2003;37:567-78.
58. Federal Register. 1997;FR 62:62243-60.
59. Federal Register. 2003;FR Final Rule:2226.

60. Ferreira-Gonzalez A, Fisher RA, Weymouth LA, Langley MR, Wolfe L, Wilkinson DS, et al. Clinical utility of a quantitative polymerase chain reaction for diagnosis of cytomegalovirus disease in solid organ transplant patients. Transplantation 1999;68:991-6.
61. Fox JD, Han S, Samuelson A, Zhang Y, Neale ML, Westmoreland D. Development and evaluation of nucleic acid sequence based amplification (NASBA) for diagnosis of enterovirus infections using the NucliSens Basic Kit. J Clin Virol 2002;24:117-30.
62. Fried MW, Shiffman ML, Reddy KR, Smith C, Marinos G, Goncales FL Jr, et al. Peginterferon alfa-2a plus ribavirin for chronic hepatitis C virus infection. N Engl J Med 2002;347:975-82.
63. Gaydos CA, Crotchfelt KA, Howell MR, Kralian S, Hauptman P, Quinn TC. Molecular amplification assays to detect chlamydial infections in urine specimens from high school female students and to monitor the persistence of chlamydial DNA after therapy. J Infect Dis 1998;177:417-24.
64. Gerna G, Baldanti F, Middeldorf J, Furione M, Zavattoni M, Lilleri D, et al. Clinical significance of expression of human cytomegalovirus pp67 late transcript in heart, lung, and bone marrow transplant recipients as determined by nucleic acid sequence-based amplification. J Clin Microbiol 1999;37:902-11.
65. Gissmann L, Wolnik L, Ikenberg H, Koldovsky U, Schnurch HG, zur Hausen H. Human papillomavirus types 6 and 11 DNA sequences in genital and laryngeal papillomas and in some cervical cancers. Proc Natl Acad Sci, USA 1983;80:560-3.
66. Gravitt PE, Peyton CL, Alessi TQ, Wheeler CM, Coutlee F, Hildesheim A, et al. Improved amplification of genital human papillomaviruses. J Clin Microbiol 2000;38:357-61.
67. Groseclose SL, Zaidi AA, DeLisle SJ, Levine WC, St Louis ME. Estimated incidence and prevalence of genital Chlamydia trachomatis infections in the United States, 1996. Sex Transm Dis 1999;26: 339-44.
68. Gunter J. Genital and perianal warts: new treatment opportunities for human papillomavirus infection. Am J Obstet Gynecol 2003;189:S3-11.
69. Hagblom P, Korch C, Jonsson AB, Normark S. Intragenic variation by site-specific recombination in the cryptic plasmid of Neisseria gonorrhoeae. J Bacteriol 1986;167:231-7.
70. Halfon P, Bourliere M, Halimi G, Khiri H, Bertezene P, Portal I, et al. Assessment of spontaneous fluctuations of viral load in untreated patients with chronic hepatitis C by two standardized quantitation methods: branched DNA and Amplicor monitor. J Clin Microbiol 1998;36:2073-5.
71. Hamilton MS, Jackson MA, Abel. Clinical utility of polymerase chain reaction testing for enteroviral meningitis. Pediatr Infect Dis J 1999;18:533-8.
72. Haubrich R, Keiser P, Kemper C, Witt M, Leedom J, Forthal D, et al. CCTG 575: a randomized, prospective study of phenotype testing versus standard of care for patients failing antiretroviral therapy [Abstract 80]. 5th International Workshop on HIV Drug Resistance and Treatment Strategies, Vol. 6. San Diego: International Medical Press Ltd., 2001:63.
73. Hawkins A, Davidson F, Simmonds P. Comparison of plasma virus loads among individuals infected with hepatitis C virus (HCV) genotypes 1, 2, and 3 by quantiplex HCV RNA assay versions 1 and 2, Roche monitor assay, and an in-house limiting dilution method. J Clin Microbiol 1997;35:187-92.
74. Henegariu O, Heerema NA, Dlouhy SR, Vance GH, Vogt PH. Multiplex PCR: critical parameters and step-by-step protocol. 1997;23:504-11.
75. Hertogs K, Bloor S, De Vroey V, van Den Eynde C, Dehertogh P, van Cauwenberge A, et al. A novel human immunodeficiency virus type 1 reverse transcriptase mutational pattern confers phenotypic lamivudine resistance in the absence of mutation 184V. Antimicrob Agents Chemother 2000;44:568-73.
76. Hirsch MS, Brun-Vezinet F, Clotet B, Conway B, Kuritzkes DR, D'Aquila RT, et al. Antiretroviral drug resistance testing in adults with human immunodeficiency virus type 1: 2003 recommendations of an international AIDS Society-USA panel. Clin Infect Dis 2003;37:113-28.
77. Hirsch MS, Conway B, D'Aquila RT, Johnson VA, Brun-Vezinet F, Clotet B, et al. Antiretrovial drug resistance testing in adults with HIV infection: implications for clinical management. International AIDS Society—USA Panel. JAMA 1998;279:1984-91.
78. Ho G, Bierman R, Beardsley L, Chang C, Burk R. Natural history of cervicovaginal papillomavirus infection in young women. N Engl J Med 1998;338:423-8.
79. Holodniy M, Rainen L, Herman S, Yen-Lieberman B. Stability of plasma human immunodeficiency virus load in VACUTAINER PPT plasma preparation tubes during overnight shipment. J Clin Microbiol 2000;38:323-6.
80. Hook EW III, Smith K, Mullen C, Stephens J, Rinehardt L, Pate MS, et al. Diagnosis of genitourinary Chlamydia trachomatis infections by using the ligase chain reaction on patient-obtained vaginal swabs. J Clin Microbiol 1997;35:2133-5.
81. Humar A, Gregson D, Caliendo AM, McGeer A, Malkan G, Krajden M, et al. Clinical utility of quantitative cytomegalovirus viral load determination for predicting cytomegalovirus disease in liver transplant recipients. Transplantation 1999;68:1305-11.
82. Humar A, Kumar D, Boivin G, Caliendo AM. Cytomegalovirus (CMV) viral load kinetics to predict recurrent disease in solid organ transplant patients with CMV disease. J Infect Dis 2002;186:829-33.

83. Ikewaki J, Ohtsuka E, Kawano R, Ogata M, Kikuchi H, Nasu M. Real-time PCR assay compared to nested PCR and antigenemia assays for detecting cytomegalovirus reactivation in adult T-cell leukemia-lymphoma patients. J Clin Microbiol 2003;41:4382-7.
84. Jackson JB, Smith K, Knott C, Korpela A, Simmons A, Piwowar-Manning E, et al. Sensitivity of the Procleix HIV-1/HCV assay for detection of human immunodeficiency virus type 1 and hepatitis C virus RNA in a high-risk population. J Clin Microbiol 2002;40: 2387-91.
85. Jagodzinski LL, Wiggins DL, McManis JL, Emery S, Overbaugh J, Robb M, et al. Use of calibrated viral load standards for group M subtypes of human immunodeficiency virus type 1 to assess the performance of viral RNA quantitation tests. J Clin Microbiol 2000;38:1247-9.
86. Jaschek G, Gaydos CA, Welsh LE, Quinn TC. Direct detection of Chlamydia trachomatis in urine specimens from symptomatic and asymptomatic men by using a rapid polymerase chain reaction assay. J Clin Microbiol 1993;31:1209-12.
87. Jonas V, Acedo M, Clarridge JE, et al. A multi-center evaluation of MTD and culture compared to clinical diagnosis. Abstract L-31. 98th General Meeting of the American Society for Microbiology, Atlanta, Ga: ASM, 1998.
88. Judson FN. Gonorrhea. Med Clin North Am 1990;74:1353-66.
89. Kahn JO, Walker BD. Acute human immunodeficiency virus type 1 infection. N Engl J Med 1998;339:32-9.
90. Kebelmann-Betzing C, Seeger K, Dragon S, Schmitt G, Moricke A, Schild TA, et al. Advantages of a new Taq DNA polymerase in multiplex PCR and time-release PCR. 1998;24:154-8.
91. Kessler HH, Santner B, Rabenau H, Berger A, Vince A, Lewinski C, et al. Rapid diagnosis of enterovirus infection by a new one-step reverse transcription-PCR assay. J Clin Microbiol 1997;35:976-7.
92. Kimberlin DW, Lakeman FD, Arvin AM, Prober CG, Corey L, Powell DA, et al. Application of the polymerase chain reaction to the diagnosis and management of neonatal herpes simplex virus disease. National Institute of Allergy and Infectious Diseases Collaborative Antiviral Study Group. J Infect Dis 1996;174:1162-7.
93. Kleiber J, Walter T, Haberhausen G, Tsang S, Babiel R, Rosenstraus M. Performance characteristics of a quantitative, homogeneous TaqMan RT-PCR test for HCV RNA. J Mol Diagn 2000;2:158-66.
94. Kolk DP, Dockter J, Linnen J, Ho-Sing-Loy M, Gillotte-Taylor K, McDonough SH, et al. Significant closure of the human immunodeficiency virus type 1 and hepatitis C virus preseroconversion detection windows with a transcription-mediated-amplification-driven assay. J Clin Microbiol 2002;40:1761-6.
95. Kornegay JR, Shepard AP, Hankins C, Franco E, Lapointe N, Richardson H, et al. Nonisotopic detection of human papillomavirus DNA in clinical specimens using a consensus PCR and a generic probe mix in an enzyme-linked immunosorbent assay format. J Clin Microbiol 2001;39:3530-6.
96. Kulasingam SL, Hughes JP, Kiviat NB, Mao C, Weiss NS, Kuypers JM, et al. Evaluation of human papillomavirus testing in primary screening for cervical abnormalities: comparison of sensitivity, specificity, and frequency of referral. JAMA 2002;288:1749-57.
97. Lakeman F, Whitley RJ. Diagnosis of herpes simplex encephalitis: Application of polyermase chain reaction to cerebrospinal fluid from brain-biopsied patients and correlation with disease. National Institute of Allergy and Infectious Diseases Collaborative Antiviral Study Group. J Infect Dis 1995;171:857.
98. Lang AM, Feris-Iglesias J, Pena C, Sanchez JF, Stockman L, Rys P, et al. Clinical evaluation of the Gen-Probe Amplified Direct Test for detection of Mycobacterium tuberculosis complex organisms in cerebrospinal fluid. J Clin Microbiol 1998;36:2191-4.
99. Larsson S, Soderberg-Naucler C, Wang FZ, Moller E. Cytomegalovirus DNA can be detected in peripheral blood mononuclear cells from all seropositive and most seronegative healthy blood donors over time. Transfusion 1998;38:271-8.
100. Lee HH, Chernesky MA, Schachter J, Burczak JD, Andrews WW, Muldoon S, et al. Diagnosis of Chlamydia trachomatis genitourinary infection in women by ligase chain reaction assay of urine. Lancet 1995;345:213-6.
101. Lee SS, Heathcote EJ, Reddy KR, Zeuzem S, Fried MW, Wright TL, et al. Prognostic factors and early predictability of sustained viral response with peginterferon alfa-2a (40KD). J Hepatol 2002;37:500-6.
102. Leung NW. Management of viral hepatitis C. J Gastroenterol Hepatol 2002;17:S146-54.
103. Ling P, Vilchez R, Keitel W, Poston D, Peng R, White Z, et al. Epstein-Barr virus DNA loads in adult human immunodeficiency virus type 1-infected patients receiving highly active antiretroviral therapy. Clin Infect Dis 2003;37:1244-9.
104. Loeffelholz MJ, Lewinski CA, Silver SR, Purohit AP, Herman SA, Buonagurio DA, et al. Detection of Chlamydia trachomatis in endocervical specimens by polymerase chain reaction. J Clin Microbiol 1992;30:2847-51.
105. Mahony J, Chong S, Jang D, Luinstra K, Faught M, Dalby D, et al. Urine specimens from pregnant and nonpregnant women inhibitory to amplification of Chlamydia trachomatis nucleic acid by PCR, ligase chain reaction, and transcription-mediated amplifica-

tion: identification of urinary substances with inhibition and removal of inhibitory activity. J Clin Microbiol 1998;36:3122-6.
106. Malm G, Forsgren M. Neonatal herpes simplex virus infections: HSV DNA in cerebrospinal fluid and serum. Arch Dis Child Fetal Neonatal Ed 1999;81:F24-9.
107. Manos MM, Ting Y, Wright DK, et al. The use of polymerase chain reaction amplification for the detection of genital human papillomaviruses. Cancer Cells 1989;7:209-14.
108. Marshall GS, Hauck MA, Buck G, Rabalais GP. Potential cost savings through rapid diagnosis of enteroviral meningitis. Pediatr Infect Dis J 1997;16:1086-7.
109. Martell M, Gomez J, Esteban JI, Sauleda S, Quer J, Cabot B, et al. High-throughput real-time reverse transcription-PCR quantitation of hepatitis C virus RNA. J Clin Microbiol 1999;37:327-32.
110. Martinot-Peignoux M, Boyer N, Le Breton V, Le Guludec G, Castelnau C, Akremi R, et al. A new step toward standardization of serum hepatitis C virus-RNA quantification in patients with chronic hepatitis C. Hepatology 2000;31:726-9.
111. Mas V, Alvarellos T, Albano S, de Boccardo G, Giraudo C, Garrett CT, et al. Utility of cytomegalovirus viral load in renal transplant patients in Argentina. Transplantation 1999;67: 1050-5.
112. Mazzulli T, Drew L, Yen-Lieberman B, Jekic-McMullen D, Kohn DJ, Isada CM, et al. Multicenter comparison of the Digene Hybrid Capture CMV DNA assay (version 2.0), the pp65 antigenemia assay, and cell culture for detection of cytomegalovirus viremia. J Clin Microbiol 1999;37:958-63.
113. Mazzulli T, Rubin RH, Ferraro MJ, D'Aquila RT, Doveikis SA, Smith BR, et al. Cytomegalovirus antigenemia: clinical correlations in transplant recipients and in persons with AIDS. J Clin Microbiol 1993;31:2824-7.
114. McCance DJ, Walker PG, Dyson JL, Coleman DV, Singer A. Presence of human papillomavirus DNA sequences in cervical intraepithelial neoplasia. Br Med J (Clin Res Ed) 1983;287:784-8.
115. McGowen K. Diagnostic tests for pertussis: culture vs. DFA vs. PCR. Clin Microbiol Newsl 2002;24:143-9.
116. McHutchison JG, Gordon SC, Schiff ER, Shiffman ML, Lee WM, Rustgi VK, et al. Interferon alfa-2b alone or in combination with ribavirin as initial treatment for chronic hepatitis C. N Engl J Med 1998;339:1485-92.
117. McOmish F, Yap PL, Dow BC, Follett EA, Seed C, Keller AJ, et al. Geographical distribution of hepatitis C virus genotypes in blood donors: an international collaborative survey. J Clin Microbiol 1994;32: 884-92.
118. Mellors JW, Kingsley LA, Rinaldo CR Jr, Todd JA, Hoo BS, Kokka RP, et al. Quantitation of HIV-1 RNA in plasma predicts outcome after seroconversion. Ann Intern Med 1995;122:573-9.
119. Mellors JW, Rinaldo CR Jr, Gupta P, White RM, Todd JA, Kingsley LA. Prognosis in HIV-1 infected predicted by the quantity of virus in plasma. Science 1996;272:1167-70.
120. Meynard J-L, Vray M, Morand-Joubert L, Race E, Descamps D, Peytavin G, et al. Phenotypic or genotypic resistance testing for choosing antiretroviral therapy after treatment failure: a randomized trial. AIDS 2002;16:727-36.
121. Middeldorp J, Sillekens P, Lunenberg J. Diagnosis of active HCMV infection: the mRNA approach. Organ Tissues 2000;2:99-107.
122. Miller V. HIV drug resistance: overview of clinical data. JAAPA 2001;6:68-72.
123. Miyada CG, Born TL. A DNA sequence for the discrimination of Neisseria gonorrhoeae from other Neisseria species. Mol Cell Probes 1991;5:327-35.
124. Moss T. International handbook of Chlamydia. UK: Polestar Wheatons Ltd, 2001.
125. Mukaide M, Tanaka Y, Katayose S, Tano H, Murata M, Hikata M, et al. Development of real-time detection direct test for hepatitis B virus and comparison with two commercial tests using the WHO international standard. J Gastroenterol Hepatol 2003;18:1264-71.
126. NCCLS. General laboratory practices GP2-A4. Clinical laboratory technical procedure manuals: approved guidelines. 4th ed. 2002.
127. NCCLS. Quantitative molecular methods for infectious diseases; approved guideline. Vol. 23 (28). Wayne, Pa: NCCLS, 2003:1-55.
128. Nigrovic LE, Chiang VW. Cost analysis of enteroviral polymerase chain reaction in infants with fever and cerebrospinal fluid pleocytosis. Arch Pediatr Adolesc Med 2000;154:817-21.
129. NIH. Management of hepatitis C: 2002. NIH Consens State Sci Statements 2002;19:1-46.
130. Nkengasong JN, Bile C, Kalou M, Maurice C, Boating E, Sasson-Moroko M, et al. Quantification of RNA in HIV Type 1 subtypes D and G by NucliSens and Amplicor Assays in Abidjan, Ivory Coast. AIDS Res Hum Retroviruses 1999;15:495-8.
131. Nolte FS. Branched DNA signal amplification for direct quantitation of nucleic acid sequences in clinical specimens. Adv Clin Chem 1998;33:201-35.
132. Nolte FS, Green AM, Fiebelkorn KR, Caliendo AM, Sturchio C, Grunwald A, et al. Clinical evaluation of two methods for genotyping hepatitis C virus based on analysis of the 5′ noncoding region. J Clin Microbiol 2003;41:1558-64.
133. Oberste MS, Maher K, Flemister MR, Marchetti G, Kilpatrick DR, Pallansch MA. Comparison of classic

and molecular approaches for the identification of untypeable enteroviruses. J Clin Microbiol 2000;38:1170-4.

134. O'Brien WA, Grovit-Ferbas K, Namazi A, Ovcak-Derzic S, Wang HJ, Park J, et al. Human immunodeficiency virus-type 1 replication can be increased in peripheral blood of seropositive patients after influenza vaccination. Blood 1995;86:1082-9.
135. Oldenberg N, Lam K, Khan M, Top B, Tacken N, McKie A, et al. Evaluation of human cytomegalovirus gene expression in thoracic organ transplant recipients using nucleic acid sequence-based amplification. Transplantation 2000;70:1209-15.
136. Palmer HM, Mallinson H, Wood RL, Herring AJ. Evaluation of the specificities of five DNA amplification methods for the detection of Neisseria gonorrhoeae. J Clin Microbiol 2003;41:835-7.
137. Parekh B, Phillips S, Granade TC, Baggs J, Hu DJ, Respess R. Impact of HIV type 1 subtype variation on viral RNA quantitation. AIDS Res Hum Retroviruses 1999;15:133-42.
138. Pasquier C, Sandres K, Salama G, Puel J, Izopet J. Using RT-PCR and bDNA assays to measure non-clade B HIV-1 subtype RNA. J Virol Methods 1999;81:123-9.
139. Pasternack R, Vuorinen P, Miettinen A. Evaluation of the Gen-Probe Chlamydia trachomatis transcription-mediated amplification assay with urine specimens from women. J Clin Microbiol 1997;35:676-8.
140. Petropoulos CJ, Parkin NT, Limoli KL, Lie YS, Wrin T, Huang W, et al. A novel phenotypic drug susceptibility assay for human immunodeficiency virus type 1. Antimicrob Agents Chemother 2000;44:920-8.
141. Podzorski RP. Molecular testing in the diagnosis and management of hepatitis C virus infection. Arch Pathol Lab Med 2002;126:285-90.
142. Poynard T, Marcellin P, Lee SS, Niederau C, Minuk GS, Ideo G, et al. Randomised trial of interferon a2b plus ribavirin for 48 weeks or for 24 weeks versus interon a2b plus placebo for 48 weeks for treatment of chronic infection with hepatitis C virus. Lancet 1998;352:1426-32.
143. Poynard T, McHutchison JG, Goodman ZD, Ling M-H, Albrecht J, for the ALGOVIRC Project Group. Is an "a la carte" combination interferon alfa-2b plus ribavirin regimen possible for the first line treatment in patients with chronic hepatitis C. Hepatology 2000;31:211-8.
144. Puolakkainen M, Hiltunen-Back E, Reunala T, Suhonen S, Lahteenmaki P, Lehtinen M, et al. Comparison of performances of two commercially available tests, a PCR assay and a ligase chain reaction test, in detection of urogenital Chlamydia trachomatis infection. J Clin Microbiol 1998;36:1489-93.
145. Ramers C, Billman G, Hartin M, Ho S, Sawyer MH. Impact of a diagnostic cerebrospinal fluid enterovirus polymerase chain reaction test on patient management. JAMA 2000;283:2680-5.
146. Razonable RR, Brown RA, Wilson JA, Groettum CM, Kremers W, Espy MJ, et al. The clinical use of various blood compartments for cytomegalovirus (CMV) DNA quantitation in transplant recipients with CMV disease. Transplantation 2002;73:968-73.
147. Rees E. The treatment of pelvic inflammatory disease. Am J Obstet Gynecol 1980;138:1042-7.
148. Regan JA, Klebanoff MA, Nugent RP. The epidemiology of group B streptococcal colonization in pregnancy. Vaginal Infections and Prematurity Study Group. Obstet Gynecol 1991;77:604-10.
149. Roberts TC, Brennan DC, Buller RS, Gaudreault-Keener M, Schnitzler MA, Sternahell KA, et al. Quantitative polymerase chain reaction to predict occurrence of symptomatic cytomegalovirus infection and assess response to ganciclovir therapy in renal transplant recipients. J Infect Dis 1998;178:626-35.
150. Ronnett BM, Manos MM, Ransley JE, Fetterman BJ, Kinney WK, Hurley LB, et al. Atypical glandular cells of undetermined significance (AGUS): cytopathologic features, histopathologic results, and human papillomavirus DNA detection. Hum Pathol 1999;30:816-25.
151. Rosenstraus M, Wang Z, Chang SY, DeBonville D, Spadoro JP. An internal control for routine diagnostic PCR: design, properties, and effect on clinical performance. J Clin Microbiol 1998;36:191-7.
152. Rotbart HA. Diagnosis of enteroviral meningitis with the polymerase chain reaction. J Pediatr 1990;117:85-9.
153. Rotbart HA. Nucleic acid detection systems for enteroviruses. Clin Microbiol Rev 1991;4:156-68.
154. Rotbart HA, Sawyer MH, Fast S, Lewinski C, Murphy N, Keyser EF, et al. Diagnosis of enteroviral meningitis by using PCR with a colorimetric microwell detection assay. J Clin Microbiol 1994;32:2590-2.
155. Rubin RH. Cytomegalovirus in solid organ transplantation. Transpl Infect Dis 2001;3:1-5.
156. Saag MS, Holodniy M, Kuritzkes DR, O'Brien WA, Coombs R, Poscher ME, et al. HIV viral load markers in clinical practice. Nature Med 1996;2:625-9.
157. Saldanha J, Lelie N, Heath A. Establishment of the first international standard for nucleic acid amplification technology (NAT) assays for HCV RNA. WHO Collaborative Study Group. Vox Sang 1999;76:149-58.
158. Schenck U, Herbert A, Solomon D, Amma NS, Collins RJ, Gupta SK, et al. Terminology. International Academy of Cytology Task Force summary. Diagnostic cytology towards the 21st century: an international expert conference and tutorial. Acta Cytol 1998;42:5-15.
159. Schlesinger Y, Tebas P, Gaudreault-Keener M, Buller RS, Storch GA. Herpes simplex virus type 2 meningi-

tis in the absence of genital lesions: improved recognition with use of the polymerase chain reaction. Clin Infect Dis 1995;20:842-8.

160. Schrag SJ, Zell ER, Lynfield R, Roome A, Arnold KE, Craig AS, et al. A population-based comparison of strategies to prevent early-onset group B streptococcal disease in neonates. N Engl J Med 2002;347: 233-9.
161. Sia IG, Wilson JA, Groettum CM, Espy MJ, Smith TF, Paya CV. Cytomegalovuris (CMV) DNA load predicts relapsing CMV infection after solid organ transplantation. J Infect Dis 2000;181:717-20.
162. Simko JP, Caliendo AM, Hogle K, Versalovic J. Differences in laboratory findings for cerebrospinal fluid specimens obtained from patients with meningitis or encephalitis due to herpes simplex virus (HSV) documented by detection of HSV DNA. Clin Infect Dis 2002;35:414-9.
163. Simmonds P, Holmes EC, Cha T, Chan SW, McOmish F, Irvine B, et al. Classification of hepatitis C virus into six major genotypes and a series of subtypes by phylogenetic analysis of the NS-5 region. J Gen Virol 1993;74:2391-99.
164. Solomon D, Schiffman M, Tarone R. Comparison of three management strategies for patients with atypical squamous cells of undetermined significance: baseline results from a randomized trial. J Natl Cancer Inst 2001;93:293-9.
165. Spector SA, Hsia K, Crager M, Pilcher M, Cabral S, Stempien MJ. Cytomegalovirus (CMV) DNA load is an independent predictor of CMV disease and survival in advanced AIDS. J Virol 1999;73:7027-30.
166. Spector SA, Wong R, Hsia K, Pilcher M, Stempien MJ. Plasma cytomegalovirus (CMV) DNA load predicts CMV disease and survival in AIDS patients. J Clin Invest 1998;101:497-502.
167. Stamm WE. Chlamydia trachomatis infections of the adult. In: Holmes KK, Sparling PF, Mardh P-A, et al, eds. Sex Transm Dis, 3rd ed. New York: McGraw-Hill, 1999:407-22.
168. Stamm WE, Guinan ME, Johnson C, Starcher T, Holmes KK, McCormack WM. Effect of treatment regimens for Neisseria gonorrhoeae on simultaneous infection with Chlamydia trachomatis. N Engl J Med 1984;310:545-9.
169. Staprans SI, Hamilton BL, Follansbee SE, Elbeik T, Barbosa P, Grant RM, et al. Activation of virus replication after vaccination of HIV-1-infected individuals. J Exp Med 1995;182:1727-37.
170. Steketee RW, Abrams EJ, Thea DM, Brown TM, Lambert G, Orloff S, et al. Early detection of perinatal human immunodeficiency virus (HIV) type 1 infection using HIV RNA amplification and detection. J Infect Dis 1997;175:707-11.
171. Stellrecht KA, Harding I, Hussain FM, Mishrik NG, Czap RT, Lepow ML, et al. A one-step RT-PCR assay using an enzyme-linked detection system for the diagnosis of enterovirus meningitis. J Clin Virol 2000;17:143-9.
172. Stramer SL. US NAT yield: where are we after 2 years? Transfus Med 2002;12:243-53.
173. Stramer SL, Caglioti S, Strong DM. NAT of the United States and Canadian blood supply [erratum appears in Transfusion 2001 Aug;41(8):1079]. Transfusion 2000;40:1165-8.
174. Stuyver L, Rossau R, Wyseur A, Duhamel M, Vanderborght B, Van Heuverswyn H, et al. Typing of hepatitis C virus isolates and characterization of new subtypes using a line probe assay. J Gen Virol 1993;74:1093-102.
175. Stuyver L, Wyseur A, Van Arnhem W, Hernandez F, Maertens G. Second-generation line probe assay for hepatitis C virus genotyping. J Clin Microbiol 1996;34:2259-66.
176. Svare EI, Kjaer SK, Worm AM, Osterlind A, Meijer CJ, van den Brule AJ. Risk factors for genital HPV DNA in men resemble those found in women: a study of male attendees at a Danish STD clinic. Sex Transm Infect 2002;78:215-8.
177. Tanaka Y, Kanda Y, Kami M, Mori S, Hamaki T, Kusumi E, et al. Monitoring cytomegalovirus infection by antigenemia assay and two distinct plasma real-time PCR methods after hematopoietic stem cell transplantation. Bone Marrow Transplant 2002;30:315-9.
178. Tedder D, Ashley R, Tyler K, Levin M. Herpes simplex virus infection as a cause of benign recurrent lymphocytic meningitis. Ann Intern Med 1994;121:334-8.
179. Tural C, Ruiz L, Holtzer C, Schapiro J, Viciana P, Gonzalez J, et al. Clinical utility of HIV-1 genotyping and expert advice—the Havana trial. AIDS 2002;16:209-18.
180. Van Der Pol B, Ferrero DV, Buck-Barrington L, Hook E III, Lenderman C, Quinn T, et al. Multicenter evaluation of the BDProbeTec ET System for detection of Chlamydia trachomatis and Neisseria gonorrhoeae in urine specimens, female endocervical swabs, and male urethral swabs. J Clin Microbiol 2001;39: 1008-16.
181. van Doorn LJ, Quint W, Kleter B, Molijn A, Colau B, Martin MT, et al. Genotyping of human papillomavirus in liquid cytology cervical specimens by the PGMY line blot assay and the SPF(10) line probe assay. J Clin Microbiol 2002;40:979-83.
182. van Doornum GJ, Schouls LM, Pijl A, Cairo I, Buimer M, Bruisten S. Comparison between the LCx Probe system and the COBAS AMPLICOR system for detection of Chlamydia trachomatis and Neisseria gonorrhoeae infections in patients attending a clinic for treatment of sexually transmitted diseases in Amsterdam, The Netherlands. J Clin Microbiol 2001;39:829-35.

CHAPTER 43

Pharmacogenetics

Gwendolyn A. McMillin, Ph.D., D.A.B.C.C., Mark W. Linder, Ph.D., and Bonny Lewis Bukaveckas, Ph.D.

The primary objective of pharmacogenetic testing is to predict how people will respond to medicines and other potentially toxic or bioactive xenobiotics based upon certain genetic characteristics. Pharmacogenetics may also help explain why an adverse drug reaction (ADR) occurred. The term pharmacogenetics has been pieced together from the words pharmacology (the study of drugs, drug action, and metabolism) and genetics (the study of how traits are inherited). Pharmacogenetic testing in a clinical setting links patient genetics (genotype) to predicted differences in the pharmacokinetics or pharmacodynamics of medications or other exogenous compounds.

Clinical pharmacogenetic test results are primarily useful for guiding medication selection and dosing. Specific dosing guidelines based on pharmacogenetic information are being developed to support the application of these test results for therapeutic drug management.[69,80,93] Such individualized pharmacotherapy is anticipated to reduce the number of ADRs, a leading cause of morbidity and mortality in the United States (see Table 43-1). For a more in-depth discussion of pharmacogenetics, the reader is referred to several excellent reviews.*

The goal of this chapter is to familiarize the clinical chemist with pharmacogenetic testing. This chapter begins with a discussion of general issues, including potential tests to offer in the clinical laboratory, choosing appropriate testing strategies, characteristics of a gene that make it a good candidate for pharmacogenetic testing, and characteristics of medications or other xenobiotics that support the need for pharmacogenetic testing. In the following sections, we provide detailed information for six well-characterized and polymorphic genes (*TPMT, CYP2D6, CYP2C19, CYP2C9, NAT1,* and *NAT2*). Variation in these genes contributes to intersubject variation in enzyme activity, kinetics, substrate specificity, and/or stability. Such variation is reflected in the ability of an individual to appropriately respond to medications that are substrates of these enzymes. This alteration in response to the medication defines the phenotype. The correlation of phenotypes and genotypes for these and several other proposed genetic targets is discussed in this chapter as well.

DEFINING PHARMACOGENETIC TARGETS AND WHAT TESTING TO CONSIDER

The response to drugs and other xenobiotics (foreign compounds absorbed by the human body) depends on many processes, such as route of administration, amount absorbed, any biotransformation (metabolism) that occurs, affinity of the parent compound and metabolite(s) for endogenous receptor(s), and the process of elimination.[40] For simplicity sake, we will use the term "drug(s)" throughout this chapter with the understanding that many principles of pharmacogenetics that apply to medications may also apply to other xenobiotics. Each process mentioned above involves several proteins that are coded from corresponding genes. Consequently, pharmacogenetic targets include any polymorphic gene that encodes for the many different proteins involved in these processes. To date, the best-studied pharmacogenetic targets are those involved in drug metabolism. Common features of pharmacogenetic tests of proven usefulness include: (1) the enzyme of interest is the primary pathway for metabolism of the drug, (2) changes in enzyme activity resulting from genetic polymorphism have a significant effect on the relationship between dose and plasma concentration, (3) the efficacy and/or toxicity of the drug correlate with changes in plasma drug concentration, and (4) the drugs affected by the pharmacogenetic variability possess a narrow therapeutic index. Further, pharmacogenetic

*References 25, 31, 35, 41, 100, 131, 134.

TABLE 43-1 Estimated Occurrence of Adverse Drug Events in the USA in 1994, in Thousands (95% confidence interval)

	ADRs in Patients While in Hospital	ADRs Responsible for Patient Admission to a Hospital	Total ADRs
All severities	3670 (2618-4596)	1547 (1033-2060)	4987 (3976-5995)
Serious	702 (635-770)	1547 (1033-2060)	2216 (1721-2711)
Fatal	63 (41-85)	43 (15-71)	106 (76-137)

Redrawn from Lazarou J, Pomeranz BH, Corey PN. Incidence of adverse drug reactions in hospitalized patients: a meta-analysis of prospective studies. JAMA 1998;279:1200-5.[75] Reproduced with the permission of the American Medical Association.

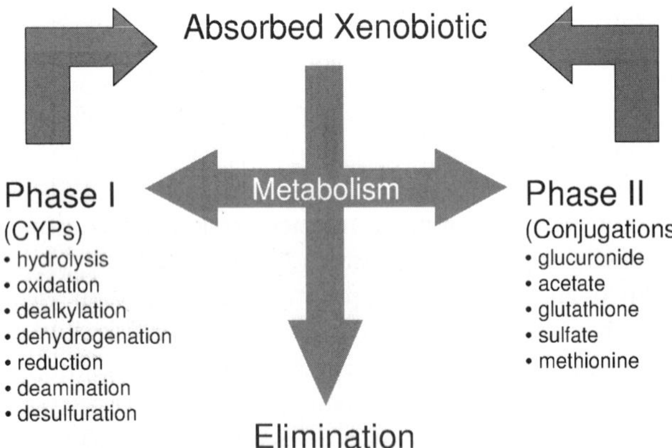

Figure 43-1 Simplified scheme of the primary metabolic reactions associated with xenobiotic handling in humans. Absorbed xenobiotics (drugs or other exogenous compounds) may be eliminated without biotransformation or be transformed into a metabolite through Phase I and/or Phase II reactions. The metabolite may be further metabolized by Phase I or Phase II reactions before elimination. Phase I reactions are primarily oxidative and are most commonly mediated by cytochrome P450 (CYP) isozymes. Phase II reactions involve conjugations to form glucuronides, acetates, and other adducts.

testing is of particular usefulness for those drugs that require a long period of time to establish efficacy or to optimize dose. Advocates of pharmacogenetics anticipate that future testing opportunities will include the ability to identify a population of nonresponders for a particular drug. Examples of drug classes likely to benefit from pharmacogenetic testing include cancer chemotherapeutics, immunosuppressants, antidepressants, antipsychotics, anticoagulants, antihypertensives, cardiac medications, and lipid-lowering therapies.

In general, drug metabolism serves to inactivate a substrate and increase water solubility of the substrate for excretion, bioactivate a substrate or prodrug (e.g., codeine and cyclophosphamide) to an active or mutagenic principle, or less commonly, extend the elimination half-life of a pharmacologically active or potentially toxic metabolite.[40,102] Metabolic reactions are often divided into Phase I and Phase II categories, as depicted in Figure 43-1.

Phase I reactions convert the parent compound into a more polar metabolite by introducing or removing a single functional group. Examples include oxidation, reduction, and hydrolysis. Most Phase I reactions are oxidative and are mediated by cytochrome P450 isozymes (CYPs). CYPs are heme-containing enzymes that are synthesized from a superfamily of *CYP* genes and are classified into families, and further into subfamilies, based on amino acid homology. The primary *CYPs* that are believed to contribute to drug metabolism are *CYP1A2, CYP2B6, CYP2C9, CYP2C19, CYP2D6, CYP2E1,* and the *CYP3A* family. All of these *CYP* families exhibit genetic variation that has been associated with clinically significant phenotypical differences caused by changes in enzyme activity, stability, and/or substrate affinity. In addition to the genetic variability, many CYP isoenzymes are susceptible to dramatic differences in expression (>1000-fold), caused in part by induction or inhibition mediated by substrates. Products of Phase I reactions may be eliminated or undergo additional modification, such as through Phase II reactions. Phase II reactions may occur independent of, or before, Phase I reactions.

Phase II enzymes are generally transferases involving enzyme-mediated conjugation with acetyl, glucuronyl, amino acid, or sulfate groups. These enzymes are not typically induced or inhibited to the same degree as CYPs. However, exhausting the substrates or cofactors for transfer, such as glutathione or acetyl-CoA, will prevent the corresponding transferase reactions from occurring.[40,102,110]

APPROACHES TO PHARMACOGENETIC TESTING

Pharmacogenetics is important to patient care because for many drugs there are interindividual differences in drug metabolism and drug response. These differences significantly alter the safety and success of therapy. Pharmacogenetic testing allows the physician to predict that a patient is likely to fail therapy or suffer an ADR before initiating therapy. This knowledge can lead to a change in drug dosage or drug selection, thus avoiding an undesired outcome.

Two major approaches are available to predict how well an individual will metabolize a medication: phenotyping

TABLE 43-2 Comparing Phenotype and Genotype Testing Strategies

	Phenotype	Genotype
Represents	"State," represents current response; may not represent inheritance	"Trait," represents inheritance; may not be consistent with the phenotype
Sensitive to gene expression	Yes	No
Sensitive to protein function	Yes	No
Requires collection of multiple specimens	Commonly	No
Requires administration of a probe drug	Commonly	No
Other limitations	Specimen instability for enzyme or other protein of interest may lead to inaccurate results	May not include all clinically relevant genes and/or alleles
	May not be appropriate for a patient who recently received a blood transfusion	Genotype to phenotype relationship (interpretation) may not be known

and genotyping. Phenotyping is accomplished by testing metabolic activity—either by administering the patient a safe drug, often called a probe drug, that is known to be metabolized by the same enzyme or pathway as the intended therapeutic drug, or alternatively, by measuring the drug metabolizing enzyme activity using peripheral blood cells as a surrogate to the metabolism of the whole patient.[89] Examples of probe drugs include dextromethorphan for assessing CYP2D6 activity and caffeine for NAT2. Examples of enzyme-based phenotyping tests that have been successfully implemented include pseudocholinesterase, for detecting individuals with susceptibility to prolonged apnea when given succinylcholine or other similar medications; thiopurine S-methyltransferase (TPMT), for detecting individuals with susceptibility to hematological toxicity with azathioprine (AZA) or 6-mercaptopurine (6-MP); and glucose-6-phosphate dehydrogenase (G6PD), for detecting susceptibility to hemolysis in response to drugs such as primaquine, sulfonamides, chloramphenicol, and vitamin K. These techniques directly measure drug metabolism phenotype and, under highly controlled circumstances, provide the most meaningful information. There are, however, several limitations to the phenotypical approach. For example, the probe compound must be easy to administer in the target population, be relatively inexpensive, and exhibit pharmacokinetics that support convenient collection of specimens from the patient. Even with these variables controlled, phenotyping may be difficult to accomplish because of other potentially confounding factors, such as diet, co-medications, recent blood transfusion, consumption of alcohol or over-the-counter medications, and disease status. The length of time required to perform the associated phenotyping assays may also complicate and compromise the value of direct phenotyping. Many enzymes are expressed in higher quantities in neonates. In a study of 60 full-term newborns, TPMT activity was >50% higher than in race-matched healthy adults, but displayed the same trimodal distribution observed in adults.[90] Thus phenotyping illustrates the "state" rather than the "trait."

Pharmacogenetics, that is genotyping, is the second major approach to predicting drug metabolism and drug response. Pharmacogenetics may be useful for predicting pharmacodynamic response by identifying inherited genetic characteristics that either account for differences in phenotype from a structural basis or are clearly associated with phenotype through rigorous clinical studies. Neither phenotyping nor pharmacogenetic testing is intended to replace the need for clinical assessments of drug response, or replace the need for therapeutic drug monitoring (TDM). Several considerations of these two testing approaches are summarized in Table 43-2. Examples of both approaches will be given throughout this chapter; however, more emphasis is given to the pharmacogenetic approaches because of the recognition of the growing evidence supporting genotyping as a superior means of classifying enzymatic capacity. That evidence includes the facts that genotyping assays are less expensive, are more reproducible between laboratories, are not subject to the intraindividual variability because of a specific set of clinical conditions or expected biological variations (i.e., hormonal fluctuations[65]) that complicate phenotyping assays, and are less invasive (i.e., a single blood sample for genotyping; several samples for phenotyping). It is estimated, for example, that genotyping of *CYP2D6* can reliably predict the phenotype 80% to 90% of the time.

Although genotyping has many advantages over phenotyping, there are limitations to genotyping that must be recognized. For example, some of the assays using target amplification are prone to false negatives because they rely on the presence or absence of a polymerase chain reaction (PCR) product. Short of sequencing the entire gene, currently available genotyping techniques cannot detect all possible variants. Because of the large amount of variation in many genes, suites of variants are screened, potentially missing some important genetic variations because the patient possesses a rare or novel polymorphism that is not detected by the screen.[108] Further, polymorphisms with unknown clinical significance may also be identified by some techniques. Extreme care must be taken to ensure that these data are not misinterpreted.

Another disadvantage of genotyping is that it may not accurately predict function of the expressed protein. Continuing to use *CYP2D6* as an example, it has been shown that patients of a single common genotype have dextromethorphan to debrisoquine ratios (metabolic phenotypes) that span a 1000- to 10,000-fold range. The precise reason for this broad range is unknown but it is probably related to individual differences in expression of the *CYP2D6* gene, inherent alternative metabolic pathways, significant interlaboratory and intraindividual variability in phenotype measurements, and possible combinations of other minor undetected genetic polymorphisms in the *CYP2D6* gene.[130]

Finally, specific interactions between the target enzyme or protein and other drugs, chemicals, or some foods can change the phenotype, such as by converting a "normal" or extensive metabolizer phenotype to a poor metabolizer phenotype. For example, grapefruit juice has been shown to inhibit CYP3A4,[57,78,105] and many antidepressant medications (e.g., tricyclic and selective serotonin reuptake inhibitors) are known to act as both substrates and inhibitors of CYP2D6.[7,110] Such drug and food interactions can have extremely important consequences for patients and can be difficult to both recognize and monitor.

CLINICAL APPLICATION OF PHARMACOGENETIC TESTING

Pharmacogenetic testing is only clinically useful when there is sufficient information to interpret the results. This information must be derived from in vivo, human studies demonstrating a clear phenotype. Many examples of this type of information can be found in the peer-reviewed literature, but most data are based on retrospective studies, and there is no single printed source in which all of this information has been collated. The Pharmacogenetics and Pharmacogenomics Knowledge Base[6] is a publicly available internet research tool developed by Stanford University with funding from the National Institutes of Health (NIH) and is part of the NIH Pharmacogenetics Research Network (PGRN), a nationwide collaborative research consortium. Its aim is to aid researchers in understanding how genetic variation among individuals contributes to differences in reactions to drugs. This regularly updated database provides genetic and clinical information derived from research studies at various medical centers in the PGRN.

Currently published dosing guidelines relate to specific combinations of pharmacogenetic markers and drugs. For example, Kirchheiner et al have published dose recommendations for 20 antidepressant medications based on single versus chronic maintenance therapy and genotypes for both *CYP2D6* and *CYP2C19*.[70] Average recommended adjustments of "standard" doses vary from 20% of the usual dose for poor metabolizers using venlafaxine, paroxetine, or desipramine to 300% of the usual dose for ultrarapid metabolizers using mianserin. Similar work suggesting specific dose ranges or adjustments based on phenotype-genotype relationships has been conducted with other substrates of these CYP isoenzymes (see CYP2D6 and CYP2C19 sections later in this chapter), AZA and 6-MP (see TPMT section of this chapter), warfarin (see CYP2C9 section of this chapter), and antipsychotics.[71]

Many ongoing clinical trials for efficacy and toxicity of new pharmaceutical products or new indications for previously developed pharmaceuticals have employed pharmacogenetic testing. Thus it is anticipated that pharmacogenetic guidelines and possibly tests will be simultaneously released to market with the pharmaceutical. In addition, medications that were previously removed from development because of adverse reactions may be reconsidered if a genetic test can be demonstrated to identify individuals at high risk for ADRs.

BEST EXAMPLES OF CLINICALLY RELEVANT PHARMACOGENETIC TARGETS

For each of six genes, *TPMT, CYP2D6, CYP2C19, CYP2C9, NAT1,* and *NAT2,* this chapter provides an overview of background information, the relationship between genotype and phenotype, unique testing methods, and clinical applications of testing.

THIOPURINE S-METHYLTRANSFERASE

TPMT is a Phase II metabolic enzyme that catalyzes the inactivation of 6-MP by S-methylation, thus preventing it from forming thioguanine nucleotides (TGN).[5,116] TPMT also affects AZA, which is a prodrug metabolized to 6-MP, as shown in Figure 43-2. Endogenous substrates for TPMT are currently unknown. AZA and 6-MP are used in the therapeutic management of a diverse range of conditions, including leukemia, rheumatic diseases, inflammatory bowel disease, and solid organ transplantation. These agents are cytotoxic, acting via incorporation of TGN into DNA. Outside of the bone marrow, these agents can be oxidatively inactivated by xanthine oxidase or methylated by TPMT. In hematopoietic tissue, however, the effect of xanthine oxidase is negligible, leaving TPMT as the only significant inactivation pathway. Thus hematopoietic tissues are susceptible to damage in cases in which TPMT activity is very low. TPMT activity is highly variable in all large populations studied to date; approximately 90% of individuals have high activity, 10% have immediate activity, and 0.3% have low or undetectable enzyme activity. This tri-modal activity is a direct result of enhanced proteasomal degradation of TPMT.[124]

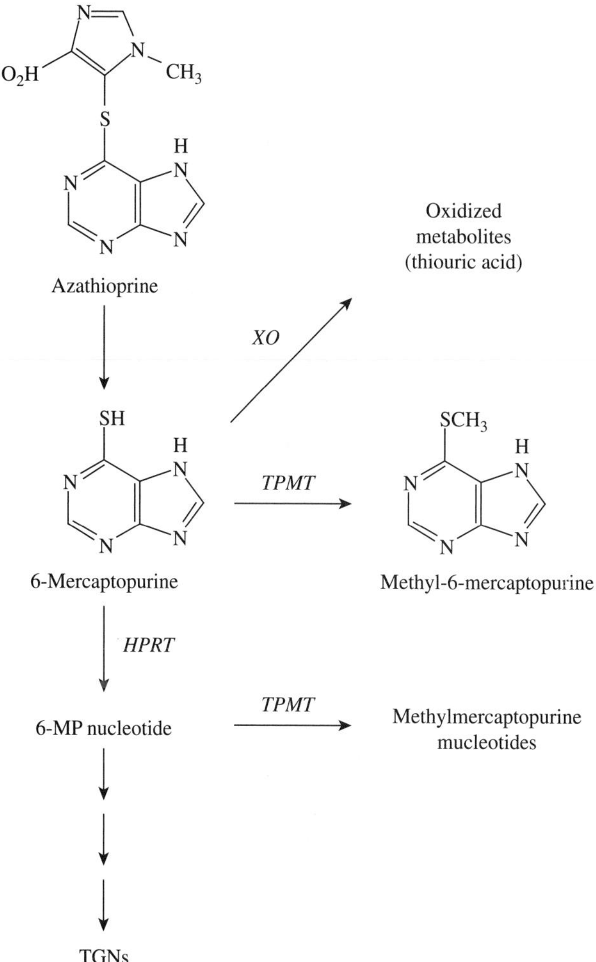

Figure 43-2 Simplified scheme of the metabolism of azathioprine and 6-mercaptopurine to 6-thioguanine nucleotides (TGNs). *TPMT,* Thiopurine S-methyltransferase; *XO,* xanthine oxidase; *HPRT,* hypoxanthine phosphoribosyltransferase. *(Redrawn from Clunie GP, Lennard L. Relevance of thiopurine methyltransferase status in rheumatology patients receiving azathioprine. Rheumatology (Oxford) 2004;43:13-8.*[23] *Reproduced by permission from Oxford University Press.)*

Numerous studies have shown that TPMT-deficient patients are at high risk for severe, and sometimes fatal, hematological toxicity.

Genotype to Phenotype

The molecular basis for variable TPMT activity has now been defined for the majority of patients.[92] TPMT activity is inherited as an autosomal co-dominant trait,[133] exhibiting genetic polymorphism in all populations studied to date. Eleven *TPMT* alleles have been identified, including nine single nucleotide polymorphisms (SNPs) leading to amino acid substitutions, *TPMT*2, *3A, *3B, *3C, *3D, *5, *6, *7, *8;* one change leading to the formation of a stop codon, *TPMT*3D;* and a change that destroys a splice site: *TPMT*4.* Three alleles, *TPMT*2, *3A,* and **3C,* account for about 95% of intermediate or low enzyme activity cases (Figure 43-3). All three alleles associated with lower enzyme activity have

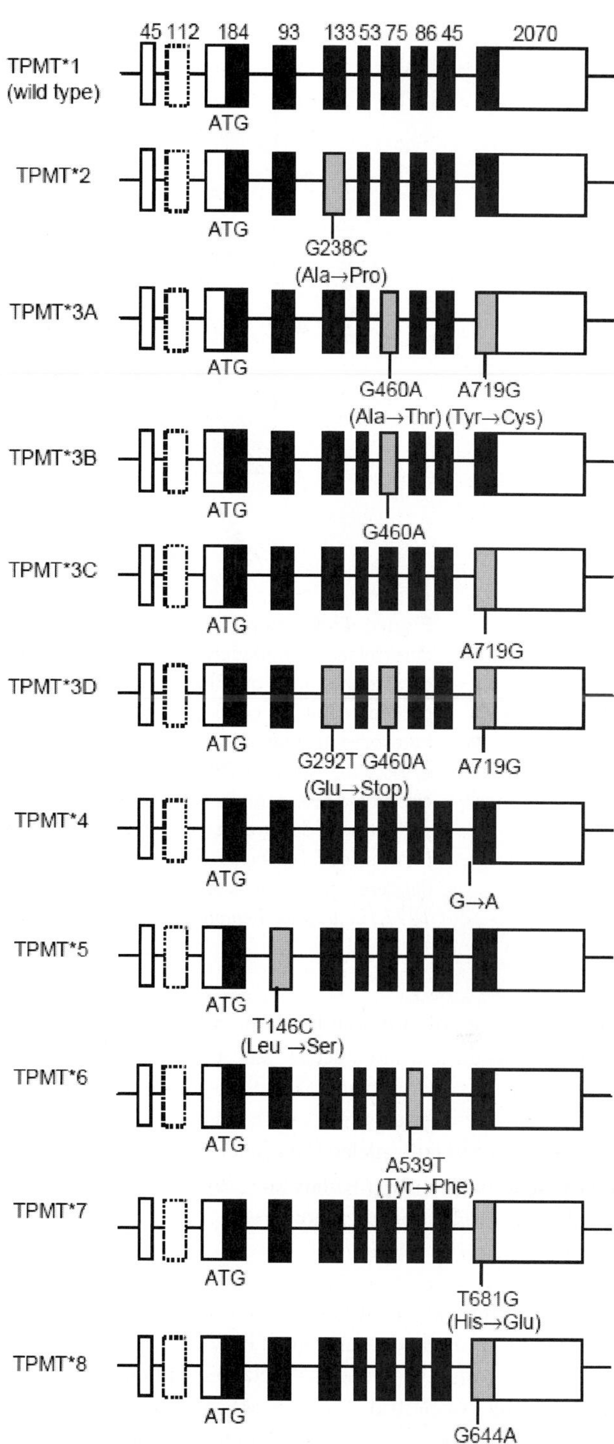

Figure 43-3 Thiopurine S-methyltransferase *(TPMT)* allele variants. Gray boxes represent mutations that result in amino acid changes. TPMT*4 is a 5′ splice site mutation for exon 10 that does not alter an amino acid. White boxes represent untranslated regions. Black boxes represent exons in the open reading frame. The dashed box represents exon 2, which was detected in 6.25% of human liver cDNAs during initial evaluation. *(From McLeod HL, Siva C. The thiopurine S-methyltransferase gene locus—implications for clinical pharmacogenomics. Pharmacogenomics 2002;3:89-98. Reproduced by permission from Future Medicine Ltd [London].)*

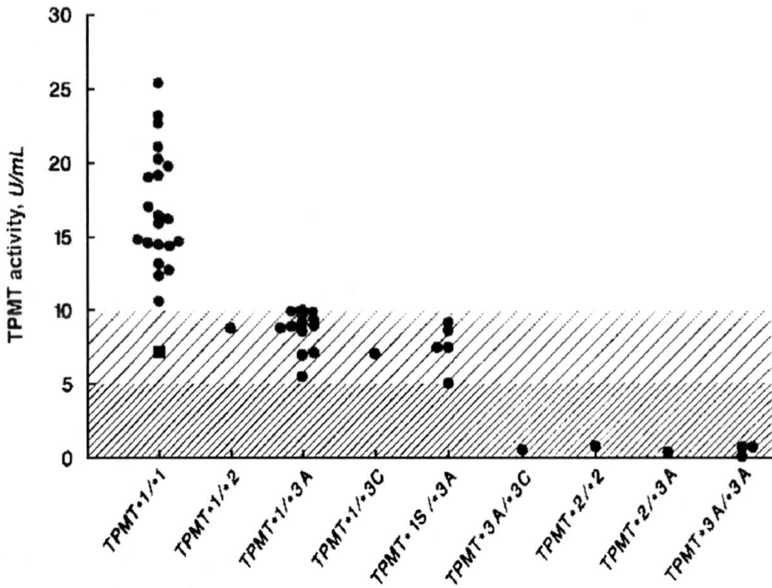

Figure 43-4 Thiopurine S-methyltransferase (TPMT) activity as related to genotypes determined by mutation-specific polymerase chain reaction methods. The heavily shaded area depicts the range of TPMT activity in erythrocytes that defines TPMT deficiency (<5 U/mL of packed red blood cells), the lightly shaded area depicts intermediate activity that defines TPMT heterozygous phenotypes (5 to 10 U/mL of packed red blood cells), and the nonshaded area depicts the range of TPMT activity in patients who have homozygous wild-type phenotypes. Black circles indicate patients with concordant genotype and phenotype; the black square indicates one patient with discordant genotype and phenotype *(TPMT*1/*1). (From Yates CR, Krynetski EY, Loennechen T, Fessing MY, Tai HL, Pui CH, et al. Molecular diagnosis of thiopurine S-methyltransferase deficiency: genetic basis for azathioprine and mercaptopurine intolerance. Ann Intern Med 1997;126:608-14. Reproduced by permission from the American College of Physicians.)*

enhanced rates of proteolysis of the alloenzymes (protein products of the variant alleles). The presence of a *TPMT* variant allele is 90% sensitive and 99% specific for predicting TPMT phenotype; patients with one wild-type allele and one of these variant alleles (i.e., heterozygous) have intermediate activity and patients inheriting two variant alleles are TPMT deficient (see Figure 43-4).[112]

Testing

TPMT testing may occur via at least three routes: biochemical phenotyping by determining TPMT activity within erythrocytes from the patient; metabolic phenotyping by determining concentrations of 6-MP and thioguanine; or genotyping. Biochemical phenotyping depends on stable enzyme activity between the times of blood collection and analytical testing. This approach is therefore challenged by storage and stability concerns and is limited to patients who have not received a blood transfusion over the weeks previous to TPMT testing. Metabolic phenotyping requires that AZA or 6-MP be administered before testing. This approach is therefore most useful for patients who have experienced an adverse event or for monitoring therapy in those for which TPMT activity is known to be impaired. *TPMT* genotype correlates well with TPMT activity in leukemia cells, as would be expected for germline mutations. By using PCR-based assays to detect the three signature mutations in these alleles, a rapid and relatively inexpensive assay may identify >90% of all variant alleles. In Caucasian populations, *TPMT*3A* is the most common variant *TPMT* allele (3.2% to 5.7% of *TPMT* alleles), although *TPMT*3C* has an allele frequency of 0.2% to 0.8% and *TPMT*2* represents 0.2% to 0.5% of *TPMT* alleles.[2,24,104] Studies in Caucasian, African, and Asian populations have revealed that the frequency of these variant *TPMT* alleles differs among various ethnic populations. East and West African populations have a frequency of variant alleles similar to Caucasians, but the variant alleles in the African populations were predominantly *TPMT*3C*.[2] Among African-Americans, *TPMT*3C* is the most prevalent allele, but *TPMT*2* and *TPMT*3A* are also found, reflecting the integration of Caucasian and African-American genes in the U.S. population.[58] In Japanese and Chinese populations, *TPMT*3C* is almost exclusively the causative variant allele.[24,73,74,84] In other Asian populations, the *TPMT*3C* is also predominant, but the *3A* and *6* alleles have also been observed in Indian and Malay children, respectively.[84]

Genotyping tests, however, may not detect TPMT deficiency in all patients, particularly those with a rare or unknown but clinically significant variant. Compound heterozygotes also present a challenge to PCR-based genetic testing in this gene. For example patients with the heterozygous genotype *TPMT*1/*3A* have a 35% risk of hematopoietic toxicity versus a 7% risk for patients with homozygous wild-type genotype. Alternatively, patients with the *TPMT*3B/*3C* genotype are TPMT-deficient and are at very high risk for thiopurine toxicity. These genotypes are impossible to distinguish when using conventional PCR genotyping.[18] The *TPMT*3B* allele is very rare (<1% of variant alleles); however, its presence can have grave clinical consequences. A haplotyping method has been published that discriminates *TPMT*1/*3A* from *TPMT*3B/*3C* using genomic DNA.[88]

Clinical Application

TPMT was the first widely used pharmacogenetic marker for individualizing drug therapy based on a patient's biochemical phenotype (erythrocyte enzyme activity) or genotype. Patients with a "low methylator" status (homozygous variant or compound heterozygote) may tolerate standard doses, but are at significantly greater risk of toxicity, often necessitating a lower dose of these medications (as low as 5% of standard doses). Prospective determination of functional TPMT status is useful for preventing mercaptopurine toxicity.[23,116] Whether TPMT testing is based on phenotype or genotype, the goal is individualized dosing, and controlled systemic exposure.[33]

An analysis of mercaptopurine therapy for childhood acute lymphocytic leukemia (ALL) found that TPMT-deficient patients tolerated full doses of mercaptopurines for only a brief period (7% of the scheduled weeks of therapy), whereas heterozygous and homozygous wild-type patients tolerated full doses for 65% and 84% of scheduled weeks of therapy during the 2½ years of treatment, respectively. The percentage of weeks in which mercaptopurine dosage had to be decreased to prevent toxicity was 2%, 16%, and 76% in wild-type, heterozygous, and homozygous variant individuals. Collectively, these studies demonstrate that the influence of *TPMT* genotype on hematopoietic toxicity is most dramatic for homozygous variant patients, but is also of clinical relevance for heterozygous individuals, which represent about 10% of patients treated with these medications.

A potentially valuable role for TPMT status testing is before intravenous AZA loading, a strategy shown to be safe in the management of Crohn's disease. Dose-related toxicities resulted in AZA discontinuation in 10% to 20% of cases, and it was estimated that over 6 months, 20% of patients would need TPMT analysis to avoid one serious adverse event. TPMT status testing before taking AZA has been modeled to be cost-effective in a variety of theoretical situations. Analysis of some recent studies suggests that by optimizing the maximum AZA dose between 0.75 and 3 mg/kg/day depending on TPMT status testing (with a drastic reduction in dosage for patients homozygous for variant *TPMT* alleles), considerable cost savings can be made by avoiding hospitalization and rescue therapy for leukopenic events.[86,126,129] Furthermore, one study reported that the median dose reduction required for TPMT-deficient patients was 90.8% (range, 50% to 94%) and median dose reduction in *TPMT* heterozygotes of 67% (range, 0% to 93%).[34] This study included only patients referred for hematopoietic toxicity. However, previous studies have reported that heterozygous patients needed only 15% to 30% dose reduction to avoid serious side effects.[109]

Although detection of *TPMT* polymorphisms is thought to prospectively identify approximately 10% of patients likely to experience dose-limiting toxicity from AZA and 6-MP therapy, toxicity is estimated to occur in 15%-28% of patients. Thus, toxicity related to thiopurine therapeutics cannot be explained by known *TPMT* polymorphisms alone. Cao and Hegele have described an inosine triphosphate (ITPA)–deficient phenotype that may provide an additional mechanism for thiopurine-related toxicity.[20] This phenotype, like TPMT deficiency, is clinically benign until a patient is exposed to a thiopurine therapeutic such as 6-MP or AZA. The ITPA deficiency phenotype is associated with a 94C>A polymorphism of *ITPA*, and approximately 25% residual red cell ITPase activity. Consequently, the metabolite 6-thio-ITP accumulates and may contribute to toxicities previously associated only with TPMT deficiency. Although currently not well characterized, determination of genotypes for *TPMT, ITPA*, and potentially other genes may form the best strategy for predicting risk of adverse reactions associated with AZA and 6-MP therapy.

Cytochrome P450 2D6 (CYP2D6)

Cytochrome P450 2D6 (CYP2D6), originally named debrisoquine hydroxylase, is a Phase I enzyme known to metabolize more than 100 drugs and environmental toxins as substrates.[42,110] Examples of drugs and drug classes metabolized by CYP2D6 are shown in Table 43-3. CYP2D6 is also inhibited by several compounds, some of which are substrates. More than 80 genetic variants have been described in the *CYP2D6* gene.[5] In general the variants can be grouped according to the resulting alterations in protein function. These groupings correlate well with the four major phenotypes described historically for CYP2D6: extensive (normal) metabolizers (EM), poor metabolizers (PM), intermediate metabolizers (IM), and ultrafast or rapid metabolizers (UM). The major coding sequence variants described result in decreased function with the exception of gene duplication, which results in increased metabolic capacity if a functional gene has been duplicated.[141] Of Caucasians, approximately 5% are UM, and 5% to 10% are PM. Only 1% to 3% of African-Americans and Asians are PM, but many are IM.

Genotype to Phenotype

The relationship between the CYP2D6 enzyme metabolic rate (phenotype) and the *CYP2D6* genotype has been extensively characterized.[1,76,98,103,111] Genetic variability accounts for the tetra-modal distribution of CYP2D6 activity described historically by the phenotypes. The rank order of

TABLE 43-3 Drug Substrates, Inhibitors, and Inducers of Cytochrome P450 Subfamilies

1A2	2B6	2C19	2C9	2D6	2E1	3A4/5/7
Substrates						
Clozapine	Buproprion	Proton pump	NSAIDs:	Beta blockers:	Acetaminophen	Macrolide
Cyclobenzaprine	Cyclophosphamide	inhibitors:	Diclofenac	S-metoprolol	Chlorzoxazone	antibiotics:
Imipramine	Efavirenz	Omeprazole	Ibuprofen	Propafenone	Ethanol	Clarithromycin
Mexiletine	Ifosfamide	Lansoprazole	Piroxicam	Timolol		Erythromycin
Naproxen	Methadone	Pantoprazole	Oral	Antidepressants:		not Azithromycin
Riluzole		Antiepileptics:	hypoglycemic	Amitriptyline		Telithromycin
Tacrine		Diazepam	agents:	Clomipramine		Antiarrhythmics:
Theophylline		Phenytoin	Tolbutamide	Desipramine		Quinidine
		Phenobarbitone	Glipizide	Imipramine		Benzodiazepines:
		Amitriptyline	Angiotensin II	Paroxetine		Alprazolam
		Clomipramine	blockers:	Antipsychotics:		Diazepam
		Cyclophosphamide	not Irbesartan	Haloperidol		Midazolam
		Progesterone	Losartan	Risperidone		Triazolam
			Candesartan	Thioridazine		Immune modulators:
			not Valsartan	Codeine		Cyclosporine
			Celecoxib	Dextromethorphan		Tacrolimus
			Fluvastatin	Flecainide		(FK506)
			Naproxen	Mexiletine		HIV protease
			Phenytoin	Ondansetron		inhibitors:
			Sulfamethoxazole	Tamoxifen		Indinavir
			Tamoxifen	Tramadol		Ritonavir
			Tolbutamide	Venlafaxine		Saquinavir
			Torsemide			Prokinetic:
			Warfarin			Cisapride
						Antihistamines:
						Astemizole
						Chlorpheniramine
						Calcium channel
						blockers:
						Amlodipine
						Diltiazem
						Felodipine
						Nifedipine
						Nisoldipine
						Nitrendipine
						Verapamil
						HMG CoA reductase
						inhibitors:
						Atorvastatin
						Cerivastatin
						Lovastatin
						not Pravastatin
						Simvastatin
						Buspirone
						Haloperidol
						Methadone
						Pimozide
						Quinine
						not Rosuvastatin
						Sildenafil
						Tamoxifen
						Trazodone
						Vincristine

TABLE 43-3 Drug Substrates, Inhibitors, and Inducers of Cytochrome P450 Subfamilies—cont'd

1A2	2B6	2C19	2C9	2D6	2E1	3A4/5/7
Inhibitors						
Cimetidine	Thiotepa	Fluoxetine	Amiodarone	Amiodarone	Disulfiram	HIV protease inhibitors:
Fluoroquinolones		Fluvoxamine	Fluconazole	Chlorpheniramine		Indinavir
Fluvoxamine		Ketoconazole	Isoniazid	Cimetidine		Nelfinavir
Ticlopidine		Lansoprazole	Ticlopidine	Clomipramine		Ritonavir
		Omeprazole		Fluoxetine		Saquinavir
		Ticlopidine		Haloperidol		Amiodarone
				Methadone		not Azithromycin
				Mibefradil		Cimetidine
				Paroxetine		Clarithromycin
				Quinidine		Diltiazem
				Ritonavir		Erythromycin
						Fluoxetine
						Fluvoxamine
						Grapefruit juice
						Itraconazole
						Ketoconazole
						Mibefradil
						Nefazodone
						Troleandomycin
						Verapamil
Inducers						
Tobacco	Phenobarbital	N/A	Rifampin	N/A	Ethanol	Carbamazepine
	Rifampin		Secobarbital		Isoniazid	Phenobarbital
						Phenytoin
						Rifabutin
						Rifampin
						St. John's wort
						Troglitazone

From Flockhart DA. Clinically relevant drug interaction table. This table is updated frequently. http://medicine.iupui.edu/flockhart/table.htm (Accessed August 30, 2004).[36] Reproduced with the permission of David A. Flockhart, M.D., Ph.D.

metabolic capacity is ultrarapid metabolizers (UM) > extensive metabolizers (EM) > intermediate metabolizers (IM) > poor metabolizers (PM), representing approximately 5% to 7%, 60%, 25%, and 10% of most populations, respectively. A summary of *CYP2D6* alleles and consequences is shown in Figure 43-5.

CYP2D6 phenotypes have historically been determined through the use of probe drugs. Urine collected at a specified time after administration of the probe drug (e.g., 8 hours) is analyzed for the parent drug and a metabolite that is primarily generated via CYP2D6. The ratio of parent and metabolite concentrations is referred to as the metabolic ratio (MR). Example parent-metabolite pairs used commonly as probe drugs for CYP2D6 include dextromethorphan/dextrorphan, debrisoquine/4-hydroxydebrisoquine, and nortriptyline/10-hydroxynortriptyline. The need to administer a probe drug and to collect urine over several hours has always limited the practical utility of patient phenotyping. Although the MR is theoretically a good indicator of enzyme expression and function at the time of the test, marked variation has been demonstrated in this phenotypical characteristic for nearly every *CYP2D6* genotype (see Figure 43-6).[22] Interpretation of MRs must consider the specificity of the probe drug for the CYP2D6 and also the elimination kinetics of the parent and metabolite.

Testing

The *CYP2D6* gene is relatively challenging to genotype because of the presence of pseudogenes and also because of the need for identification of gene dose, specifically duplications and deletions of the gene. *CYP2D6* pharmacogenetic screening protocols may detect only the most common variants. For example, testing for 7 variants in the gene is estimated to predict the CYP2D6 phenotype with >95% reliability.[81]

To separate *CYP2D6* from structurally similar pseudogenes, *CYP2D6* genotyping protocols often employ long-PCR or nested PCR strategies with a first PCR step

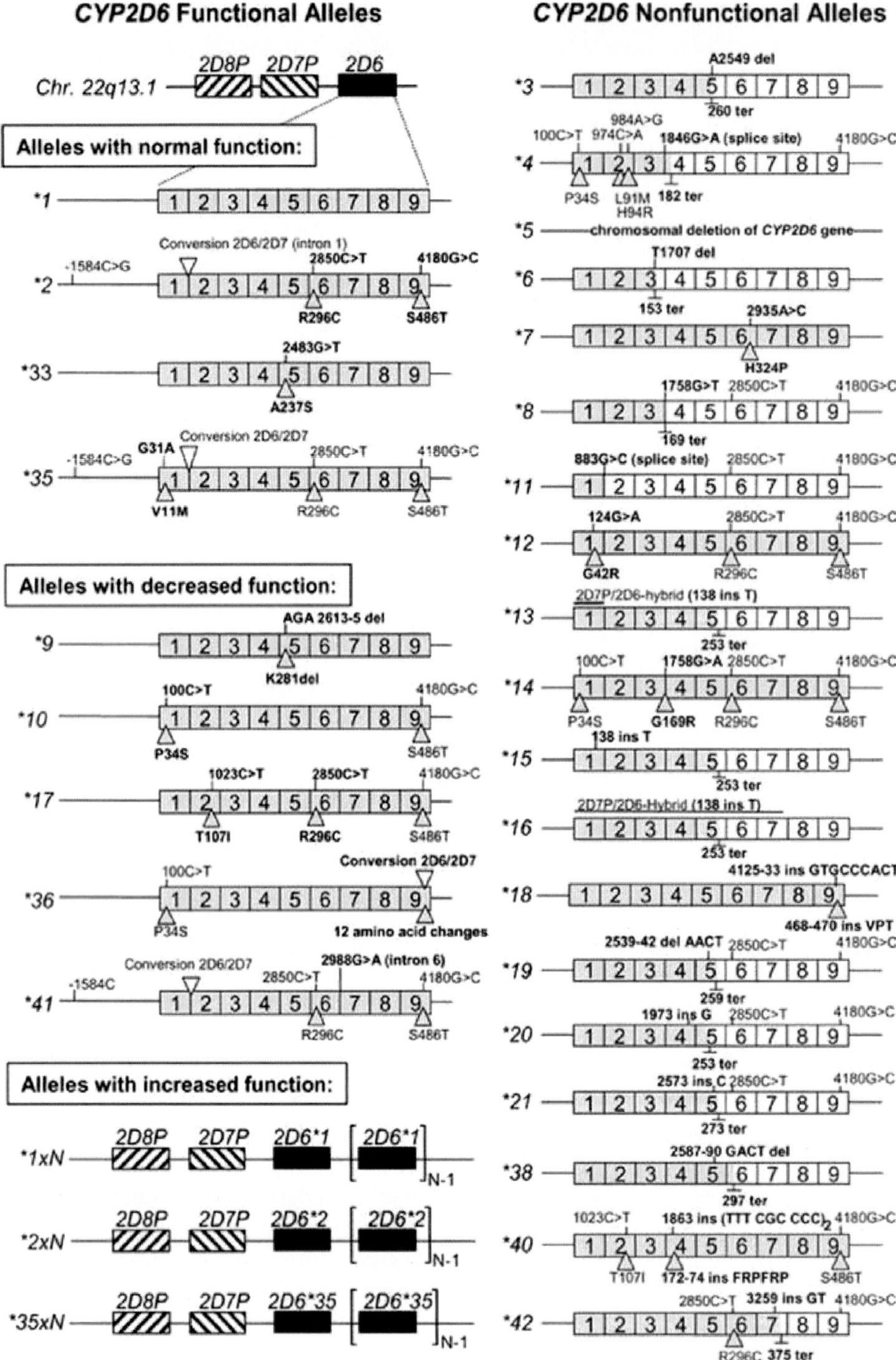

Figure 43-5 Structure of functional and nonfunctional *CYP2D6* alleles. Only alleles with available phenotypical information are shown. The 9 exons are indicated by numbered boxes with DNA polymorphisms indicated on top (*del*, deletion, *ins*, insertion). Predicted amino acid changes and translation termination *(ter)* codons are indicated below. Open reading frames are indicated by shaded boxes. Silent mutations and some promoter and intronic polymorphisms and alleles with uncertain function are not shown. *(From Zanger UM, Raimundo S, Eichelbaum M. Cytochrome P450 2D6: overview and update on pharmacology, genetics, biochemistry. Naunyn Schmiedebergs Arch Pharmacol 2004;369:23-37. Reproduced by permission from Springer.)*

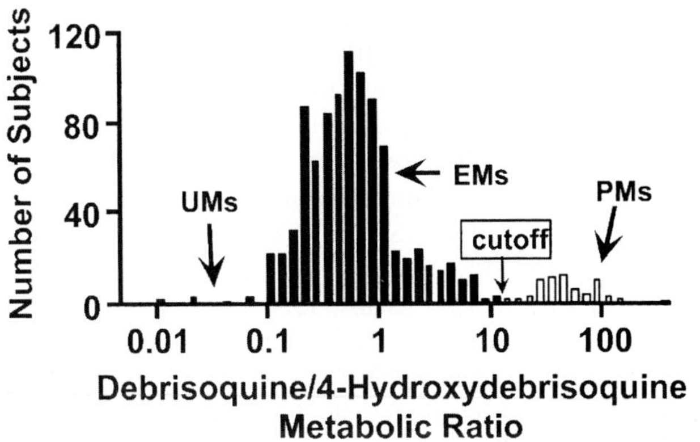

Figure 43-6 Histogram of the "debrisoquine metabolic ratio" in a typical Caucasian population. Metabolic ratios were determined from the concentrations of debrisoquine and 4-hydroxydebrisoquine (metabolite) in a urine specimen collected 8 hours after a 10 mg dose of debrisoquine. The data demonstrate a clear distinction between PM, EM, and UM phenotypes. *(From Caldwell J. Pharmacogenetics and individual variation in the range of amino acid adequacy: the biological aspects. J Nutr 2004;134:1600S-4S; discussion 30S-32S, 67S-72S. Reproduced by permission from the American Society for Nutritional Sciences.)*

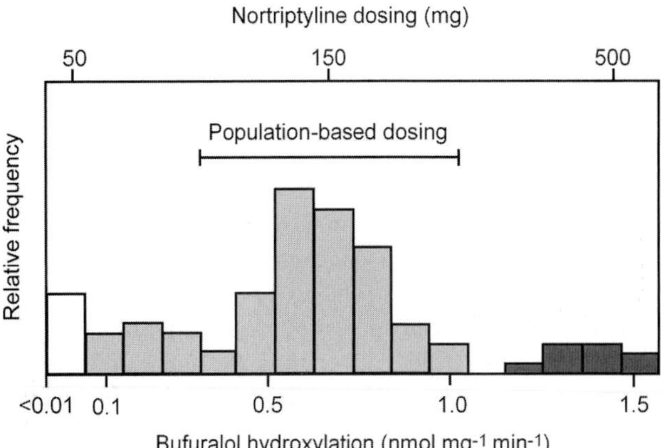

Figure 43-7 Variation in drug metabolism and nortriptyline dosing in the European population, based on cytochrome P450 CYP2D6 activity (hydroxylation of bufuralol). Within the population four phenotypes can be identified: poor metabolizers (PMs), who lack the functional enzyme; intermediary metabolizers (IMs), who are heterozygous for one functional allele or have two partially defective alleles encoding the enzyme; extensive metabolizers (EMs), who have two normal alleles; and ultrarapid metabolizers (UMs), who carry duplicated or multiduplicated functional *CYP2D6* genes. The relative frequency of these phenotypes refers to the European population as a whole. The doses of nortriptyline that are required to achieve therapeutic levels in all phenotypes are given. Despite this variation in metabolizing capability, population-based dosing is used today, and is based on the average plasma levels obtained in a given population for a given dose. *(From Ingelman-Sundberg M. Pharmacogenetics of cytochrome P450 and its applications in drug therapy: the past, present and future. Trends Pharmacol Sci 2004;25:193-200. Reproduced by permission from Elsevier.)*

designed to amplify a large *CYP2D6*-specific region.[50] Small nucleotide changes within this region, including SNPs and smaller insertions/deletions of one or a few bases, are then detected in a second amplification step either designed as a PCR-restriction fragment length polymorphism (RFLP) assay or as an allele-specific PCR without subsequent digestion.[26,38,47,111,122] By evaluating the entire gene, such as through the use of the single-strand conformation polymorphism technique described by Broly et al., both known and unknown mutations in the *CYP2D6* gene can be detected.[16,84] Other technologies used for genotyping *CYP2D6* include real-time PCR methods and microarrays.[22,56,99,101] Gene deletion events necessarily give rise to duplication or multiduplication alleles in a population. The duplicated gene can be either functional, for example *CYP2D6*1, CYP2D6*2*, or *CYP2D6*35* alleles, or nonfunctional, e.g., *CYP2D6*4*. These duplicated genes can be detected either by appropriate RFLP assays, by using one of several available long-product PCR assays, by microarray, or by real-time quantitative PCR of *CYP2D6* in relation to an internal reference gene, such as albumin.[64,82,113,143]

Clinical Applications

CYP2D6 metabolic status can be applied to prescribing of medications, which are known to be transformed by this enzyme. Such medications may be avoided entirely, or the dose can be optimized based on how CYP2D6 affects the drug. For example, many therapeutic drugs are administered as prodrugs. Prodrugs must be metabolized to the active principle to elicit the desired therapeutic effect. An example is codeine, an alkaloid obtained from opium or prepared from morphine by methylation. Codeine must be activated, through metabolism mediated primarily by CYP2D6, to morphine to produce analgesia. Therefore, a CYP2D6 PM could not activate codeine like an EM would, and may not experience analgesia with standard doses. Thus a PM may be best served clinically by selecting a different analgesic agent. An IM is likely to require higher doses of codeine than an EM, and a UM may require lower doses of codeine than an EM.

Most drugs, however, are inactivated by CYP2D6. For example, nortriptyline (NT) and other antidepressant medications are inactivated by CYP2D6. A CYP2D6 PM requires lower doses of NT than an EM to produce similar serum concentrations of active drug (see Figure 43-7). For the purpose of applying a *CYP2D6* genotype to clinical practice, homozygosity or compound heterozygosity for *CYP2D6* PM alleles is consistent with a PM phenotype. The presence of a single PM allele may lead to either an EM or an IM phenotype. Individuals with a PM phenotype have been successfully treated by reducing the dose of antidepressant medications that are inactivated by CYP2D6 by 40% to 80%.[70] Another example is provided by metoprolol succinate, used as a treatment for hypertension and angina pectoris. Therapeutic effect of this agent is proportional to serum concentrations, and striking differences in serum levels are observed with CYP2D6 PM and EM individuals following a single dose of metoprolol.

In contrast to decreased metabolism, increased metabolism of an active drug to an inactive metabolite in UMs results in subtherapeutic concentrations of active drug at standard dosages. To compensate for increased metabolism, UM subjects have been successfully treated with megadoses (twofold to twelvefold greater than the standard dose) of some drugs that are inactivated by CYP2D6 to obtain therapeutic efficacy.[70] Because most drugs act through multiple mechanisms that may or may not relate to the concentration of parent and/or metabolites, high-dose therapy may be associated with unrecognized risks. For example, potentially toxic metabolites may accumulate as a result of UM status and may lead to ADRs. Thus individuals with UM phenotypes may be best served by selecting therapeutic medications that are metabolized by an alternate (non-CYP2D6) route.[76]

Cytochrome P450 2C19 (CYP2C19)

CYP2C19 is a member of the CYP2C family, which includes CYP2C8, CYP2C9, CYP2C18, and CYP2C19 of which only *CYP2C9* and *CYP2C19* exhibit substantial genetic variability. Although substrate overlap between the family members exists, CYP2C19 is specifically associated with the 4′-hydroxylation of the S-enantiomer of the anticonvulsant mephenytoin and was originally named mephenytoin hydroxylase.[27] CYP2C19 is a Phase I enzyme for the metabolism of a number of other therapeutic drugs, including citalopram, diazepam, omeprazole, propranolol, and proguanil (see Table 43-3).[110] Like the CYP2D6 isoenzyme, specific genetic variants of *CYP2C19* lead to poor and intermediate metabolizer—PM and IM—phenotypes with respect to a number of common therapeutic drugs. In contrast to the debrisoquine polymorphism, the UM phenotype has not been characterized for this enzyme, though its existence has been postulated.

Genotype to Phenotype

At least 20 allelic variants of *CYP2C19* have been described.[5,17] The EM phenotype has historically been composed of both the homozygous and heterozygous genotypes. The PM phenotype is inherited in an autosomal recessive manner.[17] Like the *CYP2D6* polymorphisms, there are significant interethnic differences in the prevalence of the CYP2C19 PM phenotype. The PM phenotype occurs in 2% to 5% of Caucasian and Black Zimbabwean Shona populations, and 10% to 23% in Asian populations.[142]

Table 43-4 lists *CYP2C19* polymorphisms with the nucleotide change, amino acid changes, and associated enzyme activity phenotype. The principal genetic variant in PMs of S-mephenytoin is *CYP2C19*2,* arising from a 681G>A, which results in a splicing defect and essentially no enzyme activity. The second most common *CYP2C19* allele *(CYP2C19*3)* associated with the PM phenotype results from a single nucleotide substitution 636G>A, which produces a premature stop codon and no active enzyme product.[28,29,98] The allele frequency of *CYP2C19*2* is reported as 32% in East Asians and 71% in Polynesians (Vanuatu), and is approximately 15% in Caucasians and African-Americans. The allele frequency of *CYP2C19*3* is reported as 6% to 10% in East Asians, 13.3% in Polynesians, and <1% among Caucasians. Differences in the incidence of the *CYP2C19*5* polymorphism affecting the S-mephenytoin among ethnic populations have been described.[10,61] Additional alleles, *CYP2C19*4, *6, *8, *9, *10,* and **12* may also contribute to the PM phenotype or have markedly reduced activity toward S-mephenytoin.[6,138]

Testing

Genotyping tests based on PCR-amplification and restriction endonuclease digestion have been developed for detection of polymorphic *CYP2C19* variant alleles. A genotyping strategy including *CYP2C19*2, *3, *4, *5A,* and **5B* for identification of the PM phenotype was associated with a sensitivity of nearly 100% in Chinese and 92% in Caucasian populations.[61] Because the PM phenotype was thought to occur only when both alleles are affected, an initial screening approach incorporating the *CYP2C19*2* and *CYP2C19*3* alleles, with additional testing for the *CYP2C19*4, *5,* and **6* alleles for heterozygous subjects, has also been described. However, this philosophy has come into question given recent findings of the significance of heterozygosity for one inactive *CYP2C19* allele.[14] Recent advances in multiplexed PCR with multiple detection technologies and other technologies, such as pyrosequencing and arrays, will make it possible to screen simultaneously for many alleles in this gene.[107]

Clinical Applications

The proton pump inhibitor omeprazole is primarily inactivated by the CYP2C19 enzyme, and thus its metabolism is subject to this genetic polymorphism (see Figure 43-8). The homozygous variant subjects had 100% cure of upper gastrointestinal (GI) ulcers after omeprazole-based therapy versus 65% and 25% for heterozygous and homozygous wild-type patients, respectively. Studies have demonstrated greater effectiveness of single dose level omeprazole for management of *Helicobacter pylori* infection and peptic ulcer in subjects with one or more *CYP2C19* PM alleles. This is thought to be because of greater exposure to a therapeutic compound in PMs and IMs. However, using triple therapy with rabeprazole, amoxicillin, and clarithromycin, *H. pylori* antimicrobial susceptibility was shown to be a more important factor than *CYP2C19* genotype.[96] No dose adjustments have been proposed to adjust for *CYP2C19* genotype. However, gene-gene interactions may indicate a need to test for genetic variation in more than one gene to guide therapy.

TABLE 43-4 *CYP2C19* Alleles

Allele	Nucleotide Changes	Effect	Enzyme Activity	
			In vivo	**In vitro**
*CYP2C19*1A*	None		Normal	Normal
*CYP2C19*1B*	99C>T; 991A>G	I331V	Normal	
*CYP2C19*1C*	991A>G	I331V	Normal	
*CYP2C19*2A*	99C>T; **681G>A**; 990C>T; 991A>G	Splicing defect	None	
*CYP2C19*2B*	99C>T; 276G>C; **681G>A**; 990C>T; 991A>G	Splicing defect; E92D	None	
*CYP2C19*3*	**636G>A**; 991A>G; 1251A>C	Stop codon	None	
*CYP2C19*4*	**1A>G**; 99C>T, 991A>G	GTG initiation codon	None	
*CYP2C19*5A*	**1297C>T**	R433W	None	None
*CYP2C19*5B*	99C>T; 991A>G; **1297C>T**	I331V; R433W	None	
*CYP2C19*6*	99C>T; **395G>A**; 991A>G	R132Q; I331V	None	None
*CYP2C19*7*	IVS5 + 2T>A	Splicing defect	None	
*CYP2C19*8*	358T>C	W120R	None	Decr
*CYP2C19*9*	99C>T; 431G>A; 991A>G	R144H; I331V		(Decr)
*CYP2C19*10*	99C>T; 680C>T; 991A>G	P227L; I331V		Decr
*CYP2C19*11*	99C>T; 449G>A; 991A>G	R150H; I331V		
*CYP2C19*12*	99C>T; 991A>G; 1473A>C	I331V; X491C; 26 extra aa		Unstable
*CYP2C19*13*	991A>G; 1228C>T	I331V; R410C		
*CYP2C19*14*	50T>C; 99C>T; 991A>G	L17P; I331V		
*CYP2C19*15*	55A>C; 991A>G	I19L; I331V		
*CYP2C19*16*	1324C>T Existence of the *CYP2C19*2* polymorphism 681G>A on the same allele cannot be excluded	R442C		

From Human Cytochrome P450 (CYP) Allele Nomenclature Committee. CYP allele nomenclature. http://www.imm.ki.se/CYPalleles (Accessed December 5, 2004).[5] Reproduced with the permission of Sarah C. Sim, Webmaster.

Multigene studies have shown that interleukin (IL)-1β genetic polymorphism, although not an independent factor in treatment outcome, influences the impact of the *CYP2C19* genotype on the cure rate of 1-week triple therapy for *H. pylori* infections.[125]

The antimalarial prodrugs proguanil and chlorproguanil require CYP2C19-dependent bioactivation for therapeutic efficacy.[137] A clear gene-dose effect has been observed for the oxidation of proguanil to cycloguanil and 4-chlorophenyl-biguanide.[59] Clinical response has been shown to be affected in CYP2C19 PM individuals.

Currently the most common reason for genotyping *CYP2C19* is to explain inappropriate response to antidepressant medications. For example, CYP2C19 is the primary enzyme responsible for converting amitriptyline (AT) to its active metabolite NT. Monitoring serum or plasma concentrations of both AT and NT as a sum is used to guide AT therapy.[79,106] However, the utility of *CYP2C19* genotyping for this application is somewhat controversial. Using a quantitative gene dose model, it was found that *CYP2D6* but not *CYP2C19* genotyping is most useful in AT therapy based on the fact that *CYP2C19* polymorphisms alter the ratio of AT to NT, but not the sum of the two.[120] The model was derived in a Caucasian population, whereas *CYP2C19* PMs are much more common in Asian populations.[117] CYP2D6 is also thought to be more important than CYP2C19 for newer antidepressants.[46] However, genotyping *CYP2C19* becomes very important for a CYP2D6 PM and is proposed to be important for additional antidepressants such as doxepine, fluoxetine, and moclobemide.

Because of the potential overlap in substrate specificity among the CYP2C family, genotyping both *CYP2C19* and *CYP2C9* may be useful clinically as well. Optimal dosing of the anticonvulsant drug phenytoin can be predicted by testing for variation in *CYP2C9, CYP2C19,* and *MDR1,* which encodes the p-glycoprotein.[67] CYP2C9 is estimated to contribute to 90% of phenytoin metabolism, and CYP2C19 is thought to contribute to 10% of phenytoin metabolism in persons with EM phenotypes for both enzymes.[39] In patients who are CYP2C9 PM, CYP2C19 is the primary route of phenytoin elimination, and hence the importance of testing for CYP2C19 increases.[83]

Cytochrome P450 2C9 (CYP2C9)

CYP2C9 is a member of the CYP2C family, which includes CYP2C8, CYP2C9, CYP2C18, and CYP2C19—of which *CYP2C9* and *CYP2C19* exhibit substantial genetic variability. Although substrate overlap between the family members exists (see Table 43-3), CYP2C9 is specifically associated with metabolism of the sulfonylurea hypoglycemic agent tolbutamide. CYP2C9 is involved in the metabolism of approximately 16% of therapeutic compounds.[110,114] At least 12 allelic variants have been described in this gene and are shown in Table 43-5.[5]

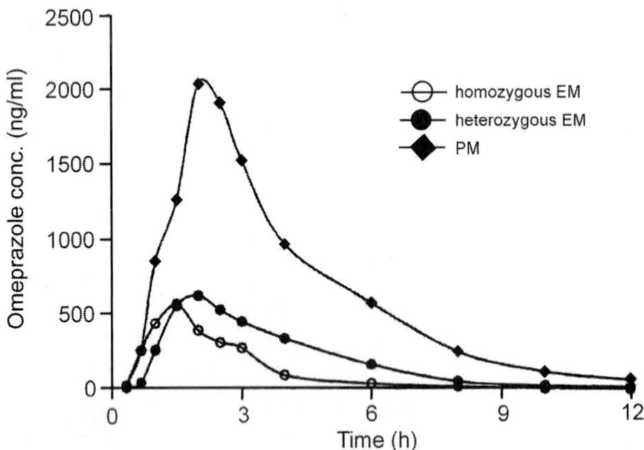

Figure 43-8 Mean plasma concentration-time profile of omeprazole after oral administration of 40 mg omeprazole (in the form of 2 × 20-mg Losec capsules) to 27 male Chinese subjects phenotyped for CYP2C19 activity with mephenytoin. Plasma concentrations of omeprazole were significantly higher in PMs (◆) than in homozygous EMs (○) or heterozygous EMs (●). In addition, the elimination half-life for omeprazole was 2.3-fold greater in PMs than in EMs ($p < 0.001$). *(From Yin OQ, Tomlinson B, Chow AH, Waye MM, Chow MS. Omeprazole as a CYP2C19 marker in Chinese subjects: assessment of its gene-dose effect and intrasubject variability. J Clin Pharmacol 2004;44:582-9. Reproduced by permission from Sage Publications, Inc.)*

Genotype to Phenotype

Two variant alleles of *CYP2C9* (*CYP2C9*2* and *CYP2C9*3*) account for most CYP2C9 PM phenotypes.[98] The allelic frequency of *CYP2C9*2* has been reported as 8% to 19% in Caucasians, and 1% to 4% in African-Americans and Canadian Native Indians. This allele has not been detected in Asians. The allelic frequency of *CYP2C9*3* has been reported as 6% to 10% in Caucasians, 1.7% to 5% in Asians, and 0.5% to 1.5% in African-Americans. Homozygosity for the *CYP2C9*3* allele is relatively rare in Caucasians (1% to 2%).[115] Studies in vitro have shown that the protein produced by the *CYP2C9*3* variant is less than 5% as efficient as the *CYP2C9*1* allozyme, whereas *CYP2C9*2* shows about 12% of *CYP2C9*1* allozyme activity in most assays. *CYP2C9*2* and *CYP2C9*3* alleles result in PM in the homozygous state, and IM phenotypes when heterozygous. Two additional alleles, found in African-Americans, have been described, *CYP2C9*5* and *CYP2C9*6*. The *CYP2C9*6* in a homozygous individual was shown to contribute to an extremely long phenytoin elimination, with a half-life approximately 5.8 times longer than *CYP2C9* extensive metabolizers.[68] The *CYP2C9*8* allele has been shown in vitro to have greater activity than the wild-type enzyme, demonstrating 175% tolbutamide hydroxylase activity of recombi-

TABLE 43-5 *CYP2C9* **Alleles**

Allele	Nucleotide Changes	Effect	Enzyme Activity	
			In vivo	In vitro
*CYP2C9*1*	None		Normal	Normal
*CYP2C9*2*	430C>T	R144C		Decr
*CYP2C9*3*	1075A>C	I359L	Decr	Decr
*CYP2C9*4*	1076T>C	I359T		
*CYP2C9*5*	1080C>G	D360E	Possibly Decr	Decr
*CYP2C9*6*	818delA	Frame shift	None	
*CYP2C9*7*	55C>A	L19I		
*CYP2C9*8*	449G>A	R150H		Incr
*CYP2C9*9*	752A>G	H251R		
*CYP2C9*10*	815A>G	E272G		
*CYP2C9*11*	1003C>T	R335W		Decr
*CYP2C9*12*	1465C>T	P489S		Decr
*CYP2C9*13*	269T>C	L90P		

From Human Cytochrome P450 (CYP) Allele Nomenclature Committee. CYP allele nomenclature. http://www.imm.ki.se/CYPalleles (Accessed December 5, 2004).[5] Reproduced with the permission of Sarah C. Sim, Webmaster.

nant wild-type (see Figure 43-9). It was previously believed that no UM phenotypes existed for the *CYP2C9* gene; however, *CYP2C9*8* may dispel that notion.[9]

Testing

There have been several published protocols for detecting variants in this gene. Many of the clinically important polymorphisms are amenable to PCR-RFLP, allele-specific primer extension (ASPE), and microarrays. Recently, multiplexed assays have been described that screen the entire gene for many variants for little additional cost above testing for a subset of alleles.[107,121]

Clinical Applications

Examples of therapeutic compounds metabolized by CYP2C9 include nonsteroidal antiinflammatory (NSAID) medications, irbesartan, naproxen, and fluvastatin (see Table 43-3). Proposed dose adjustments based on phenotype have been published for CYP2C9 drug substrates such as warfarin, glipizide, tolbutamide, and phenytoin.[55,80]

An illustration of the effects of decreased CYP2C9 activity on a therapeutic compound is the effect on anticoagulation therapy with S-warfarin. Individuals with the *CYP2C9*2* and *CYP2C9*3* polymorphisms have impaired metabolism of warfarin and thus increased plasma concentrations of the drug with standard dosing. As illustrated in Figure 43-10, standard 5 mg/day maintenance dosing of warfarin in subjects with CYP2C9 genetic variants can lead to an excessive warfarin exposure, resulting in an exaggerated anticoagulant response. The clinical impact of *CYP2C9* polymorphism includes increased risk of serious or life-threatening bleeding complications and increased time to achieve a stable INR if the dosages are not lowered to accommodate their reduced metabolizer phenotype.

Inherited impairment of CYP2C9 activity may also increase the risk for severe ADRs after NSAID use. For example, Martinez et al found that the frequency of *CYP2C9* variant alleles was higher in bleeding patients, with a significant trend to higher risk with increasing number of variant alleles ($p = 0.02$).[87]

N-Acetyl Transferases (NAT1 and NAT2)

The N-acetyl transferase (NAT) polymorphism is one of the earliest pharmacogenetic targets recognized and characterized. NATs are Phase II enzymes that catalyze the transfer of an acetyl moiety from acetyl-CoA to homocyclic and heterocyclic arylamines and hydrazines. Substrates include drugs, carcinogens, toxicants, and possibly endogenous compounds. Slow metabolizer phenotypes, which may affect up to 90% of some populations, are manifested by changes in protein expression, protein stability, and enzyme kinetics.

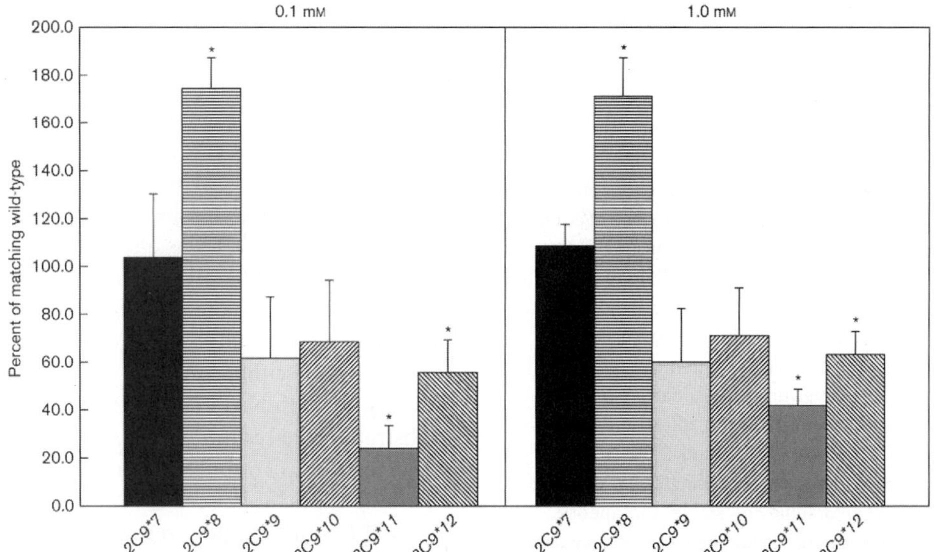

Figure 43-9 Tolbutamide hydroxylase activity of recombinant wild-type *(CYP2C9*1)* and new variant *CYP2C9* alleles. *CYP2C9* alleles were expressed in *Escherichia coli* and partially purified. For each variant allele, three individual preparations (two preparations for *CYP2C9*7*) were purified from bacteria simultaneously with wild-type. Each preparation was assayed in triplicate at high (1 mmol/L) and low (0.1 mmol/L) substrate concentrations on the same day. Values are given as a percentage of enzymatic activity of the wild-type allele. *Significantly different from *CYP2C9*1* protein activity ($P < 0.05$). *(From Blaisdell J, Jorge-Nebert LF, Coulter S, Ferguson SS, Lee SJ, Chanas B, et al. Discovery of new potentially defective alleles of human CYP2C9. Pharmacogenetics 2004;14: 527-37. Reproduced by permission from Lippincott Williams & Wilkins.)*

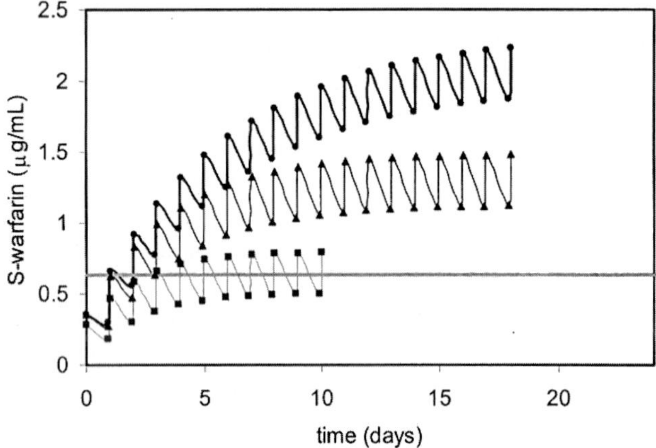

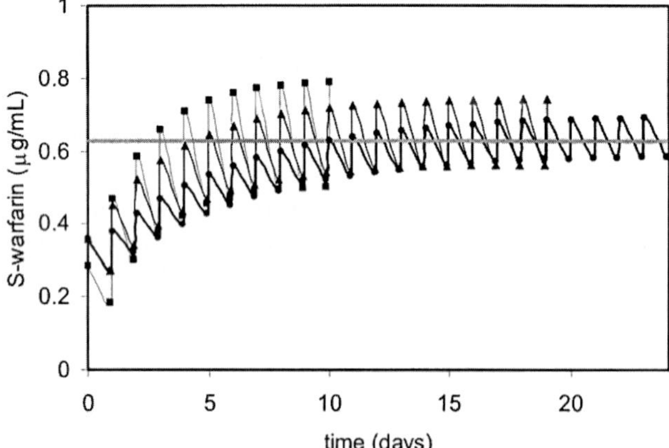

Figure 43-10 Model of warfarin dosing based on *CYP2C9* genetics. In both panels, the conventional therapeutic S-warfarin target level is shown (horizontal line) for reference. The top panel depicts a model for warfarin therapy in patients using the standard 5 mg/day dose with all genotypes. *CYP2C9**1/*1* individuals (■) on 5 mg, twice per day would attain stable and therapeutic serum S-warfarin levels (0.68 μg/mL) in approximately 4 days. *CYP2C9**1/*2* (▲) and *CYP2C9**1/*3* (●) individuals on the same 5-mg dose are modeled to attain S-warfarin serum levels that are both too high by the second day and if not adjusted would lead to overanticoagulation. *CYP2C9**1/*2* patients would stabilize at twice therapeutic serum levels after 10 to 12 days, but *CYP2C9**1/*3,* if not adjusted, would continue to rise. The bottom panel depicts serum S-warfarin level outcomes for a dosing regimen modified for genotype. All patients would be given the standard 5-mg dose twice, then switched to a *CYP2C9* genotype adjusted dose for maintenance, *CYP2C9**1/*2* receiving 3 mg and *CYP2C9**1/*3* receiving 1.5 mg. This genotype adjusted dosing could result in *CYP2C9**1/*2* and *CYP2C9**1/*3* achieving stable, therapeutic S-warfarin levels in 10 days, thereby avoiding overanticoagulation in these individuals. *(Adapted from Linder MW, Looney S, Adams JE III, Johnson N, Antonino-Green D, Lacefield N, et al. Warfarin dose adjustments based on CYP2C9 genetic polymorphisms. J Thromb Thrombolysis 2002;14:227-32. Reproduced by permission from Springer.)*

Several good reviews on the NAT polymorphisms have been published.*

Genotype to Phenotype

The first NAT polymorphism, attributed to an enzyme originally called "isoniazid transacetylase," was recognized in the 1950s with isoniazid (L-isonicotinyl hydrazide), a drug used to treat tuberculosis.[12] Population studies revealed a bimodal distribution in plasma and urine levels of the N-acetylated isoniazid metabolite. Concentration of the parent drug was highly correlated with the prevalence of toxic symptoms, including hepatotoxicity and a painful and progressive peripheral neuropathy that affected up to one third of Caucasian and African-American patients. From this initial work, patients were phenotypically described as "fast acetylators" or "slow acetylators." Slow acetylators excrete large amounts of the parent drug relative to the acetylated metabolite when compared with fast acetylators. Family studies identified a strong genetic linkage of this phenotype and suggested that the phenotype was inherited as an autosomal recessive trait.[32,132]

Studies with additional substrates for NAT demonstrated that the phenotype was not relevant to all substrates. For example, the NAT phenotype was clearly recognized for arylamines such as isoniazid, some sulfonamides, amrinone, dapsone, procainamide, caffeine, and clonazepam. The phenotype was not observed with other arylamine substrates such as p-aminobenzoate (PABA) and p-aminosalicylate (PAS). A folate catabolite, p-aminobenzoylglutamate, is the only endogenous NAT substrate proposed.[97] However, *NAT2* knock-out and *NAT1* and *NAT2* double knock-out mice do not express phenotypical abnormalities, suggesting that these enzymes are not required for development or function.[123]

In 1965 it was proposed that two isoforms of NAT, later named NAT1 and NAT2, were responsible for the differences in phenotypes observed previously. Of the two proposed isoforms, NAT2 correlated best with the isoniazid (polymorphic) phenotype.[63] It was also suggested that the fast and slow acetylator phenotypes were caused by differences in expression rather than in the enzyme kinetics. Subsequently, it was found that although most substrates exhibit higher specificity for either NAT1 or NAT2, most substrates have affinity for both NAT1 and NAT2 (Table 43-6). Nonetheless, substrates were commonly classified as monomorphic (substrates of NAT1) or polymorphic (substrates of NAT2) until the mid-1990s.

NAT1, which is now recognized to be polymorphic, is extremely unstable and therefore more difficult to study than NAT2. Because of stability differences and overlapping substrate specificity, tissue localization studies for the NATs have been challenging. It is now recognized that both NAT1 and NAT2 are expressed throughout the GI tract, and in the lung, bladder, ureter, and liver.[43,135]

*References 44, 45, 51, 95, 119, 136.

TABLE 43-6 NAT Substrates

Drugs	Potential Carcinogens or Toxicants
Aminoglutethimide	p-aminobenzoic acid (PABA)*
Amonafide	4-aminobiphenyl
Amrinone	2-aminodipyrido[1,2-a:3′2′d]-imidazole (Glu-P-2)
Caffeine	2-aminofluorene*
Clonazepam	2-amino-3,8-dimethylimidazo [4,5-f]quinoxaline (MeIQx)†
Dapsone	2-amino-3-methyl-imidazo [4,5-f]quinoline (IQ)†
Dipyrone	3-amino-1-methyl-5H-pyrido [4,3-b]indole (Trp-P-2)
Endralazine	p-aminosalicylic acid (PAS)*
Hydralazine	Benzidine
Isoniazid	3,4-dichloroaniline
Prizidilol	3,2′-dimethyl-4-aminobiphenyl
Prizidilol	B-naphthylamine
Procainamide†	p-phenetidine
Sulfonamides:†	
Sulfadiazine	o-toluidine†
Sulfadoxine	p-toluidine
Sulfamethazine	
Sulfamethoxazole	
Sulfapyridine	
Sulfasalazine	

Modified from Grant DM, Blum M, Beer M, Meyer UA. Monomorphic and polymorphic human arylamine N-acetyltransferases: a comparison of liver isozymes and expressed products of two cloned genes. Mol Pharmacol 1991;39:184-91; Grant DM, Goodfellow GH, Sugamori KS, Durette K. Pharmacogenetics of the human arylamine N-acetyltransferases. Pharmacol 2000;61:204-11; Hein DW, Doll MA, Rustan TD, Gray K, Feng Y, Ferguson RJ, et al. Metabolic activation and deactivation of arylamine carcinogens by recombinant human NAT1 and polymorphic NAT2 acetyltransferases. Carcinogenesis 1993;14:1633-8.
*Strong selectivity for NAT1 based on NAT1/NAT2 activity (nmol/min/U) ratio >300.
†Similar selectivity for NAT1 and NAT2 based on NAT1/NAT2 activity ratio <15.

There are three human NAT genes that are mapped to chromosome 8p22 and were first cloned in 1990. The *NAT1* and *NAT2* genes share 87% nucleotide sequence identity and 81% amino acid sequence identity. The third gene *NATP* is thought to be a noncoding pseudogene. Each of the NAT genes has an intronless open reading frame exon of 870 bp and codes for 290 amino acids.[11,13,127,128] Many variant alleles have been described for both NAT1 (Table 43-7) and NAT2 (Table 43-8). A consensus nomenclature was published in 1995 and updated in 2000.[4,53,128] The wild-type alleles, although somewhat arbitrary due to high population frequencies of multiple alleles, are *NAT1*3* and *NAT2*4.* For *NAT2,* former common nomenclature included M1 for *NAT2*5A,* M2 for *NAT2*6A,* and M3 for *NAT2*7A.* The *NAT2*5, *6, *7, *13,* and **14* alleles are thought to account for more than 99% of slow acetylator phenotypes. The *NAT1*10* is the most common variant *NAT1* allele in many human populations, but the phenotype-genotype relationship is not well defined. Other *NAT1* alleles that appear rare in humans produce enzymes with definitively reduced activity, and potential clinical implications include *NAT1*14, 15, 17, 19,* and *22.*[44,51,77,95,131]

The three-dimensional crystal structures of the two NAT isoenzymes have been determined. Structural studies suggest that the active catalytic site of the NATs involves three amino acids, a cysteine residue juxtaposed with histidine, and aspartate residues. The C-terminus is responsible for substrate specificity.[118] The acetylation reaction occurs through a classical two-step mechanism, where an acetyl moiety is transferred from acetyl CoA to NAT and then from NAT to the arylamine to form an arylamide. As shown in Figure 43-11, *N*-acetylation, thought to primarily generate nontoxic stable products, is mediated by both NAT1 and NAT2. *O*-Acetylation of cytochrome P450 *N*-hydroxylated products is also mediated by both NAT1 and NAT2 and is thought to generate reactive products that may spontaneously decompose to form nitrenium ions. Nitrenium ions are electrophiles that may subsequently bind covalently to intracellular nucleophiles such as DNA or proteins and be responsible for cell death, mutagenesis, or other toxicities. An intramolecular *N,O*-acetyltransfer reaction is mediated primarily by NAT1 and also may lead to reactive products. Other enzymes that may interrupt or contribute to these reactions include CYP1A2, prostaglandin H synthase, UDP-glucuronosyltransferase, and sulfotransferase.[45,136]

Testing

NAT2 slow acetylators are common in many populations: approximately 83% of Egyptians; 40% to 60% of Caucasians, Europeans, and African-Americans; 10% to 30% of Asians; and 5% of Canadian Eskimos.[48,95] *NAT1*10* allele frequency is reported high in a Japanese population (62.3%) compared with a European population (29%), but further efforts are required to fully elucidate the population frequencies of the various *NAT1* alleles currently identified.[66] Variables that affect NAT phenotyping include the substrate or probe drug used, age and disease status of the individual, medications, dietary factors such as ingestion of well-cooked meat, and lifestyle factors such as cigarette smoking or occupational exposure to NAT substrates.

The most common method of NAT1 phenotyping is to measure enzyme activity in isolated lymphocytes using PABA, PAS, or another relatively specific NAT1 substrate. However, phenotyping in vivo with a probe drug has also been performed.[52,60,94] The most common phenotyping method for NAT2 is to administer a probe drug and evaluate ratios of parent/metabolite or metabolite-A/metabolite-B concentrations. Probe drugs may include any relatively specific NAT2 substrate, the most common and safe of which is

TABLE 43-7 NAT1 Alleles

Allele	Nucleotide Changes							Amino Acid Changes	Expected Phenotype
*NAT1*3*	1095 C>A							None	Unknown
*NAT1*4*	None							None	Fast
*NAT1*5*	350, 351 G>C	497-499 G>C	884 A>G	−1 at 976	−1 at 1105			R117T, R166T, E167Q	Unknown
*NAT1*10*	1088T>A	1095C>A						None	Unknown
*NAT1*11A*	−344C>T	−40A>T	445G>A	459G>A	640T>G	−9 in 1065-90	1095C>A	V149I, S214A	Slow
*NAT1*11B*	−344C>T	−40A>T	445G>A	459G>A	640T>G	−9 in 1065-90		V149I, S214A	Slow
*NAT1*11C*	−344C>T	−40A>T	445G>A		640T>G	−9 in 1065-90	1095C>A	S214A	Slow
*NAT1*14A*	560G>A	1088T>A	1095C>A					R187Q	Slow
*NAT1*14B*	560G>A							R187Q	Slow
*NAT1*15*	559C>T							R187 Stop	Slow
*NAT1*16*	[AAA] after 1091							None	Unknown
*NAT1*17*	190C>T							R64W	Slow
*NAT1*18A*	−3 in 1065-87		1088T>A	1095C>A				None	Unknown
*NAT1*18B*	−3 in 1065-88							None	Unknown
*NAT1*19*	97C>T							R33 Stop	Slow
*NAT1*20*	402T>C							None	Unknown
*NAT1*21*	613A>G							M205V	Unknown
*NAT1*22*	725A>T							D251V	Slow
*NAT1*23*	777T>C							None	Unknown
*NAT1*24*	781G>A							E261K	Unknown
*NAT1*25*	787A>G							I263V	Unknown
*NAT1*26A*	[TAA] in 1065-90		1095C>A					None	Unknown
*NAT1*26B*	[TAA] in 1065-91							None	Unknown
*NAT1*27*	21T>G	777T>C						None	Unknown
*NAT1*28*	– [TAATAA] in 1065-90							None	Unknown
*NAT1*29*	1088T>A	1095C>A	−1 at 1025					None	Unknown

Modified from references 4, 44, 45, and 51.

TABLE 43-8 NAT2 Alleles

Allele	Nucleotide Changes				Amino Acid Changes	Expected Phenotype
*NAT2*4*	none				None	Rapid
*NAT2*5A*	341T>C	481C>T			I114T	Slow
*NAT2*5B*	341T>C	481C>T	803A>G		I114T, K268R	Slow
*NAT2*5C*	341T>C	803A>G			I114T, K268R	Slow
*NAT2*5D*	341T>C				I114T	Slow
*NAT2*5E*	341T>C	590G>A			I114T, R197Q	Slow
*NAT2*5F*	341T>C	481C>T	759C>A	803A>G	I114T, K268R	Slow
*NAT2*5G*	282C>T	341T>C	481C>T	803A>G	I114T, K268R	Slow
*NAT2*5H*	341T>C	481C>T	803A>G	859T>C	I114T, K268R, I287T	Slow
*NAT2*5I*	341T>C	411A>T	481C>T	803A>G	I114T, L137F, K268R	Slow
*NAT2*5J*	282C>T	341T>C	590G>A		I114T, R197Q	Slow
*NAT2*6A*	282C>T		590G>A		R197Q	Slow
*NAT2*6B*	590G>A				R197Q	Slow
*NAT2*6C*	282C>T	590G>A	803A>G		R197Q, K268R	Slow
*NAT2*6D*	111T>C	282C>T	590G>A		R197Q	Slow
*NAT2*6E*	481C>T	590G>A			R197Q	Slow
*NAT2*7A*	857G>A				G286E	Slow
*NAT2*7B*	282C>T	857G>A			G286E	Slow
*NAT2*10*	499G>A				E167K	Unknown
*NAT2*11A*	481C>T				None	Unknown
*NAT2*11B*	481C>T	859 del			S287 frameshift	Unknown
*NAT2*12A*	803A>G				K268R	Rapid
*NAT2*12B*	282C>T	803A>G			K268R	Rapid
*NAT2*12C*	481C>T	803A>G			K268R	Rapid
*NAT2*12D*	364G>A	803A>G			D122N, K268R	Rapid
*NAT2*13*	282C>T				None	Rapid
*NAT2*14A*	191G>A				R64Q	Slow
*NAT2*14B*	191G>A	282C>T			R64Q	Slow
*NAT2*14C*	191G>A	341T>C	481C>T	803A>G	R64W, I114T, K268R	Slow
*NAT2*14D*	191G>A	282C>T	590G>A		R64Q, R197Q	Slow
*NAT2*14E*	191G>A	803A>G			R64W, K268R	Slow
*NAT2*14F*	191G>A	341T>C	803A>G		R64W, I114T, K268R	Slow
*NAT2*14G*	191G>A	282C>T	803A>G		R64W, K268R	Slow
*NAT2*17*	434A>C				Q145P	Unknown
*NAT2*18*	845A>C				K282T	Unknown
*NAT2*19*	190C>T				R64W	Unknown

Modified from references 4, 44, 45, and 51.

caffeine. One published phenotyping method involves administration of 200 mg caffeine following an overnight fast. Urine is collected 4 and 5 hours later. The 5-hour specimen is analyzed for caffeine metabolites 5-acetylamino-6-formylamino-3-methyluracil (AFMU) and 1-methylxanthine (1X). Cutoffs for acetylator phenotypes are based on the ratio of AFMU/1X. Considering a bimodal distribution of acetylators, a ratio of less than 0.66 is used to define slow acetylators. Because a trimodal distribution has been described and may be of interest, a ratio higher than 3.0 could define "ultrarapid" acetylators; a ratio between 0.66 and 3.0 would define a classic rapid acetylator or in a trimodal distribution, an "intermediate" acetylator phenotype.[48,72]

Genotyping can predict NAT phenotype quite well, with concordance of 90% to 100% for *NAT2*. For *NAT2*, an example of the phenotype-genotype relationship published by Cascorbi et al in 1995 with a population of unrelated Germans is depicted by histogram (Figure 43-12). Only 6.7% of genotypes did not agree with the phenotypes in this study. Methods have primarily employed PCR-RFLP, but real-time PCR and other allele-specific detection methods have also been described.[8,21,37,54,95]

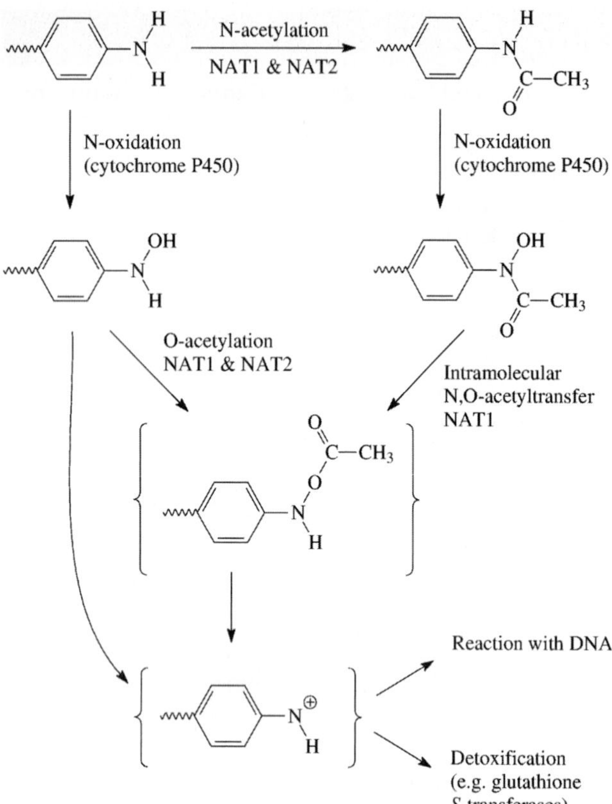

Figure 43-11 Schematic view of the role of NAT enzymes in the metabolism of aromatic amines. N-acetylation might be a detoxification reaction in a number of cases; however, after N-hydroxylation of aromatic amines (e.g., by CYP enzymes), NAT enzymes can bioactivate these intermediates by either *O*-acetylation or intramolecular *N,O*-acetyltransfer, leading to the formation of nitrenium ions, which might react with DNA or alternatively be detoxified by, for example, GST enzymes. Importantly, it is shown that a number of other biotransformation enzymes are also involved in the metabolism of aromatic amines as well. *(Redrawn from Wormhoudt LW, Commandeur JNM, Vermeulen NPE. Genetic polymorphisms of human N-acetyltransferase, cytochrome P450, glutathione-S-transferase, and epoxide hydrolase enzymes: relevance to xenobiotic metabolism and toxicity. Crit Rev Toxicol 1999;29:59-124. Reproduced by permission from Taylor and Francis, Inc.)*

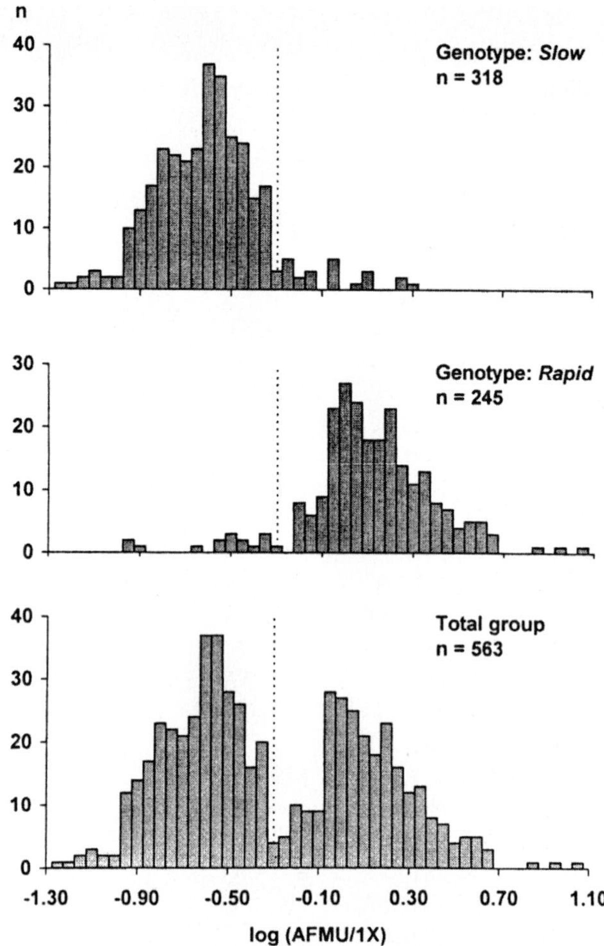

Figure 43-12 Histogram of NAT2 phenotypical activities as obtained by the caffeine test: 5 hr urine collection obtained after administration of caffeine, and analyzed for caffeine metabolite concentrations. Values represent the logarithmically transformed ratio of metabolites 5-acetylamino-6-formylamino-3-methyl-uracil (AFMU) and 1-methylxanthine (1X). From the distinct biomodal distribution an antimode of log(0.50) = −0.30 was obtained *(dotted line). (From Cascorbi I, Drakoulis N, Brockmoller J, Maurer A, Sperling K, Roots I. Arylamine N-acetyltransferase (NAT2) mutations and their allelic linkage in unrelated Caucasian individuals: correlation with phenotypical activity. Am J Hum Genet 1995;57:581-92. Reproduced by permission from the University of Chicago Press.)*

Clinical Applications

NAT status has been implicated in propensity for experiencing ADRs and, unlike the CYPs and TPMT, NAT status has been associated with risk of disease, including immunological disorders—such as rheumatoid arthritis and systemic lupus erythematous—and several cancers, particularly bladder, lung, gastric, and colorectal. NAT substrate exposure can be related to cigarette smoking, some medications, occupational exposure (cooking, dye, and rubber industries), and several environmental toxicants (see Table 43-6). NAT testing may be important for individuals at high risk of exposure to NAT substrates or in whom adverse reactions to probable NAT substrates have been experienced.

Neither genotyping nor phenotyping methods are widely available for clinical testing. However, research involving the genotyping or phenotyping of NAT polymorphisms has significantly impacted pharmacotherapy with NAT substrates and drug development. With isoniazid, the recognition of distinct phenotypical differences that led to ADRs furthered research into the pathological mechanisms. For example, the neuropathic consequences are linked to pyridoxine deficiency, which can be avoided by co-administration of pyridoxine to all patients. Because rapid acetylators are less likely to respond to the conventionally administered dose, the iso-

TABLE 43-9 Additional Pharmacogenetic Targets Being Studied

Polymorphic Gene(s)	Protein(s)	Drugs or Drug Classes Possibly Affected by Variants
ACE	Angiotensin converting enzyme	ACE inhibitors
ABCB1	MDR1, p-glycoprotein	Immunosuppressants, antiretrovirals, anticonvulsants, cardiac glycosides
ADD1	Adducin 1 (α)	Diuretics
ADRB1 and 2	β-Adrenergic receptor	β-Agonists, β-blockers
AGT and AGTR1	Angiotensinogen and receptor	Antihypertensives
ALOX5	Arachidonate 5-lipoxygenase	Leukotriene receptors, 5-lipoxygenase inhibitors
APOE	Apolipoprotein E	Statins, acetylcholinesterase inhibitors (Alzheimer's therapeutics)
BCHE	Butyrylcholinesterase	Succinylcholine
BDKRB2	Bradykinin receptor B2	ACE inhibitors
CETP	Cholesteryl ester transfer protein	Statins
COMT	Catechol O-methyltransferase	Antipsychotics
CYP1A2, 2B6, 1E, 3A	Cytochrome P450 drug metabolizing enzymes	Several; >50% of all therapeutic drugs
DRD2, 3, and 4	Dopamine receptor	Antipsychotics
ERα	Estrogen receptor α	Hormone replacement therapy
FCGR3A	FcγRIIIa receptor	Rituximab
GNB3	Guanine nucleotide binding protein	Antipsychotics, antidepressants
GRIN2B	Glutamate receptor	Antipsychotics
GST	Glutathione S-transferases	Cancer chemotherapeutics
HERG, KvLQT1, Mink, MiRP1	Ion channels involved in congenital long-QT syndrome	Antibiotics, quinidine
HLA-B	Major histocompatibility complex class I-B	Antiretrovirals
HTR2A	Serotonin (5-HTT) receptor	Antipsychotics, antidepressants
IL10	Interleukin 10	Prednisone and antivirals
LIPC	Hepatic lipase	Statins
MTHFR	5,10-Methylene-tetrahydrofolate reductase	Methotrexate
SLC6A3	Dopamine transporter	Antipsychotics, antidepressants
SLC6A4	Serotonin transporter	Antipsychotics, antidepressants
TNF	Tissue necrosis factor	Immunosuppressants, carbamazepine
TPH1	Tryptophan hydroxylase 1	Antidepressants
TYMS	Thymidylate synthase	5-Fluoruracil
UGT1A1	UDP-Glucuronosyltransferase 1A1	Irinotecan
XRCC1	DNA repair protein XRCC1	Cancer chemotherapeutics

Modified from Evans WE, McLeod HL. Pharmacogenomics—drug disposition, drug targets, and side effects. N Engl J Med 2003;348:538-49; Goldstein DB, Tate SK, Sisodiya SM. Pharmacogenetics goes genomic. Nat Rev Genet 2003;4:937-47.

niazid dosing intervals are changed from once a week to twice per week. For procainamide, determining the acetylator status is accomplished through routine therapeutic drug monitoring of the parent and metabolite, N-acetylprocainamide (NAPA). The dose of procainamide is adjusted based on the parent/metabolite ratio. In the development of amonafide, a chemotherapeutic agent inactivated by NAT conjugation, acetylator-based dosing was defined through clinical trials. Although the drug is no longer in development, it is an example of how pharmacogenetic phenomena can support individualized therapy.

Other Pharmacogenetic Targets and Future Directions

As discussed previously in this chapter, any protein for which the related gene exhibits polymorphism has potential phar-

TABLE 43-10 Pharmacogenetic Targets Involved in Xenobiotic Metabolism and Important in Cancer

Polymorphic Gene Important to Metabolism	Chemotherapeutic Drug Substrates	Carcinogen Substrates
CYP2B6	Cyclophosphamide Ifosfamide	
CYP2C9	Cyclophosphamide Ifosfamide	
CYP3A4	Teniposide Etoposide Ifosfamide Vindesine Vinblastine Vincristine Cyclophosphamide Paclitaxel Docetaxel	Aflatoxin B1 6-aminochrysene
NAT2	Amonafide	Aromatic amines Heterocyclic amines
GSTA1, GSTA2	Cyclophosphamide	Cumene hydroperoxides
GSTM1		Aflatoxin B1 epoxides Benzo[a]pyrene 4,5 oxide Trans-stilbene oxide
GSTP1	Thiotepa Cyclophosphamide Ethacrynic acid	4-nitrochinolone 1-oxide
GSTT1		Ethylene oxide Methyl chloride Dichloromethane
UGT1A1	Irinotecan	

Modified from Brockmoller J, Cascorbi I, Henning S, Meisel C, Roots I. Molecular genetics of cancer susceptibility. Pharmacology 2000;61:212-27; McLeod HL, Papageorgio C, Watters JW. Using genetic variations to optimize cancer chemotherapy. Clinical Advances in Haematology and Oncology 2003;1:107-11.

macogenetic implications. With relationship to drug metabolism, additional CYPs including *CYP1A2, CYP2B6, CYP2E1, CYP3A4*, and *CYP3A5* have also been proposed as important pharmacogenetic targets. Other Phase II enzymes that exhibit marked genetic variability among individuals, particularly the glutathione *S*-transferases, may be clinically important as well. In addition, genetic variation in alcohol dehydrogenase, catechol *O*-methyltransferase, and dihydropyrimidine dehydrogenase is important. The interrelationship of these various enzymes as major versus minor, and dependent versus independent mechanisms of metabolism for a single compound will be important to determine the most clinically useful and cost-effective pharmacogenetic testing strategy. Also important will be to gain a better understanding of haplotype relationships and the possible implications of heterozygote variants, for a single gene and combinations of related genes.

Beyond metabolism, pharmacogenetic targets that may become important to TDM and pharmacotherapeutics in general include genes that encode for any protein associated with drug handling, such as drug transporters (e.g., p-glycoprotein and lipoproteins), drug receptors (e.g., dopamine, adrenergic, and serotonin receptors) or effectors (e.g., folate metabolism and catecholamine transporters). Table 43-9 lists examples of pharmacogenetic targets not explicitly discussed in this chapter for which some genotype-to-phenotype relationship has been demonstrated.

Additional studies, particularly prospective and outcome-related, are also required to apply pharmacogenetic findings to the clinic. From an interpretive perspective, more guidelines for dose adjustments need to be established, including consideration of how the dosing recommendations are affected by co-prescribed medications and/or environmental factors. Closer integration of pharmacy professionals with clinical laboratories and clinicians will improve success in pharmacogenetic applications. Commercially available and cost-effective methods for genotyping or phenotyping are also required. The future of pharmacogenetic testing is likely to be driven most by the consumer and by the pharmaceutical providers that promote pharmacogenetic testing, such as in package labeling recommendations. Clinical trials for new pharmaceutical agents are currently considering the benefits of pharmacogenetic testing for individual products.

Complementary to, but separate from TDM, pharmacogenetics or "toxicogenetics" may apply similar concepts to the field of risk stratification, such as for cancer thought to be triggered by environmental or dietary exposure to a wide variety of xenobiotics. Shown in Table 43-10 are some of the genetic targets that have been studied with regard to risk of various cancers and also because of their role in the activation or inactivation of cancer chemotherapeutics.[15] Genes that encode for drug metabolizing enzymes are of most interest for this application as it is through these enzymes that xenobiotics become activated or inactivated. In addition to NAT1, NAT2, and the CYPs discussed previously in this chapter are the glutathione S-transferases (GSTs). At least 16 GSTs have been identified, which are divided into classes designated as Alpha (A), Kappa, Mu (M), Pi (P), Sigma, Theta (T), Zeta, and Omega. The *GSTM1* deficient trait has, for example, been associated with higher risk of lung and bladder cancer.[49] With additional study and validation of these and other genetic markers, preemployment testing to identify individuals with high susceptibility to chemical carcinogens may become important for occupational settings, such as agriculture and manufacturing.

Cancer treatments are of particular interest because of common ADRs. Current chemotherapeutic research includes the drug metabolizing enzymes dihydropyrimidine dehydrogenase (DPYD) and UDP-glucuronosyltransferase (UGT). These enzymes have significant interpatient variability in the metabolism of 5-fluorouracil (5-FU) and irinotecan, respectively.[30,91] *DPYD*2A*, the most common variant allele that leads to a nonfunctional DPYD protein, is caused by a G>A transition. The presence of this allele is correlated with severe toxicity and mortality following treatment with standard doses of 5-FU. Likewise, the *UGT1A1*28* allele has been correlated with irinotecan toxicity.[3] Such pharmacogenetic markers may prove useful for optimizing the pharmacotherapy of cancer.

The field of pharmacogenetics is currently benefiting pharmacotherapeutics by improving dose optimization tools for a select group of medications, such as AZA and 6-MP. Studies suggest that pharmacogenetics tools are potentially useful for dose selection and optimization of many clinically important drugs, particularly those with a narrow therapeutic index (e.g., cancer chemotherapeutics), those which have a narrow opportunity to exert efficacy (e.g., immunosuppressants), those which require weeks or more to determine therapeutic efficacy (e.g., antidepressants), and those which are at high risk for adverse effects and are administered chronically (e.g., lipid lowering). Pharmacogenetics also shows promise in the investigation of ADRs, including postmortem, and for assessing risk for xenobiotic-related conditions, including some cancers.

REFERENCES

1. Agundez JA, Ledesma MC, Ladero JM, Benitez J. Prevalence of CYP2D6 gene duplication and its repercussion on the oxidative phenotype in a white population. Clin Pharmacol Ther 1995;57:265-9.
2. Ameyaw MM, Collie-Duguid ES, Powrie RH, Ofori-Adjei D, McLeod HL. Thiopurine methyltransferase alleles in British and Ghanaian populations. Hum Mol Genet 1999;8:367-70.
3. Ando Y, Ueoka H, Sugiyama T, Ichiki M, Shimokata K, Hasegawa Y. Polymorphisms of UDP-glucuronosyltransferase and pharmacokinetics of irinotecan. Ther Drug Monit 2002;24:111-6.
4. Anonymous. Arylamine N-Acetyltransferase (NAT) Nomenclature. http://www.louisville.edu/medschool/pharmacology/NAT.html (Accessed December 5, 2004).
5. Anonymous. Human Cytochrome P450 (CYP) Allele Nomenclature Committee. CYP allele nomenclature. http://www.imm.ki.se/CYPalleles (Accessed December 5, 2004).
6. Anonymous. PharmGKB. The pharmacogenetics and pharmacogenomics knowledge base. http://www.pharmgkb.org (Accessed December 5, 2004).
7. Baker GB, Fang J, Sinha S, Coutts RT. Metabolic drug interactions with selective serotonin reuptake inhibitor (SSRI) antidepressants. Neurosci Biobehav Rev 1998;22:325-33.
8. Bell DA, Taylor JA, Butler MA, Stephens EA, Wiest J, Brubaker LH, et al. Genotype/phenotype discordance for human arylamine N-acetyltransferase (NAT2) reveals a new slow-acetylator allele common in African-Americans. Carcinogenesis 1993;14:1689-92.
9. Blaisdell J, Jorge-Nebert LF, Coulter S, Ferguson SS, Lee SJ, Chanas B, et al. Discovery of new potentially defective alleles of human CYP2C9. Pharmacogenetics 2004;14:527-37.
10. Blaisdell J, Mohrenweiser H, Jackson J, Ferguson S, Coulter S, Chanas B, et al. Identification and functional characterization of new potentially defective alleles of human CYP2C19. Pharmacogenetics 2002;12:703-11.
11. Blum M, Grant DM, McBride W, Heim M, Meyer UA. Human arylamine N-acetyltransferase genes: isolation, chromosomal localization, and functional expression. DNA Cell Biol 1990;9:193-203.
12. Bonicke R, Reif W. Enzymatic inactivation of isonicotinic acid hydrazide in humans and animals. Arch Exp Pathol Pharmakol 1953;220:321-33.
13. Boukouvala S, Price N, Plant KE, Sim E. Structure and transcriptional regulation of the NAT2 gene encoding for the drug-metabolizing enzyme arylamine N-acetyltransferase type 2 in mice. Biochem J 2003;375:593-602.
14. Bramness JG, Skurtveit S, Fauske L, Grung M, Molven A, Morland J, et al. Association between blood carisoprodol:meprobamate concentration ratios and CYP2C19 genotype in carisoprodol-drugged drivers: decreased metabolic capacity in heterozygous CYP2C19*1/CYP2C19*2 subjects. Pharmacogenetics 2003;13:383-8.

15. Brockmoller J, Cascorbi I, Henning S, Meisel C, Roots I. Molecular genetics of cancer susceptibility. Pharmacology 2000;61:212-27.
16. Broly F, Marez D, Sabbagh N, Legrand M, Millecamps S, Lo Guidice JM, et al. An efficient strategy for detection of known and new mutations of the CYP2D6 gene using single strand conformation polymorphism analysis. Pharmacogenetics 1995;5:373-84.
17. Brosen K, de Morais SM, Meyer UA, Goldstein JA. A multifamily study on the relationship between CYP2C19 genotype and s-mephenytoin oxidation phenotype. Pharmacogenetics 1995;5:312-7.
18. Brouwer C, Marinaki AM, Lambooy LH, Duley JA, Shobowale-Bakre M, De Abreu RA. Pitfalls in the determination of mutant alleles of the thiopurine methyltransferase gene. Leukemia 2001;15:1792-3.
19. Caldwell J. Pharmacogenetics and individual variation in the range of amino acid adequacy: the biological aspects. J Nutr 2004;134:1600S-4S; discussion 30S-32S, 67S-72S.
20. Cao H, Hegele RA. DNA polymorphisms in ITPA including basis of inosine triphosphatase deficiency. J Hum Genet 2002;47:620-2.
21. Cascorbi I, Drakoulis N, Brockmoller J, Maurer A, Sperling K, Roots I. Arylamine N-acetyltransferase (NAT2) mutations and their allelic linkage in unrelated Caucasian individuals: correlation with phenotypic activity. Am J Hum Genet 1995;57:581-92.
22. Chou WH, Yan FX, Robbins-Weilert DK, Ryder TB, Liu WW, Perbost C, et al. Comparison of two CYP2D6 genotyping methods and assessment of genotype-phenotype relationships. Clin Chem 2003;49:542-51.
23. Clunie GP, Lennard L. Relevance of thiopurine methyltransferase status in rheumatology patients receiving azathioprine. Rheumatology (Oxford) 2004;43:13-8.
24. Collie-Duguid ES, Pritchard SC, Powrie RH, Sludden J, Collier DA, Li T, McLeod HL. The frequency and distribution of thiopurine methyltransferase alleles in Caucasian and Asian populations. Pharmacogenetics 1999;9:37-42.
25. Daley AK. Related pharmacogenetics of the polymorphic metabolizing enzymes. Fundam Clin Pharmcol 2003;17:27-41.
26. Daly AK, Fairbrother KS, Andreassen OA, London SJ, Idle JR, Steen VM. Characterization and PCR-based detection of two different hybrid CYP2D7P/CYP2D6 alleles associated with the poor metabolizer phenotype. Pharmacogenetics 1996;6:319-28.
27. Daniel HI, Edeki TI. Genetic polymorphism of S-mephenytoin 4′-hydroxylation. Psychopharmacol Bull 1996;32:219-30.
28. De Morais SM, Wilkinson GR, Blaisdell J, Meyer UA, Nakamura K, Goldstein JA. Identification of a new genetic defect responsible for the polymorphism of (S)-mephenytoin metabolism in Japanese. Mol Pharmacol 1994;46:594-8.
29. de Morais SM, Wilkinson GR, Blaisdell J, Nakamura K, Meyer UA, Goldstein JA. The major genetic defect responsible for the polymorphism of S-mephenytoin metabolism in humans. J Biol Chem 1994;269: 15419-22.
30. Diasio RB, Johnson MR. The role of pharmacogenetics and pharmacogenomics in cancer chemotherapy with 5-fluorouracil. Pharmacology 2000;61:199-203.
31. Eichelbaum M, Evert B. Influence of pharmacogenetics on drug disposition and response. Clin Exp Pharmacol Physiol 1996;23:983-5.
32. Evans DAP, Manley KA, McKusick VA. Genetic control of isoniazid metabolism in man. Br Med J 1960:485-91.
33. Evans WE. Pharmacogenetics of thiopurine S-methyltransferase and thiopurine therapy. Ther Drug Monit 2004;26:186-91.
34. Evans WE, Hon YY, Bomgaars L, Coutre S, Holdsworth M, Janco R, et al. Preponderance of thiopurine S-methyltransferase deficiency and heterozygosity among patients intolerant to mercaptopurine or azathioprine. J Clin Oncol 2001;19: 2293-301.
35. Evans WE, McLeod HL. Pharmacogenomics—drug disposition, drug targets, and side effects. N Engl J Med 2003;348:538-49.
36. Flockhart DA. Clinically Relevant Drug Interaction Table. http://medicine.iupui.edu/flockhart/table.htm (Accessed August 30, 2004).
37. Fronhoffs S, Bruning T, Ortiz-Pallardo E, Brode P, Koch B, Harth V, et al. Real-time PCR analysis of the N-acetyltransferase NAT1 allele *3, *4, *10, *11, *14 and *17 polymorphism in squamous cell cancer of head and neck. Carcinogenesis 2001;22:1405-12.
38. Gaedigk A, Gotschall RR, Forbes NS, Simon SD, Kearns GL, Leeder JS. Optimization of cytochrome P4502D6 (CYP2D6) phenotype assignment using a genotyping algorithm based on allele frequency data. Pharmacogenetics 1999;9:669-82.
39. Giancarlo GM, Venkatakrishnan K, Granda BW, von Moltke LL, Greenblatt DJ. Relative contributions of CYP2C9 and 2C19 to phenytoin 4-hydroxylation in vitro: inhibition by sulfaphenazole, omeprazole, and ticlopidine. Eur J Clin Pharmacol 2001;57:31-6.
40. Gilman AG, Rall TW, Nies AS, Taylor P, eds. Goodman and Gilman's the pharmacological basis of therapeutics. Eighth ed. Elmsford, NY: Pergamon Press, 1990.
41. Goldstein DB, Tate SK, Sisodiya SM. Pharmacogenetics goes genomic. Nat Rev Genet 2003;4:937-47.
42. Gough AC, Miles JS, Spurr NK, Moss JE, Gaedigk A, Eichelbaum M, et al. Identification of the primary gene defect at the cytochrome P450 CYP2D locus. Nature 1990;347:773-6.

43. Grant DM, Blum M, Beer M, Meyer UA. Monomorphic and polymorphic human arylamine N-acetyltransferases: a comparison of liver isozymes and expressed products of two cloned genes. Mol Pharmacol 1991;39:184-91.
44. Grant DM, Goodfellow GH, Sugamori KS, Durette K. Pharmacogenetics of the human arylamine N-acetyltransferases. Pharmacol 2000;61:204-11.
45. Grant DM, Hughes NC, Janezic SA, Goodfellow GH, Chen HJ, Gaedigk A, et al. Human acetyltransferase polymorphisms. Mutation Res 1997;376:61-70.
46. Grasmader K, Verwohlt PL, Rietschel M, Dragicevic A, Muller M, Hiemke C, et al. Impact of polymorphisms of cytochrome-P450 isoenzymes 2C9, 2C19 and 2D6 on plasma concentrations and clinical effects of antidepressants in a naturalistic clinical setting. Eur J Clin Pharmacol 2004;60:329-36.
47. Griese EU, Zanger UM, Brudermanns U, Gaedigk A, Mikus G, Morike K, et al. Assessment of the predictive power of genotypes for the in-vivo catalytic function of CYP2D6 in a German population. Pharmacogenetics 1998;8:15-26.
48. Gross M, Kruisselbrink T, Anderson K, Lang N, McGovern P, Delongchamp R, et al. Distribution and concordance of N-acetyltransferase genotype and phenotype in an American population. Cancer Epidemiol Biomarkers Prev 1999;8:683-92.
49. Hayes JD, Strange RC. Glutathione S-transferase polymorphisms and their biological consequences. Pharmacology 2000;61:154-66.
50. Heim MH, Meyer UA. Genetic polymorphism of debrisoquine oxidation: restriction fragment analysis and allele-specific amplification of mutant alleles of CYP2D6. Methods Enzymol 1991;206:173-83.
51. Hein DW, Doll MA, Fretland AJ, Leff MA, Webb SJ, Xiao GH, et al. Molecular genetics and epidemiology of the NAT1 and NAT2 acetylation polymorphisms. Cancer Epidemiol Biomarkers Prev 2000;9:29-42.
52. Hein DW, Doll MA, Rustan TD, Gray K, Feng Y, Ferguson RJ, et al. Metabolic activation and deactivation of arylamine carcinogens by recombinant human NAT1 and polymorphic NAT2 acetyltransferases. Carcinogenesis 1993;14:1633-8.
53. Hein DW, Grant DM, Sim E. Update on consensus arylamine N-acetyltransferase gene nomenclature. Pharmacogenetics 2000;10:291-2.
54. Hickman D, Sim E. N-acetyltransferase polymorphism. Comparison of phenotype and genotype in humans. Biochem Pharmacol 1991;42:1007-14.
55. Higashi MK, Veenstra DL, Kondo LM, Wittkowsky AK, Srinouanprachanh SL, Farin FM, Rettie AE. Association between CYP2C9 genetic variants and anticoagulation-related outcomes during warfarin therapy. JAMA 2002;287:1690-8.
56. Hiratsuka M, Agatsuma Y, Omori F, Narahara K, Inoue T, Kishikawa Y, Mizugaki M. High throughput detection of drug-metabolizing enzyme polymorphisms by allele-specific fluorogenic 5′ nuclease chain reaction assay. Biol Pharm Bull 2000;23:1131-5.
57. Ho PC, Saville DJ, Wanwimolruk S. Inhibition of human CYP3A4 activity by grapefruit flavonoids, furanocoumarins and related compounds. J Pharm Pharm Sci 2001;4:217-27.
58. Hon YY, Fessing MY, Pui CH, Relling MV, Krynetski EY, Evans WE. Polymorphism of the thiopurine S-methyltransferase gene in African-Americans. Hum Mol Genet 1999;8:371-6.
59. Hoskins JM, Shenfield GM, Gross AS. Concordance between proguanil phenotype and CYP2C19 genotype in Chinese. Eur J Clin Pharmacol 2003;59:611-4.
60. Hughes NC, Janezic SA, McQueen KL, Jewett MAS, Castranio T, Bell DA, et al. Identification and characterization of variant alleles of human acetyltransferase NAT1 with defective function using p-aminosalicylate as an in-vivo and in-vitro probe. Pharmacogenetics 1998;8:55-66.
61. Ibeanu GC, Blaisdell J, Ghanayem BI, Beyeler C, Benhamou S, Bouchardy C, et al. An additional defective allele, CYP2C19*5, contributes to the S-mephenytoin poor metabolizer phenotype in Caucasians. Pharmacogenetics 1998;8:129-35.
62. Ingelman-Sundberg M. Pharmacogenetics of cytochrome P450 and its applications in drug therapy: the past, present and future. Trends Pharmacol Sci 2004;25:193-200.
63. Jenne JW. Partial purification and properties of the isoniazid transacetylase in human liver. Its relationship to the acetylation of p-aminosalicylic acid. J Clin Invest 1965;44:1992-2002.
64. Johansson I, Lundqvist E, Dahl ML, Ingelman-Sundberg M. PCR-based genotyping for duplicated and deleted CYP2D6 genes. Pharmacogenetics 1996;6:351-5.
65. Kashuba AD, Nafziger AN, Kearns GL, Leeder JS, Shirey CS, Gotschall R, et al. Quantification of intraindividual variability and the influence of menstrual cycle phase on CYP2D6 activity as measured by dextromethorphan phenotyping. Pharmacogenetics 1998;8:403-10.
66. Katoh T, Boissy R, Nagata N, Kitagawa K, Kuroda Y, Itoh H, et al. Inherited polymorphism in the N-acetyltransferase 1 (NAT1) and 2 (NAT2) genes and susceptibility to gastric and colorectal adenocarcinoma. Int J Cancer 2000;85:46-9.
67. Kerb R, Aynacioglu AS, Brockmoller J, Schlagenhaufer R, Bauer S, Szekeres T, et al. The predictive value of MDR1, CYP2C9, and CYP2C19 polymorphisms for phenytoin plasma levels. Pharmacogenomics J 2001;1:204-10.
68. Kidd RS, Curry TB, Gallagher S, Edeki T, Blaisdell J, Goldstein JA. Identification of a null allele of

CYP2C9 in an African-American exhibiting toxicity to phenytoin. Pharmacogenetics 2001;11:803-8.
69. Kirchheiner J, Bertilsson L, Bruus H, Wolff A, Roots I, Bauer M. Individualized medicine—implementation of pharmacogenetic diagnostics in antidepressant drug treatment of major depressive disorders. Pharmacopsychiatry 2003;36 Suppl 3:S235-43.
70. Kirchheiner J, Brosen K, Dahl ML, Gram LF, Kasper S, Roots I, et al. CYP2D6 and CYP2C19 genotype-based dose recommendations for antidepressants: a first step toward subpopulation-specific dosages. Acta Psychiat Scand 2001;104:173-92.
71. Kirchheiner J, Nickchen K, Bauer M, Wong ML, Licinio J, Roots I, et al. Pharmacogenetics of antidepressants and antipsychotics: the contribution of allelic variations to the phenotype of drug response. Mol Psychiatry 2004;9:442-73.
72. Kita T, Tanigawara Y, Chikazawa S, Hatanaka H, Sakaeda T, Komada F, et al. N-acetyltransferase 2 genotype correlated with isoniazid acetylation in Japanese tuberculous patients. Biol Pharm Bull 2001;24:544-9.
73. Kubota T, Chiba K. Frequencies of thiopurine S-methyltransferase mutant alleles (TPMT*2, *3A, *3B and *3C) in 151 healthy Japanese subjects and the inheritance of TPMT*3C in the family of a propositus. Br J Clin Pharmacol 2001;51: 475-7.
74. Kubota T, Nishida A, Takeuchi K, Iida T, Yokota H, Higashi K, et al. Frequency distribution of thiopurine S-methyltransferase activity in red blood cells of a healthy Japanese population. Ther Drug Monit 2004;26:319-21.
75. Lazarou J, Pomeranz BH, Corey PN. Incidence of adverse drug reactions in hospitalized patients: a meta-analysis of prospective studies. JAMA 1998;279:1200-5.
76. Leathart JB, London SJ, Steward A, Adams JD, Idle JR, Daly AK. CYP2D6 phenotype-genotype relationships in African-Americans and Caucasians in Los Angeles. Pharmacogenetics 1998;8:529-41.
77. Licinio J, Wong M, eds. Pharmacogenomics. The search for individualized therapies. Weinheim (Germany): Wiley-Vch, 2002.
78. Lilja JJ, Kivisto KT, Neuvonen PJ. Duration of effect of grapefruit juice on the pharmacokinetics of the CYP3A4 substrate simvastatin. Clin Pharmacol Ther 2000;68:384-90.
79. Linder MW, Keck PE Jr. Standards of laboratory practice: antidepressant drug monitoring. National Academy of Clinical Biochemistry. Clin Chem 1998;44:1073-84.
80. Linder MW, Looney S, Adams JE III, Johnson N, Antonino-Green D, Lacefield N, et al. Warfarin dose adjustments based on CYP2C9 genetic polymorphisms. J Thromb Thrombolysis 2002;14:227-32.
81. Linder MW, Valdes R Jr, Stubbins MJ, Harries LW, Smith G, Tarbit MH, et al. Pharmacogenetics in the practice of laboratory medicine. Genetic analysis of the human cytochrome P450 CYP2C9 locus. Mol Diagn 1999;4:365-79.
82. Lovlie R, Daly AK, Molven A, Idle JR, Steen VM. Ultrarapid metabolizers of debrisoquine: characterization and PCR-based detection of alleles with duplication of the CYP2D6 gene. FEBS Lett 1996;392: 30-4.
83. Mamiya K, Ieiri I, Shimamoto J, Yukawa E, Imai J, Ninomiya H, et al. The effects of genetic polymorphisms of CYP2C9 and CYP2C19 on phenytoin metabolism in Japanese adult patients with epilepsy: studies in stereoselective hydroxylation and population pharmacokinetics. Epilepsia 1998;39: 1317-23.
84. Marez D, Legrand M, Sabbagh N, Guidice JM, Spire C, Lafitte JJ, et al. Polymorphism of the cytochrome P450 CYP2D6 gene in a European population: characterization of 48 mutations and 53 alleles, their frequencies and evolution. Pharmacogenetics 1997;7:193-202.
85. Marinaki AM, Ansari A, Duley JA, Arenas M, Sumi S, Lewis CM, et al. Adverse drug reactions to azathioprine therapy are associated with polymorphism in the gene encoding inosine triphosphate pyrophosphatase (ITPase). Pharmacogenetics 2004;14:181-7.
86. Marra CA, Esdaile JM, Anis AH. Practical pharmacogenetics: the cost effectiveness of screening for thiopurine s-methyltransferase polymorphisms in patients with rheumatological conditions treated with azathioprine. J Rheumatol 2002;29:2507-12.
87. Martinez C, Blanco G, Ladero JM, Garcia-Martin E, Taxonera C, Gamito FG, et al. Genetic predisposition to acute gastrointestinal bleeding after NSAIDs use. Br J Pharmacol 2004;141:205-8.
88. McDonald OG, Krynetski EY, Evans WE. Molecular haplotyping of genomic DNA for multiple single-nucleotide polymorphisms located kilobases apart using long-range polymerase chain reaction and intramolecular ligation. Pharmacogenetics 2002;12:93-9.
89. McElroy S, Sachse C, Brockmoller J, Richmond J, Lira M, Friedman D, et al. CYP2D6 genotyping as an alternative to phenotyping for determination of metabolic status in a clinical trial setting. AAPS PharmSci 2000;2:E33.
90. McLeod HL, Krynetski EY, Wilimas JA, Evans WE. Higher activity of polymorphic thiopurine S-methyltransferase in erythrocytes from neonates compared to adults. Pharmacogenetics 1995;5:281-6.
91. McLeod HL, Papageorgio C, Watters JW. Using genetic variations to optimize cancer chemotherapy. Clinical Advances in Haematology and Oncology 2003;1:107-11.

92. McLeod HL, Siva C. The thiopurine S-methyltransferase gene locus—implications for clinical pharmacogenomics. Pharmacogenomics 2002;3:89-98.
93. Meisel C, Gerloff T, Kirchheiner J, Mrozikiewicz PM, Niewinski P, Brockmoller J, et al. Implications of pharmacogenetics for individualizing drug treatment and for study design. J Mol Med 2003;81:154-67.
94. Meisler MH, Reinke C. A sensitive fluorescent assay for N-acetyltransferase activity in human lymphocytes from newborns and adults. Clin Chim Acta 1979;1979:91-6.
95. Meyer UA, Zanger UM. Molecular mechanisms of genetic polymorphisms of drug metabolism. Annu Rev Pharmacol Toxicol 1997;37:269-96.
96. Miki I, Aoyama N, Sakai T, Shirasaka D, Wambura CM, Maekawa S, et al. Impact of clarithromycin resistance and CYP2C19 genetic polymorphism on treatment efficacy of Helicobacter pylori infection with lansoprazole- or rabeprazole-based triple therapy in Japan. Eur J Gastroenterol Hepatol 2003;15:27-33.
97. Minchin RF. Acetylation of p-amino benzoylglutamate, a folic acid catabolite, by recombinant arylamine N-acetyltransferase and U937 cells. Biochem J 1995;307:1-3.
98. Mizutani T. PM frequencies of major CYPs in Asians and Caucasians. Drug Metab Rev 2003;35:99-106.
99. Molden E, Johansen PW, Boe GH, Bergan S, Christensen H, Rugstad HE, et al. Pharmacokinetics of diltiazem and its metabolites in relation to CYP2D6 genotype. Clin Pharmacol Ther 2002;72:333-42.
100. Muller M. Pharmacogenomics and drug response. Int J Clin Pharmacol Ther 2003;41:231-40.
101. Murphy GM Jr., Pollock BG, Kirshner MA, Pascoe N, Cheuk W, Mulsant BH, Reynolds CF, III. CYP2D6 genotyping with oligonucleotide microarrays and nortriptyline concentrations in geriatric depression. Neuropsychopharmacology 2001;25:737-43.
102. Nebert DW, Dieter MZ. The evolution of drug metabolism. Pharmacology 2000;61:124-35.
103. Nelson DR, Kamataki T, Waxman DJ, Guengerich FP, Estabrook RW, Feyereisen R, et al. The P450 superfamily: update on new sequences, gene mapping, accession numbers, early trivial names of enzymes, and nomenclature. DNA Cell Biol 1993;12:1-51.
104. Otterness D, Szumlanski C, Lennard L, Klemetsdal B, Aarbakke J, Park-Hah JO, et al. Human thiopurine methyltransferase pharmacogenetics: gene sequence polymorphisms. Clin Pharmacol Ther 1997;62:60-73.
105. Paine MF, Criss AB, Watkins PB. Two major grapefruit juice components differ in intestinal CYP3A4 inhibition kinetic and binding properties. Drug Metab Dispos 2004;32:1146-53.
106. Perry PJ, Pfohl BM, Holstad SG. The relationship between antidepressant response and tricyclic antidepressant plasma concentrations: a retrospective analysis of the literature using logistic regression analysis. Clin Pharmacokinet 1987;13:381-92.
107. Pickering JW, McMillin GA, Gedge F, Hill HR, Lyon E. Flow cytometric assay for genotyping cytochrome p450 2C9 and 2C19: comparison with a microelectronic DNA array. Am J Pharmacogenomics 2004;4:199-207.
108. Pitarque M, von Richter O, Oke B, Berkkan H, Oscarson M, Ingelman-Sundberg M. Identification of a single nucleotide polymorphism in the TATA box of the CYP2A6 gene: impairment of its promoter activity. Biochem Biophys Res Commun 2001;284:455-60.
109. Relling MV, Hancock ML, Rivera GK, Sandlund JT, Ribeiro RC, Krynetski EY, et al. Mercaptopurine therapy intolerance and heterozygosity at the thiopurine S-methyltransferase gene locus. J Natl Cancer Inst 1999;91:2001-8.
110. Rendic S, Di Carlo FJ. Human cytochrome P450 enzymes: a status report summarizing their reactions, substrates, inducers, and inhibitors. Drug Metab Rev 1997;29:413-580.
111. Sachse C, Brockmoller J, Bauer S, Roots I. Cytochrome P450 2D6 variants in a Caucasian population: allele frequencies and phenotypic consequences. Am J Hum Genet 1997;60:284-95.
112. Schaeffeler E, Fischer C, Brockmeier D, Wernet D, Moerike K, Eichelbaum M, et al. Comprehensive analysis of thiopurine S-methyltransferase phenotype-genotype correlation in a large population of German-Caucasians and identification of novel TPMT variants. Pharmacogenetics 2004;14:407-17.
113. Schaeffeler E, Schwab M, Eichelbaum M, Zanger UM. CYP2D6 genotyping strategy based on gene copy number determination by TaqMan real-time PCR. Hum Mutat 2003;22:476-85.
114. Schwarz UI. Clinical relevance of genetic polymorphisms in the human CYP2C9 gene. Eur J Clin Invest 2003;33 Suppl 2:23-30.
115. Scordo MG, Aklillu E, Yasar U, Dahl ML, Spina E, Ingelman-Sundberg M. Genetic polymorphism of cytochrome P450 2C9 in a Caucasian and a black African population. Br J Clin Pharmacol 2001;52:447-50.
116. Seidman EG, Furst DE. Pharmacogenetics for the individualization of treatment of rheumatic disorders using azathioprine. J Rheumatol 2002;29:2484-7.
117. Shimoda K, Someya T, Yokono A, Morita S, Hirokane G, Takahashi S, et al. The impact of CYP2C19 and CYP2D6 genotypes on metabolism of amitriptyline in Japanese psychiatric patients. J Clin Psychopharmacol 2002;22:371-8.
118. Sim E, Pinter K, Mushtaq A, Upton A, Sandy J, Bhakta S, et al. Arylamine N-acetyltransferases: a pharmacogenomic approach to drug metabolism and

endogenous function. Biochem Soc Trans 2003;31:615-9.
119. Spielberg SP. N-acetyltransferases: pharmacogenetics and clinical consequences of polymorphic drug metabolism. J Pharmacokinet Biopharm 1996;24: 509-19.
120. Steimer W, Zopf K, Von Amelunxen S, Pfeiffer H, Bachofer J, Popp J, et al. Allele-specific change of concentration and functional gene dose for the prediction of steady-state serum concentrations of amitriptyline and nortriptyline in CYP2C19 and CYP2D6 extensive and intermediate metabolizers. Clin Chem 2004;50:1623-33.
121. Stubbins MJ, Harries LW, Smith G, Tarbit MH, Wolf CR. Genetic analysis of the human cytochrome P450 CYP2C9 locus. Pharmacogenetics 1996;6:429-39.
122. Stuven T, Griese EU, Kroemer HK, Eichelbaum M, Zanger UM. Rapid detection of CYP2D6 null alleles by long distance- and multiplex-polymerase chain reaction. Pharmacogenetics 1996;6:417-21.
123. Summerscales JE, Josephy PD. Human acetyl CoA: arylamine N-acetyltransferase variants generated by random mutagenesis. Mol Pharmacol 2004;65: 220-6.
124. Tai HL, Fessing MY, Bonten EJ, Yanishevsky Y, d'Azzo A, Krynetski EY, et al. Enhanced proteasomal degradation of mutant human thiopurine S-methyltransferase (TPMT) in mammalian cells: mechanism for TPMT protein deficiency inherited by TPMT*2, TPMT*3A, TPMT*3B or TPMT*3C. Pharmacogenetics 1999;9:641-50.
125. Take S, Mizuno M, Ishiki K, Nagahara Y, Yoshida T, Inaba T, et al. Interleukin-1beta genetic polymorphism influences the effect of cytochrome P 2C19 genotype on the cure rate of 1-week triple therapy for Helicobacter pylori infection. Am J Gastroenterol 2003;98:2403-8.
126. Tavadia SM, Mydlarski PR, Reis MD, Mittmann N, Pinkerton PH, Shear N, et al. Screening for azathioprine toxicity: a pharmacoeconomic analysis based on a target case. J Am Acad Dermatol 2000;42:628-32.
127. Vatsis KP, Martell KJ, Weber WW. Diverse point mutations in the human gene for polymorphic N-acetyltransferase. Proc Natl Acad Sci USA 1991;88:6333-7.
128. Vatsis KP, Weber WW, Bell DA, Dupret JM, Evans DAP, Grant DM, et al. Nomenclature for N-acetyltransferases. Pharmacogenetics 1995;5:1-17.
129. Veenstra DL, Higashi MK, Phillips KA. Assessing the cost-effectiveness of pharmacogenomics. AAPS PharmSci 2000;2:E29.
130. Wang SL, Lai MD, Lai ML, Huang JD. R296C and other CYP2D6 mutations in Chinese. Pharmacogenetics 1995;5:385-8.
131. Weber WW, Cronin MT. Pharmacogenetic testing. In: Meyers RA, ed. Encyclopedia of clinical analytical chemistry, Chichester, Great Britain: John Wiley & Sons Ltd, 2000.
132. Weber WW, Hein DW. Clinical pharmacokinetics of isoniazid. Clin Pharmacokinet 1979;4:401-22.
133. Weinshilboum RM, Sladek SL. Mercaptopurine pharmacogenetics: monogenic inheritance of erythrocyte thiopurine methyltransferase activity. Am J Hum Genet 1980;32:651-62.
134. West WL, Knight EM, Pradhan S, Hinds TS. Interpatient variability: genetic predisposition and other genetic factors. J Clin Pharmacol 1997;37:635-48.
135. Windmill KF, Gaedigk A, Hall PM, Samaratunga H, Grant DM, McManus ME. Localization of N-acetyltransferases NAT1 and NAT2 in human tissues. Toxicol Sci 2000;54:19-29.
136. Wormhoudt LW, Commandeur JNM, Vermeulen NPE. Genetic polymorphisms of human N-acetyltransferase, cytochrome P450, glutathione-S-transferase, and epoxide hydrolase enzymes: relevance to xenobiotic metabolism and toxicity. Crit Rev Toxicol 1999;29:59-124.
137. Wright JD, Helsby NA, Ward SA. The role of S-mephenytoin hydroxylase (CYP2C19) in the metabolism of the antimalarial biguanides. Br J Clin Pharmacol 1995;39:441-4.
138. Xiao ZS, Goldstein JA, Xie HG, Blaisdell J, Wang W, Jiang CH, et al. Differences in the incidence of the CYP2C19 polymorphism affecting the S-mephenytoin phenotype in Chinese Han and Bai populations and identification of a new rare CYP2C19 mutant allele. J Pharmacol Exp Ther 1997;281:604-9.
139. Yates CR, Krynetski EY, Loennechen T, Fessing MY, Tai HL, Pui CH, et al. Molecular diagnosis of thiopurine S-methyltransferase deficiency: genetic basis for azathioprine and mercaptopurine intolerance. Ann Intern Med 1997;126:608-14.
140. Yin OQ, Tomlinson B, Chow AH, Waye MM, Chow MS. Omeprazole as a CYP2C19 marker in Chinese subjects: assessment of its gene-dose effect and intrasubject variability. J Clin Pharmacol 2004;44: 582-9.
141. Zanger UM, Raimundo S, Eichelbaum M. Cytochrome P450 2D6: overview and update on pharmacology, genetics, biochemistry. Naunyn Schmiedebergs Arch Pharmacol 2004;369:23-37.
142. Zhou HH. CYP2C19 genotype determines enzyme activity and inducibility of S-mephenytoin hydroxylase. Clin Chim Acta 2001;313:203-8.
143. Zimmerman T, Schlenk R, Pfaff G, Lach P, Wildfeuer A. Prediction of phenotype for dextromethorphan O-demethylation by using polymerase chain reaction in healthy volunteers. Arzneimittelforschung 1995;45:41-3.

SECTION VI

Pathophysiology

CHAPTER 44

Cardiac Function

Fred S. Apple, Ph.D., and Allan S. Jaffe, M.D.

Although the heart is an efficient and durable pump, there are a variety of problems that can diminish cardiac function and lead to a variety of abnormal states. One of these problems is heart failure. It and acute ischemic heart disease are the most common diseases that rely on a biochemical diagnosis and thus will be the major focus of this chapter.[7]

The term acute myocardial infarction (AMI) is defined as an imbalance between myocardial oxygen supply and demand resulting in injury to and the eventual death of myocytes. Initially, the population of myocytes was thought fixed; however, it is now thought that the migration of stem cells has the potential at least to replace some of the damaged myocytes. When the blood supply to the heart is interrupted, "gross necrosis" of the myocardium results. Such extensive necrosis is most often associated with a thrombotic occlusion superimposed on coronary atherosclerosis. It is now apparent that the process of plaque rupture and thrombosis is one of the ways in which coronary atherosclerosis progresses and that we only recognize more severe events.[164,165] Total loss of coronary blood flow results in a clinical syndrome associated with what is known as ST segment elevation AMI (STE AMI). Partial loss of coronary perfusion if severe also can lead to necrosis as well—which is generally less severe and is known as NSTEMI (non-ST-elevation myocardial infarction), and other events of still lesser severity may be missed entirely or called angina, which can range from stable to unstable.

In the United States, approximately 700,000 patients suffer from an initial AMI annually and another 500,000 from a recurrent AMI. Coronary heart disease causes 20% of all deaths in the United States and cardiovascular diseases up to 38.5%. About 1.7 million patients are hospitalized each year in the United States with an acute coronary syndrome (ACS). Historically, most deaths caused by ischemic heart disease were acute, but as our therapeutic abilities have increased, the disease is slowly becoming a more chronic one. When deaths occur acutely, they are caused by either ventricular arrhythmias or pump dysfunction and congestive heart failure with or without cardiogenic shock. Death rates are sharply age dependent, both during hospitalization and the year following infarction. In the United States, the yearly economic burden of coronary artery disease (CAD) is in excess of $133.2 billion, more than a third of the total of $368.4 billion due to cardiovascular disease overall.

Before the advent of coronary care units, treatment of AMI was directed almost exclusively toward allowing healing of the infarct. The concept that infarctions evolve over time and that their size can be moderated led to a rethinking of this passive philosophy.[186] We now know that the reestablishment of nutritive perfusion reduces the extent of myocardial injury and is an important determinant of prognosis.[197] Today the management of AMI suggested by most guidelines is aggressive and invasively oriented in the hope of reducing the extent of the myocardial damage and thus improving prognosis.[39a,40,197] In addition, prevention is finally being recognized as a key element in the long-term treatment of patients with atherosclerosis and is included in these guidelines.

BASIC ANATOMY

The average human adult heart weighs approximately 325 g in men and 275 g in women and is 12 cm in length. The heart is a hollow muscular organ, shaped like a blunt cone, and is about the size of a human fist. It is located in the mediastinum, between the lower lobes of each lung, and rests upon the diaphragm. It is enclosed in a sac called the *pericardium.* The cardiac wall is composed of three layers: the *epicardium* (the outer most layer), a middle layer, and an inner layer called the *endocardium.* The heart has four chambers. The two upper chambers are termed the *right* and *left atria,* and the two lower chambers are termed the *right* and *left ventricles* (Figure 44-1). Under normal circumstances, the atria are compliant structures, so that intercavitary pres-

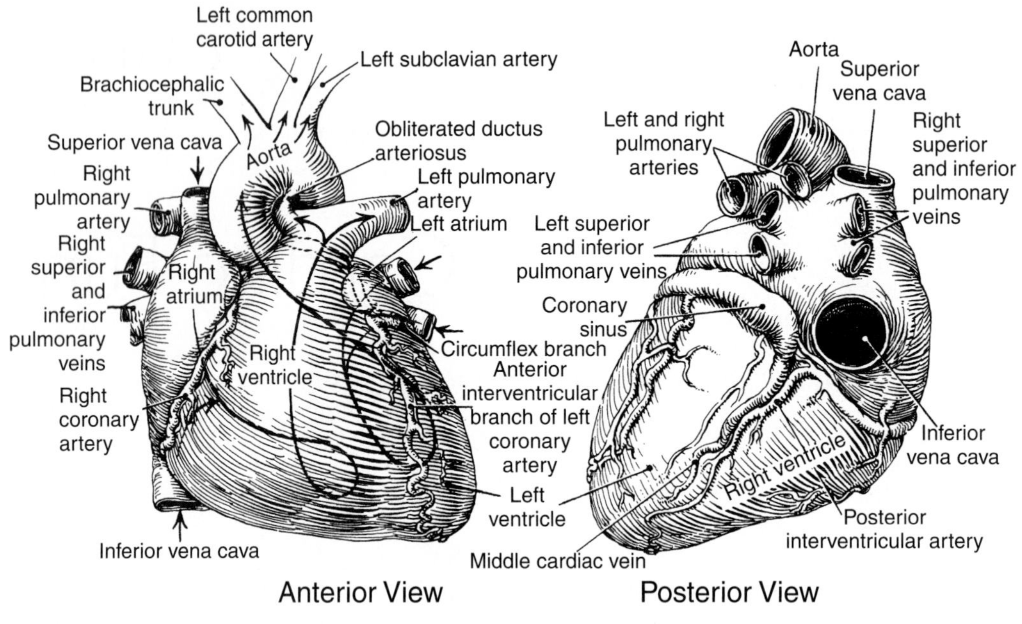

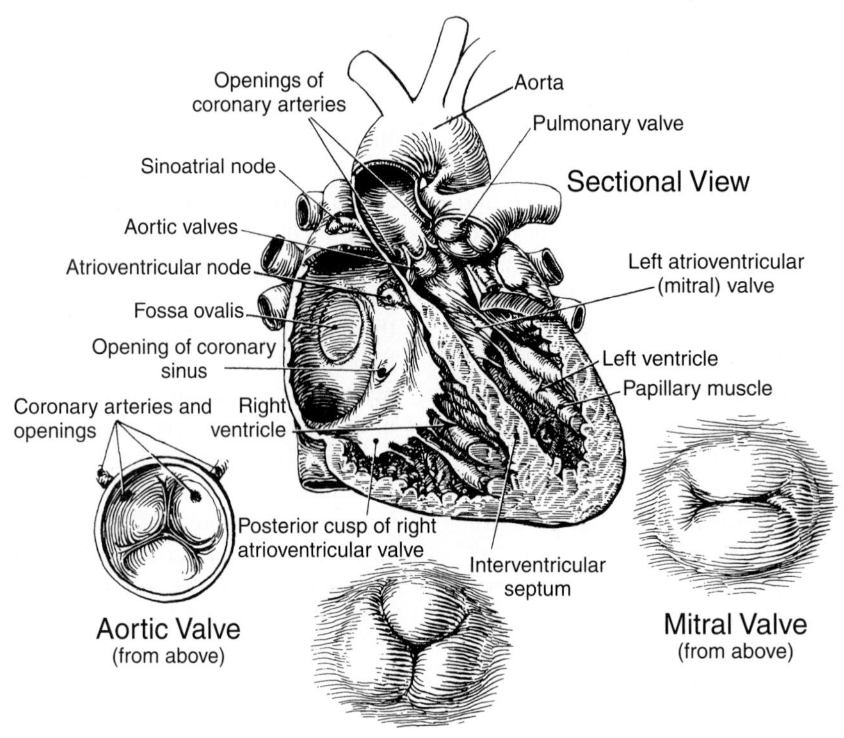

Figure 44-1 Anatomy of the heart. *(From Dorland's Illustrated Medical Dictionary, 30th ed. Philadelphia: WB Saunders Co, 2003:Panel 20.)*

sure is low. When anatomy is normal, each atrium is connected to its ventricle through an atrioventricular (AV) valve, which opens and closes (see discussion later in this chapter). The valve on the left side is called the *mitral valve* and the one on the right side, the *tricuspid valve.* The right ventricle is banana shaped and pumps blood into the *pulmonary artery* through a tri-leaflet *pulmonic valve.* The left ventricle pumps blood into the *aorta* through a tri-leaflet *aortic valve.* The ventricles, especially the left ventricle, is thicker and less compliant in keeping with its need to generate higher pressures than the right ventricle, and intercavitary pressures are much higher than in the atria. Under normal conditions, the conduction or electrical system of the heart coordinates the sequential contraction of first the atria and then the ventricles. Given they are connected, each side can effect the other. Under normal circumstances, the sequence of activation optimizes this interaction and thus the efficiency of cardiac function. The right and left coronary arteries originate from two of the three cusps of the aortic valve. They provide blood flow and thus nutritive perfusion to the heart. The largest vessels are on the epicardium and these can be accessed therapeutically fairly easily. Subsequent smaller branches divide to supply the remaining myocardium. The endocardium is the layer most susceptible to ischemia because its perfusion relies on the smallest vessels. There wall stress is greatest and opposition to flow occurs.

The myocardium contains bundles of striated muscle fibers, each of which is typically 10 to 15 μm in diameter and 30 to 60 μm in length. Work of the heart is generated by the alternating of the contraction and relaxation of these fibers. The fibers are composed of cardiac-specific contractile proteins actin and myosin, and regulatory proteins called troponins. They also contain a variety of enzymes that are vital for energy use, such as myoglobin, creatine kinase (CK), and lactate dehydrogenase (LD), some of which can be used as markers of cardiac injury.

PHYSIOLOGY

A typical cardiac cycle and the electrophysiology of the heart are discussed in this section.

CARDIAC CYCLE

A typical cardiac cycle consists of two intervals known as *systole* and *diastole* (Figure 44-2). During diastole, oxygenated blood returns from the lungs to the left atrium via the pulmonary veins and deoxygenated blood returns from other parts of the body to fill the right atrium. During this period, the AV valves are open, allowing passive filling of the ventricle. At the end of diastole, the atria contract, forcing additional blood through the AV valves and into the respective ventricles. During systole, the ventricles contract. This closes the AV valves when ventricular pressure exceeds atrial pressure and the pulmonary and aortic valves are opened when ventricular pressure exceeds the pressure in the pulmonary arteries and/or the aorta and blood flows into those conduits. During systole, a normal blood pressure in the aorta is typically 120 mm Hg, while during diastole, it falls to about 70 mm Hg. At rest, the heart pumps between 60 and 80 times per minute. Stroke volume (the amount of blood expelled with each contraction) is roughly 50 mL so cardiac output per minute is roughly 3 liters. Typically, we use values corrected for body surface area, which are usually in the range of 2.5 to 3.6 L/min/m^2. Measurements of cardiac output and ventricular filling pressures are the standards for assessing cardiac performance and function. Furthermore, therapeutic interventions in patients with heart disease are often assessed by determining cardiac output and ventricular pressures.[139]

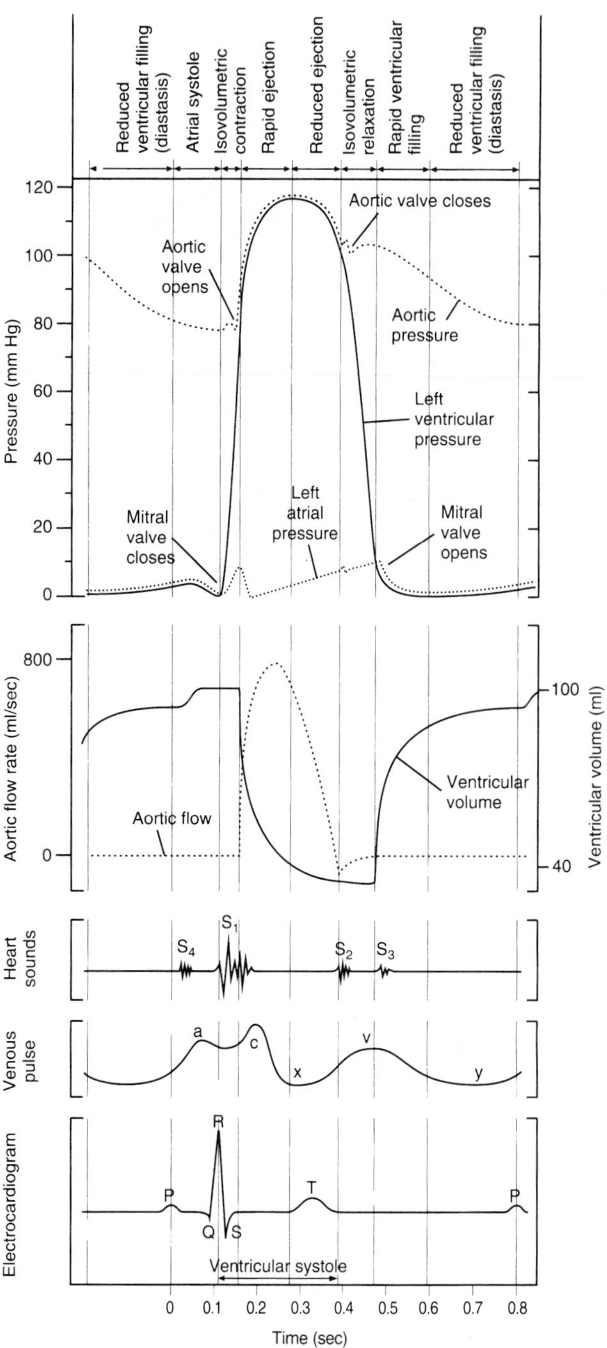

Figure 44-2 The cardiac cycle. *(From Dorland's Illustrated Medical Dictionary, 30th ed. Philadelphia: WB Saunders Co, 2003, with permission from the National Kidney Foundation.)*

CARDIAC CONDUCTING SYSTEM

The cardiac cycle is tightly controlled by the cardiac conducting system, which initiates electrical impulses and carries them, via a specialized conducting system, to the myocardium. The surface electrocardiogram (ECG) records changes in potential and is a graphic tracing of the variations in electrical potential caused by the excitation of the heart muscle and detected at the body surface.[156] Clinically, the ECG is used to identify (1) anatomic, (2) metabolic, (3)

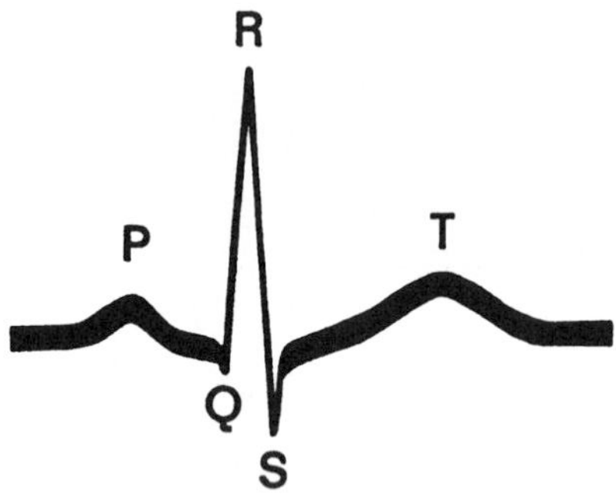

Figure 44-3 Electrocardiogram, serial tracing of a normal single heartbeat. Each beat manifests as five major waves: P, Q, R, S, and T. The QRS complex represents the ventricular contraction.

ionic, and (4) hemodynamic changes in the heart. The clinical sensitivity and specificity of ECG abnormalities are influenced by a wide spectrum of physiological and anatomical changes and the clinical situation.

Under normal circumstances, each electrical complex is similar and includes three major components (Figure 44-3): the atrial depolarization (the P wave), ventricular depolarization (the QRS complex), and repolarization (the ST segment and T wave). Atrial depolarization, which is manifested by the P wave, produces atrial contraction. Ventricular depolarization marked by the QRS complex produces contraction of the ventricles. It is composed of as many as three deflections: the Q wave, which when present is the first negative deflection; the R wave, which is the first positive deflection; and the S wave, which is a negative deflection following the R wave. On occasion, there is an R prime, which is a second positive deflection. Whether each of these occurs and their significance depends on the path of depolarization of the ventricles. Thus not every QRS complex will have discrete Q, R, and S waves. The ST segment and T wave are produced by the electrical recovery of the ventricles and their mean electrical vector is under normal circumstances concordant (i.e., in roughly the same direction) with the mean QRS vector.

A routine ECG is composed of 12 leads. Six are called limb leads (I, II, III, aVR, aVL, and aVF), because they are recorded between arm and leg electrodes, and six are called precordial or chest leads (V_1, V_2, V_3, V_4, V_5, and V_6) and are recorded across the sternum and left precordium. Each lead records the same electrical impulse but in a different position relative to the heart. Areas of pathology shown on the ECG can be localized by analyzing differences between the tracing in question and what is known to be normal in the 12 different leads.

CARDIAC DISEASE

There are many forms of cardiac disease. This chapter briefly covers congestive heart failure (CHF) and acute coronary syndromes, such as AMI. The vast number of other cardiac diseases are not discussed in depth here, because of the relatively minor role of diagnostic clinical laboratory tests in these disorders. However, the use of newer markers, such as the natriuretic peptides and the cardiac troponins, is changing that situation and is beginning to be of diagnostic utility in a number of disease states (see discussion later in this chapter).

CONGESTIVE HEART FAILURE

CHF is a condition in which there is ineffective pumping of the heart leading to an accumulation of fluid in the lungs. Typically, it results from a loss of cardiac tissue and subsequent function.[57] Medically, it is defined as the pathophysiological condition in which an abnormality of cardiac function is responsible for the failure of the heart to pump sufficient blood to satisfy the requirements of the metabolizing tissues. Encompassed in this definition are a wide spectrum of clinical conditions, ranging from (1) a primary impairment in pump function, such as might occur after a large AMI; (2) increased cardiac stiffness, which causes increases in pressure in the heart, restricts filling, and increases hydrostatic pressures behind the area of reduced compliance; and (3) situations in which peripheral demand is excessive, resulting in what is known as high output heart failure, which is defined as the inability of the heart to increase sufficiently to meet the peripheral demands for blood.

Epidemiology

In the United States, CHF is the only cardiovascular disease with an increasing incidence. The National Heart, Lung, Blood Institute estimates that current prevalence is 4.9 million Americans with CHF, with an incidence of approximately 400,000 new cases each year.[97,111] CHF is the leading cause of hospitalization in individuals 65 years and older. Current prognosis is dependent on disease severity, but overall it is poor. Five-year mortality is approximately 10% in mild CHF, 20% to 30% in moderate CHF, and up to 80% in end-stage disease.[121] These poor outcomes are not without substantial cost, estimated at $18.8 billion per year in the U.S.[95]

Currently, staging of CHF patients is with the New York Heart Association (NYHA) functional classifications I to IV. Class I patients are generally considered asymptomatic, with no restrictions on physical activity; class IV patients are often symptomatic at rest, with severe limitations on physical activity. The problem with this classification system is that much of it is based on subjective criteria. Thus patients with co-morbidities that reduce their activities are often not detected. In addition, there are many causes for dyspnea, which is the primary symptom in many of these individuals. Finally, many patients with ventricular dysfunction modify their activities to accomplish activities of daily living and thus lack overt symptoms until late in their disease. Thus patients with CHF often go undiagnosed and untreated early in their disease or are misdiagnosed because of diseases such as pulmonary disease. Initiating treatment in the more

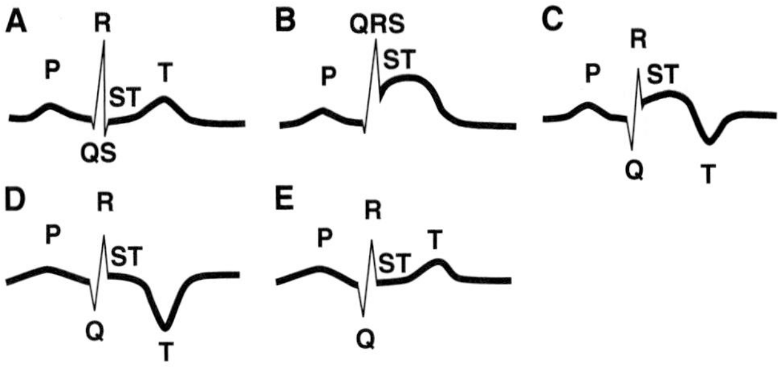

Figure 44-4 Electrocardiogram, serial tracing of a patient with an acute myocardial infarction. The sequence is **(A)** normal, **(B)** hours after infarction, the ST segment becomes elevated, **(C)** hours to days later, the T wave inverts and the Q wave becomes larger, **(D)** days to weeks later, the ST segment returns to near normal, and **(E)** weeks to months later, the T wave becomes upright again, but the large Q wave may remain.

advanced disease state is challenging (higher degree of irreversible cardiac function and patient deconditioning), more expensive (often requiring extended inpatient stay), and leaves patients with considerable morbidity on a daily basis. Obviously, misdiagnoses often lead to patient morbidity.

Clinical Manifestations

The clinical manifestations of heart failure vary considerably and depend on many factors, including the (1) clinical characteristics of the patient, (2) extent and rate at which the heart's performance becomes abnormal, (3) etiology of the heart disease, (4) concomitant co-morbidities, and (5) distribution of the abnormal cardiac function. The severity of impairment can range from mild—manifested clinically only during stress—to advanced, in which cardiac pump function is unable to sustain life without external support.

Acute Coronary Syndromes

The term acute coronary syndrome (ACS) encompasses patients who present with unstable ischemic heart disease.[40] If they have STE, they are called STE AMI (Figure 44-4). Usually, but not always, these individuals will develop Q waves on their ECGs, hence the term Q-wave MI. If they do not have STE but have biochemical criteria for cardiac injury, they are called NSTEMI and most do not develop ECG Q waves. Those who have unstable ischemia and do not manifest necrosis are designated patients with unstable angina (UA). Most of these syndromes occur in response to an acute event in the coronary artery when circulation to a region of the heart is obstructed. If the obstruction is high grade and persists, then necrosis usually ensues. Since necrosis is known to take some time to develop, it is apparent that opening the blocked coronary artery in a timely fashion can often prevent some of the death of myocardial tissue.[197] These syndromes are usually but not always associated with chest discomfort (see discussion later in this chapter).

The major cause of ACS is atherosclerosis, which contributes to significant narrowing of the artery lumen and a tendency for plaque disruption and thrombus formation.[40,164,165] Myocardial ischemia and infarction are usually segmental diseases. In up to 90% of patients with these diseases, there is a focal occlusion of only one of the three large coronary vessels or branches. The resulting impaired contractile performance of that segment occurs within seconds and is initially restricted to the affected segment(s). Myocardial ischemia and subsequent infarction usually begin in the endocardium and spread toward the epicardium.[186] The extent of myocardial injury reflects: (1) extent of the occlusion, (2) needs of the area deprived of perfusion, and (3) duration of the imbalance between coronary supply and thus substrate availability and the metabolic needs of the tissue. Irreversible cardiac injury consistently occurs in animals when the occlusion is complete for at least 15 to 20 minutes. Irreversible injury occurs maximally in the area "at risk" as supplied by the affected coronary artery. Most of the damage occurs within the first 2 to 3 hours.[186] Restoration of flow within the first 60 to 90 minutes evokes maximal salvage of tissue, but benefits are sufficient up to 4 to 6 hours to be associated with increased survival. In some situations, the restoration of coronary perfusion even later is of benefit.[197] The percentage of tissue at risk that undergoes necrosis (infarct size) depends on the amount of antegrade flow, the existing collateral flow, which is highly variable and difficult to predict, and the metabolic needs of the tissue.

In almost all instances, the left ventricle is affected by AMI. However, with right coronary and/or circumflex occlusions, the right ventricle can also be involved and there is a clinical syndrome in which the damage to the right ventricle predominates and is the major determinant of hemodynamics. Coronary thrombi will undergo spontaneous lysis, even if untreated, in about 50% of cases within 10 days. However, for patients with STE AMI, opening the vessel earlier with clot dissolving agents (thrombolysis) and/or percutaneous intervention can often save myocardium and lives (Figure 44-5).[197] Consequently, percutaneous intervention (PCI) with stenting is the preferred therapy for STE AMI. However, many hospitals cannot or do not offer urgent PCI 24 hours a day, 365 days per year. Thus clot-dissolving medications still play a major role in the treatment of these patients. In addition, it is now apparent that urgent invasive revascularization also benefits those with NSTEMI.[40] These individuals usually have only partial coronary occlusion and smaller amounts of cardiac damage acutely. However, untreated, there are often repetitive episodes that eventually damage larger amounts of myocardium, leading to increased morbidity and mortality over time. We now know that many treatments, such as newer anticoagulant, antiplatelet, and antiinflammatory agents in conjunction with coronary revascularization, save lives in this group.

The prognosis for patients with ischemia but without necrosis is far better, and there are no differences thus far described that distinguish medical from invasive therapies.

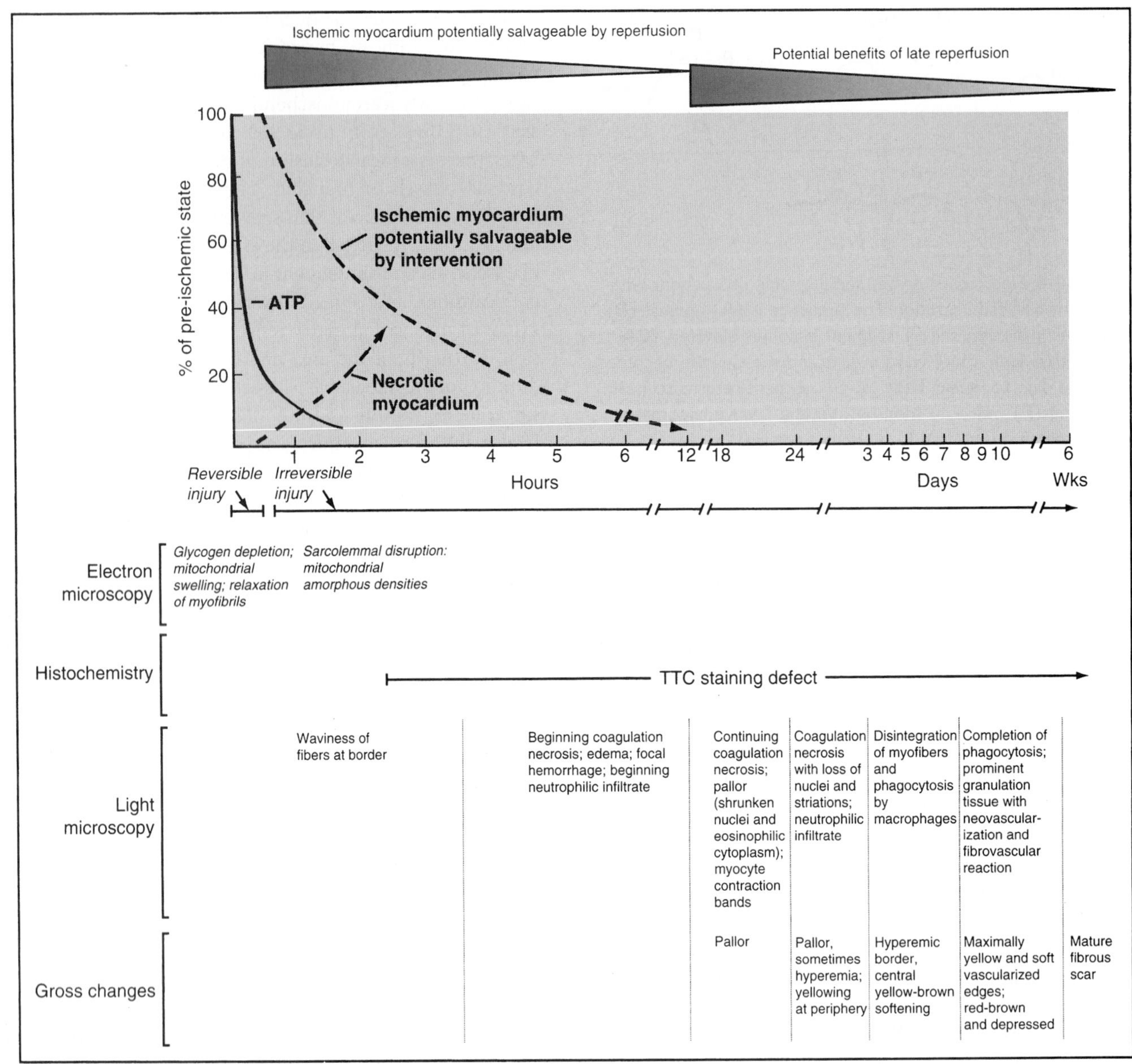

Figure 44-5 Temporal sequence of myocardial infarction. *(From Antman EM, Braunwald E. Acute myocardial infarction. In: Braunwald E, ed. Heart disease: a textbook of cardiovascular medicine, 5th ed. Philadelphia: WB Saunders Co, 1997:1189.)*

A major determinant of mortality and morbidity is the amount of myocardial damage. With STE AMI, most of it is acute whereas with NSTEMI, it may evolve because of repetitive events over many months, thus interrupting the process improves survival.

Precipitating Factors

In many patients with AMI, no precipitating factor can be identified. Studies have noted the following patient activities at the onset of AMI: (1) heavy physical exertion, 13%; (2) modest or usual exertion, 18%; (3) surgical procedure, 6%; (4) rest, 51%; and (5) sleep, 8%. If and when these activities are the trigger for infarction, the window of risk is often brief, usually only an hour or two. The severe exertion that preceded an infarction was often performed at times when the patient was fatigued or emotionally stressed. Exertion before infarction is somewhat more common among patients without preexisting angina than in patients who have had a history of angina.[200]

There are causes of infarctions other than acute atherothrombotic coronary occlusion. For example, prolonged vasospasm can induce infarction, and spontaneous dissection is becoming more commonly appreciated, especially in pregnant females.[40] Other conditions (Box 44-1) can also cause the death of cardiomyocytes and lead to a biochemical signal of myocyte damage, but these entities should not be confused with myocardial infarction.[102] Some of these injurious stimuli include (1) trauma that may precip-

BOX 44-1 Elevations of Troponins Without Overt Ischemic Heart Disease

- Trauma (including contusion, ablation, pacing, and cardioversion)
- Congestive heart failure—acute and chronic*
- Aortic valve disease and HOCM with significant LVH*
- Hypertension
- Hypotension, often with arrhythmias
- Postoperative noncardiac surgery patients who seem to do well*
- Renal failure*
- Critically ill patients, esp with diabetes, respiratory failure*
- Drug toxicity, e.g., Adriamycin, 5 FU, Herceptin, snake venoms*
- Hypothyroidism
- Coronary vasospasm, including apical ballooning syndrome
- Inflammatory diseases e.g., myocarditis, e.g., with parvovirus B19, Kawasaki disease, sarcoid, smallpox vaccination, or myocardial extension of PE
- Post PCI patients who appear to be uncomplicated*
- Pulmonary embolism, severe pulmonary hypertension*
- Sepsis*
- Burns, esp if TBSA > 30%*
- Infiltrative diseases including amyloidosis, hemochromatosis, sarcoidosis, and scleroderma*
- Acute neurologic disease, including CVA, subarachnoid bleeds*
- Rhabdomyolysis with cardiac injury
- Transplant vasculopathy
- Vital exhaustion

HOCM, Hypertrophic obstructive cardiomyopathy; *LVH,* left ventricular hypertrophy; *5 FU,* 5 fluorouracil; *PE,* pulmonary embolus; *PCI,* percutaneous coronary intervention; *TBSA,* total surface body area; *CVA,* cardiovascular accident.
*Designations imply prognostic information has been reported.

itate myocardial contusion and hemorrhage into the myocardium; (2) toxic reactions to chemotherapy agents, such as Adriamycin, or myocardial depressant substances released with sepsis; (3) heat-induced injury after cardioversion; (4) increases in wall stress with impairment of subendocardial perfusion caused by severe hypotension or hypertension; and/or (5) injury caused by catecholamine release in patients with acute neurological catastrophes. Pulmonary embolism is another common cause of biochemical elevations and is caused by right ventricular damage related to the acute increases in wall stress and reduced subendocardial perfusion.[79,123,126]

Chronobiology

There is a pronounced periodicity for the time of onset of STE AMI.[200] Often an AMI occurs in the morning hours soon after arising, a period of (1) increasing adrenergic activity, (2) increased plasma fibrinogen levels, (3) increased inhibition of fibrinolysis, and (4) increased platelet adhesiveness. Studies have demonstrated that the early morning peak in MI parallels the peak incidence of death from ischemic heart disease, occurring at about 8 AM to 9 AM There also is a second peak at approximately 5 PM. Circadian rhythms affect many physiological and biochemical parameters; the early morning hours are associated with rises in plasma catecholamines and cortisol and increases in platelet aggregability. Tissue plasminogen activator activity is low and plasminogen activator inhibitor activity is high during the early morning hours. Thus it is possible that some cyclical aspects of combined vasospastic, prothrombotic, and fibrinolytic factors, in the setting of preexisting atherosclerosis, lead to AMI.[20] NSTEMI does not exhibit this circadian rhythm.

Prognosis

STE and non-STE infarctions have distinctly different short-term prognoses. STE AMI is associated with a higher early and in-hospital mortality. It is said that mortality associated by STE AMI can occur up to 6 months post event, but the vast majority (at least two thirds) occurs during the first 30 or 40 days. It is this process that coronary recanalization seems to benefit.[5] NSTE AMI is associated with a lower acute mortality and complication rates but a longer period of vulnerability to reinfarction and death. As a result, 1- to 2-year survival rates are similar to those for transmural infarction.[40] This is why intervention has been so effective in this group.

Clinical History

The clinical history remains of substantial value in establishing a diagnosis.[40,98,197] A prodromal history of angina can be elicited in 40% to 50% of patients with AMI. Of the patients with AMI presenting with prodromal symptoms, approximately one third have had symptoms from 1 to 4 weeks before hospitalization; in the remaining two thirds, symptoms predate admission by a week or less, with one third of these patients having had symptoms for 24 hours or less.

The pain of AMI is variable in intensity; in most patients it is severe but rarely intolerable. The pain may be prolonged, up to 30 minutes. The discomfort is described as constricting, crushing, oppressing, or compressing; often the patient complains of something sitting on or squeezing the chest. Although usually described as a squeezing, choking, viselike, or heavy pain, it may also be characterized as a stabbing, knifelike, boring, or burning discomfort. The pain is usually retrosternal in location, spreading frequently to both sides of the chest, favoring the left side. Often the pain radiates down the left arm. Some patients note only a dull ache or numbness of the wrists in association with severe substernal discomfort. In some instances, the pain of AMI may begin in the epigastrium and simulate a variety of abdominal disorders, which often causes MI to be misdiagnosed as indigestion. In other patients, the discomfort of AMI radiates to the shoulders, upper extremities, neck, and jaw, again usually favoring the left side. In patients with preexisting angina, the pain of infarction usually resembles that of angina with respect to features and location. However, it is generally much more severe, lasts longer, and/or is not relieved by rest and nitroglycerin.

Older individuals, diabetics, and women often present atypically.[40,98,197] For example, in individuals older than 80 years, less than 50% of those who present with AMI will have chest discomfort. Sometimes, these patients will present with shortness of breath, fatigue, or even confusion. The pain of AMI may have disappeared by the time physicians first encounter the patient (or the patient reaches the hospital), or it may persist for a few hours.

Myocardial Changes Following Acute Myocardial Infarction

Figure 44-5 shows the temporal sequence of early biochemical, histochemical, and histological findings after the onset of AMI. On gross pathological examination, AMI can be divided into subendocardial (nontransmural) infarctions and transmural infarctions.[10] In the former, necrosis involves the endocardium, the intramural myocardium, or both without extending all the way through the ventricular wall to the epicardium. In the latter, myocardial necrosis involves the full thickness of the ventricular wall. The histological pattern of necrosis may differ: contraction band injury occurs almost twice as often in nontransmural infarctions as in transmural infarctions. Unfortunately, the pathological changes correlate poorly with clinical, ECG, and biochemical markers of necrosis, which is why those terms are no longer used clinically. It is fair to say, however, that on a statistical basis, one is more apt to have STE MI Q waves on the ECG and a larger biochemical signal when the infarction is transmural pathologically.

Ultrastructural (Electron Microscopic) Changes in Myocardium

In experimental infarction, the earliest ultrastructural changes in cardiac muscle following occlusion of a coronary artery, noted within 20 minutes by electron microscopy, consist of a reduction in the size and number of glycogen granules, intracellular edema, and swelling and distortion of the transverse tubular system, the sarcoplasmic reticulum, and the mitochondria. These early changes are partially reversible. Changes after 60 minutes of occlusion include myocardial cell swelling; mitochondrial abnormalities, such as swelling and internal disruption; development of amorphous, flocculent aggregation and margination of nuclear chromatin; and relaxation of myofibrils. After 20 minutes to 2 hours of ischemia, changes in some cells become irreversible, and there is progression of these alterations; additional changes include swollen sacs of the sarcoplasmic reticulum at the level of the A band, greatly enlarged mitochondria with few cristae, thinning and fractionation of myofilaments, disorientation of myofibrils, and clumping of mitochondria. Cells irreversibly damaged by ischemia are usually swollen, with an enlarged sarcoplasmic reticulum. Defects in the plasma membrane may appear, and the mitochondria are fragmented. Many of these changes become more intense when blood flow is restored.

Histological (Light Microscopic) Changes in Myocardium

Although it was previously believed that no light microscopic changes could be seen in infarcted myocardium until 8 hours after interruption of blood flow, in some infarcts a pattern of wavy myocardial fibers may be seen 1 to 3 hours after onset, especially at the periphery of the infarct.[10] After 8 hours, edema of the interstitium becomes evident, as do increased fatty deposits in the muscle fibers, along with infiltration of neutrophilic polymorphonuclear leukocytes and red blood cells.

By 24 hours there is clumping of the cytoplasm and loss of crossstriations, with appearance of irregular crossbands in the involved myocardial fibers. The nuclei sometimes even disappear. The myocardial capillaries in the involved region dilate, and polymorphonuclear leukocytes accumulate, first at the periphery and then in the center of the infarct. During the first 3 days, the interstitial tissue becomes edematous. Generally, on about day 4 after infarction, removal of necrotic fibers by macrophages begins, again commencing at the periphery. By day 8, the necrotic muscle fibers have become dissolved; by about 10 days, the number of polymorphonuclear leukocytes is reduced, and granulation tissue first appears at the periphery. Removal of necrotic muscle cells continues until the fourth to sixth week following infarction, by which time much of the necrotic myocardium has been removed. This process continues, along with increasing collagenization of the infarcted area. By the sixth week, the infarcted area has usually been converted into a firm connective tissue scar with interspersed intact muscle fibers.

Gross Changes in Myocardium

Gross alterations of the myocardium are difficult to identify until at least 6 to 12 hours following the onset of necrosis.[10] However, several histochemical approaches have been used to identify zones of necrosis that can be observed after only 2 to 3 hours. Initially, the myocardium in the affected region may appear pale and slightly swollen. By 18 to 36 hours after onset of the infarct, the myocardium is tan or reddish purple (because of trapped erythrocytes). These changes persist for approximately 48 hours; the infarct then turns gray and fine yellow lines, secondary to neutrophilic infiltration, appear at its periphery. This zone gradually widens and during the next few days extends throughout the infarct.

Eight to 10 days following infarction, the thickness of the cardiac wall in the area of the infarct is reduced as necrotic muscle is removed by mononuclear cells. The cut surface of an infarct of this age is yellow, surrounded by a reddish purple band of granulation tissue that extends through the necrotic tissue by 3 to 4 weeks. Over the next 2 to 3 months, the infarcted area gradually acquires a gelatinous, gray appearance, eventually converting into a shrunken, thin, firm scar that whitens and firms progressively with time. This process begins at the periphery of the infarct and gradually moves centrally. In addition, more hemorrhage is seen in the area of damage because of the use of potent thrombolytic and anticoagulant agents.

The Development and Progression of Atherosclerosis[133]

Intrinsic to the modern day understanding of ischemic heart disease and particularly why there is such intense interest in the development of markers of inflammation is the concept that atherosclerosis is a chronic inflammatory disease (see Chapter 26). The concept is that some event damages the endothelium of blood vessels, which facilitates the egress of lipid into the subendothelial space. Putative injurious stimuli include turbulent flow in a blood vessel, which could occur for example because of hypertension or a noxious metabolite from a lipid fraction. This damage tends to occur at branch points of blood vessels. Regardless of the initial stimulus, once damaged, low density lipoprotein (LDL) can cross into the vessel wall more easily in an NADPH oxidase mediated fashion. Whether minimal oxidation facilitates that egress or whether it occurs once the LDL is within the vessel wall is unclear, but a minimal degree of oxidation once in the vessel wall facilitates the egress of smooth muscle cells from the media of the vessel and macrophages that ingest cholesterol. Hence the current enthusiasm for the measurement of oxidized lipids. The process of atherosclerosis then progresses slowly with the involvement of lymphocytes, monocytes, macrophages, and smooth muscle cells. The dynamic within a given plaque may vary, but there clearly is an inflammatory milieu, in part mediated by substances like CD40 ligand, which can be measured in patients either directly or as one of the stimuli to the elaboration of C-reactive protein (CRP). Interleukins 1, 6, 8, and 18 also participate to various extents as part of this process chronically (see Chapter 22). This process also involves adherence of white blood cells to the damaged endothelial surface with subsequent degranulation and elaboration of myeloperoxidase. There also is a procoagulant component due predominantly to the presence of tissue factor, which is localized immediately under the cap of the plaque. There also is intermittent instability because of inflammatory products within the plaque that release chemicals that degrade ground substance, such as metalloproteinases. Initially the plaque expands by stretching the adventitia in a process of small ruptures with release of procoagulant and proinflammatory materials and then remodeling over time as antiinflammatory and anticoagulant and thrombolytic substances are elaborated. This process of stretching the adventitia preserves the lumen such that by the time luminal encroachment occurs, there is a very large plaque burden.[83]

A categorization of plaques has been proposed to facilitate identification of those at risk of rupture that could lead to an acute event. It is acknowledged that the propensity for a plaque to rupture probably reflects a systemic predilection rather than a local one. Thus for a given patient at risk, there likely are many plaques that are metabolically at risk of rupture at any given instance.[164,165] High risk plaques have:

1. An active inflammatory environment that may not only be intrinsic but may be stimulated additionally by systemic infections.
2. A thin fibrous cap on the endothelial surface with a large lipid core that is filled with procoagulant substances, predominantly tissue factor.
3. Endothelial denudation and fissuring because of the elaboration of metalloproteinases.
4. Local high shear stress usually because they are severe and at branch points in the vessel.

Events likely occur because of superimposed thrombosis. This can be caused by erosions on the surface of the plaque or more often because of rupture of the plaque at its edges, where the cap is thinnest and the majority of the metalloproteinases reside. If rupture induces total thrombotic occlusion, the event is usually an STE AMI. If lesser degrees of occlusion occur, an NSTE AMI or UA may ensue. One of the causes that may participate in subtotal occlusive plaque rupture involves platelets and abnormal coronary vasomotion. It is known that diseased coronary arteries respond atypically to many stimuli, often constricting rather than dilating. Since the cross sectional area of a vessel is related to the square of the radius, even modest amounts of constriction can markedly increase the extent of occlusion. Whether constriction occurs first, leading to stagnation of coronary flow and platelet aggregation on the plaque, or whether platelets stick and cause the aggregation is not certain, but these processes reinforce one another. Platelets secrete vasoconstricting substances in response to a denuded area, which expresses adhesive receptors (e.g., CAMs). This, in addition to stagnant blood flow, will cause platelets and white blood cells to adhere to the surface of the vessels. It appears likely that in many patients that platelets adhere and enhance vasoconstriction and then break off, causing small vessel emboli, sometimes in association with plaque debris and sometimes without. These processes, in addition to a reduction in flow, can lead to necrosis or at least recurrent ischemia. It is also apparent that the process that eventually leads to acute events involves a systemic propensity to platelet aggregation and inflammation since effluent flowing from the nonculprit vessel (distant from the putative coronary lesion causing the acute event) elaborates inflammatory mediators (e.g., myeloperoxidase) similar to those observed from the affected vessel. Finally, necrosis when present also stimulates acute phase reaction, including an inflammatory component.

Given this pathophysiology, many therapies are now oriented toward inhibition of thrombosis, fibrinolysis, platelet aggregation, and inflammation. Some of the same ways of assessing their efficacy are the ones used diagnostically.

Diagnosis of Acute Myocardial Infarction

Previously, the diagnosis of AMI established by the World Health Organization required at least two of the following criteria: (1) a history of chest pain, (2) evolutionary changes

BOX 44-2 Diagnosis of Acute Myocardial Infarction

Either one of the following criteria satisfies the diagnosis for an acute, evolving, or recent MI.

1. Typical rise and gradual fall (cardiac troponin) or more rapid rise and fall (CK-MB) of biochemical markers of myocardial necrosis with at least one of the following:
   a. Ischemic symptoms
   b. Development of pathological Q waves on the ECG
   c. ECG changes indicative of ischemia (ST segment elevation or depression)
   d. Coronary artery intervention (e.g., coronary angioplasty)
2. Pathological findings of an AMI

BOX 44-3 Diagnosis of Established Myocardial Infarction

1. Any one of the following criteria satisfies the diagnosis for established MI.
   a. Development of new pathologic Q waves on serial ECGs. The patient may or may not remember previous symptoms. Biochemical markers of myocardial necrosis may have normalized, depending on the length of time that has passed since the infarct developed.
   b. Pathological findings of a healed or healing MI.

on the ECG, and/or (3) elevations of serial cardiac markers. However, it was rare for a diagnosis of AMI to be made in the absence of biochemical evidence of myocardial injury. A 2000 ESC/ACC consensus conference has codified the role of markers by advocating that the diagnosis be evidence of myocardial injury based on markers of cardiac damage in the appropriate clinical situation (Box 44-2).[6] The criteria for diagnosis of an established MI are in Box 44-3. The guidelines thus recognized the reality that neither the clinical presentation nor the ECG had adequate sensitivity and specificity. This guideline does not suggest that all elevations of these biomarkers should elicit a diagnosis of AMI—only those associated with the appropriate clinical and ECG findings (see discussion later in this chapter). When elevations that are not caused by acute ischemia occur, the clinician is obligated to search for another etiology for the elevation.[21,59] The criteria suggested for use with these markers by the Biochemistry Panel of the ESC/ACC Committee are listed in Box 44-4.[103]

ECG Findings[104]

The initial ECG used to be diagnostic of AMI in about 50% of AMI patients. As the frequency of STE AMI has diminished and the diagnosis has been made with greater and greater sensitivity, this percentage has been greatly reduced. Serial tracings are helpful for STE AMI but not for what is now almost 70% of AMIs, those with NSTE AMI. The classic

BOX 44-4 ESC/ACC Recommendations for Use of Cardiac Biomarkers for Detection of Myocardial Injury and Myocardial Infarction

- Increases in biomarkers of cardiac injury are indicative of injury to the myocardium, but not an ischemic mechanism of injury
- Cardiac troponins (I or T) are preferred markers for diagnosis of myocardial injury
- Increases in cardiac marker proteins reflect irreversible injury
- Improved quality control of troponin assays is essential
- MI is present when there is cardiac damage, as detected by marker proteins (an increase above the 99th percentile of the normal range) in a clinical setting consistent with myocardial ischemia.
- For patients with an ischemic mechanism of injury, prognosis is related to the extent of troponin increases.
- If an ischemic mechanism is unlikely, other etiologies for cardiac injury should be pursued.
- Samples must be obtained at least 6 to 9 hr after the symptoms begin.
- After PCI and CABG, the significance of marker elevations and patient care should be individualized.

PCI, Percutaneous coronary intervention; *CABG,* coronary artery bypass gnaft.

ECG changes of an STE AMI are ST segment elevation, which often evolve to the development of Q waves absent intervention (see Figure 44-4). Pericarditis, some normal variants, and transient causes that may not result in myocardial injury are well described and can on occasion mimic the changes of AMI. Most NSTE AMIs present with either ST segment depression, with or without T-wave changes; T-wave changes alone; or on occasion in the absent of any ECG findings. Those with ST segment change have a substantially worse prognosis.

In some patients, the clinical history and ECG may be definitive. In others, it may not be as clear. There are many other clinical aspects that might suggest AMI as the etiology of a given biomarker elevation. For example, the finding of significant coronary obstructive lesions, especially in a pattern suggestive of recent plaque rupture, is highly suggestive.[103] At times, a positive stress test with or without imaging may be what helps make the diagnosis. However, if the clinical situation is not suggestive, other sources for cardiac injury should be sought.

Cardiac Markers

A cardiac marker is defined as a clinical laboratory test useful for detecting AMI or minor myocardial injury. They are most useful when patients have nondiagnostic ECG tracings. Patients with AMI can be categorized into four groups. First, there is the group of patients who present early to the emergency department (ED), within 0 to 4 hours after the onset of chest pain, without diagnostic ECG evidence of AMI. For laboratory tests to be clinically useful, markers of MI must be released rapidly from the heart into the circulation to provide sensitive and specific diagnostic information.

Further the analytical assays must be rapid and sensitive enough to distinguish small changes within the reference interval in serum. The second group of patients are those presenting 4 to 48 hours after the onset of chest pain, without evidence of AMI on ECG. In this group of patients, the diagnosis of AMI requires serial monitoring of both cardiac markers and ECG changes. In the third group are patients who present more than 48 hours after the onset of chest pain with nonspecific ECG changes. The ideal marker of myocardial injury in this group would persist in the circulation for several days to provide a late diagnostic time window. The shortfall of such a marker might be its inability to distinguish recurrent injury from old injury. The fourth group of patients are those who present to the ED at any time after the onset of chest pain with clear ECG evidence of AMI. In this group, detection with serum markers of myocardial injury is not necessary. Since a subgroup of these patients may qualify for thrombolytic therapy, specific and sensitive myocardial markers could be employed to monitor the success of reperfusion during the 60- to 90-minute period after therapy. Rapid assays providing early serial values followed by interpretation of the markers' patterns of appearance may assist clinicians in providing alternative or intervention therapies when thrombolytics have not been successful.

CARDIAC BIOMARKERS

Numerous biomarkers have been monitored to assess myocardial injury. Most are myocardial proteins and differ in their (1) location within the myocyte, (2) release kinetics after damage, and (3) clearance from the circulation. A number of other molecules also are thought to have potential as biomarkers.

Cardiac Troponin I and T

The contractile proteins of the myofibril include the regulatory proteins troponin. The troponins are a complex of three protein subunits, troponin C (the calcium-binding component), troponin I (the inhibitory component), and troponin T (the tropomyosin-binding component).[117,146] The subunits exist in a number of isoforms. The distribution of these isoforms varies between cardiac muscle and slow and fast twitch skeletal muscle. Only two major isoforms of troponin C are found in human heart and skeletal muscle. These are characteristic of slow and fast twitch skeletal muscle. The heart isoform is identical with the slow twitch skeletal muscle isoform. Isoforms of cardiac-specific troponin T (cTnT) and cardiac-specific troponin I (cTnI) also have been identified and are the products of unique genes.[37,60,114,129] Troponin is localized primarily in the myofibrils (94% to 97%), with a smaller cytoplasmic fraction (3% to 6%).

Cardiac troponin subunits I and T have different amino acid sequences encoded by different genes. Human cTnI has an additional post translational 31–amino acid residue on the amino terminal end compared with skeletal muscle TnI, giving it unique cardiac specificity. Only one isoform has been identified. cTnI has never been shown to be expressed in normal, regenerating, or diseased human or animal skeletal muscle.[38] Troponin T is also encoded by a different gene than encodes skeletal muscle isoforms. An 11–amino acid amino terminal residue gives this marker unique cardiac specificity. However, during human fetal development, in regenerating rat skeletal muscle, and in diseased human skeletal muscle, small amounts of cTnT are expressed as one of four identified isoforms in skeletal muscle.[9,39,199] In humans, cTnT isoform expression has been demonstrated in skeletal muscle specimens obtained from patients with muscular dystrophy, polymyositis, dermatomyositis, and end-stage renal disease.[39,153,187,199] Thus care is necessary to choose antibody pairs for cardiac assay use that do not detect the isoforms reexpressed in noncardiac tissue.

BOX 44-5 Tissue and Circulating Forms of Cardiac Troponin

1. Tissue and cytosolic
   a. TIC complex >95% myofibril
   b. TIC, IC, free I, free T <5% cytosol
2. Multiple modifications—tissue and blood
   a. C and N terminal degradation
   b. Phosphorylation
   c. Oxidation, reduction
3. Complex association/dissociation

Cardiac troponin I exists as a part of the troponin T-I-C ternary complex as a structural and regulatory component of the myofibril. A substantial body of evidence now exists that shows that following myocardial injury or because of genetic disposition, multiple forms are elaborated both in tissue and in blood. The multiple forms of cTnI are listed and described in Box 44-5.[229] These include the T-I-C ternary complex, IC binary complex, and free I. Multiple modifications of these three forms can exist, involving oxidation, reduction, phosphorylation and dephosphorylation, and both C and N terminal degradation. Figure 44-6 illustrates the detection of seven different cTnI forms in an injured human heart.[112] Figure 44-7 further demonstrates that different antibody configurations can lead to a substantially different recognition pattern depending on the selection of antibodies used to detect cTnI.[112] Figure 44-8 shows a schematic of the cTn molecule and what epitope locations are more prone to alterations and what regions are most stable.[54] The conclusions from these observations are that assays need to be developed in which the antibodies recognize epitopes in the stable region of cTnI and ideally, demonstrate an equimolar response to the different cTnI forms that do circulate in the blood.[176]

Brain Natriuretic Peptide

Brain (or B-type) natriuretic peptide (BNP) is a hormone that was originally isolated from porcine brain tissue. It has

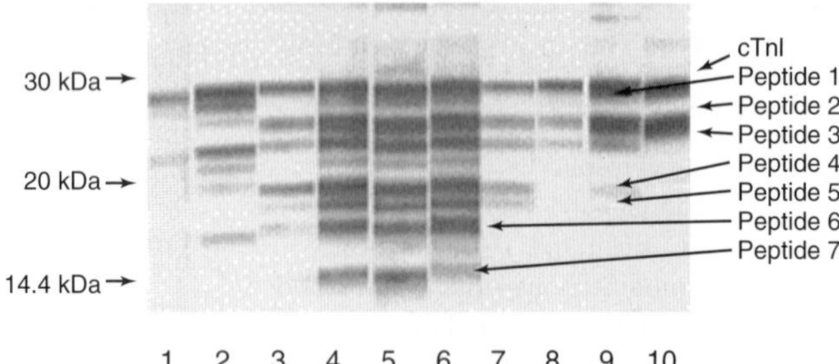

Figure 44-6 Western blot analysis of endogenous proteolytic fragments of cTnI antibodies. *(From Katrukha AG, Bereznikova AV, Filtaov VL, Esakova TV, Kolosova OV, Pettersson K, et al. Degradation of cardiac troponin I: implication for reliable immunodetection. Clin Chem 1998;44:2433-40.)*

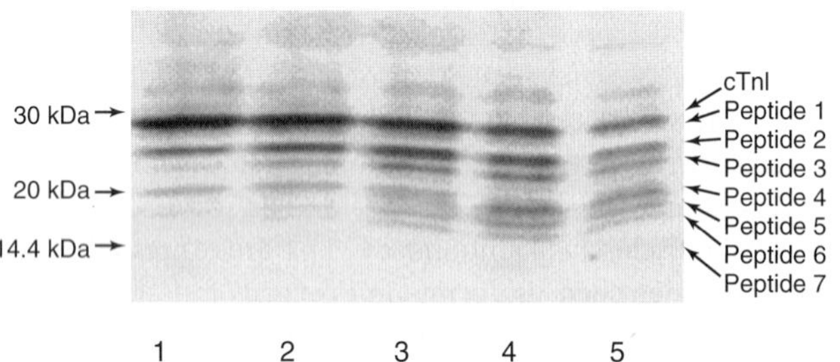

Figure 44-7 Western blot analysis of endogenous cTnI proteolysis in human heart tissue visualized with monoclonal anti-cTnI antibody. *(From Katrukha AG, Bereznikova AV, Filtaov VL, Esakova TV, Kolosova OV, Pettersson K, et al. Degradation of cardiac troponin I: implication for reliable immunodetection. Clin Chem 1998;44:2433-40.)*

biological effects similar to those of atrial natriuretic peptide (ANP) and is stored mainly in the myocardium of the cardiac ventricles. Blood levels of BNP are elevated in hypervolemic states, such as congestive heart failure and hypertension.

For the past decade, there has been increasing research of natriuretic peptides, specifically as a diagnostic marker for CHF.[173a] In November 2000, the FDA approved the first assay for detection of BNP on a point-of-care testing (POCT) platform (Biosite Triage). This effectively took BNP measurement out of the realm of research (predominant research assay, an RIA marketed by Shionogi) and provided access for monitoring BNP to the vast majority of healthcare. Since 2002, the FDA has approved the Bayer BNP, the Abbott AxSYM BNP, the Beckman Access BNP, and the Roche N-terminal proBNP (NT-proBNP) assays.

Natriuretic peptides (NP) are secreted to regulate fluid volume, blood pressure, and electrolyte balance. They have activity in both the central and peripheral nervous systems. ANP was the first described in 1981. BNP was discovered 7 years later in the porcine brain, thus the name.[232] However, in humans, while produced in the brain, the main source of circulatory BNP is the heart ventricles. Other members of the NP family include C-type natriuretic peptide (CNP) and urodilatin. Although these two hormones are not produced by myocardium, they are released with ANP and BNP in patients with volume overload, hypertension, and hyponatremia.

ANP and BNP are released in response to atrial and/or ventricular stretch from volume overload. Correspondingly,

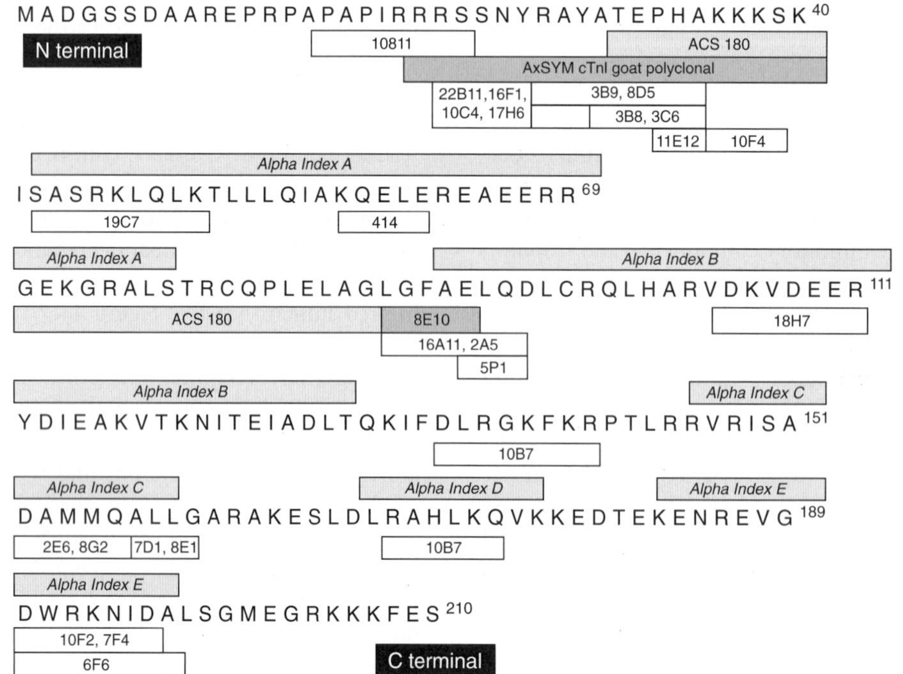

Figure 44-8 Amino acid sequence of cardiac troponin I, with identification of epitopes used by two manufacturers' cTnI assays. *(From Collinson PO, Boa FG, Gaze DC. Measurement of cardiac troponins. Ann Clin Biochem 2001;38:423-49. Figure courtesy Paul Collinson.)*

blood NPs increase in all diseases with volume overload, including renal and liver diseases, and some endocrine disorders (e.g., Cushing's disease, primary hyperaldosteronism). Thus increased NPs are not entirely specific for heart failure. NPs increase cardiac output by decreasing systemic and pulmonary vascular resistance. Additionally, the actions of NPs reduce production of renin and aldosterone by increasing renal blood flow, glomerular filtration rate (GFR), and urine output. Overall, NPs are one of the body's main tools in regulating blood pressure and volume status. They also have direct effects on the myocardial interstitium.

BNP synthesis mostly relies on gene expression and initial upregulation of mRNA.[122] Figure 44-9 illustrates the synthesis of the prepro-hormone and subsequent secretion of BNP from the cardiac myocytes. There is uncertainty whether proBNP is split in the myocyte or later in the plasma, but it is known that there is a circulating protease called corin that is capable of cleaving the NT terminal and the active BNP moiety.[210] Circulating proBNP has been documented. However, the major circulating forms are the resulting NT-proBNP, function unknown, and C-terminal BNP (physiologically active hormone). BNP is cleared via degradation by NEP (neutral endopeptidases), by receptor mediated clearance, and perhaps a bit via the kidneys, which also can secrete BNP. The NT-pro fragment is not cleared via receptor mediated mechanisms, but is thought to be predominantly cleared by the kidneys. Therefore, it will be more sensitive to changes in renal function. The majority of research on natriuretic peptides in CHF has focused on BNP and NT-proBNP.

BNP has a multiplicity of cardiac functions and is released as a counter-regulatory hormone in response to a variety of cardiac stresses but most particularly cardiac stretch. It is significantly affected by changes in volume and in cardiac performance, and among its effects are volume reduction and vasodilation. Thus this hormone is a sensitive marker for changes in ventricular physiology. BNP, like its close counterpart ANP, is released likely as a prohormone. Once in plasma, the leader sequence of 76 amino acids, known as NT-proBNP, is cleaved (see Figure 44-9) leaving the active 32–amino acid moiety to circulate.[132] Circulating concentrations of BNP are age and gender dependent.[185] In addition, they are increased in chronic heart failure and are correlated with its severity.[235] Early studies have demonstrated that BNP secretion reflects regional wall stress in the ventricles and is thus associated with adverse ventricular remodeling and poor prognosis after AMI.[173,190] It is now apparent that BNP measurements are useful in identifying patients with moderate to severe CHF, which can at times be reasonably occult,[148] and for risk stratification of CHF patients[34,100] and those who present with ACS.[64,100,159] The data suggest that this analyte provides information that is synergistic with the measurement of troponin in these settings and is especially useful for risk stratification when troponins are normal.[64,100,159] However, in contrast to troponin markers, there have yet to be differences in treatment that are known to influence prognosis when BNP is elevated. The clinical use of the enzyme-linked immunosorbent assays (ELISA), assays that measure both for the active entity and the NT-proBNP fragment will be discussed in more detail later in this chapter.

Creatine Kinase Isoenzymes and Isoforms

Three cytosolic isoenzymes (CK-3, CK-2, CK-1) and one mitochondrial isoenzyme (CK-Mt) of creatine kinase (CK) (MW 80,000 Da for all 4 isoenzymes) have been identified and are easily separated on agarose and cellulose acetate by electrophoresis (see Chapter 21).[128] Three different genes have been identified that encode for and are specific for CK-M, CK-B, and mitochondrial CK subunits.[181,196] Although CK-3 (CK-MM) is predominant in both heart and skeletal muscle, CK-2 (CK-MB) has been shown to be more specific for the myocardium, which contains 10% to 20% of its total CK activity as CK-MB, compared with amounts varying from 2% to 5% in skeletal muscle.

Numerous investigators have shown that electrophoresis of CK isoenzymes, using extended electrophoresis times or electrophoresis at higher voltages, further separates the bands of CK-MM and CK-MB.[48,224] At least three CK-MM isoforms and at least 4 CK-MB isoforms (subtypes of the individual isoenzymes) exist. The tissue isoform (gene product) of CK-MM is designated $CK\text{-}MM_3$. When this protein/enzyme is released into the circulation, a time-mediated carboxypeptidase hydrolysis of C-terminal lysine residues occurs, giving rise to at least two posttranslational products: $CK\text{-}MM_2$ and $CK\text{-}MM_1$.[180] Similarly, following release of the CK-MB tissue isoform into the circulation, carboxypeptidase cleavage of the CK-B carboxy-terminal lysine residue gives rise to a B-chain negative product and then a product devoid of lysines on both chains. There are only tiny amounts produced of the M-chain negative, B-chain positive form. Because only two forms are separated by electrophoresis (the B-chain negative, M-chain positive form co-migrates with the tissue form and the small amount of the M-chain negative, B-chain positive form migrates with the ultimate conversion product), only two forms have been

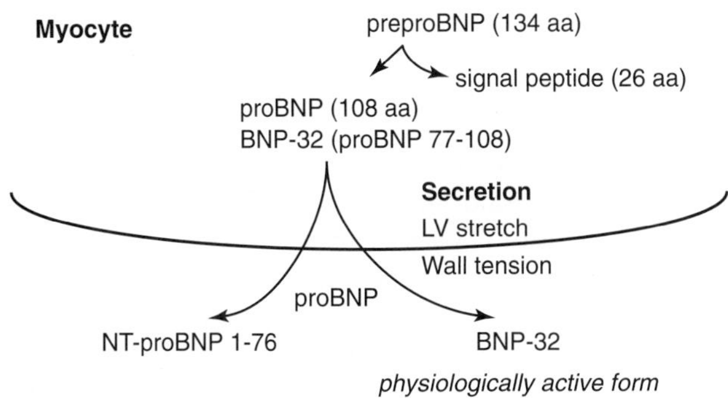

Figure 44-9 The biotransformation and release of BNP and NT-proBNP from the myocyte into the circulation (aa – amino acid).

used diagnostically and have been labeled CK-MB_2 and CK-MB_1.[35] The clearance rate of total CK activity from blood is a composite of the clearance rates of the individual isoforms.[1,2] The more prolonged half-lives are associated with the posttranslational degradation isoforms. Thus the orders of half-lives are CK-MM_1 > CK-MM_2 > CK-MM_3, and CK-MB_1 > CK-MB_2. Studies in an experimental animal model and in humans have shown that posttranslational modifications of isoforms occur in blood, are unidirectional, and do not occur in the lymphatic system or necrotic tissue.[3]

Early studies involving animal hearts or specimens obtained at autopsy from human hearts suggested a uniform distribution of CK-MB ranging from 5% to 50% of the total CK activity.[128] However, it has been shown that the proportion of CK-MB was 6% to 15% lower in the surrounding normal areas of tissue than in infarcted myocardium in humans. Further, in response to acute and chronic coronary artery occlusion in a dog model, myocardium showed twofold to threefold increases in CK-MB in both ischemic and nonischemic myocardium.[201,202] When studied more completely in humans, CK-MB concentrations ranged from 15% to 24% of total CK in myocardial tissue obtained from patients with left ventricular hypertrophy (LVH) caused by aortic stenosis, from patients with CAD without LVH, and from patients with CAD and LVH due to aortic stenosis. In contrast, patients with normal left ventricular tissue had a low percentage of CK-MB (<2%).[99] These data suggest that changes in the CK isoenzyme distribution are dynamic and occur in hypertrophied and diseased human myocardium. Diseased cells also have less total CK per cell.

Normal skeletal muscle, depending on its location, contains very little CK-MB.[128] Percentages as high as 5% to 7% have been reported, but <2% is much more common. There are some differences related to slow versus fast twitch muscle and thus to race. Severe skeletal muscle injury following trauma or surgery can lead to absolute elevations of CK-MB above the upper reference limit of CK-MB in serum. However, the percent CK-MB in serum would be low (percentages advocated vary but when comparing activity to activity, a percentage or <5% is often used and when one compares CK activity with CK-MB mass, a percentage of <2.5% is usually advocated).[128] Increases in serum total CK and CK-MB in several patient groups often present a diagnostic challenge to the clinician. Persistent elevations of serum CK-MB resulting from chronic muscle disease occur in patients with muscular dystrophy, end-stage renal disease, or polymyositis, and in healthy subjects who undergo extreme exercise or physical activities. The increase in serum CK-MB in runners, for example, may be related to the adaptation by the skeletal muscle during regular training and after acute exercise, resulting in increased CK-MB tissue concentrations.[25] The mechanism responsible for increased CK-MB in skeletal muscle following chronic muscle disease or injury is thought to be caused by the regeneration process of muscle, with reexpression of CK-MB genes similar to those found in the heart thus giving rise to increased CK-MB levels in skeletal muscle.[22,188] Thus skeletal muscle can become like heart muscle in its CK isoenzyme composition, with up to 50% CK-MB in some patients with severe polymyositis.

MYOGLOBIN

Myoglobin is an oxygen-binding protein of cardiac and skeletal muscle with a molecular mass of 17,800 Da. The protein's low molecular weight and cytoplasmic location probably account for its early appearance in the circulation following muscle (heart or skeletal) injury. There is no difference in the myoglobin protein localization in the heart versus skeletal muscle. Increases in serum myoglobin occur after trauma to either skeletal or cardiac muscle, as in crush injuries or MI.[217] Serum myoglobin methods are unable to distinguish the tissue of origin, because the proteins are identical. Even minor injury to skeletal muscle may result in elevated concentrations of serum myoglobin, which may lead to the misinterpretation of myocardial injury. Since myoglobin is cleared renally, changes in GFR will cause increases. It has a very short half life of 10 minutes in blood.

LACTATE DEHYDROGENASE ISOENZYMES

Lactate dehydrogenase (LD) (MW 180,000 Da) is localized in the cytoplasm of tissue.[227] Even though LD isoenzymes are rarely used in clinical practice anymore, for historical purposes, their biochemistry will be described here. The highest activities of LD are found in skeletal muscle, liver, heart, kidney, and red blood cells. Electrophoresis on a variety of gels and buffer media, combined with kinetic and immunological studies, has provided convincing evidence of the existence of at least five isoenzymes, composed of four subunit peptides of two distinct types, designated M (for muscle) and H (for heart). LD-1 (H_4) moves the fastest toward the anode, while LD-5 (M_4) is closest to the cathode on an electrophoretic gel. LD-1 is found in highest concentrations in the heart, kidney (cortex), and red blood cells. LD-5 is found in highest concentrations in liver and skeletal muscle. The hybrid LD isoenzymes LD-2 (H_3M), LD-3 (H_2M_2), and LD-4 (HM_3) are also found in these and several other tissues. Because LD is not a tissue-specific enzyme, it is not surprising that serum total LD is increased in a wide variety of diseases. Studies have demonstrated that activities of total LD and LD-1 increase from right to left ventricles, with the H subunit activity varying twofold between different locations of the heart.[135] As with CK-2 in skeletal muscle, the heart-specific LD-1 isoenzyme in skeletal muscle can increase twofold (from 10% to 20% of total LD activity) during a 9 week period of exercise training, with parallel decreases in LD-5.[26] Thus one must be aware that acute and chronic injury incurred during exercise training and racing, increases in serum total LD, especially LD-1 and the ratio of LD-1 to LD-2. The tissue source of these increases is likely skeletal muscle as opposed to the myocardium.[24,26]

Some tests that may potentially become helpful clinical tools as biomarkers to detect atherosclerotic processes and plaque vulnerability are listed in Boxes 44-6 and 44-7 and discussed later in this chapter.

C-Reactive Protein

CRP is an acute phase reactant initially developed to evaluate patients with infection.[179,193] It now appears that low concentrations (so called high sensitivity or hsCRP) can be a marker of the atherosclerotic process, as both chronic and acute atherosclerotic processes involve an inflammatory component (see Chapter 26). Among the ligands that can stimulate CRP are tissue necrosis factor (TNF) and interleukin 1 (IL-1), which are thought to stimulate IL-6 that then causes the elaboration of CRP from the liver (see Chapter 22). It is now clear that CRP itself can enhance the inflammatory and prothrombotic response. There are a large number of assays for hsCRP and a standard protocol for their reporting.

For primary prevention, values >3 mg/L are considered high risk. Recent data suggests that using hsCRP data with the calculated LDL is a potent way to predict risk. For risk stratification in primary prevention, the use of hsCRP routinely is not recommended by the AHA/CDC panel.[30] When used, <1 mg/L is considered low risk, 1 to 3 mg/L intermediate, and >3 mg/L high risk.

In patients who present with ACS, the initial value for hsCRP has prognostic significance. Whether it is short or long term depends on the study. In most studies, the influence of cardiac troponin measurements is the predominant short term prognostic factor and hsCRP adds to long term prognosis. However, this is not always the case. Of interest, hsCRP measurements, similar to BNP, seem to predict death but not recurrent infarction. This could be because of the effect of mortality, which can confound multivariable models, but it is different from the data in regard to cardiac troponin (see discussion later in this chapter).[107] It should be appreciated that once necrosis has occurred, hsCRP values rise and the ability to use them prognostically is attenuated.

BOX 44-6 Serological Biomarkers of Vulnerability Reflecting Metabolic and Immune Disorders

- Abnormal lipoprotein profile (high LDL, low HDL, abnormal LDL and HDL size density, Lpa)
- Nonspecific biomarkers of inflammation (hsCRP, CD40L, ICAM-1, VCAM-1, P-selectin)
- Serum biomarkers of metabolic syndrome (diabetes or hypertriglyceridemia)
- Specific biomarkers of immune activation (anti-LDL antibody, anti-HSP antibody)
- Biomarkers of lipid peroxidation (ox-LDL and ox-HDL)
- Homocysteine
- Pregnancy associated plasma protein-A
- Circulating apoptosis biomarker(s) (Fas/Fas ligand, not specific to plaque)
- ADMA/DDAH
- Circulating nonesterified fatty acids (e.g., NEFA)

hsCRP, High-sensitivity CRP; *CD40L,* CD40 ligand; *ICAM,* intracellular adhesion molecule; *VCAM,* vascular cell adhesion molecule; *MMP,* matrix metalloproteinases; *TIMP,* tissue inhibitors of MMPs; *LDL,* low-density lipoprotein; *HDL,* high-density lipoprotein; *HSP,* heat shock protein; *ADMA,* asymmetric dimethylarginine; *DDAH,* dimethylarginine dimethylaminohydrolase; and *NEFA,* nonesterified fatty acids.

BOX 44-7 Serological Biomarkers of Vulnerability Reflecting Hypercoagulability

- Markers of blood hypercoagulability (e.g., fibrinogen, D-dimer, and factor V Leiden)
- Increased platelet activation and aggregation (e.g., gene polymorphisms of platelet glycoproteins IIb/IIIa, Ia/IIa, and Ib/IX)
- Increased coagulation factors (e.g., clotting of factors V, VII, and VIII; von Willebrand factor; and factor XIII)
- Decreased anticoagulation factors (e.g., proteins S and C, thrombomodulin, and antithrombin III)
- Decreased endogenous fibrinolysis activity (e.g., reduced t-PA, increased PAI-1, certain PAI-1 polymorphisms)
- Prothrombin mutation (e.g., G20210A)
- Other athrombogenic factors (e.g., anticardiolipin antibodies, thrombocytosis, sickle cell disease, polycythemia, diabetes mellitus, hypercholesterolemia, hyperhomocysteinemia)
- Increased viscosity
- Transient hypercoagulability (e.g., smoking, dehydration, infection, adrenergic surge, cocaine, estrogens, postprandial, etc.)

t-PA, Tissue plasminogen activator; *PAI,* type 1 plasminogen activator inhibitor.

Serum Amyloid

Serum amyloid protein A is an acute phase protein, and an apolipoprotein has often been used with hsCRP in cross sectional studies. It can be synergistic with hsCRP[194] but is much less commonly used. At present, there is no standardized assay and no reference interval studies or consistent assay validations.

sCD40 Ligand

sCD40 ligand is a transmembrane protein related to TNF. It has multiple prothrombotic and proatherogenic effects. What is usually measured is the soluble form of the receptor, which has been shown to be a predictor of events after acute presentations.[218] At present, there is no standardized assay and no reference intervals studies or consistent assay validations.

Cytokines

There are a variety of stimulatory and inhibitory interleukins (TNF, IL-1, IL-6, IL-8, IL-12, IL-18) that are thought to help mediate the elaboration of CRP and the development of atherosclerosis and acute events. These cytokines either stimulate or inhibit leukocytes, often through T-cell mediated processes and effects on monocytes, which are indigenous to atherogenesis.[140] In some studies, IL-6 is more prognostic than hsCRP. These cytokines often have inhibitors and/or binding proteins that modulate their effects. At present, there are no standardized assays and no normal range studies or consistent assay validations.

Myeloperoxidase

Myeloperoxidase is released when neutrophils aggregate and thus may indicate an active inflammatory response in blood vessels. It has been shown to be elevated chronically when chronic CAD is present.[238] It is increased when patients present with ACS.[43] Initial prognostic studies were encouraging but were done without adequate consideration of other analytes and specifically cardiac troponin.[42] Accordingly, additional studies are needed. At present, there is no standardized assay and no reference interval studies or consistent assay validations.

Phospholipase A2

Phospholipase A2 (Lp PLA2) is a phospholipase associated with LDL and is thought to be an inflammatory marker. It was previously known as platelet activating factor acetyl hydrolase (PAF). It is synthesized by monocytes and lymphocytes. It is thought to cleave oxidized lipids to induce lipid fragments that are more atherogenic and that increase endothelial adhesion. There is an FDA approved assay for this analyte with obligatory normal intervals. It has been shown to be predictive of events in a primary prevention cohort even when hsCRP is present in the model, suggesting it measures something different from the acute phase reactants associated with hsCRP.[31]

Pregnancy Associated Plasma Protein A

Pregnancy associated plasma protein A (PAPP-A) is a metalloproteinase expressed when IGF is freed from inhibition. It is thought to be expressed in plaques that may be prone to rupture. The literature in this regard is mixed at present concerning its use.[18,32,143] At present, there is no standardized assay and no reference interval studies or consistent assay validations.

Oxidized LDL

Oxidized LDL has been attributed a key role in the development of atherosclerosis (see Chapter 26). Several methods have been used to measure it, but they give potentially different data. Some have correlated malondialdehyde LDL with the development of atherosclerosis and short-term events.[94] Direct identification with antibodies suggests that oxidized LDL may be released from vessels and co-localize with Lp(a) after acute events.[213]

Placental Growth Factor

Placental growth factor is an angiogenic factor related to vascular endothelial growth factor (VEGF), which stimulates smooth muscle cells and macrophages. It also increases TNF and MCP-1. There is a novel assay for this analyte that is thought to provide additional prognostic information on patients who present with ACS.[92] At present, there is no standardized assay and no reference interval studies or consistent assay validations.

Matrix Metalloproteinases

Matrix metalloproteinases (MMP) can degrade the collagen matrix in either coronary artery or myocardium. They are integral to remodeling of the coronary artery and/or the heart after acute events. Elaboration of MMP 9, a gelatinase, is thought to be important in plaque destabilization and thus some have tried to measure it as a prognostic index.[110] Other MMPs participate in the elaboration of extracellular matrix in the heart. Many of the MMPs also have inhibitors (TIMPs) that modulate their effects. At present, there are no standardized assays and no normal range studies or consistent assay validations.

Monocyte Chemotactic Protein

Monocyte chemotactic protein (MCP-1) is a chemokine that is thought to be responsible for the recruitment of monocytes into atherosclerotic plaque (see Chapter 22). It has been reported to be elevated in patients with ACS and to have long-term predictive value.[65] However, at present, there is no standardized assay and no reference interval studies or consistent assay validations.

Tumor Necrosis Factor Alpha

Tumor necrosis factor alpha (TNFα) is an inflammatory cytokine and interleukin that is involved in the genesis of sepsis, arthritis, and a variety of other inflammatory states (see Chapter 22). It also has hemodynamic effects and reduces ventricular performance. It is also a common signaling molecule. Assays for it or its receptor have been developed, but the failure of recent therapeutic trials has led to concern about how to properly interpret the high levels seen in patients with CHF and coronary heart disease.[70] At present, there are no standardized assays and no reference interval studies or consistent assay validations.

Tissue Plasminogen Activator Antigen

Tissue plasminogen activator antigen (t-PA antigen and activity) and plasminogen activator inhibitor 1 (PAI-1). t-PA is the body's physiological fibrinolytic activator. PAI-1 is its endogenous inhibitor and binds to t-PA. Inhibition of fibrinolysis has been suggested to be a reason for recurrent infarction and the fact that maximal inhibition usually occurs in the early morning hours a reason for the circadian variability of AMI.[96] It may also be the reason why diabetics have such unstable disease since the growth factor properties of insulin stimulate increases in PAI-1.[209] An accurate assessment of this system includes both and some assessment of the bound compared with free levels.

Secreted Platelet Granular Substances

Both platelet factor 4 (PF4) and beta thromboglobulin (BTG) are secreted when platelets aggregate. PF4 has a short half-life, is released by heparin, and is the cause of the antibodies that result in heparin-induced thrombocytopenia. BTG is not released by heparin and has a longer half-life. Both markers have been used to assess platelet aggregation.[87] BTG is by far the most reliable. At present, there are no standardized assays and no reference interval studies or consistent assay validations.

Isoprostanes

Isoprostanes are the end breakdown products of lipid peroxidation, and urinary levels have been used to assess the level of oxidative stress.[85,86] It is thought that oxidation of LDL is essential for the development of atherosclerosis and that HDL and other antioxidants work by antagonizing this oxidative stress. Urinary isoprostanes give one some summary assessment of this critical process. The most common ones measured are F_2-isoprostanes, but there are a large number of potential ones to measure. It does appear that they will eventually be helpful in assessing oxidative stress.

Urinary Thromboxane

Urinary thromboxane is the end metabolite of thromboxane A2, which is a measure of platelet aggregation. Urinary levels are elevated in patients with unstable coronary disease in keeping with the known participation of platelets in the pathogenesis of CAD. It is difficult to measure, and collecting urine in acute situation is at times problematic.

Adhesion Molecules

Adhesion molecules are a wide variety of molecules that can potentially be measured as a way of assessing the adherence of leukocytes and/or platelets or other adhesive proteins to the endothelial matrix.[136] Some are receptors. Some of the examples include PECAM-1 (platelet-endothelial adhesion molecule 1), P-selectin, e-selectin, and VCAM-1 (vascular cell adhesion molecule 1). At times, the receptor itself is measured but often it is a soluble portion that circulates that is the ligand. At present, there are no standardized assays and no reference interval studies or consistent assay validations.

Other Proposed Markers

Several markers of ischemia have been proposed but are yet to be validated.

Ischemia Modified Albumin

Ischemia modified albumin (IMA), measured by the albumin cobalt binding test, has been approved by the FDA for its negative predictive value in concert with a normal ECG and a normal cardiac troponin. This test relies on changes in the binding of cobalt to the albumin molecule when ischemia is present.[207] It requires additional validation of the meaning of a positive test before clinical use for ruling in ischemia.

Choline

Choline is released after stimulation by phospholipase D and has been touted as a test of prognosis in patients with chest discomfort.[61] At present, there is no standardized assay and no reference interval studies or consistent assay validations.

Unbound Free Fatty Acid

Unbound free fatty acid (uFFA) has also been touted as a marker of ischemia. Most fatty acid is bound and ischemia is thought to increase the small unbound fraction. Initial studies have reported mixed results.[4] At present, there is no standardized assay and no reference interval studies or consistent assay validations.

Nourin

Nourin I is a small protein released rapidly by "stressed myocytes." It induces changes in a variety of inflammatory cytokines and attracts neutrophils. Preliminary studies have been done attempting to validate its use.[53] At present, there is no standardized assay and no reference interval studies or consistent assay validations.

ANALYTICAL MEASUREMENT OF CARDIAC PROTEINS

The analytical techniques used to measure the most commonly used cardiac biomarkers are reviewed here. All of the initial cardiac markers were enzymes, so the earliest techniques measured the catalytic activity of the marker. Immunoassay techniques measure the mass of a marker and they are the predominant methodology used in clinical laboratory practice today. Analytically, they offer lower limits of detection, improved precision, and faster assay times, on both highly automated central laboratory platforms and POCT.

Cardiac Troponin

Methodology

Cummins and co-workers were the first to develop a radioimmunoassay to measure cTnI that used polyclonal anti-cTnI antibodies.[60] Although the assay showed approximately 2% cross-reactivity with skeletal TnI, it still had excellent clinical specificity for cardiac muscle injury. The assay was never automated or developed for commercial use. The first monoclonal ELISA, anti-cTnI antibody-based immunoassay, was described by Bodor et al.[37] This assay has less than 0.1% cross-reactivity with skeletal TnI, but it was not suited for clinical use because of the lengthy assay time. Over the past 15 years, numerous manufacturers have described the development of monoclonal antibody–based diagnostic immunoassays for the measurement of cTnI in serum.[18,54] Assay times range from 5 to 30 minutes. As shown in Table 44-1, over a dozen assays have been approved by the FDA for patient testing within the United States on central laboratory and POCT platforms. In addition to these quan-

TABLE 44-1 FDA-Approved Cardiac Troponin Assays

		Assay			
Vendor	**Instrument**	**LLD**	**99th**	**ROC**	**10% CV**
Abbott	AxSYM	0.14	0.5	2.0	0.8
Bayer	ACS	0.03	0.1	1.0	0.35
	Centaur	0.02	0.1	1.0	0.35
Beckman	Access	0.01	0.04	0.5	0.06
Biosite	Triage	0.19	0.19	0.4	0.5
Dade	RxL	0.04	0.07	0.6-1.5	0.14
	CS	0.03	0.05	0.6-1.5	0.06
DPC	Immunlite	0.1	0.2	1.0	0.6
i-STAT	i-STAT-1	0.03	0.08	ND	0.1
Ortho	Vitros	0.02	0.08	0.4	0.12
Roche	Elecsys	0.01	0.01	0.1	0.03
	Reader	0.05	<0.05	0.1	NA
Tosoh	AIA	0.06	0.06	0.31-0.64	0.06

LLD, Lower limit of detection; 99th percentile reference limit; *ROC,* receiver operator characteristic curve optimized cutoff; *10% CV,* lowest concentration to provide a total imprecision of 10%.

titative assays, several assays have been FDA approved for the qualitative determination of cTnI.

In practice, two obstacles limit the ease for switching from one cTnI assay to another. First, there is currently no primary reference cTnI material available for manufacturers to use for standardizing their assays. Second, assay concentrations fail to agree because of the different epitopes recognized by the different antibodies used. An effort has been underway since 2001 by the AACC Subcommittee on Standardization of cTnI to prepare a primary reference material.[50] In collaboration with the National Institute for Standards and Technology (NIST), two reference materials—a TIC ternary complex and an IC binary complex—have been identified. Working with NIST and the in vitro diagnostic industries, preliminary round robin studies have demonstrated that while standardization of assays remains elusive, harmonization of cTnI concentrations by different assays has been narrowed from a twentyfold difference to a twofold to threefold difference.

cTnI is present in the circulation in three forms: (1) free, (2) bound as a two-unit binary complex (cTnI-cTnC), and (3) bound as a three-unit ternary complex (cTnT-cTnI-cTnC).[113] Thus different assays do not produce equivalent concentration results, and comparisons of absolute cTnI concentrations in clinical studies cannot and should not be made. Comparisons between assay systems must view changes as relative to each assay's respective upper reference limit. Users must understand the analytical characteristics of each troponin I assay before clinical implementation.

Several adaptations of the Roche Diagnostics (Indianapolis) cTnT immunoassay have been described, resulting in an FDA-approved third-generation assay available worldwide.* Two monoclonal anticardiac troponin T antibodies are used in the third-generation assay. Skeletal muscle TnT is no longer a potential interferent, as was found in the first-generation ELISA cTnT assay.[234] In contrast to cTnI, no standardization bias exists for cTnT because the same antibodies (M11, M7) are used in both the central laboratory and POC quantitative and POC qualitative assay systems.

Surveys on cardiac troponin use have been conducted[13] but the data in the peer-reviewed literature are negligible. The distribution of cardiac troponin assays used as reported over the past several years by the College of American Pathologists surveys is listed in Table 44-2. cTnI assay usage accounts for 89% (number of vendors) and cTnT (1 vendor) for 11%. POCT assays account for approximately 10% of all testing.

In 2001, the IFCC Committee on Standardization of Markers of Cardiac Damage (C-SMCD) established recommended quality specifications for cardiac troponin assays.[176] These specifications were intended for use by the manufacturers of commercial assays and by clinical laboratories using troponin assays. The overall goal was to attempt to establish uniform criteria in order that all assays could be evaluated objectively for their analytical qualities and clinical performance. Both analytical and preanalytical factors were addressed as shown in Box 44-8. First, an adequate description of the analytical principles, method design, and assay components needs to be made. This includes the following recommendations:

*References 11, 54, 55, 77, 113, 115, 234.

TABLE 44-2 CAP Laboratory User Surveys of Cardiac Troponin Testing

Troponin Assays	1999	2000	2001	2002	2003
cTnI	2734	2870	3247	3217	3144
cTnT	107	114	193	300	308
Total	2841	2984	3440	3517	3452
POC Assays					
Percent of total	5.1%	7.1%	10.5%	14.2%	11.3%
Biosite Triage	59	93	132	137	123
Dade Stratus CS	88	119	229	206	157
Roche Cardiac T	NA	NA	NA	63	34
Qualitative Spectral	NA	—	—	96	77
Total	147	212	361	502	391

BOX 44-8 Quality Specifications—Cardiac Troponin Assays

A. Analytical Factors
1. Antibody specificity—recognize epitopes as part of molecule and equimolar for all forms
2. Influence of anticoagulants
3. Calibrate against natural form of molecule
4. Define type of material useful for dilutions
5. Demonstrate recovery and linearity of method
6. Describe detection limit and imprecision (10% CV)
7. Address inferents, i.e., rheumatoid factor, heterophile antibodies

B. Preanalytical Factors
1. Storage time and temperature conditions
2. Centrifugation effects—gel separators
3. Serum–plasma–whole blood correlations

Modified from Panteghini M, Gerhardt W, Apple FS, Dati F, Ravkilde J, Wu AH. Quality specifications for cardiac troponin assays. Clin Chem Lab Med 2001;39:174-8.

First, the antibody specificity as to what epitope locations are identified needs to be delineated. Epitopes located on the stable part of the cTnI molecule should be a priority. Further, assays need to clarify whether different cTnI forms (i.e., binary versus ternary complex) are recognized in an equimolar fashion by the antibodies used in the assay. Specific relative responses need to be described for the following cTnI forms: free cTnI, the I-C binary complex, the T-I-C ternary complex, along with oxidized, reduced, and phosphorylated isoforms of the three cTnI forms. Further, the effects of different anticoagulants on binding of cTnI need to be addressed.[76]

Second, the source of material used to calibrate cardiac troponin assays, specifically for cTnI, should be reported. Currently a cTnI standardization subcommittee of the AACC is addressing the use of several materials to develop a primary reference material that will assist in at least harmonizing cTnI concentrations across different assays.[50,113] Because antibody differences will always be present in different assays, complete standardization will never be possible for cTnI. However, for cTnT, because there is only one assay manufacturer (Roche Diagnostics), standardizing between assay generations has been consistent.

Third, assays need to describe methods used for obtaining minimal detection limits (e.g., mean plus 3 SD of 20 replicates of a zero calibrator) and total imprecision, describing at what concentration a 10% CV is attained. Preanalytical factors that should be described include the effects of storage time and temperature, glass versus plastic tubes and gel separator tubes, and the influence of anticoagulants and whole blood measurements. As more assay systems are devised for POCT, the same rigors applied to the central laboratory methodologies need to be adhered to by the POCT systems.

While clinicians and laboratorians continue to publish guidelines supporting TATs of <60 minutes for cardiac biomarkers, the largest TAT study published to date has demonstrated that TAT expectations are not being met in a large percentage of hospitals. A CAP Q probe survey study of 7020 cardiac troponin and 4368 CK-MB determinations in 159 hospitals demonstrated that the median and 90th percentile TAT for troponin and CK-MB were as follows: 74.5 minutes and 129 minutes; and 82 minutes and 131 minutes, respectively.[171] Less than 25% of hospitals were able to meet the <60 minute TAT, representing the biomarker order-to-report time. Unfortunately a separate subanalysis of just POCT systems was not reported. However, preliminary data have shown that implementation of POC cardiac troponin testing can decrease TATs to <30 minutes in cardiology critical care and short stay units.[162] These data highlight the continued necessity for laboratory services and healthcare providers to work together to develop better processes to meet a <60-minute TAT as requested by physicians.

Reference Intervals

If possible, each laboratory should determine a 99th percentile of a reference group for cardiac troponin assays with the specific assay used in clinical practice or validate the assay based on findings in the literature.[16] Further, acceptable imprecision (coefficient of variation and percent of CV) of each cardiac troponin assay (Figure 44-10) and for CK-MB mass assay has been defined as ≤10% CV at the 99th percentile reference limit.[178]

Unfortunately the majority of laboratories do not have the resources to perform adequately powered reference interval studies nor the ability to carry out NCCLS protocols to establish total imprecision criteria for every cardiac troponin assay in the marketplace. Therefore clinical laboratories have to rely upon the peer-reviewed published literature to establish reference intervals. Numerous reference studies have been carried out for specific cardiac troponin assays. When reviewing these studies, caution must be taken when comparing the findings reported in the manufacturer's FDA-approved package inserts, with the findings reported in journals because of differences in total sample size, distributions by gender and ethnicity, age ranges, and the statistic used to calculate the 99th percentile given. To date, very few in vitro diagnostic companies have published their 99th percentile cutoffs in their package inserts. There is no established guideline set by the FDA to mandate a consistent evaluation of the 99th percentile reference limit for cardiac troponins. The largest and most diverse reported reference interval study to date shows plasma (heparin) 99th percentile reference limits for eight cardiac troponin assays (seven cTnI, one cTnT) and seven CK-MB mass assays (Tables 44-3 and 44-4).[16] These studies were performed in 696 healthy adults (age range 18 to 84 years) stratified by gender and ethnicity. The data, while generally in agreement with information provided by personal communication with the manufacturer, demonstrate several issues. First, two cTnI assays show a 1.2- to 2.5-fold higher 99th percentile for males versus females. Second, two cTnI assays demonstrated a 1.1- to 2.8-fold higher 99th percentile for African Americans versus Caucasians. Third, there was a thirteenfold difference between the lowest versus the highest measured cTnI 99th percentile limit. Obviously the lack of cardiac troponin assay standardization (there is no primary reference material available) and the differences in antibody epitope recognition between assays (different assays use different antibodies) give rise to substantially discrepant results. What is generally recognized, though, as long as one understands the characteristics of an individual assay and does not attempt to compare absolute concentrations between different assays, is that clinical interpretation should be acceptable for all assays.

How to implement reference cutoffs for cardiac troponin is not clear at present. Since only one or two of the more than dozen commercially available assays can attain a total 10% CV at the 99th percentile, caution must be used in implementing a diagnostic cutoff that may potentially give

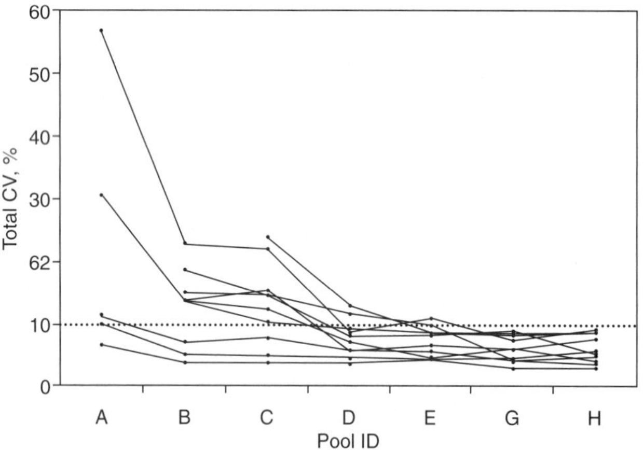

Figure 44-10 Cardiac troponin I imprecision profiles for human serum pools using different cTnI assays, with 10% CV concentration indicated by the dashed line. *(From Panteghini M, Pagani F, Yeo KT, Apple FS, Christenson RH, Dati F, et al. Evaluation of the imprecision at low range concentrations of the assays for cardiac troponin determination. Clin Chem 2004;50:327-32.)*

TABLE 44-3 Heparin-Plasma 99th Percentile Reference Limits (μg/L) by Gender and Race for FDA-Approved Cardiac Troponin Assays

	n[a]	Abbott	Beckman	Dade	OCD	Roche[b]	n[c]	Tosoh	n[d]	Bayer	n[e]	DPC
All participants	696	0.8	0.08	0.06	0.10	<0.01	473	0.07	403	0.15	281	0.21
Males	315	0.8	0.10	0.06	0.11	<0.01	223	0.07	187	0.17	115	0.21
Females	381	0.7	0.04	0.06	0.09	<0.01	250	<0.06	216	0.14	166	<0.2
P		0.739	0.034	0.985	0.017	0.534		0.521		0.441		0.219
Caucasians	400	0.8	0.07	0.04	0.11	<0.01	215	<0.06	193	0.17	166	0.21
Blacks	218	0.5	0.08[f]	0.03	0.10	<0.01	196	0.17	156	0.17	91	<0.2

[a]Number of samples tested in the Abbott, Beckman, Dade-Behring, OCD, and Roche assays.
[b]The Roche assay is the only cTnT assay on the market; all other assays are for cTnI.
[c]Number of samples tested in the Tosoh assay.
[d]Number of samples tested in the Bayer assay.
[e]Number of samples tested in the DPC assay.
[f]Significantly different ($P = 0.05$) from Caucasians based on mean concentrations.

false-positive analytical results. Many studies have addressed the total imprecision of cardiac troponin assays, including what the lowest concentration will be to attain a 10% CV. The manufacturers continue to publish package insert data, primarily based on within-run or within-day precision. Again, there is no consistent FDA specification regarding what precision value should be reported on the package insert. To better address day-to-day clinical laboratory practice, the IFCC C-SMCD has published findings demonstrating the total imprecision for 13 commercial assays, based on a 20-day NCCLS protocol.[178] None of the assays were able to experimentally achieve a 10% CV at their 99th percentile cutoff. Therefore to avoid the potential for false-positive diagnostic criteria based on cardiac troponin monitoring at the 99th percentile, a group of experts in both the laboratory medicine and cardiology communities initially endorsed the concept that until cardiac troponin assay imprecision improves at the low end, the lowest concentrations to attain a 10% CV should be used as a modified ESC/ACC diagnostic cutoff for detection of myocardial injury.[18,19,73] The ultimate goal will be to have all cardiac troponin assays attain a 10% CV at the 99th percentile reference limit. However, when using serial troponin determinations and a 99th percentile cutoff, assay imprecision differences at will misclassify less than 1% of patients ruling out for myocardial infarction. Therefore all biomarker increases above the 99th percentile should be interpreted cautiously, within the clinical context of the patient, and followed up with serial samples over a 6- to 12-hour period after presentation.[6,103]

Use of the 2000 ESC/ACC redefinition of MI consensus document, which is predicated on cardiac troponin monitor-

TABLE 44-4 Heparin-Plasma 99th Percentile Reference Limits (μg/L) by Gender and Race for FDA-Approved CK-MB Mass Assays

	n[a]	Abbott	Beckman	Dade	OCD	Roche	N[b]	Tosoh	N[c]	Bayer
All participants	696	7.6	7.9	3.9	4.07	6.96	473	5.7	403	3.28
Males	315	8.7	8.2	4.2	4.21	7.60	223	5.6	184	4.38
Females	381	4.8	5.6	3.1	2.95	4.66	250	3.6	217	1.68
P		0.0001	0.0001	0.0001	0.0001	0.0001		0.0001		0.0001
Caucasians	400	5.9	6.6	3.5	4.07	6.10	215	5.3	193	1.78
Blacks	218	9.6[d]	9.3[e]	4.2	3.97	7.27[f]	196	6.1[g]	156	4.75[h]
Other	88									

[a]Number of samples tested in the Abbott, Beckman, Dade-Behring, OCD, and Roche assays.
[b]Number of samples tested in the Tosoh assay.
[c]Number of samples tested in the Bayer assay.
[d-g]Significantly different from Caucasians based on mean concentrations:
[d]Abbott, $P < 0.0001$.
[e]P – 0.06 vs. Caucasians for Beckman.
[f]Roche, $P = 0.022$.
[g]Tosoh, $P = 0.019$.
[h]Bayer, P = 0.0001.

TABLE 44-5 Studies of CK-MB and Troponin Comparison

n	Characteristics	Positive CK-MB n (%)	Positive Troponin n (%)	% Troponin/ CK-MB
801	Acute myocardial ischemia admissions	216 (27)	289 (36)	+34%
292	Possible myocardial ischemia in emergency ward	15 (5)	34 (12)	+127%
14,777	MI discharge diagnosis plus biomarker, ECG, and pain algorithm	4157 (28)	4661 (32)	+12%
1719	All ACS admissions	373 (22)	430 (25)	+15%
80	All ACS admissions except with ECG diagnostic of MI	23 (29)	32 (40)	+39%
798	ACS admits to cardiology service	189 (23)	228 (28)	(21%)

Modified from Kojima M, Minamino N, Kangawa K, Matsuo H. Cloning and sequence analysis of cDNA encoding a precursor for rat brain natriuretic peptide. Bichem Biophys Res Commun 1989;159:1420-6.
ACS, Acute coronary syndrome.

4-6 Diagnostic Implications in 1719 Consecutive ACS Admissions Based on Cutoffs

Cutoff Conc.	cTnI+	MB+
ROC (>0.6 μg/L)	13.5% (n = 232)	17.3% (n = 298)
10% CV (≥0.4 μg/L)	17.0% (↑ 26%) (n = 293)	21.7% (↑ 25%) (n = 373)
99th (≥0.1 μg/L)	25.0% (↑ 47%) (n = 430)	21.7% (n = 373)

Dade Dimension: ROC 0.6, 10% CV 0.4, 99th 0.1 μg/L.

ing, has already demonstrated an increase in the number of MIs in (1) day-to-day clinical practice, (2) emergency departments, (3) epidemiologic departments, (4) clinical trials, (5) society, and (6) public policy.[225] Characteristics used to define a disease in one country may be interpreted differently by clinicians in another nation, thus possibly rendering comparison of cardiac disease between countries difficult but not impossible. Consequentry the AHA, the World Heart Federation Councils on Epidemiology and Prevention, the Centers for Disease Control and Prevention, and the National Heart, Lung, and Blood Institute have jointly published a statement that defines acute coronary heart disease (CHD) in epidemiology and clinical research studies.[142] This statement was based on a systematic review of evolving diagnostic strategies with the goal of developing standards for population studies of CHD. The definition of CHD cases was deemed dependent on symptoms, signs, ECG, and/or autopsy findings and biomarkers. Cardiac biomarkers, measures of myocardial necrosis, were prioritized for use as follows: cardiac troponin > CK-MB mass > CK-MB activity > CK. An adequate set of biomarkers was determined to be at least two measurements of the same biomarker at least 6 hours apart (similar to the preestablished ESC/ACC consensus). A diagnostic biomarker was, at least, one positive biomarker in an adequate set showing a rising or falling pattern in the setting of clinical ischemia and the absence of noncardiac causes of biomarker elevation. An equivocal biomarker was when only one available measurement was positive, but not in the clinical setting of ischemia or in the presence of nonischemic causes. A positive biomarker was defined as exceeding the 99th percentile or the lowest concentration at which a 10% CV can be demonstrated.

For clinical trials, to avoid the confusion of multiple centers using multiple assays, several approaches are recommended for using cardiac troponin testing.[18,167] First, all samples from trial centers should be analyzed in a core, central lab—with a precise, well-defined assay. Second, all trial centers should be provided with the same well-defined assays. Third, each center's assays should be uniformly defined using the 10% CV concentration (assay-dependent), thus not relying on local lab criteria and troponin cutoffs. Fourth, a multiple (twofold to threefold) of the 10% CV cutoff value should be used. Fifth, the degree of variability should be reported if those conducting trials decide to use cutoff values defined in earlier studies.

The advances in diagnostic technology in the development of improved low-end analytical detection of cardiac troponins have begun to impact the prevalence of acute MI detection. Increasingly, the data suggest that the more sensitive cardiac troponin tests result in greater rates of MI diagnosis and greater rates of cardiac troponin positivity compared with other markers.[124,134,142] Milder and smaller MIs will be detected. Clinical cases that were earlier classified as UA will be given a diagnosis of MI (because of an increased cardiac troponin), and now procedure-related troponin increases (i.e., following angioplasty[6,93,175]) will be labeled MI. The importance of small troponin increases has been confirmed by their association with a poor prognosis (this will be discussed later in the Risk Stratification section of this chapter). Table 44-5 demonstrates, based on several studies that compared CK-MB and cardiac troponin assays in ACS patients, that a substantial increase in the rate of MIs, ranging from 12% to 127%, was detected. In one of the studies by Lin et al, a subset (5%) of cTnI-negative, CK-MB-positive patients revealed the potentially underlying false-positive MI rate when using CK-MB as a standard for MI detection.[134] This was likely caused by release of CK-MB from skeletal muscle, in the absence of myocardial injury. Further, a subset (12%) of cTnI-positive, CK-MB-negative patients showed a subset of MIs that would not have been detected without cardiac troponin monitoring. Additional studies also have clearly demonstrated the impact of lowering diagnostic cutoff concentrations from the ROC curve, to the 10% CV value or to the 99th percentile limit. Table 44-6 contains representative data showing a 125% increase in the negative CK-MB, but a positive cardiac troponin patient group of ACS patients predicated on a changing standard of what cardiac troponin cutoff is used. Kontos et al also showed a similar incidence for increased MI, with the prevalence increasing from 7.8% using CK-MB to 28% to 195% using various lower cTnI diagnostic values.[124] All these data, taken together, support the implementation of cardiac troponin in place of, not in combination with, CK-MB.

Brain Natriuretic Peptide

Methodology

Box 44-9 shows both current assays and future assay development for BNP or NT-proBNP. Limited licensing agreements have apparently restricted BNP assay development to Shionogi (RIA, not FDA approved), Biosite (Triage POC, FDA approved), Abbott (AxSYM, FDA approved), Bayer (Centaur, FDA approved), and Beckman (Biosite assay performed on Access, FDA approved). Roche (Elecsys, FDA approved), which manufactures NT-proBNP, has (as of

TABLE 44-7 Reference Interval Concentrations for BNP and NT-proBNP Based on FDA-Approved Package Inserts

	ALL		<45		45-54		55-64		65-74		≥75	
	ng/L											
	M	F	M	F	M	F	M	F	M	F	M	F
Abbott	56	84	23	47	39	71	72	80	62	95	77	179
Bayer	54	86	29	35	32	56	38	75	67	72	121	167
Biosite	56	84	23	47	39	71	72	80	62	95	77	179
Roche	169*	251*	92	177	137	192	176	225	229	352	851	624

*<75y.

BOX 44-9 Commercially Available BNP and NT-proBNP Assays

A. BNP

1. Abbott (AxSYM)
2. Biosite (Triage)
   Licensed to Beckman (Access)
3. Shionogi (RIA)
   Licenced to Bayer (Centaur)

B. NT-proBNP

Roche (Elecsys)
Licensed to
  a. Dade Behring*
  b. DPC†
  c. Ortho-Clinical Diagnostics†

*FDA approved using same antibodies as Roche
†Same antibodies as Roche but not FDA approved.

this writing) sublicensed Dade-Behring (Dimension, FDA approved) and DPC and Ortho-Clinical Diagnostics. Characteristics of the commercial assays differ as to standardization of measurements and use of antibodies. Differential recognition of epitope regions appears to be the major determinant in BNP and NT-proBNP stability for each assay. Assays that use an antibody that recognizes the N-terminus labile region of BNP (Biosite, Beckman, Abbott) demonstrate less analyte stability at room temperature (≤4 hours) than assays that use one of their antibodies recognizing the C-terminus (Bayer). The Roche NT-proBNP antibody configuration allows for 72 hours of sample stability at room temperature. At present, reference materials are not available for either BNP or NT-proBNP, and standardization is yet to be achieved. However, for NT-proBNP, which Roche has licensed to multiple diagnostic companies, because reagents and antibody materials will be equivalent, concentrations measured between assays should be harmonized. Further information is needed to better document what NP fragments are measured in the NT-proBNP assay. For BNP, different materials have been used to calibrate different assays, and as described above, different antibody pairs are used in each assay. However, it appears that both Abbott and Bayer have set their assays to be comparable around the 100 pg/mL BNP concentration, the concentration with the largest evidence-based clinical information used for diagnostic purposes. Therefore, since neither NT-proBNP or BNP assay systems use a primary reference material to calibrate their assays, results should be reported in nanograms per liter (ng/L) concentration units and not picomoles per liter.

Stability of BNP immunoreactivity is compromised in whole blood collected in glass tubes versus plastic and siliconized tubes.[203,204] This has been described by all assay manufacturers, with 30% to 80% loss of immunoreactivity in glass after 4 to 8 hours. Further, proBNP has been shown to be more stable than its metabolized form of BNP, which is the 32–amino acid form measured by BNP immunoassays. Further studies regarding the immunoreactivity of proBNP and thus half-life differences are needed by each BNP commercial assay to better elucidate the clinical utility if any for proBNP in CHF patients. Imprecise implications also should be better understood and studied regarding different assays.[236] Quality specifications are available for BNP assays.[15A]

Reference Intervals

There are several practical issues regarding the use of serum/plasma/whole blood monitoring of BNP and NT-proBNP. First, reference intervals vary depending on which assay is used and the nature of the reference population used (Tables 44-7 and 44-8). Second, a number of clinical factors affect the BNP and NT-proBNP concentrations, most importantly age, gender, and renal function. Significant differences are observed between men and women (higher) and with increasing concentrations with age by decade, as shown in Figure 44-11. Third, for BNP and NT-proBNP,[204,210] the relative impact of these factors in relation to the degree of

TABLE 44-8 Median BNP and NT-proBNP Concentrations Versus NYSHA Classification for the Four FDA-Approved Assays*

	I		II		III		IV	
	ng/L							
	M	F	M	F	M	F	M	F
Abbott BNP	122	174	258	298	293	466	1645	1408
Biosite BNP	145	114	306	191	557	469	927	996
Bayer BNP	77	62	135	117	339	355	950	779
Roche NT-proBNP	341	337	985	725	1683	1160	1369	2088

M, Males; *F*, females.
*Data abstracted from package inserts of manufacturer's assays.

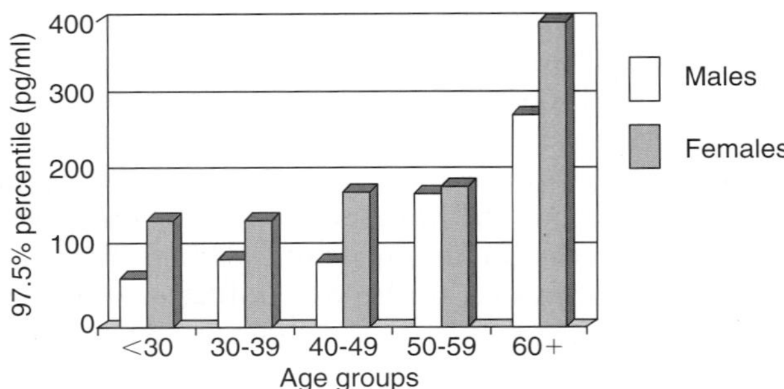

Figure 44-11 Age- and gender-related NT-proBNP concentrations in a healthy, non-CHF reference population.

left ventricle dysfunction remains a debate. When BNP concentrations are monitored in ages >60 years and reference concentrations >100 pg/mL, the cutoff that has demonstrated a high-negative predictive value (NPV) in ruling out CHF has been described. Increased NT-proBNP concentrations above 400 pg/mL in the >60 years population present the same diagnostic dilemma. For both analytes, there is an inverse relationship between values and body mass index. For NT-proBNP, establishing reference intervals has been challenging. Review of both the FDA approved U.S. package insert and the European assay package insert reveals substantial differences in what concentrations are considered normal by age and sex.

Creatine Kinase-2 and Isoforms

Methodology

CK-2 levels are measured in numerous ways.[28,233] The present discussion will concentrate on the immunoassays that use monoclonal anti-CK-2 antibodies.[107-109] Immunoassays developed in recent years have improved on the analytical and clinical sensitivity and specificity of the earlier immunoinhibition and immunoprecipitation assays. These assays now (1) measure CK-2 directly and provide mass measurements, (2) are easily automated, and (3) are rapid (≤30 minutes). This allows laboratories the ability to offer more testing services 24 hours a day, 7 days a week (24/7). This service improvement enhances the clinician's ability to triage patients from intensive to nonintensive care beds and to discharge patients who have not had an AMI. Mass assays reliably measure low CK-2 concentrations in samples with low total enzyme activity (<100 U/L) and with high total enzyme activity (>10,000 U/L). Further, no interferences from other proteins have been documented. The majority of commercially available immunoassays that use monoclonal anti-CK-2 antibodies are the same as those listed in Table 44-1 for cardiac troponin assays. Excellent concordance has been shown between mass concentration and activity assays.[68] All have detection limits of approximately 1 μg/L, are 100% specific for CK-2, and are remarkably similar in clinical performance in the diagnosis of AMI. Analytical performance, linearity, and cost may vary between assays. One of the many impacts these immunoassays provide is that serum CK-2 concentrations can be determined conveniently at almost any time of day, without additional laboratory personnel. The diagnostic cutoff is assay-dependent because of a lack of CK-2 standardization between different manufacturers. A CK-MB Standardization Subcommittee of the AACC has been successful in developing, testing, and validating a primary reference material that is commercially available to assist in harmonization.[51] If used for assay standardization, this material allows concentrations to be reported within 20% of each other. Trends documented in the College of American Pathologists surveys for CK-2 quantitation show during the past 5 to 10 years a large shift to the predominant use of monoclonal anti-CK-2 antibody-based mass assays (>80%).

At present, rarely are isoforms routinely measured in the clinical laboratory. Historically, they were widely used as a research tool, but never gained clinical acceptance. Several technologies have been applied to separate and quantitate the various CK-2 isoforms. These include isoelectric focusing, chromatofocusing, immunoblotting, anion-exchange high-performance liquid chromatography (HPLC), and electrophoresis.[29,183] Their major disadvantages have been lengthy assay time, lack of sensitivity in the very low CK range, and the inability to easily incorporate a technique into a clinical laboratory throughout a 24-hour day. A high-voltage electrophoresis procedure has been developed that provides rapid and sensitive enough results to permit CK-2 isoform measurement within the reference interval of total CK.[52]

Advances in the production of monoclonal antibodies have not provided the means for the development of rapid and sensitive immunoassays for CK-3 and CK-2 isoform quantitation.[52] Proper specimen collection and stabilization of CK-2 isoforms are essential for the correct measurement of the CK-2_2 and CK-2_1 isoforms. A progressive increase in posttranslational degradation of CK-2_2 to CK-2_1 has been observed at room temperature. Incorporation of EDTA at a final concentration of 5 to 15 mmol/L to blood has been shown to stabilize the isoform distribution.

Reference Intervals

For CK-MB, as has been recognized for years for total CK,[228] all assays demonstrate a significant 1.2- to 2.6-fold higher 99th percentile for males versus females. Further, there were four assays that showed higher, up to 2.7-fold, concentrations for African Americans versus Caucasians. These data demonstrate that clinical laboratories must consider establishing different CK-MB reference cutoffs for at least men versus women.[16,228]

MYOGLOBIN

Myoglobin has been measured in serum by RIA, latex agglutination, and two-site immunoassay based on monoclonal antibodies.[177,217] Historically, polyclonal antibody–based immunoassays, while sensitive and specific, lacked laboratory and clinical acceptance because of the lengthy assay time (2 hours). Although early latex agglutination assays provided more rapid turnaround times (30 minutes), the assays were semiquantitative. Rapid and quantitative nephelometric (15 to 30 minutes), turbidimetric[47] (2 minutes), and fluorescence (8 minutes) immunoassays[206] have been commercialized that incorporate monoclonal antibodies. Each of these techniques has good analytical performance. Immunoassay analysis times have substantially decreased with improved technology, which allows for measurements on both central laboratory and POCT. Since variability among commercial myoglobin assays exists, the IFCC C-SMCD organized an international collaborative study to identify candidate secondary reference materials. A single lyophilized, isolated human heart myoglobin material prepared in human serum was selected and has demonstrated a bias reduction between numerous commercial myoglobin assays from 32% to 13%, and established a basis for the selection of a recognized reference material.[177] Reference intervals for serum myoglobin vary according to age, race, and sex. On the average, as serum concentrations increase with age, men have higher concentrations than women, and African Americans have higher concentrations than Caucasians. For consistency with cardiac troponin and CK-MB, the 99th percentile of a reference population should be used as the reference cutoff.

LACTATE DEHYDROGENASE ISOENZYMES

The measurement of total LD has always been enzymatic (see Chapter 21). The complete spectrum of isoenzymes is determined after separation by electrophoresis. There are some inhibition techniques that measure LD-1 without separating the other isoenzymes. There also are monoclonal-based assays for determination of HBD, which consists of LD-1 and LD-2.

CLINICAL UTILITY

The ideal marker of myocardial injury should (1) provide early detection of injury, (2) provide rapid diagnosis for an acute MI, (3) serve as a risk stratification tool in ACS patients, (4) assess the success of reperfusion after thrombolytic therapy, (5) detect reocclusion and reinfarction, (6) determine the timing of an infarction and infarct size, and (7) detect procedural related perioperative MI during cardiac or noncardiac surgery. Before discussing the detailed changes in serum cardiac biomarkers following AMI, it is beneficial to review the diagnostic logic used by the ED physicians or attending clinicians (typically cardiologists) when faced with making a diagnosis. Ruling out AMI requires a test with high diagnostic specificity (preferred by the ED physician in the urgent care setting) whereas ruling in AMI requires a test with high diagnostic sensitivity (preferred by the cardiologist following admission). Diagnostic strategies often require different decision thresholds (cutoff points) for different cardiac biomarkers. It is the function of the laboratory to provide advice to physicians about cardiac biomarker characteristics. Figure 44-12 shows the classic rise and fall patterns of myoglobin, CK-MB, and cardiac troponin over a 7-day period following onset of acute MI.

Patients present to EDs or other primary care providers with a multitude of clinical signs and symptoms in which the differential diagnosis of acute myocardial infarction (AMI and heart attack) is considered. Figure 44-13 demonstrates the complete spectrum of clinical presentations of such a patient. The spectrum encompasses on one end the patient presenting with ischemia, without myocardial cell death (necrosis) or ECG alterations. The other end of the spectrum represents the patient presenting with ECG evidence of AMI indicated by an ST-elevation or Q-wave ECG finding. The entire spectrum of clinical presentations has been designated ACS. To assist in differentiating patients with AMI from non-AMI, the European Society of Cardiology/American College of Cardiology (ESC/ACC) has published consensus guidelines for the redefinition of AMI.[6,58,59,121] A cornerstone of the redefinition is predicated on cardiac biomarkers, specifically cTnI or cTnT. Boxes 44-2 to 44-4 summarize the definition of MI as defined by the ESC/ACC consensus.[6,103] The following are designated as

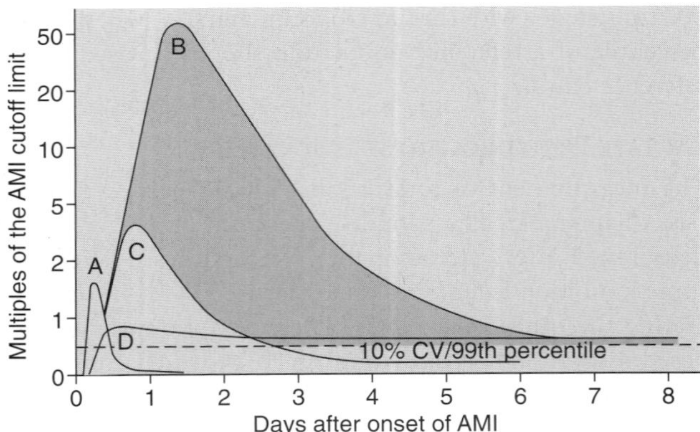

Figure 44-12 Classic rise and falling pattern of cardiac biomarkers from onset of acute myocardial infarction: **A,** myoglobin; **B,** cardiac troponin; **C,** CK-MB; **D,** cardiac troponin following minor injury.

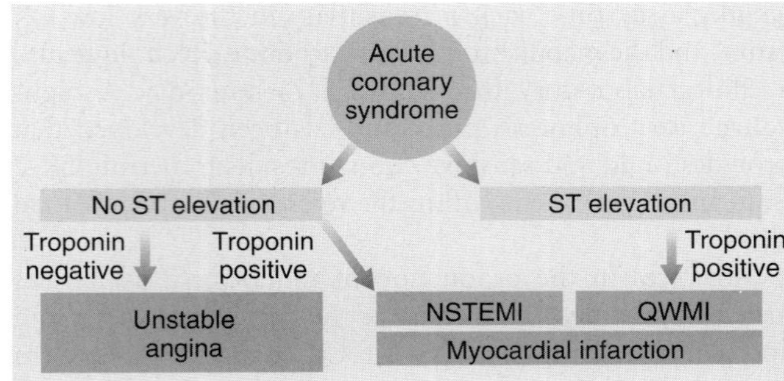

Figure 44-14 The distinction between non-ST elevation myocardial infarction and unstable angina predicated on an increased cardiac troponin in patients presenting with ischemic discomfort. *(Data from Brennan ML, Penn MS, Van Lente F, Nambi V, Shishehbor MH, Aviles RJ, et.al. Prognostic value of myeloperoxidase in patients with chest pain. N Engl J Med 2003;349:1595-604.)*

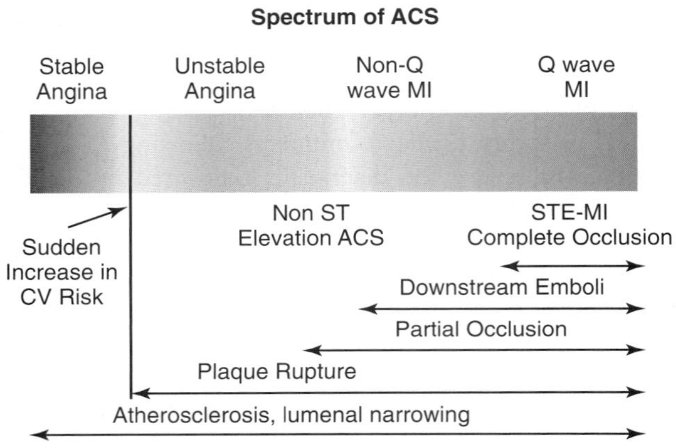

Spectrum of ACS

Stable Angina | Unstable Angina | Non-Q wave MI | Q wave MI

Sudden Increase in CV Risk

Non ST Elevation ACS

STE-MI Complete Occlusion

Downstream Emboli

Partial Occlusion

Plaque Rupture

Atherosclerosis, lumenal narrowing

Figure 44-13 Complete spectrum of acute coronary pathophysiological process from initiation of atherosclerosis to cell death. *(From Personal Communication Robert Jesse, MD.)*

biochemical indicators for detecting myocardial necrosis: (1) a maximal concentration of cTnI or cTnI exceeding the decision limit, defined as the 99th percentile of values for a reference control group, on at least one occasion during the first 24 hours after the index clinical event; (2) a maximal value of CK-MB (preferably mass) exceeding the 99th percentile of values for a reference control group on two successive samples or a maximal value exceeding twice the upper reference limit during the first hours after the index clinical event (although the consensus document states values for CK-MB should rise and fall, either a rising or falling pattern should be considered diagnostic; however, values that remain elevated without change are rarely caused by MI; and (3) in the absence of availability of a cardiac troponin or CK-MB assay, total CK greater than two times the upper reference limit may be employed. In addition to the ESC/ACC consensus document for redefining MI, the ACC/American Heart Association (AHA) guidelines for management of UA recommend monitoring cardiac troponin in ACS patients for differentiating UA (defined as when cardiac troponin is within the 99th percentile reference limit) and NSTEMI (defined as when cardiac troponin is increased above the 99th percentile reference limit), as shown in Figure 44-14.[40,42]

Several markers should no longer be used to evaluate cardiac disease. They include aspartate aminotransaminase (AST), total creatine kinase activity (CK), total lactate dehydrogenase (LD), and LD isoenzymes with the exception of hydroxyl butyrate dehydrogenase (HBD), which some clinicians use to estimate infarct size. These markers have poor specificity for the detection of cardiac injury because of their wide tissue distribution. Because total CK and CK-MB have been utilized for so many years, some laboratories may continue to measure them to allow for comparisons with cardiac troponin over time before discontinuing use of CK. In addition, the use of total CK in developing countries may be the preferred and only alternative for financial reasons. This concept is emphasized in a statement from the AHA Council on Epidemiology and Prevention regarding case definitions for acute CHD in epidemiology and clinical research studies.[142] To more accurately interpret recent trends in heart disease, specifically AMI, during the spread of new technology and a new definition of AMI predicated on cardiac troponin, the following recommendations were made: (1) simultaneous use of old biomarkers with cardiac troponin should be used to determine the effects of new biomarkers, and (2) the use of adjustment factors should be considered in databases and retrospective studies seeking to determine incidence and trends of AMI before and after cardiac troponin–derived research studies.

The cardiology recommendations imply that for clinical laboratories that cannot move as rapidly as others to implement the new cardiac troponin standard, CK-MB (preferable mass) should be used. Although it is suggested that CK-MB be used together with cardiac troponin for (1) assisting in timing of onset of myocardial injury, (2) infarct sizing, or (3) determination of reinfarction, at present there is no strong evidence to support dual testing for cTn and CK-MB. Therefore, for monitoring ACS patients to assist in clinical classification, cardiac troponin is the preferred biomarker. However, it has been observed that in practice clinicians still request CK-MB monitoring to assist in timing of patient presentation and to assist in determining a baseline value in patients with NSTE AMI who have an incidence of reinfarction of between 10% and 15%. In a recent series of cases examining in-hospital reinfarctions (extensions), CK-MB testing was of no added value. Consequently, in practice, each institution will have to weigh the cost-benefit (clinical) ratio regarding using both cardiac troponin and CK-MB testing.

For the majority of patients, blood should be obtained for testing at hospital admission (0 hours), at 6 to 9 hours, and again at 12 to 24 hours if the earlier specimens are normal and the clinical index of suspicion is high. For patients in need of an early diagnosis that will parallel a rapid triage protocol, a rapidly appearing biomarker, such as myoglobin, has been suggested to be added to serial cardiac troponin monitoring. In practice, it appears that the majority of hospitals throughout the world do not use myoglobin as an early marker. However, some early evidence suggests a potential role for multimarker testing that includes myoglobin for risk stratification in chest pain units[12,168] and for exclusion of MI.[150]

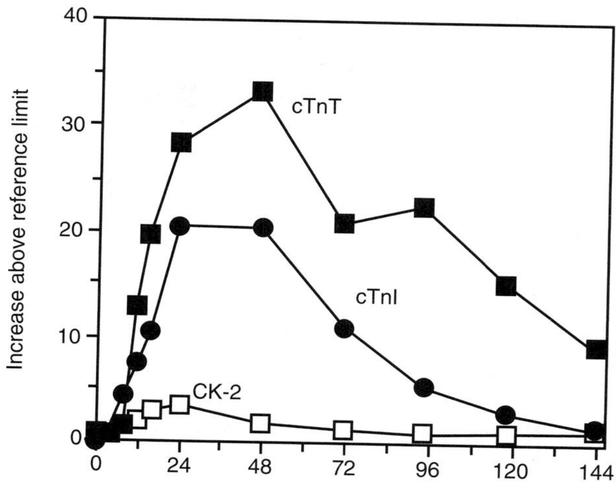

Figure 44-15 Serial serum creatine kinase-2 (CK-MB), cardiac troponin I (cTnI), and cardiac troponin T (cTnT) profiles after AMI. Cardiac markers are plotted as multiples of the upper reference limit.

GENERAL BIOMARKER OBSERVATIONS

Cardiac Troponin

Several general clinical impressions can be made regarding cardiac troponin I and T. First, the early release kinetics of both cTnI and cTnT are similar to those of CK-MB after AMI, with increases above the upper reference limit seen at 2 to 6 hours (Figures 44-12 and 44-15). The initial increase is due to the 3% to 6% cytoplasmic fraction of troponin (CK-MB is 100% cytoplasmic). Second, cTnI and cTnT can remain increased up to 4 to 14 days after AMI. The mechanism is likely the ongoing release of troponin from the 94% to 97% myofibril-bound fraction. The long interval of cardiac troponin increase is responsible for it replacing the LD isoenzyme assay in the detection of late-presenting AMI patients. Third, the very low to undetectable cardiac troponin values in serum from patients without cardiac disease (normal and healthy reference population) permit use of lower discriminator concentrations compared with CK-MB for the determination of myocardial injury. Finally, cardiac tissue specificity of cTnI and cTnT should eliminate false clinical impression of AMI in patients with increased CK-MB concentrations following skeletal muscle injuries.[21]

Numerous clinical studies involving cTnI and cTnT have been published pertaining to AMI. Several have demonstrated that the clinical sensitivity of cardiac troponin is similar to that of CK-MB during the first 48 hours after the onset of chest pain.[23,56,77,234,239] As an early marker for AMI, cardiac troponin shows a clinical sensitivity of 50% to 65% up to 6 hours after onset of chest pain.[23,44,215,234] Therefore, like CK-MB, cardiac troponin is insufficient for effective early diagnosis. This is exemplified in Figure 44-16 by ROC curve analysis.[44] However, cardiac troponin remains elevated for a much longer time after the onset of AMI (up to 4 to 10 days), giving a high clinical sensitivity (>90%) up to 4 to 7 days after AMI.[56] Clinical specificity calculations for cardiac troponin are dependent on how patients are clinically classified. Specificity will depend on whether patients with minor myocardial injury of nonischemic etiology are included with AMI patients. Typically, because of the highly analytically sensitive nature of second- and third-generation cardiac troponin assays, clinical specificity for cardiac troponin is in the 70% to 85% range.

Brain Natriuretic Peptide

Clinical laboratory testing in the setting of CHF focuses on several goals: (1) to determine the cause of diagnostic symptoms; (2) to estimate the degree of severity of CHF; (3) to estimate the risk of disease progression and risk; and (4) to screen for a less symptomatic disease. Some of the earliest observations compared BNP concentrations in CHF patients with the patient's NYSHA classification. Linear relationships with increasing BNP levels and the severity of CHF have been described for several assays, as represented in Figure 44-17 for BNP and NT-proBNP. However, substantial

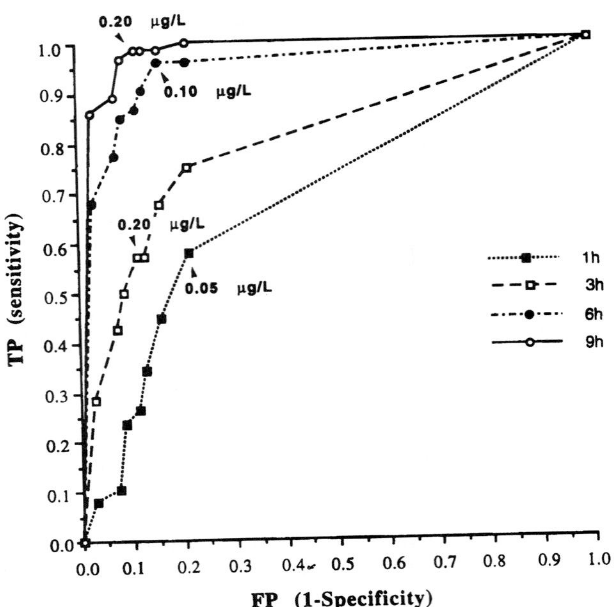

Figure 44-16 Receiver operating characteristic curves to establish the best discriminator limit for cardiac troponin T (cTnT) for predicting AMI. The number of true positives (*y*-axis) and false positives (*x*-axis) are reported in relation to time (h) after the onset of symptoms. The best discriminating point for cTnT is 0.20 µg/L at 9 hours after the onset of chest pain. *(Reprinted by permission of Elsevier Science from Burlina A, Zaninotto M, Secchiero S, Rubin D, Accorsi F. Troponin T as a marker of ischemic myocardial injury. Clin Biochem 1994;27:113-21. Copyright 1993 by Canadian Society of Clinical Chemists.)*

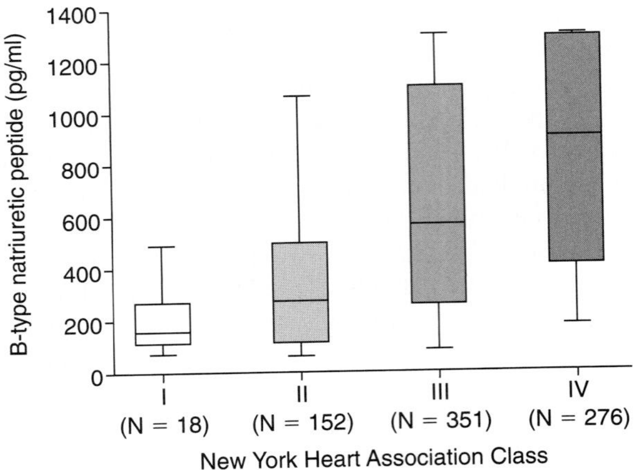

Figure 44-17 Correlation of BNP concentrations (Biosite Triage) according to NYHA classification of heart failure. *(From Maisel AS, Krishnaswamy P, Nowak RM, McCord J, Hollander JE, Duc P, et al. Rapid measurement of B-type natriuretic peptide in the emergency diagnosis of heart failure. N Engl J Med 2002;347:161-7.)*

differences in BNP and NT-proBNP concentrations are demonstrated in Table 44-8 when comparing NYSHA classes and median BNP and NT-proBNP levels from different clinical studies and assays. Very few studies have directly compared BNP and NT-proBNP measurements. The early studies have focused on the diagnostic role of BNP and NT-proBNP in patients presenting with clinical features of HF. Two large prospective, multicenter trials have evaluated the utility of plasma BNP and NT-proBNP in the initial acute evaluation of patients with CHF.

First, the largest prospective trial to date to evaluate the diagnostic value of BNP is "The Breathing Not Properly Multicenter Study," from which numerous publications have addressed multiple aspects regarding the utility of BNP monitoring.[147,151,152,157,226] In this multinational trial, more than 40% of ED clinicians showed substantial indecision regarding the diagnosis of CHF without the knowledge of BNP. Monitoring BNP was found to be an independent predictor of CHF. Using a blood BNP cutoff concentration of 100 ng/L gave a 90% clinical sensitivity and 75% clinical specificity, with an 81% accuracy. Without BNP monitoring, clinical judgment and traditional diagnostic methods demonstrated a diagnostic accuracy of only 74%. The knowledge of BNP reduced the proportion of patients in whom the clinician was uncertain of the diagnosis from 43% to 11%. These data substantiate early studies that showed that 40% to 50% of clinicians falsely diagnosed CHF in the primary care setting before the advent of BNP.[160] Figure 44-18 shows a CHF diagnosis nomogram and ROC curves that the BNP trial investigators propose to assist in the ED decision making practice, based on pre- and post-BNP testing probabilities for CHF. The second study was a randomized control trial comparing the diagnostic strategy for plasma BNP testing with clinical assessment with BNP (Figure 44-19).[152] Plasma BNP monitoring in the ED improved the treatment and evaluation of patients with early dyspnea, reducing the time to discharge and total cost of treatment. Currently, there is a general consensus that plasma BNP or NT-proBNP testing should be performed (1) to confirm the diagnosis of CHF in patients with a suspected diagnosis of CHF but presenting with ambiguous clinical features or confounding pathology etiologies, such as chronic obstructive pulmonary disease (COPD); (2) as a valuable guide to general, nonspecialist practitioners, to assist and/or improve the diagnostic accuracy for detecting HF; and (3) to assist in ruling out CHF when normal NP concentrations are found. However, other studies have shown that routine plasma BNP or NT-proBNP testing in patients with obvious CHF is not necessary and is not cost effective.[59,75]

The challenge in diagnosing CHF is that many of the presenting symptoms are nonspecific. Yet, studies have shown that there were dramatic differences in BNP of patients with dyspnea caused by cardiac failure (mean of 1076 ng/L) versus BNP in patients with dyspnea caused by noncardiac etiologies (mean of 86 ng/L).[157] ROC curves have shown that BNP had better overall accuracy than the clinician's judgment (AUC 0.97 versus 0.88), with similar findings observed for NT-proBNP.[145] It is important to remember that BNP is "not a stand-alone diagnostic test;" it must be used and

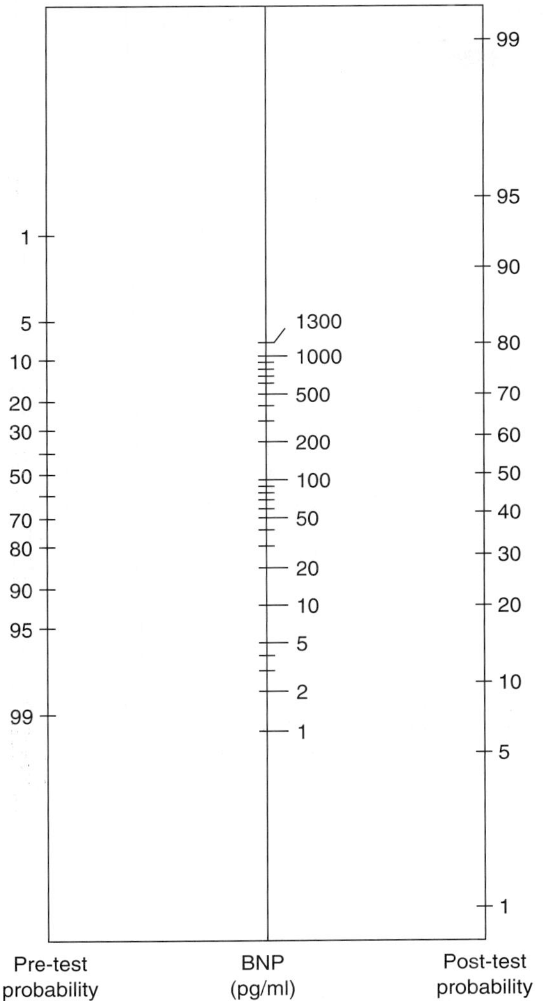

Figure 44-18 Use of BNP and clinical judgment in emergency diagnosis of CHF use a heart failure nomogram. *(From McCullough PA, Nowak RM, McCord J, Hollander JE, Herrmann HC, Steg PG, et al. B-type natriuretic peptide and clinical judgment in emergency diagnosis of heart failure: analysis from breathing not properly (BNP) multinational study. Circulation 2002;106:416-22.)*

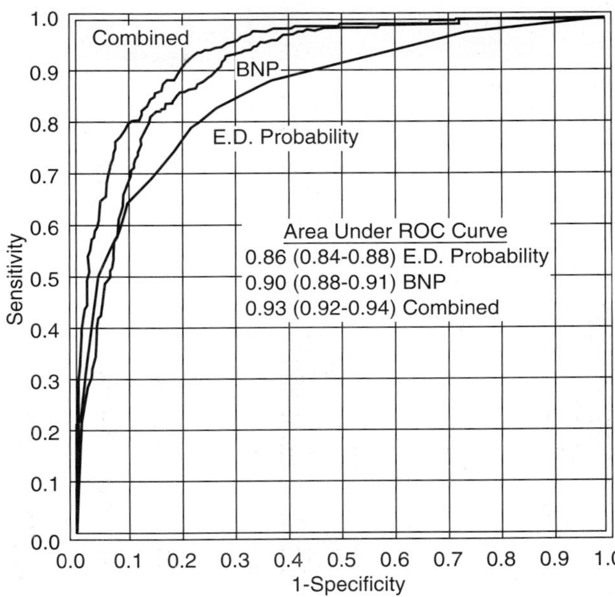

Figure 44-19 ROC curves for individual and combined estimated clinical probability for CHF diagnosis based on clinical judgment and BNP monitoring. *(From McCullough PA, Nowak RM, McCord J, Hollander JE, Herrmann HC, Steg PG, et al. B-type natriuretic peptide and clinical judgment in emergency diagnosis of heart failure: analysis from breathing not properly (BNP) multinational study. Circulation 2002;106:416-22.)*

interpreted with regard to the clinical presentation, specifically pertaining to the age and gender of the patient.[59,75]

Use of BNP for Prognosis and Risk Stratification

Results from several studies support the monitoring BNP or NT-proBNP for the risk stratification of patients with CHF, with or without a previous history. This involves patients presenting with a wide range of clinical pathologies, including CHF,[8,49,93a,222] ACS,[63,106,172,190] and noncardiac pathologies such as pulmonary embolism,[125,182] and in a general population screening with no previous history of CHF. In one analysis adjusted for several clinical factors in CHF patients, plasma BNP concentrations were shown to be more closely related to mortality than were symptoms of ejection fraction.

The evidence for risk stratification use for BNP in ACS has recently emerged. As BNP is released by intact cells, including those that are not ischemic, monitoring BNP may, in the future, provide advantages in detecting the pathophysiological consequences of ischemia and cell necrosis (infarction). Studies have demonstrated that increases in BNP concentrations following STE MI were associated with worse left ventricular (LV) systolic function, adverse ventricular remodeling over time, and a greater likelihood of death and CHF.[141,166,170,219] Further, there has been a consistent observation that increased BNP or NT-proBNP measured within the first 5 days after AMI is strongly associated with both short- and long-term risk of cardiac death. For example, BNP was monitored in 220 patients following presentation for AMI and was independently a powerful predictor of left ventricle ejection factor (LVEF), heart failure, or death in the 14-month follow-up. This suggests that BNP correlates with the amount of ventricular dysfunction present after AMI. As previously mentioned, ischemic damage is one of the major etiologies of CHF. Yet, currently it is difficult to identify patients who are at greatest risk of developing CHF following AMI. Having a reliable screening tool to identify patients at highest risk might be the initiating factor in closer follow-up, designed to reduce future morbidity and mortality.

BNP and NT-proBNP concentrations have been found to be increased in ACS patients without LV dysfunction or CHF; and monitoring levels have been demonstrated to provide important prognostic information (Table 44-9). Graded relationships between increasing plasma BNP con-

TABLE 44-9 Studies of BNP and NT-proBNP for Risk Assessment in UA/NSTEMI

Reference	Year	Study	Subjects	Marker	Follow-up	Findings
62	2001	Substudy of RCT (Opus—TIMI 16)	1698	BNP	10 months	RR 12.5 for mortality in highest vs. lowest quartile in NSTEMI, RR 7.9 for mortality in highest vs. lowest quartile in UA
109	2002	Observational	755	NT-proBNP	4 years	RR 26.6 for mortality in highest vs. lowest quartile
172	2002	Observational	405	NT-proBNP	52 months	RR 5.6 for mortality above vs. below median in NSTEMI
173	2002	Substudy of RCT (TIMI 11B)	681	NT-proBNP	6 weeks	Higher baseline biomarker levels in subjects that died (299 pmol/L) than in survivors (138 pmol/L)
159	2003	Substudy of RCT (TACTICS)	1676	BNP	6 months	Increased risk of death at 7 days (2.5% vs. 0.7%) and 6 months (8.4% vs. 1.8%) with BNP > 80 pg/mL
108	2003	Substudy of RCT (FRISC II)	775	NT-proBNP	2 years	RR 4.1 for mortality in highest tertile compared with lowest (invasive), RR 3.5 for mortality in highest tertile compared with lowest (conservative)
106	2003	Substudy of RCT (GUSTO IV)	6809	NT-proBNP	1 year	RR 10.6 for mortality in highest vs. lowest quartile

RCT, Randomized clinical trial; *RR,* relative risk.

centrations and mortality over 6 months have been demonstrated (Figure 44-20), with the OPUS-TIMI 16 trial and TACTICS-TIMI 18 trial providing the largest independent assessment of BNP as a prognostic marker in a complete spectrum of ACS patients.[64] Similar findings have also been described demonstrating that NT-proBNP are strongly associated with risk of mortality.[106,109,172] The use of BNP is synergistic with that of troponin in these patients, and in patients with a normal troponin its use may be particularly helpful. However, at present, there are no therapeutic implications to BNP elevations.

Several studies have evaluated the effects of specific therapies in decreasing the risk associated with BNP and NT-proBNP.* Data from the FRISC II study have shown a greater benefit of an invasive strategy in ACS patients in the highest tertiles of NT-proBNP (Figure 44-21).[108] Of the numerous hormonal markers that have been considered in patients with minimal symptomatic or asymptomatic LV dysfunction, BNP has repeatedly proved most useful in identifying patients with mild, asymptomatic LV dysfunction. In one representative study, only 40% of patients with BNP >56 pg/mL were free of cardiac events during a 3-year follow-up period. In contrast, 90% of those with BNP <56 pg/mL were event free. Comparing BNP levels with other commonly used parameters—such as echocardiography, 6-minute walk test, LVEF, and clinical criteria in 139 CHF patients—multivariate analysis using death as an endpoint demonstrated that BNP independently identified patients with the worst prognosis. Additionally, sustained that BNP increases have been shown to be an independent risk factor for mortality even in the face of improved LVEF and clinical symptoms. Thus, BNP objectively identified patients who were at greatest risk and required more aggressive therapy.

*References 91, 108, 118, 130, 144, 169, 189, 191, 192, 214.

Implications for Therapy

With evidence that monitoring BNP can be helpful in stratifying disease severity, whether treatments that lower BNP result in decreased morbidity and mortality has to be considered, and multicenter studies are underway to address this question. The initial data from smaller trials and pilot studies look promising. A pilot study examined BNP in patients admitted with decompensated CHF and treated with the current standard of care. BNP was monitored regularly during hospitalization (but blinded to physicians) and correlated with the following endpoints: mortality in hospital,

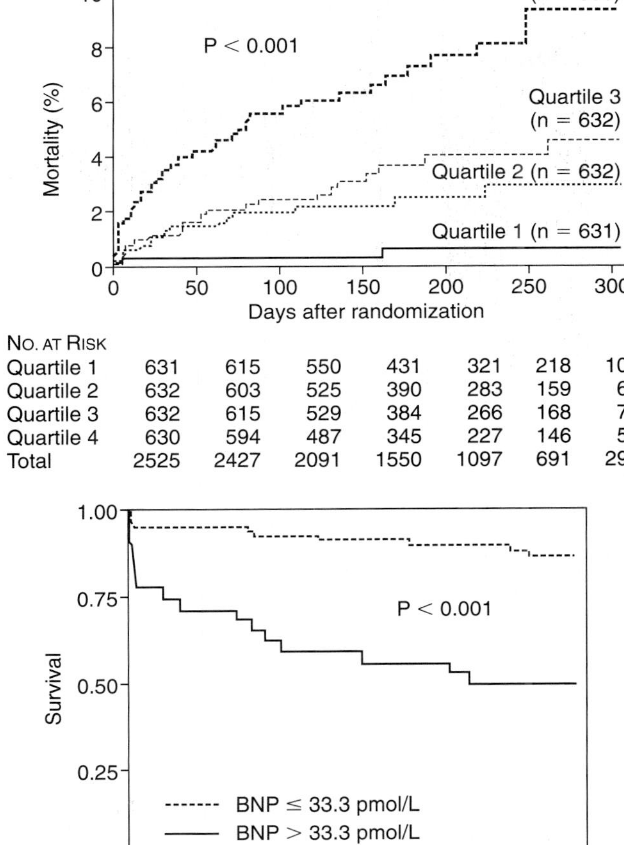

No. at Risk							
Quartile 1	631	615	550	431	321	218	104
Quartile 2	632	603	525	390	283	159	64
Quartile 3	632	615	529	384	266	168	72
Quartile 4	630	594	487	345	227	146	58
Total	2525	2427	2091	1550	1097	691	298

Figure 44-20 Risk of death for BNP and NT-proBNP in acute coronary syndrome patients according to baseline plasma concentrations. *(Panel A, from de Lemos JA, Morrow DA, Bentley JH, Omland T, Sabatine MS, McCabe CH, et al. The prognostic value of B-type natriuretic peptide in patients with acute coronary syndromes. N Engl J Med 2001;345:1014-21. Panel B, from Omland T, Persson A, Ng L, O'Brien R, Karlsson T, Herlitz J, et al. N-terminal pro-B-type natriuretic peptide and long term mortality in acute coronary syndromes. Circulation 2002;106:2913-8.)*

mortality within 30 days after admission, or readmission within 30 days. Patients whose discharge BNP fell below 500 ng/L generally did well. However, increasing BNP during hospitalization with discharge BNP greater than 1000 ng/L strongly correlated to readmission rates or death during 30-day follow-up. In a separate substudy, serial BNP concentrations were compared with changes in hemodynamics for 20 decompensated CHF patients. Patients who were felt to be responding to treatment according to a decrease in wedge pressure (51% change from baseline) experienced a significant drop in BNP compared with nonresponders (55% reduction versus 8% reduction in baseline values). There was a significant correlation between percent change in wedge pressure from baseline per hour and the percent change of BNP from baseline per hour. While outcomes of large trials are pending, BNP appears to be an objective marker that would assess response to treatment and correlate with discharge prognosis.

BNP has also been used for monitoring outpatient therapies.[118,169,189,191,192] Most CHF patients receive the same dose of angiotensin converting enzyme (ACE) inhibitors, because there is currently no objective measure of treatment efficacy. In one representative study, 20 CHF patients were randomized to receive ACE inhibitors titrated according to BNP or to standard treatment protocols for an 8-week period. In the BNP monitored group, there was a significant decrease in mean heart rate and inhibition of the renin-angiotensin-aldosterone system when compared with the empirical therapy group. Only the BNP monitored group showed significant reductions in BNP during the course of therapy. The presumption was that because BNP is a potent predictor of long-term morbidity and mortality, decreasing plasma levels were beneficial. In a similar study addressing NT-proBNP, 69 CHF patients were randomized to titrated therapy (ACE inhibitors, diuretic, and cardiac glycosides) according to plasma NT-proBNP levels or empirical therapy for up to 9 months. Those in the NT-proBNP monitored group had reduced incidence of cardiovascular death, readmission, and new episodes of decompensated CHF. These initial studies suggest that BNP and NT-proBNP are important differential tools for assessing patient status and in tailoring therapy in an outpatient basis, using BNP or NT-proBNP as an important differential tool.

Population-Based Screening

Although echocardiography is the current standard, it is not cost effective enough to be considered as a screening tool. Several studies considered the use of BNP to detect heart disease in the general population and especially those patients considered to be at high risk for CHF.[219,222] A large nonselective population-based survey recently screened more than 1200 primary care patients ages 25 to 74. It was shown that BNP was increased in some patients with asymptomatic left ventricular systolic dysfunction (LVSD). Clinical sensitivity and specificity BNP for identifying LVSD in the whole study population were 77% and 87%, respectively. When detection was restricted to LVSD in participants more than age 55, the area under the ROC curves was 0.85. However, most detection was in those with more severe disease, which often has other clinical correlations. BNP was actually disappointing in patients with mild reductions in LV performance. The accuracy of BNP as a screening tool can be optimized by targeting high-risk individuals. BNP or NT-proBNP is currently not recommended as a screening tool. However, in the Framingham cohort, there was a relationship between tertiles of BNP and long-term cardiac events and mortality even in the absence of elevations.[222]

Two additional clinical entities are worthy of a notation regarding BNP and NT-proBNP. These include obesity and

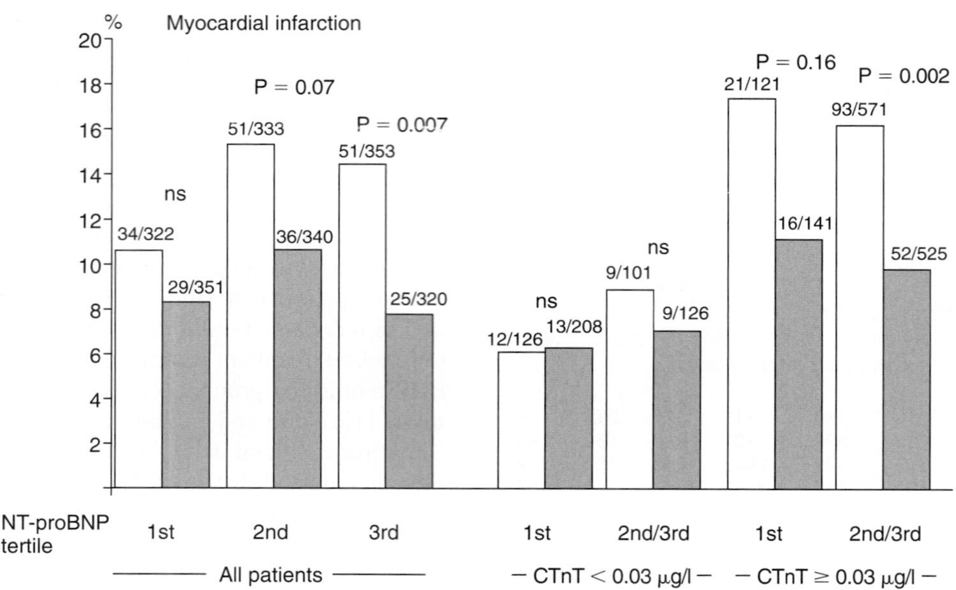

Figure 44-21 Risk of myocardial infarction in relation to the level of N-terminal pro-brain natriuretic peptide (NT-proBNP), cardiac troponin T (cTnT), and treatment strategy. *Open columns,* noninvasive strategy; *solid columns,* invasive strategy. *(From Jernberg T, Lindahl B, Siegbahn A, Andren B, Frostfeldt G, Lagerqvist B, et al. N-terminal pro-brain natriuretic peptide in relation to inflammation, myocardial necrosis, and the effect of an invasive strategy in unstable coronary artery disease. J Am Coll Cardiol 2003;42:1909-16, with permission from the American College of Cardiology Foundation.)*

renal dysfunction. Worldwide, there is an obesity epidemic.[119] Greater numbers of men and women have become obese during the past decade. Few studies have examined the relationships between BNP and NT-proBNP levels in obese patients with and without CHF. For BNP, in patients with CHF, an inverse relationship has been described between increasing body mass index (BMI; obesity) and decreasing BNP concentrations.[161] As of the writing of this chapter, similar data have not been published for NT-proBNP, although it is widely held now that NT-proBNP will manifest the same relationship to BMI as BNP. In non-CHF patients, decreasing BNP and NT-proBNP levels have been shown to correlate with decreasing BMI in conjunction with therapy.[90] The data in regard to NT-proBNP are in contrast to preliminary data that have shown that approximately 15% to 20% of asymptomatic obese patients (BMI >40) have increased NT-proBNP levels.

Regarding renal disease, the largest study to date has shown that CHF is more common in patients with advanced chronic renal disease, with BNP levels independently associated with CHF.[46] At present, however, hemodialysis appears to influence the optimum cutoff concentration for BNP and NT-proBNP in the diagnosis of CHF, with advanced stages of renal disease showing higher cutoff values.[163] BNP and NT-proBNP are secreted in a pulsatile fashion from cardiac ventricles with an approximate half-life for BNP of 22 minutes in blood, with the NT-proBNP half-life on the order of hours. While one mechanism of BNP clearance involves the renal parenchyma, the kidney is not thought to be the primary mechanism for BNP clearance, but likely a mechanism for affecting NT-proBNP clearance. Thus increases in BNP in hemodialysis patients are thought to represent both regulatory responses from the cardiac ventricle, resulting from increased wall tension, and a lack of renal clearance.

Biological Variability

As BNP and NT-proBNP become more widely used to monitor CHF patients following therapy, one investigation has questioned the usefulness of serial monitoring in assisting the success of drug therapy.[231] In this study of 11 patients with CHF, the biological variation for BNP and NT-proBNP was evaluated using four different assays. The findings indicated that a change of 130% for BNP and 90% for NT-proBNP was necessary before results of serially collected data can be considered clinically and statistically significant. For example, these findings imply that a decrease from approximately 500 ng/L to 250 ng/L would be necessary for a clinician to conclude that therapy was successful in improving CHF features. Clinicians without this knowledge may inappropriately assume that a decrease from an admission BNP value of 500 ng/L to a 24-hour postadmission value of 400 ng/L may have been a result of successful patient management. Figure 44-22 shows that in a review of 800 consecutive patients over 3 months, 75% of patients with serial BNP monitoring over 2 to 20 days did not demonstrate >100% variability.[230] These data imply the possibility of a large group of inappropriate BNP orders during the initial several days following admission for managing CHF

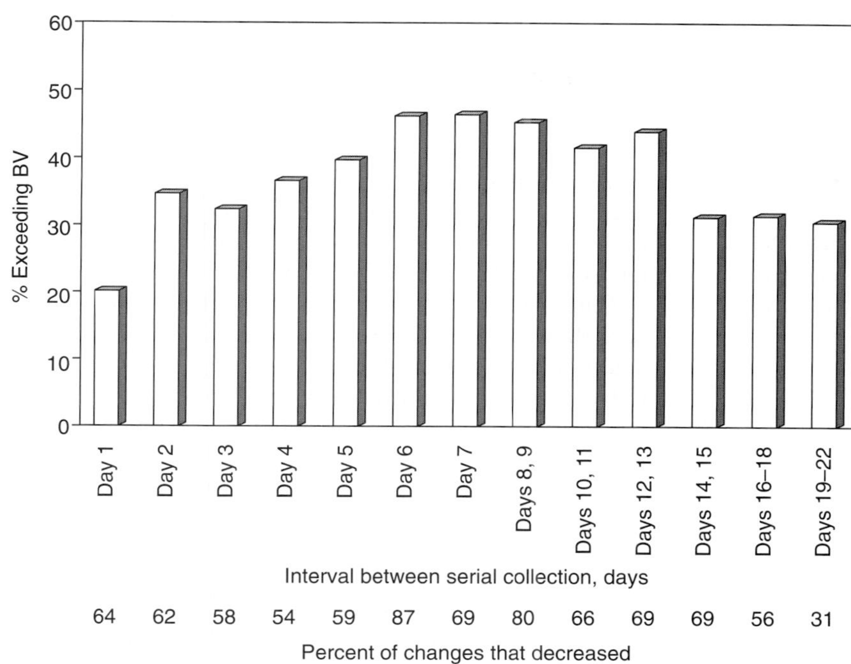

Figure 44-22 Variability of BNP concentrations by day from initial admission order, with demonstration that <50% exceed biological variability (100% change) over a 2-week time period. *(From Wu AHB, Smith A, Apple FS. Optimum blood collection intervals for B-type natriuretic peptide testing in heart failure patients. Am J Cardiol 2004;93:1562-3, with permission from Excerpta Medica.)*

patients. It has been suggested that following the admission BNP value a second BNP value be monitored within 24 hours of discharge to optimize the cost-effective role for BNP in the overall assessment of patients with CHF.

Summary

The ACC/AHA practice guidelines[40] for the evaluation and management of CHF indicate that the role of BNP in the identification of CHF patients remains to be clarified. In contrast, the ESC has incorporated monitoring BNP into their practice algorithm at the time of patient presentation alongside the clinical history, physical examination, ECG, and chest x-ray. An abnormal BNP finding would trigger an echocardiogram or other imaging modality. Several observations have been demonstrated from an overview of the evidence-based literature. First, there is an influence of age and sex in reference groups, with BNP concentrations in patients diagnosed with CHF being substantially increased (>1000 pg/mL for either BNP or NT-proBNP) compared with patients with minor increases (<400 ng/L) because of LV dysfunction without acute CHF. Second, BNP is not 100% specific for CHF. Increases have been described for other non-CHF etiologies involving filling pressure defects, including LV hypertrophy, inflammatory cardiac diseases, systemic arterial hypertension, pulmonary hypertension, acute and chronic renal failure, liver cirrhosis, and several endocrine disorders (e.g., hyperaldosteronism and Cushing's syndrome). Third, in patients with dyspnea secondary to CHF or COPD, BNP concentration is substantially different (mean >1000 ng/L [CHF] and <100 ng/L [non-CHF], respectively). Fourth, in CHF patients presenting to the ED, patients admitted trend to higher BNP concentrations (mean >500 ng/L) versus those who are discharged (mean <300 ng/L) at triage. Fifth, BNP concentrations in patients presenting with edema and in whom CHF is diagnosed trend to higher concentrations (mean >1000 ng/L) compared with non-CHF patients (mean <100 ng/L). Sixth, a survey of patients admitted to the ED with symptoms suggestive of CHF (taken early after the introduction of BNP monitoring at a county medical center) showed that the majority of orders originated from the ED (44%) and cardiology areas (45%).[243] However, after 2 years of clinician experience, there has been a shift towards a higher percentage of use by cardiology services (62%) and general medicine (17%, up from 4%), corresponding with a decrease to 20% in the ED. These findings substantiate a greater, but not necessarily more clinical, appropriate use for patient monitoring and not for diagnostic assistance. Seventh, after an AMI, BNP increases in proportion to the size of the infarction; thus investigators have explored the role of screening BNP for detection of LV dysfunction. Evidence has shown that in post-MI patients, BNP concentrations are inversely correlated with LV ejection fraction. However, there is inconclusive evidence for the role of BNP screening for asymptomatic LV dysfunction in the general population.

On the basis of the current evidence in the literature, we believe that blood BNP monitoring can be valuable in the diagnostic setting, where it will possibly improve the performance of nonspecialist clinicians in diagnosing CHF. In clinical practice, BNP monitoring can best be used as a "rule out" test for suspected cases of new CHF. It should not be a replacement for full clinical assessment, including an echocardiogram when indicated, in the presence of an increased BNP. In the presence of a normal BNP or NT-proBNP, it is highly unlikely the diagnosis will be CHF when concentrations are <100 ng/L for BNP or <400 for NT-pro-BNP. Monitoring BNP may be useful in (1) guiding therapy, (2) monitoring the course of the disease, and (3) providing useful risk stratification information. BNP has been shown to be an independent predictor of cardiovascular mortality in patients with both CHF and ACS over a 1-year period. Further, the evidence-based literature suggests that BNP or NT-proBNP monitoring may assist in identifying patients with a lower risk of readmission with the next 30 days before discharge.

CK-2

Although the measurement of CK-2 in serum has been predominantly replaced with cardiac troponin I or T, it is still a useful laboratory test for the diagnosis of AMI and recommended as an acceptable alternative to cardiac troponin.[6] The classic time versus CK-2 level (activity or mass concentration) pattern observed following the onset of chest pain in AMI is shown in Figure 44-23. An initial CK-2 rise takes 4 to 6 hours to increase above the upper reference limit. Peak levels occur at approximately 24 hours. Return to normal (baseline) takes 48 to 72 hours ($t_{1/2}$ of CK-2 is 10 to 12 hours). Factors that might affect the classic pattern include size of infarction, CK-2 composition in the myocardium, concomitant skeletal muscle injury, and reperfusion (spontaneous, following thrombolytics, or following angioplasty). The lack of tissue specificity and differentiation of increased CK-2 caused by the heart or skeletal muscle becomes important, since a normal percentage of CK-2 of total CK activity may be misleading if concomitant injury occurs in skeletal muscle coincident with an AMI. The fractional amount of CK-2 release from the heart would be obscured by the large release of total CK from skeletal muscle injury.

Clinical studies comparing CK-2 mass with activity assays have shown that CK-2 mass measurements provide earlier detection of abnormal CK-2 levels following AMI. Thus clinical sensitivity is improved without sacrificing specificity.[81] Because more than 50% of patients with AMI present to EDs with a nondiagnostic ECG, rapid and sensitive assays for the measurement of CK-2 will help clarify the diagnosis in those patients. In patients admitted to the ED, the clinical sensitivity of a single test (CK-2) result varies considerably based on time after onset of symptoms, with a range of sensitivity from 17% to 62% at 0 hours and from 92% to 100% at 3 hours after presentation.[131] This finding suggests that the traditional serial serum sampling at 0, 12, and 24 hours (which displays the classic rise-and-fall pattern of CK-2 over a 24-hour period) might be replaced with four early serum CK-2 measurements at 0, 3, 6, and 9 hours after presentation.[82]

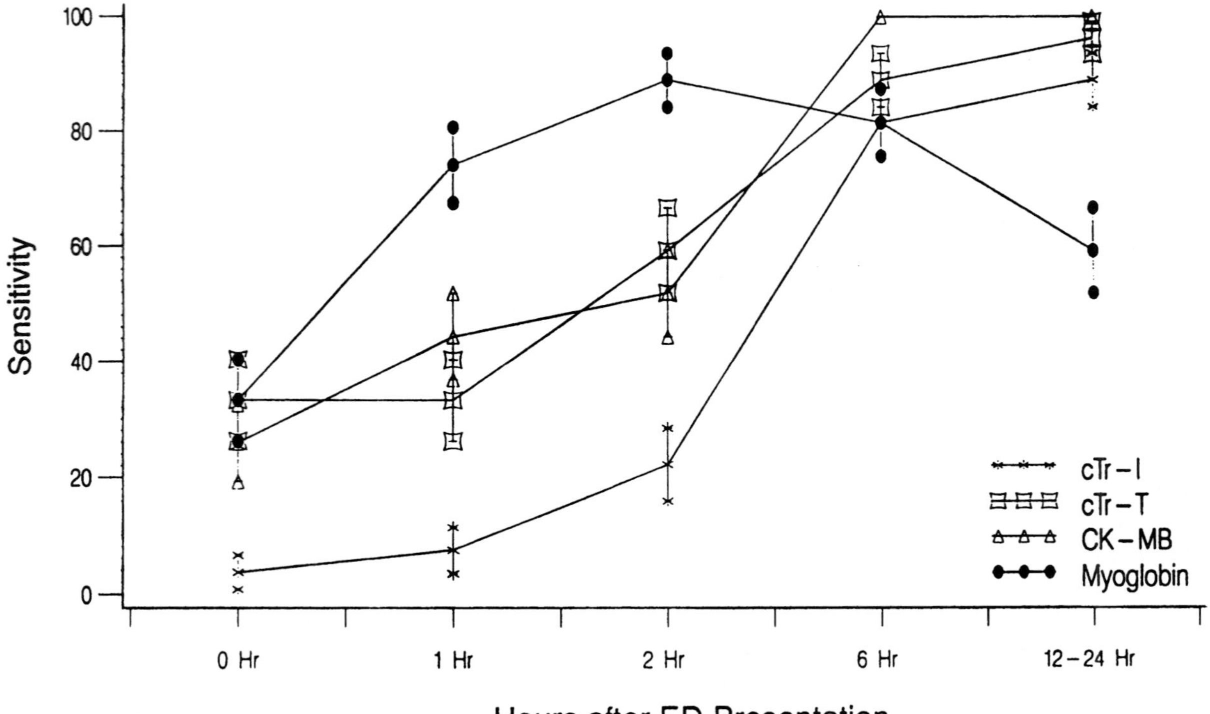

Figure 44-23 Clinical sensitivities (with 95% confidence limits) of creatine kinase-2 (CK-MB), myoglobin, and troponins I and T (cTr-I, cTr-T) for AMI as a function of time from presentation at the emergency department (ED). *(Data from Tucker JF, Collins RA, Anderson AJ, Hauser J, Kalas J, Apple FS. Early diagnostic efficiency of cardiac troponin I and cardiac troponin T for acute myocardial infarction. Acad Emerg Med 1997;4:13-21.)*

As described by the ESC/ACC consensus document on the redefinition of AMI, sampling at a minimum of 6 to 9 hours after presentation is suggested before ruling out AMI.[6] Further, CK-MB mass assays obviate the need for rapid and analytically sensitive assays to examine the small but increasing CK-2 levels in serum during the early hours after the onset of symptoms in AMI patients. The concept that it takes 4 to 6 hours for serum CK-2 levels to become elevated above the upper reference limits was derived from assays that lacked analytical sensitivity and specificity within the reference interval. The improved immunoassays are able to quantitate significant changes during the early hours after the onset of chest pain within the normal range for CK-2 to facilitate earlier AMI detection.

Clinical use of the percent relative index [%RI; %RI – (CK-2 mass/total CK activity × 100) or %CK-2 (CK-2 activity/total CK × 100)] aids in the interpretation of CK-2 concentrations for the detection of AMI. While not absolute, an increased %CK-2 or %RI points toward the heart as the source of CK-2 in serum. However, the %RI and %CK-2 should not be used for interpretation when the total CK activity remains within the reference interval, because of the potential of falsely elevated values.[36] Their use for this purpose is also compromised if there is any concomitant skeletal muscle injury, as the sensitivity for the detection of cardiac events is lost.

Myoglobin

Myoglobin is known for its excellent clinical sensitivity early after MI; however, it has not become a widely used test in clinical or laboratory practice. The majority of clinical and laboratory testing guidelines suggest a possible role for myoglobin for early myocardial detection and early monitoring. However, in general practice, the lack of tissue specificity has been its major obstacle for growth in clinical practice. The major advantage offered by myoglobin as a serum marker for early myocardial injury is that it is released earlier from damaged cells than CK-MB and cardiac troponin, allowing for earlier detection of MI.[80,84] Studies have shown that myoglobin is a very sensitive marker (90% to 100%) for AMI. As shown in Figures 44-12 and 44-23, serum concentrations of myoglobin rise above the reference interval as early as 1 hour after MI, with peak sensitivity in the range of 2 to 12 hours, suggesting that serum myoglobin reflects the early course of myocardial necrosis. Myoglobin is rapidly cleared and thus has a substantially reduced clinical sensitivity after 12 hours. If myoglobin is to have a role in detecting AMI, it must be within the first 0 to 4 hours, the time period in which CK-2 and possibly cardiac troponin are still within their reference intervals. As mentioned earlier, the measurement of serum myoglobin has not been extensively used in clinical laboratories for the routine analysis in AMI, because it has poor clinical specificity (60% to 95%), which is thought to be caused by the large quantities of myoglobin found in skeletal muscle. One attempt to improve clinical specificity involved the monitoring of carbonic anhydrase III (CA III) to assist in differentiating patients with AMI from those with skeletal muscle trauma.[216] After an AMI, serum CA III concentrations remained unchanged, while both CK-2 and myoglobin levels increased. In patients with severe skeletal muscle trauma, serum concentrations of myoglobin, CK-2, and CA III (skeletal muscle–specific) were all elevated. Therefore by using the two serum assays for myoglobin and CA III, it appears possible to distinguish between heart and skeletal muscle injury arising from numerous conditions, such as AMI, open heart surgery, vigorous exercise shock, severe renal failure, and intramuscular injections. However, if both myoglobin and CA III are elevated, one cannot rule out myocardial injury. In 2003, this concept was discussed for clinical implementation.[58] An important use of early serum myoglobin measurements following admission to EDs is their clinical utility as a negative predictor of AMI. For example, if myoglobin concentrations remain unchanged and within the reference interval on multiple, early samplings within 2 to 6 hours after the onset of chest pain, there is almost 100% certainty (99% negative predictive value) that muscle (either cardiac or skeletal) injury has not occurred recently.[80,150]

Lactate Dehydrogenase

LD isoenzymes and total LD activity are no longer measured in clinical practice.[101] For historical perspective, for patients having an AMI, serum total LD values become elevated at 12 to 18 hours after the onset of symptoms, peak at 48 to 72 hours, and return to below the upper reference limit after 6 to 10 days.[227] LD-1 rises within 10 to 12 hours, peaks at 72 to 144 hours, and returns to normal in approximately 10 days after AMI, paralleling total LD. The elevation patterns of LD-1 and total LD contrast with the elevation patterns of total CK and CK-2, which peak at 24 hours and return to below the upper reference limit within 72 hours after the onset of AMI. Because of its prolonged half-life, LD-1 is a clinically sensitive (90%) marker for infarction when used more than 24 hours after occurrence. The LD-1 increase over LD-2 in serum after AMI (the so-called flipped pattern, in which the LD-1/LD-2 ratio becomes ≥1.0) has a clinical sensitivity of about 75% in patients suspected of having sustained an AMI.[72]

GENERAL CLINICAL PRACTICE

While this chapter has reviewed the current recommendation for biomarker testing predicated on cardiac troponin at the 99th percentile or 10% CV limits, different physician groups may adhere to different principles regarding the sensitivity and specificity of a biomarker (cardiac troponin). In emergency medicine, the ED physician desires a test that will provide high specificity and not miss any possible MI patients. However, with the highly improved cardiac troponin assays in the marketplace, the 100% sensitivity that troponin assays offer demonstrates a clinical specificity of only 65% to 85%, because cardiac troponin detects myocardial injury and not just MI. This is demonstrated in Figure 44-24, which shows ROC curves of patients suggestive of ACS presenting to an inner city hospital to rule in or rule out MI for cTnI[215] and a multicenter evaluation of cTnT for assessing patients with suspected ACS.[56] The timing of serial blood draws will have a substantial influence on the changing sensitivity and specificity calculations. Because cardiac troponin detects any form of myocardial injury, nonischemic mechanisms of injury are also responsible for cardiac troponin release from the heart, causing increases in circulating cardiac troponin. Box 44-1 shows a list of potential etiologies that have been responsible for increases in nonischemic damage to the heart. Thus, whenever cardiac troponin is monitored, it is important to follow the serial pattern of a rising or a falling pattern of the biomarker, as shown in Figures 44-2 and 44-16. An increased cardiac troponin pattern that remains relatively unchanged and is not indicative of this serial trend is likely not an MI.

Strategies for the Role of Cardiac Troponin for Risk Assessment

Patients With Ischemia

In today's environment of preventive and evidence-based medicine, the use of cTnI or cTnT measured once at presentation and again at 12 to 24 hours in patients with ischemia will allow clinicians to use markers as both exclusionary and prognostic indicators. The results will assist in determining who is more at risk for AMI and death, and thereby determine who may benefit from early medical or surgical intervention. An evaluation of the majority of risk stratification studies shows that approximately 30% of all UA and NSTEMI patients present with an increased cardiac troponin level. Of these, approximately 30% (or 9% to 10% overall) have an adverse short-term (30 to 40 days) and long-term (1 to 2 years) prognosis.[93,158,175] Identifying patients at greater risk for cardiac events allows them to be treated more aggressively, with proven beneficial outcomes. There are now data that such patients benefit from the use of low molecular weight heparin, IIB/IIIA platelet antagonists, and an early invasive strategy.[33,88,137] General population screening of hospitalized patients with cTnI or cTnT is not recommended.

Numerous prospective and retrospective clinical studies have evaluated and compared the utility of measurements of cTnI, cTnT, and CK-MB (and myoglobin) for risk stratification or clinical outcomes assessment of ACS patients with possible myocardial ischemia in the ED. These studies included both single test and multitest panel situations. Patients presenting with a complaint of chest pain or other symptoms suggesting ACS have been assigned to blood sampling protocols, including only a single draw at presentation and several serial blood samplings over a 12- to 24-hour period following presentation. A large proportion of this heterogeneous ACS group are patients presenting with UA and NSTEMI. Before the redefinition of AMI by the ESC/ACC consensus document, up to 50% of UA patients progressed to AMI or cardiac death within the first year.

Studies have now demonstrated prognostic similarities between the old classification of UA patients and those with STE AMI. The use of markers is not just simply one of rapidly ruling in or ruling out AMI, but also is important for the medical management of patients with NSTEMI who are undergoing an acute coronary process (high to moderate risk patients). Therefore the goal of monitoring cardiac markers in patients suggestive of ACS with and without AMI would be to identify possible unstable coronary disease and triage to an appropriate therapy regimen. Optimal use of this strategy takes at least two blood samples for cardiac troponin. Assuming an abnormal serum cardiac troponin test is identified, this approach will allow the clinician to offer the patient alternative medical and procedural options. These include: (1) antiplatelet or antithrombic therapies, (2) percutaneous coronary interventional (PCI) procedures, (3) echocardiography, (4) a radionuclide scan, or (5) exercise stress testing to possibly identify the pathological etiology responsible for the tissue release of markers of myocardial injury.

Figure 44-25 summarizes data from a meta-analysis on this subject. Increases in cTnT or cTnI are predictive of adverse outcomes in ACS patients.[93,175] Twenty-one studies were evaluated and odds ratios (ORs) were calculated for both short-term (30 days) and long-term (5 months to 3 years) outcomes (endpoint death or nonfatal MI) in patients with and without ST-segment elevation and in UA patients. Overall, in the approximately 18,000 patients studied, at 30 days the OR for an adverse outcome was 3.4 to 1 for increased troponin. For patients with a positive troponin, the OR to have an adverse outcome in patients with UA was higher (9.3) compared with patients with ST-segment elevation (4.9) for both short- and long-term outcomes.[93] As both cTnT and cTnI offer powerful risk assessment, cardiac troponin monitoring is necessary to include in current practice guidelines—not just regarding diagnosis and management of ACS patients, but as useful risk stratification tool. This approach is supported by the new ESC, ACC, and AHA guidelines. Care must be taken, however, when evaluating individual studies pertaining to prognostic significance, because it is critical to determine the timing of sampling for cardiac marker measurements since results from a single specimen drawn at presentation may conflict with findings based on serial draws over a 24-hour period following presentation. It is recommended to draw two samples (for either cTnI or cTnT; both are not necessary) on ACS patients who do not rule in for AMI—one at presentation and one at ≥6 to 9 hours following presentation. This will allow for an increase in either cardiac troponin to occur above baseline in a patient presenting with a very recent acute coronary lesion. However, it should be noted that a normal cardiac troponin does not remove all risk. It is highly recommended that cardiac troponin results be provided to clinicians within 60 minutes with a preference toward 30 minutes (from the

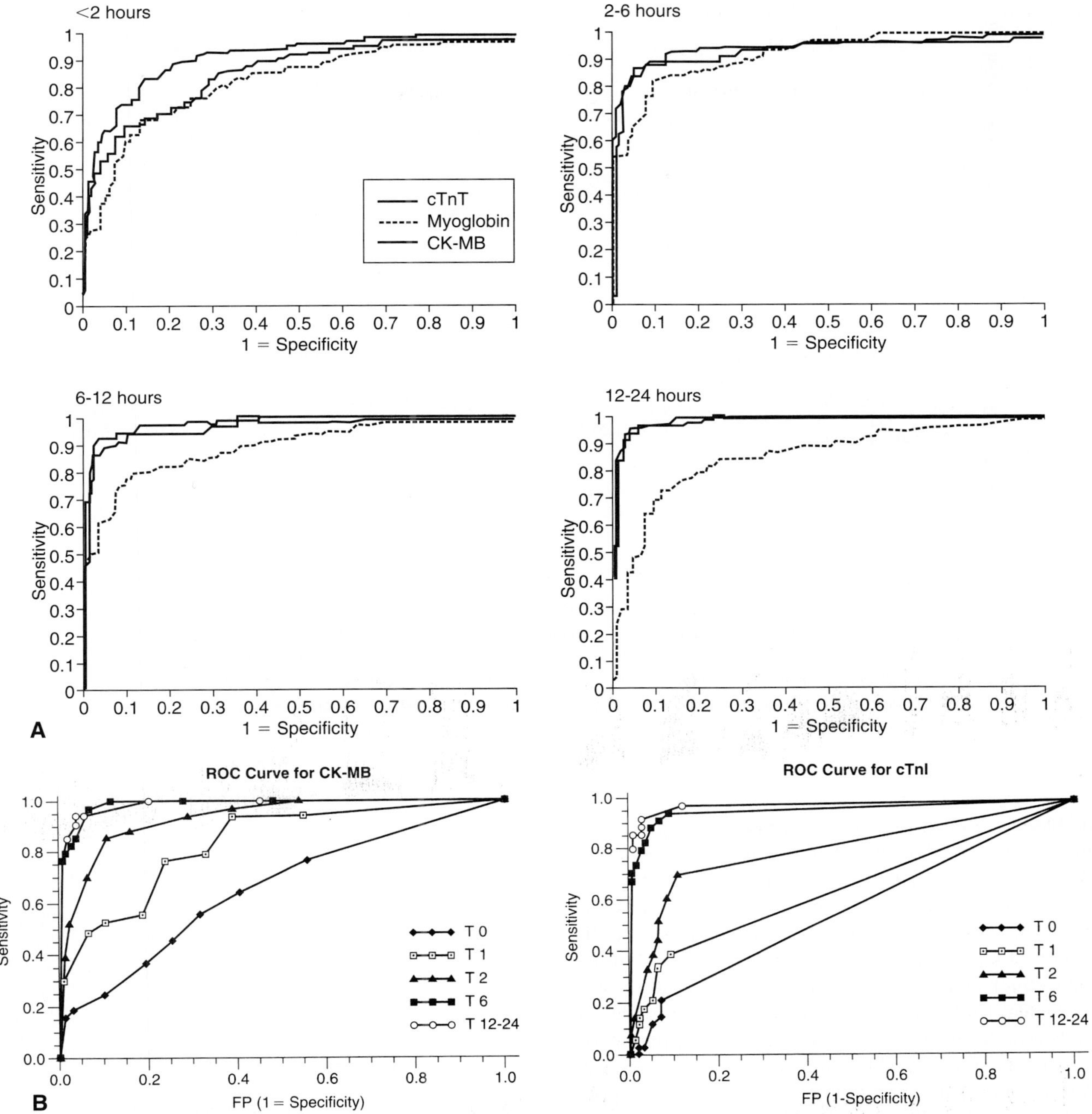

Figure 44-24 ROC curves for **A:** cTnT, CK-MB, and myoglobin and **B:** CK-MB and cTnI for diagnosis of acute myocardial infarction, according to sample time from admission (0 hours). (**A** *courtesy Collinson PO, Stubbs PJ, Kessler AC. For the multicenter evaluation of routine immunoassay of troponin T study [MERIT]. Heart 2003;89:280-6.* **B** *data from Tucker JF, Collins RA, Anderson AJ, et al. Early diagnostic efficiency of cardiac troponin I and cardiac troponin T for acute myocardial infarction. Acad Emerg Med 1997;4:13-21.*)

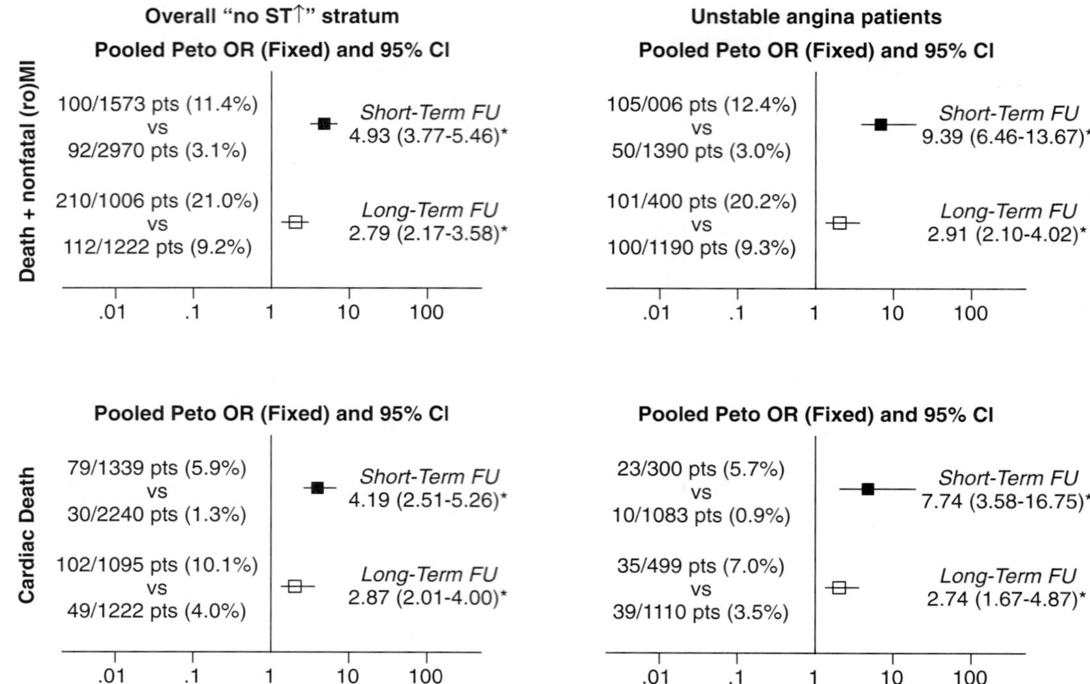

Figure 44-25 Odds ratios for death and myocardial infarction in short- and long-term follow-up among cardiac troponin–positive versus cardiac troponin–negative patients with non-ST segment elevation acute coronary syndromes, and for a subset of patients with unstable angina. *(From Ottani F, Galvani M, Nicolini FA, Ferrini D, Pozzati A, Di Pasquale G, et al. Elevated cardiac troponin levels predict the risk of adverse outcome in patients with acute coronary syndromes. Am Heart J 2000;140:917-27.)*

time blood is drawn to results reported to the physician), using either POCT[89] or central laboratory instrumentation.

For patients with an ischemic mechanism of injury for cardiac troponin increases, prognosis is related in part to the extent of the increase. An estimation of risk is useful in the selection of site of care (CCU, step-down unit, and outpatient setting) and selection of therapy, especially platelet glycoprotein IIb/IIIa inhibitors and coronary revascularization. Several large trials have demonstrated that pharmacological intervention based on an increased cardiac troponin at presentation substantially lowers the risk of death and composite MI or death, in both short- and long-term studies. Figure 44-26[41] is representative of the findings that demonstrate that death or MI is significant for all patients with increased cardiac troponin. A review of numerous trials by the ESC in ACS patient treated with GP IIb/IIIa or enoxaparin has demonstrated cost benefit of treatment and that outcomes improve by incorporating the knowledge of a cardiac troponin monitor into the management algorithm.[33,88,137,138,158] Figure 44-27 shows the reduction in risk associated with therapy in patients presenting with an increased cardiac troponin concentration.

Clinical performance of cardiac troponin assays has been shown to be strongly dependent on the analytical sensitivity and precision of measured concentrations around

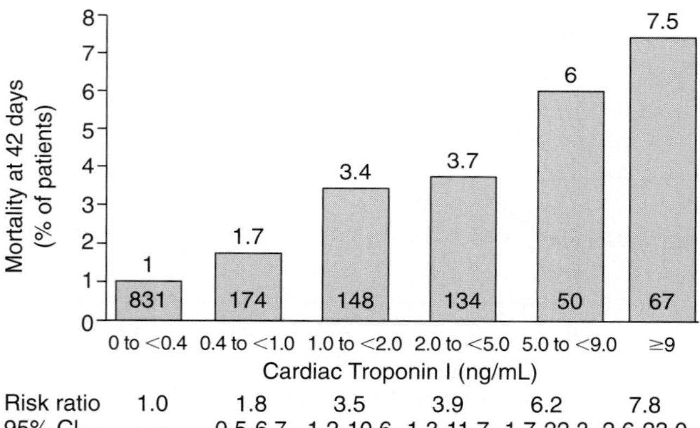

Figure 44-26 Mortality rates at 42 days according to cTnI concentrations measured at enrollment in acute coronary syndrome patients. *(Braunwald E, Antman EM, Beasley JW, Califf RM, Cheitlin MD, Hochman JS, et al. American College of Cardiology/American Heart Association Task Force on Practice Guidelines [Committee on the Management of Patients With Unstable Angina]. ACC/AHA guideline update for the management of patients with unstable angina and non-ST-segment elevation myocardial infarction—2002: summary article: a report of the American College of Cardiology/American Heart Association Task Force on Practice Guidelines [Committee on the Management of Patients With Unstable Angina]. Circulation 2002;106:1893-2000.)*

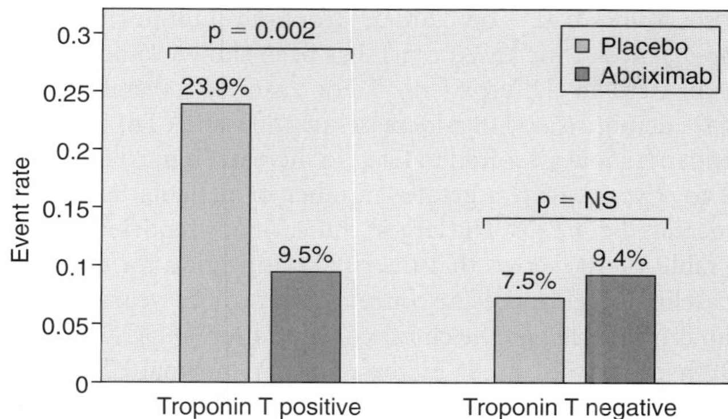

Figure 44-27 Rates of cardiac events after randomization (with or without therapy, abciximab) and during 6 months of follow-up among patients with serum cardiac troponin T concentrations above and below the diagnostic cutoff. *(Data from Hamm CW, Heeschen C, Goldmann B, Vahanian A, Adgey J, Miguel CM, et al. Benefit of ABCIXIMAB in patients with refractory unstable angina in relation to serum troponin T levels. N Engl J Med 1999;340:1623-9.)*

the 99th percentile reference limit and up to the 10% CV cutoff. Several studies have now documented that assays with lower limits of detection are able to identify more ACS patients with poor prognosis who may be candidates for early invasive procedures.[15,220] For example, in one representative study, two assays were compared and used to assess clinical performance in unstable CAD patients.[220] Although both assays showed that patients with normal cTnI levels had a significantly better prognosis than patients with increased levels, a cohort of 11% of patients (n – 98) with a poor prognosis was identified only by the assay with a lower limit of detection. Invasive treatment only reduced clinical events in the group of patients with increased cTnI. Evaluation of a first-generation cTnI assay for risk assessment between the 99th percentile and 10% CV cutoffs also may identify additional patients at risk.[15] Thus each troponin assay, I or T, needs to evaluate the stratification of patients at low-end concentrations to avoid the potential of analytical inaccuracies leading to inappropriate management decisions and therapy.

Patients With Nonischemic Presentations

Since cTnT increases can present over time (8 hours to 10 days), the timing of the myocardial injury index event can be uncertain, especially if the first troponin value is increased. The ESC/ACC consensus document recommends obtaining a CK-MB to assist in clarifying whether the event was recent (i.e., within 46 to 72 hours or later). However, there is no strong evidence to support the added testing with CK-MB. Rather, it is based on the confidence gained from years of experience using CK-MB and the concept that it might be helpful given the persistence of cardiac troponin in the blood. Following the serial rise and/or fall of cardiac troponin should differentiate an early, mid, or late evolving MI from the nonischemic, non-MI patient. For patients undergoing interventional procedures (such as PCI, stents, etc.) increases in cardiac troponin following a normal preprocedure baseline should be interpreted as indicative of myocardial injury and MI.[6,103]

For patients who undergo cardiac surgery, no cardiac biomarker is capable of differentiating injury caused by acute infarction from the injury associated with the surgical procedure itself. This is true whether CK-MB or cardiac troponin is used as a biomarker. The literature does suggest that higher blood concentrations are likely indicative of a greater amount of injury, irrespective of the mechanism. Because cardiac troponin is cardiac tissue specific (CK-MB is not), monitoring blood cardiac troponin concentrations should be superior to CK-MB. Further, it has been recommended that clinical trials, which have an extensive evidence base predicated on either CK-MB activity or mass, be transitioned toward incorporating cardiac troponin testing.[6,18,40,103,167] Additional studies are necessary for defining the appropriate application of monitoring cardiac troponin for both diagnostic and risk assessment in the cardiac surgery group. This will lend confidence to thoracic surgeons to incorporate the use of cardiac troponins over CK-MB.

Clinicians are often confronted with a clinical history of a patient without overt CAD and a low probability of myocardial ischemia. However, as a precautionary reflex, serial cardiac biomarkers, specifically cardiac troponin, are ordered. When one or two of the serial cardiac troponin concentrations come back increased, the clinician would likely be confronted with the following concerns: (1) What does this increase mean in the clinical setting of a nonischemic patient? (2) Is this a false positive, analytical finding? (3) Why was this test ordered in the first place? As cardiac troponin assays with increasing low-end analytical sensitivity have been developed and marketed, the ability to detect minor degrees of myocardial injury in a variety of clinical conditions has widened and has led to a better understanding that cardiac troponin is not just a biomarker for MI, but a sensitive biomarker for myocardial injury.* The 20% of suspected ACS patients who clinically do not rule in for MI, but display an increased cardiac troponin, represent those nonischemic pathologies in which the mechanisms of injury are well defined (such as myocarditis, blunt chest trauma, and chemotherapeutic agents), along with the unexpected finding of myocardial injury, where these patients have been shown to have increased cardiac troponin, but the mechanism of release is not clear. These observations have led to important and novel investigations involving nonischemic heart disease patients and the role for cardiac troponin as a diagnostic and prognostic tool. The highlighted conditions shown in Box 44-1 demonstrate that in addition to cardiac troponin being indicative of myocardial injury, data also have shown that an increased cardiac troponin is useful as a prognostic tool for assessing risk of death and MI. As an

*References 5, 45, 105, 120, 155, 208, 211, 221.

example (Figure 44-28), pulmonary embolism patients with an increased cTnT >0.1 µg/L were at higher risk of death (44%) during initial hospitalization compared with those with cTnT <0.1 µg/L (3%; $p < 0.001$).[154] This type of observation parallels the risk findings initially observed in ACS patients. There are now strong prognostic data in patients with pulmonary embolism, in patients with CHF, and in and postoperative vascular surgery patients. Elevations presage increased risk. In these situations, the higher the cardiac troponin, the greater the risk.

End Stage Renal Disease

Patients with end stage renal disease (ESRD) have been a subset of nonischemic patient in which risk stratification is also found based on cardiac troponin monitoring. The prevalence of increased cTnT has been shown to be greater than cTnI in these patients.[14] For example, several studies have demonstrated that increases in cTnT and cTnI in ESRD patients show a twofold to fivefold increase in mortality over 2 to 3 years, with a greater number of patients having an increased cTnT.[14,66] The largest clinical study reported to date (Table 44-10) shows that the risk stratification for death by baseline cTnT and cTnI concentration over 3 years follow-up is influenced by the cutoff concentration (ROC, 10% CV, 99th percentile) used. Increased versus normal cTnT was predictive of increased mortality using all three cutoffs for cTnT but only above the 99th percentile for cTnI. Figure 44-29 shows the respective Kaplan Meier survival curves by baseline troponin cutoffs for cTnT and cTnI. Adjusted relative risks of death associated with elevated (>99th percentile) cTnT were 3.9 for cTnT and 2.0 for cTnI. These findings may provide helpful information for decision making for the cardiologist, but may have even more of an impact on risk stratification for the nephrologist. The most important part of the evaluation is to rule out ACS. The data are similar for patients with or without renal dysfunction.[30] Any elevation of cardiac troponin is associated with increased risk. Once the presence of ACS is excluded, then attempts can be made to determine if blood pressure control, volume status, and metabolic status are optimal since it is likely they contribute to the ongoing myocardial injury. In one study, an association was found between LVH and an elevated cardiac troponin with a marked increase in risk.[66] Unfortunately, appropriate therapeutic modalities have not yet been established to address management decisions based on increased cardiac troponin values. The mechanisms responsible for the unexplained differences in elevations between cTnT and cTnI remained unexplained.[14,67,69]

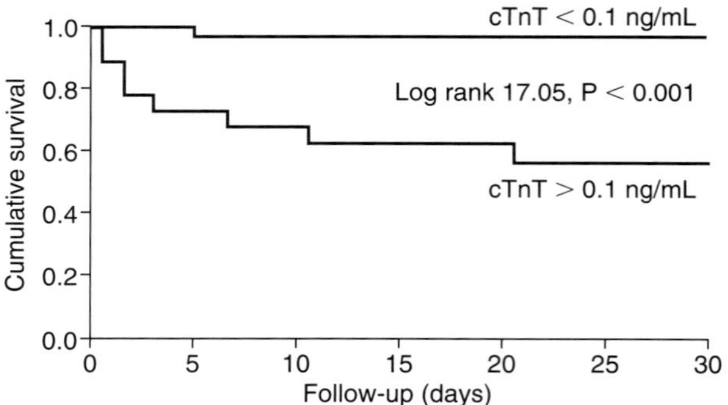

Figure 44-28 Kaplan Meier survival curves for pulmonary embolism patients without ACS based on cardiac troponin T–positive versus cardiac troponin T–negative serum samples using a cutoff concentration of 0.1 ng/mL. *(From Giannitsis E, Muller-Bardorff M, Kurowski V, Weidtmann B, Wiegand U, Kampmann M, et al. Independent prognostic value of cardiac troponin T in patients with confirmed pulmonary embolism. Circulation 2001;102:211-7.)*

TABLE 44-10 Univariate and Adjusted Relative Risks for Death by cTnT and cTnI Concentrations at Baseline

	Cumulative Mortality %					
	Normal	**Elevated**	**Univariate RR**	***P***	**Adjusted RR***	***P***
1-year follow-up						
T 0.01	3.4	19	6.2 (2.3 to 17)	<0.001	4.7 (1.7 to 13)	<0.001
I 0.10	16	25	1.8 (0.9 to 3.3)	0.10	1.8 (1.0 to 3.4)	0.08
2-year follow-up						
T 0.01	8.4	36	5.0 (2.5 to 10)	<0.001	3.9 (1.9 to 7.9)	<0.001
I 0.10	30	52	2.0 (1.3 to 3.3)	0.008	2.1 (1.3 to 3.3)	0.007
3-year follow-up						
T 0.01	8.4	51	5.5 (2.7 to 11)	<0.001	4.3 (2.1 to 8.7)	<0.001
I 0.10	44	60	2.0 (1.3 to 3.2)	0.007	2.1 (1.3 to 3.3)	0.005

RR, Relative risk.
*Adjusted for age, predraw history of coronary artery disease, and time since initial hemodialysis (<1 year, 1 to 5 years, >5 years); the number of the 733 patients with an increased troponin by cutoff (µg/L): cTnT ≥0.01, n = 601; cTnI ≥0.10, n = 45.

Clinical Utility of Cardiac Markers in Monitoring Reperfusion Following Thrombolytic Therapy

Elevations in cTnI and cTnT are highly specific for myocardial injury. However, in individuals without myocardial disease, their levels are very low to undetectable. This is in contrast to the low but measurable concentrations of CK-2 and myoglobin detected in serum from skeletal muscle turnover in patients with noncardiac-related diseases and in normal individuals. Therefore release of cTnI or cTnT from myocardium into the blood following AMI and after the washout that accompanies successful reperfusion generates an excellent signal compared with no detectable baseline levels before myocardial damage. The initial rapid release of cardiac troponin subunits I and T following successful reperfusion is most likely derived from the soluble cytosolic myocardial fraction (6% cTnT; 3% cTnI).

When an STE AMI occurs, there is a thrombus responsible for the occlusion. It can be lysed by the administration of thrombolytic agents or pushed downstream with primary angioplasty. However, this often occurs long after the anoxic myocardial tissue is irreversibly damaged. Thus to be optimally effective, reperfusion must be initiated as soon after the onset of symptoms as possible.[78]

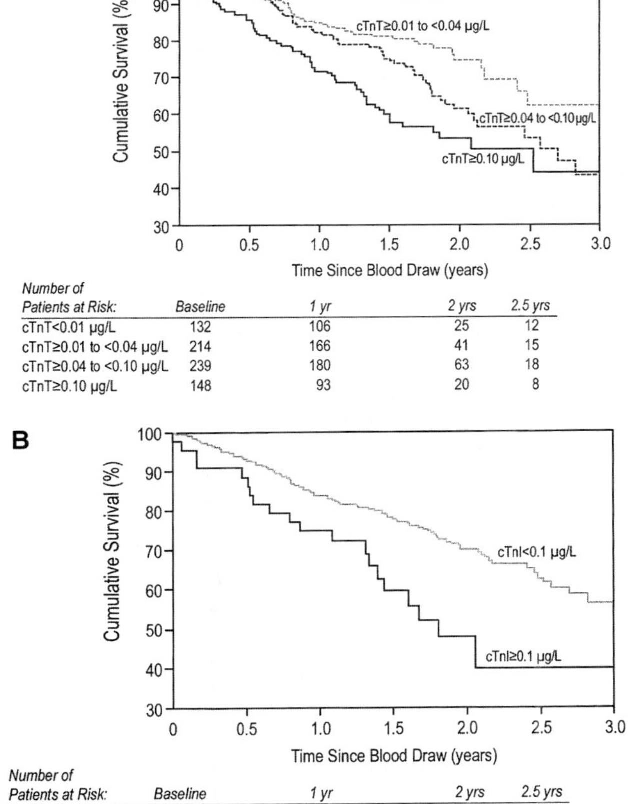

Figure 44-29 Kaplan Meier survival curves by baseline cardiac troponin cutoffs. *(From Apple FS, Murakami MM, Pearce LA, Herzog CA, et al. Predictive value of cardiac troponin I and T for subsequent death in end-stage renal disease. Circulation 2002;106:2941-5.)*

Unfortunately, reperfusion can cause tissue damage, a syndrome known as reperfusion-ischemic injury.[223] This syndrome comprises (1) membrane and microvascular damage, (2) arrhythmias, (3) myocardial stunning, (4) cell necrosis, and (5) hemorrhage. Ischemia quickly causes depletion of intracellular high-energy phosphates, such as ATP and ADP, in the endothelial cells lining the cardiac vasculature. The resulting intracellular acidosis inactivates the membrane ion pumps, causing an influx of calcium ions, which activates intracellular phospholipases, causing membrane structure disruption. Membrane disruption also permits loss of protective free radical-scavenging enzymes, such as superoxide dismutase, glutathione peroxidase, and catalase. When reperfusion occurs, the damaged endothelium attracts activated polymorphonuclear leukocytes (neutrophils) that produce oxygen free radicals that are less effectively scavenged, because of the earlier loss of the scavenging enzymes from the disrupted endothelium. The neutrophils also secrete proteases that cause microvascular damage. The membrane damage alters the cellular action potentials, resulting in cardiac arrhythmias, although these can be controlled with drug therapy. In addition, it may cause myocardial stunning and prolonged LV dysfunction after reperfusion. Thus reperfusion may increase cell necrosis. Whether this is caused by the acceleration of the death of cells already dying or by the action of free radicals killing previously healthy cells is not clear. Finally, as might be expected, the use of thrombolytic agents poses a distinct possibility of hemorrhage. Indeed the use of such agents is absolutely contraindicated in patients with evidence of recent active bleeding.

The clinical utility of cardiac biomarkers for monitoring reperfusion following thrombolytic therapy has not gained favor as a routine form of testing for determining the success or failure of reperfusion therapy.[20,27,74,116,237] It is accepted that the kinetics of myocardial protein appearance in the circulation depends on infarct perfusion. Early reperfusion causes an earlier increase above the upper reference limit and an earlier and greater enzyme peak after reperfusion. However, once the peak has occurred, there is no difference in the time of clearance of enzymes. In addition, enhanced washout identifies whether an artery is patent or closed, but cannot distinguish between normal and abnormal coronary perfusion, which is a key prognostic parameter. Further, it is difficult to assess the amount of irreversible myocardial injury by infarct sizing because of the large variability in the amount of enzyme washout that appears after reperfusion.

In practice, the laboratory becomes involved if a serum test is available as an early marker to assess successful reperfusion after AMI. With early, frequent serum sampling, it may be possible to use the rate of increase in a cardiac biomarker (cTnI, cTnT, myoglobin, and CK-2) concentration to

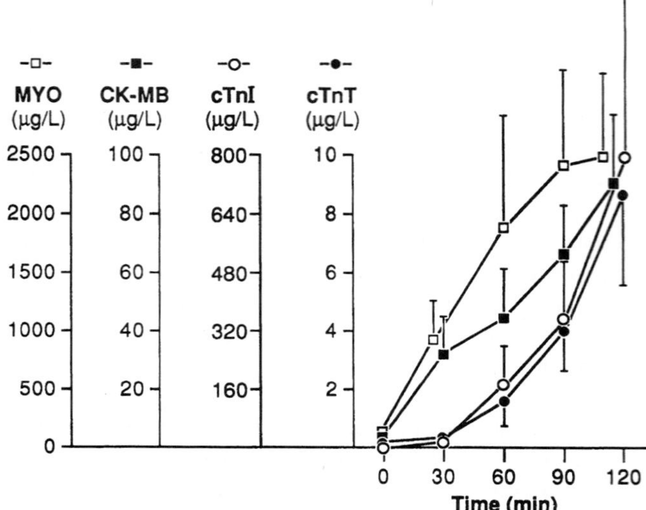

Figure 44-30 Time course (mean and standard error) of serum cardiac troponin I (cTnI), cardiac troponin T (cTnT), creatine kinase-2 (CK-MB), and myoglobin (MYO) concentrations after initiation of thrombolytic therapy in patients with TIMI Grade 3 reperfusion flow. *(From Apple FS, Sharkey SW, Henry TD. Early serum cardiac troponin I and T concentrations following successful thrombolysis for acute myocardial infarction. Clin Chem 1995;41:1197-8.)*

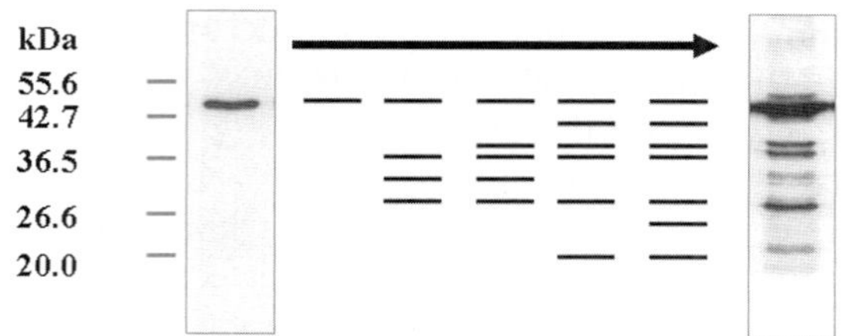

Figure 44-31 Proteomics of different disease phenotypes of cardiac troponin I associated with progression of disease. Each unique stage-specific protein change will, if detected in serum, allow disease stratification. *(Adapted courtesy J. Van Eyk.)*

determine the presence or absence of reperfusion following thrombolytic therapy as early as 30 minutes to 3 hours after the onset of chest pain in AMI. Several studies have demonstrated that (1) following thrombolytic therapy in AMI patients, greater than twofold increases in biomarkers occur within 90 minutes of reperfusion; (2) the rate of increase of biomarkers within the first 4 hours separates reperfused from nonreperfused patients; and (3) after myocardial reperfusion in AMI patients, washout of all biomarkers parallels each other (Figure 44-30). But even in this situation, a distinction between TIMI 3 (normal) and TIMI 2 (abnormal) flow is not possible.

Use of Multimarkers

There is a growing body of evidence regarding that different cardiac biomarkers provide independent and complementary information about pathophysiology, diagnostics, prognostics, and response to therapy in ACS patients. Thus it is probable that multimarker strategies or biochemical profiling may be used to characterize individual patients presenting with ACS. Two representative studies will be addressed. For example, using binary cutoffs for cTnI, BNP, and hsCRP, Sabatine et al have demonstrated 30-day mortality increases in ACS patients of twofold for one marker, fivefold for two markers, and thirteenfold for all three biomarkers.[198] In the Checkmate multicenter study,[168] a POCT system that measured cTnI, CK-MB, and myoglobin multimarker analysis identified positive patients earlier and provided a better risk stratification for 30-day mortality than the central laboratory analysis of CK-MB alone (20% versus 3%, respectively). The multimarker strategy in this study, however, was not designed for diagnostic rule in or rule out information. The addition of myoglobin to cTnI and CK-MB added one additional patient at risk for death at 30 days out of 1005 patients. Unfortunately the multimarker POCT cutoffs used were significantly lower (99th percentile) than the central laboratory assays (ROC curve) cutoff.

Figure 44-31 is a schematic that demonstrates that future proteomic research may allow for the detection of a single cTnI form (indicating recent injury) to multiple forms (indicating an older injury), thus potentially assisting in both the timing of an MI and the determination of the etiology of the injury to the myocardium.[127]

Estimation of Infarct Size

Prior studies have demonstrated the use of the integrated values for total and/or CK-MB to estimate the biochemical extent of infarction.[149,186,195] Further studies verified that the amount of cardiac damage is the primary determinant of prognosis.[71,174,205] Such determinations have been correlated with morphological infarct size. Some have used the peak CK-MB value as a surrogate for the integrated data. Reperfusion changes the release ratio (the percentage of marker that appears in the blood relative to the amount depleted from myocardium), making infarct sizing problematic in the modern era. Some, after fairly comprehensive animal experiments, have claimed that the integrated values or the 72-hour value for HBD (LD-1 and LD-2) can be used regardless of whether reperfusion occurs or not. However, there is substantial LD1 and 2 in red blood cells so that bleeding, either systemically or into the area of infarction, can lead to spurious increases in apparent infarct size. Furthermore, to date, this approach has not been compared with pathological measurements. Both experimental and patient-related data have suggested that the 72-hour troponin measurement correlates with scintigraphically determined infarct size. The data are stronger for troponin T than for I although the principles are probably similar for both analytes.

REFERENCES

1. Abendschein DR, Fontanet HL, Nohara R. Optimized preservation of isoforms of creatine kinase MM isoenzyme in plasma specimens and their rapid quantification by semi-automated chromatofocusing. Clin Chem 1990;36:723-7.
2. Abendschein D, Seacord LM, Nohara R, Sobel BE, Jaffe AS. Prompt detection of myocardial injury by assay of creatine kinase isoforms in initial plasma samples. Clin Cardiol 1988;11:661-4.
3. Abendschein DR, Morelli RL, Carlson CJ, Emilson B, Rapaport E. CK-3 isoenzyme subforms in myocardial, lymph, and blood after coronary artery occlusion. Cardiovasc Res 1984;18:690-3.
4. Adams JE, Kleinfeld A, Roe M, et al. Measurement of levels of unbound free fatty acid allows the early identification of patients with acute coronary syndromes. (abstract) Circulation 2002.
5. Adams JE 3rd, Bodor GS, Davila-Roman VG, Delmez JA, Apple FS, Ladenson JH, et al. Cardiac troponin I: a marker with high specificity for cardiac injury. Circulation 1993;88:101-6.
6. Alpert JS, Thygesen K, Antman E, Bassand JP. Myocardial infarction redefined—a consensus document of The Joint European Society of Cardiology/American College of Cardiology Committee for the redefinition of myocardial infarction. J Am Coll Cardiol 2000;36:959-9.
7. American Heart Association. Heart disease and stroke statistics—2004 update. Dallas.
8. Anand IS, Fisher LD, Chiang YT, Latini R, Masson S, Maggioni AP, et al. Changes in brain natriuretic peptide and norepinephrine over time and mortality and morbidity in the Valsartan Heart Failure Trial (Val-HeFT). Circulation 2003;107:1278-83.
9. Anderson PAW, Malouf NN, Oaleley AE, Pagani E, Allen PD. Troponin T isoform expression in humans: a comparison among normal and failing adult heart, fetal heart and adult and fetal skeletal muscle. Circ Res 1991;69:1226-33.
10. Antman EM, Braunwald E. Acute myocardial infarction. In: Braunwald E, ed. Heart disease: a textbook of cardiovascular medicine, 6th ed. Philadelphia: WB Saunders Co 2001:1114-231.
11. Antman EM, Grudzien C, Sacks DB. Evaluation of a rapid bedside assay for detection of serum cardiac troponin T. JAMA 1995;273:1279-82.
12. Apple FS, Jaffe AS. Bedside multimarker testing for risk stratification in chest pain units: the chest pain evaluation by creatine kinase-MB, myoglobin, and troponin I (CHECKMATE) study. Circulation 2001;104:e125-6.
13. Apple FS, Murakami M, Panteghini M, Christenson RH, Dati F, Mair J, et al. International survey on the use of cardiac markers. Clin Chem 2001;47: 587-8.
14. Apple FS, Murakami MM, Pearce LA, Herzog CA. Predictive value of cardiac troponin I and T for subsequent death in end stage renal disease. Circulation 2002;106:2941-5.
15. Apple FS, Murakami MM, Quist HH, Pearce LA, Wieczorek S, Wu AH. Prognostic value of the Ortho Vitros Troponin I assay in patients with symptoms of myocardial ischemia: risk stratification using ESC/ACC recommended cutoff values. Am J Clin Path 2003;120:114-20.

15A. Apple FS, Panteghini M, Ravkilde J, Mair J, Wu ABH, Tate J, et al. Quality specifications for B-type natriuretic peptide assays. Clin Chem 2005;51: 486-93.

16. Apple FS, Quist HE, Doyle PJ, Otto AP, Murakami MM. Plasma 99th percentile reference limits for cardiac troponin and creatine kinase MB mass for use with European Society of Cardiology/American College of Cardiology consensus recommendations. Clin Chem 2003;49:1331-6.
17. Apple FS, Trinity E, Steen J, Prawer S, Wu AH. BNP test utilization for CHF in community hospital practice. Clin Chim Acta 2003;328:191-3.
18. Apple FS, Wu AHB, Jaffe AS. European Society of Cardiology and American College of Cardiology guidelines for redefinition of myocardial infarction: how to use existing assays clinically and for clinical trials. Am Heart J 2002;144:981-6.
19. Apple FS, Wu AHB. Myocardial infarction redefined: role of cardiac troponin testing. Clin Chem 2001;47:377-9.
20. Apple FS. Biochemical markers of thrombolytic success. Scand J Clin Lab Invest 1999;59(suppl 230):60-6.
21. Apple FS. Tissue specificity of cardiac troponin I, cardiac troponin T, and creatine kinase MB. Clin Chim Acta 1999;284:151-9.
22. Apple FS, Billadello JJ. Creatine kinase M and B subunit mRNA levels in exercised trained rat skeletal muscle. Life Sci 1994;55:585-92.
23. Apple FS, Falahati A, Paulsen PR, Miller EA, Sharkey SW. Improved detection of minor ischemic myocardial injury with measurement of serum cardiac troponin I. Clin Chem 1997;43:2047-51.
24. Apple FS, McGue MK. Serum changes during marathon training. Am J Clin Pathol 1983;79: 716-19.
25. Apple FS, Rogers MA, Casal DC, et al. Skeletal muscle creatine kinase MB alterations in women marathon runners. Eur J Appl Physiol 1987;56:49-52.
26. Apple FS, Rogers MA. Skeletal muscle lactate dehydrogenase isozyme alterations in men and women runners. J Appl Physiol 1986;61:477-81.
27. Apple FS, Voss E, Lund L, Preese L, Berger CR, Henry TD. Cardiac troponin, CK-2, and myoglobin for the early detection of acute myocardial infarction and

monitoring of reperfusion following thrombolytic therapy. Clin Chim Acta 1995;41:13-15.
28. Apple FS. Acute myocardial infarction and coronary reperfusion: serum cardiac markers for the 1990s. Am J Clin Pathol 1992;97:217-26.
29. Apple FS. Diagnostic use of CK-3 and CK-2 isoforms for detecting myocardial infarction. Clin Lab Med 1989;9:643-54.
30. Aviles RJ, Askari AT, Lindahl B, Wallentin L, Jia G, Ohman EM, et al. Troponin T levels in patients with acute coronary syndromes, with or without renal dysfunction. N Engl J Med 2002;346:2047-52.
31. Ballantyne CM, Hoogeveen RC, Bang H, Coresh J, Folsom AR, Heiss G, et al. Lipoprotein-associated phospholipase A_2, high-sensitivity C-reactive protein, and risk for incident coronary heart disease in middle-aged men and women in the atherosclerosis risk in communities (ARIC) study. Circulation 2004;109:837-42.
32. Bayes-Genis A, Conover CA, Overgaard MT, Bailey KR, Christiansen M, Holmes DR Jr. et al. Pregnancy-associated plasma protein A as a marker of acute coronary syndromes. N Engl J Med 2001;345: 1022-9.
33. Bertrand ME, Simoons ML, Fox KA, Wallentin LC, Hamm CW, McFadden E, et al. Management of acute coronary syndromes: acute coronary syndromes without persistent ST-segment elevation. Europ Heart J 2000;21:1406-32.
34. Bettencourt P, Ferreira A, Dias P, Pimenta J, Frioes F, Martins L, et al. Predictors of prognosis in patients with stable mild to moderate heart failure. J Card Fail 2000;6:306-13.
35. Billadello JJ, Fontanet HL, Strauss AW, Abendschein DR. Characterization of MB-CK isoform conversion in vitro and in vivo in dogs. J Clin Invest 1989;83:1637-43.
36. Bilodeau L, Preese LM, Apple FS. Does low total creatine kinase activity rule out myocardial infarction? Ann Intern Med 1992;116:523-4.
37. Bodor GS, Porter S, Landt Y, Ladenson JH.Development of monoclonal antibodies for an assay of cardiac troponin-I and preliminary results in suspected cases of myocardial infarction. Clin Chem 1992;38:2203-14.
38. Bodor GS, Porterfield D, Voss EM, Smith S, Apple FS. Cardiac troponin I is not expressed in fetal and adult human skeletal muscle tissue. Clin Chem 1995;41:1710-5.
39. Bodor GS, Survant L, Voss EM, Smith S, Porterfield D, Apple FS. Cardiac troponin T composition in normal and regenerating human skeletal muscle. Clin Chem 1997;43:476-84.
39A. Braunwald E, ed. A textbook of cardiovascular medicine. 6th ed. Philadelphia: WB Saunders Co, 2001:82-128.
40. Braunwald E, Califf RM, Cannon CP, Fox KA, Fuster V, Gibler WB, et al. ACC/AHA guidelines for the management of patients with unstable angina and non-ST segment elevation myocardial infarction: executive summary and recommendations. A report of the American College of Cardiology/American Heart Association task force on practice guidelines (committee on the management of patients with unstable angina). Circulation 2000;102:1193-209.
41. Braunwald E, Antman EM, Beasley JW, Califf RM, Cheitlin MD, Hochman JS, et al. American College of Cardiology/American Heart Association Task Force on practice guidelines (Committee on the Management of Patients With Unstable Angina). ACC/AHA guideline update for the management of patients with unstable angina and non-ST-segment elevation myocardial infarction—2002: summary article: a report of the American College of Cardiology/ American Heart Association Task Force on Practice Guidelines (Committee on the Management of Patients With Unstable Angina). Circulation 2002;106:1893-2000.
42. Brennan ML, Penn MS, Van Lente F, Nambi V, Shishehbor MH, Aviles RJ, et al. Prognostic value of myeloperoxidase in patients with chest pain. N Engl J Med 2003;349:1595-604.
43. Buffon A, Biasucci LM, Liuzzo G, D'Onofrio G, Crea F, Maseri A. Widespread coronary inflammation in unstable angina. N Engl J Med 2002;347:5-12.
44. Burlina A, Zaninotto M, Secchiero S, Rubin D, Accorsi F. Troponin T as a marker of ischemic myocardial injury. Clin Biochem 1993;27:113-21.
45. Cardinale D, Sandri MT, Martinoni A, Tricca A, Civelli M, Lamantia G, et al. Left ventricular dysfunction predicted by early troponin release after high dose chemotherapy. J Am Coll Cardiol 2000;36: 517-22.
46. Cataliotti A, Malatino LS, Jougasaki M, Zoccali C, Castellino P, Giacone G, et al. Circulating natriuretic peptide concentrations in patients with end-stage renal disease: role of brain natriuretic peptide as a biomarker for ventricular remodeling. Mayo Clin Proc 2001;76:1111-9.
47. Chapelle JP, Allaf ME. Determination of myoglobin in serum by kinetic turbidimetry using the turbitime system. Clin Chem 1990;36:1193 (Abstract).
48. Chapelle JP, Heusghen C. Further heterogeneity demonstrated for serum CK isoenzyme MM. Clin Chem 1980;26:457-61.
49. Cheng V, Kazanagra R, Garcia A, Lenert L, Krishnaswamy P, Gardetto N, et al. A rapid bedside test for B-type peptide predicts treatment outcomes in patients admitted for decompensated heart failure: a pilot study. J Am Coll Cardiol 2001;37:386-91.
50. Christenson RH, Duh SH, Apple FS, Bodor GS, Bunk DM, Dalluge J, et al. Standardization of cardiac

troponin I assays: round robin performance of ten candidate reference materials. Clin Chem 2001;47: 431-7.

51. Christenson RH, Vaidya H, Landt Y, Bauer RS, Green SF, Apple FA, et al. Standardization of creatine kinase MB (CK MB) mass assays: the use of recombinant CK MB as a reference material. Clin Chem 1999;45:1414-23.
52. Christenson RH, Russell ME, Pizzo CM. Creatine kinase-MB isoforms fractionated by immunoprecipitation and quantified in a rapid analyzer. Clin Chem 1990;36:1127-33.
53. Christenson RH. Nourin: An early specific marker of cardiac ischemia. AACC Annual meeting, 2003.
54. Collinson PO, Boa FG, Gaze DC. Measurement of cardiac troponins. Ann Clin Biochem 2001;38: 423-49.
55. Collinson PO, Stubbs PJ, Kessler AC. For the multicenter evaluation of routine immunoassay of troponin T study (MERIT). Heart 2003;89: 280-6.
56. Collinson PO, Stubbs PJ, Rosalki SB. Cardiac troponin T in renal disease. Clin Chem 1995;41:1671-2.
57. Colucci WS, Braunwald E. Pathophysiology of heart failure. In: Braunwald E, ed. Heart disease: A textbook of cardiovascular medicine. 6th ed. Philadelphia: WB Saunders Co, 2001;503-614.
58. Cortina MAQ, Pituley AJ, Shin H, Liu J, Kadijevic L, Bilandzic LM, et al. Comparison of Spectral's enhanced point-of-care test for markers troponin I and myoglobin with clinical analyzers. Clin Chem 2003;49 Suppl 6:A71 (abstract).
59. Cowie MR, Jourdain P, Maisel A, Dahlstrom U, Follath F, Isnard R, et al. Clinical applications of B-type natriuretic peptide (BNP) testing. E Heart J 2003;24:1710-18.
60. Cummins B, Auckland ML, Cummins P. Cardiac specific troponin-I radioimmunoassay in the diagnosis of acute myocardial infarction. Am Heart J 1987;113:1333-44.
61. Danne O, Mockel M, Lueders C, Mugge C, Zschunke GA, Lufft H, et al. Prognostic implications of elevated whole blood choline levels in acute coronary syndromes. Am J Cardiol 2003;91:1060-7.
62. de Lemos JA, McGuire DK, Drazner MH. B-type natriuretic peptide in cardiovascular disease. Lancet 2003;362:316-22.
63. de Lemos JA, Morrow DA. Combining natriuretic peptides and necrosis markers in the assessment of acute coronary syndromes. Rev Cardiovasc Med 2003;4 Suppl 4:S37-46.
64. de Lemos JA, Morrow DA, Bentley JH, Omland T, Sabatine MS, McCabe CH, et al. The prognostic value of B-type natriuretic peptide in patients with acute coronary syndromes. N Engl J Med 2001;345: 1014-21.
65. de Lemos JA, Morrow DA, Sabatine MS, Murphy SA, Gibson CM, Antman EM, et al. Association between plasma levels of monocyte chemoattractant protein-1 and long-term clinical outcomes in patients with acute coronary syndromes. Circulation 2003;107: 690-5.
66. deFilippi C, Wasserman S, Rosanio S, Tiblier E, Sperger H, Tocchi M, et al. Cardiac troponin T and C-reactive protein for predicting prognosis, coronary atherosclerosis, and cardiomyopathy in patients undergoing long-term hemodialysis. JAMA 2003;290:353-9.
67. Diris JH, Hackeng CM, Kooman JP, Pinto YM, Hermens WT, van Dieijen-Visser MP. Impaired renal clearance explains elevated troponin T fragments in hemodialysis patients. Circulation 2004;109:23-5.
68. Eisenberg PR, Shaw D, Schaab C, Jaffe AS. Concordance of creatine kinase MB activity and mass. Clin Chem 1989;35:440-3.
69. Ellis K, Dreisbach AW, Lertora JL. Plasma elimination of cardiac troponin I in end-stage renal disease. S Med J 2001;94:993-6.
70. Feldman AM, Kadokami T, Higuichi Y, Ramani R, McTiernan CF. The role of anticytokine therapy in heart failure: recent lessons from preclinical and clinical trials? Med Clin N Am 2003;87:419-24.
71. Fishbein MC, Wang T, Matijasevic M, Hong L, Apple FS. Myocardial tissue troponins T and I: an immunohistochemical study in experimental models of myocardial ischemia. Cardiovas Path 2003;12: 65-71.
72. Galen RS, Reiffel JA, Gambino SR. Diagnosis of acute myocardial infarction: relative efficiency of serum enzyme and isoenzyme measurements. JAMA 1975;232:145-7.
73. Galvani M, Panteghini M, Ottani F, Cappelletti P, Chiarella F, Chiariello M, et al. The new definition of myocardial infarction: analysis of the ESC/ACC consensus document and reflections on its applicability to the Italian health system. Ital Heart J 2002;3: 543-57.
74. Garabedian HD, Gold HK, Yasuda T, Johns JA, Finkelstein DM, Gaivin RJ, et al. Detection of coronary artery reperfusion with CK-2 determinations during thrombolytic therapy. J Am Coll Cardiol 1988;11:729-34.
75. Gardner RS, Ozalp F, Murday AJ, Robb SD, McDonagh TA. N-terminal pro-brain natriuretic peptide: a new gold standard in predicting mortality in patients with advanced heart failure. E Heart J 2003;24:1735-43.
76. Gerhardt W, Nordin G, Herbert AK, Burzell BL, Isaksson A, Gustavsson E, et al. Troponin T and I assays show decreased concentrations in heparin plasma compared to serum: lower recoveries in early

than in late phases of myocardial injury. Clin Chem 2000;46:817-21.

77. Gerhardt W, Katus H, Ravkilde J, Hamm C, Jorgensen PJ, Peheim E, et al. S-Troponin T in suspected ischemic myocardial injury compared with mass catalytic concentrations of S-creatine kinase isoenzyme MB. Clin Chem 1991;37:1405-11.
78. Gersh BJ, Anderson JL. Thrombolysis and myocardial salvage. Circulation 1993;88:296-306.
79. Giannitsis E, Muller-Bardorff M, Kurowski V, Weidtmann B, Wiegand U, Kampmann M, et al. Independent prognostic value of cardiac troponin T in patients with confirmed pulmonary embolism. Circulation 2001;102:211-17.
80. Gibler WB, Gibler CD, Weinshenker E, Abbottsmith C, Hedges JR, Barsan WG, et al. Myoglobin as an early indicator of acute myocardial infarction. Ann Emerg Med 1987;16:851-6.
81. Gibler WB, Lewis LM, Erb RE, Makens PK, Kaplan BC, Vaughn RH, et al. Early detection of acute myocardial infarction in patients presenting with chest pain and nondiagnostic ECGs: serial CK-MB sampling in the emergency department. Ann Emerg Med 1990;19:1359-66.
82. Gibler WB, Runyon JP, Levy RC, Sayre MR, Kacich R, Hattemer CR, et al. A rapid diagnostic and treatment center for patients with chest pain in the emergency department. Ann Emerg Med 1995:25:1-8.
83. Glagov S, Weisenberg E, Zarins CK, Stankunavicius R, Kolettis GJ. Compensatory enlargement of human atherosclerotic coronary arteries. N Engl J Med 1987;316:1371-5.
84. Grenadier E, Keidar S, Kahana L, Alpan G, Marmur A, Palant A. The roles of serum myoglobin, total CK, and CK-2 isoenzymes in the acute phase of myocardial infarction. Am Heart J 1983;10:408-16.
85. Griendling KK, FitzGerald GA. Oxidative stress and cardiovascular injury: Part I: basic mechanisms and in vivo monitoring of ROS. Circulation 2003;108: 1912-6.
86. Griendling KK, FitzGerald GA. Oxidative stress and cardiovascular injury: Part II: animal and human studies. Circulation 2003;108:2034-40.
87. Gurney D, Lip GY, Blann AD. A reliable plasma marker of platelet activation: does it exist? Am J Hematol 2002;70:139-44.
88. Hamm CW, Heeschen C, Goldmann B, Vahanian A, Adgey J, Miguel CM, et al. Benefit of AXCIXIMAB in patients with refractory unstable angina in relation to serum troponin T levels. N Engl J Med 1999;340:1623-9.
89. Hamm CW, Goldmann BU, Heeschen C, Kreymann G, Berger J, Meinertz T. Emergency room triage of patients with acute chest pain by means of rapid testing for cardiac troponin T or troponin I. N Engl J Med 1997;337:1648-53.
90. Hanusch-Enserer U, Hermann KM, Cauza E, Spak M, Mahr B, Dunky A, et al. Effect of gastric banding on aminoterminal pro-brain natriuretic peptide in the morbidly obese. Obesity Res 2003;11: 695-8.
91. Hara Y, Hamada M, Shigematsu Y, Suzuki M, Kodama K, Kuwahara T, et al. Effect of beta-blocker on left ventricular function and natriuretic peptides in patients with chronic heart failure treated with angiotensin-converting enzyme inhibitor. Jpn Circ J 2000;64:365-9.
92. Heeschen C, Dimmeler S, Fichtlscherer S, Hamm CW, Berger J, Simoons ML, et al. Prognostic value of placental growth factor in patients with acute chest pain. JAMA 2004;291:435-41.
93. Heidenreich PA, Alloggiamento T, Melsop K, McDonald KM, Go AS, Hlatky MA. The prognostic value of troponin in patients with non-ST elevation acute coronary syndromes: a meta analysis. J Am Coll Cardiol 2001;38:478-85.
93a. Hermann-Arnhof KM, Hanusch-Enserer U, Kaestenbauer T, Publig T, Dunky A, Rosen HR, et al. N-terminal Pro-B-Type natriuretic peptide as an indicator of possible cardiovascular disease in severely obese individuals: Comparison with patients in different stages of heart failure. Clin Chem 2005;51:138-43.
94. Holvoet P, Mertens A, Verhamme P, Bogaerts K, Beyens G, Verhaeghe R, et al. Circulating oxidized LDL is a useful marker for identifying patients with coronary artery disease. Art Thromb Vas Bio 2001;21:844-8.
95. Horwich TB, Patel J, MacLellan WR, Fonarow GC. Cardiac troponin I is associated with impaired hemodynamics, progressive left ventricular dysfunction, and increased mortality rates in advanced heart failure. Circulation 2003;108:833-8.
96. Huber K, Christ G, Wojta J, Gulba D. Plasminogen activator inhibitor type-1 in cardiovascular disease. Status report 2001. Thromb Res 2001;103 Suppl:1S7-19.
97. Hunt SA, Baker DW, Chin MH, Cinquegrani MP, Feldman AM, Francis GS, et al. ACC/AHA Guidelines for the evaluation and management of chronic heart failure in the adult: executive summary a report of the American College of Cardiology/American Heart Association Task Force on Practice Guidelines (committee to revise the 1995 guidelines for the evaluation and management of heart failure): developed in collaboration with the International Society for Heart and Lung Transplantation; endorsed by the Heart Failure Society of America. Circulation 2001;104:2996-3007.
98. Hutter AM, Amsterdam EA, Jaffe AS. Task force 2: acute coronary syndromes: section 2b-chest discomfort evaluation in the hospital. 31st Bethesda confer-

ence. Emergency Cardiac Care J Am Coll Cardiol 2000;35:853-62.

99. Ingwall JS, Kramer MF, Fifer MA, Lorell BH, Shemin R, Grossman W, et al. The creatine kinase system in normal and diseased human myocardium. N Engl J Med 1985;313:1050-4.

100. Ishii J, Nomura M, Nakamura Y, Naruse H, Mori Y, Ishikawa T, et al. Risk stratification using a combination of cardiac troponin T and brain natriuretic peptide in patients hospitalized for worsening chronic heart failure. Am J Cardiol 2002;89:691-5.

101. Jaffe AS, Landt Y, Parvin CA, Abendschein DR, Geltman EM, Ladenson JH. Comparative sensitivity of cardiac troponin I and lactate dehydrogenase isoenzymes for diagnosing acute myocardial infarction. Clin Chem 1996;42:1770-6.

102. Jaffe AS. Elevations in cardiac troponin measurements: False false-positives. Cardiovas Toxicol 2001;1: 87-92.

103. Jaffe AS, Ravkilde J, Roberts R, Naslund U, Apple FS, Galvani M, et al. It's time for a change to a troponin standard. Circulation 2000;102:1216-20.

104. Jaffe AS, Davidenko J, Clements I. Diagnosis of acute coronary syndromes including myocardial infarction. In: Crawford MH, DiMarco JP, Paulus WJ, eds. Cardiology. 2nd ed. St Louis: Mosby 2004:311-28.

105. James P, Ellis CJ, Whitlock RM, McNeil AR, Henley J, Anderson NE. Relation between troponin T concentration and mortality in patients presenting with an acute stroke: observational study. Brit Med J 2000;320:1502-4.

106. James SK, Lindahl B, Siegbahn A, Stridsberg M, Venge P, Armstrong P, et al. N-terminal pro-brain peptide and other risk markers for separate prediction of mortality and subsequent myocardial infarction in patients with unstable coronary artery disease: a GUSTO substudy. Circulation 2003;108:275-81.

107. James SK, Armstrong P, Barnathan E, Califf R, Lindahl B, Siegbahn A, et al. Troponin and C-reactive protein have different relations to subsequent mortality and myocardial infarction after acute coronary syndrome: a GUSTO-IV substudy. J Am Coll Cardiol 2003;41:916-24.

108. Jernberg T, Lindahl B, Siegbahn A, Andren B, Frostfeldt G, Lagerqvist B, et al. N-terminal pro-brain natriuretic peptide in relation to inflammation, myocardial necrosis, and the effect of an invasive strategy in unstable coronary artery disease. J Am Coll Cardiol 2003;42:1909-16.

109. Jernberg T, Stridsberg M, Venge P, Lindahl B. N-terminal pro brain natriuretic peptide on admission for early risk stratification of patients with chest pain and no ST-segment elevation. J Am Coll Cardiol 2002;40:437-45.

110. Jones CB, Sane DC, Herrington DM. Matrix metalloproteinases: a review of their structure and role in acute coronary syndrome. Cardiovasc Res 2003;59:812-23.

111. Kalra PR, Clague JR, Bolger AP, Anker SD, Poole-Wilson PA, Struthers AD, et al. Myocardial production of C-type natriuretic peptide in chronic heart failure. Circulation 2003;107:571-3.

112. Katrukha AG, Bereznikova AV, Filatov VL, Esakova TV, Kolosova OV, Pettersson K, et al. Degradation of cardiac troponin I: implication for reliable immunodetection. Clin Chem 1998;44:2433-40.

113. Katrukha AG, Bereznikova AV, Esakova TV, Pettersson K, Lovgren T, Severina ME, et al. Troponin I is released in bloodstream of patients with acute myocardial infarction not in free form but as complex. Clin Chem 1997;43:1379-85.

114. Katus HA, Looser S, Hallermayer K, Remppis A, Scheffold T, Borgya A, et al. Development and in vitro characterization of a new immunoassay of cardiac troponin T. Clin Chem 1992;38:386-93.

115. Katus HA, Remppis A, Neumann FJ, Scheffold T, Diederich KW, Vinar G, et al. Diagnostic efficiency of troponin T measurements in acute myocardial infarction. Circulation 1991;83:902-12.

116. Katus HA, Remppis A, Scheffold T. Intracellular compartmentation of cardiac troponin T and its release kinetics in patients with reperfused and nonreperfused myocardial infarction. Am J Cardiol 1991;67:1360-7.

117. Katus HA, Scheffold T, Remppis A, Zehlein J. Proteins of the troponin complex. Lab Med 1992;23: 311-17.

118. Kawai K, Hata K, Takaoka H, Kawai H, Yokoyama M. Plasma brain natriuretic peptide as a novel therapeutic indicator in idiopathic dilated cardiomyopathy during beta-blocker therapy: a potential of hormone-guided treatment. Am Heart J 2001;141:925-32.

119. Kenchaiah S, Evans JC, Levy D, Wilson PW, Benjamin EJ, Larson MG, et al. Obesity and the risk of heart failure. N Engl J Med 2002;347:305-13.

120. Kim LJ, Martinez EA, Faraday N, Dorman T, Fleisher LA, Perler BA, et al. Cardiac troponin I predicts short term mortality in vascular surgery patients. Circulation 2002;106:2366-71.

121. Kinugawa T, Kato M, Ogino K, Osaki S, Igawa O, Hisatome I, et al. Plasma endothelin-1 levels and clinical correlates in patients with chronic heart failure. J Card Fail 2003;9:318-24.

122. Kojima M, Minamino N, Kangawa K, Matsuo H. Cloning and sequence analysis of cDNA encoding a precursor for rat brain natriuretic peptide. Bichem Biophys Res Commun 1989;159:1420-6.

123. Konstantinides S, Geibel A, Olschewski M, Kasper W, Hruska N, Jackle S, et al. Importance of cardiac troponins I and T in risk stratification of patients with acute pulmonary embolism. Circulation 2002;106: 1263-8.

124. Kontos MC, Fritz LM, Anderson FP, Tatum JL, Ornato JP, Jesse RL. Impact on the troponin standard on the prevalence of acute myocardial infarction. Am Heart J 2003;146:446-52.
125. Kruger S, Graf J, Merx MW, Stickel T, Kunz D, Hanrath P, et al. Brain natriuretic peptide predicts right heart failure in patients with acute pulmonary embolism. Am Heart J 2004;147:60-5.
126. La Vecchia L, Ottani F, Favero L, Spadaro GL, Rubboli A, Boanno C, et al. Elevation of cardiac troponin I on admission predicts in-hospital mortality in acute pulmonary embolism. Heart 2004;90:633-7.
127. Labugger R, Organ L, Collier C, Atar D, Van Eyk JE. Extensive troponin I and T modification detected in serum from patients with acute myocardial infarction. Circulation 2000;102:1221-6.
128. Lang H. Creatine kinase isoenzymes. New York: Springer-Verlag, 1981.
129. Larue C, Defacque-Lacquement H, Calzolari C, Le Nguyen D, Pau B. New monoclonal antibodies as probes for human cardiac troponin I. Mol Immunol 1992;29:271-8.
130. Latini R, Masson S, Anand I, Judd D, Maggioni AP, Chiang YT, et al. Effects of valsartan on circulating brain natriuretic peptide and norepinephrine in symptomatic chronic heart failure: the Valsartan Heart Failure Trial (Val-HeFT). Circulation 2002;106:2454-8.
131. Leung FY, Galbraith LV, Jablonsky G, Henderson AR. Re-evaluation of the diagnostic utility of serum total creatine kinase and creatine kinase-2 in myocardial infarction. Clin Chem 1989;35:1435-40.
132. Levin ER, Gardner DG, Samson WK. Natriuretic peptides. N Engl J Med 1998;339:321-8.
133. Libby P. Vascular biology of atherosclerosis: overview and state of the art. Am J Cardiol 2003;91: 3A-6A.
134. Lin JC, Apple FS, Murakami MM, Luepker RV. Rates of positive cardiac troponin I and creatine kinase MB among patients hospitalized for suspected acute coronary syndromes. Clin Chem 2004;50:333-8.
135. Lin L, Sylven C, Sotonyi P, Somogyi E, Kaijser L, Jansson E. Lactate dehydrogenase and its isoenzyme activities in different parts of the normal human heart. Cardiovasc Res 1989;23:601-6.
136. Lind L. Circulating markers of inflammation and atherosclerosis. Atherosclerosis 2003;169:203-14.
137. Lindahl B, Diderholm E, Lagerqvist B, Venge P, Wallentin L. Mechanisms behind the prognostic value of troponin T in unstable coronary artery disease: a FRISC II substudy. J Am Coll Cardiol 2001;38:979-86.
138. Lindahl B, Andren B, Ohlsson J, Venge P, Wallentin L. Noninvasive risk stratification in unstable coronary artery disease: exercise test and biochemical markers. FRISC Study Group. Am J Cardiol 1997;80:40E-4E.
139. Little WC. Assessment of cardiac function. In: Heart disease: a textbook of cardiovascular medicine. 6th ed. Braunwald E, ed. Philadelphia: WB Saunders Co, 2001:98.
140. Liuzzo G, Biasucci LM, Rebuzzi AG, Gallimore JR, Caligiuri G, Lanza GA, et al. Plasma protein acute-phase response in unstable angina is not induced by ischemic injury. Circulation 1996;94:2373-80.
141. Luchner A, Burnett JC Jr, Jougasaki M, Hense HW, Heid IM, Muders F, et al. Evaluation of brain natriuretic peptide as marker of left ventricular dysfunction and hypertrophy in the population. J Hypertens 2000;18:1121-8.
142. Luepker RV, Apple FS, Christenson RH, Crow RS, Fortmann SP, Goff D, et al. Case definitions for acute coronary heart disease in epidemiology and clinical research studies. Circulation 2003;108:2543-9.
143. Lund J, Qin QP, Ilva T, Pettersson K, Voipio-Pulkki LM, Porela P, et al. Circulating pregnancy-associated plasma protein A predicts outcome in patients with acute coronary syndrome but no troponin I elevation. Circulation 2003;108:1924-6.
144. Maeda K, Tsutamoto T, Wada A, Mabuchi N, Hayashi M, Tsutsui T, et al. High levels of plasma brain natriuretic peptide and interleukin-6 after optimized treatment for heart failure are independent risk factors for morbidity and mortality in patients with congestive heart failure. J Am Coll Cardiol 2000;36:1587-93.
145. Mair J, Hammerer-Lercher A, Puschendorf B. The impact of cardiac natriuretic peptide determination on the diagnosis and management of heart failure. Clin Chem Lab Med 2001;39:571-88.
146. Mair J, Dienstl F, Puschendorf B. Cardiac troponin T in the diagnosis of myocardial injury. Crit Rev Clin Lab Sci 1992;29:31-57.
147. Maisel AS, Krishnaswamy P, Nowak RM, McCord J, Hollander JE, Duc P, et al. Rapid measurement of B-type natriuretic peptide in the emergency diagnosis of heart failure. N Engl J Med 2002;347: 161-7.
148. Maisel AS, Krishnaswamy P, Nowak RM, McCord J, Hollander JE, Duc P, et al. Breathing not properly multinational study investigators rapid measurement of B-type natriuretic peptide in the emergency diagnosis of heart failure. N Engl J Med 2002;347: 161-7.
149. Maroko PR, Kjekshus JK, Sobel BE, Watanabe T, Covell JW, Ross J Jr, et al. Factors influencing infarct size following experimental coronary artery occlusions. Circulation 1971;43:67-82.
150. McCord J, Nowak RM, McCullough PA, Foreback C, Borzak S, Tokarski G, et al. Ninety minute exclusion of acute myocardial infarction by use of quantitative point-of-care testing of myoglobin and troponin I. Circulation 2001;104:1483-8.

151. McCullough PA, Hollander JE, Nowak RM, Storrow AB, Duc P, Omland T, et al. Uncovering heart failure in patients with a history of pulmonary disease: rationale for the early use of B-type natriuretic peptide in the emergency department. Acad Emerg Med 2003;10:1982-2004.
152. McCullough PA, Nowak RM, McCord J, Hollander JE, Herrmann HC, Steg PG, et al. B-type natriuretic peptide and clinical judgment in emergency diagnosis of heart failure: analysis from breathing not properly (BNP) multinational study. Circulation 2002;106: 416-22.
153. McLaurin MD, Apple FS, Voss EM, Herzog CA, Sharkey SW. Cardiac troponin I, cardiac troponin T, and creatine kinase MB in dialysis patients without ischemic heart disease: evidence of cardiac troponin T expression in skeletal muscle. Clin Chem 1997;43:976-82.
154. Meyer T, Binder L, Hruska N, Luthe H, Buchwald AB. Cardiac troponin I elevation in acute pulmonary embolism is associated with right ventricular dysfunction. J Am Coll Cardiol 2000;36:1632-6.
155. Miller R, Callas DD, Kahn SE, Ricchiuti V, Apple FS. Evidence of myocardial damage in mummified human tissue. JAMA 2000;284:831-2.
156. Mirvis DM, Goldberger AL. Electorcardiography. In: Braunwald E, ed. Heart disease: A textbook of cardiovascular medicine, 6th ed. Philadelphia: WB Saunders Co, 2001:744-61.
157. Morrison LK, Harrison A, Krishnaswamy P, Kazanegra R, Clopton P, Maisel A. Utility of a rapid B-natriuretic peptide assay in differentiating congestive heart failure from lung disease in patients presenting with dyspnea. J Am Coll Cardiol 2002;39:202-9.
158. Morrow DA, Cannon CP, Rifai N, Frey MJ, Vicari R, Lakkis N, Robertson DH, et al. Ability of minor elevations of troponins I and T to predict benefit from an early invasive strategy in patients with unstable angina and non-ST elevation myocardial infarction. JAMA 2001;286:2405-12.
159. Morrow DA, de Lemos JA, Sabatine MS, Murphy SA, Demopoulos LA, DiBattiste PM, et al. Evaluation of B-type natriuretic peptide for risk assessment in unstable angina/non-ST-elevation myocardial infarction: B-type natriuretic peptide and prognosis in TACTICS-TIMI 18. Journal of the Am Coll Cardiol 2003;41:1264-72.
160. Mueller C, Scholer A, Laule-Kilian K, Martina B, Schindler C, Buser P, et al. Use of B-type natriuretic peptide in and management of acute dyspnea. N Engl J Med 2004;350:647-54.
161. Mundy BJ, McCord J, Nowak RM. B-type natriuretic peptide levels are inversely related to body mass index in patients with heart failure. J Am Coll Cardiol 2003;41;suppl A:158A.
162. Murakami MM, Chung AY, Kogut ME, Apple FS. Cost effective implementation of the Stratus CS point of care cardiac troponin I testing in coronary care units. Clin Chem 2004;50:A21.
163. Murakami MM, Doyle PJ, Quist HE, Otto AP, Pearce LA, Herzog CA, et al. Risk assessment in end stage renal disease patients using cardiac troponin T and I, proBNP, and hsCRP measurements. Clin Chem 2003;49:A66 (abstract).
164. Naghavi M, Libby P, Falk E, Casscells SW, Litovsky S, Rumberger J, et al. From vulnerable plaque to vulnerable patient: a call for new definitions and risk assessment strategies: Part I. Circulation 2003;108:1664-72.
165. Naghavi M, Libby P, Falk E, Casscells SW, Litovsky S, Rumberger J, et al. From vulnerable plaque to vulnerable patient: a call for new definitions and risk assessment strategies: Part II. Circulation 2003;108:1772-8.
166. Nakamura M, Tanaka F, Yonezawa S, Satou K, Nagano M, Hiramori K. The limited value of plasma B-type natriuretic peptide for screening for left ventricular hypertrophy among hypertensive patients. Am J Hypertens 2003;16:1025-9.
167. Newby LK, Alpert JS, Ohman EM, Thygesen K, Califf RM. Changing the diagnosis of acute myocardial infarction: implications for practice and clinical investigations. Am Heart J 2002;144;957-80.
168. Newby LK, Storrow AB, Gibler WB, Garvey JL, Tucker JF, Kaplan AL, et al. Bedside multimarker testing for risk stratification in chest pain units: the chest pain evaluation by creatine kinase-MB, myoglobin, and troponin I (CHECKMATE) study. Circulation 2001;103:1832-7.
169. Ng LL, Loke I, O'Brien RJ, Squire IB, Davies JE. Plasma urotensin in human systolic heart failure. Circulation 2002;106:2877-80.
170. Nielsen OW, McDonagh TA, Robb SD, Dargie HJ.Retrospective analysis of the cost-effectiveness of using plasma brain natriuretic peptide in screening for left ventricular systolic dysfunction in the general population. J Am Coll Cardiol 2003;41:113-20.
171. Novis DA, Jones BA, Dale JC, Walsh MK; College of American Pathologists. Biochemical markers of myocardial injury test turnaround time: a College of American Pathologists Q-probe study. Arch Path Lab Med 2004;128:158-64.
172. Omland T, Persson A, Ng L, O'Brien R, Karlsson T, Herlitz J, et al. N-terminal pro-B-type natriuretic peptide and long term mortality in acute coronary syndromes. Circulation 2002;106:2913-8.
173. Omland T, Aakvaag A, Bonarjee VV, Caidahl K, Lie RT, Nilsen DW, et al. Plasma brain natriuretic peptide as an indicator of left ventricular systolic function and long term survival after acute myocardial infarction. Circulation 1996;93:1963-9.
173A. Omland T, Richards AM, Wergeland R, Vik-Mo H. B-type natriuretic peptide and long-term survival in

patients with stable coronary artery disease. Am J Card 2005;95:24-8.
174. Ooi DS, Isotalo PA, Veinot JP. Correlation of antemortem serum creatine kinase, creatine kinase-MB, troponin I, and troponin T with cardiac pathology. Clin Chem 2000;46:338-44.
175. Ottani F, Galvani M, Nicolini FA, Ferrini D, Pozzati A, Di Pasquale G, et al. Elevated cardiac troponin levels predict the risk of adverse outcome in patients with acute coronary syndromes. Am Heart J 2000;140:917-27.
176. Panteghini M, Gerhardt W, Apple FS, Dati F, Ravkilde J, Wu AH. Quality specifications for cardiac troponin assays. Clin Chem Lab Med 2001;39:174-8.
177. Panteghini M, Linsinger T, Wu AHB, Dati F, Apple FS,Christenson RH, et al. Standardization of immunoassays for measurement of myoglobin in serum. Phase I: Evaluation of candidate secondary reference materials. Clin Chim Acta 2004;341:65-72.
178. Panteghini M, Pagani F, Yeo KT, Apple FS, Christenson RH, Dati F, et al. Evaluation of the imprecision at low range concentrations of the assays for cardiac troponin determination. Clin Chem 2004;50:327-32.
179. Pearson TA, Mensah GA, Alexander RW, Anderson JL, Cannon RO 3rd, Criqui M. et al. Markers of inflammation and cardiovascular disease: application to clinical and public health practice: a statement for healthcare professionals from the centers for disease control and prevention and the American Heart Association. Circulation 2003;107:499-511.
180. Perryman MB, Knell JD, Roberts R. Carboxypeptidase-catalyzed hydrolysis of C-terminal lysine: Mechanism for in vivo production of multiple CK forms in plasma. Clin Chem 1985;30:662-5.
181. Perryman MB, Strauss AW, Olson J, Roberts R. In vitro translation of canine mitochondrial CK messenger RNA. Biochem Biophys Res Commun 1983;110:967-71.
182. Pruszczyk P, Kostrubiec M, Bochowicz A, Styczynski G, Szulc M, Kurzyna M, et al. N-terminal pro-brain natriuretic peptide in patients with acute pulmonary embolism. Eur Respir J 2003;22:649-53.
183. Puleo PR, Guadagno PA, Roberts R, Perryman MB. Sensitive, rapid assay of subforms of creatine kinase MB in plasma. Clin Chem 1989;35:1452-5.
184. Qin QP, Laitinen P, Majamaa-Voltti K. Release patterns of pregnancy associated plasma protein A (PAPP-A) in patients with acute coronary syndromes. Scand Cardiovas J 2002;36:358-61.
185. Redfield MM, Rodeheffer RJ, Jacobsen SJ, Mahoney DW, Bailey KR, Burnett JC Jr. Plasma brain natriuretic peptide concentration: impact of age and gender. J Am Coll Cardiol 2002;40:976-82.
186. Reimer KA, Lowe JE, Rasmussen MM, Jennings RB. The wavefront phenomenon of ischemic cell death: I. Myocardial infarct size vs duration of coronary occlusion in dogs. Circulation 1977;56:786-94.
187. Ricchiuti V, Apple FS. RNA expression of cardiac troponin T isoforms in diseased human skeletal muscle. Clin Chem 1999;45:2129-35.
188. Ricchiuti V, Voss EM, Ney A, Odland M, Anderson PA, Apple FS. Skeletal muscle expression of creatine kinase-B in end stage renal disease. Clin Proteomics 2004;1:161-7.
189. Richards AM, Doughty R, Nicholls MG, MacMahon S, Sharpe N, Murphy J, et al. Plasma N-terminal pro-brain natriuretic peptide and adrenomedullin: prognostic utility and prediction of benefit from carvedilol in chronic ischemic left ventricular dysfunction. Australia-New Zealand Heart Failure Group. J Am Coll Cardiol 2001;37:1781-7.
190. Richards AM, Nicholls MG, Espiner EA, Lainchbury JG, Troughton RW, Elliott J, et al. B-type natriuretic peptides and ejection fraction for prognosis after myocardial infarction. Circulation 2003;107:2786-92.
191. Richards AM, Nicholls MG, Lainchbury JG, Fisher S, Yandle TG. Plasma urotensin II in heart failure. Lancet 2002;360:545-6.
192. Richards AM, Nicholls MG, Yandle TG, Frampton C, Espiner EA, Turner JG, et al. Plasma N-terminal pro-brain natriuretic peptide and adrenomedullin: new neurohormonal predictors of left ventricular function and prognosis after myocardial infarction. Circulation 1998;97:1921-9.
193. Ridker PM. Clinical application of C-reactive protein for cardiovascular disease detection and prevention. Circulation 2003;107:363-9.
194. Ridker PM, Rifai N, Pfeffer MA, Sacks FM, Moye LA, Goldman S, et al. Inflammation, pravastatin, and the risk of coronary events after myocardial infarction in patients with average cholesterol levels. Cholesterol and Recurrent Events (CARE) Investigators. Circulation 1998;98:839-44.
195. Roberts R, Henry PD, Sobel BE. An improved basis for enzymatic estimation of infarct size. Circulation 1975;52:743-54.
196. Roman D, Billadello J, Gordon J, Grace A, Sobel B, Strauss A. Complete nucleotide sequence of dog heart CK mRNA. Proc Natl Acad Sci USA 1986;82:8394-9.
197. Ryan TJ, Antman EM, Brooks NH, Califf RM, Hillis LD, Hiratzka LF, et. al. 1999 update: ACC/AHA Guidelines for the management of patients with acute myocardial infarction: executive summary and recommendations: A report of the American College of Cardiology/American Heart Association task force on practice guidelines (committee on management of acute myocardial infarction). Circulation 1999;100:1016-30.
198. Sabatine MS, Morrow DA, deLemos JA, Gibson CM, Murphy SA, Rifai N, et al. Multimarker approach to risk stratification in non-ST-elevation acute coronary

syndromes: simultaneous assessment of troponin I, C-reactive protein, and B-type natriuretic peptide. Circulation 2002;105:1760-3.

199. Saggin L, Gorza L, Ausoni S, Schiaffino. Cardiac troponin T in developing, regenerating, and denervated rat skeletal muscle. Development 1990;110:547-54.
200. Servoss SJ, Januzzi JL, Muller JE. Triggers of acute coronary syndromes. Prog Cardiovas Dis 2002;44:369-80.
201. Sharkey SW, Elsperger KJ, Murakami M, Apple FS. Canine myocardial CK isoenzyme response to coronary artery occlusion. Am J Physiol 1989;256:H508-H514.
202. Sharkey SW, Murakami MA, Smith SA, Apple FS. Canine myocardial creatine kinase isoenzymes after chronic coronary artery occlusion. Circulation 1991;84:333-40.
203. Shimizu H, Aono K, Masuta K, Asada H, Misaki A, Teraoka H. Degradation of human brain natriuretic peptide (BNP) by contact activation of blood coagulation system. Clin Chim Acta 2001;305:181-6.
204. Shimizu H, Masuta K, Asada H, Sugita K, Sairenji T. Characterization of molecular forms of probrain natriuretic peptide in human plasma. Clin Chim Acta 2003;334:233-9.
205. Siegel RJ, Said JW, Shell WE, Corson G, Fishbein MC. Identification and localization of creatine kinase B and M in normal, ischemic and necrotic myocardium: an immunohistochemical study. J Mol Coll Cardiol 1984;16:95-103.
206. Silva DP Jr, Landt Y, Porter SE, Ladenson JH. Development and application of monoclonal antibodies to human cardiac myoglobin in a rapid fluorescence immunoassay. Clin Chem 1991;37:1356-64.
207. Singa MK, Roy D, Gaze DC. Role of "ischemia modified albumin," a new biochemical marker of myocardial ischemia, in the early diagnosis of acute coronary artery syndromes. Emerg Med J 2004;21: 29-34.
208. Smith SC, Ladenson JH, Mason JW, Jaffe AS. Elevations of cardiac troponin I associated with myocarditis. Circulation 1997;95:163-8.
209. Sobel BE. Increased plasminogen activator inhibitor-1 and vasculopathy. A reconcilable paradox. Circulation 1999;99:2496-8.
210. Stein BC, Levin RI. Natriuretic peptides: physiology, therapeutic potential and risk stratification in ischemic heart disease. Am Heart J 1998;135:914-23.
211. Stelow EB, Johari VP, Smith SA, Crosson JT, Apple FS. Propofol-associated rhabdomyolysis with cardiac involvement in adults: chemical and anatomic findings. Clin Chem 2000:46:577-81.
212. Tanaka H, Abe S, Yamashita T, Arima S, Saigo M, Nakao S, et al. Serum levels of cardiac troponin I and troponin T in estimating myocardial infarct size soon after reperfusion. Cor Art Dis 1997;8:433-9.
213. Tsimikas S, Bergmark C, Beyer RW, Patel R, Pattison J, Miller E, et al. Temporal increases in plasma markers of oxidized low-density lipoprotein strongly reflect the presence of acute coronary syndromes. J Am Coll Cardiol 2003;41:360-70.
214. Tsutamoto T, Wada A, Maeda K, Mabuchi N, Hayashi M, Tsutsui T, et al. Effect of spironolactone on plasma brain natriuretic peptide and left ventricular remodeling in patients with congestive heart failure. J Am Coll Cardiol 2001;37:1228-33.
215. Tucker JF, Collins RA, Anderson AJ, Hauser J, Kalas J, Apple FS. Early diagnostic efficiency of cardiac troponin I and cardiac troponin T for acute myocardial infarction. Acad Emerg Med 1997;4:13-21.
216. Vaananen HK, Syrjala H, Rahkila P, Vuori J, Melamies LM, Myllyla V, et al. Serum carbonic anhydrase III and myoglobin concentrations in acute myocardial infarction. Clin Chem 1990;36:635-8.
217. Vaidya H. Myoglobin. Lab Med 1992;23:306-10.
218. Varo N, de Lemos JA, Libby P, Morrow DA, Murphy SA, Nuzzo R, et al. Soluble CD40L: risk prediction after acute coronary syndromes. Circulation 2003;108:1049-52.
219. Vasan RS, Benjamin EJ, Larson MG, Leip EP, Wang TJ, Wilson PW, et al. Plasma natriuretic peptides for community screening for left ventricular hypertrophy and systolic dysfunction: the Framingham heart study. JAMA 2002;288:1252-9.
220. Venge P, Lagerqvist B, Diderholm E, Lindahl B, Wallentin L. Clinical performance of three cardiac troponin assays in patients with unstable coronary artery disease (a FRISC II substudy). Am J Cardiol 2002;89:1035-41.
221. ver Elst KM, Spapen HD, Nguyen DN, Garbar C, Huyghens LP, Gorus FK. Cardiac troponins I and T are biological markers of left ventricular dysfunction in septic shock. Clin Chem 2000;46:650-7.
222. Wang TJ, Larson MG, Levy D, Benjamin EJ, Leip EP, Omland T, et al. Plasma natriuretic peptide levels and the risk of cardiovascular events and death. N Engl J Med 2004;350:655-63.
223. Weisfeldt ML. Reperfusion and reperfusion injury. Clin Res 1987;35:13-22.
224. Wevers RA, Olthuis HP, Van Niel JC, Van Wilgenburg MG, Soons JB. A study on the dimeric structure of CK (EC 2.7.3.2). Clin Chim Acta 1977;75:377-82.
225. White HD. Things ain't what they used to be: impact of a new definition for myocardial infarction. Am Heart J 2002;144:933-7.
226. Wieczorek SJ, Wu AH, Christenson R, Krishnaswamy P, Gottlieb S, Rosano T, et al. A rapid natriuretic peptide assay accurately diagnoses left ventricular dysfunction and heart failure: a multicenter evaluation. Am Heart J 2002;144:834-9.
227. Wolf PL. LD isoenzymes in myocardial disease. Clin Lab Med 1989;9:655-65.

228. Wong ET, Cobb C, Umehara MK, Wolff GA, Haywood LJ, Greenberg T. Heterogeneity of serum creatine kinase activity among racial and gender groups of the population. Am J Clin Path 1983;79:582-6.
229. Wu AHB, Feng YJ, Moore R, Apple FS, McPherson PH, Buechler KF, et al. Characterization of cardiac troponin subunit release into serum after acute myocardial infarction and comparison of assays for troponin T and I. Clin Chem 1998;44:1198-208.
230. Wu AHB, Smith A, Apple FS. Optimum blood collection intervals for B-type natriuretic peptide testing in heart failure patients. Am J Cardiol 2004;93:1562-3.
231. Wu AHB, Smith A, Wieczorek S, Mather JF, Duncan B, White CM, et al. Biologic variation for N-terminal pro and B-type natriuretic peptides and implications for therapeutic monitoring of patients with congestive heart failure. Am J Cardiol 2003;92:628-31.
232. Wu AHB, ed. Cardiac markers: Pathology and laboratory medicine. 2nd ed., Totowa NJ: Humana Press, 2003.
233. Wu AHB, Schwartz JG. Update on creatine kinase isoenzyme assays. Diagn Clin Test 1989;27:16-9.
234. Wu AHB, Valdez R Jr, Apple FS, Gornet T, Stone MA, Mayfield-Stokes S, et al. Cardiac troponin T immunoassay for diagnosis of acute myocardial infarction. Clin Chem 1994;40:900-7.
235. Yasue H, Yoshimura M, Sumida H, Kikuta K, Kugiyama K, Jougasaki M, et al. Localization and mechanism of secretion of B-type natriuretic peptide in comparison with those of A-type natriuretic peptide in normal subjects and patients with heart failure. Circulation 1994;90:195-203.
236. Yeo KT, Wu AH, Apple FS, Kroll MH, Christenson RH, Lewandrowski KB, et al. Muticenter evaluation of the Roche NT-proBNP assay and comparison to the Biosite Triage BNP assay. Clin Chim Acta 2003;338:107-15.
237. Zabel M, Hohnloser SH, Koster W, Prinz M, Kasper W, Just H, et al. Analysis of creatine kinase, CK-2, myoglobin, and troponin T time-activity curves for early assessment of coronary artery reperfusion after intravenous thrombolysis. Circulation 1993;87: 1542-50.
238. Zhang R, Brennan ML, Fu X, Aviles RJ, Pearce GL, Penn MS, et al. Association between myeloperoxidase levels and risk of coronary artery disease.[see comment]. JAMA 2001;286:2136-42.
239. Zimmerman J, Fromm R, Meyer D, Boudreaux A, Wun CC, Smalling R, et al. Diagnostic marker cooperative study for the diagnosis of myocardial infarction. Circulation 1999;99:1671-7.

CHAPTER 45

Kidney Disease*

Michael P. Delaney, B.Sc., M.D., M.R.C.P., Christopher P. Price, Ph.D., David J. Newman, Ph.D., and Edmund Lamb, Ph.D.

The kidneys play a central role in the homeostatic mechanisms of the human body, and reduced renal function strongly correlates with increasing morbidity and mortality. Biochemical investigations, both routine and specialized, are an important part of the clinician's diagnostic armamentarium, and investigations from the nephrology wards and clinics constitute a significant element of the workload of most laboratories. The aim of this chapter is to ensure that the clinical chemist/biochemist understands the perspective of the nephrologist when dealing with laboratory investigations for patients with kidney disease. The basic anatomy and physiology of the kidneys are described as a foundation to understanding the pathophysiology of disease and the rationale for diagnostic and management strategies in kidney disease. The key analytical methods employed during the investigation of kidney disease are dealt with in Chapter 24.

ANATOMY

The kidneys form a paired organ system located in the retroperitoneal space. They extend from the level of the lower part of the 11th thoracic vertebra to the upper portion of the 3rd lumbar vertebra, with the right kidney situated slightly lower than the left. The adult kidney is about 12 cm long and weighs about 150 g in men and 135 g in women (Figure 45-1).[251] In the majority of cases, each kidney receives its blood supply from a single renal artery derived from the abdominal aorta, with the venous return along a renal vein that emerges into the vena cava. However, multiple renal arteries occur in anatomical dissection studies in 30% of cases and following angiography multiple renal arteries are observed in 20% to 27% of patients.[34]

The kidneys have both sympathetic and parasympathetic nerve supplies whose function appears to be predominantly associated with vasomotor activity. The renal lymphatic drainage includes fine lymphatics in the glomerulus, some in close proximity to the juxtaglomerular apparatus, which are associated with removal of material from the glomerular mesangial cells.[428]

Blood Supply

The renal artery divides into posterior and anterior elements, which then divide into interlobar, arcuate, interlobular, and ultimately into the afferent arterioles, which expand into the highly specialized capillary beds that form the glomerulus (Figure 45-2). These capillaries then rejoin to form the efferent arteriole that then forms the capillary plexuses and the elongated vessels (the *vasa recta*) that pass around the remaining parts of the nephron, the proximal and distal tubules, the loop of Henle, and the collecting duct, providing oxygen and nutrients and removing ions, molecules, and water, which are reabsorbed by the nephron. The efferent arteriole then merges with renal venules to form the renal veins, which emerge into the inferior vena cava.[251] The complex architecture of the intrarenal vascular tree is ordered in three dimensions in a characteristic arrangement that probably serves to distribute the blood pressure and flow appropriately to the glomeruli.

In adults, the kidneys receive approximately 25% of the cardiac output, about 90% of which supplies the renal

*This chapter is dedicated to the memory of our friend and colleague Dr. David Newman, who died during its preparation. We are grateful for data supplied by the United States Renal Data System (USRDS). The interpretation and reporting of these data are the responsibility of the authors and in no way should be seen as an official policy or interpretation of the U.S. government. We are also grateful for data supplied by the UK Renal Registry. The interpretation and reporting of these data are the responsibility of the authors and in no way should be seen as an official policy or interpretation of the UK Renal Registry.

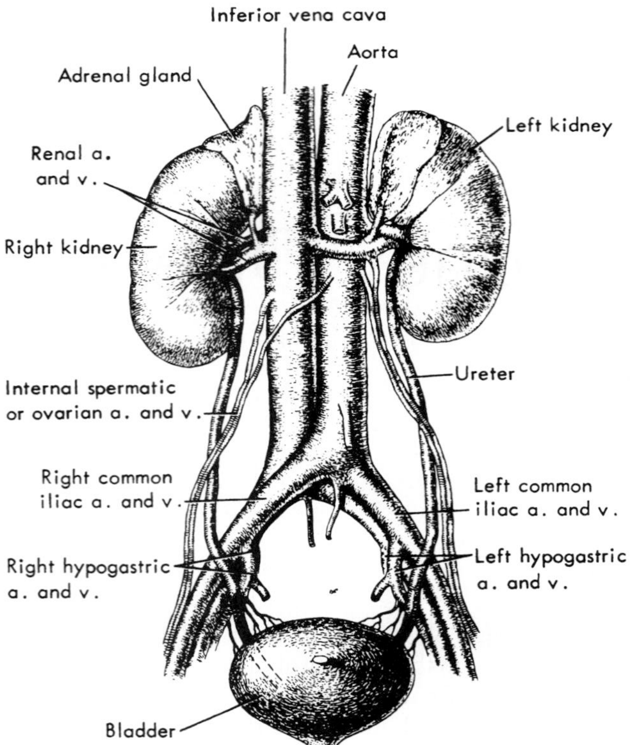

Figure 45-1 The vascular and anatomical relationships of the kidneys in man. *(From Leaf A, Cotran RS. Renal pathophysiology. 3rd ed. Oxford: Oxford University Press, 1985. Reproduced by permission of Oxford University Press.)*

cortex, maintaining the highly active tubular cells.[383] The maintenance of renal blood flow is essential to kidney function, and there is a complex array of intrarenal regulatory mechanisms that ensure that it is maintained across a wide range of systemic blood pressures (see discussion later in this chapter).[383] The renal glomerular perfusion pressure is independent of the systemic pressure between 90 and 200 mm Hg, being maintained at a constant 45 mm Hg. Renal blood flow is now rarely measured in clinical practice. Details of some of the approaches adopted for the measurement of renal blood flow may be found in the 3rd edition of this textbook.

Nephron

The functional unit of the kidney is the *nephron.* Each kidney has been reported to contain between 1 and 1.5 million nephrons, although a 1992 estimate suggests a slightly lower range, with a mean of 600,000 nephrons.[303] The number of nephrons that an individual is born with (the "nephron dose") may determine that individual's susceptibility to renal injury.

The nephron consists of a glomerulus, proximal tubule, loop of Henle, distal tubule, and collecting duct (Figure 45-2). The collecting ducts ultimately combine to develop into the renal calyces, where the urine collects before passing along the ureter and into the bladder. The kidney is divided into several lobes. The outer, darker region of each lobe, the cortex, consists of most of the glomeruli and the proximal and distal tubules. The cortex surrounds a paler inner region, the medulla, which is further divided into a number of conical areas known as the renal pyramids, the apex of which extends toward the renal pelvis, forming papillae. Medullary rays are visible striations in the renal pyramids, which connect the kidney cortex with the medulla. They are composed of descending (straight proximal) and ascending (straight distal) thick limbs of Henle and collecting ducts and associated blood vessels (the vasa recta). The central hilus is where blood vessels, lymphatics, and the renal pelvis (containing the ureter) join the kidney.

Glomerulus

The glomerulus is formed from a specialized capillary network. Each capillary develops into approximately 40 glomerular loops around 200 μm in size and consisting of a variety of different cell types supported on a specialized basement membrane (Figure 45-3, top). There are endothelial and epithelial cells that act in concert with the specialized glomerular basement membrane to form the glomerular filtration barrier, and then there are mesangial (types I and II) cells. The *capillary endothelial* cells are about 40 nm thick and are in contact with each other, but between these cells there are many circular fenestrations (pores) with diameters of between 40 and 100 nm. The fenestrations are lined with a surface coating of negatively charged glycoprotein about 12 nm thick, but allow virtually free access of plasma to the basement membrane, which forms the only continuous barrier between the capillary blood and glomerular filtrate.

The *basement membrane* (see Figure 45-3, bottom) is approximately 300 nm thick in adult humans and consists of three distinct electron-dense layers: the *lamina rara interna,* the *lamina densa,* and the *lamina rara externa.* The lamina densa consists of a close feltwork of fine, mainly type IV, collagen fibrils (each 3 to 5 nm thick) embedded in a gel-like matrix of glycoproteins and proteoglycans. This forms the main size discriminant barrier to protein passage into the tubular lumen. The other two layers of the basement membrane are rich in negatively charged polyanionic glycoproteins, such as heparin sulfate; these form the main charge discriminant barrier to the passage of proteins.

The *epithelial cells* lining Bowman's capsule (see Figure 45-3, top) are called *podocytes* and have an unusual octopus-like structure in that they have a large number of extensions or foot processes that are embedded in the basement membrane. The foot processes from adjacent podocytes are interdigitated to form filtration slits, which are covered by a loose, highly hydrated anionic mucopolysaccharide gel that is rich in sialic acid. The resulting structure is relatively impermeable to most proteins above 60 kDa, but passage of proteins is also modulated by their charge and shape.

The final cellular components of the glomerulus are the *mesangial cells,* which are found in the central part between

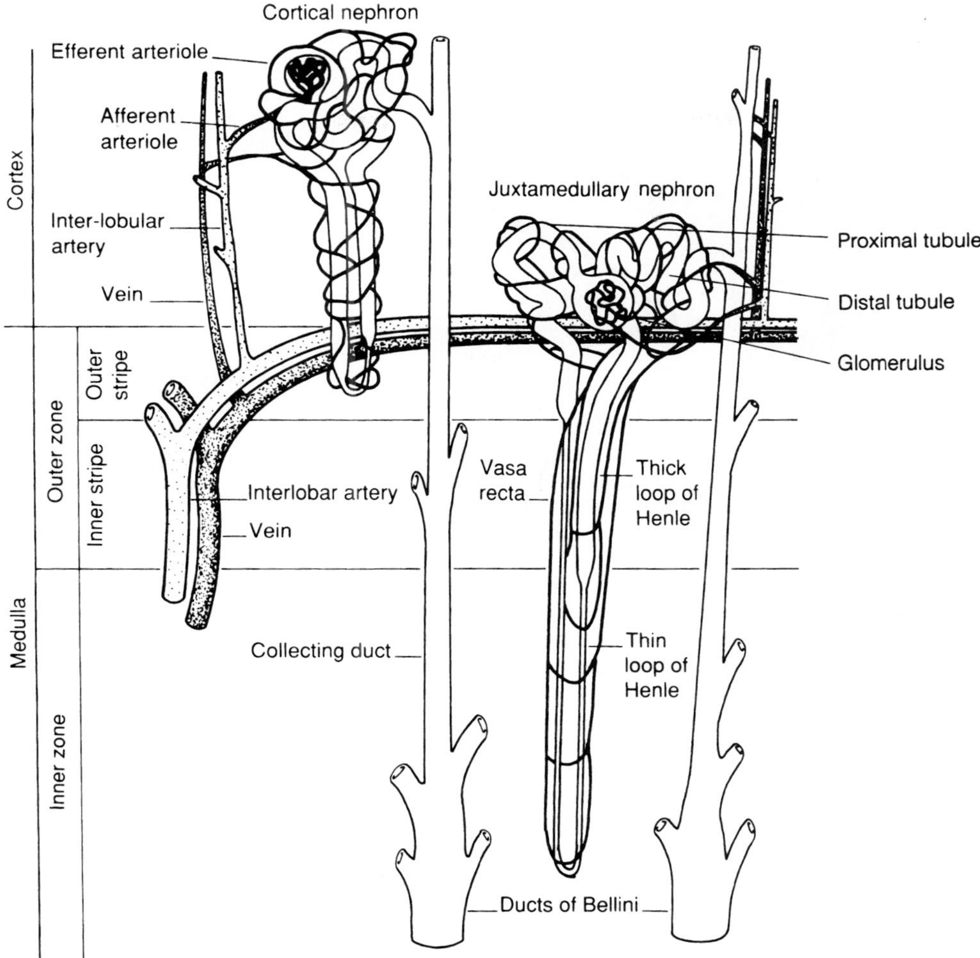

Figure 45-2 Diagrammatic representation of the nephron, the functional unit of the kidney, illustrating the anatomical and vascular arrangements. *(From Pitts RF: Physiology of the kidney and body fluids. 3rd ed. Chicago: Year Book Medical Publishers, 1974:8p.)*

and within the capillary loops suspended in a matrix that they synthesize. These cells are phagocytic and take up circulating antigen-antibody complexes that can provoke glomerulonephritis. These macromolecules are then cleared from the mesangial cells by phagocytosis and other mechanisms, such as movement by way of the glomerular stalk to the juxtaglomerular region and then via the renal lymphatics, or by regurgitation into the glomerular capillary. One view of this role of the mesangium is that it keeps the glomerular filter clear of large macromolecules, because the inner layer of the basement membrane (the lamina rara interna) is continuous with the mesangium. Mesangial cells also have characteristics of smooth muscle cells, because they are rich in myofilaments and can contract in response to a variety of stimuli (e.g., angiotensin II and arginine vasopressin). Contraction of mesangial cells can have a significant effect on the glomerular filtration rate (GFR) by reducing the available filtration surface.

Proximal Tubule

Bowman's capsule forms the beginning of the tightly coiled, proximal convoluted tubule (*pars convoluta*), which on its progress toward the renal medulla becomes straightened and is then called the *pars recta*. The human proximal tubule is about 15 mm long. The epithelial cells lining the convoluted section are cuboidal/columnar cells with a luminal brush border consisting of millions of microvilli, which enormously expand the surface area for absorption of tubular fluid. Ultrastructurally, there are three main segments, S1, S2, and S3, which consist of very different cell types (Figure 45-4). The transition from S1 to S2 is gradual and occurs in the latter part of the convoluted section. The S2 to S3 transition occurs deep within the medullary rays. The different segments are distinguished by different types of brush border, density of mitochondria, and degree of cellular interdigitation. There are also functional differences, as demonstrated by the region-specific nephrotoxicity of

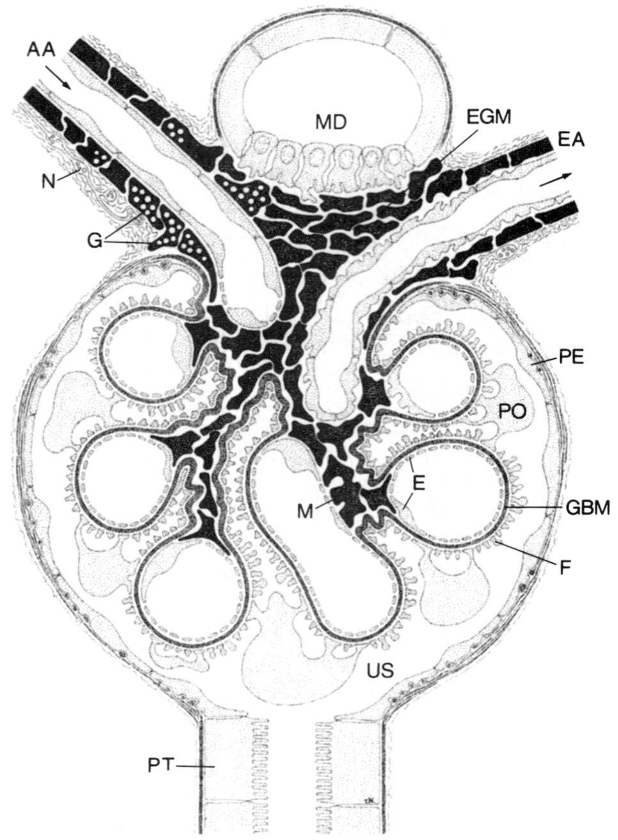

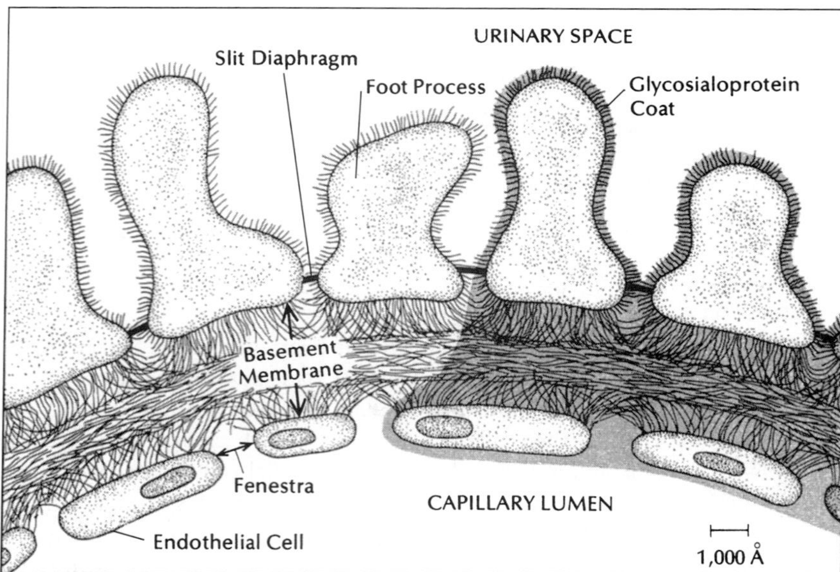

Figure 45-3 The glomerular cells and the glomerular filtration barrier. *Top,* Longitudinal section through a glomerulus and its juxtaglomerular apparatus. The capillary tuft consists of a network of specialized capillaries, which are outlined by a fenestrated endothelium (E). At the vascular pole the afferent arteriole (AA) enters, branching into capillaries immediately after its entrance; the efferent arteriole (EA) is established inside the tuft and passes through the glomerular stalk before leaving at the vascular pole. The capillary network and the mesangium are enclosed in a common compartment bounded by the glomerular basement membrane (GBM). Note that there is no basement membrane at the interface between the capillary endothelium and the mesangium. The glomerular visceral epithelium consists of highly branched podocytes (PO), which, in a typical interdigitating pattern, cover the outer aspect of the GBM. At the vascular pole, the visceral epithelium and the GBM are reflected into the parietal epithelium (PE) of Bowman's capsule, which passes over into the epithelium of the proximal tubule (PT) at the urinary pole. At the vascular pole the glomerular mesangium is continuous with the extraglomerular mesangium (EGM), which consists of extraglomerular mesangial cells and an extraglomerular mesangial matrix. The EGM and the granular cells (G) of the afferent arteriole, along with the macula densa (MD), establish the juxtaglomerular apparatus. All cells that are suggested to be of smooth-muscle origin are shown in black. *US,* Urinary space; *F,* foot processes; *N,* sympathetic nerve terminals; *M,* messenger cells. *(From Elger M, Kriz W. The renal glomerulus—the structural basis of ultrafiltration. In: Cameron JS, Davison AM, Grunfeld JP, Kerr D, Ritz E, eds. Oxford Textbook of Clinical Nephrology (vol. 1). 2nd ed. Oxford: Oxford University Press, 1998: Chapter 3.1. Reproduced by permission of Oxford University Press.) Bottom,* Glomerular capillary wall. In glomerular filtration, filtered fluid is believed to traverse the capillary wall via an extracellular route, that is, through endothelial fenestrae, basement membrane, and slit diaphragms. Circulating polyanions (e.g., albumin) are thought to be retarded by the rich distribution in inner barriers of negatively charged sialylated glycoproteins (*shaded area* in schematic diagram). *(From Brenner BM, Beeuwkes R, III. The kidney in health and disease: III. The renal circulations. Hospital Practice 1978;13:35-46.)*

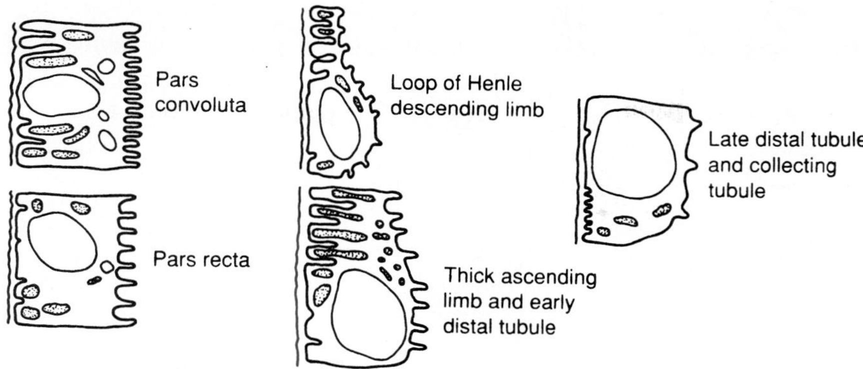

Figure 45-4 Microstructure of the proximal tubule showing the morphology of cells in the various nephron segments. In the diagram, for each cell the tubule is on the right. The cell membrane on this side is the apical, mucosal, or luminal membrane. The cell membrane on the opposite side of the cell, resting on the basement membrane (basal lamina), is the basal, serosal, or peritubular membrane. In the pars convoluta of the proximal tubule, the cells have a dense brush border (microvilli), increasing the luminal membrane surface area by a factor of about 40. Basolaterally, these cells interdigitate with each other extensively. In the pars recta, there are fewer mitochondria (suggesting that the transport functions of these cells are less well developed than those of the pars convoluta cells). The brush border is also less extensive. The cells of the descending limb of the loop of Henle are rather flat and have few interdigitations and sparse microvilli. In the thin ascending limb of the loop of Henle (not illustrated), the cells have a similar flattened appearance, but have dense interdigitations with each other. Generally the transition from the descending type of epithelium to the ascending type occurs just before the bend. The transition from the thin ascending limb to the thick ascending limb occurs abruptly at the junction of the inner and outer zones of the medulla. In most species, there are only minor differences between cells of the thick ascending limb and those of the early distal tubule. The late distal tubule and collecting tubule have a number of cell types, but the transport functions are essentially similar in both of these anatomical segments. *(From Lote CJ. Principles of renal physiology. 4th ed. London: Kluwer Academic Publishers, Chapter 2, 2000.)*

certain drugs or metals (e.g., mercury is an S3-segment–specific toxin).

The proximal tubule is the most metabolically active part of the nephron, facilitating the reabsorption of 60% to 80% of the glomerular filtrate volume—including 70% of the filtered load of sodium and chloride, most of the potassium, glucose, bicarbonate, phosphate, and sulfate—and secreting 90% of the hydrogen ion excreted by the kidney (Table 45-1).

Loop of Henle

The pars recta drains into the descending thin loop of Henle, which after passing through a hairpin loop becomes first the ascending thin limb and then the thick ascending loop. In short-looped nephrons, where there are no ascending thin limbs, the loops of Henle are situated deep in the renal medulla. The cells of the ascending thin limb are very similar to those in the descending (with little brush border, flattened and interdigitated), but there are important differences in their permeability to water and in their capability for active transport. The thick ascending limb is lined with cuboidal/columnar cells similar in size to those in the proximal tubule, but they do not possess a brush border. At the end of the thick ascending limb, near where it reenters the cortex and closely associated with the glomerulus and the efferent arteriole, there is a cluster of cells known as the *macula densa* (Figure 45-5, see discussion later in this chapter). The main role of the loop of Henle is to provide the ability to generate a concentrated urine, hypertonic with respect to plasma and with a capability that has only been demonstrated for mammalian and avian kidneys; there are several other functions (see Table 45-1).

Distal Tubule

The cells forming the distal tubule of the nephron start at the macula densa and extend to the first fusion with other tubules to form the collecting ducts. However, they have been shown to consist of three morphologically and functionally distinct segments. The first two contain similar cell types, with infoldings of the basal lamina surrounding the mitochondria. The third segment contains cells known as principal cells that have smaller infoldings and contain fewer mitochondria. All three segments have Na^+, K^+-ATPase activity. Interspersed between them are the intercalated cells, which have cytoplasmic extensions and high carbonic anhydrase activity but no Na^+, K^+-ATPase activity. Sodium

TABLE 45-1 Metabolic Functions of the Different Parts of the Nephron

	Proximal		Loop of Henle		Distal Tubule		Collecting Duct	
Molecule	**R**	**S**	**R**	**S**	**R**	**S**	**R**	**S**
Urea	+			(+)			+	
Proteins	+							
Peptides	+							
Phosphate	+							
Sulfate	+							
Organic anions			+					
Urate	+	+						
Sodium	+		+		+		+	
Chloride	+		+		+		+	
Water	+		+				+	
Potassium	+		+	(+)		+	+	
Hydrogen ion		+		+		+	+	+
Bicarbonate	+		+		+		+	+
Ammonium		+	+					+
Calcium	+		+		+		+	

R, Reabsorption; *S*, secretion; + indicates function; (+) indicates partial function.

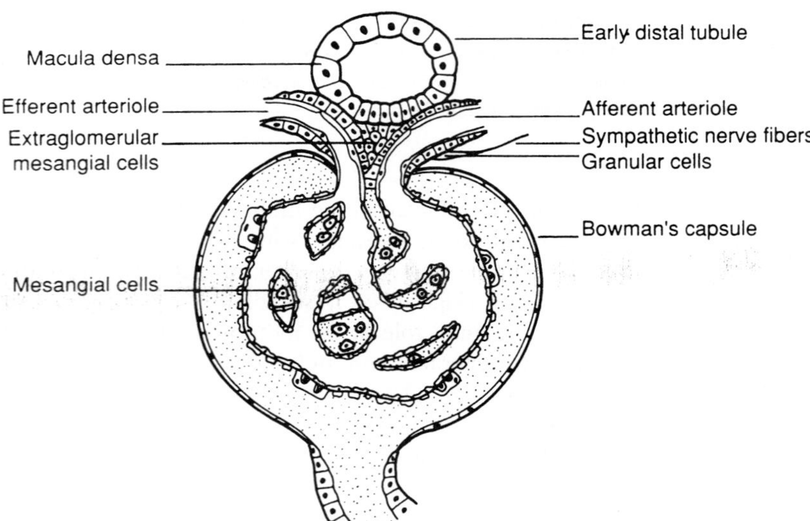

Figure 45-5 The juxtaglomerular apparatus. The beginning of the distal tubule (i.e., where the loop of Henle reenters the cortex) lies very close to the afferent and efferent arterioles, and the cells of both the afferent arteriole and the tubule show specialization. The cells of the afferent arteriole are thickened, granular (juxtaglomerular) cells and are innervated by sympathetic nerve fibers. The mesangial cells are irregularly shaped and contain filaments of contractile proteins. Identical cells are found just outside the glomerulus and are termed extraglomerular mesangial cells or Goormaghtigh cells. *(From Lote CJ. Principles of renal physiology. 4th ed. London: Kluwer Academic Publishers, 2000:Chapter 2.)*

chloride reabsorption occurs in all three; potassium secretion occurs in the first, and hydrogen ion excretion occurs in the latter two.

Collecting Duct

The collecting ducts are functionally part of the nephron, but are embryologically distinct from it and are formed from a number of distal tubules, usually about six. These are successively joined by other tubules to form ducts of Bellini, which ultimately drain into a renal calyx. The cells lining the collecting duct are cuboidal and have a less granular cytoplasm than those of the proximal tubule, although there are a number of interspersed cells with a more granular cytoplasm whose function remains uncertain.

Juxtaglomerular Apparatus

Where the ascending loop of Henle passes very close to the Bowman's capsule of its own nephron, the cells of the tubule and the afferent arteriole show regional specialization (see Figure 45-5). The tubule forms the macula densa and the arteriolar cells are filled with granules (containing renin) and are innervated with sympathetic nerve fibers. This area is called the juxtaglomerular apparatus (JGA). The JGA plays an important part in maintaining systemic blood pressure through regulation of the circulating intravascular blood volume and sodium concentration. The proteolytic enzyme renin is released primarily in response to decreased afferent arteriolar pressure and decreased intraluminal sodium delivery to the macula densa. Renin release from the macula densa is also influenced by renal cortical prostaglandins (predominantly PGI_2) and the sympathetic nervous system. The released renin then acts on the plasma protein angiotensinogen to generate angiotensin I. This is converted in the lungs by angiotensin converting enzyme (ACE) to the potent vasoconstrictor and stimulator of aldosterone release, angiotensin II (AII). The vasoconstriction and aldosterone release (with increased distal tubular sodium retention) act in concert with the other action of AII, to increase the release of antidiuretic hormone (ADH [vasopressin]) and to increase proximal tubular sodium reabsorption, intravascular volume, and pressure. AII also has an inhibitory effect on renin release as part of a negative feedback loop. Associated with the JGA are extraglomerular mesangial cells known as Goormaghtigh cells; although their function is unclear, they are thought to provide electrical coupling among themselves and to the mesangium and glomerular arterioles.[93]

Renal Interstitium

In a normal renal cortex, the interstitium is sparse (7% to 9% by volume) as the tubules lie very close together; however, a large proportion of the reabsorbed tubular fluid has to traverse a true interstitial space before entering the capillaries. The interstitium contains a variety of cells. The majority (type I) are fibroblasts, and the minority (type II) resemble lymphocytes. Subpopulations of the interstitial fibroblasts have been demonstrated using immunohistochemistry.[344]

The medullary interstitium contains a further specialized cell, the lipid-laden interstitial cells, which are arranged in a characteristic ladderlike pattern across the loops of Henle and capillaries. The extracellular space is rich in glycosaminoglycans, resulting in a gelatinous matrix that contains various poorly characterized osmolytes, osmotically active molecules that help stabilize the high osmotic gradient essential to the countercurrent mechanism involved in the generation of a hyperosmotic urine. The interstitium becomes very important in a variety of kidney diseases—and its expansion, as a consequence of, or cause of, nephron loss—plays an important part in progressive kidney disease. Interstitial expansion includes cellular infiltration and increased interstitial matrix synthesis and interstitial fibrosis.

KIDNEY FUNCTION AND PHYSIOLOGY

The major functions of the kidneys include filtration, reabsorption, and excretion. The kidneys integrate these functions to maintain homeostasis and regulate the internal milieu (Table 45-2).

TABLE 45-2 Important Components of Kidney Function

Filtration	Preparation of an Ultrafiltrate
Reabsorptive	Glucose, amino acids, electrolytes, proteins
Homeostatic	Extracellular volume, acid-base status, blood pressure, electrolytes
Metabolic	Synthetic: glutathione, glyconeogenesis, ammonia
	Catabolic: hormones, cytokines
Endocrine	Erythropoietin synthesis, activation of vitamin D

Excretory and Reabsorptive Functions

The *excretory function* of the kidneys serves to rid the body of many end products of metabolism and any excess of inorganic substances ingested in the diet. Waste products include the nonprotein nitrogenous compounds urea, creatinine, and uric acid; a number of other organic acids, including amino acids, are excreted in small quantities. Dietary intake contains a variable and usually excessive supply of sodium, potassium, chloride, calcium, phosphate, magnesium, sulfate, and bicarbonate. The efficiency of the homeostatic role in kidney function is illustrated by the way the sodium content of the body is maintained essentially constant, regardless of whether daily sodium intake is 1 or 150 mmol or more. Daily intake of water is also variable and may, on occasion, greatly exceed the minimal requirements of the body. Under such circumstances, water becomes additional waste material requiring excretion. To achieve excretion of the metabolic wastes and the ingested surpluses without disrupting homeostasis, the kidneys must exercise both their *excretory* and *reabsorptive* functions.

Mechanisms for the regulation of electrolytes, nitrogenous wastes, and organic acids are similar although not identical. For all except potassium and hydrogen ions and a few organic acids, the maximal excretory rate is limited or established by their plasma concentrations and the rate of their filtration through the glomeruli. Bulk transfer of substances from blood to glomerular filtrate determines the initial mass on which the nephron must operate to produce and excrete urine. Thus the maximal amount of substance excreted in urine does not exceed the amount transferred through the glomeruli by ultrafiltration except in the case of those substances capable of being secreted by tubular cells. Depending on the activity of the renal tubular epithelial cells and their several reabsorptive capacities, excreted amounts of urinary constituents are in general less than the amounts filtered. Because of this general behavior, for many substances a general estimate of the excretory capacity of the kidneys can be obtained by measuring either the glomerular filtration rate (GFR) or some variable that is closely related to it. The primary objective in evaluating renal excretory function is to detect quantitatively the degradation of normal capacities or the improvement of impaired ones.

Definitions

Urine is defined as a fluid excreted by the kidneys, passed through the ureters, stored in the bladder, and discharged through the urethra.[93] In health, it is sterile and clear, and has an amber color, a slightly acid pH, and a characteristic odor. In addition to dissolved compounds it contains a number of cellular fragments, complete cells, proteinaceous casts, and crystals (formed elements). Changes in these formed elements are studied using urine microscopy. Urine from a healthy individual should be clear, with a pH of about 5.0 to 6.0 and a specific gravity of about 1.024 g/mL. There is a normal turnover in tubular cells, and these are shed into the urine.

Urination, also termed *micturition,* is the discharge of urine. In normal adults adequate homeostasis is maintained with a urine output of about 500 mL/day. Alterations in urinary output are described as *anuria* (<100 mL/day), *oliguria* (<400 mL/day), or *polyuria* (>3 L/day or 50 mL/kg body weight/day).[323] The most common disorder of micturition is altered frequency, which may be associated with increased urinary volume or with partial urinary tract obstruction (e.g., in prostatic hypertrophy).

Formation of Urine—An Overview

The first step in urine formation is filtration of plasma water at the glomeruli. A net filtration pressure of about 17 mm Hg in the capillary bed of the tuft drives the filtrate through the glomerular membrane. The filtrate is called an *ultrafiltrate* because its composition is essentially the same as that of plasma, but with a notable reduction in molecules of molecular weight exceeding 15 kDa. Each nephron produces about 100 µL of ultrafiltrate per day. Overall, approximately 170 to 200 L of ultrafiltrate pass through the glomeruli in 24 hours. In the passage of ultrafiltrate through the tubules, reabsorption of solutes and water in various regions of the tubules reduces the total urine volume, which typically ranges between 0.4 and 2 L/day.

Transport of solutes and water occurs both across and between the epithelial cells that line the renal tubules. Transport is both active (energy requiring) and passive, but many of the so-called passive transport processes are dependent upon or secondary to active transport processes, particularly those involving sodium transport. All known transport processes involve receptor or mediator molecules, many of which have now been identified and characterized using molecular biological techniques. The activity of many of these molecules is regulated by phosphorylation facilitated by protein kinase C or A.[164,290] Their renal distribution has been shown to correlate with the known regional functional activities, but the same transporters, or isoforms of them,

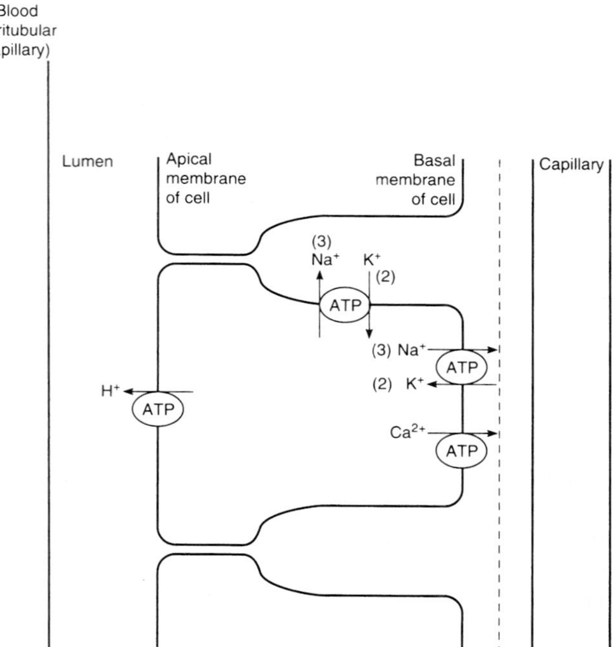

Figure 45-6 Tubular reabsorptive mechanisms: the major primary active transport processes in the proximal nephron. The renal tubular epithelium consists of a single layer of cells. At the luminal side, adjacent cells are in contact (the tight junction), whereas toward the basal side of the cells, there are gaps between adjacent cells (lateral intercellular spaces). *(From Lote CJ. Principles of renal physiology. 4th ed. London: Kluwer Academic Publishers, 2000:Chapter 4.)*

can be found in other tissues, particularly the digestive tract. There are, for instance, at least five independent proximal tubular transport processes for amino acids, including those for (1) basic amino acids plus cystine, (2) glutamic and aspartic acid, (3) neutral amino acids, (4) imino amino acids, and (5) glycine.[470] There are inherited disorders of tubular transporters, discussed later in this chapter, and a well-known generalized disorder affecting all of the transport processes, causing Fanconi syndrome.

Direct coupling of adenosine triphosphate (ATP) hydrolysis is an example of an active transport process. The most important of these in the nephron is Na^+, K^+-ATPase, which is located on the basolateral membranes of the tubuloepithelial cells (Figure 45-6). This enzymatic transporter accounts for much of renal oxygen consumption and drives more than 99% of renal sodium reabsorption. Other examples of primary active transport mechanisms are a Ca^{2+}-ATPase, an H^+-ATPase, and an H^+, K^+-ATPase. These enzymes establish ionic gradients, polarizing cell membranes and thus driving secondary transport processes.

Renal epithelial cell membranes also contain proteins that act as ion channels. For example, there is one for sodium that is closed by amiloride and modulated by hormones such as atrial natriuretic peptide (ANP). Ion channels enable much faster rates of transport than ATPases but are relatively fewer in number, approximately 100 sodium and chloride channels as against 10^7 Na^+, K^+-ATPase molecules per cell.

In the tubules, the solute composition of the ultrafiltrate is altered by the processes of reabsorption and secretion, so that the urine excreted may have a very different composition from that of the original filtrate. Different regions of the tubule have been shown to specialize in certain functions. In the proximal tubule, 60% to 80% of the ultrafiltrate is reabsorbed in an obligatory fashion, along with sodium, chloride, bicarbonate, calcium, phosphate, sulfate, and other ions. Glucose, a threshold substance,* is virtually completely reabsorbed, predominantly in the proximal tubule by a passive but sodium-dependent process that is saturated at a blood glucose concentration of about 10 mmol/L. Uric acid is also reabsorbed in the proximal tubule by a passive sodium-dependent mechanism, but there is also an active secretory mechanism. Creatinine is also secreted but only to a small extent, approximately 0.14 mmol/min. There is a well-characterized group of proton-coupled peptide transporters, some of which also transport β-lactam antibiotics, ACE inhibitors, and some of the statin group of drugs.[470]

Certain nonbiological compounds, such as phenolsulfonphthalein (PSP) and *p*-aminohippurate (PAH) are secreted by the proximal tubule and have been used for the evaluation of renal tubular secretory capacity. When blood levels of creatinine increase above normal, creatinine is secreted in this region of the nephron. In the loops of Henle, chloride and more sodium without water are reabsorbed, generating dilute urine. Water reabsorption in the more distal tubules and collecting ducts is then regulated by ADH. In the distal tubule, secretion is the prominent activity; organic ions, potassium ions, and hydrogen ions are transported from the blood in the efferent arteriole into the tubular fluid. It is also this region that secretes hydrogen ions and reabsorbs sodium and bicarbonate to aid in acid-base regulation. Paracellular (between cell) movement is driven predominantly by concentration, osmotic, or electrical gradients.

Other secretory products of the nephron are not well understood. For example, a significant proportion of normal urinary protein is formed by Tamm Horsfall glycoprotein (THG). This protein is secreted by the distal tubule and is thought to play a role in inhibiting kidney stone formation, but this has not been confirmed conclusively. The tubular epithelial cells also synthesize a vast range of growth factors and cytokines in response to a variety of stimuli that can have both autocrine and paracrine effects. All cells also secrete a range of cell adhesion molecules that are essential to cellular attachment to the tubular basement membrane.

Regulatory Function

The kidneys regulate and maintain the constant optimal chemical composition of the blood and the interstitial and intracellular fluids throughout the body. The mechanisms of differential reabsorption and secretion, located in the tubule of a nephron, are the effectors of regulation. The mechanisms operate under a complex system of control in which both extrarenal and intrarenal humoral factors participate.

Electrolyte Homeostasis

There is a complex interplay between the tubular transport systems regulating individual electrolytes. For simplicity, we have considered each electrolyte individually and have restricted our discussion to the systems of major physiological, pharmacological, and pathological significance.

Sodium

Sodium reabsorption is required for the reabsorption of water and many solutes. The proximal tubule is highly permeable to sodium, and the net flux of reabsorption from the tubular lumen is achieved against a high backflux, particularly from paracellular movement. Approximately 60% of filtered sodium is reabsorbed in the proximal tubule in an energy-dependent manner, driven by basolateral Na^+, K^+-ATPase pumps. Approximately 80% of sodium entering proximal tubular cells does so in exchange for hydrogen ion secretion, facilitated by apical sodium-hydrogen exchangers. This in turn permits bicarbonate reabsorption via carbonic anhydrases that are present in both the brush border and intracellular compartment. A variety of apical sodium co-transporters also allow for reabsorption of other organic and inorganic solutes (e.g., chloride, calcium, phosphates, bicarbonate, sulfates,[390] glucose, urea, and amino acids). Sodium transport activity is regulated by many factors, including protein kinase–dependent phosphorylation, which can increase both activity and channel numbers.

A further 30% of filtered sodium is reabsorbed in the thick ascending limb of the loop of Henle, where it is achieved by an apical, bumetanide-sensitive, 130 kDa, electroneutral, Na^+-K^+-$2Cl^-$ co-transporter (NKCC2), itself driven by a favorable inward gradient generated by the basolateral Na^+, K^+-ATPase pump (Figure 45-7). NKCC2 is a

*Certain substances, almost completely reabsorbed by the tubules when their concentrations in plasma are relatively low, appear in the urine when their plasma levels are above a certain set-point or "threshold" level. Creatinine, which is reabsorbed only minimally, is a low-threshold substance. High-threshold substances, such as glucose and amino acids (whose conservation is important to the body economy), are almost completely reabsorbed by means of specific transport systems in the tubular cells. The appearance of a high-threshold substance in the urine is evidence that the filtered load of the substance is exceeding the maximal reabsorption rate of its transport system. This may occur when the filtered load is excessive owing to elevated plasma concentration or to rapid urine flow; alternatively, the defect may be in the transport system and related to chemical inhibitors, injury to tubular epithelial cells, or genetic defects in the system. The renal threshold of a filterable compound is therefore that plasma concentration of the substance at which the tubular reabsorptive rate, operating at maximum, is not sufficiently fast to remove all of the substance from the plasma ultrafiltrate so that the substance "spills" into the urine.

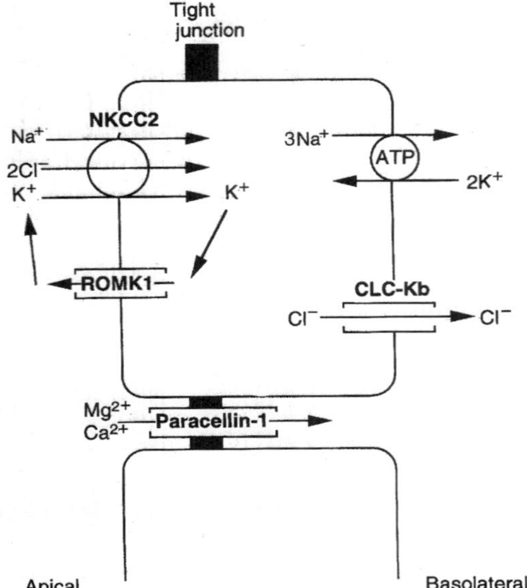

Figure 45-7 Schematic diagram showing the major pathways of solute reabsorption in the thick ascending limb of the loop of Henle. Sodium chloride is reabsorbed by the apical NKCC2 transporter. This electroneutral transport is driven by the low intracellular sodium and chloride concentrations generated by the basolateral Na^+, Ka^+-ATPase and the basolateral chloride channel CLC-Kb. The availability of potassium is rate-limiting for NKCC2, so potassium entering the cell is recycled back to the lumen via the ROMK1 potassium channel. This potassium movement is electrogenic and drives paracellular resorption of Mg^{2+} and Ca^{2+} via paracellin-1. Mutations in either NKCC2, ROMK1, or CLC-Kb cause Bartter's syndrome. Mutations in paracellin-1 lead to disruption of this paracellular pathway and the tubular disease known as hypomagnesemic hypercalciuric nephrolithiasis. *(From Sayer JA, Pearce SHS. Diagnosis and clinical biochemistry of inherited tubulopathies. Ann Clin Biochem 2001;38:459-70.)*

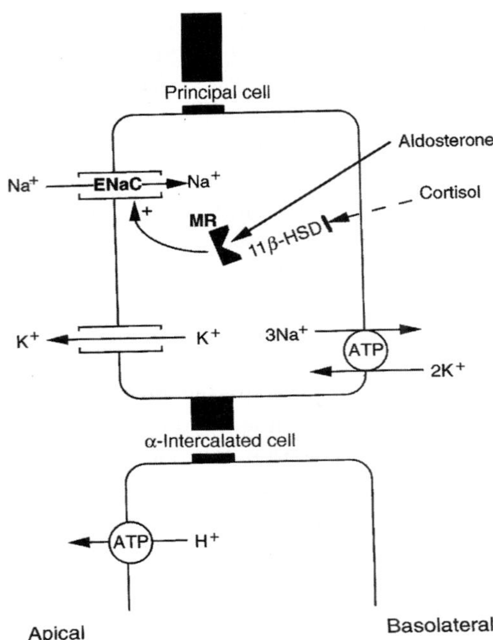

Figure 45-8 Schematic diagram showing the major pathways of solute reabsorption in the collecting duct. In principal cells, sodium reabsorption occurs through the amiloride-sensitive epithelial sodium channel (ENaC). This is influenced by the actions of aldosterone on the mineralocorticoid receptor (MR), with hyperaldosteronism producing an increase in channel activity. Cortisol, if permitted, will also bind to the MR, but a degree of specificity is maintained by 11β-hydroxysteroid dehydrogenase (11β-HSD), which inactivates cortisol to cortisone. Sodium uptake drives potassium secretion from principal cells and proton secretion from α-intercalated cells. In Liddle's syndrome, mutations lead to an increase in ENaC activity, with increased Na^+ reabsorption and consequent potassium and proton loss. In pseudohypoaldosteronism type Ia, loss of function mutations inactivates ENaC, whereas in pseudohypoaldosteronism type Ib there are MR abnormalities. Both lead to reduced sodium entry via ENaC, causing salt wasting and decreased secretion of potassium and protons. Licorice causes hypertension and a hypokalemic metabolic alkalosis by inactivating 11β-HSD, allowing cortisol to act as a mineralocorticoid. *(From Sayer JA, Pearce SHS. Diagnosis and clinical biochemistry of inherited tubulopathies. Ann Clin Biochem 2001;38:459-70.)*

kidney-specific member of a class of such channels found throughout secretory epithelia. Activation of these co-transporters appears, in part, to be a result of cell shrinkage. The distal tubule reabsorbs 5% to 8% of sodium via the thiazide-sensitive Na^+-Cl^- co-transporter (NCCT). Final sodium balance is achieved in the collecting duct via selective amiloride-sensitive, apical sodium channels (ENaCs) in exchange for potassium. ENaCs are controlled in part by the effects of aldosterone on the mineralocorticoid receptor (Figure 45-8).

Potassium

Approximately 90% of daily potassium loss occurs via renal elimination. Potassium is freely filtered across the glomerulus and normally almost completely reabsorbed in the proximal tubule. However, most regulatory mechanisms affect the loop of Henle, the distal tubule, and the collecting duct. Indeed, urinary losses can exceed filtered load, indicating the importance of distal secretion. Determinants of urinary potassium loss are dietary intake of potassium, acid-base disturbances (acidosis reduces potassium secretion and vice versa), plasma potassium concentration, circulating ADH concentration, tubular flow rate, and aldosterone secretion (enhances potassium loss and increases sodium retention).[135] Potassium ions are actively accumulated within tubular cells as a result of basolateral Na^+, K^+-ATPase activity, resulting in elevation of intracellular potassium concentration above its electrochemical equilibrium. Several types of potassium channels exist that have a range of functions: (1) maintenance of a negative resting cell membrane potential, (2) regulation of intracellular volume, (3) recycling of

K^+ across apical and basolateral membranes to supply NKCC2 and enable sodium reabsorption, and (4) K^+ secretion in the cortical collecting tubule.[25] As mentioned above, potassium is reabsorbed with sodium by the NKCC2 in the thick ascending limb of the loop of Henle, but is recycled back into the lumen by the potassium-secreting channel ROMK1. This process is electrogenic and drives paracellular reabsorption of calcium and magnesium (see Figure 45-7). ROMK1 is a pH-sensitive, membrane-spanning protein with several serine residues. At least two of these residues require phosphorylation by protein kinase A for the channel to be active.[25]

In the principal cells of the collecting duct, sodium reabsorption via ENaC is accompanied by movement of potassium into the lumen through potassium channels or a potassium chloride symporter (see Figure 45-8).

Chloride

The intracellular negative electrical potential opposes chloride entry into cells. In the early proximal tubule the main cation, sodium, is predominantly reabsorbed concomitantly with bicarbonate so that the luminal chloride concentration actually increases. There are two main reabsorption mechanisms for chloride. The first is via an antiporter in exchange for secretion of other anions (e.g., bicarbonate) or formate. The second occurs in the final two thirds of the proximal tubule. In the thick ascending limb of the loop of Henle, chloride is reabsorbed in association with sodium via NKCC2. The concentration gradient is maintained by a basolateral chloride pump, CLC-Kb (see Figure 45-7). A further chloride channel, CLC-5, is expressed at multiple sites in the nephron.[410]

Calcium

Approximately 98% of filtered calcium is reabsorbed: 65% to 75% in the proximal tubule (via a paracellular pathway), 20% to 25% in the thick ascending limb of the loop of Henle, 10% in the distal tubule, and finally small amounts in the collecting ducts.[75] This is predominantly a passive process linked to active sodium reabsorption. For example, in the thick ascending limb of the loop of Henle, paracellular calcium transport is driven by the potential difference created by ROMK1. There are also active processes, particularly in the distal tubule, that tightly regulate the final amount of calcium excreted. Here, calcium reabsorption is transcellular and is predominantly under the control of parathyroid hormone (PTH) and the calcium-sensing receptor. Following entry into the cell from the lumen via an apical epithelial active transport mechanism (ECaC1), calcium binds to calbindin-D and is delivered to the basolateral membrane. Here it is extruded by a Ca^{2+}-ATPase (PMCA1b) and a sodium-calcium exchanger (NCX1).[289] Transcription of both ECaC1 and calbindin is stimulated by calcitriol ($1,25(OH_2)D_3$), possibly synthesized locally in the distal nephron and acting in a paracrine and autocrine fashion. A functional vitamin D response element has been identified in the promoter region of the calbindin-D gene and there is a putative site in the ECaC1 gene.[289] ECaC1 is a pH-sensitive, 83 kDa protein with six transmembrane-spanning domains. Activation of the ion channel probably involves protein kinase C phosphorylation.[289] There is evidence that stimulation of the renal calcium-sensing receptor can directly affect tubular reabsorption of calcium, independent of the effects of calciotropic hormones.

Phosphate

Reabsorption of phosphate occurs predominantly in the proximal tubule and is mediated by a secondary-active transport mechanism. Three families (types I, II, and III) of sodium-dependent/phosphate co-transporters have been identified, of which the type IIa, a 640 amino acid protein located in the apical plasma membrane, is thought to be the most physiologically important. Type IIa sodium-phosphate transport is electrogenic (i.e., involves the inward flux of a positive charge), with three sodium ions and one phosphate ion (preferentially divalent) being transferred. Acute regulation of transport is primarily achieved by an alteration in the amount of type IIa protein present in the apical membrane, with longer-term changes also involving increased transcription of the protein (e.g., in response to $1,25(OH_2)D_3$). Tonic levels of type IIa in the apical membrane are thought to be high, with regulation predominantly involving internalization of the protein. Increased trafficking of the channel from the plasma membrane to the lysosomes is believed to follow both protein kinase A and C phosphorylation initiated by PTH receptor binding. Efflux of phosphate across the basolateral membrane may involve an anion exchange mechanism and/or a phosphate leak.[408]

Normally less than 20% of the filtered load of phosphate is excreted into the urine, but above a plasma phosphate concentration of approximately 1.2 mmol/L increments in urinary phosphate excretion increase linearly with the filtered load, suggesting that there is T_m (tubular maximal uptake) for phosphate.[290] Predictably the T_m for phosphate is influenced by the circulating PTH concentration and the ratio of T_m for phosphate to GFR (T_mP/GFR). T_mP/GFR has been used as a test in the differential diagnosis of hypercalcemia. Although superseded in this context by modern PTH assays, it may still be useful in the investigation of inherited disorders of tubular phosphate handling.[320]

Bicarbonate and Hydrogen Ion

The kidney plays a central role in the maintenance of acid-base homeostasis through reclamation of filtered bicarbonate and secretion of ammonium and acid. The tubular mechanisms underlying these processes are discussed in Chapter 46.

Water Homeostasis

The production of glomerular filtrate normally amounts to about 180 L/day. The unique physiology of the kidney enables approximately 99% of this to be reabsorbed in the production of a urine with variable osmolality: between 50 and 1400 mOsmol/kg/H_2O at extremes of water intake. Plasma membranes of all mammalian cells are water permeable but to variable degrees. In the kidney, different segments of the nephron show differing permeability to water, enabling the body to both retain water and produce a urine of variable concentration. This process occurs both isosmotically, in association with electrolyte reabsorption in the proximal tubule, and differentially, in the loop of Henle, distal tubule, and collecting duct in response to the action of the nonapeptide ADH. Absorption of water depends on the driving force for water reabsorption (predominantly active sodium transport) and the osmotic equilibration of water across the tubular epithelium. The generation of concentrated urine depends upon medullary hyperosmolality, which in turn requires low water permeability in some kidney segments (ascending limb of the loop of Henle), whereas in other kidney segments there is a requirement for high water permeability. In recent years our understanding of the molecular mechanisms underlying water reabsorption has increased: differing permeability and the enaction of hormonal control appear to be largely caused by the differential expression along the nephron of a family of proteins known as the aquaporins (AQP), which act as water channels.

At least 11 different mammalian AQP have now been identified, of which seven (AQP1, -2, -3, -4, -6, -7, -8) are expressed in the kidney.[299,300] Many of these also have extrarenal expression sites (e.g., AQP1 may be important in fluid removal across the peritoneal membrane). Two asparagine-proline-alanine sequences in the molecule are thought to interact in the membrane to form a pathway for water translocation. AQP1 is found in the proximal tubule and descending thin limb of the loop of Henle and constitutes almost 3% of total membrane protein in the kidney. It appears to be constitutively expressed and is present in both the apical and basolateral plasma membranes, representing the entry and exit ports for water transport across the cell, respectively. Approximately 70% of water reabsorption occurs at this site, predominantly via a transcellular (i.e., AQP1) rather than a paracellular route. Water reabsorption in the proximal tubule passively follows sodium reabsorption, so that the fluid entering the loop of Henle is still almost isosmotic with plasma.

Urinary concentration is predominantly achieved by countercurrent multiplication in the loop of Henle (Figure 45-9).[347,367] Although the descending thin limb is very permeable to water, the ascending limb and the collecting duct are not (the collecting ducts are also poorly permeable to urea). The fluid entering the loop of Henle is isotonic to plasma but is hypotonic on leaving it. The ascending limb has active sodium reabsorption driven by Na^+, K^+-ATPase with electroneutralizing transport of chloride, a combined process that can be inhibited by the so-called loop diuretics (e.g., furosemide, see discussion later in this chapter). In this section of the nephron, sodium reabsorption is not accompanied by water, creating a hypertonic medullary interstitium and facilitating water reabsorption from the anatomically adjacent descending limb. The descending limb cells are permeable to sodium chloride, which is cycled from the descending limb back to the ascending limb. The continuous flow along the loop generates an osmotic gradient at the tip of the loop that can reach 1400 mOsmol/kg/H_2O. Approximately 5% of water is reabsorbed in the loop of Henle.

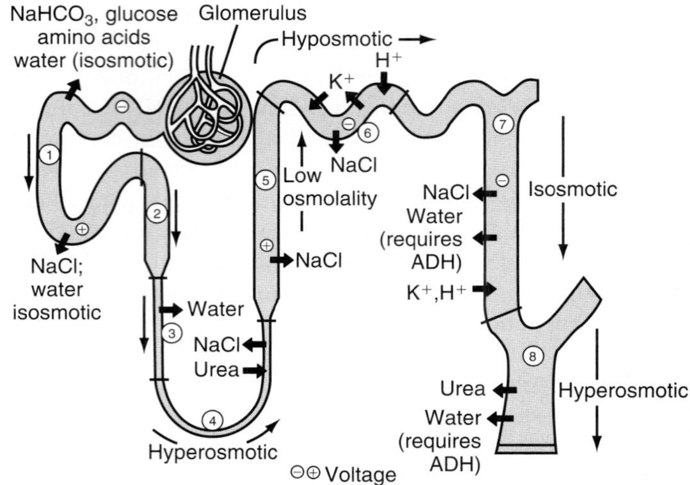

Figure 45-9 Countercurrent multiplication mechanism: schematic representation of the principal processes of transport in the nephron. In the convoluted portion of the proximal tubule *(1)*, salts and water are reabsorbed at high rates in isotonic proportions. Bulk reabsorption of most of the filtrate (65% to 70%) and virtually complete reabsorption of glucose, amino acids, and bicarbonate take place in this segment. In the pars recta *(2)*, organic acids are secreted and continuous reabsorption of sodium chloride takes place. The loop of Henle comprises three segments: the thin descending *(3)* and ascending *(4)* limbs and the thick ascending limb *(5)*. The fluid becomes hyperosmotic, because of water abstraction, as it flows toward the bend of the loop, and hyposmotic, because of sodium chloride reabsorption, as it flows toward the distal convoluted tubule *(6)*. Active sodium reabsorption occurs in the distal convoluted tubule and in the cortical collecting tubule *(7)*. This latter segment is water-impermeable in the absence of ADH, and the reabsorption of sodium in this segment is increased by aldosterone. The collecting duct *(8)* allows equilibration of water with the hyperosmotic interstitium when ADH is present. For further details, see text. *(From Burg MB: The nephron in transport of sodium, amino acids, and glucose. Hospital Practice 1978;13:100. Adapted from a drawing by A. Iselin.)*

A further 10% of water reabsorption occurs in the distal tubule, with the remainder (more than 20 L/day) being reabsorbed in the collecting ducts. Entry of water into the collecting duct cells occurs via apical AQP2 channels, with exit probably occurring via basolateral AQP3 (cortical and outer medullary collecting ducts) and AQP4 (inner medullary collecting ducts). AQP2 appears to be the primary target for ADH regulation of water reabsorption. AQP2 is stored in subapical vesicles in the collecting duct cells. In response to

ADH stimulation these vesicles are cycled through, and inserted into, the plasma membrane by a cytoskeletal, dynein-mediated, transport process. ADH stimulation occurs following binding of ADH to a V_2 receptor in the plasma membrane, which stimulates a cAMP/protein kinase A cascade resulting in phosphorylation and activation of AQP2. ADH regulates the acute cellular water-retaining response (AQP2 trafficking) and also its longer-term regulation, via a conditioning effect on AQP2 gene transcription. It is likely that there are also ADH-independent regulatory pathways of AQP2 expression. Membrane insertion of AQP2 allows water to pass into the collecting duct cells under the influence of medullary hyperosmolality. Maintenance of medullary hyperosmolality also depends upon efficient fluid removal, which is the function of the ascending vasa recta, a specialized medullary vasculature, and the close anatomical relations of all the medullary constituents (see Figure 45-2). AQP2 expression is decreased in a variety of polyuric conditions (e.g., diabetes insipidus, lithium treatment, hypokalemia, hypercalcemia, urinary obstruction) and increased in some water-retaining states (e.g., heart failure and pregnancy).[300]

ADH also increases the permeability of collecting duct cells to urea, which is the major osmotically active component of the luminal fluid in the distal tubule. Fluid of high urea concentration therefore enters the deepest layers of the medullary interstitium, passing down its concentration gradient, contributing to medullary hyperosmolality. The regulation of ADH excretion is of vital importance to fluid homeostasis. The normal plasma osmolality is maintained very tightly between 280 and 290 mOsmol/kg/H_2O and is regulated by means of specific osmoreceptors found in the anterior hypothalamus. These receptors modulate the release of ADH and also affect thirst. ADH release may also be stimulated by hypotension, hypovolemia, and vomiting independently of osmoregulation.

ENDOCRINE FUNCTION

The *endocrine functions* of the kidneys may be regarded either as primary, because the kidneys are endocrine organs producing hormones, or as secondary, because the kidneys are a site of action for hormones produced or activated elsewhere. In addition, the kidneys are a site of degradation for hormones such as insulin and aldosterone. In their primary endocrine function, the kidneys produce erythropoietin (EPO), prostaglandins and thromboxanes, renin, and $1,25(OH_2)D_3$.

Erythropoietin

Erythropoietin is a a glycoprotein hormone secreted chiefly by the kidney in the adult and by the liver in the fetus that acts on the bone marrow cells to stimulate erythropoiesis. It is an α-globulin having a molecular weight of 38 kDa. Physiologically the kidneys sense a reduction in O_2 delivery to tissues by blood and release erythropoietin, thereby stimulating the bone marrow to make more RBCs. Conversely, with a surplus of O_2 in blood traversing the kidneys, as in some forms of polycythemia, the release of erythropoietin into blood is diminished. The use of recombinant human erythropoietin (rhEPO, Epoetin) in the management of anemia of kidney disease is discussed below.

Prostaglandins and Thromboxanes

Prostaglandins and thromboxanes are synthesized from arachidonic acid by the cyclooxygenase enzyme system (see Chapter 26 for further details). This system is present in many parts of the kidney and has an important role in regulating the physiological action of other hormones on renal vascular tone, mesangial contractility, and tubular processing of salt and water. In pathophysiological circumstances, such as acute glomerulonephritis and various forms of acute renal failure, thromboxane A_2 and various prostaglandins may have a significant role in inflammation and alteration of vascular tone. The effects of nonsteroidal antiinflammatory drugs (NSAIDs) on renal prostaglandin metabolism are considered later in this chapter. The lipoxygenase pathway, which leads to formation of leukotrienes, is also present within the kidneys, although the major source of leukotrienes in inflammatory disease of the kidneys is infiltrating white cells and macrophages.

Renin

Renin is an enzyme of the hydrolase class that catalyzes cleavage of the leucine-leucine bond in angiotensinogen to generate angiotensin I.[93] The enzyme is synthesized as inactive prorenin in the kidney and released into the blood in the active form in response to various metabolic stimuli. The importance of renin in the maintenance of systemic blood pressure was discussed previously (see Juxtaglomerular Apparatus).

$1,25(OH_2)D_3$

The kidneys are primarily responsible for producing $1,25(OH_2)D_3$ from 25-hydroxycholecalciferol as a result of the action of the enzyme 25-hydroxycholecalciferol 1α-hydroxylase found in proximal tubular epithelial cells. The regulation of this system is considered in Chapter 49. The management of renal osteodystrophy is considered later in this chapter.

GLOMERULAR FILTRATION RATE

The GFR is considered to be the most reliable measure of the functional capacity of the kidneys and is often thought of as indicative of the number of functioning nephrons. As a physiological measurement, it has proved to be the most sensitive and specific marker of changes in overall renal function. Measurement of GFR is discussed in Chapter 24.

The rate of formation of the glomerular filtrate depends upon the balance between hydrostatic and oncotic forces along the afferent arteriole and across the glomerular filter. The net pressure difference must be sufficient not only to

TABLE 45-3 Summary of Factors That Influence the Glomerular Filtration Rate (See text for explanation of terminology)

	Major Influencing Factors	Effect on GFR
K_f	Increased glomerular surface area due to relaxation of mesangial cells	Increase
	Decreased glomerular surface area due to contraction of mesangial cells	Decrease
P_{GCap}	Altered renal arterial pressure	
	Afferent dilation	Increase
	Afferent constriction	Decrease
	Efferent constriction	Increase
	Efferent dilation	Decrease
P_{BC}	Increased intratubular pressure (e.g., tubular obstruction)	Decrease
Π_{GCap}	Altered plasma oncotic pressure: increased	Decrease
	Altered renal blood flow: decreased	Decrease

drive filtration across the glomerular filtration barrier but also to drive the ultrafiltrate along the tubules against their inherent resistance to flow. In the absence of sufficient pressure the lumina of the tubules will collapse. This balance of forces can be expressed as follows:

$$\text{Rate of filtration} = K_f\,((P_{GCap} + \Pi_{BC}) - (P_{BC} + \Pi_{GCap}))$$

Where
K_f = (hydraulic permeability × surface area)
P_{GCap} = glomerular-capillary hydrostatic pressure
Π_{BC} = oncotic pressure* in Bowman's capsule
P_{BC} = hydrostatic pressure in Bowman's capsule
Π_{GCap} = oncotic pressure in the glomerular capillary

As the oncotic pressure in Bowman's capsule (Π_{BC}) can be considered to be negligible (protein concentration is usually 10 to 100 mg/L), this equation becomes:

$$\text{Rate of filtration} = K_f\,(P_{GCap} - P_{BC} - \Pi_{GCap})$$

Changes in K_f can be caused by drugs and by glomerular disease, but it is also physiologically regulated. Mesangial cell contraction is thought to be the main mechanism and causes a reduction in K_f, tending to reduce GFR. Net P_{GCap} represents a balance between renal arterial pressure and afferent and efferent arteriolar resistance. Although an increase in arterial pressure will tend to increase P_{GCap}, the magnitude of the change is modulated by differential manipulation of afferent and efferent tone, which can result in minimal change to the P_{GCap}. When the renal blood flow is low, oncotic pressure can change as the plasma passes along the renal capillaries. As filtrate is removed, the oncotic pressure rises, and by the end of the capillary the net filtration rate may become zero; thus GFR falls, and this limits the amount of filtrate that can be obtained from a given volume of plasma. The average ($P_{GCap} - P_{BC} - \Pi_{GC}$) or net filtration pressure is only about 17 mm Hg. This pressure is sufficient to drive the filtration of 180 L of fluid per day only because the K_f for glomerular capillaries is several orders of magnitude greater than for nonrenal capillaries.

**Oncotic pressure* is defined in *Dorland's Illustrated Medical Dictionary* as the "osmotic pressure due to the presence of colloids in a solution.[93]"

Regulation of GFR

The factors involved in regulation of GFR are listed in Table 45-3. Autoregulation of renal blood flow and GFR is widely thought to be explained by the *myogenic theory.* This theory is based on the principle that an increase in the wall tension of the afferent arterioles, brought about by an increase in perfusion pressure, causes automatic contraction of the arteriolar smooth muscle, thus increasing resistance and keeping the flow constant despite the increase in perfusion pressure.

The *tubuloglomerular feedback mechanism,* involving the macula densa and release of the vasodilator adenosine, must also be considered. Although not fully understood, this mechanism appears to regulate GFR, with changes in renal blood flow as a secondary consequence. For individual nephrons, there is evidence that each single nephron GFR (SNGFR) is influenced by the composition of the tubular fluid in the distal tubule, which in turn is influenced by the filtration rate. The macula densa is thought to sense either the distal tubular sodium chloride content, its osmolality, or the rate at which sodium chloride is transported. The macula densa then signals the JGA via an uncertain mechanism to cause the release of adenosine and possibly AII and prostaglandins, which in turn affect vascular tone.

The result of the combination of myogenic mechanisms and tubuloglomerular feedback is that the net filtration pressure or P_{GCap} is kept reasonably constant over a very wide range of systemic arterial pressures. It should be noted that renal blood flow and GFR change across this range of systemic pressures but to a significantly smaller extent than would be predicted if these autoregulatory mechanisms were not in place.

TABLE 45-4 Factors Altering Renal Artery Tone and Renal Blood Flow

	Effect on:		Effect on:	
Factor	**Afferent Arteriole**	**Efferent Arteriole**	**RBF**	**GFR**
Adenosine	Constriction	Dilation	N	N → NE
Angiotensin II	Constriction	Constriction	N	N
Epinephrine/norepinephrine	Constriction	Constriction	N	N → NE
Antidiuretic hormone (ADH)	Constriction	Constriction	NE	N → NE
Endothelin	Constriction	Constriction	NE	N → NE
Leukotrienes	Constriction	Constriction	NE	N → NE
Thromboxane A_2	Constriction	Constriction	NE	N → NE
Prostaglandins (PGE_2, PGI_2)	Dilation	Dilation	NE	NE
Nitric oxide	Dilation	Dilation	N	N
Atrial natriuretic factor	Dilation	Constriction	N	N → P
Dopamine	—	Dilation	N	N

NE, Negligible; *N,* negative; *P,* positive; *RBF,* renal blood flow; *GFR,* glomerular filtration rate.

Other factors influencing renal blood flow are indicated in Table 45-4. The afferent and efferent arterioles are richly supplied with renal sympathetic nerves. Epinephrine acts via α-adrenergic receptors to cause constriction of both arterioles, causing a decrease in renal blood flow.

Nitric oxide (NO) has been identified as an important vasodilator produced by vascular endothelial cells. NO is synthesized from L-arginine and oxygen by nitric oxide synthetase (NOS), of which there are three isoenzymes differentially located and regulated. Within the kidney, there are eNOS (endothelial) and iNOS (inducible) isoenzymes. Activation of NOS has been shown to occur as a result of shear stress (e.g., increased arteriolar tone). There are a variety of physiological vasoconstrictors, including acetylcholine, bradykinin, endothelin, and serotonin; a rise in intracellular ionized calcium is required for the vasoconstrictors. NO synthesis is now known to play an important role in the regulation of human vascular tone and has a crucial role in control of blood pressure and kidney function.[92,143,342] It has also been found in the macula densa and has been implicated in the regulation of renin release. However, NO has an unpaired electron, and it can be oxidized by superoxide to peroxynitrite, which is further metabolized to nitrite and nitrate anions. It has been suggested that the physiological balance between superoxide and NO is important to the regulation of vascular tone.

Age and GFR

Kidney function is not constant throughout life. In utero, urine is produced by the developing fetus from about the ninth week of gestation. Nephrogenesis is complete by approximately 35 weeks gestation, although kidney function remains immature during the first 2 years of life. The kidney of the term infant receives approximately 6% of the cardiac output, compared with 25% in adults.[134] Renal vascular resistance is relatively high and the low renal blood flow is particularly directed to the medulla and inner cortex. The gradual increase in renal blood flow that occurs with increasing age is mainly directed to the outer cortex and is mediated by local neurohormonal mechanisms.[198] The GFR at birth is approximately 30 mL/min/1.73 m^2.[70] It increases rapidly during the first weeks of life to reach approximately 70 mL/min/1.73 m^2 by age 16 days.[70] Normal adult values are achieved by age 14. Tubular functions, including salt and water conservation, are also immature at birth. Birth is associated with rapid changes in kidney function, with a switch to salt and water conservation being mediated by catecholamines, the renin-angiotensin system, vasopressin, glucocorticoids, and the thyroid hormone.[70] The immaturity of the neonatal kidney contributes to the relatively common problems of water and electrolyte disturbances in infants. These disturbances are more likely to occur in premature infants, particularly those born before 35 weeks gestation.

Aging is associated with a range of structural changes in the kidney, including decreasing weight, total renal area, cortical area, and number of glomeruli.[99] The percentage of sclerotic glomeruli increases, particularly in the cortical zone.[207] These changes are paralleled by changes in the afferent and efferent arteriolar systems, with sclerosis of the cortical systems and the formation of direct channels (shunts) between the afferent and efferent arterioles in the medulla. Aging is also associated with the development of tubulointerstitial fibrosis, loss of tubular mass, and decreasing length of the proximal tubule.

Structural change is accompanied by functional changes, which in many respects are the reverse of those seen in early life. On average, GFR declines with age by approximately 1 mL/min/1.73 m^2/yr over the age of 40[9,82,439] and the rate of decline in GFR accelerates after age 65.[360] Renal blood flow also decreases with age, while the filtration fraction (i.e., GFR/renal plasma flow)[9] and renal vascular resistance[107,108] increase. Blood flow to the renal cortex would appear to be particularly affected. The higher filtration fraction of the deeper juxtamedullary glomeruli may in part explain the increase in filtration fraction with aging: this may be an adaptive response to structural change helping to preserve kidney function in the aging individual.[244] In healthy older people, renal functional reserve including the acute renal vasodilatory response to an amino acid infusion appears to be retained.[108] Tubular function, such as the ability to concentrate urine and excrete a water and salt load, is decreased and nocturnal polyuria is common. Renal salt conservation is also impaired[99] and urinary albumin excretion increases with age.[167,195]

It is not known whether these changes are the result of a normal aging process (i.e., involutional) or the result of the interplay of pathology and age. Cumulative exposure to common causes of chronic kidney disease (CKD), such as (1) atherosclerosis, (2) hypertension, (3) heart failure, (4) diabetes,[66] (5) obstructive nephropathy, (5) infection, (6) immune insult, (7) nephrotoxins such as lead,[242] and (8) dietary protein[4,46] increases with age and it is difficult to separate these effects from those of "healthy" aging. The decline in GFR with increasing age may be largely attributable to hypertension,[245,246] atherosclerosis,[207] or heart failure.[106,120] In the absence of these or other identifiable causes of kidney disease, many older subjects have stable GFR over time.

Loss of kidney function with aging appears to be heterogeneous and is not inevitable.[107,244] Kidney function may be well preserved in healthy older people and assumptions with respect to GFR based solely on age could be erroneous. Conversely, attention to the common causes of CKD could preserve function in older people.[377] What is commonly not appreciated is that kidney failure is predominantly a disease of older people. Studies from England,[103] France,[201] and Iceland (Figure 45-10)[258] have demonstrated a near exponential rise in CKD with age. The incidence of acute renal failure (ARF) also increases with age.[213]

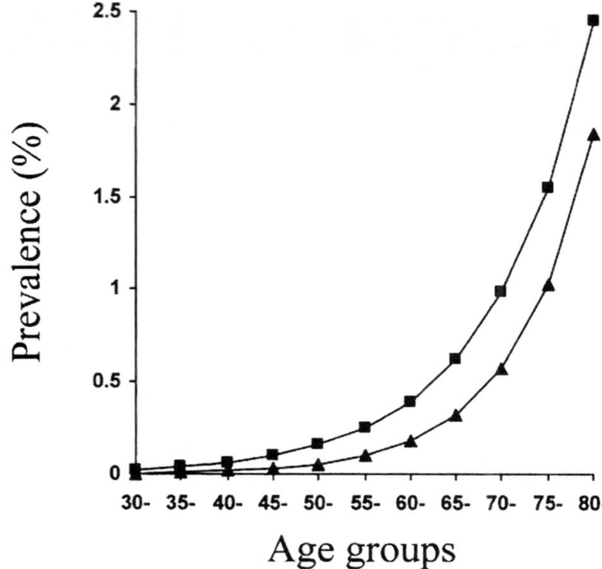

Figure 45-10 Prevalence of chronic renal failure (serum creatinine ≥150 μmol/L) in an Icelandic population according to age and sex, demonstrating the near exponential rise in prevalence with age. Curves were generated by logistic regression based on the prevalence in different age groups. Women (triangles), prevalence = $0.00016 \times 1.124^{age}$; men (squares), prevalence = $0.0016 \times 1.096^{age}$. *(Reproduced with permission from Magnason RL, Indridason OS, Sigvaldason H, Sigfusson N, Palsson R. Prevalence and progression of CRF in Iceland: a population-based study. Am J Kidney Dis 2002;40:955-63, with permission from the National Kidney Foundation.)*

Glomerular Permeability and Filtration

The glomerulus acts as a selective filter of the blood passing through its capillaries. The combination of a specialized endothelium, epithelial cell barrier, and basement membrane rich in negatively charged proteoglycans produces a filter that restricts the passage of macromolecules in a size-, charge-, and shape-dependent manner (see Figure 45-3, bottom). Various models of the basement membrane have been proposed to account for its performance; most important are the fiber-matrix and the pore theories.[36,79] It seems most likely that the fiber-matrix model is closest to reality, with fibers separated by interstices about 2 nm wide, pores not having been detected using electron microscopy. The basement membrane is a compressible filter, becoming more permeable as the applied pressure decreases and the fibers separate.[81,356]

The glomerular permeability of a molecule is expressed in terms of its glomerular sieving coefficient (GSC). Molecules smaller than approximately the molecular weight of inulin (5 kDa) are freely filtered. Therefore, inulin, urea, creatinine, glucose and electrolytes all have a GSC = 1.0. Classic experiments have used linear dextran chains of varying molecular weight and charge to study glomerular filtration characteristics. However, linear carbohydrate chains do not necessarily behave in the same manner as a globular protein of equal molecular weight or charge. For example, neutral dextran chains of 15 kDa (diameter 2.4 nm) have GSC = 1.0 whereas β_2-microglobulin (11.8 kDa, diameter 1.6 nm) has GSC = 0.7.[20] Linear molecules have higher GSC than globular proteins. Examples of the relationships between size, charge, and mass of the major urinary proteins and their glomerular handling are listed in Table 24-1.

The protein concentration in the glomerular filtrate has been measured in a number of animal models by direct glomerular puncture. The concentration of total protein found is in the range of several hundred mg/L (approximately 1% of plasma), with albumin concentrations ranging from a few hundred to less than 40 mg/L. The filtered load of protein depends on the product of the GSC and the free

TABLE 45-5 Characterization of Proteinuria

Type of Proteinuria	Causes	Examples of Proteins Seen
Glomerular	Increased glomerular permeability	Progressively increasing excretion of higher molecular weight proteins as permeability increases (e.g., albumin, IgG)
Overflow	Increased plasma concentration of relatively freely filtered protein	Bence Jones protein Lysozyme Myoglobin
Tubular	Proximal tubular damage: decreased tubular reabsorptive capacity and/or release of intracellular components (e.g., due to nephrotoxic drugs)	α_1-microglobulin β_2-microglobulin Retinol binding protein Enzymuria (e.g., *N*-acetyl-β-D-glucosaminidase, alkaline phosphatase, α-glutathione-S-transferase)
	Decreased nephron number: increased filtered load per nephron	As above
	Distal tubular damage	Tamm Horsfall glycoprotein π-glutathione-S-transferase

plasma concentration: therefore the albumin load per nephron is much greater than that of the other filtered proteins.[20,254] In general, proteins of molecular weights greater than albumin (66 kDa, diameter 3.5 nm) are retained by the healthy glomerulus and are termed high molecular weight proteins. However, lower molecular weight proteins are also retained to a significant extent.

The urinary concentration of proteins depends upon the filtered load and on the efficiency of the proximal tubular reabsorptive process. Proteins are reabsorbed by receptor-mediated, low-affinity, high-capacity processes. Megalin (600 kDa) and cubulin (460 kDa) are endocytic, multi-ligand receptors that are important in protein reabsorption.[434] Megalin belongs to the LDL-receptor family whereas cubulin is identical to the intestinal intrinsic factor-vitamin B_{12} receptor. In the kidney, both are localized in clathrin-coated pits in the apical brush border of renal proximal tubular cells and bind filtered proteins in a calcium-dependent process. Megalin appears capable of both binding and internalizing its ligands whereas the cubulin-ligand complex requires megalin to be internalized. Some proteins, such as albumin will bind to either receptor, whereas others are specific (e.g., transferrin binds to cubulin only, and retinol-binding protein (RBP) and α_1-microglobulin to megalin only). Once proteins have been internalized, they are transported by the endocytic vesicle and fuse with lysosomes. Proteolysis occurs and the resultant amino acids are released into the tubulointerstitial space across the basolateral surface of the tubular epithelial cell. The membrane vesicles are then recycled to the brush border to complete the reabsorption cycle.[272,289] In health, the reabsorptive mechanism removes 99% of the filtered protein, thus retaining most of their essential amino acid constituents for reuse.[20,144,254] Capture of filtered transport proteins is also important in conserving vitamin status (e.g., vitamin A associated with RBP). Tubular secretion of proteins also contributes to urinary total protein concentration: in particular, THG accounts for ~50% of urinary total protein. THG (200 kDa) is secreted into the tubular fluid only by the thick ascending limb and early distal convoluted tubule.[177] It is a major constituent of renal tubular casts along with albumin and traces of other proteins. The normal urinary total protein excretion is less than 150 mg/24 hours.

PROTEINURIA

The tubular reabsorptive process is saturable. Any increase in the filtered load (because of glomerular damage, increased glomerular vascular permeability [e.g., inflammatory response], or increased circulating concentration of low molecular weight proteins) or decrease in reabsorptive capacity (because of tubular damage) can result in increased urinary protein excretion (*proteinuria*). The pattern of urinary protein excretion can be used to identify the cause and to classify the proteinuria, of which there are three main types (Table 45-5).[169] Diagnostic approaches to the characterization of proteinuria are considered in Chapter 24.

Types of Proteinuria

The three main types of proteinuria are glomerular, overflow, and tubular proteinuria.

Glomerular Proteinuria

Any glomerular disease process may increase glomerular permeability as either a consequence of podocyte foot process retraction and effacement or basement membrane damage from, for example, deposition of immune complexes or increased matrix protein deposition as in diabetic nephropathy, or both.[220,309] Increased glomerular permeability increases the filtered load of all proteins, but the most characteristic feature is the increasing amounts of the higher molecular weight proteins, such as albumin excreted into the urine.[13] As permeability increases, progressively larger proteins (e.g., IgG) will be excreted in larger amounts. The relative proportion of higher to lower molecular weight proteins has been used to define selective and nonselective proteinuria (Chapter 24).

Overflow Proteinuria

The selective increase in the urinary excretion of an individual low molecular weight protein suggests that its production rate, and thus plasma concentration, has increased dramatically without concomitant glomerular or tubular damage. Examples of this are the urinary excretion of Bence Jones protein in myeloma, lysozyme in some leukemias, and myoglobin in patients with rhabdomyolysis.

Tubular Proteinuria

Tubular proteinuria occurs as a result of decreased tubular reabsorptive capacity and/or tubular damage with essentially normal glomerular permeability. Proximal tubular cells may be damaged by toxic agents (e.g., drugs and heavy metals) or by anoxia, resulting in decreased reabsorption of filtered proteins and the loss of other tubular functions (e.g., electrolyte reabsorption). Lower molecular weight proteins (e.g., RBP, α_1-microglobulin)[8] appear in relatively higher amounts in the urine than albumin, producing a so-called tubular proteinuria pattern. Albumin itself also normally undergoes extensive tubular reabsorption. Why albumin excretion is not also increased in this setting is unclear, but it has been suggested that the endocytic uptake process is mediated by receptor(s) with differing affinities for different proteins (or classes of proteins), with albumin being preferentially reabsorbed.[298] Damage to tubular epithelial cells causes not only functional disturbances but also structural change, with increased cellular turnover and cell lysis resulting in the release of both brush border (e.g., alkaline phosphatase)[302] and lysosomal enzymes (e.g., *N*-acetyl-β-D-glucosaminidase).[199] This enzymuria provides a useful means of identifying tubular damage and may give different information from that obtained by monitoring functional changes in protein reabsorption.

CKD is invariably accompanied by a decrease in the number of viable nephrons. There is a compensatory increase in glomerular filtration in the remaining glomeruli, resulting in an increased filtered load of protein per nephron. In the absence of glomerular permeability changes, this will also give a tubular protein pattern.

Leakage of various plasma proteins into the urinary space as a result of tubulointerstitial damage caused by conditions such as inflammation may also occur. This can cause hematuria and proteinuria in the absence of glomerular permeability or tubular reabsorption changes.

Investigation and Consequences of Proteinuria

Investigation for increased urinary protein excretion is mandatory in any patient with suspected kidney disease. Clinical or overt proteinuria is often detected using dipstick methods, the detection limit of which is 200 to 300 mg/L. Diagnostic approaches to the investigation of proteinuria are discussed in Chapter 24. Proteinuria above 300 mg/day is generally pathological. However, there are exceptions to this. Proteinuria can occur as a result of fever and exercise (functional) or related to posture (orthostatic).[204,265] These sporadic changes can cause interpretative difficulties when pathology is suspected. Upright posture increases protein excretion in both normal subjects and those with kidney disease. If it is postural, disappearing during recumbency and absent from early morning samples, the patient can be strongly reassured.[399] In these benign situations, the level of proteinuria rarely exceeds 1000 mg/day. Proteinuria above 1000 mg/day implies glomerular proteinuria. Glomerular proteinuria may be heavy and a mixed proteinuria with the elevation of both high and low molecular weight proteins may be observed.

It is increasingly accepted that proteinuria is not just a consequence of, but contributes directly to, progression of kidney disease. The accumulation of proteins in abnormal amounts in the tubular lumen may trigger an inflammatory reaction, which in turn may contribute to interstitial structural damage and expansion, and progression of kidney disease.* Evidence gathered from in vitro studies suggests that glomerular filtration of an abnormal amount or types of protein induces mesangial cell injury, leading to glomerulosclerosis, and that these same proteins can also have adverse effects on proximal tubular cell function.[97] Numerous studies have demonstrated that proteinuria is a potent risk marker for progression of renal disease in both nondiabetic† and diabetic[176] kidney disease. Furthermore, reducing protein excretion slows the rate of progression of proteinuric kidney disease. This has been observed in clinical trials in patients treated with angiotensin-converting enzyme (ACE) inhibitors and angiotensin II receptor blockers (ARBs), either alone or in combination.‡ These drugs reduce protein excretion by reducing intraglomerular filtration pressure and possibly by stabilizing the glomerular epithelial cell slit diaphragm proteins.[5,255] Consequently, reduction of proteinuria is an important therapeutic target.[189,209]

PATHOPHYSIOLOGY OF KIDNEY DISEASE

Despite the diverse initial causes, kidney disease that progresses to end-stage renal disease (ESRD) is a remarkably

*References 22, 33, 50, 100, 353, 373.

†References 56, 95, 190, 217, 361, 454.

‡References 19, 127, 217, 292, 317, 336, 362, 363.

monotonous process that is characterized by the relentless accumulation and deposition of extracellular matrix leading to widespread tissue fibrosis. Although correlation studies strongly suggest proteinuria to be a determinant in the progression of kidney failure, the mechanisms involved in its potential role of causing interstitial inflammation and scarring remain unresolved. Evidence gathered from in vitro studies suggests that filtration of an abnormal amount or type of protein by the damaged glomerulus may induce mesangial cell injury, leading to glomerulosclerosis, and that these same proteins can also have adverse effects on proximal tubular cell function.[97] Nephrons are lost via toxic, anoxic, or immunological injury that may initially injure the glomerulus, the tubule, or both together. Glomerular damage can involve endothelial, epithelial, or mesangial cells, and/or the basement membrane. Inflammatory stimuli are released including both cytokines and growth factors, such as transforming growth factor beta (TGF-β), interleukin-6 (IL-6), interferon-γ (INF-γ), or tissue necrosis factor-α (TNF-α); these inflammatory factors activate resident lymphocytes and macrophages and recruit additional cells from the peripheral circulation (see Chapter 22). Thus, cellular infiltration is a common but not universal finding in renal biopsy specimens. These activated cells can cause T-cell–mediated cell lysis, activation, and proliferation of interstitial fibroblasts. Fibroblast activity results in increased extracellular matrix synthesis and eventually glomerular and tubular fibrosis. The extracellular matrix expansion causes disruption of local blood flow, exaggerating regional ischemia, and a vicious cycle of inflammation, fibrosis, and cell death is propagated.

The kidneys have considerable ability to increase their functional capacity in response to injury. Thus, a significant reduction in functioning renal mass (50% to 60%) may occur before the onset of any significant symptoms or even before any major biochemical alterations appear. The most sensitive and specific measure of functional change is the GFR, which can be reduced to less than 60 mL/min/1.73 m^2 (Table 45-6) before signs and symptoms of kidney failure will be observed. This increase in workload per nephron is thought to be an important cause of progressive renal injury.[469] A well-recognized hypothesis suggests that independent of the primary renal injury, a point is reached in the decline in nephron number when further loss becomes inevitable and progressive as a consequence of a common pathway leading to interstitial fibrosis.[51,53,350] The elucidation of this common pathway is incomplete but is the focus of considerable research interest. Several animal models have been used to investigate mechanisms leading to fibrosis. It has been demonstrated that there is increased production and activity of TGF-β in glomerular disease, and this acts as a key mediator, along with angiotensin, of fibrogenesis.[40,369,464] Data support the hypothesis that during tubulointerstitial fibrosis α-smooth muscle actin-expressing mesenchymal cells might derive from the tubular epithelium via epithelial-mesenchymal transition under the influence of TGF-β.[185] Strategies to block the process of epithelial-mesenchymal transition are being explored for future therapeutic targets in CKD.[465]

Diagnosis and Screening for Kidney Disease

The patient with kidney disease generally presents to the clinician because of (1) an abnormality detected on a routine biochemical blood screen or urinalysis, (2) a symptom or physical sign, or (3) the patient has a systemic disease with a known renal involvement, such as diabetes mellitus. Effective management of the patient with kidney disease is dependent upon establishing a definitive diagnosis. Initial management includes a detailed clinical history, clinical examination, and assessment of the urinary sediment. Dipstick urinalysis allows for detection of multiple abnormalities simultaneously: clinically proteinuria and hematuria are the most important of these in suspected kidney disease. If blood cells are confirmed on repeat testing and are not associated with urine infection, then the patient should be assessed for kidney or urothelial disease. Cells may originate from the kidneys or from elsewhere in the urinary tract, including the external genitalia. Detection of urinary casts can also be performed by urine microscopy and strongly supports intrinsic renal disease. Detection of proteinuria has been discussed above. Biochemical measurements play an important role in the discovery that kidney damage has occurred and in monitoring progress and treatment. Noninvasive imaging using ultrasonography is invaluable at identifying the size and shape of the kidneys along with any evidence of obstruction. However, percutaneous kidney biopsy is routinely performed to confirm the diagnosis, guide treatment, and gain information regarding prognosis.

Classification of Kidney Failure

The terminology associated with kidney diseases has been amended and is clarified here. Previously, renal failure was divided into either *acute renal failure* (ARF) or *chronic renal failure* (CRF).[216] These terms indicate the rate at which damage occurs rather than the mechanism by which it occurs. Landmark guidelines developed in the USA by the National Kidney Foundation-Kidney Disease Outcomes Quality Initiative (NKF-K/DOQI)[295] attempt to evaluate, classify, and stratify CKD (see Table 45-6). The term "renal" has largely been replaced by "kidney" when referring to *chronic* disease since it is better understood by patients and nonspecialists. However, "acute renal failure" (ARF) remains standard nomenclature along with ESRD.

ARF is diagnosed when excretory function of the kidneys declines over hours or days. ARF is a common condition complicating 5% of hospital admissions.[172] The incidence of ARF increases with age and co-morbidity. One of the problems in identifying the true incidence and outcome of ARF is the spectrum of definitions in published studies ranging from severe (requiring dialysis) to modest increases in plasma creatinine concentrations.[172,239] In 2003, a new classification of ARF was proposed that was based on the combination of susceptibility, nature and timing of insult, biomarker response, urine output, and end-organ consequences.[278] A prospective study of the initial hospital management of ARF confirmed that in almost 40% of cases ARF was iatrogenic or preventable.[403] Intrinsic ARF can be caused by primary vascular, glomerular, or interstitial disorders. However, in the majority of cases the kidney lesion seen on histology is referred to as acute tubular necrosis (ATN). ATN is caused by ischemic or nephrotoxic injury to the kidney. In 50% of cases of hospital-acquired ARF, the cause is multifactorial. (The term "ATN" is somewhat misleading insofar as necrosis per se is seldom seen, rather tubular *damage.*)

ARF develops rapidly, and therefore its sequelae are mainly a consequence of rapid electrolyte, acid-base, and fluid imbalances that can be difficult to control. The clinical assessment of ARF should consider whether the precipitant is prerenal, intrarenal, or postrenal. The most common causes are listed in Table 45-7. ARF can arise from a variety of pathological conditions, including glomerulonephritis, interstitial nephritis,[407] and arterial, venous, or urinary tract obstruction. As indicated earlier, the most common hospital-based cause is ATN, usually as a result of severe hemodynamic disturbance or exposure to nephrotoxins. Although the pathogenesis is uncertain, there is a well-recognized clinical pattern, with anuria or oliguria and abnormalities indicating tubular dysfunction (Figure 45-11).[38] Necrosis of tubular cells need not be extensive, but there may be obstruction by tubular casts, back-leak of glomerular filtrate through gaps in the tubular epithelium caused by cellular denudation, and primary reductions in GFR caused by altered intrarenal hemodynamics, known as tubuloglomerular feedback.[232] Direct vasoconstriction of glomerular capillaries in response to ischemic insults can also occur and may be mediated by AII, endothelin,[125,451] and serotonin.[433] If the patient survives, recovery will usually occur within days or weeks following removal of the initiating event. Uncomplicated ARF has a mortality rate of 5% to 10%,[172] although ARF complicating nonrenal organ system failure in the intensive care setting is associated with mortality rates approaching 50% to 70% despite advances in dialysis treatment.[278]

The role of the clinical laboratory in the assessment and monitoring of ARF is limited to assessment of electrolyte disturbance and fluid status, as during the recovery period there is an initial polyuric phase as glomerular function recovers before tubular function recovers. This polyuric phase recedes after a few days to weeks but requires careful monitoring to enable suitable fluid and electrolyte replacement.

TABLE 45-6 Stages of Chronic Kidney Disease: Metabolic and Management Consequences

Stage	Description	GFR (mL/min/1.73 m^2)	Metabolic Consequences	Management
1	Kidney damage with normal or increased GFR	>90		Diagnosis and treatment; treatment of comorbid conditions Slowing progression CVD risk reduction
2	Mildly decreased GFR	60-89	Concentration of parathyroid hormone starts to rise (GFR 60-80)	Estimating progression
3	Moderately decreased GFR	30-59	Decrease in calcium absorption (GFR < 50); lipoprotein activity falls Malnutrition Onset of left ventricular hypertrophy Onset of anemia (erythropoietin deficiency)	Evaluating and treating complications
4	Severely reduced GFR	15-29	Triglyceride concentrations start to rise Hyperphosphatemia Metabolic acidosis Tendency to hyperkalemia	Preparation for RRT, if appropriate
5	Kidney failure	<15	Uremia/azotemia	RRT, if appropriate

Modified from National Kidney Foundation Document. Clinical practice guidelines for chronic kidney disease: evaluation, classification, and stratification. Kidney Disease Outcome Quality Initiative. Am J Kidney Dis 2002;39:S1-246.

TABLE 45-7 Causes of Acute Renal Failure

Cause	Agents
Prerenal	
Hypovolemia	Trauma, burns, surgery
Decreased effective plasma volume	Nephrotic syndrome, sepsis, shock
Decreased cardiac output	Congestive cardiac failure, pulmonary embolism
Renovascular obstruction	Atherosclerosis, stenoses
Interference with renal autoregulation	ACE inhibitors, cyclosporine
Renal	
Glomerular and small vessel disease	Aggressive glomerulonephritis (e.g., poststreptococcal, preeclampsia)
Interstitial nephritis	Infection, infiltration, drugs/toxins
Tubular lesions	Postischemic, nephrotoxins, rhabdomyolysis, Bence Jones protein, hypercalcemia
Postrenal	
Bladder outflow obstruction	Prostatism, neurogenic bladder
Ureteric obstruction	Stones, blood clots, tumors, radiotherapy, retroperitoneal fibrosis

DISEASES OF THE KIDNEY

Diseases of the kidney that are discussed in this section include (1) the uremic syndrome, (2) chronic kidney disease, (3) end-stage renal disease, (4) diabetic nephropathy, (5) hypertensive nephropathy, (6) glomerular diseases, (7) interstitial nephritis, (8) polycystic kidney disease, (9) polycystic kidney disease, (10) toxic nephropathy, (11) obstructive uropathy, (12) tubular diseases, (13) renal calculi, and (14) cystinuria. In addition, this section also includes discussions on (1) prostaglandins and NSAIDS in kidney disease, (2) monoclonal light chains and kidney disease, and (3) urinary osmolality.

THE UREMIC SYNDROME

Uremia is defined as the excess within the blood of urea, creatinine, and other nitrogenous end products of amino acid and protein metabolism that are normally excreted in the urine; it is more correctly referred to as *azotemia.*[93] The *uremic syndrome,* the terminal clinical manifestation of kidney failure, is the group of symptoms, physical signs, and abnormal findings on diagnostic studies that results from the failure of the kidneys to maintain adequate excretory, regulatory, and endocrine function. For more than 200 years, scientists have been studying the nature of uremia, but no single retained molecule has qualified for the title "uremic toxin," and many now agree that a variety of compounds are potential uremic toxins (Table 45-8). At least

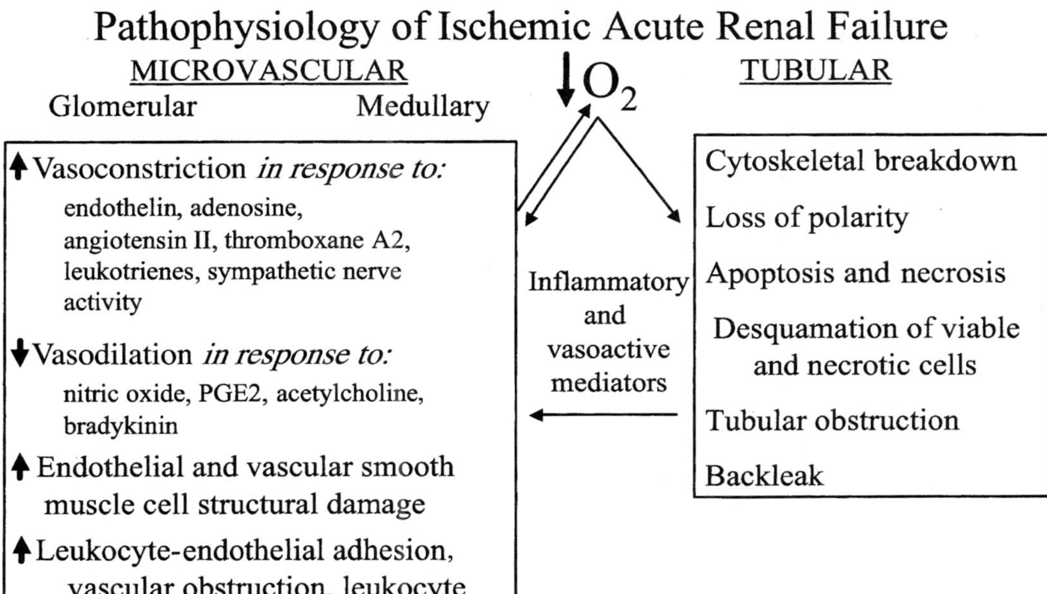

Figure 45-11 Pathogenesis of ischemic acute renal failure. Hypoxic insults cause vascular responses and tubular damage. *(From Bonventre JV, Weinberg JM. Recent advances in the pathophysiology of ischemic acute renal failure. J Am Soc Nephrol 2003;14:2199-210.)*

90 organic compounds have been retained in uremia.[11,430] Many more still unidentified solutes are possibly retained and might exert toxicity.

The classic signs of uremia include progressive weakness and easy fatigue, loss of appetite followed by nausea and vomiting, muscle wasting, tremors, abnormal mental function, frequent but shallow respirations, and metabolic acidosis. The syndrome evolves to produce stupor, coma, and ultimately death unless support is provided by dialysis or successful kidney transplantation.[341] Regulation of body fluids is impaired in patients with uremia because of failure to excrete excess ingested fluid or to cope with fluid losses caused by vomiting or diarrhea. Patients also have difficulty excreting a salt load or retaining sodium when intake is low or vascular volume inadequate. Acid excretion is impaired, as is the ability to excrete nitrogenous metabolites from dietary sources. Consequently the composition of plasma is abnormally labile in response to such factors as diet, state of hydration, gastrointestinal bleeding, vomiting, diarrhea, and intake of therapeutic drugs. In relation to the stages of kidney disease defined by NKF-K/DOQI, kidney failure is present at a level of GFR less than or equal to 15 mL/min/m^2 (Stage 5).[295] At this level there are generally signs and symptoms of uremia, or a need for renal replacement therapy (RRT).

The most characteristic laboratory findings are increased concentrations of nitrogenous compounds in plasma, such as urea nitrogen and creatinine,[325] as a result of reduced GFR and decreased tubular function. Retention of these compounds and of metabolic acids is followed by progressive hyperphosphatemia, hypocalcemia, and potentially dangerous hyperkalemia. Although most patients eventually become acidemic, respiratory compensation by elimination of carbon dioxide is extremely important. In addition, reduced endocrine function is manifested by inadequate synthesis of EPO and calcitriol, with resulting anemia and osteomalacia. Disordered regulation of blood pressure generally leads to hypertension. Biochemical characteristics of the uremic syndrome are summarized in Box 45-1.

In addition to the consequences of reduced excretory, regulatory, and endocrine function of the kidneys, the uremic syndrome has several systemic manifestations—among them pericarditis, pleuritis, disordered platelet and granulocyte function, and encephalopathy—that have been difficult to explain.

Many retained metabolites have been implicated in the systemic toxicity of the uremic syndrome. Although urea was the first of these metabolites to be identified as being increased in uremia, it does not appear to be responsible for the systemic manifestations of uremia. Urea is a 60 Da water-soluble compound that has the highest concentration of presently known uremic retention solutes in uremic plasma. Although its removal by dialysis is directly related to patient survival, the effects of urea on biological systems are not clear. Urea removal by dialysis is not necessarily representative of other molecules retained in the uremic syndrome, particularly protein bound solutes or middle molecules, such as parathyroid hormone and cystatin C.[297] Urea may be the origin of other more toxic moieties. Cyanate, produced endogenously from urea, may produce toxic effects by irreversible carbamylation of proteins.[431] Guanidine compounds, especially methylguanidine, have been implicated in toxicity of experimental renal failure, but their significance in human uremia remains to be proved. Unidentified compounds with molecular weights between 300 and 1500 Da may have a role in the pathogenesis of the clinical syndrome of uremia. However, it is more likely that the syndrome is a result of the cumulative effect of many retained compounds, which may act as toxins and may also have an effect on metabolism in general, for example through enzyme inhibition or derangement in membrane transport. The decreased ability of the kidneys to degrade or eliminate hormones may also have a role.

TABLE 45-8 Potential Uremic Toxins

Toxin	Effect
Urea	At very high concentrations (>300 mg/dL) can cause headache, vomiting, and fatigue, carbamylation of proteins
Creatinine	Possibly affects glucose tolerance and erythrocyte survival
Uric acid	Causes uremic pericarditis
Cyanate	Causes drowsiness, hyperglycemia; a breakdown product of urea, it can cause carbamylation of proteins, altering protein function
Polyols (e.g., myoinositol)	Can cause peripheral neuropathy
Phenols	Can be highly toxic as they are lipid soluble and therefore can cross cell membranes easily
Middle molecules (e.g., atrial natriuretic peptide, cystatin C, delta sleep inducing protein, IL-6, TNF-α, PTH)	CAPD patients show fewer signs of neuropathy than hemodialysis patients (many candidate molecules but none paramount)
β_2-Microglobulin	Causative agent in renal amyloid

CAPD, Continuous ambulatory peritoneal dialysis; *IL-6,* interleukin 6; *TNF-α,* tumor necrosis factor alpha; *PTH,* parathyroid hormone.

Chronic Kidney Disease

Studies established to identify the incidence, causes, and complications of CKD have largely focused on advanced disease and kidney failure. Data obtained from epidemiological surveys have been compromised by the lack of consistent surrogate markers of kidney function to identify established disease. For example, plasma creatinine, calculated creatinine clearance, and measured creatinine clearance have variously been used. The NKF-K/DOQI has published a definition of CKD in an effort to identify its early stages.[295] Early identification is essential so that adverse outcomes of CKD can be prevented or treated. CKD is defined therefore as "either kidney damage or GFR <60 mL/min/1.73 m^2 for at least 3 months." Kidney damage is defined as "pathologic abnormalities or markers of damage, including abnormalities in blood or urine tests or imaging studies."

The NKF-K/DOQI guidelines stratify CKD from stage 1 at the mild end of the spectrum to stage 5, kidney failure or GFR less than 15 mL/min/m^2. Although the cut-off levels between the stages are arbitrary, the process may allow for consistency in prevalence reporting for epidemiological studies and also focused treatment schedules for individual patients (see Table 45-6).

The incidence and major causes of CKD in the United States, United Kingdom, and Australasia have previously been identified from community-based studies and registry databases, such as the United States Renal Data System (USRDS), the United Kingdom Renal Registry Report, and the Australia and New Zealand Dialysis and Transplant Registry (ANZDATA). Similar databases are operated throughout the world. As indicated, the registry databases tend to highlight those patients that develop advanced CKD or ESRD requiring treatment with either dialysis or transplantation. The incidence of less advanced stages of CKD and those patients with ESRD that are not accepted for RRT is less clear. The prevalence of advanced CKD in the United Kingdom in the early 1990s was 132 per million population (pmp) as defined by a plasma creatinine concentration greater than 5.7 mg/dL (500 µmol/L).[212] The same study estimated that 450 pmp have a plasma creatinine greater than 3.4 mg/dL (300 µmol/L). The prevalence patterns vary around the world because of differences in (1) ethnicity, (2) incidence of diabetes and hypertension, and (3) attitudes of physicians to accept patients for treatment. The annual acceptance rate for RRT is increasing worldwide. The annual acceptance rate in the United States is 317 pmp (744 pmp in blacks)[427] and in the United Kingdom is 93 pmp.[425] The age of patients accepted for RRT is increasing, with the majority of new patients undergoing RRT within the age range of 66 to 74 years.[425]

The main causes of CKD leading to kidney failure from 1990 to 2000 in the United States are indicated in Figure 45-12. As indicated, diabetes mellitus is the largest single cause of advanced CKD and accounts for almost 45% of new dialysis patients in the United States. It is particularly prevalent among black Americans. Hypertension is the underlying diagnosis in around 25% of new dialysis patients and is also particularly prevalent among black Americans. The myriad of kidney diseases including glomerulonephritis, infections, hereditary, systemic, interstitial, obstructive, and unknown etiology account for the remainder. In the United Kingdom diabetic nephropathy as a cause of kidney failure is seen in 18% of new patients and is not increasing.[425]

Developing kidney failure is most commonly *monitored* by changes in plasma creatinine concentration and calculated estimation of GFR (see Chapter 24).[64] Obtaining a *diagnosis* relies on screening methods outlined above, and if

BOX 45-1 Biochemical Characteristics of the Uremic Syndrome

Retained Nitrogenous Metabolites
- Urea
- Cyanate
- Creatinine
- Guanidine compounds
- "Middle molecules"
- Uric acid

Fluid, Acid-Base, and Electrolyte Disturbances
- Fixed urine osmolality
- Metabolic acidosis (decreased blood pH, bicarbonate)
- Hyponatremia or hypernatremia
- Hypokalemia or hyperkalemia
- Hyperchloremia
- Hypocalcemia
- Hyperphosphatemia
- Hypermagnesemia

Carbohydrate Intolerance
- Insulin resistance (hypoglycemia may also occur)
  - Plasma insulin normal or increased
  - Delayed response to carbohydrate loading
  - Hyperglucagonemia

Abnormal Lipid Metabolism
- Hypertriglyceridemia
- Decreased high-density lipoprotein cholesterol
- Hyperlipoproteinemia

Altered Endocrine Function
- Secondary hyperparathyroidism
- Osteomalacia (secondary to abnormal vitamin D metabolism)
- Hyperreninemia and hyperaldosteronism
- Hyporeninemia
- Hypoaldosteronism
- Decreased erythropoietin production
- Altered thyroxine metabolism
- Gonadal dysfunction (increased prolactin and luteinizing hormone, decreased testosterone)

the kidney size is well maintained (>8 to 9 cm), a percutaneous renal biopsy can be obtained. This is examined using light and electron microscopy in association with immunohistochemistry and molecular biology techniques.

Establishing the differential diagnosis is important in predicting the rate of decline in kidney function and the selection of the most appropriate treatment. In some cases of aggressive glomerulonephritis, kidney failure develops over a few days or weeks, and at the other extreme diabetic nephropathy can take 10 to 15 years to reach the end stage as highlighted below. Every effort should be made to avoid an acute decline in GFR by minimizing exposure to volume depletion, intravenous radiographic contrast, selected antibacterial agents, NSAIDS and cyclo-oxygenase type 2 (COX-2) inhibitors, and urinary tract obstruction.

Management of CKD

The GFR cutoff values in the NKF-K/DOQI guidelines have been selected on limited data with respect to the relationship between complications and level of GFR. Further studies may refine these values. Nevertheless there is often a causal relationship between the burden of illness and the severity of CKD (see Table 45-6).

Rate of progression of CKD, irrespective of underlying cause, is dependent on both non-modifiable factors, such as age, sex, race, are level of kidney function at diagnosis, and modifiable characteristics, including proteinuria, blood pressure control, and smoking. The progression and treatment options for diabetic nephropathy are discussed separately below. The current discussion will focus on the optimal treatment of non-diabetic CKD.

Lowering blood pressure and reduction of proteinuria have been shown to ameliorate the progression of CKD. The Modification of Diet in Renal Disease (MDRD) Study compared the rates of decline in GFR in 840 patients with various causes of CKD to either a "usual" or "low" blood pressure goal.[217] Patients with type 1 diabetes were excluded. Outcome data suggest that the low blood pressure goal had some beneficial effect in those patients with higher levels of proteinuria.[181,217] The study supported the concept that proteinuria is an independent risk factor for progression of kidney disease. For patients with proteinuria of more than 1 g/day, the suggested target for mean blood pressure was 92 mm Hg (125/75 mm Hg).[326] This target for blood pressure is lower than the sixth report of the Joint National Committee on prevention, detection, evaluation, and treatment of high blood pressure (JNC-VI).[392] In 2002, the United Kingdom Renal Association revised the target blood pressure to 130/80 mm Hg for stable CKD and 125/75 mm Hg for progressive CKD.[422] Data from the Third National Health and Nutrition Examination Survey [NHANES III] (1988-1994) revealed that among hypertensive individuals with an elevated plasma creatinine concentration, 75% were on antihypertensive treatment and only 11% had their blood pressure reduced to lower than 130/85 mm Hg.[74]

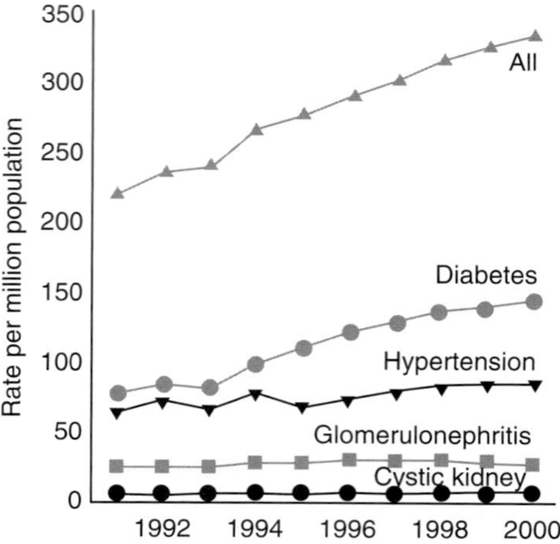

Figure 45-12 Trends in incident rates of end-stage renal disease (ESRD) by primary diagnosis. Diabetes is the primary cause of ESRD in 42% to 47% of adult dialysis patients in the United States. The overall incidence of ESRD has increased by 50% between 1991 and 2000. *(From United States Renal Data System: Excerpts from the USRDS annual data report: atlas of ESRD in the United States. Am J Kidney Dis 2003;(suppl 2) 41:50, with permission from the National Kidney Foundation.)*

ACE inhibitors are more effective than other antihypertensive drugs in slowing the rate of progression of proteinuric CKD.[127,268,362] ACE inhibitors cause a mild decrease in GFR (<10 mL/min/1.73 m^2). The development of hypotension, ARF, or severe hyperkalemia (plasma potassium concentration greater than 5.5 mEq/L) should prompt discontinuation of the drug until other causes have been excluded. Short-term studies show that ARBs have effects on blood pressure and proteinuria that are similar to ACE inhibitors. Data from a 2003 study suggest that combining the two classes of drugs can give additional benefit than either drug alone in terms of reduction in proteinuria and progression to primary end-points.[292]

Low-nitrogen (protein) diets have been advocated from the early years of treatment of severe chronic uremia.[126] The very-low-protein diets tested in the MDRD Study were of marginal benefit in these well-supervised patients with very low renal function, but are not well adhered to in practice, may lead to negative nitrogen balance, and are not recommended. Protein intake is restricted spontaneously to approximately 0.6 to 0.8 g/kg/day by uremic patients not receiving dietary advice.[182] To prevent malnutrition, patients receive professional dietary advice, with diets containing an increased proportion of first class protein and increased calorie content of up to 35 kcal/kg/day. The NHANES III has confirmed an association with reduced GFR and malnutrition in noninstitutionalized individuals studied in a cross-sectional survey of more than 5000 participants stratified according to GFR.[124]

General health measures, including cessation of cigarette smoking, should be encouraged. Complications of CKD that develop before the need for RRT are numerous (see Table 45-6) and include cardiovascular disease, bone disease, and anemia.

Cardiovascular Complications of CKD

The incidence of cardiovascular disease is sevenfold to tenfold greater in patients with CKD than in non-CKD age- and sex-matched controls.[447] By the time patients develop the need for RRT there is an approximately 17 times greater risk of cardiovascular death or nonfatal myocardial infarction than age-matched and sex-matched individuals without kidney disease.[10,113] The spectrum of cardiovascular disease studied in CKD includes (1) angina, (2) congestive heart failure, (3) myocardial infarction, (4) peripheral vascular disease, (5) stroke, and (6) transient ischemic attack. Structural heart disease, such as left ventricular hypertrophy (LVH) and valvular heart disease, is a very common sequela to CKD. Up to 75% of patients commencing dialysis have echocardiographic evidence of LVH.[109] The risk factors for cardiovascular disease in CKD are a mixture of the traditional and CKD-specific. Traditional risk factors such as diabetes, hypertension, and dyslipidemia are more likely in CKD patients.[447] In addition there are a number of other risk factors that are CKD-related (Table 45-9).

Observational studies have indicated that cardiovascular disease occurs at an early stage in CKD.[438] Thus among middle-aged men, a moderate increase in plasma creatinine concentration [>1.5 mg/dL (>130 μmol/L)] was associated with an age-adjusted relative risk of 1.5 for coronary disease and 3.0 for stroke. Reduction of GFR is associated with increased risk of composite end-points of cardiovascular death, myocardial infarction, and stroke.[263] Microalbuminuria and proteinuria have also been shown to be associated with increased risk of cardiovascular disease, cardiovascular mortality, and all-cause mortality.[2,76,437] These associations may arise because (1) CKD causes an elevated level of cardiovascular disease, (2) cardiovascular disease causes CKD, or (3) some other factor, such as diabetes and hypertension, causes both CKD and cardiovascular disease. Significantly, there are 30 times more patients with Stage 3 CKD than Stage 5 CKD.[194,427] The majority die from cardiovascular disease before they progress to kidney failure.

TABLE 45-9 Traditional and CKD-Related Risk Factors for Cardiovascular Disease in CKD

Traditional Risk Factors for Cardiovascular Disease	CKD-Related Risk Factors for Cardiovascular Disease
Older age	Extracellular fluid overload
Male gender	Left ventricular hypertrophy
White race	Proteinuria
Hypertension	Anemia
Elevated LDL cholesterol	Abnormal calcium phosphorus metabolism
Decreased HDL cholesterol	Dyslipidemia
Diabetes mellitus	MIA syndrome
Smoking	Infection
Sedentary lifestyle	Thrombogenic factors
Menopause	Oxidative stress
Family history	Elevated homocysteine
	Uremic toxins

LDL, Low-density lipoprotein; *HDL*, high-density lipoprotein; *CKD*, chronic kidney disease; *MIA*, malnutrition inflammation atherosclerosis.

Left Ventricular Hypertrophy in CKD

LVH is present in more than 70% of patients commencing dialysis.[109] In the dialysis population, LVH is an independent predictor for cardiac death that is the most common cause of death in these patients.[109,113] As indicated above, LVH is demonstrable early in the course of CKD, with the proportion of patients with LVH increasing as kidney function declines. Univariate analysis of a single-center cohort of CKD patients in Canada revealed that age, systolic blood pressure, and hemoglobin were significantly different between the groups with or without LVH.[236] For each 5 mm Hg increase in systolic BP, the risk of LVH increased by 3%. A fall in blood hemoglobin concentration of 1 g/dL increased risk of LVH by 6%. A large, prospective, multicenter study confirmed progressive increases in left ventricular mass index (LVMI) over a 12-month period, with the incidence of new LVH at 10% per year.[237] Again, lower hemoglobin levels and higher systolic blood pressures were associated with left ventricular growth. Normalizing hemoglobin concentration is possible and may have cardiovascular benefits (see discussion later in this chapter).

Anemia

The World Health Organization defines anemia as a hemoglobin of less than 13 g/dL in men and less than 12 g/dL in women.[458] It is clearly established that anemia is inevitable as CKD progresses. Therapies are available to correct anemia and therefore it is mandatory to assess a patient with CKD for anemia. The NKF-K/DOQI recommends that an estimated GFR of less than 60 mL/min/1.73 m^2 should be the cutoff value for determining presence or absence of anemia.[293] Detection is important since, left untreated, it causes many of the side effects of CKD, such as fatigue, breathlessness on exertion, intolerance to cold, and decreased exercise capacity. As indicated above, it is also a major factor in the high prevalence of cardiovascular disease in patients with CKD.

Etiology

The etiology of anemia in CKD is multifactorial. A major cause, however, is the loss of peritubular fibroblasts within the renal cortex that synthesize EPO. EPO is the glycoprotein hormone responsible for stimulating erythroid progenitor cells within the bone marrow to produce red blood cells. Failure of production leads to inappropriately low concentrations within the blood for the concomitant level of hemoglobin. Other causes of anemia include absolute or functional iron deficiency, folic acid and vitamin B_{12} deficiencies, and chronic inflammation. Red cell survival may also be reduced. Both the NKF-K/DOQI and the European Renal Association-European Dialysis Transplant Association have published algorithms for treatment of anemia in CKD and dialysis patients.[101] Treatment in Europe is targeted to achieve a hemoglobin level of 11 to 13 g/dL.

Assessment of Iron

In patients with CKD, a plasma ferritin <100 µg/L is considered to suggest iron deficiency, and a plasma ferritin of 100 to 200 µg/L in association with a transferrin saturation (TSAT) of <20% represents "functional" iron deficiency. Treatment of anemia in CKD requires adequate iron stores. Parenteral iron is the treatment of choice for absolute and functional iron deficiency since oral iron has low efficacy in CKD. Iron status is assessed by measurement of plasma ferritin and TSAT. The TSAT is calculated from the plasma iron divided by the total iron binding capacity (TIBC) and expressed as a percentage. TSAT gives an indication of iron "delivery." Ferritin is used to represent iron stores. A very high concentration of ferritin (>800 µg/L) may suggest iron overload (see Chapter 31). However, limitations with these indices exist (e.g., a high ferritin concentration is also generated by an inflammatory process and transferrin varies with nutritional state and is also influenced by inflammation). Clinical hematology laboratories may offer an automated estimate of the percentage of hypochromic red blood cells. A level above 10% is indicative of functional iron deficiency and the target is <2.5%.[101]

Treatment

Human recombinant erythropoietin (rhEPO or epoetin) is is a synthetic version of human EPO that is used to treat anemia. Following replenished iron stores and exclusion of other causes of anemia, the addition of recombinant epoetin is indicated for the treatment of CKD-related anemia. The gene for human EPO was cloned in 1985 and epoetin was introduced into clinical practice shortly afterwards.[186,455] It is effective at correcting the anemia of CKD in 90% to 95% of patients. The most common side effect is hypertension and therefore blood pressure should be well controlled before the introduction of treatment. Hypertension may develop or worsen in 23% of patients. Failure to respond to treatment requires thorough investigation for many potential causes (Box 45-2). It is estimated that 3 million patients worldwide have received treatment with epoetin. Pure red cell aplasia (PRCA) has occurred in patients treated with epoetin. This has been described in a small number of patients receiving epoetin via the subcutaneous route. In the majority of cases, neutralizing antibodies to EPO have been detected.[61] If a case of PRCA is proven, then no further recombinant erythropoietin products can be administered.

BOX 45-2 Failure to Respond to Epoetin

Iron status
Occult blood loss
Vitamin B_{12} or folate deficiency
Infection and inflammation
Inadequate dialysis
Hyperparathyroidism
Aluminum toxicity
Patient adherence
Hypothyroidism
Primary disease activity
Transplant rejection
Malignancy
Pure red cell aplasia

There are many clinical benefits of correcting anemia with epoetin therapy, including improved exercise capacity,[274] improved cognitive function,[266] better quality of life,[286,352] and increased libido. Much of the evidence derives from studies in dialysis patients. In patients with advanced CKD not yet on RRT, small nonrandomized studies have suggested that regression of LVH is possible with partial correction of anemia with epoetin.[156,334] Patients who receive epoetin consistently in the 2 years before commencement of dialysis have improved survival on dialysis compared with those who received the least consistent administration.[462] Clinical trials are ongoing to try to answer the key question of whether early normalization of anemia in CKD will translate into improved cardiovascular outcomes.

Dyslipidemia in CKD

Various dyslipidemias are associated with CKD.[270,345,447] The pattern of dyslipidemia in CKD differs from that seen in non-CKD. It is characterized by an accumulation of partly metabolized triglyceride-rich particles [predominantly very-low-density lipoprotein (VLDL) and intermediate-density lipoprotein (IDL) remnants], mainly due to abnormal lipase function.[304] This causes hypertriglyceridemia and low high-density lipoprotein (HDL) cholesterol. Although total cholesterol concentration may be normal, there is often a highly abnormal lipid subfraction profile with a predominance of atherogenic small, dense LDL particles.[10] Lipoprotein a levels are also increased in CKD. Baseline data from the Chronic Renal Impairment in Birmingham (CRIB) study have confirmed dyslipidemia in early CKD.[447] Patients had lower HDL and LDL cholesterol and higher triglyceride concentrations.

The challenge to the nephrology community is to establish whether interventions to modify the pattern of dyslipidemia with lifestyle changes and drug treatment will preserve kidney function and reduce cardiovascular morbidity and mortality. At present, there are no large, adequately controlled trials testing the hypotheses that treatment of dyslipidemia preserves kidney function. The major trials of intervention with statins [3-hydroxy-3-methylglutaryl-Co-enzyme A (HMG-CoA) reductase inhibitors] in the general population and those with established cardiovascular disease have been limited with reference to CKD, since patients with CKD are often excluded from the trials.[249,330,372] The Heart Protection Study randomly allocated 20,536 adults with coronary artery disease, occlusive disease of noncoronary arteries, or diabetes to simvastatin (40 mg) or placebo.[277] In a subgroup analysis of more than 1300 patients with plasma creatinine concentration between 1.2 mg/dL and 2.3 mg/dL (110 and 200 µmol/L), there were fewer major vascular events in the simvastatin group.

A randomized controlled trial of proteinuric CKD patients receiving ACE inhibitors and ARBs demonstrated additional benefit from treatment with atorvastatin in terms of reduction in proteinuria and progression of disease.[26] Further trials of lipid-lowering therapies in CKD are currently underway.

Homocysteine

Homocysteine is a sulfur-containing amino acid (see Chapters 20, 26 and 40). Homozygous genetic disorders (homocystinurias) result in marked hyperhomocysteinemia and are clearly associated with untimely atherothrombotic events.[288] Treatment to lower homocysteine reduces the incidence of such outcomes among these patients. Patients with CKD have an excess prevalence of mild-to-moderate hyperhomocysteinemia, which has been independently linked to the development of cardiovascular disease in observational studies.[43] In case-control studies, plasma homocysteine levels are frequently higher in patients with clinical evidence of vascular disease than those without, both in the general population and in CKD.[44] Folate, pyridoxal 5′-phosphate (PLP or "active" vitamin B_6), and vitamin B_{12} are the main vitamin cofactors and/or substrates for homocysteine metabolism (see Chapter 30). Folic acid–based B vitamin regimens, including folic acid at doses of 5 to 10 mg/day, appear to lower fasting homocysteine levels by approximately 30% to 50%.[42] There is as yet little evidence that intervention to lower homocysteine levels affects the risk of disease in the general population or in CKD patients. However, correction of folate deficiency is considered good clinical practice.

Role of Nephrologist

The role of the nephrologist in CKD is to (1) identify the cause of kidney disease, (2) treat reversible factors, (3) reduce rate of progression of CKD, and (4) deal with complications of CKD. Finally, as kidney function fails, the patient should enter an RRT program in a good general condition with suitable access for dialysis, educated and psychosocially prepared for ongoing treatment.

End-Stage Renal Disease

ESRD is an administrative term in the United States, based on the conditions for payment for healthcare by the Medicare ESRD Program, specifically the level of GFR and the occurrence of signs and symptoms of kidney failure necessitating initiation of treatment by RRT. ESRD includes patients treated by dialysis or transplantation, irrespective of the level of GFR (see later section on RRT and transplantation). The NKF-K/DOQI definition of kidney failure (stage 5) differs in two important ways from the definition of ESRD. First, not all individuals with GFR <15 mL/min/1.73 m^2 or with signs and symptoms of kidney failure are treated with RRT. However, such individuals should be considered as having kidney failure. Second, among treated patients, kidney transplant recipients have a higher mean level of GFR (usually 30 to 60 mL/min/1.73 m^2) and better average health outcomes than dialysis patients. Kidney transplant recipients should not be included in the definition of kidney failure, unless they have GFR <15 mL/min/1.73 m^2 or have resumed dialysis.

Kidney diseases or conditions that can lead to ESRD include LVH, anemia, dyslipidemias, disturbed calcium and phosphorus metabolism, and aluminum toxicity.

LVH and Anemia

In a prospective study of ESRD at three Canadian centers, of the 518 patients who survived 6 months of dialysis, 74% had echocardiographic confirmation of LVH.[109] Thirty-five percent had left ventricular dilation (LV cavity >90 ml/m^2) and 15% had systolic dysfunction (fractional shortening of less than or equal to 25%). LVH and dilation were independently associated with death at 2 years.

Anemia has both direct and indirect effects on left ventricular function and growth. Cardiac output increases because of a combination of increased cardiac preload and a reduction in afterload. Such changes lead to ventricular remodeling, with initial left ventricular dilation followed by subsequent hypertrophy. In ESRD other factors also contribute to LVH, including hypertension, volume expansion, and the metabolic consequences of uremia, to which may be added the effects of diabetes. By the time patients with diabetes reach ESRD, they are more likely to have concentric LVH, more likely to have had ischemic heart disease, and more likely to have experienced cardiac failure than nondiabetic subjects.[112]

Predictors for LVH and cardiac failure include age, hypertension, and hemoglobin concentration. In ESRD a 1 g/dL fall in hemoglobin increases the relative risk of left ventricular dilation by 1.49, left ventricular systolic dysfunction by 1.55, and death by 1.25.[110] In patients on dialysis, large observational studies have clearly shown that anemia is associated with increased mortality rates and increased hospitalization.[72,248,253,461] In hemodialysis (HD) patients hematocrit levels of 33% to 36% (corresponding to hemoglobin concentration of 11 to 12 g/dL) were associated with the lowest risk for all-cause and cardiac mortality,[253] and these patients also had the lowest risk of hospitalization.[305,461] A large randomized controlled trial has tested the hypothesis that normalization of anemia would have benefits in terms of morbidity and mortality for hemodialysis patients with New York Heart Association (NYHA) heart disease stage I-III.[24] Patients were randomized to normalization of anemia (618 patients and target hemoglobin of 14 g/dL), or to the control group (615 patients and target hemoglobin of 10 g/dL). The study was terminated early because of a nonsignificant higher risk of death in the normalization group (RR = 1.3, CI 0.09 to 1.9). Post hoc analysis revealed that although the *target* hemoglobin levels in the two groups were clearly separated, the *achieved* hemoglobin levels in the two groups were not and mortality was actually lowest in the subset of patients with the highest achieved hemoglobin level (>13 g/dL).

Dyslipidemias

The prevalence of dyslipidemias in ESRD is high. Dyslipidemias in HD patients are most often characterized by normal LDL, low HDL, and high triglycerides. In a large cross-section analysis of 1047 HD patients in the Dialysis Morbidity and Mortality Study, only 20% of patients had low risk lipid levels [i.e., LDL <130 mg/dL (3.36 mmol/L), HDL >40 mg/dL (>1.03 mmol/L), and triglycerides <150 mg/dL (<1.69 mmol/L)].[296] Low cholesterol was found to be associated with increased mortality, but this is probably a reflection of other conditions that lower cholesterol, such as inflammation and malnutrition. It is possible that other, nontraditional atherogenic lipoprotein abnormalities (e.g., lipoprotein [a] and oxidized LDL) are present in HD patients.[117,257] Similar profiles may be observed in peritoneal dialysis (PD) patients. Treatment guidelines aim to reduce LDL and triglycerides to normal levels. As indicated in the discussion of dyslipidemias in CKD, many of the data on treatment with HMG Co-A reductase inhibitors have been obtained in largely non-CKD populations.

Disturbances in Calcium and Phosphorus Metabolism

ESRD is associated with complex metabolic disturbances of divalent ion and phosphorus metabolism. Although this is commonly referred to as *renal osteodystrophy,* there has been a paradigm shift in terms of calcium, phosphate, and PTH management in patients receiving dialysis. The impetus for this change in approach has been the recognition of the importance in the previously unheralded phosphorus moiety in terms of increased risk of death in ESRD and the almost universal development of *cardiovascular calcification* that is seen in dialysis patients (discussed later in this chapter). As GFR declines, plasma phosphate concentration rises and results in a reduction in ionized calcium. The consequence of this is increased production of PTH from the parathyroid glands. The PTH-producing cells are regulated tightly through complex feedback mechanisms to maintain normocalcemia (see Chapter 49). The calcium-sensing receptor (Ca-SR) is stimulated by calcium and has an inhibitory effect on PTH production.[49] Phosphorus will directly stimulate production of PTH.[395] Elegant experiments on dogs with varying levels of induced kidney failure

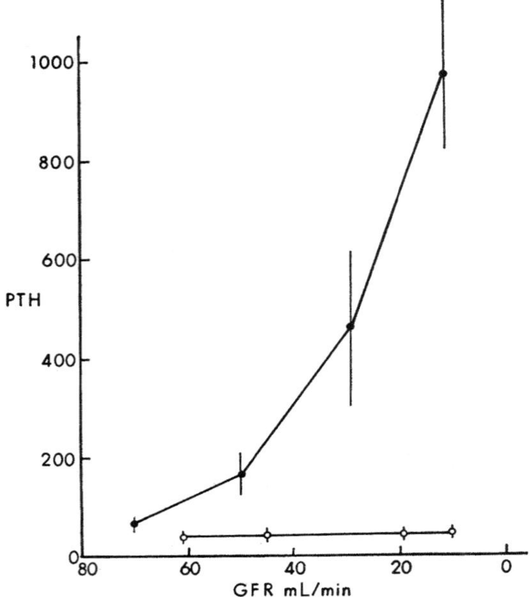

Figure 45-13 The relationship between parathyroid hormone (PTH) concentration and glomerular filtration rate (GFR) in two groups of dogs: those maintained on a normal phosphorus diet (closed circles) and those maintained on a diet containing less than 100 mg of phosphorus per day (open circles). The vertical lines represent ±1 SEM. PTH is expressed in μEq/mL. *(From Slatopolsky E, Caglar S, Pennell JP, Taggart DD, Canterbury JM, Reiss E, et al. On the pathogenesis of hyperparathyroidism in chronic experimental renal insufficiency in the dog. J Clin Invest 1971;50:492-9.)*

confirmed the rise in PTH as GFR falls. This increased production of PTH was attenuated in those animals fed a modified diet with very low levels of phosphorus[394] (Figure 45-13). In addition to hyperphosphatemia contributing to hypocalcemia, there is also reduced 1α-hydroxylation of 25-hydroxycholecalciferol (25-OH vitamin D) within the kidney. Vitamin D is required in health to increase calcium absorption from the gut and it also increases phosphorus absorption from the gut. PTH-producing cells in the parathyroid gland have receptors for vitamin D (VDR). Binding of vitamin D to the VDR inhibits PTH production. The result of these complex metabolic disturbances is secondary hyperparathyroidism. Increased secretion of PTH stimulates resorption of calcium and phosphorus from the major calcium reservoir, the bone. Problems can develop early and patients with a GFR of less than 60 mL/min/1.73 m^2 should be evaluated for these metabolic disturbances.[295] Secondary hyperparathyroidism classically causes bone changes consistent with osteitis fibrosa cystica. Bony erosions and intramedullary cysts are seen because of direct effects of PTH on osteoclasts and osteoblasts. Unchecked, this can lead to bone pain and fractures. Eventually, PTH secretion can become unhinged completely from feedback control and this autonomous production is called tertiary hyperparathyroidism. Derangements in biochemical indices include elevated plasma calcium and phosphate concentration, PTH levels more than 1000 ng/L (reference interval 10 to 60 ng/L), and elevated bone-derived alkaline phosphatase. In this setting medical treatment has failed and parathyroidectomy is required. A severe and often terminal manifestation of long-standing ESRD is calcemic uremic arteriolopathy ("calciphylaxis"). In this condition there is destruction of blood vessels because of calcium deposition and downstream necrosis of tissues, particularly the skin and adipose tissue on the legs and torso.

High concentrations of blood phosphorus are associated with increased mortality in HD patients.[31] The relative risk of death in the United States for those HD patients with plasma phosphorus greater than 6.5 mg/dL (2.10 mmol/L) is 1.27 relative to those with plasma phosphorus of 2.4 to 6.5 mg/dL (0.77 to 2.10 mmol/L). The calcium phosphorus product (calculated by multiplying concentration of calcium by concentration of phosphorus) showed a mortality trend similar to phosphorus. In at least 50% of HD patients the plasma phosphate is greater than 6.0 mg/dL (1.94 mmol/L) and in 25% of patients it is greater than 7.2 mg/dL (2.32 mmol/L). The United Kingdom Renal Association standard for pre dialysis plasma phosphate concentration is less than 5.6 mg/dL (1.8 mmol/L).[422] Strategies to reduce phosphorus levels are employed routinely in the treatment of patients on dialysis. Inorganic phosphorus measured within the blood accounts for <0.1% of total body phosphorus. The clearance of phosphorus on intermittent HD is approximately a third of that of urea and is also subject to a post dialysis rebound because of efflux from the intracellular to extracellular space. Phosphorus is present in many foods and is linearly associated with protein ingestion. The recommended daily allowance is reduced for patients on dialysis to around 800 mg. Treatment with vitamin D analogs increases gut absorption of phosphorus from 60% to 70% to almost 85%. The use of phosphate binders, taken with meals, is almost universal in dialysis patients. The binders reduce phosphorus absorption to 30% to 40%. In summary, patients on conventional dialysis are in a net positive phosphorus balance. It has been possible to normalize phosphorus balance in patients treated by daily HD.[287]

Medical treatment strategies are designed to limit phosphorus intake and normalize calcium. With the advent of vitamin D analogs it has been possible to supplement vitamin D (see Chapter 49). This has the effect of increasing plasma calcium concentration and switching off PTH production. Unfortunately the commonly used analogs, such as 1α-hydroxyvitamin D_3, also lead to increased reabsorption of calcium and phosphorus from the gut. Hyperphosphatemia has deleterious cardiovascular effects and is discussed below. Furthermore, in the setting of aggressive treatment with vitamin D analogs hypercalcemia may develop that is associated with low, suppressed, levels of PTH. Bone biopsy in this case may demonstrate very low levels of bone activity, a condition referred to as adynamic bone disease. Alternative vitamin D analogs such as paricalcitol are reported to have lower rates of hyperphosphatemia.[267,409] A further development has been the generation of calcimimetic agents that are currently being evaluated in clinical trials.[6,243] These drugs can mimic calcium directly stimulating the Ca-SR and also affect the molecular configuration of the Ca-SR to enhance the sensitivity to extracellular calcium.[243] Stimulation of the Ca-SR switches off PTH production selectively with no risk of increasing phosphorus absorption.

Aluminum Toxicity

A causative factor for renal bone disease, historically, is aluminum intoxication (see Chapter 35). Aluminum concentrations in dialysis fluids were previously high, but with modern dialysis facilities this is no longer such a problem. Dialysis patients are, however, treated intermittently with aluminum-containing phosphate binders and therefore regular monitoring of blood aluminum concentration is recommended.[422] Aluminum accumulation has been associated with deposition along the mineralization surface of the osteoid and a low-turnover form of bone disease. Aluminum accumulation may be treated by infusions of the chelating agent desferrioxamine. Aluminum intoxication may be associated with neurological disturbances characterized by dementia (dialysis dementia) and with a hypochromic microcytic anemia.

Diabetic Nephropathy

Diabetes mellitus is a state of chronic hyperglycemia sufficient to cause long-term damage to specific tissues, notably the retina, kidney, nerves, and arteries (see Chapter 25). It affects 176 million people worldwide and the World Health Organization (WHO) predicts that the prevalence of diabetes is set to double by 2030.[215,459] In the United Kingdom 3% of the population have diabetes.[421] The WHO and national diabetes agencies have approved diagnostic criteria for diabetes based on venous plasma glucose concentrations.[351]

Type 1 diabetes is due to autoimmune destruction of pancreatic islet beta cells causing loss of insulin. Type 2 diabetes is due to the combination of cellular resistance to insulin and beta cell failure. Tissue lesions are common to both types of diabetes, and chronic hyperglycemia (or a closely related metabolic abnormality) is responsible for diabetic complications including diabetic nephropathy.

Background

Diabetic nephropathy is a clinical diagnosis based on the finding of proteinuria in a patient with diabetes and in whom there is no evidence of urinary tract infection. Overt nephropathy is characterized by protein excretion greater than 0.5 g/day. This is equivalent to albumin excretion of around 300 mg/day. It is preferable to assess proteinuria as albuminuria because it is a more sensitive marker for CKD due to diabetes.[295] There has been a uniform adoption of albumin as the "criterion standard" in evaluating diabetes-related kidney damage. The NKF-K/DOQI Work Group concluded that albumin should be measured to detect and monitor kidney damage in adults. Patients with a urinary albumin excretion rate of between 30 and 300 mg/day have microalbuminuria (see Chapter 24). Diabetic nephropathy is the most common cause of ESRD in the United States and accounts for approximately 40% of incident patients onto RRT programs.[427] More than 100,000 people receiving HD in the United States have diabetes as the cause of their ESRD. Among patients who require dialysis, those with diabetes have a 22% higher mortality at 1 year and a 15% higher mortality at 5 years than patients without diabetes. Diabetic nephropathy as a cause of ESRD in the United Kingdom is seen in 18% of new patients and remains lower than that of the United States and Europe.[425] In the United States, a number of objectives have been developed for reducing threats to the health of the nation in the Healthy People 2010 report. One of the objectives (HP 2010 Objective 4.7) is to reduce the incidence rate of ESRD caused by diabetes from 145 per million population to 78 per million people by 2010.[427]

Diabetic nephropathy is clinically a very slowly developing condition, but ultrastructural evidence of glomerular damage has been found in renal biopsies taken from type 1 diabetic patients within a few years of their diagnosis.[15,66,104] In type 1 disease, early macroscopic changes include kidney enlargement and pallor. With disease progression, the kidneys become smaller. Type 2 disease is typified by variable kidney contraction because of associated ischemia. On histological examination, glomerular changes include diffuse mesangial sclerosis with accentuation of matrix and irregularly thickened basement membranes; sclerotic, acellular mesangial nodules (so-called Kimmelstiel-Wilson lesions); hyaline fibrin cap lesions around peripheral capillary loops; capsular drop lesions located within Bowman's capsule; and hyalinosis of arterioles.

Clinical progression is defined in terms of changes in urinary albumin excretion rate and decline in GFR and blood pressure (Table 45-10). In type 1 diabetes, it is unusual to develop microalbuminuria within the first 5 years of diagnosis but it can develop anytime thereafter and even after 40 years. Patients with type 1 disease and microalbuminuria will progress to overt nephropathy at an average rate of 20% over 5 years.[114] Long-term follow-up data of microalbuminuric patients confirm that 30% become normoalbuminuric and the rest remain microalbuminuric at 10 years.[58] Since the onset of type 2 diabetes is difficult to define, it is difficult to estimate the incidence of microalbuminuria, although 1% of patients in the United Kingdom have overt nephropathy at diagnosis. As albuminuria worsens and blood pressure increases, there is a relentless decline in GFR. In some patients with microalbuminuria renal lesions are already quite advanced and therefore it may be a marker of nephropathy rather than a predictor of renal structural changes.[58]

Family studies of patients with type 1 diabetes have shown that diabetic siblings of patients with nephropathy have a fourfold risk of nephropathy compared with a sibling without nephropathy. A family history of hypertension and cardiovascular disease may also increase nephropathy rates.[39] However, the best available predictor for development of nephropathy is microalbuminuria, although cellular markers are being investigated—such as increased erythrocyte Na^+/Li^+ countertransporter and overactivity of the Na^+/H^+ antiporter.[17] Considerable work has been undertaken to look for genetic linkages with the development of nephropathy in diabetes. This work has included studies of polymorphisms of the ACE and insulin genes, but as yet no clear relationship has been demonstrated.[376] Other markers of basement membrane damage have also been used to investigate dia-

TABLE 45-10 Development of Diabetic Nephropathy

Stage	Designation	Characteristics	Structural Changes	GFR (mL/min/1.73 m²)	Blood Pressure (mm Hg)
I	Hyperfunction	Hyperfiltration	Glomerular hypertrophy	>150	Normal
II	Normo-albuminuria	Normal AER	Basement membrane thickening	150	Normal
III	Incipient diabetic nephropathy	Elevated AER	AER correlates with structural damage and hypertrophy of remaining glomeruli	125	Increased
IV	Overt diabetic nephropathy	Clinical proteinuria	Advanced structural damage	<100	Hypertension
V	Uremia	End-stage renal disease	Glomerular closure	0-10	High

AER, Albumin excretion rate; *GFR*, glomerular filtration rate.

betic nephropathy, including urinary excretion of laminin, collagen IV, and fibronectin.[187,340]

Pathophysiology

Observational studies have shown that sustained poor glycemic control is associated with a greater risk for development of nephropathy in both type 1 and type 2 diabetes.[89,174-176,218,345,424] The exact mechanism for hyperglycemic tissue damage is now being elucidated and probably includes (1) glycation of proteins leading to the formation of advanced glycation end products (AGE), (2) overactivity of the polyol pathway, and (3) generation of reactive oxygen species. Polyols are sugar alcohols formed from their respective sugars under the action of aldose reductase. Glucose is preferentially shunted through the polyol pathway under hyperglycemic conditions, generating sorbitol that accumulates within cells. A key step linking glucotoxicity to cell dysfunction in diabetic nephropathy is the excess of extracellular matrix within the glomerulus and interstitium. A number of genes encoding matrix proteins in hyperglycemic conditions have been identified.[269] For example, the transcription of the gene for transforming growth factor-β (TGF-β) is stimulated by hyperglycemia, AGE, angiotensin II, and reactive oxygen species.[168,315,443] One important consequence of glucose-stimulated TGF-β is the upregulation of the insulin-independent GLUT-1 transporter in mesangial cells. Glucose is transported to the cells through GLUT-1 and metabolized mainly by the glycolytic pathway. Increased de novo synthesis of diacylglycerol results in the activation of protein kinase C and mitogen activated kinases. Activation of these enzymes can lead to stimulation of certain genes, including TGF-β. Activation of TGF-β can induce the expression of GLUT-1 and these signaling pathways induce expression of extracellular matrix proteins. The formation of AGE also generates reactive oxygen species, which can activate latent TGF-β.[269] Studies employing neutralizing anti–TGF-β antibodies have provided evidence that the prosclerotic and hypertrophic effects of high ambient glucose in cultured renal cells are largely mediated by autocrine production and activation of TGF-β.[184,471] These antibodies can reverse established nephropathy in animal models.[68,472] Furthermore, glomerular TGF-β mRNA is markedly increased in kidney biopsy specimens from patients with proven diabetic kidney disease, and blood and urine sampling across the renal vascular bed confirms net renal production of TGF-β in diabetic patients.[386] Treatment with the ACE inhibitor captopril lowers circulating TGF-β levels in patients with diabetic nephropathy.[387] The receptor for AGE has been identified (RAGE).[375] RAGE is selectively expressed in the glomerular epithelial cells (podocytes) and not the mesangial cell or glomerular endothelium.[406] Increased accumulation of AGE in diabetes engages podocyte RAGE and may lead to increased glomerular permeability.[446] Vascular hyperpermeability, a hallmark feature of diabetes, can be suppressed by inhibiting RAGE in the animal model of diabetes, the streptozotocin-treated rat.[441]

Studies of experimental diabetes in the rat suggested that hyperfiltration alone could cause glomerular changes; there are conflicting reports in humans. An increased GFR could be a predictor of progression to microalbuminuria, but is also a reflection of poor metabolic control. In the Diabetes Control and Complications Trial (DCCT) study, there was no association between hyperfiltration and subsequent development of microalbuminuria.[17] Systemic blood pressure is higher in patients with diabetes who subsequently develop microalbuminuria, although it is not clear which comes first. Tubulointerstitial fibrosis occurs in diabetic nephropathy in addition to glomerulosclerosis. Decreased GFR correlates with the interstitial expansion and the glomerular expansion.[449]

Treatment Strategies

The DCCT found in almost 1500 patients with type 1 diabetes that 9 years of intensive insulin therapy compared with conventional insulin therapy produced a 44% reduction in the development of microalbuminuria in patients with no retinopathy and a 35% reduction in patients with early retinopathy at entry.[89] The cumulative incidence of microalbuminuria was 15% and 27% in the intensively treated patients, respectively. The mean glycated hemoglobin (HbA_{1c}) was 7.2% in the intensively treated group versus 9.0% in the conventionally treated patients.

The United Kingdom Prospective Diabetes Study (UKPDS) of almost 4000 newly diagnosed type 2 diabetic patients followed for at least 10 years, showed that intensive control of blood glucose with sulfonylureas or insulin reduces the risk of diabetic nephropathy and other microvascular complications.[424] The target fasting blood glucose was 110 mg/dL (6.1 mmol/L) for the interventional group and for standard therapy was 270 mg/dL (15 mmol/L). Fasting blood sugars rose over time in both groups but mean HbA_{1c} was lower in the intervention group (7.0% compared with 7.9%). The UKPDS showed additional benefit of intensive therapy, with a 67% risk reduction on the rate of doubling of plasma creatinine at 12 years, although less than 1% of UKPDS patients developed advanced CKD.

Studies from Japan and Scandinavia have reported a lower incidence of microalbuminuria in intensively treated groups of patients with type 2 diabetes.[119,306] The American Diabetes Association Clinical Practice Recommendations target HbA_{1c} to less than 7% as the treatment goal. Additional therapy should be initiated if HbA_{1c} is above 8%.[401]

There is ongoing controversy as to whether intensive glucose therapy alone can prevent progression of incipient to overt nephropathy. Other factors, such as lowering blood pressure and blockade of ACE and AII, are important. High blood pressure accelerates the progressive increase in albuminuria in patients with initially normal urinary albumin excretion and accelerates loss of kidney function in those with overt nephropathy in type 2 diabetes.[12] A subgroup analysis of the Swedish Hypertension Optimal Trial (HOT) showed that patients with diabetes who were randomized to lower levels of blood pressure (diastolic blood pressure <90 versus <85 versus <80 mm Hg) had lower mortality and cardiovascular events than those with higher values.[150] In 1501 patients with diabetes, a 50% reduction of major cardiovascular events was seen in those targeted to a diastolic blood pressure less than 80 mm Hg as compared with 90 mm Hg. The NKF Task Force on Cardiovascular Disease has recommended a target blood pressure of less than 125/75 mm Hg in diabetic kidney disease.[235] The recent report of aggressive blood pressure control in normotensive type 2 diabetic patients reinforces this target blood pressure as appropriate in diabetes.[378]

Patients with diabetes are relatively more hypervolemic than nondiabetic patients at the same level of GFR. Therefore, it is important to emphasize reduced dietary salt intake and diuretic treatment in the management of diabetic patients with nephropathy. A low sodium diet potentiates the antihypertensive effect and antiproteinuric effect of AII blockade in type 2 diabetes.[173] Patients should be encouraged to stop smoking cigarettes since smoking increases the risk of microalbuminuria.[308] Dyslipidemias should be managed as outlined for nondiabetic proteinuric CKD.

ACE inhibitors and ARBs slow the progression of diabetic kidney disease.[47,238,282,317] A trial that was reported in 2000 confirmed that even nonmicroalbuminuric type 2 diabetic patients should be managed with ACE inhibitors or ARBs to prevent cardiovascular events.[157] In addition to lowering systemic blood pressure, such patients also have lowered glomerular capillary blood pressure and protein filtration.[158,349,468] ACE inhibitors and ARBs also reduce AII-mediated effects on glomerular permeability and cell proliferation and fibrosis[255,291] and should be incorporated into the treatment schedules of all patients with type 2 diabetes and those with type 1 diabetes and microalbuminuria. ACE inhibitors may exacerbate hyperkalemia in patients with advanced CKD and/or hyporeninemic hypoaldosteronism. In older patients with renal artery stenosis, they may cause a rapid decline in kidney function. Pooled data from large clinical trials indicated above show that only 1.5% of patients treated with ACE inhibitors or ARBs were withdrawn from trials because of hyperkalemia, and no deaths were reported as a consequence of hyperkalemia.[47,238]

To achieve the target blood pressure values, there is often a need for four to five antihypertensive agents, including ACE inhibitors and ARBs, diuretics, beta-blockers, and calcium channel blockers. There may be additional benefits from combination therapy with ACE inhibitors and ARBs.[282] Although the renal risk in diabetic nephropathy can be reduced by 20% to 40%, the fact that 70% progress suggests that novel approaches are required. Experimental strategies identified in animal models could hold the key. However, if current recommendations for management are uniformly adhered to, along with statin treatment to reduce overall cardiovascular risk, then the goal of HP 2010 Objective 4.3 may be achieved.

Hypertensive Nephropathy

Hypertension is second only to diabetes as a primary diagnosis of ESRD for incident patients commencing dialysis in the United States.[427] From 1990 to 2000, there was a 32% increase in hypertension as the primary cause of ESRD. The incidence is higher in older people and especially among the black population in the United States. Hypertension often develops as a consequence of CKD because of alterations in salt and water metabolism and activation of the sympathetic nervous and renin-angiotensin systems.[116,241] Hypertension can act as an accelerating force in the development of ESRD. As described earlier, treatment of hypertension to predefined target blood pressure values is critical to preventing the progression to ESRD.[217,326,392]

Hypertension is grouped with large vessel *renovascular disease* in the USRDS Annual Data Report database. Primary diseases of the renal arteries usually involve the origin of the renal arteries at the aorta (ostial lesions). Secondary diseases with hypertension and CKD with small-vessel and intrarenal disease are referred to as "ischemic nephropathy." There is a complex interplay between renal artery stenosis and ischemic nephropathy. Atherosclerosis accounts for greater than 90% of renal artery stenosis. The disease is progressive and may cause renal artery occlusion.[57] The prevalence increases with age and is associated with refractory hypertension, low body mass index, smoking, diabetes, and established vascular disease elsewhere. In general, as a marker of established cardiovascular disease, atheromatous renal artery stenosis is associated with a poor prognosis.[260] Diagnosis requires a high index of suspicion and is guided by radiological examination of the renal arterial anatomy. Patients who receive ACE inhibitors and ARBs may develop ARF in the setting of severe bilateral renovascular disease or severe disease to a single functioning kidney. Kidney function should be carefully monitored following the introduction of these drugs. Deterioration in kidney function following introduction of these agents should also raise the suspicion of renovascular disease. The diagnosis is important to make since radiological displacement of intraluminal stents[32] is possible and surgical repair can be performed to prolong vessel patency.[149] Patients are at risk, however, of atheroembolism following intervention.[380]

Glomerular Diseases

In many patients, significant primary glomerular disease may be recognized by the presence of distinctive clinical syndromes that result from glomerular injury. Among the more important are rapidly progressive glomerulonephritis (RPGN), the nephrotic syndrome, acute nephritis, and chronic glomerulopathies. Systemic diseases that affect glomerular structure and function include for example systemic lupus erythematosus (SLE); microscopic polyangiitis; cryoglobulinemia; bacterial endocarditis; viral infections such as those associated with hepatitis B, C, and HIV; and malignancy. Diabetes and immunoglobulin light chain mediated kidney disease are discussed separately. A discussion of all these syndromes is beyond the scope of this book. Examples serve to illustrate the use of the laboratory in their evaluation.

Primary glomerular disease presents clinically with (1) abnormalities of the urine, including proteinuria and hematuria, (2) hypertension, (3) edema, and often (4) reduced renal excretory function. Urinalysis should be ordered for patients presenting with hypertension or renal impairment or suspected of having kidney disease. Urinary casts are identified by microscopy, and red cell casts are indicative of glomerular bleeding and glomerular pathology. Specialist nephrology input is often required since histological examination of a kidney biopsy specimen, including immune reactants and electron microscopy, is usually performed to confirm the diagnosis.

Laboratory investigations performed to investigate glomerular disease and systemic disorders include (1) urinary protein excretion, (2) plasma creatinine concentration, (3) urea concentration, (4) liver function tests, (5) glucose concentration and, if myeloma is suspected, (6) serum protein electrophoresis, and (7) urinary examination for Bence Jones protein. Serological testing for the presence of autoantibodies to (1) antinuclear antigens (ANA), (2) double-stranded DNA (ds-DNA), (3) extractable nuclear antigens (ENAs), and (4) antineutrophil cytoplasmic antibody (ANCA) is performed if either SLE or systemic vasculitis is suspected. Antiglomerular basement membrane antibodies (anti-GBM) may be detected in rare cases of renal-limited anti-GBM disease (Goodpasture's disease) and pulmonary-renal syndromes (Goodpasture's syndrome). Components of the complement system can be affected (e.g., reduced levels of C3 and C4) in several conditions including SLE, infection, cryoglobulinemia, and mesangiocapillary (also referred to as membranoproliferative) glomerulonephritis. Blood cultures are taken for bacteriological examination in suspected infection.

The glomerular capillaries appear to be particularly vulnerable to immune-mediated injury, probably as a consequence of their unique function and structure. Continuous production of a protein-free filtrate across a complex capillary wall and a specialized mechanism for clearing trapped molecules through the mesangium increase the susceptibility by trapping circulating macromolecules. Deposition or generation of immune complexes can cause complement fixation and activation of lymphocytes and macrophages, all of which can mediate damage.[62] Resolution of inflammation may lead to normal tissue or kidney scarring. In some syndromes, well-characterized antigens are involved, such as the α-3 chain of type IV collagen in Goodpasture's syndrome, but in others their involvement is less clear.[219] There is evidence that environmental toxins and in particular organic solvents can increase the incidence of glomerulonephritis in Goodpasture's syndrome.[35] This might be from damage to the basement membrane lining the lung, which has some antigenic epitopes similar to those of the glomerular basement membrane. The environment plays a critical role in determining whether anti-GBM antibodies cause lung injury, since pulmonary hemorrhage only occurs in current cigarette smokers.[94]

The primary glomerulonephritides are classified morphologically according to histological analysis into subtypes with particular patterns of glomerular injury. There may be associated immune complex deposition (e.g., diffuse, focal/segmental, mesangiocapillary, and crescentic). Representative drawings from biopsy specimens from some of these conditions are shown in Figure 45-14 to show how

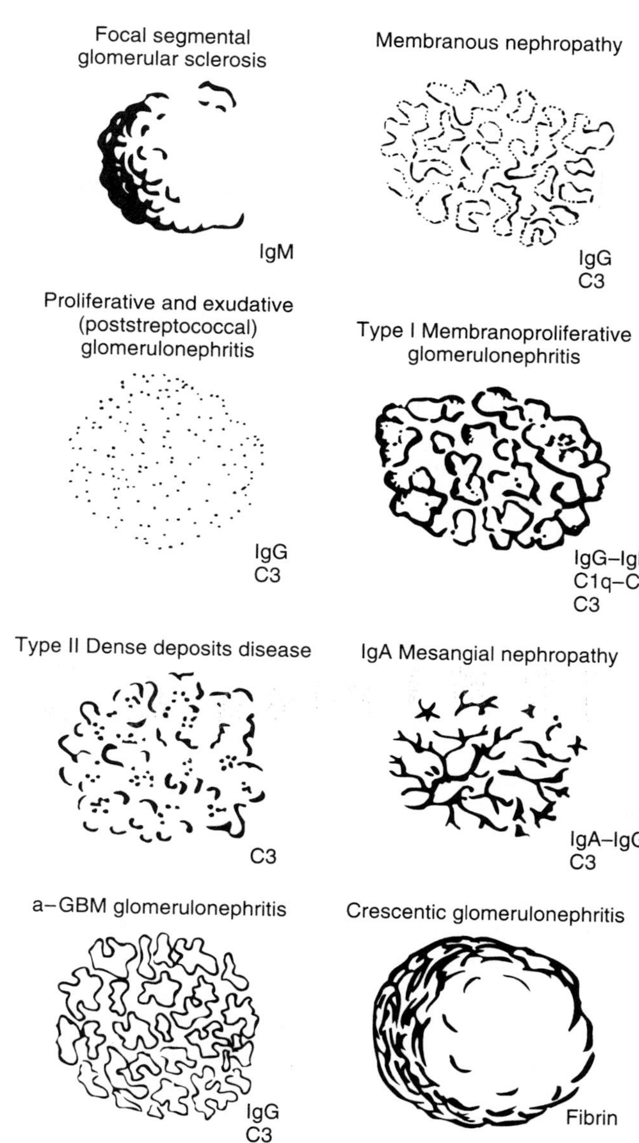

Figure 45-14 Glomerular pathology in glomerular nephritis, showing immunohistological patterns of the different types of primary glomerulonephritis. *(From Ponticelli C, Mihatsch MJ, Imbasciati E. Renal biopsy: performance and interpretation. In: Cameron JS, Davison AM, Grunfeld J-P, Kerr D, Ritz E, eds. Oxford textbook of clinical nephrology (vol. 1). 1st ed. Oxford: Oxford University Press, 1992:Chapter 1.7.2. Reproduced by permission of Oxford University Press.)*

clearly biopsy findings can distinguish different pathological conditions. However, there may be overlap in presentation, treatment, and outcome.

Glomerular diseases that are not amenable or that do not respond to treatment are chronic and often progressive. Glomerular disease eventually affects the blood supply of tubules and results in the loss of complete nephrons to produce advanced CKD and the uremic syndrome. In the United Kingdom, glomerulonephritis accounts for 13.6% of new patients to RRT in patients aged less than 65 years and 6.1% in older patients.[425] General measures to limit progression of CKD have been identified earlier and include tight blood pressure control and use of ACE inhibitors and ARBs.

IgA Nephropathy

IgA nephropathy is the most common type of glomerulonephritis worldwide. The disease tends to be slowly progressive and in 20 years 30% to 40% of patients will develop ESRD depending, as with most kidney diseases, on the degree of proteinuria and GFR at time of diagnosis and degree of interstitial fibrosis on biopsy. Biopsy findings are pathognomonic with deposition of polymeric immunoglobulin A (IgA). Up to 50% of patients exhibit elevated concentrations of plasma IgA, although diagnosis depends on kidney biopsy findings. Current treatment strategies are unsatisfactory, but involve general measures to reduce proteinuria, and prednisolone in selected cases.[335,404] Cytotoxic therapy can be considered for rapidly progressing or vasculitic IgA.[14]

Rapidly Progressive Glomerulonephritis

RPGN is a heterogeneous group of disorders characterized by a fulminant clinical course that leads to kidney failure in only weeks or a few months. These syndromes are often characterized by focal necrotizing glomerulonephritis and extracapillary crescent formation within the parietal layer of Bowman's capsules. Proliferating epithelial cells and macrophages eventually compress the glomeruli and obstruct the proximal convoluted tubules, thus severely compromising nephron function. The proliferation of epithelial cells and macrophages is in response to fibrinogen and fibrin polymers present in Bowman's space. This is a nonspecific reaction to severe glomerular injury attended by leakage of fibrinogen, activated enzymes, and macrophages out of the capillaries into Bowman's space. Crescents and deterioration in kidney function may develop rapidly.

RPGN may be classified either as idiopathic kidney disease or as a disease secondary to other conditions, such as infectious diseases, multisystem diseases, and occasionally an adverse reaction to medication. Anti-GBM antibodies may be present along the glomerular basement membrane in anti-GBM disease. Most commonly, however, there is no immunoglobulin deposition within the glomerulus (pauci-immune). Approximately 80% of patients with active pauci-immune necrotizing and crescentic glomerulonephritis have been shown to possess antineutrophil cytoplasmic antibodies (ANCA), irrespective of the presence or absence of a concomitant systemic vasculitis. This strong association has allowed serological discrimination of this type of glomerulonephritis from other types of RPGN. Wegener's granulomatosis, microscopic polyangiitis, and Churg-Strauss syndrome are small vessel vasculitides characterized by an association with ANCA.

ANCA were first reported in 1982 in patients with pauci-immune serological glomerulonephritis.[83] Three years later ANCA were detected by indirect immunofluorescence on normal human neutrophils in patients with active Wegener's granulomatosis.[429] Since 1989, two subtypes of ANCA have been described: cytoplasmic (C-ANCA) and perinuclear (P-ANCA), reflecting the patterns observed by indirect immunofluorescence microscopy using alcohol-fixed neutrophils as a substrate.[450] C-ANCA are directed toward a plasma proteinase (PR3) in neutrophil primary granules and are associated with Wegener's granulomatosis, whereas the P-ANCA target antigen is usually myeloperoxidase (MPO) and is associated with microscopic polyangiitis.[102,301] Enzyme-linked immunosorbent assays (ELISA) have been used to measure the anti-PR3 and anti-MPO antibody titers. Vasculitis or angiitis is an inflammatory reaction in the wall of any blood vessel and can have diverse clinical presentations. The exact sequence of events that triggers perivascular inflammation leading to injury is unclear, but ANCA have been identified that have at least diagnostic and prognostic usefulness. ANCA appear in the plasma of almost all patients with active and generalized disease. If unrecognized, these diseases can progress very rapidly to ESRD. However, effective treatments are available including high dose steroids, cytotoxic therapy, and plasma exchange.[205] This form of kidney disease accounts for 15% of patients presenting to specialist nephrology units for RRT and is therefore an important disease category to be aware of since, if treatment is initiated early, independent kidney function can be restored, particularly if active lesions are seen on biopsy.[154] In addition to the measurement of ANCA, C-reactive protein (CRP) may be used to monitor the acute phase reaction in active disease processes, together with tests for the general assessment of progressive kidney disease, including proteinuria.[370]

Nephrotic Syndrome

Gross changes in glomerular permeability characterize the nephrotic syndrome. The diagnostic criteria for establishing nephrotic syndrome are the presence of proteinuria (total protein >3 g/day or albumin >1.5 g/day), hypoalbuminemia, hypercholesterolemia, and finally edema. The edema was classically thought to be a consequence of the decreased intravascular oncotic pressure because of the loss of protein. However, expansion of the interstitial compartment is secondary to an accumulation of sodium in the extracellular compartment with reduced urinary sodium output, along with alterations of fluid transfer across capillary walls.[86] As shown in Figure 45-15, the proteinuria is a consequence of a reduction in the charge-selective properties of the filtration barrier, particularly the basement membrane and alter-

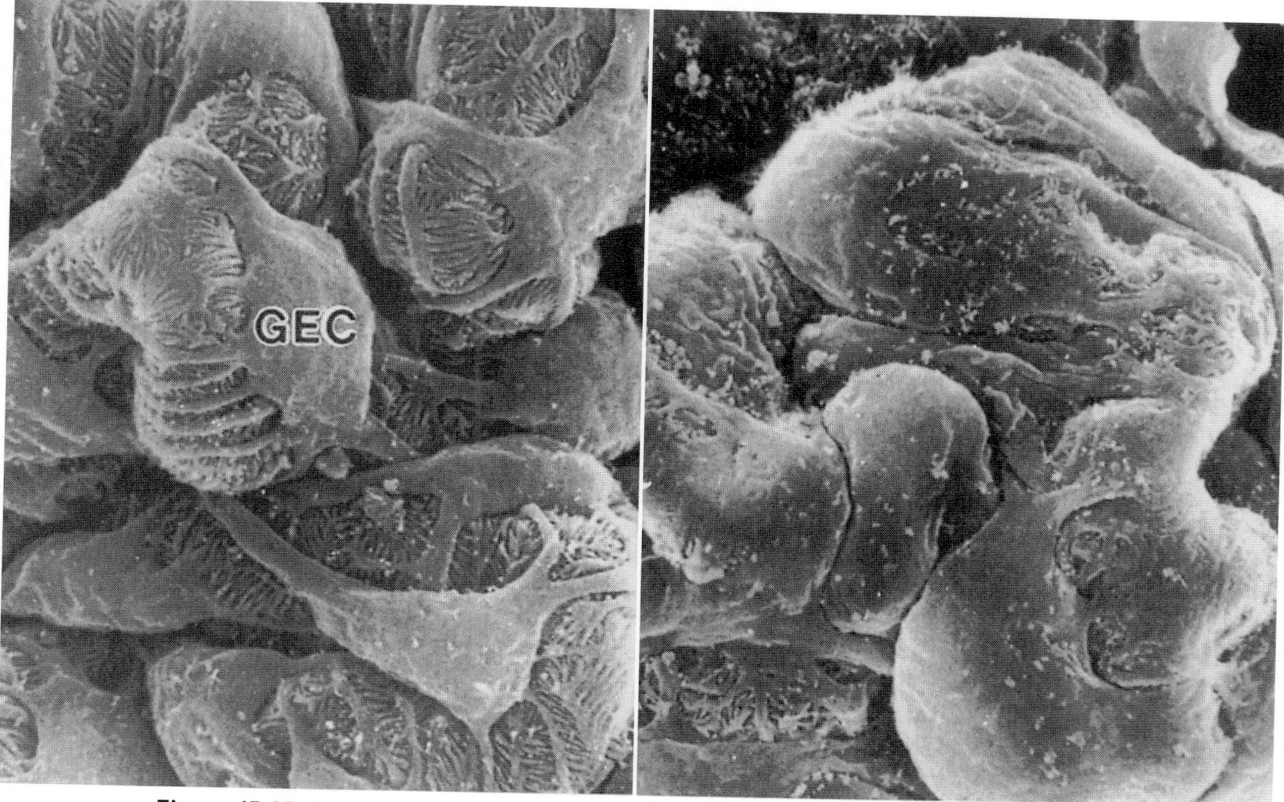

Figure 45-15 Graphic example of glomerular changes in nephrotic syndrome. Scanning electron microscopic view of glomerular epithelial podocytes from a vehicle-treated rat *(left)* and a puromycin aminonucleoside (PAN)–treated (180 mg/kg body wt) rat *(right)*. Note the extensive loss of podocyte foot processes, which occurs in response to PAN-induced nephrotic syndrome. This illustrates the major cellular changes that can occur in nephrotic syndrome. GEC, glomerular epithelial cell. *(From Ricardo SD, Bertram JF, Ryan GB: Antioxidants protect podocyte foot processes in puromycin aminonucleoside–treated rats. J Am Soc Nephrol 1994;4:1974-86.)*

ations in the slit diaphragms of interdigitating foot processes of adjacent podocytes (epithelial cells).[96,348] Nephrotic syndrome can result from a variety of causes, including minimal change nephropathy (most common in children); focal segmental glomerulosclerosis (FSGS), membranous nephropathy, which may be idiopathic or associated with carcinoma, drugs, or infection; SLE; and diabetic nephropathy. Nephrotic syndrome in children characteristically responds to steroids if associated with highly selective proteinuria (predominantly albuminuria). Following histological confirmation of the underlying cause of the nephrotic syndrome therapy is targeted to reduce proteinuria and prevent predictable complications, such as hypercholesterolemia and venous thrombosis. High dose steroids and second line therapy with cyclophosphamide and cyclosporine may be initiated for refractory disease. Repeated treatment courses are necessary in relapsing disease.

Acute Nephritic Syndrome

This disorder is characterized by the rapid onset of hematuria, proteinuria, reduced GFR, and sodium and water retention, with resulting hypertension and localized peripheral edema. Congestive heart failure and oliguria may also develop. Renal biopsy shows enlarged, inflamed glomeruli with narrowed capillary lumina.

In a number of patients with the acute nephritic syndrome, the pathological process is related to recent group A β-hemolytic streptococcal infection of the pharynx or, less commonly, the skin. Only certain strains of streptococci are capable of inducing acute nephritis. A latent period averaging about 2 weeks exists between the streptococcal infection and clinical evidence of nephritis; it is slightly longer for cutaneous than for pharyngeal-associated disease. Typical poststreptococcal glomerulonephritis is now rare in developed countries. The initial presentation usually consists of oliguria, hematuria, hypertension, and facial and hand edema, with some evidence of vascular congestion. The presentation may vary considerably from patient to patient. Percutaneous renal biopsy of patients with poststreptococcal glomerulonephritis reveals enlarged hypercellular glomeruli infiltrated by polymorphonuclear leukocytes and monocytes, usually within the mesangium or capillary lumina. Proliferation of mesangial and endothelial cells is also observed. Involvement of the kidneys is diffuse. Electron microscopy reveals deposits, presumably immune complexes, on the epithelial side of the basement membrane. Glomerular injury with damage to the glomerular basement membrane leading to a reduction in GFR is thought to be caused by activation of the inflammatory response by immune complexes.[453] Abnormal laboratory results are usually present early in the course of acute nephritis. Hematuria, gross or microscopic, and proteinuria, usually less than 3 g/day, are almost always present. Red blood cell casts are highly suggestive of glomerulonephritis. These casts are commonly present in urine but are observed only if the specimen is fresh and acidic, centrifugation is light, and sediment (after decantation) is resuspended gently. Large numbers of hyaline and granular casts are also common; waxy casts suggest a chronic process and should raise the possibility of acute exacerbation of a preexisting disease.

In patients suspected of having acute poststreptococcal glomerulonephritis, evidence of recent infection may be found in increased titers of antibodies to streptococcal extracellular products-antistreptolysin O (ASO), antihyaluronidase (AHase), and antideoxyribonuclease-B (ADNase-B). Serial measurements that document rising antibody titers against streptococcal antigens are stronger evidence of recent infection than a single determination. Most patients have moderate reductions in total hemolytic complement activity (CH_{50}) and in the C3 component of the complement cascade. Persistent and severe depression of C3 levels should suggest membranoproliferative glomerulonephritis, SLE, endocarditis, or other forms of sepsis. Although depressed levels of complement imply disease activity, they are not useful for grading the severity or determining the prognosis of the illness.

Other causes of acute nephritis are reactions to drugs, acute infection of the kidneys, systemic diseases with immune complexes such as SLE, bacterial endocarditis, and finally disease in which the antigen is unknown but possibly related to antecedent viral infections.

Primary glomerular diseases may recur following kidney transplantation and result in loss of the graft. An Australian study has confirmed a 10-year incidence of graft loss caused by recurrent glomerulonephritis as 8.4%.[48] Recurrence was the third most frequent cause of graft loss (chronic allograft nephropathy and death with a functioning graft were the most common). As compared with the average for all recipients with a primary diagnosis of glomerulonephritis, FSGS (11.8%) and mesangiocapillary glomerulonephritis type 1 (10.2%) were most likely to recur and cause graft loss. In contrast, graft loss because of recurrent IgA and pauci-immune crescentic glomerulonephritis occurred in only 2% of patients at 10 years follow-up.

Interstitial Nephritis

A variety of chemical, bacterial, and immunological injuries to the kidney cause either generalized or localized changes that primarily affect the tubulointerstitium rather than the glomerulus. This group of disorders is characterized by alterations in tubular function that, in advanced cases, may cause secondary vascular and glomerular damage. Interstitial nephritis, including chronic pyelonephritis, is the primary diagnosis, accounting for 3.8% of patients admitted onto dialysis programs in the United States.[427] In the United Kingdom the number is nearer 10%.[425] Pyelonephritis is the term associated with a bacterial infection that causes this kind of damage and is the most common of the interstitial nephritides.[411] There are both acute and chronic types of pyelonephritis, with the acute type most commonly associated with urinary tract infection. This can then develop into chronic pyelonephritis, usually as a result of a renal tract abnormality, such as abnormal urethral valves. Interstitial nephritis is also associated with proteinuria that is less severe than in glomerular disease. In addition to conventional pyelonephritis, interstitial nephritis may present in acute and chronic forms and has many causes. Acute interstitial nephritis presents with ARF and marked inflammation of the interstitium. Lymphocytes, polymorphonuclear cells, and eosinophils are prominent. The incidence is variable and depends on kidney biopsy practice. It may account for up to 7% of cases of ARF when an intrinsic kidney disease is diagnosed as opposed to purely toxic and/or ischemic acute tubular damage.[337] Higher values are likely in older people because of the increased incidence of drug reactions. A drug hypersensitivity reaction is the most common form of acute interstitial nephritis. Urinary findings may be normal or there may be low-level proteinuria and eosinophils can be seen on light microscopy. More than 100 different drugs have been implicated but NSAIDs and β-lactam antibiotics are the drugs most commonly identified.[121] Nephrotic syndrome may accompany an acute interstitial nephritis associated with NSAIDs. Treatment is directed at removing any causative agent. Steroids are used to promote early resolution of clinical course although patients can develop chronic interstitial fibrosis.[379]

Sarcoidosis is a multisystem disorder associated with chronic granulomatous interstitial nephritis. Biochemical abnormalities include hypercalcemia, hypercalciuria, and elevated serum ACE activity.[357] The condition may be effectively treated with steroids.

Polycystic Kidney Disease

Autosomal dominant polycystic kidney disease (ADPKD) is the second most common inherited monogenic disease (after familial hypercholesterolemia), with an estimated incidence of 1:1000. It is by far the most common inherited kidney disease.[118] According to data from the United Kingdom Renal Registry Report (2002), ADPKD is responsible for almost 9% of new ESRD in patients aged less than 65 years and 3.3% of incident patients over age 65.[425] The prevalence of the disease ranges from 1 in 200 to 1 in 1000 of the population, but many cases, possibly up to 50%, remain clinically undiagnosed during life. The disease causes the development of multiple kidney cysts and extrarenal cysts occurring in the liver and pancreas. About 10% of

ADPKD families have a strong family history of intracranial artery aneurysm rupture. Hypertension is an early and frequent manifestation, and gross hematuria is a common presenting symptom.

Approximately 50% of ADPKD patients develop ESRD by age 55.[118] An important clinical observation is the highly variable phenotype within families. The two major genes mutated in ADPKD, *PKD1* and *PDK2*, have been identified.[179,214,346] The most common mutation (found in 86% of cases) is the *PKD1* mutation on chromosome 16, which codes for an abnormal form of the protein polycystin (460 kDa), which has been shown to have a role in epithelial cell differentiation, regulation of cell adhesion, and apoptosis. Other mutations include the *PDK2* mutation on chromosome 4 (110 kDa) and APKD3, for which the gene product and chromosomal location remain as yet unknown.[319] *PKD2* appears to be a more slowly progressing form of the disease.[153] The median age of onset of ESRD with *PKD2* is 15 years later than *PKD1*. There is also a rare (incidence 1/20,000) autosomal recessive form of the disease that presents in childhood.

Toxic Nephropathy

A wide variety of nephrotoxins exist in the environment, many of which are associated with particular occupations. A variety of heavy metals, such as cadmium and lead, have long been known to be associated with kidney disease, often causing proximal tubular dysfunction and glomerular damage (see Chapter 35).[466] A summary of the drugs and environmental toxins known to cause kidney damage is given in Table 45-11. Both glomerular and tubulointerstitial damage result from exposure to these toxins; detection of both requires biochemical monitoring of GFR and tubular and glomerular proteinuria.

Obstructive Uropathy

Benign prostatic hypertrophy (BPH) is one of the most common types of obstructive uropathy and an almost universal finding in aging men.[276] For example, for men over 50 years, the reported prevalence of BPH varies between 50% and 75%, but there is no close relationship between the degree of enlargement and the symptoms experienced.[67] Among the most common symptoms are disorders of micturition, in particular increased frequency, and in many cases this can progress to bladder outflow obstruction. Between 10% and 40% of men with bladder outflow obstruction caused by BPH present in acute retention.[276] Approximately 5% of this group have high-pressure chronic retention of urine, which can result in upper urinary tract obstruction and consequently CKD as a result of glomerular and tubular damage. Although medical treatments are available to decrease the rate of enlargement of the prostate, resection of the enlarged gland remains the most common surgical procedure performed on men. Urinary retention can be a chronic disorder with acute exacerbations requiring bladder decompression by catheterization. If the obstruction is not removed by operation, progressive kidney injury can occur as a result of backpressure along the urinary tract. It is important to identify those patients at risk of developing CKD, because failure to remove their enlarged gland can cause ESRD. Obstruction can also occur because of kidney stones, which can cause bilateral or unilateral damage. In children severe kidney damage can be caused by vesicoureteric reflux. One of the main complications of reflux, whether caused by obstruction or by an inherited defect, is the increased incidence of urinary tract infection. When the obstruction is relieved the kidney often regains some independent function. There is a tendency to slower progression to ESRD in obstructive uropathy compared with other kidney diseases.

Tubular Diseases

Types of tubular disease discussed in this section include renal tubular acidoses and inherited tubulopathies.

Renal Tubular Acidoses

The renal tubular acidoses (RTAs) comprise a diverse group of both inherited and acquired disorders affecting either the proximal or distal tubule. They are characterized by a hyperchloremic, normal anion gap; metabolic acidosis; and urinary bicarbonate or hydrogen ion excretion inappropriate for the plasma pH. They are the result of either failure to retain bicarbonate or inability of the renal tubules to secrete hydrogen ion. Typically the GFRs in RTAs are normal, or slightly reduced, and there is no retention of anions, such as phosphate and sulfate (as opposed to the acidosis of renal failure). Before attempting to understand the pathology of these conditions, the reader should ensure a good comprehension of normal renal acid-base (and ammonia) regulation (see Chapter 46).

Classification

The classification of the RTAs is based upon the biochemical expression and region of defect rather than an understanding of the exact molecular defect. The three categories of RTA are distal (dRTA, type I); proximal (pRTA, type II); and type IV, which is secondary to aldosterone deficiency or resistance. The term "type III RTA" (mixed proximal/distal defect) has been abandoned as it is no longer considered a separate entity.[123,324]

Distal RTA (Type I). Type I dRTA occurs most often in infants (sometimes transiently) or young children, but it may also be encountered in adults, where it is more common than pRTA. Clinical features generally include a metabolic acidosis, muscle weakness, nephrocalcinosis, and urolithiasis. The defect is an inability to secrete hydrogen ions in the distal tubule in the presence of a systemic acidosis. Several subtypes may be seen: urinary pH >5.5 is a common feature.[324]

Classic (Hypokalemic, Secretory) dRTA. The molecular basis is not known, but may include defects in the H^+-ATPase or H^+, K^+-ATPase transporters. dRTA may occur in association with a wide range of conditions, including (1) an

TABLE 45-11 Drugs and Environmental Toxins Associated With the Development of Nephropathy

Drug	Toxic Action
ACE inhibitors	Drastic drop in GFR in patients with bilateral renal artery stenosis High-dose captopril can cause proteinuria
NSAIDs/COX-2 inhibitors	Drastic drop in GFR in patients with circulatory insufficiency (e.g., cardiac failure) Hypovolemia; can also cause acute and chronic interstitial nephritis
Antirheumatoid drugs	
Calcineurin inhibitors (cyclosporine and tacrolimus)	Vasoconstriction, glomerular vasculopathy, and interstitial fibrosis
Gold salts	Membranous-type picture with nephrotic syndrome (mechanism unknown)
Mercury compounds	Membranous-type picture with nephrotic syndrome (mechanism unknown)
D-penicillamine	Membranous-type picture with nephrotic syndrome (mechanism unknown)
Antitumor drugs	
Mitomycin	Hemolytic-uremic syndrome
Cisplatin	Acute tubular necrosis
Methotrexate	Intraluminal precipitation and acute tubular necrosis
Antibiotics/antifungals	
Aminoglycosides	Acute tubular necrosis and interstitial nephritis[240]
Cephalosporins	Interstitial nephritis
Penicillin G	Interstitial nephritis
Ampicillin	Interstitial nephritis
Amoxicillin	Interstitial nephritis
Amphotericin	
Lithium	Distal tubular damage with nephrogenic diabetes insipidus
Allopurinol	Interstitial nephritis
Environmental toxins	
Mercury	Glomerulonephritis
Cadmium	Chronic interstitial nephritis
Lead	Hypertension and tubulointerstitial nephritis
Chromium	Increased tubular proteins and enzymuria
Vanadium	Increased tubular proteins and enzymuria
Nickel	Increased tubular proteins and enzymuria
Solvents: dry cleaning/paints	Glomerulonephritis
Paraquat	Free radical generator: acute tubular damage

ACE, Angiotensin converting enzyme; *NSAIDs*, nonsteroidal antiinflammatory drugs.

autosomal dominant condition (more common in females); (2) a sporadic, nonfamilial disease; (3) other genetic disorders (e.g., Wilson's disease); (4) dysproteinemias (e.g., hypergammaglobulinemia, cryoglobulinemia, amyloidosis); (5) disorders of calcium metabolism (e.g., primary hyperparathyroidism); and (6) a range of autoimmune disorders (e.g., SLE, Sjögren's syndrome, primary biliary cirrhosis, thyroiditis). The pathogenesis of nephrocalcinosis and urolithiasis may be the result of decreased urinary citrate excretion secondary to cellular acidosis.

Back-Leak dRTA. Although the kidney tubule retains the ability to secrete hydrogen ions, the gradient is not maintained because of back diffusion. Typically, this occurs in association with specific drug treatments (e.g., amphotericin B).

Voltage-Dependent (Hyperkalemic) dRTA. This is due to failure to maintain an intraluminal negative potential and thus promote hydrogen (and potassium) ion secretion. This may be seen with urinary tract obstruction, sickle cell disease, and treatment with amiloride or triamterene. This condition has many features in common with type IV RTA (see discussion later in this chapter). It is frequently associated with mild to moderate CKD, and hyperkalemia is caused in part by the decreased GFR in addition to decreased potassium excretion relative to the filtered load. In contrast to classic dRTA, potassium excretion cannot be increased in response to sodium sulfate (Na_2SO_4) administration, suggesting an isolated defect in hydrogen ion secretion. However, because hydrogen ion secretion is dependent on sodium reabsorption in the distal tubules, the primary defect could also be an impairment of distal tubular sodium reabsorption.

Incomplete dRTA. This is a less severe, normokalemic form, which may represent an early stage of overt dRTA.

Some patients acidify urine at a submaximal rate, but at a rate that is generally sufficient to maintain acid-base balance. Potassium wasting, hypokalemia, and hyperchloremia are generally not present. However, when patients are stressed or are given an acid load, their ability to excrete acid and to lower urine pH is suboptimal and urinary pH may exceed 5.5.

Proximal RTA (Type II). In pRTA the primary defect is failure of proximal tubular bicarbonate reabsorption. This may occur as an isolated defect (primary or sporadic type II pRTA) that occurs chiefly in infant males and is commonly associated with growth retardation, or that produces a general Fanconi syndrome. Acquired diseases that may also produce a Fanconi syndrome and pRTA include multiple myeloma, Sjögren's syndrome, amyloidosis, heavy metal poisoning, and renal transplant rejection. Drugs that act as carbonic anhydrase inhibitors (e.g., acetazolamide and topiramate) have also produced a pRTA condition. (Note that several of these disorders and agents also cause dRTA.) In pRTA the threshold for bicarbonate reclamation is lowered (from a plasma concentration of 22 mmol/L to 15 mmol/L).[324] Once plasma bicarbonate falls below this threshold, filtered bicarbonate is reclaimed, and urinary pH will generally be <5.5. In pRTA, contrary to dRTA, nephrocalcinosis and nephrolithiasis are rarely observed but metabolic bone disease is common. Other features of the Fanconi syndrome (e.g., glycosuria, aminoaciduria, hypophosphatemia, and hypouricemia) are commonly present.

Selective Aldosterone Deficiency (Type IV RTA). In type IV RTA, there is failure of distal potassium and hydrogen ion secretion because of aldosterone deficiency or resistance. This may occur because of a range of steroid or steroid receptor synthetic defects or because of hyporeninemic hypoaldosteronism (e.g., due to diabetic nephropathy, tubulointerstitial disease, urinary obstruction, renal transplantation, or SLE). Hyperkalemia, although mild, is a usual manifestation.

Diagnosis of RTA

The finding of a hyperchloremic metabolic acidosis in a patient without evidence of gastrointestinal bicarbonate losses and with no obvious pharmacological cause should prompt suspicion of an RTA. The presence of suggestive clinical (e.g., nephrocalcinosis in dRTA) or biochemical (e.g., hypophosphatemia and hypouricemia as a result of proximal tubular wasting in pRTA) features should also be considered.

In addition to plasma electrolyte (including potassium) measurement, preliminary investigation should include measurement of urinary pH in a fresh, early morning urine sample. The finding of a urine pH > 5.5 in the presence of a systemic acidosis supports the diagnosis of dRTA, although it is not specific and will also be seen in types II and IV RTAs. If appropriate urinary acidification cannot be demonstrated, further investigation may involve assessing the kidneys' ability to excrete an acid load (ammonium chloride load test) and reabsorb filtered bicarbonate (fractional bicarbonate excretion). Further details of the conduct and interpretation of these tests may be found in the 1999 review by Penney and Oleesky.[324]

Treatment of RTA

Treatment of the RTAs is aimed at (1) correcting the biochemical disturbance and, where possible, underlying disorder, (2) improving growth in children, and (3) avoiding the development and progression of CKD. In both type I and II RTAs, bicarbonate is administered to correct the metabolic acidosis. Fludrocortisone and loop diuretics may be used to treat type IV RTA.

Inherited Tubulopathies

The inherited tubulopathies comprise a heterogeneous set of disorders often characterized by electrolyte disturbances. Most are eponymous and have been described clinically for many years. However, increased understanding of the molecular biology of tubular ion channel and transport pumps has now delineated the mechanism of disease in many of these disorders. In addition to electrolyte disturbances (particularly of potassium), general reasons to suspect a tubulopathy include a familial disease pattern, renal impairment, nephrocalcinosis, and stone formation, especially if these should present at an early age. In cases in which a diuretic-sensitive channel is affected, these disorders will clearly mimic the effects of diuretic use (see discussion later in this chapter) and exclusion of covert use of diuretics is important. Although individually uncommon or rare, an awareness of these disorders is critical for the clinical biochemist when considering the potential differential diagnoses in patients presenting with electrolyte imbalances. A brief description of these disorders follows; for more detailed information the reader is referred to the citation list, including several reviews of this subject.[321,371,374] This section should be considered in conjunction with the aforegoing description of tubular electrolyte handling (see "Electrolyte Homeostasis").

Bartter's Syndrome

This is a group of autosomal recessive disorders characterized by (1) renal salt wasting, (2) polyuria, (3) polydipsia, (4) impaired urinary concentrating ability, (5) a hyperreninemic, hypokalemic metabolic alkalosis, and (6) a mild hypomagnesemia in some patients. Biochemically the effects resemble those of loop diuretic use, but clinically the phenotype is highly variable. This arises because of the fact that the syndrome encompasses defects of three different transporters/channels in the loop of Henle. The biochemical effects are predictable from knowledge of the function of these transporters and channels (see Figure 45-7).

Mutations in the genes encoding for NKCC2 (type I) or ROMK1 (type II) are associated with the more severe phenotype, including polyhydramnios, premature birth, life-threatening salt wasting in the perinatal period, and hypercalciuria. Patients with ROMK1 defects tend to have less severe hypokalemia.

The milder ("classic," type III) Bartter's syndrome is due to defects in the basolateral pump CLC-Kb. Although the phenotype is extremely variable (neonatal, life-threatening presentations do occur), these patients typically present in the first year of life with weakness and hypovolemia and normal urinary calcium excretion. Nephrocalcinosis and kidney stone formation are not normally features.

Gitelman's Syndrome

This autosomal recessive disorder is also characterized by a hypokalemic, hyperreninemic, hypomagnesemic, metabolic alkalosis but presentation is generally much later in life than in Bartter's syndrome and hypocalciuria is typical. Clinical features include reduced blood pressure, weakness, paresthesia, tetany, fatigue, and salt craving.[16] The urinary calcium:creatinine excretion ratio can be useful in distinguishing between Gitelman's and Bartter's syndromes. The molecular defect is in the thiazide-sensitive NCCT transporter and the biochemistry can therefore mimic the effects of thiazide use (see Figure 45-7).

Liddle's Syndrome

This autosomal dominant disorder is also characterized by a hypokalemic, hypomagnesemic metabolic alkalosis but, in contrast to Bartter's and Gitelman's syndromes, there is hypertension and hyperreninism. The disease is due to activating mutations, which increase sodium transport through the ENaC channel with consequent enhanced kaliuresis (see Figure 45-8).

Pseudohypoaldosteronism Type I

This condition presents in infancy with salt wasting, hypotension, hyperkalemia, and significant hypereninism and aldosteronism. Two different molecular mechanisms are causative. Type Ia (autosomal recessive) is caused by inactivating mutations of the ENaC gene, while type Ib (autosomal dominant) is caused by mutations in the mineralocorticoid gene. In both cases, sodium loss in the collecting duct is increased with consequent retention of potassium.

Dent's Disease

Dent's disease is an X-linked condition characterized by hypercalciuria and kidney stone formation, low molecular weight proteinuria, aminoaciduria, hypophosphatemia, and rickets.[460] The disease arises from single-base change mutations, of which approximately 60 have been described, in the gene coding for the tubular chloride channel CLC-5. The exact relationship between the loss of function of this protein and the resulting Fanconi syndrome remains unclear.[410] Although X-linked, a mild form of the disease can be seen in females because of lyonization. The related syndromes (1) X-linked recessive nephrolithiasis, (2) X-linked recessive hypophosphatemic rickets, and (3) Japanese idiopathic low molecular weight proteinuria are also all related to defects in CLC-5.[410]

Phosphate Disorders

Several disorders of tubular phosphate handling have been described. The best known of these is X-linked dominant hypophosphatemic rickets (previously known as vitamin D–resistant rickets). This disorder arises because of a defect in the *PHEX* gene. A defect of the sodium-dependent/phosphate co-transporter has also been described, giving rise to autosomal recessive hereditary hypophosphatemic rickets with hypercalciuria. The molecular biology of these and other renal phosphate transport disorders has been reviewed.[408]

Other tubulopathies beyond the scope of this textbook include (1) hypomagnesemic hypercalciuric nephrocalcinosis ("congenital magnesium losing kidney"), (2) Gordon's syndrome (pseudohypoaldosteronism type II), (3) Lowe's syndrome (oculocerebral dystrophy), and (4) a series of disorders of the Ca-SR.[321,371,374]

Diuretics

Diuretics are among the most widely prescribed drugs. They are predominantly used to treat either hypertension and/or disorders associated with fluid overload. All diuretics act by interfering with tubular reabsorption of sodium and/or chloride and therefore have accompanying effects on water retention. Diuretics are taken up by tubular cells across the basolateral membrane by specific anion- (e.g., furosemide and thiazides) or cation- (e.g., amiloride and triamterene) exchangers and then secreted into the lumen by a process that has not been fully elucidated.[136] Different classes of diuretics act at different sites along the nephron. A basic understanding of these processes is helpful in understanding both the potency of different diuretic classes and their importance in the investigation of electrolyte disorders, in particular hypokalemia. Many diuretics will cause hypokalemia to some degree, depending on the potency, dose, duration of treatment, and the patient's underlying potassium balance.

Loop Diuretics

Loop diuretics act largely by blocking sodium and chloride reabsorption in the ascending limb of the loop of Henle. Since this is a site at which 30% of sodium reabsorption normally occurs, these are considered potent diuretics. Loop diuretics specifically inhibit NKCC2, and therefore also have an effect on potassium handling in the ascending limb. Consequent changes in transepithelial potential result in a direct kaliuretic effect in this region,[135] causing a hypercalciuria (see Figure 45-7). Loop diuretics also paralyze the macula densa segment, stimulating renin secretion and subsequent aldosterone release, further exacerbating the kaliuresis. Most significantly, blockage of loop sodium reabsorption results in enhanced delivery to the distal tubule, where sodium is reabsorbed in exchange for potassium secretion.[135] The affinity of loop diuretics for NKCC2 is bumetanide = torasemide > piretanide > furosemide = azosemide.[136]

Thiazide Diuretics

The benzothiadiazine group of compounds inhibit NCCT in the distal tubule. Since only 5% to 10% of sodium reabsorption occurs at this site, they are less potent than the loop diuretics but hypokalemia is still common as a result of increased sodium delivery to the collecting duct. Thiazide diuretics also have secondary effects resulting in increased calcium reabsorption.[136]

"Potassium-Sparing" Diuretics

These diuretics act by reducing sodium reabsorption in the collecting duct, and hence increasing potassium retention. Spironolactone acts as a competitive antagonist of aldosterone, blocking its stimulatory effects on sodium reabsorption via the mineralocorticoid receptor. Amiloride and triamterene both inhibit ENaC. The danger of this group of diuretics is that they can induce hyperkalemia, which is particularly likely to occur in patients with kidney disease.

Diabetes Insipidus

Primary functions of the kidney include the conservation of water and production of a concentrated urine. A range of conditions are associated with disturbances of the renal concentrating mechanism, resulting in polyuria and an inability to produce hypertonic urine. General conditions giving rise to this picture include hypercalcemia, hypokalemia, and CKD. Specifically, diabetes insipidus (DI) is due to the absence of an ADH effect, either because of impaired or failed secretion (cranial or central DI) or lack of end-organ response to ADH (nephrogenic DI). A further disorder, psychogenic polydipsia or compulsive water drinking, can also present as diabetes insipidus. These individuals may fail to concentrate urine even in response to fluid restriction or synthetic ADH as a result of medullary "washout"; sustained fluid ingestion destroys the hyperosmolality of the medulla, which may take some time to recover. The differentiation and pathology of these three conditions are discussed in Chapter 50. It should be noted that a vast diuresis can also be induced by consuming excessive fluid volumes (e.g., heavy beer drinkers).

Congenital nephrogenic diabetes insipidus is associated with defects that have now been characterized at the molecular level.[27] Most (>90%) congenital nephrogenic DI patients have mutations in the *AVPR2* gene, which codes for the ADH V_2 receptor. This results in a rise to an X-linked form of DI, with an estimated prevalence of 4 per 1 million males.[27] In <10% of cases, there is an autosomal recessive inheritance pattern caused by mutations in the *AQP2* gene. It has been suggested that measurement of the urinary excretion of AQP may be useful diagnostically.[84,300] Acquired forms of DI are more common than congenital forms. Downregulation of AQP2 has been observed in a variety of acquired forms of DI, including lithium treatment, hypokalemia, hypercalcemia, ureteric obstruction, and in animal models, chronic kidney failure.[300]

Renal Calculi

Nephrolithiasis is the diseased condition associated with the presence of renal calculi. Renal calculi, commonly termed kidney stones, occur in the renal pelvis, the ureter, or the bladder. In developed countries, bladder stones are now uncommon, as the causative factors of malnutrition and infection have been eliminated.[365] Calcification can also occur scattered throughout the parenchyma (nephrocalcinosis). Kidney stone formation is often considered to be a nutritional or environmental disease, linked to affluence, but genetic or anatomical abnormalities are also significant. Approximately 5% to 10% of the population of the western world are thought to have formed at least one kidney stone by the age of 70 years[188,365] and the prevalence of kidney stones may be increasing.[400] In both males and females, the average age of first stone formation is decreasing (Robertson WG, personal communication). For most stone types, there is a male preponderance. The passage of a stone is associated with severe pain called renal colic, which may last for 15 minutes to several hours and is commonly associated with nausea and vomiting.[452] There is some evidence that stone formation contributes to the development of CKD.[122]

Background

Chemically, urine contains many mineral salts that are present in concentrations that approach their solubility products, and the solutions are metastable. Anyone who has seen a urine sample before and after refrigeration has witnessed the consequences of this in the massive crystal deposits that form on cooling. Crystals can form spontaneously if the salt concentrations are high enough, or alternatively, preformed nuclei can provoke their formation. Human urine contains a number of promoters of stone formation and a variety of inhibitors, the concentrations of which can be influenced by dietary and metabolic factors (Figure 45-16).

Initial diagnosis and investigation of stones require radiological investigations to explore the degree of intrarenal calcification and papillary damage. Plain x-rays are undertaken at initial presentation, although it should be noted that urate and other purine stones and some cystine stones are radiolucent. An intravenous urogram or spiral computed tomography scan may be performed to establish the presence and extent of urinary tract obstruction, intrarenal reflux, and ureteric dilation. Further investigation of the patient with kidney stones or suspected of being a stone former involves analysis of blood, urine, and the stone itself, should one be obtained.[73,163]

Small stones (<5 mm in diameter) pass spontaneously in the urine as "gravel."[452] Although surgical treatment to remove large staghorn calculi may still be necessary, the most common form of treatment is ultrasonic extracorporeal shock wave lithotripsy (ESWL),[338] which can be applied to

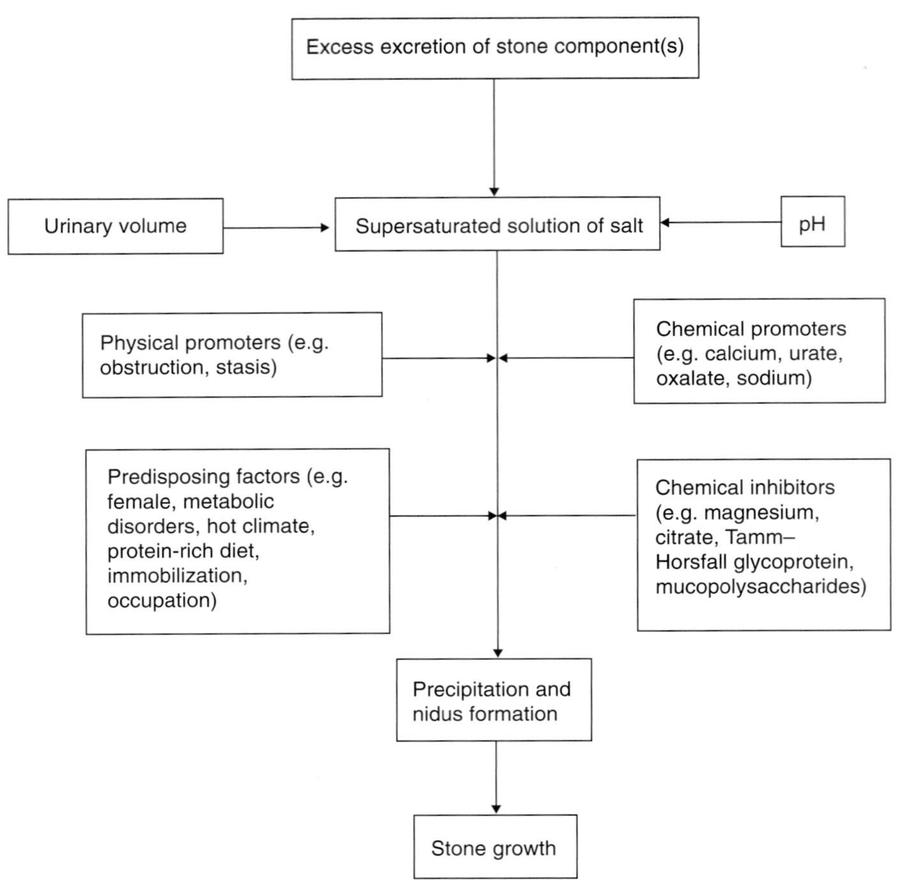

Figure 45-16 Diagrammatic representation of the interplay of factors involved in kidney stone formation. High or low pH may act as a promoter or inhibitor of stone formation depending on the stone type in question (e.g., calcium stone formation is favored by inadequate acidification while urate is less soluble in acidic urine). Controversy exists as to whether formed stones become trapped as they pass through the nephron ("free particle theory") or whether stone formation occurs at damaged sites on the tubule wall ("fixed particle theory").

stones between 5 mm and 2 cm in diameter. Although this allows noninvasive destruction of stones, the long-term sequelae of exposing the kidney to high-intensity sound waves have not been fully established.[122] Additionally, evidence is mounting that ESWL may be associated with higher recurrence rates than invasive treatment.[405] Percutaneous nephrolithotomy may be required if ESWL fails and also in the removal of cystine stones.

Following treatment and successful removal of a stone, follow-up monitoring is required, as many patients will have recurrent disease: in the absence of medical treatment the recurrence rate may be as high as 50% at 10 years.[247] The mechanisms responsible for the multiple recurrences of kidney stones in only certain individuals are not completely understood. Factors involved include (1) urine flow (fluid intake); (2) excretion of excess quantities of stone components; (3) the relative absence of a substance, or substances, in the urine that inhibit stone formation; and (4) urinary pH (see Figure 45-16). The predominant risk factor is poor hydration, a concentrated urine increasing the concentrations of the mineral salts further, predisposing to crystallization. This at least partially explains the increased incidence of kidney stone disease in hot climates, for example, in the Gulf states.

Kidney Stone Analysis

The majority of kidney stones found in the western world are composed of one or more of the following substances: (1) calcium oxalate with or without phosphate (frequency 67%), magnesium ammonium phosphate (12%); (2) calcium phosphate (8%); (3) urate (8%); (4) cystine (1% to 2%); and (5) complex mixtures of the above (2% to 3%).[365] These poorly soluble substances crystallize within an organic matrix, the nature of which is not well understood.

When available, analysis of the chemical constituents of stones may be useful in establishing the etiology and in planning rational therapy. It complements and guides metabolic investigation of the patients and may be particularly useful in identifying rare stone types (e.g., xanthine and dihydroxyadenine), artefacts (e.g., Munchausen syndrome), or drugs precipitating in the urinary tract, such as triamterene[398] and indinavir.[221] Conversely, it has been argued that stone analysis is not useful clinically,[162] since the stone material passed often does not represent the initial metabolic derangement. This is due to the phenomenon known as epitaxy, whereby nonspecific stone material, typically arising as a result of urinary tract infection (e.g., struvite), may accumulate on a preexisting "metabolic" nidus, the latter of which may not be detected during stone analysis. Clearly, for stone analysis to be useful it must be accurate. A variety of techniques have been used over the years. Traditionally, stones were crushed, solubilized, and the resulting solution analyzed (at several dilutions when appropriate) using conventional qualitative or semiquantitative chemical methods. Such techniques require relatively large amounts of stone, may miss rare and artefactual material, and analytically often perform poorly.[365] More sophisticated approaches including thermogravimetric analysis,[359] x-ray diffraction crystallography, and particularly, infrared spectroscopy[23,166] are preferred.[206] A detailed description of the infrared method is beyond the scope of this chapter; the reader is referred to descriptions in the scientific literature.[23,166,206]

Metabolic Investigation of Kidney Stone Formers

Ensuring adequate fluid intake remains the cornerstone of management of stone disease. However, specific management of disease depending on the metabolic abnormality present is also important and a treatment rationale is emerging. There have been several misconceptions about the role of diet in stone formation and optimal treatment may, at first, appear counter-intuitive; some of these paradoxes are discussed below.

Further investigation of stone formers may be guided by knowledge of the type of stone formed. However, the increasing use of lithotripsy means that there is often no stone material available for analysis. Consequently a management strategy focusing on the cause of stone formation and based upon knowledge of blood and urinary composition is useful. Although historically, metabolic investigations have often been targeted at recurrent stone formers only,[73] the increasing availability of simple assays for chemical risk factors and the health-economic burden of renal colic suggest that they are likely to become more widespread.[162,339] However, in some instances, it is not possible to demonstrate a biochemical abnormality in stone-forming individuals beyond a persistently small urine volume.

A variety of metabolic screening strategies have been proposed in stone-forming patients.* The chosen strategy should balance convenience for the patient and the laboratory against ability to intervene therapeutically. For example, although Tamm-Horsfall glycoprotein is known to inhibit stone formation, in the absence of a specific treatment, there is little merit in quantitating it. A reasonable approach would probably include measurement of plasma sodium, potassium, chloride, bicarbonate, creatinine, calcium, phosphate, and urate together with 24-hour urinary volume, pH, calcium, magnesium, phosphate, oxalate, urate, creatinine, sodium, citrate, microbiology (to exclude infection), and cystine (screening test). Some investigators have proposed complex "supersaturation indices" that combine the information obtained from these studies in a numerical index.[316,355,412] Metabolic evaluation should be undertaken at least 6 weeks after the episode of renal colic and should ideally be done on several occasions.[165] It is most informative when undertaken on an outpatient basis with patients pursuing their normal diet and lifestyle. Urinary pH and cystine should be measured on a fresh, early morning urine sample. A brief description of the role and measurement of these risk factors is given below, focusing predominantly on the investigation of calcium stone formers.

*References 73, 163, 165, 339, 365, 413.

Calcium

The majority of stones formed in the western world are composed of calcium, most commonly in association with oxalate although calcium phosphate and urate may also be present, either alone or in combination with calcium oxalate. As a consequence urinary calcium measurement has been the central investigation. However, the significant role of oxalate is increasingly appreciated and this has resulted in changes to the optimal management of hypercalciuria. As a rough guide, calcium oxalate stones tend to suggest hyperoxaluria as the main cause while calcium phosphate stones implicate hypercalciuria and/or failure to adequately acidify urine.[365] A strict definition of hypercalciuria is difficult as there is significant overlap between stone-forming and nonstone forming individuals but a cutoff of 0.1 mmol/kg body weight (4 mg/kg) is useful.[54] Excretion in excess of this is the most common metabolic abnormality seen in calcium stone formers, being observed in up to 50% of patients.

Traditionally, some investigation strategies focused on whether patients demonstrated hypercalciuria while fasting ("renal hypercalciuria") or in response to a calcium load ("absorptive hypercalciuria").[452] This classification was used as the basis of a treatment strategy in patients with absorptive hypercalciuria who have abnormally high intestinal calcium absorption compared with nonstone formers (possibly because of a relative increase in $1,25(OH)_2D_3$ concentrations and/or changes in intestinal vitamin D receptor activity). Treatment in these patients focused on dietary modification of calcium intake. Patients with renal hypercalciuria are now thought not to have a renal transport defect but to have increased turnover of skeletal calcium, although the management of such patients may involve pharmacological modification of renal calcium handling (e.g., thiazide diuretics).[452]

However, convincing evidence questions the usefulness of this classification and these therapeutic approaches. Dietary restriction of calcium is now generally regarded as ineffective, and actually counterproductive, as it results in an increase in intestinal oxalate absorption and increased risk of stone formation.[63,77] Further, patients with hypercalciuria are known to have reduced bone mineral density, and dietary calcium restriction may exacerbate a tendency to osteopenia and/or osteoporosis.[417,444]

A more useful approach is to classify hypercalciuric patients into either hypercalcemic or nonhypercalcemic causes. The former is most commonly due to primary hyperparathyroidism, which is seen in approximately 5% of stone formers. Treatment involves neck exploration and removal of the adenoma, although the risk of a stone recurring remains high for several years after parathyroidectomy.[284] Nonhypercalcemic causes of hypercalciuria constitute the majority of patients and are generally classified as idiopathic (although causes such as RTA, high sodium intake, and prolonged immobilization should be excluded). In addition to increasing fluid consumption, idiopathic hypercalciuric patients appear to benefit from a diet that is low in animal protein and sodium.[41,354] Animal protein consumption increases the production of metabolic acids, increasing urinary calcium excretion and decreasing urinary citrate (see discussion later in this chapter).[54] It also increases uric acid excretion. High sodium excretion as a result of high consumption inhibits tubular reabsorption of calcium, with a consequent increase in risk of calcium stone formation. Sodium is easily and cheaply measured in urine and represents a modifiable risk factor. Other therapeutic maneuvers that may be useful include the use of thiazide diuretics or alkaline citrate, reducing oxalate, and increasing fiber intake.[413] Some of these factors are discussed in more detail below.

Magnesium

With calcium stone disease, magnesium is an inhibitor of stone growth. Magnesium forms complexes with oxalate that are more soluble than calcium oxalate. Increased urinary magnesium therefore inhibits stone formation.[146] Administration of magnesium has been shown to reduce enteral calcium absorption and has been proposed as a treatment for idiopathic hypercalciuric stone formers.[87] However, oral magnesium supplementation may have unpleasant side effects and a positive benefit in terms of reducing stone recurrence has not been demonstrated.[413]

Urate

Some investigators believe that urate may potentiate calcium stone formation, although this perception is not universally accepted.[365] However, hyperuricosuria is common in calcium stone–forming patients, and treatment with allopurinol, thereby decreasing urate synthesis, reduces the rate of stone recurrence. Allopurinol treatment is therefore recommended for hyperuricosuric patients with calcium stone disease.[413] The formation and management of pure urate stones are discussed in Chapter 24.

Oxalate

Oxalate is an end product of metabolism, predominantly derived from breakdown of glyoxylate and glycine. Plasma concentration of oxalate is 1.0 to 2.4 mg/L (11 to 27 µmol/L) and it is excreted in the urine at a rate of 17.5 to 35.1 mg/24 hours (200 to 400 µmol/24 hours).[457] Only 10% to 15% of urinary oxalate is derived directly from dietary sources.[413] Intestinal oxalate absorption is increased when the availability of calcium in the intestine is reduced. Hyperoxaluria is a powerful promoter of calcium oxalate stone formation; indeed, it is more significant in this respect than calcium itself.[365] Hyperoxaluria may occur as a result of excessive dietary intake, because of malabsorption and/or steatorrhea (enteric hyperoxaluria) or because of an inborn error of metabolism (primary hyperoxaluria).

Enteric hyperoxaluria commonly occurs in association with inflammatory bowel diseases and may contribute to an increased incidence of stone formation in such patients.[457] Fat malabsorption contributes to the formation of calcium soaps, increasing the enteric concentration of unbound oxalate that is absorbed through the damaged bowel wall. Primary hyperoxaluria may be type 1 (glycolic aciduria) or type 2 (L-glyceric aciduria). Patients with type 1 disease present in the first decade of life with recurrent calcium oxalate nephrolithiasis. Inheritance is autosomal recessive and survival is poor. Type 2 disease is rarer and has been claimed to run a milder course, despite the passage of similarly high concentrations of urinary oxalate. The urinary excretion of oxalate may increase to 61.4 mg/day (700 µmol/day) when a diet containing an excess of oxalate-rich foods is taken and to as much as 263 mg/day (3 mmol/day) in patients with primary hyperoxaluria.

Ideally, urine for oxalate analysis should be collected into acid to prevent the crystallization of calcium oxalate crystals. This also prevents ex vivo formation of oxalate from ascorbate, a cause of factitious hyperoxaluria in individuals ingesting excessive amounts of vitamin C. A number of approaches to the measurement of urinary oxalate have been employed including high-performance liquid chromatography (HPLC), enzymatic and capillary electrophoretic methods.[159,171,233,327] The enzymatic methods employ the enzyme oxalate oxidase (EC 1.2.3.4. oxalate:oxygen oxidoreductase). With this method, the sample of urine is initially acidified to pH 1.8 (typically with 2 mmol/L HCl) to ensure complete solubilization of any calcium oxalate crystals. The oxalate is oxidized to carbon dioxide and hydrogen peroxide by oxalate oxidase, and the hydrogen peroxide is detected with horseradish peroxidase and coupled with an oxygen acceptor reagent such as 3-dimethyl aminobenzoic acid and 3-methyl-2-benzothiazolinone hydrazone to yield an indamine dye that absorbs at 590 nm. Laker and colleagues[230] have proposed a charcoal column pretreatment step to remove interferents from the urine. Petrarulo and colleagues[327] did not find this necessary. In addition, they found the method could also be used for deproteinized plasma samples. An alternative approach to the detection of hydrogen peroxide using catalase has also been described.[159] The oxalate oxidase is specific for oxalate; however, the peroxide detection reaction may suffer from interferences (e.g., turbidity in the catalase-mediated reaction, ascorbic acid, and other reducing agents in the peroxidase-mediated reaction). The choice of oxygen acceptor will determine the potential for interference from species, such as ascorbic acid.

A dietary history is important in the evaluation of calcium oxalate stone formers. Patients who are excreting large amounts of oxalate may be offered dietary advice to modify their risk of future stone formation. Foods rich in oxalate include beets, tea, spinach, sorrel, wheat bran, strawberries, rhubarb, black currants, peanuts, and chocolate.[365,413,452] Paradoxically, epidemiological evidence has actually demonstrated a protective effect of high tea consumption.[78] This has been attributed to the low bio-availability of oxalate in tea and the inhibition of tubular ADH action by caffeine. Patients may also be treated with calcium carbonate, which binds oxalate in the gut, rendering it unavailable for absorption. Alternatively, pyridoxine (vitamin B_6) may be used; this increases the catabolism of oxalate to more soluble products.[452] It should be remembered that the use of calcium-lowering diets, once favored in the treatment of calcium stone formers, increases intestinal absorption of oxalate.

Citrate

Urinary citrate inhibits stone formation by forming soluble complexes with calcium. It is present in the diet in many fruits. Excretion (typically between 116 and 926 mg/24 hours [0.6 and 4.8 mmol/24 hours] for adult males and 250 and 1160 mg/24 hours [1.3 and 6.0 mmol/24 hours] for adult females)[365] is reduced in the calcium stone–forming population.[412] Urinary citrate measurement may be of value in the assessment of stone-forming risk, particularly in the setting of distal renal tubular acidosis where the reduction in filtered bicarbonate appears to increase tubular reabsorption of citrate with consequent hypocitraturia.[147] Inadequate urinary acidification compounds the increased risk of calcium stone formation. Treatment with carbonic anhydrase inhibitors (e.g., acetazolamide[312] and topiramate[197]) mimics distal renal tubular acidosis with consequent increase in stone risk. Hypocitraturia may also be seen in malabsorption and urinary tract infection. Administration of oral alkaline citrate increases urinary citrate concentration by increasing the pH of tubular cells. It has been shown to be effective in the treatment of nephrolithiasis,[313,413] although there are side effects and compliance is poor.

Citrate is measured by gas chromatography, capillary electrophoresis,[171] or an enzyme-mediated reaction.[283] While methods using aconitase (EC 4.2.1.3) and isocitrate dehydrogenase (EC 1.1.1.42), or citrate lyase (EC 4.1.3.6) and oxaloacetate decarboxylase (EC 4.1.1.3), have been described, a method using the lyase together with malate dehydrogenase (EC 1.1.1.37) and lactate dehydrogenase (EC 1.1.1.27) is preferred. The combination of the two dehydrogenase pathways has been proposed to ensure that any oxaloacetate ion enzymatically decarboxylated is also measured. The enzyme-mediated decarboxylase pathway is less favored because of the poor stability of the enzyme. Using a reaction sequence that involves incubation of the sample with all constituents except the citrate lyase ensures that all endogenous oxaloacetate and pyruvate are removed. Analysis of serum involves a deproteinization step, while urine should be titrated to pH 8.0 before analysis. A typical incubation period is 10 to 15 minutes, and the citrate can be quantitated from the decrease in the absorbance at 340 nm.[283] A cheap, rapid, automated adaptation of this procedure, which does not require a deproteinizing step, has been described.[28]

Struvite Stones

Struvite stones (also called triple phosphate or infection stones) are composed of magnesium ammonium phosphate hexahydrate. The formation of such stones requires urinary tract infection with urea splitting organisms and such stones are therefore more common in females and in certain patient populations (e.g., paraplegics).[365] The risk of progression to CKD appears higher in patients who develop infection stones than in other forms of stone disease.[122]

CYSTINURIA

Cystinuria is an autosomal recessive condition in which there is excessive urinary excretion of cystine because of a defect in proximal renal tubular reabsorption. In the most common form of the disease there is also excess excretion of the dibasic amino acids (lysine, ornithine, and arginine). These share the same renal tubular transporter although their presence in excess in urine appears benign. More rarely, isolated cystinuria is seen. The reader should note that cystinuria should not be confused with cystinosis, which is a condition associated with intracellular accumulation of cystine but not excess urinary excretion of cystine.

The normal urinary excretion of cystine has been reported to be 4.81 to 48.1 mg/24 hours (40 to 400 µmol/24 hours).[365] Its relatively low limit of solubility, 18.0 mg/dL (1500 µmol/L),[452] is exceeded in many patients with cystinuria,[365] resulting in the formation of hexagonal crystals and, ultimately, cystine stones. Cystine stones are usually only seen in homozygotes, although there is some evidence that heterozygotes are at increased risk of stone formation.[128] Cystinuria may present at any age from infancy to old age, although presentation is most common in the second and third decades.

The finding of a cystine stone should prompt confirmation of cystinuria by urinary analysis.[365] It could be argued, however, that all stone formers should be screened for cystinuria; at least 10% of cystinurics form stones in which cystine cannot be detected, presumably because of epitaxis.[281] The index of suspicion should be increased in patients who are relatively young stone formers and in those with a positive family history. Once a cystinuric patient is diagnosed, it is important to screen all members of the family, particularly to detect affected siblings.

Cystine can be measured in urine using the cyanide-nitroprusside test,[45] thin layer chromatography, by quantitative amino acid analysis using either ion exchange or liquid chromatographic techniques[382] or mass spectrometry. In the cyanide-nitroprusside test, cystine is split into two molecules of cysteine by cyanide. Sodium nitroprusside reacts with the free sulfide groups to give a magenta color. The test is hazardous and will give false-negative results in acidified or infected urines, in patients receiving penicillamine therapy, or if the sodium nitroprusside solution is not fresh. Further, it cannot distinguish between cystine and homocystine or between heterozygote and homozygote cystinurics. It is not useful when monitoring the treatment of known cystinurics, who require quantitation of their urinary cystine output or concentration. In practice, amino acid analysis allows simultaneous quantitation of the dibasic amino acids, which may be helpful for characterizing the clinical phenotype.[382] Quantitative amino acid analysis is described in Chapter 20.

Treatment of cystinuria is aimed at maintaining cystine below its saturation point by maintaining high fluid intake, particularly at night. Other treatments include urinary alkalinization (cystine is more soluble in alkaline urine) and chelation with D-penicillamine. Quantitative analysis is an important adjunct for monitoring penicillamine therapy, which can be optimized on the basis of the free cystine versus cystine/penicillamine disulfide. Penicillamine itself may cause glomerular damage and thus regular monitoring of urinary protein excretion is also recommended.

Prostaglandins and NSAIDs in Kidney Disease

The prostaglandins are a series of C_{20} unsaturated fatty acid derivatives of cyclo-oxygenase (COX) on cell membrane arachidonic acid (see Chapter 26). The major renal vasodilatory prostaglandin is PGE_2, which is synthesized predominantly in the medulla. The major vasoconstrictor prostaglandin is thromboxane A_2, which is produced primarily within the renal cortex.[91] PGE_2 increases renal blood flow rate, inhibits sodium reabsorption in the distal nephron and collecting duct, and stimulates renin release.[91] These actions promote natriuresis and diuresis. In patients with CKD, renal PGE_2 excretion rates are 3 to 5 times higher than those in healthy subjects and therefore PGE_2 production represents a compensatory response to loss of nephron mass.[414] Vasodilatory prostaglandins are synthesized following stimulation with renal sympathetic adrenergic and AII-dependent mechanisms to offset or modulate vasoconstriction.[275] In the tubule, prostaglandins act as autocoids, exerting their effects locally, near the site of synthesis.

NSAIDs block the synthesis of COX products of arachidonic acid, which have a critical role in renal hemodynamics, control of tubular function, and renin release. It is now apparent that two isoforms of COX synthesize prostaglandins. COX-1 is a resident or constitutive form and COX-2 is an inducible form that increases with disorders of inflammation.[381] NSAIDs are nonspecific inhibitors of both COX isoforms. Analgesic nephropathy is a common cause of ESRD in a number of countries, reaching 10% in Switzerland and Australia, but is essentially a preventable condition for which biochemical monitoring has proved useful. The incidence of this disease has decreased over the last decade as awareness has improved and phenacetin was withdrawn from over-the-counter analgesic mixtures. In the United States, 1 in 5 citizens (50 million) report that they use an NSAID for an acute complaint.[448] Young healthy individuals tolerate NSAIDs well. However, older people demonstrate significant reduction of GFR within 1 week of ingestion of NSAIDs.[142] Renal blood flow, particularly within the medulla, is dependent on systemic and local production of vasodilatory prostaglandins, and analgesic-related kidney damage is seen mostly within the medulla, with late changes causing papillary necrosis and interstitial fibrosis. Hyperkalemia can develop either as a consequence of reduced GFR or secondary to hyporeninemic hypoaldosteronism.

In normal rat and dog kidney COX-2 is sparsely expressed in the macula densa, but expression is upregulated when animals are volume depleted.[152] Selective COX-2 inhibitors have been discovered but it is not known what the effects of these drugs will be on renal homeostasis. Acute interstitial nephritis has been described with COX-2 inhibitors.[160,264]

Monoclonal Light Chains and Kidney Disease

Immunoglobulin (Ig) molecules are formed in secretory B cells from polypeptide heavy (H) and light (L) chains. Disulfide bonds covalently assemble the chains. Each chain has a constant and a variable region. The heavy chains α, β, γ, δ, and ε denominate the antibody isotype and light chains include peptide molecules that are called kappa (κ) and lambda (λ). A complete Ig molecule will contain either κ or λ. The proportion of Ig containing κ versus λ is 3:2 in humans. The molecular weight of light chains is around 22.5 kDa (see Chapters 9 and 20). An excess production of light over heavy chains appears to be required for efficient Ig synthesis, resulting in the release of free light chains into the circulation. In normal individuals, the small quantity of circulating polyclonal light chains is filtered by the glomerulus and around 90% reabsorbed in the proximal tubule. The binding sites on the brush border of proximal tubule cells exhibit relative selectivity for light chains compared with albumin and lactoglobulin.[18] Light chains are then degraded by proteases and returned to the circulation. When the concentration of filtered light chains is increased, this leads to alteration in the proximal tubule cells, including prominent cytoplasmic vacuolation, loss of microvillus border, and epithelial cell exfoliation.[366]

There is evidence that light chains are directly pathogenic. The pattern of human renal injury associated with monoclonal light chains can be reproduced in mice injected intraperitoneally with large amounts of light chains isolated from patients with myeloma or light chain–associated amyloid (AL-amyloid).[223] In a rat model of multiple myeloma, spontaneously developing light chain–synthesizing tumors were transplanted to normal animals that subsequently developed crystalloid formations within phagolysosomes in proximal tubule cells.[396] Light chains can deposit in the kidney as casts, fibrils, and precipitates or crystals, giving rise to a spectrum of disease including cast nephropathy, amyloid, light chain deposition disease (LCDD), and the Fanconi syndrome. However, not all patients with a large excess production of monoclonal light chains develop disease. Other promoters including dehydration, hypercalcemia, contrast medium, and NSAIDs have been implicated.

Myeloma or multiple myeloma is a neoplastic proliferation of secretory B cells (plasma cells) that produce excess amounts of a monoclonal Ig (paraprotein), so-called M protein because of the characteristic peaks obtained from serum protein electrophoresis on agarose gel. This clonal production is associated with either an excess or pure light chain production. In multiple myeloma complete monoclonal Igs (usually IgG or IgA) are accompanied in the plasma by variable concentrations of free light chains that appear in the urine as Bence Jones proteins. Henry Bence Jones in London first described these in 1848. M proteins and light chains can be identified in the blood and/or the urine in 98% of patients with myeloma using protein electrophoresis and immunofixation. Immuneparesis, with reduction in nonparaprotein Ig, is characteristic of myeloma. The nephrotoxic potential of Bence Jones proteins has been demonstrated in elegant experiments on animal models.[397]

The incidence of myeloma is 40 new cases per million population per year.[456] Myeloma is more common in men than women and the median age at presentation is 65 years.[226] Impairment of kidney function at presentation occurs in almost 50% of patients.[85,456] Although most recover following treatment of other factors contributing to renal impairment (e.g., dehydration, hypercalcemia, infection, and nephrotoxic drugs) about 10% have severe renal involvement caused by the effects of light chains on the kidney. Severe kidney failure may be caused in myeloma following deposition of light chains within tubules in association with THG, so-called cast nephropathy (myeloma kidney). Cast nephropathy can present acutely, again precipitated by dehydration, hypercalcemia, or NSAIDs, or "de novo" in the absence of these factors. It occurs when the reabsorptive capacity of proximal tubule cells is exceeded by overproduction of light chains. In myeloma, light chain excretion can exceed 20 g/day. Casts are large and numerous and predominantly found in the distal convoluted tubule and collecting ducts, causing obstruction to urine flow. They have a hard and fractured appearance with lamination visible on histological examination of kidney biopsy specimens. Immunofluorescence confirms that casts are composed of monoclonal light chains and THG. Casts are usually stained exclusively with either anti-κ or anti-λ antibodies. At biopsy there is often an interstitial inflammatory infiltrate, and fibrosis and tubular atrophy can be extensive. Not all light chains induce cast formation. The ability of light chains to form casts is based on binding to THG, a highly glycosylated and acidic protein.[358] Light chains interfere with proximal tubule cell function and this increases delivery to the distal tubule. A specific binding site for light chains has been identified on THG, and light chains with high affinity appear to be more likely to produce obstructing intratubular casts.[178] Physico-chemical determinants of binding of light chains to THG include the isoelectric point (pI) of the light chain. Those molecules with a pI above 5.1 (above the tubular fluid pH in the distal nephron) will have a net positive charge that may promote binding via charge interaction to anionic THG (pI 3.2). Urinary alkalinization reduces binding of light chains to THG in animal models.[170] Nephrotoxicity may be determined by the ability of light chains to self-associate, leading to the formation of high molecular weight aggregates that are more likely to deposit in tissues, particularly in the setting of volume depletion.

The clinical features of myeloma include a normochromic normocytic anemia, bone pain with pathological fractures (back or chest rather than extremities), and hypercalcemia in 20% of patients. Severe kidney failure may dominate the clinical picture and 84% of patients studied retrospectively with severe renal impairment required dialysis.[183] Only 15% of these patients regained independent kidney function. Treatment has two main objectives: therapy is targeted at predisposing factors for cast nephropathy as indicated and chemotherapy is used to reduce the production of monoclonal antibodies and light chains from monoclonal plasma cells. Supportive therapy includes increased fluid intake where permissible to 3 L/day, treatment of hypercalcemia, treatment of infection, and withdrawal of NSAIDs. Anemia can be addressed by replacement with blood products or the use of epoetins. Epoetin has been demonstrated to be efficacious in a placebo-controlled study of 145 patients.[80] Skeletal complications are common in myeloma and pathological fractures occur in the setting of apparently trivial injury. There is increased osteoclastic activity mediated by interleukin (IL)-1, IL-6, TNF, and macrophage inflammatory protein-1α.[148] Biphosphonates are specific inhibitors of osteoclastic activity and have beneficial effects in myeloma.[21] Biphosphonates may exert direct antitumor effects on myeloma since they induce significant expansion of $\gamma\delta$-T cells in peripheral blood mononuclear cells, which exhibit specific cytotoxicity against myeloma cell lines in vitro.[225]

Chemotherapy can be considered as part of the urgent treatment for patients with kidney involvement in myeloma. The aim is to reduce the concentration of free light chains. Chemotherapy with alkylating agents such as melphalan, and combination treatment with cytotoxic agents and dexamethasone are the preferred initial treatment regimens and doses and schedules are adjusted depending on the level of GFR. Combination chemotherapy results in partial responses but only rarely complete remission.[3,137,256] Autologous bone marrow transplantation can be considered in some cases.[7] Estimated 5-year survival following bone marrow transplantation in one series of 200 patients was 52% compared with 12% in those patients treated with combined chemotherapy alone.

Poor prognostic features in myeloma include increased β_2-microglobulin, C-reactive protein, and lactate dehydrogenase (LD), and abnormal cytogenetics (especially deletion of 13q). Refractory disease is associated with a short survival, and treatment options include further chemotherapy and a trial of the antiangiogenesis compound thalidomide.[307,391] The rationale for thalidomide comes from the observations that prominent bone marrow vascularization occurs in myeloma and correlates with markers of poor prognosis, and that plasma levels of angiogenic cytokines are elevated in myeloma. Clinical trials of thalidomide in myeloma were first described in 1965 and more recent trials show some promise in terms of reduction of paraprotein load and 1-year survival.[391,463]

In addition to chemotherapy, plasma exchange is often used in the treatment of myeloma cast nephropathy to acutely reduce free light chain load. There is a paucity of trial data,[191,473] but one prospective study of 29 patients demonstrated an increased 1-year survival following plasma exchange treatment. However, several early deaths in the control group render the data difficult to interpret.[473] A further study of 21 patients with myeloma and ARF demonstrated advantages of plasma exchange in patients with kidney failure severe enough to require dialysis.[191] The United Kingdom Renal Association and the United Kingdom Myeloma Forum are currently recruiting almost 300 patients to a national study of plasma exchange in myeloma cast nephropathy (Myeloma Renal Impairment Trial-MERIT).

In cast nephropathy, there is glomerular filtration of *intact* light chains. Excess production of monoclonal light chains (or rarely heavy chains) can cause disorders in which *fragments* are deposited in the kidney and other tissues: AL-amyloid, LC- and HC-deposition diseases (LCDD and HCDD). The diagnosis of AL-amyloid can be suspected from the clinical findings of heavy proteinuria and serum or urinary paraprotein. However, 10% to 15% of patients with primary amyloid do not have a detectable serum or urinary paraprotein. The demonstration of a clonal excess of plasma cells on bone marrow biopsy may help with the diagnosis in those without detectable paraprotein. In AL-amyloid, fibrils derived from the variable region of light chains are deposited in the tissue. Seventy-five percent are derived from the λ-light chain. Since it is the variable region that is deposited, it is often difficult to assess with immune reactants. Only 50% of AL-amyloid cases are stainable with commercially available antisera to κ and λ. The deposits are fibrillar in nature and bind to Congo red. Amyloid fibrils also bind to serum amyloid P (SAP) component, allowing noninvasive evaluation by radiolabeled SAP scanning.[155]

The deposits in LCDD are usually composed of κ-light chains. They are granular and do not bind to Congo red, thioflavine-T, or SAP. The constant region of the light chain is typically deposited in this disorder and therefore immunostaining is strongly positive. These conditions may be associated with myeloma and other conditions leading to overproduction of monoclonal light chains, such as lymphoma. Both AL-amyloid and LCDD have a poor prognosis and the mean survival is 18 months, with 50% of patients dying from cardiac failure. Treatment options are unsatisfactory, although prednisolone and melphalan may be tried.[227,228,393] Circulating free light chains can be detected in most patients with AL-amyloid and patient outcome following treatment is improved if the concentration of free light chains can be reduced by 50%.[229]

The French Myeloma Group has published results of bone marrow or stem cell transplantation in AL-amyloid.[285] In a retrospective analysis of 21 patients treated with melphalan and stem cell transplantation, 43% died within 1 month and the remainder had a favorable outcome.

Light chains may cause tubular dysfunction, especially of the proximal tubular cells. Characteristically the light chain variable domain is resistant to degradation by proteases in lysosomes in the tubular cells. The variable domain fragments accumulate in proximal tubular cells, and clinical features include RTA and phosphate wasting.

ASSESSMENT OF RENAL CONCENTRATING ABILITY: URINARY OSMOLALITY

Urinary concentration can be quantified either by measuring specific gravity (see Chapter 24) or by measuring urinary osmolality. For most clinical purposes, measuring specific gravity is probably sufficient,[322] but urinary osmolality measurement is critical to the diagnosis and differential diagnosis of DI using the water deprivation test.

The urinary osmolality of normal individuals may vary widely, depending on the state of hydration. After excessive intake of fluids, for example, the osmotic concentration may fall as low as 50 mOsm/kg/H_2O, whereas in individuals with severely restricted fluid intake, concentrations of up to 1400 mOsm/kg/H_2O can be observed. In individuals on an average fluid intake, values of 300 to 900 mOsm/kg/H_2O are typically seen. If a random urine specimen of a patient has an osmolality of >600 mOsm/kg/H_2O (or >850 mOsm/kg/H_2O after 12 hours of fluid restriction), it can generally be assumed that the renal concentrating ability is normal.

In chronic progressive kidney disease, the concentrating ability of the tubules is diminished and in acute tubular necrosis the urinary osmolality, if there is urine output at all, approaches that of the glomerular filtrate.

For a discussion on the measurement of the urinary and plasma osmolality, readers are referred to Chapters 27 and 34.

RENAL REPLACEMENT THERAPY

RRT includes dialysis procedures such as HD, PD, continuous hemofiltration (HF), and continuous hemodiafiltration (HDF). These techniques are used to temporarily or permanently remove toxic substances from the blood when the kidneys cannot satisfactorily remove them from the circulation. In addition, kidney transplantation has also become an effective form of RRT. Extensive laboratory support is required by an RRT program (Table 45-12).

TABLE 45-12 Laboratory Support for Renal Replacement Therapy

Complications	Laboratory Tests
Acute	
Dialysis disequilibrium	Plasma electrolytes
Pyrexia	C-reactive protein
Bleeding	Clotting factors
Chronic	
Anemia	Hemoglobin, ferritin
Septicemia/peritonitis	C-reactive protein Culture and sensitivity
Malnutrition	Albumin, prealbumin
Cardiovascular disease	Lipid profiles
Amyloidosis	Serum β_2-microglobulin
Osteodystrophy	Ca^{2+}, PO^{-4}, bone alkaline phosphatase, intact PTH, aluminum
Adequacy of Dialysis	
Urea kinetic modeling (URR)	Predialysis and postdialysis urea
Weekly creatinine clearances	Predialysis and postdialysis creatinine
Peritoneal equilibration test (PET)	Plasma and dialysate creatine and glucose
Transplant Monitoring	
Immunosuppression	Trough or 2-hr whole blood cyclosporin A concentration Trough whole blood tacrolimus and rapamycin concentrations
Graft function	Serum creatinine, plasma, and urine electrolytes

BACKGROUND

In 1861, Thomas Graham Bell in Glasgow, Scotland, carried out the first dialysis experiments (and coined the term "dialysis"), separating crystalloids and colloids in a solution. Bell predicted that this technique could have medical application, but this was not realized until nearly 100 years later in the work of Willem Kolff and then Belding Scribner, who made HD a feasible treatment in the early 1960s. Since then, HD and more recently PD have extended the lives of many people, sometimes for up to 20 or 30 years.

DIALYSIS

Dialysis is the process of separating macromolecules from ions and low molecular weight compounds in solution by the difference in their rates of diffusion through a semipermeable membrane, through which crystalloids can pass readily but colloids pass very slowly or not at all. Two distinct physical processes are involved: diffusion and ultrafiltration (UF).[93]

The timing of initiation of dialysis treatment is controversial. There is debate as to whether early initiation of dialysis improves outcomes over late starters.[37,222,416] The K/DOQI 2000 Update Clinical Practice Guidelines suggest that dialysis should be started when kidney function drops below a GFR of 10.5 ml/min/1.73 m^2.[294] This is higher than the typical level in the United Kingdom. A 2002 study from Glasgow, Scotland, found no significant benefit in patient survival from earlier initiation of dialysis.[416] The calculated GFR at the beginning of dialysis was 8.3 mL/min.

Hemodialysis and Hemofiltration

HD is the most common method used to treat advanced and permanent kidney failure. Clinically, it is considered the default therapy that is utilized in the increasing numbers of patients unsuitable for other modalities of PD and kidney transplantation. Operationally, it involves connecting the patient to a hemodialyzer into which their blood flows. After filtration to remove the wastes and extra fluids, the cleansed blood is returned to the patient. It is still a complicated and inconvenient therapy requiring a coordinated effort from a healthcare team that includes the patient, nephrologist, dialysis nurse, dialysis technician, dietitian, and others.

Description

HD utilizes diffusive and convective mass transfer across a semipermeable membrane. The driving force for diffusion is the concentration gradient between blood and dialysate. Smaller solutes with larger concentration gradients give increased diffusion. The concentration gradient is maintained by using countercurrent flows and high flow rates. Heparinized blood is pumped in one direction across the membrane and the recipient fluid, the dialysate, flows at a rate of 5 to 600 mL/min in the opposite direction. Water molecules and small molecular weight molecules can cross the membrane, while larger proteins and cellular elements are retained in the vascular space. Convection is the bulk movement of solvent and dissolved solute across the membrane, down a transmembrane hydrostatic pressure gradient.

HD relies on good vascular access to the circulation of the patient to enable blood to be pumped around the extracorporeal circuit at a rate in excess of 300 mL per minute. This ability was not introduced until the 1960s. Although Kolff in Groningen Hospital in the Netherlands performed the first dialysis experiments in humans in 1943, the problem of dialysis support with long-term vascular access was not solved until Scribner developed the arteriovenous cannula in 1960. This was followed by the development of the surgically

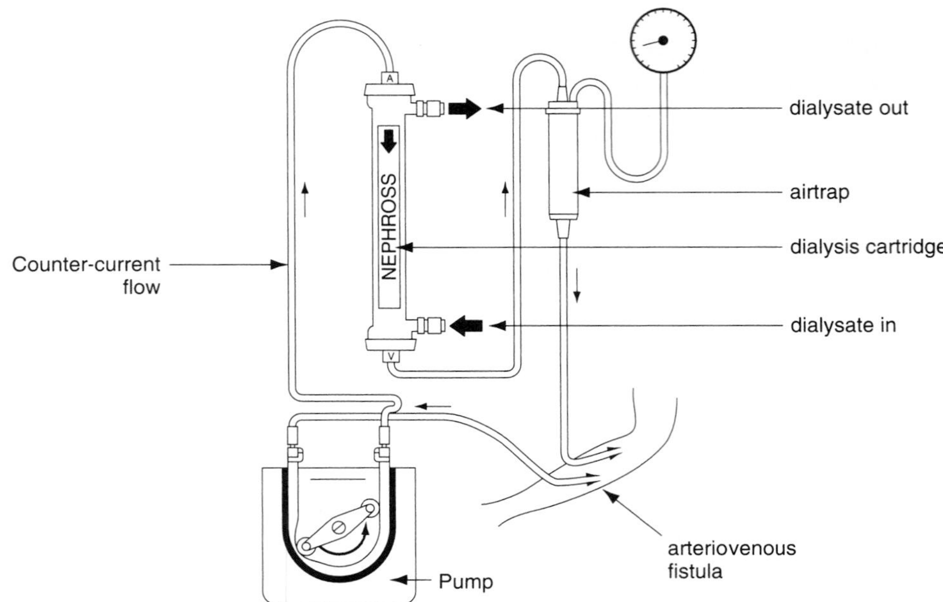

Figure 45-17 A hemodialyzer setup with inset flow diagram.

created arteriovenous fistula (AVF), introduced by Brescia and co-workers in 1966, which provided permanent vascular access. The Dialysis Outcomes Practice Patterns Study (DOPPS) has confirmed a wide variation in how dialysis is achieved throughout the world. For example, the majority of patients in Germany have an AVF as their main access, whereas in the United States a fistula is used for access in less than 30% of cases.[329] When used as a patient's first access, AVF survival is considered superior to arteriovenous grafts regarding time to first failure, and AVF survival is longer in Europe compared with the United States.

An example of a hemodialyzer is shown in Figure 45-17. The most important functional part is the dialyzer membrane. Biocompatibility of the dialyzer membrane is an essential requirement because of high surface areas and long contact times with blood. The most important physiological interactions that occur, apart from protein fouling of tubing and membranes, are complement activation and induction of cytokine release.

A variety of membranes are available with different surface areas and filtration characteristics. The oldest type of membrane was made from cuprophane and cellulose acetate; however, these have been replaced by more biocompatible synthetic membranes made from polysulfone and polyacrylonitrile. Biocompatible membranes are more rigid (allowing higher flow rates) and have higher clearances of larger molecules, such as β_2-microglobulin. By altering the applied pressure across the membrane, fluid removal by UF can be regulated, and by altering the flow rate of dialysate and blood, solute removal can be regulated. Patients are dialyzed in home-based or hospital-based units, with dialysis usually performed three times a week for sessions lasting between 3 and 5 hours. This dialysis schedule is largely empirical insofar as it reconciles adequate treatment with breaks between treatments to provide the patient with a reasonable quality of life. Approaches to increase the dose of dialysis have been explored. These include short daily HD that entails a 2- to 3-hour dialysis on 6 days per week.[271] Alternatively, slow overnight dialysis for 5 to 7 nights has been employed. These regimens have been reported to improve outcome.[271,343,420]

Conventional HD uses low-flux dialyzers, allowing diffusive but little convective solute removal. Middle molecule clearance is poor. HF is a convective treatment. Although middle molecule clearances are improved, small molecule clearance is poor. HF is used for continuous treatment in Intensive Care Units in the management of ARF. High-flux HD using biocompatible membranes allows convective and diffusive solute removal. The use of very pure water is crucial in high-flux modes, because dialysis fluid is infused directly into the bloodstream by back filtration. The Hemodialysis (HEMO) Study, a randomized clinical trial designed to determine whether increasing the dose of dialysis or using a high-flux dialyzer membrane alters major outcomes concluded that patients undergoing HD thrice weekly had no major benefit from a higher dialysis dose than that recommended by current United States guidelines or from the use of a high-flux membrane.[98]

HDF is HD in which fluid removal exceeds the desired weight loss, and fluid balance is maintained by the infusion of a sterile pyrogen-free solution. This technique offers the advantages of both HD and HF in a single therapy. The replacement fluid, previously supplied in autoclaved bags, is now generated "online" from concentrated bicarbonate and uses 20 to 30 L of water per session.[234] The result is that HDF provides 10% to 15% increase in urea clearance compared with HD and increased middle molecule clearances. Water for online preparation of substitution solution should meet common standards for dialysis water regarding chemical contaminants, but have a higher quality regarding microbiological contaminants. It should be practically free from bacteria and pyrogens (i.e., ultrapure). Dialysis water is purified using a combination of techniques, including softening and deionization, carbon adsorption, dual-pass reverse osmosis, and ultraviolet irradiation. Online HDF has been used extensively on continental Europe over the past 15 years or so. Bicarbonate is now favored over acetate as the buffer of choice in HD since it is associated with a reduction of intradialytic symptoms.

Assessment of Adequacy of Hemodialysis

The assessment of adequacy of dialysis treatment for individual patients in the clinical setting includes consideration of the patient's well-being, cardiovascular risk, nutritional status, and degree of achievable ultrafiltration. It also includes estimates of a number of laboratory parameters—such as hemoglobin, phosphate, and albumin—and clearance of the small solutes urea and creatinine. During the following discussion, the term "adequacy" will refer to small solute clearances obtained from both dialysis and residual renal function (RRF). For practical reasons, HD adequacy is calculated using urea as the small solute.

Urea kinetic modeling (UKM) is used to assess adequacy. The kinetics of urea removal during dialysis and the interdialytic regeneration of urea sessions are modeled using computer software such as Adequest (Baxter Laboratories, Deerfield, IL). The computer modeling considers duration of dialysis, RRF, total clearance predicted from the dialyzer, blood and dialysate flow rates, and fluid removal during dialysis.[132] The software then calculates K_t/V urea and protein catabolic rate. The K_t/V (defined in Table 45-13) is now the most commonly used assessment of the adequacy of dialysis. The only analytical measurements required are predialysis and postdialysis urea, duration of dialysis, and weight loss during dialysis. This technique has become more sophisticated with the development of online clearance monitoring based on conductivity variation.[224]

In practice, rather than using full UKM, the simplest calculation is the urea reduction ratio (URR). The percentage fall in plasma urea attained during a dialysis session is measured as follows:

$$\frac{\text{Predialysis [urea]} - \text{Postdialysis [urea]}}{\text{Predialysis [urea]}} \times 100\%$$

The URR does not take convective removal of urea or RRF into account. Its accuracy is lower than K_t/V measured by formal UKM, particularly at high values of URR and K_t/V.[388] Observational studies in populations of dialysis patients have shown that variations in URR are associated with major differences in mortality.[310]

TABLE 45-13 Assessment of Dialysis Adequacy

1. Urea reduction ratio (URR) = (predialysis-postdialysis urea/predialysis urea) × 100 should be >60% if dialysis is adequate.

K_t/V = 'total urea clearance/distribution volume:

$$C_t = C_0 \times e^{(-K_t/V)}$$

where

K = urea clearance
t = time of dialysis
V = volume of urea distribution
C_t = postdialysis urea
C_0 = predialysis urea

Some methods assume a constant relationship between V and body weight, which is not necessarily true in uremia.

2. Relative mortality risk for peritoneal dialysis patients (CANUSA study):

Variable	Relative Risk	
Age	1.03	For each year older
Diabetes	1.45	If present
Cardiovascular disease	2.09	If present
K_t/V	0.94	For each extra 0.1/wk
Creatinine clearance	0.93	For each extra 5 L/wk

In general, the minimum standard for HD three times a week is a K_t/V of 1.0 to 1.4. The K_t/V effectively describes the power of the dialysis session. A retrospective analysis of the National Cooperative Dialysis Study (NCDS) was the first study to identify a threshold in level of K_t/V and outcomes in HD.[252] There are several assumptions associated with the use of UKM including: (1) urea is considered to be uniformly distributed in total body water in a thoroughly mixed single pool; (2) urea is continually added to the pool by protein metabolism at a constant rate; and (3) urea is removed continuously by RRF and intermittently by dialysis following a first-order process of elimination dependent upon plasma concentration. A variety of formulas are used to calculate K_t/V, which makes the comparison of results from different institutions difficult; differences for one measurement can be as wide as 0.98 to 1.43.

Peritoneal Dialysis

Peritoneal dialysis (PD) is a type of dialysis in which dialysate is injected into the patient's peritoneal cavity with the peritoneum then employed as the dialysis membrane. It was first explored by Ganter in 1923 and initially showed poor results. The modern era of PD started in 1953, with intermittent

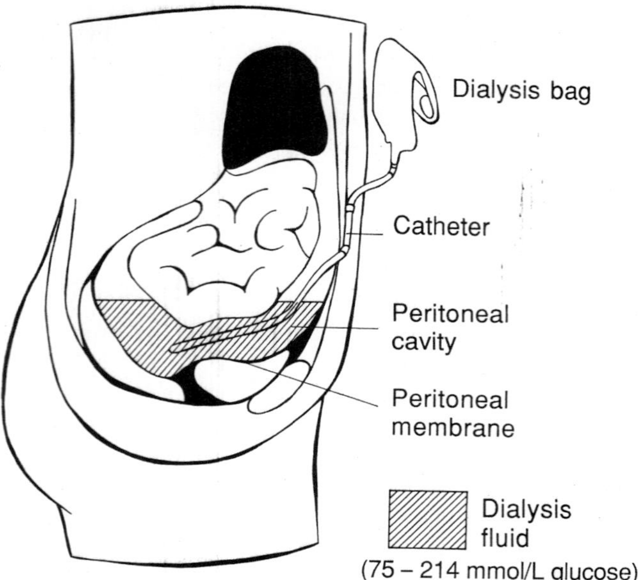

Figure 45-18 Diagrammatic sketch of peritoneal dialysis. *(Redrawn from Nolph KD. Peritoneal Anatomy and Transport Physiology. In: Maher JF, ed. Replacement of renal function by dialysis, 3rd ed. Kluwer Academic Publishers/Springer: Dordrecht, The Netherlands 1989:Chapter 23.)* To convert glucose concentration in mmol/L to mg/dL, multiply by 18.

irrigation of the peritoneal cavity with commercially prepared solutions and access achieved through a single disposable catheter (Figure 45-18). Popovich and co-workers in 1976 introduced the concept of portable equipment, and this approach developed into continuous ambulatory peritoneal dialysis (CAPD)[31]; a type of PD performed in ambulatory patients during normal activities. The percentage of incident and prevalent patients receiving PD has declined in the United States over recent years, particularly in older people. For example, between 8% to 10% of dialysis patients were treated with PD in United States in 2002.[427] Use of PD varies between countries depending on access to HD. For example, in the United Kingdom 31% of prevalent patients receive PD[425] and in Mexico 90% of patients receive PD.[318]

Description

Operationally, CAPD uses the patient's own peritoneal membrane (surface area approximately $2\,m^2$) across which fluid and solutes are exchanged between the peritoneal capillary blood and the dialysis solution placed in the peritoneal cavity. Fluid removal (UF) is achieved by using dialysis fluids containing high concentrations of dextrose acting as an osmotic agent; as the dextrose passes across the peritoneal membrane, the rate of fluid removal decreases. Conventional therapies use four daily exchanges of approximately 2 L of fluid with approximately 10 L of spent dialysate generated, including UF. RRF is critical to the success of PD since only a few milliliters per minute can contribute substantially to urea clearance and C_{Cr}, with each additional milliliter resulting in an extra 10 L of clearance per week. Practical reasons for opting for PD include (1) preservation of RRF and vascular access sites, (2) increased patient autonomy, (3) flexibility as to where the treatment can be administered, and (4) ease of self-treatment, with lower capital costs involved. The higher permeability of the peritoneal membrane provides good removal of β_2-microglobulin and may help to protect patients on PD from the development of dialysis-related amyloid. Blood pressure control and extremes of fluid shifts are not so problematic as those that occur on intermittent HD.

Automated PD (APD) is now widely available. This requires a programmable machine to regulate flow, dwell time, and drainage, and it may be performed at night. Solute clearance can be increased by leaving fluid in the peritoneum during the day and by performing an additional daytime exchange.

The main disadvantage with PD is the risk of infection causing peritonitis. Incidence rates of peritonitis have decreased over the years and the current standard from the United Kingdom Renal Association is that the peritonitis rate should be less than 1 episode per 18 patient months.[422] The immediate effect of peritonitis is to reduce UF, and repeated episodes can cause scarring and fibrosis with permanent loss of filtration. Icodextrin, a nonglucose polymer, may have some value in improving UF in patients with loss of peritoneal function. However, loss of UF in the setting of loss of RRF usually requires transfer of dialysis modality to HD.

Assessment of Adequacy in PD

A series of clinical outcome reports have demonstrated that measures of PD solute removal correlate with patient status and outcome.[231,261,384] In particular, a multicenter prospective cohort study of 680 incident CAPD patients [Canada-United States (CANUSA) Study] showed that a decrease of 0.1 in weekly urea clearance (defined by K_t/V_{urea}) was associated with a 5% increase in the relative risk of death.[71] Similarly a decrease of $5\,L/wk/1.73\,m^2$ of total creatinine clearance (C_{Cr}) was associated with a 7% increase in the risk for death. As a consequence of these studies, national guidelines from the United Kingdom,[422] Australia,[59] and the United States[294] have set standards of dialysis adequacy in terms of small solute removal. An estimate of adequacy is performed in all patients within 6 to 8 weeks of commencement of dialysis. Further studies should be performed at least annually.[422]

The role of solute removal in defining adequacy of PD is complicated by the concern that solute removal by PD may not be clinically equivalent to an equal quantitated solute removal by RRF.[90] For PD, small solute clearance targets have often been established on the assumption that peritoneal and renal clearances are equivalent and therefore additive. However, most studies that examined the relationship between small solute clearances and mortality rates noted that patient survival was directly correlated with renal clearance.[90] A prospective intervention trial reported in 2002 showed no additional benefit of increasing peritoneal clearance over the standard dialysis prescription in terms of mortality rates.[314] Additionally the value of assessing dialysis adequacy in terms of small solute removal has been questioned from the theoretical point of view, given that the relationship between these markers and the as yet unidentified "uremic toxins" is not known. This is particularly pertinent to PD, given that it provides increased clearance of larger molecules compared with HD.

In the setting of PD, the elimination of two markers has typically been used to give an assessment of dialysis adequacy. Measurements of urea in both dialysate and blood are used to generate the parameter K_t/V. This, in combination with C_{Cr}, determined using measurements of creatinine in blood, dialysate, and urine (see Chapter 24), gives an assessment of dialytic adequacy. To obtain the weekly K_t/V_{urea} requires the measurement of volume of spent dialysate and urine for a complete 24-hour period. The concentration of urea in dialysate compared with plasma is calculated (the D/P ratio). This value is multiplied by the volume of the drained effluent to give an estimate of K_t. The calculation of "V" or volume of distribution of urea is derived from an estimate of total body water (TBW).[180,440] An estimate of weekly K_t/V_{urea} is simply the daily clearance multiplied by a factor of seven. These equations are used for both peritoneal and renal clearance and the total weekly clearance obtained by addition. Measurements of urea in plasma, urine, and dialysis fluid also enable calculation of the normalized protein catabolic rate (nPCR), a marker of protein intake that may also have prognostic significance.

The calculation of C_{Cr} is based on the clearance (C) formula:

$$C = \frac{U\,(\text{or } D) \times V}{P}$$

where U is the concentration of creatinine in urine or dialysate, V is the mean daily drain volume or urine volume (measured in liters), and P is the concentration of creatinine in the plasma. The daily clearance obtained for both urine and dialysate is added together and multiplied by seven for the total weekly C_{Cr}.

Compliance with complete collections is mandatory. To avoid sampling errors in patients who infrequently void, urine is collected over a 48-hour period. The dialysate sampling requires all effluent bags in a 24-hour period to be brought to the center renal unit. This can be difficult, since the bags are heavy and bulky. In CAPD, plasma concentrations of urea and creatinine are relatively constant, and therefore blood is drawn at any convenient time for clearance determinations. In APD, blood samples are typically collected after the overnight dialysis period. Both creatinine and urea concentration can be obtained on the same sample of urine, blood, and dialysate. It is important that glucose interference in the dialysate creatinine measurement be minimized by using an enzymatic creatinine method. The limitations of creatinine and creatinine clearance measurements have been discussed in Chapter 24, but in the setting of PD adequacy assessment it particularly should be noted that it is especially compromised at low GFR because of increased tubular secretion of creatinine and decreasing accuracy of the urine collection.

An adjunct to the assessment of adequacy in PD patients is the peritoneal equilibration test (PET).[418] The PET assesses peritoneal membrane transport characteristics in terms of solute clearances and ultrafiltration. The results are used to select a dialysis regimen appropriate to the transport characteristics of the patient (e.g., high transporters may do better on short dwell APD regimens). The PET is typically undertaken at the same time as adequacy assessments in PD patients.

The measurement of adequacy is burdensome, labor intensive, and prone to multiple measurement errors. Although dialysis center nursing staff and patients may collect the necessary samples required for adequacy testing with the utmost diligence, the very complexity and number of measurements taken will cause systematic errors. Nevertheless, in the opinion of the authors of the NKF-K/DOQI Clinical Practice Guidelines for PD Adequacy, when properly performed, these measures are reproducible enough to be useful in routine clinical practice.[294] However, an alternative, simpler, method for defining dialysis adequacy would be very useful in practice.

Complications of Dialysis

A number of diseases are associated with patients on dialysis, including cardiovascular disease, hypertension, β_2-microglobulin amyloidosis, malnutrition, and others.

Cardiovascular Disease

The risk of cardiovascular disease in patients with ESRD is far greater than in the general population. Among patients treated by HD or PD, the prevalence of coronary artery disease is approximately 40% and the prevalence of LVH is approximately 75%.[109,389] Cardiovascular mortality has been estimated to be approximately 9% per year. Even after stratification by age, gender, race, and the presence or absence of diabetes, cardiovascular mortality in dialysis patients is 10 to 20 times higher than in the general population[113,368] (Figure 45-19).

Cardiovascular disease mortality, accounting for 50% of all deaths in ESRD, is defined by death caused by arrhythmias, cardiomyopathy, cardiac arrest, myocardial infarction, atherosclerotic heart disease, and pulmonary edema. Patients with ESRD should be considered in the highest risk group for subsequent cardiovascular events. Among dialysis patients, the prevalence of congestive heart failure is approximately 40%. Both coronary artery disease and LVH are risk factors for the development of heart failure. In practice, it is difficult to determine whether cardiac failure reflects left ventricular dysfunction or extracellular fluid volume overload.

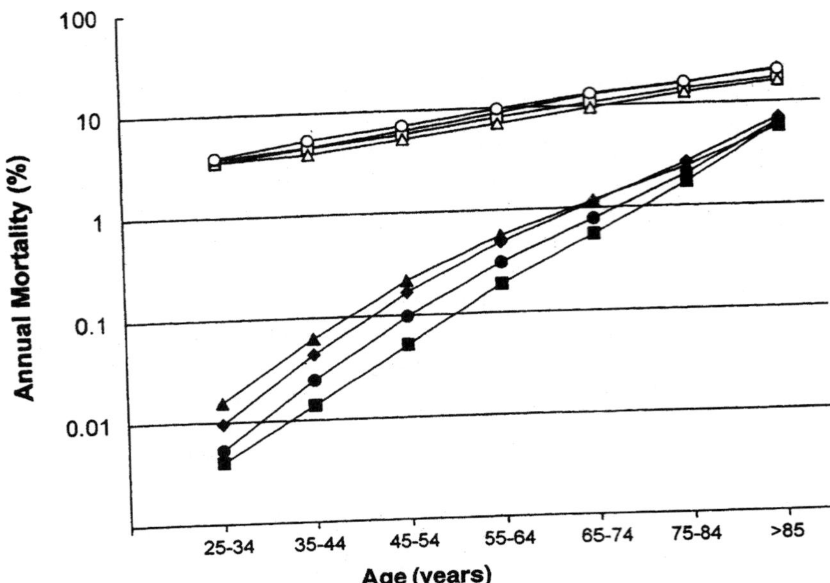

Figure 45-19 Cardiovascular disease mortality defined by death caused by arrhythmias, cardiomyopathy, cardiac arrest, myocardial infarction, atherosclerotic heart disease, and pulmonary edema in the general population (GP). Data from NCHS multiple cause of mortality data files compared with ESRD treated by dialysis. Data are stratified by age, race, and gender. *(From Foley RN, Parfrey PS, Sarnak MJ. Clinical epidemiology of cardiovascular disease in chronic renal disease. Am J Kidney Dis 1998;32 (suppl 3):S112-19, with permission from the National Kidney Foundation.)*

The risk factors for cardiovascular disease in CKD have been discussed above (and see Table 45-9). The following discussion pertains specifically to ESRD patients receiving dialysis.

Hypertension

With short hours, HD hypertension persists in many dialysis patients. Initial treatment is to ensure that excess fluid is kept to a minimum. This requires a "dry" or "target" weight to be set for the patient. The patient should reach this weight at the end of an HD session or continue at this weight during PD. The target weight is reached when there is no discernible edema and below which hypotension occurs. Blood pressure in PD patients should be below 130/80 mm Hg.[422] Standards set for HD patients are less than 140/90 mm Hg predialysis and 130/80 mm Hg postdialysis. As indicated earlier, hypertension is an early feature of CKD and its prevalence approaches 90% in patients reaching ESRD. Hypertension that is refractory to adjustments in dry weight should be treated with multiple medications, including ACE inhibitors and beta-blockers. Long-hours dialysis and salt restriction can also be considered.[65] There does, however, appear to be a U curve association of blood pressure and mortality in HD patients, with predialysis systolic blood pressure lower than 110 mm Hg also increasing risk of death.[333,467]

Dialysis Amyloid

After 10 or more years of HD, patients frequently develop carpal tunnel syndrome and evidence of amyloid deposition.[432] The main constituent of dialysis-related amyloid is β_2-microglobulin. Circulating concentrations of β_2-microglobulin can be as high as 5.0 to 10.0 mg/dL, although there is no correlation between its circulating concentration and the risk of amyloidosis. There is some suggestion that patients on CAPD are less prone to developing amyloidosis, but many still do. High-flux HD increases the removal of β_2-microglobulin and may help with symptoms. The treatment of choice is kidney transplantation.

Malnutrition

Dialysis patients with ESRD tend to have a poor appetite. Protein metabolism is also altered in the setting of chronic acidosis and low-grade inflammation. These factors in combination place patients at risk of protein and energy malnourishment. Plasma albumin is often used as a marker of malnutrition even though it is a relatively poor nutritional marker.[196,200] However, there is good evidence that the lower the plasma concentration of albumin, the worse the long-term prognosis.[110,111,310] Hypoalbuminemia is associated with increased markers of the acute phase response, such as C-reactive protein (CRP).[311,402] Persistent elevation of CRP is common in dialysis patients, and may occur in the absence of detectable infection. Episodes of peritonitis in PD patients cause significant albumin losses because of membrane leakage.

Nutritional screening is recommended in dialysis patients.[422] Such screening may involve subjective global assessment, measurement of the body mass index, a recent history of weight loss, and the measurement of albumin. An albumin concentration of <3.5 g/dL (measured by a bromocresol green method) or <3.0 g/dL (bromocresol purple method) is indicative of undernutrition.

Vascular Calcification

It has been known for more than 100 years that patients with kidney failure have vascular calcification. In 1855, Virchow noted that vascular calcification is an "ossification, and not a mere calcification."[436] Serial x-ray studies and ultrasound imaging of large arteries confirm increased calcification in patients on dialysis over many years.[130] Studies from France have linked the presence of vascular calcification with reduced survival on dialysis.[29,30,141]

Calcification of the major arteries occurs along the intimal lining of blood vessels in association with atheroma. However, in CKD there is also medial and adventitial calcification, reducing the compliance of the vessel. This can be observed by measuring pulse wave velocities along the aorta. The pulse wave velocity is increased in stiff vessels, causing the rebound pulse wave to return more quickly to the heart during the cardiac cycle. This can cause LVH.[29] Vascular calcification has also been studied in both CKD and non-CKD populations using modern sophisticated imaging. Electron-beam computed tomography acquires serial sections of the aortic arch, the coronary vessels, and the aorta. Areas of calcification can be identified and allocated a calcium score (Agatston score).[1] This approach cannot distinguish between intimal or medial calcification but, in non-CKD patients, the higher the calcium score the more predictive of stenotic vascular disease.[208,364] Dialysis patients as young as 20 years exhibit vascular calcification,[131] and the calcium scores increased rapidly within several months when the scans were repeated. The use of calcium-containing phosphate binders may be associated with increased risk of calcification, although this remains unproven.[131] The Treat to Goal Study explored the use of a noncalcium, non-aluminum containing phosphorus binder, sevelamer hydrochloride, in 200 HD patients from Europe and North America.[69] The study demonstrated a significant attenuation in the rate of calcification of vessels with sevelamer hydrochloride at 12 months. Patients were also less likely to develop hypercalcemia and had lower plasma LDL cholesterol concentration, but there was a tendency to worsening acidosis. The hope for future studies is that attenuation of vascular calcification improves patient survival.

Studies have explored the molecular pathophysiology of vascular calcification.[385,419] Mineralization-regulating proteins are deposited at sites of vascular calcification. The generation of a matrix gamma-carboxyglutamic acid (Gla) protein knockout mouse, which exhibits extensive and lethal calcification and cartilaginous metaplasia of the media of all elastic arteries, has refocused attention on the role of Gla-containing proteins in vascular calcification.[385] A number of proteins—including matrix Gla protein, osteonectin, and osteoprotegerin—are constitutively expressed by vascular smooth muscle cells in normal media but are downregulated in calcified arteries. In calcified plaques, vascular smooth muscle cells express osteoblast-like gene expression profiles as demonstrated by in situ hybridization.[419] The identification of natural inhibitors of calcification in plasma, such as human fetuin-A (AHSG; α_2-Heremans Schmid glycoprotein) and matrix-GLA protein, suggests that the vascular endothelium may be continually subjected to calcification stresses and that regulatory systems break down in uremia. A cross-sectional study in HD patients demonstrated that AHSG concentrations were significantly lower in plasma of patients on HD than in healthy controls.[211]

KIDNEY TRANSPLANTATION

Kidney transplantation is the most effective form of RRT, in terms of long-term survival and quality of life.[332] Since 1986, there have been over 340,000 organ transplants performed in the United States. On January 18, 2005, there were 60,534 patients on the waiting list for a kidney transplant in the United States alone.[423] A further 2418 were awaiting combined kidney and pancreas transplantation. In the United Kingdom, there has been a decline in the number of cadaveric donor transplants since 1992. Some of the shortfall has been addressed by increasing the supply of kidneys from live donation, with a threefold increase in the use of live donor transplants since 1992,[426] with no long-term detriment to the donor left with a single kidney. There is also evidence to suggest that the very best outcomes are achieved following preemptive live donor transplants.[262] An alternative method for organ procurement is the use of non–heartbeating donors. Although only slowly accepted as feasible, 2001-2002 data suggest good long-term outcomes.[280,442] On January 18, 2005 the waiting list for a kidney transplant in the United Kingdom was 6335. In 2004, 1,836 kidney transplants were performed in the United Kingdom.There has been a progressive decline in the proportion of the prevalent RRT stock made up by kidney transplant patients, from 51% in 1997 to 47% in 2001.[425] Only 28% of patients with ESRD were on the waiting list in 1998.[425]

Background

Joseph Murray in Boston performed the first successful transplant in 1954 when he performed a donor transplant from one twin to the other. In 1959 Dameshek and Schwartz used 6-mercaptopurine (6-MP) in place of irradiation to precondition patients for bone marrow transplantation. Calne developed this work with the introduction of a safer derivative of 6-MP called azathioprine (AZA). By 1963, maintenance AZA and corticosteroids became the standard regimen for kidney transplantation. Kidney transplant or "graft" survival with these treatment protocols was approximately 40% at 12 months. In the late 1970s to early 1980s cyclosporin A (Cy A) was introduced and has been the mainstay immunosuppressive regimen in combination with AZA and corticosteroids. Cy A–based protocols led to fewer episodes of acute rejection and improved graft survival at 12 months to 80% to 90%. Tacrolimus was introduced during the 1990s and more recently mycophenolate mofetil (MMF), sirolimus (Rapamycin), and everolimus (Ever) have been developed for use in kidney transplantation (see Chapter 33). Also, there has been marked progress on the development and use of biological agents (monoclonal or polyclonal antibodies directed against immune response cellular targets) to suppress the immune response to a graft in human transplant recipients. All these advancements have led to increases in graft and patient survival, with 1-year graft survival of approximately 90% being the rule rather than the exception.[105,140] By contrast, long-term graft survival remains a major problem, with half of the transplants failing within 12 years, usually as a result of chronic allograft nephropathy or death with a functioning graft. Data for the time interval 1988 to 1996 predict that the half-life will increase to almost 14 years for cadaveric grafts.[151]

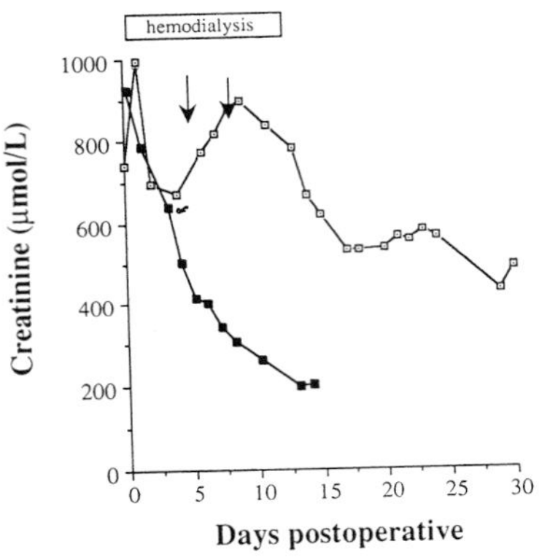

Figure 45-20 Posttransplantation biochemical profile. Open squares represent the course of a patient who experienced an early rejection episode (confirmed by biopsy, ↓) and requiring initial hemodialysis support. Solid squares represent the typical profile of an uncomplicated transplant recipient. To convert creatinine concentration in μmol/L to mg/dL, multiply by 0.011.

Preoperative Assessment

The criteria for acceptance into a transplant program differ slightly from center to center, and it is easier to consider reasons for exclusion. Candidates should not be obese (body mass index [BMI] <40 kg/m^2) and should not have (1) severe chronic lung disease, (2) inoperable ischemic heart disease, (3) active infective liver or immunological disease, (4) chronic infection (e.g., tuberculosis), (5) preexisting malignancy, or (6) lower urinary tract dysfunction. There are also two important psychological issues to be considered: the concept of organ receipt and potential difficulty in complying with immunosuppressive therapies. Age is no longer a primary issue in an otherwise healthy individual; however, only 6% of transplant recipients in the United Kingdom are over age 65.[422]

Laboratory assessment includes indicators of general operative health (e.g., electrolytes, acid-base status, clotting profile, full blood cell count, and cross-matching). In addition, full human leukocyte antigen (HLA) tissue typing is undertaken, in addition to a full screen for infectious diseases, particularly cytomegalovirus (CMV), hepatitis, herpes, and HIV status, as these infections can be activated by immunosuppressive therapy.

The donor kidney is usually placed extraperitoneally in the right or left iliac fossa. Anastomoses are constructed joining the transplant renal artery and vein to the recipient's respective iliac vessels. The ureter is joined to the bladder. The recipient native kidneys are left in situ in the majority of cases.

Postoperative Assessment

During the initial postoperative phase of 1 to 2 weeks, careful monitoring of plasma creatinine and urine output is required to monitor graft function. Most grafts produce measurable amounts of urine within a matter of hours, and this is a clear sign of a functioning graft; however, in a certain proportion, perhaps 5% to 10% of cases, there is apparently primary nonfunction. In this subgroup, continuing dialytic support is necessary. In some patients the condition resolves without treatment, but in others a percutaneous kidney biopsy may be necessary to establish whether the graft is still viable and what form of therapy should be initiated. In otherwise uncomplicated cases, the plasma creatinine concentration falls rapidly postoperatively (Figure 45-20), and consequently changes in the rate of fall of creatinine are monitored to detect early acute rejection episodes. The differential diagnosis of graft dysfunction depends on the time since the transplant. In the very early postoperative phase, this includes delayed graft function, acute vascular and cellular rejection, drug toxicity, and acute tubular damage. Relative hypotension and dehydration may also contribute. Renal artery and venous thrombosis are rare complications and ureteric obstruction can be readily diagnosed using ultrasonography. Histological examination of a transplant biopsy is necessary to aid diagnosis and adjust treatment. During acute rejection there is an interstitial cellular infiltrate, tubulitis, tubular necrosis, and a moderate or severe intimal arteritis. Unfortunately, even this approach is not completely reliable, and response or lack of it to treatment should be carefully monitored.

Immunosuppression and Therapeutic Drug Management

As mentioned earlier, the introduction of immunosuppressive drugs in the 1970s led to a vast improvement in the success rate of kidney transplantations. However, currently used drugs have potentially numerous and serious side effects. For example, treatment with prednisolone in high or prolonged doses is associated with a number of nonimmune side effects, such as development of diabetes mellitus, osteoporosis, thinning of the skin, and truncal obesity. Bone marrow suppression is the major dose-limiting side effect of treatment with azathioprine. Some side effects (infections and malignancy) reflect lack of adequate immune function and are inherent in suppressing the host immune response.

These side effects include infections such as *Pneumocystis* pneumonia and CMV, and certain malignancies such as skin cancer and lymphoma. A retrospective questionnaire study from Leeds, United Kingdom investigated 918 patients transplanted from 1967 to 1991.[250] The study demonstrated 80 different tumors in 70 patients: 42 in skin, 12 of urogenital origin, and 5 B cell lymphomas plus a number of miscellaneous tumors. In an age- and sex-matched normal population after 20 years, a 6% prevalence of cancer was observed, compared with a prevalence of 13% at 10 years and 40% at 20 years in the transplant population. Data from 2003 have shown that the prevalence of nonmelanotic skin cancer in transplant recipients at 10 years is almost 30% in the United Kingdom and 86% in Queensland, Australia.[60] These data suggest that patients receiving immunosuppressive drugs require lifelong surveillance for malignancy.

Following the introduction of Cy A in the 1980s, there was a dramatic increase in 1-year graft survival because of a reduction in the number of acute rejection episodes.[279] However, a number of important side effects have been observed. Nephrotoxicity was soon apparent in the early clinical trials[55] and remains a major clinical problem; graft biopsy may be supportive of the diagnosis if there are histological appearances of arteriolar hyalinization and glomerular ischemia leading to glomerular occlusion, and tubulointerstitial changes producing interstitial fibrosis and tubular atrophy.[138]

Clinical experience following kidney transplantation suggests that primary prophylaxis with tacrolimus results in 1-year graft and patient survival rates that are equivalent to those achieved with Cy A therapy, although with lower rates of acute rejection episodes.[129,273,328,415] Five-year follow-up data suggest improved graft survival with tacrolimus compared with Cy A.[435] Nephrotoxicity, hypertension, and post-transplant diabetes mellitus may occur and were reported commonly in the early studies.[273,328]

In 11 European centers, kidney graft recipients randomized to receive either Cy A or sirolimus as part of a triple regimen with corticosteroids and AZA had excellent graft and patient survival and incidence of acute rejection (41% and 38%).[140] Sirolimus, in contrast to Cy A, does not cause nephrotoxicity, gingival hyperplasia, or tremor. Patients treated with sirolimus have a higher incidence of thrombocytopenia, hyperlipidemia, and lymphocele formation.[203] Sirolimus and MMF have been studied in the setting of Cy A–withdrawal and Cy A–free strategies in kidney transplantation,[105,115,192,445] the hypothesis being that withdrawal or avoidance of Cy A would improve long-term outcomes, because there is no nephrotoxic stimulus. It has been shown in a multinational study to be feasible to withdraw Cy A within 3 months of transplantation.[192] Studies have also shown that sirolimus in combination with MMF is safe and associated with low rates of acute transplant rejection at 12 months.[105] These patients also received basiliximab, a monoclonal antibody to a specific target (CD 25) of T-cell activation in response to a nonidentical graft.

Cy A is insoluble and is presented for clinical use as a microemulsion. It has a narrow therapeutic window and in clinical transplantation it is important to monitor the blood level frequently. The most widely accepted practice is to monitor the "trough" blood level (C-0) just before the next dose. Accepted trough concentrations range from 100 to 200 μg/L, with higher levels for the induction phase of treatment during the first 3 months and subsequently lower maintenance levels. The trough concentration within the blood may not give a truly accurate guide to total drug exposure, since there is a wide variation in absorption over the first 2 to 4 hours following dosing.[193] This is important since most of the pharmacodynamic effects of Cy A occur within 2 hours.[145] Studies from Canada suggest that trough concentrations do not reflect clinical outcomes in terms of acute rejection rates[259] although high trough concentrations were associated with increased nephrotoxicity. A 2-hour drug (C-2) concentration correlated well with formal area under the curve (AUC) measurements and is predictive of nephrotoxicity and acute rejection episodes. In kidney transplant patients, the trough level of tacrolimus is well correlated with acute rejection episodes and nephrotoxicity.[210] Trough levels also guide sirolimus therapy.[202]

In summary, long-term graft failure is a major problem and graft loss accounts for increasing numbers of patients returning to dialysis. The most common cause, however, of graft loss is death with a functioning graft. ESRD carries a considerable burden of cardiovascular morbidity. Although some risk factors are improved following transplantation, such as volume overload and anemia, others, including dyslipidemia and hypertension, persist. The drugs used to prevent rejection can exacerbate these. The challenges to the nephrology community are complex and include increasing access to transplantation, reduction in side effects of the powerful drugs used to prevent rejection, and reduction in cardiovascular risk profiles for individual patients.

Simultaneous Pancreas-Kidney Transplantation

Patients with type 1 diabetes and stage 5 CKD with limited secondary complications of diabetes may be considered for simultaneous pancreas and kidney (SPK) transplantation. Patients tend to be younger than kidney only recipients, aged between 20 and 40 years. As of January 18, 2005, 2418 patients were awaiting combined kidney and pancreas transplantation in the United States.[423] More than 90% of pancreas transplants registered until 1996 were performed in the United States, but expertise is growing in other countries. Graft and patient survival rates have been calculated for more than 3500 recipients of an SPK transplant in the United States from 1994 to 1997 based on data reported to the United Network for Organ Sharing (UNOS) renal registry database.[52] The 1-year graft survival was 90% and patient survival around 93%. At 5 years, the graft survival was in excess of 70% and patient survival 85%. These results compare favorably with cadaveric kidney–only transplantation in diabetes. The main reason for the survival advantage of SPK over kidney-only is the fact that younger donors and recipients are selected. A separate prospective observational study has examined the impact of SPK transplant in terms of quality of life.[139] At 3 years, SPK patients report greater improvements than kidney-only recipients in physical functioning, bodily pain, general health, and perception of greater benefits to secondary complications.

The surgical technique for SPK involves whole organ pancreas transplant with the duodenal segment draining into the urinary bladder through a duodenocystostomy. The kidney is attached as usual to the iliac vessels and the donor ureter is inserted into the bladder separately. Alternatively the pancreas can be drained enterically. This distinction is important since there are metabolic consequences outlined below. Postoperatively blood glucose concentrations are monitored closely and intravenous insulin is given as necessary. Exocrine pancreatic secretion can be measured in the urine. The major fear is rejection and a number of parameters are monitored including plasma glucose, amylase, lipase, and 12- or 24-hour urinary amylase. Because of high fluid, bicarbonate, and electrolyte losses into the urine, there is an increased need for supplementation in SPK recipients although this is usually self-limiting. Hyperamylasemia is common postoperatively and may or may not signify allograft rejection. Immunosuppressive schedules will vary between centers and include induction therapy with monoclonal or polyclonal anti–T-cell agents and a combination of the drugs outlined above. Diagnosis of pancreatic rejection in the absence of a simultaneous kidney transplant is very difficult. Signs of rejection include fever, pain, hematuria, reduction of urinary amylase, and unexplained hyperglycemia. Organ scanning and biopsy are also used. However, the function of the kidney in SPK mirrors the pancreas and therefore immunosuppression can be tailored to the requirements of the kidney.

For patients with bladder drainage, enteric conversion may be required for refractory problems, such as dehydration, metabolic acidosis, chronic urethritis caused by trypsinogen activation, urinary tract infections, and recurrent reflux pancreatitis. This involves an anastomosis between the graft duodenal segment and the recipient small bowel.

REFERENCES

1. Agatston AS, Janowitz WR, Hildner FJ, Zusmer NR, Viamonte M, Detrano R. Quantification of coronary artery calcium using ultrafast computed tomography. J Am Coll Cardiol 1990;15:827-32.
2. Agewall S, Wikstrand J, Ljungman S, Fagerberg B. Usefulness of microalbuminuria in predicting cardiovascular mortality in treated hypertensive men with and without diabetes mellitus. Risk Factor Intervention Study Group. Am J Cardiol 1997;80: 164-9.
3. Alexanian R, Dimopoulos M. The treatment of multiple myeloma. N Engl J Med 1994;330:484-9.
4. Anderson S, Brenner BM. Effects of aging on the renal glomerulus. Am J Med 1986;80:435-42.
5. Anderson S, Meyer TW, Rennke HG, Brenner BM. Control of glomerular hypertension limits glomerular injury in rats with reduced renal mass. J Clin Invest 1985;76:612-19.
6. Antonsen JE, Sherrard DJ, Andress DL. A calcimimetic agent acutely suppresses parathyroid hormone levels in patients with chronic renal failure. Rapid communication. Kidney Int 1998;53:223-7.
7. Attal M, Harousseau JL, Stoppa AM, Sotto JJ, Fuzibet JG, Rossi JF, et al. A prospective, randomized trial of autologous bone marrow transplantation and chemotherapy in multiple myeloma. Intergroupe Francais du Myelome. N Engl J Med 1996;335: 91-7.
8. Ayatse JO, Kwan JT. Relative sensitivity of serum and urinary retinol binding protein and alpha-1 microglobulin in the assessment of renal function. Ann Clin Biochem 1991;28:514-16.
9. Back S-E, Ljungberg B, Nilsson-Ehle I, Borga O, Nilsson-Ehle P. Age dependence of renal function: clearance of iohexol and p-amino hippurate in healthy males. Scand J Clin Lab Invest 1989;49:641-6.
10. Baigent C, Burbury K, Wheeler D. Premature cardiovascular disease in chronic renal failure. Lancet 2000;356:147-52.
11. Bakir A, Williams RH, Shaykh M, Dunea G, Dubin A. Biochemistry of the uremic syndrome. Adv Clin Chem 1992;29:61-120.
12. Bakris GL, Williams M, Dworkin L, Elliott WJ, Epstein M, Toto R, et al. Preserving renal function in adults with hypertension and diabetes: A consensus approach. National Kidney Foundation Hypertension and Diabetes Executive Committees Working Group. Am J Kidney Dis 2000;36:646-61.
13. Ballantyne FC, Gibbons J, O'Reilly DS. Urine albumin should replace total protein for the assessment of glomerular proteinuria. Ann Clin Biochem 1993;30:101-3.
14. Ballardie FW, Roberts IS. Controlled prospective trial of prednisolone and cytotoxics in progressive IgA nephropathy. J Am Soc Nephrol 2002;13:142-8.
15. Bangstad HJ, Osterby R, Dahl-Jorgensen K, Berg KJ, Hartmann A, Nyberg G, et al. Early glomerulopathy is present in young, type 1 (insulin-dependent) diabetic patients with microalbuminuria. Diabetologia 1993;36:523-9.
16. Barakat AJ, Rennert OM. Gitelman's syndrome (familial hypokalemia-hypomagnesemia). J Nephrol 2001;14:43-7.
17. Batlle D. Clinical and cellular markers of diabetic nephropathy. Kidney Int 2003;63:2319-30.
18. Batuman V, Dreisbach AW, Cyran J. Light-chain binding sites on renal brush-border membranes. Am J Physiol 1990;258:F1259-65.

19. Beetham R, Newman D. Urinary albumin and low molecular weight protein excretion in the nephrotic syndrome—sequential studies during corticosteroid treatment. Ann Clin Biochem 1992;29:450-3.
20. Beetham R, Cattell WR. Proteinuria: Pathophysiology, significance and recommendations in clinical practice. Ann Clin Biochem 1993;30:425-34.
21. Berenson JR, Lichtenstein A, Porter L, Dimopoulos MA, Bordoni R, George S, et al. Efficacy of pamidronate in reducing skeletal events in patients with advanced multiple myeloma. Myeloma Aredia Study Group. New Engl J Med 1996;334:488-93.
22. Bertani T, Cutillo F, Zoja C, Broggini M, Remuzzi G. Tubulo-interstitial lesions mediate renal damage in adriamycin glomerulopathy. Kidney Int 1986;30: 488-96.
23. Berthelot M, Cornu G, Daudon M, Helbert M, Laurence C. Diffuse reflectance technique for infrared analysis of urinary calculi. Clin Chem 1987;33:780-3.
24. Besarab A, Bolton WK, Browne JK, Egrie JC, Nissenson AR, Okamoto DM, et al. The effects of normal as compared with low hematocrit values in patients with cardiac disease who are receiving hemodialysis and epoetin. N Engl J Med 1998;339: 584-90.
25. Bhandari S, Hunter M. Inward rectifier renal potassium channel (ROMK), the low-conductance channels for potassium secretion. Nephrol Dial Transplant 1998;13:3019-23.
26. Bianchi S, Bigazzi R, Caiazza A, Campese VM. A controlled, prospective study of the effects of atorvastatin on proteinuria and progression of kidney disease. Am J Kidney Dis 2003;41:565-70.
27. Bichet DG. Nephrogenic diabetes insipidus. Am J Med 1998;105:431-42.
28. Borland WW, Ferguson JC, Dryburgh FJ. A fast automated method for measuring serum and urine citrate. Ann Clin Biochem 1989;26:286-8.
29. Blacher J, Guerin AP, Pannier B, Marchais SJ, London GM. Arterial calcifications, arterial stiffness, and cardiovascular risk in end-stage renal disease. Hypertension 2001;38:938-42.
30. Blacher J, Safar ME, Guerin AP, Pannier B, Marchais SJ, London GM. Aortic pulse wave velocity index and mortality in end-stage renal disease. Kidney Int 2003;63:1852-60.
31. Block GA, Hulbert-Shearon TE, Levin NW, Port FK. Association of serum phosphorus and calcium x phosphate product with mortality risk in chronic hemodialysis patients: a national study. Am J Kidney Dis 1998;31:607-17.
32. Blum U, Krumme B, Flugel P, Gabelmann A, Lehnert T, Buitrago-Tellez C, et al. Treatment of ostial renal-artery stenoses with vascular endoprostheses after unsuccessful balloon angioplasty. N Engl J Med 1997;336:459-65.
33. Bohle A, Mackensen-Haen S, von-Gise H, Grund KE, Wehrmann M, Batz C, et al. The consequences of tubulo-interstitial changes for renal function in glomerulopathies. A morphometric and cytological analysis. Pathol Res Pract 1990;186:135-44.
34. Boijson E. Anomalies and malformations. In: Abrams angiography: Vascular and interventional radiology, 3rd ed. Boston: Little, Brown and Co, 1983:1217-30.
35. Bombassei GJ, Kaplan AA. The association between hydrocarbon exposure and anti-glomerular basement membrane antibody-mediated disease (Goodpasture's syndrome). Am J Ind Med 1992;21:141-53.
36. Booth JW, Lumeden CJ. Explaining glomerular pores with fiber matrices. Biophys J 1993;64:1727-34.
37. Bonomini V, Feletti C, Scolari MP, Stefoni S. Benefits of early initiation of dialysis. Kidney Int Suppl 1985;17:S57-9.
38. Bonventre JV, Weinberg JM. Recent advances in the pathophysiology of ischemic acute renal failure. J Am Soc Nephrol 2003;14:2199-210.
39. Borch-Johnsen K, Norgaard K, Hommel E, Mathiesen ER, Jensen JS, Deckert T, et al. Is diabetic nephropathy an inherited complication? Kidney Int 1992;41:719-22.
40. Border WA, Okuda S, Languino LR, Sporn MB, Ruoslahti E. Suppression of experimental glomerulonephritis by antiserum against transforming growth factor beta 1. Nature 1990;346:371-4.
41. Borghi L, Schianchi T, Meschi T, Guerra A, Allegri F, Maggiore U, et al. Comparison of two diets for the prevention of recurrent stones in idiopathic hypercalciuria. N Engl J Med 2002;346:77-84.
42. Bostom AG, Shemin D, Lapane KL, Hume AL, Yoburn D, Nadeau MR, et al. High dose-B-vitamin treatment of hyperhomocysteinemia in dialysis patients. Kidney Int 1996;49:147-52.
43. Bostom AG, Shemin D, Verhoef P, Nadeau MR, Jacques PF, Selhub J, et al. Elevated fasting total plasma homocysteine levels and cardiovascular disease outcomes in maintenance dialysis patients. A prospective study. Arterioscler Thromb Vasc Biol 1997;17:2554-8.
44. Bostom AG, Culleton BF. Hyperhomocysteinemia in chronic renal disease. J Am Soc Nephrol 1999;10: 891-900.
45. Brand E, Harris MM, Biloon S. The excretion of a cystine complex which decomposes in the urine with the liberation of free cystine. J Biol Chem 1930;86:315-31.
46. Brenner BM, Meyer TW, Hostetter TH. Dietary protein intake and the progressive nature of kidney disease. N Engl J Med 1982;307:652-9.
47. Brenner BM, Cooper ME, de Zeeuw D, Keane WF, Mitch WE, Parving H-H, et al. Effects of losartan on renal and cardiovascular outcomes in patients with

type 2 diabetes and nephropathy. N Engl J Med 2001;345:861-9.
48. Briganti EM, Russ GR, McNeil JJ, Atkins RC, Chadban SJ. Risk of renal allograft loss from recurrent glomerulonephritis. N Engl J Med 2002;347:103-9.
49. Brown EM, Gamba G, Riccardi D, Lombardi M, Butters R, Kifor O, et al. Cloning and characterization of an extracellular $Ca(2^+)$-sensing receptor from bovine parathyroid. Nature 1993;366:575-80.
50. Brunskill NJ. Albumin handling by proximal tubular cells: mechanisms and mediators. Nephrol Dial Transplant 2000;15[suppl 6]:39-40
51. Bruzzi I, Benigni A, Remuzzi G. Role of increased glomerular protein traffic in the progression of renal failure. Kidney Int Suppl 1997;62:S29-31.
52. Bunnapradist S, Cho YW, Cecka JM, Wilkinson A, Danovitch GM. Kidney allograft and patient survival in type I diabetic recipients of cadaveric kidney alone versus simultaneous pancreas kidney transplants: a multivariate analysis of the UNOS database. J Am Soc Nephrol 2003;14:208-13.
53. Burton C, Harris KP. The role of proteinuria in the progression of chronic renal failure. Am J Kidney Dis 1996;27:765-75.
54. Bushinsky DA. Recurrent hypercalciuric nephrolithiasis—does diet help? N Engl J Med 2002;346:124-5.
55. Calne RY, White DJ, Thiru S, Evans DB, McMaster P, Dunn DC, et al. Cyclosporin A in patients receiving renal allografts from cadaver donors. Lancet 1978;2:1323-7.
56. Cameron JS, Turner DR, Ogg CS, Chantler C, Williams DG. The long-term prognosis of patients with focal segmental glomerulosclerosis. Clin Nephrol 1978;10:213-18.
57. Caps MT, Perissinotto C, Zierler RE, Polissar NL, Bergelin RO, Tullis MJ, et al. Prospective study of atherosclerotic disease progression in the renal artery. Circulation 1998;98:2866-72.
58. Caramori ML, Fioretto P, Mauer M. The need for early predictors of diabetic nephropathy risk: is albumin excretion rate sufficient? Diabetes 2000;49:1399-408.
59. Caring for Australians with Renal Impairment (CARI): http://www.kidney.org.au/cari/drafts/da7.html (Accessed January 18, 2005)
60. Carroll RP, Ramsay HM, Fryer AA, Hawley CM, Nicol DL, Harden PN. Incidence and prediction of nonmelanoma skin cancer post-renal transplantation: a prospective study in Queensland, Australia. Am J Kidney Dis 2003;41:676-83.
61. Casadevall N, Nataf J, Viron B, Kolta A, Kiladjian JJ, Martin-Dupont P, et al. Pure red-cell aplasia and antierythropoietin antibodies in patients treated with recombinant erythropoietin. N Engl J Med 2002;346:469-75.
62. Cattell V: Immunopathology of glomerulonephritis. In: Age R, ed. Advanced renal medicine. Oxford: Oxford Medical, 1992:205-70.
63. Caudarella R, Rizzoli E, Buffa A, Bottura A, Stefoni S. Comparative study of the influence of 3 types of mineral water in patients with idiopathic calcium lithiasis. J Urol 1998;159:658-63.
64. Chantler C, Barrett TM. Estimation of glomerular filtration rate from plasma clearance of ^{51}chromium edetic acid. Arch Dis Child 1972;47: 613-17.
65. Charra B, Calemard E, Ruffet M, Chazot C, Terrat JC, Vanel T, et al. Survival as an index of adequacy of dialysis. Kidney Int 1992;41:1286-91.
66. Chavers BM, Bilous RW, Ellis EN, Steffes MW, Mauer SM. Glomerular lesions and urinary albumin excretion in type I diabetes without overt proteinuria. N Engl J Med 1989;320:966-70.
67. Chen JH, Pu YS, Liu SP, Chiu TY. Renal hemodynamics in patients with obstructive uropathy evaluated by duplex Doppler sonography. J Urol 1993;150:18-21.
68. Chen S, Carmen-Iglesias de la Cruz M, Jim B, Hong SW, Isono M, Ziyadeh FN. Reversibility of established diabetic glomerulopathy by anti-TGF-beta antibodies in db/db mice. Biochem Biophys Res Commun 2003;300:16-22.
69. Chertow GM, Burke SK, Raggi P. Sevelamer attenuates the progression of coronary and aortic calcification in hemodialysis patients. Kidney Int 2002;62:245-52.
70. Chevalier RL. The moth and the aspen tree: sodium in early postnatal development. Kidney Int 2001;59:1617-25.
71. Churchill D. Adequacy of dialysis and nutrition in continuous peritoneal dialysis: association with clinical outcomes. Canada-USA (CANUSA) Peritoneal Dialysis Study Group. J Am Soc Nephrol 1996;7: 198-207.
72. Collins AJ, Li S, St. Peter W, Ebben J, Roberts T, Ma JZ, et al. Death, hospitalization, and economic associations among incident hemodialysis patients with hematocrit values of 36 to 39%. J Am Soc Nephrol 2001;12:2465-73.
73. Consensus Conference. Prevention and treatment of kidney stones. JAMA 1988;260:977-81.
74. Coresh J, Wei GL, McQuillan G, Brancati FL, Levey AS, Jones C, et al. Prevalence of high blood pressure and elevated serum creatinine level in the United States: findings from the Third National Health and Nutrition Examination Survey (1988-1994). Arch Intern Med 2001;161:1207-16.
75. Costanzo LS, Windhager EE. Renal regulation of calcium balance. In: Seldin DN, Griebisch G, eds. The kidney: physiology and pathophysiology. 2nd ed. New York: Raven Press, 1992: 2375-95.

76. Culleton BF, Larson MG, Parfrey PS, Kannel WB, Levy D. Proteinuria as a risk factor for cardiovascular disease and mortality in older people: A prospective study. Am J Med 2000;109:1-8.
77. Curhan GC, Willett WC, Rimm EB, Stampfer MJ. A prospective study of dietary calcium and other nutrients and the risk of symptomatic kidney stones. N Engl J Med 1993;328:833-8.
78. Curhan GC, Willett WC, Speizer FE, Stampfer MJ. Beverage use and risk for kidney stones in women. Ann Intern Med 1998;128:534-40.
79. Curry FE, Michel CC. A fiber-matrix model of capillary permeability. Microvasc Res 1980;20:96-9.
80. Dammacco F, Castoldi G, Rodjer S. Efficacy of epoetin alfa in the treatment of anemia of multiple myeloma. Br J Hematol 2001;113:172-9.
81. Daniels BS, Hauser EB, Deen MW, Hostetter TH. Glomerular basement membrane: In vitro studies of water and protein permeability. Am J Physiol 1992;262:F919-26.
82. Davies DF, Shock NW. Age changes in glomerular filtration rate, effective renal plasma flow, and tubular excretory capacity in adult males. J Clin Invest 1950;29:496-507.
83. Davies DJ, Moran JE, Niall JF, Ryan GB. Segmental necrotising glomerulonephritis with antineutrophil antibody: Possible arbovirus aetiology? BMJ 1982;285:606.
84. Deen PM, van Aubel RA, van Lieburg AF, van Os CH. Urinary content of aquaporin 1 and 2 in nephrogenic diabetes insipidus. J Am Soc Nephrol 1996;7:836-41.
85. Defronzo RA, Humphrey RL, Wright JR, Cooke CR. Acute renal failure in multiple myeloma. Medicine (Baltimore) 1975;54:209-23.
86. Deschenes G, Feraille E, Doucet A. Mechanisms of oedema in nephrotic syndrome: Old theories and new ideas. Nephrol Dial Transplant 2003;18:454-6.
87. De Swart PMJR, Busemann Sokole E, Wilmink JM. The interrelationship of calcium and magnesium absorption in idiopathic hypercalciuria and renal calcium stone disease. J Urol 1998;159:669-72.
89. Diabetes Control and Complications Trial Research Group. The effect of intensive treatment of diabetes on the development and progression of long-term complications in insulin-dependent diabetes mellitus. N Engl J Med 1993;329:977-86.
90. Diaz-Buxo JA, Lowrie EG, Lew NL, Zhang SM, Zhu X, Lazarus JM. Associates of mortality among peritoneal dialysis patients with special reference to peritoneal transport rates and solute clearance. Am J Kidney Dis 1999;33:523-34.
91. DiBona GF. Prostaglandins and nonsteroidal anti-inflammatory drugs. Effects on renal hemodynamics. Am J Med 1986;80:12-21.
92. Dominiczak AF, Bohr DF. Nitric oxide and hypertension. Curr Opin Nephrol Hypert 1996;5:174-80.
93. Dorland's Illustrated Medical Dictionary. 30th ed. Philadelphia: WB Saunders, 2003.
94. Donaghy M, Rees AJ. Cigarette smoking and lung hemorrhage in glomerulonephritis caused by autoantibodies to glomerular basement membrane. Lancet 1983;2:1390-3.
95. D'Amico G, Minetti L, Ponticelli C, Fellin G, Ferrario F, Barbiano di Belgioioso G, et al. Prognostic indicators in idiopathic IgA mesangial nephropathy. Q J Med 1986;59:363-78.
96. D'Amico G, Bazzi C. Pathophysiology of proteinuria. Kidney Int 2003;63:809-25.
97. Eddy AA, Giachelli CM. Renal expression of genes that promote interstitial inflammation and fibrosis in rats with protein-overload proteinuria. Kidney Int 1995;47:1546-57.
98. Eknoyan G, Beck GJ, Cheung AK, Daugirdas JT, Greene T, Kusek JW, et al. Effect of dialysis dose and membrane flux in maintenance hemodialysis. N Engl J Med 2002;347:2010-19.
99. Epstein M. Aging and the kidney. J Am Soc Nephrol 1996;7:1106-22.
100. Erwin DT, Donadio JV, Holley KE. The clinical course of idiopathic membranous nephropathy. Mayo Clin Proc 1973;48:697-712.
101. European best practice guidelines for the management of anemia in patients with chronic renal failure: Working party for European best practice guidelines for the management of anemia in patients with chronic renal failure. Nephrol Dial Transplant 1999;14 Suppl 5:1-50.
102. Falk RJ, Jennette JC. Anti-neutrophil cytoplasmic autoantibodies with specificity for myeloperoxidase in patients with systemic vasculitis and idiopathic necrotizing and crescentic glomerulonephritis. N Engl J Med 1988;318:1651-7.
103. Feest TG, Mistry CD, Grimes DS, Mallick NP. Incidence of advanced chronic renal failure and the need for end stage renal replacement treatment. BMJ 1990;301:897-900.
104. Fioretto P, Steffes MW, Mauer M. Glomerular structure in nonproteinuric IDDM patients with various levels of albuminuria. Diabetes 1994;43:1358-64.
105. Flechner SM, Goldfarb D, Modlin C, Feng J, Krishnamurthi V, Mastroianni B, et al. Kidney transplantation without calcineurin inhibitor drugs: a prospective, randomized trial of sirolimus versus cyclosporine. Transplantation 2002;74:1070-6.
106. Fliser D, Franek E, Joest M, Block S, Mutschler E, Ritz E. Renal function in the elderly: impact of hypertension and cardiac function. Kidney Int 1997;51:1196-1204.
107. Fliser D, Franek E, Ritz E. Renal function in the elderly—is the dogma of an inexorable decline of renal function correct? Nephrol Dial Transplant 1997;12:1553-5.

108. Fliser D, Zeier M, Nowack R, Ritz E. Renal functional reserve in healthy elderly subjects. J Am Soc Nephrol 1993;3:1371-7.
109. Foley RN, Parfrey PS, Harnett JD, Kent GM, Martin CJ, Murray DC, et al. Clinical and echocardiographic disease in patients starting end-stage renal disease therapy. Kidney Int 1995;47:186-92.
110. Foley RN, Parfrey PS, Harnett JD, Kent GM, Murray DC, Barre PE. The impact of anemia on cardiomyopathy, morbidity, and mortality in end-stage renal disease. Am J Kidney Dis 1996;28:53-61.
111. Foley RN, Parfrey PS, Harnett JD, Kent GM, Murray DC, Barre PE. Hypoalbuminemia, cardiac morbidity, and mortality in end-stage renal disease. J Am Soc Nephrol 1996;7:728-36.
112. Foley RN, Culleton BF, Parfrey PS, Harnett JD, Kent GM, Murray DC, et al. Cardiac disease in diabetic end-stage renal disease. Diabetologia 1997;40: 1307-12.
113. Foley RN, Parfrey PS, Sarnak MJ. Clinical epidemiology of cardiovascular disease in chronic renal disease. Am J Kidney Dis 1998;32:S112-19.
114. Forsblom CM, Groop PH, Ekstrand A, Groop LC. Predictive value of microalbuminuria in patients with insulin-dependent diabetes of long duration. Brit Med J (Clinical Research Ed.) 1992;305: 1051-3.
115. Francois H, Durrbach A, Amor M, Djeffal R, Kriaa F, Paradis V, et al. The long-term effect of switching from cyclosporin A to mycophenolate mofetil in chronic renal graft dysfunction compared with conventional management. Nephrol Dial Transplant 2003;18:1909-16.
116. Freedman BI, Iskandar SS, Appel RG. The link between hypertension and nephrosclerosis. Am J Kidney Dis 1995;25:207-21.
117. Fujisawa M, Haramaki R, Miyazaki H, Imaizumi T, Okuda S. Role of lipoprotein (a) and TGF-beta 1 in atherosclerosis of hemodialysis patients. J Am Soc Nephrol 2000;11:1889-95.
118. Gabow PA. Autosomal dominant polycystic kidney disease—more than a renal disease. Am J Kidney Dis 1990;16:403-13.
119. Gaede P, Vedel P, Parving HH, Pedersen O. Intensified multifactorial intervention in patients with type 2 diabetes mellitus and microalbuminuria: the Steno type 2 randomised study. Lancet 1999;353: 617-22.
120. Galderisi M, Anderson KM, Wilson PW, Levy D. Echocardiographic evidence for the existence of a distinct diabetic cardiomyopathy (the Framingham Heart Study). Am J Cardiol 1991;68:85-9.
121. Galpin JE, Shinaberger JH, Stanley TM, Blumenkrantz MJ, Bayer AS, Friedman GS, et al. Acute interstitial nephritis due to methicillin. Am J Medicine 1978;65:756-65.
122. Gambaro G, Favaro S, D'Angelo A. Risk for renal failure in nephrolithiasis. Am J Kidney Dis 2001;37:233-43.
123. Garella S. Clinical acid base disorders. In: Cameron JS, Davison AM, Grunfeld J-P, Kerr D, Ritz E, eds. Oxford textbook of clinical nephrology, vol 2, 2nd ed. Oxford, Oxford University Press, 1992:917-66.
124. Garg AX, Blake PG, Clark WF, Clase CM, Haynes RB, Moist LM. Association between renal insufficiency and malnutrition in older adults: results from the NHANES III. Kidney Int 2001;60:1867-74.
125. Gellai M, Jugus M, Fletcher T, Nambi P, Ohlstein EH, Elliott JD, et al. Nonpeptide endothelin receptor antagonists. V: Prevention and reversal of acute renal failure in the rat by SB 209670. J Pharmacol Exp Ther 1995;275:200-6.
126. Giovannetti S, Maggiore Q. A low nitrogen diet with protein of high biological value for severe chronic uremia. Lancet 1964;i:1000-4.
127. GISEN. Randomised placebo-controlled trial of effect of ramipril on decline in glomerular filtration rate and risk of terminal renal failure in proteinuric, non-diabetic nephropathy. The GISEN Group (Gruppo Italiano di Studi Epidemiologici in Nefrologia). Lancet 1997;349:1857-63.
128. Giugliani R, Ferrari I, Greene LJ. Heterozygous cystinuria and urinary lithiasis. Am J Med Gen 1985;22:703-15.
129. Gjertson DW, Cecka JM, Terasaki PI. The relative effects of FK506 and cyclosporine on short- and long-term kidney graft survival. Transplantation 1995;60:1384-8.
130. Goldsmith DJ, Covic A, Sambrook PA, Ackrill P. Vascular calcification in long-term hemodialysis patients in a single unit: a retrospective analysis. Nephron 1997;77:37-43.
131. Goodman WG, Goldin J, Kuizon BD, Yoon C, Gales B, Sider D, et al. Coronary-artery calcification in young adults with end-stage renal disease who are undergoing dialysis. N Engl J Med 2000;342: 1478-83.
132. Gotch F. Urea kinetics modelling to guide hemodialysis therapy in adults. In: Nissenson AR, Fine RN, eds. Dialysis therapy. Philadelphia: Hanley and Belfus, 2002:117-21.
133. Gral T, Young M. Measured versus estimated creatinine clearance in the elderly as an index of renal function. J Am Geriatr Soc 1980;28:492-6.
134. Green A, Morgan I. Physiology of the newborn. In: Neonatology and clinical biochemistry. London: ACB Venture Publications, 1993:Chapter 2, 8-22pp.
135. Greger R. Why do loop diuretics cause hypokalemia? Nephrol Dial Transplant 1997;12:1799-801.
136. Greger R. New insights into the molecular mechanisms of the action of diuretics. Nephrol Dial Transplant 1999;14:536-40.

137. Gregory WM, Richards MA, Malpas JS. Combination chemotherapy versus melphalan and prednisolone in the treatment of multiple myeloma: an overview of published trials. J Clin Oncol 1992;10:334-42.
138. Griffiths MH, Crowe AV, Papadaki L, Banner NR, Yacoub MH, Thompson FD, et al. Cyclosporin nephrotoxicity in heart and lung transplant patients. Q J Med: 1996;89:751-63.
139. Gross CR, Limwattananon C, Matthees B, Zehrer JL, Savik K. Impact of transplantation on quality of life in patients with diabetes and renal dysfunction. Transplantation 2000;70:1736-46.
140. Groth CG, Backman L, Morales JM, Calne R, Kreis H, Lang P, et al. Sirolimus (rapamycin)-based therapy in human renal transplantation: similar efficacy and different toxicity compared with cyclosporine. Sirolimus European Renal Transplant Study Group. Transplantation 1999;67:1036-42.
141. Guerin AP, London GM, Marchais SJ, Metivier F. Arterial stiffening and vascular calcifications in end-stage renal disease. Nephrol Dial Transplant 2000;15:1014-21.
142. Gurwitz JH, Avorn J, Ross-Degnan D, Lipsitz LA. Nonsteroidal anti-inflammatory drug-associated azotemia in the very old. JAMA 1990;264:471-5.
143. Guyton AC. Blood pressure control-special role of the kidneys and body fluid. Science 1991;252: 1813-16.
144. Hackbarth H, Ail J-M., Gartner K, Sindermann H. Renal handling of albumin: clearance studies with bovine and rat serum albumin in conscious rats. Contrib Nephrol 1980;19:225-30.
145. Halloran PF, Helms LM, Kung L, Noujaim J. The temporal profile of calcineurin inhibition by cyclosporine in vivo. Transplantation 1999;68: 1356-61.
146. Hallson PC, Rose GA, Sulaiman S. Magnesium reduces calcium oxalate crystal formation in human whole urine. Clin Sci 1982;62:17.
147. Hamm LL. Renal handling of citrate. Kidney Int 1990;38:728-35.
148. Han JH, Choi SJ, Kurihara N, Koide M, Oba Y, Roodman GD. Macrophage inflammatory protein-1 alpha is an osteoclastogenic factor in myeloma that is independent of receptor activator of nuclear factor kappaB ligand. Blood 2001;97:3349-53.
149. Hansen KJ, O'Neil EA, Reaves SW, Craven TE, Plunk GW, Dean RH. Intraoperative duplex sonography during renal artery reconstruction. J Vasc Surg 1991;14:364-74.
150. Hansson L, Zanchetti A, Carruthers SG, Dahlof B, Elmfeldt D, Julius S, et al. Effects of intensive blood-pressure lowering and low-dose aspirin in patients with hypertension: Principal results of the Hypertension Optimal Treatment (HOT) randomised trial. HOT Study Group. Lancet 1998;351:1755-62.
151. Hariharan S, Johnson CP, Bresnahan BA, Taranto SE, McIntosh MJ, Stablein D. Improved graft survival after renal transplantation in the United States, 1988 to 1996. N Engl J Med 2000;342:605-12.
152. Harris RC, McKanna JA, Akai Y, Jacobson HR, Dubois RN, Breyer MD. Cyclooxygenase-2 is associated with the macula densa of rat kidney and increases with salt restriction. J Clin Invest 1994;94:2504-10.
153. Hateboer N, v Dijk MA, Bogdanova N, Coto E, Saggar Malik AK, San Millan JL, et al. Comparison of phenotypes of polycystic kidney disease types 1 and 2. European PKD1-PKD2 Study Group. Lancet 1999;353:103-7.
154. Hauer HA, Bajema IM, Van-Houwelingen HC, Ferrario F, Noel LH, Waldherr R, et al. Determinants of outcome in ANCA-associated glomerulonephritis: a prospective clinico-histopathological analysis of 96 patients. Kidney Int 2002;62:1732-42.
155. Hawkins PN. Serum amyloid P component scintigraphy for diagnosis and monitoring amyloidosis. Curr Opin Nephrol Hypertens 2002;11:649-55.
156. Hayashi T, Suzuki A, Shoji T, Togawa M, Okada N, Tsubakihara Y, et al. Cardiovascular effect of normalizing the hematocrit level during erythropoietin therapy in predialysis patients with chronic renal failure. Am J Kidney Dis 2000;35:250-6.
157. Heart Outcomes Prevention Evaluation Study Investigators. Effects of an angiotensin-converting-enzyme inhibitor, ramipril, on cardiovascular events in high-risk patients. N Engl J Med 2000;342: 145-53.
158. Heeg JE, de Jong PE, van der Hem GK, de Zeeuw D. Reduction of proteinuria by angiotensin converting enzyme inhibition. Kidney Int 1987;32:78-83.
159. Heinz F, Kohlbecker G. Oxalate. In: Bergmeyer HU, Bergmeyer J, Gral M, eds. Methods of enzymatic analysis. Vol 6. Weinheim, Germany: Verlag Chemie 1984:649.
160. Henao J, Hisamuddin I, Nzerue CM, Vasandani G, Hewan-Lowe K. Celecoxib-induced acute interstitial nephritis. Am J Kidney Dis 2002;39:1313-17.
161. Henderson DA. The aetiology of chronic nephritis in Queensland. Medical Journal of Australia 1958;25:196-202.
162. Henderson MJ. Stone analysis is not useful in the routine investigation of renal stone disease. Ann Clin Biochem 1995;32:109-11.
163. Henderson MJ. Renal stone disease: investigative aspects. Arch Dis Child 1993;68:160-2.
164. Herbert SC, Reeves WB, eds. Symposium on ion channels. Kidney Int 1995;48:1047-205.
165. Hess B, Hasler-Strub U, Ackermann D, Jaeger PH. Metabolic evaluation of patients with recurrent idiopathic calcium nephrolithiasis. Nephrol Dial Transplant 1997;12:1362-8.

166. Hesse A, Gergeleit M, Schuller P, Moller K. Analysis of urinary stones by computerized infrared spectroscopy. Eur J Clin Chem Clin Biochem 1989;27:639-42.
167. Hillege HL, Janssen WM, Bak AA, Diercks GF, Grobbee DE, Crijns HJ, et al. Microalbuminuria is common also in a nondiabetic, nonhypertensive population, and an independent indicator of cardiovascular risk factors and cardiovascular morbidity. J Intern Med 2001;249:519-26.
168. Hoffman BB, Sharma K, Zhu Y, Ziyadeh FN. Transcriptional activation of transforming growth factor-beta1 in mesangial cell culture by high glucose concentration. Kidney Int 1998;54:1107-16.
169. Hofmann W, Rossmuller B, Guder WG, Edel HH. A new strategy for characterizing proteinuria and hematuria from a single pattern of defined proteins in urine. Eur J Clin Chem Clin Biochem 1992;30: 707-12.
170. Holland MD, Galla JH, Sanders PW, Luke RG. Effect of urinary pH and diatrizoate on Bence Jones protein nephrotoxicity in the rat. Kidney Int 1985;27: 46-50.
171. Holmes RP. Measurement of urinary oxalate and citrate by capillary electrophoresis and indirect ultraviolet absorbance. Clin Chem 1995;41:1297-301.
172. Hou SH, Bushinsky DA, Wish JB, Cohen JJ, Harrington JT. Hospital-acquired renal insufficiency: a prospective study. Am J Med 1983;74:243-8.
173. Houlihan CA, Allen TJ, Baxter AL, Panangiotopoulos S, Casley DJ, Cooper ME, et al. A low-sodium diet potentiates the effects of losartan in type 2 diabetes. Diabetes Care 2002;25:663-71.
174. Hovind P, Tarnow L, Rossing P, Teerlink T, Stehouwer CD, Emeis JJ, et al. Progression of diabetic nephropathy: role of plasma homocysteine and plasminogen activator inhibitor-1. Am J Kidney Dis 2001;38: 1376-80.
175. Hovind P, Rossing P, Tarnow L, Smidt UM, Parving HH. Remission and regression in the nephropathy of type 1 diabetes when blood pressure is controlled aggressively. Kidney Int 2001;60:277-83.
176. Hovind P, Rossing P, Tarnow L, Smidt UM, Parving HH. Progression of diabetic nephropathy. Kidney Int 2001;59:702-9.
177. Hoyer JR, Seiler MW. Pathophysiology of Tamm-Horsfall protein. Kidney Int 1979;16:279-89.
178. Huang ZQ, Sanders PW. Localization of a single binding site for immunoglobulin light chains on human Tamm-Horsfall glycoprotein. J Clin Invest 1997;99:732-6.
179. Hughes J, Ward CJ, Peral B, Aspinwall R, Clark K, San Millan JL, et al. The polycystic kidney disease 1 (PKD1) gene encodes a novel protein with multiple cell recognition domains. Nat Genet 1995;10: 151-60.
180. Hume R, Weyers E. Relationship between total body water and surface area in normal and obese subjects. J Clin Pathol 1971;24:234-8.
181. Hunsicker LG, Adler S, Caggiula A, England BK, Greene T, Kusek JW, et al. Predictors of the progression of renal disease in the Modification of Diet in Renal Disease Study. Kidney Int 1997;51: 1908-19.
182. Ikizler TA, Greene JH, Wingard RL, Parker RA, Hakim RM. Spontaneous dietary protein intake during progression of chronic renal failure. J Am Soc Nephrol 1995;6:1386-91.
183. Irish AB, Winearls CG, Littlewood T. Presentation and survival of patients with severe renal failure and myeloma. Q J Med 1997;90:773-80.
184. Isono M, Mogyorosi A, Han DC, Hoffman BB, Ziyadeh FN. Stimulation of TGF-beta type II receptor by high glucose in mouse mesangial cells and in diabetic kidney. Am J Physiol Renal Physiol 2000;278:F830-8.
185. Iwano M, Plieth D, Danoff TM, Xue C, Okada H, Neilson EG. Evidence that fibroblasts derive from epithelium during tissue fibrosis. J Clin Invest 2002;110:341-50.
186. Jacobs K, Shoemaker C, Rudersdorf R, Neill SD, Kaufman RJ, Mufson A, et al. Isolation and characterization of genomic and cDNA clones of human erythropoietin. Nature 1985;313:806-10.
187. Jackle-Meyer I, Szukics B, Neubauer K, Metze V, Petzoldt R, Stolte H. Extracellular matrix proteins as early markers in diabetic nephropathy. Eur J Clin Chem Clin Biochem 1995;33:211-19.
188. Jaeger P. Genetic versus environmental factors in renal stone disease. Curr Opin Nephrol Hyperten 1996;5:342-6.
189. Jafar TH, Stark PC, Schmid CH, Landa M, Maschio G, Marcantoni C, et al. Proteinuria as a modifiable risk factor for the progression of non-diabetic renal disease. Kidney Int 2001;60:1131-40.
190. Jafar TH, Stark PC, Schmid CH, Landa M, Maschio G, de Jong PE, et al. Progression of chronic kidney disease: the role of blood pressure control, proteinuria, and angiotensin-converting enzyme inhibition. Ann Intern Med 2003;139:244-52.
191. Johnson WJ, Kyle RA, Pineda AA, O'Brien PC, Holley KE. Treatment of renal failure associated with multiple myeloma. Plasmapheresis, hemodialysis, and chemotherapy. Arch Intern Med 1990;150:863-9.
192. Johnson RW, Kreis H, Oberbauer R, Brattstrom C, Claesson K, Eris J. Sirolimus allows early cyclosporine withdrawal in renal transplantation resulting in improved renal function and lower blood pressure. Transplantation 2001;72:777-86.
193. Johnston A, David OJ, Cooney GF. Pharmacokinetic validation of neoral absorption profiling. Transplant Proc 2000;32:53S-56S.

194. Jones CA, McQuillan GM, Kusek JW, Eberhardt MS, Herman WH, Coresh J, et al. Serum creatinine levels in the US population: Third National Health and Nutrition Examination Survey. Am J Kidney Dis 1998;32:992-9.
195. Jones CA, Francis ME, Eberhardt MS, Chavers B, Coresh J, Enqelqau M, et al. Microalbuminuria in the US population: Third National Health and Nutrition Examination Survey. Am J Kidney Dis 2002;39: 445-59.
196. Jones CH, Newstead CG, Will EJ, Smye SW, Davison AM. Assessment of nutritional status in CAPD patients: serum albumin is not a useful measure. Nephrol Dial Transplant 1997;12:1406-13.
197. Jones MW. Topiramate—safety and tolerability. Can J Neurol Sci 1998;25:S13-15.
198. Jose PA, Fildes RD, Gomez A, Chevalier RL, Robillard JE. Neonatal renal function and physiology. Current Opinion in Pediatrics 1994;6:172-7.
199. Jung K, Mattenheimer H, Burchardt U, eds. Urinary enzymes in clinical and experimental medicine. Berlin: Springer-Verlag, 1992:p 9.
200. Jung K, Pergande M, Priem F, Becker S, Klotzek S. Rapid screening of low molecular mass proteinuria: evaluation of the first immunochemical test strip for the detection of alpha 1-microglobulin in urine. Eur J Clin Chem Clin Biochem 1993;31:683-7.
201. Jungers P, Chauveau P, Descamps-Latscha B, Labrunie M, Giraud E, Man NK, et al. Age and gender-related incidence of chronic renal failure in a French urban area: a prospective epidemiologic study. Nephrol Dial Transplant 1996;11:1542-6.
202. Kahan BD, Murgia MG, Slaton J, Napoli K. Potential applications of therapeutic drug monitoring of sirolimus immunosuppression in clinical renal transplantation. Ther Drug Monit 1995;17:672-5.
203. Kahan BD. Efficacy of sirolimus compared with azathioprine for reduction of acute renal allograft rejection: a randomised multicenter study. The Rapamune US Study Group. Lancet 2000;356: 194-202.
204. Kallmeyer JC, Miller NM. Urinary changes in ultra long-distance marathon runners. Nephron 1993;64:119-21.
205. Kamesh L, Harper L, Savage CO. ANCA-positive vasculitis. J Am Soc Nephrol 2002;13:1953-60.
206. Kasidas GP, Samuell CT, Weir TB. Renal stone analysis: why and how? Ann Clin Biochem 2003;40: In press.
207. Kasiske BL. Relationship between vascular disease and age-associated changes in the human kidney. Kidney Int 1987;31:1153-9.
208. Kaufmann RB, Sheedy PF, Maher JE, Bielak LF, Breen JF, Schwartz RS, et al. Quantity of coronary artery calcium detected by electron beam computed tomography in asymptomatic subjects and angiographically studied patients. Mayo Clin Proc 1995;70: 223-32.
209. Keane WF, Eknoyan G. Proteinuria, albuminuria, risk, assessment, detection, elimination (PARADE): A position paper of the National Kidney Foundation. Am J Kidney Dis 1999;33:1004-10.
210. Kershner RP, Fitzsimmons WE. Relationship of FK506 whole blood concentrations and efficacy and toxicity after liver and kidney transplantation. Transplantation 1996;62:920-6.
211. Ketteler M, Bongartz P, Westenfeld R, Wildberger JE, Mahnken AH, Bohm R, et al. Association of low fetuin-A (AHSG) concentrations in serum with cardiovascular mortality in patients on dialysis: A cross-sectional study. Lancet 2003;361:827-33.
212. Khan IH, Catto GR, Edward N, MacLeod AM. Chronic renal failure: factors influencing nephrology referral. Q J Med 1994;87:559-64.
213. Khan IH, Catto GR, Edward N, MacLeod AM. Acute renal failure: factors influencing nephrology referral and outcome. Q J Med 1997;90:781-5.
214. Kimberling WJ, Kumar S, Gabow PA, Kenyon JB, Connolly CJ, Somlo S. Autosomal dominant polycystic kidney disease: Localization of the second gene to chromosome 4q13-q23. Genomics 1993;18: 467-72.
215. King H, Rewers M. Global estimates for prevalence of diabetes mellitus and impaired glucose tolerance in adults. WHO Ad Hoc Diabetes Reporting Group. Diabetes Care 1993;16:157-77.
216. Klahr S. Chronic renal failure: Management. Lancet 1991;338:423-7.
217. Klahr S, Levey AS, Beck GJ, Caggiula AW, Hunsicker L, Kusek JW, et al. The effects of dietary protein restriction and blood-pressure control on the progression of chronic renal disease. Modification of Diet in Renal Disease Study Group. N Engl J Med 1994;330:877-84.
218. Klein R, Klein BE, Moss SE, Cruickshanks KJ, Brazy PC. The 10-year incidence of renal insufficiency in people with type 1 diabetes. Diabetes Care 1999;22:743-51.
219. Kluth DC, Rees AJ. Anti-glomerular basement membrane disease. J Am Soc Nephrol 1999;10:2446-53.
220. Koffler D, Agnello V, Kimkel HG. Polynucleotide immune complexes in serum and glomeruli of patients with systemic lupus erythematosus. Am J Pathol 1974;74:109-24.
221. Kohan AD, Armenakas NA, Fraccia JA. Indinavir urolithiasis: an emerging cause of renal colic in patients with human immunodeficiency virus. J Urol 1999;161:1765-8.
222. Korevaar JC, Jansen MA, Dekker FW, Jager KJ, Boeschoten EW, Krediet RT, et al. When to initiate dialysis: effect of proposed US guidelines on survival. Lancet 2001;358:1046-50.

223. Koss MN, Pirani CL, Osserman EF. Experimental Bence Jones cast nephropathy. Lab Invest 1976;34:579-91.
224. Kuhlmann U, Goldau R, Samadi N, Graf T, Gross M, Orlandini G, et al. Accuracy and safety of online clearance monitoring based on conductivity variation. Nephrol Dial Transplant 2001;16:1053-8.
225. Kunzmann V, Bauer E, Feurle J, Weissinger F, Tony HP, Wilhelm M. Stimulation of gammadelta T cells by aminobisphosphonates and induction of antiplasma cell activity in multiple myeloma. Blood 2000;96:384-92.
226. Kyle RA. Multiple myeloma: Review of 869 cases. Mayo Clin Proc 1975;50:29-40.
227. Kyle RA, Greipp PR. Primary systemic amyloidosis: comparison of melphalan and prednisone versus placebo. Blood 1978;52:818-27.
228. Kyle RA, Gertz MA, Greipp PR, Witzig TE, Lust JA, Lacy MQ, et al. A trial of three regimens for primary amyloidosis: colchicine alone, melphalan and prednisone, and melphalan, prednisone, and colchicine. N Engl J Med 1997;336:1202-7.
229. Lachmann HJ, Gallimore R, Gillmore JD, Carr-Smith HD, Bradwell AR, Pepys MB, et al. Outcome in systemic AL amyloidosis in relation to changes in concentration of circulating free immunoglobulin light chains following chemotherapy. Br J Hematol 2003;122:78-84.
230. Laker MF, Hofmann AF, Meeuse BJD. Spectrophotometric determination of urinary oxalate with oxalate oxidase prepared from moss. Clin Chem 1980;26: 827-30.
231. Lameire NH, Vanholder R, Veyt D, Lambert MC, Ringoir S. A longitudinal, five year survey of urea kinetic parameters in CAPD patients. Kidney Int 1992;42:426-32.
232. Lameire NH, Vanholder R. Pathophysiologic features and prevention of human and experimental acute tubular necrosis. J Am Soc Nephrol 2001;12 Suppl 1:S20-32.
233. Larsson L, Libert B, Asperud M. Determination of urinary oxalate by reversed-phase ion-pair high performance liquid chromatography. Clin Chem 1983;28:2272-74.
234. Ledebo I. On-line hemodiafiltration: technique and therapy. Adv Ren Replace Ther 1999;6: 195-208.
235. Levey AS, Beto JA, Coronado BE, Eknoyan G, Foley RN, Kasiske BL, et al. Controlling the epidemic of cardiovascular disease in chronic renal disease: what do we know? What do we need to learn? Where do we go from here? National Kidney Foundation Task Force on Cardiovascular Disease. Am J Kidney Dis 1998;32:853-906.
236. Levin A, Singer J, Thompson CR, Ross H, Lewis M. Prevalent left ventricular hypertrophy in the predialysis population: identifying opportunities for intervention. Am J Kidney Dis 1996;27:347-54.
237. Levin A, Thompson CR, Ethier J, Carlisle EJ, Tobe S, Mendelssohn D, et al. Left ventricular mass index increase in early renal disease: impact of decline in hemoglobin. Am J Kidney Dis 1999;34:125-34.
238. Lewis EJ, Hunsicker LG, Clarke WR, Berl T, Pohl MA, Lewis JB, et al. Renoprotective effect of the angiotensin-receptor antagonist irbesartan in patients with nephropathy due to type 2 diabetes. N Engl J Med 2001;345:851-60.
239. Liano F, Pascual J. Epidemiology of acute renal failure: a prospective, multicenter, community-based study. Madrid Acute Renal Failure Study Group. Kidney Int 1996;50:811-8.
240. Lien YH, Hansen R, Kern WF, Bangert J, Nagle RB, Ko M, et al. Ciprofloxacin-induced granulomatous interstitial nephritis and localized elastolysis. Am J Kidney Dis 1993;22:598-602.
241. Ligtenberg G, Blankestijn PJ, Oey PL, Klein IH, Dijkhorst Oei LT, Boomsma F, et al. Reduction of sympathetic hyperactivity by enalapril in patients with chronic renal failure. N Engl J Med 1999;340:1321-8.
242. Lin J-L, Lin-Tan D-T, Hsu K-H, Yu C-C. Environmental lead exposure and progression of chronic renal diseases in patients without diabetes. N Engl J Med 2003;348:277-86.
243. Lindberg JS, Moe SM, Goodman WG, Coburn JW, Sprague SM, Liu W, et al. The calcimimetic AMG 073 reduces parathyroid hormone and calcium x phosphorus in secondary hyperparathyroidism. Kidney Int 2003;63:248-54.
244. Lindeman RD. Is the decline in renal function with normal aging inevitable? Geriatr Nephrol Urol 1998;8:7-9.
245. Lindeman RD, Tobin JD, Shock NW. Association between blood pressure and the rate of decline in renal function with age. Kidney Int 1984;26: 861-8.
246. Lindeman RD, Tobin J, Shock NW. Longitudinal studies on the rate of decline in renal function with age. J Am Geriatr Soc 1985; 33:278-85.
247. Ljunghall S, Danielson BG. A prospective study of renal stone recurrences. Br J Urol 1984;56:122-4.
248. Locatelli F, Conte F, Marcelli D. The impact of hematocrit levels and erythropoietin treatment on overall and cardiovascular mortality and morbidity—the experience of the Lombardy Dialysis Registry. Nephrol Dial Transplant 1998;13:1642-4.
249. Long-Term Intervention with Pravastatin in Ischemic Disease (LIPID) Study Group. Prevention of cardiovascular events and death with pravastatin in patients with coronary heart disease and a broad range of initial cholesterol levels. N Engl J Med 1998;339:1349-57.

250. London NJ, Farmery SM, Will EJ, Davison AM, Lodge JP. Risk of neoplasia in renal transplant patients. Lancet 1995;346:403-6.
251. Lote CJ. Essential anatomy of the kidney. In: Lote CJ, ed. Principles of renal physiology, 3rd ed. London: Chapman and Hall, 1994:21-9.
252. Lowrie EG, Laird NM, Parker TF, Sargent JA. Effect of the hemodialysis prescription of patient morbidity: report from the National Cooperative Dialysis Study. N Engl J Med 1981;305:1176-81.
253. Ma JZ, Ebben J, Xia H, Collins AJ. Hematocrit level and associated mortality in hemodialysis patients. J Am Soc Nephrol 1999;10:610-19.
254. Maack T, Johnson V, Kan ST, Fiqueiredo J, Siqulem D. Renal filtration transport and metabolism of low molecular weight proteins: A review. Kidney Int 1979;16:251-70.
255. Macconi D, Ghilardi M, Bonassi ME, Mohamed EI, Abbate M, Colombi F, et al. Effect of angiotensin-converting enzyme inhibition on glomerular basement membrane permeability and distribution of zonula occludens-1 in MWF rats. J Am Soc Nephrol: Jasn 2000;11:477-89.
256. MacLennan IC, Chapman C, Dunn J, Kelly K. Combined chemotherapy with ABCM versus melphalan for treatment of myelomatosis. The Medical Research Council Working Party for Leukaemia in Adults. Lancet 1992;339:200-5.
257. Maggi E, Bellazzi R, Falaschi F, Frattoni A, Perani G, Finardi G, et al. Enhanced LDL oxidation in uremic patients: An additional mechanism for accelerated atherosclerosis? Kidney Int 1994;45:876-83.
258. Magnason RL, Indridason OS, Sigvaldason H, Sigfusson N, Palsson R. Prevalence and progression of CRF in Iceland: a population-based study. Am J Kidney Dis 2002;40:955-63.
259. Mahalati K, Belitsky P, Sketris I, West K, Panek R. Neoral monitoring by simplified sparse sampling area under the concentration-time curve: Its relationship to acute rejection and cyclosporine nephrotoxicity early after kidney transplantation. Transplantation 1999;68:55-62.
260. Mailloux LU, Napolitano B, Bellucci AG, Vernace M, Wilkes BM, Mossey RT. Renal vascular disease causing end-stage renal disease, incidence, clinical correlates, and outcomes: A 20-year clinical experience. Am J Kidney Dis 1994;24:622-9.
261. Maiorca R, Brunori G, Zubani R, Cancarini GC, Manili L, Camerini C, et al. Predictive value of dialysis adequacy and nutritional indices for mortality and morbidity in CAPD and HD patients. A longitudinal study. Nephrol Dial Transplant 1995;10:2295-305.
262. Mange KC, Joffe MM, Feldman HI. Effect of the use or nonuse of long-term dialysis on the subsequent survival of renal transplants from living donors. N Engl J Med 2001;344:726-31.
263. Mann JF, Gerstein HC, Pogue J, Bosch J, Yusuf S. Renal insufficiency as a predictor of cardiovascular outcomes and the impact of ramipril: The HOPE randomized trial. Ann Int Med 2001;134:629-36.
264. Markowitz GS, Falkowitz DC, Isom R, Zaki M, Imaizumi S, Appel GB, et al. Membranous glomerulopathy and acute interstitial nephritis following treatment with celecoxib. Clin Nephrol 2003;59: 137-42.
265. Marks MI, McLaine PN, Drummond KN. Proteinuria in children with febrile illnesses. Arch Dis Child 1970;45:250-3.
266. Marsh JT, Brown WS, Wolcott D, Carr CR, Harper R, Schweitzer SV, et al. rHuEPO treatment improves brain and cognitive function of anemic dialysis patients. Kidney Int 1991;39:155-63.
267. Martin KJ, Gonzalez EA, Gellens M, Hamm LL, Abboud H, Lindberg J. 19-Nor-1-alpha-25-dihydroxyvitamin D2 (Paricalcitol) safely and effectively reduces the levels of intact parathyroid hormone in patients on hemodialysis. J Am Soc Nephrol 1998;9:1427-32.
268. Maschio G, Alberti D, Janin G, Locatelli F, Mann JF, Motolese M, et al. Effect of the angiotensin-converting-enzyme inhibitor benazepril on the progression of chronic renal insufficiency. The Angiotensin-Converting-Enzyme Inhibition in Progressive Renal Insufficiency Study Group. N Engl J Med 1996;334:939-45.
269. Mason RM, Wahab NA. Extracellular matrix metabolism in diabetic nephropathy. J Am Soc Nephrol 2003;14:1358-73.
270. Massy ZA, Khoa TN, Lacour B, Descamps Latscha B, Man NK, Jungers P. Dyslipidaemia and the progression of renal disease in chronic renal failure patients. Nephrol Dial Transplant 1999;14:2392-7.
271. Mastrangelo F, Alfonso L, Napoli M, DeBlasi V, Russo F, Patruno P. Dialysis with increased frequency of sessions (Lecce dialysis). Nephrol Dial Transplant 1998;13 Suppl 6:139-47.
272. Maurisbach AB, Christenson EK. Functional ultrastructure of the proximal tube. In: Handbook of physiology (vol. 1): Renal physiology. Windhager EE, ed. Oxford: Oxford University Press, 1992.
273. Mayer AD, Dmitrewski J, Squifflet JP, Besse T, Grabensee B, Klein B, et al. Multicenter randomized trial comparing tacrolimus (FK506) and cyclosporine in the prevention of renal allograft rejection: A report of the European Tacrolimus Multicenter Renal Study Group. Transplantation 1997;64:436-43.
274. Mayer G, Thum J, Cada EM, Stummvoll HK, Graf H. Working capacity is increased following recombinant human erythropoietin treatment. Kidney Int 1988;34:525-8.
275. McGiff JC, Crowshaw K, Terragno NA, Lonigro AJ. Renal prostaglandins: possible regulators of the renal

actions of pressor hormones. Nature 1970;227: 1255-7.
276. McKelvie GB, Collins GN, Hehir M, Rogers AC. A study of benign prostatic hyperplasia: A challenge to British urology. Br J Urol 1993;71:38-42.
277. Medical Research Council/British Heart Foundation. Heart Protection Study of cholesterol lowering with simvastatin in 20,536 high-risk individuals: A randomised placebo-controlled trial. Lancet 2002;360: 7-22.
278. Mehta RL, Chertow GM. Acute renal failure definitions and classification: time for change? J Am Soc Nephrol 2003;14:2178-87.
279. Merion RM, White DJ, Thiru S, Evans DB, Calne RY. Cyclosporine: five years' experience in cadaveric renal transplantation. N Engl J Med 1984;310:148-54.
280. Metcalfe MS, Butterworth PC, White SA, Saunders RN, Murphy GJ, Taub N, et al. A case-control comparison of the results of renal transplantation from heart-beating and non-heart-beating donors. Transplantation 2001;71:1556-9.
281. Milliner DS. Cystinuria. Endocrinol Metab Clin North Am 1990;19:889-907.
282. Mogensen CE, Neldam S, Tikkanen I, Oren S, Viskoper R, Watts RW, et al. Randomised controlled trial of dual blockade of renin-angiotensin system in patients with hypertension, microalbuminuria, and non-insulin dependent diabetes: the candesartan and lisinopril microalbuminuria (CALM) study. BMJ 2000;321:1440-4.
283. Mollering H. Citrate. In: Bergmeyer HU, Bergmeyer J, Gral M, eds. Methods of enzymatic analysis (vol 7). Weinheim, Germany: Verlag Chemie, 1984:2.
284. Mollerup CL, Vestergaard P, Gedso Frokjaer V, Mosekilde L, Christiansen P, Blichert-Toft M. Risk of renal stone events in primary hyperparathyroidism before and after parathyroid surgery: controlled retrospective follow up study. BMJ 2002;325:807-10.
285. Moreau P, Leblond V, Bourquelot P, Facon T, Huynh A, Caillot D, et al. Prognostic factors for survival and response after high-dose therapy and autologous stem cell transplantation in systemic AL amyloidosis: a report on 21 patients. Br J Hematol 1998;101: 766-9.
286. Moreno F, Aracil FJ, Perez R, Valderrabano F. Controlled study on the improvement of quality of life in elderly hemodialysis patients after correcting end-stage renal disease-related anemia with erythropoietin. Am J Kidney Dis 1996;27:548-56.
287. Mucsi I, Hercz G, Uldall R, Ouwendyk M, Francoeur R, Pierratos A. Control of serum phosphate without any phosphate binders in patients treated with nocturnal hemodialysis. Kidney Int 1998;53: 1399-404.
288. Mudd SH, Skovby F, Levy HL, Pettigrew KD, Wilcken B, Pyeritz RE, et al. The natural history of homocystinuria due to cystathionine beta-synthase deficiency. Am J Hum Genet 1985;37:1-31.
289. Muller D, Hoenderop JG, van OS CH, Bindels RJ. The epithelial calcium channel, ECaC1: molecular details of a novel player in renal calcium handling. Nephrol Dial Transplant 2001;16:1329-35.
290. Murer H, Biber J, eds. Forefronts in nephrology: phosphates. Kidney Int 1996;49: [entire issue].
291. Nakamura T, Obata J, Kimura H, Ohno S, Yoshida Y, Kawachi H, et al. Blocking angiotensin II ameliorates proteinuria and glomerular lesions in progressive mesangioproliferative glomerulonephritis. Kidney Int 1999;55:877-89.
292. Nakao N, Yoshimura A, Morita H, Takada M, Kayano T, Ideura T. Combination treatment of angiotensin-II receptor blocker and angiotensin-converting-enzyme inhibitor in non-diabetic renal disease (COOPERATE): A randomised controlled trial. Lancet 2003;361:117-24.
293. National Kidney Foundation. K/DOQI Clinical Practice Guidelines for Anemia of Chronic Kidney Disease: Update 2000. Am J Kidney Dis 2001;37 Suppl 1 S182.
294. National Kidney Foundation. K/DOQI Clinical Practice Guidelines for peritoneal dialysis adequacy, 2000. Am J Kidney Dis 2001 (suppl 1) 37:S65-S136.
295. National Kidney Foundation. K/DOQI: Clinical practice guidelines for chronic kidney disease: evaluation, classification, and stratification. Kidney Disease Outcome Quality Initiative. Am J Kidney Dis: 2002;39:S1-246.
296. National Kidney Foundation. K/DOQI: Clinical Practice Guidelines for managing dyslipidemias in chronic kidney disease. Am J Kidney Dis 2003;41: S1-S91.
297. Newman DJ, Cystatin C. Ann Clin Biochem 2002;39:89-104
298. Nielsen S. Endocytosis in renal proximal tubules. Experimental electron microscopical studies of protein absorption and membrane traffic in isolated, in vitro perfused proximal tubules. Dan Med Bull 1994;41:243-63.
299. Nielsen S, Frokiaer J, Marples D, Kwon TH, Agre P, Knepper MA. Aquaporins in the kidney: from molecules to medicine. Physiol Rev 2002;82:205-44.
300. Nielsen S, Kwon TH, Christensen BM, Promeneur D, Frokiaer J, Marples D. Physiology and pathophysiology of the renal aquaporins. J Am Soc Nephrol 1999;10:647-63.
301. Niles JL, McCluskey RT, Ahmad MF, Arnaout MA. Wegener's granulomatosis autoantigen is a novel neutrophil serine proteinase. Blood 1989;74: 1888-93.
302. Nuyts GD, Roels HA, Verpooten GF, Bernard AM, Lauwerys RR, De Broe ME. Intestinal-type alkaline phosphatase in urine as an indicator of mercury

induced effects on the S3 segment of the proximal tubule. Nephrol Dial Transplant 1992;7:225-9.
303. Nyengaard J, Bendsten T. Glomerular number and size in relation to age, kidney weight, and body surface in normal men. Anat Rec 1992;232:194-200.
304. Oda H, Keane WF. Lipid abnormalities in end stage renal disease. Nephrol Dial Transplant 1998;13 Suppl 1:45-9.
305. Ofsthun N, Labrecque J, Lacson E, Keen M, Lazarus JM. The effects of higher hemoglobin levels on mortality and hospitalization in hemodialysis patients. Kidney Int 2003;63:1908-14.
306. Ohkubo Y, Kishikawa H, Araki E, Miyata T, Isami S, Motoyoshi S, et al. Intensive insulin therapy prevents the progression of diabetic microvascular complications in Japanese patients with non-insulin-dependent diabetes mellitus: A randomized prospective 6-year study. Diabetes Res Clin Pract 1995;28:103-17.
307. Olson KB, Hall TC, Horton J, Khung CL, Holsey HF. Thalidomide (N-phthaloylglutamimide) in the treatment of advanced cancer. Clin Pharmacol Ther 1965;6:292-7.
308. Orth SR, Ritz E, Schrier RW. The renal risks of smoking. Kidney Int 1997;51:1669-77.
309. Osterby R, Gall MA, Schmitz A, Nielsen FS, Nyberg G, Parving HH. Glomerular structure and function in proteinuric type 2 (non-insulin-dependent) diabetic patients. Diabetologia 1993;36:1064-70.
310. Owen WF, Lew NL, Liu Y, Lowrie EG, Lazarus JM. The urea reduction ratio and serum albumin concentration as predictors of mortality in patients undergoing hemodialysis. N Engl J Med 1993;329: 1001-6.
311. Owen WF, Lowrie EG. C-reactive protein as an outcome predictor for maintenance hemodialysis patients. Kidney Int 1998;54:627-36.
312. Paisley KE, Tomson CRV. Calcium phosphate stones during long-term acetazolamide treatment for epilepsy. Postgrad Med J 1999;75:427-8.
313. Pak CYC. Citrate and renal calculi. Miner Electrol Metab 1987;13:257-66.
314. Paniagua R, Amato D, Vonesh E, Correa-Rotter R, Ramos A, Moran J, et al. Effects of increased peritoneal clearances on mortality rates in peritoneal dialysis: ADEMEX, a prospective, randomized, controlled trial. J Am Soc Nephrol 2002;13:1307-20.
315. Park IS, Kiyomoto H, Abboud SL, Abboud HE. Expression of transforming growth factor-beta and type IV collagen in early streptozotocin-induced diabetes. Diabetes 1997;46:473-80.
316. Parks JH, Coward M, Coe FL. Correspondence between stone composition and urine supersaturation in nephrolithiasis. Kidney Int 1997;51:894-900.
317. Parving H-H, Lehnert H, Brochner-Mortensen J, Gomis R, Andersen S, Arner P, et al. The effect of irbesartan on the development of diabetic nephropathy in patients with type 2 diabetes. N Engl J Med 2001;345:870-8.
318. Pastan S, Bailey J. Dialysis therapy. N Engl J Med 1998;338:1428-37.
319. Paterson AD, Pei Y. Is there a third gene for autosomal dominant polycystic kidney disease? Kidney Int 1998;54:1759-61.
320. Payne RB. Renal tubular reabsorption of phosphate (T_mP/GFR): indications and interpretation. Ann Clin Biochem 1998;35:201-6.
321. Pearce SHS. Straightening out the renal tubule: advances in the molecular basis of the inherited tubulopathies. Q J Med 1998;91:5-12.
322. Penney M, Walters G. Are osmolality measurements clinically useful? Ann Clin Biochem 1987;24:566-71.
323. Penney M. Sodium, water and potassium. In: Marshall WJ, Bangert SK, eds. Clinical biochemistry. New York: Churchill Livingstone, 1995:25-60.
324. Penney MD, Oleesky DA. Renal tubular acidosis. Ann Clin Biochem 1999;36:408-22.
325. Perrone RD, Madias NE, Levey AS. Serum creatinine as an index of renal function: new insights from old concepts. Clin Chem 1992;38:1933-53.
326. Peterson JC, Adler S, Burkart JM, Greene T, Hebert LA, Hunsicker LG, et al. Blood pressure control, proteinuria, and the progression of renal disease. The Modification of Diet in Renal Disease Study. Ann Intern Med 1995;123:754-62.
327. Petrarulo M, Cerelli E, Marangella M, Cosseddu D, Vitale C, Linari F. Assay of plasma oxalate with soluble oxalate oxidase. Clin Chem 1994;40:2030-4.
328. Pirsch JD, Miller J, Deierhoi MH, Vincenti F, Filo RS. A comparison of tacrolimus (FK506) and cyclosporine for immunosuppression after cadaveric renal transplantation. FK506 Kidney Transplant Study Group. Transplantation 1997;63:977-83.
329. Pisoni RL, Young EW, Dykstra DM, Greenwood RN, Hecking E, Gillespie B, et al. Vascular access use in Europe and the United States: results from the DOPPS. Kidney Int 2002;61:305-16.
330. Plehn JF, Davis BR, Sacks FM, Rouleau JL, Pfeffer MA, Bernstein V, et al. Reduction of stroke incidence after myocardial infarction with pravastatin: The Cholesterol and Recurrent Events (CARE) study. Circulation 1999;99:216-23.
331. Popovich RP, Moncrief JW, Decherd JF, Hlavinka DJ, Bomar JB. The definition of a novel portable-wearable equilibrium peritoneal technique (abstract). Am Soc Artif Intern Organs 1976:p64.
332. Port FK, Wolfe RA, Mauger EA, Berling DP, Jiang K. Comparison of survival probabilities for dialysis patients vs cadaveric renal transplant recipients. JAMA 1993;270:1339-43.
333. Port FK, Hulbert-Shearon TE, Wolfe RA, Bloembergen WE, Golper TA, Agodoa LY, et al.

Predialysis blood pressure and mortality risk in a national sample of maintenance hemodialysis patients. Am J Kidney Dis 1999;33:507-17.
334. Portoles J, Torralbo A, Martin P, Rodrigo J, Herrero JA, Barrientos A. Cardiovascular effects of recombinant human erythropoietin in predialysis patients. Am J Kidney Dis 1997;29:541-8.
335. Pozzi C, Bolasco PG, Fogazzi GB, Andrulli S, Altieri P, Ponticelli C, et al. Corticosteroids in IgA nephropathy: A randomised controlled trial. Lancet 1999;353: 883-7.
336. Praga M, Hernandez E, Montoyo C, Andres A, Ruilope LM, Rodicio JL. Long-term beneficial effects of angiotensin-converting enzyme inhibition in patients with nephrotic proteinuria. Am J Kidney Dis 1992;20:240-8.
337. Prakash J, Sen D, Kumar NS, Kumar H, Tripathi LK, Saxena RK. Acute renal failure due to intrinsic renal diseases: Review of 1122 cases. Ren Fail 2003;25: 225-33.
338. Preminger GM. Is there a need for medical evaluation and treatment of nephrolithiasis in the "age of lithotripsy"? Semin Urol 1994;12:51-64.
339. Preminger GM. The metabolic evaluation of patients with recurrent nephrolithiasis: A review of comprehensive and simplified approaches. J Urol 1989;141:760-3.
340. Price RG, Taylor SA, Crutcher E. Assay of laminin fragments in the assessment of renal disease. Kidney Int Suppl 1994;47:S25-8.
341. Prommool S, Jhangri GS, Cockfield SM, Halloran PF. Time dependency of factors affecting renal allograft survival. J Am Soc Nephrol 2000;11:565-73.
342. Raij L, Bayki C. Glomerular actions of nitric oxide. Kidney Int 1995;48:20-32.
343. Raj DS, Charra B, Pierratos A, Work J. In search of ideal hemodialysis: Is prolonged frequent dialysis the answer? Am J Kidney Dis 1999;34:597-610.
344. Rastegar A, Kashgarian M. The clinical spectrum of tubulointerstitial nephritis. Kidney Int 1998;54: 313-27.
345. Ravid M, Brosh D, Ravid Safran D, Levy Z, Rachmani R. Main risk factors for nephropathy in type 2 diabetes mellitus are plasma cholesterol levels, mean blood pressure, and hyperglycemia. Ann Intern Med 1998;158:998-1004.
346. Reeders ST, Breuning MH, Davies KE, Nicholls RD, Jarman AP, Higgs DR, et al. A highly polymorphic DNA marker linked to adult polycystic kidney disease on chromosome 16. Nature 1985;317:542-4.
347. Reeves WB, Winters CJ, Zimniak L, Andreoli TE. Medullary thick limbs: renal concentrating segments. Kidney Int 1996;57(Suppl):S154-64.
348. Reiser J, von Gersdorff G, Simons M, Schwarz K, Faul C, Giardino L, et al. Novel concepts in understanding and management of glomerular proteinuria. Nephrol Dial Transplant 2002;17:951-5.
349. Remuzzi A, Perticucci E, Ruggenenti P, Mosconi L, Limonta M, Remuzzi G. Angiotensin converting enzyme inhibition improves glomerular size-selectivity in IgA nephropathy. Kidney Int 1991;39: 1267-73.
350. Remuzzi G, Ruggenenti P, Benigni A. Understanding the nature of renal disease progression. Kidney Int 1997;51:2-15.
351. Report of the Expert Committee on the Diagnosis and Classification of Diabetes Mellitus. Diabetes Care 1997;20:1183-97.
352. Revicki DA, Brown RE, Feeny DH, Henry D, Teehan BP, Rudnick MR, et al. Health-related quality of life associated with recombinant human erythropoietin therapy for predialysis chronic renal disease patients. Am J Kidney Dis 1995;25:548-54.
353. Risdon RA, Sloper JC, De Wardener HE. Relationship between renal function and histological changes found in renal-biopsy specimens from patients with persistent glomerular nephritis. Lancet 1968;2:363-6.
354. Robertson WG, Peacock M, Heyburn PJ, Hanes FA, Rutherford A, Clementson E, et al. Should recurrent calcium oxalate stone formers become vegetarians? Br J Urol 1979;51:427-31.
355. Robertson WG, Peacock M, Heyburn PJ, Marshall DH, Clark PB. Risk factors in calcium stone disease of the urinary tract. Br J Urol 1978;50:449-54.
356. Robinson GB, Walton HA. Glomerular basement membrane as a compressible ultra filter. Microvasc Res 1989;38:36-48.
357. Robson MG, Banerjee D, Hopster D, Cairns HS. Seven cases of granulomatous interstitial nephritis in the absence of extrarenal sarcoid. Nephrol Dial Transplant 2003;18:280-4.
358. Ronco P, Brunisholz M, Geniteau Legendre M, Chatelet F, Verroust P, Richet G. Physiopathologic aspects of Tamm-Horsfall protein: A phylogenetically conserved marker of the thick ascending limb of Henle's loop. Adv Nephrol Necker Hosp1987;16: 231-49.
359. Rose GA, Woodfine C. The thermogravimetric analysis of renal stones (in clinical practice). Br J Urol 1976;48:403-12.
360. Rowe JW, Andres R, Tobin JD, Norris AH, Shock NW. The effect of age on creatinine clearance in men: A cross-sectional and longitudinal study. J Gerontol 1976;31:155-63.
361. Ruggenenti P, Perna A, Mosconi L, Pisoni R, Remuzzi G. Urinary protein excretion rate is the best independent predictor of ESRF in non-diabetic proteinuric chronic nephropathies. Kidney Int 1998;53:1209-16.
362. Ruggenenti P, Perna A, Gherardi G, Gaspari F, Benini R, Remuzzi G. Renal function and requirement for

dialysis in chronic nephropathy patients on long-term ramipril: REIN follow-up trial. Gruppo Italiano di Studi Epidemiologici in Nefrologia (GISEN). Ramipril efficacy in nephropathy. Lancet 1998;352:1252-6.

363. Ruggenenti P, Perna A, Gherardi G, Garini G, Zoccali C, Salvadori M, et al. Renoprotective properties of ACE-inhibition in non-diabetic nephropathies with non-nephrotic proteinuria. Lancet 1999;354:359-64.

364. Rumberger JA, Simons DB, Fitzpatrick LA, Sheedy PF, Schwartz RS. Coronary artery calcium area by electron-beam computed tomography and coronary atherosclerotic plaque area. A histopathologic correlative study. Circulation 1995;92:2157-62.

365. Samuell CT, Kasidas GP. Biochemical investigations in renal stone formers. Ann Clin Biochem 1995;32: 112-22.

366. Sanders PW, Herrera GA, Galla JH. Human Bence Jones protein toxicity in rat proximal tubule epithelium in vivo. Kidney Int 1987;32:851-61.

367. Sands JM, Kokko JP. Current concepts of the countercurrent multiplication system. Kidney Int 1996;57(Suppl):S93-9.

368. Sarnak MJ. Epidemiology of cardiovascular disease in chronic renal disease. J Am Soc Nephrol 1998;9: 160A.

369. Satoh M, Kashihara N, Yamasaki Y, Maruyama K, Okamoto K, Maeshima Y, et al. Renal interstitial fibrosis is reduced in angiotensin II type 1a receptor-deficient mice. J Am Soc Nephrol 2001;12:317-25.

370. Savage CO. ANCA-associated renal vasculitis. Kidney Int 2001;60:1614-27.

371. Sayer JA, Pearce SHS. Diagnosis and clinical biochemistry of inherited tubulopathies. Ann Clin Biochem 2001;38:459-70.

372. Scandinavian Simvastatin Survival Study (4S). Randomised trial of cholesterol lowering in 4444 patients with coronary heart disease: Lancet 1994; 344:1383-9.

373. Schainuck LI, Striker GE, Cutler RE, Benditt EP. Structural-functional correlations in renal disease: Part II. The correlations. Hum Pathol 1970;1: 631-41.

374. Scheinman SJ, Guay-Woodford LM, Thakker RJ, Warnock DG. Genetic disorders of renal electrolyte transport. N Engl J Med 1999;340:1177-87.

375. Schmidt AM, Vianna M, Gerlach M, Brett J, Ryan J, Kao J, et al. Isolation and characterization of two binding proteins for advanced glycosylation end products from bovine lung which are present on the endothelial cell surface. J Biol Chem 1992;267: 14987-97.

376. Schmidt S, Ritz E. The role of angiotensin I-converting enzyme gene polymorphism in renal disease. Curr Opin Nephrol Hypertens 1996;5:552-5.

377. Schreiner GE. Prevention of renal disease and conservation of function. Am J Kidney Dis 1990;16: 360-6.

378. Schrier RW, Estacio RO, Esler A, Mehler P. Effects of aggressive blood pressure control in normotensive type 2 diabetic patients on albuminuria, retinopathy and strokes. Kidney Int 2002;61:1086-97.

379. Schwarz A, Krause PH, Kunzendorf U, Keller F, Distler A. The outcome of acute interstitial nephritis: Risk factors for the transition from acute to chronic interstitial nephritis. Clin Nephrol 2000; 54:179-90.

380. Scoble JE. Do protection devices have a role in renal angioplasty and stent placement? Nephrol Dial Transplant 2003;18:1700-3

381. Seibert K, Zhang Y, Leahy K, Hauser S, Masferrer J, Perkins W, et al. Pharmacological and biochemical demonstration of the role of cyclooxygenase 2 in inflammation and pain. Proc Natl Acad Sci U S A 1994;91:12013-17.

382. Segal S, Thier SD. Cystinuria. In: Scriver CR, Beaudet AL, Sly WS, Valle D, eds. The metabolic basis of inherited disease. New York: McGraw-Hill, 1995:3581.

383. Seldin DW, Giebisch G, eds. The kidney: physiology and pathophysiology (vol 1). 2nd ed. New York: Raven Press, 1992:943-981.

384. Selgas R, Bajo MA, Fernandez-Reyes MJ, Bosque E, Lopez-Revuelta K, Jimenez C, et al. An analysis of adequacy of dialysis in a selected population on CAPD for more than 3 years: the influence of urea and creatinine kinetics. Nephrol Dial Transplant 1993; 8:1244-53.

385. Shanahan CM, Proudfoot D, Farzaneh Far A, Weissberg PL. The role of Gla proteins in vascular calcification. Crit Rev Eukaryot Gene Expr 1998;8: 357-75.

386. Sharma K, Ziyadeh FN, Alzahabi B, McGowan TA, Kapoor S, Kurnik BR, et al. Increased renal production of transforming growth factor-beta1 in patients with type II diabetes. Diabetes 1997;46:854-9.

387. Sharma K, Eltayeb BO, McGowan TA, Dunn SR, Alzahabi B, Rohde R, et al. Captopril-induced reduction of serum levels of transforming growth factor-beta1 correlates with long-term renoprotection in insulin-dependent diabetic patients. Am J Kidney Dis 1999;34:818-23.

388. Sherman RA, Cody RP, Rogers ME, Solanchick JC. Accuracy of the urea reduction ratio in predicting dialysis delivery. Kidney Int 1995;47:319-21.

389. Silberberg JS, Barre PE, Prichard SS, Sniderman AD. Impact of left ventricular hypertrophy on survival in end-stage renal disease. Kidney Int 1989;36: 286-90.

390. Silve C. Tubular handling and regulation of sulphate. Nephrol Dial Transplant 2000;25[suppl 6]:34-5.

391. Singhal S, Mehta J, Desikan R, Ayers D, Roberson P, Eddlemon P, et al. Antitumor activity of thalidomide in refractory multiple myeloma. N Engl J Med 1999;341:1565-71.
392. Sixth report of the Joint National Committee on prevention, detection, evaluation, and treatment of high blood pressure. Arch Intern Med 1997;157: 2413-46.
393. Skinner M, Anderson J, Simms R, Falk R, Wang M, Libbey C, et al. Treatment of 100 patients with primary amyloidosis: a randomized trial of melphalan, prednisone, and colchicine versus colchicine only. Am J Med 1996;100:290-8.
394. Slatopolsky E, Caglar S, Pennell JP, Taggart DD, Canterbury JM, Reiss E, et al. On the pathogenesis of hyperparathyroidism in chronic experimental renal insufficiency in the dog. J Clin Invest 1971;50: 492-9.
395. Slatopolsky E, Finch J, Denda M, Ritter C, Zhong M, Dusso A, et al. Phosphorus restriction prevents parathyroid gland growth. High phosphorus directly stimulates PTH secretion in vitro. J Clin Invest 1996;97:2534-40.
396. Smolens P, Venkatachalam M, Stein JH. Myeloma kidney cast nephropathy in a rat model of multiple myeloma. Kidney Int 1983;24:192-204.
397. Solomon A, Weiss DT, Kattine AA. Nephrotoxic potential of Bence Jones proteins. N Engl J Med 1991;324:1845-51.
398. Sorgel F, Ettinger B, Benet LZ. The true composition of kidney stones passed during triamterene therapy. J Urol 1985;134:871-3.
399. Springberg PD, Garrett LE, Thompson AL, Collins NF, Lordon RE, Robinson RR. Fixed and reproducible orthostatic proteinuria: results of a 20-year follow-up study. Ann Intern Med 1982;97:516-19.
400. Stamatelou KK, Francis ME, Jones CA, Nyberg LM, Curhan GC. Time trends in reported prevalence of kidney stones in the United States: 1976-1994. Kidney Int 2003;63:1817-23.
401. American Diabetes Association. Position Statement. Standards of medical care for patients with diabetes mellitus. Diabetes Care 2001;24:S33-43.
402. Stenvinkel P, Heimburger O, Paultre F, Diczfalusy U, Wang T, Berglund L, et al. Strong association between malnutrition, inflammation, and atherosclerosis in chronic renal failure. Kidney Int 1999;55:1899-911.
403. Stevens PE, Tamimi NA, Al Hasani MK, Mikhail AI, Kearney E, Lapworth R, et al. Non-specialist management of acute renal failure. Q J Med 2001;94:533-40.
404. Strippoli GF, Manno C, Schena FP. An "evidence-based" survey of therapeutic options for IgA nephropathy: Assessment and criticism. Am J Kidney Dis 2003;41:1129-39.
405. Sun BY-C, Lee Y-H, Jiaan B-P, Chen K-K, Chang LS, Chen K-T. Recurrence rate and risk factors for urinary calculi after extracorporeal shock wave lithotripsy. J Urol 1996;156:903-6.
406. Tanji N, Markowitz GS, Fu C, Kislinger T, Taguchi A, Pischetsrieder M, et al. Expression of advanced glycation end products and their cellular receptor RAGE in diabetic nephropathy and nondiabetic renal disease. J Am Soc Nephrol 2000;11:1656-66.
407. Ten RM, Torres VE, Milliner DS, Schwab TR, Holley KE, Gleich GJ. Acute interstitial nephritis: immunologic and clinical aspects. Mayo Clin Proc 1988;63:921-30.
408. Tenenehouse HS, Murer H. Disorders of renal tubular phosphate transport. J Am Soc Nephrol 2003;14: 240-7.
409. Teng M, Wolf M, Lowrie E, Ofsthun N, Lazarus JM, Thadhani R. Survival of patients undergoing hemodialysis with paricalcitol or calcitriol therapy. N Engl J Med 2003;349:446-56.
410. Thakker RV. Pathogenesis of Dent's disease and related syndromes of X-linked nephrolithiasis. Kidney Int 2000;57:787-93.
411. Thomsen OF, Ladefoged J. Pyelonephritis and interstitial nephritis—clinical-pathological correlations. Clin Nephrol 2002;58:275-81.
412. Tiselius HG. Metabolic evaluation of patients with stone disease. Urol Int 1997;59:131-41.
413. Tiselius HG. Possibilities for preventing recurrent calcium stone formation: principles for the metabolic evaluation of patients with calcium stone disease. BJU Int 2001;88:158-68.
414. Toto RD. The role of prostaglandins in NSAID induced renal dysfunction. J Rheum. Suppl 1991;28:22-5.
415. Trompeter R, Filler G, Webb NJ, Watson AR, Milford DV, Tyden G et al. Randomized trial of tacrolimus versus cyclosporin microemulsion in renal transplantation. Pediatr Nephrol 2002;17:141-9.
416. Traynor JP, Simpson K, Geddes CC, Deighan CJ, Fox JG. Early initiation of dialysis fails to prolong survival in patients with end-stage renal failure. J Am Soc Nephrol 2002;13:2125-32
417. Trinchieri A, Nespoli R, Ostini F, Rovera F, Zanetti G, Pisani E. A study of dietary calcium and other nutrients in idiopathic renal calcium stone formers with low bone mineral content. J Urol 1998;159: 654-7.
418. Twardowski Z, Nolph KD, Khanna R. Peritoneal equilibration test. Perit Dial Bull 1987;7:138-147.
419. Tyson KL, Reynolds JL, McNair R, Zhang Q, Weissberg PL, Shanahan CM. Osteo/chondrocytic transcription factors and their target genes exhibit distinct patterns of expression in human arterial calcification. Arterioscler Thromb Vasc Biol 2003;23:489-94.
420. Uldall R, Ouwendyk M, Francoeur R, Wallace L, Sit W, Vas S, et al. Slow nocturnal home hemodialysis at

the Wellesley Hospital. Adv Ren Replace Ther 1996;3: 133-6.
421. United Kingdom Department of Health: http://www.doh.gov.uk/nsf/diabetes/ch1/whatisdiabetes (accessed January 18, 2005).
422. United Kingdom Renal Association. In: Treatment of adults and children with renal failure. London: Royal College of Physicians of London, 2002.
423. United Network for Organ Sharing: http://www.unos.org/data (accessed January 18, 2005).
424. UK Prospective Diabetes Study (UKPDS) Group. Intensive blood-glucose control with sulphonylureas or insulin compared with conventional treatment and risk of complications in patients with type 2 diabetes (UKPDS 33). Lancet 1998;352:837-53.
425. UK Renal Registry Report 2002; UK Renal Registry, Bristol UK.
426. UK Transplant: http://www.uktransplant.org.uk (accessed January 18, 2005).
427. U.S. Renal Data System: Excerpts from the USRDS 2002 annual data report: Atlas of end-stage renal disease in the United States. Am J Kidney Dis 2003(suppl 2)41:S1-260.
428. Vander AJ, ed. Renal physiology. 5th ed. New York: McGraw-Hill, 1995:37p.
429. Van der Woude FJ. Anticytoplasmic antibodies in Wegener's granulomatosis. Lancet 1985:425-9.
430. Vanholder R, De Smet R, Glorieux G, Argiles A, Baurmeister U, Brunet P, et al. Review on uremic toxins: classification, concentration, and interindividual variability. Kidney Int 2003;63:1934-43.
431. Vanholder R, Glorieux G, De Smet R, Lameire N. New insights in uremic toxins. Kidney Int Suppl 2003:S6-10.
432. Van Ypersele C, Crucke TB, eds. Dialysis amyloid. Oxford: OUP 1996.
433. Verbeke M, Smollich B, Van de Voorde J, de Ridder L, Lameire N. Beneficial influence of ketanserin on autoregulation of blood flow in post-ischemic kidneys. J Am Soc Nephrol 1996;7: 621-7.
434. Verroust PJ, Christensen EI. Megalin and cubulin—the story of two multipurpose receptors unfolds. Nephrol Dial Transplant 2002;17:1867-71.
435. Vincenti F, Jensik SC, Filo RS, Miller J, Pirsch J. A long-term comparison of tacrolimus (FK506) and cyclosporine in kidney transplantation: evidence for improved allograft survival at five years. Transplantation 2002;73:775-82.
436. Virchow R. Cellular pathology: as based upon physiological and pathological histology. R M De Witt: New York: 1863 (unabridged re-printing 1971): 404-408pp.
437. Wagener DK, Harris T, Madans JH. Proteinuria as a biomarker: Risk of subsequent morbidity and mortality. Environ Res 1994;66:160-72.
438. Wannamethee SG, Shaper AG, Perry IJ. Serum creatinine concentration and risk of cardiovascular disease: A possible marker for increased risk of stroke. Stroke 1997;28:557-63.
439. Watkin DM, Shock NW. Agewise standard value for C_{In}, C_{PAH}, and Tm_{PAH} in adult males. J Clin Invest 1955;34:969.
440. Watson PE, Watson ID, Batt RD. Total body water volumes for adult males and females estimated from simple anthropometric measurements. Am J Clin Nutr 1980;33:27-39.
441. Wautier JL, Zoukourian C, Chappey O, Wautier MP, Guillausseau PJ, Cao R, et al. Receptor-mediated endothelial cell dysfunction in diabetic vasculopathy. Soluble receptor for advanced glycation end products blocks hyperpermeability in diabetic rats. J Clin Invest 1996;97:238-43.
442. Weber M, Dindo D, Demartines N, Ambuhl PM, Clavien PA. Kidney transplantation from donors without a heartbeat. N Engl J Med 2002;347: 248-55.
443. Weigert C, Brodbeck K, Klopfer K, Haring HU, Schleicher ED. Angiotensin II induces human TGF-beta 1 promoter activation: similarity to hyperglycaemia. Diabetologia 2002;45:890-8.
444. Weisinger JR. New insights into the pathogenesis of idiopathic hypercalciuria: role of the bone. Kidney Int 1997;49:1507-18.
445. Weir MR, Anderson L, Fink JC, Gabregiorgish K, Schweitzer EJ, Hoehn-Saric E, et al. A novel approach to the treatment of chronic allograft nephropathy. Transplantation 1997;64:1706-10.
446. Wendt T, Tanji N, Guo J, Hudson BI, Bierhaus A, Ramasamy R, et al. Glucose, glycation, and RAGE: implications for amplification of cellular dysfunction in diabetic nephropathy J Am Soc Nephrol 2003;14:1383-95.
447. Wheeler DC, Townend JN, Landray MJ. Cardiovascular risk factors in predialysis patients: baseline data from the Chronic Renal Impairment in Birmingham (CRIB) study. Kidney Int Suppl 2003:S201-3.
448. Whelton A. Nephrotoxicity of nonsteroidal anti-inflammatory drugs: physiologic foundations and clinical implications. Am J Med 1999;106:13S-24.
449. White KE, Bilous RW. Type 2 diabetic patients with nephropathy show structural-functional relationships that are similar to type 1 disease. J Am Soc Nephrol 2000;11:1667-73.
450. Wiik A. Delineation of a standard procedure for indirect immunofluorescence detection of ANCA. APMIS Suppl 1989;6:12-13.
451. Wilhelm SM, Simonson MS, Robinson AV, Stowe NT, Schulak JA. Endothelin up-regulation and localization following renal ischemia and reperfusion. Kidney Int 1999;55:1011-18.

452. Wilkinson H. Clinical investigation and management of patients with renal stones. Ann Clin Biochem 2001;38:180-7.
453. Williams G, Mallick N. Nephropathies of systemic diseases Color atlas of renal diseases. London: Wolfe Publishing, 1994:43-80.
454. Williams PS, Fass G, Bone JM. Renal pathology and proteinuria determine progression in untreated mild/moderate chronic renal failure. Q J Med 1988;67:343-54.
455. Winearls CG, Oliver DO, Pippard MJ, Reid C, Downing MR, Cotes PM. Effect of human erythropoietin derived from recombinant DNA on the anemia of patients maintained by chronic hemodialysis. Lancet 1986;2:1175-8.
456. Winearls CG. Acute myeloma kidney. Kidney Int 1995;48:1347-61.
457. Woolfson RG, Mansell MA. Hyperoxaluria and renal calculi. Postgrad Med J 1994;70:695-8.
458. World Health Organisation. Nutritional anemia. report of a WHO scientific group. Geneva, Switzerland: WHO, 1968.
459. World Health Organisation: http://www.who.int/ncd/dia/databases4 (accessed January 18, 2005).
460. Wrong OM, Norden AGW, Feest TG. Dent's disease; a familial proximal renal tubular syndrome with low molecular weight proteinuria, hypercalciuria, nephrocalcinosis, metabolic bone disease, progressive renal failure, and a marked male predominance. Q J Med 1994;87:473-93.
461. Xia H, Ebben J, Ma JZ, Collins AJ. Hematocrit levels and hospitalization risks in hemodialysis patients. J Am Soc Nephrol 1999;10:1309-16.
462. Xue JL, St. Peter WL, Ebben JP, Everson SE, Collins AJ. Anemia treatment in the pre-ESRD period and associated mortality in elderly patients. Am J Kidney Dis 2002;40:1153-61.
463. Yakoub Agha I, Attal M, Dumontet C, Delannoy V, Moreau P, Berthou C, et al. Thalidomide in patients with advanced multiple myeloma: a study of 83 patients-report of the Intergroupe Francophone du Myelome (IFM). Hematol J 2002;3:185-92.
464. Yamamoto T, Noble NA, Miller DE, Border WA. Sustained expression of TGF-beta 1 underlies development of progressive kidney fibrosis. Kidney Int 1994;45:916-27.
465. Yang J, Liu Y. Blockage of tubular epithelial to myofibroblast transition by hepatocyte growth factor prevents renal interstitial fibrosis. J Am Soc Nephrol 2002;13:96-107.
466. Yaqoob M, Bell GM, Percy D, Finn R. Primary glomerulonephritis and hydrocarbon exposure: A case control study and literature review. Q J Med 1992;301:409-18.
467. Zager PG, Nikolic J, Brown RH, Campbell MA, Hunt WC, Peterson D, et al. "U" curve association of blood pressure and mortality in hemodialysis patients. Kidney Int 1998;54:561-9.
468. Zatz R, Dunn BR, Meyer TW, Anderson S, Rennke HG, Brenner BM. Prevention of diabetic glomerulopathy by pharmacological amelioration of glomerular capillary hypertension. J Clin Invest 1986;77:1925-30.
469. Zatz R. Hemodynamically mediated glomerular injury: the end of a 15-year-old controversy? Curr Opin Nephrol Hypertens 1996;5:468-75.
470. Zelikovic I, Chesney RW. Sodium coupled amino acid transport in renal tubules. Kidney Int 1989;36:351-9.
471. Ziyadeh FN, Sharma K, Ericksen M, Wolf G. Stimulation of collagen gene expression and protein synthesis in murine mesangial cells by high glucose is mediated by autocrine activation of transforming growth factor-beta. J Clin Invest 1994;93:536-42.
472. Ziyadeh FN, Hoffman BB, Han DC, Iglesias De La Cruz MC, Hong SW, Isono M, et al. Long-term prevention of renal insufficiency, excess matrix gene expression, and glomerular mesangial matrix expansion by treatment with monoclonal antitransforming growth factor-beta antibody in db/db diabetic mice. Proc Natl Acad Sci U S A 2000;97:8015-20.
473. Zucchelli P, Pasquali S, Cagnoli L, Ferrari G. Controlled plasma exchange trial in acute renal failure due to multiple myeloma. Kidney Int 1988;33: 1175-80.

ADDITIONAL READING

Periodicals

American Journal of Kidney Diseases http://www2.ajkd.org (Accessed January 18, 2005).
Annals of Clinical Biochemistry http://www.acb.org.uk (Accessed January 18, 2005).
Clinical Chemistry http://www.clinchem.org (Accessed January 18, 2005).
Clinical Nephrology http://www.clinnephrol.com (Accessed March 4, 2005).
Journal of the American Society of Nephrology http://www.jasn.org (Accessed January 18, 2005).
Kidney International http://www.blackwellpublishing.com (Accessed January 18, 2005).
Nephrology, Dialysis and Transplantation http://www.ndt.oupjournals.org (Accessed January 18, 2005).

USEFUL INTERNET SITES

1. American Society of Nephrology http://www.asn-online.org (Accessed January 18, 2005).
2. International Society for Nephrology http://www.isn-online.org (Accessed January 18, 2005).
3. United Kingdom Renal Association http://www.renal.org (Accessed January 18, 2005).
4. National Kidney Foundation (USA) http://www.kidney.org (Accessed January 18, 2005).

5. Hypertension, Dialysis & Clinical Nephrology http://www.hdcn.com (Accessed January 18, 2005).
6. British Renal Society http://www.britishrenal.org (Accessed January 18, 2005).

REVIEWS

Burrows-Hudson S. Chronic kidney disease: An overview. Am J Nurs 2005;105:40-9.

Cardillo M, Poli F, Barraco F, De Fazio N, Rossini G, Boschiero L, et al. Renal transplantation. Strategies to prevent organ rejection–the role of an inter-regional reference center. Contrib Nephrol 2005;146:1-10.

Chiaramonte S, Dissegna D, Ronco C.Monitoring of immunosuppressive therapy in renal transplanted patients. Contrib Nephrol 2005;146:73-86.

Greger R. New insights into the molecular mechanisms of the action of diuretics. Nephrol Dial Transplant 1999;14:536-40.

Hovind P, Rossing P, Tarnow L, Smidt UM, Parving HH. Progression of diabetic nephropathy. Kidney Int 2001;59:702-9.

Lamb EJ, O'Riordan SE, Delaney MP. Ageing and the kidney: pathology, assessment and management. Clin Chim Acta 2003;334:25-40.

Lameire N, Van Biesen W, Vanholder R. Acute renal failure. Lancet 2005;365:417-30.

Meguid El Nahas A, Bello AK. Chronic kidney disease: The global challenge. Lancet 2005;365:331-40.

National Kidney Foundation-K/DOQI. Clinical practice guidelines for chronic kidney disease: evaluation, classification, and stratification. Am J Kidney Dis 2002;39(suppl 1):S1-266.

Penney MD, Oleesky DA. Renal tubular acidosis. Ann Clin Biochem 1999;36:408-22.

Samuell CT, Kasidas GP. Biochemical investigations in renal stone formers. Ann Clin Biochem 1995;32: 112-22.

Sayer JA, Pearce SHS. Diagnosis and clinical biochemistry of inherited tubulopathies. Ann Clin Biochem 2001;38:459-70.

Tenenehouse HS, Murer H. Disorders of renal tubular phosphate transport. J Am Soc Nephrol 2003;14: 240-7.

U.S. Renal Data System. USRDS 2002 annual data report: atlas of end-stage renal disease in the United States. National Institutes of Health, National Institute of Diabetes and Digestive and Kidney Diseases. Bethesda, Md.: 2002.

Vincenti F. Chronic induction. What's new in the pipeline. Contrib Nephrol 2005;146:22-9.

CHAPTER 46

Physiology and Disorders of Water, Electrolyte, and Acid-Base Metabolism*

James Stacey Klutts, M.D., Ph.D.,
and Mitchell G. Scott, Ph.D.

Mammalian adaptation to terrestrial life has involved the development of complex physiological systems to maintain the composition of their internal milieu. These include a variety of chemical buffers and highly specialized mechanisms of the lungs and kidneys that work together to regulate water, electrolytes, and pH between the intracellular and extracellular compartments. Perturbations in the dynamic equilibria that exist for water, electrolytes, and pH may arise from external (e.g., trauma, changes in altitude, ingestion of toxic substances) or internal (e.g., normal metabolism and disease states) sources. Correction of these imbalances by buffers and the pulmonary and renal compensatory mechanisms may not always be adequate, at which time the clinical laboratory can provide valuable information for guiding therapy.

TOTAL BODY WATER—VOLUME AND DISTRIBUTION

At birth, ~75% of total body mass is water, and from roughly 1 year of age through middle age, this value is ~60% for the average male and ~55% for females. After middle age this falls to ~50%. As depicted in Figure 46-1, approximately two thirds of total body water (TBW) is distributed into the intracellular fluid (ICF) compartment, and one third exists in the extracellular fluid (ECF) compartment. The ICF and ECF compartments are physically separated by the cellular plasma membrane. The ECF may be further subdivided into the interstitial (approximately three fourths of ECF) and intravascular (approximately one fourth of ECF) fluid compartments, which are separated by the capillary endothelium. The larger blood vessels contain additional layers of smooth muscle and connective tissue but constitute a relatively small surface area for exchange compared with the capillary beds. Within the intravascular (whole blood) compartment, *plasma,* the liquid fraction, constitutes ~3.5 L for the average adult having a hematocrit of ~40% and a 5 L blood volume. Although other clinically relevant ECF compartments (e.g., cerebrospinal fluid [CSF] and urine) may be analyzed in the clinical laboratory, the majority of laboratory tests used to determine hydration status, electrolytes, and acid-base status are performed on samples from the *intravascular* (plasma, serum, or whole blood) compartment.

The minimum daily requirement for water can be estimated from renal (~1200 mL in urine) and "insensible" losses (~200 mL due to evaporation from the skin and respiratory tract). Activity, environmental conditions, and disease all have dramatic effects on daily water (and electrolyte) requirements. However, on average, an adult must take in 1.0 to 1.5 L of water daily to maintain fluid balance. Because primary regulatory mechanisms are designed to first maintain *intracellular* hydration status, uncorrected imbalances in TBW are initially reflected in the ECF compartment. Table 46-1 lists common causes and clinical

*The authors acknowledge the original contributions by Norbert W. Tietz, Elizabeth L. Pruden, Ole Siggaard-Andersen, and Jonathan W. Heusel, on which portions of this chapter are based.

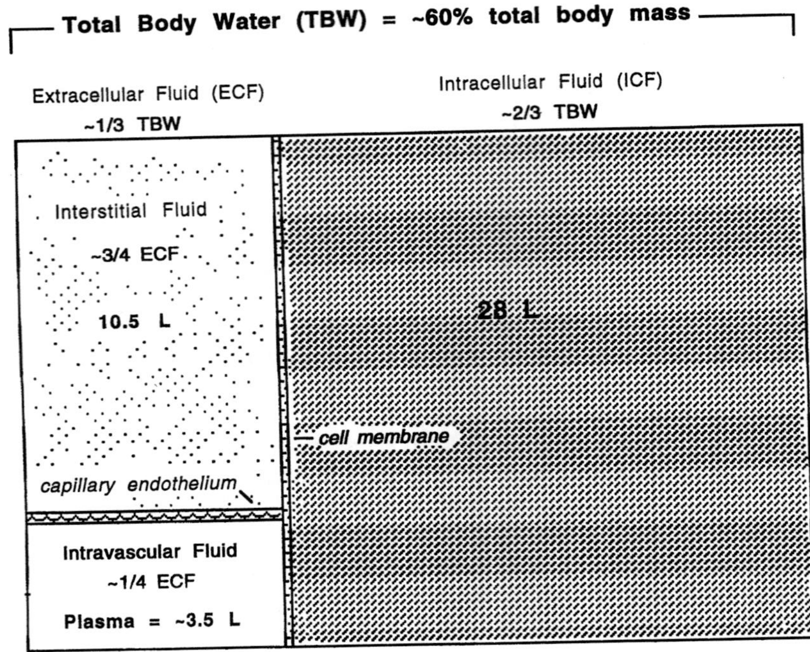

Figure 46-1 Volume and distribution of total body water. Note that the intracellular and ECF compartments (ICF and ECF, respectively) are separated by cellular plasma membranes, and within the ECF, interstitial and intravascular fluids are separated by the capillary endothelium. The volumes indicated represent water and not total volume.

TABLE 46-1 Causes and Clinical Manifestations of Changes in Extracellular Fluid (ECF) Volume

	Clinical Manifestations	Causes
ECF loss	Thirst, anorexia, nausea, lightheadedness, orthostatic hypotension, syncope, tachycardia, oliguria, decreased skin turgor and "sunken eyes," shock, coma, death	Trauma (and other causes of acute blood loss), "third-spacing" of fluid (e.g., burns, pancreatitis, peritonitis), vomiting, diarrhea, diuretics, renal or adrenal (i.e., sodium wasting) disease
ECF gain	Weight gain, edema, dyspnea (due to pulmonary edema), tachycardia, jugular venous distention, portal hypertension, esophageal varices	Heart failure, hepatic cirrhosis, nephrotic syndrome, iatrogenic (intravenous fluid overload)

manifestations of expansion and contraction of the ECF compartment.

The intravascular fluid compartment (including blood cells) represents the effective circulating or blood volume, which is the portion of the ECF perfusing the body tissues. The human body has exquisitely sensitive receptors called "baroreceptors" designed to sense both the osmotic pressure and the blood volume in the right atrium, aortic arch, and kidney. During certain pathological conditions (e.g., congestive heart failure, hepatic cirrhosis, nephrotic syndrome), the baroreceptors detect a decrease in the blood volume despite an overall expansion of the ECF. The excess fluid in the ECF compartment collects in the tissues (causing edema) and thus is not sensed by the baroreceptors. Compensatory mechanisms involve the renal retention of sodium to expand the intravascular volume, leading to a vicious cycle of fluid retention in the face of an expanding ECF compartment.

WATER AND ELECTROLYTES—COMPOSITION OF BODY FLUIDS

The major ions of body fluids are collectively called electrolytes and constitute the majority of osmotically active particles. The primary cationic (positively charged) electrolytes are sodium (Na^+), potassium (K^+), calcium (Ca^{2+}), and magnesium (Mg^{2+}), whereas the anionic (negatively charged) electrolytes include chloride (Cl^-), bicarbonate (HCO_3^-), phosphate (HPO_4^{2-}, $H_2PO_4^-$), sulfate (SO_4^{2-}), organic ions such as lactate, and negatively charged proteins. The electrolyte concentrations of the body fluid compartments are shown in Table 46-2. Na^+, K^+, Cl^-, and HCO_3^- in the plasma or serum are commonly analyzed in an *electrolyte profile,* because their concentrations provide the most relevant information about the osmotic, hydration, and pH status of the body. Although hydrogen ion (H^+) chemically is a cation, its concentration is approximately 1 million–fold

TABLE 46-2 Electrolyte and Water Composition of Body Fluid Compartments*

Component	Plasma	Interstitial Fluid	Intracellular Fluid†
Volume, H_2O	3.5 L	10.5 L	28 L (TBW = 42 L)
Na^+	142	145	12
K^+	4	4	156
Ca^{2+}	6	2-3	3
Mg^{2+}	2	1-2	26
Trace elements	1		
Total cations	155		
Cl^-	103	114	4
HCO_3^-	27	31	12
$Protein^-$	16	—	55
Organic $acids^-$	5	—	—
HPO_4^{2-}	2		
SO_4^{2-}	1		
Total anions	154		

TBW, Total body water.
*All electrolyte values are expressed in mEq/L of *fluid.* Because the H_2O content of plasma is ~90% by volume, the corresponding electrolyte concentrations in plasma water are ~10% higher. Note that the *molar concentration* of divalent ions is one-half the depicted value.
†These values are derived from skeletal muscle.

lower in plasma than the major electrolytes listed in Table 46-2 (10^{-9} mol/L vs. 10^{-3} mol/L) and thus is negligible in terms of osmotic activity. The total number of positive ions (including H^+) *must* equal that of the negative ions for electrical neutrality.

Any increase in the concentration of one anion is accompanied either by a corresponding decrease in other anions or by an increase in one or more cations or both, so total electrical neutrality is invariably maintained. Similarly, any decrease in the concentration of anions involves either a corresponding increase in other anions, or a decrease in cations, or both. In the case of polyvalent ions (e.g., Ca^{2+} or Mg^{2+}), it is important to distinguish between the substance concentration of the ion itself and the concentration of the ion charge. Thus although the concentration of total calcium ions in normal plasma is 2.5 mmol/L, the concentration of the total calcium ion *charge* is 5.0 mmol/L (also called 5 milliequivalents per liter [mEq/L]). This law of *electrical neutrality* should not be confused with acid-base neutrality (pH = 7.0, where the activity of H^+ equals the activity of OH^-).

The special nature of H^+ is discussed below in the section about acid-base physiology. The special functions of calcium, magnesium, phosphates, amino acids, iron, and the trace elements are considered separately in Chapters 20 and 30.

EXTRACELLULAR AND INTRACELLULAR COMPARTMENTS

The extracellular compartment is composed of plasma and interstitial fluid.

Plasma

Plasma, which is of main interest in discussion of water and electrolytes, generally has a volume of 1300 to 1800 mL/m^2 of body surface and constitutes approximately 5% of the body volume (~3.5 L for a 66-kg subject). Generally, total body volume is derived from body mass by using an estimated body density of 1.06 kg/L. The electrolyte composition of venous plasma is summarized in Table 46-2. The mass concentration of water in normal plasma is about 0.933 kg/L, depending on the protein and lipid content (see Electrolyte Exclusion Effect in Chapter 27). Thus a concentration of sodium in the plasma of 140 mmol/L would correspond to a molality of sodium in plasma water of 150 mmol/kg H_2O (140 mmol/L divided by 0.933 kg/L). The total weight (mass) of 1 L of plasma is about 1.026 kg; thus the total weight of solute in 1 L of plasma is about 1.026 – 0.933 = 0.093 kg. The concentration of net protein ions in plasma is ~12 mmol/L, with the charge mainly due to albumin, as the charge of globulins is negligible.[9]

Interstitial Fluid

Interstitial fluid is essentially an ultrafiltrate of blood plasma (see Figure 46-1). When all extracellular spaces except plasma are included, the volume accounts for about 26% (~17 L) of the total body volume. Plasma is separated from the interstitial fluid by the endothelial lining of the capillaries, which acts as a semipermeable membrane and allows passage of water and diffusible solutes but not compounds of large molecular mass, such as proteins. However, this "impermeability" is not absolute, as demonstrated by the varying (although low) concentration of protein in interstitial fluids. In pathological conditions causing "shock," such as bacterial sepsis, the permeability of the vascular endothelium increases dramatically, resulting in leakage of albumin, a reduction in the effective circulating volume, and hypotension. If not aggressively treated with antibiotics, intravenous fluids, and/or vasopressors, this condition can result in death secondary to decreased cerebral perfusion.

Intracellular Fluid

The exact composition of ICF is extremely hard to measure because of the relative unavailability of cells free of contamination. Although erythrocytes are easily accessible, it would be incorrect to make any generalizations based on the composition of these highly specialized cells. Data on cell composition (see Table 46-2), therefore, are considered only approximations. The volume of the ICF constitutes ~66% of the total body volume (see Figure 46-1).

Reasons for Composition Differences of Body Fluids

The composition of ICF can differ markedly from that of the ECF because of the separation of these compartments by the cell membrane. The composition differences are a consequence of both the Gibbs-Donnan equilibrium and active and passive transport of ions.

Gibbs-Donnan Equilibrium

Two solutions separated by a semipermeable membrane will establish an equilibrium so that all ions are equally distributed in both compartments provided that the solutes can move freely through the membrane. At the state of equilibrium, the total ion concentration and therefore the total concentration of osmotically active particles (osmolalities) are equal on both sides of the membrane.

If solutions on two sides of a membrane contain different concentrations of ions that cannot freely move through the membrane (e.g., proteins), distribution of the diffusible ions (e.g., electrolytes) at the steady state will be unequal, but the product of the concentrations of ions in one compartment is equal to the product of ions in the other compartment (Gibbs-Donnan law). Also the law of electrical neutrality is obeyed for both compartments. An example of the uneven distribution of an ion in two compartments with different protein content (nondiffusible ions) is the concentration of chloride ions in plasma and CSF. As a result of the increased selectivity of the blood-brain barrier against proteins, Cl^- ions are ~15% higher in CSF to establish electrical and osmotic equilibrium.[31] Calculations that demonstrate these principles can be found in the first edition of this textbook (pp. 1225-1227).[29]

Cells that contain nondiffusible protein anions can withstand only a limited and temporary difference in osmotic pressure across the cell membrane. The osmotic pressure is normally identical inside and outside the cells because the cell membrane can correct concentration differences by excluding some small ions by active, energy requiring, transport processes. If these processes cease, the cells gradually swell and eventually burst (osmotic lysis).

Distribution of Ions by Active and Passive Transport

Examination of Table 46-2 reveals that the electrolyte compositions of blood plasma and interstitial fluid (both ECFs) are similar, but their compositions differ markedly from that of ICF. The major extracellular ions are Na^+, Cl^-, and HCO_3^-, although in ICF the main ions are K^+, Mg^{2+}, organic phosphates, and protein. This unequal distribution of ions is due to an active transport of Na^+ from inside to outside the cell against an electrochemical gradient. This process requires energy supplied by the metabolic processes in the cell (e.g., glycolysis). An active sodium pump deriving its energy from adenosine triphosphate (ATP) is present in most cell membranes, frequently coupled with a transport of K^+ into the cell. The Na^+/K^+ pump is a heterodimer consisting of a catalytic transmembrane α-subunit that is about 1000 amino acid residues long, and an associated, smaller β-subunit.[13] The internal surface has a catalytic binding site for ATP and a binding site for Na^+. The external surface has a binding site for K^+. ATP phosphorylates an aspartic acid residue of the ATPase, resulting in a conformation change of the protein that ultimately triggers the expulsion of three sodium ions with a concomitant uptake of two potassium ions.[13]

In addition to the Na^+/K^+-ATPase, there is also a ubiquitous Na^+-H^+ exchanger (often referred to as an antiporter) that actively pumps H^+ out of the ICF in exchange for Na^+.[18] This exchanger is critical for maintaining intracellular pH homeostasis and volume in many cell types. At least six different isoforms of this transmembrane protein have been identified, and the regulation and tissue distribution of these differ.[18] Of particular importance is the role of this exchanger for acid-base regulation in renal tubular cells as discussed later in this chapter.

ELECTROLYTES

Homeostasis and disorders of Na^+, K^+, Cl^-, and HCO_3^- are separately considered.

Sodium

Disorders of Na^+ homeostasis can occur because of excessive loss, gain, or retention of Na^+ or because of excessive loss, gain, or retention of H_2O. It is difficult to separate disorders of Na^+ and H_2O balance because of their close relationship in establishing normal osmolality in all body water compartments. As described in detail in Chapter 45, the primary organ for regulating body water and extracellular Na^+ is the kidney. However, as a brief introduction to this section, it is important to remind the reader of the functions of healthy kidneys. In the proximal tubules, 60% to 70% of the filtered Na^+ is actively reabsorbed, with H_2O and Cl^- following passively to maintain electrical neutrality and osmotic equivalence. In the descending loop of Henle, H_2O, but not electrolytes, is passively reabsorbed because of the high osmotic strength of the interstitial fluid in the specialized environment of the renal medulla. In the ascending loop of Henle, Cl^- is reabsorbed actively, with Na^+ following. At the level of the distal tubule, the first of the two primary Na^+/H_2O regulating processes occurs. Here, aldosterone stimulates the distal tubules to reabsorb Na^+ (with water following passively) and secrete K^+ (and to a lesser extent, H^+) to maintain electrical neutrality. Aldosterone is produced by the adrenal cortex in response to the angiotensin II derived via the action of renin (see Chapter 45). The secretion of renin by renal juxtaglomerular cells is stimulated by low chloride, β-adrenergic activity, and low arteriolar pressure.[26] Thus when the kidneys are hypoperfused (as occurs when blood volume decreases or if the renal arteries are obstructed), the distal tubules, under the influence of aldosterone, reclaim Na^+. Further water regulation in the kidney occurs from the distal tubule through the collecting duct where tubular permeability to H_2O is under the influence of antidiuretic hormone (ADH) (see Chapters 45 and 50). ADH (also called vasopressin) is released by the posterior pituitary under the influence of baroreceptors in the aortic arch and hypothalamic chemoreceptors that are responsive to circulating osmolality, which is primarily a reflection of Na^+ concentration.[27] When blood volume is decreased or when plasma osmolality is increased, ADH is secreted, tubular permeability to H_2O increases, and H_2O is reabsorbed in an attempt to restore blood volume or to decrease osmolality. In contrast, when blood volume is increased or osmolality decreased, ADH secretion is inhibited, and more H_2O is excreted in the urine (diuresis).

The body's only other mechanism for restoring Na^+/H_2O homeostasis is ingestion of H_2O. Thirst is stimulated by either decreased blood volume or a hyperosmotic condition. It is important to remember that the receptors that influence renal handling of Na^+ and H_2O, and thirst, sense changes only in the intravascular blood volume and not the total ECF. Furthermore, laboratory assessment of water and electrolyte disorders is primarily made from the blood volume (plasma). As discussed in subsequent sections, the clinician must assess the status of TBW and blood volume before interpretation of laboratory values in the diagnosis of water electrolyte disorders. The physical findings and clinical manifestations of these disorders are every bit as important as laboratory values (see Table 46-1).

Hyponatremia

Hyponatremia is defined as a decreased plasma Na^+ concentration (<136 mmol/L). Hyponatremia typically manifests itself clinically as nausea, generalized weakness, and mental confusion at values <120 mmol/L, ocular palsy at <110 mmol/L, and severe mental impairment between 90 and 105 mmol/L.[25,28] The central nervous system (CNS) symptoms are primarily due to movement of H_2O into cells to maintain osmotic balance and thus swelling of CNS cells. The rapidity of the development of hyponatremia influences the concentrations of Na^+ at which symptoms develop; i.e., clinically apparent symptoms may manifest at slightly higher Na^+ concentrations (~125 mmol/L) when hyponatremia develops rapidly.[25]

Hyponatremia has occurred in the settings of hypoosmotic, hyperosmotic, and isosmotic plasma; thus the measurement (or occasionally a calculation) of plasma osmolality is an important initial step in the assessment of hyponatremia. Of these, the most common is hypoosmotic hyponatremia, since Na^+ is the primary determinant of plasma osmolality. Figure 46-2 describes an algorithm for laboratory measurements and physical examination findings in the differential diagnosis of a plasma Na^+ <135 mmol/L.

Hypoosmotic Hyponatremia

Typically when the plasma Na^+ concentration is low, the calculated or measured osmolality will also be low. This type of hyponatremia can be due to either excess loss of Na^+ (*depletional hyponatremia*) or increased ECF volume (*dilutional hyponatremia*). Differentiating these initially requires a clinical assessment of TBW and ECF volume by a history and physical examination.

Depletional hyponatremia (excess loss of Na^+) is almost always accompanied by a loss of ECF water, but to a lesser extent than the Na^+ loss. Hypovolemia is apparent in the physical examination (orthostatic hypotension, tachycardia, decreased skin turgor). Loss of isosmotic or hypertonic fluid is the cause and this can occur through renal or extrarenal losses. If urine Na^+ is low (generally <10 mmol/L), the loss is extrarenal (see Figure 46-2) because the kidneys are properly retaining filtered Na^+ in response to increased aldosterone (stimulated by the hypovolemia and hyponatremia). Causes of extrarenal loss of Na^+ in excess of H_2O include losses from the gastrointestinal tract or skin (see Figure 46-2).

Alternatively, if urine Na^+ is elevated in this setting (generally >20 mmol/L), renal loss of Na^+ is likely. Renal loss of Na^+ occurs with (1) osmotic diuresis, (2) thiazide diuretics (that inhibit reabsorption of Cl^- and Na^+ in the ascending loop), (3) adrenal insufficiency (the absence of aldosterone and cortisone prevents distal tubule reabsorption of Na^+), or (4) "potassium-sparing" diuretics such as spironolactone that block aldosterone-mediated reabsorption of Na^+ in the distal tubules. Renal loss of Na^+ in excess of H_2O can also occur in metabolic alkalosis because of prolonged vomiting, because increased renal HCO_3^- excretion is accompanied by Na^+ ions. In this case, urine sodium is elevated (>20 mmol/L), but urine chloride remains low. In proximal renal tubular acidosis (RTA), bicarbonate is lost because of a defect in HCO_3^- reabsorption and Na^+ is again co-excreted to maintain electrical neutrality.

Dilutional hyponatremia is a result of excess H_2O retention and can often be detected during the physical examination as the presence of weight gain or edema. In advanced renal failure, water is retained because of decreased filtration and H_2O excretion. However, the remaining functional

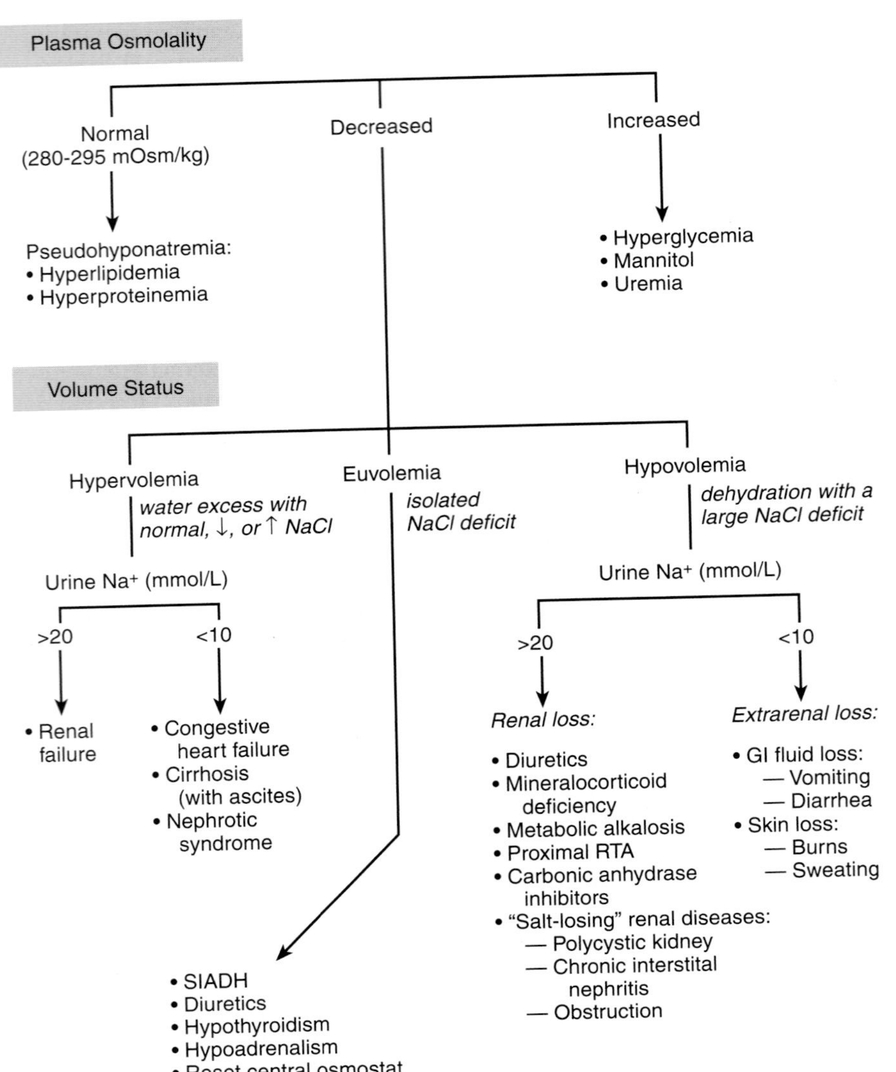

Figure 46-2 Algorithm for the differential diagnosis of hyponatremia. *(Modified from Kirkpatrick W, Kreisberg R. Acid-base and electrolyte disorders. In: Liu P, ed. Blue book of diagnostic tests. Philadelphia: WB Saunders Co, 1986:239-54.)*

nephrons will excrete excess Na^+ secondary to the increased aldosterone that is secreted in response to reduced glomerular pressure in the diseased nephrons.

When ECF is increased but the blood volume is decreased, in congestive heart failure (CHF), hepatic cirrhosis, or the nephrotic syndrome, a vicious cycle is established. The decreased blood volume is sensed by baroreceptors and results in increased aldosterone and ADH, even though ECF volume is excessive. The kidneys reabsorb Na^+ and H_2O in response to the increased aldosterone and ADH in an attempt to restore the blood volume, but this simply results in further increases in the ECF and further dilution of Na^+. It is important to note that the physical findings of congestive heart failure can be subtle, often making diagnosis difficult. Brain natriuretic peptide (BNP), a myocardial cell-derived protein, is elevated in many undiagnosed cases of heart failure.[24] As such, this hormone has become a useful marker for the diagnosis and monitoring of this disorder in patients (see Chapter 44). The release of BNP occurs in response to ventricular stretch, and the natriuretic action of the hormone suggests that one of its functions is to reduce ECF volume and thus cardiac afterload.[24] Furthermore, therapy with BNP analogs has shown promise in the treatment of CHF.[14]

In hypoosmotic hyponatremia with a normal volume status, the most common etiologies are the syndrome of inappropriate ADH (SIADH), primary polydipsia, hypothyroidism, and adrenal insufficiency (see Figure 46-2). SIADH is usually a result of ectopic or otherwise "inappropriate" ADH production arising from a variety of conditions[11] (see Chapters 45 and 50) and results in excessive H_2O retention. SIADH is often diagnosed when a urine osmolality that is greater than plasma osmolality (usually by more than >100 mOsmol/kg) is observed in the setting of hyponatremia, *but only when renal, adrenal, and thyroid functions are normal.* Hypothyroidism impairs free H_2O excretion, whereas in adrenal insufficiency, Na^+ is lost in preference to K^+ reabsorption. Finally, euvolemic hyponatremia can be found in polydipsia when water intake is greater than the renal capacity to excrete the excess H_2O. This is most often the result of psychiatric illness, but diseases that cause hypothalamic disorders, such as sarcoidosis, may also cause polydipsia by altering the thirst reflex (see Figure 46-2).

Hyperosmotic Hyponatremia

Hyponatremia occurs with an increased amount of other solutes in the ECF, causing an extracellular shift of water or intracellular shift of Na^+ to maintain osmotic balance between the ECF and ICF compartments. The most common cause of this type of hyponatremia is severe hyperglycemia. As a general rule, the Na^+ decreases ~1.6 mmol/L for every 100 mg/dL increase of glucose above 100 mg/dL. The clinical use of mannitol for osmotic diuresis can have a similar effect.

Isosmotic Hyponatremia

If the measured Na^+ concentration in plasma is decreased, but measured plasma osmolality, glucose, and urea are normal, the only explanation is pseudohyponatremia caused by the *electrolyte exclusion effect* (see Chapter 27). This occurs when Na^+ is measured by either flame emission spectrophotometry or by an indirect ion-selective electrode in patients with severe hyperlipidemia or in states of hyperproteinemia (e.g., paraproteinemia of multiple myeloma).

Hypernatremia

Hypernatremia (plasma Na^+ >150 mmol/L) is always hyperosmolar. Symptoms of hypernatremia are primarily neurological (because of intraneuronal loss of H_2O to the ECF) and include tremors, irritability, ataxia, confusion, and coma.[25] As with hyponatremia, the rapidity of the development of hypernatremia will determine the plasma Na^+ value at which symptoms occur. Acute development may cause symptoms when Na^+ reaches 160 mmol/L, although in chronic hypernatremia, overt symptoms may not occur until Na^+ exceeds 175 mmol/L. In chronic hypernatremia, the intracellular osmolality of CNS cells will increase to protect against intracellular dehydration. Because of this, rapid correction of hypernatremia can cause dangerous cerebral edema, as CNS cells will take up too much water if the ICF is hyperosmotic when normonatremia is achieved.[25]

In many cases, the symptoms of hypernatremia may be masked by underlying conditions that contributed to the development of the hypernatremia. Indeed, most cases of hypernatremia occur in patients with altered mental status or in infants, both of whom may have difficulty in rehydrating themselves despite a normal thirst reflex. Thus hypernatremia will rarely occur in an alert patient with a normal thirst response who has access to water.

In general, hypernatremia arises in the setting of (1) hypovolemia (either excessive water loss or failure to replace normal water losses), (2) hypervolemia (a net Na^+ gain in excess of water gain), or (3) normovolemia. Again, assessment of TBW status by physical examination and measurement of urine Na^+ and osmolality are important steps in establishing a diagnosis for hypernatremia (Figure 46-3).

Hypovolemic Hypernatremia

Hypernatremia in the setting of decreased ECF is caused by the renal or extrarenal loss of hypoosmotic fluid leading to dehydration. Thus once hypovolemia is established, measurement of urine Na^+ and osmolality is used to determine the source of fluid loss. Patients who have large extrarenal losses have a concentrated urine (>800 mOsmol/L) with low urine Na^+ (<20 mmol/L), reflecting the proper renal response to conserve Na^+ and water as a means to restore ECF volume. Extrarenal causes include diarrhea, skin (burns or excessive sweating), or respiratory losses coupled with failure to replace the lost water. When gastrointestinal loss is excluded, and the patient has normal mental status and access to H_2O, a hypothalamic disorder (tumor or granuloma) should be suspected, because the normal thirst response should always replace insensible water losses.[25]

Renal causes of water loss in excess of Na^+ can occur with osmotic diuresis or with thiazide diuretics coupled with decreased water intake. In the latter setting, the decreased ECF will lead to increased Na^+ reabsorption in the distal tubules, a site distal to that of the thiazide-induced inhibition of Na^+ and H_2O reabsorption. Although this increased Na^+ reabsorption will lead to hypernatremia, there will still be excess Na^+ in the urine, causing further diuresis. In the former setting, chemoreceptors sensing peripheral hypernatremia will prevent Na^+ reabsorption at the distal tubule, leading to massive diuresis and elevated urine Na^+. Therefore, in either of these settings, urine volume will be high, urine osmolality normal to low, and urine Na^+ high.

Normovolemic Hypernatremia

Hypernatremia in the presence of normal ECF volume is often a prelude to hypovolemic hypernatremia. Insensible losses through the lung or skin again must be suspected and are characterized by concentrated urine as the kidneys function to conserve water. Another cause of normovolemic hypernatremia is water diuresis, which is manifested by polyuria (see Figure 46-3). The differential for polyuria (generally defined as >3 L urine output/day) is either a water or a solute diuresis. Solute diuresis is exemplified by the osmotic diuresis of diabetes mellitus and generally is characterized by urine osmolality >300 mOsmol/L and hyponatremia (see previous discussion in this chapter). A water (or solvent) diuresis is a manifestation of diabetes insipidus (DI) and is characterized by dilute urine (osmolality <250 mOsmol/L) and slight hypernatremia.[25] DI can be either central or nephrogenic.[20] Central DI is due to decreased or total lack of ADH secretion as a result of head trauma, hypophysectomy, pituitary tumor, or granulomatous disease. Nephrogenic DI is due to renal resistance to ADH as a result of drugs (e.g., lithium, demeclocycline, amphotericin, and propoxyphene); diseases such as sickle cell anemia and Sjögren's syndrome, which affect collecting

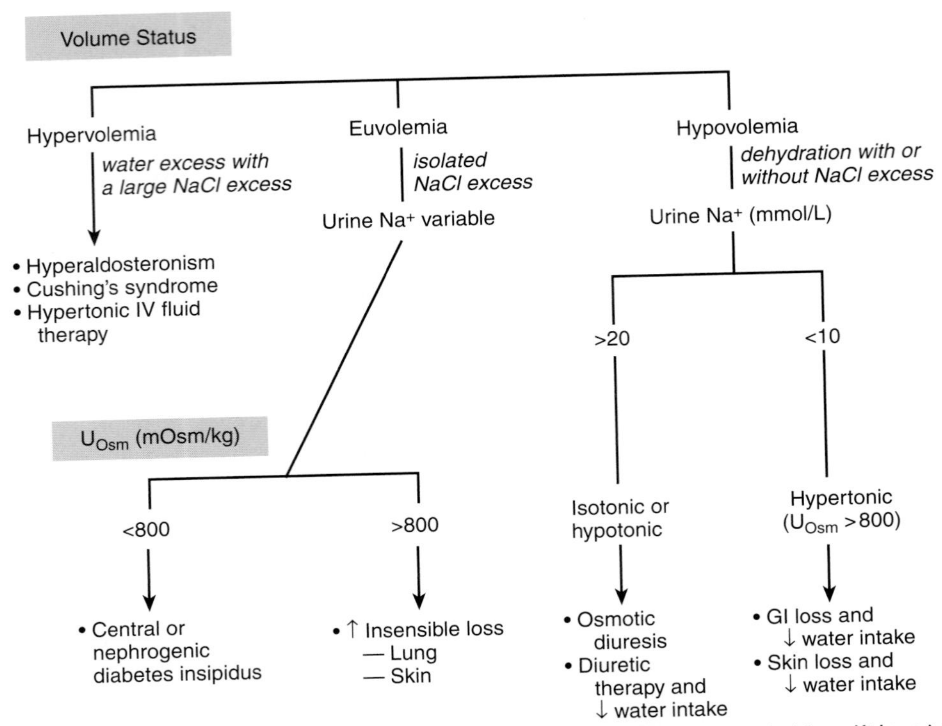

Figure 46-3 Algorithm for the differential diagnosis of hypernatremia. *(Modified from Kirkpatrick W, Kreisberg R. Acid-base and electrolyte disorders. In: Liu P, ed. Blue book of diagnostic tests. Philadelphia: WB Saunders Co, 1986:239-54.)*

duct responsiveness to ADH; or, more rarely, mutant ADH receptors.[2] Central DI is usually treated with vasopressin, whereas nephrogenic DI is treated by discontinuing the responsible drug or providing easy and frequent access to drinking water.

Hypervolemic Hypernatremia

The presence of excess TBW and hypernatremia indicates a net gain of water and Na^+, with Na^+ gain in excess of water (see Figure 46-3). This condition is commonly observed in hospital patients receiving hypertonic saline or sodium bicarbonate. Other causes of hypervolemic hypernatremia include hyperaldosteronism and Cushing's syndrome (see Chapters 24 and 51). Excess aldosterone and cortisol (which also act as ligands for the distal tubule aldosterone receptor) results in excess Na^+ and water retention. Corticosteroid therapy can have similar effects as well.

Potassium

The total body potassium of a 70 kg subject is ~3.5 mol (40 to 59 mmol/kg) of which only 1.5% to 2% is present in the ECF. Nevertheless, plasma K^+ is a relatively good indicator of total K^+ stores with only a few exceptions. Because extracellular K^+ concentrations are maintained at the expense of the intracellular supply, plasma K^+ concentration can initially be normal and belie a total body deficit of up to 200 mmol.

Disturbance of K^+ homeostasis has serious consequences. For example, decrease of extracellular K^+ (hypokalemia) is characterized by muscle weakness, irritability, and paralysis. Plasma K^+ concentrations less than 3.0 mmol/L are associated with marked neuromuscular symptoms and indicate a critical degree of intracellular depletion. At lower concentrations, tachycardia and specific cardiac conduction effects are apparent by electrocardiographic examination (flattened T waves) and can lead to cardiac arrest.[25]

Abnormally high extracellular K^+ (hyperkalemia) concentrations produce symptoms of mental confusion, weakness, tingling, flaccid paralysis of the extremities, and weakness of the respiratory muscles.[25] Cardiac effects of hyperkalemia include bradycardia and conduction defects evident on the electrocardiogram by prolonged PR and QRS intervals and "peaked" T waves. Prolonged severe hyperkalemia >7.0 mmol/L can lead to peripheral vascular collapse and cardiac arrest. There is individual variability in the concentrations of K^+ at which symptoms become apparent, but symptoms are almost always present at K^+ concentrations >6.5 mmol/L. Concentrations >10.0 mmol/L are in most cases fatal.

Hypokalemia

Causes of *hypokalemia* (plasma K^+ <3.5 mmol/L) are classified as redistribution of extracellular K^+ into ICF, or true K^+

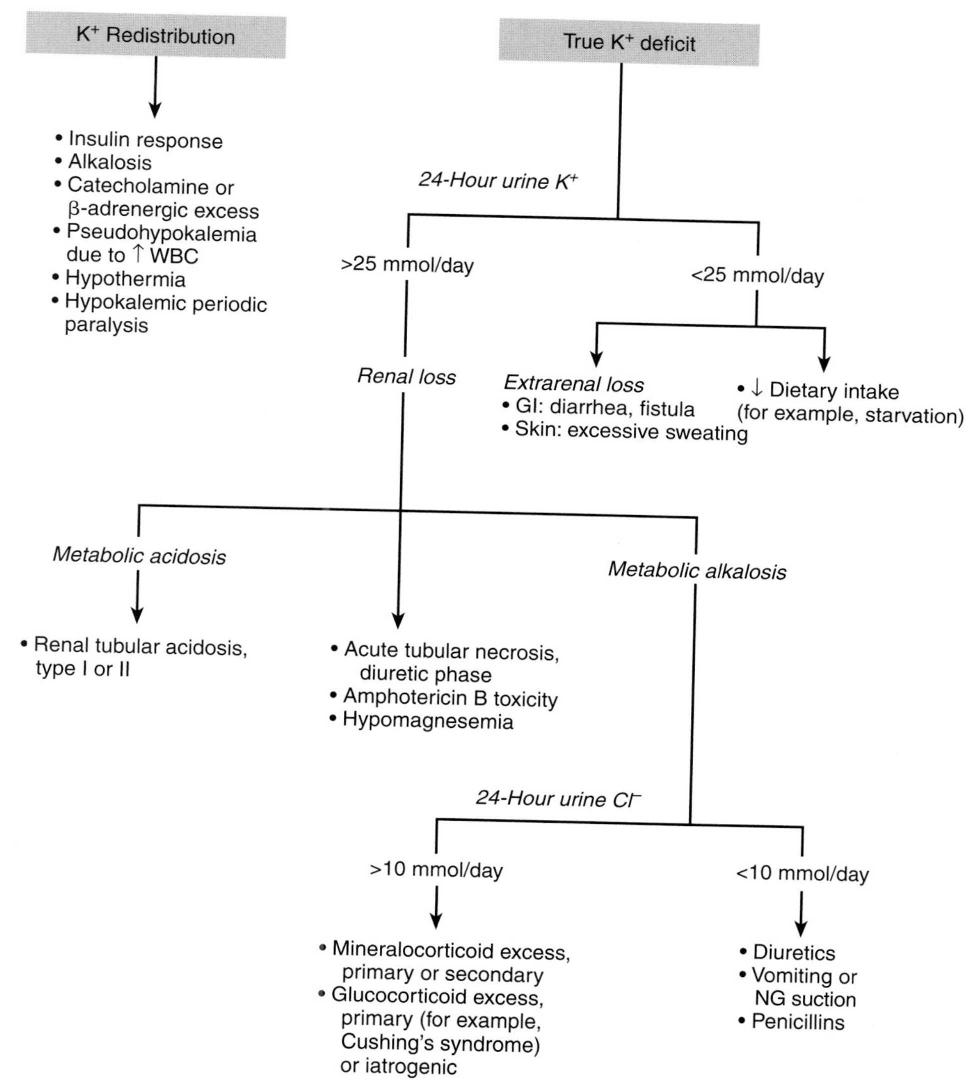

Figure 46-4 Algorithm for the differential diagnosis of hypokalemia. *(Modified from Kirkpatrick W, Kreisberg R. Acid-base and electrolyte disorders. In: Liu P, ed. Blue book of diagnostic tests. Philadelphia: WB Saunders Co, 1986:239-54.)*

deficits, as a result of either decreased intake or a loss of potassium-rich body fluids (Figure 46-4).

Redistribution

Intracellular redistribution of K^+ is illustrated by the fall in plasma K^+ that occurs following insulin therapy for diabetic hyperglycemia. The cells must take up K^+ as a consequence of glucose transport. Redistribution hypokalemia is also a feature of alkalosis, in which K^+ moves from ECF into the cells as H^+ moves in the opposite direction. In addition, the renal conservation of H^+ in the distal tubule occurs at the expense of K^+ ions. On the other hand, severe intracellular K^+ depletion may also *cause* alkalosis, as H^+ shifts intracellularly. Catecholamines and states of endogenous or pharmacological β-adrenergic excess have a similar effect. Pseudohypokalemia is a feature of acute leukemias. The elevated white blood cell count can cause a time-dependent transport of K^+ into the leukemic cells after the blood sample is drawn. Other less common causes of intracellular redistribution are listed in Figure 46-4.

True Potassium Deficit

Hypokalemia reflecting true total body deficits of K^+ can be classified into renal and nonrenal losses based on daily excretion of K^+ in the urine (see Figure 46-4). If urine excretion of K^+ is <30 mmol/day, it can be concluded that the kidneys are properly functioning and attempting to reabsorb as much K^+ as possible in the hypokalemic setting. Causes are either decreased K^+ intake or extrarenal loss of K^+-rich fluid. Situations of decreased intake include chronic starvation and postoperative intravenous fluid therapy with K^+-poor solutions. Gastrointestinal loss of K^+ occurs most commonly with diarrhea.

Urine excretion exceeding 25 to 30 mmol/day in a hypokalemic setting is inappropriate and indicates that the kidneys are the primary source of lost K^+. Renal losses of K^+ may occur during the diuretic (recovery) phase of acute tubular necrosis and during states of excess mineralocorticoid (primary or secondary aldosteronism) or glucocorticoid (Cushing's syndrome) when the distal tubules increase Na^+ reabsorption and concurrently increase K^+ excretion. Renal loss of K^+ is also caused by thiazide and loop diuretics. It is noteworthy that certain diuretics (e.g., spironolactone) are "potassium sparing," because their mechanism of action inhibits aldosterone binding. Other causes of renal loss of K^+ include the use of carbenicillin, ticarcillin, or amphotericin.[16] In addition to redistribution of K^+ into cells in an alkalotic setting, K^+ can also be lost from the kidneys in exchange for reclaimed H^+ ions. This cause of true hypokalemia will be evident by low urine Cl^- and often an alkaline urine.

Hyperkalemia

Hyperkalemia (plasma K^+ >5.0 mmol/L) is a result of (either singly or in combinations) (1) redistribution, (2) increased intake, or (3) increased retention. In addition, preanalytical conditions—such as hemolysis, thrombocytosis (>10^6/µL), and leukocytosis (>10^5/µL)—also have been known to cause marked pseudohyperkalemia as described in detail in Chapter 27 (Figure 46-5).

Redistribution

The transfer of intracellular K^+ into ECF invariably occurs in acidosis as H^+ shifts intracellularly and K^+ shifts outward to maintain electrical neutrality. As a general rule, K^+ concentrations are expected to rise 0.2 to 0.7 mmol/L for every 0.1 unit drop in pH. When the underlying cause of the acidosis is treated, normokalemia will rapidly be restored. Extracellular redistribution of K^+ may also occur in (1) dehydration, (2) shock with tissue hypoxia, (3) insulin deficiency (e.g., diabetic ketoacidosis), (4) massive intravascular or extracorporeal hemolysis, (5) severe burns, (6) tumor lysis syndrome, and (7) violent muscular activity, such as that occurring in status epilepticus. Finally, important iatrogenic causes of redistribution hyperkalemia include digoxin toxicity and β-adrenergic blockade, especially in patients with diabetes or on dialysis.[25]

Potassium Retention

When glomerular filtration or renal tubular function is decreased, hyperkalemia may be precipitated by intravenous infusion of K^+. Infusion rates in excess of 20 mmol/hr or use

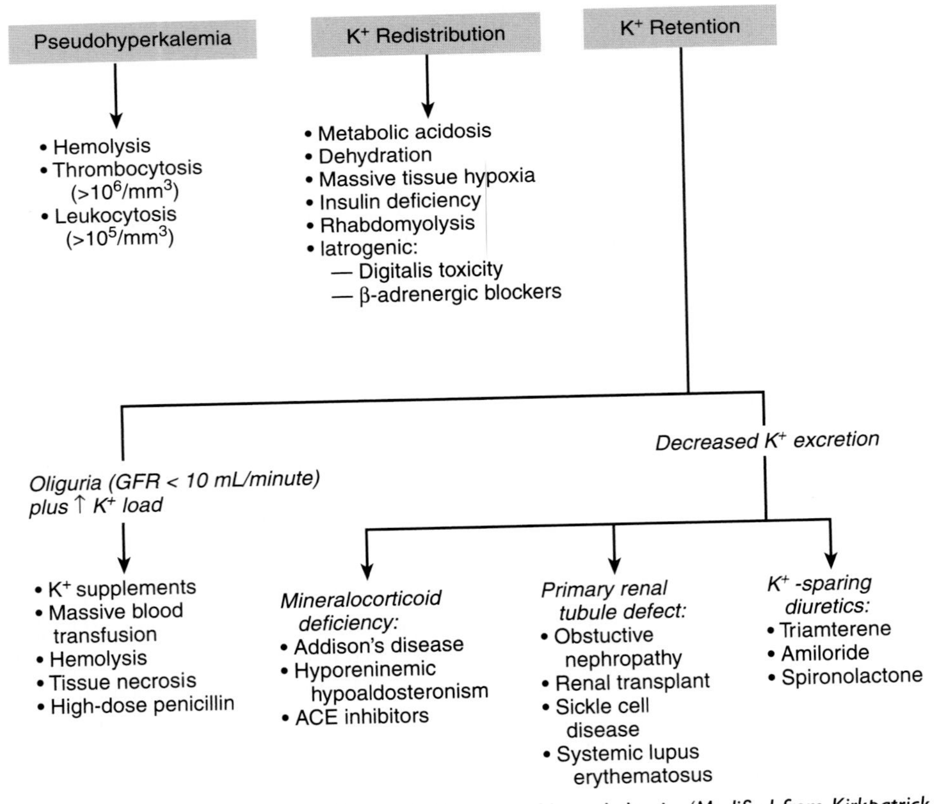

Figure 46-5 Algorithm for the differential diagnosis of hyperkalemia. *(Modified from Kirkpatrick W, Kreisberg R. Acid-base and electrolyte disorders. In: Liu P, ed. Blue book of diagnostic tests. Philadelphia: WB Saunders Co, 1986:239-54.)*

of K^+ solutions with concentrations greater than 40 mmol/L can be dangerous. When renal function is normal, overtreatment is unlikely to produce hyperkalemia because there is more than adequate renal capacity to excrete excess K^+. Indeed, in the absence of severe renal failure, hyperkalemia is seldom prolonged. Decreased excretion of K^+ in acute renal disease and end-stage renal failure (with oliguria or anuria and acidosis) are the most common causes of prolonged hyperkalemia (see Figure 46-5). Hyperkalemia occurs along with Na^+ depletion in adrenocortical insufficiency (e.g., Addison's disease) because diminished Na^+ reabsorption and concomitant decrease in Na^+-K^+ exchange results in decreased K^+ secretion. Drugs that block the production of aldosterone, such as the inhibitors of the angiotensin-converting enzyme ("ACE inhibitors," e.g., captopril) may also cause hyperkalemia. Other causes of hyperkalemia include salt-losing congenital adrenal hyperplasia and excess administration of potassium-sparing diuretics that block distal tubular K^+ secretion (e.g., triamterene and spironolactone).[12]

CHLORIDE

The chloride (Cl^-) ion is the most abundant anion in the ECF (see Table 46-2). In the absence of acid-base disturbances, Cl^- concentrations in plasma will generally follow those of Na^+. However, determination of plasma Cl^- concentration is useful in the differential diagnoses of acid-base disturbances and is essential for calculating the anion gap (see Increased Anion Gap Acidosis [Organic Acidosis] section later in this chapter). Fluctuations in serum or plasma Cl^- have little clinical consequence, but do serve as signs of an underlying disturbance in fluid and acid-base homeostasis and can be an aid in differentiating the cause of these disturbances.

Hypochloremia

In general, causes of hypochloremia will parallel those causes of hyponatremia discussed earlier. Hypochloremia is frequently observed in metabolic acidoses that are caused by increased production or diminished excretion of organic acids (e.g., diabetic ketoacidosis and renal failure). In such cases, the fraction of total anion concentration represented by Cl^- is diminished because the complementary fraction of β-hydroxybutyrate, acetoacetate, lactate, and phosphate is increased. Persistent gastric secretion and prolonged vomiting, whatever the cause, result in significant loss of Cl^- and ultimately in a hypochloremic alkalosis and depletion of total body Cl^- with corresponding retention of HCO_3^-.

Hyperchloremia

Increased plasma Cl^- concentration, like increased Na^+ concentration, occurs with dehydration, RTA, acute renal failure, metabolic acidosis associated with prolonged diarrhea and loss of sodium bicarbonate, DI, states of adrenocortical hyperfunction, and overtreatment with saline solutions. A slight rise in Cl^- concentration may also be seen in respiratory alkalosis due to the renal compensation of excreting HCO_3^-. Hyperchloremic acidosis may be a sign of severe renal tubular disease.

BICARBONATE

Total carbon dioxide (CO_2) content of plasma consists of carbon dioxide dissolved in an aqueous solution (dCO_2), CO_2 loosely bound to amine groups in proteins (carbamino compounds), HCO_3^- and vanishingly small amounts of CO_3^{2-} ions, and carbonic acid (H_2CO_3). Bicarbonate ions make up all but ~2 mmol/L of the total carbon dioxide of plasma (22 to 31 mmol/L). Measurement of the total CO_2 as part of an electrolyte profile is useful chiefly to evaluate HCO_3^- concentration in assessment of acid-base disorders.

Alterations of HCO_3^- and CO_2 dissolved in plasma are characteristic of acid-base imbalance. Its value has most significance in the context of other electrolyte values and with blood gases and pH values. The full clinical significance of the determination of total CO_2 will become apparent in the following discussion of acid-base physiology.

ACID-BASE PHYSIOLOGY

The normal human diet is almost neutral, containing only a small amount of titratable acid. However, metabolic processes in the body result in the production of relatively large amounts of carbonic, sulfuric, phosphoric, and other acids. For example, during a 24-hour period, a person weighing 70 kg disposes of about 20 mol of carbon dioxide (the volatile form of carbonic acid) through the lungs and about 70 to 100 mmol (or ~1 mmol/kg) of titratable, nonvolatile acids (mainly sulfuric and phosphoric acids) through the kidneys. These products of metabolism are transported to the lungs and kidneys via the ECF and blood without producing any appreciable change in the plasma pH and with only a minimal pH difference between arterial (pH 7.35 to 7.45) and venous (pH 7.32 to 7.38) blood. This is accomplished by the buffering capacity of blood and by respiratory and renal regulatory mechanisms.

ACID-BASE BALANCE AND ACID-BASE STATUS

A description of acid-base balance involves an accounting of the carbonic (H_2CO_3, HCO_3^-, CO_3^{2-}, and CO_2) and noncarbonic acids and conjugate bases in terms of input (intake plus metabolic production) and output (excretion plus metabolic conversion) over a given time interval. The acid-base status of the body fluids is typically assessed by measurements of total CO_2 plasma pH and PCO_2, because the bicarbonate/carbonic acid system is the most important buffering system of the plasma. Occasionally, measurement of total titratable acid or base, or other acid and base analytes (e.g., lactate and ammonia [NH_3]) is necessary to determine the etiology of an acid-base disorder.

The following clinical terms are used to describe the acid-base status. *Acidemia* is defined as an arterial blood pH <7.35 and *alkalemia* indicates an arterial blood pH >7.45. *Acidosis* and *alkalosis* refer to pathological states that lead to acidemia or alkalemia. For example, in common acid-base disorders like lactic acidosis and diabetic ketoacidosis, intermediate organic acids (lactic acid and β-hydroxybutyric acid, respectively), which are normally metabolized to carbon dioxide and water, may accumulate to a significant extent, resulting in acidemia. Additionally, more than one type of pathological process can occur simultaneously, giving rise to a mixed acid-base disturbance, in which the blood pH may be low, high, or within the reference interval. These measurements reflect a static sampling of a dynamic process involving complex interactions between multiple buffering systems and the compensatory mechanisms of the kidneys and lungs. To understand how these and other perturbations of acid-base metabolism affect human physiology, it will be necessary to examine briefly, but carefully, the concepts of acids, bases, pH, and buffers in relation to the relevant systems that function to maintain normal acid-base balance in the human body.

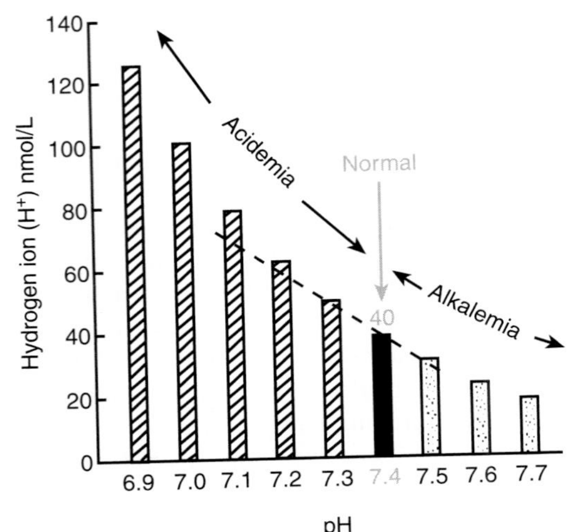

Figure 46-6 Relationship of pH to hydrogen ion concentration. **A,** *Broken line* is drawn to emphasize the (approximate) linear relationship between hydrogen ion concentration and pH over the pH range of 7.2 to 7.5. *(From Narins RG, Emmett M. Simple and mixed acid-base disorders: A practical approach. Medicine 1980;59:161-87.)* **B,** Scale for the interconversion of pH and hydrogen ion concentration.

Acid-Base Parameters—Definitions and Abbreviations

Acids are chemical substances that can donate protons (H^+ ions) in solution, and *bases* are substances that accept protons. Strong acids readily give up H^+, whereas strong bases readily accept H^+. Thus the conjugate base of a strong acid is a weak base and vice versa.

pH and pK

The pH of a solution is defined as the negative logarithm of the hydrogen ion activity ($pH = -\log aH^+$). Thus *pH is a dimensionless quantity,* such that a decrease of one pH unit represents a tenfold increase in the H^+ activity. The average pH of blood (7.40) corresponds to a hydrogen ion concentration of 4×10^{-8} mol/L = 40 nmol/L, but this assumes an activity coefficient of 1 (Figure 46-6). Potentiometric determinations of blood pH measure H^+ activity and not the H^+ concentration, although the activity is assumed to equal the concentration. The relationship between hydrogen ion activity and pH is illustrated in Figure 46-6. The relationship is inverse and obviously nonlinear. Many European centers express the acidity of blood in terms of its hydrogen ion concentration in nanomoles per liter (nmol/L). This form of expression has the advantage of avoiding logarithmic transformations when performing acid-base calculations. Even though it is consistent with how other ion concentrations are expressed, it has not gained widespread use in the United States.

The p*K* (also, p*K′* and pK_a) represents the negative logarithm of the ionization constant of a weak acid (K_a). That is, the p*K* is the pH at which an acid is half dissociated, existing as equal proportions of acid and conjugate base. Thus acids have p*K* values <7.0, whereas bases have p*K* values >7.0. The lower the p*K*, the stronger the acid, and the higher the p*K*, the stronger the conjugate base. For example, the p*K* of lactic acid is 3.5, and is 9.5 for the ammonium ion NH_4^+. The high pK for the ammonium ion indicates that this species prefers to hold onto its proton, rather than dissociating into NH_3 and H^+.

The pH of the plasma may be considered to be a function of two independent variables: (1) the PCO_2, which is regulated by the lungs and represents the acid component of the carbonic acid/bicarbonate buffer system, and (2) the concentration of titratable base (base excess or deficit, which is defined later), which is regulated by the kidneys. The plasma bicarbonate concentration is generally taken as a measure of the base excess or deficit in plasma and ECF, although it is recognized that conditions exist in which bicarbonate concentration may not accurately reflect the true base excess or deficit.

Bicarbonate and Dissolved CO_2

Bicarbonate is the second largest fraction (behind Cl^-) of plasma anions (~25 mmol/L). Conventionally, it is defined to include (1) plasma bicarbonate ion, (2) carbonate, and (3) CO_2 bound in plasma carbamino compounds (Figure 46-7). At the pH of blood, the plasma carbonate concentration is ~25 µmol/L, which is ~1/700 to 1/1000 of the total bicarbonate concentration. CO_2-bound carbamino compounds (RCNHCOOH) are 0.2 mmol/L in plasma and 1.5 mmol/L in erythrocytes. Actual bicarbonate ion concentration is not measured, but rather calculated from the Henderson-Hasselbalch equation as described below (and discussed in detail in Chapter 27). Also, as described in Chapter 27, the analyte usually measured in plasma is total CO_2, which includes bicarbonate and dissolved CO (dCO_2). The dCO_2 fraction is defined to include both the undissociated carbonic acid and physically dissolved, free CO_2. At the pH of the blood, the amount of dissolved CO_2 is 700 to 1000 times greater than the amount of carbonic acid and therefore

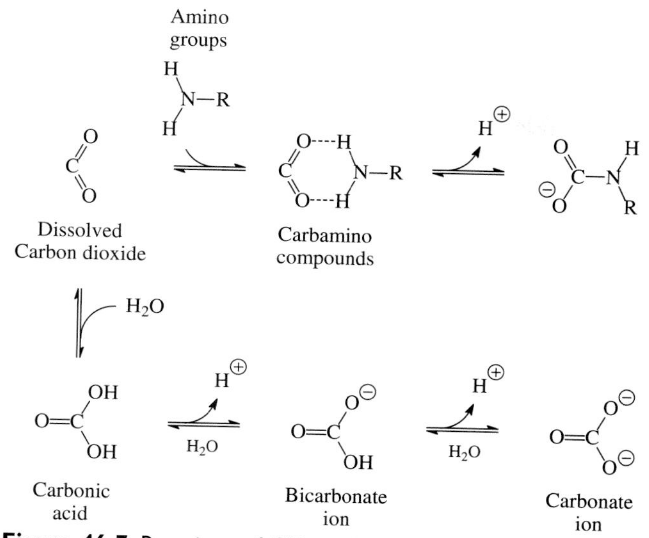

Figure 46-7 Reactions of CO_2 with water and amino groups. Hydrogen bonding is indicated by a dotted bond. The carbamino acid is fairly strong —R—NH—COOH → H^+ + R—NH—COO^-.

$cdCO_2$ is the term used to express their combined concentration. It is calculated from the solubility coefficient of CO_2 in blood at 37 °C (α = 0.0306 mmol/L per mm Hg) multiplied by the measured PCO_2 in mm Hg. Thus at a PCO_2 of 40 mm Hg, $cdCO_2$ is 1.224 mmol/L (0.0306 mmol/L × 40 mm Hg). This $cdCO_2$ value can then be used, in the Henderson-Hasselbalch equation, to calculate the total bicarbonate concentration.

Henderson-Hasselbalch Equation

The Henderson-Hasselbalch equation is described in detail in Chapter 27. However, it is important to review this equation here because it aids in understanding pH regulation of body fluids as it relates to the compensatory mechanisms of the body in acid-base disturbances. The equation derived in Chapter 27 can also be written as follows:

$$pH = 6.1 + \log \frac{cHCO_3^-}{cdCO_2}$$

where $cdCO_2$ is equal to α (0.0306 mmol/L per mm Hg) × PCO_2 and 6.1 is the apparent pK' for the carbonic acid/bicarbonate system (see Chapter 27). An alternative expression useful for approximating cH^+ in blood is:

$$cH^+ = K \times \frac{PCO_2}{cHCO_3^-}$$

where K = 24 (nmol/L) × (mmol/L) × (mm Hg^{-1}).

The average normal ratio of the concentrations of bicarbonate and dissolved carbon dioxide in plasma is 25 (mmolL)/1.25 (mmol/L) = 20/1. It follows then that any change in the concentration of either bicarbonate or dissolved CO_2 must be accompanied by a change in pH. Such changes in the ratio can occur through a change either in the numerator (the renal component) or in the denominator (the respiratory component). Clinical conditions characterized as *metabolic* disturbances of acid-base balance are classified as primary disturbances in $cHCO_3^-$. Those characterized as *respiratory* disturbances are classified as primary disturbances in $cdCO_2$. Various compensatory mechanisms attempting to reestablish the normal ratio of $cHCO_3^-/cdCO_2$ may result in changes in the bicarbonate concentration, dissolved CO_2 concentration, or both. The application of the Henderson-Hasselbalch equation to human acid-base physiology can be illustrated by a lever-fulcrum (teeter-totter) diagram (Figure 46-8).

BUFFER SYSTEMS AND THEIR ROLE IN REGULATING THE PH OF BODY FLUIDS

A buffer is a mixture of a weak acid and a salt of its conjugate base that resists changes in pH when a strong acid or base is added to the solution (see Chapter 1). If the concentrations of the acid and base components of a buffer are equal, the pH will equal the pK. Generally, buffers work best at resisting changes in pH in the interval ± one pH unit of its pK. That is, buffers work best when the ratio of acid : base is within the range of 10:1 to 1:10. Buffers are also more effective at higher concentrations, so that a 10 mmol/L buffer solution is more effective than a 1.0 mmol/L solution.

The action of buffers in the regulation of body pH can be explained by using the bicarbonate buffer system as an example. If a strong acid is added to a solution containing HCO_3^- and H_2CO_3, the H^+ will react with HCO_3^- to form more H_2CO_3 and subsequently CO_2 and H_2O. The hydrogen ions are thereby bound, and the increase in the H^+ concentration will be minimal.

$$HCO_3^- + H^+ \rightarrow H_2CO_3 \rightarrow CO_2 + H_2O$$

The buffer systems of most physiological interest in connection with regulation of the pH of body fluids are those of plasma and erythrocytes. Discussions of the most important physiological buffers follow.

Bicarbonate/Carbonic Acid Buffer System

The most important buffer of plasma is the bicarbonate/carbonic acid pair. Initially, one might not think that this buffer would be very effective because its pK is 6.1, whereas normal plasma pH is 7.4. Furthermore, the ratio of base to acid is ~20:1 in plasma, which is outside the general limits for good buffering capacity. However, the effectiveness of the bicarbonate buffer is based on its high concentration (>20 mmol/L) and on the fact that the lungs can readily dispose of or retain CO_2. In addition, the renal tubules can increase or decrease the rate of reclamation of bicarbonate from the glomerular filtrate (see Chapter 45). The importance of the high concentration becomes apparent when one considers that at normal pH, 5 mmol/L of lactate (pK ~4) generates ~5 *mmol/L* of H^+ ion, which is remarkable considering that a normal H^+ ion concentration is only 40 nmol/L.

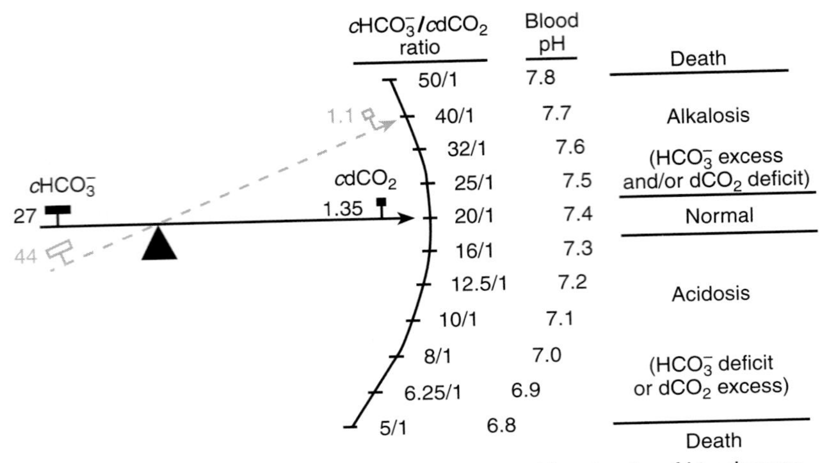

Figure 46-8 Scheme demonstrating the relation between pH and ratio of bicarbonate concentration to the concentration of dissolved CO_2. If the ratio in blood is 20 : 1 ($cHCO_3^- =$ 27 mmol/$cdCO_2$ = 1.35 mmol/L), the resultant pH will be 7.4 as demonstrated by the *solid beam*. The *dotted line* shows a case of uncompensated alkalosis (bicarbonate excess) with a bicarbonate concentration of 44 mmol/L and a $cdCO_2$ of 1.1 mmol/L. The ratio therefore is 40 : 1, and the resultant pH is 7.7. In a case of uncompensated acidosis, the pointer of the balance would point to a pH between 6.8 and 7.35, depending on the $cHCO_3^-/cdCO_2$ ratio. *(From Weisberg HF. A better understanding of anion-cation ("acid-base") balance. Surg Clin North Amer 1959;39:93-120; Snively WD, Wessner M. ABC's of fluid balance. J Ind State Med Assoc 1954;47:957-72.)*

Other nonbicarbonate buffers of blood are present at <10 mmol/L concentration.

The buffer value (β) is defined as the amount of base required to cause a change in pH of one unit. The buffer value of the bicarbonate buffer in plasma is 55.6 mmol/L. Derivation of this value is obtained by taking partial differentials of the Henderson-Hasselbalch equation, which is presented in detail in the second edition of this textbook.[30]

Phosphate Buffer System

At a plasma pH of 7.4, the ratio $cHPO_4^{2-}/cH_2PO_4^-$ is 4/1 (pK' = 6.8). The total concentration of this buffer in both erythrocytes and plasma is less than that of other major buffer systems, accounting for only about 5% of the nonbicarbonate buffer value of plasma. Organic phosphate, however, in the form of 2,3-diphosphoglycerate (present in erythrocytes in a concentration of about 4.5 mmol/L), accounts for about 16% of the nonbicarbonate buffer value of erythrocyte fluid.

The phosphate buffer reacts with acids and with bases as follows:

$$HPO_4^{\oplus\oplus} + H^{\oplus} \longrightarrow H_2PO_4^{\oplus}$$

$$H_2PO_4^{\oplus} + OH^{\ominus} \longrightarrow HPO_4^{\oplus\oplus} + H_2O$$

This system is important in the excretion of acids in the urine, as is explained in the section on renal compensatory mechanisms.

Plasma Protein Buffer System and Plasma Base Excess

The buffer value (β) of the nonbicarbonate buffers of plasma is about 7.7 mmol/L at pH 7.40 and a normal plasma protein concentration of 72 g/L. Proteins, especially albumin, account for the greatest portion (95%) of the nonbicarbonate buffer value of the plasma. The most important buffer groups of proteins in the physiological pH range are the imidazole groups of histidines (pK ~7.3). Each albumin molecule contains 16 histidines.

$$\text{Histidine residue (imidazolium, } \oplus\text{N–H)} \underset{pK = 7.3}{\rightleftharpoons} \text{Histidine residue (imidazole)} + H^{\oplus}$$

The significance of the nonbicarbonate buffers of the plasma can be illustrated when considering the chemical reactions during CO_2 equilibration:

$$CO_2 + H_2O \longrightarrow H_2CO_3 \longrightarrow HCO_3^{\ominus} + H^{\oplus}$$

$$HPr \longleftarrow H^{\oplus} + Pr^{\ominus}$$

where the HPr/Pr^- system represents all nonbicarbonate buffers. Since the purpose of this buffer system is to maintain cH^+ constant, for each molecule of HCO_3^- that is generated, one molecule of nonbicarbonate buffer base disappears. Thus in alkalosis, the cH^+ from CO_2 equilibration falls and there is a resulting excess of nonbicarbonate buffer base. As follows, there is a consumption or negative excess of this buffer base in acidosis.

Plasma base excess is defined as the initial concentration of titratable base when titrating the plasma with strong acid or base to pH (Std) = 7.4 at PCO_2 = 40 mm Hg and 37 °C. The equation for the CO_2 equilibration curve of plasma and calculation of *plasma base excess* can be written:

$$\Delta cHCO_3^-(P) = [-\beta Pr \times \Delta pH(P)] + \Delta cB'(P)$$

where $\Delta cHCO_3^-$ = actual HCO_3^- minus the standard HCO_3^- of 24.5 mmol/L, ΔpH = measured pH minus 7.40, and $\Delta cB'(P)$ is the plasma base excess.

Hemoglobin Buffer System and Whole Blood Base Excess

The buffer value (β) of the nonbicarbonate buffers of erythrocyte fluid is about 63 mmol/L at pH 7.20 for an erythrocyte hemoglobin (Fe) concentration of 21 mmol/L (33.8 g/dL). Hemoglobin accounts for the major part (53 mmol/L), with the remainder being mainly caused by 2,3-diphosphoglycerate (2,3-DPG). The imidazole groups of hemoglobin are quantitatively the most important buffer groups.

As in plasma, CO_2 equilibration of whole blood depends on the buffer value of nonbicarbonate buffers. Thus CO_2 equilibration in whole blood is dependent on hemoglobin concentration and also on pH and oxygenation status. It is possible to derive an approximate equation for whole blood CO_2 equilibration and calculation of *whole blood base excess* as follows:

$$\Delta cHCO_3^-(P) = -\beta \times \Delta pH(P) + \frac{\Delta cB'(B)}{\zeta}$$

where

$\Delta cHCO_3^-$ = measured plasma $cHCO_3^-(P)$ − 24.5 mmol/L HCO_3^-

ΔpH = measured pH − the standard pH of 7.40

$\Delta cB'(B)$ = the *whole blood base excess* (i.e., the concentration of titratable base when titrating the blood with strong acid or base to pH = 7.40 at PCO_2 [Std] and 37 °C)

$\beta = \beta_m Hb \times cHb(B) + \beta Pr$, where $\beta_m Hb$ is the molar buffer value of hemoglobin (2.3 mol/mol), $cHb(B)$ is the substance concentration of hemoglobin (Fe) in the blood (unit: mmol/L), and βPr is the buffer value of the plasma proteins (7.7 mmolL)

$\zeta = 1 - cHb(B)/c_{ref}$, where c_{ref} is an empirical parameter (43 mmol/L)

This equation for *whole blood base excess* (known as the Van Slyke equation[22,23]), together with the Henderson-Hasselbalch equation, provides the simplest algorithm for calculation of the various acid-base variables. The buffer value of HHb is slightly lower than that for O_2Hb at pH ~6.5 but higher at pH ~7.8. This is due to a decrease in the *pK* value of the "oxygen-linked" acid-base groups of Hb (C-terminal histidine and N-terminal valine) when HHb is oxygenated. When oxygenated, H^+ ions are liberated from Hb, a phenomenon called the *Haldane effect*. In a hemoglobin solution, a close relationship exists between the Bohr effect (the effect of pH on the O_2 saturation, see Chapter 27) and the Haldane effect. However, for whole blood, the rise in the concentration of titratable base, known as the Haldane coefficient for whole blood ($\Delta cB'[B]$), is only 0.3 mmol/L when oxyhemoglobin at a concentration of 1 mmol/L is converted to deoxyhemoglobin. For more detail of the interaction of the Bohr and Haldane effects, see Chapter 31 of the second edition of this textbook.[30]

Isohydric and Chloride Shift

Because of the continuous production of carbon dioxide within tissue cells, there is a concentration gradient for carbon dioxide from cells to the plasma and thus to erythrocytes. Despite this, the combination of all the buffer systems discussed previously interacts together with the Haldane effect in a phenomenon known as the isohydric Cl^- shift, which keeps the $cdCO_2$ and cH^+ (pH) essentially constant between arterial and venous blood. A small portion of the carbon dioxide entering the plasma stays as dissolved carbon dioxide, thus the slightly higher PCO_2 in venous blood. The majority reacts with water to form carbonic acid that dissociates into H^+ and HCO_3^-. The increased amount of H^+ is buffered by plasma buffers (Figure 46-9, reaction 1). Another small portion combines with the amino groups of proteins and forms carbamino compounds (Figure 46-9, reaction 2). The normal concentration of carbamino compounds in the plasma is about 0.2 mmol/L. Most of the carbon dioxide enters the erythrocytes and reacts with water to form carbonic acid. This reaction is catalyzed by the enzyme carbonic anhydrase (CA) and proceeds at a relatively high rate (Figure 46-9, reaction 3). Some CO_2 remains as dissolved CO_2 and some combines with Hb to form $HbCO_2$ (Figure 46-9, reaction 4).

The carbonic acid formed in reaction 3 initially increases the H^+ concentration. The pH change, however, is fully or partially compensated by the release of oxygen from O_2Hb, which involves the conversion of the stronger acid (O_2Hb) into a weaker acid (HHb) that then readily accepts the H^+. For each mole of O_2 released, the hemoglobin binds about 0.5 mol of H^+ ion. Furthermore, the HHb binds significantly more CO_2 in the form of carbamino-CO_2 than does oxyhemoglobin; thus an additional fraction of CO_2 is transported in this form. The oxygen released from O_2Hb moves from the erythrocytes through the plasma into the peripheral tissue cells.

The remainder of the hydrogen ions formed in reaction 3 are buffered by the nonbicarbonate buffers of the erythrocyte fluid, whereas the concentration of HCO_3^- increases to the same extent that the concentration of Hb anion falls.

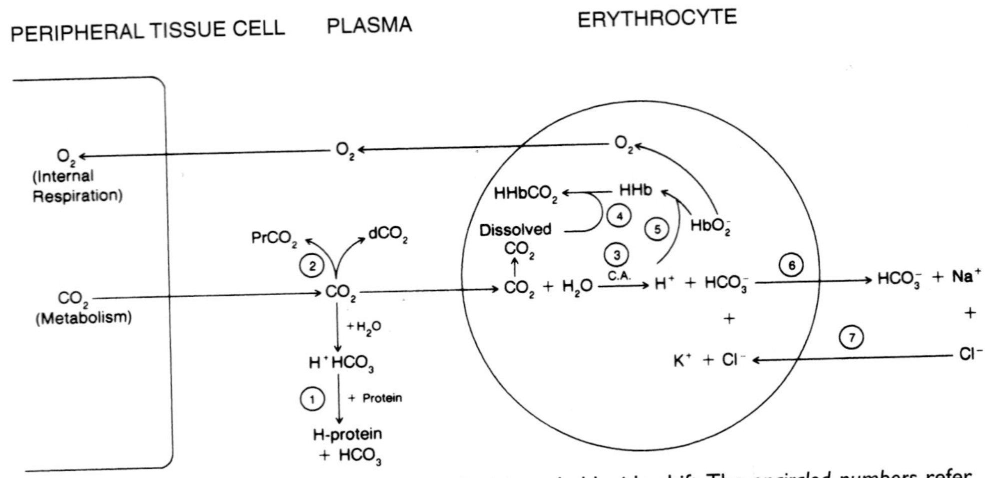

Figure 46-9 Scheme demonstrating the isohydric and chloride shift. The *encircled numbers* refer to the reactions described in the text. For details, see text.

The transformations described so far (Figure 46-9, reactions 1 through 5) are referred to as the *isohydric shift* (i.e., a shift in which the hydrogen ion concentration remains unchanged).

The equilibrium between plasma and red cells has been disturbed by the reactions described so far. The concentration of HCO_3^- has increased relatively more in the erythrocytes than in the plasma; the pH of plasma has fallen relatively more than the pH of the erythrocytes; and the nondiffusible ion concentration in the erythrocytes has fallen because of the increase in protonation of proteins and hemoglobin. The membrane potential of the erythrocytes therefore becomes less negative, and the distribution of all diffusible ions must change in accordance with the new membrane potential. The ion shifts that occur rapidly are a movement of HCO_3^- out of the erythrocytes and a movement of Cl^- into the erythrocytes to provide electrochemical balance. This shift of chloride ions is referred to as the *chloride shift* (Figure 46-9, reactions 6 and 7). As a result of these ion fluxes, the concentration of chloride in the venous plasma is about 1 mmol/L lower than that in the arterial plasma.

The HCO_3^-, the carbamino compounds, and the dissolved carbon dioxide are transported in venous blood to the pulmonary capillaries and alveoli. The comparatively low PCO_2 in the alveoli will cause a shift of carbon dioxide from the erythrocytes and the plasma into the alveoli. On the other hand, the high PO_2 in the alveoli causes a shift of oxygen into the plasma and the erythrocytes. This exchange causes a reversal of reactions 1 through 7 in Figure 46-9.

Respiratory Mechanism in the Regulation of Acid-Base Balance

In addition to supplying O_2 to tissue cells for normal metabolism, the respiratory mechanism contributes to the maintenance of normal body pH through elimination or retention of CO_2 in metabolic acidosis and alkalosis, respectively.

Respiration

Exchange of O_2 and CO_2 in the lungs between alveolar air and blood is called *external respiration,* in contrast to internal respiration occurring at the tissue level. At inspiration, contraction of the diaphragm and thoracic musculature expands intrathoracic volume and creates a fall in intrapulmonary pressure. Atmospheric air is drawn into the bronchial tree, which terminates at the alveoli. Alveoli are small saclike chambers with very thin walls in close approximation to pulmonary capillaries where the exchange of gases between alveolar air and pulmonary blood occurs. Expiration takes place passively by recoil as the elastic tissues of the lungs and chest wall rebound and the intrathoracic volume is decreased. Loss of elasticity of the lungs and destruction of the alveolar membranes are basic pathological mechanisms underlying many pulmonary diseases.

Peripheral venous blood reaches the pulmonary circulation from the right ventricle of the heart and is "arterialized" in the capillaries of the lungs by uptake of O_2 and loss of CO_2. Pulmonary venous blood then returns to the left ventricle by way of the left atrium and is pumped through the aorta to the peripheral tissues. In the capillaries of peripheral tissues, the arterial blood releases O_2 to the tissue cells and takes up CO_2. With return of blood to the lungs, the cycle is completed.

In a resting state, the respiration rate is normally 12 to 15 breaths/min. For an average-sized adult with a tidal volume (the amount of air exchanged per breath cycle) of about 0.5 L, 6 to 8 L of air is moved per minute in either direction. Physical activity increases ventilation (respiratory rate × tidal volume), i.e., the amount of air exchanged per minute. Voluntary efforts can increase the rate of ventilation 20 to 30 times over the resting concentration, but only briefly. Involuntary increases in rate and depth of respiration are regulated by the medullary respiratory center in the brain stem, which in turn is stimulated by central chemoreceptors located on the anterior surface of the medulla oblongata and by peripheral chemoreceptors located in the carotid arteries and aorta. Peripheral chemoreceptors are stimulated by a fall in pH caused by accumulation of CO_2 or by a decrease in PO_2. The central chemoreceptors are stimulated only by a decrease in pH of the CSF.

Often a patient's normal response to these chemical receptors that drive respiration is perturbed by a pathological condition in the circulatory or respiratory system. If significantly abnormal, the patient will require assisted ventilation that uses a mechanical device to provide gas mixtures intermittently via an endotracheal tube inserted through the mouth or through a tracheostomy. Gas mixtures containing different fractional compositions of O_2 and CO_2 may be administered in conjunction with assisted ventilation. A physician's adjustments of the conditions of this mechanical ventilation depend greatly on the results of blood gas and pH determinations that reflect current acid-base status.

Exchange of Gases in the Lungs and Peripheral Tissues

Diffusion of O_2 and CO_2 across alveolar and cell membranes is governed by gradients in the partial pressure of each gas (Figure 46-10). Dry air inspired at a pressure of 1 atm (760 mm Hg) consists of 21% O_2 (PO_2 ~160 mm Hg), 0.03% CO_2 (PCO_2 ~0.25 mm Hg), 78% nitrogen, and ~0.1% other inert gases. As inspired air passes over the moist mucous membranes of the upper respiratory tract, it is warmed to 37 °C, becomes saturated with water vapor, and mixes with air in the respiratory tree, resulting in partial pressures of ~150 mm Hg for O_2, 0.3 mm Hg for CO_2, ~47 mm Hg for H_2O, and 563 mm Hg for nitrogen. Further mixing with alveolar air results in partial pressures at the alveolar membrane of ~105 mm Hg for O_2, ~40 mm Hg for CO_2, and ~47 mm Hg for H_2O. Venous blood on the opposite side of the alveolar membrane contains O_2 at a partial pressure of approximately 40 mm Hg and CO_2 at approximately 46 mm Hg. Thus the gradient for O_2 is inward, toward the blood, and for CO_2, it is outward, toward the alveoli. CO_2 removal is so efficient that the PCO_2 in expired air is more than 100 times the PCO_2 in inspired air (see Figure 46-10). In the arterial blood, the PO_2 is slightly lower than in alveolar air (90 versus 105 mm Hg). This difference is due to shunting about 5% of blood through the lungs that does not equilibrate with O_2.

At the arterial end of capillaries of peripheral tissues, the PO_2 at approximately 90 mm Hg is substantially higher than the average PO_2 at the surface of the tissue cells (20 mm Hg), and the PCO_2 at ~40 mm Hg is substantially lower than that in the cells (50 to 70 mm Hg). Thus in the tissue capillary, the gradient for O_2 is inward to the cell; for CO_2 it is outward to the capillary blood. The arteriovenous difference in partial pressures is approximately 60 mm Hg for O_2 and 6 mm Hg or less for CO_2. This difference in arteriovenous PO_2 is one indicator of the efficiency of O_2 extraction in the passage of blood through the capillaries. During passage through the tissues, the concentration of total oxygen falls on average 2.3 mmol/L, whereas the concentration of total CO_2 of the blood rises about 2.0 mmol/L.

Respiratory Response to Acid-Base Perturbations

Most metabolic acid-base disorders develop slowly, within hours in diabetic ketoacidosis and months or even years in chronic renal disease. The respiratory system responds immediately to a change in acid-base status, but several hours may be required for the response to become maximal. The maximum response is not attained until both the central and peripheral chemoreceptors are fully stimulated. For example, in the early stages of metabolic acidosis, plasma pH decreases, but because H^+ ions equilibrate rather slowly across the blood-brain barrier, the pH in CSF remains nearly normal. However, because peripheral chemoreceptors are stimulated by the decreased plasma pH, hyperventilation occurs, and plasma PCO_2 decreases. When this occurs, the PCO_2 of the CSF decreases immediately because CO_2 equilibrates rapidly across the blood-brain barrier, leading to a rise in the pH of the CSF. This will inhibit the central chemoreceptors. But as plasma bicarbonate gradually falls because of acidosis, bicarbonate concentration and pH in the CSF will also fall over several hours. At this point, stimulation of respiration becomes maximal as both the central and peripheral chemoreceptors are maximally stimulated.

The reverse is true when a patient with metabolic acidosis is treated with HCO_3^-. When the pH in plasma increases as the result of HCO_3^- administration, stimulation of the peripheral chemoreceptors returns to normal. However, because of the slow equilibration of HCO_3^- between plasma and CSF, the central chemoreceptors continue to be stimulated, and the patient continues to hyperventilate, even when the blood pH has returned to normal. Respiration does not return to normal until normal acid-base balance in the CSF of the brain is restored.

Renal Mechanisms in the Regulation of Acid-Base Balance

The average pH of plasma and of the glomerular filtrate is ~7.4, whereas the average urinary pH is ~6.0, reflecting the renal excretion of nonvolatile acids produced by metabolic processes. The various functions of the kidneys respond to different alterations of acid-base status. In the case of acidosis, excretion of acids is increased and base is conserved; in alkalosis, the opposite occurs. The pH of the urine changes correspondingly and may vary in *random* specimens from pH 4.5 to 8.0. This ability to excrete variable amounts of acid or base makes the kidney the final defense mechanism against changes in body pH.

The various acids produced during metabolic processes are buffered in the ECF at the expense of HCO_3^-. Renal excre-

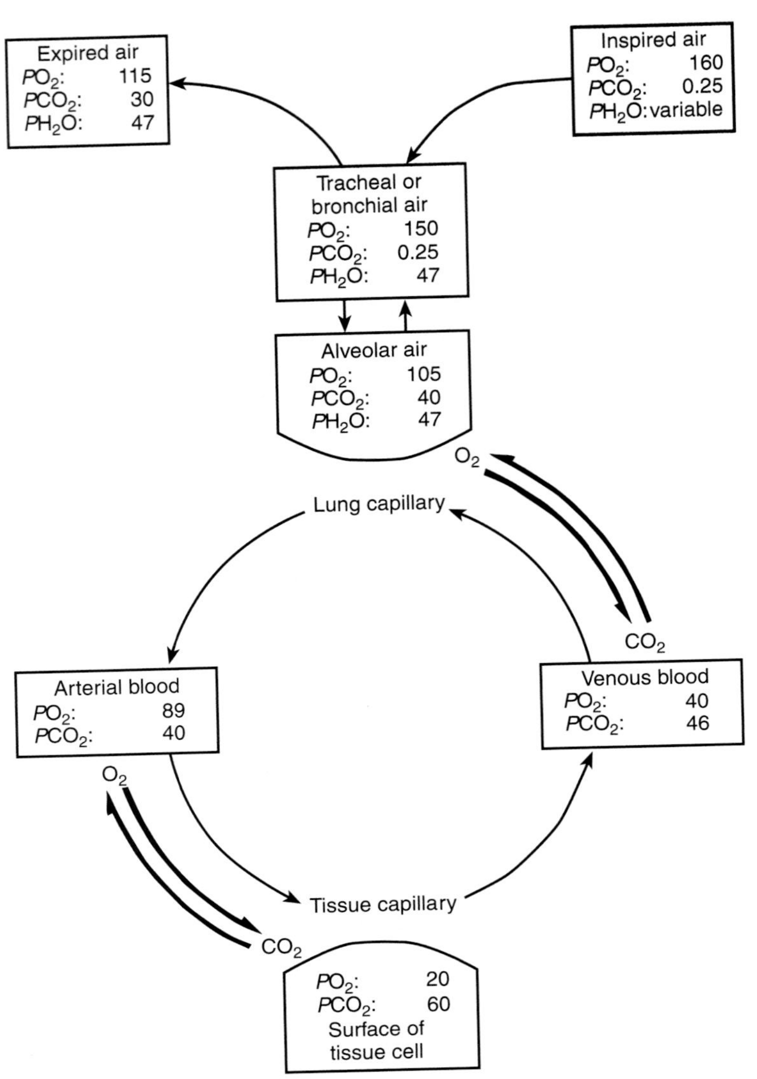

Figure 46-10 Partial pressures of oxygen and carbon dioxide in air, blood, and tissue. Values shown are approximations in mm Hg and calculated assuming a 5% shunt. *Heavy arrows* show directions of gradients. *(Modified from Tietz NW. Fundamentals of clinical chemistry, 3rd ed. Philadelphia: WB Saunders Co, 1987.)*

tion of acid and conservation of HCO_3^- occur through several mechanisms including (1) the Na^+-H^+ exchange, (2) production of ammonia and excretion of NH_4^+, and (3) reclamation of HCO_3^-.

Na^+-H^+ Exchange

Nearly all mammalian cells contain a plasma membrane ATP-hydrolyzing protein capable of exchanging sodium ions for protons—the so-called Na^+-H^+ exchanger (Figure 46-11). In 2002 it was reported that at least six isoforms of the Na^+-H^+ exchanger (NHE-1 through NHE-6) are differentially expressed in a wide variety of tissues.[18] These NHE isoforms exhibit 20% to 60% amino acid identity, with highly conserved transmembrane domains, suggesting that these domains are the sites of Na^+ and H^+ translocation.[18] In the renal tubules, NHE-1 and NHE-3 appear to be the predominant isoforms that extrude H^+ ions into the tubular fluid in exchange for Na^+ ions.

Na^+-H^+ exchange is enhanced in states of acidoses and inhibited in alkalotic states. Both NHE-1 and NHE-3 isoforms are transcriptionally upregulated in response to acidotic states. Additionally the NHE-3 isoform shows an increased V_{max} of Na^+-H^+ exchange during acidoses—a process that may be regulated by increased phosphorylation of the cytoplasmic domain. The proximal tubules, however, cannot maintain an H^+-gradient of more than ~1 pH unit whereas the distal tubules cannot maintain one of more than ~3 pH units. Thus maximum urine acidity is reached at ~pH 4.4. In Type I and Type IV RTA, this exchange process is defective and may lead to a decrease in blood pH. In Type I RTA, there is often an increase in urinary pH, but in Type IV, an additional defect in NH_3 excretion can result in normal or even decreased urine pH. Hydrogen ions of the glomerular filtrate, or those that have been transported through the Na^+-H^+ exchanger into the tubular fluid, may react with NH_3 or HPO_4^{2-} as shown in Figure 46-11 and described in the next section.

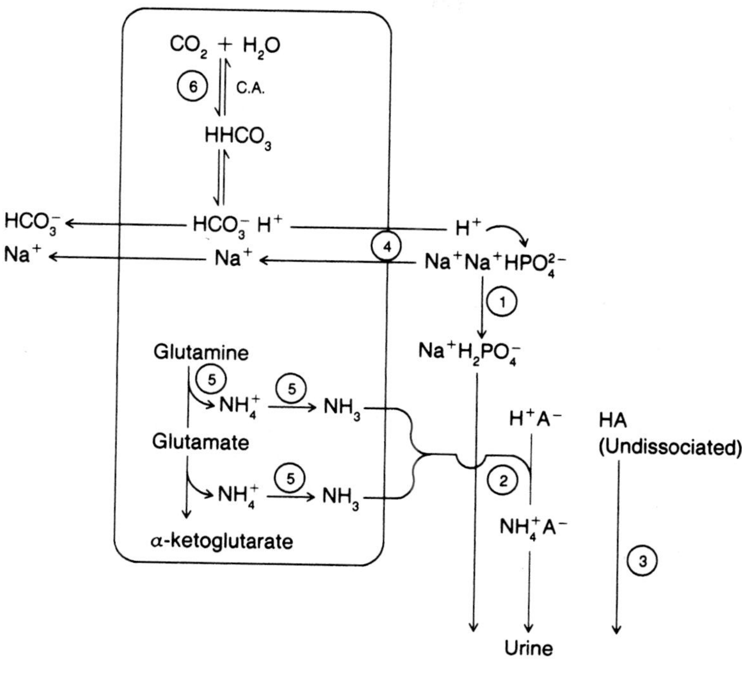

Figure 46-11 Hydrogen ion excretion, sodium hydrogen ion exchange, and ammonia production in the renal tubules. Key: *1*, conversion of HPO_4^{2-} to H_2PO_4; *2*, reaction of hydrogen ions with NH_3; *3*, excretion of undissociated acids; *4*, Na^+-H^+ exchange; *5*, NH_3 production; and *6*, synthesis of carbonic acid from CO_2.

Potassium ions compete with hydrogen ions in the renal tubular Na^+-H^+ exchanger. If the intracellular K^+ level of renal tubular cells is high, more K^+ and less H^+ are exchanged for Na^+. As a result, the urine becomes less acidic, thereby increasing the acidity of body fluids. If K^+ is depleted, more H^+ ions are exchanged for Na^+, and the urine becomes more acidic and the body fluids more alkaline. Thus hyperkalemia contributes to acidosis and hypokalemia to alkalosis. Because the body's compensatory mechanism against metabolic alkalosis is relatively ineffective, K^+ depletion alone can result in a metabolic alkalosis.

Renal Production of Ammonia and Excretion of Ammonium Ions

Renal tubular cells are able to generate ammonia from glutamine and other amino acids derived from muscle and liver cells according to the following reaction:

$$\underset{\text{Glutamine}}{H_3N^{\oplus}\text{-CH(COO}^{\ominus}\text{)-CH}_2\text{-CH}_2\text{-C(=O)NH}_2} \xrightarrow[H_2O \;\rightarrow\; NH_3]{\textit{Glutaminase}} \underset{\text{Glutamate}}{H_3N^{\oplus}\text{-CH(COO}^{\ominus}\text{)-CH}_2\text{-CH}_2\text{-C(=O)OH}} \xrightarrow[NAD^{\oplus} \;\rightarrow\; NADH + NH_4^{\oplus}]{\textit{Glutamate dehydrogenase}} \underset{\text{2-Oxoglutarate}}{O\text{=C(COO}^{\ominus}\text{)-CH}_2\text{-CH}_2\text{-C(=O)OH}}$$

$$NH_4^{\oplus} \rightleftharpoons NH_3 + H^{\oplus}$$

The ammonium ion produced dissociates into ammonia and hydrogen ions to a degree dependent on the pH (see Figure 46-11). At normal blood pH, the ratio of NH_4^+ to NH_3 is about 100 to 1. Ammonia is a gas and diffuses readily across the cell membrane into the tubular lumen, where it combines with hydrogen ions to form ammonium ions (see Figure 46-11). At the acid pH of urine, the equilibrium between NH_4^+ and NH_3 shifts markedly to the left (~10,000 to 1), strongly favoring formation of NH_4^+. The NH_4^+ formed in the tubular lumen cannot easily cross cell membranes

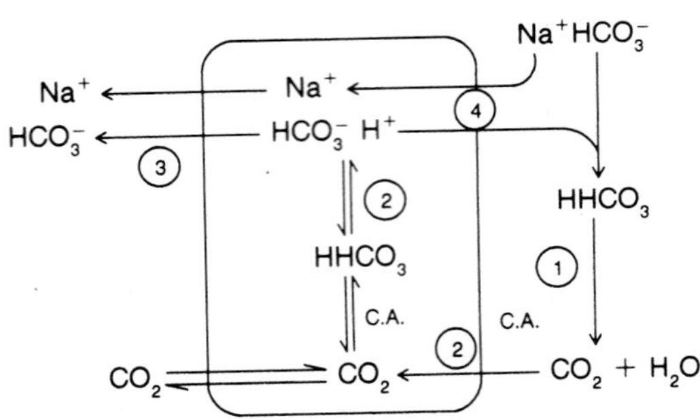

Figure 46-12 Key: *1,* Formation of CO_2 from bicarbonate in the tubular fluid; *2,* formation of H^+ and HCO_3^- from CO_2 in the tubular cell; *3,* new generation of HCO_3^-; and *4,* Na^+-H^+ exchange.

and thus is trapped in the tubular urine and excreted with anions such as phosphate, chloride, or sulfate. In normal individuals, NH_4^+ production in the tubular lumen accounts for the excretion of ~60% (30 to 60 mmol) of the hydrogen ions associated with nonvolatile acids. Finally the 2-oxoglutarate produced in this reaction is converted to bicarbonate (up to 270 mmol/day) that helps to replenish bicarbonate neutralized by metabolic acid production.

The amount of H^+ excreted bound to NH_3 can be measured as NH_4^+. The H^+ required for NH_4^+ formation may be present in the glomerular filtrate or may be generated within tubular cells by carbonic anhydrase synthesis of carbonic acid from CO_2 (see Figures 46-11 and 46-12). These hydrogen ions are secreted into the tubular lumen through the Na^+-H^+ exchangers (see Figure 46-11). In systemic acidosis, excretion accounts by far for the greatest net excretion of H^+ by the kidneys. However, the maximum rate of glutamine release and therefore of NH_3 production (~400 mmol/day) is not achieved until acidosis has persisted for 3 days. In patients with chronic Type IV RTA or with renal insufficiency, the kidneys are unable to generate sufficient NH_3 to buffer the nonvolatile acids produced, and this defect contributes significantly to the acidosis in such patients.

Excretion of H^+ as $H_2PO_4^-$

H^+ secreted into the tubular lumen by the Na^+-H^+ exchanger may also react with HPO_4^{2-} to form $H_2PO_4^-$ (see Figure 46-11). This process depends on the amount of phosphate filtered by the glomeruli and the pH of urine. Under normal physiological conditions, ~30 mmol of H^+ is excreted per day as $H_2PO_4^-$, and this amount accounts for ~90% of the titratable acidity of urine. In case of high-protein intake, phosphate production and filtration may be increased. Acidemia increases phosphate excretion and thus provides additional buffer for reaction with H^+. A decrease in the glomerular filtration rate (GFR), as observed in renal disease, may result in a decrease of $H_2PO_4^-$ excretion.

The secretion of H^+ and the subsequent reaction with $H_2PO_4^-$ allow the removal of one H^+ without any significant decrease in urinary pH. As a result, the pH gradient is not greatly affected and more H^+ can be secreted into the tubules, whereas more Na^+ is reabsorbed and conserved. The HCO_3^- formed by the action of carbonic anhydrase in the tubular cells in the process of H^+ secretion reclaims the HCO_3^- lost in buffering the body burden of ingested or produced acid.

Excretion of Other Acids

Strong acids, such as sulfuric, hydrochloric, and phosphoric, are fully ionized at the pH of urine and are excreted only after the H^+ derived from these acids reacts with a buffer base. Excretion of the anions of these acids is accompanied by the simultaneous removal of an equal number of cations, such as Na^+, K^+, or NH_4^+, to provide electrochemical balance. However, some acids, such as acetoacetic acid ($pK = 3.58$) and β-hydroxybutyric acid ($pK = 4.7$), are present in blood almost entirely in ionized form; at the acid pH frequently prevailing in urine, some are nondissociated and thus may be excreted partially as the nondissociated acid (see Figure 46-11). For example, 50% of β-hydroxybutyric acid at pH 4.7 is nonionized.

Reclamation of Filtered Bicarbonate

The unmodified glomerular filtrate has the same concentration of HCO_3^- as does plasma; however, with increasing acidification of the proximal tubular urine, the HCO_3^- concentration decreases. It is believed that these changes are triggered by the excretion of H^+ by the Na^+-H^+ exchanger mechanism, which results in a decrease in urinary pH. The H^+ excreted reacts with HCO_3^- (catalyzed by carbonic anhydrase, in the brush border of the proximal tubular cells) to form H_2CO_3 and subsequently CO_2 and H_2O (see Figure 46-12).

This increase in urinary CO_2 causes carbon dioxide to diffuse across the tubular wall into the tubular cell, where it reacts with H_2O in the presence of *cytoplasmic* carbonic anhydrase in the tubular cells to form H_2CO_3 and subsequently H^+ and HCO_3^- (see Figure 46-12). Thus reclamation of bicarbonate is in fact diffusion of CO_2 into tubular cells and its subsequent conversion to HCO_3^-. The increase in HCO_3^- helps to maintain or restore a normal pH in the general circulation. Normally, ~90% of the filtered HCO_3^- (or about 4500 mmol/day) is reclaimed in the proximal tubule, and the extent of HCO_3^- reclamation parallels Na^+ reabsorption. Thus for each H^+ secreted into the tubular fluid, one Na^+ and one HCO_3^- enter the tubular cell and return to the general circulation.

When plasma HCO_3^- concentration increases above ~28 mmol/L, the capacity of the proximal and distal tubules to reclaim is exceeded, and HCO_3^- is excreted in the urine. The process of bicarbonate reclamation is enhanced in acidosis (and decreased in alkalosis), most likely as a result of increased Na^+-H^+ exchange. In this way, the kidneys in acidosis or alkalosis support the other compensatory mechanisms to restore the normal $cHCO_3^-/cdCO_2$ ratio. Type II RTA is a decreased ability to reabsorb HCO_3^- in the proximal tubules, leading to a decrease in blood pH.

CONDITIONS ASSOCIATED WITH ABNORMAL ACID-BASE STATUS AND ABNORMAL ELECTROLYTE COMPOSITION OF THE BLOOD[6,17,25,32]

Many pathological conditions are accompanied by disturbances of the acid-base balance and electrolyte composition of the blood. These changes are usually reflected in the acid-base pattern and anion-cation composition of ECF, as measured in blood. However, results obtained on blood or plasma may not always reflect the acid-base status of the ICF.

Abnormalities of acid-base status of the blood are always accompanied by characteristic changes in electrolyte concentrations in the plasma, especially in metabolic acid-base disorders. Hydrogen ions cannot accumulate without concomitant accumulation of anions, such as Cl^- or lactate, or without exchange for cations, such as K^+ or Na^+. Consequently, electrolyte composition of blood serum or plasma is often determined along with measurements of blood gases and pH and to assess acid-base disturbances.

Acid-base disturbances are traditionally classified as (1) metabolic acidosis, (2) metabolic alkalosis, (3) respiratory acidosis, or (4) respiratory alkalosis. In simple, straight-

TABLE 46-3 Classification and Characteristics of Simple Acid-Base Disorders

	Primary Change	Compensatory Response	Expected Compensation
Metabolic			
Acidosis	↓$cHCO_3^-$	↓PCO_2	$PCO_2 = 1.5\ (cHCO_3^-) + 8 \pm 2$ PCO_2 falls by 1 to 1.3 mm Hg for each mmol/L fall in $cHCO_3^-$ Last 2 digits of pH = PCO_2 (e.g., if $PCO_2 = 28$, pH = 7.28) $cHCO_3^- + 15$ = last 2 digits of pH ($cHCO_3^- = 15$, pH = 7.30)
Alkalosis	↑$cHCO_3^-$	↑PCO_2	PCO_2 increases 6 mm Hg for each 10 mmol/L rise in $cHCO_3^-$ $cHCO_3^- + 15$ = last 2 digits of pH ($cHCO_3^- = 35$, pH = 7.50)
Respiratory			
Acidosis			
Acute	↑PCO_2	↑$cHCO_3^-$	$cHCO_3^-$ increases by 1 mmol/L for each 10 mm Hg rise in PCO_2
Chronic	↑PCO_2	↑$cHCO_3^-$	$cHCO_3^-$ increases by 3.5 mmol/L for each 10 mm Hg rise in PCO_2
Alkalosis			
Acute	↓PCO_2	↓$cHCO_3^-$	$cHCO_3^-$ falls by 2 mmol/L for each 10 mm Hg fall in PCO_2
Chronic	↓PCO_2	↓$cHCO_3^-$	$cHCO_3^-$ falls by 5 mmol/L for each 10 mm Hg fall in PCO_2

Modified from Narins RG, Gardner LB. Simple acid-base disturbances. Med Clin North Amer 1981;65:321-46.

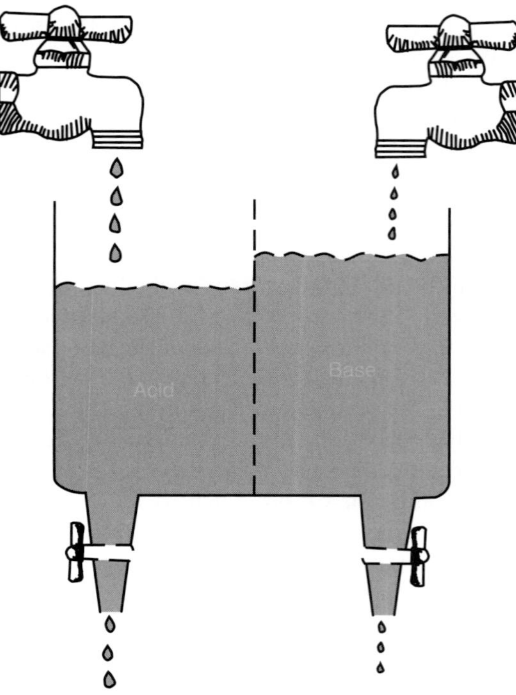

Figure 46-13 Simple depiction of the body as a two-vat system of acid and base. At equilibrium input and output from each "vat" are equal. *(From Dufour DR. Acid-base disorders. In: Dufour DR, Christenson RH, eds: Professional practice in clinical chemistry: A review. Washington DC: AACC Press, 1995:604-35.)*

forward acid-base disorders, the laboratory parameters observed for these groups are shown in Table 46-3. However, interpretation of laboratory values to classify these disorders is rarely straightforward because of compensatory responses by the respiratory and renal systems attempting to correct the imbalance.

The causes of acid-base disorders, resulting laboratory values, and compensatory responses are discussed here in the traditional categorization of these disorders. However, it is often difficult to remember which disorders fall into which categories, so it is common for mnemonic devices or tables to be used to facilitate description of these disorders. A useful and more logical approach is to realize that an acidosis can only occur as a result of one (or a combination) of three mechanisms: (1) increased addition of acid, (2) decreased elimination of acid, and (3) increased loss of base. Similarly, alkalosis occurs only by (1) increased addition of base, (2) decreased elimination of base, and (3) increased loss of acid. Dufour has illustrated this simple concept by depicting the body as a two-tank vat, one of acid and one of base, with inputs and outputs for each vat (Figure 46-13).[6] In the normal setting, these inputs and outputs are balanced; an acid-base disorder then involves a perturbation in the input or output of these body reservoirs, as discussed in the next section.

METABOLIC ACIDOSIS (PRIMARY BICARBONATE DEFICIT)

Metabolic acidosis is readily detected by decreased plasma bicarbonate (or a negative extracellular base excess), the primary perturbation in this acid-base disorder. Bicarbonate is "lost" in the buffering of excess acid. Causes include the following:

1. Production of organic acids that exceeds the rate of elimination (e.g., the production of acetoacetic acid and β-hydroxybutyric acid in diabetic acidosis and of lactic acid in lactic acidosis).
2. Reduced excretion of acids (H^+) as occurs in renal failure and some RTAs, resulting in an accumulation of acid that consumes bicarbonate.
3. Excessive loss of bicarbonate because of increased renal excretion (decreased tubular reclamation) or excessive loss of duodenal fluid (as in diarrhea). Plasma $cHCO_3^-$ falls; the fall is associated with a rise in the concentration of inorganic anions (mostly chloride) or a concomitant fall in the sodium concentration.

When any of these conditions exists, the ratio of $cHCO_3^-/cCO_2$ is decreased because of the primary decrease in bicarbonate. The resulting drop in pH stimulates a respiratory compensation via hyperventilation, which lowers PCO_2 and thereby raises the pH.

Increased Anion Gap Acidosis (Organic Acidosis)

Metabolic acidoses are classified as those associated with either an increased anion gap or a normal anion gap (Table 46-4). The concept of the *anion gap* was originally devised as a quality control rule when it was noted that if the sum of Cl^- and HCO_3^- values was subtracted from the Na^+ value ($Na^+ - [Cl^- + HCO_3^-]$), the difference, or "gap," averaged 12 mmol/L in healthy subjects.[3] This *apparent* gap is due to unmeasured anions (e.g., proteins, SO_4^{2-}, $H_2PO_4^{2-}$) that are present in plasma. Anion gap values outside the interval of 7 to 16 mmol/L suggested the possibility of an error in measurement of one of the electrolytes. However, it was also apparent that the anion gap was increased in many patients with a metabolic acidosis.[7,10] Indeed, the presence of an elevated anion gap is often the first indication of a metabolic acidosis and should be assessed in the electrolyte profiles of all patients. The gap is also slightly increased in the absence of acidosis by very low calcium, magnesium, or potassium levels because lower levels of these "unmeasured" cations will result in lower levels of anions (Figure 46-14). Conversely the gap can be artificially narrowed in settings of hypoalbuminemia (negatively charged proteins), hypergammaglobulinemia (positively charged proteins), hypercalcemia, or hypermagnesemia. Taken together, these alterations have called into question its utility according to some authors.[21,33] However, the gap in these settings is usually at the extremes of the reference intervals or only slightly outside the reference intervals.

All anion gap metabolic acidoses can be explained by one (or a combination) of eight underlying mechanisms listed

TABLE 46-4 Conditions of Metabolic Acidoses with High and Normal Anion Gaps

Etiology	Retained Acids	Other Laboratory Findings
High AG*		
Methanol toxicity	Formate	↑Osmolal gap (>15 mOsmol/kg)
Uremia of renal failure	Sulfuric, phosphoric, organic	↑BUN† and serum creatinine
Ketoacidoses		
Diabetes mellitus	Acetoacetate and β-hydroxybutyrate	↑Plasma and urine glucose
Ethyl alcohol toxicity		↑Osmolal gap (>15 mOsmol/kg)
Starvation		
Paraldehyde toxicity		
Isoniazid or iron toxicity, also ischemia	Organic, mainly lactate	Isoniazid and iron act as mitochondrial poisons
Lactic acidosis	Lactate	
Ethylene glycol toxicity	Hippurate, glycolate, oxalate	↑Osmolal gap (>15 mOsmol/kg), urine oxalate crystals
Salicylate toxicity	Salicylate, organic	Respiratory alkalosis
Normal AG		
Gastrointestinal fluid loss	A primary loss of bicarbonate	
Severe diarrhea		Hypokalemia
Pancreatitis		K^+ variable
Intestinal fistula		
Renal tubular acidoses (RTA)	Sulfuric, phosphoric, organic	
Proximal (type II) RTA		Urine pH < 5.5, with K^+ normal or low
Distal (type I) RTA		Urine pH > 5.5 with hypokalemia (usually)
Type IV RTA		Urine pH < 5.5 with hyperkalemia

*Although there is considerable variability, the anion gap is often >25 mmol/L in these conditions with the exception of uremic renal failure.
†Blood urea nitrogen (reference interval: 8 to 25 mg/dL, or ~3.0 to 9.0 mmol/L).

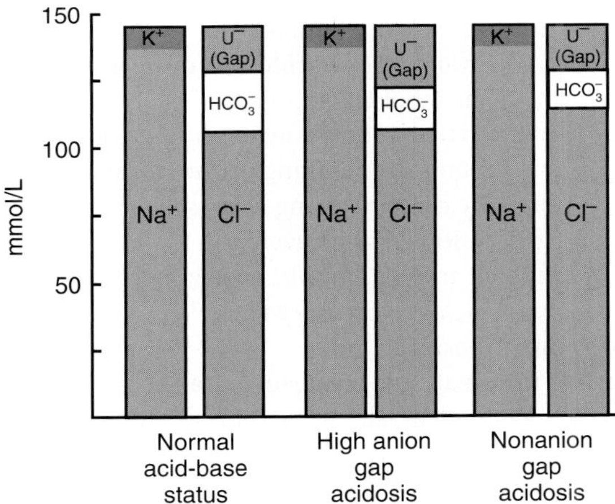

Figure 46-14 Simple "Gambelgram" depiction of normal gap, anion gap acidosis, and nonanion gap acidosis. Cations, Na^+, and K^+ are in left bar for each condition, whereas measured (Cl^- and HCO_3^-) and unmeasured (U^-) anions are in right bar for each condition.

below according to the common mnemonic device MUDPILES (see Table 46-4). The physiological basis for the anion gap in these conditions is the consumption of bicarbonate in buffering excess acid. Cl^- values remain normal when the excess acid is any other than HCl, because the lost bicarbonate is replaced by the unmeasured anions.

Methanol

Although nontoxic itself, methanol is metabolized by the liver to formaldehyde and formic acid. Accumulation of this acid leads to metabolic acidosis with a high anion gap and to clinical symptoms of optic papillitis ("snowfield" blindness), retinal edema, and ultimately blindness because of optic nerve atrophy and neurological defects that may lead to coma. Methanol and other ingested alcohols such as ethylene glycol, ethanol, and isopropanol will increase the osmolality of plasma. Thus in the presence of a high anion gap acidosis, determination of the osmolal gap (see Chapter 27) will help determine the source of the unmeasured anion[5] and suggest specific toxicological analyses.[5]

Uremia of Renal Failure

The loss of functional renal tubular mass results in decreased ammonia formation, decreased Na^+-H^+ exchange, and decreased GFR. All result in decreased acid excretion (see Chapter 45). Acidosis usually develops if GFR falls below 20 mL/min. Serum creatinine and blood urea nitrogen levels are usually elevated and are used as an estimate of the degree of renal damage or, more appropriately, as an estimate of remaining functional renal capacity.

Diabetes or Ketoacidosis

The pathogenesis of ketoacidosis is discussed in detail in Chapter 25. Ketoacids such as β-hydroxybutyrate and 2-oxoglutarate accumulate and represent the unmeasured anions. Accumulation of these "ketone bodies" causes a decrease in HCO_3^-, a normal or low serum chloride, and a high anion gap. Ketoacids also accumulate in states of starvation and alcoholic malnutrition.

Paraldehyde Toxicity

Paraldehyde toxicity may develop after chronic paraldehyde ingestion. The pathogenesis is poorly defined, but the acidosis may actually be a ketosis (nitroprusside negative) with β-hydroxybutyric acid as the main acidic product. Patients with paraldehyde toxicity have a pungent, apple-like odor to their breath.

Isoniazid, Iron, or Ischemia

These seemingly unrelated etiologies of high anion gap acidosis share a common feature: the accumulation of organic acids, with a predominance of lactic acid. Thus the "three I's" actually represent special cases in the general category of lactic acidosis, which is described next. Both isoniazid, an antimycobacterial agent commonly used in the treatment or prophylaxis of tuberculosis, and iron toxicity involve the production of toxic peroxides that act as mitochondrial poisons and interfere with normal cellular respiration. In addition, isoniazid may be hepatotoxic, leading to significant liver damage and impairment of lactate clearance.[16]

Tissue ischemia may result from many causes; in general, hypoperfusion leads to hypoxia of cells, which results in anaerobic metabolism with the attendant accumulation of organic (mainly lactic) acids. The kidneys (and brain) are especially sensitive to hypoperfusion, such that acute renal failure often is a contributing factor in the high anion gap metabolic acidosis associated with global tissue ischemia (as may occur in major trauma).

Lactic Acidosis

Lactic acid, present in blood entirely as lactate ion ($pK = 3.86$), is an intermediate of carbohydrate metabolism and is derived mainly from muscle cells and erythrocytes (see Chapter 25). It represents the end product of anaerobic metabolism and is normally metabolized by the liver. The blood lactate concentration is, therefore, affected by the rate of production and the rate of metabolism, both of which are dependent on adequate tissue perfusion. An increase in the concentration of lactate to >2 mmol/L and the associated increased H^+ is considered lactic acidosis.

Lactic acidosis caused by severe tissue hypoxia is seen in severe anemia, shock, cardiac decompensation, and pulmonary insufficiency. Severe oxygen deprivation of tissue blocks aerobic oxidation of pyruvic acid in the tricarboxylic acid cycle and results in the reduction of pyruvate to form lactate. Lactic acidosis is associated with a significant increase in the lactate/pyruvate ratio in blood. Such extreme findings signal deterioration of the cellular oxidative process and are associated with marked tachypnea, weakness, fatigue, stupor, and finally coma. Conditions at these later stages are frequently irreversible, even when treatment for acidosis and hypoxia is instituted. Examples are the irreversible, end-stage of shock; diabetic coma without ketosis; and a variety of illnesses in the terminal stage. A short-lived lactic acidosis is often observed following grand mal seizures. If the origin of lactate (e.g., seizure and hypoxic tissue) can be rectified, lactate is rapidly metabolized to CO_2, which is then eliminated if the respiratory system is intact.

Lactic acidosis is also caused by (1) drugs and toxins, such as ethanol, methanol, biguanides, isoniazid (see previous discussion), and streptozotocin; (2) acquired and hereditary defects in enzymes involved in gluconeogenesis; (3) disorders such as severe acidosis, uremia, liver failure, tumors, and seizures; (4) anesthesia; and (5) abnormal intestinal bacteria producing D-lactate (described in Chapter 25).

Alcohol taken in excess tends to prevent gluconeogenesis from lactate in the liver, because oxidation of ethanol to acetaldehyde competes for the NAD^+ that is necessary for the conversion of lactate to pyruvate. Severe acidosis, such as diabetic ketoacidosis, may suppress lactate conversion and cause a shift in the lactate-pyruvate equilibrium with the accumulation of H^+. This shift may, in part, be responsible for the lactic acidosis seen in diabetics.

Hyperventilation in lactic acidosis is more intense than in other forms of metabolic acidosis. It is believed that this is because of the participation of the respiratory center in lactic acid production and the resulting greater local acidification of the respiratory center. During exercise, lactate levels may increase significantly, from an average normal concentration of ~0.9 mmol/L to ~12 mmol/L. However, under normal conditions, the lactate is rapidly metabolized so that the "acidosis" is only transient.

Lactate in spinal fluid normally parallels blood levels. In cases of biochemical alterations in the central nervous system, however, CSF lactate values change independently of blood values. Increased CSF levels may be seen in intracranial hemorrhage, bacterial meningitis, epilepsy, and other CNS disorders.[31]

Ethylene Glycol

Ingested ethylene glycol is metabolized to glycolic and oxalic acids and other acidic metabolites. Its metabolism leads to an acidosis with high anion and osmolal gaps. Accumulation of toxic metabolites may contribute to lactic acid production that further contributes to the acidosis. Precipitation of calcium oxalate and hippurate crystals in the urinary tract may lead to acute renal failure. Clinically, patients develop a variety of neurological symptoms that may lead to coma. Some patients may develop, either singly or in combination, (1) bronchial pneumonia, (2) pulmonary edema, (3) congestive heart failure, (4) hypertension, or (5) cardiopulmonary arrest. The minimal lethal dose of ethylene glycol is ~100 mL for an average 70 kg adult.

Salicylate Intoxication

This generally occurs with blood salicylate concentrations above 30 mg/dL. Salicylate, itself an unmeasured anion, alters peripheral metabolism, leading to the production of various organic acids without dominance of any specific acid. The processes eventually result in a metabolic acidosis with a high anion gap. Salicylate also stimulates the respiratory center to increase the rate and depth of respiration, resulting in a low PCO_2, low HCO_3^-, and respiratory alkalosis (see the section entitled Respiratory Alkalosis). In adults, mixed respiratory alkalosis and metabolic acidosis are more common, whereas in children, metabolic acidosis predominates.

Normal Anion Gap Acidosis (Inorganic Acidosis)

In contrast to high anion gap acidoses, in which bicarbonate is consumed in buffering excess H^+, the cause of acidosis in the presence of a normal anion gap is the loss of bicarbonate-rich fluid from either the kidney or gastrointestinal tract. As bicarbonate is lost, more Cl^- ions are reabsorbed with Na^+ or K^+ to maintain electrical neutrality so that hyperchloremia ensues (see Figure 46-14). Normal anion gap acidosis can be divided into *hypokalemic* and *normokalemic* acidoses, which can be helpful in the differential diagnosis of this type of disorder (see Table 46-4).

Diarrhea

Diarrhea may cause acidosis as a result of loss of Na^+, K^+, and HCO_3^-. One of the primary exocrine functions of the pancreas is production of HCO_3^- to neutralize gastric contents on entry into the duodenum. If the water, K^+, and HCO_3^- in the intestine are not reabsorbed, a hypokalemic, normal anion gap metabolic acidosis will develop. The resulting hyperchloremia is due to the replacement of lost bicarbonate with Cl^- to maintain electrical balance.

Renal Tubular Acidoses, Types I and II

These syndromes are predominantly characterized by loss of bicarbonate because of decreased tubular secretion of H^+ (distal or type I RTA) or decreased reabsorption of HCO_3^- (proximal or type II RTA).[15] Because the major urine-acidifying power of the kidneys rests in the distal tubules, the proximal and distal RTAs may be differentiated by measurement of urine pH. In proximal RTA, urine pH becomes <5.5, whereas in distal RTA the distal tubules are compromised and urine pH is >5.5.[15] When distal RTA is associated with obstructive nephropathy, sickle cell disease, or systemic lupus erythematosus, hyperkalemia may be seen. Otherwise, distal RTA is usually accompanied by hypokalemia.

Carbonic Anhydrase Inhibitors

Acetazolamide is the most common drug in this class of therapeutic agents. It is infrequently used as a mild diuretic. More often, it is used for urine alkalinization and in patients suffering from open-angle glaucoma or acute mountain (altitude) sickness.[12] Inhibition of carbonic anhydrase causes wasting of Na^+, K^+, and HCO_3^- in the proximal tubules and represents a pharmacologically induced proximal RTA.

Hyperkalemic Normal Anion Gap Acidosis (Renal Tubular Acidosis Type IV)

Failure of the kidneys to synthesize renin, failure of the adrenal cortex to secrete aldosterone, and renal tubular resistance to aldosterone are the most common causes of this type of acidosis (often called type IV RTA). This inhibits Na^+ reabsorption, and both K^+ and H^+ are thus abnormally retained. The result is decreased renal ammonia formation and therefore decreased elimination of H^+. If associated with increased ECF volume, HCO_3^- reclamation in the tubules may be depressed. There is usually an associated mild renal insufficiency (elevated serum creatinine), but urine may still be acidified to a pH < 5.5. Hyperkalemia is also usually present.

Compensatory Mechanisms in Metabolic Acidosis

The buffer systems of the blood (mainly the bicarbonate/carbonic acid buffer) minimize changes in pH. In acidoses, the bicarbonate concentration decreases to give a ratio of $cHCO_3^-/cdCO_2$ of <20:1. The respiratory compensatory mechanism responds to correct the ratio with increased rate and depth of respiration to eliminate CO_2. Table 46-3 depicts expected compensation in both acidoses and alkaloses and corresponding laboratory values.

Respiratory Compensatory Mechanism

The decrease in pH in metabolic acidosis stimulates the respiratory compensatory mechanism and produces hyperventilation (Kussmaul respiration), which results in the elimination of carbonic acid as CO_2, a decrease in PCO_2 (hypocapnia), and consequently a decrease in $cdCO_2$. There is also a decrease in $cHCO_3^-$ that is smaller than that of $cdCO_2$. For example, the ratio of $cHCO_3^-/cdCO_2$ might be 16:1.28 (12:5:1) for a pH of 7.2 before compensation and 14.5:0.9 (16:1:1) for a pH of 7.30 after compensation (see Figure 46-8). As the $cdCO_2$ diminishes, the ratio of $cHCO_3^-/cdCO_2$ approaches its normal value of 20:1.

Renal Compensatory Mechanism

If possible, the kidneys respond to restore the normal pH by increased excretion of acid and preservation of base (increased rate of Na^+-H^+ exchange, increased ammonia formation, and increased reabsorption of bicarbonate). When the renal compensating mechanisms are functioning, urinary acidity and urinary ammonia are increased. The total amount of H^+ excreted may be as much as

500 mmol/day. As a result, $cHCO_3^-/cdCO_2$ will increase, for example, to 22:1.1 (20:1) for a pH of 7.40. *This is a fully compensated metabolic acidosis,* because the pH has returned to normal; however, acidosis still exists because a process that consumes HCO_3^- persists. Physiologically a normal pH suggests that the acidosis is overcompensated.

Laboratory Findings in Metabolic Acidosis

Bicarbonate concentrations have been used to empirically estimate pH and PCO_2. For pH, 15 is added to the determined bicarbonate concentration for an estimate of the decimal digits of pH. For example, a patient who has been acidotic for at least 12 to 24 hours and has a bicarbonate of 10 mmol/L (10 + 15 = 25) will have an estimated pH of 7.25. For estimating PCO_2 (mm Hg), the following formula is sometimes used:[1]

$$PCO_2 \pm 2 = 1.5(cHCO_3^-) + 8$$

For this example, the PCO_2 estimate would be 1.5(10) + 8, or 23 ± 2 (see Table 46-3). Use of this equation can have important clinical implications, because it indicates whether a given PCO_2 value is appropriate for a given degree of metabolic acidosis or if one is dealing with a mixed acid-base disorder. Another common estimator of proper compensation is that the PCO_2 will equal the last two digits of the pH. If a respiratory acidosis is superimposed on a preexisting metabolic acidosis, the PCO_2 would be higher than expected by either of these estimates.

Electrolytes are also altered depending on the cause of metabolic acidosis. In diabetic ketoacidosis, the increase in the fraction of organic acids caused by increased ketone body production is reflected by a decrease in plasma bicarbonate and sometimes in chloride. Plasma Na^+ and K^+ are also decreased because of the associated polyuria and coexcretion of these cations with acetoacetate and β-hydroxybutyrate. Furthermore, because of the high glucose, there is a dilutional effect as a result of the osmotically induced increase in vascular volume. When glucose concentration decreases following insulin treatment, water leaves the vascular compartment, and Na^+ concentration increases. Serum potassium levels, however, may be normal or even high, despite severe total body depletion of K^+; the serum level represents a balance struck between the amount of K^+ lost in the urine, the amount of K^+ shifted from cells into ECF, and the degree of dehydration.

In renal failure, organic acids, phosphate, and sulfate are increased because of retention. Chronic metabolic acidosis enhances mobilization of calcium from bone; the decrease in plasma pH increases dissociation of plasma protein-bound calcium so that more Ca^{2+} is filtered through the glomerulus and less is reabsorbed in the tubule (see also Chapter 45).

Metabolic Alkalosis (Primary Bicarbonate Excess)

Alkalosis occurs either when excess base is added to the system, base elimination is decreased, or acid-rich fluids are lost (Box 46-1). Any of these can lead to a primary bicarbonate excess, such that the ratio of $cHCO_3^-/cdCO_2$ becomes >20:1. For instance, a primary increase in bicarbonate to 48 mmol/L will alter the $cHCO_3^-/cdCO_2$ to 48:1.5 (32:1) for a pH of 7.6 (see Figure 46-8). The patient will hypoventilate to raise PCO_2 and therefore lower the pH toward normal. However, hypoxia usually prevents the patient from achieving a PCO_2 >55 mm Hg.

If the increase in pH is great enough, increased neuromuscular activity may be seen, and above pH 7.55, tetany may develop even in the presence of a normal serum total calcium concentration. The cause of the tetany is a decreased concentration of ionized calcium due to increased binding of calcium ions by protein (mainly albumin) and other anions. Measurement of Cl^- status can be helpful, as causes of metabolic alkalosis fall into Cl^- responsive, Cl^- resistant, and exogenous base categories (Box 46-1; see also Figure 46-4).

BOX 46-1 Conditions Leading to Metabolic Alkalosis

Chloride-Responsive (Urine Cl^- < 10 mmol/L)

- Contraction alkaloses
  - Prolonged vomiting or nasogastric suction
  - Pyloric or upper duodenal obstruction
  - Prolonged or abusive diuretic therapy (loop diuretics)
  - Villous adenoma
- Posthypercapnic state
- Cystic fibrosis (systemic ineffective reabsorption of Cl^-)

Chloride-Resistant (Urine Cl^- > 20 mmol/L)

- Mineralocorticoid excess
  - Primary hyperaldosteronism (adrenal adenoma or rarely, carcinoma)
  - Bilateral adrenal hyperplasia
  - Secondary hyperaldosteronism
  - Hyperreninemic hyperaldosteronism (hypertension)
  - Congenital adrenal hyperplasia (due to adrenal enzyme deficiencies in cortisol production [11β- or 17α-hydroxylase])
- Glucocorticoid excess
  - Primary adrenal adenoma (Cushing's syndrome)
  - Pituitary adenoma secreting ACTH (Cushing's disease)
  - Exogenous cortisol therapy
  - Excessive licorice ingestion
- Bartter's syndrome (defective renal Cl^- reabsorption)

Exogenous Base

- Iatrogenic
  - Bicarbonate-containing intravenous fluid therapy
  - Massive blood transfusion (sodium citrate overload)
  - Antacids and cation-exchange resins in dialysis patients
  - High-dose carbenicillin or penicillin (associated with hypokalemia)
- Milk-alkali syndrome

Cl^- Responsive Metabolic Alkalosis

Most causes of Cl^- responsive metabolic alkalosis occur as a result of *hypovolemia* (see Box 46-1). When the ECF is severely depleted, the resulting acid-base disorder is often referred to as "contraction alkalosis." Renal bicarbonate retention will occur in response to hypovolemia under the action of increased aldosterone. This also will result in increased reabsorption of Na^+ together with HCO_3^- and excretion of K^+ and H^+. The resulting hypokalemia contributes to the alkalosis, as described previously. Urine Cl^- will be <10 mmol/L as both the available Cl^- and HCO_3^- are reabsorbed with Na^+. Urine Na^+ is not useful for classifying metabolic alkalosis because there will be an obligatory loss of Na^+ when filtered HCO_3^- exceeds reclamation. Common causes of contraction alkalosis include prolonged vomiting or nasogastric suction, pyloric or upper duodenal obstruction, villous adenoma (unregulated secretion of HCl), and the use of certain diuretics. Treatment consists of replacing TBW with water and NaCl tablets or saline infusion.

Gastrointestinal Loss of HCl

Following prolonged vomiting, pyloric or high intestinal obstruction, or gastric suction, excessive loss of hydrochloric acid from the stomach and *hypovolemia* may occur. In this hypochloremic, hypovolemic setting the kidneys preferentially reabsorb Na^+ to restore volume and excess bicarbonate is reabsorbed in the absence of sufficient Cl^- to maintain electrical neutrality. In addition, H^+ and K^+ are secreted in exchange for Na^+. Urine Cl^- will be <10 mmol/L in this setting (see Figure 46-4).

Diuretic Therapy

Prolonged administration of certain diuretics has been known to cause an alkalosis that is similar to that observed in a hypovolemic setting. Most common are those acting on the ascending limb of the loop of Henle (e.g., furosemide [Lasix], bumetanide [Bumex]) that block sodium, potassium, and chloride reabsorption. The resulting increase in Na^+ concentration reaching the distal convoluted tubule, particularly when combined with activation of the renin-angiotensin-aldosterone axis, leads to increased urinary excretion of K^+ and H^+.[12] The loss of K^+ with furosemide is much greater than with thiazides. Continued abuse or unmonitored use of loop diuretics can lead to volume contraction and a contraction alkalosis. This is commonly seen among patients abusing diuretics for the purpose of weight loss.

Cl^- Resistant Metabolic Alkalosis

This condition is far less common than chloride responsive metabolic alkalosis and is almost always associated with either an underlying disease (primary hyperaldosteronism, Cushing's syndrome, or Bartter's syndrome) or with excess addition of exogenous base. In these conditions, urine Cl^- will usually be >20 mmol/L.

In states of adrenocortical excess (endogenous or pharmacological, primary or secondary) K^+ and H^+ are "wasted" by the kidneys as a consequence of the increased Na^+ reabsorption stimulated by elevated aldosterone or cortisol. The attendant hypokalemia often further contributes to the alkalosis and should be treated with replacement therapy. The resulting decreased tubular K^+ concentration stimulates NH_3 production and thus renal H^+ excretion as NH_4^+. This is accompanied by enhanced HCO_3^- reabsorption (see Figures 46-3 and 46-12). Diseases in which endogenous mineralocorticoids, glucocorticoids, or both are elevated include primary and secondary hyperaldosteronism, bilateral adrenal hyperplasia, pituitary ACTH-producing adenoma (Cushing's disease), and primary adrenal adenomas producing glucocorticoids (Cushing's syndrome) or aldosterone.

Excessive licorice ingestion may cause a form of chloride resistant alkalosis. Black licorice contains glycyrrhizic acid, which inhibits the enzyme 11-β hydroxysteroid dehydrogenase, which in turn catalyzes the conversion of cortisol to cortisone. The excess cortisol exerts a mineralocorticoid effect on the distal tubule aldosterone receptors.[8]

Finally a rare etiology of Cl^- resistant metabolic alkalosis is a genetic (autosomal recessive) defect in Cl^- reabsorption within the thick ascending limb of the loop of Henle, a condition known as Bartter's syndrome.[4]

Exogenous Base

Examples in this category include citrate toxicity following massive blood transfusion, aggressive intravenous therapy with bicarbonate solutions, and ingestion of large quantities of milk and antacids in the treatment of gastritis and peptic ulcers ("milk-alkali syndrome"). The latter is far less commonly seen since the introduction and now widespread use of H_2-receptor antagonists and proton-pump inhibitors. Finally the use of antacids and cationic exchange resins in patients with renal failure (especially those on dialysis) may result in a metabolic alkalosis.

Compensatory Mechanisms in Metabolic Alkalosis

The compensatory mechanisms for metabolic alkalosis include both respiratory compensation and, if physiologically possible, renal compensation.

Respiratory Compensatory Mechanism

The increase in pH depresses the respiratory center, causing a retention of carbon dioxide (hypercapnia), which in turn causes an increase in cH_2CO_3 and $cdCO_2$. Thus the ratio of $cHCO_3^-/cdCO_2$, which was originally increased, approaches its normal value, although the actual concentrations of both $cHCO_3^-$ and $cdCO_2$ remain increased. The respiratory response to metabolic alkalosis is erratic, and increases in PCO_2 are variable.

Renal Compensatory Mechanism

The kidneys respond to the state of alkalosis by decreased Na^+-H^+ exchange, decreased formation of ammonia, and decreased reclamation of bicarbonate. This response is blunted, however, in conditions of hypokalemia and hypovolemia.

Laboratory Findings in Metabolic Alkalosis

Blood plasma values for $cHCO_3^-$, $cdCO_2$, and PCO_2, and therefore the plasma total CO_2 concentration, are increased, and the ratio of $cHCO_3^-/cdCO_2$ is high. In uncomplicated metabolic alkalosis, the PCO_2 increases by ~6 mm Hg for each 10 mmol/L rise in $cHCO_3^-$. A higher than expected PCO_2 may indicate superimposed respiratory acidosis. The extent of increase of pH in uncompensated metabolic alkalosis can be estimated by adding 15 to the $cHCO_3^-$ to give the last two digits of the pH. If the $cHCO_3^-$ is 35 mmol/L, the estimated pH would be 7.50 (35 + 15 = 50). In cases of prolonged vomiting, Cl^- (and sometimes K^+) concentrations are low because of the loss of these ions through the vomitus. Protein values may be falsely increased owing to dehydration, and if food intake is inadequate, formation of ketone bodies may increase the organic acid fraction. In cases of excessive administration of $NaHCO_3$, Na^+ levels are increased.

In patients with adequate renal function, urinary pH values are usually increased because of the decreased excretion of acid and increased excretion of bicarbonate. Urinary ammonia values are decreased because of decreased formation of ammonia in the tubules. In K^+ depletion, H^+ is preferentially exchanged for Na^+ and the pH of the urine may be low. This is called *paradoxical aciduria.*

Respiratory Acidosis

Any condition that decreases elimination of carbon dioxide through the lungs results in an increase in PCO_2 (hypercapnia) and a primary excess of dCO_2 (respiratory acidosis). Thus respiratory acidosis only occurs by decreased elimination of CO_2. Causes of decreased CO_2 elimination (Box 46-2) are classified as acute or chronic. Alternatively, these conditions may be separated into those caused by factors that directly depress the respiratory center (such as centrally acting drugs, CNS trauma, and infections) and those that affect the respiratory apparatus or cause mechanical obstruction of the airways. Chronic obstructive pulmonary disease is the most common cause. Rebreathing, or breathing air high in CO_2 content, may also cause a high PCO_2. Increase in PCO_2 results in an increase of $cdCO_2$ (and thus H_2CO_3, which dissociates to H^+ and HCO_3^-), which in turn causes a decrease in the $cHCO_3^-/cdCO_2$ ratio (e.g., the ratio may be 28 : 1.7 (16 : 1) for a pH of ~7.30; see Figure 46-8). A doubling of PCO_2 will cause a fall in pH of about 0.23 when other factors remain constant.

BOX 46-2 Conditions Leading to Respiratory Acidosis

Factors That Directly Depress the Respiratory Center

Drugs such as narcotics and barbiturates
Central nervous system (CNS) trauma, tumors, and degenerative disorders
Infections of the CNS such as encephalitis and meningitis
Comatose states such as cerebrovascular accident due to intracranial hemorrhage
Primary central hypoventilation

Conditions That Affect the Respiratory Apparatus

Chronic obstructive pulmonary disease (most common cause)
Pulmonary fibrosis
Status asthmaticus (severe)
Diseases of the upper airways such as laryngospasm or tumor
Pulmonary infections (severe)
Impaired lung motion due to pleural effusion or pneumothorax
Adult respiratory distress syndrome
Chest wall diseases and chest wall deformities
Neurological disorders affecting the muscles of respiration

Others

Abdominal distention, as in peritonitis and ascites
Extreme obesity (pickwickian syndrome)
Sleep disorders such as sleep apnea

Compensatory Mechanisms in Respiratory Acidosis

Compensation for respiratory acidosis occurs immediately via buffers and with time via the kidneys and, if possible, the lungs.

Buffer System

Excess carbonic acid present in blood is to a great extent buffered by the hemoglobin and protein buffer systems[9] (see Figure 46-9). The buffering of CO_2 causes a slight rise in $cHCO_3^-$. Thus in the immediate posthypercapnic state, this compensation may appear as a metabolic alkalosis (see Box 46-1).

Renal Mechanism

The kidneys respond to respiratory acidosis similar to the way that they do to metabolic acidosis; namely, with (1) increased Na^+-H^+ exchange, (2) increased ammonia formation, and (3) increased reclamation of bicarbonate. In a partially compensated chronic respiratory acidosis at steady state, the plasma pH is returned about halfway toward normal as compared with the acute (uncompensated) situation. Renal compensation is not effective before 6 to 12 hours and is not optimal until 2 to 3 days. In chronic respiratory acidosis, such as occurs in patients with chronic obstructive pulmonary disease (COPD), full renal compensation may be seen even in those patients with very high PCO_2 (>50 mm Hg). However, these severe COPD patients often present with a superimposed metabolic alkalosis arising from a variety of causes, such as prolonged administration of diuretics.

Respiratory Mechanism

The increase in PCO_2 stimulates the respiratory center and results in increased pulmonary rate and depth of respiration provided that the primary defect is not in the respiratory center. The elimination of carbon dioxide through the lungs results in a decrease in $cdCO_2$, and thus the ratio of $cHCO_3^-/cdCO_2$ and pH approaches normal.

BOX 46-3 Factors Causing Respiratory Alkalosis

Nonpulmonary Stimulation of Respiratory Center
Anxiety, hysteria
Febrile states
Gram-negative septicemia
Metabolic encephalopathy (e.g., due to liver disease)
Central nervous system infections such as meningitis, encephalitis
Cerebrovascular accidents
Intracranial surgery
Hypoxia (e.g., severe anemia, high altitudes [acute condition])
Drugs and agents such as salicylates, catecholamines, and progesterone
Pregnancy, mainly third trimester (↑ progesterone?)
Hyperthyroidism

Pulmonary Disorders*
Pneumonia
Asthma
Pulmonary emboli
Interstitial lung disease
Large right to left shunt ($PCO_2 < 50$ mm Hg)
Congestive heart failure
Respiratory compensation after correction of metabolic acidosis

Others
Ventilator-induced hyperventilation

*The severe stages of some of these disorders may be associated with respiratory acidosis if elimination of CO_2 is severely impaired.

Laboratory Findings in Respiratory Acidosis

Plasma $cdCO_2$, PCO_2, $cHCO_3^-$, and therefore $ctCO_2$ are elevated in respiratory acidoses. Because of an increase in $cdCO_2$, the ratio of $cHCO_3^-/cdCO_2$ is decreased, resulting in a decreased pH. In the acute phase, $cHCO_3^-$ will increase about 1 mmol/L for each 10 mm Hg rise in PCO_2. If respiratory acidosis persists, the change will be 3.5 mmol/L, mainly as a result of renal compensation. For every 15 mm Hg increase in PCO_2, the pH changes in the *acute* phase by ~0.10 pH unit and in *chronic* conditions by slightly less than 0.05 pH unit. For example, if the PCO_2 increases acutely by 30 mm Hg, the pH drops to ~7.20. The same PCO_2 increase in a chronic condition results in a pH of ~7.31. The plasma chloride decreases as plasma bicarbonate increases. Hyperkalemia may occur but is not as predictable as in some forms of metabolic acidosis. For every 0.1 unit decrease in pH, there is generally an inverse change of 0.6 mmol/L in K^+. This increase in K^+ is mainly due to the movement of K^+ from cells into the plasma in exchange for the movement of H^+ into cells. Urinary acidity and ammonia content are increased as the kidney attempts to compensate.

RESPIRATORY ALKALOSIS

A decrease in PCO_2 (hypocapnia) and the resulting primary deficit in $cdCO_2$ (respiratory alkalosis) are caused by an increased rate or depth of respiration, or both. Therefore, the basic cause of respiratory alkalosis is excess elimination of acid via the respiratory route. Excessive elimination of carbon dioxide reduces the PCO_2 and causes an increase in the $cHCO_3^-/cdCO_2$ ratio (due to decrease in $cdCO_2$). The latter shifts the normal equilibrium of the bicarbonate/carbonic acid buffer system, reducing the hydrogen ion concentration and increasing the pH. This shift also results in a decrease in $cHCO_3^-$, which somewhat ameliorates the change in pH. Analogous to causes of respiratory acidosis, causes of respiratory alkalosis can be classified as those with a direct stimulatory effect on the respiratory center and those due to effects on the pulmonary system. These and some additional conditions underlying respiratory alkaloses are listed in Box 46-3.

Compensatory Mechanisms in Respiratory Alkalosis

The compensatory mechanisms respond to respiratory alkalosis in two stages. In the first stage, erythrocyte and tissue buffers provide H^+ ions that consume a small amount of HCO_3^-. The second stage becomes operational in prolonged respiratory alkalosis and depends on the renal compensation as described for metabolic alkalosis (decreased reclamation of bicarbonate).

Laboratory Findings in Respiratory Alkalosis

In this condition, the $cdCO_2$, PCO_2, $cHCO_3^-$, and thus the total CO_2 concentration all decrease. The ratio of $cHCO_3^-/cdCO_2$ is increased and causes an increase in pH.

During the acute phase, $cHCO_3^-$ falls by 2 mmol/L for each 10 mm Hg decrease in PCO_2 (i.e., if the PCO_2 falls by 20 mm Hg, $cHCO_3^-$ decreases by 4 mmol/L). For the same 20 mm Hg decrease in PCO_2, the $[H^+]$ will decrease by 16 nmol/L.

$$\Delta cH^+ = 0.8(\Delta PCO_2)$$

$$\Delta cH^+ = 0.8 \times 20 = 16$$

If the original cH^+ was 40 nmol/L, it would now be 24 nmol/L (40 − 16 = 24), which corresponds to a pH of 7.61 (see Figure 46-6). In chronic respiratory alkalosis, the $cHCO_3^-$ falls only ~5 mmol/L for every 10 mm Hg decrease in PCO_2 and the pH will return to near normal. Finally, individuals living at high altitudes chronically hyperventilate owing to hypoxia and have PCO_2 values lower than those seen at sea level.

REFERENCES

1. Albert MD, Dell RB, Winters RW. Quantitative displacement of acid-base equilibrium in metabolic acidosis. Ann Intern Med 1967;66:312-22.
2. Birnbaumer M. The V2 vasopressin receptor mutations and fluid homeostasis (Review). Cardiovasc Res 2001;51:409-15.

3. Bockelman HW, Cembrowski GS, Kurtycz DFI, Garber CC, Westgard JO, Weisberg HF. Quality control of electrolyte analyzers: Evaluation of the anion gap average. Amer J Clin Pathol 1984;81:219-23.
4. Chesney R. Specific renal tubular disorders. In: Goldman L, Bennett J, eds. Cecil textbook of medicine, 21st ed. Philadelphia: WB Saunders, 2000:605-10.
5. Dorwart WV, Chalmers L. Comparison of methods for calculating serum osmolality from chemical concentrations, and the prognostic value of such calculations. Clin Chem 1975;21:190-4.
6. Dufour DR. Acid-base disorders. In: Dufour R, Christenson RH, eds. Professional practice in clinical chemistry: A review. Washington DC: AACC Press, 1995:604-35.
7. Emmett M, Narins RG. Clinical use of the anion gap. Medicine 1977;56:38-54.
8. Farese RV Jr, Biglieri EG, Shackleton CH, Irony I, Gomez-Fontes R. Licorice-induced hypermineralocorticoidism. N Engl J Med 1991;325:1223-7.
9. Figge J, Rossing TH, Fencl V. The role of serum proteins in acid-base equilibria. J Lab Clin Med 1991;117:453-67.
10. Gabow PA, Kaehny WD, Fennessey PV, Goodman SI, Gross PA, Schrier RW. Diagnostic importance of an increased serum anion gap. N Engl J Med 1980;303:854-8.
11. Haycock GB. The syndrome of inappropriate secretion of antidiuretic hormone (Review). Pediatr Nephrol 1995;9:375-81.
12. Jackson E. Diuretics. In: Hardman JG, Linbird LE, eds. Goodman and Gilman's the pharmacological basis of therapeutics, 10th ed. New York: McGraw-Hill, 2001:763-7.
13. Kaplan J. Biochemistry of Na, K-ATPase (Review). Ann Rev Biochem 2002;71:511-35.
14. Keating G, Goa K. Nesiritide—a review of its use in acute decompensated heart failure (Review). Drugs 2003;63:47-70.
15. Lash JP, Arruda JAL. Laboratory evaluation of renal tubular acidosis. Clin Lab Med 1993;13:117-29.
16. MandPetri WA. Antimicrobial agents. In: Hardman JG, Linbird LE, eds. Goodman and Gilman's the pharmacological basis of therapeutics, 10th ed. New York: McGraw-Hill, 2001:1276-7.
17. Preuss HG. Fundamentals of acid-base evaluation. Clin Lab Med 1993;13:103-15.
18. Putney L, Denker S, Barber D. The changing face of the Na^+/H^+ exchanger, NHE1: structure, regulation, and cellular actions (Review). Ann Rev Pharmacol Toxicol 2002;42:527-52.
19. Ravel R, ed. Clinical laboratory medicine: Clinical application of laboratory data. 6th ed. St. Louis: Mosby-Year Book, 1995.
20. Robertson GL. Diabetes insipidus (Review). Endocrinol Metabol Clin North Amer 1995;24:549-72.
21. Salem MM, Mujais SK. Gaps in the anion gap. Arch Intern Med 1992;152:1625-9.
22. Siggaard-Andersen O. An acid-base chart for arterial blood with normal and pathophysiological reference areas. Scand J Clin Lab Invest 1971;27:239-45.
23. Siggarard-Andersen O. The Van Slyke Equation. Scand J Clin Lab Invest 1977;37(Suppl. 146):15-20.
24. Shapiro B, Chen H, Burnett J, Redfield M. Use of plasma brain natriuretic peptide concentration to aid in the diagnosis of heart failure (Review). Mayo Clin Proc 2003;78:481-6.
25. Singer G. Fluid and Electrode Management. In: Ahya SL, Flood K, Paranjothi S, Schaiff R, eds. The Washington manual of medical therapeutics, 30th ed. Philadelphia: Lippincott, Williams and Wilkins, 2001:3-75.
26. Skott O. Renin (Review). Amer J Physiol Regulatory Integrative Comp Physiol 2002;282:R937-9.
27. Thrasher TN. Baroreceptor regulation of vasopressin in renin secretion: Low pressure vs. high pressure receptors (Review). Front Neuroendocrinol 1994;15:157-96.
28. Tietz NW, ed. Clinical guide to laboratory tests, 3rd ed. Philadelphia: WB Saunders Co, 1995.
29. Tietz NW, ed. Textbook of clinical chemistry, 1st ed. Philadelphia: WB Saunders, 1986.
30. Tietz textbook of clinical chemistry. 2nd ed. Philadelphia: WB Saunders, 1994.
31. Watson MA, Scott MG. Clinical utility of biochemical analysis of cerebrospinal fluid. Clin Chem 1995;41:343-60.
32. Williamson JC. Acid-base disorders: classification and management strategies. Am Fam Physicians 1995;52:584-90.
33. Winter SD, Pearson JR, Gabow PA, Schultz AL, Lepoff RB. The fall of the serum anion gap. Arch Intern Med 1990;150:311-3.

ADDITIONAL READING

Androgué HJ, Madias NE. Hypernatremia (Review). N Engl J Med 2002;342:1493-9.

Androgué HJ, Madias NE. Hyponatremia (Review). N Engl J Med 2000;342:1581-9.

Androgué HJ, Madias NE. Management of life-threatening acid-base disorders, first of two parts (Review). N Engl J Med 1998;338:26-34. Erratum in: N Engl J Med 1998;340:247.

Androgué HJ, Madias NE. Management of life-threatening acid-base disorders, second of two parts (Review). N Engl J Med 1998;338:107-11.

Siggaard-Andersen O. The acid-base status of the blood, 4th ed. Copenhagen: Munksgaard, 1974; Baltimore: Williams & Wilkins, 1974.

CHAPTER 47

Liver Disease*

D. Robert Dufour, M.D.

The liver has a central and critical biochemical role in the metabolism, digestion, detoxification, and elimination of substances from the body. All blood from the intestinal tract initially passes through the liver, where products derived from digestion of food are processed, transformed, and stored. These include amino acids, carbohydrates, fatty acids, cholesterol, lipids, vitamins, and minerals. Most major plasma proteins (with the exception of immunoglobulins and von Willebrand factor) are either mainly or exclusively synthesized in the liver. The liver responds to multiple hormonal and neural stimuli to regulate the blood glucose concentration. Not only does it extract glucose from blood for use in generating energy, it also stores dietary glucose as glycogen for later use. The liver is also the major site for gluconeogenesis, critical for maintaining blood glucose in the fasting state. The liver is critical in lipid metabolism; not only does it extract and process dietary lipids, it is the principal site of cholesterol, triglyceride, and lipoprotein synthesis. Another major liver function is the synthesis of bile acids from cholesterol and secretion of these compounds into the bile, facilitating the absorption of dietary fat and fat soluble vitamins. The liver is also the main site of metabolism of both endogenous substances and exogenous compounds, such as drugs and toxins. This process, known as biotransformation, converts lipophilic substances to hydrophilic ones for subsequent elimination. The liver is a major site of catabolism of thyroid, steroid, and other hormones, and thus participates in regulation of plasma hormone concentrations. The liver is also involved in hormone synthesis, producing such hormones as insulin-like growth factor 1, angiotensinogen, and erythropoietin. Many of these hepatic functions may be assessed by laboratory procedures to gain insight into the integrity of the liver.

As a large organ, the liver shares with many other organs the ability to perform its functions with extensive reserve capacity. In many cases, individuals with liver disease maintain normal function despite extensive liver damage. In such cases, liver disease may only be recognized by using tests that detect injury. Most commonly, this is accomplished by measurement of plasma activities of enzymes found within liver cells released in somewhat specific patterns with different forms of injury. Chronic liver injury often involves fibrosis in the liver; detection of markers of the fibrotic process might be indicators of degree of injury. Chronic damage is often due to chronic inflammation; cytokines alter the pattern of liver protein production, allowing detection of inflammation (although not necessarily that involving the liver). Some proteins are produced in increased amounts with liver regeneration and neoplasm; such markers may be useful in detecting liver cell proliferation.

The chapter begins with a discussion of the anatomy and biochemical functions of the liver. The various disease states that involve the liver are then discussed. The chapter concludes with a discussion of use of laboratory test results in recognizing and characterizing patterns of liver injury.

ANATOMY OF THE LIVER

The liver weighs approximately 1.2 to 1.5 kg in the adult. It is located beneath the diaphragm in the right upper quadrant of the abdomen and is protected by the ribs and held in place by ligamentous attachments.

Gross Anatomy

The liver is divided into left and right anatomical lobes by the falciform ligament, an anterior extension of the peritoneal folds that connects the liver to the diaphragm and anterior abdominal wall (Figure 47-1). Two smaller lobes are found on the posterior surface (caudate lobe) and the infe-

*The author gratefully acknowledges the original contributions by Drs. Keith G. Tolman and Robert Rej upon which portions of this chapter are based.

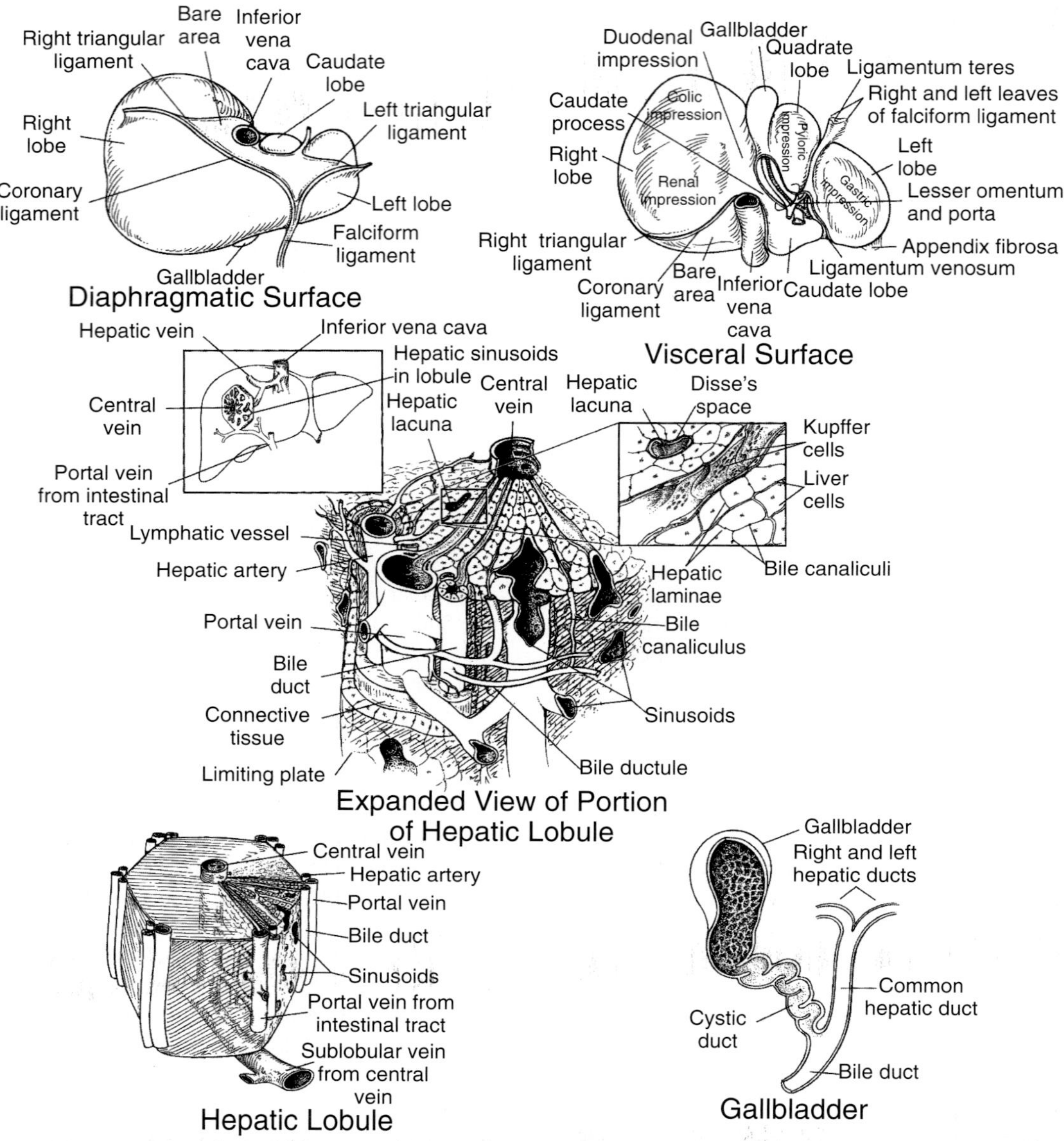

Figure 47-1 Structure of the liver. *(From Dorland's illustrated medical dictionary, 30th ed. Philadelphia: WB Saunders, 2003, plate 26.)*

rior surface (quadrate lobe) of the right lobe. Riedel's lobe is an anatomical extension of the right lobe of the liver and consists of a projection that may feel like a mobile tumor in the right abdomen.

The liver has a dual blood supply. The portal vein, which carries blood from the spleen and nutrient-enriched blood from the gastrointestinal (GI) tract, supplies approximately 70% of the blood supply, while the hepatic artery, a branch of the celiac axis, provides oxygen-enriched arterial blood. Each supplies approximately half of the oxygen reaching the liver, making it highly resistant to infarction. Ultimately, these two blood supplies merge and flow into the sinusoids that course between individual hepatocytes. The venous drainage from the liver ultimately converges into the right and left hepatic veins, which exit on the posterior surface of the liver and join the inferior vena cava near its entry into the right atrium.

The liver is covered with an anterior reflection of the peritoneum known as Glisson's capsule. Other extensions of the peritoneum form ligaments that hold the liver in place. Internal extensions of the capsule provide an internal supporting framework that divides the liver into lobules and ultimately surrounds blood vessels and nerves. One of the ligaments, the ligamentum teres, is the vestigial remnant of the umbilical vein and connects the umbilicus to the inferior border of the liver. When portal hypertension occurs, the umbilical veins may reopen, leading to venous dilation around the umbilicus (termed caput medusae).

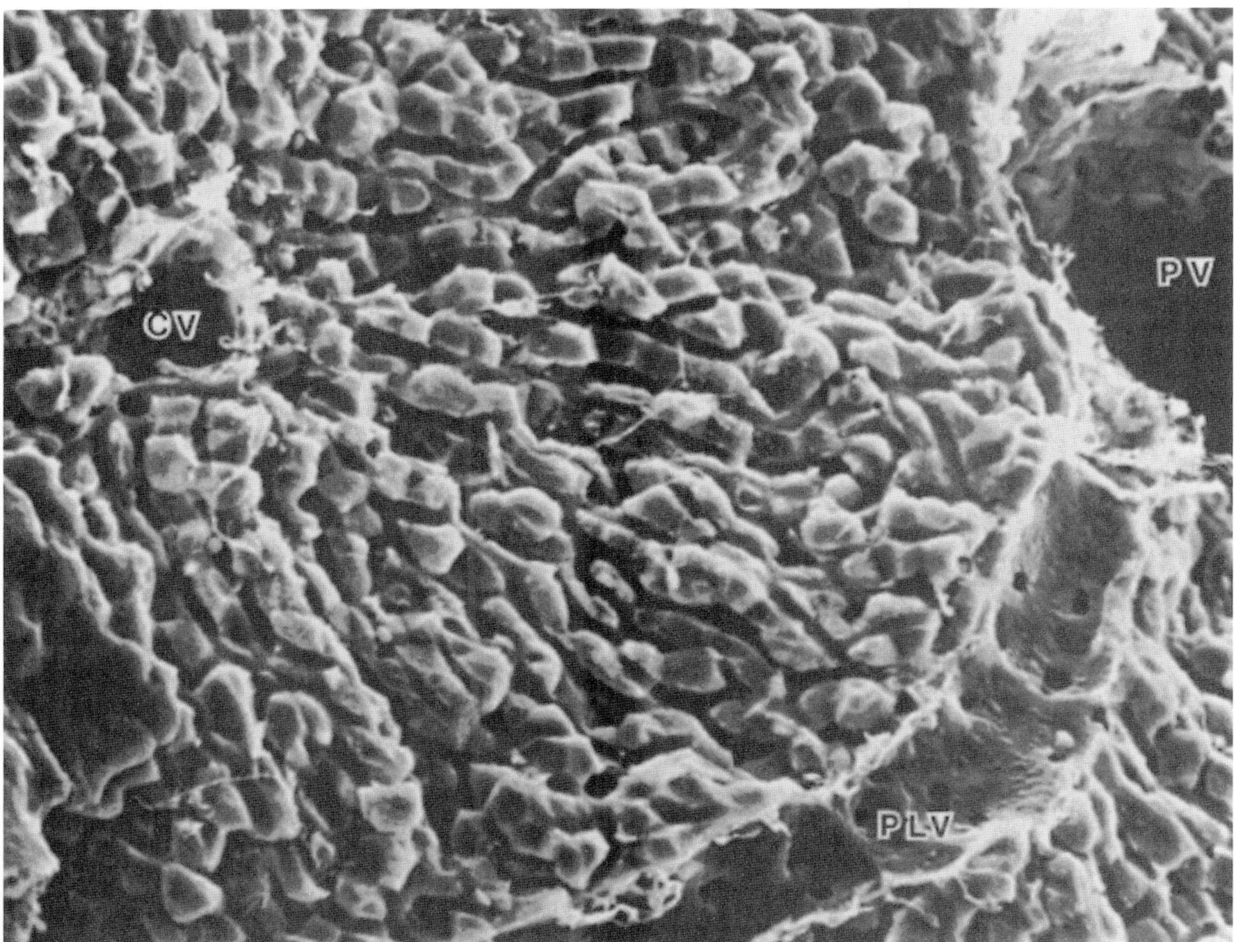

Figure 47-2 A low-magnification scanning electron micrograph depicting a portion of a liver lobule from a rat liver. *CV,* Central vein; *PV,* portal vein; *PLV,* perilobular venules. *(From Zakim O, Boyer TD. Hepatology: A textbook of liver disease, 3rd ed. Philadelphia: WB Saunders, 1996:9.)*

The nerve supply to the liver comes from the vagus and phrenic nerves and the sympathetic ganglia originating from cell bodies in the spinal cord that are located between the seventh and the tenth thoracic vertebrae. These merge to accompany the hepatic artery and bile ducts throughout the liver.

Biliary drainage originates at the bile canaliculi, grooves between adjacent hepatocytes, which form ductules that merge to form the intrahepatic bile ducts. These ultimately join to form the right and left hepatic bile ducts, which exit from the liver at the porta hepatis and merge to form the common hepatic duct. The hepatic duct is joined by the cystic duct from the gallbladder to form the common bile duct (see Figure 47-1). The common bile duct then enters the duodenum (usually with the pancreatic duct) at the ampulla of Vater. The duodenal portion of the common bile duct is surrounded by longitudinal and circular muscle fibers that form the sphincter of Oddi. This musculature relaxes when the gallbladder contracts, allowing bile to enter the duodenum; in its normally contracted state, the sphincter prevents reflux of acidic duodenal contents into the bile duct. The gallbladder, located on the undersurface of the right lobe of the liver, is the site for storage and concentration of bile, a complex mixture of bile salts and waste products. In the adult, it averages about 10 cm in length and has a capacity of 30 to 50 mL of bile. Hormonal stimuli initiated by food ingestion cause contraction of the muscular wall of the gallbladder, releasing bile salts into the intestine to facilitate digestion of fat.

Microscopic Anatomy

The functional anatomical unit of the liver is the acinus, adjacent to the portal triad, which consists of a branch of the portal vein, hepatic artery, and bile duct. Each acinus is a diamond-shaped mass of liver parenchyma that is supplied by a terminal branch of the portal vein and of the hepatic artery and drained by a terminal branch of the bile duct. The blood vessels radiate toward the periphery, forming sinusoids, which perfuse the liver and ultimately drain into the central (terminal) hepatic vein (Figure 47-2). The sinusoids are lined by fenestrated endothelial cells (allowing free filtration of blood) and phagocytic Kupffer cells (see Figure 47-1). The Kupffer cells are derived from blood monocytes. They contain lysosomes with hydrolytic enzymes that break down phagocytized foreign particles, such as bacteria. They also have immunoglobulins and complement receptors and are the main site for clearance of antigen-antibody complexes from blood. Kupffer cells secrete interleukins, tumor necrosis factor, collagenase, prostaglandins, and other factors involved in the inflammatory response (see Chapter 22).

The major functioning cells in the liver are the hepatocytes, responsible for about 70% of liver mass and performing most of the metabolic and synthetic functions of the liver. Two other cell types are found in small numbers within the liver. The stellate cells (sometimes referred to as Ito cells) are located between the endothelial lining of sinusoids and the hepatocytes within a small cleft referred to as the space of Disse. In their normal, quiescent state, stellate cells serve as a site of storage for fat soluble vitamins, particularly vitamin A. When stimulated, stellate cells are transformed both morphologically and functionally. They synthesize collagen, and are the cells responsible for fibrosis and, eventually, cirrhosis. They synthesize nitric oxide, which helps to regulate intrahepatic blood flow.

The blood supply to each acinus consists of three zones (Figure 47-3). Zone 1 is the area immediately adjacent to the portal tract and is enriched with lysosomes and mitochondria. The periphery of the acinus, zone 3, is enriched with endoplasmic reticulum, is very active metabolically, and has relatively low oxygen tension. This area is most susceptible to injury, although zone 1 appears to be involved with protecting the liver from external injury and providing a base for hepatic regeneration (by means of the oval cells of periportal bile ductules, the apparent hepatic stem cells).

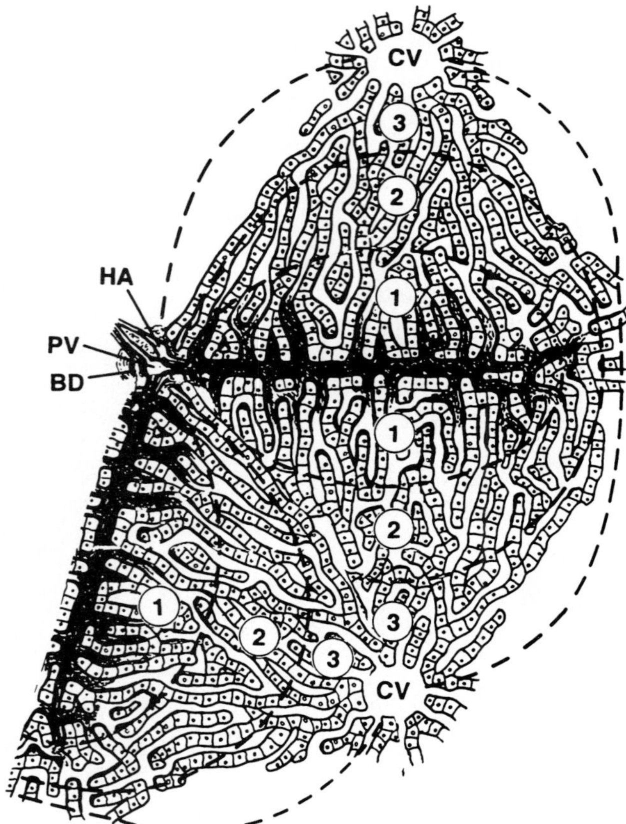

Figure 47-3 Blood supply of the simple liver acinus. *Zones 1, 2,* and *3* indicate corresponding volumes in a portion of an adjacent acinar unit. Oxygen tension and the nutrient level in the blood in sinusoids decrease from zone 1 through zone 3. *BD,* Bile duct; *HA,* hepatic artery; *PV,* portal vein; *CV,* central vein. *(From Zakim O, Boyer TD. Hepatology: A textbook of liver disease, 3rd ed. Philadelphia: WB Saunders, 1996:10.)*

ULTRASTRUCTURE OF THE HEPATOCYTE

Hepatocytes contain a well-developed organelle substructure (Figure 47-4). Mitochondria, which constitute approximately 18% of hepatocyte volume, are the site of oxidative phosphorylation and energy production. They contain enzymes involved in the citric acid cycle and β-oxidation of fatty acids. The rough endoplasmic reticulum is the site of synthesis of many proteins, including albumin, coagulation factors, enzymes (e.g., glucose-6-phosphatase), and triglycerides. The smooth endoplasmic reticulum contains microsomes that are involved with bilirubin conjugation, detoxification (cytochrome P_{450}–dependent isoenzymes), steroid synthesis, cholesterol synthesis, and bile acid synthesis. Many microsomal enzymes, including γ-glutamyl transferase, are induced by many drugs and inhibited by others. This is the site of most drug metabolism and many important drug interactions.

Peroxisomes are found near the smooth endoplasmic reticulum and contain oxidases that use molecular oxygen to modify a variety of substrates, leading to the production of hydrogen peroxide. They also contain catalase, which decomposes hydrogen peroxide. Peroxisomes also catalyze the β-oxidation of fatty acids with chain lengths from 7 to 18. Approximately 5% to 20% of the metabolism of ethanol also occurs in the peroxisomes. Lysosomes are dense organelles that contain hydrolytic enzymes that act as scavengers. Deposition of iron, lipofuscin, bile pigments, and copper occurs in the lysosomes. The Golgi apparatus lies near the canaliculus and is involved with the secretion of various substances, including bile acids and albumin.

BIOCHEMICAL FUNCTIONS OF THE LIVER

The liver is involved in a number of excretory, synthetic, and metabolic functions. Clinical laboratories perform a number of tests that are useful in the biochemical assessment of these functions.

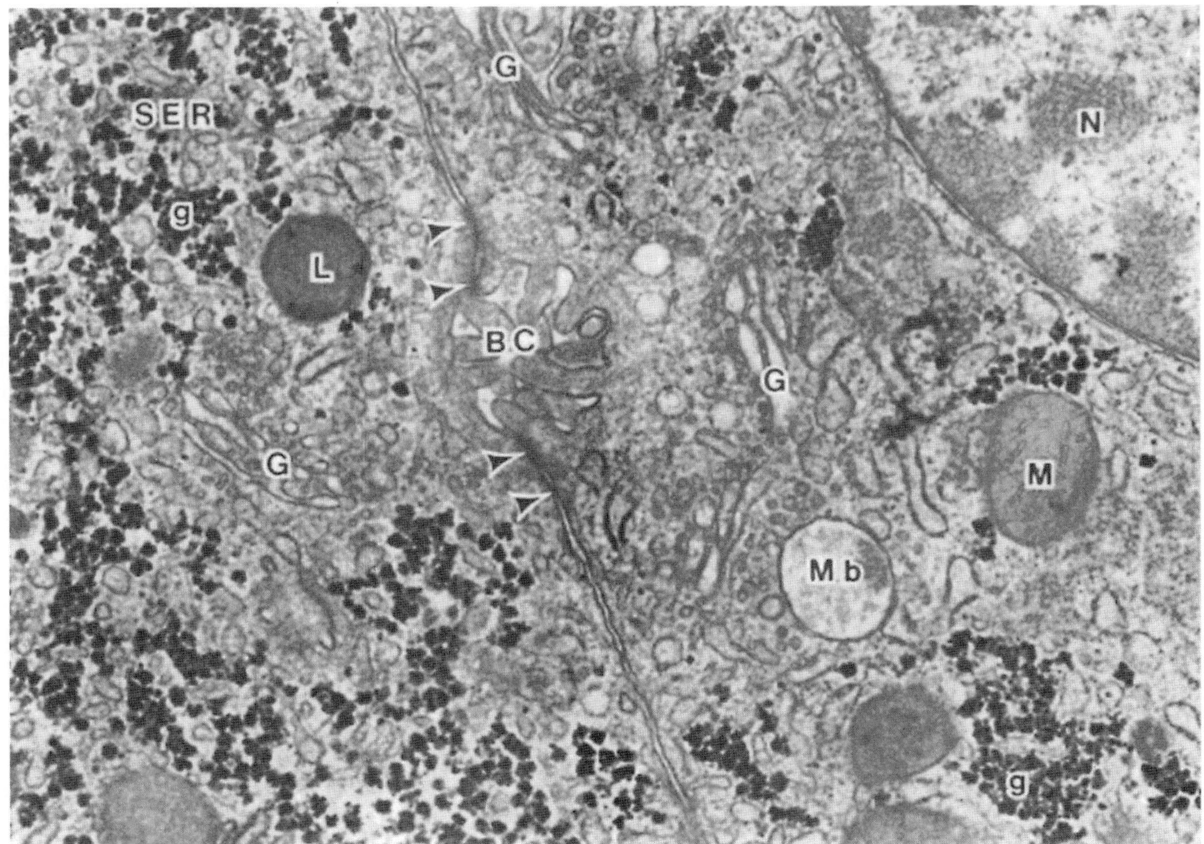

Figure 47-4 Portions of two human liver cells showing the relationship of the organelles and a typical bile canaliculus (BC). *Arrowheads* indicate light junctions. *N,* Nucleus; *M,* mitochondria; *Mb,* microbody; *G,* Golgi; *SER,* smooth endoplasmic reticulum; *L,* lysosome; *g,* glycogen. *(From Zakim O, Boyer TD. Hepatology: A textbook of liver disease, 3rd ed. Philadelphia: WB Saunders, 1996:20.)*

HEPATIC EXCRETORY FUNCTION

Organic anions of both endogenous and exogenous origin are extracted from the sinusoidal blood, biotransformed, and excreted into the bile or urine. Assessment of this excretory function provides valuable clinical information. The most frequently used tests involve the measurement of plasma concentrations of endogenously produced compounds, such as bilirubin and bile acids, and determination of the rate of clearance of exogenous compounds, such as aminopyrine, lidocaine, and caffeine.

Bilirubin

Bilirubin is the orange-yellow pigment derived from red blood cell turnover. It is extracted and biotransformed in the liver and excreted in bile and urine. The chemistry, biochemistry, and analytical methodology for bilirubin and related compounds are discussed in Chapter 31; a brief overview of factors relevant to understanding of liver disease is included here.

Bilirubin is transported from sites of production (mainly the spleen), loosely bound to albumin, in its native, unconjugated form. Bilirubin is transported across the hepatocyte membrane and is rapidly conjugated with glucuronic acid to produce bilirubin glucuronides, which are then excreted into bile by an energy-dependent process. This process is highly efficient, and bilirubin conjugates are detectable in normal plasma only using highly sensitive techniques. In the presence of bilirubin monoglucuronide, albumin (and other proteins) can be postsynthetically modified by covalent attachment to lysine residues. In the case of albumin, this produces a protein-bound form termed biliprotein or δ-bilirubin. Increases in conjugated bilirubin or δ-bilirubin are highly specific markers of hepatic dysfunction (except in the presence of rare inherited disorders impairing excretion of conjugated bilirubin, such as Dubin-Johnson syndrome). In the intestinal tract, bilirubin glucuronides are hydrolyzed and reduced by bacteria to form colorless *urobilinogens,* which undergo an enterohepatic circulation. A small fraction (2% to 5%) escapes the liver and is excreted in urine. In the colon, urobilinogens spontaneously oxidize to stool pigments stercobilin, mesobilin, and urobilin.

Deviations from normal physiology form the basis for use of laboratory tests of bilirubin metabolism to detect liver disease. Increased plasma bilirubin is typically classified as primarily indirect (an approximation of unconjugated bilirubin) or direct (an approximation of the sum of conjugated bilirubin and biliprotein). Increased indirect bilirubin indicates either overproduction of bilirubin, usually caused by hemolysis, or decreased extraction by the liver (primarily because of congenital defects involving uridine 5′-phosphate (UDP)-glucuronyl transferase). With severe liver injury, as occurs with fulminant hepatic failure and end stage cirrhosis, liver disease may cause primarily unconjugated hyperbilirubinemia. Increased urine urobilinogen occurs when there is increased bilirubin delivery to the intestinal tract (such as with hemolysis, or following recovery from hepatitis or obstruction), or decreased liver clearance, as occurs in portal hypertension.

Increased direct bilirubin generally results from functional or mechanical impairment in bilirubin excretion from the hepatocyte. Increased conjugated bilirubin is found in most cases of acute hepatitis and cholestasis (stoppage or suppression of the flow of bile); the percentage of direct bilirubin is similar in both types of liver disease.[55] Urine bilirubin is typically present in the presence of increased conjugated bilirubin. With resolution of liver disease, conjugated bilirubin is rapidly cleared, and biliprotein may become the only form present; urine bilirubin is typically absent in such circumstances. Increased conjugated bilirubin is also rarely seen with congenital defects in bilirubin excretion, such as Dubin-Johnson syndrome, and with impaired bilirubin excretion as occurs in sepsis or other acute illness.

Bile Acids

The regulation of bile acid metabolism is a major function of the liver. Alterations in bile acid metabolism are usually a reflection of liver dysfunction. Cholesterol homeostasis is in large part maintained by the conversion of cholesterol to bile acids and subsequent regulation of bile acid metabolism. Bile acids themselves provide surface-active detergent molecules that facilitate both hepatic excretion of cholesterol and solubilization of lipids for intestinal absorption. Bile acid homeostasis requires normal terminal ileum function to absorb bile acids for recirculation (enterohepatic circulation). Alterations in hepatic bile acid synthesis, intracellular metabolism, excretion, intestinal absorption, or plasma extraction are reflected in derangements in bile acid metabolism.

Chemistry

There are four major bile acids (see Figures 47-5 to 47-7). Cholic acid and chenodeoxycholic acid, the primary bile acids, are synthesized in the liver. Bacteria metabolize these primary bile acids to the secondary bile acids—deoxycholic acid and lithocholic acid, respectively. Bile acids are conjugated in the liver with the amino acids glycine or taurine. This decreases passive absorption in the biliary tree and proximal small intestine, but permits conservation through active transport in the terminal ileum. This combination of nonionic transport in the small intestine and active transport in the terminal ileum maintains the bile acid pool. This pool, along with further bile acid synthesis from cholesterol, allows for the continuous solubilization and elimination of cholesterol. Approximately 0.1 to 0.6 g of bile acids is lost in the feces daily.

Biochemistry

Synthesis of Bile Acids. The sequence of reactions involved in the synthesis of cholic acid from cholesterol is shown in Figure 47-5 and includes (1) addition of a hydroxyl group in the 7-α-position, with subsequent further hydroxylation at the 12-α-position; (2) inversion of the hydroxyl group from the 3-β-position (above the plane of the molecule) to the 3-α-position (below this plane); (3) saturation of the double bond at position 5-6; (4) loss of a 3-carbon group from the cholesterol side chain, giving rise to a 24-carbon molecule; and (5) oxidation of the C-24 carbon to a carboxyl group. The other primary bile acid formed in the liver, chenodeoxycholic acid, differs from cholic acid only by the absence of a hydroxyl group at position 12. The initial step in the synthesis of both bile acids, 7-α-hydroxylation of cholesterol, occurs under the influence of the rate-limiting enzyme 7-α-hydroxylase. The reaction is subject to feedback inhibition by bile acids returning to the liver from the ileum.

Before secretion into canaliculi, the primary bile acids are conjugated at the carboxylic acid carbon with either taurine or glycine (Figure 47-6), increasing water solubility. Through this mechanism of conjugation, four primary bile acids (cholyltaurine, cholylglycine, chenodeoxycholyltaurine, and chenodeoxycholylglycine) are formed. Conjugation decreases the pK_a values from ~6 to 4 for glycine conjugates and to 2 for taurine conjugates. Thus conjugated bile acids are in the ionized form in the relatively high pH of the intestinal lumen. In health, the glycine conjugates predominate in a ratio of approximately 3:1 to 4:1. Unconjugated (free) bile acids are not present in bile except in certain pathological states of bacterial overgrowth or ileal resection when intestinal bacteria either dehydroxylate or deconjugate the bile acids.

During passage through the small intestine and colon, both cholic acid and chenodeoxycholic acid are dehydroxylated by bacterial 7-α-dehydroxylase, giving rise to the secondary bile acids deoxycholic acid and lithocholic acid (Figure 47-7). The usual bile acid composition of normal human bile is ~38% cholate conjugates, 34% chenodeoxycholate conjugates, 28% deoxycholate conjugates, and 1% to 2% lithocholate conjugates.

Hepatic Bile Formation. Carrier-mediated active transport of bile acids across the canalicular surface generates osmotic water flow that is a major factor regulating bile formation and secretion. Transport of these organic anions also influences secretion of the remainder of the major components of bile, such as bilirubin, cholesterol, and phospholipids. There is no secretion of the latter two compounds in the absence of bile acid secretion. The influence of bile acid

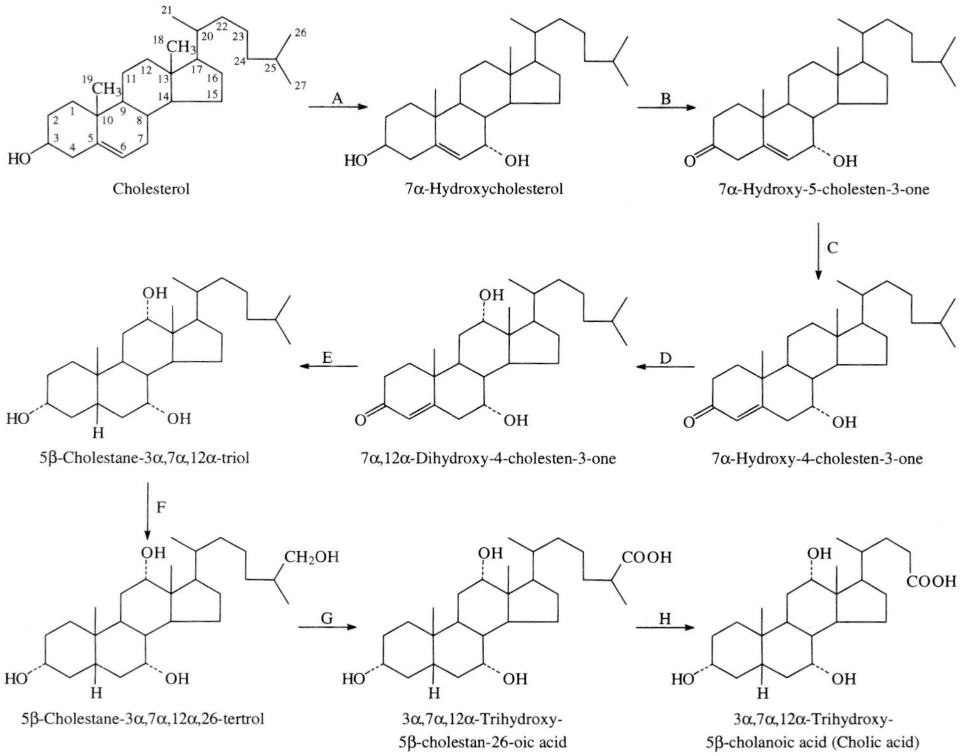

Cholesterol → A → 7α-Hydroxycholesterol → B → 7α-Hydroxy-5-cholesten-3-one → C → 7α-Hydroxy-4-cholesten-3-one → D → 7α,12α-Dihydroxy-4-cholesten-3-one → E → 5β-Cholestane-3α,7α,12α-triol → F → 5β-Cholestane-3α,7α,12α,26-tertrol → G → 3α,7α,12α-Trihydroxy-5β-cholestan-26-oic acid → H → 3α,7α,12α-Trihydroxy-5β-cholanoic acid (Cholic acid)

Figure 47-5 The biosynthetic pathways of cholesterol conversion to cholic acid. **A,** 7-α-Hydroxylation of cholesterol (addition of —OH group at position 7-α-configuration), the rate-limiting step in the biosynthetic pathway; **B,** oxidation of the 3-β-hydroxyl group (to form 3-oxo compound); **C,** isomerization of the 5-ene structure; **D,** 12-α-hydroxylation (for cholic acid only); **E,** saturation of the double bond and reduction of the 3-one group; **F,** hydroxylation of the side chain at C-26 position; **G,** side chain oxidation to cholestanoic acid; **H,** hydroxylation at C-24 and β-oxidation to reduce the length of the side chain. *(From Balistreri WF, Setchel KDR. Clinical implications of bile acid metabolism. In Silverberg M, Daum F, eds. Textbook of pediatric gastroenterology, 2nd ed. Chicago: Year Book Medical Publishers, 1988:72-89. By permission of Mosby, Inc.)*

secretion on biliary lipid excretion is a result of the ability of bile acids to solubilize cholesterol and phospholipids in an aqueous medium in mixed micelles.

Bile formation occurs by processes that are not fully defined. It takes place in canaliculi, minute passages lined by specialized modifications of the hepatocyte membrane, that ultimately unite to form bile ductules. Hepatic bile contains 5% to 15% total solids, the major component of which is bile acids. The increase in biliary water and electrolyte excretion caused by this osmotic effect represents the bile acid–dependent fraction of bile flow. Even with severe depletion of the circulating bile acid pool, as is seen with bile duct diversion, some bile flow continues. The active transport of sodium and of glutathione and bicarbonate is mediated by Na-K-ATPase, which is responsible for the bile acid-independent flow of bile (up to 40% of total flow). Hormones such as secretin increase bile flow by stimulating secretion of sodium, bicarbonate, and chloride. Hormone-dependent flow accounts for 20% to 25% of the total.

Because they possess both polar and nonpolar regions, molecules of bile acids are able to solubilize biliary lipids. Such molecules align at water-lipid interfaces and reduce surface tension, acting as detergents. In an aqueous solution, bile acids aggregate to form small polymolecular aggregates ~5 nm in diameter called *micelles.* These are capable of incorporating cholesterol and phospholipids, forming mixed micelles (Figure 47-8). Micellar solubilization of these water insoluble constituents maintains cholesterol in solution.

Physiology

Enterohepatic Circulation of Bile Acids. The body conserves the bile acid pool through a recirculating system known as the *enterohepatic circulation.* The anatomical components of the enterohepatic circulation are the liver, biliary tract, terminal ileum, and portal venous circulation.

During fasting, bile acids pass down the biliary tree to enter the gallbladder (Figure 47-9). In the gallbladder, they

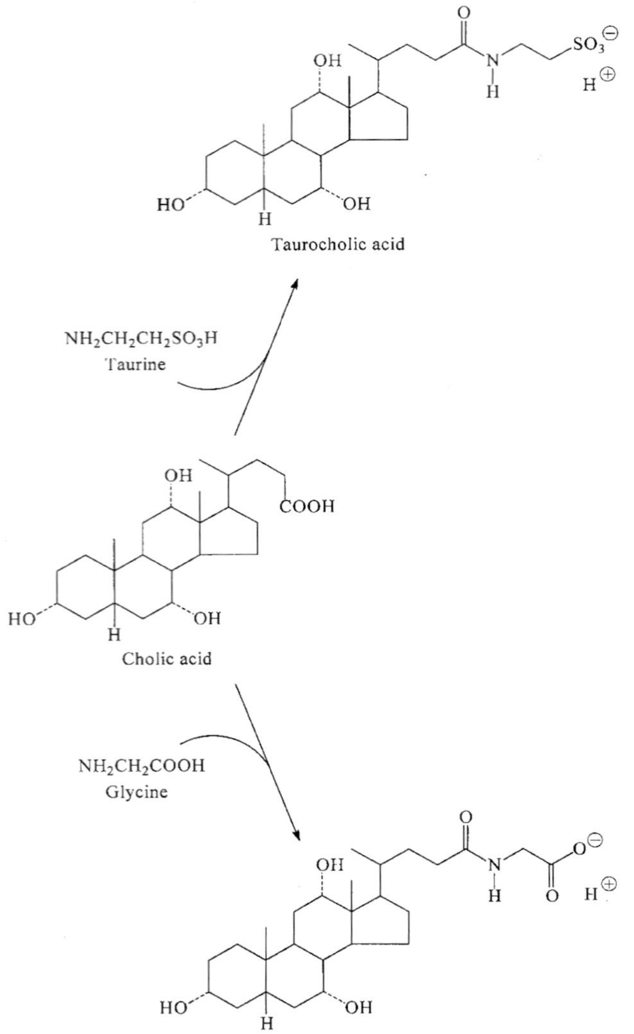

Figure 47-6 Conjugation of cholic acid with either taurine or glycine.

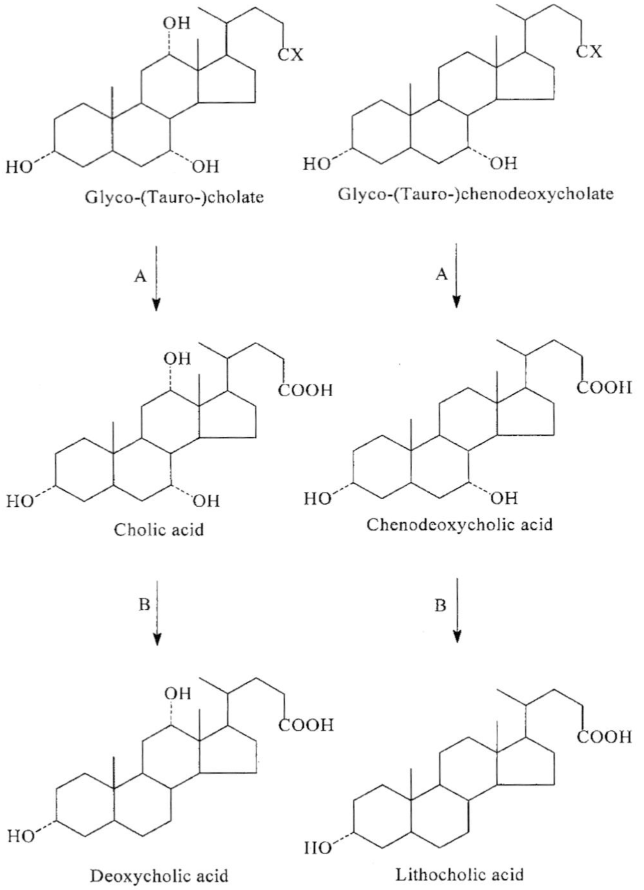

undergo a tenfold increase in concentration owing to reabsorption of water and electrolytes. After an overnight fast, 95% of the bile acid pool may be sequestered in the gallbladder. This sequestration results in low concentrations of bile acids in the intestine, portal vein, liver, and plasma.

In response to a meal, cholecystokinin is released from the intestine and causes relaxation of the sphincter of Oddi and contraction of the gallbladder (see Chapter 48). This allows a concentrated solution of micelles (consisting of bile salts, lecithin, and cholesterol) to enter the intestine. In the intestinal lumen, dietary cholesterol and the products of triglyceride digestion (predominantly free fatty acids and monoglycerides) are incorporated into mixed micelles. Micelles deliver lipolytic products to the mucosal surface. To carry out these functions, a critical micellar bile acid concentration of ~2 mmol/L is necessary.

Figure 47-7 Conversion of primary bile acids to secondary bile acids by endogenous microflora.

After delivery of lipids, bile acids are subsequently reabsorbed in the intestine by two mechanisms: active transport in the distal portion of the ileum and nonionic diffusion in the jejunum and colon.

Bile acids are carried in plasma tightly bound to protein. The concentration of bile acids in the portal vein is high but, because of the efficiency of hepatic extraction, systemic blood concentrations remain low. In a single pass through the liver, the efficiency of extraction is ~80% for cholic acid and ~60% for chenodeoxycholic acid. Hepatic extraction efficiency is unchanged over a broad range of portal bile acid concentrations.

Kinetics of Bile Acid Metabolism. Using an isotope dilution technique, the bile acid pool in normal adults has been found to average from 2 to 4 g. Steady state is reached when hepatic synthesis and fecal loss are in balance. In health, the magnitude of each process is 0.3 to 0.8 g/day. There are usually 4 to 10 enterohepatic cycles per day. Because of this recycling mechanism, the jejunal concentration of bile acids is maintained at ~5 to 10 mmol/L during the postprandial state, much higher than the critical micellar concentration of ~2 mmol/L. Between meals, with decreased entry of bile acids into the intestine, the intraluminal concentration

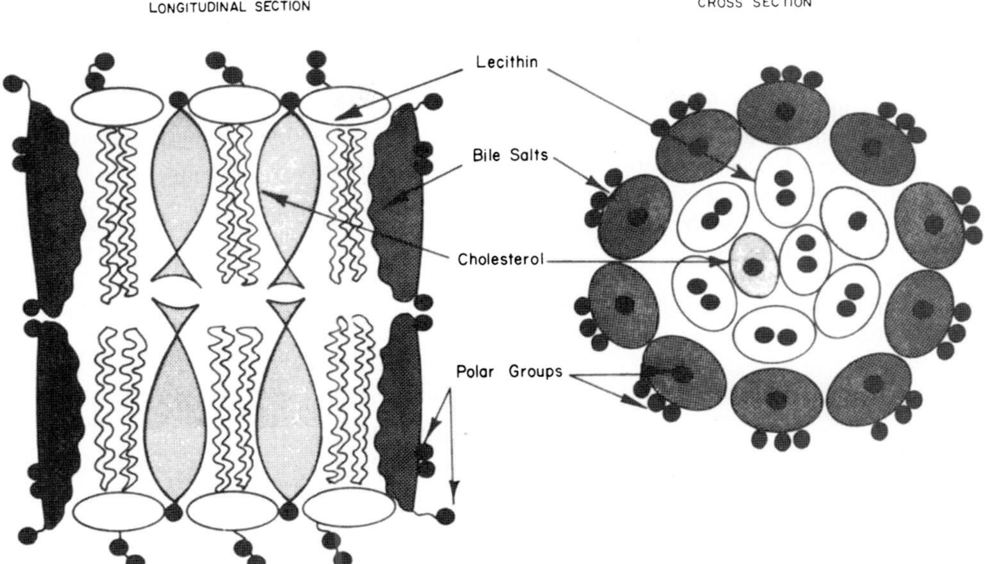

Figure 47-8 Structure of mixed micelles in bile. *(From Balistreri WF, Soloweay RD. Clinical guide to bile acid physiology and alterations in disease states. Chicago: Abbott Laboratories, 1979. Reproduction of Clinical Guide to Bile Acid Physiology and Alterations in Disease States has been granted with approval of Abbott Laboratories Inc., all rights reserved by Abbott Laboratories Inc.)*

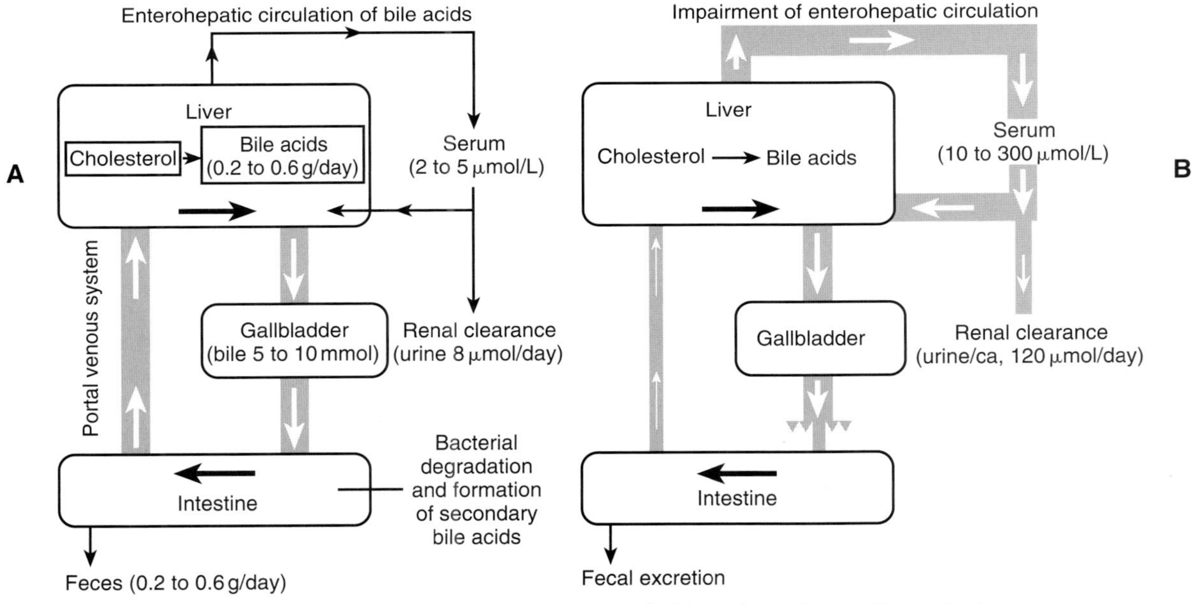

Figure 47-9 Enterohepatic circulation of bile acids. **A,** Normal circulation; **B,** impaired circulation.

decreases. Plasma bile acid concentrations depend on input from the enterohepatic circulation; therefore concentrations of total plasma bile acids will increase by 50% above fasting values 90 to 120 minutes following a meal.

Abnormalities of Bile Acid Metabolism

In view of the multiple processes involved in bile acid synthesis, conjugation, and excretion, and in their hepatic and intestinal uptake, there are several potential sites for primary or secondary disturbances (Box 47-1).

Defective Bile Acid Synthesis. Specific defects in bile acid synthesis have long been postulated. Two inborn errors of bile acid synthesis, both associated with idiopathic neonatal hepatitis, Δ^4-3-oxosteroid 5-β-reductase deficiency and 3-β-hydroxy-dehydrogenase isomerase deficiency, have been described.[37] A third disorder associated with defective bile

BOX 47-1 Disturbances in Bile Acid Metabolism

Defective Bile Acid Synthesis
- *Specific* defects in bile acid synthesis
  - Cerebrotendinous xanthomatosis
  - Intrahepatic cholestasis (familial neonatal hepatitis)
    - 3-β-hydroxysteroid dehydrogenase/isomerase deficiency
    - Δ^4-3-oxosteroid 5-β-reductase deficiency
    - C_{24} steroid: 7-α-hydroxylase deficiency
  - Peroxisomal disorders
    - Genetic diseases with a general impairment of numerous peroxisomal functions and reduced or undetectable peroxisome numbers
    - Cerebrohepatorenal (Zellweger's) syndrome
    - Infantile Refsum's disease
    - Neonatal adrenoleukodystrophy
    - Rhizomelic chondrodysplasia punctata
    - Hyperpipecolic acidemia
  - Genetic diseases with generalized impairment of peroxisomal function but normal number of peroxisomes
    - Pseudo-Zellweger's syndrome
  - Genetic diseases with a single enzyme defect and a normal number of peroxisomes
    - X-linked adrenoleukodystrophy
    - Adult Refsum's disease
    - Acatalasemia
- *Acquired* defects in bile acid synthesis (nonspecific) secondary to parenchymal liver disease (cholestasis, cirrhosis)

Abnormalities of Bile Acid Delivery to the Bowel
- Celiac sprue

Extrahepatic Bile Duct Obstruction
- Congenital biliary atresia
- Stricture
- Stone
- Carcinoma

Interruption of the Enterohepatic Circulation of Bile Acids
- External bile drainage (fistula)
- Ileojejunal exclusion for exogenous obesity or hypercholesterolemia
- Cystic fibrosis
- Contaminated small bowel syndrome (with bile acid precipitation, increased jejunal absorption, and "short circuiting")
- Entrapment of bile acids in intestinal lumen by:
  - Cholestyramine
  - Trivalent cations
  - Fiber

Bile Acid Malabsorption
- Primary bile acid malabsorption (absent or inefficient ileal active transport)
  - Intractable diarrhea (infancy)
  - Irritable bowel (adults)
- Secondary bile acid malabsorption
  - Ileal disease or resection
    - Crohn's disease
    - Ileal resection
    - Ileal bypass
    - Radiation enteritis
    - Postinfectious enteritis
  - Exogenous bile acid administration (e.g., gallstone dissolution)
  - Cystic fibrosis
- Tertiary bile acid malabsorption
  - Postcholecystectomy
  - Renal failure
  - Drugs

Defective Uptake or Altered Intracellular Metabolism
- Parenchymal disease (acute hepatitis, cirrhosis) associated with regurgitation from cells or portosystemic shunting
- Cholestasis

acid synthesis is cerebrotendinous xanthomatosis. In this disorder, chenodeoxycholic acid production is affected more than cholic acid production, and unusual metabolites, such as bile alcohols, are present in bile and feces.

In addition to *primary* defects in bile acid synthesis, *secondary* abnormalities have been noted in peroxisomal disorders, such as neonatal adrenoleukodystrophy and cerebrohepatorenal (Zellweger's) syndrome—an autosomal recessive condition associated with severe cholestasis in which side chain oxidation is impaired.

More frequently encountered are *acquired* defects in bile acid synthesis, which have been noted in liver diseases such as hepatitis and cirrhosis. In acute hepatitis, alterations of bile acid synthesis and conjugation occur because of hepatic parenchymal cell disease. In cirrhosis, there is a marked reduction in cholic acid synthesis with a low concentration of biliary deoxycholic acid. These abnormalities are due both to decreased synthesis and to portosystemic shunting. The severity of cirrhosis correlates closely with the loss of cholic acid synthetic capacity. The decreased ratio of the trihydroxy bile acid (cholic acid) to the dihydroxy bile acid (chenodeoxycholic acid) in plasma has therefore been used as a diagnostic test of liver cell dysfunction.

Abnormalities of Bile Acid Delivery to the Bowel. Decreased bile flow from intrahepatic cholestasis or extrahepatic bile duct obstruction caused by biliary atresia, stricture, stone, or carcinoma will result in bile acid retention and regurgitation from the liver cell into plasma and a decrease in delivery to the intestine. The ratio of plasma trihydroxy to dihydroxy acids increases in cholestasis.

Interruption of the Enterohepatic Circulation of Bile Acids. Approximately 95% of the bile acids that are secreted during a single enterohepatic cycle are recirculating bile acids. Therefore a significant interruption of this cycle will lead to a decrease in hepatic bile acid secretion. A negative feedback increase in bile acid synthesis can only partially compensate for the losses. Therefore resection, inflammation, or bypass of the ileum will be associated with specific clinical symptoms and disturbances of bile acid metabolism. The amount of bile acid return to the liver is reduced, and a loss of feedback inhibition results in accelerated hepatic synthesis of bile acids. The concentration of plasma cholesterol is reduced, since an increased proportion of this compound is used for bile acid synthesis. Concentrations of plasma bile acids decrease and are a reflection of ileal dysfunction, since the expected postprandial rise (due to ileal absorption of bile acids) will not be present.[37]

Disturbances of Bile Acid Metabolism in Hepatocellular Disease. Fasting plasma bile acid concentrations are elevated in hepatocellular diseases, such as hepatitis and cirrhosis. The mechanisms responsible are regurgitation of bile acids from cholestatic hepatocytes and portosystemic shunting. These defects allow the plasma concentrations to rise proportionately much higher than normal following meals, suggesting that the postprandial rise in plasma bile acids may be a sensitive test for the detection of liver disease.

Clinical Significance

Increased plasma bile acid concentrations in the fasting state suggest impaired hepatic uptake or secretion, or portosystemic shunting. Thus, such measurements may be used as a sensitive endogenous clearance test. However, a diagnosis suggested by an increase in plasma bile acid concentrations should be confirmed by standard liver function tests. In a similar manner, abnormal standard liver function tests can be confirmed as indicative of hepatic dysfunction by concomitant measurement of plasma bile acids. Plasma bile acid measurements may also be used serially to monitor patients with suspected or proven hepatic disease. However, they add little to standard tests of liver function and are now rarely used in clinical medicine.

Analytical Methodology

Analytical techniques used to quantify either total or individual bile acids in biological fluids include gas-liquid chromatography (GLC), high-performance liquid chromatography (HPLC), enzymatic assay, radioimmunoassay (RIA), enzyme-linked immunosorbent assay (ELISA), and tandem mass spectrometry (MS/MS).

Hepatic Synthetic Function

The liver has extensive synthetic capacity and plays a major role in the regulation of protein, carbohydrate, and lipid metabolism (see Chapters 20, 25, and 26). A bidirectional flux of precursors and products, such as glucose, amino acids, free fatty acids, and other nutrients, occurs across the hepatocyte membrane. Normal blood glucose concentrations are maintained during short fasts by the breakdown of hepatic glycogen and during prolonged fasts by hepatic gluconeogenesis. The primary sources of carbon atoms for gluconeogenesis are amino acids derived from muscle proteins. To a lesser extent, lactate (produced in skeletal muscle and erythrocytes) and glycerol (obtained from hydrolysis of triglycerides) also serve as substrates for gluconeogenesis. In humans, the oxidation of odd-numbered fatty acids yields propionyl-CoA, which can be converted to glucose. However, the formation of glucose in this manner is not quantitatively significant. Protein, triglyceride, fatty acid, cholesterol, and bile acid synthesis also occur within the liver.

Protein Synthesis

The liver is the primary site of the synthesis of plasma proteins (see Chapter 20). Synthesis occurs in the rough endoplasmic reticulum of the hepatocytes, followed by release into hepatic sinusoids. Although disturbances of protein synthesis occur as a consequence of impaired hepatic function, a variety of other factors also affect plasma protein concentrations. These include (1) decreased availability of amino acids (malnutrition, maldigestion, and malabsorption), (2) catabolic states (hyperthyroidism, Cushing's syndrome, burns, postsurgery recovery), (3) protein losing states (nephrotic syndrome and protein losing enteropathy), (5) actions of cytokines (decrease in transport proteins such as albumin, transferrin, and lipoproteins, but increase in inflammatory response modifiers such as α_1-antitrypsin, haptoglobin, and α_2-macroglobulin), (5) action of hormones (such as growth hormone, cortisol, estrogen, androgens, and thyroid hormones) to increase or decrease production of specific proteins, and (6) congenital deficiency states (Wilson's disease and α_1-antrypsin deficiency). In addition, the liver has a significant reserve capacity, preventing protein concentrations from decreasing unless there is extensive liver damage. In addition, many liver proteins have relatively long half-lives, such as albumin at approximately 3 weeks. For this reason, the sensitivity and specificity of protein concentrations for diagnosis of liver disease are far from ideal.

The patterns of plasma protein alterations seen in liver disease depend on the type, severity, and duration of liver injury. For example, in acute hepatic dysfunction, there is usually little change in the plasma protein profile or the total plasma protein concentration; with fulminant hepatic failure or severe liver injury, concentrations of short-lived hepatic proteins (such as transthyretin and prothrombin) will fall quickly and become abnormal, whereas proteins with longer half-lives will be unchanged. In cirrhosis, concentrations of liver-synthesized plasma proteins and immunoglobulins decrease and increase repectively. Serial determination of plasma proteins provides prognostic information; for example, a worsening of prothrombin time during acute hepatitis suggests a poor prognosis.

Plasma Proteins

Albumin. Albumin is the most commonly measured serum protein and is synthesized exclusively by the liver. The rate of synthesis varies, depending on hormonal environment, nutritional status, age, and other local factors. In inflammatory conditions. Interleukin-6 (IL-6) inhibits albumin synthesis but induces synthesis of acute phase response proteins. With liver disease, hypoalbuminemia is noted primarily in cirrhosis, autoimmune hepatitis, and alcoholic hepatitis. The mechanism is multifactorial. In cirrhosis, hepatic synthesis of albumin may be decreased, normal, or increased. Loss of albumin into ascitic fluid seems responsible for the decrease in albumin in many cases. One important consideration in measurement of albumin is the inaccuracy of dye-binding methods in patients with liver disease. Although bromcresol green measurements tend to overestimate albumin concentration at low concentrations,[290] bromcresol purple methods give falsely low values in patients with jaundice because of interference of bilirubin at the site of binding.[209]

Transthyretin. This protein has a short half-life of 24 to 48 hours, making it a sensitive indicator of current synthetic ability. Failure of transthyretin to increase is an indicator of fulminant hepatic failure in acute hepatitis and is associated with a poor prognosis.[202] It is more commonly used as a measurement of nutritional status.

Immunoglobulins. Immunoglobulins are commonly increased in cirrhosis, autoimmune hepatitis, and primary biliary cirrhosis but are normal in most other types of liver disease. IgG is increased in autoimmune hepatitis and cirrhosis; IgM is increased in primary biliary cirrhosis. IgA tends to be increased in all types of cirrhosis. None of these findings are specific, and they are seldom used in the diagnosis of liver disease.

Ceruloplasmin. This protein is decreased in Wilson's disease, cirrhosis, and many causes of chronic hepatitis, but may be increased by inflammation, cholestasis, hemochromatosis, pregnancy, and estrogen therapy. It is discussed in more detail under Wilson's disease.

α_1-Antitrypsin. This protein is the major serine protease inhibitor (serpin) in plasma, and is decreased in homozygous deficiency and cirrhosis and increased by acute inflammation. It is discussed in more detail later in this chapter under the heading for α_1-antitrypsin deficiency.

α-Fetoprotein. This protein, a normal component of fetal blood, falls to adult concentrations by 1 year of age. Mild increases are seen in patients with acute and chronic hepatitis and indicate hepatocellular regeneration. It is present at higher concentrations in hepatocellular carcinoma (HCC) and is discussed in more detail later and in Chapters 20 and 54.

Coagulation Proteins

The coagulation proteins that are synthesized in the liver are listed in Table 47-1. These proteins interact to produce a fibrin clot. Inhibitors of the coagulation system, including antithrombin, protein C, and protein S, are also synthesized in the liver. Some of the coagulation factors (II, VII, IX, and X) require vitamin K for posttranslational carboxylation within the hepatocyte. Protein C and S are also carboxylated by a vitamin K–dependent enzyme. Activated protein C in plasma inhibits coagulation by inactivating factors V and VIII. Parenchymal liver disease of sufficient severity to impair protein synthesis or obstructive liver disease sufficient to impair intestinal absorption of vitamin K is therefore a potential cause of bleeding disorders. Because of the great functional reserve of the liver, failure of hemostasis usually does not occur except in severe or long-standing liver disease.[237] Thus testing for a coagulation defect is not a screening procedure but rather a means of assessing severity and following the progress of liver disease.

TABLE 47-1 Blood Coagulation Factors

Number or Acronym	Name
I	Fibrinogen*
II	Prothrombin*†
III	Tissue factor
IV	Calcium (Ca^{2+})
V	Proaccelerin*
VI	—
VII	Proconvertin*†
VIII	Antihemophilic factor
IX	Christmas factor*†
X	Stuart-Prower factor†
XI	Plasma thromboplastin antecedent*
XII	Hageman factor*
XIII	Fibrin-stabilizing factor*
PK	Prekallikrein (Fletcher factor)*
HMWK	High molecular weight kininogen*

*Protein synthesized in liver.
†Synthesis requires vitamin K.

The prothrombin time (PT) measures activity of fibrinogen (factor I), prothrombin (factor II), and factors V, VII, and X. Since all of these factors are made in the liver and several are vitamin K dependent, a prolonged PT often indicates the presence of significant liver disease. In cholestasis, vitamin K deficiency may also cause an increase in PT. In this case, the coagulation abnormality is corrected within a few days by parenteral injection of 10 mg of vitamin K. In contrast, if PT is prolonged because of hepatocellular disease, factor synthesis is decreased and administration of vitamin K does not typically correct the problem. PT is also prolonged in some patients with liver disease because of the presence of dysfibrinogenemia, an abnormal form of fibrinogen that does not clot normally, and that may predispose to thrombosis.[158]

The method for reporting PT in liver disease remains controversial. PT measures the time to clot after exposure of plasma to tissue factor. Reagents differ in the amount of tissue factor present; in patients with coagulopathy, clotting times are more greatly prolonged when lower amounts of tissue factor are in the reagents. This makes a reagent more sensitive to clotting factor abnormalities, but makes standardization of results between laboratories difficult. The International Normalized Ratio (INR) was developed by the World Health Organization (WHO) and the International Committee on Thrombosis and Hemostasis (ICTH) for reporting the results of blood coagulation (clotting) tests. All results are standardized using the international sensitivity index (ISI) for the particular thromboplastin reagent and instrument combination used to perform the test. In practice, it requires determination of the ISI based on the slope of the relationship between prothrombin time using the reagent and that using a reference method in patients on warfarin. The INR is then calculated as:

$$\text{INR} = \left[\frac{\text{PT (patient)}}{\text{PT (geometric mean of normal)}}\right]^{\text{ISI}}$$

INR has been found to standardize interpretation of PT measurements between laboratories in those taking warfarin. Unfortunately, INR does not have the same relationship to impairment of clotting in individuals with liver disease.[224,439] The apparent explanation lies in the mechanism of clotting factor deficiency in liver disease and warfarin administration. Although liver disease inhibits synthesis of clotting factors, warfarin impairs vitamin K–dependent carboxylation, impairing the ability of the factors to bind calcium. These noncarboxylated clotting factors (termed proteins induced by vitamin K antagonists, or PIVKAs) appear to act as inhibitors of coagulation; thus when lower amounts of tissue factor are present, there is greater prolongation of clotting times.[245] In contrast, in liver disease, factor deficiency is due to impaired factor synthesis, and no PIVKAs are present (except in HCC, as discussed later in this chapter). This leads to minimal increases in PT in individuals with liver disease and underestimation of the degree of clotting impairment when reagents with low ISI are used. Although it is not clear which method of reporting PT is ideal, one study has suggested using the prothrombin index (the ratio used in calculation of INR, but without the ISI exponential).[371] However, few data exist on prothrombin indices that indicate significant impairment of coagulation.[113]

Lipid and Lipoprotein Synthesis

The liver plays a key role in the metabolism of lipids and lipoproteins (see Chapter 26). On a daily basis, approximately 33% of the fatty acids originating from adipose tissue enter the liver, where they undergo esterification into triglycerides or are oxidized. Oxidation is favored in the fasting state and esterification is favored in the nonfasting state. Excessive esterification results in "fatty liver," a disorder in which excess triglycerides are deposited in large vacuoles that displace other cellular components. Most cholesterol is endogenously synthesized in the liver. It and cholesterol of dietary origin enter the hepatic pool, where they are converted to bile acids, incorporated into lipoproteins, or used in the synthesis of liver cell membranes. The relative rates of secretion of bile acids, cholesterol, and lecithin are important factors in the pathogenesis of cholesterol gallstones.

Urea Synthesis

Patients with end-stage liver disease may have low concentrations of urea in plasma (see Chapter 45). The rate of urea excretion in urine is lower than in healthy individuals. In addition, plasma concentrations are elevated for urea precursors ammonia and amino acids. Lower specific activities are found for enzymes involved in urea synthesis. These findings suggest that patients with liver disease have an impaired ability to metabolize protein nitrogen and to synthesize urea. The rate of hepatic urea synthesis depends on exogenous intake of nitrogen and on endogenous protein catabolism. Newly synthesized urea equilibrates throughout the total body water compartment and to a large extent is excreted in urine. A small portion diffuses into the intestine, where bacterial enzymes hydrolyze urea to produce ammonia. Carbon dioxide is excreted, whereas ammonia is reabsorbed and must be recycled through the liver. Thus the rate of urea synthesis can be calculated through analysis of urinary urea excretion and the blood urea nitrogen (BUN) level if total body water and the extent of GI hydrolysis of urea can be estimated. In cirrhotic patients, the Krebs-Henseleit pathway is unable to incorporate excess ammonia nitrogen into urea.

Hepatic Metabolic Function

A recurring theme is the central importance of the liver in metabolic and regulatory pathways. The functional expression of the complex, integrated organelle structure includes the metabolism of drugs (activation and detoxification) and the disposal of exogenous and endogenous substances, such as galactose and ammonia. In addition, metabolic abnormalities due to specific, inherited enzyme deficiencies can affect the liver. A classic example is galactosemia. In this condition the congenital absence of the galactose-1-phosphate uridyltransferase enzyme allows accumulation of the toxic metabolite galactose-1-phosphate, which causes injury to the liver, brain, and kidneys.

Ammonia Metabolism

Biochemistry and Physiology

The major source of circulating ammonia is the GI tract. Plasma ammonia concentration in the hepatic portal vein is typically fivefold to tenfold higher than that in the systemic circulation. It is derived from the action of bacterial proteases, ureases, and amine oxidases on the contents of the colon and from the hydrolysis of glutamine in both the small and large intestines. Under normal circumstances, most of the portal vein ammonia load is metabolized to urea in hepatocytes in the Krebs-Henseleit urea cycle during the first pass through the liver; this process includes intramitochondrial and cytosolic enzyme-catalyzed steps (Figure 47-10).

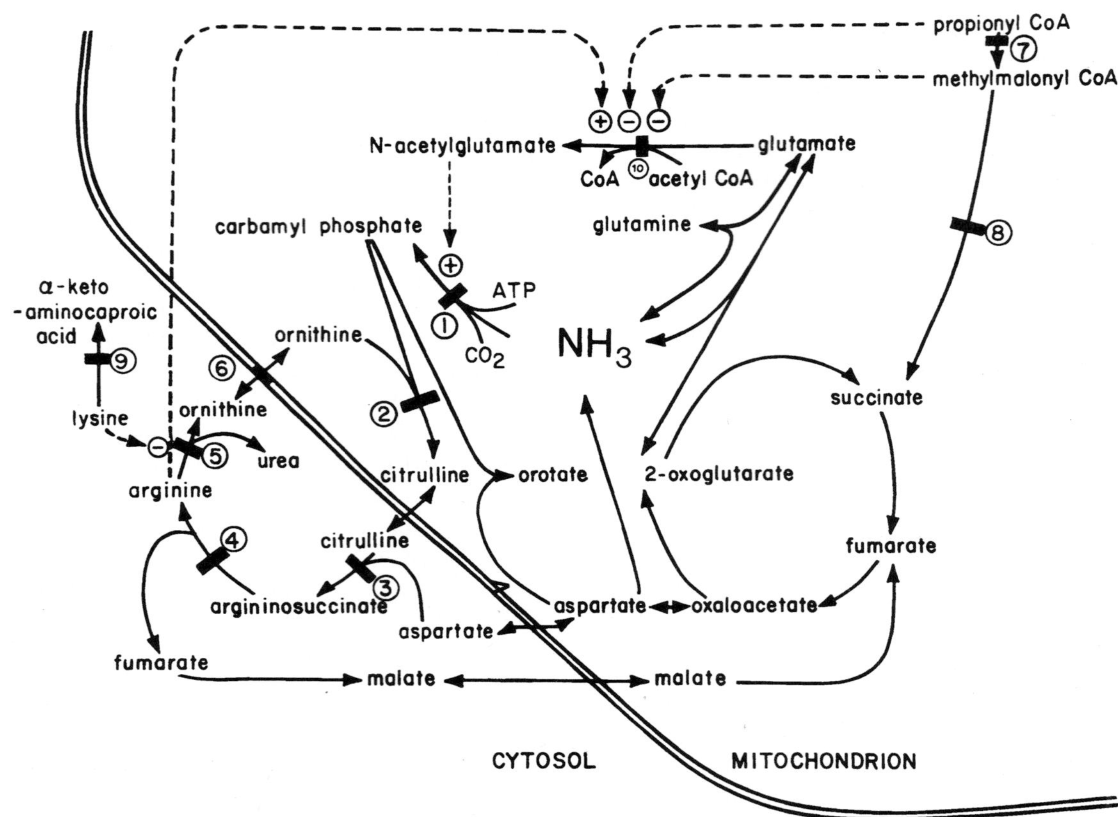

Figure 47-10 The major metabolic pathways for the use of ammonia by the hepatocyte. *Solid bars* indicate the sites of primary enzyme defects in various metabolic disorders associated with hyperammonemia: (*1*) carbamyl phosphate synthetase I, (*2*) ornithine transcarbamylase, (*3*) argininosuccinate synthetase, (*4*) argininosuccinate lyase, (*5*) arginase, (*6*) mitochondrial ornithine transport, (*7*) propionyl CoA carboxylase, (*8*) methylmalonyl CoA mutase, (*9*) L-lysine dehydrogenase, and (*10*) *N*-acetyl glutamine synthetase. *Dotted lines* indicate the site of pathway activation (+) or inhibition (–). *(From Flannery OB, Hsia YE, Wolf B. Current status of hyperammonemia syndromes. Hepatology 1982; 2:495-506.)*

Ammonia enters tissue of the central nervous system by passive diffusion. The rate of entry increases in proportion to the plasma concentration and is dependent on pH. As pH increases, the rate of entry of ammonia into the central nervous system tissue increases. This is thought to be because an increase in pH produces a shift to the right in the equilibrium

$$NH_4^{\oplus} + H_2O \rightleftharpoons NH_3 + H_3O^{\oplus}$$

that results in an increased ammonia base concentration. Ammonia crosses the blood-brain barrier membranes more readily than the ammonium ion. Given that the pK_a of ammonia is 8.9 at 37 °C, approximately 3% of blood ammonia is NH_3 at the normal physiological pH of 7.4. An increase of pH to 7.6 produces an increase in NH_3 to approximately 5% of total blood ammonia—a 67% increase in concentration.

Clinical Significance

Animal and human studies have shown that an elevated concentration of ammonia (hyperammonemia) exerts toxic effects on the central nervous system. There are several causes, both inherited and acquired, of hyperammonemia. The inherited deficiencies of urea cycle enzymes are the major cause of hyperammonemia in infants.[66] The two major inherited disorders are those involving the metabolism of the dibasic amino acids lysine and ornithine and those involving the metabolism of organic acids, such as propionic acid, methylmalonic acid, isovaleric acid, and others (see Chapter 55).

The acquired causes of hyperammonemia are advanced liver disease and renal failure. Severe or chronic liver failure (as occurs in fulminant hepatitis and cirrhosis, respectively) leads to a significant impairment of normal ammonia metabolism. Reye's syndrome, which is primarily a central nervous system disorder with minor hepatic dysfunction, is also associated with hyperammonemia. Hepatic encephalopathy, in the cirrhotic patient, is often precipitated by GI bleeding that enhances ammonia production by bacterial metabolism of the blood proteins in the colon and subsequent increases in blood ammonia concentrations. Other precipitating causes of encephalopathy include excess dietary protein, constipation, infections, drugs, or electrolyte and acid-base imbalance. Since cirrhosis is accompanied by portosystemic shunting, ammonia clearance is impaired, leading to increased concentrations of blood ammonia. Impaired renal function also causes hyperammonemia. As BUN concentration increases, more diffuses into the GI tract where is it converted to ammonia.

The fasting venous plasma ammonia concentration is useful in the differential diagnosis of encephalopathy when it is unclear if encephalopathy is of an hepatic origin. It is especially helpful in diagnosing Reye's syndrome and the inherited disorders of urea metabolism. However, it is not a useful test to use in patients with known liver disease.

Analytical Methodology

Both enzymatic and chemical methods are used to measure ammonia in body fluids. Enzymatic assay with glutamate dehydrogenase is the most frequently used method. Plasma ammonia measurement is particularly susceptible to contamination, leading to falsely elevated concentrations. Some of the common sampling problems are discussed in the third edition of this textbook.

Reference Intervals

For the enzymatic method, the reference interval is 15 to 45 μg N/dL or 11 to 32 μmol N/L. Should values in normal subjects be much higher than expected, consideration should be given to the existence and correction of sources of preanalytical error resulting from contamination.

Carbohydrate Metabolism

Because the liver is a major processor of dietary and endogenous carbohydrates, liver disease affects carbohydrate metabolism in a variety of ways (see Chapter 25). However, none of the conventional modes of evaluating carbohydrate metabolism have value in the diagnosis of liver disease. Because the liver is the major site of both glycogen storage and gluconeogenesis, hypoglycemia is a common complication in certain liver diseases, particularly Reye's syndrome, fulminant hepatic failure, advanced cirrhosis, and hepatocellular carcinoma.

Xenobiotic Metabolism and Excretion

Xenobiotics are foreign substances that are cleared and metabolized by the liver and some have been used as tests of liver function. For example, certain lipophilic substances such as bromsulfophthalein (BSP), indocyanine green (ICG), aminopyrine, caffeine, lidocaine, and rose bengal are excreted into bile as the intact parent compound, its conjugates, or both. The clearance of these xenobiotics by the liver is normally very rapid, and it is believed that uptake by hepatocytes is a carrier-mediated, active-transport process. Little, if any, is cleared by other tissue. Excretion into bile is slow. The elimination of these compounds from the bloodstream therefore depends on hepatic blood flow, patency of the biliary tree, and hepatic parenchymal function.

Dye Excretion Tests

Dye excretion tests (such as BSP and ICG clearance) were formerly used as indicators of liver disease. With the development of more sensitive and specific indicators of liver disease, dye excretion tests have become obsolete. Until the 1970s, BSP was the most frequently used dye excretion test. Because of reports of fatalities resulting from hypersensitivity and other adverse effects (nausea, syncope, headache, chills, and thrombophlebitis at the site of injection), BSP use has been discontinued. ICG clearance was used for investigation of hepatic blood flow and for predicting clearance rates of drugs that undergo first-pass clearance by the liver, such as lidocaine. Typical ICG clearance values in healthy subjects range from 6.5 to 14 mL/min/kg. ICG clearance is still occasionally used.

Drug Clearance Tests

A variety of drugs that are metabolized by the liver have been used to study the action of various P_{450} enzymes. *Aminopyrine* is demethylated to form carbon dioxide and aminoantipyrine. By using ^{14}C-labeled aminopyrine, the resulting $^{14}CO_2$ can be measured in breath as a reflection of functioning liver mass.[195] There is significant interindividual and intraindividual variation in results,[76,352] other microsomal enzyme inducing agents increase metabolism,[76] and overall diagnostic sensitivity is similar to that of other more routine laboratory tests.[331] *Caffeine* is rapidly and nearly completely absorbed from the GI tract and then undergoes N-demethylation by the hepatic mixed-function oxidase system. Caffeine clearance is altered during hepatic injury, being prolonged in both chronic hepatitis and cirrhosis.[469] A single dose of caffeine (3.5 mg/kg to a maximum dose of 200 mg, dissolved in either water, fruit juice, or milk for oral administration) is administered. This caffeine dose is equivalent to that found in one cup of brewed coffee or in one can of commercial soft drink. Blood (or salivary samples) obtained before and at timed intervals after caffeine ingestion can be analyzed by reversed-phase HPLC or immunoassay. A close correlation is found between plasma and salivary caffeine concentrations. Caffeine half-life is approximately 5.5 hours in healthy adults and 3 hours in healthy children, with clearance of approximately 2 mL/min/kg in healthy adults and 10 mL/min/kg in healthy children. Caffeine clearance correlates with the aminopyrine breath test and has similar limitations, although it is less subject to effects of variables, such as smoking and oral contraceptive use.[76] *Lidocaine* undergoes N-deethylation in the liver by cytochrome P_{450} to form monoethylglycinexylidide (MEGX); the rate of appearance of MEGX in plasma reflects hepatic lidocaine clearance. Because lidocaine is highly extracted, its clearance is flow-dependent. Thus alterations in hepatic blood flow also influence lidocaine elimination.[493] Lidocaine (1 mg/kg) is given by intravenous bolus; plasma is obtained at baseline and 15 minutes for MEGX concentration (time of plateau concentration in healthy individuals). MEGX is most commonly measured using immunoassay. Lidocaine clearance has been used to assess liver transplant function, but its use is limited by the effect of hypoperfusion (as occurs in sepsis or volume depletion).[165]

Hepatic Storage Function

Because individual cells are unable to store a sufficient supply of energy-rich carbohydrate substrates, the liver serves as the major site for their storage. For example, hepatic storage of glycogen allows the release of glucose to other tissue when the need exists (e.g., when plasma concentrations of glucose decrease). Other tissues, such as muscle and adipose tissue, store proteins and triglycerides, respectively, and are capable of adaptation. Depending on the availability of oxidizable fuels, these tissues also switch from the storage mode to the synthesis or release modes during periods of decreased carbohydrate intake.

CLINICAL MANIFESTATIONS OF LIVER DISEASE

A number of conditions are indicative of liver disease including (1) jaundice, (2) portal hypertension, (3) abnormal hepatorenal function, (4) altered drug metabolism, (5) nutritional and metabolic abnormalities, (6) disordered hemostasis, and (7) the release of enzymes into various body fluids.

Jaundice

Jaundice (or icterus) is a physical sign characterized by a yellow appearance of the skin, mucous membranes, and sclera caused by bilirubin deposition. It is the most specific clinical manifestation of hepatic dysfunction, but is not present in many individuals with liver disease (especially chronic liver disease), and may occur in states of bilirubin overproduction (such as hemolysis). Jaundice is most easily seen in the sclera of the eyes, where yellow contrasts sharply with the usual bright white color. Jaundice is usually apparent clinically when the plasma bilirubin concentration reaches 2 to 3 mg/dL (34 to 51 μmol/L), although higher concentrations may be required when fluorescent lighting is used. When bilirubin clearance from the liver to the intestinal tract is impaired (as in acute hepatitis and bile duct obstruction), it may be accompanied by acholic (gray-colored) stools. Bilirubin is the source of stercobilin, which produces the brown color of normal stool. Increases in plasma conjugated bilirubin lead to tea-colored urine, since conjugated bilirubin is water soluble. Jaundice may also be due to disorders of bilirubin metabolism. Bilirubin metabolism is discussed more fully in Chapter 31. A classification of jaundice, based on the site of altered bilirubin metabolism, is shown in Box 31-1.

Portal Hypertension

The portal circulation handles all of the venous outflow of the GI tract, the spleen, the pancreas, and the gallbladder (Figure 47-11). The portal vein is formed by the union of the splenic vein and the superior mesenteric vein. Portal flow is normally 1000 to 1200 mL/min with a pressure of 5 to 7 mm

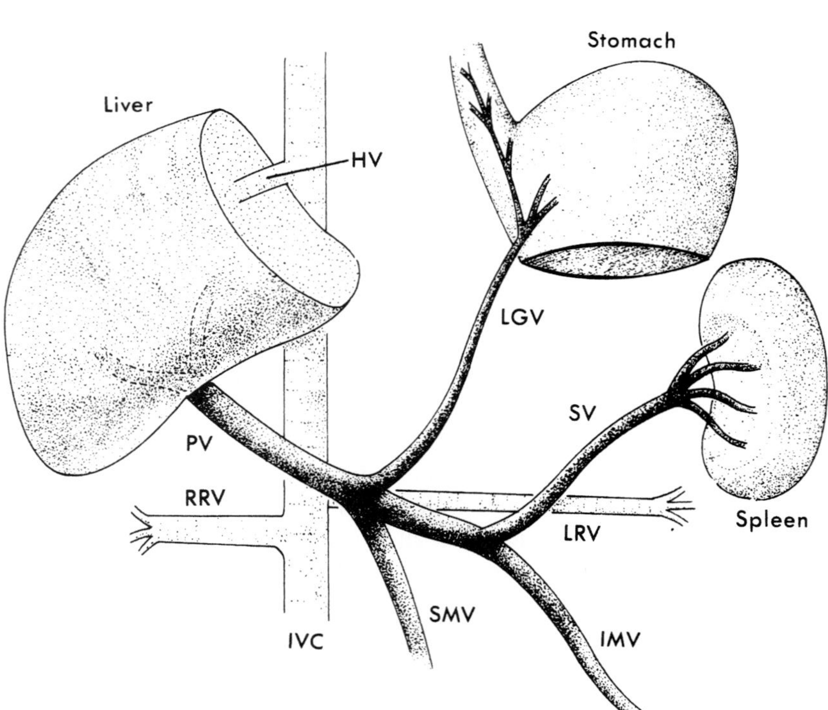

Figure 47-11 The portal-venous system. *HV*, Hepatic vein; *IVC*, inferior vena cava; *IMV*, inferior mesenteric vein; *LGV*, left gastric vein; *LRV*, left renal vein; *PV*, portal vein; *RRV*, right renal vein; *SV*, splenic vein; *SMV*, superior mesenteric vein. *(From Zakim O, Boyer TD. Hepatology: A textbook of liver disease, 3rd ed. Philadelphia: WB Saunders, 1996:721.)*

Hg. Portal hypertension occurs when there is obstruction to portal flow anywhere along its course. The causes of obstruction leading to portal hypertension are classified by site: (1) presinusoidal, (2) sinusoidal, and (3) postsinusoidal. Presinusoidal portal hypertension is most commonly caused by portal vein thrombosis or schistosomiasis but may also occur with increased portal flow, such as occurs with Felty syndrome (a combination of chronic rheumatoid arthritis, splenomegaly, leukopenia, pigmented spots on the lower extremities, and sometimes other evidence of hypersplenism, such as anemia and thrombocytopenia). Sinusoidal hypertension is most commonly caused by cirrhosis but may occur transiently with acute and chronic hepatitis or acute fatty liver. The most important cause of postsinusoidal hypertension is hepatic vein occlusion or Budd-Chiari syndrome, in which sudden obstruction or occlusion of the hepatic veins causes hepatomegaly, abdominal pain, severe ascites, mild jaundice, and eventually portal hypertension and liver failure. The most common cause of postsinusoidal hypertension is cardiac disease, most commonly congestive heart failure. Chronic congestive heart failure is usually associated with portal hypertension and ascites, and may even lead to increased activities of aminotransferases.[317] Other causes include abscesses, membranous obstruction of the vena cava, and veno-occlusive disease (as may be seen in patients following bone marrow transplantation). Although increased portal resistance is the major factor causing portal hypertension, it is often accompanied by decreased resistance to blood flow through other blood vessels, which increases blood flow through the portal veins.

When portal pressure increases, the portal venous system becomes dilated and forms collateral connections to the sys-

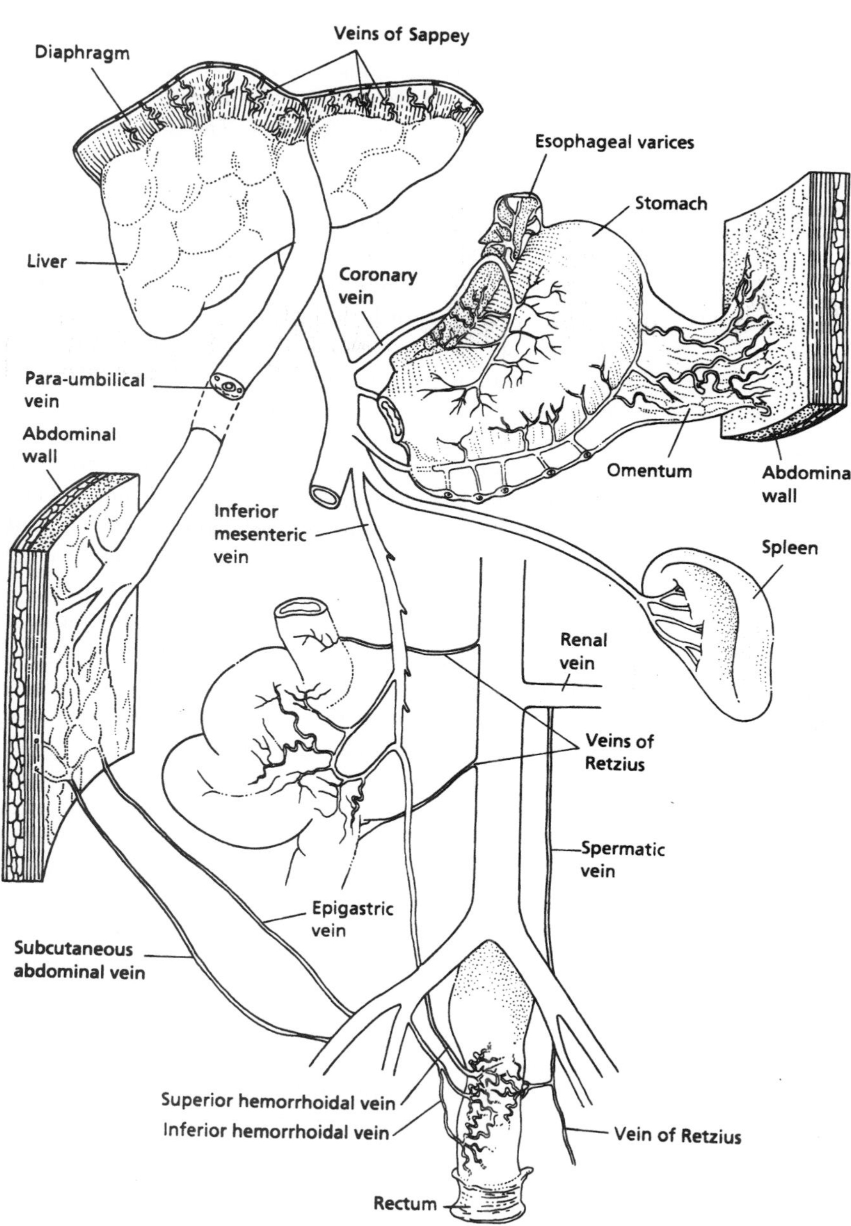

Figure 47-12 The sites of the porto-systemic collateral circulation in cirrhosis of the liver. *(From Sherlock S, Dooley J, eds. Diseases of the liver and biliary system, 9th ed. London: Blackwell Scientific Publications, 1993:134.)*

temic venous flow (Figure 47-12), leading to portosystemic shunting. Initially, this is clinically silent, but as portal hypertension worsens, it compromises many of the metabolic functions of the liver. One such abnormality is altered estrogen metabolism, increasing the ratio of estrogen to testosterone. Clinical consequences include spider telangiectasias and palmar erythema, gynecomastia (in men), and abnormal vaginal bleeding and irregular menstrual periods (in women). Impaired protein metabolic functions lead to the accumulation of ammonia and abnormal neurotransmitters, ultimately leading to hepatic encephalopathy. Because most nutrients arrive through the portal vein, synthetic functions are also impaired, leading to hypoalbuminemia (contributing to ascites), decreased clotting factors (predisposing to bleeding), and reduced thrombolytic factors, such as antithrombin (predisposing to venous thrombosis).

Bleeding Esophageal Varices

The most life-threatening consequence of portosystemic shunting is the development of varices (enlarged and tortuous veins), which can occur throughout the GI tract but are most common in the esophagus and stomach. Bleeding from varices is one of the leading causes of morbidity and mortality in patients with cirrhosis. Varices are present at the time of diagnosis of cirrhosis in about 40% of patients and develop in an additional 6% per year.[105] In general, the risk of bleeding is low until portal vein pressure exceeds 12 mm Hg.[167] The major consequences of varices are rupture and bleeding, usually presenting as hematemesis.

The treatment of portal hypertension and varices is directed at either obliterating the dilated blood vessels or reducing portal pressure. Esophageal and gastric varices can be obliterated by either sclerotherapy or banding; this treatment is typically used for active bleeding or large varices. Sclerotherapy involves the injection by endoscope of a sclerosant (a chemical irritant) into the esophageal varices. Injections are performed weekly until all of the veins are obliterated. Banding is done endoscopically and involves placing rubber bands around dilated blood vessels. Meta-analysis of published studies shows higher efficacy for banding.[252] Occasionally, emergency portacaval shunt therapy is required but is associated with a rather high mortality rate. Esophageal tamponade may be obtained with a Sengstaken-Blakemore tube. This is a four-lumen tube with an esophageal and gastric balloon, and an aspiration tube that is placed in the stomach and in the esophagus above the esophageal balloon. Such balloons are fraught with hazard and are used only in extreme emergencies.

Portal pressure may be reduced pharmacologically. Numerous studies have shown that treatment with β-adrenergic receptor blockers is highly effective in reducing likelihood of bleeding from esophageal varices, and use of β-blockers is now considered the standard of care in individuals with portal hypertension, even if varices have not been documented.[105] As with all vascular epithelium, resistance is modulated by interaction between vasodilators, such as nitric oxide, and vasoconstrictors, such as endothelins. Unfortunately, there is evidence that changes in concentrations of such mediators are different between the liver and the peripheral circulation and, in many cases, exactly opposite. It is thus difficult to simultaneously improve hepatic blood flow and reduce peripheral vasodilation, and addition of nitrates to β-blockers has shown no advantage in lowering portal venous pressure.[166] The goal of treatment is to lower portal pressure below 12 mm Hg to reduce the likelihood of bleeding[140]; this not only lowers the risk of bleeding, but also lowers the likelihood of other complications of cirrhosis and improves survival.[5]

Drugs that specifically modulate portal pressure have yet to be developed. However, it has been shown that vasopressin, nitroglycerin, and octreotide will reduce portal pressure and are useful in acutely lowering portal venous pressure in individuals with active bleeding from varices. Vasopressin is given as a continuous intravenous infusion at 0.4 IU/min. The intense vasoconstriction may lead to myocardial and gastric infarction. Because of these side effects, it is given simultaneously with nitroglycerin, which greatly reduces the vasoconstriction. The success rate in stopping bleeding is about 60% to 70%, but mortality is not reduced. Octreotide works by different mechanisms but has a similar hemodynamic effect with fewer complications. It controls bleeding in 70% to 80% of patients. Pharmacological treatment can be combined with mechanical occlusion of varices by banding or ligation.

Various surgical procedures have been employed to reduce portal pressure. All involve increasing the shunting of blood around the liver to reduce portal pressure. In the past, shunts have been primarily surgical, such as connecting the portal vein to the inferior vena cava (portacaval shunt) or the splenic vein to the renal vein (splenorenal shunt). Currently, shunts are most commonly created by placing a stent through the jugular and hepatic veins to connect to the portal vein, called transjugular intrahepatic portosystemic shunt (TIPS).[269] Since portal flow is already significantly reduced before shunting, there is usually minimal change in liver function, but often reduction in likelihood of ascites and variceal bleeding. There is an increased incidence of hepatic encephalopathy following shunts.

Ascites

Ascites is the effusion and accumulation of fluid in the abdominal cavity. Ascites is the most common clinical finding in patients with portal hypertension. Ascites itself is not life threatening, but is uncomfortable and may compromise respiration (from upward displacement of the diaphragm and compression of the lungs). It also predisposes individuals to spontaneous bacterial peritonitis, which is life threatening.

The pathogenesis of ascites is complex because of a number of simultaneously operating factors. Of these, the most important are (1) increased hydrostatic portal venous pressure, with increased resistance to flow, (2) decreased colloid osmotic (oncotic) pressure because of hypoalbuminemia, and (3) leakage from the surface of the liver of protein-enriched fluid, which increases intraperitoneal colloid pressure. The primary event is probably peripheral vasodilation due to an imbalance of vasoactive factors, including endothelins. The net effect of these forces is to shrink the central blood volume, which decreases renal perfusion and leads to sodium retention through activation of the renin-angiotensin system. The sodium retention leads to water retention, but because of the increased portal hydrostatic pressure and decreased intravascular colloid pressure, the fluid leaks into the so-called third space, causing ascites and edema.

There are many causes of ascites, and it is important to differentiate ascites secondary to portal hypertension from ascites of other causes. This is done by analyzing ascitic fluid. The feature that best distinguishes portal hypertension is an increase in the plasma to ascitic fluid albumin gradient. A gradient greater than 1.1 g/dL is diagnostic of ascites caused by portal hypertension.[12]

Ascites is managed by creating a negative sodium balance or relieving portal hypertension. A negative sodium balance is obtained by reducing sodium intake or enhancing sodium excretion with the use of diuretics or both. Because most diuretics block proximal tubular reabsorption, more sodium is available at the distal renal tubule to exchange with potassium ion. Thus patients tend to become hypokalemic and require potassium preservation either with dietary supplementation or with potassium-sparing diuretics. Ascites may be safely removed with a catheter placed percutaneously through the abdominal wall. Five or 10 liters of fluid may be drained to relieve patient discomfort or respiratory compromise. Because ascitic fluid is nutritionally enriched, repeated fluid drainage leads to significant malnutrition. Repeated paracentesis also requires plasma volume expansion to prevent renal failure; albumin is effective as an expander.[310]

Spontaneous Bacterial Peritonitis

Ascites predisposes to spontaneous bacterial peritonitis, defined as bacteremia (typically gram negative) in the absence of mechanical disruption of the bowel.[96,287] It usually presents in an individual with known cirrhosis who develops abdominal pain, fever, or leukocytosis. The diagnosis is established by examination of the ascitic fluid; greater than 250 neutrophils per microliter, or more than 500 in the absence of a positive blood culture, is considered diagnostic.[52,301] In contrast, secondary peritonitis is usually associated with higher neutrophil counts, low glucose in ascitic fluid, and high protein.[13]

Hepatic (Portosystemic) Encephalopathy

Hepatic encephalopathy is a metabolic disorder characterized by a wide spectrum of neuropsychiatric dysfunction.[69] It may occur as an acute syndrome in patients with acute hepatic failure from viral or drug-induced hepatitis or as a chronic syndrome associated with liver failure and cirrhosis. As implied by the synonym, chronic hepatic encephalopathy occurs in the setting of portosystemic shunting, usually as a result of cirrhosis.

The clinical syndrome is variable but follows a reasonably predictable course. Disturbed consciousness always occurs. It usually starts as hypersomnia and progresses to sleep reversal in which the patient tends to sleep through the day and be awake at night. This is followed by decreased spontaneous movement, apathy, and gradually increasing levels of coma. Personality changes may be conspicuous, especially in patients with chronic disease. Irritability and disturbed social behavior may follow. Intellectual deterioration occurs (but is difficult to detect in its early stages because of confabulation) and generally progresses to overt confusion. Neurological abnormalities include slurred speech, a characteristic flapping tremor called asterixis, increased muscle tone, and abnormal reflexes. Disturbed gait may ensue. In chronic encephalopathy, these changes typically fluctuate over time and follow a waxing and waning course. Acute encephalopathy progresses rapidly, often within hours, and is characterized by cerebral edema, which may result in brain stem herniation and death.[94]

The pathophysiology of hepatic encephalopathy is not completely understood but includes an increased sensitivity to dietary proteins. Ammonia concentrations are always increased with acute encephalopathy and usually increased with chronic encephalopathy. A reduction of plasma ammonia is often associated with symptomatic improvement. However, since plasma ammonia concentrations do not correlate with the severity of the encephalopathy, it has been suggested that other factors are involved.[80,451] It is now recognized that a variety of neurotransmitter systems are dysfunctional in hepatic encephalopathy, but the exact cause for the changes is not known.[16] One important contributor is the endogenous benzodiazepine agonist system, but other abnormalities must be invoked to explain all the findings.[451]

The diagnosis of hepatic encephalopathy is made on clinical grounds. Plasma ammonia concentrations are rarely helpful, either for diagnosis or for monitoring the patient's disorder; normal ammonia concentrations are helpful in excluding hepatic encephalopathy as a cause of cerebral dysfunction. An exception is a patient who presents with acute encephalopathy of unknown cause. Elevated ammonia concentrations in that situation suggest acute hepatic failure or Reye's syndrome.

Treatment is largely empirical, based on observations that intestinal bacteria and protein loads in the intestinal tract are important in the symptoms of hepatic encephalopathy.[50] Lactulose has long been recognized to reduce the symptoms in chronic hepatic encephalopathy. Antibiotic treatment with a nonabsorbable antibiotic such as neomycin reduces the number of bacteria and is especially helpful in patients with GI bleeding. Protein reduction in the diet also improves encephalopathy; reducing dietary protein to the less than 40 g/day often needed to improve symptoms may compromise nutrition. Patients with acute encephalopathy require measures to reduce intracranial pressure, such as osmotic diuretics.

Hepatorenal Syndrome

Hepatorenal syndrome (HRS) refers to decreased renal function secondary to hepatic disease; portal hypertension is a common factor in all cases of HRS developing in chronic liver disease, but HRS may also develop in acute liver failure. Although formerly thought to be a rapidly progressing, terminal event in a person with end-stage liver disease, it is now recognized that HRS falls into two major varieties.[31] Type 2 HRS is more common; it represents a slowly progressive or stable decline in renal function that is due to peripheral vasodilation and renal vasoconstriction. Type 1, or classic, HRS represents rapidly declining renal function, usually developing in a person with preexisting type 2 HRS. Type 1 HRS usually develops in the setting of an acute decrease in blood pressure, often due to spontaneous bacterial peritonitis or variceal bleeding.

The common feature in both forms of HRS is activation of the renin-angiotensin-aldosterone axis caused by intravascular volume depletion.[32] As with other forms of prerenal azotemia, HRS in the untreated patient is generally associated with increased antidiuretic hormone and with profound thirst. This leads to development of hyponatremia, hypokalemia, metabolic alkalosis, low urine sodium and high urine potassium excretion, and high urine osmolality. BUN, creatinine, and creatinine clearance are not reliable indicators of renal function in HRS.[31,116] Urea is produced by the liver and is often decreased in advanced liver disease; it is also increased after upper GI bleeding, a common cause for worsening of renal function in HRS. Creatinine production by muscle is reduced in cirrhosis, causing falsely low serum creatinine and creatinine clearance. Although cystatin-C has slightly better correlation with measured glomerular filtration rate (GFR), it is not clear that it reliably reflects renal function in cirrhotic individuals.

Treatment of HRS is best accomplished by either increasing systemic vascular resistance, as with the vasopressin analogue terlipressin, or reducing portal venous pressure, most commonly accomplished with TIPS. Both have shown promise in improving renal function in HRS.[17,247,471]

Altered Drug Metabolism

Because of the liver's central role in drug metabolism and disposition, alterations in drug metabolism may occur in patients with liver disease. In general, this is reflected in delayed metabolism such that the interval between drug doses has to be increased for drugs that are metabolized by the liver. Only patients with evidence of liver failure, such as encephalopathy, coagulopathy, or ascites, need alterations in dosing. In general, patients with liver disease are not more susceptible to drug-induced hepatotoxicity. However, patients with alcoholic liver disease who continue to consume alcohol are susceptible to liver injury from acetaminophen, even at therapeutic doses.[398]

Nutritional and Metabolic Abnormalities

The intake and disposition of nutrients in patients with chronic liver disease are altered, which subjects them to nutritional imbalance. Severe metabolic and nutritional derangements have been observed to occur in the cirrhotic patient including alterations in glucose metabolism caused by insulin resistance, and hypokalemia caused by secondary hyperaldosteronism in cirrhosis. In addition, hypoalbuminemia is frequently present because of decreased production and sinusoidal leakage of albumin in patients with portal hypertension. Also, in patients with chronic cholestasis, impaired delivery of bile salts to the duodenum results in malabsorption of lipids and fat soluble vitamins, leading to deficiencies in vitamins A, D, E, and K (see Chapters 30 and 49). Vitamin A deficiency may cause night blindness, but rarely progresses to serious visual impairment. Vitamin D deficiency causes osteopenia and, in severe cases, osteomalacia. In fact, osteopenic bone disease may be one of the most crippling results of chronic cholestatic liver disease, such as primary biliary cirrhosis.[192] Vitamin E deficiency is of little clinical significance. Vitamin K deficiency leads to hypoprothrombinemia, with easy bruising and bleeding.

Disordered Hemostasis in Liver Disease

The liver manufactures most of the clotting factors (the major exception being von Willebrand factor) and bile salts that are essential for absorption of vitamin K. The liver also clears activated clotting factors from the circulation. Thus chronic liver disease is associated with both a hemorrhagic tendency and a hypercoagulable state.[237]

The liver synthesizes fibrinogen factors V, VIII, XI, and XII, and the vitamin K–dependent factors II, VII, IX, and X. Furthermore the liver plays an important role in platelet growth and function. The vitamin K–dependent proteins contain γ-carboxy-glutamic acid. Vitamin K is necessary for the carboxylation of these proteins, which facilitate the conversion of prothrombin to thrombin. Patients with severe hepatocellular disease have decreased synthesis of the vitamin K–dependent clotting factors, especially factor VII. Furthermore, patients with cholestatic disease have decreased bile salt secretion, which is necessary for the absorption of vitamin K, leading to failure of activation of factors II, VII, IX, and X. In these patients, unlike those with hepatocellular disease, the prothrombin time can be corrected with an injection of vitamin K.

Disorders of fibrinogen also occur in the liver. For example, dysfibrinogenemia may be seen in both acute and chronic liver disease and leads to prolongation of the partial thromboplastin time.[158] Disseminated intravascular coagulation occurs with acute hepatic necrosis, presumably as a result of the release of tissue thromboplastin and defective clearance of inhibitors such as antithrombin and protein C. Thrombocytopenia may contribute to ineffective intravascular coagulation. Although commonly attributed to splenic sequestration (hypersplenism), there is evidence of antibody-mediated platelet destruction, as occurs in immune thrombocytopenic purpura.[228] Patients with chronic or severe liver disease also may be hypercoagulable because of deficiency of liver-produced inhibitors of coagulation, such as antithrombin and proteins C and S. Patients with autoimmune hepatitis may have anticardiolipin antibodies and antibodies to platelets.

ENZYMES RELEASED FROM DISEASED LIVER TISSUE

Because hepatic function is often normal in many patients with liver disease, the plasma activities of numerous cytosolic, mitochondrial, and membrane-associated enzymes are measured as they are increased in many forms of liver disease. As plasma enzyme measurements are discussed in greater detail in Chapter 21, only those factors relevant to understanding of liver disease will be summarized here.

Because the pattern and degree of elevation of enzyme activity vary with the type of liver disease, their measurement is extremely helpful in the recognition and differential diagnosis of liver damage. A number of factors govern the ability of liver enzymes to assist in diagnosis including their (1) tissue specificity, (2) subcellular distribution, (3) relative activity of enzyme activity in liver and plasma, (4) patterns of release, and (5) clearance from plasma.

Tissue Specificity

There are five enzymes that are commonly used in diagnosis of liver disease: Aspartate aminotransferase (AST; EC 2.6.1.1), alanine aminotransferase (ALT; EC 2.6.1.2), alkaline phosphatase (ALP; 3.1.3.1), and γ-glutamyl transferase (GGT; EC 2.3.2.2), are commonly used to detect liver injury, and lactate dehydrogenase (LD; EC 1.1.1.27) is occasionally used. ALT and GGT are present in several tissues, but plasma activities primarily reflect liver injury. AST is found in liver, muscle (cardiac and skeletal), and to a limited extent in red cells. LD has wide tissue distribution, and is thus relatively nonspecific. ALP is found in a number of tissues, but in normal individuals primarily reflects bone and liver sources. Thus based on tissue distribution, ALT and GGT would seem to be the most specific markers for liver injury.

Subcellular Distribution

Enzymes are found at different locations within cells. AST, ALT, and LD are cytosolic enzymes. As such, they can be released with cell injury, and appear in plasma relatively rapidly. In the case of AST and ALT, there are both mitochondrial and cytosolic isoenzymes in hepatocytes and other cells containing these enzymes. In the case of ALT, the relative amount of mitochondrial isoenzyme is small, and its plasma half-life is extremely short, making it of no diagnostic significance. In the case of AST, the mitochondrial isoenzyme represents a significant fraction of total AST within hepatocytes. In contrast, ALP and GGT are membrane-bound glycoprotein enzymes. The most important location of both enzymes is on the canalicular membrane of hepatocytes.

Relative Activity in Liver and Plasma

For cytoplasmic enzymes, the relative amount of enzyme in the liver relative to plasma is an important determinant of sensitivity. The activity of AST within hepatocytes is about twice that of ALT, although plasma activities are similar. In contrast, hepatocyte activities of LD are much lower (relative to plasma) than those of the other two enzymes, and plasma activities of LD are several times higher than those of AST and ALT. This means that there is less of an increase in LD with liver injury than occurs with AST and ALT. The relative amount of enzyme in tissue is not necessarily the same in disease; in cirrhosis and malnutrition, there are greater decreases in cytoplasmic ALT than in cytoplasmic AST.[272]

Mechanisms of Release

Several mechanisms appear to be involved in release of enzymes from hepatocytes. Cell injury is the simplest mechanism and appears to allow leakage of cytoplasmic enzymes from cells, but minimal release of other types of enzymes. Thus necroinflammatory disease leads to release of AST and ALT, and to a lesser extent LD, but not to mitochondrial isoenzyme of AST nor to release of ALP or GGT.[230] Alcohol appears to induce expression of mitochondrial AST on the surface of hepatocytes[492]; not surprisingly, alcoholic hepatitis is associated with increased plasma activities of this isoenzyme.[321,339]

The mechanism of release of membrane-bound enzymes such as GGT and ALP into the circulation is less well understood. There appears to be increased synthesis of GGT and ALP in diseased human liver.[313] How this enhanced synthesis of tissue-bound enzymes translates into increased activity in plasma is not clear. However, fragments of hepatocyte membrane rich in GGT and ALP activity have been detected in plasma of patients with cholestasis, a process that may be a result of membrane fragmentation by bile acids. Furthermore, bile acids, which are detergents, could solubilize and release GGT and ALP from plasma membranes. In vitro studies of membranes treated with bile acids demonstrate that this possibility exists.[391]

Rate of Clearance of Enzyme from Plasma

Clearance of liver enzymes from plasma occurs at variable rates. The half-life of ALT is 47 hours, of cytosolic AST, 17 hours; thus although more AST is released from liver, the much longer half-life of ALT leads to higher activities of ALT than AST in most forms of hepatocellular injury. The half-life of the liver isoenzyme of ALP has been variously reported as from 1 to 10 days; the former figure appears to correspond better to the changes seen with removal of gallstones. The half-life of GGT has been reported as 4.1 days. The mechanism by which enzymes are removed from circulation is not completely known, although receptor-mediated endocytosis by liver macrophages is likely involved.

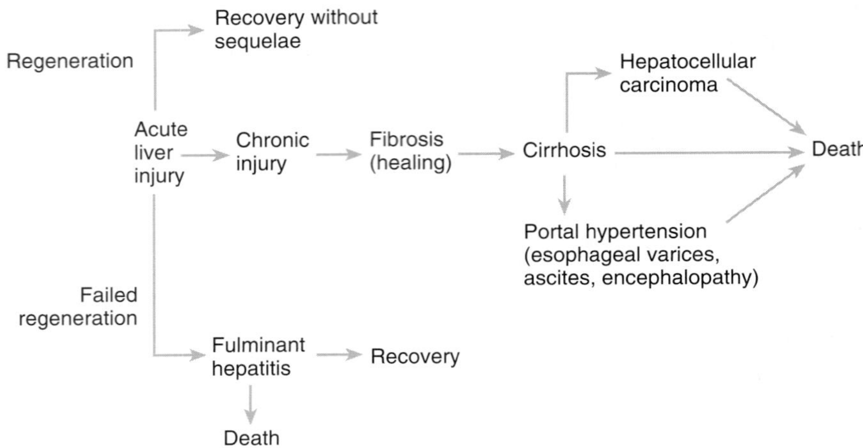

Figure 47-13 Natural history of liver disease.

DISEASES OF THE LIVER

The liver has a limited number of ways of responding to injury. Acute injury to the liver may be asymptomatic, but often presents as jaundice. The two major acute liver diseases are acute hepatitis and cholestasis. Chronic liver injury generally takes the clinical form of chronic hepatitis; its long-term complications include cirrhosis and HCC. The discussion of liver disease will focus mainly on these patterns, and a few diseases that differ from this general pattern. Because the types of disease seen in neonates differ significantly from this model, diseases of infancy are discussed separately in Chapter 31.

Mechanisms and Patterns of Injury

Cell death occurs by necrosis or apoptosis or both. The target cell determines the pattern of injury, with hepatocyte injury leading to hepatocellular disease and biliary cell injury leading to cholestasis. All cellular injury induces fibrosis as an adaptive or healing response, with the duration of injury and genetic factors determining whether cirrhosis and ultimately carcinoma occur (Figure 47-13).

Cellular necrosis occurs as the result of an injurious environment and has been referred to as "murder." It is characterized by cellular swelling with loss of membrane integrity. Toxic injury from compounds such as carbon tetrachloride, aspirin, and acetaminophen (Figure 47-14) occurs for the most part by necrosis. Apoptosis occurs as the result of accelerated programmed death in which the cell participates in its own demise and thus commits "suicide." It is characterized by cell shrinkage, with nuclear chromatin condensation and fragmentation forming apoptotic bodies. Regardless of the cause, cell death typically leads to leakage of cytoplasmic enzymes.

Laboratory tests are helpful in distinguishing the (1) pattern of injury (hepatocellular versus cholestatic), (2) chronicity of injury (acute versus chronic), and (3) severity of injury (mild versus severe). In general, the aminotransferase enzymes and ALP are used to distinguish the pattern, plasma albumin to determine the chronicity, and the PT or factor V concentration to determine the severity. At the present time, the only way to accurately detect fibrosis is by a liver biopsy.

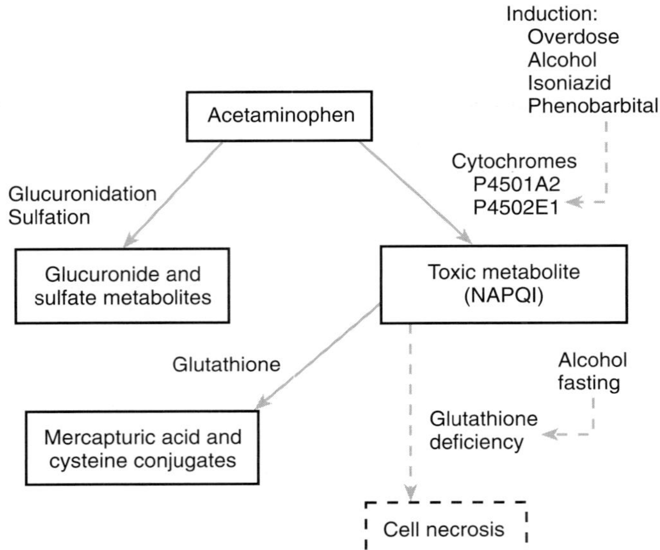

Figure 47-14 Metabolism of acetaminophen by the liver.

Disorders of Bilirubin Metabolism

Defects in bilirubin metabolism resulting in jaundice are known to occur at each step in the metabolic pathway (see Figure 31-22, Chapter 31). Disorders related to these defects are discussed in Chapter 31 (see Box 31-1)

Hepatic Viral Infection

Five viruses have been identified (A, B, C, D, E) as causes of infection that primarily targets the liver. In addition, certain other viruses may infect the liver as part of a more generalized infection, among them cytomegalovirus (CMV), Epstein-Barr virus (EBV), and herpes simplex virus (HSV).

TABLE 47-2 Types of Viral Hepatitis

	A	B	C	D	E	G
Type	RNA	DNA	RNA	Partial	RNA	RNA
Incubation period (d)	45-50	30-150	15-160	30-150	20-40	Unknown
Transmission						
Fecal-oral	Yes	No	Minimal	No	Yes	No
Household	Yes	Min	Min	Yes	Yes	No
Vertical	No	Yes	Min	Yes	No	Yes
Blood	Rare	Yes	Yes	Yes	Unknown	Yes
Sexual	No	Yes	Min	Yes	Unknown	Yes
Diagnosis	Anti-HAV IgM	HBsAg, PCR, anti-HBc IgM	Anti-HCV, PCR	Anti-HDV	Anti-HEV	Anti-HGV
Carrier state	No	Yes	Yes	Yes	Yes	Yes
Chronic hepatitis	No	10%	80%	Yes	No	No
Liver cancer	No	Yes	Yes	No	No	No
Prevention						
Vaccine	Yes	Yes	No	Yes*	No	No
Immunoglobulin	Yes	Yes	No	Yes*	No	No
Response to interferon	Not used	50%	20-45%	Yes	Not used	Yes

HAV, Hepatitis A virus; *HBsAg,* hepatitis B surface antigen; *PCR,* polymerase chain reaction; *IgM,* immunoglobulin M; *HCV,* hepatitis C virus; *HDV,* hepatitis D virus; *HEV,* hepatitis E virus; *HGV,* hepatitis G virus.
*Vaccination and passive immunization against HBV protects against HDV infection.

Several other viruses have been proposed as causes of liver injury; these include hepatitis G virus[1] (discussed below), transfusion-transmitted virus (TTV),[198] and the closely related SEN-V virus.[472] Although all three are blood borne chronic viral infections and, in the case of TTV and SEN-V, have been known to replicate in the liver, none of these viruses appear to cause acute or chronic liver injury.[332,445,481] The various hepatitis viruses are outlined in Table 47-2.

Hepatitis A Virus

Hepatitis A virus (HAV) accounts for about one fourth to one third the cases of clinical acute hepatitis in the United States and 20% to 25% worldwide. Although most commonly an infection of children and adolescents, the disease tends to be more virulent in middle-aged and older people. Most sporadic cases occur from person-to-person contact, such as occurs in children in day care centers. Epidemics have been associated with waterborne and food-borne contamination. Ingestion of raw shellfish from contaminated waters has caused both sporadic and epidemic cases. Although not as common a cause of liver infection as hepatitis B, it is more frequently associated with jaundice when occurring in adults than either hepatitis B or C; an estimated 50% to 70% of infected adults develop jaundice. In contrast, hepatitis A infection in children is rarely associated with jaundice, and thus is usually not detected clinically. The incidence of the disease is declining in the developed world with introduction of hepatitis A vaccine; complete immunization of less than half the at-risk population has been shown to reduce incidence of acute hepatitis A infection by more than 90% in areas of high endemicity.[34] Universal vaccination of infants in the United States is not currently recommended by the Centers for Disease Control and Prevention (CDC)[365]; immunization is recommended for children residing in areas with higher than average incidence of HAV, in individuals traveling to endemic areas, and in individuals who have chronic liver disease.

Hepatitis A is caused by a 27-nm RNA picornavirus. It has four capsid proteins (VP1-4), but only one serotype has been identified. The virus is not cytopathic to hepatoctyes, but causes liver injury by stimulating both cellular and humoral immune responses. Hepatitis A occurs in sporadic and epidemic forms, with an incubation period of 15 to 50 days. The clinical course of acute hepatitis A is usually that of a mild flulike illness that lasts for a few days to a few weeks. There is no chronic form of hepatitis A, but cholestasis (manifested by several weeks of jaundice and pruritus) may occur in some adults. Although a rare occurence, relapse in up to 5% of patients has been known to happen 1 to 3 months after the acute illness. It resembles the acute illness and is associated with viremia, but recovery always ensues.

Hepatitis B Virus

Hepatitis B virus (HBV) is the most common cause of acute hepatitis, and the most common chronic viral infection worldwide.[2] An estimated 350 million individuals are chronically infected with HBV, and several times as many individuals have been exposed to HBV. The frequency of chronic HBV infection varies worldwide. For example it is high in Asia and Africa but occurs rarely among those born in North America and Europe[135]; one study found that 86% of US residents with chronic HBV were actually born outside of the

United States.[241A] HBV is transmitted through body fluids, primarily by parenteral or sexual contact; it can be transmitted from mother to child, usually at or after delivery (termed vertical transmission). In parts of the world with high rates of chronic infection, much of the transmission is vertical. The residual risk from transfusion is estimated to be 1 in 600,000.[67]

Hepatitis B is caused by a 42-nm DNA virus that is a member of the hepadnavirus family. The DNA is partially double stranded, contains 3200 nucleotides, and has been cloned.[4] There are several major open reading frames. The S gene codes for HBsAg, a surface protein produced independently of and in excess of the amount needed for viral replication. The C gene encodes for HBcAg, part of the infectious core of the virus. The X gene codes for a transactivating factor that may be involved with viral replication and the development of malignancy. The precore region codes for production of the HBeAg, a protein found only in those with (but separate from) circulating viral particles. Hepadnaviruses are unusual among DNA viruses in that they reproduce from an RNA template using reverse transcriptase. Although DNA replication has a proofreading mechanism, reverse transcriptase does not; hepadnaviruses are thus prone to developing mutant strains. The significance of several mutants is described below.

Hepatitis B was first described in the 1960s by Blumberg and colleagues following discovery of a protein, termed the Australia antigen, that was initially felt to be a tumor marker for leukemia. Subsequent studies confirmed it to be a marker for a form of hepatitis initially termed serum hepatitis.[23] Later work establishrd that this was hepatitis B surface antigen (HBsAg). The complete HBV particle (Dane particle) of viral DNA consists of a core containing a number of proteins and envelope and surface proteins. The core, formed in infected cells, contains viral DNA, DNA polymerase, and core antigen (HBcAg). The surface protein (HBsAg) contains a common determinant, a, and four subdeterminants designated d, y, w, and r. The four major determinants are adw, adr, ayw, and ayr. Because the determinants breed true, they are helpful in epidemiological studies.[46] HBV species also have been classified into genotypes A-H; genotypes have less than 92% homology with other types. Although not routinely distinguished, there is evidence that genotype differences may have prognostic importance in chronic HBV infections. There are geographic differences in genotype distribution; genotype A predominates among those infected in North America, whereas genotype C is the dominant form in those infected in Asia. Genotype B is associated with a higher rate of spontaneous clearance in chronic infection,[484] slower progression of liver disease,[421] and better response to antiviral therapy[455] when compared with genotype C.

There are several mutants of HBV that may have clinical importance. The most common is due to one of a variety of mutations in the precore gene, most commonly a mutation at nucleotide 1896 that inserts a stop codon in the mRNA.[88] Mutations in the promoter region of the precore gene, particularly at nucleotides 1762 and 1764, are associated with reduced production of normal HBeAg. Such mutants are associated with undetectable HBeAg, although they are characterized by production of anti-HBe. Since HBeAg is often used as a marker of the presence of replicating virus, and anti-HBe with the absence of infectious virus, this limits utility of HBeAg testing. Precore mutants are found in the majority of individuals chronically infected with HBV in areas with high rates of infection, such as Asia and Southern Europe. In North America, it is estimated that 10% to 20% of individuals with chronic HBV infection have such precore mutants.[205] Such mutants may be present at the time of infection or may develop during the course of disease. Although initially it was thought that individuals infected with such mutants are much more likely to have severe acute infection, the high prevalence of such mutants suggests that this is not the case. Treatment with antiviral agents is equally effective in eradicating virus in the nonmutated and mutant strains. One of the most commonly used agents to treat HBV is the reverse transcriptase inhibitor lamivudine. As is true in HIV, there are specific mutations that confer resistance to antiretroviral agents. One common form involves mutations in the YMDD nucleotide binding region of the protease gene, in which substitution of isoleucine for methionine at amino acid 552 notably decreases lamivudine response.[18] Mutations can also affect other parts of the genome, and several strains with point mutations in HBsAg have also been identified. These mutants appear to be extremely rare; their major significance is that they may not be detected by immunoassays for HBsAg.[93] Rarely, infections by such mutants occur in individuals successfully immunized against HBV.[204] There is concern that such mutants may become more widespread, because their detection will be difficult and unexpected in those who have "protective" antibody titers from vaccination.[159]

Chronic infection with HBV occurs in two major forms. In the more severe form, chronic infection is associated with viral replication, reinfection of newly produced hepatocytes, and ongoing chronic inflammation (chronic hepatitis). Antiviral treatment is effective in suppressing viral replication in less than one third of such cases treated for one year; longer treatment with lamivudine increases response rate up to 60%-70%, but increases likelihood of development of resistant mutants. Individuals with ongoing viral replication have an estimated 30% risk of progression to cirrhosis over many years and have a sixtyfold increased risk of HCC (compared with those who are HBsAg negative).[477] In the less severe form, viral DNA becomes integrated into host DNA, and no viral replication occurs. Individuals with nonreplicating infection have minimal or no chronic inflammation and no risk of development of cirrhosis, but have a tenfold higher risk of development of HCC.[477]

Immunization. Hepatitis B may be prevented by either passive (hepatitis B immune globulin [HBIG]) or active (hepatitis B recombinant vaccine) immunization. Initially, vaccination was targeted toward high-risk individuals, such as (1) babies of infected mothers, (2) individuals with promiscuous sexual practices, (3) health care workers, and (4) individuals having sexual contacts with infected individuals. In the United States, current data suggest that more than 90% of children have been immunized against HBV infection; most cases of HBV seen in the United States are now occurring in those born outside the United States or in their children. The incidence of acute HBV infection fell by more than 80% after initiation of immunization.[175,301A] Since infants born to HBsAg mothers have a high risk of developing chronic HBV infection, routine prenatal testing for HBsAg is needed to identify infants at risk. Infection occurs in only about 2% of infants before birth[428]; postexposure prophylaxis (typically used in infants of HBsAg positive mothers) consisting of passive immunization with 0.06 mL/kg of HBIG and the first dose of hepatitis B vaccine within 24 hours of birth is more than 95% effective in preventing infection.[114] A universal immunization program in Taiwan, where vertical transmission of HBV was endemic, greatly reduced the death rate from HCC in young individuals.[83]

Diagnostic Tests for Hepatitis B. Hepatitis B has the largest number of diagnostic tests of any of the hepatitis viruses, which makes for a more complicated interpretation of results. Testing currently involves primarily ELISA or related techniques to measure viral antigens or antibodies, but nucleic acid–based tests are becoming more widely used.

Hepatitis B surface antigen, the most widely used marker for detecting current hepatitis B infection, is detected by kits using antibody to HBsAg. Occasionally, false positive results occur in testing, particularly during pregnancy; a neutralization assay is available. Low level reactivity (as evaluated by the ratio of the signal from the sample to that of the cutoff for distinguishing positive and negative, termed the signal:cutoff [S/C] ratio) is highly predictive of samples that fail to confirm on neutralization.[336] False negative results can occur with mutants in the surface antigen; different assays differ in their ability to detect such mutants.[93]

Antibody to the hepatitis B core antigen (anti-HBc) is the most commonly detected antibody against HBV. Two assays are usually employed: IgM and total anti-HBc. IgM anti-HBc assays typically employ a large dilution of plasma (1:100) before analysis to reduce the likelihood of positivity in individuals with chronic HBV. The total antibody assay measures both IgM and IgG antibodies. Anti-HBc appears to last longer than anti-HBs in natural infection, and is still present in 97% of previously infected individuals more than 30 years after exposure. Isolated anti-HBc is a relatively common finding, particularly in the setting of HCV co-infection, but also in immunosuppressed individuals.[460] Although this may represent a false positive result, particularly as a transient phenomenon following influenza vaccination, current guidelines on hepatitis B recommend considering individuals with isolated anti-HBc to be considered hepatitis B immune.

Antibody to the hepatitis B surface antigen (anti-HBs) is considered evidence of immunity to hepatitis B and is the only marker found in those receiving the hepatitis B vaccine. The World Health Organization has developed a standard, defined as 10 IU/mL of anti-HBs. Current guidelines suggest that immunocompetent individuals who ever achieve an anti-HBs of 10 IU/mL or greater have life-long immunity to hepatitis B.

The hepatitis Be antigen (HBeAg) and antibody to the e antigen (anti-HBe) are typically used only in the setting of chronic HBV infection. Although HBeAg typically appears at about the same time as HBsAg in acute hepatitis, it is rarely used as a marker for acute infection. In chronic infection, HBeAg is used as a marker of persistence of infectious virus; its clearance and the appearance of anti-HBe have been used as indicators of conversion to the nonreplicating state and as goals of antiviral treatment. As discussed earlier, however, conversion may also occur with development of mutations in the precore region. Although presence of HBeAg is a specific marker for presence of replicating virus, the sensitivity of antigen detection for the presence of replicating virus is less than ideal. In parts of the world where precore mutants are common, patients with negative HBeAg and positive anti-HBe require further testing using HBV DNA to clarify the status of their infection. Such testing is becoming more common even in Europe and North America, where precore mutants are relatively rare.

Hepatitis B viral DNA is now often measured using an amplification technique (see Chapter 37). Until relatively recently, non-amplified assays were used that had relatively high limits of detection (compared with assays for HIV or HCV RNA or amplified HBV DNA assays). HBV DNA was typically reported in pg/mL; this amount of HBV DNA is equivalent to 285,000 copies/mL, with assays having lower detection limits of 0.5 pg/mL to 5 to 10 pg/mL. In 2001, the World Health Organization established an international standard for HBV DNA nucleic acid amplification techniques.[384] Currently, assays using amplification, particularly PCR methods, have detection limits in the range of 100 copies/mL, although non-amplified assays are still available. It is unclear what level of HBV DNA represents clinically important viremia, but two clinical practice guidelines have adopted 100,000 copies/mL as a "clinically significant" level of viremia.[267] In a large number of "carriers" of HBV, 97% had HBV DNA below 100,000 copies/mL,[282] and 89% of individuals who failed to clear the virus with antiviral treatment had HBV DNA above 100,000 copies/mL.[87] These data supports a value of 100,000 copies/mL as a good decision point for "significant" viremia. Alternatively the likelihood of response to treatment is low in those who do not have a complete suppression of HBV DNA to less than 100,000 copies/mL after 3 months of treatment.[68] As will be discussed later, however, the evolving concept of "occult" HBV infection may require use of much lower thresholds to define "significant" viremia.

Hepatitis B mutants are usually determined by direct sequencing. A line probe method has been developed for detecting the three most common mutants causing HBeAg negative chronic infection. YMDD mutants can be detected by a number of sequencing and hybridization assays. Genotype have been determined by various methods including direct sequencing, restriction fragment length polymorphism, line probe assay, or serotype.

Hepatitis C Virus

The hepatitis C virus (HCV) was the cause of the majority of cases previously known as non-A, non-B hepatitis. It was recognized in 1989[86] and fully characterized 2 years later.[203] It is the most common cause of chronic hepatitis in North America, Europe, and Japan; it is estimated to infect approximately 170 million individuals worldwide. Although HBV infection appears to have been present for a long time, there is evidence that HCV is a more recently developing viral infection, because rates of HCV-related liver disease have been increasing in many parts of the world. Predictions are that HCV-related end stage chronic liver disease will increase twofold to threefold over the next 20 to 30 years.[109] HCV infection primarily occurs through plasma; the major risk factors are injection drug use and transfusion. For example, before the recognition of and availability of tests for HCV, the frequency of post-transfusion hepatitis (mainly due to HCV) was 3.5%[395A]; the risk of HCV transmission by transfusion was estimated at 1:2,000,000.[67] Because of its mode of spread, HCV infection is rare in children; the only common causes of pediatric infection are vertical transmission from an infected mother (estimated to occur in about 5% of infected women)[373] and, previously, transfusion of infected blood.

HCV is a single-stranded enveloped RNA virus of the flavivirus family, which includes other hepatitis viruses (yellow fever virus) and viruses that cause unrelated disease (such as West Nile virus). HCV RNA contains one reading frame (Figure 47-15). The resulting polypeptide is cleaved to core and envelope antigens and a number of nonstructural (NS) proteins, including a polymerase, a protease, and an interferon-response element. As an RNA virus, HCV is subject to a high rate of spontaneous mutation, giving rise to large numbers of variants. This results in six major genotypes (<70% nucleotide homology), along with a number of subtypes (77% to 80% homology).[62] In a chronically infected individual, there are numerous quasispecies (>90% homology) that develop over time. These quasispecies seem to be important in establishing chronic infection[143] and appear related to the fluctuating nature of chronic inflammation in chronic HCV infection.[142] Quasispecies are unique to the individual infected; those infected from a common source show different patterns of mutation.[263]

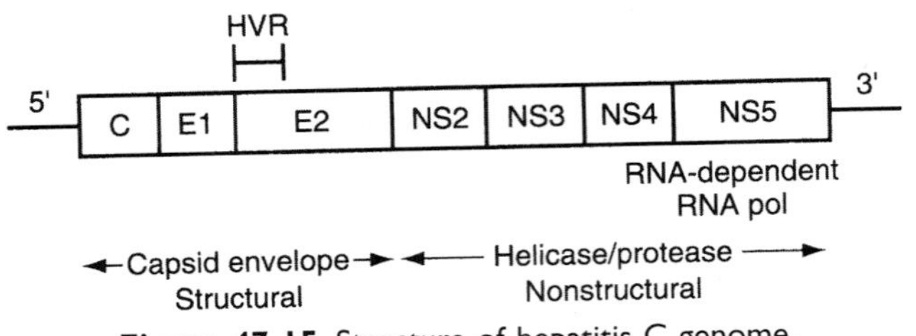

Figure 47-15 Structure of hepatitis C genome.

Chronic HCV infection is associated with evidence of chronic liver injury in most cases. Elevations in liver-associated enzymes, particularly ALT, are usually mild and fluctuate between normal and abnormal in most infected individuals. In an estimated 15% to 20% of cases, cirrhosis becomes evident an average of 20 to 30 years after exposure. HCC may develop once cirrhosis is present at an average rate of 1.5 to 3 cases per year. In North America, Europe, and Japan, HCV is the most common risk factor in development of HCC. There are a number of extrahepatic manifestations of chronic HCV infection; the most common are cryoglobulinemia and porphyria cutanea tarda. There is epidemiological evidence linking HCV to increased risk of lymphoma and type 2 diabetes mellitus.

Prevention. Prevention of hepatitis C has proven to be more difficult than with HAV and HBV. However, there has been an 80% decrease in incidence of acute HCV over the past decade, which is thought to be due to testing blood donors for HCV and to safe injection practices instituted to reduce risk of HIV infection. Vaccine development has been difficult because of the many subspecies of virus and the presence of many quasispecies with different antigenic determinants. There have been significant improvements in treatment of HCV infection, however. Treatment of acute hepatitis C with α-interferon monotherapy has been found effective in preventing chronic hepatitis in a large majority of patients in nonrandomized trials. The use of pegylated interferon and ribavirin combination therapy leads to viral eradication in about 75% of those infected with genotypes 2, 3 and 4, and almost half of those infected with genotype 1.

Diagnostic Tests for Hepatitis C. Antibody to HCV (anti-HCV) is the principal screening test for HCV exposure. The tests, using ELISA and related microparticle, chemiluminescence formats, detect the presence of antibodies to one or more HCV antigens (derived by recombinant technology from yeast cultures or through production of synthetic peptides). Although the initial assay detected only antibody to a single antigen, subsequent tests have used antigens from four different regions of the HCV genome. Second generation assays become positive an average of 12 weeks after exposure, while third generation assays become positive an average of 9 weeks after exposure. After comparison with a cutoff value, results are interpreted as positive or negative. As is true for HBsAg, samples with low S/C ratio are often false positive, whereas false positive results are rare in samples with high S/C ratio.[128,129] Current CDC recommendations suggest using an S/C ratio of <3.8 for both second and third generation ELISA assays, and an S/C ratio of <8.0 for the chemiluminescence assay, to define low positive results.[20] Samples with low S/C ratio are recommended to be confirmed, ideally using recombinant immunoblot assay (RIBA).

RIBA is a technique similar in principle to Western blot (see Chapter 5). The HCV antigens used in the anti-HCV assays are typically blotted onto a membrane as dots, and reactivity is detected after incubation with serum. Results are interpreted as negative if there is less than 1+ reactivity with any of the four antigens, indeterminate if there is 1+ or greater reactivity to only a single antigen (or to more than 1 antigen along with the nonspecific yeast marker superoxide dismutase), and positive with 1+ or greater reactivity to multiple antigens. Third generation RIBA has considerably fewer indeterminate results than second generation RIBA.

HCV RNA measurement has become the most widely used test to detect current HCV infection. Typical of RNA in general, HCV RNA is labile in whole blood, because of the action of RNAses primarily found in red blood cells. Rapid separation of serum from clot is critical for accurate measurement of HCV RNA. If serum is separated from the clot by centrifugation within 1 hour, HCV RNA does not show an appreciable decline until 6 hours after collection. If serum is physically separated from cells within 1 hour, samples are stable at room temperature for 3 days, at refrigerator temperatures for a week, and indefinitely if frozen.[111] Samples collected in EDTA, which inhibits enzyme activity, are stable for 24 hours even if plasma is not separated from red cells.[180]

Assays for HCV RNA are generally divided into qualitative and quantitative variants. An international standard for quantification of HCV RNA has been developed,[385] and quantitative HCV RNA assay results are calibrated using this standard and reported in international units per milliliter (IU/mL). The relationship between IU/mL and copies/mL differs significantly for different assays. Results expressed in IU/mL agree within 1 log in about 90% of samples, but discrepant results do occur.[405] Until recently, qualitative assays had significantly lower detection limits than quantitative assays, but some newer quantitative assays have equivalent or lower detection limits compared with qualitative assays; it is likely that qualitative assays will become obsolete as sensitive quantitative assays become commercially available. Currently the most sensitive qualitative assay involves transcription-mediated amplification (TMA); its detection limit is 5 IU/mL. A commercially available qualitative reverse transcriptase/polymerase chain reaction (rt-PCR) assay has a detection limit of 50 IU/mL. Two quantitative assays are commercially available: an rt-PCR assay with a measurement range of 500 to 500,000 IU/mL and a branched DNA (bDNA) assay with a dynamic range of 615 to 8 million IU/mL. Several other assays, available as analyte-specific reagents or offered only by reference laboratories, have lower detection limits similar to those of qualitative assays and upper detection limits similar to or higher than those of the bDNA assay.

Hepatitis C core antigen (HCV Ag) is produced by the most constant part of the HCV genome. HCV Ag is one of the major targets of antibody formation, and most HCV Ag circulates bound to antibody. HCV Ag has a similar time course to that of HCV RNA in both acute and chronic HCV infection[426]; the currently available assay for HCV Ag becomes reliably positive when HCV RNA is 20,000 IU/mL or greater.[58] In our experience with several thousand HCV RNA samples, less than 5% of untreated HCV RNA positive individuals have a viral load <20,000 IU/mL. In contrast to HCV RNA, HCV Ag is stable on storage.[427]

Hepatitis C genotype is an important parameter in determining length and intensity of antiviral therapy. Several methods are currently used to determine the infecting genotype. Although serological assays to detect antibody to specific genotypes of HCV are available, their correlation with more definitive tests is approximately 90%,[351] and a significant minority of infected individuals have antibodies to more than one genotype.[434] However, detection of viral RNA of more than one genotype is exceptionally rare. The most reliable method involves direct sequencing of regions of the genome that show characteristic patterns with specific genotypes and subtypes. Commercial assays using the 5′-untranslated region are most widely used,[377] although assays using the NS5b region are now available. A commercial line probe assay is the most widely used technique, since it is relatively simple to perform and interpret. Sequences from specific strains of HCV are immobilized on a membrane, and the pattern of banding following hybridization and addition of indicator is interpreted. The technique cannot distinguish some of the less common genotypes and occasionally has patterns that do not correspond to a specific genotype. Overall agreement with direct sequencing methods is high.[305]

Hepatitis B and C Co-infection

Approximately 2% to 10% of individuals infected with HCV are co-infected with HBV; of those with chronic HBV, 15% to 20% are also HCV positive.[99,490] The clinical and laboratory features of co-infected patients are somewhat contradictory, and differ from those in individuals infected with a single hepatitis virus. Co-infected patients have lower viral loads than do those with single infection.[98] In patients with chronic HBV who develop acute HCV infection, the likelihood of progressing to chronic HCV infection is lower.[89] These features would suggest a beneficial effect of co-infection. In contrast, patients with chronic HBV/HCV co-infection have more rapid progression to cirrhosis.[382] Patients with acute co-infection more frequently have severe acute hepatitis.[15,490] Some studies suggest that there is a high frequency of HBV DNA viral replication in the liver even in the absence of circulating HBsAg; such subclinically co-infected patients have more severe liver injury and a higher frequency of cirrhosis.[71,243] Despite some favorable findings, the outcome of hepatitis in co-infected patients seems to be worse than for those infected with only a single agent.

Hepatitis D Virus (Delta Agent)

Hepatitis D virus (HDV) is an incomplete, 36-nm RNA particle that cannot replicate on its own.[411] It is coated with HBsAg and is dependent on HBV for its activation. It is thus a satellite virus similar to that seen in plants. The D virus is a single-stranded antisense RNA virus. It is very infectious and strongly associated with intravenous drug abuse; approximately 10 million persons have been infected worldwide,[185] although the incidence is declining with the fall in incidence of HBV infection.[231] It occurs as simultaneous infection with hepatitis B (co-infection) or as superimposed infection in someone with chronic hepatitis B (superinfection). Co-infection usually runs the same time course as acute hepatitis B and HDV is spontaneously cleared as the hepatitis B resolves, but the risk of fulminant hepatitis is higher than in HBV infection alone, and mortality is higher. Superinfection typically results in chronic HDV infection, suppression of HBV DNA replication, and more rapid progression to cirrhosis. It should be suspected in a chronically infected HBV patient whose condition worsens.[476] Although traditionally diagnosed serologically by detection of anti-HDV (total or IgM) and/or HDVAg,[323] currently HDV RNA measurements are often used as evidence of current infection.[307]

Hepatitis E Virus

Hepatitis E virus (HEV) is a 34-nm, single-stranded, unenveloped RNA virus. It accounts for sporadic and epidemic hepatitis in tropical and semitropical countries and in people returning from these areas.[474] Although considered to be rare in Europe and nontropical areas of North America, it was identified in 1999 as a cause of hepatitis in the United States,[139] and HEV RNA is frequently isolated from city sewage treatment plants in such nonendemic areas.[91] It is enterically transmitted, as is HAV, and viral RNA has been detected in stool.[443] There is probably only one species. Tests to detect antibody to HEV have been developed; specificity for HEV is high only for assays detecting antibody to the open reading frame 2 (ORF2) antigen.[283] The prevalence of antibodies to HEV is high among those living in urban areas and in blood donors,[432] and HEV has been isolated from rats[227] and pigs[297]; the significance of this is unclear, although it has been speculated that HEV is a zoonotic disease.[296] The clinical course is similar to that of HAV infection in that HEV typically infects young people, has a self-limited course, and is not associated with chronicity. A peculiar feature of this disease is its virulent course in late pregnancy, with mortality generally in the range of 20% to 25%, but rates as high as 50% have been reported.[241]

Hepatitis G Virus

Hepatitis G virus (HGV), also known as GBV-C, is an RNA virus of the flavivirus family, closely related to HCV.[4] It has been found to be transmitted by the same means as HCV, although most commonly it is transmitted by plasma[220]; vertical transmission has been reported.[306] Although it has a very high infectivity rate in recipients of contaminated blood (>90%), there seem to be no adverse consequences to HGV infection.[461] In fact, although it has been called a hepatitis virus, viral RNA cannot be isolated from the liver in chronic infection.[253] Co-infection with HCV and HGV is common, but there is no effect of co-infection on prognosis in HCV.[342,479] HGV and HIV co-infection is also common[473]; individuals co-infected with HGV and HIV have lower HIV viral loads and a better prognosis than those infected with HIV alone.[258,433,435]

ACUTE HEPATITIS

Acute hepatitis refers to an acute injury directed against the hepatocytes. The injury may be mediated either directly—as occurs with certain drugs, such as acetaminophen, or with ischemia—or indirectly, as occurs with immunologically mediated injury from most of the hepatitis viruses and most drugs, including ethanol. In direct injury, there is typically a rapid rise in cytosolic enzymes, such as AST, ALT, and LD, followed by a rapid fall with rates of decline similar to known half-lives of the enzymes. With immunological injury, there is a gradual rise in cytosolic enzymes, a plateau phase, and a gradual resolution of enzyme elevation. Although jaundice is a key clinical finding in acute hepatitis, it is often absent (as discussed below under the various forms of viral infection). An increase of AST activity to greater than 200 IU/L, or of ALT activity to greater than 300 IU/L, has sensitivity and specificity of greater than 90% for acute hepatitis.[380] ALP is usually mildly elevated, and is less than three times the upper reference limit in 90% of cases of acute hepatitis.[380] Bilirubin elevation, when present, typically is predominantly direct reacting bilirubin; indirect bilirubin is higher than direct bilirubin in about 15% of cases.[55] The distribution of direct bilirubin percentage is identical in acute hepatitis and bile duct obstruction, making direct bilirubin inconsequential in the differential diagnosis of jaundice.[55] Liver synthetic function is usually well preserved in most forms of acute hepatitis. These and other features that are helpful in the differential diagnosis of acute hepatitis are summarized in Table 47-3.

The outcome of acute hepatitis is variable. In most cases, complete recovery occurs and liver regeneration leads to normal structure and function. With some viruses, failure to clear infection leads to development of chronic hepatitis. In a small percentage of cases, massive destruction of the liver leads to acute (fulminant) hepatic failure, which is associated with high mortality unless liver transplantation can occur.

Acute Viral Hepatitis

All forms of acute viral hepatitis have similar pathology and a similar clinical course. They are all diagnosed on the basis of marked elevations in aminotransferases, usually between 8 and 50 times the upper reference limits, with only slight

TABLE 47-3 Laboratory Features of Different Forms of Acute Hepatitis

Type	AST/ALT	ALP	Bilirubin	PT	Serology	Other
Viral	8-50 × URL	<3 URL	5-15 mg/dL	<15 s	Positive	
HAV					IgM anti-HAV	
HBV					HBsAg, IgM anti-HBc	
HCV					HCV RNA, ±anti-HCV	
Alcoholic	<8 × URL	>3 × URL in 25%	5-15 mg/dL	<15 s	Negative	AST > ALT
Toxic	>50 × URL	Normal	<5 mg/dL	>15 s	Negative	Toxin usually detectable; acute renal failure common
Ischemic	>50 × URL	Normal	<5 mg/dL	>15 s	Negative	Acute renal failure common
Drug induced	8-50 × URL	>3 × URL in 50%	5-15 mg/dL	<15 s	Negative	Eosinophilia, skin rash common
Autoimmune	8-50 × URL	<3 × URL	5-15 mg/dL	<15 s	Positive ANA or ASMA	Low albumin, high globulins
Wilson	8-50 × URL	Low normal or decreased	5-15 mg/dL	<15 s	Negative	Hemolytic anemia, renal failure common; low ceruloplasmin often absent

URL, Upper reference limit.

elevations in ALP and little or no effect on hepatic synthetic function. ALT is typically higher than AST because of slower clearance. Enzyme elevations typically peak before peak bilirubin occurs, and remain increased for an average of 4 to 5 weeks (longer for ALT than AST because of its longer half-life). Bilirubin elevation is variable, as discussed below. The incidence of acute viral hepatitis has declined notably since the late 1980s, with the decline reaching less than 20% of previous concentrations for both HBV and HCV by the late 1990s.[29,175,241A] The decline in incidence of these viruses seems to be caused by widespread immunization for HBV, along with reduction in risk of infection by injection drug use (thought to be related to safer injection practices following discovery of the human immunodeficiency virus) and safe sex practices. There has not been a similar decline in the overall incidence of HAV.[30] The lack of universal vaccination programs for HAV seems to explain the continued high incidence, since immunization of about half of susceptible individuals was associated with a 92% decline in incidence of HAV in one high-risk area.[34]

Acute Hepatitis A

In adults, about 70% of those with acute HAV infection develop jaundice much more commonly than with HBV or HCV. In children, acute HAV infection typically goes unrecognized and is often considered to be a viral gastroenteritis or other viral disease, since only 10% of children become jaundiced. The disease is more prolonged and serious in individuals over age 50. The specific etiological diagnosis is made with serological tests. An IgM antibody (anti-HAV IgM) appears early in the course of illness and persists for an average of 2 to 6 months; rarely, IgM antibodies may remain positive for a year or longer. The presence of IgM anti-HAV is therefore considered diagnostic of recent HAV infection. An IgG antibody (anti-HAV IgG) appears shortly after IgM antibody, and persists for many years (probably for life), inducing lifelong immunity. Total anti-HAV antibody assays detect both IgM and IgG anti-HAV. Both IgM and, subsequently, IgG anti-HAV also develop following immunization with the hepatitis A vaccine. There are no antigen tests for detection of hepatitis A in plasma. Incubation of stool samples with labeled antibodies to hepatitis A and examination with an electron microscope have been used to detect infectious viral particles in the past. Amplification techniques (usually using rt-PCR) have been used to detect virus in epidemiologic studies, but are not routinely used to diagnose infection.

Acute Hepatitis B

In most of the world, HBV is the most common cause of acute viral hepatitis. As with HAV, most infections in children are clinically silent. An estimated 30% to 50% of adolescents and adults with acute HBV infection develop jaundice. The outcome in acute HBV infection is strongly influenced by age and immune status. In healthy adolescents and adults, an estimated 1% to 3% of cases will progress to chronic infection. In a person with immunosuppression, the likelihood of chronic infection increases to 10%. Neonates infected with HBV have a 90% likelihood of chronic infection, and the risk falls gradually over the first 5 years of life.

The serological course of acute hepatitis B infection is illustrated in Figure 47-16. HBsAg is the first serological

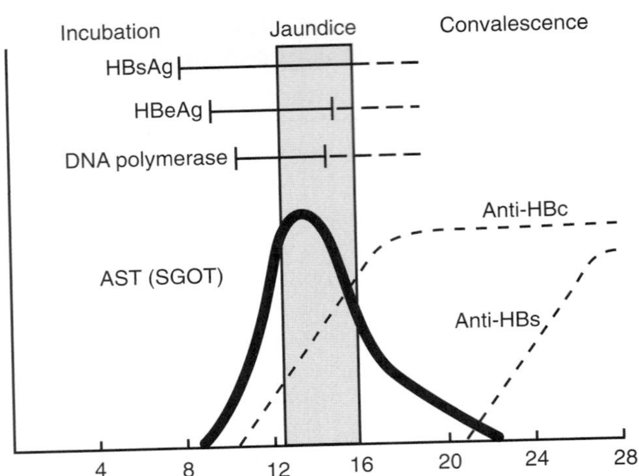

Figure 47-16 Course of acute type B hepatitis with recovery. *1*, Onset of hepatitis with jaundice 3 months after exposure; *2*, detection of hepatitis B surface antigen (HBsAg) 2 to 8 weeks after exposure, followed by appearance of its antibody (anti-HBs) 2 to 4 weeks after HBsAg is no longer detectable; *3*, detection of hepatitis Be antigen (HBeAg) shortly after appearance of HBsAg disappears (this is usually followed by the appearance of antibody to HbeAg [anti-Hbe], which persists); *4*, detection of hepatitis B core antibody (anti-HBc) at the time of onset of disease 2 to 3 months after exposure. Anti-HBc IgM will be detectable in high levels for ~5 months. *(From Balistreri WF. Viral hepatitis: Unique aspects of infection during childhood. Consultant 1984; 24:131-53.)*

marker to appear, although HBV DNA may be detectable slightly earlier. HBsAg usually appears 1 to 2 months after infection and before the onset of clinical illness, and is the last protein marker to disappear. HBV DNA replication is slower than that of HCV; doubling time averages 2 to 3 days.[462] Persistence of HBsAg for more than 6 months beyond the onset of acute hepatitis indicates chronic infection. HBeAg appears at about the same time as HBsAg; however, because it is not usually measured except in the setting of chronic HBV infection, it is usually not helpful as a marker to document acute infection. The first antibody to appear, usually coinciding with the onset of clinical evidence of hepatitis 3 to 6 months after infection, is antibody to the hepatitis B core antigen (anti-HBc). As with hepatitis A, an IgM antibody is the first to appear, and usually persists for 3 to 6 months; it is usually considered diagnostic of acute hepatitis B infection. In chronic infection, however, IgM antibody may become detectable with flares of severity of disease and is thus not completely reliable in recognizing a recent infection. The typical pattern at clinical presentation is positive serology for anti-HBc (both total and IgM), HBsAg, HBeAg (when measured), and negative anti-HBs. A small percentage of individuals have negative HBsAg and anti-HBs at the time of initial presentation, leaving IgM anti-HBc as the only commonly measured marker to be positive; this finding has been termed the "core window." With current, sensitive assays for HBsAg, it is rare to encounter individuals in the core window. Clearance of HBeAg and development of anti-HBe is the first sign of viral clearance and usually predates loss of HBsAg. Clinically, HBsAg clearance is associated with recovery from acute hepatitis and has been thought to confer lifelong immunity to HBV.

More recently, accumulating evidence indicates that HBV remains dormant in the body and HBV DNA circulates in many to most individuals who have "recovered" from acute hepatitis. This has been termed "occult" HBV infection. At the time of publication, the significance of such occult infection is unclear, as reviewed by Brechot.[59A] Several studies have demonstrated that HBV DNA is still present in low amounts, both in the plasma and liver, in most individuals who had past acute HBV infection and who were HBsAg negative and anti-HBs positive.[460,485] Viral loads are typically 100 copies/mL or lower, and it has been estimated that the number of liver cells infected may be as low as 1%. Such individuals have been shown to transmit HBV infection if their organs are used for transplantation. The significance of circulating HBV DNA to the individual infected or to others (in the absence of transplantation) seems to be minimal, however, since liver enzymes are usually normal and the circulating HBV DNA is mainly found in immune complexes.

Acute Hepatitis C

Acute HCV infection is responsible for 10% to 15% of cases of acute hepatitis in the United States; an estimated 10% to 30% of those with acute infection develop jaundice. Increased aminotransferases usually develop about 6 to 8 weeks after infection. In those cases in which clinical acute hepatitis develops, jaundice typically begins about 2 to 3 months after exposure. HCV RNA and HCV core antigen are detectable in plasma 2 to 4 weeks after initial exposure. Viremia increases rapidly (average doubling time of 17 hours), and plateaus at high viral loads (often > 10^7 IU/mL). In acute hepatitis C infection, anti-HCV is present in a little more than half of cases at the time of presentation.[39,182] IgM anti-HCV assays are not commercially available, but in contrast to HAV and HBV, IgM antibodies are encountered in both acute and chronic HCV infection, making the test useless diagnostically.[330] HCV RNA and HCV core antigen are usually both present at the time of diagnosis and viral load is often significantly elevated compared with values seen in chronic hepatitis. Diagnosis of acute HCV is likely if anti-HCV is absent but HCV RNA or core antigen is positive. Diagnosis of acute HCV is also likely if HCV RNA viral load is high and anti-HCV titer is low, or increases with time.[330,343] Viral load falls with development of antibody to one or more HCV proteins, and may become transiently negative.

Other Types of Acute Viral Hepatitis

A number of other viruses can affect the liver, causing acute hepatitis. The most common are the Epstein-Barr virus and cytomegalovirus. Features are otherwise typical of viral hepatitis, although there are often signs of systemic infection as well. Herpes simplex virus may occasionally cause severe hepatitis in adults.[235] Infection with each of these agents is more commonly associated with hepatitis in the neonatal period, where it is part of disseminated infection. Diagnosis of infection with these viruses involves serological and nucleic acid tests; none of them are specific to the liver.

Sudden outbursts of activity in individuals with chronic hepatitis B may mimic acute hepatitis. There are common situations in which an acute rise in cytoplasmic enzymes occurs, often associated with jaundice and other clinical features suggesting an acute liver disease. For example, development of an immune response that leads to clearance of either HBeAg or HBsAg is often associated with clinical and enzymatic features of acute hepatitis.[110] Recognition of this cause of the clinical picture of acute hepatitis in a person with chronic hepatitis relies on demonstration of antigen loss and antibody development, along with absence of other causes of acute hepatitis. Withdrawal of agents that suppress either the immune response (especially corticosteroids) or viral replication (particularly lamivudine),[353] or restoration of the immune system (by treatment of HIV infection)[379] has been associated with a clinical picture that mimics acute hepatitis; fulminant hepatic failure and death have been associated with these events. Diagnosis is usually dependent on clinical history.

Toxic Hepatitis

Toxic hepatitis refers to direct damage of hepatocytes by a toxin or toxic metabolite. Toxic reactions are usually predictable, and are directly related to the dose of the agent ingested. In North America and Europe, the most common cause of toxic hepatitis is acetaminophen, a widely used nonprescription pain reliever.[47] The metabolism of acetaminophen is affected by dose, induction of metabolic enzymes, and concentrations of glutathione (Figure 47-14). When a large dose of acetaminophen is ingested (average lethal dose 15 g), the metabolic pathways are overwhelmed, glutathione is depleted, and toxic intermediates accumulate and cause liver damage. When metabolic enzymes are induced (such as by ethanol) or glutathione is depleted (as occurs in alcoholics and with starvation), toxicity can occur with relatively small doses of acetaminophen (total doses of 2 to 4 g). The first laboratory abnormality to appear is an increase in PT, followed by increased activities of cytosolic enzymes. Initially, LD is often increased to higher absolute amounts than AST, and AST tends to be higher than ALT.[74] Peak activities (typically more than 100 times the upper reference limits) usually occur by 24 to 48 hours, followed by rapid clearance at rates approximating the known half-lives of the enzymes.[410] PT elevations are typical and are greater than 4 seconds above the control value in most cases.[337] Prognosis is related most closely to the prolonged increase in PT; persistent elevation of PT 4 days after ingestion is associated with a poor prognosis.[189] Other markers of risk include development of acute renal failure and presence of lactic acidosis, particularly if pH is <7.30.

Ischemic Hepatitis ("Shock Liver")

Hepatic hypoperfusion (ischemic hepatitis) is one of the most common causes of elevated cytosolic enzymes; in hospital patients, it is the cause of the majority of cases of acute hepatitis.[197,463] Ischemic hepatitis follows any cause of shock; the most common causes are septic and cardiogenic shock (sometimes termed cardiac hepatopathy).[317] Bilirubin elevations typically are minimal, and usually peak several days after enzyme activity reaches its greatest point.[130] Laboratory findings are similar to those in toxic hepatitis (including having high LD), and acute renal failure is a common complicating factor. Prognosis is primarily related to the underlying cause of hypotension[130]; individuals with prolonged elevation of bilirubin appear to have a poor prognosis.[38]

Reye's Syndrome

Acute encephalopathy in combination with fatty degeneration of the viscera was initially described by Reye and associates in Australia in 1963,[370] with nearly simultaneous case descriptions by Johnson and colleagues in the United States.[222] In the majority of these early cases, the disease was fatal. It most frequently strikes children aged 6 to 11 years and infants, although it may affect other ages. The syndrome is characterized by a prodromal, febrile viral illness (usually influenza B or varicella), followed in about a week by protracted vomiting associated with lethargy and confusion,[261] which may deteriorate rapidly into stupor and coma. At the same time, the liver enlarges, increased aminotransferases and PT develop, and ammonia increases. A PT prolonged greater than 3 seconds above normal and a plasma ammonia level greater than 100 μmol/L usually indicate a poor prognosis. Bilirubin is typically normal or only mildly increased. Other laboratory features include hypoglycemia and hyperuricemia.

Only sporadic case descriptions of Reye's syndrome were published until 1974, when 379 cases in the United States were reported to the CDC. The mortality rate in this series was 41%. The number of cases peaked in 1980 at 555.[43] At about the same time, articles began to appear linking Reye's syndrome with aspirin treatment of viral illnesses,[409] followed by a case control study strongly implicating salicylate in the pathogenesis of Reye's syndrome.[188] Although CDC guidelines recommending avoidance of aspirin in children with febrile illnesses were not published until 1985,[206] a decline in salicylate use began before this, and Reye's syndrome has again become a rare disease.

Other Causes of Acute Hepatitis

Drugs can cause liver injury by a number of mechanisms, but the most common is idiosyncratic, immune-mediated injury to hepatocytes,[265,494] characterized by elevations in

ALT or AST.[22] Cholestatic hepatitis, with increased aminotransferases and ALP, is more common in drug-induced hepatitis than with other causes of acute hepatitis. Criteria to recognize drug-induced liver disease include temporal relationship between drug exposure and onset of hepatitis; exclusion of other known causes of hepatitis; presence of extrahepatic hypersensitivity (especially skin rash, arthralgia, renal injury, and eosinophilia); development of liver injury on rechallenge; and, ideally, previously published reports of similar reactions.[279] Several standardized approaches to evaluation of possible drug-induced liver disease have been developed.[106,415] Hepatic drug reactions represent about 6% of all adverse drug reactions,[125] and about 1% of cases of acute hepatitis.[249] Although usually associated with prescription drugs, complementary and alternative products are becoming increasingly recognized as causes of acute hepatitis.[85,420] Although drug reactions typically develop soon after start of treatment, several months may elapse between initial exposure and development of acute hepatitis. Approximately 60% of cases cause severe acute hepatitis with jaundice, and fatalities can occur.[95] Serious reactions are more common in individuals who are continued on the medication.[348] In about one third of cases, liver injury becomes chronic following cessation of the drug.[22]

Some disorders that usually produce chronic hepatitis (and are discussed more fully below) may occasionally present in an acute fashion. Autoimmune hepatitis has an acute component in up to 40% of cases. Clinically, it differs from other forms of acute hepatitis in having decreased albumin, increased globulins, and a more protracted increase in aminotransferases.[97,190,358] Acute autoimmune hepatitis is diagnosed by the absence of other causes for acute hepatitis and the presence of autoimmune markers (discussed in detail under chronic hepatitis). Wilson's disease is due to deficiency of an intracellular ATPase gene,[63,429] and typically presents with neuropsychiatric findings, often associated with chronic liver injury. Wilson's disease may also present as an acute hepatitis, often associated with fulminant hepatic failure[45]; in one study, 8 out of 14 patients who had hepatic injury due to Wilson's disease had an acute presentation.[179] The classic biochemical findings of Wilson's disease are often absent (low ceruloplasmin, low plasma copper, and Kayser-Fleischer rings) or misleading (high urine copper is common to all forms of acute hepatitis) in the setting of acute Wilson's disease.[45,417] A number of additional features are often present that suggest the diagnosis, including nonimmune hemolytic anemia,[183] acute tubular necrosis, and a ratio of ALP (in IU/L) to bilirubin (in mg/dL) of <2.[45]

Differential Diagnosis of Acute Hepatitis

There are several conditions that mimic the laboratory picture of acute hepatitis. Hemolytic anemia can cause jaundice, increased LD, and slight increases in AST and ALT. In contrast to hepatitis, the increase in bilirubin is predominantly (often >80%) indirect reacting. LD activity is elevated to several times that of AST, and AST activity is usually several times that of ALT. Acute skeletal muscle injury may cause significant increases in AST and, to a lesser extent, ALT, but the ratio of AST to ALT activity is generally more than 3:1,[322A] and bilirubin is usually not elevated. Acute bile duct obstruction, particularly when caused by gallstones, can cause a picture that resembles acute hepatitis. In the early stages of obstruction, transient increases in AST and ALT are common,[414] and rarely their activities may exceed 2000 IU/L.[24,157] Increases in ALP develop more slowly than those of the aminotransferases, masking the presence of cholestasis early in the course. Increases in bilirubin are typically predominantly direct reacting, creating a presentation similar to that seen in acute hepatitis. Even if obstruction persists, aminotransferase activity falls rapidly, with AST typically returning to normal within 8 days,[350] and ALP activity gradually increases if obstruction persists. ALP activities more than 300 IU/L in this setting strongly suggest the presence of obstructive jaundice.[458] Acute biliary obstruction by gallstones is often accompanied by acute pancreatitis; increased amylase and lipase should suggest biliary tract obstruction as the cause of any liver abnormalities noted.

Once a diagnosis of acute hepatitis is established, additional laboratory testing may be required to determine the etiology. Although the incidence of acute viral hepatitis has decreased, serological studies should be performed to rule out infectious causes. A typical panel of tests would include IgM anti-HAV, HBsAg, IgM anti-HBc, anti-HCV, and HCV core antigen or HCV RNA. Marked elevations (>100 times the upper reference limits) in either AST or ALT, particularly if AST is higher than ALT, should suggest the possibility of toxic or ischemic liver injury. Minimal increases (<8 times the reference limit) in AST, with AST greater than ALT, in a patient with jaundice and leukocytosis indicates likely alcoholic hepatitis. Imaging studies of the biliary tract are appropriate to rule out obstruction in those who present with sudden onset of symptoms, especially if accompanied by right upper quadrant pain and tenderness, laboratory evidence of pancreatitis, or a history of gallstones. The presence of increased globulins and decreased albumin, or the presence of hemolytic anemia and acute renal failure, should suggest the possibility of autoimmune hepatitis or Wilson's disease, respectively.

Follow-up of Acute Hepatitis

The important uses of laboratory tests in acute hepatitis are to identify individuals with fulminant hepatic failure, document recovery, and determine clearance of any infectious agents. The most important tests in determining extent of injury are not plasma activities of cytosolic enzymes, but evidence of impaired liver function. The most important indicator of prognosis in acute hepatitis is impairment in synthetic functions of which PT is a widely accepted indicator. In acute viral or alcoholic hepatitis, PT more than 15 seconds is associated with a poor prognosis,[337] whereas in toxic hepatitis persistent elevation more than 4 days after ingestion has prognostic importance.[189] Other markers of synthetic function, such as transthyretin, or markers of hepatocyte regeneration, such as alpha-fetoprotein, have been found to predict prognosis.[202] Although hypophosphatemia is common in fulminant hepatic failure, normal phosphate concentrations in this setting have been associated with worse prognosis.[90] Cytosolic enzyme activities decrease rapidly in ischemic and toxic hepatitis or obstruction, regardless of outcome, and fall more gradually in viral and alcoholic hepatitis, but are not helpful in evaluating outcome. With both hepatitis B and C, cytosolic enzyme activities may return to normal even if viral replication persists[112,216]; serological tests are the only reliable means to evaluate resolution of infection.

Chronic Hepatitis

Chronic hepatitis is defined as a chronic inflammation of the liver that persists for at least 6 months, or signs and symptoms of chronic liver disease in the presence of elevated cytosolic enzymes.[127] It is characterized by ongoing inflammatory damage to hepatocytes, often accompanied by hepatocyte regeneration and scarring. Formerly, chronic hepatitis was subdivided into three forms (chronic persistent, chronic lobular, and chronic active) based on histological characteristics. It was recognized that individuals often had each of these "diseases" at different points in time, and often in different areas of the liver in the same biopsy. Currently, classifications describe the etiology and grade both the current severity of inflammatory injury (termed grade) and extent of fibrosis (termed stage). The importance of these findings will be discussed in detail later. The common causes of chronic hepatitis and the tests used to make a specific etiological diagnosis are listed in Table 47-4.

The clinical features of chronic hepatitis are highly variable. Most patients are asymptomatic, but nonspecific features such as fatigue, lack of concentration, and weakness may be present. Most patients are diagnosed because of an unexplained abnormality of aminotransferases or detection of positive results on a screening test for a cause of chronic hepatitis. Moderate elevations of aminotransferase activities (twofold to fivefold) are characteristic, whereas results of most other tests are normal. Normal aminotransferase activities do not rule out histological evidence of chronic hepatitis, especially in the presence of chronic viral hepatitis or nonalcoholic steatohepatitis (NASH).[124,170,308] Characteristically, ALT is elevated to a greater degree than AST,[81] although elevations in both are common; reversal of the AST:ALT ratio to greater than 1 suggests coexisting alcohol abuse or development of cirrhosis[154,215,347] (as discussed in more detail later in this chapter). Although ALT is relatively specific for the liver, skeletal muscle sources for AST and ALT should always be considered, especially in physically active young individuals.[121,251,322A] Finding persistent elevation of aminotransferase activity should lead to an evaluation for chronic hepatitis using the tests outlined in Table 47-5. A liver biopsy may be helpful in determining etiology, assessing severity, and following treatment.[25] A specific etiological diagnosis is essential because it dictates the treatment. The most common causes of chronic hepatitis are chronic HBV and HCV and NASH, but a variety of other disease processes may cause chronic hepatitis.

TABLE 47-4 Causes of Chronic Hepatitis and Diagnostic Strategies

Cause	Diagnosis
Hepatitis B	History, HBsAg, anti-HBs, anti-HBc, HBV DNA
Hepatitis C	Anti-HCV, HCV RNA by PCR
Autoimmune type 1	ANA, anti-smooth muscle antibody
Autoimmune type 2	SLA, anti-LKM$_1$
Wilson's disease	Ceruloplasmin
Drugs	History
α_1-Antitrypsin deficiency	α_1-AT phenotype
Idiopathic	Liver biopsy, absence of markers

Chronic Hepatitis B

Worldwide, HBV infection is the most important cause of chronic hepatitis. Specifically, there are approximately 350 million individuals with chronic HBV infection worldwide, with most cases found in Asia, Africa, and southern Europe.

In most circumstances, HBV is not cytopathic, as the injury results from an immune-mediated inflammatory attack against the hepatocyte. Chronic hepatitis results when the immune response is incomplete and the virus is not eliminated from infected cells. This leads to a continuing cycle of viral replication, reinfection of regenerating hepatocytes, and immune damage to newly infected cells that is inadequate to clear infection. The details are not completely understood, but it appears that in the normal circumstance, hepatocytes express surface markers (in this case, HBcAg and HLA class 1 proteins).[311] Primed lymphocytes then attack the infected hepatocytes.[84] The expression of the HLA class 1 markers is stimulated by interferon. It appears that many chronic hepatitis B patients are deficient in or have an inadequate response to interferon and, by inference, are unable to express HLA antigens that would attract an appropriate lymphocyte response.[256] The discovery of interferon deficiency led to the successful use of α-interferon (IFN alpha) therapy in chronic hepatitis B patients. The clinical presentation may be complicated by a number of extrahepatic complications, including (1) polyarteritis, (2) glomerulonephritis, (3) polymyalgia rheumatica, (4) cryoglobulinemia, (5) myocarditis, and (6) Guillain-Barré syndrome.

TABLE 47-5 Tests for Evaluating Chronic Hepatitis C Infection and Its Treatment

Time of Testing	Test	Condition	Use/Interpretation
Pretreatment	HCV viral load	Detectable	Baseline (to compare to 12 wk value)
	Genotype	2 or 3 vs other	Length of treatment (24 wk genotype 2 or 3, 48 wk if other genotype)
12 wk on treatment	HCV viral load	<2 log drop	Stop treatment (nonresponder)*
		>2 log drop	Continue treatment (on treatment responder)
24 wk on treatment†	Sensitive HCV RNA‡	Detectable	Stop treatment (nonresponder)
		Not detectable	Continue treatment (on treatment responder)
End of treatment§	Sensitive HCV RNA‡	Detectable	Nonresponder
		Not detectable	Treatment responder
24 wk after completion	Sensitive HCV RNA†	Detectable	Relapser
		Not detectable	Sustained virological responder

*Less than 3% chance of sustained virological response; some continue treatment to 24 weeks and reevaluate.
†Only done if genotype not 2 or 3.
‡Lower detection limit <50 IU/mL.
§Done at 24 weeks if genotype 2 or 3, done at 48 weeks in other genotypes; not all recommend evaluating end of treatment response.

These conditions are associated with circulating immune complexes containing HBsAg.[438] Immunocompromised patients, such as HIV-positive patients, typically have higher replication markers, less hepatic inflammation, and similar rates of survival.[233]

The natural history of chronic hepatitis B (defined by the persistence of HBsAg) varies. It is convenient to divide chronic hepatitis B infection into two basic types: replicative and nonreplicative. In the chronic replicative form, viral DNA is found in the cytoplasm of infected hepatocytes, and complete viral particles are produced and released into the circulation. In the replicating form of infection, viral loads in plasma are high (>10^5 copies/mL, often >10^8 copies/mL), and evidence of hepatocyte injury (elevated aminotransferase activity and inflammation in liver biopsy sections) is found in most cases. This variant has also been termed chronic hepatitis B. Approximately 3% to 5% of individuals with chronic replicating infection transform to the chronic, nonreplicating form yearly. In the nonreplicating form, HBV DNA becomes integrated into the host cell DNA, circulating viral load is low or undetectable, and evidence of hepatocyte injury is usually absent. This variant has also been termed HBV carrier state. Traditionally, HBeAg has been used to differentiate these two forms, with negative HBeAg and positive anti-HBe thought to indicate the nonreplicating stage of infection. As discussed earlier, however, it is common to find precore mutants of HBV that lack ability to form HBeAg. Even in individuals who were HBeAg positive in areas with low prevalence of precore mutants, loss of HBeAg may be due to development of precore mutants. Consequently, guidelines on HBV have been established that recommend measuring HBV DNA instead of HBeAg, particularly in individuals with evidence of hepatocyte injury.[135,267,447] A third variant of chronic HBV infection is termed the immunotolerant form; it is associated with HBeAg and/or high HBV viral load, but no evidence of hepatocyte injury. Immunotolerant forms of infection are common in vertically transmitted HBV for the first 2 decades of life, and in the early stages of chronic HBV infection in adults.

Although these three forms of infection represent the major variants of HBV infection, it is common for individuals to pass between the different variants. About 1% to 2% of individuals who are in the nonreplicating form will revert to the replicating form of infection. Another 1% to 2% will lose HBsAg and develop anti-HBs. Each of these transitions, along with transition from replicating to nonreplicating variants, can be associated with an acute rise in aminotransferase activities, increases in hepatocyte injury after a biopsy, and a clinical picture mimicking acute viral hepatitis.

For individuals who have chronic replicating infection, the major risk is development of cirrhosis and HCC. An estimated 30% of individuals with chronic hepatitis B will develop cirrhosis over a 20-year follow-up period. Once cirrhosis has developed, there is a 1.5% to 5% annual risk of development of HCC. Although the risk of HCC is lower in individuals with HBV infection who do not have cirrhosis, even a person in the nonreplicating stage of infection has a tenfold higher risk of HCC (compared with those who are HBsAg negative). On a worldwide basis, hepatitis B infection is the most common cause of liver cancer.

Two guidelines from the American and European hepatology societies summarize treatment recommendations.[267,447] Currently, three agents are approved for treatment of chronic HBV infection: interferon,* lamivudine, and adefovir dipivoxil.[186,277] The latter two are inhibitors of

*Interferon-alpha 2a and 2b have been extensively used and tested. Pegylated interferon is a newer formulation.

reverse transcriptase and have also been used to treat HIV infection. Other HIV treatment agents have been evaluated in research studies, but are not yet approved for use in North America or Europe. At present, only single agent therapy is used. With the low rate of response and development of lamivudine resistant mutants, trials are underway for evaluation of combination therapy, but results are generally not yet available. One large study of pegylated interferon and lamivudine found no additional benefit from combination therapy.[219A] Treatment is indicated for treatment of individuals with positive HBeAg and/or HBV DNA >10^5 copies/mL, particularly if they also have elevated ALT. Response rate is directly related to pretreatment ALT activity and is less than 10% in those with normal ALT. The goal of treatment is suppression of viral replication, detected either by undetectable HBV DNA or clearance of HBeAg and development of anti-HBe; approximately 20% to 30% of individuals treated will attain these goals. In patients who clear circulating virus, HBsAg becomes undetectable in up to a quarter of the cases.[122] This occurs almost exclusively in those with HBV DNA viral load <10^3 copies/mL.[309] Although clearance of circulating virus with interferon therapy seems to persist long term in 80% to 90% of responders, relapse is more common with lamivudine or adefovir. Even in this group who lose HBsAg and circulating HBV DNA, HBV DNA is often still detectable in liver cells.

Chronic Hepatitis C

There are approximately 170 million individuals with chronic HCV infection worldwide, with most cases found in North America, Northern Europe, and Japan. In addition, chronic infection follows acute infection much more commonly (among those exposed after age 5) among those infected with HCV than HBV.[19] There is evidence that chronic HCV infection actually develops in 50% of those with acute infection,[238,400,465] and that antibody titers decline and may become negative in those who clear infection.[374,399] Once viremia becomes established beyond 6 months after initial exposure, it essentially never resolves spontaneously; in one study of 320 patients followed serially more than 3 years, only 6 patients with end-stage liver disease lost detectable HCV RNA.[480] HCV viral load fluctuates little over time; in most individuals, viral load differs by less than 0.5 log,[177,187] and gradually increases by an average of 0.2 to 0.3 log/year.[141,328] It is estimated that approximately 20% of patients with hepatitis C will progress to cirrhosis over a period of 20 years.[397] The frequency of progression appears to be increased by age over 40 at time of infection, male gender, alcohol abuse, and immunosuppression,[276] but is less than 5% after 20 years of infection in those infected in the first 20 to 30 years of life.[238,374,399,400,465] As with HBV, the likelihood of progression to HCC is between 1.5% and 5% per year in those with cirrhosis.

The clinical picture of chronic HCV is similar to HBV in producing chronic hepatitis. In contrast to HBV, where ALT activity remains relatively constant with increases at time of seroconversion, infection with HCV is characterized by fluctuating ALT activities over time. Only about one third of those with chronic HCV have continually increased ALT, and many of these show variation in ALT activity.[126] It is common for individuals with fluctuating values to have multiple normal ALT activity values separating elevated values.[216,369] Also in contrast to HBV, individuals with continually normal ALT activity have a similar rate of response to antiviral treatment.[35]

Treatment of chronic HCV has changed from single agent treatment with interferon, with relatively low response rates, to treatment with a combination of pegylated (long-acting) interferon plus ribavirin. New agents, including protease inhibitors, have shown promise of increasing treatment response rates and providing a treatment option for those who fail interferon-based therapy. In contrast to HBV, where treatment is aimed at inhibiting viral replication, treatment of HCV is often successful in eradicating the virus. Hepatitis C viral clearance occurs in three stages; these are postulated to include clearance of circulating virus, loss of replication by cells, and clearance of infected cells. The third phase correlates best with viral clearance during treatment.[196] Several terms have been used to describe treatment response.[108] Early virological response refers to at least a 2 log decrease in viral load after 12 weeks of treatment. End of treatment response refers to undetectable HCV RNA at the end of a prescribed cours of therapy. Sustained virological response (SVR) refers to undetectable HCV RNA 6 months following completion of treatment. In those achieving SVR, long-term suppression of HCV RNA and resolution of chronic hepatitis occur in more than 99% of patients. A number of factors influence response to treatment. The most important is genotype; genotypes 2, 3, and 4 have response rates approximately twice those of other genotypes (SVR 70% to 80% versus 45%) and those infected by genotypes 2 and 3 require only 6 months of treatment rather than 12 months for other genotypes.[120] Response rates are lower in those of African ancestry, and in those at increased risk of developing fibrosis. In those who develop recurrent HCV after liver transplantation, response rate is lower and rate of progression to cirrhosis is faster than in primary infection. Table 47-5 summarizes laboratory tests used to evaluate and monitor treatment for HCV.

Nonalcoholic Fatty Liver Disease and Nonalcoholic Steatohepatitis

Ludwig first described patients who had histological features identical to alcoholic hepatitis, but who had no history of alcohol abuse and did not have AST higher than ALT.[271] He introduced the term "nonalcoholic steatohepatitis" (NASH) to describe this entity that was more common in women than men and usually was associated with diabetes and/or obesity. (Since alcohol ingestion is common in the population, and alcoholic liver disease does not occur with ingestion of less than 20 g ethanol daily, this threshold has been suggested as the maximum alcohol intake compatible with a diagnosis of nonalcoholic fatty liver disease [NAFLD]).[326] The disease can also occur in men and in those without diabetes or obesity. Although NASH represents a necroinflammatory liver disease, there is increasing recognition that fat accumulation in the liver without inflammation is also commonly found in individuals with obesity and diabetes, and those with other components of the metabolic syndrome.[278] The more encompassing term NAFLD has been introduced to include this latter form and NASH. NAFLD is defined as the presence of fat accumulation to greater than 5% to 10% of liver mass, usually recognized upon biopsy as increased cytoplasmic fat. Although ultrasound can also be used, it is insensitive to fat content less than 25% of liver mass.[408]

Current evidence suggests that accumulation of fat in NAFLD is a consequence of insulin resistance.[326] A variety of mechanisms may lead to insulin resistance, including genetic predisposition, increased concentrations of free fatty acids, and presence of cytokines such as tumor necrosis factor alpha (TNF-α). Since TNF-α is produced by fat cells, correlates with body fat, and is critical to development of insulin resistance in obesity,[446] it may be a key factor in development of NAFLD. The pathogenesis is likely to be more complicated, however, as a variety of other factors lead to increased fat accumulation in the liver, including increased carbohydrate intake, certain drugs, and mutations in lipid synthesis, but have not been associated with development of NASH.

The frequency of NAFLD is high in North America and Europe; it has been estimated that NAFLD occurs in 20% of the population and NASH in 2% to 3%; this would make NASH as common as chronic HCV as a cause of chronic liver disease. Prospective studies of patients with liver disease have confirmed that NASH is a common cause of elevated liver enzymes in an unselected population of patients referred to gastroenterologists or seen in primary care settings.[70,107,285] The frequency in obese or diabetic individuals is much higher, with NAFLD in 60% to 75% and NASH in 20% to 25%.[326,459] Although simple fat accumulation is thought to be benign, and most cases of NASH are associated with minimal fibrosis, NASH has progressed to cirrhosis in 15% of cases in the small number of published prospective studies. The frequency of cirrhosis in NASH is not well established, but there is a suggestion that NASH may be a major cause of "cryptogenic" cirrhosis, in which no underlying etiology can be determined. As weight loss develops with chronic illness, fat may disappear from the liver, leaving only fibrosis.

Laboratory diagnosis of NASH and NAFLD is not currently possible. The clinical features of NASH are nonspecific, similar to those of other causes of chronic hepatitis. Although increased activities of liver enzymes are often used to distinguish NASH from other forms of NAFLD, the degree of necroinflammatory damage is not related to elevations of AST or ALT activity, and the likelihood of significant liver damage is similar in those with normal or elevated ALT.[308]

To date, the major treatments for NAFLD have been those aimed at lowering body weight and fat content. Loss of weight is often associated with decreased ALT values; in one study, a 1% decrease in weight was associated with an 8% decrease in ALT activity.[344] The association of NAFLD with insulin resistance has suggested treatment with antidiabetic medications, particularly those that increase insulin responsiveness (such as PPAR-γ receptor agonists and metformin), but there are no conclusive studies that document safety and efficacy.

Autoimmune Hepatitis

Autoimmune hepatitis (AIH) represents a rapidly progressing form of chronic hepatitis, with up to 40%, 6-month mortality in untreated individuals[412] associated with the presence of autoimmune markers. Although typically a chronic disease, it may have an acute presentation in up to 40% of cases, as discussed earlier. It is relatively uncommon, with an annual incidence of 1.9 cases per 100,000 population,[51] but it is responsible for 3% to 6% of all liver transplants.[302,467] As with most autoimmune diseases, there is a strong female predominance. Forms of AIH can be found in all age ranges, with no racial or ethnic predilection. There are associations with specific HLA haplotypes, notably DR3 and DR4, as is true for many other autoimmune diseases. Practice guidelines on autoimmune chronic hepatitis have been developed by the American Association for the Study of Liver Diseases (AASLD).[103] Immunosuppressive treatment using prednisone, alone or in combination with azathioprine, is effective in inducing a clinical remission of disease in about 80% of cases. Since there are inherited differences in activity of thiopurine methyltransferase that affect about 10% of the population,[259] it has been recommended that pretreatment determination of enzyme activity be used to reduce the likelihood of toxicity.[194] Remission typically begins with improvement in symptoms, followed by normalization in laboratory abnormalities, and finally histological resolution.[103] Laboratory remission generally does not occur until at least 12 months of treatment, but almost always occurs by 24 months in responders. Histological remission is less common and usually requires at least 3 to 6 months longer than laboratory evidence of remission.[412] Sustained remission can persist off treatment in 80% of those with normal histology following therapy, but relapse occurs in 50% within 6 months if inflammation persists in the liver biopsy.[102]

AIH is associated with the presence of liver- and nonliver-related autoantibodies in plasma. These are helpful in diagnosis, but are not likely to be the cause of liver injury. The most important antibodies for diagnosis include antinuclear antibody (ANA), antismooth muscle antibody (ASMA), and antiliver-kidney microsomal antigen type 1 (LKM_1). A variety of other autoantibodies are found frequently in AIH, some of which are found in other disorders. A summary of the most common autoantibodies, their associations, and their molecular targets (when known) is given

TABLE 47-6 Serological Markers of Autoimmune Liver Disease

Antibody Name	Antigen target	Associations
Anti-actin	Actin	AIH type 1; more specific than ASMA, poor response to corticosteroids, early age onset
Anti-asialoglycoprotein receptor (ASGPR)	Transmembrane antigen binding protein	AIH, correlate with activity, disappear with successful treatment
Anti-liver kidney microsome (LKM_1)	Cytochrome P450 IID6	AIH type 2; seen in only 4% of U.S. cases; usually in children
Anti-liver specific cytosol (LC_1)	Enzyme (possibly formimino-transferase cyclodeaminase or argininosuccinate lyase)	AIH in younger patients, often with anti-LKM_1, primary sclerosing cholangitis; vary with activity of disease
Antimitochondrial antibody (AMA M2 type)	Dihydrolipoamide acyltransferase	Primary biliary cirrhosis
Antineutrophil cytoplasmic antibodies (p-ANCA)	Bactericidal/permeability protein, cathepsin G, lactoferrin	Primary sclerosing cholangitis (50%-70%), ulcerative colitis (50%-70%), AIH; nonspecific
Antinuclear antibody (ANA)	Multiple targets (centromere, ribonucleoproteins); may not be detected by ELISA	AIH type 1, some PSC cases
Antismooth muscle antigen (SMA)	Actin, tubulin, vimentin, desmin, skelitin	AIH type 1, seen in other autoimmune diseases in lower titers
Antisoluble liver antigen/liver pancreas (SLA)	Selenocysteine pathway protein (? serine hydroxymethyltransferase)	AIH type 3; very specific for AIH, correlate with relapse after corticosteroid withdrawal

AIH, Autoimmune hepatitis.

in Table 47-6. Tests for these autoimmune markers have typically used cell or tissue preparations studied by indirect immunofluorescence. With identification of target antigen(s) in tissue, assays have been developed to detect antibodies to these purified proteins. Such assays can be helpful in diagnosis, but the information derived from purified antigens is not always equivalent. Many laboratories currently use panels of purified antigens to detect antinuclear antibodies and many individuals with AIH are positive with tissue ANA tests, but negative using a panel of the most commonly found antinuclear antigens.[104] Antibodies to actin are the most common cause of ASMA; although they are more specific for AIH and may have stronger prognostic importance, they are less sensitive than ASMA and are not recommended for diagnostic use.[101]

Criteria for the diagnosis of AIH have been developed by an international group[223] and have been revised to improve their use.[21] The criteria include: (1) exclusion of other causes of liver injury; (2) elevation of aminotransferases with minimal increase in ALP; (3) presence of elevated immunoglobulins; positive ANA, ASMA, or anti-LKM_1, with negative antimitochondrial antibody; (4) compatible histological features; and (5) absence of intrahepatic bile duct injury. A scoring system based on these criteria has also been established; this has allowed recognition of overlap syndromes that have features of both AIH and autoimmune bile duct destruction, but is not needed in most cases to establish the diagnosis.[103]

It is controversial whether AIH should be further divided into subtypes; the international group that codified diagnostic criteria does not recommend use of subtypes,[21] but many authorities recognize three different forms. Although there may be differences in epidemiology among the different forms, there do not seem to be differences in clinical course or response to treatment. Type 1, which is the most common form and the only one seen frequently in North America, is predominantly a disease of middle-aged women. It is characterized by ASMA (found in 87% of cases) and/or ANA (found in 67% of cases); one or the other is present in nearly 100% of cases. Because of the nonspecific nature of these antibodies, titers are important in determining likelihood of AIH. In adults, positive antibodies in titers greater than or equal to a 1:80 dilution are supportive of the diagnosis, whereas lower titers are not.[21] In children, titers are typically lower than those seen in adults. Type 2 AIH, which characteristically occurs in children (although 20% occurs in adults), represents up to 20% of cases in Europe.[201] It is associated with antibodies to liver-kidney microsomal antigen 1 (anti-LKM_1) or cytochrome P450 2D6 (CYP2D6).[489] There is some cross reactivity between this antibody and certain HCV antigens, leading to positive anti-CYP2D6 in individuals with HCV infection. The epitopes recognized by anti-HCV antibodies are different from those in person with type 2 AIH.[273] Type 3 often lacks other autoimmune markers, but is positive for antibody to soluble liver antigen liver/pancreas. This antibody appears to be directed against a component in the selenocysteine pathway and has been suggested to be an enzyme.[239]

Inherited Liver Diseases Presenting as Chronic Hepatitis

Inherited liver diseases that present as chronic hepatitis include hemochromatosis, Wilson's disease, and $alpha_1$-antitrypsin (AAT) deficiency.

Hemochromatosis

Hereditary hemochromatosis (HH) is an autosomal recessive disorder of iron metabolism that results in excessive iron absorption and accumulation in tissue (see Chapter 31). The gene for HH has long been linked to chromosome 6, close to the genes for the HLA system; initially the gene was termed HLA-H. This gene has now been definitively identified and termed the HFE gene; it codes for a transmembrane protein similar to the class I MHC molecule.[149] The protein is located on the endothelial side of intestinal epithelial cells and binds transferrin-transferrin receptor complexes in some fashion, signaling a stop to iron absorption.[355] The process of iron absorption is complex.[354] At the luminal border, iron must be reduced to ferrous iron by a duodenal cytochrome enzyme termed Dcytb. Iron is then transported across the brush border by the divalent metal transporter DMT1. Iron can then be stored as ferritin, or transported across the basolateral membrane by ferroportin 1 (FP1). Iron is then oxidized by hephaestin (Hp), a transmembrane ferroxidase with 50% homology to ceruloplasmin. Ferric iron is then bound to transferrin for delivery to iron-dependent cells. The loop is completed, in the case of the duodenum, through cellular iron response proteins (IRP) that bind to iron-responsive regions (IRE) in RNA, altering translation. HFE mutations are associated with increased expression of DMT1 and FP1 in duodenal villus epithelial cells. What is not yet clear is how HFE mutations alter iron absorption, since HFE is highly expressed in crypt cells, but not in villus cells.

In North America and Europe, more than 90% of individuals with HH are homozygous for a single point mutation that inserts a tyrosine instead of cysteine at residue 282 (termed the C282Y mutation). A small percentage of cases are homozygous for a more common mutation, causing replacement of histidine with aspartate at residue 63 (H63D), or are compound heterozygotes for C282Y and H63D.[430] Homozygosity for C282Y is one of the most common genetic traits; it occurs primarily in individuals of northern European ancestry, where the gene frequency is approximately 1 in 8, and the homozygous state is found in 1 in 150 to 200.[53] It is less frequently seen in other populations; in African-Americans, the frequency is 1 in 10,000.[40] Other mutations in the HFE gene have also been linked to hemochromatosis,[49,316,418] but in some populations inherited defects in HFE have been excluded,[356] and mutations in other proteins that regulate iron absorption have been identified.[72,334,356A]

Identification of the HFE gene mutations has led to a number of screening programs for HH. These studies have confirmed the high frequency of the gene, and documented increased transferrin saturation and ferritin in most homozygous individuals.[9,48,65,341] Based on these gene frequencies, hemochromatosis should be a relatively common disease; however, it has long been considered rare. In a study from the Netherlands (an area of high prevalence of homozygous HFE mutations), the prevalence of clinically diagnosed hemochromatosis was 1.4 cases per 100,000 population before testing for the HFE gene was instituted.[304] There is no difference in the frequency of homozygosity for the C282Y mutation with increasing age through the first 70 years of life, with only a slight decrease in gene prevalence after age 80, suggesting that the gene has only a minimal effect of longevity.[42,48] In one study, in which those screened had an average age of 57 years, there was only a twofold increase in the frequency of increased liver-related enzymes or history of liver disease when compared with controls.[48] There is no difference in the frequency of symptoms linked to hemochromatosis in homozygotes when compared with those with the wild-type gene.[454] The penetrance of the gene has been estimated at only 1%.[48,289] This has led some to question whether other factors are involved in the development of the disease and whether screening for the HFE gene is advisable.[7,53] For example, excess alcohol intake is strongly linked to risk of development of cirrhosis in individuals homozygous for the C282Y mutation.[153] Practice guidelines developed by the AASLD do not advocate screening.[430]

The key clinical laboratory features of hemochromatosis are related to excess iron; iron testing is discussed in more detail in Chapter 31. Since plasma iron increases relatively rapidly after meals, it is advisable to either use fasting samples for initial testing, or confirm elevated values on a fasting sample before doing further testing for evidence of iron overload. Several studies have shown that a cutoff value of transferrin saturation (plasma iron divided by total iron binding capacity) greater than 45%, or unsaturated iron binding capacity less than 155 μg/dL (28 μmol/L) has a clinical sensitivity of close to 100% for detecting homozygous C282Y mutations.[9,341] The positive predictive value of these cutoffs for homozygous mutations ranges from 20% to 70%.[292,341] Individuals lacking HFE gene mutations typically have average transferrin saturation approximating 25%.[292,341] Plasma ferritin has been used as a test for iron overload; it is not as sensitive as plasma iron indices in most studies[9,341] and is increased by tissue injury independent of iron stores. In a large screening program in which genotype was determined, ferritin was increased above the 90th percentile of healthy individuals in only about 60% to 70% of males and females,[246] whereas transferrin saturation was above the 90th percentile in almost 80% in both genders. Individuals with both increased transferrin saturation and increased ferritin have a higher likelihood of having genetic hemochromatosis. A liver biopsy with quantification of hepatic iron has been considered the standard for diagnosis of iron overload. It is best interpreted as the hepatic iron index [liver iron {μmol/g liver (dry weight)} divided by age (y)]; values of 1.9 or over indicate excess iron. Hepatic iron index correlates well with genetic evidence of hemochromatosis, but is not as clinically sensitive as plasma tests[8,236]; guidelines suggest it has little use in diagnosis when genetic markers are available.[36,430] At present, the key to diagnosis of HH is by documentation of gene mutations in the HFE gene. This is most commonly done by PCR, but a variety of techniques are available to detect the two most common mutants. It has been reported that insignificant mutations in other regions of the normal HFE gene may prevent its amplification in vitro, leading to false interpretation of homozygosity for the abnormal gene.[117,221]

When present, clinical manifestations of hemochromatosis are variable. The classical triad of hemochromatosis consists of cirrhosis, diabetes mellitus, and bronzing of the skin. The frequency of homozygous C282Y mutations is increased in individuals with type 2 diabetes mellitus. The skin pigmentation is a result of melanin, not iron, deposition. Cardiomyopathy is another serious complication of hemochromatosis and may be the dominant clinical manifestation. With screening, it has become apparent that less classic presentations, such as abdominal pain, arthritis, and hypogonadism, are relatively common. Other endocrine problems, such as hypopituitarism and hypoparathyroidism, typically occur late in the course of disease. Although plasma iron indices are similar in men and women, clinical manifestations of hemochromatosis typically occur at a later age in women, presumably because of ongoing iron loss with menstrual bleeding.

Therapy for HH involves phlebotomy to remove excess iron and stimulate erythropoiesis to use stored iron. An average phlebotomy removes approximately 250 mg of iron. The goal of treatment is to induce iron deficiency, defined by plasma ferritin below 20 ng/mL. Phlebotomy is initially performed weekly until iron deficiency develops; this may require a year or more in individuals with advanced iron overload. Once iron deficiency has been obtained, most patients will require regular phlebotomy to maintain normal plasma iron indices.

Wilson's Disease

Wilson's disease is an autosomal recessive disorder of copper metabolism (see Chapters 20 and 30). It has a gene frequency of 1 in 200 and a disease frequency of 1 in 30,000. It is due to one of more than 200 mutations in a gene on chromosome 13 coding for a copper transporting ATPase (ATP7B).[63,429] This enzyme, found mainly in the liver, is involved in movement of copper into bile; deficiency leads to accumulation of copper in the liver and, eventually, in other tissues. Low plasma concentrations of ceruloplasmin, a copper containing enzyme made in the liver, are also characteristic of Wilson's disease. With deficiency of ATP7B, apoceruloplasmin does not gain its full complement of copper molecules before release from hepatocytes. Although originally low ceruloplasmin was thought to be the cause of Wilson's disease, apoceruloplasmin has a reduced half-life compared with the holoenzyme, leading to lower plasma concentrations.[200]

Wilson's disease usually manifests before age 30, although several patients in their 50s and 60s have been reported. For reasons that are unknown, patients usually have predominantly either the hepatic or neuropsychiatric form of the disease. In children, hepatic involvement tends to predominate,[482] whereas in adolescents and adults, the neuropsychiatric form becomes more common. The hepatic manifestations include fulminant hepatitis (as discussed earlier), but more commonly chronic hepatitis, with or without cirrhosis, is the presenting finding.[390,395] Occasionally the features mimic those of autoimmune hepatitis, with increased globulins and positive ANA.[303] Neurological findings are variable; the classic picture includes cog wheel rigidity, associated with degenerative changes in the basal ganglia on imaging studies.[419]

The classic clinical finding of increased copper deposition in the eye is the Kayser-Fleischer ring, caused by deposition of copper in Descemet membrane at limbus of the cornea. Although found in about 95% of patients with neurological or psychiatric manifestations, it is present in only about half of patients with hepatic forms of Wilson's disease[417] and is rarely present in children.[388] As mentioned earlier, hemolytic anemia and renal failure commonly accompany acute forms of Wilson's disease; hemolytic anemia may be episodic even in chronic forms of Wilson's disease.[372]

Several laboratory tests are available for diagnosis of Wilson's disease; ceruloplasmin measurement is discussed in detail in Chapter 20 and copper measurement in Chapter 30. Test results are often affected by other conditions, sometimes making diagnosis difficult. The classic findings of Wilson's disease are (1) decreased ceruloplasmin, (2) decreased total plasma copper, (3) increased plasma free (or nonceruloplasmin) copper, (4) increased urine copper excretion, and (5) increased hepatic copper content. Ceruloplasmin is a ferroxidase and typically measured either by enzymatic activity or by immunoassay. Although there has been controversy over which type is preferable, guidelines have not specified one type of assay.[127,372] Ceruloplasmin is very low in infants, gradually rises to higher than adult concentrations in early childhood, then gradually declines to adult concentrations. Use of age-appropriate reference intervals is critical for diagnosis in children. Ceruloplasmin is an acute phase protein, and its synthesis is induced by estrogen; concentrations may be falsely normal with acute illness or with high estrogen states.

Low concentrations of ceruloplasmin are seen with malnutrition, in protein losing states, and in cirrhosis of any cause. These preanalytic variables cause ceruloplasmin to have a low predictive value as a single test for Wilson's disease; in one study, the positive predictive value was only 6%.[77] Ceruloplasmin is also decreased in about 20% of heterozygous carriers of the Wilson's disease gene.[172] Because most plasma copper is bound to ceruloplasmin, total plasma copper is affected by factors that affect ceruloplasmin. Some estimate free (nonceruloplasmin) copper from total copper and ceruloplasmin as the difference between total copper (µg/dL) and [3 times ceruloplasmin (mg/dL)]; values more than 25 µg/dL suggest Wilson's disease.[164] Urine copper excretion is the most specific noninvasive test for Wilson's disease; 24 hour urine copper excretion is typically more than 100 µg/d in Wilson's disease. Unfortunately, clinical sensitivity of copper excretion appears to be only 75% to 85%.[388,417] A liver biopsy is thought to be the most reliable test for diagnosis of Wilson's disease. A copper content of >250 µg/g dry weight is fairly specific for Wilson's disease, except in the setting of chronic cholestasis, which should not cause difficulty in the differential diagnosis.[372,417]

Although genetic testing for Wilson's disease is possible, the large number of mutations, and the fact that most individuals with Wilson's disease have compound heterozygosity for two different mutations, makes genetic testing impractical for diagnostic purposes. In contrast, genetic testing of the proband is critical in determining the mutations present to allow screening of first degree relatives.[372]

Treatment of active, symptomatic Wilson's disease is aimed at increasing urine copper excretion to eliminate excess copper from tissue. The primary therapy for Wilson's disease involves chelating agents such as D-penicillamine and trientine, which is now more widely used because of its lower rate of side effects. In patients with minimal symptoms or in asymptomatic family members, zinc is used to competitively inhibit copper absorption from the intestinal tract. Lifelong therapy with one of these types of treatment is required and is usually successful in limiting further damage.

Alpha$_1$-Antitrypsin Deficiency

AAT is the most important of the serine protease inhibitors (collectively termed serpins), which include such proteins as antithrombin, plasminogen activator inhibitor, α_1-antichymotrypsin, and C_1 esterase inhibitor (see Chapter 20).[475] As its name implies, AAT inhibits trypsin, but also inhibits other proteolytic enzymes, including neutrophil-derived elastase, cathepsin G, and proteinase 3. The gene for AAT is located on chromosome 14. There are a number of genetic variants of AAT (differing by a single amino acid) that were originally classified on the basis of their electrophoretic mobility; the slowest migrating of these was termed the Z variant. Each individual has two copies of the protease inhibitor (Pi) gene, which can lead to several phenotypic variants. Some of the variants, particularly S and Z, form loop sheet polymers.[268] This leads to impaired release from the endoplasmic reticulum and hepatocytic inclusions of AAT, and reduced plasma concentrations, increased proteolytic damage to tissue, and clinical manifestations of disease. The most severe forms of disease have been associated with homozygosity for the Z variant (PiZZ), present in 1 in 1000 to 2000 individuals in Europe and North America.[208] (See Chapter 20 for additional information on AAT and its measurement.)

The major clinical manifestation of AAT deficiency is emphysema, which tends to occur at an earlier age and can occur in the absence of smoking. It is estimated that 1% of emphysema is related to AAT deficiency. In neonates, AAT deficiency is often associated with hepatitis; in one study, almost one third of infants with prolonged jaundice were found to be AAT deficient.[486] About 20% of AAT deficient infants develop hepatitis,[359] with up to 25% 1-year mortality.[207] In those who survive the first year, however, evidence of liver injury diminishes and usually resolves by age 12.[422,457] At age 18, none of 183 individuals with AAT deficiency had clinical evidence of liver disease, none had elevated procollagen III peptide, and less than 20% had elevated liver-associated enzymes.[423] These findings suggest that AAT may have minimal effects on pathogenesis of liver disease in adults.[402]

Actual data on association of AAT deficiency with liver disease in adults are somewhat contradictory. In several studies, cirrhosis was present in one third to one half of those with AAT deficiency, and HCC was present in about one third of those with cirrhosis.[138,367] The frequency was similar in those with heterozygous and homozygous presence of the PiZ variant.[367] In two studies of patients with cryptogenic liver disease, the frequency of the PiZ heterozygotes was significantly higher than found in the general population.[73,181] Two other studies, however, found a similar frequency of liver disease in those with AAT deficiency and controls.[152,312] Some evidence suggests that AAT deficiency may increase risk of liver damage from other factors. In one study, most individuals with AAT deficiency and liver injury were also positive for anti-HCV; only 11% had no other liver risk factors.[366] In those with AAT deficiency and no evidence of liver disease (usually viral related), life expectancy was no different from that in healthy controls.[366]

Estimation of AAT can be performed by protein electrophoresis, where it comprises most of the α_1-globulin band; this was the original means by which AAT deficiency was recognized.[138] AAT is quantified by a variety of techniques (see Chapter 20). AAT is an acute phase response protein; falsely normal quantitative concentrations have been reported in about 40% of PiZ heterozygotes,[199] although rarely in PiZZ homozygotes. Determination of phenotype is typically accomplished by isoelectric focusing, and has been recommended as the diagnostic test of choice in one guideline.[129]

Drug-Induced Liver Diseases

As discussed earlier, most cases of drug-induced liver disease present as acute hepatitis. Less commonly, drugs have produced a chronic liver injury, in a pattern mimicking chronic hepatitis or other chronic liver injury (chronic cholestasis and hepatic granulomas).[396] The most common drugs linked to chronic hepatitis are nitrofurantoin, methyldopa,[255] and HMG-CoA reductase inhibitors[456]; however, a large number of drugs have been associated with liver injury,[496] and herbal medications have also been linked to chronic hepatitis.[85,416] In individuals with increased activities of aminotransferases and no obvious cause, prescription drug use was significantly more likely to be present than in those with a known cause for elevated enzyme activities.[284] As with acute drug reactions, establishing drugs as the cause of chronic hepatitis is difficult[176]; temporal relationships to drug ingestion are not as clear as with acute hepatitis, and reactions can first be seen in those who have been taking the medication for many months.[265] Most chronic drug reactions resolve when administration of the drug is discontinued.[11,22]

Significance of Chronic Hepatitis

Chronic hepatitis is, in many cases, a disease with minimal consequences. As mentioned earlier, an average of 20% to 30% of individuals with chronic HBV or HCV progress to cirrhosis over a 20-year period. However, cirrhosis is the 10th leading cause of death in the United States.[133] The frequency of cirrhosis and HCC has been increasing in much of the western world,[242] thought mostly caused by the increase in cases related to HCV. The proportion of individuals with HCV with cirrhosis and HCC is expected to double over the next 20 years, and the number of deaths caused by liver disease is expected to almost triple.[109] The ability to predict which patients are at increased risk for such late complications of chronic hepatitis would allow more appropriate treatment.

Fibrosis and necroinflammatory activity are the two major components of chronic hepatitis. The extent of fibrosis (stage) is strongly related to risk of progression,[212,346,478] whereas necroinflammatory activity (grade) is correlated with progression in some,[169,286,478] but not all,[75,360,363] studies. Since ALT activity is strongly correlated with necroinflammatory activity,[288] it is also associated with risk of progression to cirrhosis in some, but not all, studies. Clinical variables are also associated with risk of progression; these include age at infection, male gender, alcohol intake, and presence of immunosuppression.[75,160,281,364]

The process of scar formation in the liver involves a number of factors, and differs in some important ways from that in other sites in the body.[14,324,394] There is increasing evidence that the process of fibrosis is reversible, even when cirrhosis is histologically present.[131,132] For example, two studies have found that successful treatment of HBV[123] and HCV[362] was associated with reversal of cirrhosis in 50% to 75% of cases. Although the principal component is type III collagen, other components include type I and type IV collagen, laminin, elastin, and fibronectin. Proteoglycans, especially hyaluronate, are also part of scar formation. Production of scar in the liver is also affected by the rate of enzymatic degradation; a variety of matrix metalloproteinases (MP) are found in areas of scar formation, and there are several tissue inhibitors of metalloproteinases (TIMP) as well.[33] MPs are involved in degradation of the normal connective tissue of the liver (a necessary prequel to fibrosis), but are also involved in breakdown and remodeling of collagen. Hepatic stellate cells are critical in this process; they produce both MP and TIMP,[44] and collagen and other matrix materials.[381] Recruitment and activation of stellate cells involves the action of a number of cytokines, particularly TGF-β, platelet derived growth factor (PDGF), and interleukin-6 (see Chapter 22).[64,280,440]

These observations led to the expectation that measurement of plasma concentrations of factors associated with scar formation would correlate with the degree of fibrosis found in the liver biopsy. There appears to be significant overlap in concentrations of such markers between individuals with cirrhosis and those with varying stages of fibrosis in chronic hepatitis.* There is also evidence that marker concentrations change with alteration in necroinflammatory activity and may actually reflect activity of disease at the time of sampling, rather than cumulative fibrosis.[442] Subsequent interest has therefore focused less on using fibrosis markers to detect progression to cirrhosis and more on identifying individuals with minimal fibrosis, who have little risk of progression to cirrhosis. Calculation of a predictive index using a combination of 5 markers (α_2-macroglobulin, apolipoprotein A_1, total bilirubin, γ-glutamyl transferase (GGT), and haptoglobin) was highly effective in predicting those persons who did not have significant fibrosis.[214,318,361] This calculation requires use of the specific assays used in the initial studies; use of kits from other manufacturers led to poor performance of the predictive index.[378] Another predictive index using age, GGT, cholesterol, and platelet count had a similarly high negative predictive value,[156] but has not been validated in other laboratories. A combination of three markers (hyaluronate, TIMP-1, and α_2-macroglobulin) also showed high specificity in detecting fibrosis, but produced indeterminate results in 20% of individuals tested.[349]

ALCOHOLIC LIVER DISEASE

Alcoholic liver disease differs clinically and biochemically from other forms of hepatitis and liver disease. It is a common cause of liver disease in the developed world but the incidence of acute alcoholic hepatitis seems to be declining in North America and Europe.[275B] Risk factors for developing alcoholic liver disease include:[161A]

1. Duration and magnitude of alcohol ingestion. Alcoholic liver disease does not occur in all individuals with chronic ethanol intake, but there is a threshold intake of 40 g/day in men and 10 g/day in women below which alcoholic hepatitis does not occur.[298] For most individuals, the risk dose is about 80 g of alcohol (200 mL of whiskey or equivalent) per day.[258A] Daily drinking appears to be riskier than intermittent drinking.

*References 154, 163, 214, 335, 357, 437.

2. Gender. In women there is a greater likelihood of progression to cirrhosis and women have reduced activities of alcohol dehydrogenase in gastric mucosa, leading to increased blood levels of alcohol.[423A]
3. Hepatitis B or C infection. Both may increase the severity in the patients who drink heavily. For example, antibodies to HCV are several times more common in individuals with alcoholic hepatitis than in alcoholics without hepatitis or in age and gender matched controls, suggesting a synergistic role for HCV.[295]
4. Genetic factors. As discussed below, inherited predisposition to alcoholism has been clearly established.
5. Nutritional status. Protein-calorie malnutrition is extremely common in alcoholics. Malnutrition may be due not only to poor intake but also to abnormal nutrient metabolism. Whereas poor nutrition may contribute to the evolution of alcoholic liver disease, adequate nutrition does not prevent its development. In fact, studies suggest that obesity may be a risk factor.

In addition, there is evidence for an immunological component in alcoholic liver disease,[161,217,242A] and there is evidence that modification of liver proteins by ethanol metabolites is involved in the pathogenesis.[6,431] Acute alcoholic hepatitis clinically is an acute febrile illness, characteristically associated with leukocytosis[294] and increased concentrations of acute phase response proteins.[184] It also causes mild increases in cytosolic enzymes; AST activity is typically more than two times that of ALT[92] and it is rare for AST to be more than eight times the upper reference limit.[294] A cholestatic form of the disease, with increases in ALP activity to greater than three times the upper reference limit, is seen in up to 20% of cases;[333] it is associated with higher mortality. Increases in bilirubin are common, and reduced liver synthesized protein concentrations are also commonly present. Increased bilirubin, decreased albumin, and prolonged PT are poor prognostic markers in alcoholic hepatitis.[174] A discriminant function [$4.6 \times (\text{PT} - \text{control PT})$] + plasma bilirubin (mg/dL)] value >32 indicates individuals with a high mortality rate,[298] and a Model for (or Mayo) End Stage Liver Disease (MELD) score more than 11 has also been found to have similar sensitivity and better specificity.[403]

Both alcoholism and susceptibility to the development of cirrhosis appear to be largely genetically determined in that only 10% to 15% of heavy consumers of alcohol develop cirrhosis. Much effort has been expended in finding specific genetic markers and it has been found that the rate of cirrhosis is much higher if a patient has a parent with alcoholic cirrhosis.[151A] Whitfield and colleagues have confirmed these findings as they have found that variation in alcohol intake is due to genetic effects.[463A,463B] In addition, genes affecting intake also affect dependence risk, but there are other genes that affect dependence alone. The predisposition may be related to different rates of alcohol elimination, which are determined by genetic polymorphism of the microsomal ethanol oxidizing system (MEOS) and alcohol dehydrogenase (ADH).[425A,463B] For example, 50% of Asians have absent alcohol dehydrogenase, leading to a flush reaction to alcohol that inhibits drinking and thus is a negative risk for alcoholism. Alternatively, heterozygotes of the acetaldehyde dehydrogenase (AADH) gene have impaired clearance of acetaldehyde, the putative toxin of alcohol, and may be at increased risk for liver injury. Two forms of alcoholism have been identified in the Stockholm Adoption Study.[408A] Type 1 has adult onset and rapid progression of dependence. Type 2 has teenage onset with recurrent social and legal problems.

Alcohol is metabolized to acetaldehyde by cytosolic ADH and the MEOS (primarily CYP 2E1—the same cytochrome P_{450}–dependent enzyme involved with acetaminophen metabolism). Acetaldehyde is subsequently metabolized to acetyl-CoA by AADH. This is further broken down to acetate, which is either converted to carbon dioxide and water or enters the citric acid cycle to be converted to fatty acids. The latter is a major mechanism for induction of fatty liver by alcohol, but acetaldehyde is probably the primary toxin. It causes most of the injury to liver cells as well as the induction of collagen synthesis leading to fibrosis and, ultimately, cirrhosis.

A large number of biochemical markers have been proposed for the detection of excessive alcohol consumption and associated liver disease.[95A,95B,151A,175A,220A,252A,253A,301B] Clinically, aminotransferase activities rarely exceed 300 U/L in acute alcoholic hepatitis, and are much lower (and frequently within reference intervals) in chronic alcoholic liver disease. Alcohol depletes vitamin B_6–dependent pyridoxal-5-phosphate, an essential precursor of aminotransferase synthesis. The AST : ALT ratio is usually greater than 2, unlike in other liver diseases, in which ALT is typically higher than AST. This has been attributed to the increased appearance of mitochondrial AST (mAST). Although mAST is elevated in serum from alcoholics, it rarely accounts for >20% of total AST activity and is unlikely to be the sole cause. The higher AST may reflect damage to other tissues that release AST but not ALT, which is confined to the liver. ALP is typically elevated about twofold but may be four- or fivefold elevated in patients with alcoholic hepatitis. Serum GGT is commonly used as a screening test for alcohol abuse. However, GGT is an inducible enzyme that is elevated by many drugs and many disease states. Thus, the clinical sensitivity of GGT for alcohol consumption is satisfactory, but it is not a specific test of chronic alcohol abuse. Ethyl esters of fatty acids have also been proposed as markers of ethanol intake.[252A] Covalent protein adducts are also formed by the liver as a result of ethanol metabolism and lipid peroxidation.[328A]

Alcohol interferes with a number of glycoconjugation reactions, perhaps as the result of acetaldehyde inhibition of hepatic glycotransferases. The isoforms of transferrin have been studied as markers of alcohol consumption, as excessive ethanol consumption results in the appearance in serum of isoforms that are carbohydrate deficient (CDT, also called hyposialyl- and asialyltransferrin).[29A,152A,175A,328B,463C,476A,479A] The use of CDT for detecting problem drinkers has been reviewed.[242B] It also has been suggested that combining markers such as CDT and GGT will increase the accuracy of identifiying problem drinkers.[83A,408B] Independent of liver function, an increased mean erythrocyte corpuscular volume, an indicator of dysfunctional production of red cells, has also been proposed as a marker of chronic ethanol consumption and is more specific than GGT.[479A]

PT may be prolonged and serum albumin decreased as the disease becomes more severe. Serum levels of procollagen type III correlate reasonably well with collagen synthesis and disease severity in chronic alcoholic liver disease. Nonspecific laboratory abnormalities reflecting the diffuse metabolic changes that occur with alcoholism include hyperuricemia, hyperlacticacidemia, hypertriglyceridemia, hypoglycemia, hyperglycemia, hypophosphatemia, hypomagnesemia, and macrocytosis. Liver biopsy is essential for determining disease severity and prognosis as well as to rule out treatable diseases such as chronic hepatitis and hemochromatosis.

The prognosis of alcoholic liver disease is better than that for other forms of liver disease, with only 10% to 15% developing cirrhosis and a much smaller fraction developing HCC.[351A] Both hepatitis B and hepatitis C appear to accelerate the course of alcoholic liver disease. The 5-y survival rate in patients with cirrhosis, jaundice, and ascites is 40% if the patient continues drinking and 60% if the patient abstains.[359A]

The primary treatment of alcoholic liver disease is abstinence from alcohol. However, new and promising approaches for drug treatment of the disease have resulted from a more extensive understanding of the neurobiological substrates of alcohol dependence, including adaptive changes in amino acid neurotransmitter systems, stimulation of dopamine and opioid peptide systems, and, possibly, changes in serotonergic activity.[27A,275A,275B] Previous studies have indicated that endogenous opioids are involved in the craving for alcohol[453A] and opioid antagonists such as naltrexone are being used to treat the disease.[73A,275A,374A,414A,453A] Currently, disulfiram, naltrexone, and acamprosate are currently the only treatments approved for the management of alcohol dependence.[275A,414A] Studies in animals have demonstrated that a diet enriched in vitamin E and saturated fatty acids reduces alcoholic liver injury by decreasing lipid peroxidation.[319A] Liver transplantation is the treatment of choice in end-stage liver disease. The results of transplantation in alcoholic liver disease are comparable to those with other forms of liver disease.[236A]

CIRRHOSIS

Cirrhosis, defined anatomically as diffuse fibrosis with nodular regeneration, represents the end stage of scar formation and regeneration in chronic liver injury. This response to injury occurs independently of the etiology and thus it is not possible, in most circumstances, to determine the cause of cirrhosis based on the histology. Classically, cirrhosis has been classified as (1) micronodular, (2) macronodular, or (3) mixed based on the histology and gross appearance of the liver. However, this is considered inadequate for etiological or prognostic purposes. Consequently, it is now more common to classify cirrhosis based on the presumed or known etiology. The common causes of cirrhosis and their therapies are listed in Table 47-7. Virtually all chronic liver diseases are known to lead to cirrhosis (see Figure 47-13), but most cases of cirrhosis occur as a result of chronic hepatitis.

TABLE 47-7 Causes and Treatment of Cirrhosis

Cause	Treatment
Viral	
Hepatitis B	Administration of α-interferon
Hepatitis C	Administration of α-interferon
Toxic	
Alcohol	Abstinence, liver transplantation
Methotraxol	Abstinence
Metabolic	
Hemochromatosis	Phlebotomy
Wilson's disease	Penicillamine
α_1-Antitrypsin deficiency	Gene therapy possible
Biliary	
Primary biliary cirrhosis	Ursodeoxycholic acid
Primary sclerosing cholangitis	Liver transplantation
Autoimmune hepatitis	Corticosteroids, azathioprine
Idiopathic	

In the early stages of transition from chronic hepatitis to cirrhosis, termed compensated cirrhosis, there may be no signs or symptoms of liver damage. Laboratory abnormalities usually appear before clinical findings such as ascites, gynecomastia, palmar erythema, and portal hypertension begin to develop. The earliest laboratory abnormalities to develop in cirrhosis are (1) fall in platelet count,[171,274] (2) increase in PT, (3) decrease in the albumin to globulin ratio to less than one,[274] and (4) increase in the AST/ALT activity ratio to greater than one.[171,274] Survival in those with compensated cirrhosis is good; 10-year survival rate in a large series was 90%.[145] As cirrhosis progresses, decompensation occurs. A variety of manifestations of portal hypertension may be present, as detailed earlier in the chapter. Jaundice is a late finding in decompensated cirrhosis. Once decompensation occurs, 10-year survival is only about 20%.[145] A variety

TABLE 47-8 Child-Pugh System for Classifying Severity of Cirrhosis

Feature	1 point	2 points	3 points
Encephalopathy	None	Grade 1-2	Grade 3-4
Ascites	None	Slight	Moderate-severe
Albumin (g/dL)	>3.5	2.8-3.5	<2.8
Prothrombin time (s prolonged)	<4	4-6	>6
Bilirubin (mg/dL)	<4	4-10	>10

Scoring: <7 points—Class A; 7-9 points—Class B; >9 points—Class C.

TABLE 47-9 The Hepatic Glycogen Storage Diseases

Type	Eponym	Enzyme Defect	Involved Tissues
0		Glycogen synthetase	Liver
I	von Gierke	Ia glucose-6-phosphatase Ib translocase for glucose 6-phosphatase Ic phosphate/pyrophosphate translocase	Liver, kidney, intestines
II	Pompe's	Lysosomal acid α-1,4 glucosidase	Most tissues
III	Cori	Amylo-1,6 glucosidase debranching enzyme	Liver, muscle, WBCs
IV	Anderson's	Amylo-1,4,1,6 trans glucosidase (branching enzyme)	Most tissue
VI	Hers'	Liver phosphorylase	Liver, WBCs
VII		Phosphorylase activation	Liver
IXa		Phosphorylase kinase	Liver, WBCs, RBCs

WBCs, White blood cells; *RBC,* red blood cells.

of staging systems have been used to predict prognosis in cirrhosis. For many years, the most common classification system was the Child-Pugh class system, summarized in Table 47-8. Currently, the MELD score [calculated as 3.8 + ln bilirubin (mg/dL) + 11.2 ln International Normalized Ratio + 9.6 ln creatinine (mg/dL) + 6.4 etiology score (0 if alcohol or obstruction, 1 for all other causes)] has been used to identify patients with advanced cirrhosis who may be candidates for liver transplantation; it appears superior to the Child-Pugh scoring system in predicting short-term survival.[57,61,155,387] Risk of death over 3 months is low in those with MELD scores below 10, intermediate in those with scores of 10 to 20, and high in those with scores above 20.[229]

Laboratory findings in cirrhosis reflect ongoing liver injury and decreased hepatic function. The most common laboratory findings in individuals with cirrhosis are summarized in Table 47-9. Activities of aminotransferases are variable in cirrhosis, and reflect activity of underlying necroinflammatory activity. If the cause of cirrhosis has been eliminated (as by abstinence from ethanol or successful treatment of viral hepatitis), aminotransferase activity is often within the reference interval. Persistence of elevation is a risk factor for development of HCC.[389] As described earlier, the ratio of AST/ALT activity is often greater than 1 in cirrhosis.[171,347,404,468] The mechanism for the change in ratio is not clear, but there appears to be a decrease in the production of ALT in cirrhotic individuals.[392] Increases in alpha fetoprotein (AFP) are common in cirrhotic patients, even in the absence of HCC.

Hepatic Glycogenoses

The glycogenoses are a group of disorders that are characterized by excessive and/or aberrant glycogen storage in various tissues. Most of these have deficient glucose production by the liver, leading to hypoglycemia. All are inherited by autosomal recessive transmission except for type IV, which is sex-linked. The hepatic glycogen storage diseases and their enzyme defects are listed in Table 47-9.

Most of these disorders are associated with growth retardation and hepatosplenomegaly. Mental development is usually normal. Hypoglycemia is a prominent feature in types I, III, and VI and needs to be treated with continuous glucose feeding of uncooked cornstarch, which results in a slow release of glucose.

The diagnosis is based on the demonstration of excess glycogen in the liver biopsy and in vitro identification of the abnormal enzyme or aberrant glycogen. Prognosis and treatment vary with each entity.

Cholestatic Liver Diseases

Cholestasis (stoppage or suppression of the flow of bile) is associated with retention of bile within the excretory system.

The term obstruction is often used inappropriately, since cholestasis can occur without mechanical obstruction to the biliary tract. Although intrahepatic cholestasis may be due to either functional or mechanical problems, extrahepatic cholestasis is always due to physical obstruction of the bile ducts by processes such as choledocholithiasis, biliary strictures, and tumors. The major cholestatic diseases are (1) mechanical obstruction of the bile ducts, (2) primary biliary cirrhosis (PBC), and (3) primary sclerosing cholangitis (PSC). Other cholestatic disorders include (1) post–bone marrow transplant cholangiopathy, (2) post–liver transplant cholangiopathy, (3) drug-induced cholestasis, (4) AIDS cholangiopathy, and (5) bilirubinostasis of acute illness. Cholestatic hepatitis, which has been discussed previously, may also cause cholestasis, but generally presents in a fashion closer to hepatitis.

The clinical consequences of prolonged cholestasis are related to the impaired biliary drainage. Deficiency of bile acids in the intestinal tract leads to malabsorption of fat and the fat soluble vitamins A, D, E, and K (see Chapters 30 and 49). Vitamin A malabsorption results in night blindness. Vitamin D malabsorption results in calcium and phosphate malabsorption, causing rickets in children and osteomalacia in adults. Vitamin K malabsorption results in deficiency of coagulation factors II, VII, IX, and X, leading to prolonged clotting times and bleeding. Lack of excretion of normal bile contents leads to their accumulation in plasma. Bile acid retention leads to increased bile acid concentrations in plasma. Although this has been historically associated with pruritus, it now appears that endogenous opioid-receptor analogues and increased serotonin are responsible.[225,226] Accumulation of cholesterol is associated with the development of an abnormal lipoprotein-X,[299,322] containing phospholipids, cholesterol, fragments of cell membrane (along with ALP),[60] and albumin; the lipid may deposit in connective tissue, producing xanthomas. Bilirubin retention leads to jaundice, dark urine, and pale stools. Increased bilirubin generally occurs only with complete obstruction and thus is more commonly seen with extrahepatic than intrahepatic cholestasis.

Laboratory features of cholestasis vary, depending on whether the process causes complete or partial impairment of biliary drainage. The common feature of all cholestatic disorders is an increase in plasma activities of canalicular enzymes, such as ALP and GGT. Because this process involves both increased synthesis of enzyme and release of enzyme from its membrane bound forms, there is generally a short lag period between the onset of cholestasis and the increase in plasma activities. In the early stages of an acute mechanical obstruction (especially from gallstones), there may be transient increases in plasma activities of liver cytosolic enzymes, such as AST and ALT. Plasma AST and ALT may exceed 400 IU/L, and in 1% to 2% of cases are more than 2000 IU/L. Even in the presence of continued obstruction, AST and ALT activity gradually decrease, and AST is typically within the reference interval within 8 to 10 days. Increases in total bilirubin typically occur only with complete extrahepatic obstruction, although they may be seen with extensive intrahepatic cholestasis. Increases in direct bilirubin are more commonly seen, and direct bilirubin has been reported to be the most sensitive functional test of the presence of cholestasis. In all forms of cholestasis, there is downregulation of the multidrug resistance transport protein 2 (MRP2), congenitally deficient in Dubin-Johnson syndrome.[436] Prolonged PT is the most commonly detected coagulation abnormality. It usually is corrected by administration of parenteral vitamin K. Increased cholesterol is a common finding in chronic cholestasis and along with increased canalicular enzymes is one of the most consistent features of cholestatic disorders. Lipoprotein-X will be included in LDL cholesterol in the Friedewald formula and in some direct LDL cholesterol methods.[150] Although lipoprotein-X is specific for cholestasis, it is not found in all individuals with cholestatic disorders.[413]

Mechanical Bile Duct Obstruction

The most common cause of cholestasis is biliary tract obstruction by space occupying lesions.[401] Extrahepatic bile duct obstruction occurs most commonly because of gallstones in the common bile duct or because of tumors in the head of the pancreas or duodenum. Other causes of extrahepatic obstruction include bile duct strictures, extrinsic compression of the bile ducts by enlarged lymph nodes, congenital biliary atresia, and PSC. Extrahepatic obstruction is commonly associated with jaundice, especially when obstruction is complete. Elevation in canalicular enzymes is common, but is not present in all cases[270]; marked increases (more than three times the upper reference limit) are more common with gallstones as a cause of obstruction.[458] Transient increases in aminotransferases are more common with choledocholithiasis than with other causes of extrahepatic obstruction.[218] Transient increases in CA 19-9 occur with bile duct obstruction[41]; this is an important consideration, as CA 19-9 is often used as a diagnostic test for pancreatic and bile duct carcinomas. A key feature of extrahepatic obstruction is dilation of more proximal and intrahepatic bile ducts, which can be visualized by imaging studies.[250]

Intrahepatic cholestasis caused by mechanical obstruction is also common, but is rarely associated with jaundice or with visibly dilated ducts on imaging studies, although it may be associated with increased direct bilirubin. Jaundice typically occurs only with lesions that are very large, or are located near the porta hepatis, where they may obstruct both hepatic ducts. Common causes of intrahepatic obstruction include (1) tumors (particularly metastases), (2) granulomatous diseases (such as sarcoidosis and tuberculosis), and (3) infiltrative processes (such as lymphoma, leukemia, and extramedullary hematopoiesis).

Primary Biliary Cirrhosis

PBC, or nonsuppurative destructive cholangitis, is an uncommon autoimmune disorder targeting intrahepatic bile ducts. Its prevalence is approximately 2 to 8 per 100,000 population in the developed world, but it is much lower in developing areas. The median age at onset is 50 years, and the female to male ratio is about 6:1. There is an association in some populations with HLA class II antigen DR8. A family history of PBC is present in 1% to 4% of cases. In up to 80% of cases, it is associated with other autoimmune processes, most commonly Sjögren syndrome[325] and hypothyroidism (which often develops before onset of PBC).[100]

The pathogenesis of PBC is not well understood. However, it is known that the destruction of the bile duct is mediated by T cells in the presence of upregulation of HLA class I antigens on hepatocytes and HLA class II antigens on biliary epithelial cells.[168] Although the target antigens of the T cells have not been identified,[450] at least 95% of patients have antimitochondrial antibodies that react against the dihydrolipoamide acyltransferase component of the pyruvate decarboxylase complex.[449] Part of this complex is found on the apical surface of biliary epithelial cells, suggesting a role for this antigen as an immune target.[314] In individuals with coexisting Sjögren syndrome, the antigen is also expressed on the surface of salivary gland cells.[441]

PBC typically presents as an asymptomatic elevation of ALP, but may present with features of cholestasis or with fatigue. Metabolic bone disease and xanthomas are common complications of PBC.[192] Occasionally, autoantibodies are detected (usually because of the presence of another autoimmune disease or because of family history of PBC) before elevation of ALP.[300] Aminotransferase activities are increased in 50% of cases, but are more than twice the upper reference limit in only 20% of cases.[266] Increased bilirubin is a late finding and is important in predicting decompensation.[248] Antibodies to mitochondria or to the recombinant pyruvate decarboxylase complex appear similar in sensitivity, although the latter are more specific.[448] A liver biopsy is not required for diagnosis in most cases, but may be helpful in those with low titer antibodies or with greater than twofold increase in aminotransferase activity.[192]

The natural history of PBC is one of slow progression to portal hypertension, often without development of cirrhosis. Medical management of PBC consists of ursodeoxycholic acid, 13 to 15 mg/kg/day, which improves symptoms but appears to have no effect on long-term survival or need for liver transplantation.[345] Although a rare complication, the relative risk of developing HCC is significantly increased in individuals with PBC.[329] Liver transplantation is the only definitive treatment, but even then, PBC may recur in the transplanted organ.[148]

Primary Sclerosing Cholangitis

PSC is a chronic inflammatory disease of the biliary tree, most commonly affecting extrahepatic bile ducts; involvement of intrahepatic ducts, either with extrahepatic involvement or as an isolated finding, is also possible.[26,491] In contrast to PBC, PSC has a male predominance and a younger median age at onset of 30 years. In 70% of patients, PSC is associated with ulcerative colitis, which usually (but not always) precedes onset of PSC. This has led to speculation that bacterial antigens in portal blood might be involved in pathogenesis of PSC.[26] An autoimmune component is likely, as 97% of patients with PSC have one or more autoantibodies present in their plasma.[27] The prevalence of PSC is similar to that of PBC, but there are geographic differences in prevalence; it is most common in Northern Europe, where PSC is the most common indication for liver transplantation.[393] There is a markedly increased prevalence of HLA antigens B8 and DR3.[464]

The clinical presentation of PSC, like that of PBC, is typically an asymptomatic patient with elevated ALP concentrations found during routine laboratory screening. Symptoms are ultimately present in most patients with PSC; the most common are pruritus and intermittent abdominal pain, but fever may also be present.[340] Treatment, either medical or surgical, may improve laboratory tests and symptoms, but does not improve long-term survival.[257,293] Transplantation is the major treatment available for end-stage PSC and has a high rate of long-term survival. Although PSC recurs after transplantation in about 20% to 35% of cases, it does not appear to affect survival.[178,452] Transplantation also appears to increase the severity of underlying ulcerative colitis, when present.[134] The major cause of death in individuals with PSC is cholangiocarcinoma, which ultimately develops in up to one third of patients.[26,491] Transplantation in the presence of cholangiocarcinoma is associated with rapid development of metastatic disease and poor survival.[10] PSC also increases the likelihood of colon carcinoma in individuals with coexisting ulcerative colitis, although the risk is not affected by liver transplantation.[466]

At the time of diagnosis, most patients with PSC have elevated ALP and other canalicular enzymes; bilirubin is typically normal, although it may increase with acute exacerbations. The diagnosis of PSC is based on the typical radiographic appearance of beading and irregularity of the bile ducts.[453] Antineutrophil cytoplasmic antibodies (ANCA) are present in approximately 50% to 80% of patients but are not specific for PSC; they are also present in PBC and autoimmune hepatitis. Typically the antibodies have an atypical perinuclear pattern, being located near the nucleus both in formalin and methanol fixed preparations. Antigens include lactoferrin, bactericidal/permeability increasing protein, and cathepsin G.[315,375,376]

Drug-Induced Cholestasis

Drugs are a common cause of cholestasis, causing about 15% of cases.[497,498] Drug reactions are especially common in older individuals, where up to 50% of individuals have increased enzymes because of medications.[497] Drugs can cause a cholestatic picture by two major mechanisms.[495,498] In some cases, only conjugated bilirubin is increased, whereas canalicular enzymes are not elevated. This picture, often seen with estrogen and anabolic steroids, appears because of inhibition of production of MRP2,[436] as discussed earlier in other cholestatic disorders. More commonly, drugs induce a cholestatic hepatitis, as discussed earlier.

Gallstones

Gallstones are solid formations in the gallbladder that are composed of cholesterol and bile salts. Although they vary in chemical composition, they generally contain a mixture of cholesterol, bilirubin, calcium, and mucoproteins. In the United States, 70% to 85% of all gallstones are predominantly cholesterol and more than 10% of the adult population is affected.

There are three major types of gallstones: (1) cholesterol gallstones, (2) pigmented gallstones, and, most common, (3) mixed gallstones. These stones form whenever bile is supersaturated with cholesterol or unconjugated bilirubin. Most gallstones are mixed cholesterol and pigment stones. For these stones or cholesterol gallstones to form, bile must be supersaturated with cholesterol. Whenever there is an increase in cholesterol or a decrease in bile acids or lecithin, bile becomes lithogenic (prone to stone formation), and cholesterol may precipitate. Factors that predispose to cholesterol hypersecretion are obesity, aging, certain drugs such as clofibrate and nicotine, and certain hormones such as estrogen. Factors that decrease bile acid secretion are terminal ileal disease and cholestatic diseases, such as PBC, PSC, and cystic fibrosis. Genetic factors also appear to be involved. Within racial groups, women are more frequently affected than men. Diet may play a role because it appears that people who ingest diets high in polyunsaturated fats have a higher incidence, whereas those with a diet high in fiber have a decreased incidence.

Pigmented gallstones are associated with conditions in which the bilirubin load is increased, such as hemolytic anemia, or when bilirubin becomes insoluble (i.e., deconjugated), such as occurs with cholestasis or chronic biliary infections.

Rare Causes of Cholestasis

A number of other disorders are associated with cholestasis. Because they occur in specific settings, they are often suggested by the clinical picture. Laboratory tests are of little help in establishing the correct diagnosis.

Cholestasis may develop following bone marrow transplantation because of a variety of factors. Acute graft-versus-host disease (GVHD) is a consequence of the infusion of allogeneic immunocompetent T-lymphoid cells into an immunocompromised host that cannot reject these cells.[210] The periductular epithelial cells are the primary targets of injury in both acute and chronic GVHD.[46,386] Clinical features of GVHD include skin rash, intestinal symptoms (nausea, vomiting, diarrhea, and abdominal pain), and cholestasis. The histological appearance is characteristic, but a liver biopsy is somewhat hazardous in these patients, and thus most patients' disorders are diagnosed on clinical grounds.

Although acute liver transplant rejection is associated with necroinflammatory changes and increases in aminotransferases, chronic rejection is often associated with cholestasis. The primary targets of immunologic injury are bile ductules and blood vessels.[115] Because of cholestasis, plasma bile acids are often increased early in the process of rejection.[219] Increased numbers of canalicular membranes are often the first evidence of rejection.[115] Although eosinophilia is common in rejection,[319] it is also a common finding in drug-induced cholestasis, and is thus not helpful in the differential diagnosis.

AIDS cholangiopathies are caused by organisms not previously known to infect the biliary tree; they have become less common with reduction in the frequency of immunosuppression because of combination antiretroviral treatment. *Cryptosporidium* is the most common organism. *Microsporidium,* cytomegalovirus, *Mycobacterium avium* complex, and *Cyclospora* have also been identified. The clinical presentation usually includes abdominal pain, diarrhea, and cholestasis manifested by threefold to tenfold elevations in plasma ALP, mild elevations in aminotransferases, and rarely jaundice. Papillary stenosis at the ampulla of Vater is present in patients with pain, and the bile ducts have features of PSC. Cholangiography is needed for the diagnosis but is only indicated in patients with pain. Brushings and biopsies at the time of cholangiography will establish the diagnosis. Treatment is primarily endoscopic. Sphincterotomy will give pain relief in approximately 70% of patients.

Hepatic Tumors

The liver is host to a wide variety of both benign and malignant primary tumors. It is also the second most common site of metastases; metastatic tumors account for 90% to 95% of all hepatic malignancies. The primary tumors may arise from many cell lines in the liver but most commonly from parenchymal and biliary epithelial cells and mesenchymal cells (Table 47-10). The two most important primary liver tumors are HCC and cholangiocarcinoma.

Hepatocellular Carcinoma

HCC is the fifth most common cancer worldwide and a leading cause of cancer death. There are wide geographic and ethnic variations in the incidence, suggesting that both host and environmental factors are involved in its etiology. For example, approximately 75% of HCC occur in Asia, with an annual incidence of HCC in China of approximately 30 cases per 100,000 males. In contrast, the average annual incidence is less than 5 cases per 100,000 males in North America. Worldwide, the incidence is twofold to threefold higher among men than it is among women.[56] The incidence of HCC has been increasing, not only in North America,[137] but in the rest of the world, thought to be caused by the increasing frequency of cirrhosis caused by HCV.[136] Although cirrhosis is present in most patients with HCC, it is absent in about 25% to 30% of cases, often in association with HBV.[59,487] More importantly the presence of cirrhosis had been recognized before diagnosis of HCC in only about one third of cases.[483,488] There are wide variations in the incidence of HCC with different etiologies of cirrhosis. For example, HCC occurs commonly in cirrhosis caused by alcohol abuse, hemochromatosis, AAT deficiency, HBV, and HCV, but is rare in that caused by autoimmune hepatitis and Wilson's disease.

In most parts of the world, the major risk factors for development of HCC are infection with HBV or HCV. In Asia, Africa, and Alaska, the major risk factor is HBV infection. The presence of HBsAg and HBeAg is associated with a relative risk of HCC of 60, whereas the presence of HBsAg with negative HBeAg was associated with a relative risk of 10.[477] It is important to note that the frequency of HCC has been reduced significantly with prevention of chronic HBV by immunization.[82,254] Once cirrhosis has developed, the rate of development of HCC is about 1.5% to 5% per year in both HBV and HCV[146,147]; the relative risk of HCC doubles in those co-infected with both viruses.[144] The mechanism of increased risk in HBV is thought to be related to integration of HBV DNA into the host genome, possibly caused by the action of the HBV X gene, which may block the activity of p53.[151,444] The mechanism of increased risk in HCC in HCV has not been identified, but may be related to ongoing injury. The risk of HCC is higher in those with cirrhosis who have elevated aminotransferases than in those with normal ALT.[191,389] Interferon, which reduces inflammation, has been found to lower the risk of HCC in HCV, both as a primary tumor[54,232,425] and as recurrences following resection of a first HCC.[211,244,407]

Aflatoxin, a product of *Aspergillus flavus* contamination of grain, has been linked to risk of HCC; although it is harmless, it is metabolized to aflatoxin 8,9-epoxide. This reactive intermediate binds to guanosine bases in DNA, leading to mutagenesis. If the formed adduct is not repaired, G to T transversion occurs in codon 249 of the *p53* gene, causing an inactivating mutation.[368] Under normal circumstances, the mutagenic aflatoxin 8,9-epoxide is rendered harmless by glutathione-S-transferase, which converts it to a glutathione conjugate, which in turn is metabolized to 1,2-dihydrodiol by epoxide hydrolase.[264] However, both detoxifying enzymes are polymorphic in humans and the mutant forms are less active. Patients with HCC are more likely to have the mutant forms of epoxide hydrolase and glutathione-S-transferase, which allows accumulation of the epoxide.[291]

The clinical presentation of HCC is variable, but usually does not occur until late in the course of disease, when the tumor is large and resection is impossible. In some cases, acute decompensation occurs in a patient with cirrhosis, but clinical presentation may include detection of a right upper quadrant mass, shock because of hemorrhage into the peritoneal cavity, or right upper quadrant pain.[119] Nonspecific signs and symptoms, such as fever, malaise, anorexia, and anemia are common, and jaundice may occur with central tumors that obstruct biliary drainage. In a small number of cases, paraneoplastic features, such as hypoglycemia, hypercalcemia (due to parathyroid hormone–related peptide [PTHrP] production) or erythrocytosis (due to erythropoietin) may be the initial presenting findings, and such paraneoplastic findings occur in up to 20% of cases, usually associated with poor prognosis.[234,275] Laboratory findings include those of cirrhosis and cholestasis, and (except for tumor markers discussed below), are nonspecific.

Because treatment is usually not possible in individuals with clinically diagnosed HCC, there has been much interest in screening high risk individuals. Currently, most professional societies have not advocated screening for HCC in Europe or North America,[327] although most practicing hepatologists perform screening in patients with cirrhosis, especially that caused by viral hepatitis.[79] Although data from some areas have suggested that screening is effective in detecting small, treatable tumors, other data have not been as supportive.

The most common screening programs have used either plasma tumor marker concentrations or tumor markers plus imaging studies. Ultrasound is typically used as the imaging modality for screening because of its low cost. The tumor marker most widely used for screening purposes is AFP; it is typically quantified using assays that measure its total

TABLE 47-10 Classification of Hepatic Tumors

Benign	Malignant
Epithelial	
Adenoma	Hepatocellular carcinoma
Bile duct adenoma	Cholangiocarcinoma
Cystadenoma	Cystadenocarcinoma
Carcinoid	Squamous carcinoma
Focal nodular hyperplasia	
Diffuse nodular hyperplasia	
Mesenchymal Tumors	
Cavernous hemangioma	Hemangiosarcoma
Fibroma	Fibrosarcoma
Leiomyoma	Leiomyosarcoma
Hematoma	Hepatoblastoma
Metastatic Tumors (Most Common Sources)	
Colon	
Pancreas	
Stomach	
Breast	
Unknown primary	
Bronchogenic	

concentration. As discussed in Chapter 54, there also are modified forms of AFP that are more specific for tumors, particularly the L3 isoform recognized by lens culinaris (lentil) lectin. Total AFP has been the most widely used tumor marker; although it appears to be relatively sensitive, elevation of AFP is common in individuals with chronic hepatitis and cirrhosis, the group at highest risk for HCC. In our experience, AFP above the upper reference limit has a positive predictive value of only 16% for HCC. Use of higher cutoff values than the upper reference limit improves clinical specificity of total AFP, at the expense of clinical sensitivity. Fewer data exist for the L3 isoform of AFP, but specificity and positive predictive value are significantly improved.[406,424] An L3 isoform more than 15% of total AFP may be associated with more aggressive and less well differentiated tumors.[240,338] Des-γ-carboxy prothrombin (DCP)—also called PIVKA-2 (factor II protein induced by vitamin K antagonists)—is the inactive form of prothrombin found in individuals taking warfarin or other vitamin K antagonists. It was first found to be increased in HCC in 1984,[262] but was not widely used until the early 1990s. Initial studies found that DCP was increased in some patients who did not have elevated AFP, but was insensitive to small HCC that might be curable.[118,162] Pretreatment with vitamin K, to eliminate other causes of increased DCP, improves specificity further.[383] More recently, DCP immunoassays with lowered detection limits have been developed and have shown increased clinical sensitivity for small HCC.[213,320] DCP is best used as an adjunct to AFP, since tumors often produce one or the other tumor marker.[28]

The treatment of HCC is dependent on the extent of the tumor. Small tumors are often treated by transplantation, which has a low rate of recurrent tumor.[193] Local techniques, such as ethanol injection, chemoembolization, and use of radio frequency ablation, are increasingly used either pretransplant or instead of transplantation.[78,173,260] Larger tumors are generally not resectable, but may be treated by chemoembolization if a single feeding vessel is identified. A novel approach to identifying micrometastases has recently been introduced using reverse transcription PCR to amplify mRNA for AFP to detect recurrence or metastasis.[470]

Tumors of the Gallbladder and Bile Ducts

Benign lesions such as papillomas or adenomas may be seen as an incidental finding at cholecystectomy; malignant disease of the gallbladder is uncommon. Cholelithiasis may be an etiological factor, as 85% of gallbladder carcinomas occur in patients with gallstones. However, fewer than 1% of patients with gallstones develop carcinoma. It has been suggested that a calcified gallbladder is especially prone to malignant transformation. Various pathological forms exist, including papillary adenocarcinoma, squamous cell carcinoma, and anaplastic tumors. These tumors usually arise in the neck of the gallbladder and spread rapidly, causing obstruction and cholestasis. Physical examination reveals a hard, tender mass in the gallbladder fossa. These lesions are particularly difficult to treat and the majority of cases are inoperable at the time of diagnosis.

Cholangiocarcinoma, or primary carcinoma of the bile ducts, can arise at any point in the biliary tree, including the small intrahepatic bile duct radicals. This lesion is typically associated with underlying liver disease, such as (1) PSC, (2) congenital cystic lesions, or (3) chronic infestation with *Clonorchis sinensis.* The clinical picture presentation is that of cholestasis, including jaundice, dark urine, tan-colored stool, and pruritus. Differentiation from other cholestatic diseases is made by visualizing the biliary tree.

DIAGNOSTIC STRATEGY

Liver function tests are useful in (1) detecting, (2) diagnosing, (3) evaluating severity, (4) monitoring therapy, and (5) assessing the prognosis of the liver disease and dysfunction. They are also useful in directing further diagnostic workup. The array of tests useful for these purposes (Table 47-11) includes measurement in plasma of total bilirubin, protein, and albumin concentrations and the activity of enzymes such as the aminotransferases (AST and ALT), ALP, lactate dehydrogenase (LD), and GGT. By using a combination of these tests, it is possible to categorize broad types of liver disease, which can then be more accurately diagnosed through disease-specific tests. An algorithm for that process is presented in Figure 47-17.

TABLE 47-11 Tests of Hepatic Function

Test	Utility
Bilirubin	Diagnosing jaundice, modest correlation with severity
Alkaline phosphatase (ALP)	Diagnosing disorders of metabolism and disorders of the newborn
Bilirubin fractionation	Diagnosing cholestasis and space-occupying lesions
Aspartate aminotransferase (AST)	Sensitive test of hepatocellular disease; AST > ALT in alcoholic disease
Alanine aminotransferase (ALT)	Sensitive and more specific test of hepatocellular disease
Albumin	Indicator of chronicity and severity
Prothrombin time (PT)	Indicator of severity of cholestasis

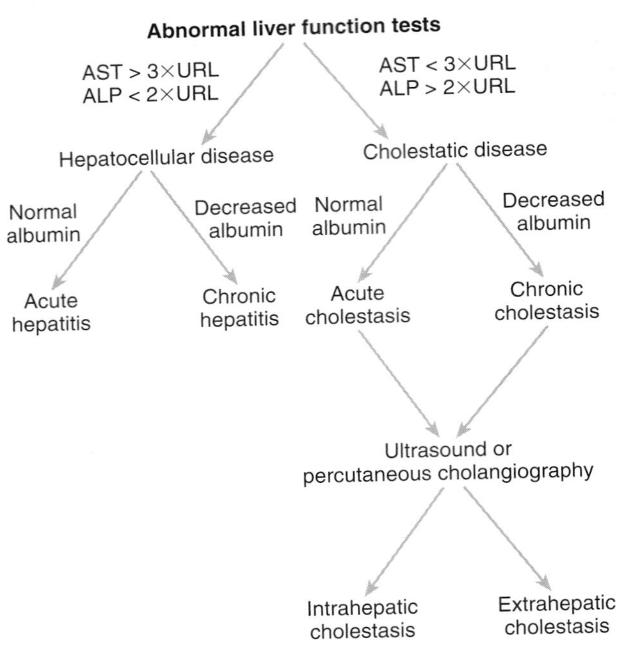

Figure 47-17 Algorithm for using abnormal liver function tests to classify and diagnose various types of liver disease. *ALP,* Alkaline phosphatase; *AST,* aspartate aminotransferase; *URL,* upper reference limit.

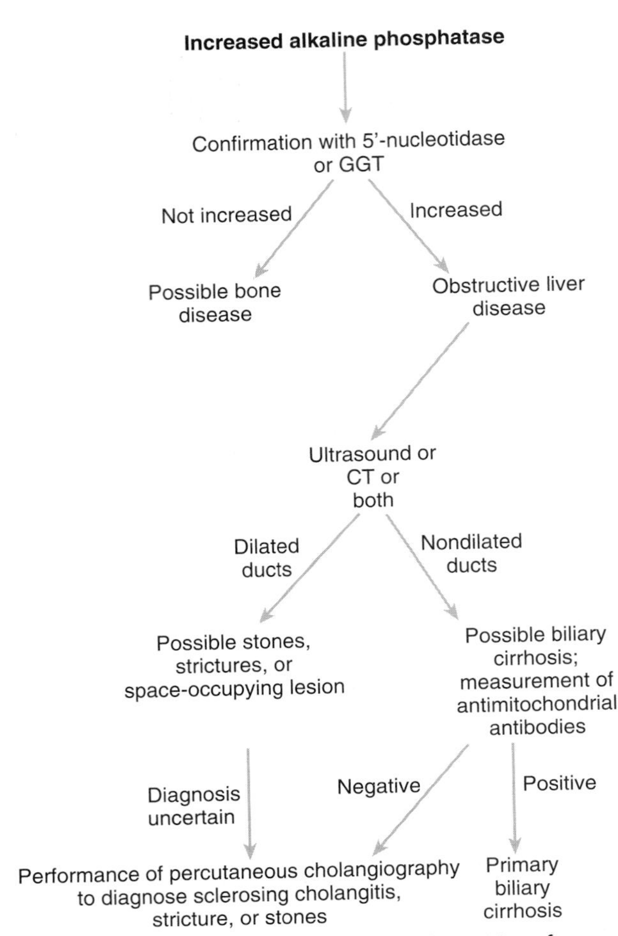

Figure 47-18 Algorithm for using elevated activities of serum alkaline phosphatase in the diagnosis of liver disease in adults.

Plasma Enzymes

In practice, the plasma aminotransferases and ALP are the most useful tests as they allow differentiation of hepatocellular disease from cholestatic disease. The importance of this distinction cannot be overstated: failure to recognize cholestatic disease caused by extrahepatic biliary obstruction will result in liver failure if the obstruction is not quickly corrected. It is also important to recognize that there may be a gray zone of mixed hepatocellular and cholestatic disease where the tests do not distinguish one disease from the other. In this case, it is wise to assume that the problem is cholestatic and rule out biliary obstruction.

Patients are occasionally seen with isolated elevations in ALP or aminotransferase enzyme activities. In practice, an isolated increase in ALP activity is difficult to interpret. In children, *benign transient hyperphosphatasemia* should always be considered. In adults, it is necessary to first confirm that the ALP is of hepatobiliary origin. This can be done by isoenzyme fractionation (see Chapter 21) or by measuring another phosphodiesterase enzyme such as 5′ nucleotidase (Figure 47-18) or by measuring GGT activities, which tend to parallel activities of ALP in cholestasis. The most important aspect of the workup is to rule out space-occupying lesions by visualizing the liver with CT, and biliary tract disease by visualizing the biliary tree with ultrasound or cholangiography.

Elevated plasma activities of AST and ALT are common in many disorders (see Chapter 21). To determine if this elevation is liver related, administration of all drugs and alcohol intake (especially if AST is higher than ALT) should be discontinued. If the elevation persists, ultrasound (looking for nonalcoholic fatty liver) and hepatitis B and C serology should be performed. More than 50% of isolated enzyme elevations of liver origin will be caused by these disorders. A liver biopsy is often needed to make a more specific diagnosis. There is no reliable test other than a liver biopsy to detect fibrosis. Plasma procollagen type III peptide has been used, but correlates better with disease activity than fibrosis.

Plasma Albumin

Plasma albumin measurements are useful in assessing the chronicity and severity of liver disease. For example, the plasma albumin concentration is decreased in chronic liver disease. However, its utility for this purpose is somewhat limited, as the plasma albumin concentration is also decreased in severe acute liver disease. Serial measurements of plasma albumin can be used to assess the severity of liver disease.

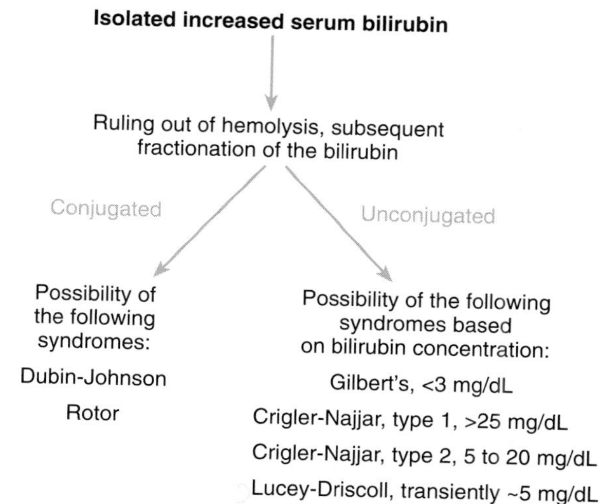

Figure 47-19 Algorithm for differentiating the familial causes of hyperbilirubinemia.

Prothrombin Time

Serial PT measurements also can be used to differentiate between cholestasis and severe hepatocellular disease. In practice, PT should be measured again after vitamin K injection, because cholestasis will cause a decrease in PT because of malabsorption of vitamin K. The patient has cholestasis if the PT corrects after vitamin K replacement (10 mg subcutaneously or intramuscularly, followed by PT measurement 4 hours later). With time, if the PT does not return to normal, the patient has severe hepatocellular disease.

Plasma Bilirubin

Serial measurement of bilirubin is helpful in measuring the severity of liver disease. Bilirubin fractionation is helpful only in jaundice of the newborn or in isolated elevations of bilirubin in the absence of other liver test abnormalities that would indicate an inherited disorder of bilirubin metabolism.

Patients are occasionally seen with isolated elevations in bilirubin concentration. In most cases, this is due to inherited disorders of bilirubin metabolism, familial hyperbilirubinemia, or hemolysis. It is not difficult to distinguish hemolysis severe enough to cause hyperbilirubinemia, because the patient with hemolysis will have many other disease manifestations. An algorithm for differentiating the familial causes of hyperbilirubinemia is presented in Figure 47-19.

REFERENCES

1. Abe K. GB virus-C/hepatitis G virus. Jpn J Infect Dis 2001;54:55-63.
2. Abe K, Edamoto Y, Park YN, Nomura AM, Taltavull TC, Tani M, et al. In situ detection of hepatitis B, C, and G virus nucleic acids in human hepatocellular carcinoma tissues from different geographic regions. Hepatology 1998;28:568-72.
3. Abe K, Hayakawa E, Sminov AV, Rossina AL, Ding X, Huy TT, et al. Molecular epidemiology of hepatitis B, C, D and E viruses among children in Moscow, Russia. Clin Virol 2004;30:57-61.
4. Abe K, Kiuchi T, Aiba N, Tran HT, Ding X, Yamaguchi M, et al. Complete nucleotide sequence of hepatitis B virus isolated from two infants with fulminant hepatitis. J Infect Dis 2003;56:38-9.
5. Abraldes J, Tarantino I, Turnes J, Garcia-Pagan J, Rodes J, Bosch J. Hemodynamic response to pharmacological treatment of portal hypertension and long-term prognosis of cirrhosis. Hepatology 2003;37:902-8.
6. Actis G, Ponzetto A, Rizzetto M, Verme G. Cell-mediated immunity to acetaldehyde in alcoholic liver disease demonstrated by leukocyte migration test. Am J Dig Dis 1978;23:883-6.
7. Adams P. Population screening for hemochromatosis—Are we finding people with a disease or a biochemical curiosity? Semin Gastrointest Dis 2002;13:89-94.
8. Adams P, Bradley C, Henderson A. Evaluation of the hepatic iron index as a diagnostic criterion for genetic hemochromatosis. J Lab Clin Med 1997;130:509-14.
9. Adams P, Kertesz A, McLaren C, Barr R, Bamford A, Chakrabarti S. Population screening for hemochromatosis: A comparison of unbound iron-binding capacity, transferrin saturation, and C282Y genotyping in 5,211 voluntary blood donors. Hepatology 2000;31:1160-4.
10. Ahrendt S, Pitt H, Nakeeb A, Klein A, Lillemoe K, Kalloo A, et al. Diagnosis and management of cholangiocarcinoma in primary sclerosing cholangitis. J Gastrointest Surg 1999;3:357-67; discussion 67-8.
11. Aithal P, Day C. The natural history of histologically proved drug induced liver disease. Gut 1999;44:731-5.
12. Akriviadis E, Kapnias D, Hadjigavriel M, Mitsiou A, Goulis J. Serum/ascites albumin gradient: Its value as a rational approach to the differential diagnosis of ascites. Scand J Gastroenterol 1996;31:814-7.
13. Akriviadis E, Runyon B. Utility of an algorithm in differentiating spontaneous from secondary bacterial peritonitis. Gastroenterology 1990;98:127-33.
14. Albanis E, Friedman S. Hepatic fibrosis. Pathogenesis and principles of therapy. Clin Liver Dis 2001;5:315-34, v-vi.
15. Alberti A, Pontisso P, Chemello L, Fattovich G, Benvegnu L, Belussi F, et al. The interaction between hepatitis B virus and hepatitis C virus in acute and chronic liver disease. J Hepatol 1995;22:38-41.

16. Albrecht J, Jones E. Hepatic encephalopathy: Molecular mechanisms underlying the clinical syndrome. J Neurol Sci 1999;170:138-46.
17. Alessandria C, Venon W, Marzano A, Barletti C, Fadda M, Rizzetto M. Renal failure in cirrhotic patients: Role of terlipressin in clinical approach to hepatorenal syndrome type 2. Eur J Gastroenterol Hepatol 2002;14:1363-8.
18. Allen M, Deslauriers M, Andrews C, Tipples G, Walters K, Tyrrell D, et al. Identification and characterization of mutations in hepatitis B virus resistant to lamivudine. Lamivudine Clinical Investigation Group. Hepatology 1998;27:1670-7.
19. Alter M, Kruszon-Moran D, Nainan O, McQuillan G, Gao F, Moyer L, et al. The prevalence of hepatitis C virus infection in the United States, 1988 through 1994. N Engl J Med 1999;341:556-62.
20. Alter M, Kuhnert W, Finelli L. Guidelines for laboratory testing and results reporting of antibody to hepatitis C virus. MMWR Morb Mortal Wkly Rep 2003;52:1-15.
21. Alvarez F, Berg P, Bianchi F, Bianchi L, Burroughs A, Cancado E, et al. International Autoimmune Hepatitis Group Report: Review of criteria for diagnosis of autoimmune hepatitis. J Hepatol 1999;31:929-38.
22. Amacher D. Serum transaminase elevations as indicators of hepatic injury following the administration of drugs. Regul Toxicol Pharmacol 1998;27:119-30.
23. Amontree J, Stuart T, Bredfeldt J. Autoimmune chronic active hepatitis masquerading as acute hepatitis. J Clin Gastroenterol 1989;11:303-7.
24. Anciaux M, Pelletier G, Attali P, Meduri B, Liguory C, Etienne J. Prospective study of clinical and biochemical features of symptomatic choledocholithiasis. Dig Dis Sci 1986;31:449-53.
25. Andriulli A, Festa V, Leandro G, Rizzetto M. Usefulness of a liver biopsy in the evaluation of patients with elevated ALT values and serological markers of hepatitis viral infection: An AIGO study. Dig Dis Sci 2001;46:1409-15.
26. Angulo P, Lindor K. Primary sclerosing cholangitis. Hepatology 1999;30:325-32.
27. Angulo P, Peter J, Gershwin M, De SC, Shoenfeld Y, Ahmed A, et al. Serum autoantibodies in patients with primary sclerosing cholangitis. J Hepatol 2000;32:182-7.
27A. Anton RF, Swift RM. Current pharmacotherapies of alcoholism: A U.S. perspective. Am J Addict 2003;12 Suppl 1:S53-68.
28. Aoyagi Y, Oguro M, Yanagi M, Mita Y, Suda T, Suzuki Y, et al. Clinical significance of simultaneous determinations of alpha-fetoprotein and des-gamma-carboxy prothrombin in monitoring recurrence in patients with hepatocellular carcinoma. Cancer 1996;77:1781-6.
29. Armstrong G, Alter M, McQuillan G, Margolis H. The past incidence of hepatitis C virus infection: Iimplications for the future burden of chronic liver disease in the United States. Hepatology 2000;31:777-82.
29A. Arndt T. Carbohydrate-deficient transferrin as a marker of chronic alcohol abuse: A critical review of preanalysis, analysis, and interpretation. Clin Chem 2001;47:13-27.
30. Armstrong G, Bell B. Hepatitis A virus infections in the United States: Model-based estimates and implications for childhood immunization. Pediatrics 2002;109:839-45.
31. Arroyo V, Gines P, Gerbes A, Dudley F, Gentilini P, Laffi G, et al. Definition and diagnostic criteria of refractory ascites and hepatorenal syndrome in cirrhosis. International Ascites Club. Hepatology 1996;23:164-76.
32. Arroyo V, Guevara M, Gines P. Hepatorenal syndrome in cirrhosis: Athogenesis and treatment. Gastroenterology 2002;122:1658-76.
33. Arthur M. Fibrogenesis II. Metalloproteinases and their inhibitors in liver fibrosis. Am J Physiol Gastrointest Liver Physiol 2000;279:G245-9.
34. Averhoff F, Shapiro C, Bell B, Hyams I, Burd L, Deladisma A, et al. Control of hepatitis A through routine vaccination of children. JAMA 2001;286:2968-73.
35. Bacon B. Treatment of patients with hepatitis C and normal serum aminotransferase levels. Hepatology 2002;36:S179-84.
36. Bacon B, Powell L, Adams P, Kresina T, Hoofnagle J. Molecular medicine and hemochromatosis: At the crossroads. Gastroenterology 1999;116:193-207.
37. Balistreri W. Fetal and neonatal bile acid synthesis and metabolism—Clinical implications. J Inherit Metab Dis 1991;14:459-77.
38. Banks J, Foulis A, Ledingham I, Macsween R. Liver function in septic shock. J Clin Pathol 1982;35:1249-52.
39. Barrera J, Bruguera M, Ercilla M, Gil C, Celis R, Gil M, et al. Persistent hepatitis C viremia after acute self-limiting posttransfusion hepatitis C. Hepatology 1995;21:639-44.
40. Barton J, Acton R. Inheritance of two HFE mutations in African Americans: Cases with hemochromatosis phenotypes and estimates of hemochromatosis phenotype frequency. Genet Med 2001;3:294-300.
41. Basso D, Fabris C, Plebani M, Del FG, Muraca M, Vilei M, et al. Alterations in bilirubin metabolism during extra- and intrahepatic cholestasis. Clin Investig 1992;70:49-54.
42. Bathum L, Christiansen L, Nybo H, Ranberg K, Gaist D, Jeune B, et al. Association of mutations in the hemochromatosis gene with shorter life expectancy. Arch Intern Med 2001;161:2441-4.

43. Belay E, Bresee J, Holman R, Khan A, Shahriari A, Schonberger L. Reye's syndrome in the United States from 1981 through 1997. N Engl J Med 1999;340:1377-82.
44. Benyon R, Arthur M. Extracellular matrix degradation and the role of hepatic stellate cells. Semin Liver Dis 2001;21:373-84.
45. Berman D, Leventhal R, Gavaler J, Cadoff E, Van TD. Clinical differentiation of fulminant Wilsonian hepatitis from other causes of hepatic failure. Gastroenterology 1991;100:1129-34.
46. Berman M, Rabin L, O'Donnell J, Gratwohl A, Graw R, Deisseroth A, et al. The liver in long-term survivors of marrow transplant—Chronic graft-versus-host disease. J Clin Gastroenterol 1980;2:53-63.
47. Bessems J, Vermeulen N. Paracetamol (acetaminophen)-induced toxicity: Molecular and biochemical mechanisms, analogues and protective approaches. Crit Rev Toxicol 2001;31:55-138.
48. Beutler E, Felitti V, Koziol J, Ho N, Gelbart T. Penetrance of 845G–>A (C282Y) HFE hereditary haemochromatosis mutation in the USA. Lancet 2002;359:211-8.
49. Beutler E, Griffin M, Gelbart T, West C. A previously undescribed nonsense mutation of the HFE gene. Clin Genet 2002;61:40-2.
50. Blei A. Diagnosis and treatment of hepatic encephalopathy. Baillieres Best Pract Res Clin Gastroenterol 2000;14:959-74.
51. Boberg K. Prevalence and epidemiology of autoimmune hepatitis. Clin Liver Dis 2002;6:347-59.
52. Boixeda D, De LD, Aller R, De AC. Spontaneous bacterial peritonitis. Clinical and microbiological study of 233 episodes. J Clin Gastroenterol 1996;23:275-9.
53. Bomford A. Genetics of haemochromatosis. Lancet 2002;360:1673-81.
54. Bonino F. Effect of interferon-a on progression of cirrhosis to hepatocellular carcinoma. A retrospective cohort study. Lancet 1998;351:1535-9.
55. Borsch G, Baier J, Glocke M, Nathusius W, Gerhardt W. Graphical analysis of laboratory data in the differential diagnosis of cholestasis: A computer-assisted prospective study. J Clin Chem Clin Biochem 1988;26:509-19.
56. Bosch F, Ribes J, Borras J. Epidemiology of primary liver cancer. Semin Liver Dis 1999;19:271-85.
57. Botta F, Giannini E, Romagnoli P, Fasoli A, Malfatti F, Chiarbonello B, et al. MELD scoring system is useful for predicting prognosis in patients with liver cirrhosis and is correlated with residual liver function: A European study. Gut 2003;52:134-9.
58. Bouvier-Alias M, Patel K, Dahari H, Beaucourt S, Larderie P, Blatt L, et al. Clinical utility of total HCV core antigen quantification: A new indirect marker of HCV replication. Hepatology 2002;36:211-8.
59. Bralet M, Regimbeau J, Pineau P, Dubois S, Loas G, Degos F, et al. Hepatocellular carcinoma occurring in nonfibrotic liver: Epidemiologic and histopathologic analysis of 80 French cases. Hepatology 2000;32:200-4.
59A. Brechot C, Thiers V, Kremsdorf D, Nalpas B, Pol S, Paterlini-Brechot P. Persistent hepatitis B virus infection in subjects without hepatitis B surface antigen: clinically significant or purely "occult"? Hepatology 2001;34:194-203.
60. Brocklehurst D. The alkaline phosphatase-lipoprotein X complex. Clin Chem 1981;27:1317-8.
61. Brown R, Kumar K, Russo M, Kinkhabwala M, Rudow D, Harren P, et al. Model for end-stage liver disease and Child-Turcotte-Pugh score as predictors of pretransplantation disease severity, posttransplantation outcome, and resource utilization in United Network for Organ Sharing status 2A patients. Liver Transpl 2002;8:278-84.
62. Bukh J, Miller R, Purcell R. Genetic heterogeneity of hepatitis C virus: Quasispecies and genotypes. Semin Liver Dis 1995;15:41-63.
63. Bull P, Thomas G, Rommens J, Forbes J, Cox D. The Wilson disease gene is a putative copper transporting P-type ATPase similar to the Menkes gene. Nat Genet 1993;5:327-37.
64. Burt A. C. L. Oakley Lecture (1993). Cellular and molecular aspects of hepatic fibrosis. J Pathol 1993;170:105-14.
65. Burt M, George P, Upton J, Collett J, Frampton C, Chapman T, et al. The significance of haemochromatosis gene mutations in the general population: Implications for screening. Gut 1998;43:830-6.
66. Burton B. Urea cycle disorders. Clin Liver Dis 2000;4:815-30, vi.
67. Bush MP, Nemo GJ. Current and emerging infectious risks of blood transfusions. JAMA 2003;289:959-62.
68. Buti M, Sanchez F, Cotrina M, Jardi R, Rodriguez F, Esteban R, et al. Quantitative hepatitis B virus DNA testing for the early prediction of the maintenance of response during lamivudine therapy in patients with chronic hepatitis B. J Infect Dis 2001;183:1277-80.
69. Butterworth R. Hepatic encephalopathy: A neuropsychiatric disorder involving multiple neurotransmitter systems. Curr Opin Neurol 2000;13:721-7.
70. Byron D, Minuk G. Clinical hepatology: Profile of an urban, hospital-based practice. Hepatology 1996;24:813-5.
71. Cacciola I, Pollicino T, Squadrito G, Cerenzia G, Orlando M, Raimondo G. Occult hepatitis B virus infection in patients with chronic hepatitis C liver disease. N Engl J Med 1999;341:22-6.
72. Camaschella C, Roetto A, Cali A, De GM, Garozzo G, Carella M, et al. The gene TFR2 is mutated in a new type of haemochromatosis mapping to 7q22. Nat Genet 2000;25:14-5.

73. Carlson J, Eriksson S. Chronic "cryptogenic" liver disease and malignant hepatoma in intermediate $alpha_1$-antitrypsin deficiency identified by a Pi Z-specific monoclonal antibody. Scand J Gastroenterol 1985;20:835-42.
73A. Carmen B, Angeles M, Ana M, Maria AJ. Efficacy and safety of naltrexone and acamprosate in the treatment of alcohol dependence: a systematic review. Addiction 2004;99:811-28.
74. Cassidy W, Reynolds T. Serum lactic dehydrogenase in the differential diagnosis of acute hepatocellular injury. J Clin Gastroenterol 1994;19:118-21.
75. Castera L, Hezode C, Roudot-Thoraval F, Bastie A, Zafrani E, Pawlotsky J, et al. Worsening of steatosis is an independent factor of fibrosis progression in untreated patients with chronic hepatitis C and paired liver biopsies. Gut 2003;52:288-92.
76. Caubet M, Laplante A, Caille J, Brazier J. [^{13}C]aminopyrine and [^{13}C]caffeine breath test: Influence of gender, cigarette smoking and oral contraceptives intake. Isotopes Environ Health Stud 2002;38:71-7.
77. Cauza E, Maier-Dobersberger T, Polli C, Kaserer K, Kramer L, Ferenci P. Screening for Wilson's disease in patients with liver diseases by serum ceruloplasmin. J Hepatol 1997;27:358-62.
78. Cha C, De MR, Blumgart L. Surgery and ablative therapy for hepatocellular carcinoma. J Clin Gastroenterol 2002;35:S130-7.
79. Chalasani N, Horlander J, Said A, Hoen H, Kopecky K, Stockberger S, et al. Screening for hepatocellular carcinoma in patients with advanced cirrhosis. Am J Gastroenterol 1999;94:2988-93.
80. Chamuleau R, Vogels B. Hyperammonaemia without portal systemic shunting does not resemble hepatic encephalopathy. Adv Exp Med Biol 1997;420:173-83.
81. Chang C, Ko Y, Liu H. Serum alanine aminotransferase levels in relation to hepatitis B and C virus infections among drug abusers in an area hyperendemic for hepatitis B. Dig Dis Sci 2000;45:1949-52.
82. Chang M, Chen C, Lai M, Hsu H, Wu T, Kong M, et al. Universal hepatitis B vaccination in Taiwan and the incidence of hepatocellular carcinoma in children. Taiwan Childhood Hepatoma Study Group. N Engl J Med 1997;336:1855-9.
83. Chang M, Chen D. Prospects for hepatitis B virus eradication and control of hepatocellular carcinoma. Baillieres Best Pract Res Clin Gastroenterol 1999;13:511-7.
83A. Chen J, Conigrave KM, Macaskill P, Whitfield JB, Irwig L. On behalf of the World Health Organization and the International Society for Biomedical Research on Alcoholism Collaborative Group. Combining carbohydrate-deficient transferrin and gamma-glutamyltransferase to increase diagnostic accuracy for problem drinking. Alcohol Alcohol 2003;38:574-82.
84. Chisari F, Ferrari C. Hepatitis B virus immunopathology. Springer Semin Immunopathol 1995;17:261-81.
85. Chitturi S, Farrell G. Herbal hepatotoxicity: An expanding but poorly defined problem. J Gastroenterol Hepatol 2000;15:1093-9.
86. Choo Q-L, Kuo G, Weiner A, Bradley D, Houghton M. Isolation of a c-DNA clone derived from a blood-borne non-A, non-B viral hepatitis genome. Science 1989;244:359-62.
87. Chu C, Hussain M, Lok A. Quantitative serum HBV DNA levels during different stages of chronic hepatitis B infection. Hepatology 2002;36:1408-15.
88. Chu C, Yeh C, Chiu C, Sheen I, Liaw Y. Precore mutant of hepatitis B virus prevails in acute and chronic infections in an area in which hepatitis B is endemic. J Clin Microbiol 1996;34:1815-8.
89. Chu C, Yeh C, Sheen I, Liaw Y. Acute hepatitis C virus (HCV) infection in chronic carriers of hepatitis B virus (HBV): The impact of underlying active HBV replication on persistence of HCV infection and antibody responses to HCV. Gut 2002;51:95-9.
90. Chung P, Sitrin M, Te H. Serum phosphorus levels predict clinical outcome in fulminant hepatic failure. Liver Transpl 2003;9:248-53.
91. Clemente-Casares P, Pina S, Buti M, Jardi R, Martin M, Bofill-Mas S, et al. Hepatitis E virus epidemiology in industrialized countries. Emerg Infect Dis 2003;9:448-54.
92. Cohen J, Kaplan M. The SGOT/SGPT ratio—An indicator of alcoholic liver disease. Dig Dis Sci 1979;24:835-8.
93. Coleman P, Chen Y, Mushahwar I. Immunoassay detection of hepatitis B surface antigen mutants. J Med Virol 1999;59:19-24.
94. Colquhoun S, Lipkin C, Connelly C. The pathophysiology, diagnosis, and management of acute hepatic encephalopathy. Adv Intern Med 2001;46:155-76.
95. Conforti A, Leone R, Ghiotto E, Velo G, Moretti U, Venegoni M, et al. Spontaneous reporting of drug-related hepatic reactions from two Italian regions (Lombardy and Veneto). Dig Liver Dis 2000;32:716-23.
95A. Conigrave KM, Saunders JB, Whitfield JB. Diagnostic tests for alcohol consumption. Alcohol 1995;30:13-6.
95B. Conigrave KM, Davies P, Haber P, Whitfield JB. Traditional markers of excessive alcohol use. Addiction 2003;98 Suppl 2:31-43.
96. Conn H, Fessel J. Spontaneous bacterial peritonitis in cirrhosis: Variations on a theme. Medicine (Baltimore) 1971;50:161-97.
97. Crapper R, Bhathal P, Mackay I, Frazer I. 'Acute' autoimmune hepatitis. Digestion 1986;34:216-25.
98. Crespo J, Lozano J, Carte B, Heras B, Cruz F, Pons-Romero F. Viral replication in patients with concomi-

tant hepatitis B and C virus infections. Eur J Clin Microbiol Infect Dis 1997;16:445-51.
99. Crespo J, Lozano J, Cruz F, Rodrigo L, Rodriguez M, San MG, et al. Prevalence and significance of hepatitis C viremia in chronic active hepatitis B. Am J Gastroenterol 1994;89:1147-51.
100. Crowe J, Christensen E, Butler J, Wheeler P, Doniach D, Keenan J, et al. Primary biliary cirrhosis: The prevalence of hypothyroidism and its relationship to thyroid autoantibodies and sicca syndrome. Gastroenterology 1980;78:1437-41.
101. Czaja A, Cassani F, Cataleta M, Valentini P, Bianchi F. Frequency and significance of antibodies to actin in type 1 autoimmune hepatitis. Hepatology 1996;24:1068-73.
102. Czaja A, Davis G, Ludwig J, Taswell H. Complete resolution of inflammatory activity following corticosteroid treatment of HBsAg-negative chronic active hepatitis. Hepatology 1984;4:622-7.
103. Czaja A, Freese D. Diagnosis and treatment of autoimmune hepatitis. Hepatology 2002;36:479-97.
104. Czaja A, Nishioka M, Morshed S, Hachiya T. Patterns of nuclear immunofluorescence and reactivities to recombinant nuclear antigens in autoimmune hepatitis. Gastroenterology 1994;107:200-7.
105. D'Amico G, Pagliaro L, Bosch J. Pharmacological treatment of portal hypertension: An evidence-based approach. Semin Liver Dis 1999;19:475-505.
106. Danan G. Causality assessment of drug-induced liver injury. Hepatology Working Group. J Hepatol 1988;7:132-6.
107. Daniel S, Ben-Menachem T, Vasudevan G, Ma C, Blumenkehl M. Prospective evaluation of unexplained chronic liver transaminase abnormalities in asymptomatic and symptomatic patients. Am J Gastroenterol 1999;94:3010-14.
108. Davis G. Monitoring of viral levels during therapy of hepatitis C. Hepatology 2002;36:S145-51.
109. Davis G, Albright JE, Cook SF, Rosenbert DM. Projecting future complications of chronic hepatitis C in the United States. Liver Transpl 2003;9:331-8.
110. Davis G, Hoofnagle J. Reactivation of chronic type B hepatitis presenting as acute viral hepatitis. Ann Intern Med 1985;102:762-5.
111. Davis G, Lau J, Urdea M, Neuwald P, Wilber J, Lindsay K, et al. Quantitative detection of hepatitis C virus RNA with a solid-phase signal amplification method: Definition of optimal conditions for specimen collection and clinical application in interferon-treated patients. Hepatology 1994;19:1337-41.
112. de FR, Meucci G, Vecchi M, Tatarella M, Colombo M, Del NE, et al. The natural history of asymptomatic hepatitis B surface antigen carriers. Ann Intern Med 1993;118:191-4.
113. Deitcher S. Interpretation of the international normalised ratio in patients with liver disease. Lancet 2002;359:47-8.
114. Delage G, Remy-Prince S, Montplaisir S. Combined active-passive immunization against the hepatitis B virus: Five-year follow-up of children born to hepatitis B surface antigen-positive mothers. Pediatr Infect Dis J 1993;12:126-30.
115. Demetris A, Adams D, Bellamy C, Blakolmer K, Clouston A, Dhillon A, et al. Update of the International Banff Schema for Liver Allograft Rejection: Working recommendations for the histopathologic staging and reporting of chronic rejection. An international panel. Hepatology 2000;31:792-9.
116. Demirtas S, Bozbas A, Akbay A, Yavuz Y, Karaca L. Diagnostic value of serum cystatin C for evaluation of hepatorenal syndrome. Clin Chim Acta 2001;311:81-9.
117. deVilliers J, Kotze M. Significance of linkage disequilibrium between C282Y and a Msel polymorphism in population screening and DNA diagnosis of hemochromatosis. Blood Cells Mol Dis 1999;25:250-2.
118. Deyashiki Y, Nishioka Y, Takahashi K, Kosaka Y, Suzuki K. Evaluation of des-gamma-carboxy prothrombin as a marker protein of hepatocellular carcinoma. Cancer 1989;64:2546-51.
119. Di BA. Epidemiology and clinical presentation of hepatocellular carcinoma. J Vasc Interv Radiol 2002;13:S169-71.
120. Di Bisceglie A, Hoofnagle J. Optimal therapy of hepatitis C. Hepatology 2002;36:S121-7.
121. Dickerman R, Pertusi R, Zachariah N, Dufour D, McConathy W. Anabolic steroid-induced hepatotoxicity: Is it overstated? Clin J Sport Med 1999;9:34-9.
122. Dienstag J, Cianciara J, Karayalcin S, Kowdley K, Willems B, Pilsek S, et al. Durability of serologic response after lamivudine treatment of chronic hepatitis B. Hepatology 2003;37:748-55.
123. Dienstag J, Goldin R, Heathcote E, Hann H, Woessner M, Stephenson S, et al. Histological outcome during long-term lamivudine therapy. Gastroenterology 2003;124:105-17.
124. Dincer D, Okten A, Kaymakoglu S, Besisik F, Demir K, Tuncer I, et al. Persistently normal alanine transaminase levels in chronic C hepatitis: What does it tell us? Hepatogastroenterology 2001;48:1397-400.
125. Dossing M, Andreasen P. Drug-induced liver disease in Denmark. An analysis of 572 cases of hepatotoxicity reported to the Danish Board of Adverse Reactions to Drugs. Scand J Gastroenterol 1982;17:205-11.
126. Dufour D R. Alanine aminotransferase variation in chronic hepatitis C infection: An analysis of 357 cases. Clin Chem 2001;47:A26-A7.
127. Dufour DR, Lott J, Nolte F, Gretch D, Koff R, Seeff L. Diagnosis and monitoring of hepatic injury. II. Rec-

ommendations for use of laboratory tests in screening, diagnosis, and monitoring. Clin Chem 2000;46:2050-68.

128. Dufour DR, Talastas M, Fernandez M, Harris B, Strader D, Seeff L. Low positive anti-hepatitis C virus enzyme immunoassay results: An important predictor of low likelihood of hepatitis C infection. Clin Chem 2003;49:479-86.
129. Dufour DR, Talastas, M, Feranndez M, Harris B. Chemiluminescence assay improves specificity of hepatitis C antibody detection. Clin Chem 2003;49:940-44.
130. Dufour DR, Teot L. Laboratory identification of ischemic hepatitis (shock liver). Clin Chem 1988;34:1287.
131. Dufour J, De Lellis R, Kaplan M. Regression of hepatic fibrosis in hepatitis C with long-term interferon treatment. Dig Dis Sci 1998;43:2573-6.
132. Dufour J, De LR, Kaplan M. Reversibility of hepatic fibrosis in autoimmune hepatitis. Ann Intern Med 1997;127:981-5.
133. Dufour M, Stinson F, Caces M. Trends in cirrhosis morbidity and mortality: United States, 1979-1988. Semin Liver Dis 1993;13:109-25.
134. Dvorchik I, Subotin M, Demetris A, Fung J, Starzl T, Wieand S, et al. Effect of liver transplantation on inflammatory bowel disease in patients with primary sclerosing cholangitis. Hepatology 2002;35:380-4.
135. EASL International Consensus Conference on Hepatitis C. Paris, 26-28, February 1999, Consensus Statement. European Association for the Study of the Liver. J Hepatol 1999;30:956-61.
136. El-Serag H. Epidemiology of hepatocellular carcinoma. Clin Liver Dis 2001;5:87-107.
137. El-Serag H, Mason A. Rising incidence of hepatocellular carcinoma in the United States. N Engl J Med 1999;340.
138. Eriksson S. Alpha 1-antitrypsin deficiency and the liver. Acta Paediatr 1994;83:444-7.
139. Erker J, Desai S, Schlauder G, Dawson G, Mushahwar I. A hepatitis E virus variant from the United States: Molecular characterization and transmission in cynomolgus macacques. J Gen Virol 1999;80:681-90.
140. Escorsell A, Bordas J, Castaneda B, Llach J, Garcia-Pagan J, Rodes J, et al. Predictive value of the variceal pressure response to continued pharmacological therapy in patients with cirrhosis and portal hypertension. Hepatology 2000;31:1061-7.
141. Fanning L, Kenny-Walsh E, Levis J, Choudhury K, Cannon B, Sheehan M, et al. Natural fluctuations of hepatitis C viral load in a homogeneous patient population: A prospective study. Hepatology 2000;31:225-9.
142. Farci P, Purcell R. Clinical significance of hepatitis C virus genotypes and quasispecies. Semin Liver Dis 2000;20:103-26.
143. Farci P, Shimoda A, Coiana A, Diaz G, Peddis G, Melpolder J, et al. The outcome of acute hepatitis C predicted by the evolution of the viral quasispecies. Science 2000;288:339-44.
144. Fattovich G. Progression of hepatitis B and C to hepatocellular carcinoma in Western countries. Hepatogastroenterology 1998;45 Suppl 3:1206-13.
145. Fattovich G, Giustina G, Degos F, et al. Morbidity and mortality in compensated cirrhosis type C: A retrospective follow-up study of 384 patients. Gastroenterology 1997;112:463-72.
146. Fattovich G, Giustina G, Degos F, Tremolada F, Diodati G, Almasio P, et al. Morbidity and mortality in compensated cirrhosis type C: A retrospective follow-up study of 384 patients. Gastroenterology 1997;112:463-72.
147. Fattovich G, Giustina G, Schalm S, Hadziyannis S, Sanchez-Tapias J, Almasio P, et al. Occurrence of hepatocellular carcinoma and decompensation in western European patients with cirrhosis type B. The EUROHEP Study Group on Hepatitis B Virus and Cirrhosis. Hepatology 1995;21:77-82.
148. Faust T. Recurrent primary biliary cirrhosis, primary sclerosing cholangitis, and autoimmune hepatitis after transplantation. Liver Transpl 2001;7:S99-108.
149. Feder J, Gnirke A, Thomas W, Tsuchihashi Z, Ruddy D, Basava A, et al. A novel MHC class I-like gene is mutated in patients with hereditary haemochromatosis. Nat Genet 1996;13:399-408.
150. Fei H, Maeda S, Kirii H, Fujigaki S, Maekawa N, Fujii H, et al. Evaluation of two different homogeneous assays for LDL-cholesterol in lipoprotein-X-positive serum. Clin Chem 2000;46:1351-6.
151. Feitelson M, Zhu M, Duan L, London W. Hepatitis B x antigen and p53 are associated in vitro and in liver tissues from patients with primary hepatocellular carcinoma. Oncogene 1993;8:1109-17.
151A. Ferguson RA, Goldberg DM. Genetic markers of alcohol abuse. Clin Chim Acta 1997;257:199-250.
152. Fisher R, Taylor L, Sherlock S. Alpha-1-antitrypsin deficiency in liver disease: the extent of the problem. Gastroenterology 1976;71:646-51.
152A. Fleming MF, Anton RF, Spies CD. A review of genetic, biological, pharmacological, and clinical factors that affect carbohydrate-deficient transferrin levels. Alcohol Clin Exp Res 2004;28:1347-55.
153. Fletcher L, Dixon J, Purdie D, Powell L, Crawford D. Excess alcohol greatly increases the prevalence of cirrhosis in hereditary hemochromatosis. Gastroenterology 2002;122:281-9.
154. Fontana R, Lok A. Noninvasive monitoring of patients with chronic hepatitis C. Hepatology 2002;36:S57-64.
155. Forman L, Lucey M. Predicting the prognosis of chronic liver disease: An evolution from child to

MELD. Mayo end-stage liver disease. Hepatology 2001;33:473-5.
156. Forns X, Ampurdanes S, Llovet J, Aponte J, Quinto L, Martinez-Bauer E, et al. Identification of chronic hepatitis C patients without hepatic fibrosis by a simple predictive model. Hepatology 2002;36: 986-92.
157. Fortson W, Tedesco F, Starnes E, Shaw C. Marked elevation of serum transaminase activity associated with extrahepatic biliary tract disease. J Clin Gastroenterol 1985;7:502-5.
158. Francis J, Armstrong D. Acquired dysfibrinogenaemia in liver disease. J Clin Pathol 1982;35:667-72.
159. Francois G, Kew M, Van DP, Mphahlele M, Meheus A. Mutant hepatitis B viruses: A matter of academic interest only or a problem with far-reaching implications? Vaccine 2001;19:3799-815.
160. Freeman A, Dore G, Law M, Thorpe M, Von OJ, Lloyd A, et al. Estimating progression to cirrhosis in chronic hepatitis C virus infection. Hepatology 2001;34:809-16.
161. French S. Alcoholic hepatitis: Inflammatory cell-mediated hepatocellular injury. Alcohol 2002;27:43-6.
161A. Friedman SL. Alcoholic liver disease, cirrhosis, and its major sequelae. In Goldman L, Bennett JC eds. Cecil textbook of medicine. 21st ed. Philadelphia: W B Saunders, 2000:804:12.
162. Fujiyama S, Morishita T, Hashiguchi O, Sato T. Plasma abnormal prothrombin (des-gamma-carboxy prothrombin) as a marker of hepatocellular carcinoma. Cancer 1988;61:1621-8.
163. Gabrielli G, Corrocher R. Hepatic fibrosis and its serum markers: A review. Dig Dis 1991;9:303-16.
164. Gaffney D, Fell G, O'Reilly D. ACP Best Practice No 163. Wilson's disease: Acute and presymptomatic laboratory diagnosis and monitoring. J Clin Pathol 2000;53:807-12.
165. Gao L, Ramzan I, Baker A. Potential use of pharmacological markers to quantitatively assess liver function during liver transplantation surgery. Anaesth Intensive Care 2000;28:375-85.
166. Garcia-Pagan J, Morillas R, Banares R, Ablbillos A, Villanueva C, Vila C, et al. Propranolol plus placebo versus propranolol plus isosorbide-5-mononitrate in the prevention of a first variceal bleed: A double-blind RCT. Hepatology 2003;37:1260-6.
167. Garcia-Tsao G, Groszmann R, Fisher R, Conn H, Atterbury C, Glickman M. Portal pressure, presence of gastroesophageal varices and variceal bleeding. Hepatology 1985;5:419-24.
168. Gershwin M, Mackay I: Primary biliary cirrhosis: Paradigm or paradox for autoimmunity. Gastroenterology 1991;100:822-33.
169. Ghany M, Kleiner D, Alter H, Doo E, Khokar F, Promrat K, et al. Progression of fibrosis in chronic hepatitis C. Gastroenterology 2003;124:97-104.
170. Gholson C, Morgan K, Catinis G, Favrot D, Taylor B, Gonzalez E, et al. Chronic hepatitis C with normal aminotransferase levels: A clinical histologic study. Am J Gastroenterol 1997;92:1788-92.
171. Giannini E, Risso D, Botta F, Chiarbonello B, Fasoli A, Malfatti F, et al. Validity and clinical utility of the aspartate aminotransferase-alanine aminotransferase ratio in assessing disease severity and prognosis in patients with hepatitis C virus-related chronic liver disease. Arch Intern Med 2003;163:218-24.
172. Gibbs K, Walshe J. A study of the caeruloplasmin concentrations found in 75 patients with Wilson's disease, their kinships and various control groups. Q J Med 1979;48:447-63.
173. Goldberg S, Ahmed M. Minimally invasive image-guided therapies for hepatocellular carcinoma. J Clin Gastroenterol 2002;35:S115-29.
174. Goldberg S, Mendenhall C, Anderson S, Garcia-Pont P, Kiernan T, Seeff L, et al. VA Cooperative Study on Alcoholic Hepatitis. IV. The significance of clinically mild alcoholic hepatitis—describing the population with minimal hyperbilirubinemia. Am J Gastroenterol 1986;81:1029-34.
175. Goldstein S, Alter M, Williams I, Moyer L, Judson F, Mottram K, et al. Incidence and risk factors for acute hepatitis B in the United States, 1982-1998: Implications for vaccination programs. J Infect Dis 2002;185:713-9.
175A. Golka K, Wiese A. Carbohydrate-deficient transferrin (CDT)–a biomarker for long-term alcohol consumption. J Toxicol Environ Health B Crit Rev 2004;7:319-37.
176. Goodman Z. Drug hepatotoxicity. Clin Liver Dis 2002;6:381-97.
177. Gordon S, Dailey P, Liver transplantation for primary sclerosing cholangitis. Liver 2000;20:97-103.
179. Gow P, Smallwood R, Angus P, Smith A, Wall A, Sewell R. Diagnosis of Wilson's disease: An experience over three decades. Gut 2000;46:415-9.
180. Grant P, Kitchen A, Barbara J, Hewitt P, Sims C, Garson J, et al. Effects of handling and storage of blood on the stability of hepatitis C virus RNA: implications for NAT testing in transfusion practice. Vox Sang 2000;78:137-42.
181. Graziadei I, Joseph J, Wiesner R, Therneau T, Batts K, Porayko M. Increased risk of chronic liver failure in adults with heterozygous $alpha_1$-antitrypsin deficiency. Hepatology 1998;28:1058-63.
182. Gretch D. Diagnostic tests for hepatitis C. Hepatology 1997;26:43S-7S.
183. Grudeva-Popova J, Spasova M, Chepileva K, Zaprianov Z. Acute hemolytic anemia as an initial clinical manifestation of Wilson's disease. Folia Med (Plovdiv) 2000;42:42-6.
184. Gupta S, Slaughter S, Akriviadis E, Valenzuela R, Deodhar S. Serial measurement of serum C-reactive

protein facilitates evaluation in alcoholic hepatitis. Hepatogastroenterology 1995;42:516-21.
185. Hadziyannis S. Review: Hepatitis delta. J Gastroenterol Hepatol 1997;12:289-98.
186. Hadziyannis S, Tassopoulos N, Heathcote E, Chang T, Kitis G, Rizzetto M, et al. Adefovir dipivoxil for the treatment of hepatitis B e antigen-negative chronic hepatitis B. N Engl J Med 2003;348:800-7.
187. Halfon P, Bourliere M, Halimi G, Khiri H, Bertezene P, Portal I, et al. Assessment of spontaneous fluctuations of viral load in untreated patients with chronic hepatitis C by two standardized quantitation methods: Branched DNA and Amplicor Monitor. J Clin Microbiol 1998;36:2073-5.
188. Halpin T, Holtzhauer F, Campbell R, Hall L, Correa-Villasenor A, Lanese R, et al. Reye's syndrome and medication use. JAMA 1982;248:687-91.
189. Harrison P, O'Grady J, Keays R, Alexander G, Williams R. Serial prothrombin time as prognostic indicator in paracetamol induced fulminant hepatic failure. BMJ 1990;301:964-8.
190. Hartleb M, Nowak A, Kajor M, Wlaszczuk P. Autoimmune LKM1 hepatitis presenting in the form of recurrent acute episodes. Am J Gastroenterol 2002;97:1267-8.
191. Hayashi K, Kumada T, Nakano S, Takeda I, Kiriyama S, Sone Y, et al. Incidence of hepatocellular carcinoma in chronic hepatitis C after interferon therapy. Hepatogastroenterology 2002;49:508-12.
192. Heathcote E. Management of primary biliary cirrhosis. The American Association for the Study of Liver Diseases practice guidelines. Hepatology 2000;31:1005-13.
193. Hemming A, Nelson D, Reed A. Liver transplantation for hepatocellular carcinoma. Minerva Chir 2002;57:575-85.
194. Heneghan M, McFarlane I. Current and novel immunosuppressive therapy for autoimmune hepatitis. Hepatology 2002;35:7-13.
195. Hepner G, Vesell E. Assessment of aminopyrine metabolism in man by breath analysis after oral administration of ^{14}C-aminopyrine. Effects of phenobarbital, disulfiram and portal cirrhosis. N Engl J Med 1974;291:1384-8.
196. Herrmann E, Lee J, Marinos G, Modi M, Zeuzem S. Effect of ribavirin on hepatitis C viral kinetics in patients treated with pegylated interferon. Hepatology 2003;37:1351-8.
197. Hickman P, Potter J. Mortality associated with ischaemic hepatitis. Aust N Z J Med 1990;20:32-4.
198. Hijikata M, Takahashi K, Mishiro S. Complete circular DNA genome of a TT virus variant (isolate name SANBAN) and 44 partial ORF2 sequences implicating a great degree of diversity beyond genotypes. Virology 1999;260:17-22.
199. Hodges J, Millward-Sadler G, Barbatis C, Wright R. Heterozygous MZ alpha 1-antitrypsin deficiency in adults with chronic active hepatitis and cryptogenic cirrhosis. N Engl J Med 1981;304:557-60.
200. Holtzman N, Gaumnitz B. Studies on the rate of release and turnover of ceruloplasmin and apoceruloplasmin in rat plasma. J Biol Chem 1970;245:2354-8.
201. Homberg J, Abuaf N, Bernard O, Islam S, Alvarez F, Khalil S, et al. Chronic active hepatitis associated with antiliver/kidney microsome antibody type 1: A second type of "autoimmune" hepatitis. Hepatology 1987;7:1333-9.
202. Horn K, Wax P, Scheider S, Martin T, Nine J, Moraca M, et al. Biomarkers of liver regeneration allow early prediction of hepatic recovery after acute necrosis. Am J Clin Pathol 1999;112:351-7.
203. Houghton M, Weiner A, Han J, Kuo G, Choo Q. Molecular biology of the hepatitis C viruses: Implications for diagnosis, development, and control of viral disease. Hepatology 1991;14:381-8.
204. Hsu H, Chang M, Ni Y, Lin H, Wang S, Chen D. Surface gene mutants of hepatitis B virus in infants who develop acute or chronic infections despite immunoprophylaxis. Hepatology 1997;26:786-91.
205. Hunt C, McGill J, Allen M, Condreay L. Clinical relevance of hepatitis B virus mutations. Hepatology 2000;31:1037-44.
206. Hurwitz E, Barrett M, Bregman D, Gunn W, Schonberger L, Fairweather W, et al. Public Health Service study on Reye's syndrome and medications. Report of the pilot phase. N Engl J Med 1985;313:849-57.
207. Hussain M, Mieli-Vergani G, Mowat A. Alpha 1-antitrypsin deficiency and liver disease: Clinical presentation, diagnosis and treatment. J Inherit Metab Dis 1991;14:497-511.
208. Hutchison D. Alpha 1-antitrypsin deficiency in Europe: Geographical distribution of Pi types S and Z. Respir Med 1998;92:367-77.
209. Ihara H, Nakamura H, Aoki Y, Aoki T, Yoshida M. Effects of serum-isolated vs synthetic bilirubin-albumin complexes on dye-binding methods for estimating serum albumin. Clin Chem 1991;37:1269-72.
210. Ikarashi Y, Matsumoto Y, Omata S, Fujiwara M. Recipient-derived T cells participate in autoimmune-like hepatic lesions induced by graft-versus-host reaction. Autoimmunity 1995;20:121-7.
211. Ikeda K, Arase Y, Saitoh S, Kobayashi M, Suzuki Y, Suzuki F, et al. Interferon beta prevents recurrence of hepatocellular carcinoma after complete resection or ablation of the primary tumor-A prospective randomized study of hepatitis C virus-related liver cancer. Hepatology 2000;32:228-32.
212. Ikeda K, Saitoh S, Suzuki Y, Kobayashi M, Tsubota A, Koida I, et al. Disease progression and hepatocellular

carcinogenesis in patients with chronic viral hepatitis: A prospective observation of 2215 patients. J Hepatol 1998;28:930-8.
213. Ikoma J, Kaito M, Ishihara T, Nakagawa N, Kamei A, Fujita N, et al. Early diagnosis of hepatocellular carcinoma using a sensitive assay for serum des-gamma-carboxy prothrombin: A prospective study. Hepatogastroenterology 2002;49:235-8.
214. Imbert-Bismut F, Ratziu V, Pieroni L, Charlotte F, Benhamou Y, Poynard T. Biochemical markers of liver fibrosis in patients with hepatitis C virus infection: A prospective study. Lancet 2001;357:1069-75.
215. Imperiale T, Said A, Cummings O, Born L. Need for validation of clinical decision aids: Use of the AST/ALT ratio in predicting cirrhosis in chronic hepatitis C. Am J Gastroenterol 2000;95:2328-32.
216. Inglesby T, Rai R, Astemborski J, Gruskin L, Nelson K, Vlahov D, et al. A prospective, community-based evaluation of liver enzymes in individuals with hepatitis C after drug use. Hepatology 1999;29:590-6.
217. Ishii K, Furudera S, Kumashiro R, Koga Y, Hamada T, Sata M, et al. Clinical and pathological features, and the mechanism of development in severe alcoholic hepatitis, especially in comparison with acute type fulminant hepatitis. Alcohol Alcohol Suppl 1993;1B:97-103.
218. Isogai M, Hachisuka K, Yamaguchi A, Nakano S. Etiology and pathogenesis of marked elevation of serum transaminase in patients with acute gallstone disease. HPB Surg 1991;4:95-105; discussion 6-7.
219. Janssen H, Lange R, Erhard J, Testa G, Malago M, Janssen P, et al. Serum bile acids in liver transplantation—Early indicator for acute rejection and monitor for antirejection therapy. Transpl Int 2001; 14:429-37.
219A. Janssen HLA, van Zonnenveld M, Senturk H, Zeuzum S, Akarca US, Cakaloglu Y, et al. Pegylated interferon alfa-2b alone or in combination with lamivudine for HbeAg positive chronic hepatitis B: A randomised trial. Lancet 2005;365:123-9.
220. Jarvis L, Davidson F, Hanley J, Yap P, Ludlam C, Simmonds P. Infection with hepatitis G virus among recipients of plasma products. Lancet 1996;348: 1352-5.
220A. Javors MA, Johnson BA. Current status of carbohydrate deficient transferrin, total serum sialic acid, sialic acid index of apolipoprotein J and serum beta-hexosaminidase as markers for alcohol consumption. Addiction 2003;98 Suppl 2:45-50.
221. Jeffrey G, Chakrabarti S, Hegele R, Adams P. Polymorphism in intron 4 of HFE may cause overestimation of C282Y homozygote prevalence in hemochromatosis. Nat Genet 1999;22:325-6.
222. Johnson G, Scurletis T, Carroll N. A study of sixteen fatal cases of encephalitis-like disease in North Carolina children. NC Med J 1963;24:464-73.
223. Johnson P, McFarlane I. Meeting report: International Autoimmune Hepatitis Group. Hepatology 1993;18:998-1005.
224. Johnston M, Harrison L, Moffat K, Willan A, Hirsh J. Reliability of the international normalized ratio for monitoring the induction phase of warfarin: Comparison with the prothrombin time ratio. J Lab Clin Med 1996;128:214-7.
225. Jones E, Bergasa N. The pruritus of cholestasis. Hepatology 1999;29:1003-6.
226. Jones E, Bergasa N. Evolving concepts of the pathogenesis and treatment of the pruritus of cholestasis. Can J Gastroenterol 2000;14:33-40.
227. Kabrane-Lazzi Y, Fine J, Elm J, Glass G, Higa H, Diwan A, et al. Evidence for widespread infection of wild rats with hepatitis E virus in the United States. Am J Trop Med Hyg 1999;61:331-5.
228. Kajihara M, Kato S, Okazaki Y, Kawakami Y, Ishii H, Ikeda Y, et al. A role of autoantibody-mediated platelet destruction in thrombocytopenia in patients with cirrhosis. Hepatology 2003;37:1267-76.
229. Kamath P, Wiesner R, Malinchoc M, Kremers W, Therneau T, Kosberg C, et al. A model to predict survival in patients with end-stage liver disease. Hepatology 2001;33:464-70.
230. Kamiike W, Fujikawa M, Koseki M, Sumimura J, Miyata M, Kawashima Y, et al. Different patterns of leakage of cytosolic and mitochondrial enzymes. Clin Chim Acta 1989;185:265-70.
231. Kao J, Chen P, Lai M, Chen D. Hepatitis D virus genotypes in intravenous drug users in Taiwan: Decreasing prevalence and lack of correlation with hepatitis B virus genotypes. J Clin Microbiol 2002;40:3047-9.
232. Kasahara A, Hayashi N, Mochizuki K, Takayanagi M, Yoshioka K, Kakumu S, et al. Risk factors for hepatocellular carcinoma and its incidence after interferon treatment in patients with chronic hepatitis C. Hepatology 1998;27:1394-402.
233. Kashala O, Mubikayi L, Kayembe K, Mukeba P, Essex M. Hepatitis B virus activation among central Africans infected with human immunodeficiency virus (HIV) type 1: Pre-s2 antigen is predominantly expressed in HIV infection. J Infect Dis 1994;169: 628-32.
234. Kassianides C, Kew M. The clinical manifestations and natural history of hepatocellular carcinoma. Gastroenterol Clin North Am 1987;16:553-62.
235. Kaufman B, Gandhi S, Louie E, Rizzi R, Illei P. Herpes simplex virus hepatitis: Case report and review. Clin Infect Dis 1997;24:334-8.
236. Kazemi-Shirazi L, Datz C, Maier-Dobersberger T, Kaserer K, Hackl F, Polli C, et al. The relation of iron status and hemochromatosis gene mutations in patients with chronic hepatitis C. Gastroenterology 1999;116:127-34.

236A. Keefe EB. Assessment of the alcoholic patients for liver transplantation: Comorbidity, outcome, and recidivism. Liver Transplant Surg 1996;2:12-20.

237. Kelly D, Summerfield J. Hemostasis in liver disease. Semin Liver Dis 1987;7:182-91.

238. Kenny-Walsh E. Clinical outcomes after hepatitis C infection from contaminated anti-D immune globulin. N Engl J Med 1999;340:1228-33.

239. Kernebeck T, Lohse A, Grotzinger J. A bioinformatical approach suggests the function of the autoimmune hepatitis target antigen soluble liver antigen/liver pancreas. Hepatology 2001;34:230-3.

240. Khien V, Mao H, Chinh T, Ha P, Bang M, Lac B, et al. Clinical evaluation of lentil lectin-reactive alpha-fetoprotein-L3 in histology-proven hepatocellular carcinoma. Int J Biol Markers 2001;16:105-11.

241. Khuroo M, Kamili S. Aetiology, clinical course and outcome of sporadic acute viral hepatitis in pregnancy. J Viral Hepat 2003;20:61-9.

241A. Kim WR, Benson JT, Therneau TM, Torgerson HA, Yawn BP, Melton LJ. Changing epidemiology of hepatitis B in a U.S. community. Hepatology 2004;39:811-6.

242. Kim W, Brown R, Terrault N, El-Serag H. Burden of liver disease in the United States: Summary of a workshop. Hepatology 2002;36:227-42.

242A. Klassen LW, Tuma D, Sorrell ME. Immune mechanisms of alcohol-induced liver disease. Hepatology 1995;22:355-7. Editorial.

242B. Koch H, Meerkerk GJ, Zaat JO, Ham MF, Scholten RJ, Assendelft WJ. Accuracy of carbohydrate-deficient transferrin in the detection of excessive alcohol consumption: A systematic review. Alcohol Alcohol 2004;39:75-85.

243. Koike K, Kobayashi M, Gondo M, Hayashi I, Osuga T, Takada S. Hepatitis B virus DNA is frequently found in liver biopsy samples from hepatitis C virus-infected chronic hepatitis patients. J Med Virol 1998;54:249-55.

244. Komorizono Y, Sako K, Yamasaki N, Hiwaki T, Sakurai K, Shibatou T, et al. Outcome of patients with hepatitis C virus-related hepatocellular carcinoma occurring after interferon therapy. Anticancer Res 2002;22:3573-8.

245. Kovacs M, Wong A, MacKinnon K, Weir K, Keeney M, Boyle E, et al. Assessment of the validity of the INR system for patients with liver impairment. Thromb Haemost 1994;71:727-30.

246. Koziol J, Ho N, Felitti V, Beutler E. Reference centiles for serum ferritin and percentage of transferrin saturation, with application to mutations of the HFE gene. Clin Chem 2001;47:1804-10.

247. Kramer L, Horl W. Hepatorenal syndrome. Semin Nephrol 2002;22:290-301.

248. Krzeski P, Zych W, Kraszewska E, Milewski B, Butruk E, Habior A. Is serum bilirubin concentration the only valid prognostic marker in primary biliary cirrhosis? Hepatology 1999;30:865-9.

249. Kshirsagar N, Karande S, Potkar C. A prospective survey of drug induced hepatotoxicity in a large hospital. Indian J Gastroenterol 1992;11:13-5.

250. Kumar M, Prashad R, Kumar A, Sharma R, Acharya S, Chattopadhyay T. Relative merits of ultrasonography, computed tomography and cholangiography in patients of surgical obstructive jaundice. Hepatogastroenterology 1998;45:2027-32.

251. Kundrotas L, Clement D. Serum alanine aminotransferase (ALT) elevation in asymptomatic US Air Force basic trainee blood donors. Dig Dis Sci 1993;38:2145-50.

252. Laine L, el-Newihi H, Migikovsky B, Sloane R, Garcia F. Endoscopic ligation compared with sclerotherapy for the treatment of bleeding esophageal varices. Ann Intern Med 1993;119:1-7.

252A. Laposata M. Fatty acid ethyl esters: Short-term and long-term serum markers of ethanol intake. Clin Chem 1997;43:1527-34.

253. Laskus T, Radkowski M, Wang L, Vargas H, Rakela J. Lack of evidence for hepatitis G virus replication in the livers of patients coinfected with hepatitis C and G viruses. J Virol 1997;71:7804-6.

253A. Legros FJ, Nuyens V, Baudoux M, Boudjeltia KZ, Ruelle J-L, Colicis J, et al. Use of capillary zone electrophoresis for differentiating excessive from moderate alcohol consumption. Clin Chem 2003;49:440-9.

254. Lee C, Ko Y. Hepatitis B vaccination and hepatocellular carcinoma in Taiwan. Pediatrics 1997;99:351-3.

255. Lee W. Drug-induced hepatotoxicity. N Engl J Med 1995;333:1118-27.

256. Lee W. Hepatitis B virus infection. N Engl J Med 1997;337:1733-45.

257. Lee Y, Kaplan M. Treatment of primary biliary cirrhosis and primary sclerosing cholangitis: Use of ursodeoxycholic acid. Curr Gastroenterol Rep 1999;1:38-41.

258. Lefrere J, Roudot-Thoraval F, Morand-Joubert L, Petit J, Lerable J, Thauvin M, et al. Carriage of GB virus C/hepatitis G virus RNA is associated with a slower immunologic, virologic, and clinical progression of human immunodeficiency virus disease in coinfected individuals. J Infect Dis 1999;179:783-9.

258A. Lelbach WK. Cirrhosis in the alcoholic and the relation to the volume of alcohol abuse. Ann NY Acad Sci 1975;252:85-108.

259. Lennard L. Clinical implications of thiopurine methyltransferase—Optimization of drug dosage and potential drug interactions. Ther Drug Monit 1998;20:527-31.

260. Liao C, Yang K, Yen M, Teng L, Duffy S, Chen T. Prognosis of small hepatocellular carcinoma treated by percutaneous ethanol injection and transcatheter

arterial chemoembolization. J Clin Epidemiol 2002;55:1095-104.

261. Lichtenstein P, Heubi J, Daugherty C, Farrell M, Sokol R, Rothbaum R, et al. Grade I Reye's syndrome. A frequent cause of vomiting and liver dysfunction after varicella and upper-respiratory-tract infection. N Engl J Med 1983;309:133-9.

262. Liebman H, Furie B, Tong M, Blanchard R, Lo K, Lee S, et al. Des-gamma-carboxy (abnormal) prothrombin as a serum marker of primary hepatocellular carcinoma. N Engl J Med 1984;310:1427-31.

263. Lin HJ, Seeff LB, Barbosa L, Hollinger FB. Occurrence of identical hypervariable region 1 sequences of hepatitis C virus in transfusion recipients and their respective blood donors: Divergence over time. Hepatology 2001;34:424-9.

264. Liu Y, Taylor J, Linko P, Lucier G, Thompson C. Glutathione S-transferase mu in human lymphocyte and liver: Rrole in modulating formation of carcinogen-derived DNA adducts. Carcinogenesis 1991;12: 2269-75.

265. Liu Z, Kaplowitz N. Immune-mediated drug-induced liver disease. Clin Liver Dis 2002;6:467-86.

266. Lohse A, zum BK, Franz B, Kanzler S, Gerken G, Dienes H. Characterization of the overlap syndrome of primary biliary cirrhosis (PBC) and autoimmune hepatitis: Evidence for it being a hepatitic form of PBC in genetically susceptible individuals. Hepatology 1999;29:1078-84.

267. Lok A, McMahon B. Chronic hepatitis B. Hepatology 2001;34:1225-41.

268. Lomas D. Loop-sheet polymerization: The mechanism of alpha$_1$-antitrypsin deficiency. Respir Med 2000;94 Suppl C:S3-6.

269. Luca A, D'Amico G, La GR, Midiri M, Morabito A, Pagliaro L. TIPS for prevention of recurrent bleeding in patients with cirrhosis: Meta-analysis of randomized clinical trials. Radiology 1999;212:411-21.

270. Lucas W, Chuttani R. Pathophysiology and current concepts in the diagnosis of obstructive jaundice. Gastroenterologist 1995;3:105-18.

271. Ludwig J, Viggiano T, McGill D, Oh B. Nonalcoholic steatohepatitis: Mayo Clinic experiences with a hitherto unnamed disease. Mayo Clin Proc 1980;55:434-8.

272. Ludwig S, Kaplowitz N. Effect of pyridoxine deficiency on serum and liver transaminases in experimental liver injury in the rat. Gastroenterology 1980;79:545-9.

273. Lunel F, Abuaf N, Frangeul L, Grippon P, Perrin M, Le CY, et al. Liver/kidney microsome antibody type 1 and hepatitis C virus infection. Hepatology 1992;16:630-6.

274. Luo J, Hwang S, Chang F, Chu C, Lai C, Wang Y, et al. Simple blood tests can predict compensated liver cirrhosis in patients with chronic hepatitis C. Hepatogastroenterology 2002;49:478-81.

275. Luo J, Hwang S, Wu J, Lai C, Li C, Chang F, et al. Clinical characteristics and prognosis of hepatocellular carcinoma patients with paraneoplastic syndromes. Hepatogastroenterology 2002;49: 1315-9.

275A. Mann K. Pharmacotherapy of alcohol dependence: A review of the clinical data. CNS Drugs 2004;18: 485-504.

275B. Mann RE, Smart RG, Govoni R. The epidemiology of alcoholic liver disease. Alcohol Res Health 2003;27:209-19.

276. Marcellin P, Asselah T, Boyer N. Fibrosis and disease progression in hepatitis C. Hepatology 2002;2002:S47-S56.

277. Marcellin P, Chang T, Lim S, Tong M, Sievert W, Shiffman M, et al. Adefovir dipivoxil for the treatment of hepatitis B e antigen-positive chronic hepatitis B. N Engl J Med 2003;348:808-16.

278. Marchesini G, Bugianesi E, Forlani G, Cerralli F, Lenzi M, Manini R, et al. Nonalcoholic fatty liver, steatohepatitis, and the metabolic syndrome. Hepatology 2003;37:917-23.

279. Maria V, Victorino R. Development and validation of a clinical scale for the diagnosis of drug-induced hepatitis. Hepatology 1997;26:664-9.

280. Marra F. Chemokines in liver inflammation and fibrosis. Front Biosci 2002;7:1899-914.

281. Martinez-Sierra C, Arizcorreta A, Diaz F, Roldan R, Martin-Herrera L, Perez-Guzman E, et al. Progression of chronic hepatitis C to liver fibrosis and cirrhosis in patients coinfected with hepatitis C virus and human immunodeficiency virus. Clin Infect Dis 2003;36: 491-8.

282. Martinot-Peignoux M, Boyer N, Colombat M, Akremi R, Pham B, Ollivier S, et al. Serum hepatitis B virus DNA levels and liver histology in inactive HBsAg carriers. J Hepatol 2002;36:543-6.

283. Mast E, Alter M, Holland P, Purcell R. Evaluation of assays for antibody to hepatitis E virus by a serum panel. Hepatitis E Virus Antibody Serum Panel Evaluation Group. Hepatology 1998;27:857-61.

284. Mathiesen U, Franzen L, Fryden A, Foberg U, Bodemar G. The clinical significance of slightly to moderately increased liver transaminase values in asymptomatic patients. Scand J Gastroenterol 1999;34:85-91.

285. Mathiesen U, Franzen L, Fryden A, Fosberg U, Bodemar G. The clinical significance of slightly to moderately increased liver transaminase values in asymptomatic patients. Scand J Gastroenterol 1999;34:85-91.

286. Mattsson L, Weiland O, Glaumann H. Application of a numerical scoring system for assessment of histological outcome in patients with chronic posttransfusion non-A, non-B hepatitis with or without antibodies to hepatitis C. Liver 1990;10:257-63.

287. Matz R, Jurmann J. Spontaneous peritonitis in cirrhosis of the liver. Lancet 1966;1:1242-3.
288. McCormick S, Goodman Z, Maydonovitch C, Sjogren M. Evaluation of liver histology, ALT elevation, and HCV RNA titer in patients with chronic hepatitis C. Am J Gastroenterol 1996;91:1516-22.
289. McCune C, Al-Jader L, May A, Hayes S, Jackson H, Worwood M. Hereditary haemochromatosis: Only 1% of adult HFEC282Y homozygotes in South Wales have a clinical diagnosis of iron overload. Hum Genet 2002;111:538-43.
290. McGinlay J, Payne R. Serum albumin by dye-binding: Bromocresol green or bromocresol purple? The case for conservatism. Ann Clin Biochem 1988;25: 417-21.
291. McGlynn K, Rosvold E, Lustbader E, Hu Y, Clapper M, Zhou T, et al. Susceptibility to hepatocellular carcinoma is associated with genetic variation in the enzymatic detoxification of aflatoxin B1. Proc Natl Acad Sci U S A 1995;92:2384-7.
292. McLaren C, McLachlan G, Halliday J, Webb S, Leggett B, Jazwinska E, et al. Distribution of transferrin saturation in an Australian population: Relevance to the early diagnosis of hemochromatosis. Gastroenterology 1998;114:543-9.
293. Meier P, Manns M. Medical and endoscopic treatment in primary sclerosing cholangitis. Best Pract Res Clin Gastroenterol 2001;15:657-66.
294. Mendenhall C. Alcoholic hepatitis. Clin Gastroenterol 1981;10:417-41.
295. Mendenhall C, Seeff L, Diehl A, Ghosn S, French S, Gartside P, et al. Antibodies to hepatitis B virus and hepatitis C virus in alcoholic hepatitis and cirrhosis: Their prevalence and clinical relevance. The VA Cooperative Study Group (No. 119). Hepatology 1991;14:581-9.
296. Meng X. Novel strains of hepatitis E virus identified from humans and other animal species: Is hepatitis E a zoonosis? J Hepatol 2000;33:842-5.
297. Meng X, Dea S, Engle R, Friendship R, Lyoo Y, Sininarumitr T, et al. Prevalence of antibodies to the hepatitis E virus in pigs from countries where hepatitis E is common or is rare in the human population. J Med Virol 1999;59:297-302.
298. Menon K, Gores G, Shah V. Pathogenesis, diagnosis, and treatment of alcoholic liver disease. Mayo Clin Proc 2001;76:1021-9.
299. Meredith J. Lipoprotein-X. Arch Pathol Lab Med 1986;110:1123-7.
300. Metcalf J, Mitchison H, Palmer J, Jones D, Bassendine M, James O. Natural history of early primary biliary cirrhosis. Lancet 1996;348:1399-402.
301. Mihas A, Toussaint J, Hsu H, Dotherow P, Achord J. Spontaneous bacterial peritonitis in cirrhosis: Clinical and laboratory features, survival and prognostic indicators. Hepatogastroenterology 1992;39:520-2.
301A. Miller J, Finelli L, Bell BP: Incidence of acute hepatitis B—United States, 1990-2002. MMWR 2004;42:1252-4.
301B. Miller PM, Anton RF. Biochemical alcohol screening in primary health care. Addict Behav 2004;29: 1427-37.
302. Milkiewicz P, Hubscher S, Skiba G, Hathaway M, Elias E. Recurrence of autoimmune hepatitis after liver transplantation. Transplantation 1999;68:253-6.
303. Milkiewicz P, Saksena S, Hubscher S, Elias E. Wilson's disease with superimposed autoimmune features: Report of two cases and review. J Gastroenterol Hepatol 2000;15:570-4.
304. Milman N, Pedersen P, a ST, Byg K, Graudal N, Fenger K. Clinically overt hereditary hemochromatosis in Denmark 1948-1985: Epidemiology, factors of significance for long-term survival, and causes of death in 179 patients. Ann Hematol 2001;80:737-44.
305. Mitchell P, Sloan L, Majewski D, Rys P, Heimgartner P, Rosenblatt J, et al. Comparison of line probe assay and DNA sequencing of 5' untranslated region for genotyping hepatitis C virus: Description of novel line probe patterns. Diagn Microbiol Infect Dis 2002;42:175-9.
306. Moaven L, Tennakoon P, Bowden D, Locarnini S. Mother-to-baby transmission of hepatitis G virus. Med J Aust 1996;165:84-5.
307. Modahl L, Lai M. Hepatitis delta virus: The molecular basis of laboratory diagnosis. Crit Rev Clin Lab Sci 2000;37:45-92.
308. Mofrad P, Contos M, Haque M, Sargeant C, Fisher R, Luketic V, et al. Clinical and histologic spectrum of nonalcoholic fatty liver disease associated with normal ALT values. Hepatology 2003;37:1286-92.
309. Mommeja-Marin H, Mondou E, Blum M, Rousseau F. Serum HBV DNA as a marker of efficacy during therapy for chronic HBV infection: Analysis and review of the literature. Hepatology 2003;2003: 1309-19.
310. Moore K, Wong F, Gines P, Bernardi M, Ochs A, Salerno F, et al. The management of ascites in cirrhosis: Report on the consensus conference of the International Ascites Club. Hepatology 2003;38:258-66.
311. Moradpour D, Wands J. Understanding hepatitis B virus infection. N Engl J Med 1995;332:1092-3.
312. Morin T, Martin J, Feldmann G, Rueff B, Benhamou J, Ropartz C. Heterozygous alpha 1-antitrypsin deficiency and cirrhosis in adults, a fortuitous association. Lancet 1975;1:250-1.
313. Moss D. Release of membrane-bound enzymes from cells and the generation of isoforms. Clin Chim Acta 1994;226:131-42.
314. Moteki S, Leung P, Dickson E, Van TD, Galperin C, Buch T, et al. Epitope mapping and reactivity of autoantibodies to the E2 component of 2-oxoglutarate dehydrogenase complex in primary biliary cir-

liver fibrosis progression in patients with chronic hepatitis C. J Hepatol 2001;34:730-9.

365. Prevention of hepatitis A through active or passive immunization: Recommendations of the Advisory Committee on Immunization Practices (ACIP). MMWR Recomm Rep 1999;48:1-37.

366. Propst T, Propst A, Dietze O, Judmaier G, Braunsteiner H, Vogel W. High prevalence of viral infection in adults with homozygous and heterozygous alpha 1-antitrypsin deficiency and chronic liver disease. Ann Intern Med 1992;117:641-5.

367. Propst T, Propst A, Dietze O, Judmaier G, Braunsteiner H, Vogel W. Alpha-1-antitrypsin deficiency and liver disease. Dig Dis 1994;12:139-49.

368. Puisieux A, Lim S, Groopman J, Ozturk M. Selective targeting of p53 gene mutational hotspots in human cancers by etiologically defined carcinogens. Cancer Res 1991;51:6185-9.

369. Puoti C, Castellacci R, Montagnese F, Zaltron S, Stornaiuolo G, Bergami N, et al. Histological and virological features and follow-up of hepatitis C virus carriers with normal aminotransferase levels: The Italian prospective study of the asymptomatic C carriers (ISACC). J Hepatol 2002;37:117-23.

370. Reye R, Morgan G, Baral J. Encephalopathy and fatty degeneration of the viscera: A disease entity in childhood. Lancet 1963;ii:249-52.

371. Robert A, Chazouilleres O. Prothrombin time in liver failure: Time, ratio, activity percentage, or international normalized ratio? Hepatology 1996;24:1392-4.

372. Roberts E, Schilsky M. A practice guideline on Wilson disease. Hepatology 2003;37:1475-92.

373. Roberts E, Yeung L. Maternal-infant transmission of hepatitis C virus infection. Hepatology 2002;36:S106-13.

374. Rodger A, Roberts S, Lanigan A, Bowden S, Brown T, Crofts N. Assessment of long-term outcomes of community-acquired hepatitis C infection in a cohort with sera stored from 1971 to 1975. Hepatology 2000;32:582-7.

374A. Rohsenow DJ. What place does naltrexone have in the treatment of alcoholism? CNS Drugs 2004;18:547-60.

375. Roozendaal C, Horst G, Pogany K, van MdWA, Kleibeuker J, Haagsma E, et al. Prevalence and clinical significance of anti-lactoferrin autoantibodies in inflammatory bowel diseases and primary sclerosing cholangitis. Adv Exp Med Biol 1998;443:313-9.

376. Roozendaal C, Van MdWA, Haagsma E, Horst G, Schwarze C, Peter H, et al. Antineutrophil cytoplasmic antibodies in primary sclerosing cholangitis: Defined specificities may be associated with distinct clinical features. Am J Med 1998;105:393-9.

377. Ross R, Viazov S, Hoffmann S, Roggendorf M. Performance characteristics of a transcription-mediated nucleic acid amplification assay for qualitative detection of hepatitis C virus RNA. J Clin Lab Anal 2001;15:308-13.

378. Rossi E, Adams L, Prins A, Bulsara M, de Boer B, Garas G, et al. Validation of the FibroTest biochemical markers score in assessing liver fibrosis in hepatitis C patients. Clin Chem 2003;49:450-4.

379. Rouanet I, Peyriere H, Mauboussin J, Terrail N, Vincent D. Acute clinical hepatitis by immune restoration in a human immunodeficiency virus/hepatitis B virus co-infected patient receiving antiretroviral therapy. Eur J Gastroenterol Hepatol 2003;15:95-7.

380. Rozen P, Korn R, Zimmerman H. Computer analysis of liver function tests and their interrelationship in 347 cases of viral hepatitis. Isr J Med Sci 1970;6:67-79.

381. Safadi R, Friedman S. Hepatic fibrosis—Role of hepatic stellate cell activation. MedGenMed 2002;4:27.

382. Sagnelli E, Coppola N, Messina V, Di Caprio D, Marrocco C, Marotta A, et al. HBV superinfection in hepatitis C virus chronic carriers, viral interaction, and clinical course. Hepatology 2002;36:1285-91.

383. Sakon M, Monden M, Gotoh M, Kobayashi K, Kanai T, Umeshita K, et al. The effects of vitamin K on the generation of des-gamma-carboxy prothrombin (PIVKA-II) in patients with hepatocellular carcinoma. Am J Gastroenterol 1991;86:339-45.

384. Saldanha J, Gerlich W, Lelie N, Dawson P, Heermann K, Heath A. An international collaborative study to establish a World Health Organization international standard for hepatitis B virus DNA nucleic acid amplification techniques. Vox Sang 2001;80:63-71.

385. Saldanha J, Lelie N, Heath A. Establishment of the first international standard for nucleic acid amplification technology (NAT) assays for HCV RNA. WHO Collaborative Study Group. Vox Sang 1999;76:149-58.

386. Sale G, Storb R, Kolb H. Histopathology of hepatic acute graft-versus-host disease in the dog. A double blind study confirms the specificity of small bile duct lesions. Transplantation 1978;26:103-6.

387. Salerno F, Merli M, Cazzaniga M, Valeriano V, Rossi P, Lovaria A, et al. MELD score is better than Child-Pugh score in predicting 3-month survival of patients undergoing transjugular intrahepatic portosystemic shunt. J Hepatol 2002;36:494-500.

388. Sanchez-Albisua I, Garde T, Hierro L, Camarena C, Frauca E, de lVA, et al. A high index of suspicion: The key to an early diagnosis of Wilson's disease in childhood. J Pediatr Gastroenterol Nutr 1999;28:186-90.

389. Sato A, Kato Y, Nakata K, Nakao K, Daikoku M, Ishii N, et al. Relationship between sustained elevation of serum alanine aminotransferase and progression

from cirrhosis to hepatocellular carcinoma: Comparison in patients with hepatitis B virus- and hepatitis C virus-associated cirrhosis. J Gastroenterol Hepatol 1996;11:944-8.

390. Schilsky M, Scheinberg I, Sternlieb I. Prognosis of Wilsonian chronic active hepatitis. Gastroenterology 1991;100:762-7.
391. Schlaeger R, Haux P, Kattermann R. Studies on the mechanism of the increase in serum alkaline phosphatase activity in cholestasis: Significance of the hepatic bile acid concentration for the leakage of alkaline phosphatase from rat liver. Enzyme 1982;28:3-13.
392. Schmidt E, Schmidt F. Progress in the enzyme diagnosis of liver disease: Reality or illusion? Clin Biochem 1990;23:375-82.
393. Schrumpf E, Boberg K. Epidemiology of primary sclerosing cholangitis. Best Pract Res Clin Gastroenterol 2001;15:553-62.
394. Schuppan D, Koda M, Bauer M, Hahn E. Fibrosis of liver, pancreas and intestine: Common mechanisms and clear targets? Acta Gastroenterol Belg 2000;63:366-70.
395. Scott J, Gollan J, Samourian S, Sherlock S. Wilson's disease, presenting as chronic active hepatitis. Gastroenterology 1978;74:645-51.
395A. Seeff L, Wright E, Zimmerman H, McCollum R. VA cooperative study of post-transfusion hepatitis, 1969-1974: Incidence and characteristics of hepatitis and responsible risk factors. Am J Med Sci 1975;270: 355-62.
396. Seeff L. Drug-induced chronic liver disease, with emphasis on chronic active hepatitis. Semin Liver Dis 1981;1:104-15.
397. Seeff L. Natural history of chronic hepatitis C. Hepatology 2002;36:S35-46.
398. Seeff L, Cuccherini B, Zimmerman H, Adler E, Benjamin S. Acetaminophen hepatotoxicity in alcoholics. A therapeutic misadventure. Ann Intern Med 1986;104:399-404.
399. Seeff L, Hollinger F, Alter H, Wright E, Cain C, Buskell Z, et al. Long-term mortality and morbidity of transfusion-associated non-A, non-B, and type C hepatitis: A National Heart, Lung, and Blood Institute collaborative study. Hepatology 2001;33:455-63.
400. Seeff L, Miller R, Rabkin C, Buskell-Bales Z, Straley-Eason K, Smoak B, et al. 45-year follow-up of hepatitis C virus infection in healthy young adults. Ann Intern Med 2000;132:105-11.
401. Sharma M, Ahuja V. Aetiological spectrum of obstructive jaundice and diagnostic ability of ultrasonography: A clinician's perspective. Trop Gastroenterol 1999;20:167-9.
402. Sharp H. Wherefore art thou liver disease associated with alpha-1 antitrypsin deficiency? Hepatology 1995;22:666-8.
403. Sheth M, Riggs M, Patel T. Utility of the Mayo End-Stage Liver Disease (MELD) score in assessing prognosis of patients with alcoholic hepatitis. BMC Gastroenterol 2002;2:2.
404. Sheth S, Flamm S, Gordon F, Chopra S. AST/ALT ratio predicts cirrhosis in patients with chronic hepatitis C virus infection. Am J Gastroenterol 1998;93:44-8.
405. Shiffman M, Ferreira-Gonzalez A, Reddy K, Sterling R, Luketic V, Stravitz R, et al. International unit standard: Implications for management of patients with chronic hepatitis C virus infection in clinical practice. Am J Gastroenterol 2003;98:1159-66.
406. Shiraki K, Takase K, Tameda Y, Hamada M, Kosaka Y, Nakano T. A clinical study of lectin-reactive alpha-fetoprotein as an early indicator of hepatocellular carcinoma in the follow-up of cirrhotic patients. Hepatology 1995;22:802-7.
407. Shiratori Y, Shiina S, Teratani T, Imamura M, Obi S, Sato S, et al. Interferon therapy after tumor ablation improves prognosis in patients with hepatocellular carcinoma associated with hepatitis C virus. Ann Intern Med 2003;138:299-306.
408. Siegelman E, Rosen M. Imaging of hepatic steatosis. Semin Liver Dis 2001;21:71-80.
408A. Sigvardsson S, Bohman M, Cloninger CR. Replication of the Stockholm adoption study of alcoholism: Confirmatory cross-fostering analysis. Arch Gen Psychiatry 1996;53:681-7.
408B. Sillanaukee P, Olsson U. Improved Diagnostic Classification of Alcohol Abusers by Combining Carbohydrate-deficient Transferrin and-Glutamyltransferase. Clin Chem 2001;47: 681-5.
409. Sillanpaa M, Makela A, Koivikko A. Acute liver failure and encephalopathy (Reye's syndrome?) during salicylate therapy. Acta Paediatr Scand 1975;64:877-80.
410. Singer A, Carracio T, Mofenson H. The temporal profile of increased transaminase levels in patients with acetaminophen-induced liver dysfunction. Ann Emerg Med 1995;26:49-53.
411. Smedile A, Rizzetto M, Gerin J. Advances in hepatitis D virus biology and disease. Prog Liver Dis 1994;12:157-75.
412. Soloway R, Summerskill W, Baggenstoss A, Geall M, Gitnick G, Elveback I, et al. Clinical, biochemical, and histological remission of severe chronic active liver disease: A controlled study of treatments and early prognosis. Gastroenterology 1972;63:820-33.
413. Soros P, Bottcher J, Maschek H, Selberg O, Muller M. Lipoprotein-X in patients with cirrhosis: Its relationship to cholestasis and hypercholesterolemia. Hepatology 1998;28:1199-205.
414. Souza M, Castro-e-Silva JO, Picinato M, Franco C, Mazzetto S, Ceneviva R, et al. Serum transaminase levels in the acute phase of chronic extrahepatic cholestasis. Braz J Med Biol Res 1990;23:995-7.

414A. Soyka M, Chick J. Use of acamprosate and opioid antagonists in the treatment of alcohol dependence: A European perspective. Am J Addict 2003;12 Suppl 1:S69-80.

415. Standardization of definitions and criteria of causality assessment of adverse drug reactions. Drug-induced liver disorders: Report of an international consensus meeting. Int J Clin Pharmacol Ther Toxicol 1990;28:317-22.

416. Stedman C. Herbal hepatotoxicity. Semin Liver Dis 2002;22:195-206.

417. Steindl P, Ferenci P, Dienes H, Grimm G, Pabinger I, Madl C, et al. Wilson's disease in patients presenting with liver disease: A diagnostic challenge. Gastroenterology 1997;113:212-8.

418. Steiner M, Ocran K, Genschel J, Meier P, Gerl H, Ventz M, et al. A homozygous HFE gene splice site mutation (IVS5+1 G/A) in a hereditary hemochromatosis patient of Vietnamese origin. Gastroenterology 2002;122:789-95.

419. Sternlieb I. Wilson's disease. Clin Liver Dis 2000;4:229-39, viii-ix.

420. Stickel F, Egerer G, Seitz H. Hepatotoxicity of botanicals. Public Health Nutr 2000;3:113-24.

421. Sumi H, Yokosuka O, Seki N, Arai M, Imazeki F, Kurihara T, et al. Influence of hepatitis B virus genotypes on the progression of chronic type B liver disease. Hepatology 2003;37:19-26.

422. Sveger T. The natural history of liver disease in alpha 1-antitrypsin deficient children. Acta Paediatr Scand 1988;77:847-51.

423. Sveger T, Eriksson S. The liver in adolescents with alpha 1-antitrypsin deficiency. Hepatology 1995;22:514-7.

423A. Svikis DS, Reid-Quinones K. Screening and prevention of alcohol and drug use disorders in women. Obstet Gynecol Clin North Am 2003;30:447-68.

424. Taketa K, Endo Y, Sekiya C, Tanikawa K, Koji T, Taga H, et al. A collaborative study for the evaluation of lectin-reactive alpha-fetoproteins in early detection of hepatocellular carcinoma. Cancer Res 1993;53: 5419-23.

425. Takimoto M, Ohkoshi S, Ichida T, Takeda Y, Nomoto M, Asakura H, et al. Interferon inhibits progression of liver fibrosis and reduces the risk of hepatocarcinogenesis in patients with chronic hepatitis C: A retrospective multicenter analysis of 652 patients. Dig Dis Sci 2002;47:170-6.

425A. Tanaka F, Shiratori Y, Yokosuka O, Imazeki F, Tsukada Y, Omata M. High incidence of ADH 2.1/ALDH 2.1 genes among Japanese alcohol dependents and patients with alcoholic liver disease. Hepatology 1996;23:234-9.

426. Tanaka E, Ohue C, Aoyagi K, Yamaguchi K, Yagi S, Kiyosawa K, et al. Evaluation of a new enzyme immunoassay for hepatitis C virus (HCV) core antigen with clinical sensitivity approximating that of genomic amplification of HCV RNA. Hepatology 2000;32:388-93.

427. Tanaka Y, Takagi K, Fujihara T, Kitsugi K, Fujiwara K, Hiramatsu K, et al. High stability of enzyme immunoassay for hepatitis C virus core antigen—Evaluation before and after incubation at room temperature. Hepatol Res 2003;26:261-7.

428. Tang J, Hsu H, Lin H, Ni Y, Chang M. Hepatitis B surface antigenemia at birth: A long-term follow-up study. J Pediatr 1998;133:374-7.

429. Tanzi R, Petrukhin K, Chernov I, Pellequer J, Wasco W, Ross B, et al. The Wilson disease gene is a copper transporting ATPase with homology to the Menkes disease gene. Nat Genet 1993;5:344-50.

430. Tavill A. Diagnosis and management of hemochromatosis. Hepatology 2001;33:1321-8.

431. Teare J, Carmichael A, Burnett F, Rake M. Detection of antibodies to acetaldehyde-albumin conjugates in alcoholic liver disease. Alcohol Alcohol 1993;28:11-6.

432. Thomas DL, Yarbough P, Vishov D, Tsarev S, Nelson K, Saah A, et al. Seroreactivity to hepatitis E virus in areas where the disease is not endemic. J Clin Microbiol 1997;35:1244-7.

433. Tillmann H, Heiken H, Knapik-Botor A, Heringlake S, Ockenga J, Wilber J, et al. Infection with GB virus C and reduced mortality among HIV-infected patients. N Engl J Med 2001;345:715-24.

434. Toyoda H, Fukuda Y, Hayakawa T, Kumada T, Nakano S, Takamatsu J, et al. Presence of multiple genotype-specific antibodies in patients with persistent infection with hepatitis C virus (HCV) of a single genotype: Evidence for transient or occult superinfection with HCV of different genotypes. Am J Gastroenterol 1999;94:2230-6.

435. Toyoda H, Fukuda Y, Hayakawa T, Takamatsu J, Saito H. Effect of GB virus C/hepatitis G virus coinfection on the course of HIV infection in hemophilia patients in Japan. J Acquir Immune Defic Syndr Hum Retrovirol 1998;17:209-13.

436. Trauner M, Meier P, Boyer J. Molecular pathogenesis of cholestasis. N Engl J Med 1998;339:1217-27.

437. Trinchet J. Clinical use of serum markers of fibrosis in chronic hepatitis. J Hepatol 1995;22:89-95.

438. Tsai J, Margolis H, Jeng J, Ho M, Chang W, Hsieh M, et al. Hepatitis B surface antigen- and immunoglobulin-specific circulating immune complexes in acute hepatitis B virus infection. Clin Immunol Immunopathol 1996;80:278-82.

439. Ts'ao C, Swedlund J, Neofotistos D. Implications of use of low international sensitivity index thromboplastins in prothrombin time testing. Arch Pathol Lab Med 1994;118:1183-7.

440. Tsukamoto H. Cytokine regulation of hepatic stellate cells in liver fibrosis. Alcohol Clin Exp Res 1999;23:911-6.

441. Tsuneyama K, Van dWJ, Nakanuma Y, Cha S, Ansari A, Coppel R, et al. Human combinatorial autoantibodies and mouse monoclonal antibodies to PDC-E2 produce abnormal apical staining of salivary glands in patients with coexistent primary biliary cirrhosis and Sjogren's syndrome. Hepatology 1994;20:893-8.
442. Tsutsumi M, Takase S, Urashima S, Ueshima Y, Kawahara H, Takada A. Serum markers for hepatic fibrosis in alcoholic liver disease: Which is the best marker, type III procollagen, type IV collagen, laminin, tissue inhibitor of metalloproteinase, or prolyl hydroxylase? Alcohol Clin Exp Res 1996;20:1512-7.
443. Turkoglu S, Lazizi Y, Meng H, Kordosi A, Dubreuil P, Crescenzo B, et al. Detection of hepatitis E virus RNA in stools and serum by reverse transcription-PCR. J Clin Microbiol 1996;34:1568-71.
444. Ueda H, Ullrich S, Gangemi J, Kappel C, Ngo L, Feitelson M, et al. Functional inactivation but not structural mutation of p53 causes liver cancer. Nat Genet 1995;9:41-7.
445. Umemura T, Yeo A, Sottini A, Moratto D, Tanaka Y, Wang R, et al. SEN virus infection and its relationship to transfusion-associated hepatitis. Hepatology 2001;33:1303-11.
446. Uysal K, Wiesbrock S, Marino M, Hotamisligil G. Protection from obesity-induced insulin resistance in mice lacking TNF-a function. Nature 1997;389:610-4.
447. Valla D, R dF, Hadengue A, Lau G, Lavanchy D, Lok A, et al. EASL international consensus conference on hepatitis B. Consensus statement (short version). J Hepatol 2003;38:533-40.
448. Van dWJ, Cooper A, Surh C, Coppel R, Danner D, Ansari A, et al. Detection of autoantibodies to recombinant mitochondrial proteins in patients with primary biliary cirrhosis. N Engl J Med 1989;320:1377-80.
449. Van dWJ, Gershwin M, Leung P, Ansari A, Coppel R. The autoepitope of the 74-kD mitochondrial autoantigen of primary biliary cirrhosis corresponds to the functional site of dihydrolipoamide acetyltransferase. J Exp Med 1988;167:1791-9.
450. Van dWJ, Shimoda S, Niho Y, Coppel R, Ansari A, Gershwin M. The role of T cells in primary biliary cirrhosis. Semin Liver Dis 1997;17:105-13.
451. Venturini I, Corsi L, Avallone R, Farina F, Bedogni G, Baraldi C, et al. Ammonia and endogenous benzodiazepine-like compounds in the pathogenesis of hepatic encephalopathy. Scand J Gastroenterol 2001;36:423-5.
452. Vera A, Moledina S, Gunson B, Hubscher S, Mirza D, Olliff S, et al. Risk factors for recurrence of primary sclerosing cholangitis of liver allograft. Lancet 2002;360:1943-4.
453. Vitellas K, Keogan M, Freed K, Enns R, Spritzer C, Baillie J, et al. Radiologic manifestations of sclerosing cholangitis with emphasis on MR cholangiopancreatography. Radiographics 2000;20:959-75; quiz 1108-9, 12.
453A. Volpicelli JR, Clay KL, Watson NT, O'Brien CP. Naltrexone in the treatment of alcoholism: Predicting response to naltrexone. J Clin Psychiatry 1995; 56: 39-44.
454. Waalen J, Felitti V, Gelbart T, Ho N, Beutler E. Prevalence of hemochromatosis-related symptoms among individuals with mutations in the HFE gene. Mayo Clin Proc 2002;77:522-30.
455. Wai C, Chu C, Hussain M, Lok A. HBV genotype B is associated with better response to interferon therapy in HBeAg(+) chronic hepatitis than genotype C. Hepatology 2002;36:1425-30.
456. Walker J. HMG CoA reductase inhibitors. Current clinical experience. Drugs 1988;36 Suppl 3:83-6.
457. Wall M, Moe E, Eisenberg J, Powers M, Buist N, Buist A. Long-term follow-up of a cohort of children with alpha-1-antitrypsin deficiency. J Pediatr 1990;116:248-51.
458. Wang C, Mo L, Lin R, Kuo J, Chang K. Rapid diagnosis of choledocholithiasis using biochemical tests in patients undergoing laparoscopic cholecystectomy. Hepatogastroenterology 2001;48:619-21.
459. Wanless I, Lentz J. Fatty liver hepatitis (steatohepatitis) and obesity: An autopsy study with analysis of risk factors. Hepatology 1990;12:1106-10.
460. Weber B, Melchior W, Gehrke R, Doerr H, Berger A, Rabenau H. Hepatitis B virus markers in anti-HBc only positive individuals. J Med Virol 2001;64:312-9.
461. Wejstal R, Norkrans G, Widell A. Chronic non-A, non-B, non-C hepatitis: Iis hepatitis G/GBV-C involved? Scand J Gastroenterol 1997;32:1046-51.
462. Whalley S, Murray J, Brown D, Webster G, Emery V, Dusheiko G, et al. Kinetics of acute hepatitis B virus infection in humans. J Exp Med 2001;193:847-54.
463. Whitehead M, Hawkes N, Hainsworth I, Kingham J. A prospective study of the causes of notably raised aspartate aminotransferase of liver origin. Gut 1999;45:129-33.
463A. Whitfield JB, Zhu G, Madden PA, Neale MC, Heath AC, Martin NG. The genetics of alcohol intake and of alcohol dependence. Alcohol Clin Exp Res 2004;28:1153-60.
463B. Whitfield JB. Alcohol dehydrogenase and alcohol dependence: Variation in genotype-associated risk between populations. Am J Hum Genet 1999;64:1147-57.
463C. Whitfield JB. Transferrin isoform analysis for the diagnosis and management of hazardous or dependent drinking. Clin Chem 2002;48:2095-6.
464. Wiencke K, Spurkland A, Schrumpf E, Boberg K. Primary sclerosing cholangitis is associated to an extended B8-DR3 haplotype including particular MICA and MICB alleles. Hepatology 2001;34: 625-30.

465. Wiese M, Berr F, Lafrenz M, Porst H, Oesen U. Low frequency of cirrhosis in a hepatitis C (genotype 1b) single-source outbreak in Germany: A 20-year multicenter study. Hepatology 2000;32:91-6.
466. Wiesner R. Liver transplantation for primary sclerosing cholangitis: Timing, outcome, impact of inflammatory bowel disease and recurrence of disease. Best Pract Res Clin Gastroenterol 2001;15:667-80.
467. Wiesner R, Demetris A, Belle S, Seaberg E, Lake J, Zetterman R, et al. Acute hepatic allograft rejection: Incidence, risk factors, and impact on outcome. Hepatology 1998;28:638-45.
468. Williams A, Hoofnagle J. Ratio of serum aspartate to alanine aminotransferase in chronic hepatitis. Relationship to cirrhosis. Gastroenterology 1988;95:734-9.
469. Wittayalertpanya S, Israsena S, Thamaree S, Tongnoppnoua P, Komolmit P. Caffeine clearance by two point analysis: A measure of liver function in chronic liver disease. Tokai J Exp Clin Med 1996;21:195-201.
470. Witzigmann H, Geissler F, Benedix F, Thiery J, Uhlmann D, Tannapfel A, et al. Prospective evaluation of circulating hepatocytes by alpha-fetoprotein messenger RNA in patients with hepatocellular carcinoma. Surgery 2002;131:34-43.
471. Wong F, Blendis L. New challenge of hepatorenal syndrome: Prevention and treatment. Hepatology 2001;34:1242-51.
472. Wong S, Primi D, Kojima H, Sottini A, Giulivi A, Zhang M, et al. Insights into SEN virus prevalence, transmission, and treatment in community-based individuals and patients with liver disease referred to a liver disease unit. Clin Infect Dis 2002;35:789-95.
473. Woolley I, Valdez H, Walker C, Landay A, Zdunek D, Hess G, et al. Hepatitis G virus RNA is common in AIDS patients' plasma but is not associated with abnormal liver function tests or other clinical syndromes. J Acquir Immune Defic Syndr Hum Retrovirol 1998;19:408-12.
474. Worm H, van der Poel C, Brandstatter G. Hepatitis E. An overview. Microbes Infect 2002;4:657-66.
475. Worrall D, Blacque O, Barnes R. The expanding superfamily of serpins: Ssearching for the real targets. Biochem Soc Trans 1999;27:746-50.
476. Wu J, Chen T, Huang Y, Yen F, Ting L, Sheng W, et al. Natural history of hepatitis D viral superinfection: Significance of viremia detected by polymerase chain reaction. Gastroenterology 1995;108:796-802.
476A. Wuyts B, Delanghe JR. The analysis of carbohydrate-deficient transferrin, marker of chronic alcoholism, using capillary electrophoresis. Clin Chem Lab Med 2003;41:739-46.
477. Yang H, Lu S, Liaw Y, You S, Sun C, Wang L, et al. Hepatitis B e antigen and the risk of hepatocellular carcinoma. N Engl J Med 2002;347:168-74.
478. Yano M, Kumada H, Kage M, Ikeda K, Shimamatsu K, Inoue O, et al. The long-term pathological evolution of chronic hepatitis C. Hepatology 1996;23:1334-40.
479. Yashina T, Favorov M, Khudyakov Y, Fields H, Znoiko O, Shkurko T, et al. Detection of hepatitis G virus (HGV) RNA: Clinical characteristics of acute HGV infection. J Infect Dis 1997;175:1302-7.
479A. Yersin B, Nicolet JF, Dercrey H, Burnier M, van Melle G, Pecoud A. Screening for excessive alcohol drinking: Comparative value of carbohydrate-deficient transferrin, gamma-glutamyltransferase and mean corpuscular volume. Arch Intern Med 1995;155:1907-11.
480. Yokosuka O, Kojima H, Imazeki F, Tagawa M, Saisho H, Tamatsukuri S, et al. Spontaneous negativation of serum hepatitis C virus RNA is a rare event in type C chronic liver diseases: Analysis of HCV RNA in 320 patients who were followed for more than 3 years. J Hepatol 1999;31:394-9.
481. Yoshida H, Kato N, Shiratori Y, Shao R, Wang Y, Shiina S, et al. Weak association between SEN virus viremia and liver disease. J Clin Microbiol 2002;40:3140-5.
482. Yuce A, Kocak N, Demir H, Gurakan F, Ozen H, Saltik I, et al. Evaluation of diagnostic parameters of Wilson's disease in childhood. Indian J Gastroenterol 2003;22:4-6.
483. Yuen M, Cheng C, Lauder I, Lam S, Ooi C, Lai C. Early detection of hepatocellular carcinoma increases the chance of treatment: Hong Kong experience. Hepatology 2000;31:330-5.
484. Yuen M, Sablon E, Yuan H, Wong D, Hui C, Wong B, et al. Significance of hepatitis B genotype in acute exacerbation, HBeAg seroconversion, cirrhosis-related complications, and hepatocellular carcinoma. Hepatology 2003;37:562-7.
485. Yuki N, Nagaoka T, Yamashiro M, Mochizuki K, Kaneko A, Yamamoto K, et al. Long-term histologic and virologic outcomes of acute self-limited hepatitis B. Hepatology 2003;37:1172-9.
486. Zakiah I, Zaini A, Jamilah B, Zawiah A. Alpha-1-antitrypsin deficiency in babies with prolonged jaundice. Malays J Pathol 1992;14:91-4.
487. Zaman S, Johnson P, Williams R. Silent cirrhosis in patients with hepatocellular carcinoma. Implications for screening in high-incidence and low-incidence areas. Cancer 1990;65:1607-10.
488. Zaman S, Johnson P, Williams R. Silent cirrhosis in patients with hepatocellular carcinoma. Implications for screening in high-incidence and low-incidence areas. Cancer 1990;65:1607-10.
489. Zanger U, Hauri H, Loeper J, Homberg J, Meyer U. Antibodies against human cytochrome P-450db1 in autoimmune hepatitis type II. Proc Natl Acad Sci U S A 1988;85:8256-60.
490. Zarski J, Bohn B, Bastie A, Pawlotsky J, Baud M, Bost-Bezeaux F, et al. Characteristics of patients with dual

infection by hepatitis B and C viruses. J Hepatol 1998;28:27-33.
491. Zein C, Lindor K. Primary sclerosing cholangitis. Semin Gastrointest Dis 2001;12:103-12.
492. Zhou S, Gordon R, Bradbury M, Stump D, Kiang C, Berk P. Ethanol up-regulates fatty acid uptake and plasma membrane expression and export of mitochondrial aspartate aminotransferase in HepG2 cells. Hepatology 1998;27:1064-74.
493. Ziebell J, Shaw-Stiffel T. Update on the use of metabolic probes to quantify liver function: Caffeine versus lidocaine. Dig Dis 1995;13:239-50.
494. Zimmerman H. Drug-induced liver disease. Drugs 1978;16:25-45.
495. Zimmerman H. Intrahepatic cholestasis. Arch Intern Med 1979;139:1038-45.
496. Zimmerman H. Hepatotoxicology: The adverse effects of drugs and other chemicals on the liver. 2nd ed. Philadelphia: JB Lippincott, 1999.
497. Zimmerman H. Drug-induced liver disease. Clin Liver Dis 2000;4:73-96, vi.
498. Zimmerman H, Lewis J. Drug-induced cholestasis. Med Toxicol 1987;2:112-60.

ADDITIONAL READING

Books & Articles

Balistreri WF, Ohi R, Todani T, Tsuchida Y. Hepatobiliary, pancreatic, and splenic disease in children: Medical and surgical management. New York: Elsevier Sciences, 1997.

Balistreri WF, Stocker JT. Pediatric hepatology. Bristol, PA: Hemisphere Publishing, 1990.

Black ER. Diagnostic strategies and test algorithms in liver disease. Clin Chem 1997;43:1555-60.

Gentilini P. New Trends in hepatology. Norwell MA: Kluwer Publishers, 1996.

Gerok W, Loginov AS, Pokrowskij VI. New trends in hepatology. 1996 Proceedings of the Falk Symposium No. 92, St. Petersburg. Norwell MA: Kluwer Publishers, 1997.

Griffiths WJ. Tandem mass spectrometry in the study of fatty acids, bile acids, and steroids. Mass Spectrom Rev 2003;22:81-152.

Hickman PE, Potter JM, Pesce AJ. Clinical chemistry and post-liver-transplant monitoring. Clin Chem 1997;43:1546-54.

Kaplowitz N. Liver and biliary disease, 2nd ed. Baltimore: Williams and Wilkins, 1996.

Lee WM, Williams R. Acute liver failure. New York: Cambridge University Press, 1996.

Lieber CS. Susceptibility to alcohol-related liver injury. Alcohol Alcohol Suppl 1994; 2:315-26.

Schiff L, Schiff ER. Diseases of the liver, 7th ed. Philadelphia: Lippincott-Raven, 1993.

Schmid R. Acute and chronic liver diseases: Proceedings of the Falk Symposium No. 87, Basel, Switzerland. Norwell MA: Kluwer Publishers, 1995.

Shaked A, Nunes FA, Olthoff KM, Lucey MR. Assessment of liver function: Pre- and peri-transplant evaluation. Clin Chem 1997;43:1539-45.

Sherlock S, Dooley J. Diseases of the liver and biliary system, 10th ed. London: Blackwell Science, 1996.

Tobler LH, Busch V. History of posttransfusion hepatitis. Clin Chem 1997;43:1487-93, 1997.

Torriani FJ, Rodriguez-Torres M, Rockstroh JK, Lissen E, Gonzalez-Garcia J, et al, APRICOT Study Group. Peginterferon Alfa-2a plus ribavirin for chronic hepatitis C virus infection in HIV-infected patients. N Engl J Med 2004;351:438-50.

Worman HJ. Molecular biological methods in diagnosis and treatment of liver diseases. Clin Chem 1997;43:1476-86.

Wu GY, Israel J. Diseases of the liver and bile ducts: Diagnosis and treatment. Totowa, NJ: Humana Press, 1998.

Zakim O, Boyer TD. Hepatology: A textbook of liver disease, 4th ed. Philadelphia: WB Saunders, 1998.

Reviews

Burroughs A, Hochhauser D, Meyer T. Systemic treatment and liver transplantation for hepatocellular carcinoma: two ends of the therapeutic spectrum. Lancet Oncol 2004;5:409-18.

Carey W. Tests and screening strategies for the diagnosis of hepatitis C. Cleve Clin J Med 2003;70 Suppl 4: S7-13.

Coleman WB. Mechanisms of human hepatocarcinogenesis. Curr Mol Med 2003;3:573-88.

Dufour R, Lott JA, Nolte FS, Gretch DR, Koff RS, Seeff LB. Diagnosis and monitoring of hepatic injury. I. Performance characteristics of laboratory tests. Clin Chem 2000;46:2027-49.

Dufour R, Lott JA, Nolte FS, Gretch DR, Koff RS, Seeff LB. Diagnosis and monitoring of hepatic injury. II. Recommendations for use of laboratory tests in screening, diagnosis, and monitoring. Clin Chem 2000;46:2050-68.

Dufour DR. Laboratory approach to acute and chronic hepatitis. MLO Med Lab Obs 2003;35:10-2, 14, 16;quiz 20-1.

Dufour R, Talastas M, Fernandez M, Harris B. Chemiluminescence assay improves specificity of Hepatitis C antibody detection. Clin Chem 2003;49:940-4.

Dufour R, Talastas M, Fernandez M, Harris B, Strader DB, Seeff LB. Low-positive anti-hepatitis C virus enzyme immunoassay results: An important predictor of low likelihood of hepatitis C infection. Clin Chem 2003;49:479-86.

Frezza EE. Therapeutic management algorithm in cirrhotic and noncirrhotic patients in primary or secondary liver masses. Dig Dis Sci 2004;49:866-71.

Harris KR, Dighe AS. Laboratory testing for viral hepatitis. Am J Clin Pathol 2002;118 Suppl:S18-25.

Higuchi H, Gores GJ. Mechanisms of liver injury: An overview. Curr Mol Med 2003;3:483-90.

Iredale JP. Cirrhosis: New research provides a basis for rational and targeted treatments. BMJ 2003;327:143-7.

Kaplan DE, Reddy KR. Rising incidence of hepatocellular carcinoma: The role of hepatitis B and C; the impact on transplantation and outcomes. Clin Liver Dis 2003;7:683-714.

Krogstad P, Martin MG. Evaluation of acute liver failure. Pediatr Infect Dis J 2003;22:831-2.

Lee WM. Acetaminophen and the U.S. Acute Liver Failure Study Group: lowering the risks of hepatic failure. Hepatology 2004;40:6-9.

Nakamoto Y, Kaneko S. Mechanisms of viral hepatitis induced liver injury. Curr Mol Med 2003;3:537-44.

Pettinati HM. Antidepressant treatment of co-occurring depression and alcohol dependence. Biol Psychiatry 2004;56:785-92.

Poon TCW, Hui AY, Chan HLY, Ang IL, Chow SM, Wong N, et al. Prediction of liver fibrosis and cirrhosis in chronic hepatitis B infection by serum proteomic fingerprinting: A pilot study. Clin Chem 2005; 51: In Press.

Rand EB, Olthoff KM. Overview of pediatric liver transplantation. Gastroenterol Clin North Am 2003;32: 913-29.

Yamaguchi F, Etoh T, Takahashi M, Misaki H, Sakuraba H, Ohshima T. A new enzymatic cycling method for ammonia assay using NAD synthetase. Clin Chim Acta 2005;352:165-73.

CHAPTER 48

Gastric, Pancreatic, and Intestinal Function*

Peter G. Hill, Ph.D., C.Chem., F.R.S.C., F.R.C.Path.

The stomach, intestinal tract, and pancreas are closely related, both anatomically and functionally, and symptoms, such as diarrhea or malabsorption, may be associated with diseases or disorders of any of these organs. It is therefore appropriate to discuss them together. Advances in imaging techniques and improvements in endoscopic procedures have led to enormous changes in the investigation of gastrointestinal (GI) and pancreatic function so that many laboratory tests, once considered important, have now been superseded.

In this chapter, the anatomy and physiology of the GI tract, and the normal processes of digestion and absorption, are briefly reviewed. Disorders of the stomach, pancreas, and intestine associated with malabsorption or diarrhea, in which the laboratory can play a role in diagnosis and monitoring, are discussed. The chapter concludes with an overview of GI regulatory peptides and neuroendocrine tumors in which GI symptoms are prominent, and with two sections presenting more integrated approaches to the problems of investigating malabsorption and diarrhea.

INTRODUCTION TO ANATOMY AND PHYSIOLOGY OF THE GASTROINTESTINAL TRACT[170]

The major organs of the GI tract include the stomach, the small and large intestines, the pancreas, and the gallbladder, all of which are involved in the digestive processes that commence with the ingestion of food and water and culminate in the excretion of feces.

Anatomy

The GI tract is a 10-meter-long tube beginning with the mouth and ending with the anus. The esophagus is about 25 cm in length and is a muscular tube connecting the pharynx to the stomach. For this chapter, the key organs are the stomach, intestines, and pancreas.

Stomach[147]

The stomach consists of three major zones: the cardiac zone, the body, and the pyloric zone (Figure 48-1). The upper cardiac zone, which includes the fundus, contains mucus-secreting surface epithelial cells, which also secrete group II pepsinogens, and several types of endocrine secreting cells. The body of the stomach contains cells or cell groups of many different types: (1) surface epithelial cells, which secrete mucus; (2) parietal (oxyntic) cells, which secrete hydrochloric acid and intrinsic factor; (3) the chief, zymogen, or peptic cells, which secrete groups I and II pepsinogens; (4) enterochromaffin cells, which secrete serotonin; and (5) several types of endocrine secreting cells. The pyloric zone is subdivided into the antrum (which is approximately the distal third of the stomach), the pyloric canal, and the sphincter. The cells of the pyloric zone secrete mucus, group II pepsinogens, serotonin, gastrin, and several other hormones but no hydrochloric acid.

Small Intestine

In the stomach, food is converted into a semi-fluid, homogeneous, gruel-like material (chyme) that passes through the pyloric sphincter into the small intestine. The small intestine consists of three parts: the duodenum, jejunum, and ileum. In the adult human, the small intestine is approximately 2 to 3 m long and decreases in cross-section as it proceeds dis-

*The author gratefully acknowledges the original contributions of Drs. A. Ralph Henderson and Alan D. Rinker, upon which a portion of this chapter is based.

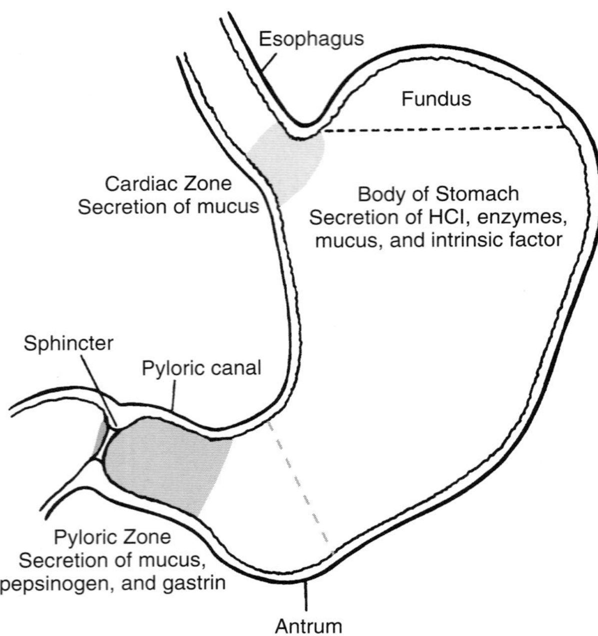

Figure 48-1 Schematic drawing of the stomach, with major zones.

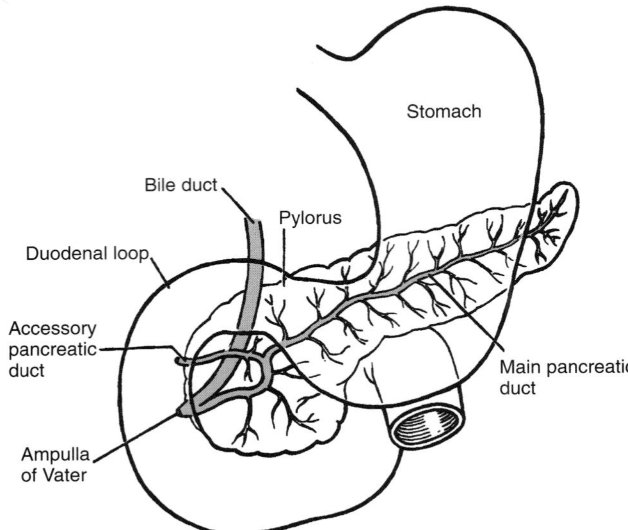

Figure 48-2 Cross-section through the pancreas.

tally. The duodenum is about 25 cm long and is the shortest and widest part of the small intestine. The jejunum and ileum comprise the remainder of the small intestine. There is no clear demarcation, but the ileum is the distal three fifths.

The wall of the small intestine consists of four layers: mucous, submucous, muscular, and serous. The internal surface of the upper small intestine contains valvulae conniventes; these are valve-like circular folds that project 3 to 10 mm into the lumen of the intestine. Covering the entire mucous surface of the small intestine are very small (1 mm) finger-like projections (villi), giving it a "velvety" appearance. The luminal surface (brush border) of each epithelial cell consists of some 600 microvilli projecting about 1 μm from the cell. The folds, villi, and microvilli together present an absorptive surface some 600 times greater than would be inferred from the length and diameter of this portion of the gut. The absorptive surface area of the small intestine is estimated to be about 250 m^2,[73] which is comparable to the area of a doubles tennis court.

Large Intestine

The large intestine is about 1.5 m in length, extending from the ileum to the anus, and includes the cecum, appendix, colon, rectum, and anal canal. The cecum is a blind pouch that begins the large intestine; it is connected to the terminal ileum via the ileocecal sphincter. The appendix is a "worm-shaped" tube connected to the blind end of the cecum. The colon is about 1 m long and is divided into the ascending, transverse, descending, and sigmoid sections. The sigmoid colon connects to the rectum, which is approximately 12 cm long. The rectum in turn connects to the anal canal, the terminal end of the large intestine.

Pancreas

The pancreas is 12 to 15 cm in length and lies across the posterior wall of the abdominal cavity. The head is located in the duodenal curve; the body and tail are directed toward the left, extending to the spleen (Figure 48-2). Pancreatic digestive enzymes, in bicarbonate-rich juice, enter the duodenum through the ampulla of Vater and the sphincter of Oddi and mix with the food bolus as it passes through the small bowel.

Phases of Digestion

The process of digestion can be conveniently subdivided into the neurogenic, gastric, and intestinal phases.

Neurogenic Phase

The neurogenic or cephalic phase is initiated by the intake of food into the mouth; the sight, smell, and taste of food stimulate the cerebral cortex and subsequently the vagal nuclei. The process is chemically mediated by acetylcholine from postganglionic parasympathetic nerve endings, which acts on gastric parietal cells. The vagus also stimulates gastric chief and parietal (oxyntic) cells to secrete pepsinogen and hydrochloric acid. (Cutting of the vagus nerve [vagotomy] decreases the volume and acidity of gastric secretion.)

The mechanism of acid secretion is still widely debated; there is, however, significant agreement that acetylcholine, histamine, and gastrin act through their respective neurocrine, paracrine, and endocrine pathways to stimulate the parietal cells, and that specific parietal cell receptors to these transmitters exist. Also, there are potentiating interactions between the mentioned secretagogues that probably occur at the parietal cell itself. Histamine has a role as a mediator or a potentiator of the actions of other secretagogues. Administration of histamine markedly increases the secretion provoked by pentagastrin or by cholinergic agonists. Histamine H_2-receptor antagonists inhibit acid secretion provoked by most types of stimulation, confirming the important role of histamine in acid secretion.

The parietal cell is transformed morphologically when acid secretion is stimulated. The tubulovesicular membranes, prominent in the resting cell, diminish, whereas there is a marked increase in the apical plasma membrane (the secretory surface of the cell) together with the appearance of long apical microvilli.

Cimetidine (Tagamet) and other H_2-receptor antagonists (such as ranitidine [Zantac] and famotidine [Pepcid]) block both the morphological transformation of the parietal cell and H^+ secretion. Proton pump inhibitors (PPIs) have a different mechanism of action. Omeprazole (a PPI) is taken up by the parietal cell and converted to an active metabolite that inactivates the parietal H^+, K^+-ATPase. Hydrogen ion secretion is inhibited until new ATPase is synthesized—a process that requires at least 24 hours.

The secretion of H^+ against a million-fold concentration gradient requires energy from the cell, and this process is coupled to H^+, K^+-ATPase. Histamine-stimulated acid secretion involves cyclic adenosine monophosphate (cAMP); cholinergic stimulation is not associated with increases in intracellular cAMP in isolated parietal cells, and this process may be mediated by changes in permeability of the cell's plasma membrane to Ca^{2+}. The latter activates a chain of events that alters the cell function in various ways. In addition to the previously mentioned mechanisms, vagal fibers to the pyloric glandular mucosa cause the release of gastrin, which also stimulates hydrochloric acid and pepsinogen secretion.

Other agents inhibiting acid secretion include somatostatin, prostaglandins, gastric inhibitory polypeptide (GIP), secretin, glucagon, vasoactive intestinal polypeptide (VIP), neurotensin, calcitonin gene-related peptide, corticotrophin-releasing factor, thyrotropin-releasing hormone, peptide YY, dopamine, and serotonin. Acid secretion is decreased in the presence of decreased amounts of circulating pituitary, adrenal, thyroid, and parathyroid hormones. Pituitary hormones are apparently essential for the maintenance of the structural integrity of the gastric mucosa and necessary for secretory function; human growth hormone may be necessary for the growth of the gastric mucosa.

Gastric Phase

When food enters the stomach, the resulting distention initiates the gastric phase of digestion, mediated by local and vagal reflexes. Hydrochloric acid release is caused by (1) direct vagal stimulation of the parietal cells; (2) local distention of the antrum and vagal stimulation of antral cells to secrete gastrin, which causes hydrochloric acid release from parietal cells; and (3) release of gastrin, stimulated by the near neutralization (pH 5-7) of gastric hydrochloric acid by ingested food entering the pyloric zone. Gastrin also stimulates antral motility, secretion of pepsinogens and of pancreatic fluid rich in enzymes, and release of a number of GI hormones (secretin, insulin, acetylcholine, somatostatin, and pancreatic polypeptide; for further information on GI hormones, see the later section of this chapter on GI Regulatory Peptides.). As a result of the acid environment, pepsinogen is rapidly converted to the active proteolytic enzyme pepsin. Food is mixed by contractions of the stomach and partially degraded by the chemical secretions of the stomach into chyme. The pylorus plays a role in emptying chyme into the duodenum by virtue of its strong musculature.

Intestinal Phase

The intestinal phase of digestion begins when the weakly acidic digestive products of proteins and lipids enter the duodenum. Many GI hormones and other regulatory peptides are released by both neural and local stimulation and act within the GI tract to regulate digestion and absorption. These are described in more detail in the section on GI Regulatory Peptides. Digestion, absorption, and storage functions are stimulated or inhibited by different hormones, creating an intricate hormonal control system that regulates the action of intestinal hormones and provides for secretion of bile acids, bicarbonate, and numerous enzymes involved in the digestion of food. In this system, the intestinal hormones secretin and VIP, for example, inhibit gastrin release and decrease the secretion of hydrochloric acid and pepsinogen; cholecystokinin (CCK; see discussion later in this chapter) binds to gastrin receptors and thus also decreases hydrochloric acid secretion. Somatostatin inhibits gastrin, secretin, CCK, and other hormones.

During the intestinal phase, carbohydrates, proteins, and fats are broken down and absorbed as described in the next section. Most nutrients, including vitamins and minerals, have been absorbed by the time the food passes from the jejunum and ileum into the large bowel. In the large intestine, water is actively absorbed, electrolyte balance is regulated, and bacterial actions take place. These processes result in the formation of feces.

PROCESSES OF DIGESTION AND ABSORPTION[52]

The total quantity of fluid absorbed each day by the gut is estimated to be about 9 L, which is composed of 2 L oral intake, 1.5 L saliva, 2.5 L gastric juice, 0.5 L bile, 1.5 L pancreatic juice, and 1 L intestinal secretions. More than 90% of this fluid is absorbed in the small intestine. The maximal absorptive capacity for fluid is probably at least 20 L. Several hundred grams of carbohydrates, about 100 g of fat, and 50 to 100 g of amino acids are absorbed daily in the small gut, but maximal absorptive capacity is believed to be at least 10 times greater. This considerable reserve capacity may compensate for mild to moderate degrees of dysfunction induced by disease processes, at least in the early phases. The efficiency of absorption is due to the unique features of the absorptive surface of the bowel and the relationship of the epithelial cells to the underlying rich vascular plexus and the lymphatic vessels.

Digestion of ingested food takes place both within the lumen of the small intestine and at the mucosal (brush border) surface. Defects of digestion may occur at one or more stages in the process. The terms maldigestion and malabsorption refer to different functional abnormalities. Maldigestion is a dysfunction of the digestive process that may occur at various sites in the GI tract. For example, hypoacidity in the stomach will reduce peptic digestion of protein; hyperacidity of the duodenum (e.g., due to overproduction of gastrin by tumor in the Zollinger-Ellison syndrome) can inactivate pancreatic enzymes; loss of brush border enzymes in the small intestine, because of any of a variety of processes, can prevent oligosaccharides and disaccharides from being further hydrolyzed; pancreatic insufficiency will reduce intraluminal enzyme activity in the small gut, causing maldigestion of fats and proteins. By contrast, malabsorption is strictly a dysfunction of the absorptive process by the small gut caused by a loss of absorptive epithelial cells caused, for example, by gluten, inflammation, infection, surgical resection, and infiltrations. A number of transport defects also lead to malabsorption of specific substances (e.g., glucose-galactose malabsorption or zinc deficiency in the congenital disorder acrodermatitis enteropathica). In clinical practice, however, the term malabsorption is often used to encompass all aspects of impaired digestion and absorption. As Figure 48-3 shows, absorption of the different nutrients proceeds at different rates and at different sites within the small bowel.

In the following three sections, the digestion and absorption of fats, carbohydrates, and proteins will be discussed separately. It must be remembered, however, that there is a complex interplay among nutrients, regulatory peptides, enzymes, gallbladder and pancreatic function, and bowel motility leading to an integrated absorptive process commencing with the ingestion of food and culminating in the excretion of feces.

Digestion and Absorption of Carbohydrates

After the action of salivary and pancreatic α-amylases on dietary starch and glycogen, the carbohydrate content of the small intestine consists of newly formed maltose; ingested monosaccharides; dietary disaccharides, such as lactose, sucrose, maltose, and trehalose; oligosaccharides, such as dextrins and maltotriose; and indigestible oligosaccharides and polysaccharides, such as cellulose, agar, and other oligosaccharide dietary fibers.

The brush border enzymes with disaccharidase and oligosaccharidase activity are listed in Table 48-1. The sucrase-isomaltase complex comprises most of the sucrase, isomaltase, and maltase (80%) activity of the small intestine. It hydrolyzes sucrose to its constituent monosaccharides, cleaves glucose from α-limit dextrins with 1,6 bonds, and hydrolyzes maltose. The activity of the complex is fourfold to fivefold greater in the jejunum than in the ileum. Changes in diet have a marked effect on the expression of the complex; starvation leads to a rapid decline in activity, which is rapidly restored on refeeding. All small intestinal saccharidases may decrease with infection or inflammation of the small bowel to the extent that carbohydrate malabsorption

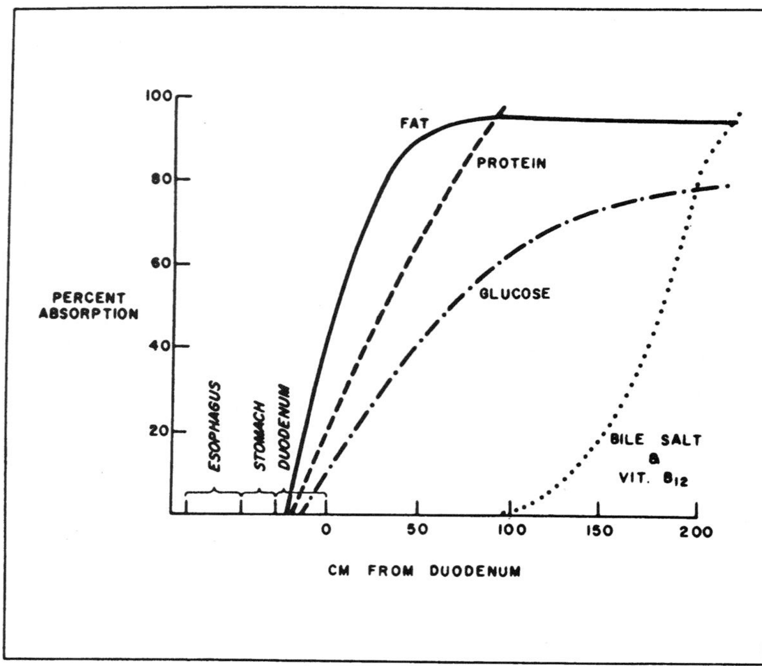

Figure 48-3 The location of small intestinal absorption. *(Modified from Morris JA, Selivanov V, Sheldon GF. Nutritional management of patients with malabsorption syndrome. Clin Gastroenterol 1983;12;463-74, based on Borgstrom B, et al. Studies of intestinal digestion and absorption in the human. J Clin Invest 1957;1521-36.)*

occurs, leading to diarrhea, flatulence, and weight loss. Paradoxically, diabetes mellitus causes a striking increase in sucrase-isomaltase activity; an increase is also observed in monosaccharide and amino acid transport. The lactase–phlorizin hydrolase complex is the only brush border enzyme able to hydrolyze lactose and is therefore essential to survival of mammals early in life.

This complex also has glycosylceramidase, β-glycosidase, and phlorizin hydrolase activities. Infectious and inflammatory diseases greatly reduce lactase–phlorizin hydrolase activity, leading to symptomatic intolerance to milk. Recovery of the enzyme activity following intestinal disease may be slow. The activity of the complex is resistant to starvation. The developmental regulation of lactase is discussed later in the section on disaccharidase deficiencies. Also present in the brush border is the α-glucosidase maltase-glucoamylase, which removes individual glucose molecules from the nonreducing end of α(1,4) oligosaccharides and disaccharides. This enzyme accounts for about 20% of the total maltase activity of the small intestine. Trehalase is also found in the brush border of the small intestine and hydrolyzes trehalose, an α(1,1) disaccharide of glucose found in yeast and mushrooms. The developmental pattern of trehalase appears to follow that of sucrase-isomaltase.

In addition to their actions on disaccharides, the brush border enzymes further hydrolyze the products of amylase action, including maltose, maltotriose, and α-limit dextrins. The brush border enzymes appear to act in an integrated manner in that there is a flow of substrate from glucoamylase and isomaltase to sucrase with the production of the monosaccharides glucose, galactose, and fructose. These monosaccharides are transported into the enterocyte by facilitative transport systems, such as the Na^+-dependent glucose (and galactose) transporter (SLGT1) and GLUT5 (one of the GLUT family of genes for monosaccharide transport), which transports fructose across the apical membrane of the enterocyte. Subsequently, absorbed glucose and fructose are transported across the basolateral membrane and out of the enterocyte and into the portal system by the GLUT2 transporter.

It is increasingly being realized that the limiting factor in carbohydrate digestion and absorption may be diffusion from the intestinal lumen to the membrane surface where the enzymes are localized. There is normally little disaccharidase activity in the luminal contents. For most oligosaccharides (with the exception of lactose), hydrolysis is rapid, and transport is the rate-limiting step in reducing the concentration of monosaccharides and the osmotic load in the gut. When the transport system is operating at its maximum rate but monosaccharide concentration is still high, inhibition of hydrolases by their monosaccharide products (i.e., product inhibition) slows hydrolytic activity, keeping monosaccharide concentrations relatively constant, thereby controlling osmotic load and water concentration in the gut. The importance of this control is evident from the consequences of intestinal disorders in which ingested disaccharide is not split and absorbed. The presence of undigested disaccharide increases fluid secretion into the gut and increases intestinal motility. Enteric bacteria ferment the unabsorbed sugars, producing hydrogen, carbon dioxide, and organic acids. Abdominal discomfort such as bloating, distention, and cramping occurs; absorption of fermentation products may lead to metabolic acidosis. In the large bowel, the presence of CO_2 and organic acids decreases pH

TABLE 48-1 Brush Border Oligosaccharidases

Enzyme or Complex	Principal Substrate(s)	Products
β-glycosidase complex:		
Lactase (EC 3.2.1.23)	Lactose	Glucose + galactose
Glycosylceramidase (EC 3.2.1.45-46) (also called phlorizin hydrolase [EC 3.2.1.62])	Galactosyl and glucosyl-β-ceramides	Galactose/glucose + ceramides
Sucrase-isomaltase complex:		
Sucrase-(maltase) (EC 3.2.1.48)	Maltose/sucrose	Glucose/fructose + glucose
Isomaltase-(maltase) (EC 3.2.1.10)	1,6-α-linkages in isomaltose and α-dextrins	Glucose
	Maltose	Glucose
Trehalase (EC 3.2.1.28)	Trehalose	Glucose
Glucoamylase complex (EC 3.2.1.20):		
Glucoamylase-(maltase)-1 and glucoamylase-(maltase)-2 (have similar substrate specificities)	1,4-α-linkages at nonreducing ends of amylose, amylopectin, glycogen, and straight chain 1,4-α-glucopyranosyl oligomers, including maltose	Glucose

From Semenza G, Auricchio S. Small intestinal disaccharidases. In: Scriver CR, Beaudet AL, Sly WS, Valle D, eds. The metabolic and molecular bases of inherited disease, 7th ed. New York: McGraw-Hill, 1995:4451-80.

and keeps the osmolality high so that water reabsorption is decreased. The result is an acidic, liquid stool. Normally, however, accumulation of monosaccharide products does not occur, because the transport system is sufficiently fast to remove them. Mucosal lactase activity is the lowest of all the disaccharidases; for lactose, the rate-limiting step in absorption is thought to be hydrolysis. Lactase activity is not increased by feeding large amounts of lactose, as is the case for maltase and sucrase. Lactase, maltase, and sucrase all show circadian rhythms in their activities; minimum and maximum activities may vary by a factor of 2.

Carbohydrate digestion is not always complete in the small intestine. Indeed, it is likely that some starch and sucrose normally pass undigested and unabsorbed into the colon. It has been estimated that colonic bacteria require 70 g of carbohydrate/day. Much of this is derived from endogenous sources, such as from glycoproteins in GI secretions, with the remainder coming from unabsorbed dietary carbohydrate and dietary fiber. Up to 15% of the carbohydrate from white bread reaches the colon, and the effects of indigestible oligosaccharides on reaching the large bowel are well known. As pointed out earlier, bacterial action creates short-chain fatty acids, which are rapidly absorbed by the colonic mucosa and are thought to provide fuel for the colonocyte. Starch and oligosaccharides are osmotically active and draw water into the gut. The colon, however, can absorb up to four times the normal colonic water load; for this reason, diarrhea is not always present in oligosaccharide malabsorption.

Digestion and Absorption of Lipids

The recommended daily dietary fat intake in Europe and North America is 70 to 95 g. Less than 5 g/24 hours is recovered in the feces, indicating the overall efficiency of the normal processes of fat digestion and absorption. Most dietary fat is in the form of long-chain triacylglycerols (triglycerides). Pancreatic lipase is quantitatively the most important hydrolytic enzyme, but the contribution of gastric lipase to overall hydrolysis should not be underestimated. Gastric lipase is secreted by the gastric mucosa and normally accounts for up to 17.5% of fatty acids released from triglycerides following a meal.[20] The enzyme has a wide pH optimum and is active in both the stomach and duodenum. This nonpancreatic lipase may have a significant role in lipid digestion when pancreatic function is impaired and in the neonatal period before pancreatic lipase activity is fully developed. A lingual lipase is also present, secreted by the tongue, but is thought not to be of much significance normally in humans.

Fats are first emulsified in the stomach by its churning action and stabilized by interaction with luminal lecithin and protein fragments. The lingual and gastric lipases do not require bile salts or cofactors to function; they have a pH optimum of 3 to 6 and their action produces 1,2-diacylglycerols and fatty acids. These products further stabilize the surface of the triglyceride emulsion and in the duodenum promote the binding of pancreatic colipase. In addition, the liberated fatty acids stimulate release of CCK from the duodenal mucosa.

Pancreatic lipase, in the presence of bile salts and colipase, acts at the oil-water interface of the triglyceride emulsion to produce fatty acids and 2-monoacylglycerols. Colipase is secreted in pancreatic juice as an inactive proenzyme, which is converted to the active form by trypsin. Other significant enzymes involved in the breakdown of fats within the intestinal lumen are cholesterol ester hydrolase, phospholipase A_2, and a nonspecific bile salt–activated lipase.

Only a small proportion of ingested triacylglycerol is completely hydrolyzed to glycerol and fatty acids. These products form micelles with bile salts and lysophosphoglycerides; the micelles convey the nonpolar lipid molecules from the lumen to the epithelial cell surface and dissociate there to produce a high concentration of monoacylglycerols, lysophosphoglycerides, and fatty acids, which are absorbed into the mucosal cell. This absorption is facilitated by a fatty acid–binding protein in the cytosol of the cell that has a high affinity for fatty acids. Within the cell, triacylglycerols are resynthesized from the absorbed 2-monoacylglycerols and fatty acids. The triacylglycerols, together with phospholipids, cholesterol and its esters, fat-soluble vitamins, and a specific apolipoprotein, are formed into chylomicrons, which are then released by exocytosis into the lymphatic system of the small bowel.

From the lymphatics, chylomicrons enter the blood stream via the thoracic duct and are distributed to the liver, adipose tissue, and other organs. Medium- and short-chain fatty acids (chain length <12 carbon atoms) in mixed triglycerides are preferentially split by lipases and pass into the aqueous phase from which they are rapidly absorbed. Medium-chain triglycerides can be absorbed without complete lipolysis and in the absence of bile. They do not require micellar solubilization and are transported from the intestinal epithelial cells predominantly via the hepatic portal vein. Figure 48-4 summarizes the processes involved in fat absorption and conditions that compromise the efficiency of one or more stages in the process of fat digestion and absorption leading to fat malabsorption.[26]

Digestion and Absorption of Proteins

The average daily dietary intake of protein in North America is about 100 g compared with an estimated requirement for adults of 50 to 70 g. In addition to dietary protein, another 50 to 60 g of protein enters the intestinal contents daily in GI secretions and from desquamated mucosal cells. Normal daily fecal loss of protein is about 10 g.

Protein digestion is initiated in the stomach by the action of pepsin in a highly acid medium. The acidity also denatures the protein, unfolding the polypeptide chains for better access by the gastric, pancreatic, and intestinal proteolytic enzymes. Additionally, the polypeptides and amino acids

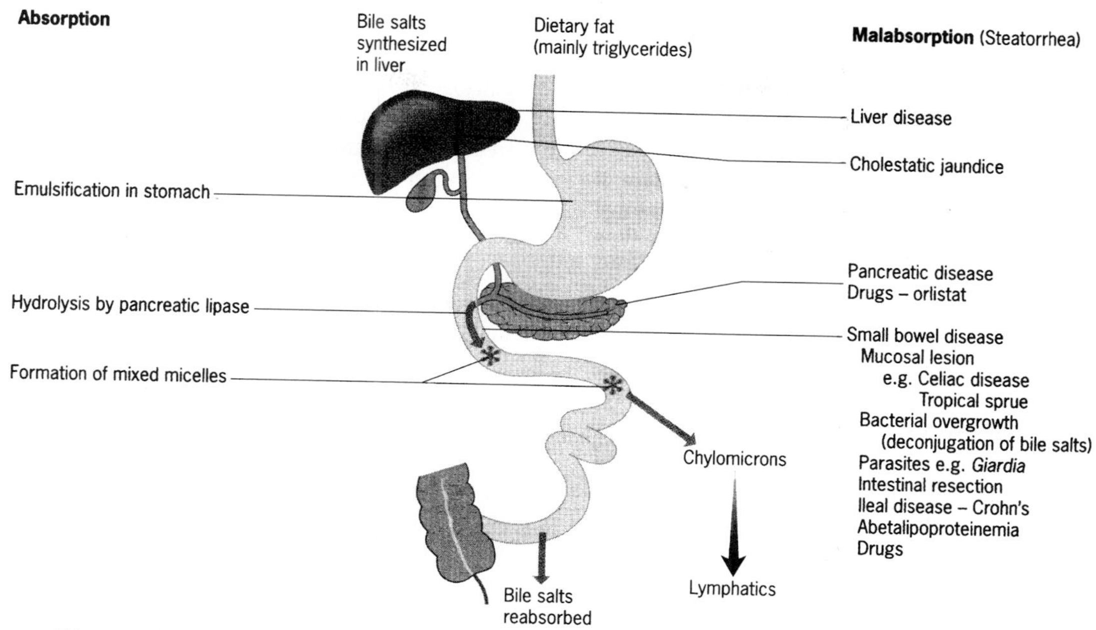

Figure 48-4 Summary of the processes involved in fat absorption and malabsorption. *(From Clark ML, Silk DB. Gastrointestinal disease. In: Kumar P, Clark M, eds. Clinical medicine, 5th ed. Edinburgh: WB Saunders, 2002:253-333.)*

produced in the stomach by the action of pepsin are potent secretagogues for the hormones that stimulate the pancreas and intestine. Stimulated pancreatic secretion contains the proenzyme forms of the proteolytic enzymes trypsin, chymotrypsin, elastase, exopeptidases, and carboxypeptidases. Proteolytic enzymes are either endopeptidases (e.g., pepsin, trypsin, chymotrypsin, and elastase), which hydrolyze peptide bonds within the polypeptide chain, or exopeptidases, which hydrolyze peptide bonds of the terminal amino acids (enzymes such as carboxypeptidase and aminopeptidase). Stimulation of the intestine by GI hormones liberates several proteolytic enzymes from the brush border. One of them, enterokinase, selectively cleaves a hexapeptide from the *N*-terminus of trypsinogen to form trypsin. Trypsin then activates more trypsin (autocatalysis) and in addition converts other pancreatic proenzymes into their active forms. The action of the pancreatic enzymes on the partly digested proteins within the lumen produces peptides, 2 to 6 amino acid residues in length, and also single amino acids. The peptides are largely hydrolyzed to single amino acids by the aminopeptidases and dipeptidases of the brush border before absorption, although some dipeptides and tripeptides are absorbed and are hydrolyzed to amino acids by cytosolic peptidases within the enterocytes. At least seven carrier systems with overlapping specificities for different amino acids are involved in transport of amino acids into the cells. Absorption of amino acids by these transport systems is faster in the jejunum than in the ileum. The amino acids pass into the underlying rich vascular plexus, drained by the portal circulation, and it is by this route that absorbed amino acids reach the liver and then the systemic circulation.

Individuals with achlorhydria or total gastrectomy have normal protein digestion and absorption as small intestinal function compensates for the lack of pepsin activity. Pancreatic and small intestinal diseases are the major causes of protein maldigestion and malabsorption. However, fecal loss of protein rarely becomes significant in pancreatic insufficiency until trypsin levels fall to about 10% of normal. Two rare disorders, trypsin deficiency and enterokinase deficiency, have far-reaching effects on efficiency of protein digestion, as would be expected from their roles in the activation of proteolytic proenzymes. Mucosal diseases may affect protein assimilation by a number of mechanisms. Reduction in number of mucosal cells decreases peptidase activity in the intestine and intestinal absorptive capacity for amino acids. Disease may increase the turnover of intestinal cells and the rate of desquamation. This cell loss, together with increased losses of plasma proteins from the damaged intestinal surface, can cause a negative nitrogen balance. Surgical resection of the intestine not only reduces the total intestinal absorptive surface but also may remove a segment of the gut that is specialized for absorption of certain nutrients (for example, resection of the distal ileum removes the active transport system for the vitamin B_{12}–intrinsic factor complex). Resection may also alter intestinal motility and lead to stasis and bacterial overgrowth that can intensify a negative nitrogen balance. There are also rare hereditary defects in amino acid transporters that produce distinct syndromes.

STOMACH: DISEASES AND LABORATORY INVESTIGATIONS

The growth in endoscopic procedures, with direct visualization of the interior of the stomach, has largely removed the need for the clinical laboratory to carry out the analysis of gastric contents. Situations remain, however, in which the laboratory continues to play a significant role in the diagnosis of gastric diseases and in monitoring the effectiveness of treatment. This section describes peptic ulcer disease and tests for *Helicobacter pylori* (*H. pylori*) and the measurement of basal acid output from the stomach.

PEPTIC ULCER DISEASE AND *HELICOBACTER PYLORI*[155,165]

Although the presence of spiral-shaped organisms in the stomach has been acknowledged for many years, it was only in 1985 that the association was described between *H. pylori* (known then as *Campylobacter pylori*) and peptic ulcer disease.[125] Most estimates suggest that the bacterium is present in the mucous layer of the stomach in half of the population of the world. In Europe 30% to 50% of adults, and in the United States at least 20% of the adult population, are infected with the organism. In all cases, colonization with *H. pylori* causes a chronic inflammatory reaction in the gastric mucosa even when direct endoscopic observation of the mucosa appears normal. Carriers of the organism are at increased risk of gastric cancer (twofold to tenfold) and peptic ulcer (threefold to tenfold).[12] Some of the increased risk is due to infection with strains of the organism that produce the cytotoxic cagA protein. About 90% of gastric cancer patients are infected with *H. pylori*, compared with 40% to 60% of age-matched controls.[139,140] In a European study comparing prevalence of *H. pylori* and gastric cancer rates in 13 countries, a significant correlation was observed between the infection rate and gastric cancer incidence and mortality.[169] It is, however, important to remember that although a large proportion of gastric cancer can be attributed to infection with *H. pylori*, only in a minority of infected subjects will the inflammatory reaction progress to gastric cancer. The current consensus is that asymptomatic subjects should not be screened for *H. pylori* infection.[123]

At least 95% of patients with duodenal ulcer disease are infected with *H. pylori*, and eradication of the organism leads to healing of the ulcer and reduction in relapse rates.[145] Eradication of *H. pylori* is now the recommended treatment for patients with duodenal or gastric ulcer who are *H. pylori*–positive. Effective combined antibiotic and acid suppression regimens (using PPIs) are available with eradication rates of about 90% after first-line treatment.[165]

H. pylori infection predominantly affects the gastric mucosa, with the antrum usually being the most densely colonized area. The reasons that a gastric mucosal infection predisposes to duodenal ulceration are complex and involve a number of pathways leading to increased acid production. Before there was an awareness of the role of *H. pylori* in the pathogenesis of peptic ulcer disease, vagotomy (surgical sectioning, or cutting, of the vagus nerve) was the mainstay of treatment as a means of reducing gastric acid output, thereby leading to an environment more conducive to healing of the ulcer.

Infection with the organism, with or without duodenal ulceration, leads to increases in both basal and meal-stimulated serum gastrin concentrations, principally due to an increase in gastrin-17.[134] Basal acid output is increased in *H. pylori*–positive subjects (see Figure 48-5), and resolves completely after successful eradication of the organism. Hypergastrinemia is believed to be only one of the mechanisms leading to increased acid output. Studies using the neuropeptide gastrin releasing peptide (GRP) suggest that impairment of inhibitory control mechanisms regulating acid production may be responsible for the increased acid output associated with *H. pylori* infection.[49] In addition to stimulating the G cells of the antrum to release gastrin, which leads to acid secretion by parietal cells, GRP also activates neuroendocrine pathways that inhibit gastric acid secretion, an effect mediated via several peptides (including cholecystokinin and secretin) that stimulate the release of the inhibitory peptide somatostatin from the gastric mucosa.

H. pylori produces urease, and hydrolysis of endogenous urea to bicarbonate and ammonia may create a more hospitable microenvironment for the survival of the organism in the stomach. Mammalian cells do not hydrolyze urea and it was only in 1984 that "gastric urease" was associated with the presence of *H. pylori*.[110] The ability of the organism to rapidly hydrolyze urea is the basis of the urea breath tests and of the direct urease tests on gastric biopsy samples.

DIAGNOSTIC TESTS FOR *H. PYLORI*

A wide range of invasive and noninvasive diagnostic tests for *H. pylori* has been described as shown in Box 48-1.

All of the tests in the "invasive" group necessitate oral gastroduodenoscopy with a biopsy of the gastric mucosa; false negative results may occur because of sampling errors, as colonization may be patchy. The antrum is the preferred biopsy site, but multiple biopsies from the anterior and posterior walls of the antrum and body of the stomach are recommended for maximum diagnostic accuracy of this group of tests. False negatives may also occur when biopsies are taken during treatment with PPIs or within 2 weeks of stopping PPI therapy. This group of drugs alters the intragastric distribution of *H. pylori* and suppresses its activity.[118] PPIs can also lead to falsely negative urea breath test results. During PPI therapy, biopsies should also be taken from the body and fundus to prevent false negatives. If PPIs cannot be withheld for at least 2 weeks before a breath test, a negative result must be interpreted with caution. Histamine H_2-receptor antagonists and antacids do not affect the tests in this way.

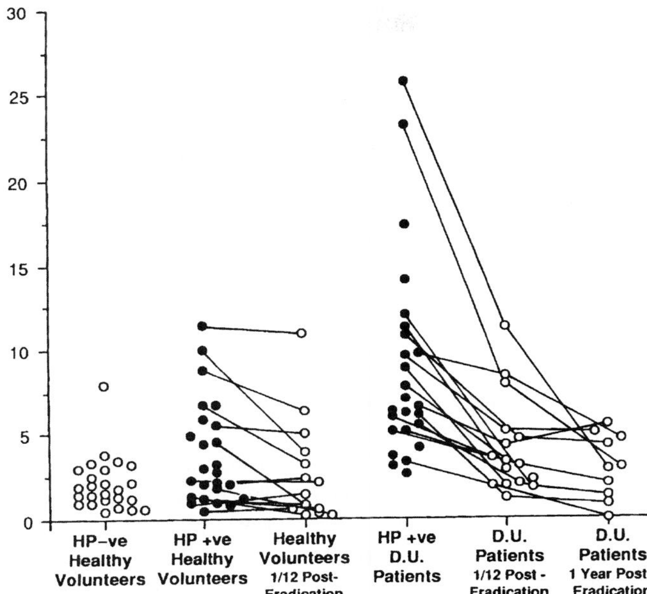

Figure 48-5 Basal acid output in healthy volunteers and patients with duodenal ulcers (DUs) of varying *H. pylori* status (●, *H. pylori* positive). Compared with *H. pylori*–negative healthy volunteers, basal acid output is increased in *H. pylori*–positive healthy volunteers ($P < 0.05$), *H. pylori*–positive patients with DUs ($P < 0.0001$), and patients with DUs 1 month after eradication ($P < 0.01$). *(From El-Omar EM, Penman ID, Ardill JES, Chittajallu RS, Howie C, McColl KEL.* H. pylori *infection and abnormalities of acid secretion in patients with duodenal ulcer disease. Gastroenterology 1995;109:681-91, with permission from the American Gastroenterological Association.)*

BOX 48-1 Diagnostic Tests for *Helicobacter pylori*

Invasive Tests—Using Gastric Mucosal Biopsy Samples

- Histology: microscopy after Giemsa or silver staining
- Histology: microscopy after immunohistochemical staining
- Direct urease test: a biopsy incubated in urea/indicator solution; visual endpoint
- Culture: incubation on suitable media for 4 to 10 days
- Polymerase chain reaction: amplification of specific DNA sequences

Noninvasive Tests—Using Breath, Blood, Saliva, or Feces

- Breath tests: rise in breath $^{14}CO_2$ or $^{13}CO_2$ after ingestion of ^{14}C- or ^{13}C-labeled urea
- Serum tests: laboratory measurement of specific IgG antibody
- Whole blood tests: point-of-care tests for specific IgG antibody
- Saliva tests: detection of specific IgG antibody
- Fecal tests: detection of specific antigen

Tests for *H. pylori* are required for diagnosis of the infection and to ascertain, in some situations, that eradication therapy has been successful. High sensitivity is required to ensure that positives are not missed; similarly, high specificity is essential to prevent inappropriate use of eradication therapy. The Maastricht 2-2000 Consensus guidelines[123] recommend a "test and treat" strategy in adults with appropriate dyspeptic symptoms under the age of 45 years using either the breath test or stool antigen test. The age limit may vary depending on local prevalence and the age distribution of gastric cancer (e.g., in the United Kingdom, testing and treatment are now recommended up to the age of 55 in patients with uncomplicated dyspepsia).[15] Successful eradication should be confirmed with the urea breath test or by a direct urease test if endoscopy is clinically indicated; the stool antigen test may be used if urea breath tests are not available. Other national guidelines confirm the urea breath test as the preferred procedure, both for initial diagnosis and for confirmation of eradication.[15,87] Testing to confirm eradication should be done at least 4 weeks after completion of the course of treatment.

Urea breath tests are simple to perform, and sensitivity and specificity are both greater than 95%. Urea labeled with either ^{14}C or ^{13}C is given orally as a drink or a capsule to swallow with water; urease from gastric *H. pylori* rapidly hydrolyzes the ingested urea to produce labeled bicarbonate, which is absorbed into the blood and exhaled as $^{14}CO_2$ or $^{13}CO_2$. The principal advantages of the ^{13}C-urea breath test over the ^{14}C-urea breath test are the simplicity of breath collection and the avoidance of the regulations and environmental issues related to the use and disposal of radioisotopes. In the ^{14}C-urea breath test, CO_2 in expired air is trapped in methanolic hyamine hydroxide as the patient exhales through a straw, which should be fitted with a one-way valve to ensure the patient does not suck the trapping solution into the mouth. A color change of an indicator (thymol blue) in the solution shows that the required quantity of CO_2 has been trapped. Scintillant is then added and $^{14}CO_2$ measured. In the ^{13}C-urea breath test, the patient blows through a straw into an empty 15 mL tube, which is then capped. $^{13}CO_2/^{12}CO_2$ ratios are compared for basal and postdose samples using isotope ratio mass spectrometry or alternative infrared measurement methods.[106,117]

In the stool test, specific *H. pylori* antigens are detected in microtiter plates coated with polyclonal antibodies. Debate continues regarding its accuracy for assessing treatment outcome; some of the variability in results between different studies appears to be caused by lack of standardization of the interval between completion of eradication therapy and stool testing.[174] However, the test is currently recommended for posteradication testing if the urea breath test is not available.[123]

Although still widely available, serological tests are no longer recommended. The systemic antibody response is variable, leading to equivocal results in some subjects; in subjects age >50 years, diagnostic accuracy is unsatisfactory. Serology cannot be used to confirm eradication because of the slow decline in antibody levels after treatment. Laboratory-based enzyme-linked immunosorbent assays (ELISA) assays and point-of-care tests are available to measure specific IgG antibodies in serum or whole blood samples. In younger subjects, the laboratory-based tests generally perform well although some have sensitivity and/or specificity of <95%. Office-based serology currently has inadequate sensitivity and specificity. Calculations based on reported diagnostic accuracy data show that when these tests are used for diagnosis, as many as 28% of those receiving eradication therapy are being treated as a result of false-positive test results.[25]

Since 1985, an enormous body of literature has accumulated on the epidemiology and transmission of *H. pylori*, on pathogenicity and host response, and on clinical outcomes and treatment options. Despite the clear link with peptic ulcer disease, the question of whether *H. pylori* causes duodenal ulceration or is just an important factor producing recurrence and chronicity continues to be raised.[13] Another interesting area is the use of gene expression studies to increase understanding of the interaction between the gastric mucosa and *H. pylori* by comparison of gene products from gastric tissue *H. pylori* and isolated strains grown in vitro.[67] It is an organism that will continue to surprise us.

Determination of Basal Acid Output[36,76,93]

The documentation of an increased basal acid output (BAO) in gastric juice provides strong evidence that a high serum gastrin concentration is caused by Zollinger-Ellison syndrome. The test is therefore used in patients with duodenal ulceration and a raised serum gastrin concentration. The test is not appropriate in patients with atrophic gastritis. Pernicious anemia, which also causes hypergastrinemia, should be excluded before assessing BAO. PPIs must be stopped for at least 14 days, and H_2-receptor antagonists for at least 3 days, before the test. *H. pylori* as a cause of increased serum gastrin should also be excluded before BAO estimation.

A basal condition, in the context of gastric analysis, is one in which the patient is at complete rest and not exposed to any visual, auditory, or olfactory stimuli. Such a condition is maintained during sleep. It is for this reason that traditionally a 12-hour overnight collection of gastric juice has been used for the determination of BAO. Such an approach has the disadvantage that the patient is exposed to significant discomfort because of the need to retain the tube overnight, while sitting upright and slightly turned to the left to prevent a loss of gastric contents into the duodenum. Close supervision throughout the entire night is necessary. A satisfactory alternative is the collection of gastric juice for 60 minutes after the patient has had a satisfactory night's sleep in a quiet separate room. After waking, the patient must remain fasting; smoking and exercise must be avoided before and during the test.

Collection of Gastric Juice

A gastric tube is inserted orally, or nasal intubation may be used if the patient has a hyperactive gag reflex. X-ray or fluoroscopic confirmation that the tip of the radio-opaque tube is in the lowest portion of the stomach is necessary. Ten or 15 minutes after the patient has become calm and adjusted to the presence of the tube, the patient is positioned with the trunk upright and inclined slightly to the left. Gastric juice is then aspirated and discarded. After checking that no further juice can be aspirated, note the time and collect and transfer to plastic bottles all gastric juice that can be aspirated over the next 60 minutes. The patient must be asked to expectorate all saliva during the collection period. The total volume of the collected juice is recorded and free acid determined by titration as described below.

Determination of Free Hydrochloric Acid in Gastric Juice

1. Measure and transfer a convenient volume of gastric juice (e.g., 5.0 to 10.0 mL) into a clean titration vessel. If the gastric juice contains food particles or mucus, centrifuge the sample or filter it through gauze.
2. Determine the pH of the gastric specimen with a pH meter. If the pH is above 3.5, no free acid is present. Such a specimen need not be titrated.
3. Titrate the sample with NaOH, 0.10 mol/L, to a pH of 3.5, using a pH meter.

Calculation:

$$\text{Free HCl (mmol/L)} = \frac{\text{mL of NaOH} \times 100}{\text{mL of gastric juice titrated}}$$

If 5 mL of gastric specimen is titrated, the calculation becomes:

$$\text{Free HCl (mmol/L)} = \text{mL of NaOH} \times 20$$

$$\text{Free HCl (mmol/hr)} = \frac{\text{mL of NaOH} \times 20 \times 60\text{min volume of gastric juice in mL}}{1000}$$

Comments and Sources of Error

Titration to a pH of 3 to 3.5 detects essentially all free hydrochloric acid. (Because HCl is the only strongly ionized acid in gastric content, this test is essentially a test for free HCl.) Titration beyond a pH of 3.5, as recommended by some, will overestimate the HCl concentration to varying degrees, depending on the composition of the gastric residue. On the other hand, titration to pH 3.5 may underestimate the amount of free H^+ secreted if some of these H^+ ions are bound to or have reacted with other constituents of gastric content. Thus no fully satisfactory procedure is available to measure accurately the true total amount of free acid secreted by the gastric mucosa.

The effectiveness of gastric aspiration may be compromised both by the position of the patient and the position of the tube in the stomach (likened to the position of a straw above or below the fluid level in a glass), by the loss of gastric fluid into the pylorus, and by regurgitation of pyloric contents into the stomach. Some evidence suggests that the exact position of the tube in the stomach does not appear to alter the recovery of gastric juice, because the stomach is not rigid and its walls contract, thus shifting the stomach contents toward the tip of the tube.

Interpretation

Gastric juice pH: if the pH is >2.5, then it is unlikely that the raised gastrin is caused by Zollinger-Ellison syndrome.

BAO: Normal: male 0 to 10.5 mmol/hr; female: 0 to 5.6 mmol/hr

Zollinger-Ellison syndrome: 15 to 100 mmol/hr, or >5 mmol/hr if there was previous acid-reducing surgery.

A level of free acid >15 mmol/hr should prompt a suspicion of gastrinoma but is not diagnostic; a level >25 mmol/hr with high serum gastrin is virtually diagnostic of Zollinger-Ellison syndrome.

Further discussion of the Zollinger-Ellison syndrome can be found in the section of this chapter on neuroendocrine tumors.

INTESTINAL DISORDERS AND THEIR LABORATORY INVESTIGATION

This section includes a discussion of celiac disease, disaccharidase deficiency, bacterial overgrowth, bile salt malabsorption, and protein-losing enteropathy and the main laboratory investigations associated with their diagnosis.

Celiac Disease (Celiac Sprue, Gluten-Sensitive Enteropathy)[53,54,124,157]

Celiac disease is sometimes called nontropical sprue, celiac sprue, or gluten-sensitive enteropathy.

Pathophysiology of Celiac Disease

Celiac disease occurs in genetically predisposed subjects as a consequence of an inappropriate T-cell–mediated immune response to the ingestion of gluten from wheat and to similar proteins in barley and rye.

The role of genetic factors in celiac disease has been recognized for many years; there is a 70% concordance for celiac disease in identical twins and typically 10% of first-degree relatives of an affected individual will also be found to have the disease. Only recently has the major genetic component been localized to the human leukocyte antigen (HLA) region of chromosome 6. Approximately 95% of subjects with celiac disease express a specific HLA heterodimer (HLA DQ2 α/β heterodimer). Most Caucasian populations have a high frequency (20% to 30%) of DQ2, but only a small minority will develop celiac disease.

The external trigger to the development of celiac disease in genetically susceptible individuals is found in gluten, which is the complex group of proteins present in wheat that form a sticky mass when dough is washed with water and the starch is removed. All of the proteins (and peptides) that are toxic to the small bowel mucosa in subjects with celiac disease contain large amounts of glutamine. The major toxic proteins of wheat are the gliadins, with homologous proteins (the hordeins and secalins) occurring in barley and rye, respectively. The gliadins are a large family of proteins accounting for about 50% of the wheat protein.

Recent evidence indicates that oats do not lead to an immune-mediated response nor to mucosal damage in subjects with celiac disease.[92] Addition of oats to the list of permitted cereals increases choice and would be welcomed by most subjects with celiac disease. However, if oats are to be introduced into the diet they must be from a reliable source to ensure no contamination from wheat, barley, or rye proteins at any stage in the process from harvesting to packaging.

The identification in 1997 of small bowel tissue transglutaminase (tTG)-2 as the auto-antigen of celiac disease[37] was a major step forward in understanding the pathogenesis of the disorder. The tissue transglutaminases are a family of calcium-dependent cytoplasmic enzymes that are released from cells during wounding. Although their physiological role is incompletely understood, they are able to catalyze the cross-linking of proteins leading to the stabilization of the wound area. Expression of the enzyme is increased during apoptosis and in active celiac disease. It selectively cross-links or deamidates protein-bound glutamine residues. Deamidation of gliadin peptides by the enzyme enhances their binding to HLA DQ2/DQ8 and increases the recognition of these peptides by gut-derived T cells from subjects with celiac disease.[158] The pathogenesis of the disease is therefore believed to involve an interaction between tissue transglutaminase and gliadin peptides in genetically susceptible individuals.

The toxic cereal proteins lead to intestinal epithelial damage, releasing tissue transglutaminase. Cross linking by the enzyme produces gliadin-gliadin or gliadin-enzyme complexes, unmasking new antigenic epitopes that bind to HLA DQ2 molecules on the antigen-presenting cells, producing an immune response by gut-derived T cells. The characteristic enteropathy is then induced by the release of interferon-γ and other proinflammatory cytokines as outlined in Figure 48-6.

A 33-mer peptide of gluten appears to be the primary initiator of the inflammatory response.[154] It is resistant to breakdown by all gastric, pancreatic, and intestinal brush-border membrane proteases, thus allowing it to reach the small intestine intact. After deamidation by tissue transglutaminase, it is a potent inducer of gut-derived human T-cell lines from patients with celiac disease. Homologs of the peptide are found in food grains that are toxic to patients with celiac disease, but are absent from nontoxic food grains. The peptide could be detoxified by exposure to a bacterial prolyl endopeptidase, suggesting a strategy for therapy of celiac disease.[154]

Increased intestinal permeability in untreated celiac disease that is reversible on withdrawal of gluten from the diet has been recognized since the early 1980s.[74] Recent evidence suggests that this may be mediated by increased expression of zonulin,[56] a protein that opens small intestinal tight junctions, or to decreased expression of intercellular epithelial cell adhesion molecules, such as Z0-1, catenin, and cadherin.[142] It is currently unclear whether these findings are

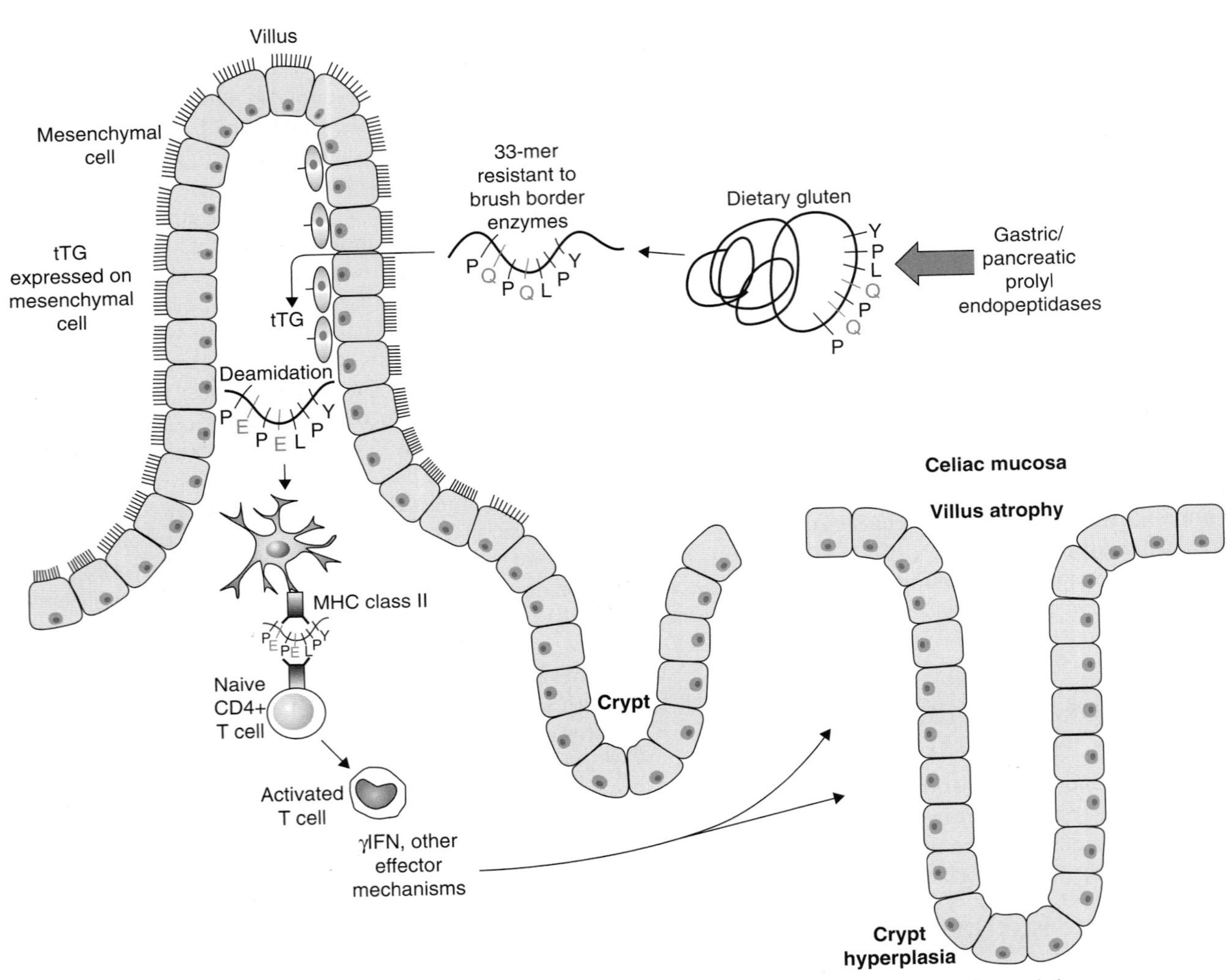

Figure 48-6 Hypothetical scheme for interaction between intestinal protein processing and the specific immune system in celiac disease. Dietary gluten is exposed to intraluminal digestive enzymes (including prolyl endopeptidases), producing stable 33-mer peptide-containing overlapping proline-rich epitopes with PQPQLPY central motif. 33-mer peptide is absorbed intact by transcellular or paracellular routes into lamina propria, and exposure to tTG results in deamidation of glutamine residues to glutamic acid. Modified peptide is presented to specific CD4+ T cells in association with HLA DQ2 or DQ8. Activated IFN-γ producing T-effector cells return to mucosa and produce characteristic villus atrophy and crypt hyperplasia. *tTG,* Tissue transglutaminase, *IFN,* interferon. *E,* glutamate, *F,* phenylalanine, *L,* leucine, *P,* proline, *Q,* glutamine, *Y,* tyrosine. *(From Mowat AM. Coeliac disease—a meeting point for genetics, immunology, and protein chemistry. Lancet 2003;361:1290-2.)*

linked to the entry of allergens into the cell and hence to the autoimmune response.

Clinical Considerations

Celiac disease is a common chronic disorder in Caucasian populations with a prevalence of about 1%.[122,181] It also occurs in northern Indian and in North African populations. It is rare in Chinese, Japanese, and African-Caribbean people. It was previously considered to be a rare disorder in North America, but recent serological and histological evidence shows that the disease has been underdiagnosed and that the prevalence is comparable, as might be expected, with that found in Europe.[55,78]

There is a wide spectrum in the clinical presentation of celiac disease, with the majority of diagnoses made in adult life. Classical celiac disease, presenting in infancy, up to the age of 2 years, with failure to thrive, abdominal distension, and diarrhea is now an uncommon presentation. The spectrum of presenting symptoms in adults has changed over the last 20 years, and frank malabsorption is now uncommon.[88,180] Most adults present now with nonspecific symptoms; mild iron deficiency is common. There is a strong association with other autoimmune disease, especially with type 1 diabetes mellitus and autoimmune thyroid disease. In type 1 diabetes, the prevalence of celiac disease is about 5% and serological screening to detect these cases has been advocated.[85] The initial presentation may be to a wide range of clinical specialties as shown in Table 48-2. To make the diagnosis there must be a high index of suspicion with an awareness of the wide range of nonspecific symptoms and easy availability of serological tests to select those patients in whom endoscopy is indicated to confirm the diagnosis.

Tests for Celiac Disease

Serological tests have played a significant role in the growing awareness of the high prevalence of the disorder, and appropriately standardized tests have high sensitivity and specificity for diagnosis and for monitoring treatment compliance with a gluten-free diet.

Table 48-3 compares the sensitivity and specificity of the four IgA-class antibodies commonly used. The antireticulin (ARA) and endomysial (EMA) antibodies are both measured by indirect immunofluorescence, ARA on rat kidney sections and EMA on monkey esophagus or human umbilical cord sections. Rat kidney sections are frequently used as one of the substrates for autoantibody profiles, and the presence of ARA indicates the need to measure antibodies with higher specificity before recommending small bowel histology for confirmation of the diagnosis. Recent evidence has confirmed that ARA and EMA are tissue type–dependent methods, which detect autoantibodies to tissue transglutaminase-2.[107]

Lack of standardization of assays for IgA-antigliadin antibodies (AGA) contributes to the variable diagnostic accuracy of this marker,[81] but sensitivity of AGA is inferior to that of EMA. In some reports, comparison of sensitivity is compromised by selection bias,[115] but most larger series in which patients have not been selected for a biopsy solely on the basis of a positive EMA result indicate that the true sensitivity for EMA is between 90% and 95% (i.e., 5% to 10% of subjects with celiac disease have a negative EMA at diagnosis). When carried out correctly, the assay has very high specificity (>99%) and laboratories should monitor their performance, as small reductions in specificity will lead to significant increase in the numbers of patients subjected

TABLE 48-2 An Indication of the Wide Range of Clinical Specialties to Which a Child or Adult With Celiac Disease May Present

Clinical Specialty	Symptoms/Manifestations
General medicine	Tired all the time
Gastroenterology	Diarrhea, flatulence, weight loss
Hematology	Anemia
Obstetrics/gynecology	Infertility
Orthopedics	Fracture, osteopenia
Dermatology	Dermatitis herpetiformis, hyperkeratosis
Neurology	Peripheral neuropathy
Rheumatology	Arthropathy
Endocrinology	Short stature, thyroid disease
Diabetes	Diarrhea, anemia

TABLE 48-3 Comparison of Serological Tests for Celiac Disease

Antibody	Method	Sensitivity	Specificity
Antireticulin antibody (R1-ARA)	Immunofluorescence on rat or mouse kidney	25%-30%	>90%
IgA-endomysial antibody	Immunofluorescence on monkey esophagus or human umbilical cord	80%-100%	>99%
IgA-antigliadin antibody	Quantitative ELISA	75%-95%	95%
IgA-antitissue transglutaminase antibody (human antigen)	Quantitative ELISA	>90%	>99%

IgA, Immunoglobulin A; *ELISA,* enzyme-linked immunosorbent assay.

TABLE 48-4 Comparison of True and False Positives and Positive Predictive Values at Different Specificities Assuming a Prevalence of Celiac Disease of 3% in the Population (n = 1000) Tested (Test Sensitivity of 95%)

Specificity	True Positives	False Positives	Positive Predictive Value
90%	29	97	0.23
95%	29	49	0.38
98%	29	19	0.60
99%	29	10	0.74
99.5%	29	5	0.85

unnecessarily to a small bowel biopsy. Table 48-4 shows the effect of test specificity on the numbers of true and false positives per 1000 subjects tested and on the positive predictive value at a disease prevalence (in the population tested) of 3%, assuming a sensitivity of 95%.

Many commercial kits are now available to measure IgA antibodies against tissue transglutaminase ("transglutaminase antibody," TGA) using human recombinant tissue transglutaminase or purified human enzyme as antigen. Lack of standardization and differences in recombinant technology (e.g., the use of eukaryotic or prokaryotic organisms to produce tTG) can lead to varying performance.[11,126] Specificity should be evaluated using a large series of samples representative of those routinely tested, and procedures should be selected on the basis of high specificity (minimum 99%) and high sensitivity (>90%). The use of TGA has advantages over EMA. Unlike EMA, which may be subject to observer bias, TGA is a quantitative procedure and does not require the use of primate tissue. It can be automated and is therefore appropriate for larger numbers of samples. This test is replacing EMA as the antibody of choice for serological testing and for assessing dietary compliance of subjects on a gluten-free diet.[16,80]

For diagnosis, current guidelines require a jejunal biopsy with the characteristic villous atrophy, increased intraepithelial lymphocytes, and hyperplasia of the crypts.[124] Wider use of serology has led to the recognition of more cases with minimal histological changes and to the use of the terms "potential" and "latent" celiac disease.[84] Patients with positive EMA or TGA are described as having potential celiac disease when the jejunal biopsy has normal villi but shows subtle changes, such as increased numbers of intraepithelial lymphocytes. It is thought that in time these patients will develop a flat mucosa. The term "latent celiac disease" is used to describe patients who have at some time had positive antibodies and a flat mucosa that recovers on a gluten-free diet, but have also been found to have a normal mucosa while on a normal diet.

TABLE 48-5 Prevalence of Hypolactasia in Adults

Racial Group	Prevalence (%)
Chinese	>90
American blacks	54-81
Asians	60-90
Greeks	60-78
North Europeans	5-30

Subjects with selective IgA deficiency (IgA <0.05 g/L, incidence about 1:600) are at greater risk of celiac disease. It is therefore important to identify these individuals rather than risk excluding the diagnosis on the basis of a negative test for IgA-class antibodies.[24] When EMA is used, total serum IgA should be measured on all samples submitted for celiac serology to identify those patients with IgA deficiency. TGA assays should be designed so that the "normal" level is distinguishable from the small proportion of subjects with *very* low levels in whom total IgA measurement is indicated to confirm or exclude IgA deficiency. When IgA deficiency is identified, IgG antibodies (IgG-EMA, IgG-TGA) should be used as serological screening tests.[23] In view of the increased risk of the disorder in IgA deficiency, a small bowel biopsy should be considered in all IgA-deficient subjects with symptoms of celiac disease.[24]

Strict adherence to a gluten-free diet leads to mucosal recovery in celiac disease and reduces the risks of bowel malignancy. TGA can be used as a marker for monitoring dietary compliance in addition to its diagnostic role.[16]

With the availability now of serological tests with high diagnostic accuracy, older tests used to investigate celiac disease should be abandoned. There is, for example, no place now in routine use for the xylose absorption test. Dual sugar tests (e.g., cellobiose and mannitol) to assess small bowel permeability have a role in research studies but as yet have not established a place in the routine diagnosis or monitoring of celiac disease. Tests of fat malabsorption are also inappropriate in the diagnosis of celiac disease although appropriate tests of pancreatic function (e.g., fecal elastase) may be indicated in patients diagnosed with celiac disease who fail to respond to a gluten-free diet.

Disaccharidase Deficiencies

The presence of the brush-border disaccharidases is essential for carbohydrate absorption, and a reduction in their activity leads to carbohydrate malabsorption and intolerance. Carbohydrate malabsorption does not always lead to clinical symptoms, but when symptoms do occur (e.g., abdominal pain, flatulence, and diarrhea) as a consequence of the malabsorption, the patient is described as having carbohydrate intolerance.

Lactose intolerance is the single most common absorptive defect in adults, with an incidence of 5% to 90% depending on the racial group, as shown in Table 48-5.

Congenital Lactase Deficiency[59]

Intestinal lactase is essential in infancy, and congenital lactase deficiency is a very rare disorder in which lactase activities in the mucosa are low or undetectable at birth. Symptoms occur as soon as milk is taken; stools have a low pH and contain glucose produced by bacterial action on undigested lactose. Absent or low intestinal lactase in the neonate, however, cannot be taken as proof of congenital deficiency, because lactase is normally the slowest of the oligosaccharidases to reach normal levels in the newborn's gut. A definitive diagnosis must be deferred until after maturation of the lactase synthesis system has occurred. In the interim, relief is dependent on adjustments of dietary composition that appear to reduce severity of symptoms. An abnormal oral lactose tolerance test obtained a few months after birth could also be caused by congenital glucose-galactose intolerance (see discussion later in this chapter); the differential diagnosis requires performance of an oral glucose tolerance test in conjunction with the lactose tolerance test.

Acquired Lactase Deficiency

Expression of the enzyme diminishes with age and by adulthood lactase levels are 10% or less of those seen in infancy. If symptoms of flatulence, abdominal discomfort, bloating, or diarrhea occur after consumption of one or two glasses of milk or of a large portion of ice cream or yogurt, lactose intolerance should be suspected. Suspicion would be increased in a subject from an ethnic group with a high incidence of lactose intolerance (see Table 48-5).

Secondary lactose intolerance may occur as a result of reduced enzyme activity following diffuse intestinal damage from infections (giardiasis, bacterial overgrowth, or viral gastroenteritis), ulcerative colitis, celiac disease, and tropical sprue. This deficiency is usually reversible following recovery from the disorder.

Sucrase-Isomaltase and Trehalase Deficiencies and Monosaccharide Malabsorption

Sucrase-isomaltase deficiency usually presents clinically in infancy when sucrose and fruit are introduced in the diet,[101] but sometimes first presents in adulthood.[133,173] The deficiency is rare in Caucasians, but more common in Eskimo groups. Deficiencies of both lactase and sucrase-isomaltase may occur secondary to other small bowel diseases (e.g., celiac disease, Crohn's disease,[172] or acute gastroenteritis). Trehalase deficiency is a rare disorder,[135] except in Greenland, where it occurs in 8% of the population.[69] It is manifested by diarrhea following the ingestion of mushrooms.

Malabsorption of monosaccharides can also cause intestinal symptoms more commonly attributed to maldigestion of disaccharides. Glucose-galactose malabsorption is also inherited as an autosomal recessive trait. Symptoms occur in the affected neonate as soon as milk (lactose) is taken, but also follow ingestion of glucose- or galactose-containing foods. Symptoms caused by fructose malabsorption occur on ingestion of fruit. This dietary intolerance is quite a different disorder from hereditary fructose intolerance in which the hepatic enzyme aldolase is defective.

BOX 48-2 Methods for Detecting Lactase Deficiency

Lactase in mucosal biopsy
Oral lactose tolerance
- Measure increase in plasma glucose
- Measure increase in plasma galactose
- Measure increase in breath H_2
- Measure increase in breath $^{13}CO_2$

Diagnostic Tests for Lactase Deficiency

Many methods have been proposed for detecting lactase deficiency (Box 48-2). Disaccharidase activities can be measured in homogenates of an intestinal biopsy.[33] These assays are rarely required for routine diagnostic purposes, but when necessary (e.g., in investigations in infancy) they must be carried out by laboratories with expertise in these tests.

Oral Lactose Tolerance Tests

Oral tolerance tests, measuring the increase in plasma glucose or galactose following the ingestion of lactose, have also been used to diagnose lactase deficiency. The usual dose of lactose is 50 g in 200 mL water, although lower doses should be used in children (2 g/kg, up to a maximum of 50 g). Multiple blood samples are collected over a 2-hour period and the peak increment in glucose (or galactose) noted. To exclude lactase deficiency, the increase above baseline for capillary plasma glucose should be >1.1 mmol/L[137] (20 mg/dL) or >1.4 mmol/L (25 mg/dL) when using venous plasma.[22] In a recent survey of laboratory practice in the United Kingdom, widely varying cut-offs were found to be in use (1.0 to 2.7 mmol/L) even with the same lactose dose.[45] Procedures using galactose[90] are probably more popular with patients, as the test dose is preceded by a gin and tonic (equivalent to 300 mg ethanol/kg body weight). However, the requirement for multiple blood samples and lack of procedural standardization suggest that these tests should be abandoned in favor of noninvasive breath-hydrogen testing.

Hydrogen is not an end-product of mammalian metabolism, and breath hydrogen is derived from bacterial metabolism in the intestinal tract.[114] Following an oral dose of lactose, the disaccharide will normally be split into its constituent monosaccharides and absorbed. With lactase deficiency, unabsorbed disaccharide will pass into the large bowel and bacterial metabolism will produce hydrogen that is absorbed into the systemic circulation and exhaled in the breath. Breath hydrogen can be measured in end-expiratory breath using laboratory or hand-held direct-reading electrochemical hydrogen monitors.

BOX 48-3 Protocol for Lactose Tolerance Test With Measurement of Breath Hydrogen

Meal before 7 PM (restriction on wheat and fiber), then fasting until test completed
Brush teeth (night and morning) or use mouthwash
Measure end-expiratory fasting breath H_2
Give lactose solution (50 g in 180 mL water)
Rinse mouth with further 20 mL water and swallow
Measure breath H_2 at 15, 30, 60, 90, and 120 min
Test can be stopped if earlier rise of >20 ppm above fasting level

Patient Preparation. Appropriate patient preparation is essential to ensure stable baseline breath hydrogen levels (see Box 48-3). Avoidance of wheat-based foods and fiber for 12 hours before the test minimizes the availability of substrates for bacterial metabolism in the large bowel. Fasting breath hydrogen is typically <5 ppm (5 μL/L) and concentrations >20 ppm (20 μL/L) may be an indication of malabsorption or bacterial overgrowth.[141] Oral hygiene before ingestion of the substrate in hydrogen breath tests minimizes the production of hydrogen by oral bacteria. Brushing of teeth or use of an antibacterial mouthwash (e.g., 1% chlorhexidine) is recommended.[128] Mouthwash containing alcohol should not be used, because this may interfere in the measurement of hydrogen. Cigarette smoke contains high hydrogen levels and smoking is therefore not permitted immediately before or during the test.

After an overnight fast, a baseline breath hydrogen level is recorded and 50 g of lactose in 180 mL water is drunk, followed by a further 20 mL of water to rinse the mouth and further reduce the possibility of an early rise in breath hydrogen from the action of oral bacteria. The dose in children should be 2 g/kg up to a maximum of 50 g. Breath hydrogen is then measured at 15, 30, 60, 90 and 120 minutes.

Interpretation. Most publications indicate that an increase in breath hydrogen of >20 ppm (20 μL/L) above the baseline fasting concentration within 2 hours of ingesting the lactose is indicative of lactose malabsorption.[129,137] However, recent data suggest that a cut-off of 10 ppm (10 μL/L) improves diagnostic sensitivity without increasing the number of false-positive test results.[97] In most patients with normal lactose absorption, breath hydrogen levels will remain at 2 to 5 ppm throughout the test. Occasionally, high levels may occur within the first 30 minutes after lactose ingestion. This may indicate either very rapid transit of lactose to the cecum or bacterial metabolism in the small bowel because of bacterial overgrowth. Repeating the breath test with lactulose or glucose as the substrate or using imaging techniques to confirm transit time will normally clarify the cause of such results.

BOX 48-4 Abnormalities of the Small Intestine Associated With Bacterial Overgrowth

Jejunal diverticuli
Crohn's disease
Autonomic neuropathy
Scleroderma (systemic sclerosis)
Pseudo-obstruction
Postgastrectomy

In lactose malabsorption, breath hydrogen is typically elevated (30 to 100 ppm, 30 to 100 μL/L) at 60 to 120 minutes after lactose ingestion. In a few subjects, the large bowel bacteria do not produce hydrogen; in such patients a normal result does not exclude lactase deficiency. Very low hydrogen when fasting and throughout the test may therefore indicate a false-negative result. Some estimates suggest that up to 10% to 13% of the population have large bowel bacteria that do not produce hydrogen,[105] although others have found the prevalence of hydrogen nonproducers to be less than 2%.[129,163] Such false negatives can be confirmed by the failure to produce hydrogen at 45 to 180 minutes after ingestion of lactulose (10 g), which is a nonabsorbable disaccharide and therefore available for bacterial metabolism in the large bowel.

A positive breath hydrogen result following ingestion of lactose may also occur in glucose-galactose malabsorption, which also causes intestinal symptoms. When necessary, glucose-galactose malabsorption can be confirmed or excluded by a breath test in which 25 g each of glucose and galactose are substituted for 50 g lactose. An increase in breath hydrogen confirms the diagnosis.

Sucrose and Trehalose Tolerance Tests

Sucrase-isomaltase deficiency can be investigated by using 50 g sucrose instead of lactose. An increase in breath hydrogen of >20 ppm (20 μL/L) within 2 hours is diagnostic. It is rarely necessary to test for trehalase deficiency, although a breath test using 25 g trehalose has been described.[3]

Bacterial Overgrowth

The proximal small intestine (duodenum and jejunum) normally contains few bacteria. Most ingested bacteria do not survive the acidic environment of the stomach and therefore few live organisms normally enter the small bowel. The motility of the jejunum prevents fecal-type organisms from progressing up into the jejunum from the cecum. The ileum normally contains some fecal-type bacteria. Colonization of the upper small bowel is described as bacterial overgrowth and usually occurs as a consequence of other abnormalities (structural or motility disorders) of the small intestine (see Box 48-4). Use of PPIs is associated with an increased risk of bacterial colonization.

TABLE 48-6 Reported Sensitivity and Specificity of Lactulose and Glucose Hydrogen Breath Tests for the Diagnosis of Bacterial Overgrowth

Substrate	Increment Over Baseline*	Sensitivity	Specificity	Reference
Glucose 50 g	≥12 ppm	93	78	Kerlin and Wong 1988
Glucose 50 g	>10 ppm	78	89	Flourie et al 1989
Glucose 50 g	≥15 ppm	90	—	Stotzer and Kilander 2000
Glucose 75 g	≥10 ppm	62	83	Corazza et al 1990
Lactulose 12 g	>10 ppm	68	44	Corazza et al 1990

*1 ppm = 1 μL/L.

The bacteria colonizing the small bowel (such as *Escherichia coli* and *Bacteroides* species) deconjugate and dehydroxylate bile salts, leading to conjugated bile salt deficiency, which causes fat malabsorption. Bacterial metabolism of vitamin B_{12} may also occur, leading to vitamin B_{12} deficiency. The clinical symptoms of bacterial overgrowth are abdominal pain, diarrhea, and steatorrhea.[108]

The diagnostic gold standard requires intubation with aspiration of jejunal contents and the demonstration of a bacterial count of $>10^7$ organisms/mL and $>10^4$ anaerobes/mL.[61] In practice, hydrogen breath tests using either lactulose or glucose as substrates are used more frequently. An alternative diagnostic approach is to use a therapeutic trial of antibiotics.

For hydrogen breath tests, patient preparation is the same as that described in the previous section for the lactose breath hydrogen test. Lactulose (usually given in a dose of 10 g in 200 mL water) is a nonabsorbable disaccharide. In a normal subject, breath hydrogen does not increase until the lactulose enters the large intestine; the time from ingestion to a rise in breath hydrogen is therefore normally an indication of small bowel transit time. In bacterial overgrowth, there is an early rise in breath hydrogen of at least 20 ppm (20 μL/L) within 30 minutes of ingestion of lactulose. The early increase is diagnostic when it can be distinguished clearly from the later colonic rise. Frequent measurements (e.g., at 5-minute intervals) are essential in the first 30 minutes, with measurements every 15 minutes thereafter for up to 3 hours.[149]

Glucose is an alternative substrate; the usual adult dose is 50 g (as monohydrate) in 250 mL water.[100,179] An increase in breath hydrogen of >12 ppm (12 μL/L) above the fasting concentration indicates bacterial overgrowth. In bacterial overgrowth, breath hydrogen usually increases within 75 minutes of ingestion of glucose and sometimes within 30 minutes. The finding of an increased fasting breath hydrogen has high specificity for bacterial overgrowth but poor sensitivity; however, a fasting breath hydrogen >15 ppm and an increment of at least 12 ppm within 2 hours of a 50 g glucose challenge is diagnostic of bacterial overgrowth.[100,141] The high fasting breath hydrogen levels, even after adequate dietary preparation, are thought to be caused by stasis of gut contents or endogenous glycoproteins being used as substrates for hydrogen production by intestinal bacteria.[141] Table 48-6 compares some of the published data for diagnostic accuracy of tests using lactulose or glucose.

Variations in gastric emptying rate and small bowel transit times are problems that limit the diagnostic accuracy of the breath hydrogen tests. In the face of an appropriate clinical picture and a negative breath hydrogen test, an alternative diagnostic approach is a therapeutic trial of appropriate antibiotics.[4]

Other tests for bacterial overgrowth have used ^{14}C-xylose or ^{14}C-glycocholic acid.[105] When there is bacterial overgrowth, the bacteria deconjugate the glycocholic acid to produce ^{14}C-glycine that is absorbed and metabolized with an increase in breath $^{14}CO_2$. As in other tests, an early rise in the marker indicates either bacterial overgrowth or rapid transit to the large bowel where the normal colonic flora release ^{14}C-glycine. These tests using radioactive isotopes have largely been replaced by hydrogen breath tests that have comparable diagnostic performance and methodological advantages.[162]

Bile Salt Malabsorption[34]

Bile acids are synthesized in the liver and pass into the lumen of the small bowel via the gallbladder. Bile acids are present in bile as taurine or glycine conjugates; as the pH of bile is slightly alkaline and contains significant amounts of sodium and potassium, most of the bile acids and their conjugates exist as salts (i.e., bile salts). In practice, the terms bile acids and bile salts are frequently used as synonyms. Their major function is to act as surface-active agents, forming micelles and facilitating the digestion of triglycerides and the absorption of cholesterol and fat-soluble vitamins. Little reabsorption of bile acids occurs in the proximal small bowel, but normally >90% are reabsorbed in the terminal ileum. They return to the liver in the portal circulation and are resecreted into the bile. This is known as the enterohepatic circulation. Less than 10% of secreted bile acids are lost in the feces, or about 0.2 to 0.6 g/day.

Bile acid malabsorption leading to chronic diarrhea occurs when there is ileal disease (e.g., Crohn's disease), or after resection of the terminal ileum; it may also occur following cholecystectomy and in some patients with irritable bowel syndrome.[160] The malabsorption of bile salts produces diarrhea by two different mechanisms. When significant bile salt depletion occurs, the deficiency of intraluminal bile salts leads to fat malabsorption and steatorrhea. More commonly, malabsorption of bile salts in the ileum leads to increased concentrations of bile salts in the colon where they alter water and electrolyte absorption. This leads to net secretion of water into the lumen and diarrhea. Bile salt malabsorption is probably an underdiagnosed condition and should be suspected in patients with unexplained chronic diarrhea.[156,171,183]

Three different procedures have been used to make a diagnosis of bile salt malabsorption—the ^{75}selenohomocholyltaurine test, measurement of serum 7α-hydroxy-4-cholesten-3-one in serum, and a therapeutic trial of bile acid sequestrants such as cholestyramine. The most widely used test involves the oral administration of the synthetic radioactive bile acid ^{75}selenohomocholyltaurine (^{75}SeHCAT). Following the dose, whole body gamma counting is carried out to estimate the basal level at 1 hour (100%). The gamma count is measured again after 7 days, when normally >15% of the administered dose is retained. Retention of <10% indicates bile salt malabsorption. Patients with <5% retention of ^{75}SeHCAT often have a good response to treatment with bile acid sequestrants.

Measurement of 7α-hydroxy-4-cholesten-3-one has been proposed as a simpler alternative to ^{75}SeHCAT. Evidence indicates that the fasting serum level of this intermediary between cholesterol and taurocholic acid reflects the activity of hepatic cholesterol 7α-hydroxylase and therefore the rate of bile acid synthesis. Bile acid malabsorption is associated with increased serum concentrations of 7α-hydroxy-4-cholesten-3-one as hepatic synthesis increases to maintain the pool of circulating bile acids.[5] A good correlation has been demonstrated between serum 7α-hydroxy-4-cholesten-3-one and results of the ^{75}SeHCAT test.[51] Two subsequent publications on patients with chronic diarrhea have documented the high sensitivity of the measurement for identifying those with bile acid–induced diarrhea.[14,151] The test has been compared with ^{75}SeHCAT and with the response to cholestyramine. The latter avoids the problems of assuming 100% sensitivity and specificity for the ^{75}SeHCAT test. Using the therapeutic response to cholestyramine as the "gold standard," the positive predictive value of serum 7α-hydroxy-4-cholesten-3-one increased to 74% (from 71%) and the negative predictive value increased to 98% (from 94%).

With the growing awareness of the likely role of bile salt malabsorption in the chronic diarrhea of a proportion of patients with irritable bowel syndrome and the therapeutic effectiveness of cholestyramine,[156,160] the measurement of serum 7α-hydroxy-4-cholesten-3-one, with its high negative predictive value, could be used to exclude bile salt malabsorption. High concentrations would be confirmed by a follow-up ^{75}SeHCAT test or a therapeutic trial with cholestyramine.

Protein-Losing Enteropathy

Loss of significant amounts of serum proteins into the bowel lumen and their passage in the feces is a consequence of a wide range of GI disorders. These may be associated with inflammation or ulceration of a segment of the small or large bowel (as in Crohn's disease and ulcerative colitis) or stomach, with diseases in which the intestinal lymphatics are obstructed or where there is elevated lymphatic pressure (e.g., lymphoma and Whipple's disease), or with disorders associated with altered immune status, such as systemic lupus erythematosus and some food allergies.

In the healthy bowel, fecal protein is largely derived from enterocytes shed from the mucosal surface and from intestinal secretions. The normal GI loss of albumin is less than 10% of albumin catabolism, representing a daily loss of less than 1% to 2% of the serum protein pool.[104] Protein loss may be greatly increased in disease. In studies using ^{51}Cr-labeled proteins, 0.1% to 0.7% of an injected dose was excreted in feces over 4 days in healthy subjects; in protein-losing enteropathies this may increase to 40%, leading to hypoalbuminemia and edema.

The diagnosis of protein-losing enteropathy should be considered in the investigation of patients with hypoalbuminemia in whom renal loss, liver disease, and malnutrition have been excluded. The classical test for the diagnosis of protein-losing enteropathy is the measurement of fecal ^{51}Cr-albumin following an intravenous injection, although it is now rarely available. Imaging techniques that seek to detect the specific site of the protein loss have also been described using either ^{99m}Tc-human serum albumin or ^{99m}Tc-dextran.

The fecal clearance of alpha-1-antitrypsin (AT) can also be used as a marker of GI protein loss. AT is a glycoprotein (MW 54,000) that is synthesized in the liver and is normally present in the serum at a concentration of about 1.5 to 2 g/L. It is a protease inhibitor and therefore resistant to degradation by proteolytic enzymes in the GI tract. The fecal clearance of AT correlates with protein loss measured by ^{51}Cr techniques ($r = 0.96$).[60] The correlation is not influenced by serum AT concentrations or by fecal weight. AT clearance can be used for both small and large bowel disease and is applicable to the evaluation of enteric protein loss in children or adults.[60,82] More recent work has confirmed these findings and also confirmed that fecal AT concentration alone does not reliably predict AT clearance (i.e., a timed fecal sample and measurement of serum AT is required).[164] An important observation is that experimentally induced diarrhea in normal subjects leads to an increased AT clearance. The mechanism is unclear but could be related to a decreased time for degradation of AT if intestinal transit time is shorter. The upper limits of the reference interval (estimated as mean + 2SD) were found to be 56 mL/day and 24 mL/day in normal subjects with and without diarrhea, respectively. In inflammatory bowel disease, AT clearance may be as high as 200 mL/day, which represents a loss of about 6 g albumin/day.[164] The AT clearance must be interpreted with caution in patients with positive fecal occult blood tests, as the blood loss might be sufficient to falsely increase the AT clearance. Measurement of fecal AT has been suggested as an alternative to fecal occult blood for the detection of colorectal cancer.[131] AT is rapidly destroyed in gastric juice (and in vitro) when the pH is below 3.0, which has meant that the test can only be used to assess protein loss distal to the pylorus.[60] However, administration of PPIs can be used to inhibit gastric acid secretion before collection of the fecal sample, thereby enabling assessment of protein loss from the stomach.[167]

A recent study evaluated the use of AT clearance as a marker of clinical relapse in patients with Crohn's disease and showed a negative predictive value of 94% for predicting relapse in the next 6 months (at a cut-off of 120 mL/day). Sensitivity was only 50% and comparable results were noted when the Bristol Simple Index score was used to predict relapse so that at present the test appears to have little clinical value in this context.[10]

AT in feces and serum can be measured most conveniently by radial immunodiffusion. Feces should be collected quantitatively, preferably for 3 days, in preweighed containers and kept refrigerated. The AT is extracted into saline before analysis. AT clearance is calculated as follows:

$$\text{AT clearance (mL/day)} = \frac{(\text{fecal weight} \times \text{fecal AT concentration})}{\text{serum AT}}$$

where fecal weight is expressed in g/day, fecal AT in mg/kg feces, and serum AT in mg/L.

THE PANCREAS: DISEASES AND ASSESSMENT OF EXOCRINE PANCREATIC FUNCTION

It will be evident from the section on processes of digestion and absorption that the pancreas plays a central role in the absorptive process for carbohydrates, fats, and proteins. Disorders of the exocrine pancreas are therefore frequently associated with GI symptoms of malabsorption or diarrhea. In this section, pediatric and adult exocrine pancreatic disorders are briefly discussed and tests for assessing exocrine pancreatic function are described. Information on exocrine pancreatic tumors can be found in the later section on GI regulatory peptides. Recent textbooks on gastroenterology or medicine have more detail on the clinical aspects of exocrine pancreatic disorders.[17,62]

BOX 48-5 The Spectrum of Pancreatic Disease in Childhood

Disorders of morphogenesis
Annular pancreas, pancreas divisum, pancreatic hypoplasia and agenesis, heterotopic pancreas
Inherited syndromes affecting the pancreas
Cystic fibrosis
Shwachman-Diamond syndrome, Johnson-Blizzard syndrome, Pearson bone marrow pancreas syndrome
Gene mutations leading to pancreatic disease
Hereditary pancreatitis; cationic trypsinogen gene mutations, trypsin inhibitor gene mutations
Pancreatic insufficiency syndrome
Isolated enzyme deficiencies, lipase, colipase, enterokinase
Pancreatic insufficiency secondary to other disorders
Celiac disease
Acquired pancreatitis in childhood
Idiopathic, traumatic, drugs, viral, metabolic, collagen vascular diseases, autoimmune, fibrosing, nutritional (tropical)

Pediatric Disorders of the Exocrine Pancreas

Pancreatic disorders in childhood have recently been reviewed[29] and are summarized in Box 48-5.

Cystic fibrosis (CF) is the most common severe autosomal recessive disease, with an estimated gene frequency in Western Europe and the United States of between 1:25 and 1:35 and a disease incidence of about 1 in 2500 to 1 in 3200. The pathogenesis and diagnosis of CF are described in Chapter 40. Pancreatic insufficiency is present at birth in 65% of infants with CF, and a further 15% develop it during infancy and early childhood. The 20% who do not develop pancreatic insufficiency have a better prognosis and develop fewer complications.

The measurement of pancreatic elastase-1 in feces (see section on noninvasive tests of exocrine pancreatic function) is considered to be a reliable test for pancreatic insufficiency in infants over the age of 2 weeks with CF and in older children at diagnosis of the disorder.[19,113,143] The test can also be used to detect the onset of pancreatic insufficiency in those previously pancreatic sufficient.

Adult Disorders of the Exocrine Pancreas

The major exocrine pancreatic disorders presenting in adult life are acute pancreatitis, chronic pancreatitis, and carcinoma of the pancreas.[62] The use of enzyme tests in the diagnosis of acute pancreatitis is discussed in Chapter 21. The etiologies of pancreatitis are given in Box 48-6.

Chronic pancreatitis is defined by irreversible pancreatic damage with histological evidence of inflammation and fibrosis leading to destruction of both endocrine and exocrine function. There are many causes of chronic pancreatitis but the major histological features are similar

BOX 48-6 Etiologies of Pancreatitis in Adults

Acute
- Gallstones
- Alcohol
- Infections, e.g., mumps, Coxsackie B
- Pancreatic tumors
- Drugs, e.g., azathioprine, estrogens corticosteroids
- Iatrogenic (e.g., postsurgical, ERCP)
- Hyperlipidemias
- Miscellaneous—trauma, scorpion bite, cardiac surgery
- Idiopathic

Chronic
- Alcohol
- Tropical (nutritional)
- Hereditary (trypsinogen and inhibitory protein defects, cystic fibrosis membrane regulator [CFTR] defects)
- Idiopathic
- Trauma
- Hypercalcemia

From Burroughs AK, Westaby D. Liver, biliary tract disease and pancreatic disease. In: Kumar P, Clark M, eds. Clinical medicine, 5th ed. Edinburgh: WB Saunders, 2002:395-404.

BOX 48-7 Pancreatic Imaging Procedures

A plain abdominal radiograph:
May show pancreatic calcification, particularly when alcohol is the etiology.

Ultrasound:
A useful screening investigation for inflammation and neoplasia. Views may be limited by overlying bowel gas.

Spiral CT:
With contrast enhancements is more reliable.

MRI scanning:
An alternative to CT. Magnetic resonance cholangiopancreatography (MRCP) gives clear definition of the pancreatic duct and the biliary tree. Gallstones (including microcalculi) may also be identified in the biliary tree using MRI/MRCP.

Endoscopic ultrasound:
Very useful for identifying distal common bile duct stones and microcalculi within the duct or within the gallbladder. Small space-occupying lesions may also be identified.

Endoscopic retrograde cholangiopancreatography (ERCP):
This has been considered a gold standard modality for defining pancreatic disease. However, with improving imaging technique, ERCP is now more likely to be restricted to therapeutic intervention.

From Burroughs AK, Westaby D. Liver, biliary tract disease and pancreatic disease. In: Kumar P, Clark M, eds. Clinical medicine, 5th ed. Edinburgh: WB Saunders, 2002:395-404.

regardless of the cause. In Western countries, the most common cause is alcohol (60% to 90% of all cases of chronic pancreatitis), although as only 5% to 15% of heavy drinkers develop the disease, there are clearly other predisposing factors (e.g., smoking, diets high in fat and protein).

The role of invasive and noninvasive tests of pancreatic exocrine tests in chronic pancreatitis has recently been reviewed.[65]

Tests of Exocrine Function of the Pancreas

The predominant exocrine functions of the pancreas are the production and secretion of pancreatic juice, which is rich in enzymes and bicarbonate. Normal pancreatic juice is colorless and odorless; it has a pH of 8.0 to 8.3 and a specific gravity of 1.007 to 1.042. The total 24-hour secretion volume may be as high as 3000 mL.[150]

A number of laboratory tests are available to measure exocrine function in the investigation of pancreatic insufficiency (most commonly caused by cystic fibrosis in children and chronic pancreatitis in adults). Tests fall into two categories, invasive and noninvasive. Invasive tests require GI intubation to collect pancreatic samples; noninvasive tests (or "tubeless tests") were developed to avoid intubation, which is uncomfortable for the patient, time-consuming, and therefore expensive. Noninvasive tests are simpler and cheaper to perform, but in general they lack the sensitivity and specificity of the invasive tests, particularly for the diagnosis of mild pancreatic insufficiency. It is important to recognize that biochemical tests have a limited clinical application in the diagnosis of pancreatic disease because of either the complexity of the invasive tests or the inadequate sensitivity and specificity for mild and moderate pancreatic disease of the noninvasive tests. Of greater importance are the imaging procedures (see Box 48-7). These techniques continue to be developed. A recent study shows that administration of secretin, causing stimulation of fluid and bicarbonate secretion, leads to anatomical changes that can be quantified by magnetic resonance cholangiopancreatography, with significant differences between normal volunteers and patients with pancreatic insufficiency.[32] In the future, it may therefore be possible to confidently diagnose pancreatic insufficiency by imaging techniques alone.

Invasive Tests of Exocrine Pancreatic Function

The main types of invasive tests are summarized in Table 48-7.

Total volume of pancreatic juice, amount or concentration of bicarbonate, and activities of pancreatic enzymes are measured in duodenal contents. The enzyme most commonly measured is trypsin, but amylase, lipase, chymotrypsin, and elastase may also be evaluated. The *Lundh test* consists of administering a standardized meal consisting of 5% protein, 6% fat, 15% carbohydrate, and 74% nonnutrient fiber. Advantages of the Lundh meal are that it provides a physiological stimulus to the pancreas and is simple to administer. However, administration of the meal prevents determination of the total enzyme and bicarbonate or secretory volume. Moreover, it provides inadequate or no stimu-

TABLE 48-7 Summary of Invasive Tests of Pancreatic Exocrine Function

Procedure	Pancreatic Stimulant	Analysis of Duodenal Contents
Lundh test	Standardized meal	Enzyme output
Secretin stimulation test	Purified or synthetic porcine secretin	Bicarbonate output
Secretin-cholecystokinin (CCK) test	Secretin as above plus CCK analogue (CCK-8 or ceruletide)	Bicarbonate and enzymes

CCK-8: Asp—Tyr(SO_3H)—Met—Gly—Trp—Met—Asp—Phe—NH_2

Ceruletide: Pyr—Gln—Asp—Tyr(SO_3H)—Thr—Gly—Trp—Met—Asp—Phe—NH_2

Figure 48-7 Comparison of amino acid sequences of CCK-8 and ceruletide.

lation in the presence of mucosal diseases, such as celiac disease, in which hormone release from the duodenal mucosa is impaired. In view of these limitations, the Lundh test is largely of historical interest.

The *secretin test* is based on the principle that secretion of pancreatic juice and bicarbonate output are related to the functional mass of pancreatic tissue. After an overnight fast, basal samples of fluid are collected from the stomach and duodenum. One clinical unit (CU) of secretin/kg body weight is administered intravenously, and duodenal fluid is collected at 15-minute intervals for at least 1 hour. Purified porcine secretin has traditionally been used for the test, but recent studies have confirmed that synthetic porcine secretin (0.2 μg/kg) gives results that are not significantly different from results with biologic secretin.[159]

Secretin stimulates the secretion of pancreatic juice and bicarbonate, but stimulation of the secretion of pancreatic enzymes is inconsistent. Addition of CCK (or a synthetic equivalent) to the secretin stimulation test provides a stimulus to the secretion of pancreatic enzymes, allowing a more complete assessment of pancreatic reserve than can be obtained with secretin alone. The functional activity of CCK resides in the C-terminal octapeptide sequence (CCK-8), and either this octapeptide or ceruletide (a synthetic decapeptide identical to the natural decapeptide cerulein) can be used to stimulate pancreatic enzyme secretion (Figure 48-7).

The procedure for the secretin-ceruletide test is similar to that described for the secretin test. Patients are required to fast overnight; they are then intubated with a gastroduodenal tube placed into the duodenum under x-ray control. After collecting basal fluid for 15 minutes, 1 U secretin/kg body weight/hr is continuously given intravenously for 2 hours; 30 mg ceruletide/kg body weight/hr is given simultaneously for the second hour. Pancreatic juice is collected during 15-minute intervals, and volume, pH, bicarbonate, and enzymes are measured.[120] Procedures and reference values are not standardized among laboratories. It is recommended that doses of secretagogues should be high enough to provide maximal pancreatic stimulation and given for at least 60 to 90 minutes to ensure better diagnostic accuracy, especially in mild pancreatic insufficiency.[65]

Noninvasive Tests of Exocrine Pancreatic Function

"For many years, gastroenterologists have searched for the holy grail of pancreatic function tests—the tubeless test."[39] Not surprisingly, a range of tests has been proposed, but none has adequate sensitivity for reliably detecting early pancreatic disease. When malabsorption is present, such tests are of value in confirming or excluding pancreatic disease. Considerable overlap often occurs between results observed in normal individuals and those found in patients with pancreatic disorders, which is mainly due to the large functional reserve of the pancreas. An estimate has been made that pancreatic insufficiency cannot clearly be demonstrated until at least 50% of the acinar cells have been destroyed. Clinical signs of pancreatic insufficiency often do not appear until the destruction of 90% of acinar tissue. In general, the noninvasive (tubeless) tests may therefore be used when investigating causes of malabsorption but have inadequate sensitivity for the diagnosis of chronic pancreatitis. Comparison between studies and of different markers is difficult because the "gold standard" may be either functional tests, which may differ in procedure and reference values,[111,120,161] or morphological assessment. In some cases a direct comparison of one noninvasive test with another has been made. Table 48-8 compares the diagnostic performance of noninvasive tests.

The principle of the *amino acid consumption test* is that stimulation of the pancreas by CCK increases the uptake of

TABLE 48-8 Diagnostic Accuracy of Noninvasive Tests for Mild, Moderate, and Severe Pancreatic Insufficiency, as Assessed by Anatomical or Functional Criteria

	Sensitivity for Pancreatic Insufficiency			
Test	**Mild**	**Moderate**	**Severe**	**Specificity**
Amino acid consumption test[71]	"... unsuitable for clinical use"			
Fecal chymotrypsin[70]	11%	54%	77%	85%
Fecal elastase-1[70]	22%	77%	100%	96%
NBT-PABA[63,138]	—	50%	70%	72%
Pancreolauryl[39,138]	<50%	50%	85%	50%
^{13}C-MCT absorption[119]	62%	—	100%	85%

amino acids from the plasma, leading to greater depletion of plasma amino acids in normal subjects compared with patients with pancreatic insufficiency. Despite initially promising results, the test is now considered unsuitable for clinical use because of low specificity.[71]

All of the other noninvasive tests are based on the reduction in the secretion of pancreatic enzymes with direct measurement of enzymes in feces (chymotrypsin or elastase) or detection of products of their catalytic reactions, after oral administration of synthetic substrates, in urine (NBT-PABA or pancreolauryl test) or in breath (^{13}C-mixed chain triglyceride breath test).

Pancreatic chymotrypsin is almost completely digested during its passage through the gut in adults, but the residual activity of the enzyme in feces is stable for several days at 20 °C. Its output in stool correlates poorly with chymotrypsin secretion in duodenal contents when both are measured after stimulation with secretin-CCK. In patients without pancreatic disease, the incidence of falsely low results is about 10% to 15% and may be due to (a) voluminous stools (>300 g/day) and thus less enzyme per gram of feces; (b) inadequate food intake; (c) partial gastrectomy or mucosal disease (e.g., celiac disease), which causes inadequate stimulation of pancreatic secretion; or (d) obstruction of the bile duct. Falsely normal results in patients with mild pancreatic insufficiency may be as high as 50%.[72] In a recent collaborative study in children, both fecal chymotrypsin and elastase showed 100% sensitivity for detecting pancreatic insufficiency in cystic fibrosis, but the specificity of chymotrypsin was lower than that of elastase in a control group of children with small intestinal diseases.[21] Most recent papers conclude that although chymotrypsin measurement is easier than elastase measurement, the latter test has significant advantages in diagnostic accuracy. The recommended procedure[98] uses a stool pretreatment stage that dissociates particle-bound chymotrypsin. The method is simple and fast and is available as a reagent kit supplied by Roche Diagnostics GmbH, Mannheim, Germany. Sample is extracted with a mixture of salts and a detergent, lauryltrimethylammonium chloride, which fully dissociates the enzyme from particles in stool. The extract is mixed with a

TABLE 48-9 Comparison of Fecal Chymotrypsin and Elastase

	Fecal Enzyme	
	Chymotrypsin	**Elastase**
10 day intraindividual variation (mean CV)	30%	15%
Loss of activity (7 days at 4 °C)	17%	2.5%
Overall diagnostic sensitivity	64%	93%
Overall diagnostic specificity	89%	93%

Loser C, Mollgaard A, Folsch UR. Faecal elastase 1: a novel, highly sensitive, and specific tubeless pancreatic function test. Gut 1996;39:580-6.

synthetic substrate, a pentapeptide of 4-nitroaniline (4-NA); the substrate is hydrolyzed by chymotrypsin to produce free 4-NA. Continuous release of 4-NA is measured photometrically at 405 nm.

Pancreatic elastase-1 is a pancreas-specific protease present in the pancreatic juice. It is not degraded during passage through the gut and concentrations in feces are fivefold to sixfold greater than those in pancreatic juice.[166] The enzyme can be determined in feces with a commercial ELISA assay that uses two monoclonal antibodies specific to the human enzyme (Schebo-Tech, Wettenberg, Germany). Treatment of patients with pancreatic enzyme supplements does not therefore interfere with the test (Figure 48-8). Table 48-9 compares chymotrypsin and elastase, indicating some of the advantages of fecal elastase measurement.

Fecal elastase-1 has been extensively evaluated both in cystic fibrosis and in adult pancreatic insufficiency. In children with cystic fibrosis, the test discriminates between those with and without pancreatic insufficiency.[70] Very low elastase-1 is seen in a wide range of *CFTR* genotypes with undetectable enzyme (<15 μg/g of stool) in most ΔF508 homozygotes.[143,178] Low fecal elastase (<200 μg/g) after 4

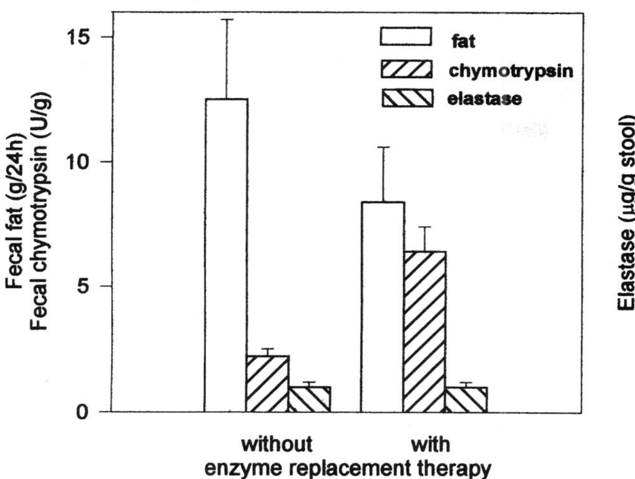

Figure 48-8 Fecal excretion (mean and SD) of chymotrypsin, fat, and immunoreactive elastase during a 24-hour collection period in 12 patients with cystic fibrosis and steatorrhea with and without enzyme replacement therapy. *(From Stein J, Jung M, Sziegoleit A, Zeuzem S, Caspary WF, Lembcke B. Immunoreactive elastase I: clinical evaluation of a new non-invasive test of pancreatic function. Clin Chem 1996;42:222-6.)*

weeks of age is indicative of pancreatic insufficiency and provides supporting evidence for a diagnosis of cystic fibrosis.[19]

The test has been evaluated in adults against the secretin-cerulein test[111,120,161] and in patients whose diagnosis of chronic pancreatitis has been made on the basis of anatomical and morphological changes detected by ultrasound and endoscopic retrograde pancreatography or computerized tomography.[40,72,127] The test is routinely carried out on a small random fecal sample, which might be expected to give inferior diagnostic accuracy to those evaluations carried out on portions of 24-hour or 72-hour fecal collections. However, with random fecal samples, specificities of 98% and 100% have been reported in healthy controls and specificities of 90% to 97% in patients with nonpancreatic GI disease. Positive results (i.e., <200 µg/g) have been reported in patients with clinical or laboratory evidence of malnutrition who also have inflammatory bowel disease or chronic diarrhea (nonpancreatic). These observations may actually be due to impaired pancreatic secretion as a consequence of malnutrition.[127] The authors also suggested that increased bacterial degradation of the enzyme might be the cause of false positives in some patients with bacterial overgrowth. Similar results have been reported in children with nonpancreatic disease; the finding of a low fecal elastase in a child with steatorrhea probably indicates coexisting pancreatic insufficiency.[21]

Measurement of pancreatic elastase-1 in feces has high sensitivity for the detection of severe and moderate chronic pancreatitis in adults. It has better sensitivity than other tests for detecting mild chronic pancreatitis and high sensitivity and high negative predictive value for discriminating between diarrhea of pancreatic and nonpancreatic origins. The test is not specific for pancreatitis and detects moderate to severe impairment of pancreatic exocrine secretion from any cause. It is considered to be the most suitable test to confirm pancreatic insufficiency in screened cystic fibrosis infants over the age of 2 weeks,[19] and as previously noted the test result is not influenced by the administration of pancreatic enzyme supplements.

The *NBT-PABA test* of pancreatic function is based on the hydrolysis, by chymotrypsin, of a synthetic tripeptide—*N*-benzoyl-l-tyrosyl-p-aminobenzoic acid. The tripeptide, variously called NBT-PABA, BTP, or bentiromide, is administered orally together with a test meal to stimulate pancreatic secretion. BTP is specifically hydrolyzed by chymotrypsin in the duodenum to release PABA, which is subsequently absorbed in the intestinal tract and metabolized in the liver to hippurate and to PABA glucuronide and PABA acetylate. These arylamines are then excreted by the kidney. In the presence of low chymotrypsin, as found in pancreatic insufficiency, less peptide is hydrolyzed, and therefore less chromogen is excreted in the urine or found in serum. Thus the amount of PABA detected in serum or urine is an indirect measure of chymotrypsin activity in duodenal content.

Test results are affected by defective intestinal absorption caused by intestinal disease or variations in transit time, by impaired hepatic conjugation caused by liver disease, and by impaired renal excretion. To compensate for these possible errors, a "control" substance (e.g., PABA) may be given on a second day, or alternatively, ^{14}C-PABA or p-aminosalicylic acid (PAS) can be given orally with the NBT-PABA. Low recovery of the control substance in the urine indicates probable decreased intestinal absorption or decreased renal excretion. About 60% (range 48% to 72%) of the orally administered dose is recovered in the urine normally. In pancreatic insufficiency, PABA excretion is significantly decreased. The result is then calculated as a "pancreatic excretion index" (PEI) as follows:

$$\text{PEI} = \frac{\text{test substance in urine} \times 100}{\text{control substance in urine}}$$

The specificity of the test was significantly improved by abandoning the nonspecific colorimetric procedures in favor of high-performance liquid chromatography (HPLC).[8,83] NBT-PABA has advantages over the pancreolauryl test in that the patient procedure can be completed in a single day; but the synthetic peptide is not now easily available, and the test has a lower diagnostic sensitivity and specificity for pancreatic insufficiency than does fecal elastase (see Table 48-8).

The *pancreolauryl test* (fluorescein dilaurate test, Temmler Pharma, Germany) is similar in its principle to the NBT-PABA test. Fluorescein dilaurate (FDL) is poorly water-soluble. It is given orally in the middle of a standard "breakfast" (50 g white bread, 20 g butter, and one cup of tea) and is specifically hydrolyzed by pancreatic cholesterol esterase, which requires bile salts for its activity. The released fluorescein is water-soluble, readily absorbed by the small intestine, conjugated in the liver, and excreted in the urine. Urine is collected for 10 hours; an adequate urinary output is imperative and is assured by a 1.5 L fluid intake during the early part of the test. The test is repeated on a second day using free fluorescein to correct for individual variability in intestinal absorption, hepatic conjugation, and urinary excretion. The urinary recovery of fluorescein is measured on a spectrophotometer each day at 492 nm after hydrolysis with 0.1 mol/L sodium hydroxide under standard conditions. A pancreatic excretion index is calculated as described for the NBT-PABA test; normal pancreatic function is indicated by PEI >30%. Pancreatic insufficiency is indicated by a PEI of <20%; values between 20% and 30% are considered inconclusive. Urines with glucose >20 g/L (2 g/dL) can give misleading results with falsely increased PEI values. Similar errors may occur when serum fluorescein is measured in samples with serum glucose >14 mmol/L (~250 mg/dL). The effect of glucose can be avoided by carrying out the hydrolysis step at 60 °C.[175]

The FDL test produces results very similar to those obtained with the PABA test, although there is now general agreement that the sensitivity is higher than that of the PABA test (see Table 48-8). Analytically, measurement of fluorescein is simple, and good agreement between laboratories has been found from external quality assessment (EQA) results for measurements of fluorescein in urine.[45] The test results can also be expressed as peak serum fluorescein concentration; high sensitivity (100%) has been reported in moderate and severe chronic pancreatitis. The serum test has poor specificity in small bowel diseases because of the influence of factors other than pancreatic enzyme hydrolysis on the absorption of fluorescein.[40] Liver diseases are associated with false-positive results because bile salts are necessary for the digestion and absorption of the FDL.

A modification of the test has been the use of mannitol as a control marker, which can then be administered together with the FDL, enabling the patient procedure to be completed within 1 day. Urine was collected from 2 to 8 hours and the ratio of fluorescein to mannitol recoveries calculated. A clear separation between healthy controls and children with cystic fibrosis was obtained regardless of whether or not they were on enzyme replacement therapy.[68]

A number of different ^{13}C breath tests have been proposed for the evaluation of fat absorption[112]; most of them assess the overall ("global") process of fat absorption and are not able to differentiate fat malabsorption from pancreatic and nonpancreatic causes.

The ^{13}C-mixed chain triglyceride test is designed as a test of intraluminal pancreatic lipase activity.[177] The substrate for the test is 1,3-distearyl,2(carboxyl-^{13}C) octanoyl glycerol, which contains long chain fatty acids in positions 1 and 3 and the ^{13}C-labeled medium chain fatty acid (octanoic acid) in position 2 (Figure 48-9). The labeled substrate is administered orally to fasting patients with a standard meal of toast and butter. Breath samples are collected over a 5-hour period, and exhaled $^{13}CO_2$ is expressed as a percentage of the administered dose. The rationale of the procedure is that before absorption or metabolism of the ^{13}C-octanoate, or ^{13}C-octanoyl monoglyceride, the stearyl groups must be hydrolyzed by the activity of pancreatic lipase. Decreased pancreatic lipase secretion will therefore lead to a reduction in the amount of ^{13}C label absorbed and subsequently metabolized to $^{13}CO_2$.

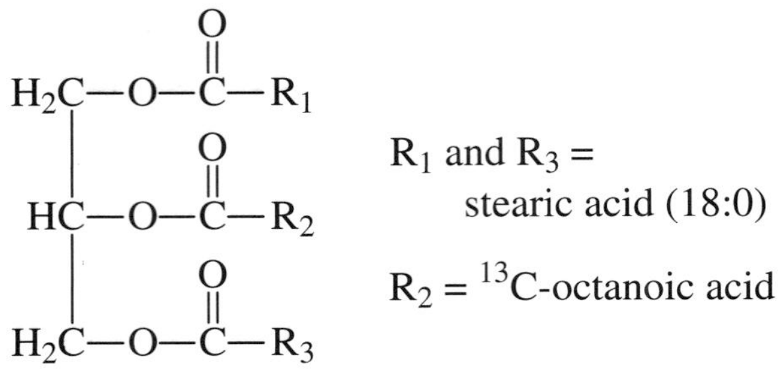

H_2C—O—C(=O)—R_1
HC—O—C(=O)—R_2
H_2C—O—C(=O)—R_3

R_1 and R_3 = stearic acid (18:0)

R_2 = ^{13}C-octanoic acid

Figure 48-9 The substrate for the ^{13}C-mixed chain triglyceride breath test: 1,3 distearyl,2(carboxyl-^{13}C) octanoyl glycerol.

In an initial assessment, a group of 25 normal control subjects were compared with 29 patients with pancreatic disease. $^{13}CO_2$ in breath (cumulative over 6 hours) was highly correlated with pancreatic lipase output (Figure 48-10). The test was superior to the estimation of fecal fat for detecting impaired pancreatic function. Sensitivity and specificity were 89% and 81%, respectively. In a later evaluation, the test was compared with results from the secretin-cerulein test, with patients categorized as having mild (n = 13) or severe (n = 13) pancreatic insufficiency.[119] Fecal elastase and chymotrypsin were also measured. Fecal elastase and the ^{13}C-mixed chain triglyceride test both detected all cases of severe pancreatic insufficiency, but sensitivity was higher for fecal elastase in those with mild disease (see Table 48-8). Similar results were obtained when cholesteryl ^{13}C-octanoate was used as a substrate for a noninvasive test of pancreatic function.[27]

The sensitivity and specificity of these tests are limited by the complexity of the processes of absorption and metabolism. The substrates are specific for pancreatic lipases and the product is absorbed independently of micelle formation, but the results of the test are affected by other factors, such as gastric emptying, mucosal absorption, hepatic metabolism, endogenous $^{13}CO_2$, and total CO_2 production.[1,43] These factors may explain the test's limited diagnostic sensitivity in mild and moderate pancreatic insufficiency and its lack of specificity in nonpancreatic GI diseases.

Fecal elastase (measured by the monoclonal antibody method) remains the test of choice as a noninvasive test for assessing pancreatic insufficiency from the perspectives of both diagnostic accuracy and patient convenience. A negative test does not exclude mild disease, and false positives in some nonpancreatic diseases and in very watery samples limit

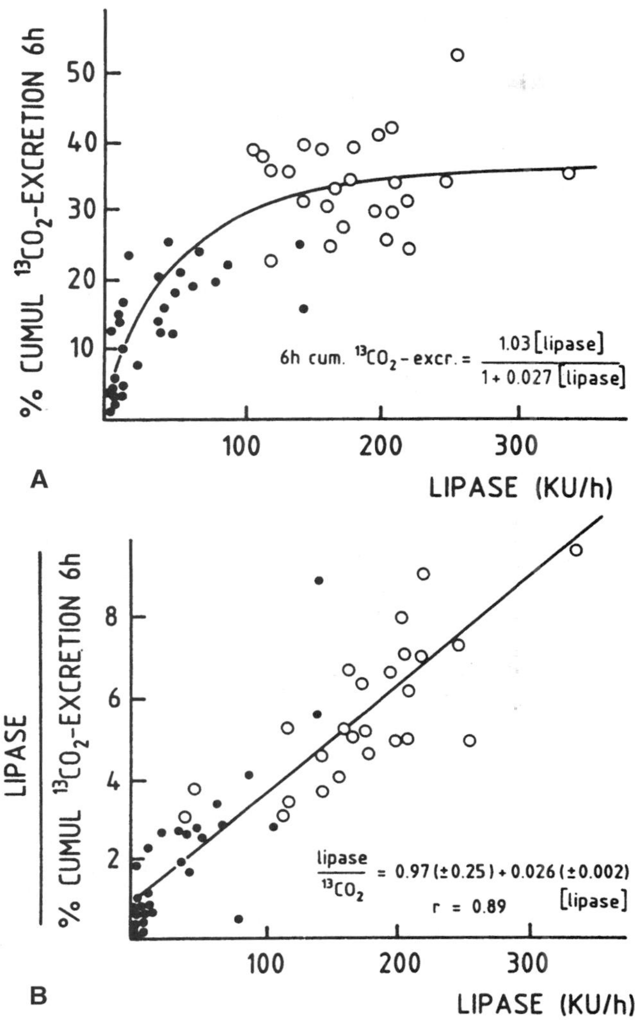

Figure 48-10 **A,** Cumulative $^{13}CO_2$ excretion (in percentage of ingested dose) 6 hours after intake of the [^{13}C]-labeled mixed triglyceride as a function of lipase activity (in kilounits per hour) in normal subjects (○) and patients with pancreatic disease (●). **B,** Linearly modified saturation curve following the relation given by the equation: Lipase/$^{13}CO_2$ = (1/A + B/A)(lipase), normal subjects (○), patients with pancreatic disease (●). *(From Vantrappen GR, Rutgeerts PJ, Ghoos YF, Hiele MI. Mixed triglyceride breath test: a noninvasive test of pancreatic lipase activity in the duodenum. Gastroenterology 1989;96:1126-34, with permission from the American Gastroenterological Association.)*

its diagnostic accuracy. A new ELISA based on polyclonal antibodies (and also called a test for "elastase 1") appears to have binding characteristics different from those of the monoclonal antibody assay and requires further evaluation.[75]

GI REGULATORY PEPTIDES

The gut is the largest endocrine organ in the body[148]; it is also a major target for many hormones, released locally and from other sites. GI regulatory peptides are released from the pancreatic islets (e.g., somatostatin) or from endocrine cells within the gut mucosa (e.g., cholecystokinin). Many of these peptides (such as VIP and somatostatin) are present in the enteric nerves and are also found in the central nervous system and have important roles in the neuroendocrine control of the gut. Although many of them (such as secretin and gastrin) fulfill the classic criteria for a hormone by acting on distant cells (see Chapter 28), others function as neurotransmitters or have local (paracrine) effects on adjacent cells. Collectively, they influence motility, secretion, digestion, and absorption in the gut. They regulate bile flow and secretion of pancreatic hormones and affect tonicity of vascular walls, blood pressure, and cardiac output.

There is a growing understanding of the role of the neuroendocrine system and gut peptides, and of the importance of the gut-hypothalamic pathway, in the normal control of food intake, and of the possibility of disorders in these mechanisms as causes of obesity.[152] The gastric peptide ghrelin and cholecystokinin act as short-term regulators of appetite and satiety. The neuropeptide $PYY_{3\text{-}36}$, a member of the neuropeptide Y family, is secreted by endocrine cells in the distal small intestine and colon in response to the ingestion of food. Recent evidence shows that infusion of $PYY_{3\text{-}36}$ to physiological plasma concentrations in humans significantly decreases appetite with a 33% reduction in food intake over 24 hours. In mice, the relevant pathway is via the arcuate nucleus of the hypothalamus.[7] $PYY_{3\text{-}36}$ is therefore a further addition to a growing list of hormones with a role in the regulation of energy balance.

Table 48-10 summarizes basic chemical characteristics of five of the major GI regulatory peptides and indicates their site of origin and major functions. More detailed descriptions of these five peptides are given below, followed by a listing of other regulatory peptides of the GI tract in Table 48-11.

CHOLECYSTOKININ[130,148]

CCK is a linear polypeptide that exists in multiple molecular forms. The first form isolated was the 33–amino acid peptide CCK-33. Other major forms are CCK-8, CCK-39, and CCK-58. In all forms, the five C-terminal amino acids are identical to those of gastrin and are necessary, together with a sulfated tyrosyl residue, for physiological activity. All of the forms of CCK are produced by enzymatic cleavage of a single 115–amino acid precursor, preprocholecystokinin.

CCK is found in the I cells of the upper small intestinal mucosa. Mixtures of polypeptides and amino acids (especially tryptophan and phenylalanine) stimulate CCK secretion, whereas pure undigested protein does not elicit a response. Secretion is also stimulated by gastric acid entering the duodenum and by fatty acids with chains of nine or more carbons, especially in the form of micelles. Circulating concentrations of CCK are therefore increased following ingestion of a mixed meal. CCK is rapidly cleared from plasma ($t_{1/2}$ = <3 min), predominantly by the kidneys. Secretion of CCK is completely inhibited after somatostatin infusion.

TABLE 48-10 Characteristics of Prominent Forms of Principal Gut Regulatory Peptides

Hormone/Peptide	Molecular Weight	No. of Amino Acids	Main Gut Localization	Principal Physiological Actions
Gastrin Family				
Cholecystokinin	3918	33 (also 385, 59)	Duodenum and jejunum Enteric nerves	Stimulates gallbladder contraction and intestinal motility; stimulates secretion of pancreatic enzymes, insulin, glucagon, and pancreatic polypeptides; has a role in indicating satiety; the C-terminal 8–amino acid peptide CCK-8 retains full activity
Little gastrin Big gastrin	2098 3839	17 34	Both forms of gastrin are found in the gastric antrum and duodenum	Gastrins stimulate the secretion of gastric acid, pepsinogen, intrinsic factor, and secretin; stimulate intestinal mucosal growth; increase gastric and intestinal motility
Secretin-Glucagon Family				
Secretin	3056	27	Duodenum and jejunum	Stimulates pancreatic secretion of HCO_3, enzymes, and insulin; reduces gastric and duodenal motility, inhibits gastrin release and gastric acid secretion
Vasoactive intestinal polypeptide (VIP)	3326	28	Enteric nerves	Relaxes smooth muscle of gut, blood, and genitourinary system; increases water and electrolyte secretion from pancreas and gut; releases hormones from pancreas, gut, and hypothalamus
Glucose-dependent insulinotropic peptide (GIP)	4976	42	Duodenum and jejunum	Stimulates insulin release; inhibits gastric acid, pepsin, and gastrin secretion; reduces gastric and intestinal motility; increases fluid and electrolyte secretion from small intestine

CCK regulates gallbladder contraction and increases small intestinal motility. It possesses the same terminal pentapeptide as gastrin, and therefore also has a mild stimulatory effect on gastric HCl and pepsinogen secretion, antral motility, and pancreatic bicarbonate secretion. Secretion of the less potent CCK results in a decreased output of HCl because CCK competes with gastrin for the receptor sites on the HCl-secreting cells. Conversely, gastrin and CCK are additive in their stimulation of the pancreas, and both increase the effect of secretin on pancreatic function. CCK also stimulates pancreatic growth, relaxes the sphincter of Oddi, and stimulates secretions from Brunner's (duodenal) glands.

CCK is also present in the brain, with highest concentrations in the cerebral cortex; its function in the CNS is unclear. It is released from the GI tract and acts as a short-term, meal-related satiety signal, thus regulating appetite. CCK is widely distributed throughout both the central and peripheral nervous systems.

GASTRIN[130,148]

Three major molecular forms of gastrin occur in blood and tissues: big gastrin (G-34), a linear polypeptide of 34 amino acids; little gastrin (G-17); and mini gastrin (G-14). In addition to these, G-71, G-52, and G-6 are present in small amounts. Gastrins originate from the cleavage of a single precursor, preprogastrin, a peptide consisting of 101 amino acids. The smallest peptide sequence of gastrin possessing biological activity is the carboxy-terminal tetrapeptide (G-4, tetrin); on a molar basis, it is only one sixth to one tenth as

TABLE 48-11 Brief Description of Other GI Regulatory Peptides

Hormone/Peptide	Major Tissue Locations in Gut	Principal Known Actions
Bombesin	Throughout the gut and pancreas	Stimulates release of CCK and gastrin
Calcitonin gene-related peptide	Enteric nerves	Unclear
Chromogranin A	Neuroendocrine cells	Secretory protein
Enkephalins	Stomach, duodenum	Opiate-like actions
Enteroglucagon	Small intestine, pancreas	
Galanin	Enteric nerves	Inhibits insulin secretion
Ghrelin	Stomach	Appetite stimulation, increases gastric emptying
Glucagon-like peptide 1	Pancreas, ileum	Increases insulin secretion
Glucagon-like peptide 2	Ileum, colon	Enterocyte-specific growth hormone
Growth factors	Throughout the gut	Cell proliferation and differentiation
Growth hormone releasing factor	Small intestine	Unclear
Leptin	Stomach	Appetite control
Motilin	Throughout the gut	Increases gastric emptying and small bowel motility
Neuropeptide Y	Enteric nerves	Regulation of intestinal blood flow
Neurotensin	Ileum	Affects gut motility; increases jejunal and ileal fluid secretion
Pancreastatin	Pancreas	Inhibits pancreatic endocrine and exocrine secretion
Pancreatic polypeptide	Pancreas	Inhibits pancreatic and biliary secretion
$PYY_{3\text{-}36}$	Colon	Inhibits food intake
Somatostatin	Stomach, pancreas	Inhibits secretion and action of many hormones
Substance P	Enteric nerves	Unclear
Trefoil peptides	Stomach, intestine	Mucosal protection and repair

potent as G-17. A synthetic pentapeptide (pentagastrin) may be used for stimulation of HCl secretion in gastric function testing.

Gastrin is produced and stored mainly by endocrine cells (G cells) of the antral mucosa and to a lesser extent by G cells of the proximal duodenum and delta cells of the pancreatic islets. After secretion, gastrin is transported by the blood through the liver to the parietal cells of the fundus of the stomach, where it stimulates the secretion of gastric acid. Gastrin also stimulates secretion of gastric pepsinogens and intrinsic factor by the gastric mucosa, release of secretin by the small intestinal mucosa, and secretion of pancreatic bicarbonate and enzymes and hepatic bile; it also increases gastric and intestinal motility, mucosal growth, and blood flow to the stomach. It is secreted in response to antral distention meals, and by amino acids, peptides, and polypeptides from partially digested proteins in the stomach. Of the free amino acids, glycine, tryptophan, and phenylalanine are the most potent stimulators. Other stimuli of gastrin include alcohol, caffeine, insulin-induced hypoglycemia, ingestion or intravenous infusion of calcium, and vagal stimulation initiated by smelling, tasting, chewing, and swallowing food.

Maximal secretion of gastrin occurs at an antral pH of 5 to 7. At pH 2.5, secretion is reduced by about 80%; maximal suppression occurs at pH 1.0. Secretion is inhibited by the direct action of acid on the G cells. This negative feedback safeguards against over-acidification by any and all stimulants.

The principal circulating form of gastrin is G-34 in healthy individuals and in patients with hypergastrinemia. Trypsin cleaves G-34 into two fragments, one of which is identical to G-17. On a molar basis, G-17 is six to eight times more potent than G-34 as a stimulant for gastric acid secretion. In the fasting state, the ratio of G-34 to G-17 is about 2:1. After meals, the concentration of G-34 doubles, but that of G-17 increases four times so that the ratio of these two forms in the circulation becomes 1:1. The half-lives of endogenous human G-17 and G-34 in the circulation are about 6 and 36 minutes, respectively; this difference probably accounts for the higher concentration of G-34 in peripheral blood of individuals in the fasting state.

SECRETIN[130]

Secretin is a linear polypeptide containing 27 amino acids and has structural similarities to glucagon, VIP, GIP, peptide histadine-isoleucine (PHI), and growth hormone-releasing hormone. The amino acid residues at 14 positions within the molecule are identical with those found in glucagon; 8 are the same as in GIP, and 9 are the same as in VIP. The intact secretin molecule is required for biological activity, and in contrast to gastrin there is no minimum active fragment.

Secretin is secreted by the mucosal granular S cells located in greatest concentration in the duodenum but present throughout the small intestine. It is released primarily on contact of the S cells with gastric HCl; however, as pancreatic juice flows into the duodenum, it neutralizes gastric acid and thereby removes one stimulus for its own secretion. Secretin is not released until the pH is lowered to at least 4.5. Below this pH, secretin release is proportional to the amount of acid entering the duodenum. A pH of <4.5 normally occurs only in the first few centimeters of the duodenum, causing little increase in plasma secretin after a normal meal. Thus secretin release after exposure of S cells to HCl may not be an important physiological stimulus. However, plasma secretin concentrations that are too low to measure may stimulate the pancreas in the presence of physiological concentrations of CCK, which is known to strongly potentiate the action of secretin. Undigested fat does not stimulate secretin release, but fatty acids with chains of 10 or more carbons are weak stimulants. Alcohol increases secretin release by stimulation of gastric acid secretion with subsequent lowering of duodenal pH rather than by a direct stimulatory effect. The half-life of secretin is about 4 minutes. The kidney is the major site of its degradation. The only known physiological inhibitor of secretin release is somatostatin.

The primary physiological role of secretin is the stimulation of the pancreas to secrete an increased volume of juice with high bicarbonate content. Other actions include stimulation of bicarbonate and water secretion from the liver and from Brunner's glands; augmentation of gallbladder contraction and increased hepatic bile flow; weak stimulation of insulin secretion (a pharmacological effect); stimulation of PTH release of pancreatic enzymes and of pepsinogen by the chief cells of the stomach; reduction of gastric and duodenal motility; reduction of the lower esophageal sphincter pressure; and promotion of pancreatic growth. Secretin inhibits normal gastrin secretion (but does not decrease serum gastrin in the Zollinger-Ellison syndrome) and therefore gastric acid secretion.

Vasoactive Intestinal Polypeptide[130]

VIP is a linear polypeptide consisting of 28 amino acids; it has structural similarities to secretin, GIP, and glucagon. VIP is present throughout the body and is found in highest concentrations in the nervous system and gut. Unlike secretin and other GI hormones, VIP is not found in the mucosal endocrine cells of the GI tract. VIP is believed to be a neurotransmitter limited to peripheral and central nervous tissue. VIP-containing nerve fibers are found throughout the GI tract from the esophagus to the colon and in all tissue layers of the gut.

Little is known about the conditions that cause VIP to be released into the circulation. There is no evidence that VIP is released during digestion, but its secretion is increased by vagal stimulation. It has a plasma half-life of about 1 minute, and most of the hormone is inactivated by a single passage through the liver.

VIP has a large number of ill-defined physiological actions, some of which are shared with other similar polypeptide hormones (secretin and GIP). It acts as a neurotransmitter in the central and autonomic nervous systems and causes vasodilation and relaxation of the smooth muscles of the circulatory and genitourinary systems and the gut. Other actions of VIP include an increase of water and electrolyte secretion from the pancreas and gut; release of hormones from the pancreas, gut, and hypothalamus; stimulation of lipolysis, glycolysis, and bile flow; and inhibition of gastrin and gastric acid secretion. Most of the actions of VIP tend to be of short duration because of its rapid degradation.

Glucose-Dependent Insulinotropic Peptide (GIP, Gastric Inhibitory Polypeptide)[130]

GIP is a linear peptide consisting of 42 amino acids. Its N-terminal end has a close resemblance to glucagon and secretin, but the C-terminal amino acid sequence of 17 residues is not common to any other known intestinal hormone.

GIP is synthesized and released by K cells located in the duodenal and jejunal mucosa. Plasma GIP is increased by oral administration of glucose, triacylglycerols, or intraduodenal infusions of solutions containing a mixture of amino acids; none of these, however, increases GIP concentrations when given intravenously. Protein ingestion does not significantly increase GIP. For food components to stimulate GIP release, they must be absorbed by the intestinal mucosa.

The biological actions of GIP include (1) stimulation of insulin secretion in the presence of hyperglycemia, (2) reduction of intestinal motility with stimulation of small intestinal fluid and electrolyte secretion, and (3) in supraphysiological concentrations, inhibition of gastric acid, pepsin, and gastrin secretion. The insulinotropic action of GIP appears to be the most important of its biological actions, and as a result, this hormone has more recently been called "glucose-dependent insulinotropic peptide" as a more accurate description of its physiological action.

Other Regulatory Peptides

Table 48-11 provides a brief description of the tissue locations and actions of other gut regulatory peptides, although the function of some of these is unclear. The growth factors belong to several families of peptides and have important roles in the control of a wide range of cell functions in the intestine.[38] The current clinical use of GI hormones/regulatory peptide measurements is in the diagnosis of neuroendocrine tumors of the pancreas and GI tract. It is likely that they will have wider applications as understanding of their functions grows (e.g., in the fields of obesity and appetite modulation).[30,31,136]

NEUROENDOCRINE TUMORS

Gastrinoma and the Zollinger-Ellison Syndrome[6,35,93]

In 1955, Zollinger and Ellison described a syndrome (Zollinger-Ellison or Z-E syndrome) consisting of fulminant peptic ulcers, massive gastric hypersecretion, and non-β-islet cell tumors of the pancreas. Hypergastrinemia, diarrhea, steatorrhea, and other endocrinopathies are frequent characteristics of this syndrome. Most cases occur between the ages of 30 and 50 years, although it has been described in patients from 7 to 90 years. It is more common in men (60% of cases) than in women. In about 25% of cases, ulcers are found beyond the first portion of the duodenum; such ulcers should always raise suspicion of Z-E syndrome. About 25% of all gastrinomas are part of the Multiple Endocrine neoplasia 1 syndrome (MEN1), which is characterized by tumors or hyperplasia in pancreatic islets and the parathyroid and pituitary glands. Fasting plasma gastrin is usually greatly increased, ranging from 2 to 2000 times normal. Concentrations more than 10 times the upper limit of normal, in the presence of gastric acid hypersecretion, are virtually diagnostic of gastrinoma. There is no correlation between the severity of the symptoms and the degree of elevation of the circulating gastrin concentration. However, the fasting plasma gastrin concentration at presentation in sporadic Z-E syndrome is associated with the size and site of the tumor and the presence of hepatic metastases and therefore has prognostic value.[9] Because management of the patient with Z-E syndrome usually requires surgical intervention, it is important to distinguish hypergastrinemia caused by gastrinoma from other conditions that may lead to similar increases in plasma gastrin.

Increased plasma gastrin occurs in hypochlorhydria or achlorhydria as a consequence of atrophic gastritis or the use of acid-suppressing drugs (e.g., histamine H_2-receptor antagonists or proton-pump inhibitors). Z-E syndrome cannot be diagnosed (or excluded) in patients taking PPIs. These drugs cause a profound reduction in gastric acid secretion and hence a large increase in plasma gastrin. *H. pylori* infection can also lead to increased plasma gastrin and to increased basal acid output, and in some cases to atrophic gastritis and high plasma gastrin.[89] Pernicious anemia and chronic atrophic gastritis associated with parietal cell antibodies are commonly associated with gastrin concentrations that overlap with those found in Z-E syndrome. Increases of plasma gastrin in chronic renal failure appear to be related to the severity of the renal failure. A direct correlation has been found between G-cell density and parathyroid function in patients with chronic renal failure, suggesting that secondary hyperparathyroidism may play a role in increasing plasma gastrin. Surgical resection or diseases of the kidneys or small intestine can cause hypergastrinemia, possibly because these are important sites of gastrin degradation or excretion.

Increased basal gastrin concentrations may be classified as "appropriate" or "inappropriate" according to their association with decreased or increased gastric acid secretion. In patients with very low or absent acid secretion and a functionally intact gastric antrum, an increase in plasma gastrin is physiologically appropriate and is expected. The increase is caused by hyperplasia of antral G cells as observed in atrophic gastritis, pernicious anemia, previous vagotomy, and renal failure. Inappropriate hypergastrinemia may be caused by gastrinoma, isolated retained antrum after gastric surgery, or primary G-cell hyperfunction.

Secretin and calcium provocation tests have been used in the past to assist in the differential diagnosis of Z-E syndrome.[64] The secretin test proved the more useful but is little used now with improved computed tomography scanning and the use of somatostatin-receptor imaging using the somatostatin analog octreotide.[109]

Measurement of Plasma Gastrin

In serum from healthy subjects, the predominant forms of gastrin are amidated G-34 and G-17. In subjects with gastrinomas, the circulating gastrins display unpredictable heterogeneity with a shift toward larger peptides. For the detection of gastrinomas, the assay should therefore be able to detect all secreted forms of gastrin to prevent false negatives.[66]

Gastrin is unstable in serum or plasma, and samples may lose up to 50% of their immunoreactivity during 48 hours at 2 °C to 8 °C, largely because of the action of proteolytic enzymes. Blood samples should be collected into a tube containing heparin as anticoagulant and aprotinin (e.g., Trasylol, 0.2 mL, 2000 KIU, in a 10 mL tube) to prevent proteolytic degradation. Samples should be mixed by inversion, transported rapidly on ice to the laboratory, and the plasma separated in a refrigerated centrifuge. The plasma should be frozen at −20 °C within 15 minutes of venipuncture. Samples collected in this way are suitable for the analysis of gastrin, VIP, pancreatic polypeptide, somatostatin, neurotensin, and chromogranins A and B.

The Watery Diarrhea Hypokalemia Achlorhydria Syndrome (Werner-Morrison Syndrome, WDHA Syndrome, VIPoma)[94]

The WDHA syndrome may be suspected in a patient producing large volumes (>1 liter/24 hours) of secretory diarrhea, with dehydration and hypokalemia. The diagnosis is confirmed by finding a high plasma VIP concentration and demonstration of the tumor by somatostatin-receptor imaging.

Other Gastrointestinal Neuroendocrine Tumors and Tumor Markers

GI neuroendocrine tumors are either endocrine pancreatic tumors or carcinoid tumors arising from enterochromaffin cells, which occur throughout the GI tract. Carcinoid tumors are discussed in Chapter 29.

Approximately two thirds of patients with tumors arising from pancreatic islet cells present with clinical syndromes associated with the excessive hormone production.[109] This group of tumors includes insulomas, gastrinomas, VIPomas, glucagonomas, and somatostatinomas. Insulinomas and glucagonomas are not usually associated with GI symptoms. Gastrinomas and VIPomas have been discussed in preceding sections. The somatostatinoma syndrome is associated with steatorrhea, gallstones, and diabetes. The remaining one third of patients with endocrine pancreatic tumors have no specific clinical symptoms associated with the tumors, which are described as nonfunctional.

The pattern of hormone and precursor production by neuroendocrine tumors is complex. Most secrete several tumor markers. Chromogranin A, a member of a family of secretory proteins, has the highest diagnostic sensitivity (94%) for endocrine pancreatic tumors, followed by pancreatic polypeptide (74%).[50] Chromogranin A is elevated in most patients and is an alternative to more specific markers in monitoring the effectiveness of surgery or drug therapy. However, as with other protein and peptide tumor markers, the epitope specificity of the antiserum has a profound effect on the diagnostic sensitivity of the assay.[109] Although chromogranin A has high sensitivity, false positives have been observed in a number of nonendocrine tumors including prostatic cancer.

INVESTIGATION OF MALDIGESTION/MALABSORPTION

This section summarizes causes of malabsorption and suggests the general laboratory approach to these disorders.

Box 48-8 summarizes the main causes of malabsorption under the three categories of (1) intraluminal disorders and malabsorption due to disorders of (2) transport into the mucosal cells, and (3) transport out of the mucosal cells.

Clinical presentation of the patient suffering from malabsorption or maldigestion classically includes the following features:

- *Evidence of general ill health.* Anorexia, weight loss, fatigue following minor effort, and dyspnea may be seen. Edema (due to hypoalbuminemia or weakness), tetany, and dehydration due to electrolyte imbalance and water loss may be present. In pancreatic exocrine insufficiency, however, hyperphagia is the rule; patients often report a very high (5000 kcal/day) food intake.
- *Isolated nutritional deficiencies.* Iron, folate, or vitamin B_{12} deficiency may manifest as anemia, which may be mild; vitamin K deficiency as a bleeding tendency; and vitamin D deficiency as bone disease. They are reflected by a variety of signs and symptoms (glossitis, pallor, dermatitis, petechiae, bruising, hematuria, muscle or bone pain, or neurological abnormalities).
- *Abdominal symptoms*, such as discomfort, distention, flatulence, and borborygmi (rumbling and gurgling sounds due to movement of gas in the intestine).
- *Watery diarrhea and possibly steatorrhe*a. In severe cases of steatorrhea (excess fat in feces), the stool is typically loose, bulky, offensive, greasy, light-colored, and difficult to flush away. Alternatively the stools may appear normal, but be more bulky or be passed with greater frequency.

Early presentation of malabsorption will, however, be more subtle than this list would indicate. There may be only a slight alteration in volume or consistency of the stool and only mild symptoms attributable to the GI tract. The patient may complain only of anorexia, fatigue, and lack of interest in daily activities. It is in these cases that the physician who suspects malabsorption on clinical grounds will rely on the laboratory to assist in the diagnosis. The initial laboratory investigations are routine tests, abnormalities of which may point to the possibility of malabsorption (e.g., blood hemoglobin concentration; mean red cell volume; serum concentrations of folate, ferritin, calcium, albumin, and alkaline phosphatase; and tests for antibodies in celiac disease [celiac serology]).

EVALUATION OF FAT ABSORPTION (FROM HILL,[79] WITH PERMISSION)

The evaluation of fat absorption or malabsorption is required in a small minority of patients being investigated for GI disorders. The British Society of Gastroenterology (BSG) guidelines[168] state that gastroenterologists should have access to such tests to ". . . assess patients with malabsorption who are proving difficult to diagnose."

BOX 48-8 Summary of Disorders Leading to Malabsorption

Disorders of intraluminal digestion:	
a. Altered gastric function	Post gastrectomy syndrome Zollinger-Ellison syndrome
b. Pancreatic insufficiency	Chronic pancreatitis Cystic fibrosis Pancreatic cancer
c. Bile acid deficiency	Disease/resection of terminal ileum Small bowel bacterial overgrowth
Disorders of transport into the mucosal cell:	
a. Generalized disorders due to reduction in absorptive surface area	Celiac disease, tropical sprue
b. Specific disorders	Hypolactasia Vitamin B_{12} in pernicious anemia Zn in acrodermatitis enteropathica
Disorders of transport out of the mucosal cell:	
a. Blockage of the lymphatics	Abdominal lymphoma Primary lymphangiectasia
b. Inherited disorders	a-β-lipoproteinemia

In a survey in 1997 of 231 hospitals in the UK,[45] fecal fat was the most widely available of all tests, with the estimated number of fecal fat measurements performed annually in the UK being 6100. Fecal fat measurement has many limitations,[86] some of which were highlighted in the 1997 survey, which must be brought to the attention of clinicians to dissuade them from placing reliance on an inherently unreliable test. In addition, dialogue with local gastroenterologists is necessary to reach consensus that the quantitative demonstration of fat malabsorption is of little value for most patients.

Limitations of Fecal Fat Measurement

The case for abandoning fecal fat measurement can be made on the grounds both of physiology and of analytical performance. The physiological problems of sample collection were convincingly demonstrated in a study in which radio-opaque pellets were administered orally (8, three times a day) for 5 days (120 total), and feces were collected for days 3 to 5.[182] Radiographic detection of 72 pellets was taken to indicate 100% recovery. In 52 patients studied, recovery ranged from 14% to 125%, and recovery was within the range 85% to 115% in only 32 of them. In 7 patients, fecal fat was normal but became abnormal after adjustment for marker recovery. Despite this evidence, few laboratories attempt to assess completeness of collection using markers.

Absorption of dietary fat is a remarkably efficient process, so that in normal health, fecal fat is largely (if not entirely) derived from endogenous rather than dietary sources.[41,77,103] Adequate dietary fat intake is therefore essential to minimize false-negative results. The BSG guidelines recommend a diet containing at least 70 g fat for 6 days.[168] In the UK only a minority of laboratories try to control (20%) or retrospectively assess (8%) fat intake.[45] Patients with steatorrhea may reduce their fat intake to control their diarrhea and despite laboratory instructions may not increase their dietary fat before and during the 72 hours of fecal collection; this will result in misleadingly low results.[41]

It is also often forgotten that diarrhea increases fecal fat excretion. In 58% of subjects with normal fat excretion, experimental induction of severe diarrhea (fecal weight >800 g/day) led to increased fecal fat (values of up to 49 mmol/day).[57] A borderline increase in fecal fat (i.e., 2 to 3 times the upper limit of normal, which is 18 mmol/day) is therefore not specific for a primary defect in fat digestion or absorption.

Available analytical performance data for fecal fat measurements in the UK also indicate that the test should now be consigned to history. Eighty-two per cent of laboratories use no internal quality control and EQA is impractical. When the titration step was assessed in an EQA exercise, between-laboratory coefficients of variation for three samples ranged from 31% to 42%.[45] Infrared spectroscopy offers the possibility of improved within- and between-laboratory precision for fecal fat measurements,[91] but does not address the problems of dietary input and sample collection, and is unlikely to be available to most laboratories.

At the end of an extensive survey of hospital laboratories in the UK, Duncan (unpublished report of the Clinical Resource and Audit Group, Scottish Office, Edinburgh 1997) concluded that ". . . the current utilization of the test, with no control of dietary fat intake, no correction for incomplete fecal collections and misgivings over analytical reliability, makes it a highly unsatisfactory investigation and probably of little clinical value."

Quantitative Demonstration of Fat Malabsorption Is Rarely Necessary

Many requests for fecal fat can be avoided or rejected by asking the requesting physician how the demonstration of fat malabsorption will help in the diagnosis of the disorder or management of the patient (see Table 48-12). In most cases it will become evident that neither fecal fat nor an alter-

TABLE 48-12 Common Situations in Which Fecal Fat May Be Requested But Is Unhelpful in Diagnosis and Management

Clinical Picture or Question	Appropriate Laboratory Response
Abdominal pain, weight loss, and diarrhea; possibly small bowel problem	Celiac serology: consider small bowel radiology
Offensive, floating, light colored stools	None (demonstrating fat malabsorption will not provide a diagnosis)
Elderly patient, weight loss, possibly malabsorption	Fat intake probably too low for fecal fat measurement; encourage use of appropriate investigations (see Table 48-13)
Pancreatic insufficiency, patient on enzyme supplements	Monitor stool consistency and clinical response (weight gain); may occasionally need to assess fat absorption
Abdominal pain, weight loss, and possibly pancreatic insufficiency	Use a specific pancreatic function test
Child, foul stool, possibly malabsorption	May sometimes need to confirm presence of fat globules in stool

From Hill PG, Ann Clin Biochem 2001;38:164-7.

TABLE 48-13 Laboratory Tests to Assess GI Function

Clinical Application	Appropriate Laboratory Investigations
Investigating diarrhea	Possible lactase deficiency: breath hydrogen after oral lactose
	Possible bacterial overgrowth: breath hydrogen after oral glucose or lactulose
	Possible laxative abuse: urine laxative screen
	Possibly induced by bile acid: ^{75}selenohomocholyltaurine whole body retention or serum 7α-hydroxy-4-cholesten-3-one
	Fecal osmotic gap; fecal Na, K
Assessing pancreatic function	Pancreolauryl test, fecal elastase
Screening for celiac disease	Tissue transglutaminase antibodies
Assessing fat absorption	^{14}C-triolein absorption (breath $^{14}CO_2$) or fecal microscopy
Other tests	Fecal α-1-antitrypsin for protein-losing enteropathy; gut hormones (gastrin)

From Hill PG, Ann Clin Biochem 2001;38:164-7.

native test for assessing fat absorption is necessary. There is no justification for assessing fat absorption for the diagnosis or management of celiac disease, and a specific pancreatic function test is more appropriate for the investigation of suspected pancreatic disease. Measuring fecal fat in patients with offensive, floating, putty-colored stools will not provide a diagnosis.

It is essential to encourage clinicians to use appropriate newer tests of GI function directed toward specific clinical situations (see Table 48-13). The availability and use of these tests will discourage the inappropriate use of fecal fat measurement.

There still remains the question, "Which test should be used when the assessment of fat malabsorption really is indicated?" Box 48-9 indicates the range of possible tests. My district hospital laboratory, serving a population of about 500,000, offers fecal microscopy and the ^{14}C-glycerol trioleate (^{14}C-triolein) fat absorption test.[176]

In the 1997 survey, performance of fecal microscopy was very poor (sensitivity 26%, specificity 64%); however, several studies have reported high sensitivity and specificity figures when compared with those derived from fecal fat measure-

BOX 48-9 Tests for Assessing Fat Absorption and Malabsorption

Measurement of fecal fat
Problems of poor recovery during sample collection (requires use of markers), inadequate dietary fat (minimum of 70 g/day), inaccurate analysis and uncertain interpretation
Butter fat test
Unreliable, poor discrimination
^{14}C-glyceryl trioleate
Sensitivity 85%, specificity 93%
Important factors to consider
Fat load (20 g) and form of "meal"
Effect of fat load on timing of peak of breath CO_2
Effect of assuming a constant CO_2 output of 9 mmol/kg/hr
Inappropriate in:
Liver, thyroid, and severe respiratory disease, diabetes, obesity, pregnancy
Mixed-chain triglyceride breath test
Valid test for pancreatic steatorrhea
Fat globules (fecal microscopy)
Need for standardized procedure

ment.[116,121] Some have argued that fecal microscopy after staining with Sudan III has advantages over fecal fat measurement, because it detects fecal triglycerides and fatty acids, which are principally of dietary origin; fecal fats include phospholipids and cholesteryl esters, which largely originate from the turnover of intestinal epithelial cells and gut bacteria.[102] There is still a need to evaluate a well-defined standardized technique for fat globules by fecal microscopy in a multilaboratory study. Meanwhile, Duncan has made several recommendations (unpublished report as above) to improve current performance related to methodology, interpretation, quality control, and adequate dietary fat before collecting fecal samples.

The ^{14}C-triolein test has been in use in my department since about 1985. The current workload is 10 to 15 patients per year from four gastroenterologists serving a population of about 500,000. In a prospective evaluation in 57 patients, the reported sensitivity was 85%, with specificity of 93% for the detection of fat malabsorption.[176] The "gold standard" for fat malabsorption was the final diagnosis made on clinical, histological, and radiological or laboratory grounds. Currently in the UK, various fat loads and procedures are used.[45] It is clear that larger fat loads (e.g., 60 g) result in significant delays in peak $^{14}CO_2$ in exhaled breath.[43] Our procedure uses a fat load of 19.3 g prepared as a palatable lemon mousse, containing protein (1.4 g) and carbohydrate (10 g). Peak $^{14}CO_2$ occurred within 6 hours in all subjects studied who had normal fat absorption. However, it must be recognized that the standard assumed CO_2 output of 9 mmol/kg/hr may lead to significant errors in the $^{14}CO_2$-triolein test because actual output varies from 5 to 12.4 mmol/kg/hr.[43]

When a similar fat load was used without the inclusion of protein and carbohydrates, peak $^{14}CO_2$ occurred later in some patients. In 53 patients in whom $^{14}CO_2$ excretion peaked within 6 hours, the sensitivity and specificity of the tests were 100% and 96%, respectively.[43] Breath samples for $^{14}CO_2$ measurement are not easily transportable, and the requirement for a scintillation counter and the administrative regulations surrounding the use of radioisotopes deter many laboratories from using the test.

With the growing interest in the application of stable isotopes, ^{13}C-substrates may replace the use of ^{14}C-triolein. A breath test using ^{13}C-mixed-chain triglycerides [1,3-distearyl, 2(carboxyl-^{13}C) octanoyl glycerol] has been used in children[2] and adults.[177] With a medium-chain fatty acid in the 2-position, the test is designed to assess intraluminal pancreatic lipase activity and is not therefore a substitute for fecal fat measurement. The ^{13}C-triolein test, using a uniformly labeled long chain triglyceride, is an alternative to fecal fat measurement.[112]

The van de Kamer method[96] for measuring fecal fat has survived for 5 decades. It really is time to give it up as a routine diagnostic test and to encourage the wider use of more specific tests for investigating disorders of GI function.

INVESTIGATION OF CHRONIC DIARRHEA

Although diarrhea is a common problem, no clear definition has existed to distinguish it from the range of stool weight, frequency, consistency, or volume that occurs in the normal population. A recent proposal, which seeks to encompass these different elements, suggests that for a Western diet, diarrhea may be defined as "the abnormal passage of loose or liquid stools more than three times daily and/or a volume of stool [with a weight] greater than 200 g/day."[171] Guidelines suggest that diarrhea may be defined as chronic when it has continued for 4 weeks; such persistence indicates the likelihood of a noninfectious cause requiring further investigation.

Several quite different mechanisms can lead to diarrhea. In carbohydrate malabsorption, the presence of unabsorbed solutes in the bowel causes an osmotic diarrhea as water enters the bowel from the tissue. By contrast, the diarrhea of most laxative abuse and in VIPomas is due to active secretion of water and electrolytes into the bowel, which is described as secretory diarrhea. Inflammatory bowel diseases (ulcerative colitis and Crohn's disease) cause diarrhea as a consequence of the inflammatory process with loss of fluid into the bowel.

Many diseases commonly thought to cause "diarrhea" in fact lead to more frequent passage of stools but not usually to an increased stool weight (or volume). Such disorders (e.g., irritable bowel syndrome) generally fall outside the scope of the definition of "chronic diarrhea." Guidelines for the management of irritable bowel syndrome are available.[95]

BOX 48-10 Causes of Chronic Diarrhea

- Colonic:
  - Colonic neoplasia
  - Ulcerative and Crohn's colitis
  - Microscopic colitis
- Small bowel:
  - Celiac disease
  - Crohn's disease
  - Other small bowel enteropathies (e.g., Whipple's disease, tropical sprue, amyloid, intestinal lymphangiectasia)
  - Bile salt malabsorption
    - Disaccharidase deficiency
    - Small bowel bacterial overgrowth
    - Mesenteric ischemia
    - Radiation enteritis
    - Lymphoma
    - Giardiasis (and other chronic infection)
- Pancreatic:
  - Chronic pancreatitis
  - Pancreatic carcinoma
  - Cystic fibrosis
- Endocrine:
  - Hyperthyroidism
  - Diabetes
  - Hypoparathyroidism
  - Addison's disease
  - Hormone secreting tumors (VIPoma, gastrinoma, carcinoid)
- Other:
  - Factitious diarrhea
  - "Surgical" causes (e.g., small bowel resection, internal fistulae)
  - Drugs
  - Alcohol
  - Autonomic neuropathy

From Thomas PD, et al. Gut 2003;52(Suppl V):Vol. 1-Vol. 15; reproduced by permission from the BMJ Publishing Group.

Box 48-10 describes the many causes of chronic diarrhea; most chronic diarrhea is due to disease of the colon in which laboratory diagnostic tests are currently of little value. A helpful algorithm for the investigation of chronic diarrhea is given in Figure 48-11.

The investigation of laxative abuse and measurement of fecal osmotic gap are described below. The other laboratory tests required for the investigation of chronic diarrhea are described in the sections above on intestinal disease, pancreatic diseases, and neuroendocrine tumors.

LAXATIVE ABUSE[42]

Surreptitious laxative abuse is an important cause of chronic diarrhea, is often overlooked, and is a diagnosis in which laboratory investigations have a significant role. It is the final diagnosis for chronic diarrhea in 15% to 26% of patients investigated in secondary or tertiary referral centers[18,46,144,146]

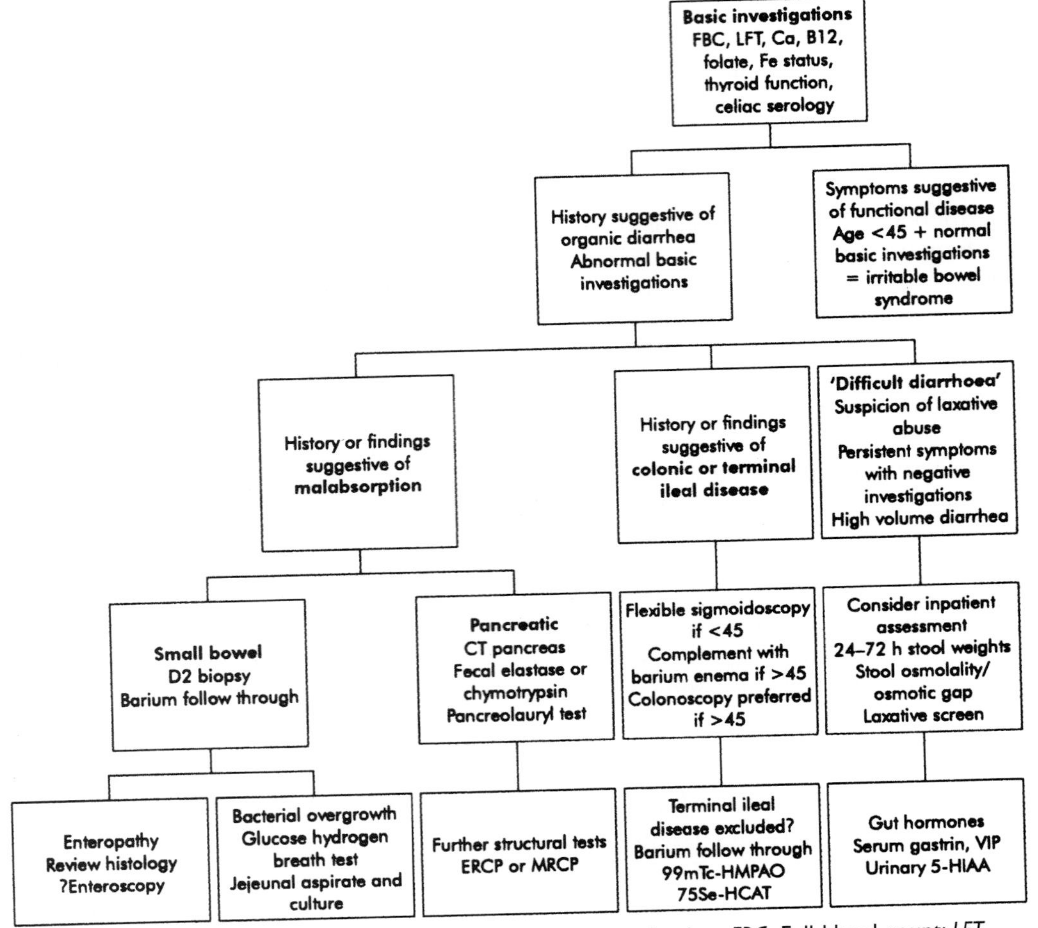

Figure 48-11 An algorithm for the investigation of chronic diarrhea. *FBC,* Full blood count; *LFT,* liver function tests; *CT,* computed tomography; *ERCP,* endoscopic retrograde cholangiopancreatography; *MRCP,* magnetic resonance cholangiopancreatography; *Tc-HMPAO,* technetium hexa-methyl-propyleneamine oxime; *75Se-HCAT,* 75Se homotaurocholate; *5-HIAA,* 5-hydroxyindoleacetic acid. *(From Thomas PD, Forbes A, Green J, Howdle P, Long R, Playford R, et al. Guidelines for the investigation of chronic diarrhoea, 2nd edition. Gut 2003;52(Suppl V):v1-v15. Used with permission of the BMJ Publishing Group.)*

and in 4% of a consecutive series of new primary care referrals to a gastroenterology clinic for evaluation of diarrhea.[46] The financial benefits of screening for laxative abuse have been established: When the diagnosis is not considered early in the investigative pathway, extensive and unnecessary investigations may occur.[18] In Munchausen syndrome by proxy, adults have administered laxatives surreptitiously to young children. A clinical diagnosis can rarely be made; no single clinical feature reliably predicts a positive test, making laboratory support essential. The main initial prerequisite for making a diagnosis of surreptitious laxative abuse is a high index of clinical suspicion,[42] followed by a request for appropriate analyses in urine and fecal samples at a time when the patient has diarrhea.

The pattern of laxative abuse has changed following legislation in several countries banning over-the-counter sales of laxatives containing phenolphthalein, which has traditionally been the most widely abused laxative. Abuse of phenolphthalein will therefore become less common, and the laxatives that will most frequently be encountered by clinical laboratories will be colonic stimulants containing bisacodyl or anthroquinones (e.g., senna, aloin, and cascara). Their absorption, metabolism, and excretion have recently been reviewed.[42] These can be detected in urine for at least 32 hours after a single dose.[184] Magnesium salts are the active ingredient of some over-the-counter laxatives and these may also be abused. The only reliable diagnostic procedure is the measurement of magnesium in fecal water. Concentrations >30 mmol/L are suggestive of magnesium-induced diarrhea.[44]

A pilot National External Quality Assurance Scheme was set up in the United Kingdom in 1996. In the light of poor overall performance highlighted by the scheme, recommendations have been made for a laxative screening service.[42]

Subsequently, thin layer chromatography (TLC) methods have been extensively evaluated to optimize the detection of laxatives.[47] The most important findings for the successful detection of laxatives by TLC were (1) the skill and experience of the operator, (2) the choice of the mobile phase (ethyl acetate:toluene:glacial acetic acid [4:16:1] and hexane:toluene:glacial acetic acid [3:1:1] gave the best results), and (3) use of high-performance TLC plates with a concentrating zone.

As for other laboratory procedures, a reliable laboratory service is essential. For such tests, false positives or false negatives may have important implications both for the patient's management and for the clinician's confidence in the laboratory. The analysis of laxatives should be regarded as part of the toxicology service, with confidence in the initial screening by TLC and ideally confirmation of positive results by mass spectrometry. Analyses should be undertaken by laboratories with appropriate expertise and ability to demonstrate good performance for these tests so as to ensure that patients with chronic diarrhea are correctly diagnosed and managed.

Fecal Osmotic (Osmolal) Gap

The osmolality of stool "water" will normally be that of serum (i.e., 290 mosm/kg), but the contribution of electrolytes and of nonelectrolytes to the total osmolality will vary depending on the cause of the diarrhea. Fecal osmotic (osmolal) gap (FOG) expresses the difference between the theoretical normal osmolality (290 mosm/kg) and the contribution of Na^+ and K^+ as follows:

$$\text{Fecal osmotic gap} = 290 - \left[2\left(\text{fecal Na}^+ + \text{K}^+\right)\right]$$

Fecal sodium and potassium can be measured in the fluid obtained by rapid centrifugation of a fecal sample. Total fecal osmolality increases significantly in unrefrigerated samples and use of the serum osmolality or 290 mosm/kg has been recommended in the above formula rather than a measurement of total fecal osmolality.[48]

Measurement of FOG enables an estimate to be made of the contribution of electrolytes or nonelectrolytes to the retention of water in the bowel and can therefore assist in distinguishing between secretory and osmotic diarrhea. In osmotic diarrhea, unabsorbed solutes lead to water retention and will thus make a larger contribution than normal to fecal osmolality; fecal sodium and potassium will therefore be present at lower concentrations than normal, leading to a larger "osmotic gap." Conversely, in secretory diarrhea, it is electrolytes that lead to water retention, and the FOG will therefore be small. FOG >50 mosm/kg is consistent with an osmotic diarrhea from carbohydrate malabsorption or magnesium-induced diarrhea[44]; by contrast FOG <50 mosm/kg suggests a secretory diarrhea, and further investigations might include a laxative screen for colonic stimulants or rarely tests for a neuroendocrine tumor.[58] A low FOG will be found in factitious diarrhea because of the addition of water to the stool; if this is suspected and if other causes are excluded, then measurement of total stool osmolality may be helpful.[99]

Measurement of creatinine can be used as an indication of contamination of the fecal sample with urine.

REFERENCES

1. Amarri S, Coward WA, Harding M, Weaver LT. Importance of measuring CO_2-production rate when using ^{13}C-breath tests to measure fat digestion. Br J Nutr 1998;79:541-5.
2. Amarri S, Harding M, Coward WA, Evans TJ, Weaver LT. ^{13}C-mixed triglyceride breath test and pancreatic enzyme supplementation in children with cystic fibrosis. Arch Dis Childhood 1997;76:349-51.
3. Arola H, Koivula T, Karvonen AL, Jokela H, Ahola T, Isokoski M. Low trehalase activity is associated with abdominal symptoms caused by edible mushrooms. Scand J Gastroenterol 1999;34:898-903.
4. Attar A, Flourie B, Rambaud JC, Franchisseur C, Ruszniewski P, Bouhnik Y. Antibiotic efficacy in small intestinal bacterial overgrowth-related chronic diarrhoea: a crossover, randomized trial. Gastroenterology 1999;117:794-7.
5. Axelson M, Bjorkhem I, Reihner E, Einarsson K. The plasma level of 7α-hydroxy-4-cholesten-3-one reflects the activity of hepatic cholesterol 7α-hydroxylase in man. Febs Lett 1991;284:216-8.
6. Barakat MT, Meeran K, Bloom SR. Neuroendocrine tumours. Endocrine-Related Cancer 2004;11:1-18.
7. Batterham RL, Cowley MA, Small CJ, Herzog H, Cohen MA, Dakin CL, et al. Gut hormone $PYY_{3\text{-}36}$ physiologically inhibits food intake. Nature 2002;418:650-4.
8. Berg JD, Chesner I, Lawson N. Practical assessment of the NBT-PABA pancreatic function test using high performance liquid chromatography determination of p-aminobenzoic acid. Ann Clin Biochem 1985;22:586-90.
9. Berger AC, Gibril F, Venzon DJ, Doppman JL, Norton JA, Bartlett DL, et al. Prognostic value of initial fasting serum gastrin levels in patients with Zollinger-Ellison syndrome. J Clin Oncol 2001;19:3051-7.
10. Biancone L, Fantini M, Tosti C, Bozzi R, Vavassori P, Pallone F. Fecal α_1-antitrypsin clearance as a marker of clinical relapse in patients with Crohn's disease of the distal ileum. Eur J Gastroenterol Hepatol 2003;15:261-6.
11. Blackwell PJ, Hill PG, Holmes GK. Autoantibodies to human tissue transglutaminase: superior predictors of coeliac disease. Scand J Gastroenterol 2002;37:1282-5.
12. Blaser MJ. Helicobacter pylori and gastric diseases. BMJ 1998;316:1507-10.
13. Boulos PB, Botha A, Hobsley M, Holton J, Oshowo AO, Tovey FI. Possible absence of Helicobacter pylori

in the early stages of duodenal ulceration. Q J Med 2002;95:749-52.
14. Brydon WG, Nyhlin H, Eastwood MA, Merrick MV. Serum 7α-hydroxy-4-cholesten-3-one and selenohomocholyltaurine (SeHCAT) whole body retention in the assessment of bile acid induced diarrhoea. Eur J Gastroenterol Hepatol 1996;8:117-23.
15. BSG guidelines <www.bsg.org.uk/clinical_prac/guidelines/dyspepsia/htm>, British Society of Gastroenterology 2002. (accessed July 2003).
16. Burgin-Wolff A, Dahlbom I, Hadziselimovic F, Petersson CJ. Antibodies against human tissue transglutaminase and endomysium in diagnosing and monitoring coeliac disease. Scand J Gastroenterol 2002;37:685-91.
17. Burroughs AK, Westaby D. Liver, biliary tract disease and pancreatic disease. In: Kumar P, Clark M, eds. Clinical medicine, 5th ed. Edinburgh: WB Saunders, 2002:395-404.
18. Bytzer P, Stokholm M, Andersen I, Klitgaard NA, de Muckadell OBS. Prevalence of surreptitious laxative abuse in patients with diarrhoea of uncertain origin. A cost benefit analysis of a screening procedure. Gut 1989;30:1379-84.
19. Cade A, Walters MP, McGinley N, Firth J, Brownlee KG, Conway SP, Littlewood JM. Evaluation of fecal pancreatic elastase-1 as a measure of pancreatic exocrine function in children with cystic fibrosis. Pediatr Pulmonol 2000;29:172-6.
20. Carriere F, Barrowman J, Verger R, Laugier R. Secretion and contribution to lipolysis of gastric and pancreatic lipases during a test meal in humans. Gastroenterology 1993;105:876-88.
21. Carroccio A, Verghi F, Santini B, Lucidi V, Iacono G, Cavataio F, et al. Diagnostic accuracy of fecal elastase 1 assay in patients with pancreatic maldigestion or intestinal malabsorption. Dig Dis Sci 2001;46:1335-42.
22. Caspary WF. Diarrhea associated with carbohydrate malabsorption. Clin Gastroenterol 1986;15:631-55.
23. Cataldo F, Lio D, Marino V, Picarelli A, Venturer A, Corazza GR. IgG_1 antiendomysium and IgG antitissue transglutaminase antibodies in coeliac patients with selective IgA deficiency. Gut 2000;47:366-9.
24. Cataldo F, Marino V, Bottaro G, Greco P, Venture A. Celiac disease and selective immunoglobulin A deficiency. J Pediatr 1997;131:306-8.
25. Churchill RD, Hill PG, Holmes GK. Breath test is better than near patient blood tests. BMJ 1998;316:1389.
26. Clark ML, Silk DB. Gastrointestinal disease. In: Kumar P, Clark M, eds. Clinical medicine, 5th ed. Edinburgh: WB Saunders, 2002:253-333.
27. Cole SG, Rossi S, Stern A, Hofmann AF. Cholesteryl octanoate breath test—preliminary studies on a new noninvasive test of human pancreatic exocrine function. Gastroenterology 1987;93:1372-80.
28. Corazza GR, Menozzi MG, Strocchi A, Rasciti L, Vaira D, Lecchini R, et al. The diagnosis of small bowel bacterial overgrowth. Gastroenterology 1990;98:302-9.
29. Couper R, Belli D, Durie P, Gaskin K, Sarles J, Werlin S. Pancreatic disorders and cystic fibrosis: working group report of the First World Congress of Pediatric Gastroenterology, Hepatology and Nutrition. J Pediatr Gastroenterol Nutr 2002;35:S213-23.
30. Cummings DE, Foster KE. Ghrelin-Leptin tango in body weight regulation. Gastroenterology 2003;124:1532-5.
31. Cummings DE, Weigle DS, Frayo RS, Breen PA, Ma MK, Dellinger EP, et al. Plasma Ghrelin levels after diet-induced weight loss or gastric bypass surgery. N Engl J Med 2002;346:1623-30.
32. Czako L, Endes J, Takacs T, Boda K, Lonovics J. Evaluation of pancreatic exocrine function by secretin-enhanced magnetic resonance cholangiopancreatography. Pancreas 2001;23:323-8.
33. Dahlquist A. Method for assay of intestinal disaccharidases. Anal Biochem 1964;7:18-25.
34. Dawson PA. Bile secretion and the enterohepatic circulation of bile acids. In: Feldman M, Friedman LS, Sleisenger MH, eds. Sleisenger and Fordtran's gastrointestinal and liver disease, 7th ed. Philadelphia: WB Saunders, 2002:1051-64.
35. Del Valle J, Scheiman JM. Zollinger-Ellison Syndrome. In: Yamada T, ed. Textbook of gastroenterology, 4th ed. Philadelphia: Lippincott Williams and Wilkins 2003:1377-94.
36. Deveney CW, Deveney KE. Zollinger Ellison Syndrome. In: Clark OH, Weber CA, eds. The surgical clinics of North America. Philadelphia: WB Saunders, 1987;67:411-22.
37. Dieterich W, Ehnis T, Bauer M, Donner P, Volta U, Riecken EO, et al. Identification of tissue transglutaminase as the autoantigen of celiac disease. Nature Med 1997;3:797-801.
38. Dignass AU, Sturm A. Peptide growth factors in the intestine. Eur J Gastroenterol Hepatol 2001;13:763-70.
39. Dimagno EP. A perspective on the use of tubeless pancreatic function tests in diagnosis. Gut 1998;43:2-3.
40. Dominguez-Munoz J, Hieronymus C, Sauerbruch T, Malfertheiner P. Fecal elastase test: evaluation of a new non-invasive pancreatic function test. Am J Gastroenterol 1995;90:1834-7.
41. Donowitz M, Kokke FT, Saidi M. Evaluation of patients with chronic diarrhea. N Engl J Med 1995;332:725-9.
42. Duncan A. Screening for surreptitious laxative abuse. Ann Clin Biochem 2000;37:1-8.
43. Duncan A, Cameron A, Stewart MJ, Russell RI. Limitations of the triolein breath test. Clin Chim Acta 1992;205:51-64.

44. Duncan A, Forrest JAH. Surreptitious abuse of magnesium laxatives as a cause of chronic diarrhoea. Eur J Gastroenterol Hepatol 2001;13:599-601.
45. Duncan A, Hill PG. A UK survey of laboratory-based gastrointestinal investigations. Ann Clin Biochem 1998;35:492-503.
46. Duncan A, Morris AJ, Cameron A, Stewart MJ, Brydon WG, Russell RI. Laxative-induced diarrhoea—a neglected diagnosis. J R Soc Med 1992;85:203-5.
47. Duncan A, Phillips IJ. Evaluation of thin-layer chromatography methods for laxative detection. Ann Clin Biochem 2001;38:64-6.
48. Duncan A, Robertson C, Russell RI. The fecal osmotic gap: technical aspects regarding its calculation. J Lab Clin Med 1992;119:359-63.
49. El-Omar EM, Penman ID, Ardill JES, Chittajallu RS, Howie C, McColl KEL. Helicobacter pylori infection and abnormalities of acid secretion in patients with duodenal ulcer disease. Gastroenterology 1995;109:681-91.
50. Eriksson B, Oberg K, Stridsberg M. Tumour markers in neuroendocrine tumours. Digestion 2000;62(suppl 1):33-8.
51. Eusufzai S, Axelson M, Angelin B, Einarsson K. Serum 7α-hydroxy-4-cholesten-3-one concentrations in the evaluation of bile acid malabsorption in patients with diarrhoea: correlation to the SeHCAT test. Gut 1993;34:698-701.
52. Farrell JJ. Digestion and absorption of nutrients and vitamins. In: Feldman M, Friedman LS, Sleisenger MH, eds. Sleisenger and Fordtran's gastrointestinal and liver disease, 7th ed. Philadelphia: WB Saunders, 2002:1715-50.
53. Farrell RJ, Kelly CP. Current concepts: celiac sprue. New Engl J Med 2002;346:180-8.
54. Farrell RJ, Kelly CP. Celiac sprue and refractory sprue. In: Feldman M, Friedman LS, Sleisenger MH, eds. Sleisenger and Fordtran's gastrointestinal and liver disease, 7th ed. Philadelphia: WB Saunders, 2002:1817-41.
55. Fasano A, Berti I, Gerarduzzi T, Not T, Colletti RB, Drago S, et al. Prevalence of celiac disease in at-risk and not-at-risk groups in the United States: a large multicenter study. Arch Intern Med 2003;163:286-92.
56. Fasano A, Not T, Wang W, Uzzau S, Berti I, Tommasini A, et al. Zonulin, a newly discovered modulator of intestinal permeability, and its expression in coeliac disease. Lancet 2000;355:1518-9.
57. Fine KD, Fordtran JS. The effect of diarrhea on fecal fat excretion. Gastroenterology 1992;102:1936-9.
58. Fine KD, Schiller LR. AGA technical review on the evaluation and management of chronic diarrhea. Gastroenterology 1999;116:1464-86.
59. Flatz G. The genetic polymorphism of intestinal lactase activity in adult humans. In: Scriver CR, Beaudet AL, Sly WS, Valle D, eds. The metabolic and molecular bases of inherited disease, 7th ed. New York: McGraw-Hill, 1995:4441-50.
60. Florent C, L'Hirondel C, Desmazures C, Aymes C, Bernier JJ. Intestinal clearance of α_1-antitrypsin. A sensitive method for the detection of protein-losing enteropathy. Gastroenterology 1981;81:777-80.
61. Flourie B, Turk J, Lemann M, Florent C, Colimon R, Rambaud JC. Breath hydrogen in bacterial overgrowth. Gastroenterology 1989;96:1225.
62. Forsmark CE. Chronic pancreatitis. In: Feldman M, Friedman LS, Sleisenger MH, eds. Sleisenger and Fordtran's gastrointestinal and liver disease, 7th ed. Philadelphia: WB Saunders, 2002:943-69.
63. Foster PN, Mitchell CJ, Robertson DRC, Hamilton I, Irving H, Kelleher J, et al. Prospective comparison of three non-invasive tests for pancreatic disease. Br Med J 1984;289:13-6.
64. Frucht H, Howard JM, Slaff JI, Wank SA, McCarthy DM, Maton PN, et al. Secretin and calcium provocative tests in the Zollinger-Ellison syndrome. Ann Intern Med 1989;111:713-22.
65. Glasbrenner B, Kahl S, Malfertheiner P. Modern diagnostics of chronic pancreatitis. Eur J Gastroenterol Hepatol 2002;14:935-41.
66. Goetze JP, Rehfeld JF. Impact of assay epitope specificity in gastrinoma diagnosis. Clin Chem 2003;49:333-4.
67. Graham JE, Peek RM, Krishna U, Cover TL. Global analysis of H. pylori gene expression in human gastric mucosa. Gastroenterology 2002;123:1637-48.
68. Green MR, Austin S, Weaver LT. Dual marker one day pancreolauryl test. Arch Dis Child 1993;68:649-52.
69. Gudmund-Hoyer E, Fenger HJ, Skovbjerg H, Kern-Hansen P, Madsen PR. Trehalase deficiency in Greenland. Scand J Gastroenterol 1988;23:775-8.
70. Gullo L, Graziano L, Babbini S, Battistini A, Lazzari R, Pezzilli R. Fecal elastase 1 in children with cystic fibrosis. Eur J Pediatr 1997;156:770-2.
71. Gullo L, Pezzilli R, Ventrucci M. Diagnostic value of the amino acid consumption test in pancreatic diseases. Pancreas 1996;12:64-7.
72. Gullo L, Ventrucci M, Tomassetti P, Migliori M, Pezzilli R. Fecal elastase 1 determination in chronic pancreatitis. Dig Dis Sci 1999;44:210-3.
73. Guyton AC, Hall JE. Human physiology and mechanisms of disease, 6th ed. Philadelphia: WB Saunders, 1997.
74. Hamilton I, Cobden I, Rothwell J, Axon AT. Intestinal permeability in coeliac disease: the response to gluten withdrawal and single dose gluten challenge. Gut 1982;23:202-10.
75. Hardt PD, Hauenschild A, Nalop J, Marzeion AM, Porsch-Ozcurumez M, Luley C, et al. The commercially available ELISA for pancreatic elastase 1 based on polyclonal antibodies does measure an as yet

unknown antigen different from purified elastase 1. Z Gastroenterol 2003;41:903-6.

76. Henderson AR, Rinker AD. Gastric, pancreatic and intestinal function. In: Burtis CA, Ashwood ER, Tietz NW, Williams A, eds. Tietz textbook of clinical chemistry 3rd ed. Philadelphia: WB Saunders, 1998:1271-1327.
77. Hernell O. Assessing fat malabsorption. J Paediatr 1999;135:407-9.
78. Hill I, Fasano A, Schwartz R, Counts D, Glock M, Horvath K. The prevalence of celiac disease in at-risk groups of children in the United States. J Pediatr 2000;136:86-90.
79. Hill PG. Faecal fat: time to give it up. Ann Clin Biochem 2001;38:164-7.
80. Hill PG, Forsyth JM, Semeraro D, Holmes GK. IgA antibodies to human tissue transglutaminase: audit of routine practice confirms high diagnostic accuracy. Scand J Gastroenterol 2004;39:1078-82.
81. Hill PG, Thompson SP, Holmes GKT. IgA anti-gliadin antibodies in adult celiac disease. Clin Chem 1991;37:647-50.
82. Hill RE, Comm B, Herez A, Corey ML, Gilday DL, Eng B, et al. Fecal clearance of alpha-1-antitrypsin: a reliable measure of enteric protein loss in children. J Pediatr 1981;99:416-8.
83. Hoek FJ, Van den Bergh FAJTM, Klein Elhorst JT, Meijer JL, Timmer E, Tytgat GNJ. Improved specificity of the PABA test with p-aminosalicylic acid (PAS). Gut 1987;28:468-73.
84. Holmes GKT. Potential and latent coeliac disease. Eur J Gastroenterol Hepatol 2001;13:1057-60.
85. Holmes GKT. Screening for coeliac disease in type 1 diabetes. Arch Dis Child 2002;87:495-9.
86. Holmes GKT, Hill PG. Do we still need to measure faecal fat? BMJ 1988;296:1552-3.
87. Howden CW, Hunt RH. Guidelines for the management of Helicobacter pylori infection. Am J Gastroenterol 1998;93:2330-8.
88. Howdle PD, Losowsky MS. Coeliac disease in adults. In: Marsh MN, ed. Coeliac disease. Oxford: Blackwell, 1992:49-80.
89. Huang SM, Lin HH, Hsu YH. Extreme hypergastrinaemia caused by atrophic gastritis and Helicobacter pylori infection—a case report. Hepatogastroenterology 2001;48:1215-6.
90. Isokoski M, Jussila A, Sarna S. A simple screening method for lactose malabsorption. Gastroenterology 1972;62:28-32.
91. Jakobs BS, Volmer M, Swinkels DW, Hofs MTW, Donkervoort S, Joostings MMJ, et al. New method for faecal fat determination by mid-infrared spectroscopy, using a transmission cell: an improvement in standardization. Ann Clin Biochem 2000;37:343-9.
92. Janatuinen EK, Kemppainen TA, Julkunen RJ, Kosma VM, Maki M, Heikkinen M, et al. No harm from five year ingestion of oats in coeliac disease. Gut 2002;50:332-5.
93. Jensen RT. Gastrinoma. In: O'Shea D, Bloom SR, eds. Baillieres clinical gastroenterology. London: Bailliere Tindall, 1996;10:603-43.
94. Jensen RT. Endocrine neoplasms of the pancreas. In: Yamada T, ed. Textbook of gastroenterology, 4th ed. Philadelphia: Lippincott Williams and Wilkins, 2003:2108-46.
95. Jones J, Boorman B, Cann P, Forbes A, Gomborone J, Heaton K, et al. Guidelines for the management of the irritable bowel syndrome. British Society of Gastroenterology 2000. http://www.bsg.org.uk/pdf_word_docs/man_ibd.pdf (accessed July 2003).
96. van de Kamer JH, Ten Huinink BH, Weyers HA. Rapid method for the determination of fat in feces. J Biol Chem 1949;177:347-55.
97. Karcher RE, Truding RM, Stawick LE. Using a cutoff of <10 ppm for breath hydrogen testing: a review of 5 years' experience. Ann Clin Lab Sci 1999; 29:1-8.
98. Kaspar P. Chymotrypsin in stool. In: Bergmeyer HU, Bergmeyer J, Grassl M, eds. Methods of enzymatic analysis, Vol 5, 3rd ed. Weinheim: Verlag Chemie, 1984:109-18.
99. Katz SL, McGee P, Geist R, Durie P. Factitious diarrhea: a case of watery deception. J Pediatr Gastroenterol Nutr 2001;33:607-9.
100. Kerlin P, Wong L. Breath hydrogen testing in bacterial overgrowth of the small intestine. Gastroenterology 1988;95:982-8.
101. Kerner JA. Formula allergy and intolerance. Gastroenterol Clin North Am 1995;24:1-25.
102. Khouri MK, Huang G, Shiau YF. Sudan stain of fecal fat: new insight into an old test. Gastroenterology 1989;96:421-7.
103. Khouri MK, Huang G, Shiau YF. Dietary fat intake, 72-h excretion and Sudan stain for fecal fat. Gastroenterology 1989;97:550-3.
104. Kim KE. Protein losing enteropathy. In: Feldman M, Friedman LS, Sleisenger MH, eds. Sleisenger and Fordtran's gastrointestinal and liver disease, 7th ed. Philadelphia: WB Saunders, 2002:446-52.
105. King CE, Toskes PP. Comparison of the 1-gram [^{14}C]Xylose, 10-gram Lactulose-H_2, and 80-gram Glucose-H_2 breath tests in patients with small intestine bacterial overgrowth. Gastroenterology 1986;91:1447-51.
106. Koletzko S, Haisch M, Seeboth I, Braden B, Hengels K, Koletzko B, Hering P. Isotope-selective non-dispersive infrared spectrometry for detection of *Helicobacter pylori* infection with ^{13}C-urea breath test. Lancet 1995;345:961-2.
107. Korponay-Szabo IR, Laurila K, Szondy Z, Halttunen T, Szalai Z, Dahlbom I, et al. Missing endomysial and

reticulin binding of coeliac antibodies in transglutaminase 2 knockout tissues. Gut 2003;52:199-204.
108. Kumar PJ, Clark ML. Malabsorption and Weight Loss. In: Bloom S, ed. Practical gastroenterology. London: Martin Dunitz, 2002:371-82.
109. Lamberts SWJ, Hofland LJ, Nobels FRE. Neuroendocrine tumor markers. Frontiers in Neuroendocrinol 2001;22:309-39.
110. Langenberg ML, Tytgat GNJ, Schipper MEI, Rietra PJGM, Zanen HC. *Campylobacter*-like organisms in the stomachs of patients and healthy individuals. Lancet 1984;i:1348.
111. Lankisch PG, Schmidt I, Konig H, Lehnick D, Knollman R, Lohr M, et al. Faecal elastase 1: not helpful in diagnosing chronic pancreatitis associated with mild to moderate exocrine pancreatic insufficiency. Gut 1998;42:551-4.
112. Lembcke B, Braden B, Caspary WF. Exocrine pancreatic insufficiency: accuracy and clinical value of the uniformly labelled ^{13}C-hiolein breath test. Gut 1996;39;668-74.
113. Leus J, Van Biervliet S, Robberecht E. Detection and follow up of exocrine pancreatic insufficiency in cystic fibrosis: a review. Eur J Pediatr 2000;159:563-8.
114. Levitt MD. Production and excretion of hydrogen gas in man. N Engl J Med 1969;281:122-7.
115. Lijmer J, Heisterkamp S, Bonsel GJ, Prins MH, van der Meulen JHP, et al. Empirical evidence of design-related bias in studies of diagnostic tests. JAMA 1999;282:1061-6.
116. Lip-Bin T, Stopard M, Anderson S, Grant A, Quantrill D, Wilkinson RH, et al. Assessment of fat malabsorption. J Clin Pathol 1983;36:1362-6.
117. Logan RPH, Dill S, Bauer FE, Walker MM, Hirschl AM, Gummett PA, et al. The European ^{13}C-urea breath test for the detection of *Helicobacter pylori.* Eur J Gastroenterol Hepatol 1991;3:915-21.
118. Logan RPH, Walker MM, Misiewicz JJ, Gummett PA, Karim QN, Baron JH. Changes in intragastric distribution of *Helicobacter pylori* during treatment with omeprazole. Gut 1995;36:12-6.
119. Loser C, Brauer C, Aygen S, Hennemann O, Folsch UR. Comparative clinical evaluation of the ^{13}C-mixed triglyceride breath test as an indirect test of pancreatic function. Scand J Gastroenterol 1998;33:327-34.
120. Loser C, Mollgaard A, Folsch UR. Faecal elastase 1: a novel, highly sensitive, and specific tubeless pancreatic function test. Gut 1996;39:580-6.
121. Luk GD. Screening for steatorrhea. Gastroenterology 1979;77:205-6.
122. Maki M, Mustalahti K, Kokkonen J, Kulmala P, Haapalahti M, Karttunen T, et al. Prevalence of celiac disease among children in Finland. N Engl J Med 2003;348:2517-24.
123. Malfertheiner P, Megraud F, O'Morain C, Hungin AP, Jones R, Axon A, et al. Current concepts in the management of Helicobacter pylori infection—the Maastricht 2-2000 Consensus Report. Aliment Pharmacol Ther 2002;16:167-80.
124. Marsh MN, ed. Coeliac disease. Oxford: Blackwell, 1992.
125. Marshall BJ, McGechie DB, Rogers PA, Glancy RJ. Pyloric Campylobacter infection and gastroduodenal disease. MJA 1985;142:439-44.
126. Martini S, Mengozzi G, Aimo G, Giorda L, Pagni R, Guidetti CS. Comparative evaluation of serologic tests for celiac disease diagnosis and follow-up. Clin Chem 2002;48:960-3.
127. Masoero G, Zaffino C, Laudi C, Lombardo L, Rocca R, Gallo L, et al. Fecal pancreatic elastase 1 in the work up of patients with chronic diarrhea. Int J Pancreatol 2000;28:175-9.
128. Mastropaolo G, Rees WDW. Evaluation of the hydrogen breath test in man: definition and elimination of the early hydrogen peak. Gut 1987;28:721-5.
129. Metz G, Blendis LM, Jenkins DJA. H_2 breath test for lactase deficiency. N Engl J Med 1976;294:730.
130. Miller LJ. Gastrointestinal hormones and receptors. In: Yamada T, ed. Textbook of gastroenterology, 4th ed. Philadelphia: Lippincott Williams and Wilkins, 2003:48-77.
131. Moran A, Radley S, Neoptolomos J, Jones AF, Asquith P. Detection of colorectal cancer by faecal α_1-antitrypsin. Ann Clin Biochem 1993;30:28-33.
132. Morris JA, Selivanov V, Sheldon GF. Nutritional management of patients with malabsorption syndrome. Clin Gastroenterol 1983;12;463-74.
133. Muldoon C, Maguire P, Gleeson F. Onset of sucrase-isomaltase deficiency in late adulthood. Am J Gastroenterol 1999;94:2298-9.
134. Mulholland G, Ardill JES, Fillmore D, Chittajallu RS, Fullarton GM, McColl KEL. Helicobacter pylori—related hypergastrinaemia is due to a selective increase in gastrin G17. Gut 1993;34:757-61.
135. Murray IA, Coupland K, Smith JA, Ansell ID, Long RG. Intestinal trehalase activity in a UK population: establishing a normal range and the effect of disease. Br J Nutr 2000;83:241-5.
136. Neary NM, Small CJ, Bloom SR. Gut and mind. Gut 2003;52:918-21.
137. Newcomer AD, McGill DB, Thomas PJ, Hofmann AF. Prospective comparison of indirect methods for detecting lactase deficiency. N Engl J Med 1975;293:1232-5.
138. Niederau C, Grendell JH. Diagnosis of chronic pancreatitis. Gastroenterology 1985;88:1973-95.
139. Nomura A, Stemmermann GN, Chyou P-H, Kato I, Perez-Perez GI, Blaser MJ. Helicobacter pylori infection and gastric carcinoma among Japanese Americans in Hawaii. N Engl J Med 1991;325:1132-6.
140. Parsonnet J, Friedman GD, Vandersteen DP, Chang Y, Vogelman JH, Orentreich N, et al. Helicobacter pylori

infection and the risk of gastric carcinoma. N Engl J Med 1991;325:1127-31.
141. Perman JA, Modler S, Barr RG, Rosenthal P. Fasting breath hydrogen concentration: normal values and clinical application. Gastroenterology 1984;87: 1358-63.
142. Perry I, Iqbal T, Cooper B. Intestinal permeability in coeliac disease. Lancet 2001;358:1729-30.
143. Phillips IJ, Rowe DJ, Dewar P, Connett GJ. Faecal elastase 1; a marker of exocrine pancreatic insufficiency in cystic fibrosis. Ann Clin Biochem 1999;36:739-42.
144. Phillips S, Donaldson L, Geisler K, Pera A, Kochar R. Stool composition in factitial diarrhea: a 6-year experience with stool analysis. Ann Intern Med 1995;123:97-100.
145. Rauws EAJ, Tytgat GNJ. Cure of duodenal ulcer associated with eradication of H. pylori. Lancet 1990;335:1233-5.
146. Read NW, Kerjs GJ, Read MG, Santa Ana CA, Morawski SG, Fordtran JS. Chronic diarrhea of unknown origin. Gastroenterology 1980;78:264-71.
147. Redel CA. Anatomy of the stomach. In: Feldman M, Friedman LS, Sleisenger MH, eds. Sleisenger and Fordtran's gastrointestinal and liver disease, 7th ed. Philadelphia: WB Saunders, 2002:675-80.
148. Rehfeld JF. The new biology of gastrointestinal hormones. Physiol Rev 1998;78:1087-108.
149. Rhodes JM, Middleton P, Jewell DP. The Lactulose hydrogen breath test as a diagnostic test for small-bowel bacterial overgrowth. Scand J Gastroenterol 1979;14:333-6.
150. Rinderknecht H, Renner IG, Douglas AP, Adham NF. Profiles of pure pancreatic secretions obtained by direct pancreatic duct cannulation in normal healthy human subjects. Gastroenterology 1978;75:1083-9.
151. Sauter GH, Munzing W, von Ritter C, Paumgartner G. Bile acid malabsorption as a cause of chronic diarrhea: diagnostic value of 7α-hydroxy-4-cholesten-3-one in serum. Dig Dis Sci 1999;44:14-9.
152. Schwartz MW, Morton GJ. Keeping hunger at bay. Nature 2002;418:595-7.
153. Semenza G, Auricchio S. Small intestinal disaccharidases. In: Scriver CR, Beaudet AL, Sly WS, Valle D, eds. The metabolic and molecular bases of inherited disease, 7th ed. New York: McGraw-Hill, 1995: 4451-80.
154. Shan L, Molberg O, Parrot I, Hausch F, Filiz F, Gray GM, et al. Structural basis for gluten intolerance in celiac sprue. Science 2002;297:2275-9.
155. Shiotani A, Graham D. Pathogenesis and therapy of gastric and duodenal ulcer disease. Med Clin N Am 2002;86:1447-66.
156. Smith MJ, Cherian P, Raju GS, Dawson BF, Mahon S, Bardhan KD. Bile acid malabsorption in persistent diarrhoea. J R Coll Physicians Lond 2000;34:448-51.
157. Sollid LM. Coeliac disease: dissecting a complex inflammatory disorder. Nat Rev Immunol 2002;2:647-55.
158. Sollid LM, Scott H. New tool to predict celiac disease on its way to the clinics. Gastroenterology 1998;115:1584-94.
159. Somogyi L, Cintron M, Toskes PP. Synthetic porcine secretin is highly accurate in pancreatic function testing in individuals with chronic pancreatitis. Pancreas 2000;21:262-5.
160. Spiller RC. Postinfectious irritable bowel syndrome. Gastroenterology 2003;124:1662-71.
161. Stein J, Jung M, Sziegoleit A, Zeuzem S, Caspary WF, Lembcke B. Immunoreactive elastase 1: clinical evaluation of a new non-invasive test of pancreatic function. Clin Chem 1996;42:222-6.
162. Stotzer PO, Kilander AF. Comparison of the 1-gram ^{14}C-D-xylose breath test and the 50-gram hydrogen glucose breath test for diagnosis of small intestinal bacterial overgrowth. Digestion 2000;61:165-71.
163. Strocchi A, Corazza G, Ellis CJ, Gasbarrini G, Levitt MD. Detection of malabsorption of low doses of carbohydrate: accuracy of various breath H_2 criteria. Gastroenterology 1993;105:1404-10.
164. Strygler B, Nicar M, Santangelo WC, Porter JL, Fordtran JS. α_1-Antitrypsin excretion in stool in normal subjects and in patients with gastrointestinal disorders. Gastroenterology 1990;99:1380-7.
165. Suerbaum S, Michetti P. Medical progress: Helicobacter pylori infection. (Review Article). N Engl J Med 2002;347:1175-86.
166. Sziegoleit A, Linder D. Studies on the sterol-binding capacity of human pancreatic elastase. Gastroenterology 1991;100:768-74.
167. Takeda H, Nishise S, Furukawa M, Nagashima R, Shinzawa H, Takahas T. Fecal clearance of alpha-1-antitrypsin with lansoprazole can detect protein losing gastropathy. Dig Dis Sci 1999;44:2313-8.
168. Tests for malabsorption. BSG guidelines in gastroenterology. London: British Society of Gastroenterology, 1996.
169. The EUROGAST Study Group. An international association between Helicobacter pylori infection and gastric cancer. Lancet 1993;341:1359-62.
170. Thibodeau GA, Patton KT. Anatomy and physiology 5th ed. St Louis: Mosby 2003.
171. Thomas PD, Forbes A, Green J, Howdle P, Long R, Playford R, et al. Guidelines for the investigation of chronic diarrhoea, 2nd edition. Gut 2003;52(Suppl V):v1-v15.
172. von Tirpitz C, Kohn C, Steinkamp M, Geerling I, Maier V, Möller P, et al. Lactose intolerance in active Crohn's disease: clinical value of duodenal lactase analysis. J Clin Gastroenterol 2002;34:49-53.
173. Treem WR. Congenital sucrase-isomaltase deficiency. J Pediatr Gastroenterol Nutr 1995;21:1-14.

174. Trevisani L, Sartori S. The accuracy of the Helicobacter pylori stool antigen test in diagnosing H. pylori in treated patients. Eur J Gastroenterol Hepatol 2002;14:89.
175. Trewick AL. Glucose interference in the pancreolauryl test. Ann Clin Biochem 1998;38:274-8.
176. Turner JM, Lawrence S, Fellows IW, Johnson I, Hill PG, Holmes GKT. ^{14}C-triolein absorption: a useful test in the diagnosis of malabsorption. Gut 1987;28:694-700.
177. Vantrappen GR, Rutgeerts PJ, Ghoos YF, Hiele MI. Mixed triglyceride breath test: a noninvasive test of pancreatic lipase activity in the duodenum. Gastroenterology 1989;96:1126-34.
178. Wallis C, Leung T, Cubitt D, Reynolds A. Stool elastase as a diagnostic test for pancreatic function in children with cystic fibrosis. Lancet 1997;350:1001.
179. Watts D, Brydon G, Crichton S, Ghosh S. Glucose hydrogen breath test in the investigation of diarrhoea. Gut 2000;46(suppl II):A23.
180. West J, Palmer BP, Holmes GKT, Logan RFA. Trends in clinical presentation of adult coeliac disease: a 25-year prospective study. Gut 2001;48(Suppl I): A78.
181. West J, Logan RFA, Hill PG, Lloyd A, Lewis S, Hubbard R, et al. Seroprevalence, correlates, and characteristics of undetected coeliac disease in England. Gut 2003;52:960-5.
182. West PS, Levin GS, Griffin GE, Maxwell JD. Comparison of simple screening tests for fat malabsorption. BMJ 1981;282:1501-4.
183. Williams AJK, Merrick MV, Eastwood MA. Idiopathic bile acid malabsorption—a review of clinical presentation, diagnosis and response to treatment. Gut 1991;32:1004-6.
184. de Wolff FA, de Haas EJM, Verweij M. A screening method for establishing laxative abuse. Clin Chem 1981;27:914-7.

CHAPTER 49

Mineral and Bone Metabolism

David B. Endres, Ph.D., and Robert K. Rude, M.D.

Among the multitude of homeostatic processes in the body, one of the most tightly controlled is the metabolism of calcium. This tight control is necessary because calcium has critical roles in intracellular signaling, at the plasma membrane of cells, and in control of function of extracellular proteins, such as those in the coagulation cascade. The body's handling of extracellular calcium is closely intertwined with that of phosphate and to a somewhat lesser extent of magnesium. It is also intricately connected with the active cellular processes in bone, which is the body's storehouse of calcium and a metabolically and functionally important system in its own right.

In this chapter, after an overview of bone and mineral metabolism, we discuss the clinical chemistry of calcium, phosphate, and magnesium; the hormones regulating these minerals; the major disorders of bone; and the clinical use of markers of bone formation and degradation. A goal of the chapter is to provide, in one place, a view of these highly interrelated topics.

OVERVIEW OF BONE AND MINERAL

The main functions of bone are (1) mechanical, for locomotion; (2) protective, for organs; and (3) metabolic, as a reserve for minerals, especially calcium and phosphate. Bones are composed of cortical and trabecular bone. Cortical (compact) bone is 80% to 90% mineralized by volume and constitutes 80% of the skeleton. Its function is primarily mechanical and protective. Trabecular bone constitutes the remaining 20% of the skeleton. Trabecular (cancellous or spongy) bone, which is 15% to 25% mineralized, is more metabolically active.

Bone is composed primarily of an extracellular mineralized matrix with a smaller cellular fraction. The organic matrix is primarily type I collagen (90%) with lesser amounts of a large number of noncollagenous proteins including osteocalcin. The organic matrix is mineralized by the deposition of inorganic calcium and phosphate in small, imperfect hydroxyapatite crystals with lesser amounts of carbonate, magnesium, sodium, potassium, and various ions. *Osteoclasts* and *osteoblasts*, the two main types of bone cells, are located on surfaces undergoing bone resorption and formation, respectively. Osteoclasts resorb bone, whereas osteoblasts participate in the synthesis of new bone.

Continuous turnover or *remodeling* of bone occurs, enabling bone to repair damage and adjust strength. Bone remodeling does not occur at random, but instead in discrete packets known as *bone remodeling units*. Bone resorption and bone formation are coupled. The remodeling cycle can be divided into activation, resorption, reversal, formation, and resting phases (Figure 49-1). Circulating osteoclast precursors are recruited, proliferate, and fuse to form osteoclasts. These giant multinucleated cells resorb bone by producing hydrogen ions to mobilize minerals and lysosomal enzymes to digest the organic matrix. Deep foldings of their plasma membrane (ruffled border) are in contact with the bone surface, forming the osteoclastic bone-resorbing compartment. After resorption ceases, a cement line is deposited in the resorption cavity, probably by mononucleated cells. Stromal lining cells differentiate to osteoblasts. Osteoblasts form bone by synthesizing the organic matrix, including type I collagen, and participating in the mineralization of the newly synthesized matrix. Remodeling is followed by a quiescent phase. An estimated 10% to 30% of the skeleton is remodeled each year.

Bone growth and turnover are influenced by the metabolism of calcium, phosphate, and magnesium and a number of hormones, the primary ones being parathyroid hormone (PTH) and 1,25-dihyroxyvitamin D (1,25[OH]$_2$D). In addition, a large number of other hormones and factors are

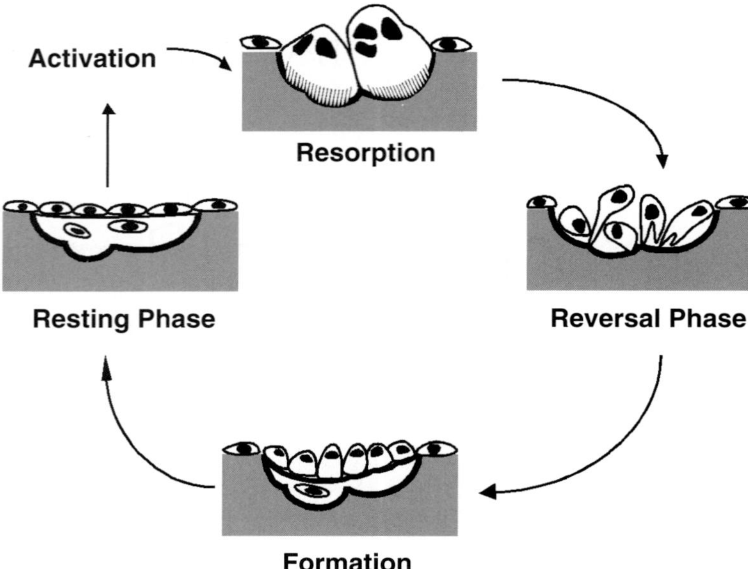

Figure 49-1 Bone remodeling. The bone remodeling sequence includes activation, reversal, formation, and resting phases. Reproduced from Baron R 2003 General Principles of Bone Biology. In: Favus M (ed.) *The Primer on the Metabolic Bone Diseases and Disorders of Mineral Metabolism*, 5th ed. American Society for Bone and Mineral Research, Washington DC, USA, pp. 1–8 with permission of the American Society for Bone and Mineral Research.

involved in the regulation of bone formation and resorption, including thyroid hormones, estrogens, androgens, cortisol, insulin, growth hormone, insulin-like growth factors (IGF-I and IGF-II), transforming growth factor β (TGF-β), fibroblast growth factor (FGF), and platelet-derived growth factor (PDGF). A number of cytokines, including interleukin (IL)-1, -4, -6 and -11; macrophage and granulocyte/macrophage colony-stimulating factors; and tumor necrosis factor (TNFα) alter bone remodeling primarily by stimulating resorption.

Recently, two products of the osteoblast have been identified that appear to be the final common pathway in coordinating osteoblast and osteoclast activity.[70,255] The first, receptor activator of nuclear factor-κB (RANK) ligand, binds to a receptor on osteoclast progenitor cells and increases osteoclast differentiation and activity. The second, osteoprotegerin (OPG), serves as a decoy receptor for RANK ligand. When OPG binds to RANK ligand, the osteoclast-stimulation activity is prevented. The relative ratios of these two molecules determine bone turnover.

Significant research progress has increased our understanding of bone and mineral metabolism and the pathophysiology of associated disorders. At the same time, improvements in technology have allowed laboratories to expand their role from measuring total calcium, phosphate, and magnesium to measuring other analytes, such as free (ionized) calcium, intact PTH, vitamin D metabolites, and calcitonin. An aging population is accelerating this trend and increasing the need for determining other analytes, such as biochemical markers of bone resorption (collagen cross-links [deoxypyridinoline and telopeptides]) and bone formation (osteocalcin and bone alkaline phosphatase [BAP]) and parathyroid hormone-related protein (PTHrP).

Bone contains nearly all of the calcium (99%), most of the phosphate (85%), and much of the magnesium (55%) of the body. The concentrations of calcium, phosphate, and magnesium in plasma are dependent on the net effect of bone mineral deposition and resorption, intestinal absorption, and renal excretion. PTH and 1,25-dihydroxyvitamin D are the principal hormones regulating these three processes.

CALCIUM

Calcium is the fifth most common element, and the most prevalent cation, in the body. An average human body contains approximately 1 kg (24.95 mol) of calcium. Calcium is found in three main compartments: the skeleton, soft tissues, and extracellular fluid (Table 49-1).[23,41] The skeleton contains 99% of the body's calcium, predominantly as extracellular crystals of unknown structure with a composition approaching that of hydroxyapatite $[Ca_{10}(PO_4)_6(OH)_2]$. Soft tissues and extracellular fluid contain about 1% of the body's calcium.

Biochemistry and Physiology

In blood, virtually all of the calcium is in the plasma, which has a mean normal calcium concentration of approximately 9.5 mg/dL (2.38 mmol/L). Calcium exists in three physiochemical states in plasma (Table 49-2), of which approxi-

TABLE 49-1 Distribution of Calcium, Phosphate, and Magnesium in the Body

Tissue	Calcium	Phosphate	Magnesium
Skeleton	99%	85%	55%
Soft tissues	1%	15%	45%
Extracellular fluid	<0.2%	<0.1%	1%
Total	1000 g (25 mol)	600 g (19.4 mol)	25 g (1.0 mol)

Modified from Aurbach GD, Marx SJ, Speigel AM. Parathyroid hormone, calcitonin, and the calciferols. In: Wilson JD, Foster DW, eds. Williams textbook of endocrinology, 8th ed. Philadelphia: WB Saunders, 1992:1397-476.

TABLE 49-2 Physiochemical States of Calcium, Phosphate, and Magnesium in Normal Plasma

	Approximate Percent of Total		
State	Calcium	Phosphate	Magnesium
Free (ionized)	50	55	55
Protein-bound	40	10	30
Complexed	10	35	15
Total (mg/dL)	8.6-10.3	2.5-4.5	1.7-2.4
(mmol/L)	2.15-2.57	0.81-1.45	0.70-0.99

Modified from Marshall RW. Plasma fractions. In: Nordin BEC, ed. Calcium, phosphate and magnesium metabolism. London: Churchill Livingstone, 1976:162-85.

mately 50% is free (ionized), 40% is bound to plasma proteins, and 10% is complexed with small anions.

The free calcium fraction is the biologically active form. Its concentration in plasma is tightly regulated by the calcium-regulating hormones PTH and 1,25-dihydroxyvitamin D.

About 80% of protein-bound calcium is associated with albumin,[189,314] with the remaining 20% associated with globulins. Because calcium binds to negatively charged sites on proteins, its binding is pH dependent. Alkalosis leads to an increase in negative charge and binding and a decrease in free calcium; conversely, acidosis leads to a decrease in negative charge and binding and an increase in free calcium. In vitro, for each 0.1-unit change in pH, approximately 0.2 mg/dL (0.05 mmol/L) of inverse change occurs in the serum free calcium concentration. In some patients with multiple myeloma, the high concentrations of serum globulin may bind sufficient calcium to produce an increase in the total serum calcium concentration.

Complexed calcium, about 10%, is complexed with small diffusible inorganic and organic anions, including bicarbonate, lactate, phosphate, and citrate.

Calcium can be redistributed among the three plasma pools, acutely or chronically, by alterations in the concentration of protein and small anions, changes in pH, or changes in the quantities of free calcium and total calcium in the serum (Figure 49-2).

Physiologically, calcium is classified as either intracellular or extracellular. The skeleton is a major reservoir for providing calcium for both the extracellular and intracellular pools. Intracellular calcium has key roles in many important physiological functions, including muscle contraction, hormone secretion, glycogen metabolism, and cell division.[23,449] The intracellular concentration of calcium in the cytosol of unstimulated cells is $<10^{-6}$ to 10^{-7} mol/L or lower, which is less than 1/1000 of that in the extracellular fluid (10^{-3} mol/L).

Extracellular calcium provides calcium ion for the maintenance of intracellular calcium, bone mineralization, blood coagulation, and plasma membrane potential. Calcium stabilizes the plasma membranes and influences permeability and excitability. A decrease in the serum free calcium concentration causes increased neuromuscular excitability and tetany; an increased concentration reduces neuromuscular excitability.

Clinical Significance

Disorders of calcium metabolism are separated into those causing hypocalcemia and hypercalcemia.

Hypocalcemia

Low total serum calcium (hypocalcemia) may be due to either a reduction in the albumin-bound calcium, the free fraction of calcium, or both (Box 49-1).[23,41,485] Hypoalbuminemia is the most common cause of pseudohypocalcemia (decreased total and normal free calcium) because 1 g/dL of albumin binds approximately 0.8 mg/dL of calcium. Common clinical conditions associated with low serum

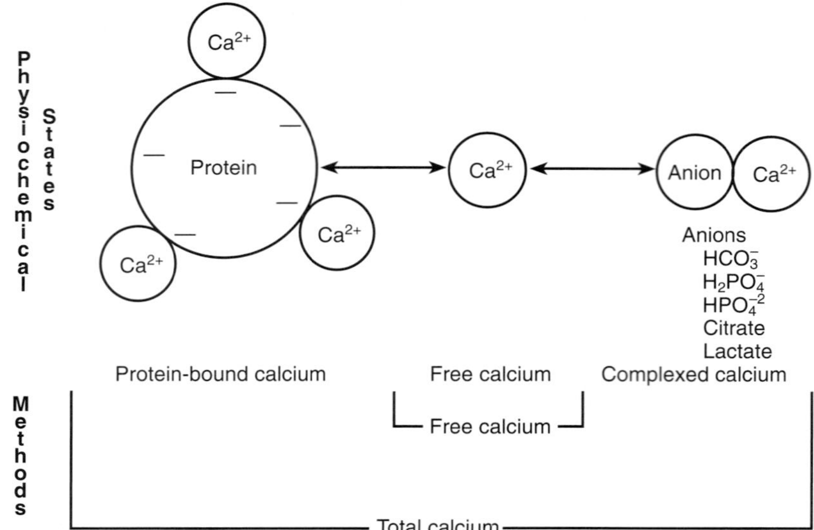

Figure 49-2 Equilibria and determinations of calcium in serum. Calcium can move among three physiochemical pools: (1) free calcium, (2) protein-bound calcium, and (3) calcium complexed with inorganic and organic anions. Methods for determining total calcium measure all three pools, whereas methods for determining free calcium measure only that pool.

BOX 49-1 Differential Diagnosis of Hypocalcemia

Hypoalbuminemia
Chronic renal failure
Magnesium deficiency
Hypoparathyroidism
Pseudohypoparathyroidism
Osteomalacia and rickets due to vitamin D deficiency or resistance
Acute hemorrhagic and edematous pancreatitis
Healing phase of bone disease of treated hyperparathyroidism, hyperthyroidism, and hematological malignancies (hungry bone syndrome)

albumin include chronic liver disease, nephrotic syndrome, congestive heart failure, and malnutrition.

Common causes of hypocalcemia are chronic renal failure and hypomagnesemia. In chronic renal failure, hypoproteinemia, hyperphosphatemia, low serum 1,25(OH)$_2$D (reduced synthesis because of inadequate renal mass), and/or skeletal resistance to PTH contribute to hypocalcemia. Magnesium deficiency, as discussed in a later section of this chapter, impairs PTH secretion and causes PTH end-organ resistance.

Other causes of low serum calcium are less common.[415] Hypoparathyroidism is due most commonly to parathyroid gland destruction during neck surgery (90%), and less commonly is idiopathic. Pseudohypoparathyroidism is biochemically similar to hypoparathyroidism; however, these patients have inherited resistance to PTH and elevated concentrations of PTH.[331] The molecular basis for the most common form, pseudohypoparathyroidism type I (Albright's hereditary osteodystrophy), is a reduction in guanine nucleotide regulatory complex, Ns, in the adenylate cyclase complex.

Acute symptomatic hypocalcemia may be seen in hospitalized patients for various reasons. Rapid remineralization of bone after surgery for primary hyperparathyroidism (hungry bone syndrome), treatment for hyperthyroidism, or treatment for hematological malignancy may result in hypocalcemia. Acute hemorrhagic or edematous pancreatitis is frequently complicated by hypocalcemia. Vitamin D deficiency may also be associated with hypocalcemia because of impaired intestinal absorption of calcium and skeletal resistance to PTH. Osteomalacia and rickets are discussed in a later section of this chapter.

Clinically, hypocalcemia most commonly presents with neuromuscular hyperexcitability, such as tetany, paresthesia, and seizures. A rapid fall in the serum calcium also may be associated with hypotension and electrocardiographic abnormalities.

The initial laboratory evaluation is directed toward the assessment of renal function and measurement of serum albumin and magnesium concentrations. Serum intact PTH concentrations are low or inappropriately normal in hypoparathyroidism and elevated in pseudohypoparathyroidism. Vitamin D deficiency is characterized by low serum 25(OH)D, high PTH (secondary hyperparathyroidism), and high serum alkaline phosphatase (ALP).

For symptomatic hypocalcemia, calcium may be administered intravenously. If hypocalcemia is secondary to hypoparathyroidism or pseudohypoparathyroidism, vitamin D and oral calcium supplements are administered.

An unusual and treatment-resistant form of symptomatic hypocalcemia is seen in patients treated with large amounts of burn cream that contains polyethylene glycols. The glycols are absorbed and metabolized to dicarboxylic acids that bind calcium. Patients develop markedly increased total calcium and decreased free calcium, along with a metabolic acidosis and increased serum osmolality from the glycols.

BOX 49-2 Differential Diagnosis of Hypercalcemia

- Primary hyperparathyroidism
  - Adenoma, hyperplasia, carcinoma
  - Familial
  - Multiple endocrine neoplasia type I with pituitary and pancreatic tumors
  - Multiple endocrine neoplasia type II with medullary thyroid carcinoma and pheochromocytoma
- Malignancy
  - With skeletal involvement
    - Direct tumor erosion of the bone
    - Local tumor production of bone-resorbing agents
  - No skeletal involvement (humoral hypercalcemia of malignancy)
    - Parathyroid hormone–related protein
    - Growth factor(s) (tumor growth factor, epidermal growth factor, platelet-derived growth factor)
  - Hematological malignancy
    - Cytokines (interleukin-1, tumor necrosis factor, lymphotoxin)
    - 1,25-Dihydroxyvitamin D (lymphoma)
  - Coexistent primary hyperparathyroidism
- Other endocrine disorders
  - Hyperthyroidism
  - Hypothyroidism
  - Acromegaly
  - Acute adrenal insufficiency
  - Pheochromocytoma
- Familial hypocalciuric hypercalcemia
- Idiopathic hypercalcemia of infancy
- Vitamin overdose
  - Vitamin D
  - Vitamin A
- Granulomatous diseases
  - Sarcoidosis
  - Tuberculosis
  - Berylliosis
  - Coccidioidomycosis
- Renal failure
  - Chronic renal failure
  - Acute renal failure—diuretic phase
  - Post–renal transplantation
- Chlorothiazide diuretics
- Lithium therapy
- Milk-alkali syndrome
- Hyperalimentation regimens
- Immobilization
- Increased serum proteins
  - Hemoconcentration
  - Hyperglobulinemia due to multiple myeloma

Hypercalcemia

Hypercalcemia is commonly encountered in clinical practice[23,41] and results when the flux of calcium into the extracellular fluid compartment from the skeleton, intestine, or kidney is greater than the efflux. For example, when excessive resorption of bone mineral occurs in malignancy, hypercalciuria develops. When the capacity of the kidney to excrete filtered calcium is exceeded, hypercalcemia develops. Hypercalcemia can be caused by increased intestinal absorption (vitamin D intoxication), increased renal retention (thiazide diuretics), increased skeletal resorption (immobilization), or a combination of mechanisms (primary hyperparathyroidism).

Common and many of the uncommon etiologies of hypercalcemia are listed in Box 49-2. Primary hyperparathyroidism is the most common cause in outpatients, whereas malignancy is the most common cause in hospitalized patients. Together, these two disorders account for 90% to 95% of all cases of hypercalcemia.

Primary hyperparathyroidism is characterized by excessive secretion of PTH that results in hypercalcemia.[491] It is most often due to a solitary adenoma (80% to 85% of cases), less frequently (about 15%) due to chief cell hyperplasia involving all glands, and rarely due to parathyroid carcinoma (<1%).

Greater than 80% of hyperparathyroid patients are relatively free of symptoms on presentation because of the early detection of this disorder by the widespread use of chemistry panels, including calcium.[393] The most common signs and symptoms of hypercalcemia are nonspecific and related to the neuromuscular system. They include fatigue, malaise, and weakness with mild hypercalcemia (calcium <12 mg/dL); depression, apathy, and inability to concentrate may be present at higher concentrations. Hypercalcemia may induce mild nephrogenic diabetes insipidus with thirst, polydipsia, and polyuria. Renal colic caused by kidney stones can result from chronic hypercalcemia and hypercalciuria. Nephrocalcinosis can lead to slowly developing renal failure. Osteoporosis is more common than osteitis fibrosa. The majority of patients with primary hyperparathyroidism (>60%) are postmenopausal women.

Primary hyperparathyroidism is diagnosed by laboratory studies. Hypercalcemia should be documented by measuring total calcium and serum albumin, or ideally free calcium, on more than one occasion before initiating further testing. Measurement of intact PTH (with concomitant measurement of calcium) is the most sensitive and specific test for parathyroid function and is central to the differential diagnosis of hypercalcemia. Serum $1,25(OH)_2D$ is usually in the upper half of the reference interval or increased in primary hyperparathyroidism, as PTH stimulates its production. By contrast, $1,25(OH)_2D$ (like PTH) is low-normal or suppressed in nonparathyroid hypercalcemia, except in sarcoidosis, other granulomatous diseases, and certain lymphomas in which the pathological tissues contain the 25-hydroxyvitamin D-1α-hydroxylase required to produce $1,25(OH)_2D$.

PTH increases the renal clearance of bicarbonate and phosphate. In hyperparathyroidism, a mild hyperchloremic metabolic acidosis may be observed whereas in nonparathyroid hypercalcemia, a mild hypochloremic metabolic alkalosis may be observed. Although hypophosphatemia is often seen in hyperparathyroidism, the measurement of serum phosphate is of limited value because hypophosphatemia is also found in hypercalcemic cancer patients.

Patients with primary hyperparathyroidism with signs or symptoms of hypercalcemia should undergo parathyroid surgery. If the patient is asymptomatic, guidelines have been established recommending surgery over monitoring depending on the serum calcium concentration, creatinine clearance, urine calcium, and bone density.[42]

Hypercalcemia occurs in 10% to 20% of individuals with cancer. Tumors most commonly cause hypercalcemia by producing PTHrP, which is secreted into the circulation and stimulates bone resorptions and/or by invasion of the bone by metastatic tumor, which produces local factors that stimulate bone resorption. PTHrP binds to the PTH receptor and is the principal mediator of humoral hypercalcemia of malignancy (HHM). Cytokines such as lymphotoxin, interleukin-1, tumor necrosis factor, and PTHrP appear to be important mediators of hypercalcemia in multiple myeloma and other hematological malignancies. Some lymphomas associated with acquired immunodeficiency syndrome or HTLV I infections cause hypercalcemia by producing $1,25(OH)_2D$. It is estimated that 5% of patients with hypercalcemic cancer have coexisting primary hyperparathyroidism.

Signs and symptoms of hypercalcemia are often evident in patients with hypercalcemia due to malignancy, because the serum calcium increases rapidly and often reaches concentrations higher than those usually seen in primary hyperparathyroidism. Lethargy, obtundation, nausea, and vomiting are additional symptoms.

Laboratory test selection is similar to that in suspected hyperparathyroidism, with the addition of PTHrP in some individuals with HHM. In specific instances (for example, lymphoma), measurement of $1,25(OH)_2D$ may be useful.

Therapies are directed toward treating the malignancy, decreasing the serum calcium concentration by saline diuresis, and decreasing osteoclastic resorption (bisphosphonates, calcitonin, etc.). Steroids are useful in reducing intestinal absorption of calcium in $1,25(OH)_2D$-mediated hypercalcemia.

Measurement of Calcium

The methods most widely used for quantifying calcium measure either free (ionized) calcium or total calcium. The term *ionized calcium* is a misnomer because all plasma or serum calcium is ionized whether or not it is associated with protein or small anions by ionic binding. Throughout this chapter, we use the term *free calcium*, analogous to free hormones (e.g., free thyroxine or free testosterone).

Free calcium is considered the best indicator of calcium status, because it is biologically active and tightly regulated by PTH and $1,25(OH)_2D$. Although the measurement of free calcium is clinically more useful, it has not replaced the measurement of total calcium. Although an ion-specified electrode (ISE) method is available on large chemistry analyzers from one manufacturer, the ISE has not been implemented in a way to measure free calcium. Nonetheless, free calcium determinations have assumed increasing importance, because of the availability of improved analyzers (that typically measure free calcium, other electrolytes, blood gases, hemoglobin, and glucose) and more convenient methods for specimen handling. They are recommended for all requests for calcium apart from chemistry panels, because of the consequences of delayed treatment and the cost of working-up patients with misleading total calcium results.[67]

Adjusted or Corrected Total Calcium

The recognition that serum proteins, particularly albumin, and organic and inorganic ions affect total calcium concentrations has resulted in the concept of adjusting or correcting serum total calcium concentrations. Although various calculations have been proposed for adjusting total calcium results to correct for alterations in total protein, albumin, globulin, pH, anion gap, bicarbonate, and other calcium-complexing ions,[283,409] only adjustments based on albumin are widely used. The term "adjusted calcium" may be preferable to the more widely used "corrected calcium," because "corrected" may suggest the result has been corrected because of an error.

Adjusted calcium is calculated from total calcium and albumin by first calculating a correction factor by multiplying the deviation of plasma albumin from the mean of its reference interval by the slope of the regression of total calcium against albumin. The following equation is often seen in textbooks, but fails to consider the lack of harmonization of albumin and calcium methods, and differences in patient populations:

$$\text{Corrected total calcium (mg/dL)} = \text{Total calcium (mg/dL)} + 0.8(4 - \text{albumin [g/dL]})$$

Evidence suggests that it is inappropriate to adjust calcium data in one laboratory with equations derived in other laboratories.[20,283] Laboratories can establish their own equations for correcting total calcium by determining the slope of the regression of total calcium against albumin and the mean of their albumin reference interval in selected or unselected groups of patients and normal persons.[20,283,533,562,602] This is especially important if the laboratory is reporting corrected calcium, a practice that may be more common outside the United States. Because regression equations vary between individuals and among groups of patients in different physiological and pathological states,

BOX 49-3 Factors Altering the Distribution Between Protein-Bound, Complexed, and Free Calcium and Compounding the Interpretation of Total Calcium

Factors Altering Protein Binding of Calcium
- Altered concentration of albumin or globulins
- Abnormal proteins
- Heparin
- pH
- Free fatty acids
- Bilirubin
- Drugs
- Temperature

Factors Altering Complex Formation
- Citrate
- Bicarbonate
- Lactate
- Phosphate
- Pyruvate and β-hydroxybutyrate
- Sulfate
- Anion gap

mathematical corrections are only approximations. Some factors complicating the interpretation of total calcium and limiting the effectiveness of these equations are pH effects on calcium binding to protein, variation in binding kinetics, free and albumin-bound fatty acids,[621] substances and drugs that are bound by albumin, unusual quantities or types of serum proteins, heparin, and anions complexing calcium (Box 49-3).

Corrections have been applied with some success in patients who have liver disease and low concentrations of protein, but less successfully in patients with renal failure.[297] Their value in hypercalcemia and in specimens with increased proteins because of venous occlusion has been questioned.[283] Several studies have questioned the value of adjusting total calcium values,[319,533,562,602] and one[319] showed that adjusted calcium results were no better than total calcium in predicting free calcium. Equations that are derived for a specific patient group, such as patients with liver disease, may be better than no correction in that group of patients.

When possible, mathematical adjustments or corrections should be replaced by direct determination of free calcium by ISE.

Measurement of Total Calcium

Many methods have been used historically to measure total calcium.[7,252,283,469,597] Today, only photometric, ISE, and occasionally atomic absorption spectrophotometry methods are routinely used by clinical laboratories for the measurement of serum and urine total calcium. According to the College of American Pathologists Comprehensive Chemistry Survey, in 2004 approximately 79% of participating clinical laboratories used photometric methods (35% arsenazo III and 44% cresolphthalein complexone) and 20% of laboratories used ISE methods for total serum calcium.

ISEs for the measurement of total calcium were introduced more recently than photometric methods. The specimen is acidified to convert protein-bound and complexed calcium to free calcium before measurement of calcium by ISE. Calcium ISEs are discussed later in this chapter.

Photometric and atomic absorption spectrophotometric methods for measuring the total calcium in serum and plasma are described and discussed below.

Photometric Methods

Total calcium is most frequently measured by spectrophotometry using metallochromic indicators or dyes. Of the metallochromic indicators that change color on selectively binding calcium, *o*-cresolphthalein complexone (CPC) (3′,3″-bis[[bis-(carboxymethyl)amino]-methyl]-5′,5″-dimethylphenolphthalein) (Figure 49-3) and arsenazo III are most widely used. These methods, although less accurate and reproducible than atomic absorption spectrophotometry, have been easier to automate on chemistry analyzers.

o-Cresolphthalein Complexone Method. In alkaline solution, the metal-complexing dye CPC forms a red chromophore with calcium, which is usually measured at a wavelength between 570 and 580 nm.[118,220,299,347,539] The sample is diluted with acid to release protein-bound and complexed calcium. Organic base, most often diethylamine, 2-amino-2-methyl-1-propanol, or 2-ethylaminoethanol, is added to buffer the reaction and to produce an alkaline pH.[185,384] Interference by magnesium ions can be reduced by (1) the addition of 8-hydroxyquinoline (see Figure 49-3); buffering the reaction mixture to near pH 12; and (3) measurement of the absorbance near 580 nm.[118,220,592] Urea may be added to reduce the turbidity of lipemic specimens and enhance complex formation.[220,299] The use of cyanide has been questioned.[107,159] Ethanol or other organic solvents may be included to reduce blank absorbance.[347] Calcium forms both 1:1 and 2:1 complexes with CPC, with the 1:1 complex predominating at lower concentrations.[122] Because the 1:1 complex has a lower molar absorptivity, calibration curves are nonlinear at low calcium concentrations. Multipoint calibration of CPC methods has been recommended. Linearity may be improved by adding sodium acetate.[124] Temperature is carefully controlled, because the reaction is temperature-sensitive.

Arsenazo III Method. Arsenazo III (1,8-dihydroxynaphthalene-3,6-disulfonic acid-2,7-bis[azo-2]-phenylarsonic acid)* (see Figure 49-3), at mildly acidic pH, has much higher affinity for calcium than magnesium. A reaction pH of about 6 is commonly used. Imidazole has been used to buffer the reaction. The solution must be thoroughly

*References 29, 326, 378, 386, 417, 504.

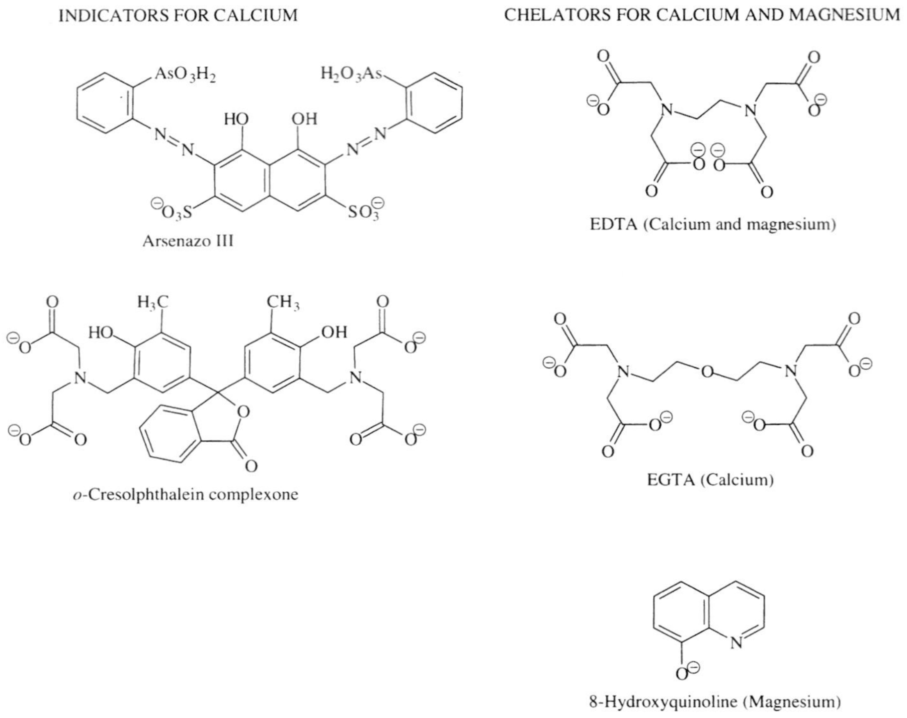

INDICATORS FOR CALCIUM

Arsenazo III

o-Cresolphthalein complexone

CHELATORS FOR CALCIUM AND MAGNESIUM

EDTA (Calcium and magnesium)

EGTA (Calcium)

8-Hydroxyquinoline (Magnesium)

Figure 49-3 Metallochromic indicators for calcium and chelators for calcium and magnesium.

buffered, because the spectral properties of arsenazo III are dependent on pH. Binding of calcium to arsenazo III can be influenced by buffer and sodium concentration.[29] Interference from most biological pigments is reduced by measuring the calcium-dye complex near 650 nm. Citrate has been reported to cause negative interference with the Vitros dry-slide technique.[33,214] Clinically significant interference may be noted in patients receiving citrated blood or blood products. Unlike CPC, a reagent that has limited stability when used as a single reagent, arsenazo III reagent is stable.

Atomic Absorption Spectrometry Methods

The National Committee for Clinical Laboratory Standards (NCCLS) has approved a method using atomic absorption spectrophotometry (AAS) as a reference method for measuring total serum calcium.[398] This method has been compared with isotope dilution-mass spectrometry (ID-MS), the definitive method for total serum calcium developed by the National Institute of Standards and Technology. The reference method is reported to have an accuracy of 100 ± 2%, compared with 100 ± 0.2% for ID-MS.[93] Although AAS can provide better accuracy and precision for total serum calcium than the widely used photometric methods, it is used by only a few laboratories. It should continue to be used for validating new total calcium methods.

In this method, the specimen is first diluted 1 to 50 with a solution of lanthanum-HCl ($LaCl_3$, 10 mmol/L; HCl, 50 mmol/L) and then aspirated into an air-acetylene flame, where the ground state calcium atoms absorb incident light from a calcium hollow-cathode lamp (422.7 nm). The amount of light absorbed is measured by a phototube or detector after the 422.7-nm resonance line is isolated with the monochromator. Absorbance is directly proportional to the number of ground state calcium atoms in the flame. Detailed procedures[68,93,446,598] for the determination of total calcium in serum and reviews[68,469] of this method have been published.

Dilution with lanthanum-HCl reduces interference from protein, phosphate, citrate, sulfate, and other anions. Phosphate causes the greatest interference because calcium-phosphate complexes are not dissociated readily by the air-acetylene flame. Lanthanum-HCl dissociates complexes, ensuring that all fractions of calcium (free, protein-bound, and complexed) are measured. Dilution effectively reduces the viscosity, which can also interfere by reducing the aspiration rate and atomization of the specimen.

The effect of the three major cations, Na^+, K^+, and Mg^{2+}, is offset by their inclusion in calibrators at normal serum concentrations. An automated diluter is recommended because the imprecision (expressed as the coefficient of variation [CV]) for measurements of total calcium should be less than 1.5% and preferably less than 1%. A serum-based calibrator with calcium concentration determined by ID-MS is available commercially.

Strontium may be included in the diluent to be used as an internal standard with double-beam spectrophotometers.[446] The signal from calcium is referenced to the simultaneously measured strontium signal, thereby reducing variability caused by fluctuations in the flame and atomization rate.

Specimen Requirements

Serum and heparinized plasma are the preferred specimens. Citrate, oxalate, and ethylene diamine tetraacetic acid (EDTA) anticoagulants should not be used for the spectrophotometric methods, because they interfere by forming complexes with calcium. Total calcium measurements are not affected by storage provided the loss of water associated with prolonged refrigerator or freezer storage is prevented (by use of tightly capped containers designed for such storage). Co-precipitation of calcium with fibrin (for example, in heparinized plasma) or lipids has been reported with storage or freezing.[112,223] Plastic[238] and glass may adsorb calcium from dilute solutions during storage.

Interferences

Hemolysis, icterus, lipemia,[221,222] paraproteins, and magnesium have been reported to interfere either positively or negatively with photometric methods. Many methods use bichromatic analysis or multiwavelength corrections, or blanking to reduce interference. Lipemic specimens should be ultracentrifuged before analysis. Although hemolysis can cause a negative error because red blood cells contain lower concentrations of calcium than does serum, more significant errors may be caused by the spectral interference of hemoglobin. Depending on the method, hemoglobin has been reported to produce either negative or positive interference.[103,121] In photometric methods, if hemolyzed specimens must be analyzed, blanking with ethylene glycol-*O,O′*-bis(2-aminoethyl)-*N,N,N′,N′*-tetraacetic acid (EGTA)-treated serum is suggested. Individual instruments and methods should be evaluated for their susceptibility to interference from magnesium, hemoglobin, bilirubin, turbidity, and other interferents.

Care should be taken in handling specimens, calibrators, and solutions to prevent contamination with calcium. Any glassware or plastic ware that is reused should be washed with dilute hydrochloric acid (HCl), followed by distilled water, to eliminate calcium contamination. Corks should not be used because they can contaminate specimens with calcium.[532]

How the patient is prepared and the specimen is obtained can have a significant effect on both free and total calcium measurements. For information on these preanalytical effects, the reader is directed to a later section in this chapter on the subject and to Box 49-4.

BOX 49-4 Preanalytical Factors in Measurement of Serum Total or Free Calcium

In Vivo

Tourniquet use and venous occlusion
Changes in posture: 10% to 12% increase of total calcium and 5% to 6% increase of free calcium on standing
Exercise
Hyperventilation
Fist clenching
Alimentary status
Alterations in protein binding (see Box 49-3)
Alterations in complex formation (see Box 49-3)

In Vitro

Inappropriate anticoagulants
Dilution with liquid heparin
Interfering levels of heparin
Contamination with calcium
- Corks, glassware, tubes

Specimen handling
- Alterations in pH (free calcium)
- Adsorption or precipitation of calcium

Spectrophotometric interference
- Hemolysis, icterus, lipemia

Measurement of Free (Ionized) Calcium (See also Chapter 27.)

Analyzers using ISEs capable of providing immediate whole-blood determinations of free calcium, electrolytes, and blood gases are now widely available.* The free calcium analyzer consists of a system of pumps under microprocessor control that transport calibration solutions, samples, and wash solutions through a measuring cell containing calcium ion-selective, reference, and pH electrodes. Sensitive potentiometers measure the voltage difference between the calcium or pH and reference electrodes for calibrating solutions or samples. A microprocessor calibrates the system and calculates calcium concentration and pH. Most instruments simultaneously measure the actual free calcium and pH at 37 °C.

Calcium ISEs contain a calcium-selective membrane, which encloses an inner reference solution of calcium chloride often containing saturated silver chloride (AgCl) and physiological concentrations of sodium chloride and potassium chloride (KCl) and an internal reference electrode.* The reference electrode, usually of Ag/AgCl, is immersed in this inner reference solution.

Modern calcium ISEs use liquid membranes containing the ion-selective calcium sensor dissolved in an organic liquid trapped in a polymeric matrix. Neutral carriers (for example, ETH 1001) are the most commonly used calcium sensors, followed by ion exchangers, such as organophosphate sensors (Figure 49-4). Neutral carrier membranes contain an uncharged calcium-selective organic molecule, such as ETH 1001, dissolved in a plasticizer and trapped in a polyvinyl chloride membrane. These molecules have a favorable stearic and electrostatic pocket or site for selectively binding calcium. Ion exchangers or negatively

*References 67, 81, 230, 469, 515, 559, 567.

*References 67, 81, 332, 416, 469, 559, 567.

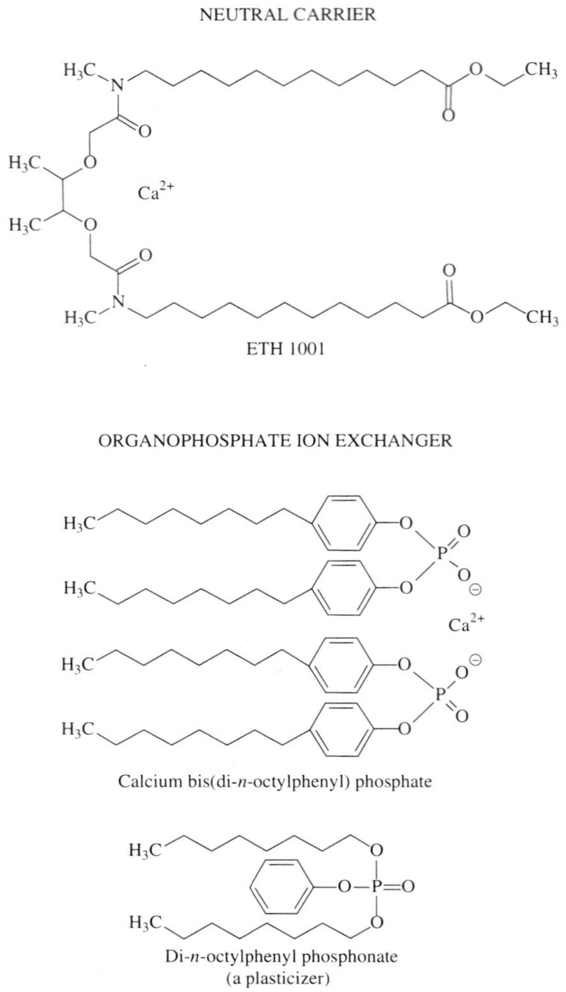

NEUTRAL CARRIER

ETH 1001

ORGANOPHOSPHATE ION EXCHANGER

Calcium bis(di-*n*-octylphenyl) phosphate

Di-*n*-octylphenyl phosphonate
(a plasticizer)

Figure 49-4 Free calcium sensors.

charged carrier membranes are calcium salts, usually calcium bis(di-*n*-octylphenyl) phosphate dissolved in di-*n*-octylphenyl phosphonate and trapped in a polyvinyl chloride membrane.

The electrochemical cell is completed by the external reference electrode, an Ag/AgCl or calomel electrode, which is in contact with the specimen by a liquid/liquid junction or salt bridge of KCl or sodium formate. The potential difference across the cell is logarithmically related to the activity of free calcium ions in the sample by Nernst's equation. By convention, free calcium is converted from activity to concentration with its activity coefficient, which is itself dependent on ionic strength.

Temperature affects electrode response and the extent of calcium binding by protein and small anions. Most free calcium analyzers adjust and maintain samples at 37 °C, thereby ensuring that results are physiologically relevant for the majority of patients.

Carryover has been minimized with the use of flush solutions containing 5.0 mg/dL (1.25 mmol/L) of free calcium, by using the leading edge of the specimen to clean the fluid path, or by purging with air.[81] Significant carryover is noted only at extremely low or high concentrations of free calcium.

The International Federation of Clinical Chemistry and Laboratory Medicine (IFCC) has recommended a reference method for free calcium.[85]

Interferences

Because ISEs measure ion activity, they are affected by the ionic strength of a specimen. Free calcium analyzers and calibrators are optimized for specimens of serum, plasma, or whole blood. Because the ionic strength of these fluids is primarily a result of Na^+ and Cl^-, calibrators are usually prepared in buffer and NaCl with a final ionic strength of 160 mmol/kg.[56,81,123,515] Although the range of Na^+ and Cl^- concentrations usually observed in serum or plasma does not cause a clinically significant error in the measurement of free calcium, significant errors can occur with other specimens unless the matrices and ionic strength of the calibrators and samples are matched closely.

Modern electrodes have a high selectivity for calcium over Na^+, K^+, Mg^{2+}, H^+, and Li^+.[81,567] At normal concentrations, these cations have little effect on the accuracy of free calcium measurements. Wide variations in the concentration of Na^+ and high concentrations of Mg^{2+} and Li^+ may influence the apparent concentration of free calcium. Electrodes are quite insensitive to H^+, with insignificant interference between pH 5 and 9.

Many physiological anions, including protein, phosphate, citrate, lactate, sulfate, and oxalate, form complexes with calcium ions. Although these anions reduce the concentration of free calcium by complex formation, they do not directly interfere with the measurement of the calcium that is free. Protein deposits on the electrode may act as a divalent cation exchanger, resulting in positive interference with high concentrations of Mg^+.[81] Older electrodes were sensitive to the concentration of protein in the sample. The newer electrodes use a dialysis membrane or neutral carrier to reduce or eliminate this protein effect.[81,370,416,428,559] Investigators disagree about whether the relationship between free calcium and protein concentration is a consequence of Donnan's equilibrium or a protein effect. With current electrodes, the effect is less than +0.02 mmol/L for 1 g/dL (10 g/L) of protein. Regular instrument maintenance and protein removal are reported to minimize this interference.

Chemicals may interfere in the measurement of free calcium. Anionic surfactants and ethanol have been reported to affect the calcium-selective membrane.

Effect of pH

The binding of calcium by protein and small anions is influenced by pH in vitro and in vivo.[81,559] Albumin, with up to 30 binding sites for calcium,[189,314] accounts for approximately 80% of the protein-bound calcium. Increasing the pH of a specimen in vitro increases the ionization and negative charge on albumin and other proteins, leading to an increase

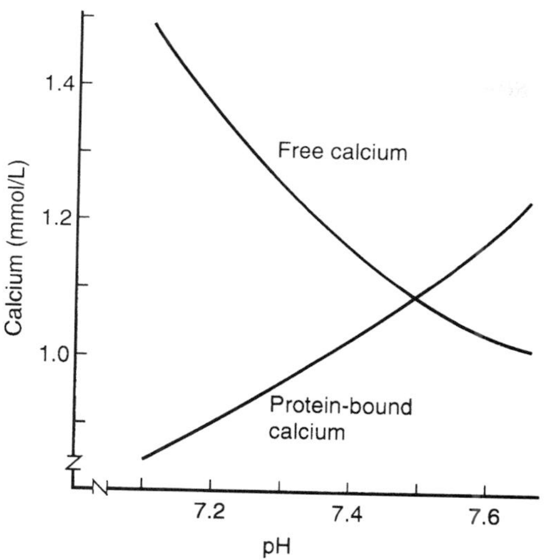

Figure 49-5 Effect of pH on free and protein-bound calcium.

in protein-bound calcium and a decrease in free calcium. Decreasing pH in vitro decreases ionization and negative charge, decreasing protein-bound calcium and increasing free calcium. Free calcium changes by about 5% for each 0.1-unit change in pH (Figure 49-5).

Because of this inverse relationship between free calcium and pH, specimens must be analyzed at the patient's pH in vivo, requiring that all specimens be handled to prevent alterations in pH.

Specimen Requirements

Preanalytical considerations, including specimen collection and handling, are particularly important for free calcium. Specimens for free calcium must be collected and handled to minimize alterations in pH and free calcium by (1) loss of CO_2 and (2) metabolism by blood cells. Free calcium may be measured in heparinized whole blood, heparinized plasma, or serum. For the majority of laboratories in which specimens are analyzed within minutes of sampling using blood gas analyzers, heparinized whole blood is preferable since it reduces processing time and the required specimen volume and avoids the alteration in pH associated with centrifugation. All syringes and evacuated tubes should be filled completely, kept tightly sealed, and handled anaerobically to prevent the loss of CO_2 and the increase in pH that occurs when specimens are exposed to air. Specimens should also be handled to prevent a decrease in pH caused by the production of lactic acid by glycolysis, by erythrocytes, and by white blood cells. The NCCLS has published guidelines for free calcium specimen collection and handling.[400]

Ideally, whole blood specimens should be analyzed within 15 to 30 minutes of sampling, although free calcium is reported to be stable in whole blood specimens for at least 1 hour at room temperature and for 4 hours at 4 °C.* If specimens cannot be analyzed within minutes, they can be collected in an ice-water slurry to minimize metabolism, but plasma K^+ concentrations may be significantly increased because of the inhibition of ATPase. One study[187] reported that K^+ was significantly increased after 1 hour at 4 °C, the earliest time investigated; no change was apparent for any other analytes for as long as 2 hours at 4 °C.

If analysis cannot be completed within 30 to 60 minutes at room temperature, then serum may be the optimal specimen because of elimination of the anticoagulant and microclots and its greater stability. Serum specimens should be collected in evacuated gel tubes.[324,570] The tubes should be filled completely and centrifuged to form an effective barrier between the serum and the clot with its cellular elements. Once centrifuged, specimens are stable for hours at 25 °C and for days at 4 °C, provided the tube remains sealed. Free calcium has been reported to be less stable in specimens from both acidotic and nonacidotic patients with uremia.[408]

The practice of using aerobic specimens for the measurement of free calcium should be abandoned because of the widespread availability of blood gas analyzers measuring free calcium and the use of evacuated gel tubes by reference laboratories. In the past, specialized free calcium analyzers equilibrated aerobic specimens with a carbon dioxide (5.3 kPa) air mixture to adjust their pH to near 7.4 (7.2-7.6), and then mathematically corrected the free calcium to pH 7.4, using an algorithm relating free calcium and pH.[81,188,559] In the event that aerobic free calcium results are corrected to pH 7.4 after equilibration with a mixture of CO_2 and air, only the free calcium at pH 7.4 should be reported with appropriate identification. The normalized or adjusted free calcium at pH 7.4 has been reported to accurately reflect the free calcium status of normal persons and individuals without acid-base disturbances.[81,559,561] However, aerobic handling of specimens with correction of the free calcium to pH 7.4 has been increasingly criticized.[81,494,558,594] The free calcium value at pH 7.4 may be misleading in patients with respiratory and metabolic alkalosis or acidosis.[408] Furthermore, aerobic handling of specimens has been associated with irreversible precipitation of calcium-phosphate complexes and a decrease in free calcium in some specimens having a high total calcium and phosphate content or a high pH (pH > 7.9).[559]

Effects of Anticoagulants

Because citrate, oxalate, and EDTA bind calcium and significantly reduce free calcium, heparin is the only acceptable anticoagulant for free calcium determinations. However, heparin, a polyanion, significantly lowers free calcium at the concentrations (30 to 100 U/mL or more) found in many conventional blood gas syringes (Table 49-3).[86,402,495,496,567] In addition, the use of liquid heparin should be avoided; it can result in errors in free calcium because of dilution, as well as high and variable concentrations of heparin.

A number of commercially available syringes containing lyophilized heparin are suitable for free calcium-determinations: (1) electrolyte-balanced or calcium-titrated heparin

*References 57, 81, 498, 559, 560, 570.

TABLE 49-3 Effect of Heparin on Free Calcium

Specimen	Heparin (U/mL)	Free Calcium (mg/dL)	(mmol/L)
Serum	0	5.00	1.25
Plasma	44 (Ca-heparin)	4.96	1.24
Plasma	29 (Na-heparin)	4.84	1.21
Plasma	100 (Na-heparin)	3.76	0.94
Whole blood	44 (Ca-heparin)	5.08	1.27
Whole blood	19 (Na-heparin)	5.04	1.26
Whole blood	100 (Na-heparin)	3.88	0.97

Modified from Toffaletti J. Ionized calcium. In: Pesce AJ, Kaplan LA, eds. Methods in clinical chemistry. St. Louis: CV Mosby, 1987:1010-20.

syringes (final concentration of 40 to 50 U/mL); (2) very low heparin syringes with heparin in an inert filler, providing a final heparin concentration of 2 to 3 U/mL; and (3) lithium-zinc heparin syringes.[572] With electrolyte-balanced or calcium-titrated heparin syringes, the heparin is titrated with calcium so that the free calcium is not significantly altered over most observed concentrations (3.6 to 6.4 mg/dL [0.9 to 1.6 mmol/L]); however, some bias may be apparent at very low and high free calcium concentrations. Electrolyte-balanced heparin may also produce a bias in specimens with pathologically low protein concentrations.[350] In the very low heparin syringes that contain 2 to 3 U/mL of heparin dispersed in a puff of inert proprietary material, the puff allows the heparin to be accurately dispensed during manufacturing and rapidly dissolve with proper mixing, providing effective anticoagulation. A blend of lithium and zinc heparins has been reported to eliminate the heparin interference in free calcium measurements.[322,548,574] In addition, lithium-zinc heparin did not alter total calcium, unlike electrolyte-balanced or calcium-titrated heparin. Three-milliliter syringes containing a total of 50 U of a 1:1 blend of lithium and zinc heparins did not alter results of any general chemistry tests except total magnesium, which was increased by 0.19 mg/dL (0.08 mmol/L). In no instance should the individuals obtaining the blood specimen add additional liquid heparin to heparinized syringes.

Most evacuated collection tubes, when filled completely, contain concentrations of heparin (15 U/mL) that only slightly decrease free calcium.[568] Specific brands of syringes, evacuated tubes, and heparin should be carefully evaluated. It is important that all syringes and tubes be filled completely to minimize dilution and/or heparin effects.

Calibrators and Quality Controls

Various calibration solutions are used by manufacturers for free calcium analyzers. The buffers in which these calibrations are prepared may have an effect on the liquid junction potential and calcium binding; however, it is usually corrected for by the instrument software.[81] Until reference solutions are available, it is best to use the calibrators provided by the instrument manufacturer.

Aqueous quality control materials are commercially available for free calcium. Because simple aqueous controls may not reliably detect changes in performance with patient specimens, serum-based quality control materials should be used daily.[198,573] Serum-based controls may be prepared by acidifying serum with 10 μL of 1 mol/L HCl and leaving it exposed in the refrigerator for 1 week to remove carbon dioxide. The pH is then adjusted to 7.4, and the serum is aliquoted and frozen. Alternatively, serum-based controls can be equilibrated with carbon dioxide before their analysis.

Patient Preparation and Sources of Preanalytical Error for Total and Free Calcium Measurements

Patient preparation and the manner of specimen collection can significantly alter the results of total and free calcium determinations (see Box 49-4).[81,230,469,498,559]

A common and important source of preanalytical error in the measurement of calcium is the increase in total, but not free, calcium concentration associated with tourniquet use and venous occlusion during sampling.[461,469] Errors of 0.5 to 1.0 mg/dL (0.12 to 0.25 mmol/L) in total calcium may result because of the increase in protein-bound calcium caused by the efflux of water from the vascular compartment during stasis. Only small and clinically insignificant increases in free calcium have been reported with venous stasis. If a tourniquet is required, it should be applied just before sampling and released as soon as possible.

Fist clenching or other forearm exercise should be avoided before phlebotomy, because forearm exercise causes a decrease in pH (lactic acid production) and an increase in free calcium. The NCCLS and IFCC have published recommendations on blood collection.[86,399]

Changes in posture cause fluid shifts within 10 minutes and thus alter the concentration of cells and large molecules, including albumin and total calcium (as part of it is protein-bound) in the vascular compartment. Standing decreases intravascular water and increases the total calcium concentration by 0.2 to 0.8 mg/dL (0.05 to 0.20 mmol/L), whereas a much smaller effect has been reported for free calcium.* One partial explanation (along with hypoalbuminemia) for the mild hypocalcemia observed in many hospital patients may be the hemodilution associated with recumbency.

Most other preanalytical factors are less likely to lead to confusion. Prolonged immobilization and bed rest[250,540] can decrease bone density and increase total and free calcium. Hyperventilation and exercise decrease and increase the concentration of free calcium, respectively, because of changes in serum pH.[81,461,469] Both serum free calcium and calcium excretion are lower during the night.[95] Food ingestion has been reported to have various effects, but usually causes a mild increase in serum calcium. Ingestion of calcium salts may increase serum calcium. Hemolysis can alter free calcium because of dilution and alterations in pH and binding (see previous discussion under Interferences). Prolonged contact with blood cells may decrease plasma calcium.

Reference Intervals for Total and Free Calcium in Serum and Plasma

Total Calcium

The reference interval for serum and plasma is usually defined by an upper limit of 10.1 to 10.3 mg/dL (2.54 to 2.57 mmol/L) and a lower limit between 8.6 and 8.8 mg/dL (2.15 to 2.20 mmol/L). Although higher upper limits of 10.5 to 11.0 mg/dL (2.62 to 2.74 mmol/L) have been used by some laboratories, it is now appreciated that these concentrations are inappropriately high.[283]

Adults: 8.6 to 10.2 mg/dL (2.15 to 2.55 mmol/L)

An analytical goal, or quality specification, for between-day imprecision, expressed as the CV, is 0.9% or less based on within-person biological variation.[192] Current methods are capable of achieving a between-day CV of 1.5% or less.

Free Calcium

The reference interval established by the author at LAC+USC Medical Center using whole blood is representative of free calcium reference intervals:

Adults: 4.6 to 5.3 mg/dL (1.15 to 1.33 mmol/L).

Because of the dependence of free calcium on pH, it is recommended that pH be measured and reported with all free calcium determinations. This will assist the laboratory and physician in identifying specimens in which inappropriate preanalytical handling has led to an in vitro change in pH. Correction of the free calcium to pH 7.4 may be inappropriate and confusing to the physician.

Whole blood specimens develop a liquid-junction potential different from that of serum or plasma because of the presence of erythrocytes.[81,416,559] A positive bias that is directly proportional to the hematocrit has been reported. In addition, free calcium values have been reported to differ among capillary blood, venous blood, and serum samples because of differences in pH. Therefore, reference intervals should be determined by each laboratory using the local instrument, specimen type, and collection protocol and reference subjects representative of their patient population.

Physiological Variation in Calcium

Calcium has been reported to vary with age, gender, and season and during pregnancy.[469] Total and free calcium have been reported both to decline modestly and to remain unchanged in the elderly.[522] We were unable to find an age-related decline or a gender-related difference in either total or free calcium values in a healthy ambulatory group of men and women residing in the Southwest.[171] During pregnancy, the total calcium declines in parallel with serum albumin, whereas free calcium is unchanged.[132,434] The fetal circulation is relatively hypercalcemic, as evidenced by higher total and free calcium in cord blood than in maternal serum. Calcium concentrations decline after birth in healthy term neonates during the first few days, but soon rise to concentrations slightly greater than those observed in adults.[89,349,484,593]

Interpretation of Total and Free Calcium Results

Calcium status is more accurately determined by measuring free calcium, the tightly regulated, biologically active species.* Interpretation of total serum calcium value is complicated by its association with protein and inorganic and organic ions.[230,283,469] Interpretation of free calcium concentration is less complicated, provided the specimen has been properly obtained, handled, and analyzed. Disagreement between free and total calcium (abnormal total calcium and normal free calcium, or vice versa) values occurs in a high percentage of specimens.[319,533,562,602] One study[562] of 1213 patients suspected of having calcium disorders found disagreement between free calcium and total calcium or corrected calcium values in 18% and 31% of patients, respectively.

Free calcium is far more useful than total calcium determination in hospital patients, especially those undergoing major surgery (Figure 49-6) who have received citrated blood or platelets, heparin, bicarbonate, intravenous solutions, or calcium.† Alterations in blood pH and temperature further reduce the usefulness of total calcium assay in these patients. Rapid measurement of free calcium, blood gases, and potassium permits maintenance of good cardiac function during liver transplant operations and other major operations such as those in which cardiopulmonary bypass is used. Free calcium is more useful than total calcium determination in patients in intensive care because of abnormal protein concentrations and putative circulating factors that alter calcium binding to albumin. Abnormally low free calcium is frequently found in critically ill patients.[25,99,620] A study at one hospital[67] where free calcium has replaced total calcium determinations found that 41% of free calcium concentrations were abnormal in inpatients. Of these, 31% were

*References 81, 230, 275, 460, 469, 559.

*References 67, 87, 232, 311, 358, 567, 571.
†References 81, 87, 232, 283, 469, 559.

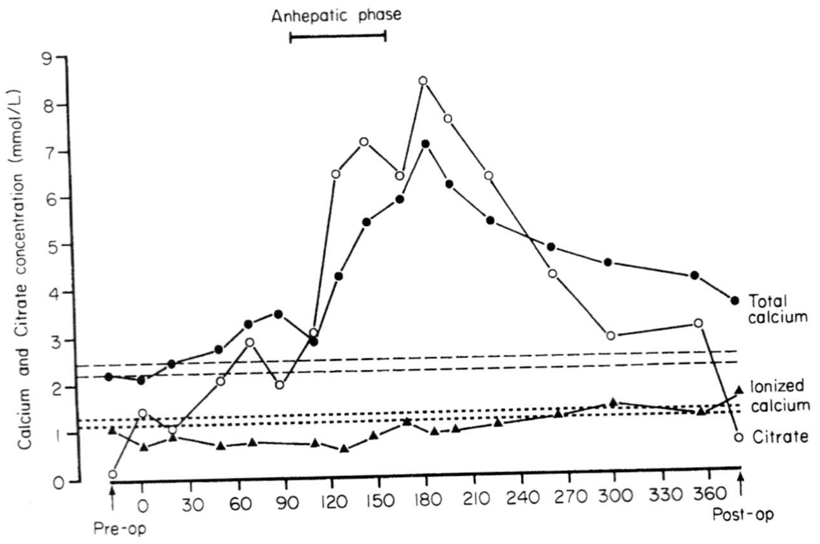

Figure 49-6 Free calcium (▲), total calcium (●), and citrate (○) concentration in a patient undergoing liver transplantation. The reference intervals are indicated by the upper (total calcium) and lower (free calcium) sets of dashed horizontal lines. The reference interval for citrate is 0.03 to 0.15 mmol/L. *(From Gray TA, Paterson CR. The clinical value of ionized calcium assays. Ann Clin Biochem 1988;25:210-9.)*

below and 10% were above the reference interval. The recovery room, surgical intensive care unit, renal transplantation ward, medical intensive care unit, and medical oncology unit had the highest percentages of abnormal values.

Bone and mineral disorders are common in patients with renal disease. Therapy and calcium metabolism of these patients are best evaluated with the determination of free calcium because of alterations in protein, pH, protein binding of calcium, and calcium complexes with organic and inorganic anions. Total and adjusted calcium concentrations are often invalid when compared with free calcium measurements.[87,88,155,297]

Free calcium has proved to be more useful than total calcium in the diagnosis of hypercalcemia.[69,320,323,376] Patients with subsequently surgically proven primary hyperparathyroidism more often have increases of free calcium than of total calcium (Figure 49-7). Free calcium is more sensitive than total calcium in detecting hypercalcemia associated with malignancy, as may be expected in patients who frequently have decreased serum albumin. Less commonly, paraproteins produced in myeloma may bind calcium, complicating the interpretation of total or corrected calcium measurements.

In neonates, the assay of free calcium rather than total calcium is recommended because of its speed and the ability to use small capillary specimens, and because of its greater validity in the presence of hyperphosphatemia, alterations in pH, and the persistence of alpha fetoprotein after birth.[87,232,310,593]

Urinary Calcium

Normal men and women excrete up to 300 mg (7.49 mmol) of calcium per day on a diet with unrestricted calcium content and up to 200 mg/day (4.99 mmol/d) on a calcium-restricted diet (500 mg [12.48 mmol] dietary calcium per day or less for several days).

The reference interval for urinary calcium (UCa) for spot fasting or timed specimens collected after an overnight fast is less than 0.16 mg/100 mL (<0.04 mmol/L) of glomerular filtrate (GF), calculated by the following equation[74]:

$$\text{UCa (mg/100mL GF)} = \frac{(\text{UCa [mg/dL]}) \times (\text{Serum creatinine [mg/dL]})}{\text{Urinary creatinine (mg/dL)}}$$

The amount of calcium excreted into the urine reflects intestinal absorption, skeletal resorption, and renal tubular filtration and reabsorption.[74] Under fasting conditions, the intestinal and renal components are relatively fixed, and calcium excretion (milligrams per 100 mL of GF) in the fasting state is used to assess the skeletal component. A value exceeding 0.16 mg/100 mL (>0.04 mmol/L) of GF usually implies an increase in osteoclastic bone resorption. This test is useful in assessing renal stone disease and high-turnover osteoporosis.

Calcium salts, such as calcium oxalate, precipitate in urine specimens during and after collection. Specimens may be collected in a container containing acid to prevent calcium salt precipitation. A commonly used acid is HCl, 6 mol/L, with 20 to 30 mL added to the container for a 24-hour collection (1 to 2 mL for a random specimen). The safety of the patient and the patient's family in handling such a container may be a concern. The measured urinary calcium concentration must be corrected for the dilution by the acid solution when the urinary volume is low. The specimen should be kept well mixed during collection. Specimens collected without acid should be acidified and allowed to stand for 1 hour before thorough remixing and aliquoting. Some have questioned the ability of postcollection acidification to redissolve all of the calcium salts with or without heating.[230]

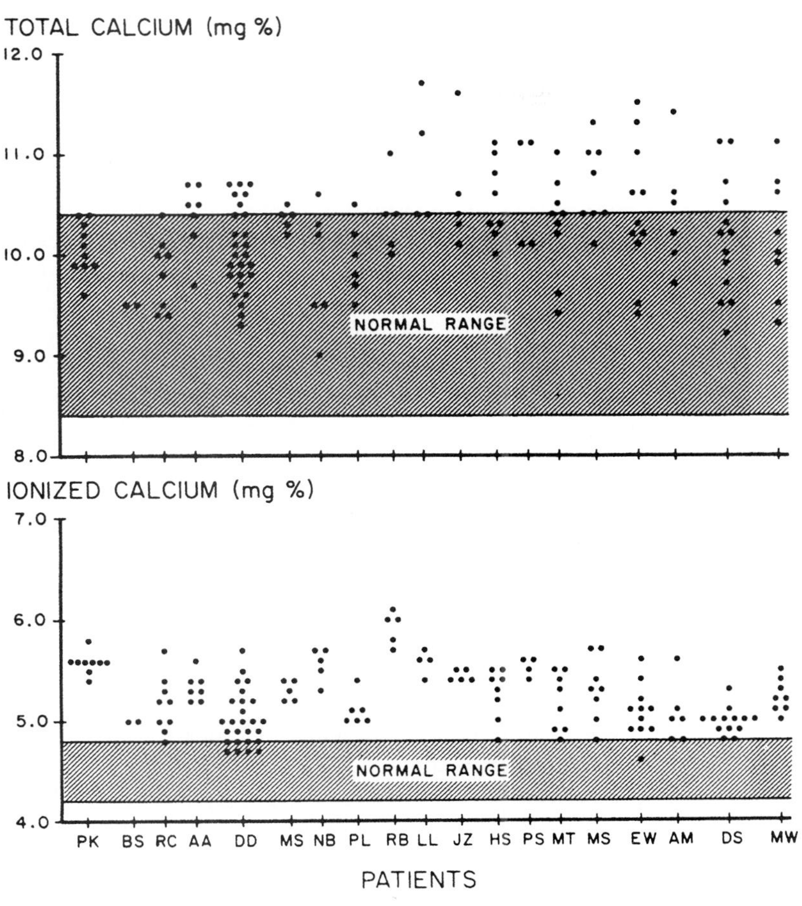

Figure 49-7 Concurrent total and free calcium in patients with primary hyperparathyroidism and intermittent total hypercalcemia. Shaded areas represent the normal reference intervals. *(From McLeod MK, Monchik JM, Martin HF. The role of ionized calcium in the diagnosis of subtle hypercalcemia in symptomatic primary hyperparathyroidism. Surgery 1984;95:667-73.)*

PHOSPHATE

An adult has approximately 600 g (19.4 mol) of phosphorus in inorganic and organic phosphates, of which about 85% is in the skeleton and the rest principally in soft tissue (see Table 49-1).[41,308]

Biochemistry and Physiology

Plasma contains both inorganic and organic phosphate, but only inorganic phosphate is measured. Inorganic phosphate exists as both the monovalent ($H_2PO_4^-$) and divalent (HPO_4^{2-}) phosphate anions. The ratio of $H_2PO_4^-$ to HPO_4^{2-} is pH-dependent and varies from approximately 1:1 in acidosis to 1:4 at pH 7.4 and 1:9 in alkalosis. Approximately 10% of the phosphate in serum is protein-bound; 35% complexed with sodium, calcium, and magnesium; and the remainder, or 55%, is free (see Table 49-2). The organic phosphate esters are located primarily within the cellular elements of blood.

Inorganic phosphate is a major component of hydroxyapatite in bone, thereby playing an important role in the structural support of the body and providing phosphate for the extracellular and intracellular pool.

In the soft tissue, most phosphate is cellular. Although both inorganic and organic phosphate are present in cells, most is organic and incorporated into nucleic acids, phospholipids, phosphoproteins, and "high-energy" compounds involved in metabolism.[618] ATP and other phosphates, such as creatine phosphate, are involved in many energy-intensive physiological functions, such as muscle contractility, neurological function, and electrolyte transport. Phosphate is also an essential element of cyclic nucleotides (such as cyclic AMP) and nicotinamide-adenine dinucleotide phosphate (NADP). It is important for the activity of several enzymes including adenylate cyclase, 25-hydroxyvitamin-D-1α-hydroxylase, and those involved in the production of 2,3-diphosphoglycerate (which regulates the oxygen affinity of hemoglobin). Intracellular phosphate is therefore involved in the regulation of intermediary metabolism of proteins, fats, and carbohydrates, and in gene transcription and cell growth.

Clinical Significance

Disorders of phosphate metabolism are separated into those causing hypophosphatemia and hyperphosphatemia.

Hypophosphatemia

Hypophosphatemia, defined as the concentration of inorganic phosphate in the serum below the normal reference

BOX 49-5 Common Causes of Hypophosphatemia and Phosphate Depletion

- Intracellular shift
  - Glucose
    - Oral or intravenous
    - Hyperalimentation
  - Insulin
  - Respiratory alkalosis
- Lowered renal phosphate threshold
  - Primary or secondary hyperparathyroidism
  - Renal tubular defects
    - Familial hypophosphatemia
    - Fanconi's syndrome
- Decreased net intestinal phosphate absorption
  - Increased loss
    - Vomiting
    - Diarrhea
    - Phosphate binding antacids
  - Decreased absorption
    - Malabsorption syndrome
    - Vitamin D deficiency
- Intracellular phosphate loss
  - Acidosis
    - Ketoacidosis
    - Lactic acidosis

interval, usually less than 2.5 mg/dL (<0.81 mmol/L), is relatively common in hospitalized patients (approximately 2%). Hypophosphatemia is not necessarily associated with intracellular phosphate depletion. Hypophosphatemia may be present when cellular concentrations are normal, and cellular phosphate depletion may exist when serum concentrations are normal or even high.

Hypophosphatemia or phosphate depletion may be caused by (1) a shift of phosphate from extracellular to intracellular spaces, (2) renal phosphate wasting, (3) decreased intestinal absorption, and (4) loss from intracellular phosphate.[308,618] Box 49-5 lists the commonly encountered causes of hypophosphatemia and phosphate depletion.

A shift of phosphate from extracellular fluid to intracellular fluid is a common cause of hypophosphatemia. A major etiology of low serum phosphate is carbohydrate-induced stimulation of insulin secretion, which increases the transport of glucose and phosphate into insulin-sensitive cells, where it is incorporated into sugar phosphates and ATP. Oral or intravenous carbohydrate and injected insulin decrease serum phosphate. Refeeding of malnourished individuals creates an anabolic state, causing an intracellular shift of phosphate. Respiratory alkalosis leads to an increase in intracellular pH, which activates phosphofructokinase and accelerates glycolysis, causing a shift of phosphate into the cell.

Renal phosphate wasting may also cause hypophosphatemia. Any cause of excessive PTH secretion (primary and secondary hyperparathyroidism) lowers the renal phosphate threshold and may result in hypophosphatemia and phosphate depletion. The renal phosphate threshold is also lowered in Fanconi's syndrome, X-linked hypophosphatemic rickets, and tumor-induced osteomalacia.

Hypophosphatemia and phosphate depletion may result from inadequate intestinal phosphate absorption. Patients taking aluminum- or magnesium-containing antacids may develop hypophosphatemia, because these antacids bind phosphate in the intestine, rendering it nonabsorbable. The hypophosphatemia observed in patients with malabsorption may be more closely related to their secondary hyperparathyroidism than to malabsorption of phosphate. Because phosphate is abundant in most foods, dietary deprivation is not usually a cause of phosphate depletion in patients with normal intestinal function and an adequate diet.

Intracellular phosphate may be lost in acidosis as a result of the catabolism of organic compounds within the cell. Diabetic ketoacidosis is associated initially with high-normal to increased serum phosphate. Treatment of the ketosis and acidosis with insulin and intravenous fluids, however, results in a rapid reduction in the serum phosphate concentration. Consequently, patients being treated for diabetic ketoacidosis may have both intracellular phosphate depletion and hypophosphatemia.

The clinical manifestations of serum phosphate depletion depend on the length and degree of the deficiency. Moderate hypophosphatemia of 1.5 to 2.4 mg/dL (0.48 to 0.77 mmol/L) is usually not associated with clinical signs and symptoms (unless chronic, when osteomalacia or rickets develops). Plasma concentrations less than 1.5 mg/dL (0.48 mmol/L) may produce clinical manifestations. Because phosphate is necessary for the formation of ATP, glycolysis and cellular function are impaired by low intracellular phosphate concentrations. Muscle weakness, acute respiratory failure, and decreased cardiac output may occur in phosphate depletion. At very low serum phosphate (<1 mg/dL or <0.32 mmol/L), rhabdomyolysis may occur. Phosphate depletion in erythrocytes decreases erythrocyte 2,3-diphosphoglycerate, which causes tissue hypoxia because of increased affinity of hemoglobin for oxygen. Severe hypophosphatemia (serum phosphate concentration <0.5 mg/dL [<0.16 mmol/L]) may result in hemolysis of the red blood cells. Mental confusion and frank coma also may be secondary to the low ATP and tissue hypoxia. If hypophosphatemia is chronic, impaired mineralization of bone produces rickets in children and osteomalacia in adults.

Treatment of hypophosphatemia depends on the degree of hypophosphatemia and the presence of symptoms. Patients with moderate hypophosphatemia may require only treatment of the underlying disorder or oral phosphate supplementation. In patients with marked symptoms of hypophosphatemia, particularly if respiratory muscle weakness is present, parenteral administration of phosphate may be indicated.

BOX 49-6 Common Causes of Hyperphosphatemia

- Decreased renal phosphate excretion
  - Decreased glomerular filtration rate
    - Renal failure, chronic and acute
  - Increased tubular reabsorption
    - Hypoparathyroidism
    - Pseudohypoparathyroidism
    - Acromegaly
    - Disodium etidronate
- Increased phosphate intake
  - Oral or intravenous administration
  - Phosphate-containing laxatives or enemas
- Increased extracellular phosphate load
  - Transcellular shift
    - Lactic acidosis
    - Respiratory acidosis
    - Untreated diabetic ketoacidosis
  - Cell lysis
    - Rhabdomyolysis
    - Intravascular hemolysis
    - Cytotoxic therapy
    - Leukemia
    - Lymphoma

Hyperphosphatemia

Common causes of hyperphosphatemia are listed in Box 49-6.

Hyperphosphatemia is usually secondary to the inability of the kidneys to excrete phosphate.[308] In acute or chronic renal failure, a decrease in glomerular filtration rate (GFR) reduces the renal excretion of phosphate, resulting in hyperphosphatemia. Moderate increases of serum phosphate occur in individuals with low PTH (hypoparathyroidism), PTH resistance (pseudohypoparathyroidism), or acromegaly (increased growth hormone) caused by an increased renal phosphate threshold. Growth hormone is responsible for the increased renal phosphate threshold and higher phosphate concentrations observed in children. EDTA therapy has also been associated with hyperphosphatemia.

Increased intake and a shift of phosphate from the tissues into the ECF are also causes of hyperphosphatemia. Excessive oral, rectal, or intravenous phosphate administration for the treatment of phosphate depletion is a common cause of hyperphosphatemia. Release of phosphate because of cell breakdown in cases of rhabdomyolysis, intravascular hemolysis, or chemotherapy of certain malignancies may cause hyperphosphatemia. Hyperphosphatemia may also be associated with acidosis, a consequence of the hydrolysis of intracellular organic phosphate-containing compounds, with the release of phosphate into the plasma.

The clinical manifestations of hyperphosphatemia depend on the rate of onset. A rapid increase in serum phosphate may be associated with hypocalcemia. Therefore, symptoms may include tetany, seizures, and hypotension. Long-term hyperphosphatemia may be associated with secondary hyperparathyroidism, osteitis fibrosa, and soft-tissue calcification of the kidneys, blood vessels, cornea, skin, and periarticular tissue.

Therapy for hyperphosphatemia is directed toward correcting the cause of the high serum phosphate. In renal failure and in hypoparathyroidism, dietary restriction of phosphate and agents that bind phosphate in the intestine (calcium carbonate and others) are useful in lowering the serum phosphate concentrations.

Measurement of Phosphate

All widely used methods for serum inorganic phosphate are based on the reaction of phosphate ions with ammonium molybdate to form a phosphomolybdate complex[203] that is then measured by a spectrophotometer.

$$7H_3PO_4 + 12(NH_4)_6Mo_7O_{24} \cdot 4H_2O \rightarrow$$
$$7(NH_4)_3[PO_4(MoO_3)_{12}] + 51NH^{+4} + 51OH^- + 33H_2O$$

The colorless phosphomolybdate complex is measured directly by ultraviolet absorption (340 nm), or reduced to molybdenum blue and measured at 600 to 700 nm.[21,252] An acid pH is necessary for the formation of complexes but must be controlled, because both complex formation and reduction of molybdate are dependent on pH. A less acidic pH can result in spontaneous reduction of molybdate. The rate of complex formation is also influenced by protein concentration. Solubilizing agents are used to prevent protein precipitation. Measurement of unreduced complexes has several advantages, including simplicity, speed, and stability.[16,129,601] Disadvantages include the greater interference of hemolysis, icterus, and lipemia at 340 nm. Approximately 70% of laboratories participating in the College of American Pathologists Comprehensive Chemistry Survey in 2004 used a direct UV procedure, with most of the others using a reduced photometric method.

Many reducing agents have been used for producing the blue phosphomolybdate complex, including aminonaphtholsulfonic acid, stannous chloride, methyl-*p*-aminophenol sulfate, ferrous ammonium sulfate, ascorbic acid, and *N*-phenyl-*p*-phenyldiamine (semidine) HCl.[21,252] Each of these reagents appears to have some individual advantage, such as increased stability, increased color stability, lower detection limit, or reduced hydrolysis of organic esters. Ferrous sulfate and especially ascorbic acid have often been used for biological specimens containing organic esters, because they cause less breakdown of labile phosphate esters. Aminonaphtholsulfonic acid has been widely used but is unstable, tends to precipitate, and requires careful timing because color continues to increase for several hours. With this reagent, color formation is increased with heating. Stannous chloride provides greater color intensity. Hydrazine has been added to stannous chloride to stabilize the reagent and improve the linearity. Methyl-*p*-aminophenol sulfate is acid-tolerant, allowing for a one-component acid-molybdate reagent. A method using semidine HCl was published as a "Selected Method" by the American Association for Clinical Chemistry.[203]

Phosphate concentrations have been determined by a number of other procedures, including the vanadate-molybdate and enzymatic methods. Vanadate and molybdate form a yellow complex with phosphate at acid pH, but the method tends to overestimate inorganic phosphate because of hydrolysis of organic esters.[252] Enzymatic methods do not have this problem, because they are performed at a neutral pH that does not hydrolyze organic esters. A number of enzymatic methods have been described, including those using the following enzymes: (1) glycogen phosphorylase, phosphoglucomutase, and glucose-6-phosphate dehydrogenase, with monitoring of the formation of the reduced form of nicotinamide-adenine dinucleotide phosphate (NADPH)[506]; (2) purine nucleoside phosphorylase and xanthine oxidase, with measurement of hydrogen peroxide (H_2O_2) with peroxidase and a chromogenic substrate[3]; and (3) sucrose phosphorylase, phosphoglucomutase, and glucose-6-phosphate dehydrogenase, with measurement of the formation of the reduced form of nicotinamide-adenine dinucleotide (NADH).[556]

Specimen Requirements

Serum and heparinized plasma are the preferred specimens for the measurement of phosphate. Concentrations of inorganic phosphate are about 0.2 to 0.3 mg/dL (0.06 to 0.10 mmol/L) lower in heparinized plasma than in serum.[321] Anticoagulants such as citrate, oxalate, and EDTA interfere with formation of the phosphomolybdate complex.

Inorganic phosphate in whole blood specimens may either decrease or increase with time, depending on the type of specimen, the storage temperature, and the duration of storage.[318] Phosphate concentrations in plasma or serum are increased by prolonged storage with cells at room temperature or 37 °C. Hemolyzed specimens are unacceptable because erythrocytes contain high concentrations of organic phosphate esters, which can be hydrolyzed to inorganic phosphate during storage. Inorganic phosphate increases by 4 to 5 mg/dL (1.29 to 1.61 mmol/L) per day in hemolyzed specimens stored at 4 °C, more rapidly at room temperature or 37 °C. Glucose phosphate, creatine phosphate, and other organic phosphates may also be hydrolyzed by assay conditions, resulting in overestimation of inorganic phosphate concentrations.

Phosphate is considered to be stable in separated serum for days at 4 °C and for months when frozen, provided evaporation and lyophilization are prevented.

Interferences

Depending on the method used, positive or negative interference has been noted with hemolyzed, icteric, and lipemic specimens.[221,222] Mannitol,[156] fluoride, and monoclonal immunoglobulins[438] have also been reported to interfere. Glassware should be properly cleaned and rinsed because phosphate is a common component of many detergents.

Reference Intervals

Phosphate is often referred to as "phosphorus," a practice that is inaccurate and misleading because only phosphate, not elemental phosphorus, circulates in blood and is measured. This practice originated because results are reported as milligrams per deciliter of phosphorus, rather than phosphate. When results are reported in molar units (as in SI), the numerical results and reference intervals are the same for phosphorus and phosphate, but confusion occurs when results are reported in mg/dL.

In adults, the reference interval for serum phosphate is 2.5 to 4.5 mg of phosphorus/dL (0.81 to 1.45 mmol/L). In children, it is 4.0 to 7.0 mg phosphorus/dL (1.29 to 2.26 mmol/L).

Serum phosphate concentrations are about 50% higher in infants than in adults and decline throughout childhood,[227] a consequence of the ability of growth hormone to increase the renal phosphate threshold. Serum phosphate is unchanged in elderly women but decreases in elderly men.[171,522] During pregnancy, serum phosphate decreases.[216]

Because a diurnal variation[95,120,298,436] in serum phosphate has been reported, fasting morning specimens are recommended (Figure 49-8). Concentrations are higher in the afternoon and evening. Serum phosphate concentrations are influenced by dietary intake and meals and increased by exercise.

Urinary phosphate varies with age, muscle mass, renal function, PTH, the time of day, and other factors. Urinary excretion of phosphate varies widely with diet and is essentially equivalent to dietary intake. On a nonrestricted diet, the reference interval for urinary phosphate is 0.4 to 1.3 g/day (12.9 to 42.0 mmol/day).

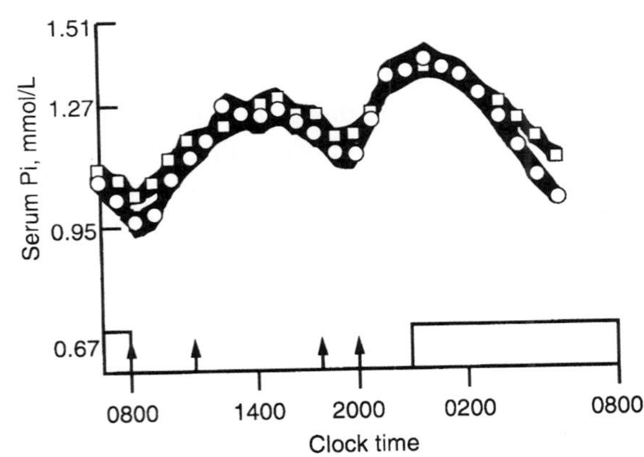

Figure 49-8 Diurnal variation of serum phosphate in men (○) and women (□). Meals and snacks are indicated by arrows; the bar indicates recumbent posture. *(From Calvo MS, Eastell R, Offord KP, Bergstralh EJ, Burritt MF. Circadian variation in ionized calcium and intact parathyroid hormone: evidence for gender differences in calcium homeostasis. J Clin Endocrinol Metab 1991;72:69-76, © The Endocrine Society.)*

Urine should be collected in 6 mol/L HCl, 20 to 30 mL for a 24-hour specimen, to avoid precipitation of phosphate complexes. Simultaneous measurement of phosphate and creatinine in serum and urine with fasting morning spot or 1- to 2-hour timed collections permits calculation of the renal phosphate threshold ($TmPO_4$/GFR). The clearance of phosphate divided by creatinine clearance can be plotted on a nomogram, and the $TmPO_4$/GFR determined.[36,541] This index expresses phosphate reabsorption as a function of both serum phosphate concentration and GFR and is more useful than urinary phosphate excretion.

MAGNESIUM

Magnesium is the fourth most abundant cation in the body and the second most prevalent intracellular cation.[487,490] The total body magnesium content is approximately 25 g (1.03 mol), of which about 55% resides in the skeleton (see Table 49-1). One third of skeletal magnesium is exchangeable and is thought to serve as a reservoir for maintaining extracellular magnesium concentration. About 45% of magnesium is intracellular.

BIOCHEMISTRY AND PHYSIOLOGY

The concentration of magnesium in cells is approximately 1 to 3 mmol/L (2.4 to 7.3 mg/dL). In general, the higher the metabolic activity of a cell, the higher its magnesium content. Within the cell, most of the magnesium is bound to proteins and negatively charged molecules; 80% of cytosolic magnesium is bound to ATP, and MgATP is the substrate for numerous enzymes. The nucleus, mitochondria, and endoplasmic reticulum contain significant amounts of magnesium. Approximately 0.5% to 5.0% of the total cellular magnesium is free. Transport of magnesium across the cellular membrane is regulated by a specific magnesium transport system.

Extracellular magnesium accounts for about 1% of the total body magnesium content. About 55% of magnesium is free, 30% is associated with proteins (primarily albumin), and 15% is complexed with phosphate, citrate, and other anions (see Table 49-2).

Magnesium is a cofactor for more than 300 enzymes in the body.[487,490] It is required for enzyme substrate formation (for example, MgATP). In addition, magnesium is an allosteric activator of many enzyme systems. Examples of enzymes that require magnesium for action include adenylate cyclase, Na^+-K^+-adenosine triphosphate (ATPase), Ca^{2+}-ATPase, phosphofructokinase, and creatine kinase. The guanine nucleotide regulatory proteins Gs and Gi require magnesium for activity. Magnesium is important in oxidative phosphorylation, glycolysis, cell replication, nucleotide metabolism, and protein biosynthesis.

Reducing the serum magnesium concentration decreases the threshold of axonal stimulation and increases nerve conduction velocity. Magnesium also influences the release of neurotransmitter at the neuromuscular junction by competitively inhibiting the entry of calcium in the presynaptic nerve terminal. Reducing the serum magnesium concentration results in increased neuromuscular excitability.

CLINICAL SIGNIFICANCE

Disorders of magnesium metabolism are separated into those causing hypomagnesemia/magnesium deficiency and hypermagnesemia.

Hypomagnesemia/Magnesium Deficiency

Hypomagnesemia is common in hospitals.[487,490] Ten percent of the patients admitted to city hospitals and as many as 65% of patients in intensive care units may be hypomagnesemic. Moderate or severe magnesium deficiency is usually due to losses of magnesium from the gastrointestinal (GI) tract or kidneys (Box 49-7).

GI, vomiting, and nasogastric suction may deplete body stores of magnesium as upper GI fluids contain approxi-

BOX 49-7 Differential Diagnosis of Magnesium Deficiency

- Gastrointestinal disorders
  - Prolonged nasogastric suction
  - Malabsorption syndromes
  - Extensive bowel resection
  - Acute and chronic diarrhea
  - Intestinal and biliary fistulas
  - Protein-calorie malnutrition
  - Acute hemorrhagic pancreatitis
  - Primary hypomagnesemia (neonatal)
  - Renal loss
  - Chronic parenteral fluid therapy
  - Osmotic diuresis
    - Glucose (diabetes mellitus)
    - Mannitol
    - Urea
  - Hypercalcemia
  - Alcohol
  - Drugs
    - Diuretics (furosemide, ethacrynic acid)
    - Aminoglycosides
    - Cisplatin
    - Cyclosporine
    - Amphotericin B
    - Cardiac glycosides
    - Pentamidine
- Metabolic acidosis (starvation, ketoacidosis, alcoholism)
- Renal diseases
  - Chronic pyelonephritis, interstitial nephritis, and glomerulonephritis
  - Diuretic phase of acute tubular necrosis
  - Postobstructive nephropathy
  - Renal tubular acidosis
  - Post–renal transplantation
- Primary hypomagnesemia
- Phosphate depletion

mately 0.5 mmol/L of magnesium. More commonly, magnesium deficiency is associated with losses from the lower intestine. Diarrhea may result in marked losses of magnesium; therefore, acute diarrheal states, regional enteritis, and ulcerative colitis are frequently complicated by magnesium deficiency. Because magnesium is most efficiently absorbed from the distal small bowel, malabsorption and bypass surgery for obesity are also associated with magnesium malabsorption.

Excessive urinary losses of magnesium from the kidneys are important causes of magnesium deficiency. Clinically important causes include alcohol, diabetes mellitus (osmotic diuresis), loop diuretics (furosemide), and aminoglycoside antibiotics. Increased sodium excretion (parenteral fluid therapy) and increased calcium excretion (hypercalcemic states) also result in renal magnesium wasting.

Because magnesium deficiency is usually secondary to another disease process or to a therapeutic agent, the features of the primary disease process may complicate or mask magnesium deficiency. Neuromuscular hyperexcitability with tetany and seizures may be present. These symptoms and signs may also be due to hypocalcemia, and magnesium deficiency is a common cause of hypocalcemia. Magnesium deficiency impairs PTH secretion and causes resistance to PTH in the kidneys and bone.

One of the more serious complications of magnesium deficiency is cardiac arrhythmias. Premature atrial complexes, atrial tachycardia and fibrillation, ventricular premature complexes, ventricular tachycardia, and ventricular fibrillation may be associated with magnesium deficiency. These effects may be partly caused by the hypokalemia, renal wasting, and intracellular depletion of potassium caused by hypomagnesemia.

Although extracellular magnesium accounts for only about 1% of total body magnesium, and plasma magnesium concentrations correlate poorly with total body magnesium, determination of serum magnesium is the most widely used test to assess magnesium deficiency. Hypomagnesemia is often transient and not an indication of magnesium deficiency. Conversely, intracellular magnesium depletion and magnesium deficiency may exist despite a normal serum magnesium concentration. Consequently, hypocalcemia, hypokalemia, neuromuscular hyperirritability, and cardiac arrhythmias should alert one to the possible presence of magnesium deficiency. Other tests less commonly used include the magnesium tolerance test and measurements of intracellular magnesium (e.g., in red blood cell, lymphocyte, or skeletal muscle).[487]

Acute symptomatic magnesium deficiency is usually treated with parenteral magnesium; mild depletion may be treated with oral magnesium.

Hypermagnesemia

Magnesium intoxication is not a frequently encountered clinical problem, although mild to moderate elevation in the serum magnesium concentration may be noted in as many as 12% of hospital patients.[385,490] Symptomatic hypermagnesemia is almost always casued by excessive intake, resulting from the administration of antacids, enemas, and parenteral fluids containing magnesium (Box 49-8). The majority of these patients have concomitant renal failure, thereby limiting the ability of the kidneys to excrete excess magnesium. Magnesium is a standard therapy for pregnancy-induced hypertension (preeclampsia and eclampsia) and may cause magnesium intoxication in mothers and their neonates.

Depression of the neuromuscular system is the most common manifestation of magnesium intoxication. Deep tendon reflexes disappear at a serum magnesium above 5 to 9 mg/dL [2.06 to 3.70 mmol/L], whereas depressed respiration and apnea, caused by voluntary muscle paralysis, may occur at serum magnesium concentrations greater than 10 to 12 mg/dL (4.11 to 4.94 mmol/L). Higher concentrations may result in cardiac arrest. Somnolence, hypotension, nausea, vomiting, and cutaneous flushing may also be seen. Hypermagnesemia induces a decrease in the serum concentration of calcium, presumably because of the inhibition of both PTH secretion and end-organ action of PTH by magnesium.

The possibility of magnesium intoxication should be anticipated in patients receiving magnesium, especially those with renal failure. Replacement therapy should be discontinued in patients with mildly to moderately increased serum magnesium. Higher serum concentrations are used in treatment of preeclampsia and eclampsia. Since calcium acutely antagonizes the toxic effects of magnesium, patients with severe magnesium intoxication may be treated with intravenous calcium. If necessary, peritoneal dialysis or hemodialysis against a low-dialysis magnesium bath effectively lowers the serum magnesium concentration.

BOX 49-8 Causes of Hypermagnesemia

- Excessive intake
  - Orally (usually in the presence of chronic renal failure)
    - Antacids
    - Cathartic
  - Rectally
    - Purgation
  - Parenterally
    - Treatment of pregnancy-induced hypertension
    - Treatment of magnesium deficiency
- Renal failure
  - Chronic (usually with administration of magnesium)
    - Antacid
    - Cathartic
    - Enema
    - Infusion
    - Dialysis
  - Acute
    - Rhabdomyolysis
- Familial hypocalciuric hypercalcemia
- Lithium ingestion

Measurement of Total Magnesium

Serum magnesium has been measured by various techniques including fluorometry, flame emission spectroscopy, and atomic absorption spectrometry (AAS).[252,590,606] Today, photometric methods are most commonly used by clinical laboratories, although AAS,[363] considered the reference method, is also used by a few laboratories.

Photometric Methods

Several metallochromic indicators or dyes change color on selectively binding magnesium and have been used to measure it in biological samples.[252,590,606] According to the College of American Pathologists Comprehensive Chemistry Survey for 2004, calmagite and methylthymol blue were each used by 26% of laboratories for magnesium determinations, followed by a formazan dye (23%), magon/xylidyl blue (15%), chlorophosphonazo III (7%), and arsenazol (2%).

Calmagite (1-[1-hydroxy-4-methyl-2-phenylazo]-2-naphthol-4-sulfonic acid) (Figure 49-9), a metallochromic indicator, forms a colored complex with magnesium in alkaline solution, which is measured at 530 to 550 nm.[1,335,503,590] A specific calcium-chelating agent, EGTA (see Figure 49-3), is added to reduce interference by calcium. Reagents may include potassium cyanide (to prevent formation of heavy metal complexes) and polyvinylpyrrolidone and surfactants to reduce interference from protein and lipemia.

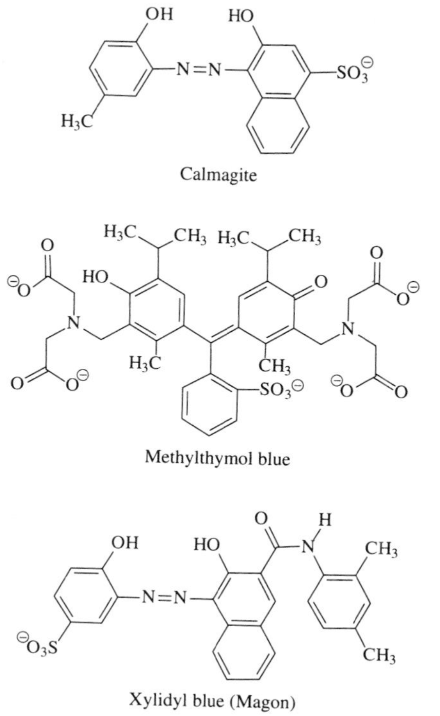

Calmagite

Methylthymol blue

Xylidyl blue (Magon)

Figure 49-9 Metallochromic indicators for magnesium.

Methylthymol blue (see Figure 49-9) forms a blue complex with magnesium, which is measured around 600 nm.[606] EGTA is added to reduce interference by calcium.

A formazan dye (1,5-bis[3,5-dichloro-2-hydroxyphenyl]-3-formazan carbonitrile) forms a complex with magnesium at alkaline pH, which has been measured at 630 nm by thin-film reflectance photometry.[569] *N,N'*-[1,2-ethanediylbis[oxy-2,1-phenylene]bis(N-carboxymethyl)] glycine is used to chelate calcium. This thin-film reflectance method shows relatively little interference from icteric, lipemic, and hemolyzed specimens. Elevated calcium concentrations cause a measurable but small overestimation.

Magon, or xylidyl blue (1-azo-2-hydroxy-3-[2,4-dimethylcarboxanilido]-naphthalene-1'-[2-hydroxybenzene]) (see Figure 49-9), binds magnesium in alkaline solution, causing a spectral shift and forming a red complex.[28,83,131,357] The absorbance has most often been measured around 600 nm. Calcium and protein interferences are reduced by EGTA and dimethyl sulfoxide, respectively.

Atomic Absorption Spectrometry

As with calcium, AAS methods provide greater accuracy and precision for magnesium measurements than do photometric methods; however, they are not frequently used for routine determination of magnesium by clinical laboratories. AAS is used as a reference method for magnesium.

Magnesium is determined by AAS after diluting the specimen 1:50 with a solution of lanthanum-HCl to eliminate interference from anions, including phosphate and protein and metal oxides.[363,606] The dilution also reduces viscosity, ensuring that the aspiration rates for aqueous calibrators and specimens are comparable. The specimen is aspirated into an air-acetylene flame, in which the ground state magnesium ions absorb light from a magnesium hollow cathode lamp (285.2 nm). Absorption at 285.2 nm is directly proportional to the number of ground state magnesium atoms in the flame. Electrothermal atomic absorption methods have also been described for serum, urine, and other fluids.

Other Methods

Flame emission, fluorometric, and enzymatic methods have also been used to measure magnesium. Flame emission spectroscopy is not a good method for magnesium because of its poor emission at low temperature and interference by large concentrations of sodium, potassium, and phosphate. A number of fluorometric methods have used calcein or 8-hydroxyquinoline. Enzymatic methods[549,578] have been developed with hexokinase or other enzymes that use Mg^{2+}-ATP as a substrate. The rate of this reaction is dependent on the concentration of magnesium in the sample. Coupling hexokinase to glucose-6-phosphate dehydrogenase allows the reaction to be monitored at 340 nm with the formation of NADPH. A simple one-step reaction using stabilized isocitrate dehydrogenase has been reported.[197,545] This enzyme is activated by magnesium and produces NADPH.

MEASUREMENT OF FREE (IONIZED) MAGNESIUM

Instruments for the measurement of free magnesium in whole blood, plasma, or serum are available commercially.* These instruments use ISEs with neutral carrier ionophores, including ETH 5220, ETH 7025, or a proprietary ionophore. Current ionophores or electrodes have insufficient selectivity for magnesium over calcium. Free calcium is simultaneously determined and used chemometrically with the signal from the magnesium electrode to calculate free magnesium concentrations.

Comparisons of instruments for free magnesium determinations have been reported.† Electrodes are warranted by the manufacturer for as little as a couple days to several months. Differences in measured free magnesium were apparent between analyzers, mainly because of interference from free calcium. Further improvements in ISEs and instruments for free magnesium would improve performance and increase the availability of these determinations.

Decreased total magnesium is a common finding in hospital patients.[487,490] Magnesium salts are frequently administered to patients for antiarrhythmic, vasomotor, and neuronal actions and to patients with preeclampsia, myocardial infarctions, and ischemic heart disease. Monitoring of free magnesium concentrations has been suggested,[524] as both low and high concentrations can be life threatening.

Discordance between total and free magnesium measurements has been reported in selected patient populations, including those with cardiovascular disorders, diabetes mellitus, alcoholism, migraine headaches, asthma, renal transplants, head trauma, and in pregnant women.[10,615] Interferences, such as that from thiocyanate, in measurement of free magnesium may explain some of these discrepencies. Free magnesium determinations may be helpful in others of these disorders and in critically ill patients and during cardiopulmonary bypass, preeclampsia, neonatal distress, and therapy with a number of drugs.[310,311,501,502,615]

Specimen Requirements

Serum and heparinized plasma are the preferred specimens for measuring magnesium. Zinc heparin, lithium-zinc heparin, and some of the newer heparins developed for free calcium determinations should be avoided because they significantly increase magnesium.[574,603] Other anticoagulants, such as citrate, oxalate, and EDTA, are not acceptable because they form complexes with magnesium. Storage of serum for days at 4 °C and for months frozen does not affect measured concentrations of total magnesium provided evaporation of the specimen is prevented.

Serum or plasma must be separated from the clot or red blood cells as soon as possible to prevent an increase in serum magnesium because of cell leakage. Because erythrocytes contain higher concentrations of magnesium than serum or plasma, hemolyzed specimens are unacceptable. Interference by icterus or lipemia depends on the method and can be decreased by use of bichromatic analysis or blanking with EDTA.[221,222,335,374] Lipemic specimens should be ultracentrifuged.

Urine specimens should be collected in acid (e.g., HCl, 20 to 30 mL of 6 mol/L for a 24-hour specimen) to prevent precipitation of magnesium complexes. As with calcium, if acid must be added after collection, the entire specimen must be acidified, warmed, and mixed thoroughly before a sample is removed for analysis. Collection of the specimen in acid to prevent precipitation is recommended.

Factors that alter free calcium concentration by altering the distribution of calcium between free, protein-bound, and complexed pools can also alter free magnesium concentration.[98,524] Therefore specimens should be handled anaerobically to prevent loss of CO_2 and analyzed without delay to prevent changes in pH because of metabolism. As with free calcium, high concentrations of heparin should be avoided. Certain silicones or other tube additives, thiocyanate (smokers and diet), and zinc heparin interfere with free magnesium determinations.[98,457,468,524]

REFERENCE INTERVALS FOR TOTAL AND FREE MAGNESIUM

For adults, the reference interval for serum magnesium is 1.7 to 2.4 mg/dL (0.66 to 1.07 mmol/L).[139,422] Magnesium concentrations in erythrocytes are approximately three times those of serum. Conversion factors for the units used to express magnesium concentration are given below:

$$\text{mmol/L} = \text{mEq/L} \times 0.5 = \text{mg/dL} \times 0.41$$
$$\text{mEq/L} = \text{mmol/L} \times 2 = \text{mg/dL} \times 0.82$$
$$\text{mg/dL} = \text{mEq/L} \times 1.22 = \text{mmol/L} \times 2.43$$

The reference interval for free magnesium is instrument-dependent; a typical range for the Nova Biomedical CRT is listed below:

0.45 to 0.60 mmol/L

HORMONES REGULATING MINERAL METABOLISM

PTH and 1,25-dihydroxyvitamin D are the primary hormones regulating bone and mineral metabolism. Calcitonin has pharmacological actions, but a physiological role has not been established in adults. PTHrP is the principal mediator of humoral hypercalcemia of malignancy.

PARATHYROID HORMONE

PTH is synthesized and secreted by the parathyroid glands; usually two superior and two inferior, located bilaterally on or near the thyroid gland capsule.[612] The glands are composed of chief and oxyphil cells; the chief cells synthesize, store, and secrete PTH.

*References 11-13, 176, 361, 483, 497, 585.

†References 9, 10, 98, 102, 273, 274, 456.

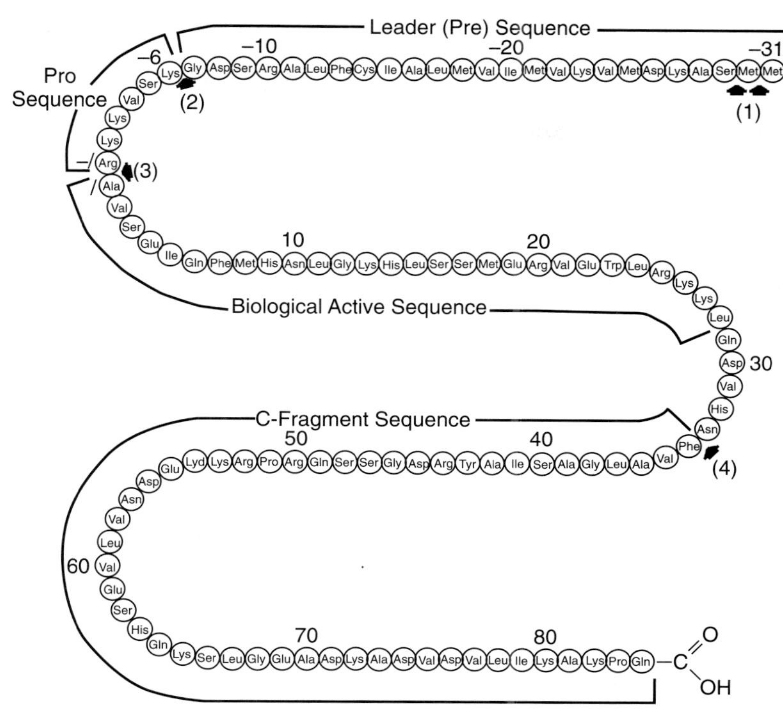

Figure 49-10 Amino acid sequence of preproparathyroid hormone. Arrows indicate the sites of cleavage by proteases to remove the N-terminal methionines (*1*), the leader (pre) sequence (*2*), and the pro sequence (*3*), producing intact PTH (1-84). Cleavage at position 4 produces inactive carboxyl (C)-terminal fragments. *(From Habener JF, Rosenblatt M, Potts JT Jr. Parathyroid hormone: Biochemical aspects of biosynthesis, secretion, action, and metabolism. Physiol Rev 1984;64:985-1053.)*

Biochemistry and Physiology

The concentration of PTH in plasma is determined by its synthesis and secretion by the parathyroids and its metabolism and clearance by the liver and kidneys. PTH acts directly on bone and kidney, and indirectly on intestine to regulate the concentration of calcium and phosphate in plasma.

Synthesis and Secretion

PTH is synthesized as a precursor, pre-pro-PTH, of 115 amino acids (Figure 49-10).[437] The amino(N)-terminal hydrophobic "pre" or leader sequence (25 amino acids) is involved in transporting PTH across the endoplasmic reticulum membrane into the cisternae. Both the "pre" and N-terminal "pro" (6 amino acids) are enzymatically cleaved during intracellular processing and before packaging in the Golgi apparatus. After processing, intact PTH (84 amino acids, molecular weight of 9425) is secreted, stored, or degraded intracellularly. Unlike proinsulin, proPTH does not appear to be secreted or to circulate in measurable concentrations.

Classical biological activity resides in the first third or N-terminal region of intact PTH. Synthetic PTH(1-34) is at least as potent as intact PTH(1-84) at interacting with the PTH/PTHrP receptor (type 1 PTH receptor) and stimulating calcemic, phosphaturic, and other biological responses in kidney and bone. Oxidation of the methionine residues at position 8 or 18 results in loss of biological activity. PTH contains a large number of basic amino acids. The middle portion of the molecule is quite immunogenic because of its hydrophobicity and species specificity.

The concentration of free calcium in blood or extracellular fluid is the primary acute physiological regulator of PTH synthesis, metabolism, and secretion.[76,435,437] Free calcium is sensed by a calcium-sensing receptor in the plasma membrane of parathyroid cells; this receptor activates intracellular events leading to release of free calcium from intracellular stores and the opening of plasma membrane calcium channels.[104] An increase in extracellular free calcium inhibits PTH synthesis and secretion and increases PTH metabolism, whereas a decrease has the opposite effect. An inverse sigmoidal relationship exists between PTH secretion and free calcium (Figure 49-11). Maximal secretion and suppression are attained with mild hypocalcemia and mild hypercalcemia, respectively. The midpoint of this relationship, or set-point, is the calcium concentration at which PTH secretion is half maximal. Set-points appear to vary somewhat from individual to individual and may be altered by physiological or pathological processes.

$1,25(OH)_2D$, phosphate, and magnesium also influence the synthesis and secretion of PTH.[76,435,437] $1,25(OH)_2D$ interacts with vitamin D receptors in the parathyroid glands to chronically suppress PTH synthesis by suppressing PTH gene transcription and therefore secretion. Hyperphosphatemia and hypophosphatemia increase and decrease PTH synthesis and secretion, respectively. Magnesium probably does not play an important role in PTH secretion except at the extremes of magnesium concentration. Chronic severe hypomagnesemia, such as that occurring in alcoholism, has been associated with impaired PTH secretion, whereas acute hypomagnesemia may stimulate secretion. Hypermagne-

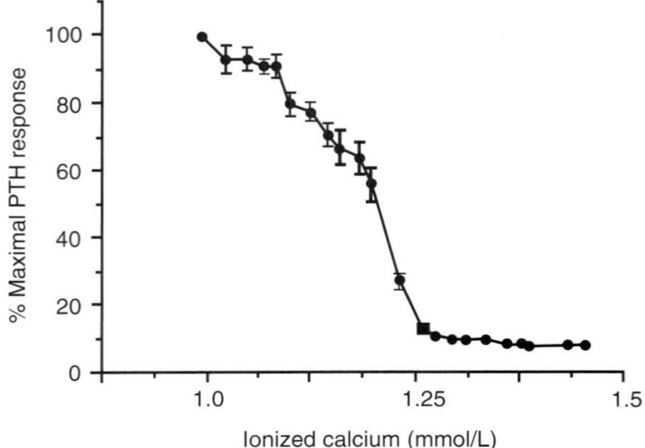

Figure 49-11 Regulation of intact PTH secretion by calcium in normal humans. Calcium and EDTA were infused to demonstrate the sigmoidal relationship between PTH secretion and free calcium. *(From Brown EM. Extracellular Ca^{2+} sensing, regulation of parathyroid cell function, and role of Ca^{2+} and other ions as extracellular (first) messengers. Physiol Rev 1991;71:371-411.)*

semia suppresses PTH secretion via the calcium-sensing receptor, although not as effectively as calcium.

Biological Actions

PTH influences both calcium and phosphate homeostasis directly through its actions on both bone and kidney and indirectly on the intestine through $1,25(OH)_2D$.[72,401,437,541] PTH exerts its actions by interacting with PTH/PTHrP receptors located in the plasma membrane of target cells. This interaction initiates a cascade of intracellular events, including the generation of cyclic adenosine monophosphate (cAMP), activation of kinases, phosphorylation of proteins, increased entry of calcium and intracellular calcium, stimulated phospholipase C activity with generation of diacylglycerol and phosphoinositide-activated enzyme and transport systems, and secretion of lysosomal enzymes.[437,541]

In the kidneys, PTH (1) induces 25-hydroxyvitamin D-1α-hydroxylase, increasing the production of $1,25(OH)_2D$, which stimulates intestinal absorption of both calcium and phosphate, (2) increases calcium reabsorption in the distal convoluted tubule of the nephron, (3) decreases reabsorption of phosphate by the proximal tubule, and (4) inhibits Na^+-H^+ antiporter activity, which favors a mild hyperchloremic metabolic acidosis in hyperparathyroid states.

The effects of PTH on bone are complex, as evidenced by its stimulation of bone resorption or bone formation, depending on the concentration of PTH and the duration of exposure. Chronic exposure to high concentrations of PTH leads to increased bone resorption. PTH acts directly by altering the activity or numbers of osteoblasts and indirectly on osteoclasts. Bone resorption, a prompt effect, is important for the maintenance of calcium homeostasis, whereas delayed effects are important for extreme systemic needs and skeletal homeostasis.

Integration of the direct effects of PTH on bone and kidney, and the indirect effects on intestine through $1,25(OH)_2D$, result in alterations in calcium and phosphate concentrations in serum and urine. In serum, total and free calcium are increased, but the concentration of phosphate is decreased. In urine, inorganic phosphate and cAMP concentrations are increased. Urinary calcium is usually increased because the larger filtered load of calcium (deriving from bone resorption and intestinal calcium absorption) overrides increased tubular reabsorption of calcium. In the absence of disease, the increase in serum calcium reduces PTH secretion through a negative-feedback loop, maintaining homeostasis.

Metabolism and Circulating Heterogeneity

PTH circulates as biologically active intact hormone and as carboxyl (C)-terminal fragments containing the midregion and C-terminal amino acids, but lacking the biologically active amino(N)-terminal region. Its heterogeneity is a consequence of (1) the secretion of both intact hormone and C-terminal fragments by the parathyroids, (2) peripheral metabolism of intact hormone by liver and kidney to C-terminal fragments, and (3) renal clearance of intact hormone and C-terminal fragments (Figure 49-12).[127,130,437] In the parathyroids, secretion of intact PTH is increased by hypocalcemia and greatly reduced or absent in hypercalcemia, whereas secretion of C-terminal fragments persists in hypercalcemia.[127,173,437] Biologically active intact PTH is rapidly cleared from plasma (half-life < 5 minutes) by metabolism to C-terminal fragments by the liver and kidneys and clearance of intact PTH by the kidneys.[437,509] Peripheral metabolism appears to inactivate intact hormone without releasing measurable concentrations of biologically active N-terminal fragments.[73,437]

Circulating immunoreactive PTH is composed primarily of “inactive” C-terminal fragments and secondarily of intact hormone (see N-terminal-Truncated-Fragments and Second Generation Intact PTH Methods for a discussion of N-terminal-truncated fragments measured by first generation intact PTH immunoassays). Although the exact length of circulating C-terminal fragments is uncertain, fragments consisting of the middle and carboxyl regions of the molecule (e.g., amino acids 34-84, 36-84) have been most frequently reported. These fragments are devoid of the N-terminal region and classical PTH biological activity and were considered to be inactive degradation products. However, recent reports have identified C-terminal PTH receptors in bone cells and have suggested that these fragments may affect the maturation and biological activity of these cells. C-terminal fragments are cleared by glomerular filtration and normally have a half-life of less than 1 hour. Their half-life and circulating concentration are increased significantly in individuals with impaired renal function. Generally, 5% to 25% of the total immunoreactive PTH is

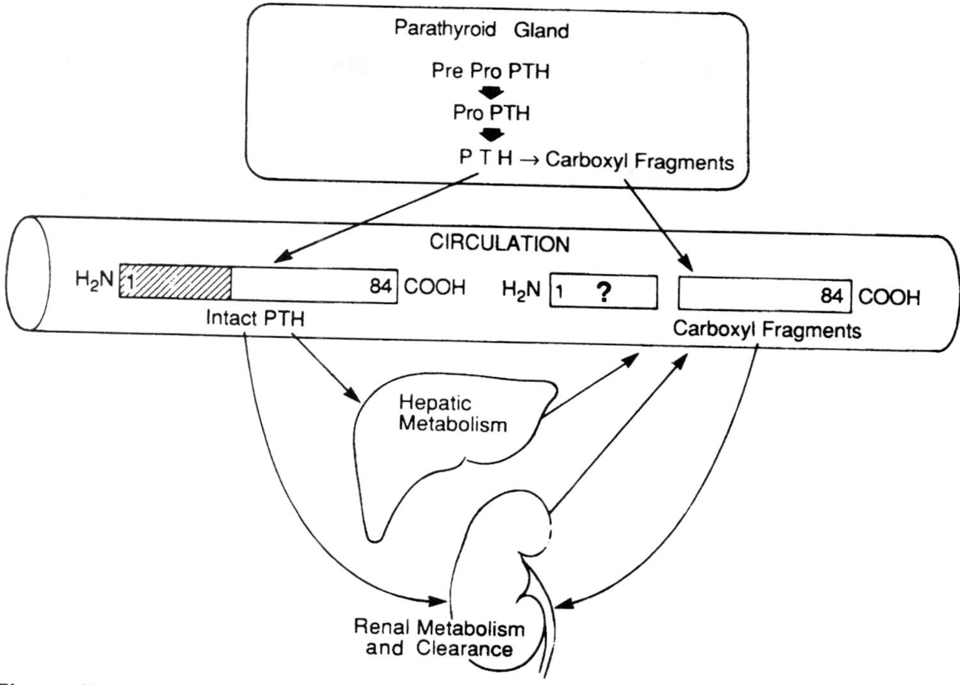

Figure 49-12 Secretion, metabolism, clearance, and circulating forms of PTH. Both intact PTH and inactive fragments containing the middle and carboxyl (C)-terminal amino acids are secreted by the parathyroid glands. These inactive fragments are also produced by peripheral metabolism of intact PTH by the liver and kidneys. Carboxyl fragments are cleared by the kidneys by glomerular filtration. The half-life and concentration of intact hormone are small compared with those of inactive fragments. *(From Endres DB, Villanueva R, Sharp CF Jr, Singer FR. Measurement of parathyroid hormone. Endocrinol Metab Clin North Am 1989;18:611-29.)*

intact hormone, and 75% to 95% is C-terminal fragments.[172,437,509] The relative concentrations of intact hormone and fragments vary with physiology and pathology.

Clinical Significance

Determination of PTH is useful in the differential diagnosis of both hypercalcemia and hypocalcemia for assessing parathyroid function in renal failure and for evaluating parathyroid function in bone and mineral disorders (see Calcium, Clinical Significance, Hypocalcemia, and Hypercalcemia; Metabolic Bone Diseases; and Interpretation of PTH Results).

Measurement of PTH

Noncompetitive immunoassays are now widely used for the measurement of intact PTH.[167,411] The low concentration of intact hormone and high concentrations of C-terminal fragments presented too great a challenge for competitive immunoassays.[172,509] Competitive immunoassays, primarily radioimmunoassays (RIAs), including those recognizing the midregion, C-terminal, N-terminal, and other sequences (Figure 49-13), have largely been discontinued because of their limited specificity and/or sensitivity. Midregion and C-terminal methods: (1) measure primarily C-terminal fragments, which are present in much higher concentrations than is biologically active intact hormone, the species regulated by free calcium; (2) often provide a poor indication of parathyroid function, because the measured concentration is dependent on peripheral metabolism and glomerular filtration of the fragments[437]; (3) are difficult to interpret in patients with impaired renal function (PTH can be falsely elevated, up to 30 times the upper limit of normal, in dialysis patients without secondary hyperparathyroidism)[18]; and (4) are not suppressed in nonparathyroid hypercalcemia and are often falsely modestly elevated.[173] N-terminal PTH RIAs were an attempt to overcome the limitations of assays measuring C-terminal fragments. These competitive immunoassays lacked the sensitivity required to measure intact PTH in patients with normal or modestly elevated concentrations.

Fortunately the following advances permitted the development of noncompetitive methods for intact PTH: (1) the determination of the amino acid sequence of human (h)PTH; (2) increased understanding of the secretion, metabolism, clearance, and circulating forms of PTH; and (3) the synthesis of hPTH, fragments of hPTH, and analogues of fragments for use as immunogens, tracers, and calibrators, for characterization of antiserum and antibody specificity, and for affinity purification of antibodies.

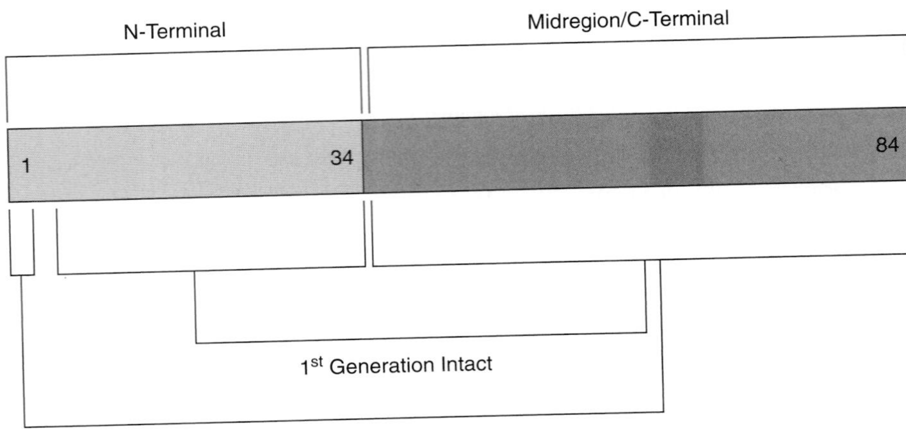

Figure 49-13 Schematic representation of PTH immunoassays including first and second generation noncompetitive intact immunoassays and midregion/C-terminal and N-terminal competitive methods. The approximate location of the peptide regions recognized by the antibodies of the four classes of methods is indicated. *(Modified from Jüppner H, Potts JT Jr. Immunoassays for the detection of parathyroid hormone. J Bone Miner Res 2002;17:N81-86.)*

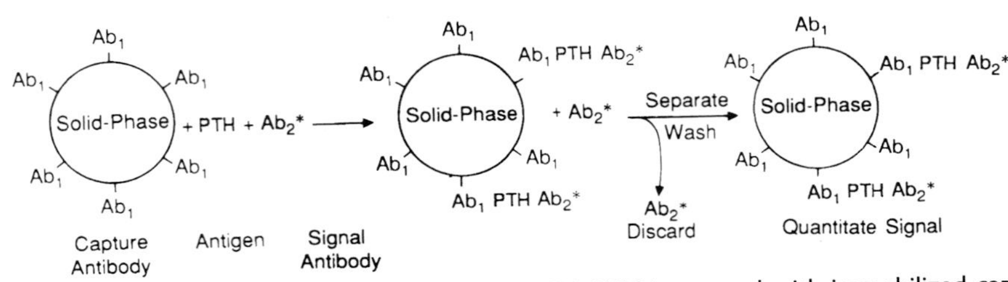

Figure 49-14 Noncompetitive immunoassay for PTH. PTH is reacted with immobilized capture antibody (Ab_1) against one antigenic determinant and a labeled signal antibody (Ab_2*) against a second antigenic determinant. PTH forms a bridge between the two antibodies, producing a "sandwich" or ternary complex. Both antibodies are added in excess, ensuring that all PTH reacts and is measured. Free signal antibody is separated, and the solid-phase antibody-PTH-labeled antibody complexes are quantified with an appropriate detection system. The signal increases with increasing concentrations of PTH. *(Modified from Endres DB, Villanueva R, Sharp CF Jr, Singer FR. Measurement of parathyroid hormone. Endocrinol Metab Clin North Am 1989;18:611-29.)*

Noncompetitive Methods for Intact PTH

Noncompetitive (also known as two-site, sandwich, labeled antibody, or immunometric methods) (see Chapter 9) require two antibodies capable of simultaneously binding PTH (Figure 49-14): (1) a capture antibody immobilized to a solid phase, and (2) a signal or reporter antibody labeled with a measurable substance or an enzyme changing the concentration (substrate or product) of a measurable substance. Unlike competitive immunoassays, with noncompetitive methods, both antibodies are added in excess, ensuring that all analyte is measured. After formation of the ternary complex or sandwich, excess labeled antibody is removed by washing before quantification of complexes. Noncompetitive immunoassays provide increased sensitivity, specificity, reproducibility, and convenience.[167,411]

For intact PTH, the capture antibody is most often directed against the carboxyl or middle region of the molecule (for example, amino acid sequences 39 to 84,[196,414] 44 to 68[78], 44 to 84, or 78 to 84[344]) and the signal antibody against the N-terminal amino acid sequence (1 to 34).[78,196,344,414] A few methods have reversed this, using capture antibodies against the N-terminal amino acid sequence (1 to 34,[55,62] 26 to 32, or 1 to 38[47]) and signal antibodies against the middle or C-terminal amino acid sequence (44 to 68,[62] 55 to 64, or 53 to 68).[47,55] With the latter, a higher concentration of signal antibody is required because of the high concentration of inactive fragments relative to intact hormone, potentially adversely impacting sensitivity by increasing the blank (signal in the absence of intact PTH). The specificity of these noncompetitive methods depends on the sequence specificity of the antibodies used. The methods described above do not measure classical C-terminal fragments lacking the N-terminal amino acid sequence (1-34).

Antibodies may be either monoclonal or polyclonal antibodies purified by affinity chromatography to produce sequence-specific antibodies. Affinity-purified polyclonal antibodies have been most widely used, particularly for the signal antibody, because of the difficulty of producing high-affinity monoclonal antibodies against PTH, although some success has been reported.[62,77,343,344,413]

Capture antibodies have been noncovalently bound or covalently attached to a variety of solid phases, including polystyrene beads,[196,414] plastic tubes,[55,62] paramagnetic particles, microparticulate cellulose,[47,78] and sepharose.[344]

Signal antibodies have most often been radiolabeled (for *immunoradiometric* assays [IRMA]) with (^{125}I)[47,62,196,344,414] or labeled with a chemiluminescent (for *immunochemiluminometric* assays [ICMA]) compound, such as acridinium ester,[55,77] or an enzyme (enzyme-linked immunosorbent assay [ELISA] or enzyme immunoassay [EIA]), such as ALP, converting a substrate (1,2-dioxetane phosphate) to a chemiluminescent product.

As of 2004, the College of American Pathologists Interlaboratory Survey listed five manufacturers as providing first generation noncompetitive immunoassays for intact PTH. Most of these commercially available methods are on fully automated immunoassay analyzers using chemiluminescence detection including ALP with 1,2-dioxetane phosphate, acridinium ester, or electrochemiluminescence (ruthenium chelate). Signal antibody is less commonly radiolabeled with ^{125}I.

N-Terminal-Truncated PTH and Second Generation Intact PTH Methods

More recently, evidence has been presented for circulating N-terminal-truncated fragment(s) (also called non-[1-84]PTH and PTH[7-84]), containing all but a few of the N-terminal amino acids. The fragment(s) were identified by immunoassay with first generation noncompetitive methods for intact PTH after fractionation of extracts of plasma from hyperparathyroid patients and normal subjects by high-performance liquid chromatography (HPLC).[75,328] Although its exact length is unknown, the fragment(s) migrate before PTH(1-84) and just ahead of PTH(7-84). N-terminal-truncated PTH concentration accounts for averages of 20% and 50% of "intact" PTH in normal subjects and patients with chronic renal failure, respectively. Furthermore the relative concentration of N-terminal-truncated PTH increased with hypercalcemia and decreased with hypocalcemia. Like C-terminal fragments, N-terminal-truncated PTH originates from both secretion by the parathyroids and peripheral metabolism of intact hormone.[404]

First generation, noncompetitive methods for intact PTH cross-react with N-terminal-truncated fragment(s) overestimating the concentration of biologically active, intact PTH. Using synthetic PTH(7-84), cross-reactivity of 40% to 160% has been reported for first generation methods.[202,328] These findings have stimulated the development of a few second generation methods for intact PTH, using N-terminal antibodies that do not cross-react with synthetic PTH (7-84) (Figure 49-13). These second generation methods, which do not recognize N-terminal-truncated fragments, have been referred to as "bio-intact PTH, PTH(1-84)," "whole PTH," or "CAP" (cyclase-activating PTH). We prefer the term "second generation intact PTH" assays, but because of its convenience we will also use PTH(1-84) to distinguish these methods from first generation intact PTH methods that recognize both intact hormone and N-terminal-truncated PTH. This terminology avoids the implication that these immunoassays measure only biologically active hormone.

One method uses antibodies against PTH(1-4) and even requires the presence of the most N-terminal amino acid, as evidenced by its failure to recognize PTH(2-34).[202] As of 2004, three second generation methods from two manufacturers were listed on the College of American Pathologists Interlaboratory Survey.

Recent studies have suggested that N-terminal-truncated PTH may be biologically active. Synthetic PTH(7-84), used as the available representative of N-terminal-truncated PTH, decreased serum calcium; antagonized the calcemic, phosphatemic, and phosphaturic effects of intact PTH in thyroparathyroidectomized animals; and was bound by a C-terminal PTH receptor distinct from the PTH/PTHrP receptor.[405,531]

Since first generation methods for intact PTH measure N-terminal-truncated PTH, they overestimate the concentration of biologically intact hormone. The degree of overestimation will be method-dependent, but intact PTH is 50% higher on average than PTH(1-84) in patients with primary hyperparathyroidism or end-stage renal disease.[202]

The inability of first generation intact PTH methods to accurately measure biologically active intact hormone may explain why intact PTH is not a reliable indicator of bone turnover in dialysis patients.[356] PTH often fails to distinguish patients with low-, normal-, and high-turnover bone disease. Furthermore, treatment of patients to suppress intact PTH to normal or near normal frequently results in adynamic bone disease. Recently the PTH(1-84)/N-terminal-truncated fragment ratio has been proposed for evaluating bone turnover in renal osteodystrophy based on the ability of PTH(7-84) to antagonize the biological activity of intact PTH and preliminary experimental evidence for the predictive value of this ratio.[383] The ratio is calculated after measuring intact PTH (first generation) and PTH(1-84) (second generation) and calculating the N-terminal-truncated fragments by subtracting PTH(1-84) from intact PTH. Additional studies are required as subsequent studies were unable to substantiate the greater clinical utility of measuring both PTH(1-84) and intact PTH and calculating this ratio to assess bone turnover in renal osteodystrophy.[114,356,500A]

Even second generation intact PTH assays may not be absolutely specific for intact PTH as evidenced by a recent report demonstrating an amino-terminal form of PTH distinct from intact hormone and the N-truncated fragment. This form represented approximately 20% of the intact PTH measured with a second generation intact PTH method. The clinical implications of this form have not yet been established.[125A]

Specimen Requirements

Specimen requirements may depend on the specific method; however, serum or EDTA plasma is generally preferred. After separation, serum or plasma should be frozen if the analysis is delayed. Lower concentrations of PTH are observed in serum incubated at room temperature for more than a few hours or after one to several days at 4 °C.[330,403,450,492,613] PTH has been reported to be more stable in EDTA plasma, a probable consequence of reduced proteolytic activity.

Reference Intervals

Reference intervals for PTH vary with the method. Typical reference intervals are:

Intact PTH (First Generation): 10 to 65 pg/mL (1.1 to 6.8 pmol/L)

PTH(1-84) (Second Generation): 6 to 40 pg/mL (0.6 to 4.2 pmol/L)

Interpretation of PTH concentrations should consider the patient's calcium concentration at the time of sampling.[329]

The upper limit of the reference interval for PTH may be inappropriately high because of the prevalence of vitamin D insufficiency and mild secondary hyperparathyroidism in the reference group. Significantly lower intervals have been established for these methods by excluding individuals with vitamin D insufficiency (see section on vitamin D, reference intervals).[534]

Intact PTH concentrations vary with age and are low or normal during pregnancy,[132,200,272,500] lower in fetuses and umbilical cord blood, and increased during the first few days of life,[424,484,499,500] in response to neonatal hypocalcemia. Concentrations in children and adolescents are reportedly similar, if not identical, to those in adults.[499] In healthy adults, circulating concentrations of intact PTH increase with age.[171,522]

Intact PTH is reported to be secreted in a pulsatile fashion with an overall circadian rhythm characterized by a nocturnal rise.[95,242,301,342] Measurement of PTH on more than one occasion should assist in preventing misinterpretation of parathyroid status because of episodic secretion.

Interpretation of PTH Results

PTH is the most important test for the differential diagnosis of hypercalcemia. Intact PTH is elevated in the majority of patients with primary hyperparathyroidism (see Figure 39-15)[78,168,173,414] and below normal or in the lower half of the reference interval in most patients with nonparathyroid hypercalcemia including hypercalcemia-associated malignancy.[78,173,414] In patients with stable hypercalcemia, PTH in the upper half of the reference interval is inappropriately high and suggestive of primary hyperparathyroidism. Whenever possible, PTH specimens should be obtained before therapy for hypercalcemia, because PTH

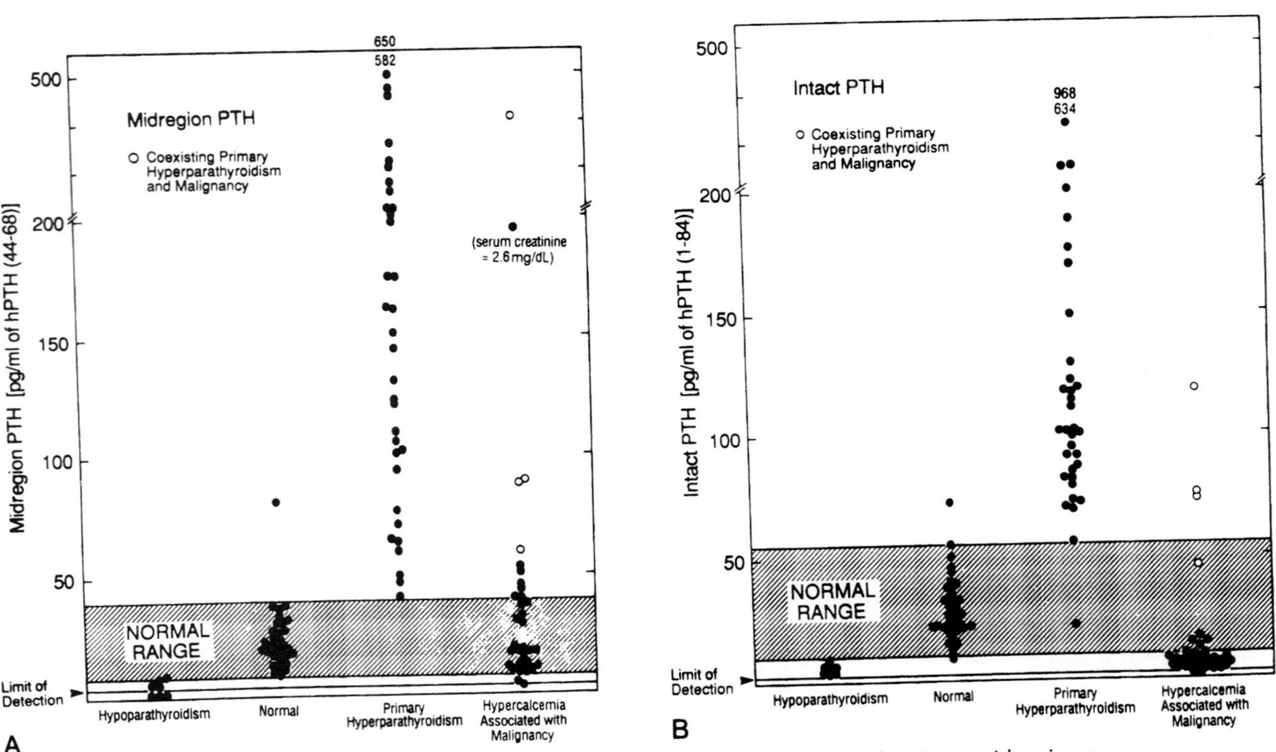

Figure 49-15 Midregion **(A)** and intact **(B)** PTH in normal subjects and patients with primary hyperparathyroidism, hypercalcemia associated with malignancy, and hypoparathyroidism. *(From Endres DB, Villanueva R, Sharp CF Jr, Singer FR. Measurement of parathyroid hormone. Endocrinol Metab Clin North Am 1989;18:611-29.)*

secretion may be stimulated by declining serum calcium.[193] Increased PTH in patients with hypercalcemia and malignancy suggests coexisting hyperparathyroidism and malignancy,[488] since ectopic PTH production appears to be extremely rare.[412] Hypercalcemia in malignancy is usually associated with bony metastases and/or production of PTHrP. PTHrP does not cross-react in any of the PTH immunoassays that have been evaluated. According to a recent study, PTH(1-84) is more sensitive in diagnosing primary hyperparathyroidism.[526] PTH(1-84) and intact PTH were elevated in 96% and 73% of 56 patients with primary hyperparathyroidism, respectively.

Intraoperative determination of intact PTH is useful for assessing the completeness of parathyroidectomy and facilitating minimally invasive parathyroid surgery, thereby improving cost-effectiveness and cosmetic outcomes.[100] PTH is measured just before the incision and again at 10 minutes after resection of the hyperfunctioning parathyroid tissue. A decline of 50% or more is usually considered indicative of the removal of all hyperfunctioning tissue. In contrast to patients with solitary parathyroid adenomas, interpretation of results in patients with multiglandular disease is more complicated. Preoperative or intraoperative PTH may also be useful for localization of hyperfunctioning parathyroid tissue by sampling multiple veins from the cervical and mediastinal regions. PTH(1-84) may decrease more rapidly and completely than intact PTH after removal of hyperfunctioning tissue.[617]

Subnormal or low normal PTH is observed in the majority of patients with hypoparathyroidism (see Figure 49-15); such concentrations are inappropriately low for patients with hypocalcemia.[62,78,173] The apparently detectable concentrations observed in many patients with hypoparathyroidism or nonparathyroid hypercalcemia may be a result of the imprecision of methods at low concentrations, a nonspecific serum (ligand-free matrix) effect, and/or measurement of N-terminal-truncated PTH.[130] More rigorous assessment of the limit of detection[407] of PTH immunoassays and use of PTH(1-84) methods may show that concentrations are undetectable in these patients.

In secondary hyperparathyroidism, PTH is increased before total or free calcium becomes abnormally low, a consequence of homeostatic mechanisms for maintenance of serum calcium. Consequently, PTH is more sensitive than calcium for identifying secondary hyperparathyroidism.

In patients with end-stage renal disease, measurement of PTH is helpful in assessing parathyroid function, in estimating bone turnover, and in improving management. Patients with high-turnover bone disease because of secondary hyperparathyroidism (advanced osteitis fibrosa) have the highest concentrations of PTH, whereas patients with low-turnover, adynamic bone disease, including osteomalacia, have the lowest concentrations (Figure 49-16).* Intermediate concentrations are seen in low-turnover adynamic (aplastic) disease and early osteitis fibrosa. Considerable overlap in intact PTH concentrations is apparent among the various forms of renal osteodystrophy. In dialysis patients, cut-points ("decision levels") of less than 100 or 150 pg/mL and greater than 250 to 300 pg/mL have been suggested for distinguishing patients with low-turnover and high-turnover bone disease, respectively. A reasonable therapeutic goal for intact PTH (first generation) concentrations is two to four times the upper limit of the reference interval to prevent parathyroid-suppressed, adynamic, and hyperparathyroid bone diseases.[340,595]

Parathyroid status is usually determined by measuring PTH on predialysis specimens, because various factors, including changes in serum calcium and the type of dialysis membrane, affect PTH secretion and clearance.[126,317] Comparison of predialysis and postdialysis specimens has been suggested for determining acute parathyroid responsiveness to alterations in serum calcium concentrations.[155,433,589]

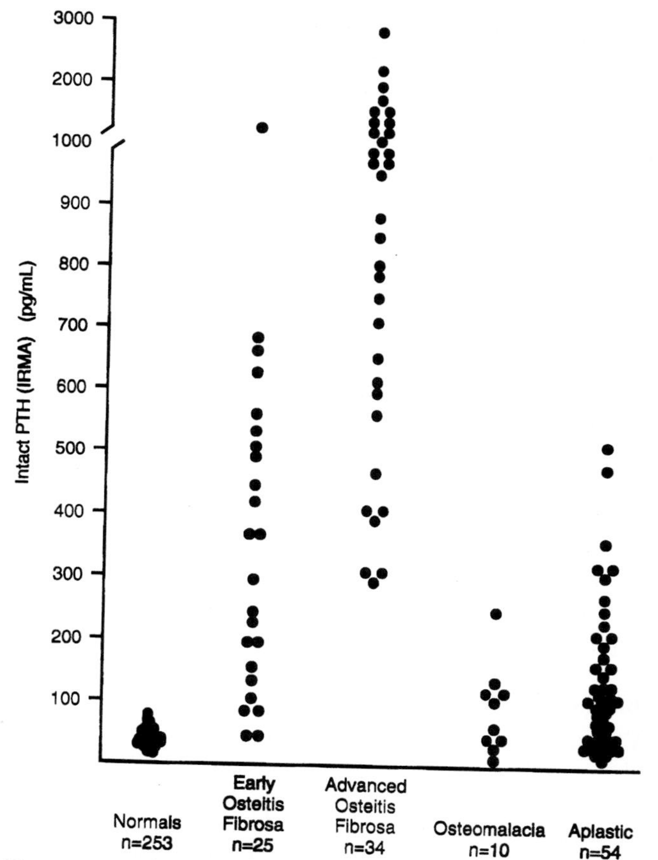

Figure 49-16 Intact PTH in assessing parathyroid function in end-stage renal disease. Dialysis patients were separated into those with early and advanced osteitis fibrosa, osteomalacia, and aplastic disease by quantitative histomorphometric analysis of undecalcified bone biopsies. *(From Segre GV, Sherrard DJ, Pandian MR, et al. Intact PTH (IRMA) II: New applications to issues in parathyroid hormone and mineral metabolism. San Juan Capistrano, Calif: Nichols Institute, 1989.)*

*References 18, 115, 340, 447, 510, 589, 595.

It is likely that PTH(1-84) will more accurately assess parathyroid status and bone turnover and guide therapy in patients with end-stage renal disease[356,383] (see N-Terminal Truncated PTH and Noncompetitive Methods for PTH(1-84). The therapeutic targets for intact PTH (two to four times the upper limit of normal) will need to be revised for PTH(1-84).

Noncompetitive immunoassays for intact PTH or PTH(1-84) must have high concentrations of the C-terminal antibody to avoid underestimating PTH in dialysis patients with secondary hyperparathyroidism who have high concentrations of C-terminal fragments. Absence of interference can be assessed by confirming that specimens from dialysis patients with the highest concentrations of PTH dilute in a parallel fashion.[46,154] Alternatively, recovery can be determined by adding a known amount of intact PTH to these specimens.

PTH concentrations may be altered in hyperthyroidism, in hypothyroidism, and with lithium carbonate treatment. PTH is decreased and inversely correlated with T3 concentrations in hyperthyroid patients. Serum PTH increases in patients who become hypothyroid after radioactive iodine treatment, and decreases with replacement therapy,[194,375,481] changes apparently mediated by serum calcium. Chronic lithium carbonate therapy has been reported to increase parathyroid gland size and circulating intact PTH.[354]

One remaining but uncommon use for PTH methods measuring C-terminal fragments is the analysis of fluid from suspected parathyroid cysts. Parathyroid cyst fluid appears to contain primarily inactive fragments of PTH, not intact hormone.[43]

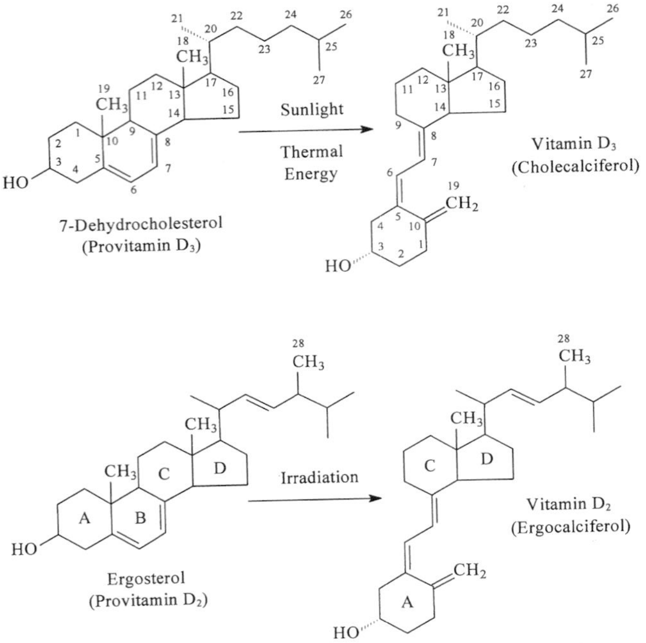

Vitamin D and Its Metabolites

Vitamin D is produced endogenously by exposure of skin to sunlight, and is absorbed from foods containing or supplemented with vitamin D. Vitamin D is metabolized to its biologically active form, 1,25-dihydroxyvitamin D (1,25[OH]$_2$D), a hormone regulating calcium and phosphate metabolism. Deficiency of vitamin D results in impaired formation of bone, because of a mineralizing defect, producing rickets in children and osteomalacia in adults.

Biochemistry and Physiology

Vitamin D and its metabolites may be categorized as either cholecalciferols or ergocalciferols (Figure 49-17). Cholecalciferol (vitamin D$_3$) is the parent compound of the naturally occurring family and is produced in the skin from 7-dehydrocholesterol on exposure to the ultraviolet B portion of sunlight.[257,258] Latitude, season, aging, sunscreen use, and skin pigmentation influence production of vitamin D$_3$ by the skin. Vitamin D$_2$ (ergocalciferol), the parent compound of the other family, is manufactured by irradiation of ergosterol produced by yeasts. Vitamin D$_2$ differs from vitamin D$_3$ by the double bond between carbon 22 and carbon 23 and a methyl group on carbon 24. When vitamin D or its metabolites are written without a subscript, both families are included.

Figure 49-17 Structure of vitamin D$_3$ (cholecalciferol) and vitamin D$_2$ (ergocalciferol) and their precursors. 7-Cholecalciferol is produced in the skin from 7-dehydrocholesterol on exposure to sunlight. Ergocalciferol is produced commercially by irradiation of ergosterol. *(Modified from Holick MF, Adams JS. Vitamin D metabolism and biological function. In: Avioli LV, Krane SM, eds. Metabolic bone disease, 2nd ed. Philadelphia: WB Saunders, 1990:155-95.)*

Only a few foods, primarily fish liver oils, fatty fish, egg yolks, and liver, naturally contain significant amounts of vitamin D.[257,258,410] Consequently, before foods were supplemented with vitamin D$_2$ or vitamin D$_3$, most vitamin D in the body was produced by synthesis in skin. In North America, a considerable fraction of vitamin D is acquired by ingestion of fortified foods (some cereals, bread products, and milk) or vitamin D supplements. The recommended daily allowance is 400 IU (10 μg).

Metabolism, Regulation, and Transport

Vitamin D$_2$ and vitamin D$_3$ are metabolized to 25-hydroxyvitamin D [25(OH)D] by vitamin D-25-hydroxylase, a cytochrome P450 enzyme, in liver (Figure 49-18).[146,257,258,458] The concentration of 25(OH)D in serum is approximately 10 to 65 ng/mL (25 to 162 nmol/L) (Table 49-4). The half-life of circulating 25(OH)D is 2 to 3 weeks. At physiological concentrations, 25(OH)D is biologically inactive.

25(OH) D$_2$ and 25(OH)D$_3$ are metabolized to 1,25-dihydroxyvitamin D (1,25[OH]$_2$D), the biologically active hormone, by 25(OH)D-1α-hydroxylase, a cytochrome P450 enzyme, in kidney and placenta (see Figure 49-18). Normal circulating concentrations are approximately 15 to 60 pg/mL

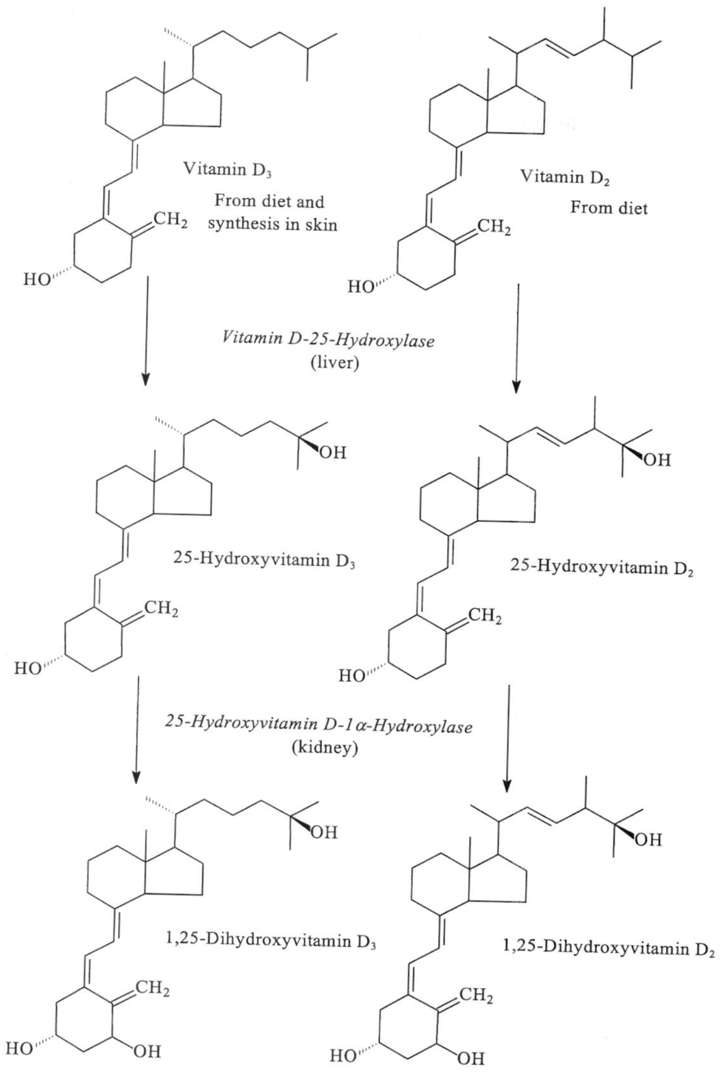

Figure 49-18 Metabolism of vitamin D. Vitamin D_2 and vitamin D_3 are enzymatically hydroxylated to 25-hydroxyvitamin D in the liver and 1,25-dihydroxyvitamin D by the kidneys. 1,25-Dihydroxyvitamin D_2 and 1,25-dihydroxyvitamin D_3 are the biologically active forms of vitamin D.

TABLE 49-4 Vitamin D and Its Metabolites in Plasma

Compound	Concentration	Free (%)	Half-Life
Vitamin D (ng/mL)	<0.2-20	—	1-2 days
(nmol/L)	<0.5-52		
25-Hydroxyvitamin D (ng/mL)	10-65	0.03	2-3 wk
(nmol/L)	25-162		
1,25-Dihydroxyvitamin D (pg/mL)	15-60	0.4	4-6 hr
(pmol/L)	36-144		

(36 to 144 pmol/L), about 1/1000 that of 25(OH)D (Table 49-4). The half-life of $1,25(OH)_2D$ is 4 to 6 hours.

Circulating concentrations of $1,25(OH)_2D$ are tightly regulated, primarily by PTH, phosphate, calcium, and $1,25(OH)_2D$.[146,147,257,258,458] PTH and hypophosphatemia increase the synthesis of $1,25(OH)_2D$ by increasing 25(OH)D-1α-hydroxylase, whereas hypocalcemia acts indirectly by stimulating the secretion of PTH. Hypercalcemia, hyperphosphatemia, and $1,25(OH)_2D$ reduce 25(OH)D-1α-hydroxylase and $1,25(OH)_2D$. $1,25(OH)_2D$ also induces 25(OH)D-24-hydroxylase, an enzyme producing 24,25-dihydroxyvitamin D ($24,25[OH]_2D$), the most prevalent dihydroxylated vitamin D in serum. The activity of this enzyme may reduce the formation of biologically active $1,25(OH)_2D$.

Vitamin D, 25(OH)D, and $1,25(OH)_2D$ are bound in the circulation to vitamin D–binding protein (DBP), a specific, high-affinity transport protein also known as *group-specific component*.[119,257,258] In humans, DBP contains 458 amino acid residues and has a molecular weight of 51 335. DBP is synthesized by the liver and circulates in great excess (at about 400 mg/L), with fewer than 5% of the binding sites normally occupied. Vitamin D and its metabolites are bound with the following preference: $25(OH)D > 1,25(OH)_2D >> $ vitamin D. Only 0.03% of 25(OH)D and 0.4% of $1,25(OH)_2D$ are normally free in plasma (Table 49-4). DBP concentrations are increased in pregnancy and with estrogen therapy and are decreased in nephrotic syndrome.

Biological Actions of 1,25-Dihydroxyvitamin D

$1,25(OH)_2D$ helps to maintain calcium and phosphate in serum by its actions on intestine, bone, kidney, and the parathyroids. In the small intestine, $1,25(OH)_2D$ stimulates calcium absorption, primarily in the duodenum, and phosphate absorption by the jejunum and ileum.[146,147,257,258,458] At high concentrations, $1,25(OH)_2D$ increases bone resorption by inducing monocytic stem cells in bone marrow to differentiate into osteoclasts and by stimulating osteoblasts to produce cytokines and other factors influencing osteoclast activity. By stimulating osteoblasts, it also increases the circulating concentration of ALP and the noncollagenous bone protein osteocalcin (also called bone Gla protein, or BGP, because it contains γ-carboxyglutamic acid or Gla). In the kidneys, $1,25(OH)_2D$ inhibits its own synthesis and stimulates its metabolism. $1,25(OH)_2D$ also acts directly on the parathyroids to inhibit the synthesis and secretion of PTH. $1,25(OH)_2D$ exerts its actions by associating with a specific nuclear vitamin D receptor, analogous to the steroid receptors for androgens, estrogens, and corticosteroids (see Chapters 43 and 45).

Clinical Significance

Determination of vitamin D is useful in the differential diagnosis of hypocalcemia, hypercalcemia, or hypercalciuria and for evaluating vitamin D status in health and in bone and mineral disorders (see Calcium, Clinical Significance, Hypocalcemia, and Hypercalcemia; and Metabolic Bone Diseases). Only the measurements of 25(OH)D and $1,25(OH)_2D$ have proven clinical value.* Routine clinical determination of vitamin D, $24,25(OH)_2D$, or other metabolites is not indicated at this time.

Vitamin D nutritional status is determined best by the measurement of 25(OH)D (Box 49-9), rather than vitamin D because (1) 25(OH)D is the main circulating form of vitamin D (see Table 49-4), (2) 25(OH)D varies less, day-to-day, with exposure to sunlight and diet intake[256,258] because of its longer half-life, (3) and the measurement of 25(OH)D is relatively easy compared with the more technically complicated methods for vitamin D.[110,267,269] Groups at higher risk for developing nutritional vitamin D deficiency include breast-fed infants, strict vegetarians who abstain from eggs and milk, individuals of color, and the elderly.

BOX 49-9 Abnormal Circulating Levels of 25(OH)D

Decreased 25(OH)D
- Inadequate exposure to sunlight
- Inadequate dietary vitamin D
- Vitamin D malabsorption
- Severe hepatocellular disease
- Increased catabolism (e.g., drugs, such as anticonvulsants)
- Increased loss (nephrotic syndrome)

Increased 25(OH)D (hypercalcemia)
- Vitamin D or 25(OH)D intoxication

25(OH)D is useful in evaluating hypocalcemia, vitamin D status, bone disease, and other disorders of mineral metabolism. Circulating concentrations of 25(OH)D may be decreased by (1) reduced availability of vitamin D, (2) inadequate conversion of vitamin D to 25(OH)D, (3) accelerated metabolism of 25(OH)D, and (4) urinary loss of 25(OH)D with its transport protein. Reduced availability of vitamin D occurs with inadequate exposure to sunlight, dietary deficiency, malabsorption syndromes, or gastric or small bowel resection. Severe hepatocellular disease has been associated with inadequate conversion of vitamin D to 25(OH)D. Drugs such as phenytoin, phenobarbital, and rifampin induce drug-metabolizing enzymes that accelerate the metabolism of vitamin D and its metabolites. Serum 25(OH)D concentrations may be reduced in patients with nephrotic syndrome because of the urinary loss of DBP and 25(OH)D. Measurement of 25(OH)D has limited value in hypercalcemia. Its most common use in hypercalcemia is in confirming intoxication after ingestion of large amounts of vitamin D or 25(OH)D[587]; 25(OH)D concentration is typically greater than 100 ng/mL (250 nmol/L) in such patients.

Measurement of $1,25(OH)_2D$ is useful in detecting inadequate or excessive hormone production in the evaluation of hypercalcemia, hypercalciuria, hypocalcemia, and bone and mineral disorders (Box 49-10). Because activated macrophages convert 25(OH)D to $1,25(OH)_2D$, serum concentrations of $1,25(OH)_2D$ are often increased in sarcoidosis, tuberculosis, other granulomatous diseases. Rarely is lymphoma associated with increased concentrations of $1,25(OH)_2D$.[4] Concentrations of $1,25(OH)_2D$ are elevated in vitamin D–dependent rickets type II and in $1,25(OH)_2D$ intoxication, and may be elevated in primary hyperparathyroidism. Patients with primary hyperparathyroidism and

*References 22, 113, 257, 258, 458, 541.

BOX 49-10 Abnormal Levels of 1,25(OH)$_2$D

Decreased 1,25(OH)$_2$D
- Renal failure
- Hyperphosphatemia
- Hypomagnesemia
- Hypoparathyroidism
- Pseudohypoparathyroidism
- Vitamin D–dependent rickets, type I
- Hypercalcemia of malignancy

Increased 1,25(OH)$_2$D
- Granulomatous diseases
- Primary hyperparathyroidism
- Lymphoma
- 1,25(OH)$_2$D intoxication
- Vitamin D–dependent rickets, type II

high concentrations of 1,25(OH)$_2$D appear to be more prone to developing hypercalciuria and renal stones. Reduced concentrations of 1,25(OH)$_2$D are observed in patients with renal failure, hypercalcemia of malignancy, hyperphosphatemia, hypoparathyroidism, pseudohypoparathyroidism, type I vitamin D–dependent rickets, hypomagnesemia, nephrotic syndrome, and severe hepatocellular disease. Measurement of 1,25(OH)$_2$D is not useful in confirming intoxication with vitamin D or 25(OH)D, because 1,25(OH)$_2$ concentrations may be low, normal, or elevated.

Measurement of Vitamin D Metabolites

Specific and sensitive assays have been developed for vitamin D, 25(OH)D, and 1,25(OH)$_2$D.[261] 25(OH)D and 1,25(OH)$_2$D assays should measure D$_2$ and D$_3$ metabolites equally (with "equimolar" reactivity), since both D$_2$ and D$_3$ are metabolized to produce biologically active 1,25(OH)$_2$D. Separate measurement of the D$_2$ and D$_3$ forms does not necessarily distinguish dietary and endogenous sources of vitamin D, as food is supplemented with D$_3$ and D$_2$.[257]

Most assays for 25(OH)D and 1,25(OH)$_2$D contain two or three of the following steps: (1) deproteinization or extraction, (2) purification, and (3) quantification. Deproteinization or extraction frees the metabolites from DPB and may partially purify the metabolites. Purification steps, most often column chromatography, separate the various forms of vitamin D, lipid, and interfering substances. The method of quantification depends on the metabolite being measured.

Extraction and Deproteinization

Before the advent of commercially available methods, it was common to use two-phase, liquid-liquid partition with organic solvents and solvent mixtures, including methylene chloride, hexane, diethyl ether, ethanol/chloroform/water, methylene chloride/methanol, hexane/isopropanol, and cyclohexane/ethyl acetate.[108,169,288,555] Ethanol and methanol were also used to free 25(OH)D from DBP when measuring 25(OH)D.[108,288]

Today, the most widely used commercially available methods use acetonitrile to deproteinize the specimen and to denature DBP, thereby freeing vitamin D metabolites.[261] A method using immunoextraction for 1,25(OH)$_2$D has also been reported.[260,261,278]

Column Chromatography

The differences in their polarities, because of the number of hydroxyl groups, have been used to separate vitamin D and its metabolites. With three hydroxyl groups, 1,25(OH)$_2$D is more polar than 25(OH)D, with two hydroxyls, which is more polar than vitamin D, with one hydroxyl group.

Extracts have been purified by chromatography on minicolumns of silica, silicic acid, Sephadex LH-20, hydroxyalkoxypropyl Sephadex LH-20 (Lipidex 5000), celite, alumina, or some other absorbents.* Solid-phase extraction using octadecyl (C$_{18}$)-silica was widely used for measuring 1,25(OH)$_2$D.† The most popular method[459] used both a reversed-phase C$_{18}$-silica minicolumn and a normal-phase silica minicolumn to separate vitamin D metabolites. This method was modified by eliminating the silica cartridge and using "phase switching" with a single nonend-capped C$_{18}$OH cartridge.[259]

Measurement of 25-Hydroxyvitamin D

Serum 25(OH)D has been measured by CPBA, competitive immunoassay (RIA, EIA, ICMA), or UV absorption after separation by HPLC. Determination by HPLC with UV absorption requires the appropriate HPLC equipment (see Chapter 6), more specialized training, and a larger sample. Most clinical laboratories measuring 25(OH)D have chosen the more familiar competitive immunoassays or CPBA. These assays are relatively easy to perform, use widely available reagents, and require only a small specimen. Although assays do not have difficulty in recognizing supranormal concentrations of 25(OH)D, measurement of subnormal and low normal concentrations is more difficult, requiring well-validated methods free from interference.

Radioimmunoassay. Development of an antiserum with equimolar cross-reactivity for 25(OH)D$_2$ and 25(OH)D$_3$ permitted the development of a competitive immunoassay (RIA) for 25(OH)D.[261,266] Previous antisera did not equally cross-react with D$_2$ and D$_3$ forms,[65] limiting their clinical usefulness. This antiserum was raised against a bovine serum albumin (BSA) conjugate of a vitamin D analogue lacking the side chain (23,24,25,26,27-pentanor vitamin D-C[22]carboxylic acid). A radioiodinated tracer was subsequently developed using a vitamin D analogue (3-aminopropyl derivative of vitamin D-C[22]-amide) and Bolton-Hunter reagent.[265] Samples and calibrators are

*References 5, 169, 247, 268, 288, 309, 348, 575.
†References 169, 263, 288, 293, 462, 575.

deproteinized with acetonitrile and analyzed directly without chromatography. Although the antiserum also recognizes 24,25$(OH)_2D$, 25,26$(OH)_2D$, and 25(OH)D-26,23-lactone, 25(OH)D results are comparable with HPLC because of the much lower concentration of these metabolites. RIA is reported to be less sensitive to interfering substances in serum extracts than CPBA using DBP. A second RIA has been approved by the Food and Drug Administration (FDA) for the measurement of 25(OH)D; however, this method does not appear to have equimolar cross-reactivity for 25$(OH)D_2$ and 25$(OH)D_3$.[262] Automated, nonisotopic immunoassays (even with pretreatment) for 25(OH)D are needed to increase the availability of 25(OH)D determinations.

Competitive Protein-Binding Assays with Vitamin D–Binding Protein. Before the development of immunoassays, 25(OH)D was measured primarily with CPBA with DBP as the specific binder, and with tritiated 25$(OH)D_3$ (>100 Ci/mmol) as tracer.[290,372,508] Rat serum, diluted approximately 1:50 000 (v/v), provides a convenient source of DBP. Assays based on DBP measure both 25$(OH)D_2$ and 25$(OH)D_3$. Assays that do not chromatographically isolate 25(OH)D measure other metabolites, including 25$(OH)D_3$-23,26-lactone, 24,25$(OH)_2D$, 25,26$(OH)_2D$, and to a lesser extent vitamin D, overestimating 25(OH)D by about 10% in normal individuals. It is important to verify that assays respond equally to 25$(OH)D_2$ and 25$(OH)D_3$. Serum extracts may contain other substances that cross-react in nonchromatographic assays using DBP, increasing the apparent concentration of 25(OH)D.* 25(OH)D concentrations are reported to be significantly higher when measured by CPBA when compared with RIA or HPLC.[338] An automated chemiluminescent assay is available for measuring 25(OH)D using DBP.[406]

HPLC and Ultraviolet Absorption. HPLC methods for 25(OH)D have used normal-phase chromatography on silica, reversed-phase chromatography on C_{18}-silica, or a combination of the two followed by quantification by UV absorption at 254 or 265 nm.† Most methods have required both extraction and preparative chromatography before HPLC. More recently, methods without preparative chromatography have been developed using gradient or isocratic reversed-phase HPLC and with photodiode-array UV detection.[14,580] A specimen of 0.5 to 1.0 mL is required because of the limited sensitivity of UV detection. Although HPLC methods allow 25$(OH)D_2$ and 25$(OH)D_3$ to be separated, independent determination is not of routine clinical value. HPLC is useful for validating the accuracy of immunoassays and CPBAs.

Measurement of 1,25-Hydroxyvitamin D

1,25$(OH)_2D$ circulates at approximately 1/1000 the concentration of 25(OH)D and at significantly lower concentrations than other dihydroxylated metabolites, greatly complicating its determination in serum. The most widely used methods require extraction, chromatography, and quantification by radioreceptor assay (RRA) or RIA. RRAs have been widely used because of the high specificity of the vitamin D receptor (VDR) for 1,25$(OH)_2D$, whereas antisera have been less specific. The most widely used RRA and RIA are described and discussed in the following section.

Radioreceptor Assay. A flow diagram for the extraction, purification, and radioreceptor assay of 1,25$(OH)_2D$[259,261,459] is shown in Figure 49-19. Specimens (1 mL of serum or plasma) are deproteinized with acetonitrile, alkalinized and diluted, and applied to a $C_{18}OH$ cartridge (solid-phase extraction). After washing with water and methanol/water (70:30), 25(OH)D and 24,24$(OH)_2D$ are eluted with hexane/methylene chloride (90:10) and discarded. The column is washed with hexane/isopropanol (99:1), before the elution of 1,25$(OH)_2D$ with hexane/isopropanol (95:5). The fraction containing 1,25$(OH)_2D$ is evaporated, rehydrated, and assayed using an RRA with VDR from calf thymus. A nonequilibrium, delayed addition of tracer (5000 cpm of tritiated 1,25$[OH]_2D_3$) is used to lower the detection limit (2 to 5 pg/mL [4.8 to 12 pmol/L] with 1 mL of serum), followed by separation of bound and free tracer with dextran-treated charcoal. Recovery of the extraction, chromatographic, and other preparative procedures is monitored with a small amount of tritiated 1,25$(OH)_2D_3$.

This method is a substantial improvement over earlier methods using VDR from chick intestine. Calf thymus provides an unlimited, more reproducible source of VDR with several advantages over chick intestinal VDR.[270,287,459] Thymus receptor recognizes 1,25$(OH)_2$ D_2 and 1,25$(OH)_2D_3$ equally, unlike chick intestinal receptor, which underestimates the concentration of 1,25$(OH)_2$ D_2. VDR from thymus appears to be less sensitive than that from intestine to lipid and other nonspecific interferences extracted from serum, eliminating the need for extensive purification, including preparative HPLC. Patients treated with dihydrotachysterol may have falsely elevated concentrations of 1,25$(OH)_2D$ when measured with chick intestinal receptor, but not with the thymus receptor assay.[554]

Radioimmunoassay. Before the development of the method described below, RIAs were not widely used in the United States because previous antisera: (1) did not reliably measure vitamin D status, since they discriminated between 1,25$(OH)_2D_2$ and 1,25$(OH)_2D_3$, and (2) cross-reacted with other vitamin D metabolites to a much greater extent than VDR requiring more extensive sample purification, including preparative HPLC.[63,111,139,233,261]

The RIA described below is more convenient than the RRA for 1,25$(OH)_2D$[261,264] because a radioiodinated tracer eliminates the need for liquid scintillation, and the antiserum eliminates the need to prepare VDR from calf thymus. The RIA uses a previously developed antiserum[191] with 1% to 2% cross-reactivity with the more abundant, non-1-hydroxylated vitamin D metabolites and a ^{125}I-labeled tracer prepared from 1,25$(OH)_2$-24,25,26,27, tetranor-

*References 65, 96, 169, 336, 367, 605.

†References 80, 116, 285, 286, 288, 293, 309, 396, 508, 521, 547, 551.

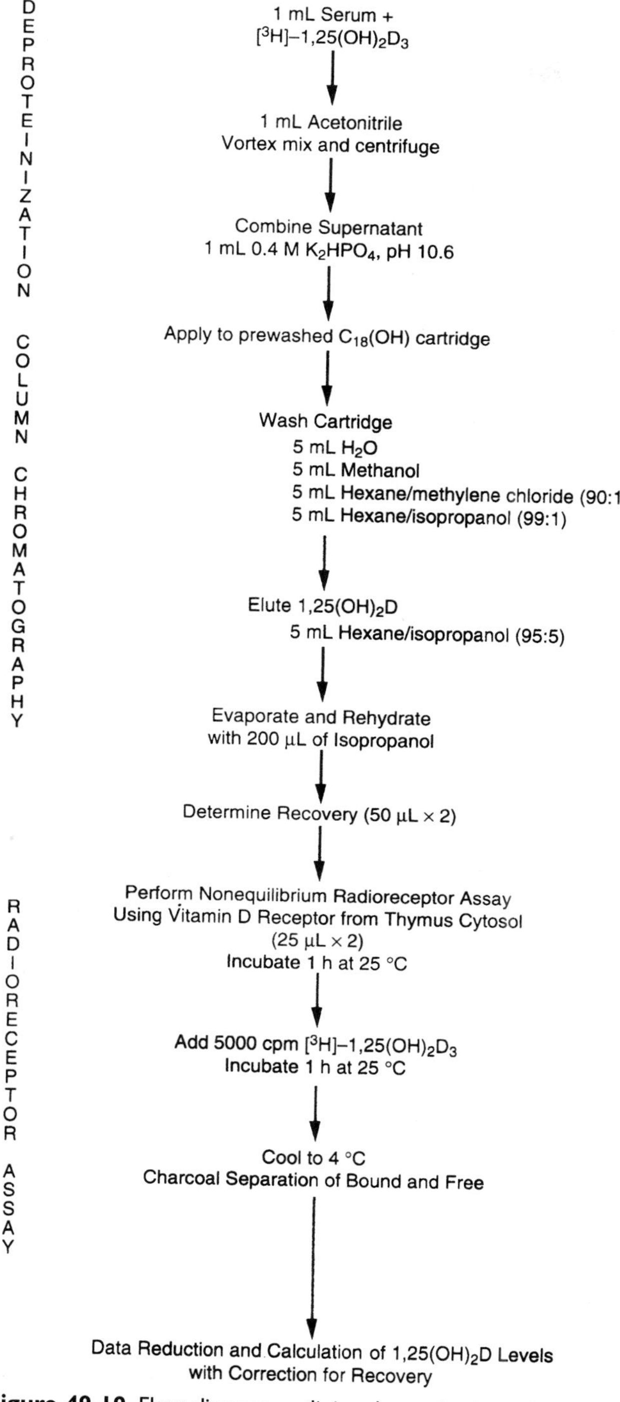

Figure 49-19 Flow diagram outlining determination of 1,25-dihydroxyvitamin D using a single-column extraction and purification method and a nonequilibrium radioreceptor assay with vitamin D receptor from calf thymus.

C(23)-carboxylic acid and radiolabeled Bolton-Hunter reagent. Before analysis, specimens are deproteinized with acetonitrile, oxidized with sodium metaperiodate, and purified using C_{18}-OH and silica cartridges. Sodium metaperiodate is necessary to eliminate interference by $24,24(OH)_2D$ and $25,26(OH)_2D$ by oxidizing them to their aldehyde and ketone forms, which are easily removed by chromatography. A silica column was added to the single C_{18}-OH cartridge used with the radioreceptor assay to reduce interference in the RIA. With this RIA, $1,25(OH)_2D_2$ is about 70% as potent as $1,25(OH)_2D_3$. Recovery of individual samples is not determined, although calibrators are prepared in a stripped serum base and treated identically to samples. The method does cross-react (13% to 25%) with a number of 1-hydroxylated metabolites, including $1,24,25(OH)_3D$, $1,25,26(OH)_3D$, and $1,25(OH)_2D$-26,23-lactone. $1,25(OH)_2D$-26,23-lactone is a significant metabolite with a concentration of 0% to 30% of $1,25(OH)_2D_3$. A modification of this method using a single C_{18}-OH "extra clean" cartridge is commercially available.[153]

Another commercially available RIA has been developed that uses selective immunoextraction of $1,25(OH)_2D$.[260,261,278] This method is reported to have greater cross-reactivity with the 1-hydroxylated metabolites, including 1,25-dihydroxyvitamin D_3-26,23-lactone[260,261] and calcipotriol,[278] which is used for treating psoriasis. Apparent concentrations of $1,25(OH)_2D$ are significantly higher with this method than the RRA in patients with hypoparathyroidism receiving vitamin D treatment, patients with biliary atresia, vitamin D–intoxicated subjects, and some normal specimens.[261]

Troubleshooting Vitamin D Assays

Methods requiring extraction and chromatography should be monitored for recovery of the vitamin D metabolites of interest and for solvent or column blanks. For the RRA assay, recovery is monitored and the final result is corrected for losses by the addition of a small, known amount of tritiated $1,25(OH)_2D_3$ before extraction of specimens. Care must be taken to ensure that D_2 and D_3 metabolites are recovered equally, providing a total measurement of 25(OH)D or 1,25(OH)D. Solvents, chromatographic materials, and cartridges may contain substances that interfere with quantification of vitamin D metabolites by CPBA, RIA, and RRA or UV absorption after HPLC, resulting in an overestimation of vitamin D metabolites. Any interferences can be monitored by treating a water blank identically to the specimens. Undetectable concentrations of vitamin D in this blank verify the absence of positive interference.

Calibrators for vitamin D assays should be prepared from stock solutions whose concentration and purity are checked by UV spectrophotometry.[270] Stock solutions are suitable if the ratio of the absorbance at 264 to 228 nm is greater than or equal to 1.5. Stock solutions are adjusted using a molar extinction coefficient of 18,200 L/mol/cm for vitamin D_3 metabolites at 264 nm. Tracers used for recovery must be pure to determine recovery accurately. Both calibrators and tracers may be purified by HPLC.

Specimen Requirements

Serum is typically used for measuring vitamin D metabolites, although plasma is generally acceptable for assays using extraction and chromatography. Once separated from the clot, serum is relatively stable at both room temperature and 4 °C; however, specimens should be frozen if the analysis is delayed.[339] Vitamin D metabolites in serum or plasma do not appear to be sensitive to light and do not require special handling in the laboratory.

Reference Intervals

Reference intervals for vitamin D are method-dependent, but representative ones are:

25(OH)D: 10 to 65 ng/mL (25 to 162 nmol/L)

$1,25(OH)_2D$: 15 to 60 pg/mL (36 to 144 pmol/L)

The lower limit of the reference range for 25(OH)D of 10 to 15 ng/mL (25 to 37 nmol/L) has been increasingly criticized as inappropriately low. Although a decision level for vitamin D insufficiency has not been determined, concentrations of less than 20 to 30 ng/mL (50 to 75 nmol/L) are associated with increased PTH[352,534] and reduced calcium absorption.[248] The recent NHANES III study reported an unexpectedly high prevalence of vitamin D insufficiency.[94,346] For example, vitamin D insufficiency (25 (OH)D <20 ng/mL [50 nmol/L]) was exceedingly common during the winter in adult (30 years and older) Caucasian men (15%) and women (30%) living in the South. Vitamin D insufficiency was most common in Blacks, with the prevalence in Hispanics between Caucasians and Blacks.

Circulating concentrations of 25(OH)D are increased by exposure to sunlight and show seasonal variation, with the highest concentrations in summer or fall and the lowest concentrations in winter or spring.[522] Concentrations are influenced by latitude, sunscreen use, and skin pigmentation.[257,258] Serum 25(OH)D concentrations of 100 ng/mL (250 nmol/L) are not uncommon in lifeguards.

Concentrations of vitamin D metabolites vary with age and are increased in pregnancy.[216,454] Concentrations of $1,25(OH)_2D$ are higher in pregnancy and in children than adults, with the highest concentrations occurring during periods of greatest growth.[6,360,373,476,536] Although 25(OH)D and $1,25(OH)_2D$ concentrations have been reported to decrease with age, this decline may be a consequence of poor nutrition, reduced exposure to sunlight, and declining health. Concentrations of these metabolites have been unchanged with age in studies limited to healthy and active subjects.[162,418]

CALCITONIN

Calcitonin is secreted by the parafollicular or C cells, which arise from the neural crest and are distributed throughout the thyroid gland. These cells are included in the APUD (*a*mine *p*recursor *u*ptake and *d*ecarboxylation) family, which explains the association of medullary thyroid carcinoma (a tumor of the C cells) and other tumors of the APUD family in multiple endocrine neoplasia type-2A and -2B (MEN-2A and MEN-2B). Release of calcitonin is stimulated by calcium, and it has been used pharmacologically as an inhibitor of bone resorption.

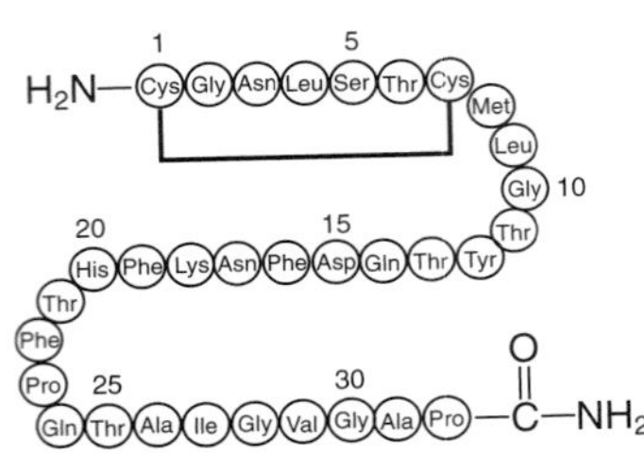

Figure 49-20 Amino acid sequence of calcitonin.

Biochemistry and Physiology

Calcitonin is a 32–amino acid peptide (MW = 3418) with an N-terminal disulfide bond linking cysteine residues 1 and 7 and a C-terminal proline-amide (Figure 49-20). The C-terminal portion of the molecule, with its proline-amide residue, the disulfide bond between residues 1 and 7, and the methionine residue at position 8 are necessary for biological activity. The amino-terminal amino acids are highly conserved; five of the first nine amino acids are identical in all species. In humans, porcine calcitonin is 1/10 as active as human calcitonin, whereas salmon calcitonin is 10 times more potent.

The physiological control of calcitonin secretion is incompletely understood. Calcium appears to be the most important secretagogue; an increase in serum calcium increases calcitonin. In some animals, a number of other factors, including the hormones gastrin, cholecystokinin, glucagon, and secretin, can stimulate calcitonin secretion; the physiological role of these hormones in humans is uncertain.

Pharmacological doses of calcitonin reduce serum calcium and phosphate concentration primarily by inhibiting osteoclastic bone resorption. Recognition of this pharmacological effect has resulted in the use of salmon and human calcitonin to reduce bone resorption in patients with Paget's disease and osteoporosis and as a treatment for hypercalcemia in diseases associated with increased bone resorption. Pharmacological doses of calcitonin also decrease the renal tubular reabsorption of calcium and phosphate.

Despite these pharmacological effects, the physiological role of calcitonin in adults is uncertain. No apparent alterations in bone or mineral metabolism are evident in humans with calcitonin deficiency or excess. Calcitonin may be important during periods of calcium stress in fetuses or young children or during pregnancy or lactation, as evidenced by the higher concentrations observed during these physiological states.

Multiple forms of circulating calcitonin have been reported in normal individuals and patients with medullary thyroid carcinoma (MTC) or nonthyroidal malignancies.* Much of the immunoreactive calcitonin generally migrates as larger forms rather than with monomeric calcitonin. A

*References 30, 151, 224, 390, 486, 528, 566.

sulfoxide of the monomer, dimers, glycosylated forms, and precursors have been proposed to explain this heterogeneity.[30,279,528,566]

Clinical Significance

MTC occurs as a sporadic disease and as part of the syndromes of MEN-2A, MEN-2B, and familial MTC (FMTC).[8,71,150,381] MEN-2A and MEN-2B are autosomal dominant inherited multiglandular syndromes with age-related penetrance and variable expression. All forms of MTC combined account for 5% to 10% of thyroid malignancies. Sporadic MTC is believed to comprise approximately 75% of all MTC. The routine measurement of serum calcitonin in nodular thyroid diseases assists in detecting unsuspected sporadic MTC.[158,421,463] With the advent of genetic testing for MEN-2A, MEN-2B, and FMTC, calcitonin is primarily used for diagnosing sporadic MTC or the index case in familial MTC or for monitoring MTC.

In approximately 95% of individuals with MEN-2A, MEN-2B, and FMTC, mutations are identified with genetic testing of the coding sequence of the *RET* proto-oncogene transmembrane tyrosine kinase receptor.* Genetic testing provides the most sensitive and specific method for detection of the disorder in family members of the index case; and unlike calcitonin monitoring, it does not require annual testing. Genetic testing is also justified in sporadic cases of MTC, as 5% to 10% carry germline *RET* mutations.

Many patients with MTC have increased basal concentrations of calcitonin (after biological penetrance), but provocative testing using calcitonin secretagogues increases the sensitivity of detecting MTC and C-cell hyperplasia.[27,296,530,599] Calcium,[489] pentagastrin,[219] or a combination of calcium and pentagastrin[530,599] have been the most commonly used agents for stimulating calcitonin secretion. Specificity is also increased with provocative testing.[54] Minimally increased concentrations that are not stimulated after provocative testing should be questioned. Resolution may require the use of other provocative agents, confirmation that a proper stimulation test was conducted (e.g., determination of serum calcium when calcium is used as the stimulant), or the use of different methods for measuring calcitonin. The effectiveness of surgery is often monitored by serial measurement of basal and, preferably, stimulated calcitonin concentrations.[565,600] Increased calcitonin concentrations are generally believed to be indicative of persistent or recurrent disease, although many of these patients remain asymptomatic for years.

Calcitonin concentrations are increased in various nonthyroidal cancers (Box 49-11). Although increased calcitonin is most often associated with tumors arising from tissues derived from the neural crest, it may also be increased in other malignancies. These include intestinal, bronchial, and gastric carcinoids; carcinoma of the lung, especially oat-cell or small-cell carcinoma; melanoma and pheochromocytoma; and pancreatic and breast carcinoma.[135,391,507,591]

Elevated concentrations of calcitonin or increased responsiveness to stimulation have also been reported in acute and chronic renal failure, hypercalcemia, hypergastrinemia and other gastrointestinal disorders, pulmonary disease, and severe illness.[32,135,604]

*References 8, 71, 134, 150, 199, 381, 600.

BOX 49-11 Increased Circulating Levels of Calcitonin

C-cell hyperplasia
Medullary thyroid carcinoma
Nonthyroidal cancers
  Oat-, small-cell carcinomas
  Other malignancies
Acute and chronic renal failure
Hypercalcemia
Hypergastrinemia and other gastrointestinal disorders
Pulmonary disease

Measurement of Calcitonin

Measurement and interpretation of serum calcitonin are complicated by the heterogeneity circulating of calcitonin and large differences in the sensitivity and specificity of calcitonin immunoassays.

Radioimmmoassays

Historically, calcitonin was measured primarily by RIA. Using RIA, the upper limit of the normal reference interval varied from 20 to 1000 pg/mL (ng/L) or more.[135,249] Differences in assay sensitivity, sensitivity to matrix effects and specificity, and the heterogeneity of calcitonin probably explain these differences. Basal calcitonin concentrations in normal individuals have generally been less than 100 pg/mL (ng/L) with the newer and more sensitive, homologous RIAs. Normal concentrations of less than 50 pg/mL (ng/L) have been reported by investigators with certain RIAs or after concentration and partial purification of specimens using affinity chromatography with immobilized calcitonin antiserum before RIA.[614]

Upper reference limits of 20 and 25 pg/mL (ng/L) for women and men, respectively, have been reported using a highly sensitive RIA with detection limit of 3 pg/mL (ng/L).[170,430] Other investigators reported normal concentrations of less than 20 pg/mL (ng/L) using preparative chromatography on silica columns to extract and partially purify calcitonin from 15 to 20 mL of plasma.[53]

Noncompetitive Immunoassays

More recently, noncompetitive immunoassays (IRMA, ELISA, and ICMA) have been reported for calcitonin.* Com-

*References 235, 390, 431, 516, 517, 596, 608, 622.

pared with earlier RIAs, these methods provide improved sensitivity and specificity for the diagnosis of MTC.* With most noncompetitive methods, basal concentrations of calcitonin in normal individuals are less than 10 to 20 pg/mL (ng/L). Investigations of two-site assays indicate that they may also recognize multiple forms of immunoreactive calcitonin.[390,608]

Automated noncompetitive chemiluminescent (ICMA) methods have recently been reported using acridinium ester or ALP with 1,2-dioxetane phosphate.

Reference Intervals

The basal and pentagastrin-stimulated reference intervals for normal men, women, and athyroidal patients for a sensitive, noncompetitive chemiluminescent method are listed below[174]:

Basal concentrations of serum calcitonin:

Men:	<8.8 pg/mL (ng/L)
Women:	<5.8 pg/mL (ng/L)
Athyroidal:	<0.5 pg/mL (ng/L)

Provocative testing

Pentagastrin†

Normals:	<30 pg/mL (ng/L) (N = 20)
Athyroidal:	<0.5 pg/mL (ng/L) (N = 10)

Reference intervals for calcitonin are dependent on the method. Basal and stimulated (calcium and pentagastrin) ranges should be determined for normal individuals and athyroidal individuals, by gender, for each method.

Gender, age, growth, pregnancy, lactation, and ingestion of food have been reported to influence calcitonin concentrations in normal individuals. Most investigators[170,249] have observed higher concentrations of basal and stimulated calcitonin in men than in women. The effect of age is less certain, as basal and stimulated concentrations have been reported both to decline and to remain unchanged with age.[137,430,563] Higher concentrations have been reported during pregnancy and lactation[525] and in children and infants.[51,306] Food ingestion has been reported both to increase and to have little effect on the concentration of circulating calcitonin.[53,518]

Parathyroid Hormone–Related Protein

PTHrP was discovered in 1987 by investigators studying the mechanism by which certain cancers produce humoral hypercalcemia of malignancy (HHM).‡

Biochemistry and Physiology

PTHrP is derived from a gene on chromosome 12 that is distinct from the PTH gene on chromosome 11. Three isoforms of 139, 141, and 173 amino acids are predicted by alternative messenger RNA (mRNA) splicing (Figure 49-21). The N-terminal end of the molecule shows close homology to PTH (8 of the first 13 amino acids being identical). The remainder of the PTHrP molecule shows little homology with PTH. The PTH-like activity of PTHrP is contained within the N-terminal amino acids (PTHrP[1-36]).

The common N-terminal explains the ability of PTHrP to interact with the PTH/PTHrP receptor, mimicking the biological actions of PTH in classic target tissues, including bone and kidney. Like PTH, PTHrP causes hypercalcemia and hypophosphatemia and increases urinary cyclic AMP. However, when compared with patients with primary hyperparathyroidism, patients with PTHrP-induced hypercalcemia have lower concentrations of 1,25$(OH)_2$D and more typically have metabolic alkalosis (instead of hyperchloremic metabolic acidosis), reduced distal tubular calcium reabsorption, and reduced and uncoupled bone formation.

The multitude of basic residues in PTHrP suggests that it may undergo extensive posttranslational processing.[419] Forms of PTHrP containing the following amino acids have been detected in serum: (1) PTHrP(1-36) measured by N-terminal assays, (2) PTHrP containing N-terminal and midregion amino acids measured with noncompetitive immunoassays against PTHrP(1-74 or 1-86), (3) midregion fragments, beginning at position 38 and extending 70 to 80 amino acids, measured with midregion assays, and (4) carboxyl fragments, beginning at position 107, measured with antiserum directed against PTHrP(109 to 138). Midregion and carboxyl forms may exert biological actions distinct from the PTH-like actions associated with the N-terminal region.

Besides its endocrine role in the pathophysiology of HHM, PTHrP appears to participate in normal physiology by acting locally on cells or tissue as an autocrine or paracrine factor.[353,419,432] PTHrP is widely expressed in most normal tissues of fetuses and adults.[315,448,579] Although it is unlikely that the low circulating concentrations of PTHrP have a significant effect on calcium homeostasis in normal adults, PTHrP may exert endocrine effects on calcium homeostasis during fetal life and lactation.[535] Breast milk contains high concentrations of PTHrP. Examination of the physiological effects of PTHrP identifies several themes: (1) PTHrP regulates transepithelial calcium transport; (2) PTHrP is a potent, smooth muscle relaxant; (3) PTHrP regulates growth, differentiation, and development; and (4) PTHrP's role in many tissues is unknown.

Clinical Significance

Hypercalcemia associated with malignancy is the second most common cause of hypercalcemia. This frequent paraneoplastic syndrome is believed to occur primarily through

*References 27, 235, 296, 390, 431, 596.

†Gender-based provocative intervals are preferable because of the differences in basal and stimulated calcitonin between men and women. Because pentagastrin is not readily available in the US, studies are needed to define gender-based ranges for the more widely used calcium stimulation tests.

‡References 90, 92, 353, 364, 389, 420, 542, 546, 616.

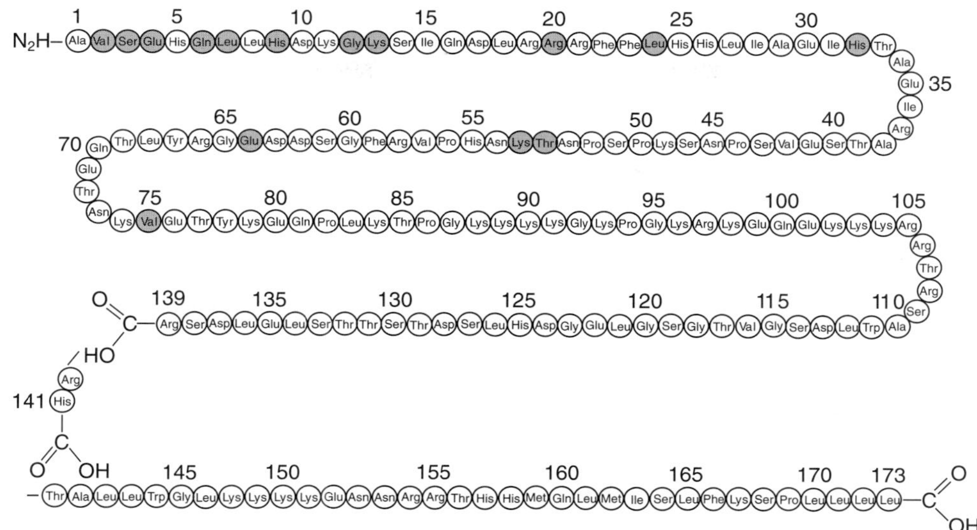

Figure 49-21 Amino acid sequence of PTHrP. Although the exact length of circulating PTHrP is unknown, proteins of 139, 141, and 173 amino acids have been predicted from alternative splicing events. The black circles show amino acids that are identical in PTH and PTHrP. *(Modified from Hendy GN, Goltzman D. Parathyroid hormone-like peptide. In: Endocrinology and metabolism inservice, Vol 9. Washington, DC: American Association for Clinical Chemistry, 1991:9-24.)*

two mechanisms: HHM and local osteolysis. Patients with HHM account for approximately 75% to 80% of patients with hypercalcemia associated with malignancy. HHM is common in patients with squamous (lung, head and neck, esophagus, cervix, vulva, and skin), renal, bladder, and ovarian carcinomas. Hypercalcemia due to skeletal metastases and local osteolysis are common in breast cancer and multiple myeloma, lymphomas, and other hematological malignancies. The hypercalcemia of a subset of lymphomas (human T-cell leukemia virus-1) appears to be caused by HHM. Breast carcinomas may cause hypercalcemia by HHM and/or skeletal metastases with local osteolysis. It is now well established that PTHrP is the principal mediator of HHM. After being secreted by tumors, PTHrP circulates and acts on its target tissues (skeleton and kidney) as an endocrine hormone causing hypercalcemia.

PTHrP determinations are usually considered investigational, because HHM nearly always occurs in advanced disease when the diagnosis is obvious. The need for PTHrP determinations may increase if it becomes important in prognosis,[577] selection of therapy, or monitoring.

Measurement of PTHrP

A number of competitive immunoassays have been used for measuring PTHrP in sera from patients with HHM. For example, N-terminal (PTHrP[1-34]), midregion (PTHrP [37-67, 37-74]), and C-terminal (PTHrP[109-138]) competitive RIAs have been developed.* Of the competitive immunoassays, the N-terminal assays have been used most widely. Affinity chromatography with immobilized antisera against PTHrP,[82] reversed-phase chromatography,[294] and other purification techniques have been used to improve the sensitivity and specificity of these competitive RIAs. C-terminal assays are elevated in patients with renal insufficiency.[91]

More sensitive and noncompetitive immunoassays (IRMAs) have also been developed.* Currently available assays use antibodies against PTHrP (sequences 37-74, 1-40, 1-40, 1-34, 1-40, and so on) as capture antibodies. Their radiolabeled signal antibodies are against PTHrP (sequences 1-36, 60-72, 57-80, 37-67, 50-83, and so on), respectively. The limit of detection for these assays is reported to be from 0.1 to 1.0 pmol/L.

Specimen Requirements

PTHrP is unstable in serum and plasma at 4 °C and at room temperature unless collected in the presence of protease inhibitors.[195,276,330,422] A combination of aprotinin, leupeptin, pepstatin, and EDTA provides the greatest protection.[422] In general, specimens should be collected with protease inhibitors and kept on ice. Serum or plasma should be promptly separated from the clot and/or cells and frozen.

Reference Intervals

PTHrP: 1.3 pmol/L or less.

PTHrP concentrations in normal persons are dependent on both the assay and specimen collection. Concentrations

*References 45, 82, 90, 91, 251, 294, 452.

*References 82, 90, 195, 277, 422, 451, 452.

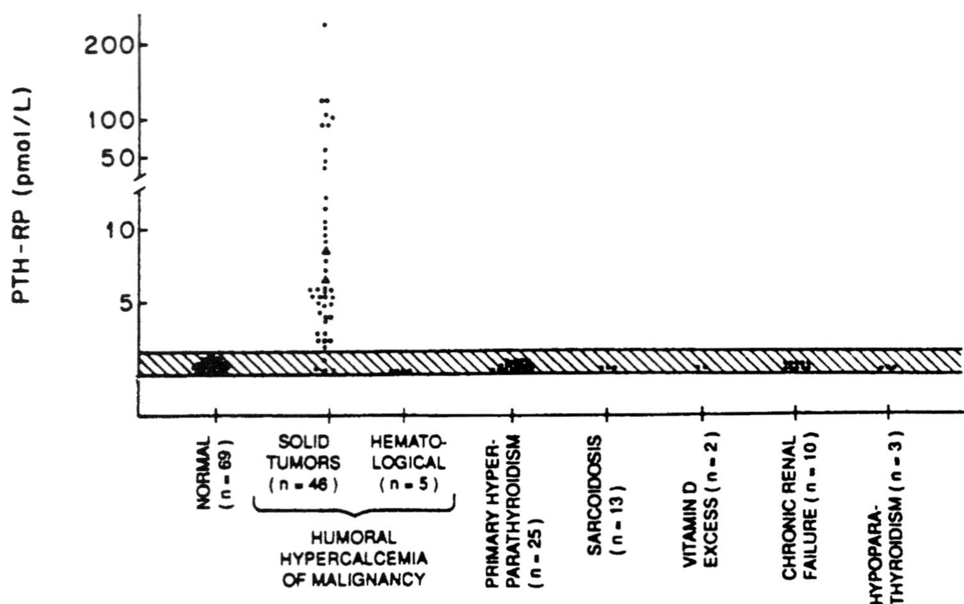

Figure 49-22 PTHrP in normal subjects and patients with malignancies and other disorders. Hatched area indicates the normal reference interval. *(Adapted from Pandian MR, Morgan CH, Carlton E, Segre GV. Modified immunoradiometric assay of parathyroid hormone-related protein: clinical application in the differential diagnosis of hypercalcemia. Clin Chem 1992;38:282-88.)*

in normal individuals range from undetectable to up to 5 pmol/L.* With sensitive noncompetitive immunoassays, concentrations of up to approximately 1 to 2 pmol/L have been reported in normal subjects.† PTHrP is reported to be detectable in approximately 50% to 80% of healthy individuals with the most sensitive methods.[90,195,422,452]

Interpretation

PTHrP is increased in 50% to 90% of patients with hypercalcemia associated with malignancy (Figure 49-22).‡ In addition to squamous cell carcinomas of the lung, head and neck, esophagus, cervix, skin, and other sites, concentrations have been elevated in a wide variety of malignancies, irrespective of their source or histology. Increased concentrations of PTHrP have been found in breast, renal, bladder, and ovarian carcinomas. Concentrations are elevated in a number of endocrine malignancies with hypercalcemia, including pheochromocytoma and islet carcinomas. PTHrP is elevated in hypercalcemic patients with adult T-cell lymphomas/leukemia and B-cell lymphoma.[277] PTHrP concentrations have been less frequently elevated in patients with hypercalcemia and other hematological malignancies (e.g., multiple myeloma).

PTHrP is undetectable or normal in most, but not all, patients with malignancy not associated with hypercalcemia.* Increased concentrations of PTHrP have been reported to precede hypercalcemia in some patients with malignancy. Concentrations are normal in patients with primary hyperparathyroidism, hypoparathyroidism, miscellaneous causes of hypercalcemia, and chronic renal failure (with noncompetitive methods).

*References 82, 91, 251, 294, 422, 451.
†References 90, 91, 195, 422, 451, 452.
‡References 82, 91, 92, 251, 294, 422, 451, 616.

INTEGRATED CONTROL OF MINERAL METABOLISM

The metabolism of calcium is linked intimately with that of phosphate (Figure 49-23).[23,41] The homeostatic mechanisms are directed principally toward the maintenance of normal extracellular calcium and phosphate concentrations, which sustain the extracellular and intracellular processes and provide substrate for skeletal mineralization. The parathyroid gland responds to a decrease in free calcium concentration within seconds. During a time of calcium deprivation, the increase in serum PTH rapidly alters both renal and skeletal metabolism.

Renal Handling of Calcium and Phosphate

Of the approximately 10 g (250 mmol) of calcium filtered by the kidneys each day, 65% is reabsorbed in the proximal tubule. Calcium reabsorption here is closely linked to sodium and is independent of PTH. Approximately 10% to

*References 82, 91, 251, 294, 422, 451.

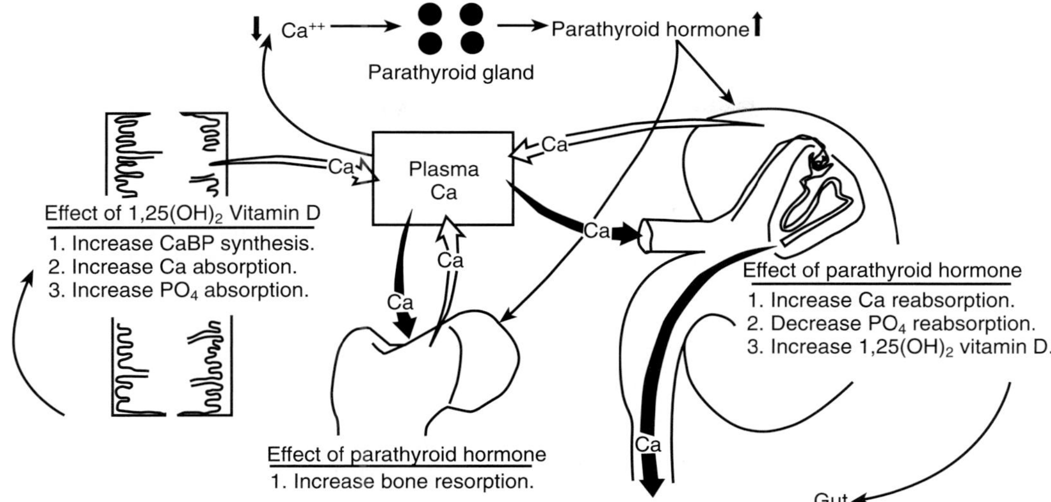

Figure 49-23 Integrated control of mineral metabolism. *CaBP,* Calcium-binding protein.

20% of calcium is reclaimed in the thick ascending loop of Henle and 5% to 10% in the distal convoluted tubule. PTH enhances calcium reabsorption at the distal tubule, presumably through a cyclic AMP mechanism. A small portion of filtered calcium, about 5%, is reabsorbed in the collecting duct via a PTH-independent mechanism.

In contrast to the calcium-conserving effect of PTH on the kidneys, PTH increases renal phosphate excretion at the proximal tubule by directly lowering the renal phosphate threshold. Approximately 6.5 g (210 mmol) of phosphate is filtered by the kidneys each day. Normally, 85% to 90% is reabsorbed by the renal tubules (proximal and distal convoluted tubule). PTH is one of the most important factors regulating the renal phosphate threshold and hence the serum phosphate concentration.

Intestinal Absorption of Calcium and Phosphate

PTH also increases intestinal calcium absorption by increasing $1,25(OH)_2D$. PTH is a major trophic factor for renal 25(OH)D-1α-hydroxylase. It increases the conversion of 25(OH)D to the active vitamin D metabolite, $1,25(OH)_2D$. Calcium is absorbed principally in the duodenum, although it can also be absorbed by the distal small bowel and colon. About 30% of a daily calcium intake of 1 g (25 mmol) is absorbed. Approximately 100 mg (2.5 mmol) of calcium is secreted into gut lumen by intestinal secretion; therefore net calcium absorption is 200 mg (5.0 mmol)/day. Calcium is absorbed by passive diffusion and by an active transport system. It is estimated that passive diffusion accounts for absorption of about 10% of ingested calcium per day. Active calcium absorption in the duodenum is under the control of $1,25(OH)_2D$. This vitamin D metabolite increases the intestinal cell synthesis of a calcium-binding protein (CaBP), which enhances the net absorption of ingested calcium.

Dietary phosphate intake is usually 1.2 to 1.4 g (39 to 45 mmol)/day, nearly twice the recommended intake, of which approximately 60% to 70% is absorbed, principally in the jejunum. As with calcium, both passive and active transport systems exist; $1,25(OH)_2D$ is the principal regulator of the active transport of phosphate. PTH-stimulated synthesis of $1,25(OH)_2D$ thus offsets the phosphaturic effect of PTH. The prevailing serum phosphate concentration also modulates renal 25(OH)D-1α-hydroxylase. Phosphate depletion or hypophosphatemia stimulates formation of $1,25(OH)_2D$ by the kidneys. In general, at pharmacological concentrations, calcitonin has the opposite effect of PTH. It is unclear, however, if calcitonin has any physiological role in mineral homeostasis in adult humans.

Bone Metabolism

PTH also has an acute effect on the skeleton. Acutely, PTH decreases osteoblastic collagen synthesis, but osteoclastic bone resorption increases, with a net increase of mineral (calcium and phosphate) release from bone into the ECF. PTH is able to act directly on osteoblasts by interacting with their PTH receptors. The effect of PTH on osteoclasts appears to be indirect, through local mediators produced by the osteoblast (e.g., RANK ligand and OPG) or released from the bone matrix (e.g., TGF-β). Prolonged calcium deprivation results in enhanced recruitment of osteoclasts and an increased number of mature osteoclasts, which continue to resorb bone, releasing calcium and phosphate and bone matrix peptides such as pyridinium collagen cross-links. Prolonged exposure to PTH eventually also increases osteoblast activity, thus increasing markers of bone formation such as ALP and osteocalcin.

Magnesium

Magnesium is efficiently absorbed in the intestinal tract (most efficiently in the distal small bowel). During normal dietary magnesium intake, approximately 30% to 40% of magnesium is absorbed. Magnesium is absorbed by both active and passive transport.

No hormone or factor has been described as regulating magnesium homeostasis. About 25% to 35% of filtered magnesium is passively reabsorbed in the proximal convoluted tubule, where reabsorption is linked closely to sodium and calcium transport. The major site of active reabsorption is the thick ascending loop of Henle, where 60% to 75% of magnesium is reabsorbed. During times of magnesium deprivation, magnesium essentially disappears from the urine (<0.5 mmol/day). The renal threshold for magnesium is close to the filtered load. When magnesium intake is excessive, any amount greater than this maximum is excreted.

METABOLIC BONE DISEASES

Metabolic bone diseases result from a partial uncoupling or imbalance between bone resorption and formation. Decreased bone mass, or *osteopenia,* is more common than abnormal increases of bone mass. The most prevalent metabolic bone diseases are osteoporosis, osteomalacia and rickets, and renal osteodystrophy. Osteoporosis, the most prevalent metabolic bone disease in developed countries, is characterized by loss of bone mass, microarchitectural deterioration of bone tissue, and increased risk of fracture. Rickets and osteomalacia, which are more common in the less-developed countries, are characterized by defective mineralization of bone matrix. Renal osteodystrophy is a complex condition that develops in response to abnormalities of the endocrine and excretory functions of the kidneys. These three metabolic bone diseases and Paget's disease, a localized bone disease, are discussed below followed by laboratory markers of bone metabolism.

OSTEOPOROSIS

Osteoporosis is the most prevalent metabolic bone disease in the United States and results in 1.5 million fractures each year.[24,464] Osteoporosis is associated with an increased risk for vertebral, hip, and distal forearm fractures. At age 50, women have a lifetime fracture risk (any of the above three sites) of about 40%. Men have a lifetime fracture risk of approximately one third that of women. Since trabecular bone turns over at five to seven times the rate of cortical bone, fractures of bones that are predominantly trabecular (vertebra and distal forearm) occur earlier in life. One third of women older than 65 years suffer vertebral crush fractures. Vertebral crush fractures can occur acutely and result in disabling pain and discomfort. Long-term complications include immobility and loss of height. Secondary problems include protuberant abdomen, chronic constipation, and loss of self-esteem. Fractures of bone with more cortical bone (proximal femur or hip) occur later in life. For women, the lifetime risk of hip fracture is 15%. The mortality rate accompanying hip fracture may be as high as 20%. Twenty-five percent of the survivors are confined to long-term care in nursing homes. The cost of medical care for osteoporosis was estimated to be $17 billion in 2001.

Peak bone mass is normally attained by 30 years of age and decreases after 35 to 45 years of age in both men and women. The amount of bone attained during growth is an important determinant of whether clinical osteoporosis develops later in life. Exercise and adequate nutrition play important roles in attaining and maintaining skeletal mass. During early adult life, bone formation is coupled to bone resorption so that bone mass remains stable. Aging is a major risk factor, because after 35 to 40 years of age bone resorption slightly exceeds bone formation so that approximately 1% of the skeletal mass is lost per year. In women, the decrease in sex steroids at menopause accelerates bone loss (postmenopausal osteoporosis) to about 2% per year. Osteoporosis is usually due to either inadequate bone formation during growth or a pathophysiological process that impairs osteoblastic bone formation or increases bone resorption. Osteoporosis is most commonly encountered in postmenopausal women. Advanced age, female gender, and sex steroid deficiency are prominent risk factors. Other risk factors include a family history of osteoporosis, alcohol abuse, smoking, and chronic diseases.

After decreased bone mass is documented by bone mass measurements, the diagnostic work-up is directed at determining the cause (Box 49-12). Most often the cause is attributed to age ("senile" osteoporosis), postmenopausal osteoporosis, or both, but it may be secondary to chronic diseases, drug therapies, or other causes. If osteoporosis is inconsistent with age or gender (such as in a middle-aged man or a premenopausal woman), laboratory testing should be performed to exclude other secondary causes of osteoporosis including hyperthyroidism, Cushing's syndrome, hypogonadism, primary hyperparathyroidism, and multiple myeloma. Chronic excess of thyroid hormone, cortisol, or PTH may cause osteoporosis. Long-standing hyperthyroidism or excessive thyroid hormone replacement increases bone resorption more than formation leading to osteoporosis. Cortisol markedly decreases bone formation and causes an increase in bone resorption. Patients with Cushing's syndrome may have severe osteoporosis. More commonly, patients receiving glucocorticoid therapy for diseases like asthma and rheumatoid arthritis may have disabling osteoporosis. Hyperparathyroidism occurs most commonly in postmenopausal women and may lead to osteoporosis. Multiple myeloma not uncommonly presents with vertebral crush fractures, and osteoporosis must be considered in these patients.

Bone markers are used to assess bone turnover (resorption or formation) in patients with osteoporosis. This testing is useful for identifying osteoporotic individuals with elevated bone resorption and for predicting and assessing the response to therapy. Markers of bone resorption include collagen cross-links (N-telopeptide, deoxypyridinoline, or C-telopeptide). Because bone resorption and formation are coupled, markers of bone formation (BAP and serum osteo-

BOX 49-12 Causes of Osteoporosis

Failure to develop normal skeletal mass during growth and development because of poor nutrition or inadequate exercise
Endocrine deficiency or excess
- Estrogen or testosterone deficiency
- Cushing's syndrome
- Hyperthyroidism
- Hyperparathyroidism

Immobilization or weightlessness
Hematological malignancies (multiple myeloma)
Inherited defects of collagen synthesis (osteogenesis imperfecta)
Systemic mastocytosis
Heparin therapy
Rheumatoid arthritis
Idiopathic juvenile osteoporosis

calcin) are also increased in high-turnover osteoporosis. Elevated markers of bone turnover indicate increased bone formation and/or resorption, but are not diagnostic of osteoporosis. They are best used to monitor therapy for osteoporosis; a 30% or greater decrease in a bone marker suggests efficacy of therapy. Serial bone mass measurements are made every 1 to 3 years during therapy; bone mass changes slowly and the imprecision of the measurements allows detection of only relatively large changes. The measurements are nonetheless considered useful in monitoring therapy.[284]

Prevention of osteoporosis is an important goal. Adequate nutrition and exercise during growth allow achievement of optimal bone mass. High calcium intake (1000 [24.9 mmol] to 1500 mg [37.4 mmol]/day), adequate vitamin D (400 to 800 U/day), and a regular exercise program are helpful in preventing osteoporosis. Calcium supplements slow the loss of cortical bone but are less effective in preventing trabecular bone loss.

Treatment of osteoporosis depends on the cause. In secondary osteoporosis, treatment is directed at the underlying condition. Most therapies for the treatment of postmenopausal osteoporosis are directed at decreasing osteoclastic bone resorption. Antiresorptive therapies include bisphosphonates (alendronate and risedronate), estrogen replacement, selective estrogen receptor modulators (raloxifene), and calcitonin (nasal spray or injection). The FDA has recently approved recombinant hPTH(1-34) (injection), the first approved therapy for stimulating bone formation.

Osteomalacia and Rickets

Osteomalacia and rickets are caused by a mineralization defect during bone formation, resulting in an increase in osteoid, the unmineralized organic matrix of bone.[24] Defective mineralization produces rickets in children and osteomalacia in adults. Osteomalacia or rickets is usually due to either vitamin D deficiency or phosphate depletion.

The causes of decreased 25[OH]D and $1,25(OH)_2D$ are listed in Boxes 49-9 and 49-10, respectively.[245] Vitamin D deficiency may be secondary to dietary deprivation and/or inadequate exposure to sunlight, vitamin D malabsorption, disorders of vitamin D metabolism, or end-organ resistance to the action of vitamin D. In spite of the supplementation of milk, bread, and some cereals with vitamin D, vitamin D insufficiency may be common in the United States.[94,346] Breast-fed infants, the elderly, strict vegetarians, and individuals with darker skin pigmentation are at increased risk. Although clinical osteomalacia caused by vitamin D deficiency appears to be uncommon in the United States, the prevalence of subclinical or mild osteomalacia in the overall population is unknown. Subclinical osteomalacia may coexist with osteoporosis in elderly patients with poor diets and little exposure to sunlight. Vitamin D deficiency may develop in patients with malabsorption caused by postgastrectomy syndrome, small bowel disease (e.g., celiac sprue), hepatobiliary disease, or pancreatic insufficiency.

Vitamin D resistance is rare. Vitamin D–dependent rickets type I is an inherited defect in 25(OH)D-1α-hydroxylase causing impaired formation of $1,25(OH)_2D$. The disease is manifested in infancy and can be treated with physiological doses of $1,25(OH)_2D$. Vitamin D–dependent rickets type II is an inherited disorder characterized by very high serum concentrations of $1,25(OH)_2D$. This syndrome is due to resistance to $1,25(OH)_2D$, secondary to defects in the $1,25(OH)_2D$ receptor.

Osteomalacia and rickets may also occur because of phosphate depletion. The most common cause of rickets in the United States is hypophosphatemic osteomalacia (also known as *hypophosphatemic vitamin D–resistant rickets* and *vitamin D–resistant rickets*).[243] This disorder is an X-linked dominant inherited trait characterized by renal phosphate wasting. Tubular phosphate wasting can also occur sporadically in adults and as part of Fanconi syndrome. Certain rare mesenchymal tumors may also produce a phosphaturic factor (phosphatonin or FGF-23), resulting in renal phosphate wasting and osteomalacia.

Drugs have also been associated with osteomalacia. Anticonvulsants increase the hepatic catabolism of vitamin D metabolites, and produce end-organ resistance. Phosphate-binding antacids used for treatment of peptic ulcer disease cause osteomalacia by preventing the intestinal absorption of phosphate. Etidronate treatment (e.g., of Paget's disease, osteoporosis, or hypercalcemia of malignancy) can cause a mineralization defect and result in osteomalacia.

Clinical manifestations of rickets and osteomalacia are a consequence of the defect in mineralization. Rachitic manifestations include bowing of the extremities, short stature, costochondral-junction swelling, indentation of the lower ribs, and flattening of the skull. In adults, bone pain is the most common symptom, and stress fractures and frank skeletal fractures may occur. X-rays show classic findings in rickets, such as cupping and fraying of the epiphyseal and diaphyseal ends of the long bone. Pseudofractures are common in adults.

Laboratory findings in rickets and osteomalacia include an increased serum ALP, with other alterations in bone and mineral metabolism dependent on the cause and severity of the disorder. ALP is usually increased because of the increased osteoblastic activity associated with producing unmineralized osteoid. Calcium may be low-normal or low in vitamin D deficiency depending on the severity of the disease. Phosphate may be normal or low, but falls with the development of secondary hyperparathyroidism. The serum calcium and PTH concentrations are usually normal in renal tubular defects of phosphate transport. Vitamin D nutrition may be assessed by the determination of serum 25(OH)D. Renal phosphate defects can be best assessed by determination of the renal phosphate threshold.

Treatment of rickets and osteomalacia is dictated by the etiology of the disorder.[243] Nutritional rickets and osteomalacia are healed by treatment with physiological doses of vitamin D, whereas higher doses may be required in malabsorption. Adequate dietary intakes of calcium and phosphorus are critical during therapy. Renal phosphate-wasting syndromes require frequent, pharmacological administration of oral phosphorus.

Paget's Disease

Paget's disease is a localized disease of bone characterized by osteoclastic bone resorption, followed by replacement of bone in a chaotic fashion.[529] It may affect one or several bones. Paget's disease is common, affecting up to 4% of people older than 40 years. The cause of Paget's disease is unknown, although a viral cause has been suggested by its late onset, spotty involvement, and inclusions that resemble viral nucleocapsids in the nuclei of osteoclasts from patients with Paget's disease. A family history of Paget's disease is reported by 20% to 30% of patients.

The signs and symptoms of Paget's disease depend on which skeletal site is affected; the skull, femur, pelvis, and vertebrae are affected most commonly. In the majority of affected individuals in the United States, the disease is diagnosed from radiographs or laboratory tests (ALP) performed for another reason. In more extensive disease, localized bone pain and increased warmth may occur in or over the affected bone. Advanced disease can produce deformities such as skull enlargement and bowing of the weight-bearing bones (femur and tibia). Complications of deformed bone include arthritic symptoms, nerve compression, deafness, spinal nerve compression and, in rare cases, osteogenic sarcoma.

Laboratory and other findings include increased markers of bone turnover, and abnormal radiographs and bone scans. The most common finding leading to the diagnosis of Paget's disease is increased serum ALP (up to tenfold). Increases in markers of bone resorption (N-telopeptide, deoxypyridinoline, and C-telopeptide) reflect the osteoclastic nature of this disease. Bone markers may be useful in diagnosis and therapeutic monitoring. Radiological examination demonstrates the characteristic findings of Paget's disease: lytic areas in the sites of active osteoclastic bone resorption and thickened, expanded, and sclerotic areas in the site where osteoblasts have formed woven bone. The bone scan is the most sensitive test for detecting small, early lesions.

Therapy is directed at decreasing osteoclastic bone resorption. Bisphosphonates (alendronate, risedronate, pamidronate, and etidronate) and calcitonin are effective in decreasing bone pain, serum ALP, and markers of bone resorption. Patients may occasionally need surgery for skeletal deformity that limits mobility or for arthritic changes, fractures, or nerve compression.

Renal Osteodystrophy

Renal osteodystrophy includes all of the disorders of bone and mineral metabolism associated with chronic renal failure.[113,229,256] The renal bone diseases include both high-turnover bone disease (osteitis fibrosa or secondary hyperparathyroidism) and low-turnover bone disease (osteomalacia and adynamic bone disease). Quantitative histomorphometric analysis of bone biopsies, measurement of bone formation by double tetracycline labeling, and special stains are often necessary to correctly diagnose patients with osteitis fibrosa, osteomalacia, adynamic bone disease, and mixed bone disease of renal osteodystrophy.

Osteitis fibrosa (hyperparathyroid bone disease) is the most common high-turnover bone disease. This disorder is caused by the high concentrations of serum PTH in secondary hyperparathyroidism. Secondary hyperparathyroidism is a consequence of the hypocalcemia associated with hyperphosphatemia and $1,25(OH)_2D$ deficiency. Hyperphosphatemia is a result of the kidneys' inability to excrete phosphate. $1,25(OH)_2D$ deficiency results from the inability of the kidneys to synthesize $1,25(OH)_2$ because of decreased renal mass and suppression of 25(OH)D-1α-hydroxylase activity by high concentrations of phosphate. Deficiency of $1,25(OH)_2D$ leads to reduced intestinal absorption of calcium and reduced inhibition of PTH secretion by $1,25(OH)_2D$. Skeletal resistance to PTH also contributes to the hypocalcemia and secondary hyperparathyroidism.

Low-turnover bone diseases include osteomalacia and adynamic (also known as aplastic) bone diseases. Osteomalacia and adynamic bone disease are distinguished by the extent of unmineralized bone matrix or osteoid: osteoid is increased in osteomalacia and normal or low in adynamic bone disease. Osteomalacia in chronic renal failure may reflect vitamin D deficiency because of the decreased renal synthesis of $1,25(OH)_2D$ (see Osteomalacia and Rickets) or aluminum-related disease. In the 1970s and 1980s, aluminum intoxication was a significant contributing factor to the development of osteomalacia and adynamic bone disease. Aluminum intoxication was commonly caused by aluminum contamination of dialysis water and by the therapeutic use of oral aluminum-containing antacids to reduce serum phosphate by binding phosphate and preventing its intestinal absorption. The inability of patients with renal failure to excrete aluminum leads to high concentrations in serum (see Chapter 35) and deposition in bone, inhibiting bone cell function and bone mineralization. Aluminum-related disease is less common today because of the reduced use of aluminum-containing antacids and the use of effective means to decrease the concentrations of aluminum in dialysis water. Other causes of adynamic renal bone disease include calcium supplementation, excessive vitamin D administration, treatment of hyperparathyroidism, advanced age and osteoporosis, diabetes, corticosteroid therapy, and immobilization. Today, oversuppression of parathyroid function (produced by the use of oral calcium carbonate to control hyperphosphatemia and treatment with vitamin D and dialysate solutions containing high calcium to control hyperparathyroidism) is believed to be the main cause of adynamic renal bone disease.

Amyloid deposition may be noted in bone and in other tissues. It is thought to result from the reduced degradation of β_2-microglobulin by the kidneys. The amyloid in renal failure is primarily composed of β_2-microglobulin. The fraction of patients with amyloidosis increases with the duration of dialysis therapy; 70% to 80% of patients have clinical features of amyloidosis after 10 or more years of hemodialysis. Amyloidosis may coexist with either high-turnover or low-turnover bone disease.

Bone pain is the most common complaint of patients with renal osteodystrophy. The weight-bearing bones are the site of most discomfort, with leg and hip pain and back pain being common. If the patient is a growing child, skeletal deformities may result, with bowing of the extremities, kyphoscoliosis, and slipped femoral epiphyses. Extracellular calcification is also commonly found in the periarticular areas, in the medial layer of arteries, and as calcification of internal organs (lungs, heart muscle, and other tissue).

Biochemical findings in chronic renal failure may include hyperphosphatemia and hypocalcemia. PTH may be increased and $1,25(OH)_2D$ decreased. Serum ALP is increased in patients with either hyperparathyroidism or osteomalacia. Because magnesium is cleared by the kidney, modest elevations (2 to 4 mg/dL) are common, especially in those taking magnesium-containing antacids.

Early management of renal failure calls for dietary restriction of phosphate and administration of phosphate-binding agents. Calcium supplements added to the diet to prevent secondary hyperparathyroidism may also serve as phosphate binders. Administration of $1,25(OH)_2D$ or other active forms of vitamin D enhances intestinal calcium absorption and may also act directly on the parathyroid gland to reduce PTH secretion. Ultimately, dialysis or renal transplantation may be necessary.

TABLE 49-5 Markers of Bone Resorption

Marker	Method
Telopeptides	
N-telopeptide (NTx)	ELISA, ICMA
C-telopeptide (CTx)	ELISA, electrochemiluminescence
Pyridinium cross-links	
Free deoxypyridinoline	ELISA, ICMA
Free pyridinoline and deoxypyridinoline	ELISA
Total deoxypyridinoline and pyridinoline	HPLC
Tartrate-resistant acid phosphatase	Enzyme inhibition, immunoassay
Hydroxyproline	HPLC, photometric

BOX 49-13 Markers of Bone Formation

Bone alkaline phosphatase
Osteocalcin (Bone Gla protein, BGP)
Procollagen type I propeptides

BIOCHEMICAL MARKERS OF BONE TURNOVER

The development of methods to measure serum and urinary markers of bone turnover has been stimulated by a greater understanding of bone metabolism, increasing awareness of bone diseases—particularly osteoporosis—and the approval of new drugs for treating osteoporosis and other metabolic bone diseases.* Biochemical markers of bone turnover can be separated into markers of bone resorption (Table 49-5), which are produced by osteoclasts during bone resorption, and markers of bone formation, which are produced by osteoblasts during bone formation (Box 49-13).

More recently, methods have been developed for the measurement of osteoprotegerin and RANK ligand, proteins synthesized by the osteoblast and influencing osteoclast formation, activation, and bone resorption. Additional studies are required to determine the roles of RANK ligand and osteoprotegerin as markers of bone turnover.[255,557]

Selection and interpretation of biochemical markers of bone resorption and formation, for osteoporosis and other metabolic diseases, are complicated by preanalytical, analytical, and postanalytical considerations. Bone markers measure the overall rate of bone resorption or formation.

*References 3, 97, 106, 149, 208, 209, 236, 282, 291, 300, 313, 345, 397, 511, 512, 514, 610.

They cannot identify the type of bone or the location of the bone with the altered formation or resorption. In bone disorders in which bone resorption and formation are coupled and dramatically altered, either class of marker will identify changes in bone turnover.

Biochemical markers of bone resorption and formation have a number of potential uses* including (1) monitoring the effectiveness of therapy, (2) selection of patients for therapy, (3) prediction of bone loss, and (4) prediction of fracture risk. Of these, bone markers are currently most used for monitoring the effectiveness of therapy. Effective antiresorptive therapy is followed by a significant reduction in resorption markers within few weeks, normally reaching a plateau within 3 to 6 months. Markers of bone formation respond more slowly, usually reaching a plateau at 6 to 12 months. Depending on the antiresorptive therapy and the bone marker, effective therapy is associated with a bone marker reduction of 20% to 80%.

In contrast to many bone diseases, osteoporosis is often characterized by modest alterations in bone turnover, and thus only small changes may occur during therapy. A period of 1 to 3 years must pass before measurements of bone mass (for example, dual energy x-ray absorptiometry) can identify statistically significant changes in bone mass during therapy. Measurements of bone markers provide earlier assessments of bone resorption and/or formation. Because most current therapies are antiresorptive and resorption markers respond more quickly to these therapies, resorption markers have received the greatest attention.

In addition to their use in metabolic bone disease, markers of bone turnover are potentially useful tools in diagnosing and monitoring metastatic bone disease.[2,117,149,190] As with metabolic bone disease, there is more evidence supporting the use of resorption markers in monitoring therapy. Additional studies are required to determine the ultimate clinical utility of bone markers in metastatic bone disease.

Preanalytical and Analytical Variables

Preanalytical and analytical variables significantly reduce the usefulness of measurements of markers of bone formation and resorption. The long-term, within-individual variability of urine markers is generally higher (15% to 60%) than that of serum markers (5% to 10%).[31,218,345,550,586]

Bone marker concentrations in urine and serum vary with the time of day because of the diurnal variation of bone resorption and formation.[58,160,161,505] Because of the nocturnal peak in bone turnover, most bone markers peak in the early morning hours (4 AM to 8 AM) and reach their nadir in the afternoon (1 PM to 11 PM). The amplitude of this variation is greatest for resorption markers, with nadir values averaging 70% of peak values. Consequently, specimens should be collected at a specific time of day to minimize the impact of diurnal variability on between-specimen comparisons. For urinary markers, collection of the second morning void is often recommended. Compared with other bone markers, BAP does not demonstrate much diurnal variation because of its long half-life in serum.

Concentrations of urinary resorption markers are usually normalized by dividing by the urinary creatinine concentration. The variability (within- and between-method) of creatinine measurements, within-subject variability in urinary creatinine, and creatinine's dependence on muscle mass contribute to the overall variability of urinary resorption markers.

Markers of Bone Resorption

Bone resorption markers are listed in Box 49-5. N- and C-telopeptides of type I collagen (NTx and CTx) and deoxypyridinoline are most frequently measured. Other markers include serum tartrate-resistant acid phosphatase (TRAP) and hydroxyproline. Bone resorption markers, apart from TRAP, were initially measured in urine. More recently, methods using serum have been developed for a number of these analytes including N- and C-telopeptides.

Telopeptides and Pyridinium (Deoxypyridinoline and Pyridinoline) Cross-Links

Type I collagen accounts for approximately 90% of the organic matrix of bone. Type I collagen, a triple helix of two identical α-1(I) chains and a slightly different α-2(I) chain, is synthesized as a precursor, type I procollagen, containing both N- and C-terminal extensions.[482]

Each chain contains approximately 1000 amino acids and has a molecular weight of approximately 140,000. Procollagen undergoes extensive intracellular posttranslational processing, including hydroxylation of proline and lysine residues, glycosylation, and formation of intrachain and interchain disulfide bonds and the triple helix. After it is secreted, procollagen is converted to collagen during extracellular processing with the enzymatic removal of N- and C-terminal propeptides (procollagen peptides).

Type I collagen molecules spontaneously assemble into immature fibrils with limited tensile strength, then mature by the formation of intramolecular and intermolecular covalent bonds or cross-links.[473] Lysyl oxidase deaminates the ε-amino group of specific lysines or hydroxylysines to produce active aldehydes. Three amino acid side chains react to form a trivalent amino acid containing the 3-hydroxypyridinium ring. The following two nonreducible cross-links have been identified.

1. Deoxypyridinoline (lysyl pyridinoline) formed by the reaction of two hydroxylysine side chains and one lysine side chain
2. Pyridinoline (hydroxylysyl pyridinoline) formed by the reaction of three hydroxylysine side chains

These prominent pyridinium cross-links stabilize mature collagen chains within the extracellular matrix in fibrous

*References 141, 143, 144, 208, 209, 303, 379, 453, 538, 610.

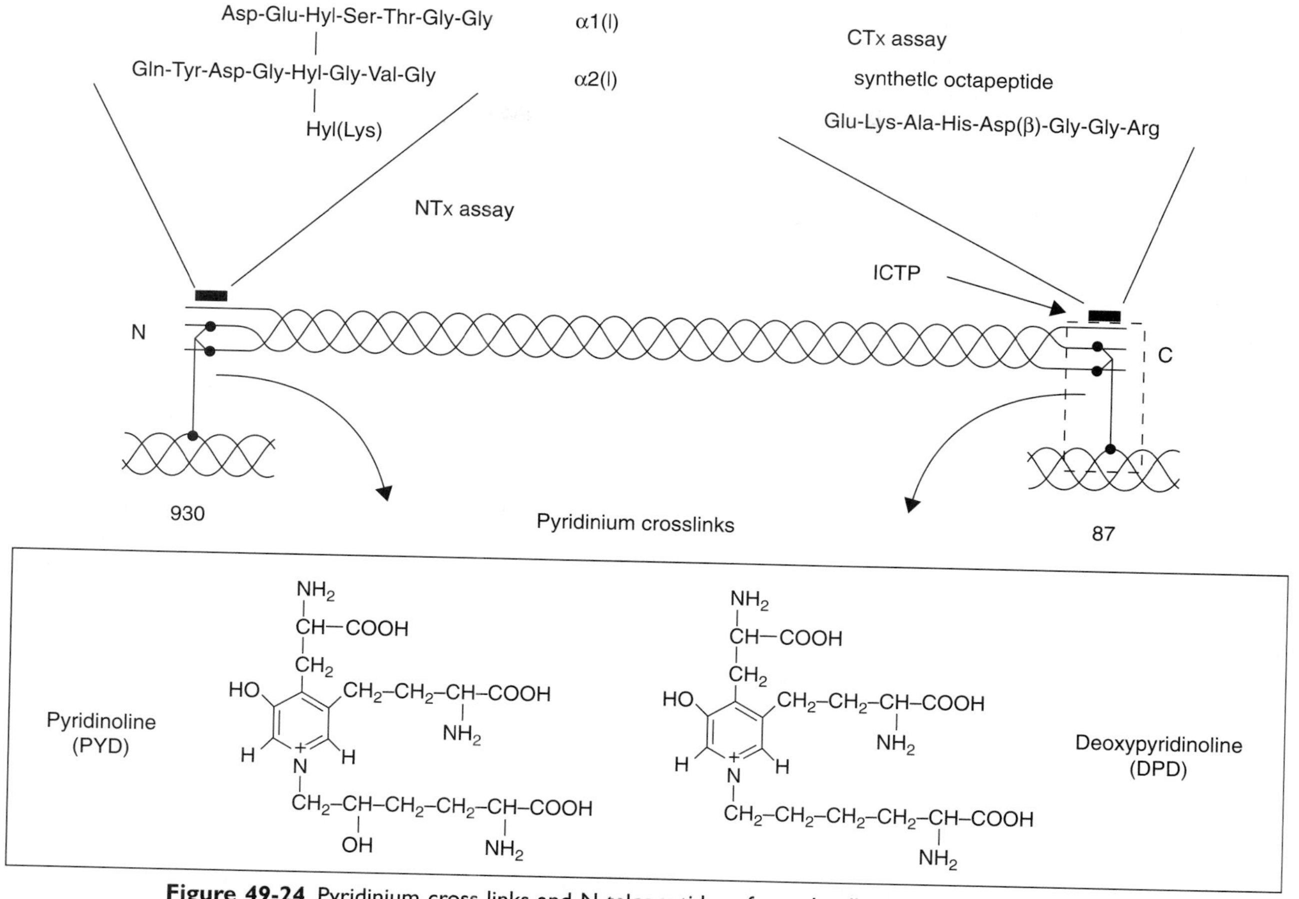

Figure 49-24 Pyridinium cross-links and N-telopeptides of type I collagen. Cross-links occur at two intermolecular sites in the collagen fibril: (1) two N-telopeptides are linked to a helical site at residue 930, and (2) two C-telopeptides are linked to helical residue 87. The location and amino acid sequence of the N-telopeptide (NTx) and the C-telopeptide (CTx) and the structures of the free pyridinium cross-links (pyridinoline and deoxypyridinoline) are shown. *ICTP,* C-terminal telopeptide of type I collagen. *(From Robins SP. Biochemical markers of bone metabolism. CPD Bulletin Clin Biochem 1999;1:116-21.)*

collagen and most mature connective tissues, with the notable exception of skin.

Intermolecular cross-linking sites have been located that form the pyridinium cross-links in type I collagen (Figure 49-24). Two N-telopeptide sites are linked to the helical site at amino acid 930 (N-telopeptide) or two C-telopeptides are linked to the helical site amino acid 87 (C-telopeptide).

Deoxypyridinoline (DPD) (Figure 49-24) is a more sensitive and specific marker of bone resorption than pyridinoline (PYD):* DPD is found in significant quantities only in bone, dentine, ligaments, and aorta, whereas PYD is more widespread, occurring in hard connective tissues with high levels in cartilage. Because of the large mass of the skeletal system, bone is usually the major source for both PYD and DPD. Neither substance is present in significant quantities in skin.

*References 35, 97, 177, 180, 206, 282.

DPD is a sensitive and specific marker of bone resorption because:

1. It is formed during collagen maturation, not biosynthesis, and originates only as a breakdown product of mature matrix.
2. It does not appear to be metabolized before excretion in urine.
3. Bone is the major source of DPD.
4. It does not appear to be absorbed from the diet.

Pyridinium cross-links (DPD and PYD) and telopeptides containing these cross-links are released into the circulation by hydrolysis of type I collagen during bone resorption and excreted in urine.

Clinical Significance of Telopeptides and Deoxypyridinoline

Elevated concentrations of telopeptides and DPD have been reported in osteoporosis, Paget's disease, metastatic bone disease, primary and secondary hyperparathyroidism, hyperthyroidism, and other diseases with increased bone resorption.* When postmenopausal women are compared with premenopausal controls, telopeptides are usually increased more than other markers of resorption and formation.[163,211,213,441]

Inhibition of bone resorption with pharmacological agents leads to a decrease in telopeptides and DPD. Treatment of postmenopausal women or osteoporotics with bisphosphonates or estrogen replacement therapy decreases bone resorption markers. Although markers of bone formation are also decreased because of coupling, reductions are delayed and not as great as those observed for markers of bone resorption. Response to antiresorptive therapy is generally greatest with telopeptides, intermediate with total DPD, and lowest with free DPD.[210,292]

In patients with Paget's disease treated with bisphosphonates, N-telopeptide was suppressed more than total or free DPD or hydroxyproline and best predicted the outcome of therapy.[15,50,210,425]

Measurement of Telopeptides and Pyridinium Cross-Links

NTx, CTx, and DPD are most frequently used to measure bone resorption. Methods are commercially available for the measurement of NTx and CTx in serum and urine and deoxypyridinoline in urine (see Table 49-5).

N-Telopeptide. NTx in urine is measured with a commercially available ELISA. It uses a monoclonal antibody against the NTx fraction of normal adolescent urine.[241] The antibody recognizes a conformational epitope of the cross-linked α_2(I)N-telopeptide containing the sequence QYDGKGVG, which is a product of osteoclastic proteolysis. It does not recognize a precursor that is not cross-linked, but does measure other types of cross-links (pyrrolic). Its freedom from cross-reactivity with precursors that are not cross-linked ensures that only collagen degradation is measured. Measurement of NTx may provide increased specificity for bone because DPD cross-links involve primarily the α_2(I) chain, whereas the α_1(I) predominates in other tissue, and two thirds of the DPD cross-links in bone collagen are at the NTx site, whereas one third are at the CTx site. In this assay, microtiter plates are coated with a urinary peptide conjugate. Samples or calibrators are added, followed by the NTx monoclonal antibody. After incubation and washing, bound antibody is quantified by adding goat antimouse IgG conjugated to horseradish peroxidase. A modification of this method is also available on an automated immunoassay analyzer using an EIA with chemiluminescence detection.

More recently, this method has been adapted for the measurement of NTx in serum.[109,217] The use of serum eliminates the need to measure urine creatinine to correct for urine concentration and significantly reduces the within-subject day-to-day variation in NTx measurements.

*References 15, 50, 52, 97, 145, 441, 472, 477, 513, 582, 583.

C-Telopeptide. Unlike the NTx assay, which used the NTx from adolescent urine as the immunogen, CTx immunoassays used an antibody against a synthetic fragment of the CTx corresponding to residues 15C to 22C (EKAHDGGR) of the α_1(I) chain of type I collagen.[61] This region includes the cross-linking hydroxylysine at residue 16C. Several methods have been developed for measuring CTx in urine and serum. The most widely used methods recognize the β-isomer, formed during aging of bone by the transfer of the peptide backbone from the α-carboxyl group to the β-carboxyl group. This ensures that the measured CTx is from mature collagen, not precursors, and reflects bone resorption. All methods require the C-terminal amino acid to be a free arginine (R). CTx is measured in urine with an ELISA using a polyclonal rabbit antibody. Microtiter plates are coated with the synthetic peptide, followed by incubation with samples or calibrators and rabbit antibody against the 8–amino acid synthetic fragment. After washing, bound antibody is quantified by addition of peroxidase-conjugated goat antirabbit IgG. CTx is measured in serum using two monoclonal murine antibodies.[60,429,479] With two α_1(I) chain telopeptides in each collagen molecule, the use of two antibodies directed against the β-isomer ensures that only the β/β forms are measured. A modification of this method is now available on an automated immunoassay analyzer using electrochemiluminescence detection.[204]

Another group of investigators has reported an RIA for the C-terminal telopeptide of type I collagen (ICTP) in serum.[467] Rabbit antibodies were raised against a cross-linked C-telopeptide of type I collagen produced by collagenase digestion of human bone. This method is relatively insensitive to changes in bone resorption in osteoporosis, but does detect increases in myeloma and metastatic bone disease. This appears to be because of the metabolism of the epitope recognized by this assay by cathepsin K, an enzyme likely to be responsible for collagen resorption in osteoporosis.

Pyridinium Cross-links (Deoxypyridinoline and Pyridinoline). DPD and PYD were originally measured by HPLC (see Table 49-5). Today, DPD is measured primarily by immunoassay using automated analyzers (EIA with chemiluminescence detection and ICMA) or manual ELISA. Unlike most HPLC methods, which measure total DPD and total PYD, the immunoassays for DPD or DPD/PYD measure primarily free but not peptide-bound forms. In urine, approximately 40% of the PYD and DPD is free and 60% is protein-bound.

Comparisons of free and total DPD and PYD suggest that the ratio of free to total pyridinolines varies with physiology, pathophysiology, and treatment.[163,210,292] Total DPD has been reported to be increased more than free DPD in individuals with disorders involving increased bone resorption (postmenopausal women, osteoporosis, Paget's disease, and hyperthyroidism). Furthermore, short-term bisphosphonate treatment of patients with Paget's disease or osteoporosis reduced the total, but not the free, DPD, whereas estrogen treatment of postmenopausal women decreased both.

Immunoassays. A number of immunoassays[97,206,282] have been developed to measure DPD and PYD. One commercially available ELISA measures both PYD and DPD with equimolar cross-reactivity.[225,520] Of greater interest for monitoring bone resorption is the commercially available ELISA that measures DPD but not PYD.[475] This method, a competitive ELISA, uses a streptavidin-coated microtiter plate and biotinylated deoxypyridinoline as the solid phase. Sample or calibrator and the monoclonal antibody against DPD are added and incubated. After washing, a second antibody, goat antimouse IgG conjugated to ALP, is added. Bound antibody-antibody-enzyme conjugate is measured after addition of *p*-nitrophenyl phosphate.

More recently, automated immunoanalyzer methods for DPD have become commercially available. The most widely used is a solid-phase, competitive EIA with chemiluminescence detection. The solid-phase antibody is incubated with serum or calibrator and ALP conjugated to DPD. After washing, the antibody-antigen-enzyme complexes are determined after the addition of substrate.

High-Performance Liquid Chromatography. DPD and PYD can be measured by HPLC with fluorescence detection.* Because about 60% of the pyridinolines in urine are contained in peptides, most methods use acid hydrolysis to generate free amino acids. The hydrolysate is fractionated by column chromatography on cellulose CF-1 before resolution of the pyridinolines by reversed-phase chromatography. Because the pyridinolines are highly polar at acid pH, ion-pairing agents have been used to increase their retention by reversed-phase columns. Although most methods have used gradient elution, simpler isocratic methods have been described.[281,334] Fluorometric detection is used to quantify these naturally occurring fluorescent pyridinium compounds. The lack of synthetic calibrators, controversy over the molar fluorescence yield of pyridinolines, and the variability of acid hydrolysis have been suggested as factors contributing to the differences observed between laboratories.[178,474]

Specimen Requirements. DPD and telopeptides are relatively stable in urine.[48,215] Exposure to UV light, but not laboratory lighting, decreased DPD and PYD. Free pyridinolines were especially vulnerable to UV lighting. It is recommended that prolonged exposure to light and exposure to direct sunlight be avoided.

Peak urinary excretion of pyridinolines occurs at about 5 AM to 8 AM, reflecting the nocturnal peak in bone turnover. Urinary pyridinolines reach a nadir between 2 PM and 11 PM.[58,160,161,505]

Both timed and random urine tests have been used for pyridinolines and telopeptides. Although early studies used 24-hour urine samples, timed or early-morning voided urine have also been used. A second-morning void, collected by 10 AM, is most commonly recommended. For monitoring, specimens should be collected at the same time as the baseline specimen.

Within-subject biological variation of bone markers has been reported to be (coefficients of variation) 5% to 60%.[31,218,550,586]

Reference Intervals. Appropriate reference intervals for telopeptides and DPD depend on the reason for ordering the test. For osteoporotic women, results are usually compared with those for healthy premenopausal women. Representative reference intervals for NTx, CTx, and DPD are listed below[614A]:

Test	Premenopausal Women	Men
N-telopeptide		
Serum, nmol BCE/L	8.7-19.8	10.7-22.9
Urine, μmol BCE/mol creatinine	10-110	11-103
C-telopeptide		
Serum,* ng/L	≤573	≤584
Urine (mg/mol creatinine)	220 (128)†	249 (128)†
Deoxypyridinoline, Free (μmol/mol creatinine)	3.0-7.4	2.3-5.4

*CTx by automated immunoassay with electrochemiluminescence detection
†Mean (SD)

Concentrations of collagen cross-links are influenced by age and gender. Concentrations are markedly higher in children, with the highest concentrations observed during early infancy and adolescence, periods of rapid bone growth. In adults, concentrations of collagen cross-links are relatively constant between the ages of 30 and 45, but increase significantly after menopause in women. For women, adult reference intervals are usually based on normally cycling premenopausal women (with normal menstrual cycle and normal follicle-stimulating hormone), 30 to 45 years of age. Age-related increases have also been reported in men.

Tartrate-Resistant Acid Phosphatase

During bone resorption, osteoclasts produce and secrete an acid phosphatase. The activity of this TRAP has been measured using a number of methods. Unfortunately, most methods failed to distinguish between the osteclastic TRAP (isoform 5b) and other TRAPs (isoform 5a) found in plasma.[443] In addition, instability of the enzyme and association of the enzyme with α_2-macroglulin have complicated

*References 44, 97, 177, 179, 206, 282, 583.

the development of methods. Immunoassays have also been developed for measuring TRAP using antibodies raised against TRAP obtained from spleen cells of patients with hairy cell leukemia, human cord plasma, and recombinant TRAP.[105,312,443] More recently, two approaches have been used to measure TRAP 5b: (1) a kinetic method measuring enzyme activity of TRAP 5b using fluoride inhibition of TRAP 5b and heparin inhibition of TRAP 5a,[394] and (2) an immunoassay using monoclonal antibody for TRAP 5b.[239,240] Although the initial investigations of these new methods for TRAP 5b are encouraging, limited data are currently available regarding the clinical performance of these methods.

Urinary Hydroxyproline

Hydroxyproline is found mainly in collagens, where it accounts for about 13% of the total amino acid content and is derived from proline by posttranslational hydroxylation.[35,140,175,470] About 10% of hydroxyproline released during collagen catabolism is excreted in urine, mainly as small dialyzable peptides. Although assays have been reported for free hydroxyproline and hydroxyproline in dialyzable and nondialyzable peptides in urine and serum, methods for total urinary hydroxyproline have been more commonly used.[140,175,470,581,607] Hydroxyproline is released from peptides by acid hydrolysis. Early photometric assays involved oxidation of hydroxyproline to pyrrole, followed by reaction with Ehrlich's reagent (4-dimethylaminobenzaldehyde).[34,302,445] Ion-exchange chromatography before analysis and other modifications have been advocated to reduce interference by urinary components and improve assay specificity.[231] Sensitive and specific reversed-phase HPLC methods have been described. They use photometric or fluorometric precolumn derivatizing agents, including dabsyl and dansyl chloride, phenylisothiocyanate, *o*-phthalaldehyde, 4-chloro-7-nitrobenzofurazan, 9-fluorenylmethyl chloroformate, and *N,N*-diethyl-2,4-dinitro-5-fluoroaniline.[133,426,455]

Urinary hydroxyproline is not specific for either bone turnover or bone resorption for a number of reasons, including: (1) other tissues, including muscle and skin, and the C1q fraction of complement contain a significant proportion of the body's collagen[140]; (2) a significant percentage of collagen is degraded during synthesis and maturation, including N-terminal and C-terminal propeptides (procollagen peptides); and (3) its concentration is altered by various diseases and other factors, including diet. With the availability of more sensitive and specific markers of bone resorption, hydroxyproline is not routinely used to assess bone turnover or bone resorption.[97,206]

Markers of Bone Formation

Bone formation markers are listed in Box 49-13. BAP and osteocalcin are most frequently measured. Procollagen peptides are less frequently measured. Bone formation markers are measured in serum or plasma.

Bone Alkaline Phosphatase

ALP is found in many tissues, including bone, liver, intestine, kidney, and placenta (see Chapter 21). Four different genes code for the tissue-nonspecific, intestinal, placental, and germ-cell (placental-like) isoenzymes.[97,244,442] The ALPs from liver, bone, and kidney are isoforms of the same gene product, the tissue-nonspecific gene. These tissue-specific isoforms are produced by tissue-specific posttranslational processing (e.g., glycosylation) of the gene product.

ALP determined by usual biochemical panels reflects total serum concentrations and does not distinguish the source of the isoenzyme (i.e., liver, bone, or some other source). Clinicians must therefore rely on other markers of liver or other organ function or a more tissue-specific determination of ALP to assess the source of ALP. In normal individuals, ALP originates primarily from liver and bone. The bone isoenzyme is the marker of bone formation and is found in osteoblasts.

Clinical Significance

BAP is increased in metabolic bone diseases, including osteoporosis, osteomalacia and rickets, hyperparathyroidism, renal osteodystrophy, and thyrotoxicosis, and in individuals with acromegaly, bony metastases, glucocorticoid excess, Paget's disease, and other disorders with increased bone formation.*

The measurement of BAP has several advantages over osteocalcin measurement. Because of its relatively long half-life in vivo (1 to 3 days), it is relatively unaffected by diurnal variation. BAP is more stable in vitro and does not require special specimen handling. BAP is more useful in individuals with impaired renal function because it is not cleared by glomerular filtration.

Of current biochemical markers, total ALP or BAP provides the highest clinical sensitivity and specificity in the diagnosis and monitoring of Paget's disease.[15] Although total ALP is most often used, BAP is more sensitive than total ALP in mild Paget's disease. Osteocalcin is relatively insensitive and less useful than BAP in Paget's disease. Total ALP is not useful in metabolic bone diseases with mild elevations of BAP.

Measurement of BAP may be misleading in patients with liver disease, severe osteomalacia, or increased concentrations of $1,25(OH)_2D$. BAP may be misleading in liver disease because of the cross-reactivity of current methods with liver ALP. In severe osteomalacia, BAP may be markedly increased without an increase in bone mineralization because of a mineralizing defect.[553] Because 1,25-dihydroxyvitamin D regulates the synthesis of BAP and osteocalcin, both of these markers may be misleading in patients treated with calcitriol and in patients with abnormal concentrations of this hormone.

*References 97, 106, 136, 236, 289, 316, 345, 397, 512, 514.

Measurement of Bone Alkaline Phosphatase

BAP measurement methods have used heat inactivation, chemical inhibition, electrophoresis, isoelectric focusing, lectin precipitation and chromatography, HPLC, and other approaches, singly and in combination. Conventional electrophoresis provides qualitative, not quantitative, detection because of the overlapping migration of isoforms and isoenzymes. Heat inactivation and chemical inhibition with urea, l-phenylalanine, l-homoarginine, or levamisole have been used with some success. Internal standards of ALP isoenzymes have been used to increase assay precision.[182,184]

Wheat germ agglutinin (WGA), a lectin, has been used to measure BAP by affinity chromatography, affinity electrophoresis, or differential precipitation of isoforms.[17,84,228,371] Some methods have used a combination of techniques to improve specificity. These classic measurements for BAP are usually technically complicated and labor-intensive, imprecise, insensitive, and inaccurate. Of these techniques, heat denaturation and WGA precipitation have been used most frequently. Heat denaturation has been criticized because of its irreproducibility or variability.[305] WGA precipitation has been criticized because WGA does not precipitate all BAP from pagetic sera or from the SaOS-2 osteosarcoma cell line and fails to completely separate bone and liver activity.[305]

Several immunoassays have been reported for BAP.* Two immunoassays are commercially available; both use monoclonal antibodies against BAP from SaOS-2 cells. One immunoassay is an IRMA using two monoclonal antibodies, a capture antibody and a radioiodinated signal antibody, reacting preferentially with BAP.[79,205,253,254,316] This two-site immunoassay measures the mass of BAP in ng/mL (μg/L). Subsequently an immunoenzymatic method was developed by replacing the signal antibody with the direct measurement of the activity of immobilized BAP.[79] A modification of this method is available on an automated immunoassay analyzer using a chemiluminescent assay. The other assay uses a single monoclonal antibody against BAP.[181,226] Microtiter plates are coated with this antibody and used to separate BAP from other isoforms and isoenzymes. After immunoseparation, the activity (U/L) of BAP is determined with a *p*-nitrophenyl phosphate substrate.

The analytical and clinical performance of these BAP immunoassays have been characterized in a series of articles.† Unfortunately, current immunoassays are not completely specific for BAP and exhibit 7% to 17% cross-reactivity with ALP from liver.[79,444] It has been difficult to exactly determine cross-reactivity for the liver isoform because of limitations of existing preparations and an incomplete understanding of the exact nature of the circulating isoforms. BAP immunoassays provide greater sensitivity and specificity for bone formation than does the measurement of total ALP. Current methods for BAP are not reliable in patients with liver disease with increased concentrations of the liver isoform.

*References 79, 97, 157, 181, 205, 206, 226, 253, 254, 316, 325.
†References 66, 79, 183, 316, 423, 444, 584, 609, 611.

Osteocalcin [Bone Gla Protein (BGP)]

1 Tyr	Leu	Tyr	Gln	5 Trp	Leu	Gly	Ala	Pro	10 Val
11 Pro	Tyr	Pro	Asp	15 Pro	Leu	**Gla**	Pro	Arg	20 Arg
21 **Gla**	Val	Cys	**Gla**	25 Leu	Asn	Pro	Asp	Cys	30 Asp
31 Glu	Leu	Ala	Asp	35 His	Ile	Gly	Phe	Gln	40 Glu
41 Ala	Tyr	Arg	Arg	45 Phe	Tyr	Gly	Pro	49 Val	

Figure 49-25 Amino acid sequence of osteocalcin. A disulfide bond formed between cysteines in positions 23 and 29 stabilizes two antiparallel α-helical structures representing 40% of the overall structure. Three glutamyl residues at positions 17, 21, and 24 can be carboxylated in a posttranslational, vitamin K–dependent, enzymatic step producing γ-carboxyglutamyl (Gla) residues.

Reference Intervals

Normal concentrations of BAP are approximately 5 to 20 ng/mL (μg/L) with the IRMA[205,423,609,611] and 11.6 to 29.6 and 15.0 to 41.3 U/L for premenopausal women and men, respectively, with the immunoabsorption assay.[226,609,611] For the automated chemiluminescent immunoenzymatic method, the 95th percentile limit is reported to be 14.3 and 20.1 ng/mL for premenopausal women and men, respectively. Serum concentrations of BAP are influenced by age and gender. Concentrations are higher in men and increase with age in both men and women, consistent with the age-related increase in bone turnover. Children have much higher concentrations, especially during growth spurts.

Osteocalcin

Osteocalcin (OC) is the major and most thoroughly characterized noncollagenous protein in human bone (Figure 49-25).* This protein, previously referred to as bone Gla protein (BGP), accounts for approximately 1% of the total protein in human bone. It is a small protein of 49 amino acids with a molecular weight of 5669.

OC is considered to be a marker of bone formation because during bone formation 10% to 30% of the OC synthesized by osteoblasts is released into the circulation. However, OC, especially OC fragments, may also be liberated during bone resorption and measured by some

*References 97, 208, 236, 237, 327, 333, 440, 512, 514.

methods. Its synthesis is stimulated by 1,25$(OH)_2$D. OC is cleared by the kidneys. The half-life of circulating OC is approximately 5 minutes.

OC contains three specific glutamyl residues at amino acid positions 17, 21, and 24, which may be converted to γ-carboxyglutamyl residues by a posttranslational, vitamin K–dependent enzymatic carboxylation. This unique carboxylated amino acid binds calcium ions and is found in various proteins involved in blood coagulation and in calcium transport, deposition, and homeostasis. Undercarboxylated OC, which has been reported in serum in some conditions, may be related to decreased bone density and may respond to administration of vitamin K. Although OC binds calcium and hydroxyapatite, its physiological role is unknown.

Immunochemical and chromatographic studies have demonstrated considerable heterogeneity for circulating OC in normal individuals and patients with osteoporosis, chronic renal failure, and Paget's disease.* This heterogeneity may be a result of proteolytic hydrolysis of susceptible peptide bonds involving arginine residues at positions 19-20 and 43-44. Peptides containing amino acids 1-19, 20-43, 45-49, 1-43, and 20-49 can be produced by hydrolysis of one or two of these bonds.

Sequence-specific competitive and noncompetitive immunoassays have been developed and used to measure OC and fragments of OC.[212] Intact OC accounts for about 35% of immunoreactivity in normal subjects, 45% in patients with osteoporosis, and 25% in patients with chronic renal failure (CRF). The N-terminal/midregion fragment, possibly 1-43, accounted for 30% of immunoreactivity in normal subjects and osteoporotics and 50% in patients with CRF. Other fragments were present at considerably lower concentrations than 1-43. All specimens were collected in tubes containing agar-agar, placed on ice, promptly separated, and frozen at −80 °C to minimize proteolysis.

Intact OC appears to be rapidly hydrolyzed when serum is incubated at room temperature, and more slowly at 4 °C.[49,212] At room temperature, immunoreactivity measured with the intact assay had declined by about 20% at 3 hours, whereas immunoreactivity with the assay measuring both intact hormone and the 1-43 fragment was unchanged. This N-terminal/midregion fragment may be released by osteoblasts during bone formation and produced in vivo in the circulation and in vitro during specimen handling by proteolysis of intact OC.

Clinical Significance

OC is increased in metabolic bone diseases with increased bone or osteoid formation, including osteoporosis, osteomalacia and rickets, hyperparathyroidism, renal osteodystrophy, and thyrotoxicosis, and in individuals with fractures, acromegaly, and bony metastases.* OC is decreased in hypoparathyroidism, hypothyroidism and growth hormone deficiency, and during estrogen replacement therapy and treatment with glucocorticoids, bisphosphonates, and calcitonin.

OC concentrations may be misleading in several situations.[553] Concentrations may be increased in patients with impaired renal function without an increase in bone formation, since OC is cleared by the kidneys. OC may increase during bed rest without an increase in bone formation. Serum OC may not reflect bone formation in patients treated with 1,25$(OH)_2$D or those with abnormalities in this hormone since OC is regulated by 1,25$(OH)_2$D.

Measurement of Osteocalcin

Many different immunoassays have been developed for OC since the first assay was reported in 1980.† The first immunoassays for human OC were competitive RIAs using bovine OC as immunogen and radioiodinated tracer. Because of the complete homology between amino acids 20 to 49 of bovine and human OC, the majority of antisera were directed against the C-terminal of OC. Consequently, these methods measured both intact OC and OC fragments containing the C-terminal region. Others developed antisera against ovine OC, with its complete homology with human OC between amino acids 11 and 49,[427] purified intact human OC,[552] or synthetic fragments of human OC.[101] Competitive immunoassays have also used enzyme[439,440,478,576] and chemiluminescent[295] labels. Monoclonal antibodies against bovine and human OC have also been used in competitive immunoassays.[439,440,576]

More recently, noncompetitive methods have been developed for measuring human OC. These immunoassays use monoclonal antibodies and affinity-purified polyclonal antisera against synthetic peptides of human OC or intact human or bovine OC.‡ Many antibody pairs have been reported including capture [and signal] antibodies, respectively, against amino acid sequences 12-33 [and 34-49], 43-49 [and 5-13], 25-37 [and 5-13], 20-43 [and 7-19], 1-19 [and 20-49], and 1-12 [and 15-30 or 38-49]. These noncompetitive methods have used signal antibodies labeled with radioactivity (IRMA), enzymes (EIA/ELISA), or chemiluminescent compounds (ICMA).

Noncompetitive methods measuring intact OC and especially those measuring both intact OC plus the N-terminal/midregion (1-43) fragment are of particular interest.[49,212,480] These assays do not measure smaller fragments of OC, which is an advantage, since fragments might be produced during bone resorption. OC concentrations are more stable when measured with assays recognizing both

*References 97, 206, 212, 327, 333, 440, 512, 514, 576.

*References 97, 206, 236, 333, 395, 440, 470, 512, 514.

†References 64, 97, 236, 327, 333, 440, 512, 514, 576.

‡References 49, 97, 138, 152, 271, 369, 382, 440, 480.

intact hormone (1-49) and the N-terminal/midregion (1-43) since this fragment is produced in vitro by hydrolysis of intact OC.

The circulating concentration of OC measured in normal subjects varies widely among methods and laboratories.[97,152,369,440,576] One study reported that *mean* values for normal individuals ranged from 3 to 27 ng/mL (μg/L). This variability may be a consequence of differences in antisera specificity and sensitivity, and in the purity, potency, and immunoreactivity of OC calibrators.[142] Another important source of variation between methods may be their dependence on or independence of calcium concentration in the assay.[576] Calcium binding to γ-carboxyglutamyl residues induces a conformational change in OC. Although EDTA is added to some assays to eliminate this effect, other assays require the addition of calcium.

Antiserum specificity and the heterogeneity of circulating OC are probably the primary reasons for differences observed between methods.[49,212] Depending on antiserum specificity, methods may measure intact OC or fragments containing the N-terminal, C-terminal, or midregion amino acids or some combination of these forms. These fragments may be produced during bone formation or resorption, in the circulation, or in vitro during preanalytical handling. The development of two-site methods and greater knowledge of OC metabolism should provide a basis for greater standardization of these measurements.

Specimen Requirements

Serum is the most widely used specimen for the measurement of OC; heparinized plasma can be used with some methods. The stability of OC in samples is method-dependent. Decreases in OC immunoreactivity of 50% to 70% after 6 to 24 hours at room temperature and 40% to 80% after 2 weeks at 4 °C have been reported.[26,49,212] Trasylol,[26] mixed protease inhibitors,[212] and collection on ice[49,212] improve the stability of OC with some but not all methods. Serum OC concentrations are more stable with methods measuring both intact OC and the N-terminal/midregion fragment (1-43). Concentrations were unchanged after 3 hours at room temperature and after 24 hours at 4 °C.[49,212]

Specimen stability should be determined and collection and handling optimized for each method. Unless proven unnecessary, specimens should be collected on ice, separated within 1 hour, and immediately frozen. Freeze-thaw cycles should be avoided. The use of EDTA plasma and/or protease inhibitors should be evaluated.

Reference Intervals

Methods for OC are not harmonized as illustrated by the reference intervals listed below[614A]:

	ng/mL (μg/L)
IRMA	
Children	
6-9.9 y	40.2-108
10-13.9 y	35.8-166
14-17.9 y	
Males	27.8-194
Females	16.3-68.7
Adult male	11.3-35.4
Adult female	7.2-27.9
ICMA	
Adult male	1.1-7.2
Adult female	
Premenopausal	0.5-7.0

OC concentrations are influenced by age, gender, and diurnal variation.[97,333,440,470] Concentrations are higher in children, with the highest concentrations observed during periods of rapid growth. Males have somewhat higher concentrations of OC. OC concentrations have been reported to increase, decrease, or remain unchanged with advancing age, a probable consequence of the heterogeneity of circulating OC and differences in immunoassay specificity. OC concentrations are generally increased during menopause. OC exhibits a diurnal variation with a nocturnal peak, dropping by as much as 50% to a morning nadir. OC concentrations are increased in individuals with renal failure.

Procollagen Peptides (Collagen Propeptides)

Type I collagen is synthesized as a precursor, procollagen, containing both N- and C-terminal extensions.* These extensions, or propeptides, are cleaved from type I procollagen during collagen formation. Collagen propeptides are a marker of bone formation. Several immunoassays have been developed to measure the N-terminal (PINP)[337] and C-terminal (PICP)[377,380,527] propeptides.

Because type I collagen is also the major matrix of several other tissues, collagen propeptides are not as sensitive or specific for bone formation as osteocalcin or BAP. Measurement of procollagen peptides may be helpful for assessing bone formation in patients treated with 1,25-dihydroxyvitamin D or in patients with abnormal concentrations of this hormone when osteocalcin and BAP may be misleading.

REFERENCES

1. Abernethy MH, Fowler RT. Micellar improvement of the calmagite compleximetric measurement of magnesium in plasma. Clin Chem 1982;28:520-2.

*References 97, 136, 140, 208, 236, 380, 470.

2. Abildgaard N, Brixen K, Kristensen JE, Eriksen EF, Nielsen JL, Heickendorff L. Comparison of five biochemical markers of bone resorption in multiple myeloma: elevated pre-treatment levels of S-ICTP and U-Ntx are predictive of early progression of the bone disease during standard chemotherapy. Br J Hematol 2003;120:235-42.
3. Adam A, Boulanger J, Azzouzi M, Ers P. Colorimetric versus enzymatic determination of serum phosphorus. Clin Chem 1984;30:1724-5.
4. Adams JS. Vitamin D metabolite-mediated hypercalcemia. Endocrinol Metab Clin North Am 1989;18:765-78.
5. Adams JS, Clemens TL, Holick MF. Silica Sep-Pak preparative chromatography of vitamin D and its metabolites. J Chromatogr 1981;226:198-201.
6. Aksnes L, Aarskog D. Plasma concentrations of vitamin D metabolites in puberty: effect of sexual maturation and implications for growth. J Clin Endocrinol Metab 1982;55:94-101.
7. Alexander RL Jr. Evaluation of an automatic calcium titrator. Clin Chem 1971;17:1171-5.
8. Alsanea O, Clark OH. Familial thyroid cancer. Curr Opin Oncol 2001;13:44-51.
9. Altura BT, Bertschat F, Jeremias A, Ising H, Altura BM. Comparative findings on serum IMg^{2+} of normal and diseased human subjects with Nova and Kone ISE's for Mg^{2+}. Scand. J Clin Lab Invest Suppl 1994;54:217:77-81.
10. Altura BT, Burack JL, Cracco RQ, Galland L, Handwerker SM, Markell MS. Clinical studies with the Nova ISE for IMg^{2+}. Scand J Clin Lab Invest Suppl 1994;217:53-67.
11. Altura BT, Dell'Orfano K, Yeh Q. A new ion selective electrode for ionized magnesium in whole blood, plasma and serum. Clin Chem 1991;37:948 (abstract).
12. Altura BT, Shirey TL, Young CC. A new method for rapid determination of ionized Mg^{2+} in whole blood, serum and plasma. Methods Find Exp Clin Pharmacol 1992;14:297-304.
13. Altura BT, Shirey TL, Young CC. Characterization of a new ion selective electrode for ionized magnesium in whole blood, plasma, serum and aqueous samples. Scand J Clin Lab Invest 1994;54(Suppl. 217): 21-36.
14. Alvarez JC, De Mazancourt P. Rapid and sensitive high-performance liquid chromatographic method for the simultaneous determination of retinol, α-tocopherol, 25-hydroxyvitamin D_3 and 25-hydroxyvitamin D_2 in human plasma with photodiode-array ultraviolet detection. J Chromatogr 2001;755:129-35.
15. Alvarez L, Guanabens N, Peris P. Discriminative value of biochemical markers of bone turnover in assessing Paget's disease. J Bone Miner Res 1995;10: 458-65.
16. Amador E, Urban J. Simplified serum phosphorus analyses by continuous-flow ultraviolet spectrophotometry. Clin Chem 1972;18:601-4.
17. Anderson DJ, Branum EL, O'Brien JF. Liver- and bone-derived isoenzymes of alkaline phosphatase in serum as determined by high-performance affinity chromatography. Clin Chem 1990;36:240-6.
18. Andress DL, Endres DB, Maloney NA. Comparison of parathyroid hormone assays with bone histomorphometry in renal osteodystrophy. J Clin Endocrinol Metab 1986;63:1163-9.
19. Armitage EK. Parathyrin (parathyroid hormone): metabolism and methods of assay. Clin Chem 1986;32:418-24.
20. Ashby JP, Wright DJ, Rinsler MG. The adjusted serum calcium concept: a reappraisal. Ann Clin Biochem 1986;23:533-7.
21. Atkinson A, Gatenby AD, Lowe AG. The determination of inorganic orthophosphate in biological systems. Biochim Biophys Acta 1973;320:195-204.
22. Audran M. The physiology and pathophysiology of vitamin D. Mayo Clin Proc 1985;60:851-66.
23. Aurbach GD, Marx SJ, Speigel AM. Parathyroid hormone, calcitonin and the calciferols. In: Wilson JD, Foster DW, eds. Williams textbook of endocrinology, 8th ed. Philadelphia: WB Saunders, 1992: 1397-476.
24. Aurbach GD, Marx SJ, Spiegel AM. Metabolic bone disease. In: Wilson JD, Foster DW, eds. Williams textbook of endocrinology, 8th ed. Philadelphia: WB Saunders, 1992:1477-517.
25. Baldwin TE, Chernow B. Hypocalcemia in the ICU: coping with the causes and consequences. J Crit Illness 1987;2:9-16.
26. Banfi G, Daverio R. In vitro stability of osteocalcin. Clin Chem 1994;40:833-4.
27. Barbot N, Calmettes C, Schuffenecker I, Saint-Andre JP. Pentagastrin stimulation test and early diagnosis of medullary thyroid carcinoma using an immunoradiometric assay for calcitonin: comparison with genetic screening in hereditary medullary thyroid carcinoma. J Clin Endocrinol Metab 1994;78:114-20.
28. Barbour HM, Davidson W. Studies on measurement of plasma magnesium: application of magon dye method to the "Monarch" centrifugal analyzer. Clin Chem 1988;34:2103-5.
29. Bauer PJ. Affinity and stoichiometry of calcium binding by arsenazo III. Anal Biochem 1981;110: 61-72.
30. Baylin SB, Wieman KC, O'Neil JA, Roos BA. Multiple forms of human tumor calcitonin demonstrated by denaturing polyacrylamide gel electrophoresis and lectin affinity chromatography. J Clin Endocrinol Metab 1981;53:489-97.
31. Beck-Jensen JE, Kollerup G, Sorensen HA. A single measurement of biochemical markers of bone

turnover has limited utility in the individual person. Scand J Clin Lab Invest 1997;57:351-9.

32. Becker KL, Nash D, Silva OL. Increased serum and urinary calcitonin levels in patients with pulmonary disease. Chest 1981;79:211-6.
33. Beilby J, Randall A. Variable citrate interference in arsenazo III dye assays of total calcium in serum. Clin Chem 1990;36:824-5.
34. Bergman I, Loxley R. The determination of hydroxyproline in urine hydrolysates. Clin Chim Acta 1970;27:347-9.
35. Bettica P, Moro L, Robins SP. Bone resorption markers galactosyl hydroxylysine, pyridinium crosslinks, and hydroxyproline compared. Clin Chem 1992;38:2313-18.
36. Bijovet OL. Phosphate homeostasis. In: Avioli LV, Krane SM, eds. Metabolic bone disease. New York: Academic Press, 1977:49-83.
37. Bikle DD, Gee E, Halloran BP. Assessment of the free fraction of 25-hydroxyvitamin D in serum and its regulation by albumin and the vitamin D-binding protein. J Clin Endocrinol Metab 1986;63:954-9.
38. Bikle DD, Gee E, Halloran B, Haddad JG. Free 1,25-dihydroxyvitamin D levels in serum from normal subjects, pregnant subjects and subjects with liver disease. J Clin Invest 1984;74:1966-71.
39. Bikle DD, Halloran BP, Gee E. Free 25-hydroxyvitamin D levels are normal in subjects with liver disease and reduced total 25-hydroxyvitamin D levels. J Clin Invest 1986;78:748-52.
40. Bikle DD, Siiteri PK, Ryzen E, Haddad JG. Serum protein binding of 1,25-dihydroxyvitamin D: A reevaluation by direct measurement of free metabolite levels. J Clin Endocrinol Metab 1985;61:969-75.
41. Bilezikian JP. Calcium and bone metabolism. In: Becker KL, ed. Principles and practice of endocrinology and metabolism. Philadelphia: JB Lippincott, 1990:398-569.
42. Bilezikian JP, Potts JT Jr, Fuleihan Gel-H, Kleerekoper M, Neer R, Peacock M, et al. Summary statement from a workshop on asymptomatic primary hyperparathyroidism: a perspective for the 21st century. J Bone Miner Res 2002;17 Suppl 2:N2-11.
43. Birnbaum J, Van Herle AJ. Immunoheterogeneity of parathyroid hormone in parathyroid cysts: diagnostic implications. J Endocrinol Invest 1989;12:831-6.
44. Black D, Duncan A, Robins SP. Quantitative analysis of the pyridinium crosslinks of collagen in urine using ion-paired reversed-phase high-performance liquid chromatography. Anal Biochem 1988;169:197-203.
45. Blind E. Humoral hypercalcemia of malignancy: role of parathyroid hormone-related protein. Recent Results Cancer Res 1994;137:20-43.
46. Blind E, Raue F, Reichel H. Validity of intact plasma parathyrin measurements in chronic renal failure as determined by two-site immunoradiometric assays with N- or C-terminal capture antibodies. Clin Chem 1992;38:2345-7.
47. Blind E, Schmidt-Gayk H, Armbruster FP, Stadler A. Measurement of intact human parathyrin by an extracting two-site immunoradiometric assay. Clin Chem 1987;33:1376-81.
48. Blumsohn A, Colwell A, Naylor K, Eastell R. Effect of light and γ-irradiation on pyridinolines and telopeptides of type I collagen in urine. Clin Chem 1995;41:1195-7.
49. Blumsohn A, Hannon R, Eastell R. Apparent instability of osteocalcin in serum as measured with different commercially available immunoassays. Clin Chem 1995;41:318-9.
50. Blumsohn A, Naylor KE, Assiri AMA, Eastell R. Different responses of biochemical markers of bone resorption to bisphosphonate therapy in Paget's disease. Clin Chem 1995;42:1592-8.
51. Body JJ, Chanoine JP, Dumon JC, Delange F. Circulating calcitonin levels in healthy children and subjects with congenital hypothyroidism from birth to adolescence. J Endocrinol Metab 1993;77:565-7.
52. Body JJ, Delmas PD. Urinary pyridinium cross-links as markers of bone resorption in tumor-associated hypercalcemia. J Clin Endocrinol Metab 1992;74:471-5.
53. Body JJ, Heath H III. Estimates of circulating monomeric calcitonin: physiological studies in normal and thyroidectomized man. J Clin Endocrinol Metab 1983;57:897-903.
54. Body JJ, Heath H III. "Nonspecific" increases in plasma immunoreactive calcitonin in healthy individuals: discrimination from medullary thyroid carcinoma by a new extraction technique. Clin Chem 1984;30:511-14.
55. Bohler U, Bind E, Vogel G, Hitzler W, Flentje D, Schmidt-Gayk H. Two-site immunochemiluminometric assay of intact human parathyrin in serum with use of a tracer peptide purified by reversed-phase high-performance liquid chromatography. Clin Chem 1989;35:215-22.
56. Boink ABT, Buckley BM, Cristiansen TF, Covington AK, Maas A, Mueller-Plathe O, et al. Reference method for determination of ionized calcium in serum, plasma or whole blood. In: Maas AHJ, ed. Methodology and clinical applications of ion selective electrodes. Copenhagen: International Federation of Clinical Chemistry, 1986:39-61.
57. Boink ABT, Buckley BM, Christiansen TF, Covington AK, Maas A, Mueller-Plathe O, et al. Recommendations on blood sampling, transport and storage for the determination of the substance concentration of ionized calcium. In: Maas AHJ, ed. Methodology and clinical applications of ion selective electrodes.

Copenhagen: International Federation of Clinical Chemistry, 1986:81-8.
58. Bollen A-M, Martin MD, Leroux BG, Eyre DR. Circadian variation in urinary excretion of bone collagen cross-links. J Bone Miner Res 1995;10:1885-90.
59. Bonde M, Fledelius C, Qvist P, Christiansen C. Coated-tube radioimmunoassay for C-telopeptides of type I collagen to assess bone resorption. Clin Chem 1996;42:1639-44.
60. Bonde M, Garnero P, Fledelius C, Qvist P, Delmas PD, Christiansen C. Measurement of bone degradation products in serum using antibodies reactive with an isomerized form of an 8 amino acid sequence of the C-telopeptide of type I collagen. J Bone Miner Res 1997;12:1028-34.
61. Bonde M, Qvist P, Fledelius C, Riis BJ, Christiansen C. Immunoassay for quantifying type I collagen degradation products in urine evaluated. Clin Chem 1994;40:2022-5.
62. Bouillon R, Coopmans W, Degroote DEH, Radoux D, Eliard PH. Immunoradiometric assay of parathyrin with polyclonal and monoclonal region-specific antibodies. Clin Chem 1990;36:271-6.
63. Bouillon R, DeMoor P, Baggiolini EG, Uskokovic MR. A radioimmunoassay for 1,25 dihydroxycholecalciferol. Clin Chem 1980;26:562-7.
64. Bouillon R, Vanderschueren D, Van Herck E, Nielsen HK, Bex M, Heyns W, et al. Homologous radioimmunoassay of human osteocalcin. Clin Chem 1993;38:2055-60.
65. Bouillon R, Van Herck E, Jans I, Tan BK, Van Baelen H, De Moor P. Two direct (nonchromatographic) assays for 25-hydroxyvitamin D. Clin Chem 1984;30:1731-6.
66. Bouman AA, Scheffer PG, Ooms ME, Lips P, Netelenbos C. Two bone alkaline phosphatase assays compared with osteocalcin as a marker of bone formation in healthy elderly individuals. Clin Chem 1995;41:196-9.
67. Bowers GN Jr, Brassad C, Sena SF. Measurement of ionized calcium in serum with ion-selective electrodes: a mature technology that can meet the daily service needs. Clin Chem 1986;32:1437-44.
68. Bowers GN Jr, Rains TC. Measurement of total calcium in biological fluids: flame atomic absorption spectrometry. Methods Enzymol 1988;158:302-19.
69. Boyd JC, Lewis JW, Slatopoksky E, Ladenson JH. Parathyrin measured concurrently with free and total calcium in the differential diagnosis of hypercalcemia. Clin Chem 1981;27:574-9.
70. Boyle WJ, Simonet WS, Lacey DL. Osteoclast differentiation and activation. Nature 2003;423:337-42.
71. Brandi ML, Gagel RF, Angeli A, Bilezikian JP, Beck-Peccoz P, Bordi C, et al. Consensus guidelines for diagnosis and therapy of MEN type 1 and type 2. J Clin Endocrinol Metab 2001;86:5658-71.
72. Bringhurst FR. Calcium and phosphate distribution, turnover, and metabolic actions. In: DeGroot LJ, ed. Endocrinology, 3rd ed., Vol. 2. Philadelphia: WB Saunders, 1995:1015-43.
73. Bringhurst FR, Stern AM, Yotts M, Mizrahi N, Segre GV, Potts JT Jr. Peripheral metabolism of PTH: fate of biologically active amino terminus in vivo. Am J Physiol 1988;255:E886-93.
74. Broadus AE. Nephrolithiasis. In: Felig P, Baxter JD, Broadus AE, Frohman LA, eds. Endocrinology and metabolism. New York: McGraw-Hill Book Co, 1981:1119-72.
75. Brossard J-H, Cloutier M, Roy L, Lepage R, Gascon-Barre M, D'Amour P. Accumulation of a non-(1-84) molecular form of parathyroid hormone (PTH) detected by intact PTH assay in renal failure: importance in the interpretation of PTH values. J Clin Endocrinol Metab 1996;81:3923-9.
76. Brown EM. Extracellular Ca^{2+} sensing regulation of parathyroid cell function, and role of Ca^{2+} and other ions as extracellular (first) messengers. Physiol Rev 1991;71:371-411.
77. Brown RC, Aston JP, St John A, Woodhead JS. Comparison of poly- and monoclonal antibodies as labels in a two-site immunochemiluminometric assay for intact parathyroid hormone. J Immunol Methods 1988;109:139-44.
78. Brown RC, Aston JP, Weeks I, Woodhead JS. Circulating intact parathyroid hormone measured with a two-site immunochemiluminometric assay. J Clin Endocrinol Metab 1987;65:407-14.
79. Broyles DL, Nielsen RG, Bussett EM, Lu WD, Mizrahi IA, Nunnelly PA, et al. Analytical and clinical performance and characteristics of tandem-MP ostase, a new immunoassay for serum bone alkaline phosphatase. Clin Chem 1998;44:2139-47.
80. Bruton J, Wray HL, Dawson E, Butler V. 25-Hydroxyvitamin D_2 and 25-hydroxyvitamin D_3 as measured by liquid chromatography and by competitive protein binding. Clin Chem 1985;31:783-4.
81. Buckley BM, Russell LJ. The measurement of ionized calcium in blood plasma. Ann Clin Biochem 1988;25:447-65.
82. Budayr AA, Nissenson RA, Klein RF. Increased serum levels of parathyroid hormone-like protein in malignancy associated with hypercalcemia. Ann Intern Med 1989;111:807-12.
83. Burcar PJ, Boyle AJ, Mosher RE. Spectrophotometric determination of magnesium in blood serum using magon. Clin Chem 1964;10:1028-38.
84. Burlina A, Plebani M, Secchiero S, Zaninotto M, Sciacovelli L. Precipitation method for separating and quantifying bone and liver alkaline phosphatase isoenzymes. Clin Biochem 1991;24:417-23.
85. Burnett RW, Christiansen TF, Covington AK, Fogh-Andersen N, Kulpmann WR, Lewenstam A,

et al. IFCC recommended reference method for the determination of the substance concentration of ionized calcium in undiluted serum, plasma or whole blood. Clin Chem Lab Med 2000;38:1301-14.

86. Burnett RW, Covington AK, Fogh-Anderson N, Kulpman WR, Maas AH, Muller-Plathe, et al. Recommendations on whole blood sampling, transport, and storage for simultaneous determination of pH, blood gases, and electrolytes. J Int Fed Clin Chem 1994;6:115-20.
87. Burrit MF. Electrolytes and blood gases (ionized calcium). Anal Chem 1993;65:409R-11R.
88. Burritt MF, Pierides AM, Offord KP. Comparative studies of total and ionized calcium values in normal subjects and patients with renal disorders. Mayo Clin Proc 1980;55:606-13.
89. Burritt MF, Slockbower JM, Forsman RW, Offord KP, Bergstralh EJ, Smithson WA. Pediatric reference intervals for 19 biologic variables in healthy children. Mayo Clin Proc 1990;65:329-36.
90. Burtis WJ. Parathyroid hormone-related protein: structure, function, and measurement. Clin Chem 1992;38:2171-83.
91. Burtis WJ, Brady TG, Orloff JJ, Ersbak JB, Warrell RP Jr, Olson BR, et al. Immunochemical characterization of circulating parathyroid hormone-related protein in patients with humoral hypercalcemia of cancer. N Engl J Med 1990;322:1106-12.
92. Burtis WJ, Wu TL, Insogna KL, Stewart AF. Humoral hypercalcemia of malignancy. Ann Intern Med 1988;108:454-6.
93. Cali JP, Mandel J, Moore L, Young DS. A referee method for the determination of calcium in serum. NBS Special Publication 1972;260-236: 1-121.
94. Calvo MS. Prevalence of vitamin D insufficiency in Canada and the United States: importance to health status and efficacy of current food fortification and dietary supplement use. Nutrition Reviews 2003;61:107-13.
95. Calvo MS, Eastell R, Offord KP, Bergstralh EJ, Burritt MF. Circadian variation in ionized calcium and intact parathyroid hormone: evidence for sex differences in calcium homeostasis. J Clin Endocrinol Metab 1991;72:69-76.
96. Calvo M, Ena JM. Relations between vitamin D and fatty acid binding properties of vitamin D-binding protein. Biochem Biophys Res Comun 1989;163: 14-17.
97. Calvo MS, Eyre DR, Gundberg CM. Molecular basis and clinical application of biological markers of bone turnover. Endocr. Rev, 1996;17:333-68.
98. Cao Z, Tongate C, Elin RJ. Evaluation of AVL988/4 analyzer for measurement of ionized magnesium and ionized calcium. Scand J Clin Lab Invest 2001;61: 389-94.
99. Cardenas-Rivero N, Chernow B, Stoiko MA, Nussbaum SR, Todres ID. Hypocalcemia in critically ill children. J Pediatr 1989;114:946-51.
100. Carter AB, Howanitz PJ. Intraoperative testing for parathyroid hormone: a comprehensive review of the use of the assay and the relevant literature. Arch Pathol Lab Med 2003;127:1424-42.
101. Catherwood BD, Marcus R, Madvig P, Cheung AK. Determinants of bone gamma-carboxyglutamic acid-containing protein in plasma of healthy aging subjects. Bone 1985;6:9-13.
102. Cecco SA, Hristova EN, Rehak NN, Elin RJ. Clinically important intermethod differences for physiologically abnormal ionized magnesium results. Am J Clin Pathol 1997;108:564-9.
103. Chan K-M, Arriaga C, Landt M, Smith CH, Ng RH. Interference by hemolysis with various methods for total calcium and its correction by trichloroacetic acid precipitation. Clin Chem 1983;29:1497-500.
104. Chattopadhyay N, Mithal A, Brown E. The calcium-sensing receptor: a window into the physiology and pathophysiology of mineral ion metabolism. Endocr Rev 1996;17:289-307.
105. Cheung CK, Panesar NS, Haines C, Masarei J, Swaminathan R. Immunoassay of tartrate-resistant acid phosphatase in serum. Clin Chem 1995;41: 679-86.
106. Christiansen C, Hassager C, Riis BJ. Biochemical markers of bone turnover. In: Avioli LV, Krane SM, eds. Metabolic bone disease, 3rd ed. San Diego: Academic Press, 1998;313-26.
107. Clark WL, Baginski ES, Marie SS, Zak B. Spectrophotometric study of a direct determination of serum calcium. Microchem J 1975;20:22-32.
108. Clarke AD, Rowbury CS. Removal of lipids before liquid chromatography of vitamin D in serum. Clin Chem 1985;31:657-8.
109. Clemens JD, Herrick M, Singer F, Eyre DR. Evidence that serum NTx (collagen type 1 N-telopeptides) can act as an immunochemical markers of bone resorption. Clin Chem 1997;43:2058-63.
110. Clemens TL, Adams JS, Nolan JM, Holick MF. Measurement of circulating vitamin D in man. Clin Chim Acta 1982;121:301-8.
111. Clemens TL, Hendy GN, Papapoulos SE, Fraher LJ, Care AD, O'Riordan JL. Measurement of 1,25-dihydroxycholecalciferol in man by radioimmunoassay. Clin Endocrinol (Oxf) 1979;11:225-34.
112. Coburn JW, Massry SG, Gordon S, Rubini M. Spurious hypocalcemia in patients undergoing maintenance hemodialysis. Am J Clin Pathol 1969;52:572-6.
113. Coburn JW, Slatopolsky E. Vitamin D, parathyroid hormone, and renal osteodystrophy. In: Brenner BM, Rector FC Jr, eds. The kidney, 4th ed. Philadelphia: WB Saunders, 1991:2213-305.

114. Coen G, Bonucci E, Ballanti P, Balducci A, Calabria S, Nicolai GA, et al. PTH 1-84 and PTH "7-84" in the noninvasive diagnosis of renal bone disease. Am J Kidney Dis 2002;40:348-54.
115. Cohen-Solal ME, Sebert J-L, Boudailliez B, Marie A, Moriniere P, Gueris J, et al. Comparison of intact, midregion, and carboxy terminal assays of parathyroid hormone for the diagnosis of bone disease in hemodialysed patients. J Clin Endocrinol Metab 1991;73:516-24.
116. Coldwell RD, Trafford DJH, Makin HLJ. Improved chromatographic determination of 25-hydroxyvitamins D_2 and D_3. Clin Chem 1985;31:1919-20.
117. Coleman RE. The clinical use of bone resorption markers in patients with malignant bone disease. Cancer 2002;94:2521-33.
118. Connerty HV, Briggs AR. Determination of serum calcium by means of orthocresolphthalein complexone. Am J Clin Pathol 1966;45:290-6.
119. Cooke NE, Haddad JG. Vitamin D binding protein (Gc-globulin). Endocr Rev 1989;10:294-307.
120. Cornelisson G. Broadly pertinent chronobiology methods quantify phosphate dynamics (chronome) in blood and urine. Clin Chem 1992;38:329-33.
121. Corns CM. Interference by haemoglobin with cresolphthalein complexone method for serum calcium measurement. Ann Clin Biochem 1990;27:152-5.
122. Corns CM, Ludman CJ. Some observations on the nature of the calcium-cresolphthalein complexone reaction and its relevance to the clinical laboratory. Ann Clin Biochem 1987;24:345-51.
123. Covington AK, Ferra MIA. Calculation of single ion activities in solutions simulating blood plasma. In: Maas AHJ, ed. Methodology and clinical applications of ion selective electrodes. Copenhagen: International Federation of Clinical Chemistry, 1986:239-47.
124. Cowley DM, Mottram BM, Haling NB, Sinton TJ. Improved linearity of the calcium cresolpthalein-complexone reaction with sodium acetate. Clin Chem 1986;32:894-5.
125. Curley IR, Wheeler MH, Aston JP, Brown RC, Weeks I, Woodhead JS. Studies in patients with hyperparathyroidism using a two-site immunochemiluminometric assay for circulating intact (1-84) parathyroid hormone. Surgery 1987;102:926-31.
125A. D'Amour P, Brossard J-H, Rousseau L, Roy L, Gao P, Cantor T. Amino-terminal form of parathyroid hormone (PTH) with immunologic similarities to hPTH(1-84) is overproduced in primary and secondary hyperparathyroidism. Clin Chem 2003;49:2037-44.
126. D'Amour P, Jobin J, Hamel L, L'Ecuyer N. iPTH values during hemodialysis: role of ionized calcium, dialysis membranes and iPTH assays. Kidney Int 1990;38:308-14.
127. D'Amour P, Labelle F, Lacavalier L, Plourde V, Harvey D. Influence of serum calcium concentration on circulating molecular forms of PTH in three species. Am J Physiol 1986;251:E680-7.
128. D'Orazio P, Bowers GN Jr. Design and preliminary performance characteristics of a newly proposed reference cell for ionized calcium in serum. Clin Chem 1992;38:1332-9.
129. Daly JA, Ertingshausen G. Direct method for determining inorganic phosphate in serum with Centrifichem. Clin Chem 1972;18:263-5.
130. Daugaard H, Egfjord M, Olgaard K. Influence of calcium on the metabolism of intact parathyroid hormone by isolated perfused rat kidney and liver. Endocrinology 1990;126:1813-20.
131. Davidson W, Barbour HM. Determination of urine magnesium using the magon method on the "Monarch" centrifugal analyser. Ann Clin Biochem 1990;27:595-6.
132. Davis OK, Hawkins DS, Rubin LP, Posillico JT, Brown EM, Schiff I. Serum parathyroid hormone in pregnant women determined by an immunoradiometric assay for intact PTH. J Clin Endocrinol Metab 1988;67:850-2.
133. Dawson CD, Jewell S, Driskell WJ. Liquid-chromatographic determination of total hydroxyproline in urine. Clin Chem 1988;34:1572-4.
134. Decker RA, Peacock ML, Borst MJ, Sweet JD, Thompson NW. Progress in genetic screening of multiple endocrine neoplasia type 2A: is calcitonin testing obsolete? Surgery 1995;118:257-64.
135. Deftos LJ. The thyroid gland in calcium and skeletal metabolism. In: Avioli LV, Krane SM, eds. Metabolic bone disease, 2nd ed. Philadelphia: WB Saunders, 1990:702-29.
136. Deftos LJ. Bone protein and peptide assays in the diagnosis and management of skeletal disease. Clin Chem 1991;37:1143-8.
137. Deftos LJ, Weisman MH, Williams GW, Karpf DB, Frumar AM, Davidson BJ, et al. Influence of age and sex on plasma calcitonin in human beings. N Engl J Med 1980;302:1351-3.
138. Deftos LJ, Wolfert RL, Hill CS, Burton DW. Two-site assays of bone gla protein (osteocalcin) demonstrate immunochemical heterogeneity of the intact molecule. Clin Chem 1992;38:2318-21.
139. DeLeenheer AP, Bauwens RM. Radioimmunoassay for 1,25-dihydroxyvitamin D in serum and plasma. Clin Chem 1985;31:142-6.
140. Delmas PD. Biochemical markers of bone turnover for the clinical assessment of metabolic bone disease. Endocrinol Metab Clin North Am 1990;19:1-18.
141. Delmas PD. Markers of bone turnover for monitoring osteoporosis with antiresorptive drugs. Osteoporosis Int 2000;S6:S66-76.

142. Delmas PD, Christiansen C, Mann KG, Price PA. Bone Gla protein (osteocalcin) assay standardization report. J Bone Miner Res 1990;5:5-11.
143. Delmas PD, Eastell R, Garnero P, Seibel MJ, Stepan J. The use of biochemical markers of bone turnover in osteoporosis. Osteoporosis Int 2000;Suppl 6:S2-17.
144. Delmas PD, Hardy P, Garnero P, Dain M. Monitoring individual response to hormone replacement therapy with bone markers. Bone 2000;26:553-60.
145. Delmas PD, Schlemmer A, Gineyts E, Riis B, Christiansen C. Urinary excretion of pyridinoline crosslinks correlates with bone turnover measured on iliac crest biopsy in patients with vertebral osteoporosis. J Bone Miner Res 1991;6:639-44.
146. DeLuca HF. The vitamin D story: a collaborative effort of basic science and clinical medicine. FASEB J 1988;2:224-36.
147. DeLuca HF, Krisinger J, Darwish H. The vitamin D system: 1990. Kidney Int 1990;38:S-2-8.
148. Demers LM. New biochemical markers for bone disease: is it a breakthrough? (editorial). Clin Chem 1992;38:2169-70.
149. Demers LM. Bone markers in the management of patients with skeletal disease. Cancer 2003;97: 874-9.
150. Demers LM, Spencer CA, eds. Laboratory support for the diagnosis and monitoring of thyroid disease. Thyroid 2003;13:1-126.
151. Dermody WC, Rosen MA, Ananthaswamy R, McCormick WM, Levy AG. Characterization of the major forms of human calcitonin in tissue and serum. J Clin Endocrinol Metab 1981;52: 1090-8.
152. Diaz Diego EM, Guerrero R, de la Piedra C. Six osteocalcin assays compared. Clin Chem 1994;40:2071-7.
153. Dihydroxyvitamin D, 1,25-^{125}I Kit. DiaSorin, Stillwater, MN, 2002.
154. Dilena BA, White GH. Interference with the measurement of intact parathyrin in serum from renal dialysis patients. Clin Chem 1989;35:1543-4.
155. Dilena BA, White GH. Assessing acute parathyroid responsiveness in hemodialysis patients by measuring intact parathyrin in pre- and post-dialysis serum. Clin Chem 1991;37:1216-20.
156. Donhowe JM, Freier EF, Wong ET, Steffes MW. Factitious hypophosphatemia related to mannitol therapy. Clin Chem 1981;27:1765-9.
157. Duda RJ Jr, O'Brien JF, Katzman JA, Peterson JM, Mann KG, Riggs BL. Concurrent assays of circulating bone gla-protein and bone alkaline phosphatase: effects of sex, age, and metabolic bone disease. J Clin Endocrinol Metab 1988;66:951-7.
158. Dunn JT. When is a thyroid nodule a sporadic medullary carcinoma? (editorial). J Clin Endocrinol Metab 1994;78:824-5.
159. Earl RE, Feld RD. Cyanide is not needed in the cresolphthalein complexone determination of serum calcium. Clin Chem 1982;28:1730.
160. Eastell R, Calvo MS, Burrit MF, Offord KP, Russell RG, Riggs BL. Abnormalities in circadian patterns of bone resorption and renal calcium conservation in type I osteoporosis. J Clin Endocrinol Metab 1992;74:487-94.
161. Eastell R, Mallinak N, Weiss S, Ettinger M, Pettinger M, Cain D, et al. Biological variability of serum and urinary N-telopeptide of type I collagen in postmenopausal women. J Bone Miner Res 2000;15:594-8.
162. Eastell R, Yergey AL, Vierira NE, Cedel SL, Kumar R, Riggs BL. Interrelationship among vitamin D metabolism, true calcium absorption, parathyroid function, and age in women: evidence of an age-related intestinal resistance to 1,25-dihydroxyvitamin D action. J Bone Miner Res 1991;6:125-32.
163. Ebeling PR, Atley LM, Guthrie JR, Burger HG, Dennerstein L, Hopper JL, et al. Bone turnover markers and bone density across the menopausal transition. J Clin Endocrinol Metab 1996;81:3366-71.
164. Elin RJ. Assessment of magnesium status. Clin Chem 1987;33:1965-70.
165. Elin RJ. Magnesium metabolism in health and disease. Dis Mon 1988;34:161-219.
166. Elin RJ. Magnesium: the fifth but forgotten electrolyte. Am J Clin Pathol 1994;102:616-22.
167. Endres DB. Which parathyrin assay is really best for clinical use? Clin Chem 1991;37:1466-7.
168. Endres DB. Hypercalcemia and parathyroid disorders. Curr Opin Rheumatol 1992;4:383-8.
169. Endres DB, Adams JS. Vitamin D and metabolites. In: Favus MJ, ed. Primer on the metabolic bone diseases and disorders of mineral metabolism. Kelseyville, Calif.: American Society for Bone and Mineral Research, 1990:70-3.
170. Endres DB, Cornell ME, Nelson JC, Cantor TL. Calcitonin in normal individuals with a sensitive, specific radioimmunoassay. Calcif Tissue Int 1984;36:476.
171. Endres DB, Morgan CH, Garry PJ, Omdahl JL. Age-related changes in serum immunoreactive parathyroid hormone and its biological action in healthy men and women. J Clin Endocrinol Metab 1987;65:724-31.
172. Endres DB, Villanueva R, Sharp CF Jr, Singer FR. Measurement of parathyroid hormone. Endocrinol Metab Clin North Am 1989;18:611-29.
173. Endres DB, Villanueva R, Sharp CF Jr, Singer FR. Immunochemiluminometric and immunoradiometric determinations of intact and total immunoreactive parathyrin: performance in the differential diagnosis of hypercalcemia and hypoparathyroidism. Clin Chem 1991;37:162-8.
174. Engelbach M, Gorges R, Forst T, Pfutzner A, Dawood R, Heerdt S, et al. Improved diagnostic methods in

the follow-up of medullary thyroid carcinoma by highly specific calcitonin measurements. J Clin Endocrinol Metab 2000;85:1890-4.
175. Epstein S. Serum and urinary markers of bone remodeling: assessment of bone turnover. Endocr Rev 1988;9:437-49.
176. Eugster R, Rusterholz B, Schmid A, Spichiger UE, Simon W. Characterization procedure for ion-selective electrode assays of magnesium activity in aqueous solutions of physiological composition. Clin Chem 1993;39:855-9.
177. Eyre DR. Collagen cross-linking amino acids. Methods Enzymol 1987;144:115-39.
178. Eyre DR. New biomarkers of bone resorption, (editorial). J Clin Endocrinol Metab 1992;74:470A-C.
179. Eyre DR, Koob TJ, Van Ness KP. Quantitation of hydroxypyridinium crosslinks in collagen by high-performance liquid chromatography. Anal Biochem 1984;137:380-8.
180. Eyre DR, Paz MA, Gallop PM. Cross-linking in collagen and elastin. Annu Rev Biochem 1984;53:717-48.
181. Farley J, Baylink DJ. Skeletal alkaline phosphatase activity in serum. Clin Chem 1995;41:1551-3.
182. Farley JR, Hall SL, Herring S, Libanati C, Wergedal JE. Reference standards for quantification of skeletal alkaline phosphatase activity in serum by heat inactivation and lectin precipitation. Clin Chem 1993;39:1878-84.
183. Farley JR, Hall SL, Ilacas D, Orcutt C, Miller BE, Hill CS, Baylink DJ. Quantification of skeletal alkaline phosphatase in osteoporotic serum by wheat germ agglutinin precipitation, heat inactivation and a two-site immunoradiometric assay. Clin Chem 1994;40:1749-59.
184. Farley JR, Kyeyune-Nyombi E, Tarbaux NM, Hall SL, Strong DD. Alkaline phosphatase activity from human osteosarcoma cell line SaOS-2: an isoenzyme standard for quantifying skeletal alkaline phosphatase activity in serum. Clin Chem 1989;35:223-9.
185. Fischl J, Schwartz F. Modified "calcium base reagent" for simultaneous determination of serum calcium and inorganic phosphate with the "Autoanalyzer." Clin Chem 1972;18:1430-1.
186. Fitzpatrick CP, Pardue HL. Simultaneous determinations of liver- and bone-type alkaline phosphatase by curve-fitting of inhibition kinetic data: I. Development and evaluation of an absorbance-based method. Clin Chem 1992;38:238-46.
187. Fleisher M, Gladstone M, Crystal D, Schwartz MK. Two whole-blood multi-analyte analyzers evaluated. Clin Chem 1989;35:1532-5.
188. Fogh-Anderson N. Ionized calcium analyzer with built-in pH correction. Clin Chem 1981;27:1264-7.
189. Fogh-Anderson N, Bjerrum PJ, Siggaard-Anderson O. Ionic binding, net charge, and Donnan effect of human serum albumin as a function of pH. Clin Chem 1993;39:48-52.
190. Fohr B, Dunstan CR, Seibel MJ. Markers of bone remodeling in metastatic bone disease. J Clin Endocrinol Metab 2003;88:5059-75.
191. Fraher LJ, Adami S, Clemens TL, Jones G, O'Riordan JL. Radioimmunoassay of 1,25-dihydroxyvitamin D_2 in man. Clin Endocrinol (Oxf) 1983;18:151-65.
192. Fraser CG. The application of theoretical goals based on biological variation data in proficiency testing. Arch Pathol Lab Med 1988;112:404-15.
193. Fraser WD, Logue FC, Gallacher SJ, O'Reilly DS, Beastall GH, Ralston SH, et al. Direct and indirect assessment of the parathyroid response to pamidronate therapy in Paget's disease of bone and hypercalcemia of malignancy. Bone Miner 1991;12:113-21.
194. Fraser WD, Logue FC, MacRitchie K, Wilson RM, Gray HW, Beastall GH, et al. Intact parathyroid hormone concentration and cyclic AMP metabolism in thyroid disease. Acta Endocrinol 1991;124:652-7.
195. Fraser WD, Robinson J, Lawton R, Durham B, Gallacher SJ, Boyle IT, et al. Clinical and laboratory studies of a new immunoradiometric assay of parathyroid hormone-related protein. Clin Chem 1993;39:414-19.
196. Frolich M, Walma ST, Paulson C, Papapoulos SE. Immunoradiometric assay for intact human parathyroid hormone: characteristics, clinical application and comparison with a radioimmunoassay. Ann Clin Biochem 1990;27:69-72.
197. Fujita T, Kawakami Y, Kohda S, Takata S, Sunahara Y, Arisue K. Assay of magnesium in serum and urine with use of only one enzyme, isocitrate dehydrogenase ($NADP^+$). Clin Chem 1995;41:1302-5.
198. Fyffe JA. Serum-based controls for calcium ion-selective electrodes. Clin Chem 1986;32:1790-1.
199. Gagel RF. Multiple endocrine neoplasia type II and familial medullary thyroid carcinoma: impact of genetic screening on management. Cancer Treat Res 1997;89:421-41.
200. Gallacher SJ, Fraser WD, Owens OJ, Dryburgh FJ, Logue FC, Jenkins A, et al. Changes in calciotrophic hormones and biochemical markers of bone turnover in normal pregnancy. Eur J Endocrinol 1994;131:369-74.
201. Gallagher JC, Riggs BL, Jerpbak CM, Arnaud CD. The effect of age on serum immunoreactive parathyroid hormone in normal and osteoporotic women. J Lab Clin Med 1980;95:373-85.
202. Gao P, Scheibel S, D'Amour PD, John MR, Rao SD, Schmidt-Gayk H, et al. Development of a novel immunoradiometric assay exclusively for biologically active whole parathyroid hormone 1-84: implications for improvement of accurate assessment of parathyroid function. J Bone Miner Res 2001;16:605-14.

203. Garber CC, Miller RC. Revision of the 1963 semidine HCl standard method for inorganic phosphorous. Clin Chem 1983;29:184-8.
204. Garnero P, Borel O, Delmas PD. Evaluation of a fully automated serum assay for C-terminal cross-linking telopeptide of type I collagen in osteoporosis. Clin Chem 2001;47:694-702.
205. Garnero P, Delmas PD. Assessment of the serum levels of alkaline phosphatase with a new immunoradiometric assay in patients with metabolic bone disease. J Clin Endocrinol Metab 1993;77:1046-53.
206. Garnero P, Delmas PD. Measurements of biochemical markers: methods and limitations. In: Bilezikian JP, Raisz LG, Rodan GA, eds. Principles of bone biology. San Diego: Academic Press, 1996:1277-91.
207. Garnero P, Delmas PD. New developments in biochemical markers for osteoporosis. Calcif Tissue Int 1996;59:S2-S9.
208. Garnero P, Delmas PD. Biochemical markers of bone turnover in osteoporosis. In: Marcus R, Feldman D, Kelsey J, eds. Osteoporosis, 2nd ed. San Diego: Academic Press, 2001;459-77.
209. Garnero P, Delmas PD. Evaluation of risk of osteoporotic fracture. In: Principles of bone biology, 2nd ed. San Diego: Academic Press, 2002;1291-301.
210. Garnero P, Gineyts E, Arbault P, Christiansen C, Delmas PD. Different effects of bisphosphonates and estrogen therapy on free and peptide-bound bone cross-links excretion. J Bone Miner Res 1995;10:641-9.
211. Garnero P, Gineyts E, Riou JP, Delmas PD. Assessment of bone resorption with a new marker of collagen degradation in patients with metabolic bone disease. J Clin Endocrinol Metab 1994;79:780-5.
212. Garnero P, Grimaux M, Seguin P, Delmas P. Characterization of immunoreactive forms of human osteocalcin in vivo and in vitro. J Bone Miner Res 1994;9:255-64.
213. Garnero P, Shih WJ, Gineyts E, Karpf DB, Delmas PD. Comparison of new biochemical markers of bone turnover in late postmenopausal osteoporotic women in response to alendronate treatment. J Clin Endocrinol Metab 1994;79:1693-700.
214. Gawoski JM, Walsh D. Citrate interference in assays of total calcium in serum. Clin Chem 1989;35:2140-1.
215. Gerrits MI, Thijssen JHH, van Rijn HJM. Determination of pyridinoline and deoxypyridinoline in urine, with special attention to retaining their stability. Clin Chem 1995;41:571-4.
216. Gertner JM, Coustan DR, Kliger AS, Mallette LE, Ravin N, Broadus AE. Pregnancy as state of physiologic absorptive hypercalciuria. Am J Med 1986;81:451-6.
217. Gertz BJ, Clemens JD, Holland SD, Yuan W, Greenspan S. Application of a new serum assay for type I collagen cross-linked N-telopeptides: assessment of clinical changes in bone turnover with and without alendronate treatment. Calcif Tiss Int 1998;63:102-6.
218. Gertz BJ, Shao P, Hanson DA, Quan H, Harris ST, Genant HK, et al. Monitoring bone resorption in early postmenopausal women by an immunoassay for cross-linked collagen peptides in urine. J Bone Miner Res 1994;9:135-42.
219. Gharib H, Kao PC, Heath H III. Determination of silica-purified plasma calcitonin for the detection and management of medullary thyroid carcinoma: comparison of two provocative tests. Mayo Clin Proc 1987;62:373-8.
220. Gitelman HJ. An improved automated procedure for the determination of calcium in biological specimens. Anal Biochem 1967;18:521-31.
221. Glick MR, Ryder KW. Analytical systems ranked by freedom from interferences. Clin Chem 1987;33:1453-8.
222. Glick MR, Ryder KW, Jackson SA. Graphical comparisons of interferences in clinical chemistry instrumentation. Clin Chem 1986;32:470-5.
223. Goldsmith MW, Parry DJ. An investigation into the mechanism of the in vitro fall in rabbit plasma calcium which follows intravenous heparin injection. Clin Chim Acta 1968;19:429-38.
224. Goltzman D, Tischler AS. Characterization of the immunochemical forms of calcitonin released by a medullary thyroid carcinoma in tissue culture. J Clin Invest 1978;61:449-58.
225. Gomez B Jr, Ardakani S, Evans BJ, Merrell LD, Jenkins DK, Kung VT. Monoclonal antibody assay for free urinary pyridinium cross-links. Clin Chem 1996;42:1168-75.
226. Gomez B Jr, Ardakani S, Ju J, Jenkins D, Cerelli MJ, Daniloff GY, et al. Monoclonal antibody assay for measuring bone-specific alkaline phosphatase in serum. Clin Chem 1995;41:1560-6.
227. Gomez P, Coca C, Vargas C, Acebillo J, Martinez A. Normal reference intervals for 20 chemical variables in healthy infants, children and adolescents. Clin Chem 1984;30:407-12.
228. Gonchoroff DG, Branum EL, O'Brien JF. Alkaline phosphatase isoenzymes of liver and bone are incompletely resolved by wheat-germ-lectin affinity chromatography. Clin Chem 1989;35:29-32.
229. Goodman WG, Coburn JW, Slatopolsky E, Salusky IB. Renal osteodystrophy in adults and children. In: Favus MJ, ed. Primer on the metabolic bone diseases and disorders of mineral metabolism. Philadephia: Lippincott Williams & Wilkins, 1999:347-63.
230. Gosling P. Analytical reviews in clinical biochemistry: Calcium measurement. Ann Clin Biochem 1986;23:146-56.
231. Goverde BC, Veenkamp FJN. Routine assay of total urinary hydroxyproline based on resin-catalyzed hydrolysis. Clin Chim Acta 1972;41:29-40.

232. Gray TA, Paterson CR. The clinical value of ionized calcium assays. Ann Clin Biochem 1988;25:210-9.
233. Gray TK. Radioimmunoassay for 1,25-dihydroxycholecalciferol. Clin Chem 1983;29:196-200.
234. Griffiths WC, Camara PD, Rosner M, Lev R, Brooks EM. Prevalence and properties of the intestinal alkaline phosphatase identified in serum by cellulose acetate electrophoresis. Clin Chem 1992;38:507-11.
235. Guilloteau D, Perdrisot R, Calmettes C, Baulieu JL, Lecomte P, Kaphan G, et al. Diagnosis of medullary carcinoma (MCT) of the thyroid by calcitonin assay using monoclonal antibodies: criteria for the pentagastrin stimulation test in hereditary MCT. J Clin Endocrinol Metab 1990;71:1064-7.
236. Gundberg CM. Biochemical markers of bone formation. Clin Lab Med 2000;489-501.
237. Gundberg CM. Osteocalcin. In: Eastell R, Baumann M, Hoyle NR, Wieczorek L., eds. Bone markers: biochemical and clinical perspectives. London: Martin Dunitz, 2001:65-72.
238. Hall RA, Whitehead TP. Adsorption of serum calcium by plastic sample cups. J Clin Pathol 1970;23:323-6.
239. Halleen JM, Alatalo SL, Janckila AJ, Woitge HW, Seibel MJ, Vaananen HK. Serum tartrate-resistant acid phosphatase 5b is a specific and sensitive marker of bone resorption. Clin Chem 2001;47:597-600.
240. Halleen JM, Alatalo SL, Suominen H, Woitge HW, Seibel MJ, Vaananen HK. Tartrate-resistant acid phosphatase 5b, a novel serum marker of bone resorption. J Bone Miner Res 2000;15:1337-45.
241. Hanson DA, Weis MAE, Bollen A-M, Maslan SL, Singer FR, Eyre DR. A specific immunoassay for monitoring human bone resorption: quantitation of type I collagen cross-linked N-telopeptides in urine. J Bone Miner Res 1992;7:1251-8.
242. Harms H-M, Kaptaina U, Kulpmann WR, Brabant G, Hesch RD. Pulse amplitude and frequency modulation of parathyroid hormone in plasma. J Clin Endocrinol Metab 1989;69:843-51.
243. Harrell RM, Lyles KW, Harrelson JM, Friedman NE, Drezner MK. Healing of bone disease in X-linked hypophosphatemic rickets/osteomalacia. J Clin Invest 1985;75:1858-68.
244. Harris H. The human alkaline phosphatases: what we know and what we don't know. Clin Chim Acta 1989;186:133-50.
245. Haussler MR, McCain TA. Basic and clinical concepts related to vitamin D metabolism and action. N Engl J Med 1977;297:974-83, 1041-50.
246. Hawker CD. Parathyroid hormone: radioimmunoassay and clinical interpretation. Ann Clin Lab Sci 1975;5:383-98.
247. Hay AWM, Jones G. The elution profile of vitamin D_2 metabolites from LH_2O columns. Clin Chem 1979;25:473-5.
248. Heaney RP, Dowell S, Hale C, Bendich A. Calcium absorption varies within the reference range for serum 25-hydroxyvitamin D. J Am Coll Nutr 2003;22:142-6.
249. Heath H III, Body JJ, Fox J. Radioimmunoassay of calcitonin in normal human plasma: problems, perspectives and prospects. Biomed Pharmacother 1984;38:241-5.
250. Heath H III, Earll JM, Schaaf M, Piechocki JT, Li TK. Serum ionized calcium during bed rest in fracture patients and normal men. Metabolism 1972;21:633-40.
251. Henderson JE, Shustik C, Kremer R, Rabbani SA, Hendy GN, Goltzman D. Circulating concentrations of parathyroid hormone-like peptide in malignancy and in hyperparathyroidism. J Bone Miner Res 1990;5:105-13.
252. Henry RJ. Inorganic ions. In: Henry RJ, ed. Clinical chemistry: principles and techniques. New York: Harper & Row, 1964:345-421.
253. Hill C, Cerrito M, Grafstein E, Rao S, Wolfert R. Development of the BAP Tandem-R assay for the specific detection of bone alkaline phosphatase in human serum. Clin Chem 1991;37:1019.
254. Hill CS, Wolfert RL. The preparation of monoclonal antibodies which react preferentially with human bone alkaline phosphatase and not liver alkaline phosphatase. Clin Chim Acta 1989;186:315-20.
255. Hofbauer LC, Heufelder AE. Role of receptor activator of nuclear factor-kappaB ligand and osteoprotegerin in bone cell biology. J Mol Med 2001;79:243-53.
256. Holick MF. Vitamin D and the kidney. Kidney Int 1987;32:912-29.
257. Holick MF. Vitamin D: Photobiology, metabolism and clinical applications. In: DeGroot LJ, ed. Endocrinology, 3rd ed, Vol. 2. Philadelphia: WB Saunders, 1995:990-1014.
258. Holick MF, Adams JS. Vitamin D metabolism and biological function. In: Avioli LV, Krane SM, eds. Metabolic bone disease, 2nd ed. Philadelphia: WB Saunders, 1990:155-95.
259. Hollis BW. Assay of circulating 1,25-dihydroxyvitamin D involving a novel single-cartridge extraction and purification procedure. Clin Chem 1986;32:2060-3.
260. Hollis B. 1,25-Dihydroxyvitamin D_3-26,23-lactone interferes in determination of 1,25-dihydroxyvitamin D by RIA after immunoextraction. Clin Chem 1995;41:1313-14.
261. Hollis B. Detection of vitamin D and its major metabolites. In: Feldman DD, Glorieux FH, Pike JW, eds. Vitamin D. New York: Academic Press, 1997:587-606.
262. Hollis B. Comparison of commercially available ^{125}I-based RIA methods for the determination of circulat-

ing 25-hydroxyvitamin D. Clin Chem 2000;46: 1657-61.

263. Hollis BW, Frank NE. Solid phase extraction system for vitamin D and its major metabolites in human plasma. J Chromatogr 1985;343:43-9.
264. Hollis BW, Kamerud JQ, Kurkowski A, Beaulieu J, Napoli JL. Quantification of circulating 1,25-dihydroxyvitamin D by radioimmunoassay with a 125-I-labeled tracer. Clin Chem 1996;42: 586-92.
265. Hollis BW, Kamerud JQ, Selvaag SR, Lorenz JD, Napoli JL. Determination of vitamin D status by radioimmunoassay with an ^{125}I-labeled tracer. Clin Chem 1993;39:529-33.
266. Hollis BW, Napoli JL. Improved radioimmunoassay for vitamin D and its use in assessing vitamin D status. Clin Chem 1985;31:1815-9.
267. Hollis BW, Ross BA, Lambert PW. Vitamin D in plasma: quantitation by a nonequilibrium ligand binding assay. Steroids 1981;37:609-19.
268. Horst RL, Littledike ET, Riley JL, Napoli JL. Quantitation of vitamin D and its metabolites and their plasma concentration in five species of animals. Anal Biochem 1981;116:189-203.
269. Horst RL, Reinhardt TA, Beitz DC, Littledike ET. A sensitive competitive protein binding assay for vitamin D in plasma. Steroids 1981;37:581-91.
270. Horst RL, Reinhardt TA, Hollis BW. Improved methodology for the analysis of plasma vitamin D metabolites. Kidney Int 1990;38:S28-35.
271. Hosada K, Yamaji T, Baylink D. Simultaneous sandwich enzyme immunoassay for the measurement of human osteocalcin using antibodies against synthetic peptides. Clin Chem 1989;35:1208-9.
272. Hosking DJ. Calcium homeostasis in pregnancy. Clin Endocrinol 1996;45:1-6.
273. Hristova EN, Cecco S, Niemela JE, Rehak NN, Elin RJ. Analyzer-dependent differences in results for ionized calcium, ionized magnesium, sodium and pH. Clin Chem 1995;41:1649-53.
274. Huijgen HJ, Sanders R, Cecco SA, Rehak NN, Sanders GT, Elin RJ. Serum ionized magnesium: comparison of results obtained with three instruments. Clin Chem Lab Med 1999;37:465-70.
275. Husdan H, Rapoport A, Locke S. Influence of posture on the serum concentration of calcium. Metabolism 1973;22:787-97.
276. Hutchesson ACJ, Hughes SV, Bowden SJ, Ratcliffe WA. In vitro stability of endogenous parathyroid hormone-related-protein in blood and plasma. Ann Clin Biochem 1994;31:35-9.
277. Ikeda K, Ohno H, Hane M, Yokoi H, Okada M, Honma T. Development of a sensitive two-site immunoradiometric assay for parathyroid hormone-related peptide: evidence for elevated levels in plasma from patient with adult T-cell leukemia/lymphoma and B-cell lymphoma. J Clin Endocrinol Metab 1994;79:1322-7.
278. Iqbal SJ, Whittaker P, Bourke J, Mumford R, Huthinson P, Le Van LW. Possible interference with calcipotriol on new IDS RIA for 1,25-dihydroxyvitamin D. Clin Chem 1996;42:112-3.
279. Jacobs JW, Lund PK, Potts JT Jr, Bell NH, Habener JF. Procalcitonin is a glycoprotein. J Biol Chem 1981;256:2803-7.
280. Jacobson MA, Gambertoglio JG, Aweeka FT, Causey DM, Portale AA. Foscarnet-induced hypocalcemia and effects of foscarnet on calcium metabolism. J Clin Endocrinol Metab 1991;72:1130-5.
281. James IT, Perrett D, Thompson PW. Rapid assay for hard tissue collagen cross-links using isocratic ion-pair reversed-phase liquid chromatography. J Chromatogr 1990;525:43-57.
282. James IT, Walne AJ, Perrett D. The measurement of pyridinium crosslinks: a methodological overview. Ann Clin Biochem 1996;33:397-420.
283. Johnson KR, Mascall GC, Howarth AT. Differential laboratory diagnosis of hypercalcemia. Crit Rev Clin Lab Sci 1984;21:51-97.
284. Johnston CC, Melton LJ, Lindsay R, Eddy DM. Clinical indications for bone mass measurement. J Bone Miner Res 1989;4(Suppl. 2):1-28.
285. Jones G. Assay of vitamins D_2 and D_3, and 25-hydroxyvitamins D_2 and D_3 in human plasma by high-performance liquid chromatography. Clin Chem 1978;24:287-98.
286. Jones G. Ternary solvent mixtures for improved resolution of hydroxylated metabolites of vitamin D_2 and vitamin D_3 during high-performance liquid chromatography. J Chromatogr 1980;221:27-37.
287. Jones G, Byrnes B, Palma F, Segev D, Mazur Y. Displacement potency of vitamin D_2 analogs in competitive protein-binding assays for 25-hydroxyvitamin D_3, 24,25-dihydroxyvitamin D3 and 1,25-dihydroxyvitamin D_3. J Clin Endocrinol Metab 1980;50:773-5.
288. Jones G, Seamark DA, Trafford DJH, Makin HLJ. Vitamin D: cholecalciferol, ergocaliferol and hydroxylated metabolites. Chromatogr Sci 1985;30:73-129.
289. Jones RG, Dyson EH, Cook JA, Forbes MA, Cooper EH. The use of a two-site immunoradiometric assay for bone alkaline phosphatase in the investigation of renal bone disease. Clin Chem 1991;37:1067.
290. Jonger MJM, Van Ginkel FC, van der Vijgh WJF, Kuiper S, Netelenbos JC, Lips P. An international comparison of vitamin D metabolite measurements. Clin Chem 1984;30:399-403.
291. Kallner A, Woloszczuk W, Holzel W. Biochemical markers for bone diseases: current status and future trends. In: Proceedings of the 6th Bergmeyer conference, IFCC master discussion: improving the clinical value of laboratory data. Scand J Clin Lab Invest 57(Suppl. 227):1-127, 1997.

292. Kamel S, Brazier M, Neri V, Picard C, Samson L, Desmet G, Sebert JL. Multiple molecular forms of pyridinoline cross-links excreted in human urine evaluated by chromatographic and immunoassay methods. J Bone Miner Res 1995;10:1385-92.
293. Kao PC, Heser DW. Simultaneous determination of 25-hydroxy- and 1,25-dihydroxyvitamin D from a single sample by dual-cartridge extraction. Clin Chem 1984;30:56-61.
294. Kao PC, Klee GG, Taylor RL, Heath H III. Parathyroid hormone-related peptide in plasma of patients with hypercalcemia and malignant lesions. Mayo Clin Proc 1990;65:1399-407.
295. Kao PC, Riggs BL, Schryver PG. Development and evaluation of an osteocalcin chemiluminoimmunoassay. Clin Chem 1993;39:1369-74.
296. Kaplan MM, Stall GM, Cummings T, MacAulay A, MacAulay A, Motte P, Wolfe HJ, et al. High-sensitivity serum calcitonin assays applied to screening for thyroid C-cell disease in multiple endocrine neoplasia type 2A. Henry Ford Hosp Med J 1992;40:227-31.
297. Kelly PM, Bending MR, Barron JL. Comparison of serum calcium fractions during hemodialysis and peritoneal dialysis. Ann Clin Biochem 1987;24:585-90.
298. Kemp GJ, Blumsohn A, Morris BW. Circadian changes in plasma phosphate concentration, urinary phosphate excretion and cellular phosphate shifts. Clin Chem 1992;38:400-2.
299. Kessler G, Wolfman M. An automated procedure for the simultaneous determination of calcium and phosphorus. Clin Chem 1964;10:686-703.
300. Khosla S, Kleerekoper M. Biochemical markers of bone turnover. In: Favus MJ, ed. Primer on the metabolic bone diseases and disorders of mineral metabolism, 4th ed. Philadelphia: Lippincott, Williams & Wilkins, 1999:128-33.
301. Kitamura N, Shigeno C, Shiomi K, Lee K, Ohta S, Sone T, et al. Episodic fluctuation in serum intact parathyroid hormone concentration in men. J Clin Endocrinol Metab 1990;70:252-63.
302. Kivirikko KI, Laitinen O, Prockop DJ. Modification of a specific assay for hydroxyproline in urine. Anal Biochem 1967;19:249-55.
303. Klee G, Kopher R, Brown D, Schousboe J. Biochemical markers for bone turnover in osteoporosis. Technology assessment report, Institute for Clinical Systems Improvement, 2001, http://www.icsi.org/knowledge/detail.asp?catID=107&itemID=267. Accessed 7 February 2005.
304. Klee GG, Preissner CM, Schryver PG, Taylor RL, Kao PC. Multisite immunochemiluminometric assay for simultaneously measuring whole-molecule and amino-terminal fragments of human parathyrin. Clin Chem 1992;38:628-35.
305. Klein G, Bodenmuller H. Standards required for quantification of skeletal alkaline phosphatase. Clin Chem 1996;42:480-2.
306. Klein GL, Wadington EL, Collins ED, Catherwood BD, Deftos LJ. Calcitonin levels in sera of infants and children: relations to age and periods of bone growth. Calcif Tissue Int 1984;36:635-8.
307. Knochel JP. The pathophysiology and clinical characteristics of severe hypophosphatemia. Arch Intern Med 1977;137:203-20.
308. Knochel JP, Jacobson HR. Renal handling of phosphorus in health and disease. In: Brenner BM, Rector EC Jr, eds. The kidney, 3rd ed, Vol. 1. Philadelphia: WB Saunders, 1986:619-62.
309. Koshy KT. Chromatography of vitamin D_3 and metabolites. Adv Chromatogr 1982;20:83-138.
310. Kost GJ. New whole blood analyzers and their impact on cardiac and critical care. Crit Rev Clin Lab Sci 1993;30:153-202.
311. Kost GJ, Hague C. The current and future status of critical care testing and patient monitoring. Am J Clin Pathol 1995;104(4 Suppl. 1):S2-S17.
312. Kraenzlin ME, Lau KHW, Liang L, Freeman TK, Singer FR, Stepan J, et al. Development of an immunoassay for serum osteoclastic tartrate resistant acid phosphatase. J Clin Endocrinol Metab 1990;71:442-51.
313. Kraenzlin ME, Seibel MJ. Measurement of biochemical markers of bone resorption. In: Seibel MJ, Robins SP, Bilezikian, eds. Dynamics of bone and cartilage metabolism. San Diego: Academic Press, 1999:411-26.
314. Kragh-Hansen U, Vorum H. Quantitative analyses of the interaction between calcium ions and human serum albumin. Clin Chem 1993;39:202-8.
315. Kramer S, Reynolds FH Jr, Castillo M, Valenzuela DM, Thorikay M, Sorvillo JM. Immunological identification and distribution of parathyroid hormone-like protein polypeptides in normal and malignant tissues. Endocrinology 1991;128:1927-37.
316. Kress BC. Bone alkaline phosphatase: methods of quantitation and clinical utility. J Clin Ligand Assay 1998;21:139-48.
317. Kudlac H, Fielding AM, Williams AJ. Effect of hemodialysis membrane type on parathyroid hormone removal. Miner Electrolyte Metab 1994;20:245-9.
318. Ladenson JH. Nonanalytical sources of variation in clinical chemistry results. In: Sonnenwirth AC, Jarett L, eds. Gradwohl's clinical laboratory methods and diagnosis, 8th ed., Vol. II. St Louis: CV Mosby, 1980:149-92.
319. Ladenson JH, Lewis JW, Boyd JC. Failure of total calcium corrected for protein, albumin and pH to correctly assess free calcium status. J Clin Endocrinol Metab 1979;46:986-93.

320. Ladenson JH, Lewis JW, McDonald JM, Slatopolsky E, Boyd JC. Relationship of free and total calcium in hypercalcemic conditions. J Clin Endocrinol Metab 1978;48:393-7.
321. Ladenson JH, Tsai LM, Michael JM, Kessler G, Joist JH. Serum versus heparinized plasma for eighteen common chemistry tests. Am J Clin Pathol 1974;62:545-52.
322. Landt M, Hortin GL, Smith CH, McClellan A, Scott MG. Interference in ionized calcium measurements by heparin salts. Clin Chem 1994;40:565-70.
323. Larsson L, Ohman S. Serum ionized calcium and corrected total calcium in borderline hyperparathyroidism. Clin Chem 1978;24:1962-5.
324. Larsson L, Ohman S. Effect of silicone-separator tubes and storage time on ionized calcium in serum. Clin Chem 1985;31:169-70.
325. Lawson GM, Katzmann JA, Kimlinger TK, O'Brien JF. Isolation and preliminary characterization of a monoclonal antibody which interacts preferentially with the liver enzyme of human alkaline phosphatase. Clin Chem 1985;31:381-5.
326. Leary NO, Pembroke A, Duggan PF. Single stable reagent (Arsenazo III) for optically robust measurement of calcium in serum and plasma. Clin Chem 1992;38:904-8.
327. Lee AJ, Hodges S, Eastell R. Measurement of osteocalcin. Ann Clin Biochem 2000;37:432-46.
328. Lepage R, Roy L, Brossard J-H, Rousseau L, Dorais C, Lazure C, et al. A non-(1-84) circulating parathyroid hormone (PTH) fragment interferes significantly with intact PTH commercial assay measurements in uremic samples. Clin Chem 1998; 44:805-9.
329. Lepage R, Whittom S, Bertrand S, Bahsali G, D'Amour P. Superiority of dynamic over static reference intervals for intact, mid-molecule, and C-terminal parathyrin in evaluating calcemic disorders. Clin Chem 1992;38:2129-35.
330. Levin GE, Nisbet JA. Stability of parathyroid hormone-related protein and parathyroid hormone at room temperature. Ann Clin Biochem 1994;31: 497-500.
331. Levine MA, Spiegel AM. Pseudohypoparathyroidism. In: DeGroot LJ, ed. Endocrinology, 3rd ed, Vol. 2. Philadelphia: WB Saunders, 1995:1136-50.
332. Lewenstam A. Design and pitfalls of ion selective electrodes. Scand J Clin Lab Invest 1994;54:11-9.
333. Lian JB, Gundberg CM. Osteocalcin: Biochemical considerations and clinical applications. Clin Orthop Rel Res 1988;226:267-91.
334. Lichy A, Macek J, Adam M. Determination of hydroxylysylpyridinoline in tissues and urine by high-performance liquid chromatography. J Chromatogr 1991;563:153-7.
335. Liedtke RJ, Kroon G. Automated calmagite complexi-metric measurement of magnesium in serum, with sequential addition of EDTA to eliminate endogenous interference. Clin Chem 1984;30:1801-4.
336. Lindback B, Berlin T, Bjorkhem I. Three commercial kits and one liquid-chromatographic method evaluated for determining 25-hydroxyvitamin D_3 in serum. Clin Chem 1987;33:1226-7.
337. Linkhart SG, Linkhart TA, Taylor AK, Wergedal JE, Bettica P, Baylink DJ. Synthetic peptide-based immunoassay for amino-terminal propeptide of type I procollagen: application for evaluation of bone formation. Clin Chem 1993;39:2254-8.
338. Lips P, Chapuy MC, Dawson-Hughes B, Pols HA, Holick MF. An international comparison of serum 25-hydroxyvitamin D measurements. Osteoporos Int 1999;9:394-7.
339. Lissner D, Mason RS, Posen S. Stability of vitamin D metabolites in human blood serum and plasma. Clin Chem 1981;27:773-4.
340. Llach F, Hervas J, Cerezo S. The importance of dosing intravenous calcitriol in dialysis patients with severe hyperparathyroidism. Am J Kidney Dis 1995;26: 845-51.
341. Lo CW, Paris PW, Clemens TL, Nolan J, Holick MF. Vitamin D absorption in healthy subjects and in patients with intestinal malabsorption syndromes. Am J Clin Nutr 1985;42:644-9.
342. Logue FC, Fraser WD, O'Reilly DStJ, Beastall GH. The circadian rhythm of intact parathyroid hormone (1-84) and nephrogenous cyclic adenosine monophosphate in normal men. J Endocrinol 1989;121:R1-3.
343. Logue FC, Perry B, Biggart EM, Chapman RS, Beastall GH. Production and characterization of monoclonal antibodies to parathyroid hormone (1-34). J Immunol Methods 1991;137:159-66.
344. Logue FC, Perry B, Chapman RS, Milne I, James K, Beastall GH. A two-site immunoradiometric assay for PTH(1-84) using N and C terminal specific monoclonal antibodies. Ann Clin Biochem 1991;28:160-6.
345. Looker AC, Bauer DC, Chestnut CH III, Gundberg CM, Hochberg MC, Klee G, et al. Clinical uses of biochemical markers of bone remodeling: current status and future directions. Osteoporosis Int 2000;11: 467-80.
346. Looker AC, Dawson-Hughes B, Calvo MS, Gunter EW, Sahyoun NR. Serum 25-hydroxyvitamin D status of adolescents and adults in two seasonal populations from NHANES III. Bone 2002;30:771-7.
347. Lorentz K. Improved determination of serum calcium with 2-cresolphthalein complexone. Clin Chim Acta 1982;126:327-34.
348. Lu J, Endres D, Mueller J, Broughton A. Development and evaluation of an accurate, sensitive method for

the determination of serum 25-hydroxyvitamin D. Clin Chem 1982;28:1592.

349. Lynch RE. Ionized calcium: pediatric perspective. Pediatr Clin North Am 1990;37:373-89.
350. Lyon ME, Guajardo M, Laha T, Malik S, Henderson PJ, Kenny MA. Electrolyte balanced heparin may produce a bias in the measurement of ionized calcium concentration in specimens with abnormally low protein concentration. Clin Chim Acta 1995;233:105-13.
351. MacIntyre I. Calcitonin: physiology, biosynthesis, secretion, metabolism and mode of action. In: DeGroot LJ, ed. Endocrinology, 3rd ed, Vol. 2. Philadelphia: WB Saunders, 1995:978-89.
352. Malabanan A, Veronikis IE, Holick MF. Redefining vitamin D deficiency. Lancet 1998;351(9105):805-6.
353. Mallette LE. The parathyroid polyhormones: new concepts in the spectrum of peptide hormone action. Endocr Rev 1991;12:110-7.
354. Mallette LE, Khouri K, Zengotita H, Hollis BW, Malini S. Lithium treatment increases intact and midregion parathyroid hormone and parathyroid volume. J Clin Endocrinol Metab 1989;68:654-60.
355. Mallette LE, Tuma SN, Berger RE, Kirkland JL. Radioimmunoassay for the middle region of human parathyroid hormone using an homologous antiserum with a carboxy-terminal fragment of bovine parathyroid hormone as radioligand. J Clin Endocrinol Metab 1982;54:1017-24.
356. Malluche HH, Mawad H, Truba D, Monier-Faugere MC. Parathyroid hormone assays—evolution and revolutions in the care of dialysis patients. Clin Nephrol 2003;59:313-8.
357. Mann CK, Yoe JH. Spectrophotometric determination of magnesium with 1-azo-2-hydrozy-3-(2,4-dimethylcarbox-anilido)-napthalene-1′-(2-hydroxybenzene). Anal Chim Acta 1957;16:155-60.
358. Mann SW, Buckley BM, Roberts KD, Green A. Changes in plasma ionized calcium concentration during pediatric cardiopulmonary bypass surgery. Ann Clin Biochem 1988;25:226-7.
359. Marcus R. Laboratory diagnosis of primary hyperparathyroidism. Endocrinol Metab Clin North Am 1989;18:647-58.
360. Markestad T. Plasma concentrations of 1,25-dihydroxyvitamin D, 24,25-dihydroxyvitamin D, and 25,26-dihydroxyvitamin D in the first year of life. J Clin Endocrinol Metab 1983;57:755-9.
361. Marsoner HJ, Spichiger UE, Ritter C, Sachs C, Ghahramani M, Offenbacher H, et al. Measurement of ionized magnesium with neutral carrier ISE's: progress and results with the AVL 988-4 magnesium analyzer. Scand J Clin Lab Invest 1994;54(Suppl. 217):45-51.
362. Martens MFWC, van Hoek MJC, Walchli R, Gamse R, Rosmalen FMA. The first radioimmunoassay for monitoring human bone resorption: quantitation of type I collagen cross-linked N-telopeptides in urine. J Bone Miner Res 1994;9:S335.
363. Martin MT, Shapiro R. Atomic absorption spectrometry of magnesium. Methods Enzymol 1988;158: 365-70.
364. Martin TJ, Allan EH, Caple IW, Care AD, Danks JA, Diefenbach-Jagger H. Parathyroid-related protein: isolation, molecular cloning, and mechanism of action. Recent Prog Horm Res 45:467-506.
365. Martin TJ, Moseley JM. Calcitonin. In: Avioli LV, Krane SM, eds. Metabolic bone disease, 2nd ed. Philadelphia: WB Saunders, 1990:131-54.
366. Marx ST, Sharp ME, Krudy A, Rosenblatt M, Mallette LE. Radioimmunoassay for the middle region of human parathyroid hormone: studies with a radioiodinated synthetic peptide. J Clin Endocrinol Metab 1981;53:76-84.
367. Mason RS, Posen S. Some problems associated with assay of 25-hydroxycalciferol in human serum. Clin Chem 1977;23:806-10.
368. Mass AHJ. IFCC reference methods and materials for measurement of pH, gases and electrolytes in blood. Scand J Clin Invest 1993;53(Suppl. 214):83-94.
369. Masters PW, Jones RG, Purves DA, Cooper EH, Cooney JM. Commercial assays for serum osteocalcin give discordant results. Clin Chem 1994;40:358-63.
370. Masters PW, Payne RB. Comparison of hypertonic and isotonic reference electrode junctions for measuring ionized calcium in whole blood: a clinical study. Clin Chem 1993;39:1082-5.
371. Mattiazzo M, Ramasamy I. Wheat germ lectin affinity electrophoresis of serum alkaline phosphatase with commercially available gels. Clin Chem 1993;39: 1404-7.
372. Mayer E, Schmidt-Gayk H. Interlaboratory comparison of 25-hydroxyvitamin D determination. Clin Chem 1984;30:1199-204.
373. Mayne PD, Kovar IZ. Calcium and phosphorus metabolism in the premature infant. Ann Clin Biochem 1991;28:131-42.
374. McCoy S, Maclaren NK, Gudat JC. Bilirubin interferes in the aca determination of Mg^{2+} in serum. Clin Chem 1983;29:1309.
375. McGowan DM, Vaswani A, Shperling I. Coexisting hyperparathyroidism with thyrotoxicosis. J Endocrinol Invest 1991;14:305-10.
376. McLeod MK, Monchik JM, Martin HF. The role of ionized calcium in the diagnosis of subtle hypercalcemia in symptomatic primary hyperparathyroidism. Surgery 1984;95:667-73.
377. Melkko J, Niemi S, Risteli L, Risteli J. Radioimmunoassays of the carboxylterminal propeptides of human type I procollagen. Clin Chem 1990;36: 1328-32.

378. Michaylova V, Ilkova P. Photometric determination of micro amounts of calcium with arsenazo III. Anal Chim Acta 1971;53:194-8.
379. Miller PD, Baran DT, Bilezikian JP, Greenspan SL, Lindsay R, Riggs BL, et al. Practical clinical application of biochemical markers of bone turnover: consensus of an expert panel. J Clin Densitom 1999;2:323-42.
380. Mintz KP, Mann KG. Detection of procollagen biosynthesis using peptide-specific antibodies. Matrix 1990;10:186-99.
381. Modigliani E, Franc B, Niccoli-sire P. Diagnosis and treatment of medullary thyroid carcinoma. Bailliere's Best Pract Res Clin Endocrinol Metab 2000;14: 631-49.
382. Monaghan DA, Power MJ, Fottrell PF. Sandwich enzyme immunoassay of osteocalcin in serum with use of an antibody against human osteocalcin. Clin Chem 1993;39:942-7.
383. Monier-Faugere MC, Geng Z, Mawad H, Friedler RM, Gao P, Cantor TL, Malluche HH. Improved assessment of bone turnover by PTH-(1-84)/large C-PTH ratio in ESRD patients. Kidney Inter 2001;60:1460-8.
384. Moorehead WR, Biggs HG. 2-Amino-2-methyl-1-propanol as the alkalizing agent in an improved continuous-flow cresolphthalein complexone procedure for calcium in serum. Clin Chem 1974;20:1458-60.
385. Mordes JP, Wacker WEC. Excess magnesium. Pharmacol Rev 1978;29:273-300.
386. Morgan BR, Artiss JD, Zak B. Calcium determination in serum with stable arsenazo III and triglycerides clearing. Clin Chem 1993;39:1608-12.
387. Moro L, Gazzarrini C, Crivellari D, Galligioni E, Talamini R, de Bernard B. Biochemical markers for detecting bone metastases in patients with breast cancer. Clin Chem 1993;39:131-4.
388. Moro L, Gazzarrini C, Modricky C, Rovis L, de Bernard B, Galligioni E. High predictivity of galactosyl-hydroxylysine in urine as an indicator of bone metastases from breast cancer. Clin Chem 1990;36:772-4.
389. Moseley JM, Gillespie MT. Parathyroid hormone-related protein. Crit Rev Clin Lab Sci 1995;32: 299-343.
390. Motte P, Vauzelle P, Gardet P, Ghillani P, Caillou B, Parmentier C, et al. Construction and validation of a sensitive and specific assay for serum mature calcitonin using monoclonal antipeptide antibodies. Clin Chim Acta 1988;174:35-54.
391. Mulder H, Hackeng WHL, Silberbusch J, den Ottolander GJ, van der Meer C. Value of serum calcitonin estimation in clinical oncology. Br J Cancer 1981;43:786-92.
392. Mundy GR. Hypercalcemia of malignancy revisited. J Clin Invest 1988;82:1-6.
393. Mundy GR, Cove DH, Fisken R. Primary hyperparathyroidism: Changes in the pattern of clinical presentation. Lancet 1980;1:1317-20.
394. Nakanishi M, Yoh K, Miura T, Ohasi T, Rai SK, Uchida K. Development of a kinetic assay for band 5b tartrate-resistant acid phosphatase activity in serum. Clin Chem 2000;46:469-73.
395. Nakatsuka K, Miki T, Nishizawa Y, Iba K, Morii H. Two-site immunoradiometric assay for circulating bone gla-protein in end-stage renal disease. J Bone Miner Res 1990;5(Suppl. 2):S235.
396. Napoli JL, Koszewski NJ, Horst RL. Isolation and identification of vitamin D metabolites. Methods Enzymol 1986;123:127-40.
397. Naylor KE, Eastell R. Measurement of biochemical markers of bone formation. In: Seibel MJ, Robins SP, Bilezikian, eds. Dynamics of bone and cartilage metabolism. San Diego: Academic Press, 1999:401-10.
398. NCCLS. Proposed summary of methods and materials credentialed by the NRSCL council, RS9-P-Calcium. Wayne, Pa, 1989.
399. NCCLS. Gas preanalytical considerations: specimen collection, calibration, and controls; approved guideline, C27-A-Blood. Wayne, Pa, 1993.
400. NCCLS. Ionized calcium determinations: precollection variables, specimen choice, collection, and handling; approved guideline, 2nd ed, C31-A2. Wayne, Pa, 2001.
401. Neer RM. Calcium and inorganic phosphate homeostasis. In: DeGroot LJ, ed. Endocrinology, 2nd ed, Vol. 2. Philadelphia: WB Saunders, 1989:927-53.
402. Nelson N, Ohman S, Larsson L. Effect of hematocrit and added heparin on ionized calcium in capillary blood samples from neonates. Clin Chem 1989;35:486-8.
403. Newman DJ, Ashby JP. Clinical and laboratory evaluation of a two-site immunoradiometric assay for intact parathyroid hormone. Ann Clin Biochem 1988;25:654-60.
404. Nguyen-Yamamoto L, Rousseau L, Brossard J-H, Lepage R, Gao P, Cantor T, et al. Origin of parathyroid (PTH) fragments detected by intact-PTH assays. Eur J Endocrinology 2002;147:123-31.
405. Nguyen-Yamamoto L, Rousseau L, Brossard J-H, Lepage R, D'Amour P. Synthetic carboxylterminal fragments of PTH decreased ionized calcium concentration in rats by acting on a receptor different from the PTH/PTHrP receptor. Endocrinolgy 142:1386-92.
406. Nichols Advantage 25-hydroxyvitamin D (25-OH-D). Nichols Institute Diagnostics, San Clemente, Calif, 2003.
407. Nicoloff JT, Spencer CA. Clinical review 12: the use and misuse of the sensitive thyrotropin assays. J Clin Endocrinol Metab 1990;71:553-8.
408. Nikolakakis NI, DeFrancisco AM, Rodger RSC, Gaiger E, Goodship TH, Ward MK. Effect of storage

on measurement of ionized calcium in uremic patients. Clin Chem 1985;31:287-9.

409. Nordin BEC, Need AG, Hartley TF, Philcox JC, Wilcox M, Thomas DW. Improved method for calculating calcium fractions in plasma: reference values and effect of menopause. Clin Chem 1989;35:14-7.
410. Norman AW, ed. Vitamin D: the calcium homeostatic steroid hormone. New York: Academic Press, 1979.
411. Nussbaum SR. Immunometric assays of parathyrin in the diagnosis of hypercalcemic individuals. Clin Chem 1991;37:142-3.
412. Nussbaum SR, Gaz RD, Arnold A. Hypercalcemia and ectopic secretion of parathyroid hormone by an ovarian carcinoma with rearrangement of the gene for parathyroid hormone. N Engl J Med 1990;323:1324-8.
413. Nussbaum SR, Lin CS, Potts JT, Rosenthal AS, Rosenblatt M. Development of monoclonal antibodies against parathyroid hormone: genetic control of the immune response to human PTH. Methods Enzymol 1985;109:625-38.
414. Nussbaum SR, Zahradrik RJ, Lavigne JR, Brennan GL, Nozawa-Ung K, Kim LY. Highly sensitive two-site immunoradiometric assay of parathyrin, and its clinical utility in evaluating patients with hypercalcemia. Clin Chem 1987;33:1364-7.
415. Nusyrowitz ML, Frame B, Kolb FO. The spectrum of the hypoparathyroid states: a classification based on physiological principles. Medicine 1976;55:105-19.
416. Oesch U, Ammann D, Simon W. Ion-selective membrane electrodes for clinical use. Clin Chem 1986;32:1448-59.
417. Ohnishi ST. Characterization of the murexide method: dual-wavelength spectrophotometry of cations under physiological conditions. Anal Biochem 1978;85:165-79.
418. Omdahl JL, Garry PJ, Hunsaker LA, Hunt WC, Goodwin JS. Nutritional status in a healthy elderly population: Vitamin D. Am J Clin Nutr 1982;36:1225-33.
419. Orloff JJ, Reddy D, De Papp AE, Soifer NE, Stewart AF. Parathyroid hormone-related protein as a prohormone: posttranslational processing and receptor interactions. Endocr Rev 1994;15:40-60.
420. Orloff JJ, Wu TL, Stewart AF. Parathyroid hormone-like proteins: biochemical responses and receptor interactions. Endocr Rev 1989;10:476-95.
421. Pacini F, Fontanelli M, Fugazzola L, Elisei R, Elisei R, Romei C, Di Coscio G, et al. Routine measurement of serum calcitonin in nodular thyroid diseases allows the preoperative diagnosis of unsuspected sporadic medullary thyroid carcinoma. J Clin Endocrinol Metab 1994;78:826-9.
422. Pandian MR, Morgan CH, Carlton E, Segre GV. Modified immunoradiometric assay of parathyroid-related protein: clinical application in the differential diagnosis of hypercalcemia. Clin Chem 1992;38:282-8.
423. Panigrahi K, Delmas PD, Singer F, Ryan W, Reiss O, Fisher R, et al. Characteristics of a two-site immunoradiometric assay for alkaline phosphatase in serum. Clin Chem 1994;40:822-8.
424. Papantoniou NE, Papapetrou PD, Antsaklis AJ, Kontoleon PE, Mesogitis SA, Aravantinos D. Circulating levels of immunoreactive parathyroid hormone-related protein and intact parathyroid hormone in human fetuses and newborns. Eur J Endocrinol 1996;134:437-42.
425. Papapoulos SE, Frolich M. Prediction of the outcome of Paget's disease of bone with bisphosphonates from short-term changes in the rate of bone resorption. J Clin Endocrinol Metab 1996;81:3993-7.
426. Paroni R, De Vecchi E, Fremo I, Arcelloni C, Diomede L, Magni F, et al. Total urinary hydroxyproline determined with rapid and simple high-performance liquid chromatography. Clin Chem 1992;38:407-11.
427. Pastoureau P, Delmas PD. Measurement of serum bone Gla-protein (BGP) in humans with an ovine BGP-based radioimmunoassay. Clin Chem 1990;36:1620-4.
428. Payne RB, Jones DP. Protein interferes with ionized calcium measurement at the reference electrode liquid junction. Ann Clin Biochem 1987;24:400-7.
429. Pedersen BJ, Ravn P, Bonde M. Type I collagen C-telopeptide degradation products as bone resorption markers. J Clin Ligand Assay 1998;21:118-27.
430. Pedrazzoni M, Mantovani M, Ciotti G, Girasole G, Pioli G, Palummeri E. Calcitonin levels in normal women of various ages evaluated with a new sensitive radioimmunoassay. Horm Metab Res 1988;20:118-9.
431. Perdrisot R, Bigorgne JC, Guilloteau D, Jallet P. Monoclonal immunoradiometric assay of calcitonin improves investigation of familial medullary thyroid carcinoma, Clin Chem 1990;36:381-3.
432. Philbrick WM, Wysolmerski JJ, Galbraith S, Holt E, Holt E, Orloff JJ, et al. Defining the roles of parathyroid hormone-related protein in normal physiology. Physiol Rev 1996;76:127-73.
433. Pietila K, Morsky P, Pasternack A, Mustonen J, Koivula T. Intact parathyroid hormone, ionized calcium and calcium infusion test in the evaluation of hyperparathyroidism in chronic renal failure. Nephron 1987;47:284-9.
434. Pitkin RM. Calcium metabolism in pregnancy and the perinatal period: a review. Am J Obstet Gynecol 1985;151:99-109.
435. Pocotte SL, Ehrenstein G, Fitzpatrick LA. Regulation of parathyroid hormone secretion. Endocr Rev 1991;12:291-301.
436. Portale AA, Halloran BP, Morris RC Jr. Dietary intake of phosphorus modulates the circadian rhythm in serum concentration of phosphorus: implications for

the renal production of 1,25-dihydroxyvitamin D. J Clin Invest 1987;80:1147-54.

437. Potts JT Jr, Bringhurst FR, Gardella T, Nussbaum SR, Segre GV, Kronenberg HM. Parathyroid hormone: physiology, chemistry, biosynthesis, secretion, metabolism and mode of action. In: DeGroot LJ, ed. Endocrinology, 3rd ed, Vol. 2. Philadelphia: WB Saunders, 1995:920-66.

438. Poupon-Fleuret C, Chapuis-Cellier C. Monoclonal immunoglobulin interferences in measurement of serum inorganic phosphate with a new modified reagent. Clin Chem 1996;42:1298-300.

439. Power MJ, Fottrell PF. Solid-phase enzymoimmunoassay for osteocalcin in human serum or plasma, with use of monoclonal antibody. Clin Chem 1989;35:2087-92.

440. Power MJ, Fottrell PF. Osteocalcin: diagnostic methods and clinical applications. Crit Rev Clin Lab Sci 1991;28:287-335.

441. Prestwood KM, Pilbeam CC, Burleson JA, Woodiel FN, Delmas PD, Deftos LJ, et al. The short term effects of conjugated estrogen on bone turnover in older women. J Clin Endocrinol Metab 1994;79:366-71.

442. Price CP. Multiple forms of human serum alkaline phosphatase: detection and quantitation. Ann Clin Biochem 1993;30:355-72

443. Price CP, Kirwan A, Vader C. Tartrate-resistant acid phosphatase as a marker of bone resorption. Clin Chem 1995;41:641-3.

444. Price CP, Milligan TP, Darte C. Direct comparison of performance characteristics of two immunoassays for bone isoforms of alkaline phosphatase in serum. Clin Chem 1997;43:2052-7.

445. Prockop DJ, Undenfriend S. A specific method for the analysis of hydroxyproline in urine. Anal Biochem 1960;1:228-39.

446. Pybus J, Feldman FJ, Bowers GN Jr. Measurement of total calcium in serum by atomic absorption spectrophotometry with use of a strontium internal reference. Clin Chem 1970;16:998-1007.

447. Qi Q, Monier-Faugere MC, Geng Z, Malluche HH. Predictive value of serum parathyroid hormone levels for bone turnover in patients on chronic maintenance dialysis. Am J Kidney Dis 1995;26:622-31.

448. Ralston SH, Danks J, Hayman J, Fraser WD, Stewart CS, Martin TJ. Parathyroid hormone-related protein of malignancy: immunohistochemical and biochemical studies in normal and hypercalcemic patients with cancer. J Clin Pathol 1991;44:472-6.

449. Rasmussen H. The calcium messenger systems. N Engl J Med 1986;314:1094-1101, 1164-70.

450. Ratcliffe WA, Heath DA, Ryan M, Jones SR. Performance and diagnostic application of a two-site immunoradiometric assay for parathyrin in serum. Clin Chem 1989;35:1957-61.

451. Ratcliffe WA, Norbury S, Heath DA, Ratcliffe JG. Development and validation of an immunoradiometric assay of parathyrin-related protein in unextracted plasma. Clin Chem 1991;37:678-85.

452. Ratcliffe WA, Norbury S, Stott RA, Heath DA, Ratcliffe JG. Immunoreactivity of plasma parathyrin-related peptide: three region-specific radioimmunoassays and a two-site immunoradiometric assay compared. Clin Chem 1991;37:1781-7.

453. Ravn P, Thompson DE, Ross PD, Christiansen C. Biochemical markers for prediction of 4-year response in bone mass during bisphosphonate treatment for prevention of postmenopausal osteoporosis. Bone 2003;33:150-8.

454. Reddy GS, Norman AW, Willis DM, Goltzman D, Guyda H, Solomon S, et al. Regulation of vitamin D metabolism in normal human pregnancy. J Clin Endocrinol Metab 1983;56:363-70.

455. Reed P, Holbrook IB, Gardner MLG, McMurray JR. Simple, optimized liquid-chromatographic method for measuring total hydroxyproline in urine evaluated. Clin Chem 1991;37:285-90.

456. Rehak NN, Cecco SA, Niemela JE, Hristova EN, Elin RJ. Linearity and stability of the AVL and Nova magnesium and calcium ion-selective electrodes. Clin Chem 1996;42:880-7.

457. Rehak NN, Cecco SA, Niemela JE, Elin RJ. Thiocyanate in smokers interferes with the Nova magnesium ion-selective electrode. Clin Chem 1997;43:1595-600.

458. Reichel H, Koeffler HP, Norman AW. The role of the vitamin D endocrine system in health and disease. N Engl J Med 1989;320:981-91.

459. Reinhardt TA, Horst RL, Orf JW, Hollis BW. A microassay for 1,25-dihydroxyvitamin D not requiring high performance liquid chromatography: Application to clinical studies. J Clin Endocrinol Metab 1984;58:91-8.

460. Renoe BW, McDonald JM, Ladenson JH. Influence of posture on free calcium and related variables. Clin Chem 1979;25:1766-9.

461. Renoe BW, McDonald JM, Ladenson JH. The effects of stasis with and without exercise on free calcium, various cations and related parameters. Clin Chim Acta 1980;103:91-100.

462. Rhodes CJ, Claridge PA, Trafford PJH, Makin HLJ. An evaluation of the use of Sep-Pak C_{18} cartridges for the extraction of vitamin D_3 and some of its metabolites from plasma and urine. J Steroid Biochem 1983;19:1349-54.

463. Rieu M, Lame MC, Richard A, Lissak B, Lissak B, Sambort B, et al. Prevalence of sporadic medullary thyroid carcinoma: the importance of routine measurement of serum calcitonin in the diagnosis and evaluation of thyroid nodules. Clin Endocrinol (Oxf) 1995;42:453-60.

464. Riggs BL. Overview of osteoporosis. West J Med 1991;154:63-77.
465. Riggs BL, Hodgson SF, O'Fallon WM, Chao EY, Wahner HW, Muhs JM, et al. Effect of fluoride treatment on the fracture rate in postmenopausal women with osteoporosis. N Engl J Med 1990;322:802-9.
466. Riis BJ. Biochemical markers of bone turnover in diagnosis and assessment of therapy. Am J Med 1991;91(Suppl. 5B):64S-68S.
467. Risteli J, Elomaa I, Novamo A, Risteli L. Radioimmunoassay for the pyridinoline cross-linked carboxyterminal telopeptide of type I collagen: a new marker of bone degradation. Clin Chem 1993;39:635-40.
468. Ritter C, Ghahramani M, Marsoner HJ. More on the measurement of ionized magnesium in whole blood. Scand J Clin Lab Invest 1996;56(Suppl 224):275-80.
469. Robertson WG, Marshall RW. Calcium measurements in serum and plasma: total and ionized. CRC Crit Rev Clin Lab Sci 1979;11:271-304.
470. Robey PA, Termine JD. Biochemical markers of metabolic bone disease. In: Avioli LV, Krane SM, eds. Metabolic bone disease, 2nd ed. Philadelphia: WB Saunders, 1990:244-63.
471. Robins SP. An enzyme-linked immunoassay for the collagen cross-link pyridinoline. Biochem J 1982;207:617-20.
472. Robins SP, Black D, Paterson CR, Reid DM, Duncan A, Seibel MJ. Evaluation of urinary hydroxypyridinium crosslinks measurements as resorption markers in metabolic bone disease. Eur J Clin Invest 1991;21:310-15.
473. Robins SP, Brady JD. Collagen cross-linking and metabolism. In: Bilezikian JP, Raisz LG, Rodan GA, eds. Principles of bone biology, 2nd ed, Vol. 1. San Diego: Academic Press, 2002:211-23.
474. Robins SP, Duncan A, Wilson N, Evans BJ. Standardization of pyridinium crosslinks pyridinoline and deoxypyridinoline, for use as biochemical markers of collagen degradation. Clin Chem 1996;42:1621-26.
475. Robins SP, Woitge H, Hesley R, Ju J, Seyedin S, Seibel MJ. Direct enzyme-linked immunoassay for urinary deoxypyridinoline as a specific marker for measuring bone resorption. J Bone Miner Res 1994;9:1643-9.
476. Rosen JF, Chesney RW. Circulating calcitriol concentrations in health and disease. J Pediatr 1983;103: 1-17.
477. Rosen RH, Dresner-Pollak R, Moses AC, Rosenblatt M, Zeind AJ, Clemens JD, et al. Specificity of urinary excretion of crosslinked N-telopeptide of type I collagen as a marker of bone turnover. Calcif Tissue Int 1994;54:26-9.
478. Rosenquist C, Bonde M, Fledelius C, Qvist P. A simple enzyme-linked immunosorbent assay for human osteocalcin. Clin Chem 1994;40:1258-64.
479. Rosenquist C, Fledelius C, Christgau S, Pedersen BJ, Bonde M, Qvist P, et al. Serum crosslaps one step ELISA. First application of monoclonal antibodies for measurement in serum of bone-related degradation products from C-terminal telopeptides of type I collagen. Clin Chem 1998;44:2281-9.
480. Rosenquist C, Qvist P, Bjarnason N, Christiansen C. Measurement of a more stable region of osteocalcin in serum by ELISA with two monoclonal antibodies. Clin Chem 1995;41:1439-45.
481. Ross DS, Nussbaum SR. Reciprocal changes in parathyroid hormone and thyroid function after radioiodine treatment of hyperthyroidism. J Clin Endocrinol Metab 1989;68:1216-9.
482. Rossert J, de Crombrugghe B. Type I collagen. In: Bilezikian JP, Raisz LG, Rodan GA, eds. Principles of bone biology, 2nd ed, Vol. 1. San Diego: Academic Press, 2002:189-210.
483. Rouilly M, Rusterholz B, Spichiger UE, Simon W. Neutral ionophore-based selective electrode for assaying the activity of magnesium in undiluted blood. Clin Chem 1990;36:466-9.
484. Rubin LP, Posillico JT, Anast CS, Brown EW. Circulating levels of biologically active and immunoreactive intact parathyroid hormone in human newborns. Pediatr Res 1991;29:201-7.
485. Rude RK. Hypocalcemia, and hypoparathyroidism. In: Kassirer JP, ed. Current therapy in internal medicine, 3rd ed. Philadelphia: BC Decker, 1991: 1386-90.
486. Rude RK, Matsumoto S, Singer FR. Heterogeneity of immunoreactive calcitonin in extracts of medullary thyroid carcinoma. Miner Electrolyte Metab 1982;7:292-7.
487. Rude RK, Oldham SB. Disorders of magnesium metabolism. In: Cohen RD, Lewis B, Alberti KGMM, Denman AM, eds. The metabolic and molecular basis of acquired disease, Vol. 1. London: Bailliere Tindall, 1990:1124-48.
488. Rude RK, Sharp CF Jr, Fredericks RS, Oldham SB, Elbaum N, Link J, et al. Urinary and nephrogenous adenosine-3′,5′-monophosphate in hypercalcemia of malignancy. J Clin Endocrinol Metab 1981;52: 765-71.
489. Rude RK, Singer FR. Comparison of serum calcitonin levels after a 1-minute calcium injection and after pentagastrin injection in the diagnosis of medullary thyroid carcinoma. J Clin Endocrinol Metab 1977;44:980-3.
490. Rude RK, Singer FR. Magnesium deficiency and excess. Annu Rev Med 1981;32:245-59.
491. Rude RK, Singer FR. Primary hyperparathyroidism. In: Conn RB, ed. Current diagnosis, 8th ed. Philadelphia: WB Saunders, 1991:859-63.
492. Russell D, Henley R. The stability of parathyroid hormone in blood and serum specimens at 4 degrees C and at room temperature. Ann Clin Biochem 1995;32:216-7.

493. Ryan MF. The role of magnesium in clinical biochemistry: an overview. Ann Clin Biochem 1991;28:19-26.
494. Sachs C, Chaneac M, Rabouine P, Kindermans C, Dechaux M. Inadequate algorithm: a cause for "incorrect pH 7.4 correction" in ionized calcium analyzers. Scand J Clin Lab Invest 1989;49:561-5.
495. Sachs CH, Rabouine PH, Chaneac M, Kindermans C, Dechaux M, Falch-Christiansen T. Preanalytical errors in ionized calcium measurements induced by the use of liquid heparin. Ann Clin Biochem 1991;28:167-73.
496. Sachs CH, Rabouine PH, Chaneac M, Kindermans C, Dechaux M. In vitro evaluation of a heparinized blood sampler for ionized calcium measurement. Ann Clin Biochem 1991;28:240-4.
497. Sachs CH, Ritter CH, Puaud AC, Ghahramani M, Kindermans C, Marsoner H. Measurements of ionized magnesium in blood. Clin Chem 1991;37:945.
498. Sachs C, Thode J. Preanalytical errors in ionized calcium determination in blood: a review for a subsequent recommendation for sampling. In: Maas AHJ, ed. Methodology and clinical applications of ion selective electrodes. Copenhagen: International Federation of Clinical Chemistry, 1986:259-70.
499. Saggese G, Baroncelli GI, Bertelloni S. Determination of intact parathyrin by immunoradiometric assay evaluated in normal children and in patients with various disorders of calcium metabolism. Clin Chem 1991;37:1999-2001.
500. Saggese G, Baroncelli GI, Bertelloni S, Cipolloni C. Intact parathyroid hormone levels during pregnancy in healthy term neonates and in hypocalcemic preterm infants. Acta Paediatr Scand 1991;80:36-41.
500A. Salusky IB, Goodman WG, Kuizon BD, Lavigne JR, Zahranik RJ, Gales B, et al. Similar predictive value of bone turnover using first and second-second generation immunometric PTH assays in pediatric patients treated with peritoneal dialysis. Kidney Int 2003;63:1801-8.
501. Sanders GT, Huijgen HJ, Sanders R. Magnesium in disease: a review with special emphasis on the serum ionized magnesium. Clin Chem Lab Med 1999;37:1011-33.
502. Saris N-EL, Mervaala E, Karppanen H, Khawaja JA, Lewenstam A. Magnesium: an update on physiological, clinical and analytical aspects. Clin Chim Acta 2000;294:1-26.
503. Savory J, Margrey KS, Shipe JR Jr, Savory MG, Margrey MH, Mifflin TE, et al. Stabilization of calmagite reagent for automated measurement of magnesium in serum and urine. Clin Chem 1985;31:487-8.
504. Scarpa A, Brinkley FJ, Tiffert T, Dubyak GR. Metallochromic indicators of ionized calcium. Ann NY Acad Sci 1978;307:86-112.
505. Schlemmer A, Hassager C, Jensen SB, Christiansen C. Marked diurnal variation in urinary excretion of pyridinium cross-links in premenopausal women. J Clin Endocrinol Metab 1992;74:476-80.
506. Schultz DW, Passonneau JV, Lowry OH. An enzymatic method for the measurement of inorganic phosphate. Anal Biochem 1967;19:300-14.
507. Schwartz KE, Wolfsen AR, Forster B, Odell WD. Calcitonin in nonthyroidal cancer. J Clin Endocrinol Metab 1979;49:438-44.
508. Seamark DA, Trafford DJH, Makin HLJ. The estimation of vitamin D and its metabolites in human plasma. J Steroid Biochem 1981;14:111-23.
509. Segre GV, Potts JT Jr. Differential diagnosis of hypercalcemia. In: DeGroot LJ, ed. Endocrinology, 3rd ed, Vol. 2. Philadelphia: WB Saunders, 1995: 1075-93.
510. Segre GV, Sherrard DJ, Pandian MR, et al. Intact PTH (IRMA) II: new applications to issues in parathyroid hormone and mineral metabolism. Nichols Institute, San Juan Capistrano, Calif, 1989.
511. Seibel MJ. Molecular markers of bone metabolism in parathyroid disease. In: Bilezikian JP, ed. The parathyroids, 2nd ed. San Diego: Academic Press, 2001: 399-409.
512. Seibel MJ. Biochemical markers of bone remodeling. Endocrinol Metab Clin North Am 2003;32:83-113.
513. Seibel MJ, Gartenberg F, Silverberg SJ, Ratcliffe A, Robins SP, Bilezikian JP. Urinary hydroxypyridinium cross-links of collagen in primary hyperparathyroidism. J Clin Endocrinol Metab 1992;74:481-6.
514. Seibel MJ, Robins SP, Bilezikian JP. Markers of bone metabolism. In: Becker KL, ed. Principles and practice of endocrinology and metabolism, 3rd ed. Philadelphia: Lippincott Williams & Wilkins, 2001:548-57.
515. Sena SF, Bowers GN Jr. Measurement of ionized calcium in biological fluids: ion-selective electrodes method. Methods Enzymol 1988;158:320-34.
516. Seth R, Motte P, Kehely A, Wimalawansa SJ, Wimalawansa SJ, Self CH, et al. A sensitive and specific two-site enzyme-immunoassay for human calcitonin using monoclonal antibodies. J Endocrinol 1988;119:351-7.
517. Seth R, Motte P, Kehely A, Wimalawansa SJ, Wimalawansa S, Self CH, et al. The development of a two-site enzyme immunometric assay (EIA) for calcitonin and its application in the measurement of hormone in normal subjects, MTC patients and postmenopausal women. Horm Metab Res 1989; 21:3-5.
518. Sethi R, Kukreja SC, Bowser EN, Hargis GK, Henderson WJ, Williams GA. Effect of meal on serum parathyroid hormone and calcitonin: possible role of secretin. J Clin Endocrinol Metab 1983;56: 549-52.

519. Severini G, Aliberti LM, Di Giovannandrea R. Diagnostic aspects of alkaline phosphatase: separation of isoenzymes in normal and pathological human serum by high-performance liquid chromatography. J Chromatogr 1991;563:147-52.
520. Seyedin SM, Kung VT, Daniloff YN, Hesley RP, Gomez B, Nielsen LA, et al. Immunoassay for urinary pyridinoline: the new marker of bone resorption. J Bone Miner Res 1993;8:635-41.
521. Shepard RM, DeLuca HF. Determination of vitamin D and its metabolites in plasma. Methods Enzymol 1980;67:393-413.
522. Sherman SS, Hollis BW, Tobin JD. Vitamin D status and related parameters in a healthy population: the effects of age, sex and season. J Clin Endocrinol Metab 1990;71:405-13.
523. Shirey TL. Critical care profiling for informed treatment of severely ill patients. Am J Clin Pathol 1995;104(Suppl 1):S79-87.
524. Shirey TL. Importance and interpretation of ionized magnesium (iMg) activity in acutely and chronically ill patients. Nova Biomedical, Waltham, Mass, 2001.
525. Silva OL, Titus-Dillon P, Becker KL, Snider RH, Moore CF. Increased serum calcitonin in pregnancy. J Natl Med Assoc 1981;73:649-52.
526. Silverberg SJ, Gao P, Brown I, LoGerfo P, Cantor TL, Bilezikian JP. Clinical utility of an immunoradiometric assay for parathyroid hormone (1-84) in primary hyperparathyroidism. J Clin Endocrinol Metab 2003;88:4725-30.
527. Simon LS, Krane SM, Wortman PD, Krane IM, Kovitz KL. Serum levels of type I and III procollagen fragments in Paget's disease of bone. J Clin Endocrinol Metab 1984;58:110-20.
528. Singer FR, Habener JF. Multiple immunoreactive forms of calcitonin in human plasma. Biochem Biophys Res Commun 1974;61:710-16.
529. Singer FR, Wallach S, eds. Paget's disease of bone: clinical assessment, recent and future therapy. New York: Elsevier, 1991.
530. Sisson JC, Gross MD, Frietas JE, Jackson CE, England BG. Combining provocative agents of calcitonin to detect medullary carcinoma of the thyroid. Henry Ford Hosp Med J 1981;29:75-80.
531. Slatopolsky E, Finch J, Clay P, Martin D, Sicard G, Singer G, et al. A novel mechanism for skeletal resistance in uremia. Kidney Int 2000;58:753-61.
532. Smith FE, Reinstein H, Braverman LE. Cork stoppers and hypercalcemia. N Engl J Med 1965;272:787-8.
533. Sorva A, Elfving S, Pohja P, Tilvis RS. Assessment of calcaemic status in geriatric hospital patients: serum ionized calcium versus albumin-adjusted total calcium. Scand J Clin Lab Invest 1988;48:489-94.
534. Souberbielle JC, Cormier C, Kindermans C, Gao P, Cantor T, Forette F, Baulieu EE. Vitamin D status and redefining serum parathyroid hormone reference range in the elderly. J Clin Endocrinol Metab 2001;86;3086-90.
535. Sowers MF, Hollis BW, Shapiro B, Randolph J, Janney CA, Zhang D, et al. Elevated parathyroid hormone-related peptide associated with lactation and bone density loss. JAMA 1996;276:549-54.
536. Specker BL, Tsang RC. Vitamin D in infancy and childhood: factors determining vitamin D status. Adv Pediatr 1986;33:1-22.
537. Steindel SJ, Heard NV. Critical values. Q-Probes 92-04. Northfield, Ill: College of American Pathologists, 1992.
538. Stephan JJ. Clinical utility of bone markers in the evaluation and follow-up of osteoporotic patients: why are the markers poorly accepted by clinicians. J Endocrinol Invest 2003;26:458-63.
539. Stern J, Lewis WHP. The colorimetric estimation of calcium in serum with o-cresolphthalein complexone. Clin Chim Acta 1957;2:576-80.
540. Stewart AF, Adler M, Byers CM, Segre GV, Broadus AE. Calcium homeostasis in immobilization: an example of resorptive hypercalciuria. N Engl J Med 1982;306:1136-40.
541. Stewart AF, Broadus AE. Mineral metabolism. In: Felig P, Baxter JD, Broadus AE, Frohman LA, eds. Endocrinology and metabolism, 2nd ed. New York: McGraw-Hill Book Co, 1987:1317-453.
542. Stewart AF, Broadus AE. Clinical review 16: parathyroid hormone-related proteins: coming of age in the 1990s. J Endocrinol Metab 1990;71:1410-4.
543. Stewart AF, Horst R, Deftos LJ, Cadman EC, Lang R, Broadus AE. Biochemical evaluation of patients with cancer-associated hypercalcemia. N Engl J Med 1980;303:1377-83.
544. Stewart AF, Insogna KL, Broadus AE. Malignancy-associated hypercalcemia. In: DeGroot LJ, ed. Endocrinology. 3rd ed, Vol. 2. Philadelphia: WB Saunders, 1995:1061-74.
545. Stone M, Chowdrey PE, Maill P, Price CP. Validation of an enzymatic total magnesium determination based on activation of modified isocitrate dehydrogenase. Clin Chem 1996;42:1474-7.
546. Strewler GJ. The parathyroid hormone-related protein. Endocrinol Metab Clin North Am 2000;29:629-45.
547. Stryd RP, Gilbertson TJ. Some problems in development of a high-performance liquid chromatographic assay to measure 25-hydroxyvitamin D_2 and 25-hydroxyvitamin D_3 simultaneously in human serum. Clin Chem 1978;24:927-30.
548. Swanson JR, Heeter C, Limbocker M, Sullivan M. Bias of ionized calcium results from blood gas syringes. Clin Chem 1994;40:669-70.
549. Tabata M, Kido T, Totani M, Murachi T. Direct spectrophotometry of magnesium in serum after reaction

with hexokinase and glucose-6-phosphate dehydrogenase. Clin Chem 1985;31:703-5.
550. Takahashi M, Kawana K, Nagano A. Biological variability of biochemical markers of bone turnover in healthy women. Endocr Res 2002;28:257-64.
551. Tanaka Y, DeLuca HF, Ikekawa N. High-pressure liquid chromatography of vitamin D metabolites and analogs. Methods Enzymol 1980;67:370-85.
552. Taylor AK, Linkhart SG, Mohan S, Baylink DJ. Development of a new radioimmunoassay for human osteocalcin: evidence for a midmolecule epitope. Metabolism 1988;37:872-7.
553. Taylor AK, Lueken SA, Libanatic C, Baylink DJ. Biochemical markers of bone turnover for the clinical assessment of bone metabolism. Rheum Dis Clin North Am 1994;20:589-607.
554. Taylor A, Norman ME. 1,25$(OH)_2$D levels in dihydrotachysterol-treated patients: influence on 1,25$(OH)_2$D assays. J Bone Miner Res 1987;2:567-70.
555. Taylor GA, Peacock M, Pelc B, Brown W, Holmes A. Purification of plasma vitamin D metabolites for radioimmunoassay. Clin Chim Acta 1980;108:239-46.
556. Tedokon M, Suzuki K, Kayamori Y, Fujita S, Katayama Y. Enzymatic inorganic phosphate with use of sucrose phosphorylase and phosphoglucomutase. Clin Chem 1992;38:512-5.
557. Terpos E, Szydlo R, Apperley JF, Hatjiharissi E, Politou M, Meletis J, et al. Soluble receptor activator of nuclear factor kB ligand-osteoprotegerin ratio predicts survival in multiple myeloma: proposal for a novel prognostic index. Blood 2003;102:1064-9.
558. Thode J. Actual ionized calcium and pH in blood collected in capillary or evacuated tubes. Scand J Clin Lab Invest 1986;46:89-93.
559. Thode J. Ionized calcium and cyclic AMP in plasma and urine. Scand J Clin Lab Invest 1990;50(Suppl. 197):13-45.
560. Thode J, Fogh-Anderson N, Aas F, Siggaard-Andersen O. Sampling and storage of blood for determination of ionized calcium. Scand J Clin Lab Invest 1985;45:131-8.
561. Thode J, Holmegaard N, Transbol I, Fogh-Andersen N, Siggaard-Andersen O. Adjusted ionized calcium (at pH 7.4) and actual ionized calcium (at actual pH) in capillary blood compared for clinical evaluation of patients with disorders of calcium metabolism. Clin Chem 1990;36:541-4.
562. Thode J, Juul-Jorgensen B, Bhatia HM, Kjaerulf-Nielsen M, Bartels PD, Fogh-Andersen N, Siggaard-Andersen O. Comparison of serum total calcium, albumin-corrected total calcium and ionized calcium in 1213 patients with suspected calcium disorders. Scand J Clin Lab Invest 1989;49:217-23.
563. Tiegs RD, Body JJ, Barta JM, Heath H III. Secretion and metabolism of monomeric human calcitonin: effects of age, sex, and thyroid damage. J Bone Miner Res 1986;1:339-49.
564. Tietz NW, ed. Clinical guide to laboratory tests. 3rd ed. Philadelphia, WB Saunders, 1995.
565. Tisell LE, Dilley WG, Wells SA Jr. Progression of postoperative residual medullary carcinoma as monitored by plasma calcitonin levels. Surgery 1996;119:34-9.
566. Tobler PH, Tschopp FA, Dambacher MA, Born W, Fischer JA. Identification and characterization of calcitonin forms in plasma and urine of normal subjects and medullary carcinoma patients. J Clin Endocrinol Metab 1983;57:749-54.
567. Toffaletti J. Ionized calcium. In: Pesce AJ, Kaplan LA, eds. Methods in clinical chemistry. St. Louis: CV Mosby, 1987:1010-20.
568. Toffaletti J. Use of novel preparations of heparin to eliminate interference in ionized calcium measurement: have all the problems been solved. Clin Chem 1994;40:508-9.
569. Toffaletti J, Abrams B, Bird C, Schwing M. Clinical validation of an automated thin-film reflectance method for measurement of magnesium in serum and urine. Magnesium 1988;7:84-90.
570. Toffaletti J, Blosser N, Kirvan K. Effects of storage temperature and time before centrifugation on ionized calcium in blood collected in plain vacutainer tubes and silicone-separator (SST) tubes. Clin Chem 1984;30:553-6.
571. Toffaletti J, Christenson RH, Mullins S, Harris RE. Relationship between serum lactate and ionized calcium in open-heart surgery. Clin Chem 1986;32:1849-53.
572. Toffaletti J, Ernst P, Hunt P, Abrams B. Dry electrolyte-balanced heparinized syringes evaluated for determining ionized calcium and other electrolytes in blood. Clin Chem 1991;37:1730-3.
573. Toffaletti J, Lee KM. Preparation and use of serum-based material as control and calibrator in evaluating ion-selective electrodes for calcium. Clin Chem 1985;31:1349-52.
574. Toffaletti J, Thompson T. Effects of blended lithium-zinc heparin on ionized calcium and general chemistry tests. Clin Chem 1995;41:328-9.
575. Traba M, Navarro A, Marin C, et al. A comparative study of 25-hydroxyvitamin D_3 separation in human serum. In: Norman AW, Schaefer K, Herrath DV, Grigoleit H-G, eds. Vitamin D, chemical, biochemical and clinical endocrinology of calcium metabolism, New York: W de Gryter, 1982:805-7.
576. Tracy RP, Andrianorivo A, Riggs BL, Mann KG. Comparison of monoclonal and polyclonal antibody-based immunoassays for osteocalcin: a study of sources of variation in assay results. J Bone Miner Res 1990;5:451-61.
577. Truong NU, deB Edwardes MD, Papavasiliou V, Goltzman D, Kremer R. Parathyroid hormone-related

peptide and survival of patients with cancer and hypercalcemia. Am J Med 2003;115:115-21.
578. Tsang WM, Howell MJ, Miller AL. A simple enzymic method for the measurement of magnesium in serum and urine on a centrifugal analyzer. Ann Clin Biochem 1988;25:162-8.
579. Tsuchihashi T, Yamaguchi K, Miyake Y, Otsubo K, Nagasaki K, Honda S, et al. Parathyroid hormone-related protein in tumor tissues obtained from patients with humoral hypercalcemia of malignancy. JNCI 1990;82:40-4.
580. Turpeinen U, Hohenthal U, Stenman U-H. Determination of 25-hydroxyvitamin D. Clin Chem 2003;49:1521-4.
581. Turpeinen U, Pomoell U-M. Liquid chromatography of free hydroxyproline in serum. Clin Chem 1985;31:1710-2.
582. Uebelhart D, Gineyts EC, Chapuy MC, Delmas PD. Urinary excretion of pyridinium crosslinks: a new marker of bone resorption in metabolic bone disease. Bone Miner 1990;8:87-96.
583. Uebelhart D, Schlemmer A, Johansen JS, Gineyts E, Christiansen C, Delmas PD. Effect of menopause and hormone replacement therapy on the urinary excretion of pyridinium cross-links. J Clin Endocrinol Metab 1991;72:367-73.
584. Van Hoof VO, Martin M, Blockx P, Prove A, Van Oosterom A, Couttenye MM, et al. Immunoradiometric method and electrophoretic system compared for quantifying bone alkaline phosphatase in serum. Clin Chem 1995;41:853-7.
585. Van Ingen HE, Huijgen HJ, Kok WT, Sanders TB. Analytical evaluation of Kone Microlyte determination of ionized magnesium. Clin Chem 1994;40:52-5.
586. Vesper HW, Demers LM, Eastell R, Garnero P, Kleerekoper M, Robins SP, et al. Assessment and recommendations on factors contributing to preanalytical variation of urinary pyridinoline and deoxypyridinoline. Clin Chem 2002;48:220-35.
587. Vieth R. The mechanisms of vitamin D toxicity. Bone Miner 1990;11:267-72.
588. Vieth R. Simple method for determining specific binding capacity of vitamin D-binding protein and its use to calculate the concentration of "free" 1,25-dihydroxyvitamin D. Clin Chem 1994;40:435-41.
589. Voigts A, Felsenfeld AJ, Andress D, Llach F. Parathyroid hormone and bone histology: response to hypocalcemia in osteitis fibrosa. Kidney Int 1984;25:445-52.
590. Wacker WEC. Measurement of magnesium in human tissues and fluids: a historical perspective. Magnesium 1987;6:61-4.
591. Wallach SR, Royston I, Taetle R, Wohl H, Deftos LJ. Plasma calcitonin as a marker of disease activity in patients with small cell carcinoma of the lung. J Clin Endocrinol Metab 1981;53:602-6.
592. Walmsley TA, Fowler RT. Optimum use of 8-hydroxyquinoline in plasma calcium determinations. Clin Chem 1981;27:1782.
593. Wandrup J. Critical analytical and clinical aspects of ionized calcium in neonates. Clin Chem 1989;35:2027-33.
594. Wandrup J, Kacir C, Hyltoft-Petersen P. Ionized calcium and acid-base status in arterial and venous whole blood during general anaesthesia. Scand J Clin Lab Invest 1988;48:115-22.
595. Wang M, Hercz G, Sherrard DJ, Maloney NA, Maloney NA, Segre GV, et al. Relationship between intact 1-84 parathyroid hormone and bone histomorphometric parameters in dialysis patients without aluminum toxicity. Am J Kidney Dis 1995;26:836-44.
596. Weissel M, Kainz H, Tyl E, Ogunyemi E, Woloszczuk W. Clinical evaluation of new assays for determination of serum calcitonin concentrations. Acta Endocrinol (Copenhagen)1991;124:540-4.
597. Weissman EB, Pragay DA, Bishop C. Evaluation of the Corning 940 calcium titrator for use with serum or urine. Clin Chem 1975;21:264-7.
598. Welch MW, Hamar DW, Fettman MJ. Method comparison for calcium determination by flame atomic absorption spectrophotometry in presence of phosphate. Clin Chem 1990;36:351-54.
599. Wells SA Jr, Baylin SB, Linehan WM, Farrell RE, Cox EB, Cooper CW. Provocative agents and the diagnosis of medullary carcinoma of the thyroid gland. Ann Surg 1978;188:139-41.
600. Wells SA Jr, Donis-Keller H. Current perspectives on the diagnosis and management of patients with multiple endocrine neoplasia type 2 syndromes. Endocrinol Metab Clin North Am 1994;23:215-8.
601. Wentz PW, Savory J, Cross RE. Improved method for measurement of inorganic phosphate in serum with a centrifugal analyzer. Clin Chem 1976;22:257-60.
602. White TF, Farndon JR, Conceicao SC, Laker MF, Ward MK, Kerr DN. Serum calcium status in health and disease: a comparison of measured and derived parameters. Clin Chim Acta 1986;157:199-214.
603. Wilhite TR, Smith CH, Landt M. Interference of zinc heparin anticoagulant in determination of plasma magnesium. Clin Chem 1994;40:848-9.
604. Williams ED. Medullary carcinoma of the thyroid. In: DeGroot LJ, ed. Endocrinology, 3rd ed. Vol. Philadelphia: WB Saunders, 1995:855-70.
605. Williams MH, VanAlstyne EL, Galbraith RM. Evidence of a novel association of unsaturated fatty acids with Gc (vitamin D-binding protein). Biochem Biophys Res Commun 1988;153:1019-24.
606. Wills MR, Sunderman FW, Savory J. Methods for the estimation of serum magnesium in clinical laboratories. Magnesium 1986;5:317-27.
607. Wilson PS, Kleerekoper M, Bone H, Parfitt AM. Urinary total hydroxyproline measured by HPLC:

comparison of spot and timed urine collections. Clin Chem 1990;36:388-9.
608. Wimalawansa SJ, Bailey F. Validation, role in perioperative assessment, and clinical applications of an immunoradiometric assay for human calcitonin. Peptides 1995;16:307-12.
609. Withold W, Schulte U, Reinauer H. Method for determination of bone alkaline phosphatase activity: analytical performance and clinical usefulness in patients with metabolic bone disease and malignant bone diseases. Clin Chem 1996;42:210-7.
610. Woitge HW, Seibel MJ. Risk assessment for osteoporosis II: biochemical markers of bone turnover: bone resorption indices. Clin Lab Med 2000:503-25.
611. Woitge HW, Seibel MJ, Ziegler R. Comparison of total and bone-specific alkaline phosphatase in patients with nonskeletal disorders or metabolic bone disease. Clin Chem 1996;42:1796-804.
612. Wolfe HJ. The anatomy of the parathyroids. In: DeGroot LJ, ed. Endocrinology, 2nd ed, Vol. 2. Philadelphia: WB Saunders, 1989:844-7.
613. Wood PJ. The measurement of parathyroid hormone. Ann Clin Biochem 1992;29:11-21.
614. Wright DR, Voelkel EF, Tashjian AH Jr. Measurement of human calcitonin by affinity chromatography and radioimmunoassay. In: Abraham GE, ed. Handbook of radioimmunoassay. New York: Marcel Dekker, 1977:391-423.
614A. Wu A, ed. Tietz clinical guide to laboratory tests, 4th ed. St Louis, Elsevier, In Press.
615. Wu C, Kenny M. Circulating total and ionized magnesium after ethanol ingestion. Clin Chem 1996;42:625-9.
616. Wysolmerski JJ, Broadus AE. Hypercalcemia of malignancy: the central role of parathyroid hormone-related protein. Annu Rev Med 1994;45: 189-200.
617. Yamashita H, Gao P, Noguchi S, Cantor T, Uchino S, Watanabe S, et al. Role of cyclase activating parathyroid hormone (1-84 PTH) measurements during parathyroid surgery: potential improvement of intraoperative PTH assay. Ann Surg 2002;236: 105-11.
618. Yu GC, Lee DB. Clinical disorders of phosphorus metabolism. West J Med 1987;147:569-76.
619. Zaidi M, Moonga BS, Beves PJR, Bascal ZA, Breimer LH. The calcitonin gene peptides: biology and clinical relevance. CRC Crit Rev Clin Lab Sci 1990;28: 109-74.
620. Zaloga GP, Chernow B. Hypocalcemia in critical illness. JAMA 1986;256:1924-9.
621. Zaloga GP, Willey S, Tomasic P, Chernow B. Free fatty acids alter calcium binding: a cause for misinterpretation of serum calcium values and hypocalcemia in critical illness. J Clin Endocrinol Metab 1987;64: 1010-4.
622. Zink A, Blind E, Raue F. Determination of serum calcitonin by immunometric two-site assays in normal subjects and patients with medullary thyroid carcinoma. Eur J Clin Chem Clin Biochem 1992;30: 831-5.

ADDITIONAL READING

Avioli LV, Krane SM, eds. Metabolic bone disease, 3rd ed. San Diego: Academic Press, 1998:811pp.
Becker KL, ed. Principles and practice of endocrinology and metabolism, 3rd ed. Philadelphia: Lippincott Williams & Wilkins, 2001:2477pp.
Bilezikian JP, Marcus R, Levine MA, eds. The parathyroids: basic and clinical concepts, 2nd ed. San Diego: Academic Press, 2001:881pp.
Bilezikian JP, Raisz LG, Rodan GA, eds. Principles of bone biology, 2nd ed. San Diego: Academic Press, 2002:1696pp.
DeGroot LJ, Jamison LJ, eds. Endocrinology, 4th ed. Philadelphia: WB Saunders, 2001:1775pp.
Eastell R, Baumann M, Hoyle N, Wieczorek L, eds. Bone markers: biochemical and clinical perspectives. London: Martin Dunitz, 2001:252pp.
Endres DB, ed. Biochemical Markers of Bone Metabolism, J Clinical Ligand Assay 1998;21:92-170.
Favus MJ, ed. Primer on the metabolic bone diseases and disorders of mineral metabolism, 5th ed. New York: Raven Press, 2003.
Larsen PE, Kronenberg HM, Melmed S, Polonsky KS, eds. Williams textbook of endocrinology. 10th ed., Philadelphia: WB Saunders, 2003:1927pp.
Marcus R, Feldman D, Kelsey J, eds. Osteoporosis, 2nd ed. San Diego: Academic Press, 2001:1672pp.
Masssry SG, Coburn JW, Hruska K, Langman C, Malluche H, Martin K, et al. National Kidney Foundation K/DOQI Guidelines for Bone Metabolism and Disease in Chronic Kidney Disease 2003, http://www.kidney.org/professionals/kdoqi/guidelines_bone/index.htm.
Seibel MJ, Robins SP, Bilezikian JP, eds. Dynamics of bone and cartilage metabolism. San Diego: Academic Press, 1999:672pp.

CHAPTER 50

Pituitary Function*

Laurence M. Demers, Ph.D., F.A.C.B., D.A.B.C.C., and Mary Lee Vance, M.D.

The pituitary gland (*hypophysis*) regulates the endocrine system by integrating chemical signals from the brain with feedback from the concentration of hormones in the circulation to stimulate intermittent hormone release from target endocrine glands.[124] Historically, because it is intimately involved in the regulation of growth, development, thyroid function, adrenal function, gonadal function, and water and salt homeostasis, the pituitary has been called the "master endocrine organ."[106,124,127] It consists of two lobes of differing embryonic origin, the *anterior lobe* or *adenohypophysis* and the *posterior lobe* or *neurohypophysis*.

The adenohypophysis secretes growth hormone (GH), prolactin (PRL), thyrotropin (TSH), adrenocorticotropin (ACTH), follicle-stimulating hormone (FSH), and luteinizing hormone (LH), all of which are proteins or peptides (see Table 28-1 in Chapter 28). It also secretes β-lipotropin (β-LPH) and a number of smaller peptides of undetermined significance.[45] Vasopressin (also known as antidiuretic hormone [ADH]) and oxytocin are produced in the hypothalamus and are carried through the neurohypophyseal nerve axons to the neurohypophysis. Thus the neurohypophysis is not a discrete endocrine organ, but rather functions as a reservoir for these two hormones.

Of the six major hormones from the adenohypophysis, GH and PRL act primarily on diffuse target tissue, with TSH ACTH, and the gonadotropins (LH and FSH) acting primarily on specific target endocrine glands (i.e., the thyroid gland, adrenal cortex, and gonads, respectively). These peptide hormones originating from the pituitary and related hormones elaborated by the placenta during pregnancy can be classified based on their molecular structure and biochemical evolution.

*The authors gratefully acknowledge the contributions of Ronald J. Whitley, A. Wayne Meikle, and Nelson B. Watts, on which portions of this chapter are based.

ANATOMY

The pituitary gland (hypophysis) is located at the base of the skull (Figure 50-1) in a bone cavity called the *sella turcica* (Turkish saddle). The gland is small—1 cm or less in height and width and weighs approximately 500 mg. As discussed previously, the gland is anatomically divided into the anterior (adenohypophysis) and the posterior (neurohypophysis) lobes. A third lobe (the intermediate lobe) is present in most vertebrates and in the human fetus; this lobe is rudimentary in the adult human.

Arterial blood reaches the pituitary gland via the superior hypophyseal artery, a branch of the internal carotid artery. Venous blood is supplied through a venous portal system that originates in the median eminence of the hypothalamus and ends in sinusoidal capillaries of the pituitary gland. This venous system is known as the *hypothalamic-hypophyseal portal system*. This system carries neurosecretory hormones from the hypothalamus to the adenohypophysis. These hypothalamic factors stimulate or inhibit the release of hormones from the adenohypophysis. Retrograde flow from the adenohypophysis to the median eminence of the hypothalamus is also believed to occur. With upstream flow, pituitary hormones can reach the hypothalamus and influence hypothalamic function through a *short feedback loop*.

Historically, cells of the human anterior pituitary lobe have been categorized into three specific types based on their staining reaction in histological sections: (1) acidophils (approximately 40% of the cells) that stain with acidic dyes; (2) basophils (about 10% of the cells) that stain with basic dyes; and (3) chromophobes (the remaining 50% of the cells) that do not stain with either acidic or basic dyes. Using modern techniques of immunohistochemistry and electron microscopy, five types of cells have been identified: (1) somatotropes that secrete GH; (2) mammotropes that secrete PRL; (3) thyrotrophs that secrete TSH; (4) gonadotropes, single cells that secrete both gonadotropins,

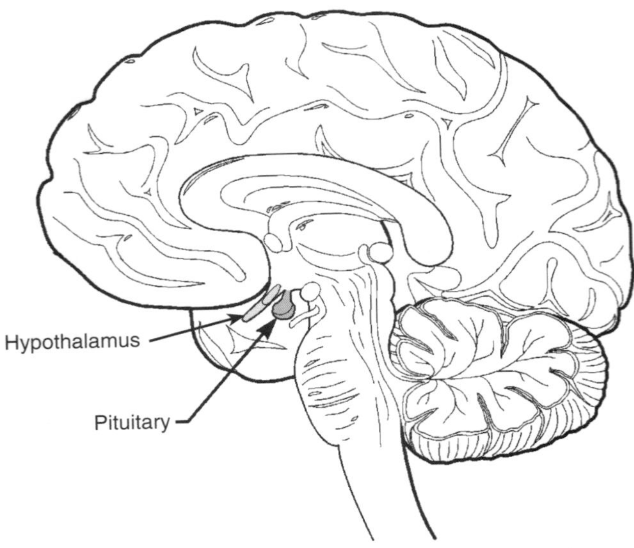

Figure 50-1 Location of pituitary and hypothalamus in the brain.

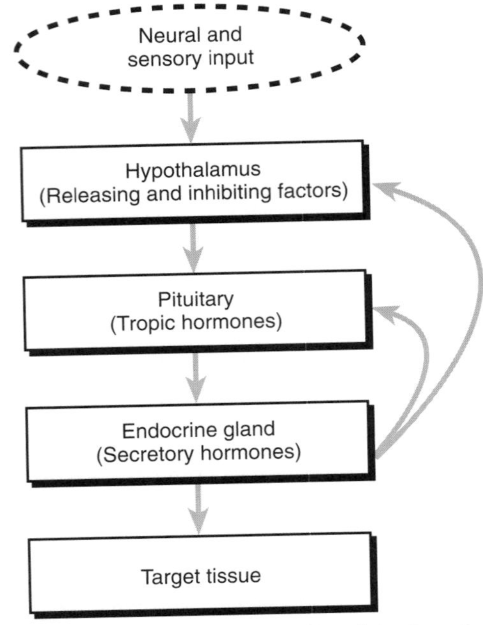

Figure 50-2 Functional interrelationship of the hypothalamus, pituitary, and endocrine glands.

LH and FSH; and (5) corticotropes that secrete both ACTH and β-LPH.

ADENOHYPOPHYSIS

The adenohypophysis and the individual hormones produced by it are discussed in this section, which concludes with a discussion of the assessment of the anterior pituitary lobe reserve.

Regulation of Function

Secretion of hormones from the anterior lobe of the pituitary gland is controlled by the hypothalamus, which manufactures small peptides known as *releasing* or *inhibitory factors* (Figure 50-2). These substances qualify as hormones because they are transported in the blood stream and produce a specific effect on the activities of a distal target tissue; however, they were initially called *releasing* or *inhibitory factors,* and these terms are still in use today. Several different hypothalamic hormones have been characterized including: (1) corticotropin-releasing hormone (CRH),[65] (2) thyrotropin-releasing hormone (TRH), (3) GH-releasing hormone (GH-RH), (4) somatostatin (also called somatotropin release-inhibiting factor [SRIF]), (5) gonadotropin-releasing hormone (Gn-RH, also called *luteinizing hormone-releasing hormone*), and (6) PRL-inhibiting factor (PIF) that is actually the neurotransmitter dopamine. In addition, Gn-RH stimulates the secretion of FSH and LH. However, a separate and distinct releasing factor for FSH has not yet been established, although negative feedback control of this gonadotropin is affected by inhibin, a peptide of gonadal origin. The principal hypothalamic hormones and their chemical nature and action are summarized in Table 50-1.

TABLE 50-1 Neurotransmitter Effect on Hormonal Secretions by the Anterior Lobe of the Pituitary Gland

	Secretion Stimulated by	Secretion Inhibited by
ACTH	Serotonin Acetylcholine Endorphins	GABA
TSH	Norepinephrine	Dopamine Serotonin Endorphins
PRL	Norepinephrine Endorphins	Dopamine
GH	Dopamine Norepinephrine Serotonin Endorphins	
Gonadotropins	Norepinephrine Acetylcholine GABA	Serotonin Dopamine Endorphins

The hypothalamic peptides, in contrast to some pituitary tropic hormones such as the gonadotropins, are not entirely species specific. Porcine Gn-RH and TRH have been shown to have an effect in humans. The availability of highly purified and synthetic releasing hormones has important diagnostic and therapeutic implications. CRH, GH-RH, Gn-RH, and TRH have all been used to test for pituitary hormone reserve. In addition, pulsatile Gn-RH administration is used to initiate puberty and to induce ovulation or spermatogenesis. Alternately, Gn-RH antagonists that inhibit the action of endogenous Gn-RH are used to treat patients with precocious puberty, endometriosis, uterine fibroids, and prostate carcinoma. GH-RH is yet another hypothalamic peptide that is used to treat patients with GH deficiency caused by hypothalamic disease.

The neurons that elaborate hypophysiotropic hormones are themselves influenced by hypothalamic neurotransmitters, such as dopamine, norepinephrine, serotonin, acetylcholine, and endorphins. These neurotransmitters also modify the secretory activity of anterior pituitary hormones (see Table 50-1). Indeed basal and episodic secretion, diurnal rhythm, and nocturnal release of pituitary hormones are all considered to be secondary to central nervous system events that are mediated through hypothalamic hormones.

In addition to higher center regulation of the hypothalamic-pituitary axis by classic neurotransmitters, such as dopamine, there is an advancing body of evidence showing that chemical mediators released by inflammatory cells (cytokines)[4] participate in altering the control mechanisms associated with the neuroendocrine axis (see Chapter 22).[48,56,77] Modulation of the feedback loop between the hypothalamic-pituitary-adrenal axis by cytokines, such as interleukin 1 (IL-1) and IL-6, released as a result of infection or stress has been shown to diminish the immune system.[26] The concept of a hypothalamic-pituitary-adrenal-immune axis has been evolving for some time, and now substantial evidence is available to support the concept that cytokines do modulate the responsiveness of the hypothalamic-pituitary-adrenal axis under certain physiological response situations, such as infection or stress.[108]

The functional relationship that exists between the pituitary gland and its target organs is based on the principle of feedback control, which is primarily negative between the blood concentration of circulating hormones and the pituitary gland and hypothalamus (Figure 50-3). The effect of negative feedback is typically opposite to that of the initial stimulus. For example, an elevated concentration of cortisol (initial stimulus) diminishes the synthesis and release of CRH, resulting in decreased secretion of ACTH and, ultimately, reduced secretion of cortisol (final response). Conversely a diminished concentration of cortisol in the blood triggers release of CRH from the hypothalamus; this causes enhanced synthesis and release of ACTH. Increased blood concentrations of ACTH in turn stimulate the adrenal cortex to produce more cortisol. The importance of such feedback control lies in the maintenance of an optimal concentration of hormones in the blood under a fluctuating variety of circumstances. Although hormones such as thyroxine, cortisol, estradiol, progesterone, and testosterone interact with hypothalamic receptors to control the release of hypothalamic hormones, studies indicate that these secretory products directly modulate the response of pituitary cells to their respective releasing hormones. For example, progesterone and testosterone suppress the response of gonadotropin-producing cells to Gn-RH, whereas small doses of estradiol potentiate this response. In addition to the "long" feedback loops comprising pituitary, hypothalamic, and target gland hormones, a "short" feedback loop exists by which pituitary hormones can directly act on the hypothalamus to modify their own secretion (see Figure 50-3).

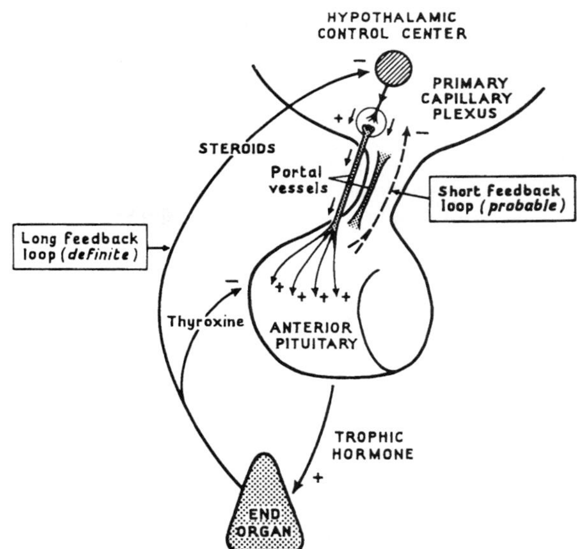

Figure 50-3 Control of anterior pituitary function. *(Modified from Catt KJ. Pituitary function. Lancet 1970;1:827-31.)*

Growth Hormone and Insulin-like Growth Factors

The most abundant hormone produced by the adenohypophysis is GH. Insulin-like growth factors (IGFs) I and II are polypeptides with considerable sequence and functional similarity to insulin.

Biochemistry

GH is a single-chain polypeptide with a molecular mass of 21,500 Da that contains 191 amino acids and two intramolecular disulfide bridges. It is structurally similar to PRL and to the placental hormone chorionic somatomammotropin (hCS, placental lactogen), with which it has overlapping biological effects. Many consider GH, PRL, and hCS to have descended from a common single primordial peptide.

GH is synthesized by the somatotropic (acidophilic) cells of the adenohypophysis and is stored within intracellular granules. During the daytime hours, the plasma concentration of GH in normal adults remains stable and relatively low (<2 ng/mL), with several secretory "spikes" occurring approximately 3 hours after meals and after exercise. In contrast, during the evening hours, adults and children show a marked rise in GH secretory activity ~90 minutes after the onset of sleep; GH concentrations reach a peak value during the period of deepest sleep. This pattern of GH secretion

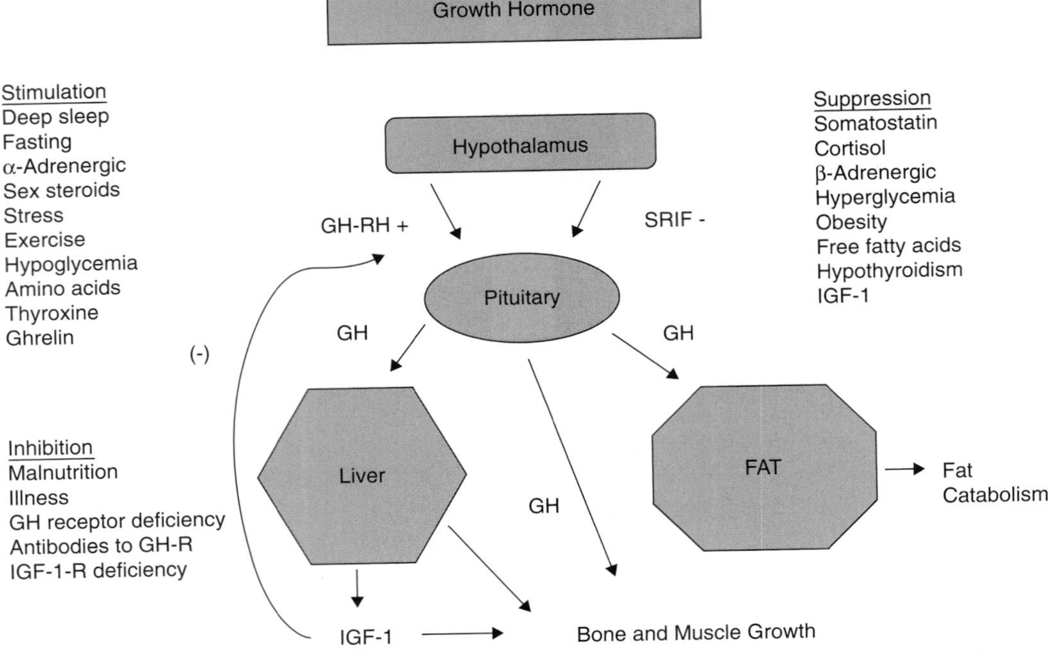

Figure 50-4 The regulatory feedback loop of the hypothalamic-pituitary-growth hormone axis. Growth hormone-releasing hormone (GH-RH) acts on the pituitary to produce GH. GH acts on the liver to produce IGF-1, which together with GH modulates bone and muscle growth and differentiation. GH also has a catabolic effect on fat tissue. IGF-1 has a negative feedback effect on GH-RH and GH secretion, and SRIF attenuates the effects of GH-RH on the pituitary.

may be important to anabolic and repair processes and for proper skeletal growth.

Regulation of Growth Hormone Secretion

The release of GH appears to be controlled by two hypothalamic factors secreted into the portal system circulation from nerve terminals in the median eminence. One of these factors is GH-RH, which stimulates GH release; the other is SRIF (somatotropin release-inhibitory factor), which inhibits GH release. (SRIF is also found in the delta cells of the pancreatic islets and in many other sites in the digestive tract; it has important effects on gastrointestinal hormone secretion and causes inhibition of insulin and glucagon release.) The hypothalamic influence on GH release appears to be predominantly inhibitory through the action of SRIF (Figure 50-4). The evidence for this comes from a twist of nature where damage to the hypothalamic-pituitary connection (e.g., resulting from pituitary stalk section and lesions of the median eminence) is followed by a dramatic decrease in both basal and provoked GH release. Release of these two hypothalamic factors is in turn influenced by higher centers of the brain. Thus different stimuli, such as exercise, physical and emotional stress, hypoglycemia, increased circulating amino acid concentrations (particularly arginine), and hormones such as testosterone, estrogens, and thyroxine, can evoke an increase in GH secretion (see Figure 50-4). In the presence of abnormally high concentrations of glucocorticoids, GH secretion is suppressed. In addition, the concentration of GH in the circulation is thought to influence the release of hypothalamic hormones through the short feedback loop. Other hypothalamic hormones, such as TRH and Gn-RH, do not affect GH release in normal subjects but may provoke GH release in patients with acromegaly.

Isolation and discovery of ghrelin support another control system for GH release in addition to GH-RH and SRIF. Ghrelin is a small 28 amino acid (AA) peptide released from neuroendocrine cells in the gastric mucosa that binds to the GH secretagogue receptor to induce the secretion of both GH-RH and GH itself. Ghrelin also induces food intake and the development of obesity.

Physiological Actions

Growth Hormone

The overall effect of GH is to promote growth in soft tissue, cartilage, and bone. This action results from stimulation of protein synthesis that is partly induced by an increase in amino acid transport through cell membranes. The effects of GH on bone and muscle are exerted both directly and through the effects of IGFs that are produced primarily in the liver and other tissue (e.g., bone) under the influence of GH. The increased growth of soft tissue and the skeleton is accompanied by changes in electrolyte metabolism, including a positive nitrogen and phosphorus balance, a rise in plasma phosphorus concentrations, and a fall in blood urea nitrogen and amino acid concentrations. Additional responses to GH include increased intestinal absorption of calcium and decreased urinary excretion of sodium and potassium. The metabolic changes are most likely a result of the increased uptake of these ions by growing tissue. GH has other effects on intermediary metabolism. GH stimulates the uptake of nonesterified fatty acids by muscle and accelerates the mobilization and metabolism of fat from adipose tissue to the liver. Acutely, GH causes a decrease in blood glucose concentrations; however, chronic GH excess stimulates hepatic glycogenolysis and antagonizes the effect of insulin on glucose uptake by peripheral cells (see Metabolism of Carbohydrates, Chapter 25) leading to an increase in blood glucose concentrations. GH and insulin induce growth in a similar manner, because both have protein anabolic effects and stimulate the transport of amino acids into peripheral cells. Their respective effects on glucose homeostasis, however, oppose each other. Most growth-promoting GH effects are delayed rather than immediate and are exerted primarily through IGF-I.

Insulin-Like Growth Factors[110]

The first GH-dependent growth factor to be isolated was termed *sulfation factor*, because of its ability to enhance the incorporation of sulfate into cartilage. However, this substance had other effects on cartilage, including the stimulation of deoxyribonucleic acid (DNA) and ribonucleic acid synthesis and collagen formation. Initially, this factor and other peptides with similar biological activities that are stimulated by GH were called *somatomedins*. Later this term was changed to *insulin-like growth factor* because of the peptides' structural similarities to insulin.

The most important of the IGFs is IGF-I. In addition to its growth-promoting effects on cartilage, IGF-I also shows insulin-like activity in other tissue. IGF-I increases glucose oxidation in adipose tissue and stimulates glucose and amino acid transport into diaphragmatic muscle and heart muscle. Synthesis of collagen and proteoglycans is enhanced by IGF-I, which also has positive effects on calcium, magnesium, and potassium homeostasis. The insulin-like effects of this growth factor have been ascribed in part to its structural similarity to insulin. Unlike most other peptide hormones, IGFs circulate in blood complexed to specific plasma-binding proteins. Six major IGF-binding proteins have been identified in human plasma.[110] Insulin-like growth factor binding protein (IGFBP)-3, a glycosylated binding protein, complexes >75% of the circulating IGF-I. The concentration of this binding protein is GH dependent and provides for a circulating reserve pool of IGF-I. Dissociation of the IGFs from the binding proteins occurs before passage through capillary membranes and entrance into dense tissue, such as cartilage.

Plasma concentrations of immunoreactive IGF-I rise during childhood and achieve adult concentrations by the time of puberty. During puberty, IGF-I concentrations can be two to three times the adult concentration. During adolescence, IGF-I concentrations show a gradual decline, reaching a steady state in the third decade of life. IGF-I concentrations are increased as expected in patients with acromegaly[85] and are reduced in GH deficiency states and in many other forms of growth retardation, hypothyroidism, chronic illness, nutritional deficiency, and liver disease.

Clinical Significance

Clinically important states of GH excess or deficiency are relatively uncommon and often difficult to diagnose.[101,131] GH concentrations vary widely under normal circumstances, so the measurement of GH under random conditions is not generally considered useful. A single GH measurement cannot be used to distinguish normal fluctuations from the low or high concentrations that are seen in various disease states. GH measurements are best determined as part of dynamic testing that involves the use of pharmacological or physiological provocative stimuli to stimulate or suppress GH release.[37]

In contrast to GH, a single measurement of IGF-I is considered an accurate reflection of IGF-I production.[100] Serum concentrations of IGF-I are influenced by age, degree of sexual maturation, and nutritional status. As mentioned previously, IGF-I concentrations are low in states of GH deficiency but also in patients with acute or chronic protein or caloric deprivation.

Growth Hormone Excess

Excess GH production is associated with eosinophilic or chromophobe adenomas[21] of the pituitary gland; these tumors are sufficiently large to be demonstrated using computed tomography or magnetic resonance imaging in approximately 75% of patients. Prolonged exposure to GH excess causes an overgrowth of the skeleton and soft tissue. This occurs most commonly in adults and is known as *acromegaly*.[31,135] When GH excess is seen before long-bone growth is complete, the condition is called *pituitary gigantism*. With pituitary gigantism, in addition to the overgrowth of bone and soft tissue particularly evident in the face and extremities, there is a striking acceleration of linear growth. In severe or advanced cases of GH excess, the diagnosis can be made on the basis of physical appearance alone; however, the physical changes are often subtle and gradual, so that a high degree of clinical suspicion is needed to make an early diagnosis. The reversibility of the tissue changes depends largely on the duration of the disease. In addition to the soft-tissue changes, acromegaly may cause severe disability or death from cardiac or neurological sequelae. The most important requirement for the diagnosis of acromegaly is the demonstration of inappropriate and excessive GH secretion.[88]

GH-secreting pituitary tumors account for most of the cases of acromegaly. Patients who have pituitary tumors that produce GH are frequently shown to release GH in response to other hypothalamic peptides (TRH and Gn-RH) that under normal circumstances do not elicit a release of GH. On occasion, pituitary tumors that produce excess amounts of both GH and PRL are observed. Few cases of acromegaly, however, are due to GH-RH hypersecretion by tumors.

As many as 10% of patients with active acromegaly have random serum GH concentrations that fall within the normal reference interval.[88] Essentially, all patients with acromegaly have an abnormal response to oral glucose (see Box 50-1). Patients with acromegaly typically show either no change in their basal concentration of GH or demonstrate a paradoxical increase in GH[36]; normal individuals, on the other hand, show suppression of GH concentrations to <1 ng/mL after the oral ingestion of glucose.

BOX 50-1 Protocol for Glucose Suppression of Growth Hormone Test

Rationale Normal subjects show suppression of serum GH concentrations after oral administration of glucose; subjects with acromegaly fail to show this suppression.

Procedure The test should be performed after an overnight fast with the patient maintained at bed rest. After a baseline blood specimen is collected for GH measurement, a solution of 75 g of glucose is given orally; serum GH is measured again on specimens collected 60 and 120 minutes later.

Interpretation Serum GH concentrations in normal individuals fall to <2 ng/mL; subjects with acromegaly fail to show this suppression and sometimes show a paradoxical increase in GH concentration. Patients with liver disease, uremia, or heroin addiction may have false-positive results with this test (failure to suppress serum GH concentrations after oral glucose load).

GH, Growth hormone.

Serum IGF-I concentrations are elevated in active acromegaly (Figure 50-5). IGF-I concentrations often correlate better with the clinical severity of acromegaly than with glucose-suppressed or basal GH concentrations.[27]

Growth Hormone Deficiency States and Growth Retardation

Children who have inadequate GH production or a GH receptor defect do not grow normally. GH deficiency may be (1) congenital or acquired; (2) idiopathic or caused by anatomical damage to the pituitary gland or hypothalamus; or (3) caused by isolated or associated deficiencies of other pituitary hormones. In one reversible GH deficiency state known as *psychosocial dwarfism,* environmental stress has been shown to inhibit pituitary and hypothalamic function, leading to GH suppression and growth retardation. Children with this disorder show clinical and chemical evidence of growth deficiency when first evaluated but usually have normal pituitary function after a few days of hospital stay. GH deficiency is not a common cause of growth retardation; about one half of the children evaluated for growth retardation have no specific organic cause. About 15% of children with growth retardation have endocrine problems, and approximately one half of these (about 8% of all children with short stature) have GH deficiency. However, children with growth retardation or dwarfism with no clear explanation should at least be screened for GH deficiency. With the availability of recombinant GH for therapeutic use, many children with short stature are now being selectively treated with GH to advance their growth pattern to closer toward normal.

GH deficiency in adults is probably the most common demonstrable abnormality in patients with large pituitary

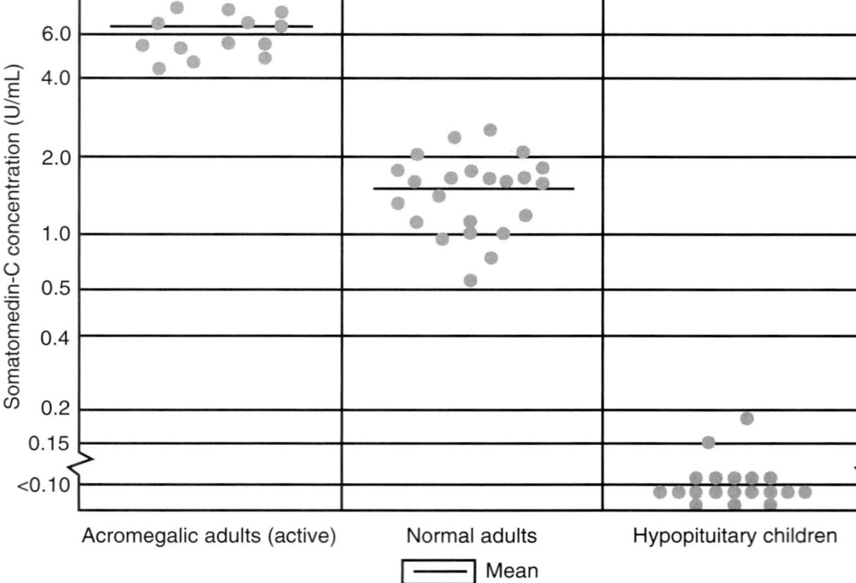
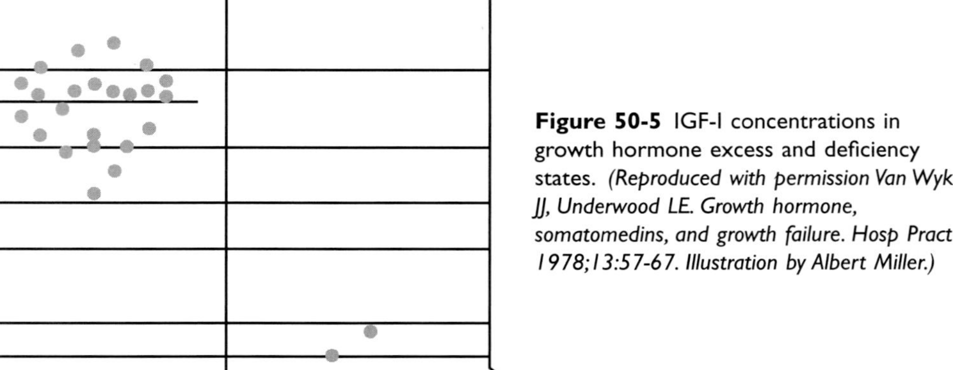

Figure 50-5 IGF-I concentrations in growth hormone excess and deficiency states. *(Reproduced with permission Van Wyk JJ, Underwood LE. Growth hormone, somatomedins, and growth failure. Hosp Pract 1978;13:57-67. Illustration by Albert Miller.)*

adenomas[21] or patients who have undergone pituitary irradiation; GH deficiency in adults can lead to premature mortality, abnormal body composition, impaired serum lipids, decreased bone density with an increase in fracture risk, and overall, an impaired quality of life. Thus GH replacement therapy is an important clinical intervention in GH-deficient adults and considered the standard of care.

Insensitivity to GH results in growth failure despite normal or increased serum GH concentrations. Patients who have familial short stature and high serum GH or low serum IGF-I concentrations[72] probably represent many different defects in genetic coding for the GH receptor that result in the absence of or defective GH receptors. In affected individuals, exogenous GH fails to produce any appreciable metabolic changes or to promote growth. In normal individuals, the basal concentration of GH is usually low, and the half-life of circulating GH is rather brief (~20 minutes). Moreover, GH is secreted by the pituitary gland in short pulses or bursts. Thus assays of GH performed on a single random or fasting specimen may not distinguish patients with abnormally low concentrations from healthy subjects who have GH values at the low end of normal. When evaluating GH reserve, provocative tests are frequently used to sort out a true deficiency. Although a normal GH response to a provocative test is a strong indication for the absence of GH deficiency, no single test can be considered diagnostic in this situation; as many as 30% of subjects with normal GH secretion fail to show the expected elevation in serum GH in response to a specific provocative stimulus at any given time. For this reason, to diagnose GH deficiency as a cause of growth retardation, it is necessary to demonstrate that the serum concentration of GH remains low after the use of at least two different provocative stimuli.[37,78] The definition of subnormal responses, however, is arbitrarily defined and assay dependent. In general a GH response >7 to 10 ng/mL after stimulation is considered normal.

A number of physiological and pharmacological circumstances provoke GH release. Some of these are presented in Table 50-2 and Figure 50-4. In one simple screening test, the patient performs 20 minutes of vigorous exercise, and then a sample is obtained for a GH measurement (Box 50-2).[62] Taking advantage of the known rise in the concentration of GH that occurs with deep sleep, a sample may be obtained 60 to 90 minutes after the onset of sleep.[80] The obvious limitation of this approach is that the patient must be in the hospital or a clinical research center for testing. The infusion of insulin[103] (Box 50-3) and arginine[86,96] (Box 50-4) are the standard pharmacological stimuli used to test for GH release; protocols for their use are well established and standardized. Other medications used to stimulate GH release

TABLE 50-2 Stimuli for Growth Hormone Release

Test	Test Conditions and Dosages	Time of Peak Growth Hormone Release	References
Exercise	20 min of vigorous exercise	20 min after exercise has begun	62
Sleep	Sample drawn 1 hr after the onset of deep sleep (stage III or IV); EEG documentation if possible	Usually 1 hr after onset of deep sleep, coincident with onset of stage III or IV sleep	80
Arginine*†	Arginine hydrochloride, 0.5 g/kg body weight, given intravenously over a 30-min period	60-120 min	87, 96
Insulin*†‡	Regular insulin, 0.1-0.15 U/kg, IV push (severe hypoglycemia may result, and a physician should be in constant attendance)	45-75 min	103
Glucagon†	0.03 mg/kg IM or subcutaneously (not to exceed 1 mg)	120-180 min	114
L-Dopa	0.5 g/1.73 m^2, usually given with lunch (responses may be improved by giving priming doses of L-dopa, 0.25 g/1.73 m^2, for 1 or more days before the test)	30-120 min	38
Clonidine	0.15 mg/m^2	90 min	46
Diazepam	0.15 mg/kg, orally	60 min	70
Pentagastrin	IV infusion, 1.5 mg/kg/hr	75 min	38

EEG, Electroencephalography; *IV*, intravenous; *IM*, intramuscular.
*Sequential administration of arginine and insulin may reduce the need for additional testing.[98]
†Propranolol, 0.75 mg/kg (20 to 40 mg orally), given 30 to 60 minutes before glucagon, insulin, or arginine may enhance a normal response.[97]
‡Insulin, TRH, and Gn-RH can be given as a "cocktail" to evaluate GH, ACTH, TSH, PRL, LH, and FSH in a single test period.[113]

BOX 50-2 Protocol for the Exercise Stimulation Test for Growth Hormone

Rationale Brisk exercise normally causes an increase in serum GH concentrations.

Procedure The test is best performed in the morning after an overnight fast, but may be done at any time. Vigorous physical exercise (running or calisthenics) is performed for 20 minutes. A venous blood specimen for determination of GH is drawn immediately after termination of exercise.

Interpretation If the serum GH concentration is >7 ng/mL, GH deficiency is unlikely. An intermediate response (3 to 6 ng/mL) should be considered suspect and further testing performed if clinically warranted. A subnormal response is not diagnostic for GH deficiency and should be confirmed with a second provocative test.

GH, Growth hormone.

BOX 50-3 Protocol for the Insulin-Induced Hypoglycemia Stimulation Test (Insulin Tolerance Test)

Rationale The stress of insulin-induced hypoglycemia triggers the release of GH and ACTH from the pituitary gland in normal subjects. GH response is measured directly; cortisol is measured as the indication of ACTH response.

Procedure The test is done after an overnight fast with the patient at bed rest. An indwelling needle or IV line is inserted. Sampling is begun after a 30-minute rest period. Baseline samples are drawn for determination of glucose, GH, and cortisol. Regular insulin, 0.1 to 0.15 units/kg body weight, is injected intravenously. Samples are then obtained at 30, 60, and 90 minutes for glucose, GH, and cortisol determinations. To be confident that an adequate stress has been applied, the patient must become symptomatic (exhibit sweating or tremor), or the glucose concentration must fall to <40 mg/dL (2.2 mmol/L). Additional IV insulin may be given if this has not occurred by 30 minutes, in which case sampling should be prolonged by 30 minutes. The physician should be in attendance throughout the test, and 50% dextrose for IV administration should be kept on hand to be used in the event of severe hypoglycemic reaction and after adequate hypoglycemia has been documented. The test is contraindicated in patients with seizure disorders, ischemic heart disease, or cardiovascular insufficiency.

Interpretation The serum cortisol concentration should increase to a peak value of >20 µg/dL (550 nmol/L). Serum GH concentration should rise to a peak value of >10 ng/mL. No response or inadequate responses may be due to pituitary hormone deficiency or to a hypothalamic lesion.

GH, Growth hormone; *ACTH,* adrenocorticotropin.

BOX 50-4 Protocol for the Arginine Stimulation Test for Growth Hormone

Rationale In normal subjects, IV administration of arginine hydrochloride stimulates GH release.

Procedure The test should be done after an overnight fast with the patient maintained at bed rest. Arginine hydrochloride, 0.5 g/kg body weight, is infused intravenously over 30 minutes. Blood samples are drawn for determination of GH before the infusion is started and 30, 60, and 90 minutes after the infusion is begun.

Interpretation The GH concentration should rise at least threefold above the baseline value to a peak value >10 ng/mL. A subnormal response is seen in GH-deficient subjects. A subnormal GH response is not diagnostic for GH deficiency and should be confirmed with a second provocative test.

GH, Growth hormone.

include glucagon. GH-RH administration intravenously has also been used to test for pituitary GH reserve directly to distinguish between a hypothalamic or a pituitary-based defect in GH release.

As expected, IGF-I concentrations are low in patients with GH deficiency and growth failure (see Figure 50-5). Patients with growth failure caused by other endocrine diseases or by nonendocrine organic diseases can also have low circulating concentrations of IGF-I; thus a low concentration of IGF-I is not a specific indication of GH deficiency. The presence of a normal concentration of IGF-I, however, does rule out severe GH deficiency.

Measurement of Growth Hormone in Blood and Urine

Bioassays, receptor assays, and immunoassays are used to measure GH.[100A] Most bioassays assess GH activity by analyzing a variety of growth-related metabolic changes in hypophysectomized rats or in cell cultures. A relatively simple and convenient bioassay, the *Nb2 cell assay,* uses cultures of GH-sensitive rat lymphoma cells.[123] These bioassays are used primarily for calibrating GH reference materials or for comparing the biological potency and immunoreactivity of GH fragments and synthetic peptides. Receptor assays have also been applied to the measurement of GH, but their use has been limited to research applications.

Binding assays that use specific GH antibodies are preferred for routine laboratory use. For many years, serum concentrations were measured by radioimmunoassay (RIA) using reagents provided by the United States National Hormone and Pituitary Program (NHPP; http://www.humc.edu/hormones/), which was formerly known as the National Pituitary Agency. Today a variety of isotopic and nonisotopic assays are commercially available. Many use polyclonal antibodies produced in rabbits or in guinea pigs against purified pituitary preparations of the unmodified, monomeric hormone. However, an increasing number of

GH assays now use mouse monoclonal antibodies, and some of these assays are able to discriminate GH variants. Most procedures use recombinant-derived GH for labeling with a tracer and calibration material. The latter is usually prepared gravimetrically and verified by comparison with an international reference preparation (IRP), such as the World Health Organization's (WHO's) international standard, IRP 80/505 human growth hormone recombinant (hGHr), which has a potency of 3.3 IU/mg of r-hGH, or other standard preparations, such as WHO IRP 66/217 or 88/624. The assay diluent, however, can vary considerably from one assay to another and is a potential source of bias; some commercial kits use phosphate-buffered saline, and others use horse, calf, or human serum.

Sensitive immunometric assays that use excess labeled antibodies in noncompetitive formats have been developed for measuring GH.[126] Several of these two-site "sandwich" assays are commercially available. Most are immunoradiometric assays (IRMAs) that are based on the use of two monoclonal antibodies directed at different antigenic sites on the GH molecule; one of the antibodies is labeled with ^{125}I, the so-called signal antibody, and the other antibody referred to as the capture antibody is anchored to a solid phase separation system. These isotopic methods for measuring GH are, however, gradually being replaced with assays that employ monoclonal antibodies coupled to either a nonisotopic enzyme,[130] a chemiluminescence tagged antibody, or a fluorescent[122] label. The detection limit of these immunometric assays ranges from 0.1 to 0.5 μg/L.

Problems

Human GH is not a single molecular species but is present in the pituitary gland and in the circulation as a heterogenous mixture of structural isoforms.[11,111,120] Normally the human gene for GH directs the synthesis of a monomeric 22-kDa protein that accounts for 75% of the GH found in the circulation. In addition to this predominant form, however, approximately 10% of GH from human pituitaries is present in plasma as a 20-kDa protein. This smaller form lacks amino acid residues 32 to 46 and is probably a product of posttranslational processing. Fractionation of serum by gel filtration also reveals the presence of aggregates and oligomers of GH. These large molecules are often referred to as "big" and "big-big" forms. The big forms are predominantly dimers of the monomeric hormone, whereas the big-big forms are mainly complexes formed by GH and its serum-binding protein. All of these GH variants are antigenic; in normal plasma, 75% of immunoreactive GH consists of monomeric forms, 18% are present in dimeric forms, and 7% in oligomeric forms.

Analytically the presence of GH variants in serum often leads to problems with quantitation and to discrepancies among the results given by different assays.[55] The use of (1) different antibodies, (2) different calibration materials, (3) different labels, and (4) different assay diluents further increases the complexity of GH measurements. For example, immunometric assays using monoclonal antibodies tend to give lower GH estimates than polyclonal RIAs and may not recognize some forms of the hormone.[107] Discordant results have also been noted among immunometric assays. One commercial IRMA, for example, detects the 20-kDa variant of GH, whereas another IRMA does not[25]; the dimeric form of GH interferes with some immunometric kits but not with others.[19] Variations in assay performance can also be attributed to the inappropriate use of serum proteins from animal sources in buffer diluents.[41] In addition, the calibrators used in most GH assays are derived from pituitary extracts and thus may not reflect the concentrations and types of GH variants present in the specimen being assayed. However, the use of recombinant standards for GH has improved this problem and it has been suggested that the 22-kDa form of GH be used to establish uniformity of results between methods.

Variations in GH isoform detection can seriously affect the interpretation of GH stimulation tests when using different GH assays. For example, one assay may indicate an adequate amount of GH following a stimulation test, whereas another might give a low estimate of the GH concentration that could lead to misclassification of a child as GH deficient. It is important therefore that cutoff values and reference intervals be established separately for each method proposed for routine use to prevent misinterpretation and a misdiagnosis.[8] Moreover, particular care should be taken when comparing serum GH values obtained using different immunoassay systems.

Most GH assays are performed with serum specimens, but the highly sensitive immunometric assays have been modified to allow for direct measurement of GH in untreated urine.[40,47] Because the concentration of GH in urine is only 0.1% of that in serum, conventional RIAs usually require preliminary extraction and concentration procedures.

Specimen Collection and Storage

The preferred specimen is serum; plasma with ethylenediaminetetraacetic acid (EDTA) or heparin added to prevent coagulation may also be used, but values are method dependent. Serum specimens should be stored at 2 °C to 8 °C if they are not to be tested within 8 hours. If they must be stored for long periods, serum samples should be frozen at −20 °C or colder.

Reference Intervals

The following intervals are based on a competitive RIA technique that is calibrated against the WHO IRP 80/505 for r-hGH.

	μg/L
Basal	2-5
Insulin tolerance test	>10
Arginine	>7.5
L-Dopa	>7.5

Comments

A single basal or random concentration of GH provides little diagnostic information. Secretion of GH by the pituitary gland is both episodic and pulsatile, and transient concentrations of up to 40 ng/mL have been observed in normal, healthy subjects. Serum concentrations are rather low between pulses in healthy individuals, and some immunoassays may not be able to distinguish patients with abnormally low values from healthy subjects who have values that happen to fall in the low-normal reference interval. In some individuals, spontaneous GH secretion is better monitored using a continuous withdrawal pump or by drawing specimens for GH assay every 20 to 30 minutes over a 12- to 24-hour period. To interpret meaningful GH concentrations, a number of provocative tests have been established to stimulate or suppress GH release. The insulin tolerance test, which produces a transient hypoglycemia to provoke GH release, is the most common stimulation test used to assess adequacy of GH secretion.

Measurement of Insulin-Like Growth Factors

IGFs are measured in plasma or serum by a variety of methods including in vitro bioassay, radioreceptor assay, or immunoassay techniques.[71] Most bioassays measure the sum of IGF-I and IGF-II bioactivity using rabbit chondrocytes, chick pelvic cartilage, or porcine rib cartilage.[111] Such assays are relatively imprecise, insensitive, and often not specific.

The original immunoassays for IGF-I (somatomedin C) were based primarily on double-antibody methods under equilibrium or nonequilibrium conditions and on the use of ^{125}I-labeled tracers.[111] Purified preparations of IGF-I isolated from human serum generally serve as calibrators, although recombinant IGF-I is now available and used in some procedures. The IGF-I standards are calibrated against the WHO preparation IGF-I 87/518. To remove interfering IGF-binding proteins, most assays preextract serum specimens by a variety of methods, such as gel filtration, acid-ethanol precipitation, cryoprecipitation, C18 Sep-Pak column extraction, or reversed-phase chromatography.[20] Direct (no extraction) procedures are also available, but extraction methods prevent complex problems associated with the presence of carrier proteins and serum proteases. Moreover, extraction procedures better discriminate GH-deficient patients from age-matched controls. Commercial RIA, IRMA, and assays that employ chemiluminescence signaling are available for measuring IGF-I, usually with minimal cross-reactivity to IGF-II (0% to 3%).[64,118] A typical IRMA procedure calls for incubating extracted serum specimens with two different monoclonal antibodies either for 3 hours at room temperature or overnight (16 to 18 hours) at 2 °C to 8 °C. The signal antibody is labeled with ^{125}I, and the capture antibody is attached to the inner walls of plastic test tubes or free in solution. Interassay coefficients of variation for most methods range between 5% and 10% across a wide analytical range. It is important to establish age-related reference interval for IGF-I because of the marked differences in concentrations that exist between adults and children.

Immunoassays for IGF-II complement the measurement of IGF-I. Together they provide better identification of GH-deficient children. The IGF-II assay, like that for IGF-I, is best performed after the removal of high molecular weight binding proteins. Adding excess IGF-I to each tube[16] can block interference from smaller IGF-binding proteins; the use of highly specific antisera ensures negligible cross-reactivity with related molecules, such as IGF-I and insulin. Single measurements of IGF-binding protein 3 (IGFBP-3), the major protein carrier of IGFs in circulation, can also provide additional information for the determination of GH deficiency. This protein can be quantitated in unextracted plasma by RIA using rabbit antihuman IGFBP-3; cross-reactivity with other binding proteins is <0.2%.[17]

Specimen Collection and Storage

Serum or plasma (with heparin or EDTA added to prevent coagulation) can be used depending on the assay method. Samples should be centrifuged within 1 hour of collection and stored frozen at −20 °C or colder until assay. It is recommended that storage before assay under these conditions not exceed 30 days. Some procedures use dried whole blood or serum collected on filter paper.[89]

Reference Intervals

Published intervals for IGF-I differ because of variations in methods and calibration. The values listed on p. 1977 are expressed in nanograms per milliliter of synthetic peptide; dividing by 220 converts IGF-I values to units per milliliter, where one unit is arbitrarily defined as the amount of IGF-I in a pool of normal adult human sera.[39]

IGF-I concentrations are highly age dependent. For the care of adolescent patients, reference values are based on Tanner stage and chronological age. (Tanner staging is a classification of pubertal development based on the manifestation of secondary sex characteristics; many hormones involved in adolescent growth are more closely related to Tanner stages than to chronological age.[134]) By comparison, IGF-II concentrations are relatively unaffected by differences in maturity. A typical adult reference interval for IGFBP-3 is 0.9 to 4.0 mg/L.[90]

Prolactin

Prolactin (PRL) is a hormone secreted by special cells of the adenohypophysis. It stimulates and sustains lactation in postpartum mammals, the mammary glands having been prepared by other hormones, including estrogens, progesterone, growth hormone, corticosteroids, and insulin. It also stimulates formation of "milk" in the crop sac of birds, such as pigeons and doves (an action formerly used for bioassay), is luteotropic in certain mammals, and has many other

IGF-I (ng/mL)[125]

By Chronological Age			By Tanner Stage		
Age (yr)	Males (ng/mL)	Females (ng/mL)	Stage	Males (ng/mL)	Females (ng/mL)
1-2	31-160	11-206	1	215 ± 71	225 ± 83
3-6	16-288	70-316	2	320 ± 137	410 ± 84
7-10	136-385	123-396	3	475 ± 176	492 ± 180
11-12	136-440	191-462	4	500 ± 135	505 ± 155
13-14	165-616	286-660	5	500 ± 135	505 ± 155
15-18	134-836	152-660			
19-25	202-433	231-550			
26-85	135-449	135-449			

IGF-I (ng/mL)[125]

Prepubertal children	334-642
Pubertal children	245-737
Adults	288-736
GH deficiency	51-299

effects, including essential roles in the maintenance of immune system functions. It is called also *lactogen, lactotropin, luteotropin, mammotropin,* and *galactopoietic, lactation, lactogenic,* or *luteotropic hormone.*

Biochemistry

The structure of PRL is similar to that of GH in that the human gene for PRL located on chromosome 6 arose from a single common ancestral gene, which gave rise to not only PRL but to GH and placental lactogen-related peptides. PRL contains 199 amino acids and has three intramolecular disulfide bridges. Its molecular mass is 22,000 Da. It is secreted by the pituitary lactotroph cells, which are acidophilic. PRL circulates in the blood in different forms; monomeric PRL, 23 kDa (referred to as little PRL), dimeric PRL, 48 to 56 kDa (so-called big PRL), and polymeric forms of PRL >100 kDa (called "big-big" PRL). The monomeric form is considered the most bioactive of the different forms found in the circulation and demonstrates the greatest response to TRH, the hypothalamic releasing factor that stimulates the pituitary to release PRL. The relative number and PRL content of lactotroph cells are increased in women during pregnancy and also found elevated in fetal pituitary glands. The increase in the number of lactotroph cells during pregnancy is the result of the elevated concentration of circulating estrogens present in pregnancy.

Secretion of PRL, as for other hormones released by the anterior lobe of the pituitary gland, falls under hypothalamic control. PRL is unique, however, among the adenohypophyseal hormones in that the primary control of its secretion is inhibitory rather than stimulatory (Figure 50-6). Dopamine is believed to be the principal PIF that tonically regulates PRL secretion by binding to the D2 receptors on pituitary lactotrophs. Other factors, such as endothelin-1 and transforming growth factor β1, can also inhibit PRL release. In contrast, TRH is a potent PRL releasing factor (PRF) and stimulates PRL secretion within minutes when injected intravenously into human subjects. TRH, however, is not the only PRF, because hypothalamic extracts cause PRL release even when the TRH content has been inactivated or removed. Factors such as vasoactive intestinal peptide, epidermal growth factor, and estrogen also stimulate PRL release. The regulation of PRL is not altered in experiments with anti-TRH antibody, and suckling, which causes a sharp rise in plasma PRL, does not affect TSH secretion. Thus these other PRFs play an important role in PRL secretion. As with other adenohypophyseal hormones, the release of PRL is episodic and varies predictably during the day, with lowest concentrations found at midday and highest values shortly after the onset of deep sleep. The major physiological stimulus for PRL release is suckling, and maternal plasma PRL concentrations increase within minutes after the initiation of breast-feeding. Following labor and delivery, PRL concentrations remain elevated longer when the newborn is breast-fed. Other stimuli induce PRL release, probably through suppression of dopamine releasing the pituitary from its inhibitory effects; stress is one of these stimuli. ACTH concentrations, which are also increased with stress, can cause an elevation in plasma PRL values. Plasma hyperosmolality is yet another stimulus for PRL release, whereas hypoosmolar conditions induce a decrease in plasma PRL concentrations. Whether this effect is stress related or is associated with the role of PRL in the control of osmolality has not been established. Finally an important influence on PRL regulation appears to be exerted by PRL itself by way of a short feedback loop between the pituitary and hypothalamus. PRL participates in negative feedback to control its own release by increasing the concentration of tyrosine hydroxylase activity in the neurons that produce dopamine. Short-

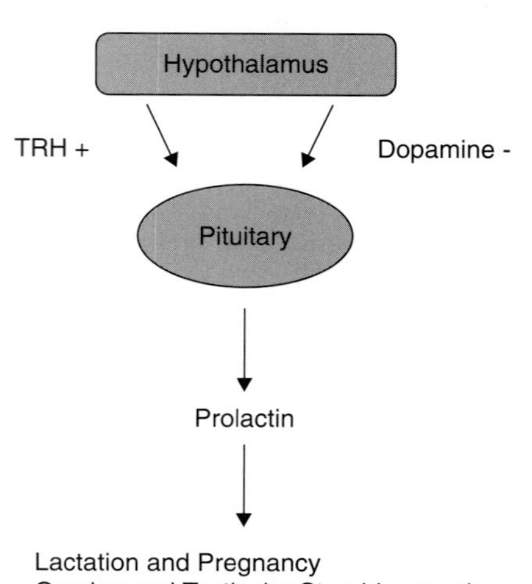

Figure 50-6 Regulatory control of PRL release. TRF along with a variety of other factors stimulates the release of PRL from the pituitary. Dopamine and other factors are inhibitory to PRL release.

feedback-loop inhibition of Gn-RH secretion by PRL has also been suggested as the reason for the inhibition of gonadotropin secretion that occurs in women who are nursing and in patients with PRL-secreting adenomas of the pituitary gland.

Physiological Action

The principal hormone that controls the initiation and maintenance of lactation is PRL. However, for an appropriate expression of PRL action, breast tissue requires priming by estrogens, progestins, corticosteroids, thyroid hormone, and insulin. PRL induces ductal growth, development of the breast lobular alveolar system, and the synthesis of specific milk proteins, including casein and γ-lactalbumin. PRL has effects on the immune system[138] and is important in the control of osmolality and various metabolic events, including the metabolism of subcutaneous fat, carbohydrate metabolism, calcium and vitamin D metabolism, fetal lung development, and steroidogenesis. This last function may be related to its antigonadotropic effect.

PRL, like other pituitary hormones, binds to a specific receptor on the cell membrane of its target organs (breast, adrenal, ovaries, testes, prostate, kidney, and liver). However, the exact intracellular mechanism of PRL action is not known. It has been suggested that PRL regulates the transport of lipoproteins in the adrenal gland, ovary, and testis to ensure a constant supply of low-density lipoprotein cholesterol for steroidogenesis. In addition, PRL promotes the synthesis of enzymes of the adrenal androgen pathway, thus facilitating the conversion of pregnenolone to dehydroepiandrosterone and dehydroepiandrosterone sulfate (see Adrenocortical Steroids, Chapter 51). PRL can also stimulate the enzyme 3-β-ol-dehydrogenase in the gonads, resulting in increased testosterone production and ovarian steroid biosynthesis, particularly the synthesis of progesterone.

Clinical Significance

When assays for PRL became routinely available in the early 1970s, it became apparent that patients with elevations in PRL were observed more frequently than previously thought in clinical practice.[67,99] However, PRL deficiency does not appear to have clinical significance except as an additional test of pituitary function in patients already known to have pituitary disease.

Hyperprolactinemia is the most common hypothalamic-pituitary disorder encountered in clinical endocrinology.[66] PRL concentrations also may be elevated in women who have only subtle alterations of fertility, such as (1) anovulation with or without menstrual irregularity, (2) amenorrhea and galactorrhea, or (3) galactorrhea alone. PRL excess in men is frequently manifested as oligospermia or impotence or both. In addition, men with PRL-secreting pituitary adenomas more often present with macroadenomas and visual field disturbances as a result of a larger tumor pressing on the optic chiasm. Men do not have the subtle reminder of an irregular menstrual period that can frequently expose a microadenoma in women. Elevated PRL concentrations are observed in as many as 30% of patients with polycystic ovarian syndrome and patients with clinically silent pituitary adenomas. Other causes of PRL elevation are shown in Box 50-5 and Figure 50-6 and should be kept in mind when evaluating patients who present with an elevated concentration of PRL. There is no reliable

BOX 50-5 Causes of Prolactin Elevation

Chronic renal failure
Pregnancy
Breast stimulation or chest wall trauma
Primary hypothyroidism
Empty sella syndrome
Pituitary adenoma (microadenoma or macroadenoma)
- "Nonsecretory"
- With galactorrhea and amenorrhea or oligospermia

Idiopathic
Drugs
- Dopaminergic-blocking agents: phenothiazines, butyrophenones, benzamides (metoclopramide, sulpiride)
- Dopamine-depleting agents: α-methyldopa, reserpine
- Noncatecholamine-dependent agents: TRH, estrogens
- H_2-receptor blocking agents: cimetidine
- Tricyclic antidepressants

Hypothalamic etiologies

stimulation or suppression test as with other pituitary hormones to distinguish tumor from nontumor causes of PRL elevation.

Basal gonadotropin concentrations are low in most patients with hyperprolactinemia; most studies suggest that PRL inhibits the release of Gn-RH, resulting in a state of functional hypogonadotropism. Other pituitary function tests are usually normal in patients with hyperprolactinemia, except in individuals with very large tumors. It has been reported that the usual nocturnal increase in PRL is blunted in patients with pituitary adenomas and hyperprolactinemia but not in normal subjects or patients with the empty sella syndrome. A ratio of greater than 1:2 in night-to-day PRL is considered normal. The extent of PRL elevations in patients with PRL-secreting pituitary adenomas is generally greater than is seen with other nonadenoma causes of a PRL elevation. However, none of the laboratory approaches used to evaluate a prolactinoma is sufficiently definitive to differentiate hyperprolactinemia from nonpituitary causes from that caused by pituitary disease.

If a borderline elevation of PRL is found, it is advisable to repeat the measurement on at least two other occasions, taking care to obtain the specimen with minimal excitement or stress to the patient, no trauma, no breast stimulation, and in the morning; the patient should also not be on any medication that could stimulate PRL release.

Clinically, medications that can stimulate PRL release are the single most common cause for creating a biochemical picture of a prolactinoma in an otherwise healthy individual. When a significant elevation of PRL is confirmed, a careful history must be recorded to rule out the possibility that medications are not the cause for the elevation in PRL. A significant list of medications has been identified that have spuriously elevated PRL concentrations in an otherwise normal individual. In addition to estrogens, dopamine receptor blockers, such as the phenothiazines, and dopamine antagonists, such as metoclopramide and domperidone used to treat gastrointestinal diseases, produce a significant elevation in PRL release. A number of psychiatric drugs also cause elevations in PRL concentrations, including haloperidol and resperidol. In addition, antihypertensive agents, such as beta blockers and calcium channel blockers, and antihistamines, such as cimetidine and ranitidine, are associated with modest elevations in PRL. TSH measurements should be considered in patients suspected of a prolactinoma to rule out primary hypothyroidism, a thyroid condition associated with elevations in PRL. Imaging of the pituitary gland with computed tomography or magnetic resonance imaging is usually performed as part of the clinical work-up for a suspected prolactinoma. Most patients with PRL concentrations >200 μg/L have a PRL-secreting tumor; many large prolactinomas are associated with PRL concentrations of >1000 μg/L. Most patients with a prolactinoma fail to show a further increase in PRL after TRH stimulation; however, the same is true for most patients with hyperprolactinemia from other causes. Unless a pituitary tumor can be demonstrated by computed tomography or magnetic resonance imaging, the diagnosis of a PRL-secreting microadenoma (<10 mm in diameter) is one of exclusion. Because 50% of PRL-secreting microadenomas are too small to be seen using neuroradiological techniques, delineating the distinction between a small pituitary tumor, PRL-cell hyperplasia, and idiopathic hyperprolactinemia may not be possible without surgical intervention.

Finding an elevated PRL concentration in a patient with a pituitary tumor does not establish a cause-and-effect relationship. Usually a PRL concentration in excess of 200 ng/mL is sufficient evidence to strongly suspect a PRL-secreting pituitary tumor. However, "pseudoprolactinomas" do occur and are large nonsecretory tumors that press on the pituitary stalk, disrupting the normal inhibitory flow of dopamine from the hypothalamus, resulting in modest elevations in PRL concentrations (typically between 50 and 200 μg/L). It is particularly important to recognize this distinction when deciding on treatment, because PRL-secreting macroadenomas (>10 mm in diameter) usually decrease in size with medical therapy, but "pseudoprolactinomas" do not. (Even though PRL concentrations usually decrease with bromocriptine treatment, pseudoprolactinomas often continue to grow in size.) In patients with pituitary macroadenomas, a PRL concentration <200 μg/L usually indicates the presence of a pseudoprolactinoma, and a PRL concentration >500 μg/L suggests a true PRL-producing tumor. On occasion patients will present with macroprolactinemia, a condition associated with elevated circulatory concentrations of the polymeric forms of PRL with a molecular mass in excess of 100 kDa.

Polymeric forms of PRL lack biological activity; thus none of the sequelae associated with an elevated PRL concentration (sexual dysfunction and galactorrhea) are present. In addition, macroprolactinemia is not associated with either negative or positive feedback effects at the concentration of the hypothalamus, and macroprolactin has not been found in pituitary tissue or cerebrospinal fluid. Thus macroprolactinemia appears confined to the vascular compartment and appears to be due to an atypical complexing of the different isoforms of PRL in the circulation. Macroprolactinemia, although not causative of symptoms associated with an elevated PRL, is troublesome for the clinician and laboratory in terms of interference in standard PRL immunoassays. In one report, almost 20% of patients who presented for a clinical work-up for prolactinoma had hyperprolactinemia attributable to the presence of macroprolactin. Although the prevalence of macroprolactinemia was approximately 1.5% in the population studied, the report suggested that macroprolactinemia is more common than previously realized. Thus clinical laboratories must have a mechanism in place to rule out the presence of a macroprolactinemia early in the work-up of the suspected prolactinoma patients.[122A] Measurement of the recovery of serum PRL following precipitation of the macroprolactin in the sample with polyethylene glycol (PEG) is the most common laboratory approach to look for the presence of macroprolactin.[125A] Gel-filtration chromatography has also been used to separate out the PRL isoforms, but the PEG approach is more practical and appears to effectively expose macroprolactinemia in patients without a pituitary prolactinoma in that PEG can precipitate out most of the isoforms not monomeric in size (>50 kDa).

Measurement of Prolactin

Before immunoassays for PRL became widely available, PRL concentrations were estimated using impractical bioassays based on the growth-promoting action of PRL using the pigeon crop sac or the rat mammary gland, both of which also measure effects of GH and human placental lactogen.[57,92] More sensitive and specific in vitro bioassays for PRL used a mitogenic responsive Nb2 cell line derived from a rat lymphoma.[123] Receptor assays have also been used for measuring PRL; in these assays, lactogenic activity is determined by the ability of specimens to inhibit the binding of radioiodinated hormone to membrane-bound receptors.[117] In general, bioassays and radioreceptor assays for PRL are too impractical, insensitive, and nonspecific for routine use; thus they have been restricted for evaluating PRL bioreactivity when immunoassay results appear to be at variance with the clinical effects of the hormone.

The early development of reliable immunoassays for PRL was hampered by extensive cross-reactivity of the antibodies used and the lack of purified human PRL calibrators. To minimize such problems, heterologous systems in which the hormones used for immunization and labeling were derived from different species were used.[57] As purified human PRL became more readily available, homologous competitive-binding immunoassays were developed for the specific determination of PRL in microliter volumes of serum or plasma specimens.[119] Initially, RIA was the predominant method for measuring PRL. These RIA methods used conventional liquid phase double-antibody techniques to separate antibody-bound and free fractions; others sped up the separation step by using a modified double-antibody approach (e.g., PEG-assisted double-antibody separation, solid phase-linked antibody, or magnetizable solid phase-linked second-antibody techniques).

Performance characteristics of PRL immunoassays varied from one procedure to another.[59] When selecting an RIA method, it was desirable that the method use reagents of human origin, have a wide analytical range linear from 5 to 200 μg/L, show a 50% displacement point in the upper normal reference interval (10 to 20 μg/L), and not be affected by GH concentrations.[6] Because most immunoassays for PRL have an upper limit of measurement of 200 μg/L, a 2× dilution should be performed with results in the 180 to 200 μg/L range and greater to produce an accurate result. Patients with a macroadenoma can have PRL concentrations in the thousands and could be missed if the sample is not diluted properly. The final and absolute concentration reported is an important determinant of the type of clinical management the patient will receive and whether surgical or medical therapy is indicated. For most PRL RIAs, the interlaboratory coefficient of variation ranges from about 5% to 10% at 50 μg/L; the detection limit, defined as the 95% confidence limit at the zero calibrator, is approximately 1 to 3 μg/L; and the cross-reactivity with GH <1%.

Two-site immunometric or "sandwich" assays that made use of two or more antibodies directed at different parts of the PRL molecule were next to be developed. As with other two-site IRMA assays, the capture antibody is attached to a solid phase separation system and the second or signal antibody is labeled with a detection molecule (e.g., radioisotope,[83] enzyme,[18,82,121] fluorophor,[63] or chemiluminescence tag[69]). In some assays, the capture antibody is attached to the wall of test tubes, plastic beads, microtiter plates, ferromagnetic particles, or glass-fiber paper. Other assays have used the strep-avidin approach that couples biotin to the signal antibody with avidin linked to a solid phase. Most of the current immunometric assays for PRL have been adapted to fully automated immunoassay systems. Compared with the older traditional RIA methods, these automated immunometric assays for PRL generally achieve lower detection limits (0.2 to 1.0 μg/L) and improved precision (interlaboratory coefficients of variation of <8% at all concentrations), and have superior specificity (<0.05% cross-reactivity with GH).

Comparison of PRL results yielded by different immunoassay methods, however, provides evidence of considerable variation. Some of these discrepancies relate to the molecular heterogeneity of the different PRL isoforms found in the circulation as previously discussed. All of the isoforms identified possess immunoreactivity, with the monomeric PRL representing more than 75% of the total, big PRL <20%, and big-big PRL <5%.[120] A glycosylated form of the monomeric hormone (G-PRL) predominates in the serum of normal subjects; in hyperprolactinemia and pregnancy, the ratio of G-PRL to PRL decreases. In competitive immunoassay methods, some antisera do not recognize the high molecular weight variants and others, particularly at high PRL concentrations. Immunometric assays tend to give lower estimates of PRL concentration than do competitive immunoassays or bioassays and may not recognize some forms of the hormone. G-PRL, for example, is significantly underestimated in many immunoassays by 50% to 70%.

In view of the fluctuation in the proportion of PRL variants with different molecular masses and immunoreactivities, PRL procedures should be calibrated against reference materials with known international unit potency, such as the WHO first IRP 75/504, the second international standard (IS) 83/562, or the third IS 84/500 (http://www.nibsc.ac.uk). Without such calibration, PRL results expressed in mass units cannot be compared from assay to assay. Despite the heterogeneity of PRL, immunoassays correlate well with bioassays and remain the standard method of measurement in routine practice.

Specimen Collection and Storage

Serum is the specimen of choice for the PRL assay. No special handling procedures are necessary, and samples can be stored at 4 °C for 24 hours. Freezing is preferred when analysis is to be delayed a day or two for maintaining long-term stability. Specimens should be collected 3 to 4 hours after the subject has awakened, because PRL concentrations rise rapidly during sleep and peak in the early morning hours. Emotional stress, exercise, ambulation, and the ingestion of protein all produce a modest elevation in PRL concentrations; thus specimens should be collected after an overnight fast when the patient is resting. Because PRL is secreted episodically, multiple sampling techniques may be advantageous (e.g., pooling equal volumes of sera from specimens drawn at 6- to 18-minute intervals). Blood specimens can also be collected by finger puncture, spotted on filter paper, and stored in air-tight plastic bags. PRL in blood spots is stable for 1 week at room temperature.[10]

Reference Intervals

Representative values using an IRMA are as follows[125]:

		μg/L
Cord blood		45-539
Children		
Tanner stage		
1	Male	<10
	Female	3.6-12
2-3	Male	<6.1
	Female	2.6-18
4-5	Male	2.8-11
	Female	3.2-20
Adults	Male	3.0-14.7
	Female	3.8-23.0
Pregnancy, third trimester		95-473

Comments

Data on reference intervals for a large pediatric population have been published.[28] In view of PRL heterogeneity, there is a strong case for expressing assay results in international units rather than in mass units. Most reagent manufacturers supply a conversion factor for this purpose.

Corticotropin (Adrenocorticotropin) and Related Peptides

Corticotropin is a peptide hormone secreted by the adenohypophysis, one of the derivatives of pro-opiomelanocortin (POMC); it acts primarily on the adrenal cortex, stimulating its growth and the secretion of corticosteroids. Its production is increased during times of stress. It is also known as adrenocorticotropic hormone, ACTH, corticotrophin, adrenocorticotrophin, and adrenocorticotropin.

Biochemistry

Corticotropin and related peptides originate from a large precursor molecule of MW 31 kDa, called POMC. As shown in Figure 50-7, processing of POMC to smaller peptides takes place in both the anterior and intermediate lobes of the pituitary gland (the latter is vestigial in humans except during fetal life and at the end of pregnancy). In the anterior lobe of the pituitary gland, enzymes hydrolyze POMC to β-LPH and a 22-kDa fragment known as *pro-ACTH*. This latter peptide is further processed to ACTH (1-39, a peptide consisting of 39 amino acids) and to a 16-kDa peptide, pro-γ-melanotropin (pro-MSH). β-LPH in turn is cleaved to two smaller peptides, β-endorphin and γ-LPH. Both β-LPH and β-endorphin are released with ACTH from the anterior lobe of the pituitary gland, but only about one third of the β-LPH is converted to β-endorphin. In contrast the intermediate lobe (when present) fully processes β-LPH to β-endorphin, cleaving pro-α-melanotropin (MSH) to α-melanotropin (α-MSH), and splitting ACTH to α-MSH and a corticotropin-like intermediate-lobe peptide. These smaller peptides are found in the human fetus, but only trace amounts exist in the adult human pituitary gland. The changes observed in skin pigmentation in several endocrine diseases (e.g., with adrenal insufficiency) are most likely due to the α-MSH activity of excess ACTH.

In addition to β-endorphin, β-LPH contains the amino acid sequence of another endogenous opioid, *met-enkephalin*. However, this peptide is not the product of β-LPH breakdown, but rather arises from a precursor molecule known as *pro-enkephalin*. Pro-enkephalin is widely distributed in neurons throughout the brain and spinal cord. Some pro-enkephalin is found in the pituitary gland, but most is localized in the catecholamine-synthesizing cells of the adrenal medulla and is co-released with epinephrine and norepinephrine. In the medulla, pro-enkephalin gives rise to met-enkephalin (Tyr-Gle-Gle-Phe-Met) and leu-enkephalin (Tyr-Gle-Gle-Phe-Leu) and to larger opioid peptides. A third family of endogenous opioid peptides is derived from *prodynorphin*, a prohormone stored primarily in the poste-

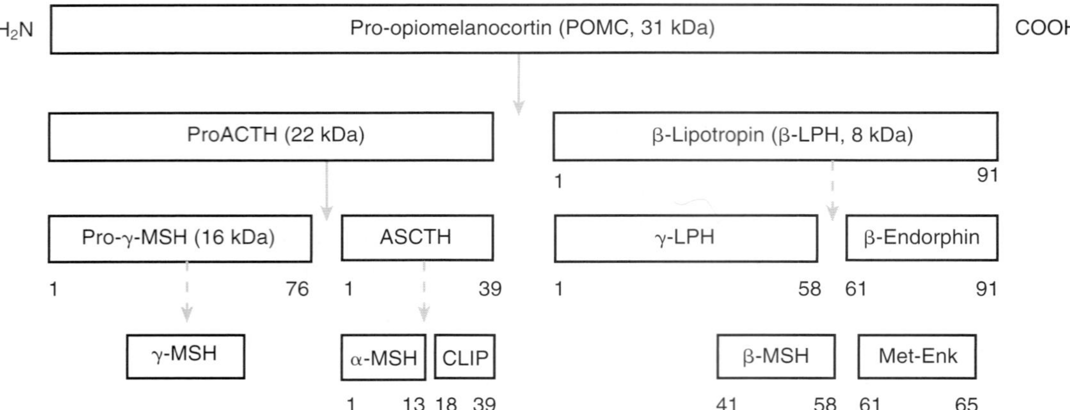

Figure 50-7 Diagrammatic representation of POMC and its precursor relationship to ACTH, β-LPH, α- and β-MSH, and the endorphins.

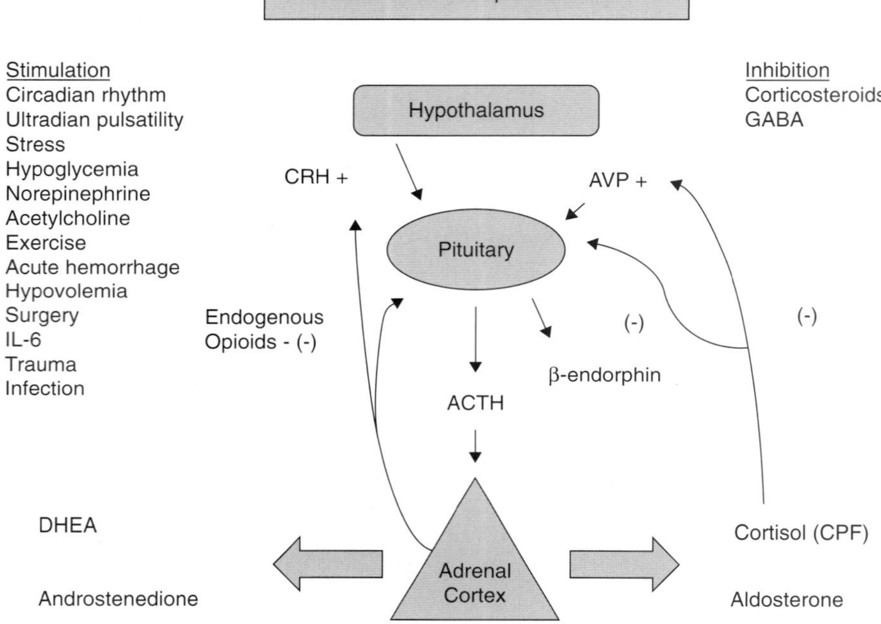

Figure 50-8 The regulatory feedback loop of the hypothalamic-pituitary-adrenal axis. CRH under the influence of neural factors and other modifiable factors that control its pulsatile and circadian secretion acts on the pituitary to produce hormone (ACTH). ACTH in turn stimulates the adrenal gland to form cortisol, aldosterone, dehydroepiandrosterone (DHEA), and androstenedione. Corticosteroids and gamma amino butyric acid (GABA) are inhibitory to CRH and ACTH release, and AVP stimulates ACTH release.

rior lobe of the pituitary gland where it is co-released with vasopressin.

Regulation of Adrenocorticotropin Secretion

Regulation of the secretion of ACTH is described in detail in Chapter 51 and is shown in Figure 50-8. Many variables affect the secretion of ACTH, which is both pulsatile and circadian in nature. Thus the regulation of pituitary secretion of ACTH by the hypothalamus and higher centers is complex. This complex control underscores the importance of the neuroendocrine regulation of stress homeostasis. Cortisol is the major negative feedback hormone for the tonic inhibition of CRH and ACTH release; however, endogenous opioids such as met-enkephalin and β-endorphin formed by the adrenal glands have a down regulatory effect on the hypothalamic-pituitary-ACTH axis as well.

Clinical Significance

Because ACTH synthesis originates from the POMC precursor peptide, its production by the pituitary is closely tied to the secretion of endogenous opiate peptides, such as β-endorphin. The physiological effects of endogenous opiates include (1) sedation, (2) an increased threshold of pain, and (3) autonomic regulation of respiration, blood pressure, and heart rate. These peptides are also involved in modifying endocrine responses to stress and water balance and may play a role in the regulation of reproduction and the immune system. Gonadotropin secretion by the pituitary is under some form of inhibitory control by opioid peptides as evidenced by the effects of β-endorphin analogues on the pulse frequency and amplitude of pituitary LH release. In contrast, β-endorphin antagonists such as naloxone can elicit an increase in the amount and pattern of gonadotropin secretion. ACTH secretion is similarly down regulated by endogenous opioid peptides, and naloxone causes an increase in plasma ACTH concentrations. No diseases, however, have been clearly associated with disordered metabolism of opioid peptides, but changes in their plasma concentrations may accompany other disorders, such as Cushing's disease and depression (increased β-endorphin concentrations)[33] or pheochromocytoma (increased enkephalin concentrations).[136] Altered concentrations of opioids in cerebrospinal fluid may reflect disorders such as chronic pain syndromes, schizophrenia, and depression.

Measurement of ACTH

ACTH has been measured by bioassay, receptor assay, or immunoassay. Most bioassays are based on the effects of ACTH on adrenocortical cells (e.g., the stimulation of steroidogenesis or depletion of ascorbic acid). Responses are usually observed in the adrenal glands of hypophysectomized animals in situ or in isolated adrenal cells in vivo.[94] In general these bioassays are expensive and difficult to perform and are limited to research laboratories. Receptor assays use solubilized binding proteins obtained from normal or neoplastic adrenocortical cells.[74] Only biologically active ACTH is measured, and a 10-pg/mL detection limit has been reported in unextracted plasma. These assays have limited application in the clinical laboratory partly because of the complexity and lability of receptor preparations.

Binding assays that use specific ACTH antibodies are more common than either bioassays or receptor assays. In one of the earliest RIAs, ACTH in unextracted patient specimens competed with radioiodinated hormone for a limited number of antibody binding sites. After a 5- to 7-day incubation period, separation was achieved using either chromatoelectrophoresis or precipitation with talc.[15] Other competitive binding immunoassays have been described for ACTH; they differ in the choice of radiolabel tracer (^{125}I is preferred), separation system (e.g., charcoal adsorption, PEG, or second-antibody precipitation), antisera (e.g., N-terminal or C-terminal specificity), or the need to extract ACTH before assay.[91] Individual immunoassay components (anti-ACTH antisera and ACTH calibrators) and complete reagent test kits continue to be readily available commercially. Most use polyclonal antisera directed at a segment of the biologically active N-terminal portion of the molecule. As expected, these antisera react with intact ACTH (amino acids 1-39) and with ACTH fragments (amino acids 1-24) and precursor molecules, such as POMC and pro-ACTH.[133]

The concentration of ACTH in plasma is normally very low (about 5 to 80 pg/mL in morning specimens). Because most competitive RIAs use antibodies of modest affinity, such procedures that directly measure ACTH in unextracted plasma are usually unable to quantitate low or even low-normal concentrations with confidence (detection limit >15 pg/mL). Various approaches have been used to decrease the ACTH method lower limit of detection. For example, preliminary extraction of 1 to 5 mL of plasma (e.g., by adsorption of ACTH to glass particles, cation-exchange chromatography, and C18 Sep-Pak chromatography) concentrates the specimen and removes nonspecific plasma protein interferences that might otherwise inhibit antigen-antibody binding. Other enhancements include increasing the primary antibody incubation time to several days and using sequential addition of reagents (e.g., preincubate the patient specimen with antibody for 30 minutes before adding the tracer).[50] These maneuvers, however, often add to the complexity of ACTH assays and are less precise and more time consuming than other methods.

Immunometric assays for ACTH that use labeled monoclonal antibodies in noncompetitive formats have also been developed.[42] In these assays, two monoclonal antibodies are directed at different sites on the ACTH molecule (e.g., the N-terminal and C-terminal regions). In terms of assay detection limit, simplicity, and speed, these "two-site sandwich" immunometric assays can detect relatively low ACTH concentrations (1 to 4 pg/mL) with reasonable certainty and are able to distinguish true low from low-normal specimens.[139] Monoclonal immunometric assays also show improved analytical specificity for intact ACTH, but in some cases, they may be too specific and may fail to recognize biologically active and clinically relevant precursors and fragments.[104] Less specific ACTH immunoassays are sometimes used to detect the presence of these peptide fragments in patients with cancer-related syndromes (e.g., ectopic ACTH Cushing's syndrome); a two-site IRMA has also been developed for measuring ACTH precursors in plasma.[30] A direct (unextracted) immunoradiometric test kit for ACTH is commercially available that uses a polyclonal antibody–monoclonal antibody sandwich of the ACTH molecule. The monoclonal antibody is radiolabeled with ^{125}I for detection. A nonisotopic time-resolved immunofluorometric method has also been reported.[34] ACTH assays also have been developed on automated immunoassay platforms using immunochemiluminescence (ICMA)-based methods. These methods are much more precise than the manual methods (coefficients of variation [CVs] <8%) and provide more laboratories with the opportunity to measure ACTH. The enhanced sensitivity of the ICMA methods makes it possible to distinguish low-normal from genuinely depressed concentrations, thus the newer ACTH methods make it possible to measure ACTH at both low and high concentrations.

Numerical results from different ACTH immunoassays may be difficult to compare because of differences in calibration. At present, laboratories and manufacturers of commercial kits usually calibrate their assays against ACTH preparations obtained from research centers, such as human purified ACTH 1-39 (MRC 74/555, 6.2 IU per 25 μg) supplied by the National Institute for Biological Standards and Control (United Kingdom) or synthetic ACTH 1-39 (4.71 IU per 50 μg) supplied by the United States National Hormone and Pituitary Program (NHPP; http://www.humc.edu/hormones/), which was formerly known as the National Pituitary Agency. For comparison purposes, the calibrators used in a particular assay system must be clearly defined.

Specimen Collection and Storage

Proper precautions must be taken in the collection, transportation, and storage of specimens. ACTH is easily oxidized, strongly adsorbs to glass surfaces, and can be rapidly degraded by plasma proteases into immunoreactive fragments during freezing and thawing of the specimen. Factors that influence plasma ACTH, such as prior administration of corticosteroids, time of day at which the specimen is taken (diurnal variation), and stress from a poorly performed venipuncture, must be taken into account. To minimize these problems, it is usually recommended that blood specimens be collected into prechilled polystyrene (plastic) tubes containing EDTA, immediately placed on ice, and centrifuged at 4 °C. Some laboratories also recommend the use of protease inhibitors, such as aprotinin (Trasylol). The supernatant is then transferred to another plastic tube and stored at −20 °C or colder. To protect the ACTH molecule further, antioxidants such as mercaptoethanol may also be used. Immediately before setting up the ACTH assay, frozen specimens should be thawed and centrifuged to remove any fibrin clots, which can interfere with the assay system.

Reference Intervals

Representative values using an IRMA are as follows:

REFERENCE INTERVALS—IRMA METHOD[125]

Adults	0800-0900 hr	8-25 ng/L
	2400 hr (supine)	<10 ng/L

Measurement of Endogenous Opioid Peptides

Beta-endorphin is a frequently measured opioid peptide. Immunoassay is the method of choice for the analysis of plasma β-endorphin. Both RIAs and direct IRMAs[51] have been developed for this purpose. Commercial reagent kits are widely available, and many commercial reference laboratories offer β-endorphin assays. The concentrations of β-endorphin are usually very low to undetectable in normal subjects, and it may be necessary to use extraction procedures to detect meaningful concentrations in plasma. The specificity of commercial antibodies for β-endorphin relative to β-LPH varies widely; in some immunoassays, 50% cross-reactivity is seen with β-LPH. With polyclonal antibodies, results may be spuriously high owing to cross-reactivity with serum immunoglobulin G (e.g., in patients with immunoglobulin G myeloma).[53]

The preferred specimen is plasma with EDTA as the anticoagulant. A typical adult reference interval for specimens collected between 6 AM and 10 AM is 16 to 48 pg/mL (5 to 30 pmol/L).[125]

The measurement of met-enkephalin in plasma is difficult because of its very short half-life (2.5 minutes at 37 °C). Even if blood is immediately chilled on ice and centrifuged under refrigeration, about 50% of the enkephalin is lost unless the specimen is collected with 23 mmol/L of citric acid.[1] Commercial kits for met-enkephalin measurements have been developed, and antienkephalin antibodies are available.

GONADOTROPINS (FOLLICLE-STIMULATING HORMONE, LUTEINIZING HORMONE)

Follicle-stimulating hormone (FSH) is synthesized in the adenohypophysis, and (1) stimulates the growth and maturation of ovarian follicles, (2) stimulates estrogen secretion, (3) promotes the endometrial changes characteristic of the first portion (proliferative phase) of the mammalian menstrual cycle, and (4) stimulates spermatogenesis in the male. It is also called *follitropin*. Luteinizing hormone (LH) is also synthesized in the adenohypophysis and acts with FSH to promote ovulation and secretion of androgens and progesterone. It instigates and maintains the second (secretory) portion of the mammalian estrus and menstrual cycle. In females it is concerned with corpus luteum formation, and in males it stimulates the development and functional activity of testicular Leydig cells. LH is also called *interstitial cell-stimulating hormone* and *lutropin*.

Biochemistry

The glycoprotein hormones of the pituitary (LH, FSH, and TSH) and of the placenta (chorionic gonadotropin [CG]; see Chapter 54) are composed of two peptide chains (usually referred to as α- and β-subunits), each with carbohydrate substituent groups attached. The carbohydrate moiety, which accounts for 15% to 31% of the molecular weight, includes fucose, mannose, galactose, glucosamine, galactosamine, and sialic acid. The α-subunits of these hormones are similar to one another and are interchangeable. For example, the hybrid molecule made up of the α-subunit of TSH and the β-subunit of LH possesses LH activity. The β-subunits display greater differences in amino acid sequences among the various hormones that confer hormonal and immunological specificity. Isolated α-subunits are devoid of biological activity. Isolated β-subunits may have slight intrinsic biological activity, but full activity is attained when α- and β-subunits are recombined. This suggests that the presence of both α- and β-subunits is important for specific receptor recognition, and that the β-subunit is responsible for eliciting the specific biological response. The availability of specific antisera for β-subunits has led to the development of RIA methods targeted for the specific measurements of these structurally similar glycoprotein hormones (see discussion of CG, Chapter 54).

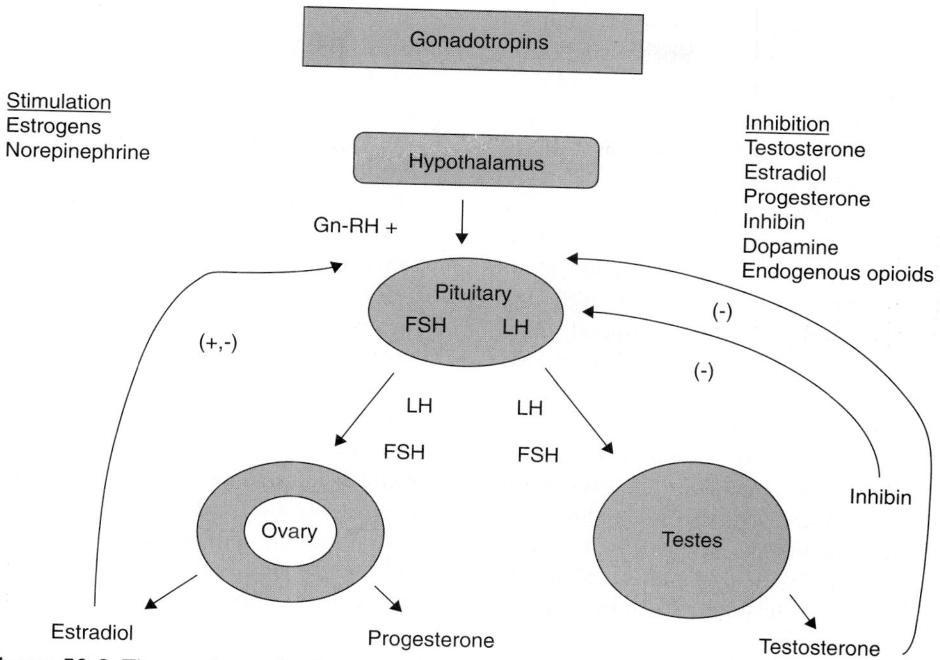

Figure 50-9 The regulatory feedback loop of the hypothalamic-pituitary-gonadal axis. Neural and sensory input from the brain elicits the release of Gn-RH. Gn-RH in turn stimulates the synthesis and release of the gonadotropins FSH and LH, which act on the gonads (ovary and testes) to elicit the ripening and ovulation of the ovary and steroidogenesis (estradiol and progesterone) in the female and spermatogenesis and testosterone production in the male. Inhibin formed by the ovaries and testes along with estradiol and testosterone negatively feeds back to the hypothalamic-pituitary axis to modulate Gn-RH, FSH, and LH release.

The gonadotropic cells of the anterior lobe of the pituitary gland secrete FSH (MW 30 kDa) and LH (MW 32 kDa). In males, LH has in the past been referred to as *interstitial cell–simulating hormone*. Because these two hormones control the functional activity of gonads, they are grouped together under the generic term *gonadotropins*. The regulation of gonadotropin secretion in males and females is shown in Figure 50-9. Pituitary gonadotropin secretion comes under the classic feedback system characteristic of higher centers of control. Estrogen and inhibin regulate LH and FSH secretion, respectively, in the female, and testosterone and inhibin regulate LH and FSH release in the male.

Physiological Action

In females, FSH stimulates the growth of ovarian follicles and, in the presence of LH, promotes secretion of estrogens by the maturing follicles. LH in females causes ovulation and release of the ovum from the ovarian follicle, which has previously ripened under the influence of FSH, and causes luteinization of the ruptured follicle to form the corpus luteum. The corpus luteum then secretes both progesterone and estradiol under the influence of pulsatile LH release. In males, FSH stimulates spermatogenesis by the germ cells in the testes, and LH is responsible for the production of testosterone by the Leydig cells of the testes.

Regulation and Clinical Significance

Regulation of LH and FSH secretion and its clinical significance in reproductive endocrinology are discussed in Chapter 53.

Measurement of Luteinizing Hormone, Follicle-Stimulating Hormone, and Free α-Subunits

Methods for assaying gonadotropins have evolved from bioassays and receptor assays to immunoassays that make use of radioactive and nonisotopic labels. Early in vivo bioassays were based on the direct effects of gonadotropins on the rat ovary, such as depletion of ascorbic acid (by LH) or augmentation of ovarian weight (by FSH).[76] These methods were insensitive and lacked the necessary specificity and precision to measure LH and FSH in small volumes of serum; consequently, they were mainly applied to the assay of urine concentrates. Most bioassays developed in recent years for gonadotropins have gravitated to in vitro techniques. The LH method, for example, measures testosterone synthesis by dispersed rat Leydig cells in response to gonadotropin stimulation.[35] Cultured rat granulosa cells secreting estradiol are used to measure FSH activity in serum.[61] Bioassay methods are still in use today but are primarily tools used in research laboratories investigating the mechanism of action of gonadotropins. Immunoassays have replaced bioassays and receptor assays for gonadotropin measurements in the routine clinical laboratory. A number of different immunoassay methods have been developed for determining FSH and LH in blood and urine, and reliable commercial kits are widely available.[112] RIA steps are similar to those described for other protein hormones. Assays performed by sequential saturation analysis generally give better sensitivity at low hormone concentrations than equilibrium type assays. In a typical delayed addition procedure, specimens, calibrators, and controls are incubated with rabbit antisera for 5 to 7 hours at 4 °C, although some assays require incubation for only 30 minutes at 37 °C. During this time, a significant proportion of LH or FSH becomes bound to the relevant antibody. ^{125}Iodine-labeled hormone is then added, and during a second incubation period (e.g., 16 to 24 hours at 4 °C or 1 hour at room temperature), the label binds to unoccupied binding sites on the antibody. Separation of antibody-bound from free hormone is usually accomplished by precipitation with a second (double) antibody. Inclusion of a high molecular weight polymer, such as PEG, can significantly reduce the incubation time for complete precipitation. Alternatively the second antibody can be coupled to a solid phase support that is centrifuged or sedimented with gravitation. The concentration of gonadotropins in the sample is determined by comparing radioactivity in the specimen tubes with the calibration curve prepared with known concentrations of the relevant gonadotropin. RIAs for LH and FSH are capable of detecting hormone concentrations to a sensitivity of about 1.0 and 0.5 IU/L, respectively. For specimens containing 5 IU/L or more of FSH or LH, between-run CVs average 5% to 10%.[13]

A small number of methods allow for simultaneous determination of FSH and LH in a single assay tube. Double-label RIAs using ^{57}Co-labeled LH and ^{125}I-labeled FSH as tracers are available as commercial kits. Following separation, each radioisotope is determined in the bound fraction by dual isotope counting or by repeat counting. A simultaneous immunofluorometric assay of LH and FSH, based on the use of the fluorescent lanthanides Eu^{3+} and Tb^{3+}, has also been described; each is detected with a time-resolved fluorometer.[54]

The antibodies used in the older RIAs for LH and FSH cross-reacted with each other and with structurally similar glycoprotein hormones, such as TSH and hCG. Assay specificity significantly improved when antisera were produced against the purified beta subunits of both LH and FSH. Currently, most RIAs for FSH show <1% cross-reactivity with LH, TSH, or hCG, or with their free α- or β-chains. In contrast, some RIAs for LH do show cross-reactivity with hCG (10% to 25%), such that LH estimates are invalid in pregnant women or individuals with hCG-secreting tumors.[13] Interference from high blood concentrations of TSH in untreated hypothyroid patients can also produce elevations in LH concentrations.

The introduction of two-site immunometric assays significantly improved the method for gonadotropin measurements. A number of LH and FSH "sandwich" assays became available for manual and automated instrument applications. In some commercial kits, the first antibody is immobilized on test tubes or plastic beads; in others, the antibody is attached to magnetic particles or glass-fiber paper. Multiple signal molecules are associated with the second antibody, including radioisotopes, enzymes,[43,75] fluorophors,[68] and chemiluminescent[79,116] molecules. The analytical advantages of these immunometric assays are significant. For example, hCG interference in LH assays has essentially been eliminated (<0.008% cross-reactivity), better assay precision has resulted (between-assay CVs of <10%), and improvements in assay sensitivity have been realized (detection limits of <0.2 IU/L).[5,13,115] The latter are especially important for use in the evaluation of prepubertal children and patients with hypothalamic disorders when LH concentrations are barely detectable.

The calibration of gonadotropin hormone assays is a difficult task,[24] because producing calibrators that are identical to the analytes found in clinical specimens is confounded by the fact that LH and FSH are not single chemical entities but rather are mixtures of closely related compounds. The earliest reference material used for this purpose was the second IRP for Human Menopausal Gonadotropins. This material was prepared from the urine of postmenopausal women and contained high concentrations of LH and FSH. Because of alterations during metabolism and excretion, however, this urinary calibrator is not appropriate for serum measurements and has been replaced by material derived from the human pituitary gland. Partially purified pituitary extracts, such as the first and second IRPs for FSH and/or LH, were available for many years but have recently been replaced by highly purified pituitary preparations that have high biological potency and low potential for contamination with cross-reacting glycoproteins and their subunits (Table 50-3). Most manufacturers of immunoassay kits for LH and FSH use one or more pituitary reference materials for standardizing their working calibrators. Recombinant gonadotropin calibrators are now available (Table 50-3) that are expected to obviate the problems associated with reference materials isolated from pituitary glands.

Despite enormous improvements in assay design and calibration, discrepancies in results are still obtained when using different immunoassay systems (notably those for LH)[60,129,133]; results can differ by more than 50% even when calibrated with the same reference preparation. The most likely explanation lies with the epitope specificity of the antibodies used in each method. In addition, many glycosylation isoforms exist in patient specimens, and different assays may recognize them differently depending on the antibodies used.[55] In the case of LH, immunometric assays that use monoclonal antibodies give considerably lower values than RIAs that use polyclonal antibodies. This difference is partly a result of the greater specificity of the monoclonal antibodies, which recognize only a subset of LH isoforms and epitopes. Other factors, however, also contribute to method-

TABLE 50-3 Reference Materials for Luteinizing Hormone and Follicle-Stimulating Hormone*

Reference Material	Code No.	Preparation Date	LH Potency	FSH Potency
Second IRP-HMG	—	1964	40	40
First IRP-FSH/LH	69/104	1969	60‡	20†
First IRP-LH	68/40	1974	77‡	—
Second IRP-FSH/LH	78/549	1980	25‡	10‡
First IS-FSH	83/575	1986	—	80§
Second IS-LH	80/552	1988	35‖	—
FSH, human, recombinant for immunoassay	92/510	1997	–	60
FSH, human, urinary (urofollitropin), for bioassay	92/512	1995	—	121
FSH and LH human, urinary for bioassay	98/704	2000	70	72
LH, bovine, for immunoassay	98/566	1985	0.025	—

IRP, International reference preparation; *HMG,* human menopausal gonadotropin; *FSH,* follicle-stimulating hormone; *LH,* luteinizing hormone; *IS,* international standard.

*Information obtained from the World Health Organization Web Page (http://www9.who.int/vaccines/biologicals/KEnd.pdf). Unless otherwise noted, biological potencies were estimated by bioassay and are expressed in International Units (IU) per ampoule.

†In terms of second IRP-HMG, potency is expressed in IU per milligram of an LER-907 preparation.

‡In terms of 69/104.

§In terms of 78/549.

‖In terms of 68/40.

dependent bias, such as differences in calibration procedures and assay matrix.

Several immunoassays have been described for quantifying the free α-subunit of pituitary glycoprotein hormones in serum. As expected, monoclonal antibody–based IRMAs of free α-subunits are more sensitive and specific than are conventional polyclonal RIAs. For example, the free α-subunit IRMA described by Grover and colleagues[49] showed negligible cross-reactivity with intact pituitary glycoprotein hormones (<0.001%) and had adequate sensitivity to detect these subunits in normal nonpregnant individuals and in patients with hormone-secreting tumors (detection limit ~10 ng/L).

Specimen Collection and Storage

Serum is the preferred specimen for gonadotropin measurements; hemolyzed, lipemic, or icteric specimens should not be used. Both hormones are stable for 8 days at room temperature and for 2 weeks at 4 °C; for longer periods, the serum specimen should be stored frozen at or below −20 °C. Because of episodic, circadian, and cyclic variations in the secretion of gonadotropins, a meaningful clinical evaluation of these hormones may require determinations in pooled blood specimens, multiple serial blood specimens, or timed urine specimens. Urine specimens should not contain preservatives; storage at or below −20 °C is recommended.

Reference Intervals

Expected values in serum using a sensitive ("third-generation") immunochemiluminometric assay are as follows[125]:

	LH (IU/L)	FSH (IU/L)
Males, 23-70 yr	1.2-7.8	1.4-15.4
Females		
Follicular phase	1.7-15.0	1.4-9.9
Midcycle peak	21.9-56.6	0.2-17.2
Luteal phase	0.6-16.3	1.1-9.2
Postmenopausal	14.2-52.3	19.3-100.6

	LH (mIU/hr)	FSH (mIU/hr)
Prepubertal	3-97	10-160
Pubertal	20-1800	18-1330
Adult female	190-3350	120-1490
Adult male	550-2500	190-1700

Measurement of Urinary Gonadotropins

Clinically, the pulsatile and episodic release of gonadotropins make a single blood concentration of FSH or LH difficult to interpret. In normal adults, the concentrations of gonadotropins in blood, particularly LH, have been known to differ as much as threefold between samples taken from the same individual 20 minutes apart. In addition, the concentrations in blood with most immunoassays for FSH or LH can often reach the sensitivity limits of the blood assay in normal adults. In the prepubertal child, most blood assays cannot measure normal concentrations because of the low concentration usually encountered in the prepubertal period.

To prevent the problems associated with inadequate detection limits with most blood gonadotropin assays in children and to minimize the episodic secretion of FSH or LH, urine assays have become popular as a means of concentrating the urine sample to improve the detection limits and to integrate the pulsatility of secretion by collecting a urine specimen over a 3-hour period.[112] The kidney essentially integrates the pulsatile secretion over that time period, and the urine can be concentrated eightyfold using an acetone precipitation method to extract the gonadotropins from urine thereby enhancing the sensitivity of the method. Many pediatric endocrinologists favor the urine assay when working up young patients who are suspected of having a pubertal disorder of gonadotropin secretion. Consequently the concentrations of urine FSH and LH are easily detectable in normal prepubertal children when compared with the undetectable concentrations observed in these same normal children when using a blood assay for gonadotropins.

Clinically the measurement of urine FSH and LH using a timed collection (usually 3 hours) allows for integration of the marked pulsatility that occurs with gonadotropin secretion, improves method sensitivity (fiftyfold decrease in detection limit over the serum method), and facilitates the measurement of gonadotropins in young children suspected of a gonadotropin disorder or to test for constitutional delay in adolescence during the latter transition period of puberty.

Thyrotropin

Thyrotropin is a glycoprotein hormone synthesized in the adenohypophysis that promotes the growth of, sustains, and stimulates the hormonal secretion of the thyroid gland. It is also called thyroid-stimulating hormone (TSH).

Biochemistry

With a molecular weight of 26.6 kDa, TSH is secreted by the thyrotroph cells of the anterior lobe of the pituitary gland. TSH is a heterodimer, glycoprotein hormone consists of two noncovalently linked α- and β-subunits with the α-subunit chemically similar to the α- subunits of LH, FSH, and hCG. TSH stimulates the growth and vascularity of the thyroid gland; stimulates the growth of thyroid follicular cells; and promotes a number of the steps in thyroid hormone synthesis, including the uptake of iodine, organification of iodine on to tyrosine, the coupling of tyrosines, and the proteolytic release of stored thyroid hormone from thyroglobulin stores.

Regulation, Clinical Significance, and Methodology

The regulation of TSH secretion, its clinical significance, and methods for determining TSH are discussed in detail in Chapter 52.

Assessment of Anterior Pituitary Lobe Reserve

Evaluation of endocrine function is an important part of the management of patients with pituitary tumors.[14,22] Detection of hormone deficiencies before and after treatment and recognition of hormone-producing tumors are the two objectives of testing of pituitary function in patients with pituitary tumors.[32]

The assessment of anterior and posterior pituitary lobe function in patients with pituitary tumors is important in the identification of clinically significant hormone deficiency states caused by the tumor itself and for the reevaluation of patients after pituitary surgery or irradiation to detect hormone deficiencies that occur as a result of invasive treatment. Testing of pituitary function is usually performed under basal conditions but can be performed under provocative conditions to bring out subtle or mild deficiencies that are observed with disorders of the adrenal gland, thyroid, or gonads. Evaluation of pituitary reserve for GH or PRL is usually unnecessary in adult patients because deficiencies of these hormones are not believed to be clinically important.

The lowered detection limits of the newer two-site immunoassays for the measurement of pituitary hormones now make it possible to distinguish an abnormally low value from the lower end of the normal reference interval. Although assessment of a particular aspect of pituitary function should also include clinical signs and symptoms of hormone deficiency and the measurement of hormones secreted by the pertinent endocrine gland (e.g., T_4, cortisol, and testosterone), the newer, ultrasensitive assays for TSH, FSH, LH, and ACTH allow for an accurate distinction of a true low result from low normal. A scheme for testing of pituitary reserve is listed in Box 50-6.

BOX 50-6 Method of Assessment of Pituitary Reserve

A. Before Pituitary Surgery
- Adrenal glands: measurement of morning serum cortisol concentration or cosyntropin stimulation test
- Thyroid gland: ultrasensitive determination of TSH
- Gonads: sex hormone determinations (estradiol in women and testosterone in men) and gonadotropins

B. Shortly After Pituitary Surgery (2 to 4 days After Surgery)
- Adrenal glands: morning serum cortisol concentration
- Thyroid gland: deferred
- Gonads: deferred

C. One Month After Pituitary Surgery
- Adrenal glands: cosyntropin stimulation test
- Thyroid gland: ultrasensitive determination of TSH concentration
- Gonads: sex hormone determinations (estradiol in women and testosterone in men)

TSH, Thyroid-stimulating hormone.

Hypothalamic-Pituitary-Adrenal Axis

A normal morning serum cortisol concentration is usually adequate evidence that the hypothalamic-pituitary-adrenal axis is intact and functioning properly. On occasion, however, the *Synacthen stimulation test* is used when the morning cortisol results are low or equivocal (<5 µg/dL) or when there is a strong clinical suspicion of adrenal insufficiency (see Table 51-1). This provocative test is performed by obtaining a baseline blood specimen for cortisol followed by the intravenous (IV) administration of 250 µg of Synacthen (a potent analogue of ACTH). Specimens for cortisol are then obtained at 30 and 60 minutes after IV administration of the synthetic ACTH. A peak value for plasma cortisol of >18 µg/dL is considered a normal response to ACTH administration.

Results of tests of the entire hypothalamic-pituitary-adrenal axis, such as the *insulin tolerance test* (also called the *insulin-induced hypoglycemia stimulation test;* see Box 50-3), occasionally are abnormal in patients who have a normal morning cortisol concentration, a normal response to exogenous ACTH, and no signs of adrenal insufficiency. Although an abnormality in these sensitive tests suggests some diminution of ACTH reserve, the clinical significance of such impairment in this setting is not clear. These tests should be reserved for patients who are strongly suspected of having adrenal insufficiency or whose morning cortisol concentration or response to ACTH has been found to be abnormal. Standard protocols for the performance and interpretation of these tests have been published. These tests involve some patient risk and discomfort and should be performed only under the direct supervision of an experienced physician.

Measurement of ACTH in blood collected either at baseline or after stimulation with insulin adds little to the utility of the above tests and is not generally recommended. In fact, in patients who have undergone pituitary surgery, it takes some time before the cortisol negative feedback loop to ACTH secretion is normalized. ACTH and cortisol measurements after administration of CRH are potentially a direct test of pituitary ACTH reserve. However, the insulin-induced hypoglycemia test is currently the definitive test of ACTH and/or cortisol reserve. This test, however, is contraindicated in patients with a history of coronary heart disease, seizure disorder, and general debility.

Hypothalamic-Pituitary-Thyroid Axis

When the serum free thyroxine concentration (FT_4) or ultrasensitive TSH result is normal, the hypothalamic-pituitary-thyroid axis is assumed to be intact. If primary hypothyroidism is suspected clinically, however, a single measurement of a basal TSH concentration may be sufficient to confirm the diagnosis. In patients with a history of pituitary disease and secondary hypothyroidism, the serum TSH concentration is frequently normal; thus in this situation, an FT_4 concentration is the better test to gauge normality of the hypothalamic-pituitary-thyroid axis. On occasion a TRH *stimulation test* is used to distinguish hypothalamic dysfunction from pituitary disease. This test is accomplished by drawing a blood specimen for measurement of baseline TSH concentrations, administering 500 µg of TRH intravenously, and collecting additional specimens for TSH measurements at 30, 45, and 60 minutes after IV injection. A normal response to TRH is a fivefold to tenfold increase in the serum TSH concentrations within 60 minutes after TRH administration. An impaired response in a patient with a low serum FT_4 concentration indicates a pituitary abnormality, whereas a delayed peak (at 45 or 60 minutes) suggests hypothalamic dysfunction. A blunted response is observed in patients with hyperthyroidism. With the availability of better third-generation tests for TSH (see Chapter 52), the TRH stimulation test is now rarely used.

Hypothalamic-Pituitary-Gonadal Axis

History and physical examination are extremely helpful in evaluating the status of the hypothalamic-pituitary-gonadal axis, particularly in women during their reproductive years.[3,81] Normal menstrual cycles are usually indicative of an intact hypothalamic-pituitary-gonadal axis in reproductive-age women. Baseline laboratory assessment for hypothalamic-pituitary-gonadal dysregulation should include measurement of serum gonadotropins (LH and FSH) and sex steroids (estradiol in females and testosterone in males). Provocative testing of this axis with Gn-RH and measurements of FSH and LH (Box 50-7) are useful in selected patients. These tests, however, can be unreliable in differentiating pituitary disorders from hypothalamic

BOX 50-7 Protocol for the Gonadotropin-Releasing Hormone (Gn-RH) Stimulation Test for Luteinizing Hormone (LH) and Follicle-Stimulating Hormone (FSH) Reserve

Rationale The hypothalamic releasing hormone Gn-RH stimulates release of both LH and FSH in normal individuals. Subnormal responses are seen in some patients with pituitary or hypothalamic disorders. However, the magnitude of LH and FSH response to Gn-RH is usually predictable from the basal LH and FSH concentrations. This test may be useful in patients in whom the clinical picture and basal gonadotropin measurements are inconclusive.

Procedure The test may be performed without regard for previous feeding or time of day. After baseline specimens are obtained for LH or FSH determination, or both, 100 µg Gn-RH is given intravenously. Samples for LH or FSH determination, or both, should be drawn every 15 to 30 minutes for 1 to 2 hours.

Interpretation LH response should increase by threefold to tenfold. The FSH response is of lesser magnitude (usually a 1.5- to 3-fold increase). The peak responses for both LH and FSH occur between 15 and 30 minutes. Patients with pituitary disorders may have normal, diminished, or absent responses. In patients with hypothalamic disorders, the response may be exaggerated, normal, diminished, or absent.

dysfunction; thus the physician is usually dependent on an accurate determination of gonadotropins and sex steroids along with clinical judgment.

Preoperative Endocrine Testing: A Simple Approach

Initial Assessment

Pituitary reserve is almost never compromised in patients with small pituitary tumors, so testing is usually limited to patients with large tumors or specific clinical indications (see Box 50-6, *A*). For most patients with large pituitary tumors, in addition to history and physical examination, an adequate evaluation of endocrine function before surgery can be performed based on laboratory measurements of serum PRL, TSH, LH, FSH, sex steroids (testosterone in males and estradiol in females), serum sodium, and results of a morning serum cortisol or ACTH stimulation test.

After Pituitary Surgery

The optimum time for retesting endocrine function after pituitary surgery is not generally known (see Box 50-6, *B*). At the M.S. Hershey Medical Center (Hershey, Pa.), the following protocol is used (Figure 50-10):

"Stress" steroid coverage with hydrocortisone is administered immediately before, during, and after surgery. If adrenal function is normal before surgery, steroid coverage is usually stopped on the second or third postoperative day and a morning blood sample for plasma cortisol concentration is obtained 24 hours later. If the morning plasma cortisol concentration is 5 μg/dL or less, ACTH deficiency is likely and steroid coverage is reinstituted and continued after discharge from the hospital. If the plasma cortisol concentration is 10 μg/dL or greater, the hypothalamic-pituitary-adrenal axis is presumed to be normal and steroid coverage is no longer mandated. Patients with a morning plasma cortisol concentration between 5 and 10 μg/dL should either have normal adrenal function confirmed with provocative testing (i.e. metyrapone test) or should be started back on hydrocortisone coverage.

Follow-Up Testing After Pituitary Surgery

It is advisable to wait until 1 month after surgery to evaluate thyroid function (measurement of TSH concentration) and gonadal function (measurement of testosterone concentration in males and estradiol concentration in females; see Box 50-6, *C*). Early treatment of thyroid and gonadal deficiencies is not critical, and misleading test results might be obtained in the early postoperative period. Adrenal function should be reassessed with an ACTH stimulation test 1 month after surgery, even if pituitary function was subnormal soon after surgery; ACTH deficiency after pituitary surgery is often transient. Periodic clinical follow-up and laboratory assessment should be tailored to the individual patient's circumstances.

After pituitary irradiation, patients should be evaluated every six months with an FT_4 and TSH measurement, sex steroid determination, and ACTH stimulation testing.

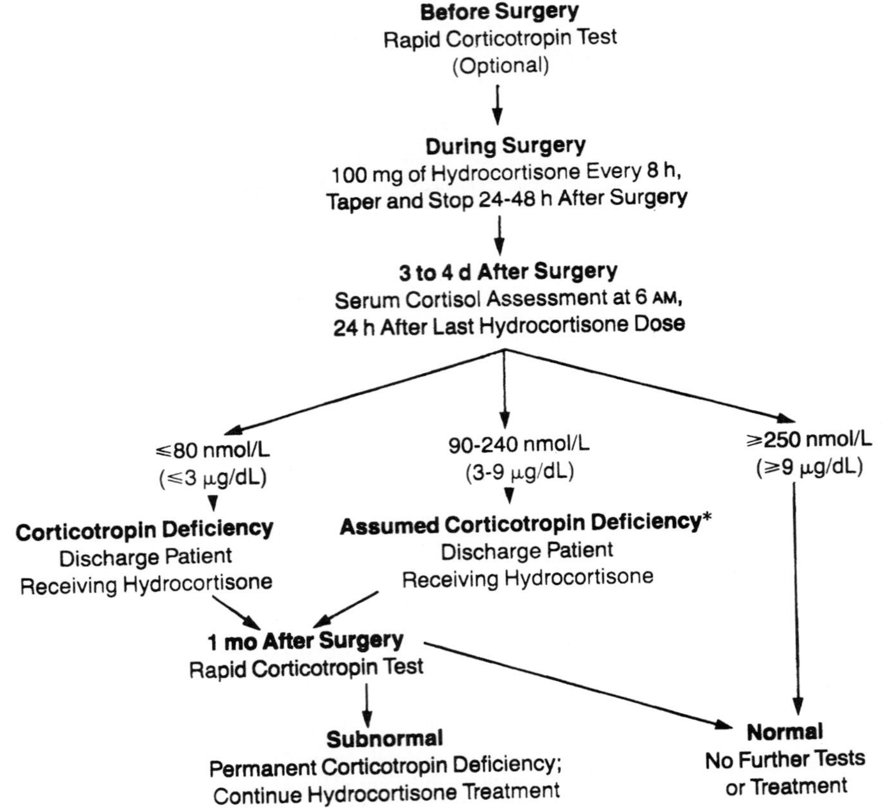

Figure 50-10 Algorithm for evaluation of the hypothalamic-pituitary-adrenal axis after transsphenoidal pituitary surgery. *(From Watts NB, Tindall GT. Rapid assessment of corticotropin reserve after pituitary surgery. JAMA 1988;259:708-11. Copyright 1988, American Medical Association. Used with permission.)*

NEUROHYPOPHYSIS

The neurohypophyseal system is composed of neural tissue and neurons of the supraoptic and paraventricular nuclei of the hypothalamus. These neurons are located in and travel through the median eminence and pituitary stalk, with the nerve endings projecting to the posterior lobe of the pituitary gland. The cell bodies of these neurons synthesize and secrete *oxytocin* and arginine vasopressin (AVP); the latter is also called *antidiuretic hormone (ADH)*. Oxytocin and AVP are nonapeptides (MW 1080 Da) consisting of a cyclic hexapeptide and a three–amino acid side chain. Most mammals secrete vasopressin and oxytocin, with the exception of the pig and hippopotamus, in which lysine vasopressin (contains lysine rather than arginine in position 8) is released. The structure of oxytocin is similar to that of AVP (Figure 50-11) but with isoleucine rather than phenylalanine at position 3 and leucine instead of arginine at position 8.

ARGININE VASOPRESSIN

AVP is formed by neuronal cells of hypothalamic nuclei and stored in the neurohypophysis. In humans, it contains arginine at position 8. (In pigs, lysine is found at position 8.) AVP stimulates contraction of the muscles of capillaries and arterioles, raising blood pressure; promotes contraction of the intestinal musculature, increasing peristalsis; exerts contractile influence on the uterus; and has a specific effect on the epithelial cells of renal collecting tubules, augmenting resorption of water independently of solutes to cause concentration of urine and dilution of blood serum. Its rate of secretion is regulated chiefly by the osmolarity of the plasma.

Biochemistry

AVP is synthesized as part of a large precursor molecule (preprovasopressin) in conjunction with a specific neurophysin-binding protein; the latter serves as a carrier protein for it during axonal transport and storage. Oxytocin is also synthesized as part of a preprohormone along with a separate neurophysin-binding protein. These molecular complexes are packaged into secretory granules that migrate down the nerve axons for 12 to 14 hours before reaching the posterior pituitary lobe for storage. Release of the neurohypophyseal hormones into the portal circulation occurs via calcium-dependent exocytosis on nerve cell stimulation. When a stimulus for secretion of either vasopressin or oxytocin occurs, the stimulus acts on the appropriate magnicellular cell body in the hypothalamus, sending an action potential down the long axon to the posterior pituitary, causing an influx of calcium and the release of hormone from neurosecretory granules. At the physiological pH of plasma, AVP and oxytocin circulate mainly in unbound forms.

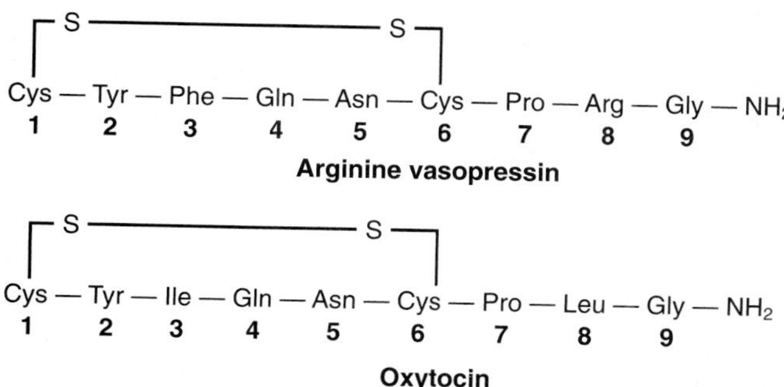

Figure 50-11 The amino acid sequence of AVP and oxytocin.

Regulation of Secretion

The tonicity (osmolality) of blood falls largely under direct control of vasopressin secretion. Osmoreceptors located in cell bodies in or near the magnicellular nuclei of the hypothalamus respond to changes in plasma osmolality. As little as a 2% increase in extracellular fluid osmolality can cause shrinkage of osmoreceptor cells with stimulation of AVP release from the posterior pituitary lobe (Figure 50-12). A plasma osmolality above 280 mOsm/kg is considered the osmotic threshold for AVP release.

Besides the osmoreceptor mechanism of vasopressin release, the physiological regulation of vasopressin secretion also involves a pressure-volume mechanism that is distinct from the osmotic sensor. AVP release is regulated by baroreceptors that respond to alterations in blood volume. For example, a reduction in plasma volume or arterial pressure,

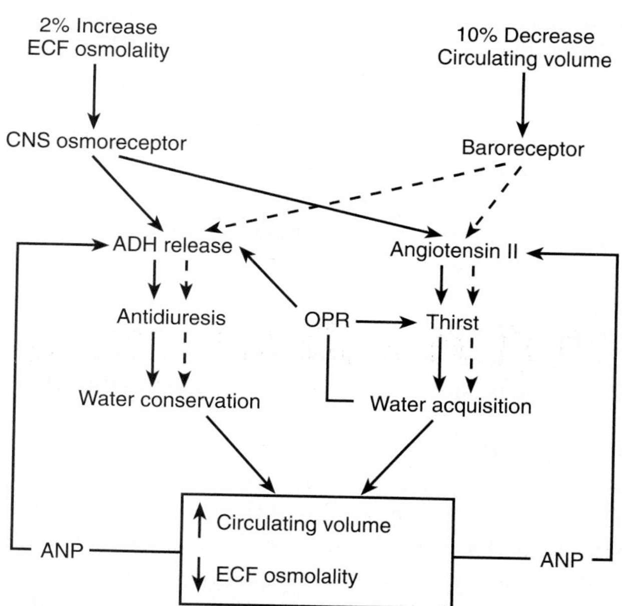

Figure 50-12 Key elements in water homeostasis. *Solid lines* indicate osmotically stimulated pathways, and *dashed lines* indicate volume-stimulated pathways. The *dotted lines* indicate negative feedback pathways. Abbreviations: *ANP,* atrial natriuretic peptide; *AVP,* arginine vasopressin; *CNS,* central nervous system; *ECF,* extracellular fluid; *OPR,* oropharyngeal reflex. *(From Reeves W, Andreoli T. The posterior pituitary and water metabolism. In: Wilson JD, Foster DW, eds. Williams textbook of endocrinology, 8th ed. Philadelphia: WB Saunders Co, 1992:312.)*

or both, stimulates vasopressin secretion. Other nonosmotic stimuli for AVP release include pain, stress, sleep, exercise, and chemical agents such as catecholamines, angiotensin II, opiates, prostaglandins, anesthetics, nicotine, and barbiturates. An increase in plasma volume or a decrease in plasma osmolality was previously thought to inhibit the release of AVP directly. It now seems likely that atrial natriuretic peptide provides some negative feedback for vasopressin release. Agents such as alcohol, phenytoin, and glucocorticoids can inhibit vasopressin release, leading to a water diuresis and physiological dehydration.

The thirst center is regulated by many of the same factors that determine AVP release. This center has a higher set point than the osmoreceptors and responds to osmolalities above 290 mOsm/kg. Responses involving AVP, thirst, and the kidney are coordinated in a complex scheme to maintain plasma osmolality in healthy individuals within a narrow range (284 to 295 mOsm/kg).

Physiological Actions

The major physiological function of vasopressin is the control of water homeostasis at the concentration of the kidney through the regulation of water permeability in the collecting tubules and ascending limb of Henle's loop (see Chapter 45). These effects, which are mediated through the adenylate cyclase system, allow the kidney to reabsorb water and concentrate urine. A further action of AVP is expressed by the "pressin" part of its name.[44] When released in sufficient quantity, AVP induces a generalized vasoconstriction that leads to a rise in arterial blood pressure. AVP is believed to play an important role in the maintenance of arterial blood pressure during blood loss. Release of vasopressin into the pituitary portal system also augments the action of CRH in stimulating the release of ACTH from the adenohypophysis. However, AVP does not appear to affect the release of other anterior pituitary hormones.

Clinical Significance

Disorders of AVP activity have been divided into hypofunction (diabetes insipidus) and hyperfunction (syndrome of inappropriate antidiuretic hormone secretion [SIADH]).

Polyuric States

Deficient production or action of vasopressin results in polyuria caused by the failure of the renal tubules to reabsorb solute-free water.[9] Under normal circumstances, urine output is largely dependent on fluid intake; thus an arbitrary limit for normal urine output cannot be defined. When urine output is >2.5 L/day, an investigation is usually indicated; with complete deficiency of AVP, urine output may approach 1 L/hr. If the thirst response is normal, increased ingestion of fluid (polydipsia) will follow. If access to water is not restricted, plasma osmolality and serum electrolytes will usually remain normal.

Polyuric states are divided into three main categories: (1) deficient AVP production (hypothalamic diabetes insipidus [HDI]), (2) deficient AVP action on the kidney (nephrogenic diabetes insipidus [NDI]), and (3) excessive water intake (psychogenic polydipsia). An osmotic diuresis may also produce polyuria and polydipsia. Uncontrolled diabetes mellitus with a high glucose load to the kidney is a common cause of an osmotic diuresis.

Hypothalamic Diabetes Insipidus. This is also called *neurogenic, central,* or *cranial diabetes insipidus.* HDI is caused by a failure of the pituitary gland to secrete normal amounts of AVP in response to osmoregulatory factors. Increased fluid intake promoted by thirst mechanisms prevents severe dehydration. When the thirst center is also abnormal, severe dehydration can occur. Destruction of 80% of vasopressin-secreting neurons is required to produce HDI; injury to the neurohypophysis may cause a transient diabetes insipidus. The incidence of HDI is about 1 in 25,000 people. In 30% of patients, HDI occurs without apparent cause; other cases are associated with neoplastic diseases, neurological surgery, head trauma, ischemic or hypoxic disorders, granulomatous diseases, infections, or autoimmune disorders. A hereditary form of the disorder is transmitted as an autosomal dominant trait, and the vasopressin gene defect responsible for this disorder has been identified. The genetic abnormality has been described at the concentration of the preprohormone for vasopressin, preventing normal cleavage of the signal peptide at the carboxy terminus of preprovasopressin. Although rare, diabetes insipidus can present in pregnancy as a result of high circulating activities of the enzyme cysteine aminopeptidase (vasopressinase) that inactivates vasopressin. The etiology of this phenomenon has not been delineated, but is believed to be a result of placental release of vasopressinase.

Nephrogenic Diabetes Insipidus. Failure of the kidney to respond to normal or increased concentrations of AVP can cause NDI. In the majority of these patients, AVP is incapable of stimulating cyclic adenosine monophosphate (cAMP) formation. Two causes have been described for this disorder: (1) mutation in the vasopressin receptor and (2) mutations in the aquaporin-2 water channels. The vasopressin receptor mutation form of NDI is an X-chromosome–linked disorder that mostly affects males. Females are more likely to have the aquaporin-2 water channel gene defect on chromosome 12,q12-13, which produces an autosomal recessive disease. Acquired forms of NDI may be caused by metabolic disorders (hypokalemia, hypercalcemia, and amyloidosis), drugs (lithium, demeclocycline, and barbiturates), and renal diseases (polycystic disease and chronic renal failure). NDI may also be seen in the absence of these factors (idiopathic).

Psychogenic or Primary Polydipsia. A chronic, excessive intake of water suppresses AVP secretion and produces hypotonic polyuria. The polyuria and polydipsia are usually not as sustained as in HDI or NDI; nocturnal polyuria also is less frequent. Psychogenic factors are most commonly associated with this disorder, but hypothalamic disease affecting the thirst center may be a cause. Drugs also can affect the thirst center and result in primary polydipsia.

BOX 50-8 Diagnosis of Diabetes Insipidus

1. Document polyuria (urine volume >2.5 L/day) and exclude glycosuria. If desired, creatinine excretion can be measured as an estimate of completeness of urine collections; substances that influence ADH secretion should be avoided (e.g., nicotine, alcohol, and caffeine). If plasma osmolality is ≥295 mOsm/kg or if serum sodium concentration ≥145 mmol/L, primary polydipsia is unlikely; proceed with the overnight water deprivation test (Box 50-9) or the hypertonic saline infusion test (Box 50-10).
2. Overnight water deprivation test (Box 50-9): If the ratio of urine to plasma osmolality is <1.5 at the end of the test, primary polydipsia is unlikely. Measure plasma and urine osmolalities and plasma ADH concentrations at the end of the test; use these relationships to differentiate normal, nephrogenic, or hypothalamic diabetes insipidus, and psychogenic polydipsia. If urine osmolality is ≤400 mOsm/kg at the end of the test, give 5 U of aqueous vasopressin subcutaneously. If urine osmolality increases ≥10%, hypothalamic diabetes insipidus is probable; if urine osmolality does not increase, nephrogenic diabetes insipidus is highly probable.
3. Hypertonic saline infusion test (Box 50-10): Plot plasma osmolality versus plasma ADH concentration.

ADH, Antidiuretic hormone.

Diagnostic Studies. A differential diagnosis of polyuric states can be made using measurements of plasma and urine osmolality and plasma AVP concentrations; a recommended strategy is shown in Box 50-8.

The classic approach to the diagnosis of polyuric disorders is the *overnight water deprivation test* usually conducted in a hospital setting because of immediate concerns of profound hypotension and possible death (Box 50-9).[87,102] If access to water is denied, patients with HDI or NDI cannot conserve free water and thus show weight loss, hypernatremia, and an increase in plasma osmolality; urine osmolality remains low and is often less than that of plasma. Once urine osmolality is stabilized, aqueous vasopressin is given subcutaneously, and urine osmolality is measured 60 minutes later. An increase in urine osmolality of >10% suggests HDI, whereas failure to increase urine osmolality after vasopressin injection supports the diagnosis of NDI. Most patients with psychogenic polydipsia usually have a normal urine osmolality after water deprivation, but some of these patients can fail to produce concentrated urine unless water deprivation is prolonged. When psychogenic polydipsia is suspected, the patient should be given a minimum of 1 L of normal saline IV to reestablish the renal medullary concentrating gradient so that the patient can respond appropriately to AVP.

Measurements of AVP in plasma or urine can also be used to establish the correct diagnosis in difficult cases (Figure 50-13). After water deprivation, patients with HDI have low or inappropriately normal plasma vasopressin concentrations relative to a high plasma osmolality or low urine osmolality; patients with NDI have high plasma concentrations of vasopressin when plasma osmolality exceeds 300 mOsm/kg and low urine osmolality; and patients with primary polydipsia have normal concentrations of vasopressin relative to their plasma osmolality.[12] Because AVP concentrations discriminate best when plasma osmolality is high, vasopressin can also be measured after hypertonic saline is administered to the patient (Box 50-10); this saline infusion test is usually not needed unless results of the water deprivation test are inconclusive.

BOX 50-9 Protocol for the Overnight Water Deprivation Test

Rationale Dehydration provides a strong stimulus for ADH release, which can be assessed indirectly by measuring urine osmolality or directly by measuring plasma ADH. If urine remains hyposmolal during water deprivation, the administration of ADH helps differentiate HDI from NDI.

Procedure This test can be conducted if the plasma osmolality is <295 mOsm/kg. The patient is weighed at 22:00 at which time plasma and urine specimens are collected for the determination of sodium and osmolality. No oral intake is allowed until the test is terminated. Care is taken to ensure that the patient's body weight does not decrease by more than 5% during the test. Beginning at 6:00, the patient is weighed again. Urine is collected hourly for measurement of volume and determination of osmolality. When urine osmolality is stable (a change of ≤30 mOsm/kg for 2 consecutive hours, which usually takes 8 to 12 hours to occur), specimens are collected for plasma osmolality (and plasma ADH, if desired). Five units of aqueous vasopressin (ADH) are given subcutaneously, and urine osmolality is measured 1 hour later. The test is then terminated.

Interpretation Normal individuals will lose 3% or less of body weight, will not develop an elevated serum sodium or plasma osmolality, and will produce a concentrated urine (osmolality ≤400 mOsm/kg) with no further increase in urine osmolality after ADH administration. Patients with HDI show an increase in plasma osmolality and serum sodium; their urine will be less concentrated than normal (≤400 mOsm/kg, but often less than plasma) and plasma ADH concentrations will not rise normally; and urine osmolality will increase by 10% or greater after ADH administration. Patients with NDI show plasma and urine osmolalities that are similar to those of patients with HDI during water dehydration; however, they show high ADH concentrations as the plasma osmolality exceeds 300 mOsm/kg. Also, they will not show a significant increase in urine osmolality after ADH injection. In patients with psychogenic polydipsia, normal responses may be seen; however, the period of water deprivation may need to be prolonged. Measuring plasma ADH in response to hypertonic saline (see Box 50-11) may be needed if the diagnosis remains unclear.

ADH, Antidiuretic hormone; *HDI*, hypothalamic diabetes insipidus; *NDI*, nephrogenic diabetes insipidus.

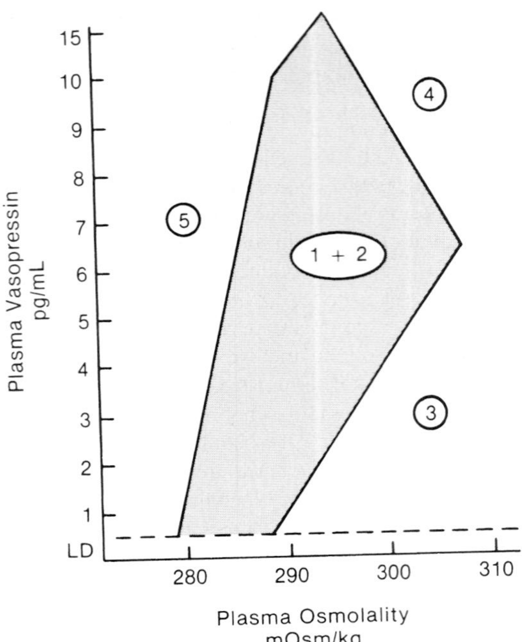

Figure 50-13 Retention of plasma vasopressin to osmolality. *Regions 1 and 2* represent the normal reference interval and values seen in subjects with psychogenic polydipsia. *Region 3* indicates central diabetes insipidus, *Region 4* is NDI, and *Region 5* is SIADH. LD denotes the lowest detectable plasma vasopressin correlation with this assay. *(Modified and abstracted from Zerbe RL, Robertson GL. A comparison of plasma vasopressin measurements with a standard indirect test in the differential diagnosis of polyuria. N Engl J Med 1981;305:1539-46.)*

BOX 50-10 Protocol for the Saline Infusion Test for Diabetes Insipidus

Rationale An increase in plasma osmolality is a strong stimulus for release of ADH. The administration of hypertonic saline intravenously will produce a hyperosmolal state, causing a rise in plasma ADH concentration. Plasma ADH concentration can be plotted against plasma osmolality and compared with a nomogram.

Procedure An intravenous infusion of 3% saline is begun at a minimum rate to maintain flow; two baseline blood specimens are drawn 15 minutes apart for plasma osmolality and ADH determination. The rate of saline infusion is then adjusted to 0.1 mL/kg/min and maintained with an infusion pump for 2 hours. Blood specimens are collected for plasma osmolality and ADH measurement every 15 minutes during this 2-hour period.

Interpretation Normal subjects show a plasma ADH that is >7 pg/mL when plasma osmolality is ≥310 mOsm/kg.

ADH, Antidiuretic hormone.

Syndrome of Inappropriate Antidiuretic Hormone Secretion (SIADH)

The autonomous, sustained production of AVP in the absence of known stimuli for its release is called SIADH. In this syndrome, plasma AVP concentrations are "inappropriately" increased relative to a low plasma osmolality and to a normal or increased plasma volume. SIADH may be the result of one of several factors: production of vasopressin by a malignancy (such as a small cell carcinoma of the lung), the presence of acute and chronic diseases of the central nervous system, pulmonary disorders, or a side effect of certain drug therapies. In addition, as many as 10% of patients undergoing pituitary surgery have a transient SIADH approximately 8 to 9 days after surgery (when the patient is at home), which responds to water restriction (2 to 3 days) and resolves without recurrence. In SIADH, a primary excess of AVP, coupled with unrestricted fluid intake, promotes increased reabsorption of free water by the kidney. The result is a decreased urine volume and an increased urine sodium concentration and urine osmolality. As a consequence of water retention, these patients become modestly volume expanded. The increase in intravascular volume causes hemodilution accompanied by dilutional hyponatremia and a low plasma osmolality. Volume expansion also decreases renal sodium reabsorption and thus further increases the urine sodium concentration.

The most common cause of hyponatremia in hospital patients is SIADH.[2] However, other disorders can cause dilutional hyponatremia and must be differentiated from SIADH. These conditions include (1) congestive heart failure, (2) renal insufficiency, (3) nephrotic syndrome, (4) liver cirrhosis, and (5) hypothyroidism. Excessive administration of hypotonic fluids and treatment with drugs that stimulate AVP (e.g., chlorpropamide, vincristine, clofibrate, carbamazepine, nicotine, phenothiazines, and cyclophosphamide) can cause dilutional hyponatremia as well. Hyponatremia may also occur from renal or extrarenal sodium losses (depletional hyponatremia) as a result of vomiting, diarrhea, excessive sweating, diuretic abuse, salt-losing nephropathy, or mineralocorticoid deficiency.

The clinical manifestations of hyponatremia are nonspecific; weakness and apathy occur in mild cases, and central nervous system changes (lethargy, coma, and seizures) are present in more severe cases. No signs or symptoms are specific for SIADH. History, physical examination, and routine laboratory test results often suggest that hyponatremia is dilutional or depletional.

Measurements of sodium and osmolality in blood and urine, combined with a clinical assessment of volume status, usually permit the appropriate differential diagnosis of hyponatremic conditions (Box 50-11). The typical patient with SIADH has a hyposmolar plasma (<270 mOsm/kg), a urine osmolality that is slightly greater than that of plasma, and a urine sodium concentration that is inappropriately elevated (~40 to 80 mmol/L). Patients with dilutional hyponatremia resulting from excess water intake have a hypotonic plasma, an unremarkable urine sodium concentration (<20 mmol/L), and a dilute urine (a urine osmolality that is less than that of plasma). Patients with depletional

BOX 50-11 Diagnosis of Syndrome of Inappropriate Antidiuretic Hormone (SIADH)

Document plasma hypoosmolality (≤275 mOsm/kg) and hyponatremia (sodium concentration of ≤130 mmol/L). Use history, physical examination, and appropriate laboratory tests to exclude cardiac, hepatic, renal, thyroid, or adrenal failure; and the effects of pituitary surgery, diuretic therapy, or medications known to stimulate ADH release. (SIADH cannot be diagnosed unless these factors are corrected.) Measure the urine sodium concentration and osmolality. Urine osmolality greater than plasma osmolality and without correspondingly low urine sodium concentration (usually >60 mmol/L) indicates that SIADH is probable. If further tests seem to be indicated: (1) Perform water loading test (Box 50-12). Use with caution. Normal results exclude SIADH. (2) Measure plasma ADH and plasma renin concentrations. SIADH is characterized by high ADH concentration and low renin concentration. If plasma ADH and renin concentrations are both low, a primary defect in renal water excretion is present.

ADH, Antidiuretic hormone; *SIADH,* syndrome of inappropriate antidiuretic hormone.

BOX 50-12 Protocol for the Water Loading Test for Syndrome of Inappropriate Antidiuretic Hormone (SIADH)

Rationale An excess of ADH leads to hyponatremia, because it interferes with the ability of the kidneys to excrete a water load normally. This test is useful if SIADH is suspected in a patient with normal or near-normal serum sodium and plasma osmolality or in a patient with "reset osmostat." This test should not be performed in patients who are already significantly hyponatremic because of the danger that the water load will worsen the hyponatremia.

Procedure The test is started in the morning 2 hours after the patient has eaten a light breakfast. Plasma and urine osmolalities are measured. The patient is given water to drink (20 mL/kg) over a 15- to 30-minute period; lightly salted crackers may be given with the water if needed. The patient is kept in a recumbent position, and specimens are taken hourly for the next 4 hours for assessment of plasma and urine osmolality. Total urine output is measured.

Interpretation Plasma osmolality should decrease by ≥5 mOsm/kg, and urine osmolality should drop to ≤100 mOsm/kg, with 90% or more of the water load excreted in 4 hours. SIADH is characterized by excretion of <90% of the water load and by urine osmolality that remains at >100 mOsm/kg. Plasma ADH may be measured at 90 or 120 minutes after the water loading to confirm the diagnosis. Subnormal responses are seen with glucocorticoid deficiency, hypothyroidism, and renal diseases.

ADH, Antidiuretic hormone; *SIADH,* syndrome of inappropriate antidiuretic hormone.

hyponatremia caused by extrarenal sodium loss have hypotonic plasma, a low urine sodium concentration (usually <20 mmol/L), and a urine osmolality that is greater than that of plasma; patients with depletional hyponatremia caused by impaired renal conservation of sodium have similar results except that their urine sodium concentrations are elevated.

If the cause for mild hyponatremia remains unclear after the above tests are performed, a water-loading test may be performed (Box 50-12). This test is potentially dangerous in patients with severe hyponatremia and should not be performed if the serum sodium concentration is <130 mmol/L. Patients with SIADH have impaired excretion of the water load and fail to dilute their urine. Measurements of vasopressin in plasma are not usually needed to make a diagnosis of SIADH, but basal values would be expected to be inappropriately high relative to plasma hyposmolality. Interpretations of plasma vasopressin concentrations are sometimes complicated, because values are often within the physiological reference interval or are undetectable.[93]

Measurement of Arginine Vasopressin

Numerous immunoassays for measuring AVP in plasma or urine have been described.[58] However, their routine clinical application has been hampered because of method complexity and lack of assay sensitivity and specificity. With most plasma assays, a preliminary extraction procedure is required, not only to concentrate the minute amount of hormone that is present in the specimen, but also to remove nonspecific interfering substances.

Procedures for extracting and concentrating AVP from biological fluids often involve the use of solvents such as acetone, petroleum ether, or ethanol.[23] Alternatively, column chromatography using octadecyl silica (C_{18}) columns is an efficient purification technique.[7,132,137] Although a few nonisotopic immunoassays have been developed for ADH,[52,128] most clinical laboratories use some variant of an RIA; complete test kits or individual components (antivasopressin antisera and vasopressin labeled with ^{125}I) are available commercially. Most RIAs are of the delayed-addition type; this nonequilibrium approach provides better sensitivity than equilibrium assays at low hormone concentrations. Separation of bound and free ligand is commonly achieved using second-antibody precipitation techniques.

In the method described by Crawford and Gyory,[29] plasma samples (0.5 mL) are acidified, extracted through C18 Sep-Pak cartridges, and evaporated to dryness. The concentrated specimen is then reconstituted with buffer and incubated with rabbit antivasopressin antisera for 26 to 30 hours at 5 °C. During this time, essentially all the endogenous vasopressin binds to the antibody. Radioactive ^{125}I-labeled vasopressin is subsequently added, and the mixture is incubated for an additional 16 hours at 5 °C. An antirabbit antibody-coated cellulose suspension is used to precipitate the antibody-bound hormone immunologically. The detection limit of this method is 0.1 pg per tube (0.45 ng/L or 0.42 pmol/L). The between-run CV is 7.6% to

11.3% at concentrations ranging from 3 to 10 ng/L (2.8 to 9.3 pmol/L).

Specimen Collection and Storage

Blood specimens for AVP are collected into prechilled tubes containing EDTA as an anticoagulant. Most procedures recommend that specimens be delivered to the laboratory on ice and centrifuged at 4 °C within 30 minutes of collection. The plasma is then removed and stored or shipped frozen at −20 °C until analysis is performed. Random urine specimens are collected without preservatives; alternatively, complete 24-hour urine specimens may be collected in 10 mL of 6 mol/L hydrochloric acid.[95] Significant deterioration of both hormones occurs with prolonged storage.

Reference Intervals

The plasma concentration of AVP in healthy adults (ages 24 to 42 years) with normal water intake and normal physical activity is 0.35 to 11.94 ng/L (0.32 to 11.80 pmol/L).[52] For best interpretation of results, plasma AVP values should be correlated with serum or plasma osmolality[125]:

AVP		
ng/L	**pmol/L**	**Osmolality mOsm/kg**
<1.5	<1.4	270-280
<2.5	<2.3	280-285
1-5	0.9-4.6	285-290
2-7	1.9-6.5	290-295
4-12	3.7-11.1	295-300

The reference interval for AVP in a random urine specimen is reported to be 1 to 112 pg/mL.[90]

OXYTOCIN

Oxytocin is a nonapeptide secreted by the magnicellular neurons of the hypothalamus and stored in the neurohypophysis along with AVP. It promotes uterine contractions and milk ejection and contributes to the second stage of labor.

Regulation of Secretion

The primary stimulus for oxytocin release is suckling. Stimulation of tactile receptors located around the nipples of the breasts initiates an action potential that propagates along afferent nerve fibers through the spinal cord and midbrain to the hypothalamus. The cell bodies in the paraventricular nucleus are then stimulated, resulting in the episodic release of oxytocin. Stretch receptors in the uterus and possibly in the vaginal mucosa may also initiate action potentials in afferent nerve fibers that ultimately stimulate the release of oxytocin from the neurohypophysis. Estrogens enhance the response of oxytocin to these stimuli. The influence of other parts of the brain on the release of oxytocin has been reported; emotional stress, for instance, inhibits lactation.

Physiological Actions

Oxytocin is present in males and females, but its physiological effects are known only for females. Oxytocin stimulates contraction of the uterine myometrium only in the estrogen-primed uterus and can activate the smooth muscles associated with milk letdown with nursing. Thus the effects of oxytocin appear limited to events of parturition and lactation. Oxytocin has been used as a therapeutic agent to induce labor, but the physiological mechanism whereby it induces uterine contractions remains obscure. There is some evidence to show that oxytocin can stimulate prostaglandin production, which may be the vehicle through which myometrial contractility is enhanced. There is evidence indicating that oxytocin may affect the central nervous system and thus modulate human behavior.[84] Progestins are believed to counteract the actions of oxytocin.

Measurement of Oxytocin

Numerous immunoassays for measuring oxytocin in plasma or urine have been described.[58] However, their routine clinical application has been limited because of a lack of physiological relevance to human reproductive disorders and because of a lack of easy-to-use immunoassays with acceptable sensitivity and specificity. With most plasma assays, a preliminary extraction procedure with column chromatography is required, not only to concentrate the minute amount of hormone that is present in the specimen, but also to remove nonspecific interfering substances.

Specimen Collection and Storage

Blood specimens for oxytocin are collected into prechilled tubes containing EDTA as an anticoagulant. Most procedures recommend that specimens be delivered to the laboratory on ice and centrifuged at 4 °C within 30 minutes of collection. The plasma is then removed and stored frozen at −20 °C until analysis is performed. Random urine specimens are collected without preservatives; alternatively, complete 24-hour urine specimens may be collected in 10 mL of 6 mol/L hydrochloric acid.[95] Significant deterioration of both hormones occurs with prolonged storage.

Reference Intervals

Oxytocin values are quantified relative to the bioassay potency of a synthetic reference preparation. Plasma results are reported as microunits per milliliter (1 μU is equivalent to 2 pg of synthetic oxytocin):

	Oxytocin μU/mL[73]
Males	1.1-1.9
Females	
Nonpregnant	1.0-1.8
Second stage of labor	3.1-5.3

REFERENCES

1. Aloya V, Shaker S, Van Loon G. Stabilization of methionine-enkephalin in human and rat blood. Life Sci 1986;39:21-8.
2. Anderson R, Chung H, Kluge R, Schrier RW. Hyponatremia: a prospective analysis of its epidemiology and the pathogenic role of vasopressin. Ann Intern Med 1985;102:164-8.
3. Apter D. Development of the hypothalamic-pituitary-ovarian axis. Ann NY Acad Sci 1997;816:9-21.
4. Arzt E, Stalla GK. Cytokines: autocrine and paracrine roles in the anterior pituitary. Neuroimmunomodulation 1996;3:28-34.
5. Ashby C: Lutropin assays: analytical and clinical expectations. Endocrinology and metabolism in-service training and continuing education, Washington DC: American Association for Clinical Chemistry 1991;9:3-6.
6. Ashby D. Prolactin. In: Pesce A, Kaplan L, eds. Methods in clinical chemistry. St Louis: Mosby, 1987:258-65.
7. Badola F, Benedict C. Rapid, simplified radioimmunoassay of arginine-vasopressin and atrial natriuretic peptide in plasma. Clin Chem 1988;34:970-3.
8. Banfi G, Marinelli M, Casari E, Murone M, Bonini P. Isotopic and nonisotopic assays for measuring somatotropin compared: re-evaluation of cutoff value in provocative tests. Clin Chem 1991;37:273-6.
9. Bartter FC, Delea SC. Diabetes insipidus: Its nature and diagnosis. Lab Management 1982; 20:23.
10. Bassett F, Gross B, Eastman C. Radioimmunoassay of prolactin in blood spotted on filter paper. Clin Chem 1986;32:854.
11. Baumann G. Growth hormone binding proteins and various forms of growth hormone: implications for measurements. Acta Paediatr Scand Suppl 1990;370:72-80.
12. Baylis, P, Gaskill M, Robertson G. Vasopressin secretion in primary polydipsia and cranial diabetes insipidus. Quart J Med NS 1981;50:345-58.
13. Beastall G, Ferguson K, O'Reilly D, Seth J, Sheridan B. Assays for follicle stimulating hormone and luteinizing hormone: Guidelines for the provision of a clinical biochemistry service. Ann Clin Biochem 1987;24:246-62.
14. Benbow SJ, Foy P, Jones B, Shaw D, MacFarlane IA. Pituitary tumours presenting in the elderly: Management and outcome. Clin Endocrinol 1997;46:657-60.
15. Berson S, Yalow R: Radioimmunoassay of ACTH in plasma. J Clin Invest 1968;47:2725-57.
16. Blum W, Ranke W, Bierich RR. A specific radioimmunoassay for insulin-like growth factor II: The interference of IGF binding proteins can be blocked by excess IGF-I. Acta Endocrinol 1988;18:374-80.
17. Blum W, Ranke M, Kietzmann K, Gauggel E, Zeisel HJ, Bierich JR. A specific radioimmunoassay for the growth hormone (GH)-dependent somatomedin binding protein: Its use for diagnosis of GH deficiency. J Clin Endocrinol Metab 1990;70:1292-8.
18. Bodner J, Klein L, Baar J, Bogacz, Strarup-Barnes I, Necklaws E, et al. Quantitation of human prolactin in an automated immunoassay. Clin Chem 1990;36:1100.
19. Bowsher R, Apathy J, Ferguson A, Riggin RM, Henry DP. Cross-reactivity of monomeric and dimeric biosynthetic human growth hormone in commercial immunoassays. Clin Chem 1990;36:362-6.
20. Breier B, Gallaher B, Gluckman P. Radioimmunoassay for insulin-like growth factor-I: Solutions to some potential problems and pitfalls. J Endocrinol 1991;128:347-57.
21. Buatti JM, Marcus RB Jr. Pituitary adenomas: Current methods of diagnosis and treatment. Oncology 1997;11:791-6.
22. Bulatov AA, Martynov AV, Grigor'ian AL, Komolov IS. Molecular forms of human growth hormone and prolactin, secreted by cultured pituitary tumor cells. Biokhimiia 1995;60:1637-46.
23. Camps J, Martinez-Vea A, Perez-Arjuso R. Radioimmunoassay for arginine-vasopressin in cold ethanol extracts of plasma. Clin Chem 1983;29:882-4.
24. Canadian Society of Clinical Chemists: Canadian Society of Clinical Chemists position paper: Standardization of selected polypeptide hormone measurements. Clin Biochem 1992;25:415-24.
25. Celniker AC, Chen AB, Wert RM Jr, Sherman BM. Variability in the quantitation of circulating growth hormone using commercial immunoassays. J Clin Endocrinol Metab 1989;68:469-76.
26. Chryssikopoulos A. The relationship between the immune and endocrine systems. Ann N Y Acad Sci 1997;816:83-93.
27. Clemmons DR, Van Wyk JJ, Ridgway EC, Kliman B, Kjellberg RN, Underwood LE. Evaluation of acromegaly by radioimmunoassay of somatomedin-C. N Engl J Med 1979;301:1138-42.
28. Cook J, Hicks J, Godwin I. Pediatric reference ranges for prolactin. Clin Chem 1992;38:959.
29. Crawford G, Gyory A. Measuring arginine vasopressin in children and babies. Clin Chem 1990;36:1689.
30. Crosby S, Steward M, Ratcliff J, White A. Direct measurement of the precursors of adrenocorticotropin in human plasma by two-site immunoradiometric assay. J Clin Endocrinol Metab 1988;67:1272-8.
31. Daughaday WH, Cryer PE. Growth hormone hypersecretion and acromegaly. Hosp Pract 1978;13: 75-80.
32. Davies MJ, Howlett TA. A survey of the current methods used in the UK to assess pituitary function. J R Soc Med 1996;89:159P-64P.

33. Dean B, Kolavcic M, Tizian L, Harrison L. Should plasma beta-endorphin be measured in patients with disorders of the hypothalamic-pituitary-adrenal axis? Clin Chem 1986;32:895.
34. Dodson S, White A, Hoadley M, Lovgren T, Ratcliffe J. Measurement of corticotropin in unextracted plasma: comparison of a time-resolved immunofluorometric assay and an immunoradiometric assay, with use of the same monoclonal antibodies. Clin Chem 1987;33:1747-51.
35. Dufau M, Pock R, Neubauer A, Catt KJ. In vitro bioassay of LH in human serum: The rat interstitial cell testosterone (RICT) assay. J Clin Endocrinol Metab 1976;42:958-69.
36. Earll JM, Sparks LL, Forsham PH. Glucose suppression of serum growth hormone in the diagnosis of acromegaly. JAMA 1967;201:628-30.
37. Eddy RL, Gilliland PF, Ibarra JD Jr, McMurry JF Jr, Thompson JQ. Human growth hormone release: Comparison of provocative test procedures. Am J Med 1974;56:179-85.
38. Eddy RL, Jones AL, Chakmakjian ZH, Silverthorne MC. Effects of levodopa (L-dopa) on human hypophyseal tropic hormone release. J Clin Endocrinol Metab 1971;33:709-12.
39. Endocrine Sciences: Pediatric Laboratory Services, Tarzana, Calif, 1988.
40. Evans A, Wood P. Development of an assay for human growth hormone in urine using commercially available reagents. Ann Clin Biochem 1989;26:353-7.
41. Felder R, Hall R, Martha P, Bauler G, Hellman P, Wills MR, et al. Influence of matrix on concentrations of somatotropin in serum with commercial immunoradiometric assays. Clin Chem 1989;35:1423-6.
42. Findling J, Engeland W, Raff H. The use of immunoradiometric assay for the measurement of ACTH in human plasma. Trends Endocrinol Metab 1990;1:283-7.
43. Ford K, Baker H, Br J. Automated enzyme immunoassay for lutropin with the Abbott Imx™ Analyzer. Clin Chem 1989;35:2333-5.
44. Gavras H. Role of vasopressin in clinical hypertension and congestive cardiac failure: interaction with the sympathetic nervous systems. Clin Chem 1991;37:1828-30.
45. Ghigo E, Arvat E, Muccioli G, Camanni F. Growth hormone-releasing peptides. Eur J Endocrinol 1997;136:445-60.
46. Gid-Ad I, Topper E, Laron Z. Oral clonidine as a growth hormone stimulation test. Lancet 1979;2:278-80.
47. Girard J, Fisher-Wasels T. Measurement of urinary growth hormone: A noninvasive method to assess growth hormone status. Horm Res 1990;33:12-18.
48. Givalois L, Dornand J, Mekaouche M, Solier MD, Bristow AF, Ixart G, et al. Temporal cascade of plasma concentration surges in ACTH, corticosterone, and cytokines in endotoxin-challenged rats. Am J Physiol (United States) 1995;267:R164-R170.
49. Grover J, Griffin J, Odell W. Ultrasensitive, specific, two-antibody immunoradiometric assay that detects free alpha subunits of glycoprotein hormones in blood of nonpregnant humans. Clin Chem 1991;37:2069-75.
50. Gupta MK, Kolar T, Sheeler LR. Development and evaluation of a highly sensitive and specific radioimmunoassay for measurement of adrenocorticotropin concentrations in plasma. Clin J Med 1988;55:365-9.
51. Han C, Mokhtri A, Brennan G, Li J, Hutchison S, Hill C. et al. Development of an immunoradiometric assay for direct measurement of intact beta-endorphin. Clin Chem 1992;38:1082.
52. Hashida S, Tanaka K, Yamamoto N, Uno T, Yamaguchi K, Ishikawa E. Detection of one attomole of [Arg8]-vasopressin by novel noncompetitive enzyme immunoassay. J Biochem 1991;110:486-92.
53. Hashimoto T, Miyabo S, Nishibu M, Matsubara F, Migita S. Interference of immunoglobulins in the radioimmunoassay of human β-endorphin. J Clin Chem Clin Biochem 1990;28:937-41.
54. Hemmila I, Holttinen S, Pettersson K, Lovgren T. Double-label time-resolved immunofluorometry of lutropin and follitropin in serum. Clin Chem 1987;33:2281-3.
55. Howanitz J. Review of the influence of polypeptide hormone forms of immunoassay results. Arch Pathol Lab Med 1993;117:369-72.
56. Imura H, Fukata J, Mori T. Cytokines and endocrine function: An interaction between the immune and neuroendocrine systems. Clin Endo 1991;35:107-15.
57. Jacobs L. Prolactin. In: Jaffe BM, Behrman H, eds. Methods of hormone radioimmunoassay. New York: Academic Press Inc, 1979.
58. Jaffe BM, Behrman HR, eds. Methods of hormone radioimmunoassay. New York: Academic Press Inc., 1979.
59. Jeffcoate SL, Bacon RR, Beastall GH, Diver MJ, Franks S, Seth J, et al. Assays for prolactin: Guidelines for the provision of a clinical biochemistry service. Ann Clin Biochem 1986;23:638-51.
60. Jeffcoate S. What are we measuring in gonadotropin assays? Acta Endocrinol (Copenh) 1988;288:28-30.
61. Jia XC, Kessel B, Yen SS, Tucker EM, Hsueh AJ. Serum bioactive follicle-stimulating hormone during the human menstrual cycle and in hyper- and hypo-gonadotropic states: Application of a sensitive granulosa cell aromatase bioassay. J Clin Endocrinol Metab 1986;62:1243-9.

62. Johnsonbaugh RE, Bybee DE, Georges LP. Exercise tolerance test: Single-sample screening technique to rule out growth hormone deficiency. JAMA 1978;240:664-6.
63. Kahan I, Papanastasiou-Dimandi A, D'Costa M, Diamandis E. A time-resolved immunofluorometric assay for the measurement of prolactin in serum. Clin Chem 1988;34:1226.
64. Kahn S, Savjani G, Mukherje A. A rapid extraction and IRMA for insulin-like growth factor-I (somatomedin-C) with use of monoclonal antibodies. Clin Chem 1988;34:1223-4.
65. Karalis K, Muglia LJ, Bae D, Hilderbrand H, Majzoub JA. CRH and the immune system. J Neuroimmunol 1997;2:131-6.
66. Kaye TB. Hyperprolactinemia. Causes, consequences, and treatment options. Postgrad Med 1996;99:265-8.
67. Keye WR Jr, Chang RJ, Wilson CB, Jaffe RB. Prolactin-secreting pituitary adenomas: III. Frequency and diagnosis in amenorrhea-galactorrhea. JAMA 1980;244:1329-32.
68. Khosrari M, Morton R, Diamandis E. Sensitive, rapid procedure for time-resolved immunofluorometry of lutropin. Clin Chem 1988;34:1640-4.
69. Kilroy J, Zhou A, Gaumond G, Provuncher G, Ling E. An automated chemiluminescence immunoassay for human prolactin. Clin Chem 1991;37:935.
70. Koulu M, Lammintausta R, Kangas L, Dahlstrom S. The effect of methysergide, pimozide and sodium valproate on the diazepam-stimulated growth hormone secretion in man. J Clin Endocrinol Metab 1979;48:119-22.
71. Krywicki RF, Yee D. The insulin-like growth factor family of ligands, receptors, and binding proteins. Breast Cancer Res Treat (Netherlands) 1992;22: 7-19.
72. Laron Z, Pertzelan A, Karp M. Administration of growth hormone to patients with familial dwarfism with high plasma immunoreactive growth hormone. J Clin Endocrinol Metab 1971;33:332-42.
73. Leake RD, Weitzman RE, Glatz TH, Fisher DA. Plasma oxytocin concentrations in men, nonpregnant women, and pregnant women before and during spontaneous labor. J Clin Endocrinol Metab 1981;53:730-3.
74. Lefkowitz P, Roth J, Paston I. Radioreceptor assay of adrenocorticotropic hormone: New approach to assay of polypeptide hormones in plasma. Science 1970;170:633-5.
75. Leung K, Dawson S, Rugg J. A rapid automated radial partition immunoassay for the measurement of human lutropin. Clin Chem 1988;34:1221.
76. Licht P, Papkoff H, Farmer SW, Muller CH, Tsui HW, Crews D. Evolution of gonadotropin structure and function. Recent Prog Horm Res 1977;33: 169-248.
77. Lilly MP, Gann DS. The hypothalamic-pituitary-adrenal-immune axis. A critical assessment Arch Surg (United States) 1992;127:1463-74.
78. Lin T, Tucci JR. Provocative tests of growth hormone release. A comparison of results with seven stimuli. Ann Intern Med 1974;80:464-9.
79. Ling E, Schubert W, Yannoni C. An automated chemiluminescence immunoassay for human follicle stimulating hormone. Clin Chem 1991;37:935.
80. Mace JC, Gotlin RW, Beck P. Sleep-related human growth hormone release, a test of physiologic growth hormone secretion in children. J Clin Endocrinol Metab 1972;34:339-41.
81. Magiakou MA, Mastorakos G, Webster E, Chrousos GP. The hypothalamic-pituitary-adrenal axis and the female reproductive system. Ann N Y Acad Sci 1997;816:42-56.
82. Mahmood N, Srebro S, McCarthy N, Brotherton M, Hunter T, DeMarco C. Rapid automated determination of total prolactin on the Stratus analyzer. Clin Chem 1989;35:1095.
83. Mansbach L, Kolz K, Giga M. Development of a solid phase prolactin immunoradiometric assay. Clin Chem 1988;34:1224.
84. McCarthy MM, Altemus M. Central nervous system actions of oxytocin and modulation of behavior in humans. Mol Med Today 1997;3:269-75.
85. Melmed S. Unwanted effects of growth hormone excess in the adult. J Pediatr Endocrinol Metab, 9 Suppl 1996;3:369-74.
86. Merimee TJ, Rabinowitz D, Fineberg SE. Arginine-initiated release of human growth hormone: Factors modifying the response in normal man. N Engl J Med 1969;280:1434-8.
87. Miller M, Dalakos T, Moses AM, Fellerman H, Streeten DH. Recognition of partial defects in antidiuretic hormone secretion. Ann Intern Med 1970;73:721-9.
88. Mimbs RB, Bethune JE. Acromegaly with normal fasting growth hormone concentration but abnormal growth hormone regulation. Ann Intern Med 1974;81:781-4.
89. Mitchell ML, Hermos RJ, Schoepfer A, Orson JM. Reference ranges for insulin-like growth factor-I in healthy children and adolescents, determined with filter-paper blood specimens. Clin Chem 1990;36:2138-9.
90. Nichols Institute Diagnostics: Test catalog. San Clemente, Calif: Nichols Institute Diagnostics, 1992.
91. Nicholson WE, Davis DR, Sherrell BJ, Orth DN. Rapid radioimmunoassay for corticotropin in unextracted human plasma. Clin Chem 1984;30:259-65.
92. Nicoll C. Bioassay of prolactin: Analysis of the pigeon crop sac response to local prolactin injection by an objective and quantitative method. Endocrinology 1967;80:641-55.

93. Ober K. Diabetes insipidus. Crit Care Clin 1991;7: 109-23.
94. Orth D. Adrenocorticotropic hormone (ACTH). In: Jaffe BM, Behrman H, eds. Methods of hormone radioimmunoassay, 2nd ed. New York: Academic Press Inc, 1979:245-83.
95. Panzail A, Signorini C, Ferari R, Albertini A. Direct determination of arginine-vasopressin in urine. Clin Chem 1990;36:384-5.
96. Parker ML, Hammond JM, Daughaday WH. The arginine provocative test: An aid in the diagnosis of hyposomatotropism. J Clin Endocrinol Metab 1967;27:1129-36.
97. Parks JS, Amrhein JA, Vaidya V, Moshang T Jr, Bongiovanni AM. Growth hormone response to propranolol-glucagon stimulation: A comparison with other tests of growth hormone reserve. J Clin Endocrinol Metab 1973;37:85-92.
98. Penney R, Blizzard RM, Davis WT. Sequential arginine and insulin tolerance tests. J Clin Endocrinol Metab 1969;29:1499-501.
99. Pepperell RJ. Prolactin and reproduction. Fertil Steril 1981;35:267-74.
100. Phillips LS, Vassilopoulou-Sellin R. Somatomedins (in two parts). N Engl J Med 1980;302:371-80, 438-46.
100A. Popii V, Baumann G. Laboratory measurement of growth hormone. Clin Chim Acta 2004;350:1-16.
101. Preece MA. Making a rational diagnosis of growth-hormone deficiency. J Pediatr 1997;131:S61-S64.
102. Price JD, Lauener RW. Serum and urine osmolality in the differential diagnosis of polyuric states. J Clin Endocrinol Metab 1966;26:143-8.
103. Rabkin MT, Frantz AG. Hypopituitarism: A study of growth hormone and other endocrine functions. Ann Intern Med 1966;64:1197-207.
104. Raff H, Findling J. A new immunoradiometric assay for corticotropin evaluated in normal subjects and patients with Cushing's syndrome. Clin Chem 1989;35:596-600.
105. Rappaport E, Olander C, Steffes M. Radioimmunoassay of human somatotropin. Clin Chem 1979;25: 800-6.
106. Reeves WB, Andreoli TE. The posterior pituitary and water metabolism. In: Wilson JD, Foster DW, eds. Williams textbook of endocrinology, 8th ed. Philadelphia: WB Saunders, 1992:311-56.
107. Reiter EO, Morris AH, MacGillivray MH, Weber D. Variable estimates of serum growth hormone concentrations by different radioassay systems. J Clin Endocrinol Metab 1988;66:68-71.
108. Renner U, Pagotto U, Arzt E, Stalla GK. Autocrine and paracrine roles of polypeptide growth factors, cytokines and vasogenic substances in normal and tumorous pituitary function and growth: A review. Eur J Endocrinol 1996;135:515-32.
109. Rosano TG, Demers LM, Hillam R, Dybas MT, Leinung M. Clinical and analytical evaluation of an immunoradiometric assay for corticotropin. Clin Chem 1995;41:961-1064.
110. Rosenfeld RG, Gargosky SE. Assays for insulin-like growth factors and their binding proteins: Practicalities and pitfalls. J Pediatr (United States) 1996;128:S52-S57.
111. Rudd B. Growth, growth hormone and the somatomedins: An historical perspective and current concepts. Ann Clin Biochem 1991;28:542-55.
112. Santner SJ, Santen RJ, Kulin HE, Demers LM. A model for validation of radio-immunoassay kit reagents: Measurement of follitropin and lutropin in blood and urine. Clin Chem 1981;27:1892-5.
113. Sato T, Inoue M, Masuyama T, Suzuki Y, Izumisawa A. Simultaneous evaluation of the pituitary reserve of GH, TSH, ACTH, and LH in children. J Clin Endocrinol Metab 1974;39:595-9.
114. Sawin CT, Mitchell ML. A comparison of response of serum growth to glucagon and vasopressin. Metabolism 1970;19:898-903.
115. Seth J, Hanning I, Al-Sadie R, Bacon RRA, Hunter WM. The UK external quality assurance scheme (EQAS) for FSH, LH and prolactin—the past decade. Clin Chem 1990;36:1003.
116. Shellum C, Klee G. A sensitive, specific immunochemiluminometric assay for luteinizing hormone in serum and urine. Clin Chem 1991;37:1038-9.
117. Shiu R, Kelly P, Friesen H. Radioreceptor assay for prolactin and other lactogenic hormones. Science 1973;180:968-71.
118. Silbergeld A, Jaber L, Lilos P, Laron Z. A comparison of IGF-I concentrations measured by two commercially available radioimmunoassays. Acta Endocrinol 1988;119:333-8.
119. Sinha YN, Selby FW, Lewis UJ, VanderLaan WP. A homologous radioimmunoassay for human prolactin. J Clin Endocrinol Metab 1973;36:509-16.
120. Smith C, Norman M. Prolactin and growth hormone: Molecular heterogeneity and measurement in serum. Ann Clin Biochem 1990;27:542-50.
121. Spencer DH, Dilly K, Jackson R, Price JA, Vallejo R. A totally automated immunoenzymetric prolactin assay designed for the Affinity™ system. Clin Chem 1990;36:1100.
122. Strasburger L, Barnard G, Toldo L, Zarmi B, Zadik Z, Kowarski A, et al. Somatotropin as measured by a two-site time-resolved immunofluorometric assay. Clin Chem 1989;35:913-17.
122A. Suliman AM, Smith TP, Gibney J, McKenna TJ. Frequent misdiagnosis and mismanagement of hyperprolactinemic patients before the introduction of macroprolactin screening: Application of a new strict laboratory definition of macroprolactinemia. Clin Chem 2003;49:1504-9.

123. Tanaka T, Shiu RP, Gout PW, Beer CT, Noble RL, Friesen HG. A new sensitive and specific assay for lactogenic hormones: Measurement of prolactin and growth hormones in human serum. J Clin Endocrinol Metab 1980;51:1058-63.
124. Thorner MO, Vance ML, Horvath E, Kovacs K. The anterior pituitary. In: Wilson JD, Foster DW, eds. Williams textbook of endocrinology, 8th ed. Philadelphia: WB Saunders, 1992:221-310.
125. Tietz N, ed. Clinical guide to laboratory tests, 3rd ed. Philadelphia: WB Saunders Co, 1995.
125A. Toldy E, Locsei Z, Szabolcs I, Goth MI, Kneffel P, Szoke D, et al. Macroprolactinemia: The consequences of a laboratory pitfall. Endocrine 2003;22:267-73.
126. Underwood LE, ed. Human growth hormone: Progress and challenges. New York: Marcel Dekker Inc, 1988.
127. Underwood LE, Van Wyk JJ. Normal and aberrant growth. In: Wilson JD, Foster DW, eds. Williams textbook of endocrinology, 8th ed. Philadelphia: WB Saunders, 1992:1079-138.
128. Uno T, Uehara K, Motomatsu K, Ishikawa E, Kato K. Enzyme immunoassay for arginine vasopressin. Experientia 1982;38:786-7.
129. Vermes I, Bonte HA, v d Sluijs Veer G, Schoemaker J. Interpretations of five monoclonal immunoassays of lutropin and follitropin: Effects of normalization with WHO standards. Clin Chem 1991;37:415-21.
130. Vieira J, Lombardi M, Nishida S. Monoclonal antibody-based immunoenzymometric assay for serum human growth hormone. Braz J Med Biol Res 1990;23:293-6.
131. Vierhapper H, Nowotny P, Czech T, Bieglmayer C, Raber W, Waldhausl W. How (not) to diagnose growth hormone deficiency in adults: Stimulated serum concentrations of growth hormone in healthy subjects and in patients with pituitary macroadenomas. Metabolism 1997;46:680-3.
132. Watabe T, Tanaka K, Kumagae M, Itoh S, Takeda F, Morio K, et al. Hormonal responses to insulin-induced hypoglycemia in man. J Clin Endocrinol Metab 1987;65:1187-91.
133. Wheeler M, D'Souza A, Horn A. Evaluation of test kits for gonadotropins. Lancet 1989;ii:616-17.
134. Whitley R. Tanner stages in adolescent medicine. Endocrinology and metabolism in-service training and continuing education, Washington DC: American Association for Clinical Chemistry 1990;9: 3-4.
135. Wong NA, Ahlquist JA, Camacho-Hubner C, Goodwin CJ, Dattani M, Marshall NJ, et al. Acromegaly or chronic renal failure: A diagnostic dilemma. Clin Endocrinol 1997;46:221-6.
136. Young E. Endogenous opioid peptides in neuroendocrine regulation. Endocrinology and metabolism in-service training and continuing education, Washington DC: American Association for Clinical Chemistry 1990;8:7-13.
137. Ysewijn-Van Brussel K, De Leenheer A. Development and evaluation of a radioimmunoassay of arg8-vasopressin, after extraction with Sep-Pak C_{18}. Clin Chem 1985;31:861-3.
138. Yu-Lee LY. Molecular actions of prolactin in the immune system. Proc Soc Exp Biol Med 1997;215: 35-52.
139. Zahradnik R, Brennan G, Hutchison JS, Odell WD. Immunoradiometric assay of corticotropin with use of avidin-biotin separation. Clin Chem 1989;35: 804-7.

ADDITIONAL READING

Reviews

Abellan R, Ventura R, Pichini S, Pascual JA, Pacifici R, Di Carlo S, et al. Evaluation of immunoassays for the measurement of insulin-like growth factor-I and procollagen type III peptide, indirect biomarkers of recombinant human growth hormone misuse in sport. Clin Chem Lab Med 2005;43:75-85.
Bidlingmaier M, Wu Z, Strasburger CJ. Doping with growth hormone. J Pediatr Endocrinol Metab 2001;14:1077-83.
Brabant G. Insulin-like growth factor-I: Marker for diagnosis of acromegaly and monitoring the efficacy of treatment. Eur J Endocrinol 2003;148 Suppl 2:S15-20.
Christiansen JS. Growth hormone and body composition. J Pediatr Endocrinol Metab 1996;9 Suppl 3:365-8.
Clarke IJ. Two decades of measuring GnRH secretion. Reprod Suppl 2002;59:1-13.
Conrad P, Potter D. Human growth hormone and the temptations of biomedical enhancement. Sociol Health Illn 2004;26:184-215.
Dieterich KD, Lehnert H, De Souza EB.Corticotropin-releasing factor receptors: An overview. Exp. Clin. Endocrinol. Diabetes 1997;105:65-82.
Dyke PC 2nd, Tobias JD. Vasopressin: Applications in clinical practice. J Intensive Care Med 2004;19:220-8.
Johnson RW, Arkins S, Dantzer R, Kelley KW. Hormones, lymphohemopoietic cytokines and the neuroimmune axis. Comp Biochem Physiol A Physiol 1997;116:183-201.
Kalia V, Jadhav AN, Bhutani KK. Luteinizing hormone estimation. Endocr Res 2004;30:1-17.
Levy A. Pituitary disease: Presentation, diagnosis, and management. J Neurol Neurosurg Psychiatry 2004;75 Suppl 3:iii47-52.
Popii V, Baumann G. Laboratory measurement of growth hormone. Clin Chim Acta 2004;350:1-16
Shimon I, Melmed S. Genetic basis of endocrine disease: Pituitary tumor pathogenesis. J Clin Endocrinol Metab 1997;82:1675-81.

Simard M. The biochemical investigation of Cushing syndrome. Neurosurg Focus 2004;16:E4.

Vignozzi L, Vannelli GB, Morelli A, Mancina R, Marini M, Ferruzzi P, et al. Identification, characterization and biological activity of oxytocin receptor in the developing human penis. Mol Hum Reprod 2005; [Epub ahead of print].

Wood P. Growth hormone: Its measurement and the need for assay harmonization. Ann Clin Biochem 2001;38:471-82.

Books

DeGroot LJ Jameson JL, eds. Endocrinology, 4th ed. Philadelphia: WB Saunders Co, 2003:3048 pp.

Dickson RB, Salomon DS. Hormones and growth factors in development and neoplasia. New York: John Wiley & Sons, 1998.

Greenspan FS, Gardner DG. Basic & clinical endocrinology, 7th ed. New York: McGraw-Hill/Appleton & Lange, 2003:1100pp.

Martin ME. Dictionary of endocrinology and related biomedical sciences. Oxford: Oxford University Press, 1995.

Moore WT, Eastman RC. Diagnostic endocrinology, 2nd ed. St Louis: Mosby-Year Book, 1996.

Shlomo M, Conn PM. Endocrinology: Basic & clinical principles, 2nd ed. Totowa, NJ: Humana Press, 2005.

Thakker RV. Molecular genetics of endocrine disorders. New York: Chapman & Hall, 1997.

Von Werder K. Pituitary adenomas: From basic research to diagnosis and therapy. New York: Elsevier Science, 1996.

Wieman ME. Disease of the pituitary: Diagnosis and treatment. Totowa, NJ: Humana Press, 1997.

Williams RH, Wilson JD. Williams textbook of endocrinology, 10th ed. Philadelphia: WB Saunders Co, 2003.

CHAPTER 51

The Adrenal Cortex*

Laurence M. Demers, Ph.D., F.A.C.B., D.A.B.C.C.

An adrenal gland lies at the upper pole of each human kidney. Each gland is pyramidal in shape, is approximately 2 to 3 cm in width, 4 to 6 cm long, 1 cm thick, and weighs approximately 4 g, regardless of age, weight, or gender.[135] Each gland consists of a yellow, outer cortex and a gray, inner medulla. Beneath the capsule of the outer cortex lies the zona glomerulosa that constitutes approximately 15% of the cortex. The next layer is the zona fasciculata that comprises about 75% of the cortex with large and lipid-laden cells. The innermost zone is the zona reticularis that contains irregular looking cells with little lipid content. The cells of the adrenal cortex synthesize steroid hormones, which are discussed in this chapter, and the cells of the adrenal medulla synthesize catecholamines, such as dopamine, norepinephrine, and epinephrine aromatic amines, which have important consequences for blood pressure regulation. The catecholamines and their function are discussed in Chapter 29.

The human adrenal cortex secretes three major classes of *steroid* hormones that possess a wide range of physiological functions. These include the glucocorticoids, the mineralocorticoids, and the adrenal androgens. This chapter begins with a section on general steroid biochemistry, followed by a discussion of the clinical and biological functions of the steroid hormones produced by the adrenal cortex.

GENERAL STEROID CHEMISTRY

Chemical Structure

Steroids are hormones that contain the cyclopentanoperhydrophenanthrene nucleus as the backbone structure (Figure 51-1). The three six-sided rings (A, B, and C) constitute the phenanthrene nucleus, to which is attached the (D) or cyclopentane ring. The prefix "perhydro" refers to the saturation of the compound with hydrogen atoms. This class of compounds includes such natural products as sterols (e.g., cholesterol), bile acids (e.g., cholanic acid), sex hormones (e.g., estrogens and androgens), vitamin D, and the corticosteroids. The steroid hormones contain up to 21 carbon atoms (C_{21} steroids), numbered as shown in Figure 51-1. The carbon atoms composing the rings and the hydrogen atoms attached to them are not usually written into the structure unless it is necessary to draw special attention to configuration. Furthermore, in all naturally occurring steroid hormones, the projected solid line from the carbon atom at position 10 or 13 usually designates the presence of an angular (CH_3) group, unless otherwise indicated.

Steroids are three-dimensional molecules with their constituent atoms lying in different planes—such spatial arrangements give rise to *isomers.* The direction of the hydrogen atoms, of the substituents, and of the side chain plays a much more important role in the distinction of various isomers of the steroid compounds than does the relative position of the carbon atoms in the rings. Thus the isomers resulting from fusion of two rings are decided on the basis of the spatial relationship between the hydrogen atoms or the substituents at common carbon atoms. When rings A and B are fused, two isomers are possible, depending on whether the hydrogen atom at C-5 and the methyl group at C-10 are on the same or the opposite side of the plane of the rings. If the hydrogen atom points in the same direction as that of the angular methyl group at C-10, the compound is said to be in the *cis* or *normal* form. If, however, they are on the opposite sides, the compound is said to be in the *trans* or *allo* form. Although rings A and B may be either *cis* or *trans,* the rings B-C and C-D have the *trans* configuration in all naturally occurring steroid hormones.

The two methyl groups attached to C-10 and C-13 lie above the plane of the molecule and are customarily the points of reference for describing the spatial orientation of

*The author gratefully acknowledges the contribution of Ronald J. Whitley on which portions of this chapter are based.

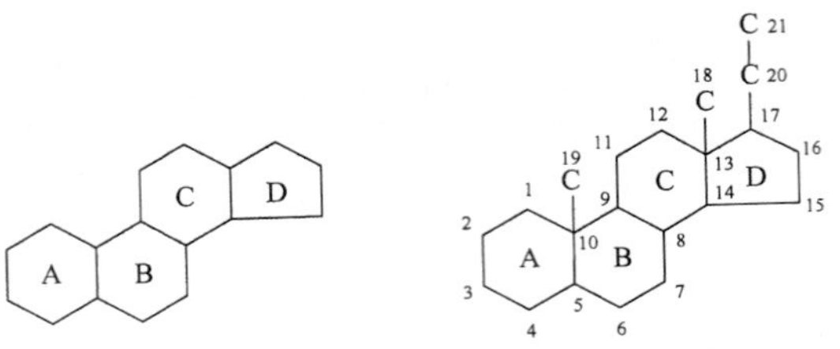

Cyclopentanoperhydrophenanthrene

Figure 51-1 Common features and numbering system of steroids.

cis-

Hydrogen atom and methyl group are on the same side (above the plane of the paper: 5β-isomer.)

trans-

Hydrogen atom is on the opposite side (below the plane of the paper: 5α-isomer.)

Figure 51-2 Fusion of rings A and B and their isomerism in naturally occurring steroids.

other substituents in the steroid nucleus. Depending on which side of the molecule that substituents are attached relative to these two methyl groups, they are said to have either an α- or β-orientation (Figure 51-2). For example, when substituents are on the same side as the two methyl groups, they are said to possess a β-*configuration,* which is indicated by a solid line (—) joining the substituents to the appropriate carbon atoms in the nucleus. Substituents on the opposite side are attached by a broken line (— — —) to denote an α-*configuration.* In the structures shown in Figure 51-2, when the hydrogen substituent at C-5 is *cis,* the isomer is the 5β-isomer, and when it is *trans,* the isomer is accordingly the 5α-isomer. Similarly the substituents at C-3, C-11, C-17, or any other carbon atoms are indicated as either α- or β-configuration, depending on their spatial orientation relative to these methyl groups (C-10 and C-13).

The different steroids containing the cyclopentanoperhydrophenanthrene nucleus differ from one another by the introduction of double bonds between certain pairs of carbon atoms, by the introduction of substituents for the hydrogen atoms, or by the addition or deletion of a specific type of side chain. On the basis of such structural characteristics, the steroidal compounds are classified as derivatives of certain parent hydrocarbons, namely, *estrane* (for estrogens), *androstane* (for androgens), and *pregnane* (for corticosteroids and progestins). Chemically, estranes are C_{18} compounds that lack one methyl group at C-10, androstanes are C_{19} compounds that possess 5α- or 5β-configuration, and pregnanes are C_{21} compounds that have a β-oriented, ethyl side chain ($—CH_2—CH_3$) attached to C-17. Further discussion of the chemistry of estranes and androstanes is presented in more detail in Chapter 53.

The prefix *allo-* is a term used to describe the stereoisomerism of the hydrogen atom at C-5. When the configuration differs at any other carbon atom, the prefix *epi-* is used (e.g., androsterone possesses a 3α-hydroxyl group, and epiandrosterone a 3β-hydroxyl group; testosterone possesses a 17β-hydroxyl group, and epitestosterone a 17α-hydroxyl group).

To describe a compound with chemical nomenclature, a variety of other suffixes and prefixes are used. The suffix *-ane* indicates a fully saturated compound (e.g., pregn*ane*); *-ene,* the presence of one double bond (e.g., pregn*ene*); *-diene,* two double bonds; and *-triene,* three double bonds; the terminal "e" is omitted before a vowel (e.g., -4-en-β3-ol). The position of the double bond is indicated by the number of the carbon atom from which it originates, and it is understood to terminate at the next higher carbon atom (e.g., "4-ene" means that a double bond lies between C-4 and C-5). However, when an alternative is possible, as in a double bond originating at C-8 in the estrane nucleus that can terminate at C-9 or C-14, the number of the carbon atom at which the bond ends is written in parentheses. Thus a double bond at C-8 terminating at C-14 is designated as "8(14)-ene." A formerly used prefix for a double bond is the symbol Δ, with a superscript indicating the position of the double bond (e.g., Δ^5). An alcohol (—OH substituent of the nucleus) is indicated by the suffix *-ol* (two alcohol groups as *-diol,* three as *-triol,* etc.), or by the prefix *hydroxy-* or *oxy-* (*dihydroxy-* for two, *trihydroxy-* for three, etc.). Ketones (=CO) are identified by the suffixes *-one* for one keto group, *-dione* for two keto groups, and so on, or by the prefix *oxo-* (Table 51-1).

In naming a compound containing double bonds, hydroxyl groups, and ketones, priorities are given to the use of suffixes and prefixes. Thus hydroxyl groups are indicated by the prefix followed by the suffixes for other substituents. Accordingly the systematic name of dehydroepiandrosterone is written as 3β-hydroxy-androst-5-en-17-one. Note that to denote the bond of unsaturation, the first part of the parent hydrocarbon is followed by the position of the bond and the suffix (e.g., androst-5-en). If the prefix Δ for unsaturation is chosen, then suffixes for both the hydroxyl and the ketone groups are used (e.g., Δ^5-androsten-3β-ol-17-one). When only one kind of substituent is present, the use of a suffix is customary (e.g., pregnanediol [5β-pregnane-3α, 20α-diol] and androstenedione [androst-4-ene-3,17-dione]).

The utility of the *systematic name* of a compound lies in the information that it provides about the parent compound, the position of bond unsaturation, and the nature, position, and orientation of substituents. The *trivial name,* as the term suggests, conveys little or no information about the chemical origin and characteristics of a compound (e.g., cortisol, progesterone, and testosterone). The trivial and systematic names of some of the important steroid hormones are given in Table 51-2.

TABLE 51-1 Common Suffixes and Prefixes for Steroids

Suffix or Prefix	Definition
Suffix	
-al	Aldehyde group
-ane	Saturated hydrocarbon
-ene	Unsaturated hydrocarbon
-ol	Hydroxyl group
-one	Ketone group
Prefix	
hydroxy- (oxy-)	Hydroxyl group
keto- (oxo-)	Ketone
deoxy- (desoxy-)	Replacement of hydroxyl group by hydrogen
dehydro-	Loss of two hydrogen atoms from adjacent carbon atoms
dihydro-	Addition of two hydrogen atoms
cis-	Spatial arrangement of two substituents on the same side of the molecule
trans-	Spatial arrangement of two substituents on opposite sides of the molecule
α-	Substituent that is *trans* to the methyl group at C-10
β-	Substituent that is *cis* to the methyl group at C-10
epi-	Isomeric in configuration at any carbon atom except at the junction of two rings
Δn-	Position of unsaturated bond

TABLE 51-2 Trivial and Systematic Names of Some Important Steroid Hormones

Trivial Name	Systematic Name
Aldosterone	11β-21-Dihydroxy-3,20-dioxopregn-4-en-18-al
Androstenedione	Androst-4-ene-3,11,17-trione
Androsterone	3α-Hydroxy-5α-androstan-17-one
Cortisol	11β,17,21-Trihydroxypregn-4-ene-3,20-dione
Dehydroepiandrosterone	3β-Hydroxyandrost-5-en-17-one
Estradiol-17β	Estra-1,3,5(10)-triene-3,17β-diol
Estriol	Estra-1,3,5(10)-triene-3,16α,17β-triol
Estrone	3-Hydroxyestra-1,3,5(10)-trien-17-one
Etiocholanolone	3α-Hydroxy-5β-androstan-17-one
Pregnanediol	5β-Pregnane-3α,20α-diol
Progesterone	Pregn-4-ene-3,20-dione
Testosterone	17β-Hydroxy-androst-4-en-3-one
Urocortisol (tetrahydro F)	3α,11β,17,21-Tetrahydroxy-5β-pregnan-20-one

In addition to the usual suffixes and prefixes just discussed, a few special prefixes are usually used for the semitrivial names of the compounds. Thus the prefix *dehydro-* is used to indicate the loss of two hydrogen atoms from adjacent carbon atoms with the formation of a double bond (e.g., dehydroepiandrosterone). The prefix *dihydro-* or *tetrahydro-* indicates the addition of two or four hydrogen atoms to the molecule, respectively, as in dihydrocortisol and tetrahydrocortisol. The replacement of a hydroxyl group by hydrogen (COH CH) is denoted by the prefix *deoxy-* (or *desoxy-* [e.g., 11-deoxycorticosterone]).

Steroid nomenclature is officially defined by the International Union of Pure and Applied Chemistry (IUPAC).

Biochemistry

Human steroid hormones are synthesized primarily from cholesterol in the adrenal glands and gonads. In most cases, cholesterol is made available from the circulation in the form of low-density lipoprotein cholesterol (LDL). The uptake of LDL takes place by way of specific cell surface LDL receptors on the adrenal gland surface that internalize the cholesterol moiety, releasing it as substrate for steroidogenesis; however, all steroidogenic cells are capable of de novo synthesis from acetyl coenzyme A.[43] To ensure a continuous supply of free cholesterol for steroid synthesis, lipoprotein cholesterol uptake is coordinated with intracellular cholesterol synthesis and with the mobilization of intracellular cholesteryl ester pools. When the rate of cholesterol uptake exceeds the rate of steroidogenesis, intracellular cholesterol synthesis is suppressed, and cholesterol in excess of cellular needs is esterified and stored for future use.

The initial rate limiting step in the transport of intracellular cholesterol to sites of steroidogenesis is mediated by a steroidogenic acute regulatory protein (StAR) that is regulated by adrenocorticotropic hormone (ACTH).

The nature and quantity of steroid hormones produced by the adrenal glands and gonads are different. The difference is inherent in the degree of activity of certain enzyme systems. For example, the enzymes 11β-hydroxylase and 21-hydroxylase, present only in the adrenal glands, synthesize steroids characteristic of the adrenal glands. Similarly the ovaries and the testes contain enzymes that synthesize the male and female sex hormones (see Chapter 53).

TABLE 51-3 The Genes, Chromosomal Location, and Common Names of the Adrenal Steroidogenic Enzymes

Enzyme Name	Gene	Chromosome Location
11-Aldosterone synthase	CYP11B2	8q24.3
Cholesterol side-chain cleavage (SCC, desmolase)	CYP11A1	15q23-q24
17α-Hydroxylase/17,20 lyase	CYP17	10q24.3
21-Hydroxylase	CYP21A2	6p21.3
β-Hydroxylase	CYP11B1	8q24.3
3β-Hydroxysteroid dehydrogenase (3β-HSD)	HSD3B2	1p13.1

Biosynthesis

Enzymes participating in the biosynthesis of steroid hormones are broadly classified as (1) hydroxylases, (2) lyases, (3) dehydrogenases, and (4) isomerases.

Hydroxylases

These enzymes are all cytochrome P-450 enzymes[175] and catalyze the substitution of the hydroxyl group (—OH) for hydrogen (—H). For example, 21-hydroxylase (also known as "P-450_{C21}") introduces a hydroxyl group at C-21. Similarly, 11β-hydroxylase (P-450_{C11}) introduces a hydroxyl group at the β-position of C-11. The required cofactors are nicotinamide-adenine dinucleotide phosphate (NADP) and molecular oxygen; the reaction is irreversible. The hydroxylation is carried out in conjunction with an electron transport system that consists of NADPH → flavoprotein → nonheme iron protein → cytochrome P-450 → oxygen. Cytochrome P-450 couples with specific hydroxylases for the introduction of an atom of oxygen into the steroid molecule.

Lyases

Enzymes with lyase activity are required for cleavage of the side chain. Previously, it was thought that three distinct enzymes, including a 20,22-lyase, participated in the conversion of cholesterol to pregnenolone. However, it is now known that a single cholesterol side-chain cleavage enzyme (P-450_{SCC}) catalyzes the complete reaction.[87] This enzyme is located within mitochondria and participates in an electron shuttle system where the oxidation and hydroxylation of the different adrenal steroids takes place. The C_{21} steroid hormones are transformed to C_{19} steroid hormones by the 17,20-lyase activity of P-450_{C17}, a microsomal enzyme that also catalyzes the hydroxylation of C-17.

Dehydrogenases

This group of enzymes catalyzes the transfer of hydrogen within the steroid structure (oxidation and reduction). The reaction is in general reversible. The cofactor is either the oxidized or reduced form of nicotinamide-adenine dinucleotide $(NAD)^+$ or $NADP^+$, depending on the direction of the reaction. Examples include 3β-hydroxysteroid dehydrogenase, 11β-hydroxysteroid dehydrogenase, 17β-hydroxysteroid dehydrogenase, Δ^5-3β-hydroxysteroid dehydrogenase, and 3α-hydroxysteroid dehydrogenase.

Isomerases

Isomerases catalyze the migration of a double bond. The most important enzyme of this group that is involved in steroidogenesis is Δ^5-*ketosteroid isomerase* ($\Delta^{4,5}$isomerase). The concerted action of Δ^5-3β-hydroxysteroid dehydrogenase and Δ^5-ketosteroid isomerase on pregnenolone produces progesterone through the oxidation of the 3β-hydroxyl group and the migration of a double bond from Δ^5 to Δ^4.

Chromosomes and Genes

The chromosomes and genes responsible for the adrenal steroidogenic enzymes have been identified. Table 51-3 depicts the current nomenclature and chromosome localization for the genes that regulate these enzymes.

Metabolism

The liver is the major site of steroid metabolism. The kidney and the gastrointestinal tract, however, also both carry out important metabolic transformation of steroids.

In addition to using acetate and cholesterol, some steroidogenic tissues produce hormones by converting steroid intermediates that originate from other sources. For example, ovarian granulosa cells can convert androgens produced in thecal cells to estrogens. Some target tissues, such as the prostate, can also convert the circulating form of a steroid to a more potent and bioactive form, which then exerts its effects within the cells. For example, the prostate contains a 5α-reductase that converts testosterone to its biologically more potent form, dihydrotestosterone. Another example of this is the conversion of the adrenal androgen precursor, dehydroepiandrosterone (DHEA), to estrone in fat tissue by way of the aromatase enzyme.

Important biochemical steps for neutralizing the potent biological activity of hormones and facilitating their rapid elimination from the systemic circulation include (1) the introduction of an additional hydroxyl group (e.g., estradiol to estriol); (2) dehydrogenation (e.g., testosterone to androstenedione); (3) reduction of a double bond (e.g., cortisol to dihydrocortisol); and (4) conjugation of an essential hydroxyl group or groups with a chemical moiety, such as glucuronic acid (e.g., testosterone to testosterone glucuronide). The conjugation of these hormones and their metabolites with sulfuric or glucuronic acid is, by far, the most efficient single metabolic process for their excretion in the urine. Almost all steroid metabolites are excreted as water-soluble glucuronides or sulfates.

ADRENOCORTICAL STEROIDS

The human adrenal cortex secretes a number of steroid hormones that are involved with a wide range of metabolic processes from three discrete anatomical zones; the *zona fasciculata*, the *zona reticularis*, and the *zona glomerulosa*.

General Biochemistry

Steroids isolated from the adrenal glands include the *corticosteroids* and adrenal androgens. Their chemical structure and how they are synthesized and transported are discussed in this section.

Chemical Structure

The *corticosteroids* include the *glucocorticoids* and *mineralocorticoids:* they are physiologically and quantitatively the most important group of adrenal steroids.[122] The structural formula of some of the most significant biologically active corticosteroids are shown in Figure 51-3; their trivial and systematic names are listed in Table 51-2. These compounds all possess a Δ^4-3-keto group (unsaturated double bond between C-4 and C-5 and a keto group at C-3); a side-chain hydroxyl substitution at C-17 in the β-position (above the plane of the paper); and, with the exception of 11-deoxycortisol (compound S) and 11-deoxycorticosterone (DOC), an oxygen function (keto or β-hydroxyl) at C-11. Cortisone and hydrocortisone (cortisol) also have a 17α-hydroxyl group (below the plane of the paper). Corticosteroids show maximal structural specificity. Structural alterations, especially the reduction of the Δ^4-3-keto group, render them biologically inactive. The major corticosteroids—cortisol and aldosterone—are secreted by the adrenal glands at the rate of approximately 25 mg/day and 200 μg/day, respectively.[169]

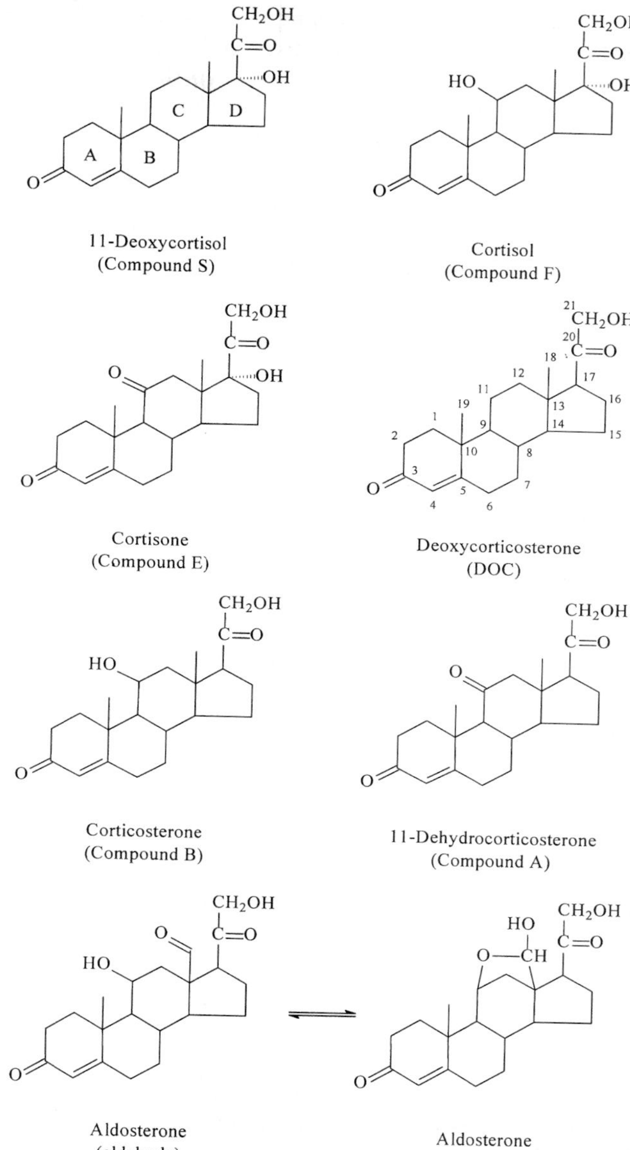

Figure 51-3 Structural formulas and trivial names of some biologically active corticosteroids. Note alphabetical ring system and the numerical system for 21 carbon atoms.

Glucocorticoids

Cortisol is the major glucocorticoid synthesized from cholesterol in the zona fasciculata and reticularis of the human adrenal cortex. Cortisol has major effects on carbohydrate, protein, and lipid metabolism. The influence of *glucocorticoids* on carbohydrate metabolism (Figure 51-4) includes promotion of gluconeogenesis through the activation of key enzymes in this pathway, including phosphoenolpyruvate carboxykinase and glucose-6-phosphatase, increased deposition of liver glycogen through the activation of glycogen synthase and inhibition of glycogen phosphorylase, and a reduction in glucose use and uptake by peripheral tissues, such as muscle and fat. The increase in gluconeogenesis is also due to an increase in muscle protein breakdown and an inhibition of amino acid uptake and protein synthesis in peripheral tissues (muscle, skin, and bone). Glucocorticoids also affect fat metabolism with an activation in lipolysis and the release of free fatty acids into the circulation; when present in excess, glucocorticoids cause a central distribution of fat to the face, neck, and trunk. Glucocorticoids can also stimulate adipocyte differentiation and promote lipogenesis through the activation of enzymes such as lipoprotein lipase and increased messenger ribonucleic acid (mRNA) expression for leptin.

Circulating glucocorticoids have other clinically important effects (see Figure 51-4), such as antiinflammatory effects and a suppression of the immune system. Consequently, glucocorticoids are used therapeutically to treat inflammatory conditions such as rheumatoid arthritis.[169]

Inhibition of the normal immune response results from a gradual destruction of lymphoid tissue, followed by a decline in antibody production and a decrease in the numbers of eosinophils, basophils, and lymphocytes. The reduction in T-lymphocyte counts by glucocorticoids can occur acutely as a result of the redistribution of these cells from the intravascular space to the spleen, lymph nodes, and bone marrow. Thus an increase in the neutrophil count is commonly observed after glucocorticoid administration. The major suppressive effects of glucocorticoids on the inflammatory response and the immune system appear to be through the modulation of cytokine production via an inhibition of nuclear factor kappa B (NF-κB) expression and nuclear translocation. Cytokines released from immunocompetent cells mediate both the acute and chronic phases of inflammation and participate in the control of the immune response (see Chapter 22).

For example, cytokines such as interleukin (IL)-1, IL-2, IL-6, tumor necrosis factor (TNF), interferon-γ, and granulocyte-macrophage colony-stimulating factor (GMCSF) released from white blood cells with activation of the inflammatory response are inhibited by the glucocorticoid's antiinflammatory and immunosuppressive effects (Figure 51-5). Cytokines, such as IL-1, IL-6, and TNF have also been shown to directly stimulate the hypothalamic-pituitary-adrenal (HPA) axis as part of the link that exists between the neuroendocrine system and the immune system. Thus activated immunocompetent cells that produce cytokines suppress the immune response partly through glucocorticoids and the HPA (see Chapter 50). Inhibition of the immune response by exogenous glucocorticoids can sometimes be helpful, as is the case in organ transplant and graft recipients. Suppression of the immune response for any prolonged period of time, however, can render the patient more susceptible to infection.[26]

Glucocorticoids also have antiallergic properties, as a result of and by an inhibition of the synthesis of histamine by mast cells and basophils. Of the naturally occurring corticosteroids, only cortisol and corticosterone possess glucocorticoid activity, with cortisol the most effective. Cortisone and 11-dehydrocorticosterone lack direct glucocorticoid activity, but have potential glucocorticoid activity because they can be metabolized to cortisol and corticosterone, respectively.[135]

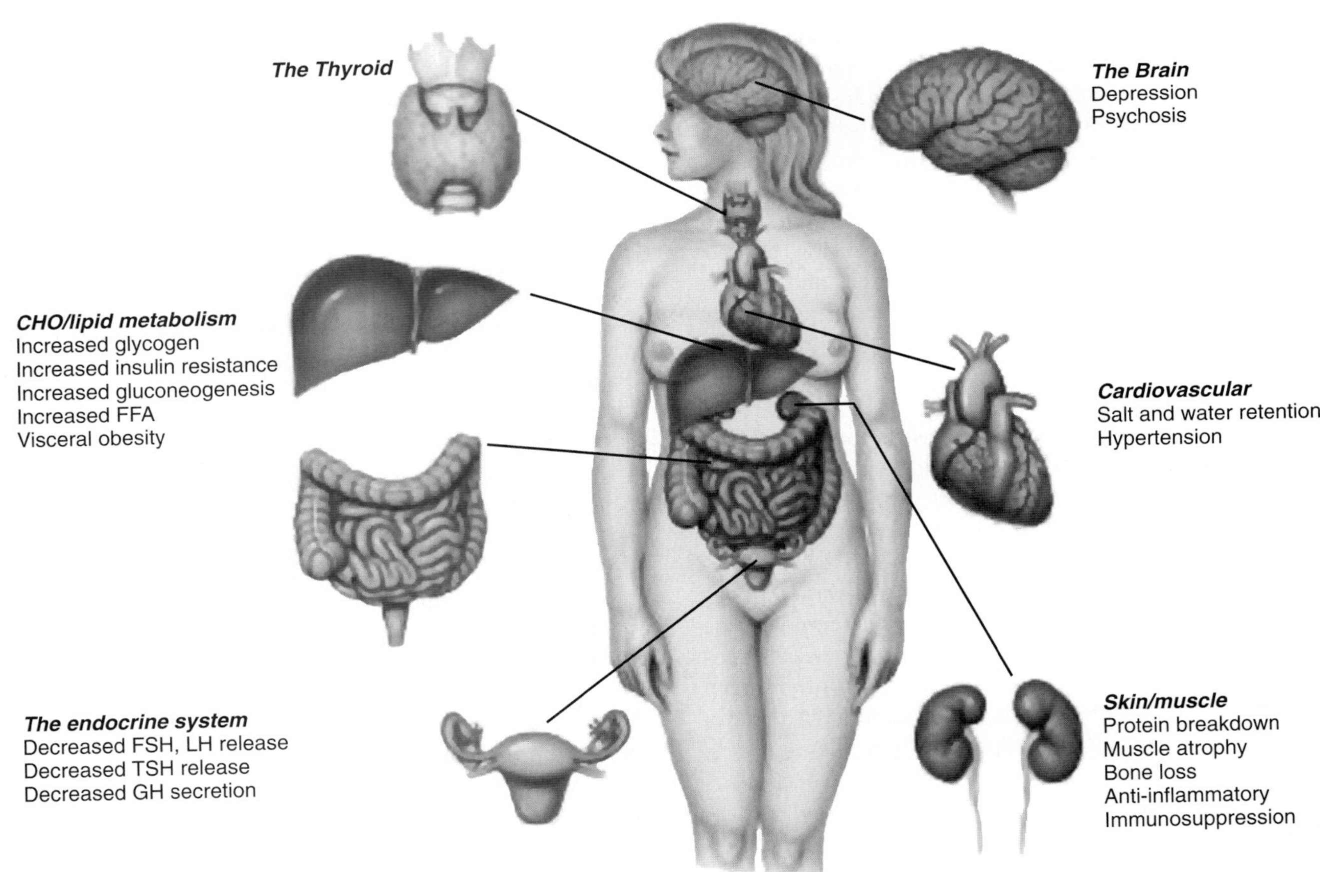

Figure 51-4 Principal effects of glucocorticoids on major organ systems in the human.

Mineralocorticoids

Mineralocorticoid refers to those steroids that regulate salt homeostasis (sodium conservation and potassium loss) and extracellular fluid volume.[6,30,38] Aldosterone is the most potent naturally occurring mineralocorticoid and is synthesized exclusively in the zona glomerulosa region of the adrenal cortex. This zone uniquely contains the enzyme aldosterone synthase, an obligatory enzyme in the synthetic pathway to aldosterone. Other adrenocortical steroids that have mineralocorticoid properties with varying degrees of potency include DOC, 18-hydroxy-DOC, corticosterone, and cortisol. A large number of analogues with mineralocorticoid and glucocorticoid activity have been synthesized; some are actually more potent than those that occur naturally (Table 51-4).

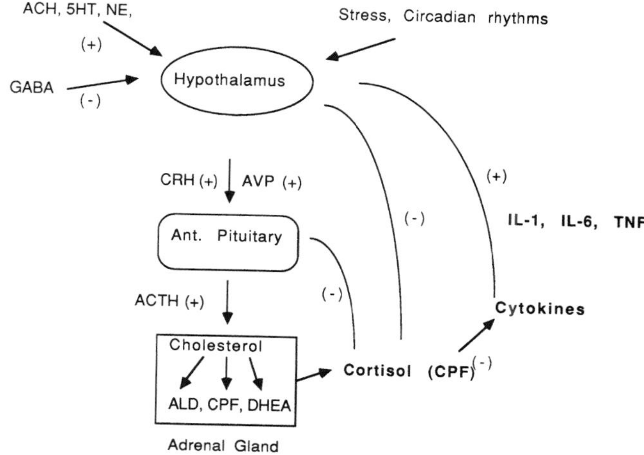

Figure 51-5 Positive and negative factors that affect the HPA axis. Note positive effects of the cytokines on HPA that link an activation of the immune system to the neuroendocrine axis. *ACH,* Acetylcholine; *ACTH,* adrenocorticotropic hormone; *ALD,* aldosterone; *AVP,* arginine vasopressin; *CPF,* cortisol; *CRH,* corticotropin-releasing hormone; *DHEA,* dehydroepiandrosterone; *GABA,* γ-aminobutyric acid; *5HT,* 5-hydroxytryptamine; *IL,* interleukin; *NE,* norepinephrine; *TNF,* tumor necrosis factor.

Adrenal Androgens[140]

In addition to the corticosteroids, the adrenal glands also secrete androgens, progesterone, and estrogen, all of which are produced by the gonads as well. Adrenal androgens are synthesized in the zona fasciculata and/or reticularis from the precursor substrate 17α-hydroxypregnenolone. The adrenal androgens include DHEA, androstenedione, and testosterone (Figure 51-6). DHEA and its sulfated derivative, DHEA sulfate (DHEA-S), are the most important adrenal androgens found in the circulation and are present in the highest concentration. The adult adrenal secretes approximately 6 to 8 mg/day of DHEA, 8 to 16 mg/day of DHEA-S, 1.5 mg/day of androstenedione, and 0.05 mg/day of testosterone. The amount of DHEA and/or DHEA-S produced is second only to that of cortisol among the adrenal steroids released daily into the circulation; these amounts account for about 50% of DHEA and more than 90% of DHEA-S that circulates in plasma. The adrenal glands also produce small amounts of the estrogens estradiol and estrone and insignificant amounts of progesterone and other precursor steroids on a daily basis.[154,189]

Steroidogenesis[169]

Cortisol Biosynthesis

Cortisol is synthesized from pregnenolone by two pathways in the fasciculata and reticularis zones of the adrenal gland. For simplicity, only one pathway is shown in Figure 51-6. The enzyme 17α-hydroxylase and the enzyme complex Δ^5-3β-hydroxysteroid dehydrogenase: Δ^5-ketosteroid isomerase located in the endoplasmic reticulum will synthesize 17α-hydroxyprogesterone from either 17α-hydroxypregnenolone or progesterone. Hydroxylation of this compound by the

TABLE 51-4 Relative Potencies of Corticosteroids

Corticosteroid	Glucocorticoid Activity	Mineralocorticoid Activity
Aldosterone	0.1	400
Corticosterone	0.2	2
Cortisol	1	1
Cortisone	0.7	0.7
Dexamethasone*	50-150	2
11-Deoxycorticosterone	0	20
Fludrocortisone*	10	400
6α-Methylprednisolone*	5	0.5
Prednisolone*	4	0.7
Prednisone*	4	0.7
Triamcinolone*	3	0

*Synthetic.

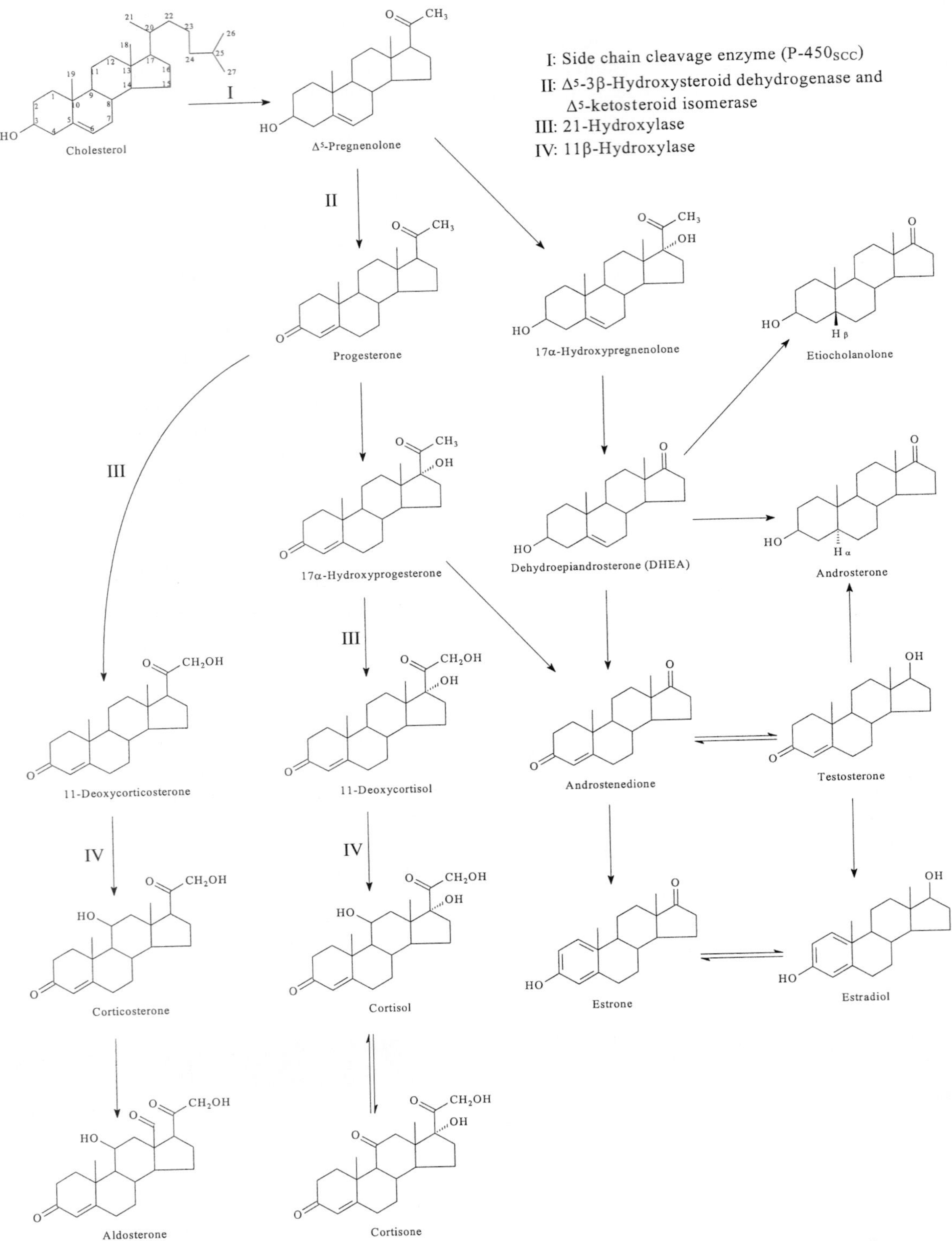

Figure 51-6 Biosynthesis of corticosteroids. Roman numerals I (side-chain cleavage enzyme), II (3-β-ol dehydrogenase and/or Δ^4 isomerase), III (21-hydroxylase), and IV (IIβ-hydroxylase) indicate sites of major blocks that cause adrenogenital syndromes. *(Copyright 1959 CIBA Pharmaceutical Co. Division of CIBA-GEIGY Corp. Reproduced, with permission, from* The CIBA Collection of Medical Illustrations *by Netter FH. All rights reserved.)*

21-hydroxylase enzyme at the 21α-position forms 11-deoxycortisol, which is then converted to cortisol by an 11β-hydroxylase enzyme located in the mitochondria.[135]

Synthesis of Mineralocorticoids

Aldosterone is the principal mineralocorticoid and is uniquely synthesized in the zona glomerulosa region of the adrenal cortex (see Figure 51-6). This layer lacks the 11β-hydroxylase enzyme required for cortisol synthesis, but it uniquely contains aldosterone synthase, the enzyme complex that catalyzes the formation of aldosterone from corticosterone. Although ACTH stimulates aldosterone production in the zona glomerulosa from progesterone and corticosterone,[169] the major control mechanism for the transformation of corticosterone to aldosterone in this region of the adrenal cortex is the renin-angiotensin system. Renin is an enzyme sensitive to the concentration of sodium in the plasma water perfusing the kidney that is released into the circulation when the sodium concentration in the perfusate declines. A decrease in perfusion pressure to the juxtaglomerular apparatus in the kidney and a negative sodium balance are the primary stimuli for renin release.

Other important regulatory factors that modulate aldosterone biosynthesis either directly or indirectly by affecting the renin-angiotensin system include the adrenergic and dopaminergic systems and the circulating concentrations of sodium and potassium. The renin-angiotensin system is affected by alterations in the adrenergic system by increasing epinephrine release and by changes in blood volume and glomerular blood flow. ACTH attains a more prominent role in the control of aldosterone secretion when the renin-angiotensin system is suppressed.

The zona glomerulosa also secretes 18-hydroxycorticosterone, a precursor steroid in the aldosterone biosynthetic pathway. This steroid also has mineralocorticoid properties, but is usually present in the circulation in extremely low concentrations. Mineralocorticoids are also synthesized in the zona fasciculata; DOC is the most potent, but corticosterone and cortisol also have weak mineralocorticoid activity. All of these steroids are synthesized as products of the glucocorticoid pathway.

Synthesis of Adrenal Androgens

The zona fasciculata and zona reticularis produce and secrete 17α-hydroxypregnenolone, the main precursor of the adrenal androgens. A microsomal 17α-hydroxylase/C-17,20-lyase ($P\text{-}450_{C17}$) enzyme converts 17α-hydroxypregnenolone to DHEA, which is then converted to DHEA-S by a sulfokinase. 17α-Hydroxyprogesterone can also be converted to androstenedione by this same 17α-hydroxylase/C-17, 20-lyase enzyme. Androstenedione is also derived from DHEA through the action of the 3β-hydroxysteroid dehydrogenase:Δ^5-ketosteroid isomerase complex. DHEA-S and DHEA are the most abundant adrenal-derived androgens.[20]

The adrenal cortex also secretes small quantities of the estrogenic steroids (C_{18} steroids).[185] However, 17β-estradiol and estrone are largely derived from the gonads and from peripheral conversion of testosterone and androstenedione by the aromatase enzyme located in other tissues, such as fat and the liver.

Circulating Forms

Steroid hormones circulate in blood either as free hormones or bound to carrier proteins, such as α_2-globulin corticosteroid-binding globulin (CBG), albumin, or sex hormone-binding globulin (SHBG).[198] Some steroids are conjugated to glucuronide or sulfate and thus circulate independent of a protein carrier. The excretion of steroids occurs via the kidneys or gastrointestinal tract, where they can be reabsorbed. CBG, albumin, and SHBG are produced by the liver (see Chapter 20). CBG and SHBG concentrations are increased by estrogens and in some patients with hepatitis and reduced by glucocorticoids, testosterone, and in patients with liver and kidney disease. At physiological concentrations, about 90% to 98% of steroid hormones circulate bound to a carrier protein, usually with high affinity for a binding globulin, such as CBG and SHBG. At higher physiological concentrations, albumin, which has a high capacity but low affinity for steroids, becomes a more important transport medium for steroids. When a steroid has low affinity for a "carrier protein," 60% to 70% of the steroid circulates bound principally to albumin.[198] Some steroids, such as aldosterone, have a relatively high affinity for CBG, but CBG is not a major carrier protein because cortisol, corticosterone, and 17α-hydroxyprogesterone far exceed the concentration of aldosterone. Similarly, testosterone and dihydrotestosterone circulate primarily bound to SHBG in men, whereas estradiol, despite high binding affinity for SHBG, is bound largely to albumin because its concentration is low relative to that of testosterone. DHEA-S and DHEA circulate primarily bound to albumin, and neither CBG nor SHBG is important in the transport of these adrenal androgens. Prednisolone is the only synthetic glucocorticoid with high binding affinity for CBG, whereas dexamethasone, methylprednisolone, and triamcinolone acetonide are primarily bound to albumin.[198]

One function of both CBG and SHBG is to serve as a circulating storage reserve for steroid hormones and to protect steroid hormones from inactivation. The binding constant for steroids with their respective binding globulins is relatively close to that of the tissue receptor. The biologically active fraction of steroid hormones is still somewhat controversial. There is general agreement that the free fraction and the albumin-bound fraction are readily available for steroid receptor uptake by tissue. This is sometimes referred to as the bioavailable steroid or as the free and weakly bound steroid. Steroids specifically bound to CBG or SHBG are considered to be biologically unavailable because of their high binding affinity to these carrier proteins.[9,61,177] This concept of hormone availability, however, is continuously being challenged. Some tissue have plasma membrane receptors that can bind the carrier protein–hormone complex. SHBG bound to dihydrotestosterone can activate the membrane signaling mechanism in prostate cells, increasing cyclic adenosine monophosphate (cAMP) formation and mitogenesis.[151] In addition, CBG and SHBG may have a function in tissues that have receptors for cortisol or dihydrotestosterone, respectively. Thus sex steroid hormones appear to act on tissue through two distinct structures, steroid receptors and R_{SHBG}. It has now been suggested that crosstalk occurs between membrane receptors and intranuclear receptors as part of the steroid mechanism of action. The measurement of SHBG-bound steroids may be an important part of interpreting steroid concentrations in states of deficiency and excess.

Metabolism

The liver is the principal site for the transformation and conjugation of steroid hormones, largely through the enriched presence of the cytochrome P-450 metabolizing enzyme systems; however, the kidneys also play an important role in steroid metabolism. Approximately 90% of conjugated steroids released by the liver are excreted by the kidney and about 50% of secreted cortisol appears in the urine as tetrahydrocortisol (THF) and tetrahydrocortisone (THE). Many tissues contain the necessary enzymes that can activate steroids or render them biologically inactive.[135] Cortisol, for example, is metabolized to cortisone through the activity of 11β-hydroxysteroid dehydrogenase; this change renders this steroid incapable of binding to the glucocorticoid receptor. The liver, however, can convert cortisone back to cortisol, which is biologically active. 17α-Hydroxyprogesterone can be metabolized to 11-DOC, a relatively potent mineralocorticoid in nonsteroid-synthesizing tissue. Androgens such as DHEA and androstenedione can be converted to testosterone in fat tissue and then to dihydrotestosterone in tissues containing the 5α-reductase enzyme. The aromatase enzyme converts testosterone and androstenedione to estradiol and estrone, respectively, in tissues such as fat and the liver. Even sulfated and glucuronidated steroids can be activated by the action of the enzymes sulfatase and β-glucuronidase.[209] Macrophages, for example, can convert DHEA-S to DHEA, which alters cytokine production by associated T lymphocytes. Testosterone is a potent androgen in muscle, a tissue that has little 5α-reductase activity. In skin and prostate tissue, with high Δ^4-5α-reductase activity, testosterone is a prohormone for dihydrotestosterone, the active androgen in these tissues.[58,204] Thus considerable metabolism of steroids takes place outside of their original site of synthesis.

Cortisol

An understanding of the metabolism of cortisol is important in interpreting tests designed to evaluate alterations in cortisol production rates and disorders of adrenal function.[135] Less than 2% of cortisol is excreted unchanged in the urine. As a result of its tight binding to CBG, cortisol is metabolized slowly ($t_{1/2} \sim 100$ minutes). In the liver, metabolism of cortisol involves reduction of the double bond between C-4 and C-5 by Δ^4-5β- or Δ^4-5α-reductase to form dihydrocortisol or dihydrocortisone. Further metabolism of cortisol and cortisone produces THF and THE, respectively, which are in turn metabolized to the cortoic acids, cortol, and cortolone (Figure 51-7). A minor metabolite of cortisol is 6β-cortisol, which appears unconjugated in the urine. More than 95% of the metabolites of cortisol and cortisone are conjugated by the liver; glucuronidation at the 3α-hydroxyl position is favored over the other hydroxyl groups, and the 21-hydroxyl group is favored for sulfations; glucuronide metabolites are more abundant than sulfated steroids.

Androgens

Adrenal androgens also have a complex metabolic fate; DHEA-S is formed in the adrenal cortex or by sulfokinases in the liver and kidney from DHEA and excreted by the kidney.[129] DHEA and DHEA-S can be metabolized by 7α- and 16α-hydroxylases. 17β-Reduction of both compounds forms Δ^4-5-androstenediol and its sulfate. Androstenedione can be metabolized to androsterone after 3α- and 5α-reduction. 5β-Reduction results in the formation of etiocholanolone (see Figure 51-7). These metabolites are conjugated to glucuronides and sulfates, which are then excreted in the urine.

Factors Affecting Metabolism

Liver, kidney, and thyroid disease affect the secretion and metabolism of the adrenal steroids. Other factors affecting these processes include stress, age, estrogen therapy, nutrition, and drugs.

Liver Disease

Chronic liver disease reduces cortisol clearance and the production of urinary metabolites. Cortisol concentrations are elevated by acute ingestion of alcohol. Individuals with alcoholic cirrhosis have normal to elevated basal cortisol concentrations, blunted circadian rhythms, and prolonged clearance rates.

Kidney Disease

In patients with chronic renal failure, plasma concentrations of total and free cortisol and ACTH are usually normal. Plasma-conjugated metabolites of cortisol are elevated, and renal excretion, as expected, is reduced. ACTH stimulation (4 hours) produces normal to slightly exaggerated responses of cortisol, DHEA-S, and aldosterone and normal responses of DHEA-S and androstenedione.

Thyroid Disease

Hypothyroidism reduces and hyperthyroidism increases both the secretion and metabolism of cortisol without substantially affecting its blood concentrations. Thyroid hormone alters 11β-hydroxysteroid dehydrogenase activity

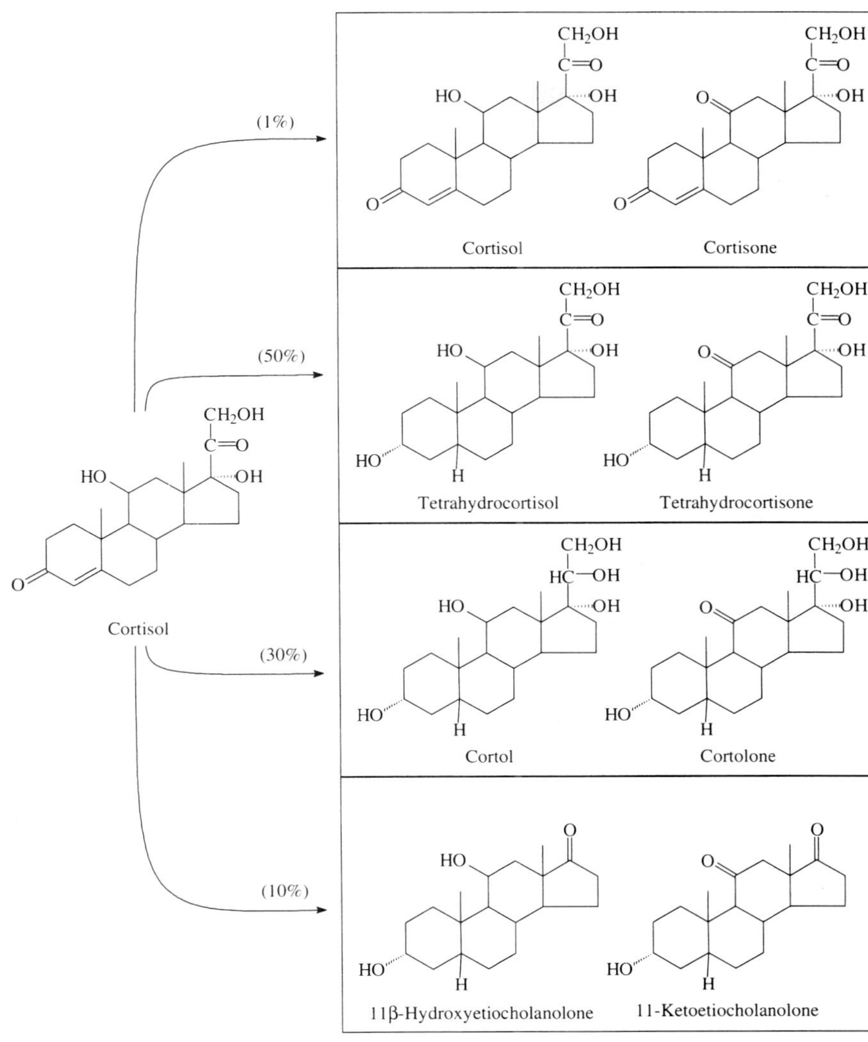

Figure 51-7 Schematic drawing of the major urinary metabolites of cortisol showing the approximate extent of conversion and the metabolites as determined by different methods. *(From James VHT, Landon J. In: Recent advances in endocrinology, 8th ed. Boston: Little, Brown & Co Inc, 1968.)*

that converts cortisol to cortisone. In hyperthyroidism, 11-ketometabolites, tetrahydrocortisone, and cortolones are favored; in hypothyroidism, tetrahydrocortisol and cortols predominate. Hypothyroidism decreases the concentrations of DHEA and DHEA-S. 5α-Reductase activity is reduced, which leads to the formation of more androsterone relative to etiocholanolone.

Stress

Acute stress from trauma or illness elevates the concentrations of both adrenal glucocorticoids, cortisol and corticosterone, and the adrenal androgens DHEA and DHEA-S. Chronic illness elevates plasma cortisol concentrations but suppresses DHEA, DHEA-S, and androstenedione concentrations.

Age

The newborn produces more cortisone than cortisol. A few days after birth, cortisol production predominates in a pattern similar to that of adults. Neonates lack 5α-reductases and have deficient glucuronyl transferase and therefore produce more 6β-hydroxylated metabolites of cortisol than adults.[134] Circulating concentrations of cortisol and CBG remain constant after the neonatal period. In old age, both the production and metabolic clearance rates of cortisol are about 25% lower than in younger adults. Urinary excretion of cortisol and other 17-hydroxyl metabolites decreases with age, but ACTH stimulation of cortisol remains normal in the elderly.

Age and familial factors in both men and women influence both plasma adrenal androgens (DHEA and DHEA-S). Adrenal androgen secretion starts to rise about the age of 9, peaks at about age 25, and declines after age 30.[170] In the seventh decade of life, the adrenal androgen concentrations fall to prepubertal concentrations. Thus in the elderly, the circadian variation in plasma DHEA is relatively blunted and dissociated from the circadian variation in cortisol. The adrenal contribution of serum androstenedione declines with age.[108] DHEA and DHEA-S responses to stimulation with exogenous ACTH are decreased in the elderly, but the androstenedione response is minimally affected.[108,141]

Estrogen Therapy

Estrogens increase the plasma concentrations of CBG and thus markedly influence total cortisol blood concentrations. The concentration of free cortisol is unaffected; the clearance of cortisol and its production rate and concentrations of urinary metabolites are subnormal with estrogen therapy.

Nutrition

Obesity elevates the urinary conjugated metabolites of cortisol thus erroneously suggesting the diagnosis of Cushing's syndrome. The measurement of urinary free cortisol, which is not influenced by obesity, is therefore recommended when screening for Cushing's syndrome. Plasma concentrations of total and free cortisol and urinary free cortisol excretion rates in obesity are all normal.[174] Dexamethasone suppression of adrenal function is also normal. However, cortisol responses to exogenous ACTH are increased, suggesting adrenocortical hyperplasia. Obesity also can elevate the adrenal androgens DHEA and DHEA-S and androstenedione production and clearance rates.[41,152] Plasma concentrations of these steroids are elevated in obese children during pubertal development but not in obese adults.

Starvation is associated with a decrease in both the production and clearance rates of cortisol. In patients with anorexia nervosa, despite reductions in urinary excretion of cortisol metabolites, plasma concentrations and urinary excretion of cortisol may be elevated.[135] The responses of cortisol to dexamethasone are blunted in many patients with anorexia nervosa, but cortisol responses to ACTH in these patients are normal.

Drugs

Hepatic mixed-function oxidases are induced by many drugs, including phenytoin, phenobarbital, mitotane, aminoglutethimide, and rifampin. In addition, 6β-hydroxylase and other drug-metabolizing pathways that metabolize cortisol and other steroids are increased by a number of drugs. Urinary excretion rates of cortisol metabolites are reduced, but plasma cortisol concentrations and urinary free excretion rates of cortisol are not affected. The metabolism of synthetic glucocorticoids, prednisolone, and dexamethasone is markedly increased by drugs that induce the hepatic hydroxylase enzyme systems. Dexamethasone suppression test results and metyrapone test results are also altered. Knowledge of the patient's drug history is important for the proper interpretation of tests that validate the integrity of the pituitary-adrenal axis.

The Hypothalamic-Pituitary-Adrenal Cortical Axis

Secretion of adrenal glucocorticoids and androgens is regulated by ACTH (see Chapter 50), which in turn is under the control of the hypothalamic peptide, corticotropin-releasing hormone (CRH).[169,211] The pituitary gland also has been found to secrete a separate hormonal factor that specifically regulates adrenal androgen production.[141] This substance, called cortical androgen-stimulating hormone, has been identified as a glycopeptide in human pituitary extracts and shows sequence homology to an 18–amino acid *N*-terminal component of pro-opiomelanocorticotropin, the precursor peptide of ACTH and of melanocyte-stimulating hormone. The HPA relationships in health and in various adrenal disorders are depicted in Figure 51-8.

Regulation of Adrenal Hormones

Adrenocorticotropic Hormone Secretion

Biorhythms and other physiological events in the brain result in episodic and circadian secretion of CRH from the hypothalamus. This in turn elicits similar circadian variation in ACTH release.[50,76,135] Secreted ACTH then stimulates cortisol production, which provides negative feedback inhibition to the CRH-ACTH axis.[169] The secretion of CRH, a 41–amino acid peptide, is modulated by neuroendocrine, physical, and emotional factors.[169] Besides CRH, other circulating factors can have an influence on the secretory dynamics of ACTH release. Antidiuretic hormone from the

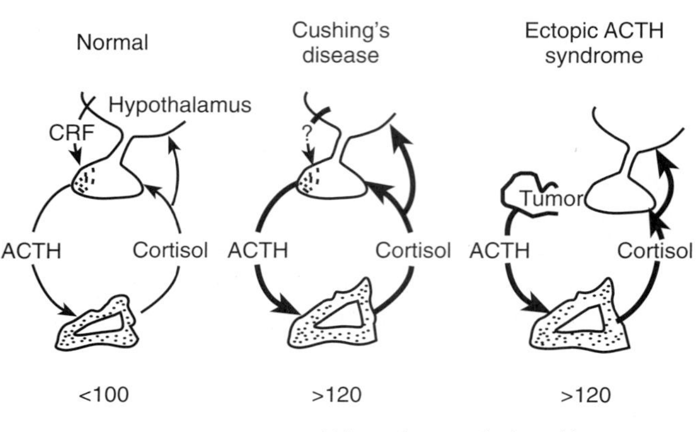

Figure 51-8 HPA under normal conditions and in various adrenal disorders. *ACTH*, Adrenocorticotropic hormone; *CRF*, corticotropin-releasing factor. *(From Lipsett MB, Odell WD, Rosenberg LE. Humoral syndromes associated with nonendocrine tumors. Ann Intern Med 1964;61:733. Copyright 1964, American Medical Association.)*

posterior pituitary and other peptides (angiotensin II, activin, cytokines, opiates, and somatostatin) and catecholamines influence the secretion of ACTH from the adenohypophysis.[46,156]

The circadian rhythm of ACTH secretion under normal wake and sleep cycles produces higher cortisol concentrations in the morning between 0400 and noon and lower concentrations in late evening and early morning.[135] The magnitude of the morning cortisol concentration is affected by familial and genetic factors.[109]

Trauma, fever, surgery, hypoglycemia, alcohol ingestion, uncontrolled diabetes, and nutritional deprivation, including that associated with anorexia nervosa, are physical stresses that elevate plasma cortisol concentrations and alter the circadian rhythm.[169] Major depression and severe anxiety are psychological stresses that also elevate plasma cortisol concentrations. ACTH secretion in response to minor stresses is inhibited by the administration of exogenous glucocorticoids. Major stress responses such as surgery, however, result in cortisol secretion unresponsive to glucocorticoid suppression. Cortisol secretion is suppressed by glucocorticoids in lesser forms of stress, such as minor surgery, exercise, or hypoglycemia.

Prolonged suppression of ACTH by administration of glucocorticoids causes atrophy of the adrenal cortex.[135] The degree of atrophy is related to the duration and magnitude of suppression of ACTH secretion. With prolonged intense suppression, recovery of the HPA axis can take several days to a few months.

Cortisol Secretion

ACTH has both trophic and steroidogenic effects on the adrenal cortex and is under negative feedback control from nonprotein-bound cortisol.[169] ACTH binds to a G protein–coupled, melanocortin-2 receptor at the membrane of each adrenocortical cell with signal transduction mediated via cAMP. Cortisol is secreted within a few minutes after a rise in serum ACTH through a StAR-mediated increase in cholesterol delivery to the desmolase enzyme located in the inner mitochondrial membrane. Chronic exposure to ACTH results in increased synthesis of all steroidogenic enzymes through gene activation at the nuclear concentration. Deficiency of ACTH results in atrophy of the zona fasciculata and zona reticularis. With atrophy of the adrenal cortex from various causes and reduced cortisol synthesis and release, plasma ACTH concentrations rise. Other modifying factors such as age, various diseases, estrogen therapy, nutrition, general illness, and drugs also affect cortisol secretion. Both hypertrophy and hyperplasia of the adrenal cortex occur in response to chronic exposure to ACTH. The trophic response to ACTH can be reproduced by cAMP stimulation of insulin-like growth factor-II rather than cAMP directly.[135]

The proinflammatory cytokines including IL-1, IL-6, and TNFα also increase cortisol secretion through an increase in pituitary ACTH secretion as part of the important immune-endocrine interaction that occurs with disease and infection (see Chapter 22).

Adrenal Androgen Secretion

The adrenal cortex secretes DHEA (~4 mg/day), DHEA-S (10 mg/day), androstenedione (1.5 mg/day), and testosterone (0.05 mg/day) as components of the adrenal androgen pathway. ACTH partially regulates adrenal androgen production in adults; both DHEA and androstenedione are secreted in conjunction with cortisol.[141] Adrenal androgen production begins to rise in late childhood about the age of 9 just months before the onset of puberty, reaches a peak in the third decade of life, and then gradually decreases, reaching low concentrations again in advanced age.[20] Glucocorticoid therapy also suppresses the secretion of adrenal androgens.[106,141] The secretion of cortisol and adrenal androgens, however, can be dissociated, particularly in children, adolescents, and the elderly. The explanation for the dissociation is unclear, although it lends credence to the suggestion that an independent factor from the pituitary gland, such as cortical androgen-stimulating hormone, can stimulate adrenal androgen production independent of ACTH.[141] In young children, the low adrenal androgen concentrations are not further suppressed by glucocorticoid therapy.

Aldosterone Secretion

The primary control mechanism for the secretion of aldosterone involves the renin-angiotensin system although potassium and to a lesser extent ACTH can also promote secretion of aldosterone from the zona glomerulosa. *Renin* is a proteolytic enzyme synthesized and stored in specialized cells, the *juxtaglomerular epithelial cells,* located along the terminal part of the afferent arterioles of the renal glomeruli.[6,121] These specialized cells constitute part of the juxtaglomerular apparatus. Upon stimulation of the juxtaglomerular apparatus, renin is released into the circulation, where it hydrolyzes its substrate, angiotensinogen, to produce a decapeptide known as *angiotensin I.* Angiotensinogen is a globulin synthesized in the liver. Angiotensin I is then rapidly converted to an octapeptide, *angiotensin II,* by a circulating *angiotensin-converting enzyme,* which is found in abundance in the lung. Angiotensin II is a potent vasoconstrictor and stimulates the cells of the zona glomerulosa to produce aldosterone. Angiotensin II stimulates aldosterone secretion by increasing the transcription of CYP11B2, the gene responsible for aldosterone synthase through common intracellular signaling pathways. Potassium, on the other hand, stimulates aldosterone synthesis and release through a membrane depolarization effect that opens up calcium channels in adrenal cells to activate cell signaling mechanisms such as phospholipase C, leading to an increase in aldosterone synthase synthesis and release. The primary stimuli for renin release are a decrease in renal arteriolar pressure, oncotic pressure, and an increase in sympathetic drive to the macula densa of the juxtaglomerular apparatus and a negative sodium balance. Stimulation of renin release and aldosterone secretion under different physiological and pathological conditions is discussed later. ACTH also increases aldosterone secretion. However, the size and function of the zona glomerulosa are affected primarily by the renin-angiotensin system and potassium. Hyperplasia results when concentrations of angiotensin II or K^+, or both, are elevated, and atrophy occurs with a deficiency of angiotensin II or with defects in its actions.

Testing the Functional Status of the Adrenal Cortex

Concentrations of hypothalamic and anterior pituitary peptides and adrenal glucocorticoids are measured accurately and at low concentrations in body fluids using immunoassay and instrumental methods. Relying on basal hormone concentrations for confirming adrenocortical dysfunction, however, can be problematic because of the episodic and circadian secretion of the hormones that regulate the HPA axis. For example, some individuals have an abnormality of the HPA axis, but still maintain basal cortisol and ACTH secretion within the reference interval of the normal population. Dynamic testing of the HPA axis helps define abnormalities that are not reflected in basal hormone secretion.

Corticosteroid Function

Basal Peptide and Steroid Hormone Concentrations

Episodic secretion and circadian variation limit the clinical diagnostic accuracy of basal serum cortisol concentrations. Serum cortisol concentrations are highest in the early morning hours and varies from 5 to 25 µg/dL between 0400 and 1200 hours. Late afternoon values are about half the morning concentrations and are frequently less than 5 µg/dL between 2200 and 0200 hours. Serum cortisol combined with plasma ACTH improves the diagnostic accuracy of basal values.

Urinary free cortisol obtained from a 24-hour urine collection is an integrated measure of plasma free cortisol and eliminates the circadian influence on cortisol secretion. Urine free cortisol measurements are therefore considered to be the best screening test for hyperadrenocorticism. The urinary free cortisol excretion rate in normal subjects falls between 20 and 80 µg/day (Figure 51-9). The measurement of urinary 17-hydroxycorticosteroid excretion rates for determining adrenocortical hyperfunction is no longer recommended because of problems with method sensitivity and specificity.

Mineralocorticoid and adrenal androgen secretion is also circadian and episodic in nature, but the dynamic swings in concentrations are not as pronounced as with cortisol. It is usually recommended, however, that blood samples for adrenal steroids be collected in the 0700 to 1000 hour time frame for consistency in result interpretation.

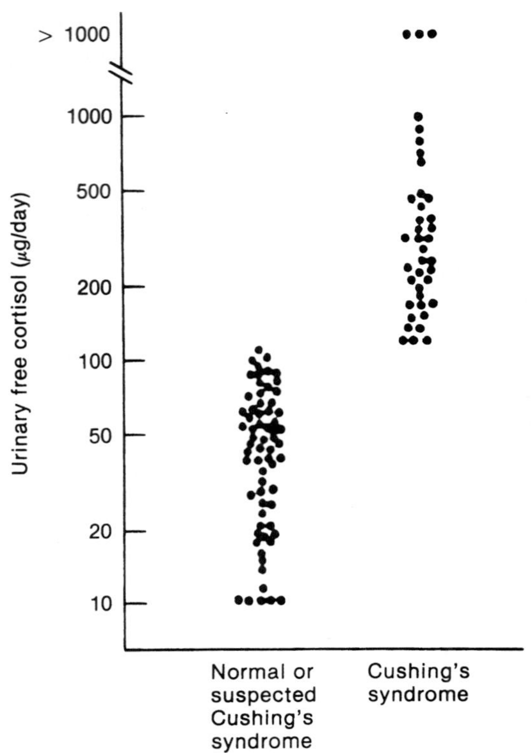

Figure 51-9 Urinary free cortisol excretion in normal individuals with Cushing's syndrome. *(From Burke CW, Beardwell CG. Cushing's syndrome. An evaluation of the clinical usefulness of urinary free cortisol measurements in screening for Cushing's syndrome. Q J Med 1973;42:1175.)*

Stimulation Tests of Adrenal Function

Provocative stimulation tests are useful in documenting hyposecretion of adrenocortical hormones.[135] A specific stimulus is applied, and the release of a given hormone is measured in a specific time frame. *ACTH stimulation tests,* sometimes referred to as the cosyntropin test, are designed to document the functional capacity of the adrenal glands to synthesize cortisol (Boxes 51-1 and 51-2). In healthy individuals, the administration of exogenous ACTH rapidly increases the secretion of cortisol by twofold to threefold within 60 minutes of the applied stimulus. This functional response may be impaired either by adrenal atrophy, caused by a chronic deficiency of ACTH, or by primary destruction of the adrenal cortex. The biologically active 1-24 amino acid sequence of human ACTH has been synthesized and is available as tetracosactrin (Synacthen). This compound is a potent stimulant for cortisol secretion and has a very brief half-life and minimal antigenicity. A peak plasma cortisol concentration >20 µg/dL (525 nmol/L) within 60 minutes of the intravenous administration of Synacthen is defined as a normal response.

A direct and selective test of pituitary gland function is the *CRH stimulation test* (Box 51-3).[93] Injection of ovine CRH stimulates ACTH secretion in normal subjects within

BOX 51-1 Protocol for the Rapid Adrenocorticotropic Hormone (ACTH) (Synacthen) Test

Rationale The administration of ACTH to normal subjects results in a rapid rise in the serum cortisol concentration. Patients with adrenal destruction (Addison's disease) show no change in serum cortisol concentration after ACTH administration. Patients with atrophy of the adrenal cortex caused by exogenous glucocorticoid treatment or dysfunction of the pituitary gland or hypothalamus may show a slight rise in serum cortisol concentration, but not one of normal magnitude.

Procedure A baseline blood sample is drawn for determination of serum cortisol concentration; then 250 μg of Synacthen (1-24 ACTH) is given intramuscularly or intravenously. Further samples for serum cortisol determination are drawn 30 and 60 minutes after injection.

Interpretation A peak serum cortisol concentration of >20 μg/dL is a normal response. The peak value is more important than the incremental change. The incremental change may not be seen in patients who are tested at times of stress, when their adrenal output of cortisol is already maximally stimulated by endogenous ACTH.

BOX 51-2 Protocol for the Multiple-Day Adrenocorticotropic Hormone (ACTH) Stimulation Test

Rationale Multiple-day ACTH stimulation testing for assessment of adrenal cortex function is required occasionally to evaluate adrenal cortisol responsiveness. A common situation is the diagnosis of adrenal insufficiency, which is treated with glucocorticosteroids before establishment of an etiology. Prolonged ACTH stimulation is also used to distinguish primary from secondary and/or tertiary causes of adrenal insufficiency.

Procedure ACTH gel, 80 U/day, is injected for 3 days. This is followed by a standard 8-hour infusion of ACTH (250 μg of Synacthen over 8 hours). Urinary free cortisol and serum cortisol are measured daily.

Interpretation Serum cortisol values more than 20 μg/dL exclude primary adrenal insufficiency. Glucocorticoid withdrawal would be required before assessing secondary or tertiary adrenal insufficiency in such cases. Little or no increase in cortisol secretion is seen in primary adrenal failure even over successive days. A progressive staircase rise is seen over 2 to 3 days in adrenal insufficiency caused by pituitary or hypothalamic disease or steroid concentration suppression. Little or no response is also seen in congenital adrenal hyperplasia (CAH) caused by 21- and 17-hydroxylase deficiencies.

BOX 51-3 Protocol for the Corticotropin-Releasing Hormone (CRH) Stimulation Test

Rationale Exogenous CRH stimulates the secretion of ACTH from the anterior pituitary gland in normal subjects. Cortisol concentration is an indicator of ACTH response.

Procedure Synthetic ovine CRH (preferred) or human CRH (1 μg/kg body weight) is administered intravenously in bolus form at either 0900 or 2000 hours. Blood samples for cortisol and ACTH assays are collected 15 minutes and immediately before and 5, 15, 30, 60, 120, and 180 minutes after CRH injection.

Interpretation In normal subjects, plasma ACTH concentrations peak 30 minutes after CRH injection (80 ± 7 pg/mL at 0930 hr; 29 ± 2.6 pg/mL at 2030 hr), and serum cortisol peaks at 60 minutes (13 ± 1 μg/dL at 1000; 17 ± 0.7 μg/dL at 2100 hr). Patients with pituitary ACTH deficiency (secondary adrenal insufficiency) have decreased ACTH and cortisol responses. Patients with hypothalamic disease have prolonged ACTH responses and subnormal cortisol responses. Most patients with Cushing's syndrome caused by adrenal tumors or nonendocrine ACTH-producing tumors do not respond to CRH. Most patients with Cushing's syndrome respond with a normal or excessive increase in ACTH. Responses are usually normal in patients with depression.

60 to 180 minutes; glucocorticoids inhibit this effect. The use of this test is in the differential diagnosis of adrenocortical hyperfunction and hypofunction. This test is also used in the differential diagnosis of endogenous Cushing's syndrome and to distinguish secondary from tertiary ACTH deficiency.[42]

A variation of the CRH stimulation test measures ACTH in blood samples drawn from the inferior petrosal sinus (IPS) both to document the presence of a pituitary microadenoma and to determine on which side of the pituitary the microadenoma is located. Blood samples are collected from both right and left IPS veins and from a peripheral vein before and 2, 5, and 10 minutes after the intravenous administration of ovine CRH (1 μg/kg body weight) over 20 to 60 seconds. The ratio of the IPS concentration to peripheral venous concentration of plasma ACTH is used to predict the location of excess corticotropin secretion. As shown in Figure 51-10, the maximum ratio is >3 in patients with pituitary Cushing's syndrome and <3 in those with the likelihood of an ectopic ACTH syndrome or an adrenal tumor. Some endocrinologists claim that IPS sampling is the best test for distinguishing ACTH-dependent forms of Cushing's syndrome when performed in the setting of prolonged hypercortisolism. ACTH concentrations are suppressed in patients with primary adrenal tumors compared with those with either Cushing's syndrome or the ectopic ACTH syndrome.

To test the integrity of the pituitary-adrenal axis, other indirect tests of ACTH secretion rely on the adrenal response

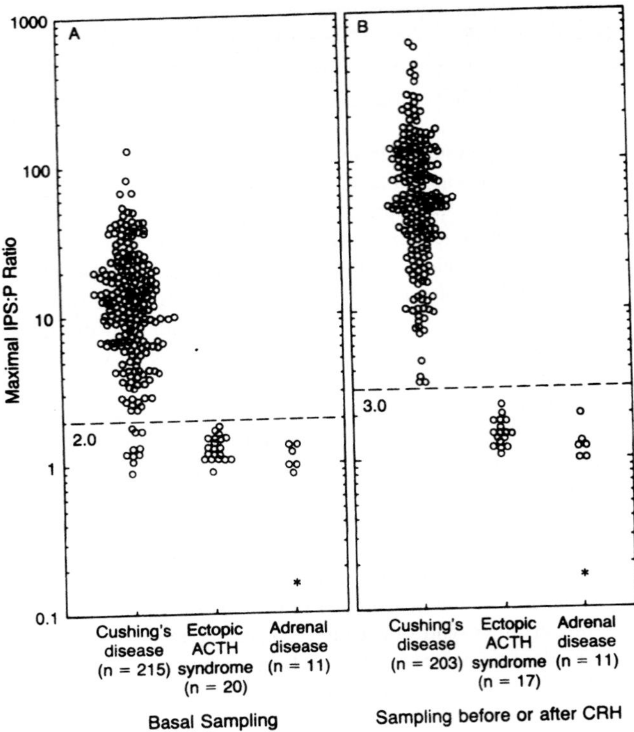

Figure 51-10 Inferior petrosal sinus-to-peripheral venous (IPS: P) plasma ACTH ratios in patients with Cushing's syndrome during basal sampling (*panel A*) and either during basal sampling or 2 or 5 minutes after ovine corticotropin-releasing hormone (oCRH) administration (*panel B*). During basal sampling, the maximum ratio was ≥2.0 in 205 of 215 patients with confirmed Cushing's syndrome and <2.0 in 20 patients with ectopic ACTH syndrome and 11 patients with adrenal Cushing's syndrome. All of the 203 patients who had confirmed Cushing's syndrome and who received oCRH had a maximum IPS:P ratio >3.0 in one of the basal sample sets or in one of the post-oCRH sample sets, whereas all of the 17 patients with ectopic ACTH syndrome and the 11 patients with adrenal Cushing's syndrome who received oCRH had a ratio <3.0. The *asterisks* represent five patients in whom immunoreactive ACTH was undetectable in peripheral plasma before and after oCRH administration. *(From Oldfield EH, Doppman JL, Nieman LK, Chrousos GP, Miller DL, Katz DA, et al. Petrosal sinus sampling with and without corticotropin-releasing hormone for the differential diagnosis of Cushing's syndrome. N Engl J Med 1991;325:897-905.)*

to maneuvers that stimulate endogenous ACTH release. In the *insulin-induced hypoglycemia stimulation test,* insulin is given to stimulate the release of CRH through hypoglycemia, and plasma ACTH or cortisol concentrations are evaluated for an increase (see Box 50-3; Chapter 50). This test involves risks and should be performed only with an experienced physician in attendance.

A less risky indirect test of HPA axis function involves the administration of metyrapone, an inhibitor of the 11β-hydroxylase enzyme that converts 11-deoxycortisol to cortisol. In normal individuals, the fall in the plasma cortisol concentration that accompanies the metyrapone-induced enzyme block stimulates pituitary ACTH release, and adrenal steroid precursors then accumulate to the point of the enzyme block. Under normal circumstances, 11-deoxycortisol (compound S), the steroid substrate for the 11β-hydroxylase enzyme, increases fortyfold to eightyfold within 3 hours after metyrapone administration. The lack of an increase suggests primary adrenal failure. Several protocols have been designed for *metyrapone stimulation testing;* one that is simple and relatively safe for outpatient testing is described in Box 51-4.

BOX 51-4 Protocol for the Overnight Single-Dose Metyrapone Stimulation Test

Rationale Metyrapone inhibits 11β-hydroxylase, the enzyme that catalyzes the step immediately preceding cortisol synthesis. As the blood concentration of cortisol falls, the negative feedback effect is diminished, causing release of ACTH from the pituitary gland. The stimulatory effect of ACTH on the adrenal cortex leads to a rise in 11-deoxycortisol, the compound immediately preceding cortisol in the biosynthetic pathway.

Procedure Metyrapone (30 mg/kg body weight) is given orally at midnight with milk or a snack (to delay absorption). At 0800 hours the following morning, blood is drawn for determination of 11-deoxycortisol, cortisol, and ACTH concentrations.

Interpretation In normal subjects, 11-deoxycortisol increases from <1 μg/dL to >7 μg/dL after metyrapone stimulation, and ACTH values exceed 150 pg/mL. No response or impaired response may be seen in pituitary or hypothalamic disease combined with inadequate enzyme blockade (plasma cortisol >3 μg/dL) or with Cushing's syndrome caused by adrenal tumors or nonendocrine ACTH-secreting tumors. Exaggerated responses may be seen in pituitary Cushing's syndrome.

Suppression Tests

Suppression tests are used to document hypersecretion of the adrenocortical hormones.[135] In normal individuals, an elevation in the blood concentration of cortisol inhibits ACTH release from the pituitary gland. This results in decreased production of cortisol and other adrenal steroids from the adrenal cortex. The integrity of this feedback mechanism can be tested by administering a potent glucocorticoid, such as dexamethasone, and judging suppression of ACTH secretion by measuring serum or urine cortisol concentrations. A number of *dexamethasone suppression tests* are available for clinical use (Boxes 51-5 through 51-8). A low dose of dexamethasone is used initially to document true hypersecretion of cortisol.[207] Patients with Cushing's syndrome of any cause will fail to suppress their cortisol secretion overnight with a low dose of dexamethasone. Higher doses of dexamethasone given over 48 hours are then used to establish the differential diagnosis of an ACTH-secreting pituitary adenoma as distinct from an ectopic ACTH source. A >50% suppression of plasma cortisol in comparison with

BOX 51-5 Protocol for the Overnight Low-Dose Dexamethasone Suppression Test

Rationale Dexamethasone, a cortisol analogue, suppresses ACTH and cortisol production in normal subjects but not in patients with Cushing's syndrome.

Procedure One milligram of dexamethasone is given orally at 2300 or midnight. Blood is drawn for determination of serum cortisol at 0800 hours on the next morning.

Interpretation In normal subjects, serum cortisol concentration is suppressed to 2 μg/dL or less after administration of 1 mg of dexamethasone. Most patients with Cushing's syndrome do not show adequate suppression, and 0800 hours cortisol concentrations are usually >10 μg/dL. Serum cortisol >2 μg/dL may also be seen in cases of stress, obesity, infection, acute or chronic illness, alcohol abuse, severe depression, oral contraceptive use, pregnancy, estrogen therapy, failure to take the dexamethasone, or treatment with phenytoin or phenobarbital (enhancement of dexamethasone metabolism).

BOX 51-6 Protocol for the Multiple Low-Dose Dexamethasone Suppression Test

Rationale Normal subjects show lowering of serum and urinary free cortisol concentrations under the conditions of low-dose dexamethasone suppression. Patients with excess cortisol production regardless of etiology usually show persistent elevation of cortisol under these conditions.

Procedure Twenty-four-hour urine samples are collected daily for 4 consecutive days. Dexamethasone, 0.5 mg, is given orally every 6 hours starting at 0800 hours on day 2 (for a total of 8 doses). Free cortisol, 17-hydroxycorticosteroids, and creatinine are measured in each 24-hour urine sample. Other measurements include serum cortisol determinations on day 1 (at 0800 hours and 2000 hours) to look for diurnal variation and on day 5 (at 0800 hours).

Interpretation Normal subjects have suppressed serum and urinary free cortisol concentrations on day 4 to <50% of baseline values; serum cortisol at 2000 hours on day 1 should be one third of the value at 0800 hours. Patients with Cushing's syndrome usually do not show diurnal rhythmicity and do not show suppression with low-dose dexamethasone. Those patients taking phenytoin or phenobarbital, or both, metabolize dexamethasone more rapidly than do normal subjects and may not show suppression.

the original basal result defines a positive response. Patients with an ectopic ACTH-producing tumor will fail to suppress with high-dose dexamethasone. Abnormal suppression of cortisol by dexamethasone has been observed in patients with depression, severe stress, uncontrolled diabetes mellitus, or anorexia nervosa; with estrogen administration, and in subjects receiving medications, such as phenytoin, that induce the hepatic enzyme systems that can metabolize the dexamethasone.

BOX 51-7 Protocol for the Multiple High-Dose Dexamethasone Suppression Test

Rationale Patients with Cushing's syndrome caused by an ACTH-producing pituitary adenoma usually show suppression of cortisol with high-dose dexamethasone. Patients with Cushing's syndrome from other causes (adrenocortical adenoma, adrenocortical carcinoma, or ectopic production of ACTH) usually do not demonstrate any change in cortisol concentration.

Procedure Twenty-four-hour urine collections are obtained daily for 4 days for free cortisol and 17-hydroxycorticosteroid determinations. Dexamethasone, 2.0 mg orally every 6 hours, is begun at 0800 hours on day 2 and continued for eight doses. Free cortisol and creatinine are measured in each 24-hour urine sample. Other measurements include plasma cortisol at 0800 hours and 2000 hours on day 1 to look for diurnal variation and at 0800 hours on day 5.

Interpretation Patients with Cushing's syndrome caused by an ACTH-secreting pituitary adenoma usually show (1) suppression of urinary free cortisol and 17-hydroxycorticosteroid excretion ≥50% of baseline by day 4; (2) lack of diurnal variation in plasma cortisol; and (3) plasma cortisol ≤10 μg/dL at 0800 hours on day 5.

BOX 51-8 Protocol for the High-Dose Overnight Dexamethasone Suppression Test

Rationale The rationale for this test is similar to the rationale for the multiple high-dose dexamethasone suppression test (see Box 51-7).

Procedure Dexamethasone, 4 mg, is given orally at 2300 and 2400 hours. Blood is drawn for determination of plasma cortisol at 0700 hours or 0800 hours the next morning or 8 to 9 hours after dexamethasone is given.

Interpretation Most patients with Cushing's syndrome show a suppression of baseline cortisol concentration of at least 50%. If suppression is <50%, the test should be repeated with 8 to 24 mg of dexamethasone.

Mineralocorticoid Function

Basal Peptide and Steroid Hormone Concentrations

Concentrations of adrenal mineralocorticoids (e.g., aldosterone and DOC) and factors of the renin-angiotensin system (e.g., renin) are routinely measured in body fluids by various immunoassay and instrument-based methods.[6] Aldosterone, like cortisol, is secreted episodically, with the highest circulating concentrations at about the time of awakening and the lowest concentrations shortly after sleep onset; aldosterone concentrations, however, are only modestly stimulated by ACTH secretion.[119] In healthy subjects, a low-sodium diet, maintaining an upright posture, and use of diuretics all increase plasma aldosterone concentrations, whereas a high-sodium diet and lying in the supine position decrease aldosterone secretion. Standardized procedures for obtaining blood and urine specimens are required for proper interpretation of test results.[6] It is also useful to interpret the aldosterone concentrations along with a urinary sodium determination because salt intake can profoundly influence the aldosterone concentration. The aldosterone concentration is inversely proportional to the urinary sodium concentration.

Unlike aldosterone, plasma renin is often measured in terms of its enzymatic activity, although immunometric-based mass assays for renin have become available. *Plasma renin activity* (PRA) is gauged by the generation of angiotensin I, which is measured using immunoassay techniques, and renin mass assays directly measure renin using monoclonal antibodies targeted to the renin enzyme itself. Renin release is controlled by many physiological factors. Low-sodium diets, maintaining an upright posture, and use of diuretic medications increase renin release and should be controlled or eliminated before testing of the renin-angiotensin-aldosterone axis.[21] Because plasma renin activities also vary with sodium balance, it is helpful to interpret ambulatory PRA with urinary sodium excretion. An inverse relationship is found, allowing the identification of low-, normal-, and high-plasma renin groups from a nomogram (Figure 51-11). Age, estrogen therapy, and diabetes mellitus without renal failure affect plasma renin results. Patients older than age 55 and those with diabetes have PRA results that are about 50% of normal. Estrogen causes an increase in the hepatic synthesis of angiotensinogen, thereby increasing the endogenous substrate concentration for the renin enzyme. This causes an inappropriately elevated renin activity for the urinary sodium concentration. A number of medications affect plasma renin activities. Angiotensin converting enzyme (ACE) inhibitors, beta blockers, spironolactone, and nonsteroidal antiinflammatory agents lead the list of drugs that can alter plasma renin.

Even when time of sampling, posture, drug intake, and diet are controlled, it is often difficult to identify disorders of mineralocorticoid secretion on the basis of basal hormone concentrations alone. A variety of dynamic tests have therefore been developed to help document hypersecretion or hyposecretion of aldosterone and renin.

Stimulation Tests

The renin-angiotensin-aldosterone system responds to electrolyte balance. Sodium excretion and extracellular fluid volume are inversely associated with plasma renin and aldosterone concentrations.[21] The sodium-to-creatinine ratio in a urine specimen can be used as a marker for the sodium volume status. Procedures for stimulating the renin-angiotensin system are based on volume-depletion maneuvers, such as sodium restriction, upright posture, or diuretic administration.[6,64] In the *furosemide stimulation test,* oral or intravenous furosemide (40 to 80 mg) is administered, followed by 4 hours of upright posture (Box 51-9). This test does not require hospitalization, special diets, or prolonged standing, although it works better when a diet with normal salt intake is maintained. The normal response to this diuretic is a twofold to threefold rise in plasma renin.

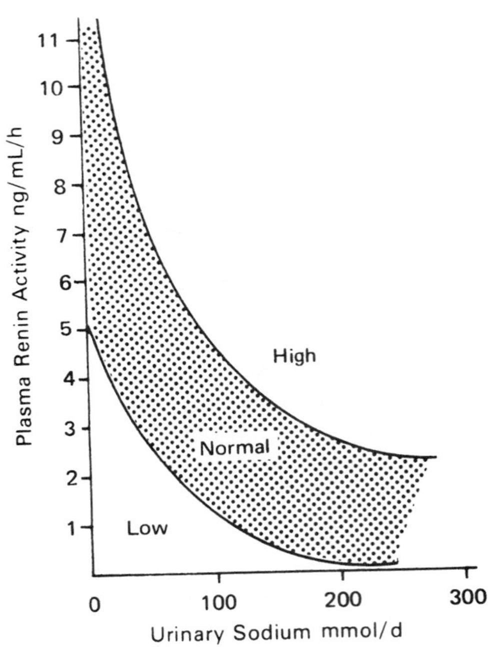

Figure 51-11 PRA correlated to urinary sodium excretion. *(From Laragh JH, Sealey J, Brunner HR. The control of aldosterone secretion in normal and hyperactive man: Abnormal renin and aldosterone patterns in low renin hypertension. Am J Med 1972;53:649.)*

BOX 51-9 Protocol for the Furosemide Stimulation Test

Rationale PRA varies with the state of hydration and sodium intake. The administration of furosemide, a potent diuretic, provides a stimulus to increase plasma renin secretion.

Procedure Furosemide (Lasix; Hoechst-Roussel Pharmaceuticals, Somerville, NJ), 40 to 80 mg, is given orally after an overnight fast. The subject is maintained in an upright posture (sitting, standing, or walking) throughout the test. Blood is drawn for the determination of PRA before and 4 hours after furosemide administration.

Interpretation Responses must be defined for the assay technique used. Patients with renin-dependent forms of hypertension (e.g., renovascular hypertension) show values that are approximately five times normal. Stimulated responses are also seen in patients with high-renin essential hypertension, pheochromocytoma, and Bartter's syndrome. Patients with hypertension from mineralocorticoid excess (e.g., primary aldosteronism) usually have PRA below the concentration of assay sensitivity. Patients with hyporeninemic hypoaldosteronism usually have low concentrations of plasma renin and low aldosterone concentrations. Figure 51-17 shows typical responses.

Another simple and convenient stimulation test consists of sodium restriction and upright posture. A low-salt diet containing less than 20 mmol/day of sodium is administered for 3 to 5 days; urine is collected for creatinine and sodium measurements until equilibrium with the new diet is established. At that point, a plasma renin activity is obtained after 2 hours of standing. A normal response is a twofold to threefold increase in plasma renin output.

Suppression Tests

Mineralocorticoid suppression tests have been designed that are based on salt loading.[31] For example, saline infusions, oral salt loading, or mineralocorticoid administration have been used to suppress the secretion of aldosterone by the adrenal gland. In normal individuals, acute expansion of the plasma volume with salt increases renal perfusion, suppresses renin release, and decreases aldosterone secretion. In the *saline suppression test,* isotonic saline is infused intravenously for 4 hours, after which plasma aldosterone concentration and renin activity are measured.[4,6] Aldosterone concentrations normally fall to <5 ng/dL (<140 pmol/L), and PRA is suppressed (Box 51-10). This test should not be performed if hypertension is severe or if cardiac failure is present. Administration of fludrocortisone, a synthetic mineralocorticoid, produces a comparable suppression of aldosterone secretion (see *fludrocortisone suppression test;* Box 51-11). Fludrocortisone should be administered with caution in patients with hypokalemia and heart or renal failure. An alternate suppression test uses the ACE inhibitor *captopril.*[95] This test is recommended when risks from volume overload preclude the use of other procedures. Captopril essentially inhibits the conversion of angiotensin I to angiotensin II, removing the angiotensin II stimulus to aldosterone secretion. Plasma aldosterone is measured, while the patient is sitting, before and 2 to 3 hours after the oral administration of 25 mg of captopril. Healthy subjects suppress plasma aldosterone to <15 ng/dL (410 pmol/L).

Adrenal Androgen Function

Stimulation Tests

The responses of adrenal androgen secretion to ACTH stimulation are variable. Plasma DHEA and androstenedione increase threefold to fourfold after 90 minutes of stimulation with ACTH (10 µg/m^2). DHEA-S, on the other hand, increases 30% to 50% with ACTH administration. ACTH stimulation studies are not considered useful in evaluating hypoandrogenic disorders.[141]

Suppression Tests

Overnight suppression using dexamethasone produces small changes in adrenal androgen concentrations compared with those of cortisol. Dexamethasone, 0.75 mg, administered at midnight for several days reliably suppresses adrenal androgen concentrations measured in blood. Tissue stores of these androgens may account in part for the delay in the response.[106,135]

DISORDERS OF THE ADRENAL CORTEX

Thomas Addison first reported on hypofunction of the adrenal cortex in 1855.[124] However, it has only been in the last 60 years that many of the disease states that are associated with abnormal adrenal function have been discovered and studied. In general, diseases of this organ are classified as resulting from either hypofunction or hyperfunction of the adrenal cortex.

Hypofunction of the Adrenal Cortex

Adrenal Insufficiency[74,92]

Adrenal insufficiency is a rare disorder with a prevalence of only 4 to 11 cases per 100,000 population; if untreated it is fatal. The disorder is classified as primary,[195] secondary, or tertiary. *Primary adrenal insufficiency,* also known as

BOX 51-10 Protocol for the Saline Suppression Test

Rationale Rapid volume expansion with intravenous saline should suppress plasma aldosterone in normal subjects but not in patients with primary aldosteronism.

Procedure Care must be taken to ensure that the subject is not hypokalemic before starting the test. The subject is awakened at 0600 hours and kept in an upright posture for 2 hours. Blood is drawn for determination of plasma aldosterone at 0800 hours. The subject then assumes a supine position, and 2 L of isotonic saline, 0.9 g/dL, is infused over a 4-hour period. Blood is drawn for plasma aldosterone determination at noon.

Interpretation Normal subjects show a plasma aldosterone concentration of 5 ng/dL (140 pmol/L) or less after saline infusion. Concentrations >10 ng/dL are usually seen in patients with autonomously functioning aldosterone-secreting tumors.

BOX 51-11 Protocol for the Fludrocortisone Suppression Test

Rationale Fludrocortisone, a potent mineralocorticoid, suppresses aldosterone production in normal subjects but not in subjects with primary aldosteronism.

Procedure Hypokalemia must be corrected before starting this test and serum potassium monitored during the test. Fludrocortisone, 0.1 mg every 6 hours, is given for 3 days. Plasma is collected for aldosterone determination after a standing position has been maintained for 2 hours (for baseline measurement) and at the end of fludrocortisone administration. Twenty-four-hour urine collections for measurement of aldosterone are obtained 1 day before fludrocortisone administration is started and on day 3 of the test course.

Interpretation Normal subjects show suppression of plasma aldosterone to <4 ng/dL (111 pmol/L); urine aldosterone is ≤20 µg/day on day 3.

Addison's disease, results from progressive destruction or dysfunction of the adrenal glands by a local disease process or systemic disorder (Box 51-12). Worldwide, infectious diseases are the most common cause of primary adrenal insufficiency and include tuberculosis, fungal infections (histoplasmosis and cryptococcosis), and cytomegalovirus infections. Autoimmune adrenalitis accounts for more than 70% of cases reported in the Western world, with adrenal autoantibodies noted in more than 75% of cases. The adrenal glands are atrophic, with loss of cortical cells but an intact medulla. Almost 50% of patients with autoimmune adrenalitis have an associated autoimmune disease with autoimmune thyroid disease the most common.

Because the entire cortex is affected in primary adrenal insufficiency, all classes of adrenal steroids are deficient.[135] The onset of clinical manifestations is usually gradual, and the degree and severity of symptoms depend on the extent of adrenal failure. In early or mild expressions of primary adrenal insufficiency, hypofunction may not be evident unless the patient is under stress. Complete glucocorticoid deficiency can manifest in a variety of ways, including fatigue, weakness, weight loss, gastrointestinal disturbances, and postprandial hypoglycemia. Mineralocorticoid deficiency leads to dehydration with hypotension, hyponatremia, and hyperkalemia. Excessive pituitary release of ACTH and related precursor peptides, unchecked by the negative feedback system, may cause hyperpigmentation of the skin and mucous membranes through the action of melanocyte-stimulating hormone on melanocytes.

BOX 51-12 Causes of Primary Adrenal Insufficiency

Autoimmune disease
- Sporadic
- Polyglandular autoimmune syndrome type I (Addison's disease, candidiasis, hypoparathyroidism, and primary gonadal failure)
- Polyglandular autoimmune syndrome type II (Addison's disease, primary hypothyroidism, primary hypogonadism, diabetes, and pernicious anemia)

Granulomatous disease
- Tuberculosis, histoplasmosis, sarcoidosis, fungal infections, and cytomegalovirus

Neoplastic infiltration
- Amyloid
- Hemochromatosis

Adrenoleukodystrophies
Congenital adrenal hypoplasia
ACTH resistance syndromes
HIV
Abdominal irradiation
Bilateral adrenalectomy
Intraadrenal hemorrhage: infection (caused by meningococci, *Pseudomonas*)
Anticoagulants

Measurement of basal ACTH and cortisol concentrations along with the ACTH stimulation test (see Box 51-1) is recommended if primary adrenal insufficiency is suspected from the patients' clinical history and symptoms. Basal plasma ACTH concentrations >150 pg/mL with serum cortisol concentrations <10 µg/dL are diagnostic of adrenal insufficiency (Figure 51-12). A subnormal cortisol response in the ACTH stimulation test supports the diagnosis of primary adrenal insufficiency (Figure 51-13). A normal cortisol response to ACTH stimulation establishes that the adrenal cortex is capable of releasing cortisol in a normal fashion. A subnormal response to ACTH stimulation suggests the diagnosis of secondary or tertiary adrenal failure.

In *secondary* and *tertiary adrenal insufficiency* (Table 51-5), inadequate cortisol production may be due to destructive processes in the hypothalamic-pituitary that result in a decreased ability to secrete ACTH (secondary) or CRH (tertiary).[135,169] However, the most common cause of tertiary insufficiency is chronic pharmacological administration of glucocorticoids that suppress CRH synthesis. This leads to a decrease in both ACTH release and cortisol secre-

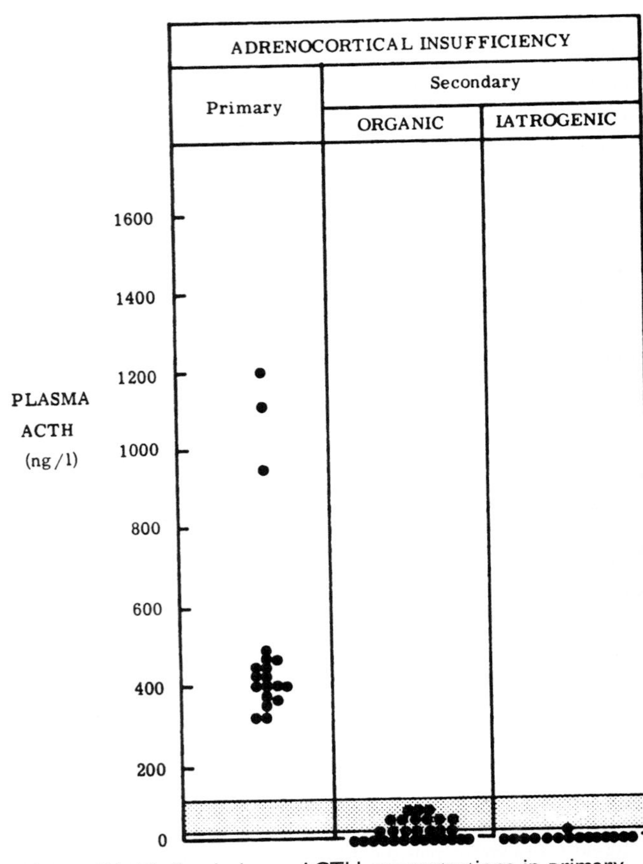

Figure 51-12 Basal plasma ACTH concentrations in primary and secondary adrenocortical insufficiency. *(From Irvine WJ, Toft AD, Feek CM. Addison's disease. In: James VHT, ed. The adrenal gland. New York: Raven Press, 1979:131.)*

tion. The clinical features of secondary and tertiary adrenal insufficiency are similar to those of primary insufficiency, except that hyperpigmentation is not present and hypotension is less severe; mineralocorticoid deficiency and ACTH excess are not seen in secondary or tertiary adrenal insufficiency. The ACTH stimulation test is also used to determine adrenal insufficiency in patients with secondary and tertiary adrenal insufficiency. When results are abnormal, however, the ACTH stimulation test cannot identify the cause of adrenal failure. Mild to moderate dysfunction of ACTH secretion may go undetected. Some patients with partial ACTH deficiency maintain sufficient ACTH to prevent adrenal atrophy, but are unable to augment ACTH secretion in response to stress or hypoglycemia.[135,169] In these cases, pituitary ACTH reserve can be investigated with either a metyrapone (see Box 51-4) or insulin-induced hypoglycemia test (see Box 50-3; Chapter 50). Neither test, however, should be performed if primary adrenal insufficiency is suspected. Subnormal responses to these tests suggest that pituitary ACTH release is inadequate, thus supporting a diagnosis of secondary or tertiary adrenal insufficiency. Basal ACTH and cortisol concentrations are often not useful for establishing the diagnosis of secondary adrenal insufficiency. Episodic secretion and circadian variation of both ACTH and cortisol can result in values in normal subjects that overlap with those with secondary or tertiary adrenal insufficiency. An elevated basal plasma ACTH in a patient with an abnormal response to acute ACTH stimulation suggests primary adrenal failure, whereas a low ACTH value and subnormal response to the Synacthen stimulation test suggest a hypothalamic or pituitary disorder.

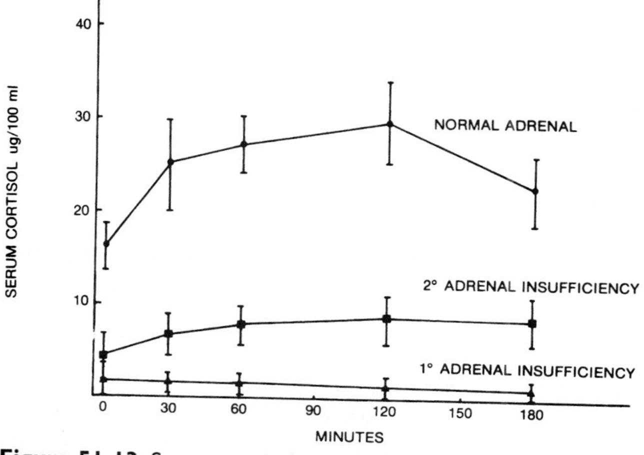

Figure 51-13 Serum cortisol response to 0.25 mg of cosyntropin (ACTH) in nine normal individuals (normal adrenal), eight patients with hypopituitarism (secondary adrenal insufficiency), and seven patients with Addison's disease (primary adrenal insufficiency). *(From Spechart P, Nicoloff J, Bethune J. Screening for adrenocortical insufficiency with cosyntropin [synthetic ACTH]. Arch Intern Med 1971;128:761. Copyright 1971, American Medical Association.)*

The multiple-day ACTH stimulation test is used to distinguish between primary and secondary or tertiary causes of adrenal insufficiency (see Box 51-2). It is particularly useful when patients have been receiving glucocorticoid therapy. In primary adrenal insufficiency, the damaged adrenal glands do not respond even with several days of repeated ACTH stimulation. Patients with secondary or tertiary adrenal insufficiency usually have an inadequate or absent cortisol response at first because the adrenal glands have been unstimulated for some time and steroidogenesis needs priming. Eventually, a delayed or staircase response is seen, indicating reactivation of the normal steroidogenic

TABLE 51-5 Adrenocortical Insufficiency

		Adrenal Insufficiency		
	Normal	**Primary**	**Secondary**	**Tertiary**
Screening Tests				
Plasma ACTH (0800 hours)	10-85 pg/mL	Increased	Normal or decreased	Normal or decreased
Serum cortisol (0800 hours)	5-23 μg/dL	Decreased	Normal or decreased	Normal or decreased
Challenge Tests				
Rapid ACTH stimulation (see Box 51-1) Peak cortisol	>20 μg/dL	<20 μg/dL	Any	Any
Overnight metyrapone test (see Box 51-4) Plasma 11-deoxycortisol Plasma ACTH	>7 μg/dL >150 pg/mL	Not indicated Not indicated	<7 μg/dL <150 pg/mL	<7 μg/dL <150 pg/mL
CRH stimulation test (see Box 51-3) Plasma ACTH	Not indicated	Not indicated	Decreased response	Increased response

ACTH, Adrenocorticotropic hormone; *CRH*, corticotropin-releasing hormone.

TABLE 51-6 Syndromes of Hypoaldosteronism

Entity	Mechanisms	Comments
Addison's disease	Diffuse destruction of adrenal cortex including the zona glomerulosa	
Heparin treatment	Direct effect of heparin therapy	Usually after prolonged treatment
After resection of aldosterone-producing adenoma	Suppression of aldosterone secretion in normal cortical tissue by adenoma with delayed recovery after surgery	Can be prevented by spironolactone treatment before surgery
Hyperreninemic hypoaldosteronism	Selective injury to the renal zona glomerulosa during hypotensive episodes in critically ill patients	Cortisol secretion is intact; presents with hyperkalemia in intensive care unit patients
Congenital adrenal hyperplasia with methyloxidase type II defect	Enzymatic block in the conversion of 18-OHβ corticosterone to aldosterone	
Pseudohypoaldosteronism	Decreased responsiveness to aldosterone caused by mineralocorticoid receptor defect	Aldosterone concentrations are higher
Hyporeninemic hypoaldosteronism	Low renin secondarily decreasing aldosterone secretion	Seen in diabetic and older patients with mild renal failure

pathways. This test, however, is not used as frequently in this situation because of the availability of better and sensitive ACTH immunoassays that more accurately determine ACTH concentrations at baseline. In primary adrenal insufficiency, the ACTH concentration is disproportionately elevated compared with the plasma cortisol concentration.

The CRH stimulation test (see Box 51-3) can be used to differentiate tertiary from secondary adrenal insufficiency.[131] Those with tertiary disease show an elevation in ACTH with CRH administration, whereas those with secondary disease show only minimal changes in ACTH concentrations.

Although subnormal basal plasma concentrations of DHEA-S occur in primary, secondary, and tertiary forms of adrenal insufficiency, measurement is of little value in the diagnosis of adrenal insufficiency; low concentrations of adrenal androgens are normally observed in children and in the elderly. Patients with human immunodeficiency virus (HIV) infection have been shown to have reduced concentrations of DHEA-S.[108] DHEA-S concentrations are usually determined in the management of women with hirsutism or in patients suspected of having adrenal tumors.[202]

Measurement of adrenal autoantibodies has been shown to be useful in evaluating patients suspected of adrenal insufficiency. Antibodies against the 21-hydroxylase enzyme have been used in this regard.

Hypoaldosteronism

Deficient aldosterone production occurs in conditions other than Addison's disease (Table 51-6).[6] Isolated aldosterone deficiency[190] accompanied by normal cortisol production is seen in patients with (1) inadequate production of renin by the kidney, which leads to secondary aldosterone deficiency (hyporeninemic hypoaldosteronism); (2) inherited enzyme defects in aldosterone biosynthesis; and (3) acquired forms of primary aldosterone deficiency (heparin therapy and postsurgery). The resulting metabolic changes are hyperkalemia and hyponatremia, often with a hypochloremic acidosis. Mild or moderate volume depletion, often with postural or unprovoked hypotension, may also occur. Hyporeninemic hypoaldosteronism can be established by demonstrating failure of both plasma renin and aldosterone to increase in response to furosemide stimulation or upright posture (see Box 51-9).[6] This disorder is more common in older patients and in individuals with diabetes mellitus. A high-renin form has been observed less frequently than the hyporenin form.

Patients with primary adrenal insufficiency usually also have aldosterone deficiency. Most endocrinologists, however, do not conduct tests to confirm aldosterone deficiency in these patients.

Hyperfunction of the Adrenal Cortex

Hyperfunction of the adrenal cortex produces clinical syndromes of glucocorticoid excess, mineralocorticoid excess, and androgen excess.[99,111,135]

Corticosteroid Excess (Cushing's Syndrome)[16,128]

In 1912 Harvey Cushing first described a 23-year-old woman with hirsutism, obesity, and amenorrhea and called it a polyglandular syndrome with pituitary involvement. Cushing's syndrome is the result of autonomous, excessive production of cortisol leading to classic symptoms characteristic of this disorder.[135,169] The clinical picture includes truncal obesity, moon face, hypertension, hirsutism,

TABLE 51-7 Incidence of Clinical Manifestations in Cushing's Syndrome

Clinical Manifestation	Incidence (%)
Obesity	90
Hypertension	85
Hyperglycemia and decreased glucose tolerance	80
Menstrual and sexual dysfunction	76
Hirsutism, acne, plethora	72
Striae, atrophic skin	67
Weakness, proximal myopathy	65
Osteoporosis	55
Easy bruisability	55
Psychiatric disturbances	50
Edema	46
Polyuria, polyphagia	16
Ocular changes and exophthalmos	8

TABLE 51-8 Causes of Spontaneous Cushing's Syndrome

Underlying Disorder	Incidence (%)
ACTH dependent	
Cushing's disease	68
Ectopic ACTH-secreting tumor	15
ACTH independent	
Adenoma	5
Carcinoma	3
Nodular adrenal hyperplasia	9
Adrenocortical rest tumor	<1

ACTH, Adrenocorticotropic hormone.

hypokalemic metabolic alkalosis, carbohydrate intolerance, disturbance of reproductive function, and neuropsychiatric symptoms (Table 51-7). Frequently the cause is iatrogenic, caused by excessive exogenous steroid therapy. Endogenous disorders that cause hypersecretion of cortisol and Cushing's syndrome are classified either as *ACTH dependent* or *ACTH independent* (Table 51-8). Cushing's disease is the pituitary-dependent form of Cushing's syndrome that accounts for 70% of the cases seen in clinical practice. In Cushing's disease, hypersecretion of ACTH by a pituitary microadenoma is the primary defect that leads to bilateral adrenal hyperplasia and cortisol overproduction. In the ectopic ACTH syndrome, nonendocrine tumors (e.g., lung, gut, ovarian, and carcinoid tumors) develop the ability to secrete ACTH, resulting in adrenal hyperplasia, unregulated cortisol secretion, and suppression of pituitary ACTH activity. In the form of Cushing's syndrome associated with primary adrenal disease, such as adrenocortical adenoma[85] or carcinoma (see Table 51-8), increased secretion of cortisol suppresses both CRH synthesis and ACTH secretion, and atrophy of nontumorous adrenal tissue results. Multiple endocrine neoplasia type 1 (MEN 1) and type 2 (MEN 2) also are causes of Cushing's syndrome. MEN 1 results in Cushing's syndrome through ACTH hypersecretion from a pituitary microadenoma or from an ectopic ACTH-secreting tumor of the pancreas or medullary thyroid.

Screening Tests for Cushing's Syndrome

Cushing's syndrome is an uncommon disorder but many of the usual signs and symptoms of this syndrome are seen in patients with normal adrenal function. The initial diagnosis of Cushing's syndrome, particularly in mild or early disease, rests on laboratory evidence of excessive and autonomous cortisol production.[135,144,169] Two simple screening tests are available for detecting Cushing's syndrome (Table 51-9). One is the measurement of 24-hour urinary free cortisol. Under normal circumstances, <2% of the secreted cortisol appears in urine as free cortisol. In general, a 24-hour urinary free cortisol concentration <100 μg/day excludes the diagnosis of Cushing's syndrome, and concentrations >120 μg/day suggest the diagnosis of Cushing's syndrome (see Figure 51-9). The diagnostic accuracy is more than 90% when the test is properly performed.[17] An elevated excretion rate documents overproduction of cortisol. However, improper timing of the urine specimen (>24 hours), concomitant use of a diuretic, high salt intake, depression, and stress can cause false-positive test results.[135] Urine cortisol measurements do not establish the diagnosis; an abnormal result should be followed by repeat or provocative testing.

Another reliable and convenient screening test for Cushing's syndrome is the overnight low-dose dexamethasone suppression test (1 mg at midnight) with measurement of serum cortisol (suppressed to <5 μg/dL [140 nmol/L]) at 0800 hours the following morning (see Box 51-5). A multiple low-dose test is sometimes also used (see Box 51-6). A diagnostic accuracy of 90% has been achieved with the simultaneous measurement of both cortisol and dexamethasone, although this approach is rarely used.[17,135] The measurement of dexamethasone assesses the resistance of the HPA axis to suppression. Incorrect dosing and alterations in clearance of dexamethasone are detected by measuring dexamethasone; thus both false-negative and false-positive suppression test results can be identified.

Examining the circadian rhythm of cortisol secretion can also be used to screen for Cushing's syndrome. The morning to night difference is lost in patients with Cushing's syndrome so that the nocturnal concentrations are inappropriately raised from normal.

Differential Diagnosis of Cushing's Syndrome

The screening tests discussed above suggest endogenous Cushing's syndrome. More definitive testing should then be

TABLE 51-9 Differential Diagnosis in Cushing's Syndrome

	Normal	Cushing's Syndrome	Adrenal Tumor	Ectopic ACTH Syndrome
Screening Tests				
Urinary free cortisol	<100 μg/day	>120 μg/day	>120 μg/day	>120 μg/day
Overnight dexamethasone suppression test (see Box 51-5)				
Serum cortisol (0800h)	<3 μg/dL	>10 μg/dL	>10 μg/dL	>10 μg/dL
Differential Diagnostic Tests				
Plasma ACTH (0800 h)	10-85 pg/mL	40-260 pg/mL	<10 pg/mL	Normal to greatly elevated
Serum cortisol (0800 h)	5-23 μg/dL	Normal	Normal or elevated	Normal or elevated
High-dose overnight dexamethasone suppression test (see Box 51-8)				
Serum cortisol (0800 h)	50% suppression	Most suppress	Fail to suppress	Fail to suppress
CT or MRI				
Of adrenal glands	−	−	+	−
Of pituitary gland	−	+	−	−
Of other locations	−	−	−	+
CRH stimulation test (see Box 51-3) with IPS venous sampling				
Ratio of ACTH in IPS vein to that in peripheral vein	Not indicated	>3	<3	<3

ACTH, Adrenocorticotropic hormone; *CRH,* corticotropin-releasing hormone; *CT,* computed tomography; *IPS,* inferior petrosal sinus; *MRI,* magnetic resonance imaging.

performed to determine the source of the overproduction of cortisol when observed with screening tests (see Table 51-9). Plasma ACTH concentrations are low in patients with adrenal tumors and normal or moderately elevated in patients with Cushing's syndrome and macronodular hyperplasia. The plasma concentrations of ACTH are very often markedly elevated in patients with nonendocrine ACTH-secreting tumors (Figure 51-14) because the normal negative feedback loop does not respond in this situation. Plasma ACTH concentrations >300 pg/mL are usually suggestive of a nonendocrine ACTH-secreting tumor.

High-dose dexamethasone suppression testing (see Boxes 51-7 and 51-8) is useful to differentiate Cushing's syndrome caused by adrenal tumors and nonendocrine ACTH-secreting tumors from pituitary Cushing's disease.[135,169] Some patients with Cushing's disease have false-negative test results with low-dose dexamethasone suppression. False-negative test results can be assessed by administering either 1.0 mg (low dose) or 8 mg (high dose) of dexamethasone at midnight (overnight dexamethasone suppression test). Serum is collected at 0800 hours for the measurement of cortisol. In patients with adrenal tumors and, with a few exceptions, in those patients with nonendocrine ACTH-secreting tumors, suppression does not occur after high-dose dexamethasone administration. Most patients with macronodular hyperplasia do not show normal suppression on high-dose testing with either the overnight or multiple-dose tests. They usually have measurable concentrations of ACTH. With high-dose testing, <10% of patients with Cushing's disease fail to show some degree of suppression, although most show only 50% to 60% suppression.[17] False-positive results have occurred in patients with accelerated clearance of dexamethasone as in patients receiving hepatic enzyme–inducing drugs, such as phenytoin. In these patients, measurements of plasma dexamethasone can be useful to gauge the effective blood concentration.

The CRH stimulation test (see Box 51-3) produces exaggerated ACTH or cortisol responses, or both, in about 90% of patients with Cushing's disease.[93,135,169] Poor responses occur in patients with adrenal tumors and in most patients with nonendocrine ACTH-secreting tumors (usually those having elevated basal concentrations of plasma ACTH). Patients with depression and anorexia nervosa usually do not exhibit exaggerated responses of ACTH to CRH injections. CRH testing has no major advantage over the high-dose dexamethasone suppression test. If the cause of Cushing's syn-

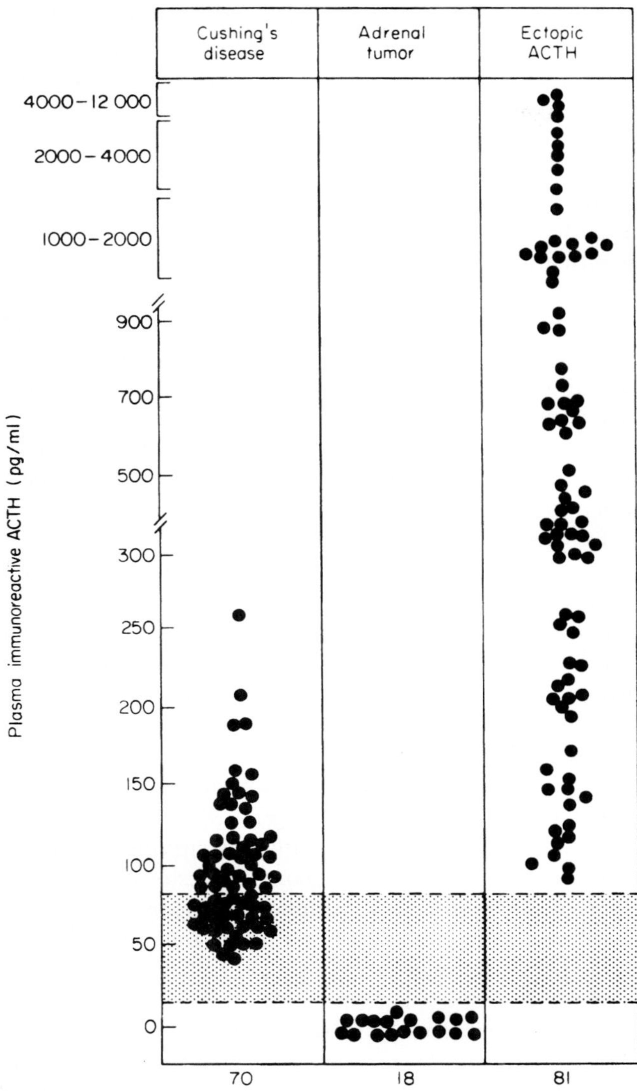

Figure 51-14 Basal plasma ACTH concentrations in patients with spontaneous Cushing's syndrome. *(From Scott AP. Pituitary adrenocorticotrophin and the melanocyte stimulating hormones. In: Parsons JA, ed. Peptide hormones. Baltimore: University Park Press, 1979.)*

drome is uncertain, measurement of ACTH from inferior petrosal vein specimens before and after CRH stimulation can be helpful. When ACTH concentrations in petrosal vein specimens are similar to those of simultaneously obtained peripheral vein plasma specimens, the diagnosis of a nonpituitary source of the ACTH is then considered. In virtually all patients with ectopic production of ACTH, the ratio of ACTH concentrations between the IPS and a peripheral venous concentration is <1.4:1. In contrast patients with Cushing's disease have a ratio >3.0. Unilateral elevation of petrosal vein ACTH, however, does not always predict which side of the pituitary the tumor is hypersecreting ACTH.[131]

BOX 51-13 Tests for Anatomical Localization of Defects in Cushing's Syndrome

Pituitary Studies
CT; MRI; selective venous sampling for ACTH measurements (inferior petrosal sinus venous to peripheral venous ratios)

Adrenal Studies
CT; selective arteriography; selective venography; selective venous sampling for cortisol measurement

Ectopic ACTH Production
Conventional radiography, ultrasonography, CT to look at sites of suspected neoplasms

ACTH, Adrenocorticotropic hormone; *CT,* computed tomography; *MRI,* magnetic resonance imaging.

Adrenal androgens and plasma DHEA-S are measured in the differential diagnosis of hirsutism without Cushing's syndrome.[37,135] In patients with Cushing's syndrome, plasma DHEA-S concentrations are usually normal or moderately elevated (plasma DHEA-S ~5 µg/mL). Those patients with an adrenal adenoma usually have low age-adjusted concentrations of DHEA-S. The concentrations for plasma DHEA-S in patients with nonendocrine ACTH-secreting tumors range from normal to elevated. In patients with congenital adrenal hyperplasia (CAH), adrenal androgens suppress normally with the administration of 0.75 mg of dexamethasone for 2 to 3 weeks, but suppression does not occur in those patients with adrenal tumors and nonendocrine ACTH-secreting tumors.

In addition to suppression and stimulation testing, methods of anatomical localization, listed in Box 51-13, should be used to document the diagnosis of Cushing's syndrome. Computed tomography (CT) of the adrenal glands has been helpful in localizing adrenal tumors, macronodular hyperplasia, and bilateral hyperplasia of the adrenal glands. CT in combination with magnetic resonance imaging (MRI) of the pituitary gland can help detect pituitary microadenomas.[24,135]

Conditions That Mimic Cushing's Syndrome

Alcohol abuse has been known to induce a "pseudo-Cushing's syndrome" that mimics the clinical and biochemical features of the actual disease.[135,169] The abnormalities are all reversible once alcohol abuse by the patient is eliminated. The clinician must therefore use considerable judgment in detecting the cause of Cushing's syndrome before therapy.[35,194] HIV, anorexia nervosa, and depression are associated with elevated serum cortisol concentrations, and patients with these disorders may have positive low-dose, overnight dexamethasone suppression tests. However, the clinical features of patients with HIV and anorexia nervosa are not typical of those with Cushing's syndrome. Measurement of urinary free cortisol and plasma cortisol with the dexamethasone suppression test improves the predictive value in the diagnosis of both Cushing's syndrome and depression.[107]

Obese patients have also presented with clinical features that mimic true Cushing's syndrome. Truncal obesity, striae, and the excretion of elevated concentrations of 17-hydroxysteroids are features of Cushing's syndrome that occur in normal, obese subjects. Urinary free cortisol, however, is normal in the obese individual and can effectively differentiate normal subjects from those with true Cushing's syndrome.

Congenital Adrenal Hyperplasia (Adrenogenital Syndrome)[126]

The biosynthesis of cortisol and aldosterone from cholesterol requires the action of specific enzymes in the adrenal cortex for the chemical modification and introduction of the different functional groups.[112,176,199,200] CAH is characterized by the congenital absence or deficiency of one or more of the biosynthetic enzymes that lead to cortisol biosynthesis.[113] As noted in Figure 51-6, a defect or deficiency in any one or all of the four key enzymes of adrenocorticoid biosynthesis can occur. As a result, cortisol biosynthesis is impaired, leading to a compensatory increase in ACTH release. ACTH then stimulates steroid biosynthesis to the point of the enzyme block. Enzyme defects therefore cause hyperplasia of the adrenal cortex and accumulation of intermediate compounds proximal to the block with shunting of the substrate toward the adrenal androgen pathway. Measurements of the specific precursor steroids in blood are useful for identifying the specific enzyme defect and for monitoring response to cortisol replacement therapy.[199,200]A partial block may cause either marked or subtle clinical manifestations, whereas a complete enzyme block can be incompatible with life. The closer the enzyme block is to the final cortisol product, the less life threatening are the symptoms caused by compensatory action by the elevated precursor steroids.

The term CAH is used to denote the congenital presentation of this disorder (usually at birth) and the adrenocortical hyperplasia that results from the compensatory ACTH response to cortisol deficiency. "Adrenogenital syndrome" is also used to describe this disorder in that it affects the genitalia and secondary sex characteristics of the newborn. In girls, particularly, the diagnosis of CAH in the neonatal period is commonly suggested first by the observed presence of ambiguous genitalia. In boys the abnormality may not be suspected until signs of precocious puberty or accelerated growth are present. Because aldosterone production can be compromised with accumulation and diversion of intermediate steroids to other pathways, hypertension and salt wasting may also be present. The adrenogenital syndrome is recognized with increased frequency in adults, with affected people presenting with subtle abnormalities at the time of puberty that go unrecognized. In adult women, the clinical presentation may be indistinguishable from the polycystic ovary syndrome (PCOS) or idiopathic hirsutism.[8,213]

Deficiency of the 21-hydroxylase enzyme (Figure 51-15; see also Figure 51-6) is the most common form of CAH, with more than 90% of cases caused by 21-hydroxylase deficiency.[199,200] The incidence in Western societies ranges from 1 in 5000 to 1 in 15,000 live births. An elevation in 17α-hydroxyprogesterone is characteristic of this enzyme defect. The concentrations of several other steroids are increased in the circulation of patients with 21-hydroxylase deficiency. These include progesterone, 17α-hydroxypregnenolone, and pregnenolone. The adrenal androgens, DHEA-S and DHEA, are also elevated in patients with this enzyme defect. An increase in plasma androstenedione and testosterone occurs primarily as a result of the peripheral conversion of precursor adrenal androgens by the liver. There are several variants of 21-hydroxylase deficiency: a simple virilizing form, a salt-wasting form, and a late-onset form. The simple virilizing form is associated with 21-hydroxylase enzyme deficiency occurring only in the zona fasciculata, and the major clinical manifestation is virilization caused by the increase in adrenal androgen secretion. The salt-wasting form extends

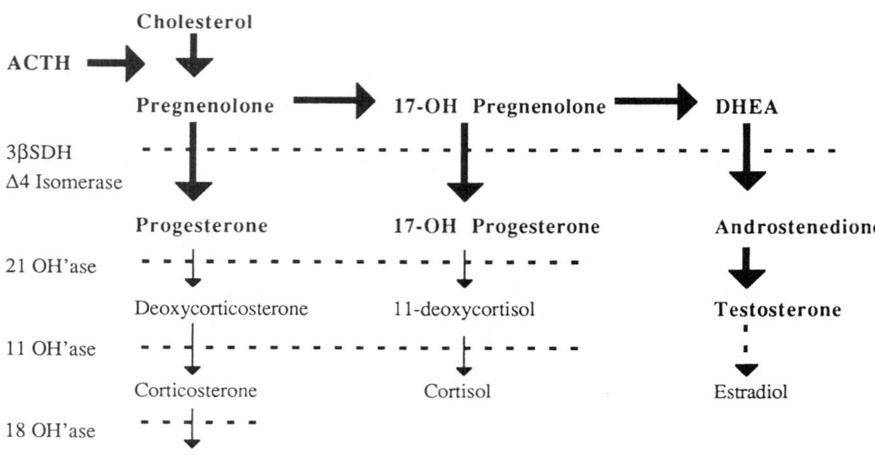

Figure 51-15 Formation of steroids in patients with adrenogenital syndrome caused by 21-hydroxylase deficiency. Bold lettering indicates steroids that are found elevated in the circulation. *ACTH,* Adrenocorticotropic hormone; *3βSDH,* 3β-hydroxysteroid dehydrogenase.

to the zona glomerulosa and includes a deficiency in aldosterone leading to salt wasting and hypotension. Late-onset 21-hydroxylase deficiency is associated with mild to moderate hirsutism in women in early adulthood that commonly masquerades as PCOS, with primary or secondary amenorrhea and anovulation as major characteristics. Plasma testosterone and androstenedione and basal and ACTH-stimulated 17α-hydroxyprogesterone concentrations are elevated in these individuals. Plasma 3α-androstanediol glucuronide, a metabolite of tissue androgens, is also elevated in most patients with this enzyme deficiency. Males can develop enlarged testes because of ectopic adrenal tissue that rests within the testes and responds to the ACTH compensatory increase. The ACTH stimulation test with the measurement of 17-hydroxyprogesterone (see Box 51-1) is useful in identifying heterozygotes for this condition and exposing patients with acquired forms of 21-hydroxylase deficiency.

A deficiency *of 11β-hydroxylase* is the second most common form of CAH, with an incidence of 1 per 100,000 births, and is associated with manifestations of virilization, elevated concentrations of plasma androstenedione and DHEA-S, and hypertension. The mineralocorticoid-induced hypertension is caused by an elevation of DOC; 11-deoxycortisol concentrations are markedly raised in subjects with this enzyme defect.[199,200] The major distinguishing characteristic of this disorder from 21-hydroxylase deficiency, besides the elevated plasma concentrations of 11-deoxycortisol, is hypertension elicited by the salt retention caused by increased concentrations of DOC. A deficiency of 3β-*hydroxysteroid dehydrogenase-isomerase* has been reported and leads to an elevation in the ratio of 17α-hydroxypregnenolone to that of 17α-hydroxyprogesterone and to an increased ratio of DHEA to androstenedione. In severe forms of this rare disorder, female infants have pseudohermaphroditism, and male infants present with incomplete masculinization. Patients with this disorder usually present in early infancy with complete adrenal insufficiency including salt wasting. A late-onset form has also been reported in patients with premature pubarche with hirsutism, acne, and menstrual irregularities.[13,138,199,200,213] The diagnosis is made by demonstrating an increased ratio of pregnenolone and 17-hydroxypregnenolone to progesterone and 17-hydroxyprogesterone, respectively.

A reduction in the conversion of 17-hydroxypregnenolone to DHEA and of 17-hydroxyprogesterone to androstenedione results from a deficiency of *C-17,20-lyase/17α-hydroxylase.* A defect of this enzyme complex in the gonads of genetic females results in pubertal failure, and a defect in genetic males causes pseudohermaphroditism. The synthesis of cortisol, androgens, and estrogens is decreased, and the production of progesterone, corticosterone, and DOC is increased. In the complete form, hypertension and hyperkalemia with a lack of sexual development are observed in girls, whereas male pseudohermaphroditism is seen in boys. The diagnosis is usually made at the time of puberty when patients present with hypogonadism in association with hypertension and hypokalemia.

Concentrations of all classes of steroid hormones are low when a deficiency of the cholesterol side-chain cleavage enzyme is present. This disorder is extremely rare; few affected children survive infancy, and sexual differentiation is absent in boys.

The effectiveness of a treatment program for CAH is judged on the basis of the presence or absence of normal linear growth, normal sexual development, and suppression of abnormal blood and urine steroid concentrations into the normal range with exogenous cortisol. With virilizing congenital hyperplasia caused by either 21-hydroxylase deficiency or 11α-hydroxylase deficiency, excess DHEA and androstenedione from the adrenal glands is converted to testosterone in peripheral tissue; plasma testosterone values within the reference interval of the adult male are commonly encountered in infants diagnosed with CAH. With effective treatment, suppression of plasma testosterone to <0.2 ng/mL is achieved. Most pediatric endocrinologists use cortisol replacement therapy in these patients with measurement of the elevated steroid just proximal to the enzyme block and with androstenedione concentrations. Increases in androstenedione are an early indicator of inadequate steroid replacement.

Adrenal Tumors[171]

Plasma DHEA-S, DHEA, androstenedione, and testosterone concentrations are elevated in patients with virilizing adrenal adenomas and Cushing's syndrome. The plasma concentrations of DHEA also may be elevated in women with virilizing ovarian tumors. CT scans along with MRI are useful in differentiating the sites of the tumors.[37,169] Aldosterone-secreting adenomas referred to as Conn's syndrome are typically small microadenomas found in the zona glomerulosa that hypersecrete aldosterone, producing the syndrome characterized by low renin hypertension.

Adrenal carcinomas are rare, with an incidence of only 1 per million population, and may cause only virilization and not the typical features of Cushing's syndrome. Women are more commonly affected than men in a 2.5:1 ratio. Plasma DHEA-S, DHEA, and androstenedione concentrations are markedly elevated in patients with adrenal carcinoma along with raised concentrations of cortisol. The concentrations of DHEA-S can often exceed 10 μg/mL in patients presenting with adrenal carcinoma and are usually diagnostic of this malignancy. High-dose glucocorticoids do not suppress the elevated androgen concentrations.[37,169]

Feminizing adrenocortical carcinomas are also rare.[37,169] They result in elevation of plasma DHEA-S, DHEA, androstenedione, estrone, and estradiol concentrations. Serum cortisol concentrations may be normal or elevated in those patients with Cushing's syndrome. Gynecomastia and sexual dysfunction occur in men and precocious pseudopuberty in women. Steroid hormone production fails to decrease normally after treatment with dexamethasone.

TABLE 51-10 Differential Diagnosis of Hyperaldosteronism

	Plasma Renin	Plasma Aldosterone	Blood Pressure	Serum Potassium
Primary aldosteronism	Low	High	High	Low
Secondary hypertension				
Edematous disorder	High	High	Normal	Low
Malignant hypertension	High	High	High	Low
Renovascular hypertension	Normal or high	Normal or high	High	Normal or low
Renin-secreting tumors	High	High	High	Normal or low
CAH (11- and 17-hydroxylase deficiency)	Low	Low	High	Low
Cushing's syndrome	Normal or low	Normal or low	High	Low
Liddle's syndrome	Low	Low	High	Low
Bartter's syndrome	High	High	Normal or low	Low
Licorice ingestion	Low	Low	High	Low
Low-renin essential hypertension	Low	Normal or low	High	Normal
Ingestion of exogenous mineralocorticoids	Low	Low	High	Low

CAH, Congenital adrenal hyperplasia.

Nonfunctioning Adrenocortical Tumors

Approximately 2% of the population have an adrenal tumor; most of these tumors are nonfunctioning and are sometimes called incidentalomas. They are found when CT scans of the abdomen are performed that can easily detect tumors 1 cm in diameter or 5 g in weight. No virilizing tumors smaller than 1 cm in diameter have been reported. Carcinomas are usually more than 30 g in weight.[37,169]

Mineralocorticoid Excess (Hyperaldosteronism)[28,133]

Hyperaldosteronism, commonly referred to as Conn's syndrome, is a syndrome associated with hypersecretion of the major mineralocorticoid, aldosterone.[6,64] In *primary aldosteronism,*[90,132,193,196] excessive aldosterone production originates from within the adrenal gland; in *secondary aldosteronism,* a stimulus outside the adrenal gland activates the renin-angiotensin system. The interaction of renin, angiotensin, and aldosterone is important in the regulation of extracellular fluid volume, blood pressure, and the balance of sodium and potassium ions. A change in one of these variables leads to changes in the others.

Control of renin release from the kidney is influenced by (1) specialized cells in the distal convoluted tubules called the macula densa function as chemoreceptors for the concentration of sodium delivered to the distal tubules; (2) juxtaglomerular cells functioning as mini pressure transducers sense the renal perfusion pressure in the kidney; (3) the sympathetic nervous system that feeds the kidney and catecholamine release; and (4) humoral factors such as potassium, atrial natriuretic peptides, and angiotensin II. All of these influences are involved in the normal control of salt and water balance and with diseases of the kidney. Secondary events that disturb the normal equilibrium of renin release are much more common than primary abnormalities of renin secretion (Table 51-10). For example, a decrease in effective plasma volume or mean arterial pressure with sudden blood loss leads to release of renin from juxtaglomerular cells of the kidneys; more angiotensin I and angiotensin II are formed, and an increased production of aldosterone by the adrenal glands occurs. This results in retention of water and sodium, an increase in extracellular volume, and a decrease in the serum potassium ion concentration. This state of secondary aldosteronism is commonly present in patients with congestive heart failure, nephrotic syndrome, cirrhosis of the liver, other hypoproteinemic states, or conditions of chronic depletion of plasma volume.

Secondary hyperaldosteronism is suspected in patients with volume depletion, edema, and hypokalemic alkalosis. Measurements of renin activities and aldosterone concentrations are seldom needed in these cases. Their measurements are invaluable, however, in the investigation of primary disturbances in the renin-angiotensin-aldosterone system, in the assessment of renal artery stenosis, and in the genesis and maintenance of arterial hypertension.

Primary Aldosteronism

Primary aldosteronism was first described by Conn in 1955 and is characterized by an elevated plasma concentration of aldosterone along with hypertension and hypokalemia.[4,6] Because $<1\%$ of hypertensive patients have primary aldosteronism, indications that should lead to further evaluation include hypokalemia that is unprovoked by diuretics or the lack of response to conventional antihypertensive drug treatment. Overproduction of aldosterone may be due to an

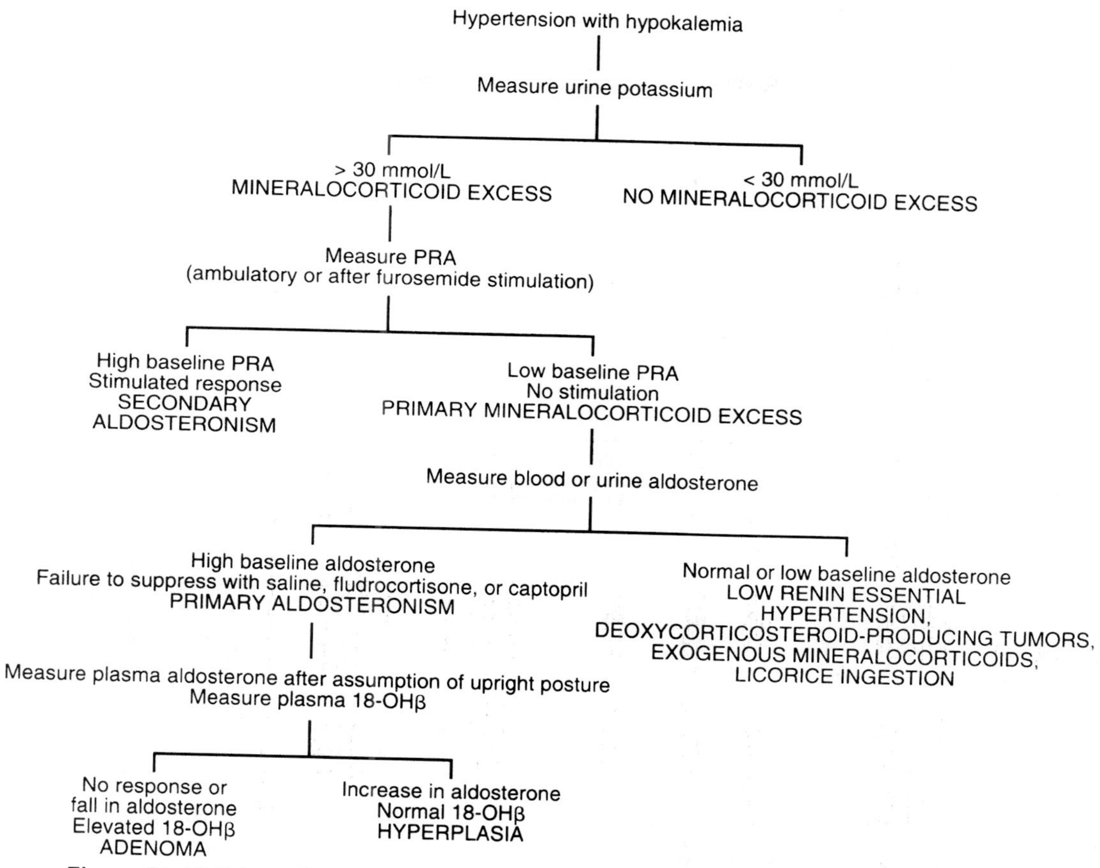

Figure 51-16 Scheme for the laboratory work-up of suspected aldosteronism causing hypertension. *PRA,* plasma renin activity; *18-OH,* 18-hydroxycorticosterone.

autonomous and inappropriate secretion of aldosterone by an adenoma of one adrenal gland (*aldosterone-producing adrenal adenoma* [APA] or *Conn's syndrome*), hyperplasia of aldosterone-producing cells in both glands (*idiopathic adrenal hyperplasia* [IAH]), an aldosterone-producing adrenal carcinoma, or a rare familial condition known as *glucocorticoid-suppressible aldosteronism.* The clinical features of primary aldosteronism are generally related to the consequences of aldosterone overproduction. Increased retention of sodium through the effects of aldosterone on the renal tubular handling of sodium, expansion of extracellular fluid volume, and increased tubular secretion of potassium and hydrogen ions reflect the cardinal manifestations of primary aldosteronism. Hypokalemia and metabolic alkalosis result as a consequence of a progressive renal depletion of body potassium. As a consequence of sodium retention, there is a modest expansion of extracellular fluid volume and an increase in arterial blood pressure.

Laboratory Diagnosis of Primary Aldosteronism

Hypokalemia is the key clinical finding that primary aldosteronism may be present in a patient with diastolic hypertension.[5] To confirm the diagnosis, it is necessary to demonstrate (1) hyposecretion of renin that is not appropriately corrected during volume depletion, and (2) hypersecretion of aldosterone that fails to suppress appropriately during volume expansion. Figure 51-16 shows a suggested scheme for evaluating patients with suspected mineralocorticoid excess.

Most patients with autonomous aldosterone overproduction are hypokalemic, but most patients with hypokalemia do not have primary aldosteronism. In hyperaldosteronism, urinary potassium excretion is inappropriately high, and a random urine potassium >30 mmol/L is usually indicative of primary aldosteronism or some type of mineralocorticoid excess condition. If hypokalemia can be shown to be due to nonrenal potassium loss, the diagnosis of aldosteronism does not need to be considered further.[4,6,64]

In primary aldosteronism, low renin activity and high aldosterone concentration are expected. Many other factors, however, influence the secretion of renin and aldosterone, and these factors must be recognized and understood before testing. Because drugs such as ACE inhibitors, beta blockers, and spironolactone alter renin release, patients should be withdrawn from these medications for several weeks before determining the plasma aldosterone/plasma renin activity

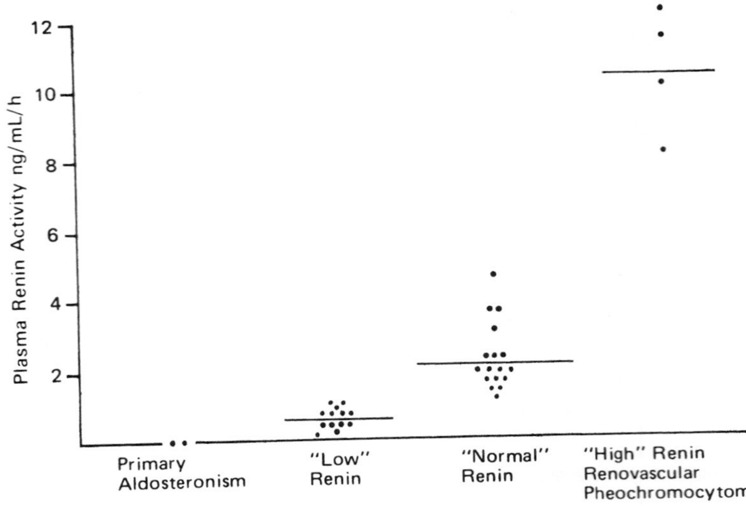

Figure 51-17 PRA 5 hours after the oral administration of 60 mg of furosemide. *(From Wallach L, Nyari I, Dawson K. Stimulated renin: A screening test for hypertension. Ann Intern Med 1975;82:27.)*

ratio. When working up patients with suspected primary aldosteronism, it is helpful, for example, to compare the ambulatory PRA activity with sodium excretion or to stimulate renin production with a potent diuretic such as furosemide (Figure 51-17). A high PRA activity could be due to secondary aldosteronism (e.g., renovascular hypertension or pheochromocytoma). A low value, on the other hand, suggests primary aldosteronism or low-renin hypertension. The latter may be caused by exogenous or endogenous mineralocorticoids that mimic the action of aldosterone, producing an expansion in plasma volume, hypertension, and hypokalemia. The use of an ACE inhibitor such as captopril has also been employed for the diagnosis of primary aldosteronism. In individuals who are normotensive or have essential hypertension, acute inhibition of ACE decreases angiotensin-mediated aldosterone production, and the autonomous aldosterone production from an aldosterone-producing adenoma is unaffected by the ACE inhibitor.

The determination of plasma renin responsiveness, however, is not sufficient to diagnose primary aldosteronism because suppressed PRA also occurs in about 25% of patients with essential hypertension. Primary aldosteronism can be differentiated from other hypermineralocorticoid states on the basis of inappropriate secretion of aldosterone. The demonstration of an elevated concentration of aldosterone in blood or urine in a patient with an unequivocally suppressed PRA concentration (a plasma aldosterone/plasma PRA ratio >50) is presumptive evidence of primary aldosteronism. Because hypokalemia has a suppressive effect on aldosterone secretion, the potassium deficit should be replaced before aldosterone measurements are done. To establish aldosterone autonomy, the clinician may attempt to suppress aldosterone production with rapid volume expansion[68] (see Box 51-10), with a potent mineralocorticoid (see Box 51-11),[5] or as mentioned with captopril. Failure of aldosterone to be suppressed using these maneuvers confirms a diagnosis of primary aldosteronism.

Once the diagnosis of primary aldosteronism is established, it is necessary to distinguish between APA and bilateral IAH. This differentiation is vital because most patients with adrenal adenomas respond well to surgical removal of the tumor, whereas patients with adrenal hyperplasia do not and are managed medically. Localization using imaging techniques[67] can be helpful (spiral CT scans,[3,52,165] ultrasonography, and adrenal scanning with NP-59 [^{131}I-6β-iodomethyl-19-norcholesterol]) and adrenal venography with or without selective adrenal venous sampling for aldosterone measurements to determine whether the right or left adrenal is hypersecreting aldosterone when the tumors are too small to be detected by imaging techniques. A number of biochemical clues can help with the differential diagnosis. Aldosterone hypersecretion and plasma renin suppression are usually greater with adrenal adenomas. After sodium depletion or after 2 to 4 hours of upright posture, patients with APA usually show no change or a paradoxical fall in plasma aldosterone, whereas patients with IAH typically show a rise in plasma aldosterone (presumably because the hyperplastic glands are sensitive to small increments in PRA).[48] Elevated plasma concentrations of aldosterone precursor substrates, such as 18-hydroxycorticosteroid (>85 ng/dL), are observed in most patients with APA but not in those with IAH (see Figure 51-16).

A small percentage of patients with APA or IAH respond to dexamethasone treatment with a normalization of their blood pressure and correction of their biochemical abnormalities.[39] Dexamethasone treatment should be attempted before surgery, particularly in young patients, or when the normal fall in plasma aldosterone concentration after salt depletion and standing does not occur, and no unilateral lesion is seen on radiographs. Also, a trial treatment of *spironolactone*, an aldosterone antagonist, usually normalizes

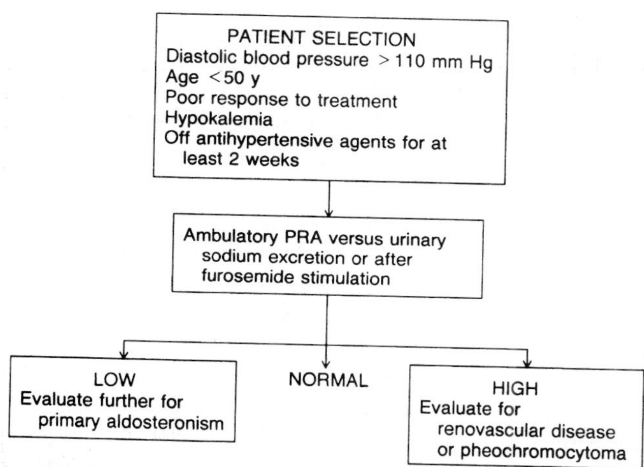

Figure 51-18 Screening with PRA in hypertension. *(From Watts NB, Keffer JH. Practical endocrine diagnosis, 3rd ed. Philadelphia: Lea & Febiger, 1982. Used with permission.)*

BOX 51-14 Protocol for the Differential Renal Vein Renin Test

Rationale In renovascular hypertension, PRA is higher in the renal vein on the involved side.

Procedure The patient should be on a low-sodium, high-potassium diet and receiving a diuretic for 3 days before the procedure. Under fluoroscopic guidance, percutaneous catheterization is performed, and blood samples are obtained from both renal veins and the inferior vena cava for determination of PRA.

Interpretation Various criteria have been suggested for interpretation. A ratio of PRA (affected side to unaffected side) that is >1.5 suggests functionally significant renovascular disease.

blood pressure in patients who are likely to have a good response to surgery.

Other Causes of Adrenal Mineralocorticoid Excess

Adrenocortical carcinomas have been found to produce excess mineralocorticoid and cause hypertension with hypokalemia.[6,37] Either aldosterone or DOC, or both, may be produced in excess. Mineralocorticoid concentrations do not respond to glucocorticoid therapy or alterations in salt status. CT scans are helpful; adrenal carcinomas are usually large tumors that weigh more than 30 g; aldosterone-secreting adenomas are usually much smaller. Finding low plasma renin activity and aldosterone concentration under circumstances that should cause an elevation (furosemide stimulation or upright posture) would support the diagnosis (see Figure 51-17).

Other unusual conditions that suggest aldosterone excess or deficiency but are not connected to the renin-angiotensin-aldosterone system[163] include *Liddle's syndrome* (pseudohyperaldosteronism),[86] which resembles primary aldosteronism clinically, but aldosterone production is low and hypertension is absent; and *Bartter's syndrome,*[201] which involves a prostaglandin-mediated renal potassium wasting and renal chloride handling defect, in which both aldosterone concentrations and renin activities are elevated. In renal tubular acidosis and pseudohypoaldosteronism, the clinical picture of hypoaldosteronism is seen concurrent with greater-than-normal concentrations of aldosterone.

Plasma Renin in Renovascular Hypertension

Used as a screening test, an elevated plasma renin activity after furosemide stimulation or when correlated with urinary sodium excretion[78] can suggest renal artery stenosis as the cause of the hypertension (Figure 51-18). If there is arteriographic evidence for renal artery stenosis, measurement of plasma renin in specimens obtained from selective renal vein catheterization can be helpful in predicting the response to surgical correction of the renal vascular lesion or nephrectomy. Lateralization of renin in the renal vein to the radiographically involved side, especially after sodium depletion, is also predictive of a good response to surgery in 90% of cases (Box 51-14).[104] Comparing renin activity in the renal artery with that in the renal vein can make a further distinction.[188]

ANALYTICAL METHODOLOGY

Many different types of methods have been used to measure steroids in body fluids.[2A] Earlier methods included photometric and fluorometric methods.[25,91] However, they have been replaced by immunoassays* and methods based on some type of a separation step, such as capillary electrophoresis,[158,159] gas chromatography (GC),[32,208] liquid chromatography (LC),[66,120] high-performance liquid chromatography (HPLC),[120] or mass spectrophotometry (MS) interfaced with either gas (GC/MS)† or liquid (LC/MS)[23,166,184] chromatographs. These techniques are discussed in more detail in Chapters 6, 7, and 9. For routine, high-volume measurements, immunoassay is still the most widely used method because of the widespread availability of automated instruments that include immunoassays in their repertoire of analytical methods (see Chapter 9).[11,147] Many high-volume clinical laboratories, however, are now routinely using LC/MS and/or liquid chromatography/tandem mass spectrometry (LC-MS/MS)[77A,99A,176A] methods for the measurement of urinary cortisol and cortisone.

Choice of Specimen

Steroids are now measured in urine, blood, and saliva specimens.

*References 2, 57, 60, 63, 77, 94, 123, 147, 150.
†References 18, 53, 54, 137, 178, 180, 187, 210.

Urine

Although the urinary excretion of a hormone, or its metabolites, or both does not account for the total amount of hormone secreted by the gland, it usually represents a good approximation of the amount secreted during the period of urine collection. Thus urinary assays provide a good estimate of the secretory activity of the adrenal gland. However, factors such as incompleteness of collection, altered renal function with renal disease, and the contribution by more than one gland to the total excretion pool of the same hormone or hormones (e.g., adrenal glands and gonads both contribute to the concentration of androstenedione) warrant special attention in the interpretation of urinary values. Analyses of total urinary metabolites have further shortcomings because they reflect only a fraction of the active steroid hormones that are metabolized through different pathways; the quantity and the nature of these metabolites may, in turn, depend not only on the pathological condition but on the intake of drugs and on diet. Other arguments against urinary assay of metabolites include the time and inconvenience encountered in the collection of 24-hour urine specimens. Urine assays, however, do have their place in the determination of free hormones. Urinary free cortisol and the measurement of urinary free estradiol, estrone, and testosterone have been shown to provide clinical information that reflects the production rates of these steroids.

Blood

The determination of steroids in blood has now been the accepted routine for determining the secretion rates of steroids from the endocrine organs that produce them. Immunoassays along with chromatographic methods have been developed that efficiently determine all of the clinically relevant steroids found in the circulation. In addition, because endocrine testing is founded on provocative testing (stimulation and suppression tests), blood samples for rapid dynamic testing are more convenient to obtain than urine and reflect a more relevant point in time to the patient's endocrine status. The determination of steroids in plasma, however, still has its limitations because of the rapid fluctuations and pulsatility that occur in the secretion of hormone concentrations during the day; thus a single plasma sample is representative only of the concentration that existed at the time of sampling. Therefore the measurement of some steroids, such as free cortisol, using timed urine collections still has value.

There is no experimental evidence that steroid hormone concentrations in serum are different from those in plasma. However, rapid separation of red blood cells in the specimen is important because red blood cells at room temperature can alter plasma concentrations of active steroid hormones; red blood cells degrade estradiol to estrone and cortisol to cortisone, and they can adsorb testosterone.

Saliva

In general most steroids of clinical interest can be measured in saliva.[191] For some steroids, such as cortisol, estriol, and progesterone, the measurement of the salivary concentration appears to be a reliable indicator of the free concentration in plasma. For others (e.g., testosterone, 17-hydroxyprogesterone, estradiol, and aldosterone) the clinical usefulness of salivary measurements has not yet been fully established.

It has been suggested that measurement of salivary steroids reflects the free (nonprotein-bound) steroid fraction in blood and may provide information similar to that derived from measurement of urinary free steroids.[139,148] The measurement of both cortisol and progesterone has been determined in saliva. Salivary sampling protocols are advantageous in that they allow for frequent and easy collection of samples by noninvasive, stress-free techniques. Salivary sample testing is particularly helpful when assessing hormone concentrations in children who may be averse to a needle stick. The measurement of steroids in saliva also obviates the difficulties of ensuring the completeness of a 24-hour urine collection. Patients find little difficulty in salivating directly into disposable tubes and can provide an adequate volume in ~10 minutes. Assays of samples collected at 1- to 2-hour intervals during waking hours provide an accurate assessment of baseline endocrine concentrations. Because smaller aliquots (500 μL) can be collected at 15- or even 10-minute intervals, salivary samples could well be more useful than either plasma or urine samples with short-term dynamic testing protocols. The possibilities and pitfalls of salivary hormone assays have been further discussed by Vining and McGinley.[191]

Free Versus Bound Steroids

The measurement of steroid hormones in a free state distinct from a protein-bound state may be advantageous under certain situations. When alterations in the binding proteins that carry the bulk of steroids in the circulation occur, the interpretation of the total circulating concentration of that particular steroid may be significantly influenced. In addition, it is the free hormone that binds to the steroid receptor and elicits the biochemical effect; thus knowledge of the free hormone concentration is desirable in a number of clinical situations. The concept of measuring free hormones has been in the literature for a number of years with the documented clinical utility of urinary free cortisol. Other applications include the measurement of free and weakly bound testosterone in the clinical work-up of the patient presenting with hirsutism.[139]

Hydrolysis, Extraction, and Separation

Although steroid hormones differ greatly in their physiological effects in the body, the assay procedures used for their measurement have many similarities. One or more of the following general steps may be required before final quantitation: (1) hydrolysis, (2) extraction, (3) purification, and (4) separation. Note, however, that with techniques such as HPLC and with specific immunoassay methods, steps such as hydrolysis, extraction, purification, and separation are frequently unnecessary for routine clinical measurement of steroids. Improvements in antibody specificity have been the most important advance in the routine measurement of steroids, obviating the need for a purification step before immunoassay for steroids such as aldosterone, cortisol, progesterone, testosterone, and estradiol. There are still those, however, who believe that chromatography-based methods are preferable for specificity and accuracy reasons for urine steroid measurements. LC, LC-mass spectrometry (LC-MS), and LC-MS/MS methods have been developed and applied to the measurement of urinary free cortisol and other steroid hormones.

Hydrolysis

Steroid hormones are present in blood both protein bound and in a free state and excreted in the urine primarily as water-soluble conjugates of glucuronic (glucosiduronic) acid and sulfuric acid. When total concentrations (unconjugated plus conjugated forms) of a steroid hormone or its metabolites are determined, the hydrolysis of ester linkages is an obligatory step. Two general types of procedures are available, namely, acid hydrolysis and enzymatic hydrolysis. In *acid hydrolysis,* an aliquot of a 24-hour urine sample is boiled, usually with reflux, in the presence of a specified concentration of mineral acid for a specified length of time (10 to 60 minutes). For *enzymatic hydrolysis,* a portion of a 24-hour urine specimen or an aliquot of plasma is adjusted with buffer to the optimum pH for the enzyme used; after the addition of an adequate amount of the necessary hydrolytic enzymes, *β-glucuronidase* (to hydrolyze glucuronates [glucosiduronates]) and *sulfatase* (to hydrolyze sulfate conjugates), the test sample is incubated for 18 to 72 hours at a specified temperature, such as 45 °C.

Technically, acid hydrolysis is often preferred (except for acid-labile hormones), because the process offers simplicity and speed and usually results in complete hydrolysis regardless of the nature of conjugates. Enzymatic hydrolysis requires special attention to factors such as optimal concentration and type of enzyme, pH, temperature, and duration of incubation. In addition, the possible presence of enzyme inhibitors, which vary in amount and nature with different specimens, may affect the completeness of hydrolysis. In spite of potential problems, enzymatic hydrolysis is used for plasma analysis of steroids that are labile in strong acid solution (e.g., pregnanetriol and corticosteroids), and because it prevents interference from substances that are produced by acid hydrolysis. Enzymatic hydrolysis, for example, has been used successfully to determine the urine concentration of estrone and the plasma concentration of estrone sulfate in postmenopausal women.

Extraction

After hydrolysis, deconjugated steroids become sparingly soluble in aqueous solution. Thus when an immiscible organic solvent in which steroids are highly soluble is added to the hydrolyzed sample and shaken, most of the steroids are extracted into the organic layer. Repeating the extraction process with a fresh volume of the organic solvent increases the recovery of the steroid extracted. The same procedure is followed for the assay of unconjugated steroid hormones in plasma or serum. Note that addition of an organic solvent to the plasma denatures the binding proteins. Thus the extracted steroid represents both protein-bound and unbound fractions.

Selection of the organic solvent is based on the polarity of the steroid hormone to be measured. The nonpolar tetracyclic ring system is common to all steroids, but the polarity increases as the number of oxygen groups (ketone and hydroxyl groups) and double bonds increase. Steroids with one or two oxygens (e.g., androgens and estrogens) are of low polarity; a good solvent for their extraction is a relatively nonpolar solvent, such as diethyl ether. Similarly, steroids with three or more oxygen groups (e.g., corticosteroids and their metabolites) are quite polar; for their extraction, polar organic solvents such as chloroform, dichloromethane, or ethyl acetate are more suitable.

The relative solubility of substances in two immiscible solvents is used not only for the extraction process but for the separation and purification of substances (partition chromatography). The ratio of the concentration of a substance in a nonpolar phase to the concentration of the same compound in the polar phase is known as the *partition coefficient* (K) (see Chapter 6). Substances with high K values will remain in the nonpolar phase, and substances with low K values will preferentially move into the polar phase. In the extraction process, the solvent system is composed of an organic solvent (a relatively nonpolar phase) and the hydrolyzed urine or plasma (polar phase). Steroids with high Ks are consequently extracted into the organic layer. A better recovery of polar compounds (e.g., urinary corticosteroids and estriol) from the polar phase can be conveniently achieved by adding ammonium sulfate or sodium chloride before extraction. The addition of inorganic salts increases the K by decreasing the solubility of the steroid in the aqueous solution.

Purification and Separation

Although a proper choice of solvent improves the selectivity of extraction, a large number of closely related steroids, chromogenic substances, and other nonspecific materials are also extracted with the steroids. Removal of such contaminants, especially those that will interfere in the final estimation, is important when the antibody specificity used to measure the steroid is relatively low. With high specificity and high affinity antibodies, this becomes less of an issue and is now more the rule than the exception.

When the need arises to purify the steroid, the *solvent partition method* is the simplest and most suitable method for the clinical laboratory. It is widely used for preliminary purification and separation of steroid compounds of interest. The basic principle is the same as that for extraction. Steroids and other urinary impurities contained in the organic solvent are treated with weakly basic solutions (e.g., sodium bicarbonate and sodium carbonate). By virtue of their greater solubility, strongly acidic components partition into the basic aqueous layer. The separation of neutral and phenolic steroids is achieved in a similar manner. Because of the acidic nature of the phenolic steroids (estrogens), they are readily extracted from an organic phase with an aqueous solution of sodium hydroxide. After the pH of the alkaline solution is lowered, estrogens are reextracted with a suitable solvent (e.g., diethyl ether) and are processed further for final estimation. Most often the organic extract is washed to neutrality with water to ensure complete removal of alkali, which if allowed to remain might interfere in the subsequent work-up of the extract.

The degree of purification and separation needed before quantitative measurement depends on the method used for final quantitation. For example, if the final mode of estimation is a chemical reaction that is very specific for an individual steroid or for a group of steroids, further purification of the steroid extract may be omitted. In fact many of the older photometric assays for steroid hormones (e.g., urinary 17-ketosteroids) were performed on crude extracts. Similarly, with many immunoassays using highly specific antisera, the quantitation is frequently carried out without prior purification with organic extracts. Although such determinations may yield adequate information for most clinical purposes, specific measurement of an individual steroid or group of steroids may occasionally necessitate further purification and separation of the extract. Various techniques are available for this purpose. For detailed descriptions of the theory and application of these methods to steroid analysis, the reader is referred to Dorfman.[25] These methods are based on physical techniques such as countercurrent distribution, paper and column-partition chromatography, column and thin-layer adsorption chromatography, gel filtration using LH-20, GC, GC/MS, LC/MS-MS, or HPLC. Celite microcolumn chromatography is still used by many laboratories to purify and separate steroid hormones (estrone and dihydrotestosterone) before immunoassay quantitation.[118,155] Nonpolar steroids elute with low concentrations of ethyl acetate in iso-octane; more polar steroids elute as the ethyl acetate/iso-octane concentration ratio increases.

Specific Methods

Measurement of Cortisol in Blood and Urine

Approximately 90% of the circulating cortisol is bound to plasma proteins, primarily to an α-globulin known as *CBG* or *transcortin*. There is also weak binding to albumin. The exact function of these carrier proteins is still unknown, but it has been suggested that they represent a circulating storage source of hormone and protection of the steroid from inactivation and conjugation in the liver or filtration by the kidney. The concentration of CBG in the plasma rises with hyperestrogenic states, including pregnancy, and with the use of oral contraceptives; thus there is a concomitant increase of total cortisol in serum under these conditions. However, because the amount of free cortisol remains normal, there are no untoward phenotypic effects suggestive of hypercortisolism.

Although methods involving organic solvent extraction or protein precipitation will estimate both free and protein-bound cortisol in the circulation, immunoassay-based methods that determine cortisol directly from serum have essentially replaced all extraction-based methods for routine cortisol measurements save for urine free cortisol methods. Historically, four general methods have been used for the quantitative estimation of total blood cortisol concentrations in the clinical laboratory. These are the Porter-Silber color reaction method modified for plasma,[125,146] the use of sulfuric acid–induced fluorescence,[70,103] HPLC methods, or immunoassay. In general, HPLC and immunoassay are now used in both clinical laboratories and reference laboratories for the quantitative determination of cortisol in serum or urine.

Chromatographic Methods

Several types of chromatographic methods have been used to measure cortisol including GC,[32,208] LC,[59,66,88,120,183] HPLC,[102,120,130] and gas and liquid chromatography coupled to mass spectrophotometry (GC/MS* and LC/MS[23,166,184]). In addition, methods based on capillary electrophoresis have become available.[75,158,159] All of these methods easily distinguish cortisol from other steroids and steroid metabolites. However, most of them are labor intensive, have low throughput capabilities, and require considerable processing of the sample before analysis. For example, most HPLC methods require preanalytical extraction of cortisol from the specimen, with either solid-phase columns[184] or liquid-liquid extraction[94] followed by reversed-phase and normal-phase chromatography and detection using native fluorescence or ultraviolet absorption.[45,82,142] HPLC methods have the advantage of being able to separate all relevant steroids with one chromatography step, but for the practical reasons already cited are not widely used for routine purposes. Cortisol assays based on isotope dilution combined with GC/MS are widely recognized as reference procedures and are often used to validate routine methods.† In most GC/MS methods, cortisol is extracted from plasma and converted to its methoxime-trimethylsilyl derivative; deuterated cortisol is used as an internal standard.

*References 18, 53, 54, 137, 159, 178, 180, 187, 210, 214.

†References 40, 143, 178, 179, 180, 187.

Immunoassay

In practice, immunoassays are the easiest and most common methods used for cortisol measurements in serum and urine and are widely available in most clinical laboratories on different semiautomated and automated systems.[11,147,203]

Principle

A large number of cortisol immunoassays* have been developed using different types of antibodies[91]; processing schemes[215]; labels (both isotopic[2,60,117] and nonisotopic[63]); and measurement principles, including beta and gamma counting,[2,60] photometry,[77,84,114] fluorometry,[62,65,83,197] and chemiluminescence.[89,100,172,212] Many immunoassay methods have employed antibodies produced in animals immunized with a variety of different cortisol derivatives conjugated to protein. Antisera raised against cortisol-21-hemisuccinate and cortisol-3-carboxymethyloxime conjugates have proved quite suitable and are widely used for direct immunoassays that require no sample extraction. Specific monoclonal cortisol antibodies have also been produced using hybridoma techniques.

As mentioned earlier, most cortisol immunoassays performed in clinical laboratories are direct assays and require no initial extraction of steroids from the specimen. In these direct assays, cortisol is quantitatively displaced from endogenous binding proteins by protein-binding agents, such as 8-anilino-1-naphthalene-sulfonic acid (ANS) or salicylate, by low pH or by heat treatment.[56] The efficiency of steroid displacement by protein-binding agents, such as ANS, may be influenced by the concentration of binding protein present in the specimen. For example, the amount of ANS that is adequate for plasma obtained from normal men and nonpregnant women may be insufficient to displace cortisol from CBG in pregnancy, when CBG concentrations are elevated. Furthermore, the concentration of ANS required for complete displacement may reduce specific binding of the steroid to the antiserum.

In situations where a lower detection limit is required and highly specific antisera are not available, cortisol is first extracted from serum before measurement.[94,150] The extraction is performed in a manner similar to that for urine specimen extractions (see discussion later in this chapter).[12] An important advantage of the direct assays is their superior precision compared with assays involving extraction. In part this may reflect the variability inherent in manual extraction techniques. In general, however, with the high specificity of the antibodies available today and with the use of very sensitive nonisotopic techniques, such as chemiluminescence and fluorescence, the quantitative measurement of cortisol in blood and urine is now relatively straightforward.

*References 11, 57, 80, 123, 147, 150.

Methods

Isotopic Methods. The tracer most widely used in radioimmunoassay methods for total cortisol is ^{125}I. A variety of formats have been used for the different cortisol radioimmunoassays. Some use a solid-phase first antibody to capture the cortisol, whereas others use a liquid-liquid format. Solid-phase antibodies have been chemically or physically attached to the inner or outer surfaces of test tubes, beads, or magnetizable particles. In antibody-coated tube assays, the cortisol antibody is immobilized onto the inner wall of polyethylene tubes. Test specimens and calibrators are incubated with ^{125}I-labeled cortisol in these tubes; the contents of the tubes are aspirated or decanted; and the radioactivity remaining in the tubes (^{125}I-labeled cortisol bound to antibody) is counted. This relatively quick and simple procedure does not require a centrifugation step.

Other commercial radioimmunoassay kits for serum cortisol use liquid phase double-antibody separations or solid-phase antibody suspensions. In double-antibody systems, a second antibody is used to precipitate the primary antibody, and after centrifugation and aspiration of the supernatant, the antibody-bound tracer is counted. Solid-phase suspension systems for cortisol use antibodies bound to small solid-phase particles that remain suspended in the reaction medium, thus exposing a large surface area for antibody-antigen binding and obviating the need for mixing. The suspended particles are separated by centrifugation, the supernatant is aspirated, and the bound radioactivity of the precipitate is counted.

Almost all commercial radioimmunoassay methods for serum cortisol show some cross-reactivity with prednisolone. Because prednisone is converted to prednisolone in vivo, these kits cannot be used to analyze specimens from patients on prednisone therapy. The degree of cross-reactivity with 11-DOC, corticosterone, and prednisone varies from 1% to 5%; these cross-reactions are antiserum dependent.[29] When high plasma concentrations of 11-DOC are found (such as in 11β-hydroxylase deficiency or after administration of metyrapone), preliminary extraction with carbon tetrachloride to remove this steroid is usually indicated.

In general, direct radioimmunoassays for serum cortisol are precise, sensitive, and show a high degree of correlation with reference methods such as GC/MS. According to the College of American Pathologists Ligand Assay Survey,[14] interlaboratory imprecision of the different commercial radioimmunoassay methods (expressed as coefficients of variation [CVs]) is under ±10% for serum cortisol concentrations in the range of 10 to 40 μg/dL (280 to 1100 nmol/L). Most of these radioimmunoassay methods show little bias and give results that are close to target values. Radioimmunoassay, however, is not routinely performed in clinical laboratories because of the emergence of reasonably accurate and precise nonisotopic methods for serum and urine cortisol.

Nonisotopic Methods. Most automated and semiautomated methods rely on nonisotopic labels for the quantitative measurement of cortisol. Most of these methods use enzymes such as horseradish peroxidase, alkaline phosphatase, or β-galactosidase as cortisol labels; enzyme activity is commonly determined using photometric,[77,84,114] fluorescent,[62,65,83,197] or chemiluminescent substrates.[100,172,212] Immunoassays for cortisol that use fluorescence[22,69] and chemiluminescence[89] labels are the most common methods in use today. Both heterogeneous (separation required) and homogeneous (nonseparation) methods have been developed. An example of the former is the radial partition immunoassay for cortisol.[10] In this automated assay, serum cortisol, freed from its binding proteins by ANS, competes with alkaline phosphatase–labeled cortisol for antibody binding sites on a borosilicate paper matrix. A washing procedure radially elutes unbound material while concomitantly allowing the bound enzyme to catalyze substrate cleavage. Homogeneous assays, such as fluorescence polarization immunoassay[101] and the cloned enzyme donor immunoassay[15] for cortisol, eliminate the need to separate bound and free fractions. Most immunoassay methods for cortisol are available on fully automated immunoassay systems.[11,203,147]

Specimen Collection and Storage

Serum or plasma (with heparin as an anticoagulant) can be used. No special handling procedures are necessary, and specimens may be stored refrigerated overnight at 2 °C to 8 °C. Freezing is preferred for long-term stability. Urinary free cortisol is determined on a 24-hour urine collection with or without boric acid preservative. If collected without preservative, the specimen should be refrigerated between collections and an aliquot frozen immediately after completion of the 24-hour collection.

Reference Intervals

Representative values of total cortisol (free and bound) in *serum* assayed by immunoassay are as follows:

	μg/dL	nmol/L
Cord blood[34]	5-17	138-469
Infant (1-7 days)[34]	2-11	53-304
Child (1-16 yr)[34]		
0800 hours	3-21	83-580
Adult[181]		
0800 hours	5-23	138-635
1600 hours	3-16	83-441
2000 hours	<50% of 0800 hours values	<50% of 0800 hours values

Comments

Blood cortisol concentrations parallel those of ACTH, with episodic and diurnal concentrations observed throughout the day. The blood concentration at 2000 hours is normally <50% of the concentration obtained at 0800 hours. Increased cortisol secretion is observed in patients with stress, after glucocorticoid therapy, and in pregnancy, states of depression, hypoglycemia, and hyperthyroidism. In adults there is no significant dependence of cortisol values on age or sex. The half-life of cortisol in the circulation is ~100 minutes. In the newborn period, a transient rise in cortisol occurs immediately after delivery; this is followed by a decline to a concentration below that of umbilical cord blood at 12 to 48 hours and then by an increase that stabilizes at about 1 week of age. Renal failure has little effect on serum cortisol, except that retained metabolites can cross-react in some direct assays and thus cause a significant overestimate of cortisol concentrations. Extraction of the sample with dichloromethane usually overcomes this interference. Celite chromatography has also been used to "clear" the sample of possible interference before immunoassay measurements are carried out in renal failure patients. Urine free cortisol results are influenced by a number of factors, including completeness of the 24-hour urine collection, the subject's hydration state, and renal disease.

Measurement of Free Cortisol in Blood, Urine, and Saliva

Free or unbound cortisol represents the biologically active form of the circulating hormone, and its concentration is practically independent of alterations of its transport proteins. Various methods have been developed for estimating the *free fraction in serum,* but these assays are technically demanding, expensive, and not in general use.[7,149] The measurement of *urine free cortisol* comes closest to providing an estimate of the free hormone concentration.[9] As mentioned previously, approximately 2% of cortisol is excreted into the urine in a free form, and its measurement has been shown to be of use as a screening test for cortisol hypersecretion.[136] However, β-hydroxycortisol has been reported to interfere with the immunoassay of free cortisol in urine.[80]

Free cortisol can also be measured in other body fluids, such as saliva.[71] The measurement of free cortisol in *saliva* is a practical and convenient approach to assessing the free hormone.[79,115] Salivary cortisol measurements accurately reflect the concentration of nonprotein-bound cortisol in blood (probably because of the absence of substantial amounts of transcortin or albumin in saliva), and its concentration is independent of salivary flow rate. Most immunoassay kits for total serum cortisol can be used for the measurement of cortisol in saliva[123]; extraction is not required because saliva contains virtually no cortisol-binding proteins or other cortisol metabolites. The preferred method for handling saliva samples before assaying them for their cortisol content is to quick freeze the sample on collection. With thawing and centrifugation, the glycoproteins in saliva precipitate, leaving behind a clear fluid that can then be analyzed.

Principle

Most immunoassays for total serum cortisol can be used for the measurement of urinary free cortisol after appropriate *extraction* of the urine specimen. Preliminary extraction of free cortisol before measurement is usually required because of the large number of cortisol metabolites and conjugates in urine that cross-react with the cortisol antibody in the assay. Because most interfering substances are more soluble than cortisol in urine, the cortisol can be extracted with an organic solvent such as dichloromethane or ethyl acetate. Usually the sample is thoroughly mixed with the organic solvent in a ratio of ~1:5, the layers are allowed to separate, and the aqueous layer is removed. An aliquot of the organic layer containing the free cortisol is transferred to a separate tube, evaporated to dryness, and redissolved in a buffered solution. This solution can then be used as the unknown sample in the assay described for serum cortisol. Adding a known quantity of cortisol to an aliquot of the specimen and then extracting the spiked sample along with an aliquot of specimen to which no standard has been added can be used to monitor extraction efficiency. Extraction efficiency of cortisol is calculated from the difference in measured cortisol between the two samples divided by the known amount of cortisol added to one of the samples. The calculation of the amount of cortisol in an extracted sample must take into account the dilution with organic solvent and the extraction efficiency. Spiking the original sample with radiolabeled cortisol and determining recovery by counting the sample following the procedural steps can also determine extraction efficiency.

Immunoassay of unextracted urine is feasible with selected antisera, although reference values usually have a higher upper limit than those for extracted methods.[115] Even with solvent extraction of urine, most commercial assays for cortisol are subject to interference and show a wide range of imprecision (CV of ±15% to 25%). Chromatographic procedures, such as HPLC, are more specific than immunoassays for urine cortisol measurement and may be an attractive alternative for some laboratories.[10,59]

Urine Specimens. A complete 24-hour urine specimen is collected with 10 g of boric acid to maintain the urine pH below 7.5. Urine should be refrigerated during the collection period. After measuring the total volume, a thoroughly mixed aliquot (~10 mL) is stored frozen at −20 °C. Care should be taken to ensure an appropriately timed, complete 24-hour collection because an incorrectly timed sample is the largest source of error with this method. Free cortisol determinations on randomly collected urines are discouraged because of the variation and pulsatile characteristic of cortisol secretion.

Salivary Specimens. Cortisol is stable in saliva for 1 week at 4 °C and for 4 months when stored frozen. Freezing of specimens is recommended because it leads to precipitation of salivary glycoproteins and leaves a nonviscous liquid for pipetting.[115]

Reference Intervals

The following are representative values for free cortisol excreted per 24 hours in *urine:*

	μg/day	nmol/day	Method
Child			
1-10 yr	2-27	6-74	Radioimmunoassay (extracted)[110]
2-11 yr	1-21	3-58	HPLC[127]
11-20 yr	5-55	14-152	Radioimmunoassay (extracted)[110]
12-16 yr	2-38	6-105	HPLC[127]
Adult	20-90	55-248	Radioimmunoassay (extracted)[47]
	75-270	207-745	Radioimmunoassay (unextracted)[47]

Representative values for free cortisol in *serum* (equilibrium dialysis and/or immunochemiluminometric assay)[127] and *saliva* (radioimmunoassay)[148] of adults are as follows:

Serum	μg/dL	nmol/L
0800 hours	0.6-1.6	17-44
1600 hours	0.2-0.9	6-25
Saliva	**ng/mL**	**nmol/L**
0700 hours	1.4-10.1	4-28
2200 hours	0.7-2.2	2-6

Comments

Disadvantages of urine methods include incomplete collection owing to patient error and impaired excretion caused by renal disease. Concomitant measurement of urinary creatinine excretion allows assessment of the completeness of the collection. Salivary cortisol measurement is practical and convenient to assess cortisol secretion in ambulatory patients who can provide multiple specimens that can be stored in a freezer between clinic visits. Morning salivary cortisol concentration is decreased in adrenal insufficiency; evening values are increased in Cushing's syndrome.[135]

Measurement of Aldosterone in Blood and Urine

Simple and reliable immunoassay methods for measuring aldosterone in blood and urine[60] are readily available. These methods differ primarily in the specificity of the anti-aldosterone antibodies. Most direct radioimmunoassay methods for plasma aldosterone use antisera generated against an aldosterone-3-monooxime-bovine serum albumin (BSA) conjugate, and use an ^{125}I-labeled ligand and ANS at pH 3.6 to displace aldosterone from plasma-binding proteins.[56]

Principles

A variety of commercial immunoassay kits are available for the determination of plasma and urine aldosterone.[153,161] The differences in these kits lie in the specificity of the antibodies used and the method used to achieve separation of bound from free aldosterone. Some methods use either a solid-phase first antibody,[164] an accelerated liquid-phase second antibody,[105] a solid-phase second antibody, dextran-coated charcoal, or a polyethylene glycol precipitant. Most assay procedures for urinary total aldosterone are similar to those for plasma except that urine is acid hydrolyzed before assay.[60]

The cross-reactivity of commercial aldosterone antisera with other steroids (e.g., DOC and corticosterone) is relatively low (<0.01%). Nevertheless, the concentration of these other steroids can sometimes be quite high, requiring the partial isolation of aldosterone before assay. Unconjugated plasma aldosterone can be extracted with an organic solvent and then purified with celite column chromatography; tritiated aldosterone is often added to each specimen to correct for procedural losses. In urine, interfering unconjugated steroids are first extracted using an organic solvent such as ethyl acetate or methylene chloride, and then the aldosterone conjugate is hydrolyzed with acid. The free aldosterone thus formed is extracted into the same solvent, the solvent is evaporated, and the radioimmunoassay is performed on the dried extract after reconstitution in an assay buffer. The need for preliminary purification depends on the diagnostic kit being used and the type of patient being evaluated. For example, specificity is not a significant concern in hypertensive adults without adrenal disease, whereas greater specificity may be needed for children, patients with adrenal disease, and pregnant women.

Several nonisotopic enzyme immunoassays have been developed for serum and urinary aldosterone using both monoclonal and polyclonal antibodies generated against aldosterone.[44,160] These assays use either immobilized antigen (aldosterone-protein complexes) or immobilized anti-aldosterone antibodies. A chemiluminescence-based immunoassay for direct measurement of aldosterone in serum has also been described.[173] In this competitive assay, the specimen is incubated for 2 hours at room temperature with a rabbit antialdosterone antibody, an isoluminol-labeled aldosterone conjugate, and paramagnetic particles coated with a second antibody. After separation and washing, the samples are incubated with sodium hydroxide for 30 minutes at 60 °C and then placed into a luminometer for a 5-second reading time. The minimum concentration of aldosterone that can be distinguished from the zero calibrator is 1 ng/dL (0.03 nmol/L), which is comparable with the detection limits of most radioimmunoassay methods. A shelf life of several years for the chemiluminescent label makes this an attractive method. Recent application of the aldosterone assay to an automated immunoassay platform will make this assay more accessible to routine clinical laboratories.

Specimen Collection and Storage

Plasma (preserved with heparin, ethylenediaminetetraacetic acid [EDTA], or citrate) or serum can be used. If an upright blood specimen is to be collected, the subject should be in an upright position (standing or seated) for at least 2 hours before collection. Specimens should be stored frozen in an airtight container and are stable for up to 2 years at −20 °C. For urine assays, a complete 24-hour urine specimen is collected with boric acid as a preservative. Fifty percent acetic acid should also be added to the urine collection to achieve a pH between 2.0 and 4.0. Specimens should not be acidified with strong mineral acids, such as hydrochloric acid. Urine should be refrigerated during collection; aliquots are stored frozen at −20 °C. It is recommended that a urine sodium test also be performed to facilitate the interpretation of the aldosterone result.

Reference Intervals

The serum, plasma, or urine concentration of aldosterone depends on the patient's salt intake and posture at the time of collection. The following serum values are based on a morning specimen collected from subjects on a normal salt diet and in an upright position for at least 2 hours[181]:

	ng/dL	nmol/L
Cord blood	0-200	1.11-5.54
Premature infants	19-141	0.53-3.91
Full-Term infants		
3 days	7-184	0.19-5.10
1 wk	5-175	0.03-4.85
1-12 mo	5-90	0.14-2.49
Children		
1-2 yr	7-54	0.19-1.50
2-10 yr	3-35	0.08-0.97 (supine)
	5-80	0.14-2.22 (upright)
10-15 yr	2-22	0.06-0.61 (supine)
	4-48	0.11-1.33 (upright)
Adults	3-16	0.08-0.44 (supine)
	5-30	0.14-0.83 (upright)

The following aldosterone concentrations excreted per 24 hours in urine have been reported[34]:

	μg/day	nmol/day	μg/g Creatinine
Newborns, 1-3 days	0.5-5	1-14	20-140
Prepubertal children, 4-10 yr	1-8	3-22	4-22
Adults	3-19	8-51	1.5-20

Measurement of 11-Deoxycortisol in Blood

With clinical evidence of an adrenal enzyme deficiency, it is customary to determine the steroid concentration just proximal to the suspected enzyme block. In the case of 21α-hydroxylase deficiency, the measurement of 17-hydroxyprogesterone documents the enzyme deficiency. Similarly, 11-deoxycortisol measurements will confirm a 11β-hydrolyase block. A number of biosynthetic precursors of both cortisol and aldosterone can be measured by immunoassay, either directly or after sample extraction, or chromatography, or both. Other examples include pregnenolone, 17-hydroxypregnenolone, corticosterone, and DOC.

In practice the measurement of serum or plasma 11-deoxycortisol (compound S) is used to document an 11β-hydroxylase deficiency or as part of the metyrapone stimulation test. Because metyrapone inhibits the 11β-hydroxylase enzyme, a fortyfold to eightyfold increase in plasma 11-deoxycortisol is observed in patients with normal pituitary-adrenal reserve. Consequently, immunoassay methods for 11-deoxycortisol in metyrapone test specimens need not be highly sensitive. In these patients, a corresponding drop in serum cortisol is observed. A failure to demonstrate an increase in 11-deoxycortisol to at least 4 μg/dL suggests either an inadequate pituitary ACTH reserve or primary adrenal failure.

Principle

Radioimmunoassay methods for the direct determination of plasma 11-deoxycortisol are available.[56,145] Antiserum raised against 11-deoxycortisol-3-carboxymethyloxime-BSA has provided appropriate specificity with minimal cross-reactivity against other adrenal steroids. Some radioimmunoassay methods still include an extraction step, or column chromatography, or both.[19,60] In one commercial kit,[29] plasma specimens are extracted with hexane and/or ethyl acetate and then assayed. Antibody-bound and free steroid fractions are separated using a double-antibody technique and polyethylene glycol precipitation. The principal interfering steroid in this kit is 17-hydroxyprogesterone (4% cross-reactivity). A few nonisotopic methods for measuring 11-deoxycortisol in serum have been described, but these procedures are not widely used.[1] Most radioimmunoassays for 11-deoxycortisol are appropriately sensitive and specific enough for use with the metyrapone test and for assessing the possibility of an 11-hydroxylase deficiency.

Reference Intervals

Representative values for 11-deoxycortisol in serum are as follows[181]:

	ng/dL	nmol/L
Cord blood	295-554	9-16
Children and adults	20-158	0.6-4.6

Measurement of 17-Hydroxyprogesterone in Blood

Measurement of serum or plasma 17-hydroxyprogesterone, a C_{21} steroid, is primarily used for the rapid diagnosis of CAH caused by the congenital absence or deficiency of the 21-hydroxylase enzyme. In classic CAH caused by 21-hydroxylase deficiency, 17-hydroxyprogesterone concentrations are several hundred times the upper limit of normal. This test is also used to monitor the effectiveness of cortisol replacement therapy in CAH patients. Measurements of 17-hydroxyprogesterone are also determined as part of the clinical work-up of women who present with hirsutism or infertility, either of which may be due to adult-onset 21-hydroxylase deficiency. This test is sometimes used after ACTH stimulation to distinguish classic affected, nonclassic affected, and heterozygote carrier individuals with the 21-hydroxylase deficiency gene.

Principle

Direct radioimmunoassays for 17-hydroxyprogesterone are available that use highly specific antibodies against 17-hydroxyprogesterone-3-carboxymethyloxime-BSA with sufficient affinity and specificity to permit direct assay of small volumes of serum, plasma, saliva, and even amniotic fluid. In addition, high–specific activity radioiodinated tracers[27,51,192] and nonisotopic labels have been used to construct enzyme immunoassays with photometric, fluorescent, and chemiluminescent substrates.[96,182] Fluorescence-based immunoassays using fluorescein or streptavidin-europium labels[33,206] and a chemiluminescence assay using an isoluminol derivative label have been described.[73] These direct assays are available in kit form[81] commercially and are convenient and simple to perform. Some are marketed with liquid calibrators. Separation of free and antibody-bound fractions is often achieved using a solid-phase coated tube or liquid-phase double-antibody methods. Despite the use of highly specific antisera, most direct assays are subject to some interference by cross-reacting substances present in neonatal and infant plasma specimens.[98] These substances increase the apparent 17-hydroxyprogesterone concentration, thereby reducing the discrimination between normal individuals and those with congenital disease. Some of the steroids that cause this interference have been identified.[205] Direct assays appear to function satisfactorily with specimens from children, adolescents, and young adults (ages 90 days to 21 years). However, for the analysis of specimens from premature neonates and infants aged 3 to 90 days, some form of extraction is recommended. Elevated results obtained by direct methods should be confirmed by reassay using an extraction method. On occasion amniotic fluid specimens are submitted for the in utero diagnosis of 21-hydroxylase deficiency in certain high-risk pregnancies. Amniotic fluid samples should be extracted before the radioimmunoassay is performed.

Specimen Collection and Storage

The preferred specimen for 17α-hydroxyprogesterone is serum; plasma with EDTA as an anticoagulant may also be used. Specimens can be stored at 4 °C for up to 4 days or at −20 °C for up to 1 month. Specimens can be obtained from infants by heel puncture and collected in capillary tubes or on filter paper. Dried blood specimens are stable and easily transported and thus are ordinarily obtained for purposes of screening neonates for CAH.

Reference Intervals

The following serum values are representative of expected normal values for 17-hydroxyprogesterone[34]:

	ng/dL	nmol/L
Cord blood	900-5000	27.3-151.5
Premature	26-568	0.8-17.0
Newborn, 3 days	7-77	0.2-2.7
Prepubertal child	3-90	0.1-2.7
Puberty		
Tanner stage		
1. Male	3-90	0.1-2.7
Female	3-82	0.1-2.5
2. Male	5-115	0.2-3.5
Female	11-98	0.3-3.0
3. Male	10-138	0.3-4.2
Female	11-155	0.3-4.7
4. Male	29-180	0.9-5.4
Female	18-230	0.5-7.0
5. Male	24-175	0.7-5.3
Female	20-265	0.6-8.0
Adults		
Male	27-199	0.8-6.0
Female		
Follicular phase	15-70	0.4-2.1
Luteal phase	35-290	1.0-8.7
Pregnancy[186]	200-1200	6.0-36.0
Post-ACTH	<320	<9.6
Postmenopausal	70	<2.1

Measurement of Renin and Angiotensin I

The activity of the renin-angiotensin-aldosterone system is usually assessed in the clinical laboratory by measuring plasma renin activity and aldosterone concentrations. Most of the polyclonal antibodies used measure angiotensin I and are unable to distinguish between active renin and inactive prorenin. This can lead to an overestimation of renin activity and cause problems with interpretation in patients with low renin activities. However, a sensitive immunoradiometric mass assay specific for physiologically active renin has been developed using monoclonal antibodies.[168] This assay uses two monoclonal antibodies: one specifically recognizes renin but prorenin only minimally, and the other sees prorenin only with the use of the renin inhibitor remikiren. This approach may resolve the problems noted with earlier immunoassay methods for the direct determination of renin mass.

Most clinical laboratories measure PRA using an enzyme kinetic assay in which angiotensin I is formed by the action of renin on its substrate, angiotensinogen.[161,162] Angiotensin I is measured before and after a timed incubation period. The amount of angiotensin I generated from its endogenous substrate can also be quantitated using nonisotopic methods (e.g., enzyme immunoassay,[29,55,157] HPLC,[72] and fluorescence polarization[97]), but in general these approaches have not been put to large-scale use.

To obtain the maximum rate of renin activity, saturating amounts of the renin substrate, angiotensinogen, should be present in the reaction system. In most procedures, however, the only substrate provided is that present in the test plasma, and its concentration can be quite variable. According to some investigators, PRA is best estimated when the plasma specimen is incubated with an excess of exogenous renin substrate prepared from nephrectomized human subjects, oxen, or sheep. This type of assay is usually known as a plasma renin concentration assay rather than PRA assay. Unfortunately the measured renin depends on the source and concentration of the renin substrate. Synthetic peptides that resemble the *N*-terminal portion of angiotensinogen have also been used as renin substrates, but these substances can be hydrolyzed by nonspecific plasma proteases.

Several radioimmunoassays for angiotensin I and angiotensin II in native plasma have been reported, but most of them do not appear to differ significantly in their essential characteristics. Like steroid hormones, angiotensin I and angiotensin II are poor immunogens because of their small molecular size. Therefore they must be conjugated to proteins, such as albumin, hemocyanin, or succinylated polylysine, for the production of antisera. Polyclonal antisera are seldom strictly specific, and samples usually contain cross-reacting decapeptide, heptapeptide, and hexapeptide congeners of the angiotensins. In addition, plasma can continue to produce or destroy angiotensins during the assay and may contain materials that affect the assay by interfering with the antigen-antibody reaction or by binding to angiotensin itself. Isolation of angiotensin from the sample before assay has been found to minimize these problems. Acetone, methanol, ethanol, and Fuller's earth have all been used for this purpose. Other chromatographic procedures for separating and purifying the different forms of angiotensin, such as HPLC, have also been used.[49] Problems regarding cross-reactivity and interference are best eliminated by using sensitive and specific antisera.

Angiotensin II, the active peptide of the renin-angiotensin system, is the most difficult component of the renin cascade to measure accurately. Most immunoassay methods are unable to detect the very low concentrations in blood, and interfering peptides or degradation products must be removed before radioimmunoassay. An additional chromatographic separation step is usually required to distinguish angiotensin II from other angiotensins. However, monoclonal antibodies with high affinity and specificity have been produced against angiotensin II and used to develop a direct radioimmunoassay; as little as 0.8 fmol of angiotensin II in 2 mL of plasma has been detected in the presence of angiotensin I.[167]

Sealey[162] and Freedlender and Goodfriend[36] have reviewed the special problems encountered in the preparation of plasma specimens for radioimmunoassay of angiotensins. Angiotensins are very labile peptides in plasma and can be generated in vitro in untreated plasma even in the frozen state. Therefore great care must be taken in the collection and storage of specimens for angiotensin assays,[49] including special attention to the inactivation of the cleavage enzymes, angiotensinases.

A number of commercial kits are available for determining PRA[161,162]; the basic elements of these procedures are summarized in the following sections. With continued improvements and availability of the immunometric assay methods for determining renin mass, renin activity assays will likely be replaced by the direct mass assays for the routine assessment of plasma renin.

Principle

PRA is defined as the rate of angiotensin I produced from the substrate angiotensinogen by the enzyme renin in a patient's plasma. PRA is expressed in nanograms of angiotensin I generated per milliliter of plasma per hour and is determined by measuring angiotensin I after incubation of plasma at 37 °C and then subtracting the amount of baseline angiotensin I in a control plasma aliquot kept at 4 °C.

Specimen Collection and Storage

A blood sample is drawn into a lavender-top vacutainer tube containing EDTA. After centrifugation to sediment cells, the plasma is removed and frozen at −20 °C or lower. Plasma for PRA can be stored frozen up to 1 month before assay. Freeze-thaw cycles should be avoided because of the possible activation of prorenin. At the time of collection, blood should not be chilled or placed on ice because irreversible cryoactivation of prorenin can occur, leading to falsely high estimates of PRA. Serum or plasma collected into another anticoagulant can also be used as long as EDTA is added (3 mmol/L, final concentration) before the angiotensin I generation step. It should be recognized, however, that prorenin is more likely to cryoactivate in serum than in plasma. Uncentrifuged blood is stable at room temperature for up to 6 hours without significant accumulation of angiotensin I. Hemolyzed specimens should not be used because red blood cells contain angiotensinases. Heparin should be avoided as an anticoagulant for this reason. The use of EDTA is preferred for PRA because it not only acts as an anticoagulant but also inhibits the ACE and other hydrolytic enzymes that break down angiotensin.

Factors such as time of day, posture, salt intake, and diuretic or other drug use should be properly documented for appropriate interpretation of test results. The patient should be ambulatory for 2 hours before blood collection. A 24-hour urine specimen for sodium is collected on the day before the renin test to reference the result to salt intake. Specimens with high renin activity can generate considerable amounts of angiotensin I before and during storage even at −20 °C. This will not affect results, however, because angiotensin I is determined before and after the incubation step. An angiotensinase enzyme inhibitor is used in the reaction system to prevent further metabolism of angiotensin I. The buffering of plasma samples is also important because any change in pH alters the generation of angiotensin I at 37 °C. Most PRA assays use a pH that is optimum for the renin enzyme (5.7 to 6.3). The baseline angiotensin I concentration obtained at 4 °C is subtracted from the angiotensin I concentration generated after 60 to 90 minutes of incubation at 37 °C. The time of incubation varies depending on the sensitivity of the angiotensin I antiserum and the amount of renin activity. Most assays use an incubation period of 60 minutes with satisfactory results, but the time of incubation can be extended to improve the sensitivity of the assay. Subtracting the baseline angiotensin I value normalizes the result to endogenous angiotensin I concentrations, but this can be a source of error particularly when renin activity is low. Some investigators ignore the blank when the baseline angiotensin I result exceeds the generated angiotensin I concentration.[162]

Angiotensin I Generation

Angiotensin I is generated using the following procedure:

1. Thaw frozen specimens in front of a fan for a few minutes until they are at room temperature. Do not thaw frozen specimens in a refrigerator.
2. Add one or more of the following inhibitors to thawed plasma: phenylmethyl sulfonyl fluoride, 8-hydroxyquinoline sulfate, dimercaprol, and neomycin (see Comments section for explanation of the use of inhibitors).
3. Add the maleate generation buffer (pH 6.0) to each plasma specimen.
4. Divide the plasma mixture into four aliquots.
5. Incubate two aliquots for 60 to 90 minutes at 37 °C (see Comments section for discussion of choice of period of incubation) and store the other two aliquots at 4 °C.
6. At the end of the incubation period, chill the aliquots in an ice bath at 4 °C.
7. The incubated and nonincubated aliquots are then assayed for angiotensin I. Incubated plasma represents the endpoint of renin activity, whereas the 4 °C plasma represents renin activity at baseline.
8. Renin activity is then calculated as nanograms of angiotensin I produced per milliliter of plasma per hour of incubation, adjusting for the volume of plasma, the time of incubation, and the difference in angiotensin I concentrations between the incubated and nonincubated samples.

Comments

Phenylmethyl sulfonyl fluoride added to thawed plasma inhibits angiotensinases that can cleave the generated angiotensin I but are unaffected by metal chelators.

The other inhibitors help retard proteolysis and bacterial growth.

Plasma specimens must be buffered. Otherwise, the pH will increase during enzymatic incubation at 37 °C, in which case the rate of angiotensin I generation will decrease owing to a shift in the kinetics and to the destruction of renin above pH 8. Thus assays use a buffer near the pH optimum of renin (5.7 to 6.3).

Reference Intervals

Reference intervals for PRA vary depending on salt intake, posture, and certain medications. For adults on a normal sodium diet, a reference interval of 0.7 to 3.3 ng of angiotensin I/mL/hr has been reported.[181] Sodium intake, posture, hydration state, and other factors that can affect renin activity should be noted. For example, a low-sodium diet and upright posture increase renin activities in normal individuals. High renin values may also be seen in patients receiving diuretics (volume and sodium depletion) or estrogen-containing medications (stimulation of hepatic synthesis of angiotensinogen).[116] Most antihypertensive drugs alter PRA, and such drugs should be discontinued 1 to 2 weeks before the test is performed. Only stimulated PRA values (e.g., after furosemide stimulation) are of practical value in evaluating hypertensive patients.

Plasma renin activity decreases gradually with age in both men and women. In women, renin activity is increased during the luteal phase of the menstrual cycle and in pregnancy.

REFERENCES

1. Al-Ansari A, Massoud M, Perry L, Smith DS. Polarization fluoroimmunoassay of 11-deoxycortisol in serum and saliva. Clin Chem 1983;29:1803-5.
2. Abraham GE, ed. Radioassay systems in clinical endocrinology. New York: Marcel Dekker Inc, 1981.

2A. Andrew R. Clinical measurement of steroid metabolism. Best Pract Res Clin Endocrinol Metab 2001;15:1-16.

3. Baer L, Sommers SC, Krakoff LR, Newton MA, Laragh JH. Pseudoprimary aldosteronism. Circ Res 1970;27(Suppl1):203-16.
4. Baxter JD, Perloff D, Hsuch W, Bigleria EG. The endocrinology of hypertension. In: Felig P, ed. Endocrinology and metabolism, 2nd ed. New York: McGraw-Hill, 1987:693-772.
5. Biglieri EG, Stockigt JR. A preliminary evaluation for primary aldosteronism. Arch Intern Med 1970;126:1004-7.
6. Biglieri EG, Kater CE. Mineralocorticoids. In: Greenspan FS, Forsham PH, eds. Basic and clinical endocrinology, 3rd ed. East Norwalk, Conn: Appleton & Lange, 1992:310-25.
7. Brien T. Free cortisol in human plasma. Horm Metab Res 1980;12:643-50.
8. Can BR. Disorders of the ovary and female reproductive tract. In: Wilson JD, Foster DW. Williams textbook of endocrinology. Philadelphia: WB Saunders Co, 1992:733-798.
9. Canalis E, Reardon G, Caldarella A. A more specific, liquid-chromatographic method for free cortisol in urine. Clin Chem 1982;28:2418-20.
10. Castillo M, Linne A, Soto A. A radial partition immunoassay for cortisol. Clin Chem 1984;30:1042.
11. Chan DW, ed. Immunoassay automation: An updated guide to systems. San Diego: Academic Press, 1995.
12. Chattoraj SC, Turner AK, Pinkus JL, Charles D. The significance of urinary free cortisol and progesterone in normal and anencephalic pregnancy. Am J Obstet Gynecol 1976;124:848-54.
13. Chrousos GP, Loriaux DL, Mann D, Cutler GB. Late-onset 21-hydroxylase deficiency is an allelic variant of congenital adrenal hyperplasia characterized by attenuated clinical expression and different HLA haplotype associations. Horm Res 1982;16:193-200.
14. College of American Pathologists. Ligand assay series I survey, set K/KN-A. Skokie, Ill: College of American Pathologists, 1997.
15. Collinsworth W, Padgett R, Keller C. Multicenter evaluation of CEDIA cortisol on Boehringer Mannheim/Hitachi analyzers. Clin Chem 1992;38:1077.
16. Contreras P, Araya V: Cushing's syndrome: Review of a national caseload. Rev Med Chil 1995;123:350-62.
17. Crapo L. Cushing's syndrome: A review of diagnostic tests. Metabolism 1979;28:955-77.
18. De Brabandere VI, Thienpont LM, Stockl D, De Leenheer AP. Three routine methods for serum cortisol evaluated by comparison with an isotope dilution gas chromatography-mass spectrometry method. Clin Chem 1995;41:1781-3.
19. Demers L, Ebright L, Derck D. Improved radioimmunoassay for 11-deoxycortisol (compound S) in plasma. Clin Chem 1979;25:1704-7.
20. Demers LM. Biochemistry and laboratory measurement of androgens in women. In: Redmond GP, ed. Androgenic disorders. New York: Raven Press, 1995:21-34.
21. Demers LM, Sampson EJ, Hayes AH. Plasma renin activity and plasma and urine aldosterone: A normal range study by radioimmunoassay. Clin Biochem 1976;9:243-6.
22. Diamandis E, Bhayana V, Conway K, Reichstein E, Papanastasiou-Diamandis, A. A time-resolved fluoroimmunoassay of cortisol in serum: A rapid non-isotopic assay. Clin Chem 1988;34:1216.
23. Dodds HM, Taylor PJ, Cannell GR, Pond SM. A high-performance liquid chromatography-electrospray-tandem mass spectrometry analysis of cortisol and metabolites in placental perfusate. Anal Biochem 1997;247:342-7.

24. Doppman JL. Adrenal imaging. In: Besser M, Burger HG, Jameson JL, eds. Endocrinology, 3rd ed. Philadelphia: WB Saunders Co, 1995:1711-32.
25. Dorfman RI, ed. Methods in hormone research, Vol I. 2nd ed. New York: Academic Press, 1968.
26. Durant S, Duval D, Homo-Delarche F. Factors involved in the control of fibroblast proliferation by glucocorticoids: A review. Endocr Rev 1986;7:254-69.
27. Dyas J, Read GF, Guha-Maulik T, Hughes IA, Riad-Fahmy D. A rapid assay for 17α-OH progesterone in plasma, saliva and amniotic fluid using a magnetisable solid-phase antiserum. Ann Clin Biochem 1984;21:417-24.
28. Edwards CR. Primary mineralocorticoid excess syndromes. In: Besser M, Burger HG, Jameson JL, eds. Endocrinology, 3rd ed. Philadelphia: WB Saunders Co, 1995:1775-803.
29. Edwards L, ed. Product guide for radioassays and non-isotopic ligand assays. Clin Chem 1983;29: 889-986.
30. Ehrlich EN, Friedman AL, Shenker Y. Hormonal regulation of electrolyte and water metabolism. In: Besser M, Burger HG, Jameson JL, eds. Endocrinology, 3rd ed. Philadelphia: WB Saunders Co, 1995:1685-710.
31. Ehrlich EN, Friedman AL, Shenker Y. Hormonal regulation of electrolyte and water metabolism. In: DeGroot LJ, ed. Endocrinology. Philadelphia: WB Saunders Co, 1995:1685-710.
32. Eik-Nes KB, Horning EC. Gas phase chromatography of steroids. New York: Springer-Verlag, 1968.
33. El-Gamal B, Eremin S, Smith D, Landon J. Development of a direct fluoroimmunoassay for serum levels of 17-hydroxyprogesterone. Ann Clin Biochem 1988;25:35-41.
34. Endocrine Sciences: Pediatric laboratory services. Tarzana, Calif: Endocrine Sciences, 1988.
35. Fernandez-Real JM, Ricart-Engel W, Simo R. Preclinical Cushing's syndrome: Report of three cases and literature review. Horm Res 1994;41:230-5.
36. Freedlender AE, Goodfriend TL: Renin and the angiotensins. In: Jaffe BM, Behrman HR, eds. Methods of hormone radioimmunoassay. New York: Academic Press, 1979:889-907.
37. Freeman DA. Steroid hormone-producing tumors in man. Endocr Rev 1986;7:204-20.
38. Funder JW, Krozowski Z, Myles K, Sato A, Sheppard KE, Young M. Mineralocorticoid receptors, salt, and hypertension. Recent Prog Horm Res 1997;52:247-62.
39. Ganguly A. New insights and questions about glucocorticoid-suppressible hyperaldosteronism. Am J Med 1982;72:851-4.
40. Gaskell S, Sieckmann L. Mass-spectrometric determination of serum cortisol: Comparison of data from two independent laboratories. Clin Chem 1986;32:536-8.
41. Grenman S, Ronnemaa T, Irjala K, Kailhola HL, Gronroos M. Sex steroid, gonadotropin, cortisol, and prolactin levels in healthy, massively obese women: Correlation with abdominal fat cell size and effect of weight reduction. J Clin Endocrinol Metab 1986;63:1257-61.
42. Grossman A. Corticotropin-releasing hormone: Basic physiology and clinical applications. In: DeGroot LJ, ed. Endocrinology. Philadelphia: WB Saunders Co, 1995:341-54.
43. Gwynne JT, Strauss JF III: The role of lipoprotein in steroidogenesis and cholesterol metabolism in steroidogenic glands. Endocr Rev 1982;3:299-329.
44. Hanquez C, Urios P, Desfosses B, Samake H, Lince E, Rajkowski KM, et al. A competitive microtitre plate enzyme immunoassay for plasma aldosterone using a monoclonal antibody. J Steroid Biochem 1988;31: 939-45.
45. Hariharan M, Naga S, VanNoord T, Kindt EK. Simultaneous assay of corticosterone and cortisol in plasma by reversed-phase liquid chromatography. Clin Chem 1992;38:346-52.
46. Hashimoto K, Suemaru S, Takao T, Sugawara M, Hattori T, Kageyama J, et al. Human corticotropin-releasing factor plus lysine vasopressin test during glucocorticoid therapy. J Clin Invest 1988;82:13-6.
47. Healthcare Corp. Package insert for clinical assays gammacoat [125I] cortisol radioimmunoassay kit. Cambridge, Mass: Healthcare Corp, 1990.
48. Herf SM, Teates DC, Tegtmeyer CJ, Vaughan ED Jr, Ayers CR, Carey RM. Identification and differentiation of surgically correctable hypertension due to primary aldosteronism. Am J Med 1979;67:397-402.
49. Hermann K, Ganten D, Unger T, Bayer C, Lang RE. Measurement and characterization of angiotensin peptides in plasma. Clin Chem 1988;34:1046-51.
50. Hermus AR, Pieters GF, Pesman GJ, Smals AG, Benraad TJ, Kloppenborg PW. ACTH and cortisol responses to ovine corticotrophin-releasing factor in patients with primary and secondary adrenal failure. Clin Endocrinol (Oxf) 1985;22:761-9.
51. Hofman L, Klaniecki J, Smith E. Direct solid-phase radioimmunoassay for screening 17-hydroxyprogesterone in whole-blood samples from newborns. Clin Chem 1985;31:1127-30.
52. Hogan MJ, McRae J, Schambelan M, Biglieri EG. Location of aldosterone-producing adenomas with 131-I-19-iodocholesterol. N Engl J Med 1976;294:410-4.
53. Hsu FF, Wang L, Bier DM. Determination of cortisol in human plasma by gas chromatography/negative ion chemical ionization/mass spectrometry. Anal Biochem 1994;216:401-5.
54. Hubbard WC, Bickel C, Schleimer RP. Simultaneous quantitation of endogenous levels of cortisone and cortisol in human nasal and bronchoalveolar lavage

fluids and plasma via gas chromatography-negative ion chemical ionization mass spectrometry. Anal Biochem 1994;221:109-17.

55. Hubl W, Haussig K, Hofmann F, Buchner M, Rohde W, Dorner G. Enzyme immunoassay and radioimmunoassay for plasma AI activity. Endokrinologie 1981;77:330-40.
56. Hunter WM, Corrie JET, eds. Immunoassays for clinical chemistry. Edinburgh: Churchill Livingstone, 1978.
57. Hunter WM, Corrie JET, eds. Immunoassays for Clinical Chemistry. 2nd ed. Edinburgh: Churchill Livingstone, 1983.
58. Imperato-Mcginley J, Guerrero T, Peterson RE. Steroid 5 α reductase deficiency in man: An inherited form of male pseudohermaphroditism. Science 1974;186:1213-5.
59. Inoue S. Simultaneous high-performance liquid chromatographic determination of 6 beta-hydroxycortisol and cortisol in urine with fluorescence detection and its application for estimating hepatic drug-metabolizing enzyme induction. J Chromatogr B Biomed Appl 1994;661:15-23.
60. Jaffe BM, Behrman HR, eds. Methods of Hormone Radioimmunoassay. New York: Academic Press, 1979.
61. Jerkunica I, Sophianopoulos J, Sgoutas D. Improved ultrafiltration method for determining unbound cortisol in plasma. Clin Chem 1980;26:1734-7.
62. Jonsson KB. A new fluorometric assay for determination of osteoblastic proliferation: Effects of glucocorticoids and insulin-like growth factor-I. Calcif Tissue Int 1997;60:30-6.
63. Joshi U. Non-isotopic immunoassays for the estimation of steroid hormones. In: Pal SB, ed. Immunoassay technology, Vol 1. Berlin: Walter de Gruyter & Co, 1985.
64. Kaplan NM. Endocrine hypertension. In: Wilson JD, Foster DW. Williams textbook of endocrinology. Philadelphia: WB Saunders Co, 1992:707-31.
65. Kapsner K, Cyr M, Smith D. Fluorometric enzyme immunoassay for the determination of cortisol for use on the Kallestad immunoassay analyzer. Clin Chem 1990;36:1162.
66. Kautsky MP, ed. Steroid analysis by HPLC. New York: Marcel Dekker Inc, 1981.
67. Kehlet H, Blichert-Toft M, Hancke S, Pedersen JF, Kristensen JK, Efsen F, et al. Comparative study of ultrasound, 131-I-19-iodocholesterol scintigraphy, and aortography in localizing adrenal lesions. Br Med J 1976;2:665-7.
68. Kem DC, Weinberger MH, Mayes DM, Nugent CA. Saline suppression of plasma aldosterone in hypertension. Arch Intern Med 1971;128:380-6.
69. Khosravi M, Morton R, Reichstein E. Strepavidin as a universal carrier of haptens: Applications to immunoassays of cortisol by time-resolved fluorometry. Clin Chem 1990;36:1097.
70. Khveshchuk PF. Analysis of glucocorticoids in biological objects using spectrofluorometry. Klin Lab Diagn 1995;4:33-5.
71. Kiess W, Meidert A, Dressendorfer RA, Schriever K, Kessler U, Konig A, et al. Salivary cortisol levels throughout childhood and adolescence: Relation with age, pubertal stage, and weight. Pediatr Res 1995;37:502-6.
72. Klickstein L, Wintroub B. Separation of angiotensins and assay of angiotensin-generating enzymes by high-performance liquid chromatography. Anal Biochem 1982;120:146-50.
73. Klingler W, Staedt P, Haupt O. Luminescence and radioimmunoassay of 17α-hydroxyprogesterone in small samples. Fresenius A Anal Chem 1984;317:721-2.
74. Kong MF, Jeffcoate W. Eighty-six cases of Addison's disease. Clin Endocrinol 1994;41:757-61.
75. Koutny LB, Schmalzing D, Taylor TA, Fuchs M. Microchip electrophoretic immunoassay for serum cortisol. Anal Chem 1996;68:18-22.
76. Krieger DT, Ganong WF. ACTH and related peptides: Structure, regulation, and action. Ann NY Acad Sci 1977;297:205-19.
77. Kronkvist K, Lovgren U, Svenson J, Edholm LE, Johansson G. Competitive flow injection enzyme immunoassay for steroids using a post-column reaction technique. J Immunol Methods 1997;200:145-53.

77A. Kushnir MM, Rockwood AL, Nelson GJ, Terry AH, Meikle AW. Liquid chromatography-tandem mass spectrometry analysis of urinary free cortisol. Clin Chem 2003;49:965-967.

78. Laragh JH, Sealey J, Brunner HR. The control of aldosterone secretion in normal and hypertensive man: Abnormal renin-aldosterone patterns in low renin hypertension. Am J Med 1972;53:649-63.
79. Laudat MH, Cerdas S, Fournier C, Guiban D, Guilhaume B, Luton JP. Salivary cortisol measurement: A practical approach to assess pituitary-adrenal function. J Clin Endocrinol Metab 1988;66:343-8.
80. Lee C. 6 beta-hydroxycortisol interferes with immunoassay of urinary free cortisol. Clin Chem 1996;42:1290-1.
81. Lee A, Ellis G. Serum 17α-hydroxyprogesterone in infants and children as measured by a direct radioimmunoassay kit. Clin Biochem 1991;24:505-11.
82. Lensmeyer G, Carlson I, Wiebe D, DeVos D. Determination of cortisol (C), cortisone (CN), corticosterone (CC), prednisone (P), and prednisolone (PL) in serum with solid reversed-phase extraction and high performance liquid chromatography (HPLC). Clin Chem 1992;38:945.

83. Lentjes EG. Free cortisol in serum assayed by temperature-controlled ultrafiltration before fluorescence polarization immunoassay. Clin Chem 1993;39: 2518-21.
84. Letellier M, Levesque A, Daigle F, Grant A. Performance evaluation of automated immunoassays on the Technicon Immuno 1 system. Clin Chem 1996;42:1695-701.
85. Li JT, Shu SG, Chi CS. Aldosterone-secreting adrenal cortical adenoma in an 11-year-old child and collective review of the literature. Eur J Pediatr 1994;153: 715-7.
86. Liddle GW, Bledsoe T, Coppage WS. A familial renal disorder simulating primary aldosteronism but with negligible aldosterone secretion. Trans Assoc Am Physicians 1963;76:199-213.
87. Lieberman S, Prasad V. Heterodox notions on pathways of steroidogenesis. Endocr Rev 1990;11: 469-93.
88. Lin CL. Urinary free cortisol and cortisone determined by high performance liquid chromatography in the diagnosis of Cushing's syndrome. J Clin Endocrinol Metab 1997;82:151-5.
89. Lindstrom L, Meurling L, Lovgren T. The measurement of serum cortisol by a solid-phase chemiluminescence immunoassay. J Steroid Biochem 1983;16:577-80.
90. Lo CY, Tam PC, Kung AW, Lam KS, Wong J. Primary aldosteronism: Results of surgical treatment. Ann Surg 1996;224:125-30.
91. Loraine JA, Bell ET, eds. Hormone assays and their clinical application, 4th ed. Edinburgh: Churchill Livingstone, 1976.
92. Loriaux DL, McDonald WJ. Adrenal insufficiency. In: Besser M, Burger HG, Jameson JL, eds. Endocrinology, 3rd ed. Philadelphia: WB Saunders Co, 1995:1731-40.
93. Loriaux DL, Nieman L. Corticotropin-releasing hormone testing in pituitary disease. Endocrinol Metab Clin North Am 1991;20:363-70.
94. Lovgren U, Johansson M, Kronkvist K, Edholm LE. Sample pretreatment for immunochemical techniques using micellar liquid chromatography for separation of corticosteroids. J Chromatogr B Biomed Appl 1995;672:33-44.
95. Luderer JR, Demers LM, Harrison TS, Hayes AH. Converting enzyme inhibition with captopril in patients with primary hyperaldosteronism. Clin Pharmacol Ther 1982;31:305-11.
96. Maeda M, Arakawa H, Tsuji A, Yamagami Y, Isozaki A, Takahashi T. et al. Enzyme-linked immunosorbent assay for 17α-hydroxyprogesterone in dried blood spotted on filter paper. Clin Chem 1987;33:761-4.
97. Maeda H, Nakayama M, Iwaoka D, Sato T. Assay of angiotensin I by fluorescence polarization method. Adv Exp Med Biol 1979;120A:203-11.
98. Makela S, Ellis G. Nonspecificity of a direct 17α-hydroxyprogesterone radioimmunoassay kit when used with samples from neonates. Clin Chem 1988;34:2070-5.
99. Malchoff DM, Malchoff CD. Glucocorticoid resistance. In: Besser M, Burger HG, Jameson JL, eds. Endocrinology, 3rd ed. Philadelphia: WB Saunders Co, 1995:1770-4.
99A. Marsden D, Larson CA. Emerging role for tandem mass spectrometry in detecting congenital adrenal hyperplasia, Clin Chem 2004;50:467-8.
100. Martin J, Brett G, Thompson W. Measurements of cortisol with a non-radioactive immunoassay based on enhanced luminescence. Clin Chem 1988;34:1217.
101. Martinus J, Klein L, Fino J, Shipchandler M, Wang P. A fluorescence polarization immunoassay (FPIA) for the quantitation of cortisol. Clin Chem 1985;31:956.
102. Mason SR. Fluorimetric detection of serum corticosterone using high-performance liquid chromatography. J Chromatogr 1992;581:267-71.
103. Mattingly D. A simple fluorimetric method for the estimation of free 11-hydroxycorticoids in human plasma. J Clin Pathol 1962;15:374-9.
104. Maxwell MH, Marks LS, Lupu AN, Cahill PJ, Franklin SS, Kaufman JJ. Predictive value of renin determinations in renal artery stenosis. JAMA 1977;238: 2617-20.
105. Mehra M, Etemtindong N. Direct radioimmunoassay for serum aldosterone using specific antisera. Clin Chem 1986;32:1165, 1986.
106. Meikle AW, Odell WD. Effect of short- and long-term dexamethasone on 3α-androstanediol glucuronide in hirsute women. Fertil Steril 1986;46:227-31.
107. Meikle AW. Dexamethasone suppression test: Usefulness of simultaneous measurement of plasma cortisol and dexamethasone. Clin Endocrinol (Oxf) 1982;16:401-8.
108. Meikle AW, Daynes RA, Araneo BA. Adrenal androgen secretion and biologic effects. Endocrinol Metab Clin North Am 1991;20:381-400.
109. Meikle AW, Stringham JD, Woodward MG, Bishop DT. Heritability of variation of plasma cortisol levels. Metabolism 1988;37:514-7.
110. Meites S, ed. Pediatric clinical chemistry, 2nd ed. Washington DC: AACC Press, 1981.
111. Melby JC, Azar ST. Hypoaldosteronism and mineralocorticoid resistance. In: Besser M, Burger HG, Jameson JL, eds. Endocrinology, 3rd ed. Philadelphia: WB Saunders Co, 1995:1804-12.
112. Migeon CJ, Donohoue PA. Congenital adrenal hyperplasia caused by 21-hydroxylase deficiency: Its molecular basis and its remaining therapeutic problems. Endocrinol Metab Clin North Am 1991;20: 277-96.
113. Mikhail G. Hormone assays and the gynecologist. Fertil Steril 1976;27:229-37.

114. Mindicino H, Struve G, Hutchins J, Schwarzberg M. Technicon cortisol assay: A fully automated direct immunoassay for the determination of cortisol in human serum. Clin Chem 1990;36:1097-8.
115. Moore A, Aitken R, Burke C, Gaskell S, Groom G, Holder G, et al. Cortisol assays; Guidelines for the provision of a clinical biochemistry service. Ann Clin Biochem 1985;22:435-54.
116. Morgan L, Pipkin FB, Kalsheker N. Angiotensinogen: Molecular biology, biochemistry and physiology. Int J Biochem Cell Biol 1996;28:1211-22.
117. Morineau G. Radioimmunoassay of cortisone in serum, urine, and saliva to assess the status of the cortisol-cortisone shuttle. Clin Chem 1997;43: 1397-407.
118. Morineau G, Gosling J, Patricot MC, Soliman H, Boudou P, al Halnak A, et al. Convenient chromatographic prepurification step before measurement of urinary cortisol by radioimmunoassay. Clin Chem 1997;43:786-93.
119. Mortensen RM, Williams GH, Funder JW, Marver D. Aldosterone action. In: Besser M, Burger HG, Jameson JL, eds. Endocrinology, 3rd ed. Philadelphia: WB Saunders Co, 1995:1668-84.
120. Mueller HW, Eitel J. Quality control in the determination of cortisol in plasma/serum by using, on every sample, two different three-step separation methods including ultrafiltration, restricted-access high-performance liquid chromatography and reversed-phase high-performance liquid chromatography, and contrasting results to immunoassays. J Chromatogr B Biomed Appl 1996;678:137-50.
121. Mulrow PJ. Adrenal renin: Regulation and function. Front Neuroendocrinol 1992;1:47-60.
122. Munck A, Naray-Fejes-Toth A, Miesfeld RL. Glucocorticoid action. In: Besser M, Burger HG, Jameson JL, eds. Endocrinology, 3rd ed. Philadelphia: WB Saunders Co, 1995:1642-67.
123. Nahoul K, Patricot MC, Bressot N, Penes MC, Revol A. Measurement of salivary cortisol with four commercial kits. Ann Biol Clin (Paris) 1996;54: 75-82.
124. Nelson DH. A historical overview of the adrenal cortex. In: Besser M, Burger HG, Jameson JL, eds. Endocrinology, 3rd ed. Philadelphia: WB Saunders Co, 1995:1627-9.
125. Nelson D, Samuels L. A method for the determination of 17-hydroxycorticosteroids in blood: 17-Hydroxycorticosterone in the peripheral circulation. J Clin Endocrinol Metab 1952;12:519-26.
126. New MI. Congenital adrenal hyperplasia. In: Besser M, Burger HG, Jameson JL, eds. Endocrinology, 3rd ed. Philadelphia: WB Saunders Co, 1995:1813-34.
127. Nichols Institute Reference Laboratories. Test catalog. San Juan Capistrano, Calif, Nichols Institute Reference Laboratories, 1992.
128. Nieman LK, Cutler GB Jr. Cushing's syndrome. In: Besser M, Burger HG, Jameson JL, eds. Endocrinology, 3rd ed. Philadelphia: WB Saunders Co, 1995:1741-69.
129. Odell W, Parker J. Control of adrenal androgen secretion. In: Genazzani AR. Adrenal androgens. New York: Raven Press, 1980:27-42.
130. Okumura T. Column-switching high-performance liquid chromatographic system with a laser-induced fluorimetric detector for direct, automated assay of salivary cortisol. J Chromatogr B Biomed Appl 1995;670:11-20.
131. Oldfield EH, Doppman JL, Nieman LK, Chrousos GP, Miller DL, Katz DA, et al. Petrosal sinus sampling with and without corticotropin-releasing hormone for the differential diagnosis of Cushing's syndrome. N Engl J Med 1991;325:897-905.
132. Opocher G, Rocco S, Carpene G, Armanini D, Mantero F. Primary hyperaldosteronism. Minerva Endocrinol 1995;20:49-54
133. Opocher G, Schiavi F, Conton P, Scaroni C, Mantero F. Clinical and genetic aspects of phaeochromocytoma. Horm Res 2003;59 Suppl 1: 56-61.
134. Orentreich N, Brind JL, Rizer RL, Vogelman JH. Age changes and sex differences in serum dehydroepiandrosterone sulfate levels throughout adulthood. J Clin Endocrinol Metab 1984;59:551-5.
135. Orth DN, Kovacs WJ, DeBold CR. The adrenal cortex. In: Wilson JD, Foster DW. Williams textbook of endocrinology. Philadelphia: WB Saunders Co, 1992:489-620.
136. Palermo M, Shackleton CH, Mantero F, Stewart PM. Urinary free cortisone and the assessment of 11 beta-hydroxysteroid dehydrogenase activity in man. Clin Endocrinol 1996;45:605-11.
137. Palermo M, Gomez-Sanchez C, Roitman E, Shackleton CH. Quantitation of cortisol and related 3-oxo-4-ene steroids in urine using gas chromatography/mass spectrometry with stable isotope-labeled internal standards. Steroids 1996;61: 583-9.
138. Pang S, Softness B, Sweeney WJ, New MI. Hirsutism, polycystic ovarian disease and ovarian 17-ketosteroid reductase deficiency. N Engl J Med 1987;316: 1295-301.
139. Pardridge W, Demers LM. Bioavailable testosterone in salivary glands. Clin Chem 1991;37:139-40.
140. Parker LN. Adrenal androgens. In: Besser M, Burger HG, Jameson JL, eds. Endocrinology, 3rd ed. Philadelphia: WB Saunders Co, 1995:1836-52.
141. Parker LN. Control of adrenal androgen secretions. Endocrinol Metab Clin 1991;20:401-22.
142. Patel S, Lott J. Cortisol. In: Pesce A., Kaplan L, eds. Methods in clinical chemistry. St Louis: CV Mosby, 1987:224-31.

143. Patterson DG, Patterson MB, Culbreth PH, Fast DM, Holler JS, Sampson EJ, et al. Determination of steroid hormones in a human-serum reference material by isotope dilution-mass spectrometry: A candidate definitive method for cortisol. Clin Chem 1984;30:619-26.
144. Perry LA, Grossman AB. The role of the laboratory in the diagnosis of Cushing's syndrome. Ann Clin Biochem 1997;34:345-59.
145. Perry L, Al-Dujaili E, Edwards C. A direct radioimmunoassay for 11-deoxycortisol. Steroids 1982;39:115-28.
146. Porter CC, Silber RH. A quantitative color reaction for cortisone and related 17,21-dihydroxy-20-ketosteroids. J Biol Chem 1950;185:201-7.
147. Price CP, Newman DJ. Principles and practice of immunoassay. New York: Stockton Press, 1996.
148. Riad-Fahmy D, Read GF, Walker RF, Griffiths K. Steroids in saliva for assessing endocrine function. Endocr Rev 1982;3:367-95.
149. Robin P, Predine J, Milgrom E. Assay of unbound cortisol in plasma. J Clin Endocrinol Metab 1977;46:277-83.
150. Rodriguez ML, McConnell I, Lamont J, Campbell J, FitzGerald SP. Generic immunoassay of corticosteroids with minimum pre-treatment of urine samples. Analyst 1994;119:2631-4.
151. Rosner W, Hryb DJ, Khan MS, Nakhla AM, Romas NA. Sex hormone binding globulin binding to cell membranes and generation of a second messenger. J Androl 1992;13:101-6.
152. Samojlik E, Kirschner MA, Silber D, Schneider G, Ertel NH. Elevated production and metabolic clearance rates of androgens in morbidly obese women. J Clin Endocrinol Metab 1984;49:949-54.
153. Sampson EJ, Derck DD, Demers LM. Comparison of two radioimmunoassay kits for aldosterone determination. Clin Biochem 1976;9:216-21.
154. Santen RJ. Male hypogonadism. In: Yen SSC, Jaffe RB, eds. Reproductive endocrinology. Philadelphia: WB Saunders Co, 1992:739-94.
155. Santen RJ, Demers LM, Harvey H, Santner S, Sanders S, Lipton A. Inhibition of aromatase with 16949A in postmenopausal women. J Clin Endocrinol Metab 1989;68:99-107.
156. Sapolsky R, Rivier C, Yamamoto G, Plotsky P, Vale W. Interleukin-1 stimulates the secretion of hypothalamic corticotropin-releasing factor. Science 1987;238:522-4.
157. Scharpe S, Verkerk R, Sasmito E, Theeuws M. Enzyme immunoassay for angiotensin I and renin. Clin Chem 1987;33:1774-7.
158. Schmalzing D, Nashabeh W, Fuchs M. Solution-phase immunoassay for determination of cortisol in serum by capillary electrophoresis. Clin Chem 1995;41: 1403-6.
159. Schmalzing D, Nashabeh W, Yao XW, Mhatre R, Regnier FE, Afeyan NB. Capillary electrophoresis-based immunoassay for cortisol in serum. Anal Chem 1995;67:606-12.
160. Schwartz F, Hadas E, Harnik M, Solomon B. Enzyme-linked immunosorbent assays for determination of plasma aldosterone using highly specific polyclonal antibodies. J Immunoassay 1990;11: 215-34.
161. Sealey J, Campbell G, Preibisz J. Hormone assays: Renin, aldosterone, peripheral vein, and urinary assays. In: Laragh J, Brenner B, eds. Hypertension: pathophysiology, diagnosis, and management. New York: Raven Press, 1990:1443-60.
162. Sealey J. Plasma renin activity and plasma prorenin assays. Clin Chem 1991;37:1811-9.
163. Sebastian A, Hulter HN, Kurtz I, Maher T, Schambelan M. Disorders of distal nephron function. Am J Med 1982;72:289-307.
164. Shami S, Ziering S. Solid-phase no extraction aldosterone RIA. Clin Chem 1984;30:1049.
165. Sheaves R. Relative value of computed tomography scanning and venous sampling in establishing the cause of primary hyperaldosteronism. Eur J Endocrinol 1996;134:308-13.
166. Shibasaki H, Furuta T, Kasuya Y. Quantification of corticosteroids in human plasma by liquid chromatography-thermospray mass spectrometry using stable isotope dilution. J Chromatogr B Biomed Appl 1997;692:7-14.
167. Simon D, Romestand B, Huang H, Badouaille G, Fehrentz JA, Pau B, et al. Direct, simplified, and sensitive assay for angiotensin II in plasma extracts performed with a high-affinity monoclonal antibody. Clin Chem, 1992;38:1963-7.
168. Simon D, Hartmann DJ, Badouaille G, Caillot G, Guyenne TT, Corvol P, et al. Two-site direct immunoassay for active renin. Clin Chem 1992;38:1959-62.
169. Simpson ER, Waterman MR. Steroid hormone biosynthesis in the adrenal cortex and its regulation by adrenocorticotropin. In: Besser M, Burger HG, Jameson JL, eds. Endocrinology, 3rd ed. Philadelphia: WB Saunders Co, 1995:1630-41.
170. Sizonenko PC, Paunier L. Hormonal changes in puberty: III. Correlation of plasma dehydroepiandrosterone, testosterone, FSH, and LH with stages of puberty and bone age in normal boys and girls and in patients with Addison's disease or hypogonadism or with premature or late adrenarche. J Clin Endocrinol Metab 1975;41:894-904.
171. Sloan DA, Schwartz RW, McGrath PC, Kenady DE. Diagnosis and management of adrenal tumors. Curr Opin Oncol 1996;8:30-6.
172. Smith C, Kapsner K. A heterogeneous competitive assay for cortisol using magnetic microparticles and

enzyme chemiluminescence. Clin Chem 1992;38:1085.

173. Stabler T, Siegel A. Chemiluminescence immunoassay of aldosterone in serum. Clin Chem 1991;37:1987-9.
174. Streeten DH, Stevenson CT, Dalakos TG, Nicholas JJ, Dennick LG, Fellerman H. The diagnosis of hypercortisolism: Biochemical criteria differentiating patients from lean and obese normal subjects and from females on oral contraceptives. J Clin Endocrinol Metab 1969;29:1191-211.
175. Stryer L. Biochemistry. 4th ed. New York: W H Freeman, 1995.
176. Styne DM, Grumbach MM. Disorders of puberty in the male and female. In: Yen SSC, Jaffe RB, eds. Reproductive endocrinology. Philadelphia: WB Saunders Co, 1992:511-54.
176A. Taylor RL, Machacek D, Singh RJ. Validation of a high-throughput liquid chromatography-tandem mass spectrometry method for urinary cortisol and cortisone. Clin Chem 2002;48:1511-19.
177. Tenover JS, Matsumoto AM, Plymate SR, Bremner WJ. The effects of aging in normal men on bioavailable testosterone and luteinizing hormone secretion: Response to clomiphene citrate. J Clin Endocrinol Metab 1987;65:1118-26.
178. Thienpont LM, De Brabandere VI, Stockl D, De Leenheer AP. Candidate reference method for determining serum cortisol based on isotope dilution-gas chromatography/mass spectrometry using heptafluorobutyrilation as derivatization method. Anal Biochem 1996:234:204-209.
179. Thienpont L, Siekmann L, Lawson A, Colinet E, De Leenheer A. Development, validation, and certification by isotope dilution gas chromatography-mass spectrometry of lypholized human serum reference materials for cortisol (CRM 192 and 193) and progesterone (CRM 347 and 348). Clin Chem 1991;37:540-6.
180. Thienpont LM, Van Nieuwenhove B, Stockl D, Reinauer H, De Leenheer AP. Determination of reference method values by isotope dilution-gas chromatography/mass spectrometry: A five years' experience of two European reference laboratories. Eur J Clin Chem Clin Biochem 1996;34:853-60.
181. Tietz NW, ed. Clinical guide to laboratory tests. 3rd ed. Philadelphia: WB Saunders Co, 1995.
182. Tsuji A, Maeda M, Arakawa H, Shimizu S, Ikegami T, Sudo Y, et al. Fluorescence and chemiluminescence enzyme immunoassays of 17α-hydroxyprogesterone in dried blood spotted on filter paper. J Steroid Biochem 1987;28:33-40.
183. Turpeinen U, Markkanen H, Valimaki M, Stenman UH. Determination of urinary free cortisol by HPLC. Clin Chem 1997;43:1386-91.
184. van der Hoeven RA, Hofte AJ, Frenay M, Irth H, Tjaden UR, van der Greef J, et al. Liquid chromatography-mass spectrometry with on-line solid-phase extraction by a restricted-access C18 precolumn for direct plasma and urine injection. J Chromatogr A 1997;762:193-200.
185. Van Thiel DH, Loriaux DL. Evidence for an adrenal origin of plasma estrogens in alcoholic men. Metabolism 1978;28:536-41.
186. Vanderbilt University Medical Center: Pathology Laboratory Services. Nashville, Tenn, Vanderbilt University Medical Center, 1991.
187. Varelis P, Smythe GA, Hodgson D, Lazarus L. Measurement of urinary free cortisol by stable isotope dilution mass spectrometry using a new cortisol derivative. J Chromatogr B Biomed Appl 1994;660:151-9.
188. Vaughan ED, Buhler FR, Laragh JH. Renovascular hypertension: Renin measurements to indicate hypersecretion and contralateral suppression, estimate renal plasma flow, and score for surgical curability. Am J Med 1973;55:402-14.
189. Veldhuis JD. The hypothalamic-pituitary-testicular axis. In: Yen SSC, Jaffe RB, eds. Reproductive endocrinology. Philadelphia: WB Saunders Co, 1992:409-60.
190. Veldhuis JD, Melby JC. Isolated aldosterone deficiency in man: Acquired and inborn errors in the biosynthesis or action of aldosterone. Endocr Rev 1981;2:495-517.
191. Vining R, McGinley R. The measurement of hormones in saliva: Possibilities and pitfalls. J Steroid Biochem 1987;27:81-94.
192. Wallace AM, Beastall GH, Cook B, Currie AJ, Ross AM, Kennedy R, et al. Neonatal screening for congenital adrenal hyperplasia: A program based on a novel direct radioimmunoassay for 17-hydroxyprogesterone in blood spots. J Endocrinol 1986;108:299-308.
193. Webb JC, Bayliss P. Pregnancy complicated by primary aldosteronism. South Med J 1997;90:243-5.
194. Weber A, Trainer PJ, Grossman AB, Afshar F, Medbak S, Perry LA, et al. Investigation, management and therapeutic outcome in 12 cases of childhood and adolescent Cushing's syndrome. Clin Endocrinol 1995;43:19-28.
195. Webster JB, Bell KR. Primary adrenal insufficiency following traumatic brain injury: A case report and review of the literature. Arch Phys Med Rehabil 1997;78:314-8.
196. Weingartner K, Gerharz EW, Bittinger A, Rosai J, Leppek R, Riedmiller H. Isolated clinical syndrome of primary aldosteronism in a patient with adrenocortical carcinoma: Case report and review of the literature. Urol Int 1995;55:232-5.
197. Weller RA. Comparison of fluorescent polarization immunoassay and radioimmunoassay in measuring cortisol levels in prepubertal depressed children. Am J Psychiatry 1992;149:1395-6.

198. Westphal U. Steroid protein interactions. Monogr Endocrinol 1985;27:356-66.
199. White PC, New MI, Dupont B. Congenital adrenal hyperplasia, part 1. N Engl J Med 1987;316:1519-24.
200. White PC, New MI, Dupont B. Congenital adrenal hyperplasia, part 2. N Engl J Med 1987;316:1580-6.
201. White MG. Bartter's syndrome: A manifestation of renal tubular defects. Arch Intern Med 1972;129:41-7.
202. Wild RA, Applebaum-Bowden D, Demers LM, Bartholomew M, Landis JR, Hazzard WR, et al. Lipoprotein lipids in women with androgen excess: Independent associations with elevated insulin and androgens. Clin Chem 1990;36:283-9.
203. Wild D. The immunoassay handbook. London: Stockton Press, 1994.
204. Wilson JD, George FW, Griffin JE. The hormonal control of sexual development. Science 1981;211:1278-84.
205. Wong T, Shackleton CH, Covey TR, Ellis G. Identification of the steroids in neonatal plasma that interfere with 17α-hydroxyprogesterone in radioimmunoassays. Clin Chem 1992;38:1830-7.
206. Wong T, McLaurin J, Makela S, Makela SK, Eleftherios E. Development of a time-resolved fluorescence immunoassay for 17α-hydroxyprogesterone. Clin Chem 1990;36:1150.
207. Wood PJ, Barth JH, Freedman DB, Perry L, Sheridan B. Evidence for the low dose dexamethasone suppression test to screen for Cushing's syndrome: Recommendations for a protocol for biochemistry laboratories. Ann Clin Biochem 1997;34:222-9.
208. Wotiz HH, Chattoraj SC. The role of gas-liquid chromatography in steroid hormone analysis. J Chromatogr Sci 1973;11:167-74.
209. Wright BE, Porter JR, Browne ES, Svec F. Antiglucocorticoid action of dehydroepiandrosterone in young obese Zucker rats. Int J Obes 1992;16:579-83.
210. Wudy SA, Homoki J, Wachter UA, Teller WM. Diagnosis of the adrenogenital syndrome caused by 11β-hydroxylase deficiency using gas chromatographic-mass spectrometric analysis of the urinary steroid profile. Dtsch Med Wochenschr 1997;122:3-11.
211. Yamamoto T, Fukuyama J, Hasegawa K, Sugiura M. Isolated corticotropin deficiency in adults. Report of 10 cases and review of literature. Arch Intern Med 1992;152:1705-12.
212. Yatscoff RW, Chapelsky L, Morrish D. Analytical and clinical evaluation of an automated cortisol assay on the ACS: 180. Clin Biochem 1996;29:315-9.
213. Yen SSC. Chronic anovulation caused by peripheral endocrine disorders. In: Yen SSC, Jaffe RB, eds. Reproductive endocrinology. Philadelphia: WB Saunders Co, 1992:576-630.
214. Yergey AL, Teffera Y, Esteban NV, Abramson FP. Direct determination of human urinary cortisol metabolites by HPLC/CRIMS. Steroids 1995;60:295-8.
215. Yeung JH, Wong JK, Park BK. Development of a screening method for anti-6 beta-hydroxycortisol antibody using an enzyme-linked immunosorbent assay (ELISA) and its applications. Methods Find Exp Clin Pharmacol 1997;19:79-86.

ADDITIONAL READING

Bruce SS, Bruce JN. Harvey Cushing, neurosurgical pioneer. Curr Surg 2005;62:138-40.

Burry LD, Wax RS. Role of corticosteroids in septic shock. Ann Pharmacother 2004;38:464-72. Epub 2004 Jan 23.

Cleland SJ, Reid JL. The renin-angiotensin system and the heart: A historical review. Heart 1996;76(Suppl 3):7-12.

Clow A, Thorn L, Evans P, Hucklebridge F. The awakening cortisol response: Methodological issues and significance. Stress 2004;7:29-37.

Dallman MF, la Fleur SE, Pecoraro NC, Gomez F, Houshyar H, Akana SF. Minireview: Glucocorticoids—food intake, abdominal obesity, and wealthy nations in 2004. Endocrinology 2004;145:2633-8. Epub 2004 Mar 24.

De Kloet ER. Hormones and the stressed brain. Ann N Y Acad Sci 2004;1018:1-15.

Dieterich KD, Lehnert H, De Souza EB. Corticotropin-releasing factor receptors: An overview. Exp Clin Endocrinol Diabetes 1997;105:65-82.

Fenske M. How much "urinary free cortisol" is really cortisol during water diuresis in healthy individuals? Clin Chem 2004;50:1102-4.

Franchimont D. Overview of the actions of glucocorticoids on the immune response: A good model to characterize new pathways of immunosuppression for new treatment strategies. Ann N Y Acad Sci 2004;1024:124-37.

Garcia C, Biller BM, Klibanski A. The role of the clinical laboratory in the diagnosis of Cushing syndrome. Am J Clin Pathol 2003;120 Suppl:S38-45.

Griffiths WJ. Tandem mass spectrometry in the study of fatty acids, bile acids, and steroids. Mass Spectrom Rev 2003;22:81-152.

Harvey PW, Healing G, Rees SJ, Everett DJ, Cockburn A. Glucocorticosteroid interactions with natural toxins: A mini review. Nat Toxins 1994;2:341-6.

Helin K, Stoll M, Meffert S, Stroth U, Unger T. The role of angiotensin receptors in cardiovascular diseases. Ann Med 1997;29:23-9.

Holst JP, Soldin OP, Guo T, Soldin SJ. Steroid hormones: relevance and measurement in the clinical laboratory. Clin Lab Med 2004;24:105-18.

Ito N, Ito T, Paus R. The human hair follicle has established a fully functional peripheral equivalent of the hypothamalic-pituitary-adrenal-axis (HPA). Exp Dermatol 2005;14:158.

Kiraly SJ, Ancill RJ, Dimitrova G. The relationship of endogenous cortisol to psychiatric disorder: A review. Can J Psychiatry 1997;42:415-20.

Lopez JA, Kleinschmidt-Demasters Bk B, Sze CI, Woodmansee WW, Lillehei Silent corticotroph adenomas: Further clinical and pathological observations. Hum Pathol 2004;35:1137-47.

Maes M, Mommen K, Hendrickx D, Peeters D, D'Hondt P, Ranjan R, et al. Components of biological variation, including seasonality, in blood levels of TSH, TT3, FT4, PRL, cortisol and testosterone in healthy volunteers. Clin Endocrinol 1997;46:587-98.

Nieman LK. Dynamic evaluation of adrenal hypofunction. J Endocrinol Invest 2003;26(7 Suppl):74-82.

Nylen ES, Muller B. Endocrine changes in critical illness. J Intensive Care Med 2004;19:67-82.

Pascoe L, Curnow KM. Genetic recombination as a cause of inherited disorders of aldosterone and cortisol biosynthesis and a contributor to genetic variation in blood pressure. Steroids 1995;60:22-7.

Provost PR, Tremblay Y. Genes Involved in the Adrenal Pathway of Glucocorticoid Synthesis are Transiently Expressed in the Developing Lung. Endocrinology 2005 Jan 27; [Epub ahead of print].

Schimmer BP. The 1994 Upjohn award lecture: Molecular and genetic approaches to the study of signal transduction in the adrenal cortex. Can J Physiol Pharmacol 1995;73:1097-107.

Schwartz GL, Turner ST. Screening for Primary Aldosteronism in Essential Hypertension: Diagnostic Accuracy of the Ratio of Plasma Aldosterone Level to Plasma Renin Activity. Clin Chem 2005;51:386-94.

Shimada K, Mitamura K, Higashi T. Gas chromatography and high-performance liquid chromatography of natural steroids. J Chromatogr A 2001;935:141-72.

Sidhu S, Sywak M, Robinson B, Delbridge L. Adrenocortical cancer: Recent clinical and molecular advances. Curr Opin Oncol 2004;16:13-8.

Simard M. The biochemical investigation of Cushing syndrome. Neurosurg Focus 2004;15;16:E4.

Sokoll LJ, Wians FH Jr, Remaley AT. Rapid intraoperative immunoassay of parathyroid hormone and other hormones: A new paradigm for point-of-care testing. Clin Chem 2004;50:1126-35. Epub 2004 Apr 29.

Sonino N, Boscaro M, Fallo F. Pharmacologic management of Cushing syndrome: New targets for therapy. Treat Endocrinol 2005;4:87-94.

Speiser PW. Improving neonatal screening for congenital adrenal hyperplasia. J Clin Endocrinol Metab 2004;89:3685-6.

Talbot JA, Kane JW, White A. Analytical and clinical aspects of adrenocorticotrophin determination. Ann Clin Biochem 2003;40:453-71.

van der Kamp HJ, Wit JM. Neonatal screening for congenital adrenal hyperplasia. Eur J Endocrinol 2004;151 Suppl 3:U71-5.

Vaughan ED Jr. Diseases of the adrenal gland. Med Clin North Am 2004;88:443-66

Watterberg KL. Adrenocortical function and dysfunction in the fetus and neonate. Semin Neonatol 2004;9: 13-21.

Yeager MP, Guyre PM, Munck AU. Glucocorticoid regulation of the inflammatory response to injury. Acta Anaesthesiol Scand 2004;48:799-813.

Young EA, Altemus M. Puberty, ovarian steroids, and stress. Ann N Y Acad Sci 2004;1021:124-33.

CHAPTER 52

The Thyroid: Pathophysiology and Thyroid Function Testing*

Laurence M. Demers, Ph.D., F.A.C.B., D.A.B.C.C., and Carole Spencer, Ph.D.

The *thyroid* is a butterfly-shaped gland located in the front of the neck just above the trachea that weighs approximately 15 to 20 grams in the adult human. The fully developed thyroid gland in a human is composed of two lobes connected by a thin band of tissue, the *isthmus,* which gives the gland the appearance of a butterfly. The gland is closely attached to the trachea in the anterior aspect of the neck. Each lobe measures ~2.0 to 2.5 cm in thickness and width and ~4.0 cm in length. The isthmus measures ~2.0 cm in length and width and ~0.5 cm in thickness.

The secretory units of the thyroid gland are follicles that consist of an outer layer of epithelial cells. These cells rest on a basement membrane and enclose an amorphous material called *colloid.* Colloid is mainly composed of thyroglobulin (an iodinated glycoprotein) and small quantities of iodinated thyroalbumin. The follicles are embedded in stromal tissue, which contains blood vessels and autonomic nerve fibers. Increased activity of the gland is characterized by a decrease in the quantity of colloid with subsequent reduction of follicular volume; the lining cells become columnar and may even proliferate into the colloid. During decreased glandular activity, the follicles enlarge because of the accumulation of colloid and the flattening of follicular cells. The cytoplasm of the follicular cells has a microtubular network, and microvilli that extend from the apices of these cells into the colloid. The important reactions of thyroid hormone synthesis, such as iodination and the initial phase of hormone secretion (colloid resorption), are believed to take place at or near the apical surface of the cell. Thyroid follicular cells, like cells of other endocrine glands, have a prominent endoplasmic reticulum.

The thyroid gland also contains another type of cell known as *parafollicular* or *C cells.* These cells have been shown to produce the polypeptide hormone *calcitonin* (see Chapter 49). These cells never border the follicular lumen but are confined within the follicular basement lamina or exist in clusters in the interfollicular spaces.

*The authors gratefully acknowledge the original contributions of R. J. Whitly on which portions of this chapter are based.

THYROID HORMONES

CHEMISTRY

The thyroid gland secretes two hormones, thyroxine (3,5,3′,5′-L-tetraiodothyronine) and triiodothyronine (3,5,3′-L-triiodothyronine), which are commonly known as T_4 and T_3, respectively (Table 52-1). In addition, the thyroid gland secretes small amounts of biologically inactive 3,3′,5′-L-triiodothyronine (reverse T_3 [rT_3]) and minute quantities of monoiodotyrosine (MIT) and diiodotyrosine (DIT), which are precursors of T_3 and T_4. The structures of these compounds are shown in Figure 52-1.

Approximately 40% of the secreted T_4 is deiodinated by peripheral tissues by enzyme deiodinases to yield T_3, and about 45% is deiodinated to yield rT_3. Therefore, with a normal T_4 production of ~100 nmol (80 μg) daily, approximately 40 nmol (26 μg) of T_3 and 45 nmol (29 μg) of rT_3 are produced by peripheral deiodination. From the esti-

TABLE 52-1 Nomenclature and Abbreviations for Thyroid Tests

Hormone Concentration	
Total thyroxine	T_4
Total triiodothyronine (3,5,3′-triiodothyronine)	T_3
Free thyroxine*	FT_4
Free triiodothyronine*	FT_3
Thyrotropin (thyroid-stimulating hormone)	TSH
Reverse T_3 (3,3′,5′-triiodothyronine)	rT_3
Estimates of Free Hormone Fraction	
Free T_4 fraction†	% FT_4
Free T_3 fraction†	% FT_3
Thyroid hormone binding ratio‡	THBR
Estimates of Free Hormone Concentration	
Free T_4 estimate [$T_4 \times$ % FT_4]	FT_4E
Free T_3 estimate [$T_3 \times$ % FT_3]	FT_3E
Free T_4 index [$T_4 \times$ THBR]	FT_4I
Free T_3 index [$T_3 \times$ THBR]	FT_3I
T_4/TBG ratio	T_4/TBG
Free T_4 estimate (by immunoassay)§	FT_4E
Serum Binding Proteins	
Thyroxine-binding globulin	TBG
Thyroxine-binding prealbumin (transthyretin)	TBPA
Tests for Autoimmune Thyroid Disease	
Antithyroglobulin antibodies	TgAb
Antimicrosomal antibodies	TMAb
Antithyroid peroxidase antibodies	TPO Ab
TSH receptor antibodies	TRAb
Other Hormones and Thyroid-Related Proteins	
Thyrotropin-releasing hormone	TRH
Thyroglobulin	Tg
Calcitonin	CT

*Measured by "direct" immunoassay of a dialysate (or ultrafiltrate) of undiluted serum.
†Measured by equilibrium dialysis (or ultrafiltration) of diluted serum containing tracer T_4 or T_3.
‡Derived from T_3 or T_4 "uptake" methods (see text for details).
§Measured by two-step or analog (one-step) assays.

Figure 52-1 Structure of thyroid hormones and their precursors. *MIT,* Monoiodotyrosine; *DIT,* diiodotyrosine; rT_3, 3,3′,5′-L-triiodothyronine; T_3, 3,5,3′-L-triiodothyronine; T_4, 3,5,3′,5′-L-tetraiodothyronine.

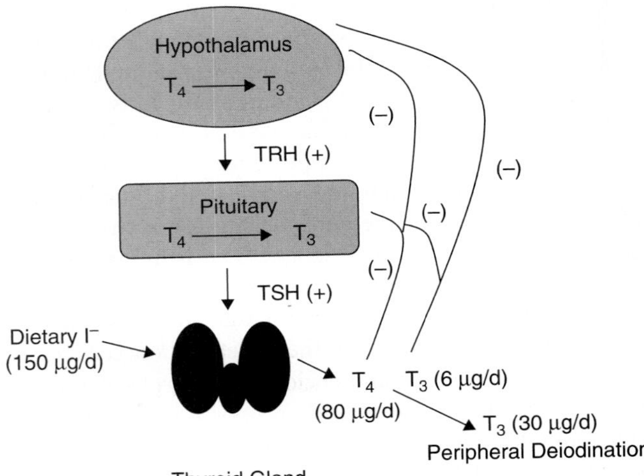

Figure 52-2 Hypothalamic-pituitary-thyroid axis—hormone synthesis dependent on dietary intake of 150 µg of iodine per day. T_4 major thyronine secreted from thyroid gland with T_3 coming predominantly from peripheral deiodination.

mated daily production rates for T_3 (30 µg) and rT_3 (30 µg), it is evident that in a euthyroid state at least 85% of T_3 production and essentially all of rT_3 production are accounted for by peripheral deiodination of T_4 rather than by direct secretion by the thyroid gland (Figure 52-2). T_3 is four to five times more potent in biological systems than T_4. Because one third of all T_4 is converted to T_3 during the course of its metabolism, T_4 is considered to be a prohormone without any intrinsic biological activity.

Biological Function

Thyroid hormones have many important biological effects.[13] A major function is their control of the basal metabolic rate and calorigenesis through increased oxygen consumption in tissue via the effects of thyroid hormone on membrane

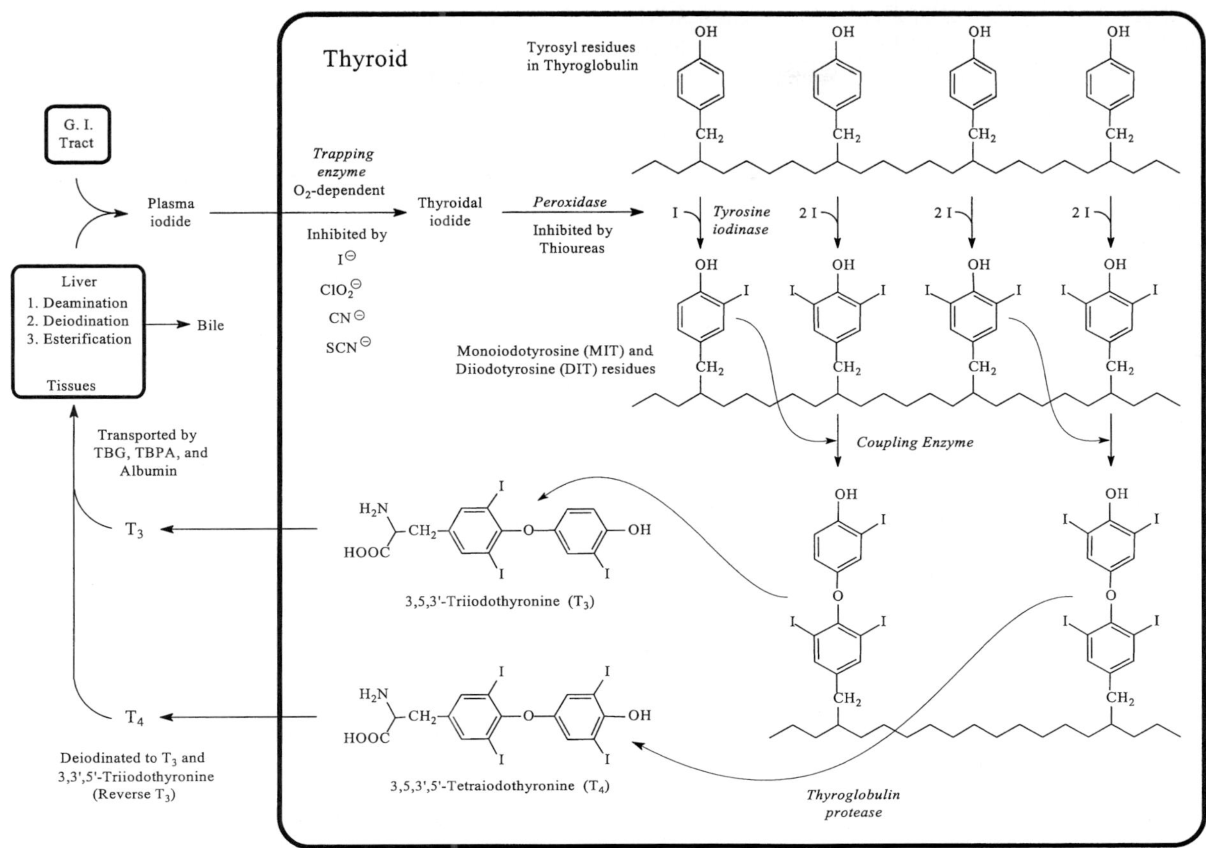

Figure 52-3 Formation and secretion of thyroid hormone. Iodine transport into the gland is inhibited by anions such as thiocyanate (SCN^-), perchlorate (ClO^{-4}), and pertechnetate (TcO_4^{-1}). The oxidation and organic binding of iodide to thyroglobulin are blocked by thioureas, sulfonamides, and high concentrations of iodide. *(Modified from Berger S, Quinn JL. Thyroid function. In: Tietz NW, ed. Fundamentals of clinical chemistry, 2nd ed. Philadelphia: WB Saunders Co, 1976:585.)*

transport (cycling of Na^+/K^+-ATPase with increased synthesis and consumption of adenosine triphosphate) and enhanced mitochondrial metabolism (stimulation of mitochondrial respiration and oxidative phosphorylation). Thyroid hormones are indispensable for neural development, normal growth, and sexual maturation in mammals. Other actions include stimulation of adrenergic activity with increased heart rate and myocardial contractility, stimulation of protein synthesis and carbohydrate metabolism, increased synthesis and degradation of cholesterol and triglycerides, increased requirement for vitamins, increased calcium and phosphorus metabolism, and enhanced sensitivity of adrenergic receptors to catecholamines. These effects are typically magnified in patients with hyperthyroidism and subdued in patients with hypothyroidism.

BIOCHEMISTRY

The biosynthesis of thyroid hormones involves the trapping of circulating iodide (iodide transport) by the thyroid gland, the incorporation of iodine into tyrosine, and the coupling of iodinated tyrosyl residues to form the thyronines (T_4 and T_3) within the protein backbone of the thyroglobulin protein in the follicular lumen. Endocytosis followed by proteolytic cleavage of thyroglobulin releases the iodothyronines into the circulation. A schematic outline of iodine metabolism, with emphasis on the formation and secretion of thyroid hormones, is shown in Figure 52-3.

Dietary iodine is the basic element involved in the synthesis of thyroid hormones; it is normally ingested in the form of iodide. Iodide transport to the follicles is the first and rate-limiting step in the synthetic process. The follicular cells of the thyroid concentrate iodide to some 30 to 40 times the normal plasma concentration by means of an energy-dependent pump mechanism. Upon stimulation of the gland by the pituitary hormone thyroid-stimulating hormone (TSH; MW 30 kDa; also called *thyrotropin*), or with blockade of iodide uptake by antithyroid drugs such as propylthiouracil or methimazole, the glandular iodide concentration can reach 800 times the plasma iodide concentration. Other anions are attracted to the thyroid gland and can act as competitive inhibitors of iodide uptake and transport. Two clinically useful anions are pertechnetate

TcO_4^{-1} and perchlorate (ClO^{-4}). The ability of perchlorate to inhibit iodide transport is the basis for its use in the so-called perchlorate-discharge test used to detect defects in thyroid gland–binding and uptake of iodide. The use of radioactive pertechnetate is also the basis for thyroid gland imaging studies used to evaluate patients with suspected thyroid disease. The salivary glands, gastric mucosa, placenta, ciliary body of the eye, choroid plexus, and mammary glands are also capable of transporting iodide against a concentration gradient, but this uptake does not come under the influence of TSH. The physiological significance of this extrathyroidal iodide-concentrating mechanism is not well understood.

Iodide is oxidized at or near the thyroid gland membrane to a more reactive iodine, probably as the free radical of iodine, I•; within seconds, the active iodine is bound to tyrosine molecules attached to a thyroidal protein called *thyroglobulin* (Tg; 660 kDa). Tg is also synthesized within the follicular cells of the gland before being secreted into the follicular lumen by exocytosis. The enzyme responsible for the oxidation and binding of iodide (organification) is thyroid peroxidase (TPO); hydrogen peroxide accepts the electron. Initially, monoiodotyrosine and diiodotyrosine (MIT and DIT) molecules are formed (see Figure 52-3). Two DIT molecules then undergo an oxidative condensation with the release of an alanine residue for the formation of T_4, which is still in peptide linkage to Tg. Similarly, T_3 is produced from the coupling of MIT and DIT. A small amount of rT_3 is also formed, probably by condensation of DIT and MIT. The condensation reaction is an aerobic, energy-requiring reaction, and like oxidation and binding, is considered to be catalyzed by TPO. Iodide thus bound to tyrosine residues can no longer be discharged by thiocyanate, perchlorate, or other inhibitors of iodide transport.

The synthesis of T_3, T_4, DIT, and MIT in Tg molecules occurs mainly at the follicular cell–colloid interface but also within the colloid. Tg is present in highest concentrations within the colloid, where it is stored. The follicular cells engulf colloid globules by endocytosis; these globules then merge with lysosomes in the follicular cell. Lysosomal proteases break the peptide bonds between iodinated residues and Tg, and T_4, T_3, DIT, and MIT are released into the cytoplasm of the follicular cell. T_4 and T_3 diffuse into the systemic circulation after their liberation from Tg. DIT and MIT are deiodinated by an intracellular microsomal iodotyrosine dehalogenase. The freed iodide is then reused for thyroid hormone synthesis.

Each step in the synthesis of thyroid hormones is regulated by pituitary TSH. TSH stimulates the "iodide pump," Tg synthesis, and colloidal uptake by follicular cells. TSH also regulates the rate of proteolysis of Tg for the liberation of T_4 and T_3 is also regulated by TSH. In addition, TSH induces an increase in the size and number of the thyroid follicular cells. Prolonged TSH stimulation leads to increased vascularity and eventual hypertrophic enlargement of the thyroid gland (goiter).

Metabolism

Metabolism of T_4 to T_3 and the transport of these two thyroid hormones in the blood are discussed later in this section. The degradative metabolism of T_3 and T_4 occurs by oxidative deamination, which produces pyruvic acid analogues that are ultimately converted to thyroacetates by a decarboxylation reaction. These analogues have some residual biological activity, but there is no evidence that they are physiologically significant. In the liver, T_3 and T_4 are conjugated to form sulfates and glucuronides. These conjugates enter the bile and pass into the intestine. Thyroid hormone conjugates are hydrolyzed, and some are reabsorbed (enterohepatic circulation) or excreted in the stools. The amounts of thyroidal substances in the urine are very small, and urinary assays to measure these substances have little clinical value. For a thorough discussion of thyroid metabolism, secretion, and synthesis, the reader is referred to a chapter by Larsen and Ingbar.[115]

Physiology

A tightly controlled feedback system exists between the thyroid gland, the hypothalamus, and the pituitary gland (Figure 52-2).[113] The function of these three glands is closely integrated, resulting in thyroid hormone concentrations in blood being maintained within certain limits in the face of large changes in basal metabolism and physiological need for thyroid hormone. Thyrotropin-releasing hormone (TRH), a tripeptide, is produced in the hypothalamus. TRH acts on the pituitary thyrotropes to stimulate both the synthesis and release of TSH.[92] TSH in turn controls the thyroid gland and the synthesis and release of thyroid hormones. TSH also controls the size and number of thyroid follicular cells. A rise in the thyroid hormone concentration elicits an inhibitory effect on the pituitary response to TRH (negative feedback). Conversely, a fall in thyroid hormone concentrations causes an increase in both TRH and TSH secretion (positive feedback).

Free (unbound) T_4 is the primary secretory product of the normal thyroid gland. T_4 is progressively degraded by deiodination and ether-link cleavage to form its intrinsic thyronine and tyrosine core molecules. Only 5′ deiodination of T_4 is an activation step and leads to the production of a metabolically active metabolite (T_3). All other deiodinations are inactivating. The T_4 deiodination cascade to form T_3, rT_3, MIT, and DIT derivatives is catalyzed by three types of selenodeiodinase enzymes (Type 1, Type 2, and Type 3). T_4 to T_3 conversion is catalyzed by both Type 1 and 2 deiodinases. These enzymes coexist in the same tissue, but generally have different tissue distributions (hepatic versus nonhepatic, Type 1 versus Type 2, respectively). In hypothyroid and euthyroid conditions, circulating T_3 is primarily derived from Type 2 enzymes, whereas when T_4 substrate is high (i.e., hyperthyroidism) T_3 production is primarily derived from Type 1 enzymes. Type 3 deiodinases that catalyze the inner-ring deiodination of T_4 to produce metabolically inert rT_3 are considered important for controlling the amount of maternal thyroid hormone delivered to the developing fetus (see Figure 52-3). Type 1 deiodinase activity is inhibited during acute or chronic stress or illness and with a number of medications. Inhibition of Type 1 deiodinase activity causes a decrease in circulating T_3 secondary to decreased production and an increase in rT_3 secondary to reduced clearance; however the total T_4 concentration remains essentially unchanged.

When released by the thyroid gland, T_4 and T_3 are carried in the circulation bound to carrier proteins. These carrier proteins (T_4-binding globulin [TBG], T_4-binding prealbumin [TBPA], and albumin) bind 99.97% of T_4 and 99.7% of T_3. Thus only a very small fraction of each of these hormones circulates unbound and is free for biological activity. The largest concentration of protein-bound hormone acts as a reservoir for T_4 to maintain a constant concentration of free T_4 (FT_4). Because of the wide variation in the concentration of T_4-binding proteins, even under normal circumstances, there is a wide variation in total T_4 concentrations among euthyroid individuals (i.e., those having normal thyroid function). Total T_3 concentrations also vary with alterations in the concentration of the binding proteins, although to a lesser degree than T_4 concentrations. Common situations in which the thyroid hormone-binding protein concentrations are increased or decreased are shown in Box 52-1. When relying on the measurement of total thyroid hormone concentrations to diagnose thyroid hormone excess or deficiency states, knowledge of possible changes in binding proteins can be extremely important. The measurement of FT_4, however, obviates this need since free hormone concentrations are independent of the binding protein concentration.

BOX 52-1 Alterations in the Concentration or Affinity of Thyroid Hormone-Binding Proteins

Increases in:

A. TBG concentration (or affinity)
   1. Genetic (inherited) causes
   2. Nonthyroidal illness (HIV infection, infectious and chronic active hepatitis, estrogen-producing tumors, acute intermittent porphyria)
   3. Normal physiology (pregnancy, newborn)
   4. Drug use (oral contraceptives, estrogens, tamoxifen, methadone)

B. Prealbumin concentration

C. Albumin binding (familial dysalbuminemic hyperthyroxinemia)

D. T_4 binding by antibodies (autoimmune thyroid disease, hepatocellular carcinoma)

Decreases in:

A. TBG concentration
   1. Genetic (inherited) determination
   2. Nonthyroidal illness (major illness or surgical stress, nephrotic syndrome)
   3. Drug use (androgens, anabolic steroids, large doses of glucocorticoids)

B. TBG binding capacity (drugs bound to TBG such as salicylates and phenytoin)

C. Prealbumin concentration

THYROID DYSFUNCTION

Hypothyroidism and hyperthyroidism are the two primary pathological conditions that involve the thyroid glands.[6] Laboratory testing of thyroid hormones is used to diagnose and document the presence of thyroid disease, a condition that often presents with vague and subtle symptoms. Accurate measurement of thyroid hormone concentrations is key to the proper diagnosis of thyroid gland dysfunction.[169,216]

HYPOTHYROIDISM

Hypothyroidism is defined as a deficiency in thyroid hormone secretion and action.[44] It is a common disorder that occurs in mild or severe forms in 2% to 15% of the population.[164] Women are afflicted more often than men, and both sexes are affected more frequently with increasing age. Clinical symptoms can range from the obvious and easy-to-recognize lethargy, fatigue, and cold intolerance to more subtle, subclinical disease with general symptoms that escape detection. Figure 52-4 depicts the constellation of physiological events associated with decreased thyroid hormone availability. *Myxedema* is a severe form of hypothyroidism in which there is accumulation of mucopolysaccharides in the skin and other tissues, leading to a thickening of facial features and a doughy induration of the skin.[84] *Cretinism* is the term used to describe severe hypothyroidism that develops in the newborn period.

Many structural or functional abnormalities of the thyroid gland can lead to thyroid hormone deficiency (Box 52-2). Primary hypothyroidism is frequently caused by diseases or treatments that directly destroy thyroid tissue or interfere with thyroid hormone biosynthesis. Secondary hypothyroidism occurs as a result of pituitary or hypothalamic disease and/or disorders.

Primary Hypothyroidism

Primary goitrous hypothyroidism results when the synthesis of T_4 and T_3 is impaired, either because of some extrinsic factor or because of an intrinsic, inherited defect in thyroid hormone biosynthesis. As a result, the positive feedback loop causes compensatory thyroid enlargement (goiter) through the hypersecretion of TRH and TSH. Primary nongoitrous hypothyroidism is characterized by loss or atrophy of thyroid tissue, resulting in decreased production of thyroid hormones despite maximum stimulation by TSH. Hashimoto's thyroiditis is the most frequent cause of primary hypothyroidism in developed countries where iodine intake is sufficient. Worldwide, iodine deficiency is the most common cause of goitrous hypothyroidism. The

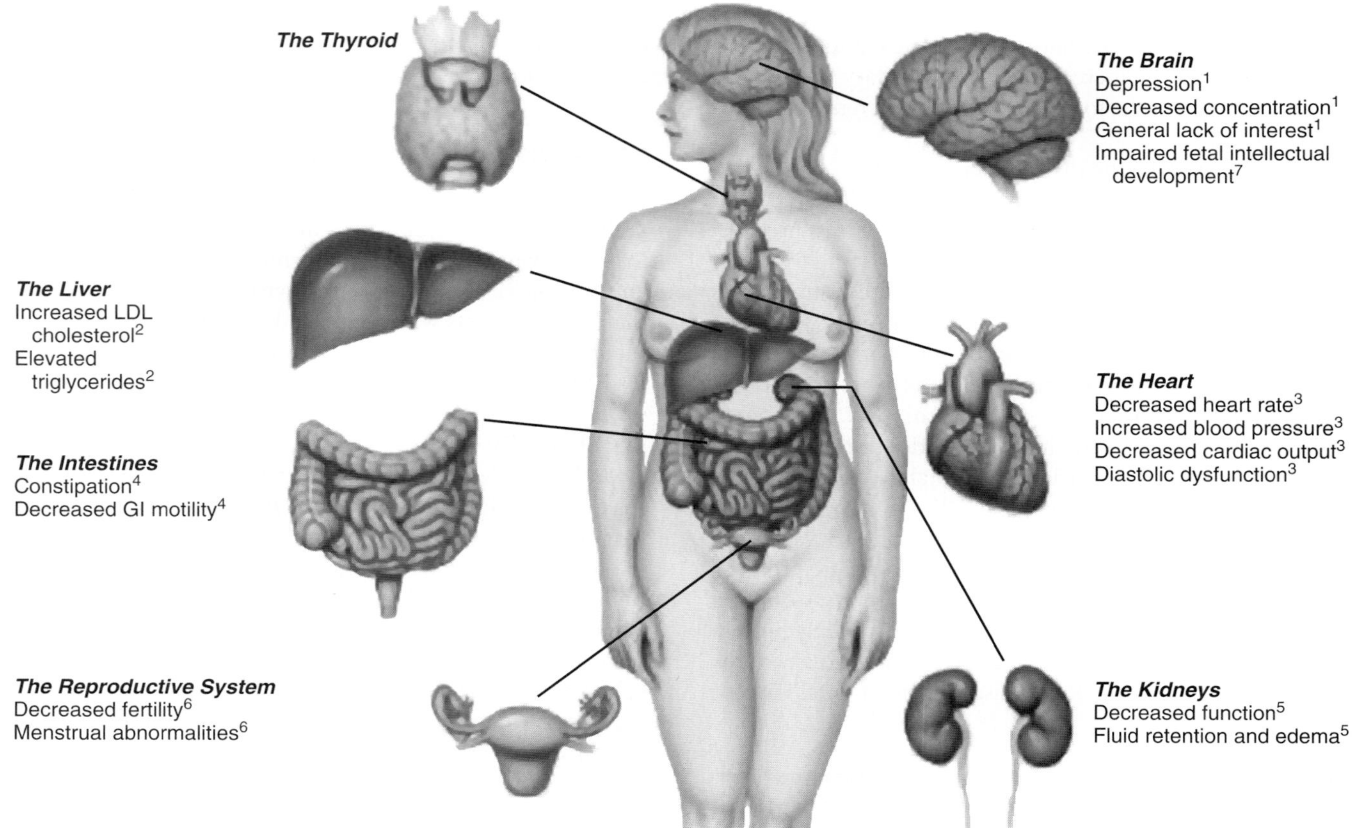

Figure 52-4 The clinical effects of hypothyroidism on different organ systems.

most common cause of nongoitrous hypothyroidism is surgical removal or radioablation of the thyroid gland in the treatment of Graves' disease. Primary hypothyroidism is frequently associated with circulating antithyroid antibodies and may coexist with other diseases in which autoantibodies are found. In addition, primary hypothyroidism may be one manifestation of an autoimmune syndrome of polyglandular endocrine failure.[221]

Reduced concentrations and availability of T_4 and T_3 lead to hypersecretion of pituitary TSH and marked elevations in serum TSH concentrations. The elevated concentration of TSH is an important laboratory finding, particularly in the early detection of thyroid failure. In mild or subclinical hypothyroidism, thyroid hormone concentrations can remain within the normal reference interval, but the TSH concentration is elevated. The etiology of primary hypothyroidism is usually determined on the basis of a good history, a physical examination, and the tests for circulating thyroid autoantibodies.

Congenital hypothyroidism that is recognized at birth may be caused by the complete absence of the thyroid gland (athyreosis) itself or can occur secondary to defects in thyroid hormone synthesis. This disorder occurs once in every 3500 to 4000 live births, and early treatment with thyroid hormone replacement is critical if irreversible neurological damage is to be prevented.[41,45,64,116] Screening programs for congenital hypothyroidism have been established in almost all developed countries of the world.[77,112] Initially North American programs used a two-tiered laboratory approach in which an initial T_4 measurement is obtained followed by a measurement of TSH in specimens with low T_4 values. In most programs, T_4 is measured in blood eluted from a filter paper spot collected from the newborn infant using a heel stick. Floating cutoff values are set high enough to preclude false-negative results. In general, when T_4 results are outside the lower 10th to 20th percentile of the normal distribution, a TSH measurement on another specimen from the same filter paper spot is then performed. In most instances, the diagnosis of congenital hypothyroidism in the neonate can be made at this time; in some cases, further testing is needed on follow-up. Alternatively European and Japanese programs favor screening by means of TSH mea-

BOX 52-2 Causes of Hypothyroidism

Primary (Thyroidal) Hypothyroidism

A. Loss of functional tissue
   1. Chronic lymphocytic (Hashimoto's) thyroiditis
   2. Radiation injury to the neck (I-131 therapy, radiotherapy)
   3. Postoperative hypothyroidism (neck surgery)
   4. Thyroid gland dysgenesis, developmental defects (neonatal)
B. Infiltrative disease of the thyroid
   1. Viral infections
   2. Bacterial infections
C. Defects in thyroid hormone synthesis
   1. Congenital biosynthetic defects
   2. Endemic iodine deficiency
   3. Drug-induced defects (lithium, glucocorticoids, iodine, propranolol)
   4. Idiopathic primary hypothyroidism (TSH receptor defect)
   5. Antithyroid agents (propylthiouracil [PTU])
   6. Thyroiditis with autoantibodies

Hypothyrotropic (Secondary) Hypothyroidism

A. Pituitary disease—TSH deficiency
B. Hypothalamic disease—TRH deficiency

Peripheral Resistance to Thyroid Hormones

BOX 52-3 Causes of Hyperthyroidism

Common Causes of Thyroid Hyperfunction*

A. Diffuse toxic hyperplasia (Graves' disease)
B. Toxic multinodular goiter (Plummer's disease)
C. Toxic solitary adenoma

Less Common Causes of Thyroid Hyperfunction†

A. Acute or subacute thyroiditis (viral or bacterial etiology)
   1. Hashimoto's (autoimmune) thyroiditis
   2. De Quervain's thyroiditis (subacute)
   3. Lymphocytic thyroiditis (painless, subacute)
B. TSH-secreting pituitary tumor
C. Thyroid carcinoma (papillary, follicular, anaplastic)
D. Postpartum thyroiditis
E. HCG-secreting trophoblastic tumor
F. Iodine-induced hyperthyroidism
G. Iatrogenic thyrotoxicosis factitia
H. T_3 toxicosis
I. Drug-induced thyrotoxicosis (amiodarone)
J. Ectopic thyroid tissue (struma ovarii, thyroid carcinoma metastases)

*Associated with increased radioactive iodine uptake, except iodine induced.
†Associated with decreased radioactive iodine uptake.

surements followed by T_4 determinations on infants with TSH values elevated above 20 mIU/L.* Many newborn screening programs in the United States have switched or are considering a switch to the first TSH approach.

Primary hypothyroidism is easily treated by the daily administration of oral thyroxine.[185] During initial treatment, serum FT_4 concentrations adjust quickly, but TSH concentrations remain high. Because the pituitary is slow to register acute changes in thyroid hormone status ("pituitary lag"), 4 to 8 weeks may be needed for serum TSH values to reach a new steady state after dose adjustments. Periodic monitoring of serum TSH, one to three times a year, is recommended to help maintain clinical euthyroidism and a serum TSH concentration within normal limits.[173] Excessive treatment with oral T_4 should be avoided to minimize the risk of accelerated bone resorption and/or atrial fibrillation.

Secondary Hypothyroidism

Secondary hypothyroidism (central thyroid disease) occurs as a result of pituitary or hypothalamic diseases that produce a deficiency in either TSH, TRH, or both. Isolated TSH deficiency is rare, and most patients with secondary hypothyroidism also have other pituitary hormone deficiencies as well (panhypopituitarism). With secondary hypothyroidism, the serum concentration of thyroid hormone is low, but TSH concentrations are either low or within the normal reference interval. When T_4 and TSH concentrations are both low, a TRH test may offer some benefit. In patients who have destructive lesions of the pituitary gland that result in TSH deficiency, no TSH response is expected with exogenous TRH administration. In patients with hypothalamic abnormalities that affect TRH and TSH release, the peak TSH response to TRH may be normal, but is generally delayed until 45 or 60 minutes after the TRH administration rather than after the usual time of 20 to 30 minutes.

*The reader should note that "U" had been reserved by chemists for the international unit of enzyme activity. However, U is often used to mean a unit of TSH concentration as defined by the WHO. To avoid confusion with enzyme activity units, "IU" and "int units" are used in this chapter to refer to the units of TSH concentration.

HYPERTHYROIDISM

Hyperthyroidism is defined as a hypermetabolic condition caused by excessive production of thyroid hormones.[44] This disorder is caused by a number of conditions resulting from excess availability of thyroid hormones (Box 52-3).[14,96] Some clinicians prefer the general term *thyrotoxicosis* rather than hyperthyroidism to define the hypermetabolic state associated with increased amounts of thyroid hormone in the circulation. Figure 52-5 depicts the metabolic changes associated with increased availability of thyroid hormone. Causes of thyrotoxicosis are divided into two types: (1) those associated with frank hyperthyroidism and increased production and secretion of thyroid hormones from the gland, and (2) those that are not. In North America, the most

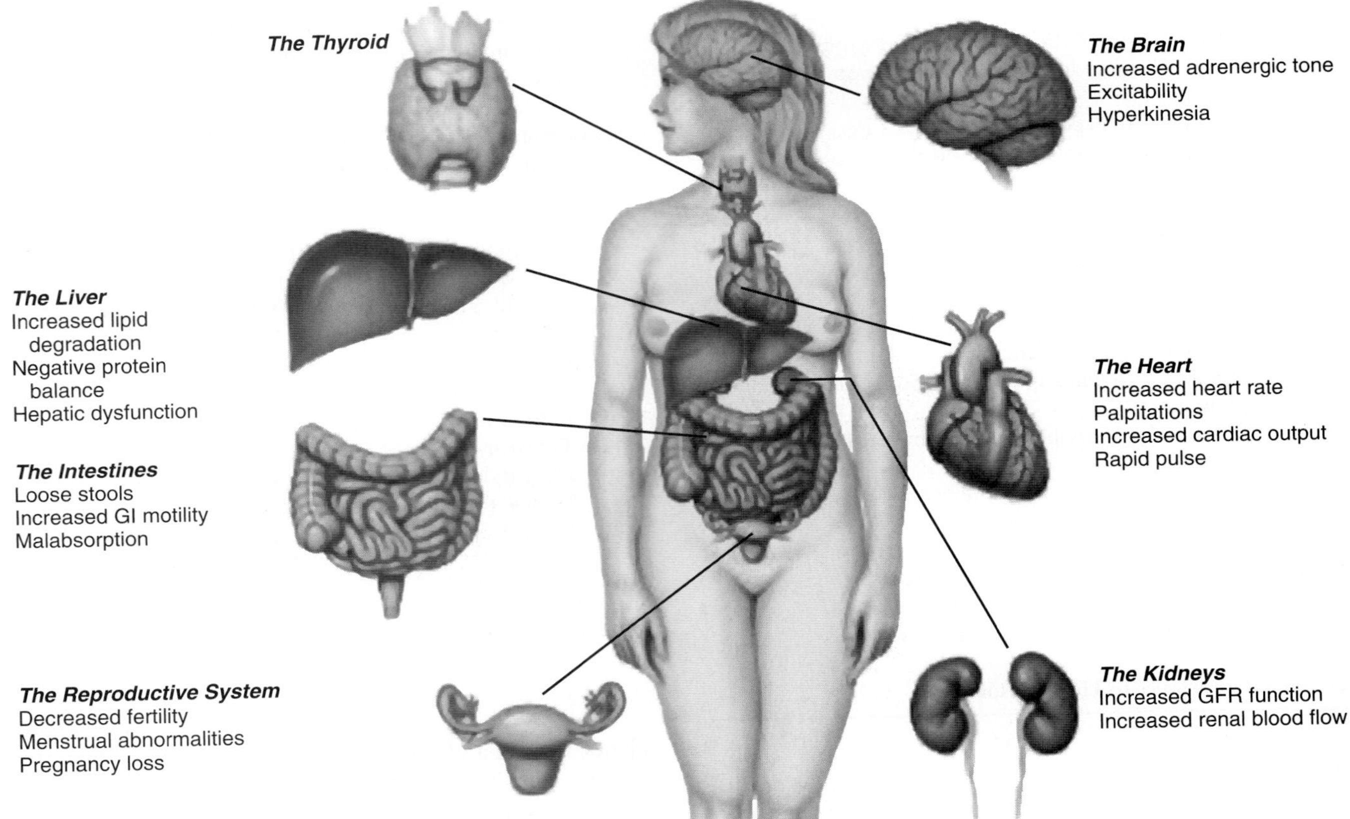

Figure 52-5 The clinical effects of hyperthyroidism on different organ systems.

common cause of thyrotoxicosis due to hyperthyroidism is Graves' disease, an autoimmune disorder that affects 0.4% of the U.S. population; its etiology involves the development of an IgG antibody against the thyroid TSH receptor, resulting in overproduction of T_4 and T_3 by the thyroid gland. Overproduction of thyroid hormones can also result from autonomous production by solitary or multiple thyroid nodules, from a toxic solitary adenoma, or from excessive TSH secretion by pituitary tumors (rare). Less common causes of hyperthyroidism include acute and subacute thyroiditis caused by viral or bacterial infections that affect the thyroid gland itself, producing increased leakage of stored hormone from the gland as a result of inflammatory changes and white cell infiltration. New hormone synthesis can be decreased due to suppression of TSH secretion by the hormone excess. Other secondary causes of hyperthyroidism include exogenous intake (thyrotoxicosis factitia) of thyroid hormone, iodide ingestion in excess, thyroid carcinoma, and drug-induced thyrotoxicosis with medications such as amiodarone.

The prevalence of hyperthyroidism is fairly low in the general population (0.3% to 0.6%) and women are more prone to developing hyperthyroidism than men, with the ratio of females to males with Graves' disease being 5:1. Hyperthyroidism is often easier to diagnose on clinical observations than is hypothyroidism (Box 52-4). In some patients with hyperthyroidism, particularly individuals older than 60 years of age, the diagnosis may not be self-evident, and symptoms may be dismissed or attributed to stress or other causes. The biochemical picture of primary hyperthyroidism shows increases in T_4 and T_3, with a TSH suppressed to undetectable concentrations, except in those rare cases in which hyperthyroidism is mediated by TSH itself (e.g., TSH-secreting pituitary adenoma or pituitary resistance to thyroid hormones). Patients with hyperthyroidism typically have serum TSH concentrations less than 0.05 mIU/L. A serum TSH within the euthyroid reference interval almost always eliminates the diagnosis of hyperthyroidism.

When the TSH concentration is suppressed, the serum FT_4 concentration should be measured and will be elevated in most cases of hyperthyroidism. Finding a low TSH concentration and an elevated FT_4 concentration is usually sufficient to establish the diagnosis of hyperthyroidism. If the TSH concentration is low but the FT_4 concentration is

BOX 52-4 Symptoms of Hyperthyroidism and Hypothyroidism

Hyperthyroidism
- Weight loss
- Fatigue
- Nervousness
- Palpitations
- Rapid pulse
- Menstrual irregularities
- Heat intolerance
- Increased sweating
- Diarrhea
- Restlessness
- Tremor
- Muscle weakness
- Eye changes (Graves' disease)
- Variable gland enlargement

Hypothyroidism
- Weight gain
- Easy fatigue
- Lethargy
- Cold intolerance
- Hair loss
- Constipation
- Depression
- Slow reflexes
- Slower heart beat
- Hoarseness/deepening of voice
- Dry, patchy skin
- Elevated cholesterol
- Puffy eyes
- Menstrual irregularities
- Muscle weakness/cramps

within the normal reference interval, a T_3 measurement should be performed, because serum T_3 concentration is often elevated to a greater degree than is T_4 in the early phases of Graves' disease and in some patients with solitary or multinodular toxic goiters (so-called T_3 thyrotoxicosis). A persistently suppressed serum TSH concentration in the face of normal concentrations of serum T_3 and FT_4 could signify "subclinical hyperthyroidism," a defined biochemical entity with few or subtle clinical symptoms. Because only the free fraction of T_3 is biologically active, the estimation of a free T_3 (FT_3) is helpful to compensate for variations in binding proteins. A number of medications and acute and chronic illnesses cause a transient lowering of T_3 concentrations. In patients with nonthyroidal illnesses (NTIs), an early diagnosis of hyperthyroidism may not be possible until the other illness has resolved.

Occasionally, increases in serum concentrations of T_4 and T_3 will occur as a result of the ingestion of large quantities of exogenous thyroid hormones or to the release of thyroid hormones as a result of damage to the thyroid parenchyma associated with subacute thyroiditis or chronic lymphocytic thyroiditis. The increase in T_4 and T_3 concentrations may be associated with clinical findings that suggest true hyperthyroidism. This diagnostic dilemma, however, can be resolved by finding a low radioactive iodine uptake (percent of orally administered radioactive iodine taken up by the gland at 6 or 24 hours) that accompanies these nontoxic forms of hyperthyroidism. In most cases of thyroiditis, the condition is self-limited and will resolve without residual thyroid function abnormalities.

Until sensitive TSH assays became available, the most conclusive test for hyperthyroidism was the TRH stimulation test. Patients with high concentrations of circulating thyroid hormone have an active negative feedback loop that blocks the release of TSH from the pituitary gland. In a patient with vague but suggestive symptoms of hyperthyroidism and T_4 or T_3 concentrations that are not clearly elevated, failure of the TSH concentration to rise after TRH administration establishes the diagnosis of hyperthyroidism. The TRH test is rarely used for the diagnosis of hyperthyroidism now that sensitive TSH assays are able to distinguish the profoundly suppressed TSH concentrations in true hyperthyroidism from the mild transient depressed TSH concentrations that occur in patients with other nonthyroidal conditions, such as an acute or chronic illness. Patients with a nonthyroidal illness will often have a suppressed TSH but the concentration is still detectable with current TSH methodology. Treatment strategies for hyperthyroidism include (1) administration of antithyroid drugs, (2) radioiodine ablation, and (3) surgical removal of the thyroid gland itself. Treatment is typically designed to decrease thyroid hormone production or inhibit peripheral conversion of T_4 to T_3.[185] At the time treatment is initiated, measurements of serum FT_4 are recommended every few weeks until symptoms abate and serum values normalize; continuous monitoring for recurrence of hyperthyroidism is suggested two or three times a year after successful therapy.[173] Because the pituitary gland is suppressed in hyperthyroidism, measurement of the concentration of serum TSH is not a good monitor of thyroid status in the immediate period following the start of antithyroid therapy. In fact, TSH concentrations remain suppressed for months after the patient becomes clinically euthyroid. Ablation of thyroid tissue or overtreatment with antithyroid drugs sometimes leads to clinical hypothyroidism and an increase in serum TSH; surveillance for hypothyroidism in previously treated hyperthyroid patients must continue for the life of the patient and can best be monitored with a serum TSH.

Nonthyroidal Illness

Many disorders are associated with thyroid hormone excess or deficiency in the absence of definable thyroid disease. These states of euthyroid hyperthyroxinemia or euthyroid hypothyroxinemia often result from alterations in the concentration of thyroid hormone–binding proteins, the actions

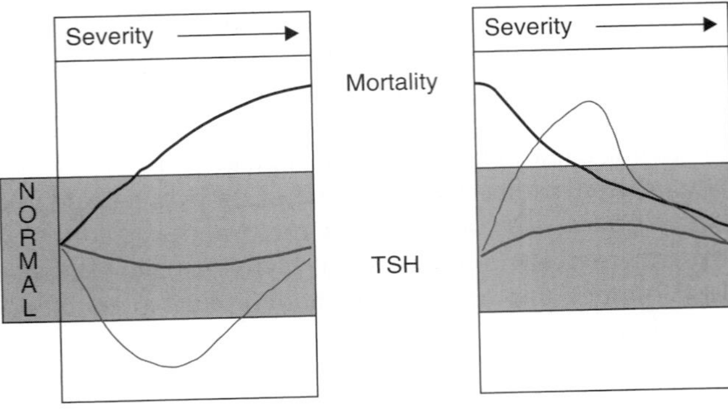

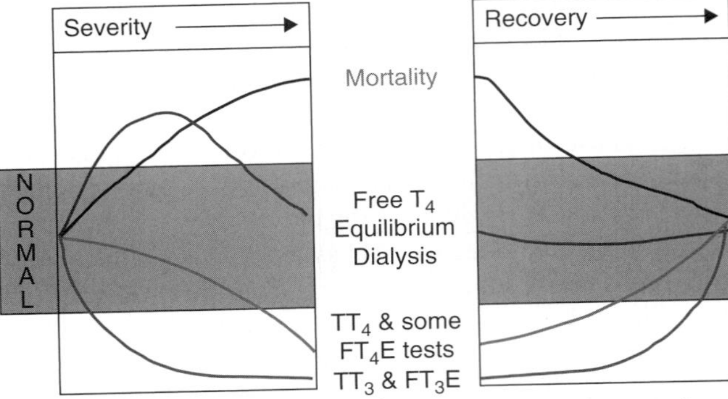

Figure 52-6 The spectrum of thyroid hormone concentrations with illness.

of certain drugs, the effects of acute and chronic NTIs, or peripheral resistance to thyroid hormones.

A progressive spectrum of thyroid test result anomalies accompanies NTIs in euthyroid patients (the "euthyroid sick syndrome")[25,135,201,219] (Figure 52-6 and Box 52-5). The earliest and most common changes that occur are a reduction in the serum concentrations of total and free T_3, sometimes to extremely low concentrations, and an elevation in the serum concentration of rT_3 (the "low T_3 state"). These changes have been ascribed to a block in the 5′deiodinases that convert T_4 to T_3 in peripheral tissue. Acute and chronic nutritional problems, poorly controlled diabetes mellitus, and drugs such as hydrocortisone and beta blockers can also inhibit this conversion.

Declining concentrations of total T_4 may also be seen in NTIs; however, FT_4 concentrations, determined by immunoassay and by equilibrium dialysis, usually remain within the normal reference interval or are found to be mildly elevated. This disparity between falling total T_4 values and normal, or even elevated, free T_4 concentrations may be caused by decreases in serum concentrations of thyroid hormone–binding proteins, changes in binding properties induced by circulating inhibitors and drugs, or both. Unfortunately, some methods for estimating FT_4, such as the one-step immunoassays, may provide artifactually low results in euthyroid patients with increasing severity of chronic illness.

BOX 52-5 Effects of Acute and Chronic Illness on Thyroid Function

Reduced peripheral conversion of T_4 to T_3
Increased production of rT_3
Reduced production of thyroid hormone–binding proteins
Circulating inhibitors of thyroid hormone binding
Mild elevation of serum TSH during recovery phase
Mild depression of serum TSH during acute phase

Conversely, some methods give artifactually high results in some circumstances, such as IV heparin administration.

Serum TSH concentrations are usually normal in euthyroid sick patients, but may be mildly to moderately depressed during the acute phase of NTI or slightly elevated during recovery from a severe illness.[75] Causes of these transient abnormal TSH concentrations are not fully understood but may relate to the effects of endogenous or exogenous hormones, such as glucocorticoids or dopamine, which independently suppress pituitary TSH secretion, altered nutrition, or altered biological activity of immunoreactive TSH.[7]

As patients recover from NTIs, many of the thyroid test abnormalities revert to normal. Total T_4 concentrations will be corrected first followed by a rise in T_3. Serum TSH may also transiently rebound to high concentrations for several days or weeks before returning to normal. Thus, in NTI, abnormal thyroid function test results do not necessarily indicate the presence of thyroid disease, but may demonstrate adaptations to the catabolic state. Conversely, paradoxically normal values may be seen in patients with thyroid disease as a result of medications or nonthyroidal illness per se. Assessments of thyroid function in ill patients are best postponed until the illness resolves, unless a diagnosis would affect patient outcome.

Hypothyroidism Versus Euthyroid Sick Syndrome

The most common dilemma presented by the thyroid test result aberrancy seen with the euthyroid sick syndrome occurs when hypothyroidism is suspected in an ill patient. Total and FT_3 concentrations are expected to be low in nonthyroidal illness and should not be measured for this purpose. If the total or FT_4 concentration is normal, hypothyroidism is unlikely; however, a reduced total T_4 and a slightly subnormal FT_4 estimate may be seen in extremely ill euthyroid patients. Serum TSH is probably the best single test to distinguish between euthyroid sick syndrome and hypothyroidism (in the absence of suspected pituitary or hypothalamic disease or medications, such as dopamine or glucocorticoids). A clear elevation of the TSH concentration (>20 mIU/L) would indicate hypothyroidism. Lesser TSH elevations may be seen transiently in euthyroid sick syndrome patients during recovery. Increasing the upper limit of the TSH reference limit to 8 or 12 mUL in critical illness has been suggested to improve the specificity for hypothyroidism with minor loss of sensitivity.[40] Dopamine or glucocorticoids also suppress pituitary TSH release and may result in a normal TSH concentration in a hypothyroid patient. If the question of hypothyroidism in acutely ill patients cannot be resolved with TSH and FT_4 testing, measurement of rT_3 may help (rT_3 being low in hypothyroidism [either primary or secondary] and normal or high in euthyroid subjects). Documentation of a normal serum cortisol may help distinguish euthyroid sick syndrome patients from those with hypothalamic or pituitary hypothyroidism.

Hyperthyroid Versus Euthyroid Sick Syndrome

As many as 3% of hospitalized patients on admission have subnormal TSH values often associated with the acute phase of illness or with glucocorticoid or dopamine therapy. With more sensitive TSH assays, most (~75%) hyperthyroid patients have profoundly low TSH values (less than 0.01 mIU/L) compared with critically ill euthyroid patients with only mild transient suppression of TSH in the 0.05 to 0.1 mIU/L range.

Effect of Drugs

A number of medications have been shown to alter thyroid function and thyroid function tests.[38,186,202] Few drugs are associated with the development of clinically significant thyroid disease (amiodarone may be an exception), but difficulty in the interpretation of thyroid function tests results when patients are placed on medications that affect thyroid function testing. In general, drugs do not interfere chemically with the assays for thyroid hormones or TSH. The medications most likely to affect TSH concentrations are glucocorticoids and dopamine (reduced TSH concentrations) and amiodarone (increased TSH concentrations). The most commonly encountered variations in thyroid hormone measurements induced by medications are reduced peripheral conversion of T_4 to T_3 or altered binding of T_4 and T_3 to carrier proteins. Some of the medications that affect thyroid function tests are shown in Table 52-2.

Diagnosis of Thyroid Dysfunction

Laboratory tests most commonly used to evaluate patients for thyroid gland dysfunction are listed in Table 52-1. Familiarity with normal physiology and with pathophysiology is important if these tests are to be properly used and selected. However, it is important to note that normal serum thyroid hormone concentrations do not exclude thyroid disease, and abnormal thyroid tests do not always indicate thyroid disease. Diffuse or nodular thyroid enlargement, for example, may be seen in euthyroid patients.[111]

The clinical signs and symptoms of thyroid hormone excess or deficiency are generally vague and nonspecific (see Box 52-4). Therefore when hypothyroidism or hyperthyroidism is suspected, confirmation with laboratory tests is generally required. Guidelines for the selection of appropriate laboratory tests for thyroid function have been published by professional organizations such as the American Thyroid Association (www.thyroid.org),[69A,185,204] the National Academy of Clinical Biochemistry[37,173] (www.nacb.org), and the Royal College of Physicians in London.[220,214] Several algorithms have been published for thyroid function testing, including an algorithm used in a large hospital in Detroit.[58] For a thorough discussion of the diagnosis and treatment of thyroid disease, the reader is referred to general endocrine texts[13,39,115] or reviews on specific topics, such as cardiac disease,[170] disturbances in menstruation,[104] fetal disorders,[63] general thyroid disease,[7,217] hypothyroidism,[45,68,123,224] hyperthyroidism,[78,117,118,174,177] mood disorders,[56] and pregnancy.[17,71,91,137,140]

Historically, thyroid testing was performed stepwise, with the initial step being either a total serum T_4 measurement or a free thyroxine estimate (FT_4E) using, for example, the FT_4 index. Total T_4 measures both bound and free hormone and reflects thyroid hormone production; however, changes in the concentration or affinity of serum thyroid hormone–binding proteins affect total T_4 concentrations without changing the free, active hormone ("abnormal" total T_4 test results in the absence of thyroid disease). Mild changes in serum binding proteins, such as those induced by pregnancy or estrogen therapy, can be corrected with an indirect estimate of FT_4 by immunoassay (FT_4E); extreme binding protein abnormalities, however, can give artifactual FT_4E results. Elevated protein concentrations tend to produce an overestimation of the FT_4E result, whereas low protein concentrations produce an underestimation of the FT_4 value. For patients with primarily TBG abnormalities, an FT_4E provides more reliable diagnostic information than does a total T_4 value alone. If necessary, in some circumstances when equivocal results are obtained, the FT_4 concentration may be measured directly using equilibrium dialysis methods.

Total T_4 and FT_4E measurements are not ideal indicators of thyroid status, in part because of the effects of variations in serum binding protein concentrations, but also because T_3 is the biologically active and most potent form of thyroid hormone and because the relationships between these hormones (T_4 and T_3) are not always predictable. In patients with hyperthyroidism, T_3 is usually elevated to a greater extent than T_4 because it is derived from two sources: increased thyroidal secretion of T_3 and increased peripheral conversion of T_4 to T_3. The measurement of total T_3 is sometimes a useful adjunct test in patients suspected of hyperthyroidism. However, because T_3 concentrations fluctuate rapidly in response to stress and other nonthyroidal factors, T_3 concentrations are low not only in hypothyroidism, but also in many other conditions. Thus the routine measurement of total T_3 is not a good screening test of thyroid status.

The serum concentration of TSH reflects the integrated action of thyroid hormones at the concentration of one of its target tissues—the pituitary cells that secrete TSH. Thus measurement of TSH is more reliable in the diagnosis of

TABLE 52-2 Effects of Some Drugs on Tests of Thyroid Function

Cause	Drug	Effect
Inhibit TSH secretion	Dopamine	$\downarrow T_4$; $\downarrow T_3$; $\downarrow$ TSH
	L-dopa	
	Glucocorticoids	
	Somatostatin	
Inhibit thyroid hormone synthesis or release	Iodine	$\downarrow T_4$; $\downarrow T_3$; $\uparrow$ TSH
	Lithium	
Inhibit conversion of T_4 to T_3	Amiodarone	$\downarrow T_3$; $\uparrow rT_3$; $\downarrow, \leftrightarrow, \uparrow T_4$ and FT_4; $\leftrightarrow, \uparrow$ TSH
	Glucocorticoids	
	Propranolol	
	Propylthiouracil	
	Radiographic contrast agents	
Inhibit binding of T_4/ T_3 to serum proteins	Salicylates	$\downarrow T_4$; $\downarrow T_3$; $\downarrow FT_4E, \leftrightarrow, \uparrow FT_4$; $\leftrightarrow$ TSH
	Phenytoin	
	Carbamazepine	
	Furosemide	
	Nonsteroidal antiinflammatory agents	
	Heparin (in vitro effect)	
Stimulate metabolism of iodothyronines	Phenobarbital	$\downarrow T_4$; $\downarrow FT_4$; $\leftrightarrow$ TSH
	Phenytoin	
	Carbamazepine	
	Rifampicin	
Inhibit absorption of ingested T_4	Aluminum hydroxide	$\downarrow T_4$; $\downarrow FT_4$; $\uparrow$ TSH
	Ferrous sulfate	
	Cholestyramine	
	Colestipol	
	Iron sucralfate	
	Soybean preparations	
	Kayexalate	
Increase in concentration of T_4 binding proteins	Estrogen	$\uparrow T_4$; $\uparrow T_3$; $\leftrightarrow FT_4$; $\leftrightarrow$ TSH
	Clofibrate	
	Opiates (heroin, methadone)	
	5-Fluorouracil	
	Perphenazine	
Decrease in concentration of T_4 binding proteins	Androgens	$\downarrow T_4$; $\downarrow T_3$; $\leftrightarrow FT_4$; $\leftrightarrow$ TSH
	Glucocorticoids	

Data from Smallridge RD. Chapter 33: Thyroid function tests. In: Becker KL, ed. Principles and practice of endocrinology and metabolism. 7th ed. Philadelphia: JB Lippincott, 1995:299-306; Stockigt JR. Thyroid hormone changes in critical illness: The sick euthyroid "syndrome." Diag Endo Metab 1997;15:39-46.

$\downarrow$ reduced serum concentration; $\uparrow$ increased serum concentration; $\leftrightarrow$ no change.

thyroid gland dysfunction than is the measurement of thyroid hormone concentrations themselves. Pituitary TSH secretion is exquisitely sensitive to circulating thyroid hormone concentrations; in fact, a twofold change in FT_4 can elicit a 100-fold change in the serum TSH concentration.[99,190] This reciprocal log-linear relationship, shown in Figure 52-7, explains why some patients may have normal concentrations of FT_4 or FT_3, or both, and few clinical signs or symptoms of thyroid dysfunction, but may have TSH concentrations that are abnormally high or low. Not all such "subclinical" thyroid disease warrants treatment, but detection of mild changes in thyroid function may be important for some patients.

In the past, clinical use of TSH measurements was limited by the inability of most immunoassays to differentiate the lower limit of normal from abnormally low concen-

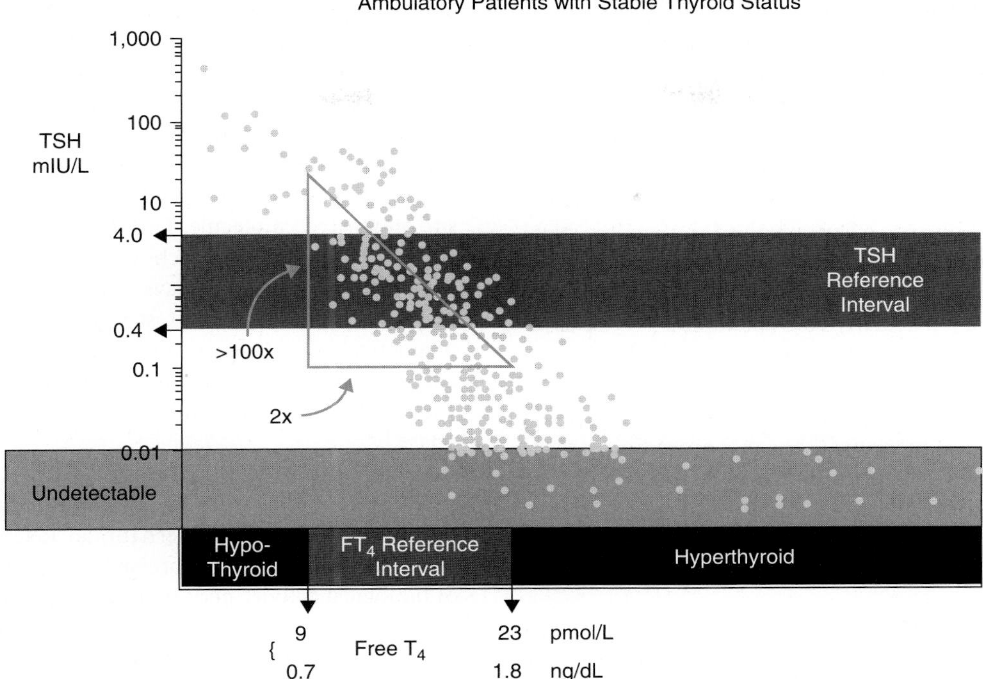

Figure 52-7 The log-linear relationship between TSH and FT_4. A twofold change in TSH is associated with an approximate 100-fold change in circulating FT_4 concentrations. *(Modified from Spencer CA, LoPresti JS, Patel A, Guttler RB, Eigen A, Shen D, et al. Applications of a new chemiluminometric thyrotropin assay to subnormal measurement. J Clin Endocrinol Metab 1990;70:453-60. Copyright 1990, The Endocrine Society.)*

trations. Improvements in assay technique have led to the availability of so called third generation high sensitive TSH assays that distinguish low from normal concentrations. These new assays have altered the approach to thyroid function testing. Instead of screening for thyroid disease with an FT_4E test, a sensitive TSH assay is now the accepted initial screening test of thyroid function in ambulatory patients; TSH concentrations are elevated in hypothyroidism and low in hyperthyroidism. FT_4 testing can be ordered in a reflex fashion when the TSH concentration is abnormally high or low (Figure 52-8). This TSH-centered strategy for the initial evaluation of thyroid function has proven to be both cost-effective and medically efficient.[8,192]

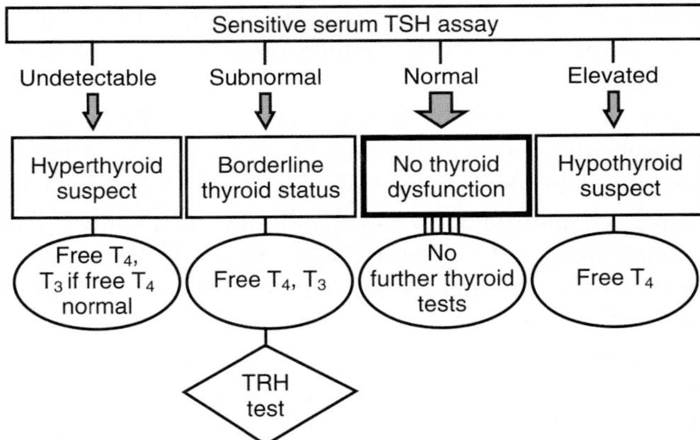

Figure 52-8 Strategies for thyroid diagnosis using a sensitive TSH assay as the initial step. *(Modified from Klee GG, Hay ID. Assessment of sensitive thyrotropin assays for an expanded role in thyroid function testing: Proposed criteria for analytic performance and clinical utility. J Clin Endocrinol Metab 1987;3:461-71. Copyright 1987, The Endocrine Society.)*

ANALYTICAL METHODS

As the laboratory assessment of thyroid disease has been refined through the wide-scale availability of improved techniques and commercial kits, some confusion in terminology has developed. Table 52-1 is a review of the nomenclature for tests of thyroid hormones and thyroid-related proteins in serum. Guidelines for the classification of various thyroid tests have been further described in a special report of the American Thyroid Association.[114]

Almost all laboratory tests for thyroid function are commercially available in kit form and on automated immunoassay platforms. The following is a brief description of tests that are considered useful for the evaluation of thyroid status. With space limitations, literature citations are representative, but not inclusive. For detailed descriptions of methods, refer to original reports or to the documentation accompanying commercial products.

Determination of Thyroid-Stimulating Hormone in Blood

The measurement of TSH was originally based on bioassays such as the stimulation of colloid droplet formation in the guinea pig thyroid gland and the release of labeled thyroidal iodide into mouse blood.[32] These early in vivo bioassays, however, were of limited sensitivity and precision and were not applicable to the measurement of TSH in unfractionated serum. Most TSH bioassays have involved the in vitro stimulation of thyroid cyclic adenosine monophosphate (cAMP) or adenylate cyclase activity. The rat FRTL-5 thyroid cell line is an example of a particularly convenient and precise assay system.[211] Unfortunately, such methods require purification and concentration of TSH from serum before assay. Sensitive detection of TSH in unfractionated serum is possible using a cytochemical bioassay,[158] but this procedure is technically difficult and time-consuming. At present, immunoassay is the procedure of choice for the measurement of serum TSH in the clinical laboratory.

Principle

The first immunological assay for TSH was based on the cross-reaction of human and bovine TSH in a hemagglutination inhibition test;[121] however, this method was too insensitive for clinical purposes. Immunoassay measurement of serum TSH concentration did not become a routine test until the purified pituitary hormone became available for immunization and iodination.

Radioimmunoassay

The traditional radioimmunoassay (RIA) for TSH was based on competition between endogenous and radiolabeled hormone for binding sites on a limited amount of antibody. Separation of antibody-bound and free radioligands was conveniently performed by double-antibody precipitation (enhanced by the addition of polyethylene glycol) or by using a solid-phase, second-antibody procedure. The amount of labeled TSH bound to the antibody was inversely related to the amount of unlabeled TSH present in the serum specimen.

The determination of serum TSH by RIA proved very valuable in assessing the elevated TSH values in primary hypothyroidism. However, because these assays could only detect 1 mU of TSH per liter, most conventional RIAs could not distinguish normal values from the subnormal values associated with hyperthyroidism.

Immunometric Assays

Immunometric methods based on chemiluminescence are capable of measuring TSH at concentrations required to accurately detect the low concentrations of serum TSH found in patients with true hyperthyroidism or the suppressed concentrations found in patients with nonthyroidal illnesses. These sensitive methods resulted from the application of the immunometric sandwich configuration, in which a serum TSH molecule forms a bridge between two or more distinct anti-TSH antibodies. The first antibody (of monoclonal origin) is often directed at the specific TSH beta subunit and is anchored to a solid-phase separation system. This antibody is present in excess and selectively immunoextracts the majority of TSH molecules from the serum specimen. Bound hormone is then quantitated using a second TSH antibody (of either monoclonal or polyclonal origin) that is directed against a distinctly different antigenic site on the TSH molecule. This detection antibody is labeled with a signal molecule such as a luminescent molecule. In some immunometric assays, the separation antibody is attached to plastic beads, test tube walls, microtiter plates, magnetizable particles, or glass fiber paper (see Chapters 9 and 11). Another variation is to attach biotin to the antibody and separate the TSH complex using avidin linked to a solid phase.[152]

Assay results for TSH are customarily calibrated against a reference preparation of TSH (e.g., the World Health Organization's Second International Reference Preparation [2nd IRP] 80/558) and expressed as milliinternational units of biological activity per liter of serum (mIU/L). In contrast to the inverse dose-response curve found in RIA, immunometric assays have a positive dose-response curve, with higher concentrations of signal corresponding to higher concentrations of TSH. High-dose hook effects are rarely found. Immunometric assays offer not only improved sensitivity for TSH measurement, but also rapid turnaround time and a wider linear measurement range as compared with traditional RIA methods.

Immunometric assays for TSH are available commercially as manual kit procedures or for use on automated systems. For practical reasons, nonisotopic methods dominate the market and have replaced radioactive tracer methods in most routine laboratories. The majority of immunometric TSH assays label the detection antibody with chemiluminescent labelled molecules[52,138,160]; other labels include peroxidase or alkaline phosphatase and sensitive photometric[42,66] and fluorescent[42,66,154,168] molecules. Other assays are based on the use of fluorescent labels using europium chelates[95,162]; chemiluminescent compounds such as acridinium esters[109] or ruthenium[87]; or bioluminescent molecules such as recombinant aequorin.[165]

To distinguish immunometric TSH assays from less sensitive RIAs, descriptive terms such as "sensitive," "highly sensitive," "ultrasensitive," and "supersensitive" have been used, generating much confusion as to the exact meaning of these terms. In 1991, a Nomenclature Committee of the American Thyroid Association recommended that the *functional detection limit* of serum TSH assays be determined on the basis of low-end interassay precision characteristics.[80] Further, the committee recommended that precision at the lower reporting limit should optimally be 10% to 15% and preferably <20%. At present, functional sensitivity is defined as the lowest concentration of TSH at which an interassay coefficient of variation of 20% can be achieved.[171,195] This functional detection limit encompasses both analytical and

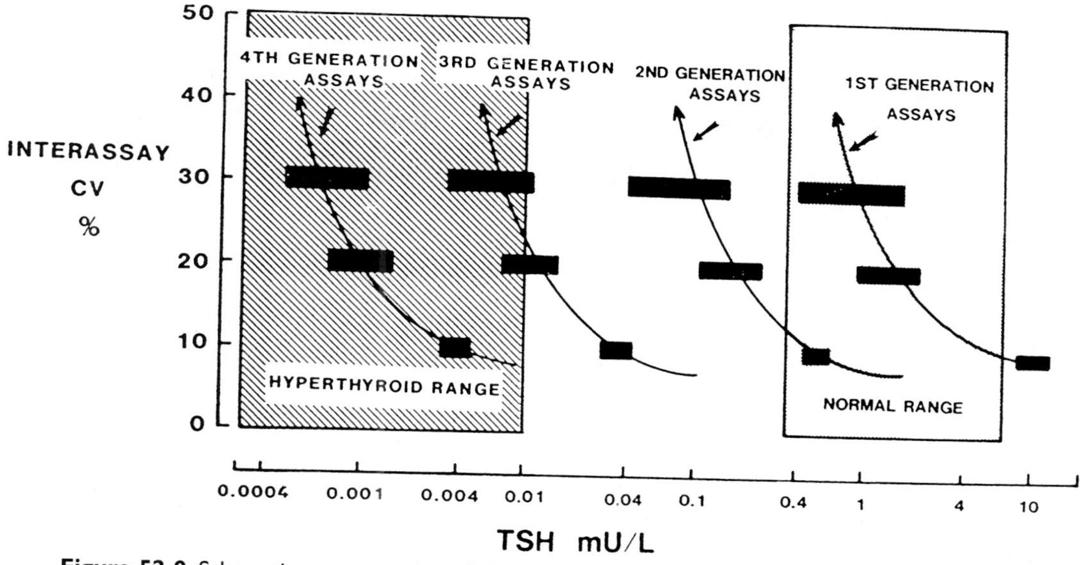

Figure 52-9 Schematic representation of the generation system of nomenclature for TSH assays based on interassay precision (% coefficient of variation). Each generation represents a tenfold improvement in functional sensitivity (20% interassay coefficient value). The black bars denote the 95% confidence limits of measurement at different TSH concentrations. *(Modified from Nicoloff JT, Spencer CA. The use and misuse of sensitive thyrotropin assays. J Clin Endocrinol Metab 1990;71:553-8.)*

biological variations and ensures that the measured TSH concentration is different from zero. Some manufacturers claim a detection limit for their assays that is based on intraassay precision of duplicates of the zero calibrator (i.e., the least detectable concentration). Unfortunately, this detection limit is sometimes overly optimistic. However, the American Thyroid Association has determined that only TSH assays with third generation functional sensitivity can be used as first line thyroid tests.[111A]

A "generational" classification based on functional sensitivity has been suggested to describe improvements in TSH assays[153,190] (Figure 52-9). Each generation of assay represents one log improvement in its detection limit. First generation RIAs typically had a functional detection limit of 1 to 2 mIU/L. The subsequent immunometric assays had about a tenfold improvement in their functional detection limit (0.1 to 0.2 mIU/L) and are considered second generation TSH assays. Second generation assays can reliably distinguish normal from hyperthyroid (or hypothyroid) values in ambulatory patients; however, they have limited value for distinguishing mildly subnormal values (0.02 to 0.1 mIU/L) from the very low values (<0.01 mIU/L) that are typical of thyrotoxicosis.

Third generation immunometric assays have been developed for TSH measurements that have enhanced precision at even lower detection limits. Most of these assays use chemiluminescence-based technologies and have a functional detection limit of less than 0.02 mIU/L. Fourth generation assays having a functional detection limit of 0.001 to 0.002 mIU/L range also have been developed.[196]

Different approaches have been used to implement chemiluminescence-based assays.[132] For example, one assay configuration consists of a polystyrene tube coated with a monoclonal capture antibody and a polyclonal detection antibody conjugated with an acridinium ester; this ester emits a flash of light on treatment with hydrogen peroxide and sodium hydroxide.[193] Another approach uses an antibody-coated tube, a polyclonal antibody conjugated to alkaline phosphatase, and an adamantyl dioxetane phosphate ester as substrate; on dephosphorylation, the substrate decomposes and emits a sustained glow of light.[15] Cross-reactivity of this TSH assay with luteinizing hormone, follicle-stimulating hormone, human chorionic gonadotropin, or the free beta-subunit of glycoprotein hormones is less than 0.001%.

Third and fourth generation assays provide the lower limit of detection needed to distinguish mildly subnormal TSH values (such as those seen in euthyroid hospital patients with a nonthyroidal illness) from the profoundly low values of frank hyperthyroidism. In addition, these assays appear to be helpful in subclassifying hyperthyroid patients according to the degree of TSH suppression, monitoring thyroid cancer patients on thyroxine who require complete suppression of TSH, and judging the adequacy of thyroid hormone replacement in hypothyroid patients.[82,191] However, not all chemiluminescent assays are capable of consistently achieving the detection limit of third generation assays.[194] Clinical laboratories should establish their own detection limit using human sera and clinically relevant patient samples.[173]

Specimen Collection and Storage

Serum or plasma is used for the measurement of TSH and the thyroid hormones, with serum free of hemolysis and lipemia preferred. Specimens are stable for 5 days at 2 °C to 8 °C and for at least 1 month when stored frozen. For newborn screening, whole blood is collected by heel puncture 48 to 72 hours after birth.

Reference Intervals

Secretion of TSH occurs in a circadian fashion: highest concentrations prevail at night between 0200 and 0400 hours, and lowest concentrations occur between 1700 and 1800 hours. Low-amplitude oscillations also occur throughout the day.[60] The nocturnal increase in TSH is lost in critical illness and after surgery. TSH surges immediately after birth, peaking at 30 minutes at 25 to 160 mIU/L; values decline back to cord blood concentrations by 3 days and reach adult values in the first weeks of life. There are no significant sex or race differences. Euthyroid serum TSH concentrations are log-Gaussian or log-normal in distribution; reference intervals should be evaluated logarithmically to achieve accurate estimates of the lower limit of normal.

Expected values using a third generation immunochemiluminometric assay are as follows:[209]

	mIU/L
Prematures, 28-36 wk (1st week of life)	0.7-27.0
Cord blood (>37 wk)	2.3-13.2
Children	
Birth to 4 days	1.0-39.0
2-20 wk	1.7-9.1
21 wk-20 yr	0.7-64.0
Adults	
21-54 yr	0.4-4.2
55-87 yr	0.5-8.9
Pregnancy	
First trimester	0.3-4.5
Second trimester	0.5-4.6
Third trimester	0.8-5.2

Determination of Thyroxine in Serum

Indirect Methods

Serum total T_4 concentrations were initially determined indirectly, using methods that measured the amount of iodine in a protein precipitate of serum (protein-bound iodine, PBI).[5] In addition to hormonal iodine, the PBI tests also measured iodoproteins, iodotyrosines, inorganic iodine, and thyroglobulin. More specific T_4 procedures involved the measurement of hormonal iodine in either a butanol extract of a serum protein precipitate (butanol-extractable iodine) or in a purified fraction of serum (T_4 by column).[128] These methods were useful because the iodine in T_4 normally accounts for 80% to 90% of all iodine in serum. Both butanol extraction and ion-exchange column chromatography selectively separate iodothyronines from other organic iodine compounds. Nevertheless, these methods were relatively nonspecific and rarely used. In some research centers, however, the PBI test is still used to assess patients with iodine-induced thyroid disease or thyroid dyshormonogenesis or as a method to diagnose thyroiditis.

Competitive Protein-Binding Assays

More sensitive and direct methods for the measurement of total serum T_4, known collectively as *competitive protein-binding assays,* were popular for many years.[146] These methods were based on the competition between labeled and unlabeled T_4 for a limited number of protein-binding sites. The specific binding protein used in the majority of these assays was TBG, which was usually obtained from pooled human sera. Anion-exchange resins were often used to separate free and bound hormone fractions. Competitive protein-binding methods, however, required a time-consuming step to extract T_4 from serum before the assay. Although these methods were free from interference by nonhormonal iodine, they were subsequently replaced by more sensitive and specific immunoassay methods.

Instrument-Based Methods

Electron capture gas chromatography,[157] high-performance liquid chromatography,[79] and isotope dilution tandem mass spectrometry[139,188A] have been used for measuring T_4 in human serum. The latter method has been suggested as a reference method for assay of T_4 in serum.[139] In this technique, tritium-labeled T_4 is added to a fixed amount of serum. T_4 is then extracted from the serum, derivatized, and subjected to combined gas chromatography–mass spectrometry.

Immunoassays

In general, most clinical laboratories assay total T_4 with competitive immunoassays performed on automated platforms. Many T_4 immunoassays use high-affinity antibodies produced against an albumin-T_4 conjugate. These polyclonal antisera are quite specific and are able to distinguish among molecules differing by only one atom (e.g., T_3 and T_4). Tg has sometimes been used as an immunogen, because it contains T_4 (and T_3) as part of its structure. Monoclonal antibodies against T_4 have also been developed.

Immunoassays of total T_4 measure both free and protein-bound thyroxine. Accurate measurement of total endogenous hormone therefore requires dissociation of T_4 from its serum transport proteins, because 99.97% of T_4 circulates tightly bound to TBG, albumin, and TBPA. Binding of T_4 to albumin is usually not a concern, because the association constant of T_4 for antibody (usually 10^9 L/mol or greater) is several orders of magnitude higher than that of T_4 for albumin (~1.6×10^6 L/mol). However, binding constants for T_4 with TBG and TBPA are high (2×10^{10} L/mol and 2×10^8 L/mol, respectively). Binding of T_4 to TBPA is overcome by the use of barbital buffers, because barbital ions selectively inhibit this binding. Various blocking agents are used to inhibit binding of T_4 to TBG with 8-anilino-1-naphthalene-sulfonic (ANS) acid being the agent of choice, although salicylate, thimerosal (Merthiolate), and phenytoin are also used. These blocking agents effectively displace T_4 from TBG without affecting its binding characteristics with antibody. In some assays, proportional bias has been attributed to incomplete release of T_4 from serum binding proteins.[150]

Isotopic Methods

Radioactive iodine (e.g., ^{125}I) has been widely used as a signal to follow and measure the distribution of T_4 between unbound and antibody-bound fractions. Before the advent of nonisotopic assays, many reliable commercial RIA kits were used. These RIA kits differed primarily in their approach to separation of free and bound labeled T_4 fractions. Some separation methods used protein precipitation with ammonium sulfate or polyethylene glycol. Others used a double-antibody technique with polyethylene glycol to hasten and enhance separation. A majority, however, used a solid-phase technique with T_4-specific antibody chemically or physically bound to beads, magnetizable particles, or tubes. The latter two modes simplified the procedure by eliminating the centrifugation step for separation of bound and free labeled components.

The older RIA kit procedures required about 1 hour incubation either at room temperature or at 37 °C. Overall, a batch of 20 patient specimens, 2 or 3 controls, and 6 calibrators (each in duplicate) required less than 3 hours to process. Sample volumes per test were small (about 25 μL). Interassay reproducibility, expressed as a coefficient of variation, was typically ±7% at a T_4 concentration of 3.8 μg/dL (50 nmol/L); cross-reactivity of T_3 was about 5% at the 50% displacement concentration. The detection limit of these assays (defined as mean minus 2 standard deviations [SD] of the zero calibrator) was approximately 0.4 μg/dL (5 nmol/L). This limit of detection was not sufficient to measure T_4 directly in dialysates or ultrafiltrates of serum. Highly sensitive T_4 RIAs that have a detection limit of 0.8 pg per tube or 0.16 ng/dL of dialysate were eventually developed.

Nonisotopic Methods

Considerable effort was expended in the development of alternative technologies that did not require the use and measurement of radioactivity. A number of nonisotopic assays for T_4 were subsequently developed commercially for use on fully automated immunoassay systems or for use with existing chemistry analyzers. According to a 2002 College of American Pathologists Ligand Assay Survey,[29] more than 95% of laboratories now use a nonisotopic T_4 method. A variety of different labels were used to construct these nonisotopic assays. Enzymes such as horseradish peroxidase, alkaline phosphatase, and β-D-galactosidase were the most widely used in conjunction with fluorescent and chemiluminescence-based molecules.

Enzyme immunoassays that require physical separation of free and bound T_4 are generally based on principles analogous to those of conventional RIAs except that enzyme activity rather than radioactivity is measured. Most enzyme immunoassays use labeled T_4 as antigen. An assortment of photometric, fluorescent, and luminescent substrates have been used to monitor the enzyme activity of the antibody-bound fraction.

Like radioassays, heterogeneous enzyme assays for T_4 make extensive use of solid-phase separation systems. Some methods immobilize the T_4 antibody on plastic surfaces (e.g., polystyrene beads, test tubes, and microwells) so that bound and free analyte are conveniently separated by decanting and washing. For example, one automated assay uses test tubes that contain polystyrene beads coated with a monoclonal T_4 capture antibody.[2] T_4 in the specimen, liberated from binding proteins by ANS, competes with a T_4–alkaline phosphatase conjugate for a limited number of binding sites on the bead. After washing off the unbound label, the catalytic activity of the bound enzyme is estimated using a chemiluminescent substrate (adamantyl dioxetane phenylphosphate ester). This combination of an enzyme label and a chemiluminescent end point has been applied to other automated T_4 procedures.[70,178] An antibody-coated tube enzyme immunoassay has also been used with T_4 using a peroxidase-T_4 conjugate and a photometric substrate.[206]

Several enzyme immunoassays attach T_4 antibodies to ferromagnetic particles so that free and bound T_4 can be separated magnetically. For example, one fully automated enzyme immunoassay system uses plastic cups that contain magnetic beads coated with a specific T_4 antibody.[212] Endogenous T_4, displaced from its binding proteins by ANS, competes with T_4 labeled with alkaline phosphatase for a limited number of binding sites on the immobilized antibody. The magnetized beads are washed to remove unbound enzyme-labeled T_4 and are then incubated with a fluorogenic substrate. The amount of enzyme-labeled T_4 that binds to the beads is inversely proportional to the T_4 concentration in the test specimen.

Homogeneous enzyme immunoassays have also been developed for serum T_4 determination. These procedures are rapid and simple to use and have also been applied to several major automated instruments.[107] For example, the enzyme-multiplied immunoassay technique (EMIT) for T_4 measurement uses glucose-6-phosphate dehydrogenase covalently linked to T_4 as the enzyme label.[124] Binding of T_4-specific antibody to this label reduces enzyme activity, perhaps as a result of steric or allosteric inhibition As the concentration of unlabeled T_4 increases, less enzyme-labeled hormone is bound by the antibody. As a result, the catalytic activity of the unbound enzyme conjugate increases in direct proportion to the amount of T_4 in the specimen. The indicator reaction involves oxidation of glucose-6-phosphate with simultaneous reduction of nicotinamide-adenine dinucleotide (oxidized form; NAD+) to nicotinamide-adenine dinucleotide (reduced form; NADH). The rate of increase of absorbance at 340 nm is related to T_4 concentration by means of a calibration curve. Separation of free from antibody-bound labeled hormone is not required in this assay, because the latter is inactive.

The cloned enzyme donor immunoassay (CEDIA) technique for T_4 measurement is based on the use of inactive fragments of β-galactosidase called *enzyme acceptor* (EA) and *enzyme donor* (ED).[83] In this method, T_4 in a serum sample competes with ED-labeled T_4 for a limited number of anti-T_4 binding sites. As the concentration of unlabeled T_4 increases, less ED-labeled T_4 binds to the antibody and more reassociates with EA to form an active enzyme. The catalytic activity of the holoenzyme increases in proportion to the amount of T_4 in the sample. This method has been adapted for use on on routine chemistry analyzers.[31]

Fluorescent probes are an attractive alternative to the use of radiolabels, especially because additional substrates are not required to monitor changes in fluorescence. Both heterogeneous (separation required) and homogeneous (nonseparation) fluorescence methods have been described for the measurement of T_4 in serum. An example of the latter is the very popular fluorescence polarization immunoassay.[19,179] In this automated system, fluorescein-labeled T_4 and T_4 in patient specimens compete for binding sites on a T_4 antibody. Polarized excitation light (485 nm) is used to induce fluorescence of the tracer. The emitted light (525 to 550 nm) is also polarized, but the degree of polarization is inversely related to the rate of rotation of the tracer in solution. Polarization of fluorescence of the tracer is therefore very dependent on its effective size. For tracer bound to antibody, the polarization is higher, because the complex is hundreds of times larger than the free tracer. Thus the observed polarization is inversely proportional to the concentration of T_4 present in the specimen. Interassay precision, expressed as a coefficient of variation, is 6% at a T_4 concentration of 4.0 μg/dL (52 nmol/L); cross-reactivity of T_3 is less than 10%. The detection limit, defined as mean minus 2 SD of the zero calibrator, is approximately 1.9 μg/dL (25 nmol/L). Unlike RIA methods, in which each batch of patient specimens required two or three controls and six calibrators (each in duplicate), the fluorescence polarization method needs only a single sample of control tested once every 24 hours each day of use. Once a T_4 calibration is stored, samples may be tested without further calibration unless a new lot of reagent is used.

Heterogeneous fluorescent immunoassays for T_4 based on lanthanide rare earth ions and time-resolved fluorescence were also developed.[43] The use of europium chelates as fluorescent probes is particularly attractive because of their extraordinarily long Stoke's shifts and long fluorescence decay times. Thus the sharp emission peak of europium (613 nm) can be easily separated from scattering caused by excitation light (340 nm) or by interfering substances in serum (400 to 600 nm). In a typical assay, T_4 present in serum specimens competes with europium-labeled T_4 for a limited number of binding sites on T_4-specific monoclonal antibodies. Separation of antibody-bound and free antigen is effected by using a second antibody directed against mouse immunoglobulin G that is coated to the surface of microwells. After incubation and washing, the europium ions are dissociated from the bound phase, converted into a highly fluorescent chelate, and measured in a specially designed fluorometer with time-resolution capability. The fluorescence signal is inversely proportional to the amount of T_4 in the specimen. Because counting times for each specimen are extremely short, a rapid throughput of specimens is allowed. An interesting variant of this technique involves the attachment of biotin to a monoclonal T_4 antibody and streptavidin coupled to a europium chelate.

The feasibility and advantages of using chemiluminescence molecules as direct labels for T_4 immunoassays were subsequently recognized, and fully-automated, random-access analyzers using this signaling system are now widely used to measure total and FT_4 by immunoassay. In one system,[119] endogenous T_4 competes with T_4 coupled to paramagnetic particles for binding with a mouse monoclonal antibody labeled with acridinium ester. After a brief incubation, the magnetized particles are washed to remove the unbound label; the bound fraction is then quantitated in a luminometer after the addition of hydrogen peroxide to initiate the chemiluminescence reaction.

A different immunoassay for T_4 uses electrochemiluminescence as the detection system.[46] This technology uses a ruthenium tris(bipyridyl) complex as the reporter molecule, which, in the presence of tripropylamine, participates in an electrochemiluminescent reaction that is triggered by the application of an electrical potential at two electrodes. Serum T_4, which is set free by ANS, competes with biotin-labeled T_4 for a $Ru(bpy)_3^{2+}$-labeled anti-T_4 polyclonal antibody. The complex of labeled antibody and biotinylated T_4 is captured by streptavidin-coated paramagnetic particles. The reaction mixture is then drawn into a flow cell where the particles are fixed to an electrode surface by application of a magnetic field. A voltage is applied, and the resulting electroluminescence is measured. This automated system requires only 15 μL of sample; interassay precision, expressed as coefficient of variation, is generally found to be ±3% to 6% in the clinical range. Calibration is performed using two calibrators, and the onboard stability of reagents is 4 weeks.

Particle-enhanced immunoassays involving turbidimetric measurements have been described for T_4 in serum. These homogeneous assays are based on competition between the T_4 in the sample and a T_4-ficoll conjugate for binding sites on a specific monoclonal antibody coupled to microparticles. The rate of agglutination is determined turbidimetrically by measuring the absorbance change at 600 nm. Automated systems using this method have been developed.[73]

Dry-chemistry immunoassay systems that require no liquid reagents and no sample pretreatment have also been developed for T_4.[35,155] One system uses a thin-film multilayer test module consisting of three distinct layers coated on a plastic base. The serum specimen first spreads through a topcoat layer, which contains an agent (phenoxy naphthalene sulfonic acid) to displace T_4 from its binding proteins. The unbound T_4 then passes through an iron oxide screen layer into a signal layer, where the hormone competes with and displaces rhodamine-labeled T_4 from the binding sites of an immobilized T_4 antibody. The unbound fluorescent-labeled T_4 diffuses into the opaque screening layers above, where it cannot be seen by the optical detection system. The fluorescent signal of the antibody-bound fraction is measured by front-surface fluorimetry and is inversely proportional to the concentration of T_4 in the serum specimen.

Specimen Collection and Storage

Serum is the preferred specimen for the measurement of T_4; plasma with ethylenediaminetetraacetic acid (EDTA) or heparin as anticoagulant is also used. However, plasma tends to form fibrin clots after freezing and thawing; these clots may interfere mechanically with an assay, especially in an automated system. Gel barrier tubes have no apparent adverse effect on T_4 concentrations. T_4 in serum is quite stable; storage of serum specimens at room temperature up to 7 days shows no appreciable loss of T_4. However, serum specimens are best stored at 2 °C to 8 °C if they will not be tested within 24 hours. If longer periods of storage are necessary, freezing the specimens is recommended. Frozen specimens are stable for at least 30 days. Repeated freezing and thawing of the specimens should be avoided. Hemolysis and lipemia have no significant effect on most T_4 immunoassays; however, grossly hemolyzed specimens should be avoided, because hemolysis may dilute the sample and cause a false decrease in the T_4 concentration. Turbid samples should be centrifuged before testing. Immunoassay procedures are not affected by organic dyes and inorganic iodine compounds. However, radioactive materials can interfere with RIA methods. Patients undergoing therapy for a thyroid disorder should stop treatment 1 month before sampling if a true baseline is to be established. T_4 autoantibodies interfere with some immunoassays for T_4 in that they can produce artificially low or high results, depending on the method.[218]

Specimens have been obtained from infants by heel puncture; such specimens also are collected in capillary tubes or on filter paper. Dried blood specimens are stable and easily transported and are ordinarily obtained for purposes of screening neonates for congenital hypothyroidism.[135A] When this collection technique is used, a one-eighth-inch dot is punched out from the blood-saturated paper and is extracted into the buffer before performing the T_4 assay. It is best to avoid touching the filter paper or exposing it to extreme heat or light.

Reference Intervals[209]

	µg/dL	nmol/L
Cord	7.4-13.0	95-168
Children		
1-3 days	11.8-22.6	152-292
1-2 wk	9.8-16.6	126-214
1-4 mo	7.2-14.4	93-186
4-12 mo	7.8-16.5	101-213
1-5 yr	7.3-15.0	94-194
5-10 yr	6.4-13.3	83-172
10-15 yr	5.6-11.7	72-151
Adults (15-60 yr)		
Males	4.6-10.5	59-135
Females	5.5-11.0	65-138
Adults >60 yr	5.0-10.7	65-138
Newborn screen (whole blood)		
1-5 days	>7.5	>97
6 days	>6.5	>84

Comments

By itself, the concentration of total T_4 does not provide adequate clinical information; an FT_4E test should be determined along with the total T_4 measurement to compensate for binding protein effects. Cord blood T_4 concentrations are lower in preterm than in full-term neonates, and they correlate positively with birth weight in full-term infants. At birth, serum total T_4 concentrations are higher in neonates because of the maternal estrogen-induced increase in serum TBG; FT_4 values are near adult concentrations. Total T_4 values rise abruptly in the first few hours after birth and decline gradually until the age of 15. Males experience a gradual decline in T_4 production as they mature sexually; females do not.

Reference intervals for newborns should be developed by each laboratory that provides screening for neonatal hypothyroidism. Imprecision of the T_4 assay is handled on a daily basis, usually by setting floating cutoffs to include false-positive results and to preclude false-negative results.[94]

Based on biological information, analytical performance goals have been recommended for thyroid hormone assays.[173] When a total T_4 assay is used to rule in or rule out disease, the suggested goals for maximum bias and imprecision (calculated as a percent coefficient of variation) are ±2.9% and ±5.7%, respectively. When the assay is used for monitoring changes in an individual over time, bias and imprecision goals are ±1.3% and ±2.6%, respectively.

Determination of Triiodothyronine in Serum

Older Methods

T_3 has been measured using a variety of chemical reactions, but such chemical methods are generally too insensitive or impractical for measuring the low T_3 concentrations present in serum. In the 1960s, competitive protein-binding assays were introduced for the measurement of T_3, with TBG serving as a natural binding protein; prior isolation of T_3 from serum (e.g., by extraction of iodothyronines with a cation-exchange resin, followed by separation of T_3 and T_4 using paper chromatography) was required to increase assay performance.[198]

Immunoassay

Direct measurement of T_3 by immunoassay has been made possible by the production of T_3-specific antibodies. Unlike T_4 antiserum, high-titer, specific T_3-antiserum is seldom obtained by immunization of rabbits with naturally occurring Tg. Good-quality antiserum, however, has been produced using T_3-enriched Tg, T_3-human serum albumin (HSA), or T_3-bovine serum albumin (BSA) conjugates.[23] Monoclonal T_3 antibodies have also been produced using hybridoma technologies.

Isotopic Methods

Numerous commercial kits have been introduced for measuring serum total T_3 concentrations. Procedures are similar to those described for T_4 except that an ^{125}I-T_3 tracer and T_3-specific antibody are used. Liquid-phase separation systems, such as those using charcoal adsorption, polyethylene glycol, and double-antibody precipitation, are not used as often as solid-phase systems (e.g., those using antibody-coated tubes or magnetizable particles). As with the T_4 methods, ANS is frequently used to release T_3 from its serum binding proteins without disturbing the binding of T_3 to antibody. A typical calibration curve ranges from 25 to 800 ng/dL; values for unknown specimens are obtained from the curve by interpolation.

Nonisotopic Methods

Nonisotopic assays similar to those described for serum T_4 have been applied to the measurement of T_3. Many of these procedures have been developed for use on fully automated immunoassay systems,[97] and some are compatible with chemistry analyzers. Many commercial methods use peroxidase or alkaline phosphatase to label T_3 antigens or T_3 antibodies; enzyme activity is commonly determined using a variety of sensitive photometric,[105,120] fluorescent,[3,142] or chemiluminescent[36] substrates. Immunoassays for T_3 that use fluorescent[156] and chemiluminescent labels[30] are also available and, as with T_4 assays, chemiluminescence-based assays on automated platforms have become the rule rather than the exception. Both heterogeneous (separation required) and homogeneous methods have been described.[98,166] An example of the former is the microparticle enzyme immunoassay for T_3.[74] In this automated system, serum T_3 binds to anti–T_3-coated microparticles, forming an antibody-antigen complex that is then separated by a glass-fiber matrix. An alkaline phosphatase–labeled T_3 conjugate, which forms a sandwich with the T_3 bound to the glass fiber, is added. A fluorescent product is formed when the enzyme substrate, 4-methylumbelliferyl phosphate, reacts with the enzyme label. Values obtained with this enzyme immunoassay are generally higher than those obtained with RIA methods.

Specimen Collection and Storage

Serum is the preferred specimen; plasma with EDTA or heparin as anticoagulant may also be used. However, gel tubes should be avoided for T_3 measurements due to possible contaminating chemicals in the gel that can cause a false elevation in results. Serum specimens once collected are best stored at 2 °C to 8 °C if they will not be tested within 24 hours. If longer periods of storage are necessary, freezing the specimens is recommended. Frozen specimens are stable for at least 30 days. Repeated freezing and thawing of the specimens should be avoided. Turbid samples should be centrifuged before testing. Specimen volume per test is usually 50 to 100 µL.

Reference Intervals

The reference intervals for T_3 may vary from one procedure and reference population to another. Each laboratory should establish its own reference intervals. Expected values using an RIA method are as follows.[209]

	ng/dL	nmol/L
Cord (>37 wk)	5-141	0.08-2.17
Children		
1-3 days	100-740	1.54-11.40
1-11 mo	105-245	1.62-3.77
1-5 yr	105-269	1.62-4.14
6-10 yr	94-241	1.45-3.71
11-15 yr	82-213	1.26-3.28
Adolescents		
16-20 yr	80-210	1.23-3.23
Adults		
20-50 yr	70-204	1.08-3.14
50-90 yr	40-181	0.62-2.79
Pregnancy[33]		
First trimester	81-190	1.25-2.93
Second and third trimesters	100-260	1.54-4.00

Comments

Different T_3 immunoassays may show unexplained discrepancies between values for the same sera. Results from interlaboratory quality assurance schemes also demonstrate a higher analytical variance for T_3 than for T_4 methods. Many factors have been suggested as accounting for these disparities, such as the lower quantity of T_3 in sera, differences in antisera cross-reactivity, protein interferences, and different assay limits of detection.[223]

Typical coefficients of variation for interassay performance are ±5% to 7%; assay detection limit is approximately 10 ng/dL. Most T_3 immunoassays have negligible cross-reactivity with T_4 (<0.12%), thus permitting direct measurement of T_3 in serum specimens regardless of the fact that T_3 concentrations are 100-fold lower than are T_4 concentrations. T_3 autoantibodies interfere with some assays, producing low or high results (depending on the method).

Performance goals for bias and precision have been suggested for T_3.[173] When a total T_3 assay is used for diagnostic applications, the suggested goals for maximum bias and imprecision (expressed as percent coefficient of variation) are ±5.7% and 11.5%, respectively. When the assay is used for therapeutic applications, bias and imprecision goals are ±2.6% and 5.2%, respectively. The major clinical roles for total T_3 measurements are in the diagnosis and monitoring of hyperthyroid patients with suppressed TSH and normal FT_4 concentrations ("T_3-thyrotoxicosis"); T_3 measurements have only a limited role in euthyroid and hypothyroid patients.[102]

Determination of Reverse Triiodothyronine (rT_3) Using Radioimmunoassay

The rT_3 molecule (3,5,5′ triiodothyronine) is biologically inert. A number of radioimmunoassay methods for rT_3 measurement have been published.[65] Antisera for rT_3 are generally obtained by immunizing rabbits using rT_3 conjugates with HSA or BSA.[22] The antisera are usually devoid of significant cross-reactivity with T_2 or T_3; cross-reaction with T_4 varies between 0.01 and 0.15%.[136] Like T_3 and T_4, rT_3 also binds with TBG, TBPA, and albumin in serum. The binding of rT_3 to serum proteins has been overcome by the use of an ethanol extract of serum or by the addition of ANS to the serum in a manner similar to that described for T_3 and T_4.[24] Separation of free and antibody-bound hormone is often achieved using a second antibody (e.g., anti-rabbit γ-globulin) procedure with precipitation accelerated with polyethylene glycol.

Although commercial assays for direct serum analysis of rT_3 are available, kit procedures are not as convenient as are those for other thyroid hormones and no rT_3 method has been adapted to an automated platform because this measurement has no recognized diagnostic value. In comparison with the reference method described by Chopra,[22] the typical kit procedure is relatively fast; it requires a 3-hour incubation at room temperature, followed by polyethylene glycol precipitation and centrifugation. The entire procedure requires less than 6 hours to perform.

Specimen Collection and Storage

Serum is the preferred specimen; plasma with EDTA or heparin as anticoagulant may also be used. Serum specimens are best stored at 2 °C to 8 °C if they will not be tested within 24 hours. If longer periods of storage are necessary, freezing the specimens is recommended. Frozen specimens are stable for at least 30 days. Repeated freezing and thawing of the specimens should be avoided. Turbid samples should be centrifuged before testing. Amniotic fluid obtained by amniocentesis or by transmembrane aspiration at delivery may also be analyzed for rT_3. The amniotic fluid should be clear. To avoid debris and other cellular particles, centrifugation of the fluid for 15 minutes at 900 ×g is suggested. Specimens are stable for 1day at 2 °C to 8 °C and for up to 3 months when frozen. Amniotic fluid contaminated with hemolyzed blood should not be used.

Reference Intervals [209]

	ng/dL	nmol/L
Cord blood (>37 wk)	130-300	2.00-4.62
Children		
1 day	83-194	1.28-2.99
2 days	107-209	1.65-3.22
3 days	102-166	1.57-2.56
1 mo-20 yr	10-35	0.15-0.54
Adult	10-28	0.15-0.43
Maternal serum (15-40 wk)[209]	11-33	0.17-0.51
Amniotic fluid (17-22 wk)[209]	163-599	2.51-9.22

Comments

Reverse T_3 in serum is present almost entirely as a result of its generation from T_4 in peripheral tissues by 5-deiodinases. The concentration of serum rT_3 is lower than that of T_3 because of the faster metabolic clearance of rT_3. Serum rT_3 concentrations are elevated at birth, but decrease to stable values by about the fifth day of life. Reverse T_3 in amniotic fluid decreases with increasing gestational age. The use of reverse T_3 in patients with the euthyroid sick syndrome has fallen out of favor with the recognition that rT_3 is not always elevated in illness. Specifically, renal failure is associated with low rT_3 concentrations.

Determination of Free Thyroid Hormones

T_4 and T_3 circulate in the blood as equilibrium mixtures of free and protein-bound hormones. Thus changes in the concentration or affinity of TBG or other transport proteins profoundly affect the total hormone concentration in serum. Alternatively the steady-state concentration of the free hormone is independent of these binding protein variations and remains almost constant.

The interaction between free thyroid hormones and their binding proteins (TBPs) conforms to a reversible binding equilibrium that is described by the following mass action relationship:

$$[FT_4] \times [TBP] = K \times [T_4{:}TBP]$$

where

$[FT_4]$ = concentration of free T_4 in serum
$[TBP]$ = concentration of unoccupied binding sites on TBP
K = association constant
$[T_4{:}TBP]$ = concentration of T_4-occupied binding sites on TBP

The relationship among these entities has important diagnostic implications. A primary increase in either [FT_4] or [TBP] drives this reaction to the right, increasing serum [T_4:TBP]. Because 99.97% of the total T_4 is bound to TBP, the value of [T_4:TBP] is considered equivalent to that of total T_4. Hyperthyroidism produces a primary increase in FT_4, whereas estrogens and idiopathic or genetic conditions may produce a primary increase in TBP. In both cases, [T_4:TBP] increases, but in the former, the patient is ill and requires treatment; in the latter, the patient is euthyroid. Likewise a low serum [T_4:TBP] may be due to a primary decrease in [FT_4] or to a primary decrease in [TBP]. It is therefore clinically important to differentiate between changes in [T_4:TBP] that are due to primary changes in [FT_4] (e.g., hyperthyroidism or hypothyroidism) and those that are due to primary changes in [TBP].

Numerous methods have been developed for assessing the concentrations of FT_4 and FT_3 in serum. These methods include direct assays that currently serve as reference methods and indirect assays that are more widely available for general laboratory use. The following section describes the principles of these methods and offers some guidelines for their use. The theoretical basis, analytical validity, and clinical utility of these methods have been discussed.[47,48,50] Special reports from the Nomenclature Committee of the American Thyroid Association,[80] the National Academy of Clinical Biochemistry,[173] and the NCCLS also review some of the issues and concerns regarding free thyroid hormone measurements.

Direct Reference Methods

Direct measurement of FT_4 and FT_3 in serum presents a considerable technical challenge as free hormone concentrations are exceedingly low in normal serum. For example, they are approximately 0.03% of the total serum T_4 and 0.3% of the total serum T_3 concentrations, respectively. Consequently assays for them must be capable of measuring subpicomole amounts. Theoretically the most reliable methods for measuring FT_4 and FT_3 in serum employ equilibrium dialysis and ultrafiltration techniques that physically separate free hormone from protein-bound hormone before direct measurement of the free fraction with a sensitive T_4 or T_3 immunoassay. Only minimal dilution of serum specimens is allowed, because dilution alters the binding of drugs, free fatty acids, and other substances to serum proteins, thus disturbing the equilibrium between bound and free hormone.

Historically, direct procedures were too cumbersome, time-consuming, and expensive for use in a routine clinical laboratory. The introduction of very sensitive immunoassays for T_4 and T_3 combined with improvements in the dialysis or ultrafiltration of undiluted serum has allowed direct measurement of free thyroid hormones. Thus *direct equilibrium dialysis* and *ultrafiltration* methods are available for FT_4 measurement.[149,210]

Principles

Direct Equilibrium Dialysis. In this method, undiluted serum specimens are dialyzed for 16 to 18 hours at 37 °C in a reusable dialysis chamber.[149] The dialysis buffer provides for minimal changes in the serum matrix. The dialysate is then analyzed directly using a sensitive RIA. The range of reportability is 2 to 128 ng/L (2.6 to 165 pmol/L), and the interassay coefficient of variation is approximately ±7%.

Ultrafiltration. The second method is an ultrafiltration procedure for FT_4 determination in serum that is significantly less time-consuming than dialysis.[210] In this method, the serum specimen is adjusted to pH 7.4, incubated for 20 minutes at 37 °C (to achieve equilibrium of the binding at this temperature), and then applied to an ultrafiltration device for centrifugation for 30 minutes at 37 °C and 2000 ×g (using a fixed-angle rotor). Subsequently the ultrafiltrate is analyzed for T_4. Variable protein leakage in ultrafiltration devices continues to hamper commercialization of this method.

Specimen Collection and Storage

Serum is the preferred specimen; plasma with EDTA or heparin as anticoagulant may also be used. Serum specimens are best stored at 2 °C to 8 °C if they will not be tested within 24 hours. If longer periods of storage are necessary, freezing the specimens is recommended. Frozen specimens are stable for at least 30 days. Repeated freezing and thawing of the specimens should be avoided. Turbid samples should be centrifuged before testing.

Reference Intervals

Expected values for FT_4 using direct equilibrium dialysis are as follows:[209]

	ng/dL	pmol/L
Newborns (1-4 days)	2.2-5.3	28.4-68.4
Children (2 wk-20 yr)	0.8-2.0	10.3-25.8
Adults (21-87 yr)	0.8-2.7	10.3-34.7
Pregnancy		
First trimester	0.7-2.0	9.0-25.7
Second and third trimesters	0.5-1.6	6.4-20.6

Comments

FT_4 assays based on direct equilibrium dialysis or ultrafiltration measure free hormone without the need for total hormone measurements. These methods are unaffected by either variations in serum binding proteins or thyroid hormone autoantibodies. However, IV heparin administration can cause spurious elevations in FT_4 determined by these techniques as a consequence of in vitro generation of free fatty acids. Mean values obtained in euthyroid healthy subjects are reported to be slightly higher when using ultrafiltration methods than when using equilibrium dialysis.[210,222]

Analytical performance goals have been recommended for free thyroid hormone assays.[102,150,173] When an FT_4 assay is used to rule in or rule out disease, the suggested goals for maximum bias and imprecision (calculated as percent coefficient of variation) are ±3.8% and 7.7%, respectively. When the assay is used for monitoring changes in an individual over time, bias and imprecision goals are ±2.4% and ±4.8%, respectively.

Indirect Methods for Estimating Free Thyroid Hormones

Most routine immunoassay methods for determining FT_4 and FT_3 concentrations in serum are estimates. These approaches are often more convenient and less expensive than reference methods, and most are available commercially in kit form and on automated immunoassay instruments. Two test strategies are used for estimating the concentrations of free hormones: "indirect" index methods and "direct" immunoassays.

Unlike direct reference assays, indirect index methods use two separate tests to estimate the free hormone concentration: a total serum T_4 (or T_3) measurement and an assessment of either the serum TBG concentration or the fraction of T_4 (or T_3) that is free in serum; the latter is traditionally derived using equilibrium tracer dialysis or "T uptake" methods. Results of these tests are then combined mathematically to give estimates of the free hormone concentration. Indirect index-based methods have essentially fallen out of favor in deference to the direct immunoassay methods.

Direct two-step and one-step immunoassays estimate free hormone concentrations by using antibody extraction techniques. Although it is often claimed or implied that these immunoextraction assays measure FT_4 or FT_3 directly, virtually all methods do so indirectly by relating test results to extracted serum calibrators with free hormone values that have been independently measured using reference methods (e.g., direct equilibrium dialysis/RIA). Further, studies have shown that all of the free hormone estimate methods on current instrument platforms are binding protein dependent to some extent.[217A]

Free Hormone Fraction by Indirect Equilibrium Tracer Dialysis

Several isotopic methods have been used to accurately estimate the free hormone fraction, including equilibrium tracer dialysis,[90,199] ultrafiltration,[189] Sephadex chromatography,[188] and polyacrylamide gel filtration.[134] However, these techniques are very cumbersome and time consuming for routine clinical use and, with the exception of equilibrium tracer dialysis, have found little practical application. Unfortunately the free hormone fraction as estimated in normal sera by equilibrium tracer dialysis varies substantially among laboratories. Methodological difficulties include the presence of residual impurities in the tracer, the temperature and duration of dialysis, the adsorption of tracer by components of the dialysis system, and the in vitro generation of free fatty acids.[80]

Principle. Test serum is enriched with very small quantities of radioiodine-labeled T_4, which quickly distributes between free and bound T_4 to approximate the distribution of endogenous hormone. The fraction of labeled hormone that dialyzes through a semipermeable membrane is then measured. The method of Ingbar and coworkers[90] consists of a double dialysis procedure. In the first dialysis, the serum-radioactive T_4 mixture is dialyzed against phosphate buffer (pH 7.4) overnight at 37 °C. The dialysate (i.e., the part that passes through the semipermeable membrane) contains both free radiolabeled thyroxine and labeled inorganic iodide and other contaminating iodinated compounds generally present in commercial preparations of radioiodine-labeled T_4. The second dialysis is used to remove these contaminants. In this procedure, a mixture of the first dialysate and pooled plasma is dialyzed against phosphate buffer containing an anion exchange resin. The resin adsorbs only the radioactive contaminants and thereby maintains an effective diffusion gradient for impurities until all are removed. Because the binding proteins in the pooled plasma possess a high affinity for T_4, little if any radioactive T_4 is available for diffusion and adsorption by the resin. All radioactivity that remains within the dialysis bag is considered to be the FT_4.

The method of Sterling and Brenner[199] simplified the FT_4 method significantly by replacing the second dialysis step with a precipitation procedure. It involves dialysis of the serum-radioactive T_4 mixture against phosphate buffer as described previously and precipitation of the radioactive T_4 in the dialysate with magnesium chloride after addition of carrier T_4. This method is often called the *magnesium precipitation method,* and the method of Ingbar and coworkers[90] is called the *resin dialysis technique.* Values of % FT_4 are calculated according to the following formula:

$$\%\,FT_4 = \frac{C_o}{C_i} \times 100$$

where C_o is the counts per minute of dialysate-magnesium precipitate, and C_i is the counts per minute per milliliter of dialysate.

Specimen Collection and Storage. Serum is the preferred specimen; plasma with EDTA or heparin as anticoagulant may also be used. Serum specimens are best stored at 2 °C to 8 °C if they will not be tested within 24 hours. If longer periods of storage are necessary, freezing the specimens is recommended. Frozen specimens are stable for at least 30 days. Repeated freezing and thawing of the specimens should be avoided. Turbid samples should be centrifuged before testing.

Reference Intervals. Reference values for % FT_4 range between 0.02% and 0.04% of total hormone concentration. Because T_3 is less firmly bound by TBG than is T_4, the dialyzable fraction of T_3 is appreciably greater (by almost 10 times) than that of T_4. Thus the reference interval for % FT_3 is 0.2% to 0.4%.

Calculation of Free Hormone Estimates

Principle. The free hormone fraction, as measured by dialysis or ultrafiltration of diluted serum containing tracer

T_4 or T_3, is multiplied by the respective total hormone concentration to obtain indirect estimates of FT_4 or FT_3:

$$FT_4E = \text{Total } T_4 \times \% FT_4$$

$$FT_3E = \text{Total } T_3 \times \% FT_3$$

Reference Intervals. The expected calculated values for FT_4 and FT_3 using equilibrium tracer dialysis are as follows:

FT_4E[52]

	ng/dL	pmol/L
Cord	1.7-4.0	22-52
Newborn	2.6-6.3	34-81
Adult	0.8-2.3	10-30

FT_3E[33]

	pg/dL	pmol/L
Cord	15-391	0.2-6.0
Child and adult	210-440	3.2-6.8
Pregnancy	200-380	3.1-5.9

Free Hormone Fraction by Uptake Methods (Thyroid Hormone–Binding Ratio)

The THBR is derived from a version of the T_3 or T_4 uptake test. Uptake tests are used to estimate the number of unoccupied (unsaturated) thyroid hormone binding sites on serum proteins. This information is important because variations in total thyroid hormone concentrations in blood, as discussed previously, have resulted from changes in binding protein concentrations. Values obtained by uptake methods are expressed as a THBR, which is directly proportional to the free hormone fraction (within limits). Measurement of THBR, in conjunction with a total hormone concentration, is a clinically useful indirect method for calculating the FT_4 (or FT_3) index. The index approach is particularly useful in patients with nonthyroidal illness in whom FT_4 immunoassay methodologies are unreliable. Specifically, TT_4 measurement is more diagnostically useful in such patients provided that values are interpreted in accord with the severity of illness in the patient that is indirectly reflected by abnormalities in THBR.

Isotopic Methods

Many different radioactive tracer methods have been used for estimating the unsaturated thyroid hormone binding capacity. The simplest is the T_3 *uptake test.* Traditionally, this test is performed by measuring the distribution of radiolabeled T_3 between serum binding proteins and a solid-phase binding material. In a typical assay, a diluted sample of patient serum is allowed to equilibrate with a trace amount of ^{125}I-T_3 and the secondary binder. A portion of the radioactive T_3 binds to empty binding sites on serum proteins, principally TBG, and the remainder attaches to the solid matrix. At the end of a specific incubation period, the reactants are separated, and the proportion of radioactivity bound by the solid matrix (the "uptake") is measured. The amount of T_3 tracer bound to the secondary binder varies inversely with the number of unoccupied TBG binding sites in the serum specimen and directly with the free fraction of T_4 and T_3.

In the original T_3 uptake test, red blood cells were used to remove labeled hormone not tightly bound to TBG.[76] To minimize methodological difficulties, erythrocytes were replaced with an ion-exchange resin, either in granular form or impregnated in a sponge.[28] The test then became known as the *resin T_3* uptake test. Many solid-phase materials have subsequently been used, including charcoal, talc, macroaggregated albumin, or immobilized T_3 antibody. Many of these secondary binders are incorporated in commercial kit methods.

Radiolabeled T_3 is used more often than is labeled T_4 because of its relatively low affinity for TBG compared with T_4, which leads to higher uptake values and better discrimination between normal and abnormal test results. In addition, radioactive T_3 fills the unoccupied binding sites on TBG but does not displace any bound T_4. Under most circumstances, the use of labeled T_3 to approximate the free fraction of T_4 does not introduce serious errors, because T_3 and T_4 are both predominantly bound by TBG and occupy virtually the same binding sites. Major problems are encountered, however, when some factor changes the binding affinity for T_4 but not for T_3. For example, in abnormal binding protein states (i.e., NTI) differential abnormalities in protein binding of T_3 versus T_4 may occur, rendering a T_3 uptake an inappropriate approach for calculating an FT_4I.

T_3 uptake values are customarily expressed as matrix-bound counts divided by the total counts added (typical euthyroid reference interval: 25% to 37%). This calculation, however, is theoretically unsound and has led to problems of interpretation, particularly when serum TBG concentrations are very high or very low. Instead the uptake value should be expressed as the matrix-bound counts divided by the counts that remain bound to serum proteins (typical euthyroid reference interval: 33% to 50%). This result corresponds more closely to the mass action law and is more linearly related to the free hormone fraction over a wide range of values.

Several uptake kits are commercially available. T_3 uptake values for individual subjects depend on specific assay conditions such as incubation time and temperature, quantity and avidity of the binding material, and specific activity and choice of the label. To compensate for variations in uptake values, the percent uptake for each unknown should be determined by comparison with a calibrator, reference material, or euthyroid reference serum of known percent uptake. Almost all commercial assays determine the percent uptake directly from the radioactivity (in cpm) taken up on the secondary binder:

$$\% \text{ uptake} = \frac{\text{cpm (patient)}}{\text{cpm (calibrator)}} \times \% \text{ uptake (calibrator)}$$

Nonisotopic Methods

T_4 and T_3 uptake assays that use nonisotopic tracers have been developed and are available on most automated immunoassay instruments. Some methods use enzymes to label T_4 or T_3; different photometric, fluorescent, and luminescent substrates are available for monitoring the enzyme activity. Direct labeling of T_4 or T_3 antigens with fluorophores or chemiluminescence molecules is the most popular. These nonisotopic methods are generically named "uptake" assays, regardless of whether T_4 or T_3 is used as the labeled analogue. The competitive binder commonly used in many of these assays is a T_4 antibody bound to a solid phase. Some methods probe the total binding capacity of all thyroid hormone–binding proteins, but most estimate the concentration of unoccupied TBG binding sites. As mentioned, these T-uptake assays have essentially been replaced by the use of free hormone estimate assays to compensate for the variations in protein binding that affect total hormone assays.[57]

Some enzyme immunoassays for uptake do not require separation of the reactants. In the homogenous EMIT assay, a serum sample is incubated with a known amount of exogenous T_4, which binds to available sites on TBPs:

$$T_4 \text{ (exogenous)} + \text{TBP} \rightleftharpoons \text{TBP}: T_4 + T_4 \text{ (residual)}$$

Residual T_4 is the the amount of T_4 that remains unbound and competes with the T_4 linked to glucose-6-phosphate dehydrogenase (T_4-E) for anti-T_4 antibody binding sites:

$$T_4 + T_4\text{-E (active)} + \text{Ab} \rightleftharpoons \text{Ab}: T_4 + \text{Ab}: T_4\text{-E (inactive)}$$

Binding of antibody to T_4-E decreases enzyme activity. The unbound T_4-enzyme conjugate, on the other hand, is active and catalyzes the oxidation of glucose-6-phosphate with simultaneous reduction of NAD+ to NADH. The rate of increase of absorbance at 340 nm is inversely proportional to the number of unsaturated TBP binding sites. Test results are expressed as percent of T uptake using a calibration curve or a mathematical function. Manual and automated versions of this assay are commercially available.[161,184]

Another homogenous immunoassay for T_4 uptake, based on CEDIA technology, uses the two inactive fragments EA and ED of β-galactosidase. In this assay, serum TBPs compete with EA for binding to an ED-T_4 conjugate. As the concentration of unsaturated TBPs increases, less ED-T_4 reassociates with EA to form the active enzyme:

$$\text{TBP} + \text{EA} + \text{ED-}T_4 \rightleftharpoons \text{ED-}T_4\text{:TBP} + \text{EA:ED-}T_4$$

The catalytic activity of the holoenzyme is inversely proportional to the concentration of unoccupied TBP binding sites and directly related to the percent T uptake. This assay has also been adapted for use on automated instruments.[85,103]

Several heterogenous enzyme immunoassays are commercially available for THBR assessment. In one competitive assay, a fixed excess of unlabeled T_4 is added to the serum specimen and binds to vacant sites on TBPs. The remaining unbound T_4 competes with an alkaline phosphatase–T_4 reagent for a limited number of binding sites on anti-T_4 polyclonal antibody immobilized on magnetic beads. As the concentration of unoccupied TBPs increases in serum, less unlabeled T_4 is available to compete with enzyme-labeled T_4 for antibody binding sites, and vice versa. Steric and molecular changes prevent enzyme-labeled T_4 from combining with endogenous serum proteins, and only unlabeled T_4 binds to TBPs. After washing to remove unbound components, the magnetic beads are incubated with a fluorogenic substrate. The enzyme activity measured in this assay (i.e., the fluorescence that is produced) changes in a direction opposite to the amount of radioactivity measured in the classic T_3-uptake test and is therefore directly proportional to the concentration of unoccupied TBP binding sites in the patient's serum but inversely related to the percent uptake.

Fluorescent and luminescence molecules have replaced radiolabels in the T-uptake test,[143] and both heterogenous and homogenous methods have been described. An example of the latter is the popular fluorescence polarization immunoassay for T uptake.[180] In this competitive assay, fluorescein-labeled T_4 is added to the serum specimen and binds to TBG and TBPA. As the number of T_4-binding sites increases, more labeled T_4 is bound. As a result, the degree of polarization of the protein-bound tracer increases, because this complex is larger than the free tracer. Specified quantities of T_4 antibody in a buffered protein matrix are used as calibrators. The observed polarization is directly proportional to the total serum TBP binding capacity and inversely related to percent T uptake. Test results are usually reported in "T-uptake units," but may be mathematically transformed into percent T-uptake equivalents. This method reflects the total number of binding sites rather than the concentration of unoccupied binding sites.[205]

To improve the understanding of THBR tests from different laboratories, the Committee on Nomenclature of the American Thyroid Association has recommended that uptake results for individual patients be normalized to those of a control serum (or reference serum pool) obtained from euthyroid patients who have normal quantities of TBPs.[114] The quotient of these results is proportional to the free fraction of T_4 or T_3 in serum and is properly known as the THBR:

$$\text{THBR} = \frac{\% \text{ uptake (patient serum)}}{\% \text{ uptake (reference serum)}}$$

A value of 1.0 indicates that the two values are identical. Some laboratories prepare their own normal reference serum pool, stored frozen at −70 °C in small aliquots, to analyze in every assay run. This enables the laboratory to maintain consistency in T-uptake values in case of changes in assay procedure or kit components. Other laboratories determine a mean uptake value for their own local reference populations to use in calculating the THBR. Terms such as "T_3-resin uptake" or "T_3 uptake" are a continuing source of confusion and should be avoided.

Unfortunately, different laboratories calculate THBR either as being directly or indirectly related to TBG concentration and this causes laboratories and physicians confusion.

Specimen Collection and Storage. The preferred specimen is serum. Specimens may be stored at 4 °C for 1 week or at −20 °C for 30 days. Repeated freezing and thawing, mixing using a vortex mixer, or vigorous agitation of serum specimens should be avoided, because such treatment causes denaturation of proteins. The use of hemolyzed or lipemic specimens is also not recommended.

Reference Intervals. Although centered on a ratio of 1.0, reference values for THBR may differ by method and by local population. Each laboratory therefore should establish its own reference intervals. The following values are representative:[209]

	THBR
Cord	0.75-1.05
Children	
1-3 days	0.90-1.40
1-2 wk	0.85-1.15
1-4 mo	0.75-1.05
1-15 yr	0.88-1.12
Adult	0.83-1.15
>50 yr	
Male	0.87-1.11
Female	0.80-1.04
Pregnancy (last 5 mo)	0.68-0.87

Comments. In hyperthyroidism, more binding sites—and in hypothyroidism, fewer binding sites—on TBG are occupied by T_4. As a result, the THBR is high in hyperthyroidism and low in hypothyroidism. In cases of decreased and increased TBG (see Box 52-1), the THBR is high and low, respectively. Deviations of THBR and total T_4 in the same direction from normal (i.e., a concordant variance) suggest an abnormality in thyroid hormone production; a discordant variance suggests a primary change in the concentration or affinity of circulating TBG (Table 52-3).

Calculation of Free T_4 and T_3 Indexes

The THBR assay is not designed to be used as an independent and isolated test for thyroid disease. It is useful only when combined with a measurement of total T_4 (or T_3) concentration to calculate an FT_4 or FT_3 index.

Principle

The calculation of an FT_4 index is based on the equilibrium relationship that exists between bound [TBP:T_4] and FT_4:

TABLE 52-3 Diagnostic Utility of THBR and FT_4 Index

Clinical Condition	Total T_4	THBR	FY_4I
Euthyroid	N	N	N
Hyperthyroid	↑	↑	↑
Hypothyroid	↓	↓	↓
Increased TBH	↑	↓	N
Decreased TBH	↓	↑	N

N, Normal; ↑, increase; ↓, decrease.

$$[FT_4] + [uTBP] \underset{}{\overset{K}{\rightleftharpoons}} [TBP{:}T_4]$$

Here, [uTBP] represents unsaturated (unoccupied) binding sites on TBPs, and *K* represents the equilibrium constant for the interaction. This interaction can also be expressed by the mass action equation:

$$K = \frac{[TBP{:}T_4]}{[FT_4] \times [uTBP]}$$

Rearranging,

$$K[FT_4] = \frac{[TBP{:}T_4]}{K[uTBP]}$$

Because more than 99.97% of the total T_4 circulating in blood is protein bound, the term [TBP:T_4] is essentially replaced by the total T_4 concentration. Also, because [uTBP] (the concentration of unoccupied TBP binding sites) varies inversely with the THBR, then

$$K \times [FT_4] = [T_4] \times \frac{1}{[uTBP]} = [T_4] \times \text{THBR}$$

If FT_4I is defined as $K \times [FT_4]$, then

$$FT_4I = [T_4] \times \text{THBR}$$

The FT_3 index is calculated similar to the FT_4 index, as $T_3 \times$ THBR, and is used in the same way as an estimate of FT_3. In general, the FT_3 index offers no advantage over the FT_4 index and is used less frequently in clinical practice.

Reference Intervals

Reference intervals for FT_4 and FT_3 indices are derived in two ways: (1) directly from matched total T_4 (or T_3) and THBR results obtained from a sufficiently large number of euthyroid individuals or (2) indirectly by calculation from reference intervals established for total T_4 (or T_3) and THBR. In the latter case, the lower limit of the FT_4 index is calculated by multiplying the lower limit of the THBR interval and the lower limit of the T_4 interval; the upper limit of the FT_4 index interval is obtained by multiplying the upper limit of the THBR interval and the upper limit of the T_4 interval. Estimates based on calculation may yield a broader reference interval for FT_4 and FT_3 indices than the first approach.

Reference intervals are numerically close to the normal intervals for total T_4 or T_3. Most automated immunoassay analyzers are capable of performing the THBR and total T_4 tests with online calculation of the FT_4 index. Theoretically, because the calculated indices are products of T_4 or T_3 concentrations and a ratio, they have concentration units. However, to avoid confusion with serum T_4 or T_3, the free hormone index units are usually omitted or termed "index units." Typical values are as follows:[52]

	FT_4 INDEX	
	µg/dL	nmol/L
Cord	6.0-13.2	77-170
Infant		
1-3 days	9.9-17.5	128-226
1 wk	7.5-15.1	97-195
1-12 mo	5.0-13.0	65-168
Children		
1-10 yr	5.4-12.8	70-165
Pubertal child and adult	4.2-13.0	54-168

Comments

A number of pseudonyms for the FT_4 index have appeared in the literature and in commercial kits; this has led to some confusion. Effective thyroxine ratio, T-7, and T-12 are only a few examples. Such terms are now archaic and should not be used.

Unlike direct FT_4 methods, index methods measure both the serum total T_4 and the FT_4 fraction and have the advantage that they can define whether an abnormal FT_4 estimate is due to abnormal hormone production or to abnormal protein binding.

An FT_4 index is sometimes directly calculated using the percentage T uptake:

$$FT_4I = \text{Total } T_4\ (\mu g/dL) \times \frac{\%\ \text{T uptake}}{100}$$

$FT_4I = \text{Total } T_4\ (mg/dL) \times \%\ \text{T uptake}/100$

Typical reference intervals are 1.5 to 4.4. Calculations using THBR are preferred.[114]

Calculation of T_4/TBG and T_3/TBG Ratios

Measurements of serum TBG concentration have been used in the diagnosis of thyroid disease in two ways. The most common approach is to calculate a T_4:TBG or T_3:TBG ratio.[18] Such indices are derived from mass action equations and are used to approximate FT_4 or FT_3 concentrations. These ratios correlate variably with FT_4 or FT_3 concentrations and are particularly useful in sera with altered TBG concentrations; however, they may fail to compensate for TBG variants with reduced T_4 affinity or for abnormal albumin binding. The reference interval for T_4:TBG ratios is 3.8 to 4.5 when the reference intervals for total T_4 and TBG are 4.5 to 12.5 µg/dL and 1.2 to 2.8 mg/dL, respectively.

Measurements of TBG also have been used to derive values for FT_4 or FT_3 by calculation. Assuming TBG is the major determinant of thyroid hormone binding, serum concentrations of TBG and total T_4 (or T_3), together with the association constant for the binding of T_4 (or T_3) to TBG, are used to calculate values of the free hormone. In most cases, these calculated values correlate well with those directly determined.

Direct Immunoassay Methods

Immunoassays of various designs for estimating free thyroid hormones using antibody extraction techniques have been developed.[48,122] These assays are subdivided as either *sequential two-step assays* or *simultaneous one-step ("analogue") assays.* Each procedure involves the direct incubation of serum with a specific anti-T_4 or anti-T_3 antibody, during which thyroid hormones reach a new equilibrium with all of the binders present. A slight decrease in free hormone concentration occurs, but is insignificant if the antibody sequesters less than 5% of the total amount of hormone present in the specimen. Thus the amount of immunoextracted T_4 or T_3 closely approximates the undisturbed free hormone concentration that preexists in serum at equilibrium.

Two-Step Immunoassays. These methods use two processing steps. In the first step, the serum specimen is incubated briefly with specific solid-phase antibody. Under standard conditions of temperature and incubation time, a percentage of the total thyroid hormone proportional to the original FT_4 or FT_3 concentration is extracted and bound by the antibody. After thorough washing to remove serum proteins and other interfering substances, a second step estimates the remaining unoccupied (vacant) antibody binding sites by back titration with labeled T_4 or T_3. Excess label is then washed away from the solid-phase antibody, and the quantity of bound tracer is compared with a calibration curve generated from secondary calibrators that have had target values assigned to them by a reference method. The amount of labeled hormone retained by the antibody is inversely related to the free hormone concentration in the test specimen.

The key feature of this two-step method is that the labeled hormone is physically prevented from interacting with serum binding proteins. This ensures that antibody binding of tracer is governed solely by the free hormone concentration and not by changes in thyroid hormone–binding proteins. Test results obtained with two-step methods correlate well with those obtained by reference methods across a wide range of clinical disorders.

A sequential two-step immunoassay for FT_4 was first introduced commercially in 1979.[34] Subsequently, a number of manual and automated procedures have become available for FT_4 and FT_3. The earliest kit methods used radioactive labels and antibody-coated tubes or microbeads, but automated systems are now available that use nonisotopic tracers and a variety of solid-phase formats.[20] One two-step FT_4 method involves the application of serum to glass-fiber paper on which the clinical specimen reacts with preimmobilized anti-T_4 antibody.[187] After a 2-minute incubation period, an alkaline phosphatase–labeled T_4 conjugate binds to unoccupied antibody binding sites and at the same time washes out the protein-bound T_4 fraction. After a second incubation (3 minutes), excess unbound conjugate is washed from the filter paper by radial elution. A fluorogenic substrate for the enzyme is also included in the wash solution to initiate the enzyme reaction. Enzyme activity of the bound conjugate is measured by front-faced fluorimetry and is inversely related to the concentration of FT_4 in the sample.

Two-step microparticle capture immunoassays have been developed to fully automate the measurement of free thyroid hormones.[12,89] In one type of FT_4 assay, FT_4 is first immunoextracted from serum using polyclonal anti–T_4-coated latex microparticles; T_4 bound to serum proteins does not react with the antibody. An aliquot of the reaction mixture is then transferred to a glass fiber matrix that irreversibly captures the T_4–anti-T_4–microparticle complex; washing removes any serum materials not bound to the solid phase. In the second back-titration step, the remaining unoccupied antibody binding sites are reacted with a T_3–alkaline phosphatase conjugate; serum binding proteins are not available for binding to this enzyme conjugate. Excess unbound enzyme conjugate is removed by washing followed by addition of the substrate, 4-methylumbelliferyl phosphate, to the matrix cell. The concentration of the fluorescent product varies inversely with the amount of FT_4 in the serum. A T_3–alkaline phosphatase conjugate is used in this assay system rather than a T_4 conjugate because of its lower affinity for the anti-T_4 antibody. Although the T_3 conjugate possesses the ability to bind to vacant anti-T_4 sites on the microparticles, this enzyme label does not displace or dislodge FT_4 already bound to the microparticles. The detection limit of this assay (defined as mean minus 2 SD of the zero calibrator) is approximately 0.4 ng/dL. Interassay reproducibility, expressed as coefficient of variation, is typically ±3% to 6% over a concentration range of 0.6 to 3.5 ng/dL (8 to 45 pmol/L); cross-reactivity with FT_3 is less than 0.5%.

One-Step Immunoassays. These methods are widely used for direct estimation of FT_4 or FT_3 and are known as one-step or "hormone analogue" immunoassays. These single-step techniques are usually subdivided into formats relying on labeled hormone analogue and solid-phase antibody or those relying on labeled antibody and solid-phase hormone analogue. Both approaches use structurally modified analogues of thyroid hormones that, in theory, retain the ability to compete with free hormone for binding to specific anti-T_4 or anti-T_3 antibodies but are chemically restricted from interacting with thyroid hormone–binding proteins in the serum specimen. Unlike two-step methods, analogue assays rely on simultaneous rather than sequential back-titration of unoccupied antibody-binding sites. For one-step methods to succeed, the hormone analogue should not displace T_4 (or T_3) from binding proteins; binding of the hormone analogue by serum proteins must be either totally absent or essentially insignificant.

Labeled-Analogue Methods. In a typical one-step RIA for FT_4, endogenous free hormone and a ^{125}I-labeled T_4 analogue compete for solid-phase antibody binding sites in the presence of serum protein; the amount of labeled analogue bound by the specific antibody is inversely related to the amount of FT_4 in the specimen.[106] Test results are expressed relative to secondary serum calibrators that have been independently calibrated using equilibrium dialysis or ultrafiltration techniques. A number of one-step RIAs have been developed and are commercially available.

The chemical composition of the labeled hormone analogues used in commercial kits is proprietary. However, it has been speculated that some analogue tracers are produced by altering the alanine side chain of the iodothyronine molecule, thus hindering the binding of TBG and TBPA. Unfortunately, most of these synthetic analogue tracers bind significantly to serum proteins, particularly albumin, resulting in inaccurate free hormone measurements when the albumin in patient specimens differs from that in the assay calibrators. Attempts have been made to limit albumin binding by using chemical blockers to saturate albumin binding sites. However, some of these blockers also displace T_4 from TBG, thereby disrupting the equilibrium between free and protein-bound hormone during the assay and making these modified assays TBG-dependent.

It is known that the presence in serum of an abnormal amount of any substance affecting analogue binding—such as endogenous antibody, nonesterified fatty acids, or certain anions—greatly distorts assay results.[50,51] If analogue binding to protein is greater in the serum sample than in the calibrators, as in dysalbuminemia or with T_4 autoantibodies, then less analogue tracer is available to compete for the assay antibody, thus giving a falsely high FT_4 estimate. Conversely, if analogue binding to protein is less in the sample than in the calibrators, e.g., increased binding of albumin by nonesterified fatty acids or decreased serum albumin concentration, then FT_4 estimates are falsely low.[200]

Techniques involving nonradioactive conjugates that claim to reduce some of these problems have been introduced. For example, one-step enzyme immunoassays for FT_4 in which a T_4-peroxidase conjugate competes with FT_4 for a solid-phase antibody have been described.[108] A chemiluminescence system based on similar principles involves the use of a T_4-acridinium ester conjugate that competes with free hormone for binding sites on antibodies immobilized on paramagnetic particles.[110] Manufacturers claim that these conjugates are insignificantly bound by serum-binding proteins. A number of automated immunoassay systems based on single-step, labeled-analogue methods are commercially available for estimating both FT_4 and FT_3 concentrations.

Labeled-Antibody Method. Most one-step immunoassays use labeled analogues of T_4 or T_3. Alternatively a number of labeled antibody methods have also been developed in which the distribution of a labeled antibody between exogenous

TABLE 52-4 Free Thyroxine Measurements in Common Conditions Affecting Thyroid-Binding Proteins

Clinical Condition	Direct Equilibrium Dialysis/RIA*	Other Index Methods	Two-Step Methods	Analogue Methods
Near Normal Concentration of Serum Binding Proteins				
Hypothyroidism	L	L	L	L
Hyperthyroidism	H	H	H	H
Hyperestrogenism	N	N	N	N
Abnormal Concentration of Serum Binding Proteins				
TBG excess	N	H	N	L, N, or H
TBG deficiency	N	L	N	L, N, or H
Dysalbuminemia	N	N-H†	N	H
Hypoalbuminemia	N	N	N	N-L
T_4 autoantibody	N	H	N	H
Low T_4 NTI	H	L	N-L	L
High T_4 NTI	N-H	N-H	N-H	H

From Hay ID, Bayer MF, Kaplan MK, et al: American Thyroid Association Assessment of current free thyroid hormone and thyrotropin measurement and guidelines for future clinical assays. Clin Chem 1991;37:2002-8.
L, Low; *H,* high; *N,* normal; *NTI,* nonthyroidal illness.
*Methods involving minimal dilution.
†Normal when determined with labeled T_4, high when with labeled T_3.
Note: The National Academy of Clinical Biochemistry practice guidelines for the use of thyroid tests for the diagnosis and monitoring of thyroid disease was published in Thyroid 2003;13:1-126 and is also available on the NACB web site www.nacb.org.

solid-phase hormone and free hormone reflects the free hormone concentration.[26,27,181] This assay design is similar to the labeled-analogue principle except that unoccupied antibody-binding sites are identified by their absorption from the reaction mixture onto a hormone analogue coupled to a solid support. Linking of T_4 or T_3 to the solid phase creates a macroanalogue with a reduced interaction with serum proteins.[49,159] These labeled-antibody assays are claimed to be more reliable than labeled-analogue methods and to be less sensitive to major protein modifications or progressive dilution of serum.

Reference Intervals.[33] Expected values using a one-step immunochemiluminometric assay are as follows: for FT_4, 0.8 to 2.3 ng/dL (10 to 30 pmol/L); for FT_3, 230 to 420 pg/dL (3.5 to 6.5 pmol/L).

Selection and Use of Tests for Measuring Free Thyroid Hormones

Estimates of FT_4 and FT_3 generally give results in healthy subjects, hyperthyroid and hypothyroid patients, and patients with only mild binding protein abnormalities that are comparable with those of reference methods such as direct equilibrium dialysis and RIA assays. In these individuals, the selection of a specific FT_4 or FT_3 measurement method can be based on factors such as technical convenience, turnaround time, commercial availability, and cost. In certain clinical conditions, free hormone estimate methods may give abnormal results that differ from the generally normal values obtained using direct reference methods. These abnormalities, summarized in Table 52-4 and discussed later, are commonly encountered in euthyroid patients who show significant changes in T_4 or T_3 binding to serum proteins. In these situations, the selection of appropriate FT_4 or FT_3 estimate methods should be based more on their analytical and diagnostic reliability than on the ease of performance and cost.

Unfortunately, FT_4 and FT_3 estimate methods have been found to be unreliable in a number of situations. One of these is familial dysalbuminemic hyperthyroidism, an inherited disorder in which a normally minor component of serum albumin is increased. This variant albumin binds T_4 with abnormally high affinity, but its avidity for T_3 is not comparably increased. Although total T_4 concentrations are usually high, patients with familial dysalbuminemic hyperthyroidism are clinically euthyroid, and free hormone concentrations are normal as measured by reference methods and by most two-step immunoassays. However, if tracer T_3 is used to estimate the FT_4 fraction, the resin uptake and THBR results are normal, and the calculated FT_4 index is falsely increased. (In contrast, uptake methods using T_4 tracers provide more accurate THBR and FT_4 index values.) One-step immunoassays likewise give high FT_4 estimates owing to the binding of the T_4 analogue to the variant albumin. Test results similar to those in familial dysalbuminemic hyperthyroidism are also obtained from patients with circulating T_4 autoantibodies or when T_4 binding by prealbumin is increased.

In addition, FT_4 and FT_3 estimate methods are not reliable when used in patients with congenital TBG excess or deficiency. Patients with these conditions are clinically euthyroid, and their FT_4 and FT_3 concentrations are normal as determined by direct reference methods and two-step immunoassays. Index methods and one-step analogue immunoassays, however, yield abnormal results. For example, in the case of TBG excess, total serum concentrations of T_4 and T_3 are increased, and the THBR is low. However, the THBR is not linearly related to the free fraction of T_4 or T_3 at extremes of the free fraction range. Accordingly, the THBR cannot be reduced as much as the free fraction, and the calculated FT_4 index is abnormally high.

Another situation in which free hormone estimates may be unreliable is in the assessment of critically ill patients who are believed to be euthyroid (i.e., have a nonthyroidal illness). For example, serum FT_4 concentrations in nonthyroidal illness patients with low total T_4 values are usually normal or high by reference methods, whereas most FT_4 or FT_3 estimates give low values, although some consistently provide normal results. Distinguishing severe nonthyroidal illness from true hypothyroidism presents a difficult analytical challenge. This is why the current NACB guidelines recommend the use of TT_4 in preference to current FT_4E tests.

Estimates of FT_4 or FT_3 may be profoundly affected by medications that compete with T_4 or T_3 for binding to serum proteins. With reference methods that use undiluted serum, the free hormone concentration may rise and eventually return to a new steady state in the presence of T_4- or T_3-displacing drugs. In contrast, most estimates of FT_4 or FT_3 use diluted serum in which the drug competitor declines before the free hormone declines. Consequently the hormone-displacing effect of the drug also decreases, leading to a major underestimation of the true FT_4 concentration.

Rigorous evaluation of free thyroid hormone methods is required before new assays are placed into clinical service.[80] Performance data on analytical accuracy should be obtained not only on serum from patients with thyroid dysfunction but also in serum from patients with binding protein abnormalities. Effects of drugs that compete for hormone binding sites on serum proteins should also be evaluated. Moreover, adequate assessment requires an examination of the effects of progressive sample dilution. In theory, the free concentration of T_4 and T_3 should not decrease with dilution until about 20% of the bound ligand is dissociated. In the case of T_4, this decrease occurs at a dilution of about 1:1000 (1:100 for T_3). Near constancy of assay results in the face of progressive serum dilution is widely accepted as the classic test of FT_4 (or FT_3) validity.[47,148,225] In practice, many methods demonstrate lower than predicted free hormone concentrations with dilution.

Determination of Thyroxine-Binding Globulin and Other Thyroid Hormone–Binding Proteins

TBG is the thyroid hormone–binding protein having the greatest affinity for T_4. As such, it is very important in regulating the concentration of the FT_4 hormone. Estrogen-induced TBG excess and congenital TBG deficiency are the most significant TBG abnormalities that affect the interpretation of thyroid function test results (see Box 52-1).

Principle

TBG is measured indirectly in terms of its T_4-binding capacity or preferably by the direct determination of the protein concentration of TBG. Tests based on binding capacity are usually performed by adding to the test serum a mixture of unlabeled and radiolabeled T_4 in a concentration sufficient to saturate all the binding sites on the TBG. Binding to T_4-binding prealbumin (transthyretin, TBPA) can be blocked by carrying out the reaction in a barbital buffer; the excess (unbound) T_4 is removed with dextran-coated charcoal that also strips T_4 from albumin and other weak binders. The fraction of radioactivity associated with the supernatant is then multiplied by the amount of T_4 added to the serum to give the T_4-binding capacity for TBG (units: μg T_4/dL). In normal adult sera, the binding capacity for TBG ranges from 16 to 24 μg T_4/dL. Although this assay is relatively specific for TBG (i.e., TBPA and albumin do not react appreciably), various drugs or abnormal thyroid hormone binders may interfere by inhibiting T_4 binding, thus giving artificially low values for TBG.

Direct measurement of the protein concentration of TBG by immunoassay is more widely used because it is technically less complex and offers increased precision and immunospecificity. A typical RIA measures the competition between endogenous TBG and ^{125}I-labeled TBG for binding with a limited quantity of TBG antisera.[69] After incubation, bound and free fractions are separated using either a polyethylene glycol precipitant or a mixture of polyethylene glycol and second antibody. Commercial kits based on both isotopic and nonisotopic formats are available. One competitive chemiluminescence enzyme immunoassay for TBG makes use of peroxidase-labeled TBG and TBG antibody, which is captured by a solid-phase second antibody.[133] The bound conjugate is measured by enhanced luminescence after the addition of luminol and hydrogen peroxide. The dynamic range of the assay is 5 to 80 mg/L, and the interassay imprecision is less than ±10% at three concentrations. In healthy adults, the reference interval is 12 to 28 mg/L. Automated nonisotopic immunoassays for TBG are also available, such as the procedure based on the principle of enhanced microparticle turbidimetry.[73] In this test, the rate of agglutination of serum TBG and a solid-phase TBG antibody is determined by measuring the absorbance change at 600 nm.

TBG tests that use labeled T_4 have also been developed. In one commercial assay, a two-site IRMA or "sandwich" assay is used.[207] TBG antibody bound to glass particles is added in excess to the patient specimen and binds virtually all the endogenous TBG present. ^{125}I-T_4 is then added; it binds to the TBG, forming an anti-TBG-TBG-^{125}I-T_4 sandwich. After a short 15-minute incubation period at room temperature, the precipitate is collected by centrifugation and its radioactivity is counted. Test values are interpreted from a calibration curve run simultaneously with the patient specimens. Unlike the typical RIA procedure, radioactivity in this IRMA method is directly proportional to the amount of TBG present in the specimen. Patients with molecular variants of TBG may have discordant results, but the assay is not affected by excess thyroxine or phenytoin.[147]

Individual TBPs have been measured using electrophoresis to assess binding of radioactive T_4.[101] In this procedure, excess unlabeled T_4 and radiolabeled T_4 are added to the test specimen to saturate the binding of TBG. Total T_4 is determined on this enriched serum, which is then subjected to electrophoresis. Radioactivity bound to the individual protein bands (albumin, prealbumin, and TBG) is counted, and the fraction associated with each band is calculated. The fractional radioactivity is then multiplied by the total T_4 concentration in the T_4-enriched serum to give the T_4-binding capacity of each particular protein. Binding capacity of TBG for T_4 in normal serum generally ranges from 10 to 25 μg/dL of prealbumin for T_4 from 49 to 70 μg/dL, and of albumin for T_4 from 12 to 34 μg/dL.

The major application of this electrophoretic method is the identification of patients with euthyroid hyperthyroxinemias or euthyroid hypothyroxinemias.[81] This assay distinguishes abnormalities in the concentration of normal T_4-binding proteins from abnormal binding proteins with altered affinities for T_4. Congenital and drug-induced elevations (or deficiencies) of TBG are examples of the former. Anti-T_4 antibodies and unusual forms of albumin and prealbumin are examples of the latter.

Specimen Collection and Storage

Serum is the preferred specimen; plasma with EDTA or heparin as anticoagulant may also be used. Serum specimens are best stored at 2 °C to 8 °C if they will not be tested within 24 hours. If longer periods of storage are necessary, freezing the specimens is recommended. Frozen specimens are stable for at least 30 days. Repeated freezing and thawing of the specimens should be avoided. Turbid samples should be centrifuged before testing.

Determination of Thyroglobulin

Tg is a large glycoprotein having a molecular weight of 660 kDa that is stored in the follicular colloid of the thyroid gland. It functions as a propeptide for the intrathyroidal synthesis of T_4 and T_3. It is made by the follicular cells and secreted into the follicular lumen where it is iodinated, after which its iodinated tyrosyl moieties form T_4 and T_3. Thyroglobulins are then taken up by endocytosis into the follicular cells, where T_4 and T_3 are liberated by proteolysis, followed by release into the extracellular fluid and thence to the bloodstream.

Principle

Traditionally, circulating concentrations of Tg have been measured using double-antibody immunoassays.[213] Commercial RIA kits based on sequential addition techniques have been developed for routine use. These methods involve the preliminary incubation of serum with primary antibody. After a number of hours (2 to 72), the Tg tracer is added and allowed to compete for antibody binding sites. The longer the preincubation the more sensitive the method. Separation of bound from free Tg is then accomplished by precipitation with a second antibody.

Two-site immunometric assays have also been developed for Tg. These assays are based on the use of two or more monoclonal antibodies directed to different portions of the Tg molecule. One of the antibodies is attached to a signal molecule, such as a radioisotope, enzyme, or chemiluminescent molecule, and the other to a solid support, such as polystyrene beads or magnetic microbeads.[160,175,226] Another variation is to attach biotin to the antibody and separate the Tg complex using avidin linked to a solid phase.[86,93] Commercial kits based on these techniques are available. Compared to RIAs, these immunometric assays have the advantage of shorter incubation times, a larger working range, a more stable labeled antibody reagent, longer shelf life, and potential for automation. Interassay reproducibility, expressed as a coefficient of variation, is typically less than ±6% at the optimal dose range but can rise to >15% at the extremes of the curve. Limit of detection, derived from the 20% coefficient of variation point of the interassay precision profile, is 0.5 to 1.0 ng/mL.[93] Most current immunometric assays are calibrated using a Tg reference preparation developed by the Community Bureau of Reference. Use of this standard reduces interassay variability somewhat to around 30%, a value that is threefold higher than the within-person variability.[197] The high between-method variability precludes switching between methods during long-term monitoring of patients.

A major difficulty in most immunoassays for Tg is interference due to endogenous anti-Tg antibodies that are present in about 15% to 35% of thyroid cancer patients. Interference effects can be substantial, causing either an overestimation or an underestimation of the true value. With newer immunometric assays, this effect is an underestimation. It is crucial that all serum samples be screened for the presence of anti-Tg with a sensitive immunoassay.[125] When detected, the concentration of such antibodies should be reported, and a warning issued to clinicians to interpret the serum Tg value with caution. Some laboratories assess the impact of anti-Tg interference by measuring the recovery of known amounts of Tg added to patient sera.[55,172,208] If Tg recovery is high (90% to 110%), then significant autoantibody interference may be absent. The reliability of recovery studies, however, has been disputed and is currently discouraged by the NACB.[197] A multisite immunoradiometric assay (IRMA) also has been reported to measure serum Tg with minimal interference from anti-Tg autoantibodies (TgAb).[127] This assay uses five different monoclonal antibodies directed against antigenic regions on the Tg molecule that are not recognized by most anti-TgAb. Four of these antibodies are coupled to polystyrene tubes, and the fifth is coupled to radioiodine. Unfortunately, this approach has not been found to overcome TgAb interference.

Other technical problems, such as heterophilic antibody (HAMA) interference, may limit the clinical value of Tg measurements. Recommendations regarding approaches to standardization, precision, limits of detection, and hook effects have been suggested.[196] Serum Tg values obtained by different methods are usually not interchangeable, and the same assay should be used to perform serial serum Tg measurements in a patient. When a change in method is made, the laboratory should define performance characteristics of the new method and validate its clinical utility before implementing the method for patient care.

Specimen Collection and Storage

Serum is the preferred specimen; plasma with EDTA or heparin as anticoagulant may also be used. Serum specimens are best stored at 2 °C to 8 °C if they will not be tested within 24 hours. If longer periods of storage are necessary, freezing the specimens is recommended. Frozen specimens are stable for at least 30 days. Repeated freezing and thawing of the specimens should be avoided. Turbid samples should be centrifuged before testing.

Reference Interval

The reference interval for Tg in euthyroid individuals ranges from a lower limit of 0.5 to 3 to an upper limit of 20 to 42 ng/mL (3 to 42 μg/L), depending on the method.[131,209] For athyreotic patients not receiving T_4, replacement therapy should have undetectable serum Tg irrespective of TSH status. Tg concentrations are elevated in the neonate and decrease significantly during the first 2 years of life.

Comments

Tg is primarily used as a tumor marker in patients carrying a diagnosis of differentiated thyroid carcinoma (DTC). Although serum Tg is elevated in patients with thyroid cancer, including thyroid follicular and papillary carcinoma, elevations are also are seen in nonneoplastic conditions such as thyroid adenoma, subacute thyroiditis, Hashimoto's thyroiditis, and Graves' disease. Serum Tg concentrations are not increased in patients with medullary thyroid carcinoma. Serial measurement of Tg is most useful in detecting recurrence of DTC following surgical resection or radioactive iodine ablation.[111] Tg determination is used as an adjunct to ultrasound and ^{134}I scanning. Assessment of serum Tg also aids in the management of infants with congenital hypothyroidism. All patients with hyperthyroidism should have elevated Tg; low concentrations of Tg may be an indication that thyrotoxicosis factitia is present.

Determination of Antithyroid Antibodies

Increased circulating concentrations of antithyroid antibodies are found in a variety of thyroid disorders and in other autoimmune diseases and certain malignancies. These autoantibodies are directed against several thyroid and thyroid hormone antigens, including Tg (TgAb), thyroid peroxidase (TPOAb), thyroidal microsomal antigen, the TSH receptor (TRAb), a non-Tg colloid antigen, TSH, T_4, and T_3. Of these antibodies, TPOAb is most commonly used in evaluating thyroid autoimmune diseases, whereas TgAb is used for detecting interference with Tg measurement.

Antithyroglobulin Antibodies

Tg antibodies are directed against the Tg protein, a major constituent of thyroid colloid. Several different techniques have been used to detect and quantify TgAb in peripheral blood. These include passive hemagglutination, the agar gel diffusion precipitin technique, immunofluorescence of tissue sections, enzyme-linked immunosorbent assay (ELISA), radioassay techniques, and chemiluminescence-based immunometric assays.

Principle

In the tanned erythrocyte hemagglutination method, an aliquot of patient serum is mixed with erythrocytes that have been treated with tannic acid and then coated with purified human Tg. When antibodies in the patient's serum combine with Tg antigen bound to erythrocytes, agglutination of the erythrocytes occurs. The use of Tg-coated erythrocytes makes this agglutination reaction much more sensitive than a simple antigen-antibody reaction. Several commercial kits are available for measuring anti-Tg antibodies in serum. A commonly used one is based on the passive hemagglutination method of Boyden.[11] In this system, turkey red blood cells coated with Tg are agglutinated by the specific antibody, yielding a smooth carpet of cells at the bottom of a microtiter well. Lack of agglutination is indicated by the settling of the cells into a compact ring or button. Before testing, patient sera are deactivated at 56 °C for 30 minutes. Heating is important for inactivation of complement and TBG, which otherwise would interfere with the assay.

Serial dilutions of the patient's serum are used to establish a Tg antibody titer. The reported result is the highest dilution that causes agglutination. Titers are usually considered negative at a less than 1:10 dilution ratio. This hemagglutination test is not highly specific, and about 5% to 10%

of the normal population may have a low titer of Tg antibodies with no symptoms of disease, an incidence that is higher in women and that increases with age. Reactivity occurs more frequently in Hashimoto's thyroiditis (>85% of patients) and Graves' disease (>30% of patients); titers greater than 1 : 1600 are common. Positive responses are also seen in patients with idiopathic myxedema (>75% of cases), but antibody titers are generally lower. Weakly positive tests may also be found in patients with nontoxic goiter, thyroid cancer, and pernicious anemia; in these patients, antibody titers are not found with any greater frequency than in an unselected population.

Agglutination tests are being rapidly replaced by more sensitive immunoassays that can be automated. Radioimmunoassays, ELISA, and chemiluminescence-based immunoassays have been all been developed for measuring both Tg and TPO antibodies.[144] Several commercial kits and automated methods are currently available, including systems based on Tg-coated cells, particles, magnetic beads, microtiter plates, or tubes and chemiluminescence automated instruments. These methods correlate well with agglutination tests and are generally more sensitive and more specific for thyroid autoimmune diseases. Some assays allow identification of subclasses of Tg antibodies; the clinical significance of these subclasses, however, is not known.

In a typical IRMA,[1] Tg antibodies in diluted serum specimens bind to human Tg in coated test tubes. After incubation for 1 hour at 37 °C, the tubes are washed and ^{125}I-labeled protein A is added. After another 1 hour of incubation at 37 °C, the supernatants are washed again and the radioactivity counted. The amount of bound radioactivity in each tube is directly proportional to the amount of anti-Tg antibody present. Interassay precision is about 3% at 36 U/mL.

A nonisotopic ELISA method in which serum specimens are added to microtiter wells coated with human Tg is also available.[176] In this method, antibody binding is assessed using a peroxidase-conjugated anti-IgG/*o*-phenylenediamine system. An automated two-step fluorescent enzyme immunoassay has been reported.[183] In this assay, Tg is immobilized on magnetic beads, and anti-human IgG mouse monoclonal antibody is labeled with alkaline phosphatase; 4-methylumbelliferyl phosphate is used as the substrate. IRMA and ELISA both have similar detection limits (approximately 3 to 5 U/mL). A considerably more sensitive radioassay has been reported in which diluted serum is incubated with ^{125}I-labeled Tg to allow formation of antigen-antibody complexes[9]; these complexes are then precipitated by adding solid-phase protein A. Its detection limit is reported to be approximately 0.2 U/mL.

Specimen Collection and Storage

The preferred specimen for testing is serum, which should be kept frozen if the test is not performed on the day that the blood is drawn. Repeated freezing and thawing must be avoided.

Reference Interval

Assessment of a normal reference interval for anti-Tg antibodies is controversial, mainly due to the fact that Tg autoantibodies have been found in individuals without apparent thyroid disease. Variable reference intervals have been reported, depending on whether a random population was sampled or a population without active or previous thyroid disease. Thyroglobulin antibodies follow a logarithmic normal distribution and are usually expressed as units per milliliter with reference to the MRC 1st IRP for Thyroglobulin Autoantibody 65/93. As with TPOAb, TgAb methods fall into two classes. Class 1 methods have a lower numeric detection limit (<2 IU/ml) and report that normal individuals should not have antibody detected. Class 2 methods have a higher numeric detection limit (>10 IU/mL) and report a "normal range.[33]"

Comments

The measurement of TgAb adds little diagnostic information over and above TPOAb measurement for diagnosing autoimmune thyroid disease.[85A] However, measurement of TgAb is needed to identify sera with autoantibodies that may interfere with serum Tg measurements in patients being managed for treatment of thyroid carcinoma.

Antimicrosomal/Antithyroid Peroxidase Antibodies

Principle

Antimicrosomal antibodies are directed against a protein component of thyroid cell microsomes. These autoantibodies are measured using complement fixation, immunofluorescence of tissue sections, passive hemagglutination, ELISA techniques, or radioassay methods. The tanned erythrocyte agglutination method uses cells that have been coated with microsomal antigen isolated from human hyperplastic thyroid glands. This semiquantitative procedure is simple, and commercial kits are available. Reactivity occurs in nearly all adult patients with Hashimoto's thyroiditis and in about 85% of patients with Graves' disease. Low titers, however, may be seen in 5% to 10% of normal asymptomatic individuals. Hemagglutination tests for TgAb and TPOAb are often performed together. Of the two, the result of the one for TPOAb is more frequently positive for thyroid autoimmune disease and usually is in higher concentration. This is particularly the case in patients younger than 20 years.

Procedures for the more sensitive ELISA and radioassays are similar to those previously described for anti-Tg antibodies; a number of quantitative commercial kits are available. A combined micro-ELISA for simultaneous measurement of TgAb and TPOAb antibodies in a single test has also been described.[151] Microsomal antibody concentrations are usually expressed in units per milliliter with reference to the MRC IRP for Microsomal Autoantibody 66/387. The mean TPOAb activity, measured with an IRMA kit, is 280 ± 60 IU/mL in normal sera.[129]

The enzyme TPO is now recognized as the principal and possibly only autoantigenic component of thyroid microsomes. Assays based on TPO itself are preferred for routine clinical use in the management of patients with suspected autoimmune disease of the thyroid. Performance of antimicrosomal antibody assays is complicated by the limited availability of human thyroid tissue, the presence of irrelevant thyroid antigens and autoantibodies, and the contamination of microsome preparations with Tg.[53] These complications seem to have been eliminated by using TPO as the antigen.

Purification of TPO by affinity chromatography or production by recombinant techniques has led to the development of assays for anti-TPO antibodies based on RIA or chemiluminescence-based immunometric techniques.[59,61] These procedures provide greater sensitivity and specificity than passive hemagglutination assays for microsomal antibodies in detecting, confirming, and monitoring autoimmune thyroid disorders[126,129] and are more suitable for screening or high-volume testing. The immunometric assay of Ruf and coworkers,[167] for example, is based on competitive inhibition of the binding of radioiodinated TPO to an anti-TPO monoclonal antibody coated onto plastic tubes. This assay is rapid (only one 2-hour incubation period is involved), easy to perform, and available as a commercial kit. The design of the assay ensures specific measurement with minimal interference from Tg or TgAb. Manual and automated nonisotopic immunoassays for anti-TPO are also available[81,86,183]; detection limits range from 0.3 to 2 U/mL.

Reference Interval

The normal reference interval for TPOAb is controversial. With sensitive assays, low concentrations of TPOAb may be detected in some healthy individuals without thyroid disease. There is a high prevalence of anti-TPO antibodies in the elderly.[203] However, longitudinal studies suggest that the presence of TPOAb is a risk factor for autoimmune thyroid dysfunction. TPO antibody concentrations are usually expressed as units per milliliter with reference to the MRC Standard 66/387. With a competitive IRMA, the mean TPOAb activity in normal sera is 69 ± 15 U/mL (SEM).[129] Using a sensitive chemiluminescence assay, values are less than 2 U/mL.[33]

Comments

Detectable concentrations of TPOAb are observed in nearly all patients with Hashimoto's thyroiditis and idiopathic myxedema and in the majority of patients with Graves' disease. These antibodies have also been demonstrated in the sera of patients with type I insulin-dependent diabetes mellitus. The frequency of detectable TPOAb antibodies observed in nonimmune thyroid disease is similar to that observed in a normal population.[53]

Thyrotropin-Receptor Antibodies

Thyrotropin-receptor antibodies are a group of related immunoglobulins that bind to thyroid cell membranes at or near the TSH-receptor site. These antibodies are frequently found in the sera of patients with Graves' disease or other thyroid autoimmune disorders. In general, these antibodies demonstrate substantial heterogeneity; some cause thyroid stimulation, whereas others have no effect or decrease thyroid secretion by blocking the action of TSH. At present, these abnormal immunoglobulins cannot be differentiated by chemical or immunological methods; rather, their presence is demonstrated using radioreceptor assays or bioassays with cAMP as the endpoint.

The first indication that autoantibodies to the TSH receptor might play a role in the pathogenesis of Graves' disease came with the discovery of long-acting thyroid stimulator (LATS) in the serum of some patients. The estimation of LATS using in vivo bioassay is important historically.[67] In a modification of the LATS assay, the so-called *LATS protector assay,* antibody binding to a thyroid homogenate prevents the expected inhibition of the standard LATS response.[72] This indirect assay is more sensitive than the direct LATS assay, but is cumbersome and seldom used in laboratories today.

The direct radioreceptor assay assesses the capacity of immunoglobulins to inhibit the binding of labeled TSH to its receptors in human or animal thyroid membrane preparations. Such antibodies are usually designated *thyrotropin-binding inhibitory immunoglobulins* (TBII). In this method, originally described by Shewring and Rees-Smith,[182] detergent-solubilized porcine TSH receptors and ^{125}I-labeled TSH are used. The ability of a purified fraction of serum immunoglobulins to displace ^{125}I-labeled TSH from the receptors is measured.[16] This method, available as a commercial kit, detects more than 85% of patients with Graves' disease and requires only 2 to 3 hours to perform.[130] Normal immunoglobulin G concentrates do not produce significant displacement of labeled TSH from the TSH receptor (<10% inhibition). This method detects all TSH receptor antibodies but cannot distinguish whether the antibodies stimulate the TSH receptor to cause hyperthyroidism or block the TSH receptor to cause hypothyroidism. Measurement of TBII is mainly used in pregnant women with present or past Graves' disease to assess the risk of fetal or neonatal thyrotoxicosis occurring secondary to transplacental passage of maternal antibodies.[21,60,138]

In vitro bioassays assess the capacity of immunoglobulins to stimulate functional activity of the thyroid gland, such as adenylate cyclase stimulation, cAMP formation, colloid mobilization, or iodothyronine release. Such antibodies are often referred to as *thyroid-stimulating immunoglobulins* (TSIs). Measuring the increase in cAMP concentration has been accomplished using human thyroid slices, frozen human thyroid cells in culture, or a cloned line of thyroid follicular cells (FRTL-5).[102,215] The last of these has greatly facilitated TSI measurements, and assays for TSIs can be performed in 1 day. In this test, the cell line is grown to confluency and then deprived of TSH. The thyroid cells then become very sensitive to stimulation by immunoglobulin G preparations from patients with Graves' disease. These immunoglobulins mimic the effect of TSH, activating adenylate cyclase. Cyclic AMP is subsequently released into the surrounding medium and assayed. The effect of stimulation is expressed as a percentage of basal activity; the range in normal serum is 70% to 130%. TSIs are present in 95% of patients with untreated Graves' disease. In addition to being a highly sensitive and specific indicator of Graves' disease, TSI measurement is also used for following the course of therapy and predicting relapse and remission.[59,145] However, the marginal clinical value of this test in individual patients together with its relatively high cost suggests that TSI may not be the ideal measure for the diagnosis and management of Graves' hyperthyroidism.[60]

REFERENCES

1. Antithyroglobulin Antibody IRMA Test (package insert). Dana Point, CA: Kronus Inc, 1987.
2. Babson AL, Olson DR, Palmieri T, Ross AF, Becker DM, Mulqueen PJ. The Immulite assay tube: A new approach to heterogenous ligand assay. Clin Chem 1991;37:1521-2.
3. Bahar I, Kana A, Woodring C, Lekousi S, Inbar S, Metzmann E. Rapid self-contained immunoassay for total T3. Clin Chem 1991;37:940.
4. Baqui M, Botero D, Gereben B, Curcio C, Harney JW, Salvatore D, et al. Human type 3 iodothyronine selenodeiodinase is located in the plasma membrane and undergoes rapid internalization to endosomes. J Biol Chem 2003;278:1206-11.
5. Barker SB, Humphrey MJ, Solely MH. The clinical determination of protein-bound iodine. J Clin Invest 1951;30:55-62.
6. Barzel US. Thyroid disease after the sixth decade. Curr Ther Endocrinol Metab 1997;6:134-7.
7. Beck-Peccoz P, Persani L. Variable biological activity of thyroid-stimulating hormone. Eur J Endocrinol 1994;131:331-40.
8. Becker DV, Bigos ST, Gaitan E, Morris JC 3rd, Rallison ML, Spencer CA, et al. Optimal use of blood tests for assessment of thyroid function. JAMA 1993;269:2736-7
9. Beever K, Bradbury J, Phillips D, McLachlan SM, Pegg C, Goral A, et al. Highly sensitive assays of autoantibodies to thyroglobulin and to thyroid peroxidase. Clin Chem 1989;35:1949-54.
10. Bianco AC, Salvatore D, Gereben B, Berry MJ, Larsen PR. Biochemistry, cellular and molecular biology, and physiological roles of the iodothyronine selenodeiodinases. Endocr Rev 2002;23:38-89.
11. Boyden SV. Adsorption of proteins on erythrocytes treated with tannic acid and subsequent hemagglutination by antiprotein sera. J Exp Med 1951;93:107-20.
12. Brandt D, Forsythe C, Babik D, Gates RC, Eng KK, Figard SD, et al. Quantitation of free 3,5,3′-L-triiodothyronine on the Abbott IMx analyzer. Clin Chem 1990;36:1079.
13. Braverman LE, Utigen RD, eds. Werner and Ingbar's the thyroid. A fundamental and clinical text, 7th ed. Philadelphia: Lippincott-Raven, 1996.
14. Braverman LE. Evaluation of thyroid status in patients with thyrotoxicosis. Clin Chem 1996;42: 174-8.
15. Bronstein I, Voyta JC, Thorpe GH, Kricka LJ, Armstrong G. Chemiluminescent assay of alkaline phosphatase applied in an ultrasensitive enzyme immunoassay of thyrotropin. Clin Chem 1989;35:1441-6.
16. Brown R, Kertiles L, Kleinmann R. Choice of immunoglobin G purification method in assays for antibodies to the thyrotropin receptor. Clin Chem 1986;32:2034-9.
17. Browne-Martin K, Emerson CH. Postpartum thyroid dysfunction. Clin Obstet Gynecol 1997;40:90-101.
18. Burr WA, Evans SE, Lee J. The ratio of thyroxine to thyroxine-binding globulin in the assessment of thyroid function. Clin Endocrinol 1979;11:333-42.
19. Chan D, Fowler M, Castillo A, Neidulski E, Painter P. Evaluation of AxSYM total T_4. Clin Chem 1994;40:1096.
20. Chen I, Sperling M. Estimation of free thyroxine by automated immunoassay systems. Endocrinology and Metabolism In-Service Training and Continuing Education Program. Washington, DC: AACC Press 1992;10:3-5.
21. Cho BY, Shong MH, Yi KH, Lee HK, Koh CS, Min HK. Evaluation of serum basal thyrotropin levels and thyrotropin receptor antibody levels and thyrotropin receptor antibody activities as prognostic markers for discontinuation of antithyroid drug treatment in patients with Graves' disease. Clin Endocrinol 1992;36:585-90.
22. Chopra IJ. A radioimmunoassay for measurement of 3,3′,5′-triiodothyronine (reverse T_3). J Clin Invest 1974;54:583-92.
23. Chopra IJ. Radioimmunoassay of iodothyronines. In: Abraham GE, ed. Handbook of radioimmunoassay. New York: Marcel Dekker Inc, 1977:679.
24. Chopra IJ. Thyroid function tests: thyroxine and reverse triiodothyronine measurements. In: Abraham GE, ed. Radioassay systems in clinical endocrinology. New York: Marcel Dekker Inc, 1981:101-15.
25. Chopra IJ. Clinical review 86: Euthyroid sick syndrome: is it a misnomer? J Clin Endocrinol Metab 1997;82:329-34.

26. Christofides ND, Sheehan CP. Enhanced chemiluminescence labeled-antibody immunoassay (Amerlite-MAB) for free thyroxine: Design, development, and technical evaluation. Clin Chem 1995;41:12-23.
27. Christofides N, Sheehan C, Midgley J. One-step labeled-antibody assay for measuring free thyroxin. I. Assay development and validation. Clin Chem 1992;38:11-8.
28. Clark F, Horn D. Assessment of thyroid function by the combined use of the serum protein-bound iodine and resin uptake of ^{131}I-triiodothyronine. J Clin Endocrinol Metab 1965;25:39-45.
29. College of American Pathologists. Ligand assay series I survey, set K-A. Skokie IL, 2002.
30. Comeau L, Pianan U, Leo-Mensah T, Huntress MA, Hudson T. An automated chemiluminescent immunoassay test for total triiodothyronine. Clin Chem 1991;37:941.
31. Concepcion J, Carino C, Johnson F, Klonizcii W, Worthy TE. Application of the Microgenics CEDIA T4 LC MAb assay to the Olympus AU5200. Clin Chem 1994;40:1133A.
32. Condliffe P, Weintraub B. Pituitary thyroid-stimulating hormone and other thyroid-stimulating substances. In: Gray C, James V, eds. Hormones in blood. Vol 3. London: Academic, 1979:499-574.
33. Corning Nichols Institute Reference Manual. San Juan Capistrano, CA, 1996.
34. Crandell R, Sherrill S, Parsons G. Free T_4 measurement in antibody coated tubes. Clin Chem 1979;25:1080.
35. Danielson S, Warren K, Birecree J, Fyles J, Hermann S, Ponticello N, et al. Measurement of total thyroxine in serum using a thin-film slide enzyme immunoassay. Clin Chem 1994;40:1024A.
36. Datta P, Sundarapandyan K, Becker D. An automated chemiluminescent assay for total triiodothyronine (TT3) on the Immulite. Clin Chem 1991;37:1021.
37. Davey RX, Clarke MI, Webster AR. Thyroid function testing based on assay of thyroid-stimulating hormone: Assessing an algorithm's reliability. Med J Aust 1996;164:329-32.
38. Davies PH, Franklyn JA. The effects of drugs on tests of thyroid function. Eur J Clin Pharmacol 1991;40:439-51.
39. DeGroot LJ, Larsen PR, Hennemann G, eds. The thyroid and its diseases. 6th ed. New York: Churchill Livingstone, 1996.
40. DeGroot LJ, Mayor G. Admission screening by thyroid function tests in an acute general care teaching hospital. Am J Med 1992;93:558-64.
41. Delange F. Neonatal screening for congenital hypothyroidism: results and perspectives. Horm Res 1997;48:51-61.
42. Della-Puca R, Dayal S, Schwarzberg M, Dayal S, Schwarzberg M, Struve G, et al. Technicon high sensitivity human thyrotropin (TSH) assay: improved adaptation to the fully automated Immunolite system. Clin Chem 1991;37:1032.
43. Diamandis EP, Christopoulos TK. Immunological assays based on time-resolved fluorometry with lanthanide chelates as labels. Endocrinology and Metabolism In-Service Training and Continuing Education Program. Washington, DC: AACC Press 1992;10:9-19.
44. Dorland's illustrated medical dictionary. 30th ed. Philadelphia: WB Saunders, 2003.
45. Dussault JH. Screening for congenital hypothyroidism. Clin Obstet Gynecol 1997;40:117-23.
46. Eckert B, Blaut M, Holzderber M, Lenz H, Angermaier L, Franken N, et al. Electrochemiluminescent immunoassay for thyroxin and thyroxin binding capacity using the random-access analyzer Elecsys. Clin Chem 1995;41:S53.
47. Ekins R. Validity of free thyroxin immunoassays. Clin Chem 1987;33:2137-52.
48. Ekins R. Measurement of free hormones in blood. Endocr Rev 1990;11:5-46.
49. Ekins R. Free triiodothyronine in nonthyroidal illness [Letter]. Clin Chem 1994;40:162-3.
50. Ekins R. The free hormone hypothesis and measurement of free hormones. Clin Chem 1992;38:1289-93.
51. Ekins R. Free hormone measurement (in two parts). Endocrinology and Metabolism In-Service Training and Continuing Education Program. Washington, DC: AACC Press 1993;11:149-57, 181-91.
52. Endocrine Sciences: Pediatric Laboratory Services. Tarzana, CA, 1992.
53. Endres D. Antithyroid peroxidase antibodies (antimicrosomal antibodies) in thyroid disease. Endocrinology and metabolism on-service training and continuing education program. Washington, DC: AACC Press 1991;10:3-5.
54. Enebo DJ, Rossow KL, Werness PG. An improved automated immuno-chemiluminometric third generation hTSH assay for the ACCESS immunoassay system. Clin Chem 1996;42:S170.
55. Erali M, Bigelow RB, Meikle AW. ELISA for thyroglobulin in serum: recovery studies to evaluate autoantibody interferences and reliability of thyroglobulin values. Clin Chem 1996;42:766-70.
56. Esposito S. The thyroid axis and mood disorders: Overview and future prospects. Psychopharmacol Bull 1997;33:205-17.
57. Faix JC, Rosen HN, Valazquez FR. Indirect estimation of thyroid hormone-binding proteins to calculate free thyroxine index: comparison of nonisotopic methods that use labeled thyroxine ("T-Uptake"). Clin Chem 1995;41:41-7.

58. Feldkamp C, Carey J. An algorithmic approach to thyroid function testing in a managed care setting: 3-year experience. Am J Clin Pathol 1996;105:11-6.
59. Feldt-Rasmussen U. Analytical and clinical performance goals for testing autoantibodies to thyroperoxidase, thyroglobulin, and thyrotropin receptor. Clin Chem 1996;42:160-3.
60. Feldt-Rasmussen U, Schleusener H, Carayon P. Meta-analysis evaluation of the impact of thyrotropin receptor antibodies on long term remission after medical therapy of Graves' disease. J Clin Endocrinol Metab 1994;78:98-102.
61. Finke R, Bogner U, Kotulla P, Schleusener H. Anti-TPO antibody determinations using different methods. Exp Clin Endocrinol 1994;102:145-50.
62. Fisher DA. Physiological variations in thyroid hormones: physiological and pathophysiological considerations. Clin Chem 1996;42:135-9.
63. Fisher DA. Fetal thyroid function: Diagnosis and management of fetal thyroid disorders. Clin Obstet Gynecol 1997;40:16-31.
64. Fisher DA, Foley BL. Early treatment of congenital hypothyroidism. Pediatrics 1989;83:785-9.
65. Fitzgibbon RJ, ed. Clinical laboratory reference. 22nd ed. Supplement to Medical Laboratory Observer. Montvale, NJ: Medical Economics, July, 1995.
66. Franken N, Lenz H, Maier L, Kessler A. Sensitive, fully mechanized TSH enzyme immunoassay using strepavidin/biotin technology. Clin Chem 1991;37: 1035.
67. Furth ED, Rathbun M, Postillico J. A modified bioassay for the long-acting thyroid stimulator (LATS). Endocrinology 1969;85:592-3.
68. Gaitan E. Primary hypothyroidism. Curr Ther Endocrinol Metab 1997;6:94-8.
69. Gershengorn MC, Larsen PR, Robbins J. Radioimmunoassay for serum thyroxine-binding globulin: Results in normal subjects and in patients with hepatocellular carcinoma. J Clin Endocrinol Metab 1976;42:907-11.
69A. Gharib H, Tuttle RM, Baskin HJ, Fish LH, Singer PA, McDermott MT. Subclinical thyroid dysfunction: A joint statement on management from the American Association of Clinical Endocrinologists, the American Thyroid Association, and the Endocrine Society. J Clin Endocrinol Metab 2005;90:581-5; discussion 586-7.
70. Giles AF, Charles SA, DeVriendt JK, et al. Amerlite assays for total T4, T3, and T3 uptake. Clin Chem 1986;32:1160.
71. Glinoer D. The regulation of thyroid function in pregnancy: Pathways of endocrine adaptation from physiology to pathology. Endocr Rev 1997;18: 404-33.
72. Gorden P, Weintraub B. Radioreceptor and other functional hormone assays. In: Wilson JD, Foster DW, eds. Williams textbook of endocrinology. 8th ed, Philadelphia: WB Saunders, 1992:1647-61.
73. Greene H, Hwang D, Hutchins J, Johnson A. Technicon thyroxine and thyroid binding globulin: Two fully automated immunoassays for the determination of total thyroxine and TBG in human serum. Clin Chem 1990;36:1082.
74. Groskopf W, Hsu S, Sohn L. A fully automated assay for total T_3 utilizing the Abbott Imx™ analyzer. Clin Chem 1988;34:1210.
75. Hamblin PS, Dyer SA, Mohr VS, Le Grand BA, Lim CF, Tuxen DV, et al. Relationship between thyrotropin and thyroxine changes during recovery from severe hypothyroxinemia of critical illness. J Clin Endocrinol Metab 1986;62:717-22.
76. Hamolsky M, Stein M, Freedberg A. The thyroid hormone-plasma protein complex in man. II. A new in vitro method for study of "uptake" of labeled hormonal components by human erythrocytes. J Clin Endocrinol Metab 1957;17:33-44.
77. Hannon WH, Therrell BL. Laboratory methods for detecting congenital hypothyroidism. In: Therrell BL, ed. Laboratory methods for neonatal screening. Washington, DC: American Public Health Association, 1993:139-54.
78. Hashizume K. Hyperthyroidism. Curr Ther Endocrinol Metab 1997;6:71-6.
79. Hay I, Annesley T, Jiang N, Gorman C. Simultaneous determination of D- and L-thyroxine in human serum by liquid chromatography with electrochemical detection. J Chromatogr 1981;226:383-90.
80. Hay ID, Bayer MF, Kaplan MK, Klee GG, Larsen PR, Spencer CA. American Thyroid Association assessment of current free thyroid hormone and thyrotropin measurement and guidelines for future clinical assays. Clin Chem 1991;37:2002-8.
81. Hay ID, Klee GG. Thyroid dysfunction. Endocrinol Metab Clin North Am 1988;17:473-509.
82. Hay ID, Klee GG. Linking medical needs and performance goals: clinical and laboratory perspectives on thyroid disease. Clin Chem 1993;39:1519-24.
83. Henderson DR, Friedman SB, Harris JD, Manning WB, Zoccoli MA. CEDIA™: A new homogeneous immunoassay system. Clin Chem 1986;32:1637-41.
84. Hierholzer K. Myxedema. Kidney Int Suppl 1997;59:S82-S89.
85. Hollander L, Klonizchii W, Young K, Mellies J, Scalici M, Lynch B. Application and evaluation of CEDIA™: T4 and T-uptake to the Roche Cobas Mira. Clin Chem 1988;34:1209.
85A. Hollowell JG, Staehling NW, Flanders WD, Hannon WH, Gunter EW, Spencer CA, et al. Serum TSH, T(4), and thyroid antibodies in the United States population (1988 to 1994): National Health and Nutrition Examination Survey (NHANES III). J Clin Endocrinol Metab 2002;87:489-99.

86. Hoyle NR. The development and performance of three new immunoassays for serum thyroglobulin and serum autoantibodies to thyroglobulin and thyroid peroxidase. Clin Chem 1993;39:1258A.
87. Hoyle NR, Eckert B, Kraiss S. Electrochemiluminescence: Leading-edge technology for automated immunoassay analyte detection. Clin Chem 1996;42: 1576-8.
88. Huang SA, Dorfman DM, Genest DR, Salvatore D, Larsen PR. Type 3 iodothyronine deiodinase is highly expressed in the human uteroplacental unit and in fetal epithelium. J Clin Endocrinol Metab 2003;88: 1384-8.
89. IMx Free T_4. Abbott Laboratories: Application manual. Abbott Park, Ill, 1990.
90. Ingbar SH, Braverman LE, Dawber NA, Lee GY. A new method for measuring the free thyroid hormone in human serum and an analysis of the factors that influence its concentration. J Clin Invest 1965;44:1679-89.
91. Inzucchi SE. Hyperthyroidism in pregnancy. Curr Ther Endocrinol Metab 1997;6:312-7.
92. Jackson IM. Thyrotropin-releasing hormone. N Engl J Med 1982;306:145-55.
93. Jain A, Hutchison J, Hoang A, Blad D, Kiang JJ, Spencer C. Chemiluminescent immunometric assay of thyroglobulin in serum. Clin Chem 1995; 41:S74.
94. Jewell SE, Slazyk WJ, Smith SJ, Hannon WH. Sources of imprecision in laboratories screening for congenital hypothyroidism: Analysis of nine years of performance data. Clin Chem 1989;35: 1701-5.
95. Kaihola HL, Irjala K, Viikari J, Nanto V. Determination of thyrotropin in serum by time-resolved fluoroimmunoassay evaluated. Clin Chem 1985;31:1706-9.
96. Kannan CR, Seshadri KG. Thyrotoxicosis. Dis Mon 1997;43:601-77.
97. Katz P, Bellet N, Leos M, Chan D, Morgon R, Lingenfelter D, et al. CEDIA™: Total T3, an automated homogenous enzyme-immunoassay for serum total T3. Clin Chem 1991;37:936.
98. Keffer JH. Preanalytical considerations in testing thyroid function. Clin Chem 1996;42:125-34.
99. Keller C, Novotny M, Ramp S, Brashear J, Brandt D, Abbott K. A rapid, sensitive assay for human thyroid-stimulating hormone (hTSH) on the Abbott IMx automated immunoassay system. Clin Chem 1988;34:1208.
100. Ki MR, Gupta MK, Hoogwerf B, Faiman C. Evaluation and validation of a microassay for cAMP measurement on detecting thyroid stimulating antibodies using FRTL-5 cells. Clin Chem 1995; 41:S40.
101. Klee G, Meek R, Dodge L, Gharib H. Polyacrylamide electrophoresis assay for measuring serum thyroxine-binding proteins. Clin Chem 1988;34:1213.
102. Klee GC. Clinical usage recommendations and analytic performance goals for total and free triiodothyronine measurements. Clin Chem 1996;42: 155-9.
103. Klonizchii W, Kowalik K, Worthy T. Application of the Microgenic CEDIA™: T_4MAb and TU assays on the Olympus Reply. Clin Chem 1992;36:1148.
104. Koutras DA. Disturbances of menstruation in thyroid disease. Ann N Y Acad Sci 1997;816:280-4.
105. Kozwich D, Davis G, Sockol C. Development of a total triiodothyronine enzyme immunoassay in microtiter format. Clin Chem 1991;37:1040.
106. Kubasik NP, Lundberg PA, Brodows RG, Hallauer GD, Same DG, Lindstedt G, et al. Free thyroxin by radioimmunoassay: Evaluation of a new direct method involving a radiolabeled thyroxin analog. Clin Chem 1983;29:1781-6.
107. Kung C, Wong E, Hefner A, Greenquist A. Syva Emit 2000 thyroxine assay. Clin Chem 1993;39: 1238A.
108. Kunst A, Seidenschwarz E, Burk H, Schauer S, Haug H, Lehmann P, et al. New one-step enzyme immunoassay for free thyroxin. Clin Chem 1988;34:1830-3.
109. Kwiatkowski M, Long L, Seery J, Blake D, Travis K. An automated chemiluminescence immunoassay test for thyroid stimulating hormone (TSH). Clin Chem 1990;36:1078.
110. Kwiatkowski M, Long L, Sickel M. An automated chemiluminescence immunoassay test for free thyroxine (FT_4). Clin Chem 1990;36:1078.
111. Ladenson PW. Optimal laboratory testing for diagnosis and monitoring of thyroid nodules, goiter, and thyroid cancer. Clin Chem 1996;42:183-7.
111A. Ladenson PW, Singer PA, Ain KB, Bagchi N, Bigos ST, Levy EG, et al. American Thyroid Association guidelines for detection of thyroid dysfunction. Arch Intern Med 2000;160:1573-5.
112. LaFranchi S. American Academy of Pediatrics. American Thyroid Association. Newborn screening for congenital hypothyroidism: Recommended guidelines. Thyroid 1993;3:257-63.
113. Larsen PR. Thyroid-pituitary interaction. N Engl J Med 1982;306:23-32.
114. Larsen PR, Alexander NM, Chopra IJ, Hay ID, Hershman JM, Kaplan MM, et al. Revised nomenclature for tests of thyroid hormones and thyroid-related proteins in serum. J Clin Endocrinol Metab 1987;64:1089-94.
115. Larsen PR, Davies TR, Schlumberger M, Hay ID. The thyroid gland. In: Larsen PR, Kronenberg HM, Melmed S, Polonsky KS, eds. Williams textbook of

endocrinology. 10th ed. Philadelphia: WB Saunders, 2003:331-491.

116. Laudo-Pardos C. Current status of the treatment with thyroid hormones. An Med Interna 1996;13: 555-61.
117. Lazarus JH. Hyperthyroidism. Lancet 1997;349: 339-43.
118. Lazarus JH. Use of radioiodine in the management of hyperthyroidism in the UK: Development of guidelines. Thyroid 1997;7:229-31.
119. Leo-Mensah A, Piran U, Blick M, Edgeworth D, Hayes E, Simonaitis R, et al. An automated chemiluminescence immunoassay test for total thyroxin. Clin Chem 1991;37:942.
120. Letellier M, Levesque A, Daigle F. Performance evaluation of automated immunoassays on the Technicon Immuno I system. Clin Chem 1996;42:1695-701.
121. Liewendahl K. Assessment of thyroid status by laboratory methods: Developments and perspectives. Scand J Clin Lab Invest Suppl 1990;201:83-92.
122. Liewendahl K. Thyroid function tests: Performance and limitations of current methodologies. Scand J Clin Lab Invest 1992;52:435-45.
123. Lindsay RS. Hypothyroidism. Lancet 1997;349:413-7.
124. Madsen K, Schulkamp K, Bellet N. Homogeneous enzyme immunoassay for the measurement of serum or plasma thyroxine. Clin Chem 1986;32:1163.
125. Mariotti S, Barbesino G, Caturegli P, Marino M, Manetti L, Pacini F, et al. Assay of thyroglobulin in serum with thyroglobulin autoantibodies: An unobtainable goal? J Clin Endocrinol Metab 1995;80: 468-72.
126. Mariotti S, Caturegli P, Piccolo P, Barbesino G, Pinchera A. Antithyroid peroxidase autoantibodies in thyroid diseases. J Clin Endocrinol Metab 1990;71:661-9.
127. Marquet PY, Daver A, Sapin R, Bridgi B, Muratet JP, Hartmann DJ, et al. Highly sensitive immunoradiometric assay for serum thyroglobulin with minimal interference from autoantibodies. Clin Chem 1996;42:258-62.
128. Masen JM. A simplified procedure for serum butanol extractable iodine. Am J Clin Pathol 1967;48:561-7.
129. Massart C, Guilhem I, Gibassier J, Allannic H, Nicol M. Comparison of thyroperoxidase and microsomal antibody assays in sera from patients with Graves' disease. Clin Chem 1991;37:1777-80.
130. Massart C, Hody B, Mouchel L, Edan G, Nicol M. Assays for thyrotropin-receptor binding and thyroid-stimulating antibodies in sera from patients with Graves' disease. Clin Chem 1986;32:1332-5.
131. Mayo Medical Laboratories: 1997 test catalog. Rochester, MN.
132. McCapra F, Watmore D, Sumun F, Patel A, Beheshti I, Ramakrishnan K, et al. Luminescent labels for immunoassay—from concept to practice. J Biolumin Chemilumin 1989;4:51-8.
133. McCormack G, Faix J. Evaluation of chemiluminescent enzyme immunoassay for thyroid binding globulin (TBG) and comparison of T4/TBG ratio with free thyroxin index. Clin Chem 1990;36:1149.
134. McDonald LJ, Robin NI, Siegel L. Free thyroxine in serum as estimated by polyacrylamide gel filtration. Clin Chem 1978;24:652-6.
135. McIver B. Euthyroid sick syndrome: An overview. Thyroid 1997;7:125-32.
135A. Mei JV, Alexander JR, Adam BW, Hannon WH. Use of filter paper for the collection and analysis of human whole blood specimens. J Nutr 2001;131:1631S-6S.
136. Meinhold H, Visser T. International survey of the radioimmunological measurement of serum reverse triiodothyronine. Clin Chim Acta 1980;105:343-50.
137. Mestman JH. Hyperthyroidism in pregnancy. Clin Obstet Gynecol 1997;40:45-64.
138. Mestman HH, Goodwin M, Montoro MM. Thyroid disorders in pregnancy. Endocrin Metab Clin North Am 1995;24:41-71.
139. Moller B, Falk O, Bjorkhem I. Isotope dilution-mass spectrometry of thyroxin proposed as a reference method. Clin Chem 1983;29:2106-10.
140. Montoro MN. Management of hypothyroidism during pregnancy. Clin Obstet Gynecol 1997;40: 65-80.
141. Moore P, Layte K, Aslam M, Martin JK. One-step immunometric assay for thyroid stimulating hormone (TSH) based on enhanced luminescence. Clin Chem 1989;35:1149.
142. Morejon C, Soto A, Timmons P, Delgado J, Singh P, Ni WC, et al. Radial partition immunoassay for triiodothyronine. Clin Chem 1988;34:1213.
143. Morello A, Schubert L, Piran U, Riordan B, Silbert D, Hudson T. An automated chemiluminescence immunoassay test for T-uptake. Clin Chem 1991; 37:941.
144. Mori T, Kriss JP. Measurements by competitive binding radioassay of serum antimicrosomal and antithyroglobulin antibodies in Graves' disease and other thyroid disorders. J Clin Endocrinol Metab 1971;33:688-98.
145. Morris JC 3rd, Hay ID, Nelson RE, Jiang NS. Clinical utility of thyrotropin-receptor antibody assays: Comparison of radioreceptor and bioassay methods. Mayo Clin Proc 1988;63:707-17.
146. Murphy BEP. The determination of thyroxine by competitive protein-binding analysis, employing an anion-exchange resin and radiothyroxine. J Lab Clin Med 1965;66:161-7.
147. Nelson J, Linarelli L, Pandian M. Discordant RIA results for thyroxin-binding globulin (TBG): A new

indicator of variant TBG molecules with decrease affinity for thyroxin. Clin Chem 1989;35:1257-8.

148. Nelson JC, Nayak SS, Wilcox B. Variable underestimates by serum free thyroxine (T_4) immunoassays of free T_4 concentrations in simple solutions. J Clin Endocrinol Metab 1994;79:1371-5.
149. Nelson J, Tomei R. Direct determination of free thyroxin in undiluted serum by equilibrium dialysis/radioimmunoassay. Clin Chem 1988;34: 1737-44.
150. Nelson JC, Wilcox RB. Analytical performance of free and total thyroxine assays. Clin Chem, 1996;42:146-54.
151. Ng M, Rajna A, Khalid B. Enzyme immunoassay for simultaneous measurement of autoantibodies against thyroglobulin and thyroid microsome in serum. Clin Chem 1987;33:2286-8.
152. Nichols Institute Diagnostics: Allegro highly sensitive TSH kit (package insert). San Juan Capistrano, CA, 1991.
153. Nicoloff JT, Spencer CA. The use and misuse of sensitive thyrotropin assays. J Clin Endocrinol Metab 1990;71:553-8.
154. Novotny M, Bogacz J, Peters TK, Mallas T, LaFoe M, Isom L, et al. Development of an automated random/continuous access microparticle enzyme immunoassay (MEIA) for the determination of hTSH on the Abbott AxSYM automated immunoassay system. Clin Chem 1996;42:S180.
155. Olive C. PB Diagnostic OPUS™ immunoassay system. J Clin Immunoassay 1991;14:126-32.
156. Papanastasiou-Diamandi A, Khosravi M. Total triiodothyronine (T_3) measurement in serum by time-resolved fluorescence immunoassay. Clin Chem 1991;37:1029.
157. Peterson B, Hanson R, Giese R, Karger B. Picogram analysis of free triiodothyronine and free thyroxine in serum by equilibrium dialysis and electron capture gas chromatography. J Chromatogr 1976;126: 503-16.
158. Peterson V, Smith B, Hall R. A study of thyroid stimulating activity in human serum with the highly sensitive cytochemical bioassay. J Clin Endocrinol Metab 1975;41:199-202.
159. Piketty ML, d'Herbomez M, Le Guillouzic D, Lebtahi R, Cosson E, Dumont A, et al. Clinical comparison of three labeled-antibody immunoassays for free triiodothyronine. Clin Chem 1996;42:933-41.
160. Preissner C, Klee G, Krco C. Nonisotopic "sandwich" immunoassay of thyroglobulin in serum by the biotin-streptavidin technique: Evaluation and comparison with an immunoradiometric assay. Clin Chem 1988;34:1794-8.
161. Rehkemper C, Fisher C, DeLaurentis M, et al. EMIT™ serum thyroid hormone uptake assay for use on the Cobas MIRA™ and Cobas Bio analyzers. Clin Chem 1989;35:1141.
162. Reichstein E, Morton R, Diamandis E. A sensitive assay for TSH with time-resolved fluorescence and monoclonal antibodies. Clin Chem 1988;34: 1216.
163. Reichstein E, Yachera E, Holt R, et al. An automated chemiluminescent high sensitivity TSH assay for the Immulite. Clin Chem 1991;37:1028.
164. Ridgway EC. Modern concepts of primary thyroid gland failure. Clin Chem 1996;42:179-82.
165. Rigl CT, Rivera HN, Patel MT, et al. Bioluminescence immunoassays for human endocrine hormones based on Aqualite™, a calcium-activated protoprotein. Clin Chem 1995;41:1363-4.
166. Robins B, Stoilov I. Development of a fluorescence polarization assay for total T_3. Clin Chem 1995; 41:S75.
167. Ruf J, Czarnocka B, Ferrand M, et al. Novel routine assay of thyroperoxidase autoantibodies. Clin Chem 1988;34:2231-4.
168. Rugg J, Flaa C, Dawson S, et al. Automated quantification of thyrotropin by radical partition immunoassay. Clin Chem 1988;34:118-22.
169. Rusterholtz A. Interpretation of diagnostic laboratory tests in selected endocrine disorders. Nurs Clin North Am 1996;31:715-24.
170. Saadi H. Clinical implications of the interaction between hypothyroidism and the cardiovascular system. Cleve Clin J Med 1997;64:93-8.
171. Sadler WA, Murray LM, Turner JG. What does "Functional Sensitivity" mean? Clin Chem 1996;42: 2051-2.
172. Sapin R, Gasser F, Chambron J. Recovery determination in 600 sera analyzed for thyroglobulin with a recently commercialized IRMA kit. Clin Chem 1992;38:1920-1.
173. Sawin CT, ed. Laboratory support for the diagnosis and monitoring of thyroid disease. Washington, DC: National Academy of Clinical Biochemistry, standards of laboratory practice monograph, 1996.
174. Schilling JS. Hyperthyroidism: diagnosis and management of Graves' disease. Nurse Pract 1997; 22:72.
175. Schlumberger M, Fragu P, Lumbroso J, et al. A new immunoradiometric assay (IRMA) system for thyroglobulin measurement in the follow-up of thyroid cancer patients. Eur J Nucl Med 1991;18: 153-7.
176. Schumdt C, McLachlan S, Matheson J, et al. An enzyme-linked immunoassay for thyroid microsomal antibodies. J Immunol Methods 1982;55: 155-68.
177. Schweizer I. Primary hyperthyroidism 1996. Schweiz Med Wochenschr 1997;127:243-53.
178. Sekiya K, Saito Y, Ikegami T, et al. Fully automated analyzer for chemiluminescent enzyme immunoassay. In: Stanley PE, Kricka LJ, eds. Bioluminescence and

chemiluminescence: Current status. Chichester England:Wiley, 1991:123-6.

179. Sellers D, Franklin M, Behling R, et al. A fully automated FPIA T_4 assay for the Abbott IMx™; Clin Chem 1988;34:1208.
180. Sellers D, Kashik M, Behling R. A fully automated FPIA T-uptake assay for the Abbott IMx™; Clin Chem 1988;34:1209-10.
181. Sheehan C, Christofides N. One-step, labeled-antibody assay for measuring free thyroxin: II. Performance in a multicenter trial. Clin Chem 1992;38:19-25.
182. Shewring G, Rees-Smith B. An improved radioreceptor assay for TSH receptor antibodies. Clin Endocrinol 1982;17:409-17.
183. Shimada H, Nada T, Kanai A. Sensitive assay for anti-thyroglobulin autoantibody (TgAb) on the AIA-series of immunoassay analyzers. Clin Chem 1996;42:S168.
184. Siefring G, Stille D, Schulkamp K. Performance of revised thyroxine uptake methods on the DuPont aca™ discrete clinical analyzer. Clin Chem 1991;37:936-7.
185. Singer PA, Cooper DS, Levy EG, et al. Treatment guidelines for patients with hyperthyroidism and hypothyroidism. JAMA 1995;273:808-12.
186. Smallridge RD. Chapter 33: Thyroid function tests. In: Becker KL, ed. Principles and practice of endocrinology and metabolism. 7th ed. Philadelphia: JB Lippincott, 1995:299-306.
187. Smith D, Soto A, Chivite J, Gil P, Singh P, Ni WC. Radial partition immunoassay for free thyroxine. Clin Chem 1987;33:885.
188. Snyder SM, Cavalieri RR, Ingbar SH. Simultaneous measurement of percentage free thyroxine and triiodothyronine: Comparison of equilibrium dialysis and Sephadex chromatography. J Nucl Med 1976;17:660-4.
188A. Soldin OP, Hilakivi-Clarke L, Weiderpass E, Soldin SJ. Trimester-specific reference intervals for thyroxine and triiodothyronine in pregnancy in iodine-sufficient women using isotope dilution tandem mass spectrometry and immunoassays. Clin Chim Acta 2004;349:181-9.
189. Sophianopoulos JA, Jerkunica I, Sgoutas DS. A rapid ultrafiltration method for the measurement of free thyroxine (FT_4) or free triiodothyronine (FT_3) in serum. Clin Chem 1979;25:1080-1.
190. Spencer CA. Thyroid profiling for the 1990s: Free T_4 estimate or sensitive TSH measurement. J Clin Immunoassay 1989;12:82-9.
191. Spencer CA. Strategy for use of serum thyrotropin vs. free thyroxin measurement in thyroid testing. Endocrinology and Metabolism In-Service Training and Continuing Education Program. Washington, DC: AACC 1991;10:9-17.
192. Spencer C, LoPresti J, Middlesworth LV, et al. Screening for thyroid dysfunction: Which test is best [In Reply]. JAMA 1993;270:2297-8.
193. Spencer CA, LoPresti JS, Patel A, et al. Applications of a new chemiluminometric thyrotropin assay to subnormal measurement. J Clin Endocrinol Metab 1990;70:453-60.
194. Spencer CA, Takeucho M, Kazarosyn M, et al. Interlaboratory/intermethod differences in functional sensitivity of immunometric assays for thyrotropin (TSH): Impact on reliability of measurement of subnormal concentration. Clin Chem 1995;41:367-74.
195. Spencer CA, Takeucho M, Kazarosyan M. Current status and performance goals for serum thyrotropin (TSH) assays. Clin Chem 1996;42:140-5.
196. Spencer CA, Schwarzbein D, Guttler RB, et al. TRH stimulation test responses employing third and fourth generation TSH assays. J Clin Endocrinol Metab 1993;76:494-8.
197. Spencer CA, Takeucho M, Kazarosyan M. Current status and performance goals for serum thyroglobulin assays. Clin Chem 1996;42:164-73.
198. Sterling K, Bellabarba D, Newman E, Brenner M. Determination of triiodothyronine concentration in human serum. J Clin Invest 1969;48:1150-8.
199. Sterling K, Brenner MA. Free thyroxine in human serum: simplified measurement with the aid of magnesium precipitation. J Clin Invest 1966;45:153-63.
200. Stockigt JR. Chapter 18: Serum thyrotropin and thyroid hormone measurements and assessment of thyroid hormone transport. In Braverman LE, Utiger RD, eds. Werner and Ingbar's the thyroid. 7th ed. Philadelphia: Lippincott-Raven, 1996:377-96.
201. Stockigt JR. Guidelines for diagnosis and monitoring of thyroid disease: Nonthyroiodal illness. Clin Chem 1996;42:183-7.
202. Stockigt JR. Thyroid hormone changes in critical illness: the sick euthyroid "syndrome." Diag Endo Metab 1997;15:39-46.
203. Sundbeck G, Eden S, Jagenburg R, Lundberg PA, Lindstedt G. Prevalence of serum antithyroid peroxidase antibodies in 85-year-old women and men. Clin Chem 1995;41:707-12.
204. Surks MI, Chopra IJ, Mariash CN. American Thyroid Association guidelines for use of laboratory tests in thyroid disorders. JAMA 1990;263:1529-32.
205. Symons RG, Vining RF. An evaluation of a fluorescence polarization immunoassay of thyroxin and thyroxin-uptake. Clin Chem 1985;31:1342-8.
206. T_4 Enzymun-Test™; (package insert). Boehringer Mannheim Corp, Indianapolis.
207. TBG RIA procedure (package insert). Corning Medical, Corning Glass Works, Medfield, MA.
208. Thyroglobulin RIA Test, Technical Bulletin. Vol 2. No 3. Dana Point, CA: Kronus Inc.

209. Tietz N, ed. Clinical guide to laboratory tests. 3rd ed. Philadelphia: WB Saunders, 1995.
210. Tikanoja S, Liewendahl R. New ultrafiltration method for free thyroxin compared with equilibrium dialysis in patients with thyroid dysfunction and nonthyroidal illness. Clin Chem 1990;36:800-4.
211. Tokuda Y, Kasagi K, Lida Y, et al. Sensitive, practical bioassay of thyrotropin, with the use of FRTL-5 thyroid cells and magnetizable solid-phase-bound antibodies. Clin Chem 1988;34:2360-4.
212. TOSOH Corporation: A1A-pack T_4. Tokyo, Japan, Analyte Application Manual, 1990.
213. Van Herle AJ, Uller RP, Matthews NI, et al. Radioimmunoassay for measurement of thyroglobulin in human serum. J Clin Invest 1973;52:1320-7.
214. Vanderpump M, Ahlquist JA, Franklyn JA, Clayton RN. Consensus statement for good practice and audit measures in the management of hypothyroidism and hyperthyroidism. Br Med J 1996;313:539-44.
215. Vitti P, Rotella CM, Valente WA, et al. Characterization of the optimal stimulatory effects of Graves' monoclonal and serum immunoglobulin G on adenosine 3′,5′-monophosphate production in FRTL5 thyroid cells: A potential clinical assay. J Clin Endocrinol Metab 1983;57:782.
216. Vogiatzi MG. Frequency and necessity of thyroid function tests in neonates and infants with congenital hypothyroidism. Pediatrics 1997;100:E6.
217. Wang C. The epidemiology of thyroid disease and implications for screening. Endocrinol Metab Clin North Am 1997;26:189-218.
217A. Wang R, Nelson JC, Weiss RM, Wilcox RB. Accuracy of free thyroxine measurements across natural ranges of thyroxine binding to serum proteins. Thyroid 2000;10:31-9.
218. Ward G, Mckinnon L, Badrick T, Hickman PE. Heterophilic antibodies remain a problem for the immunoassay laboratory. Am J Clin Pathol 1997;108:417-21.
219. Wartofsky L, Burman KD. Alterations in thyroid function in patients with systemic illness: The "euthyroid sick syndrome." Endocr Rev 1982;3:164-217.
220. Weetman AP. Hypothyroidism: screening and subclinical disease. Brit Med J 1997;314:1175-8.
221. Whitley RJ. Polyglandular autoimmune syndromes: disorders affecting multiple endocrine glands. Endocrinology and Metabolism In-Service Training and Continuing Education Program. Washington, DC: AACC Press 1994;12:41-7.
222. Wilcox P, Nelson J. Time course of pH regulation in free thyroxin determinations in serum. Clin Chem 1991;37:1298-9.
223. Witherspoon L, Shuler S, Baird F, et al. Measurement of triiodothyronine (T_3) by RIA compared to automated systems. Clin Chem 1992;38:954.
224. Woeber KA. Subclinical thyroid dysfunction. Arch Intern Med 1997;157:1065-8.
225. Zucchelli GC, Pilo A, Chiesa MR, Masini S. Systematic differences between commercial immunoassays for free thyroxine and free triiodothyronine in an external quality assessment program. Clin Chem 1994;40:1956-61.
226. Zucchelli G, Pilo A, Prontera C, et al. Evaluation of a luminescence immunoassay for the measurement of human thyroglobulin. Clin Chem 1990;36:1083.

ADDITIONAL READING

Books

Braverman LE. Diseases of the thyroid, 2nd ed. Totowa, NJ: Humana Press, 2003:395 pp.

Braverman LE. Werner and Ingbar's the thyroid: A fundamental & clinical text. 7th ed. Philadelphia: Lippincott-Raven Publishers, 1996.

Falk SA. Thyroid disease: Endocrinology, surgery, nuclear medicine, and radiotherapy. 2nd ed. Philadelphia: Lippincott-Raven Publishers, 1997.

Schmid KW, Bocker W. Thyroid pathology. Current topics in pathology. Vol 91. New York: Springer-Verlag, 1996.

Sing-Yung W, Visser TJ. Thyroid hormone metabolism: Molecular biology and alternate pathways. Boca Raton: CRC Press, 1994.

Weetman AP, Grossman A, Born GV, et al. Pharmacotherapeutics of the thyroid gland. New York: Springer-Verlag, 1997.

Papers

Baloch Z, Carayon P, Conte-Devolx B, Demers LM, Feldt-Rasmussen U, et al. Guidelines Committee, National Academy of Clinical Biochemistry. Laboratory medicine practice guidelines. Laboratory support for the diagnosis and monitoring of thyroid disease 2003;13:3-126.

Caldwell KL, Maxwell CB, Makhmudov A, Pino S, Braverman LE, et al. Use of inductively coupled plasma mass spectrometry to measure urinary iodine in NHANES 2000: Comparison with previous method. Clin Chem 2003;49:1019-21.

Demers LM, Spencer CA. Laboratory medicine practice guidelines: Laboratory support for the diagnosis and monitoring of thyroid disease. Clin Endocrinol (Oxf) 2003;58:138-40; Thyroid 2003;13:1-126.

Gharib H, Tuttle RM, Baskin HJ, Fish LH, Singer PA, McDermott MT. Subclinical thyroid dysfunction: A joint statement on management from the American Association of Clinical Endocrinologists, the American Thyroid Association, and the Endocrine Society. J Clin Endocrinol Metab 2005;90:581-5; discussion 586-7.

Hollowell JG, Lafranchi S, Smallridge RC, Spong CY, Haddow JE, Boyle CA. 2004 where do we go from here?-Summary of working group discussions on thyroid function and gestational outcomes. Thyroid 2005;15:72-6.

Hollowell JG, Staehling NW, Flanders WD, Hannon WH, Gunter EW, Spencer CA, et al. Serum TSH, T(4), and thyroid antibodies in the United States population (1988 to 1994): National Health and Nutrition Examination Survey (NHANES III). J Clin Endocrinol Metab 2002;87:489-99.

Mazzaferri EL, Robbins RJ, Spencer CA, Braverman LE, Pacini F, et al. A consensus report of the role of serum thyroglobulin as a monitoring method for low-risk patients with papillary thyroid carcinoma. Clin Endocrinol Metab 2003;88:1433-41.

Midgley JEM. Direct and indirect free thyroxine assay methods: Theory and practice. Clin. Chem 2001;47:1353-63.

Pearce EN, Braverman LE. Hyperthyroidism: Advantages and disadvantages of medical therapy. Surg Clin North Am 2004;84:833-47.

Pinchera A. Subclinical thyroid disease: To treat or not to treat? Thyroid 2005;15:1-2.

Rawlins ML, Roberts WL. Performance characteristics of six third-generation assays for thyroid-stimulating hormone. Clin Chem 2004;50:2338-44. Epub 2004 Oct 7.

Spencer CA. Challenges of serum thyroglobulin (Tg) measurement in the presence of Tg autoantibodies. J Clin Endocrinol Metab 2004;89:3702-4.

CHAPTER 53

Reproductive Related Disorders*

Shannon Haymond, Ph.D.,
and Ann M. Gronowski, Ph.D.

Reproductive endocrinology encompasses the hormones of the hypothalamic-pituitary-gonadal axis, and the adrenal glands (see Chapters 50 and 51). These hormones are crucial for proper reproductive function, and include gonadotropin-releasing hormone (GnRH), luteinizing hormone (LH), follicle-stimulating hormone (FSH), and a multitude of sex steroids. The sex steroids are synthesized by the ovaries, testes, and adrenal glands, and are responsible for the manifestation of primary and secondary sex characteristics. Steroids that feminize are classified as estrogens; those that masculinize are known as androgens. Discussed in this chapter are (1) male reproductive biology, (2) female reproductive biology, (3) infertility, and (4) analytical methodology.

MALE REPRODUCTIVE BIOLOGY

ANATOMY

The male reproductive anatomy includes the penis, two testes, and a system of exocrine glands whose secretions form the seminal fluid. The exocrine glands consist of the two bulbourethral glands (Cowper's glands), two seminal vesicles, and the prostate. The bilateral ducts that connect this system and transport sperm and seminal fluid are the epididymis, the vas deferens, and the ejaculatory duct, which enters the urethra.

The function of the testes is to synthesize both sperm and androgens. The mature testis contains a structured network of tightly packed seminiferous tubules. The lumina of the seminiferous tubules are lined by maturing germ cells and Sertoli cells (Figure 53-1). Sertoli cells play a crucial role in sperm maturation and secrete *inhibin*, a glycoprotein that inhibits the pituitary secretion of FSH.[130] Surrounding the seminiferous tubules are the interstitial Leydig cells, which are responsible for the production of testicular androgens. Testosterone is essential for sperm maturation and the complex endocrine feedback mechanism between Sertoli cells, Leydig cells, maturing sperm, the anterior pituitary, and the hypothalamus (Figure 53-1).

HYPOTHALAMIC-PITUITARY-GONADAL AXIS

GnRH is a decapeptide that is synthesized in the hypothalamus and transported to the anterior pituitary gland, where it stimulates the release of both FSH and LH (see Figure 53-1; see also Chapter 50).

In adult men, GnRH and thus LH and FSH are secreted in pulsatile patterns. A circadian rhythm is present, with higher concentrations found in the early morning hours and lower concentrations in the late evening.[342] LH acts on Leydig cells to stimulate the conversion of cholesterol to pregnenolone and in turn the synthesis of testosterone. The exact role of FSH is not yet clear; however, it is known that FSH acts on Sertoli cells to stimulate gametogenesis and the synthesis and release of inhibin. Sex steroids and inhibin together provide negative feedback control of LH and FSH secretion, respectively (see Figure 53-1). LH secretion is inhibited by testosterone and its metabolites, estradiol and dihydrotestosterone (DHT).[330] FSH may be elevated in disorders in which Sertoli cell numbers (and hence inhibin concentrations) are reduced. Likewise, a reduction in the number of Leydig cells (and hence testosterone secretion) leads to an elevation of LH concentration.

*The authors gratefully acknowledge the original contribution of R. J. Whitley, A. W. Meikle, and N. B. Watts, on which portions of this chapter are based.

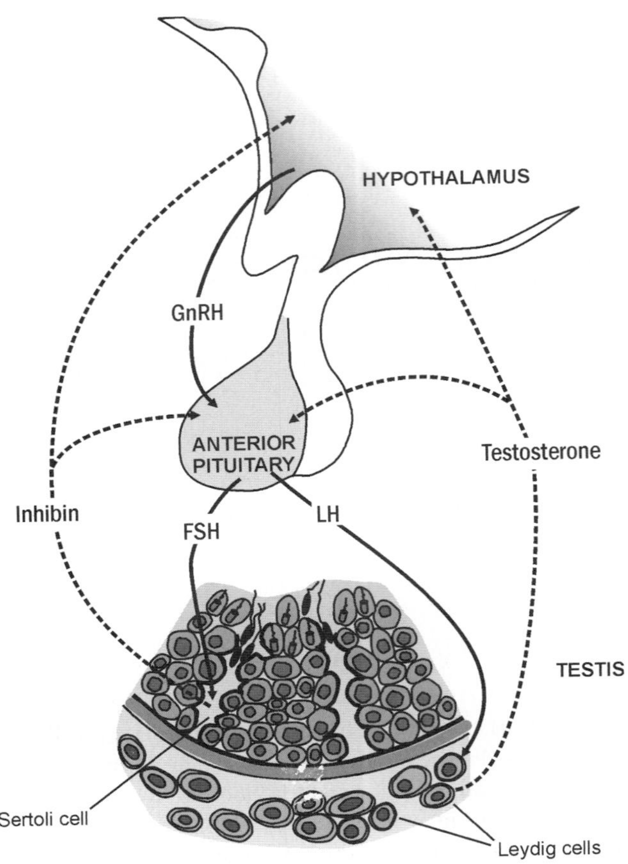

Figure 53-1 Summary of the endocrine control of the testis. *Dashed lines* indicate inhibitory effects, and *solid lines* stimulatory effects. *FSH,* Follicle-stimulating hormone; *GnRH,* gonadotropin-releasing hormone; *LH,* luteinizing hormone.

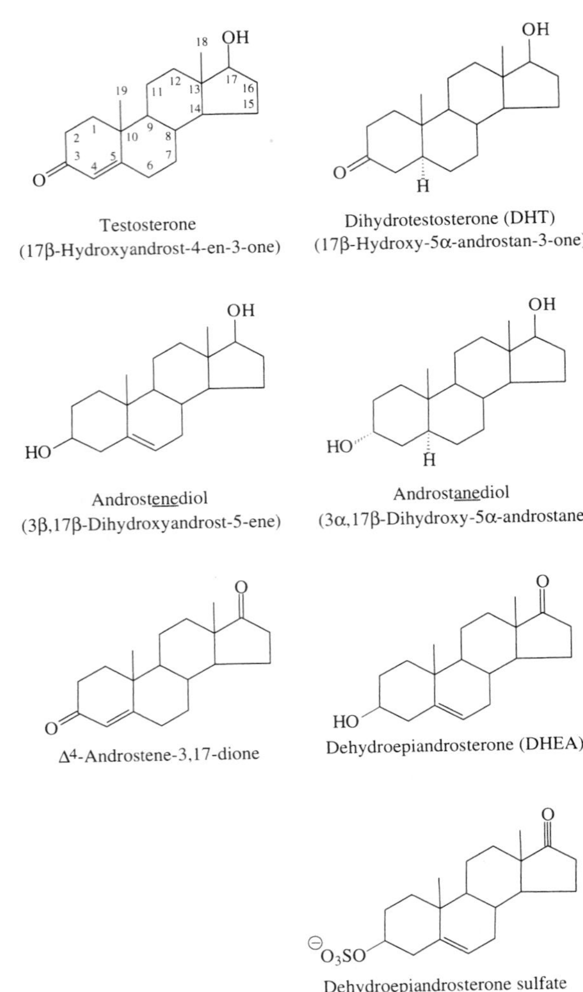

Figure 53-2 Chemical structure of androgens.

ANDROGENS

Function

Androgens are a group of C_{19} steroids (Figure 53-2) that cause masculinization of the genital tract and the development and maintenance of male secondary sex characteristics.[162,367] They also contribute to muscle bulk, bone mass, libido, and sexual performance in men. Testosterone is the main androgen secreted by the Leydig cells of the testes, and its production increases during puberty. Women produce about 5% to 10% as much testosterone as do men.

Testosterone directly affects some aspects of secondary sex development, such as deepening of the voice, increase of muscle mass, and libido. It also has indirect effects in tissue with high 5α-reductase activity, where it serves as a prehormone for formation of DHT (Figure 53-3). Other androgens secreted by the adrenal glands include dehydroepiandrosterone (DHEA), dehydroepiandrosterone sulfate (DHEA-S), androstenedione, and androstenediol and by the gonads androstenedione and DHEA. These steroids can be metabolized to testosterone and DHT in target tissue.[162,367] The mean androgen production rates in men are testosterone, 7 mg/day; androstenedione, 1.4 mg/day; and DHT, 0.3 mg/day. In women androgen production rates are as follows: testosterone, 0.25 mg/day; androstenedione, 3.4 mg/day (cycling) and 1.6 mg/day (menopausal); DHT, 0.056 mg/day.[374]

Biochemistry and Physiology

Biosynthesis of Testosterone

The synthesis of androgens begins with the mobilization of cholesterol from depots of cholesterol esters stored in lipid droplets in the cytoplasm. The cholesterol in these droplets may be derived from lipoprotein cholesterol or de novo synthesis.[97,141] Cholesterol released from the lipid droplets migrates to the inner mitochondrial membrane, where pregnenolone formation occurs by the action of the cholesterol side-chain cleavage enzyme. The conversion of cholesterol to pregnenolone appears to be the rate-limiting step in testosterone synthesis.[130,318] The pathway for testosterone formation is shown in Figure 53-4, with the preferred pathway defined by heavy arrows.

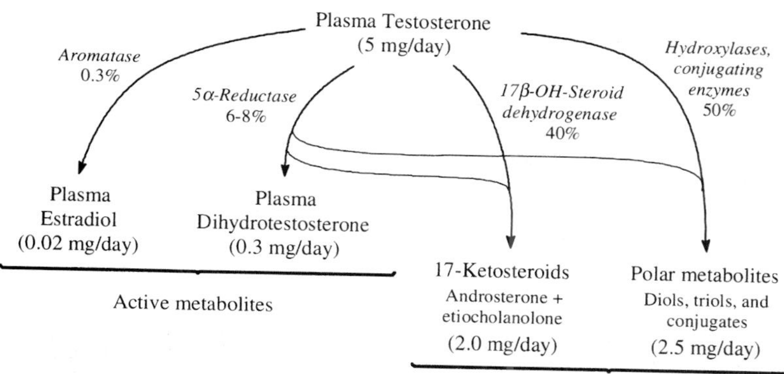

Figure 53-3 Pathways of peripheral metabolism of plasma testosterone. Testosterone can be metabolized either to active metabolites or to excretory metabolites. *(From Griffin JE, Wilson JD. The testis. In: Bondy PK, Rosenberg LE, eds. Metabolic control and disease. 8th ed. Philadelphia: WB Saunders Co, 1980:1535-78.)*

Androgen Transport in Blood

Testosterone and DHT circulate in plasma either free (approximately 2% to 3%) or bound to plasma proteins. The binding proteins include the specific sex hormone-binding globulin (SHBG) and nonspecific proteins such as albumin. SHBG is an α-globulin that has low capacity for steroids, but binds with very high affinity ($Ka = 1 \times 10^8$ to 1×10^9), whereas albumin has high capacity but low affinity ($Ka = 1 \times 10^4$ to 1×10^6.[318] SHBG has the highest affinity for DHT and lowest for estradiol. In men, testosterone circulates bound 44% to 65% to SHBG and 33% to 50% to albumin, whereas in women, testosterone is bound 66% to 78% to SHBG and 20% to 30% to albumin.[248,255]

For years, it was believed that the free fraction of testosterone represented the biologically active fraction. However, it is now thought that dissociation of protein-bound testosterone also occurs within a capillary bed. In studies of tissue delivery in vivo, nearly all of the albumin-bound testosterone was available for tissue uptake.[255] Therefore, the *bioavailable testosterone* is equal to about 35% of the total, or the free plus the albumin-bound.[130] The albumin-bound fraction is referred to as the "non–SHBG-bound" fraction or *weakly bound* fraction.

Testosterone and SHBG exhibit rhythmic variations in their circulating concentrations. Testosterone concentrations peak at approximately 0400 to 0800 hours and nadir concentrations occur at between 1600 and 2000 hours.[293,340] Daily variations in SHBG concentrations are similar to those of other proteins and albumin in serum, with major changes related to posture.[340] Concentrations of SHBG are elevated with hyperthyroidism and in hypogonadal men.[130]

Metabolism of Testosterone

Circulating testosterone serves as a precursor for the formation of two types of active metabolites (see Figure 53-3). Through the actions of 5α-reductase, 6%-8% of testosterone is converted to DHT. Alternatively, testosterone and androstenedione can be converted to estrogens (~0.3%) through aromatase.[130] DHT is formed in androgen target tissues, such as the skin and prostate, whereas aromatization occurs in many tissues. Peripheral aromatization occurs primarily in adipose tissue (of both men and women) because of the high concentration of aromatase in this tissue. The rate of extraglandular aromatization therefore increases with body fat.[130]

Dihydrotestosterone is metabolized to 3α-androstanediol (see Figure 53-4) and 3α-androstanediol glucuronide. These metabolites have been used as markers of DHT production in peripheral tissues. Serum concentrations of 3α-androstanediol glucuronide or 3α-androstanediol reflect the production of DHT in peripheral tissue such as skin.[154,206] However, DHT may also arise from precursors other than testosterone. The reduction in serum 3α-androstanediol glucuronide concentrations in patients treated with glucocorticoids that suppress adrenal glucocorticoid and androgen production supports this conclusion.[223]

The main excretory metabolites of androstenedione, testosterone, and DHEA are shown in Figure 53-5. Except for epitestosterone, these catabolites constitute a group of steroids known as *17-ketosteroids* (17-KSs). These metabolites are excreted primarily in the urine (>90%), with approximately half as 17-KSs, and half as diols, triols, conjugates, and other polar compounds.[130]

Male Reproductive Development

Fetal

During early embryogenesis, the fetus possesses the genital ducts for both the female and male reproductive tracts—mullerian and wolffian ducts, respectively. The mullerian ducts have the potential to differentiate into the fallopian tubes, uterus, and upper part of the vagina of the female reproductive tract. The wolffian ducts differentiate into the vas deferens, epididymis, and seminal vesicles of the male reproductive tract. In male fetuses, testosterone is responsible for maintaining the wolffian ducts and for virilization of the urogenital sinus and external genitalia. Mullerian inhibiting substance (MIS) is responsible for the regression of the mullerian ducts.[130] MIS is the earliest known secretory product of the Sertoli cells in the fetal testis. Mutations in the gene for MIS, or its receptor, are responsible for the lack

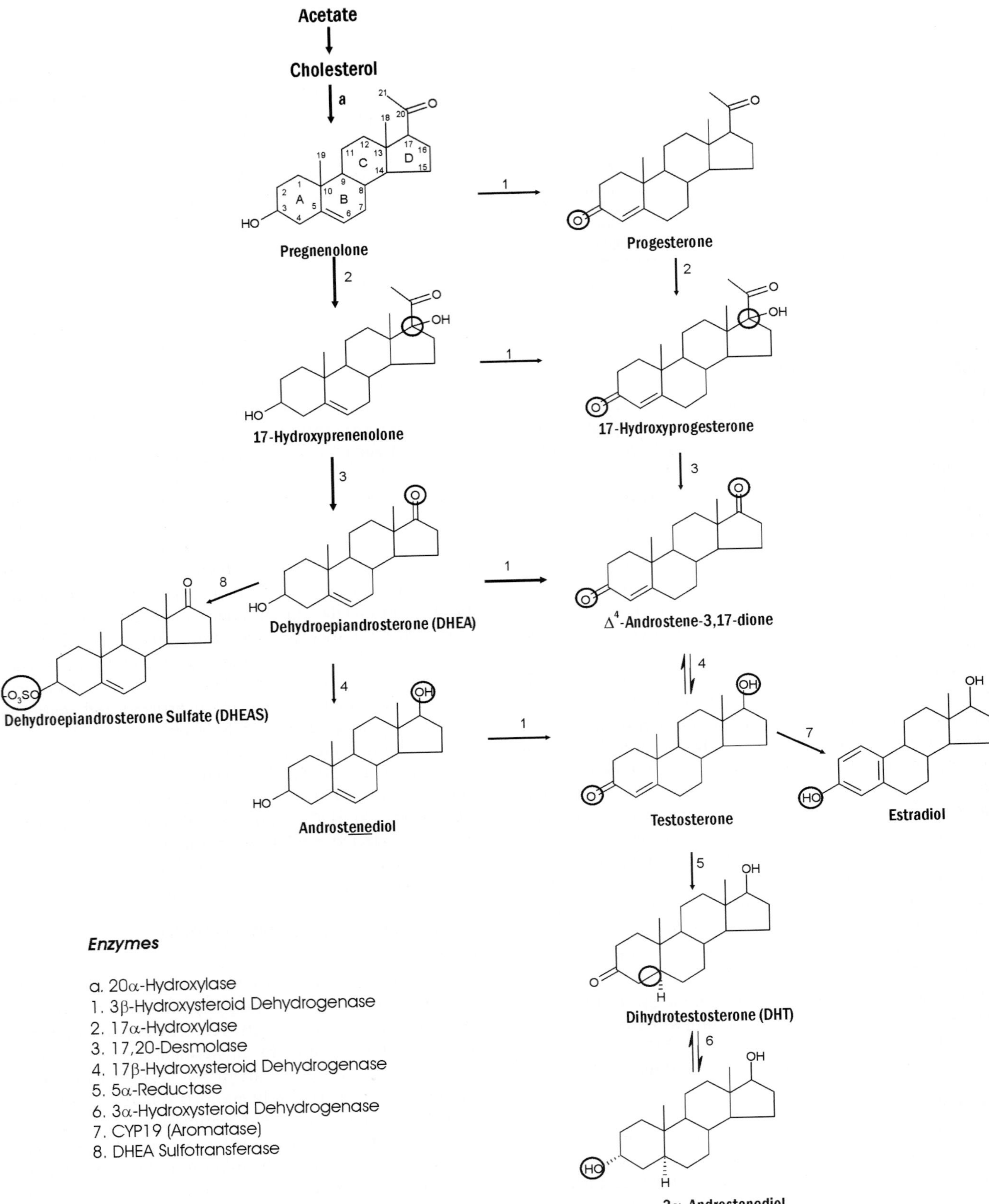

Figure 53-4 Biosynthesis of androgens (adrenal glands and testis). The *heavy arrows* indicate the preferred pathway. The *enclosed area* represents the site of chemical change.

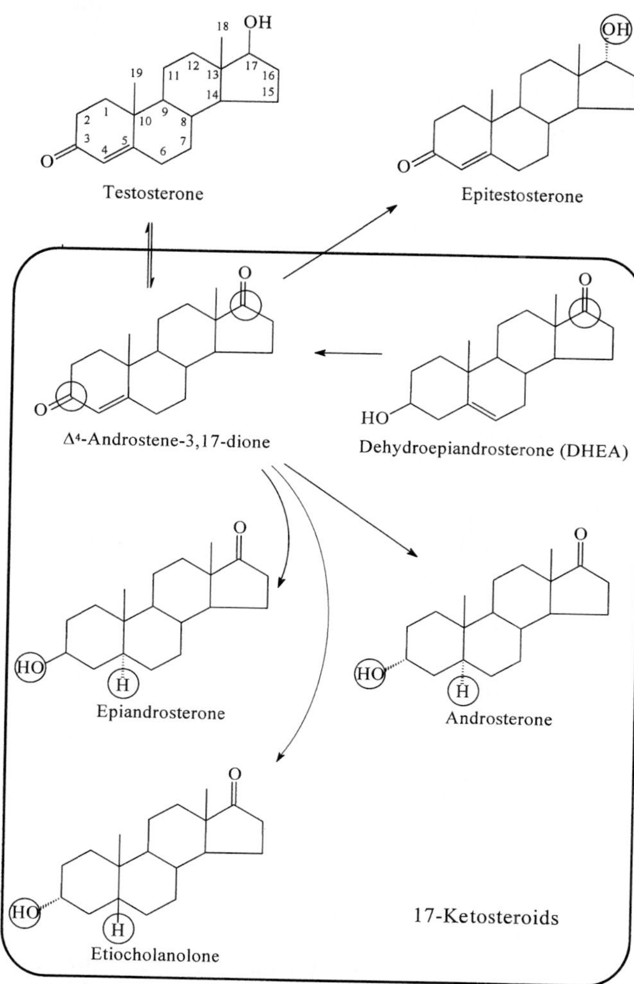

Figure 53-5 Catabolism of $C_{19}O_2$ androgens. The *circled area* represents the site of chemical change.

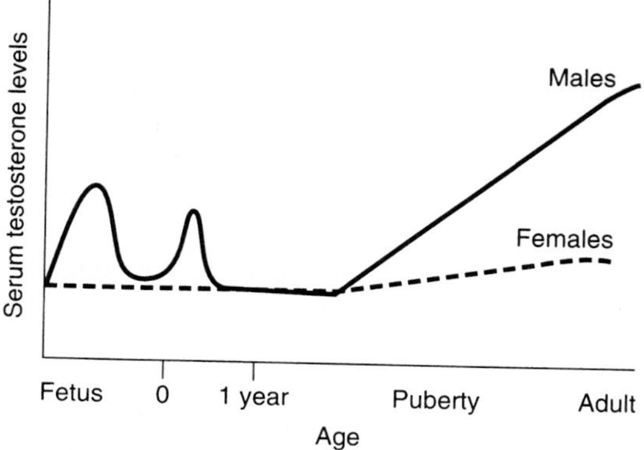

Figure 53-6 Schematic drawing of the changes in male and female total serum testosterone throughout life. *(From Wheeler MJ. The determination of bio-available testosterone. Ann Clin Biochem 1995;32:353-7.)*

of regression of the mullerian ducts in patients with persistent mullerian duct syndrome.[114] For normal male sexual development to occur, there must be production of MIS and testosterone, conversion of testosterone to DHT, and functioning androgen receptors.[162,367] A microphallus (<2.5 cm fully stretched length) at birth can be caused by lack of testosterone or DHT, or defective androgen receptors. In the male embryo, the production of testosterone by the testes, and the concentration of plasma testosterone, start to rise by the second month of gestation and peak at 12 weeks at approximately 5.5 nmol/L.[357] A high concentration is maintained until it decreases late in gestation (see Figure 53-6).[357,367]

Several enzyme defects will cause a deficiency of testosterone production during fetal development. These include *20α-hydroxylase (cholesterol 20,22-desmolase) deficiency,* which prevents conversion of cholesterol to pregnenolone and results in congenital lipoid adrenal hyperplasia, so named because the adrenals are large and filled with lipoid material.[189] Affected male fetuses have female or ambiguous genitalia. Urinary 17-KSs are completely absent.[167,189] This disorder causes severe salt wasting and can be fatal if not treated early.

When the condition of *17α-hydroxylase deficiency* occurs, the production of cortisol and sex steroids (except for progesterone) is impaired and the production of mineralocorticoids increased (see Figure 51-4, Chapter 51).[189] With this deficiency, plasma concentrations of corticosterone, 11-deoxycorticosterone, progesterone, and pregnenolone are elevated. Boys exhibit pseudohermaphroditism and deficiency in development of secondary sex characteristics.

Boys with *17β-hydroxysteroid dehydrogenase deficiency* fail to form testosterone from androstenedione, androstenediol from DHEA, or estradiol from estrone in a normal manner (see Figure 53-4). At puberty, plasma concentrations of testosterone and DHT are low, and plasma androstenedione and estrone are elevated in those individuals.[312]

Postnatal

At birth, the concentration of testosterone is only slightly higher in boys than in girls. Shortly after birth, the concentration of testosterone increases, remains elevated for about 3 months, and then falls to baseline again by 1 year (<1 nmol/L). The concentration of androgens remains low, although higher in boys than in girls, until puberty (see Figure 53-6).[130]

Puberty

Concentrations of androstenedione, DHEA, and DHEA-S begin to increase as early as 6 to 7 years of age, several years before maturation of the hypothalamic-pituitary-gonadal axis. The onset of puberty is associated with nocturnal surges in LH and, to a lesser extent, FSH secretion. The overall changes associated with puberty reflect the theory that the hypothalamic-pituitary system becomes less sensitive to feedback inhibition by circulating androgens, resulting in higher androgen concentrations. Androgen secretion during puberty appears to be necessary for normal bone density and is associated with a fall in high-density lipoprotein concentrations, and an increase in hematocrit. On average, puberty is completed between the ages of 16 and 19.[130]

Andropause

Increased life expectancy has generated interest in aging-related health problems and among those is the gradual decrease in gonadal function in men after the age of 50. The aging process in men leads to the physiological lowering of androgens including testosterone. Because it parallels the changes observed in the aging female during menopause, this state has been referred to as andropause.[230,319,328] The clinical presentation of andropause is symptomatic or asymptomatic, with symptoms including decreased well-being, energy levels, and sexual function. Unlike its female counterpart, andropause does not result in universal or absolute loss of gonadal function and the process is much more gradual, progressing over several decades. Thus alternate names such as androgen decline in the aging male (ADAM) or partial androgen deficiency in the aging male (PADAM) have been suggested to describe this biochemical and physiological state.[229]

Age-related decreases in testicular androgen production are primarily caused by a decline in the number of Leydig cells.[143,238,355] Both total and free testosterone concentrations decrease with age on average 3.2 ng/dL (0.11 nmol/L) per year.[143] The mean testosterone concentration at 80 years old is approximately 60% of that at 20 to 50 years.[344] Testosterone concentrations are affected by a number of factors—namely, age, obesity, time of day, and binding protein concentrations (albumin and SHBG). Free (or bioavailable) testosterone measurements of morning specimens are considered the most accurate indicator of androgenicity and are therefore the preferred laboratory test in the diagnosis of andropause.[346] Androgen replacement therapy is available as a form of treatment when indicated by severity of symptoms along with low circulating concentrations of bioavailable testosterone (typically <4 nmol/L).[78,230,319,328] There is considerable uncertainty regarding the long-term effects of androgen replacement therapy on the prostate. Specifically, the role of exogenous testosterone in the pathogenesis of benign prostatic hyperplasia and prostate cancer has not been determined.

Male Reproductive Abnormalities

There are a number of abnormalities that can affect the male reproductive system before birth, in childhood, or in adulthood. For the purposes of this chapter, they have been divided into categories of (1) hypogonadotropic hypogonadism, (2) hypergonadotropic hypogonadism, (3) defects in androgen action (Box 53-1), (4) impotence, and (5) gynecomastia. The effects of these abnormalities on infertility are discussed later in this chapter.

BOX 53-1 Male Reproductive Abnormalities

Hypogonadotropic Hypogonadism

- Panhypopituitarism (congenital or acquired)
- Hypothalamic syndrome (acquired or congenital)
  - Structural defects (neoplastic, inflammatory, and infiltrative)
  - Prader-Willi syndrome
  - Laurence-Moon-Biedl syndrome
- GnRH deficiency (Kallmann's syndrome)
- Hyperprolactinemia (prolactinoma or drugs)
- Malnutrition and anorexia nervosa
- Drug-induced suppression of luteinizing hormone (androgens, estrogens, tranquilizers, antidepressants, antihypertensives, barbiturates, cimetidine, GnRH analogs, and opiates)

Hypergonadotropic Hypogonadism

- Acquired (irradiation, mumps orchitis, castration, and cytotoxic drugs)
- Chromosome defects
  - Klinefelter's syndrome (47, XXY) and mosaics
  - Autosomal and sex chromosomes, polyploidies
  - True hermaphroditism
- Defective androgen biosynthesis
  - 20α-Hydroxylase (cholesterol 20,22-desmolase) deficiency
  - 17,20-Lyase deficiency
  - 3β-Hydroxysteroid dehydrogenase deficiency
  - 17α-Hydroxylase deficiency
  - 17β-Hydroxysteroid dehydrogenase deficiency
- Testicular agenesis
- Selective seminiferous tubular disease
- Miscellaneous
  - Noonan's syndrome (short stature, pulmonary valve stenosis, hypertelorism, and ptosis)
  - Streak gonads
  - Myotonia dystrophica
  - Acute and chronic diseases

Defects in Androgen Action

- Complete androgen insensitivity (*testicular feminization*)
- Incomplete androgen sensitivity
  - Androgen receptor defects
  - 5α-Reductase deficiency

GnRH, Gonadotropin-releasing hormone.

Hypogonadotropic Hypogonadism

Male hypogonadism is a condition caused by a decreased function of the testes that can lead to retardation of sexual development if manifested early in life. The disorder can be classified as *hypo*gonadotropic or *hyper*gonadotropic.

Hypogonadotropic hypogonadism occurs when defects in the hypothalamus or pituitary prevent normal gonadal stimulation. Causative factors include congenital or acquired panhypopituitarism, hypothalamic syndromes, GnRH deficiency, hyperprolactinemia, malnutrition or anorexia, and iatrogenic causes. These abnormalities are all associated with decreased testosterone and gonadotropin concentrations.

Kallmann's syndrome is the most common form of hypogonadotropic hypogonadism and results from a deficiency of GnRH in the hypothalamus during embryonic development.[136] It is characterized by hypogonadism and anosmia (loss of the sense of smell) in male or female patients, and is inherited as an autosomal dominant trait with variable penetrance.[46,293] This syndrome arises from a defect in the migration of GnRH neurons to the hypothalamus. The pituitary disorders may be characterized by isolated gonadotropin deficiency or may be combined with growth hormone deficiency. Patients with the isolated disorder display sexual infantilism and long arms and legs; those with the combined deficiency do not have long arms and legs. These patients must be distinguished from those with growth delay. In all of these patients, LH, FSH, and testosterone concentrations are lower than normal. However, heterogeneity exists in the degree of gonadotropin deficiency, and hence urinary concentrations of LH, FSH, and testosterone have been shown to vary between affected patients (FSH: 10 to 500 mIU/hr; LH: 10 to 700 mIU/hr; testosterone: 5 to 60 ng/dL).[293]

Hypergonadotropic Hypogonadism

Hypergonadotropic hypogonadism arises from a primary gonadal disorder. Patients with primary testicular failure have elevated concentrations of LH and FSH and decreased concentrations of testosterone. Causes for primary hypogonadism include testicular damage such as from irradiation, disease, or drugs; chromosomal defects; enzymatic defects in androgen synthesis; testicular agenesis; and seminiferous tubular disease, among other miscellaneous causes. Aging is also associated with gonadal failure, which occurs in about 20% of men older than 60 years of age who exhibit defects both in primary Leydig cell function and in abnormal secretion of gonadotropins in response to GnRH (see earlier section on andropause).[34,293,330]

Defects in Androgen Action

The most common and severe defect in androgen action is *testicular feminization syndrome.* These individuals have female habitus and develop breast tissue; however, the vagina ends in a blind pouch and male testes are present. This disorder is thought to arise from a defect in the androgen receptor. Circulating concentrations of testosterone in these patients are the same as or greater than in normal men.[167] Testosterone can serve as a substrate for further estrogen formation, which may account for the elevated estrogen concentrations in these individuals.[167] Concentrations of LH are also increased, presumably because of the resistance of the hypothalamic-pituitary system to androgen inhibition.

Males with *5α-reductase deficiency* also have ambiguous genitalia.[367] If the deficiency remains undiagnosed before puberty, patients have an increase in muscle mass, voice change, and enlargement of the phallus; however, they lack normal male-pattern hair growth, and their prostate gland remains small. There is evidence that DHT formation is deficient in the tissue of the urogenital tract in these patients.[167]

In patients with cryptorchidism or ambiguous genitalia, the identification of abdominal gonads is essential for proper diagnosis and treatment. Measurement of plasma MIS has been advocated for detecting the presence of testicular tissue.[114,194,228] However, this test is not yet commercially available. The best indication for the use of MIS measurement is as a first approach to the differentiation between cryptorchidism and anorchidism in boys with a normal phenotype but undescended testes. Mean plasma MIS concentration in anorchid patients was 0.8 ng/mL, compared with 48.2 ng/mL in patients with normal testes.[194] MIS concentrations are also elevated in boys with delayed puberty and partial androgen insensitivity. Other reports suggest that inhibin B may be used as a basal serum marker for the presence and function of testicular tissue in boys with nonpalpable testicles.[4,134,186] Kubini and co-workers found that boys with anorchia have undetectable serum inhibin B concentrations.[186] Boys with severe testicular damage or gonadal dysgenesis also have undetectable or very low concentrations of inhibin B, whereas normal serum inhibin B concentrations are observed for boys with abdominal "normal" testes.[186]

Impotence

Impotence is the persistent inability to develop or maintain a penile erection that is sufficient for intercourse and ejaculation in 50% or more of attempts.[185,293] A wide variety of organic and psychological abnormalities may cause changes in sexual drive and the ability to have an erection or to ejaculate. Psychogenic impotence is the most common diagnosis. Other causes include vascular disease, diabetes mellitus, hypertension, uremia, neurologic disease, hypogonadism, hyperthyroidism and hypothyroidism, neoplasms, and drugs. The physician must pursue a careful evaluation of the possible psychological factors, neuropathy, or vascular abnormalities that may be interfering with proper sexual function. If no obvious explanation for impotence can be found, measurements of morning serum testosterone, LH, and thyroid-stimulating hormone concentrations have been suggested.[128,293] Elevated gonadotropin concentrations indicate primary hypogonadism. Total and even free testosterone concentrations may be within normal reference intervals, yet still may be subnormal for a given patient if found in the presence of elevated LH or FSH. Hyperprolactinemia is an infrequent cause of impotence but should be considered in unusual situations.

Sildenafil (Viagra) was approved by the FDA in April 1998 for use as an oral therapeutic agent for male erectile dysfunction.[25,26,147,233,296] It has been found to be a selective inhibitor of phosphodiesterase 5 (PDE5).[26] A high-performance liquid chromatography (HPLC) method for sildenafil has been reported.[65] Cialis and Levitra are other PDE5 inhibitors that are used to treat male erectile dysfunction (http://www.erectile-dysfunction-impotence.org/).

Gynecomastia

Gynecomastia is the benign growth of glandular breast tissue in men and is a common finding in males of varied ages.[33,120,217] Gynecomastia is associated with an increase in the estrogen/androgen ratio. There are three distinct periods of life with which gynecomastia is commonly associated. First, transient gynecomastia can be found in 60% to 90% of all newborns because of high estrogen concentrations that cross the placenta. The second peak occurs during puberty in 50% to 70% of normal boys. It is usually self-limited and may be caused by low serum testosterone, low DHT, or a high estrogen/androgen ratio. The last peak is found in the adult population, most frequently 50- to 80-year-old men. This gynecomastia may be due to testicular failure, resulting in an increased estrogen/androgen ratio, or to increased body fat, resulting in increased peripheral aromatization of testosterone to estradiol.[33,120,217]

Gynecomastia may also develop because of iatrogenic causes[334] or hyperthyroidism.[120] Finally, germinal cell or nonendocrine tumors that produce human chorionic gonadotropin (hCG), and estrogen-producing tumors of the adrenal glands, the testes, or the liver can cause gynecomastia. hCG can stimulate testicular aromatase activity and estrogen production.[120] In cases of striking gynecomastia in which history and physical examination point to no specific disorder, measurements of hCG, plasma estradiol, testosterone, and LH concentrations are appropriate.[33] It is important to note that prolactin plays an important role in *galactorrhea* (milk production), but only an indirect role in gynecomastia.

FEMALE REPRODUCTIVE BIOLOGY

Anatomy

The female reproductive system consists of a vagina, a uterus, and the bilateral fallopian tubes and ovaries. The ovaries are located on either side of the uterus in close proximity to the fallopian tubes. They function as both the producers of ova and the secretors of the sex hormones progesterone and estrogens.

Every healthy female neonate possesses approximately 400,000 primordial follicles, each containing an immature ovum. During the reproductive life span of an adult woman, 300 to 400 follicles will reach maturity.[112,127] A single mature follicle is produced during each normal menstrual cycle at approximately day 14 (Figure 53-7). Surrounding the oocyte of the mature follicle are three distinct cell layers: the *theca externa*, the *theca interna*, and the *granulosa cells.* The theca interna cells are the primary source of androgens, which are transported to adjacent granulosa cells, where they are aromatized to estrogens.[46]

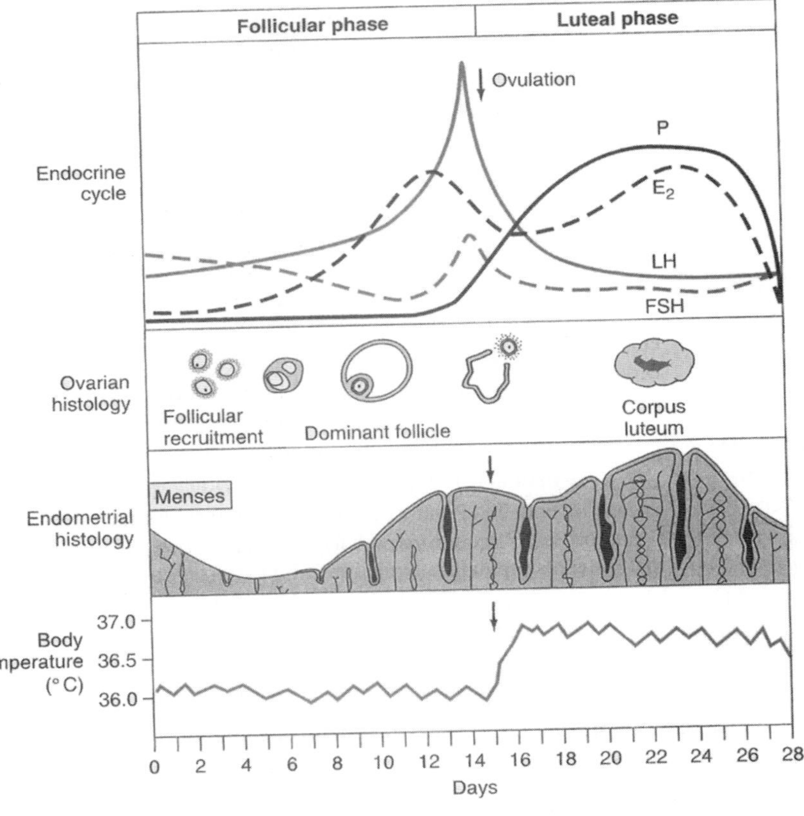

Figure 53-7 The hormonal, ovarian, endometrial, and basal body temperature changes throughout the normal menstrual cycle. *(From Carr BR, Bradshaw KD. Disorders of the ovary and female reproductive tract. In Braunwald E, Fauci A, Kasper D, Hauser SL, Longo DL, Jameson JL, eds. Harrison's principles of internal medicine. 15th ed. New York: McGraw-Hill Co, 2001:2158.)*

The mature follicle undergoes ovulation by the process of rupture, thereby releasing the oocyte into the proximity of the fallopian tubes. The follicle then fills with blood to form the corpus hemorrhagicum. The granulosa and theca cells of the follicle lining quickly proliferate to form lipid-rich luteal cells, replacing the clotted blood and forming the *corpus luteum* (yellow body). The luteal cells produce estrogen and progesterone. If fertilization and pregnancy occur, the corpus luteum persists and continues to produce estrogen and progesterone. If no pregnancy occurs, the corpus luteum regresses and is eventually replaced by scar tissue.

The fallopian tubes arise from the uterus and extend toward the ovaries. They convey the sperm upward from the uterine cavity and provide the site for fertilization of the oocyte. The fertilized egg is transported back along the fallopian tubes to the uterine cavity. The uterine cavity is lined by the endometrium. The endometrium undergoes cyclical changes in preparation for implantation and pregnancy. During the luteal phase, the endometrial lining increases in thickness and vascularity; during menstruation, the endometrium is shed (Figure 53-7).

Hypothalamic-Pituitary-Gonadal Axis

In adult women, a tightly coordinated feedback system exists between the hypothalamus, anterior pituitary, and ovaries to orchestrate menstruation. FSH serves to stimulate follicular growth and LH stimulates ovulation and progesterone secretion from the developing corpus luteum (see Figure 53-8). These actions are discussed in greater depth later in this chapter.

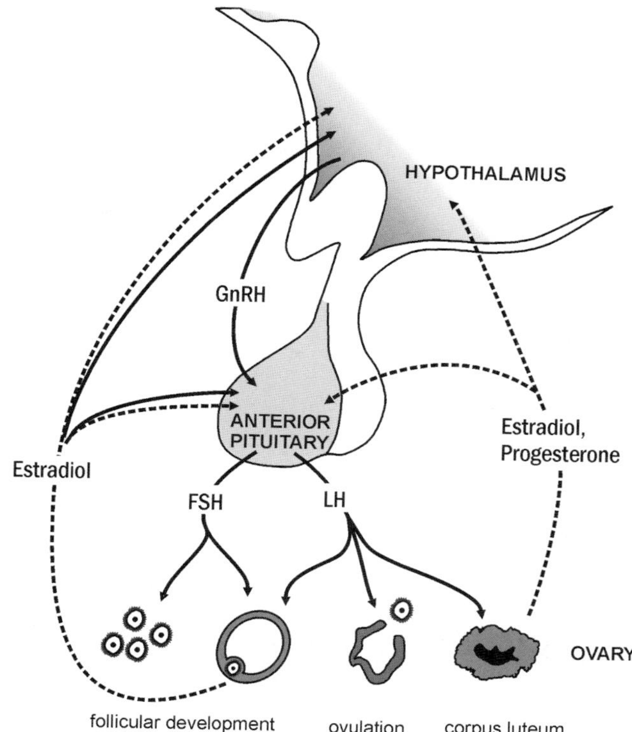

Figure 53-8 Summary of the endocrine control and changes in ovary and endometrium during the menstrual cycle. *Dashed lines* indicate inhibitory effects, and *solid lines* stimulatory effects. *FSH,* Follicle-stimulating hormone; *GnRH,* gonadotropin-releasing hormone; *LH,* luteinizing hormone.

Estrogens

Function

Estrogens are sex hormones that are responsible for the development and maintenance of the female sex organs and female secondary sex characteristics. In conjunction with progesterone, they also participate in the regulation of the menstrual cycle and breast and uterine growth, and in the maintenance of pregnancy.

Estrogens affect calcium homeostasis and have a beneficial effect on bone mass. They decrease bone resorption, and in prepubertal girls estrogen accelerates linear bone growth and results in epiphyseal closure.[130] Long-term estrogen depletion is associated with loss of bone mineral content, an increase in stress fractures, and postmenopausal osteoporosis.[180]

Estrogens also have well established effects on plasma proteins that influence endocrine testing. They increase concentrations of SHBG, corticosteroid-binding globulin, and thyroxine-binding globulin.[255,356] Hence, boys and girls have comparable concentrations of SHBG, but adult men have SHBG concentrations that are about one half those of adult women. Concentrations of plasma proteins that bind copper and iron are also elevated in response to estrogen, as are those of high-density and very high-density lipoproteins. The rise in very high-density lipoprotein concentrations and the increase in lipogenesis in the liver may cause triglyceride elevation. In addition, estrogens are believed to play a preventive role in coronary heart disease.[131]

Chemistry

The names and structural formulas of some of the important estrogens are shown in Figure 53-9. Structurally, estrogens are derivatives of the parent hydrocarbon *estrane,* which is an 18-carbon molecule with an aromatic ring A and a methyl group at C-13.[46,373] Estrogens possess a phenolic hydroxyl group at C-3, which gives the compounds acidic properties, do not possess a methyl group at C-10 (as do androgens), and may possess a ketone (estrone) or hydroxyl group (estradiol) at C-17 and frequently at C-16 (estriol). The phenolic ring A and the oxygen function at C-17 are essential for biological activity. Substituents at other positions in the molecule diminish feminizing potency. For example, estriol that contains a hydroxyl group at C-16 possesses very little biological activity.

Biochemistry and Physiology

Estrogen Biosynthesis

In normal women, most estrogens are secreted by the ovarian follicles and the corpus luteum, and during pregnancy by the placenta. Adrenals and testes are also believed

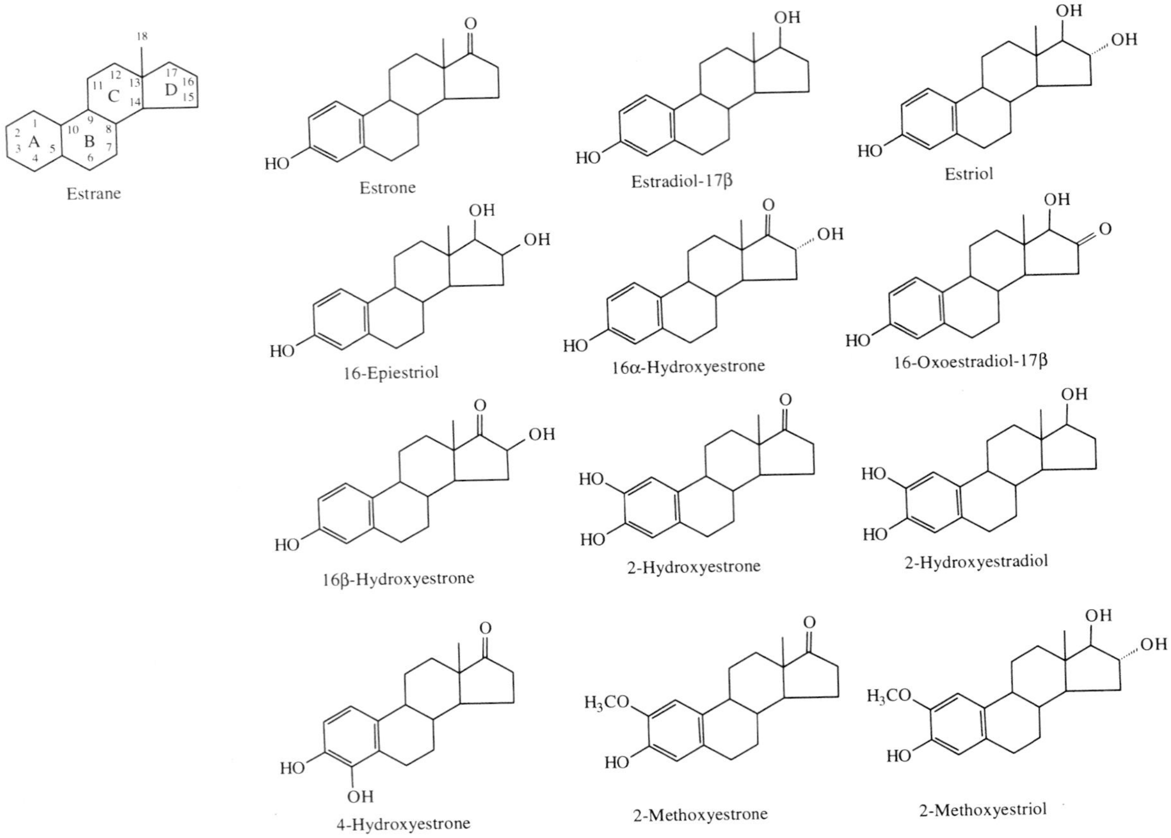

Estrane
Estrone
Estradiol-17β
Estriol
16-Epiestriol
16α-Hydroxyestrone
16-Oxoestradiol-17β
16β-Hydroxyestrone
2-Hydroxyestrone
2-Hydroxyestradiol
4-Hydroxyestrone
2-Methoxyestrone
2-Methoxyestriol

Figure 53-9 Structural formulas of important estrogens.

to secrete minute quantities of estrogens. The ovary follows the same steroidogenic pathway as do the other steroid-producing organs.[46,373] In vivo and in vitro studies indicate that acetate, cholesterol, progesterone, and testosterone can all serve as precursors of estrogens. The normal human ovary produces all three classes of sex steroids—estrogens, progestins, and androgens; however, estradiol and progesterone are its primary secretory products. Unlike the testis, the ovary possesses a highly active aromatase system that rapidly converts androgens such as testosterone to estrogens. Unlike the adrenal cortex, the normal ovary lacks both the 21-hydroxylase and the 11β-hydroxylase enzymes, and therefore cannot produce glucocorticoids and mineralocorticoids.[46,373] More than 20 estrogens have been identified, but only 17β-estradiol (also denoted as *E2*) and estriol (also denoted as *E3*) are routinely measured clinically. The most potent estrogen secreted by the ovary is 17β-estradiol. Because it is derived almost exclusively from the ovaries, its measurement is often considered sufficient to evaluate ovarian function.

The biochemical pathway illustrating the aromatization of testosterone to estradiol and androstenedione to estrone is shown in Figure 53-10. Steroidogenesis and its regulation during the menstrual cycle have been discussed in detail by Channing and associates.[54] The role of estrogens in normal and abnormal menstrual cycles is described later in this chapter.

Estrogens are also produced by peripheral aromatization of androgens, primarily androstenedione. In healthy men and women, ~1% of the secreted androstenedione is converted to estrone.[46,373] Although the ovaries of postmenopausal women do not secrete estrogens, these women have significant blood concentrations of estrone originating from the peripheral conversion of adrenal androstenedione. Because a major site of this conversion is adipose tissue, estrone increases in obese postmenopausal women, sometimes yielding enough estrogen to produce bleeding.[46,373,376] The significance of extraglandular estrogen production in health and disease has been discussed at length by Siiteri and MacDonald.[305]

Biosynthesis of Estriol During Pregnancy

Research has shown that biosynthesis of estrogens differs qualitatively and quantitatively in pregnant women compared with nonpregnant ones. In pregnant women, the major source of estrogens is the placenta, whereas in nonpregnant women, the ovaries are the main site of synthesis.[46,373,376] In contrast to the microgram quantities secreted

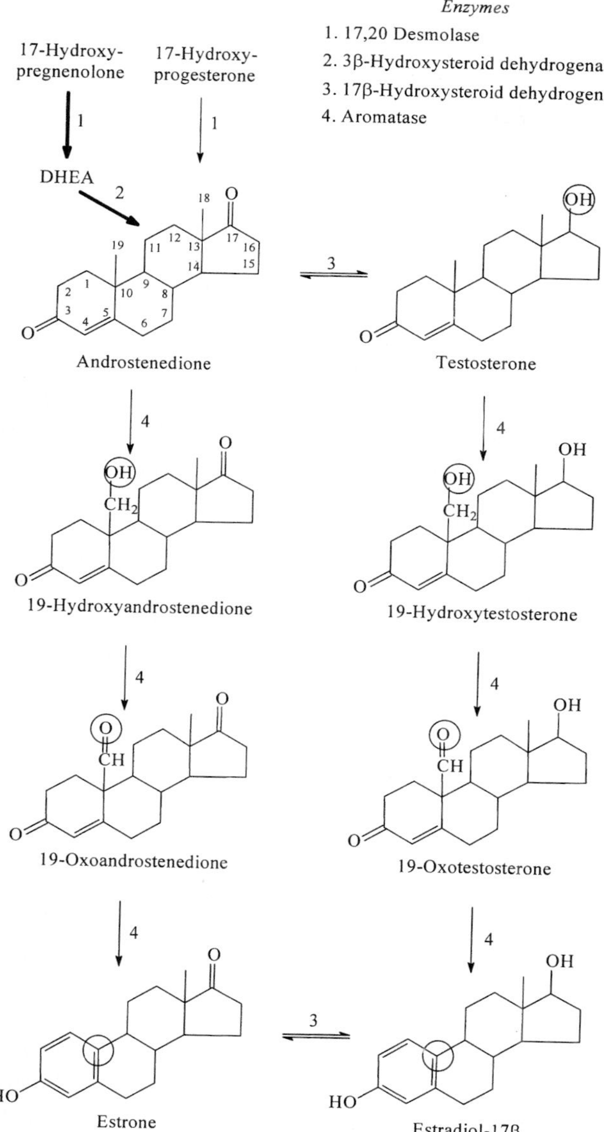

Figure 53-10 Biosynthesis of estrogens. *Heavy arrows* indicate the Δ5-3β-hydroxy pathway. The *circled area* represents the site of chemical change. See Figure 53-5 for the early synthetic steps.

by nonpregnant women, the amount of estrogen secreted during pregnancy increases to milligram amounts. The major estrogen secreted by the ovary is estradiol, whereas the major product secreted by the placenta is estriol. Estriol is formed in the placenta by sequential desulfurylation and aromatization of plasma DHEA-S. Except during pregnancy, measurements of estriol have little clinical value, because in nonpregnant women estriol is derived almost exclusively from estradiol (see also Chapter 54).

Estriol is the predominant hormone of late pregnancy. Maternal estriol is almost entirely (~90%) derived from fetal and placental sources. It is first detected during the 9th gestational week and gradually increases during the first and second trimesters. Plasma and salivary estriol concentrations peak approximately 3 to 5 weeks before labor and delivery.[125] This characteristic surge in estriol has been observed for term, preterm, and postterm pregnancies. Some reports have suggested utility in the measurement of salivary estriol in the prediction of risk for spontaneous preterm birth.[124,148-150,187,219] This test has a high negative predictive value but low positive predictive value. Currently, the American College of Obstetrics and Gynecologists does not suggest measuring salivary estriol concentrations except for research purposes.[2] Details regarding the techniques used to determine serum and salivary estriol concentrations are discussed in the section on analytical methods.

Serum estriol measurements are commonly used as part of the "triple" or "quad" maternal screens for Down syndrome–affected fetuses (see Chapter 54). On average, unconjugated estriol is 0.72 times less than normal (median value at 16 weeks: 0.30 to 1.50 μg/L) when fetal Down syndrome is present.[43,222,329,349]

Estrogen Transport in Blood

Greater than 97% of circulating estradiol is bound to plasma proteins. It is bound specifically and with high affinity to SHBG and nonspecifically to albumin.[248,318] SHBG concentrations are increased by estrogens and therefore are higher in women than in men. They are also increased during pregnancy, oral contraceptive use, hyperthyroidism, and administration of certain antiepileptic drugs, such as Dilantin. SHBG concentrations may decrease in hypothyroidism, obesity, or androgen excess. In women, estradiol circulates bound 40% to 60% to SHBG and 40% to 60% to albumin. SHBG has a higher affinity for testosterone than estradiol; therefore in men, estradiol circulates 20% to 30% bound to SHBG and 70% to 80% bound to albumin.[248,255] Only 2% to 3% of total estradiol circulates in the free form. In contrast, estrone and estrone sulfate circulate bound almost exclusively to albumin. As with testosterone, both the free and albumin-bound fractions of estradiol are thought to be biologically available,[255] but measurement of this fraction has not been shown to be clinically important.

In the normal, nonpregnant woman, estradiol is produced at the rate of 100 to 300 μg/day.[46,305,373] The production of estrone ranges from 100 to 200 μg/day. Diurnal variation of blood estrone concentrations occurs in postmenopausal women, presumably reflecting the variation in the androstenedione precursor that originates in the adrenal glands. However, no such diurnal rhythms have been demonstrated for estradiol.

Metabolism of Estrogens

In the normal course of estrogen metabolism (Figure 53-11), estradiol is believed to form a reversible redox system with estrone. Normally, blood estrone concentrations parallel estradiol concentrations throughout the menstrual cycle, but at one third to one half their magnitude.[261] Estrone is

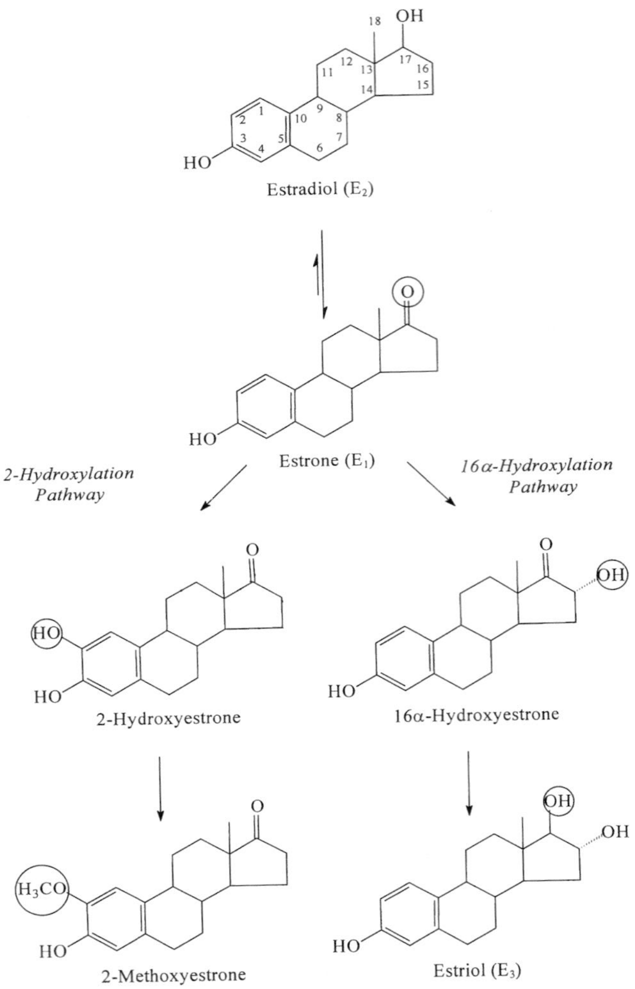

Figure 53-11 Main pathways of estradiol metabolism in humans. The *circled area* represents the site of chemical change.

then metabolized along two alternative pathways: the *2-hydroxylation pathway* leads to the formation of catechol estrogens (2-hydroxyestrone, 2-hydroxyestradiol, and 2-hydroxyestriol and their corresponding methoxy derivatives), and the *16α-hydroxylation pathway* leads predominantly to the formation of estriol.[46,373] The direction of estradiol metabolism depends on the pathophysiological state. For example, obesity and hypothyroidism are associated with an increase in estriol formation, whereas low body weight and hyperthyroidism are associated with the formation of catechol estrogens.[46] Although assays for catechol estrogen measurement are available,[56,220] they have no known current clinical value.

As is the case for other steroids, the liver is the primary site for the inactivation of estrogens. The main biochemical reactions are hydroxylation, oxidation, reduction, and methylation. Conjugation with glucuronic or sulfuric acid, which imparts more water solubility to these steroids and thus allows them to be eliminated rapidly through the kidney, is the final step in the metabolic process. Catechol estrogens, in addition, can bind covalently with protein through *o*-quinone or *o*-semiquinone intermediates.

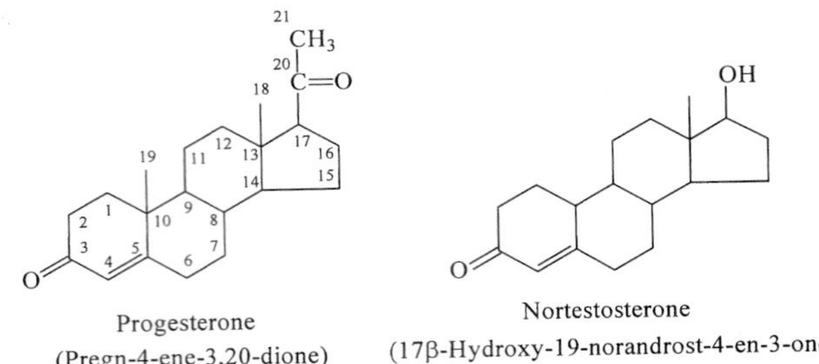

Figure 53-12 Structural formulas of progesterone and 19-nortestosterone.

PROGESTERONE

Progesterone, like the estrogens, is a female sex hormone. In conjunction with estrogens, it helps to regulate the accessory organs during the menstrual cycle.[373,376] This hormone is especially important in preparing the uterus for the implantation of the blastocyst and in maintaining pregnancy. In nonpregnant women, progesterone is secreted mainly by the corpus luteum. During pregnancy, the placenta becomes the major source of this hormone. Minor sources are the adrenal cortex in both sexes and the testes in men.

Chemistry

The structural formula of progesterone, a C_{21} compound, is shown in Figure 53-12. Like the corticosteroids and testosterone, progesterone (pregn-4-ene-3,20-dione) contains a keto group (at C-3) and a double bond between C-4 and C-5 (Δ^4); both structural characteristics are essential for progestational activity. The two-carbon side chain (CH_3CO) on C-17 is not thought to be important for its physiological action. Indeed the synthetic compound 19-nortestosterone (see Figure 53-12) and its derivatives, which are widely used as oral contraceptives, are more potent progestational agents than progesterone itself.

Biochemistry and Physiology

Biosynthesis

Biosynthesis of progesterone in ovarian tissue is believed to follow the same path from acetate to cholesterol through pregnenolone as it does in the adrenal cortex (see Chapter 51).[46,373,375] In luteal tissue, however, low-density lipoprotein cholesterol is thought to serve as the preferred precursor despite the potential of the corpus luteum to synthesize progesterone de novo from acetate.[306] Initiation and control of luteal secretion of progesterone are regulated by LH and FSH.[46,320,373]

Transport

Progesterone does not have a specific plasma-binding protein, but like cortisol is bound to corticosteroid-binding globulin. Reported concentrations for plasma free progesterone vary from 2% to 10% of total concentrations, and the percentage of unbound progesterone remains constant throughout the normal menstrual cycle.[115] The production rate of progesterone during the luteal phase reaches as high as 30 mg/day, whereas the production rate of progesterone by the placenta during the third trimester of pregnancy is ~300 mg/day.

Metabolism

The important metabolic events leading to inactivation of progesterone are reduction and conjugation. The main metabolic pathway for the metabolism of progesterone is shown in Figure 53-13.

Metabolites of progesterone may be classified into three groups based on the degree of reduction:

1. ***Pregnanediones.*** The C4-5 double bond is reduced, producing two compounds: pregnanedione (hydrogen atom at C-5 is in β-orientation) and allopregnanedione (hydrogen atom at C-5 is in α-orientation).
2. ***Pregnanolones.*** The keto group at C-3 is reduced, producing hydroxyl groups in α- or β-orientation. However, most urinary pregnanolones exist in the α-configuration.
3. ***Pregnanediols.*** The keto group at C-20 is also reduced. As in the previous case, metabolites containing the 20-hydroxyl group in α-orientation are quantitatively more important. In fact, urinary measurement of pregnanediol (5β-pregnane-3α,20α-diol) can be used as an index of endogenous production of progesterone, because this metabolite is quantitatively very significant and its concentration correlates with most clinical conditions.

Reduced metabolites are eventually conjugated with glucuronic acid and excreted as water-soluble glucuronides.

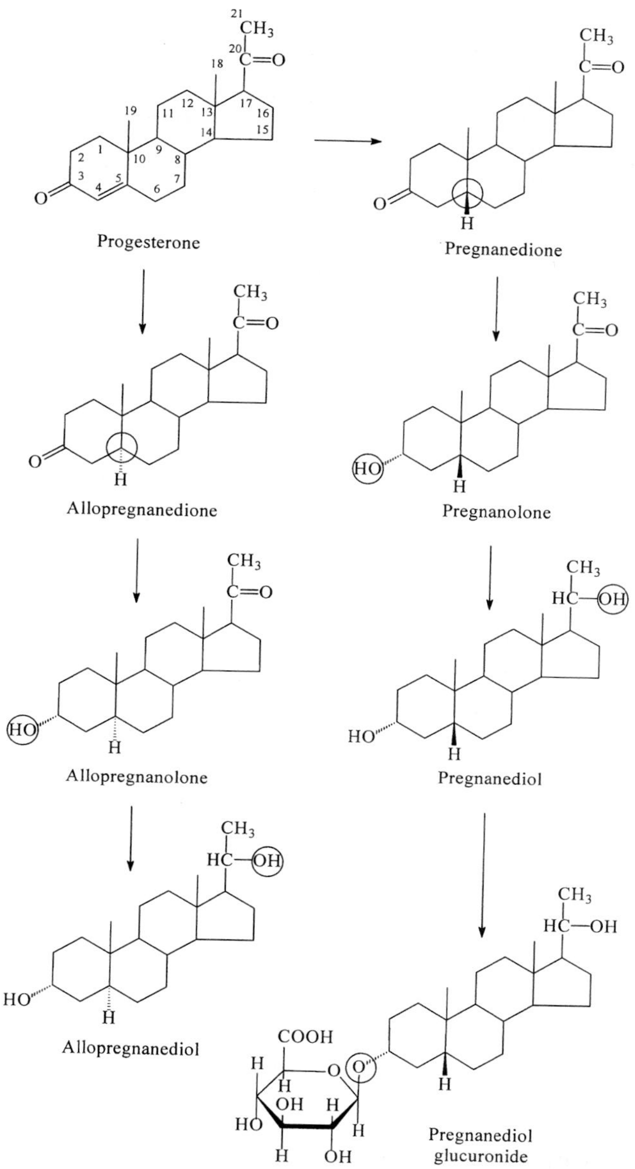

Progesterone → Pregnanedione; Progesterone → Allopregnanedione → Allopregnanolone → Allopregnanediol; Pregnanedione → Pregnanolone → Pregnanediol → Pregnanediol glucuronide

Figure 53-13 Metabolism of progesterone. The *circled area* represents the site of chemical change.

Female Reproductive Development

Fetal

In the genotypic female, lack of testosterone and MIS causes regression of the wolffian ducts and maintenance of the mullerian ducts, thus forming the female reproductive tract.[46,114] Gonadotropin activity in utero is suppressed because of high concentrations of circulating estrogens derived from the mother.[46,373]

Postnatal

When the placenta separates, concentrations of fetal sex steroids drop abruptly. Serum estradiol in neonates decreases to basal concentrations within 5 to 7days after birth and persists at this concentration until puberty. The negative feedback action of steroids is now removed, and gonadotropins are released. Postnatal peaks of LH and FSH are measurable for a few months after birth, peaking at 2 to 5 months and then dropping to basal concentrations.

During childhood, circulating concentrations of sex steroids and gonadotropins are low and are similar for both sexes. However, in patients with hypogonadism (Turner's syndrome), LH and FSH concentrations are higher than in normal children.[46,373] Pituitary response to exogenous GnRH stimulation parallels the endogenous secretion rates of LH and FSH. In children younger than 2 years of age, LH and FSH production increases dramatically in response to exogenous GnRH administration.[110] From then until about age 10, the responses are less than during the first 2 years. At the peripubertal stage, LH concentrations rise to more than 15 IU/L in both boys and girls, a response comparable with that in adults.[46,373] FSH response parallels that of LH, but is lesser in magnitude.

Puberty

The transition from sexual immaturity appears to begin with a diminished sensitivity of the pituitary gland or hypothalamus, or both, to the negative feedback effect of the sex steroids. The mechanism for this change is unclear. As puberty approaches, nocturnal secretion of gonadotropins occurs. Concentrations for LH, FSH, and gonadal steroids rise gradually over several years before stabilizing at adult concentrations, when full sexual maturity is reached. In girls, puberty is considered precocious if the onset of pubertal development (secondary sex characteristics) occurs before the age of 8 (see later section on precocious puberty), and delayed if there has been no development by the age of 13 or if menarche has not occurred by age 16.5.[69,227] Current literature reports that the median age of menarche in the United States is 12.43 years, which is 0.34 years earlier than reported in 1973.[60,213] This study also found that the median age at menarche of non-Hispanic black (12.06 years) girls is significantly earlier than that of non-Hispanic white (12.55 years) and Mexican-American (12.25 years) girls.[60]

Adrenarche precedes puberty by a few years. In girls, the rise in adrenal androgen concentrations (DHEA, DHEA-S, and androstenedione) begins at 6 to 7 years.[256] This rise in adrenal androgen concentrations lasts until late puberty. A cortical androgen-stimulating hormone may contribute to the rise of adrenal androgens at puberty in both sexes.[256] In girls, puberty is associated with rises in estrogen secretion by the ovary in response to gonadotropin concentrations that increase in response to GnRH.[30,46,307] Estrogen secretion by the ovary increases and causes enlargement of the uterus and breasts. In the breast, estrogen enhances growth of ducts; progesterone augments this effect. As the breast develops, estrogen also increases adipose tissue around the lactiferous duct system and contributes to the further enlargement of breast tissue.[46,373] The alveoli shift to a secretory pattern under the influence of progesterone.

Female Reproductive Abnormalities

Female Pseudohermaphroditism

In pseudohermaphroditism, the gonadal sex varies from the genital sex. The female pseudohermaphrodite is an individual who is genetically female but whose phenotypic characteristics are, to varying degrees, male. In neonates with a 46 XX karyotype and ambiguous genitalia, *congenital adrenal hyperplasia* (CAH) should be considered. CAH is a family of autosomal recessive disorders of adrenal steroidogenesis (see Chapter 51). Each disorder has a specific pattern of hormonal abnormalities resulting in deficiency or excess of androgens. The molecular genetics of CAH are discussed in detail in several reviews.[68,156,157,189,360] In female fetuses, exposure to androgens before the 12th week of gestation causes ambiguous genitalia; after 13 weeks, it results in clitoral enlargement.[46,293] Because androgen excess occurs before the 12th week of gestation in those with CAH, ambiguous genitalia are almost always present. Only deficiencies of 21-hydroxylase and 11β-hydroxylase are predominantly virilizing disorders. Deficiency of 3β-hydroxysteroid dehydrogenase is rare, but when present, affected girls may exhibit virilization.

Diagnosis of *21-hydroxylase deficiency* can be made in infants and children with excess excretion of urinary 17-KSs and pregnanetriol (a metabolite of 17-hydroxyprogesterone; see Chapter 51) and an elevated concentration of plasma 17-hydroxyprogesterone and androstenedione.[136,157,241] However, sick and premature infants may have elevated concentrations of 17-hydroxyprogesterone and androstenedione.[136,157] An elevation of 17-hydroxyprogesterone concentrations in early infancy (>3000 ng/dL) confirms the diagnosis of this disorder.[136,350] Additionally, molecular diagnostic testing is now available for detection of the mutations that account for a majority (80% to 90%) of 21-hydroxylase deficiency cases.[315]

An *11β-hydroxylase deficiency* is confirmed by finding elevated plasma concentrations of 11-deoxycortisol and deoxycorticosterone, increased concentrations of their metabolites in urine, and their suppression by glucocorticoid therapy (see Chapter 51). Plasma renin activity and aldosterone concentrations are low in this deficiency.[136,189,259]

Elevated plasma concentrations of 17-hydroxypregnenolone, DHEA, and DHEAS are found in patients with *3β-hydroxysteroid dehydrogenase deficiency* (see Chapter 51). Plasma concentrations of 17-hydroxyprogesterone may be elevated due to peripheral conversion of 17-hydroxypregnenolone. The ratio of 17-hydroxypregnenolone to 17-hydroxyprogesterone is strikingly elevated in these patients.[136,189,252]

Precocious Puberty

Precocious puberty is the development of secondary sexual characteristics in girls less than 8 years old and boys less than 9 years old.[276] In 1999, the Lawson Wilkins Pediatric Society issued new recommendations to lower the age standards at which puberty should be considered precocious from 8 to 7 in white girls and to 6 in black girls.[173] The new recommendations were met with criticism because they are based solely on a single epidemiological study performed by Herman-Giddens and collaborators in 1997.[151] Many argue that the decreased age standards will result in underdiagnosis of this condition.[197,225,278]

Despite the debate over the age of onset, pediatric endocrinologists agree that it is important to distinguish between benign advanced pubertal conditions and true precocious puberty.* Early puberty is manifested by the appearance of secondary sexual characteristics such as premature thelarche (premature breast development), premature adrenarche (premature sexual hair development), or phallic enlargement. When presented as isolated cases, these secondary sexual characteristics are not considered to be pathological as none progresses to full-blown puberty, nor are they associated with increased rates of bone growth and maturation. However, if a child has at least two signs of puberty and also demonstrates increased rates of bone growth and

*References 48, 166, 182, 192, 196, 224.

maturation, the many causes of true precocious puberty must be considered.[224]

Precocious puberty is classified as GnRH dependent or independent.[48,166,182,224] GnRH-dependent precocious puberty (also called central precocious puberty) is due to precocious activation of the hypothalamic-pituitary-gonadal axis. In girls, the cause is most commonly idiopathic (90%); however, idiopathic cases account for less than 10% of central precocious puberty in boys. Central nervous system tumors can also cause central precocious puberty, the most common being hypothalamic hamartomas. Neurofibromatosis has been also reported to lead to GnRH-dependent precocious puberty.

GnRH-independent precocious puberty (also called pseudoprecocious puberty) refers to precocious sex steroid secretion that is independent of pituitary gonadotropin release. CAHs is a common cause of pseudoprecocious puberty. Classic forms of CAH present with virilization, growth acceleration, and accelerated bone maturation. Nonclassical or late-onset forms usually present in childhood or adolescence with premature adrenarche and acne. In fact, 5% to 10% of children presenting with premature adrenarche have late-onset adrenal hyperplasia. Tumors of the adrenal gland, ovaries, and testes that secrete androgens or estrogens may result in GnRH-independent precocious puberty. Males exhibiting signs of puberty around age 2 are characteristic of testotoxicosis, a familial male-limited form of precocious puberty. This autosomal dominant disorder is due to activating mutations affecting LH receptors. The McCune-Albright syndrome is due to a point mutation in the G protein associated with gonadotropin receptors, which causes the gonads to function as if both the FSH and LH receptors are constitutively activated. Although this mutation results in GnRH-independent precocious puberty in both sexes, it is most common in girls. Precocious puberty combined with polyostotic fibrous dysplasia and café-au-lait pigmentation are hallmarks for McCune-Albright syndrome. Severe hypothyroidism is also associated with GnRH-independent precocious puberty, likely due to the intrinsic FSH activity of high circulating concentrations of TSH. Unlike the other causes, hypothyroid-induced precocious puberty is associated with skeletal and growth delay.

Diagnosis of precocious puberty is based on (1) clinical presentation, (2) a thorough pubertal history, (3) bone age determinations, and (4) laboratory tests to assess gonadotropin concentrations and response to exogenous GnRH.* The GnRH stimulation test is the gold standard for diagnosis of GnRH-dependent precocious puberty. Pubertal responses of LH and FSH to GnRH stimulation are considered diagnostic of precocious puberty when the chronological age is inappropriate for the hormone response. The GnRH stimulation test is also used to monitor the effectiveness of GnRH agonist therapy.[190,288,289] Typically, an IV bolus of exogenous GnRH is administered followed by a single measurement (at 40 to 45 minutes) or serial measurements of LH and FSH concentrations.* A predominant LH response correlates with a pubertal pattern and cutoffs vary depending on the assay, with sex differences noted. A typical pubertal response is characterized by a rise in LH ≥8 IU/L after IV administration of 100 μg GnRH.[227] In girls, peak LH/FSH ratios >0.66 to 1.0 have also been proposed to be diagnostic of central precocious puberty.[247,348] Highly sensitive fluorometric[37] and chemiluminetric[240] immunoassays are now available for measuring basal LH concentrations. Basal LH concentrations can be used instead of the GnRH stimulation test for diagnosis of central precocious puberty. A fluorometric assay resulting in a basal concentration of LH >0.6 IU/L in either sex indicates a pubertal pattern and is consistent with precocious puberty. Values <0.6 IU/L can occur with any form of precocious puberty and require follow-up with a GnRH stimulation test.[37] A similar pattern is observed for the immunochemiluminometric assays using a cutoff of 0.3 IU/L.[239,240]

Response to exogenous GnRH is suppressed and LH and FSH concentrations are low in individuals with GnRH-independent precocious puberty. The diagnosis of GnRH-independent precocious puberty must exclude nonclassical adrenal hyperplasia (NCAH). Basal 17-hydroxyprogesterone concentrations of early morning samples can be used to screen for 21-OH-deficient NCAH. A basal 17-hydroxyprogesterone concentration <200 ng/L (<6.0 nmol/L) almost always rules out 21-OH-deficient NCAH. Patients with intermediate (200 to 500 ng/dL) basal 17-hydroxyprogesterone concentrations should undergo an ACTH stimulation test to confirm the presence of a 21-OH-deficient NCAH. Such a test is done by measuring the 17-hydroxyprogesterone response to ACTH stimulation. An exaggerated response is expected in cases of NCAH. Although controversial, current guidelines use a 17-hydroxyprogesterone diagnostic cutoff of >1000 ng/dL (>30 nmol/L).[242] Some argue that the cutoff should be raised to >1500 ng/dL (>45 nmol/L) or >2000 ng/dL (>60 nmol/L), as the value of 30 nmol/L was set before the availability of molecular genotyping, and studies have indicated that several nonaffected carriers exhibit 17-hydroxyprogesterone concentrations above 30 nmol/L.[7,8,10]

The therapy for precocious puberty is dependent upon the presenting symptoms and underlying causes.[182,192,196,224,257] Isolated premature thelarche or adrenarche does not require therapy. Patients with premature thelarche should be followed for 3 to 6 months and require further evaluation for precocious puberty. Cases of premature adrenarche should be evaluated for NCAH and/or polycystic ovary syndrome (PCOS) in girls with determined insulin resistance. GnRH-dependent precocious puberty is

*References 48, 166, 182, 192, 196, 224.

*References 53, 100, 166, 183, 195, 239, 240.

treated using GnRH agonists to inhibit normal gonadotropin release, thereby slowing pubertal progression. The therapy for GnRH-independent precocious puberty is determined by the underlying cause.

Estrogens and Breast Cancer

Suspicions of estrogen-based etiologies in the development of human breast cancer result from both epidemiological and experimental observations.[99A,159,211,233A] Early menarche and later natural menopause are associated with increased risk of breast cancer. A two-stage mechanism has been postulated: (1) initiation of a precancerous state by ovarian activity during the early reproductive years, and (2) continuation of ovarian activity in later years as a promoting influence on already initiated tumor cells. Ovarian estrogen has been assumed to be the causative factor, as the administration of estrogen negates the protective effects of early oophorectomy. Moreover, treatment of men with estrogen for prostatic cancer or after transsexual operations is also associated with an increased risk of breast cancer.

Low risk for breast cancer has consistently been connected with high parity. Increased risk is associated with early menarche, late (>30 years) first full-term pregnancy, and late menopause. Pregnancy occurring before age 25 to 30 years has a protective effect.

According to the theory, the relative concentrations of individual estrogen fractions (estrone, estradiol, and estriol) produced in the first decade or so after puberty are important determinants of a woman's lifetime risk of breast cancer.[63] In particular, pregnancy at a young age is associated with both favorable estrogen fraction ratios and decreased risk. Further discussion of the role of estrogen in the genesis of breast cancer is found in monographs and review articles.[62,144-146,175,176,204]

The rationale for using endocrine therapy in women with breast carcinoma is based on the fact that estrogen stimulates biochemical processes in cells of the uterus, pituitary gland, hypothalamus, and breast that normally contain the estrogen receptor. A reduction in circulating estrogen concentrations would be expected to decrease the biochemical activity of these cells. Approximately one third of women with metastatic breast carcinoma obtain an objective remission after various types of endocrine therapy directed at lowering their estrogen concentrations. Such therapy includes oophorectomy, hypophysectomy, and adrenalectomy (ablative therapy), and administration of antiestrogens, androgens, and aromatase inhibitors (additive therapy).[22,42,188,274]

Cytoplasmic estrogen receptors are important prognostic indicators and are now routinely measured in samples of breast tissue after surgical removal of the tumor. Sixty percent of patients with carcinoma of the breast have tumors that are estrogen receptor positive. Approximately two thirds of patients with estrogen receptor–positive tumors respond to endocrine therapy; 95% of the patients with estrogen receptor–negative tumors fail to respond. Therefore, the greater the estrogen receptor content of the tumor, the higher the response rate to endocrine therapy and lower incidence of recurrence.

Normal Menstrual Cycle

During a normal menstrual cycle, there is a closely coordinated interplay of feedback effects between the hypothalamus, the anterior lobe of the pituitary gland, and the ovaries. In addition, there are cyclic hormone changes that lead to functional and structural changes in the ovaries (follicle maturation, ovulation, and corpus luteum development), uterus (preparation of the endometrium for possible implantation of the fertilized ovum), cervix (to permit transport of sperm), and vagina (see Figure 53-7).[46,373,376]

Phases

The menstrual cycle is measured beginning with day 1 as the first day of menstrual bleeding. Each cycle consists of a follicular and a luteal phase.

Follicular Phase

The *follicular phase,* the initiation of follicular growth, actually begins during the last few days of the previous luteal phase and terminates at ovulation (see Figure 53-7). During the early part of the follicular phase, concentrations of FSH are elevated, but decline up until ovulation (Figure 53-7).[46] LH secretion begins to increase around the middle of the follicular phase. Just before ovulation, estrogen secretion by the follicle increases dramatically, which positively stimulates the hypothalamus and triggers the LH surge. The LH surge is a reliable predictor of ovulation, with the onset of the surge occurring 24 to 36 hours and the peak occurring 10 to 12 hours before ovulation.[46] Ovulation occurs around day 14 of the menstrual cycle.

Luteal Phase

The *luteal phase* is the last half of the cycle and is characterized by increasing production of progesterone and estrogen from the corpus luteum with consequent gradual lowering of LH and FSH concentrations. Progesterone reaches a peak of approximately 8 mg/day at about 8 days postovulation. If ovulation does not occur, the corpus luteum fails to form, and a cyclical rise in progesterone is subnormal. If pregnancy occurs, hCG maintains the corpus luteum and progesterone continues to rise. In the absence of conception, the corpus luteum resolves and results in a decrease in estrogen and progesterone concentrations and a breakdown of the endometrium. The average duration of menstrual flow is 4 to 6 days and average menstrual blood loss is 30 mL.[46]

Role of Individual Hormones

To explain further the intricacies of the normal menstrual cycle, the fluctuations of each major hormone are discussed separately in the following sections with regard to control and effects (see also Figures 53-7 and 53-14).

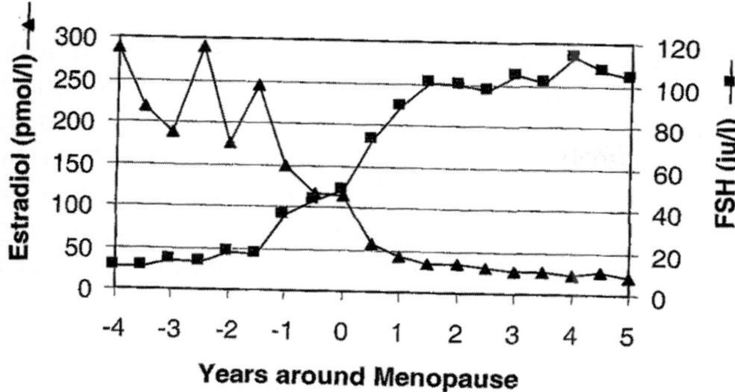

Figure 53-14 Geometric means for FSH and estradiol in relation to the final menstrual period (FMP). The horizontal axis represents time (yr) with respect to the FMP (0); negative (positive) numbers represent time before (after) the FMP. *(From Burger HG, Dudley EC, Hopper JL, Groome N, Guthrie JR, Green A, et al. Prospectively measured levels of serum follicle-stimulating hormone, estradiol, and the dimeric inhibins during the menopausal transition in a population-based cohort of women. J Clin Endocrinol Metab 1999;84:4025-30; Figure 1A.)*

Gonadotropin-Releasing Hormone

Gonadotropin-releasing hormone triggers the surge of LH that precedes ovulation.[46,373,376] There appear to be two separate feedback centers in the hypothalamus: a tonic negative feedback center in the basal medial hypothalamus and a cyclical positive feedback center in the anterior regions of the hypothalamus. Low concentrations of estradiol, such as those that are present during the follicular phase, affect the negative feedback center, whereas high concentrations of estradiol, such as are seen just before the midcycle LH peak, trigger the positive feedback center. Progesterone, in combination with estrogen, affects the negative feedback center in the luteal phase. GnRH is released in a pulsatile fashion and has a self-priming effect; the first dose potentiates the effect of subsequent doses. The magnitude of the LH response to GnRH increases steadily through the follicular phase and is greatest at the time of the preovulatory surge of LH, after which it declines again.

Follicle-Stimulating Hormone

A few days before day 1 of the cycle, FSH shows a slight but important peak (see Figure 53-7), probably triggered by a fall in estradiol concentration that briefly eliminates the negative feedback effect.[46,373,376] This peak of FSH initiates the growth and maturation of a cohort of ovarian follicles. LH and FSH release are pulsatile throughout the cycle. As estrogen is released from the growing follicles, FSH concentrations fall again and remain low through the follicular phase. By days 5 to 7, a single follicle is selected for further growth. The effect of FSH on the maturing follicle is increased through estradiol-induced changes in FSH receptors. FSH, aided by estradiol, acts on the cells of the follicle to increase responsiveness of LH receptors by the time of midcycle surge. FSH and LH receptors respond with an increase either in their number or in their affinity for corresponding gonadotropin. There is a rise in FSH at midcycle that is triggered by progesterone. The function of this peak is not entirely known, but is thought to stimulate plasminogen activator and increase granulosa cell LH receptors.[46] During the luteal phase, FSH is suppressed by negative feedback from estradiol until a lesser FSH peak, occurring near the end of the cycle, starts off the follicular maturation of the next cycle.

Luteinizing Hormone

Luteinizing hormone secretion is suppressed in the follicular phase by negative feedback from estradiol.[46,373,376] As estradiol production by the developing follicle increases, the effect of estradiol on the positive feedback center becomes important. Increasing release of GnRH from the hypothalamus and increasing sensitivity of the anterior lobe of the pituitary gland to GnRH result in the midcycle surge of LH. Ovarian follicle receptors for LH, sensitized by FSH and estradiol, transmit the stimulus to enhance differentiation of the theca cell and the production of progesterone by the developing corpus luteum. LH production is suppressed during the luteal phase by negative feedback from progesterone combined with estradiol, but a low concentration of LH is probably necessary to prolong corpus luteum function.

Estradiol

Estradiol production by the ovary falls near the end of a cycle, but begins to increase again under the influence of FSH (see Figure 53-7).[46,373,376] Estradiol enhances the FSH effect on a maturing follicle through changes in FSH receptors of the follicular cells, but suppresses pituitary FSH and LH release during the follicular phase through negative feedback. Before the midfollicular phase, estrogen concentrations are <50 pg/mL, but rise rapidly as the follicle matures. Estradiol production increases, reaching a midcycle peak between 250 and 500 pg/mL.[318] Estradiol concentrations fall off abruptly after ovulation, but rise again as the corpus luteum forms, reaching concentrations of approximately 125 pg/mL during the luteal phase.[318] Progesterone produced by the corpus luteum, combined with estrogen, exerts a negative effect on the hypothalamus and anterior lobe of the pituitary gland. As a result, LH and FSH secretion is suppressed again during the luteal phase. Estradiol is essential for the development of proliferative endometrium and is synergistic with progesterone for the development of the changes in the endometrium that initiate shedding; the decrease in negative feedback from estradiol on the anterior lobe of the pituitary gland triggers the FSH surge that begins the development of an ovarian follicle for the next cycle.

Changes in androgen production also occur during the menstrual cycle, with a peak at midcycle. Estradiol is not the only estrogen produced; estrone secretion, mainly from peripheral sources, also increases throughout the cycle. Estrogen and progesterone have visible effects on vaginal cytology and cervical mucus, and progesterone elevates body temperature (as discussed later).

Progesterone

Progesterone is not produced in significant amounts until the midcycle LH surge and ovulation. LH enhances theca cell differentiation and progesterone production, which increase by a factor of 10 to 20, to a maximum about 8 days after the midcycle peak of LH. Progesterone is thought to stimulate the ovulatory peak of FSH and promote the growth of secretory endometrium, which is necessary for implantation of the fertilized ovum.[46]

OVULATION

An intricate interplay of endocrine events contributes to follicular maturation. Growth of ovarian follicles appears to be continuous. How an individual follicle is singled out for each menstrual cycle is not known. The late-cycle peak of FSH is likely important in this process. Once a follicle has been stimulated, estradiol production causes that specific follicle to be more receptive to effects from FSH. The high concentration of estradiol just before midcycle is responsible for triggering the positive feedback in the hypothalamus that leads to the midcycle LH surge. The precise cause of ovulation is not known, but ovulation occurs 1 to 24 hours after the LH peak. After ovulation, LH is suppressed by progesterone and estradiol, but the effect of LH is increased on the corpus luteum.[46,320,373,376] In the event of successful fertilization and implantation, corpus luteum function is sustained by hCG produced by the trophoblastic cells of the developing embryo. hCG has high molecular homology to LH and is capable of binding and stimulating LH receptors. Otherwise, the declining concentration of estradiol leads to regression of the corpus luteum and to the late-cycle FSH peak that starts the process again.

IRREGULAR MENSES

In a normal ovulatory menstrual cycle, menstruation occurs every 28 days on average. Normal women display considerable variation in cycle length that varies from 25 to 30 days.[46] Amenorrhea, the absence of menstrual bleeding, is traditionally categorized as either primary (women who have never menstruated) or secondary (women in whom menstruation is present for a variable time and then ceases). Amenorrhea is a relatively common disorder, with an estimated prevalence of 5% in the general population and as high as 8.5% in an unselected adolescent postpubescent population.[215]

Primary Amenorrhea

Primary amenorrhea (Box 53-2) is defined as a failure to establish spontaneous periodic menstruation by the age of 16 regardless of whether secondary sex characteristics have developed.[69,178,221] About 40% of phenotypic females who have primary amenorrhea (nearly always associated with absence of development of secondary sex characteristics) have *Turner's syndrome* (55 X karyotype) or *pure gonadal dysgenesis* (either 46 XX or XY karyotype).[46,375] *Mullerian duct agenesis* or *dysgenesis* with absence of the vagina or uterus is the second most common manifestation, and the third most common is *testicular feminization* (androgen receptor deficiency and normal or elevated plasma testosterone concentrations if the patient is past puberty and is karyotype XY).

A *17α-hydroxylase deficiency* is a rare form of CAH that is associated with delayed puberty, primary amenorrhea, and hypertension. These patients have a 46 XX karyotype with elevated gonadotropins, low sex steroids, hypertension, and hypokalemia (see Chapter 51).[69,189]

Another rare cause of amenorrhea is the so-called *resistant ovary syndrome.* This primary hypogonadal condition is associated with increased concentrations of plasma FSH and LH, and ovaries that contain predominantly primordial follicles. It is thought to arise from a defect in FSH receptors.[46] This disorder can be diagnosed only by examination of an ovarian biopsy specimen, which will exhibit functioning ovarian follicles despite the presence of amenorrhea. Ovulation can sometimes be induced in these patients with administration of high doses of gonadotropins.

As discussed earlier, *Kallmann's syndrome* involves hypogonadotropic hypogonadism associated with anosmia or hyposmia and is caused by a defect in the formation and migration of GnRH neurons. Sexual infantilism is the prominent manifestation and primary amenorrhea is common.[46,375] Finally, delayed pubertal development also should be considered.

Secondary Amenorrhea

Secondary amenorrhea is defined as an absence of periodic menstruation for at least 6 months in women who have previously experienced menses, or for 12 months in a woman with prior oligomenorrhea.[70,178,221,270,352] *Oligomenorrhea* is infrequent menstruation, occurring less than nine times per year.[279] With a few exceptions, the causes of primary and secondary amenorrhea overlap (see Box 53-2). Pregnancy is the most common cause of secondary amenorrhea and must be considered first and ruled out.[178,221,352] Elevated prolactin, either iatrogenic or induced by a prolactin-secreting tumor, can result in oligomenorrhea or amenorrhea.[178,221,352] About one third of women with no obvious cause of amenorrhea have elevated prolactin concentrations.[178] It is thought that hyperprolactinemia inhibits the release of LH and FSH.[184] Both hyperthyroidism and hypothyroidism are associated with a variety of menstrual disorders because of their effect on metabolism and interconversion of androgens and estrogens.[178,221,373]

Often it is helpful to separate patients with secondary amenorrhea into those with and without signs of hirsutism and androgen excess.

BOX 53-2 Causes of Amenorrhea

Primary Amenorrhea
- Lower tract defects
  - Vaginal aplasia
  - Imperforate hymen
  - Congenital vaginal atresia
- Uterine disorders
  - Congenital absence of the uterus
  - Endometritis
  - Mullerian agenesis (Mayer-Rokitansky-Kuster-Hauser syndrome)
- Ovarian disorders
  - XO gonadal and X dysgenesis and variants
  - XX gonadal dysgenesis
  - Turner's syndrome
  - Testicular feminization syndrome
  - 17-Hydroxylase deficiency of the ovaries and adrenal glands
  - Autoimmune oophoritis
  - Resistant ovary syndrome
  - Polycystic ovary syndrome
- Adrenal disorders (congenital adrenal hyperplasia)
- Thyroid disorders (hypothyroidism)
- Pituitary-hypothalamic disorders
  - Hypopituitarism
  - Constitutional delay in the onset of menses (physiological)
  - Nutritional disorders
  - Kallmann's syndrome

Secondary Amenorrhea
- Pregnancy/lactation
- Uterine disorders
  - Posttraumatic uterine synechiae (Asherman's syndrome)
  - Progestational agents
- Ovarian disorders
  - Polycystic ovary syndrome (hypothalamic)
  - Ovarian tumors
  - Premature ovarian failure (idiopathic, autoimmune, injury)
  - Antimetabolite therapy
- Adrenal disorders
  - Late-onset adrenal hyperplasia
  - Cushing's syndrome
  - Virilizing adrenal tumors
  - Adrenocorticoid insufficiency
- Thyroid disorders
  - Hypothyroidism
  - Hyperthyroidism
- Pituitary disorders
  - Acquired hypopituitarism (trauma, tumors, Sheehan's syndrome, lymphocytic hypophysitis)
  - Physiological or pathological hyperprolactinemia
- Hypothalamic disorders
  - Tumors and infiltrative diseases
  - Nutritional disorders
  - Hypophysitis
  - Excessive exercise
  - Stress
- Iatrogenic
  - Antipsychotics (phenothiazines, haloperidol, clozapine, pimozide)
  - Antidepressants (tricyclics, monoamine oxidase inhibitors)
  - Antihypertensives (calcium channel blockers, methyldopa, reserpine)
  - Drugs with estrogenic activity (digitalis, flavonoids, marijuana, oral contraceptives)
  - Drugs with ovarian toxicity (busulfan, chlorambucil, cisplatin, cyclophosphamide, fluorouracil)

Androgen Excess

A patient with androgen excess can present with variable degrees of excess hair on the face, chest, abdomen, and thighs, acne, and obesity. Amenorrhea caused by androgen excess can be due to adult-onset CAH, corticotropin-dependent Cushing's syndrome, or PCOS.

Some individuals with 21-hydroxylase deficiency do not manifest any developmental abnormalities or salt wasting, but they present with signs of androgen excess. This clinical syndrome, referred to as *nonclassic, adult-onset,* or *late-onset CAH,* may be indistinguishable from PCOS (see also Chapter 50).[7,80,116]

PCOS occurs in about 5% to 10% of premenopausal women and is thought to be caused by a hypothalamic disorder.[46,126,316,377] PCOS is clinically defined by hyperandrogenism with chronic anovulation in women without underlying disease of the adrenal or pituitary glands.[116,201] This syndrome is characterized by infertility, hirsutism, obesity (in approximately half of those affected), and various menstrual disturbances ranging from amenorrhea to irregular vaginal bleeding (Table 53-1). Although this syndrome is associated with polycystic ovaries, this has not been considered essential for the diagnosis. The name is actually a misnomer, as the ovaries are covered with follicles not cysts. Women with PCOS have a greater frequency of both hyperinsulinemia and insulin resistance.[98,116,202,260,317] As a result, acanthosis nigricans (dark pigmentation of the spiny layer of the skin) is sometimes present in obese women with PCOS.[99] Relatively low FSH concentrations and disproportionately high LH concentrations are common in PCOS. Serum androstenedione and testosterone concentrations (total and free concentrations) are elevated, with mean concentrations 50% to 150% higher than normal.[19,46,116] PCOS patients have substantial estrogen production because of the peripheral conversion of androgens to estrogens. The anovulation is caused by continuous estrogen stimulation of the endometrium. This chronic stimulation may predispose these patients to endometrial cancer.[116] There has been some attempt to link PCOS to *leptin,* a hormone that is secreted by adipocytes and thought to play a role in regulating food

TABLE 53-1 Clinical Features of the Polycystic Ovary Syndrome

Clinical Feature	Frequency (%)
Hirsutism	65
Acne	26
Obesity	37
Infertility	48
Amenorrhea	35
Oligomenorrhea	42
Regular menstrual cycle	20

Data were compiled from three studies. Two used ultrasonography as the primary method of diagnosis, one used ovarian histology. Total $N = 1935$. Modified from Franks S. Polycystic ovary syndrome. N Engl J Med 1995;333.

intake and metabolism.[39] Animals that lack leptin are infertile, and leptin injection increases gonadotropin secretion and restores fertility.[15,58] However, literature suggests that leptin concentrations are normal in patients with PCOS.[45] In a 2001 report, Veldhuis and collaborators note that although the serum leptin concentrations were the same in PCOS patients and controls, the pattern of leptin secretion was abnormal in girls with PCOS.[343]

Ovarian hyperthecosis, a nonneoplastic lesion of the ovary characterized by the presence of islands of luteinized thecal cells in the ovarian stroma, is sometimes confused with PCOS. The features that distinguish it from PCOS include higher concentrations of testosterone, androstenedione, and DHT derived from ovarian secretion. Thus there is greater androgenization than is usually observed in patients with PCOS. Estrone secretion is greater, and both LH and FSH concentrations are either reduced or less than normal. Insulin resistance and hyperinsulinism are present to a greater degree than in PCOS. Finally, patients with ovarian hyperthecosis fail to ovulate when treated with an antiestrogen, such as clomiphene citrate.[377]

Hirsutism and Virilization

Hirsutism is defined as the excessive growth of terminal hair in women and children in a distribution similar to that occurring in postpubertal men.[6,275,287] True hirsutism, which is androgen responsive, has to be distinguished from hypertrichosis, which is excessive growth of vellus or non–androgen-responsive hair. Vellus is fine, downy hair, which is usually unpigmented, whereas terminal hairs are thick and found in androgen-responsive areas of the skin.[280,287] Growth of vellus hair diffusely over the trunk and face is either familial or drug induced, and can be treated only by mechanical hair removal or withdrawal of the inducing drug. Women with androgen-dependent hirsutism either have exposure to excess androgens or have a heightened sensitivity to normal circulating concentrations of androgen. As a consequence, the vellus follicles develop into terminal hair follicles in the areas of androgen-sensitive skin.

BOX 53-3 Causes of Hirsutism

Ovarian
- Severe insulin resistance
- Hyperthecosis, hilus cell or stromal cell hyperplasia
- Androgen-producing ovarian tumors
- Menopause

Adrenal
- Classical congenital hyperplasia
  - 21-Hydroxylase deficiency
  - 11-Hydroxylase deficiency
  - 3β-Hydroxysteroid dehydrogenase deficiency
- Adult or attenuated adrenal hyperplasia
- Androgen-producing adrenal tumors

Familial Hirsutism

Endocrine Disorders
- Polycystic ovary syndrome
- Hyperprolactinemia
- Acromegaly
- Cushing's syndrome

Idiopathic Hirsutism (includes increased skin sensitivity to androgens)

Iatrogenic
- Androgens
- Dilantin
- Diazoxide
- Minoxidil
- Streptomycin
- Cyclosporine
- Danazol
- Metyrapone
- Phenothiazides
- Progestogens (19-norsteroid derivatives)

Causes of hirsutism are listed in Box 53-3. The estimated prevalence for idiopathic hirsutism ranges from 6% to 50% of women evaluated for hirsutism depending on the definition.[9,44,287,291] Typically, idiopathic hirsutism is defined by normal physical and laboratory findings in hirsute women. However, Azziz and collaborators report that the prevalence of idiopathic hirsutism changes drastically whether or not factors such as ovulatory function and androgen concentrations are considered.[9] It is thought that an increased sensitivity of the hair follicle to normal circulating androgens causes the excess hair growth.[287] Nonneoplastic forms of hirsutism are slow to progress and usually manifest at the time of puberty, when circulating concentrations of androgens increase, or after a period of weight gain, or when oral contraceptives have been stopped.[275] A rapid onset of hirsutism suggests an iatrogenic cause, or if associated with virilization, a neoplastic source of androgens. The most common cause of androgen hypersecretion in women is PCOS, with a reported 70% to 80% of hirsute women affected with this disorder.[291] The hyperandrogenism usually arises from both ovaries and the adrenal glands (for more on PCOS, see previous section). Late-onset CAH (see Chapter 51), acromegaly, hyperprolactinemia, menopause (see also section on menopause, later in this chapter), and adrenocorticotropic hormone (ACTH)–dependent Cushing's syndrome can also cause hirsutism.

Virilization is characterized by clitoral hypertrophy, deepening of the voice, temporal hair recession, baldness, increased libido, decreased body fat, and menstrual irregularities or amenorrhea. Hirsutism is usually associated with normal or slightly elevated serum androgens, whereas virilization is associated with marked increases in ovarian or adrenal androgen production.[46]

The role of the laboratory in evaluation of women for hirsutism and virilization is discussed in a later section on tests for the evaluation of amenorrhea in this chapter.

Other Factors

Many other factors or conditions will cause secondary amenorrhea. They include disorders of the ovary, uterus, pituitary, and hypothalamus, and drugs.

Disorders of the ovary such as premature ovarian failure (POF) and loss of ovarian function can cause amenorrhea. *POF* has been defined as failure of ovarian estrogen production occurring in a hypergonadotropic state at any age between menarche and age 40.[46,70,178,352] If the patient is younger than 25 years of age, karyotyping should be performed to rule out the presence of a variety of chromosomal abnormalities involving duplications or absence of the X chromosome or presence of a Y chromosome. Patients present with symptoms of hypoestrogenism, including hot flashes and high gonadotropin concentrations. Autoimmune disorders have been associated with 20% to 40% of cases of POF that result in destruction of the ovary and in amenorrhea.[46,70,178,352] These patients also may have antibodies to other endocrine and nonendocrine tissue. Other causes for ovarian failure include oophorectomy, cystic degeneration, trauma, infection, or interference with blood supply. In rare patients, there may be evidence of ovarian resistance to gonadotropins.[46,353]

Secondary amenorrhea also is caused by uterine failure. The patient with a uterine problem is normal hormonally, but does not menstruate. *Asherman's syndrome,* or intrauterine adhesions, is the most common outflow-tract abnormality that causes amenorrhea. Endometrial damage may occur in response to a dilatation and curettage and to infections of the endometrium.[70,178] Pituitary dysfunction can cause secondary amenorrhea. This is most often caused by intrinsic pituitary tumors. However, Sheehan's syndrome and pituitary apoplexy can also result in hormone deficiency. Empty sella syndrome has been reported in 4% to 16% of patients with amenorrhea and galactorrhea.[178]

Hypothalamic dysfunctions consist of those disorders that disrupt the frequency or amplitude of GnRH. Rarely, this can be caused by a lesion or tumor. However, most commonly, disruption occurs in response to psychological stress, depression, severe weight loss, anorexia nervosa, or strenuous exercise.[70,178] A syndrome known as the *female athletic triad* has also been described. This syndrome is prevalent in women who exercise vigorously, and is associated with amenorrhea, disordered eating, and osteoporosis. Competitive long-distance runners, gymnasts, and professional ballet dancers appear to be at highest risk. Although the mechanism for the disturbance is unclear, the symptoms and laboratory profiles are similar to those of other forms of hypothalamic amenorrhea. LH and FSH concentrations are normal or low, and estradiol concentrations are low. As a result of the chronic low estrogen, bone mineral content is low and the incidence of stress fractures is increased.[70,215]

Several tumors of the ovary, pituitary gland, and adrenal glands occur in combination with amenorrhea.[46,209,339,375] The amenorrhea may be confused with pregnancy if the tumors produce hCG. Choriocarcinomas of the uterus or ovary may produce large amounts of hCG that can cause hyperthyroidism because of the slight thyrotropic action of hCG. Granulosa–theca cell tumors are usually associated with estrogen secretion that results in amenorrhea and irregular menses and, rarely, excessive androgen with associated virilization.[46,375]

Many drugs can also produce amenorrhea (see Box 53-2), particularly phenothiazines and other psychotropic drugs such as haloperidol, pimozide, or clozapine.[178] The phenothiazine-induced amenorrhea is usually associated with hyperprolactinemia and galactorrhea. Drugs affecting the normal pathway of dopamine secretion can produce amenorrhea by decreasing the secretion of norepinephrine. Because norepinephrine is important in controlling the synthesis and secretion of GnRH, any alteration in its synthesis or secretion has resulted in menstrual abnormalities.[70,184] Amenorrhea may follow the discontinuation of contraceptive steroids, so-called *post-pill amenorrhea.* Contraceptive steroids have a suppressive effect on the pituitary that sometimes persists after medication has been discontinued. In most women, menses resumes within 6 months after discontinuation of oral contraceptives.[70]

Tests for the Evaluation of Amenorrhea

Evaluation of Primary Amenorrhea

When puberty is delayed in a girl, measurement of serum gonadotropins is useful for diagnostic purposes. Low concentrations may indicate pituitary failure, whereas concentrations elevated into the postmenopausal interval indicate definite gonadal failure.[46,268,375] In the latter case, chromosome studies are indicated. In the former case, pituitary function testing and radiography may be helpful. Patients with short stature without Turner's syndrome but with primary amenorrhea may have multiple deficiencies of pituitary hormone secretion. In these patients, a craniopharyngioma or pituitary tumor should be suspected.

The diagnosis of *17α-hydroxylase deficiency* is made when (1) serum progesterone is greater than 3 ng/mL; (2) 17α-hydroxyprogesterone is <0.2 ng/mL; (3) aldosterone is low; and (4) an elevated 11-deoxycorticosterone concentration exists. Plasma concentrations of 11-deoxycortisol, testosterone, estradiol, and DHEA-S are also low. This diagnosis is confirmed with an *ACTH stimulation test.* After baseline progesterone and 17α-hydroxyprogesterone are measured, 0.25 mg of ACTH is administered. Diagnosis is made if serum concentrations of progesterone are significantly elevated and 17α-hydroxyprogesterone concentrations are unchanged at 60 minutes after ACTH administration.[69,250]

Many causes of secondary amenorrhea have also caused primary dysfunction. These disorders are discussed in the following section. Often, delayed puberty is not caused by specific organic disease, but is simply an unusual outcome of the spectrum of maturation.

Evaluation of Secondary Amenorrhea

In the evaluation of women with amenorrhea, a careful history and physical examination in those who are otherwise normal usually leads to determination of the correct cause. The history should define the complete description of the menstrual patterns; the presence or absence of galactorrhea; hot flashes; symptoms of hypothyroidism; hirsutism; prior surgery of the abdomen, pelvis, or uterus; trauma; medications; nutritional history; patterns of exercise; previous contraceptive use; changes in weight; stress; and chronic diseases. The physical examination should determine the visual fields, thyroid size and function, cushingoid appearance, galactorrhea, hirsutism, abdominal masses, pelvic masses, clitoral enlargement, and evidence of malnutrition. Serum or urine β-hCG should be measured to rule out pregnancy. Because both hypothyroidism and hyperprolactinemia can cause amenorrhea, they are easily excluded by measuring serum thyroid-stimulating hormone and prolactin concentrations.

A 24-hour urine sample for cortisol measurement or an overnight dexamethasone suppression test is performed in those patients suspected of having Cushing's syndrome (see Chapter 51). Based on the preliminary assessment, computed tomography of the sella should be performed in patients with evidence of pituitary or hypothalamic disease. A GnRH stimulation test with measurement of LH and FSH concentrations in those patients with gonadotropin deficiency assists in differentiating hypothalamic disease from pituitary disease. For diagnosis of PCOS, see the later section on the laboratory evaluation of hirsutism/virilization.

Progesterone Challenge

When the cause of amenorrhea is unclear after the initial assessment, relative estrogen status should be determined. Serum estradiol is measured or a *progesterone challenge* performed.[46,375] Women with an estrogen-primed uterus have withdrawal vaginal bleeding after treatment with oral progestin (medroxyprogesterone acetate; Provera), 30 mg daily for 3 days, or 10 mg daily for 5 to 10 days, or 100 to 200 mg of progesterone in oil given intramuscularly. If estrogen concentrations are adequate, and the outflow tract is intact, menstrual bleeding should occur within a week of treatment. In patients with withdrawal bleeding, the plasma estradiol concentration is usually >40 pg/mL.[46,70] Measurement of serum estradiol can be made instead of the progesterone challenge, but is not preferred because estrogen concentrations fluctuate throughout the day, and withdrawal bleeding is an indication of a normal outflow tract.

If bleeding fails to occur after progestin challenge, then additional laboratory tests are indicated. LH and FSH should be measured to localize the problem to the follicle, pituitary, or hypothalamus. High gonadotropin concentrations and low estrogen indicate the ovarian follicle is not responding to the gonadotropin stimulation. A single measurement of LH or FSH >50 mIU/mL is a reliable indicator of ovarian failure. Because of the association of POF with thyroid, parathyroid, or adrenal insufficiency secondary to autoimmune disease, it has been suggested that patients younger than age 35 should be screened for thyroid antibodies.[70] The differential diagnosis for evaluation of amenorrhea is listed in Table 53-2. As indicated by the clinical presentation, special additional testing may be required.

If the patient demonstrates withdrawal bleeding after the progesterone challenge test, this indicates that the ovaries are producing sufficient estrogen to cause endometrial proliferation and there is no anatomical obstruction. Most of these women have a history of oral contraceptive use, stress, weight loss, or excessive exercise.

Laboratory Evaluation of Hirsutism/Virilization

The two most important screening tests used in the evaluation of women for hirsutism and virilization are the measurements of serum total or free testosterone and DHEA-S.[46,280] Elevation of DHEA-S concentrations suggests an adrenal origin of androgens, whereas elevations in testosterone suggest either an adrenal or ovarian source. Unless the history is suspect, neoplastic disease is unlikely if the serum testosterone concentration is <2 ng/mL, the DHEA-S concentration is <700 μg/dL, or the 17-KS concentrations are <30 mg/day.[46,116,287] Regardless of the source of the excess androgen production, the androstanediol glucuronide concentration is elevated in more than 90% of women with hirsutism, because it is a marker of excessive DHT production in skin. Because concentrations of SHBG can be decreased in hirsute women, there has been some debate over whether total testosterone or bioavailable testosterone (free and weakly bound testosterone) is more clinically informative in diagnosing hirsutism. The reader is directed to a review by Wheeler that discusses many of these issues.[357]

TABLE 53-2 Differential Diagnosis of Amenorrhea

Causes	FSH	LH	Estrogen (E_2)	Uterine Bleeding After Progesterone
Hypothalamic				
CNS—hypothalamic dysfunction				
Idiopathic	N	N	N	+
Secondary to medications	N	N	N	+
Secondary to stress	N	N	N	+
CNS—hypothalamic dysfunction or failure due to exercise	↓ or N	↓ or N	↓ or N	±
CNS—hypothalamic dysfunction or failure due to weight loss				
Simple weight loss	↓ or N	↓ or N	↓ or N	±
Anorexia nervosa	↓	↓	↓	–
CNS—hypothalamic failure				
Lesions	↓	↓	↓	–
Idiopathic	↓	↓	↓	–
CNS—hypothalamic-adreno-ovarian dysfunction (polycystic ovary syndrome) or hyperandrogen chronic anovulation	N	↑	N	+
Pituitary				
Destructive lesions (Sheehan's syndrome)	↓	↓	↓	–
Tumor	↓	↓	↓	–
Ovarian				
Premature ovarian failure	↑	↑	↓	–
Loss of ovarian function (oophorectomy, infection, cystic degeneration)	↑	↑	↓	–
Uterine				
Uterine synechiae (Asherman's syndrome)	N	N	N	–

From Davajan V, Kletzky OA. Amenorrhea. In: Mishell DR, Davajan V, Lobo RA, eds. Infertility, contraception and reproductive endocrinology. 3rd ed. Boston: Blackwell Scientific Publications, 1991:373.

FSH, Follicle-stimulating hormone; *LH,* luteinizing hormone; *CNS,* central nervous system; *N,* value within normal reference interval; ↓, value below normal reference interval; ↑, value above normal reference interval; (↑, >25 mlU/mL, less than menopausal level; ±, positive or negative bleeding response to progesterone).

Patients with PCOS usually have estradiol concentrations >40 pg/mL and therefore exhibit a positive progesterone stimulation test. The diagnosis of PCOS can be confirmed with laboratory determinations of serum testosterone, DHEA-S, LH, and FSH. LH concentrations are frequently elevated, and FSH concentrations are disproportionately normal or low. It has been suggested that a ratio of LH to FSH >2.5 indicates the presence of PCOS.[46,287] The total testosterone concentration is modestly elevated in 40% to 60% of patients.[46,287] In women with normal testosterone concentrations, free testosterone is usually elevated.[287] Concentrations of DHEA-S are usually normal or slightly elevated.

Morning plasma 17α-hydroxyprogesterone concentrations are measured to evaluate *nonclassical* or *late-onset*

21-hydroxylase deficiency (NCAH, see Chapter 51). A concentration <200 ng/dL (<6.1 nmol/L) excludes this diagnosis, and a concentration >1500 ng/dL (>30 nmol/L) in nonpregnant women is confirmatory. When basal concentrations of between 200 and 1500 ng/dL are found, an ACTH stimulation test should be performed. NCAH typically has a 17α-hydroxyprogesterone concentration of >1500 ng/dL, and classical CAH has a response more than 2000 ng/dL.[227,275,280] Patients with attenuated forms of CAH usually have normal concentrations of FSH and LH. About one half have elevated testosterone and androstenedione concentrations.[376] Most of these patients also have increased concentrations of DHEA-S, and more than 90% have supranormal concentrations of androstanediol glucuronide.[223,253]

Menopause

Menopause is defined as the permanent cessation of menstruation resulting from loss of ovarian follicular activity.[273] The ovaries fail to produce adequate amounts of estrogen and inhibin and, as a result, gonadotropin production increases in a continued attempt to stimulate the ovary (see Figure 53-14). The mean age of menopause in the United States is 51, but this age varies considerably.[35,46,129,168] Ovarian failure may occur at any age, but menopause before age 40 is considered premature.[70]

Hormonal changes begin about 5 years before the actual menopause, as the response of the ovary to gonadotropins begins to decrease, and menstrual cycles become increasingly irregular.[129,168,314] The term "perimenopausal" refers to the time interval from the onset of these menstrual irregularities to menopause itself. This transition phase can last from 2 to 8 years.[129,314] At this time, FSH concentrations increase and estradiol concentrations decrease, whereas LH and progesterone concentrations remain unchanged, indicating that the menstrual cycles are ovulatory. As estrogen continues to decline, there is an associated decrease in prolactin concentrations. The decrease in estrogen concentrations gives rise to vasomotor instability and "hot flashes."

After menopause, the ovary continues to produce androgens, particularly testosterone and androstenedione, as a result of increased LH concentrations. In addition, the adrenal gland continues to secrete androgens. The resulting decrease in the estrogen/androgen ratio is the cause of hirsutism often seen in postmenopausal women.[168] Prolonged estrogen deficiency results in increased resorption and bone remodeling, leading to accelerated bone loss and osteoporosis in postmenopausal women. Estrogen replacement therapy reduces bone loss and has been reported to reduce fracture risk by half.[129,168] The issue of hormone replacement treatment for menopausal symptoms, osteoporosis, various cardiac problems, and other disorders has received a great deal of attention. Data from several studies concerning the benefits and risks have changed ideas about indications and contraindications.[72,123,294] There is no single, reliable hormonal marker of menopause status for a given woman. Physicians should diagnose menopausal status based on menstrual history and age without relying on laboratory test results.[20,40]

It is important to note that with the advent of highly sensitive immunoassays for the measurement of serum and urine β-hCG concentrations, it has been occasionally observed that postmenopausal women have slightly elevated β-hCG concentrations (typically >5 but <25 IU/L).[5,14,28,193] These results may cause confusion when the concentrations are above the detection limit defined for a positive pregnancy test. Although this phenomenon is not associated with pregnancy, these results are not false positives as they are routinely confirmed by alternate methods.

INFERTILITY

Ninety percent of healthy couples practicing unprotected intercourse can expect to conceive within 1 year, and 95% will be successful within 2 years. *Infertility* is defined as the inability to conceive after 1 year of unprotected intercourse.[16,46,347] It is estimated that 25% of couples will experience an episode of infertility during their reproductive life.[171] Primary infertility refers to couples or patients who have had no previous successful pregnancies. Secondary infertility encompasses patients who have previously conceived, but are currently unable to conceive. Both types of infertility generally share common causes.

Infertility problems often arise as a result of hormonal dysfunction of the hypothalamic-pituitary-gonadal axis. Measurement of peptide and steroid hormones in the serum is therefore an essential aspect of the evaluation of infertility. This section focuses on the hormonal and biochemical aspects of evaluating infertility.

Male Infertility

Causative Factors

It has been reported that ~50% of infertility problems are male in origin.[109,312] However, male infertility often goes undetected, because low sperm count or abnormal sperm motility, combined with normal female reproductive function, merely results in delayed conception. Most infertile men (80%) will not have a definable cause and are said to have so-called "idiopathic impaired sperm function."[321] In about 20% of cases, a cause can be determined.[321] A study at Monash University Infertility Clinic in Australia indicated that primary testicular failure accounted for 11% of male patients seen; 8.5% had genital tract obstruction, 0.5% had hypothalamic-pituitary disease, and less than 1% had coital disorders or abnormal sperm.[13,321] A list of the most common male infertility factors is given in Box 53-4.

Many of the endocrine disorders that result in male infertility have been discussed earlier in this chapter in the section on male reproductive abnormalities. Testosterone is essential for normal sperm development. Therefore, any disorder that results in hypogonadism (and hence low testosterone concentrations) results in infertility. Among the causes are both hypogonadotropic and hypergonadotropic hypogo-

BOX 53-4 Male Infertility Factors

Endocrine Disorders
- Hypothalamic dysfunction (Kallmann's syndrome)
- Pituitary failure (tumor, radiation, surgery)
- Hyperprolactinemia (drug, tumor)
- Exogenous androgens
- Thyroid disorders
- Adrenal hyperplasia
- Testicular failure

Anatomic
- Congenital absence of vas deferens
- Obstructed vas deferens
- Congenital abnormalities of ejaculatory system
- Varicocele
- Retrograde ejaculation

Abnormal Spermatogenesis
- Unexplained azoospermia
- Chromosomal abnormalities
- Mumps orchitis
- Cryptorchidism
- Chemical or radiation exposure

Abnormal Motility
- Absent cilia (Kartagener's syndrome)
- Antibody formation

Psychosocial
- Unexplained impotence
- Decreased libido

Modified from Morell V. Basic infertility assessment. Primary Care 1997;24:195-204.

nadism. The most common cause of hypothalamic hypogonadism is *congenital idiopathic hypogonadotropic hypogonadism* (IHH) or its variant, Kallmann's syndrome (see earlier section on male reproductive abnormalities).[242] An adult-onset form of IHH has been recognized as a potentially treatable form of male infertility.[235] Ten men with postpubertal development of sexual dysfunction, low serum testosterone, and a pulsatile secretion of LH were compared with 24 cases of classic GnRH deficiency and 29 normal control subjects. The decreased serum GnRH concentrations in the adult-onset group were similar to those in the classic cases of IHH. Men with adult-onset IHH had larger mean testicular volumes and serum testosterone concentrations (78 ± 34 versus 49 ± 20 ng/dL) than classic cases of IHH. Treatment with GnRH successfully reversed hypogonadism and restored fertility in each of five men who accepted therapy.[235]

Pituitary insufficiency or failure can also cause infertility and is primarily caused by adenomas, but can also be caused by trauma, infiltration, metastases, or hemochromatosis. Hyperprolactinemia is a cause of secondary testicular dysfunction.[130] Prolactin excess likely causes hypogonadism by impairing GnRH release. It also leads to underandrogenization and impotence (see earlier section on impotence). Pituitary adenomas and drugs such as anxiolytics, antihypertensives, serotonergics, and histamine H_2 receptor antagonists will increase serum prolactin.[372]

Other endocrine causes of infertility include exogenous androgens, thyroid disorders, adrenal hyperplasia, and testicular failure. Gynecomastia or obesity in the infertile male may signify elevated concentrations of estrogen and possibly testicular feminization syndrome (see earlier section on male reproductive abnormalities).[109]

Antibodies to sperm surface antigens are a well-documented cause of infertility. They can decrease motility, cause agglutination, and be responsible for failure of sperm to penetrate human ova.[338] Antibodies arise from autoimmune processes that can be initiated by infection, trauma, obstruction, cryptorchidism, and cancer.[109,243] Immunosuppressive therapy has shown little to no benefit.

Among the other causes of male infertility are anatomical abnormalities, abnormal spermatogenesis, abnormal motility, and psychosocial causes. A list of drugs that can affect male reproductive function is given in Table 53-3.

Evaluation of Male Infertility

An initial evaluation of male infertility should include a detailed history and physical examination with special emphasis on the reproductive organs for evidence of proper androgenization. The history must include prescribed medications, recreational and performance-enhancing drug and alcohol use, systemic illnesses, and potential toxin exposure. A sexual history should include sexual technique and frequency of intercourse. Issues of potency must be distinguished from those of infertility or subfertility.

The laboratory evaluation of male infertility is separated into three main components: (1) the semen analysis, (2) endocrine parameters, and (3) immunological parameters. A basic approach to the diagnosis of male factor infertility is shown in Figure 53-15.

Evaluation of Semen

Semen Analysis. The semen analysis measures ejaculate volume, pH, sperm count, motility, and forward progression. Semen should be analyzed within 1 hour after collection. Although the semen analysis is not a test for infertility, it is considered the most important laboratory test in the evaluation of male fertility. Controversy exists as to what constitutes a "normal" semen profile. With the exception of the *azoospermic* male (defined as no sperm in the ejaculate), the lines between fertility and infertility are blurred, and are intimately associated with the status of the female partner's reproductive function. However, clinical studies of infertile men and World Health Organization (WHO) guidelines have helped establish limits of adequacy (Table 53-4).[109,362]

TABLE 53-3 Drugs and Chemicals Affecting Male Reproductive Function

Drug/Chemical	Effect
Alcohol	Depression of testicular production and increase in peripheral metabolism of testosterone, independent of liver disease
Amebicides	Toxic to testes in animals and humans
Antihypertensives	Depression of libido and potency
Arsenic	Replacement of phosphorus in DNA synthesis
Aspirin	Inhibition of prostaglandins in seminal fluid
Busulfan	Radiomimetic
Chlorambucil	Azoospermia
Colchicine	Arrests cell division in metaphase
Cyclophosphamide	Depression of spermatogenesis
Diethylstilbestrol (in utero)	Small testes, poor semen quality
Lead poisoning	Oligospermia, poor motility, abnormal sperm forms
Marijuana	Depression of sperm count and testosterone
Medroxyprogesterone	Male pill, reversible
Methotrexate	Mutagenic
Monoamine oxidase inhibitors	Decreased sperm count
Nicotine	Depression of sperm motility and density
Nitrofurantoin	Interference with carbohydrate metabolism in germinal epithelium leading to arrest at spermatocyte stage (dose related, reversible)
Phenytoin sodium	Depression of follicle-stimulating hormone levels
Spironolactone	Decreased testosterone concentrations
Sulfasalazine	Depression of sperm counts, reversible
Testosterone	Germinal atrophy by suppressing luteinizing hormone and decreasing intratesticular testosterone
Triethylenemelamine	Radiomimetic

From Caldemone AA. Evaluation of the infertile or subfertile male. Urol Clin North Am 1981;8:17.

Sperm Function. Functional tests have yet been established that can unequivocally predict the fertilizing capacity of spermatozoa. However, detailed methods describing the analysis of sperm function exist in the current literature.[109] These methods attempt to measure the functions of sperm necessary for fertilization. For a sperm to be successful, it must be able to (1) reach the ova through directed motility, (2) undergo capacitation, (3) fuse with the oocyte membrane, and (4) be incorporated into the oocyte cytoplasm.[109] The postcoital test (as described in the later section on evaluation of female infertility) is the most widely used measure of sperm adequacy. The WHO has accepted and offered guidelines for the postcoital test and the sperm-mucus penetration test.[362] The sperm-mucus penetration test evaluates the ability of sperm to travel through a vaginal mucus sample obtained from either the female partner or a donor. This test is no longer performed on a routine basis and the reader is referred to an earlier edition of this chapter for a complete description of this procedure.[133] Other tests such as the hypo-osmotic swelling test, hamster oocyte penetration test, and acrosome reaction test are still considered experimental and have not gained universal acceptance.[243]

Evaluation of Obstruction. Analysis of specific semen parameters has proven useful in the evaluation of male reproductive tract obstruction. Testosterone produced after administration of hCG causes the seminal vesicles, epididymis, and prostate to increase the volume of ejaculate. An appropriate increase in serum testosterone without change in the ejaculate volume may indicate mechanical blockage. Absence or decrease in specific biochemical markers such as acid phosphatase and citric acid (from prostate), fructose, and prostaglandins (from seminal vesicles) aids in determining the location of blockage.[121] Low seminal glucosidase concentrations, in the presence of testes of normal size and consistency, normal semen volume, and normal serum FSH, have also been used as an indication of obstruction (usually in the epididymis) or congenital bilateral absence of the vas deferens (a condition associated with mutations of the cystic fibrosis gene).[105]

Evaluation of Endocrine Parameters

Serum testosterone should be measured especially when the patient history or physical examination suggests deficient development of secondary sex characteristics. Patients with borderline or suppressed testosterone concentrations are

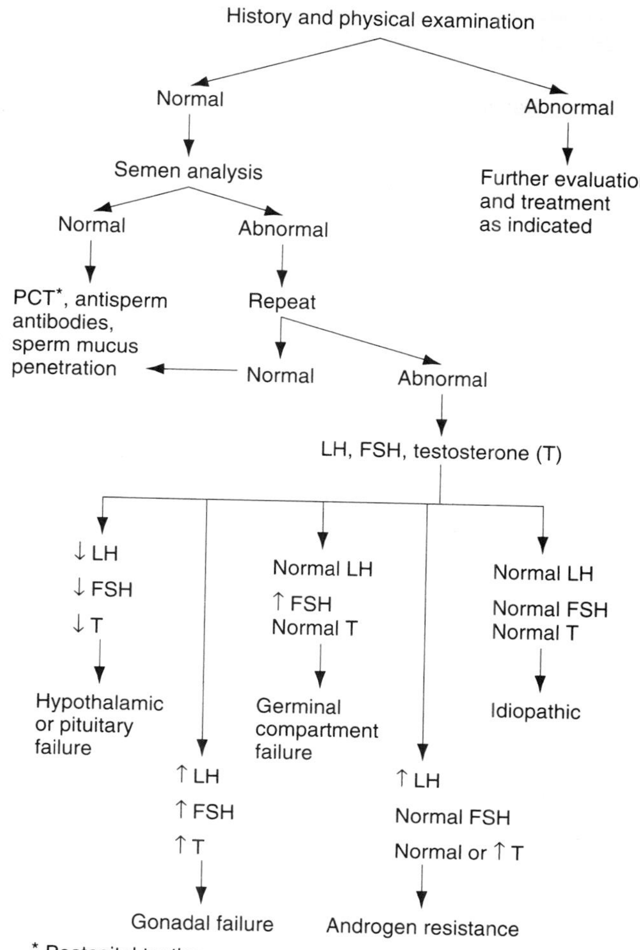

Figure 53-15 Algorithm for the evaluation of male infertility. *FSH,* Follicle-stimulating hormone; *LH,* luteinizing hormone; *T,* testosterone.

TABLE 53-4 Normal Seminal Fluid Values

Parameter	Value
Ejaculate volume	>2 mL*
Sperm density	>20 million/mL*
Total sperm count	>40 million/ejaculate*
Motility	>50% with forward progression or >25% with rapid progression within 60 min of ejaculation*
Morphology	>30% normal*
pH	7.2-8.0*
Color	Gray-white-yellow
Liquefaction	Within 40 min
Fructose	>1200 μg/mL
Acid phosphatase	100-300 μg/mL
Citric acid	>3 mg/mL
Inositol	>1 mg/mL
Zinc	>75 μg/mL
Magnesium	>70 μg/mL
Prostaglandins ($PGE_1 + PGE_2$)	30-200 μg/mL
Glycerylphosphorylcholine	>650 μg/mL
Carnitine	>250 μg/mL
Glucosidase	>20 mU per ejaculate

From Glezerman M, Bartoov B. Semen analysis. In: Insler V, Lunenfeld B, eds. Infertility: male and female. 2nd ed. New York: Churchill Livingstone, 1993:285-315.
*Values from World Health Organization: laboratory manual for the examination of human semen and semen-cervical mucus penetration. 3rd ed. Cambridge, UK: Cambridge University Press, 1992.

evaluated with an *hCG stimulation test.* With this test, an injection of 5000 IU hCG is administered intramuscularly following collection of a basal, early morning testosterone sample. Serum testosterone is measured 72 hours later. Hypogonadal men show a depressed testosterone rise in response to this challenge. A doubling of testosterone concentration over baseline is consistent with normal Leydig cell function. Failure to increase testosterone >150 ng/dL indicates primary hypogonadism.[170]

Hypergonadotropic Hypogonadism. Follicle-stimulating hormone measurement is indicated in men with sperm counts of less than 5 to 10 million/mL. Elevated concentrations of FSH indicate Sertoli cell dysfunction and, in azoospermic men, primary germinal cell failure, Sertoli-cell–only syndrome, or genetic conditions such as Klinefelter's syndrome.[122] Elevated FSH (>120 mIU/mL) in the setting of decreased testosterone (<200 ng/dL) and oligospermia indicate primary testicular failure or "andropause" (see previous section on andropause).

Hypogonadotropic Hypogonadism. Decreased concentrations of testosterone (<200 ng/dL) and decreased concentrations of FSH (<10 mIU/mL) are suggestive of hypogonadotropic hypogonadism. Administering GnRH may help to distinguish between gonadal insufficiency caused by pituitary versus hypothalamic failure. Because the pituitary is sensitive to sex steroids for appropriate gonadotropin secretion, patients with long-standing hypogonadism should be given exogenous testosterone for 1 week before the GnRH stimulation test. One approach to this test involves the intravenous injection of 100 μg of GnRH with measurement of FSH and LH concentrations at 0, 30, 60, 120, and 180 minutes after injection. Results of the GnRH test are classified as follows. An increase in serum gonadotropins ≥10 mIU/mL over baseline is normal. If there is little to no increase in gonadotropins, pituitary disease is likely. Patients with hypothalamic disease will demonstrate a delayed but significant increase ≥7 mIU/mL within 180 minutes.[170]

Evaluation of Immunological Parameters

The method of measurement of antisperm antibodies is identical for male or female infertility evaluation. Agglutination, immobilization, enzyme-linked immunosorbent assays, radioimmunoassays (RIA), and immunofluorescent assays are available.[47,140] The immunobead technique is the most widely used and is reported to have excellent clinical sensitivity (97.5%) and acceptable clinical specificity (66%).[47] In this technique, a polyacrylamide bead is coated with a rabbit antihuman antibody. This binds to antibodies that are either already present on human sperm, or present after incubation of sperm with the appropriate fluid (cervical mucus or serum). Beads that bind sperm are microscopically detected. This technique allows determination of percentage of human sperm bound, the immunoglobulin isotype, and the location of antibody binding (head, midpiece, or tail).[38,47] The practice of testing for antisperm antibodies is not recommended.[365] Although antisperm antibodies are associated with infertility, the concentration at which these decrease fertility is unknown.

Female Infertility

Causative Factors

Factors that contribute to female infertility are shown in Box 53-5. Ovulatory disorders (including ovarian and hormonal causes) account for approximately 30%, pelvic factors (including tubal, cervical, and uterine disease) account for approximately 50%, and immunological factors are implicated in approximately 5% of infertility cases.[46] This section focuses primarily on the ovulatory and immunological factors, where the laboratory plays an important role.

Ovulatory Factors

Ovulatory dysfunction manifests itself in the presence or absence of normal menses, making it difficult to diagnose. Metabolic diseases of many kinds can effect ovulatory function, including ones that result in androgen excess. PCOS, which results in androgen excess, is the most common cause of anovulation and has been discussed in detail earlier in the chapter. In women with hirsutism, CAH should be considered. A 21-hydroxylase deficiency or 3-β-hydroxysteroid deficiency may be present in up to 26% of cases.[254] Ovulatory dysfunction can also be secondary to liver or thyroid disorders.

As with male infertility, hypogonadism (hypergonadotropic or hypogonadotropic) also results in female infertility. Causes of hypergonadotropic hypogonadism include POF, gonadal dysgenesis, resistant ovary syndrome, menopause, and luteal phase deficiency. Causes of hypogonadotropic hypogonadism include pituitary or hypothalamic insufficiency and hyperprolactinemia. Many of these pathological states have been discussed in the earlier section on irregular menses.

Ovulation with inadequate luteinization and reduced progesterone secretion during the luteal phase has been termed *luteal phase deficiency*. The contribution of luteal insufficiency to infertility is controversial. It is manifested by a short luteal phase, in which the interval between LH peak and the onset of menses is ≥10 days, or a normal length luteal phase with reduced progesterone secretion.[46] An inadequate luteal phase and deficit of progesterone lead to poor proliferation of the endometrium and therefore an unsuitable environment for the early embryo.[46,376] Luteal dysfunction is believed to cause infertility in 5% of infertile women. It can be found periodically in 30% of women, and is not considered to contribute to infertility unless diagnosed twice in separate cycles.[347]

BOX 53-5 Female Infertility Factors

Ovarian or Hormonal Factors
- Metabolic disease
  - Thyroid
  - Liver
  - Obesity
  - Androgen excess
  - Polycystic ovarian syndrome
- Hypergonadotropic hypogonadism
  - Menopause
  - Luteal phase deficiency
  - Gonadal dysgenesis
  - Premature ovarian failure (autoimmune, cytotoxic chemotherapy, tumor)
  - Resistant ovary syndrome
- Hypogonadotropic hypogonadism
  - Hyperprolactinemia (tumor, drugs)
  - Hypothalamic insufficiency (Kallmann's syndrome)
  - Pituitary insufficiency (tumor, necrosis, thrombosis, stress, exercise, anorexia)

Tubal Factors
- Occlusion or scarring
- Salpingitis isthmica nodosa
- Infectious salpingitis

Cervical Factors
- Stenosis
- Inflammation or infection
- Abnormal mucus viscosity

Uterine Factors
- Leiomyomata
- Congenital malformation
- Adhesions
- Endometritis or abnormal endometrium

Psychosocial Factors
- Decreased libido
- Anorgasmia

Iatrogenic

Immunological (Antisperm Antibodies)

Modified from Morell V. Basic infertility assessment. Primary Care 1997;24:195-204.

Immunological Factors

Antisperm antibodies contribute to female infertility and may be present in female serum, in cervical mucus, or in seminal fluid. Their role in female infertility remains contentious. Some cases of infertility, especially when associated with an abnormal postcoital test, are found in the presence of a high percentage of sperm-binding antibodies.[38] The percentage of total binding and the region of binding (head, midpiece, or tail) appear to play a role in infertility and specifically in the ability of the sperm to bind the ovum in vitro.[38] However, one prospective study of 235 infertile couples examined pregnancy rates over time and found no correlation of serum antisperm antibodies between couples who achieved pregnancy and those who did not.[101] Cervical mucus and semen antisperm antibodies were not measured in this study. Methods for antisperm antibody measurement are described in the earlier section on evaluation of male infertility.

Evaluation of Female Infertility

The initial evaluation of female infertility should include a detailed history and physical examination, including a Papanicolaou cervical and vaginal smear with appropriate cervical and endocervical cultures, a search for tubal patency and endometriosis or adhesions, and assessment of ovulation and adequate luteal function.[160,171] After obvious treatable abnormalities have been excluded, a menstrual history indicates further endocrine evaluation and a postcoital test helps to determine coital sufficiency (Figure 53-16; see also earlier section on irregular menses).

Postcoital Test

The postcoital test is a quick assessment of multiple factors affecting fertility; however, opinions vary regarding its clinical utility. The test is scheduled around the time of the LH surge. A sterile speculum examination is performed 9 to 24 hours (based on WHO guidelines) after intercourse. A sample of endocervical mucus is aspirated and placed onto a glass slide with two coverslips. Mucus with adequate estrogen stimulation appears clear and thin and forms a thread 6 cm or greater in length when the coverslips are separated from the slide. This represents a positive "spinnbarkeit," which is defined as the formation of a thread by mucus from the cervix uteri when spread onto a glass slide and drawn out by a cover glass; the time at which it can be drawn to the maximum length usually precedes or coincides with the time of ovulation.[96] When examined under the microscope, mucus air dried under the second coverslip forms a fernlike pattern when adequate estrogen is present. Before the mucus has dried, greater than 20 motile sperm per high-power field should be visualized (WHO recommended cutoff).[246] A normal test result suggests coital sufficiency, probable ovulation, "nonhostile" cervical mucus, and a normal male fertility test.[347] Predictive values vary from nearly 50% chance of conception within 1 year with an optimal test to 15% chance of conception if the test is abnormal.[102]

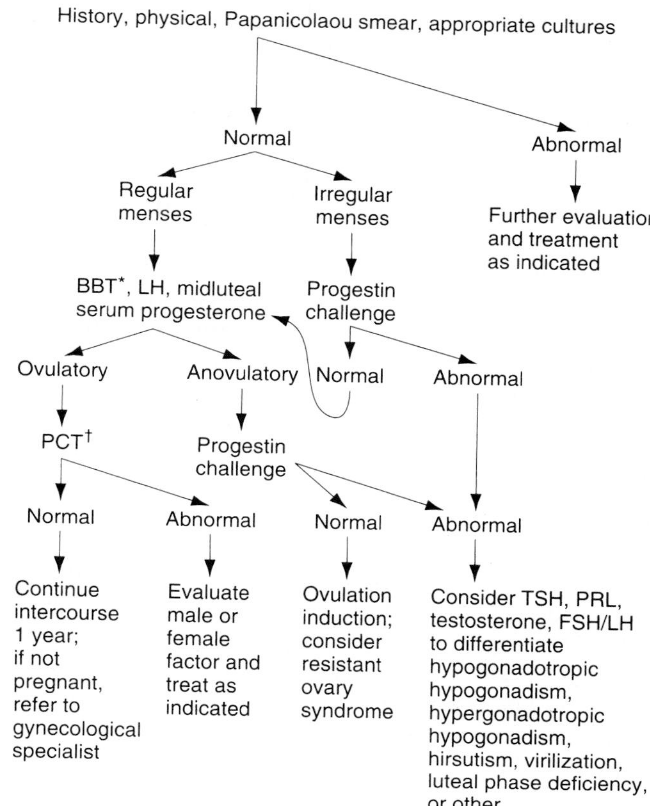

Figure 53-16 Algorithm for the evaluation of female infertility. *FSH,* Follicle-stimulating hormone; *LH,* luteinizing hormone; *PRL,* prolactin; *TSH,* thyroid-stimulating hormone.

Evaluation of Ovulation

Current laboratory tests do not confirm ovum release. However, the measurement of midluteal plasma progesterone does indicate that a corpus luteum was formed. Other methods, such as basal body temperature and evaluation of LH surge, have also been used to detect or predict ovulation.

Progesterone Measurement. Serum progesterone measurement is the primary assay used for the evaluation of ovulation.[171,297] It is important to note that an increase in the progesterone concentration indicates that a corpus luteum has been formed, but cannot confirm that the egg was actually released. Beginning immediately after ovulation, serum progesterone concentrations rise, and peak within 5 to 9 days during the midluteal phase (days 21 to 23).[297] If ovulation does not occur, the corpus luteum fails to form and the expected cyclical rise in progesterone concentration is subnormal. If pregnancy occurs, hCG stimulates the corpus luteum and progesterone production continues to rise. Midluteal progesterone concentrations of >10 ng/mL indicate normal ovulation; concentrations <10 ng/mL suggest anovulation, inadequate luteal phase progesterone production, or inappropriate timing of sample collection.[365]

Basal Body Temperature. Basal body temperature charts have long been accepted as simple and cost-effective indicators of ovulation. Ovulation is associated with a rapid rise in body temperature, by 0.5 °F, which persists through the luteal phase. The rise in temperature is due to the increased progesterone concentration. However, like progesterone, the rise in body temperature is evident only retrospectively and therefore does not predict imminent ovulation in a way helpful for timing intercourse.

Measurement of the Luteinizing Hormone Surge. Luteinizing hormone appears in the urine just after the serum LH surge and 24 to 36 hours before ovulation. Measurement of LH does not confirm the presence of ovulation or provide insight as to the etiology of anovulation, but rather indicates when ovulation should occur and can provide a guide with which to time intercourse. Methods for laboratory measurement of LH are given in Chapter 51.

Monoclonal technology has led to the use of *home LH kits* that not only provide accurate information as to the timing of ovulation but may reduce stress and costs associated with infertility programs because these tests are performed at home and are comparatively inexpensive.[191] Most home ovulation kits consist of a "dipstick" that uses a two-site, double monoclonal enzyme-linked immunoassay. Urine is applied to the test pad and capillary action draws the fluid across the pad. LH in the urine is first bound to an anti-LH antibody that is coupled to an enzyme conjugate, or colloidal gold. The LH-antibody complex then migrates to a region coated with a second anti-LH antibody. Once bound to this site, the substrate-enzyme reaction or colloidal gold complexes result in a color change that is proportional to the amount of LH present. A reference region is provided. A test result that matches or is darker in color than the reference region is considered a positive result, indicating that the LH surge is occurring. The tests effectively predict ovulation in 70% of women.[103] In some studies, these tests are said to be more reliable than laboratory plasma analysis, and the results are easily read by patients.[66,285] In one study of 26 normal women, home LH kits had a 92% positive predictive value for ovulation to occur within 48 hours of a positive urine LH screen.[226]

Evaluation of Endocrine Parameters

Hypergonadotropic Hypogonadism. Primary ovarian failure is indicated by repeatedly elevated basal FSH concentrations (>30 IU/L) or a single elevation of >40 IU/L. These patients are hypoestrogenic (estradiol <20 IU/L)[297] and do not respond to a progestin challenge (see earlier section on evaluation of secondary amenorrhea). Basal serum FSH can be used as an indicator of relative ovarian age. Figure 53-17 shows the relationship between rising serum FSH and the reduced rate of successful pregnancy. A precipitous drop occurs at concentrations >20 IU/L.

Luteal phase deficiency is diagnosed when the time between ovulation and menses is 10 days or less. The most specific diagnostic information may be gained from an

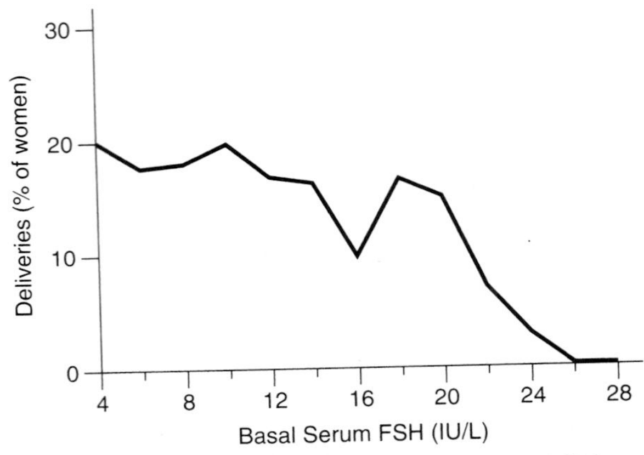

Figure 53-17 The relationship between increasing follicle-stimulating hormone (FSH) concentrations and decreased percentage of successful pregnancies. *(From Jones H, Toner JP. The infertile couple. N Engl J Med 1993;329:1710-5. Copyright © 1993 Massachusetts Medical Society. All rights reserved.)*

endometrial biopsy obtained on day 26 of a 28-day cycle.[354] If peak progesterone concentrations are repetitively below 10 ng/mL, the diagnosis of luteal phase deficiency does not require an endometrial biopsy. Decreased progesterone production is presumed to be responsible, but this may follow insufficient follicular phase FSH secretion, abnormal LH surge, or other endocrine abnormalities.[313] Some studies show luteal phase deficiency to be no more prevalent in infertile women than in normal women.[309,353] Other studies have shown an association with an increased risk of infertility, ectopic pregnancy, and spontaneous abortion.[21,139] Luteal phase dysfunction may also be secondary to excess androgen production, which suppresses follicle development. Prolactin excess may also contribute to the development of this disorder.[320]

Hypogonadotropic Hypogonadism. In hypogonadotropic hypogonadism, serum estradiol concentrations are <40 pg/mL (110 pmol/L) and therefore there is no withdrawal bleeding with a progestin challenge.[284] Decreased LH (<10 IU/L) and decreased FSH (<10 IU/L) are also present.[297] Hyperprolactinemia also causes hypergonadotropic hypogonadic infertility. The upper limit of normal plasma prolactin in an amenorrheic, hypoestrogenic, nonpregnant woman is 400 to 500 mIU/mL (20 to 25 ng/mL). If estrogen status is normal, maximum prolactin concentrations vary from 600 to 800 mIU/mL (30 to 40 ng/mL).[198] Thyroid-stimulating hormone should be measured to exclude hypothyroidism. Prolactin concentrations can be elevated in patients with PCOS and those taking medications such as antidepressants, cimetidine, and methyldopa. Radiographic imaging of the pituitary is indicated to rule out pituitary adenomas or empty sella syndrome.

Assessing Ovarian Reserve. Women in their mid to late 30s and early 40s with infertility constitute the largest portion of the total infertility population. These women are also at an increased risk for pregnancy loss. This reflects a diminished ovarian reserve as a result of follicular depletion and a decline in oocyte quality. As women age, serum FSH concentrations in the early follicular phase begin to increase. It has been suggested that this is caused by a decline in the number of small follicles secreting inhibin B.

Basal serum FSH and estradiol measurements have been the screening test of choice for assessing ovarian reserve. The rise in basal FSH is an excellent indicator of ovarian aging. In general, day 3 FSH concentrations >20 to 25 IU/L are considered to be elevated and associated with poor reproductive outcome.[181] Concomitant measurement of serum estradiol adds to the predictive power of an isolated FSH determination. Basal estradiol concentrations >75 to 80 pg/mL are associated with poor outcome.[203]

Inhibin B is produced by the developing follicles, and concentrations peak during the follicular phase. Concentrations of inhibin B have been used in conjunction with serum FSH and estradiol to assess ovarian function. Because inhibin is produced by gonadal tissue, it is thought to be a more direct marker of gonadal activity and ovarian reserve than pituitary hormones. In addition, cycle day 3 inhibin B concentrations may demonstrate a decrease before day 3 FSH concentrations.[300]

Seifer and colleagues reported that women undergoing in vitro fertilization (IVF) with day 3 inhibin B concentration <45 pg/mL had a pregnancy rate of 7% and spontaneous abortion rate of 33% as compared with pregnancy rate of 26% and abortion rate of 3% in women with day 3 inhibin B concentrations of >45 pg/mL.[299] Women who have diminished ovarian reserve should be counseled regarding options such as oocyte donation or adoption.

Assisted Reproduction

Couples with a multitude of infertility problems, including unidentified causes and persistent infertility despite standard treatments, may benefit from assisted reproductive techniques. Standard initial therapy consists of ovulation induction and artificial insemination for at least 6 months before progressing to more expensive and exotic techniques.

The laboratory plays an important role in the process of ovulation induction. The principle involves administration of gonadotropins to stimulate follicular growth followed by hCG to stimulate ovulation. Clinical, laboratory, and ultrasound monitoring of the treatment cycle is necessary to (1) determine the dose and length of therapy, (2) determine when or whether to administer hCG, and (3) obtain an adequate ovulatory response while avoiding hyperstimulation.[298]

Assisted reproductive techniques involve procedures that deliver a concentrated sperm sample directly to the uterus (artificial insemination), or procedures that acquire fertile ova using laparoscopic or ultrasonographic techniques and assisting fertilization in the laboratory (in vitro fertilization) or in the fallopian tubes using either gamete intrafallopian transfer or zygote intrafallopian transfer.[232] In vitro fertilization then requires embryo transfer back into the uterus. Gamete intrafallopian transfer places unfertilized ova and sperm directly into the fallopian tube, whereas zygote intrafallopian transfer involves placing the fertilized zygote into the fallopian tube. The latest successful techniques include direct ovum fertilization using micropipette penetration of the zona pellucida and introduction of the sperm or direct intracytoplasmic injection of the sperm.[303] These procedures provide hope to even the azoospermic man for whom testicular aspiration may yield a few nonmotile sperm.

ANALYTICAL METHODOLOGY

Many methods are available for measuring reproductive hormones in body fluids. Methods for the reproductive protein hormones are discussed in Chapter 50. Methods for the reproductive steroid hormones are discussed in the following sections.

Measurement of Total Testosterone in Blood

Circulating testosterone comprises three different forms or pools: a non–protein-bound or "free" form, a weakly bound form, and a tightly bound form. The weakly bound form is associated with albumin and the tightly bound form with SHBG (also known as testosterone/estradiol-binding globulin). The term *total testosterone* refers to serum measurements of (1) free testosterone, (2) albumin-bound testosterone, and (3) SHBG-bound testosterone. Bioavailable testosterone includes circulating free testosterone and albumin-bound testosterone.[130] Testosterone bound to SHBG is not biologically active, whereas the free form is available for target cells. Albumin-bound testosterone is also available to target tissue, because testosterone can dissociate from the albumin carrier and rapidly diffuse into target cells.[130]

Methodology

Early methods for measuring serum or plasma testosterone using fluorometry, double-isotope derivative, electron-capture gas-liquid chromatography, and competitive protein binding assays have been largely replaced by immunoassays that use specific antisera.[179,208] A 2002 CAP survey from the College of American Pathologists (CAP) reports that enzyme (nonisotopic) immunoassays have replaced RIAs as the most widely used technique for measuring the concentration of circulating testosterone (both protein-bound and non–protein-bound forms).[64] Individual immunoassay methods differ mainly in the mode of sample preparation, in the quality of antisera used, and in the nature of the steroid-protein conjugate used to generate the antiserum.[165] Gas chromatography combined with mass spectrometry (GC-MS) remains the reference method for testosterone measurement and is often used to assess the bias of routine immunoassay methods.[95,108,110] It has been suggested that liquid chromatography-tandem mass spectrometry (LC-

MS/MS) may become the clinical method of choice for measuring low testosterone concentrations.[350A]

Direct (no extraction required) immunoassay methods have been reported for the determination of testosterone in serum or plasma.[161,179] The steroid must be displaced from its binding proteins (albumin and SHBG). The results of the assay depend on the effectiveness of the displacement. Methods used to release testosterone from the endogenous binding proteins include use of salicylates or surfactants, pH alterations, temperature changes, and competing steroids such as estrone or estradiol. Most of the direct immunological methods use antisera generated against a C_{19} testosterone-protein conjugate.[165] Several commercial assay kits for direct assay of testosterone are available. These kits are classified into two types: RIA and automated, nonisotopic immunoassay. Many single-step kits employ antibody-coated tubes or magnetic particles for added convenience, eliminating the need for centrifugation. Liquid- or solid-phase double-antibody methods have also been introduced.

Fully automated immunoassays incorporating analogs labeled with enzymes, and fluorescent- or chemiluminescent-signaling molecules have been described and are commercially available for routine use.[29,165,292,358] The advantages of the newer, nonisotopic immunoassay formats include (1) faster results, (2) smaller sample size, and (3) the elimination of radioactive reagents. For adult male patients, these assays have demonstrated good precision and recovery, and agreement with GC-MS–validated pools and established RIA methods.[110,292,358] However, there is some question regarding the utility of such assays for female and prepubertal subjects.[111,152,325,358,363] The testosterone is low in these subjects and measurements compare poorly with mass spectrometry methods.[325,350A,363] The accuracy of immunoassay combined with extraction is uncertain.[152]

The preferred tracer in commercially available RIA kits for labeled testosterone is ^{125}I. The size of the iodinated group and the site of linkage may greatly affect assay affinity and specificity. Some methods use solvent extraction or chromatography, or both, to remove interferences from other steroids and some drugs. These preliminary steps also permit concentration of the sample when low concentrations of testosterone are expected. Like automated assays, manual RIA assays perform better at higher concentrations, with questionable utility in female and prepubertal subjects.[27,95]

Direct assays for total testosterone may produce spuriously high results, especially at low concentrations. In particular, some samples collected from women give concentrations within the reference interval for men when direct assays are used, but yield concentrations within the normal reference interval for women if extraction methods are used.[111,165,358,359] Similar interferences have been reported in the direct measurement of testosterone in infants.[118] During the first 3 weeks postpartum, testosterone concentrations measured by a direct assay were 3.8-fold greater than those measured after purification. These differences were most prominent in the first week of life, although some persisted through the first 2 months. This lack of accuracy is serious and may result in misdiagnosis and inappropriate treatment. Overestimations of testosterone concentrations by some direct methods are thought to be caused by the presence of a water-soluble cross-reacting substance(s).[264] Alternatively, the presence of endogenous antibodies that recognize the labeled testosterone analogs may cause falsely elevated concentrations.[337]

The validity of assay results is best proved by tests for parallelism of the response curves for both calibrators and randomly selected samples from male and female subjects of various ages. In addition, comparison of extraction/chromatography immunoassays should be validated by comparison with mass spectrometry methods.[152] Direct immunoassays should not be used for female and prepubertal subjects, especially infants. These groups should be tested using an extraction immunoassay or an LC-MS/MS assay. It is important to note that both types of direct immunoassay demonstrate problems with functional sensitivity for low concentrations. Each lab should determine the low-end detection limit of their assay despite manufacturer claims.

Regardless of immunoassay type, almost all testosterone antisera show some degree of cross-reactivity with DHT (typically 3% to 5%), but show negligible cross-reactivity with other androgens. Assays that use antisera generated against the C-19 position give maximum analytical specificity with respect to endogenous steroids. However, cross-reactions with 19-norsteroids that are used in contraceptive preparations have caused a problem. In most clinical situations, estimation of testosterone without prior separation of DHT is permitted because plasma concentrations of DHT are only 10% to 20% of those for testosterone. Moreover, testosterone and DHT are the two most important androgens in the systemic circulation; even when a method measures the concentrations of both of them, clinically useful information about the total androgen load is obtained. However, if specific estimation of testosterone concentration is required, then chromatographic separation of testosterone and DHT before immunoassay is usually necessary to obtain consistently reliable results.[169]

Specimen Collection and Storage

Either serum or heparinized plasma is used to measure total or free testosterone. Testosterone is subject to a diurnal variation, reaching a peak concentration between 0400 hours and 0800 hours. Therefore, morning specimens are preferred. Specimens are stable for a week (men) or 3 days (women) refrigerated and for up to 1 year frozen at 20 °C.[85,163] No steroids, thyroid, ACTH, estradiol, or gonadotropin medications should be given for 48 hours before sample collection.[92,138] Most assays are standardized for serum or heparinized plasma. Other anticoagulants such as ethylenediaminetetraacetic acid (EDTA) may give different values. In certain RIA assays, presence of EDTA appears to cause a 10% decrease in total testosterone concentrations.[85]

TABLE 53-5 Reference Intervals for Total Testosterone in Serum

	ng/dL	nmol/L
Prepubertal Levels		
1-5 mo, Male	1-177	0.03-6.14
Female	1-5	0.03-0.17
6-11 mo, Male	2-7	0.07-0.24
Female	2-5	0.07-0.17
1-5 yr, Male	2-25	0.07-0.87
Female	2-10	0.07-0.35
6-9 yr, Male	3-30	0.10-1.04
Female	2-20	0.07-0.69
Pubertal Levels (Tanner Stage)		
1, Male	2-23	0.07-0.80
Female	2-10	0.07-0.35
2, Male	5-70	0.17-2.43
Female	5-30	0.17-1.04
3, Male	15-280	0.52-9.72
Female	10-30	0.35-1.04
4, Male	105-545	3.64-18.91
Female	15-40	0.52-1.39
5, Male	65-800	9.19-27.76
Female	10-40	0.35-1.39
Adult Levels		
Male	260-1000	9-34.72
Female	15-70 (higher at mid-cycle peak)	0.52-2.43

From Quest Diagnostics/Nichols Institute. The Corning Endocrine Manual. Capistrano, CA: Quest Diagnostics/Nichols Institute, 1996; Tietz NW, ed. Clinical guide to laboratory tests. 3rd ed. Philadelphia: WB Saunders Co, 1995.

Reference Intervals

Reference intervals for total testosterone in serum are listed in Table 53-5.[261,336] Reference concentrations for total testosterone in other body fluids are listed in Chapter 56 and elsewhere.[336]

Comments

Estimation of SHBG in serum is sometimes very useful for interpreting blood concentrations of testosterone.[301] Procedures for measuring SHBG have been reviewed elsewhere.[281] Two types of assays are generally available: (1) binding assays, in which the quantity of a radiolabeled androgen bound to SHBG is measured; and (2) specific immunoassays for the SHBG protein. Commercial kits for SHBG determination are available. Serum concentrations measured using a solid-phase immunoenzymometric assay vary from 10 to 80 nmol/L in men and 20 to 130 nmol/L in nonpregnant women.[218] When measured using an RIA, SHBG concentrations vary from 6 to 44 nmol DHT bound per liter in men, and from 8 to 85 nmol DHT bound per liter in women.[261] Interference by SHBG has been reported to occur in a number of direct RIAs for testosterone[23,216]; the use of extraction techniques, however, abolishes the influence of SHBG.

Measurement of Free and Weakly Bound Testosterone in Blood

In cases in which SHBG concentrations are altered, such as in women, aging men, and illness, measurements of free or bioavailable testosterone are believed to be better reflections of androgen status. An excellent review of various methods used to measure this fraction of testosterone is available.[357]

Several methods are available for determining the concentrations of the free or bioavailable forms of testosterone in serum or plasma: (1) estimation of the free testosterone fraction by equilibrium dialysis or ultrafiltration; (2) estimation of the free hormone using a direct ("analog tracer") immunoassay; (3) estimation of the combined free and weakly bound ("bioavailable") testosterone fractions by selective precipitation of the tightly bound form; (4) calculation of androgen index using indices that reflect ratios of the testosterone pools; and (5) calculation of free and weakly bound testosterone concentrations by mathematical modeling.[308,346,357] The last approach uses mass action equations to calculate free and weakly bound testosterone concentrations from the concentrations of total testosterone, SHBG, and albumin, and from the association constants for the binding of testosterone to the two binding proteins.

Equilibrium Dialysis/Ultrafiltration

Only a small fraction (1% to 2%) of unconjugated testosterone exists freely (non–protein bound) in serum or plasma. None of the conventional assay methods, including RIA, is sufficiently sensitive to quantify the free steroid directly in a protein-free ultrafiltrate of plasma. Instead, the free steroid is estimated in plasma by adding a known amount of radiolabeled compound to the sample and allowing labeled and unlabeled compounds to reach equilibrium in their competition for the same binding sites on the proteins. Bound and free radiolabeled fractions are then separated and the ratio of free labeled to total labeled compound is determined. At equilibrium, this ratio is taken as a measure of the free testosterone fraction. An estimate of serum free testosterone can then be calculated by multiplying the free testosterone fraction by the total testosterone concentration.

Methodological Principle

In the equilibrium dialysis/ultrafiltration method for determining free testosterone in blood, a sample is first equilibrated with radioactive testosterone. Free steroid is then separated from bound steroid by filtration through an anisotropic, hydrophilic ultrafiltration membrane. The driving force for ultrafiltration is provided by centrifugation at 1000 to 2000 ×g. Filtrate containing free steroid collects in the filtrate cup, whereas protein-bound steroid remains above the filter. Radioactivity in the filtrate is a measure of

TABLE 53-6 Reference Intervals for Free Testosterone in Serum

	pg/mL	pmol/L	Free Fraction (% of Total)
Children			
6-9 yr, Male	0.1-3.2	0.3-11.1	0.9-1.7
Female	0.1-0.9	0.3-3.1	0.9-1.4
10-11 yr, Male	0.6-5.7	2.1-19.8	1.0
Female	1.0-5.2	3.5-18.0	1.0-1.9
12-14 yr, Male	1.4-156	4.9-541	1.3-3.0
Female	1.0-5.2	3.5-18.0	1.0-1.9
15-17 yr, Male	80-159	278-552	1.8-2.7
Female	1.0-5.2	3.5-18.0	1.0-1.9
Adults			
Male	50-210	174-729	1.0-2.7
Female	1.0-8.5	3.5-29.5	0.5-1.8

From Quest Diagnostics/Nichols Institute. The Corning Endocrine Manual. Capistrano, CA: Quest Diagnostics/Nichols Institute, 1996; Tietz NW, ed. Clinical guide to laboratory tests. 3rd ed. Philadelphia: WB Saunders Co, 1995.

the free testosterone fraction. A detailed procedure for the equilibrium dialysis method is included in the previous edition of this chapter.[133]

Reference Intervals

Reference intervals for free testosterone and percent free testosterone in serum are listed in Table 53-6 and in Chapter 56.[261,336] These concentrations compare favorably with those obtained when using membrane ultrafiltration and gel filtration methods. Equilibrium dialysis is considered the reference method for determining free testosterone in serum.

Comments

Most problems with this procedure have involved tracer impurities and the separation of bound and free labeled fractions. Several separation techniques have been used, including equilibrium dialysis, membrane ultrafiltration, and steady-state gel filtration. Their deficiencies include a requirement for a large sample volume, the need for complicated correction of sample volume changes that occur during the separation, and difficulties of collecting and measuring radioactivity in numerous fractions of each sample. Equilibrium dialysis has been used most often in the past, but serious errors often arise from the sample dilution required by this method.[345] Symmetrical dialysis of undiluted samples is reported to be less susceptible to tracer contamination and dilution effects.[322] Ultrafiltration also appears to overcome these problems and to obviate errors caused by dilution.[142]

Direct Immunoassay

Several RIA procedures are commercially available for the direct estimation of free testosterone.[179,231,286,357,368] These assays use a labeled derivative (analog) of testosterone that, in theory, retains the ability to react with exogenous antitestosterone antibodies, but is restricted from interacting with testosterone-binding proteins in the serum sample. The analog method is claimed to have a significant advantage as a screening test for investigating androgen excess in women,[364] although others have found free androgen index to be a better indicator.[357]

The advantages of RIA analog methods include a small sample requirement, relatively rapid results, an easy procedure, and the option to measure free testosterone without having to measure total testosterone.[179,231,346,368] Thus the RIA analog assays are the most commonly used method for determining free testosterone. Although there is reportedly good correlation between the values obtained by RIA and equilibrium dialysis, the RIA assays are grossly inaccurate, underestimating free testosterone concentrations by many fold.[231,282,283,346] One study in females revealed that free testosterone concentrations obtained by two different analog assays were 15% to 35% and 25% to 30% of those obtained by ultrafiltration.[137] The calculated free testosterone is considered more reliable than the RIA method.

Selective Precipitation

Measurement of bioavailable testosterone has been estimated by selective precipitation of SHBG with ammonium sulfate. In this technique, aliquots of serum or plasma are first incubated with tritiated testosterone. Testosterone bound to SHBG is then precipitated with 50% ammonium sulfate. The samples are centrifuged, and aliquots of the supernatant containing the free and albumin-bound testosterone (also known as *non–SHBG-bound testosterone*) are counted. The percentage of tritiated label not bound to SHBG is subsequently multiplied by the total testosterone concentration to give the bioavailable testosterone.[357] The amount of bioavailable testosterone has also been measured directly, by RIA, in the supernatants of plasma after ammonium sulfate precipitation and solvent extraction.[75] An indirect method using a commercially available enzyme immunoassay has been described for measuring bioavailable testosterone.[71] Alternatively, the fraction of testosterone not bound to SHBG has also been estimated by a technique that involves saturating SHBG binding sites with 5α-DHT, the natural steroid bound with highest affinity by SHBG; the non–protein-bound fraction is subsequently measured in treated and untreated samples by centrifugal ultrafiltration dialysis[258] or semiautomated equilibrium dialysis.[17] The reference intervals for bioavailable testosterone in serum are listed in Table 53-7.

Androgen Index

This index is a ratio of testosterone and SHBG multiplied by 100 to give concentrations similar to measured free testos-

TABLE 53-7 Reference Intervals for Bioavailable Testosterone in Serum

	ng/dL	nmol/L	% of Total
Adult men	66-417	2.29-14.5	12.3-63.0
Adult women	0.6-5.0	0.02-0.17	2.4-12.9

From Quest Diagnostics/Nichols Institute. The Corning Endocrine Manual. Capistrano, CA: Quest Diagnostics/Nichols Institute, 1996; Tietz NW, ed. Clinical guide to laboratory tests. 3rd ed. Philadelphia: WB Saunders Co, 1995.

terone concentrations.[357] Although this is only an indicator of free testosterone, some have found it to be useful in the evaluation of hirsutism.[236] Other reports have indicated that the free androgen index is not a reliable parameter of free testosterone because of its variation as a function of SHBG concentration.[174,231,346]

Mathematical Modeling

Methods based on mathematical modeling use algorithms to derive non–SHBG-bound testosterone. SHBG has been shown to be highly correlated with the percentage of free testosterone. Using this relationship, an algorithm is used to calculate percent free testosterone from the SHBG concentration. The calculated percent free value is then multiplied by total testosterone to obtain the concentration of free testosterone. For example, the algorithm used by Nanjee and Wheeler is:[236]

$$\%\ \text{Free testosterone} = 6.11 - 2.38 \log \text{SHBG} \times 10^{-9}$$

More complex calculations have been used to calculate the concentration of free testosterone that are based on the law of mass action. For example, Vermeulen and co-workers derived the following calculation of the concentration of free testosterone from the measurement of the concentrations of total testosterone and SHBG:[346]

$$FT = \frac{T - ((K_A)(C_A) + 1)(FT)}{(K_T)(SHBG) - (K_T)(T) + ((K_A)(C_A)+1)(K_T)(FT)}$$

where

FT = Concentration of free testosterone (mol/L)

T = Concentration of total testosterone (mol/L)

K_T = Association constant of SHBG for T (suggested value = 1×10^9 L/mol)

SHBG = Concentration of SHBG (mol/L)

K_A = Association constant of albumin for T (suggested value = $3.0 - 3.6 \times 10^4$ L/mol)

C_A = Concentration of albumin (MW = 69,000 Da)

Solving this equation for FT yields a quadratic equation* in the form:

$$Ax^2 + Bx + C = 0$$

*The authors acknowledge the assistance of Curtis Parvin, Washington University and Jim Boyd, University of Virginia in solving the quadratic equation.

Assuming x = FT, the formula for the positive x would be:

$$x = FT = \frac{-B + \sqrt{B^2 - 4AC}}{2A}$$

where

$A = [(K_A)(C_A) + 1]K_T$

$B = (K_A)(C_A) + (K_T)(SHBG) - (K_T)(T) + 1$

$C = -T$

Although complex, these calculations have demonstrated a very good correlation (both linearity and value agreement) with equilibrium dialysis measurements and are considered a reliable indicator of free testosterone.[346] The reader is directed to other references for further details on this method.[311,375] Conditions resulting in abnormal plasma protein concentrations, such as nephrotic syndrome, cirrhosis, and pregnancy require adjustments in the assumption for albumin concentration.

Measurement of Testosterone in Saliva

Salivary testosterone concentration correlates with free testosterone concentrations in plasma and has been advocated as an indicator of androgen status.[244] In a multicenter evaluation that examined nine different laboratories using various RIA methods with and without extraction, good correlation was found between laboratories despite widely varying methods.[67] Reference intervals of 4 to 14 ng/dL[267] and 2 to 6 ng/dL[163] have been reported for testosterone in saliva of men. Measurement of salivary testosterone in women has been less reliable, with no consensus on salivary concentrations available.[237,267,304,357] However, one commercial laboratory reports a reference interval of 0.5 to 1.8 ng/dL for women.[163] An enzyme immunoassay method for determination of testosterone concentration in saliva has been described and evaluated in female specimens.[304]

Measurement of Testosterone Precursors and Metabolites in Blood

Several biosynthetic precursors and metabolites of testosterone have been measured using specific immunoassays (either directly or after sample extraction), chromatography, or both. Examples include DHT, 3α-androstanediol glucuronide,[263] androstenedione,[335] and DHEA. DHT is a product of testosterone, produced in androgen-sensitive tissues, and is a potent androgen. 3α-Androstanediol glucuronide is a metabolite of DHT and provides a marker of peripheral disorders of androgen action and formation, particularly hirsutism. Patients with hirsutism of either idiopathic nature or secondary to PCOS have elevated 3α-androstanediol glucuronide concentrations. Androstenedione is a product of 17α-hydroxyprogesterone and DHEA and is the immediate precursor of testosterone. Circulating concentrations have been found increased in several pathological disorders, such as CAH, adrenal tumors, and polycystic ovarian disease.

TABLE 53-8 Reference Intervals for Dihydrotestosterone, 3α-Androstanediol Glucuronide, and Androstenedione in Serum

	ng/dL	nmol/L
Dihydrotestosterone		
Adult men	30-85	1.03-2.92
Adult women	4-22	0.14-0.76
Children (prepubertal)	<3	<0.10
3α-Androstenediol Glucuronide		
Adult men	260-1500	5.5-32
Adult women	60-300	1.3-6.4
Children (prepubertal)	10-60	0.2-1.3
Androstenedione		
Adults	75-205	2.6-7.2
Postmenopausal	82-275	3.0-9.6
Children (prepubertal)	<5	<0.2
Pubertal Levels (Tanner Stage)		
1, Male	5-55	0.2-1.9
Female	10-35	0.3-1.2
2, Male	10-100	0.3-3.49
Female	15-120	7.8-4.2
3, Male	25-85	0.9-3.0
Female	40-170	1.4-5.9
4, Male	20-85	0.7-3.0
Female	25-195	0.9-6.8
5, Male	50-250	1.7-8.7
Female	70-200	2.4-7.0

From Quest Diagnostics/Nichols Institute. The Corning Endocrine Manual. Capistrano, CA: Quest Diagnostics/Nichols Institute, 1996; Tietz NW, ed. Clinical guide to laboratory tests. 3rd ed. Philadelphia: WB Saunders Co, 1995.

Reference intervals for these analytes in serum are listed in Table 53-8[261,336] and in Chapter 56.

Measurement of Dehydroepiandrosterone and Its Sulfate

Measurements of DHEA or its sulfated conjugate, DHEA-S, in serum and plasma are important to investigations of adrenal androgen production, such as the assessment of hyperplasia, adrenal tumors, adrenarche, delayed puberty, or hirsutism. DHEA-S in circulation originates primarily from the adrenal glands, although in men some may be derived from the testes; none is produced by the ovaries. DHEA is secreted almost entirely by the adrenal glands.

DHEA concentrations exhibit a circadian rhythm that reflects the secretion of ACTH and also varies during the menstrual cycle. DHEA-S concentrations do not exhibit a circadian rhythm because of their longer circulating half-life.[250] Concentrations in serum are increased in cord blood and drop precipitously at birth. Concentrations in premature infants are in general much higher than those in full-term infants. Pregnancy and oral contraceptives induce a modest reduction and glucocorticoids a marked decrease. Patients with PCOS often have elevated concentrations of DHEA-S, suggesting an adrenal androgen contribution to the defect in this disorder. Concentrations of DHEA-S are also elevated in CAH and with adrenocortical tumors (concentrations higher with adrenal carcinoma than with adrenal adenomas),[250] whereas concentrations are not elevated in women with virilizing ovarian tumors. Glucocorticoid administration for several days suppresses concentrations in patients with adrenal hyperplasia. DHEA is commercially available in health food stores; therefore increased serum concentrations may be caused by exogenous use.

Methodology

Immunoassay is the method of choice for measurements of DHEA and DHEA-S. Other methods include gas-liquid chromatography,[107] double-isotope derivative methods,[119] and competitive protein-binding assays.[34,36,277] The latter actually measures 5-androstenediol derivatives and uses SHBG as a naturally occurring binding protein. A reference method based on high-performance liquid chromatography-mass spectrometry has been used for independent evaluation of routine methods.[302] Immunoassays for DHEA-S demonstrate significant cross-reactivity with DHEA, androstenedione, and androsterone, yet the relative concentrations of these steroids cause a minimal effect on assay performance.

Radioimmunoassay

Analysis of DHEA-S in serum or plasma is routinely performed using direct RIA; neither extraction nor chromatography is required in most methods. In the direct procedures of Buster and Abraham[41] and Cattaneo and co-workers,[52] plasma samples are assayed with an antibody generated against DHEA-3-hemisuccinate coupled to albumin. This antiserum completely cross-reacts with unconjugated DHEA, but only minimally with androstenedione. Because of the presence of relatively large amounts of DHEA-S, this steroid has been measured directly in plasma by diluting out interfering steroids that are present in relatively low concentration.

A variety of commercial RIA kits are available for measuring DHEA-S in serum or plasma. In one procedure (Coat-a-count; Diagnostic Products Corp.), ^{125}I-labeled DHEA-S competes with DHEA-S in the patient sample for sites on antibody-coated tubes.[82] After incubation for 30 minutes at 37 °C, separation of bound from free DHEA-S is achieved by simply decanting. This solid-phase kit is equipped with protein-based calibrators having DHEA-S concentrations ranging from 5 to 1000 μg/dL (0.14 to 27 μmol/L). The assay detects as little as 2.1 μg/dL (0.05 μmol/L). Intraassay and interassay coefficients of variation are less than ± 7% at concentrations ranging from 204 to 761 μg/dL (5.5 to 20.5 μmol/L). The antiserum is stated to be highly specific for DHEA-S, with very low cross-reactivity to other compounds, including DHEA (0.08%). Bilirubin, protein, and hemolysis have no clinically significant effects on the assay. Supraphysiological concentrations of free fatty acids and lipids, however, interfere with the procedure. Discordance has been reported among different RIA methods for DHEA-S, and in several disorders the presence of interfering DHEA-like steroids in serum has been confirmed.[55]

Nonisotopic Immunoassay

Nonisotopic methods have also been described. For example, a homogeneous (nonseparation) fluorescence polarization immunoassay for DHEA-S that uses a rabbit polyclonal antibody and a DHEA-fluorescein tracer is available.[135] The measured polarization is inversely related to DHEA-S concentration. This fully automated system has a dynamic range of 1 to 1000 μg/dL (0.03 to 27 μmol/L), and interassay coefficients of variation are less than ± 10% over a broad concentration interval (25 to 1000 μg/dL; 0.7 to 27 μmol/L). Assay time is about 15 minutes for a single sample and 30 minutes for 20 samples.

A heterogeneous solid-phase enzyme immunoassay for DHEA-S is commercially available.[87] This method uses horseradish peroxidase as enzyme label, rabbit anti-DHEA-S-coated microtiter wells, and tetramethylbenzidine as substrate. The assay is stated to have a lower limit of detection of 15 ng/dL (40.6 nmol/L). An automated method employing chemiluminescent detection of alkaline phosphatase–labeled conjugate has been described. This assay reported a lower limit of detection of 2 μg/mL (54.0 nmol/L).

Specimen Collection and Storage

Serum or plasma (preserved with EDTA) is suitable for DHEA or DHEA-S immunoassays.[163,261] No steroids, ACTH, estradiol, or gonadotropin medications should be given for 48 hours before sample collection.[163] Early morning collection, before 1030 hours, is preferred for DHEA.[218,261] Refrigerated samples (4 °C to 8 °C) are stable for up to 14 days, those frozen at −20 °C are stable for >1 years.[92,138,378]

Reference Intervals

Reference intervals for serum concentrations of DHEA-S and DHEA are listed in Table 53-9.[163,336]

Comments

Enzyme immunoassay and RIA kits for the measurement of salivary DHEA and DHEA-S are commercially available for research purposes.[90,290] Analysis of DHEA by immunoassay usually requires pretreatment of serum samples, because the serum concentration of DHEA is 1000-fold lower than that of DHEA-S. Several extraction and chromatographic procedures have been suggested for this purpose. Celite is the preferred adsorbent, and dichloromethane and ethyl acetate are common choices for extraction solvents. Commercial RIA kits using solid-phase separation techniques and ^{125}I-

TABLE 53-9 Reference Intervals for Dehydroepiandrosterone Sulfate and Unconjugated Dehydroepiandrosterone in Serum

		μg/dL	μmol/L
Dehydroepiandrosterone Sulfate			
Children			
1-5 d,	Male	12-254	0.3-6.9
	Female	10-248	0.3-6.7
1 mo-5 yr,	Male	1-41	0.03-1.1
	Female	5-55	0.1-1.5
6-9 yr,	Male	2.5-145	0.07-3.9
	Female	2.5-140	0.07-3.8
10-11 yr,	Male	15-115	0.4-3.1
	Female	15-260	0.4-7.0
12-17 yr,	Male	20-555	0.5-15.0
	Female	20-535	0.5-14.4
Pubertal levels (Tanner Stage)			
1, Male		5-265	0.1-7.2
Female		5-125	0.1-3.4
2, Male		15-380	0.4-10.3
Female		15-150	0.4-4.0
3, Male		60-505	1.6-13.6
Female		20-535	0.5-14.4
4, Male		65-560	1.8-15.1
Female		35-485	0.9-13.1
5, Male		165-500	4.4-13.5
Female		75-530	2.0-14.3
Adults			
Male			
18-30 yr		125-619	3.4-16.7
31-50 yr		59-452	1.6-12.2
51-60 yr		20-413	0.5-11.1
61-83 yr		10-285	0.3-7.7
Female			
18-30 yr		45-380	1.2-10.3
31-50 yr		12-379	0.8-10.2
Postmenopausal		30-260	0.8-7.0
		ng/dL	**nmol/L**
Dehydoepiandrosterone, Unconjugated			
Children			
6-9 yr, Male		13-187	0.45-6.49
6-9 yr, Female		18-189	0.62-6.55
10-11 yr, Male		31-205	1.07-7.11
10-11 yr, Female		112-224	3.88-7.77
12-14 yr, Male		83-258	2.88-8.95
12-14 yr, Female		98-360	3.40-12.5
Adult			
Male		180-1250	6.25-43.4
Female		130-980	4.51-34.0

From Quest Diagnostics/Nichols Institute. The Corning Endocrine Manual. Capistrano, CA: Quest Diagnostics/Nichols Institute, 1996; Tietz NW, ed. Clinical guide to laboratory tests. 3rd ed. Philadelphia: WB Saunders Co, 1995.

labeled DHEA are widely available for convenient measurement of serum concentrations. A typical kit method can detect as little as 3 ng/dL (0.1 nmol/L) of DHEA.[81] Cross-reactivity of antisera with related steroids is relatively low, with some exceptions (androstenediol, about 6%; androstenedione, about 2%; and testosterone, about 1%). Interextraction precision, expressed as a coefficient of variation, is less than ± 12% at a DHEA concentration of 120 ng/dL (4.1 nmol/L).

Measurement of 17-Ketosteroids in Urine

The 17-KSs are metabolites of precursors secreted by the adrenal glands, the testes, and to some extent the ovaries. In men, approximately one third of the total urinary 17-KSs represent metabolites of testosterone secreted by the testes, whereas most of the remaining two thirds are derived from the steroids produced by the adrenal glands. In women, who normally excrete smaller quantities than men, the total 17-KS concentrations are derived almost exclusively from the adrenal glands.

The bulk of the urinary 17-KSs consists of androsterone, epiandrosterone, etiocholanolone, DHEA, 11-keto- and 11β-hydroxyandrosterone, and 11-keto- and 11β-hydroxyetiocholanolone. DHEA and 11-oxygenated 17-KSs are produced only by the adrenal glands, whereas the others also arise from precursors (androstenedione and testosterone) elaborated by the gonads. Thus the main purpose of measuring these steroid metabolites is to assess adrenal androgen production.

Decreased concentrations of 17-KSs usually are found in men with primary hypogonadism (Klinefelter's syndrome and castration), in secondary hypogonadism (panhypopituitarism), and in women with pituitary hypoadrenalism (Addison's disease). *Increased concentrations* are found in patients with testicular tumors (interstitial cell tumor and chorioepithelioma), adrenal hyperplasia, and adrenal carcinoma, and in some women with hirsutism.

All 17-KSs are not androgens, and not all androgens are 17-KSs. DHEA and androstenedione are 17-KSs with only weak androgenic properties, and etiocholanolone is a 17-KS with no androgenic effects. The potent androgens, testosterone and DHT, are not 17-KSs. A specific measurement of testosterone and DHT in blood is required to evaluate the production of these androgens. The measurement of DHEA-S in blood serves as a more convenient marker for adrenal androgen production than does urinary 17-KS excretion both because a 24-hour urine collection is not required, and because of the many drugs that interfere with the 17-KS assay.[207] For these reasons, many clinicians now prefer to have concentrations for plasma DHEA-S to interpret rather than those for urinary 17-KS.

Methodology

Several chemical methods are available for estimating the concentration of total 17-KSs in urine. Final quantitation in some of these methods is based on the color reaction originally described by Zimmerman. The method described by Sobel and co-workers[310] has been shown to be adequate for routine clinical use. In this procedure, acid cleavage of glucuronic and sulfuric acid conjugates of 17-KSs is followed by extraction, washing with alkali, and finally color development. Estrone, which is an "acidic" 17-KS, is removed by alkali treatment because of its phenolic nature, and thus is eliminated before the photometric reaction of the remaining "neutral" 17-KS fraction. The color formation is based on the reaction of 17-KS with *m*-dinitrobenzene in alcoholic potassium hydroxide to produce a reddish-purple color with maximum absorption at 520 nm.[214] Marlow has demonstrated that the development of color depends on the presence of an active methylene group adjacent to a carbonyl group.[214] When the ketone group is situated at other positions (e.g., Δ^4-3-keto in testosterone, progesterone, and cortisol), the color development is less intense and the absorption maximums differ. Quantitation is carried out by comparison of the optical absorbance obtained with the sample with that obtained with a known amount of pure calibrator, such as DHEA. For specific analytical details, the interested reader is referred to the first edition of this textbook.[57] The reference interval for the urinary excretion of 17-KSs is 10 to 25 mg/day (35 to 87 μmol/day) in men and 6 to 14 mg/day (21 to 49 μmol/day) in women.[336] Various drugs interfere with the 17-KS assay. Agents that produce a positive interference include chlorpromazine, ethinamate, meprobamate, nalidixic acid, penicillin, phenaglycodol, and spironolactone. Agents that produce a negative interference include chlordiazepoxide, progestational agents, propoxyphene, and reserpine.[250]

Measurement of Anabolic Steroids

Exogenous steroids such as testosterone and DHT that are used to improve athletic performance are a challenge to detect and measure for the laboratory. The ratio of testosterone to epitestosterone, its 17α-epimer, has been used for detection of testosterone abuse. A ratio of testosterone to epitestosterone >6 : 1 suggests exogenous testosterone use and further testing should be performed for confirmation.[50] Others have suggested a ratio of testosterone to LH in the urine as an indication of testosterone doping. Detailed studies of these ratios are available.[177] GC-MS remains the most widely used method for screening and confirmation. For additional information regarding methods, the reader is directed to reviews on the subject.[3,32,49,50,51]

Measurement of Estrogens in Blood

Methodology

Both chromatographic and immunoassay methods are used to measure estrogens in blood.

Chromatographic Methods

GC-MS methods associated with isotope dilution provide the most accurate and reliable measurement of estradiol.[77,303,332,371] The main steps in these reference methods are solvent extraction, chromatographic fractionation, and chemical derivatization before instrumental analysis. Validation of routine methods by this technique has become important in many external quality assurance programs. For routine purposes, these chemical and physical methods have been largely replaced by immunoassays, which are easier and faster than chromatographic methods.

Immunoassay

Immunoassays consist of both indirect (extraction required) and direct (no extraction required) methods. The most common antigen used to prepare antibodies for estradiol assays is estradiol-6-(*O*-carboxymethyl)oxime conjugated to bovine serum albumin.[265] Cross-reactivity with other C_{18} steroids is usually minimal as the 3- and 17-hydroxyl groups are left free. A 2002 CAP survey confirms that direct enzyme immunoassays have largely replaced RIAs for routine measurement of estradiol concentrations. The limitations of automated, nonisotopic immunoassays will be discussed later in this section. Evaluation of estrogen concentrations in men, postmenopausal women, and children requires use of more sensitive RIAs. Many of the early immunoassays used organic solvents for selective extraction of estradiol from serum. This step not only removes estradiol from endogenous binding proteins but also removes other compounds that interfere with the method.

To measure estradiol directly without extraction and chromatography, the steroid must be displaced from its binding proteins. The displacing agents used in commercial methods are often not disclosed, but in some systems effective displacement is achieved by adding 8-anilino-1-naphthalene sulfonic acid (ANS) or a large excess of a competing steroid such as DHT to the sample.[265]

A number of direct RIA kit methods are commercially available for measuring serum estradiol.[76,265] Assay conditions used in these kits vary, with sample volumes ranging from 25-200 μL and incubation times of 45 to 190 minutes. One of the simplest kits available (Coat-a-count; Diagnostic Products Corp.) is a simple two-step assay that requires only the pipetting of an aliquot of sample into an antibody-coated tube followed by a single 3-hour incubation at room temperature; no centrifugation is necessary.[83] This kit is equipped with human serum-based calibrators that have estradiol concentrations ranging from 20 to 3600 pg/mL (0.07 to 13.20 nmol/L); intraassay and interassay precision across a range of estradiol concentrations is less than ±9%.

Bilirubin, hemolysis, and lipemia do not affect this assay, but free fatty acids have significant effects on it. Cross-reacting steroids in samples from neonates have also caused interference. Some direct assays exhibit interference from SHBG, resulting in overestimation of estradiol concentrations at low SHBG concentrations and in underestimation at high concentrations. There has also been a report of an unknown water-soluble interfering substance, which caused falsely increased estradiol results in a variety of direct assays.[199] This interferant is removed by simple extraction with an organic solvent.

Caution should also be exercised when assaying samples from subjects who are receiving oral contraceptives or estrogen replacement therapy because cross-reacting steroids may cause elevated results. Most notably, cross-reactivity with estrone is as high as 10% for some assays, but much lower (<1%) in others. This is likely due to a difference in the specificity of the antibody used for estradiol. Similar effects have been observed for metabolites conjugated at the 3 position, like estrone-3-sulfate and estrone-3-glucuronide.[153,200]

A number of nonisotopic immunoassays for estradiol have been developed and adapted for use on fully automated immunoassay systems. All are heterogeneous assays (separation step needed), but most are direct assays and do not require preliminary extraction. Most procedures offer the convenience of solid-phase separation methods. For routine clinical applications, the greatest experience is with enzyme immunoassays. Most commercial enzyme immunoassays use horseradish peroxidase or alkaline phosphatase to label estradiol antigens; enzyme activity is determined using a variety of photometric,[31,132,200] fluorescent,[11,12,269,271] or chemiluminescent substrates.[158]

Immunoassays using fluorescent labels[18] (e.g., europium chelates and time-resolved fluorescent immunoassay) and chemiluminescent labels[29,73] have also been described. England and co-workers describe a semiautomated "ultrasensitive" chemiluminescent immunoassay for estradiol.[104] This method is reportedly capable of accurately measuring low concentrations (<50 pmol/L) of estradiol observed in perimenopausal and postmenopausal women, healthy men, and children. Taieb and co-workers compared the detection limits and functional sensitivities for nine automated estradiol immunoassays.[323] They concluded that the functional sensitivities, defined as the lowest concentration of analyte that can be measured with a run-to-run imprecision of 20%, were 2- to 4-fold higher than the detection limits of the tests. It is also important to note that none of the assays analyzed in this study had the functional sensitivity required for the evaluation of serum estradiol measurements in men, menopausal women, and children.[93] The functional sensitivities ranged from 5.5 to 46 pg/mL (20 to 169 pmol/L). These assays have been optimized for clinical applications, such as the monitoring of ovarian stimulation in which high estradiol concentrations are expected. A comparison of two direct immunoassay methods for measuring serum estradiol concentration revealed that such assays are useful during monitoring in vitro fertilization progress, but that the values obtained depend on the method used.[324] The authors suggest that, until estradiol assays are better standardized, reference intervals and cutoff points used as clinical decision criteria must be evaluated and modified, if necessary, for each assay.

Specimen Collection and Storage

Serum or plasma (with EDTA or heparin as anticoagulant) is used. Samples should be centrifuged and separated within

24 hours. Samples may be stored refrigerated for 24 hours or frozen for up to 1 year.[92,138,378] Estradiol concentrations are increased in liver cirrhosis, and oral contraceptives have been found to alter concentrations.[163] No steroid, ACTH, gonadotropin, or estradiol medications should be given within 48 hours of sample collection.[163]

Reference Intervals

Reference intervals for serum concentrations of estradiol and estrone are listed in Table 53-10, in Chapter 56, and elsewhere.[163,336]

TABLE 53-10 Reference Intervals for Estradiol and Estrone in Serum

	pg/mL	pmol/L
Estradiol		
Children		
1-5 yr, Male	3-10	11-37
Female	5-10	18-37
6-9 yr, Male	3-10	11-37
Female	5-60	18-220
10-11 yr, Male	5-10	18-37
Female	5-300	18-1100
12-14 yr, Male	5-30	18-110
Female	25-410	92-1505
15-17 yr, Male	5-45	18-165
Female	40-410	147-1505
Adult men	10-50	37-184
Adult women		
Early follicular phase	20-150	73-550
Late follicular phase	40-350	147-1285
Midcycle	150-750	550-2753
Luteal phase	30-450	110-1652
Postmenopausal	≤20	≤73
Pubertal levels (Tanner Stage)		
1, Male	3-15	11-55
Female	5-10	18-37
2, Male	3-10	11-37
Female	5-115	18-422
3, Male	5-15	18-55
Female	5-180	18-660
4, Male	3-40	11-147
Female	25-345	92-1267
5, Male	15-45	55-165
Female	25-410	92-1505
Estrone		
Male	15-65	55-240
Female		
Early follicular phase	15-150	55-555
Late follicular phase	100-250	370-925
Luteal phase	15-200	55-740
Postmenopausal	15-55	55-204

From Quest Diagnostics/Nichols Institute. The Corning Endocrine Manual. Capistrano, CA: Quest Diagnostics/Nichols Institute, 1996; Tietz NW, ed. Clinical guide to laboratory tests. 3rd ed. Philadelphia: WB Saunders Co, 1995.

Measurement of Estriol

Measurement of estriol has little clinical value, except during pregnancy (see Chapter 54), because in nonpregnant women estriol is derived almost exclusively from estradiol. Both RIA and nonisotopic immunoassay methods for estriol measurement in serum and plasma are commercially available. The RIA methods employ both double-antibody and coated-tube technologies using ^{125}I-labeled estriol conjugate.[89,91] The manufacturers claim that the reportable range for these assays is ~0.1 to 30 ng/mL. Competitive enzyme immunoassays are also commercially available. Chemiluminescent detection via an alkaline phosphatase–labeled conjugate has been described.[86] Additionally, an enzymatic method based on biotin-streptavidin binding that photometrically monitors the turnover of horseradish peroxidase in the presence of tetramethylbenzidine (TMB) is available.[88] A 2002 CAP survey reports that automated enzymatic immunoassay methods account for the majority of unconjugated estriol measurements, with <30% performed by RIA.[64]

Specimen Collection and Storage

Estriol serum or plasma specimens are stable at room temperature for 24 hours, and can be refrigerated for 2 days and frozen at −20 °C for up to 1 year.[138] Patients should not be fasting before specimen collection.

Comments

Estrone determinations are limited to diagnosis of postmenopausal bleeding and the menstrual dysfunction caused by extraglandular estrone production. Normally, blood estrone concentrations parallel estradiol concentrations throughout the menstrual cycle, but at slightly lower concentrations. For a specific analysis of estrone, the interested reader is directed to other references.[61,94]

Measurement of Estrogens in Urine

Several chemical methods for urinary estrogen determination have been described.[208] In most, detection is carried out by either fluorometry or photometry. When heated with sulfuric acid, estrogens form an orange-yellow color with intense yellowish-green fluorescence. Such acid-induced fluorescence is sufficiently sensitive to permit detection of as little as 0.005 μg of estrogens. However, nonspecific fluorescence and a number of other variables—such as length of exposure of acid and steroids to elevated temperatures, the amount of water added, and the presence or absence of solvents—are sources of analytical difficulty in using fluorometry for routine analysis. Of the photometric methods available, the *Kober reaction* is best known. For details on this reaction, the reader is directed to the second edition of this book.[361]

Total and fractionated urinary estrogens have been quantitated by RIA after hydrolysis or enzymatic digestion of estrogen glucuronides; analytical specificity for estradiol, estrone, and estradiol is attained by performing a celite chromatograph step before the RIA. A time-resolved fluoroimmunoassay for unconjugated estrogens in urine has been proposed as an alternative to RIA and to the fluorometric assay of total estrogen.[333] Several nonradioactive enzyme immunoassays for urinary estrone conjugates have been described.[59,234,245]

Measurement of Estrogens in Saliva

Measurement of steroids in saliva is noninvasive and suitable for the collection of frequent samples.[205,262] Serial monitoring of estradiol has been used for clinical diagnosis and treatment of infertile women with anovulatory cycles, during in vitro fertilization, or when monitoring hormone replacement therapy of postmenopausal women. Because salivary concentrations of estradiol closely reflect the free fraction of the steroid in plasma, the concentration in saliva is only 1% to 2% of the concentration in blood (1 to 36 pmol/L in nonpregnant women). Hence this requires a sensitive assay for accurate measurement.

Methodology

In general, kits for the measurement of estradiol in saliva are not commercially available. However, Tamate and coworkers have reported the use of a direct enzyme immunoassay that shows promise for the measurement of salivary estradiol.[327] This assay uses monoclonal anti–estradiol-coated microtiter plates and an estradiol-peroxidase conjugate. No extraction is required. These authors reported a salivary estradiol peak of 15 to 31 pmol/L in the preovulatory phase and from 9 to 33 pmol/L in the midluteal phase. Lu and co-workers have described a double-antibody RIA using ^{125}I-labeled estradiol conjugate for the determination of salivary estradiol.[210]

Specimen Collection and Storage

Saliva should be collected after thoroughly rinsing the mouth and frozen immediately. Freezing may help to break down mucin and give a more fluid specimen. Samples are thawed and then centrifuged to remove debris, and can be heat treated at 56 °C for 2 hours to reduce interference by the saliva matrix.

Reference Intervals

Reference intervals for salivary concentrations of estradiol have been reported to be 20 to 70 pg/dL in men and 50 to 300 pg/dL in women.[163]

Comment

Assays for the measurement of estradiol are reported to be highly reagent dependent.[267]

Measurement of Progesterone in Blood

Measurement of progesterone in serum or plasma is considered to be the most reliable technique to assess its rate of production.

Methodology

Double–isotope derivative methods[370] and competitive protein-binding assays[79] have been applied to the measurement of serum progesterone, but require extensive purification of the steroid and are labor intensive. Gas chromatography procedures using flame ionization, electron capture, or nitrogen detection have been used to improve the accuracy of progesterone analysis.[36,79] These methods also are time consuming and often require solvent extraction, chromatography, and derivatization before the steroid can be quantitated. GC-MS has been recommended as a reference method for progesterone determination. The method of Thienpont and associates[331] makes use of heptafluorobutyric ester derivatives and 19-$^2H_3$-progesterone as internal standards.

For routine measurement of progesterone in the clinical laboratory, immunoassays using steroid-specific antibodies are preferred. Initial immunoassays for serum progesterone measurement used organic solvents to remove the steroid from endogenous binding proteins, such as corticosteroid-binding globulin and albumin. Direct (nonextraction) measurement of progesterone in serum or plasma is considered the method of choice for routine applications. A number of different antigens have been used to prepare antisera for progesterone assays. Cross-reactivity is most prominent with 5α-pregnanediol, ranging from 6% to 11%. Both RIA and nonisotopic immunoassays are available for measuring progesterone. A 2002 CAP survey reports that enzyme immunoassays account for the majority of progesterone assays used today.[64]

Radioimmunoassay Methods

Most RIA procedures for progesterone use antibodies generated against a progesterone-11α-hemisuccinate conjugated to bovine serum albumin. Other points on the steroid molecule (e.g., C-3, C-6, C-7, and C-20) have also have been used to link carrier proteins. Some of the antisera produced with these conjugates may cross-react with other C_{21}-corticosteroids present in the sample. If these corticosteroids become a problem, a simple solvent extraction or chromatographic purification procedure before immunoassay can be conducted.[54] Fortunately, these interfering steroids are much more polar than is progesterone. The use of a nonpolar solvent, such as petroleum ether or hexane, quantitatively extracts progesterone, whereas the polar corticosteroids remain mostly in the serum sample.

Historically, tritiated progesterone was the label of choice, but various ^{125}I radioligands have since become more widely used because of the convenience and cost saving of γ-over β-counting. In particular, ^{125}I-labeled progesterone-glucuronyl-tyramine yields satisfactory assays with a number of different progesterone antisera.[369] Other iodinated derivatives of progesterone have also been prepared and combined with antisera from several sources to produce homologous and heterologous bridge systems with variable sensitivity and specificity. In general, poor sensitivity is observed in homologous systems, because the common structural features of both the immunogen and the tracer result in the latter having a much higher affinity than the analyte for the antibody. A variety of procedures have been used to separate the free and antibody-bound radioligand fractions. Dextran-coated charcoal is the conventional separation technique for assays using tritiated labels. Double-antibody and solid-phase separation methods are preferred for assays using radioiodine.

A number of direct RIA kits are simple to perform, rapid, precise, accurate, and commercially available.[272,369] Most of these kits use either 8-anilino-1-naphthalene sulfonic acid or danazol to displace progesterone from binding proteins. One of the simplest direct kits (Coat-a-count; Diagnostic Products Corp.) uses antibody-coated tubes, two pipetting steps, and a single 3-hour incubation at room temperature.[84] This kit includes serum-based calibrators having progesterone concentrations ranging from 0.1 to 40 ng/mL (0.3 to 127 nmol/L).

Direct RIAs for progesterone have been reported to give quantitative recovery of both exogenous progesterone added to serum and patient serum.[266] Assay accuracy, however, is affected by the nature of the matrix used in preparing the calibrators. For progesterone assays, satisfactory accuracy may be achieved by using pooled sera for men who have progesterone concentrations <0.3 ng/mL (<1 nmol/L). The precision of direct assays is superior to that of extraction assays. Both intraassay and interassay coefficients of variation are below ±10%.

Nonisotopic Immunoassays

Several nonisotopic immunoassays are available on fully automated immunoassay systems. Most of these nonisotopic assays measure progesterone directly without extraction. All are heterogeneous assays and require separation of free and antibody-bound fractions. Enzymes appear to be the most widely used nonradioactive label. Alkaline phosphatase and horseradish peroxidase coupled to progesterone or antiprogesterone antibodies are particularly popular. An assortment of photometric,[155,200,341] fluorescent,[113,272,366] and luminescent[29,212] substrates are available for monitoring the enzyme activity of the antibody-bound fraction. Direct time-resolved fluoroimmunoassays for progesterone have also been described.[74,172]

Although automated immunoassays are less labor intensive than RIAs and yield results in less time without the need for radioactivity, these assays do not have adequate functional sensitivity for applications involving low progesterone concentrations (i.e., men, postmenopausal women, and children). Taieb and co-workers analyzed the detection limits and functional sensitivities for eight automated progesterone methods.[323] They reported that the functional sensitivities (0.32 to 1.43 nmol/L) were from 2- to 4-fold higher than the manufacturer-stated detection limit (0.19 to 0.48 nmol/L). Automated progesterone assays have been optimized for use in in vitro fertilization protocols as a rapid, cost effective way to evaluate ovarian stimulation and monitor ovulation.

TABLE 53-11 Reference Intervals for Progesterone in Serum

	ng/dL	nmol/L
Prepubertal child (1-10 yr)	7-52	0.2-1.7
Adult man	13-97	0.4-3.1
Adult woman		
Follicular phase	15-70	0.5-2.2
Luteal phase	200-2500	6.4-79.5
Pregnant woman		
First trimester	725-4400	23.0-139.9
Second trimester	1950-8250	62.0-262.4
Third trimester	6500-22 900	206.7-728.2

From Quest Diagnostics/Nichols Institute. The Corning Endocrine Manual. Capistrano, CA: Quest Diagnostics/Nichols Institute, 1996; Tietz NW, ed. Clinical guide to laboratory tests. 3rd ed. Philadelphia: WB Saunders Co, 1995.

Plasma concentrations of 17α-hydroxyprogesterone are measured to evaluate 21-hydroxylase deficiency. For specific methods regarding this analyte, the reader is referred to a review by Wallace.[350]

Specimen Collection and Storage

Serum or plasma (with heparin or EDTA as anticoagulant) has been used, but should be separated within 24 hours.[163] The patient need not be fasting, and no special handling procedures are necessary.[1,84] Samples can be stored refrigerated for up to 3 days at 4 °C to 8 °C or for up to 1 year at 20 °C.[92,138,378] Patients should not be on any corticosteroid, ACTH, estrogen, or gonadotropin medication for at least 48 hours before specimen collection.[163]

Reference Intervals

Reference intervals for serum concentrations of progesterone are listed in Table 53-11[336] and in Chapter 56.

Measurement of Progesterone in Saliva

Serial sampling of progesterone has been used to (1) investigate luteal defects in women with undefined infertility, (2) monitor the return of fertility after parturition, and (3) assess the bioavailability of oral progesterone.[24,164,205] Several have advocated the use of early-morning saliva for measuring 17-hydroxyprogesterone to aid in the diagnosis of CAH.[251,379] Salivary progesterone concentrations are in general thought to reflect free "unbound" progesterone in the blood,[351] although Evans reported that the amount of progesterone transported into saliva is not determined exclusively by the unbound concentration in plasma and cautioned against the direct correlation between the saliva and serum unbound fraction.[106]

Methodology

Both RIA and enzyme immunoassay methodologies have been applied to the determination of progesterone in saliva. Although sample extraction procedures are often necessary to eliminate protein influences,[117] direct methods are favored in routine laboratories and have been described.[210,249,326] Rigorous standardization of sample collection and preparation is important for obtaining meaningful results for clinical purposes.[295]

Specimen Collection and Storage

Saliva specimens should be collected after a thorough mouth rinsing, centrifuged to remove debris, and frozen immediately. Samples can be heat treated at 56 °C for 2 hours to reduce interference by saliva matrix.

Reference Intervals

Salivary progesterone measurements are not widely commercially available, and no standardized reference intervals exist. However, the reference concentration for salivary concentrations of progesterone in men is reported to be <0.5 ng/dL.[163] In women, the reported reference intervals are 0.5 to 4.0 ng/dL in the follicular phase and 6 to 12 ng/dL in the luteal phase.[163]

REFERENCES

1. Abbott Laboratories. Package insert for progesterone on AxSym. Abbott Park, Ill: Abbott Laboratories, 1996.
2. ACOG Practice Bulletin. Assessment of risk factors for preterm birth. Clinical management guidelines for obstetrician-gynecologists. No. 31, October 2001. (Replaces Technical Bulletin No. 206, June 1995; Committee Opinion No. 172, May 1996; Committee Opinion No. 187, September 1997; Committee Opinion No. 198, February 1998; and Committee Opinion No. 251, January 2001). Obstet Gynecol 2001;98:709-16.
3. Aguilera R, Becchi M, Casabianca H, Hatton CK, Catlin DH, Starcevic B, et al. Improved method of detection of testosterone abuse by gas chromatography/combustion/isotope ratio mass spectrometry analysis of urinary steroids. J Mass Spectrom 1996;31:169-76.
4. Andersson AM, Skakkebaek NE. Serum inhibin B levels during male childhood and puberty. Mol Cell Endocrinol 2001;180:103-7.
5. Armstrong EG, Ehrlich PH, Birken S, Schlatterer JP, Siris E, Hembree WC, et al. Use of a highly sensitive and specific immunoradiometric assay for detection of human chorionic gonadotropin in urine of normal, nonpregnant, and pregnant individuals. J Clin Endocrinol Metab 1984;59:867-74.
6. Azziz R. The evaluation and management of hirsutism. Obstet Gynecol 2003;101:995-1007.
7. Azziz R, Dewailly D, Owerbach D. Clinical review 56: nonclassic adrenal hyperplasia: Current concepts. J Clin Endocrinol Metab 1994;78:810-5.
8. Azziz R, Hincapie LA, Knochenhauer ES, Dewailly D, Fox L, Boots LR. Screening for 21-hydroxylase-deficient nonclassic adrenal hyperplasia among hyperandrogenic women: A prospective study. Fertil Steril 1999;72:915-25.
9. Azziz R, Waggoner WT, Ochoa T, Knochenhauer ES, Boots LR. Idiopathic hirsutism: An uncommon cause of hirsutism in Alabama. Fertil Steril 1998;70:274-8.
10. Bachega TA, Brenlha EM, Billerbeck AE, Marcondes JA, Madureira G, Arnhold IJ, et al. Variable ACTH-stimulated 17-hydroxyprogesterone values in 21-hydroxylase deficiency carriers are not related to the different CYP21 gene mutations. J Clin Endocrinol Metab 2002;87:786-90.
11. Bahar I, Case A, Jackson M. Rapid self-contained immunoassay for estradiol. Clin Chem 1992;38:954.
12. Baker HN, Massei MK, Ramp SK, Trach P, Strarup I, Garner W, et al. Development of a fully automated immunoassay for estradiol on the Abbott IMx™ automated immunoassay system. Clin Chem 1991;37:1036.
13. Baker HWG, Burger HG, DeKretser DM, Hudson B. Relative incidence of etiologic disorders in male infertility. In: Santen RJ, Swerdloff RS, eds. Male reproductive dysfunction. New York: Marcel Dekker Inc, 1986:341-78.
14. Bandi ZL, Schoen I, Waters M. An algorithm for testing and reporting serum choriogonadotropin at clinically significant decision levels with use of "pregnancy test" reagents. Clin Chem 1989;35:545-51.
15. Barash IA, Cheung CC, Weigle DS, Ren H, Kabigting EB, Kuijper JL, et al. Leptin is a metabolic signal to the reproductive system. Endocrinology 1996;137:3144-7.
16. Barbieri RL. Infertility. In: Yen SSC, Jaffe RB, Barbieri RL, eds. Reproductive endocrinology: Physiology, pathophysiology, and clinical management. 4th ed. Philadelphia: WB Saunders Co, 1999:562-93.
17. Barini A, Liberale I, Menini E. Simultaneous determination of free testosterone and testosterone bound to non-sex-hormone-binding globulin by equilibrium dialysis. Clin Chem 1993;39:938-41.
18. Barnard G, Kohen F. Idiometric assay: noncompetitive immunoassay for small molecules typified by the measurement of estradiol in serum. Clin Chem 1990;36:1945-50.
19. Barontini M, Garcia-Rudaz MC, Veldhuis JD. Mechanisms of hypothalamic-pituitary-gonadal

disruption in polycystic ovarian syndrome. Arch Med Res 2001;32:544-52.
20. Bastian LA, Smith CM, Nanda K. Is this woman perimenopausal? JAMA 2003;289:895-902.
21. Batista MC, Cartledge TP, Zellmer AW, Merino MJ, Nieman LK, Loriaux DL, et al. A prospective controlled study of luteal and endometrial abnormalities in an infertile population. Fertil Steril 1996;65: 495-502.
22. Benson JR, Pitsinis V. Update on clinical role of tamoxifen. Curr Opin Obstet Gynecol 2003;15: 13-23.
23. Bodlaender P. No SHBG interference with the "Coat-A-Count Total Testosterone" direct RIA kit. Clin Chem 1990;36:173.
24. Bolaji II, Tallon DF, Meehan FP, O'Dwyer EM, Fottrell PF. The return of postpartum fertility monitored by enzyme-immunoassay for salivary progesterone. Gynecol Endocrinol 1992;6:37-48.
25. Boolell M, Allen MJ, Ballard SA, Gepi-Attee S, Muirhead GJ, Naylor AM, et al. Sildenafil: An orally active type 5 cyclic GMP-specific phosphodiesterase inhibitor for the treatment of penile erectile dysfunction. Int J Impot Res 1996;8:47-52.
26. Boolell M, Gepi-Attee S, Gingell JC, Allen MJ. Sildenafil, a novel effective oral therapy for male erectile dysfunction. Br J Urol 1996;78:257-61.
27. Boots LR, Potter S, Potter D, Azziz R. Measurement of total serum testosterone levels using commercially available kits: High degree of between-kit variability. Fertil Steril 1998;69:286-92.
28. Borkowski A, Puttaert V, Gyling M, Muquardt C, Body JJ. Human chorionic gonadotropin-like substance in plasma of normal nonpregnant subjects and women with breast cancer. J Clin Endocrinol Metab 1984;58:1171-8.
29. Bouma S, Worobec S, Baker A, Dubler R, Frias E, Ginsburg S, et al. Performance of automated chemiluminescent paramagnetic microparticle immunoassays for estradiol, progesterone, and testosterone on the Abbott i200 system. Clin Chem 1997;43:S171.
30. Bourguignon JP. Linear growth as a function of age at onset of puberty and sex steroid dosage: Therapeutic implications. Endocr Rev 1988;9:467-88.
31. Bouve J, De Boever J, Leyseele D, Bosmans E, Dubois P, Kohen F, et al. Direct enzyme immunoassay of estradiol in serum of women enrolled in an in vitro fertilization and embryo transfer program. Clin Chem 1992;38:1409-13.
32. Bowers LD. Analytical advances in detection of performance-enhancing compounds. Clin Chem 1997;43:1299-304.
33. Braunstein GD. Gynecomastia.[comment]. [Review]. N Engl J Med 1993;328:490-5.
34. Bremner WJ, Vitiello MV, Prinz PN. Loss of circadian rhythmicity in blood testosterone levels with aging in normal men. J Clin Endocrinol Metab 1983;56: 1278-81.
35. Brenner PF, Mishell DR. Menopause. In: Mishell DR, Davajan V, Lobo RA, eds. Infertility, contraception and reproductive endocrinology. Boston: Blackwell Scientific Publications, 1993:241-53.
36. Breuer H, Hamel D, Kruskemper H, eds. Methods of hormone analysis. New York: John Wiley & Sons Inc, 1976.
37. Brito VN, Batista MC, Borges MF, Latronico AC, Kohek MB, Thirone AC, et al. Diagnostic value of fluorometric assays in the evaluation of precocious puberty. J Clin Endocrinol Metab 1999;84:3539-44.
38. Bronson R, Cooper G, Rosenfeld D. Sperm antibodies: their role in infertility. [Review] [78 refs]. Fertil Steril 1984;42:171-83.
39. Brzechffa PR, Jakimiuk AJ, Agarwal SK, Weitsman SR, Buyalos RP, Magoffin DA. Serum immunoreactive leptin concentrations in women with polycystic ovary syndrome. J Clin Endocrinol Metab 1996;81:4166-69.
40. Burger HG, Dudley EC, Hopper JL, Groome N, Guthrie JR, Green A, et al. Prospectively measured levels of serum follicle-stimulating hormone, estradiol, and the dimeric inhibins during the menopausal transition in a population-based cohort of women. J Clin Endocrinol Metab 1999;84:4025-30.
41. Buster JE, Abraham GE. Radioimmunoassay of plasma dehydroepiandrosterone sulfate. Anal Lett 1972;5:543-51.
42. Buzdar A. Anastrozole as adjuvant therapy for early-stage breast cancer: Implications of the ATAC trial. Clin Breast Cancer 2003;4 Suppl 1:S42-8.
43. Canick JA, Knight GJ, Palomaki GE, Haddow JE, Cuckle HS, Wald NJ. Low second trimester maternal serum unconjugated oestriol in pregnancies with Down's syndrome. Br J Obstet Gynaecol 1988;95: 330-3.
44. Carmina E. Prevalence of idiopathic hirsutism. Eur J Endocrinol 1998;139:421-3.
45. Caro JF. Leptin is normal in PCOS, an editorial about three "negative" papers. J Clin Endocrinol Metab 1997;82:1685-6.
46. Carr BR. Disorders of the ovary and female reproductive tract. In: Williams RH, Foster DW, Kronenberg HM, Larsen PR, Wilson JD, eds. Williams textbook of endocrinology. 9th ed. Philadelphia: WB Saunders, 1998:751-817.
47. Carson SA, Reiher J, Scommegna A, Prins GS. Antibody binding patterns in infertile males and females as detected by immunobead test, gel-agglutination test, and sperm immobilization test. Fertil Steril 1988;49:487-92.
48. Cassio A, Cacciari E, Zucchini S, Balsamo A, Diegoli M, Orsini F. Central precocious puberty: Clinical and imaging aspects. J Pediatr Endocrinol Metab 2000;13 Suppl 1:703-8.

49. Catlin DH, Cowan DA, de la Torre R, Donike M, Fraisse D, Oftebro H, et al. Urinary testosterone (T) to epitestosterone (E) ratios by GC/MS. I. Initial comparison of uncorrected T/E in six international laboratories. J Mass Spectrom 1996;31:397-402.
50. Catlin DH, Hatton CK, Starcevic SH. Issues in detecting abuse of xenobiotic anabolic steroids and testosterone by analysis of athletes' urine. Clin Chem 1997;43:1280-8.
51. Catlin DH, Murray TH. Performance-enhancing drugs, fair competition, and Olympic sport. JAMA 1996;276:231-7.
52. Cattaneo S, Forti G, Fiorelli G, Barbieri U, Serio M. A rapid radioimmunoassay for determination of dehydroepiandrosterone sulphate in human plasma. Clin Endocrinol 1975;4:505-12.
53. Cavallo A, Richards GE, Busey S, Michaels SE. A simplified gonadotrophin-releasing hormone test for precocious puberty. Clin Endocrinol (Oxf) 1995;42:641-6.
54. Channing CP, Schaerf FW, Anderson LD, Tsafriri A. Ovarian follicular and luteal physiology. In: Greep RO, ed. Reproductive physiology III. Baltimore: University Park Press, 1980:117.
55. Chasalow FI, Blethen SL, Duckett D, Zeitlin S, Greenfield J. Serum levels of dehydroepiandrosterone sulfate as determined by commercial kits and reagents. Steroids 1989;54:373-83.
56. Chattoraj SC, Turner AK, Pinkus JL, Charles D. The significance of urinary free cortisol and progesterone in normal and anencephalic pregnancy. Am J Obstet Gynecol 1976;124:848-54.
57. Chattoraj SC, Watts NB. Endocrinology. In: Tietz NW, ed. Textbook of clinical chemistry. Philadelphia: WB Saunders Co, 1986:1091-4.
58. Chehab FF, Lim ME, Lu R. Correction of the sterility defect in homozygous obese female mice by treatment with the human recombinant leptin. Nat Genet 1996;12:318-20.
59. Chen C, Malone KE, Prunty J, Daling JR. Measurement of urinary estrogen metabolites using a monoclonal enzyme-linked immunoassay kit: Assay performance and feasibility for epidemiological studies. Cancer Epidemiol Biomarkers Prev 1996;5:727-32.
60. Chumlea WC, Schubert CM, Roche AF, Kulin HE, Lee PA, Himes JH, et al. Age at menarche and racial comparisons in US girls. Pediatrics 2003;111:110-3.
61. Ciotti PM, Franceschetti F, Bulletti C, Jasonni VM, Bolelli GF. Rapid and specific RIA of serum estrone sulfate with selective solid phase extraction. J Steroid Biochem 1989;32:473-4.
62. Clemons M, Goss P. Estrogen and the risk of breast cancer. N Engl J Med 2001;344:276-85.
63. Cole P, MacMahon B. Oestrogen fractions during early reproductive life in the aetiology of breast cancer. Lancet 1969;1:604-6.
64. College of Pathologists. Y-C Ligands (special) survey 2002. Northfield, Ill: College of American Pathologists; 2002. Report.
65. Cooper JD, Muirhead DC, Taylor JE, Baker PR. Development of an assay for the simultaneous determination of sildenafil (Viagra) and its metabolite (UK-103,320) using automated sequential trace enrichment of dialysates and high-performance liquid chromatography. J Chromatogr B Biomed Sci Appl 1997;701:87-95.
66. Corsan GH, Blotner MB, Bohrer MK, Shelden R, Kemmann E. The utility of a home urinary LH immunoassay in timing the postcoital test. Obstet Gynecol 1993;81:736-8.
67. Dabbs JM, Jr, Campbell BC, Gladue BA, Midgley AR, Navarro MA, Read GF, et al. Reliability of salivary testosterone measurements: A multicenter evaluation. Clin Chem 1995;41:1581-4.
68. Dacou-Voutetakis C, Maniati-Christidi M, Dracopoulou-Vabouli M. Genetic aspects of congenital adrenal hyperplasia. J Pediatr Endocrinol Metab 2001;14 Suppl 5:1303-8; discussion 17.
69. Davajan V, Kletzky OA. Primary amenorrhea: phenotypic female external genitalia. In: Mishell DR, Davajan V, Lobo RA, eds. Infertility, contraception and reproductive endocrinology. 3rd ed. Boston: Blackwell Scientific Publications, 1993:356-71.
70. Davajan V, Kletzky OA. Secondary amenorrhea without galactorrhea or androgen excess. In: Mishell DR, Davajan V, Lobo RA, eds. Infertility, contraception and reproductive endocrinology. 3rd ed. Boston: Blackwell Scientific Publications, 1993:372-95.
71. Davies R, Collier C, Raymond M, Heaton J, Clark A. Indirect measurement of bioavailable testosterone with the Bayer Immuno 1 system. Clin Chem 2002;48:388-90.
72. Davison S, Davis SR. Hormone replacement therapy: Current controversies. Clin Endocrinol (Oxf) 2003;58:249-61.
73. De Boever J, Kohen F, Usanachitt C, Vandekerckhove D, Leyseele D, Vandewalle L. Direct chemiluminescence immunoassay for estradiol in serum. Clin Chem 1986;32:1895-900.
74. Dechaud H, Bador R, Claustrat F, Desuzinges C, Mallein R. New approach to competitive lanthanide immunoassay: Time-resolved fluoroimmunoassay of progesterone with labeled analyte. Clin Chem 1988;34:501-4.
75. Dechaud H, Lejeune H, Garoscio-Cholet M, Mallein R, Pugeat M. Radioimmunoassay of testosterone not bound to sex-steroid-binding protein in plasma. Clin Chem 1989;35:1609-14.

76. DeChene N, McNamara B, Breglio S. A simple and sensitive solid phase radioimmunoassay for estradiol. Clin Chem 1992;38:951.
77. Dehennin L. Estradiol-17 beta determined in plasma by gas chromatography-mass spectrometry with selected ion monitoring of mixed silyl ether-perfluoroacyl ester derivatives and use of various stable-isotope-labeled internal standards. Clin Chem 1989;35:532-6.
78. Demers LM. Andropause: an androgen deficiency state in the ageing male. Expert Opin Pharmacother 2003;4:183-90.
79. Demetriou J. Progesterone. In: Pesce A, Kaplan L, eds. Methods in clinical chemistry. St Louis: CV Mosby Co, 1987:253-7.
80. Dewailly D. Nonclassic 21-hydroxylase deficiency. Semin Reprod Med 2002;20:243-8.
81. Diagnostic Products Corp. Package insert for Coat-A-Count DHEA kit. Los Angeles: Diagnostic Products Corp, 1992.
82. Diagnostic Products Corp. Package insert for Coat-A-Count DHEA-SO4 kit. Los Angeles, CA: Diagnostic Products Corp, 1997.
83. Diagnostic Products Corp. Package insert for Coat-A-Count estradiol (no extraction) kit. Los Angeles: Diagnostic Products Corp, 1997.
84. Diagnostic Products Corp: Package insert for Coat-A-Count progesterone kit. Los Angeles: Diagnostic Products Corp, 1997.
85. Diagnostic Products Corp. Package insert for Coat-A-Count testosterone kit. Los Angeles: Diagnostic Products Corp, 1997.
86. Diagnostic Products Corp: Package insert for Immulite unconjugated estriol kit. Los Angeles: Diagnostic Products Corp, 2003.
87. Diagnostic Systems Laboratories: Package insert for DSL-10-3500 Active DHEA-S EIA kit. Webster, Tex: Diagnostic Systems Laboratories, 2001.
88. Diagnostic Systems Laboratories: Package insert for DSL-10-3700-1 Active ultra-sensitive unconjugated estriol EIA kit. Webster, Tex.: Diagnostic Systems Laboratories, 2003.
89. Diagnostic Systems Laboratories: Package insert for DSL-1400 ultra-sensitive unconjugated estriol RIA kit. Webster, Tex.: Diagnostic Systems Laboratories, 2003.
90. Diagnostic Systems Laboratories: Package insert for DSL-2700-S DHEA-S-7 (saliva) RIA kit. Webster, Tex.: Diagnostic Systems Laboratories, 2000.
91. Diagnostic Systems Laboratories: Package insert for DSL 3700 Active ultra-sensitive unconjugated estriol RIA kit. Webster, Tex.: Diagnostic Systems Laboratories, 2003.
92. Diver MJ, Hughes JG, Hutton JL, West CR, Hipkin LJ. The long-term stability in whole blood of 14 commonly-requested hormone analytes. Ann Clin Biochem 1994;31(Pt 6):561-5.
93. Diver MJ, Nisbet JA. Warning on plasma oestradiol measurement. Lancet 1987;2:1097.
94. Dobson H, Dean PD. Radioimmunoassay of oestrone, oestradiol-17alpha and -17 beta in bovine plasma during the oestrous cycle and last stages of pregnancy. J Endocrinol 1974;61:479-86.
95. Dorgan JF, Fears TR, McMahon RP, Aronson Friedman L, Patterson BH, Greenhut SF. Measurement of steroid sex hormones in serum: a comparison of radioimmunoassay and mass spectrometry. Steroids 2002;67:151-8.
96. Dorland's illustrated medical dictionary. 30th ed. Philadelphia: WB Saunders Co, 2003.
97. Dufau ML, Winters CA, Hattori M, Aquilano D, Baranao JL, Nozu K, et al. Hormonal regulation of androgen production by the Leydig cell. J Steroid Biochem 1984;20:161-73.
98. Dunaif A. Insulin resistance in polycystic ovarian syndrome. Ann N Y Acad Sci 1993;687:60-4.
99. Dunaif A, Green G, Phelps RG, Lebwohl M, Futterweit W, Lewy L. Acanthosis Nigricans, insulin action, and hyperandrogenism: clinical, histological, and biochemical findings. J Clin Endocrinol Metab 1991;73:590-5.
99A. Dunn BK, Wickerham DL, Ford LG. Prevention of hormone-related cancers: Breast cancer. J Clin Oncol 2005;23:357-67.
100. Eckert KL, Wilson DM, Bachrach LK, Anhalt H, Habiby RL, Olney RC, et al. A single-sample, subcutaneous gonadotropin-releasing hormone test for central precocious puberty. Pediatrics 1996;97:517-9.
101. Eggert-Kruse W, Christmann M, Gerhard I, Pohl S, Klinga K, Runnebaum B. Circulating antisperm antibodies and fertility prognosis: a prospective study. Hum Reprod 1989;4:513-20.
102. Eimers JM, te Velde ER, Gerritse R, van Kooy RJ, Kremer J, Habbema JD. The validity of the postcoital test for estimating the probability of conceiving. Am J Obstet Gynecol 1994;171:65-70.
103. Elkind-Hirsch K, Goldzieher JW, Gibbons WE, Besch PK. Evaluation of the OvuSTICK urinary luteinizing hormone kit in normal and stimulated menstrual cycles. Obstet Gynecol 1986;67:450-3.
104. England BG, Parsons GH, Possley RM, McConnell DS, Midgley AR. Ultrasensitive semiautomated chemiluminescent immunoassay for estradiol. Clin Chem 2002;48:1584-6.
105. ESHRE Capri Workshop: Infertility revisited: The state of the art today and tomorrow. Hum Reprod 1996;11:1179-807.
106. Evans JJ. Progesterone in saliva does not parallel unbound progesterone in plasma. Clin Chem 1986;32:542-4.
107. Fehér T, Bodrogi L, Fehér K, Poteczin E. Gas chromatographic determination of free and solvalysable

dehydroepiandrosterone. Chromatographia 1977;10: 86-91.
108. Finlay EM, Gaskell SJ. Determination of testosterone in plasma from men by gas chromatography/mass spectrometry, with high-resolution selected-ion monitoring and metastable peak monitoring. Clin Chem 1981;27:1165-70.
109. Fisch H, Lipshultz LI. Diagnosing male factors of infertility. [Review]. Arch Path Lab Med 1992;116: 398-405.
110. Fisch H, Laor E, Lipshultz LI. Simplified gonadotropin-releasing hormone (GnRH) stimulation test. Urology 1990;36:260-3.
111. Fitzgerald RL, Herold DA. Serum total testosterone: immunoassay compared with negative chemical ionization gas chromatography-mass spectrometry. Clin Chem 1996;42:749-55.
112. Forabosco A, Sforza C, De Pol A, Vizzotto L, Marzona L, Ferrario VF. Morphometric study of the human neonatal ovary. Anat Rec 1991;231:201-8.
113. Ford K, Caplan DE, Tobias DD, Turn JE, Osikowicz E. Automated direct enzyme immunoassay of progesterone on the Abbott IMx analyzer. Clin Chem 1990;36:1099.
114. Forest MG. Serum mullerian inhibiting substance assay—a new diagnostic test for disorders of gonadal development. N Engl J Med 1997;336:1519-21.
115. Fotherby K. Progesterone II. Clinical aspects. In: Gray CH, James VHT, eds. Hormones in blood. 3rd ed. London: Academic Press Ltd, 1979:439-91.
116. Franks S. Polycystic ovary syndrome. [Comment] [erratum appears in N Engl J Med 1995 Nov 23; 333(21):1435]. [Review]. N Engl J Med 1995;333: 853-61.
117. Fulton A, Chan S, Coleman G. Effect of salivary proteins on binding curves of three radioimmunoassay kits: Amerlex-M progesterone, Amerlex cortisol, and Biodata testosterone. Clin Chem 1989;35:641-4.
118. Fuqua JS, Sher ES, Migeon CJ, Berkovitz GD. Assay of plasma testosterone during the first six months of life: importance of chromatographic purification of steroids. Clin Chem 1995;41:1146-9.
119. Gandy H, Peterson R. Measurement of testosterone and 17-ketosteroids in plasma by the double isotope dilution derivative technique. J Clin Endocrinol 1975;4:505-12.
120. Glass AR. Gynecomastia. Endocrinol Metab Clin North Am 1994;23:825-37.
121. Glezerman M, Bartoov B. Semen analysis. In: Insler V, Lunenfeld B, eds. Infertility: Male and female. New York: Churchill Livingstone, 1993:285-315.
122. Glezerman M, Lunenfeld B. Diagnosis of male infertility. In: Insler V, Lunenfeld B, eds. Infertility: Male and female. 2nd ed. New York: Churchill Livingstone, 1993:317-22.
123. Gnatuk CL. The controversy over estrogen replacement therapy: An update on clinical trials. Curr Womens Health Rep 2002;2:89-94.
124. Goffinet F, Maillard F, Fulla Y, Cabrol D. Biochemical markers (without markers of infection) of the risk of preterm delivery. Implications for clinical practice. Eur J Obstet Gynecol Reprod Biol 2001;94:59-68.
125. Goodwin TM. A role for estriol in human labor, term and preterm. Am J Obstet Gynecol 1999;180:S208-13.
126. Gordon CM. Menstrual disorders in adolescents. Excess androgens and the polycystic ovary syndrome. Pediatr Clin North Am 1999;46:519-43.
127. Gougeon A, Ecochard R, Thalabard JC. Age-related changes of the population of human ovarian follicles: increase in the disappearance rate of non-growing and early-growing follicles in aging women. Biol Reprod 1994;50:653-63.
128. Govier FE, McClure RD, Kramer-Levien D. Endocrine screening for sexual dysfunction using free testosterone determinations. J Urol 1996;156:405-8.
129. Greendale GA, Lee NP, Arriola ER. The menopause. Lancet 1999;353:571-80.
130. Griffin JE, Wilson JD. Disorders of the testes and male reproductive tract. In: Williams RH, Foster DW, Kronenberg HM, Larsen PR, Wilson JD, eds. Williams textbook of endocrinology. 9th ed. Philadelphia: WB Saunders Co, 1998:819-75.
131. Grodstein F, Stampfer M. The epidemiology of coronary heart disease and estrogen replacement in postmenopausal women. Prog Cardiovasc Dis 1995;38:199-210.
132. Grol M, Stock W, Ebert C. Fully automated steroid determination on the immuno-analyzer ES 300: Development and performance of a new direct highly sensitive enzyme immunoassay for serum estradiol. Clin Chem 1991;37:1027.
133. Gronowski AM, Landau-Levine M. Reproductive Endocrine Function. In: Burtis CA, Ashwood ER, eds. Tietz Textbook of Clinical Chemistry. 3rd ed. Philadelphia: WB Saunders, 1999:1601-41.
134. Groome NP, Evans LW. Does measurement of inhibin have a clinical role? Ann Clin Biochem 2000;37(Pt 4):419-31.
135. Groskopf WR, Necklaws E, Osikowicz E. An automated FPIA for DHEAS using the Abbott IMx analyzer. Clin Chem 1991;37:937.
136. Grumbach MM, Conte FA. Disorders of sex differentiation. In: Williams RH, Foster DW, Kronenberg HM, Larsen PR, Wilson JD, eds. Williams textbook of endocrinology. 8th ed. Philadelphia: WB Saunders Co, 1998:1303-425.
137. Gruschke A, Kuhl H. Validity of radioimmunological methods for determining free testosterone in serum. Fertil Steril 2001;76:576-82.
138. Guder W, Narayanan H, Wisser H, Zawata B. List of analytes preanalytical variables. In: Guder W,

Narayanan H, Wisser H, Zawata B, eds. Samples: from the patient to the laboratory: The impact of preanalytical variables on the quality of laboratory results. Germany: Git Verlag, GmBH, 1996:1-48.
139. Guillaume AJ, Benjamin F, Sicuranza B, Deutsch S, Spitzer M. Luteal phase defects and ectopic pregnancy. Fertil Steril 1995;63:30-3.
140. Haas GG Jr, D'Cruz OJ, DeBault LE. Comparison of the indirect immunobead, radiolabeled, and immunofluorescence assays for immunoglobulin G serum antibodies to human sperm. Fertil Steril 1991;55:377-88.
141. Hall PF. Testicular steroid synthesis: Organization and regulation. In: Knobil E, Neill JD, eds. The physiology of reproduction. New York: Raven Press, 1988:975-98.
142. Hammond GL, Nisker JA, Jones LA, Siiteri PK. Estimation of the percentage of free steroid in undiluted serum by centrifugal ultrafiltration-dialysis. J Biol Chem 1980;255:5023-6.
143. Harman SM, Metter EJ, Tobin JD, Pearson J, Blackman MR. Longitudinal effects of aging on serum total and free testosterone levels in healthy men. Baltimore Longitudinal Study of Aging. J Clin Endocrinol Metab 2001;86:724-31.
144. Harris JR, Lippman ME, Veronesi U, Willett W. Breast cancer (1). [Review]. N Engl J Med 1992;327: 319-28.
145. Harris JR, Lippman ME, Veronesi U, Willett W. Breast cancer (2). [Review]. N Engl J Med 1992;327:390-98.
146. Harris JR, Lippman ME, Veronesi U, Willett W. Breast cancer (3). [Review]. N Engl J Med 1992;327:473-80.
147. Hawton K. Integration of treatments for male erectile dysfunction. Lancet 1998;351:7-8.
148. Hedriana HL, Munro CJ, Eby-Wilkens EM, Lasley BL. Changes in rates of salivary estriol increases before parturition at term. Am J Obstet Gynecol 2001;184:123-30.
149. Heine RP, McGregor JA, Dullien VK. Accuracy of salivary estriol testing compared to traditional risk factor assessment in predicting preterm birth. Am J Obstet Gynecol 1999;180:S214-8.
150. Heine RP, McGregor JA, Goodwin TM, Artal R, Hayashi RH, Robertson PA, et al. Serial salivary estriol to detect an increased risk of preterm birth. Obstet Gynecol 2000;96:490-7.
151. Herman-Giddens ME, Slora EJ, Wasserman RC, Bourdony CJ, Bhapkar MV, Koch GG, et al. Secondary sexual characteristics and menses in young girls seen in office practice: A study from the Pediatric Research in Office Settings network. Pediatrics 1997;99:505-12.
152. Herold DA, Fitzgerald RL. Female testosterone immunoassays: Better than a guess? Clin Chem 2003;49:1250-1.
153. Hershlag A, Zinger M, Lesser M, Scholl G, Bjornson L. Is chemiluminescent immunoassay an appropriate substitution for radioimmunoassay in monitoring estradiol levels? Fertil Steril 2000;73:1174-8.
154. Horton R, Lobo R, Hawks D. Androstanediol glucuronide in plasma, a marker of androgen action in men and women. Clin Res 1982;30:491A.
155. Hoyle N, Ebert C. Fully automated determination on the immunoanalyzer ES 300: Performance of serum progesterone and testosterone assays. Clin Chem 1991;37:1020.
156. Hughes I. Congenital adrenal hyperplasia: phenotype and genotype. J Pediatr Endocrinol Metab 2002;15 Suppl 5:1329-40.
157. Hughes IA. Congenital adrenal hyperplasia: 21-hydroxylase deficiency in the newborn and during infancy. Semin Reprod Med 2002;20:229-42.
158. Hughes J, Weston S, Montague D, Summers M, Shepard H, Shepard B. Enhanced luminescence immunoassay for estradiol. Clin Chem 1989;35: 1149.
159. Hulka BS. Epidemiologic analysis of breast and gynecologic cancers. Prog Clin Biol Res 1997;396: 17-29.
160. Hull MG, Glazener CM, Kelly NJ, Conway DI, Foster PA, Hinton RA, et al. Population study of causes, treatment, and outcome of infertility. Br Med J (Clin Res Ed) 1985;291:1693-7.
161. Hunter WM, Corrie JET, eds. Immunoassays for clinical chemistry. 2nd ed. Edinburgh: Churchill Livingstone, 1983.
162. Imperato-McGinley J, Guerrero L, Gautier T, Peterson RE. Steroid 5alpha-reductase deficiency in man: An inherited form of male pseudohermaphroditism. Science 1974;186:1213-15.
163. Inter Science Institute. Current unique and rare endocrine assays. Inglewood, Calif: Inter Science Institute, 1997.
164. Ishikawa M, Sengoku K, Tamate K, Takaoka Y, Kane M, Fottrell PF. The clinical usefulness of salivary progesterone measurement for the evaluation of the corpus luteum function. Gynecol Obstet Invest 2002;53:32-7.
165. Ismail AA, Astley P, Cawood M, Short F, Wakelin K, Wheeler M. Testosterone assays: guidelines for the provision of a clinical biochemistry service. Ann Clin Biochem 1986;23:135-45.
166. Iughetti L, Predieri B, Ferrari M, Gallo C, Livio L, Milioli S, et al. Diagnosis of central precocious puberty: Endocrine assessment. J Pediatr Endocrinol Metab 2000;13 Suppl 1:709-15.
167. Jaffe RB. Disorders of sexual development. In: Yen SSC, Jaffe RB, Barbieri RL, eds. Reproductive endocrinology: physiology, pathophysiology, and clinical management. 4th ed. Philadelphia: WB Saunders Co, 1999:363-87.
168. Jaffe RB. Menopause and aging. In: Yen SSC, Jaffe RB, Barbieri RL, eds. Reproductive endocrinology: Physi-

ology, pathophysiology, and clinical management. 4th ed. Philadelphia: WB Saunders Co, 1999:301-62.

169. Jaffe RB, Behrman HR, eds. Methods of hormone radioimmunoassay. New York: Academic Press Inc, 1979.
170. Jialal I, Winter WE, Chan DW, eds. Handbook of diagnostic endocrinology. Washington, DC: AACC Press, 1999.
171. Jones HW Jr, Toner JP. The infertile couple. N Engl J Med 1993;329:1710-15.
172. Kakabakos SE, Khosravi MJ. Direct time-resolved fluorescence immunoassay of progesterone in serum involving the biotin-streptavidin system and the immobilized-antibody approach. Clin Chem 1992;38:725-30.
173. Kaplowitz PB, Oberfield SE. Reexamination of the age limit for defining when puberty is precocious in girls in the United States: implications for evaluation and treatment. Drug and therapeutics and executive committees of the Lawson Wilkins Pediatric Endocrine Society. Pediatrics 1999;104:936-41.
174. Kapoor P, Luttrell BM, Williams D. The free androgen index is not valid for adult males. J Steroid Biochem Mol Biol 1993;45:325-6.
175. Kelsey JL, Gammon MD. Epidemiology of breast cancer. Epidemiol Rev 1990;12:228-40.
176. Key TJ, Verkasalo PK, Banks E. Epidemiology of breast cancer. Lancet Oncol 2001;2:133-40.
177. Kicman AT, Brooks RV, Collyer SC, Cowan DA, Nanjee MN, Southan GJ, et al. Criteria to indicate testosterone administration. Br J Sports Med 1990;24:253-64.
178. Kiningham RB, Apgar BS, Schwenk TL. Evaluation of amenorrhea. Am Fam Physician 1996;53:1185-94.
179. Klee GG, Heser DW. Techniques to measure testosterone in the elderly. Mayo Clin Proc 2000;75 Suppl:S19-25.
180. Kleerekoper M, Sullivan JM. Osteoporosis as a model for the long-term clinical consequences of the menopause. Prog Cardiovasc Dis 1995;38:181-8.
181. Klein J, Sauer MV. Assessing fertility in women of advanced reproductive age. Am J Obstet Gynecol 2001;185:758-70.
182. Klein KO. Precocious puberty: Who has it? Who should be treated? J Clin Endocrinol Metab 1999;84:411-4.
183. Klein KO, Baron J, Colli MJ, McDonnell DP, Cutler GB Jr. Estrogen levels in childhood determined by an ultrasensitive recombinant cell bioassay. J Clin Invest 1994;94:2475-80.
184. Kletzky OA, Davajan V. Hyperprolactinemia. In: Mishell DR, Davajan V, eds. Infertility, contraception and reproductive endocrinology. 3rd ed. Boston: Blackwell Scientific Publications, 1993:372-95.
185. Korenman SG. Sexual function and dysfunction. In: Williams RH, Foster DW, Kronenberg HM, Larsen PR, Wilson JD, eds. Williams textbook of endocrinology. 9th ed. Philadelphia: WB Saunders Co, 1998:927-38.
186. Kubini K, Zachmann M, Albers N, Hiort O, Bettendorf M, Wolfle J, et al. Basal inhibin B and the testosterone response to human chorionic gonadotropin correlate in prepubertal boys. J Clin Endocrinol Metab 2000;85:134-8.
187. Lachelin GC, McGarrigle HH. A comparison of saliva, plasma unconjugated and plasma total oestriol levels throughout normal pregnancy. Br J Obstet Gynaecol 1984;91:1203-9.
188. Lake DE, Hudis C. Aromatase inhibitors in breast cancer: an update. Cancer Control 2002;9:490-8.
189. Laue L, Rennert OM. Congenital adrenal hyperplasia: molecular genetics and alternative approaches to treatment. Adv Pediatr 1995;42:113-43.
190. Lawson ML, Cohen N. A single sample subcutaneous luteinizing hormone (LH)-releasing hormone (LHRH) stimulation test for monitoring LH suppression in children with central precocious puberty receiving LHRH agonists. J Clin Endocrinol Metab 1999;84:4536-40.
191. Leader LR, Russell T, Clifford K, Stenning B. The clinical value of Clearplan home ovulation detection kits in infertility practice. Aust N Z J Obstet Gynaecol 1991;31:142-4.
192. Lebrethon MC, Bourguignon JP. Management of central isosexual precocity: Diagnosis, treatment, outcome. Curr Opin Pediatr 2000;12:394-9.
193. Lee CL, Iles RK, Shepherd JH, Hudson CN, Chard T. The purification and development of a radioimmunoassay for beta-core fragment of human chorionic gonadotrophin in urine: Application as a marker of gynaecological cancer in premenopausal and postmenopausal women. J Endocrinol 1991;130:481-9.
194. Lee MM, Donahoe PK, Silverman BL, Hasegawa T, Hasegawa Y, Gustafson ML, et al. Measurements of serum mullerian inhibiting substance in the evaluation of children with nonpalpable gonads. N Engl J Med 1997;336:1480-6.
195. Lee PA. Laboratory monitoring of children with precocious puberty. Arch Pediatr Adolesc Med 1994;148:369-76.
196. Lee PA. Central precocious puberty. An overview of diagnosis, treatment, and outcome. Endocrinol Metab Clin North Am 1999;28:901-18, xi.
197. Lee PA, Kulin HE, Guo SS. Age of puberty among girls and the diagnosis of precocious puberty. Pediatrics 2001;107:1493.
198. Lenton EA, Sulaiman R, Sobowale O, Cooke ID. The human menstrual cycle: Plasma concentrations of prolactin, LH, FSH, oestradiol and progesterone in conceiving and non-conceiving women. J Reprod Fertil 1982;65:131-9.

199. Leung YS, Dees K, Cyr R, Schloegel I, Kao PC. Falsely increased serum estradiol results reported in direct estradiol assays. Clin Chem 1997;43:1250-1.
200. Levesque A, Letellier M, Dillon PW, Grant A. Analytical performance of Bayer Immuno 1 estradiol and progesterone assays. Clin Chem 1997;43:1601-9.
201. Lewis V. Polycystic ovary syndrome. A diagnostic challenge. Obstet Gynecol Clin North Am 2001;28:1-20.
202. Lewy VD, Danadian K, Witchel SF, Arslanian S. Early metabolic abnormalities in adolescent girls with polycystic ovarian syndrome. J Pediatr 2001;138:38-44.
203. Licciardi FL, Liu HC, Rosenwaks Z. Day 3 estradiol serum concentrations as prognosticators of ovarian stimulation response and pregnancy outcome in patients undergoing in vitro fertilization. Fertil Steril 1995;64:991-4.
204. Lippman ME. Endocrine-responsive cancers. In: Williams RH, Foster DW, Kronenberg HM, Larsen PR, Wilson JD, eds. Williams textbook of endocrinology. 9th ed. Philadelphia: WB Saunders Co, 1998:1675-92.
205. Lipson SF, Ellison PT. Comparison of salivary steroid profiles in naturally occurring conception and nonconception cycles. Hum Reprod 1996;11:2090-6.
206. Lobo RA, Goebelsmann U, Horton R. Evidence for the importance of peripheral tissue events in the development of hirsutism in polycystic ovary syndrome. J Clin Endocrinol Metab 1983;57:393-7.
207. Lobo RA, Paul WL, Goebelsmann U. Dehydroepiandrosterone sulfate as an indicator of adrenal androgen function. Obstet Gynecol 1981;57:69-73.
208. Loraine JA, Bell ET, eds. Hormone assays and their clinical application. 4th ed. Edinburgh: Churchill Livingstone, 1976.
209. Loriaux DL, Malinak LR, Noall MW. The contribution of plasma dehydroepiandrosterone sulfate to testosterone in a virilized patient with an arrhenoblastoma. J Clin Endocrinol Metab 1970;31:702-4.
210. Lu Y, Bentley GR, Gann PH, Hodges KR, Chatterton RT. Salivary estradiol and progesterone levels in conception and nonconception cycles in women: Evaluation of a new assay for salivary estradiol. Fertil Steril 1999;71:863-8.
211. Lupulescu A. Estrogen use and cancer incidence: a review. Cancer Invest 1995;13:287-95.
212. Mabbett S, McIntyre A, Thompson W, Montague D. Development of an enhanced luminescence immunoassay for progesterone. Clin Chem 1989;35:1149.
213. MacMahon B. Age at menarche, United States. Series 11. Washington, DC: National Center for Health Statistics, Vital and Health Statistics, 1973. Report No. 133NCHS. DHEW Publ. No. (HRA) 74-1615.
214. Marlow HW. Groups involved in the Zimmermann and Kober reactions. J Biol Chem 1950;183:167-71.
215. Marshall LA. Clinical evaluation of amenorrhea in active and athletic women. [Review]. Clin Sports Med 1994;13:371-87.
216. Masters AM, Hahnel R. Investigation of sex-hormone binding globulin interference in direct radioimmunoassays for testosterone and estradiol.[Comment]. Clin Chem 1989;35:979-84.
217. Mathur R, Braunstein GD. Gynecomastia: pathomechanisms and treatment strategies. Horm Res 1997;48:95-102.
218. Mayo Medical Laboratories: Interpretive handbook. Rochester, Minn: Mayo Medical Laboratories, 1997.
219. McGregor JA, Jackson GM, Lachelin GC, Goodwin TM, Artal R, Hastings C, et al. Salivary estriol as risk assessment for preterm labor: A prospective trial. Am J Obstet Gynecol 1995;173:1337-42.
220. McGuinness BJ, Power MJ, Fottrell PF. Radioimmunoassay of 2-hydroxyestrone in urine. Clin Chem 1994;40:80-5.
221. McIver B, Romanski SA, Nippoldt TB. Evaluation and management of amenorrhea. Mayo Clin Proc 1997;72:1161-9.
222. Meier C, Huang T, Wyatt PR, Summers AM. Accuracy of expected risk of Down syndrome using the second-trimester triple test. Clin Chem 2002;48:653-5.
223. Meikle AW, Odell WD. Effect of short- and long-term dexamethasone on 3 alpha-androstanediol glucuronide in hirsute women. Fertil Steril 1986;46:227-31.
224. Merke DP, Cutler GB Jr. Evaluation and management of precocious puberty. Arch Dis Child 1996;75:269-71.
225. Midyett LK, Moore WV, Jacobson JD. Are pubertal changes in girls before age 8 benign? Pediatrics 2003;111:47-51.
226. Miller PB, Soules MR. The usefulness of a urinary LH kit for ovulation prediction during menstrual cycles of normal women. Obstet Gynecol 1996;87:13-17.
227. Miller WL, Styne DM. Female puberty and its disorders. In: Yen SSC, Jaffe RB, Barbieri RL, eds. Reproductive endocrinology: Physiology, pathophysiology, and clinical management. 4th ed. Philadelphia: WB Saunders Co, 1999:388-412.
228. Misra M, MacLaughlin DT, Donahoe PK, Lee MM. Measurement of Mullerian inhibiting substance facilitates management of boys with microphallus and cryptorchidism. J Clin Endocrinol Metab 2002;87:3598-602.
229. Morales A, Heaton JP, Carson CC III. Andropause: A misnomer for a true clinical entity. J Urol 2000;163:705-12.

230. Morales A, Tenover JL. Androgen deficiency in the aging male: when, Who, and how to investigate and treat. Urol Clin North Am 2002;29:975-82.
231. Morley JE, Patrick P, Perry HM III. Evaluation of assays available to measure free testosterone. Metabolism 2002;51:554-9.
232. Morrell V. Basic infertility assessment. Primary Care Women's Health 1997;24:195-204.
233. Mulhall J. Sildenafil: a novel effective oral therapy for male erectile dysfunction. [Letter; comment.]. Br J Urol 1997;79:663-4.
233A. Muti P. The role of endogenous hormones in the etiology and prevention of breast cancer: The epidemiological evidence. Recent Results Cancer Res 2005;166:245-56.
234. Munro CJ, Stabenfeldt GH, Cragun JR, Addiego LA, Overstreet JW, Lasley BL. Relationship of serum estradiol and progesterone concentrations to the excretion profiles of their major urinary metabolites as measured by enzyme immunoassay and radioimmunoassay. Clin Chem 1991;37:838-44.
235. Nachtigall LB, Boepple PA, Pralong FP, Crowley WF Jr. Adult-onset idiopathic hypogonadotropic hypogonadism—a treatable form of male infertility. N Engl J Med 1997;336:410-15.
236. Nanjee MN, Wheeler MJ. Plasma free testosterone—Is an index sufficient? Ann Clin Biochem 1985;22 (Pt 4):387-90.
237. Navarro MA, Alia P, Ruiz R, Valles A, Orozco P. Relationship between blood levels of sex hormone binding globulin, testosterone levels in blood and saliva and body morphology in premenopausal women. Medicina Clinica 1996;106:405-8.
238. Neaves WB, Johnson L, Porter JC, Parker CR Jr, Petty CS. Leydig cell numbers, daily sperm production, and serum gonadotropin levels in aging men. J Clin Endocrinol Metab 1984;59:756-63.
239. Neely EK, Hintz RL, Wilson DM, Lee PA, Gautier T, Argente J, et al. Normal ranges for immunochemiluminometric gonadotropin assays. J Pediatr 1995;127:40-6.
240. Neely EK, Wilson DM, Lee PA, Stene M, Hintz RL. Spontaneous serum gonadotropin concentrations in the evaluation of precocious puberty. J Pediatr 1995;127:47-52.
241. New MI. Antenatal diagnosis and treatment of congenital adrenal hyperplasia. Curr Urol Rep 2001;2: 11-8.
242. New MI, Lorenzen F, Lerner AJ, Kohn B, Oberfield SE, Pollack MS, et al. Genotyping steroid 21-hydroxylase deficiency: hormonal reference data. J Clin Endocrinol Metab 1983;57:320-6.
243. Nieschlag E. Care for the infertile male. [Review]. Clin Endocrinol 1993;38:123-33.
244. Obminski Z, Stupnicki R. Comparison of the testosterone-to-cortisol ratio values obtained from hormonal assays in saliva and serum. J Sports Med Phys Fitness 1997;37:50-5.
245. O'Connor KA, Brindle E, Holman DJ, Klein NA, Soules MR, Campbell KL, et al. Urinary estrone conjugate and pregnanediol 3-glucuronide enzyme immunoassays for population research. Clin Chem 2003;49:1139-48.
246. Oei SG, Keirse MJ, Bloemenkamp KW, Helmerhorst FM. European postcoital tests: Opinions and practice. Br J Obstet Gynaecol 1995;102:621-4.
247. Oerter KE, Uriarte MM, Rose SR, Barnes KM, Cutler GB Jr. Gonadotropin secretory dynamics during puberty in normal girls and boys. J Clin Endocrinol Metab 1990;71:1251-8.
248. O'Malley B, Strott CA. Steroid hormones: metabolism and mechanism of action. In: Yen SSC, Jaffe RB, Barbieri RL, eds. Reproductive endocrinology: Physiology, pathophysiology, and clinical management. 4th ed. Philadelphia: WB Saunders Co, 1999:110-33.
249. O'Rorke A, Kane MM, Gosling JP, Tallon DF, Fottrell PF. Development and validation of a monoclonal antibody enzyme immunoassay for measuring progesterone in saliva. Clin Chem 1994;40:454-8.
250. Orth DN, Kovacs WJ. The adrenal cortex. In: Williams RH, Foster DW, Kronenberg HM, Larsen PR, Wilson JD, eds. Williams textbook of endocrinology. 9th ed. Philadelphia: WB Saunders, 1998: 517-664.
251. Otten BJ, Wellen JJ, Rijken JC, Stoelinga GB, Benraad TJ. Salivary and plasma androstenedione and 17-hydroxyprogesterone levels in congenital adrenal hyperplasia. J Clin Endocrinol Metab 1983;57:1150-4.
252. Pang S. Congenital adrenal hyperplasia owing to 3 beta-hydroxysteroid dehydrogenase deficiency. Endocrinol Metab Clin North Am 2001;30:81-99, vi-vii.
253. Pang S, Wang M, Jeffries S, Riddick L, Clark A, Estrada E. Normal and elevated 3 alpha-androstanediol glucuronide concentrations in women with various causes of hirsutism and its correlation with degree of hirsutism and androgen levels. J Clin Endocrinol Metab 1992;75:243-8.
254. Pang SY, Lerner AJ, Stoner E, Levine LS, Oberfield SE, Engel I, et al. Late-onset adrenal steroid 3 beta-hydroxysteroid dehydrogenase deficiency. I. A cause of hirsutism in pubertal and postpubertal women. J Clin Endocrinol Metab 1985;60:428-39.
255. Pardridge WM. Serum bioavailability of sex steroid hormones. Clin Endocrinol Metab 1986;15:259-78.
256. Parker LN. Control of adrenal androgen secretion. Endocrinol Metab Clin North Am 1991;20:401-21.
257. Partsch CJ, Sippell WG. Treatment of central precocious puberty. Best Pract Res Clin Endocrinol Metab 2002;16:165-89.
258. Pearce S, Dowsett M, Jeffcoate SL. Three methods compared for estimating the fraction of testosterone

and estradiol not bound to sex-hormone-binding globulin. Clin Chem 1989;35:632-5.

259. Peter M. Congenital adrenal hyperplasia: 11Beta-hydroxylase deficiency. Semin Reprod Med 2002;20:249-54.
260. Plosker SM. Polycystic ovary syndrome and insulin resistance. Med Health R I 2003;86:12-5.
261. Quest Diagnostics/Nichols Institute. The Corning Endocrine Manual. Capistrano, CA: Quest Diagnostics/Nichols Institute, 1996.
262. Quissell DO. Steroid hormone analysis in human saliva. Ann NY Acad Sci 1993;694:143-5.
263. Rao J, Savjani G, Petersen JR. Radioimmunoassay kit for the quantitative measurement of androstanediol glucuronide in unextracted serum. Clin Chem 1991;37:1049.
264. Ratcliffe WA. Direct (non-extraction) serum assays for steroids. In: Hunter WM, Corrie JET, eds. Immunoassays for clinical chemistry. Edinburgh: Churchill Livingstone, 1983:401-9.
265. Ratcliffe WA, Carter GD, Dowsett M, Hillier SG, Middle JG, Reed MJ. Oestradiol assays: Applications and guidelines for the provision of a clinical biochemistry service. Ann Clin Biochem 1988; 25(Pt 5):466-83.
266. Ratcliffe WA, Corrie JE, Dalziel AH, Macpherson JS. Direct ^{125}I-radioligand assays for serum progesterone compared with assays involving extraction of serum. Clin Chem 1982;28:1314-18.
267. Read GF. Status report on measurement of salivary estrogens and androgens. Ann NY Acad Sci 1993;694:146-60.
268. Rebar RW. Practical evaluation of hormonal status. In: Yen SSC, Jaffe RB, Barbieri RL, eds. Reproductive endocrinology: Physiology, pathophysiology, and clinical management. 4th ed. Philadelphia: WB Saunders Co, 1999:709-48.
269. Regan J, Mahmood N, Alvarez W, Gamble J, Sissors D, Knez R, et al. Automated quantification of estradiol by readial partition immunoassay. Clin Chem 1991;37:936.
270. Reindollar RH, Novak M, Tho SP, McDonough PG. Adult-onset amenorrhea: A study of 262 patients. Am J Obstet Gynecol 1986;155:531-43.
271. Reinsberg J, Jost E. Analytical performance of the fully automated AxSYM estradiol assay. Clin Chem Lab Med 2000;38:51-5.
272. Reinsberg J, Jost E, van der Ven H. Performance of the fully automated progesterone assays on the Abbott AxSYM and the Technicon Immuno 1 analyser compared with the radioimmunoassay Progesterone MAIA. Clin Biochem 1997;30: 469-71.
273. Research on the menopause in the 1990s. Technical report. Geneva, Switzerland: World Health Organization, 1996. Report No. Scr 866.
274. Riggs BL, Hartmann LC. Selective estrogen-receptor modulators—mechanisms of action and application to clinical practice. N Engl J Med 2003;348:618-29.
275. Rittmaster RS. Hirsutism. Lancet 1997;349:191-5.
276. Rogol A, Blizzard RM. Variations and disorders of pubertal development. In: Kappy MS, Blizzard RM, Migeon CJ, eds. Wilkins' The diagnosis and treatment of endocrine disorders in childhood and adolescence. 4th ed. Springfield, Ill: Charles C Thomas, 1994: 857-917.
277. Rosenfield RL. A competitive protein binding method for the measurement of unconjugated and sulfate-conjugated dehydroepiandrosterone in peripheral plasma. Steroids 1971;17:689-96.
278. Rosenfield RL, Bachrach LK, Chernausek SD, Gertner JM, Gottschalk M, Hardin DS, et al. Current age of onset of puberty. Pediatrics 2000;106:622-3.
279. Rosenfield RL, Barnes RB. Menstrual disorders in adolescence. Endocrinol Metab Clin North Am 1993;22:491-505.
280. Rosenfield RL, Lucky AW. Acne, hirsutism, and alopecia in adolescent girls. Clinical expressions of androgen excess. Endocrinol Metab Clin North Am 1993;22:507-32.
281. Rosner W. Measurement of TeBG in biological fluids: evolution and problems. In: Forest M, Pugeat M, eds. Binding proteins of steriod hormones. London: John Libby Eurotext, 1986:207-14.
282. Rosner W. Errors in the measurement of plasma free testosterone. J Clin Endocrinol Metab 1997;82:2014-5.
283. Rosner W. An extraordinarily inaccurate assay for free testosterone is still with us. J Clin Endocrinol Metab 2001;86:2903.
284. Rowe PJ, Comhaire FH, Hargreave TB, Mellows HJ. WHO manual for the standardizing investigation of the infertile couple. Cambridge: Cambridge University Press, 1993.
285. Rudy EB, Estok P. Professional and lay interrater reliability of urinary luteinizing hormone surges measured by OvuQuick test. J Obstet Gynecol Neonatal Nurs 1992;21:407-11.
286. Said El Shami A, Ito T, Durham A. First solid-phase radioimmunoassay for free testosterone by the analog method. Clin Chem 1985;31:910.
287. Sakiyama R. Approach to patients with hirsutism. West J Med 1996;165:386-91.
288. Salerno M, Di Maio S, Gasparini N, Mariano A, Macchia V, Tenore A. Central precocious puberty: A single blood sample after gonadotropin-releasing hormone agonist administration in monitoring treatment. Horm Res 1998;50:205-11.
289. Salerno M, Di Maio S, Tenore A. Monitoring therapy for central precocious puberty. Pediatrics 2002;110:1255; author reply 55.
290. Salimetrics. Package insert for salivary DHEA EIA kit. State College, Pa: Salimetrics, 2003.

291. Sanchez LA, Knochenhauer ES, Gatlin R, Moran C, Azziz R. Differential diagnosis of clinically evident hyperandrogenism: Experience with over 1000 consecutive patients. Fertil Steril 2001;76:S111.
292. Sanchez-Carbayo M, Mauri M, Alfayate R, Miralles C, Soria F. Elecsys testosterone assay evaluated. Clin Chem 1998;44:1744-6.
293. Santen RJ. The testis: function and dysfunction. In: Yen SSC, Jaffe RB, Barbieri RL, eds. Reproductive endocrinology: Physiology, pathophysiology, and clinical management. 4th ed. Philadelphia: WB Saunders Co, 1999:632-68.
294. Santoro NF, Col NF, Eckman MH, Wong JB, Pauker SG, Cauley JA, et al. Therapeutic controversy: hormone replacement therapy—where are we going? J Clin Endocrinol Metab 1999;84:1798-812.
295. Schramm W, Smith RH, Craig PA, Paek SH, Kuo HH. Determination of free progesterone in an ultrafiltrate of saliva collected in situ. Clin Chem 1990;36: 1488-93.
296. Schultheiss D, Stief CG, Truss MC, Jonas U. [Pharmacological therapy in erectile dysfunction-current standards and new viewpoints]. Wien Med Wochenschr 1997;147:102-4.
297. Scott MG, Ladenson JH, Green ED, Gast MJ. Hormonal evaluation of female infertility and reproductive disorders. Clin Chem 1989;35:620-9.
298. Seibel MM. Ovulation induction with follicle-stimulating hormone. In: Seibel MM, ed. Infertility: A comprehensive text. 2nd ed. Stamford, Conn: Appleton & Lange, 1997:525-36.
299. Seifer DB, Lambert-Messerlian G, Hogan JW, Gardiner AC, Blazar AS, Berk CA. Day 3 serum inhibin-B is predictive of assisted reproductive technologies outcome. Fertil Steril 1997;67:110-4.
300. Seifer DB, Scott RT Jr, Bergh PA, Abrogast LK, Friedman CI, Mack CK, et al. Women with declining ovarian reserve may demonstrate a decrease in day 3 serum inhibin B before a rise in day 3 follicle-stimulating hormone. Fertil Steril 1999;72:63-5.
301. Selby C. Sex hormone binding globulin: Origin, function and clinical significance. Ann Clin Biochem 1990;27:532-41.
302. Shackleton CH, Kletke C, Wudy S, Pratt JH. Dehydroepiandrosterone sulfate quantification in serum using high-performance liquid chromatography/mass spectrometry and a deuterated internal standard: a technique suitable for routine use or as a reference method. Steroids 1990;55:472-8.
303. Shane JM. Evaluation and treatment of infertility. Clin Adv Pediatr Symp 1993;45:2-32.
304. Shirtcliff EA, Granger DA, Likos A. Gender differences in the validity of testosterone measured in saliva by immunoassay. Horm Behav 2002;42:62-9.
305. Siiteri PK, MacDonald PC. Role of extraglandular estrogen in human endocrinology. In: Greep RO, Astwood EB, Geiger SR, eds. Handbook of physiology. Baltimore: Waverly Press Inc, 1973:615-29.
306. Simpson ER. Initiation of parturition, prevention of prematurity. In: MacDonald PC, Hasselmeyer EC, eds. Report of the fourth Ross conference on obstetric research. Columbus, Ohio: Ross Laboratories, 1983:94.
307. Sizonenko PC, Paunier L. Hormonal changes in puberty III: correlation of plasma dehydroepiandrosterone, testosterone, FSH, and LH with stages of puberty and bone age in normal boys and girls and in patients with Addison's disease or hypogonadism or with premature or late adrenarche. J Clin Endocrinol Metab 1975;41:894-904.
308. Smith S. Free testosterone. Endocrinology and metabolism in-service training and continuing education. Vol. 11. Washington, DC: American Association for Clinical Chemistry, 1993:59-62.
309. Smith SK, Lenton EA, Landgren BM, Cooke ID. The short luteal phase and infertility. Br J Obstet Gynaecol 1984;91:1120-2.
310. Sobel C, Golub OJ, Henry RJ, Jacobs SL, Basu GK. Study of the Norymberski methods for determination of 17-ketogenic steroids (17-hydroxycorticosteroids) in urine. J Clin Endocrinol Metab 1958;18:208-21.
311. Sodergard R, Backstrom T, Shanbhag V, Carstensen H. Calculation of free and bound fractions of testosterone and estradiol-17 beta to human plasma proteins at body temperature. J Steroid Biochem 1982;16:801-10.
312. Sokol RZ, Swerdloff RS. Male infertility: diagnosis and medical management. In: Aiman J, ed. Infertility: diagnosis and management. New York: Springer-Verlag, 1984:185-210.
313. Soules MR, McLachlan RI, Ek M, Dahl KD, Cohen NL, Bremner WJ. Luteal phase deficiency: Characterization of reproductive hormones over the menstrual cycle. J Clin Endocrinol Metab 1989;69:804-12.
314. Soules MR, Sherman S, Parrott E, Rebar R, Santoro N, Utian W, et al. Executive summary: Stages of reproductive aging workshop (STRAW). Fertil Steril 2001;76:874-8.
315. Speiser PW. Molecular diagnosis of CYP21 mutations in congenital adrenal hyperplasia: implications for genetic counseling. Am J Pharmacogenomics 2001;1:101-10.
316. Stafford DE, Gordon CM. Adolescent androgen abnormalities. Curr Opin Obstet Gynecol 2002;14:445-51.
317. Stanciu IN, Pitale S, Prinz RA, Jakate S, Webb G, Steiner D, et al. Insulinoma presenting with hyperandrogenism: A case report and a literature review. J Intern Med 2003;253:484-9.
318. Stanczyk FZ. Steroid hormones. In: Mishell DR, Davajan V, Lobo RA, eds. Infertility, contraception and reproductive endocrinology. 3rd ed. Boston: Blackwell Scientific Publications, 1993:53-76.

319. Stas SN, Anastasiadis AG, Fisch H, Benson MC, Shabsigh R. Urologic aspects of andropause. Urology 2003;61:261-6.
320. Strauss JF, Coutifaris C. The endometrium and myometrium: Regulation and dysfunction. In: Yen SSC, Jaffe RB, Barbieri RL, eds. Reproductive endocrinology: Physiology, pathophysiology, and clinical management. 4th ed. Philadelphia: WB Saunders Co, 1999:218-56.
321. Swerdloff RS, Overstreet JW, Sokol RZ, Rajfer J. UCLA conference. Infertility in the male. Ann Intern Med 1985;103:906-19.
322. Swinkels LM, Ross H, Benraad TJ. A symmetric dialysis method for the determination of free testosterone in human plasma. Clin Chem Acta 1978;165:341-9.
323. Taieb J, Benattar C, Birr AS, Lindenbaum A. Limitations of steroid determination by direct immunoassay. Clin Chem 2002;48:583-5.
324. Taieb J, Benattar C, Diop R, Birr AS, Lindenbaum A. Use of the Architect-i2000 estradiol immunoassay during in vitro fertilization. Clin Chem 2003;49:183-6.
325. Taieb J, Mathian B, Millot F, Patricot M-C, Mathieu E, Queyrel N, et al. Testosterone measured by 10 immunoassays and by isotope-dilution gas chromatography-mass spectrometry in sera from 116 men, women, and children. Clin Chem 2003;49:1381-95.
326. Tallon DF, Gosling JP, Buckley PM, Dooley MM, Cleere WF, O'Dwyer EM, et al. Direct solid-phase enzyme immunoassay of progesterone in saliva. Clin Chem 1984;30:1507-11.
327. Tamate K, Charleton M, Gosling JP, Egan D, Ishikawa M, Fottrell PF, et al. Direct colorimetric monoclonal antibody enzyme immunoassay for estradiol-17 beta in saliva. Clin Chem 1997;43:1159-64.
328. Tan RS, Culberson JW. An integrative review on current evidence of testosterone replacement therapy for the andropause. Maturitas 2003;45:15-27.
329. Tanski S, Rosengren SS, Benn PA. Predictive value of the triple screening test for the phenotype of Down syndrome. Am J Med Genet 1999;85:123-6.
330. Tenover JS, Dahl KD, Hsueh AJ, Lim P, Matsumoto AM, Bremner WJ. Serum bioactive and immunoreactive follicle-stimulating hormone levels and the response to clomiphene in healthy young and elderly men. J Clin Endocrinol Metab 1987;64:1103-8.
331. Thienpont L, Siekmann L, Lawson A, Colinet E, De Leenheer A. Development, validation, and certification by isotope dilution gas chromatography-mass spectrometry of lyophilized human serum reference materials for cortisol (CRM 192 and 193) and progesterone (CRM 347 and 348). Clin Chem 1991;37:540-6.
332. Thienpont LM, Verhaeghe PG, Van Brussel KA, De Leenheer AP. Estradiol-17 beta quantified in serum by isotope dilution-gas chromatography-mass spectrometry: reversed-phase C18 high-performance liquid chromatography compared with immunoaffinity chromatography for sample pretreatment. Clin Chem 1988;34:2066-9.
333. Thomas CM, van den Berg RJ, Segers MF, Geelen LM, Hollanders JM, Doesburg WH, et al. Time-resolved fluoroimmunoassay for unconjugated estrogen in urine: Comparison with a fluorometric assay for total estrogen and application in an in vitro fertilization program. Clin Chem 1990;36:1774-8.
334. Thompson DF, Carter JR. Drug-induced gynecomastia. Pharmacotherapy 1993;13:37-45.
335. Thomson S, Wallace AM, Cook B. A 125I-radioimmunoassay for measuring androstenedione in serum and in blood-spot samples from neonates. Clin Chem 1989;35:1706-12.
336. Tietz NW, ed. Clinical guide to laboratory tests. 3rd ed. Philadelphia: WB Saunders Co, 1995.
337. Torjesen PA, Bjoro T. Antibodies against [^{125}I] testosterone in patient's serum: a problem for the laboratory and the patient. Clin Chem 1996;42:2047-8.
338. Tsukui S, Noda Y, Fukuda A, Matsumoto H, Tatsumi K, Mori T. Blocking effect of sperm immobilizing antibodies on sperm penetration of human zonae pellucidae. J In Vitro Fert Embryo Transf 1988;5:123-8.
339. Tulchinsky D, Chopra IJ. Estrogen-androgen imbalance in patients with hirsutism and amenorrhea. J Clin Endocrinol Metab 1974;39:164-9.
340. Valero-Politi J, Fuentes-Arderiu X. Daily rhythmic and non-rhythmic variations of follitropin, lutropin, testosterone, and sex-hormone-binding globulin in men. Eur J Clin Chem Clin Biochem 1996;34:453-62.
341. Vallejo R, Cananaugh A, Price J, Lawruk T, Parente M, Simon F, et al. Development of an enzyme immunoassay for the direct measurement of serum progesterone using monoclonal antibodies. Clin Chem 1988;34:1162.
342. Veldhuis JD. The male hypothalamic-pituitary-gonadal axis. In: Yen SSC, Jaffe RB, Barbieri RL, eds. Reproductive endocrinology: Physiology, pathophysiology, and clinical management. 4th ed. Philadelphia: WB Saunders Co, 1999:622-31.
343. Veldhuis JD, Pincus SM, Garcia-Rudaz MC, Ropelato MG, Escobar ME, Barontini M. Disruption of the synchronous secretion of leptin, LH, and ovarian androgens in nonobese adolescents with the polycystic ovarian syndrome. J Clin Endocrinol Metab 2001;86:3772-8.
344. Vermeulen A, Kaufman JM. Ageing of the hypothalamo-pituitary-testicular axis in men. Horm Res 1995;43:25-8.

345. Vermeulen A, Stoica T, Verdonck L. The apparent free testosterone concentration, an index of androgenicity. J Clin Endocrinol Metab 1971;33:759-67.
346. Vermeulen A, Verdonck L, Kaufman JM. A critical evaluation of simple methods for the estimation of free testosterone in serum. J Clin Endocrinol Metab 1999;84:3666-72.
347. Viniker DA. Investigations for infertility management. In: Viniker DA, ed. Practical guide to reproductive medicine. New York: Parthenon Publishing Group Ltd, 1997:93-110.
348. Wacharasindhu S, Srivuthana S, Aroonparkmongkol S, Shotelersuk V. A cost-benefit of gnRH stimulation test in diagnosis of central precocious puberty (CPP). J Med Assoc Thai 2000;83:1105-11.
349. Wald NJ, Densem JW, Smith D, Klee GG. Four-marker serum screening for Down's syndrome. Prenat Diagn 1994;14:707-16.
350. Wallace AM. Analytical support for the detection and treatment of congenital adrenal hyperplasia. Ann Clin Biochem 1995;32(Pt 1):9-27.
350A. Wang C, Catlin DH, Demers LM, Starcevic B, Swerdloff RS. Measurement of total serum testosterone in adult men: Comparison of current laboratory methods versus liquid chromatography-tandem mass spectrometry. J Clin Endocrinol Metab 2004;89:534-43.
351. Wang DY, Knyba RE. Salivary progesterone: relation to total and non-protein-bound blood levels. J Steroid Biochem 1985;23:975-9.
352. Warren MP. Clinical review 77: Evaluation of secondary amenorrhea. J Clin Endocrinol Metab 1996;81:437-42.
353. Wentz AC. Diagnosing luteal phase inadequacy. Fertil Steril 1982;37:334-5.
354. Wentz AC, Kossoy LR, Parker RA. The impact of luteal phase inadequacy in an infertile population. Am J Obstet Gynecol 1990;162:937-43.
355. Wespes E, Schulman CC. Male andropause: Myth, reality, and treatment. Int J Impot Res 2002;14 Suppl 1:S93-8.
356. Westphal U. Steroid protein interactions. In: Gross F, Labhart A, Mann T, al e, eds. Monographs on endocrinology. Berlin: Springer-Verlag, 1986:211-19.
357. Wheeler MJ. The determination of bio-available testosterone. [Review]. Ann Clin Biochem 1995;32:345-57.
358. Wheeler MJ, D'Souza A, Matadeen J, Croos P. Ciba Corning ACS:180 testosterone assay evaluated. Clin Chem 1996;42:1445-9.
359. Wheeler MJ, Shaikh M, Jennings RD. An evaluation of 13 commercial kits for the measurement of testosterone in serum and plasma. Ann Clin Biochem 1986;23(Pt 3):303-9.
360. White PC. Genetic diseases of steroid metabolism. [Review]. Vitam Horm 1994;49:131-95.
361. Whitley RJ, Meikle AW, Watts NB. Endocrinology. In: Burtis CA, Ashwood ER, eds. Textbook of clinical chemistry. 2nd ed. Philadelphia: WB Saunders Co, 1994:1091-4.
362. WHO: Laboratory manual for the examination of human semen and semen-cervical mucus penetration. 4th ed. Cambridge: Cambridge University Press, 1999.
363. Wians FH Jr, Stuart J. Ciba Corning ACS:180 direct total testosterone assay can be used on female sera. Clin Chem 1997;43:1466-8.
364. Wilke TJ, Utley DJ. Total testosterone, free-androgen index, calculated free testosterone, and free testosterone by analog RIA compared in hirsute women and in otherwise-normal women with altered binding of sex-hormone-binding globulin. Clin Chem 1987;33:1372-5.
365. Williams C, Giannopoulos T, Sherriff EA. ACP best practice No. 170. Investigation of infertility with the emphasis on laboratory testing and with reference to radiological imaging. J Clin Pathol 2003;56:261-7.
366. Wilson DH, Groskopf W, Hsu S, Caplan D, Langner T, Baumann M, et al. Rapid, automated assay for progesterone on the Abbott AxSYM analyzer. Clin Chem 1998;44:86-91.
367. Wilson JD, George FW, Griffin JE. The hormonal control of sexual development. Science 1981;211:1278-84.
368. Winters SJ, Kelley DE, Goodpaster B. The analog free testosterone assay: Are the results in men clinically useful? Clin Chem 1998;44:2178-82.
369. Wood P, Groom G, Moore A, Ratcliffe W, Selby C. Progesterone assays: guidelines for the provision of a clinical biochemistry service. Ann Clin Biochem 1985;22(Pt 1):1-24.
370. Woolever C, Goldfien A. A double isotope derivative method for plasma progesterone assay. Int J Appl Radiat Isot 1963;14:163-71.
371. Wu H, Ramsay C, Ozaeta P, Liu L, Aboleneen H. Serum estradiol quantified by isotope dilution-gas chromatography/mass spectrometry. Clin Chem 2002;48:364-6.
372. Yazigi RA, Quintero CH, Salameh WA. Prolactin disorders. Fertil Steril 1997;67:215-25.
373. Yeh J, Adashi EY. The ovarian life cycle. In: Yen SSC, Jaffe RB, Barbieri RL, eds. Reproductive endocrinology: Physiology, pathophysiology, and clinical management. 4th ed. Philadelphia: WB Saunders Co, 1999:153-90.
374. Yen SSC. Chronic anovulation caused by peripheral endocrine disorders. In: Yen SSC, Jaffe RB, Barbieri RL, eds. Reproductive endocrinology: Physiology, pathophysiology, and clinical management. 4th ed. Philadelphia: WB Saunders Co, 1999:479-515.
375. Yen SSC. Chronic anovulation due to cns-hypothalamic-pituitary dysfunction. In: Yen SSC, Jaffe

RB, Barbieri RL, eds. Reproductive endocrinology: Physiology, pathophysiology, and clinical management. 4th ed. Philadelphia: WB Saunders Co, 1999: 516-61.

376. Yen SSC. The human menstrual cycle: neuroendocrine regulation. In: Yen SSC, Jaffe RB, Barbieri RL, eds. Reproductive endocrinology: Physiology, pathophysiology, and clinical management. 4th ed. Philadelphia: WB Saunders Co, 1999:191-217.
377. Yen SSC. Polycystic ovary syndrome: (Hyperandrogenic Chronic Anovulation). In: Yen SSC, Jaffe RB, Barbieri RL, eds. Reproductive endocrinology: Physiology, pathophysiology, and clinical management. 4th ed. Philadelphia: WB Saunders Co, 1999:436-78.
378. Young D. Effects of preanalytical variables on clinical laboratory tests. Washington: AACC Press, 1993.
379. Zerah M, Ueshiba H, Wood E, Speiser PW, Crawford C, McDonald T, et al. Prevalence of nonclassical steroid 21-hydroxylase deficiency based on a morning salivary 17-hydroxyprogesterone screening test: A small sample study. J Clin Endocrinol Metab 1990;70:1662-7.

ADDITIONAL READING

Textbooks

Brinkworth M. Andrology: Male reproductive health and dysfunction. New York: Springer-Verlag, 1997.

Gronowski AM. Handbook of clinical laboratory testing during pregnancy. Totowa, NJ: Humana Press, 2004.

Jones RE. Human reproductive biology, 2nd ed. San Diego: Academic Press, 1997.

Lobo RA, Mishell DR, Davajan V. Mishell's textbook of infertility, contraception and reproductive endocrinology. Malden, Mass: Blackwell Science, 1997.

Rainsbury PA, Viniker DA. Practical guide to reproductive medicine. Pearl River, NY: Parthenon Publishing Group, 1997.

Runnebaum B, Rabe T. Gynecological endocrinology and reproductive medicine. New York: Springer-Verlag, 1997.

Yen SSC. Reproductive endocrinology. Philadelphia: WB Saunders Co, 1998.

Reviews

Andrew R. Clinical measurement of steroid metabolism. Best Pract Res Clin Endocrinol Metab 2001;15:1-16.

Bowers LD. Abuse of performance-enhancing drugs in sport. Ther Drug Monit 2002;24:178-81.

Giese RW. Measurement of endogenous estrogens: Analytical challenges and recent advances. J Chromatogr A 2003;1000:401-12.

Griffiths WJ. Tandem mass spectrometry in the study of fatty acids, bile acids, and steroids. Mass Spectrom Rev 2003;22:81-152.

Holst JP, Soldin OP, Guo T, Soldin SJ. Steroid hormones: relevance and measurement in the clinical laboratory. Clin Lab Med 2004;24:105-18.

Kazlauskas R, Trout G. Drugs in sports: Analytical trends. Ther Drug Monit 2000;22:103-9.

Klee GG, Heser DW. Techniques to measure testosterone in the elderly. Mayo Clin Proc 2000;75 Suppl:S19-25.

Lucassen A, Watson E. Family history of breast cancer. BMJ 2005;330(7481):26.

Meuleman EJ, van Lankveld JJ. Hypoactive sexual desire disorder: An underestimated condition in men. BJU Int 2005;95:291-6.

O'Connor DB, Archer J, Wu FC. Effects of testosterone on mood, aggression, and sexual behavior in young men: A double-blind, placebo-controlled, cross-over study. J Clin Endocrinol Metab 2004;89:2837-45.

Osborne CK, Schiff R. Estrogen-receptor biology: Continuing progress and therapeutic implications. J Clin Oncol 2005;23:1616-22.

Pugh PJ, Jones RD, West JN, Jones TH, Channer KS. Testosterone treatment for men with chronic heart failure. Heart 2004;90:446-7.

van de Kerkhof DH, de Boer D, Thijssen JH, Maes RA. Evaluation of testosterone/epitestosterone ratio influential factors as determined in doping analysis. J Anal Toxicol 2000;24:102-15.

CHAPTER 54

Clinical Chemistry of Pregnancy

Edward R. Ashwood, M.D., and George J. Knight, Ph.D.

The clinical laboratory has an important role in managing pregnancy.[19] In contrast to most clinical situations, when treating an expectant mother, a physician must simultaneously care for more than one patient. The health of the mother and her fetus are intertwined, each affecting the other; thus pregnancy management must consider both. This chapter reviews the biology of pregnancy and discusses laboratory tests used to detect, evaluate, and monitor pregnancy, both normal and abnormal. These include common tests, such as chorionic gonadotropin (CG), hematocrit, blood type, and glucose tolerance testing; screening tests, such as the "quad test" (alpha fetoprotein [AFP], CG, unconjugated estriol [uE_3], and dimeric inhibin A [DIA]); and esoteric tests, such as fetal lung maturity tests and amniotic fluid bilirubin examination.

HUMAN PREGNANCY

To appreciate the role of laboratory tests in pregnancy health care, it is necessary to understand fundamental topics, such as conception, embryo development, fetal growth, the role of the placenta, the importance and composition of amniotic fluid, maternal adaptation to pregnancy, and functional maturation of the fetus.

Conception, Embryo, and Fetus

Normal human pregnancy lasts approximately 40 weeks, as measured from the first day of the last normal menstrual period, a date commonly represented by the abbreviations LMP or LNMP. The anticipated date of birth of an infant is commonly referred to as the *expected date of confinement*, or EDC. During pregnancy, a woman undergoes dramatic physiological and hormonal changes. When talking with patients, physicians customarily divide pregnancy into three time intervals called *trimesters*, each of which is slightly longer than 13 weeks. By convention, the first trimester, 0 to 13 weeks, begins on the first day of the last menses.

Ovulation occurs on approximately the 14th day of the regular menstrual cycle (see Chapter 53). If conception occurs, the ovum is fertilized, usually in the fallopian tube, and becomes a *zygote*, which is then carried down the tube into the uterus. The zygote divides, becoming a *morula*. After 50 to 60 cells are present, the morula develops a cavity, the primitive *yolk sac*, and thus becomes a *blastocyst*, which implants into the uterine wall about 5 days after fertilization. The cells on the exterior wall of the blastocyst, *trophoblasts*, synergistically invade the uterine endometrium and develop into chorionic villi, creating the placenta. Trophoblasts can be subdivided into syncytiotrophoblasts and cytotrophoblasts, depending on location and cellular morphology.

At this stage, the product of conception is referred to as an *embryo*. A cavity called the *amnion* forms and enlarges with the accumulation of *liquor amnii*, commonly referred to as *amniotic fluid*. Nourished by the placenta and protected by the amniotic fluid, an embryo undergoes rapid cell division, differentiation, and growth. From combinations of three primary cell types, *ectoderm*, *mesoderm*, and *endoderm*, organs begin to form, a process called *organogenesis*. At 10 weeks, an embryo has developed most major structures and is now referred to as a *fetus*. At 13 weeks, the fetus weighs approximately 13 g and is 8 cm long.

During the second trimester, 13 to 26 weeks, rapid fetal growth occurs. By the end of the second trimester, the fetus weighs approximately 700 g and is 30 cm long. Many fetal organs begin to mature. The third trimester, 26 to 40 weeks, is the period in which fetal organs complete their prenatal maturation. During this trimester, the growth rate decelerates. At the end of the third trimester, the fetus weighs approximately 3200 g and is about 50 cm long. *Term* is the interval from 37 to 42 weeks. Normal labor, rhythmic uterine contractions, and birth occur during this period.

PLACENTA

The placenta and umbilical cord are the primary link between the fetus and mother. The placenta grows throughout pregnancy and is normally delivered through the birth canal immediately after birth of the infant.

Function

The placenta keeps the maternal and fetal circulation systems separate, nourishes the fetus, eliminates fetal wastes, and produces hormones vital to pregnancy. It is composed of large collections of fetal vessels called *villi*, which are surrounded by intervillous spaces in which maternal blood flows. For substances to move from maternal circulation to fetal circulation, they must cross through the trophoblasts and several membranes. The transfer of any substance depends largely on the concentration gradient between the maternal and fetal circulatory systems, the presence or absence of circulating binding proteins, the lipid solubility of the substance, and the presence of facilitated transport, such as ion pumps or receptor-mediated endocytosis (Box 54-1). The placenta is an effective barrier to the movement of large proteins and hydrophobic compounds bound to plasma proteins. Maternal IgG crosses the placenta via receptor-mediated endocytosis. Because of its long half-life, maternally produced IgG protects a newborn for the first 6 months of life. Antibody assays with low limits of detection may be positive in infants up to age 18 months.

Placental Hormones

The placenta produces several protein and steroid hormones (Figure 54-1). The major protein hormones are CG and placental lactogen (PL). The steroids include progesterone, estradiol, estriol, and estrone. The placenta secretes most of its products into the maternal circulation; only small amounts reach the fetal circulation. Close proximity of the maternal blood vessels to the site of placental hormone production may explain some of this preferential accumulation of hormones in the maternal blood circulation. Generally, hormone production by the placenta increases in proportion to the increase in placental mass. Therefore concentrations of hormones derived from the placenta, such as PL, increase in maternal peripheral blood as the placenta increases in size; CG, which peaks at the end of the first trimester, is an exception.

BOX 54-1 Normal Placental Transport

No Transport
- Most proteins
- Thyroid hormones
- Maternal IgM, IgA
- Maternal and fetal erythrocytes

Limited Passive Transport
- Unconjugated steroids
- Steroid sulfates
- Free fatty acids

Passive Transport
- Molecules up to 5000 Da having lipid solubility
- Oxygen
- Carbon dioxide
- Sodium and chloride
- Urea
- Ethanol

Active Transport Across Cell Membranes
- Glucose
- Many amino acids
- Calcium

Receptor-Mediated Endocytosis
- Maternal IgG
- Insulin
- Low-density lipoprotein

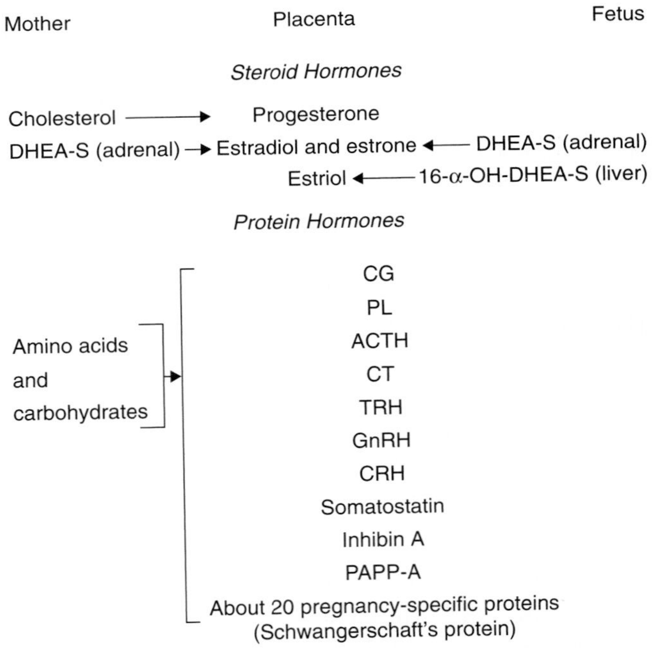

Figure 54-1 Schematic representation of steroid and protein hormone production by the placenta. *DHEA-S,* Dehydroepiandrosterone sulfate; *CG,* chorionic gonadotropin; *PL,* placental lactogen; *ACTH,* adrenocorticotropic hormone; *TRH,* thyroid-stimulating hormone; *CT,* chorionic thyrotropin; *GnRH,* gonadotropin-releasing hormone; *CRH,* corticotropin-releasing hormone; *PAPP-A,* pregnancy associated plasma protein-A.

Chorionic Gonadotropin

One of the most important placental hormones is CG. CG stimulates the ovary to produce progesterone which, in turn, prevents menstruation thereby protecting the pregnancy. The chemistry, biochemistry, and methods for CG are discussed in the section on laboratory tests later in this chapter.

Placental Lactogen

PL, also known as human placental lactogen (hPL) and human chorionic somatomammotropin (hCS), is a single polypeptide chain of 191 amino acids having two intramolecular disulfide bridges and a molecular mass of 22,279 Da. The structure of PL is exceptionally homologous (96%) with growth hormone (GH) and less so with prolactin (67%). Not surprisingly, PL has potent growth and lactogenic properties. Five genes on chromosome 17 compose a gene family that codes for both GH and PL.[246] PL production has been localized by immunofluorescence studies to the syncytiotrophoblast cells of the placenta. The increase in maternal serum PL concentration with advancing gestational age is directly correlated with the increasing mass of placental tissue and of functional syncytiotrophoblast tissue.[289] The placental secretion near term is 1 to 2 g/day, the largest of any known human hormone.

From the physiological point of view, PL has many biological activities, including lactogenic, metabolic, somatotropic, luteotropic, erythropoietic, and aldosterone-stimulating effects. Either directly or in synergism with prolactin, PL has a significant role in preparing the mammary glands for lactation. The many metabolic activities of PL closely resemble those of GH, including inhibition of glucose uptake, enhanced lipolysis leading to increased mobilization of free fatty acids, and enhancement of nitrogen retention. Because glucose is the primary energy substrate for a fetus, it has been suggested that the glucose-sparing action of PL may be a strategy to direct maternal metabolism toward greater use of fat for the mother's requirements, thereby sparing maternal glucose for fetal use. Rare normal pregnancies have been reported in which there was a complete absence of PL. Although PL was used in the past to evaluate fetal well-being, currently no apparent clinical reason exists to measure PL.[92]

Placental Steroids

The placenta produces a wide variety of steroid hormones, including estrogen and progesterone. Phenomenal amounts of estrogens are produced at term. The chemistry of these steroids is described in Chapter 53. Maternal cholesterol is the main precursor for placental progesterone production. Biosynthesis of estrogens by the placenta differs from that of the ovaries because the placenta has no 17α-hydroxylase. Thus each of the estrogens—estrone (E_1), estradiol (E_2), and estriol (E_3)—must be synthesized from C_{19} intermediates that already have a hydroxyl group at position 17. In nonpregnant women, the ovaries secrete 100 to 600 μg/day of estradiol, of which about 10% is metabolized to estriol. During late pregnancy, the placenta produces 50 to 150 mg/day of estriol and 15 to 20 mg/day of estradiol and estrone. The secretion of estrogens and progesterone throughout pregnancy ensures appropriate development of the endometrium, uterine growth, adequate uterine blood supply, and preparation of the uterus for labor. Although measurement of estriol in the third trimester was used in the past to assess fetal well-being, many obstetricians consider this practice obsolete.[93] Estriol measurements at 16 to 18 weeks gestational age are useful in predicting fetal trisomy 21 and 18 (see later discussion on maternal serum screening for fetal defects).

AMNIOTIC FLUID

Throughout intrauterine life, the fetus lives within a fluid-filled compartment. The amniotic fluid provides a medium in which a fetus can readily move; it cushions a fetus against possible injury and helps maintain a constant temperature. This fluid is a dynamic medium whose volume and chemical composition are controlled within relatively narrow limits.

Volume and Dynamics

The volume of amniotic fluid increases progressively until 34 weeks of gestation, when it decreases slightly through the 40th week and then more sharply declines until the 42nd week.[268] The volume is 200 to 300 mL at 16 weeks, 400 to 1400 mL at 26 weeks, 300 to 2000 mL at 34 weeks, and 300 to 1400 mL at 40 weeks. The volume at any given moment is a function of several interrelated fluid fluxes. Direct measurements in primates and indirect measurements in humans have been used to derive a mathematical model of amniotic fluid volume.[211] At term, total fluid fluxes into and out of the amniotic cavity are large (~60 mL/hr) and result in complete exchange of the amniotic fluid volume twice per day. Gross unidirectional fluid volume shifts occur episodically: into the amniotic cavity by fetal urination and out of the cavity by fetal swallowing. These unidirectional shifts begin at the end of the first trimester and increase linearly until approximately 30 weeks. Fetal swallowing and urination then exponentially increase, peaking at term at about 1000 mL/day. Bidirectional water exchanges—so-called intramembranous fluxes—occur across the following surfaces: (1) placenta (mother-fetus), (2) umbilical vessels, through the substance of the umbilical cord (fetus–amniotic fluid), (3) fetal skin (fetus–amniotic fluid), and (4) fetal membranes (amniotic fluid–mother). These exchanges increase in a linear fashion throughout pregnancy. At term, they are approximately 400 mL/day. The fetal tracheobronchial tree is filled with amniotic fluid, and measurements in fetal lambs demonstrate a net flux of 50 to 80 mL/day of fluid up the trachea from the lungs. Although this is a small volume, flux is important in terms of transporting surfactant produced by the fetal lungs into the amniotic fluid.

Pathological decreases and increases of amniotic fluid volume are encountered frequently in clinical practice.

TABLE 54-1 Composition of Amniotic Fluid (Mean Values)

Component	Gestational Age (Wk) 15	25	40
Sodium, mmol/L	136	138	126
Potassium, mmol/L	3.9	4.0	4.3
Chloride, mmol/L	111	109	103
Bicarbonate, mmol/L	16	18	16
Urea nitrogen, mg/dL (mmol urea/L)	11 (3.9)	11 (3.9)	18 (6.4)
Creatinine, mg/dL (μmol/L)	0.8 (71)	0.9 (80)	2.2 (194)
Glucose, mg/dL (mmol/L)	47 (2.6)	39 (2.2)	32 (1.8)
Uric acid, mg/dL (mmol/L)	4.0 (0.24)	5.7 (0.34)	10.4 (0.61)
Total protein, g/dL (g/L)	0.5 (5)	0.8 (8)	0.3 (3)
Bilirubin, mg/dL (μmol/L)	0.13 (2.2)	0.14 (2.4)	0.04 (0.7)
Osmolality, mOsm/kg H_2O	272	272	255

From Benzie RJ, Doran TA, Harkins JL, Owen VM, Porter CJ. Composition of the amniotic fluid and maternal serum in pregnancy. Am J Obstet Gynecol 1974;119:798-810.

Intrauterine growth retardation and anomalies of the fetal urinary tract, such as bilateral renal agenesis or obstruction of the urethra, are associated with *oligohydramnios*, an abnormally low amniotic fluid volume. Increased fluid volume is known as *hydramnios* (also termed *polyhydramnios*). Conditions associated with hydramnios are as diverse as maternal diabetes mellitus, severe Rh isoimmune disease, fetal esophageal atresia, multifetal pregnancy, anencephaly, and spina bifida.

Composition

Early in gestation, the composition of the amniotic fluid resembles a complex dialysate of the maternal serum. As a fetus grows, the amniotic fluid changes in several ways (Table 54-1). Most notably, the sodium concentration and osmolality decrease and the concentrations of urea, creatinine, and uric acid increase.[34] The activities of many enzymes in amniotic fluid have been studied with respect to both gestational age and fetal status but have not been found to be clinically useful. The major lipids of interest are the phospholipids, whose type and concentrations reflect fetal lung maturity (discussed further later). Numerous steroid and protein hormones are also present in amniotic fluid.[348] Concentrations of androgens and estrogens have been measured in futile attempts to predict fetal sex. The rare syndrome of congenital adrenal hyperplasia (CAH) has been diagnosed antenatally by measuring 17-hydroxyprogesterone and pregnanetriol in the amniotic fluid near term.[171] Measurements of thyroid-stimulating hormone (TSH) and thyroxine in amniotic fluid may be useful in cases of fetal thyroid disease.[298] No other diagnostic uses for amniotic fluid hormone measurements are in common use. Prostaglandins E_1, E_2, $F_{1\alpha}$, and $F_{2\alpha}$ all are found in low concentrations in amniotic fluid and increase gradually during pregnancy. PGE_2 and $PGF_{2\alpha}$ concentrations are very high during active labor.[103] Attempts to demonstrate an acute rise in PGE_2 or $PGF_{2\alpha}$ immediately before the onset of labor, at the initiation of parturition, have been unsuccessful.

Early in pregnancy, there is little or no particulate matter in the amniotic fluid. By 16 weeks of gestation, large numbers of cells are present, having been shed from the surfaces of the amnion, skin, and tracheobronchial tree. These cells have proved to be of great utility in antenatal diagnosis. As pregnancy continues to progress, scalp hair and *lanugo* (fine hair on the body of the fetus) are also shed into the fluid and contribute to its turbidity. The production of surfactant particles in the lung, termed *lamellar bodies*, greatly increases the haziness of the fluid, which can be demonstrated by attempting to read newsprint through a clear tube containing amniotic fluid. At term, the amniotic fluid contains gross particles of *vernix caseosa*, the oily substance composed of sebum and desquamated epithelial cells covering the fetal skin.

Normal fetuses do not defecate during pregnancy. If severely stressed, a fetus may pass stool that is called *meconium*. This heterogeneous material contains many bile pigments and therefore stains the amniotic fluid green. Meconium-stained amniotic fluid is a sign of fetal stress.

Maternal Adaptation

During pregnancy a woman undergoes dramatic physiological and hormonal changes. The large amounts of estrogens, progesterone, PL, and corticosteroids produced during pregnancy affect various metabolic, physiological, and endocrinological systems. An increase in resistance to angiotensin, a predominance of lipid metabolism over glucose use, and an increased synthesis by the liver of thyroid- and steroid-binding proteins, fibrinogen, and other proteins are characteristic of pregnancy. As a result of such changes, many of the laboratory reference intervals for nonpregnant patients are not appropriate for pregnant patients. Lockitch[204] is the editor of the most comprehensive handbook of reference intervals in normal pregnancy. Her study group included 29 pregnant subjects who had over 70 analytes tested from 16 weeks to term and also postpartum. Mean values for selected tests expressed as a percentage of control means are presented in Table 54-2.

Hematological Changes

Maternal blood volume increases during pregnancy by an average of 45%. Plasma volume increases more rapidly than red blood cell mass; therefore, despite augmented erythropoiesis, the hemoglobin concentration, erythrocyte count, and hematocrit decrease during normal pregnancy. Hemoglobin concentrations at term average 12.6 g/dL, compared with 13.3 g/dL for the nonpregnant state. The leukocyte count varies considerably during pregnancy, from 4000 to 13,000/μL. During labor and puerperium (the interval immediately after delivery), leukocyte counts may be markedly elevated.

The concentrations of several blood coagulation factors are increased during pregnancy. Plasma fibrinogen increases approximately 65%, from 275 to 450 mg/dL; the increase contributes to the increase in sedimentation rate. Other clotting factors also increase, including factors VII, VIII, IX, and X. Prothrombin and factors V and XII do not change, whereas factors XI and XIII decrease slightly. Even though the platelet count remains unchanged in most women and the prothrombin time and activated partial thromboplastin time shorten slightly (see Table 54-2), pregnancy increases the risk of thromboembolism up to five times that of nonpregnant women.

Chemical Changes

During pregnancy, the electrolytes show little change, but there is approximately a 40% increase in serum triglycerides, cholesterol, phospholipids, and free fatty acids. Plasma albumin is decreased to an average of 3.4 g/dL in late pregnancy; plasma globulin concentrations increase slightly. Several of the plasma transport proteins increase markedly, including thyroxine-binding globulin (TBG), cortisol-binding globulin (CBG), and sex hormone-binding globulin (SHBG). Serum cholinesterase activity is reduced, whereas alkaline phosphatase activity in serum triples, mainly because of an increase in very heat-stable alkaline phosphatase of placental origin. Delivery can markedly increase creatine kinase.

Renal Function

Pregnancy increases the glomerular filtration rate (GFR) to about 170 mL/min/1.73 m^2 by 20 weeks, and therefore increases the clearance of urea, creatinine, and uric acid. The concentrations of these three analytes are therefore slightly decreased in serum for much of the pregnancy. As term approaches, GFR begins to return to nonpregnant values. Urea and creatinine concentrations rise slightly during the last 4 weeks. During this time, tubular reabsorption of uric acid increases dramatically, which increases serum uric acid compared with the nonpregnant state. Glucosuria, up to 1000 mg/day, may be present owing to increased GFR, which presents more fluid to the tubules and therefore lowers the renal glucose threshold. Protein loss in the urine can increase to up to 300 mg/day.

Endocrine Changes

The action of progesterone prevents menses and thus allows pregnancy to continue. In early pregnancy, the progesterone is produced by the corpus luteum of the maternal ovary in response to CG. In later stages the placenta directly produces enough progesterone to maintain the pregnancy.

Throughout pregnancy the plasma parathyroid hormone (PTH) is increased by approximately 40%, with almost no change in the plasma free ionized calcium fraction, thus suggesting a new set-point for the secretion of PTH. Calcitonin does not increase predictably during pregnancy, whereas 1,25-dihydroxyvitamin D is increased during pregnancy and promotes increased intestinal calcium absorption. These changes permit the transfer of large amounts of calcium to the developing fetus.

The elevated estrogen concentration stimulates increased hepatic production of CBG. The hepatic clearance of cortisol decreases. Thus, the absolute plasma concentrations of both total and free cortisol are several times higher during pregnancy. The diurnal rhythm of cortisol, higher in the morning and lower in the evening, is maintained. Increased plasma aldosterone and deoxycorticosterone concentrations are also observed.

Increasing estrogen concentrations throughout pregnancy increase the secretion of prolactin up to tenfold. Conversely, the high estrogen concentrations during pregnancy suppress the secretion of luteinizing hormone (LH) and follicle-stimulating hormone (FSH) below the detection limit. Baseline concentrations of other pituitary hormones such as TSH remain nearly unchanged (see Table 54-2), but the growth hormone (GH) response to provocative stimuli is blunted.

Although normal pregnancy is a euthyroid state, many changes occur in thyroid function. The high concentrations of TBG raise the concentration of total thyroxine (T_4) and triiodothyronine (T_3), but a slight decrease in free T_4 concentration occurs during the second and third trimesters. A slight reciprocal increase in TSH was reported by Lockitch.[204] Thyroglobulin is significantly increased, especially in the third trimester.[138] Very few (less than 0.2%) pregnant individuals develop hyperthyroidism, and hypothyroidism is very rare.[54] Postpartum thyroid dysfunction is common and is frequently unrecognized. The fetal thyroid-pituitary axis functions independently from the mother's axis in most cases. However, if the mother has preexisting Graves' disease (hyperthyroidism caused by autoantibodies that stimulate the thyroid) those antibodies can cross the placenta and cause hyperthyroidism in the fetus. If the mother has anti-TSH autoantibodies, the infant can develop transient hypothyroidism.[204]

TABLE 54-2 Mean Serum and Plasma Laboratory Values During Normal Pregnancies Expressed as a Percentage of the Nonpregnant Mean

	Time of Gestation		
Analyte	**12 wk**	**32 wk**	**Term**
Sodium	97	98	97
Potassium	95	95	100
Bicarbonate	85	85	81
Chloride	98	100	99
Urea nitrogen	77	63	77
Creatinine	71	74	81
Fasting glucose	98	94	94
Bilirubin, unconjugated	56	67	78
Albumin	93	78	78
Protein	92	83	83
Uric acid	68	92	120
Calcium	98	94	97
Free ionized calcium	99	101	102
Parathyroid hormone, intact	—	—	140
1,25-Dihydroxyvitamin D	—	—	400
Phosphate	108	97	96
Magnesium	92	87	87
Alkaline phosphatase	90	203	347
Creatine kinase	87	86	135
α_1-Antitrypsin	129	174	191
Transferrin	105	160	170
Cholesterol	100	144	156
HDL-cholesterol	121	119	130
LDL-cholesterol	80	118	146
Fasting triglycerides	141	300	349
Iron	112	94	94
Iron-binding capacity	95	139	144
Transferrin saturation	136	68	64
Zinc protoporphyrin	107	109	144
Ferritin	81	33	59
Thyroxine	103	107	100
Triiodothyronine	100	121	121
Free thyroxine	98	72	74
Thyroxine-binding globulin	114	155	182
Thyroid-stimulating hormone	111	122	139
Cortisol	111	301	309
Aldosterone	—	—	1500
Prolactin	—	—	800
Hemoglobin	95	90	96
Hematocrit	94	91	97
Leukocyte count	144	167	240
Prothrombin time	99	97	97
Activated partial thromboplastin time	95	91	93
Platelet count	98	96	100
Fibrinogen	119	154	165

Data from Lockitch G, ed. Handbook of diagnostic biochemistry and hematology in normal pregnancy, Boca Raton, Fla: CRC Press, 1993.
HDL, High-density lipoprotein; *LDL*, low-density lipoprotein.

Functional Development of the Fetus

The fetal organs mature during the third trimester but not at the same rate. This section reviews the lung, liver, kidneys, and blood development of the fetus.

Lungs and Pulmonary Surfactant

In normal air-breathing lungs, a substance called *pulmonary surfactant* coats the alveolar epithelium and responds to alveolar volume changes by reducing the surface tension in the alveolar wall during expiration. Surfactant is needed because the surface tension is an inverse function of the radius of the airway. Thus small alveoli have a higher collapsing force than larger alveoli. Surfactant opposes the force and keeps the small alveoli from collapsing. Specialized alveolar cells called *type II granular pneumocytes* synthesize pulmonary surfactant and package it into laminated storage granules called *lamellar bodies.*[169,299] These storage granules are 1 to 5 μm in diameter and contain phospholipids, cholesterol, and protein.[245] Production starts as early as 20 weeks gestation,[299] but adequate amounts do not accumulate until about 36 weeks. Exudation of pulmonary fluid (via the trachea) and fetal breathing movements transport the lamellar bodies into the amniotic fluid. The internal structure of the particles rearranges into a formation described as *tubular myelin* by those using electron microscopy.[169] The newborn lung contains 100 times more surfactant per cm^3 than the adult lung. The excessive surfactant is needed at birth as the newborn transforms from breathing water to breathing air. The surfactant overcomes the surface tension produced in water-filled alveoli that are admitting air for the first time.

Pulmonary surfactant is a complex mixture of lipids and proteins, and less than 5% is composed of carbohydrates. Most of the lipid is phospholipid, and the majority of that is lecithin (phosphatidylcholine).[53] Unlike lecithin from other organs, pulmonary lecithin has two saturated fatty acids, usually palmitoyl groups. Other lipids present are phosphatidylglycerol (PG), phosphatidylinositol (PI), and phosphatidylethanolamine (see Chapter 26). Sphingomyelin is present in very small amounts (~2%). The protein fraction of lamellar bodies is approximately 4% and is composed of four surfactant-specific proteins, SP-A, SP-B, SP-C, and SP-D.[160,256]

The type II pneumocytes synthesize phosphatidylcholine in a fashion quite different from that in other cells. Most other cells synthesize phosphatidylserine from cytidine diphosphate diacylglycerol and serine. The phosphatidylserine is then decarboxylated to yield phosphatidyl ethanolamine. The final step is the successive donation of three methyl groups via S-adenosylmethionine to form phosphatidylcholine. The pulmonary biosynthetic pathway is shown in Figure 54-2. The enzyme choline phosphotransferase forms PC directly from cytidine diphosphocholine and diacylglycerol. Phosphatidylinositol formation peaks at about 35 weeks. As PI decreases in concentration, PG begins to increase.

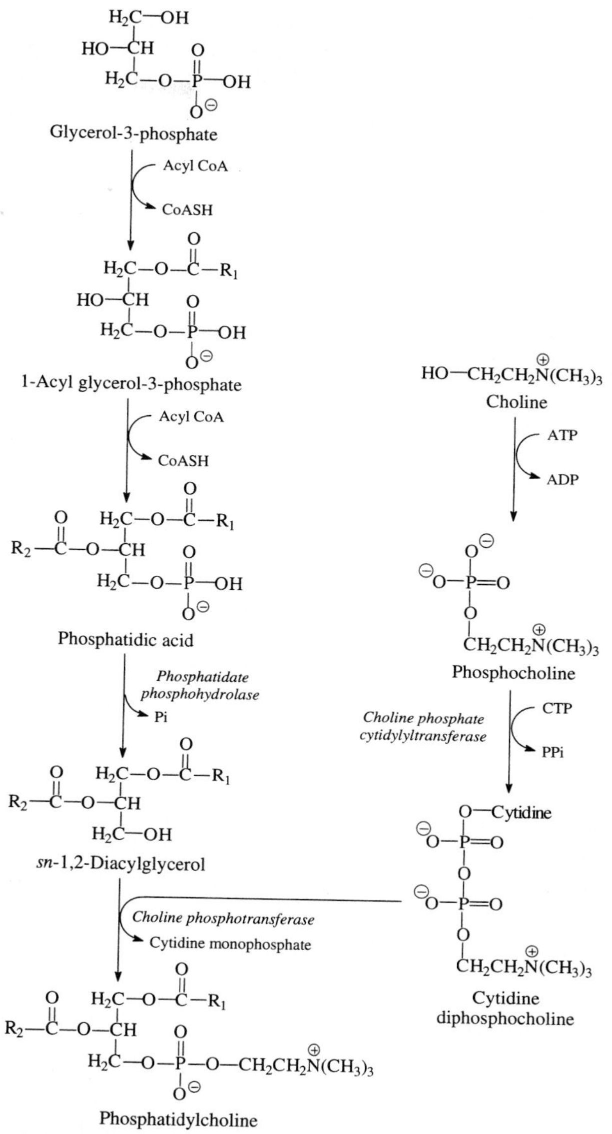

Figure 54-2 The biosynthetic pathway for phosphatidylcholine in type 2 pneumocytes.

Liver

Hematopoiesis occurs in the liver during the first two trimesters and transfers to the fetal bone marrow during the third trimester. The liver is also responsible for production of specific proteins (such as albumin and clotting factors), metabolism and detoxification of many compounds, and secretion of substances such as bilirubin. A clinically useful protein produced by the liver is AFP. Detoxification and bilirubin secretion mechanisms are immature until late in pregnancy and even in the first few months after birth. Thus premature infants often have high serum bilirubin concentrations and metabolize drugs poorly.

Kidneys

Toward the end of the first trimester the fetal kidneys begin to produce urine, which is the main component of amniotic fluid. The early nephrons cannot produce concentrated urine, and pH regulation is also limited. Complete maturation occurs after birth. Although kidneys are not required for fetal survival, amniotic fluid is required for proper lung development. Thus newborns without kidneys die of pulmonary failure.

Fetal Blood Development

Fetal blood is produced first by the embryonic yolk sac, then by the liver, and finally by the fetal bone marrow. The yolk sac produces three embryonic hemoglobins: Portland ($\zeta_2\varepsilon_2$), Gower-1 ($\zeta_2\varepsilon_2$), and Gower-2 ($\alpha_2\varepsilon_2$). These normal embryonic hemoglobins are of little importance in clinical chemistry because they are present in fetal blood only in the first trimester.

With the switch of erythropoiesis to the fetal liver and spleen, fetal hemoglobin (Hb F) production begins. Hb F consists of two α- and two γ-chains ($\alpha_2\gamma_2$). Small amounts of adult hemoglobin, Hb A ($\alpha_2\beta_2$), are also produced, but Hb F predominates during the remainder of fetal life.

As the fetal bone marrow begins red cell production, Hb A production increases. At birth, fetal blood contains 75% Hb F and 25% Hb A. Hb F production rapidly diminishes during the first year of postnatal life. In normal adults, less than 1% of hemoglobin is Hb F. The difference between fetal and adult hemoglobin is very significant. Hb F has a higher affinity for oxygen than does Hb A. Thus in the placenta, oxygen is released from the maternal Hb A, diffuses into the chorionic villi, and binds to the fetal Hb F. In addition, 2,3-diphosphoglycerate (2,3-DPG) does not bind Hb F and therefore cannot decrease its affinity for oxygen.

MATERNAL AND FETAL HEALTH ASSESSMENT

Individuals who desire optimum health care during pregnancy should consult their physicians before conception.[11,244] Unfortunately, 49% of pregnancies in the United States are unintended—higher for unmarried women.[162] Preconception evaluation should include a medical, reproductive, and family history; physical examination; and laboratory tests. Hematocrit, blood type and Rh compatibility, erythrocyte antibody screen, Papanicolaou smear, urinalysis, rubella titer, rapid plasma reagin test, gonococcal culture, cystic fibrosis carrier status,[146] human immunodeficiency virus (HIV) antibody,[12] and hepatitis B surface antigen[7] are recommended. Depending on demographic risks, genetic testing for disorders such as Tay-Sachs disease, thalassemia, and sickle cell disease may be offered. A careful diet history is warranted. Folic acid supplementation should be recommended to reduce the risk of neural tube defects.[218]

Most individuals consult a physician a few days after a missed menses if they suspect they might be pregnant. Many laboratory tests are useful for managing normal and abnormal pregnancies. A pregnancy test result is positive (meaning that the test can detect a CG concentration of about 25 IU/L) in about half of pregnant females at the beginning of the missed menses—at about 2 weeks after conception. Screening for fetal neural tube defects and Down syndrome should be offered to all pregnant patients. Until 2002 screening was recommended at 16 to 18 weeks of gestation,[14,10] but Down syndrome screening can be performed as early as 10 weeks.[337] Glucose tolerance testing should be performed at 24 to 28 weeks. Some physicians screen patients for preterm labor risk at 24 to 30 weeks. Although PL and estriol measurements were used previously to predict fetal well-being, both tests are now obsolete for this purpose.[92,93] Maternal observation and recording of fetal movements,[8] ultrasound examination, and tests that monitor the fetal heart rate during random uterine contractions or fetal movement are the currently accepted methods for monitoring fetal well-being.

CLINICAL SPECIMENS

Many different samples are available for clinical laboratory analysis before and during pregnancy. These include paternal serum and blood; maternal serum, blood, and urine; amniotic fluid obtained by amniocentesis[92,297] or from pools of fluid in the vagina after rupture of the fetal membranes; chorionic villi; fetal blood obtained by percutaneous umbilical blood sampling; and fetal tissue obtained by biopsy.[97]

The technique of amniocentesis is described in Chapter 2. Additional information can be found in the section on tests for evaluating fetal lung maturity later in this chapter.

A small sample of placental tissue, or chorionic villi, can be obtained with a catheter between 9 and 12 weeks gestation. Chorionic villi specimens can be used to identify the fetal chromosomes (the karyotype), determine enzyme levels, or detect specific gene mutations. This procedure can be performed earlier in pregnancy than can amniocentesis, but has a rate of higher fetal loss.

DIAGNOSIS AND DATING OF PREGNANCY

The most important aspects of pregnancy management are detection of pregnancy and establishing accurate estimates of fetal age. Obstetricians measure the length of pregnancy in terms of *weeks*, not trimesters. The most useful test for pregnancy is the CG test.

Qualitative tests for CG in blood or urine are primarily used for the confirmation of pregnancy. Urine CG tests usually suffice to diagnose normal pregnancy when it has progressed beyond the first week after the first missed period. However, qualitative serum pregnancy tests can detect pregnancy earlier, and quantitative serum tests can help reveal problems in early pregnancy.

To establish accurate dates, obstetricians rely on menstrual history, physical examination, fetal heart tones, ultrasonography, and CG concentration or detection. In the first 8 weeks of pregnancy, the CG concentration in maternal serum rises geometrically (Figure 54-3). Detectable amounts (~5 IU/L) are present 8 to 11 days after conception, which is in the third week of pregnancy as measured from the LMP.[198] Concentrations in approximately half of pregnant women

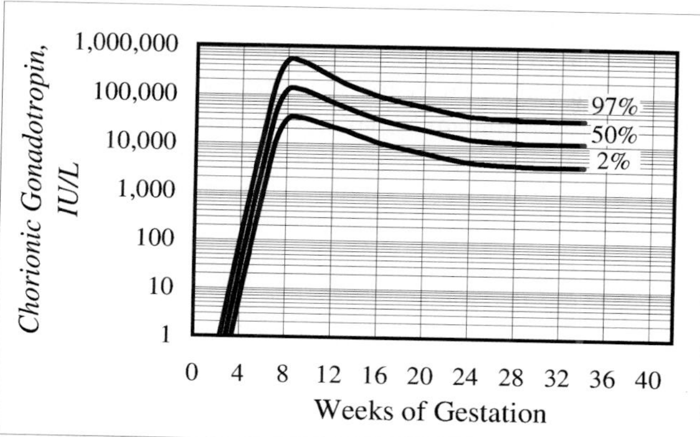

Figure 54-3 Concentration of chorionic gonadotropin (CG) in maternal serum as a function of gestational age. Lines represent the 2nd, 50th, and 97th percentiles. The maternal serum values from 14 to 25 weeks are medians calculated from 24,229 pregnancies from testing performed at ARUP Laboratories Inc. from January to October 1997. *(Redrawn from Ashwood ER. Evaluating health and maturation of the unborn: the role of the clinical laboratory. Clin Chem 1992;38:1523-1529. Permission granted from Clin Chem.)*

reach 25 IU/L on the first day of their missed period. The peak concentration occurs at about 8 to 10 weeks and is about 100,000 IU/L. Subsequently CG concentrations start to decline in serum and urine, and by the end of the second trimester a 90% reduction from peak concentration has usually occurred. In the first trimester, maternal serum CG is about 96% to 98% intact, 1% to 3% β-subunit, and 0% to 1% α-subunit. During the second trimester, subunit synthesis becomes unbalanced and the serum distribution shifts to 92% to 98% intact, 1% to 7% α-subunit, and 0% to 1% β-subunit.[247] Concentrations are approximately constant during the third trimester, with the predominant species being intact CG. The presence of twins approximately doubles CG concentrations.[328]

COMPLICATIONS OF PREGNANCY

Although most pregnancies progress without problems, complications can arise in the mother, placenta, or fetus.

Abnormal Pregnancies

Conditions arising primarily in the mother include ectopic pregnancy, hyperemesis gravidarum, preeclampsia, HELLP syndrome (hemolysis, elevated liver enzymes, and low platelet counts in association with preeclampsia), liver diseases, Graves' disease, and hemolytic disease of the newborn. The clinician must distinguish abnormal changes in laboratory tests from the normal physiological changes induced by pregnancy (see Table 54-2). Notably, total bilirubin, 5′-nucleotidase, γ-glutamyltransferase (GGT), alanine aminotransferase (ALT), and aspartate aminotransferase (AST) are unchanged in mothers with a normal pregnancy.

Ectopic Pregnancy and Threatened Abortion

When a fertilized egg implants in a location other than the body of the uterus, the condition is called an *ectopic pregnancy.* Most abnormal implantations occur in the fallopian tube but they can also occur in the abdomen, although this is rare. Tubal rupture and hemorrhage are common serious complications of ectopic pregnancy. About 25% of individuals with an ectopic pregnancy have three classic symptoms: lower abdominal pain, vaginal bleeding, and an adnexal mass.[288] Of all individuals with these symptoms, about 15% have an ectopic pregnancy and a smaller percentage have incomplete or complete spontaneous abortion. In the United States from 1990 to 1999, there were 11.8 pregnancy-related deaths per 100,000 live births—6% caused by ectopic pregnancy.[78] Even though the risk of maternal death decreased during this time period, a patient has about a 0.5% chance of dying from an ectopic pregnancy.[142] Management of ectopic pregnancy can be surgical (by laparoscopy) or medical (with intramuscular administration of methotrexate).[16] Early detection and proper management of ectopic pregnancy are the most effective means of preventing maternal morbidity and mortality. Some have suggested that asymptomatic women at high risk for ectopic pregnancy should be screened using ultrasound and laboratory tests.[57]

Ultrasound examination and quantitative measurements of serum CG can be useful in identifying women with ectopic pregnancies or abnormal intrauterine pregnancies. These conditions frequently produce abnormal CG concentrations and slow rates of increase.[48] In addition, progesterone measurements can be helpful either individually or in combination with CG.

Kadar and colleagues[177] reported in 1981 that ultrasonography should detect a gestational sac in the uterus of all patients having CG concentrations greater than 6500 IU/L. They termed this concentration the "discriminatory zone." The threshold has now decreased several times because of improvements in ultrasonographic resolution and the introduction of endovaginal ultrasound. The current cutoff is as low as 1500 IU/L, but has a sensitivity of only 42% and specificity of 81% for the detection of ectopic pregnancy when no gestational sac is found in the uterus.[187] In 1994, Kadar and colleagues[175] concluded that the CG concentration should not be used to predict a gestational sac if the gestational age is known with confidence. The best predictor is an accurate gestational age. Failure to detect a gestational sac by sonography 24 days or more after conception is presumptive evidence of an ectopic pregnancy.

Romero and colleagues[277] reported that in 184 patients with ectopic pregnancies, CG concentrations ranged from 0 to 200,000 IU/L, with a geometric mean of about 1000 IU/L. Concentrations of CG depend on the size and viability of the trophoblastic tissue. In about 1% of patients with an ectopic pregnancy, the CG is undetectable using serum tests capable of measuring concentrations as low as 5 IU/L. Qualitative serum tests with limits of detection of about 50 IU/L can be very useful for rapid determination of pregnancy in this clinical setting.[197] To distinguish further between the various possibilities, serial testing of CG may be very helpful. In normal intrauterine pregnancy, a rapid increase in CG follows. During the second through fifth weeks, the CG doubles in about 1.5 days. After 5 weeks of gestation, the doubling time gradually lengthens to 2 to 3 days.[263] Before 7 weeks, calculation of the slope of log(CG) versus time in days is useful for identifying normal pregnancies.[176] At least two CG determinations should be obtained from specimens collected 1 to 7 days apart. The log-linear slope, Δlog(CG)/Δ time (in log(IU/L)/day), is greater than 0.11 in the vast majority of normal pregnancies. In cases of ectopic pregnancies or spontaneous abortions, the slope is usually less than 0.11, and the CG concentrations often decrease.

Serum progesterone concentration is often low in mothers with abnormal pregnancies.[269] In a study[98] of asymptomatic women less than 8 weeks from their last menses, a serum progesterone less than 6 ng/mL predicted an abnormal pregnancy outcome with 81% confidence, but the average serum progesterone in nonviable pregnancies was 10 ng/mL. For women with clinical symptoms of abnormal pregnancy, measurement of both CG and progesterone is more predictive of abnormal pregnancy than a single CG measurement. In a large outcome study, 97% of the patients with CG $<$3000 IU/L and progesterone $<$12.6 ng/mL had an abnormal pregnancy outcome, whereas those with CG $>$3000 IU/L or progesterone $>$12.6 ng/mL had a normal pregnancy.[241] McCord and associates[214] reported that for women at risk for ectopic pregnancy, a progesterone cutoff of 17.5 ng/mL detected 92% of the ectopic cases (clinical sensitivity), but had a very poor clinical specificity of about 14%. They concluded that patients with progesterone greater than 17.5 ng/mL needed no additional laboratory tests. Finally, in symptomatic patients, Stewart and colleagues[304] reported a sensitivity of 99% and specificity of 65% when using the Δlog(CG)/Δtime $>$0.14 to distinguish normal intrauterine pregnancy from ectopic pregnancy combined with inevitable abortion. A progesterone cutoff above 8 ng/mL had a sensitivity of 81% and a specificity of 88%.

Liver Disease

There are a number of liver disorders unique to pregnancy.[186] These include hyperemesis gravidarum, cholestasis of pregnancy, fatty liver of pregnancy, preeclampsia and eclampsia, and the HELLP syndrome. These disorders must be distinguished from the normal physiological changes of pregnancy (see Table 54-2). Significant changes normally seen in pregnancy include a dilutional decrease in serum albumin and elevation of alkaline phosphatase (from the placenta). Total bilirubin, 5′-nucleotidase, GGT, ALT, and AST are unchanged. Changes in these analytes reflect hepatobiliary disease.

Hyperemesis Gravidarum

Hyperemesis gravidarum is characterized by nausea and vomiting and, in severe cases, dehydration and malnutrition. It typically occurs in the first trimester. When hyperemesis is severe enough to cause dehydration, abnormal liver enzyme values—usually less than four times the upper reference limit—are seen in approximately 50% of patients.[340] Mild hyperbilirubinemia may occur. However, significant liver disease does not occur, and liver biopsy results are normal. Low-birth-weight babies are common, especially for women who develop malnutrition.

Cholestasis of Pregnancy

Cholestasis of pregnancy usually occurs in the third trimester and is manifested clinically by diffuse pruritus and, in 20% to 60% of patients, jaundice. The typical features of cholestasis, including pale stools and dark urine, are present and last until delivery. Women who experience cholestasis while taking oral contraceptives will usually develop cholestasis of pregnancy. Serum bilirubin rarely exceeds 5 mg/dL. Alkaline phosphatase is typically two to four times the upper reference limit. Aminotransferase enzyme concentrations are mildly elevated. There may be an elevated prothrombin time because of vitamin K malabsorption. Although some clinicians order serum bile acids in this setting, this test is rarely necessary for diagnosis. The condition itself is benign, but is associated with an increased risk of premature birth and fetal death. It recurs with subsequent pregnancies.[271]

Fatty Liver of Pregnancy

Fatty liver of pregnancy occurs in 1 in 7000 pregnancies and is characterized by accumulation of microvesicular fat in the liver.[65] Although the exact cause is unknown, this disorder occurs more often in women who have a fetus affected with a mitochondrial fatty acid oxidation disorder, long chain 3-hydroxyacyl-CoA dehydrogenase deficiency (LCHAD).[318] The disease typically occurs at week 37 and is manifested clinically by the rapid onset of malaise, nausea, vomiting, and abdominal pain. Mild elevations in aminotransferase enzyme concentrations occur, with the AST elevation typically greater than the ALT elevation but both less than six times the upper reference limit. The serum bilirubin is usually greater than 6 mg/dL. Life-threatening hypoglycemia may occur.[275] Hyperuricemia, presumably from tissue destruction and renal failure, is characteristic. Liver histology shows acute fatty infiltration with little necrosis or inflammation. The fat is microvesicular and pericentral in the cell, similar to what is seen in Reye's syndrome. If untreated, fulminant hepatic failure with hepatic encephalopathy ensues. Treatment is immediate termination of the pregnancy, at which time rapid recovery usually occurs. Infant and maternal mortality is approximately 20%. Recurrence in subsequent pregnancies is very rare.

Preeclampsia and Eclampsia

Preeclampsia is characterized by hypertension, proteinuria, and edema, usually occurring late in the second trimester or early in the third trimester. The cause is unclear, but research suggests that increased circulating soluble fms-like tyrosine kinase 1 (sFlt-1) may have a role.[200]

It is related to abnormal endothelial reactivity that leads to intravascular deposition of fibrin with subsequent end-organ damage.[276] Most maternal deaths are due to central nervous system complications, but the liver may also be the target of injury. The injury to the liver is ischemic. Modest elevations in ALT and AST occur, typically 4 to 10 times the upper reference limit. Hepatic complications, including hemorrhage, infarction, and fulminant hepatic failure, may occur and necessitate early delivery.

HELLP Syndrome

The HELLP syndrome occurs in 0.1% of pregnancies. The most prominent features are thrombocytopenia and disseminated intravascular coagulation (DIC). Most cases occur between the 27th and 36th weeks of pregnancy, but it also may occur postpartum. Women typically present with epigastric or right upper quadrant pain, malaise, nausea, vomiting, and headache.[212,282] Jaundice occurs in 5% of patients. Lactate dehydrogenase (LD) concentrations may be very high, and ALT and AST are usually 2 to 10 times upper reference limits. Treatment is delivery. The postpartum management of the patient may require plasmapheresis or organ transplantation. Recurrence rates are 3% to 27%.

Non–Pregnancy-Related Liver Disease in Pregnancy

Pregnancy does not preclude the acquisition or aggravation of non–pregnancy-related liver disease. Thus cholestasis during pregnancy may reflect the presence of hepatotoxicity from drugs, primary biliary cirrhosis, Dubin-Johnson syndrome, or cholelithiasis (see Chapter 47). Abdominal ultrasound, endoscopic retrograde cholangiography, or liver biopsy may be necessary to exclude these conditions.

Viral hepatitis occurs with the same frequency in pregnancy as would be expected in a comparable age group.[280] It is manifested by malaise, nausea, vomiting, dark urine, and mild fever. AST and ALT are virtually always greater than 10 times the upper reference limit and usually greater than 20 times the upper reference limit. The prognosis, with the exception of hepatitis E and herpes simplex, is the same as in nonpregnant women. Hepatitis E, an enteric infection occurring in India, Africa, the Middle East, and Central America, has a mortality rate of 15% to 20% in the pregnant patient.[190] Herpes simplex hepatitis, usually accompanied by oral or vulvar vesicles, has a mortality rate of 43%.[183] Distinguishing features include a mild bilirubin elevation and marked aminotransferase elevations. Liver biopsy is usually required for diagnosis and demonstrates typical intranuclear inclusions and the other usual features of viral hepatitis. Antiviral therapy greatly improves the prognosis.

Women who acquire hepatitis B late in pregnancy or who are chronic carriers are likely to transmit the disease to their babies. This is especially so if the mother is HBeAg positive (see Chapter 47). The outcome in the infant varies from fulminant hepatitis (rare and usually in anti-HBe-positive mothers) to mild hepatitis to chronic hepatitis (the usual outcome in 90% of chronically infected woman). All pregnant women should be screened for hepatitis B with HBsAg.[7] If positive, their babies should be immunized with hepatitis B immune globulin and hepatitis B vaccine. Babies born to hepatitis C–positive mothers usually have the passively transmitted antibody for several months, but transmission of active hepatitis is unusual.[311] Because there is no known treatment for the newborn, screening is not recommended for hepatitis C virus infection.

Differential Diagnosis

It is often difficult to distinguish the various liver diseases of pregnancy from each other and from naturally occurring liver diseases. Acute fatty liver is suggested when nausea, vomiting, and abdominal pain are followed by jaundice, and encephalopathy occurs in the presence of a small or normal-sized liver. The white blood cell count is usually elevated above 15,000 cells/μL and ALT levels are typically four to six times the upper reference limit. Hypoalbuminemia, hyperuricemia, hypoglycemia, and DIC are typical. Hepatic ultrasound and computed tomography (CT) will usually demonstrate fatty liver when present. In preeclampsia and the HELLP syndrome, the liver is usually enlarged, ALT levels are usually lower, and bilirubin levels are mildly elevated or normal. Hyperuricemia is uncommon. Marked elevations in aminotransferase enzyme levels suggest hepatic infarction or viral hepatitis. Liver biopsy may be needed to differentiate non–pregnancy-related causes of liver disease, but should not be used to differentiate acute fatty liver from preeclampsia or HELLP syndrome because the treatment is the same for all of these conditions—delivery of the infant.[219]

Effect of Pregnancy on Preexisting Liver Disease

Conception and full-term parturition do not usually occur in women who have cirrhosis. However, liver disease is not a reason for termination. The hypervolemia associated with pregnancy may aggravate cirrhosis and predispose to bleeding from esophageal varices.[49]

Autoimmune chronic hepatitis is usually associated with amenorrhea, but pregnancy may occur after treatment to remission with corticosteroids. The steroids should be continued during the pregnancy. Pregnancy should be avoided in patients being treated with azathioprine.

Neonatal Graves' Disease

The fetal thyroid-pituitary axis functions independently from the mother's axis in most cases. However, if the mother has preexisting Graves' disease (see Chapter 52), her autoantibodies can cross the placenta and stimulate the fetal thyroid gland. Thus the fetus can develop hyperthyroidism. Measurement of thyrotropin-binding inhibitory immunoglobulins (TBII) is useful for assessing risk of fetal or neonatal Graves' disease.

Hemolytic Disease of the Newborn

Hemolytic disease of the newborn (HDN) is a fetal hemolytic disorder caused by maternal antibodies directed against antigen on fetal erythrocytes. Commonly used synonyms for this disorder are *isoimmunization disease*, *Rh isoimmune disease*, *Rh disease*, or *D isoimmunization.* Any of a large number of erythrocyte surface antigens Rh(CDE), A, B, Kell, Duffy, Kidd, and others may be responsible for isoimmune hemolysis. When severe, the disorder is known as *erythroblastosis fetalis* and is life threatening to fetus and newborn. The most common cause of severe disease is sensitization of a D-negative woman. The amount of bilirubin in the amniotic fluid is useful for determining the severity of the disease. Pioneering work by Bevis[37-40] uncovered the association between amniotic fluid bilirubin and D isoimmunization. Liley[201] extended this work by noting an association between gestational age, severity of the disease, and bilirubin concentration.

Rh Blood Groups

Two genes, *RhD and RhCE*, encode for erythrocyte membrane proteins that are antigenic. Both are located on chromosome 1p about 30 kb apart. Approximately 15% of Caucasians, 5% of Africans, and less than 1% of Asians are RhD-negative. The most prevalent RhD-negative allele appears to be a deletion.[27] Exon 5 of *RhCE* has two common polymorphisms producing *E* or *e* antigen. Exon 2 of *RhCE* has two common polymorphisms producing *C* or *c* antigen.

Etiology

Sensitization, or production of a maternal antibody, may occur in response to blood transfusion or a pregnancy in which the fetus has a blood cell antigen that the mother lacks. Although the fetal and maternal blood compartments are generally considered to be separate during normal gestation, small numbers of fetal erythrocytes are continually gaining access to the maternal circulation. This antigenic challenge is sufficient in some women to provoke an antibody response. Substantially larger antigenic exposures may result from those disruptions in the integrity of the fetal compartment that accompany spontaneous or induced abortion, ectopic pregnancy, or delivery of an infant. The larger the fetomaternal hemorrhage, the more likely it is that the mother will respond to the challenge by developing an antibody. Other antigens of the Rh system—C, c, E, e—may stimulate antibody formation, but appear to be less than one one thousandth as potent.

The IgG produced is actively transported across the placenta into the fetus. When a sensitized woman is pregnant with an RhD-positive fetus, the antibodies cause destruction of the fetal erythrocytes. Furthermore, during pregnancy or at the time of delivery, repeat exposure to RhD-positive erythrocytes causes an augmented response, resulting in higher antibody titers. This augmented response is responsible for the frequent observation that subsequent pregnancies are frequently more severely affected than earlier ones.

The pathophysiology of isoimmune hemolysis is the same for all antigens. The differences in severity of disease are due to differences in the expression of the antigen on the surface of the cells, the intrinsic immunogenicity of the antigen, and peculiarities of the immune response of the mother. Destruction of the fetal erythrocytes, which is the central problem, produces several other problems. Fetal anemia imposes an extra burden on the fetal heart to provide adequate oxygen supply to fetal tissues. Anemia stimulates the fetal marrow and extramedullary erythropoiesis in the liver and spleen to replace the destroyed erythrocytes. Extramedullary erythropoiesis destroys hepatocytes and leads to decreased production of serum albumin and decreased oncotic pressure in the intravascular space.

These changes, when severe, lead to congestive heart failure and generalized fetal edema, with ascites and pleural and pericardial effusions. When the fetal condition has deteriorated to this degree, it is referred to as *hydrops fetalis* and carries a very grave prognosis. The edema and effusions are readily observable by ultrasonographic examination. When these changes are observed and there is no therapeutic intervention, intrauterine demise follows in a relatively short time.

If a fetus survives, the newborn will encounter a number of problems. In utero, the placenta and mother perform the functions of respiration and removal of bilirubinoid pigments resulting from hemolysis. Newborns must assume these functions for themselves in the presence of hydrops. The lungs are edematous, and pleural effusions and ascites physically restrict their ability to expand. The damaged liver is unable to conjugate and excrete bilirubin adequately. When bilirubin accumulates in the blood to excessive concentrations, it passes through the blood-brain barrier to deposit in the brain and destroy brain cells. This form of brain damage is termed *kernicterus.* Thus, although kernicterus was not a concern in the fetus, it is a significant concern in these sick newborns. A severely erythroblastotic baby can be one of the most challenging problems in a neonatal intensive care unit.

Prophylaxis

An anti-RhD immune globulin, RhoGAM (Ortho Clinical Diagnotics, Raritan, N.J.), has been used in the United States since 1968,[46] and other similar products were introduced in 1971 and later. A 300 μg dose is administered intramuscularly to a mother potentially exposed to 15 mL or less of RhD-positive fetal erythrocytes following abortion, fetomaternal hemorrhage, amniocentesis, chorionic villi sampling, or delivery.[13] Use of RhD immunoglobulin has been responsible for the dramatic reduction in the incidence of HDN. In addition to recognized fetomaternal hemorrhage, undetected transplacental fetomaternal bleeding during an apparently normal pregnancy can lead to antepartum sensitization. This would not be prevented by immediate postpartum administration of RhD immunoglobulin; therefore antepartum administration at 28 weeks of gestation is recommended for RhD-negative women. Despite this immune prophylaxis, a small number of sensitized pregnancies continue to occur.

Clinical Management of Sensitized Mothers

To identify sensitized women, an alloantibody screen is performed at the first prenatal visit.[222] If an antibody to an erythrocyte antigen is identified, the titer is determined.[9] The critical anti-RhD titer depends on the laboratory, usually 1:8 to 1:32, although studies of critical titer are quite disparate.[144] For all sensitized women, the paternal erythrocyte phenotype is determined. If the father is RhD-negative, then no follow-up studies are required. If he is D-positive, then his Rh phenotypic zygosity is estimated (genotyping will most likely be used in the future). If the paternal Rh genotype is likely heterozygous for D, then the Rh D status of the fetus needs to be determined.[222] Amniotic fluid is collected by amniocentesis for fetal RhD genotyping by polymerase chain reaction (PCR). To guard against a false negative caused by a paternal RhD gene rearrangement (occurring in about 1.5% of Caucasians), the father can also be genotyped. A frequent occurrence in those of African ancestry is an RhD pseudogene; the patient is RhD-negative by serology, but RhD-positive on genotype. If the fetus is RhD-genotype-positive, the mother (who is RhD-negative serologically) should be tested for RhD genotype. In the United Kingdom, laboratories have begun to offer fetal Rh genotyping using cell-free fetal DNA that circulates in maternal blood (see Chapter 36).[123]

For sensitized mothers with an at-risk fetus, serial titers are performed on maternal serum every month until 24 weeks gestation, then every 2 weeks thereafter. If a critical titer anti-D is detected, then ultrasound Doppler measurements are used to determine the peak velocity of blood flow in the fetal middle cerebral artery. Higher velocity is a strong indicator of fetal anemia. In addition, amniocentesis is performed to assess the bilirubin concentration in amniotic fluid.

Liley noted that the degree of hemolysis in sensitized pregnancies could be assessed by measuring the absorbance of bilirubinoid pigments in amniotic fluid and classifying the results into three zones based on gestational age.[201] The procedure was originally called ΔOD_{450},[201] a term still used by most clinicians. The preferred clinical chemistry term is ΔA_{450}. This method is described later in this chapter in the section entitled Laboratory Tests. Serial testing is indicated every 10 to 14 days. If the ΔA_{450} rises or plateaus at about the 80th percentile of zone 2 on the Liley curve, fetal blood sampling is indicated. Ultrasound-guided umbilical blood sampling is performed to determine fetal blood type, hematocrit, antibody screen, reticulocyte count, and total bilirubin. Intrauterine intravascular blood transfusion can be performed if indicated. If fetal pulmonary maturation has occurred (usually 35 weeks or greater), delivery is indicated.

Trophoblastic Disease

Serum CG determinations are very useful for monitoring patients with germ cell–derived neoplasms or other CG-producing tumors, such as lung carcinoma. The use of CG in these diseases is discussed in Chapter 23.

Fetal Anomalies

Open neural tube defects, Down syndrome, and trisomy 18 (discussed separately below) are fetal anomalies that are partially detectable by maternal serum screening. However, because of the large number of pregnancies screened, and the interest in other fetal conditions and their possible association with abnormal maternal serum analyte concentrations, a wealth of associations between rarer conditions and screening results has been published. These findings are never diagnostic and are reported rarely by the screening laboratory. In certain circumstances, however, the healthcare provider may determine a need for more extensive medical evaluation.

Neural Tube Defects

Neural tube defects are serious abnormalities that occur early in embryonic development. By 19 days after fertilization, the area that is to form the central nervous system (brain and spinal cord) has differentiated into a plate of cells. The flat plate then rolls up, and its edges fuse into a hollow neural tube that drops into the embryo to develop just underneath what will become the skin of the back. Neural tube formation is normally complete 4 weeks after fertilization. Failure of neural tube fusion leads to permanent developmental defects of the brain or spinal cord or both. These defects are called *anencephaly*, *meningomyelocele* (which is commonly called *spina bifida*), and *encephalocele*. Although there are many heterogeneous causes, about 90% fall into the classification of multifactorial inheritance.[165] Folic acid deficiency is clearly associated with increased frequency of neural tube closure defects.[326] The cause in these cases may be derangement of homocysteine metabolism caused by the folate deficiency.[302] Estimates attribute 70% or more of all neural tube defects to folate deficiency.[334] Since 1997, grain products in the United States and Canada have been fortified with 140 µg folic acid/100 g,[124] but the amount added is unlikely to be sufficient to reduce the birth prevalence by more than about 30%, the reduction that is commonly reported in observational trials.[253] Organizations such as the March of Dimes are conducting vigorous campaigns to educate women of the need for folic acid supplementation before becoming pregnant, as recommended by the Centers for Disease Control and Prevention.[67] Most vitamin supplements contain the 400 µg of folic acid recommended daily by authorities.[226]

The birth prevalence of open neural tube defects varies with factors such as geographic location (higher in the Eastern United States, lower in the West), race (lower in African-Americans), ethnicity (higher in Scotch-Irish), family history (higher with prior births of affected individuals),[83] and maternal weight (higher in obese women).[290,339] An average figure for the United States is 1 open neural tube defect per 1000 pregnancies (about 1 in 2000 for each indi-

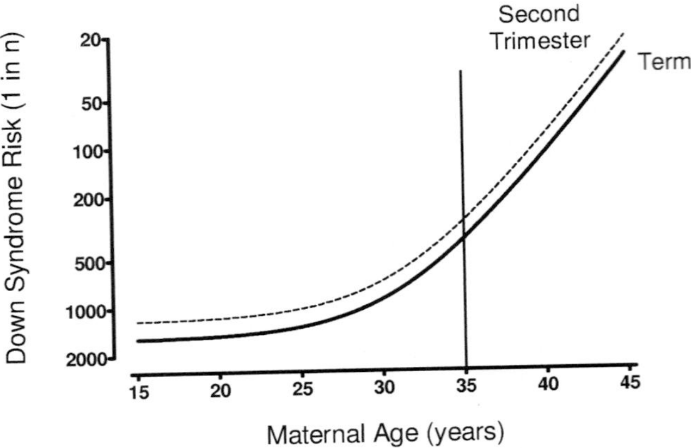

Figure 54-4 The relationship of maternal age and the risk of having a pregnancy affected with Down syndrome. *Dotted line,* Second trimester risk; *solid line,* term risk. *Vertical line* at age 35 is the cutoff used for selecting women at increased risk based on maternal age.

vidual defect). Almost all cases of anencephaly and about 95% of meningomyeloceles are open, with no overlying skin, and therefore are in direct communication with the amniotic fluid. Thus the fetal serum proteins normally present in amniotic fluid at low concentrations gain access in large quantities to the amniotic fluid. The elevated amniotic fluid AFP concentration leads to increased amounts in the maternal circulation. Only open neural tube defects are detected by maternal serum AFP screening, and approximately 90% of these can be detected using maternal serum AFP testing.[330]

Down Syndrome

Down syndrome is the most common serious disorder of the autosomal chromosomes, occurring in 1 in 800 live births. An extra copy of the long arm region q22.1 to q22.3 of chromosome 21 results in a phenotype consisting of moderate to severe mental retardation, hypotonia, congenital heart defects, and flat facial profile. The autosome is the smallest chromosome, making up about 1.7% of the human genome. Most often an affected child has three copies of chromosome 21 (i.e., trisomy 21), but 5% of cases are caused by translocations and 1% of cases are mosaics. The risk increases slowly up to age 30 and then steadily increases as maternal age advances (see Figure 54-4).[168] At 25 years of age, the risk at birth is about 1 in 1000; at age 40 it is 1 in 90.

Trisomy 18

Trisomy 18 (Edwards syndrome) is caused by a nondisjunction event during meiosis that results in a fetus having an extra copy of chromosome 18. Although it occurs in only 1 in 8000 births, it is probably the most common chromosome defect at the time of conception. The dramatic change in prevalence is due to the very high fetal loss rate both before 8 weeks (~80%) and during the second and third trimesters (~70%). Approximately 25% of affected fetuses have meningomyelocele (spina bifida) or omphalocele. There is a high cesarean section rate for undiagnosed cases.[249] Following birth, half of the infants die within the first 5 days and 90% die within 100 days.[64]

Preterm Delivery

The leading cause of neonatal morbidity and mortality in the United States is preterm delivery, with 300,000 to 500,000 cases each year.[5] Infants born before 37 weeks gestation often develop *respiratory distress syndrome* (RDS) and are usually of low birth weight (<2500 g). Some are of very low birth weight (<1500 g). According to the National Center for Health Statistics,[228] in 1993 7.2% of all U.S. live-born infants were low birth weight and 1.3% were very low birth weight. Most of these infants will spend time in intensive care units at a cost of up to $3500 per day.

The cause of preterm labor is unknown, but recent evidence in a mouse model indicates that a maternal serum surfactant protein, SP-A, may trigger labor.[82] Fetal fibronectin and cervical ultrasound have proven value for evaluating patients suspected of having preterm labor. The fetal fibronectin test is described later in the section entitled Laboratory Tests. Use of salivary estriol,[161] corticotropin-releasing hormone,[199] and interleukin-6[140] for preterm labor prediction is being investigated.

Fetal Lung Maturity

RDS, also called *hyaline membrane disease,* is the most common critical problem encountered in clinical management of preterm newborns. The worldwide incidence of RDS is 1% of live births and 10% to 15% of live preterm births (<37 weeks or <2500 g).[232] The risk of RDS is affected strongly by the gestational age at the time of birth: 1% at 37 weeks, 20% at 34 weeks, and 60% at 29 weeks.[120] In 2000 RDS killed just over 1000 infants in the United States.[220] Affected infants require supplemental oxygen and mechanical ventilation to remain properly oxygenated. The disorder is caused by a deficiency of *pulmonary surfactant.* In normal lungs, surfactant coats the alveolar epithelium and responds to alveolar volume changes by reducing the surface tension in the alveolar wall during expiration. When the quantity of surfactant is deficient, many of the alveoli collapse on expiration and thereby overinflate the remaining airways. This process is known as *focal atelectasis.* The lungs become progressively noncompliant, and blood flowing through the capillary beds of collapsed alveoli fails to oxygenate. During the first few hours of life, affected infants develop tachypnea with or without cyanosis, nasal flaring, expiratory grunting, and intercostal retractions. The disease exacerbates during the next few days and is usually worse on the third or fourth day of life. Infants at risk for developing RDS can be treated with intratracheal administration of exogenous surfactant immediately at birth.[157]

Very rarely, respiratory distress in a term newborn can be caused by a mutation in the gene encoding for SP-B.[238] This condition, termed congenital alveolar proteinosis, is often

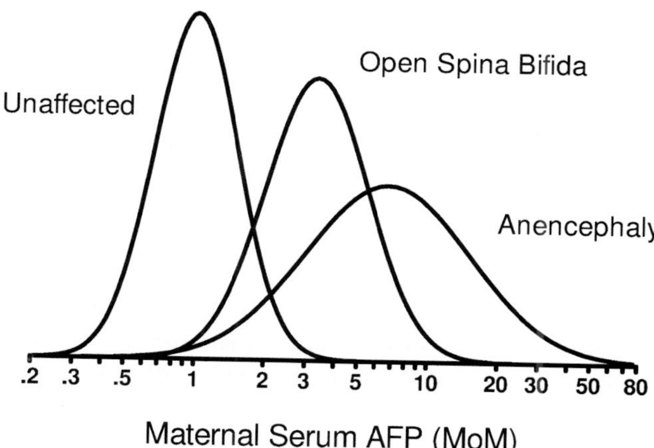

Figure 54-5 Distribution of maternal serum alpha fetoprotein (AFP) measurements in unaffected pregnancies, and pregnancies affected with open spina bifida or anencephaly.

fatal. There is a significant derangement in lamellar body production in these cases. A study of the genetic variation suggests that there may be mild, nonfatal cases of this disorder.[106]

MATERNAL SERUM SCREENING FOR FETAL DEFECTS

In the early 1970s, Brock and colleagues demonstrated increased AFP concentrations in amniotic fluid of mothers carrying fetuses affected with an open neural tube defect (e.g., anencephaly, open spina bifida).[52] Subsequently, it was shown that AFP concentrations were increased in maternal serum (in the second trimester) as well.[50] The concentrations in serum in affected and unaffected pregnancies overlapped considerably, however, indicating that maternal serum AFP would be useful only as an initial screening test to identify women at high risk for having an affected fetus (Figure 54-5). These women would then need to be referred for diagnostic procedures (e.g., high resolution ultrasound and, if indicated, amniocentesis for measurement of AFP and acetylcholinesterase in amniotic fluid) to determine if the fetus had an open neural tube defect. A large collaborative study conducted in the United Kingdom in 1977 showed that maternal serum AFP screening for open neural tube defects in the second trimester of pregnancy was feasible, and the final report provided estimates of screening performance in terms of detection and false-positive rates.[330] A family history of neural tube defects in either parent increases the risk that the fetus is affected by fivefold to fifteenfold, but more than 90% of all infants with neural tube defects are born to unsuspecting parents who have no recognized risk factor for the disorder.[130,316] Maternal serum AFP testing thus provided a screening method available to all women to identify pregnancies at high risk or to estimate the numerical risk of having a fetus with an open neural tube defect.[329] In the 1980s, the use of maternal serum AFP to screen for open neural tube defects became a standard of care in the United States. The American College of Obstetricians and Gynecologists,[10,14] the American Society of Human Genetics,[15] and the American Academy of Pediatrics[3] have issued official statements supporting its use.

In 1984, a major expansion of biochemical prenatal screening became possible when an association between second trimester maternal serum AFP and fetal Down syndrome was reported.[217] Maternal serum AFP concentrations are about 25% lower in Down syndrome than in unaffected pregnancies. Significantly the association was found to be independent of maternal age.[91] Before this discovery, the only available screening test for Down syndrome involved asking a woman her age. If she would be 35 years or older at the time of delivery, she would be offered amniocentesis and fetal karyotyping. Down syndrome screening using maternal age is based on the well-documented increase in risk for having a baby with Down syndrome as maternal age increases (see Figure 54-3). At the time, about 20% of Down syndrome cases occurred in the 5% of women who were 35 years of age or older at the time of delivery. The independence of maternal serum AFP measurements and maternal age established that it was possible to offer a screening method to younger women, in whom most cases of Down syndrome occur. Maternal serum AFP screening for Down syndrome also introduced the concept of using risk, rather than analyte concentration, as the screening variable for identifying high-risk women.[91] Subsequently a large collaborative study established the effectiveness of maternal serum AFP screening in younger women.[235]

The discovery that a protein produced in pregnancy could be altered in the presence of a fetal chromosomal defect stimulated a search for other substances in pregnancy serum that would have predictive value. Of the many that were examined, two emerged as sufficiently discriminatory and independent to be useful additions in screening for Down syndrome in the second trimester. Unconjugated estriol (uE_3),[61] a product of the fetoplacental unit, is also about 25% lower in pregnancies with Down syndrome. In contrast, concentrations of CG were found to be about twice as high.[44] In 1988, a method was proposed for combining maternal age with measurements of these three analytes (the triple test) into a single Down syndrome risk estimate.[331] As with AFP screening, risk, rather than the analyte values themselves, is the screening variable. The triple test was projected to detect 60% of Down syndrome pregnancies by identifying 5% of all pregnant women as having a screen-positive test result (performance based on pregnancies being dated via LMP). The utility of the triple test was confirmed in 1992 by two intervention trials.[149,259] A fourth analyte, DIA, appears to be a useful addition to the triple test, increasing the detection rate by 8% to 10%.[154] This "quadruple test" is becoming more common and the results of two intervention trials confirm its performance advantage.[31,336] A recent external proficiency testing survey conducted by the Foundation for Blood Research and the College of American Pathologists found that approximately 25% of participating laboratories now offer the quadruple test.[81] Other combinations of second trimester screening tests have been advocated,[210,333] but have not received wide acceptance.

A further expansion of prenatal screening was found to be possible with the discovery that fetal trisomy 18 has a distinctive triple-test pattern that is different from the Down syndrome pattern.[62] In trisomy 18 pregnancies, the AFP and uE_3 concentrations are low, but the CG concentrations are also very low. This is in contrast to Down syndrome, in which the CG measurements are high. Thus few trisomy 18 pregnancies are likely to receive high Down syndrome risk estimates. The initial report[62] included an algorithm that used fixed cutoffs to identify women at high risk of fetal trisomy 18; that algorithm was subsequently validated in an intervention trial.[251] Subsequently, an improved method for trisomy 18 screening was published that used risk as the screening variable as had become standard practice for Down syndrome.[32,122,249]

Clinical Application of Prenatal Screening

Before 2003, most obstetricians offered amniocentesis for fetal karyotype determination to all mothers who would be 35 years of age or older at the time of birth. However, the risk for Down syndrome calculated using biochemical tests is more accurate than the use of maternal age alone, and it is now common practice to offer maternal serum screening to women of all ages. It may be prudent, however, to continue to offer the option of amniocentesis to women age 35 and older, because amniocentesis is still considered by some to be the standard of care. In recent years, the proportion of pregnant women who are 35 years of age or older increased from 5% to 14% of the total, and about half (up from 20%) of all Down syndrome cases occur in this group.[184] If all of these women were to undergo amniocentesis, 1 in every 180 would be found to have a Down syndrome pregnancy. In contrast, the second trimester quadruple test can detect 75% to 80% of Down syndrome cases with only 5% to 6% of women having a positive screening test when the screening is applied to pregnant women of all ages.[154] Approximately 1 in every 50 mothers who are classified as being at high risk will be found to have a fetus with Down syndrome.[149]

Maternal serum screening using the triple test sometimes produces a pattern of low results for AFP, CG, and uE_3.[62] Using an algorithm specifically designed to assign patient-specific risk for trisomy 18, 60% of affected pregnancies can be detected with a false-positive rate of about 0.3%.[249] Among women with a second trimester trisomy 18 risk of 1:100 or greater, 1 in 16 will have a pregnancy affected with trisomy 18.

Multiple of the Median

Understanding the published literature and clinical screening applications requires an understanding of the statistic used to normalize analyte values, the multiple of the median (MoM). The initial step in calculating a MoM is to develop a set of median values for each week (or day) of gestation using the laboratory's own assay values measured on the population to be screened. Individual test results are then expressed as MoM by dividing each individual test result by the median for the relevant gestational week. This convention was originally developed as a means of taking into account the large differences among centers in AFP assay values seen in the 1977 U.K. collaborative study.[330] Converting assay results to MoM units also compensates for the steadily rising AFP concentration in maternal serum during the second trimester and the corresponding decrease in AFP values in amniotic fluid, allowing a single statistic to be used for expressing results. Subsequently, it was found that MoM values could also be adjusted to take into account other factors (e.g., maternal weight and maternal race) that materially affect analyte values.[151] The MoM is now universally used as a common currency for converting analyte values into an interpretative unit and is also the starting point for calculating risks for neural tube defects, Down syndrome, and trisomy 18.[249,329,331]

Neural Tube Defect Screening Using Maternal Serum Alpha Fetoprotein

Population-based prenatal screening began in the late 1970s with the use of maternal serum AFP measurements to identify women at increased risk of carrying a fetus with an open neural tube defect.[330] Although a patient-specific risk can be used when screening for open neural tube defects,[329] nearly all laboratories define a screen-positive result as AFP at or above a fixed MoM cutoff. Optimal screening is between 16 and 18 completed weeks of gestation, a time when the distributions of results for affected and unaffected pregnancies are maximally different and there is adequate time for follow-up studies. Screening at 15 weeks is acceptable, but at 14 weeks or earlier, screening for open neural tube defects is difficult to justify.[330,334] The two most commonly used AFP MoM cutoffs in the United States are 2.0 and 2.5 MoM, yielding initial screen-positive rates of 3% to 5%, and 1% to 3%, respectively. The observed rates are more likely to be at the lower end of the cited ranges if many pregnancies are dated by ultrasound. This improvement is a result of the finding that increased AFP values attributable to underestimated gestational age, fetal demise, and twin gestation will usually have been identified. The lower initial positive rate at 2.5 MoM is associated with a reduced detection rate for open spina bifida: 70% to 75% as compared with 80% to 85% at 2.0 MoM.[94,330] A recent survey found that 52% of laboratories in the United States use a 2.5 MoM cutoff, 30% use a 2.0 MoM, and the remainder use a cutoff in between these two values.[60]

Follow-up Testing for Women With Screen-Positive Results

Women who have a positive screening test result for open neural tube defects are usually referred for genetic counseling and further testing. Some programs may ask for a second sample for moderately elevated results (2.0 to 3.0 MoM) to repeat the test. If the result for the second AFP test is not elevated, the woman is considered to be screen-negative. If the result is still elevated, the patient is referred for further testing. After genetic counseling to explain the test results, to provide more information about the disorder, and to describe the risks and benefits of further testing, a low resolution ultrasound examination may be offered as a way to verify gestational age and to identify other possible reasons for the increased AFP test results (e.g., recent fetal demise and twins). Patients having an unexplained high maternal serum AFP result can then be offered amniocentesis for measurement of amniotic fluid AFP and acetylcholinesterase (AChE), high resolution ultrasound, or both.

Compared with maternal serum, amniotic fluid AFP concentrations in pregnancies affected with open neural tube defects are far more separated from unaffected pregnancies.[327] However, amniotic fluid AFP measurements are not by themselves diagnostic because of false-positive results. If the amniotic fluid is contaminated with even a small amount of fetal blood, as many as 2% to 3% of the results can be falsely positive.[327] All abnormal amniotic fluid AFP results must be confirmed by measurement of amniotic fluid AChE. The combination of amniotic fluid AFP and AChE is virtually diagnostic for an open neural tube defect.[270,327]

High resolution ultrasound can almost always confirm a chemical diagnosis of a neural tube defect. Anencephaly is readily identifiable, and ultrasound diagnosis of open spina bifida is considerably enhanced by the presence of two cranial signs (fruit signs) resulting from the Arnold-Chiari malformation associated with this defect.[104,236] The first sign is a "pinched" skull in the frontal region resulting in a "lemon" shape compared with the normal egg shape. The second sign is a reduction in the transverse diameter of the cerebellum leading to the two cerebellar hemispheres assuming a bow shape, the "banana sign." Ultrasound diagnosis of open neural tube defects is now so reliable that it is often used for diagnosis in women with elevated maternal serum AFP without waiting for amniotic fluid measurements.

Down Syndrome Screening Using Multiple Biochemical Tests

The most common combination of second trimester maternal serum biochemical tests used to screen for Down syndrome in the United States is the triple test (maternal age in combination with AFP, uE_3, and CG measurements).[80] Many laboratories are offering DIA measurements to form the quadruple test.[81] Measurements of each analyte are made on a single serum sample (the same one used for open neural tube defect screening) and the results in mass units are converted to MoM for the appropriate week (or day) of gestation. This MoM value is then adjusted for other variables, such as maternal weight and race. Patient-specific Down syndrome risks are then calculated using the adjusted MoM values along with the woman's maternal age at delivery employing an algorithm that uses overlapping multivariate Gaussian distributions. The prior odds based on age are then multiplied by this likelihood ratio to assign the final patient-specific Down syndrome risk. This final risk, rather than the analyte values themselves, is the screening variable upon which clinical decisions are made.

The detection and false-positive rates achievable depend on many factors including (1) the test combination chosen, (2) the risk cutoff chosen, (3) the method of dating used to establish gestational age, and (4) the maternal ages of the women being tested. Table 54-3 summarizes the impact of these factors in a hypothetical cohort of women having the maternal age distribution found in the United States in 2000.[154] In the United States, many laboratories use the triple test (AFP, uE_3, CG) and a cutoff equivalent to the risk of a 35-year-old woman (1:270 in the second trimester or 1:350 at term). At this risk cutoff and with use of the date of the

TABLE 54-3 Estimated Down Syndrome Detection Rates (DR), False-Positive Rates (FPR), and Odds of Being Affected Given a Positive Result (OAPR) at Three Risk Cutoff Values for Selected Combinations of Maternal Serum Marker and Two Methods of Dating

SECOND TRIMESTER		DR (%)		FPR (%)		OAPR (1:n)	
Risk Cutoff (term)	Maternal Age and Serum Markers	LMP	US	LMP	US	LMP	US
150 (200)	AFP, uE_3, CG	61	67	3.6	3.7	43	40
	AFP, uE_3, CG, DIA	68	71	2.8	2.9	30	29
190 (250)	AFP, uE_3, CG	65	70	4.6	4.7	51	49
	AFP, uE_3, CG, DIA	71	74	3.5	3.7	36	36
270 (350)	AFP, uE_3, CG	70	74	6.6	6.5	69	64
	AFP, uE_3, CG, DIA	75	78	5.0	5.1	48	48

LMP, Gestation age estimated from last menstrual period; *US*, gestational age estimated from ultrasound measurements; *AFP*, alpha fetoprotein; *uE_3*, unconjugated estriol; *CG*, chorionic gonadotropin; *DIA*, dimeric inhibin A.

LMP to estimate gestational age, the triple test yields an initial positive rate of 6.6% and a detection rate of 70%. If pregnancies are dated by ultrasound, the detection rate increases to 74% and the screen-positive rate declines slightly to 6.5%. Some laboratories choose instead a risk cutoff to obtain an initial positive rate of about 5% (4.6% in the table with LMP dating). This lower rate occurs at a second trimester screening cutoff that corresponds to a 1:190 risk (1:250 risk at term) and is associated with a detection rate of 65%. If DIA measurements are added to the triple test, the detection rate increases to about 78%, and the initial positive rate decreases to 5.1% (LMP dating at a risk cutoff of a 35-year-old woman). The table demonstrates how the choices of test combination and risk cutoff affect the detection and screen-positive rates.

Follow-up Testing for Women With Screen-Positive Results

Women who have a positive screening test result for Down syndrome are usually referred for genetic counseling and further testing. After counseling, a low-resolution ultrasound examination may be offered as a way to verify gestational age and to identify other possible reasons for the positive test result. One of the most common reasons for increased Down syndrome risk is overestimated gestational age. Up to one third of women with positive Down syndrome screening results who are dated by the last menstrual period will be found to be too early in their pregnancies for reliable screening (less than 15 weeks) or reclassified as low risk after ultrasound revision of gestational age.[149] Women who are still at increased risk after the ultrasound examination should be offered amniocentesis to obtain fetal cells for karyotyping. Although some second trimester ultrasound findings are associated with Down syndrome (e.g., nuchal fold and shortened femur and humeral length), these findings are not diagnostic.[296] The only way to diagnose Down syndrome is via fetal karyotype. However, the benefits of accurately diagnosing a chromosome abnormality early in gestation must be weighed against the potential for harming a normal fetus during amniocentesis. This invasive procedure carries a small but real risk of harming the fetus or causing spontaneous abortion. Even amniocentesis performed by an experienced obstetrician using ultrasonography for guidance has a procedure-related rate of fetal loss of about 1 in 200.[297] Given that about 1 in 50 women with an unexplained screen-positive test result (high risk) will have a fetus with a chromosome abnormality, the offer of the invasive procedure is reasonable.

Trisomy 18 Screening Using Multiple Tests

Trisomy 18 is the least common of the three disorders considered for second trimester maternal serum screening. It is also the one that is least compatible with life. For these reasons, justification of a screening program exclusively devoted to the prenatal identification of trisomy 18 is difficult. However, given that the serum analytes are already being measured to screen for Down syndrome and open neural tube defects, adding an additional interpretation of these analytes to quantify the risk of fetal trisomy 18 might be warranted. However, since the birth prevalence of trisomy 18 is one tenth that of Down syndrome,[249] the percentage of women identified as screen-positive must be correspondingly lower than that for Down syndrome. A risk-based algorithm showed that at a second trimester risk cutoff of 1:100, 60% of trisomy 18 pregnancies could be identified, with about 0.5% of women having an initial positive screen. This algorithm will identify 1 trisomy 18 fetus for every 16 amniocenteses that result from the program.[249] Risk for trisomy 18 is also based on multivariate overlapping Gaussian distributions, with the appropriate parameters being used for the affected population. Women with a risk higher than a specified cutoff are referred for genetic counseling and further testing.

Follow-up Testing for Women With Screen-Positive Results

In contrast to the screening protocols for open neural tube defects and Down syndrome, a dating ultrasound is not recommended as the first step after a finding of increased risk of trisomy 18. The trisomy 18 pattern of low AFP, low uE_3, and low CG is not consistent with incorrect gestational dating, and the direct offer of amniocentesis is warranted.[122,251] A high proportion of fetuses with trisomy 18 will have abnormal but nondiagnostic second trimester ultrasound findings (e.g., heart defects and clenched fists).[28]

Establishing Assay-Specific and Population-Specific Median Values

One of the most important responsibilities of the prenatal screening laboratory is to establish kit-specific and population-specific median values for each analyte used in screening or to show that median values obtained from another source are appropriate. Relatively small errors in median values can have a disproportionate impact on both the accuracy of the calculated risk and the number of women identified as screen-positive. Values measured on the same patients and the same proficiency testing samples can differ among methods by 5% to 200% depending on the analyte measured.[81] Median values are therefore not directly transferable between reagent sets from different methods. Median values can also differ among laboratories even when the same methodology is employed. This difference is caused by such factors as the method and reliability of gestational dating, race, maternal weight, and even apparently subtle differences in assay instrumentation, or changes in manufacturer's lot numbers of reagents or calibrators.[116]

Median values must be routinely monitored and updated as necessary. Median values provided in package inserts for AFP are not acceptable for many of the reasons given above. It has been recommended that median values be established using at least 100 values for 15 through 20 weeks of gestation. In practice, however, obtaining 100 serum samples for each gestational week is very difficult even for large laboratories, because most specimens are now routinely collected between 16 and 18 weeks gestation (the optimum time for open neural tube defect screening). Given these constraints, the following strategies are recommended for obtaining reliable median values, categorized according to whether a laboratory is implementing a screening test for the first time or is updating an existing set of median values.

Two alternatives are available when a laboratory is establishing median values for the first time. The optimal method is to obtain measurements on 300 to 500 patient specimens using the assay selected for screening. Establishing that all of these samples come from unaffected singleton pregnancies is not necessary because the prevalence of conditions that produce abnormal values (e.g., twins, fetal demise, and open fetal defects) is small and will have minimal impact.[150] The data are used to derive median values for each completed week of gestation. Appropriate weighted regression analysis can then be used to fit the observed data. The regression equation is used to predict "smoothed" medians for each week of gestation. Measurements of AFP and uE_3 increase by a constant proportion—about 10% to 15% per week for AFP and 20% to 25% per week for uE_3 measurements. A log-linear model best fits this relationship (i.e., the log of the measurements [y-axis] is regressed against gestational age [x-axis]). Usually the median value is found at each completed week and regressed against the average gestational age for that week. This technique helps reduce the effect of outliers. Weighting takes into account the reliability of these summary estimates and is usually based on the square root of the number of samples observed at each week. The regression model for CG versus gestational age fits an exponential model similar to that used for radioactive decay. Measurements of DIA are relatively flat, but experience has shown that a quadratic model fits the data well, with a minimum found between 16 and 18 weeks gestation. Table 54-4 provides data for these four tests along with the weighted regression equation and resulting smoothed medians. The AFP and uE_3 medians increase 11% and 23% per week, respectively. Figures 54-6 to 54-9 are graphical representations of the data in Table 54-4, and the legends contain the respective median regression equation. Although laboratories cannot use these medians to interpret their own assay results, they can use the observed median concentrations for each analyte (plus weeks and N) to verify their ability to compute regressed median concentrations.

Figure 54-10 shows the relative gestational age effects on the four tests. Each test is assigned a 100% relative value for the median at 15 completed weeks of gestation. If the median values increase, the line will have a positive slope. The test that is least influenced by gestational age is DIA. The

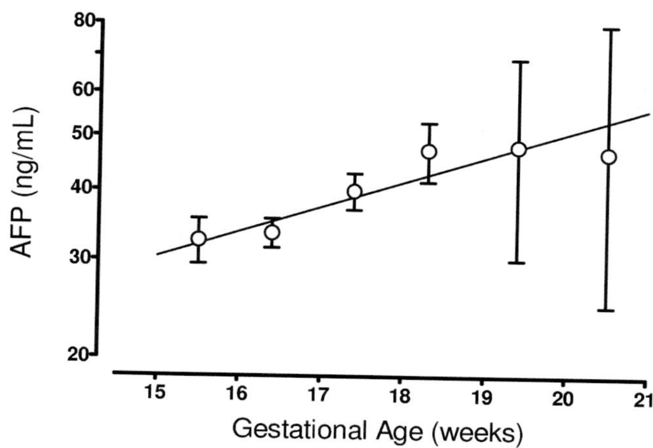

Figure 54-6 Computation of median values for maternal serum alpha fetoprotein (AFP) in the second trimester. The observed average gestational age from Table 54-4 is plotted on the horizontal axis and the median of that week's AFP measurements on the vertical logarithmic axis. The thin vertical lines represent the 95% confidence intervals of the medians. The line represents the results of a linear regression analysis of log AFP versus age weighted by the square root of the number of samples. The equation of that line in completed weeks is median $AFP = 10^{0.04465 \times (weeks) + 0.8334}$. The corresponding equation for day-specific medians is median $AFP = 10^{0.006378 \times (days) + 0.8142}$.

TABLE 54-4 Observed and Regressed Median Values for Four Second Trimester Down Syndrome Analytes

Week of Gestation	Mean GA	Number Studied	AFP (ng/mL)		uE_3 (ng/mL)		CG (IU/mL)		DIA (pg/mL)	
			Obs	Reg	Obs	Reg	Obs	Reg	Obs	Reg
15	15.5	79	32.6	31.8	0.56	0.57	34.9	35.3	175	171
16	16.4	183	33.6	35.3	0.68	0.71	28.4	27.7	164	170
17	17.4	94	40.0	39.1	0.92	0.87	23.3	22.1	179	176
18	18.3	29	47.4	43.4	1.21	1.08	15.5	17.9	191	188
19	19.4	8	48.2	48.0	1.31	1.33	17.0	14.8	210	207
20	20.5	4	47.0	53.2	1.30	1.64	13.0	12.5	227	233
Average or total	16.7	397								

GA, Gestational age; *AFP*, alpha fetoprotein; *uE_3*, unconjugated estriol; *CG*, chorionic gonadotropin; *DIA*, dimeric inhibin A; *Obs*, observed median; *Reg*, regressed median.

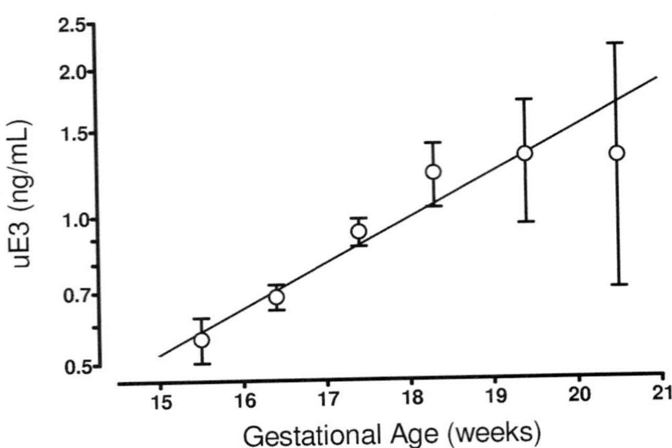

Figure 54-7 Computation of median values for maternal serum unconjugated estriol (uE_3) in the second trimester. The observed average gestational age from Table 54-4 is plotted on the horizontal axis and the median of that week's uE_3 measurements on the vertical logarithmic axis. The thin vertical lines represent the 95% confidence intervals of the medians. The line represents the results of a linear regression analysis of log uE_3 versus age weighted by the square root of the number of samples. The equation of that line in completed weeks is median $uE_3 = 10^{0.09165 \times (\text{weeks}) - 1.618}$. The corresponding equation for day-specific medians is median $uE_3 = 10^{0.01309 \times (\text{days}) - 1.657}$.

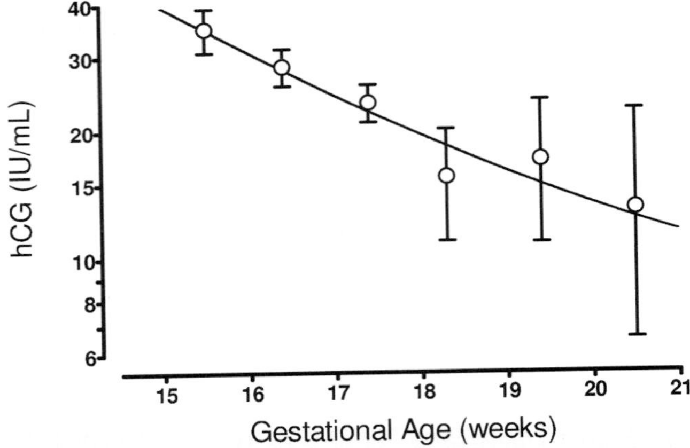

Figure 54-8 Computation of median values for maternal serum chorionic gonadotropin (CG) in the second trimester. The observed average gestational age from Table 54-4 is plotted on the horizontal axis and the median of that week's CG measurements on the vertical logarithmic axis. The thin vertical lines represent the 95% confidence intervals of the medians. The line represents the results of a nonlinear regression analysis weighted by the square root of the number of samples. The equation of that curve in completed weeks is CG median $= 39.69 \times e^{-0.3001 \times (\text{weeks}-14)} + 5.93$. The corresponding equation for day-specific medians is CG median $= 45.14 \times e^{-0.04287 \times (\text{days})} + 5.93$.

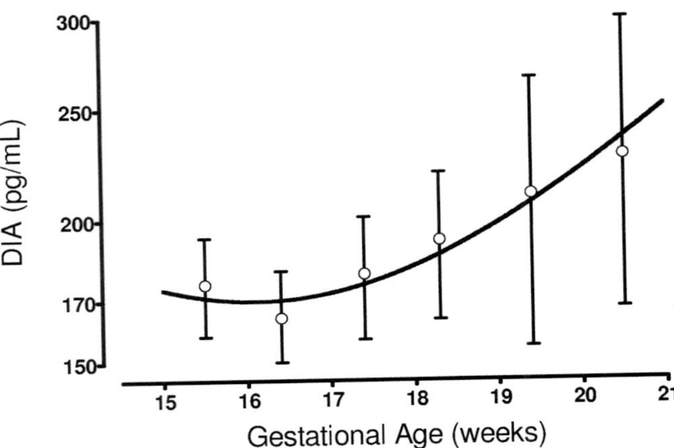

Figure 54-9 Computation of median values for maternal serum dimeric inhibin A (DIA) in the second trimester. The observed average gestational age from Table 54-4 is plotted on the horizontal axis and the median of that week's DIA measurements on the vertical logarithmic axis. The thin vertical lines represent the 95% confidence intervals of the medians. The line represents the results of a quadratic regression analysis weighted by the square root of the number of samples. The equation of that curve in completed weeks is DIA median $= 3.404 \times \text{weeks}^2 - 106.7 \times \text{weeks} + 1005.7$. The corresponding equation for day-specific medians is DIA median $= 0.06947 \times \text{days}^2 - 15.66 \times \text{days} + 1052$.

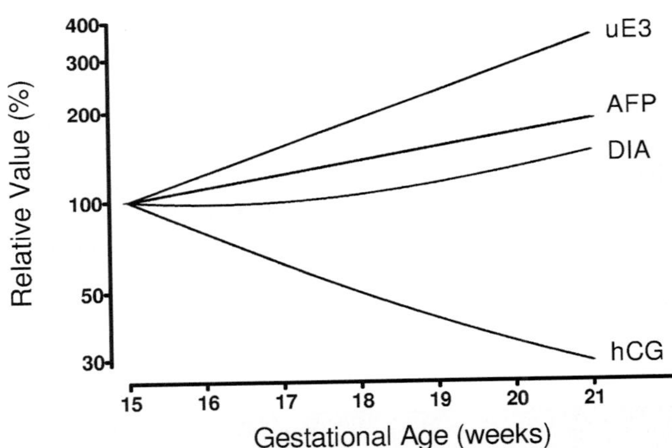

Figure 54-10 A comparison of the associations between gestational age and the four second trimester maternal serum markers for Down syndrome. For each of the analytes, the median at 15 weeks gestation has been assigned a value of 100%. Each subsequent median is represented as a percentage of that initial median. The marker that has the weakest association with gestational age is dimeric inhibin A (DIA). The strongest associations are found for unconjugated estriol (uE_3) and chorionic gonadotropin (CG). The association between gestational age and alpha fetoprotein (AFP) is intermediate.

TABLE 54-5 Observed and Regressed Day-Specific Medians for Unconjugated Estriol During the 17th Week of Gestation

Gestational Age (Week, day)	Number of Observations	uE_3 (ng/mL) Observed	Regressed
16,0	195	0.67	0.68
16,1	225	0.69	0.70
16,2	228	0.71	0.72
16,3	219	0.76	0.74
16,4	186	0.78	0.76
16,5	191	0.80	0.79
16,6	175	0.78	0.81

strongest association with gestational age is found for uE_3 and CG measurements. This association indicates that errors in dating will have the greatest impact on these two tests.

Some laboratories use "day-specific" medians rather than weekly medians (i.e., a different median value is used for each day of pregnancy). Although individual pregnancies cannot be reliably dated to within 1 day, there is a consistent day-by-day change in analyte concentrations if a group of pregnant women is observed. Table 54-5 shows the observed and regressed medians for uE_3 for a group of ultrasound-dated women in their 17th week of gestation. The observed median levels clearly increase during that week. The regressed median for 16 weeks, 0 days, is quite different from the median for 16 weeks, 6 days. If weekly medians were to have been used instead, all of these samples would have been interpreted against a single median—about 0.74 ng/mL (0.74 μg/L).

The second method is an acceptable alternative. The laboratory must identify an established laboratory that is willing to share its reliable median values. Then, 25 to 50 specimens are assayed at each laboratory. These specimens are selected so that their results span the analytical measurement range. The two sets of values can then be compared using linear regression analysis (after appropriate transformations) to establish the relationship between the two assays. The regression equation can then be applied to the reliable set of median values to derive a set of medians appropriate for the laboratory. These median values can be used temporarily until values from 300 to 500 patients are available for the analysis provided earlier.

Laboratories must update existing median values in several situations. Significant differences in values on the same patient specimens are common when using either a new lot of the reagents or reagents from a different manufacturer. In this situation, the relationship between the new and old methods can be established by regression analysis of values measured on the same patient specimens as described in the second method in the previous paragraph. If a periodic adjustment is required, the laboratory should carefully choose the characteristics of the population to be used (e.g., race, method of dating, and time period) and verify that the assay has been providing consistent results over the time period of interest. This can be done by routinely monitoring the median MoM over time (epidemiological monitoring) as discussed in more detail later in this chapter. The resulting data are then analyzed as indicated in the first method described previously.

Adjustments for Factors That Influence Analyte Measurements

Prenatal screening for both open neural tube defects and Down syndrome is optimized when each woman's analyte concentration is compared with other women (the reference group) who are "similar" to her in many respects.[151] In addition to gestational age, this "similarity" extends to other factors that have been shown to affect the analyte concentrations, including maternal weight, race, insulin-dependent diabetes (IDD), and multiple pregnancy. Taking into account these factors increases the accuracy of the interpretation. These factors are taken into account by dividing the patient's MoM value by a factor corresponding to the ratio of the MoM values found in those without the factor to the MoM values in those with the factor. A meta-analysis of the data supporting the following recommendations has been published.[151]

Maternal Weight

As maternal weight increases, the average concentration of analyte values decreases, perhaps because a fixed amount of analyte is diluted in an increased maternal blood volume. For example, heavier women have, on average, lower AFP values and are less likely than lighter weight women to be screen-positive for neural tube defects. Without taking maternal weight into account, screening is less effective in heavier women because their MoM values are inappropriately low. The importance of adjusting AFP MoM values for weight is reinforced by recent studies showing that heavier women have a twofold to threefold increased risk for open spina bifida.[339] The weight effect is also significant for CG and DIA, but less so for uE_3 (Figure 54-11). Maternal weight is taken

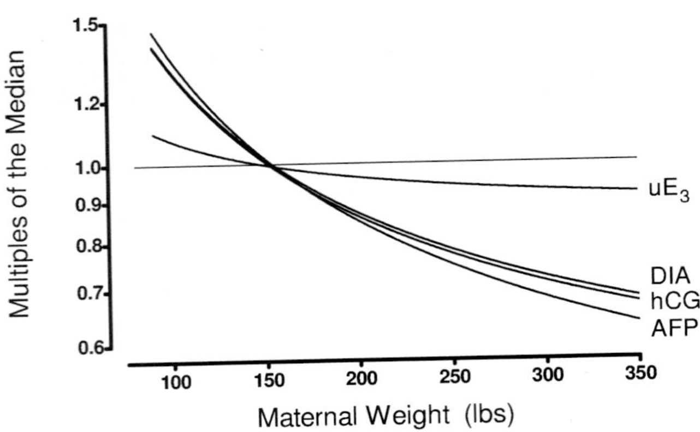

Figure 54-11 The relationship of AFP, uE_3, CG, and DIA (expressed as multiples of the median [MoM]) and maternal weight. The horizontal line at 1.0 MoM is the value found for a woman of average weight.

into account by adjusting each woman's MoM values by a factor corresponding to the expected MoM value in Figure 54-11 for average women with her weight. These factors are empirically derived from the screened population in a manner that is similar to deriving median analyte concentrations for each gestational age. Optimally, each laboratory should derive its own maternal weight adjustment factors for each analyte, because the average maternal weight may differ from that seen in other laboratories. These adjustment factors should be applied only over the maternal weight range in which they have been shown to be appropriate. For example, if few or no data are available to derive adjustment factors for women weighing more than 350 pounds, then the laboratory should be careful in extrapolating factors to these women from data on women of lower weight. Laboratories should limit the range of adjustment using upper (and lower) truncation limits. If a woman's weight is outside these limits, adjustment should be applied as if the woman were at the respective limit. An effective model for all analytes is a linear reciprocal model. Maternal weights are stratified into weight groups and regressed against the reciprocal of maternal weight. This model and its application have been described in detail elsewhere.[151,233] Although not routine, some screening programs have implemented separate weight adjustments for selected racial groups because of systematic differences in maternal weight. Although this would theoretically improve performance, there is little evidence that the increased complexity and propensity for error are warranted. Obesity is associated with a threefold to fourfold increase in risk for open neural tube defects.[290,339] There is no reported association between maternal weight and Down syndrome.

Maternal Race

African-American women have maternal serum AFP and CG concentrations that are 10% to 15% higher than those found in Caucasian women.[151] Adjustment for this difference can be accomplished in two ways. The first approach is to calculate an MoM value for African-American women using medians derived from the Caucasian population, and then to divide the resulting MoM by a factor corresponding to the ratio between values in the two populations (i.e., 1.10 to 1.15). For example, if an African-American woman has a maternal serum AFP MoM of 1.60 calculated using median values from the Caucasian population, her adjusted MoM is 1.45 (1.60 ÷ 1.10). The second approach is to calculate a separate set of medians using values measured on the African-American population. uE_3 and DIA do not appear to differ in these two populations. Only limited data are available for other racial/ethnic groups and therefore routine adjustments are not generally performed. Although there is little evidence that the age-specific birth prevalence of Down syndrome differs by race, there is strong evidence that the birth prevalence of open neural tube defects in African-American women is half or less that of Caucasian women from the same geographic region.[142A] Thus at any given maternal serum AFP MoM, an African-American woman has half the risk of a Caucasian woman of having a pregnancy affected by an open neural tube defect. Some programs have addressed this "disparity" by moving the cutoff higher for African-American women. For example, the risk for the Caucasian woman at 2.0 MoM is similar to that for the African-American woman at 2.5 MoM. However, programs that do this must acknowledge that the detection rate (and false-positive rate) will be lower in the population with the higher screening cutoff. Limited information is available on the AFP concentrations in African-American women with an open neural tube defect, but what is published indicates that screening in this population should be equally effective.

Insulin-Dependent Diabetes

Maternal serum AFP values in women who have IDD before pregnancy have been reported to be systematically lower by about 20%.[151] This difference is taken into account by dividing the computed MoM value in women with IDD by 0.8, the ratio of maternal serum AFP values found in the two populations. After adjustment, the proportion of women with IDD at or above any given MoM cutoff should be approximately equal to that found in the general population. It is not possible to define the associated detection rate for open neural tube defects because no large series of maternal serum AFP measurements in IDD women with a fetus affected with an open neural tube defect have been published. In a recent study, the expected lowering of maternal serum AFP concentrations in pregnant women with IDD was not observed.[284] Because these women are now carefully monitored to help ensure appropriate blood glucose concentrations, it is speculated that this tight control might account for the finding of no effect.

It has been recommended that in locations where women with IDD are carefully monitored to maintain glucose control, adjustment of maternal serum AFP is no longer warranted.[284] This recommendation poses a dilemma for screening laboratories. In the absence of this detailed patient information, the screening program must determine whether or not routine adjustment of maternal serum AFP levels for IDD status is warranted.

There is no compelling evidence that the rate of Down syndrome births in women with IDD is substantially different from that in the general population.[172] However, there is evidence that birth prevalence of open neural tube defects is higher by up to a factor of 5.[1] Thus at a given AFP MoM concentration, women with IDD are at a substantially higher risk of open neural tube defects than the general population. This can be taken into account by lowering the AFP MoM cutoff from, for example, 2.0 to 1.5.

Current information suggests that maternal serum AFP concentrations are not altered among women with gestational diabetes, even if insulin is subsequently required later in pregnancy.

In women with IDD, uE_3 and CG MoMs are on average 8% and 7% lower, respectively, than in nondiabetic women.[151] These differences are small, and whether or not they are taken into account will have little impact on the resulting Down syndrome risk. The impact of IDD on DIA results is more variable, ranging from 0.91 MoM to 1.17 MoM (weighted average of 1.06 MoM), and adjustment is not yet warranted.[337A]

Twin Pregnancy and Open Neural Tube Defect

Maternal serum AFP concentrations in twin pregnancies are about twice the concentration found in singleton pregnancies (i.e., 2.0 MoM).[151] Among singleton pregnancies with open spina bifida, the median serum AFP MoM is about 3.5.[330] Thus the expected maternal serum AFP in the average twin pregnancy affected with open spina bifida might be around 4.5 MoM (1.0 MoM contributed by the unaffected fetus and 3.5 MoM from the fetus with open spina bifida). Screening performance in twin pregnancies will therefore not be as effective as in singleton pregnancies since the AFP distributions are less separated. Although most affected twin pregnancies are discordant for open neural tube defects, if both twins are affected (seen in about 5% of affected twin pregnancies), screening performance can be expected to approach that in singleton pregnancies.

Twin Pregnancy and Down Syndrome Screening

Calculation of Down syndrome risk requires that the distribution of analyte values for all tests in both unaffected and affected pregnancies be known. These distributions are well defined for AFP, uE_3, CG, and DIA in singleton pregnancies, and thus reliable risks can be calculated. The distributions of these analytes also are available for twin pregnancy unaffected by Down syndrome; the average MoMs in unaffected twin pregnancy for AFP, uE_3, CG, and DIA are about 2.0, 1.7, 1.9, and 2.0, respectively.[151] Fewer data are available for concentrations of these analytes in twin pregnancies affected with Down syndrome. A further complication is that in approximately one third of pregnancies, both twins will be affected (monozygotic), and in two thirds of pregnancies, only one twin will be affected (dizygotic). Screening will be less effective when only one twin is affected. Another difficulty is that the prevalence of Down syndrome is not well defined in twin pregnancies. Based on the rate of monozygotic and dizygotic twins, the prevalence of Down syndrome would be predicted to be 1.67 times higher in twin pregnancies. Published data indicate that the prevalence in twin pregnancies is actually similar to that found in singleton pregnancies.[110]

Given these limitations, calculation of only an approximate risk (sometimes called a pseudorisk) for twin pregnancy is possible.[234] This is accomplished by dividing the MoM value for each analyte by the corresponding average found in the unaffected twin pregnancy. The twin pregnancy risk is computed in the same way as for singleton pregnancies. The same risk cutoff used to identify women with singleton pregnancies is used to identify women with twin pregnancies as being screen positive.

This twin screening protocol will: (1) correctly rank the pregnancies from highest to lowest risk, and (2) yield a screen-positive rate similar to the rate found for singleton pregnancies at any given screening cutoff. The Down syndrome pseudorisk, however, may not be correct, and it is recommended that this risk not be routinely reported. Screen-positive women with twin pregnancies can be informed that their test results place them in a high-risk group, but that their actual risk is uncertain. Interpretation of risk for triplets and higher gestations is not recommended because of the limited data available. Additional factors that need to be considered when offering such screening are the increased difficulty and fetal loss associated with multiple needle insertions necessary during amniocentesis, and the loss of the unaffected twin should an affected twin be identified and selectively terminated.[117]

Other Tests and Combinations of Tests

Several other maternal serum analytes have been reported to be associated with Down syndrome in second trimester maternal serum, including the free alpha and free beta subunits of CG[44,210,333] and β1-glycoprotein[29] and DIA.[154,344] Of these, only DIA has been shown to provide any significant advantage in combination with the triple test. Two analytes found in maternal urine have been investigated as tests for Down syndrome screening. Early studies reported that urinary gonadotropin peptide, a metabolite of CG, had the best screening performance of any proposed test (80% for a 5% false-positive rate).[60,87] These early studies have not been confirmed.[88,170] Attention has now turned to another urinary analyte, invasive trophoblast antigen or ITA (also called hyperglycosylated CG). One study reported a detection rate of 79% for a 5% false-positive rate,[73] while another reported less favorable results.[89] A recent retrospective study concluded that serum ITA could effectively replace CG or free CGβ in a multianalyte panel.[252] A large prospective study is currently underway to determine the screening performance in routine practice.

Down Syndrome Screening in the First Trimester of Pregnancy

Most screening programs recommend testing mothers between 16 and 18 weeks gestation, but will accept specimens collected from 15 to 20 weeks or later. Screening pregnancies after 20 weeks gestation allows little time for further testing and increases the difficulty of decision-making for the couple. Attention is now being focused on moving Down syndrome screening to the first trimester of pregnancy (at 10 to 13 weeks of gestation). Both ultrasound findings and serum tests have been identified for first trimester application. First trimester values of maternal serum pregnancy associated plasma protein-A (PAPP-A) are low and free CGβ values elevated in cases of Down syndrome.[126] In combination with maternal age, these two serum tests yield a detection rate of 60% at a 5% false-positive rate.[155] This screening performance is inferior to quadruple test screening in the second trimester.[154] Ultrasound measurements of nuchal translucency (NT), the subcutaneous space between the skin and cervical spine, have been shown to be increased in fetuses with Down syndrome.[237,307] Increased NT measurements are also a nonspecific finding for many fetal structural abnormalities, and therefore are only useful as a screening test.[248] NT measurements alone can detect 60% or more of the Down syndrome cases at a 5% screen positive rate, making NT the best single screening test described to date.[335]

Neither ultrasound findings nor serum tests in the first trimester have sufficient predictive power to be used alone. In 1997, it was estimated that a combination of NT and serum tests (the combined test) could detect 85% of Down syndrome at a 5% false-positive rate. If confirmed, this would be the best Down syndrome screening test available.[335] The combined test is widely available in Europe and is being increasingly offered in the United States. Although first trimester screening would have obvious advantages, it also has limitations. To be reliable, NT measurements must be performed at specialized referral centers that employ sonographers who have undergone rigorous training and participate in on-going quality control programs. Routine office ultrasound is unsuitable for obtaining this measurement. Therefore access for women in rural areas will be limited. If first trimester diagnostic testing is to be performed, it will have to include chorionic villus sampling (CVS). CVS is less safe than amniocentesis performed in the second trimester of pregnancy,[58] and may not be readily available. Several studies have shown that Down syndrome fetuses with increased NT and low PAPP-A are spontaneously aborted at a higher rate than for those with normal NT measurements.[248] Thus the real screening performance may be lower than expected,[86,90] and many Down syndrome fetuses identified in the first trimester will spontaneously abort in the absence of screening. If screening for Down syndrome were to be moved to the first trimester, routine screening for open neural tube defects using maternal serum AFP would still need to be performed, as such screening is not effective in the first trimester.[330,334] Lastly, NT measurements are likely to be expensive in the United States, as first trimester ultrasound examinations are not routine, and third party payers may be reluctant to pay. Despite these shortcomings, first trimester screening is a recommended option on the condition that appropriate diagnostic testing is available locally.[6]

Combining First and Second Trimester Screening into a Single Integrated Test

An innovative approach to combining the best of the first and second trimester tests has been proposed that avoids most of the limitations of stand-alone first trimester screening—the integrated test.[338] With this approach, measurements of NT and PAPP-A are made in the first trimester but not interpreted or acted upon until the second trimester. In the second trimester, a second serum is drawn and a quadruple test performed. Results from all six tests (NT, PAPP-A, AFP, uE_3, CG, and DIA) are combined into a single risk estimate for interpretation in the second trimester. It is projected that this approach could detect 85% of Down syndrome cases with only a 1% false-positive rate. A recent study (SURUSS) involving results from 47,507 pregnancies at multiple centers obtained results consistent with this estimate.[337]

Reporting Individual Results

The maternal serum screening report should contain the following information: the concentrations and MoM values of the measured analytes, the Down syndrome risk estimate (along with risks for other abnormalities such as trisomy 18), an interpretation as either screen-positive or screen-negative, and an interpretation of the information that includes possible further actions. The physician-provided information should include specimen collection date, identification as a first or second specimen, date of LMP or gestational age by ultrasound, maternal birth date (or age), relevant family history, number of fetuses (if known), maternal race, and the presence or absence of maternal diabetes requiring insulin therapy.

Calculating Individualized Patient-Specific Risks With Use of Biochemical Measurements

Calculating an individualized risk (patient-specific risk) for any given condition is accomplished by multiplying the *a priori* risk for that condition by a likelihood ratio that is calculated using the woman's analyte measurements (i.e., patient risk = *a priori* risk × likelihood ratio). This basic equation is used to calculate patient-specific risk for neural tube defects, Down syndrome, trisomy 18, or any other condition in which the distributions of tests for the unaffected and affected population have been defined. The *a priori* risk is obtained from large epidemiological studies that ascertain the prevalence for the condition under consideration. For example, a woman's age is used to define her *a priori* risk for having a fetus with Down syndrome. The likelihood ratio is determined by calculating the ratio of the heights of the affected and unaffected overlapping population distributions for any specified MoM value. When multiple tests are used, a single likelihood ratio is calculated using the overlapping distributions for each test but with the correlation between the tests taken into account. Complete details for calculating risks are available on this book's accompanying Evolve Web site, found at http://evolve.elsevier.com/Tietz/textbook/.*

Use of Epidemiological Monitoring in Quality Control

In prenatal screening the interpretative unit for each analyte is the MoM, which takes into account variables such as gestational age, maternal weight, race, and IDD. Expressing these results in MoMs allows the calculation of a patient-specific risk for Down syndrome. One of the most common causes of poor laboratory performance is the use of incorrect median values, either because those values are inappropriate for the kit being used or because systematic shifts in the assay values have occurred. Poor performance can also occur when a kit is nonspecific or relatively inaccurate. Ensuring that median values (and by extension the MoM values) are accurate is one of the most important responsibilities of the screening laboratory. The following discussions are adapted from Knight and Palomaki,[184] a publication that discusses in detail the process of epidemiological monitoring.

Definition of Epidemiologic Monitoring

A powerful method for evaluating and monitoring the appropriateness of medians is epidemiologic monitoring. This process involves gathering data from the screened population to allow calculation of the detection rate (proportion of affected pregnancies with positive test results) and the false-positive rates (proportion of unaffected pregnancies with a positive test result). These rates can then be compared with expectations. Obtaining a detection rate is difficult because complete ascertainment of all pregnancy outcomes is required, and it can take years before a sufficient number of affected pregnancies occurs to achieve reliable estimates. In practice, the false-positive rate is used for epidemiologic monitoring because a reliable estimate can be calculated in a short time and it is not necessary to have outcome information. For prenatal screening, the false-positive rate is defined as the proportion of women with test results falling at or above a specified AFP MoM (for open neural tube defect screening), or with a Down syndrome risk at or above the specified risk cutoff (Down syndrome screening). However, these rates are not actually false-positive rates, because a few of the screen-positive individuals are actually true-, rather than false-, positive results (i.e., they do have an affected fetus). For this reason, the term initial positive rate (IPR) has been suggested, because it more accurately describes what is being calculated. The IPR can be used to assess whether medians are appropriate, since it will be shifted upward or downward if medians are incorrect for the population being screened. Further, once the IPR is shown to be within acceptable limits, continuous monitoring can help detect shifts in assay values.

Epidemiologic Monitoring of Open Neural Tube Defect Screening

In maternal serum AFP screening for open neural tube defects, the IPR is the proportion of women with values above the specified MoM cutoff. For most screening programs, the two most commonly used screening cutoffs are 2.0 and 2.5 MoM; these cutoffs produce IPRs of 3% to 5% and 1% to 3%, respectively. When new medians are implemented, the IPR can be used to determine if the medians are appropriate by comparing the expected with the actual IPRs. If the IPR falls outside the expected range, it is possible that the medians are incorrect for the assay being used or for the population being screened (assuming that the AFP assay is known to be reliable). For example, if the IPR at a cutoff of 2.5 MoM is 5%, median values may be too low. Thus more women will have results above the 2.5 MoM cutoff.

Once the IPR is shown to be within an acceptable range, ongoing monitoring of this rate serves as a check on shifts in assay calibration caused by changes in kit lots, reagent deterioration, poor technical performance, and other factors. Simultaneous monitoring of the IPR and the results of quality control samples can facilitate identification of shifts in assay values. If, for instance, the IPR at a 2.5 AFP MoM cutoff increases from 2% to 4%, and at the same time some or all of the values of quality control (QC) samples shift significantly upward by 10% or more, the change is consistent with an upward shift in assay calibration. The IPR increases when the assay values increase because individual AFP values are interpreted by using medians generated from data gathered in the past. In the example given above, it may be necessary to calculate new medians or adjust existing median values to take into account the assay shift.

It is difficult to provide an absolute rule as to how large a change in the IPR is sufficient to warrant recomputing medians as factors other than the assay can affect the IPR. For example, a significant increase in the number of pregnancies dated by ultrasound will reduce the IPR, because incorrectly dated pregnancies will be identified before the AFP test is done. However, consider that an upward shift in AFP values of just 10% can increase the IPR by more than 50% (e.g., from 2% to 3%) with little gain in detection. In effect, more interventions (ultrasound examinations or amniocenteses or both) will be required to detect each case of neural tube defect. Therefore if a change in the IPR of 50% or more occurs simultaneously with an identifiable shift in assay values of 10% or more, medians need to be recalcu-

*References 86A, 91A, 116A, 150A, 160A, 184A, 225A, 239A, 271A, 332A, 332B, 333A, 335A.

lated. Laboratories may wish to have stricter warning limits (e.g., shifts of 25% or more in the IPR occurring simultaneously with a change of 7% or more in quality control samples). In applying these rules, enough values should be used to ensure that a reliable IPR can be calculated (generally 300 to 500 values will ensure reliability) and that observed changes are statistically significant. Further the change should be persistent and occur over several kit lots. Otherwise the laboratory may be tracking random error. IPR values can also be calculated using a moving window to improve reliability. For example, consider a laboratory that screens 300 women per month. In addition to calculating a monthly IPR, the lab could calculate a cumulative 3-month moving window (i.e., each month, the current month's data are added and the oldest month is dropped). The actual time period for both the individual and a cumulative moving window will be determined by how many samples are screened per unit time by any given laboratory.

Epidemiological Monitoring of Down Syndrome Screening

In screening for Down syndrome, the IPR is the proportion of women with a risk at or above the risk cutoff. In contrast to neural tube defect screening, the IPR for Down syndrome screening is influenced by each of the analytes used in the risk calculation. Therefore monitoring the IPR does not provide information on which assay(s) might be responsible when an inappropriate IPR is obtained. Consequently, it is necessary to individually monitor each assay separately. Individual monitoring of each assay can be accomplished according to the following rationale. When individual MoM values are calculated for each patient using gestational age–specific medians, MoM values can be analyzed collectively without regard for the gestational week. If the medians are appropriate, the resulting distribution of MoM values will have a grand median MoM of 1.00. The center of the distribution is typically expressed as the median, rather than as the mean, because MoM distributions are not Gaussian on the linear scale.

The initial application of the grand MoM is to ensure that when medians are first implemented they are appropriate for the assay and population being screened. This is accomplished by calculating the grand MoM using values from 300 to 500 individuals screened after the new set of medians is implemented. The grand MoM should be 1.00, within statistical limits. A convenient approach is to plot the grand MoM values on a graph, facilitating the detection of trends. The IPR observations can also be plotted on the same graph. If the IPR begins to trend in either a positive or negative direction, the grand MoM for each assay can be examined to determine if one of the analytes is paralleling the IPR change. If a significant change in one of the assays has occurred, corrective action should be taken (e.g., recalculating medians). For example, suppose the IPR shows a significant upward trend (e.g., from 6% to 9%), and over the same time period the median MoM of the uE_3 assay significantly decreases (e.g., from 1.03 to 0.91). Since decreasing uE_3 values are associated with increasing risk for fetal Down syndrome, it is possible that the change in the uE_3 assay is responsible for the increase in the IPR. The next step would be to examine quality control specimen values to determine if a corresponding downward shift in values has occurred. If a shift has occurred, it may be necessary to recalculate and implement a new set of uE_3 medians using data collected after the time when the change in the uE_3 assay occurred (or apply an adjustment factor to the old medians). A simultaneous change in two assays can complicate monitoring, because the IPR might not change if the shift in one analyte value increases risk and the other analyte decreases risk. Simultaneous monitoring is therefore recommended of the IPR and the median MoM for each analyte. When interpreting median MoM values, rates should be calculated only when enough patient values are available (typically, 300 to 500 samples) to ensure a statistically reliable rate. Further, a single IPR or median MoM that deviates from the expected one should serve as only a warning to examine quality control data more closely.

Laboratories need to have an action limit in place to determine how much variability is to be allowed in the grand MoM. To do this, consider the impact on the Down syndrome detection rate and the IPR of a 10% downward shift in the uE_3 values (grand MoM of 0.90). This can be simulated by recalculating MoM values after assay values are artificially shifted down by 10%, followed by mathematical modeling of the detection rate and associated IPR. Such an assay shift effectively changes the MoM for any given sample, because current assay values are interpreted using reference data collected in the past. When uE_3 values shift downward by 10%, the detection rate increases only slightly from 59% to 62%. However, the IPR increases from 4.8% to 6.7%, a 40% increase. Thus what might be viewed as a small shift in assay values has a large impact on the IPR, with little corresponding gain in detection. Similar but somewhat smaller effects are seen when considering similar shifts in AFP and CG measurements. The relatively large changes in the IPR with relatively small shifts in assay values are some of the primary reasons for closely monitoring assays to ensure that the amniocentesis referral rate is maintained within reasonable limits. Given these facts, screening laboratories should consider, as a minimum, a consistent deviation of 10% from 1.00 MoM (range 0.90 to 1.10) as important. Laboratories may wish to consider setting up more strict warning limits, such as 7% (assuming this percentage is based on sufficient numbers of samples to yield statistically significant results). With this limit, median MoM values outside the range of 0.93 to 1.07 MoM would be considered sufficiently deviate to warrant further investigation to determine if a problem exists.

Although the IPR for laboratories screening for Down syndrome using multiple tests is generally between 5% and 10% in an unselected pregnancy population, it may be affected by various factors (other than incorrect medians), including the number of tests used, the screening cutoff chosen, and the maternal age distribution of the screened population. For example, if screening is being applied primarily to older women, the IPR will be substantially higher because older women are collectively more likely to be screen-positive because of their higher age-specific risks. For example, if the triple test is being used to screen women of age 35 and older at a term risk cutoff of 1 : 250, approximately 25% of women will be screen-positive.[153] The method of gestational dating will also affect the IPR. Laboratories with a high percentage of pregnancies dated by the first day of the LMP will have a higher IPR than do laboratories where most gestational ages have been provided from ultrasound measurements.[149]

External Proficiency Testing

All laboratories performing prenatal screening must participate in an external proficiency testing program that distributes unknown specimens that reflect the concentrations of analytes found near the middle of the second trimester of pregnancy. These programs also evaluate the laboratory's ability to convert analyte values into an MoM using the laboratory's own median values, to make screening recommendations, to adjust for variables that influence analyte values, and to calculate patient-specific risks. Two such external proficiency testing programs for prenatal screening are currently available in the United States. The Foundation for Blood Research and the CAP sponsor a joint program (FBR/CAP Maternal Screening Survey FP) serving approximately 300 laboratories. Five serum and two amniotic fluid proficiency samples are distributed three times each year. The FBR/CAP program also has a special topic in each distribution that allows FP Survey participants to obtain CME/CEU credits. New York State also has an external proficiency testing program that is required for laboratories serving New York State residents. Five serum and five amniotic fluid samples are distributed three times each year. Neither survey includes first trimester serum tests (free beta CG and PAPP-A). The Foundation for Blood Research also sponsors an amniotic fluid AFP/AChE proficiency testing program for diagnostic laboratories. Five amniotic fluid samples are distributed three times each year.

LABORATORY TESTS

In this section of the chapter, we review methods for measurements of CG, AFP, uE_3, DIA, fetal fibronectin, and amniotic fluid bilirubin, and six tests for fetal lung maturity.

CHORIONIC GONADOTROPIN

Measurement of CG can be used to detect pregnancy and its abnormalities (e.g., ectopic and molar pregnancies), to screen for Down syndrome and trisomy 18, and to monitor the course of a patient with a CG-producing cancer. Because CG has these diverse uses, many assays are used, including qualitative urine and serum kits and quantitative serum assays. Cole has published reviews of CG methods.[72,77]

This hormone is commonly called "human chorionic gonadotropin" and often abbreviated hCG or HCG. This term and its abbreviations should be abandoned because the adjective "human" is superfluous.[229] Nonetheless, when communicating with clinicians (at least in the United States), hCG is the preferable term to avoid misunderstanding.

Chemistry

CG is a glycoprotein containing a protein core with branched carbohydrate side chains that usually terminate with sialic acid. The hormone is a heterodimer composed of two nonidentical, noncovalently bound glycoprotein subunits, alpha (α) and beta (β). When the CG dimer is dissociated, the hormone activity is lost. However, a major part of the original activity is restored by equimolar recombination of the two subunits.

The CG carbohydrate composition changes as pregnancy progresses. At the time of implantation in normal pregnancies, more than 80% of immunoreactive CG is a large molecular mass form (Mr 41,000 to 42,000) called hyperglycosylated CG (H-CG).[240] Later in pregnancy, a 36,000 to 37,000 molecular mass form predominates. The CGα subunit contains 92 amino acids, two carbohydrate side chains, and five disulfide bridges. The molecular weight of the α-subunit is estimated to be 14,900 of which 10,200 is the protein component. CGβ consists of 145 amino acids and has six carbohydrate side chains and six disulfide bridges. The molecular mass of CGβ is estimated to be 23,000. Thus the heterodimer has a molecular weight of approximately 37,900 and has a higher carbohydrate proportion than any other human hormone.

In maternal serum, CG can be in many forms, including unmodified CG dimer with differing oligosaccharides and forms modified by varying degrees of degradation. In a normal pregnancy, differences in oligosaccharides produce seven charge isomers with isoelectric points from pH 3.8 to pH 4.7.[75] Serum enzymes cleave peptide bonds in CGβ at position 44-45 (and, after prolonged incubation, at 51-52) to form nicked CG (CGn).[180] The nicking inactivates the hormone and also reduces ability to bind some CG antibodies. Other nicking sites are at β44-45, β47-48, and α70-71.[42,229] Both free CGα (fCGα) and free CGβ (fCGβ) are found in the serum, along with nicked free forms (e.g., fCGβn). In the second trimester, more than 99% of CG is the dimer form; only a small amount circulates as free β-subunit.[152] The C-terminal portion of fCGβ can be cleaved to create a core fragment of CGβ (CGβcf), which is composed of two pieces of the β-subunit, residues 6-40 and residues 55-92, held together by disulfide bridges.[41] CGβcf has a molecular mass of 13,000.

Urine contains predominantly CGβcf and to a lesser degree unmodified CG and CGn. Clearance occurs both in the liver and through the kidneys and varies for the different CG forms. Hepatic clearance[342] is approximately 2 mL/min/m^2, and renal clearance is approximately 0.4 mL/min/m^2; thus early morning urine specimens have CG concentrations comparable with those in serum. A study using highly specific immunoassays for CG, CGβ, and CGα found that the disappearance after term pregnancy was triphasic.[188] The rapid, medium, and slow half-lives were, respectively: CG, 3.6, 18, and 53 hours; CGβ, 1.0, 23, and 194 hours; and CGα, 0.63, 6, and 22 hours.

Biochemistry

CG is synthesized in the syncytiotrophoblast cells of the placenta. Minute amounts are also made in the pituitary of men and nonpregnant women, and, like many other pituitary hormones, it is secreted in a pulsatile fashion.[242] A single gene located on chromosome 6 encodes the α-subunit of all four glycoprotein hormones (TSH, LH, FSH, and CG). Chromosome 19 contains a family of seven genes that encode the CGβ subunit, though only three appear to be active.[265] Separate messenger RNAs are transcribed from the respective genes, and the α- and β-subunits are translated from each. The subunits spontaneously combine in the rough endoplasmic reticulum and are then continuously secreted into the maternal circulation.

Synthesis of CGβ peaks at about 8 to 10 weeks, but production of the α-subunit continues to increase and appears to be a function of the mass of the placenta. The production of CGβ in the syncytiotrophoblasts may be under paracrine control of gonadotropin-releasing hormone (GnRH) produced in cytotrophoblasts. Studies suggest that the cytotrophoblasts produce inhibin, which stimulates CG production.[257] The number of cytotrophoblasts peaks at about the same time the CGβ production peaks.

Extensive homology exists between the peptide portions of CGβ and LHβ subunits. Investigators have proposed that a single deletion in the ancestral LHβ gene lengthened the subunit from 115 amino acids to 145 amino acids; 80% of the first 115 amino acids in both β-subunits are identical, but 20 additional amino acid residues are unique in CGβ.[310]

Physiology

CG stimulates the corpus luteum in the ovary to make progesterone during the first weeks of pregnancy. The placenta makes inadequate amounts of progesterone during this time. No specific receptor for CG is known; it binds to and activates the LH receptor in cells of the corpus luteum in the maternal ovary. Species other than primates and horses use LH for this function. The glycation of the α-subunit has a dominant role[283] in signal transduction, an increase in intracellular cyclic adenosine monophosphate (cAMP). The cAMP increase in turn stimulates the production of progesterone, a steroid that prevents menses and thus facilitates the pregnancy. CG binds weakly to TSH receptors in the maternal thyroid; thus CG concentrations greater than 1 million IU/L are thyrotropic.

CG Assays

Many assay techniques have been used for determining CG. All modern techniques use immunoassay. Vaitukaitis and colleagues took advantage of the uniqueness of CGβ to produce the first specific assay for CG, which used polyclonal antibodies raised against the β-subunit.[323] Since then, highly specific monoclonal antibodies have been produced that recognize only epitopes on the last 30 amino acid residues of the CGβ. Many of these have low affinity. Highly specific monoclonal antibodies having high affinity have been produced that bind to unique epitopes in the first 115 amino acids.[59] These antibodies are the most frequently used in assays that measure CG.

Bioassays, receptor assays, and agglutination inhibition assays are obsolete for detecting pregnancy. The historical bioassays are interesting because they exploit the physiological effect of CG. A further discussion of bioassay[66,68,114,286] and agglutination inhibition assays[313] is available on the Evolve site that accompanies this book.

Qualitative CG Tests

In the United States, about 30 urine or serum point-of-care CG tests and 25 home tests are available. The FDA web site[321] lists the products under device codes LCX, DHA, JHI, JHJ, and LFS.

Home test kit assays are the most commonly used pregnancy tests in the United States. Purchased without a prescription, these tests are simple and can be performed by a woman in the privacy of the home. One third of females who suspect they may be pregnant use home kits.[173] Most kits provide a single test and use an enzyme immunometric or immunochromatographic strategy to measure urine CG. Butler et al[56] have evaluated 15 home pregnancy tests. Detection limits vary from 6.3 to 50 IU/L,[56] although the manufacturers' claims vary from 25 to 100 IU/L. The tests require from 1 to 5 minutes to perform. Some poorly detect H-CG (ITA), which makes them less sensitive tests of early pregnancy.

Although the techniques used are straightforward, consumers do make more mistakes performing these tests than do trained laboratory professionals.[164] An extensive evaluation[102] of the commercial use of home test kits in France revealed that only 11 of 27 home-use tests performed by experienced technologists were as accurate as claimed. When the 11 tests were further evaluated by a group of female lay individuals, the clinical specificity ranged from 77% to 100% and the clinical sensitivity ranged from 31% to 100% even with samples at two times the claimed detection limit of the test. The high number of false-negative results was attributed to difficulty understanding the literature that accompanied the test. In the United States, the FDA has established guidelines evaluating manufacturers' submissions of home test pregnancy kits for approval.

First-morning specimens are preferred for qualitative point-of-care urine pregnancy tests because they are concentrated and contain abundant CG. Almost all tests use immunochromatography. Urine applied to the device is absorbed into a nitrocellulose bed. The CG is concentrated into a narrow band as the urine migrates. A dye-labeled anti-CG antibody in the device binds to the migrating CG and passes through a zone having solid phase capture antibody to CG. The appearance of a colored line indicates a positive test. Positive controls are usually an integral component of these devices—immobilized CG works well. Falsely positive results occur in 1% of tests because of the presence in urine of interfering substances such as proteins, drugs, bacteria, erythrocytes, or leukocytes. False-negative results can occur because some tests do not detect CG below 100 IU/L, even though most claim a detection limit below this concentration.[76] About half of these qualitative tests will be positive on the day after the first missed menstrual period. Denaturation of the CG antiserum caused by high temperature, pH extremes, or old reagents may also yield false-negative results. The simplicity and speed with which the results are obtained make these tests valuable for pregnancy confirmation, but they may miss the diagnosis of a very early or abnormal pregnancy. Qualitative *serum* assays are available and tend to be more reliable than urine assays, because urine CG concentrations can vary considerably.

Quantitative Laboratory Test Kits

Serum is used for quantitative CG assays. Blood specimens are collected into suitable tubes without anticoagulants, allowed to clot at room temperature, and centrifuged to obtain clear serum. If testing is to be delayed beyond 1 week, serum should be stored at −20 °C. As with most biological materials, repeated freezing and thawing of the specimen should be avoided. Serum specimens showing gross hemolysis, gross lipemia, or turbidity may give false results. Cole and Kardana[74] describe the five common strategies for measuring CG among 10 CG immunoassays: anti-CGβ RIA, anti-CGβ : anti-CGβ sandwich, anti-CGβ : anti-CGα sandwich, anti-CGβ C terminal : anti-CGβ sandwich, and anti-CG : anti-CGβ sandwich. The sandwich techniques used either immunoradiometric assay (IRMA) or immunoenzymometric assay (IEMA) for detection of CG. The specificity of quantitative serum assays varies considerably.[72] Most of the differences are attributed to differences in antibody recognition of the various forms of CG, nicked, β-subunit, H-CG, and other fragments present in serum. The lowest detectable concentration of these assays is 1 to 2 IU/L. Typical between-run imprecision (CV) is 10% to 15% at 10 IU/L, 6% to 15% at 30 IU/L, and 7 to 12% at 150 IU/L.[243]

Assay Methods for Second Trimester Screening

Almost all commercially available CG kits are high-sensitivity assays designed to measure concentrations from 2 to 1000 IU/L. Consequently, existing CG assays can be used for second trimester screening without modification. It is only necessary for laboratories to select an appropriate serum dilution so that measurements fall within the range of the calibration curve. A serum dilution of 1 : 200 to 1 : 500 is suitable for most assays. The vast majority of prenatal screening laboratories use automated immunometric assays for measuring CG. Such assays are available from Abbott Laboratories (Abbott Park, Ill.), Bayer (Medfield, Mass.), Beckman Coulter (Fullerton, Calif.), Diagnostic Products (Los Angeles), and Perkin Elmer (Norwalk, Conn.).

Calibrating CG Assays

Calibration of CG assays depends on standardized reference materials provided by the World Health Organization (WHO). The first material was released in 1938 by WHO and was designated the First International Standard (1st IS). This crude urine preparation was highly contaminated with biologically inactive CG fragments. In 1964, WHO released a product with higher potency, the Second International Standard (2nd IS, 61/6). Although the 2nd IS had higher biological activity per weight of protein, it too was contaminated with biologically inactive hormone. In addition, it also contained CGβ that reacted in some but not all immunoassays for CG. In 1978, WHO released the First International Reference Preparation (1st IRP, 75/537) of CG from the highly pure National Institutes of Health preparation, CR119. To avoid confusion, the 1st IRP was later renamed the Third International Standard (3rd IS). WHO released the 4th IS (75/589) in 1999, which is essentially identical to the 3rd IS. Results obtained from methods calibrated to each of these materials are not the same and cannot be directly compared. On a weight basis, the 2nd IS has about half the biological potency of the 3rd IS. Thus 160 ng of the 2nd IS has the same activity (1 IU) as 80 ng of the 3rd IS. Therefore tests calibrated against the 2nd IS have approximately half the value (in international units per liter [IU/L]) of tests calibrated against the 3rd IS. Most CG immunoassays are calibrated against the 3rd IS. Nonetheless, many of the CG results reported in the literature since 1972 are based on assays calibrated to the 2nd IS.

Because the 3rd and 4th IS contain about 5% nicked CG and other CG contaminants, highly pure CG materials have been prepared.[42] These preparations are designated *reference reagents* (RR) and contain CG (99/688), CGn (99/642), CGβ (99/650), CGβn (99/692), CGβcf, and CGα (99/720). The impact of using RR for assay calibration and harmonization is under study.

In spite of a common calibrator, assays calibrated using the 1st IRP/3rd IS still yield significant differences in CG values on the same specimens.[81] Therefore CG median values calculated for second trimester serum screening are not transferable and should be considered method-specific. CG measurements in early pregnancy are generally expressed as IU/L or international units per milliliter. A typical CG concentration at 16 weeks is approximately 30,000 IU/L, and many screening laboratories express CG concentrations in international units per milliliter (e.g., 30,000 IU/L is expressed as 30 IU/mL) (see Figure 54-8). A simple alternative is to use kilo-international units per liter, consistent with the international system for SI units, in which concentrations are expressed per liter.

Specimen Collection and Handling

Serum specimens can be obtained from fasting or nonfasting women by standard phlebotomy techniques. CG is stable in maternal serum and can be shipped at ambient temperature and stored at 4 °C to 8 °C for 1 week.[152]

Specificity of CG Assays

Modern CG immunoassays should have little or no cross-reactivity with LH. Testing of serum samples with high physiological LH concentrations can be used to ascertain that this hormone does not significantly influence the CG results. Serum from postmenopausal women is a convenient source of specimens with high LH. The assay should be designed so that low concentrations of CG are detected and false-positive values caused by LH interference are minimized.

Clinical Significance

Measurement of CG can assist in the diagnosis and dating of pregnancy, identifying ectopic pregnancies and other abnormalities, managing certain neoplasms, and predicting the risk of Down syndrome and trisomy 18. Each of these clinical uses was discussed earlier in this chapter. Typical values during pregnancy are shown in Figure 54-3.

ALPHA FETOPROTEIN

Measurement of AFP in maternal serum and amniotic fluid is used extensively throughout the United States and the United Kingdom for prenatal detection of some serious fetal anomalies. Use of AFP in nonpregnant patients for monitoring certain cancers is described in Chapter 23.

Chemistry

A fetal protein having α-electrophoretic motility was discovered in 1956 by Bergstrand and Czar.[35] Gitlan subsequently named this substance *α-fetoprotein.*[195] This glycoprotein has a molecular weight of ~70,000. The gene, located within q11-22 on chromosome 4, is part of a family of genes that also codes for albumin and vitamin D–binding protein (also called group-specific component and Gc globulin).[159] The protein is composed of carbohydrate and a single polypeptide chain containing 591 amino acids. The complete amino acid sequence has been determined.[136] The carbohydrate composition varies depending on the organ of synthesis, length of gestation, and source of the specimen (fetal serum versus amniotic fluid),[100] Although determination of the carbohydrate content does not appear to be useful diagnostically in the setting of pregnancy, it may be useful in the diagnosis of hepatocellular carcinoma.[266] The heterogeneity can be demonstrated by electrophoresis and dissimilar binding to various lectins, such as concanavalin A.

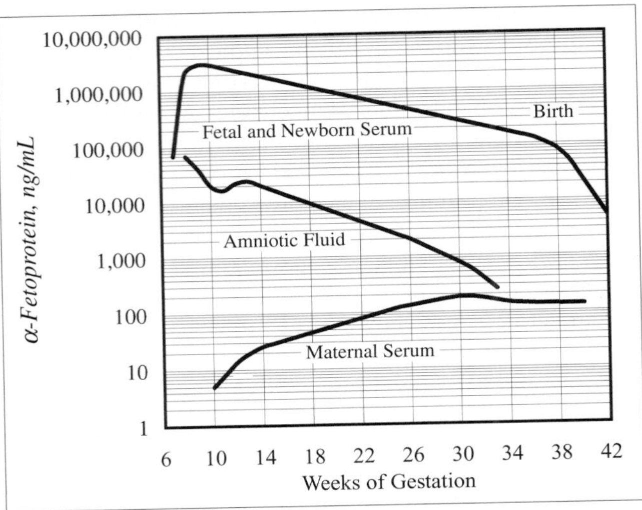

Figure 54-12 Concentrations of alpha fetoprotein (AFP) in fetal and newborn serum, maternal serum, and amniotic fluid. The maternal serum values are medians calculated from 24,232 pregnancies and the amniotic fluid values are medians calculated from 1544 pregnancies from testing performed at ARUP Laboratories Inc. from January to October 1997. The fetal serum values are from Gitlan.[137] The newborn serum values are from Wu et al.[349]

Biochemistry

AFP is produced initially by the fetal yolk sac in small quantities and then in larger quantities by the fetal liver as the yolk sac degenerates. Trace amounts are also produced in the fetal gut and kidneys. Early in embryonic life, this protein has a high concentration in fetal serum, reaching about one tenth the concentration of albumin. Maximal concentration in the fetal serum, approximately 3 million μg/L, is reached at about 9 weeks gestation. The concentration then declines steadily to about 20,000 μg/L at term (Figure 54-12).[137] The increase and decrease in concentration of AFP in the amniotic fluid roughly parallel those in the fetal serum but the concentration is two to three orders of magnitude lower (~15,000 μg/L at 16 weeks gestation). The relationship with respect to maternal serum concentration is slightly more complicated because of several factors, including fetal-maternal transfer, the rapid growth of the fetus, the relatively constant size of the mother, the maternal clearance of the protein, and variation of the volume of distribution in the mother with maternal weight. AFP is first detectable (~5 μg/L) in maternal serum at about the 10th week of gestation. The concentration increases about 15% per week to a peak of approximately 180 μg/L at about 25 weeks. A typical 16-week concentration is approximately 35 μg/L (see Figure 54-6).[150] The concentration in maternal serum then subsequently declines slowly until term. After birth, the maternal serum AFP rapidly decreases to less than 2 μg/L. In an infant, serum AFP declines exponentially to reach adult concentrations by the 10th month of life.[349]

The distribution of serum AFP concentrations in a population of pregnant mothers is Gaussian after logarithmic transformation.[330] Factors that affect the concentration of AFP in maternal serum include gestational age, maternal weight, the presence of insulin-dependent maternal diabetes mellitus, maternal race, the number of fetuses present, fetal renal disorders that cause proteinuria, and fetal structural anomalies.

Amniotic fluid AFP has been measured as early as 8 weeks.[341] It rapidly decreases to its lowest point at 11 weeks, then increases to reach a second maximum at 13 weeks. The concentration then falls in a log-linear fashion until 25 weeks, when the decline steepens. Several studies have shown that AChE used in combination with amniotic fluid AFP can aid in the detection of open neural tube defects from 13 to 25 weeks of pregnancy.[84]

Methods for Determining Alpha Fetoprotein

Although AFP was traditionally measured by RIA, newer methods use IEMA or chemiluminescent immunoassay (CIA) because of their lower detection limits, better precision, speed, avoidance of radioactivity, and ease of automation.[43] Most laboratories in the United States measure AFP by use of automated systems available from Abbott Laboratories (Abbott Park, Ill.), Bayer (Medfield, Mass.), Beckman Coulter (Fullerton, Calif.), Diagnostic Products (Los Angeles), and Perkin Elmer (Norwalk, Conn.). Judging from the results of proficiency testing sponsored by the Foundation for Blood Research and College of American Pathologists (Survey FP), all of these systems perform satisfactorily.[81]

Calibration

Although two essentially equivalent international standards (WHO Reference Preparation for AFP [72-225] and British Standard [72-227])—both calibrated in international units—are available, most laboratories in the United States report AFP in nanograms per milliliter (i.e., micrograms per liter). The relationship between nanograms and international units usually is given as 1.21 ng = 1 IU, but conversion factors may vary by manufacturer, perhaps reflecting differences in the carbohydrate content of the respective calibrators.[152]

Specimen Collection and Handling

Serum specimens can be obtained from nonfasting women by standard phlebotomy techniques. AFP is very stable in maternal serum and can be shipped at ambient temperature and stored at 4 °C to 8 °C for 1 week or at −20 °C for years.[152]

Clinical Significance

Maternal serum and amniotic fluid AFP are useful tests for detecting some serious fetal anomalies. Maternal serum AFP is elevated in 85% to 95% of cases of fetal open neural tube defect[330] and is low in about 30% of cases of fetal Down syndrome.[91,217] Because maternal serum screening for fetal defects involves multiple tests, this subject was discussed earlier under Maternal Serum Screening for Fetal Defects.

Measuring Amniotic Fluid Alpha Fetoprotein

Amniotic fluid AFP is measured using the same immunoassays as for maternal serum AFP after a suitable dilution (usually 1:50 to 1:200). Results can be expressed in micrograms per milliliter, micrograms per liter, or kilo IU per liter, and most laboratories use mass units. AFP in amniotic fluid is less stable than in serum. Leaving samples at room temperature for prolonged periods, such as might occur during processing for chromosome analysis, can result in degradation of amniotic fluid AFP. Refrigeration of amniotic fluid can compromise the chromosome analysis. Therefore a portion of the collected fluid should be placed in the refrigerator as soon as possible after collection. Samples sent to reference labs can be shipped for next day delivery at ambient temperature or on ice packs if the outside temperature is high. The presence of fetal blood in amniotic fluid samples can increase AFP results, and laboratories should note the presence of blood on the report. In the event of an increased amniotic fluid AFP result (usually above 2.0 or 2.5 MoM), the laboratory should test for the presence of fetal blood. Laboratories that measure amniotic fluid AFP need to establish medians for each week between 13 and 25 weeks of gestation. A method has been published that allows extrapolation to 13 weeks using data from 14 to 25 weeks.[250] Medians from ARUP Laboratories Inc. (Salt Lake City) are shown graphically in Figure 54-12.

Measuring Amniotic Fluid Acetylcholinesterase

AChE is an essential confirmatory test for all fluids with elevated amniotic fluid AFP. Normal amniotic fluid contains a group of nonspecific cholinesterases referred to as pseudocholinesterase (PChE). Cerebrospinal fluid contains high concentrations of the neural enzyme AChE, and in cases of fetal open neural tube defects (and in about 80% of cases with defects of the abdominal wall), fluid leaks from the open lesion and allows AChE to enter the amniotic fluid.

The usual technique for identification of AChE is fractionation by polyacrylamide gel electrophoresis followed by incubation of the gel with the substrate acetylcholine and copper ions. AChE migrates more rapidly than PChE and appears as a distinct white precipitate band below the PChE band. That the second band is AChE is documented by inhibition of the enzyme activity in the band by the specific AChE inhibitor 1,5-bis(4-allyldimethylammoniumphenyl) pentan-3-one dibromide—BW284C51. No method is available commercially; laboratories develop their own assay systems using published methodology.[51,148] Enzyme immunoassay using a monoclonal antibody specific for neurally derived AChE has also been used.[239]

UNCONJUGATED ESTRIOL

Measurement of urinary and serum estriol (E_3), once used to assess fetal well-being, is no longer recommended for that

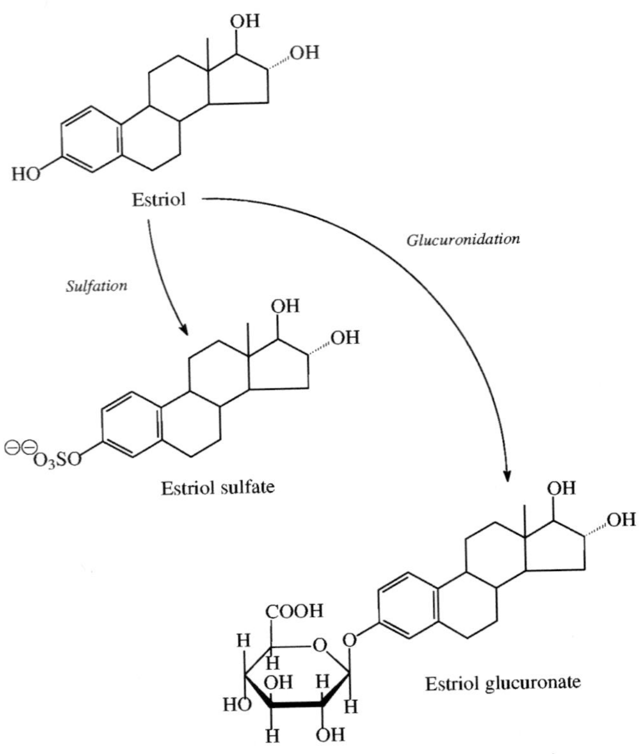

Figure 54-13 The forms of estriol present in maternal serum. Glucuronidation and sulfation can also occur at the other hydroxyl positions.

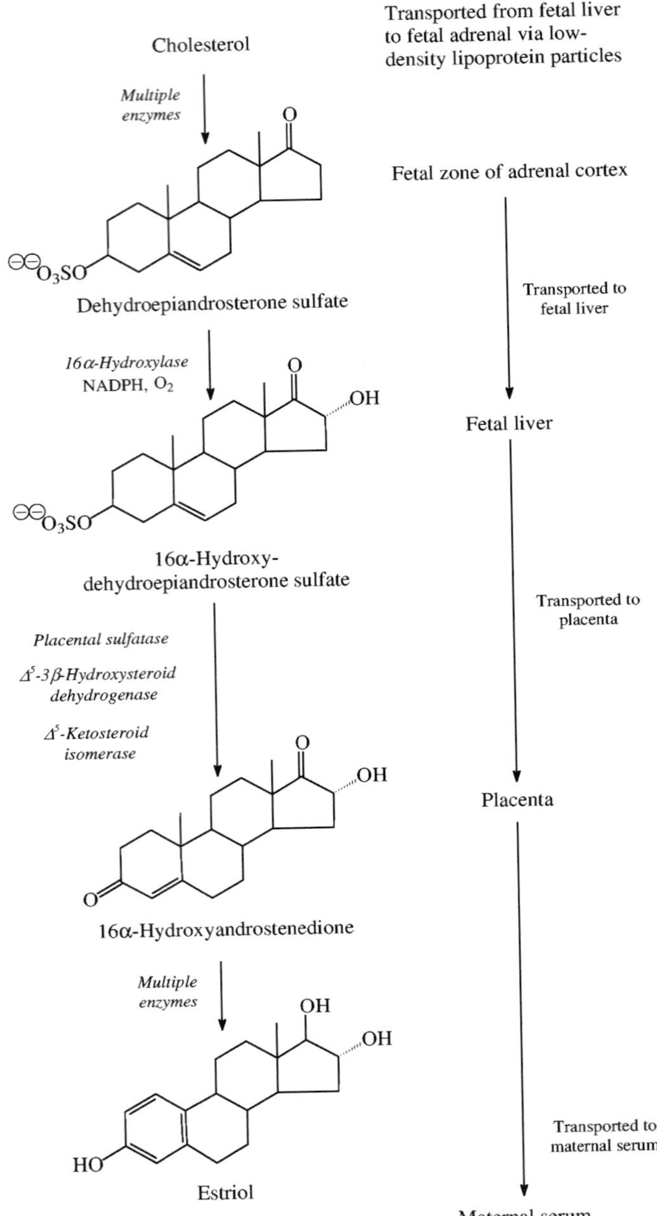

Figure 54-14 The biosynthetic pathway for estriol during pregnancy.

purpose.[93] Measurement of unconjugated estriol (uE_3) is now used routinely by most United States laboratories that provide screening for Down syndrome. This steroid, rather than total estriol (unconjugated plus conjugated estriol), is the most specific of the estrogens for identifying a fetus with Down syndrome.

Chemistry

Estriol, as its name implies, is an estrogen with three hydroxyl groups (at positions 3, 16, and 17). Its systematic name is 1,3,5(10)-estriene-3,16-α,17-β-triol. Although present in nonpregnant patients in very low concentrations, during late pregnancy this estrogen predominates. Only a minor amount (~9%) of the hormone circulates in plasma unconjugated and, because of its low solubility, this form is strongly bound to SHBG. The majority exists as conjugates of glucuronate and sulfate (Figure 54-13). The conjugation occurs in the maternal liver, makes the hormone more soluble and, thus, permits renal clearance.

Biochemistry

Estriol is produced in very large amounts during the last trimester of pregnancy. The biosynthetic pathway requires three organs to be fully functioning: fetal adrenal, fetal liver, and placenta (Figure 54-14). The fetal adrenal cortex possesses a unique zone for the production of steroids. The demand for estriol is so great that the fetal adrenal is massive compared with that of an adult. The fetal zone accounts for approximately 80% of the adrenal weight. The fetal adrenal avidly binds low-density lipoprotein to take in cholesterol, which is converted to two major steroid intermediates: pregnenolone sulfate and dehydroepiandrosterone sulfate (DHEAS). These intermediates are secreted into the fetal circulation. The fetal liver, possessing 16α-hydroxylase, converts DHEAS to 16α-hydroxy-DHEAS, which is secreted back into the fetal circulation. Finally the placenta synthesizes estriol from 16α-hydroxy-DHEAS. Approximately 90% of maternal serum estriol is derived from this pathway. A

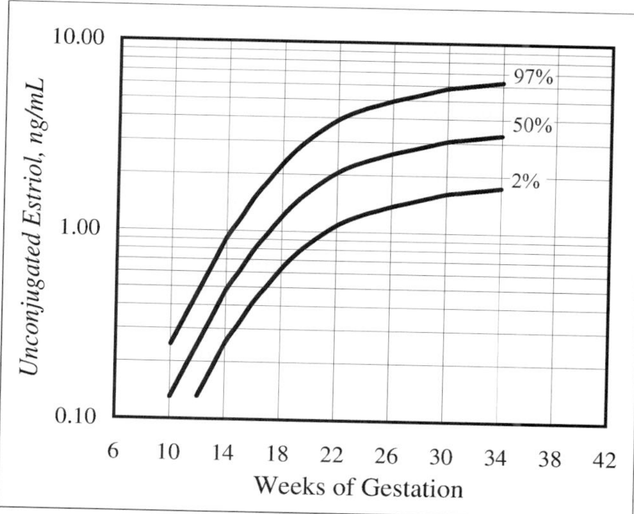

Figure 54-15 Concentration of unconjugated estriol (uE_3) in maternal serum as a function of gestational age. Lines represent the 2nd, 50th, and 97th percentiles. The maternal serum values from 14 to 25 weeks are medians calculated from 11,309 pregnancies from testing performed at ARUP Laboratories Inc. from January to October 1997.

minor amount is made using precursors from the maternal ovary. The relationship of maternal serum uE_3 to gestational age in the second trimester is log-linear, increasing at a rate of 20% to 25% per gestational week[150] (Figure 54-15). The concentrations typical for the second trimester of pregnancy are 0.70 to 2.50 μg/L, depending on the assay used. Serum concentrations of estriol conjugates are fivefold to tenfold higher than serum concentrations of uE_3 during pregnancy.

Methods for Determining Unconjugated Estriol

Concentrations of estrone, estriol-3-sulfate, and estriol-3-glucuronide up to 1000 ng/mL cross-react less than 0.03% in current assays.

The determination of uE_3 is made difficult by its low concentration. Until 2002, uE_3 was measured by ultrasensitive RIA methods (primarily the assay available from Diagnostic Systems Laboratories [DSL, Webster, Tex.]) that have been clinically validated extensively by case-control and intervention studies. More recently, nonisotopic assays have become available, usually as part of automated systems. The correlation between these methods and the RIA methods is generally low, ($r^2 \sim 0.8$), and most have not been clinically validated. Many laboratories have switched to nonisotopic methods because of the convenience of a common platform for measuring uE_3 and other screening tests. Ideally, screening laboratories should not use these nonisotopic assays until they have been clinically validated using known cases of Down syndrome and unaffected pregnancies or they have shown good agreement with validated assays after conversion to MoM. A recent publication shows that the nonisotopic method manufactured by Beckman Coulter (Fullerton, Calif.) yields screening performance that is equivalent to a previously validated RIA.[209] Other nonisotopic assays are available from Bayer (Medfield, Mass.), Diagnostic Products (Los Angeles), and Perkin Elmer (Norwalk, Conn.). Values obtained with the various uE_3 assays vary widely as judged using the Foundation for Blood Research/CAP proficiency testing Survey FP.[81] Conversion to MoM reduces the between-method differences, but uE_3 is still the most variable of the screening analytes.

Calibration

Assays for uE_3 are calibrated by use of chemically pure estriol. Estriol values can be reported in mass units (nanograms per milliliter or micrograms per liter) or SI units (nanomoles per liter). The equation for converting mass to SI units is 1 nmol/L = 3.47 ng/mL = 3.47 μg/L. Although pure uE_3 is available for calibrating uE_3 assays, commercial kits yield values on clinical specimens that can differ by factors of 2 to 3.

Specimen Collection and Handling

Maternal serum specimens can be obtained from nonfasting women by standard phlebotomy techniques. uE_3 is the least stable of the four analytes currently used for screening, and consequently, requirements for collection, storage, and shipment are dictated by this analyte. The uE_3 concentration increases in blood at room temperature and at 4 °C, because the conjugated forms can spontaneously deconjugate to form the parent hormone.[152] Therefore collected blood should be allowed to clot and then serum should be removed promptly. If serum separator tubes are used, specimens should be centrifuged promptly after collection. Shipment of whole blood is not preferred. If whole blood is shipped through the mail, next day delivery is essential. uE_3 is stable in serum for up to 7 days at 2 °C to 4 °C (unpublished data, Foundation for Blood Research, Woman and Infant's Hospital, and ARUP Laboratories). The concentration of uE_3 increases when sera have been stored for more than 4 days at room temperature.

Clinical Significance

Any disruption in the biosynthetic pathway will lead to very low maternal serum uE_3. Conditions that cause disruption include fetal anencephaly, placental sulfatase deficiency, fetal death, chromosome abnormalities, molar pregnancy, and Smith-Lemlit Opitz syndrome (SLOS).[47,314] Placental sulfatase deficiency presents in the infant as X-linked ichthyosis. It is present in approximately 1 in every 2000 males. Because of the lack of uE_3, the mother often has delayed onset of labor. The cesarean section rate is significantly higher in these mothers. SLOS is a serious, rare birth defect that is the result of an inborn error in cholesterol metabolism, 7-dehydrosterol-7-reductase deficiency. Down syndrome leads to a modest decrease in uE_3. Screening for Down syndrome is now the most common application of uE_3 measurements.[332]

Dimeric Inhibin A

Inhibins are members of the transforming growth factor β (TGFβ) superfamily of proteins. Inhibin forms include inhibin A and B, and activin A, B, and AB. As described in Chapter 53, inhibin is a negative feedback regulator of FSH secretion in both males and females. The placenta produces large quantities of inhibin A that completely suppress FSH.

Chemistry

Inhibins are proteins consisting of dimers of dissimilar subunits (α and β) linked by disulfide bridges (Table 28-1). The β-subunit occurs in two closely related forms (β_A and β_B), leading to two types of dimeric inhibin (dimeric inhibin A, $\alpha\beta_A$ and dimeric inhibin B, $\alpha\beta_B$). The mature form of inhibin, which has a molecular mass of approximately 30,000, is produced by cleavage of larger precursor forms. Precursor forms are relatively less bioactive than the mature forms. In follicular fluid and serum, mature inhibins, precursors of inhibins (particularly the processed form of the free α-subunit, pro-αC), and intermediate molecules of varying molecular weight are present.[312] Another group of related molecules, the activins, are dimers consisting of just the β-subunits. They are also found in biological fluids. Of the two forms of inhibin and the many related molecules found in serum, only DIA has been shown to provide sufficient discrimination to be useful for Down syndrome screening.[194]

Biochemistry

Inhibins, and the closely related activins, are proteins that suppress or stimulate follicle-stimulating hormone secretion. Inhibins are secreted by granulosa cells of the ovary and by the Sertoli cells of the testis. Inhibin A and inhibin B have distinctive profiles during the human menstrual cycle. Inhibin A rises from 10 to 20 ng/L in the follicular phase of pregnancy to a maximum of 40 to 60 ng/L. Inhibin B is maximal in the midfollicular phase, with a peak at ovulation (about 60 ng/L) before decreasing to basal levels in the luteal phase. In postmenopausal women, the concentrations of both forms of inhibin are below 5 ng/L.[207] Men secrete inhibin B, but do not appear to produce inhibin A. Inhibin A is produced by the fetoplacental unit beginning in early pregnancy. DIA concentrations exhibit a complex pattern during the course of pregnancy, rising to a peak at 8 to 10 weeks of gestation, declining to a minimum at 17 weeks of pregnancy, and then resuming to slowly increase at term (see Figure 54-9). Unlike the other screening tests, average inhibin levels change relatively little from 15 to 20 weeks gestation. A typical value at 17 weeks gestation is 175 ng/L (175 pg/mL).

Assay Methods for DIA

Inhibin assays used for Down syndrome screening must measure only dimeric inhibin A and not the free α-subunits and the precursors of higher molecular weight, which also circulate in blood. The original inhibin assays (ELISA or RIA) used antibodies directed against epitopes on the α-subunit and measured all forms of inhibin, including precursors. These assays are referred to as total inhibin or immunoreactive inhibin assays. Highly specific assays using monoclonal antibodies are available that measure only dimeric inhibin A. Specific DIA assays provide better screening performance than the nonspecific total inhibin assays.[194] The widely used DIA method from Diagnostic Systems Laboratories (Webster, Tex.) has been clinically validated[185] and performs well in the Foundation for Blood Research/College of American Pathologists Maternal Survey FP.[81]

Typical values in the second trimester of pregnancy range from 50 to 400 pg/mL (50 to 400 ng/L), as shown in Figure 54-9.

Specimen and Sampling Handling

Serum specimens can be obtained from nonfasting women by standard phlebotomy techniques. DIA is stable in maternal serum and can be shipped at ambient temperature and stored at 4 °C to 8 °C for 1 week.

Clinical Significance

In addition to the usefulness of DIA as a predictor of Down syndrome risk discussed previously, inhibin A and B measurements have found applications in ovarian cancer monitoring, disorders of ovulation, early detection of viable pregnancy following in vitro fertilization, and evaluation of male infertility.[194,272]

Fetal Fibronectin

Determining the risk of preterm labor would help clinicians manage those at high risk more aggressively and thereby lower the incidence of preterm delivery. In 1991, fetal fibronectin concentration in cervical and vaginal secretions was proposed as a test to aid in predicting preterm delivery.[206]

Fibronectin is a term for a family of ubiquitous adhesive glycoproteins that cross-link to collagen to bind cells together. These proteins are found on cell surfaces and in plasma and amniotic fluid. The fetus has a unique fibronectin that is defined by a monoclonal antibody, FDC-6, which recognizes the epitope defined by α-*N*-acetylgalactosamine linked to threonine in a hexapeptide sequence (Val-Thr-His-Pro-Gly-Tyr), the IIICS domain.[213] When labor begins and the cellular adhesion between the placenta and the uterine wall is disrupted, the concentration of fetal fibronectin in cervical and vaginal secretions increases. Mothers with more than 50 ng/mL (50 μg/L) of fetal fibronectin in these secretions during the second and third trimesters have a higher risk for preterm delivery. The majority of patients with results >50 ng/mL will, however, repair any placental disruption and successfully continue the pregnancy.[141]

Assay Method

In the past, Adeza Biomedical Corp. (Sunnyvale, Calif.) offered an enzyme-linked immunosorbent assay (ELISA) for fetal fibronectin that used a 96-well microtiter plate format and took 2 hours to complete. In 1995 the FDA approved the use of this test in symptomatic women; in 1997 screening asymptomatic women was approved. Currently, two rapid tests are available. The one that is available in the United States is a membrane immunoassay, using a solid phase polyclonal goat anti-fFN antibody and an enzyme-labeled monoclonal anti-fFN, FDC-6 detection antibody. The specimen is obtained by collecting cervical or vaginal mucus with a Dacron polyester swab. The fully saturated swab contains approximately 150 μL of fluid. The swab is placed into 750 μL of buffer, creating a 1:5 dilution. An aliquot of the specimen is added to the cassette containing the antibodies. The color development is measured using the Adeza TLi_{IQ}^{TM} analyzer.

Asymptomatic Patients

In screening asymptomatic women, testing should take place sometime between 24 and 30 weeks gestation. Women with a positive result (>50 ng/mL) are at a twofold to fourfold higher risk for preterm delivery. A negative test following a positive test lowers the risk, and a second subsequent negative test returns the risk to baseline.[141] Among asymptomatic women, positive fFN results have a likelihood ratio of 4.01 (95% confidence interval 2.93 to 5.49) for predicting birth before 34 weeks' gestation. For negative fFN results, the corresponding likelihood ratio is 0.78 (0.72 to 0.84).[167]

Symptomatic Patients

The symptoms of preterm labor include regular uterine contractions, low back pain, lower abdominal cramping, and vaginal bleeding and increased vaginal discharge. Among symptomatic women, positive fFN results have a likelihood ratio of 5.42 (95% confidence interval 4.36 to 6.74) for predicting delivery before 34 weeks' gestation or within the next 7 days. For negative fFN results, the corresponding likelihood ratio is 0.25 (0.20 to 0.31).[167] Those patients with a negative test can safely return home, because they have only a ~1% chance of delivering in 1 week.[254]

AMNIOTIC FLUID BILIRUBIN (ΔA_{450})[201]

The concentration of bilirubin in amniotic fluid is generally too low (~0.01 to 0.03 mg/dL; 0.17 to 0.51 μmol/L) to be measured by standard photometric techniques, but the determination can be done rapidly, accurately, and directly by absorption spectrophotometry. The maximal absorbance of bilirubin is at 450 nm. In the absence of significant amounts of bilirubin, the absorbance spectrum for the amniotic fluid between 365 and 550 nm defines a nearly exponential curve (Figure 54-16). On log-linear axes, the height of the curve at 450 nm above the straight line is linearly proportional to the concentration of bilirubin in the amniotic fluid. This is the difference in absorbance at 450 nm (ΔA_{450}), which is still occasionally referred to as ΔOD_{450} in the clinical literature. There is normally a small amount of bilirubin in amniotic fluid, and this amount changes with gestational age (Figure 54-17). To interpret properly the ΔA_{450}, it is necessary to know the gestational age. The procedural details are available on the Evolve site that accompanies this book.

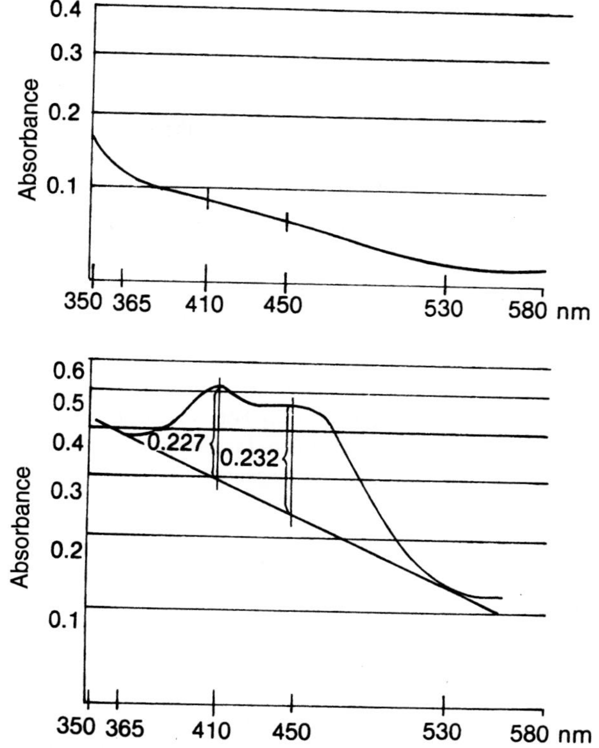

Figure 54-16 A, Normal amniotic fluid. Note near linearity of the curve when plotted on log-linear graph. **B,** Amniotic fluid showing the bilirubin peak at 450 nm and the oxyhemoglobin peak at approximately 410 nm. Note the baseline drawn between linear parts of the curve, from 530 and 365 nm.

Interpretation

Interpretation of ΔA_{450} depends on knowing the gestational age of the pregnancy (see Figure 54-17). Values that fall into Liley's bottom zone (Figure 54-17) are considered to represent an unaffected or very mildly affected fetus. Values in the middle zone are still compatible with a minimally affected fetus, but as values rise within this zone, it is increasingly likely that a fetus is suffering moderate to marked hemolysis. Depending on the trend with time and the clinical circumstances, some clinicians recommend intervention when ΔA_{450} has climbed 85% up in the middle zone. Values in the top zone (zone III) denote severe disease. Without intervention, a fetus with values in the top zone will most likely die.[201]

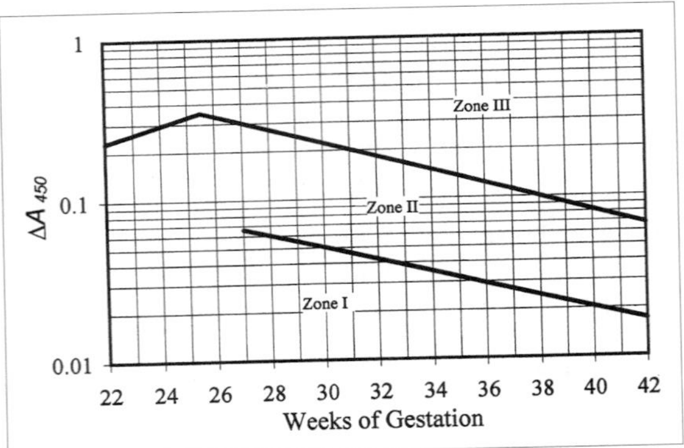

Figure 54-17 Liley's three-zone chart (with modification) for interpretation of amniotic fluid ΔA_{450}. For explanation of the three zones, see text. *(Modified from Liley AW. Liquor amnii analysis in the management of the pregnancy complicated by rhesus sensitization. Am J Obstet Gynecol 1961;82:1359-70.)*

Contamination of an amniotic fluid specimen with fetal blood from an affected fetus with a high serum bilirubin level could introduce a substantial error, the magnitude of which cannot accurately be predicted. Blood contamination of amniotic fluid should be obvious from the red color and the presence of erythrocytes in the pellet after centrifugation. It is important to minimize hemolysis of the erythrocytes in such samples (by rapid processing) as the hemoglobin will interfere in the test. A Kleihauer-Betke (or other) test should be performed on the erythrocytes to establish their origin. The Kleihauer-Betke test uses an acid solution to elute the hemoglobin A, but not hemoglobin F, from erythrocytes fixed on a glass slide. Thus under microscopic examination, maternal cells appear as ghosts, and fetal cells appear red. If the erythrocytes are largely fetal, this should be kept in mind when interpreting the fluid results. If the amniotic fluid remaining within the amniotic cavity has been contaminated with blood by traumatic amniocentesis, these erythrocytes lyse and contaminate the fluid with hemoglobin and bilirubinoid pigments. It takes 2 to 3 weeks for these pigments to be cleared and for the fluid to return to the original state. Both mathematical corrections and choloform extraction can be used for bloody specimens (see the Evolve site that accompanies this book).[127]

In a pregnancy with twins within separate sacs, the individual sacs must be sampled. Inadvertent sampling of maternal urine is always a possibility,[202] although the risk of this error is reduced when using ultrasonography.

Occasionally, during monitoring of a sensitized pregnancy, delivery seems imminent and a large dose of glucocorticoids is administered to stimulate fetal lung maturation. If the patient is not delivered and if amniocentesis is repeated within 2 to 4 days of the steroid course, the ΔA_{450} is lowered relative to the level found immediately before the steroid administration.[63] Further observation and amniocenteses show that the ΔA_{450} returns to the previous level or higher within a week. It seems doubtful that this phenomenon represents a decrease in hemolysis; instead, it may be an artifact, possibly caused by acute changes in amniotic fluid volume.

Meconium staining of amniotic fluid increases the ΔA_{450} with a broad and variable peak at 400 to 415 nm.[202] There is no way to compensate quantitatively for meconium contamination. Clearance of meconium from a single episode of passage into the amniotic fluid requires about 3 weeks.

Tests for Evaluating Fetal Lung Maturity

Fetal lung maturity (FLM) tests help a clinician decide whether the best perinatal survival will be achieved in utero or in the nursery. The most common situation in which a fetal lung maturity test is ordered is before repeat cesarean delivery when the age of gestation is somewhat uncertain. Another major indication is anticipated early delivery because of some medical or obstetrical indication, such as preterm labor, premature rupture of the membranes, worsening maternal hypertension, severe renal disease, intrauterine growth retardation, or fetal distress. Results indicating immaturity of the fetal lungs might cause postponement of elective delivery or prompt active intervention with tocolytics to suppress preterm labor. Pharmacological administration of corticosteroids before birth accelerates pulmonary maturation and can prevent RDS.[4] If delivery of an infant is inevitable, transfer to a tertiary health care center is appropriate.

Numerous tests of amniotic fluid for FLM have been proposed.[216] Some of these, such as creatinine determination,[101] urea measurement,[2] or the lipid staining characteristics of cells, correlate with gestational age but do not measure lung maturation. Tests that measure lamellar bodies directly or indirectly, the surfactant they contain, or the biophysical property of surfactant are the most useful for evaluating FLM. Six methods that measure pulmonary surfactant are presented in detail: the lecithin/sphingomyelin (L/S) ratio, DSPC, phosphatidylglycerol, foam stability, fluorescence polarization (both commercial and noncommercial assays), and lamellar body counts. Since 1994, the CAP has offered a proficiency testing survey for FLM methods. Table 54-6 lists the number of laboratories that reported using each of the methods in recent surveys by the CAP. The number of laboratories performing methods requiring thin-layer chromatography (L/S ratio and phosphatidylglycerol) has decreased, while the number of laboratories using commercial fluorescence polarization has dramatically increased.

Other surfactant-based tests include those that measure turbidity at either 400 nm or 650 nm.[285,300] These tests measure the effect of light scattering by lamellar bodies suspended in the amniotic fluid. An absorbance greater than 0.15 at 650 nm is claimed to indicate lung maturity. Unfortunately, the absorbance of amniotic fluid is affected not only by light scattering but also by substances that absorb light. Use of these rapid techniques has been discouraged.[264] Dubin modified amniotic fluid absorbance by measuring the dif-

TABLE 54-6 Number of Laboratories Performing Fetal Lung Maturity Testing, by Method: College of American Pathologists Proficiency Testing Survey (2001-2004)

Method	YEAR			
	2001	2002	2003	2004
TDx FLM II	427	462	470	469
Phosphatidylglycerol (AmnioStat-FLM)	421	447	401	43*
Phosphatidylglycerol (thin-layer chromatography)	113	110	103	87
Lecithin/sphingomyelin ratio	142	138	122	97
Fluorescence polarization (NBD-PC)	10	9	7	9

*In late 2003 through 2004, Irvine Scientific was unable to provide AmnioStat-FLM reagents to laboratories.

ferential absorbance of amniotic fluid when mixed with water versus glycerol.[111] He coined the term refractive index-matched anomalous diffraction (RIMAD). This technique measures just the absorbance caused by light scattering and can be used to predict the particle density of the lamellar bodies. A prospective clinical outcome study reported that RIMAD has clinical sensitivity and specificity as good as fluorescence polarization.[274] Addition of as little as 25 µL of erythrocytes, however, causes significant interference.

Surfactant proteins (SP-A and SP-B) have been evaluated as potential fetal lung maturity tests, but the results are disappointing.[178,267]

The American College of Obstetricians and Gynecologists issued an educational bulletin on the assessment of fetal lung maturity in 1996.[5] Readers may want to carefully read that bulletin, because many obstetricians rely on it.

Standards of laboratory practice for FLM testing[20] have been published that make several recommendations regarding specimen collection, handling, centrifugation, and mixing. Hospital laboratories should offer a rapid test, such as fluorescence polarization, phosphatidylglycerol, or foam stability index (FSI). These should be available daily on both a routine and emergency basis. Requests for L/S ratios and lung profiles may be sent to a reference laboratory. Analysts should communicate the results of any FLM test immediately to the ordering location, because the patient's status may be changing and the information might assist with management of labor.

Collection and Handling of Amniotic Fluid for Fetal Lung Maturity Assessment

Before the details of individual methods are given, details of the specimen and specimen handling are described. These topics are common to many methods.

Specimen

Amniotic fluid is obtained by transabdominal amniocentesis usually during real-time sonographic visualization. The clinician should try to avoid traversing the placenta, but will sometimes fail. In a multifetal pregnancy, there are usually separate sacs. Each individual sac should be sampled. Fluid may be obtained by transvaginal puncture of the bulging membranes, but it should not be grossly contaminated with vaginal secretions as might occur with aspiration of a vaginal pool after spontaneous rupture of the membranes. Vaginal pool specimens are rarely adequate for testing. Clinicians should seriously consider amniocentesis in patients with ruptured membranes.[20] Bedside ultrasound examination will often locate a pocket of amniotic fluid that can be tapped without endangering the fetus.

Whenever possible, the fluid should be tested immediately. If there is to be a delay of a few hours, the fluid should be refrigerated at 4 °C.[287] The total phospholipid content of amniotic fluid does not change significantly during at least a week of storage.[324] If testing will be delayed longer than 1 week (e.g., fluids kept for research studies), fluids should be stored frozen at −20 °C or −70 °C. Immediately before testing the fluid, it should be gently inverted 20 times to obtain a uniform suspension. At least 2 minutes on a test tube rocker is recommended.[20]

Specimen Handling

Most procedures for measuring fetal lung maturity include a centrifugation step to remove debris. Careful attention to technique is needed to obtain reproducible results. Any centrifugation removes some pulmonary surfactant from the specimen. Accidentally prolonged centrifugation can reduce recovery of the phospholipids to less than 50%.[244] For best results, the specimen should be well mixed, lightly centrifuged, decanted, and mixed again.

1. Invert the amniocentesis collection tube 20 times or place it on a tube rocker for 2 to 5 minutes. Transfer the entire contents to a clear test tube.
2. Note the condition of the specimen: uncontaminated, bloody, meconium stained, xanthochromic, or obviously contaminated with mucus. Blood and meconium interfere with most tests. The report of the result should always list any contaminates seen.
3. For tests other than the Abbott fluorescence polarization method (which uses filtered fluid) and the lamellar body count, centrifuge the fluid for 2 minutes at 400 ×g.
4. Decant the supernatant into a new test tube.

Before transfer of any aliquot from the new tube, mix it well by inverting 20 times or placing it on a tube rocker for at least 2 minutes. When not mixing, keep the specimen on wet ice.

Fluorescence Polarization Fetal Lung Maturity Tests[26,125,309]

The TDx FLM II fluorescence polarization technique is the most commonly used quantitative method, as judged by enrollment in the CAP Fetal Lung Maturity proficiency test survey (see Table 54-6). This rapid test has better precision than the L/S ratio.[295] The test was originally described in 1976 by Shinitzky and colleagues, who used diphenylhexatriene (DPH) as the fluorescent dye. Although the DPH test is predictive of FLM, many laboratories had difficulty working with this dye, because it is an easily oxidized compound that absorbs UV light. The UV fluorescence polarimeter instrument, the FELMA, was difficult to maintain. These disadvantages prevented widespread use of DPH fluorescence polarization in clinical laboratories. Tait and associates[309] improved the technique by using a more stable fluorescent dye, NBD-PC, and a commercial polarimeter, the Abbott TDx. Russell[278] developed a commercial version of the assay using a slightly different dye, PC-16. The first generation TDx FLM was replaced with the second generation TDx FLM II in 1995. This transition lowered the results approximately 4%.[260]

The commercial version is calibrated with solutions containing phospholipid and albumin in various ratios, expressed as milligrams of surfactant per gram albumin. The vast majority of laboratories performing fluorescence polarization testing for FLM use the commercial version of the assay (see Table 54-6). The NBD-PC method is described on the Evolve site that accompanies this book for those laboratories that are willing to prepare the reagents and perform the calculations required for interpretation.

Fluorescence polarization is a dimensionless ratio with values from 0.000 to 0.500 for dilute solutions containing fluorescing compounds (see Chapter 3).[193] Polarization (P) measures the rotational diffusion of the fluorophore relative to its fluorescent half-life. If the half-life is short compared with the rate of rotational diffusion, P will be high. In contrast, if molecular rotation is faster than the excited state decay, then P will be low. Shinitzky proposed that for amniotic fluid, lower polarization values reflected a decrease in the microviscosity of surfactant phospholipids. The fluidity of these phospholipids paralleled the change in lipid composition with maturation of the fetal lungs.[295] This mechanism is incorrect for the NBD-PC method. NBD-PC binds to albumin and to surfactant; thus the resulting polarization is a function of the surfactant/albumin ratio.[22]

TDx FLM II Method

The commercial fluorescence polarization test, TDx FLM II (Abbott Laboratories, Abbott Park, Ill.), has an analytical measurement range of 0 to 160 mg surfactant/g albumin. Uncentrifuged amniotic fluid is used for this method. If specimens have been accidentally centrifuged, the surfactant can be resuspended before testing.[145] Approximately 1 mL of amniotic fluid is passed through a glass filter before testing on the TDx analyzer. The TDx FLM II assay uses 25 μL of filtered amniotic fluid. Imprecision (CV) is 4% to 5% at both 20 and 115 mg/g.

Although studies of the first-generation test[166,279,303,347] recommended a maturity cutoff of 70 mg phospholipid/g of albumin or greater, the second-generation decision limits are different; values less than or equal to 39 mg/g are considered immature, those greater than or equal to 55 mg/g mature, and others (40 to 54 mg/g) intermediate. Several clinical outcome studies of the first-generation test suggested that the upper cutoff could be lowered without impacting the sensitivity for RDS.[17,163,303] Similar studies of the TDx FLM II show that ≥45 mg/g can be used as a cut point, which will improve the assay specificity to 85% while maintaining sensitivity for clinically significant RDS at 95% to 100%.[119,182]

Several investigators have recommended that TDx FLM II be interpreted as a function of gestational age.[179,261] Instead of changing the decision limits for each gestational age, the authors recommend reporting the RDS risk for a given TDx FLM II result at a specific gestational age. The calculated risks, however, will vary with the tested population.[147] The outcome studies were conducted at tertiary hospitals that handle high-risk obstetrical cases. Thus use of these risk models is best restricted to those settings. If the risk calculations are used at hospitals that care for low-risk obstetrical populations, the risks are overestimated.

Most twins are delivered preterm and many suffer from preterm complications. If those complications are excluded, twins have the same RDS incidence as do singletons matched for gestational age.[132] After 31 weeks' gestation, however, the average TDx FLM II results from twin pregnancies are 22 mg/g higher than those from singleton pregnancies.[215] Sampling both sacs is recommended when testing before 32 weeks' gestation.[345]

Several studies have concluded that diabetes does not affect the reference values of TDx FLM II.[105,203]

NBD-PC Fluorescence Polarization Method

The NBD-PC method, also called FPol, is described in detail on the Evolve site that accompanies this book. The specimen is amniotic fluid that has been centrifuged at 400 ×g for 2 minutes. Results are expressed using artificial units of millipolarization (P × 1000, mP). The analytical measurement range is 150 to 350 mP. No calibrators are used, but use of a Triton ×100 control assures that the temperature is correct and that the dye is not degraded. Comparison of the TDx FLM II and the NBD-PC assay reveals, as expected, a strong nonlinear, inverse correlation:[21,24]

$$\text{TDx FLM II (in mg/g)} = -139.5 \ln(\text{FPol in mP}) + 817$$

An NBD-PC fluorescence polarization value of less than 260 mP is considered mature, values between 260 and 290 mP are considered transitional, and values greater than

290 are considered immature.[69,308] Using 260 mP as the cutoff, this test has a clinical sensitivity of 94% and a clinical specificity of 84%. The supplemental use of the L/S ratio for those patients with transitional results is of little benefit. The 260 mP cutoff is appropriate for high-risk pregnancies. In the setting of a patient who needs a cesarean section at term, when there is no penalty for delaying delivery, a cutoff of 230 mP is more appropriate.

If there is less than 0.5% blood in the amniotic fluid, the results are not affected. Contamination with more than this amount tends to increase low results and decrease high results.[309] Results that are clearly mature (<230 mP) or immature (>290 mP) are reliable for predicting fetal lung status. Results between these values cannot be interpreted.

Because of improved pregnancy management, very few infants with RDS are born to women with diabetes. Thus exact estimates of clinical sensitivity and specificity are not available in this clinical setting. The predictive value of a mature status in a patient with diabetes mellitus appears to be equivalent to that in a patient without diabetes.[69] The diabetes studies that used the commercial TDx FLM II test imply that diabetes mellitus does not affect the medical decision limit of NBD-PC fluorescence polarization.[105,203]

Determination of Lecithin/Sphingomyelin Ratio and Saturated Phosphatidylcholine[315]

The major surface-active component of the lung surfactant is DSPC, which represents 85% of the total lecithins. Its concentration in amniotic fluid tends to rise with increasing gestational age. The majority of the DSPC in amniotic fluid comes from the fetal lungs via tracheal effluent. The concentration of DSPC in amniotic fluid can be measured directly and correlated with FLM, or its concentration can be related to another lipid, sphingomyelin, and that ratio used to predict lung maturity. Although sphingomyelin is a minor component of pulmonary surfactant, it is ubiquitously distributed in cell membranes, especially those of erythrocytes, and is also found in plasma. Nearly all of the sphingomyelin in amniotic fluid is derived from non-lung sources; thus it has no role in the surfactant system in the lungs. The concentration of lecithin relative to sphingomyelin, the L/S ratio, tends to rise with increasing gestational age. This is not a uniform gradual increase; a rather sudden increase occurs at 34 to 36 weeks of gestation and correlates with the development of fetal lung maturity.[139]

Although the majority of laboratories use a commercially available method for L/S determination (Fetal-Tek, Helena Laboratories, Beaumont, Tex.), some continue to use methods developed in their own laboratories (the so-called "home brew" methods). Because there are many techniques, laboratories should be very careful when establishing medical decision limits. Some methods measure all phosphatidylcholine species, both saturated and unsaturated. Different staining methods will differentially stain phosphatidylcholine compared with the biological internal standard, sphingomyelin. The CAP proficiency testing program for FLM tests has shown a steady decline in the number of laboratories performing this test, from 234 in 1994 to 97 in 2004 (see Table 54-6).

Methodological details of both L/S ratio and DSPC procedures are given on the Evolve site that accompanies this book. The procedures described there should not be considered definitive or representative.[53,301,315]

Interpretation

The original maturity decision limit for the L/S ratio was 2.0 or greater.[319,320] Most laboratories use a method that omits the acetone precipitation step, which will produce slightly higher values. A conservative reference interval for lung maturity is an L/S ratio of 2.5 or greater. About 1% of babies delivered within 24 hours of obtaining an L/S ratio of greater than 2.5 can be expected to develop RDS; thus 99% of babies predicted to be mature will in fact be mature. Almost half of the infants with L/S ratios between 1.5 and 2.5, however, will not develop RDS. Thus in contrast to the high degree of reliability of a prediction of maturity, only one third of the babies predicted to be immature will in fact develop RDS.

Before the use of tight glycemic control during pregnancy, babies of diabetic mothers more frequently developed RDS.[273] A number of investigators have reported that infants of diabetic mothers more frequently develop RDS despite mature L/S ratios,[85] but other studies have reported no delay in lung maturity for infants of diabetic mothers.[133,306] In poorly controlled diabetic cases, both maturation delay[262] and lack of delay[223] have been reported. Although no RDS outcome studies exist, other studies of well-controlled diabetic mothers report no effect in the relationship between L/S ratio and gestational age.[223,36] For this reason, separate reference intervals are not recommended for well-controlled diabetic pregnancies.[20]

For multifetal pregnancies, separate specimens should be analyzed for each fetus. Infrequently, more than one fetus shares an amniotic fluid cavity. In such a case, a mature result is less predictive of maturity, because it represents a mixture of pulmonary surfactant from multiple fetuses. In the case of twins, the smaller is more likely to develop RDS than the larger.[225]

Serum has a large concentration of lecithin and sphingomyelin. The serum ratio varies between 1.5 and 2.0, depending on the individual. The values of blood-contaminated specimens therefore tend to be drawn into that range from either higher or lower values. A high L/S ratio in the presence of even substantial blood contamination can safely be interpreted as reflecting mature lungs.[135] Similarly, contaminated samples with very low ratios clearly reflect immature lungs. Borderline values of bloody specimens cannot be interpreted, because they may represent either very immature values falsely elevated or mature values falsely depressed. Various effects of meconium contamination have been reported, including some evidence that the L/S ratio may be changed in the absence of contamination that is visible to the eye.[325] The chromatograms of fluids heavily contaminated with meconium are not interpretable.

Vaginal contamination of specimens obtained from a pool of fluid that has been present in the vagina for a relatively brief period does not affect either test.[109,258]

L/S ratio results show considerable differences among laboratories. For proficiency testing samples LM-09 and LM-10 from the CAP, the reported CVs were 26% (at mean L/S = 4.46) and 27% (at 2.31), respectively.[79]

Phosphatidylglycerol

The determination of PG is a commonly used qualitative method used to assess FLM in the United States. Measurement of PG was classically performed by thin-layer chromatography. It could be performed alone or in combination with other amniotic fluid phospholipids. The later test was known as a *lung profile* since its introduction in the early 1970s.[22] Although thin-layer chromatography is still offered by some reference and hospital laboratories, most hospital laboratories use a rapid slide method for qualitative PG detection. Several enzyme-based tests for quantitative PG have also been published, but none is widely used.[18,131,174,227]

The exact role of PG in lung surfactant is unclear.[55] Many claim that the appearance of PG in the amniotic fluid indicates the final biochemical maturation of surfactant,[156,191] but PG can be found in measurable quantities in amniotic fluid as early as 32 weeks,[129] and its presence in small quantities does not necessarily imply that the fetal lungs are mature.[95,129,221] The concentration of PG in amniotic fluid increases with gestational age. Most thin-layer chromatography techniques are positive when PG exceeds about 2 μmol/L. At this cutoff, results indicating maturity are almost always correct, but results indicating immaturity are frequently wrong.

AmnioStat-FLM

Most laboratories that offer PG testing use a qualitative rapid agglutination test (AmnioStat-FLM, Irvine Scientific, Santa Ana, Calif.) that uses less than 0.5 mL of amniotic fluid.[115,134,281] The protocol is as follows: 25 μL of amniotic fluid is mixed with 25 μL of a lecithin-cholesterol ethanol solution; 250 μL of phosphate buffer is added and mixed; 10 μL of this mixture is placed on a glass slide and mixed with 25 μL of an anti-PG reagent. Agglutination occurs in the presence of PG and is compared with three controls. Results are reported as negative, low-positive (0.5 to 2 μg/mL [0.5 to 2 mg/L]), or high-positive (2 μg/mL [2 mg/L] or greater). RDS rarely develops in an infant from a mother with a high-positive PG determined by AmnioStat. Although Irvine Scientific was unable to provide AmnioStat reagents to laboratories for much of 2004, it recently resumed production.

Interpretation

Several clinical outcome studies using AmnioStat have been reported.* Although positive PG results are about 99% predictive of maturity, negative results are highly unpredictive (RDS develops in about 25% of cases with a negative PG, depending on the population) and are therefore not useful clinically. A positive PG result is very useful in low-risk pregnancies that require cesarean section. Determination of PG is also useful for specimens contaminated with blood or meconium. PG is not found in either blood or meconium, and therefore results are not affected by the presence of either of these contaminants.[33,121]

Many clinicians rely on PG whenever they need to assess FLM in a diabetic patient.[113,318] No modern studies support this practice. In normal pregnancies, PG is detected by thin-layer chromatography (TLC) or AmnioStat-FLM at approximately 35 weeks' gestation. In diabetic patients, regardless of glycemic control, PG is detected about 1.5 weeks later.[96,223,320] Many diabetic patients will deliver term infants unaffected by RDS before any PG is detected.[262] The diabetic status of the patient does not affect the method of detection.[281]

Determination of the Lung Profile[191,192]

This method for assessing FLM was invented by Marie Kulovich and Louis Gluck in the early 1970s. Although it is still offered by some reference laboratories, most hospital laboratories have substituted newer techniques. The details of the procedure are available on the Evolve site that accompanies this book. The pattern of L/S ratio, phosphatidylinositol (PI), and PG are used to determine the status of fetal pulmonary maturation.

Foam Stability Index[292]

Many laboratories used a commercial version of this test, called Lumadex, FSI Fetal Lung Maturity Test (Beckman Instruments, Fullerton, Calif.), which was introduced in 1982.[205,291] Beckman Instruments discontinued this test in 1997. The procedure is described on the Evolve site that accompanies this book.

When pulmonary surfactant is present in amniotic fluid in sufficient concentrations, the fluid is able to form a highly stable surface film that can support bubbles. Other substances in the fluid, including proteins, bile salts, and salts of free fatty acids, are also capable of forming stable bubbles, but they can be removed from the film by ethanol, which competes with the other substrates for a position in the surface film.[71] The test makes use of the principle that more surfactant activity is necessary to support a stable foam as the fraction of ethanol in the mixture is increased.[291-294] Therefore a fixed volume of undiluted amniotic fluid is mixed with increasing volumes of ethanol, and the largest fraction of ethanol in which the amniotic fluid is still capable

*References 121, 128, 134, 158, 208, 317, 343.

of supporting a foam is determined. The highest fraction of ethanol at which a positive reading is obtained is the FSI.

Interpretation

An FSI value of 0.47 or greater is interpreted as mature. In two studies, a combined total of 270 fetuses with an FSI of 0.47 or greater was reported, two of which developed RDS. In 110 fetuses with an FSI of 0.46 or less, 44 (40%) developed RDS. Thus the test appears to have more false predictions of immaturity than the L/S ratio or surfactant/albumin ratio. Tubes and stoppers must be clean and free of detergents to prevent false-positive readings. The final concentration of the ethanol is critical. Ethanol is hygroscopic; therefore careful attention must be paid to its preparation and storage. The test should be conducted at 20 °C to 25 °C.[181] Specimens contaminated with either blood or meconium tend to give a falsely mature result.

Lamellar Body Counts[25]

Lamellar bodies avidly scatter light, producing a haziness in mature amniotic fluid.[111] These particles can be counted directly using the platelet channel of most whole blood cell counters. This technique is termed lamellar body count (LBC).[23,112] LBC is a direct reflection of surfactant concentration in amniotic fluid, in contrast to L/S ratio and TDx FLM II, which are ratios. Fetal urination lowers LBC, but does not affect results of the other two methods.

Lamellar bodies have a broad size distribution, ranging from 0.2 to 10 fL.[25] The whole blood cell counters used during the development of the LBC method used a size gate from 2 to 20 fL. Therefore only a portion of lamellar bodies are counted in these instruments.

Centrifugation of amniotic fluid can be omitted.[20,113] Mixing is critical—two minutes is recommended on a tube rocker or at least 20 inversions immediately before analysis.[230] Typical LBC results are from 0 to 150,000/μL. A detailed procedure is available on the Evolve site that accompanies this book.

Because of different platelet identification algorithms, counts will be lower or higher on different instruments. Instruments that use similar algorithms (for example, the resistive pulse instruments, Coulter Gen-S, Cell-dyn 3500, and Sysmex XE-2100) have high correlation but poor agreement.[305] The proportional bias was from −32% to +76% among these instruments. The Advia 120, a flow cytometer that uses a different platelet algorithm, did not correlate with the resistive pulse counters, but has been shown to predict FLM using a modified algorithm.[70] The imprecision (CV) is typically 6% to 8% at an LBC of 35,000/μL.[143]

Specimens containing mucus produce erratic results.[230] More than 1% contamination with blood initially increases LBC because of the addition of platelets, but lamellar bodies are trapped in any clots that occur thus lowering the LBC by up to 20%.[230] Moderate meconium contamination (A_{390} up to 0.5) increases LBC by 5000/μL or less.[112]

Interpretation

The maturity decision cutoff varies from 19,000 to 60,000/μL. Typically 35,000/μL is used,[230] but this is affected strongly by the instrument used. All clinical outcomes studies* have reported that LBC has high sensitivity (95% to 100%) but low specificity (about 70%) for prediction of RDS. A recent meta-analysis[346] reported that at a fixed sensitivity of 95%, the LBC specificity was 80%, whereas the L/S ratio specificity was 70%.

No studies of diagnostic accuracy exist for diabetic mothers. An assay comparison study of LBC, L/S ratio, and PG reported good agreement among the tests for 90 diabetic subjects with no cases of RDS.[107]

REFERENCES

1. Adams MJ, Windham GC, James LM, Greenberg F, Clayton-Hopkins JA, Reimer CB, et al. Clinical interpretation of maternal serum alpha-fetoprotein concentrations. Am J Obstet Gynecol 1984;148: 241-54.
2. Almeida OD Jr, Kitay DZ. Amniotic fluid urea nitrogen in the prediction of respiratory distress syndrome. Am J Obstet Gynecol 1988;159:465-8.
3. American Academy of Pediatrics Committee on Genetics: Maternal serum α-fetoprotein screening. Pediatrics 1991;88:1282-3.
4. American College of Obstetricians and Gynecologists. Antenatal corticosteroid therapy for fetal maturation. ACOG Committee Opinion No. 147. Washington, DC: American College of Obstetricians and Gynecologists, 1994.
5. American College of Obstetricians and Gynecologists. Assessment of fetal lung maturity. ACOG Educational Bulletin No. 230. Washington, DC: American College of Obstetricians and Gynecologists, 1996.
6. American College of Obstetricians and Gynecologists. First-Trimester screening for fetal aneuploidy. ACOG Committee Opinion No. 296. Washington, DC: American College of Obstetricians and Gynecologists, 2004.
7. American College of Obstetricians and Gynecologists. Guidelines for hepatitis B virus screening and vaccination during pregnancy. ACOG Committee Opinion No. 111. Washington, DC: American College of Obstetricians and Gynecologists, 1992.
8. American College of Obstetricians and Gynecologists. Home uterine activity monitoring. ACOG Committee Opinion No. 172. Washington, DC: American College of Obstetricians and Gynecologists, 1996.
9. American College of Obstetricians and Gynecologists. Management of isoimmunization in pregnancy. ACOG Educational Bulletin No. 227. Washington,

*References 23, 30, 45, 99, 108, 112, 118, 143, 196, 231, 255.

DC: American College of Obstetricians and Gynecologists, 1996.
10. American College of Obstetricians and Gynecologists. Maternal serum screening. ACOG Educational Bulletin No. 228. Washington, DC: American College of Obstetricians and Gynecologists, 1996.
11. American College of Obstetricians and Gynecologists. Preconceptional care. ACOG Technical Bulletin No. 205. Washington, DC: American College of Obstetricians and Gynecologists, 1995.
12. American College of Obstetricians and Gynecologists. Prenatal and perinatal human immunodeficiency virus testing: expanded recommendations. ACOG Committee Opinion No. 304. Washington, DC: American College of Obstetricians and Gynecologists, 2004.
13. American College of Obstetricians and Gynecologists. Prevention of D isoimmunization. ACOG Technical Bulletin No. 147. Washington, DC: American College of Obstetricians and Gynecologists, 1990.
14. American College of Obstetricians and Gynecologists. Professional liability implications of AFP tests. Professional liability alert. Washington, DC: American College of Obstetricians and Gynecologists, 1985.
15. American Society of Human Genetics. Policy statement for maternal serum alpha-fetoprotein screening programs and quality control for laboratories performing maternal serum and amniotic fluid alpha-fetoprotein assays. Am J Hum Genet 1987;40: 75-82.
16. Ander DS, Ward KR. Medical management of ectopic pregnancy: the role of methotrexate. J Emerg Med 1997;15:177-82.
17. Apple FS, Bilodeau L, Preese LM, Benson P. Clinical implementation of a rapid, automated assay for assessing fetal lung maturity. J Reprod Med 1994;39:883-887.
18. Artiss JD, Epstein E, Kiechle FL, Zak B. Enzyme reagents for measurement of phospholipids of amniotic fluid. Ann Clin Lab Sci 1985;15:488-94.
19. Ashwood ER. Evaluating health and maturation of the unborn: the role of the clinical laboratory. Clin Chem 1992;38:1523-9.
20. Ashwood ER. Standards of laboratory practice: evaluation of fetal lung maturity. Clin Chem 1997;43:1-4.
21. Ashwood ER. Markers of fetal lung maturity. In Gronowski AM, ed. Handbook of clinical laboratory testing during pregnancy. Totowa, NJ: Humana Press, 2004:55-70.
22. Ashwood ER, Chamberlain BV. Binding of fluorescent phosphatidylcholine in amniotic fluid. Obstet Gynecol 1988;71:370-4.
23. Ashwood ER, Oldroyd RG, Palmer SE. Measuring the number of lamellar body particles in amniotic fluid. Obstet Gynecol 1990;75:289-2.
24. Ashwood ER, Palmer SE, Lenke RR. Rapid fetal lung maturity testing: commercial versus NBD-phosphatidylcholine assay. Obstet Gynecol 4992;81:1048-53.
25. Ashwood ER, Palmer SE, Taylor JS, Pingree SS. Lamellar body counts for rapid fetal lung maturity testing. Obstet Gynecol 1993;81:619-24.
26. Ashwood ER, Tait JF, Foerder CA, Benedetti TJ. Improved fluorescence polarization assay for use in evaluating fetal lung maturity: III. Retrospective clinical evaluation and comparison with the lecithin/sphingomyelin ratio. Clin Chem 1986;32: 260-4.
27. Avent ND. Molecular biology of the Rh blood group system. J Pediatr Hematol Oncol 2001;23: 394-402.
28. Bahado-Singh RO, Choi SJ, Oz U, Mendilcioglu I, Rowther M, Persutte W. Early second-trimester individualized estimation of trisomy 18 risk by ultrasound. Obstet Gynecol 2003;101:463-8.
29. Bartels I, Lindemann A. Maternal levels of pregnancy-specific beta 1-glycoprotein (SP-1) are elevated in pregnancies affected by Down's syndrome. Hum Genet 1988;80:46-8.
30. Beinlich A, Fischass C, Kaufmann M, Schlosser R, Dericks-Tan JS. Lamellar body counts in amniotic fluid for prediction of fetal lung maturity. Arch Gynecol Obstet 1999;262:173-80.
31. Benn PA, Fang M, Egan JF, Horne D, Collins R. Incorporation of inhibin-A in second-trimester screening for Down syndrome. Obstet Gynecol 2003;101:451-4.
32. Benn PA, Leo MV, Rodis JF, Beazoglou T, Collins R, Horne D. Maternal serum screening for fetal trisomy 18: a comparison of fixed cutoff and patient-specific risk protocols. Obstet Gynecol 1999;93:707-11.
33. Benoit J, Merrill S, Rundell C, Meeker CI. Amniostat-FLM: an initial clinical trial with both vaginal pool and amniocentesis samples. Am J Obstet Gynecol 1986;154:65-8.
34. Benzie RJ, Doran TA, Harkins JL, Owen VM, Porter CJ. Composition of the amniotic fluid and maternal serum in pregnancy. Am J Obstet Gynecol 1974;119:798-810.
35. Bergstrand CG, Czar B. Paper electrophoretic study on human fetal serum proteins with demonstration of a new protein fraction. Scand J Clin Lab Invest 1957;9:277-86.
36. Berkowitz K, Reyes C, Saadat P, Kjos SL. Fetal lung maturation. Comparison of biochemical indices in gestational diabetic and nondiabetic pregnancies. J Reprod Med 1997;42:793-800.
37. Bevis DCA. Composition of liquor amnii in haemolytic disease of newborn. Lancet 1950;2:443.
38. Bevis DCA. The antenatal prediction of haemolytic disease of the newborn. Lancet 1952;1:395-8.

39. Bevis DCA. The composition of liquor amnii in haemolytic disease of the newborn. J Obstet Gynaecol Br Emp 1953;60:244-51.
40. Bevis DCA. Blood pigments in haemolytic disease of the newborn. J Obstet Gynaecol Br Emp 1956;63: 68-75.
41. Birken S, Armstrong EG, Kolks MA, Cole LA, Agosto GM, Krichevsky A, et al. Structure of the human chorionic gonadotropin β-subunit fragment from pregnant urine. Endocrinology 1988;123:572-83.
42. Birken S, Berger P, Bidart JM, Weber M, Bristow A, Norman R, et al. Preparation and characterization of new WHO reference reagents for human chorionic gonadotropin and metabolites. Clin Chem 2003;49:144-54.
43. Bock JL. Current issues in maternal serum alpha-fetoprotein screening. Am J Clin Pathol 1992;97: 541-54.
44. Bogart MH, Pandian MR, Jones OW. Abnormal maternal serum chorionic gonadotropin levels in pregnancies with fetal chromosome abnormalities. Prenat Diagn 1987;7:623-30.
45. Bowie LJ, Shammo J, Dohnal JC, Farrell E, Vye MV. Lamellar body number density and the prediction of respiratory distress. Am J Clin Pathol 1991;95: 781-6.
46. Bowman J. Thirty-five years of Rh prophylaxis. Transfusion 2003;43:1661-6.
47. Bradley LA, Canick JA, Palomaki GE, Haddow JE. Undetectable maternal serum unconjugated estriol levels in the second trimester: risk of perinatal complications associated with placental sulfatase deficiency. Am J Obstet Gynecol 1997;176:531-5.
48. Braunstein GD, Karow WG, Gentry WC, Rasor J, Wade ME. First-trimester chorionic gonadotropin measurements as an aid in the diagnosis of early pregnancy disorders. Am J Obstet Gynecol 1978;131:25-32.
49. Britton RC. Pregnancy and esophageal varices. Am J Surg 1982;143:421.
50. Brock DJH, Bolton AE, Monaghan JM. Prenatal diagnosis of anencephaly through maternal serum-alpha fetoprotein measurement. Lancet 1973;2(7835):923-4.
51. Brock DJH, Hayward C. Gel electrophoresis of amniotic fluid acetylcholinesterase as an aid to the prenatal diagnosis of fetal defects. Clin Chim Acta 1980;108:135-41.
52. Brock DJH, Sutcliffe RG. Alpha-fetoprotein in the antenatal diagnosis of anencephaly and spina bifida. Lancet 1972;2(7770):197-9.
53. Brown LM, Duck-Chong CG. Methods of evaluating fetal lung maturity. In Batsakis J, Savory J, eds. Critical reviews in clinical laboratory science. Boca Raton, Fla: CRC Press, 1982:84-159.
54. Burrow GN. The management of thyrotoxicosis in pregnancy. N Engl J Med 1985;313:562-5.
55. Bustos R, Kulovich MV, Gluck L, Gabbe SG, Evertson L, Vargas C, et al. Significance of phosphatidylglycerol in amniotic fluid in complicated pregnancies. Am J Obstet Gynecol 1979;133:899-903.
56. Butler SA, Khanlian SA, Cole LA. Detection of early pregnancy forms of human chorionic gonadotropin by home pregnancy test devices. Clin Chem 2001;47:2131-6.
57. Cacciatore B, Stenman UH, Ylostalo P. Early screening for ectopic pregnancy in high-risk symptom-free women. Lancet 1994;343:517-8.
58. The Canadian Early and Mid-trimester Amniocentesis Trial (CEMAT) Group. Randomised trial to assess safety and fetal outcome of early and midtrimester amniocentesis. Lancet 1998;351:242-7.
59. Canfield RE, O'Connor JF, Chen Y, et al. The clinical utility of the measurement of urinary hCG and its fragments. In Bellet D, Bidart JM, eds. Structure-function relationship of gonadotropins. Serono Symposia Publications, Vol 65. New York: Raven Press, 1989:297-311.
60. Canick JA, Kellner LH, Saller DN Jr, Palomaki GE, Walker RP, Osathanondh R. Second-trimester levels of maternal urinary gonadotropin peptide in Down syndrome pregnancy. Prenat Diagn 1995;15: 739-44.
61. Canick JA, Knight GJ, Palomaki GE, Haddow JE, Cuckle HS, Wald NJ. Low second trimester maternal serum unconjugated oestriol in pregnancies with Down's syndrome. Br J Obstet Gynaecol 1988;95: 330-3.
62. Canick JA, Palomaki GE, Osathanondh R. Prenatal screening for trisomy 18 in the second trimester. Prenat Diagn 1990;10:546-8.
63. Caritis SN, Mueller-Heubach E, Edelstone DI. Effect of betamethasone on analysis of amniotic fluid in the rhesus-sensitized pregnancy. Am J Obstet Gynecol 1977;127:529-32.
64. Carter PE, Pearn JH, Bell J, Martin N, Anderson NG. Survival in trisomy 18: life tables for use in genetic counselling and clinical paediatrics. Clin Genet 1985;27:59-61.
65. Castro MA, Fassett MJ, Reynolds TB, Shaw KJ, Goodwin TM. Reversible peripartum liver failure: a new perspective on the diagnosis, treatment, and cause of acute fatty liver of pregnancy, based on 28 consecutive cases. Am J Obstet Gynecol 1999;181: 389-95.
66. Catt KJ, Dufau ML, Tsuruhara J. Radioligand-receptor assay of luteinizing hormone and chorionic gonadotropin. J Clin Endocrinol Metab 1972;34: 123-32.
67. Centers for Disease Control and Prevention. Recommendations for the use of folic acid to reduce the number of cases of spina bifida and other neural tube defects. MMWR 1992;41(RR14):1-7.

68. Chayen J, Daly JR, Loveridge N, Bitensky L. The cytochemical bioassay of hormones. Recent Prog Horm Res 1976;32:33-79.
69. Chen C, Roby PV, Weiss NS, Wilson JA, Benedetti TJ, Tait JF. Clinical evaluation of the NBD-PC fluorescence polarization assay for prediction of fetal lung maturity. Obstet Gynecol 1992;80:688-92.
70. Chapman JF, Ashwood ER, Feld R, Wu AH. Evaluation of two-dimensional cytometric lamellar body counts on the ADVIA 120 hematology system for estimation of fetal lung maturation. Clin Chim Acta 2004;340:85-92.
71. Clements JA, Platzker ACG, Tierney DF, Hobel CJ, Creasy RK, Margolis AJ, et al. Assessment of the risk of the respiratory-distress syndrome by a rapid test for surfactant in amniotic fluid. N Engl J Med 1972;286:1077-81.
72. Cole LA. Immunoassay of human chorionic gonadotropin, its free subunits, and metabolites. Clin Chem 1997;43:2233-43.
73. Cole LA, Shahabi S, Oz UA, Bahado-Singh RO, Mahoney MJ. Hyperglycosylated human chorionic gonadotropin (invasive trophoblast antigen) immunoassay: a new basis for gestational Down syndrome screening. Clin Chem 1999; 45:2109-19.
74. Cole LA, Kardana A. Discordant results in human chorionic gonadotropin assays. Clin Chem 1992;38:263-70.
75. Cole LA, Kardana A, Birken S. The isomers, subunits and fragments of hCG. In Bellet D, Bidart JM, eds. Structure-function relationship of gonadotropins. Serono Symposia Publications, Vol 65. New York: Raven Press, 1989:59-79.
76. Cole LA, Khanlian SA, Sutton JM, Davies S, Rayburn WF. Accuracy of home pregnancy tests at the time of missed menses. Am J Obstet Gynecol 2004;190: 100-5.
77. Cole LA, Shahabi S, Butler SA, Mitchell H, Newlands ES, Behrman HR, et al. Utility of commonly used commercial human chorionic gonadotropin immunoassays in the diagnosis and management of trophoblastic diseases. Clin Chem 2001;47: 308-15.
78. Chang J, Elam-Evans LD, Berg CJ, Herndon J, Flowers L, Seed KA, et al. Pregnancy-related mortality surveillance—United States, 1991-1999. MMWR Surveill Summ 2003;52:1-8.
79. College of American Pathologists. CAP surveys, lung maturity survey, set LM-C. Northfield, Ill: College of American Pathologists, 1995.
80. College of American Pathologists. CAP surveys, maternal screening survey, set FP-A. Northfield, Ill: College of American Pathologists, 2000.
81. College of American Pathologists. CAP surveys, maternal screening survey, set FP-A. Northfield, Ill: College of American Pathologists, 2003.
82. Condon JC, Jeyasuria P, Faust JM, Mendelson CR. Surfactant protein secreted by the maturing mouse fetal lung acts as a hormone that signals the initiation of parturition. Proc Natl Acad Sci USA 2004;101:4978-83.
83. Crandall BF. Prenatal screening for the detection of neural tube defects. In: Essentials of prenatal diagnosis. JL Simpson, S Elias, eds. New York: Churchill Livingstone 1993:253-74.
84. Crandall BF, Chua C. Risks for fetal abnormalities after elevated and moderately elevated AFAFPs. Prenat Diagn 1997;17:837-41.
85. Cruz AC, Buhi WC, Birk SA, Spellacy WN. Respiratory distress syndrome with mature lecithin/sphingomyelin ratios: diabetes mellitus and low Apgar scores. Am J Obstet Gynecol 1978;126:78-82.
86. Cuckle H. Down syndrome fetal loss rate in early pregnancy. Prenat Diagn 1999;19:1177-9.
86A. Cuckle H. Improved parameters for risk estimation in Down's syndrome screening. Prenat Diagn 1995;15:1055-7.
87. Cuckle HS, Iles RK, Chard T. Urinary beta-core human chorionic gonadotrophin: a new approach to Down's syndrome screening. Prenat Diagn 1994;14:953-8.
88. Cuckle HS, Canick JA, Kellner LH. Collaborative study of maternal urine beta-core human gonadotrophin screening for Down syndrome. Prenat Diagn 1999;19:911-7.
89. Cuckle HS, Shahabi S, Sehmi IK, Jones R, Cole LA. Maternal urine hyperglycosylated hCG in pregnancies with Down syndrome. Prenat Diagn 1999;19:918-20.
90. Cuckle HS, Sehmi IK, Jones RG, Mason G. Low maternal serum PAPP-A and fetal viability. Prenat Diagn 1999;19:787-92.
91. Cuckle HS, Wald NJ, Lindenbaum RH. Maternal serum alpha-fetoprotein measurement: a screening test for Down syndrome. Lancet 1984;1(8383): 926-9.
91A. Cuckle HS, Wald NJ, Thompson SG. Estimating a woman's risk of having a pregnancy associated with Down's syndrome using her age and serum alpha-fetoprotein level. Br J Obstet Gynaecol 1987;94: 387-402.
92. Cunningham FG, MacDonald PC, Gant NF. Techniques to evaluate fetal health. In Williams obstetrics. 18th ed. Norwalk, Conn: Appleton & Lange, 1989:277-305.
93. Cunningham FG, MacDonald PC, Gant NF. The placental hormones. In Williams obstetrics. 18th ed. Norwalk, Conn: Appleton & Lange, 1989:67-85.
94. Cunningham GC, Tompkinison DG. Cost and effectiveness of the California triple marker prenatal screening program. Genet Med 1999;1:199-206.
95. Cunningham MD, Desai NS, Thompson SA, Greene JM. Amniotic fluid phosphatidylglycerol in

diabetic pregnancies. Am J Obstet Gynecol 1978;131: 719-24.

96. Cunningham MD, McKean HE, Gillispie DH, Greene JW. Improved prediction of fetal lung maturity in diabetic pregnancies: a comparison of chromatographic methods. Am J Obstet Gynecol 1982;142: 197-204.
97. D'Alton ME, DeCherney AH. Prenatal diagnosis. N Engl J Med 1993;328:114-20. [Editorial].
98. Daily CA, Laurent SL, Nunley WCJ. The prognostic value of serum progesterone and quantitative β-human chorionic gonadotropin in early human pregnancy. Am J Obstet Gynecol 1994;171:380-3.
99. Dalence CR, Bowie LJ, Dohnal JC, Farrell EE, Neerhof MG. Amniotic fluid lamellar body count: a rapid and reliable fetal lung maturity test. Obstet Gynecol 1995;86:235-9.
100. Dallaire L, Belanger L, Smith CJP, Kelleher PC. Origin of amniocentesis-induced rises of alpha-fetoprotein concentrations in maternal serum. Br J Obstet Gynaecol 1980;87:856-9.
101. Darling RE, Zlatnik FJ. Comparison of amniotic fluid optical density, L/S ratio and creatinine concentration in predicting fetal pulmonary maturity. J Reprod Med 1985;30:460-4.
102. Daviaud J, Fournet D, Ballongue C, Guillem GP, Leblanc A, Casellas C, et al. Reliability and feasibility of pregnancy home-use tests: laboratory validation and diagnostic evaluation by 638 volunteers. Clin Chem 1993;39:53-9.
103. Dawood MY. Hormones in amniotic fluid. Am J Obstet Gynecol 1977;128:576-83.
104. de Courcy-Wheeler RH, Pomeranz MM, Wald NJ, Nicolaides KH. Small fetal transverse cerebellar diameter: a screening test for spina bifida. Br J Obstet Gynaecol 1994;101:904-5.
105. Del Valle GO, Adair CD, Ramos EE, Gaudier FL, Sanchez-Ramos L, Morales R. Interpretation of the TDx-FLM fluorescence polarization assay in pregnancies complicated by diabetes mellitus. Am J Perinatol 1997;14:241-4.
106. deMello DE, Nogee LM, Heyman S, Krous HF, Hussain M, Merritt TA, et al. Molecular and phenotypic variability in the congenital alveolar proteinosis syndrome associated with inherited surfactant protein B deficiency. J Pediatr 1994;125: 43-50.
107. DeRoche ME, Ingardia CJ, Guerette PJ, Wu AH, LaSala CA, Mandavilli SR. The use of lamellar body counts to predict fetal lung maturity in pregnancies complicated by diabetes mellitus. Am J Obstet Gynecol 2002;187:908-2.
108. Dilena BA, Ku F, Doyle I, Whiting MJ. Six alternative methods to the lecithin/sphingomyelin ratio in amniotic fluid for assessing fetal lung maturity. Ann Clin Biochem 1997;34:106-8.
109. Dombroski RA, Mackenna J, Brame RG. Comparison of amniotic fluid lung maturity profiles in paired vaginal and amniocentesis specimens. Am J Obstet Gynecol 1981;140:461-4.
110. Doyle PE, Beral V, Botting B, Wale CJ. Congenital malformations in twins in England and Wales. J Epidemiol Community Health 1991;45:43-8.
111. Dubin SB. Determination of lamellar body size, number density, and concentration by differential light scattering from amniotic fluid: physical significance of A_{650}. Clin Chem 1988;34:938-43.
112. Dubin SB. Characterization of amniotic fluid lamellar bodies by resistive-pulse counting: relationship to measures of fetal lung maturity. Clin Chem 1989;35:612-6.
113. Dubin SB. Assessment of fetal lung maturity. Practice parameter. Am J Clin Pathol 1998;110:723-32.
114. Dufau ML, Mendelson CR, Catt KJ. A highly sensitive in vitro bioassay for luteinizing hormone and chorionic gonadotropin: testosterone production by dispersed Leydig cells. J Clin Endocrinol Metab 1974;39:610-3.
115. Eisenbrey AB, Epstein E, Zak B, McEnroe RJ, Artiss JD, Kiechle FL. Phosphatidylglycerol in amniotic fluid: comparison of an "ultrasensitive" immunologic assay with TLC and enzymatic assay. Am J Clin Pathol 1989;91:293-7.
116. Erickson JA, Ashwood ER, Gin CA. Evaluation of a dimeric inhibin-A assay for assessing fetal Down syndrome: establishment, comparison, and monitoring of median concentrations for normal pregnancies. Arch Pathol Lab Med 2004;128: 415-20.

116A. Evans MI, Chik L, O'Brien JE, Chin B, Dvorin E, Ayoub M, et al. MOMs (multiples of the median) and DADs (discriminant aneuploidy detection): improved specificity and cost-effectiveness of biochemical screening for aneuploidy with DADs. Am J Obstet Gynecol 1995;172:1138-47.

117. Evans MI, Berkowitz RL, Wapner RJ, Carpenter RJ, Goldberg JD, Ayoub MA, et al. Improvement in outcomes of multifetal pregnancy reduction with increased experience. Am J Obstet Gynecol 2001;184:97-103. Comment in: Am J Obstet Gynecol 2001;184:1041-3 and Am J Obstet Gynecol 2002;186:596-7; author reply 597.
118. Fakhoury G, Daikoku NH, Benser J, Dubin NH. Lamellar body concentrations and the prediction of fetal pulmonary maturity. Am J Obstet Gynecol 1994;170:72-6.
119. Fantz CR, Powell C, Karon B, Parvin CA, Hankins K, Dayal M, et al. Assessment of the diagnostic accuracy of the TDx-FLM II to predict fetal lung maturity. Clin Chem 2002;48:761-5.
120. Farrell PM, Avery ME. Hyaline membrane disease. Am Rev Respir Dis 1975;111:657-88.

121. Farquharson J, Jamieson EC, Berry E, Buchanan R, Logan RW. Assessment of the AmnioStat-FLM immunoagglutination test for phosphatidylglycerol in amniotic fluid. Clin Chim Acta 1986;156:271-7.
122. Feuchtbaum LB, Currier RJ, Lorey FW, Cunningham GC. Prenatal ultrasound findings in affected and unaffected pregnancies that are screen-positive for trisomy 18: the California experience. Prenat Diagn 2000;20:293-9.
123. Finning K, Martin P, Daniels G. A clinical service in the UK to predict fetal Rh (Rhesus) D blood group using free fetal DNA in maternal plasma. Ann N Y Acad Sci 2004;1022:119-23.
124. Food and Drug Administration. Food standards: amendment of standards of identity for enrichment of grain products to require addition of folic acid. Federal Register 1996;61:8781-97.
125. Foerder CA, Tait JF, Franklin RW, Ashwood ER. Improved fluorescence polarization assay for use in evaluating fetal lung maturity: II. Analytical evaluation and comparison with the lecithin/sphingomyelin ratio. Clin Chem 1986;32:255-9.
126. Forest JC, Masse J, Moutquin JM. Screening for Down syndrome during first trimester: a prospective study using free beta-human chorionic gonadotropin and pregnancy-associated plasma protein A. Clin Biochem 1997;30:333-8.
127. Foster K, Moore J, Hankins K, Parvin CA, Gronowski AM. Effect of blood contamination on delta 450 bilirubin measurement: an in vitro comparison of two corrective methods. Clin Chem 2004;50:1420-2.
128. Francoual J, Cohen H, Benattar C, Papiernik E, Leluc R. Phosphatidylglycerol in amniotic fluid. Value of rapid determination using an immunologic technic. J Gynecol Obstet Biol Reprod (Paris) 1985;14:879-82.
129. Freer DE, Statland BE, Sher G. Quantitation of disaturated phosphatidylcholine and phosphatidylglycerol in amniotic fluid by fluorescence diminution: methodology and clinical results. Clin Chem 1979;25:960-8.
130. Frey L, Hauser WA. Epidemiology of neural tube defects. Epilepsia 2003;44 Suppl 3:4-13.
131. Fried AM, Loh FK, Umer MA, Dillon KP, Kryscio R. Echogenicity of fetal lung: relation to fetal age and maturity. Am J Roentgenol 1985;145:591-4.
132. Friedman SA, Schiff E, Kao L, Kuint J, Sibai BM. Do twins mature earlier than singletons? Results from a matched cohort study. Am J Obstet Gynecol 1997;176:1193-6.
133. Gabbe SG, Lowensohn RI, Mestman JH, Freeman RK, Goebelsmann U. Lecithin/sphingomyelin ratio in pregnancies complicated by diabetes mellitus. Am J Obstet Gynecol 1977;128:757-60.
134. Garite TJ, Yabusaki KK, Moberg LJ, Symons JL, White T, Itano M, et al. A new rapid slide agglutination test for amniotic fluid phosphatidylglycerol: laboratory and clinical correlation. Am J Obstet Gynecol 1983;147:681-6.
135. Gibbons JM, Huntley TE, Corral AG. Effect of maternal blood contamination on amniotic fluid analysis. Obstet Gynecol 1974;44:657-60.
136. Gibbs PE, Zielinski R, Boyd C, Dugaiczyk A. Structure, polymorphism, and novel repeated DNA elements revealed by a complete sequence of the human α-fetoprotein gene. Biochemistry 1987;26:1332-43.
137. Gitlan D. Normal biology of alpha-fetoprotein. Ann N Y Acad Sci 1975;259:7-16.
138. Glinoer D, de Nayer P, Bourdoux P, Lemone M, Robyn C, van Steirteghem A, et al. Regulation of maternal thyroid during pregnancy. J Clin Endocrinol Metab 1990;71:276-87.
139. Gluck L, Kulovich MV. Lecithin/sphingomyelin ratios in amniotic fluid in normal and abnormal pregnancy. Am J Obstet Gynecol 1973;115:539-46.
140. Goepfert AR, Goldenberg RL, Andrews WW, Hauth JC, Mercer B, Iams J, et al. The preterm prediction study: association between cervical interleukin 6 concentration and spontaneous preterm birth. National Institute of Child Health and Human Development Maternal-Fetal Medicine Units Network. Am J Obstet Gynecol 2001;184:483-8.
141. Goldenberg RL, Mercer BM, Iams JD, Moawad AH, Meis PJ, Das A, et al. The preterm prediction study: patterns of cervicovaginal fetal fibronectin as predictors of spontaneous preterm delivery. Am J Obstet Gynecol 1997;177:8-12.
142. Goldner TE, Lawson HW, Zhisen X, Atrash HK. Surveillance for ectopic pregnancy—United States, 1970-1989. Morbid Mortal Weekly Rep 1994;42:73-85.
142A. Greenberg F, James LM, Oakley GP Jr. Estimates of birth prevalence rates of spina bifida in the United States from computer-generated maps. Am J Obstet Gynecol 1983;145:570-3.
143. Greenspoon JS, Rosen DJ, Roll K, Dubin SB. Evaluation of lamellar body number density as the initial assessment in a fetal lung maturity test cascade. J Reprod Med 1995;40:260-6.
144. Grenache DG. Hemolytic disease of the newborn. In Gronowski AM, ed. Handbook of clinical laboratory testing during pregnancy. Totowa, NJ: Humana Press, 2004:219-43.
145. Grenache DG, Parvin CA, Gronowski AM. Preanalytical factors that influence the Abbott TDx Fetal Lung Maturity II assay. Clin Chem 2003;49:935-9.
146. Grody WW, Cutting GR, Klinger KW, Richards CS, Watson MS, Desnick RJ. Subcommittee on cystic fibrosis screening, accreditation of genetic services committee, ACMG. American College of Medical

Genetics. Laboratory standards and guidelines for population-based cystic fibrosis carrier screening. Genet Med 2001;3:149-54.
147. Gronowski AM, Parvin CA. Prediction of risk for respiratory distress syndrome using gestational age and the TDx FLM II assay. Am J Obstet Gynecol 2003;189:1511-2.
148. Haddow JE, Morin ME, Holman MS, Miller WA. Acetylcholinesterase and fetal malformations: modified qualitative technique for diagnosis of neural tube defects. Clin Chem 1981;27:61-3.
149. Haddow JE, Palomaki GE, Knight GJ, Williams J, Pulkkinen A, Canick JA, et al. Prenatal screening for Down's syndrome with use of maternal serum markers. N Engl J Med 1992;327:588-93.
150. Haddow JE, Palomaki GE, Knight GJ, Canick JA. Variables which influence levels of AFP, uE3, and hCG and/or risk for Down syndrome. Foundation for Blood Research handbook. Vol. II: screening for Down syndrome. Scarborough, Me: Foundation for Blood Research, 1998: section 19;19-1 to 19-34 (see www.fbr.org, accessed February 13, 2005).
150A. Haddow JE, Palomaki GE, Knight GJ, Canick JA. Principles of prenatal screening for Down's syndrome: combining multiple biochemical markers and maternal age. Foundation for Blood Research handbook. Vol. II: screening for Down syndrome. Scarborough, Me: Foundation for Blood Research, 1998: section 20:20-1 to 20-38 (see www.fbr.org, accessed February 13, 2005).
151. Haddow JE, Palomaki GE, Knight GJ, Canick JA. Variables which influence levels of AFP, uE3, and hCG and/or risk for Down syndrome. Foundation for Blood Research handbook Vol II: screening for Down syndrome. Scarborough, Me: Foundation for Blood Research, 1998: section 21; 21-1 to 21-48 (see www.fbr.org, accessed February 13, 2005).
152. Haddow JE, Palomaki GE, Knight GJ, Canick JA. Laboratory considerations in multiple marker screening. Foundation for Blood Research handbook. Vol II: Screening for Down syndrome. Scarborough, Me: Foundation for Blood Research, 1998:section 22; 22-1 to 22-49. (see www.fbr.org, accessed February 13, 2005).
153. Haddow JE, Palomaki GE, Knight GJ, Cunningham GC, Lustig MS, Boyd PA. Reducing the need for amniocentesis in women age 35 years and older with serum markers for screening. N Engl J Med 1994;330:1114-18.
154. Haddow JE, Palomaki GE, Knight GJ, Foster DL, Neveux LM. Second trimester screening for Down's syndrome using maternal serum dimeric inhibin A. J Med Screen 1998;5:115-19.
155. Haddow JE, Palomaki GE, Knight GJ, Williams J, Miller WA, Johnson A. Screening of maternal serum for fetal Down's syndrome in the first trimester. N Engl J Med 1998;338:955-61.
156. Hallman M, Kulovich M, Kirkpatrick E, Sugarman RG, Gluck L. Phosphatidylinositol and phosphatidylglycerol in amniotic fluid: indices of lung maturity. Am J Obstet Gynecol 1976;125: 613-17.
157. Hallman M, Merritt TA, Jarvenpaa AL, Boynton B, Mannino F, Gluck L, et al. Exogenous human surfactant for treatment of severe respiratory distress syndrome: a randomized prospective clinical trial. J Pediatr 1985;106:963-9.
158. Halvorsen PR, Gross TL. Laboratory and clinical evaluation of a rapid slide agglutination test for phosphatidylglycerol. Am J Obstet Gynecol 1985;151: 1061-6.
159. Harper ME, Dugaiczyk A. Linkage of the evolutionarily-related serum albumin and α-fetoprotein genes within q11-22 of human chromosome 4. Am J Hum Genet 1983;35:565-72.
160. Hawgood S, Clements JA. Pulmonary surfactant and its apoproteins. J Clin Invest 1990;86:1-6.
160A. Hecht CA, Hook EB. Rates of Down's syndrome at livebirth by one-year maternal age intervals in studies with apparent close to complete ascertainment in populations of European origin: a proposed revised rate schedule for use in genetic and prenatal screening. Am J Med Genet 1996;62: 376-85.
161. Heine RP, McGregor JA, Goodwin TM, Artal R, Hayashi RH, Robertson PA, et al. Serial salivary estriol to detect an increased risk of preterm birth. Obstet Gynecol 2000;96:490-7.
162. Henshaw SK. Unintended pregnancy in the United States. Fam Plann Perspect 1998;30:24-9.
163. Herbert WNP, Chapman JF, Schnoor MM. Role of the TDx FLM assay in fetal lung maturity. Am J Obstet Gynecol 1993;168:808-12.
164. Hicks JM, Iosefsohn M. Reliability of home pregnancy-test kits in the hands of laypersons. N Engl J Med 1989;320:320-1. Erratum in: N Engl J Med 1989;321:193.
165. Holmes LB, Driscoll SG, Atkins L. Etiologic heterogeneity of neural-tube defects. N Engl J Med 1976;294:365-9.
166. Holt JA, Ryan DF, Russell JC, et al. Automated rapid assessment of surfactant and fetal lung maturity. Lab Med 1990;21:359-66.
167. Honest H, Bachmann LM, Gupta JK, Kleijnen J, Khan KS. Accuracy of cervicovaginal fetal fibronectin test in predicting risk of spontaneous preterm birth: systematic review. BMJ 2002;325:301.
168. Hook EB, Cross PK, Schreinemachers DM. Chromosomal abnormality rates at amniocentesis and in liveborn infants. JAMA 1983;249:2034-8.

169. Hook GER, Gilmore LB, Tombropoulos EG, Fabro SE. Fetal lung lamellar bodies in human amniotic fluid. Am Rev Respir Dis 1978;117:541-50.
170. Isozaki T, Palomaki GE, Bahado-Singh RO, Cole LA. Screening for Down syndrome pregnancy using beta-core fragment: prospective study. Prenat Diagn 1997;17:407-13.
171. Jeffcoate TN, Fliegner JR, Russell SH, Davis JC, Wade AP. Diagnosis of the adrenogenital syndrome before birth. Lancet 1965;2(7412):553-5.
172. Janssen PA, Rothman I, Schwartz SM. Congenital malformations in newborns of women with established and gestational diabetes in Washington State, 1984-91. Paediatr Perinat Epidemiol 1996;10:52-63.
173. Jeng LL, Moore RM Jr, Kaczmarek RG, Placek PJ, Bright RA. How frequently are home pregnancy tests used? Results from the 1988 National Maternal and Infant Health Survey. Birth 1991;18:11-13.
174. Jones GW, Ashwood ER. Enzymatic measurement of phosphatidylglycerol in amniotic fluid. Clin Chem 1994;40:518-25.
175. Kadar N, Bohrer M, Kemmann E, Shelden R. The discriminatory human chorionic gonadotropin zone for endovaginal sonography: a prospective, randomized study. Fertil Steril 1994;61:1016-20.
176. Kadar N, Bohrer M, Kemmann E, Shelden R. A prospective, randomized study of the chorionic gonadotropin-time relationship in early gestation: clinical implications. Fertil Steril 1993;60:409-12.
177. Kadar N, DeVore G, Romero R. Discriminatory hCG zone: its use in the sonographic evaluation for ectopic pregnancy. Obstet Gynecol 1981;58:156-61.
178. Kaneko K, Shimizu H, Arakawa H, Ogawa Y. Pulmonary surfactant protein A in sera for assessing neonatal lung maturation. Early Hum Dev 2001;62:11-21.
179. Kaplan LA, Chapman JF, Bock JL, Santa Maria E, Clejan S, Huddleston DJ, et al. Prediction of respiratory distress syndrome using the Abbott FLM-II amniotic fluid assay. Clin Chim Acta 2002;326:61-8.
180. Kardana A, Cole LA. Polypeptide nicks cause erroneous results in assays of human chorionic gonadotropin free β-subunit. Clin Chem 1992;38:26-33.
181. Keniston RC, Noland GL, Pernoll ML. The effect of blood, meconium, and temperature on the rapid surfactant test. Obstet Gynecol 1976;48:442-6.
182. Kesselman EJ, Figueroa R, Garry D, Maulik D. The usefulness of the TDx/TDxFLx fetal lung maturity II assay in the initial evaluation of fetal lung maturity. Am J Obstet Gynecol 2003;188:1220-2.
183. Klein NA, Mabie WC, Shaver DC, Latham PS, Adamec TA, Pinstein ML, et al. Herpes simplex virus hepatitis in pregnancy: two patients successfully treated with acyclovir. Gastroenterology 1991;100:239-44.
184. Knight GJ, Palomaki GE. Epidemiologic monitoring of prenatal screening for neural tube defects and Down syndrome. Clin Lab Med 2003;23:531-51.
184A. Knight GJ, Palomaki GE, Neveux LM, Fodor KK, Haddow JE. hCG and the free beta-subunit as screening tests for Down's syndrome. Prenat Diagn 1998;18:235-45.
185. Knight GJ, Palomaki GE, Neveux LM, Haddow JE, Lambert-Messerlian GM. Clinical validation of a new dimeric inhibin-A assay suitable for second trimester Down's syndrome screening. J Med Screen 2001;8:2-7.
186. Knox TA, Olans LB. Liver disease in pregnancy. N Engl J Med 1996;335:569-76.
187. Kohn MA, Kerr K, Malkevich D, O'Neil N, Kerr MJ, Kaplan BC. Beta-human chorionic gonadotropin levels and the likelihood of ectopic pregnancy in emergency department patients with abdominal pain or vaginal bleeding. Acad Emerg Med 2003;10:119-26.
188. Korhonen J, Alfthan H, Ylostalo P, Veldhuis J, Stenman UH. Disappearance of human chorionic gonadotropin and its alpha- and beta-subunits after term pregnancy. Clin Chem 1997;43:2155-63.
189. Kornman LH, Morssink LP, Wortelboer MJM, Beekhuis JR, De Wolf BT, Pratt JJ, et al. Maternal urinary β-core hCG in chromosomally abnormal pregnancies in the first trimester. Prenat Diagn 1997;17:135-9.
190. Krawczynski K, Hepatitis E. Hepatology 1993;17:932-41.
191. Kulovich MV, Gluck L. The lung profile: II. Complicated pregnancy. Am J Obstet Gynecol 1979;135:64-70.
192. Kulovich MV, Hallman MB, Gluck L. The lung profile: I. Normal pregnancy. Am J Obstet Gynecol 1979;135:57-63.
193. Lakowicz JR. Fluorescence polarization. In: Principles of fluorescence spectroscopy. New York: Plenum Press, 1983:111-53.
194. Lambert-Messerlian GM, Canick JA, Palomaki GE, Schneyer AL. Second trimester levels of maternal serum inhibin A, total inhibin, alpha inhibin precursor, and activin in Down's syndrome pregnancy. J Med Screen 1996;3:58-62.
195. Lau HL, Linkins SE. Alpha-fetoprotein. Am J Obstet Gynecol 1976;124:533-53.
196. Lee IS, Cho YK, Kim A, Min WK, Kim KS, Mok JE. Lamellar body count in amniotic fluid as a rapid screening test for fetal lung maturity. J Perinatol 1996;16:176-80.
197. LeMaistre A, Bracey A, Katz A, Wu HB. Role of qualitative choriogonadotropin assays in diagnosis of ectopic pregnancy. Clin Chem 1987;33:1908-10.
198. Lenton EA, Neal LM, Sulaiman R. Plasma concentrations of human chorionic gonadotropin from the

time of implantation until the second week of pregnancy. Fertil Steril 1982;37:773-8.
199. Leung TN, Chung TK, Madsen G, McLean M, Chang AM, Smith R. Elevated mid-trimester maternal corticotrophin-releasing hormone levels in pregnancies that delivered before 34 weeks. Br J Obstet Gynaecol 1999;106:1041-6.
200. Levine RJ, Maynard SE, Qian C, Lim KH, England LJ, Yu KF, et al. Circulating angiogenic factors and the risk of preeclampsia. N Engl J Med 2004;350:672-83.
201. Liley AW. Liquor amnii analysis in the management of the pregnancy complicated by rhesus sensitization. Am J Obstet Gynecol 1961;82:1359-70.
202. Liley AW. Errors in the assessment of hemolytic disease from amniotic fluid. Am J Obstet Gynecol 1963;86:485-94.
203. Livingston EG, Herbert WN, Hage ML, Chapman JF, Stubbs TM. Use of the TDx-FLM assay in evaluating fetal lung maturity in an insulin-dependent diabetic population. The Diabetes and Fetal Maturity Study Group. Obstet Gynecol 1995;86:826-9.
204. Lockitch G, ed. Handbook of diagnostic biochemistry and hematology in normal pregnancy. Boca Raton, Fla: CRC Press, 1993.
205. Lockitch G, Wittmann BK, Snow BE, Campbell DJ. Prediction of fetal lung maturity by use of the Lumadex-FSI test. Clin Chem 1986;32:361-3.
206. Lockwood CJ, Senyei AS, Dische MR, Casal D, Shah KD, Thung SN, et al. Fetal fibronectin in cervical and vaginal secretions as a predictor of preterm delivery. N Engl J Med 1991;325:669-74.
207. Lockwood GM, Muttukrishna S, Ledger WL. Inhibins and activins in human ovulation, conception and pregnancy. Hum Reprod Update 1998;4:284-95.
208. Lockitch G, Wittmann BK, Mura SM, Hawkley LC. Evaluation of the Amniostat-FLM assay for assessment of fetal lung maturity. Clin Chem 1984;30:1233-7.
209. MacRae AR, Gardner HA, Allen LC, Tokmakejian S, Lepage N. Outcome validation of the Beckman Coulter access analyzer in a second-trimester Down syndrome serum screening application. Clin Chem 2003;49:69-76.
210. Macri JN, Kasturi RV, Krantz DA, Cook EJ, Moore ND, Young JA, et al. Maternal serum Down syndrome screening: free β-protein is a more effective marker than human chorionic gonadotropin. Am J Obstet Gynecol 1990;163:1248-53.
211. Mann SE, Nijland MJ, Ross MG. Mathematic modeling of human amniotic fluid dynamics. Am J Obstet Gynecol 1996;175:937-44.
212. Martin JN Jr, Blake PG, Perry KG Jr, McCaul JF, Hess LW, Martin RW. The natural history of HELLP syndrome: patterns of disease progression and regression. Am J Obstet Gynecol 1991;164:1500-13.
213. Matsuura H, Greene T, Hakomori SI. An alpha-N-acetylgalactosaminylation at the threonine residue of a defined peptide sequence creates the oncofetal peptide epitope in human fibronectin. J Biol Chem 1989;264:10472-6.
214. McCord ML, Muram D, Buster JE, Arheart KL, Stovall TG, Carson SA. Single serum progesterone as a screen for ectopic pregnancy: exchanging specificity and sensitivity to obtain optimal test performance. Fertil Steril 1996;66:513-6.
215. McElrath TF, Norwitz ER, Robinson JN, Tanasijevic MJ, Lieberman ES. Differences in TDx fetal lung maturity assay values between twin and singleton gestations. Am J Obstet Gynecol 2000;182:1110-2.
216. Menashe M, Finci Z, Milwidsky A, Mayer M. Amniotic fluid protease activity, protease inhibitory activity, and fetal lung maturity. Am J Perinatol 1987;4:68-71.
217. Merkatz IR, Nitowsky HM, Macri JN, Johnson WE. An association between low maternal serum α-fetoprotein and fetal chromosomal abnormalities. Am J Obstet Gynecol 1984;148:886-94.
218. Milunsky A, Jick H, Jick SS, Bruell CL, MacLaughlin DS, Rothman KJ, et al. Multivitamin/folic acid supplementation in early pregnancy reduces the prevalence of neural tube defects. JAMA 1989;262:2847-52.
219. Minakami H, Takahashi T, Tamada T. Should routine liver biopsy be done for the definite diagnosis of acute fatty liver of pregnancy? Am J Obstet Gynecol 1991;164:1690-1.
220. Miniño AM, Arias E, Kochanek KD, Murphy SL, Smith BL. Deaths: final data for 2000. National vital statistics reports. Vol 50, No 15. Hyattsville, Md: National Center for Health Statistics, 2002.
221. Mitnick MA, DeMarco B, Gibbons JM. Amniotic fluid phosphatidylglycerol and phosphatidylinositol separated by stepwise-development thin-layer chromatography. Clin Chem 1980;26:277-81.
222. Moise KJ Jr. Management of rhesus alloimmunization in pregnancy. Obstet Gynecol 2002;100:600-11. Review. Erratum in: Obstet Gynecol 2002;100:833
223. Moore TR. A comparison of amniotic fluid fetal pulmonary phospholipids in normal and diabetic pregnancy. Am J Obstet Gynecol 2002;186:641-50.
224. Moos MK, Cefalo RC. Preconceptional health promotion: a focus for obstetric care. Am J Perinatol 1987;4:63-7.
225. Morales WJ, O'Brien WF, Knuppel RA, Gaylord S, Hayes P. The effect of mode of delivery on the risk of intraventricular hemorrhage in nondiscordant twin gestations under 1500 g. Obstet Gynecol 1989;73:107-10.
225A. Morris JK, Wald NJ, Mutton DE, Alberman E. Comparison of models of maternal age-specific risk for Down's syndrome live births Prenat Diagn 2003;23:252-8.

226. Moss AJ, Levy AS, Kim I, Park YK. Use of vitamin and mineral supplements in the United States: current users, types of products, and nutrients: advance data, No 174. Hyattsville, Md: National Center of Health Statistics, 1989.
227. Muneshige A, Okazaki T, Quirk JG, MacDonald PC, Nozaki M, Johnston JM. A rapid and specific enzymatic method for the quantification of phosphatidylcholine, disaturated phosphatidylcholine, and phosphatidylglycerol in amniotic fluid. Am J Obstet Gynecol 1983;145:474-80.
228. National Center for Health Statistics: Health, United States-1995. Hyattsville, Md: Public Health Service, 1996:90.
229. National Committee for Clinical Laboratory Standards. Choriogonadotropin testing: nomenclature, reference preparations, assay performance, and clinical application, approved guideline. NCCLS document, I/LA 10-A. NCCLS: Wayne Pa, 1996.
230. Neerhof MG, Dohnal JC, Ashwood ER, Lee IS, Anceschi MM. Lamellar body counts: a consensus on protocol. Obstet Gynecol 2001;97:318-20.
231. Neerhof MG, Haney EI, Silver RK, Ashwood ER, Lee IS, Piazze JJ. Lamellar body counts compared with traditional phospholipid analysis as an assay for evaluating fetal lung maturity. Obstet Gynecol 2001;97:305-9.
232. Nelson GH, McPherson JC Jr. Respiratory distress syndrome in various cultures and a possible role of diet. In Nelson GH, ed. Pulmonary development: transition from intrauterine to extrauterine life. New York: Marcel Dekker Inc, 1985:159-78.
233. Neveux LM, Palomaki GE, Larrivee DA, Knight GJ, Haddow JE. Refinements in managing weight adjustment for interpreting prenatal screening results. Prenat Diagn 1996;16:1115-9.
234. Neveux LM, Palomaki GE, Knight GJ, Haddow JE. Multiple marker screening for Down syndrome in twin pregnancies. Prenat Diagn 1996;16:29-34.
235. New England Regional Genetics Group Prenatal Collaborative Study of Down Syndrome Screening: Combining maternal serum α-fetoprotein measurements and age to screen for Down syndrome in pregnant women under age 35. Am J Obstet Gynecol 1989;160:575-81.
236. Nicolaides KH, Campbell S, Gabbe SG, Guidetti R. Ultrasound screening for spina bifida: cranial and cerebellar signs. Lancet 1986;2(8498):72-4.
237. Nicolaides KH, Azar G, Byrne D, Mansur C, Marks K. Fetal nuchal translucency: ultrasound screening for chromosomal defects in first trimester of pregnancy. BMJ 1992;304:867-9.
238. Nogee LM, Garnier G, Dietz HC, Singer L, Murphy AM, deMello DE, et al. A mutation in the surfactant protein B gene responsible for fatal neonatal respiratory disease in multiple kindreds. J Clin Invest 1994;93:1860-3.
239. Norgaard-Pedersen B, Hangaard J, Bjerrum OJ. Quantitative enzyme antigen immunoassay of acetylcholinesterase in amniotic fluid. Clin Chem 1983;29:1061-4.
239A. Norgaard-Pederson, Larsen SO, Arends J, Svenstrup B, Tabor A. Maternal serum markers in screening for Down's syndrome. Clin Genet 1994;37:35-43.
240. O'Connor JF, Ellish N, Kakuma T, Schlatterer J, Kovalevskaya G. Differential urinary gonadotrophin profiles in early pregnancy and early pregnancy loss. Prenat Diagn 1998;18:1232-40.
241. O'Leary P, Nichols C, Feddema P, Lam T, Aitken M. Serum progesterone and human chorionic gonadotropin measurements in the evaluation of ectopic pregnancy. Aust NZ J Obstet Gynaecol 1996;36:319-23.
242. Odell WD, Griffin J. Pulsatile secretion of human chorionic gonadotropin in normal adults. N Engl J Med 1987;317:1688-91.
243. Ooi DS, Perkins SL, Claman P, Muggah HF. Serum human chorionic gonadotropin levels in early pregnancy. Clin Chim Acta 1989;181:281-92.
244. Oulton M. The role of centrifugation in the measurement of surfactant in amniotic fluid. Am J Obstet Gynecol 1979;135:337-43.
245. Oulton M, Martin TR, Faulkner GT, Stinson D, Johnson JP. Developmental study of a lamellar body fraction isolated from human amniotic fluid. Pediatr Res 1980;14:722-8.
246. Owerbach D, Rutter WJ, Martial JA, Baxter JD, Shows TB. Genes for growth hormone, chorionic somatomammotropin, and growth hormone-like gene on chromosome 17 in humans. Science 1980;209:289-92.
247. Ozturk M, Bellet D, Manil L, Hennen G, Frydman R, Wands J. Physiological studies of human chorionic gonadotropin (hCG), αhCG, and βhCG as measured by specific monoclonal immunoradiometric assays. Endocrinology 1987;120:549-58.
248. Pajkrt E, Mol BW, Bleker OP, Bilardo CM. Pregnancy outcome and nuchal translucency measurements in fetuses with a normal karyotype. Prenat Diagn 1999;19:1104-8.
249. Palomaki GE, Haddow JE, Knight GJ, Wald NJ, Kennard A, Canick JA, et al. Risk-based prenatal screening for trisomy 18 using alpha-fetoprotein, unconjugated oestriol and human chorionic gonadotropin. Prenat Diagn 1995;15:713-23.
250. Palomaki GE, Knight GJ, Haddow JE. Calculating amniotic fluid alpha-fetoprotein median values in the first trimester. Prenat Diagn 1993;13:887-9.
251. Palomaki GE, Knight GJ, Haddow JE, Canick JA, Saller DN Jr, Panizza DS. Prospective intervention

trial of a screening protocol to identify fetal trisomy 18 using maternal serum alpha-fetoprotein, unconjugated oestriol, and human chorionic gonadotropin. Prenat Diagn 1992;12:925-30.

252. Palomaki GE, Neveux LM, Knight GJ, Haddow JE, Pandian R. Maternal serum invasive trophoblast antigen (hyperglycosylated hCG) as a screening marker for Down syndrome during the second trimester. Clin Chem 2004;50:1804-8.
253. Palomaki GE, Williams J, Haddow JE. Comparing the observed and predicted effectiveness of folic acid fortification in preventing neural tube defects. J Med Screen 2003;10:52-3.
254. Peaceman AM, Andrews WW, Thorp JM, Cliver SP. Fetal fibronectin as a predictor of preterm birth in patients with symptoms: a multicenter trial. Am J Obstet Gynecol 1997;177:13-18.
255. Pearlman ES, Baiocchi JM, Lease JA, Gilbert J, Cooper JH. Utility of a rapid lamellar body count in the assessment of fetal maturity. Am J Clin Pathol 1991;95:778-80.
256. Persson A, Chang D, Crouch E. Surfactant protein D is a divalent cation-dependent carbohydrate-binding protein. J Biol Chem 1990;265:5755-60.
257. Petraglia F, Sawchenko P, Lim AT, Rivier J, Vale W. Localization, secretion, and action of inhibin in human placenta. Science 1987;237:187-9.
258. Phillippe M, Acker D, Torday J, Schiff I, Frigoletto FD. The effects of vaginal contamination on two pulmonary phospholipid assays. J Reprod Med 1982;27:283-6.
259. Phillips OP, Elias S, Shulman LP, Andersen RN, Morgan CD, Simpson JL. Maternal serum screening for fetal Down syndrome in women less than 35 years of age using α-fetoprotein, hCG, and unconjugated estriol: a prospective 2-year study. Obstet Gynecol 1992;80:353-8.
260. Pinette MG. Prediction of risk for respiratory distress syndrome using gestational age and the TDx-FLM II assay [reply]. Am J Obstet Gynecol 2003;189:1513-4.
261. Pinette MG, Blackstone J, Wax JR, Cartin A. Fetal lung maturity indices—a plea for gestational age-specific interpretation: a case report and discussion. Am J Obstet Gynecol 2002;187:1721-2.
262. Piper JM, Langer O. Does maternal diabetes delay fetal pulmonary maturity? Am J Obstet Gynecol 1993;168:783-6.
263. Pittaway DE, Reish RL, Wentz AC. Doubling times of human chorionic gonadotropin increase in early viable intrauterine pregnancies. Am J Obstet Gynecol 1985;152:299-302.
264. Plauche WC, Faro S, Wycheck J. Amniotic fluid optical density: relationship to L:S ratio, phospholipid content, and the desquamation of fetal cells. Obstet Gynecol 1981;58:309-13.
265. Policastro P, Ovitt CE, Hoshina M, Fukuoka H, Boothby MR, Boime I. The β subunit of human chorionic gonadotropin is encoded by multiple genes. J Biol Chem 1983;258:11492-9.
266. Poon TC, Mok TS, Chan AT, Chan CM, Leong V, Tsui SH, et al. Quantification and utility of monosialylated alpha-fetoprotein in the diagnosis of hepatocellular carcinoma with nondiagnostic serum total alpha-fetoprotein. Clin Chem 2002;48:1021-7.
267. Pryhuber GS, Hull WM, Fink I, McMahan MJ, Whitsett JA. Ontogeny of surfactant proteins A and B in human amniotic fluid as indices of fetal lung maturity. Pediatr Res 1991;30:597-605.
268. Queenan JT, Thompson W, Whitfield CR, Shah SI. Amniotic fluid volumes in normal pregnancies. Am J Obstet Gynecol 1972;114:34-8.
269. Radwanska E, Frankenberg J, Allen E. Plasma progesterone levels in normal and abnormal early pregnancy. Fertil Steril 1978;30:398-402.
270. Rasmussen-Loft AG, Nanchahal K, Cuckle HS, Wald NJ, Hulten M, Leedham P, et al. Amniotic fluid acetylcholinesterase in the prenatal diagnosis of open neural tube defects and abdominal wall defects: a comparison of gel electrophoresis and a monoclonal antibody immunoassay. Prenat Diagn 1990;10:449-59.
271. Reyes H. The spectrum of liver and gastrointestinal disease seen in cholestasis of pregnancy. Gastroenterol Clin North Am 1992;21:905-21.
271A. Reynolds TM, Penney MD. The mathematical basis of multivariate risk screening with special reference to screening for Down's syndrome associated pregnancy. Ann Clin Biochem 1990;27:452-8.
272. Risbridger GP, Schmitt JF, Robertson D. Activins and inhibins in endocrine and other tumors. Endocr Rev 2001;22:836-58. Review.
273. Robert MF, Neff RK, Hubbell JP, Taeusch HW, Avery ME. Association between maternal diabetes and the respiratory-distress syndrome in the newborn. N Engl J Med 1976;294:357-60.
274. Rohlfs EM, Chaing SH, Chapman JF. Analytical and clinical evaluation of refractive index-matched anomalous diffraction (RIMAD) for assessment of fetal lung maturation. Clin Chem 1996;42:1861-8.
275. Rolfes DB, Ishak KG. Acute fatty liver of pregnancy: a clinicopathologic study of 35 cases. Hepatology 1985;5:1149-58.
276. Rolfes DB, Ishak KG. Liver disease in toxemia of pregnancy. Am J Gastroenterol 1986;81:1138-4.
277. Romero R, Kadar N, Copel JA, Jeanty P, DeCherney AH, Hobbins JC. The effect of different human chorionic gonadotropin assay sensitivity on screening for ectopic pregnancy. Am J Obstet Gynecol 1985;153:72-4.
278. Russell JC. A calibrated fluorescence polarization assay for assessment of fetal lung maturity. Clin Chem 1987;33:1177-84.

279. Russell JC, Cooper CM, Ketchum CH, Torday JS, Richardson DK, Holt JA, et al. Multicenter evaluation of TDx test for assessing fetal lung maturity. Clin Chem 1989;35:1005-10.
280. Rustgi VK, Hoofnagle JH. Viral hepatitis during pregnancy. Semin Liver Dis 1987;7:40-6.
281. Saad SA, Fadel HE, Fahmy K, Nelson GH, Moustafa M, Davis HC. The reliability and clinical use of a rapid phosphatidylglycerol assay in normal and diabetic pregnancies. Am J Obstet Gynecol 1987;157:1516-20.
282. Sabai BM. The HELLP syndrome (hemolysis, elevated liver enzymes, and low platelets): much ado about nothing? Am J Obstet Gynecol 1990;162:311-6.
283. Sairam MR, Bhargavi GN. A role for glycosylation of the α subunit in transduction of biological signal in glycoprotein hormones. Science 1985;229:65-7.
284. Sancken U, Bartels I. Biochemical screening for chromosomal disorders and neural tube defects (NTD): is adjustment of maternal alpha-fetoprotein (AFP) still appropriate in insulin-dependent diabetes mellitus (IDDM)? Prenat Diagn 2001;21:383-6.
285. Sbarra AJ, Michlewitz H, Selvaraj RJ, Mitchell GW Jr, Cetrulo CL, Kelley EC Jr, et al. Correlation between amniotic fluid optical density and LS ratio. Obstet Gynecol 1976;48:613-5.
286. Schneck P. Selmar Aschheim (1878-1965) and Bernhard Zondek (1891-1966)—on the fate of 2 Jewish physicians and researchers at the Berlin Charite Hospital. Z Arztl Fortbild Qualitatssich 1997;91:187-94.
287. Schwartz DB, Engle MJ, Brown DJ, Farrell PM. The stability of phospholipids in amniotic fluid. Am J Obstet Gynecol 1981;141:294-8.
288. Schwartz RO, Di Pietro DL. β-hCG as a diagnostic aid for suspected ectopic pregnancy. Obstet Gynecol 1980;56:197-203.
289. Sciarra JJ, Sherwood LM, Varma AA, Lundberg WB. Human placental lactogen (HPL) and placental weight. Am J Obstet Gynecol 1968;101:413-6.
290. Shaw GM, Velie EM, Schaffer D. Risk of neural tube defect-affected pregnancies among obese women. JAMA 1996;275:1093-6.
291. Sher G, Statland BE. Assessment of fetal pulmonary maturity by the Lumadex foam stability index test. Obstet Gynecol 1983;61:444-9.
292. Sher G, Statland BE, Freer DE. Clinical evaluation of the quantitative foam stability index test. Obstet Gynecol 1980;55:617-20.
293. Sher G, Statland BE, Freer DE, Kraybill EN. Assessing fetal lung maturation by the foam stability index test. Obstet Gynecol 1978;52:673-7.
294. Sher G, Statland BE, Knutzen VK. Diagnostic reliability of the lecithin/sphingomyelin ratio assay and the quantitative foam stability index test: results of a comparative study. J Reprod Med 1982;27:51-5.
295. Shinitzky M, Goldfisher A, Bruck A, Goldman B, Stern E, Barkai G, et al. A new method for assessment of fetal lung maturity. Br J Obstet Gynaecol 1976;83:838-44.
296. Shipp TD, Benacerraf BR. Second trimester ultrasound screening for chromosomal abnormalities. Prenat Diagn 2002;22:296-307.
297. Simpson JL. Genetic counseling and prenatal diagnosis. In Gabbe SG, Niebyl JR, Simpson JL, eds. Obstetrics: normal and problem pregnancies. 2nd ed. New York: Churchill Livingstone, 1991:269-98.
298. Singh PK, Parvin CA, Gronowski AM. Establishment of reference intervals for markers of fetal thyroid status in amniotic fluid. J Clin Endocrinol Metab 2003;88:4175-9.
299. Snyder JM, Mendelson CR, Johnston JM. The morphology of lung development in the human fetus. In: Nelson GH, ed. Pulmonary development: transition from intrauterine to extrauterine life. New York: Marcel Dekker Inc, 1985:19-46.
300. Spellacy WN, Buhi WC, Cruz AC, Gelman SR, Kellner KR, Birk SA. Assessment of fetal lung maturity: a comparison of the lecithin/sphingomyelin ratio and the tests of optical density at 400 and 650 nm. Am J Obstet Gynecol 1979;134:528-31.
301. Spillman T, Cotton DB, Lynn SC, Bretaudiere JP. Influence of phospholipid saturation on classical thin-layer chromatographic detection methods and its effect on amniotic fluid lecithin/sphingomyelin ratio determinations. Clin Chem 1983;29:250-5.
302. Steegers-Theunissen RP, Boers GH, Blom HJ, Nijhuis JG, Thomas CM, Borm GF, et al. Neural tube defects and elevated homocysteine levels in amniotic fluid. Am J Obstet Gynecol 1995;172:1436-41.
303. Steinfeld JD, Samuels P, Bulley MA, Cohen AW, Goodman DB, Senior MB. The utility of the TDx test in the assessment of fetal lung maturity. Obstet Gynecol 1992;79:460-4.
304. Stewart BK, Nazar-Stewart V, Toivola B. Biochemical discrimination of pathologic pregnancy from early, normal intrauterine gestation in symptomatic patients. Am J Clin Pathol 1995;103:386-90.
305. Szallasi A, Gronowski AM, Eby CS. Lamellar body count in amniotic fluid: a comparative study of four different hematology analyzers. Clin Chem 2003;49:994-7.
306. Tabsh KM, Brinkman CR 3rd, Bashore RA. Lecithin: sphingomyelin ratio in pregnancies complicated by insulin-dependent diabetes mellitus. Obstet Gynecol 1982;59:353-8.
307. Taipale P, Hiilesmaa V, Salonen R, Ylostalo P. Increased nuchal translucency as a marker for fetal chromosomal defects. N Engl J Med 1997;337:1654-8.
308. Tait JF, Foerder CA, Ashwood ER, Benedetti TJ. Prospective clinical evaluation of an improved fluo-

rescence polarization assay for predicting fetal lung maturity. Clin Chem 1987;33:554-8.

309. Tait JF, Franklin RW, Simpson JB, Ashwood ER. Improved fluorescence polarization assay for use in evaluating fetal lung maturity: I. Development of the assay procedure. Clin Chem 1986;32:248-54.
310. Talmadge K, Vamvakopoulos NC, Fiddes JC. Evolution of the genes for the β subunits of human chorionic gonadotropin and luteinizing hormone. Nature 1984;307:37-40.
311. Thaler MM, Park CK, Landers DV, Wara DW, Houghton M, Veereman-Wauters G, et al. Vertical transmission of hepatitis C virus. Lancet 1991;338(8758):17-8.
312. Thirunavukarasu P, Stephenson T, Forray J, Stanton PG, Groome N, Wallace E, et al. Changes in molecular weight forms of inhibin A and pro-alpha C in maternal serum during human pregnancy. J Clin Endocrinol Metab 2001;86:5794-804.
313. Tietz NW. Comparative study of immunologic and biologic pregnancy tests in early pregnancy. Obstet Gynecol 1965;2:197-200.
314. Tint GS, Irons M, Elias ER, Batta AK, Frieden R, Chen TS, et al. Defective cholesterol biosynthesis associated with the Smith-Lemli-Opitz syndrome. N Engl J Med 1994;330:107-13.
315. Torday J, Carson L, Lawson E. Saturated phosphatidylcholine in amniotic fluid and prediction of respiratory-distress syndrome. N Engl J Med 1979;301:1013-8.
316. Toriello HV, Higgins JV. Occurrence of neural tube defects among first-, second-, and third-degree relatives of probands: results of a United States study. Am J Med Genet 1983;15:601-6.
317. Towers CV, Garite TJ. Uselessness of the phosphatidylglycerol assay for prediction of lung maturity [reply]. Am J Obstet Gynecol 1989;161:1419.
318. Treem WR. Mitochondrial fatty acid oxidation and acute fatty liver of pregnancy. Semin Gastrointest Dis 2002;13:55-66.
319. Tsai MY, Cain M, Josephson MW. Improved thin-layer chromatography of disaturated phosphatidylcholine in amniotic fluid. Clin Chem 1981;27: 239-42.
320. Tsai MY, Shultz EK, Williams PP, Bendel R, Butler J, Farb H, et al. Assay of disaturated phosphatidylcholine in amniotic fluid as a test of fetal lung maturity: experience with 2000 analyses. Clin Chem 1987;33:1648-51.
321. U.S. Food and Drug Administration. Center for Devices and Radiological Health. Device listing. http: accessdata.fda.gov/scripts/cdrh/cfdocs/cfRL/Listing. cfm (Accessed November 2003).
322. U.S. Food and Drug Administration. Center for Devices and Radiological Health. Guidance for Over-the-Counter (OTC) Human Chorionic Gonadotropin (hCG) 510(k)s. http: fda.gov/cdrh/ode/guidance/ 1172.html (Accessed November 2003).
323. Vaitukaitis JL, Braunstein GD, Ross GT. A radioimmunoassay which specifically measures human chorionic gonadotropin in the presence of luteinizing hormone. Am J Obstet Gynecol 1972;113:751-8.
324. van Voorst tot Voorst EJGM. Effects of centrifugation, storage, and contamination of amniotic fluid on its total phospholipid content. Clin Chem 1980;26:232-4.
325. Wagstaff TI, Whyley GA, Freedman G. Factors influencing the measurement of the lecithin/sphingomyelin ratio in amniotic fluid. J Obstet Gynaecol Br Commonw 1974;81:264-77.
326. Wald N. Folic acid and the prevention of neural tube defects. Ann NY Acad Sci 1993;678:112-29.
327. Wald N, Cuckle H, Nanchahal K. Amniotic fluid acetylcholinesterase measurement in the prenatal diagnosis of open neural tube defects. Second report of the Collaborative Acetylcholinesterase Study. Prenat Diagn 1989;9:813-29.
328. Wald N, Cuckle H, Wu TS, George L. Maternal serum unconjugated oestriol and human chorionic gonadotropin levels in twin pregnancies: implications for screening for Down's syndrome. Br J Obstet Gynaecol 1991;98:905-8.
329. Wald NJ, Cuckle HS. Estimating an individual's risk of having a fetus with open spina bifida and the value of repeat alpha-fetoprotein testing. J Epidemiol Community Health 1982;36:87-95.
330. Wald NJ, Cuckle H, Brock JH, Peto R, Polani PE, Woodford FP. Maternal serum-alpha-fetoprotein measurement in antenatal screening for anencephaly and spina bifida in early pregnancy. Report of U.K. collaborative study on alpha-fetoprotein in relation to neural-tube defects. Lancet 1977;1(8026):1323-32.
331. Wald NJ, Cuckle HS, Densem JW, Nanchahal K, Royston P, Chard T, et al. Maternal serum screening for Down's syndrome in early pregnancy. BMJ 1988;297:883-7. Erratum in: BMJ 1988;297:1029.
332. Wald NJ, Cuckle HS, Densem JW, Nanchahal K, Canick JA, Haddow JE, et al. Maternal serum unconjugated oestriol as an antenatal screening test for Down's syndrome. Br J Obstet Gynaecol 1988;95: 334-41.
332A. Wald NJ, Densem JW, George L, Muttukrishna S, Knight PG. Prenatal screening for Down's syndrome using inhibin-A as a serum marker. Prenat Diagn 1996;16:143-53. Erratum in: Prenat Diagn 1997;17:285-90.
332B. Wald NJ, Densem JW, George L, Muttukrishna S, Knight PG, Watt H, et al. Inhibin-A in Down's syndrome pregnancies: revised estimate of standard deviation. Prenat Diagn 1997;17:285-90.
333. Wald NJ, Densem JW, Smith D, Klee GG. Four-marker serum screening for Down's syndrome. Prenat Diagn 1994;14:707-16.

333A. Wald NJ, Hackshaw A. Alternative methods of estimating risk and determining detection and false-positive rates. In: Wald NJ, Leck I, eds. Antenatal and neonatal screening. Oxford, England: Oxford University Press, 2000:34-5.
334. Wald NJ, Hackshaw A, Stone R, Densem J. Serum alpha-fetoprotein and neural tube defects in the first trimester of pregnancy. MRC Vitamin Study Research Group. Prenat Diagn 1993;13:1047-50.
335. Wald NJ, Hackshaw AK. Combining ultrasound and biochemistry in first-trimester screening for Down's syndrome. Prenat Diagn 1997;17:821-9.
335A. Wald NJ, Hackshaw AK, George LM. Assay precision of serum alpha fetoprotein in antenatal screening for neural tube defects and Down's syndrome. J Med Screen 2000;7:74-7. Erratum in: J Med Screen 2000;7:168.
336. Wald NJ, Huttly WJ, Hackshaw AK. Antenatal screening for Down's syndrome with the quadruple test. Lancet 2003;361:835-6.
337. Wald NJ, Rodeck C, Hackshaw AK, Chitty L, Mackinson AM. First and second trimester screening for Down's syndrome: the results of the Serum, Urine and Ultrasound Screening Study (SURUSS). J Med Screen 2003;10:56-104.
337A. Wald NJ, Watt HC, George L. Maternal serum inhibin-A in pregnancies with insulin-dependent diabetes mellitus: implications for screening for Down's syndrome. Prenat Diagn 1996;16:923-6.
338. Wald NJ, Watt HC, Hackshaw AK. Integrated screening for Down's syndrome based on tests performed during the first and second trimester. N Engl J Med 1999;341:461-7.
339. Waller DK, Mills JL, Simpson JL, Cunningham GC, Conley MR, Lassman MR, et al. Are obese women at higher risk for producing malformed offspring? Am J Obstet Gynecol 1994;170:541-8.
340. Wallstedt A, Reily CA, Shaver D, et al. Prevalence and characteristics of liver dysfunction in hyperemesis gravidarum. Clin Res 1990;38:970A.
341. Wathen NC, Campbell DJ, Kitau MJ, Chard T. Alpha-fetoprotein levels in amniotic fluid from 8 to 18 weeks of pregnancy. Br J Obstet Gynaecol 1993;100:380-2.
342. Wehmann RE, Nisula BC. Metabolic and renal clearance rates of purified human chorionic gonadotropin. J Clin Invest 1981;68:184-94.
343. Weinbaum PJ, Richardson D, Schwartz JS, Gabbe SG. Amniostat FLM: a new technique for detection of phosphatidylglycerol in amniotic fluid. Am J Perinatol 1985;2:88-92.
344. Wenstrom KD, Owen J, Chu DC, Boots L. Elevated second-trimester dimeric inhibin A levels identify Down syndrome pregnancies. Am J Obstet Gynecol 1997;177:992-6.
345. Whitworth NS, Magann EF, Morrison JC. Evaluation of fetal lung maturity in diamniotic twins. Am J Obstet Gynecol 1999;180:1438-41.
346. Wijnberger LD, Huisjes AJ, Voorbij HA, Franx A, Bruinse HW, Mol BW. The accuracy of lamellar body count and lecithin/sphingomyelin ratio in the prediction of neonatal respiratory distress syndrome: a meta-analysis. BJOG 2001;108:583-8.
347. Wong SS, Schenkel O, Qutishat A. Strategic utilization of fetal lung maturity tests. Scand J Clin Lab Invest 1996;56:525-32.
348. Wu CH, Mennuti MT, Mikhail G. Free and protein-bound steroids in amniotic fluid of midpregnancy. Am J Obstet Gynecol 1979;133:666-72.
349. Wu JT, Roan Y, Knight JA. Serum AFP levels in normal infants: their clinical and physiological significance. In: J Mizejewski G, Porter IH, eds. Alpha-fetoprotein and congenital disorders. Orlando, Fla: Academic Press, 1985:111-21.

ADDITIONAL READING

Cunningham FG, ed. Williams obstetrics, 20th ed. New York: McGraw-Hill, 2001.
Gabbe SG, Niebyl JR, Simpson JL, eds. Obstetrics: normal and problem pregnancies, 4th ed. New York: Churchill Livingstone, 2002.
Gronowski AM, ed. Handbook of clinical laboratory testing during pregnancy. Totowa, NJ: Humana Press, 2004.
Lockitch G, ed. Handbook of diagnostic biochemistry and hematology in normal pregnancy. Boca Raton, Fla: CRC Press, 1997.
Quilligan EJ, Zuspan FP, eds. Current therapy in obstetrics and gynecology, 5th ed. Philadelphia: WB Saunders, 2000.

CHAPTER 55

Inborn Errors of Amino Acid, Organic Acid, and Fatty Acid Metabolism*

Piero Rinaldo, M.D., Ph.D., Sihoun Hahn, M.D., Ph.D., and Dietrich Matern, M.D.

With increasing frequency, inborn errors of metabolism (IEM) are recognized to be the underlying cause of clinical manifestations that are encountered in all venues of medicine from the fetus to the geriatric patient.[39,52,122] To adequately support the care of these patients, a new discipline has gradually developed, one that differs from a conventional clinical chemistry laboratory in the extent of interpretation that is necessary to make its results meaningful to the clinician. In the United States, this field is called *clinical biochemical genetics,* and is defined by the American College of Medical Genetics as the laboratory discipline that covers the biochemical diagnosis of IEM by metabolite and enzymatic analysis of physiological fluids and tissue and is concerned with (1) the evaluation and diagnosis of patients and families with inherited metabolic disease; (2) monitoring of treatment; and (3) distinguishing heterozygous carriers from noncarriers.[125]

Until recently, the practice of biochemical genetics was confined to a few academic centers in which services were driven by specific research interests. Although these laboratories made seminal contributions to our understanding of IEM and provided diagnostic services that were otherwise not available, in most cases they had limited capacity and slow turnaround time.[110] These and other factors contributed to a progressive decline of interest, research funding, and enrollment of young physicians and scientists in accredited training programs[136] to the point that biochemical genetics was deemed obsolete in anticipation of the predominance that nucleic acid–based diagnostics was forecast to have after the completion of the Human Genome Project. To date, however, the appreciation that irreplaceable information is derived by the biochemical analysis of proteins and small molecules has sparked a renewed interest in this discipline both at the clinical and research levels, a rebound also driven by the introduction of tandem mass spectrometry (MS/MS; see Chapter 7) into newborn screening programs (Figure 55-1) and the consequent surge of laboratory services needed for confirmatory testing and follow-up purposes.[24,27,78,140,145]

BIOCHEMICAL DIAGNOSIS

Although the diagnosis of a specific IEM is with a few exceptions strictly a laboratory process, two basic patterns of acute clinical presentation, called "intoxication" and "energy deficiency," are informative clinical elements that should not be overlooked in the anticipation of a laboratory diagnosis.[118] A clinical picture of the intoxication type is found when a newborn or infant experiences a trigger event and rapidly becomes comatose after a symptom-free period. Alternatively the absence of a symptom-free period is more indicative of an energy deficiency type of neurological distress. In both cases, the failure to respond to symptomatic therapy and a rapid deterioration of the patient's general status are typical manifestations. Organic acidemias, urea cycle disor-

*The authors gratefully acknowledge the contributions by Robert H. Christenson and Hassan M. E. Azzazy on which portions of this chapter are based.

ders, and a few other disorders of amino acid metabolism are classic examples of endogenous intoxication. Fatty acid oxidation (FAO) disorders may present with a combination of intoxication and energy deficiency manifestations.[111]

Once a clinical suspicion has been raised, a basic set of routine laboratory tests (blood electrolytes and gases, glucose, ammonia, lactate, and urine ketones) is strongly recommended as the first level of laboratory evaluation. General guidelines for diagnostic orientation on the basis of the outcome of these tests are shown in Table 55-1 and discussed in greater detail elsewhere.[108,118] Recognition of informative patterns, for example hypoglycemia without ketonuria in medium-chain acyl-CoA dehydrogenase (MCAD) and other FAO disorders, could expedite the implementation of appropriate therapeutic measures independently of the turnaround time of specialized laboratory investigations. Obviously, deviations from established patterns (such as ketonuria in MCAD deficiency)[99,107] or unexpected combinations[143] should not be overlooked considering the unpredictable role that genetic, dietary, and environmental factors may play in individual cases.

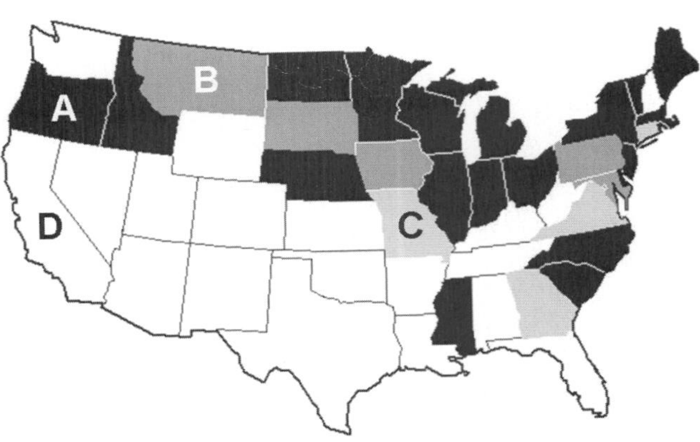

Figure 55-1 Current status of newborn screening in the United States for disorders of amino acid, organic acid, and fatty acid metabolism by tandem mass spectrometry. **A** *(black)*: active program, screening required by the state or ongoing universal pilot. **B** *(dark grey)*: program not mandated, testing of selected populations or limited pilot programs. **C** *(light grey)*: testing mandated but not implemented. **D** *(white)*: no MS/MS screening. Georgia, Michigan, New York, and Virginia screen for only one disorder by MS/MS, Connecticut and Maryland for two. *(Data obtained from National Newborn Screening & Genetic Resource Center web site [http://genes-r-us.uthscsa.edu/resources/newborn/screenstatus.htm, updated Nov 11, 2003].)*

In addition to the traditional role of investigating symptomatic patients, biochemical genetics is evolving into a discipline with a major focus on early diagnosis and prevention of morbidity and mortality.[112] Prenatal diagnosis and particularly newborn screening are obvious examples of this trend; postmortem screening enables genetic counseling and testing of at-risk relatives, thereby preventing morbidity and mortality in other affected but still undiagnosed, or unborn, family members.[9] Hopefully the need to provide a metabolic autopsy in the future will decline in parallel to the expansion of newborn screening programs.[102]

Prenatal Diagnosis

Despite constant progress in medical treatment, most IEM result in severe morbidity and inevitable mortality in early life. As these disorders typically follow an autosomal recessive mode of inheritance, the recurrence risk in subsequent pregnancies is 25%. Genetic counseling of parents consists of a balanced assessment of (1) familial risk factors (parental consanguinity and ethnic origin), (2) risk of pregnancy loss as a consequence of the sampling procedure (0.5% to 1% by chorionic villus sampling [CVS], 0.5% by amniocentesis), (3) risk of maternal complications,[114] and (4) the potential fallacy of "experimental" procedures yielding uninformative results because of limited prior experience.[112]

Methods used for prenatal diagnosis of IEM have different requirements in terms of timing, sample collection, and options for independent confirmation. CVS is performed at 10 to 12 weeks of gestational age, has a higher risk of fetal loss, and entails the occurrence of artifactual results caused by contamination with maternal tissue, which has made this

TABLE 55-1 Typical Outcome of Routine Laboratory Investigations in Disorders of Amino Acid, Fatty Acid, and Organic Acid Metabolism

	Organic Acidurias	Fatty Acid Oxidation Disorders	Urea Cycle Disorders	MSUD	NKHG
Neurological distress	I	I/ED	I	I	I
Metabolic acidosis	+++	–	+	+	–
Ketonuria (ketone bodies)	+++	–	–	+	–
Hyperammonemia	+	+	+++	–	–
Hypoglycemia (fasting)	+	+++	–	–	–
Lactic acidemia	++	+	–	–	–

ED, Energy deficiency; *I*, intoxication type of neurological distress (see text); *MSUD*, maple syrup urine disease; *NKHG*, nonketotic hyperglycinemia. +, possibly present; ++, frequently present; +++, typically present with high diagnostic significance; –, not typically present.

approach very unreliable in specific disorders (e.g., methylmalonic acidemia). Amniocentesis is performed later in pregnancy (16 to 19 weeks) and provides both amniocytes and amniotic fluid to be used for independent and complementary diagnostic methods. Reliance on separate tests based on independent methods performed by laboratories with adequate prior experience is strongly encouraged to avoid the occurrence of either incorrect or inconclusive results. For example, Figure 55-2 shows the results obtained by analysis of an amniotic fluid specimen from a pregnancy at risk for methylmalonic acidemia (*cblC* complementation group).[139] The finding of elevated concentrations of methylmalonic acid, propionylcarnitine, and homocysteine using different MS/MS methods provides strong biochemical evidence of an affected fetus. However, validation of these results by assay of [^{14}C]-propionate fixation and cobalamin uptake in cultured amniocytes remains an essential part of the recommended diagnostic process. When a multianalyte approach is not possible, at least two separate laboratories should perform the same test independently to minimize the risk of incorrect results.[8] The major advantages of direct metabolite analysis in amniotic fluid are the independence from tissue expression and a rapid turnaround time.

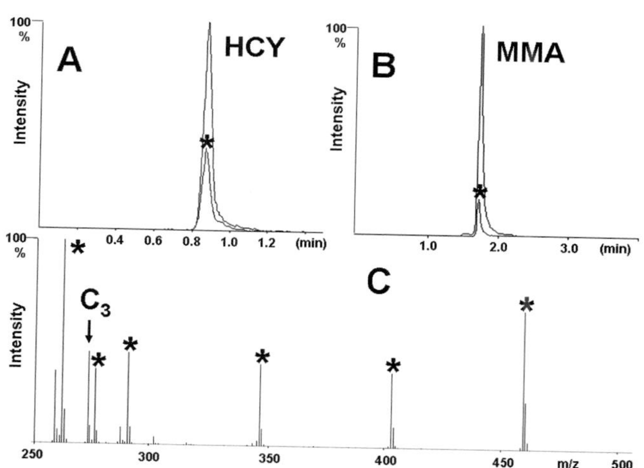

Figure 55-2 Multi-analyte approach to the prenatal diagnosis of methylmalonic acidemia (*cblC* complementation group) by metabolite analysis in cell-free supernatant of amniotic fluid collected at 16 weeks of gestational age. The symbol * marks internal standards. **A,** Determination of total homocysteine by LC-MS/MS (selected reaction monitoring, SRM, transition m/z 136 to m/z 90 and m/z 140 to m/z 94 for the d_4-labeled internal standard).[74] The concentration of total homocysteine was 15.7 μmol/L (0.7 to 2.0 μmol/L). **B,** Determination of methylmalonic acid by LC-MS/MS (SRM, transition m/z 231 to m/z 119 and m/z 234 to m/z 122 for the d_3-labeled internal standard).[73] The concentration of methylmalonic acid was 8.7 μmol/L, the reference interval for 16 to 19 weeks of gestational age is 0.2 to 0.7 μmol/L. **C,** Determination of propionylcarnitine by LC-MS/MS (parent of m/z 85 scan, the $[M+H]^+$ ion of C3 is m/z 274, m/z 277 for the internal standard). The concentration was 5.6 μmol/L (1.5 to 1.8 μmol/L), the C3/C4 ratio was 6.9 (0.9 to 2.6).

Newborn Screening

More than 4 million babies are born in the United States every year. Newborn screening has become an important and effective component of preventive medicine, allowing detection of treatable disorders before irreversible clinical symptoms manifest themselves. Originally instituted in the 1960s for the early detection of phenylketonuria (PKU), newborn screening programs have gradually added assays for other disorders over the years. There is, however, a striking level of discrepancy in the scope of programs offered by states even in the same region, a reality that seems to be driven more by political decisions than scientific evidence and expert opinions.[33] This situation has received even greater scrutiny since MS/MS has dramatically expanded the number of IEM detectable in neonatal blood spots, notably by performance of a single multiplex analysis of acylcarnitine and amino acid profiles.[24,78] The inclusion of these disorders as a whole in newborn screening panels has been controversial, because with few exceptions their incidence, natural history, prospective screening experience, and effectiveness of treatment have not been defined yet.[50] However, cautionary concerns often underestimate the complex differential diagnosis that is required for any abnormal metabolites detected in amino acid, organic acid, and acylcarnitine profiles.[24,101] Actively developing tools for proper confirmatory testing and differential diagnosis of all detectable IEM seems more reasonable than debating the exclusion of one or more rare conditions that are detected anyway, at no additional cost, and could be misinterpreted as "false positives" of a better known condition. Finally, because some inborn errors of amino acid, organic acid, and fatty acid metabolism are undetectable by MS/MS analysis of amino acids and acylcarnitines, a negative newborn screening outcome should not be regarded as a blanket exclusion of metabolic disorders in patients presenting with unexplained clinical manifestations at any age.

Evaluation of Symptomatic Patients

When a patient with acute metabolic decompensation is brought to medical attention, the utmost consideration should be given to the immediate collection of urine and blood samples. Specimens collected even after a partial recovery may not reveal diagnostic abnormalities otherwise detectable, or more easily detectable, under acute conditions. Any volume of urine (stored at −20 °C with no preservatives, or even a wet diaper brought to the emergency room) and plasma/serum (~0.5 mL, stored at −20 °C) are adequate to perform specialized tests. Quantitative profiling of amino acids, carnitine, acylcarnitines, and fatty acids in plasma, organic acids, and acylglycines in urine is the method of choice to reach a biochemical diagnosis of these disorders. Alternatively a blood spot on filter paper could provide enough material for one or more of the investigations described in this chapter. In case of death, collection of body fluid and tissue should be secured according to available protocols.[22,115]

As already stated, the extent of interpretation that is necessary to make results meaningful to the clinician is the defining characteristic of biochemical genetics as a laboratory discipline. An interpretive report of complex organic acid, amino acid, and acylcarnitine metabolite profiles should include the following elements: (1) an overview of positive and negative results (e.g., ketotic versus nonketotic dicarboxylic aciduria, and presence or absence of alloisoleucine in specimens with elevated concentrations of branched-chain amino acids); (2) quantitative determination in comparison to age-matched reference values; (3) a list of possible diagnoses with correlation with available clinical information; (4) clinical and laboratory criteria of differential diagnosis; (5) recommendations for additional biochemical testing and in vitro confirmatory studies (enzyme assay and molecular analysis); (6) name and means to contact investigators able to provide such studies at times available only on a research basis; and (7) a phone number to reach the laboratory director who is familiar with the report in case the referring physician has additional questions.

Postmortem Screening

In view of the high mortality rate that is associated with acute episodes of metabolic decompensation, it is not surprising that sudden death has been sporadically associated with a few inborn errors of amino acid, organic acid, and energy metabolism, such as (1) fumaric acidemia, (2) methylmalonic acidemia, (3) glutaric acidemia type I, (4) biotinidase deficiency, (5) glycogenoses, and (6) disorders of the mitochondrial oxidative phosphorylation pathway. Despite these anecdotal reports, these disorders are unlikely to have a significant role among the metabolic causes of sudden death. Conversely, the number of cases affected with a FAO disorder who were recognized either postmortem or after the diagnosis of an affected sibling has soared in the last few years.[9,17] Based on these observations, experts postulate that FAO disorders might be responsible for up to 5% of children who die suddenly and unexpectedly from birth to 5 years of age, particularly with evidence of acute infection.[16]

Figure 55-3 shows a flow chart for the postmortem evaluation of sudden and unexpected death that is centered on the analysis of acylcarnitines in blood and bile spots.[111] Blood and bile could be conveniently collected on a single filter paper card, one identical to those used for newborn screening, which can be shipped at room temperature once properly dried. Both specimens should be collected to detect patients who may have only mild blood abnormalities when carnitine is depleted (Figure 55-4). In cases with a higher level of suspicion, an effort should be made to collect and freeze a specimen of liver[16] and a skin biopsy,[71] which could be analyzed only if needed to reduce cell culture workload.[44]

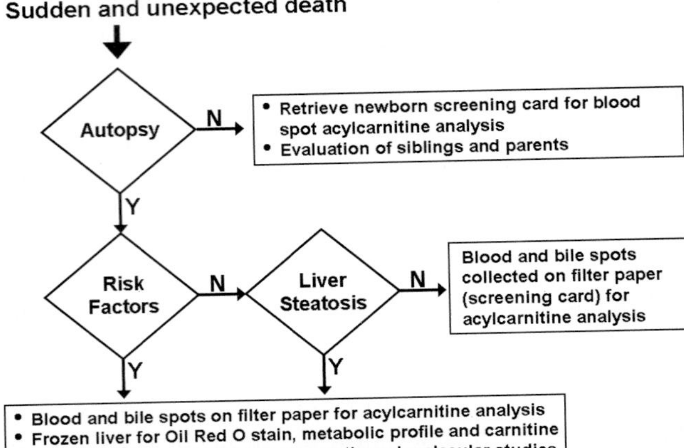

Figure 55-3 Protocol for the postmortem screening of FAO disorders. *(From Rinaldo P, Matern D, Bennett MJ. Fatty acid oxidation disorders. Ann Rev Physiol 2002;64:477-502.)*

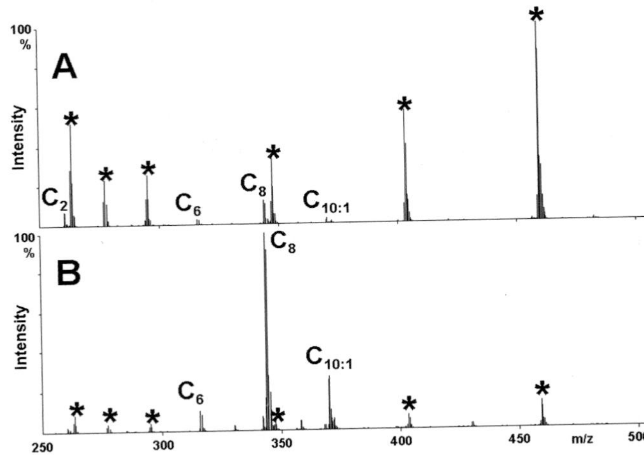

Figure 55-4 Postmortem diagnosis of MCAD deficiency by acylcarnitine analysis of blood and bile collected at autopsy. The patient was a 3-year-old, previously healthy child who had symptoms of a viral respiratory tract infection. He was a compound heterozygote for the common 985A>G mutation and another mutation. The symbol * marks the internal standards, same amount added to both specimens. **A,** Blood acylcarnitine profile. The concentrations of acetylcarnitine (C2), hexanoylcarnitine (C6), octanoylcarnitine (C8), and decenoylcarnitine (C10:1) were 2.8, 0.3, 1.4, and 0.3 μmol/L, respectively (for reference intervals see Table 55-8). **B,** Bile acylcarnitine profile (after 10× dilution). The concentrations of C2, C6, C8, and C10:1 were 52.8, 73.1, 665.6, and 181.3 μmol/L, respectively (for reference intervals see Table 55-8). The bile/blood C8 ratio was 475. In postmortem urine, hexanoylglycine was also markedly elevated (69.6 mmol/mol creatinine; reference interval 0.1 to 1.3).

BOX 55-1 Factors That Increase the Risk of an Underlying Metabolic Disorder in Cases of Sudden Unexpected Death

Family history of sudden infant death syndrome (SIDS) or other sudden, unexplained deaths at any age
Family history of Reye's syndrome
Maternal complications of pregnancy (acute fatty liver of pregnancy, HELLP syndrome, others)
Lethargy, vomiting, fasting in the 48 hours before death
Macroscopic findings at autopsy
  Fatty infiltration of the liver and/or other organs
  Dilated or hypertrophic cardiomyopathy
Allegation of child abuse (not trauma, physical harm)
Autopsy evidence of infection that routinely would not represent a life-threatening event

HELLP, Hemolysis, elevated liver enzymes, low platelets.

Although fatty infiltration of the liver and/or other organs (e.g., heart and kidneys) is a common observation in FAO disorders, the finding of macroscopic steatosis should not be used as the only criterion in deciding whether to investigate a possible underlying FAO disorder during the postmortem evaluation of a case of sudden death. Special attention should be paid to the risk factors listed in Box 55-1, and allegations of child abuse should also be fully investigated to avoid any recurrence of a tragic miscarriage of justice,[49] with the exception of obvious cases of trauma or physical harm. The frozen liver and skin biopsy could be discarded at a later time without further testing when a credible cause of death has been established, but could otherwise be crucial to reach a proper diagnosis and conclusive confirmation in vitro. If parental permission to perform an autopsy is not granted, an attempt should be made to retrieve leftover specimens that may still be available in a hospital setting. If death occurs at home, retrieval of any unused portion of the blood spots collected for newborn screening could be arranged via a written request submitted to the state laboratory, as long as the storage period, ranging from only a few weeks to indefinitely, had not expired already in the state where the patient was born.[95]

DISORDERS OF AMINO ACID METABOLISM

The concentrations of individual amino acids in physiological fluids reflect a balance between (1) intestinal uptake, (2) anabolic use by the liver, (3) the synthesis and turnover of the body's structural proteins, and (4) integrity of renal functions (filtration and tubular reabsorption). Any interference or unusual event in the metabolism, growth, or replication of the body's cells and tissues that affects protein and amino acid metabolism could be accompanied by either accumulation or excessive losses of one or more amino acids.[121]

Inborn errors of amino acid metabolism will manifest themselves at anytime in a person's life, but most become evident in infancy and early childhood. Affected patients may have failure to thrive, neurological symptoms, digestive problems, locomotor retardation, and a wide spectrum of laboratory findings. If not diagnosed promptly and treated properly, these disorders can result in poor growth, mental retardation, and death.[13]

Table 55-2 shows a summary of known disorders of amino acid metabolism and transport, including information about their incidence, major clinical features and biochemical patterns, availability of prenatal diagnosis and newborn screening, and association with sudden unexpected death. Several of these disorders are discussed next.

CLASSIC PHENYLKETONURIA AND OTHER HYPERPHENYLALANINEMIAS

Phenylalanine is an essential amino acid. Dietary intake in excess of anabolic needs is converted to tyrosine by phenylalanine hydroxylase and further degraded via a ketogenic pathway (Figure 55-5). A primary or cofactor-related defect of phenylalanine hydroxylase activity causes accumulation of phenylalanine, phenylketones, and phenylamines.[14,119] Several distinct forms of hyperphenylalaninemia exist (see Table 55-2); all are inherited as autosomal recessive traits. They have a collective prevalence of 1:10,000 to 1:20,000 live births, with classic PKU being the most common entity and GTP cyclohydrolase I the rarest one. Together with congenital hypothyroidism and galactosemia, hyperphenylalaninemias are the only IEMs that are screened for at birth in all of the United States and their territories.

Although vomiting may be an early symptom severe enough to be misdiagnosed as pyloric stenosis, patients with classic PKU are clinically silent at birth and neurological manifestations typically do not become evident until a few months of age. To avoid missing a PKU case, infants should not be screened until at least 24 hours after birth. Although a delayed diagnosis is an exceptionally rare event for properly screened newborns, the consequences are severe. PKU infants may lose about 50 points in their adult IQ if left untreated until the end of the first year of life. Those who are diagnosed even later require institutional care because of severe mental retardation and hyperactivity. Other common findings in untreated patients include fair skin and blue eyes, microcephaly, prominent maxilla with widely spaced teeth, enamel hypoplasia, and growth retardation. Some have a seborrheic or eczematous skin rash, which progressively attenuates with age. Although there are no consistent neurological findings, most infants are hypertonic with increased deep tendon reflexes. About one fourth of children have seizures, and more than 50% have abnormal electroencephalographic (EEG) findings.

The criteria for a biochemical diagnosis of untreated classic PKU are: (1) a plasma phenylalanine level above 20 mg/dL (1.2 mmol/L) (Figure 55-6, *A*); (2) a phenylalanine/tyrosine ratio >3; (3) increased urinary levels of metabolites of phenylalanine (i.e., phenylpyruvic and 2-hydroxyphenylacetic acids); and (4) a normal concentration of the cofactor

Text continued on p. 2217

TABLE 55-2 Clinical and Laboratory Characteristics of Disorders of Amino Acid Metabolism

Common Name	OMIM No.	Enzyme/Transport Defect	Incidence (USA)	Major Clinical Features	Complication of Pregnancy (Maternal, Fetal)
Disorders of Aromatic Amino Acid Metabolism					
Classical phenylketonuria (PKU)	261600	Phenylalanine hydroxylase	>1:25,000	Mental retardation, fair complexion and pigmentation	Congenital anomalies of fetus born to affected mother
Defect of biopterin cofactor biosynthesis	233910	GTP cyclohydrolase I	<1:100,000	Progressive mental retardation, seizures, muscle tone abnormalities	Affected patients unlikely to reach reproductive age
Defect of biopterin cofactor biosynthesis	261640	6-Pyruvoyltetrahydropterin synthase	<1:100,000	Progressive mental retardation, seizures, muscle tone abnormalities	Affected patients unlikely to reach reproductive age
Defect of biopterin cofactor regeneration	261630	Dihydropterin reductase (DHPR)	<1:100,000	Progressive mental retardation, spasticity, dystonia, myoclonus	Affected patients unlikely to reach reproductive age
Defect of biopterin cofactor regeneration	126090	Pterin-4a-carbinolamine dehydratase	<1:100,000	Transient muscle tone abnormalities	/
Tyrosinemia type I	276700	Fumarylacetoacetase	<1:100,000	Cirrhosis, hepatocellular carcinoma, rickets, renal disease	/
Tyrosinemia type II	276600	Tyrosine aminotransferase	<1:100,000	Corneal ulcers, keratosis on palms and soles	/
Tyrosinemia type III	276710	4-Hydroxyphenylpyruvate dioxygenase	<1:100,000	Prematurity, anecdotal reports of mild developmental delay	/
Hawkinsinuria	140350	Unknown	<1:100,000	Failure to thrive, reported asymptomatic cases	/
Disorders of Branched Chain Amino Acid Metabolism					
Maple syrup urine disease (MSUD IA, IB, II)	248600	Branched chain ketoacid dehydrogenase complex	<1:100,000 (1:378 Mennonite)	Hypotonia, lethargy, seizures, coma	/
E3 deficiency	246900	Dihydrolipoyl dehydrogenase (E3)	<1:100,000	Failure to thrive, hypotonia, developmental delay, seizures, coma	/
Disorders of Sulfur Amino Acid Metabolism					
Hypermethioninemia	250850	Methionine adenosyltransferase	<1:100,000	Fetid breath, demyelination	/
Homocystinuria	236200	Cystathionine beta-synthase	<1:100,000	Mental retardation, ectopia lentis, skeletal anomalies	/
Cystathionuria	219500	Cystathionase	>1:75,000	Mental retardation in some cases, possible ascertainment bias	/

OMIM, Online Mendelian Inheritance in Man (www.ncbi.nlm.nih.gov/entrez/query.fcgi?db=OMIM); *NBS,* newborn screening; *5-HIAA,* 5-hydroxyindoleacetic acid; *HVA,* homovanillic acid; *RFLP,* restriction fragment length polymorphism.

Modality of Acute Episodes	Major Biochemical Marker(s)	Prenatal Diagnosis	NBS in the US (% Births)	Sudden Unexpected Death
Increased incidence of pyloric stenosis	Phenylalanine (B), phenylpyruvic (U), phenyllactic (U), 2-OH phenylacetic (U)	Possible by DNA analysis	51/51 states (100%)	/
Hyperthermia	Phenylalanine (B), low neopterin and biopterin (U), low 5-HIAA and HVA (CSF)	Possible by DNA analysis, AF metabolites	Secondary target (PKU)	/
/	Phenylalanine (B), high neopterin, low biopterin (U), low 5-HIAA, HVA (CSF)	Possible by DNA analysis, AF metabolites	Secondary target (PKU)	/
/	Phenylalanine (B), high biopterin (U), low 5-HIAA, HVA (CSF)	Possible by DNA analysis, AF metabolites	Secondary target (PKU)	/
/	Phenylalanine (B), high neopterin and primapterin (U)	/	Secondary target (PKU)	/
Acute liver failure, porphyria-like neurological crisis	Tyrosine (B), succinylacetone (U), 4-OH phenylpyruvic, 4-OH phenyllactic (U)	RFLPs	16/51 states (24%)	/
Photophobia	Tyrosine (B), 4-OH phenylpyruvic, 4-OH phenyllactic (U)	/	Secondary target (TYR-I)	/
/	Tyrosine (B), 4-OH phenylpyruvic, 4-OH phenyllactic (U)	/	Secondary target (TYR-I)	/
Metabolic acidosis	2-Cystenyl-1,4-dihydrocyclohexenylacetate (U), pyroglutamic (U)	/	Not available	/
Acidosis, ketotic hypoglycemia, pancreatitis	Branched chain amino acids (B), allo isoleucine (B), 2-keto and 2-OH acids (U)	Possible by DNA analysis	30/51 states (54%)	Anecdotal reports
Lactic acidosis, ketotic hypoglycemia	Branched chain amino acids (B), allo isoleucine (B), lactic and pyruvic (B,U), 2-keto glutaric 2-keto 2-OH acids (U)	Possible by DNA analysis	Secondary target (MSUD)	/
/	Methionine (B), methionine sulfoxide (B,U)	/	Secondary target (HCY)	/
Mitral valve prolapse, thomboembolism	Homocysteine and methionine (B,U)	Possible by DNA analysis, AF metabolites	28/51 states (47%)	/
/	Cystathionine (B,U)	/	Not available	/

Continued.

TABLE 55-2 Clinical and Laboratory Characteristics of Disorders of Amino Acid Metabolism—*Continued*

Common Name	OMIM No.	Enzyme/Transport Defect	Incidence (USA)	Major Clinical Features	Complication of Pregnancy (Maternal, Fetal)
Sulfite oxidase deficiency	272300	Sulfite oxidase	<1 : 100,000	Mental retardation, seizures, ectopia lensis, dysmorphic features, muscle tone abnormalities	/
Urea Cycle Disorders					
N-Acetylglutamate synthase deficiency	237310	N-Acetylglutamate synthase	<1 : 100,000	Encephalopathy	/
CPS deficiency	237300	Carbamoylphosphate synthetase	<1 : 100,000	Lethargy, hypothermia, apnea	/
OTC deficiency (X-linked)	311250	Ornithine transcarbamylase	>1 : 50,000	Lethargy, hypothermia, apnea	Hyperammonemia in pregnancy and post-partum period (heterozygote females)
Citrullinemia	603470	Argininosuccinate synthase	>1 : 75,000	Lethargy, hypothermia, apnea	/
Citrullinemia type II (citrin deficiency)	603471	Argininosuccinate synthase (liver), citrin (citrulline transport)	<1 : 100,000	Cholestatic jaundice, hepatic steatosis and siderosis, psychiatric symptoms	/
Argininosuccinic acidemia	207900	Argininosuccinate lyase	<1 : 100,000	Trichorrexis nodosa	/
Argininemia	207800	Arginase	<1 : 100,000	Progressive spasticity, mental retardation	/
HHH syndrome	238970	Mitochondrial ornithine transporter	<1 : 100,000	Mental retardation, seizures, pyramidal signs, compromised sense of vibration	/
Miscellaneous Disorders of Amino Acid Metabolism					
Nonketotic hyperglycinemia	605899, 238300 238310 238330	Glycine cleavage system (P, H, T, L proteins)	<1 : 100,000	Lethargy, seizures, myoclonic jerks, hypotonia, hiccups	/
Gyrate atrophy of the retina	258870	Ornithine aminotransferase	<1 : 100,000	Myopia, night blindness, progressive loss of peripheral vision	/
Carnosinemia	212200	Carnosinase	<1 : 100,000	Mental retardation, myoclonic seizures, possible ascertainment bias	/
Hyperprolinemia type I	239500	Proline oxidase	<1 : 100,000	Renal disease, likely ascertainment bias	/
Hyperprolinemia type II	239510	Delta 1 Pyrroline-5-carboxylate dehydrogenase	<1 : 100,000	Mental retardation, seizures in early life	/
Histidinemia	235800	Histidine ammonia lyase	>1 : 25,000	Mental retardation, speech delay, possible ascertainment bias	/

Modality of Acute Episodes	Major Biochemical Marker(s)	Prenatal Diagnosis	NBS in the US (% Births)	Sudden Unexpected Death
Neurological deterioration	S-sulfocysteine and taurine (B,U)	Enzyme assay in CVS, AF sulfocysteine	Not available	/
Hyperammonemia	Glutamine, alanine (B), low citrulline (B)	Not reported	Not available	/
Hyperammonemia	Glutamine, alanine (B), low citrulline, arginine (B)	Possible by DNA analysis	2/51 states (5%)	/
Hyperammonemia	Orotic (U), glutamine, alanine (B), low citrulline, arginine (B)	Possible by DNA analysis	Not available	/
Hyperammonemia	Citrulline (B), orotic (U)	Possible by DNA analysis, AF citrulline	20/51 states (32%)	/
Hyperammonemia	Citrulline (B), orotic (U)	Not reported	Secondary target (CIT)	/
Hyperammonemia	Argininosuccinic (B,U)	Possible by DNA analysis, AF argininosuccinic	20/51 states (32%)	/
Hyperammonemia (uncommon)	Arginine (B, CSF)	Not reported but possible by DNA analysis	15/51 states (22%)	/
Hyperammonemia, episodic vomiting	Ornithine (B,U), homocitrulline (U)	Not reported but possible by DNA analysis	13/51 states (16%)	/
Neurological deterioration	Glycine (B,CSF), CSF/plasma ratio >0.09	Enzyme assay in CVS, DNA analysis if mutations known	7/51 states (8%)	/
/	Ornithine (B), low LYS, GLU, GLN (B)	Enzyme assay in CVS/amniocytes, DNA analysis if mutations known	Secondary target (HHH)	/
/	Carnosine (B,U), homocarnosine (CSF)	Not reported	Not available	/
/	Proline (B,U)	Not applicable	Not available	/
/	Proline (B,U), Pyrroline 5-carboxylic (U)	Not reported	Not available	/
/	Histidine (B)	Not reported	Not available	/

Continued.

TABLE 55-2 Clinical and Laboratory Characteristics of Disorders of Amino Acid Metabolism—*Continued*

Common Name	OMIM No.	Enzyme/Transport Defect	Incidence (USA)	Major Clinical Features	Complication of Pregnancy (Maternal, Fetal)
Disorders of Amino Acid Membrane Transport					
Cystinuria	220100	Absorption of cystine and dibasic amino acids in renal tubule and GI tract	>1:25,000	Nephrolithiasis	/
Lysinuric protein intolerance	222700	Absorption of lysine and cationic amino acids in renal tubule and GI tract	<1:100,000	Protein intolerance, organomegaly, osteoporosis, interstitial lung disease, variable mental retardation	Severe hemorrhages, toxemic crisis (affected mothers)
Hartnup disease	234500	Absorption of neutral amino acids in renal tubule and GI tract	>1:50,000	Ataxia, seizures, photodermatitis (pellagra-like)	/
Iminoglycinuria	242600	Absorption of proline, hydroxyproline, and glycine in renal tubule	<1:100,000	Benign phenotype, anecdotal reports of mental retardation	/

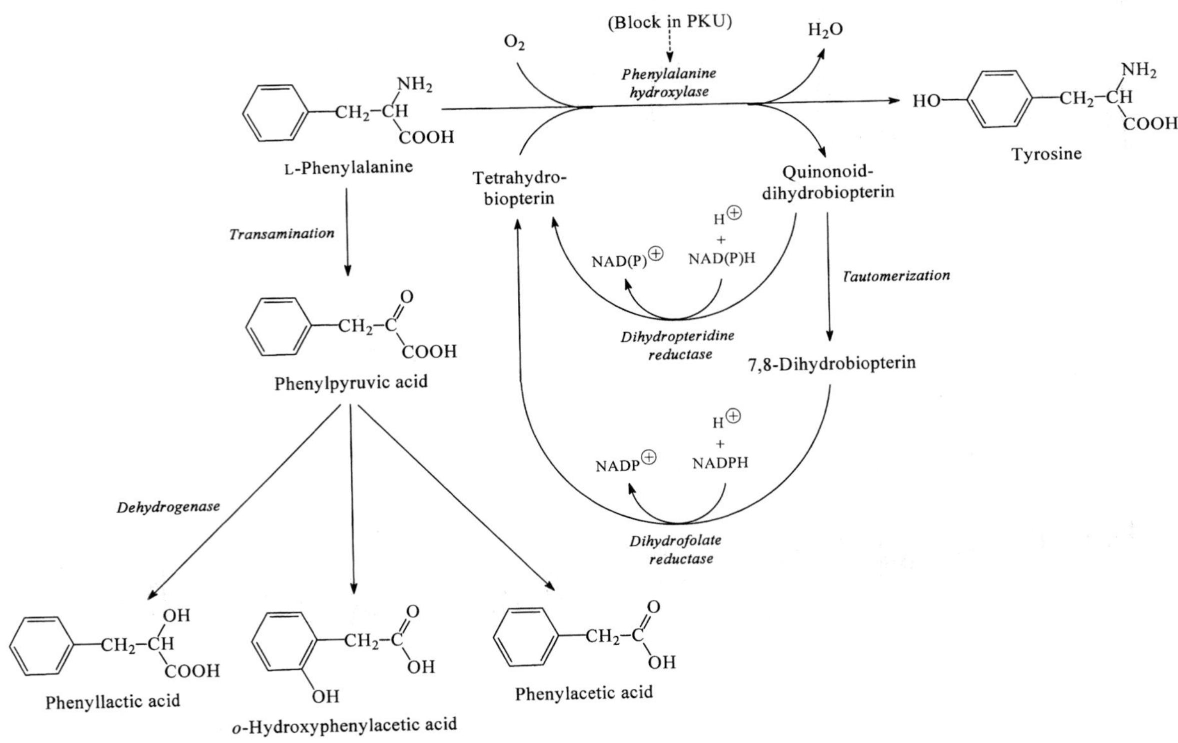

Figure 55-5 Metabolic pathway of phenylalanine.

Modality of Acute Episodes	Major Biochemical Marker(s)	Prenatal Diagnosis	NBS in the US (% Births)	Sudden Unexpected Death
Obstructive uropathy	Cystine, lysine, ornithine, arginine (U)	Not recommended	Not available	/
Attacks of stupor and asterixis	Lysine (U), orotic (U), mild elevation of GLN, ALA, CIT, others (B)	Linkage analysis	Not available	Reported after alcohol ingestion
Psychotic episodes	Hyperexcretion of ALA, SER, THR, VAL, LEU, ILE, PHE, TYR, TRP, HIS, GLN, ASN (U)	Not reported	Not available	/
/	Proline, hydroxyproline, glycine (U)	Not reported	Not available	/

tetrahydrobiopterin (BH_4). In vitro assay of enzyme catalytic activity and genotyping are not commonly applied in clinical practice, making the biochemical phenotype a de facto conclusive diagnosis immediately followed by dietary treatment. The goal of therapy is to sustain growth and keep serum phenylalanine concentrations below an appropriate-for-age threshold to minimize the occurrence of neurological damage.[106] Frequent monitoring is critical, because excessive restriction may lead to phenylalanine and tyrosine deficiency, the latter requiring exogenous supplementation.

Dietary treatment should be started as soon as possible and ideally before 2 weeks of age.[103] Although a less strict dietary regimen is possible after 6 years of age, some forms of restriction are necessary indefinitely because central nervous system (CNS) damage has been described after discontinuation of treatment beyond childhood.[6] Pregnant women with PKU who are not on a low phenylalanine diet and have phenylalanine levels >360 μmol/L (6 mg/dL) have higher risks of either spontaneous abortion or the birth of offspring with microcephaly, congenital heart defects, facial dysmorphism, and developmental delay caused by the teratogenic effect of phenylalanine.[63,69]

In about 2% of cases, hyperphenylalaninemia is due to a deficiency of either biosynthesis or recycling of BH_4, the cofactor of phenylalanine hydroxylase and related enzymes (see Figure 55-5).[62] These infants could be diagnosed with PKU at first, but they deteriorate neurologically despite adequate dietary control. BH_4 is a cofactor for phenylalanine, tyrosine, and tryptophan hydroxylases. The latter two enzymes are involved in the synthesis of the neurotransmitters dopamine and serotonin. BH_4 is also a cofactor for nitric oxide synthase, which catalyzes the generation of nitric oxide from arginine. All patients with hyperphenylalaninemia should be routinely tested to rule out the possibility of a cofactor deficiency.[96]

Four enzyme deficiencies leading to BH_4 deficiency have been reported (see Table 55-2). 6-Pyruvoyltetrahydropterin synthase (6-PTS) is found in approximately 50% of all cases. They are clinically indistinguishable from classic PKU when detected by newborn screening, but progressively deteriorate with loss of head control, hypertonia, drooling, swallowing difficulties, and myoclonic seizures around 3 months of age. Plasma phenylalanine levels could be as high as those in classic PKU or in the range of benign hyperphenylalaninemia (<1.0 mmol/L). Measurement of urinary neopterin and biopterin provides a tool for the differential diagnosis among these disorders.[14]

Infants with benign hyperphenylalaninemia are occasionally identified because of a moderately elevated blood concentration of phenylalanine. These patients have a partial deficiency of phenylalanine hydroxylase with residual enzyme activity up to 35% of normal subjects. Although detected by neonatal screening, they remain healthy without dietary treatment once the possibility of an underlying cofactor deficiency has been ruled out.

Tyrosinemia Type 1

Tyrosine derives from the breakdown of dietary or tissue proteins or through the hydroxylation of the essential amino acid phenylalanine. Hepatorenal tyrosinemia (tyrosinemia type I, TYR-I) is an autosomal recessive disease caused by a deficiency of the enzyme fumarylacetoacetase (Figure 55-7),

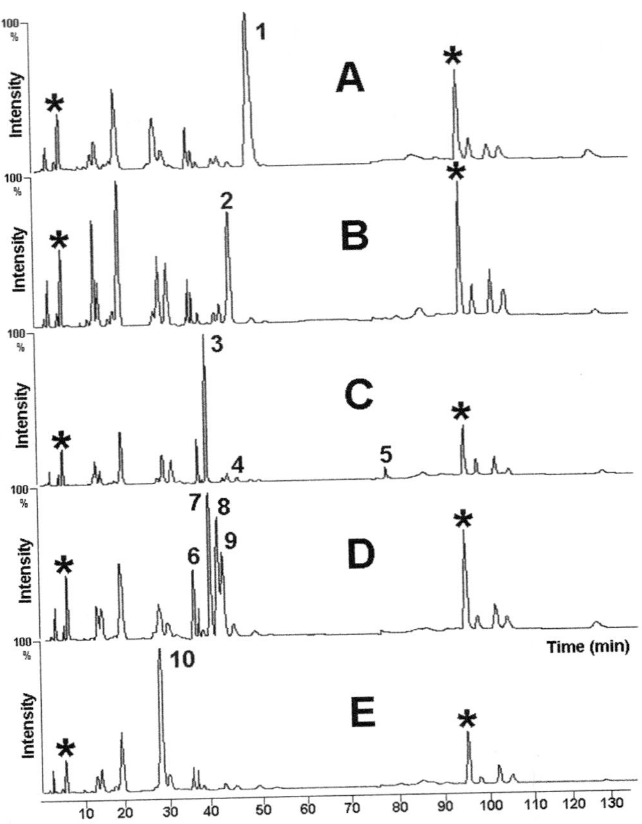

Figure 55-6 Plasma amino acid profiles by ion-exchange chromatography. **A,** Phenylketonuria (16 day old), phenylalanine 1550 μmol/L. **B,** Tyrosinemia type I (10 day old), tyrosine 696 μmol/L. **C,** Homocystinuria (8 year old), methionine 885 μmol/L, free homocysteine 38 μmol/L. **D,** Maple syrup urine disease (6 month old), valine 194 μmol/L, allo-isoleucine 693 μmol/L, isoleucine 636 μmol/L, leucine 418 μmol/L. **E,** Nonketotic hyperglycinemia (3 days old), glycine 1624 μmol/L. For age-matched reference intervals see Shapira et al.[12] **Peak legend:** *1,* Phenylalanine; *2,* tyrosine; *3,* methionine; *4,* mixed disulfide; *5,* free homocysteine; *6,* valine; *7,* allo-isoleucine; *8,* isoleucine; *9,* leucine, *10,* glycine. The symbol * marks the internal standards glucosaminic acid (retention time 6 minutes) and aminoethylcysteine (retention time 97 minutes), signal abundance is normalized on the intensity of the latter.

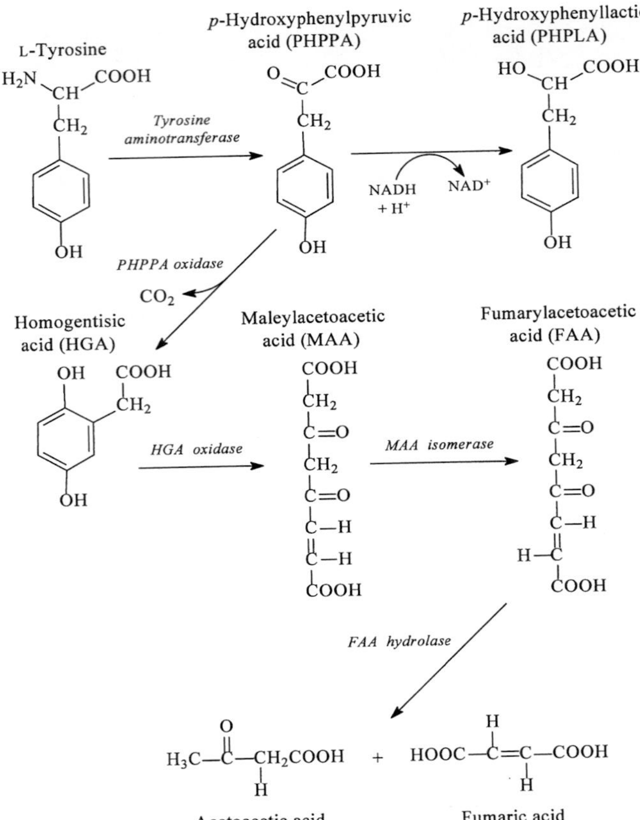

Figure 55-7 Metabolic pathway of tyrosine.

which is expressed primarily in the liver and renal proximal tubule.[90] The incidence of TYR-I is approximately 1 in 100,000, with well known clustering of cases in Scandinavia and the Lac-St. Jean region of Quebec (Canada). In the United States, screening for TYR-I is not offered in 35 states, with a cumulative number of births corresponding to 76% of all babies born each year (see Table 55-2). Under these circumstances, a clinical encounter with an undiagnosed and acutely ill patient is a realistic possibility in most pediatric gastroenterology practices. Symptoms are highly variable and include (1) acute liver failure, (2) cirrhosis, (3) hepatocellular carcinoma, (4) renal Fanconi syndrome, (5) glomerulosclerosis, and (6) crises of peripheral neuropathy that mimic acute intermittent porphyria caused by an accumulation of 5-aminolevulinic acid.[89]

An elevated concentration of tyrosine in plasma (Figure 55-6, *B*) is an expected finding of TYR-I but lacks specificity. A biochemical diagnosis is based instead on the detection in urine of succinylacetone (4,6-dioxaneheptanoic acid), the by-product of fumarylacetoacetic acid, which is the intermediate immediately upstream of the enzyme defect.[58] Absence of this metabolite in a patient with elevated plasma tyrosine and a urinary pattern of tyrosyluria (elevated excretions of 4-hydroxy phenyllactic acid, 4-hydroxy phenylpyruvic acid, and N-acetyltyrosine) points to any of several alternative causes, including other inherited disorders (tyrosinemia type II and type III, hypertyrosinemia of the premature, gluconeogenesis disorders, galactosemia, fructosemia, peroxisomal disorders) and acquired conditions (hepatitis, dietary load of aromatic amino acids, and overgrowth of intestinal flora). However, there have been rare instances when a patient with a diagnosis of TYR-I confirmed by DNA analysis does not excrete succinylacetone (Figure 55-8), suggesting that genotyping should still be pursued in patients with strongly suggestive clinical manifestations but no accumulation of succinylacetone.

NTBC (2-(2-nitro-4-trifluoro-methylbenzoyl)-1,3-cyclohexanedione) is a chemical initially developed as a herbicide. Animal studies show that NTBC is an inhibitor of

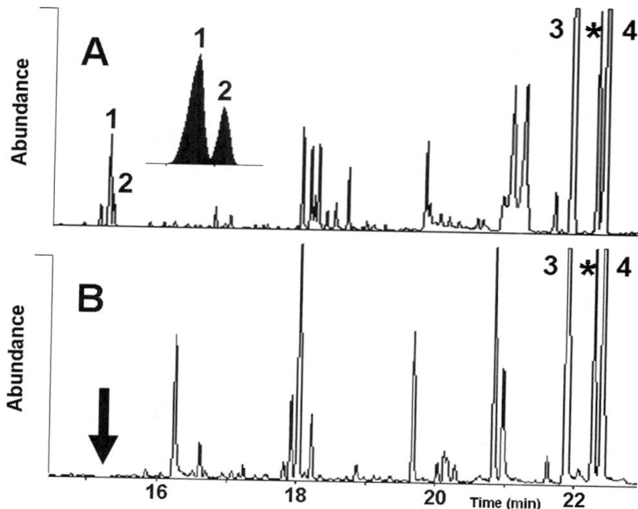

Figure 55-8 Partial urine organic acid profiles (15-23 minute portion of a 33 minute run) of two patients with tyrosinemia type I. **A,** Acutely ill patient with markedly elevated excretion of succinylacetone, pre-NTBC treatment. The insert shows the selected ion chromatogram of the $[M-15]^+$ ion of succinylacetone O-TMS-oxime TMS ester, m/z 212; **B,** Fifteen month old patient, succinylacetone was not detected by either total ion current (*arrow*) or selected ion chromatogram in three different urine specimens. This patient was later shown to be compound heterozygote for the French Canadian common splice mutation (IVS12+5G>A) and another previously unreported mutation. **Peak legend:** *1,* Succinylacetone (oxime, peak I); *2,* succinylacetone (oxime, peak II); *3,* 4-hydroxy phenyllactic acid; *4,* 4-hydroxy phenylpyruvic acid (oxime). The symbol * marks the internal standard (pentadecanoic acid), signal abundance is normalized to the intensity of the internal standard peak.

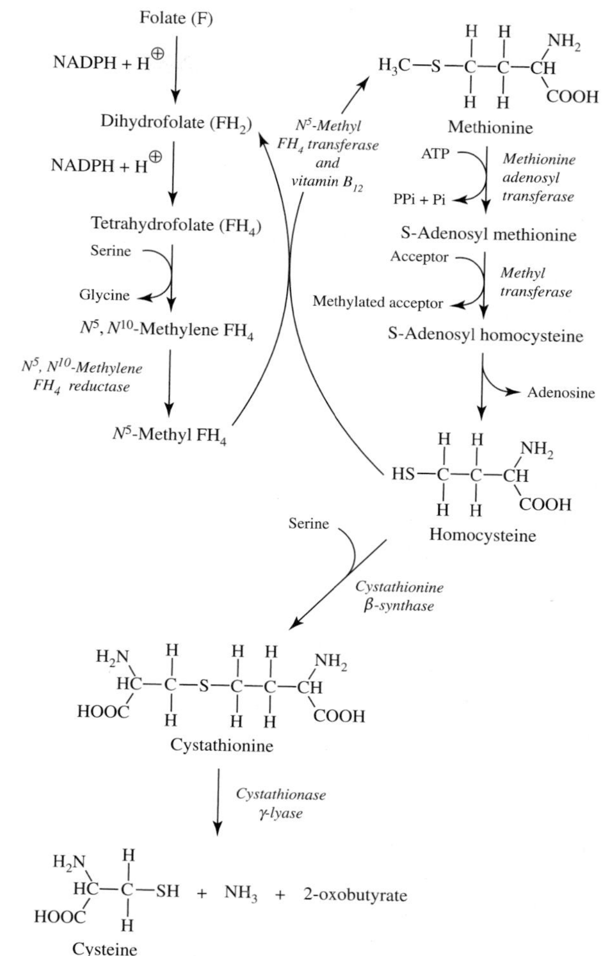

Figure 55-9 Biochemical pathways of the conversion of methionine to homocysteine and cysteine.

4-hydroxyphenylpyruvate dioxygenase, an enzyme of the tyrosine pathway located upstream of fumarylacetoacetate hydrolase. Pharmacological doses of NTBC virtually prevent the synthesis of succinylacetone and have become the treatment of choice for TYR-I in combination with dietary restriction and liver transplantation.[70]

Homocystinuria

Methionine, homocysteine, and cysteine are linked by the methylation cycle and transsulfuration pathway (Figure 55-9).[91] Conversion of methionine into homocysteine proceeds via the formation of S-adenosyl intermediates including S-adenosylmethionine, the methyl group donor in a wide range of transmethylation reactions. Homocysteine is further condensed with serine by cystathionine β-synthase to form cystathionine.

A defect of cystathionine β-synthase is an autosomal recessive disorder with an incidence of approximately 1:350,000 live births. In the United States, screening for homocystinuria is not offered in 23 states, corresponding to 53% of all babies born each year (see Table 55-2). Clinical manifestations are nonspecific at first and may include failure to thrive and developmental delay. A diagnosis is usually delayed 3 years or more if newborn screening is not available.[92] Ophthalmological problems include downward dislocation of the lens, myopia, and glaucoma; retinal detachment and degeneration, and optic atrophy and zonal cataracts may develop later in life. Osteoporosis is common after childhood when patients, as in Marfan syndrome, tend to be tall, with thinning and elongation of long bones near puberty. Besides mental retardation found in more than half of patients, neurological manifestations include seizures, abnormal EEG, and psychiatric disturbances. Thromboembolic episodes are common and involve both large and small vessels, especially in the brain, and constitute the major cause of morbidity and mortality. Thrombosis of carotid or renal arteries is a frequent cause of death.

The biochemical phenotype of homocystinuria is characterized by increased plasma concentrations of methionine, free homocysteine and cysteine-homocysteine disulfide, together with low cystine (Figure 55-6, *C*).[40] Determination of total homocysteine after treatment of the sample with reducing agents is useful because 80% of homocysteinyl moieties are bound to protein. The differential diagnosis of hyperhomocysteinemia includes (1) remethylation defects, (2) 5,10-methylene-tetrahydrofolate reductase deficiency, (3) 5-methyl-tetrahydrofolate-homocysteine-methyltransferase deficiency, and (4) defects of cytosolic cobalamin metabolism. There are at least six distinct defects in cobalamin metabolism, designated as *cblC, cblD, cblE, cblF, cblG,* and *cblH.*[139] Patients with *cblC, cblD,* and *cblF* defects have methylmalonic aciduria in addition to homocystinuria, because formation of both adenosylcobalamin and methylcobalamin is impaired.

The methylenetetrahydrofolate reductase enzyme reduces 5,10-methylenetetrahydrofolate to form 5-methyltetrahydrofolate, which provides methyl groups necessary for homocysteine remethylation to methionine. The severity of the enzyme defect and of clinical symptoms varies considerably. Completely absent enzyme activity results in neonatal apneic episodes, myoclonus leading to coma, and death, whereas partial deficiency may result in mental retardation and seizures. Premature cardiovascular disease or peripheral neuropathy could be the only manifestation. A common polymorphism (677C>T) is associated with enzyme thermal lability and mild elevation of homocysteine in the presence of folate insufficiency, implicating a risk for both vascular disease[61] and neural tube defects.[88]

Maple Syrup Urine Disease

Leucine, isoleucine, and valine are the three essential branched-chain amino acids. They undergo decarboxylation by branched-chain α-ketoacid dehydrogenase, a complex enzyme that requires thiamine pyrophosphate as a coenzyme (see Chapter 30).[29] This complex is composed of four subunits, $E_1\alpha$, $E_1\beta$, E_2, and E_3. The E_3 subunit is shared by two other dehydrogenases, pyruvate dehydrogenase and α-ketoglutarate dehydrogenase. A defect on any component of the complex causes maple syrup urine disease (MSUD), an autosomal recessive disorder with an incidence of approximately 1:250,000 live births. In the United States, screening for MSUD is not offered in 21 states, corresponding to 46% of all babies born per year. About 75% of affected patients suffer from a severe classical form and the remainder from intermediate or intermittent forms.

Babies with classical MSUD present with poor feeding and vomiting during the first week of life followed by lethargy and coma within a few days. Hypertonia, rigidity, and severe opisthotonus are often interpreted as signs of general sepsis and CNS infection. Seizure and hypoglycemia are also common. At a more advanced stage, neurovegetative dysregulation with respiratory distress, bradycardia, and hypothermia may appear. Routine laboratory work is only remarkable for severe metabolic acidosis, and death rapidly ensues in untreated patients.

In some patients, symptoms appear after a symptom-free period of 1 year or more, occasionally in adolescence or even adulthood. Vomiting, ataxia, lethargy, and even coma characterize intermittent episodes of acute decompensation. Once they recover, patients return to a normal status with no obvious sequelae. Such episodes are triggered by catabolic stress, infections, or increased protein intake, and are associated with laboratory findings that are indistinguishable from neonatal-onset MSUD. Finally a chronic, progressive form of MSUD has also been described with (1) persistent anorexia, (2) chronic vomiting, (3) failure to thrive, (4) hypotonia, and (5) osteoporosis. Most patients remain undiagnosed until the occurrence of an acute neurological crisis.

A diagnosis of MSUD is suspected when a patient's urine, sweat, and particularly ear wax have the characteristic odor of maple syrup. At the bedside, mixing urine with a solution of 2,4-dinitrophenylhydrazine (DNPH) is a simple and rapid test to confirm a clinical suspicion,[12] a practical alternative to quantitative amino acid analysis if the latter is not available on site. Eventually, plasma amino acid analysis must be performed to show marked elevation of leucine (usually the prominent amino acid), isoleucine, and valine plus the pathognomonic presence of L-alloisoleucine (Figure 55-6, *D*). L-Alloisoleucine is a stereoisomer derived through stepwise racemization and keto-enol tautomerization of (2*S*) 2-keto-3-methylvaleric acid to its (2*R*) enantiomer, followed by transamination.[83] The 2-keto acids, the substrates immediately upstream of the enzyme block, are responsible for the positive DNPH test, and their respective hydroxy analogues are detectable by urine organic acid analysis after stabilization of the 2-keto groups via oximation. An elevated excretion of 2-hydroxyisovaleric acid could be the most informative finding in asymptomatic patients with intermediate and intermittent MSUD.

Cornerstones of treatment are dietary restriction of branched-chain amino acids and high dose thiamine, the latter showing responsiveness in cases with mild and/or intermittent presentations. Acute episodes are life threatening and require aggressive treatment; peritoneal dialysis may be necessary because renal clearance of the toxic metabolites is poor.[59]

Urea Cycle Defects

Enzymes of the urea cycle regulate the disposal of the amino groups removed by transamination and deamination of amino acids before their carbon skeleton is metabolized to gluconeogenic (most amino acids) or ketogenic precursors (leucine and lysine), or both (isoleucine, phenylalanine, tyrosine, and tryptophan). Disorders described in this pathway include (1) carbamylphosphate synthase (CPS) deficiency, (2) X-linked ornithine transcarbamylase (OTC) deficiency, (3) argininosuccinate synthase (ASS) deficiency (citrullinemia), (4) argininosuccinate lyase (AL) deficiency, and (5) arginase deficiency (argininemia).[18] The inclusion of these disorders in newborn screening programs varies from 2 to 20 U.S. states (5% to 32% of births) and is summarized in Table 55-2 (see also Figure 24-2, p. 802).

Patients with urea cycle defects may present at any age. In the neonatal period, a variable but usually brief interval is

followed by the clinical manifestations of hyperammonemia: poor feeding, vomiting, lethargy or irritability, coma and not infrequently death when cases are not properly diagnosed and aggressively treated. In infancy, the symptoms are similar to the neonatal period, but less severe and more variable. Neurological abnormalities also include ataxia and irritability. These patients are often misdiagnosed as having gastrointestinal disorders, food allergies, behavioral problems, or nonspecific hepatitis. In children and adults, chronic neurological problems are characterized by (1) learning difficulties, (2) mental retardation, (3) behavioral problems, and (4) cyclic vomiting, which occasionally deteriorates to acute decompensation with severe encephalopathy.[93] Arginase deficiency differs by the frequent absence of hyperammonemia and a clinical picture of spastic diplegia frequently diagnosed as cerebral palsy.

The dominant laboratory findings are hyperammonemia and respiratory alkalosis, even though the clinical reliability of the latter has been questioned.[7] Plasma amino acids and urine orotic acid levels are necessary for a differential diagnosis.[18] High glutamine and alanine concentrations are typical, but not diagnostic for these disorders, reflecting an imbalance of the intracellular nitrogen pool. However, if the concentration of citrulline is low or undetectable, the overall profile is consistent with either OTC deficiency or CPS deficiency. These two have been differentiated by testing orotic acid in urine, which is elevated only in OTC deficiency. A more than twentyfold increase of the citrulline concentration indicates a defect at the level of argininosuccinic synthase, a condition commonly known as citrullinemia. A twofold to fivefold elevation of plasma citrulline in the presence of argininosuccinic acid in urine is indicative of argininosuccinase deficiency, but could also be indicative of other conditions (e.g., pyruvate carboxylase deficiency).

Acute hyperammonemia should be treated promptly as a medical emergency. A variety of conjugating agents (benzoate, phenylacetate, phenylbutyrate) are used to deplete the nitrogen pool via excretion of their glycine and glutamine conjugates.[72] Citrulline and/or arginine supplementation are used to provide substrates to the urea cycle downstream of specific blocks; neomycin and lactulose reduce the production of ammonia by intestinal bacteria. If these therapies along with the reversal of catabolism fail to effectively reduce blood ammonia within hours, dialysis (hemodialysis or peritoneal dialysis) must be instituted.

Nonketotic Hyperglycinemia

The large endogenous pool of glycine is maintained by dietary intake (3 to 5 g per day) and synthesis from serine, and provides approximately a fourth of the amino acid residue incorporated in major structural proteins. Glycine is also a precursor in the synthesis of purines, glutathione, creatine, and porphyrins. The enzyme glycine *N*-acyltransferase forms glycine conjugates of many acyl-CoA species that accumulate in the mitochondrial matrix in disorders of organic acid and fatty acid metabolism.[45] Glycine is catabolized by the glycine cleavage system, a four peptide complex (protein P, H, T, and L) attached to the inner membrane of mitochondria in liver, brain, kidney, and placenta. One carbon is converted to carbon dioxide, the other is transferred to tetrahydrofolate to from hydroxymethyltetrahydrofolate, which may either react with another mole of glycine to produce serine or form methyltetrahydrofolate, which serves as a methyl donor.

Nonketotic hyperglycinemia (NKHG) is a severe condition caused, in most cases, by a defect of either the T or P protein of the glycine cleavage system. In the newborn period, poor feeding, failure to suck, lethargy, and profound hypotonia rapidly progress to coma and death, which occur during the first few days of life. Intractable seizures and hiccups are common. The EEG pattern is characteristic with bursts of high complex waves of 1 to 3 seconds arising periodically from a hypoactive background, called burst-suppression pattern.[77] In infantile NKHG, symptoms, usually seizures, develop after 6 months of age. Late onset NKHG is a poorly defined entity reported only in a few patients with progressive spastic paraparesis, optic atrophy, and choreoathetoid movements. In the United States, screening NKHG is included in 7 state programs, corresponding to 8% of all babies born each year.

A key element that should raise the suspicion of NKHG is the finding of uninformative routine laboratory investigations in a child with progressing neurological symptoms. Plasma and CSF amino acid analysis reveal a high concentration of glycine (plasma>1000 μmol/L; CSF >30 μmol/L) with no other notable abnormalities (Figure 55-6, *E*), and urine organic acids are unremarkable. The calculated CSF: plasma glycine concentration ratio (NKHG: >0.09, reference intervals: <0.04) is critical in the differential diagnosis of this condition,[128] but caution should be used to avoid measuring the ratio when the plasma and CSF specimens were not collected simultaneously (no more than 1 hour apart). Contamination of CSF with blood could increase the concentration of glycine, but when it occurs, other unrelated amino acids are also elevated.

No effective treatment is known. Drugs that counteract the effect of glycine on neuronal cells, such as strychnine, diazepam, and dextromethorphan, could bring mild benefits in milder forms of the condition. Ketamine, an anesthetic blocker of the N-methyl-D-aspartate (NMDA) receptor channel, brought a partial improvement of neurological symptoms and EEG findings in some patients, but their developmental milestones were delayed.

DISORDERS OF ORGANIC ACID METABOLISM

Organic acids are water-soluble compounds containing one or more carboxyl groups and other functional groups (-keto, -hydroxy), which are intermediate metabolites of all major groups of organic cellular components: amino acids, lipids, carbohydrates, nucleic acids, and steroids. Organic acidurias are a biochemically heterogeneous group of inborn errors of metabolism biochemically characterized by the accumulation of either (1) metabolites, which are not present under physiological conditions, from the activation of alternative pathways in response to the loss of function of a specific gene product, or (2) pathological amounts of normal metabolites.[26,48,68,127]

Table 55-3 shows a summary of known disorders of organic acid metabolism, including information about their incidence, major clinical features and biochemical patterns, availability of prenatal diagnosis and newborn screening, and association with sudden unexpected death. The incidence of individual inborn errors of organic acid metabolism varies from 1:10,000 to >1:1,000,000 live births. All possible disease entities included, the incidence of conditions in which informative organic acid profiles could be detected in urine is likely to approach 1:1000 live births.

The biochemical diagnosis of individual organic acidemias ultimately relies on urine organic acid analysis by gas chromatography-mass spectrometry (GC-MS).[43] Detection, positive identification, and eventually quantitation of pathognomonic organic acids by GC-MS could be available in a matter of hours if the analysis is performed at a local laboratory. Otherwise, results from a referral laboratory should be available within 24 hours for an urgent case. Informative profiles may not always be detected in disorders in which the excretion of diagnostic metabolites depends on the residual activity of the defective enzyme, the dietary load of precursors, and the anabolic status of a patient.

Several selected disorders of organic acid metabolism are discussed below.

Disorders of Propionate Metabolism

Propionyl-CoA is an intermediary product in the metabolism of four essential amino acids (isoleucine, valine, threonine, and methionine), the aliphatic side-chain of cholesterol, pyrimidines (uracil and thymine), and the final product of the β-oxidation of odd-chain fatty acids. Under normal circumstances, propionyl-CoA first is converted by a biotin-dependent carboxylase to methylmalonyl-CoA, then to succinyl-CoA by an adenosylcobalamin-dependent mutase, leading to oxidation in the tricarboxylic acid cycle.[38] Primary or secondary defects of these two enzymes were among the first organic acidurias to be discovered, and their natural history has been characterized perhaps better than any other inborn error of organic acid metabolism.

Propionic acidemia (PA) and methylmalonic acidemia (MMA) are panethnic disorders, but their combined incidence varies considerably, with estimates ranging from 1:2000 to 1:5000 (Saudi Arabia) to 20 times lower. However, there is a general consensus that many patients with this disorder die undiagnosed, being masked by a variety of catastrophic processes (sepsis and intraventricular hemorrhage).[97] In the United States, screening for these disorders by means of MS/MS detection of propionylcarnitine is not offered in 31 states, corresponding to 69% of all babies born each year. Curiously the state of Missouri has mandated screening for PA only.

Patients with PA and MMA typically are born at term with no pregnancy complications and present with an intoxication type of picture after hours or even days without apparent symptoms. Prominent manifestations include vomiting, hypotonia, lethargy, apnea, hypothermia, and rapid onset of coma. Routine laboratory investigations show severe metabolic acidosis and ketonuria (a finding of critical significance never to be overlooked in the newborn period); lactic acidemia, hypoglycemia, and hyperammonemia are often present[118]; the latter could be so severe as to direct the diagnostic work-up toward a urea cycle defect and not include urine organic acid analysis. Similarly, neutropenia caused by growth inhibition of myeloid progenitors is a common finding that in many cases is attributed to a primary immunodeficiency. Acute and chronic pancreatitis have also been observed in several patients with methylmalonic acidemia and other inborn errors of branched-chain amino acid metabolism.[60]

Hyperglycinemia is found when samples from affected patients are analyzed for plasma amino acids. In addition, the urine organic acid profile from a sample from an acutely affected individual could reveal lactic aciduria, ketonuria, and a large number of propionate metabolites, particularly 3-hydroxypropionic acid and 2-methylcitric acid. The glycine conjugates propionylglycine and tiglylglycine could be markedly elevated, and the latter could be confused with 3-methylcrotonylglycine (Figure 55-10), a distinction that is critical for the correct differential diagnosis between PA and multiple carboxylase deficiency. The presence or absence of methylmalonic acid is the main difference between PA and MMA (Figure 55-11, *A* and *B*). Although this is an easy distinction in most cases, a relatively small excretion of methylmalonic acid is actually possible in early stages of an acute episode,[109] and other factors may also lead to an incorrect differential diagnosis between these disorders.[34,35] In plasma, the concentration of propionylcarnitine is markedly elevated in PA and MMA caused by either one of the apoenzyme defects, and marginal elevations could be observed in patients with a coenzyme defect (various *cbl* complementation groups).

Patients who survive the initial event have developmental delay, hypotonia or hypertonia, and variable cognitive and neurological sequelae that are linked to the number and severity of acute episodes. Early detection seems to improve the prognosis; treatment is based on restriction of precursor amino acid intake, carnitine, and cofactors—biotin or cobalamin—as indicated.

Isovaleric Acidemia

Isovaleric acidemia (IVA) is a disorder of leucine catabolism caused by a deficiency of isovaleryl-CoA dehydrogenase. Since the initial report 40 years ago, IVA has been the main focus of the work of Dr. Kay Tanaka, one of the pioneers and arguably most productive contributors to our current

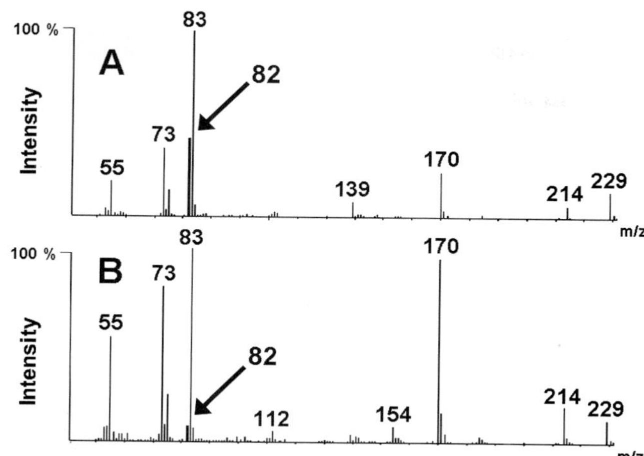

Figure 55-10 Electron impact positive ion mass spectra of isomeric acylglycines detected by GC/MS analysis of organic acid trimethylsilyl (TMS) derivatives. **A,** 3-Methylcrotonylglycine mono-TMS ester (leucine metabolism). **B,** Tiglylglycine mono-TMS ester (isoleucine metabolism). As their retention times are relatively close in most chromatographic systems, proper differentiation between the two compounds is best achieved by evaluation of the fragment ion at m/z 82 *(arrow)* which is prominent in the spectrum of 3-methylcrotonylglycine but not tiglylglycine.

understanding of inborn errors of organic acid metabolism. His seminal work on IVA was particularly significant for the first application of GC-MS to the study of an IEM, and for the recognition and later complete characterization of a previously unknown enzyme on the basis of the biochemical phenotype found in patients with an inherited defect at that level.[129] In the United States, screening by means of MS/MS detection of isovalerylcarnitine is not offered in 35 states, corresponding to 69% of all babies born each year.

The clinical presentation of the neonatal form is similar to disorders of propionate metabolism. One revealing feature of this IEM is the characteristic odor of "sweaty feet." This feature is difficult to miss, but occasionally is absent or attributed to other causes. In practice, the diagnosis is confirmed by the specific pattern of excretion of organic acids with isovalerylglycine accumulating as the major by-product followed by 3-hydroxyisovaleric acid (Figure 55-11, *C*). In plasma, C5-acylcarnitine is elevated, but is actually a mixture of isovalerylcarnitine and 2-methylbutyrylcarnitine derived from leucine and isoleucine degradation, respectively.[79] Also the differential diagnosis has been further complicated by another C5 isomer, pivaloylcarnitine, which is formed in patients treated with antibiotics containing pivalic acid.[1] Initially, it was thought that IVA was an easily recognizable disorder at any clinical stage because of the magnitude of accumulation of isovalerylglycine and isovalerylcarnitine. However, this has been recently questioned by a number of cases detected by newborn screening in which several infants had much milder, even intermittent accumulation of

Text continued on p. 2230

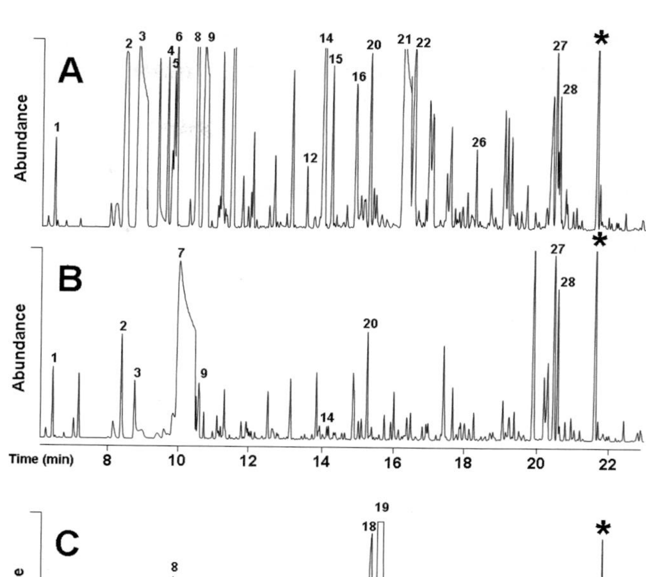

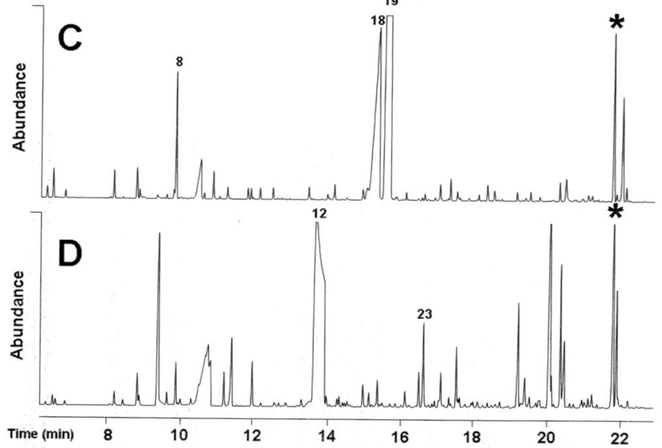

Figure 55-11 Partial urine organic acid profiles (7-22 minute portion of a 33 minute run). **A,** Propionic acidemia (acute episode). **B,** Methylmalonic acidemia. **C,** Isovaleric acidemia. **D,** Glutaric acidemia type I. **Peak legend** (only metabolites directly related to the chosen disorders): *1,* Lactic acid; *2,* 3-hydroxy propionic acid; *3,* 3-hydroxy butyric acid; *4,* 2-methyl 3-hydroxy butyric acid; *5,* acetoacetic acid (peak I); *6,* 3-hydroxy valeric acid; *7,* methylmalonic acid; *8,* 3-hydroxy valeric acid; *9,* acetoacetic acid (peak II); *10,* ethylmalonic acid; *11,* isobutyrylglycine (di-TMS); *12,* glutaric acid; *13,* 2-methylbutyrylglycine (di-TMS); *14,* propionylglycine (di-TMS); *15,* 3-methylglutaconic acid (peak I); *16,* 3-methylglutaconic acid (peak II); *17,* 3-hydroxy adipic lactone; *18,* isovalerylglycine (di-TMS); *19,* isovalerylglycine (mono-TMS); *20,* adipic acid; *21,* tiglylglycine (di-TMS); *22,* tiglylglycine (mono-TMS); *23,* 3-hydroxy glutaric acid; *24,* octenedioic acid; *25,* 3-hydroxy adipic acid; *26,* suberic acid; *27,* methylcitric acid (peak I); *28,* methylcitric acid (peak II); *29,* decenedioic acid (multiple isomers); *30,* 3-hydroxy octanedioic acid; *31,* 3-hydroxy suberic acid; *32,* sebacic acid; *33,* 3-hydroxy decenedioic acid; *34,* 3-hydroxy sebacic acid; *35,* 3-hydroxy dodecadienoic acid (C12:2); *36,* 3-hydroxy dodecenedioic acid; *37,* 3-hydroxy dodecanedioic acid; *38,* 3-hydroxy tetradecadienoic acid (C14:2); *39,* 3-hydroxy tetradecenedioic acid; *40,* 3-hydroxy tetradecanedioic acid. The symbol * marks the internal standard (pentadecanoic acid), signal abundance is normalized to the intensity of the internal standard peak. Note: The peak legend also applies to Figure 54-12.

TABLE 55-3 Clinical and Laboratory Characteristics of Disorders of Organic Acid Metabolism

Common Name	OMIM No.	Enzyme/Transport Defect	Incidence (USA)	Major Clinical Features	Complication of Pregnancy (Maternal, Fetal)
Disorders of Propionate Metabolism and Related Cofactors					
Propionic acidemia	232000, 232050	Propionyl-CoA carboxylase (subunit alpha, beta)	>1 : 75,000	Failure to thrive, developmental delay, hypotonia, neutropenia	/
Multiple carboxylase deficiency	253270	Holocarboxylase synthase	<1 : 100,000	Alopecia, perioral skin erosions, hearing loss, developmental delay, hypotonia, seizures, breathing problems	/
Methylmalonic acidemia (mut 0 and mut–)	251000	Methylmalonyl-CoA mutase	>1 : 75,000	Failure to thrive, anorexia, developmental delay, hypotonia	/
Methylmalonic acidemia (cblA)	251100	Mitochondrial cobalamin reductase	<1 : 100,000	Failure to thrive, anorexia, developmental delay, hypotonia	/
Methylmalonic acidemia (cblB)	251110	Cob(I)alamin transferase	<1 : 100,000	Failure to thrive, anorexia, developmental delay, hypotonia	/
Methylmalonic acidemia (cblC and cblD)	277400	Methylfolate-H(4) methyltransferase; methylmalonyl-CoA isomerase	<1 : 100,000	Failure to thrive, developmental delay, hypotonia, megaloblastic anemia, hemolytic uremic syndrome	/
Methylmalonic acidemia (cblF)	277380	Lysosomal release	<1 : 100,000	Failure to thrive, developmental delay, hypotonia	/
Methylmalonic acidemia (cblH)	606169	Synthesis of adenosylcobalamin	<1 : 100,000	Failure to thrive, developmental delay, hypotonia	/
Other Disorders of Branched Chain Amino Acid Metabolism					
Isovaleric acidemia	243500	Isovaleryl-CoA dehydrogenase	<1 : 100,000	Episodic vomiting, lethargy, coma, sweaty feet odor	/
3-Methylcrotonyl glycinuria	210200	3-Methylcrotonyl-CoA carboxylase	>1 : 75,000	Episodic vomiting, lethargy, coma	/
3-Methylglutaconic aciduria	250950	3-Methylglutaconyl-CoA hydratase	<1 : 100,000	Speech defect, mental retardation, hypertonia, spasticity	/

OMIM, Online Mendelian Inheritance in Man (www.ncbi.nlm.nih.gov/entrez/query.fcgi?db=OMIM); *NBS,* newborn screening; *MMA,* methylmalonic acid; *GLY,* glycine; *tHey,* total homocysteine.

Modality of Acute Episodes	Major Biochemical Marker(s)	Prenatal Diagnosis	NBS in the US (% Births)	Sudden Unexpected Death
Dehydration, ketoacidosis, hyperammonemia	GLY, propionylcarnitine (B), methylcitric, 3-OH propionic, propionylglycine, tiglylglycine (U)	Enzyme assay in amniocytes, methylcitric, propionylcarnitine (AF)	20/51 states (31%)	Anecdotal reports
Dehydration, ketoacidosis, lactic acidemia	Lactic C5-OH acylcarnitine (B), 3-OH isovaleric, 3-methylcrotonyl glycine, 3-OH propionic, methylcitric, lactate, tiglylglycine (U)	Enzyme assay in amniocytes, methylcitric C3 C5-OH acylcarnitines (AF)	13/51 states (22%)	Anecdotal reports
Dehydration, ketoacidosis	GLY, MMA, propionylcarnitine (B), MMA, methylcitric, 3-OH propionic, propionylglycine (U)	Enzyme assay in amniocytes, MMA, methylcitric, propionylcarnitine (AF)	19/51 states (29%)	Anecdotal reports
Dehydration, ketoacidosis	GLY, MMA, propionylcarnitine (B), MMA, methylcitric, 3-OH propionic, propionylglycine (U)	Enzyme assay in amniocytes, MMA, methylcitric, propionylcarnitine (AF)	19/51 states (29%)	/
Dehydration, ketoacidosis	GLY, MMA, propionylcarnitine (B), MMA, methylcitric, 3-OH propionic, propionylglycine (U)	Enzyme assay in amniocytes, MMA, methylcitric, propionylcarnitine (AF)	19/51 states (29%)	/
Dehydration, ketoacidosis	GLY, MMA, tHcy, propionylcarnitine (B), MMA, methylcitric, 3-OH propionic, propionylglycine (U)	Enzyme assay in amniocytes, MMA, HCY, methylcitric, propionylcarnitine (AF)	19/51 states (29%)	/
/	MMA (B,U)	Enzyme assay in amniocytes, MMA (AF)	Secondary target (MMA)	/
Dehydration, ketoacidosis	GLY, MMA, propionylcarnitine (B), MMA, methylcitric, 3-OH propionic, propionylglycine (U)	Enzyme assay in amniocytes, MMA, methylcitric, propionylcarnitine (AF)	Secondary target (MMA)	/
Dehydration, ketoacidosis	Isovalerylcarnitine (B), 3-OH isovaleric, isovalerylglycine (U)	Enzyme assay in amniocytes, isovalerylcarnitine, isovalerylglycine (AF), DNA analysis	20/51 states (31%)	/
Dehydration, ketoacidosis	C5-OH acylcarnitine (B), 3-OH isovaleric, 3-methylcrotonylglycine (U)	Enzyme assay in amniocytes, isovalerylcarnitine, isovalerylglycine (AF), DNA analysis	19/51 states (29%)	/
Hypoglycemia, acidosis	C5-OH acylcarnitine (B), 3-OH isovaleric, 3-methylglutaconic, 3-methylglutaric (U)	Enzyme assay in amniocytes, 3-OH isovaleric, 3-methylglutaconic acid (AF)	9/51 states (13%)	/

Continued.

TABLE 55-3 Clinical and Laboratory Characteristics of Disorders of Organic Acid Metabolism—*Continued*

Common Name	OMIM No.	Enzyme/Transport Defect	Incidence (USA)	Major Clinical Features	Complication of Pregnancy (Maternal, Fetal)
3-Hydroxy-3-methylglutaric aciduria	246450	3-Hydroxy-3-methylglutaryl-CoA lyase	<1 : 100,000	Episodic vomiting, hypotonia, hypoglycemia, metabolic acidosis, hepatomegaly	/
2-Methylbutyrylglycinuria	600301	2-Methylbutyryl-CoA dehydrogenase	<1 : 100,000 (1 : 500 Hmong)	Developmental delay, seizures, progressive muscle weakness. Lack of symptoms also possible.	/
2-Methyl-3-hydroxybutyric aciduria	203750	2-Methyl-3-hydroxybutyryl-CoA dehydrogenase	<1 : 100,000	Progressive loss of mental and motor skills	/
Beta-ketothiolase deficiency	203750	Beta-ketothiolase	<1 : 100,000	Episodic vomiting, lethargy, hypotonia, mental retardation, speech problems	/
Isobutyrylglycinuria	Pending	Isobutyryl-CoA dehydrogenase	<1 : 100,000	Anemia, dilated cardiomyopathy	/
3-Hydroxyisobutyric aciduria	Pending	3-Hydroxyisobutyryl-CoA dehydrogenase or methylmalonic semialdehyde dehydrogenase	<1;100,000	Congenital anomalies, short stature, hypotonia	/
Methylmalonic aciduria (atypical)	248360	Methylmalonic semialdehyde	<1 : 100,000	Developmental delay	/
Miscellaneous Disorders of Organic Acid Metabolism					
Alkaptonuria	203500	Homogentisic dioxygenase	<1 : 100,000	Arthritis, ochronosis	/
Biotinidase deficiency	253260	Biotinidase	>1 : 75,000	Alopecia, periorificial skin rash, conjunctivitis, developmental delay, hypotonia	/
4-OH butyric aciduria	271980	Succinic semialdehyde dehydrogenase	<1 : 100,000	Developmental delay, ataxia, hypotonia, seizures, hyperkinetic behavior	/
Canavan disease	271900	N-aspartoacylase	<1 : 100,000 (1 : 5,000 Ashkenazi)	Hypotonia, developmental delay, macrocephaly, optic atrophy, seizures, progressive neurological degeneration	/

RFLP, Restriction fragment length polymorphism; *NAA,* N-acetylaspartic acid.

Modality of Acute Episodes	Major Biochemical Marker(s)	Prenatal Diagnosis	NBS in the US (% Births)	Sudden Unexpected Death
Hypoglycemia, acidosis	C5-OH acylcarnitine (B), 3-OH isovaleric, 3-methylglutaconic, 3-OH-3-methylglutaric (U)	Association with Down syndrome and VATER syndrome	19/51 states (29%)	/
Hypothermia, hypoglycemia, acidosis	C5 acylcarnitine (B), 2-methylbutyrylglycine (U)	Enzyme assay in amniocytes, C5 acylcarnitine, 2-methylbutyrylglycine (AF)	11/51 states (22%)	/
Acidosis	C5-OH acylcarnitine (B), 2-methyl-3-OH-butyric acid, tiglylglycine (U)	Not reported	1/51 states (<1%)	/
Ketoacidosis, seizures	C5-OH acylcarnitine (B), 2-methyl-3-OH-butyric acid, 2-methylacetoacetic, tiglylglycine (U)	Immunoblotting, RFLP	19/51 states (29%)	/
/	C4 acylcarnitine (B), isobutyrylglycine inconsistently elevated (U)	Not reported	11/51 states (22%)	/
Dehydration, ketoacidosis	3-OH isobutyric, 2-ethylhydracrylic (U)	3-OH isobutyric (AF)	Not available	Anecdotal reports
/	NORMAL propionylcarnitine (B), MMA (U)	Not reported	Secondary target (MMA)	/
Heart valvulitis	Homogentisic (U)	/	Not available	/
Ketoacidosis (early in life)	Biotinidase (B), 3-OH isovaleric (U)	Enzyme assay in amniocytes	30/51 states (50%)	Anecdotal reports
/	4-OH butyric acid (U)	Enzyme assay in CVS, 4-OH butyric acid (AF)	Not available	/
/	NAA (U)	Enzyme assay in amniocytes/CVS, NAA (AF), DNA analysis	Not available	/

Continued.

TABLE 55-3 Clinical and Laboratory Characteristics of Disorders of Organic Acid Metabolism—*Continued*

Common Name	OMIM No.	Enzyme/Transport Defect	Incidence (USA)	Major Clinical Features	Complication of Pregnancy (Maternal, Fetal)
Ethylmalonic encephalopathy	602473	Unknown (*ETHE1* gene)	<1 : 100,000	Hypotonia, spastic tetraparesis, petechiae, orthostatic acrocyanosis, diarrhea	/
Glutaric acidemia type I	231670	Glutaryl-CoA dehydrogenase	>1 : 75,000 (1 : 500 Amish)	Macrocephaly, hypotonia, abnormal movements, frontotemporal atrophy, basal ganglia lesions	/
Glyceroluria (X-linked)	307030	Glycerol kinase	<1 : 100,000	Failure to thrive, episodic vomiting, developmental delay, bone fractures	/
Hyperoxaluria type I	259900	Alanine:glyoxylate aminotransferase	<1 : 100,000	Urolithiasis, nephrocalcinosis, renal failure	/
Hyperoxaluria type II	260000	D-Glyceric dehydrogenase	<1 : 100,000	Urolithiasis, hematuria, urinary tract infections, rarely nephrocalcinosis and renal failure	/
2-Ketoadipic aciduria	Pending	2-Ketoadipic dehydrogenase	<1 : 100,000	Developmental delay possible. Lack of symptoms also possible	/
Malonic acidemia	248360	Malonyl-CoA decarboxylase	<1 : 100,000	Short stature, cardiomyopathy, GI symptoms, hypotonia, developmental delay	/
Pyroglutamic aciduria	266130	Glutathione synthase	<1 : 100,000	Mental retardation, ataxia, spastic tetraparesis, seizures	/
Mevalonic aciduria	251170	Mevalonate kinase	<1 : 100,000	Failure to thrive, developmental delay, ataxia, hypotonia, hepatosplenomegaly, skin rashes, diarrhea	/

EMA, Ethylmalonic acid; *SCAD,* short-chain acyl-CoA dehydrogenase deficiency.

Modality of Acute Episodes	Major Biochemical Marker(s)	Prenatal Diagnosis	NBS in the US (% Births)	Sudden Unexpected Death
Lactic acidosis	C4 C5 acylcarnitines (B), EMA, isobutyrylglycine, 2-methylbutyrylglycine (U)	Not reported	Likely to be misdiagnosed as SCAD or GA-II	Frequent
Encephalopathy	C5-DC acylcarnitine (B,U), glutaric, 3-OH glutaric (U)	Enzyme assay in amniocytes, glutaric (AF), DNA analysis	20/51 states (31%)	Anecdotal reports
Acidosis, Reye-like illness, adrenal insufficiency	Pseudo-hypertriglyceridemia (B), glycerol (B, U)	Enzyme assay in amniocytes, DNA analysis	Not available	/
Vomiting, acidosis, uremia	Oxalic glycolic (U)	Enzyme assay of fetal liver biopsy, DNA analysis	Not available	/
/	Oxalic glyceric (U)	Not reported	Not available	/
/	2-Ketoadipic, 2-OH adipic, 2-aminoadipic (U)	Not reported	Not available	/
Hypoglycemia, acidosis	C3-DC acylcarnitine (B), malonic, methylmalonic, 3-methylglutaconic (U)	Not reported	7/51 states (13%)	/
Acidosis, hemolytic anemia, neutropenia	Pyroglutamic (U)	Enzyme assay in amniocytes/CVS, pyroglutamic (AF), DNA analysis	8/51 states (9%)	/
Hyper IgD and periodic fever	Mevalonic, mevalonolactone (U)	Enzyme assay in amniocytes, mevalonic (AF)	Not available	/

diagnostic metabolites. Treatment with a low protein diet and glycine (250 mg/kg/day) and carnitine (50 mg/kg/day) supplements allows for a good prognosis, but acute episodes of metabolic decompensation could be life threatening at any age.

Glutaric Acidemia Type I

Glutaric acidemia type I (GA-I) results from an inherited defect in glutaryl-CoA dehydrogenase, an enzyme involved in the degradation of lysine and tryptophan. Affected individuals present with very severe but preventable neurological consequences and unpredictable variability of the biochemical phenotype. Characteristic clinical findings are macrocephaly and frontal bossing, sometimes present at birth, and the sudden onset of an encephalopathic episode usually before 3 years of age. Brain imaging of affected individuals demonstrates frontotemporal atrophy, and after a crisis the characteristic sequelae of acute striatal degeneration and shrinkage of the caudate and nucleate nuclei of the basal ganglia. Hypotonia, abnormal movements, seizures, hypoglycemia, and hepatomegaly have also been associated with acute events. In the United States, screening for GA-I by means of MS/MS detection of glutarylcarnitine is not offered in 31 states, corresponding to 69% of all babies born each year.

The classic biochemical phenotype consists of massive glutaric aciduria with increased concentrations of glutarylcarnitine in plasma. Increased concentrations of glutarylglycine are inconsistently detected in humans, even though it is readily detected in the GA-I mouse knockout model.[65] The typical pattern in urine and plasma is abnormal and many cases present with minimal excretion of metabolites and normal plasma acylcarnitines. Evaluation of glutarylcarnitine and glutarylglycine in urine could aid in the interpretation of inconclusive findings. It is not known what impact this variability may have on the sensitivity and specificity of newborn screening for GA-I by acylcarnitine analysis, but false-negative results are likely to occur.

Ethylmalonic Encephalopathy

Ethylmalonic encephalopathy (EE) is an autosomal recessive disorder originally reported in Italian families.[20] EE patients described thereafter have been of Mediterranean[42] or Arabic[98] descent, with a few exceptions.[142] The first group of patients to be reported presented with (1) neonatal hypotonia, (2) progressive pyramidal dysfunction, (3) mental retardation, (4) orthostatic acrocyanosis with distal swelling, (5) chronic diarrhea, (6) recurrent petechiae, and (7) abnormal brain MRI, showing symmetrical lesions of the caudate and lenticular nuclei. Other manifestations later recognized in additional patients are retinal lesions and hematuria. In addition to persistent lactic acidemia, blood metabolite profiles include elevated C4 (predominantly isobutyryl-) and C5 acylcarnitine (2-methylbutyryl-) species. In urine, excretion of high concentrations of ethylmalonic acid is the most consistent finding, in association with elevated excretion of

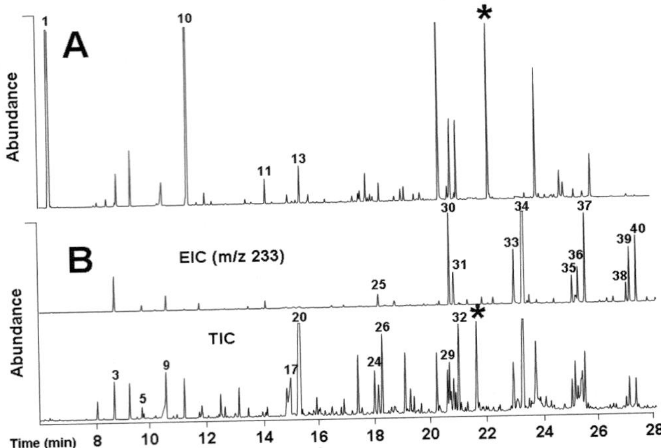

Figure 55-12 Partial urine organic acid profiles (7-28 minute portion of a 33 minute run). **A,** Ethylmalonic encephalopathy. **B,** LCHAD deficiency. The top section shows the extracted ion chromatogram (EIC) of m/z 233, the signature fragment of 3-hydroxy acid TMS-esters. Peak legend as in Figure 55-8. The symbol * marks the internal standard (pentadecanoic acid), signal abundance (total ion current, TIC) is normalized on the intensity of the internal standard peak. EIC abundance was set arbitrarily for better graphic display.

isobutyrylglycine, 2-methylbutyrylglycine, and other C4-C6 glycine esters (Figure 55-12, *A*). Ethylmalonic acid derives from either the carboxylation of butyryl-CoA, in disorders of β-oxidation of short-chain fatty acids, or from 2-ethylmalonic-semialdehyde, the final product of the R-pathway catabolism of isoleucine.[75]

Although the combination of these findings is indicative of a generalized impairment of multiple mitochondrial acyl-CoA dehydrogenase enzymes, extensive studies have failed to unveil the specific underlying defect. However, the gene locus of EE was identified in 2004,[132] but the function of the gene product, a mitochondrial protein, remains to be elucidated. It is likely that this discovery will lead to a better understanding of the natural history of the disorder, and possibly uncover evidence that its incidence could have been significantly underestimated, because the biochemical phenotype was incorrectly attributed to other metabolic disorders, particularly defects of the mitochondrial electron transfer flavoprotein pathway.

DISORDERS OF FATTY ACID OXIDATION

Long-chain fatty acids are involved in a wide variety of cellular processes, including (1) phospholipid synthesis, (2) protein posttranslational modifications, (3) cell signaling, (4) membrane permeability, and (5) transcription control.[36] Yet the most critical function is to sustain energy production during fasting or periods of higher energy demands via mitochondrial β-oxidation. Once mobilized from adipose tissue, fatty acids are taken up by liver and muscle cells via an active transport system.[10] After activation to their respective coenzyme A (CoA) esters by ATP-dependent acyl-CoA

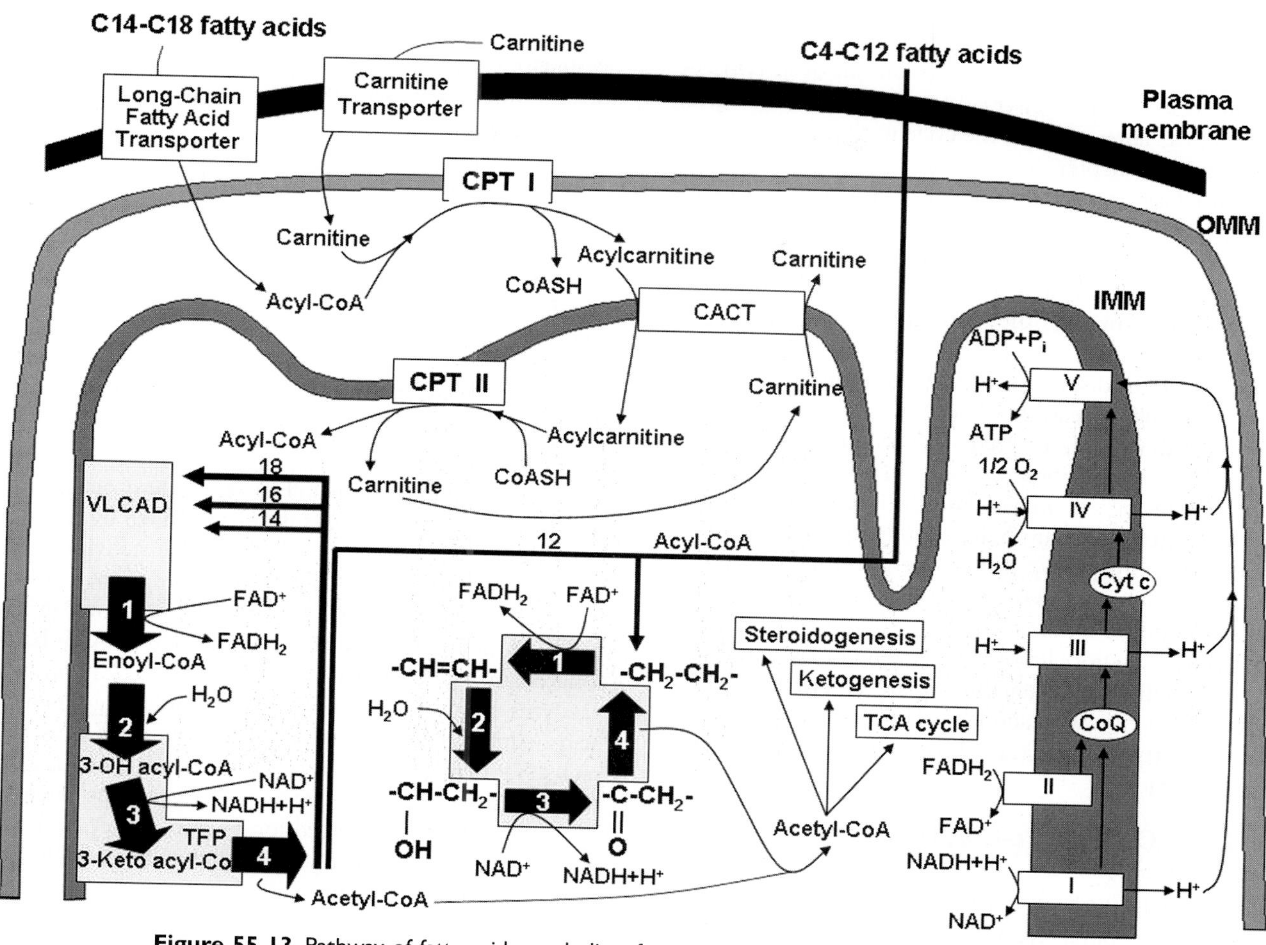

Figure 55-13 Pathway of fatty acid metabolism from the transport of long-chain fatty acids and carnitine across the plasma membrane to the production of acetyl-CoA. Medium- and short-chain fatty acids do not require an active transport mechanism to reach the mitochondrial matrix. Enzymes of the carnitine cycle (CPT I, CACT, and CPT II) shuttle long-chain fatty acids across the mitochondrial membranes. The fatty acid β-oxidation spiral includes (1) an FAD-dependent acyl-CoA dehydrogenase step followed by (2) a 2,3-enoyl-CoA hydratase reaction, (3) the NAD-dependent 3-hydroxyacyl-CoA dehydrogenase step, (4) and the thiolase cleavage reaction. Oxidation of long-chain fatty acids (membrane-bound enzymes) and medium-/short-chain fatty acids (matrix) is shown separately. Reducing equivalents ($FADH_2$ and $NADH+H^+$) are directed to the oxidative phosphorylation pathway (*right*). *CACT,* Carnitine:acylcarnitine translocase; *CPT,* carnitine palmitoyltransferase; *IMM,* inner mitochondrial membrane; *OMM,* outer mitochondrial membrane; *TCA,* tricarboxylic acid; *TFP,* trifunctional protein; *VLCAD,* very-long chain acyl-CoA dehydrogenase. *(From Rinaldo P, Matern D, Bennett MJ. Fatty acid oxidation disorders. Ann Rev Physiol 2002;64:477-502.)*

synthetases, fatty acids are transported into mitochondria by a series of three membrane-bound enzymes that temporarily convert the acyl-CoA into an acylcarnitine species before delivering a reconstituted fatty acyl-CoA into the inner mitochondrial space (Figure 55-13).[84] Medium- and short-chain fatty acids enter the mitochondria independently of the so-called carnitine cycle and are activated within the mitochondrial matrix by different acyl-CoA synthetases.

Enzymes with affinity for long-chain species of fatty acids are associated with the inner mitochondrial membrane while the enzymes responsible for the metabolism of medium- and short-chain species are located within the mitochondrial matrix. Fatty acids are oxidized to their final product, acetyl-CoA, in a cyclic fashion, which consists of four sequential reactions mediated by highly homologous enzymes.[37] These enzymes are characterized by their affinity for substrates of decreasing chain length, hence the common nomenclature using prefixes, such as very long-chain, long-chain, medium-chain, and short-chain. The catalytic activities of these enzymes are FAD-dependent acyl-CoA dehydrogenase, enoyl-CoA hydratase, NAD-dependent L-3-hydroxyacyl-CoA dehydrogenase, and ketoacyl-CoA thiolase, respectively, and in sequential order (Figure 55-13). Each cycle of the pathway produces a molecule of acetyl-CoA and a fatty acid with two fewer carbons. Under physiological conditions, the latter reenters the cycle until it is completely consumed (see Chapter 26). In the muscle, acetyl-CoA is directly used as energy substrate for the citric acid cycle, whereas in the liver it constitutes the building block for the synthesis of ketone bodies (acetoacetic acid and D-3-hydroxy butyric acid), which serve as fuels for production of energy in other tissues when the supply of glucose is depleted (see Chapter 25).

Inherited FAO disorders represent a rapidly expanding class of metabolic diseases.[111] Symptoms may appear at any age, from birth to adult life, frequently leading to life-threatening episodes of metabolic decompensation after a period of inadequate caloric intake and/or intercurrent illness. Typical manifestations are hypoketotic hypoglycemia, liver disease, cardiomyopathy, and sudden death. Table 55-4 shows a summary of known disorders of fatty acid transport and mitochondrial oxidation, including information about their incidence, major clinical features and biochemical patterns, availability of prenatal diagnosis and newborn screening, and association with sudden and unexpected death.

Selected fatty acid oxidation disorders are discussed in the following sections.

Very Long-Chain Acyl-CoA Dehydrogenase Deficiency

Very-long-chain acyl-CoA dehydrogenase (VLCAD) deficiency is an autosomal recessive condition. In the mid 1980s, patients with VLCAD deficiency were initially described as having long-chain acyl-CoA dehydrogenase (LCAD) deficiency.[47] However, without exception, once the VLCAD protein was identified,[5] affected patients were shown to have no detectable VLCAD protein by immunoblot analysis[141] or to harbor disease-causing mutations in the VLCAD gene.[123]

VLCAD catalyzes the first step of the fatty acid β-oxidation spiral. The severity of the phenotype appears to correlate with specific genotypes.[4] The most severe phenotype manifests early in life and is associated with nonsense mutations resulting in complete loss of enzyme activity. Morbidity and mortality are significant because of involvement of multiple organ systems, in particular liver and heart, resulting in recurrent metabolic crises and cardiomyopathy.[81] Patients carrying missense mutations or with single amino acid deletions permitting some residual enzyme activity are at high risk of metabolic decompensation with nonketotic hypoglycemia and a Reye's-like syndrome (see Chapter 47) triggered by increased energy demands (prolonged fasting, fever, etc.). As patients become older, the phenotype switches from a more hepatic presentation to muscle weakness. Some patients are able to sustain metabolic stress during childhood and do not present until adulthood with exercise-induced myopathy and rhabdomyolysis.

Laboratory indicators during acute episodes include hypoketotic hypoglycemia and creatine kinase elevations. Urine organic acid analysis is nonspecific with hypoketotic dicarboxylic aciduria. Acylcarnitine analysis is most informative, revealing a characteristic profile with elevated levels of saturated and unsaturated C14 to C18 carnitine esters, the predominant species being tetradecenoylcarnitine (C14:1) (Figure 55-14, *F*).[85] The diagnosis is confirmed by specific enzyme assay or fatty acid oxidation in vitro, by probing in fibroblast cultures,[116] or by molecular genetic analysis of the VLCAD gene.

Trifunctional Protein and Long-Chain 3-Hydroxy Acyl-CoA Dehydrogenase Deficiencies

The trifunctional protein (TFP) is a hetero-octamer containing four α- and four β-subunits encoded by two different genes.[21] The α-subunit harbors the activities of the second and third step of fatty acid β-oxidation, long-chain enoyl-CoA hydratase (LCEH) and long-chain 3-hydroxy acyl-CoA dehydrogenase (LCHAD). The β-subunit harbors long-chain 3-ketoacyl-CoA dehydrogenase (LCKAT), which catalyzes the last step in β-oxidation of long-chain fatty acids. Although mutations in either gene may cause complete TFP deficiency,[57,138] a few mutations in the α-subunit cause isolated LCHAD deficiency.[54] A genotype-phenotype correlation has also emerged for TFP deficiency, with residual enzyme activity being associated with a milder, later onset phenotype. Patients with late onset TFP deficiency present with a progressive peripheral neuropathy and episodic rhabdomyolysis.[124] While the phenotype of both disorders includes all the symptoms expected in an FAO disorder, patients with LCHAD/TFP deficiencies may also develop pigmentary retinitis and a peripheral neuropathy, whose pathophysiology remains obscure. In addition, many patients are born prematurely and small for gestational age.[80]

Patients with isolated LCHAD deficiency have a reduction in LCHAD activity with normal LCEH and LCKAT activities.[56] The most common cause of isolated LCHAD deficiency is the 1528G>C mutation that changes a glutamate to a glutamine residue (E474Q) in the active site of the α-subunit of the LCHAD gene.[53] The replacement of the acidic residue with a neutral amide amino acid is thought to involve the NAD^+-binding site of the enzyme and subsequently results in an isolated reduction of LCHAD activity without affecting the activities of LCEH and LCKAT.

Another feature that was thought to be specific to LCHAD deficiency was the observation that approximately 20% of patients were born following pregnancies complicated with maternal liver disease, in particular acute fatty liver of pregnancy (AFLP)[52] and the syndrome of hemolysis, elevated liver enzymes, and low platelets (HELLP).[126] However, several other FAO disorders have meanwhile been implicated as possible triggers of maternal liver disease during pregnancy.[111]

The biochemical diagnosis of TFP/LCHAD is based on the finding of hypoketotic C6-C10 dicarboxylic aciduria and

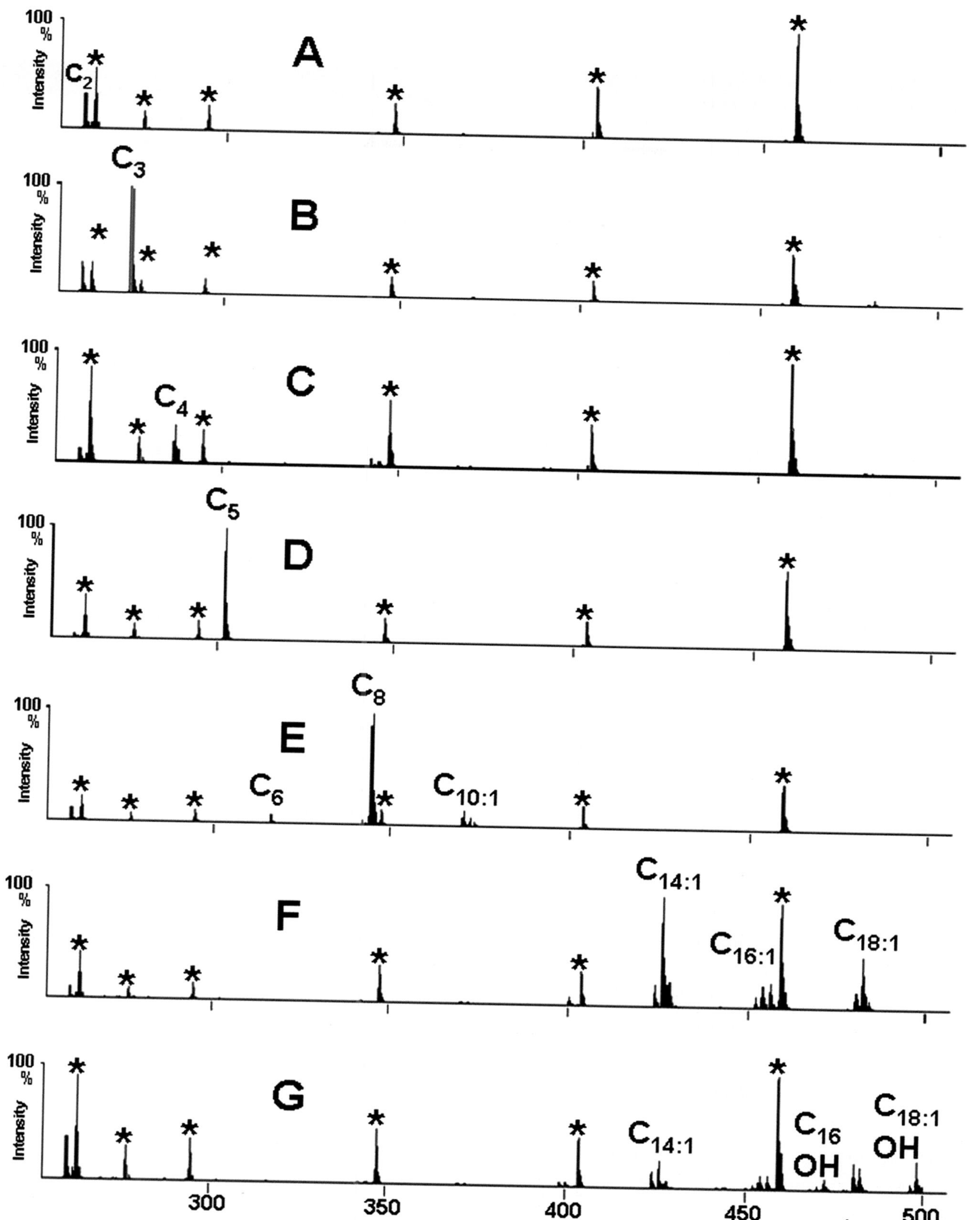

Figure 55-14 Plasma profiles of plasma acylcarnitine butyl-ester derivatives. **A,** Normal control. **B,** Propionic acidemia. **C,** Short-chain acyl-CoA dehydrogenase deficiency. **D,** Isovaleric acidemia. **E,** Medium-chain acyl-CoA dehydrogenase deficiency. **F,** Very long-chain acyl-CoA dehydrogenase deficiency. **G**, Long-chain L-3-hydroxy acyl-CoA dehydrogenase deficiency. The symbol * marks internal standards: [$^2H_3$]-acetylcarnitine (m/z 263); [$^2H_3$]-propionylcarnitine (m/z 277); [$^2H_7$]-butyrylcarnitine (m/z 295); [$^2H_3$]-octanoylcarnitine (m/z 347); [$^2H_3$]-dodecanoylcarnitine (m/z 403); [$^2H_3$]-palmitoylcarnitine (m/z 459).

TABLE 55-4 Clinical and Laboratory Characteristics of Fatty Acid Oxidation Disorders

Common Name	OMIM No.	Enzyme/Transport Defect	Incidence (USA)	Major Clinical Features	Complication of Pregnancy (Maternal, Fetal)
Long-chain fatty acid uptake defect	603376	/	<1:100,000	Liver disease	/
Carnitine uptake defect	212140	Carnitine transporter	<1:100,000	Hypoglycemia, cardiomyopathy	/
CPT-I deficiency (liver and muscle types)	255120 600528 601987	Carnitine palmitoyl transferase I	<1:100,000	Liver disease, hypotonia, renal tubular acidosis	AFLP
Translocase deficiency	212138	Carnitine acylcarnitine translocase	<1:100,000	Cardiomyopathy, liver disease	Pre-eclampsia
CPT-II deficiency	600649 600650	Carnitine palmitoyl transferase II	<1:100,000	Cardiomyopathy, liver disease, congenital anomalies. Adult onset myopathy.	/
VLCAD deficiency	201475	Very long-chain acyl-CoA dehydrogenase	>1:75,000	Spectrum from early onset cardiomyopathy, coma, liver disease to adult onset myopathy	/
LCHAD deficiency	600890	Long-chain 3-hydroxyacyl-CoA dehydrogenase	>1:75,000	Cardiomyopathy, liver disease, retinopathy, peripheral neuropathy	AFLP, HELLP syndrome, preeclampsia, placental floor infarction
TFP deficiency	600890 143450	Trifunctional protein	<1:100,000	Cardiomyopathy, liver disease, retinopathy, peripheral neuropathy	AFLP, HELLP syndrome
Glutaric acidemia type II	231680 130410 231675	Electron transfer flavoprotein (ETF), ETF ubiquinone oxidoreductase	<1:100,000	Cardiomyopathy, liver disease, congenital anomalies. Adult onset myopathy.	/
MCAD deficiency	201450	Medium-chain acyl-CoA dehydrogenase	>1:25,000	Liver disease	HELLP syndrome
M/SCHAD deficiency	601609	Medium/short-chain 3-hydroxyacyl-CoA dehydrogenase	<1:100,000	Liver disease	/
MCKAT deficiency	602199	Medium-chain 3-ketoacyl-CoA thiolase	<1:100,000	Cardiomyopathy, liver disease	/
SCAD deficiency	201470	Short-chain acyl-CoA dehydrogenase	>1:50,000	Developmental delay, hypotonia, seizures	AFLP, HELLP syndrome
SCHAD deficiency	601609	Short-chain 3-hydroxyacyl-CoA dehydrogenase	<1:100,000	Hypoglycemia, liver disease	/
Dienoyl-CoA reductase deficiency	222745	Dienoyl-CoA reductase	<1:100,000	Myopathy	/

OMIM, Online Mendelian Inheritance in Man (www.ncbi.nlm.nih.gov/entrez/query.fcgi?db=OMIM); *NBS*, newborn screening; *AFLP*, acute fatty liver of pregnancy; *HELLP syndrome*, hemolysis, elevated liver enzymes, and low platelet count.

Modality of Acute Episodes	Major Biochemical Marker(s)	Prenatal Diagnosis	NBS in the US (% Births)	Sudden Unexpected Death
Acute liver failure	Low long-chain fatty acids (Liver)	Not reported	Not available	Anecdotal reports
Fasting intolerance, hypoketotic hypoglycemia	Low free carnitine (B)	Enzyme assay in amniocytes, DNA analysis	1/51 states (2%)	Frequent
Fasting intolerance, hypoketotic hypoglycemia	High free carnitine (B)	Enzyme assay in amniocytes/CVS and molecular genetics	12/51 states (16%)	Frequent
Fasting intolerance, hypoketotic hypoglycemia	C16/C18 acylcarnitines (B)	Enzyme assay in amniocytes, DNA analysis	15/51 states (25%)	Frequent
Fasting/exercise/cold intolerance, myoglobinuria	C16/C18 acylcarnitines (B)	Enzyme assay in amniocytes, DNA analysis	8/51 states (29%)	Not reported
Hypoketotic hypoglycemia, myoglobinuria	C14:1 acylcarnitine (B)	Enzyme assay in amniocytes, DNA analysis	20/51 states (32%)	Frequent
Hypoketotic hypoglycemia, myoglobinuria	C16-OH/C18-OH acylcarnitines (B); C6-C14 3-OH dicarboxylic acids (U)	Enzyme assay in amniocytes, DNA analysis	21/51 states (31%)	Frequent
Hypoketotic hypoglycemia, myoglobinuria	C16-OH/C18-OH acylcarnitines (B); C6-C14 3-OH dicarboxylic acids (U)	Enzyme assay in amniocytes, DNA analysis	15/51 states (25%)	Frequent
Fasting intolerance, hypoketotic hypoglycemia	C4 to C18 acylcarnitines (B); C5-C10 dicarboxylics, ethylmalonic, C4-C8 acylglycines (U)	Enzyme assay in amniocytes, glutaric C4 C5 acylcarnitines (AF), DNA analysis	18/51 states (29%)	Frequent
Fasting intolerance, hypoketotic hypoglycemia	C6, C8 and C10 acylcarnitines (B); hexanoylglycine, suberylglycine, phenylpropionylglycine (U)	Enzyme assay in amniocytes, DNA analysis	29/51 states (53%)	Frequent
Fasting intolerance, hypoketotic hypoglycemia	C6-C10 3-OH fatty acids (B)	DNA analysis	1/51 states (2%)	Anecdotal reports
Fasting intolerance, hypoketotic hypoglycemia	C6-C12 dicarboxylic acids (U)	Not reported	3/51 states (5%)	Anecdotal reports
Hypoglycemia	Butyrylcarnitine (B); ethylmalonic methylsuccinic butyrylglycine (U)	Enzyme assay in amniocytes, DNA analysis	28/51 states (51%)	Anecdotal reports
Ketotic hypoglycemia	Ketosis 3-OH fatty acids (B); 3-OH dicarboxylic acids (U)	Not reported	3/51 states (4%)	Frequent
/	2-trans,4-cis-decadienoylcarnitine	Not reported	5/51 states (8%)	Not reported

C6-C14 3-hydroxydicarboxylic aciduria (Figure 55-11, *F*) with prominent unsaturated species, and elevated plasma concentrations of C16-OH and C18-OH acylcarnitine species (Figure 55-14, *G*). These metabolites could not be found in specimens collected when patients are clinically asymptomatic.

Medium-Chain Acyl-CoA Dehydrogenase Deficiency

MCAD deficiency is responsible for the initial dehydrogenation of acyl-CoAs with a chain length between 4 and 12 carbon atoms. First reported in 1982, MCAD deficiency is frequently diagnosed in previously healthy children who present with hypoketotic hypoglycemia, vomiting, and lethargy triggered by a common illness, which quickly progress to coma and death. Hepatomegaly and acute liver disease are often present. Affected individuals typically present between 3 and 24 months of age; later presentation, even into adulthood, is possible.[15,105] The prognosis is excellent once the diagnosis is established and frequent feedings are instituted to avoid any prolonged period of fasting. It is unfortunate that only half of the babies born in the United States are currently screened for this disorder.

Early diagnosis is crucial, because MCAD deficiency is a potentially lethal disease, documented by the fact that up to at least 20% of undiagnosed patients die during their first metabolic decompensation.[51] A common missense mutation (985A>G; K304E) has been identified in Caucasians of Northern European descent,[82] which results in reduced production of an unstable protein.

A defect of the MCAD enzyme leads to accumulation of medium-chain fatty acids, which are conjugated with either carnitine or glycine.[113] Analysis of plasma acylcarnitines by MS/MS reveals accumulation of C6 to C10 acylcarnitine species, with prominent concentration of octanoylcarnitine (Figure 55-14, *E*).[135] A potential pitfall of acylcarnitine analysis in the diagnosis of MCAD deficiency and other FAO disorders is the possibility that patients with secondary carnitine deficiency may not have a significant elevation of C6-C10 acylcarnitine concentrations.[30] Hexanoylglycine, phenylpropionylglycine, and suberylglycine are consistently detected in urine of asymptomatic patients and represent the most sensitive and specific markers of the disease, but are frequently overlooked by standard organic acid analysis. Proper detection of acylglycines at concentrations of excretion below 10 mmol/mol creatinine requires a different derivatization process (methylation or butylation) and quantitation using stable-isotope labeled internal standards.[113] A biochemical diagnosis of MCAD deficiency is confirmed by measurement of the activity of the MCAD enzyme in fibroblasts and other tissues and by molecular genetic testing of the *ACADM* gene; both test methods have been used for prenatal diagnosis.

Detection of C6-C10 acylcarnitines in neonatal blood spots by MS/MS is the basis for newborn screening of MCAD deficiency.[23] Identification of numerous patients by newborn screening has led also to the discovery of patients with only mild biochemical abnormalities and significant residual enzyme activity in vitro.[2,3,144] Whether patients with such genotypes will remain asymptomatic, even during times of increased energy demands, remains to be determined either by long-term follow-up or by carefully conducted fasting challenges.

Short-Chain Acyl-CoA Dehydrogenase Deficiency

First reported in 1984, 133 individuals with short-chain acyl-CoA dehydrogenase (SCAD) deficiency present with a surprising variety of clinical phenotypes, ranging from catastrophic illness in the neonatal period to adult onset of skeletal myopathy.[11] Hypotonia, developmental delay, and seizures are relatively common findings,[32] underscoring the need of a metabolic work-up in patients presenting with nondescriptive phenotypes,[19] and also the benefits that universal newborn screening could bring to patients with this and many other IEM by reducing the length and costs of the medical odyssey many of them endure.

When the first step of the β-oxidation of butyryl-CoA is impaired, alternative metabolism takes place via carboxylation to ethylmalonic acid (EMA) mediated by propionyl-CoA carboxylase and conjugation with carnitine and glycine. The most useful biochemical markers of SCAD deficiency are therefore EMA and butyrylglycine in urine, and butyrylcarnitine in plasma (Figure 55-14, *C*). However, these findings still require a complex differential diagnosis. Butyrylcarnitine is measured by MS/MS together with isobutyrylcarnitine as total C4-species, and the two could be easily confused or misinterpreted.[64,98] The corresponding glycine conjugates, however, are readily separated and measured by GC-MS.[20,142]

EMA aciduria may be associated with several other inherited and acquired conditions, including (1) glutaric acidemia type II (some cases are actually labeled to have ethylmalonic adipic aciduria),[76] (2) disorders of the intramitochondrial flavin adenine dinucleotide pathway,[41] (3) mitochondrial respiratory chain disorders,[28,67] and (4) ethylmalonic encephalopathy.[20] Jamaican vomiting sickness (due to ingestion of unripe ackee fruit containing the poison hypoglycin A)[130] and ifosfamide treatment[66] represent two additional causes of ethylmalonic aciduria.

In vitro confirmation of SCAD deficiency is also challenging and should include both biochemical and molecular genetic studies. Fibroblasts have been used to first assess fatty acid oxidation of palmitate in whole cells and/or the specific SCAD activity using butyryl-CoA as substrate, followed by SCAD gene sequencing. However, while several pathogenic mutations have been identified, molecular genetic testing for SCAD deficiency may reveal only two SCAD gene variants, 625G>A (G185S) and 511C>T (R147W),[31,46] which occur in the homozygous or compound heterozygous state in 7% of the United States population.[94] Among patients with mild to moderate EMA aciduria, these variants are over-represented[31]; some patients with biochemical evidence of SCAD deficiency do not carry any other SCAD gene mutations.[32]

In vitro studies have shown that these variants compromise SCAD activity because of abnormal protein folding and thermolability, respectively.[100] In general, the two common variants are believed to confer disease susceptibility in combination with other genetic and environmental factors.

ANALYTICAL CONSIDERATIONS

Diagnosis of the disorders discussed above requires the analysis of amino acids, organic acids, and acylcarnitines. Further details of such analytical procedures are available on this book's accompanying Evolve site, found at http://evolve.elsevier.com/Tietz/textbook/. Here, we briefly describe the assay principles.

Analysis of Amino Acids

Amino acids are quantitatively measured in plasma, urine, and CSF using a variety of techniques, which include capillary electrophoresis, gas-liquid chromatography, reversed phase high performance liquid chromatography (HPLC),[131] ion-exchange liquid chromatography,[121] and MS/MS (see Chapters 5, 6, 7, and 20).[25] Currently, ion exchange chromatography analysis of amino acids is the most widely used method to identify defects of amino acid metabolism. Screening methods, such as thin layer chromatography, that do not result in positive identification of all amino acids of clinical interest lead to errors and should be considered obsolete.

Ion Exchange Liquid Chromatography

Several amino acid analyzers are commercially available. With such analyzers, the sample is applied to a column of ion-exchange resin. Buffers of varying pH and ionic strength are pumped through the column at a constant rate. The individual amino acids are retained on the resin depending on their affinity to the resin. The eluate from the column is mixed with ninhydrin reagent, heated to 135 °C for color development, and monitored with a flow cell photometer at 440 nm (for imino acids) and at 570 (for amino acids). The sum of the absorbances at 440 and 570 is interfaced to a commercial software that stores, calculates, and prints the concentrations of the amino acids in reference to an internal standard. Peak identification is based on retention time, absolute and relative to the nearest internal standard; the 570/440 area ratio; and eventually spiking with the standard solution. Amino acids are quantified by comparing area peak ratios with those of an internal standard.

Sample Requirements

Fasting plasma (heparin) is the preferred specimen type. In newborns and infants blood should be collected immediately before the next scheduled feeding. Serum is generally derived from blood left to clot at room temperature, a process that leads to artifacts from deamination, loss of sulfur-containing amino acids due to protein binding, conversion of arginine to ornithine by red blood cell arginase, and release of oligopeptides. Hemolyzed specimens show higher concentrations of amino acids that are found in higher concentration in blood cells (taurine, aspartic acid, and glutamic acid).

Analysis of urine is indicated for the diagnosis of disorders affecting renal transport of one or more amino acids. Urine collection should avoid fecal contamination and the addition of preservatives. Although a 24-hour collection (kept refrigerated during collection) is necessary in a few clinical circumstances, it is rarely needed during the diagnostic work-up of a patient and should be avoided when a patient is acutely ill, especially when of pediatric age. Urine creatinine is used for normalization and the concentration ratio to creatinine is widely used in clinical practice. One potential problem could be encountered in the evaluation of patients with unrecognized disorders of creatine metabolism[55,117,137] in whom a low creatinine excretion leads to quantitative results suggestive of a general amino aciduria that is out of proportion with the magnitude of changes observed by visual inspection of the chromatogram. Cerebrospinal fluid (CSF) must be collected free of blood contamination.

Reference Intervals

Reference intervals for urine and plasma amino acids are listed in Table 56-2, Chapter 56.

Analysis of Organic Acids

Capillary gas chromatography-mass spectrometry is being used to separate and measure the trimethylsilyl (TMS) ethers of organic acids. A capillary GC column is used that contains an immobilized nonpolar stationary phase. Organic acids are detected by electron impact (EI) mass spectrometry performed in the scan mode m/z 50 to m/z 550 to obtain mass spectra. Identification is by comparison to a library of spectra generated by analysis of pure standard compounds integrated by published spectra, when applicable.

Sample Preparation

Organic acids (OA) are extracted from urine by liquid-liquid extraction. A volume of a random urine specimen corresponding to 0.25 mg of creatinine is used. For analysis, urine samples normalized to creatinine concentration are first mixed with the internal standard solution (100 μL). Then 2.5 mL of ethyl acetate are added and mixed vigorously before centrifugation for 1 minute. After transfer evaporation, organic acids present in the dry residue are converted to their corresponding TMS ethers by addition of 100 μL of BSTFA/1%TMCS, and allowed to react in a heating block for 30 minutes at 80 °C. After cooling at room temperature, specimens are analyzed.

Reference Intervals

Age-matched reference intervals of selected organic acids and acylglycines are listed in Table 55-5.

TABLE 55-5 Reference Intervals of Selected Organic Acids and Acylglycines in Urine (mmol/mol Creatinine)

Age Groups	0-1 Month	1-6 Months	6 Months-5 Years	>5 Years
Acetylaspartic acid*	nd-13	nd-13	nd-13	nd-13
cis-Aconitic acid	5-31	10-97	10-97	3-44
Adipic acid	9-37	9-37	nd-15	nd-5
Azelaic acid	nd-1	nd-1	nd-1	nd-1
Butyrylglycine*	0.1-2	0.1-2	0.1-2	0.1-2
trans-Cinnamoylglycine*	0.1-8	0.1-8	0.1-8	0.1-8
Citric acid	nd-1045	104-268	0-656	87-639
Dodecanedioic acid*	nd-0.05	nd-0.05	nd-0.05	nd-0.05
Ethylmalonic acid*	0.4-17	0.4-17	0.4-17	0.4-17
Fumaric acid	10-45	4-45	1-27	2-4
Glutaric acid*	0.5-13	0.5-13	0.5-13	0.5-13
Glyceric acid*	nd-39	nd-184	nd-70	0-60
Glycolic acid*	nd-62	nd-104	3-121	nd-166
Glyoxylic acid*	nd-13	0-16	nd-7	nd-9
Hexadecanedioic acid*	nd-0.4	nd-0.4	nd-0.4	nd-0.4
Hexanoylglycine*	0.1-1.2	0.1-1.2	0.1-1.2	0.1-1.2
Homogentisic acid	nd-10	nd-10	nd-10	nd-10
Homovanillic acid*	nd-22	nd-22	nd-8	nd-7
3-Hydroxy butyric acid	nd-5	nd-5	nd-5	nd-10
2-Hydroxy glutaric acid	nd-15	nd-15	nd-15	nd-15
5-Hydroxy indoleacetic acid*	nd-12	nd-12	nd-12	nd-9
4-Hydroxy phenyllactic acid	nd-50	nd-10	nd-10	nd-10
4-Hydroxy phenylpyruvic acid	nd-20	nd-5	nd-5	nd-5
Isobutyrylglycine*	nd-9	0-9	0-9	0-9
Isocitric acid	0-368	0-67	0-77	16-99
Isovalerylglycine*	0.2-10	0.2-10	0.2-10	0.2-10
2-Ketoglutaric acid	22-567	63-552	36-103	41-82
Lactic acid	46-348	57-346	21-38	20-101
Malic acid	0-52	8-73	4-57	17-47
2-Methylbutyrylglycine*	0.2-5	0.2-5	0.2-5	0.2-5
Methylmalonic acid*	nd-3.6	nd-3.6	nd-3.6	nd-3.6
Methylsuccinic acid*	0-12	0-12	0-12	0-12
Octanoylglycine*	0.1-1.2	0.1-1.2	0.1-1.2	0.1-1.2
Orotic acid	1.4-5.3	1.0-3.2	0.5-3.3	0.4-1.2
Oxalic acid*	51-931	7-567	7-352	nd-187
3-Phenylpropionylglycine*	nd-0.6	nd-0.6	nd-0.6	nd-0.6
Pimelic acid	nd-1	nd-1	nd-1	nd-1
Pyroglutamic acid	nd-61	nd-61	nd-61	nd-61
Pyruvic acid	24-123	8-90	3-19	6-9
Sebacic acid	3-16	3-16	nd-8	nd-8
Suberic acid	4-20	4-20	nd-8	nd-8
Suberylglycine*	nd-5.4	nd-5.4	nd-5.4	nd-5.4
Succinic acid	35-547	34-156	16-118	29-87
Tetradecanedioic acid*	nd-0.40	nd-0.40	nd-0.40	nd-0.40
Uracil*	nd-32	nd-32	nd-21	nd-17
Uric acid*	359-2644	359-2644	185-1134	199-1034
Vanilylmandelic acid*	nd-15	nd-10	nd-7	nd-5

nd, Not detected.
*Measured using a stable isotope-labeled internal standard.
TIC detection limit: 0.1 mmol/mol creatinine.
SIM detection limit (with stable isotope labeled internal standard): 0.01 mmol/mol creatinine.

TABLE 55-6 Acylcarnitine Reference Intervals in Plasma

		0-7 Days (N = 143)		8 Days-7 Years (N = 2677)		>7 Years (N = 834)	
		Median	5-95%ile	Median	5-95%ile	Median	5-95%ile
		(μmol/L)					
Acetylcarnitine	C2	8.37	2.82-19.67	10.45	4.70-33.66	8.45	3.29-25.72
Acrylylcarnitine	C3:1	0.01	0.00-0.03	0.01	0.00-0.03	0.01	0.00-0.03
Propionylcarnitine	C3	0.34	0.07-1.85	0.49	0.17-1.27	0.45	0.17-1.49
Iso-/Butyrylcarnitine	C4	0.27	0.13-0.70	0.31	0.16-0.74	0.30	0.15-1.05
Tiglylcarnitine	C5:1	0.01	0.00-0.06	0.01	0.00-0.05	0.02	0.00-0.10
Isovaleryl/2-CH_3 butyrylcarnitine	C5	0.15	0.04-0.42	0.15	0.05-0.44	0.14	0.06-0.51
3-OH butyrylcarnitine	C4-OH	0.04	0.01-0.15	0.04	0.01-0.29	0.03	0.01-0.19
Hexanoylcarnitine	C6	0.05	0.01-0.49	0.06	0.02-0.20	0.05	0.02-0.21
3-OH isovalerylcarnitine	C5-OH	0.03	0.01-0.15	0.02	0.01-0.07	0.02	0.01-0.19
Heptanoylcarnitine	C7	0.01	0.00-0.05	0.01	0.00-0.04	0.01	0.00-0.06
3-OH hexanoylcarnitine	C6-OH	0.02	0.00-0.07	0.02	0.01-0.06	0.02	0.00-0.07
Octenoylcarnitine	C8:1	0.18	0.03-0.45	0.19	0.06-0.53	0.19	0.06-0.72
Octanoylcarnitine	C8	0.16	0.08-1.40	0.15	0.08-0.41	0.16	0.08-0.45
Malonylcarnitine	C3-DC	0.03	0.01-0.08	0.03	0.01-0.09	0.04	0.01-0.17
Decadienoylcarnitine	C10:2	0.03	0.01-0.07	0.02	0.01-0.07	0.02	0.01-0.11
Decenoylcarnitine	C10:1	0.09	0.03-0.41	0.12	0.04-0.37	0.14	0.03-0.46
Decanoylcarnitine	C10	0.10	0.02-0.51	0.13	0.04-0.44	0.14	0.03-0.58
Methylmalonylcarnitine	C4-DC	0.01	0.00-0.03	0.01	0.00-0.03	0.01	0.00-0.06
3-OH decenoylcarnitine	C10:1-OH	0.03	0.01-0.11	0.02	0.01-0.05	0.03	0.01-0.11
Glutarylcarnitine (3-OH C10)	C5-DC	0.02	0.00-0.11	0.02	0.00-0.06	0.02	0.00-0.12
Dodecenoylcarnitine	C12:1	0.04	0.01-0.29	0.05	0.01-0.19	0.06	0.01-0.21
Dodecanoylcarnitine	C12	0.07	0.02-0.33	0.07	0.03-0.18	0.06	0.02-0.18
3-OH dodecenoylcarnitine	C12:1-OH	0.02	0.00-0.07	0.01	0.00-0.05	0.02	0.00-0.08
3-OH dodecanoylcarnitine	C12-OH	0.02	0.00-0.08	0.01	0.00-0.03	0.01	0.00-0.04
Tetradecadienoylcarnitine	C14:2	0.03	0.01-0.12	0.03	0.01-0.12	0.03	0.01-0.12
Tetradecenoylcarnitine	C14:1	0.05	0.01-0.39	0.05	0.01-0.23	0.05	0.01-0.24
Tetradecanoylcarnitine	C14	0.04	0.01-0.23	0.03	0.01-0.10	0.02	0.01-0.12
3-OH tetradecenoylcarnitine	C14:1-OH	0.02	0.01-0.08	0.02	0.01-0.05	0.02	0.01-0.07
3-OH tetradecanoylcarnitine	C14-OH	0.01	0.00-0.06	0.01	0.00-0.03	0.01	0.00-0.04
Hexadecenoylcarnitine	C16:1	0.04	0.01-0.24	0.03	0.01-0.10	0.03	0.01-0.09
Hexadecanoylcarnitine	C16	0.17	0.05-0.67	0.10	0.04-0.23	0.09	0.04-0.21
3-OH hexadecenoylcarnitine	C16:1-OH	0.01	0.00-0.30	0.01	0.00-0.05	0.01	0.00-0.04
3-OH hexadecanoylcarnitine	C16-OH	0.01	0.00-0.08	0.01	0.00-0.03	0.01	0.00-0.03
Octadecadienoylcarnitine	C18:2	0.04	0.01-0.12	0.05	0.02-0.16	0.06	0.02-0.15
Octadecenoylcarnitine	C18:1	0.12	0.03-0.38	0.13	0.05-0.35	0.14	0.04-0.33
Octadecanoylcarnitine	C18	0.04	0.01-0.20	0.05	0.02-0.11	0.05	0.02-0.10
3-OH octadecadienoylcarnitine	C18:2-OH	0.01	0.00-0.04	0.01	0.00-0.02	0.01	0.00-0.02
3-OH octadecenoylcarnitine	C18:1-OH	0.01	0.00-0.04	0.01	0.00-0.03	0.01	0.00-0.03
3-OH octadecanoylcarnitine	C18-OH	0.01	0.00-0.03	0.01	0.00-0.02	0.01	0.00-0.02

TABLE 55-7 Acylcarnitine Reference Intervals in Urine

		0-7 Days (N = 20)		8 Days-7 Years (N = 20)		>7 Years (N = 20)	
		Mean	Range	Mean	Range	Mean	Range
		(mmol/mol Creatinine)					
Acetylcarnitine	C2	1.13	0.19-2.92	4.30	0.07-16.46	0.35	0.04-1.26
Acrylylcarnitine	C3:1	0.02	0.00-0.06	0.01	0.00-0.04	0.00	0.00-0.00
Propionylcarnitine	C3	0.06	0.01-0.20	0.23	0.01-1.20	0.02	0.00-0.06
Iso-/Butyrylcarnitine	C4	0.14	0.02-0.36	0.79	0.02-2.74	0.10	0.01-0.29
Tiglylcarnitine	C5:1	0.05	0.01-0.14	0.10	0.00-0.34	0.01	0.00-0.03
Isovaleryl/2-CH_3 butyrylcarnitine	C5	0.09	0.00-0.25	0.39	0.00-1.53	0.03	0.00-0.07
3-OH butyrylcarnitine	C4-OH	0.03	0.01-0.06	0.09	0.00-0.26	0.01	0.00-0.03
Hexanoylcarnitine	C6	0.03	0.01-0.06	0.05	0.00-0.16	0.01	0.00-0.04
3-OH isovalerylcarnitine	C5-OH	0.09	0.00-0.19	0.17	0.01-0.52	0.02	0.01-0.05
Benzoylcarnitine	BZC	0.02	0.00-0.05	0.11	0.01-0.37	0.01	0.00-0.04
Heptanoylcarnitine	C7	0.02	0.00-0.06	0.04	0.00-0.15	0.00	0.00-0.01
3-OH hexanoylcarnitine	C6-OH	0.02	0.01-0.06	0.08	0.00-0.32	0.00	0.00-0.01
Octenoylcarnitine	C8:1	0.12	0.01-0.36	0.84	0.02-4.30	0.09	0.01-0.23
Octanoylcarnitine	C8	0.26	0.02-0.82	0.14	0.01-0.61	0.02	0.00-0.05
Malonylcarnitine	C3-DC	0.10	0.02-0.22	0.13	0.01-0.50	0.02	0.00-0.04
Decadienoylcarnitine	C10:2	0.04	0.00-0.09	0.17	0.01-0.48	0.03	0.01-0.08
Decenoylcarnitine	C10:1	0.05	0.01-0.13	0.24	0.01-0.65	0.03	0.01-0.07
Decanoylcarnitine	C10	0.03	0.01-0.08	0.04	0.00-0.21	0.01	0.00-0.02
Methylmalonylcarnitine	C4-DC	0.14	0.03-0.25	0.15	0.02-0.57	0.02	0.01-0.05
3-OH decenoylcarnitine	C10:1-OH	0.12	0.01-0.25	0.08	0.01-0.26	0.01	0.00-0.03
Glutarylcarnitine (3-OH C10)	C5-DC	0.14	0.03-0.31	0.13	0.01-0.37	0.03	0.01-0.06
Dodecenoylcarnitine	C12:1	0.01	0.00-0.03	0.03	0.00-0.07	0.00	0.00-0.01
Dodecanoylcarnitine	C12	0.05	0.01-0.10	0.05	0.00-0.19	0.01	0.00-0.02
Adipoylcarnitine	C6-DC	0.17	0.04-0.40	0.19	0.01-0.81	0.03	0.00-0.13
3-OH dodecenoylcarnitine	C12:1-OH	0.07	0.01-0.25	0.07	0.00-0.27	0.01	0.00-0.03
3-OH dodecanoylcarnitine	C12-OH	0.05	0.01-0.12	0.05	0.00-0.16	0.01	0.00-0.01
Tetradecadienoylcarnitine	C14:2	0.12	0.01-0.55	0.01	0.00-0.02	0.00	0.00-0.00
Tetradecenoylcarnitine	C14:1	0.05	0.00-0.24	0.05	0.00-0.21	0.01	0.00-0.01
Tetradecanoylcarnitine	C14	0.05	0.01-0.11	0.09	0.00-0.39	0.01	0.00-0.02
3-OH tetradecenoylcarnitine	C14:1-OH	0.04	0.01-0.10	0.04	0.00-0.14	0.01	0.00-0.01
3-OH tetradecanoylcarnitine	C14-OH	0.03	0.01-0.07	0.03	0.00-0.09	0.00	0.00-0.02
Hexadecenoylcarnitine	C16:1	0.01	0.00-0.03	0.01	0.00-0.04	0.00	0.00-0.00
Hexadecanoylcarnitine	C16	0.05	0.01-0.13	0.05	0.00-0.18	0.01	0.00-0.02
3-OH hexadecenoylcarnitine	C16:1-OH	0.32	0.00-2.06	0.01	0.00-0.02	0.00	0.00-0.00
3-OH hexadecanoylcarnitine	C16-OH	0.05	0.00-0.24	0.01	0.00-0.05	0.00	0.00-0.00
Octadecadienoylcarnitine	C18:2	0.08	0.00-0.37	0.01	0.00-0.02	0.00	0.00-0.00
Octadecenoylcarnitine	C18:1	0.01	0.00-0.03	0.01	0.00-0.02	0.00	0.00-0.00
Octadecanoylcarnitine	C18	0.01	0.00-0.02	0.01	0.00-0.05	0.00	0.00-0.00
3-OH octadecadienoylcarnitine	C18:2-OH	0.01	0.00-0.02	0.00	0.00-0.01	0.00	0.00-0.00
3-OH octadecenoylcarnitine	C18:1-OH	0.01	0.00-0.03	0.01	0.00-0.03	0.00	0.00-0.00
3-OH octadecanoylcarnitine	C18-OH	0.01	0.00-0.03	0.01	0.00-0.02	0.00	0.00-0.00

TABLE 55-8 Acylcarnitine Reference Intervals in Postmortem Blood and Bile Dried Spots

		BLOOD (N = 448)		BILE (N = 525)	
		Median	5-95%ile	Median	5-95%ile
		(μmol/L)			
Acetylcarnitine	C2	73.87	23.55-181.22	87.34	20.44-245.72
Acrylylcarnitine	C3:1	0.03	0.01-0.12	0.07	0.02-0.30
Propionylcarnitine	C3	2.95	0.55-8.01	2.07	0.36-8.10
Iso-/Butyrylcarnitine	C4	4.24	0.79-14.49	1.81	0.50-5.75
Tiglylcarnitine	C5:1	0.07	0.02-0.21	0.13	0.03-0.53
Isovaleryl/2-CH_3 butyrylcarnitine	C5	0.65	0.18-1.73	0.85	0.19-2.90
3-OH butyrylcarnitine	C4-OH	1.97	0.35-6.25	0.65	0.12-2.26
Hexanoylcarnitine	C6	0.61	0.12-1.58	0.56	0.12-3.31
3-OH isovalerylcarnitine	C5-OH	0.28	0.10-0.74	0.22	0.06-0.67
Heptanoylcarnitine	C7	0.05	0.01-0.14	0.12	0.03-0.75
3-OH hexanoylcarnitine	C6-OH	0.14	0.03-0.45	0.16	0.03-0.59
Octenoylcarnitine	C8:1	0.16	0.03-0.48	2.56	0.18-36.01
Octanoylcarnitine	C8	0.35	0.19-1.02	0.63	0.19-6.46
Malonylcarnitine	C3-DC	0.12	0.03-0.32	0.22	0.04-0.96
Decadienoylcarnitine	C10:2	0.03	0.01-0.08	0.26	0.03-3.93
Decenoylcarnitine	C10:1	0.05	0.01-0.15	0.58	0.06-11.80
Decanoylcarnitine	C10	0.09	0.02-0.37	0.35	0.05-6.47
Methylmalonylcarnitine	C4-DC	0.29	0.09-0.81	0.30	0.06-0.92
3-OH decenoylcarnitine	C10:1-OH	0.05	0.02-0.14	0.18	0.04-1.97
Glutarylcarnitine (3-OH C10)	C5-DC	0.07	0.02-0.21	0.18	0.04-1.53
Dodecenoylcarnitine	C12:1	0.03	0.01-0.13	0.30	0.03-13.50
Dodecanoylcarnitine	C12	0.17	0.07-0.61	0.49	0.08-7.40
3-OH dodecenoylcarnitine	C12:1-OH	0.04	0.01-0.11	0.24	0.04-4.86
3-OH dodecanoylcarnitine	C12-OH	0.04	0.01-0.18	0.28	0.03-2.28
Tetradecadienoylcarnitine	C14:2	0.06	0.01-0.26	0.36	0.04-9.49
Tetradecenoylcarnitine	C14:1	0.07	0.02-0.30	0.30	0.03-12.49
Tetradecanoylcarnitine	C14	0.14	0.04-0.47	0.25	0.04-3.81
3-OH tetradecenoylcarnitine	C14:1-OH	0.04	0.01-0.10	0.15	0.03-2.60
3-OH tetradecanoylcarnitine	C14-OH	0.03	0.01-0.08	0.11	0.02-1.15
Hexadecenoylcarnitine	C16:1	0.07	0.02-0.28	0.15	0.03-2.73
Hexadecanoylcarnitine	C16	0.53	0.10-1.74	0.42	0.09-3.39
3-OH hexadecenoylcarnitine	C16:1-OH	0.06	0.02-0.24	0.24	0.04-1.45
3-OH hexadecanoylcarnitine	C16-OH	0.04	0.01-0.12	0.27	0.03-1.48
Octadecadienoylcarnitine	C18:2	0.18	0.03-0.55	0.22	0.03-2.93
Octadecenoylcarnitine	C18:1	0.53	0.11-1.69	0.38	0.07-3.75
Octadecanoylcarnitine	C18	0.43	0.12-1.34	0.36	0.06-2.13
3-OH octadecadienoylcarnitine	C18:2-OH	0.03	0.01-0.08	0.09	0.01-0.55
3-OH octadecenoylcarnitine	C18:1-OH	0.04	0.01-0.11	0.10	0.02-1.01
3-OH octadecanoylcarnitine	C18-OH	0.03	0.01-0.10	0.07	0.00-0.66

ANALYSIS OF ACYLCARNITINES

Acylcarnitines are quantified by MS/MS, with their profiles playing a critical role in every clinical application of biochemical genetics: prenatal diagnosis, newborn screening, evaluation of symptomatic patients, and postmortem screening. As with other complex metabolic profiles, it is critical to complement analytical proficiency with in-depth interpretation of results and informative reporting.

Electrospray Tandem Mass Spectrometry

With electrospray ionization tandem mass spectrometry (ESI-MS/MS), the liquid sample is introduced into the ion source through a capillary tube and exposed to a strong electric field and a counter flow of nitrogen gas, which in combination produce the electrospray (see Chapter 7). The solvent evaporates and eventually desorption of charged ions occurs into the mass analyzer. ESI occurs under atmospheric pressure, allowing efficient ionization, whereas the mass analyzers operate at very low pressure. The combination is possible by introducing the ions into the analyzers through a very small orifice (<1 mm) and using powerful vacuum pumps.

A data file is generated for all ions with precursors of m/z 85 within a mass range of m/z 250 to m/z 500. Profiling of acylcarnitines as $[M+H]^+$ molecular ions allows identification, automated calculation of quantitative and semiquantitative concentrations for each acylcarnitine species against the internal standards, and comparison with age-appropriate reference intervals.

Sample Requirements

Carnitine and its esters are physiologically present in all biological fluids. For diagnostic purposes, acylcarnitines were first measured in urine[87] until plasma/serum became the preferred specimen types in diagnostic settings[86,135] and blood dried on filter paper for newborn screening.[23] However, urinalysis could be valuable in the investigation of patients with inconclusive/borderline urine organic acid and plasma acylcarnitine profiles, and useful in the selection of further in vitro investigations. Bile is analyzed postmortem in the evaluation of cases of sudden and unexpected death.[104] Cell-free supernatant of amniotic fluid is used for the prenatal diagnosis of selected IEM.[114,134] All sample types, with the exception of blood and bile spots dried on filter paper, which can be sent at room temperature, should be kept frozen until analysis. Long-term storage at room temperature causes progressive losses; degradation of short-chain acylcarnitines happens faster than long-chain species.

Reference Intervals

Acylcarnitine reference intervals are listed for plasma in Table 55-6, for urine in Table 55-7, and for postmortem blood and bile in Table 55-8. The last two are calculated as the 5 to 95 percentile range of all postmortem cases previously investigated in our laboratory.

REFERENCES

1. Abdenur JE, Chamoles NA, Guinle AE, Schenone AB, Fuertes AN. Diagnosis of isovaleric acidaemia by tandem mass spectrometry: false positive result due to pivaloylcarnitine in a newborn screening programme. J Inherit Metab Dis 1998;21:624-30.
2. Albers S, Levy HL, Irons M, Strauss AW, Marsden D. Compound heterozygosity in four asymptomatic siblings with medium-chain acyl-CoA dehydrogenase deficiency. J Inherit Metab Dis 2001;24:417-8.
3. Andresen BS, Dobrowolski SF, O'Reilly L, Muenzer J, McCandless SE, Frazier DM, et al. Medium-chain Acyl-CoA dehydrogenase (MCAD) mutations identified by MS/MS-based prospective screening of newborns differ from those observed in patients with clinical symptoms: identification and characterization of a new, prevalent mutation that results in mild MCAD deficiency. Am J Hum Genet 2001;68:1408-18.
4. Andresen BS, Olpin S, Poorthuis BJ, Scholte HR, Vianey-Saban C, Wanders R, et al. Clear correlation of genotype with disease phenotype in very-long-chain acyl-CoA dehydrogenase deficiency. Am J Hum Genet 1999;64:479-94.
5. Aoyama T, Ueno I, Kamijo T, Hashimoto T. Rat very-long-chain acyl-CoA dehydrogenase, a novel mitochondrial acyl-CoA dehydrogenase gene product, is a rate-limiting enzyme in long-chain fatty acid beta-oxidation system. cDNA and deduced amino acid sequence and distinct specificities of the cDNA-expressed protein. J Biol Chem 1994;269:19088-94.
6. Azen C, Koch R, Friedman E, Wenz E, Fishler K. Summary of findings from the United States Collaborative Study of children treated for phenylketonuria. Eur J Pediatr 1996;155:S29-32.
7. Bachmann C, Colombo JP. Acid-base status and plasma glutamine in patients with hereditary urea cycle disorders. In: Soeters PB, Wilson JHP, Meijer AJ, eds. Advances in ammonia metabolism and hepatic encephalopathy, 1st ed. Amsterdam: Elsevier, 1988:72-8.
8. Bennett MJ, Gibson KM, Sherwood WG, Divry P, Rolland MO, Elpeleg ON, et al. Reliable prenatal diagnosis of Canavan disease (aspartoacylase deficiency): comparison of enzymatic and metabolite analysis. J Inherit Metab Dis 1993;16:831-6.
9. Bennett MJ, Rinaldo P. The metabolic autopsy comes of age. Clin Chem 2001;47:1145-6.
10. Berk PD, Stump DD. Mechanisms of cellular uptake of long chain free fatty acids. Mol Cell Biochem 1999;192:17-31.
11. Bhala A, Willi SM, Rinaldo P, Bennett MJ, Schmidt-Sommerfeld E, Hale DE. The emerging clinical and biochemical picture of short-chain acyl-CoA dehydrogenase deficiency. J Pediatr 1995;126:910-5.
12. Blau N, Blaskovics ME, Duran M. Simple tests in urine and blood. In: Blau N, Blaskovics ME, Duran M, Gibson KM, eds. Physician's guide to the laboratory diagnosis of metabolic diseases, 2nd ed. Berlin: Springer, 2003:3-10.
13. Blau N, Duran M, Blaskovics ME, Gibson KM. Physician's guide to the laboratory diagnosis of metabolic disease, 2nd ed. Berlin: Springer, 2003.
14. Blau N, Thöny B, Cotton RGH, Hyland K. Disorders of tetrahydrobiopterin and related biogenic amines. In: Scriver CR, Beaudet AL, Valle D, Sly WS, Childs B, Kinzler KW, et al, eds. The metabolic & molecular bases of inherited disease, 8th ed. New York: McGraw-Hill, 2001:1725-76.
15. Boles RG, Boesel C, Rinaldo P. Sudden death beyond SIDS. Pediatr Pathol Lab Med 1996;16:691-3.
16. Boles RG, Buck EA, Blitzer MG, Platt MS, Cowan TM, Martin SK, et al. Retrospective biochemical

screening of fatty acid oxidation disorders in postmortem livers of 418 cases of sudden death in the first year of life. J Pediatr 1998;132:924-33.
17. Bove KE. The metabolic crisis: a diagnostic challenge. J Pediatr 1997;131:181-2.
18. Brusilow SW, Horwich AL. Urea cycle enzymes. In: Scriver CR, Beaudet AL, Valle D, Sly WS, Childs B, Kinzler KW, et al, eds. The metabolic & molecular bases of inherited disease, 8th ed. New York: McGraw-Hill, 2001:1909-63.
19. Buist NRM, Dulac O, Bottiglieri T, Gärtner J, Rinaldo P, Wolf NI. Metabolic evaluation of infantile epilepsy: summary recommendations of the Amalfi group. J Child Neurol 2002;17 (Suppl. 3):3S98-3S102.
20. Burlina AB, Dionisi-Vici C, Bennett MJ, Gibson KM, Servidei S, Bertini E, et al. A new syndrome with ethylmalonic aciduria and normal fatty acid oxidation in fibroblasts. J Pediatr 1994;124:79-86.
21. Carpenter K, Pollitt RJ, Middleton B. Human liver long-chain 3-hydroxyacyl-coenzyme A dehydrogenase is a multifunctional membrane-bound beta-oxidation enzyme of mitochondria. Biochem Biophys Res Commun 1992;183:443-8.
22. Chace DH, DiPerna JC, Mitchell BL, Sgroi B, Hofman LF, Naylor EW. Electrospray tandem mass spectrometry for analysis of acylcarnitines in dried postmortem blood specimens collected at autopsy from infants with unexplained cause of death. Clin Chem 2001;47:1166-82.
23. Chace DH, Hillman SL, Vanhove JLK, Naylor EW. Rapid diagnosis of MCAD deficiency—quantitative analysis of octanoylcarnitine and other acylcarnitines in newborn blood spots by tandem mass spectrometry. Clin Chem 1997;43:2106-13.
24. Chace DH, Kalas TA, Naylor EW. Use of tandem mass spectrometry for multianalyte screening of dried blood specimens from newborns. Clin Chem 2003;49:1797-817.
25. Chace DH, Millington DS, Terada N, Kahler SG, Roe CR, Hofman LF. Rapid diagnosis of phenylketonuria by quantitative analysis for phenylalanine and tyrosine in neonatal blood spots by tandem mass spectrometry. Clin Chem 1993;39:66-71.
26. Chalmers RA, Lawson AM. Organic acids in man—analytical chemistry, biochemistry, and diagnosis of the organic acidurias. London: Chapman and Hall, 1982.
27. Charrow J, Goodman SI, McCabe ERG, Rinaldo P. Tandem mass spectrometry in newborn screening. Genet in Med 2000;2:267-9.
28. Christensen E, Brandt NJ, Schmalbruch H, Kamieniecka Z, Hertz B, Ruitenbeek W. Muscle cytochrome c oxidase deficiency accompanied by a urinary organic acid pattern mimicking multiple acyl-CoA dehydrogenase deficiency. J Inherit Metab Dis 1993;16:553-6.
29. Chuang DT, Shih VE. Branched chain organic acidurias. In: Scriver CR, Beaudet AL, Valle D, Sly WS, Childs B, Kinzler KW, et al, eds. The metabolic & molecular bases of inherited disease, 8th ed. New York: McGraw-Hill, 2001:1971-2005.
30. Clayton PT, Doig M, Ghafari S, Meaney C, Taylor C, Leonard JV, et al. Screening for medium chain acyl-CoA dehydrogenase deficiency using electrospray ionisation tandem mass spectrometry. Arch Dis Child 1998;79:109-15.
31. Corydon MJ, Gregersen N, Lehnert W, Ribes A, Rinaldo P, Kmoch S, et al. Ethylmalonic aciduria is associated with an amino acid variant of short chain acyl-coenzyme A dehydrogenase. Pediatr Res 1996;39:1059-66.
32. Corydon MJ, Vockley J, Rinaldo P, Rhead WJ, Kjeldsen M, Winter V, et al. Role of common gene variations in the molecular pathogenesis of short-chain acyl-CoA dehydrogenase deficiency. Pediatr Res 2001;49:18-23.
33. Cunningham G. The science and politics of screening newborns. N Engl J Med 2002;346:1084-5.
34. de Almeida IT, Duran M, Silva MF, Portela R, Cabral A, Tasso T, et al. Mild form of methylmalonic aciduria misdiagnosed as propionic acidaemia during a ketotic crisis. J Inherit Metab Dis 1991;14:259-62.
35. Duran M, Ketting D, Wadman SK, Trijbels JM, Bakkeren JA, Waelkens JJ. Propionic acid, an artefact which can leave methylmalonic acidemia undiscovered. Clin Chim Acta 1973;49:177-9.
36. Dutta-Roy AK. Cellular uptake of long-chain fatty acids: role of membrane-associated fatty-acid-binding/transport proteins. Cell Mol Life Sci 2000;57:1360-72.
37. Eaton S, Bartlett K, Pourfarzam M. Mammalian mitochondrial beta-oxidation. Biochem J 1996;320:345-57.
38. Fenton WA, Gravel RA, Rosenblatt DS. Disorders of propionate and methylmalonate metabolism. In: Scriver CR, Beaudet AL, Valle D, Sly WS, Childs B, Kinzler KW, et al, eds. The metabolic & molecular bases of inherited disease, 8th ed. New York: McGraw-Hill, 2001:2165-93.
39. Finsterer J, Jarius C, Eichberger H, Jaksch M. Phenotype variability in 130 adult patients with respiratory chain disorders. J Inherit Metab Dis 2001;24:560-76.
40. Fowler B, Jakobs C. Post- and prenatal diagnostic methods for the homocystinurias. Eur J Pediatr 1998;157:S88-93.
41. Frerman FE, Goodman SI. Defects of the electron transfer flavoprotein and electron transfer flavoprotein-ubiquinone oxidoreductase: glutaric acidemia type II. In: Scriver CR, Beaudet AL, Valle D, Sly WS, Childs B, Kinzler KW, et al, eds. The metabolic & molecular bases of inherited disease, 8th ed. New York: McGraw-Hill, 2001:2357-65.

42. Garcia-Silva MT, Ribes A, Campos Y, Garavaglia B, Arenas J. Syndrome of encephalopathy, petechiae, and ethylmalonic aciduria. Pediatr Neurol 1997;17: 165-70.
43. Goodman SI, Markey SP. Diagnosis of organic acidemias by gas chromatography-mass spectrometry. New York: Alan R. Liss, 1981.
44. Gray RGF, Ryan D, Green A. The cryopreservation of skin biopsies—a technique for reducing workload in a cell culture laboratory. Ann Clin Biochem 1995;32:190-2.
45. Gregersen N, Kolvraa S, Mortensen PB. Acyl-CoA: glycine N-acyltransferase: in vitro studies on the glycine conjugation of straight- and branched-chained acyl-CoA esters in human liver. Biochem Med Metab Biol 1986;35:210-8.
46. Gregersen N, Winter VS, Corydon MJ, Corydon TJ, Rinaldo P, Ribes A, et al. Identification of four new mutations in the short-chain acyl-CoA dehydrogenase (SCAD) gene in two patients: one of the variant alleles, 511C->T, is present at an unexpectedly high frequency in the general population, as was the case for 625G->A, together conferring susceptibility to ethylmalonic aciduria. Hum Mol Genet 1998;7: 619-27.
47. Hale DE, Stanley CA, Coates PM. The long-chain acyl-CoA dehydrogenase deficiency. Prog Clin Biol Res 1990;321:303-11.
48. Hoffman GF, Feyh P. Organic acid analysis. In: Blau N, Blaskovics ME, Duran M, Gibson KM, eds. Physician's guide to the laboratory diagnosis of metabolic diseases, 2nd ed. Berlin: Springer, 2003:27-44.
49. Hoffman M. Scientific sleuths solve a murder mystery. Science 1991;254:931.
50. Holtzman NA. Expanding newborn screening. How good is the evidence? JAMA 2003;290:2606-8.
51. Iafolla AK, Thompson RJ Jr., Roe CR. Medium-chain acyl-coenzyme A dehydrogenase deficiency: clinical course in 120 affected children. J Pediatr 1994;124:409-15.
52. Ibdah JA, Bennett MJ, Rinaldo P, Zhao Y, Gibson B, Sims HF, et al. A fetal fatty-acid oxidation disorder as a cause of liver disease in pregnant women. N Engl J Med 1999;340:1723-31.
53. Ijlst L, Ruiter JP, Hoovers JM, Jakobs ME, Wanders RJ. Common missense mutation G1528C in long-chain 3-hydroxyacyl-CoA dehydrogenase deficiency. Characterization and expression of the mutant protein, mutation analysis on genomic DNA and chromosomal localization of the mitochondrial trifunctional protein alpha subunit gene. J Clin Invest 1996;98:1028-33.
54. Ijlst L, Wanders RJ, Ushikubo S, Kamijo T, Hashimoto T. Molecular basis of long-chain 3-hydroxyacyl-CoA dehydrogenase deficiency: identification of the major disease-causing mutation in the alpha-subunit of the mitochondrial trifunctional protein. Biochim Biophys Acta 1994;1215:347-50.
55. Item CB, Stockler-Ipsiroglu S, Stromberger C, Muhl A, Alessandri MG, Bianchi MC, et al. Arginine:glycine amidinotransferase deficiency: the third inborn error of creatine metabolism in humans. Am J Hum Genet 2001;69:1127-33.
56. Jackson S, Bartlett K, Land J, Moxon ER, Pollitt RJ, Leonard JV, et al. Long-chain 3-hydroxyacyl-CoA dehydrogenase deficiency. Pediatr Res 1991;29:406-11.
57. Jackson S, Kler RS, Bartlett K, Briggs H, Bindoff LA, Pourfarzam M, et al. Combined enzyme defect of mitochondrial fatty acid oxidation. J Clin Invest 1992;90:1219-25.
58. Jakobs C, Dorland L, Wikkerink B, Kok RM, de Jong AP, Wadman SK. Stable isotope dilution analysis of succinylacetone using electron capture negative ion mass fragmentography: an accurate approach to the pre- and neonatal diagnosis of hereditary tyrosinemia type I. Clin Chim Acta 1988;171:223-31.
59. Jouvet P, Poggi F, Rabier D, Michel JL, Hubert P, Sposito M, et al. Continuous venovenous haemodiafiltration in the acute phase of neonatal maple syrup urine disease. J Inherit Metab Dis 1997;20: 463-72.
60. Kahler SG, Sherwood WG, Woolf D, Lawless ST, Zaritsky A, Bonham J, et al. Pancreatitis in patients with organic acidemias. J Pediatr 1994;124: 239-43.
61. Kang SS, Passen EL, Ruggie N, Wong PW, Sora H. Thermolabile defect of methylenetetrahydrofolate reductase in coronary artery disease. Circulation 1993;88:1463-9.
62. Kaufman S. Phenylketonuria and its variants. Adv Hum Genet 1983;13:217-97.
63. Koch R, Friedman E, Azen C, Hanley W, Levy H, Matalon R, et al. The international collaborative study of maternal phenylketonuria: status report 1998. Eur J Pediatr 2000;159:S156-S60.
64. Koeberl DD, Young SP, Gregersen N, Vockley J, Smith WE, Benjamin DK Jr., et al. Rare disorders of metabolism with elevated butyryl- and isobutyryl-carnitine detected by tandem mass spectroscopy newborn screening. Pediatr Res 2003;7:219-23.
65. Koeller DM, Woontner M, Crnic LS, Kleinschmidt-DeMasters B, Stephens J, Hunt EL, et al. Biochemical, pathologic and behavioral analysis of a mouse model of glutaric acidemia type I. Hum Mol Genet 2002;11:347-57.
66. Kupfer A, Aeschlimann C, Wermuth B, Cerny T. Prophylaxis and reversal of ifosfamide encephalopathy with methylene-blue. Lancet 1994;343:763-4.
67. Lehnert W, Ruitenbeek W. Ethylmalonic aciduria associated with progressive neurological disease and partial cytochrome c oxidase deficiency. J Inherit Metab Dis 1993;16:557-9.

68. Lehotay DC, Clarke JT. Organic acidurias and related abnormalities. Crit Rev Clin Lab Scie 1995;32: 377-429.
69. Lenke RR, Levy HL. Maternal phenylketonuria and hyperphenylalaninemia. An international survey of the outcome of untreated and treated pregnancies. N Engl J Med 1980;303:1202-8.
70. Lindstedt S, Holme E, Lock EA, Hjalmarson O, Strandvik B. Treatment of hereditary tyrosinaemia type I by inhibition of 4-hydroxyphenylpyruvate dioxygenase. Lancet 1992;340:813-7.
71. Lundemose JB, Kolvraa S, Gregersen N, Christensen E, Gregersen M. Fatty acid oxidation disorders as primary cause of sudden and unexpected death in infants and young children: an investigation performed on cultured fibroblasts from 79 children who died aged between 0-4 years. Mol Pathol 1997;50: 212-7.
72. Maestri NE, Brusilow SW, Clissold DB, Bassett SS. Long-term treatment of girls with ornithine transcarbamylase deficiency. N Engl J Med 1996;335:855-9.
73. Magera MJ, Helgeson JK, Matern D, Rinaldo P. Methylmalonic acid measured in plasma and urine by stable-isotope dilution and electrospray tandem mass spectrometry. Clin Chem 2000;46:1804-10.
74. Magera MJ, Lacey JM, Casetta B, Rinaldo P. Method for the determination of total homocysteine in plasma and urine by stable isotope dilution and electrospray tandem mass spectrometry. Clin Chem 1999;45:1517-22.
75. Mamer OA, Tjoa SS, Scriver CR, Klassen GA. Demonstration of a new mammalian isoleucine catabolic pathway yielding an R series of metabolites. Biochem J 1976;160:417-26.
76. Mantagos S, Genel M, Tanaka K. Ethylmalonic-adipic aciduria. In vivo and in vitro studies indicating deficiency of activities of multiple acyl-CoA dehydrogenases. J Clin Invest 1979;64:1580-9.
77. Markand ON, Garg BP, Brandt IK. Nonketotic hyperglycinemia: electroencephalographic and evoked potential abnormalities. Neurology 1982;32:151-6.
78. Matern D. Tandem mass spectrometry in newborn screening. Endocrinologist 2002;12:50-7.
79. Matern D, He M, Berry SA, Rinaldo P, Whitley CB, Madsen PP, et al. Prospective diagnosis of 2-methylbutyryl-CoA dehydrogenase deficiency in the Hmong population by newborn screening using tandem mass spectrometry. Pediatrics 2003;112:74-8.
80. Matern D, Schehata BM, Shekhawa P, Strauss AW, Bennett MJ, Rinaldo P. Placental floor infarction complicating the pregnancy of a fetus with long-chain 3-hydroxyacyl-CoA dehydrogenase (LCHAD) deficiency. Mol Genet Metab 2001;72:265-8.
81. Mathur A, Sims HF, Gopalakrishnan D, Gibson B, Rinaldo P, Vockley J, et al. Molecular heterogeneity in very-long-chain acyl-CoA dehydrogenase deficiency causing pediatric cardiomyopathy and sudden death. Circulation 1999;99:1337-43.
82. Matsubara Y, Narisawa K, Miyabayashi S, Tada K, Coates PM. Molecular lesion in patients with medium-chain acyl-CoA dehydrogenase deficiency. Lancet 1990;335:1589.
83. Matthews DE, Ben-Galim E, Haymond MW, Bier DM. Alloisoleucine formation in maple syrup urine disease: isotopic evidence for the mechanism. Pediatr Res 1980;14:854-7.
84. McGarry JD, Brown NF. The mitochondrial carnitine palmitoyltransferase system. From concept to molecular analysis. Eur J Biochem 1997;244:1-14.
85. Millington DS, Chace DH. Carnitine and acylcarnitines in metabolic disease diagnosis and management. In: Desiderio DM, eds. Mass spectrometry: clinical and biomedical applications, New York: Plenum Press, 1992:299-318.
86. Millington DS, Norwood DL, Kodo N, Roe CR, Inoue F. Application of fast atom bombardment with tandem mass spectrometry and liquid chromatography/mass spectrometry to the analysis of acylcarnitines in human urine, blood, and tissue. Anal Biochem 1989;180:331-9.
87. Millington DS, Roe CR, Maltby DA. Application of high resolution fast atom bombardment and constant B/E ratio linked scanning to the identification and analysis of acylcarnitines in metabolic disease. Biomed Mass Spectrom 1984;11:236-41.
88. Miner SE, Evrovski J, Cole DE. Clinical chemistry and molecular biology of homocysteine metabolism: an update. Clin Biochem 1997;30:189-201.
89. Mitchell G, Larochelle J, Lambert M, Michaud J, Grenier A, Ogier H, et al. Neurologic crises in hereditary tyrosinemia. N Engl J Med 1990;322:432-7.
90. Mitchell GA, Grompe M, Lambert M, Tanguay RM. Hypertyrosinemia. In: Scriver CR, Beaudet AL, Valle D, Sly WS, Childs B, Kinzler KW, et al, eds. The metabolic & molecular bases of inherited disease, 8th ed. New York: McGraw-Hill, 2001:1777-805.
91. Mudd SH, Levy HL, Krauss JP. Disorders of transsulfuration. In: Scriver CR, Beaudet AL, Valle D, Sly WS, Childs B, Kinzler KW, et al, eds. The metabolic & molecular bases of inherited disease, 8th ed. New York: McGraw-Hill, 2001:2007-56.
92. Mudd SH, Skovby F, Levy HL, Pettigrew KD, Wilcken B, Pyeritz RE, et al. The natural history of homocystinuria due to cystathionine beta-synthase deficiency. Am J Hum Genet 1985;37:1-31.
93. Myers JH, Shook JE. Vomiting, ataxia, and altered mental status in an adolescent: late-onset ornithine transcarbamylase deficiency. Am J Emerg Med 1996;14:553-7.
94. Nagan N, Kruckeberg KE, Tauscher AL, Snow Bailey K, Rinaldo P, Matern D. The frequency of short-chain acyl-CoA dehydrogenase gene variants in the US

population and correlation with the C(4)-acylcarnitine concentration in newborn blood spots. Mol Genet Metab 2003;78:239-46.
95. National Newborn Screening Report—2000. National Newborn Screening and Genetics Resource Center, Austin, TX, 2003.
96. Naylor EW, Ennis D, Davidson AG, Wong LT, Applegarth DA, Niederwieser A. Guanosine triphosphate cyclohydrolase I deficiency: early diagnosis by routine urine pteridine screening. Pediatrics 1987;79:374-8.
97. Nyhan WL, Ozand PT. Propionic acidemia and methylmalonic acidemia. In: Nyhan WL, Ozand PT, eds. Atlas of metabolic diseases. London: Chapman & Hall Medical, 1998:4-23.
98. Ozand PT, Rashed M, Millington DS, Sakati N, Hazzaa S, Rahbeeni Z, et al. Ethylmalonic aciduria: an organic acidemia with CNS involvement and vasculopathy. Brain Dev 1994;16:12-22.
99. Patel JS, Leonard JV. Ketonuria and medium-chain acyl-CoA dehydrogenase deficiency. J Inherit Metab Dis 1995;18:98-9.
100. Pedersen CB, Bross P, Winter VS, Corydon TJ, Bolund L, Bartlett K, et al. Misfolding, degradation and aggregation of variant proteins—the molecular pathogenesis of short chain acyl-CoA dehydrogenase (SCAD) deficiency. J Biol Chem 2003;278: 47449-58.
101. Pitt JJ, Eggington M, Kahler SG. Comprehensive screening of urine samples for inborn errors of metabolism by electrospray tandem mass spectrometry. Clin Chem 2002;48:1970-80.
102. Pollitt RJ, Leonard JV. Prospective surveillance study of medium chain acyl-CoA dehydrogenase deficiency in the UK. Arch Dis Child 1998;79:116-9.
103. Prince AP, McMurray MP, Buist NR. Treatment products and approaches for phenylketonuria: improved palatability and flexibility demonstrate safety, efficacy and acceptance in US clinical trials. J Inherit Metab Dis 1997;20:486-98.
104. Rashed MS, Ozand PT, Bennett MJ, Barnard JJ, Govindaraju DR, Rinaldo P. Inborn errors of metabolism diagnosed in sudden death cases by acylcarnitine analysis of postmortem bile. Clin Chem 1995;41:1109-14.
105. Raymond K, Bale AE, Barnes CA, Rinaldo P. Medium-chain acyl-CoA dehydrogenase deficiency: sudden and unexpected death of a 45 year old woman. Genet in Med 1999;1:293-4.
106. Recommendations on the dietary management of phenylketonuria. Report of medical research council working party on phenylketonuria. Arch Dis Child 1993;68:426-7.
107. Rinaldo P. Fatty acid transport and mitochondrial oxidation disorders. Seminars in Liver Disease 2001;21:489-500.
108. Rinaldo P. Laboratory diagnosis of inborn errors of metabolism. In: Suchy FJ, Sokol RJ, Balistreri WF, eds. Liver disease in children. Philadelphia: Lippincott Williams & Wilkins, 2001:171-84.
109. Rinaldo P, Barachino A, Poletto M, Alba C, Chiandetti L, Zacchello F. Acute metabolic decompensation in methylmalonic acidosis: time sequence in the urinary excretion pattern of precursor organic acids and their major metabolites. Perspect Inherit Metab Dis 1987;7:57-70.
110. Rinaldo P, Hahn SH, Matern D. Clinical biochemical genetics in the XXI century. Acta Paediatr Scand 2004;93:22-6.
111. Rinaldo P, Matern D, Bennett MJ. Fatty acid oxidation disorders. Ann Rev Physiol 2002;64:477-502.
112. Rinaldo P, Matern D. Biochemical diagnosis of inborn errors of metabolism. In: Rudolph CD, Rudolph AM, Hostetter MK, Lister G, Siegel NJ, eds. Rudolph's Pediatrics, 21st ed. New York: McGraw-Hill, 2003:578-83.
113. Rinaldo P, O'Shea JJ, Coates PM, Hale DE, Stanley CA, Tanaka K. Medium-chain acyl-CoA dehydrogenase deficiency. Diagnosis by stable-isotope dilution measurement of urinary n-hexanoylglycine and 3-phenylpropionylglycine. N Engl J Med 1988;319:1308-13.
114. Rinaldo P, Studinski AL, Matern D. Prenatal diagnosis of disorders of fatty acid transport and mitochondrial oxidation. Prenat Diagn 2001;21:52-4.
115. Rinaldo P, Yoon HR, Yu C, Raymond K, Tiozzo C, Giordano G. Sudden and unexpected neonatal death: a protocol for the postmortem diagnosis of fatty acid oxidation disorders. Sem Perinatol 1999;23: 204-10.
116. Roe DS, Vianey-Saban C, Sharma S, Zabot MT, Roe CR. Oxidation of unsaturated fatty acids by human fibroblasts with very-long-chain acyl-CoA dehydrogenase deficiency: aspects of substrate specificity and correlation with clinical phenotype. Clin Chim Acta 2001;312:55-67.
117. Salomons GS, van Dooren SJM, Verhoeven NM, Marsden D, Schwartz C, Cecil KM, et al. X-linked creatine transporter defect: an overview. J Inherit Metab Dis 2003;26:309-18.
118. Saudubray JM, Nassogne MC, de Lonlay P, Touati G. Clinical approach to inherited metabolic disorders in neonates: an overview. Semin Neonatol 2002;7:3-15.
119. Scriver CR, Kaufman S. Hyperphenylalaninemia: phenylalanine hydroxylase deficiency. In: Scriver CR, Beaudet AL, Valle D, Sly WS, Childs B, Kinzler KW, et al, eds. The metabolic & molecular bases of inherited disease, 8th ed. New York: McGraw-Hill, 2001: 1667-724.
120. Shapira E, Blitzer MG, Miller JB, Affrick DK. Biochemical genetics: a laboratory manual. New York: Oxford University Press Inc, 1989.

121. Slocum RH, Cummings JG. Amino acid analysis of physiological samples. In: Hommes FA, eds. Techniques in diagnostic human biochemical genetics, New York: Wiley-Liss, 1991:87-126.
122. Smeitink JAM. Mitochondrial disorders: clinical presentation and diagnostic dilemmas. J Inherit Metab Dis 2003;26:199-207.
123. Souri M, Aoyama T, Orii K, Yamaguchi S, Hashimoto T. Mutation analysis of very-long-chain acyl-coenzyme A dehydrogenase (VLCAD) deficiency: identification and characterization of mutant VLCAD cDNAs from four patients. Am J Hum Genet 1996;58:97-106.
124. Spiekerkoetter U, Sun B, Khuchua Z, Bennett MJ, Strauss AW. Molecular and phenotypic heterogeneity in mitochondrial trifunctional protein deficiency due to beta-subunit mutations. Hum Mutat 2003;21: 598-607.
125. Standards and guidelines for clinical genetics laboratories, 3rd ed. American College of Medical Genetics, 2002.
126. Strauss AW, Bennett MJ, Rinaldo P, Sims HF, O'Brien LK, Zhao Y, et al. Inherited long-chain 3-hydroxyacyl-CoA dehydrogenase deficiency and a fetal-maternal interaction cause maternal liver disease and other pregnancy complications. Sem Perinatol 1999;23: 100-12.
127. Sweetman L. Organic acid analyis. In: Hommes FA, eds. Techniques in diagnostic human Biochemical Genetics, New York: Wiley-Liss, 1991:143-76.
128. Tada K. A block in glycine cleavage reaction as a common mechanism in ketotic and nonketotic hyperglycinemia. Pediatr Res 1974;8:721-3.
129. Tanaka K. Isovaleric acidemia: personal history, clinical survey and study of the molecular basis. Prog Clin Biol Res 1990;321:273-90.
130. Tanaka K, Ikeda Y. Hypoglycin and Jamaican vomiting sickness. Prog Clin Biol Res 1990;321: 167-84.
131. Terrlink T, van Leeuwen PA, Houdijk A. Plasma amino acids determined by liquid chromatography within 17 minutes. Clin Chem 1994;40: 245-9.
132. Tiranti V, D'Adamo P, Briem E, Ferrari G, Mineri R, Lamantea E, et al. Ethylmalonic encephalopathy is caused by mutations in ETHE1, a gene encoding a mitochondrial matrix protein. Am J Hum Genet 2004;74:239-52
133. Turnbull DM, Bartlett K, Stevens DL, Alberti KG, Gibson GJ, Johnson MA, et al. Short-chain acyl-CoA dehydrogenase deficiency associated with a lipid-storage myopathy and secondary carnitine deficiency. N Engl J Med 1984;311:1232-6.
134. Van Hove JL, Chace DH, Kahler SG, Millington DS. Acylcarnitines in amniotic fluid: application to the prenatal diagnosis of propionic acidaemia. J Inherit Metab Dis 1993;16:361-7.
135. Van Hove JL, Zhang W, Kahler SG, Roe CR, Chen YT, Terada N, et al. Medium-chain acyl-CoA dehydrogenase (MCAD) deficiency: diagnosis by acylcarnitine analysis in blood. Am J Hum Genet 1993;52:958-66.
136. Velazquez A. The rise and fall and (urgently needed) rebirth of metabolic medicine. Mol Genet Metab 2002;76:252-5.
137. Von Figura K, Hanefeld F, Isbrandt D, Stocker-Ipsiroglu S. Guanidinoacetate methyltransferase deficiency. In: Scriver CR, Beaudet AL, Valle D, Sly WS, Childs B, Kinzler KW, et al, eds. The metabolic & molecular bases of inherited disease, 8th ed. New York: McGraw-Hill, 2001:1897-908.
138. Wanders RJ, Ijlst L, Poggi F, Bonnefont JP, Munnich A, Brivet M, et al. Human trifunctional protein deficiency: a new disorder of mitochondrial fatty acid beta-oxidation. Biochem Biophys Res Commun 1992;188:1139-45.
139. Watkins D, Rosenblatt DS. Cobalamin and inborn errors of cobalamin absorption and metabolism. Endocrinologist 2001;11:98-104.
140. Wilcken DE, Wilcken B, Dudman NP, Tyrrell PA. Homocystinuria: the effects of betaine in the treatment of patients not responsive to pyridoxine. N Engl J Med 1983;309:448-53.
141. Yamaguchi S, Indo Y, Coates PM, Hashimoto T, Tanaka K. Identification of very-long-chain acyl-CoA dehydrogenase deficiency in three patients previously diagnosed with long-chain acyl-CoA dehydrogenase deficiency. Pediatr Res 1993;34:111-3.
142. Yoon HR, Hahn SH, Ahn YM, Jang SH, Shin YJ, Lee EH, et al. Therapeutic trial in the first three Asian cases of ethylmalonic encephalopathy: response to riboflavin. J Inherit Metab Dis 2001;24:870-3.
143. Zammarchi E, Filippi L, Novembre E, Donati MA. Biochemical evaluation of a patient with a familial form of leucine-sensitive hypoglycemia and concomitant hyperammonemia. Metabol Clin Exp 1996;45:957-60.
144. Zschocke J, Schulze A, Lindner M, Fiesel S, Olgemoller K, Hoffmann GF, et al. Molecular and functional characterisation of mild MCAD deficiency. Hum Genet 2001;108:404-8.
145. Zytkovicz TH, Fitzgerald EF, Marsden D, Larson CA, Shih VE, Johnson DM, et al. Tandem mass spectrometric analysis for amino, organic, and fatty acid disorders in newborn dried blood spots: a two-year summary from the New England Newborn Screening Program. Clin Chem 2001;47:1945-55.

SECTION VII

Appendix

CHAPTER 56

Reference Information for the Clinical Laboratory*

William L. Roberts, M.D., Ph.D., Gwendolyn A. McMillin, Ph.D., D.A.B.C.C., Carl A. Burtis, Ph.D., and David E. Bruns, M.D.

CONTENTS

*The authors gratefully acknowledge the contributions of Pennell C. Painter, June Y. Cope, and Jane L. Smith upon which portions of this chapter are based.

TABLE 56-1 Reference Intervals and Values

The results of laboratory tests have little practical utility until clinical studies have ascribed various states of health and disease to intervals of values. Reference intervals are useful because they attempt to describe the typical results found in a defined population of apparently healthy people. Different methods may yield different values, depending on calibration and other technical considerations. Hence, different reference intervals and results may be obtained in different laboratories. Variability among methods is particularly characteristic of methods that use antibodies to detect the material of interest and when results are reported as relative units of activity. Values from apparently "healthy" and diseased people may overlap significantly. Therefore reference intervals, although useful as a guideline for clinicians, should not be used as absolute indicators of health and disease (see Chapter 16). The reference intervals presented in this chapter are for **general informational purposes only.** Guidelines for defining and determining reference intervals have been discussed in Chapter 16 and published in the 2000 NCCLS C28-A2 guideline (How to Define and Determine Reference Intervals in the Clinical Laboratory; Approved Guideline—Second Edition.) As stated in several chapters in this textbook, individual laboratories should generate their own set of reference intervals.

Where both exist, reference intervals are listed in both conventional and international units and are for adults in the fasting state unless otherwise stated. Values for other age groups, when included, are clearly identified. Most of the values listed were obtained from chapters in this book. Some were extracted from Tietz NW. *Clinical guide to laboratory tests,* 3rd ed. Philadelphia: WB Saunders, 1995 and Burtis CA, Ashwood ER. *Tietz textbook of clinical chemistry,* 3rd ed. Philadelphia: WB Saunders, 1999. For several of the specific proteins, reference intervals—obtained after calibration of the analytical system with the international protein reference RPPHS/CRM-470—are listed in Chapter 20. Additional intervals can be found in Wu AH, ed. *Tietz clinical guide to laboratory tests,* 4th ed. Philadelphia: WB Saunders, In Press.

A valuable source for reference intervals for older methods is http://cclnprod.cc.nih.gov/dlm/testguide.nsf/ (Accessed February 19, 2005).

For convenience and to preserve space, we have used standard abbreviations commonly used in laboratory medicine. Less common abbreviations and some nonstandard abbreviations are given below:

Amf	Amniotic fluid
CSF	Cerebrospinal fluid
EDTA	Ethylenediaminetetraacetic acid
F^-	Fluoride ion
F^-/Ox	Fluoride ion & oxalate
Hep	Heparin
Occup. exp.	Occupational exposure
Ox	Oxalate
P	Plasma
Plt	Platelets
RBC	Red blood cells
S	Serum
Sal	Saliva
U	Urine
WB	Whole blood

TABLE 56-1 Reference Intervals and Values—*Continued*

Analyte	Specimen	Condition	Reference Intervals: Conventional Units	Conversion Factor	SI Units
Acetaldehyde			mg/dL		µmol/L
	WB (F^-/Ox)		<0.2	22.7	<4.5
		Occup. exp.	<0.5		<11.4
		Toxic	1-2		22.7-45.4
Acetylaspartic acid					mmol/mol creatinine
		U			<14
Acetylcarnitine					µmol/L
	P	0-7 days			2.82-19.67
		8 days-7 yr			4.70-33.66
		>7 yr			3.29-25.72
					µmol/L
	WB spots				23.55-181.22
	Bile spots				20.44-245.72
					mmol/mol creatinine
	U	0-7 days			0.19-2.92
		8 days-7 yr			0.07-16.46
		>7 yr			0.04-1.26
α_1-Acid glycoprotein			mg/dL		g/L
	S	Adult (20-60 yr)	50-120	0.01	0.5-1.2
cis-Aconitic acid					mmol/mol creatinine
	U	0-1 mo			5-31
		1-6 mo			10-97
		6 mo-5 yr			10-97
		>5 yr			3-44
Acrylylcarnitine					µmol/L
	P	0-7 days			0.00-0.03
		8 days-7 yr			0.00-0.03
		>7 yr			0.00-0.03
					µmol/L
	WB spots				0.01-0.12
	Bile spots				0.02-0.30
					mmol/mol creatinine
	U	0-7 days			0.00-0.06
		8 days-7 yr			0.00-0.04
		>7 yr			0.00-0.00
Adipic acid					mmol/mol creatinine
	U	0-6 mo			9-37
		6 mo-5 yr			<16
		>5 yr			<6
Adipoylcarnitine					mmol/mol creatinine
	U	0-7 days			0.04-0.40
		8 days-7 yr			0.01-0.81
		>7 yr			0.00-0.13

Continued

TABLE 56-1 Reference Intervals and Values—*Continued*

Analyte	Specimen	Condition	Reference Intervals: Conventional Units	Reference Intervals: Conversion Factor	Reference Intervals: SI Units
Adrenocorticotropic hormone			pg/mL		pmol/L
	P, EDTA	Cord	50-570	0.22	11-125
		Newborn	10-185		2.2-41
		Adult (0800-0900)	<120		<26
		Adult (24 hr, supine)	<85		<19
Alanine			mg/dL		μmol/L
	P	Premature, 1 day	2.44-4.24	112.2	274-476
		Newborn, 1 day	2.10-3.65		236-410
		1-3 mo	1.19-3.71		134-416
		2-6 mo	1.58-3.68		177-413
		9 mo-2 yr	0.88-2.79		99-313
		3-10 yr	1.22-2.71		137-305
		6-18 yr	1.72-4.85		193-545
		Adult	1.87-5.88		210-661
	U, 24 h		mg/day		μmol/day
		10 days-7 wk	4.1-9.3	11.2	46-104
		3-12 yr	9.1-39.2		102-439
		Adult	7.9-48.3		88-541
			μmol/g creatinine		μmol/mol creatinine
		0-1 mo	554-2957	0.113	62.6-334.1
		1-6 mo	613-2874		59.3-324.8
		6 mo-1 yr	428-2064		48.4-233.2
		1-2 yr	389-1497		44.0-169.2
		2-3 yr	255-1726		28.8-195.0
β-Alanine			mg/dL		μmol/L
	P		<0.44	112.2	<49
			<0.26		<29
			mg/d		μmol/d
	U, 24	3-16 yr	<3.8	11.2	<42
		Adult	<8.3		<93
			mg/g creatinine		mmol/mol creatinine
			11	1.27	14
Alanine aminotransferase (ALT, SGPT) IFCC, 37 °C	S		U/L		μkat/L
		Adult male	<45	0.017	<0.77
		Adult female	<34		<0.58
Albumin			g/dL		g/L
	S	0-4 days	2.8-4.4	10	28-44
		4 days-14 yr	3.8-5.4		38-54
		14-18 yr	3.2-4.5		32-45
		Adult (20-60 yr)	3.5-5.2		35-52
		60-90 yr	3.2-4.6		32-46
		>90 yr	2.9-4.5		29-45
			mg/day		mg/day
	U, 24 hr		3.9-24.4	1	3.9-24.4
			mg/dL		mg/L
	CSF, lumbar		17.7-25.1	10	177-251
Aldolase			U/L		μkat/L
	S	Child			
		10-24 mo	10-40		0.17-0.68
		25 mo-16 yr	5-20		0.09-0.34
		Adult	2.5-10.0	0.017	0.04-0.13

TABLE 56-1 Reference Intervals and Values—*Continued*

			Reference Intervals			
Analyte	**Specimen**	**Condition**	**Conventional Units**	**Conversion Factor**		**SI Units**
Aldosterone			ng/dL			nmol/L
	S	Cord blood	40-200	0.0277		1.11-5.54
		Premature infants	19-141			0.53-3.91
		Full-term infants				
		3 days	7-184			0.19-5.10
		1 wk	5-175			0.03-4.85
		1-12 mo	5-90			0.14-2.49
		1-2 yr	7-54			0.19-1.50
		2-10 yr (supine)	3-35			0.08-0.97
		2-10 yr (upright)	5-80			0.14-2.22
		10-15 yr (supine)	2-22			0.06-0.61
		10-15 yr (upright)	4-48			0.11-1.33
		Adults				
		(supine)	3-16			0.08-0.44
		(upright)	7-30			0.19-0.83
	U, 24 hr		μg/day		nmol/d	μg/g creatinine
		Newborns (1-3 days)	0.5-5	2.77	1-14	20-140
		Prepubertal children 4-10 yr	1-8		3-22	4-22
		Adults	3-19		8-51	1.5-20
Aluminum			μg/L			μmol/L
	S, P		<5.51	0.0371		<0.2
		Patients on hemodialysis	20-550			0.74-20.4
		Al medication	<30			<1.11
	U		5-30			0.19-1.11
Ammonia nitrogen	P (Hep)		μg N/dL			μmol N/L
		Newborn	90-150	0.714		64-107
		0-2 wk	79-129			56-92
		>1 mo	29-70			21-50
		Adult	15-45			11-32
	U, 24 h		mg N/day			mmol N/day
		Infant	560-2900	0.0714		40-207
		Adult	140-1500			10-107
Amylase	S		U/L			μkat/L
IFCC, 37 °C		Adult	28-100	0.017		0.48-1.70
3α-Androstanediol glucuronide			ng/dL			nmol/L
	S	Child, prepubertal	10-60	0.0213		0.2-1.3
		Adult, M	260-1500			5.5-32
		Adult, F	60-300			1.3-6.4
Androstenedione			ng/dL			nmol/L
	S	Child, prepubertal	<5	0.0349		<0.2
		Adults	75-205			2.6-7.2
		Adult, F postmenopausal	82-275			3.0-9.6
Antidiuretic hormone (ADH)	P, EDTA	mOsm/kg	ng/L			pmol/L
		270-280	<1.5	0.926		<1.4
		280-285	<2.5			<2.3
		285-290	1-5			0.9-4.6
		290-294	2-7			1.9-6.5
		295-300	4-12			3.7-11.1

Continued

TABLE 56-1 Reference Intervals and Values—*Continued*

Analyte	Specimen	Condition		Conventional Units (Reference Intervals)	Conversion Factor (Reference Intervals)	SI Units (Reference Intervals)
Antimony				μg/dL		nmol/L
	P (Hep)			0.014-0.090	82.1	1.15-7.39
				μg/L		nmol/L
	U			<10	8.21	<82.1
				mg/L		μmol/L
		Toxic		>1		>8.21
α_1-Antitrypsin	S			mg/dL		g/L
		Adult (20-60 yr)		90-200	0.01	0.9-2.0
Apolipoprotein A-1				mg/dL		g/L
	S	4-5 yr	M	109-172	0.01	1.09-1.72
			F	104-163		1.04-1.63
		6-11 yr	M	111-177		1.11-1.77
			F	110-166		1.10-1.66
		12-19 yr	M	99-165		0.99-1.65
			F	105-180		1.05-1.80
		20-29 yr	M	105-173		1.05-1.73
			F	111-209		1.11-2.09
		30-39 yr	M	105-173		1.05-1.73
			F	110-189		1.10-1.89
		40-49 yr	M	103-178		1.03-1.78
			F	115-195		1.15-1.95
		50-59 yr	M	107-173		1.07-1.73
			F	117-211		1.17-2.11
		60-69 yr	M	111-184		1.11-1.84
			F	120-205		1.20-2.05
		>69 yr	M	109-180		1.09-1.80
			F	118-199		1.18-1.99
Apolipoprotein B				mg/dL		g/L
	S	4-5 yr	M	58-103	0.01	0.58-1.03
			F	58-104		0.58-1.04
		6-11 yr	M	56-105		0.56-1.05
			F	57-113		0.57-1.13
		12-19 yr	M	55-110		0.55-1.10
			F	53-119		0.53-1.19
		20-29 yr	M	59-130		0.59-1.30
			F	59-132		0.59-1.32
		30-39 yr	M	63-143		0.63-1.43
			F	70-132		0.70-1.32
		40-49 yr	M	71-152		0.71-1.52
			F	75-136		0.75-1.36
		50-59 yr	M	75-160		0.75-1.60
			F	75-168		0.75-1.68
		60-69 yr	M	81-156		0.81-1.56
			F	75-173		0.75-1.73
		>69 yr	M	73-152		0.73-1.52
			F	79-168		0.79-1.68
Arginine				mg/dL		μmol/L
	P	Premature, 1 day		0.17-1.57	57.4	10-90
		Newborn, 1 day		0.38-1.53		22-88
		1-3 mo		0.38-1.30		22-74
		2-6 mo		0.98-2.47		56-142
		9 mo-2 yr		0.19-1.13		11-65
		3-10 yr		0.40-1.50		23-86
		6-18 yr		0.77-2.26		44-130
		Adult		0.37-2.40		21-138

TABLE 56-1 Reference Intervals and Values—*Continued*

Analyte	Specimen	Condition	Reference Intervals: Conventional Units	Conversion Factor	SI Units
Arginine—*cont'd*					
	U, 24 h		mg/day		µmol/day
		10 days-7 wk	<1.2	5.74	<7
		3-12 yr	<5.1		<29
		Adult	<50.2		<288
			mg/g creatinine		mmol/mol creatinine
		Adult	0-4	0.65	0-2.7
Arsenic	WB (Hep)		µg/L		µmol/L
			2-23	0.0133	0.03-0.31
		Chronic poisoning	100-500		1.33-6.65
		Acute poisoning	600-9300		7.98-124
	U, 24 hr		µg/day		µmol/day
			5-50		0.07-0.67
Ascorbic acid (see Vitamin C)					
Asparagine	P		mg/dL		µmol/L
		1-3 mo	0.08-0.44	75.7	6-33
		3 mo-6 yr	0.95-1.90		72-144
		6-18 yr	0.42-0.82		32-62
		Adult	0.40-0.91		30-69
	U, 24 h		mg/day		µmol/day
		Adult	4.5-13.2	7.57	34-100
			mg/g creatinine		mmol/mol creatinine
		Adult	2-10	0.86	1.8-8.6
Aspartate aminotransferase (AST, SGOT) IFCC, 37 °C	S		U/L		µkat/L
		Adult male	<35	0.017	<0.60
		Adult female	<31		<0.53
Aspartic acid	P		mg/dL		µmol/L
		Premature, 1 day	0-0.39	75.1	0-30
		Newborn, 1 day	<0.21		<16
		1-3 mo	0-0.15		0-8
		9 mo-2 yr	<0.12		<9
		19 mo-10 yr	<0.27		<20
		6-18 yr	<0.19		<14
		Adult	<0.32		<24
	U, 24 h		mg/day		µmol/day
		3-12 yr	<5.1	7.51	<38
		Adult	<26.2		<197
			mg/g creatinine		mmol/mol creatinine
		Adult	0-4	0.85	0.1-3.7
Azelaic acid	U				mmol/mol creatinine
					<1.1
Benzoylcarnitine	U				mmol/mol creatinine
		0-7 days			0.00-0.05
		8 days-7 yr			0.01-0.37
		>7 yr			0.00-0.04
Beryllium	U, 24 hr		µg/L		µmol/L
		Negative	None detected	0.111	None detected
		Toxic	>20		>2.22

Continued

TABLE 56-1 Reference Intervals and Values—*Continued*

Analyte	Specimen	Condition	Reference Intervals: Conventional Units	Conversion Factor	SI Units
Bilirubin			mg/dL		μmol/L
Total	S	Cord (premature)	<2.0	17.1	<34.2
		Cord (full term)	<2.0		<34.2
		0-1 day (premature)	1.0-8.0		17-187
		0-1 day (full term)	2.0-6.0		34-103
		1-2 days (premature)	6.0-12.0		103-205
		1-2 days (full term)	6.0-10.0		103-171
		3-5 days (premature)	10.0-14.0		171-240
		3-5 days (full term)	4.0-8.0		68-137
		Adult	0-2.0		0-34
	U		Negative		Negative
	Amf	28 wk	<0.075		<1.28
			$\Delta A_{450} < 0.048$		
		40 wk	<0.025		<0.43
			$\Delta A_{450} < 0.02$		
Conjugated	S		0.0-0.2		0.0-3.4
Biotin	WB	Healthy			0.5-2.20 nmol/L
		Deficiency			<0.5 nmol/L
BNP (See Table 44-5, Chapter 44.)					
Butyrylglycine					mmol/mol creatinine
	U				0.1-2.0
Cadmium	WB (Hep)		μg/L		nmol/L
		Nonsmokers	0.3-1.2	8.897	2.7-10.7
		Smokers	0.6-3.9		5.3-34.7
			μg/L		μmol/L
	U, 24 hr	Toxic range	100-3000		0.9-26.7
Calcitonin	S, P		pg/mL		ng/L
		Men	<8.8	1.0	<8.8
		Women	<5.8		<5.8
		Athyroidal	<0.5		<0.5
Calcium, ionized (free)	S, P (Hep)		mg/dL		mmol/L
		Adults	4.6-5.3	0.25	1.15-1.33
Calcium, total	S, P (Hep)		mg/dL		mmol/L
		Adults	8.6-10.2	0.25	2.15-2.55
β-Carotene	S		μg/dL		μmol/L
HPLC			10-85	0.0186	0.19-1.58
Cancer antigen 15-3			U/mL		kU/L
	S		<30	1.0	<30
Cancer antigen 19-9			U/mL		kU/L
	S		<37	1.0	<37
Cancer antigen 27.29			U/mL		kU/L
	S		<37.7	1.0	<37.7
Cancer antigen 50			U/mL		kU/L
	S		<14-20	1.0	<14-20
Cancer antigen 72-4			U/mL		kU/L
	S		<6	1.0	<6
Cancer antigen 125			U/mL		kU/L
	S		<35	1.0	<35

TABLE 56-1 Reference Intervals and Values—*Continued*

Analyte	Specimen	Condition	Reference Intervals: Conventional Units	Conversion Factor	SI Units
Cancer antigen 242			U/mL		kU/L
	S		<20	1.0	<20
Cancer antigen 549			U/mL		kU/L
	S		<11	1.0	<11
Carbon dioxide, partial pressure			mm Hg		kPa
PCO_2	WB, arterial (Hep)	Newborn	27-40	0.133	3.59-5.32
		Infant	27-41		3.59-5.45
		Adult M	35-48		4.66-6.38
		Adult F	32-45		4.26-5.99
Carbon dioxide, total (tCO_2)			mEq/L		mmol/L
	Cord blood		14-22	1.0	14-22
	P, S	Adult	23-29		23-29
		>60 yr	23-31		23-31
		>90 yr	20-29		20-29
	P, Capillary	Premature, 1 wk	14-27		14-27
		Newborn	13-22		13-22
		Infant	20-28		20-28
		Child	20-28		20-28
		Adult	22-28		22-28
	Whole blood				
	Arterial		19-24		19-24
	Venous		22-26		22-26
Carbon monoxide	WB (EDTA)		% HbCO		HbCO Fraction
		Nonsmokers	0.5-1.5	0.01	0.005-0.015
		Smokers			
		1 pack-2 packs/day	4-5		0.04-0.05
		>2 packs/day	8-9		0.08-0.09
		Toxic	>20		>0.20
		Lethal	>50		>0.5
Carcinoembryonic antigen (CEA)			ng/mL		μg/L
	S	Nonsmokers	<3	1.0	<3
		Smokers	<5		<5
Catecholamines					
Epinephrine	P	Adults	pg/mL		pmol/L
		Supine (30 min)	<50	5.46	<273
		Sitting (15 min)	<60		<328
		Standing (30 min)	<90		<491
Norepinephrine	P	Adults	pg/mL		pmol/L
		Supine (30 min)	110-410	5.91	650-2423
		Sitting (15 min)	120-680		709-4019
		Standing (30 min)	125-700		739-4137
Dopamine	P	Adults	pg/mL		pmol/L
		Supine (30 min)	<87	6.53	<475
		Sitting (15 min)	<87		<475
		Standing (30 min)	<87		<475
Epinephrine	U, 24 hr		μg/day		nmol/day
		0-1 yr	0-2.5	5.46	0-14
		1-2 yr	0-3.5		0-19
		2-4 yr	0-6.0		0-33
		4-7 yr	0.2-10		1-55
		7-10 yr	0.2-10		1-55

Continued

TABLE 56-1 Reference Intervals and Values—*Continued*

Analyte	Specimen	Condition	Reference Intervals: Conventional Units	Conversion Factor	SI Units
Catecholamines—*cont'd*					
		10-15 yr	0.5-20		3-109
		>15 yr	0.5-20		3-109
Norepinephrine	U, 24 hr		µg/day		nmol/day
		0-1 yr	0-10	5.91	0-59
		1-2 yr	1-17		6-100
		2-4 yr	4-29		24-171
		4-7 yr	8-45		47-266
		7-10 yr	13-65		77-384
		10-15 yr	15-80		89-473
		>15 yr	15-80		89-473
Dopamine	U, 24 hr		µg/day		nmol/day
		0-1 yr	0-85	6.53	0-555
		1-2 yr	10-140		65-914
		2-4 yr	40-260		261-1697
		4-7 yr	65-400		424-2612
		7-10 yr	65-400		424-2612
		10-15 yr	65-400		424-2612
		>15 yr	65-400		424-2612
Ceruloplasmin			mg/L		g/L
	P	Cord (term)	50-330	0.001	0.050-0.33
		Birth-4 mo	150-560		0.15-0.56
		5-6 mo	260-830		0.26-0.83
		7-36 mo	310-900		0.31-0.90
		4-12 yr	250-450		0.25-0.45
		13-19 yr (male)	150-370		0.15-0.37
		13-19 yr (female)	220-500		0.22-0.50
		Adult (male	220-400		0.22-0.40
		Adult (female) no contraceptive	250-600		0.25-0.60
		Adult (female) contraceptives (estrogen)	270-660		0.27-0.66
		Adult, pregnant female	300-1200		
			mg/dL		g/L
	S	Adult (20-60 yr)	20-60	0.01	0.2-0.6
Chloride (Cl)			mEq/L		mmol/L
	S, P	Cord	96-104	1.0	96-104
		Premature	95-110		95-110
		0-30 days	98-113		98-113
		Adult	98-107		98-107
		>90 yr	98-111		98-111
			mEq/day		mmol/day
	U, 24 hr	Infant	2-10		2-10
		Child <6 yr	15-40		15-40
		6-10 yr			
		M	36-110		36-110
		F	18-74		18-74
		10-14 yr			
		M	64-176		64-176
		F	36-173		36-173
		Adult	110-250		110-250
		>60 yr	95-195		95-195
	Sweat (iontophoresis)		mEq/L		mmol/L
		Normal	5-35		5-35
		Marginal	30-70		30-70
		Cystic fibrosis	60-200		60-200

TABLE 56-1 Reference Intervals and Values—*Continued*

Analyte	Specimen	Condition		Conventional Units	Conversion Factor	SI Units
				Reference Intervals		
Cholesterol				mg/dL 5th-95th percentile		mmol/L 5th-95th percentile
	S	0-4 yr	M	114-203	0.0259	2.96-5.26
			F	112-200		2.90-5.18
		5-9 yr	M	125-189		3.23-4.89
			F	131-197		3.39-5.10
		10-14 yr	M	124-204		3.21-5.29
			F	125-205		3.24-5.31
		15-19 yr	M	118-191		3.06-4.95
			F	119-208		3.08-5.39
		20-24 yr	M	118-212		3.06-5.49
			F	121-237		3.14-6.14
		25-29 yr	M	130-234		3.37-6.06
			F	130-231		3.37-5.99
		30-34 yr	M	142-258		3.68-6.68
			F	133-227		3.45-5.87
		35-39 yr	M	147-267		3.81-6.92
			F	139-249		3.60-6.45
		40-44 yr	M	150-260		3.89-6.74
			F	146-259		3.78-6.71
		45-49 yr	M	163-275		4.22-7.12
			F	148-268		3.83-6.94
		50-54 yr	M	156-274		4.04-7.10
			F	163-281		4.22-7.28
		55-59 yr	M	161-280		4.17-7.25
			F	167-294		4.33-7.61
		60-64 yr	M	163-287		4.22-7.43
			F	172-300		4.46-7.77
		65-69 yr	M	166-288		4.30-7.46
			F	167-291		4.33-7.54
		>69 yr	M	144-265		3.73-6.87
			F	173-280		4.48-7.25
	Coronary heart disease risk					
	Child	Desirable		<170		<4.4
		Borderline high		170-199		4.40-5.15
		High		>199		>5.15
	Adult	Desirable		<200		<5.18
		Borderline high		200-239		5.18-6.19
		High		>239		>6.19
Cholinesterase (37 °C)				U/L		μkat/L
	S	Male		40-78	0.017	0.68-1.33
		Female		33-76		0.56-1.29
Chorionic gonadotropin intact molecule				mIU/mL		IU/L
	S	Male & nonpregnant female		<5.0	1.0	<5.0
		Female				
		Pregnancy (weeks of gestation)				
		4 wk		5-100		5-100
		5 wk		200-3000		200-3000
		6 wk		10,000-80,000		10,000-80,000
		7-14 wk		90,000-500,000		90,000-500,000

Continued

TABLE 56-1 Reference Intervals and Values—*Continued*

Analyte	Specimen	Condition	Conventional Units	Conversion Factor	SI Units
			Reference Intervals		
Chorionic gonadotropin intact molecule—*cont'd*					
		15-26 wk	5000-80,000		5000-80,000
		27-40 wk	3000-15,000		3000-15,000
			Values based on the Second International Standard for CG.		
		Trophoblastic disease	>100 000		>100 000
	U		Negative		Negative
			One half of pregnancies are detected on the first day of the missed menstrual period		One half of pregnancies are detected on the first day of the missed menstrual period
Chromium			μg/L		nmol/L
	WB (Hep)		0.7-28.0	19.23	14-538
	S		0.1-0.2		2-3
			μg/day		nmol/day
	U, 24 hr		0.1-2.0		1.9-38.4
			μg/L		nmol/L
	RBC		20-36		384-692
Chymotrypsin (37 °C)	F		12 U/g stool	1	12 U/g stool
trans-Cinnamoylglycine					mmol/mol creatinine
	U				0.1-8.0
Citric acid					mmol/mol creatinine
	U	0-1 mo			<1046
		1-6 mo			104-268
		6 mo-5 yr			0-656
		>5 yr			87-639
Cobalt			μg/L		nmol/L
	S		0.11-0.45	16.97	1.9-7.6
	U		1-2		17.0-34.0
			μg/kg		nmol/kg
	RBC		16-46		272-781
Complement C3	S		mg/dL		g/L
		Adult (20-60 yr)	90-180	0.01	0.9-1.8
Complement C4	S		mg/dL		g/L
		Adult (20-60 yr)	10-40		0.1-0.4
Copper	S		μg/dL		μmol/L
		Birth 6 mo	20-70	0.157	3.14-10.99
		Deficiency	<30		<5
		6 yr	90-190		14.13-29.83
		12 yr	80-160		12.56-25.12
		Adult			
		Male	70-140		10.99-21.98
		Female	80-155		12.56-24.34
		Deficiency	50		8
		Pregnancy, at term	118-302		18.53-47.41
		Blacks	Blacks 8-12% higher		Blacks 8-12% higher
	U, 24 h	Adults	<60 μg/24 g	0.0157	1.0 μmol/ 24 h
		Wilson's disease	>200 μg/24 hr		>3 μmol/24 h

TABLE 56-1 Reference Intervals and Values—*Continued*

Analyte	Specimen	Condition	Conventional Units	Conversion Factor	SI Units
Cortisol, free					
	S		μg/dL		nmol/L
		0800 hr	0.6-1.6	27.6	17-44
		1600 hr	0.2-0.9		6-25
			ng/mL		nmol/L
	Sal?	0700 hr	1.4-10.1	2.76	4-30
		2200 hr	0.7-2.2		2-6
			μg/day		nmol/day
	U, 24 hr	Child			
		1-10 yr	2-27		6-74
		2-11 yr	1-21		3-58
		11-20 yr	5-55		14-152
		12-16 yr	2-38		6-105
		Adult			
		Extracted	20-90		55-248
		Unextracted	75-270		207-745
Cortisol, total			μg/dL		nmol/L
	S	Cord blood	5-17	27.6	138-469
		Infant (1-7 days)	2-11		55-304
		Child (1-16 yr)			
		0800 hr	3-21		83-580
		Adult			
		0800 hr	5-23		138-635
		1600 hr	3-16		83-441
		2000 hr	<50% of 0800 values		<50% of 0800 values
CKMB, Mass (See Table 44-4, Chapter 44.)					
C-Reactive protein (CRP)	S		mg/dL		mg/L
		Adult (20-60 yr)	<0.5	10	<5
CRP (High-sensitivity)	S		mg/L		mg/L
		American males	0.3-8.6	1.0	0.3-8.6
		White American males	0.2-12.3		0.2-12.3
		African American males	0.1-8.2		0.1-8.2
		Mexican American males	0.2-6.3		0.2-6.3
		European males	0.3-8.6		0.3-8.6
		Japanese males	<7.8		<7.8
		American females	0.2-9.1		0.2-9.1
		European females	0.3-8.8		0.3-8.8
Creatine kinase (CK) IFCC, 37 °C	S		U/L		μkat/L
		Male	46-171	0.017	0.78-2.90
		Female	34-145		0.58-2.47
Creatine kinase isoenzymes	S	Fraction 2 (MB)	<5.0 μg/L	1.0	<5.0 μg/L
		Relative index MB/Total CK	<3.9%	0.01	<0.039 Fractional activity
Creatine kinase isoforms	S		% Total activity		Fractional activity
		$CK\text{-}3_1$	42-75	0.01	0.42-0.75
		$CK\text{-}3_2$	18-51		0.18-0.51
		$CK\text{-}3_3$	2-14		0.02-0.14

Continued

TABLE 56-1 Reference Intervals and Values—*Continued*

Analyte	Specimen	Condition	Reference Intervals: Conventional Units	Conversion Factor	SI Units
Creatinine					
Enzymatic	S		mg/dL		μmol/L
		0-1 yr	0.04-0.33		4-29
		2-5 yr	0.04-0.45		4-40
		6-9 yr	0.20-0.52		18-46
		10 yr	0.22-0.59		19-52
		Adult male	0.62-1.10		55-96
		Adult female	0.45-0.75		40-66
Jaffe	S		mg/dL		μmol/L
		Cord	0.6-1.2	88.4	53-106
		Newborn (1-4 days)	0.3-1.0		27-88
		Infant	0.2-0.4		18-35
		Child	0.3-0.7		27-62
		Adolescent	0.5-1.0		44-88
		18-60 yr			
		Male	0.9-1.3		80-115
		Female	0.6-1.1		53-97
		60-90 yr			
		Male	0.8-1.3		71-115
		Female	0.6-1.2		53-106
		>90 yr			
		Male	1.0-1.7		88-150
		Female	0.6-1.3		53-115
Jaffe, manual	U, 24 hr		mg/kg/day		μmol/kg/day
		Infant	8-20	8.84	71-177
		Child	8-22		71-194
		Adolescent	8-30		71-265
		Adult			
		Male	14-26		124-230
		Female	11-20		97-177
Creatinine clearance (see Glomerular filtration rate)					
C-Telopeptide	S		ng/L		ng/L
		Men	<1009	1.0	<1009
		Premenopausal women	<574		<574
			mg/mol creatinine		mg/mol creatinine
	U	Men	0-505		0-505
		Premenopausal women	0-476		0-476
Cyanide	WB (Ox)		mg/L		μmol/L
		Nonsmokers	<0.2	38.5	<7.7
		Smokers	<0.4		<15.4
		Nitroprusside therapy	Up to 100 without toxicity		Up to 3850
		Toxic	>1		>38.5
Cystine			mg/dL		μmol/L
	S	Premature, 1 day	0.54-1.02	83.3	45-85
		Newborn, 1 day	0.43-1.01		36-84
		1-3 mo	0.15-1.15		13-96
		2-6 mo	0.64-0.97		53-81
		3-10 yr	0.54-0.92		45-77
		6-18 yr	0.43-0.70		36-58
		Adult	0.40-1.40		33-117

TABLE 56-1 Reference Intervals and Values—*Continued*

Analyte	Specimen	Condition	Conventional Units	Conversion Factor	SI Units
			REFERENCE INTERVALS		
Cystine—*cont'd*					
	U, 24 hr		mg/day		μmol/day
		10 days-7 wk	2.16-3.37	8.33	18-28
		3-12 yr	4.9-30.9		41-257
		Adult	<38.1		<317
			mg/g creatinine		mmol/mol creatinine
		Adult	2-14	0.94	1.9-13.1
Decadienoylcarnitine	P				μmol/L
		0-7 yr			0.01-0.07
		>7 yr			0.01-0.11
					μmol/L
	WB spots				0.01-0.08
	Bile spots				0.03-3.93
					mmol/mol creatinine
	U	0-7 days			0.00-0.09
		8 days-7 yr			0.01-0.48
		>7 yr			0.01-0.08
Decanoylcarnitine	P				μmol/L
		0-7 days			0.02-0.51
		8 days-7 yr			0.04-0.44
		>7 yr			0.03-0.58
					μmol/L
	WB spots				0.02-0.37
	Bile spots				0.05-6.47
					mmol/mol creatinine
	U	0-7 days			0.01-0.08
		8 days-7 yr			0.00-0.21
		>7 yr			0.00-0.02
Decenoylcarnitine	P				μmol/L
		0-7 days			0.03-0.41
		8 days-7 yr			0.04-0.37
		>7 yr			0.03-0.46
					μmol/L
	WB spots				0.01-0.15
	Bile spots				0.06-11.80
					mmol/mol creatinine
	U	0-7 days			0.01-0.13
		8 days-7 yr			0.01-0.65
		>7 yr			0.01-0.07
Dehydroepiandrosterone, unconjugated	S		ng/dL		nmol/L
		Children			
		6-9 yr, M	13-187	0.0347	0.45-6.49
		6-9 yr, F	18-189		0.62-6.55
		10-11 yr, M	31-205		1.07-7.11
		10-11 yr, F	112-224		3.88-7.77
		12-14 yr, M	83-258		2.88-8.95
		12-14 yr, F	98-360		3.40-12.5
		Adult			
		M	180-1250		6.25-43.4
		F	130-980		4.51-34.0

Continued

TABLE 56-1 Reference Intervals and Values—*Continued*

Analyte	Specimen	Condition	Reference Intervals: Conventional Units	Conversion Factor	SI Units
Dehydroepiandrosterone sulfate			μg/dL		μmol/L
	S	Children			
		1-5 days, M	12-254	0.027	0.3-6.9
		1-5 days, F	10-248		0.3-6.7
		1 mo-5 yr, M	1-41		0.03-1.1
		1 mo-5 yr, F	5-55		0.1-1.5
		6-9 yr, M	2.5-145		0.07-3.9
		6-9 yr, F	2.5-140		0.07-3.8
		10-11 yr , M	15-115		0.4-3.1
		10-11 yr, F	15-260		0.4-7.0
		12-17 yr, M	20-555		0.5-15.0
		12-17 yr, F	20-535		0.5-14.4
		Pubertal levels, tanner stage			
		1 M	5-265		0.1-7.2
		1 F	5-125		0.1-3.4
		2 M	15-380		0.4-10.3
		2 F	15-150		0.4-4.0
		3 M	60-505		1.6-13.6
		3 F	20-535		0.5-14.4
		4 M	65-560		1.8-15.1
		4 F	35-485		0.9-13.1
		5 M	165-500		4.4-13.5
		5 F	75-530		2.0-14.3
		Adults			
		18-30 yr, M	125-619		3.4-16.7
		18-30 yr, F	45-380		1.2-10.3
		31-50 yr, M	5-532		1.6-12.2
		31-50 yr, F	12-379		0.8-10.2
		51-60 yr, M	20-413		0.5-11.1
		61-83 yr, M	10-285		0.3-7.7
		Postmenopausal F	30-260		0.8-7.0
11-Deoxycortisol			ng/dL		nmol/L
	S	Cord blood	295-554	0.0289	9-16
		Children and adults	20-158		0.6-4.6
Deoxypyridinoline			μmol/mol creatinine		μmol/mol creatinine
	U	Men	2.3-5.4		2.3-5.4
			1.0		
		Premenopausal women	3.0-7.4		3.0-7.4
Dihydrotestosterone			ng/dL		nmol/L
	S	Child, prepubertal	<3	0.0344	<0.10
		Adult, M	30-85		1.03-2.92
		Adult, F	4-22		0.14-0.76
Dodecanedioic acid					mmol/mol creatinine
	U				<0.06
Dodecanoylcarnitine					μmol/L
	P	0-7 days			0.02-0.33
		8 days-7 yr			0.03-0.18
		>7 yr			0.02-0.18
					μmol/L
	WB spots				0.07-0.61
	Bile spots				0.08-7.40

TABLE 56-1 Reference Intervals and Values—*Continued*

Analyte	Specimen	Condition	Reference Intervals: Conventional Units	Reference Intervals: Conversion Factor	Reference Intervals: SI Units
Dodecanoylcarnitine—*cont'd*					
					mmol/mol creatinine
	U	0-7 days			0.01-0.10
		8 days-7 yr			0.00-0.19
		>7 yr			0.00-0.02
Dodecenoylcarnitine					µmol/L
	P	0-7 days			0.01-0.29
		8 days-7 yr			0.01-0.19
		>7 yr			0.01-0.21
					µmol/L
	WB spots				0.01-0.13
	Bile spots				0.03-13.50
					mmol/mol creatinine
	U	0-7 days			0.00-0.03
		8 days-7 yr			0.00-0.07
		>7 yr			0.00-0.01
Dopamines	P, S	Normotensive adults	pg/mL		nmol/L
L-Dopa (L-Dodecenoylcarnitine)			1042-2366	0.0051	5.3-12.0
DOPAC (3,4-dihydroxyphenylacetic acid)			674-2636	0.0059	4.0-15.7
DHPG (3,4-dihydroxyphenylglycol)			797-1208	0.0059	4.7-7.1
DU-PAN-2			U/mL		kU/L
			<401	1.0	<401
Estradiol			pg/mL		pmol/L
	S	Children			
		1-5 yr, M	3-10	3.69	11-37
		1-5 yr, F	5-10		18-37
		6-9 yr, M	3-10		11-37
		6-9 yr , F	5-60		18-220
		10-11 yr, M	5-10		18-37
		10-11 yr, F	5-300		18-1100
		12-14 yr, M	5-30		18-110
		12-14 yr, F	24-410		92-1505
		15-17 yr, M	5-45		18-165
		12-17 yr, F	40-410		147-1505
		Adults			
		M	10-50		37-184
		F			
		Early follicular phase	20-150		73-550
		Late follicular phase	40-350		147-1285
		Midcycle	150-750		550-2753
		Luteal phase	30-450		110-1652
		Postmenopausal	<21		<74
		Pubertal levels, Tanner stage			
		1, M	3-15		11-35
		1, F	5-10		18-37
		2, M	3-10		11-37
		2, F	5-115		18-422

Continued

TABLE 56-1 Reference Intervals and Values—*Continued*

			Reference Intervals		
Analyte	**Specimen**	**Condition**	**Conventional Units**	**Conversion Factor**	**SI Units**
Estradiol—*cont'd*					
		3 M	5-15		18-55
		3, F	5-180		18-660
		4, M	3-40		11-147
		4, F	25-345		92-1267
		5, M	15-45		55-165
		5, F	25-410		92-1505
Estriol, free (unconjugated, uE_3)			ng/mL		nmol/L
	S	Males & nonpregnant females	<2.0	3.47	<6.9
		Pregnancy (weeks of gestation)			
		16	0.30-1.05		1.04-3.64
		18	0.63-2.30		2.19-7.98
		34	5.3-18.3		18.4-63.5
		35	5.2-26.4		18.0-91.6
		36	8.2-28.1		28.4-97.5
		37	8.0-30.1		27.8-104.0
		38	8.6-38.0		29.8-131.9
		39	7.2-34.3		25.0-119.0
		40	9.6-28.9		33.3-100.3
	Amf	Pregnancy (weeks of gestation)			
		16-20	1.0-3.2		3.5-11
		20-24	2.1-7.8		7.3-27
		24-28	2.1-7.8		7.3-27
		28-32	4.0-13.6		14-47
		32-36	3.6-15.5		12-54
		36-38	4.6-18.0		16-62
		38-40	5.4-19.8		19-69
Estriol, total (E_3)			ng/mL		nmol/L
	S	Pregnancy (weeks of gestation)			
		34	38-140	3.47	132-486
		35	31-140		108-486
		36	35-330		121-1145
		37	45-260		156-902
		38	48-350		167-1215
		39	59-570		205-1978
		40	95-460		330-1596
			µg/day		nmol/day
	U, 24 hr	Male	1.0-11.0	3.47	3.5-38.2
		Female			
		Follicular phase	0-15.0		0-52.0
		Ovulatory phase	13.0-54.0		45.1-187.4
		Luteal phase	8.0-60.0		27.8-208.2
		Postmenopausal	0-11.0		0-38.2
		Pregnancy			
		1st Trimester	0-800		0-2776
		2nd Trimester	800-12,000		2776-41,640
		3rd Trimester	5000-50,000		17,350-173,500
			ng/mL		nmol/L
	Amf	Weeks of gestation			
		21-32	5-50		17-174
		33-35	90-240		312-833
		36-41	150-213		521-739

TABLE 56-1 Reference Intervals and Values—*Continued*

Analyte	Specimen	Condition	Conventional Units	Conversion Factor	SI Units
			Reference Intervals		
Estrone	S		pg/mL		pmol/L
		Male	15-65	3.69	55-240
		Female			
		Early follicular phase	15-150		55-555
		Late follicular phase	100-250		370-925
		Luteal phase	15-200		55-740
		Postmenopausal	15-55		55-204
Ethanol	WB (Ox)		mg/dL		mmol/L
		Impairment	50-100	0.217	11-22
		Depression of CNS	>100		>21.7
		Fatalities reported	>400		>86.8
Ethylmalonic acid	U				mmol/mol creatinine 0.4-17
Ferritin	S		ng/mL		µg/L
		Newborn	25-200	1.0	25-200
		1 mo	200-600		200-600
		2-5 mo	50-200		50-200
		6 mo-15 yr	7-140		7-140
		Adult			
		Male	20-250		20-250
		Female	10-120		10-120
α-Fetoprotein (AFP)	S		mg/L		g/L
		Fetal, 1st trimester	200-400	0.01	2.0-4.0
		Cord blood	<5		<0.05
			ng/mL		µg/L
		Child, 1 yr	<30	1.0	<30
		Adult (85% of population)	<8.5		<8.5
		Adult (100% of population)	<15		<15
	Maternal serum	Weeks of gestation	ng/mL (Median)		µg/L (Median)
		14	25.6		25.6
		15	29.9		29.9
		16	34.8		34.8
		17	40.6		40.6
		18	47.3		47.3
		19	55.1		55.1
		20	64.3		64.3
		21	74.9		74.9
	S	Tumor marker	ng/mL		µg/L
		Early marker	10-20		10-20
		Cancer	>1000		>1000
	Amf		µg/mL (Median)		mg/L (Median)
		Weeks of gestation			
		15	16.3		16.3
		16	14.5		14.5
		17	13.4		13.4
		18	12.0		12.0
		19	10.7		10.7
		20	8.1		8.1

Continued

TABLE 56-1 Reference Intervals and Values—*Continued*

Analyte	Specimen	Condition	Reference Intervals: Conventional Units	Conversion Factor	SI Units
Fluoride	S		mg/L 0.2-3.2	52.6	μmol/L 10.5-168
Folate			μg/L		nmol/L
	S		2.6-12.2	2.265	6.0-28.0
	Erythrocyte		103-411		237-948
	S Deficiency		<1.4		<3.2
	Erythrocyte deficiency		<110		<252
Follicle-stimulating hormone (FSH)			mIU/mL		IU/L
	S	Males (23-70 yr)	1.4-15.4	1.0	1.4-15.4
		Female			
		Follicular phase	1.4-9.9		1.4-9.9
		Midcycle peak	0.2-17.2		0.2-17.2
		Luteal phase	1.1-9.2		1.1-9.2
		Postmenopausal	19.3-100.6		19.3-100.6
Fructosamine	S	Child	5% below adult levels		
		Adult	205-285 μmol/L	1.0	205-285 μmol/L
Fumaric acid					mmol/mol creatinine
	U	0-1 mo			10-45
		1-6 mo			4-45
		6 mo-5 yr			1-27
		>5 yr			2-4
Glomerular filtration rate (endogenous)			mL/min/1.73 m^2		mL/sec/m^2
	S or P and U	Males			
		17-24 yr	93-131	0.00963	0.90-1.26
		25-34 yr	78-146		0.75-1.41
		35-44 yr	74-138		0.71-1.33
		45-54 yr	74-129		0.72-1.24
		55-64 yr	69-122		0.67-1.18
		65-74 yr	61-114		0.59-1.10
		78-84 yr	52-102		0.50-0.98
		Females			
		40-49 yr	65-123		0.63-1.19
		50-59 yr	58-110		0.56-1.06
		60-69 yr	50-111		0.48-1.07
		70-79 yr	46-105		0.44-1.01
		80 + yr	48-85		0.46-0.82
Glucagon			ng/L		ng/L
	P (Hep or EDTA)	Adult	70-180	1.0	70-180
	Amf	Midgestation	23-63		23-63
		Term	41-193		41-193
Glucose	S, fasting		mg/dL		mmol/L
		Cord	45-96	0.0555	2.5-5.3
		Premature	20-60		1.1-3.3
		Neonate	30-60		1.7-3.3
		Newborn			
		1 day	40-60		2.2-3.3
		>1 day	50-80		2.8-4.5
		Child	60-100		3.3-5.6
		Adult	74-100		4.1-5.6

TABLE 56-1 Reference Intervals and Values—*Continued*

Analyte	Specimen	Condition	Conventional Units	Conversion Factor	SI Units
			REFERENCE INTERVALS		
Glucose—*cont'd*					
		>60 yr	82-115		4.6-6.4
		>90 yr	75-121		4.2-6.7
	WB (Hep)	Adult	65-95		3.5-5.3
	CSF	Infant, child	60-80		3.3-4.5
		Adult	40-70		2.2-3.9
	U		1-15		0.1-0.8
	U, 24 hr		<0.5 g/day	5.55	<2.8 mmol/day
Glucose-6-phosphate dehydrogenase (G-6-PD) In erythrocytes WHO & ICSH	WB (ACD, EDTA, or Hep)		7.9-16.3 U/g Hb	64.5	510-1050 U/mmol Hb
			230-470 U/10^{12} RBC	10^{-3}	0.23-0.47 nU/RBC
			2.69-5.53 U/mL RBC	1.0	2.69-5.53 kU/L RBC
Glutamic acid			mg/dL		µmol/L
	P	Premature, 1 day	0-1.98	68.0	0-135
		Newborn, 1 day	0.29-1.57		20-107
		6 mo-3 yr	0.28-1.47		19-100
		3-10 yr	0.34-3.68		23-250
		6-18 yr	0.10-0.96		7-65
		Adult	0.21-2.82		14-192
	U, 24 hr		mg/day		µmol/day
		10 days-7 wk	0.3-1.5	6.80	2-10
		Adult	<33.8		<230
			mg/g creatinine		mmol/mol creatinine
		Adult	2-6	0.77	1.5-4.7
Glutamine	P		mg/dL		µmol/L
		3 mo-6 yr	6.93-10.89	68.5	475-746
		6-18 yr	5.26-10.80		360-740
		Adult	5.78-10.38		396-711
	U, 24 hr		mg/day		µmol/day
		10 days-7 wk	12.4-25.8	6.85	85-177
		3-12 yr	20.4-113.7		140-779
		Adult	43.8-151.8		300-1040
			mg/g creatinine		mmol/mol creatinine
		Adult	2-78	0.77	2-60
γ-Glutamyltransferase IFCC, 37 °C	S		U/L		µkat/L
		Male	<55	0.017	<0.94
		Female	<38		<0.65
Glutaric acid					mmol/mol creatinine
	U				0.5-13
Glutarylcarnitine (3-OH C10)					µmol/L
	P	0-7 days			0.00-0.11
		8 days-7 yr			0.00-0.06
		>7 yr			0.00-0.12
					µmol/L
	WB spots				0.02-0.21
	Bile spots				0.04-1.53

Continued

TABLE 56-1 Reference Intervals and Values—*Continued*

Analyte	Specimen	Condition	Reference Intervals: Conventional Units	Conversion Factor	SI Units
Glutarylcarnitine (3-OH C10)—*cont'd*					mmol/mol creatinine
	U	0-7 days			0.03-0.31
		8 days-7 yr			0.01-0.37
		>7 yr			0.01-0.06
Glycated hemoglobin (HbA_{1c})	WB (EDTA, Hep, or Ox)		% Total Hb 4.0-6.0 (NGSP)		Hb Fraction 4.0-6.0
Glyceric acid					mmol/mol creatinine
	U	0-1 mo			<40
		1-6 mo			<185
		6 mo-5 yr			<71
		>5 yr			<61
Glycine			mg/dL		μmol/L
	P	Premature 1 day	0-7.57	133.3	0-1010
		Newborn 1 day	1.68-3.86		224-514
		1-3 mo	0.79-1.67		106-222
		2-6 mo	1.31-2.22		175-296
		9 mo-2 yr	0.42-2.31		56-308
		3-10 yr	0.88-1.67		117-223
		6-18	1.18-2.27		158-302
		Adult	0.90-4.16		120-554
			mg/day		μmol/day
	U, 24 hr	10 days-7 wk	14.6-59.2	13.3	194-787
		3-12 yr	12.4-106.8		165-1420
		Adult	59.0-294.6		785-3918
			mg/g creatinine		mmol/mol creatinine
		Adult	12-108	1.51	18.2-163
Glycolic acid					mmol/mol creatinine
	U	0-1 mo			<63
		1-6 mo			<105
		6 mo-5 yr			3-121
		>5 yr			<167
Glyoxylic acid					mmol/mol creatinine
	U	0-1 mo			<14
		1-6 mo			<17
		6 mo-5 yr			<8
		>5 yr			<10
Growth hormone	S		ng/mL		μg/L
		Basal	2-5	1.0	2-5
		Insulin tolerance test	>10		>10
		Arginine	>7.5		>7.5
		L-Dopa	>7.5		>7.5
Haptoglobin	S		mg/dL		g/L
		Children	20-160	0.01	0.2-1.6
		Adult (20-60 yr)	30-200		0.3-2.0
Heptanoylcarnitine					μmol/L
	P	0-7 days			0.00-0.05
		8 days-7 yr			0.00-0.04

TABLE 56-1 Reference Intervals and Values—*Continued*

Analyte	Specimen	Condition	Reference Intervals: Conventional Units	Reference Intervals: Conversion Factor	Reference Intervals: SI Units
Heptanoylcarnitine—*cont'd*					
		>7 yr			0.00-0.06
					μmol/L
	WB spots				0.01-0.14
	Bile spots				0.03-0.75
					mmol/mol creatinine
	U	0-7 days			0.00-0.06
		8 days-7 yr			0.00-0.15
		>7 yr			0.00-0.01
Hexadecanedioic acid					mmol/mol creatinine
	U				<0.5
Hexadecanoylcarnitine					μmol/L
	P	0-7 days			0.05-0.67
		8 days-7 yr			0.04-0.23
		>7 yr			0.04-0.21
					μmol/L
	WB spots				0.10-1.74
	Bile spots				0.09-3.39
					mmol/mol creatinine
	U	0-7 days			0.01-0.13
		8 days-7 yr			0.00-0.18
		>7 yr			0.00-0.02
Hexadecenoylcarnitine					μmol/L
	P	0-7 days			0.01-0.24
		8 days-7 yr			0.01-0.10
		>7 yr			0.01-0.09
					μmol/L
	WB spots				0.02-0.28
	Bile spots				0.03-2.73
					mmol/mol creatinine
	U	0-7 days			0.00-0.03
		8 days-7 yr			0.00-0.04
		>7 yr			0.00-0.00
Hexanoylcarnitine					μmol/L
	P	0-7 days			0.01-0.49
		8 days-7 yr			0.02-0.20
		>7 yr			0.02-0.21
					μmol/L
	WB spots				0.12-1.58
	Bile spots				0.12-3.31
					mmol/mol creatinine
	U	0-7 days			0.01-0.06
		8 days-7 yr			0.00-0.16
		>7 yr			0.00-0.04
Hexanoylglycine					mmol/mol creatinine
	U				0.1-1.2

Continued

TABLE 56-1 Reference Intervals and Values—*Continued*

Analyte	Specimen	Condition		Conventional Units (Reference Intervals)	Conversion Factor	SI Units
High-density lipoprotein cholesterol (HDL-C)				mg/dL 5th-95th percentile		mmol/L 5th-95th percentile
	S	5-9 yr	M	38-75	0.0259	0.99-1.94
			F	36-73		0.93-1.89
		10-14 yr	M	37-74		0.96-1.92
			F	37-70		0.96-1.82
		15-19 yr	M	30-63		0.78-1.63
			F	35-74		0.91-1.92
		20-24 yr	M	30-63		0.78-1.63
			F	33-79		0.86-2.05
		25-29 yr	M	31-63		0.81-1.63
			F	37-83		0.96-2.15
		30-34 yr	M	28-63		0.73-1.63
			F	36-77		0.94-2.00
		35-39 yr	M	29-62		0.75-1.61
			F	34-82		0.88-2.13
		40-44 yr	M	27-67		0.70-1.74
			F	34-88		0.88-2.28
		45-49 yr	M	30-64		0.78-1.66
			F	34-87		0.88-2.26
		50-54 yr	M	28-63		0.73-1.63
			F	37-92		0.96-2.39
		55-59 yr	M	28-71		0.73-1.84
			F	37-91		0.96-2.36
		60-64 yr	M	30-74		0.78-1.92
			F	38-92		0.99-2.39
		65-69 yr	M	30-75		0.78-1.95
			F	35-96		0.91-2.49
		>69 yr	M	31-75		0.80-1.95
			F	33-92		0.86-2.39
	ATP III classification			mg/dL		g/L
	S	Low		<40	0.01	<0.40
		High		>59		>0.59
Histidine				mg/dL		µmol/L
	P	Premature, 1 day		0.16-1.40	64.5	10-90
		Newborn, 1 day		0.76-1.77		49-114
		1-3 mo		0.66-1.30		43-83
		2-6 mo		1.49-2.12		96-137
		9 mo-2 yr		0.37-1.74		24-112
		3-10 yr		0.37-1.32		24-85
		6-18 yr		0.99-1.64		64-106
		Adult		0.50-1.66		32-107
	U, 24 hr			mg/day		µmol/day
		10 days-7 wk		16.0-38.6	6.45	103-249
		3-12 yr		47.4-199.2		306-1285
		Adult		72.9-440.8		470-2843
				mg/g creatinine		mmol/mol creatinine
		Adult		1-141	0.73	1-103
Homocysteine, total				µmol/L		µmol/L
	S, P	Folate supplemented diet				
		<15 yr		<8	1.0	<8
		15-65 yr		<12		<12

TABLE 56-1 Reference Intervals and Values—*Continued*

Analyte	Specimen	Condition	Reference Intervals: Conventional Units	Conversion Factor	SI Units
Homocysteine, total—*cont'd*					
		>65 yr	<16		<16
		No folate supplementation			
		<15 yr	<10		<10
		15-65 yr	<15		<15
		>65 yr	<20		<20
Homogentisic acid	U				mmol/mol creatinine
					<11
Homovanillic acid (HVA)	U, 24 hr		mg/day		µmol/day
		3-6 yr	1.4-4.3	5.49	8-24
		6-10 yr	2.1-4.7		12-26
		10-16	2.4-8.7		13-48
		16-83	1.4-8.8		8-48
	U		mg/g creatinine		mmol/mol creatinine
		0-6 mo	<40	0.571	<23
		6 mo-5 yr	<10		<6
		3-6 yr	5.4-15.5		3.4-9.6
		6-10 yr	4.4-11.5		2.7-7.1
		10-16 yr	3.3-10.3		2.0-6.4
3-Hydroxybutyric acid	U				mmol/mol creatinine
		0-5 yr			<6
		>5 yr			<11
3-Hydroxybutyrylcarnitine	P				µmol/L
		0-7 days			0.01-0.15
		8 days-7 yr			0.01-0.29
		>7 yr			0.01-0.19
					µmol/L
	WB spots				0.35-6.25
	Bile spots				0.12-2.26
	U				mmol/mol creatinine
		0-7 days			0.01-0.06
		8 days-7 yr			0.00-0.26
		>7 yr			0.00-0.03
3-Hydroxydecenoylcarnitine	P				µmol/L
		0-7 days			0.01-0.11
		8 days-7 yr			0.01-0.05
		>7 yr			0.01-0.11
					µmol/L
	WB spots				0.02-0.14
	Bile spots				0.04-1.97
	U				mmol/mol creatinine
		0-7 days			0.01-0.25
		8 days-7 yr			0.01-0.26
		>7 yr			0.00-0.03
3-Hydroxydodecanoylcarnitine	P				µmol/L
		0-7 days			0.00-0.08
		8 days-7 yr			0.00-0.03
		>7 yr			0.00-0.04

Continued

TABLE 56-1 Reference Intervals and Values—*Continued*

Analyte	Specimen	Condition	Reference Intervals: Conventional Units	Conversion Factor	SI Units
3-Hydroxydodecanoylcarnitine—*cont'd*					µmol/L
	WB spots				0.01-0.18
	Bile spots				0.03-2.28
					mmol/mol creatinine
	U	0-7 days			0.01-0.12
		8 days-7 yr			0.00-0.16
		>7 yr			0.00-0.01
3-Hydroxydodecenoylcarnitine					µmol/L
	P	0-7 days			0.00-0.07
		8 days-7 yr			0.00-0.05
		>7 yr			0.00-0.08
					µmol/L
	WB spots				0.01-0.11
	Bile spots				0.04-4.86
					mmol/mol creatinine
	U	0-7 days			0.01-0.25
		8 days-7 yr			0.00-0.27
		>7 yr			0.00-0.03
3-Hydroxyhexadecanoylcarnitine					µmol/L
	P	0-7 days			0.00-0.08
		8 days-7 yr			0.00-0.03
		>7 yr			0.00-0.03
					µmol/L
	WB spots				0.01-0.12
	Bile spots				0.03-1.48
					mmol/mol creatinine
	U	0-7 days			0.00-0.24
		8 days-7 yr			0.00-0.05
		>7 yr			0.00-0.00
3-Hydroxyhexadecenoylcarnitine					µmol/L
	P	0-7 days			0.00-0.30
		8 days-7 yr			0.00-0.05
		>7 yr			0.00-0.04
					µmol/L
	WB spots				0.02-0.24
	Bile spots				0.04-1.45
					mmol/mol creatinine
	U	0-7 days			0.00-2.06
		8 days-7 yr			0.00-0.02
		>7 yr			0.00-0.00
3-Hydroxyhexanoylcarnitine					µmol/L
	P	0-7 days			0.00-0.07
		8 days-7 yr			0.01-0.06
		>7 yr			0.00-0.07
					µmol/L
	WB spots				0.03-0.45
	Bile spots				0.03-0.59
					mmol/mol creatinine
	U	0-7 days			0.01-0.06
		8 days-7 yr			0.00-0.32
		>7 yr			0.00-0.01

TABLE 56-1 Reference Intervals and Values—*Continued*

Analyte	Specimen	Condition	Conventional Units	Conversion Factor	SI Units
			REFERENCE INTERVALS		
2-Hydroxyglutaric acid	U				mmol/mol creatinine
					<16
5-Hydroxyindolacetic acid	P		ng/L		nmol/L
			5.2-13.4	5.23	27-70
	U		mg/g creatinine		mmol/mol creatinine
		0-5 yr	<21	0.592	<13
		>5 yr	<16		<10
3-Hydroxyisovalerylcarnitine	P				µmol/L
		0-7 days			0.01-0.15
		8 days-7 yr			0.01-0.07
		>7 yr			0.01-0.19
					µmol/L
	WB spots				0.10-0.74
	Bile spots				0.06-0.67
	U				mmol/mol creatinine
		0-7 days			0.00-0.19
		8 days-7 yr			0.01-0.52
		>7 yr			0.01-0.05
3-Hydroxyoctadecadienoylcarnitine	P				µmol/L
		0-7 days			0.00-0.04
		8 days-7 yr			0.00-0.02
		>7 yr			0.00-0.02
					µmol/L
	WB spots				0.01-0.08
	Bile spots				0.01-0.55
	U				mmol/mol creatinine
		0-7 days			0.00-0.02
		8 days-7 yr			0.00-0.01
		>7 yr			0.00-0.00
3-Hydroxyoctadecanoylcarnitine	P				µmol/L
		0-7 days			0.00-0.03
		8 days-7 yr			0.00-0.02
		>7 yr			0.00-0.02
					µmol/L
	WB spots				0.01-0.10
	Bile spots				0.00-0.66
	U				mmol/mol creatinine
		0-7 days			0.00-0.03
		8 days-7 yr			0.00-0.02
		>7 yr			0.00-0.00
3-Hydroxyoctadecenoylcarnitine	P				µmol/L
		0-7 days			0.00-0.04
		>7 days			0.00-0.03
					µmol/L
	WB spots				0.01-0.11
	Bile spots				0.02-1.01
	U				mmol/mol creatinine
		0-7 days			0.00-0.03
		8 days-7 yr			0.00-0.03
		>7 yr			0.00-0.00

Continued

TABLE 56-1 Reference Intervals and Values—*Continued*

Analyte	Specimen	Condition	Conventional Units	Conversion Factor	SI Units
			REFERENCE INTERVALS		
4-Hydroxyphenyllactic acid					mmol/mol creatinine
	U	0-1 mo			<51
		>1 mo			<11
4-Hydroxyphenylpyruvic acid					mmol/mol creatinine
	U	0-1 mo			<21
		>1 mo			<6
17-Hydroxyprogesterone			ng/dL		nmol/L
		Cord blood	900-5000	0.03	27.3-151.5
		Premature	26-568		0.8-17.0
		Newborn, 3 days	7-77		0.2-2.7
		Prepubertal child	3-90		0.1-2.7
		Puberty			
		Tanner stage			
		1. Male	3-90		0.1-2.7
		Female	3-82		0.1-2.5
		2. Male	5-115		0.2-3.5
		Female	11-98		0.3-3.0
		3. Male	10-139		0.3-4.2
		Female	11-155		0.3-4.7
		4. Male	29-180		0.9-5.4
		Female	18-230		0.5-7.0
		5. Male	24-175		0.7-5.3
		Female	20-26		0.6-8.0
		Adults			
		Male	27-199		0.8-6.0
		Female			
		Follicular phase	15-70		0.4-2.1
		Luteal phase	35-290		1.0-8.7
		Pregnancy[186]	200-1200		6.0-36.0
		Post-ACTH	<320		<9.6
		Postmenopausal	<70		<2.1
Hydroxyproline			mg/dL		μmol/L
	P	Premature, 1 day	0-1.56	76.3	0-120
		6-18 yr (M)	<0.66		<50
		6-18 yr (F)	<0.58		<44
		Adult (M)	<0.55		<42
		Adult (F)	<0.45		<34
			mg/day		μmol/day
	U, 24 hr	Adult	<1.4	7.63	<11
			μg/g creatinine		mmol/mol creatinine
		Adult	19-36	0.863	16-31
3-Hydroxytetradecanoylcarnitine					μmol/L
	P	0-7 days			0.00-0.06
		8 days-7 yr			0.00-0.03
		>7 yr			0.00-0.04
					μmol/L
	WB spots				0.01-0.08
	Bile spots				0.02-1.15
					mmol/mol creatinine
	U	0-7 days			0.01-0.07
		8 days-7 yr			0.00-0.09
		>7 yr			0.00-0.02

TABLE 56-1 Reference Intervals and Values—*Continued*

Analyte	Specimen	Condition	Reference Intervals: Conventional Units	Conversion Factor	SI Units
3-Hydroxytetradecenoylcarnitine					
	P				μmol/L
		0-7 days			0.01-0.08
		8 days-7 yr			0.01-0.05
		>7 yr			0.01-0.07
					μmol/L
	WB spots				0.01-0.10
	Bile spots				0.03-2.60
					mmol/mol creatinine
	U	0-7 days			0.01-0.10
		8 days-7 yr			0.00-0.14
		>7 yr			0.00-0.01
Immunoglobin A			mg/dL		g/L
	S	Neonate (4 days)	0-2.2	0.01	0.0-0.02
		Adult (20-60 yr)	70-400		0.7-4.0
		Adult (>60 yr)	90-410		0.9-4.1
	CSF		0.0-0.6		0.0-0.006
	Saliva		≈11		≈0.11
Immunoglobulin D			mg/dL		g/L
	S	Adult (20-60 yr)	0-8	0.01	0.0-0.08
Immunoglobulin E					
	S	Adult (20-60 yr)	0-160 IU/mL	1	0-160 kIU/L
			0-380 ng/mL[*]	1	0-380 μg/L
Immunoglobin G			mg/dL		g/L
	S	Newborn (4 days)	700-1480	0.01	7.0-14.8
		Adult (20-60 yr)	700-1600		7.0-16.0
		Adult (>60 yr)	600-1560		6.0-15.6
	CSF		0-5.5		0-0.055
Immunoglobin M			mg/dL		g/L
	S	Newborn (4 days)	5-30	0.01	0.05-0.30
		Adult (20-60 yr)	40-230		0.4-2.3
		Adult (>60 yr)	30-360		0.3-3.6
	CSF		0.0-1.3		0.0-0.013
Inhibin-A			pg/mL		ng/L
	S	Males	1.0-3.6	1.0	1.0-3.6
		Females (Cycling; days of cycle)			
		Early follicular phase (−14 to −10 days)	5.5-28.2		5.5-28.2
		Midfollicular phase (−9 to −4 days)	7.9-34.5		7.9-34.5
		Late follicular phase (−3 to −1 days)	19.5-102.3		19.5-102.3
		Midcycle (Day 0)	49.9-155.5		49.9-155.5
		Early luteal (1 to 3 days)	35.9-132.7		35.9-132.7
		Midluteal (4 to 11)	13.2-159.6		13.2-159.6
		Late luteal (12 to 14 days)	7.3-89.9		7.3-89.9
		IVF-peak levels	354.2-1690.0		354.2-1690.0
		PCOS-ovulatory	5.7-16.0		5.7-16.0
		Postmenopausal	1.0-3.9		1.0-3.9

Continued

TABLE 56-1 Reference Intervals and Values—*Continued*

Analyte	Specimen	Condition	Conventional Units	Conversion Factor	SI Units
			REFERENCE INTERVALS		
Inhibin-A—*cont'd*	S, Maternal	Pregnancy (wk)	pg/mL (Median)		ng/L (Median)
		15	174		174
		16	170		170
		17	173		173
		18	182		182
		19	198		198
		20	222		222
Insulin	S		µIU/mL		pmol/L
		Adult	2-25	6.95	12-150
Insulin-like growth factor I	S		ng/mL		µg/L
		1-2 yr			
		Male	31-160	1.0	31-160
		Female	11-206		11-206
		3-6 yr			
		Male	16-288		16-288
		Female	70-316		70-316
		7-10 yr			
		Male	136-385		136-385
		Female	123-396		123-396
		11-12			
		Male	136-440		136-440
		Female	191-462		191-462
		13-14 yr			
		Male	165-616		165-616
		Female	286-660		286-660
		15-18 yr			
		Male	134-836		134-836
		Female	152-660		152-660
		19-25 yr			
		Male	202-433		202-433
		Female	231-550		231-550
		Adult (25-85 yr)			
		Male	135-449		135-449
		Female	135-449		135-449
Insulin-like growth factor II	S		ng/mL		µg/L
		Child			
		Prepubertal	334-642	1.0	334-642
		Pubertal	245-737		245-737
		Adult	288-736		288-736
		GH deficiency	51-299		51-299
Iron	It is advised that a laboratory independently define its own reference intervals. (See Chapter 31.)				
Isobutyrylcarnitine					µmol/L
	P	0-7 days			0.13-0.70
		8 days-7 yr			0.16-0.74
		>7 yr			0.15-1.05
					µmol/L
	WB spots				0.79-14.49

TABLE 56-1 Reference Intervals and Values—*Continued*

Analyte	Specimen	Condition	Reference Intervals: Conventional Units	Conversion Factor	SI Units
Isobutyrylcarnitine—*cont'd*					
	Bile spots				0.50-5.75
					mmol/mol creatinine
	U	0-7 days			0.02-0.36
		8 days-7 yr			0.02-2.74
		>7 yr			0.01-0.29
Isobutyrylglycine					mmol/mol creatinine
	U				<10
Isocitric acid					mmol/mol creatinine
	U	0-1 mo			0-368
		1-6 mo			0-67
		6 mo-5 yr			0-77
		>5 yr			16-99
Isoleucine			mg/dL		µmol/L
	P	Premature, 1 day	0.26-0.78	76.3	20-60
		Newborn, 1 day	0.35-0.69		27-53
		1-3 mo	0.59-0.95		45-73
		2-6 mo	0.50-1.61		38-123
		9 mo-2 yr	0.34-1.23		26-94
		3-10 yr	0.37-1.10		28-84
		6-18 yr	0.50-1.24		38-95
		Adult	0.48-1.28		37-98
			mg/day		µmol/day
	U	10 days-7 wk	Trace-0.4	7.62	Trace-3
		3-12 yr	2-7		15-53
		Adult	5-24		38-183
			mg/g creatinine		mmol/mol creatinine
		Adult	1-5	0.86	0.8-4.4
Isovaleryl glycine acid					mmol/mol creatinine
	U				0.2-10
Isovaleryl/2-CH3 butyrylcarnitine					µmol/L
	P	0-7 days			0.04-0.42
		8 days-7 yr			0.05-0.44
		>7 yr			0.06-0.51
					µmol/L
	WB spots				0.18-1.73
	Bile spots				0.19-2.90
					mmol/mol creatinine
	U	0-7 days			0.00-0.25
		8 days-7 yr			0.00-1.53
		>7 yr			0.00-0.07
2-Ketoglutaric acid					mmol/mol creatinine
	U	0-1 mo			22-567
		1-6 mo			63-552
		6 mo-5 yr			36-103
		>5 yr			41-82

Continued

TABLE 56-1 Reference Intervals and Values—*Continued*

				Reference Intervals		
Analyte	**Specimen**	**Condition**		**Conventional Units**	**Conversion Factor**	**SI Units**
L-lactate				mg/dL		mmol/L
	WB (Hep)	At bed rest				
		Venous		5-12	0.111	0.56-1.39
		Arterial		3-7		0.36-0.75
	CSF	Child		16-17		1.78-1.88
	U, 24 hr	Adult		496-1982 mg/day	0.0111	5.5-22 mmol/day
						mmol/mol creatinine
		0-1 mo				46-348
		1-6 mo				57-346
		6 mo-5 yr				21-38
		>5 yr				20-101
	Gastric fluid			Negative		Negative
Lactate dehydrogenase (LD) Total L → P IFCC, 37 °C				U/L		μkat/L
	S	24 mo-12 yr		180-360	0.017	2.1-3.7
		12-60 yr		125-220		3.1-6.1
Lead				μg/dL		μmol/L
	WB (Hep)	Child		<25	0.0483	<1.21
		Adult		<25		<1.21
		Toxic		>99		>4.78
				μg/L		μmol/L
	U, 24 hr			<80		<0.39
Leucine				mg/dL		μmol/L
	P	Premature, 1 day		0.26-1.58	76.3	20-120
		Newborn, 1 day		0.62-1.43		47-109
		1-3 mo		10.58-2.14		44-164
		9 mo-2 yr		0.59-2.03		45-155
		3-10 yr		0.73-2.33		56-178
		6-18 yr		1.03-2.28		79-174
		Adult		0.98-2.29		75-175
	U, 24 hr			mg/day		μmol/day
		10 days-7 wk		0.9-2.0	7.624	7-15
		3-12 yr		3-11		23-84
		Adult		2.6-8.1		20-62
				mg/g creatinine		mmol/mol creatinine
		Adult		0-8	0.86	0-6.8
Lipase, 37 °C				U/L		μkat/L
	S	Adult		<38	0.017	<0.65
Low-density lipoprotein cholesterol (LDL-C)				mg/dL 5th-95th percentile		mmol/L 5th-95th percentile
	S	5-9 yr	M	63-129	0.0259	1.63-3.34
			F	68-140		1.76-3.63
		10-14 yr	M	64-133		1.66-3.44
			F	68-136		1.76-3.52
		15-19 yr	M	62-130		1.61-3.37
			F	59-137		1.53-3.55
		20-24 yr	M	66-147		1.53-3.81
			F	57-159		1.48-4.12
		25-29 yr	M	70-165		1.81-4.27
			F	71-164		1.84-4.25
		30-34 yr	M	78-185		2.02-4.79
			F	70-156		1.81-4.04

TABLE 56-1 Reference Intervals and Values—*Continued*

Analyte	Specimen	Condition		Reference Intervals	
			Conventional Units	Conversion Factor	SI Units
Low-density lipoprotein cholesterol (LDL-C)—*cont'd*					
		35-39 yr M	81-189		2.10-4.90
		F	75-172		1.94-4.45
		40-44 yr M	87-186		2.25-4.82
		F	74-174		1.92-4.51
		45-49 yr M	97-202		2.51-5.23
		F	79-186		2.05-4.82
		50-54 yr M	89-197		2.31-5.10
		F	88-201		2.28-5.21
		55-59 yr M	88-203		2.28-5.26
		F	89-210		2.31-5.44
		60-64 yr M	83-210		2.15-5.44
		F	100-224		2.59-5.81
		65-69 yr M	98-210		2.54-5.44
		F	92-221		2.39-5.73
		>69 yr M	88-186		2.28-4.82
		F	96-206		2.49-5.34
	Risk coronary heart disease		mg/dL		mmol/L
		Optimal	<100	0.0259	<2.59
		Near/above optimal	100-129		2.59-3.34
		Borderline high	130-159		3.37-4.12
		High	160-189		4.15-4.90
		Very high	>189		>4.90
L/S Ratio	Amf		Ratio		Ratio
		State of fetal maturity			
		Immature	<1.5	1.0	<1.5
		Transitional	1.6-2.4		1.6-2.4
		Mature	>2.5		>2.5
		Diabetic	>2.5		>2.5
Luteinizing hormone (LH)			mIU/mL		IU/L
		Males (23-70 yr)	1.2-7.8	1.0	1.2-7.8
		Female			
		Follicular phase	1.7-15.0		1.7-15.0
		Midcycle peak	21.9-56.6		21.9-56.6
		Luteal phase	0.6-16.3		0.6-16.3
		Postmenopausal	14.2-52.3		14.2-52.3
Lysine			mg/dL		µmol/L
	P	Premature, 1 day	1.01-4.53	68.5	70-310
		Newborn, 1 day	1.66-3.93		114-269
		1-3 mo	0.54-2.46		37-169
		9 mo-2 yr	0.66-2.10		45-144
		3-10 yr	1.04-2.20		71-151
		6-18 yr	1.58-3.40		108-233
		Adult	1.21-3.47		83-238
	U, 24 hr		mg/day		µmol/day
		10 days-7 wk	5.7-10.9	6.85	39-75
		3-12 yr	9.3-93.7		64-642
		Adult	3.1-153.0		21-1048
			mg/g creatinine		mmol/mol creatinine
		Adult	4-12	0.77	3.2-9.2
α_2-Macroglobulin	S		mg/dL		g/L
		Adult (20-60 yr)	130-300	0.01	1.3-3.0

Continued

TABLE 56-1 Reference Intervals and Values—*Continued*

			REFERENCE INTERVALS		
Analyte	**Specimen**	**Condition**	**Conventional Units**	**Conversion Factor**	**SI Units**
Magnesium AAS			mg/dL		mmol/L
	S	Newborn, 2-4 days	1.5-2.2	0.4114	0.62-0.91
		5 mo-6 yr	1.7-2.3		0.70-0.95
		6-12 yr	1.7-2.1		0.70-0.86
		>12 yr	1.6-2.6		0.66-1.07
	U, 24 hr		6.0-10.0 mEq/L	0.5	3.0-5.0 mmol/L
Magnesium, free	S		mmol/L		mmol/L
			0.45-0.60	1.0	0.45-0.60
Malic acid					mmol/mol creatinine
	U	0-1 mo			0-52
		1-6 mo			8-73
		6 mo-5 yr			4-57
		>5 yr			17-47
Malonylcarnitine					μmol/L
	P	0-7 days			0.01-0.08
		8 days-7 yr			0.01-0.09
		>7 yr			0.01-0.17
					μmol/L
	WB spots				0.03-0.32
	Bile spots				0.04-0.96
					mmol/mol creatinine
	U	0-7 days			0.02-0.22
		8 days-7 yr			0.01-0.50
		>7 yr			0.00-0.04
Manganese			μg/L		nmol/L
	WSB (Hep)		5-15	18.0	90-270
	S		0.5-1.3		9-24
	U, Collect in metal free container		0.5-9.8		9.1-178
					>182
		Toxic conc.	>19		>342
Mercury			μg/L		nmol/L
	WB (EDTA)		0.6-59	4.99	3.0-294.4
	U, 24 hr		<20		<99.8
		Toxic conc.	>150		>748.5
		Lethal conc.	>800		>3992
Metanephrines					
Free					
Normetanephrine	S, P		pg/mL		nmol/L
		Hypertensive adults	24-145	0.0054	0.13-0.79
		Nomotensive adults	18-101		0.10-0.55
		Normotensive children	22-83		0.12-0.45
Metanephrine	S, P		pg/mL		nmol/L
		Hypertensive adults	12-72	0.0050	0.06-0.37
		Nomotensive adults	12-67		0.06-0.34
		Normotensive children	10-95		0.05-0.48

TABLE 56-1 Reference Intervals and Values—*Continued*

Analyte	Specimen	Condition	Conventional Units	Conversion Factor	SI Units
Metanephrines—*cont'd*					
Total					
Normetanephrine	S, P		pg/mL		nmol/L
		Hypertensive adults	755-5623	0.0054	4.1-30.7
		Nomotensive adults	624-3041		3.4-16.6
		Normotensive children	851-2398		4.7-13.1
Metanephrine	S, P		pg/mL		nmol/L
		Hypertensive adults	327-2042	0.0050	1.7-10.4
		Nomotensive adults	328-1837		1.7-9.3
		Normotensive children	380-1995		1.9-10.1
Metanephrines (total)					
Metanephrine	U, 24 hr		μg/day		nmol/day
		0-3 mo	5.9-37	5.07	130-188
		4-6 mo	6.1-42		31-213
		7-9 mo	12-41		61-210
		10-12 mo	8.5-101		43-510
		1-2 yr	6.7-52		34-264
		2-6 yr	11-99		56-501
		6-10 yr	54-138		275-701
		10-16 yr	39-242		200-1231
		Adult	74-297		375-1506
Metanephrine	U		μg/g creatinine		mmol/mol creatinine
		0-3 mo	202-708	0.574	116-407
		4-6 mo	156-572		89-328
		7-9 mo	150-526		86-302
		10-12 mo	148-651		85-374
		1-2 yr	40-526		23-302
		2-6 yr	74-504		42-289
		6-10 yr	121-319		69-183
		10-16 yr	46-307		26-176
Normetanephrine	U, 24 hr		μg/day		nmol/day
		0-3 mo	47-156	5.46	257-852
		4-6 mo	31-111		171-607
		7-9 mo	42-109		230-595
		10-12 mo	23-103		127-562
		1-2 yr	32-118		175-647
		2-6 yr	50-111		274-604
		6-10 yr	47-176		255-964
		10-16 yr	53-290		289-1586
		Adult	105-354		573-1933
Normetanephrine	U		μg/g creatinine		mmol/mol creatinine
		0-3 mo	1535-3355	0.617	947-2070
		4-6 mo	737-2194		454-1354
		7-9 mo	592-1046		365-645
		10-12 mo	271-1117		167-689
		1-2 yr	350-1275		216-787
		2-6 yr	104-609		64-376
		6-10 yr	103-452		63-279
		10-16 yr	96-411		59-254
Methanol			mg/L		mmol/L
	WB (F^-/Ox)		<1.5	0.0312	<0.05
		Toxic	>200		>6.24

Continued

TABLE 56-1 Reference Intervals and Values—*Continued*

			Reference Intervals		
Analyte	**Specimen**	**Condition**	**Conventional Units**	**Conversion Factor**	**SI Units**
Methanol—*cont'd*					
	U	Occup. exp.	<50 ppm		<1.56 mmol/L
	Breath		0.8		0.03
		Occup. exp.	2.5		0.08
Methemoglobin (MetHb)			g/dL		μmol/L
	WB (EDTA, Hep, or ACD)		0.06-0.24	155	9.3-37.2
			% of total HB		Mass fraction of total HB
			0.04-1.52	0.01	0.0004-0.0152
Methionine			mg/dL		μmol/L
	P	Premature, 1 day	0.38-0.66	67.7	25-45
		Newborn, 1 day	0.13-0.61		9-41
		1-3 mo	0.05-0.57		3-39
		2-6 mo	0.24-0.73		16-49
		9 mo-2 yr	0.04-0.43		3-29
		3-10 yr	0.16-0.24		11-16
		6-18 yr	0.24-0.55		16-37
		Adult	0.09-0.60		6-40
			mg/day		μmol/day
	U, 24 hr	10 days-7 wk	0.1-1.9	6.70	0.7-13
		3-12 yr	3-14		20-95
		Adult	<9.1		<63
			mg/g creatinine		mmol/mol creatinine
		Adult	0-9.5	0.76	0-7.2
2-Methylbutyrylglycine					mmol/mol creatinine
	U				0.2-5
Methylmalonic acid					mmol/mol creatinine
	U				<3.7
Methylmalonylcarnitine					μmol/L
	P	0-7 yr			0.00-0.03
		8 days-7 yr			0.00-0.03
		>7 yr			0.00-0.06
					μmol/L
	WB spots				0.09-0.81
	Bile spots				0.06-0.92
					mmol/mol creatinine
	U	0-7 days			0.03-0.25
		8 days-7 yr			0.02-0.57
		>7 yr			0.01-0.05
Methylsuccinic acid					mmol/mol creatinine
	U				0-12
β_2-Microglobulin			mg/dL (mean)		mg/L (mean)
	S	Neonates	0.30	10	3.0
		0-59 yr	0.19		1.9
		60-69 yr	0.21		2.1
		>70 yr	0.24		2.4

TABLE 56-1 Reference Intervals and Values—*Continued*

Analyte	Specimen	Condition	Conventional Units	Conversion Factor	SI Units
			Reference Intervals		
Molybdenum			µg/L		nmol/L
	S		0.1-3.0	10.42	1.0-31.3
	U, 24 hr		40-60 µg/day		416-625 nmol/day
Mucinlike carcinoma-associated antigen (MCA)			U/mL		kU/L
	S		<14	1.0	<14
Niacin			mg/day		µmol/day
	U, 24 hr		2.4-6.4	7.30	17.5-46.7
Nickel			µg/L		nmol/L
	S or P (Hep)		0.14-1.0	17	2.4-17.0
	WB		1.0-28.0		17-476
			µg/day		nmol/day
	U, 24 hr		0.1-10		2-170
N-Telopeptide (BCE = bone collagen equivalents)			nmol BCE/L		nmol BCE/L
	S	Men	5.4-24.2		5.4-24.2
		Premenopausal women	6.2-19.0		6.2-19.0
			nmol BCE/ mmol creatinine		nmol BCE/mmol creatinine
	U	Men	3-63		3-63
		Premenopausal women	5-65		5-65
Nuclear matrix protein 22 (NMP-22)			U/mL		kU/L
		S	<10	1.0	<10
Octadecadienoylcarnitine					µmol/L
	P	0-7 days			0.01-0.12
		8 days-7 yr			0.02-0.16
		>7 yr			0.02-0.15
					µmol/L
	WB spots				0.03-0.55
	Bile spots				0.03-2.93
					mmol/mol creatinine
	U	0-7 days			0.00-0.37
		8 days-7 yr			0.00-0.02
		>7 yr			0.00-0.00
Octadecanoylcarnitine					µmol/L
	P	0-7 days			0.01-0.20
		8 days-7 yr			0.02-0.11
		>7 yr			0.02-0.10
					µmol/L
	WB spots				0.12-1.34
	Bile spots				0.06-2.13
					mmol/mol creatinine
	U	0-7 days			0.00-0.03
		8 days-7 yr			0.00-0.02
		>7 yr			0.00-0.00
Octadecenoylcarnitine					µmol/L
	P	0-7 days			0.03-0.38
		8 days-7 yr			0.05-0.35
		>7 yr			0.04-0.33

Continued

TABLE 56-1 Reference Intervals and Values—*Continued*

			Reference Intervals		
Analyte	**Specimen**	**Condition**	**Conventional Units**	**Conversion Factor**	**SI Units**
Octadecenoylcarnitine—*cont'd*					µmol/L
	WB spots				0.11-1.69
	Bile spots				0.07-3.75
					mmol/mol creatinine
	U	0-7 days			0.00-0.03
		8 days-7 yr			0.00-0.03
		>7 yr			0.00-0.00
Octanoylcarnitine					µmol/L
	P	0-7 days			0.08-1.40
		8 days-7 yr			0.08-0.41
		>7 yr			0.08-0.45
					µmol/L
	WB spots				0.19-1.02
	Bile spots				0.19-6.46
					mmol/mol creatinine
	U	0-7 days			0.02-0.82
		8 days-7 yr			0.01-0.61
		>7 yr			0.00-0.05
Octanoylglycine					mmol/mol creatinine
	U				0.1-1.2
Octenoylcarnitine					µmol/L
	P	0-7 days			0.03-0.45
		8 days-7 yr			0.06-0.53
		>7 yr			0.06-0.72
					µmol/L
	WB spots				0.03-0.48
	Bile spots				0.18-36.01
					mmol/mol creatinine
	U	0-7 days			0.01-0.36
		8 days-7 yr			0.02-4.30
		>7 yr			0.01-0.23
Orotic acid					mmol/mol creatinine
	U	0-1 mo			1.4-5.3
		1-6 mo			1.0-3.2
		6 mo-5 yr			0.5-3.3
		>5 yr			0.4-1.2
Osteocalcin			ng/mL		µg/L
	S	Adult male	3.0-13.0	1.0	3.0-13.0
		Adult female			
		Premenopausal	0.4-8.2		0.4-8.2
		Postmenopausal	1.5-11.0		1.5-11.0
Oxalic acid					mmol/mol creatinine
	U	0-1 mo			51-931
		1-6 mo			7-567
		6 mo-5 yr			7-352
		>5 yr			<188

TABLE 56-1 Reference Intervals and Values—*Continued*

Analyte	Specimen	Condition	Reference Intervals: Conventional Units	Conversion Factor	SI Units
Oxygen, partial pressure (PO_2)			mm Hg		kPa
	Cord blood				
	Arterial		5.7-30.5	0.133	0.8-4.0
	Venous		17.4-41.0		2.3-5.5
	WB, arterial				
		Birth	8-24		1.06-3.19
		5-10 min	33-75		4.39-9.96
		30 min	31-85		4.12-11.31
		1 hr	55-80		7.32-10.64
		1 day	54-95		7.18-12.64
		2 days-60 yr	83-108		11.04-14.36
		>60 yr	>80		>10.64
		>70 yr	>70		>9.31
		>80 yr	>60		>7.98
		>90 yr	>50		>6.65
Oxygen, saturation (sO_2)	WB, arterial		Percent saturation		Fraction saturation
		Newborn	40-90	0.01	0.40-0.90
		Thereafter	94-98		0.94-0.98
Oxytocin	P, EDTA		μU/mL		mU/L
		Males	1.1-1.9	1.0	1.0-1.9
		Females			
		Nonpregnant	1.0-1.8		1.0-1.8
		Second stage of labor	3.2-5.3		3.2-5.3
Pantothenic acid (Vitamin B_3)	WB		344-583 μg/L	0.0046	1.57-2.66 μmol/L
	U, 24 hr		1-15 mg/day	4.53	5-68 μmol/day
Parathyroid hormone, intact	S		pg/mL		ng/L
			10-65	1.0	10-65
Parathyroid hormone, (1-84)	S		pg/mL		ng/L
			6-40	1.0	6-40
Parathyroid hormone related peptide (PTHrP)	S		pmol/L		pmol/L
			<1.4		1.4
pH (37 °C)	WB, arterial		pH		pH
		Cord blood			
		Arterial	7.18-7.38	1.0	7.18-7.38
		Venous	7.25-7.45		7.25-7.45
		Newborn			
		Premature, 48 hr	7.35-7.50		7.35-7.50
		Full term			
		Birth	7.11-7.36		7.11-7.36
		5-10 min	7.09-7.30		7.09-7.30
		30 min	7.21-7.38		7.21-7.38
		1 hr	7.26-7.49		7.26-7.49
		1 day	7.29-7.45		7.29-7.45
		Children, adults			
		Arterial	7.35-7.45		7.35-7.45
		Venous	7.32-7.43		7.32-7.43
		Adults			
		60-90 yr	7.31-7.42		7.31-7.42
		>90 yr	7.26-7.43		7.26-7.43

Continued

TABLE 56-1 Reference Intervals and Values—*Continued*

Analyte	Specimen	Condition	Reference Intervals: Conventional Units	Conversion Factor	SI Units
Phenylalanine			mg/dL		µmol/L
	WB on filter paper		<2.1	60.5	<122
	P	Premature	2.0-7.5		121-454
		Newborn	1.2-3.4		73-205
		Phenylketonuric 2-3 days	>4.5		>272
		Phenylketonuric untreated	15-30		907-1815
		Adult	0.8-1.8		48-109
			mg/day		µmol/day
	U, 24 hr	10 days-7 wk	1.2-1.7	6.05	7-10
		3-13 yr	4.0-17.5		24-106
		Adult	<16.5		<100
			mg/g creatinine		mmol/mol creatinine
		Adult	2-10	0.68	1.3-6.9
3-Phenylpropionylglycine					mmol/mol creatinine
	U				<0.7
Phosphate	S, P (Hep)		mg/dL		mmol/L
		Children	4.0-7.0	0.323	1.29-2.26
		Adults	2.5-4.5		0.81-1.45
	U, 24 hr		g/day		mmol/day
		Adults	0.4-1.3	32.3	12.9-42.0
Phosphatase, acid tartrate resistant 37 °C	S		U/L		µkat/L
		Children	3.4-9.0	0.017	0.05-0.15
		Adult	1.5-4.5		0.03-0.08
Phosphatase, alkaline IFCC, 37 °C			U/L		µkat/L
	S	4-15 Y (Male)	54-369	0.017	0.91-6.23
		4-15 Y (Female)	54-369		0.91-6.23
		20-50 (Male)	53-128		0.90-2.18
		20-50 (Female)	42-98		0.71-1.67
		≥60 yr (Male)	56-119		0.95-2.02
		≥60 yr (Female)	53-141		0.90-2.40
Phosphatase, alkaline (bone specific, by immunoabsorption)			U/L		U/L
	S	Men	15.0-41.3	1.0	15.0-41.3
		Premenopausal women	11.6-29.6		11.6-29.6
Phosphatase, alkaline isoenzymes					
Percentage of Total Activity	<1 yr	1-15 yr	Adult	Pregnant women	Postmenopausal women
Biliary	3-6	2-5	1-3	1-3	0-12
Liver	20-34	22-34	17-35	5-17	17-48
Bone	20-30	21-30	13-19	8-14	8-21
Placental	8-19	5-17	13-21	53-69	7-15
Renal	1-3	0-1	0-2	3-6	0-2
Intestinal	0-2	0-1	0-1	0-1	0-1
Fraction activity	<1 yr	1-15 yr	Adult	Pregnant women	Postmenopausal women
Biliary	0.3-0.06	0.02-0.05	0.01-0.03	0.01-0.03	0.0-0.12
Liver	0.20-0.34	0.22-0.34	0.17-0.35	0.05-0.17	0.17-0.48
Bone	0.20-0.30	0.21-0.30	0.13-0.19	0.08-0.14	0.08-0.21
Placental	0.08-0.19	0.05-0.17	0.13-0.21	0.53-0.69	0.07-0.15
Renal	0.01-0.03	0.0-0.01	0.0-0.02	0.03-0.06	0.0-0.02
Intestinal	0.0-0.02	0.0-0.01	0.0-0.01	0.0-0.01	0.0-0.01

TABLE 56-1 Reference Intervals and Values—*Continued*

Analyte	Specimen	Condition	Reference Intervals: Conventional Units	Conversion Factor	SI Units
Pimelic acid	U				mmol/mol creatinine <1.1
Porphobilinogen	U, 24 hr		mg/L <2.26	4.42	µmol/L <10
Porphyrins, total	U, 24 hr				nmol/L 20-320
	Feces				nmol/L g dry wt 10-200
	Erythrocytes				µmol/L erythrocytes 0.4-1.7
Potassium (K)	S		mEq/L		mmol/L
		Premature cord	5.0-10.2	1.0	5.0-10.2
		Premature, 48 hr	3.0-6.0		3.0-6.0
		Newborn cord	5.6-12.0		5.6-12.0
		Newborn	3.7-5.9		3.7-5.9
		Infant	4.1-5.3		4.1-5.3
		Child	3.4-4.7		3.4-4.7
		Adults	3.5-5.1		3.5-5.1
	P (Hep)	Male	3.5-4.5		3.5-4.5
		Female	3.4-4.4		3.4-4.4
	U, 24 hr		mEq/day		mmol/day
		6-10 yr			
		M	17-54		17-54
		F	8-37		8-37
		10-14 yr			
		M	22-57		22-57
		F	18-58		18-58
		Adult	25-125		25-125
Progesterone	S		ng/dL		nmol/L
		Prepubertal child	7-52	0.0318	0.2-1.7
		Adult M	13-97		0.4-3.1
		Adult F			
		Follicular phase	15-70		0.5-2.2
		Luteal phase	200-2500		6.4-79.5
		Pregnant F			
		First trimester	725-4400		23.0-139.9
		Second trimester	1950-8250		62.0-262.4
		Third trimester	6500-22,900		206.7-728.2
Proinsulin	S		pmol/L 1.1-6.9	1.0	pmol/L 1.1-6.9
Prolactin	S		ng/mL		µg/L
		Cord blood	45-539	1.0	45-539
		Children, Tanner stage I			
		Male	<10		<10
		Female	3.6-12		3.6-12
		Children, Tanner stage 2-3			

Continued

TABLE 56-1 Reference Intervals and Values—*Continued*

Analyte	Specimen	Condition	Conventional Units	Conversion Factor	SI Units
			REFERENCE INTERVALS		
Prolactin—*cont'd*					
		Male	<6.1		<6.1
		Female	2.6-18		2.6-18
		Children, Tanner stage 4-5			
		Male	2.8-11		2.8-11
		Female	3.2-20		3.2-20
		Adult			
		Male	3.0-14.7		3.0-14.7
		Female	3.8-23.0		3.8-23.0
		Pregnancy, third trimester	95-473		95-473
Proline			mg/dL		µmol/L
	P	Premature, 1 day	0.92-4.36	86.9	80-380
		Newborn, 1 day	1.23-3.18		107-277
		1-3 mo	0.89-3.73		77-325
		9 mo-2 yr	0.59-2.13		51-185
		3-10 yr	0.78-1.70		68-148
		6-18 yr	0.67-3.72		58-324
		Adult	1.17-3.86		102-336
	U, 24 hr		mg/day		µmol/day
		10 days-7 wk	3.2-11.0	8.69	28-96
		3-12 yr	Trace		Trace
		Adult	Trace		Trace
			µmol/g creatinine		µmol/mol creatinine
		0-1 mo	70-2300	0.113	7.91-259.9
		1-6 mo	<600		<67.8
		6 mo-1 yr	<300		<33.9
		1-2 yr	<270		<30.5
		2-3 yr	<220		<24.9
Propionylcarnitine					µmol/L
	P	0-7 days			0.07-1.85
		8 days-7 yr			0.17-1.27
		>7 yr			0.17-1.49
	WB spots				0.55-8.01
	Bile spots				0.36-8.10
					mmol/mol creatinine
	U	0-7 days			0.01-0.20
		8 days-7 yr			0.01-1.20
		>7 yr			0.00-0.06
Prostate specific antigen (PSA)			ng/mL		µg/L
	S	Males			
		40-49 yr	0-2.5	1.0	0-2.5
		50-59 yr	0-3.5		0-3.5
		60-69 yr	0-4.5		0-4.5
		70-79 yr	0-6.5		0-6.5
Protein, total			g/dL		g/L
	S	Cord	4.8-8.0	10	48-80
		Premature	3.6-6.0		36-60
		Newborn	4.6-7.0		46-70
		1 wk	4.4-7.6		44-76
		7 mo-1 yr	5.1-7.3		51-73
		1-2 yr	5.6-7.5		56-75
		>2 yr	6.0-8.0		60-80

TABLE 56-1 Reference Intervals and Values—*Continued*

Analyte	Specimen	Condition	Conventional Units	Conversion Factor	SI Units
			REFERENCE INTERVALS		
Protein, total—*cont'd*					
		Adult, ambulatory	6.4-8.3		64-83
		Adult, recumbent	6.0-7.8		60-78
		>60 yr	Lower by ≈0.2		Lower by ≈2.0
			mg/dL		mg/L
	U, 24 hr	Adult	1-14		10-140
		Excretion	mg/day		g/day
		Adult	<100	0.001	<0.1
		Pregnancy	<150		<0.15
			mg/dL		g/L
	CSF	Premature	15-130	10	150-1300
		Full term newborn	40-120		400-1200
		<1 mo	20-80		200-800
		>1 mo	15-40		150-400
		Ventricular fluid	5-15		50-150
		Cisternal fluid	15-25		150-250
			g/dL		g/L
	Amf	Early pregnancy	0.2-1.7		2.0-17.0
		Late pregnancy	0.175-0.705		1.8-7.1
Pyroglutamic acid					mmol/mol creatinine
	U				<62
Pyruvic acid			mg/dL		µmol/L
	WB, arterial	Adult	0.2-0.7	0.114	0.02-0.08
	WB, venous	Adult	0.3-0.9		0.03-0.10
	CSF	Adult	0.5-1.7		0.06-0.19
	U, 24 hr	Adult			<1.1 mmol/day
					mmol/mol creatinine
	U	0-1 mo			24-123
		1-6 mo			8-90
		6 mo-5 yr			3-19
		>5 yr			6-9
Retinol binding protein (RBP)			mg/dL		g/L
	S	Birth	1.1-3.4	0.01	0.011-0.034
		6 mo	1.8-5.0		0.018-0.05
		Adult	3.0-6.0		0.03-0.06
Reverse triiodothyronine (rT_3)			ng/dL		nmol/L
	S	Cord (>37 wk)	130-300	0.0154	2.00-4.62
		Children			
		1 day	83-194		1.28-2.99
		2 days	107-209		1.65-3.22
		3 days	102-166		1.57-2.56
		1 mo-20 yr	10-35		0.15-0.54
		Adult	10-28		0.15-0.43
		Maternal serum (15-40 wk)	11-33		0.17-0.51
		Amniotic serum (17-22 wk)	163-599		2.51-9.22
Riboflavin (Vitamin B_2)			µg/dL		nmol/L
	S		4-24	26.6	106-638
	Erythrocytes		10-50		266-1330
	U		>80 µg/g creatinine	0.3	>24 µmol/mol creatinine
	U, 24 hr		>100 µg/day	2.66	>266 nmol/L

Continued

TABLE 56-1 Reference Intervals and Values—*Continued*

Analyte	Specimen	Condition	Reference Intervals: Conventional Units	Conversion Factor	SI Units
Sebacic acid					mmol/mol creatinine
	U	0-1 mo			3-16
		1-6 mo			3-26
		>6 mo			<9
Selenium			μg/L		μmol/L
	S		<8.0 (deficiency)	0.0127	<0.10 (deficiency)
		Neonates	16-71		0.2-0.9
		<2 yr	40-103		0.5-1.3
		2-4 yr	55-134		0.7-1.7
		4-16	63-160		0.8-2.0
		Adults	58-234		0.74-2.97
	WB (Hep)		7-160		0.09-2.03
	U, 24 hr	Toxic conc.	>400		>5.08
Serine			mg/dL		μmol/L
	P	Newborn, 1 day	0.99-2.55	95.2	94-243
		1-3 mo	0.8-1.60		76-152
		9 mo-2 yr	0.35-1.34		33-128
		3-10 yr	0.83-1.18		79-112
		6-18 yr	0.75-1.90		71-181
		Adult	0.68-2.03		65-193
	U, 24 hr		mg/day		μmol/day
		10 days-7 wk	6.2-24.7	9.52	59-235
		3-12 yr	16.3-56.7		155-540
		Adult	13.6-145.7		129-1387
			mg/g creatinine		mmol/mol creatinine
		Adult	0-47	1.08	0-50.8
Serotonin			ng/mL		nmol/L
	WB		50-200	5.68	280-1140
			ng/10^9 platelets		nmol/10^9 platelets
	WB		88-1230	0.00568	0.5-7.0
			ng/mL		nmol/L
	S		30-200	5.68	170-1140
			μg/day		nmol/day
	U, 24 hr		60-167		340-950
			μg/g creatinine		μmol/mol creatinine
	U		38-101	0.653	25-66
			ng/mL		nmol/L
	CSF		1.0-2.1	5.68	5.7-12.0
			ng/10^9 platelets		nmol/10^9 platelets
	Platelet-rich serum		370-970	0.00568	2.07-5.55
			ng/10^9 platelets		nmol/10^9 platelets
	Isolated platelets		154-1086		0.88-6.16
			ng/mL		nmol/L
	Platelet poor plasma		0-3.60	5.68	0-12.9
Sodium (Na)			mEq/L		mmol/L
		Premature cord	116-140	1.0	116-140
		Premature, 48 hr	128-148		128-148
		Newborn cord	126-166		126-166
		Newborn	133-146		133-146
		Infant	139-146		139-146
		Child	138-145		138-145
		Adult	136-145		136-145

TABLE 56-1 Reference Intervals and Values—*Continued*

Analyte	Specimen	Condition	Conventional Units	Conversion Factor	SI Units
Sodium (Na)—*cont'd*					
		>90 yr	132-146		132-146
	U, 24 hr	6-10 yr	mEq/day		mmol/L
		M	41-115		41-115
		F	20-69		20-69
		10-14 yr			
		M	63-177		63-177
		F	48-168		48-168
		Adult			
		M	40-220		40-220
		F	27-287		27-287
Suberic acid					mmol/mol creatinine
	U	0-6 mo			4-20
		>6 mo			<9
Suberylglycine					mmol/mol creatinine
	U				<5.5
Succinic acid					mmol/mol creatinine
	U	0-1 mo			35-547
		1-6 mo			34-156
		6 mo-5 yr			16-118
		>5 yr			29-87
Testosterone, bioavailable	S		ng/dL		nmol/L
		Adult, M	66-417	0.0347	2.29-14.5
		Adult, F	0.6-5.0		0.02-0.17
Testosterone, free	S		pg/mL		pmol/L
		Cord, M	5-22	3.47	17.4-76.3
		Cord, F	4-19		13.9-55.5
		Newborn, 1-15 days, M	1.5-31.0		5.2-107.5
		Newborn, 1-15 days, F	0.5-2.5		1.7-8.7
		1-3 mo, M	3.3-8.0		11.5-62.5
		1-3 mo, F	0.1-1.3		0.3-4.5
		3-5 mo, M	0.7-14.0		2.4-48.6
		3-5 mo, F	0.3-1.1		1.0-3.8
		5-7 mo, M	0.4-4.8		1.4-16.6
		5-7 mo, F	0.2-0.6		0.7-2.1
		6-9 yr, M	0.1-3.2		0.3-11.1
		6-9 yr, F	0.1-0.9		0.3-3.1
		10-11 yr, M	0.6-5.7		2.1-19.8
		10-11 yr, F	1.0-5.2		3.5-18.0
		12-14 yr, M	1.4-156		4.9-541
		12-14 yr, F	1.0-5.2		3.5-18.0
		15-17 yr, M	80-159		278-552
		15-17 yr, F	1.0-5.2		3.5-18.0
		Adult, M	50-210		174-729
		Adult, F	1.0-8.5		3.5-29.5
Testosterone, total			ng/dL		nmol/L
	S	Cord, M	13-55	0.0347	0.45-1.91
		Cord, F	5-45		0.17-1.56
		Premature, M	37-198		1.28-6.87
		Premature, F	5-22		0.17-0.76

Continued

TABLE 56-1 Reference Intervals and Values—*Continued*

Analyte	Specimen	Condition	Conventional Units (Reference Intervals)	Conversion Factor (Reference Intervals)	SI Units (Reference Intervals)
Testosterone, total—*cont'd*					
		Newborn, M	75-400		2.6-13.9
		Newborn, F	20-64		0.69-2.22
		Prepubertal child			
		1-5 mo M	1-177		0.03-6.14
		1-5 mo F	1-5		0.03-0.17
		6-11 mo M	2-7		0.07-0.24
		6-11 mo F	2-5		0.07-0.17
		1-5 yr M	2-25		0.07-0.87
		1-5 yr F	2-10		0.07-0.35
		6-9 yr M	3-30		0.10-1.04
		6-9 yr F	2-20		0.07-0.69
		Puberty, Tanner stage			
		1, M	2-23		0.07-0.80
		1, F	2-10		0.07-0.35
		2, M	5-70		0.17-2.43
		2, F	5-30		0.17-1.04
		3, M	15-280		0.52-9.72
		3, F	10-30		0.35-1.04
		4, M	105-545		3.64-18.91
		4, F	15-40		0.52-1.39
		5, M	65-800		9.19-27.76
		5, F	10-40		0.35-1.39
		Adult M	260-1000		9-34.72
		Adult F	15-70		0.52-2.43
Tetradecadienoylcarnitine					μmol/L
	P				0.01-0.12
					μmol/L
	WB spots				0.01-0.26
	Bile spots				0.04-9.49
					mmol/mol creatinine
	U	0-7 days			0.01-0.55
		8 days-7 yr			0.00-0.02
		>7 yr			0.00-0.00
Tetradecanedioic acid					mmol/mol creatinine
	U				<0.5
Tetradecanoylcarnitine					μmol/L
	P	0-7 days			0.01-0.23
		8 days-7 yr			0.01-0.10
		>7 yr			0.01-0.12
					μmol/L
	WB spots				0.04-0.47
	Bile spots				0.04-3.81
					mmol/mol creatinine
	U	0-7 days			0.01-0.11
		8 days-7 yr			0.00-0.39
		>7 yr			0.00-0.02
Tetradecenoylcarnitine					μmol/L
	P	0-7 days			0.01-0.39
		8 days-7 yr			0.01-0.23
		>7 yr			0.01-0.24
					μmol/L
	WB spots				0.02-0.30

TABLE 56-1 Reference Intervals and Values—*Continued*

Analyte	Specimen	Condition	Conventional Units	Conversion Factor	SI Units
			Reference Intervals		
Tetradecenoylcarnitine—*cont'd*					
	Bile spots				0.03-12.49 mmol/mol creatinine
	U	0-7 days			0.00-0.24
		8 days-7 yr			0.00-0.21
		>7 yr			0.00-0.01
Thallium			μg/L		nmol/L
	WB (Hep)		<5	4.89	<24.5
			mg/L		μmol/L
		Toxic	0.1-8.0		0.5-390
			μg/L		nmol/L
	U, 24 hr		<2.0		<9.8
			mg/L		μmol/L
		Toxic	1.0-20.0		4.9-97.8
Thiocyanate			mg/dL		μmol/L
	S	Nonsmokers	<0.4	172.4	<69
		Smokers	<1.2		<207
		Nitroprusside therapy	0.6-2.9		103-500
		Toxic	>5		>862
Threonine			mg/dL		μmol/L
	P	Premature, 1 day	1.14-3.98	84.0	95-335
		Newborn, 1 day	1.36-3.99		114-335
		1-3 mo	0.75-2.67		64-224
		2-6 mo	2.27-4.33		191-364
		3-10 yr	0.50-1.13		42-95
		6-18 yr	0.88-2.40		74-202
		Adult	0.94-2.30		79-193
	U, 24 hr		mg/day		μmol/day
		10 days-7 wk	1.5-11.9	8.40	13-100
		3-12 yr	10.1-29.6		85-249
		Adult	14.3-46.7		120-392
			mg/g creatinine		mmol/mol creatinine
		Adult	0-28	0.95	0-27
Thyroglobulin (Tg)			ng/mL		μg/L
	S	Adult euthyroid	3-42	1.0	3-42
		Athyroidic patient	<5		<5
Thyrotropin			μIU/mL		mIU/L
(thyroid-stimulating hormone)	S	Premature, 28-36 wk	0.7-27.0	1.0	0.7-27.0
(TSH)		Cord blood (>37 wk)	2.3-13.2		2.3-13.2
		Children			
		Birth-4 days	1.0-39.0		1.0-39.0
		2-20 wk	1.7-9.1		1.7-9.1
		21 wk-20 yr	0.7-64.0		0.7-64.0
		Adults			
		21-54 yr	0.4-4.2		0.4-4.2
		55-87 yr	0.5-8.9		0.5-8.9
		Pregnancy			
		First trimester	0.3-4.5		0.3-4.5
		Second trimester	0.5-4.6		0.5-4.6
		Third trimester	0.8-5.2		0.8-5.2
	Whole blood (heel puncture)	Newborn screen	<20		<20

Continued

TABLE 56-1 Reference Intervals and Values—*Continued*

Analyte	Specimen	Condition	Reference Intervals: Conventional Units	Conversion Factor	SI Units
Thyroxine-binding globulin (TBG)			mg/dL		mg/L
	S	Cord	3.6-9.6	10	36-96
		Children			
		4-12 mo	3.1-5.6		31-56
		1-5 yr	2.9-5.4		29-54
		5-10 yr	2.5-5.0		25-50
		10-15 yr	2.1-4.6		21-46
		Adult			
		Male	1.2-2.5		12-25
		Female	1.4-3.0		14-30
		Female (oral contraceptive)	1.5-5.5		15-55
Thyroxine (T_4)			μg/dL		nmol/L
	S	Cord	7.4-13.1	12.9	95-168
		Children			
		1-3 days	11.8-22.6		152-292
		1-2 wk	9.9-16.6		126-214
		1-4 mo	7.2-14.4		93-186
		4-12 mo	7.8-16.5		101-213
		1-5 yr	7.3-15.0		94-194
		5-10 yr	6.4-13.3		83-172
		1-15 yr	5.6-11.7		72-151
		Adults (15-60 yr)			
		Males	4.6-10.5		59-135
		Females	5.5-11.0		65-138
		>60 yr	5.0-10.7		65-138
		Newborn screen			
		1-5 day	>7.5		>97
		6 days	>6.5		>84
Thyroxine, free (FT_4)			ng/dL		pmol/L
	S	Newborns (1-4 days)	2.2-5.3	12.9	28.4-68.4
		Children (2 wk-20 yr)	0.8-2.0		10.3-25.8
		Adults (21-87 yr)	0.8-2.7		10.3-34.7
		Pregnancy			
		First trimester	0.7-2.0		9.0-25.7
		Second and third trimester	0.5-1.6		6.4-20.6
Thyroxine, free index (FT_4I)			μg/dL		nmol/L
	S	Cord	6.0-13.2	12.9	77-170
		Infants			
		1-3 days	9.9-17.5		128-226
		1 wk	7.5-15.1		97-195
		1-12 mo	5.0-13.0		65-168
		Children			
		1-10 yr	5.4-12.8		70-165
		Pubertal child & adult	4.2-13.0		54-168
Tiglylcarnitine					μmol/L
	P	0-7 days			0.00-0.06
		8 days-7 yr			0.00-0.05
		>7 yr			0.00-0.10

TABLE 56-1 Reference Intervals and Values—*Continued*

Analyte	Specimen	Condition		Conventional Units	Conversion Factor	SI Units
				REFERENCE INTERVALS		
Tiglylcarnitine—*cont'd*						
						μmol/L
	WB spots					0.02-0.21
	Bile spots					0.03-0.53
						mmol/mol creatinine
	U	0-7 days				0.01-0.14
		8 days-7 yr				0.00-0.34
		>7 yr				0.00-0.03
Transferrin	S			mg/dL		g/L
		Newborn		117-250	0.01	1.17-2.5
		20-60 yr		200-360		2.0-3.6
		>60 yr		160-340		1.6-3.4
Transketolase, erythrocyte	Erythrocytes			0.75-1.30 U/g Hb	64.53	48.4-83.9 kU/mol Hb
Transthyretin (prealbumin)	S			mg/dL		g/L
		Adult (20-60 yr)		20-40	0.01	0.2-0.4
Triglycerides				mg/dL 5th-95th percentile		mmol/L 5th-95th percentile
	S	0-4 yr	M	29-99	0.0113	0.33-1.12
			F	34-112		0.39-1.27
		5-9 yr	M	28-85		0.32-0.96
			F	32-126		0.36-1.43
		10-14 yr	M	33-111		0.38-1.26
			F	39-120		0.44-1.36
		15-19 yr	M	38-143		0.43-1.62
			F	36-126		0.41-1.43
		20-24 yr	M	44-165		0.50-1.87
			F	37-168		0.42-1.90
		25-29 yr	M	45-204		0.57-2.31
			F	42-159		0.48-1.80
		30-34 yr	M	46-253		0.52-2.86
			F	40-163		0.45-1.84
		35-39 yr	M	52-316		0.59-3.57
			F	40-205		0.45-2.32
		40-44 yr	M	56-318		0.63-3.60
			F	45-191		0.51-2.16
		45-49 yr	M	56-279		0.64-3.16
			F	44-223		0.50-2.52
		50-54 yr	M	63-313		0.71-3.54
			F	53-223		0.60-2.52
		55-59 yr	M	60-261		0.68-2.95
			F	59-279		0.67-3.16
		60-64 yr	M	56-240		0.64-2.71
			F	57-256		0.65-2.90
		65-69 yr	M	54-256		0.61-2.90
			F	56-260		0.64-2.94
		>69 yr	M	63-239		0.71-2.70
			F	60-289		0.68-3.27
	Recommended cutoff points			mg/dL		mmol/L
		Normal		<150	0.0113	<1.70
		High		150-199		1.70-2.25

Continued

TABLE 56-1 Reference Intervals and Values—*Continued*

Analyte	Specimen	Condition	Reference Intervals: Conventional Units	Conversion Factor	SI Units
Triglycerides—*cont'd*					
		Hypertriglyceridemic	200-499		2.26-5.64
		Very high	>499		>5.64
Triiodothyronine (T_3), free			pg/dL		pmol/L
	S	Cord	15-391	0.0154	0.2-6.0
		Child & adult	210-440		3.2-6.8
		Pregnancy	200-380		3.1-5.9
Triiodothyronine (T_3), total			ng/dL		nmol/L
	S	Cord (>37 wk)	5-141	0.0154	0.08-2.17
		Children			
		1-3 days	100-700		1.54-11.40
		1-11 mo	105-245		1.62-4.14
		1-5 yr	105-269		1.45-3.71
		6-10 yr	94-241		1.26-3.28
		11-15 yr	82-213		
		Adolescents			
		16-20 yr	80-210		1.23-3.23
		Adults			
		20-50 yr	70-204		1.08-4.14
		50-90 yr	40-181		0.62-2.79
		Pregnancy			
		First trimester	81-190		1.25-2.93
		Second & third trimesters	100-260		1.54-4.00
Troponins (See Table 44-3, Chapter 44.)					
Tryptophan			mg/dL		μmol/L
	P	Premature, 1 day	0-1.23	49.0	0-60
		Newborn, 1 day	<1.37		<67
		1-16 yr	0.49-1.61		24-79
		>16 yr	0.41-1.94		20-95
			mg/day		μmol/day
	U, 24 hr	Adult	5-39	4.90	25-191
			mg/g creatinine		mmol/mol creatinine
		Adult	<30	0.55	<16.5
Tumor-associated trypsin inhibitor (TATI)			ng/mL		μg/L
	S		3-21	1.0	3-21
	U		7-51		7-51
Tyrosine			mg/dL		mmol/L
	P	Premature, 1 day	0-5.79	55.2	0-320
		Newborn, 1 day	0.76-1.79		42-99
		1-3 mo	0.54-2.42		30-134
		2-6 mo	1.30-3.91		72-216
		9 mo-2 yr	0.20-2.21		11-122
		3-10 yr	0.56-1.29		31-71
		6-18 yr	0.78-1.59		43-88
		Adult	0.40-1.58		22-87
			mg/day		μmol/day
	U, 24 hr	10 days-7 wk	4.0-7.2	5.52	22-40
		3-12 yr	7.2-30.4		40-168
		Adult	12.0-55.1		66-304
			mg/g creatinine		mmol/mol creatinine
		Adult	0-23	0.62	0-14.2

TABLE 56-1 Reference Intervals and Values—*Continued*

Analyte	Specimen	Condition	Reference Intervals: Conventional Units	Conversion Factor	SI Units
Uracil					mmol/mol creatinine
	U	0-6 mo			<33
		6 mo-5 yr			<22
		>5 yr			<18
Urea nitrogen	S		mg/dL		mmol/L
		Cord	21-40	0.357	7.5-14.3
		Premature (1 wk)	3-25		1.1-8.9
		Newborn	4-12		1.4-4.3
		Infant/child	5-18		1.8-6.4
		Adult	6-20		2.1-7.1
		Adult >60 yr	8-23		2.9-8.2
			g/day		mol/day
	U, 24 hr		10-20	0.0357	0.43-0.71
Uric acid	S		mg/dL		mmol/L
Phosphotungstate		Adult			
		Male	4.4-7.6	0.059	0.26-0.45
		Female	2.3-6.6		0.13-0.39
		>60 yr			
		Male	4.2-8.0		0.25-0.47
		Female	3.5-7.3		0.20-0.43
Uricase		Child	2.0-5.0		0.12-0.32
		Adult			
		Male	3.5-7.2		0.21-0.42
		Female	2.6-6.0		0.15-0.35
	U, 24 hr		mg/day		mmol/L
		Purine-free diet			
		Male	<420	0.0059	<2.48
		Female	Slightly lower		Slightly lower
		Low-purine diet			
		Male	<480		<2.83
		Female	<400		<2.36
		High-purine diet	<1000		<5.90
		Average diet	250-750		1.48-4.43
	U				mmol/mol creatinine
		0-1 mo			359-2644
		1-6 mo			359-2644
		6 mo-5 yr			185-1134
		>5 yr			199-1034
Valine			mg/dL		µmol/L
	P	Premature, 1 day	0.34-2.70	85.5	30-230
		Newborn, 1 day	0.94-2.88		80-246
		1-3 mo	1.13-3.41		96-292
		9 mo-2 yr	0.67-3.07		57-262
		3-10 yr	1.50-3.31		128-283
		6-18 yr	1.83-3.37		156-288
		Adult	1.65-3.71		141-317
			mg/day		µmol/day
	U	10 days-7 wk	1.4-3.2	8.55	12-27
		3-12 yr	1.8-6.0		15-51
		Adult	2.5-11.9		21-102
			mg/g creatinine		mmol/mol creatinine
		Adult	2-6	0.97	1.9-5.9

Continued

TABLE 56-1 Reference Intervals and Values—*Continued*

Analyte	Specimen	Condition	Reference Intervals: Conventional Units	Conversion Factor	SI Units
Vanillylmandelic acid (VMA)	U, 24 hr		mg/day		μmol/day
		3-6 yr	1-2.6	5.05	5-13
		6-10 yr	2.0-3.2		10-16
		10-16	2.3-5.2		12-26
		16-83	1.4-6.5		7-33
	U		mg/g creatinine		mmol/mol creatinine
		0-1 mo	<27	0.571	<16
		1-6 mo	<19		<11
		6 mo-5 yr	<13		<8
		3-6 yr	4.0-10.8		2.3-6.2
		6-10 yr	4.0-7.5		2.3-4.3
		10-16 yr	3.0-8.8		1.7-5.0
Vitamin A	S		μg/dL		μmol/L
		1-6 yr	20-40	0.0349	0.70-1.40
		7-12 yr	26-49		0.91-1.71
		13-19 yr	26-72		0.91-2.51
		Adult	30-80		1.05-2.8
Vitamin B_1 (Thiamine diphosphate)	WB		90-140 nmol/L	1.0	90-140 nmol/L
	Erythrocytes		280-590 ng/g Hb	0.146	40.3-85.0 μmol/mol Hb
Vitamin B_2 (See Riboflavin)					
Vitamin B_6	P (EDTA)		ng/mL		nmol/L
			5-30	4.046	20-121
		Deficiency	<5		<20.2
Vitamin B_{12}			ng/L		pmol/L
	S		206-678	0.733	151-497
		Acceptable (WHO)	>201		>147
		Deficiency (WHO)	<150		<110
Vitamin C (ascorbic acid)			mg/dL		μmol/L
	S		0.4-1.5	56.78	23-85
		Deficiency	<0.2		<11
	Leukocyte		20-53 μg/10^8 leukocytes	0.057	1.14-3.01 fmol/10^8 leukocytes
		Deficiency	<10 μg/10^8 leukocytes		<0.57 fmol/10^8 leukocytes
Vitamin D	S		ng/mL		nmol/L
25(OH)D			10-65	2.50	25-162
			pg/mL		pmol/L
$1,25(OH)_2D$			15-60	2.4	36-144
Vitamin E	S		mg/dL		μmol/L
		Premature neonates	0.1-0.5	23.2	2.3-11.6
		Children	0.3-0.9		7-21
		Teenagers	0.6-1.0		14-23
		Adults	0.5-1.8		12-42
Vitamin K	S		ng/mL		nmol/L
			0.13-1.19	2.22	0.29-2.64
Zinc			μg/dL		μmol/L
	S		80-120	0.153	12-18
		Deficiency	<30		<5
	U, 24 hr		0.2-1.3 mg/24 hr	15.3	3-21 μmol/24 hr

[*] 1 IU = 2.4 ng.

TABLE 56-2 Therapeutic and Toxic Levels of Drugs

Therapeutic drug monitoring and detection of drug overdose have become increasingly important aspects of the laboratory's role in patient care. The information given for the drugs in this table has been gathered from published sources. Because knowledge and drug measurement methodologies are continuously improving, it may be necessary to supplement the information given here with information obtained from other sources as it becomes available. Reliable drug analysis information depends on a well coordinated sample collection, assay methodology characteristics, and patient-associated considerations such as age, disease state, concomitant drug administration, and clinical procedures that the patient may have undergone. In practice, each organization should have its own set of therapeutic and toxic levels for the drugs it measures.

Many tests for therapeutic drugs require careful timing between administration and sample collection if the measured drug level is to be of optimal use clinically. Therapeutic and toxic intervals for which definitive limits do not exist have been omitted from the table. Drugs are listed by their chemical or generic name, followed by a commercial brand of the drug (where appropriate).

For convenience and to preserve space, we have used standard abbreviations commonly used in laboratory medicine. Less common abbreviations and some nonstandard abbreviations are given below.

Abbreviation	Term
EDTA	Ethylenediaminetetraacetic acid
Hep	Heparin
Occup. exp.	Occupational exposure
P	Plasma
Prem	Premature
S	Serum
Therap	Therapeutic
U	Urine
WB	Whole blood

References
Johannessen SI, Battino D, Berry DJ, Bialer M, Kramer G, Tomson T, et al. Therapeutic drug monitoring of the newer antiepileptic drugs. Ther Drug Monit 2003;25:347-63.
Kelly P, Kahan BD. Review: metabolism of immunosuppressant drugs. Curr Drug Metab 2002;3:275-87.
Schulz M, Schmoldt A. Therapeutic and toxic blood concentrations of more than 800 drugs and other xenobiotics. Pharmazie 2003;58:447-74.
Tietz NW. Clinical guide to laboratory tests, 3rd ed. Philadelphia: WB Saunders, 1995.
Physicians Desk Reference, 59th ed. Montvale: Thomson, 2005.
Drug Information Handbook, 11th ed. Hudson: Lexi-Comp, 2003.

Continued

TABLE 56-2 Therapeutic and Toxic Levels of Drugs—*Continued*

Drug	Specimen	Status	Reference Interval: Conventional Units	Reference Interval: Conversion Factor	Reference Interval: SI Units
Acetaminophen (Tylenol)	S or P (Hep or EDTA)		μg/mL	6.62	μmol/L
		Therap	10-30		66-199
		Toxic			
		4 hr after dose	>200		>1324
		12 hr after dose	>50		>132
Amikacin (Amikin)	S or P (EDTA)		μg/mL	1.71	μmol/L
		Therap			
		Peak	25-35		43-60
		Trough			
		Less severe infections	1-4		1.7-6.8
		Severe infections	4-8		6.8-13.7
		Toxic			
		Peak	>35		>60
		Trough	>10		>17
Aminocaproic acid (Amicar)	S or P (Hep or EDTA)		μg/mL	0.00762	mmol/L
		Therap			
		Trough	100-400		0.8-3.0
Amiodarone (Cordarone)	S or P (Hep or EDTA)		μg/mL	1.55	μmol/L
		Therap	1.0-2.0		1.5-3.1
		Toxic	>3.5		>5.4
Amitriptyline (Elavil)	S or P (Hep or EDTA)		ng/mL	3.61	nmol/L
		Therap	80-250		289-903
		Toxic	>500		>1805
Amobarbital (Amytal)	S		μg/mL	4.42	μmol/L
		Therap	1-5		4-22
		Toxic	>10		>44
Amoxapine (Asendin)	S or P (Hep or EDTA)		ng/mL	3.19	nmol/L
		Therap	200-600		638-1914
		Toxic	>600		>1914
Amphetamine	S or P (Hep or EDTA)		ng/mL	7.40	nmol/L
		Therap	20-30		148-222
		Toxic	>200		>1480
Bromide as bromine	S		μg/mL	0.0125	mmol/L
		Therap	750-1500		9.4-18.7
		Toxic	>1250		>15.6
Bupropion (Wellbutrin, Zyban)	S or P (Hep or EDTA)		ng/mL	4.17	nmol/L
		Therap	25-100		104-417
		Toxic	>100		>417
Caffeine	S or P (Hep or EDTA)		μg/mL	5.15	μmol/L
		Therap	8-14		41-72
		Toxic	>20		>103

TABLE 56-2 Therapeutic and Toxic Levels of Drugs—*Continued*

Drug	Specimen	Status	Conventional Units (Reference Interval)	Conversion Factor (Reference Interval)	SI Units (Reference Interval)
Carbamazepine (Tegretol)	S or P (Hep or EDTA)		μg/mL	4.23	μmol/L
		Therap	4-12		17-51
		Toxic	>15		>63
Carbamazepine-10,11-epoxide (Tegretol metabolite)	S		μg/mL	3.97	
		Therap	0.4-4		1.6-15.9
		Toxic	>8		>31.8
Carbenicillin (Geopen)	S or P (Hep or EDTA)		μg/mL	2.64	μmol/L
		Therap	Dependent on minimum inhibition conc. of specific organism		Same
		Toxic	>250 (neurotoxicity)		>660
Chloral hydrate (Noctec) as trichloroethanol	S		μg/mL	6.69	μmol/L
		Therap	2-12		13-80
		Toxic	>20		>134
Chloramphenicol (Chloromycetin)	S or P (Hep or EDTA)		μg/mL	3.09	μmol/L
		Therap	10-25		31-77
		Toxic	>25		>77
		Gray baby syndrome	>40		>124
Chlordiazepoxide (Librium)	S or P (Hep or EDTA)		ng/mL	0.0033	μmol/L
		Therap	700-1000		2.3-3.3
		Toxic	>5000		>16.7
Chlorpromazine (Thorazine)	S or P (Hep or EDTA)		ng/mL	3.14	nmol/L
		Therap			
		Adult	50-300		157-942
		Child	40-80		126-251
		Toxic	>750		>2355
Cimetidine (Tagamet)	S or P (Hep or EDTA)		μg/mL	3.96	μmol/L
		Therap			
		Trough	0.5-1.2		2.0-5.0
		Toxic	>1.3		>5.1
Ciprofloxacin	S		μg/mL	3.02	μmol/L
		Therap			
		Peak (oral dose)	0.5-1.5		1.51-4.53
		Peak (IV dose)	<5.0		<15.1
		Toxic	>5.0		>15.1
Clonazepam (Klonopin)	S or P (Hep or EDTA)		ng/mL	3.17	nmol/L
		Therap	15-60		48-190
		Toxic	>80		>254
Clonidine (Catapres)	S or P (Hep or EDTA)		ng/mL	4.35	nmol/L
		Therap	1.0-2.0		4.4-8.7
Clorazepate (Tranxene)	S or P (Hep or EDTA)		μg/mL	3.01	μmol/L
		Therap (as desmethyldiazepam)	0.12-1.0		0.36-3.01

Continued

TABLE 56-2 Therapeutic and Toxic Levels of Drugs—*Continued*

Drug	Specimen	Status	Reference Interval: Conventional Units	Conversion Factor	SI Units
Clozapine (Clozaril)	S or P		ng/mL	3.06	nmol/L
	(Hep or EDTA)	Therap	100-600		306-1836
		Toxic	>900		>2754
Cocaine			ng/mL	3.3	nmol/L
	S or P	Toxic	>1000		3300
	(Hep or EDTA)				
	U	Toxic	>1000		>3300
Codeine	S		ng/mL	3.34	nmol/L
		Therap	10-100		33-334
		Toxic	>200		>668
Cyclosporine A (Sandimmune)	WB (EDTA)	Therap	ng/mL	0.832	nmol/L
		12 hr after dose	100-400		83-333
		24 hr after dose	100-200		83-166
		Toxic	>400		>333
Delavirdine (Rescriptor)			μg/mL	1.80	μmol/L
	S	Therap			
		Trough	3-8		5.4-14.4
		Peak	14-16		25.2-28.8
		Toxic	>16		>28.8
Desipramine (Norpramin)	S or P				
	(Hep or EDTA)		ng/mL	3.75	nmol/L
		Therap	75-300		281-1125
		Toxic	>400		>1500
Diazepam (Valium)	S or P		ng/mL	0.0035	μmol/L
	(Hep or EDTA)	Therap	100-1000		0.35-3.51
		Toxic	>5000		>17
Didanosine (DDL, Videx, Dideoxyinosine)	S		μg/mL	4.23	μmol/L
		Therap			
		Trough	0.1-0.3		0.4-1.2
		Peak	0.7-1.5		3.0-6.4
		Toxic	>1.5		>6.4
Digitoxin	S or P		ng/mL	1.31	nmol/L
	(Hep or EDTA)	Therap	20-35		26-46
	≥8 hr after dose	Toxic	>45		>59
Digoxin (Lanoxin)	S or P		ng/mL	1.28	nmol/L
	(Hep or EDTA)	Therap			
	(≥12 hr after dose)		0.5-1.5		0.64-1.92
		Toxic			
		Adult	>2.0		>2.6
		Child	>3.0		>3.8
Diphenylhydantoin (see Phenytoin)					

TABLE 56-2 Therapeutic and Toxic Levels of Drugs—*Continued*

Drug	Specimen	Status	Reference Interval: Conventional Units	Conversion Factor	SI Units
Disopyramide (Norpace)	S or P (Hep or EDTA)		μg/mL	2.95	μmol/L
		Therap			
		Arrhythmias			
		Atrial	2.0-5.0		5.9-14.8
		Ventricular	3.3-7.5		9.7-22.1
		Toxic	>7		>20.6
Doxepin (Sinequan, Adapin)	S or P (Hep or EDTA)		ng/mL	3.58	nmol/L
		Therap	150-250		537-895
		Toxic	>500		>1790
Efavirenz (Sustiva)	S		μg/mL	3.16	μmol/L
		Therap	0.5-2.9		1.6-9.2
		Toxic	>2.9		>9.2
Ephedrine (Ectasule)	S		μg/mL	6.05	μmol/L
		Therap	0.05-0.10		0.3-0.6
		Toxic	>2		>12.1
Ethchlorvynol (Placidyl)	S or P (Hep or EDTA)		μg/mL	6.92	μmol/L
		Therap	2-8		14-55
		Toxic	>20		>138
Ethosuximide (Zarontin)	S or P (Hep or EDTA)		μg/mL	7.08	μmol/L
		Therap	40-100		283-708
		Toxic	>150		>1062
Felbamate (Felbatol)	S or P (Hep or EDTA)		μg/mL	4.20	μmol/L
		Therap	40-100		168-420
		Toxic	>120		>504
Fenoprofen (Nalfon)	P (EDTA)		μg/mL	4.12	μmol/L
		Therap	20-65		82-268
Flecainide (Tambocor)	S or P (Hep or EDTA)		μg/mL	2.41	μmol/L
		Therap	0.2-1.0		0.5-2.4
		Toxic	>1.0		>2.4
Fluoxetine (Prozac)	S		ng/mL	3.23	nmol/L
		Therap	90-1150		291-3715
Flurazepam (Dalmane)	S or P (EDTA)		μg/mL	2.58	μmol/L
		Toxic	>0.2		>0.5
Gabapentin (Neurontin)	S or P (Hep or EDTA)		μg/mL	5.84	μmol/L
		Therap	2-12		12-70
		Toxic	>12		>70
Gentamicin (Garamycin)	S or P (EDTA)		μg/mL	2.09	μmol/L
		Therap			
		Peak			
		Less severe infections	5-8		10.5-16.7
		Severe infections	8-10		16.7-20.9

Continued

TABLE 56-2 Therapeutic and Toxic Levels of Drugs—*Continued*

			Reference Interval		
Drug	**Specimen**	**Status**	**Conventional Units**	**Conversion Factor**	**SI Units**
Gentamicin (Garamycin)—*cont'd*					
		Trough			
		Less severe infections	<1		<2
		Moderate infections	<2		<4
		Severe infections	<4		<8
		Toxic			
		Peak	>10		>21
		Trough	>2		>4
Glutethimide (Doriden)	S		μg/mL	4.60	μmol/L
		Therap	2-6		9-28
		Toxic	>5		>23
Haloperidol (Haldol)	S or P		ng/mL	2.66	nmol/L
	(Hep or EDTA)	Therap	1-10		2.7-26.6
Hydromorphone (Dilaudid)	S		ng/mL	3.50	nmol/L
		Therap	1-3		4-10.5
		Toxic	>100		>350
Ibuprofen (Motrin)	S or P		μg/mL	4.85	μmol/L
	(EDTA)	Therap	10-50		49-243
		Toxic	>100		>485
Imipramine (Tofranil)	S or P		ng/mL	3.57	nmol/L
	(Hep or EDTA)	Therap	150-250		536-893
		Toxic	>500		>1785
Indinavir (Crixivan)	S or P		μg/mL	1.41	μmol/L
	(Hep or EDTA)	Therap			
		Trough	>0.1		>0.14
		Peak	8-10		11.3-14.1
		Toxic	>10		>14.1
Isoniazid (Hyzyd, Nydrazid)	S or P		μg/mL	7.29	μmol/L
	(Hep or EDTA)	Therap	1-7		7-51
		Toxic	>20		>146
Kanamycin (Kantrex)	S or P		μg/mL	2.06	μmol/L
	(EDTA)	Therap			
		Peak	25-35		52-72
		Trough			
		Less severe infections	1-4		2-8
		Severe infections	4-8		8-17
		Toxic			
		Peak	>35		>72
		Trough	>10		>21

TABLE 56-2 Therapeutic and Toxic Levels of Drugs—*Continued*

Drug	Specimen	Status	Reference Interval: Conventional Units	Conversion Factor	SI Units
Lamivudine (Epivir; Epivir-HBV, 3TC)	S		μg/mL	4.36	μmol/L
		Therap			
		Trough	0.1-1.0		0.5-4.4
		Peak	1.4-1.8		6.1-7.9
		Toxic	>5		>21.8
Lamotrigine (Lamictal)	S or P (Hep or EDTA)		μg/mL	3.91	μmol/L
		Therap			
		Trough	1-2		3.9-7.8
		Peak	5-8		19.6-31.3
		Toxic	>10		>39.1
Levetiracetam (Keppra)	S or P (Hep or EDTA)		μg/mL	5.88	μmol/L
		Therap			
		Trough	3-34		18-200
		Peak	10-63		59-371
		Toxic	>63		>371
Lidocaine (Xylocaine)	S or P (Hep or EDTA) ≥45 min following bolus dose		μg/mL	4.27	μmol/L
		Therap	1.5-6.0		6.4-26
		Toxic			
		CNS, cardiovascular depression	6-8		26-34
		Seizures, obtundation, decreased cardiac output	>8		>34
Lithium (Eskalith)	S or P (Hep or EDTA)		mEq/L	1.0	mmol/L
		Therap	0.6-1.2		0.6-1.2
		Toxic	>2		>2
Lorazepam (Ativan)	S or P (Hep or EDTA)		ng/mL	3.11	nmol/L
		Therap	50-240		156-746
Lysergic acid diethylamide (LSD)			ng/mL	3.09	nmol/L
	P (EDTA)	After hallucinogenic dose	5-9		15-28
	U	After hallucinogenic dose	1-50		3-155
Maprotiline (Ludiomil)	S or P (Hep or EDTA)		ng/mL	3.60	nmol/L
		Therap	200-600		720-2160
		Toxic	>600		>2160
Meperidine (Demerol)	S or P (Hep or EDTA)		μg/mL	4.04	μmol/L
		Therap	0.4-0.7		1.6-2.8
		Toxic	>1		>4.0
Mephobarbital (Mebaral)	S or P (Hep or EDTA)		μg/mL	4.06	μmol/L
		Therap	1-7		4.1-28.4
		Toxic	>15		>60.9

Continued

TABLE 56-2 Therapeutic and Toxic Levels of Drugs—*Continued*

Drug	Specimen	Status	Reference Interval: Conventional Units	Conversion Factor	SI Units
Meprobamate (Equanil)	S		μg/mL	4.58	μmol/L
		Therap	6-12		28-55
		Toxic	>60		>275
Methadone (Dolophine)	S or P		ng/mL	0.00323	μmol/L
	(Hep or EDTA)	Therap	100-400		0.32-1.29
		Toxic	>2000		>6.46
Methamphetamine	S		μg/mL	6.70	μmol/L
(Desoxyn)		Therap	0.01-0.05		0.07-0.34
		Toxic	>0.5		>3.35
Methaqualone	S or P		μg/mL	4.00	μmol/L
(Quaalude)	(Hep or EDTA)	Therap	2-3		8-12
		Toxic	>10		>40
Methotrexate	S or P		μmol/L	1.00	μmol/L
	(Hep or EDTA)	Toxic			
		1-2 wk after low-dose therapy	>0.2		>0.2
		24 hr after high-dose therapy	≥5		≥5
		48 hr after high-dose therapy	≥0.5		≥0.5
		72 hr after high-dose therapy	≥0.05		≥0.05
Methsuximide	S		μg/mL	5.29	μmol/L
(N-desmethyl		Therap	0.01-0.04		0.053-0.212
methsuximide)		Toxic	>0.04		>0.212
(Celontin)					
Methyldopa (Aldomet)	P (EDTA)		μg/mL	4.73	μmol/L
		Therap	1-5		4.7-23.7
		Toxic	>7		>33
Methyprylon (Noludar)	S		μg/mL	5.46	μmol/L
		Therap	8-10		43-55
		Toxic	>50		273
Mexiletine (Mexitil)	S or P		μg/mL	4.64	μmol/L
	(Hep or EDTA)	Therap	0.7-2.0		3.2-9.3
		Toxic	>2.0		>9.3
Morphine	S or P		ng/mL	3.50	nmol/L
	(Hep or EDTA)	Therap	10-80		35-280
		Toxic	>200		>700
Mycophenolate mofetil	S or P		μg/mL	3.12	μmol/L
as mycophenolic acid	(EDTA)	Therap	1.0-3.5		3.1-10.9
(CellCept)		Toxic	>12		>37.5
N-Acetylprocainamide	S or P		μg/mL	3.61	μmol/L
(Pronestyl)	(Hep or EDTA)	Therap	4-30		14-108
		Toxic	>30		>108

TABLE 56-2 Therapeutic and Toxic Levels of Drugs—*Continued*

			REFERENCE INTERVAL		
Drug	**Specimen**	**Status**	**Conventional Units**	**Conversion Factor**	**SI Units**
Nefazodone (Serzone)	S or P		ng/mL	2.13	μmol/L
	(Hep or EDTA)	Therap	25-2500		53-5325
		Toxic	>2500		>5325
Nelfinavir (Viracept)	S		μg/mL	1.51	μmol/L
		Therap	1-3		1.5-4.5
		Toxic	>3		>4.5
Nevirapine (Viramune)	S		μg/mL	3.76	μmol/L
		Therap			
		Trough	3-8		11.3-30.1
		Peak	10-15		37.6-56.4
		Toxic	>15		>56.4
Netilmicin (Netromycin)			μg/mL	2.10	μmol/L
		Therap			
		Peak			
		Less severe infections	5-8		10-17
		Severe infections	8-10		17-21
		Trough			
		Less severe infections	<1		<2
		Moderate infections	<2		<4
		Severe infections	<4		<8
		Toxic			
		Peak	>10		>21
		Trough	>2		>4
Normethsuximide (Celontin)	S or P		μg/mL	4.92	μmol/L
	(Hep or EDTA)	Therap	10-40		49-197
		Toxic	>40		>197
Nortriptyline (Aventyl)	S or P		ng/mL	3.80	nmol/L
	(Hep or EDTA)	Therap	50-150		190-570
		Toxic	>500		>1900
Olanzapine (Zyprexa)	S or P		ng/mL	3.20	nmol/L
	(Hep or EDTA)	Therap	10-1000		32-3200
		Toxic	>1000		>3200
Oxazepam (Serax)	S or P		μg/mL	3.49	μmol/L
	(Hep or EDTA)	Therap	0.2-1.4		0.70-4.9
Oxcarbazepine (Trileptal) monitored as the monohydroxy metabolite (MHD)	S or P		μg/mL	3.97	μmol/L
	(EDTA)	Therap			
		Trough	6-10		24-40
		Peak	<40		<159
		Toxic	>40		>159

Continued

TABLE 56-2 Therapeutic and Toxic Levels of Drugs—*Continued*

			Reference Interval		
Drug	**Specimen**	**Status**	**Conventional Units**	**Conversion Factor**	**SI Units**
Oxycodone (Percodan)	S		ng/mL	3.17	nmol/L
		Therap	10-100		32-317
		Toxic	>200		>634
Paraldehyde	S or P		µg/mL	7.57	µmol/L
	(Hep or EDTA)	Therap			
		Sedation	10-100		76-757
		Anesthesia	>200		>1514
		Toxic	>200		>1514
		Lethal	>500		>3785
Paroxetine (Paxil; Paxil CR)	S or P (EDTA)		ng/mL	3.04	nmol/L
		Therap	30-70		91-213
		Toxic	>70		>213
Pentazocine (Talwin)	S or P		µg/mL	7.57	µmol/L
	(Hep or EDTA)	Therap	0.05-0.2		0.4-1.5
		Toxic	>1.0		>7.6
	U	Toxic	>3.0		>22.7
Pentobarbital (Nembutal)	S or P		µg/mL	4.42	µmol/L
	(Hep or EDTA)	Therap			
		Hypnotic	1-5		4-22
		Therap coma	20-50		88-221
		Toxic	>10		>44
Phenacetin	P (EDTA)		µg/mL	5.58	µmol/L
		Therap	1-30		6-167
		Toxic	50-250		279-1395
Phencyclidine (Sernylan)	S or P		ng/mL	4.11	nmol/L
	(Hep or EDTA)	Toxic	>90		>370
		Lethal	>500		>2055
Phenobarbital (Luminal)	S or P		µg/mL	4.31	µmol/L
	(Hep or EDTA)	Therap			
		Children	15-35		65-151
		Adults	20-40		86-173
		Toxic			
		Slowness, ataxia, nystagmus	35-80		151-345
		Coma, with reflexes	65-117		280-504
		Coma, without reflexes	>100		>431
Phensuximide (including parent molecule and N-desmethyl metabolites)	P (EDTA)		µg/mL	5.71	µmol/L
		Therap	40-60		228-343
Phenylbutazone (Butazolidin)	S or P		µg/mL	3.08	µmol/L
	(Hep or EDTA)	Therap	50-100		154-308
		Toxic	>100		>308

TABLE 56-2 Therapeutic and Toxic Levels of Drugs—*Continued*

			Reference Interval		
Drug	**Specimen**	**Status**	**Conventional Units**	**Conversion Factor**	**SI Units**
Phenytoin (Dilantin)	S or P		µg/mL	3.96	µmol/L
	(Hep or EDTA)	Therap	10-20		40-79
		Toxic	>20		>79
Primidone (Mysoline)	S or P		µg/mL	4.58	µmol/L
	(Hep or EDTA)	Therap	5-12		23-55
		Toxic	>15		>69
Procainamide (Pronestyl)	S or P		µg/mL	4.23	µmol/L
	(Hep or EDTA)	Therap	4-12		17-51
		Toxic	>10		>42
Propafenone (Rythmol)	S or P		µg/mL	2.93	µmol/L
	(EDTA)	Therap	0.5-2.0		1.5-5.9
		Toxic	>2		>5.9
Propoxyphene (Darvon)	P (EDTA)		µg/mL	2.95	µmol/L
		Therap	0.1-0.4		0.3-1.2
		Toxic	>0.5		>1.5
Propranolol (Inderal)	S or P		ng/mL	3.86	nmol/L
	(Hep or EDTA)	Therap	20-100		77-386
Protriptyline (Vivactil)	S or P		ng/mL	3.80	nmol/L
	(Hep or EDTA)	Therap	70-260		266-988
		Toxic	>500		>1900
Ritonavir (Norvir)	S		µg/mL	1.39	µmol/L
		Therap			
		Trough	1-6		1.4-8.4
		Peak	8-14		11.1-19.5
		Toxic	>14		>19.5
Quetiapine (Seroquel)	S or P (EDTA)		mg/L	2.58	µmol/L
		Therap	0.1-1.0		0.26-2.6
		Toxic	>2		5.16
Quinidine	S or P		µg/mL	3.08	µmol/L
	(Hep or EDTA)	Therap	2-5		6.2-15.4
		Toxic	>6		>18.5
Salicylates as salicylic acid	S or P		µg/mL	0.00727	mmol/L
	(Hep or EDTA)	Therap			
		Analgesia, antipyresis	<100		<0.72
		Antiinflammatory	150-300		1.09-2.17
		Toxic	>100		>0.72
		Lethal, 24+ hrs after a dose or with chronic ingestion	>500		>3.62

Continued

TABLE 56-2 Therapeutic and Toxic Levels of Drugs—*Continued*

Drug	Specimen	Status	Reference Interval: Conventional Units	Conversion Factor	SI Units
Saquinavir (Fortovase; Invirase)	S		μg/mL	1.49	μmol/L
		Therap			
		Trough	0.05-0.2		0.07-0.30
		Peak	0.5-2.5		0.75-3.73
		Toxic	>2.5		>3.73
Secobarbital (Seconal)	S		μg/mL	4.20	μmol/L
		Therap	1-2		4.2-8.4
		Toxic	>5		>21.0
Sirolimus (Rapamune, Rapamycin)	WB (EDTA)		ng/mL	1.10	nmol/L
		Therap	3-20		3.3-22
		Toxic	>20		>22
Sertraline (Zoloft)	S		ng/mL	3.27	nmol/L
		Therap			
		Trough	20-50		65-164
		Peak	100-200		327-654
		Toxic	>500		>1635
Sulfonamides (all)	S or P		mg/mL	5.81	mmol/L
	(Hep or EDTA)	Therap	5.0-15.0		29.1-87.2
		Toxic	>20.0		116.2
Tacrolimus (FK 506, Prograf)	WB (EDTA)		ng/mL	1.30	nmol/L
		Therap	3-20		3.9-26.0
		Toxic	>25		>32.5
Theophylline	S or P		μg/mL	5.55	μmol/L
	(Hep or EDTA)	Therap			
		Broncodilator	8-20		44-111
		Prem apnea	6-13		33-72
		Toxic	>20		110
Thiopental (Pentothal)	S or P		μg/mL	4.13	μmol/L
	(Hep or EDTA)	Hypnotic	1-5		4-21
		Coma	30-100		124-413
		Anesthesia	7-130		29-536
		Toxic	>10		>41
Thioridazine (Mellaril)	S or P		μg/mL	2.70	μmol/L
	(Hep or EDTA)	Therap	1.0-1.5		2.7-4.1
		Toxic	>10		>27
Tiagabine (Gabitril)	S		ng/mL	2.66	nmol/L
		Therap			
		Trough	5-35		14-93
		Peak	110-520		293-1383
		Toxic	>520		>1383
Tobramycin (Nebcin)	S or P		μg/mL	2.14	μmol/L
	(Hep or EDTA)	Therap			
		Peak			
		Less severe infections	5-8		11-17

TABLE 56-2 Therapeutic and Toxic Levels of Drugs—*Continued*

Drug	Specimen	Status	Reference Interval: Conventional Units	Conversion Factor	SI Units
Tobramycin (Nebcin)—*cont'd*					
		Severe infections	8-10		17-21
		Trough			
		Less severe infections	<1		<2
		Moderate infections	<2		<4
		Severe infections	<4		<9
		Toxic			
		Peak	>10		>21
		Trough	>2		>4
Tocainide (Tonocard)	S or P (Hep or EDTA)		µg/mL	5.61	µmol/L
		Therap	6-15		34-84
		Toxic	>15		>84
Tolbutamide (Orinase)	S		µg/mL	3.70	µmol/L
		Therap	90-240		333-888
		Toxic	>640		>2368
Topiramate (Topamax)	S		µg/mL	2.95	µmol/L
		Therap			
		Trough	2-4		6-12
		Peak	9-12		27-36
		Toxic	>12		>36
Trazodone (Desyrel)			ng/mL	2.68	nmol/L
		Therap	800-1600		2144-4288
Trimipramine (Surmontil)	S or P (Hep or EDTA)		ng/mL	3.40	nmol/L
		Therap	100-300		340-1020
		Toxic	>300		>1020
Valproic acid (Depakene)	S or P (Hep or EDTA)		µg/mL	6.93	µmol/L
		Therap	50-100		346-693
		Toxic	>100		>693
Vancomycin (Vancocin)	S or P (Hep or EDTA)		µg/mL	0.690	µmol/L
		Therap			
		Peak	20-40		14-28
		Trough	5-10		3-7
		Toxic	>80		>55
Venlafaxine (Effexor)	S or P (Hep or EDTA)		ng/mL	3.61	nmol/L
		Therap	70-250		253-903
		Toxic	>250		>903
Warfarin (Coumadin)	S or P (Hep or EDTA)		µg/mL	3.24	µmol/L
		Therap	1-10		3-32
		Toxic	>10		>32
Zalcitabine (ddC, Hivid, 2′,3′-dideoxycytidine)	S or P (Hep or EDTA)		ng/mL	4.73	nmol/L
		Therap	5-25		24-119
		Toxic	>25		>119

Continued

TABLE 56-2 Therapeutic and Toxic Levels of Drugs—*Continued*

			Reference Interval		
Drug	**Specimen**	**Status**	**Conventional Units**	**Conversion Factor**	**SI Units**
Zidovudine (AZT, Retrovir, azidodeoxythymidine)	S or P (Hep or EDTA)		μg/mL	3.74	μmol/L
		Therap	0.02-1.2		0.08-4.49
		Toxic	>1.2		>4.49
Zonisamide (Zonegran)			μg/mL	4.71	μmol/L
		Therap	10-30		47-141
		Toxic	>30		>141

TABLE 56-3 Critical Values

Critical values, also known as panic or alert values, are laboratory results that indicate a life-threatening situation for the patient. Because of their critical nature, urgent notification of a critical value to the appropriate healthcare professional is necessary. Table 56-3 has been adapted from extensive national surveys. The median or average critical limit determined by these surveys is shown. In practice, each organization should have its own set of critical limits and physician notification policy.

Test	Units	Lower Limit	Upper Limit	Comments
Blood Gases				
pH		7.2	7.6	
PCO_2	mm Hg	20	70	Arterial, capillary
PO_2	mm Hg	40	—	Arterial, capillary
PO_2 (children)	mm Hg	45	125	Arterial
PO_2 (newborn)	mm Hg	35	90	Arterial
Chemistry				
Albumin (children)	g/dL	1.7	6.8	Serum or plasma
Ammonia (children)	μmol/L	—	109	Plasma
Bilirubin (newborn)	mg/dL	—	15	Serum or plasma
Calcium	mg/dL	6.0	13	Serum or plasma
Calcium (children)	mg/dL	6.5	12.7	Serum or plasma
Calcium, ionized	mmol/L	0.75	1.6	Plasma
Carbon dioxide, total	mmol/L	10	40	Serum or plasma
Chloride	mmol/L	80	120	Serum or plasma
Creatinine	mg/dL	—	5.0	Serum or plasma
Creatinine (children)	mg/dL	—	3.8	Serum or plasma
Glucose	mg/dL	40	450	Serum or plasma
Glucose (children)	mg/dL	46	445	Serum or plasma
Glucose (newborn)	mg/dL	30	325	Serum or plasma
Glucose, CSF	mg/dL	40	200	CSF
Glucose, CSF (children)	mg/dL	31	—	CSF
Lactate	mmol/L	—	3.4	Plasma
Lactate (children)	mmol/L	—	4.1	Plasma
Magnesium	mg/dL	1.0	4.7	Serum or plasma
Osmolality	mOsm/kg	250	325	Serum or plasma
Phosphorus	mg/dL	1.0	8.9	Serum or plasma
Potassium	mmol/L	2.8	6.2	Serum or plasma
Potassium (newborn)	mmol/L	2.8	7.8	Serum or plasma
Protein (children)	g/dL	3.4	9.5	Serum or plasma
Protein, CSF (children)	mg/dL	—	188	CSF
Sodium	mmol/L	120	160	Serum or plasma
Urea nitrogen	mg/dL	—	80	Serum or plasma
Urea nitrogen (children)	mg/dL	—	55	Serum or plasma
Uric acid	mg/dL	—	13	Serum or plasma
Uric acid (children)	mg/dL	—	12	Serum or plasma
Hematology				
Hematocrit				
Adult	%	20	60	First report only
Newborn	%	33	71	
Hemoglobin				
Adult	g/dL	7	20	First report only
Newborn	g/dL	10	22	

Continued

TABLE 56-3 Critical Values—*Continued*

Test	Units	Lower Limit	Upper Limit	Comments
WBC				
Adult	$\times 10^3/\mu L$	2.0	30	First report only
Children	$\times 10^3/\mu L$	2.0	43	
Platelets	$\times 10^3/\mu L$	40	1000	
Blasts	Any seen (first report only)			
Drepanocytes	Presence of sickle cells or aplastic crisis			
Coagulation				
Fibrinogen	mg/dL	100	800	
Prothrombin time	s	—	30	
Partial thromboplastin time	s	—	78	
Urinalysis				
Microscopic	Presence of pathological crystals (urate, cysteine, leucine, or tyrosine)			
Chemical	Strongly positive glucose and ketones			
Cerebrospinal fluid				
WBC (0-1 yr)	Cells per μL	—	>30	
WBC (1-4 yr)	Cells per μL	—	>20	
WBC (5-17 yr)	Cells per μL	—	>10	
WBC (>17 yr)	Cells per μL	—	>5	
Malignant cells, blasts, or microorganisms		Any	Applies to other sterile body fluids	

References
Emancipator K. Critical values: ASCP practice parameter. Am J Clin Path 1997;108:247-53.
Hortin GL, Csako G. Critical values, panic values, or alert values? Am J Clin Pathol 1998;109:496-8.
Howanitz PJ, Steindel SJ, Heard NV. Laboratory critical values policies and procedures: a College of American Pathologists Q-probes study in 623 institutions. Arch Pathol Lab Med 2002;126:663-9.
Kost GJ. Critical limits for urgent clinician notification at US medical centers. JAMA 1990;263:701-7.
Kost GJ. Critical limits for emergency clinician notification at United States children's hospitals. Pediatrics 1991;88:597-603.
Kost GJ. Using critical limits to improve patient outcome. Med Lab Observ 1993;23:22-7.
Kost GJ. The significance of ionized calcium in cardiac and critical care. Availability and critical limits at U. S. medical centers and children's hospitals. Arch Pathol Lab Med 1993;117:890-6.
Tillman J, Barth JH; ACB National Audit Group. A survey of laboratory 'critical (alert) limits' in the UK. Ann Clin Biochem 2003;40:181-4.

Index

A

Page numbers followed by "f" refer to illustrations; page numbers followed by "t" refer to tables; page numbers followed by "b" refer to boxes.

F

G

J

K

L

O

W

X

Y

Z